P9-DHS-724

HARRISON'S

PRINCIPLES OF INTERNAL MEDICINE

TWELFTH EDITION

K. Stenn
Yale University

EDITORS OF PREVIOUS EDITIONS

T. R. Harrison, Editor-in-Chief,
Editions 1, 2, 3, 4, 5

W. R. Resnik, Editor,
Editions 1, 2, 3, 4, 5

M. M. Wintrobe,
Editor, Editions 1, 2, 3, 4, 5
Editor-in-Chief, Editions 6, 7

G. W. Thorn,
Editor, Editions 1, 2, 3, 4, 5, 6, 7
Editor-in-Chief, Edition 8

R. D. Adams,
Editor, Editions 2, 3, 4, 5, 6, 7, 8, 9, 10

P. B. Beeson,
Editor, Editions 1, 2

I. L. Bennett, Jr.,
Editor, Editions 3, 4, 5, 6

E. Braunwald,
Editor, Editions 6, 7, 8, 9, 10
Editor-in-Chief, Edition 11

K. J. Isselbacher,
Editor, Editions 6, 7, 8, 10, 11
Editor-in-Chief, Edition 9

R. G. Petersdorf,
Editor, Editions 6, 7, 8, 9, 11
Editor-in-Chief, Edition 10

J. D. Wilson,
Editor, Editions 9, 10, 11

J. B. Martin,
Editor, Editions 10, 11

A. S. Fauci,
Editor, Edition 11

HARRISON'S

PRINCIPLES OF INTERNAL MEDICINE

TWELFTH EDITION

Editors

JEAN D. WILSON, M.D.
Professor of Internal Medicine, The University of Texas Southwestern Medical Center, Dallas

EUGENE BRAUNWALD, A.B., M.D., M.A. (Hon.), M.D. (Hon.)
Hersey Professor of the Theory and Practice of Physic, Harvard Medical School; Chairman, Department of Medicine, Brigham and Women's Hospital, Boston

KURT J. ISSELBACHER, A.B., M.D.
Mallinckrodt Professor of Medicine, Harvard Medical School; Director, Cancer Center, Massachusetts General Hospital, Boston

ROBERT G. PETERSDORF, A.B., M.D., M.A. (Hon.), D.Sc. (Hon.), M.D. (Hon.), L.H.D. (Hon.)
President, Association of American Medical Colleges, Washington, D.C.

JOSEPH B. MARTIN, M.D., Ph.D., F.R.C.P.(C), M.A. (Hon.)
Professor of Neurology and Dean, School of Medicine, University of California at San Francisco, San Francisco

ANTHONY S. FAUCI, M.D.
Director, National Institute of Allergy and Infectious Disease; Chief, Laboratory of Immunoregulation; Director, Office of AIDS Research, National Institutes of Health, Bethesda

RICHARD K. ROOT, M.D.
Professor of Medicine and Associate Dean for Clinical Education, School of Medicine, University of California at San Francisco, San Francisco

McGRAW-HILL, Inc.
Health Professions Division
New York St. Louis San Francisco Colorado Springs
Auckland Bogotá Caracas Hamburg Lisbon London
Madrid Mexico Milan Montreal New Delhi Paris
San Juan São Paulo Singapore Sydney Tokyo Toronto

HARRISON'S
PRINCIPLES OF INTERNAL MEDICINE
Twelfth Edition

Copyright © 1991, 1987, 1983, 1980, 1977, 1974, 1970, 1966, 1962, 1958 by McGraw-Hill, Inc. All rights reserved. Copyright 1954, 1950 by McGraw-Hill, Inc. All rights reserved. Copyright renewed 1978 by Maxwell Myer Wintrobe and George W. Thorn. Printed in the United States of America. Except as permitted under the United States Copyright Act of 1976, no part of this publication may be reproduced or distributed in any form or by any means, or stored in a data base or retrieval system, without the prior written permission of the publisher.

1 2 3 4 5 6 7 8 9 0 DOW DOW 9 8 7 6 5 4 3 2 1 0

Foreign Editions
FRENCH (Eleventh Edition)—Flammarion, © 1988
GERMAN (Tenth Edition)—Schwabe and Company, Ltd., © 1986
GREEK (Eleventh Edition)—Parissianos, © 1990
ITALIAN (Twelfth Edition)—McGraw-Hill Libri Italia S.r.l. © 1992 (est.)
JAPANESE (Tenth Edition)—Hirokawa, © 1985
PORTUGUESE (Eleventh Edition)—Editora Guanabara Koogan, S.A., © 1988
SPANISH (Twelfth Edition)—McGraw-Hill/Interamericana de Espana, © 1991 (est.)

This book was set in Times Roman by Monotype Composition Company. The editors were J. Dereck Jeffers and Stuart D. Boynton. The indexer was Irving Tullar; the production supervisor was Robert Laffler; the designer was Marsha Cohen; R. R. Donnelley & Sons Company was printer and binder.

Library of Congress Cataloging-in-Publication Data

Harrison's principles of internal medicine—12th ed./editors, Jean D. Wilson . . . [et al.]
p. cm.
Also issued in 2 v.
Includes bibliographical references.
ISBN 0-07-070890-8 (1-vol. ed.)—ISBN 0-07-079749-8 (2-vol. set), 0-07-070891-6 (vol. 1), 0-07-070892-4 (vol. 2)
1. Internal medicine. I. Harrison, Tinsley Randolph, Date. II. Wilson, Jean D., Date. III. Title: Principles of internal medicine.
[DNLM: 1. Internal Medicine. WB 115 P957]
RC46.H333 1991
616—dc20
DLC
for Library of Congress 90-5814
CIP

A salute to Raymond D. Adams by the editors of Harrison's

We dedicate this twelfth edition of *Harrison's Principles of Internal Medicine* to Raymond D. Adams. Dr. Adams joined the Harrison's editorial board for preparation of the second edition, which was published in 1954. Together with the other members of the editorial board at the time, Tinsley R. Harrison, William R. Resnik, Maxwell M. Wintrobe, George W. Thorn, and Paul B. Beeson, he established *Harrison's* as a serious competitor in the field.

Ray Adams left an indelible mark on the textbook with his first contributions. He advocated what was to become the chief feature of the book, namely, the use of the introductory chapters to discuss symptoms and signs—the "Cardinal Manifestations of Disease." He argued forcibly for including diseases of the nervous system as a major component. He developed over time a systematic syndromic approach to understanding diseases of the nervous system that came to be the foundation for teaching a substantial portion of the emerging community of academic neurologists in the United States. With the assistance of his able collaborator, Maurice Victor, and other members of the neurological staff at the Massachusetts General Hospital, the section on neurology became a major instrument for teaching several generations of medical students and house officers. Because of the way that he formulated neurology as an essential component of medicine, he has had an equally important impact on the training of internists. At times the arguments over how much neurology to include in a textbook of general medicine became thunderous, leading Tinsley Harrison on one occasion to suggest (only half-facetiously) that the title be changed to *The Principles of Internal Medicine and Details of Neurology*.

The syndromic approach to diseases that affect the nervous system arose from Ray Adams' enormous personal experience with patients, an experience that continues to the present day. A complete exposition of this approach has now appeared in four editions of *Principles of Neurology*, written with Maurice Victor.

Raymond Adams was graduated from Duke University Medical School. With support from a Rockefeller fellowship he trained with James Ayer and Charles Kubik in neurology at the Massachusetts General Hospital and with Eugen Kahn in psychiatry at Yale. He returned to Boston to Harvard's service at the City Hospital as head of the Neuropathology Laboratory in 1939 where, over the course of the next decade, he made major contributions in studies of neurosyphilis, meningitis, muscle disease, and the effects of alcohol on the nervous system. He became Bullard Professor of Neuropathology at Harvard Medical School and chief of the Neurology Service at the Massachusetts General Hospital in 1951 and continued in these positions until 1978. During those years he created the leading neurological service in the country and participated in the training of a generation of academic leaders who would populate many of the university chairs of neurology in the United States and elsewhere. During this time he contributed a series of landmark studies on clinicopathologic correlations of diseases affecting the nervous system. He produced some of the first evidence for autoimmune disease of the brain and made major contributions to the understanding of developmental diseases of the nervous system. He is an expert neuropathologist and a fine neuropsychiatrist. It is difficult to find a topic in neurology that has not been advanced by the scholarship of Ray Adams.

To those who have studied under Dr. Adams and to those who have worked with him in the development of *Harrison's*, he has always been a wise and congenial colleague who demanded excellence of himself and expected it of others. His generosity, wisdom, and creativity have meant much to us, and we affectionately dedicate this volume to him.

NOTICE

Medicine is an ever-changing science. As new research and clinical experience broaden our knowledge, changes in treatment and drug therapy are required. The editors and the publisher of this work have checked with sources believed to be reliable in their efforts to provide information that is complete and generally in accord with the standards accepted at the time of publication. However, in view of the possibility of human error or changes in medical sciences, neither the editors, nor the publisher, nor any other party who has been involved in the preparation or publication of this work warrants that the information contained herein is in every respect accurate or complete. Readers are encouraged to confirm the information contained herein with other sources. For example and in particular, readers are advised to check the product information sheet included in the package of each drug they plan to administer to be certain that the information contained in this book is accurate and that changes have not been made in the recommended dose or in the contraindications for administration. This recommendation is of particular importance in connection with new or infrequently used drugs. Readers should also consult their own laboratories for normal values.

ABBREVIATED CONTENTS

CONTENTS

Section 2: Disorders of immune-mediated injury

Section 3: Disorders of the joints

PART ELEVEN
HEMATOLOGY AND ONCOLOGY

Section 1: Clotting disorders

Section 2: Disorders of the hematopoietic system

Section 3: Neoplastic diseases

PART FIFTEEN ENVIRONMENTAL AND OCCUPATIONAL HAZARDS

COLOR PLATES *After page 402*

LIST OF CONTRIBUTORS

ITAMAR B. ABRASS, M.D.
Professor of Medicine and Head, Division of Gerontology and Geriatric Medicine, University of Washington School of Medicine, Seattle

ELIAS ABRUTYN, M.D.
Professor and Assistant Chairman, Department of Medicine, Medical College of Pennsylvania; Associate Chief, Medical Service, Veterans Administration Medical Center, Philadelphia

RAYMOND D. ADAMS, B.A., M.A., M.D., M.A. (Hon.), D.Sc. (Hon.), M.D. (Hon.)
Bullard Professor of Neuropathology, Emeritus, Harvard Medical School; Consultant Neurologist and formerly Chief of Neurology Service, Massachusetts General Hospital; Emeritus Director, Eunice K. Shriver Research Center, Boston; Médicin Adjoint, L'Hôpital Cantonale de Lausanne, Lausanne

JOHN ADAMSON, M.D.
President, The New York Blood Center, New York

SETH L. ALPER, M.D., Ph.D.
Instructor in Medicine, Harvard Medical School; Section of Molecular Medicine and Nephrology, Beth Israel Hospital, Boston

ROBERT J. ANDERSON, M.D.
Professor of Medicine, University of Colorado Health Sciences Center, Denver

JACK P. ANTEL, M.D.
Professor and Chairman, Department of Neurology and Neurosurgery, McGill University; Neurologist-in-Chief, Montreal Neurological Institute and Hospital, Montreal

BARRY G.W. ARNASON, M.D.
Raymond Professor and Chairman, Department of Neurology, and Director of Brain Research Institute, University of Chicago Pritzker School of Medicine, Chicago

ARTHUR K. ASBURY, M.D.
Ruth Wagner Van Meter and J. Ray Van Meter Professor of Neurology, University of Pennsylvania School of Medicine and Hospital of the University of Pennsylvania, Philadelphia

K. FRANK AUSTEN, M.D.
Theodore Bevier Bayles Professor of Medicine, Harvard Medical School; Chairman, Department of Rheumatology and Immunology, Brigham and Women's Hospital, Boston

ROBERT AUSTRIAN, M.D., D.Sc. (Hon.)
Professor Emeritus and Chairman, Department of Research Medicine, University of Pennsylvania School of Medicine, Philadelphia

BERNARD M. BABIOR, M.D., Ph.D.
Head, Division of Biochemistry, Department of Molecular and Experimental Medicine, and Member, Division of Hematology and Oncology, Department of Medicine, Scripps Clinic and Research Foundation, La Jolla

KAMAL F. BADR, M.D.
Assistant Professor of Medicine, Vanderbilt University School of Medicine, Nashville

DONALD S. BAIM, M.D.
Associate Professor of Medicine, Harvard Medical School; Director of Invasive Cardiology, Beth Israel Hospital, Boston

M. FLINT BEAL, M.D.
Associate Professor, Harvard Medical School; Assistant Neurologist, Massachusetts General Hospital, Boston

ARTHUR L. BEAUDET, M.D.
Investigator, Howard Hughes Medical Institute; Professor of Pediatrics and Cell Biology, Baylor College of Medicine, Boston

JOHN E. BENNETT, M.D.
Head, Clinical Mycology Section, National Institute of Allergy and Infectious Diseases, National Institutes of Health, Bethesda

MICHAEL S. BERNSTEIN, M.D.
Fellow, Department of Medicine, University of California, San Francisco

DAVID R. BICKERS, M.D.
Professor and Chairman, Department of Dermatology, Case Western Reserve University School of Medicine; Director, Department of Dermatology, University Hospitals of Cleveland, Cleveland

EDWIN L. BIERMAN, M.D.
Professor of Medicine and Head, Division of Metabolism, Endocrinology, and Nutrition, University of Washington School of Medicine, Seattle

ALAN L. BISNO, M.D.
Professor of Medicine, University of Miami School of Medicine; Chief, Medical Service, Veterans Administration Medical Center, Miami

JEAN BOLOGNIA, M.D.
Assistant Professor of Dermatology, Department of Dermatology, Yale University School of Medicine, New Haven

WALTER G. BRADLEY, M.D.
Chairman and Professor of Neurology, University of Vermont College of Medicine; Chairman, Department of Neurology, University Health Center, Burlington

DAVID L. BRAFF, M.D.
Professor of Psychiatry, University of California at San Diego; Director of Psychiatry, U.C.S.D. Medical Center, San Diego

KENNETH D. BRANDT, M.D.
Professor of Medicine and Head, Rheumatology Division, Indiana University School of Medicine; Director, Indiana University Specialized Center of Research in Osteoarthritis, Indianapolis

EUGENE BRAUNWALD, A.B., M.D., M.A. (Hon.), M.D. (Hon.)
Hersey Professor of the Theory and Practice of Physic, Harvard Medical School; Chairman, Department of Medicine, Brigham and Women's Hospital, Boston

IRWIN M. BRAVERMAN, M.D.
Professor of Dermatology, Department of Dermatology, Yale University School of Medicine, New Haven

BARRY M. BRENNER, B.S., M.D., M.A. (Hon.)
Samuel A. Levine Professor of Medicine, Harvard Medical School; Senior Physician and Director, Renal Division, Brigham and Women's Hospital, Boston

KENNETH R. BRIDGES, M.D.
Assistant Professor of Medicine, Harvard Medical School; Brigham and Women's Hospital, Boston

KAREN THATCHER BRITTON, M.D., Ph.D.
Associate Professor of Psychiatry, School of Medicine, University of California at San Diego, La Jolla

MARTIN M. BROWN, M.A., M.D., M.R.C.P.
Senior Lecturer in Neurology, St. Georges Hospital Medical School, London

MICHAEL S. BROWN, M.D.
Paul J. Thomas Professor, Department of Molecular Genetics, The University of Texas Southwestern Medical Center, Dallas

ROBERT H. BROWN, Jr., M.D., D.Phil.
Assistant Professor, Harvard Medical School; Associate Neurologist, Massachusetts General Hospital, Boston

H. FRANKLIN BUNN, M.D.
Professor of Medicine, Harvard Medical School; Senior Physician and Director, Hematology Research, Brigham and Women's Hospital, Boston

RONALD M. BURDE, M.D.
Professor and Chairman, Department of Ophthalmology, Ophthalmologist and Neuroophthalmologist, Albert Einstein College of Medicine, New York

JOHN BUTLER, M.D.
Professor of Medicine, University of Washington School of Medicine, Seattle

ROBERT N. BUTLER, M.D.
Chairman, Brookdale Professor of Geriatrics and Adult Development, Ritter Department of Geriatrics and Adult Development, The Mount Sinai Medical Center, New York

ALFRED E. BUXTON, M.D.
Associate Professor of Medicine, University of Pennsylvania School of Medicine; Director, Clinical Electrophysiology Laboratory, Hospital of the University of Pennsylvania, Philadelphia

EDWIN C. CADMAN, M.D.
Ensign Professor of Medicine and Chairman, Department of Medicine, Yale University Medical School, New Haven

CHARLES B. CARPENTER, M.D.
Professor of Medicine, Harvard Medical School; Director, Laboratory of Immunogenetics and Transplantation, Brigham and Women's Hospital, Boston

CHARLES C.J. CARPENTER, M.D.
Professor of Medicine, Brown University; Physician-in-Chief, The Miriam Hospital, Providence

BRUCE R. CARR, M.D.
Professor, Department of Obstetrics and Gynecology and Cecil and Ida Green Center for Reproductive Biology Sciences, The University of Texas Southwestern Medical Center, Dallas

EDWIN H. CASSEM, M.D.
Associate Professor of Psychiatry, Harvard Medical School; Acting Chief, Psychiatric Service, Massachusetts General Hospital, Boston

AGUSTIN CASTELLANOS, M.D.
Professor of Medicine, University of Miami School of Medicine; Director, Clinical Electrophysiology, Jackson Memorial Hospital, Miami

VERNE S. CAVINESS, Jr., M.D., Ph.D.
Joseph and Rose Kennedy Professor of Child Neurology and Mental Retardation, Harvard Medical School; Interim Chief, Neurology Service, and Chief, Child Neurology, Massachusetts General Hospital, Boston

RICHARD CHAMPLIN, M.D.
Associate Professor of Medicine and Director, Leukemia/Bone Marrow Transplant Service, School of Medicine, University of California at Los Angeles

KEITH H. CHIAPPA, M.D.
Associate Professor of Neurology, Harvard Medical School; Director, EEG and Evoked Potentials Unit of the Clinical Neurophysiology Laboratory and Department of Neurology, Massachusetts General Hospital, Boston

JOHN S. CHILD, M.D.
Professor of Medicine, School of Medicine, University of California at Los Angeles; Associate Chief, Division of Cardiology, and Director, Adult Cardiac Imaging and Hemodynamics Laboratories, UCLA Medical Center, Los Angeles

WALLACE A. CLYDE, Jr., M.D.
Professor of Pediatrics and Microbiology, University of North Carolina School of Medicine; Attending Physician, North Carolina Memorial Hospital, Chapel Hill

FREDRIC L. COE, M.D.
Professor of Medicine and Physiology and Chief, Nephrology Program, University of Chicago Pritzker School of Medicine, Chicago

ALAN S. COHEN, M.D.
Chief of Medicine and Director, Thorndike Memorial Laboratory; Conrad Wesselhoeft Professor of Medicine, Boston University School of Medicine, Boston

HARVEY R. COLTEN, M.D.
Professor and Chairman, Department of Pediatrics, Washington University School of Medicine; St. Louis Children's Hospital, St. Louis

WILSON S. COLUCCI, M.D.
Associate Professor of Medicine, Harvard Medical School; Associate Physician, Brigham and Women's Hospital, Boston

PATRICIA C. COME, M.D.
Associate Professor of Medicine, Harvard Medical School; Harvard Community Health Plan, West Roxbury

MAX D. COOPER, M.D.
Investigator, Howard Hughes Medical Institute; Professor of Medicine, Pediatrics, and Microbiology and Director, Division of Developmental and Clinical Immunology, University of Alabama at Birmingham, Birmingham

RICHARD A. COOPER, M.D.
Professor of Medicine, Executive Vice-President and Dean, Medical College of Wisconsin, Milwaukee

LAWRENCE COREY, M.D.
Professor of Laboratory Medicine and Microbiology and Head, Virology Division, University of Washington School of Medicine, Seattle

MARK A. CREAGER, M.D.
Assistant Professor of Medicine, Harvard Medical School; Director, Noninvasive Vascular Laboratory, Division of Vascular Medicine and Atherosclerosis, Brigham and Women's Hospital, Boston

RONALD G. CRYSTAL, M.D.
Chief, Pulmonary Branch, National Heart, Lung and Blood Institute, National Institutes of Health, Bethesda

JOHN J. CUSH, M.D.
Assistant Professor, Department of Internal Medicine, The University of Texas Southwestern Medical Center, Dallas

CHARLES A. CZEISLER, Ph.D., M.D.
Associate Professor of Medicine, Harvard Medical School; Associate Physician, Brigham and Women's Hospital; Director, Center for Circadian and Sleep Disorders, Boston

DAVID C. DALE, M.D.
Professor of Medicine, University of Washington School of Medicine, Seattle

THOMAS M. DANIEL, M.D.
Professor of Medicine, Case Western Reserve University, Cleveland

GILBERT H. DANIELS, M.D.
Associate Professor of Medicine, Harvard Medical School; Physician, Massachusetts General Hospital, Boston

ROBERT B. DAROFF, M.D.
Gilbert W. Humphrey Professor and Chairman, Case Western Reserve University School of Medicine; Director, Department of Neurology, University Hospitals of Cleveland; Neurology Service, Cleveland Veterans Administration Medical Center, Cleveland

JOHN R. DAVID, M.D.
John LaPorte Given Professor and Chairman, Department of Tropical Public Health, Harvard School of Public Health; Chief, Division of Tropical Medicine, Brigham and Women's Hospital, Boston

KENNETH DAVIS, M.D.
Professor of Radiology, Harvard Medical School; Director of Neuroradiology, Massachusetts General Hospital, Boston

MARC A. DICHTER, M.D., Ph.D.
Professor of Neurology, University of Pennsylvania School of Medicine, Philadelphia

JULES L. DIENSTAG, M.D.
Associate Professor of Medicine, Harvard Medical School; Associate Physician, Gastrointestinal Unit, Massachusetts General Hospital, Boston

ROBERT G. DLUHY, M.D.
Associate Professor of Medicine, Harvard Medical School; Associate Program Director of the Clinical Research Center, Brigham and Women's Hospital, Boston

RAPHAEL DOLIN, M.D.
Professor of Medicine, Microbiology and Immunology, and Head, Infectious Diseases Unit, University of Rochester School of Medicine and Dentistry, Rochester

DANIEL B. DRACHMAN, M.D.
Professor of Neurology and Neurosciences and Director, Neuromuscular Unit, The Johns Hopkins University School of Medicine, Baltimore

JEFFREY M. DRAZEN, M.D.
Professor of Medicine, Harvard Medical School; Chief, Pulmonary Division, Brigham and Women's and Beth Israel Hospitals, Boston

HENRY J. DURIVAGE, Pharm.D.
Associate Research Scientist and Director of Clinical Research, Section of Medical Oncology, Department of Internal Medicine, Yale University School of Medicine, New Haven

JOHANNA T. DWYER, D.Sc., R.D.
Professor of Medicine and Community Health, Tufts University School of Medicine; Senior Scientist, USDA Human Nutrition Research Center on Aging, Tufts University; Director, Frances Stern Nutrition Center, New England Medical Center Hospital, Boston

VICTOR J. DZAU, M.D.
William G. Irwin Professor and Chief, Division of Cardiovascular Medicine, Stanford University School of Medicine; Stanford University Hospital, Stanford

KENNETH H. FALCHUK, M.D.
Associate Professor of Medicine, Harvard Medical School; Physician, Brigham and Women's Hospital, Boston

ANTHONY S. FAUCI, M.D.
Director, National Institute of Allergy and Infectious Diseases, and Chief, Laboratory of Immunoregulation, and Director, Office of AIDS Research, National Institutes of Health, Bethesda

MURRAY J. FAVUS, M.D.
Professor of Medicine, University of Chicago Pritzker School of Medicine, Chicago

BERNARD N. FIELDS, M.D.
Adele Lehman Professor of Microbiology and Molecular Genetics, and Professor of Medicine and Chairman, Department of Microbiology and Molecular Genetics, Harvard Medical School, Boston

STUART C. FINCH, M.D.
Professor of Medicine, Robert Wood Johnson Medical School, University of Medicine and Dentistry of New Jersey, Camden

J. STEPHEN FINK, M.D.
Assistant Professor, Harvard Medical School; Assistant Neurologist, Massachusetts General Hospital, Boston

ADAM FINN, M.D.
Lecturer in Immunology, Institute of Child Health; Honorary Senior Registrar, The Hospital for Sick Children, London

DANIEL W. FOSTER, M.D.
Donald W. Seldin Distinguished Chair in Internal Medicine and Chairman, Department of Internal Medicine, The University of Texas Southwestern Medical Center, Dallas

MICHAEL M. FRANK, M.D.
Chief, Laboratory of Clinical Investigation, National Institute of Allergy and Infectious Diseases, National Institutes of Health, Bethesda

STANLEY D. FREEDMAN, M.D.
Head, Division of Infectious Diseases, Scripps Clinic and Research Foundation; Clinical Professor of Medicine, University of California at San Diego, La Jolla

BISHARA J. FREIJ, M.D.
Assistant Professor of Pediatrics, Division of Infectious Diseases, Department of Pediatrics, Georgetown University School of Medicine, Washington, D.C.

MICHAEL FREISSMUTH, M.D.
Instructor, Department of Pharmacology, University of Vienna

HARVEY M. FRIEDMAN, M.D.
Associate Professor, Department of Medicine, University of Pennsylvania School of Medicine, Philadelphia

LAWRENCE S. FRIEDMAN, M.D.
Associate Professor of Medicine and Vice Chairman of the Department of Medicine, Division of Gastroenterology and Hepatology, Thomas Jefferson University Hospital, Philadelphia

PAUL J. FRIEDMAN, M.D.
Professor of Radiology, University of California, San Diego

WILLIAM F. FRIEDMAN, M.D.
J.H. Nicholson Professor of Pediatric Cardiology and Executive Chairman, Department of Pediatrics, School of Medicine; UCLA Medical Center, Los Angeles

LAWRENCE A. FROHMAN, M.D.
Professor of Medicine, Director of Division of Endocrinology and Metabolism, University of Cincinnati College of Medicine, Cincinnati

JOHN I. GALLIN, M.D.
Director, Intramural Research Program, National Institute of Allergy and Infectious Diseases, National Institutes of Health, Bethesda

ROBERT C. GALLO, M.D.
Chief, Laboratory of Tumor Cell Biology, National Cancer Institute, National Institutes of Health, Bethesda

DONALD E. GANEM, M.D.
Associate Professor of Medicine and Microbiology, Division of Infectious Disease, Department of Medicine, University of California, San Francisco

PIERCE GARDNER, M.D.
Professor of Medicine and Associate Dean for Academic Affairs, School of Medicine, State University of New York at Stony Brook, Stony Brook

MARC B. GARNICK, M.D.
Associate Clinical Professor of Medicine, Dana-Farber Cancer Institute, Harvard Medical School; Vice President for Clinical Development, Genetics Institute, Cambridge

JAMES L. GERMAN III, M.D.
Professor (Genetics), Department of Pediatrics, Cornell University Medical College; Senior Investigator and Director, Laboratory of Human Genetics, The New York Blood Center, New York

ELOISE R. GIBLETT, M.D.
Executive Director Emeritus, Puget Sound Blood Center, Seattle

BRUCE C. GILLILAND, M.D.
Associate Dean for Clinical Affairs, University of Washington School of Medicine, Seattle

J. CHRISTIAN GILLIN, M.D.
Professor of Psychiatry, University of California at San Diego, and Director of U.C.S.D. Mental Health Research Center; Director of U.C.S.D. Fellowship in Psychopharmacology and Psychobiology, La Jolla

ALFRED G. GILMAN, M.D., Ph.D.
Raymond and Ellen Willie Professor of Molecular Neuropharmacology and Chairman, Department of Pharmacology, The University of Texas Southwestern Medical Center, Dallas

SID GILMAN, M.D.
Professor and Chairman, Department of Neurology, The University of Michigan Medical Center, Ann Arbor

RICHARD J. GLASSOCK, M.D.
Professor of Medicine, School of Medicine, University of California at Los Angeles; Chairman, Department of Medicine, Harbor-UCLA Medical Center, Torrance

ROBERT M. GLICKMAN, M.D.
Herrman L. Blumgart Professor of Medicine, Harvard Medical School; Physician-in-Chief, Beth Israel Hospital, Boston

DAVID W. GOLDE, M.D.
Professor of Medicine and Chief, Division of Hematology/Oncology, School of Medicine, University of California, Los Angeles

STEPHEN E. GOLDFINGER, M.D.
Associate Dean, Department of Continuing Education, and Associate Professor of Medicine, Harvard Medical School; Physician, Gastrointestinal Unit, Massachusetts General Hospital, Boston

PAUL GOLDHABER, D.D.S.
Dean and Professor of Periodontology, Harvard School of Dental Medicine, Boston

LEE GOLDMAN, M.D.
Professor of Medicine, Harvard Medical School; Vice-Chairman, Department of Medicine, Brigham and Women's Hospital; Chief, Division of Clinical Epidemiology, Brigham and Women's and Beth Israel Hospitals, Boston

JOSEPH L. GOLDSTEIN, M.D.
Paul J. Thomas Professor and Chairman, Department of Molecular Genetics, The University of Texas Southwestern Medical Center, Dallas

RAJ K. GOYAL, M.D.
Rabb Professor of Medicine, Harvard Medical School; Chief, Division of Gastroenterology, Beth Israel Hospital, Boston

JOHN W. GRAEF, M.D.
Associate Clinical Professor of Pediatrics, Harvard Medical School; Director, The Lead/Toxicology Clinic, The Children's Hospital, Boston

IGOR GRANT, M.D.
Professor and Acting Chairman, Department of Psychiatry, School of Medicine, University of California at San Diego, La Jolla

HARRY B. GREENBERG, M.D.
Professor of Medicine, Microbiology, and Immunology and Chief, Gastroenterology Division, Stanford University School of Medicine, Stanford

NORTON J. GREENBERGER, M.D.
Peter T. Bohan Professor and Chairman, Department of Medicine, University of Kansas School of Medicine, Kansas City

BRUCE M. GREENE, M.D.
Professor of Medicine, and Director, Division of Geographic Medicine, Department of Medicine, University of Alabama at Birmingham, Birmingham

JOHN S. GREENSPAN, Ph.D.
Professor and Chairman, Division of Oral Biology, University of California School of Dentistry, San Francisco Medical Center, San Francisco

JAMES E. GRIFFIN III, M.D.
Professor of Internal Medicine, The University of Texas Southwestern Medical Center, Dallas

J. McLEOD GRIFFISS, M.D.
Professor of Laboratory Medicine and Medicine, University of California San Francisco; Chief of Microbiology, Veterans Administration Medical Center, San Francisco

ROBERT C. GRIGGS, M.D.
Edward A. and Alma Vollertsen Rykenboer Professor of Neurophysiology, Professor of Neurology and Medicine, and Chairman, Department of Neurology, University of Rochester School of Medicine and Dentistry, University of Rochester Medical Center, Rochester

WILLIAM GROSSMAN, M.D.
Dana Professor of Medicine, Harvard Medical School; Chief, Cardiovascular Division, Beth Israel Hospital, Boston

JOHN H. GROWDON, M.D.
Associate Professor of Neurology, Harvard Medical School; Associate Neurologist and Director, Memory Disorders Unit, Massachusetts General Hospital, Boston

VLADIMIR C. HACHINSKI, M.D.
Richard and Beryl Ivey Professor and Chairman, Department of Clinical Neurological Sciences, University of Western Ontario, University Hospital, London, Ontario

BEVRA H. HAHN, M.D.
Chief of Rheumatology, University of California, Los Angeles

ROBERT I. HANDIN, M.D.
Associate Professor of Medicine, Harvard Medical School; Director, Hematology Division, Brigham and Women's Hospital, Boston

H. HUNTER HANDSFIELD, M.D.
Professor of Medicine, University of Washington School of Medicine; Director, Sexually Transmitted Disease Control Program, Seattle-King County Department of Public Health, Seattle

DONALD G. HARTER, M.D.
Senior Scientific Officer and Director, HHMI-NIH Research Scholars Program, Howard Hughes Medical Institute, Bethesda; Clinical Professor of Neurology, George Washington University School of Medicine and Health Sciences, Washington, D.C.

BARTON F. HAYNES, M.D.
Frederick M. Hanes Professor of Medicine and Chief, Division of Rheumatology and Immunology, Duke University School of Medicine, Durham

STEVEN C. HEBERT, M.D.
Associate Professor of Medicine, Harvard Medical School; Associate Physician, Brigham and Women's Hospital, Boston

CRAIG HENDERSON, M.D.
Associate Professor of Medicine, Harvard Medical School; Division of Medical Oncology, Dana-Farber Cancer Institute, Boston

FRED J. HENDLER, M.D., Ph.D.
Associate Professor of Medicine and Biochemistry, University of Louisville School of Medicine; James Graham Brown Cancer Center, Division of Hematology/Oncology, Louisville; Consulting Physician, Veterans Administration Medical Center, Dallas

FREDERICK P. HEINZEL, M.D.
Associate Professor of Medicine, Division of Infectious Disease, Department of Medicine, University of California, San Francisco

CHARLES B. HIGGINS, M.D.
Professor of Radiology and Chief, Magnetic Resonance Imaging, University of California School of Medicine, San Francisco

RAYMOND L. HINTZ, M.D.
Professor of Pediatrics and Head, Division of Pediatric Endocrinology, Stanford University School of Medicine, Stanford

MARTIN S. HIRSCH, M.D.
Associate Professor of Medicine, Harvard Medical School; Associate Physician, Infectious Diseases Unit, Massachusetts General Hospital, Boston

JAN V. HIRSCHMANN, M.D.
Associate Professor of Medicine, University of Washington School of Medicine; Assistant Chief, Medical Service, Seattle Veterans Administration Medical Center, Seattle

FRED HOCHBERG, M.D.
Associate Professor of Neurology, Harvard Medical School; Neurologist, Massachusetts General Hospital, Boston

PAUL D. HOEPRICH, M.D.
Professor of Medicine, Section of Medical Myocology, Division of Infectious and Immunologic Diseases, School of Medicine, University of California, Davis

GARY S. HOFFMAN, M.D.
Senior Investigator, Laboratory of Immunoregulation, National Institute of Allergy and Infectious Diseases, National Institutes of Health, Bethesda

JOHN H. HOLBROOK, M.D.
Professor of Internal Medicine, University of Utah School of Medicine, Salt Lake City

MICHAEL F. HOLICK, M.D., Ph.D.
Professor of Medicine, Chief of Endocrinology, and Director of the Clinical Research Center, Boston University School of Medicine, Boston

KING K. HOLMES, M.D., Ph.D.
Director, Center for AIDS and Sexually Transmitted Diseases; Professor of Medicine, University of Washington School of Medicine, Seattle

RANDALL K. HOLMES, M.D., Ph.D.
Professor and Chairman, Department of Microbiology, and Associate Dean for Academic Affairs, Uniformed Services University of the Health Sciences, Bethesda

THOMAS H. HOSTETTER, M.D.
Professor of Medicine, University of Minnesota School of Medicine; Director, Division of Renal Disease, University Hospital, Minneapolis

LYN J. HOWARD, B.M., D.Ch., F.R.C.P.
Professor of Medicine and Associate Professor of Pediatrics, and Head, Division of Clinical Nutrition, Albany Medical College, Albany

GARY W. HUNNINGHAKE, M.D.
Professor of Internal Medicine and Director, Pulmonary and Critical Care Medicine, University of Iowa College of Medicine, Iowa City

SIDNEY H. INGBAR, M.D., D.Sc. (Deceased)
Former William Bosworth Castle Professor of Medicine, Harvard Medical School; former Director, Thorndike Laboratory, Beth Israel Hospital, Boston

ROLAND H. INGRAM, JR., M.D.
Professor and Vice-Chairman of Medicine, University of Minnesota Medical School; Chief of Medicine, Hennepin County Medical Center, Minneapolis

KURT J. ISSELBACHER, A.B., M.D.
Mallinckrodt Professor of Medicine, Harvard Medical School; Director, Cancer Center, Massachusetts General Hospital, Boston

RICHARD JACOBS, M.D., Ph.D.
Associate Clinical Professor of Medicine, Division of Infectious Disease, Department of Medicine, University of California, San Francisco

MARK E. JOSEPHSON, M.D.
Robinette Professor of Medicine (Cardiovascular Diseases), University of Pennsylvania School of Medicine; Chief, Cardiovascular Section, Hospital of the University of Pennsylvania, Philadelphia

LEWIS L. JUDD, M.D.
Director, National Institute of Mental Health, Rockville

LEE M. KAPLAN, M.D., Ph.D.
Assistant Professor of Medicine, Harvard Medical School; Assistant in Medicine, Gastrointestinal Unit, Massachusetts General Hospital, Boston

DENNIS L. KASPER, M.D.
William Ellery Channing Professor of Medicine, Harvard Medical School; Chief, Infectious Disease Division, Beth Israel Hospital, Boston

SATISH KATHPALIA, M.D.
Assistant Professor of Medicine, University of Chicago Pritzker School of Medicine; Attending Physician, Michael Reese Hospital and Medical Center, Chicago

DONALD KAYE, M.D.
Professor and Chairman, Department of Medicine, The Medical College of Pennsylvania, Philadelphia

WILLIAM N. KELLEY, M.D.
Professor of Medicine and Dean, School of Medicine, University of Pennsylvania, Philadelphia

GERALD T. KEUSCH, M.D.
Professor of Medicine, Tufts University School of Medicine; Chief, Division of Geographic Medicine and Infectious Diseases, New England Medical Center Hospital, Boston

MICHAEL B. KIMMEY, M.D.
Assistant Professor of Medicine and Director of Therapeutic Endoscopy, Division of Gastroenterology, University of Washington School of Medicine, Seattle

LOUIS V. KIRCHHOFF, M.D., M.P.H.
Assistant Professor of Medicine, Department of Internal Medicine, University of Iowa College of Medicine; Staff Physician, Veterans Administration Medical Center, Iowa City

J. PHILLIP KISTLER, M.D.
Associate Professor of Neurology, Harvard Medical School; Associate Neurologist, Massachusetts General Hospital, Boston

JOSEPH J. KLIMEK, M.D.
Associate Professor of Medicine, University of Connecticut Health Center; Acting Director, Department of Medicine, Hartford Hospital, Hartford

JAMES P. KNOCHEL, M.D.
Professor of Internal Medicine, The University of Texas Southwestern Medical Center; Chairman, Department of Medicine, Presbyterian Hospital, Dallas

HOWARD K. KOH, M.D.
Associate Professor of Dermatology, Medicine, and Public Health, Boston University Schools of Medicine and Public Health, Boston

WILLIAM J. KOVACS, M.D.
Assistant Professor of Medicine, Division of Endocrinology, Vanderbilt University School of Medicine, Nashville

KAREN KOVALOV-ST. JOHN, M.D.
Rheumatology Fellow, Indiana University School of Medicine, Indianapolis

STEPHEN M. KRANE, M.D.
Persis, Cyrus, and Marlow B. Harrison Professor of Medicine, Harvard Medical School; Physician and Chief, Arthritis Unit, Massachusetts General Hospital, Boston

J. THOMAS LAMONT, M.D.
Professor of Medicine, Boston University School of Medicine; Chief, Section of Gastroenterology, The University Hospital, Boston

LEWIS LANDSBERG, M.D.
Professor of Medicine, Harvard Medical School; Chief, Division of Endocrinology and Metabolism, Beth Israel Hospital, Boston

H. CLIFFORD LANE, M.D.
Deputy Clinical Director, National Institute of Allergy and Infectious Diseases, National Institutes of Health, Bethesda

PAUL N. LANKEN, M.D.
Associate Professor of Medicine, University of Pennsylvania School of Medicine; Medical Director, Medical Intensive Care Unit, Hospital of the University of Pennsylvania, Philadelphia

THOMAS J. LAWLEY, M.D.
Professor and Chairman, Department of Dermatology, Emory University School of Medicine, Atlanta

ALEXANDER R. LAWTON III, M.D.
Professor of Pediatrics and Microbiology, Division of Pediatrics, Immunology, and Rheumatology, Vanderbilt University School of Medicine, Nashville

J. MICHAEL LAZARUS, M.D.
Associate Professor of Medicine, Harvard Medical School; Physician, Brigham and Women's Hospital, Boston

ROBERT LEBOVICS, M.D.
Chief, Otolaryngology/Head, Neck Surgery, National Institute on Deafness and Other Communication Disorders, National Institutes of Health, Bethesda

NORMAN G. LEVINSKY, M.D.
Wade Professor and Chairman, Department of Medicine, Boston University School of Medicine; Physician-in-Chief and Director, Evans Memorial Department of Clinical Research, University Hospital, Boston

CHRISTOPHER H. LINDEN, M.D.
Assistant Professor of Medicine, University of Massachusetts Medical School; Director, Regional Poisoning Treatment Center, Worcester, Massachusetts

PETER E. LIPSKY, M.D.
Director, Harold C. Simmons Arthritis Research Center; Professor, Department of Internal Medicine, The University of Texas Southwestern Medical Center, Dallas

RICHARD M. LOCKSLEY, M.D.
Associate Professor of Medicine and Chief, Division of Infectious Disease, Department of Medicine, University of California, San Francisco

HARVEY F. LODISH, Ph.D.
Professor, Department of Biology, Massachusetts Institute of Technology; Member, Whitehead Institute for Biomedical Research, Cambridge

DAN L. LONGO, M.D.
Director, Biological Response Modifiers Program, Division of Cancer Treatment, National Cancer Institute-Frederick Cancer Research Facility, Frederick

FREDERICK H. LOVEJOY, Jr., M.D.
Professor of Pediatrics, Harvard Medical School; Associate Physician-in-Chief, The Children's Hospital, Boston

SHEILA A. LUKEHART, Ph.D.
Research Associate Professor, Department of Medicine, Division of Infectious Diseases, University of Washington School of Medicine, Seattle

ROB ROY MacGREGOR, M.D.
Professor of Medicine and Chief of Infectious Diseases Division, Department of Medicine, University of Pennsylvania School of Medicine, Philadelphia

RAYMOND MACIEWICZ, M.D.
Associate Professor of Neurology, Harvard Medical School; Associate Neurologist, Massachusetts General Hospital, Boston

JON T. MADER, M.D.
Professor of Medicine, Division of Infectious Diseases, Department of Internal Medicine, The University of Texas Medical Branch, Galveston

HENRY J. MANKIN, M.D.
Edith M. Ashley Professor of Orthopedic Surgery, Harvard Medical School; Chief, Orthopedic Services, Massachusetts General Hospital, Boston

FRANCIS E. MARCHLINSKI, M.D.
Associate Professor of Medicine, University of Pennsylvania School of Medicine; Director, Arrhythmia Evaluation Center, Hospital of the University of Pennsylvania, Philadelphia

JOSEPH B. MARTIN, M.D., Ph.D., F.R.C.P.(C), M.A.(Hon.)
Professor of Neurology and Dean, School of Medicine, University of California, San Francisco

JOEL B. MASON, M.D.
Assistant Professor of Medicine, Tufts University School of Medicine; Scientist, USDA Human Nutrition Research Center on Aging, Tufts University, Boston

HENRY MASUR, M.D.
Deputy Chief, Critical Care Medicine, Clinical Center, National Institutes of Health, Bethesda

ROBERT J. MAYER, M.D.
Associate Professor of Medicine, Harvard Medical School; Division of Medical Oncology, Dana-Farber Cancer Institute, Boston

JOHN D. McCONNELL, M.D.
Assistant Professor of Urology, The University of Texas Southwestern Medical Center, Dallas

GEORGE H. McCRACKEN, Jr., M.D.
Professor of Pediatrics and Chief, Division of Infectious Diseases, Department of Pediatrics, The University of Texas Southwestern Medical Center, Dallas

E. R. McFADDEN, Jr., M.D.
Argyl J. Beams Professor of Medicine and Director, Airway Disease Center, Case Western Reserve University School of Medicine, Cleveland

JAMES E. McGUIGAN, M.D.
Professor of Medicine and Chairman, Department of Medicine, University of Florida College of Medicine, Gainesville

NANCY K. MELLO, Ph.D.
Professor of Psychology, Department of Psychiatry (Neuroscience), Harvard Medical School, Boston; Co-Director, Alcohol and Drug Abuse Research Center, McLean Hospital, Belmont

JERRY R. MENDELL, M.D.
Professor of Neurology, Ohio State University College of Medicine, Columbus

JOHN MENDELSOHN, M.D.
Winthrop Rockefeller Chair in Medical Oncology and Chairman, Department of Medicine, Memorial Sloan-Kettering Cancer Center, New York

JACK H. MENDELSON, M.D.
Professor of Psychiatry (Neuroscience), Harvard Medical School, Boston; Co-Director, Alcohol and Drug Abuse Research Center, McLean Hospital, Belmont

URS A. MEYER, M.D.
Professor of Pharmacology and Chairman, Department of Pharmacology, Biocenter of the University of Basel, Basel, Switzerland

EDGAR L. MILFORD, M.D.
Associate Professor of Medicine, Harvard Medical School; Associate Physician, Brigham and Women's Hospital, Boston

RICHARD A. MILLER, M.D.
Assistant Professor of Medicine, University of Washington School of Medicine; Chief, Infectious Disease Division, Seattle Veterans Administration Medical Center, Seattle

JOHN D. MINNA, M.D.
Chief, NCI-Navy Medical Oncology Branch, National Cancer Institute, National Institutes of Health; Professor of Medicine, Uniformed Services University for the Health Sciences, Naval Hospital, Bethesda

JAY P. MOHR, M.D.
Sciarra Professor of Clinical Neurology, College of Physicians and Surgeons of Columbia University Neurological Institute, New York

STEPHEN A. MORSE, MSPH, Ph.D.
Director, Division of Sexually Transmitted Diseases Laboratory Research, Centers for Disease Control, Atlanta

KENNETH M. MOSER, M.D.
Professor of Medicine, School of Medicine, University of California at San Diego; Director, Pulmonary and Critical Care Division, U.C.S.D. Medical Center, La Jolla

ARNOLD M. MOSES, M.D.
Professor of Medicine and Director, Clinical Research Center, State University of New York Health Science Center; Chief, Endocrinology Section, Veterans Administration Medical Center, Syracuse

HARALAMPOS M. MOUTSOPOULOS, M.D.
Professor and Head of Medicine, Department of Internal Medicine, University of Ioannina Medical School, Ioannina, Greece

HENRY W. MURRAY, M.D.
Professor of Medicine, Cornell University School of Medicine; Chief, Infectious Diseases, The New York Hospital-Cornell Medical Center, New York

ROBERT J. MYERBURG, M.D.
Professor of Medicine and Physiology and Director, Division of Cardiology, University of Miami School of Medicine, Miami

LEE M. NADLER, M.D.
Associate Professor of Medicine, Harvard Medical School; Division of Tumor Immunology, Dana-Farber Cancer Institute, Boston

THEODORE E. NASH, M.D.
Medical Officer, Laboratory of Parasitic Diseases, National Institute of Allergy and Infectious Diseases, National Institutes of Health, Bethesda

LAURENCE NEEDLEMAN, M.D.
Assistant Professor of Radiology, Jefferson Medical College, Philadelphia

PAUL NEIMAN, M.D.
Professor of Medicine and Adjunct Professor of Pathology, University of Washington School of Medicine; Fred Hutchinson Cancer Research Center, Seattle

HAROLD C. NEU, M.D.
Professor of Medicine and Pharmacology and Chief, Division of Infectious Diseases, College of Physicians and Surgeons, Columbia University, New York

JOHN A. OATES, M.D.
Professor and Chairman, Department of Medicine, Vanderbilt University School of Medicine; Physician-in-Chief, Vandberbilt University Hospital, Nashville

JERROLD M. OLEFSKY, M.D.
Professor of Medicine and Head, Division of Endocrinology and Metabolism, School of Medicine, University of California at San Diego, La Jolla

STUART H. ORKIN, M.D.
Leland Fikes Professor of Pediatric Medicine, Harvard Medical School; Children's Hospital, Boston

ROBERT A. O'ROURKE, M.D.
Charles Conrad Brown Distinguished Professor of Medicine, University of Texas Health Science Center at San Antonio; Chief of Cardiology, University of Texas Health Science Center Teaching Hospitals, San Antonio

THOMAS D. PALELLA, M.D.
Associate Professor of Internal Medicine and Chief, Division of Rheumatology, University of Michigan Medical School, Ann Arbor

DARWIN L. PALMER, M.D.
Professor of Medicine and Chief, Division of Infectious Disease, University of New Mexico School of Medicine, Albuquerque

JOSEPH E. PARRILLO, M.D.
James B. Herrick Professor of Medicine, Rush Medical College; Chief, Section of Cardiology, Chief, Section of Critical Care Medicine, Medical Director, Rush Heart Institute, Rush-Presbyterian-St. Luke's Medical Center, Chicago

RICHARD C. PASTERNAK, M.D.
Assistant Professor of Medicine, Harvard Medical School; Director, Coronary Care Unit, Beth Israel Hospital, Boston

PETER L. PERINE, M.D.
Professor and Director, Division of Tropical Public Health, Uniformed Services University of the Health Sciences, Bethesda

ROBERT G. PETERSDORF, M.D.
President, Association of American Medical Colleges; Clinical Professor of Medicine, Georgetown University School of Medicine, Washington, D.C.

ELIOT A. PHILLIPSON, M.D.
Professor of Medicine, University of Toronto; Physician-in-Chief, Mount Sinai Hospital, Toronto

DAVID J. PIERSON, M.D.
Professor of Medicine, University of Washington School of Medicine; Medical Director of Respiratory Care, Harborview Medical Center, Seattle

JAMES J. PLORDE, M.D.
Professor of Medicine, Departments of Laboratory Medicine and Microbiology, University of Washington School of Medicine; Chief, Microbiology Laboratory, Seattle Veterans Administration Hospital, Seattle

STANLEY A. PLOTKIN, M.D.
Professor of Pediatrics and Microbiology, University of Pennsylvania; Chair, Division of Infectious Diseases, The Children's Hospital of Philadelphia, Philadelphia

FRANCIS A. PLUMMER, M.D., F.R.C.P.(C)
Associate Professor, Department of Medical Microbiology, University of Manitoba, Winnipeg

DANIEL K. PODOLSKY, M.D.
Associate Professor of Medicine, Harvard Medical School; Chief, Gastrointestinal Unit, Massachusetts General Hospital, Boston

JOHN T. POTTS, Jr., M.D.
Jackson Professor of Clinical Medicine, Harvard Medical School; Chief of the General Medical Service, Massachusetts General Hospital, Boston

LAWRIE W. POWELL, M.D.
Professor of Medicine, University of Queensland; Physician, Royal Brisbane Hospital, Brisbane, Australia

DARWIN J. PROCKOP, M.D., Ph.D.
Professor and Chairman, Department of Biochemistry, Jefferson Medical College of Thomas Jefferson University; Director, Department of Biochemistry, Jefferson Institute of Molecular Medicine, Philadelphia

AMY PRUITT, M.D.
Assistant Professor of Neurology, Harvard Medical School; Associate Neurologist, Massachusetts General Hospital, Boston

PAUL G. RAMSEY, M.D.
Associate Professor and Associate Chairman, Department of Medicine, University of Washington School of Medicine, Seattle

JOEL M. RAPPEPORT, M.D.
Professor of Medicine, Yale University School of Medicine; Director, Bone Marrow Transplantation Program, Yale New Haven Hospital, New Haven

C. GEORGE RAY, M.D.
Professor, Departments of Pathology and Pediatrics, College of Medicine, The University of Arizona Health Sciences Center, Tucson

RICHARD C. REICHMAN, M.D.
Associate Professor of Medicine, Microbiology, and Immunology, The University of Rochester Medical Center, Rochester

HERBERT Y. REYNOLDS, M.D.
J. Lloyd Huck Professor of Medicine and Chairman, Department of Medicine, The Pennsylvania State University College of Medicine; University Hospital, The Milton S. Hershey Medical Center, Hershey

STUART RICH, M.D.
Associate Professor of Medicine and Chief, Section of Cardiology, University of Illinois College of Medicine, Chicago

EDWARD P. RICHARDSON JR., M.D.
Bullard Professor of Neuropathology, Harvard Medical School; Senior Neurologist, Massachusetts General Hospital, Boston

GARY S. RICHARDSON, M.D.
Instructor in Medicine, Harvard Medical School; Associate Physician, Brigham and Women's Hospital, Boston

HAL B. RICHERSON, M.D.
Professor of Internal Medicine and Director, Allergy-Immunology Division, University of Iowa College of Medicine, Iowa City

JAMES M. RICHTER, M.D.
Assistant Professor of Medicine, Harvard Medical School; Chief, Gastrointestinal Clinic, Massachusetts General Hospital, Boston

S. CRAIG RISCH, M.D.
Professor of Psychiatry and Director of Clinical Research Programs, Emory University, Atlanta

R. PAUL ROBERTSON, M.D.
Professor of Medicine, Director of Clinical Research Center, and Director, Diabetes Center, University of Minnesota, Minneapolis

ALLAN R. RONALD, M.D.
H. E. Sellers Professor and Head, Department of Medicine, The University of Manitoba, Winnipeg

RICHARD K. ROOT, M.D.
Professor of Medicine, Department of Medicine, and Associate Dean for Clinical Education, School of Medicine, University of California, San Francisco

ALLAN H. ROPPER, M.D.
Associate Professor of Neurology, Harvard Medical School; Associate Neurologist and Director of Neurological/Neurosurgical Intensive Care Unit, Massachusetts General Hospital, Boston

IRWIN H. ROSENBERG, M.D.
Professor of Medicine, Nutrition, and Physiology, Tufts University School of Medicine; Director, USDA Human Nutrition Research Center on Aging, Tufts University, Boston

LEON E. ROSENBERG, M.D.
Dean and C.N.H. Long Professor of Human Genetics, Medicine, and Pediatrics, Yale University School of Medicine, New Haven

DANIEL ROTROSEN, M.D.
Bacterial Diseases Section, National Institute of Allergy and Infectious Diseases, National Institutes of Health, Bethesda

JODI ROY, M.S., R.D.
Frances Stern Nutrition Center, New England Medical Center Hospital, Boston

ARTHUR H. RUBENSTEIN, M.D.
Professor and Chairman, Department of Medicine, University of Chicago Pritzker School of Medicine, Chicago

JEREMY N. RUSKIN, M.D.
Associate Professor of Medicine, Harvard Medical School; Director of Cardiac Arrhythmia Service, Massachusetts General Hospital, Boston

ARTHUR I. SAGALOWSKY, M.D.
Professor of Urology and Director of Renal Transplantation, The University of Texas Southwestern Medical Center, Dallas

JAY P. SANFORD, M.D.
President and Dean, Uniformed Services University of the Health Sciences, Bethesda

DENNIS R. SCHABERG, M.D.
Professor of Internal Medicine, The University of Michigan Medical School, Ann Arbor

I. HERBERT SCHEINBERG, M.D.
Professor of Medicine and Head, Division of Genetic Medicine, Albert Einstein College of Medicine; Attending Physician, Hospital of the Albert Einstein College of Medicine, New York

ALAN L. SCHILLER, M.D.
Irene Heinz Given and John LaPorte Given Professor and Chairman of Pathology, The Mount Sinai School of Medicine, New York

R. NEIL SCHIMKE, M.D.
Professor of Pediatrics and Internal Medicine and Director, Division of Metabolism, Endocrinology, and Genetics, The University of Kansas College of Health Sciences, Kansas City

RUDI SCHMID, M.D., Ph.D.
Professor of Medicine and Associate Dean, University of California, San Francisco

ROBERT T. SCHOOLEY, M.D.
Associate Professor of Medicine, Harvard Medical School; Assistant Physician, Infectious Disease Unit, Department of Medicine, Massachusetts General Hospital, Boston

ROBERT W. SCHRIER, M.D.
Professor and Chairman, Department of Medicine, University of Colorado School of Medicine, Denver

JOHN S. SCHROEDER, M.D.
Professor of Medicine, Cardiology Division, Stanford University School of Medicine; Stanford University Medical Center, Stanford

MARC A. SCHUCKIT, M.D.
Professor of Psychiatry, School of Medicine, University of California at San Diego; Director, Alcohol Research Center, San Diego Veterans Administration Medical Center, La Jolla

PETER H. SCHUR, M.D.
Professor of Medicine, Department of Rheumatology, Brigham and Women's Hospital, Boston

DAVID S. SEGAL, Ph.D.
Professor of Psychiatry, School of Medicine, University of California at San Diego, La Jolla

JULIAN L. SEIFTER, M.D.
Assistant Professor of Medicine, Harvard Medical School; Associate Physician, Brigham and Women's Hospital, Boston

ANDREW P. SELWYN, M.D.
Associate Professor of Medicine, Harvard Medical School; Director of Cardiac Catheterization, Brigham and Women's Hospital, Boston

BHAGWAN T. SHAHANI, M.B., B.S.
Associate Professor of Neurology, Harvard Medical School; Associate Neurologist, Massachusetts General Hospital, Boston

GORDON C. SHARP, M.D.
Department of Medicine, Division of Immunology and Rheumatology, University of Missouri-Columbia School of Medicine, Columbia

ELIZABETH M. SHORT, M.D.
Director, Division of Biomedical Research and Faculty Development, American Association of Medical Colleges, Washington, D.C.

WILLIAM SILEN, M.D.
Johnson and Johnson Professor of Surgery, Harvard Medical School; Surgeon-in-Chief, Beth Israel Hospital, Boston

FRED E. SILVERSTEIN, M.D.
Professor of Medicine, Director, Gastrointestinal Endoscopy, Division of Gastroenterology, University of Washington School of Medicine, Seattle

THOMAS L. SLAMOWITZ, M.D.
Vice Chairman of Ophthalmology and Associate Professor of Ophthalmology and Neuroophthalmology, Albert Einstein College/Montefiore Medical Center, New York

JAMES B. SNOW, Jr., M.D.
Director, National Institute on Deafness and Other Communication Disorders, National Institutes of Health, Bethesda

ARTHUR SOBER, M.D.
Associate Professor of Dermatology, Harvard Medical School; Associate Chief of Dermatology, Massachusetts General Hospital, Boston

FRANK E. SPEIZER, M.D.
Professor of Medicine, Harvard Medical School; Co-Director, Channing Laboratory, Brigham and Women's Hospital, Boston

WALTER E. STAMM, M.D.
Professor of Medicine, University of Washington School of Medicine; Head, Division of Infectious Diseases, Harborview Medical Center, Seattle

ALLEN C. STEERE, M.D.
Professor of Medicine and Chief, Division of Rheumatology, Department of Medicine, Tufts University School of Medicine, Boston, Massachusetts

ROBERT S. STERN, M.D.
Associate Professor of Dermatology, Harvard Medical School; Beth Israel Hospital, Boston

CHARLES F. STEVENS, M.D., Ph.D.
Professor of Molecular Neurobiology, Salk Institute, La Jolla

GENE H. STOLLERMAN, M.D.
Professor of Medicine, Boston University School of Medicine; Clinical Director, Bedford Division of The Geriatric Research, Educational, and Clinical Center, Veterans Administration Medical Center, Bedford

DAVID H.P. STREETEN, M.B., D. Phil, F.R.C.P.
Professor of Medicine and Head, Section of Endocrinology, State University of New York Upstate Health Science Center, Syracuse

NEIL A. SWANSON, M.D.
Professor of Dermatology, Otolaryngology, and Surgery (Plastic), Division of Plastic Surgery, Oregon Health Sciences University, Portland

ROBERT A. SWERLICK, M.D.
Department of Dermatology, Emory University School of Medicine, Atlanta

RUP TANDAN, M.D., M.R.C.P.
Assistant Professor, Department of Neurology, University of Vermont College of Medicine, Burlington

JOEL D. TAUROG, M.D.
Assistant Professor, The University of Texas Southwestern Medical Center; Southwestern Medical School, Dallas

E. DONNALL THOMAS, M.D.
Professor of Medicine, University of Washington School of Medicine; Member, Fred Hutchinson Cancer Research Center, Seattle

PHILLIP P. TOSKES, M.D.
Professor of Medicine and Chief, Division of Gastroenterology, University of Florida College of Medicine, Gainesville

MARVIN TURCK, M.D.
Professor of Medicine, University of Washington School of Medicine, Seattle

DAVID VALLE, M.D.
Professor of Pediatrics and Molecular Virology and Genetics, Johns Hopkins University School of Medicine; Investigator, Howard Hughes Medical Institute, Baltimore

MAURICE VICTOR, M.D.
Professor of Medicine (Neurology), Dartmouth Medical School, Hanover

DAVID C. WAAGNER, M.D.
Assistant Professor of Pediatrics, Department of Pediatrics, The University of Texas Health Sciences Center, Houston

JAMES F. WALLACE, M.D.
Professor of Medicine, University of Washington School of Medicine; Associate Physician-in-Chief, University Hospital, Seattle

PETER D. WALZER, M.D.
Associate Professor of Medicine, University of Cincinnati College of Medicine; Chief, Infectious Disease Service, Cincinnati Veterans Administration Medical Center, Cincinnati

JACK R. WANDS, M.D.
Associate Professor of Medicine, Harvard Medical School; Molecular Hepatology Laboratory, Cancer Center, Massachusetts General Hospital, Charlestown

LEONARD WARTOFSKY, M.D.
Professor of Medicine and Physiology, Uniformed Services University of the Health Sciences, Bethesda; Chief of Endocrinology and Metabolism, Walter Reed Army Medical Center, Washington, D.C.

STEVEN E. WEINBERGER, M.D.
Associate Professor of Medicine, Harvard Medical School; Clinical Director, Pulmonary Unit, Beth Israel Hospital, Boston

NICHOLAS J. WHITE, M.D., M.R.C.P.
Tropical Medicine Unit, Nuffield Department of Clinical Medicine, Oxford University, England; Faculty of Tropical Medicine, Mahidol University, Bangkok, Thailand

RICHARD J. WHITLEY, M.D.
Professor of Pediatrics, Microbiology, and Medicine, Department of Pediatrics, School of Medicine, The University of Alabama at Birmingham, Birmingham

GRANT R. WILKINSON, M.D.
Professor of Pharmacology, Vanderbilt University School of Medicine, Nashville

GORDON H. WILLIAMS, M.D.
Professor of Medicine, Harvard Medical School; Chief, Endocrine-Hypertension Division, Brigham and Women's Hospital, Boston

LEWIS T. WILLIAMS, Jr., M.D., Ph.D.
Associate Professor of Medicine, University of California at San Francisco School of Medicine; Cardiovascular Research Institute, Howard Hughes Medical Institute, San Francisco

JEAN D. WILSON, M.D.
Professor of Internal Medicine, The University of Texas Southwestern Medical Center, Dallas

BRUCE U. WINTROUB, M.D.
Professor and Chairman, Department of Dermatology, University of California, San Francisco

SHELDON M. WOLFF, M.D.
Endiocott Professor and Chairman, Department of Medicine, Tufts University School of Medicine; New England Medical Center, Boston

ALASTAIR J.J. WOOD, M.B., Ch.B., F.R.C.P. (Edin)
Professor of Medicine and Professor of Pharmacology, Vanderbilt University School of Medicine; Attending Physician, Vanderbilt University Hospital, Nashville

THEODORE E. WOODWARD, M.D.
Professor of Medicine Emeritus, University of Maryland School of Medicine, Baltimore

SHIRLEY H. WRAY, M.D., Ph.D., F.R.C.P.
Associate Professor of Neurology, Harvard Medical School; Director, Unit for Neurovisual Disorders, Department of Neurology, Massachusetts General Hospital, Boston

JOSHUA WYNNE, M.D.
Professor of Internal Medicine and Chief, Division of Cardiology, Wayne State University School of Medicine; Chief, Section of Cardiology, Harper Grace Hospitals, Detroit

KIM B. YANCEY, M.D.
Department of Dermatology, Uniformed Services University of the Health Sciences, Bethesda

JAMES B. YOUNG, M.D.
Associate Professor of Medicine, Harvard Medical School; Associate Physician, Beth Israel Hospital, Boston

PREFACE

In the twelfth edition of *Harrison's Principles of Internal Medicine* the editors have again attempted to incorporate the latest advances in the biology, pathophysiology, diagnosis, and treatment of disease and simultaneously to build appropriate bridges between the basic sciences and clinical medicine and emphasize the advances in medical science while retaining those facts which, while not new, remain clinically useful. Although in a preface we cannot describe all of the new and extensively updated parts of the eleventh edition, we would like to call the reader's attention to several of these:

"Introduction to Clinical Medicine" contains articles on the practice of medicine, clinical reasoning, cost awareness in medicine, and geriatric medicine.

"The Biological Basis of Disease," Part One, has been expanded and given added emphasis as the text's first major topic. It focuses on disorders affecting multiple organ systems, especially genetic diseases and disturbances of the immune system. The section provides more detailed coverage of cell growth and regulation with new chapters on normal cell growth and growth factors and on cell membranes and their receptors.

Now Part Two, "Cardinal Manifestations of Disease" remains a mainstay of this edition and serves as a comprehensive introduction to clinical medicine. Major patient symptoms, reviewed by organ system, are correlated with specific disease states—the basis of differential diagnosis. The twelfth edition contains new or rewritten chapters on chills and fever, visual disturbances, assessment of patients with disorders of cognition, disorders of sleep and circadian rhythm, prevention of cardiovascular collapse and death, and management of the resuscitated patient. The section on skin disease has been completely reorganized.

Part Three, "Clinical Pharmacology," and Part Four, "Nutrition," also have been reorganized. Chapters on clinical pharmacology review the fundamentals of clinical pharmacokinetics and individualized drug therapy. Up-to-date coverage of the physiology and pharmacology of the autonomic nervous system explores its key role in many disease states and the various ways in which drugs interact with this system. Included here as well is a new chapter on cyclic AMP and cellular messengers that work through G proteins.

Coverage of nutrition in clinical medicine encompasses nutritional requirements, the assessment of nutritional status, eating disorders such as anorexia nervosa, bulimia, and obesity, vitamin deficiency and excess, and disturbances in trace element metabolism. New discussions are featured on diet therapy and enteral and parenteral nutrition.

A primarily etiologically oriented review, Part Five, "Infectious Disease," details the latest approaches to the diagnosis, prevention, and treatment of bacterial, viral, and fungal infections and parasitic infestations. A new section focusing on commonly encountered clinical syndromes reviews septicemia and septic shock, infectious endocarditis, localized infections and abscesses, acute infectious diarrheal diseases, sexually transmitted diseases, pelvic inflammatory disease, acute urinary tract infections, infectious arthritis and osteomyelitis, and animal bite and scratch infections. Chapters on the treatment of bacterial, viral, mycotic, and parasitic infections have been grouped together and follow the section on the syndromic approach to infectious diseases.

In addition, a new chapter, "Infectious Diseases and the New Biology," accompanies major updates on host-microbe interactions, immunization, diphtheria, tetanus, botulism, meningococcal infections, salmonella infections, shigellosis, *Haemophilus* infections, cholera, Lyme disease, human retroviruses, Epstein-Barr virus, cytomegalovirus infection, leishmaniasis, trypanosomiasis, and filariasis.

"Disorders of the Organ Systems," the core of *Harrison's*, encompass Parts Six through Fourteen and include succinct accounts of the pathophysiology of major diseases—with emphasis on disease manifestations, diagnostic procedures, differential diagnosis, and treatment strategies. This comprehensive review of organ system disorders includes new chapters on therapeutic applications of cardiac catheterization, mechanical ventilatory support, endocrine tumors of the gastrointestinal tract and pancreas, cancer chemotherapy, breast cancer, benign and malignant skin lesions, gastrointestinal and pancreatic tumors, cognitive disorders, disorders of sleep and circadian rhythm, paraneoplastic diseases that affect the central nervous system, myasthenia gravis, and disorders of phosphorus and magnesium metabolism. Of particular note, the chapter on the acquired immunodeficiency syndrome has been expanded and revised to provide in-depth understanding of all aspects of this disease.

In the twelfth edition the comprehensive review of organ system disorders is complemented by a series of new chapters highlighting the impact of cellular and molecular biology on the understanding of cardiovascular, pulmonary, hematologic, renal, and neurologic disease. The impact of newer imaging techniques on diagnoses is described in chapters on the use of such techniques in diseases of the cardiovascular, pulmonary, hepatobiliary, and central nervous systems.

Finally Part Fifteen is an expanded and reorganized section on "Environmental and Occupational Hazards."

In organizing this edition of *Harrison's* the editors faced the special problem of the dual systems of laboratory nomenclature within the United States. Since July of 1988 virtually all medical journals throughout the world have utilized the International System (SI) of units for clinical laboratory values whereas most hospital laboratories in the United States use the conventional system of laboratory nomenclature. The net consequence is that the student of medicine uses one system in reading medical literature and another in dealing with patients. This dual system will probably be in operation for the indefinite future, and consequently we have decided to use both systems in the text, listing the SI units first and the conventional units in parentheses for all measurements except blood pressure, which is given only in millimeters of mercury, and for those measurements in which the numbers are the same for both systems (mmol/L or meq/L for sodium). In most instances the interconversion between SI and conventional units is straightforward. In other cases, however, the best way to convert from one system to the other is not always clearcut since there are different ways to express values in both. It is imperative that each reader consult his own laboratory for normal values. Perhaps the greatest potential danger inherent in the existence of the two systems is in the interpretation of plasma glucose and plasma calcium, but caution should be observed in the interpretation of all laboratory values.

In view of the requirements for continuing education for licensure and relicensure and of the emphasis on certification and recertification, a revision of the *PreTest Self-Assessment and Review* will appear with this edition. *PreTest Self-Assessment and Review* consists of several hundred questions based upon the textbook, along with answers and explanations for the answers. In addition, the *Companion Handbook* that was pioneered for the eleventh edition for use as a supplement to the text will be revised and updated.

One of the strengths of *Harrison's* is the close-knit relationships among the editors. Dr. Richard K. Root, Professor of Medicine and Associate Dean for Clinical Education at the University of California, San Francisco, worked together with Robert G. Petersdorf to edit the infectious disease coverage of the twelfth edition. We welcome Dr. Root as a valuable member of the editorial group.

We also wish to express our appreciation to our many associates and colleagues who as experts in their fields have helped us with constructive criticism and helpful suggestions: Raymond D. Adams, Carmen Allegra, Julian L. Ambrus, Jr., W. French Anderson, David

W. Bilheimer, Homer Boushey, George A. Bray, Barry M. Brenner, Neil A. Breslau, Michael S. Brown, William J. Burke, Harold A. Chapman, Allen W. Cheever, William W. Chin, Fred Cohen, Shaun Coughlin, George T. Curlin, Pat O. Daley, Richard T. Davey, Jr., Gregory J. Dehmer, Victor J. Dzau, Judith Falloon, Robert Fishman, Daniel W. Foster, Stephen Friend, Joseph L. Goldstein, Mark R. Green, James E. Griffin, Donald H. Harter, Jane E. Henney, Gary Hoffman, Allan Hunter, Steve Hyman, Roland H. Ingram, Jr., Seigo Izumo, Michael Jenike, Stephanie L. James, T. Scott Johnson, William S. Jordan, Jr., Lewis L. Judd, Robert E. Kalina, Robert Katzman, Joyce V. Kelly, Jeff Klein, Joseph A. Kovacs, Thomas J. Lawley, Robert S. Lebovics, John Leddy, Kenneth Luskey, James D. Marsh, Michael Matthay, Dale E. McFarlin, Steve McPhee, John Mendelsohn, John Mills, Eva J. Neer, Arthur W. Niehnuis, Frederick P. Ognibene, Steve Perkins, Dorothy Perloff, Stephen Petersdorf, Michael A. Polis, Herbert Y. Reynolds, William O. Robertson, Mark Rosenblum, Burton D. Rose, Daniel Rotrosen, Eugene H. Rubin, Walter Rubin, Kenneth Sack, Steven Schnittman, Christine E. Seidman, Julian Seifter, James H. Shelhamer, Gordon Strewler, Anthony F. Suffredini, Martin Tauber, Mark Taubman, Steven E. Weinberger, J. Woodrow Weiss, Scott Weiss, J.B. West, Peggy Wintroub, Daniel T. Wright, and Charles F. Zormuski.

This book could not have been edited without the dedicated help of our coworkers in the editorial offices of the individual editors. We are especially indebted to Patricia A. Clougherty, Hilda Gardner, Christy K. Gonzales, Brenda H. Hennis, Ann London, Joyce McKinney, Lucy A. Renzi, Kathryn A. Saxon, S. Horatio Slawson, Sandra Taylor, and Betsy Zickler.

Finally, we need to say a word of thanks to our colleagues at McGraw-Hill, J. Dereck Jeffers, Editor-in-Chief, and Stuart Boynton, Development Editor. They are an effective team who gave the editors constant encouragement and were of enormous help in the efforts involved in bringing this edition to fruition.

THE EDITORS

INTRODUCTION TO CLINICAL MEDICINE

1 THE PRACTICE OF MEDICINE

THE EDITORS

WHAT IS EXPECTED OF THE PHYSICIAN The practice of medicine combines both science and art. The role of science in medicine is clear. Technology based on science is the foundation for the solution to many clinical problems; the dazzling advances in biochemical methodology and in biophysical imaging techniques that allow access to the remotest recesses of the body are the products of science. So too are the therapeutic maneuvers which increasingly are a major part of medical practice. Yet skill in the most sophisticated application of laboratory technology or the use of the latest therapeutic modality alone does not make a good physician. The ability to extract from a mass of contradictory physical signs and from the crowded computer printouts of laboratory data those items that are of crucial significance, to know in a difficult case whether to "treat" or to "watch," to determine when a clinical clue is worth pursuing or when to dismiss it as a "red herring," and to estimate in any given patient whether a proposed treatment entails a greater risk than the disease are all involved in the decisions which the clinician, skilled in the practice of medicine, must make many times each day. This combination of medical knowledge, intuition, and judgment is termed the *art of medicine*. It is as necessary to the practice of medicine as a sound scientific base.

The editors of the first edition of this book defined what is expected of the physician. Their words ring as true now as they did then.

No greater opportunity, responsibility, or obligation can fall to the lot of a human being than to become a physician. In the care of the suffering he needs technical skill, scientific knowledge, and human understanding. He who uses these with courage, with humility, and with wisdom will provide a unique service for his fellow man, and will build an enduring edifice of character within himself. The physician should ask of his destiny no more than this; he should be content with no less.

Tact, sympathy and understanding are expected of the physician, for the patient is no mere collection of symptoms, signs, disordered functions, damaged organs, and disturbed emotions. He is human, fearful, and hopeful, seeking relief, help and reassurance. To the physician, as to the anthropologist, nothing human is strange or repulsive. The misanthrope may become a smart diagnostician of organic disease, but he can scarcely hope to succeed as a physician. The true physician has a Shakespearean breadth of interest in the wise and the foolish, the proud and the humble, the stoic hero and the whining rogue. He cares for people.

THE PATIENT-PHYSICIAN RELATIONSHIP It may be trite to emphasize that physicians need to approach patients not as "cases" or "diseases" but as individuals whose problems all too often transcend the complaints which bring them to the doctor. Most patients are anxious and frightened. Often they go to great ends to convince themselves that illness does not exist, or unconsciously they set up elaborate defenses to divert attention from the real problem that they perceive to be serious or life-threatening. Some patients use illness to gain attention or to serve as a crutch to extricate themselves from an emotionally stressful situation; some even feign physical illness. Whatever the patient's attitude, the physician needs to consider the terrain in which an illness occurs—in terms not only of the patients themselves but also of their families and social backgrounds. All too often medical workups and records fail to include essential information about the patient's origins, schooling, job, home and family, hopes and fears. Without this knowledge it is difficult for the physician to gain rapport with the patient or to develop insight into the patient's illness. Such a relationship must be based on thorough knowledge of the patient and on mutual trust and the ability to communicate with one another.

The direct, one-to-one patient-physician relationship which traditionally has characterized the practice of medicine is changing, primarily because of the changing setting in which medicine is being practiced. Often the management of the individual patient requires the active participation of a variety of trained professional personnel as well as several physicians. In most instances, health care is a team effort. The patient can benefit greatly from such collaboration, but it is the duty of the primary physician to guide the patient through an illness. To carry out this increasingly difficult task, this physician must have some familiarity with the techniques, skills, and objectives of specialist physicians as well as colleagues in the fields allied to medicine. In giving the patient an opportunity to receive all the benefits of the important advances of science, the primary physician must, in the last analysis, retain responsibility for the major decisions concerning diagnosis and treatment.

Increasingly, patients are cared for by groups of physicians, clinics, hospitals, or health-maintenance organizations (HMOs) rather than by individual independent practitioners. There are many potential advantages in the use of such organized medical groups, but there are also drawbacks, the chief of which is a loss of the concept of a physician who is primarily and continuously responsible for the patient. It is essential, even in the group setting, that each patient have a physician who has an overview of the patient's problems and who maintains familiarity with the patient's reaction to his or her illness, to the drugs given, and to the challenges of daily living that the patient faces. Moreover, because a number of physicians may, at any one time, contribute to the care of a particular patient, accurate and detailed medical records are essential to patient care.

The modern hospital poses a particularly intimidating environment for most patients. Lying in a bed surrounded by air jets, buttons, and lights; invaded by tubes and wires; beset by the numerous members of the health care team—nurses, nurses' aides, physicians' assistants, social workers, technologists, physical therapists, medical students, house officers, attending and consulting physicians, and many others; transported to special laboratories and x-ray chambers replete with machines with blinking lights and strange sounds, it is little wonder that patients lose their sense of reality. In fact, the physician is often the only tenuous link between the patient and the real world. A strong personal relationship with the physician is essential in order to sustain the patient in such a stressful situation.

Many influences in contemporary society have the potential of leading to the impersonalization of medical care. Some of these have been mentioned already and include (1) vigorous efforts to reduce the escalating costs of health care; (2) the increasing reliance on technologic advances and computerization for many aspects of diagnosis and treatment; (3) the increased geographic mobility of both patients and physicians; (4) the growing number of "closed-system" arrangements, such as health maintenance organizations, in which the patient has little if any choice in selecting a physician; (5) the need for more than a single physician to be involved in the care of most patients who are seriously ill; and (6) an increasing reliance by patients on legal means to express their disappointments with the health care system (i.e., by malpractice litigation). Given these changes in the medical care system, maintaining the humane aspects of medical care and the empathetic qualities of the physician is a particular challenge. It is now more important than ever that the physician consider each patient to be a unique individual deserving of humane treatment, regardless of personal or financial circumstances.

The American Board of Internal Medicine has defined humanistic qualities as encompassing integrity, respect, and compassion. Availability, the expression of sincere concern, the willingness to take the time to explain all aspects of the patient's illness, and an attitude of being nonjudgmental with patients who have lifestyles, attitudes, and values different from those of the physician and which he or she may in some instances even find repugnant are just a few of the characteristics of the humane physician. Every physician will, at times, be challenged by patients who evoke strongly negative (and occasionally strongly positive) emotional responses. Physicians should be alert to their own reactions to such patients and situations and consciously monitor and control their behavior so that the patients' best interests remain the principal motivation for their actions at all times.

The famous statement of Dr. Francis Peabody is even more relevant today than when delivered more than a half century ago:

The significance of the intimate personal relationship between physician and patient cannot be too strongly emphasized, for in an extraordinarily large number of cases both the diagnosis and treatment are directly dependent on it. One of the essential qualities of the clinician is interest in humanity, for the secret of the care of the patient is in caring for the patient.

CLINICAL SKILLS History taking The written history of an illness should embody all the facts of medical significance in the life of the patient. If the history is recorded in chronologic order, recent events should be given the most attention. Likewise, if a problem-oriented approach is used, the problems that are clinically dominant should be listed first. Ideally, the narration of symptoms or problems should be in the patient's own words. However, few patients have sufficient powers of observation or recall to give a history without some guidance from the physician, who must be careful not to suggest the answers to the questions being posed. Often a symptom which has concerned a patient has little significance, while a seemingly minor complaint may be of considerable importance. Therefore, the physician must be constantly alert to the possibility that any event related by the patient, however trivial or apparently remote, may be the key to the solution of the medical problem.

An informative history is more than an orderly listing of symptoms. Something is always gained by listening to patients and noting the way in which they talk about their symptoms. Inflections of voice, facial expression, and attitude may betray important clues to the meaning of the symptoms to the patient. In listening to the history, the physician discovers not only something about the disease but also something about the patient.

With experience, the pitfalls of history taking become apparent. What patients relate for the most part consists of subjective phenomena colored by past experience. Patients obviously differ widely in their responses to the same stimuli and in their coping mechanisms. Their attitudes are variably influenced by fear of disability and death and by concern over the consequences of their illness to their families. Sometimes the accuracy of the history is affected by language or sociologic barriers, by failing intellectual powers that interfere with recall, or by disorders of consciousness that make them unaware of their illness. It is not surprising, then, that even the most careful physician may at times despair of collecting factual data and be forced to proceed with evidence that represents little more than an approximation of the truth. It is in obtaining the history that the physician's skill, knowledge, and experience are most clearly in evidence.

The family history serves several functions. First, in rare single-gene defects a positive family history of a similarly affected individual or a history of consanguinity may have important diagnostic implications. Second, in diseases of multifactorial etiology that have a familial aggregation, it may be possible to identify patients at risk for disease and to intervene prior to development of overt manifestations. For example, recent weight gain may be a more ominous development in a woman who has a family history of diabetes than in one who does not. In certain situations the family history has major implications for preventive medicine. When a diagnosis of a hereditary condition known to predispose to cancer is made, it is the physician's obligation to follow up this possibility carefully in the patient, to survey the family, and to educate them about the need for long-term follow-up.

However accurate and complete, the medical history does much more than provide facts of critical importance. The very act of taking the history provides the physician with the opportunity to establish or enhance the unique bond that is the basis for the critically important patient-physician relationship. An effort should be made to place the patient at ease, regardless of the circumstances of the encounter. The patient should, at some point, have the opportunity to tell his or her own story of the illness without frequent interruption and, when appropriate, should receive expression of interest, encouragement, and empathy from the physician. It is often enlightening to develop an appreciation of the patient's own perception of the illness, the patient's expectations of the physician and the medical care system, and the financial and social implications of the illness to the patient. The confidentiality of the patient-physician relationship should be emphasized, and the patient should be given the opportunity to identify those aspects of the history which he or she wishes not to be disclosed to anyone else.

Physical examination Physical signs are the objective and verifiable marks of disease and represent solid, indisputable facts. Their significance is enhanced when they confirm a functional or structural change already suggested by the patient's history. At times, the physical signs may be the only evidence of disease, especially when the history has been inconsistent, confused, or lacking altogether.

The physical examination should be performed methodically and thoroughly, with due regard for the patient's comfort and modesty. Although attention has often been directed by the history to the diseased organ or part of the body, the examination must extend from head to toe in an objective search for abnormalities. Unless the examination procedure is systematic, important parts of it may be omitted, a common error even among the most skilled clinicians. The results of the examination, like the details of the history, should be recorded at the time they are elicited, not hours later when they are subject to the distortions of memory. Many inaccuracies stem from the careless practice of writing or dictating notes long after the examination has been concluded. Skill in physical diagnosis is acquired with experience, but it is not merely technique that determines success in eliciting signs. The detection of a few scattered petechiae, a faint diastolic murmur, or a small mass in the abdomen is not a question of keener eyes and ears or more sensitive fingers but of a mind alert to these findings. Skill in physical diagnosis reflects a way of thinking more than a way of doing. Physical findings are subject to change. Just because the examination is normal on one occasion does not guarantee that this will be the case on subsequent examinations. Likewise, abnormal findings may disappear in the course of illness. It is important, therefore, to repeat the physical examination as frequently as the clinical situation warrants.

Laboratory tests The increase in the number and availability of laboratory tests has resulted in increasing reliance on these studies in the solution of clinical problems. It is essential, however, to bear in mind the limitations of such procedures, which by virtue of their impersonal quality and complexity often gain an aura of authority regardless of the fallibility of the tests themselves, of the individuals doing or interpreting them, or of their instruments. More importantly, the accumulation of laboratory data cannot relieve the physician from the responsibility of careful observation and study of the patient. Physicians also must weigh carefully the hazards and the expense involved in the laboratory procedures they order. Moreover, laboratory tests are rarely ordered and reported singly. Rather, they are produced as "batteries." Some laboratories now perform batteries of 24 and even 40 tests. The various combinations of laboratory tests are often useful. For example, they may provide the clue to such nonspecific symptoms as generalized weakness and increased fatigability by revealing abnormalities of hepatic function together with elevated levels of serum IgG which, in turn, would suggest the diagnosis of chronic liver disease. Sometimes a single abnormality, such as an elevated serum calcium, points to a specific disease, such as hyperparathyroidism.

The thoughtful use of screening tests should not be confused with indiscriminate laboratory testing. The use of screening tests is based on the fact that a group of laboratory determinations can be carried out conveniently on a single specimen of blood at relatively low cost. Biochemical measurements, together with simple laboratory examinations such as blood count, urinalysis, and sedimentation rate, often provide the major clue to the presence of a pathologic process. At the same time the physican must learn to evaluate occasional abnormalities among the screening tests that may not necessarily connote significant disease. There is nothing more wasteful and unproductive than an in-depth workup following a report of an isolated laboratory abnormality in a patient who is otherwise well. Among the more than 40 tests that are performed on many patients, one is often slightly abnormal. If there is no suspicion of an underlying illness, the test is ordinarily repeated to ensure that the abnormality does not represent a laboratory error. If the abnormality is confirmed it is important to distinguish a minor one (less than two standard deviations) from a major one (more than two standard deviations). Even in the case of the latter, the decision of whether to proceed with further workup is a test of the physician's clinical judgment.

Imaging techniques The past two decades have seen the arrival of ultrasonography, a variety of scans that employ isotopes to visualize organs heretofore inaccessible, computed tomography with its varying permutations, magnetic resonance imaging, and position emission tomography. Aside from opening up new diagnostic vistas, this new technology benefits patients because it has frequently supplanted invasive techniques that require surgical biopsy or the insertion of tubes, wires, or catheters into the body—procedures that are often painful and sometimes risky. While the enthusiasm for noninvasive technology is understandably justified, all too often the results of these tests have not been validated properly before they are disseminated as clinical dogma. Moreover, the expense entailed in performing these imaging tests is often substantial and is not always considered when ordering them. There is no question that computed tomography has led to new insights into the problem of adrenal tumors, just as routine measurement of calcium caused a redefinition of hyperparathyroidism. Nevertheless, these examinations should be used judiciously, preferably in lieu of, not in addition to, the invasive maneuvers they are meant to replace.

THE DIAGNOSIS OF DISEASE Clinical diagnosis requires both aspects of logic—analysis and synthesis—and the more difficult the clinical problem, the more important is a logical approach to it. Such an approach requires that the physician list carefully each problem suggested by the symptoms and physical and laboratory findings and seek answers to each. Most physicians attempt consciously or unconsciously to fit a given problem into one of a series of syndromes. *The syndrome is a group of symptoms and signs of disordered function, related to one another by means of some anatomic, physiologic, or biochemical peculiarity.* It embodies a hypothesis concerning the deranged function of an organ, organ system, or tissue. Congestive heart failure, Cushing's syndrome, and dementia are examples. In congestive heart failure, dyspnea, orthopnea, cyanosis, dependent edema, engorged neck veins, pleural effusion, rales, and hepatomegaly are known to be connected by a single pathophysiologic mechanism—insufficiency of the cardiac pump mechanism. In Cushing's syndrome, moon facies, hypertension, diabetes mellitus, and osteoporosis are recognized effects of excess glucocorticoids acting on many target organs. In dementia, deterioration of memory, incoherent thinking, impaired language functions, visual-spatial disorientation, and faulty judgment are related to destruction of the association areas of the cerebrum.

A syndrome usually does not identify the precise cause of an illness, but it narrows the number of possibilities and often suggests certain special clinical and laboratory studies. The derangements of each organ system in humans are reducible to a relatively small number of syndromes. The diagnosis is simplified greatly if a clinical problem conforms neatly to a well-defined syndrome, because only a few diseases need to be considered in the differential diagnosis. In contrast, the search for the cause of an illness that does not conform to a syndrome is more difficult because a much greater number of diseases have to be considered. Even here an orderly approach which proceeds from symptom to sign to laboratory findings will usually result in the diagnosis.

CARING FOR THE PATIENT Patient care begins with the development of a personal relationship between the patient and the physician. In the absence of a sense of trust and confidence on the part of the patient, the effectiveness of most therapeutic measures is diminished. In many instances, when there is confidence in the physician, reassurance is the best treatment and is all that is needed. Likewise, in those cases that do not lend themselves to easy solutions and for which no effective treatment is available, a feeling on the part of the patient that the physician is doing all that is possible is one of the most important therapeutic measures that can be provided. An important aspect of clinical decision making and patient care involves the "quality of life," a subjective assessment of what each patient values most. Such an assessment requires detailed, sometimes intimate knowledge of the patient, which can usually be obtained only through deliberate, unhurried, and often repeated conversation. In situations where complete freedom from signs and symptoms of disease is impossible, enhancement of the quality of life is the major goal of therapy.

Drug therapy With each succeeding year, more drugs are released, every one with the hope and the promise that it is an improvement over its predecessor. Although the pharmaceutical industry must be given most of the credit for advances in drug therapy, it is also true that many new drugs have only a marginal advantage over the agents they are aimed to replace. The barrage of new information with which practitioners are deluged does little to provide a clear picture of clinical pharmacology; on the contrary, to most physicians new drugs are confusing. With some exceptions, however, the approach to a new drug should be one of caution. Unless the new agent is established beyond doubt to be a real advance, it is wiser to use well-tested and well-established agents which are efficacious and whose safety is well established.

Iatrogenic disorders An iatrogenic disorder occurs when the deleterious effects of a therapeutic or diagnostic regimen produce pathology independent of the condition for which the regimen is given. No matter what the clinical situation, it is the responsibility of the physician to use powerful therapeutic measures wisely, with due regard to their action, potential dangers, and cost. Every medical procedure, whether diagnostic or therapeutic, has the potential for harm, but it would be impossible to afford the patient the benefits of modern scientific medicine if reasonable steps in diagnosis and therapy were withheld because of possible risks. "Reasonable" implies that the physician has weighed the pros and cons of a procedure and has concluded that it is advisable or essential for the relief of discomfort or the cure or amelioration of disease. For example, the use of glucocorticoids to arrest progressive systemic lupus erythematosus may produce Cushing's syndrome. In this instance, the benefits usually exceed the untoward side effects. However, much harm can result when the deleterious effects of a procedure or a drug exceed any possible advantages that might have been anticipated. Examples include the dangerous or fatal drug reactions that occasionally follow the use of antibiotics given for trivial respiratory infections, the gastric hemorrhage or perforation caused by glucocorticoid administration for mild arthritis, or the occurrence of fatal hepatitis that may follow needless transfusions of blood or plasma.

But the harm that a physician can do to a patient is not limited to the imprudent use of medication or procedures. Equally important are ill-considered or unjustified remarks. Many a patient has developed a cardiac neurosis because the physician ventured a grave prognosis on the basis of a misinterpreted noninvasive cardiac examination. Not only the treatment itself but the physician's words and behavior are capable of causing injury.

The physician must never become so absorbed in the disease as to forget the patient who is its victim. As the science of medicine advances, it is all too easy to become so fascinated by the manifestations of disease that the ailing person's fears and concerns about suffering and death, job and family, the cost of medical care, and the specter of economic insecurity are disregarded. Treatment of a patient consists of more than the dispassionate confrontation of a disease. It embodies also the exercise of warmth, compassion, and understanding.

Informed consent In an era of rapidly advancing technology, patients will require diagnostic and therapeutic procedures that are painful and that pose some risk. These include all surgical procedures, e.g., biopsies of tissues, endoscopy, radiographic maneuvers involving the insertion of catheters, and many others. In most hospitals and clinics, patients undergoing such procedures are required to sign a form consenting to them. More important, however, is the notion that the patient must understand clearly the risk entailed in these procedures; this is the definition of *informed consent*. It is incumbent upon the physician to explain to the patient, in a clearly understandable fashion, the procedures which he or she faces. By doing this conscientiously much of the dread of the unknown that is inherent in hospitalization will be mitigated.

Accountability Throughout the world physicians, once licensed to practice medicine, have not had to account for their actions except to their peers. In the United States, however, during the past two decades, there have been increasing demands for physicians to account for the way in which they practice medicine by meeting certain standards prescribed by federal and state governments. The hospitalization of patients whose health care is reimbursed by the government (Medicare and Medicaid) and other third parties is subjected to utilization review. This means that the physician must defend the cause for and duration of a patient's hospitalization if it falls outside certain "average" standards. In some instances a second opinion is necessary before a patient can have elective surgery. The purpose of these regulations is to contain spiraling health care costs. It is likely that this type of review will be extended to all phases of medical practice and will alter the practice of medicine even more profoundly.

Physicians also may be expected to give account of their continuing competence by mandatory continuing education, patient record audit, recertification by examination (time-limited certification), or relicensing. While these measures probably enhance the physician's factual knowledge, there is no evidence that they have a similar effect on the quality of practice.

Cost-effectiveness in medical care As the cost of medical care continues to rise, it has become necessary to establish stringent priorities in the expenditure of money for health care. In some instances, preventive measures offer the greatest return for the expenditure; outstanding examples include vaccination, immunization, reduction in accidents and occupational hazards, improved environmental control, and biochemical screening of newborns. For example, the detection of phenylketonuria by newborn screening may result in a net saving of many thousands of dollars.

As resources become more and more constrained, it will be necessary to weigh the justification of performing costly operations that provide only a limited life expectancy against the pressing need for more primary care for those persons who do not have adequate access to medical services. At the level of the individual patient it is important to minimize costly hospital admissions as far as possible, if total health care is to be provided at a cost that most can afford. This, of course, implies and depends upon a close cooperative effort between patients, their physicians, their employers, third-party carriers, and government, along with constant surveillance of those types of procedures that can be conducted safely and effectively on an ambulatory basis. Equally important in reducing total health care expenditures is the need for individual physicians to monitor both the cost and effectiveness of the drugs they prescribe. In the last analysis the medical profession should provide leadership and guidance to the public in matters of cost control, and physicians must take this responsibility seriously without being or seeming to be self-serving. It is important, however, that the socioeconomic aspects of health care delivery not be permitted to interfere with the concern of physicians for the welfare of their patients. The patient must be able to rely on the individual physician as his or her principal advocate in matters of health care.

Research and teaching The title "doctor" is derived from the Latin *docere,* "to teach," and the physician should share information and medical knowledge with others and be willing to teach what he or she has learned to colleagues as well as to students of medicine and related professions. The practice of medicine is dependent on the sum total of medical knowledge, which in turn is based on an unending chain of scientific discovery, clinical observation, analysis, and interpretation. Advances in medicine depend on the acquisition of new information, i.e., on research, which must often involve patients; improved medical care requires the transmission of this information. As part of broader societal responsibilities, the physician should encourage patients to participate in ethical and properly approved clinical investigations if they do not impose undue hazard, discomfort, or inconvenience.

Incurability and death No problem is more distressing than that presented by the patient with an incurable disease, particularly when premature death is inevitable. What should the patient and family be told, what measures should be taken to maintain life, and how is death to be defined?

Although some would argue otherwise, there is no ironclad rule that the patient must immediately be told "everything," even if the patient is an adult and the head of a family. How much the patient is told should depend upon the patient's ability and capacity to deal with the possibility of imminent death; often this capacity grows with time and, whenever possible, gradual rather than abrupt disclosure is the best strategy. This decision may also take into consideration the patient's religious beliefs, financial and business status, and to some extent the wishes of the family. The patient must be given an opportunity to talk with the physician and ask questions. Patients may find it easier to share their feelings about death with their physician, who is likely to be more objective and less emotional than family members.

One thing is certain; it is not for you to don the black cap and, assuming the judicial function, take hope away from any patient . . . hope that comes to us all.

William Osler

Even when the patient directly inquires, "Doctor, am I dying?" the physician must attempt to determine whether this is a request for information, a demand for reassurance, or even an expression of hostility. Most would agree that only open communication between the patient and the physician can resolve these questions and guide the physician in what to say and how to say it.

The physician should provide or arrange for emotional, physical, and spiritual support and must be compassionate, unhurried, and open. Pain should be adequately controlled, human dignity maintained, and isolation from family avoided. The last two in particular tend to be overlooked in hospitals, where the intrusion of life-sustaining apparatus can so easily detract from attention to the whole person and concentrate instead on the life-threatening disease. The physician must also prepare to deal with guilt feelings on the part of the family when a member becomes gravely or hopelessly ill. It is important for the doctor to reassure the family that everything possible has been done.

The President's Committee for the Study of Ethical Problems in Medicine defined death as (1) irreversible cessation of circulatory and respiratory function or (2) irreversible cessation of all functions of the entire brain, including the brainstem. Clinical and electroencephalographic criteria permit the reliable diagnosis of cerebral death. According to the criteria adopted by the staff of the Massachusetts General Hospital and the Harvard Committee on Brain Death, death occurs when all signs of receptivity and responsivity are absent, including all brainstem reflexes (pupillary reactions, ocular movement, blinking, swallowing, breathing), and the electroencephalogram is isoelectric. Occasionally, intoxications and metabolic disorders may simulate this state; hence the diagnosis requires expert evaluation. Under the aforementioned circumstances, to continue with heroic, highly costly supportive measures merely for the purpose of preserving cardiac function is against the best interests of patient, family, and society. In such instances, the dilemma of continuing care could be avoided if the medical profession, in accord with social sanction, can be brought to redefine life and death by these criteria.

A practice that has proved acceptable in many settings is as follows:

1 The diagnosis of brain death, based on the above criteria, should be corroborated by another physician and confirmed by clinical examination and EEG, repeated one or more times.
2 The family should be informed of the irreversibility of brain function but should not be requested to ratify the decision whether the medical treatment should be discontinued. An exception to this limited decision-making power of the family might apply where the patient has directed the family that he or she wishes them to make the decision.
3 The physician, after consultation with a professional colleague, may withdraw supportive measures, assuming that nothing more can be offered.
4 The possibility that such patients may become sources of organs for grafting should not enter into the aforementioned decisions, although prior to the cessation of heart action the family may be asked whether this would be their wish, or the family may suggest that organs be used for this purpose.

"Do not resuscitate" orders and cessation of therapy When carried out in a timely and expert manner, cardiopulmonary resuscitation is often useful in the prevention of sudden, unexpected death. However, unless there are reasons to the contrary it should not be carried out when it merely prolongs life in a patient with terminal, incurable disease. The decision not to resuscitate a patient and decisions about the intensity of therapy and, indeed, whether or not treatment is to be delivered at all to patients who are incurably and terminally ill must be reviewed frequently and must take into consideration any unexpected changes in the patient's condition. These decisions must also take into account both the underlying medical condition and the wishes of the patient or, if these cannot or have not been ascertained directly, those of a close relative or other surrogate who can be relied upon to transmit the patient's feelings and to be guided by the patient's best interests. The issues involving death and dying are among the most difficult in medicine. In approaching them rationally and consistently, the physician must combine the art and the science of medicine.

2 QUANTITATIVE ASPECTS OF CLINICAL REASONING

LEE GOLDMAN

The process of clinical reasoning is poorly understood but is based upon factors such as experience and learning, inductive and deductive reasoning, interpretation of evidence that itself varies in reproducibility and validity, and intuition that often is difficult to define. In an effort to improve clinical reasoning, a number of attempts have been made to analyze quantitatively the many factors involved, including defining the cognitive approaches that clinicians apply to difficult problems, devising computerized decision support systems that are designed to emulate certain features of decision making, and applying decision theory to understand how judgments should be reached. While each of these approaches has advanced the understanding of the diagnostic process, all have practical and/or theoretical problems that limit their direct applicability to the care of the individual patient.

Nevertheless, these preliminary attempts to apply the rigor and logic inherent in the quantitative method have provided significant insights into the process by which clinical reasoning is accomplished, have identified ways in which the process may be improved, and have made it possible to minimize certain features of the workup that are not cost-effective. Thus, while clinical reasoning cannot be reduced to probabilities or numbers, attempts at quantitative analysis of the process may improve the ways in which the problems of individual patients are approached and solved.

In a simplified model, quantitative clinical reasoning includes five phases. The *first* consists of an investigation of the chief complaint through key questions that are included in the history of the present illness (Table 2-1). These questions are supplemented by the past medical history and by a physical examination that emphasizes detailed investigation of potential key organ systems. In the *second* phase, the physician may select from an array of diagnostic tests, each with its own accuracy and usefulness for investigating the possibilities raised in the differential diagnosis. Since each test has its costs, and some entail risk and discomfort as well, the physician must ask whether the history and physical examination are sufficiently diagnostic before ordering tests. *Third*, the clinical data must be integrated with test results to estimate the likelihood of conditions in the differential diagnosis. *Fourth*, the comparative risks and benefits of further diagnostic and therapeutic options must be weighed to reach a recommendation for the patient. In the *fifth* and final phase, this recommendation is presented to the patient, and after appropriate discussion of the options, a therapeutic plan is initiated. Each of the five steps in this simplified model of the clinical reasoning process can be analyzed individually.

HISTORY AND PHYSICAL EXAMINATION It originally had been assumed that physicians begin investigating a patient's chief complaint by obtaining a comprehensive history, which includes many if not most of the questions included in a full review of systems, and by performing an all-inclusive physical examination. However, experienced clinicians begin to form hypotheses based on the chief complaint and on the responses to initial questioning, and they ask further questions in a sequence that allows them to evaluate the initial

TABLE 2-1 Phases of clinical reasoning and decision making

1	Investigation of the complaint by means of clinical examination (history and physical examination)
2	Ordering of diagnostic tests, each with its own intrinsic accuracy and usefulness
3	Integration of clinical findings with test results to assess diagnostic probabilities
4	Weighing of comparative risks and benefits of alternative courses of action
5	Determination of patient's preferences and development of a therapeutic plan

hypotheses and, if necessary, shorten or amend the list of possibilities. Only a limited number of diagnostic hypotheses can be entertained at any one time, and information is used to build a case for or against the most likely. In such a way, high-priority questions are selected from the almost limitless number that might be asked, and these specific questions are incorporated into the history of the present illness. Often, a key response, such as a history of melena, will be selected, a list of potential explanations for it will be formulated, and this list will then be trimmed, based on the response to more probing questions, so that a principal diagnosis can be selected and then tested. This process, termed *iterative hypothesis testing*, is an efficient approach to diagnosis and is preferable to attempts to gather every conceivable piece of information prior to formulating a differential diagnosis.

Advocacy of iterative hypothesis testing does not argue against the need for a systematic, thorough, and complete history of the present illness, past medical history, review of systems, family history, social history, and physical examination. For example, if a patient presents with abdominal pain, the physician should gather information regarding its location and quality as well as the factors that precipitate and/or relieve it. The physician then asks questions relating to the diagnoses that may be suspected based on the response to the initial questions. If the pain is suggestive of pancreatitis, the clinician would ask about alcohol intake, the use of thiazide diuretics or glucocorticosteroids, symptoms suggestive of concomitant gallbladder disease, a family history of pancreatitis, and questions aimed at uncovering the possibility of a posterior penetrating ulcer. Alternatively, if the discomfort seems more typical of reflux esophagitis, a different sequence of questions would be triggered. The use of iterative hypothesis testing encourages the physician to elicit detailed information in high-yield areas, without forgoing a systematic and thorough approach to the patient. Findings on the history and physical examination should influence each other. The history focuses the physical examination on certain organs, and findings on physical examination should encourage more detailed review of certain systems.

As physicians proceed through this reasoning process with both the history and physical examination, a variety of issues may influence the accuracy of the decision-making process. First is the potential for some historical information or physical findings to be poorly reproducible, either because the patient's responses vary or because different physicians elicit information differently or vary in the way they interpret the answers. The careful use of clear, and when possible, precise questions can increase the reproducibility and validity of the medical history, but still cannot eliminate all variability.

When assessing the reproducibility of findings on the physical examination, two observers frequently agree that an uncommon abnormality such as an enlarged spleen is not present but agree less often when one of them thinks that it is present in a patient in whom it would not usually be expected. This principle can best be demonstrated by understanding that some agreement always occurs by chance, and the likelihood of chance agreement is higher if the finding is either very common or very uncommon. For example, if two physicians each consider 90 percent of patients to be abnormal in some manner, such as having a systolic heart murmur, they will agree 81 percent of the time by chance alone. In some studies of the reproducibility of common signs and symptoms, such as an enlarged liver, actual agreement rates have not been substantially better than chance. Disagreement rates may be reduced by emphasizing physical examination skills during medical training, by looking for other correlative physical findings, and by learning how physical findings correlate with the results of diagnostic tests. Therefore, when a clinician notes an unexpected and somewhat subjective abnormality for which there may be a high rate of interobserver disagreement, such as an unexpectedly enlarged spleen, other abnormalities that may often be associated with it, such as hepatomegaly or lymphadenopathy, should be sought to increase the likelihood that the spleen would be expected to be abnormal. In some situations, ordering a diagnostic test, such as a liver and spleen scan, to assess the finding more objectively should be considered if the test is sufficiently reliable.

These comments about the factors that limit the reproducibility and validity of the medical history and physical examination do not denigrate their critical importance in clinical reasoning. Rather, they emphasize that care and diligence in the application of these skills are necessary. For example, careful auscultation of the heart during various bedside maneuvers (see Chap. 175) has been shown to be remarkably accurate in determining the cause of systolic murmurs.

When physicians use the history and the physical examination to arrive at a diagnosis, they are rarely certain of it. Therefore, it would be better to assess the likelihood of the diagnosis in terms of probabilities. All too frequently, this probability is not expressed as an actual percentage but rather in such terms as "nearly always," "commonly," "sometimes," or "rarely." Since different physicians may assign different probabilities to the same terms, these imprecise words frequently lead to major misunderstandings among physicians or between the physician and the patient. Physicians should be as rigorous and quantitative as possible in their assessments, and when feasible, a quantitative expression of probability should be used. For example, rather than saying that it is unlikely that a radiographic pattern is indicative of a carcinoma of the colon, it would be preferable, if possible, to provide a more precise indication of the probability of carcinoma with this radiographic pattern. A 10 to 15 percent probability of carcinoma may be interpreted as "unlikely," but from a clinical perspective usually warrants further evaluation because of the serious consequences of missing a potentially resectable tumor.

Although such quantitative estimates would be desirable, they usually are not available in practice. Even experienced physicians often are unable to estimate accurately the likelihood of particular conditions. There is a tendency to overestimate the likelihood of relatively uncommon conditions, and physicians are especially poor at quantifying probabilities that are very high or very low. For example, a physician may not know whether the probability of bacterial meningitis or of another disease that could be diagnosed by a lumbar puncture in a patient with a severe headache is 1 in 20 or 1 in 2000. In both situations, the probability is low, but the decision as to whether a lumbar puncture should be performed may depend on this estimate.

As was emphasized in Chap. 1, the history and physical examination have other important purposes. They allow the physician to evaluate the emotional status of the patient and to understand how the present problems fit into the context of the patient's social and family life, and they encourage the development in the patient of confidence in the physician, which is so necessary for reaching an agreement on the coming plan of action.

DIAGNOSTIC TESTS: INDICATIONS, ACCURACY, AND USEFULNESS A diagnostic test should be ordered for specified clinical indications, be sufficiently accurate to be efficacious for such indications, and be the least expensive and/or risky of the available efficacious tests. No diagnostic test is totally accurate, and physicians often have difficulty interpreting test results. It is therefore critical to understand several commonly used terms in test analysis and epidemiology, including prevalence, sensitivity, specificity, positive predictive value, and negative predictive value (Table 2-2).

Although reports of the accuracies of diagnostic tests are commonly expressed in terms of positive and negative predictive values, these calculated values are dependent on the prevalence of the disease in the population being studied (Table 2-3). A test with a particular sensitivity and specificity has different positive and negative predictive values when used in groups of patients that have different prevalences of disease. For example, a mildly abnormal alkaline phosphatase level in a young adult with a known lymphoma suggests hepatic involvement by the tumor, i.e., it is likely to be a *true positive*, while the same alkaline phosphatase level as part of a routine screening battery of blood tests in an asymptomatic person of the same age is

TABLE 2-2 Definitions of commonly used terms in epidemiology and decision making

	Disease state	
Test result	Present	Absent
Positive	a (true positive)	b (false positive)
Negative	c (false negative)	d (true negative)

Prevalence (prior probability)	= (a+c)/(a+b+c+d)	= all patients with the disease/all patients tested
Sensitivity	= a/(a+c)	= true-positive test results/all patients with the disease
Specificity	= d/(b+d)	= true-negative test results/all patients without the disease
False-negative rate	= c/(a+c)	= false-negative test results/all patients with the disease
False-positive rate	= b/(b+d)	= false-positive test results/all patients without the disease
Positive predictive value	= a/(a+b)	= true-positive test results/all positive test results
Negative predictive value	= d/(c+d)	= true-negative test results/all patients with negative results
Overall accuracy	= (a+d)/(a+b+c+d)	= true-positive + true-negative test results/all tests

unlikely to be due to tumor, i.e., in this setting it is more likely to be a *false positive*.

Although the sensitivity and specificity of a test do not depend on the prevalence (or percentage of patients being tested who have the disease), they do depend on the spectrum of patients in whom the test is being evaluated. For example, a technetium pyrophosphate scintiscan for diagnosing myocardial infarction (Chap. 189) will appear to have a nearly perfect sensitivity and specificity if the diseased population has a history typical of myocardial infarction, electrocardiographic changes of transmural infarction, and clear-cut elevations of the MB isoenzyme of creatine kinase (CK) and the nondiseased population is composed of normal medical students. If, however, without changing the prevalence of disease in the population being tested, the spectrum of the diseased and nondiseased patients is altered by including patients with other characteristics, i.e., if the population of patients with myocardial infarction were composed principally of those with non-Q-wave infarctions and small or borderline elevations of CK-MB, while the population without acute infarction included patients with old infarcts and unstable angina pectoris, the sensitivity and specificity would change dramatically. In the latter situation, the sensitivity and specificity of the technetium pyrophosphate scintiscan are not only lower than in the first example, because the spectrum of diseased and nondiseased patients has been changed, but, more importantly, they are so low that the test has little clinical value. This example also demonstrates the methodologic problems encountered when applying data from one study to a different type of patient or when pooling data from studies of different subsets of patients.

In some situations, uncertainty about the sensitivity and specificity of the test in the type of patient being assessed may limit its clinical value. Since the physician rarely knows (or can know) the population on which every test which is ordered has been standardized, the results provide information that is far less decisive than usually thought. Furthermore, it may be quite difficult to distinguish random laboratory errors from test results that might be falsely positive or negative because of coexistence of a process that can affect the test, such as the finding of an elevated level of CK in a patient who has undergone strenuous exercise and is being evaluated for chest pain.

Because no single value or cutoff point of an individual test can be expected to have both a perfect sensitivity and a perfect specificity, it is often necessary to determine which value or cutoff point is the most appropriate to guide decision making. A graph (Fig. 2-1) of the test's *receiver operating characteristic curve*, which displays the inevitable trade-off between emphasizing a high sensitivity, such as defining an exercise electrocardiogram as abnormal if it shows ≥0.5 mm of ST-segment depression, versus emphasizing a high specificity, such as defining an exercise electrocardiogram as abnormal only if it shows ≥2.0 mm of ST-segment depression, can help the clinician understand the implications of various definitions of a "positive" test result. Such a graph demonstrates that different definitions of normal versus abnormal may be appropriate depending on whether one wishes to rule in the disease via a positive result on a test that has a high specificity or to exclude the disease via a negative result on a test that has a high sensitivity. Different tests may have different sensitivities and specificities, and better tests may have both a higher sensitivity and a higher specificity than poorer tests.

TABLE 2-3 How the positive and negative predictive values of the same test vary depending on the prior probability of disease

INTERPRETATION OF THE TEST RESULT WHEN 10% OF THE PATIENTS BEING TESTED HAVE THE DISEASE (PRIOR PROBABILITY = 10%)

1,000,000 patients

	With the disease		Without the disease	
Prior probability	0.10		0.90	
	100,000 with the disease		900,000 without the disease	
Test with sensitivity 90% specificity 95%	90,000 + test result (true positive)	10,000 − test result (false negative)	45,000 + test result (false positive)	855,000 − test result (true negative)

The probability of disease in a patient with a positive test result (positive predictive value) = 90,000/135,000 = 67%
The probability of no disease in a patient with a negative test result (negative predictive value) = 855,000/865,000 = 99%

INTERPRETATION OF THE TEST RESULT WHEN 50% OF THE PATIENTS BEING TESTED HAVE THE DISEASE (PRIOR PROBABILITY = 50%)

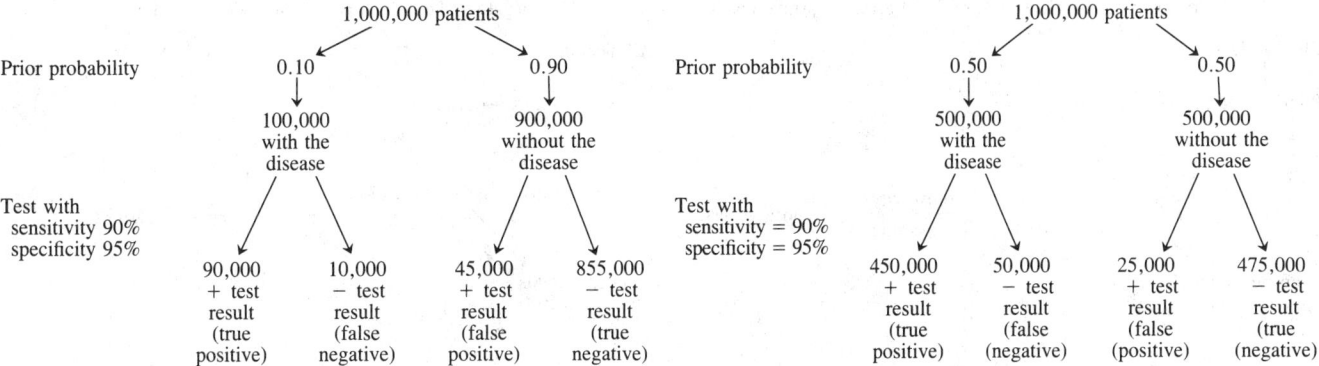

1,000,000 patients

	With the disease		Without the disease	
Prior probability	0.50		0.50	
	500,000 with the disease		500,000 without the disease	
Test with sensitivity = 90% specificity = 95%	450,000 + test result (true positive)	50,000 − test result (false (negative)	25,000 + test result (false (positive)	475,000 − test result (true (negative)

The probability of disease in a patient with a positive test result (positive predictive value) = 450,000/475,000 = 95%
The probability of no disease in a patient with a negative test result (negative predictive value) = 475,000/525,000 = 90%

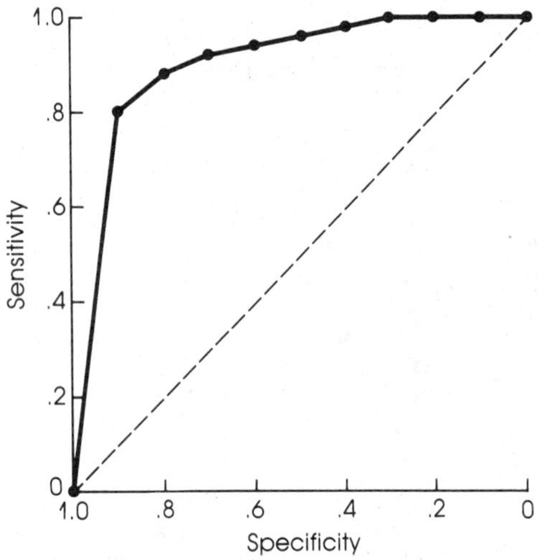

FIGURE 2-1 The inherent trade-off between sensitivity and specificity. For any diagnostic test, an increase in sensitivity will be associated with a decline in specificity. The closer this curve comes to the upper-left-hand corner, the more useful the test; the closer to the broken line, the less useful it is. When deciding on the cutoff between normal versus abnormal, one must determine what sensitivity and specificity are most useful clinically.

One example of a sensitive test is an M-mode echocardiogram to exclude severe aortic stenosis in adults: the sensitivity of this relatively inexpensive test for aortic stenosis is close to 100 percent, and a normal aortic valve echogram virtually excludes the diagnosis of severe aortic stenosis in the adult. Unfortunately, this sensitive test is not very specific, and many patients who have abnormal aortic valves on echocardiogram do not have severe aortic stenosis and require further testing (e.g., with Doppler echocardiography and perhaps cardiac catheterization) to establish the diagnosis (Chap. 188). A common example of a reasonably specific test would be an electrocardiogram to diagnose acute myocardial infarction. While the precise specificity depends on the spectrum of patients being tested, the presence of new ST-segment elevations exceeding 1.0 mm in two or more electrically contiguous leads in patients who present to an emergency room with prolonged acute chest pain consistent with myocardial ischemia is sufficiently specific, i.e., sufficiently unlikely to be a false positive, that admission to an intensive care unit is virtually always recommended. However, this test is not sensitive, and if admission to the unit were restricted to patients with this electrocardiographic finding, almost half of patients with myocardial infarctions presenting to hospital emergency rooms would be missed.

To optimize the clinical value of a diagnostic test, it is helpful to obtain local experience with it; oftentimes, its value will differ from that reported in the literature. Reports of the efficacy of a test should emphasize its accuracy when compared to an independent standard, and the test must be evaluated in a spectrum of patients with varying severities of the disease in question and in patients who have conditions that are part of the same differential diagnosis. The reproducibility of the test should be known, and the "normal limits" of the test should be clear and appropriate. In some instances, the test or procedure required to establish the validity of a diagnostic test is so risky that only a skewed sample of patients are included in a study, as, for example, in the analysis of the usefulness of the abdominal CT scan in patients with suspected pancreatic carcinoma. If patients with "negative" CT scan results never come to laparotomy or postmortem examination, neither the sensitivity nor specificity of the CT scan for pancreatic carcinoma can be assessed. In such situations, an estimated value of the diagnostic test may be inaccurate because it has not been validated.

INTEGRATION OF CLINICAL DATA AND TEST RESULTS Although, as we have seen, neither clinical data nor test results may be entirely accurate, the integration of the two can lead to better diagnostic predictions than either alone. By knowing the probability that the patient has a particular condition before a test is performed (the prior, or pretest, probability), and by knowing the sensitivity and the specificity of the test, the posttest probability can be calculated. A common mathematical technique for integrating clinical data and a test result is the odds-likelihood form of Bayesian analysis (Table 2-4). A pretest probability can be expressed as odds (as in a horse race for example) and multiplied by the likelihood ratio (which is the sensitivity of the test divided by 1 minus the specificity of the test) to yield the posttest odds, which may be transformed back into a posttest probability. This approach can be employed in any situation in which the physician can use clinical findings to estimate a pretest diagnostic probability and integrate this with the result as well as the sensitivity and specificity of the diagnostic test. Many clinical situations may be so complex that it is not practical to estimate the prior probabilities of all likely diagnoses or to know the sensitivities and specificities of each of the tests that might be performed individually or in sequence. Nevertheless, attempts in this direction will stimulate critical thinking, expose uncertainties, and generate ideas for original investigations or a review of past experiences to

TABLE 2-4 Example of the use of Bayesian analysis to integrate the pretest probability with the test result to calculate a posttest probability

Example 1: Prior probability of disease = 25%; a test with a sensitivity (true-positive rate) of 90% and a specificity of 80% (which implies a false-positive rate of 20%) gives a positive result

Clinical data
↓
Prior probability → prior odds
25% 1:3

$$\frac{0.90}{0.20} \leftarrow \frac{\text{sensitivity*}}{(1-\text{specificity})\dagger} \leftarrow \text{positive test}$$

Posttest odds

$$(1{:}3) \times \frac{0.90}{0.20} = 4.5{:}3$$

Posttest probability

$$\frac{4.5}{7.5} = 60\%$$

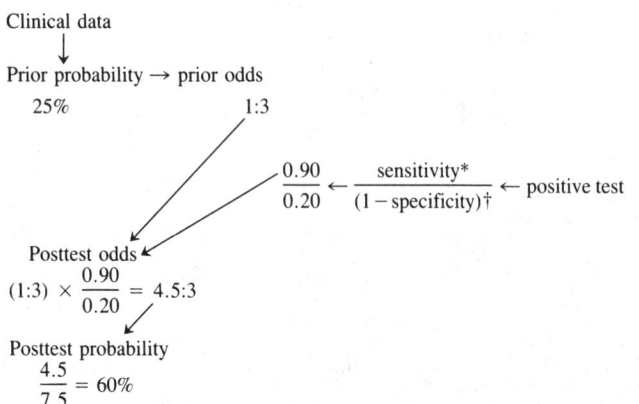

Example 2: Same pretest probability and test, but now the test gives a negative result. Here the true-negative rate would be 80% and the false negative rate (which is 1 − sensitivity) would be 10%.

Clinical data
↓
Prior probability → prior odds
25% 1:3

$$\frac{0.10}{0.80} \leftarrow \frac{(1-\text{sensitivity})\ddagger}{\text{specificity}\,\S} \leftarrow \text{negative test}$$

Posttest odds

$$(1{:}3) \times \frac{0.10}{0.80} = 0.125{:}3 = 1{:}24$$

Posttest probability

$$\frac{1}{25} = 4\%$$

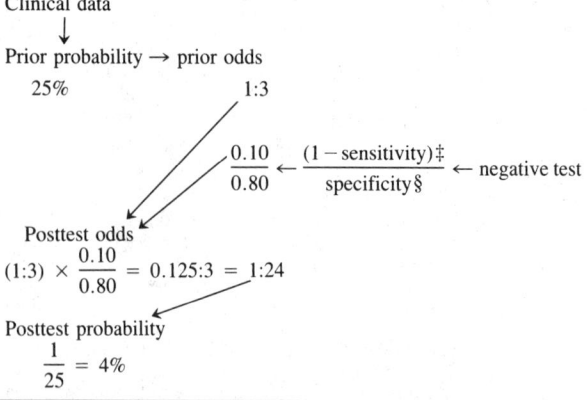

* Sensitivity = probability of a positive test result in a patient with the disease
† (1 − Specificity) = probability of a positive test result in a patient without the disease
‡ (1 − sensitivity) = probability of a negative test result in a patient with the disease.
§ Specificity = probability of a negative test result in a patient without the disease.

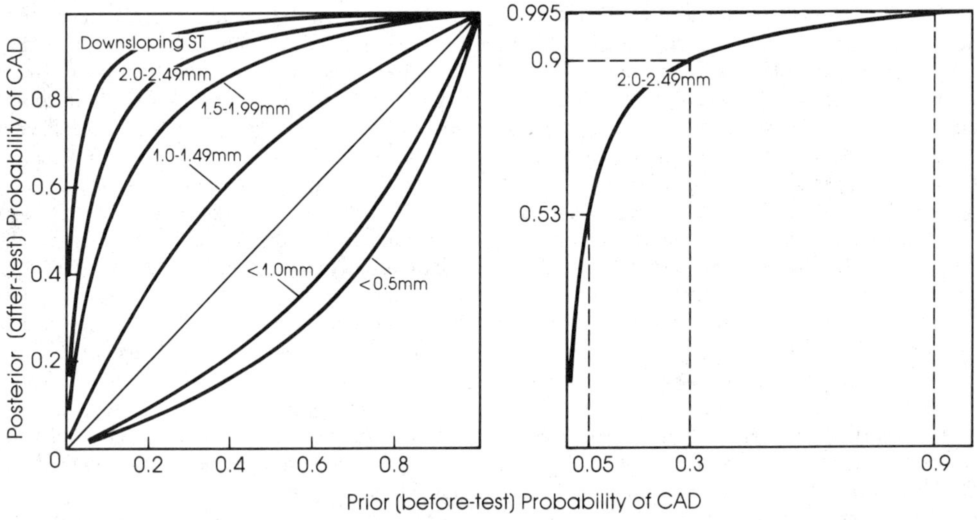

FIGURE 2-2 How the exercise tolerance test affects the probability of coronary artery disease. The before-test probability of coronary artery disease (CAD) will be modified by the result of the exercise electrocardiogram to yield a after-test probability of CAD. Note that the finding of <1 mm of ST depression will reduce the probability of CAD, whereas ≥ 1 mm of ST depression will increase the probability. For example, if a patient with a before-test probability of CAD of 90 percent (about that of a middle-aged man with typical anginal symptoms) had 2 to 2.49 mm on ST depression on exercise testing, the after-test probability of CAD would be 99.5 percent. In contrast the same exercise test result in a patient with 30 percent before-test probability of CAD (about that of a patient with atypical anginal symptoms) would yield an after-test probability of about 90 percent. In an asymptomatic patient, with a before-test probability of about 5 percent, the same exercise test result would yield an after-test probability of 53 percent. Thus, the same test yields different after-test probabilities in patients with different before-test probabilities. *(Adapted, with permission of the New England Journal of Medicine, from RD Rifkin, WB Hood, Bayesian analysis of electrocardiographic exercise stress testing. N Engl J Med 297:684, 1977.)*

facilitate the application of Bayesian analysis to the integration of clinical data and laboratory tests.

The results of Bayesian analyses often can be expressed in graphic form, such as the value of exercise electrocardiograms for predicting the presence of coronary artery disease (Fig. 2-2; also see Chap. 190). This series of curves also demonstrates how to consider a test whose result may be in the "gray zone" rather than clearly positive or clearly negative.

One of the key assumptions inherent in most such analyses is that the correlation between the pretest probability and the test result is no greater than expected by chance. If the diagnostic test simply duplicates information that has already been obtained by the clinical examination, it will not have any additional benefit for predicting whether or not the disease is present. For example, in trying to determine whether or not a patient with carcinoma of the colon has hepatic metastases, the finding of jaundice on physical examination should be a strong predictor. The degree of hyperbilirubinemia can also be measured, but the bilirubin level in a patient with clinical jaundice does not add substantial *independent* information to that obtained by a careful physical examination. When integrating a diagnostic test with clinical information, the test is helpful only when it adds incremental information to what can be inferred based on the history and physical examination and on prior less costly or less risky diagnostic tests. If a diagnostic test (such as a retrograde cholangiogram in the patient with hyperbilirubinemia) provides information that cannot be inferred directly, it is less likely that its results are associated with pretest probabilities to an extent greater than would be expected by chance.

A diagnostic test has an impact on the evaluation of a specific patient only if it changes the diagnostic probability to the extent that the new probability dictates a change in the diagnostic strategy or therapeutic plans or if the test serves as part of a sequence of tests that moves the probability across such a threshold. An example is a patient suspected of having a pulmonary embolism, with an estimated probability of 50 percent based on clinical data alone. A "low probability" pulmonary ventilation-perfusion scan may reduce the probability of pulmonary embolism, but if the goal is to exclude pulmonary embolism with the highest possible degree of certainty, a pulmonary angiogram would be required (Chap. 213).

Because diagnostic tests oftentimes do not provide important new information even when their results are accurate, several questions should be considered in deciding when to order diagnostic tests. First, how likely is the disease in question? Second, what would be the clinical consequences if the diagnosis were missed or if the patient were mistakenly treated for a disease that is not present? Third, what is the likelihood that the diagnostic test will change the probability sufficiently to have an effect on either diagnosis or therapy? The physician should consider the probabilities, the risks, the likelihood and costs of obtaining new information, and the adverse consequences of delay, because observation and follow-up are always among the available diagnostic options.

Since the establishment of valid diagnostic probabilities is a cornerstone to clinical reasoning, accumulated clinical experience, often in the form of computerized data banks, has been used to generate statistical approaches for improving diagnostic predictions. In such research, it is common to begin by identifying individual factors that have a univariate correlation with the diagnosis in question. Then, these univariate correlates may be included in a multivariate analysis to determine which of them are significant independent predictors of the diagnosis. Some analyses may identify the important predictive factors and then assign them "weights," which can be transformed to calculate a probability. Alternatively, the analysis may result in a limited number of categories of patients, each with a discrete probability of the diagnosis.

These quantitative approaches to the estimation of various diagnostic probabilities, which are often termed "prediction rules," are especially helpful if they are in a format that is readily usable by the clinician and if they have been validated prospectively on a sufficient number and spectrum of patients. For example, by carefully defining the key historical questions, findings on physical examination, and electrocardiographic abnormalities that might predict the probability of acute myocardial infarction among emergency department patients with chest pain, a protocol was devised and shown in prospective validation testing to have the same sensitivity as physicians for identifying infarction and at the same time to have a significantly higher specificity.

For such prediction rules to be useful to the clinician, they must be derived from relevant patient populations and use tests that are reproducible and readily available, so that the results can be extrapolated to local medical practice. Since only a minority of published prediction rules have adhered to rigid criteria as to the number and spectrum of patients examined and their prospective validation, most are not yet suitable for routine clinical application. Furthermore, many prediction rules cannot evaluate the probability of each of the diagnoses or outcomes that the clinician must consider.

COMPARING RISKS AND BENEFITS: DECISION ANALYSIS Inherent in the concept that probabilities can guide decision making is the assumption that one can arrive at a reasonable threshold by knowing the relative risks (or costs) and benefits of various options and deciding at what probability this ratio changes to favor an alternative strategy. Decision analysis is an organized process for evaluating such situations and identifies the key issues and problems.

One problem with applying decision-analysis techniques to difficult clinical problems is that the decision analysis is no better than the data on which it is based. In some instances, an attempted decision analysis of a complex clinical problem may yield no more information than that the critical data required for the analysis are missing and that more research in the field needs to be performed. In addition, when clinicians are uncertain about diagnostic or therapeutic strategies, formal analyses may indicate that the differences in outcome among various strategies are very small. In such cases, the formal analysis may have such inherent error that it is not dependable. Even when decision analysis is potentially helpful, it may not be feasible to complete the detailed estimations and calculations within the time constraints of bedside decision making. Nevertheless, the value of the analytic approach to decision making is that it integrates available data, mandates rigorous thinking, and exposes areas of uncertainty or ignorance.

Decision analysis depicts graphically two types of issues in the decision-making process: first, the decisions (or choices) available to the physician and second, the probabilities of all of the events that may result from each decision. To illustrate how this process works, a decision analysis of whether to biopsy the brain, treat, or wait in suspected herpes encephalitis (Chap. 135) may be considered. Figure 2-3 depicts the decision tree for this problem. The square box or "node" labeled A indicates a decision that the physician must make. The circular nodes, labeled B through I, indicate where different outcomes, each of which has an estimatable probability, could occur. In this analysis, the initial choices were to treat with vidarabine (a relatively toxic drug), not to treat with vidarabine, or to perform a brain biopsy and use its results to guide the treatment decision. The use of vidarabine may or may not result in complications of therapy, and a biopsy itself may or may not be associated with a complication.

Each of the possible outcomes for a patient is typically assigned a "utility," which is the relative preference for the outcome, where 1.0 is a perfect outcome and 0 is the worst possible outcome. Each terminal branch of the decision tree is assigned the utility corresponding to its outcome, and the "expected value" of each terminal branch is calculated by multiplying its probability by its utility. To calculate the "expected value" of each of the three possible courses of action (see Fig. 2-3, node A), the expected values of each of the terminal branches that originate from it would be summed. The preferred course of action is the one which, when all possible outcomes are considered, yields the highest expected value, which is the sum of the product of the probability multiplied by the utility for each of its possible outcomes.

In performing any decision analysis, the relevant probabilities must be known or estimated, a process that sometimes requires guesswork. Next, utilities could be assigned to each of these outcomes. A major practical limitation of decision analysis is the subjective judgment often required to estimate utilities. It is also difficult to adjust future years of life for their quality in any numerical fashion, for example, in considering how drug toxicity or the disability resulting from disease or treatment lowers the quality of future years of life.

The results and usefulness of a decision analysis depend on the probabilities and utilities that are used in the calculation, and it is imperative for decision analyses to include a *sensitivity analysis*, in which various estimates for each probability are included in the analysis to determine if the conclusions would be changed. For example, in the analysis in Fig. 2-3, some range of probabilities must be assumed for vidarabine toxicity, for serious complications of brain biopsy, and for the likelihood of false-positive or false-negative biopsy results. The authors of this particular analysis concluded that waiting, i.e., neither treating nor performing a biopsy, was the preferable course of action when the likelihood of herpes encephalitis is less than 3 percent. At probabilities between 3 and 42 percent, the analysis favored brain biopsy, but at probabilities above

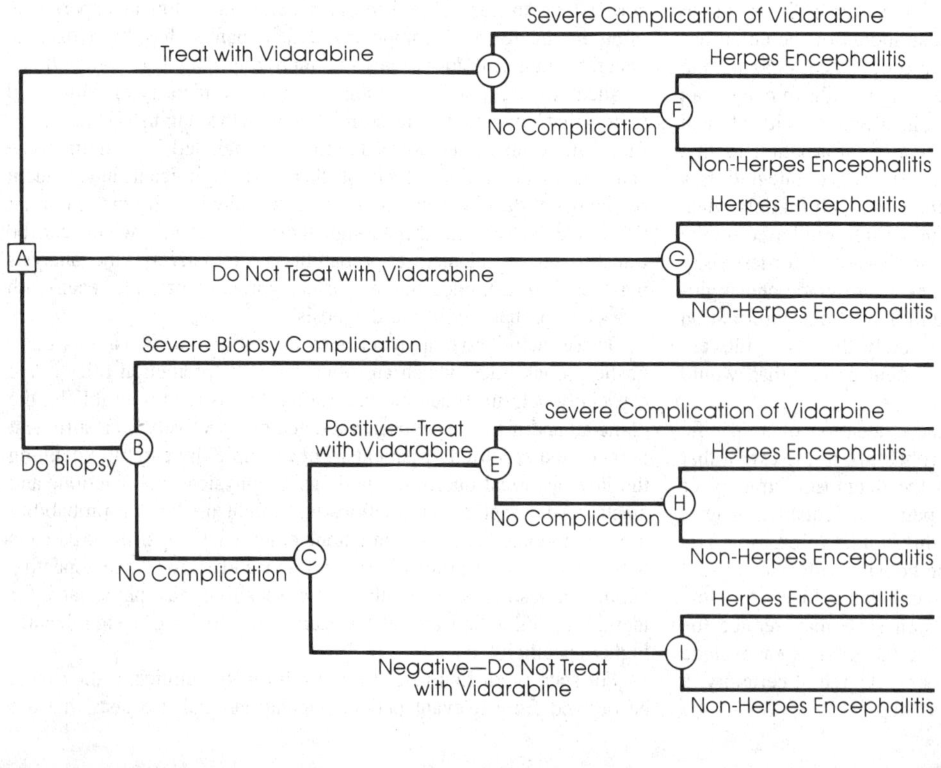

FIGURE 2-3 Decision tree for diagnosis and treatment of suspected herpes simplex encephalitis. The square node represents the decision point, and the round nodes denote chance events. See text for details. *(Reprinted with permission from M Barza, SG Pauker, The decision to biopsy, treat, or wait in suspected herpes encephalitis, Ann Intern Med 92:644, 1980.)*

42 percent, it favored immediate treatment with vidarabine. However, it is uncommon for any patient to have substantially greater than a 42 percent probability of herpes encephalitis, and hence it would be unusual for empiric vidarabine treatment ever to be preferred over brain biopsy. The authors demonstrated that these conclusions did not change when they varied the assumptions about the probabilities of several relevant events. If the conclusions of an analysis were altered by relatively minor changes in the assumptions on which it was based, the analysis would not be sufficiently reliable to become the basis for decision making.

Decision analysis sometimes demonstrates a clear and dramatic advantage with one particular option. In other circumstances, there may be little difference between two options; either option may be reasonable, or secondary issues that cannot be taken into account in the formal analysis, such as the patient's feelings about taking risks or the recent local experience with particular interventions, should be the final determinants in the decision. Physicians who perform a decision analysis therefore must determine the probabilities of each of the possible events by reviewing the pertinent patient experience at their own institution or practice, or by reviewing the pertinent literature. Even when the outcome of the analysis seems clear, the physician or the patient may believe that the situation in question is an exception to the rule. Furthermore, even the best analyses, like all clinical intuition, are based on assumptions that may be open to debate.

In the preceding example, the management of an individual patient with possible herpes encephalitis, decision analysis indicated the preferred strategy in terms of outcome but did not consider the costs at which such benefits might be achieved. In determining health policy, a formal cost-effectiveness analysis can be performed to determine how many dollars must be spent to achieve a unit of benefit, often defined as a life saved, a year of life saved, or a quality-adjusted year of life saved, in which the years are adjusted to take into account the quality of life during that time. For example, in 1990 dollars, 1 year of in-center hemodialysis can be estimated to cost about $30,000 to $35,000 per quality-adjusted year of life saved; this figure includes only the direct medical costs and not indirect costs related to issues such as time lost or travel, or any benefits in terms of a patient's ability to work. In some situations, the ability of the patient to maintain gainful employment may offset some or all of the direct medical expenses.

Although many analyses are now expressed in terms of cost-effectiveness, where dollars spent are compared to lives or years of life gained, some studies have utilized cost-benefit analyses in which a dollar value is placed on the life that is saved. For example, an analysis of the rubella vaccination, which attempted to place a dollar value on the vaccine's ability to prevent the congenital rubella syndrome and the resulting expenses, concluded that the optimal national policy would be to vaccinate all females at age 12.

ETHICS AND PATIENT INPUT In both quantitative and non-quantitative clinical reasoning, the physician must consider ethical issues as well as the patient's values and preferences. While a detailed discussion of these issues is beyond the scope of this chapter, it is important to emphasize that patients' preferences for alternate therapies may not agree with the preferences that the physicians propose on the basis of their own clinical judgment or the results of a decision-analysis approach. For example, many patients with carcinoma of the larynx may prefer radiation therapy, with a lower cure rate but a higher likelihood of maintaining speech, to extirpative surgery. It is imperative that physicians assess those characteristics of life that the patient prizes most (the elusive "quality of life") prior to basing controversial decisions solely on quantitative approaches, the physicians' own subjective impressions of the likely medical benefits, their own personal preferences, or their assumptions about the patient's preferences. Therefore, the final plan should reflect an agreement between a well-informed patient and a sympathetic physician who has detailed knowledge of the relevant medical issues and of the impact of the various possible outcomes on the specific patient.

REFERENCES

CASSIRER JP: Diagnostic reasoning. Ann Intern Med 110:893, 1989

ELSTEIN AS et al: *Medical Problem Solving. An Analysis of Clinical Reasoning.* Cambridge, Harvard University, 1978

GOLDMAN L et al: A computer protocol to predict myocardial infarction in emergency department patients with chest pain. N Engl J Med 318:797, 1988

LEMBO NJ et al: Bedside diagnosis of systolic murmurs. N Engl J Med 318:1572, 1988

MCNEIL BJ et al: Speech and survival: Trade offs between quality and quantity of life in laryngeal cancer. N Engl J Med 305:982, 1981

RANSOHOFF DF, FEINSTEIN AR: Problems of spectrum and bias in evaluating the efficacy of diagnostic tests. N Engl J Med 299:926, 1978

ROBERTS SD et al: Cost-effective care of end-stage renal disease: A billion dollar question. Ann Intern Med 92:243, 1980

SACKETT DL et al: *Clinical Epidemiology: A Basic Science for Clinical Medicine.* Boston, Little, Brown, 1985

SCHOENBAUM SC et al: Benefit-cost analysis of rubella vaccination policy. N Engl J Med 294:303, 1976

WEINSTEIN MC, FINEBERG HV: *Clinical Decision Analysis.* Philadelphia, Saunders, 1980

3 COST AWARENESS IN MEDICINE

LEE GOLDMAN

COSTS OF HEALTH CARE IN THE UNITED STATES

Health care expenditures in the United States are now about $600 billion per year. Through the 1980s, these expenditures rose at a rate of more than 10 percent per year, which exceeded the rates of inflation and of growth in the gross national product (GNP). As a consequence, the percentage of the GNP that is spent on health care increased from about 7 percent in 1970 to 9 percent in 1980 and is expected to be nearly 12 percent in 1990. As a percentage of the GNP, medical care expenditures in the United Kingdom are about five percentage points lower than in the United States. In Canada, expenditures as a percentage of GNP were similar to the United States until about 1970 but now are more than two percentage points lower.

The reasons for the increase in health care costs are multifactorial. The aging of the population and the availability of new diagnostic and therapeutic advances have increased the demand for health care. Furthermore, between 1970 and 1986, the supply of physicians in the United States increased from about 150 to 200 per 100,000 population. This increase in physicians provided Americans with easier access to medical services but raised concerns that a possible oversupply of physicians in portions of the country could contribute to an excessive escalation in costs. The costs of care are especially influenced by decisions regarding hospital admission and surgery, and by decisions affecting the use of intensive care units, life-sustaining treatments, and long-term care facilities. Efforts at cost-containment have attempted to identify unnecessary services, such as routine preoperative electrocardiograms in healthy young patients, or situations in which extraordinary expenses occur, such as in the last 6 months of life. Although some services may represent "fat" in the health care system, it is likely that any future reduction in unnecessary care may be more than counterbalanced in costs by growth in the number and age of the population and by continued advances in technology.

Despite these rising costs, an estimated 37 million Americans, or about 15% of the population, do not have health care insurance of any kind, even though nearly half are in households in which someone is employed. This lack of insurance coverage and access to health care is often blamed for the fact that the United States, despite its high expenditures on health care, ranks twentieth in the world in infant mortality and is not in the top ten in life expectancy.

HEALTH INSURANCE Traditional fee-for-service insurance reimburses the hospital and the physician for services rendered, but frequently does not cover preventive care. Even when insurance provides coverage for a service, the patient may be responsible for an initial "deductible" and a copayment, which is usually a fixed percentage of the entire amount charged.

Patients who must pay such out-of-pocket charges for some of their medical care seek less care than those whose care is fully covered by insurance. In the working poor this may result in reduced utilization of services and in an increase in the prevalence of serious disease. When adults of all socioeconomic classes lose health insurance coverage, they may use fewer medical services; as a result, their health status tends to decline.

Most alternatives to traditional fee-for-service medical care require enrolled persons to prepay a fixed premium, which, except when a relatively small copayment is required, usually covers acute, chronic, and preventive medical services, and sometimes covers medications and other health care needs. Prepaid plans have varying organizational and financial structures. Early on in their development, staff-model HMOs were among the most popular formats. In this model, groups of salaried physicians practiced physically together in one or a few central facilities to provide prepaid care. In recent years, Independent Practice Associations (IPAs) have shown the most rapid growth. IPAs provide prepaid care to the patient by contracting with office-based practitioners who agree to see patients on a prenegotiated fee schedule. To balance the normal fee-for-service incentives and control utilization, IPAs employ various forms of administrative controls and review. The rate of hospitalization can be reduced among enrollees in HMOs, and HMOs have been among the leaders in attempts to reduce hospital costs and lengths-of-stay.

REIMBURSEMENT OF HOSPITALS AND PHYSICIANS In 1983 Medicare introduced a system of prospective reimbursement using diagnosis-related groups (DRGs), whereby hospitals were paid a predetermined sum based on the patient's principal diagnosis, procedures, complications, and comorbidities regardless of the costs or charges that were actually generated by the hospital stay (Table 3-1). This reimbursement system was designed to reward hospitals for being more efficient, and hospitals could actually be paid more than their costs. In the first few years after the introduction of the DRG system, many hospitals, and especially the large teaching hospitals, reported substantial operating surpluses. In response, Medicare kept the rate of annual increase in reimbursement below the rate of increase in hospital costs, and the extra payments for teaching hospitals were reduced. By 1986, as many as one-third of all U.S. hospitals reported negative operating balances for Medicare patients. While the prospective reimbursement system has undoubtedly stimulated efficiency, it has also raised concerns about the practice of discharging patients prematurely or transferring them to other institutions if the projected cost of caring for them exceeds the expected reimbursement.

Since the introduction of federal prospective reimbursement, the number of inpatient hospital days has decreased. This reduction has been accompanied by a marked increase in ambulatory services, including a shift to the outpatient arena of services that previously were delivered only on an inpatient basis. This shift should lower the cost of delivering an individual unit of service, such as the cost of a breast biopsy, but the overall cost of medical care will rise if, for example, the breast biopsy is performed on an ambulatory basis *and* the inpatient resources that the breast biopsy patient would have used are now consumed by new services such as the treatment of a cancer patient with bone marrow transplantation.

TABLE 3-1 Example of diagnosis-related groups (DRGs) for prospective payment by medicare

DRG no.	Name	Approximate average Medicare reimbursement for a large urban teaching hospital in 1989, $
89	Simple pneumonia and pleurisy with complications or comorbid conditions	5,000
121	Acute myocardial infarction with complications, discharged alive	6,500
148	Major small or large bowel procedure with complications or comorbid conditions	13,000
156	Coronary artery bypass surgery with catheterization on same admission	22,000

SOURCE: Prospective Payment Assessment Commission.

TABLE 3-2 Physician reimbursement: Traditional fee for service versus the relative value scale

Average Medicare reimbursement, 1986*	Method of calculating reimbursement: Traditional fee for service, $†	Relative value scale, $‡
Office visit, limited service, established patient	19	24
Initial hospital consultation, comprehensive service	81	86
Repair of inguinal hernia	503	233
Coronary artery bypass, three grafts	3652	1936

* Average relative value scale reimbursement assumes same total amount of dollars is available to reimburse the sum of all Medicare physician services.
† Defined as individual physician's customary fee for service, limited to a prevailing fee by third party insurers.
‡ Defined as service-specific reimbursement based on the resource inputs required to perform a service, including the physician's work involved and specialty differences in practice expenses and costs related to training.
SOURCE: Hsiao WC et al: *A National Study of Resource-Based Relative Value Scales for Physician Services: Final Report to the Health Care Financing Administration, No. 17-C-98795/1-03*. Boston, Harvard University School of Public Health, 1988.

Physician payment Methods of physician payment have also been questioned. Physician reimbursement in the United States, whether by Medicare or by private insurers, has traditionally been a direct payment based on the doctor's "usual and customary" fee. In recent years, the rate of annual increase in fees has been fixed by the payor, so that relative payments really reflect fee patterns from a decade or more ago. Because of concerns that this traditional approach had led to inequities in reimbursement and especially to underreimbursement for nonprocedural tasks such as office visits, recent analyses have considered the resource inputs of physicians' services, including time, intensity, practice costs, and the investment in training, to propose a new and fairer approach to physician reimbursement. This new proposal, which has been termed the *Relative Value Scale* (Table 3-2), is based upon the concept that payment rates for medical services should, as with other economic "goods," reflect the costs of producing those services. Using this approach, results to date suggest that procedural tasks are currently reimbursed at rates exceeding those of nonprocedural tasks that require comparable time, skill, and experience. The suggested new relative rates are similar to current fee schedules in Canada.

Proponents of changes in the reimbursement system hope that more equitable pay for cognitive tasks will reduce the incentive to perform procedures and increase the incentive for physicians to spend more time with patients, including time for discussion of issues such as health screening, health promotion, and disease prevention. Opponents of a change in the physician reimbursement system argue, among other issues, that changes in the reimbursement system may limit access and fail to take into account the extent to which patients may value some services more than others. Regardless of the outcome of this ongoing debate, the physician's diagnostic and therapeutic recommendations should be guided by the goal of providing maximal welfare for the patient, tempered by an awareness of the relative cost that must be incurred to reap this benefit.

Control of health care costs Two different approaches have been suggested to control health care costs: regulation and competition. Regulations, such as per diem rate setting, attempt to control costs by setting and enforcing practice or reimbursement standards. Other regulatory means of attempting to reduce costs include mandatory second opinions prior to elective hospitalization or surgery, but such programs usually do not save more than the costs of administration of the programs themselves. It is vital that physicians work closely with third-party payors, government agencies and commissions, and regulatory bodies such as the Joint Commission on Accreditation of Health Care Organizations that have assumed increasing responsibilities for setting reimbursement rates and for determining performance standards and conditions for payment.

The competitive approach encourages hospitals and providers to bid in a free-market atmosphere, in which consumers will presumably make rational choices based on the perceived cost and quality of the available alternatives. Insurance plans that utilize deductibles and copayments reflect this approach. It has also been proposed that physicians who practice inexpensively should be rewarded financially, but if physicians are paid to perform fewer services, the quality of care may suffer.

The reimbursement system differs in different countries. In the United Kingdom, for example, the National Health Service insurance program covers hospital and physician reimbursement on a non-fee-for-service basis, although patients can pay privately for services outside of the system. Patients often must endure long delays for nonemergency procedures. In Canada, hospitals are paid an annual lump sum, and most physicians are paid on a fee-for-service basis via a fee schedule that is negotiated between the medical societies and the provincial governments. Private insurance, by law, can cover only services such as long-term care and dental care that are not covered by public insurance. New technology has diffused less rapidly in Canada, and the rates at which many procedures are performed are lower, but may not be less optimal, than in the United States. In Canada, delays for elective services have not been a major problem, life expectancy is higher than in the United States, and the prestige and relative income of physicians is analogous to those in the United States.

COSTS AND COST-EFFECTIVENESS

The costs of medical care include direct costs, such as the salaries of health personnel, and indirect costs, such as utilities, maintenance, and mortgage payments. Some costs are fixed, i.e., they do not vary with the volume of services provided, and other costs are variable, i.e., they depend on volume. For example, consider a situation in which a new instrument to perform a blood chemistry test costs $1000 and will last for 1 year. Also assume that each individual chemical analysis has an incremental cost of $10 in reagents, personnel time, and other resource inputs. If the laboratory utilizes the instrument to analyze 100 specimens in a year, the average cost per specimen is $20 ($10 each in fixed and variable costs), but if it analyzes 10,000 specimens, the average cost per specimen is $10.10 ($0.10 in fixed costs and $10.00 in variable costs) because the fixed costs are spread over more specimens.

The charges for medical services do not necessarily correspond to the true costs of providing the services. This is in part because the costs are difficult to measure and in part because charges are usually fixed regardless of volume while costs vary with volume. Most analyses of cost and cost-effectiveness in medicine are based on charges rather than on true costs.

The net costs for a health care program include the costs of providing the program, costs that are generated by adverse side effects of treatment, and costs for treating disease that would not have occurred if the patient had not lived longer as a result of the original treatment. From these costs, the savings in health care, rehabilitation, or custodial costs due to prevention or alleviation of disease are subtracted to determine the net cost. For example, consider a program to perform mammography in women over age 40. The program would have its own direct costs related to advertising, screening, mammography, physician visits, breast biopsy, etc. Some women would have false-positive mammograms and would receive unnecessary breast biopsies. Other women would live longer as a result of early diagnosis and treatment of breast cancer, but they might develop other illnesses, such as coronary disease, in the interim. If they developed conditions such as Alzheimer's disease, the custodial costs might be substantial. However, these costs would be countered by savings from hospitalizations for advanced cancer and by a potential increase in productive wage-earning years.

In all analyses of costs, it is important to consider *when* the costs will be incurred and *when* the effects in health benefits may be realized. Present dollars or health benefits are considered to have greater worth than a promise of future dollars or health benefits for several reasons. Other events may intercede so that a projected future cost or benefit may never occur, and there is always the possibility that money spent now will not achieve the desired effect at some time in the future. Furthermore, another illness may intervene, or there might be better ways to spend the money in the future. The principle by which future dollars and benefits are less highly valued than known immediate costs and benefits is termed *discounting*. It is independent of monetary inflation. By this concept it is preferable to spend $1000 today to prevent someone from dying today than it is to spend $1000 today in the expectation that someone will not die ten years from now.

It is unusual for any program simultaneously to achieve the greatest possible benefit and have the lowest possible cost. Instead, one usually either determines the desired benefit and then finds the lowest cost needed to achieve it or determines the resources available and then finds the greatest possible benefit that can be achieved.

Analyses of cost-effectiveness commonly examine the ratio of cost to effectiveness, i.e., the number of dollars required to save a life or a year of life. Such analyses are relevant to medicine because interventions only rarely both save lives and reduce costs. Hence, it is important to estimate the tradeoff of costs for gains in health. Two strategies with the same ratio may have quite different absolute costs and absolute benefits. For example, a program that saves 100 lives for $100,000 has the same cost effectiveness ratio as one that saves 1000 lives for $1,000,000, but the absolute costs and absolute benefits vary ten-fold. The choice between these two programs may depend on how much money is available to spend. In assessing any program, it is important to measure incremental costs and effects rather than average costs and effects. For example, consider two programs to reduce death from lung cancer. If, on average, program A costs $100,000,000 to save 100,000 years of life (average of $1000 per year of life) and program B costs $200,000,000 to save 100,100 years of life (about $2000 per year of life), the *incremental* cost of program B versus program A is $1,000,000 per year of life saved.

SOCIETAL ISSUES IN COSTS It is rare to find a medical intervention, such as measles vaccination programs, that both saves lives and reduces overall costs because the savings from disease prevention more than outweigh the expenses of the treatment itself. More commonly, medical practices that are truly of benefit also cause an associated increase in medical care costs. Among the more cost-effective examples is coronary artery bypass surgery in patients with left main coronary artery disease, which costs about $6000 per year of life saved.

The shift of services from the inpatient to the outpatient setting or from the hospital to the home generally reduces the expense of delivery of that aspect of medical care. For example, home dialysis is less expensive than dialysis in an outpatient center, which in turn is less expensive than dialysis in a hospital. Similarly, the administration of parenteral nutrition and intravenous antibiotics at home as well as home care for patients with the acquired immunodeficiency syndrome have greatly reduced the need for hospitalization for conditions in which skilled nursing care is otherwise not required. However, a byproduct of this strategy is an increased percentage of severely ill hospital inpatients, who require more intensive and expensive care than the less sick patients who otherwise might have occupied hospital beds.

To date, society has been reluctant to make ethical decisions regarding the amount of cost appropriate for any particular net benefit. Neither medicine nor society is accustomed to placing a dollar value on a life or a year of life. In many analyses, however, the annual costs of approximately $30,000 to $35,000 (in 1990 dollars) for renal dialysis for 1 year of useful life have been used as a benchmark of how much the United States is willing to spend to save a year of life, because such a program is supported with tax dollars and presumably is a reasonable reflection of national priorities.

The physician has a unique responsibility. On the one hand, the physician must serve as an advocate for the individual patient and recommend the course of action most likely to be beneficial to the patient. The overriding nature of the patient-physician relationship is the cornerstone of humane medical care. On the other hand, physicians must understand the costs as well as the benefits of medical interventions so that they can choose from among the wide range of options. The physician must serve as the advocate for providing the best options to the individual patient and should know which options are of little or no value or are more likely to do harm than good. The physician must, with the assistance and consent of the patient and the family, set priorities for the patient's management within any limits or restrictions imposed by society; such limits may be expressed, for example, in a finite number of dollars available for the treatment of a specific illness. In addition, physicians have a broad role in determining health costs. Individually and through various professional organizations, physicians have a responsibility to help set national priorities, based on their appreciation of the finite resources available for health care and their knowledge of the relative benefits and costs of various diagnostic and therapeutic options in particular types of patients.

HEALTH SCREENING Screening refers to the performance of a medical evaluation and/or diagnostic tests in asymptomatic persons in the hope that early diagnosis may lead to improved outcome. For such persons it was initially assumed that a periodic health examination, often accompanied by multiphasic diagnostic testing, is beneficial. However, there is no definitive information regarding the value of such an approach and even less information regarding which aspects yield results that are worth the costs incurred. In fact, there is no universally accepted approach to screening in the asymptomatic adult, given the uncertainties about the benefits and cost-effectiveness of each intervention. Nevertheless, the recommendations in Table 3-3 represent a reasonable set of guidelines for the periodic health assessment of asymptomatic adults.

Another issue in screening concerns the choice of which routine tests to perform in a patient who is about to undergo an operation or who is admitted to the hospital. For example, routine preoperative chest radiography is not indicated in persons without signs, symptoms, or risk factors for pulmonary or cardiac disease. Routine preoperative electrocardiography is generally recommended in any person with cardiac signs or symptoms and in men over age 40 and women over age 50, because of the age-related increase in asymptomatic cardiac disease and the likelihood that the preoperative tracing may be helpful for comparison, should any cardiac problems arise during the perioperative period. In these situations, appropriate tests must be performed to investigate specific symptoms and signs. In terms of screening tests for asymptomatic conditions, those tests and procedures that have not been performed under the guidelines in Table 3-3 normally should be performed while the patient is under medical care.

HEALTH PROMOTION AND DISEASE PREVENTION Health promotion and disease prevention require investment of time, energy, and resources, in the hope that the yield in terms of improved health warrants this investment. Unfortunately, there is limited information on the effectiveness of health promotion and disease prevention efforts. Interventions that result in a specified *relative* reduction in adverse outcomes have a greater *absolute* effect in higher-risk populations. For example, the same relative reduction in serum cholesterol will be of greater absolute benefit in persons with higher serum cholesterol levels or other unfavorable risk factors. In general, interventions to alter risk factors have a diminishing effect as risk factors decrease in severity.

Both patients and society commonly expect physicians to play a leadership role in health promotion and disease prevention. Patients expect and desire their physicians to make recommendations regarding physical activity, diet, and other lifestyle issues, and physicians often fail in this regard. If physicians do not become involved, patients seek advice elsewhere, risking the possibility that fads or other erroneous sources may influence their choices.

When physicians become actively involved in health promotion, patients respond frequently and make appropriate behavior changes. For example, a physician's encouragement to increase physical activity, especially if combined with explicit suggestions, is likely to

TABLE 3-3 Guidelines for preventive medical services*

	Age of person		
	19–39 years	40–64 years	65+ years
History	Every 1 to 3 years†: diet; physical activity; tobacco, alcohol, drugs; sexual practices	Same as 19–39 years	Every year: same as 19–39 years; and also functional status and symptoms of transient ischemia attacks
Exam	Every 1 to 3 years: height, weight, blood pressure High risk: oral cavity, thyroid, breast, testes, skin	Every 1 to 3 years: height, weight, blood pressure, breast High risk: oral cavity, thyroid, skin, carotids	Every year: as for 40–64 years and also hearing and visual acuity High risk: as for 40–64 years (but every year)
Laboratory	Pap smear (every 1 to 3 years), total cholesterol	Pap smear every 1 to 3 years, mammogram (every 1 to 2 years after age 50), total cholesterol	Mammogram (every 1 to 2 years until age 75), thyroid indices (women), dipstick urinalysis, total cholesterol
	High risk: fasting glucose, rubella antibodies, VDRL, urinalysis, chlamydia testing, gonorrhea culture, HIV testing, hearing, PPD, EKG, mammogram, colonoscopy	High risk: fasting glucose, VDRL, urinalysis, chlamydia testing, gonorrhea culture, HIV testing, hearing, PPD, EKG, fecal occult blood/sigmoidoscopy/colonoscopy, bone mineral content	High risk: fasting glucose, PPD, EKG, Pap smear (every 1 to 3 years), fecal occult blood/sigmoidoscopy/colonoscopy
Special counseling	Injury prevention, dental health High risk: hemoglobin testing, skin protection from ultraviolet light	Injury prevention, dental health, skin protection from ultraviolet light, discussion of aspirin therapy in men and estrogen replacement in women	As for 40 to 64 years and also glaucoma testing
Immunizations	Tetanus-diphtheria booster every 10 years	As for 19 to 39 years except not measles-mumps-rubella	Tetanus-diphtheria booster (every 10 years) influenza (every year), pneumococcal
	High risk: hepatitis B, pneumococcal, influenza (every year), measles-mumps-rubella		High risk: hepatitis B

* Except for the visit itself, the frequency is at clinical discretion unless otherwise specified.
† With counseling for any high-risk behaviors.
SOURCE: Adapted from U.S. Preventive Services Task Force (Guide to Clinical Preventive Services, Maryland: Williams and Wilkins, 1989), whose official report lists full details, including the definition of high-risk situations.

lead to changes in behavior so that the time spent by the physician appears to be cost-effective. Advice by a physician that a patient should lose weight or discontinue smoking is successful in only a small minority of cases, but it is an excellent first step toward health promotion and disease prevention (Chap. 373).

Programs in the workplace or in schools can commonly achieve weight losses of 2 to 5 kg at a cost of about $10 to $30 per kilogram lost. Despite high attrition rates, group approaches, such as Weight Watchers, can also produce similar weight losses at similar costs. A physician's advice is about as effective as these programs, and it is often the physician's advice that stimulates patients to try other interventions.

Physician-directed dietary interventions commonly lower the serum cholesterol level by as much as 10 percent. Drug treatment may be more effective but is more expensive. For example, treatment with cholestyramine in men costs more than $50,000 per year of life saved except in very high risk persons. Treatment strategies for hypertension are more cost-effective; the approximate cost of screening and treating hypertension, given the average medication compliance rates, ranges from about $10,000 per year of life saved for a patient with a diastolic blood pressure of 105 mmHg or higher to about $20,000 for a person with a diastolic blood pressure of 95 to 104 mmHg.

Immunizations, including pneumococcal and influenza vaccination in elderly and high-risk patients, are effective ways to reduce disease and its associated costs. Guidelines for immunizations in adults are indicated in Table 3-3 (see also Chap. 84).

DIAGNOSTIC TESTING As detailed in Chap. 2, diagnostic tests are valuable only to the extent that they provide new, *incremental* information that cannot be obtained less expensively from the history, physical examination, or other less expensive tests. Although these tests may often be of psychological benefit in reassuring the patient or the physician, they commonly generate redundant information, often result in a needless expense, and may entail risk. For example, in the evaluation of left ventricular function, the physician must decide whether a two-dimensional echocardiogram is sufficient or whether the more precise but more expensive measurement by radionuclide ventriculography is worthwhile. The physician faces analogous choices when deciding whether to obtain both an abdominal ultrasound examination and an abdominal computed tomogram or, in a different case, whether computed tomography and magnetic resonance imaging of the head are both required.

Ideally, each test should be ordered in sequence only to the extent that it is expected to add to the data available. However, this iterative approach can be expensive in hospitalized patients, where the sequencing of tests may lead to delays in scheduling and performing them. In these situations, the expense of the additional days of waiting may more than offset the savings from possibly avoiding a particular test. Usually, careful consideration of the problem by a physician is one of the most cost-effective ways to evaluate the patient. Expert consultation may be more cost-effective and helpful than ordering more diagnostic tests. Although interventions designed to reduce test utilization have met with variable success, those that have been successful have generally included educational components, full endorsement by locally respected leaders, and frequent reinforcement.

TREATMENT CHOICES In choosing among various treatments, physicians try to enhance the likelihood of an optimal outcome. It is important to consider whether an equivalent outcome could be achieved at a lower cost. For example, generic medications may be substituted for more expensive brand-name counterparts. Similarly, outcome is not usually compromised by interventions designed to encourage the use of less expensive antibiotic regimens. Endorsement by the medical profession of restricted indications for procedures such as pacemaker implantation and tonsillectomy have led to decreased utilization without any detectable reduction in life expectancy or quality of life. Whenever possible, diagnostic and therapeutic options should be subjected to strict evaluation of both benefit and cost-effectiveness, and physicians have responsibility to assist in such evaluations and to learn from their results.

INDIVIDUALIZATION

As already stated, the physician has a moral and legal responsibility to serve as the advocate for the patient, within the limits set by society. This requires an individual approach to the patient and an understanding of how the available resources of the health care system can best be applied to the person and the problem at hand. Nevertheless, the physician and the patient must recognize that expensive medicine is not necessarily better medicine.

Special consideration revolves around the use of expensive procedures in medical care, such as liver, heart, and bone marrow transplantation. In these situations, the limited availability of donors makes it necessary to choose the best possible recipients from among a wide range of potential candidates and to "ration." Although rationing is not pleasant, physicians have often responded well in situations with limited resources. For example, when faced with a reduction in intensive care unit availability, physicians are usually successful at maintaining normal admission rates for patients who most require intensive care so that little if any adverse effects occur in those excluded from intensive care.

There is marked variability in the rates at which various procedures are performed in different geographic areas, even though there are no obvious differences in the types or ages of patients. For example, the rates of prostatectomy vary markedly in different parts of New England. To date, little difference in health care outcomes can be detected despite wide differences in the rates of various procedures. These variations may in part be related to patients' preferences and in part to differing beliefs among physicians regarding optimal medical care choices. When the records of patients who have undergone such procedures are reviewed to determine how the indications for their procedure compared to the standards recommended by experts, a substantial proportion of procedures are deemed inappropriate. However, so far there is no close correlation between the percentage of cases deemed inappropriate and the rate at which the procedure is performed in a given location. There is no definitive evidence that high rates of performance can be equated with a high rate of unnecessary use.

The variations in rates of utilization, the proportion of cases in which some procedures seem not to be necessary, and the ability of physicians to respond to situations in which rationing is necessary suggest that in many situations the quality of medical care and the likelihood of a favorable outcome can be maintained while lowering costs. Society, with the input of physicians, must exercise this role without compromising the physician's responsibility to the individual patient.

REFERENCES

CHASSIN MR et al: Does inappropriate use explain geographic variations in the use of health care services? A study of three procedures. JAMA 258:2533, 1987

DETSKY AS et al: The effectiveness of a regulatory strategy in containing hospital costs. N Engl J Med 309:151, 1983

DRUMMOND M et al: Health economics: An introduction for clinicians. Ann Intern Med 107:88, 1987

ENTHOVEN A, KRONICK R: A consumer-choice health plan for the 1990s. Universal health insurance in a system designed to promote quality and economy. N Engl J Med 320:29, 94, 1989

EVANS RG et al: Controlling health expenditures—the Canadian reality. N Engl J Med 320:571, 1989

FUCHS VR: The "competition revolution" in health care. Health Aff (Millwood) 7(3):5, 1988

GOLDBERGER AL, OKONSKI M: Utility of the routine electrocardiogram before surgery and on general hospital admission. Ann Intern Med 105:552, 1986

GOLDMAN L: Cost-effective strategies in cardiology, in *Heart Disease*, 3d ed, E Braunwald (ed). Philadelphia, Saunders, 1988, pp 1680–92

GUTERMAN S et al: The first three years of Medicare prospective payment: An overview. Health Care Financ Rev 9:67, 1988

HSIAO WC et al: Special Report. Results and policy implications of the resource-based relative-value study. N Engl J Med 319:881, 1988

ROBINSON JC, LUFT HS: Competition, regulation and hospital costs, 1982 to 1986. JAMA 260:2676, 1988

RUSSELL LB, MANNING CL: The effect of prospective payment on Medicare expenditures. N Engl J Med 320:439, 1989

SCHROEDER SA: Strategies for reducing medical costs by changing physicians' behavior. Int J Technol Assess Health Care 3:39, 1987
WEINSTEIN MC, STASON WB: Foundations of cost effectiveness analysis for health and medical practices. N Engl J Med 296:716, 1977
WENNBERG JE et al: Are hospital services rationed in New Haven or over-utilised in Boston? Lancet 1:1185, 1987

4 THE CHALLENGE OF GERIATRIC MEDICINE

ROBERT N. BUTLER

INTRODUCTION Since the beginning of this century, industrialized countries have witnessed an unprecedented increase in the absolute number and relative proportion of older persons.[1] In 1900, the average life expectancy in the United States was 47 years, and only 4 percent of the population was over 65 years of age; today's average life expectancy is 75, and 12.2 percent of Americans are over 65.

A 28-year gain in average life expectancy is quite extraordinary; in fact, it nearly equals those years of life expectancy gained between the bronze age (approximately 3000 B.C.) and 1900. This is a social achievement, not a consequence of biologic evolution. It is a function not only of medical science, but of socioeconomic progress, sanitation, and better nutrition. Approximately 80 percent of this gain is a result of marked reductions of maternal, childhood, and infant mortality rates; about 20 percent has been gained from base age 65, due to effective prevention, management, or control of hypertension, diabetes, and other chronic as well as acute diseases. It is estimated that the control of heart disease could add another 10 years of life, and the conquest of cancer could add a little more than 2 years.

These sudden, dramatic demographic changes have demanded rapid adaptation. For comparative purposes, one might note that the industrialized world is still adapting to the industrial scientific revolution initiated in the 1730s. Efforts are still underway to adapt to the separation of the family from the workplace, pollution, despoilation of the environment, and urbanization. Therefore, it should not be surprising that time is required to adjust to the major demographic changes of population aging, which, in fact, is a consequence of the industrial revolution itself. The development of social security systems and medical and health insurance in industrialized nations such as the United States, Japan, and those in Europe illustrates these social adjustments.

The development of geriatrics, particularly in Great Britain and Scandinavia, and in some measure in Japan and less so in the United States, also reflects response to current demographic trends. Demographic, epidemiologic, and socioeconomic issues have forced attention upon research into aging and encouraged new forms of health service delivery for older persons.

DEMOGRAPHICS OF AGING The dramatic rise in the number and proportion of older persons as an extraordinary historic event is important. Medicine and public health, having had their parts to play in this new, unprecedented demographic change, have assumed some of the responsibilities to help deal with the resulting challenges. In 1987, the total U.S. elderly population was 29.8 million, 12.2 percent of the country's total population. Life expectancy at age 65 increased by only 2.4 years between 1900 and 1960, but since 1960 it has increased by another 2.7 years. In 1987, those persons reaching age 65 could expect, on the average, to live another 16.9 years—18.6 years for females and 14.8 years for males.

The gradually increasing number and proportion of older persons are only partly explained by a rise in longevity; they are also due to an increased birth rate in the 1920s and after World War II. The aging of the pre-1920s group, along with the decline in the birth rate during the mid-1960s, has contributed to an increased proportion of older persons and to the rise of the median age of the U.S. population from 27.9 years in 1970 to 32.1 in 1987.

Should current fertility and immigration levels remain stable in the United States, only the over-55 age group will experience significant growth in the next century. This is apt to occur in two stages: through the year 2000, the proportion of those aged 55 and over will remain relatively stable, at approximately one in five; by 2010, due to the aging of the "baby boomers," it will rise dramatically. Over one-fourth of the U.S. population will be 55 and over, and one in seven will be at least 65. These figures will rise to one in three and one in five, respectively, by 2030 (Fig 4-1).

Since 1960, life expectancy at age 85 has increased 24 percent. Next to the baby boomer population, the 85-plus age group is growing most rapidly. Moreover, the number of centenarians has increased from 15,000 in 1980 to 25,000 in 1986 and is expected to surpass 100,000 by the year 2000. This increase in the very old makes it likely that the elderly themselves will have at least one surviving parent. Indeed, the twentieth century has seen the rise of the multigenerational family; four- and five-generation families are becoming more common. According to 1982 data, the most recent figures available from the National Center for Health Statistics, approximately 2.2 million caregivers with an average age of 57 (72 percent of whom are females) provide unpaid assistance to 1.6 million noninstitutionalized older disabled persons.

A distinct difference in life expectancy exists between the sexes. Women outlive men by an average of 6.8 years. The proportion of men to women within elderly age groups declines with age. In 1987, the over-65 group had 17.7 million women and only 12.1 million men, or 146 women for every 100 men. The upper-age ranges saw an even more marked difference. For every 100 men in the 65-to-69 age group, there were 120 women; for those 85 and over, the number of women rose to 256 for every 100 men.

This sex difference in mortality accounts for most older men being married and most older women widowed; there are at least three times as many widows as widowers. In 1988, only 23.7 percent of noninstitutionalized men aged 75 and older were widowed, compared with 66.1 percent of women in this same age group, making older women more likely to end up living alone for a longer period of time and, as a group, the ones who are especially confronted with the challenge of aging.

Diseases and accidents account for approximately 75 percent of this distinction between the sexes. In the United States, the higher male mortality rate is a result of coronary artery disease, lung cancer and emphysema associated with tobacco intake, industrial accidents and exposure to toxic chemicals, motor vehicle and other accidents, suicide, and cirrhosis of the liver. Further research is needed to determine to what extent the other 25 percent is due to differences in life-style, life stress, hormonal status, genetic make-up, immune function, and other factors.

The risk of institutionalization at age 65 is the subject of debate. Some believe that no more than 20 percent of those who live past 65 years will enter, even briefly, an institution of any kind (e.g., chronic-care hospital, home for the aged, nursing home, foster home); other projections suggest an estimated figure of closer to 40 percent. However, only 5 percent of the elderly are institutionalized at any one time. These residents tend to be very old, female, and white. Nearly 84 percent of nursing home residents are without a spouse, compared to 45 percent of the noninstitutionalized elderly. In addition, only 63 percent of older nursing-home residents have children, compared to 81 percent of the elderly living in the community.

Before 1980, most older people lived in inner-city and rural areas; since that time, however, more of the 65-and-over population has resided in the suburbs than the central cities.

EPIDEMIOLOGY OF AGING In the United States, changes in behavior during this century have resulted in different causes of death.

[1]Although age 75 is the conventional definition of a geriatric patient, age 65 is used throughout this chapter (unless noted otherwise) to designate entry into old age, for this is when many people retire and one becomes eligible for such social entitlements as Medicare.

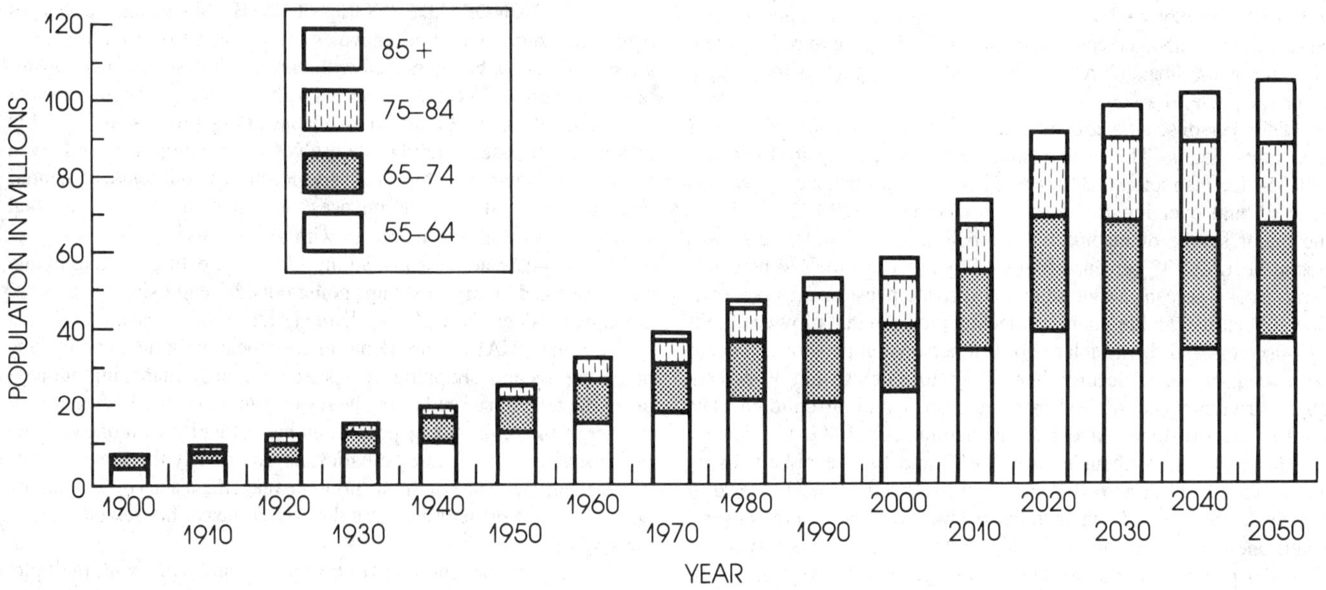

FIGURE 4-1 Population 55 years and over by age: 1900 to 2050. (*Source: CM Teuber, Current Population Reports ser. P-23, no. 128; and G Spencer, Current Population Reports ser. P-25, no. 952.*)

In 1900, heart disease was the fourth leading cause of death, but since 1910 it has remained in the number one position. Cancer was not even among the top five causes of death until 1930, when it became number three; it has been in the number two spot since 1950. Stroke was the fifth leading cause of death from 1900 to 1930, but since 1950 it has been in third place. Accidents were not among the top five until 1950, when they became, and remain, the fourth leading cause of death. Lung disease has been the fifth leading cause of death since 1986. Since 1985, the number of suicides has increased among all age groups, but the most dramatic increase has occurred in the 75-to-84-year category.

Together, heart disease, cancer, and stroke account for 75 percent of all deaths among the elderly, 20 percent of doctor visits, 30 percent of hospital days, and 50 percent of bed-ridden days. Stroke, the third leading cause of death for this group, has been decreasing over the past 30 years, perhaps due to improved control of hypertension and better management and rehabilitation.

The average length of an older person's hospital stay has been declining, from 14.2 days in 1968 to 8.6 days in 1987. (For those under 65, the average stay is 5.4 days.) In part, this decline is a result of changing hospital regulations (DRGs), although a decrease in hospital stay occurred even prior to these changes. Most older persons are admitted to a hospital because of acute episodes of a chronic condition. In 1985, circulatory diseases accounted for 31 percent of admissions, digestive diseases for 12 percent, respiratory diseases for 11 percent, and neoplasms for 10 percent.

It is obvious that the older one gets, the more likely that illness will occur. Yet most elderly persons are in reasonably good health and able to function independently. Although acute conditions have become less frequent, chronic conditions, single and multiple, are common among the elderly, especially women. Arthritis is probably the number one, everyday quality-of-life medical problem of old age and produces immense morbidity. Although it results in relatively few deaths and only 2 percent of hospital days, it accounts for 16 percent of the days spent in bed, nearly as much as for heart disease. In fact, arthritis, hypertension, and hearing impairment, respectively, are the top three chronic conditions of the elderly.

SOCIOECONOMICS OF AGING Negative attitudes toward older persons are common throughout U.S. culture, including the medical profession. In the latter, such prejudice probably reflects the sense of helplessness that physicians feel when required to respond to the complex needs of the older patient, coupled with the discomfort engendered by the reality of aging and proximity to dying and death. Misconceptions and prejudices about aging must be refuted and overcome; for example, age itself does not produce senility, lack of productivity, or loss of sexual desire and ability.

Many older persons prefer to retire and do not seek work. Almost two-thirds of retirees leave the work force before age 65, largely for health reasons. There has been a steady decline in work-force participation rates. In 1900 the average male spent a little over one year, or 3 percent of his life, in retirement or in other activities outside the work force; by 1980, however, he spent 19 percent of his 70 years in retirement, or 13.6 years. In 1950, almost half of all men aged 65 and over were in the labor force; by 1987, this figure had fallen to 16 percent. Labor force participation of older women has varied only slightly: 10 percent in 1950 compared with approximately 7.4 percent in 1987. Part-time work is favored by the working public of all ages and is deemed desirable during retirement by many older persons who view their health positively.

The increase of eligibility for Social Security from age 65 to age 67, to be phased in by the year 2027, and the elimination of mandatory retirement may have only minimal impact on increasing the number of older persons in the work force, even though an estimated worker shortage is predicted in the 1990s and the next century, particularly in the service industries. Already some U.S. businesses are seeking to mainstream, hire, or rehire older workers.

Some are afraid that the increasingly older population will become unaffordable, lead to stagnation of society's productive and economic growth, and generate intergenerational conflict. While there is an increasing number of retirees compared to nonretirees, the combined total of the dependent group, defined as the young (below 18) plus the old (above 60), has decreased since 1900 and is expected to continue to decline until early into the next century, depending on immigration, when it will then begin to rise. Although working-age Americans support the young and the old, our birth rate is below the zero population growth, helping to offset the increasing number of the aged.

The support ratio has become a political issue. It has been argued that the support of the old is on the backs of the young, especially in the federal outlay of funds. However, while it is true that entitlements for the elderly are primarily supported by federal publicly funded programs, the young are supported primarily by the community, state, and private funds in the form of taxes for public education. In any case, survey data (e.g., the Louis Harris polls) show that the young, and not just the old, favor entitlements for the old. This is due partly to the fact that the young understand that they, too, will one day be old. Furthermore, such entitlements directly benefit the middle-aged children of the old by helping to relieve them of some of the financial responsibilities for their parents they might otherwise have to assume.

Older persons, as a group, enjoy a lower socioeconomic status than other adults. The median income of the elderly in 1987 was $11,854 for men and $6734 for women. Families headed by persons aged 65 and over reported a median income of $20,813. In 1986, the major source of income for older families and individuals was Social Security (35 percent), followed by asset income (24 percent), earnings (24 percent), and public and private pensions (15 percent). Social Security is a life-course protection program that provides funds for survivors and the disabled, not just persons on pensions. Indeed, 60 percent of Social Security benefits go to retirees, and 40 percent go to surviving widows and to more than 3 million children. The poverty level of older Americans is alarming. In 1987, the poverty threshold for elderly couples was $6872 and for the elderly living alone, $5447 ($132 and $104 per week, respectively). One-third of elderly Americans had total incomes below 150 percent of the poverty level; one-fifth had incomes below 125 percent of the poverty level.

Older people living alone have special problems. They tend to be aged 75 and above and are at greater risk for institutionalization. Low-income elderly are in poorer health and are more likely to suffer from chronic illness and to be functionally impaired than higher income elderly. Three-fifths of the elderly living on less than $104 per week live alone. Two-thirds of this group are widows, the primary victims of poverty among the aged.

Although older persons spend 67 percent of their income on housing (including utilities), food, and medical care, compared to 49 percent spent by younger households, one of their greatest expenditures is health care. The average per capita expenditure for acute medical care for an older person was approximately $3500 in 1987, and one-third of all the near-poor elderly were forced into poverty by medical expenses. Direct out-of-pocket health costs for the elderly average 15 percent of their income, the same amount as before Medicare and Medicaid were enacted.

According to 1984 data from the Health Care Financing Administration, Medicare covered 49 percent of all personal health care expenses for older persons. Medicare primarily provides for acute care services; care provided by hospitals accounts for 69 percent of health care. In 1984, the program paid 75 percent of hospital costs and 58 percent of physician service costs. Although spending for home health care has grown dramatically, it accounts for only 3.3 percent of Medicare benefit payments. Five percent of the elderly do not have Medicare. Since its enactment, Medicare's deductible and co-insurance requirements have increased, as has the premium. Medicaid, the federal/state program that is the principal source of financing nursing home care, accounts for 42 percent of all expenditures for nursing home care; however, only one in three older persons officially below the poverty line actually qualifies for Medicaid.

The Old Age and Survivors Insurance Trust Fund of the Social Security system is in close actuarial balance: during the next 75 years there will be no problems of insolvency. In contrast, it is estimated that the Medicare Trust Fund will be in trouble shortly after the turn of the century. The provision of new financing of long-term care is a critical issue. Some progress has been made in resolving the problem. Pending legislation reflects the government's concern with rising long-term care costs. Many large private insurers have become interested in testing and marketing long-term care, and coverage is becoming more comprehensive, inexpensive, and readily available. Several major employers, including the federal government, have been investigating long-term care insurance for their employees, and corporations are developing various programs to help workers care for aging relatives. As the elderly population continues to grow, so, too, will the need for long-term care services, both home and institutional. More pressure then will be brought to bear upon Medicaid and alternative sources of financing. Deciding the balance between private and public sectors is a major challenge for the future.

EVALUATION OF ELDERLY INDIVIDUALS Many biologic changes over time, such as altered enzymes indicating hepatic malfunction, are now found to be connected with chronic disease and alcoholism, rather than normal aging. Numerous pathophysiologic alterations that had been attributed to the unavoidable aging process are actually results of disease, lending themselves to amelioration and even prevention. Notable examples are arteriosclerosis and senile dementia, once feared most as consequences of aging. It is also true that vulnerability to disease increases with age.

Personal-care activities—bathing, dressing, eating, getting in and out of bed and chairs, walking, going outside, and using the toilet—are known as *activities of daily living* (ADLs). *Instrumental activities of daily living* (IADLs) are home-management activities, and include preparing meals, shopping for personal items, managing money, using the telephone, and doing heavy or light housework. About one-quarter of the 65-and-over population has difficulty with one or more of the seven personal-care activities; approximately the same number has difficulty with one of the six home-management activities. Walking poses the most difficulty among the ADLs, heavy housework among the IADLs.

The geriatric patient tends to be aged 75 and over, with multiple, complex, interacting psychosocial and physical pathology, both acute and chronic. A person may enter a hospital with a kidney problem and, as a consequence of sophisticated care, leave with improved kidney function, but may barely be able to walk for numerous other reasons. To provide comprehensive care, what is required is not just a nephrologist or internist, but a team consisting of a nurse, social worker, psychiatrist, and/or neuropsychologist, among others, who are concerned with why such patients cannot walk, whether they are depressed, and how they will be able to cope outside the hospital.

The National Institutes of Health Consensus Conference defined an assessment and evaluation method that is particularly suited to older patients. It is a multidisciplinary team approach that looks at a patient functionally rather than in terms of specific organs, systems, and diseases. The American College of Physicians also argues that patients aged 75 and older need to be tested for baseline function. Geriatric assessment uncovers, describes, and explains the multiple problems of older patients, their resources and strengths, and their need for services; a coordinated care plan is then developed to focus on possible interventions. The functional assessment identifies problems that may require more detailed assessment by other medical and nonmedical professionals, including audiologists, clinical psychologists, dentists, nutritionists, occupational and physical therapists, podiatrists, and pharmacists. The assessment process provides the physician with reliable information about the patient's true ability to function independently in the community. It also identifies nonmedical issues with which a patient may need help, such as Medicaid eligibility, or community facilities with which both patient and physician may be unfamiliar, such as Meals on Wheels or respite for the caregiver. The physician also may gain insight into the patient's wishes about ultimate life support.

Numerous in-patient studies support the effectiveness of this interdisciplinary approach to management and evaluation. A Veterans Administration study revealed reduced hospital stays, less rehospitalization, and decreased mortality and morbidity rates for groups that had comprehensive assessments and received the services that were needed. Team-oriented outpatient geriatric assessment provides a promising way to deliver high-quality, satisfying care to the elderly, besides possibly decreasing health care costs.

Geriatrics requires integration throughout medicine. It need not be a practice specialty. Rather, every primary care and specialty physician must have adequate training and knowledge in the principles of geriatrics. Attention must be paid to the functional and geriatric assessment and to these interdisciplinary approaches. The definition of geriatrics implies a broad perspective that integrates all aspects of medicine, not internal medicine alone. To achieve this integration, geriatric medicine must develop the resources to pioneer innovations in diagnosis and care and to concentrate on age-related research.

REFERENCES

American College of Physicians: Comprehensive functional assessment for elderly patients. Ann Intern Med 109:70, 1988

Birren JE et al: *Human Aging I: A Biological and Behavioral Study*. Public Health Service Publication No. 986. Washington, DC, US Government Printing Office, 1963, reprinted 1971 and 1974

Brody JA, Schneider EL: Diseases and disorders of aging: An hypothesis. J Chron Dis 39:871, 1986

Butler RN: An overview of research on aging and the status of gerontology today. Milbank Mem Fund Q 61:351, 1983

———: The relation of extended life to extended employment since the passage of Social Security in 1935. Milbank Mem Fund Q 61:420, 1983

Commonwealth Fund Commission: Medicare's poor: Filling the gaps in medical coverage for low-income elderly Americans. New York, The Commonwealth Fund, 1987

———: Old, alone and poor: A plan for reducing poverty among elderly people living alone. New York, The Commonwealth Fund, 1987

Granick S, Patterson RD (eds): *Human Aging II: An Eleven Year Biomedical and Behavioral Study*. US Public Health Service Monograph No. (HSM) 71-9037, 1971. Reprinted 1976

Hazzard WR et al (eds): *Principles of Geriatric Medicine and Gerontology*, 2d ed. New York, McGraw-Hill, 1990

NIH Consensus Development Panel. National Institutes of Health Consensus Development Conference Statement: Geriatric assessment methods for clinical decision-making. J Am Geriatr Soc 36:342, 1988

Rodin J: Aging and health: Effects of the sense of control. Science 233:1271, 1986

Rowe JW, Kahn RL: Human aging: Usual and successful. Science 237:143, 1987

Rubenstein LZ et al: Effectiveness of geriatric evaluation unit: A randomized clinical trial. N Engl J Med 311:1664, 1984

———: The Sepulveda VA geriatric evaluation unit: Data on four-year outcomes and predictors of improved patient outcomes. J Am Geriatr Soc 32:503, 1984

US Senate Special Committee on Aging, American Association of Retired Persons, Federal Council on the Aging, and US Administration on Aging: Aging America: Trends and projections, 1987–88. Washington, DC, U.S. Department of Health and Human Services, LR 3377 (188) D12198

Williams ME et al: How does the team approach to outpatient geriatric evaluation compare with traditional care: A report of a randomized controlled trial. J Am Geriatr Soc 35:1071, 1987

PART ONE THE BIOLOGICAL BASIS OF DISEASE

section 1 Genetics

5 GENETIC ASPECTS OF DISEASE

JOSEPH L. GOLDSTEIN / MICHAEL S. BROWN

GENETIC PRINCIPLES

More than one-fifth of the proteins (and hence genes) in each human being exist in a form that differs from the one present in the majority of the population. This remarkable genetic variability, or polymorphism, among "normal" people accounts for much of the normal variation in body traits such as height, intelligence, and blood pressure. These genetic differences also determine the ability of each individual to meet environmental challenges, including those that produce disease. All human diseases can be considered to result from an interaction between an individual's unique genetic makeup and the environment. In certain diseases, the genetic component is so overwhelming that it expresses itself in a predictable manner without a requirement for extraordinary environmental challenges. Such diseases are termed *genetic disorders.*

MOLECULAR BASIS OF GENE EXPRESSION All hereditary information is transmitted from parent to offspring through the inheritance of deoxyribonucleic acid (DNA). DNA is a linear polymer composed of purine and pyrimidine bases whose sequence ultimately determines the sequence of amino acids in every protein made by the body. The four types of bases in DNA are arranged in groups of three, each triplet forming a code word, or codon, that signifies a particular amino acid. A *gene* represents the total sequence of bases in DNA that specifies the amino acid sequence of a single polypeptide chain of a protein molecule.

Genetic information encoded in the DNA of the chromosomes is first transcribed into a *ribonucleic acid* (RNA) copy. During transcription the ribose nucleotides align themselves along the DNA according to base-pairing rules. Thus, adenine of DNA pairs with uridine of RNA, cytosine pairs with guanine, thymine pairs with adenine, and guanine pairs with cytosine. The ribose bases are joined together by RNA polymerase. The resulting *RNA transcript* forms the template for translation into the amino acid sequence of a protein. Figure 5-1 shows the DNA and mRNA code words for each of the amino acids in protein.

Figure 5-2 illustrates a schematic diagram of the genetic control of protein synthesis in higher organisms, including humans. The DNA of most genes is fragmented into discrete coding regions (exons) separated by noncoding regions (introns or intervening sequences). The *coding regions* contain the bases that specify the sequence of amino acids in the polypeptide chain. The *intervening sequences* are composed of bases that act as spacers between the coding regions; they are not translated into protein. The transcription of DNA produces a faithful copy of the entire gene sequence; thus, the RNA transcript

FIGURE 5-1 The genetic code.

Second nucleotide

First nucleotide	**A** or *U*			**G** or *C*			**T** or *A*			**C** or *G*			Third nucleotide
A or *U*	**AAA**	*UUU*	Phe	**AGA**	*UCU*	Ser	**ATA**	*UAU*	Tyr	**ACA**	*UGU*	Cys	**A** or *U*
	AAG	*UUC*		**AGG**	*UCC*		**ATG**	*UAC*		**ACG**	*UGC*		**G** or *C*
	AAT	*UUA*	Leu	**AGT**	*UCA*		**ATT**	*UAA*	Stop	**ACT**	*UGA*	Stop	**T** or *A*
	AAC	*UUG*		**AGC**	*UCG*		**ATC**	*UAG*		**ACC**	*UGG*	Trp	**C** or *G*
G or *C*	**GAA**	*CUU*	Leu	**GGA**	*CCU*	Pro	**GTA**	*CAU*	His	**GCA**	*CGU*	Arg	**A** or *U*
	GAG	*CUC*		**GGG**	*CCC*		**GTG**	*CAC*		**GCG**	*CGC*		**G** or *C*
	GAT	*CUA*		**GGT**	*CCA*		**GTT**	*CAA*	Gln	**GCT**	*CGA*		**T** or *A*
	GAC	*CUG*		**GGC**	*CCG*		**GTC**	*CAG*		**GCC**	*CGG*		**C** or *G*
T or *A*	**TAA**	*AUU*	Ile	**TGA**	*ACU*	Thr	**TTA**	*AAU*	Asn	**TCA**	*AGU*	Ser	**A** or *U*
	TAG	*AUC*		**TGG**	*ACC*		**TTG**	*AAC*		**TCG**	*AGC*		**G** or *C*
	TAT	*AUA*		**TGT**	*ACA*		**TTT**	*AAA*	Lys	**TCT**	*AGA*	Arg	**T** or *A*
	TAC	*AUG*	Met	**TGC**	*ACG*		**TTC**	*AAG*		**TCC**	*AGG*		**C** or *G*
C or *G*	**CAA**	*GUU*	Val	**CGA**	*GCU*	Ala	**CTA**	*GAU*	Asp	**CCA**	*GGU*	Gly	**A** or *U*
	CAG	*GUC*		**CGG**	*GCC*		**CTG**	*GAC*		**CCG**	*GGC*		**G** or *C*
	CAT	*GUA*		**CGT**	*GCA*		**CTT**	*GAA*	Glu	**CCT**	*GGA*		**T** or *A*
	CAC	*GUG*		**CGC**	*GCG*		**CTC**	*GAG*		**CCC**	*GGG*		**C** or *G*

Note: The DNA codons appear in boldface type; the complementary RNA codons are in italics. A = adenine, C = cytosine, G = guanine, T = thymine, U = uridine (replaces thymine in RNA). In RNA, adenine is complementary to thymine of DNA; uridine is complementary to adenine of DNA; cytosine is complementary to guanine, and vice versa. "Stop" = termination. The amino acids are abbreviated as follows:

Ala = alanine	*Cys = cysteine*	*His = histidine*	*Met = methionine*	*Thr = threonine*
Arg = arginine	*Gln = glutamine*	*Ile = isoleucine*	*Phe = phenylalanine*	*Trp = tryptophan*
Asn = asparagine	*Glu = glutamic acid*	*Leu = leucine*	*Pro = proline*	*Tyr = tyrosine*
Asp = aspartic acid	*Gly = glycine*	*Lys = lysine*	*Ser = serine*	*Val = valine*

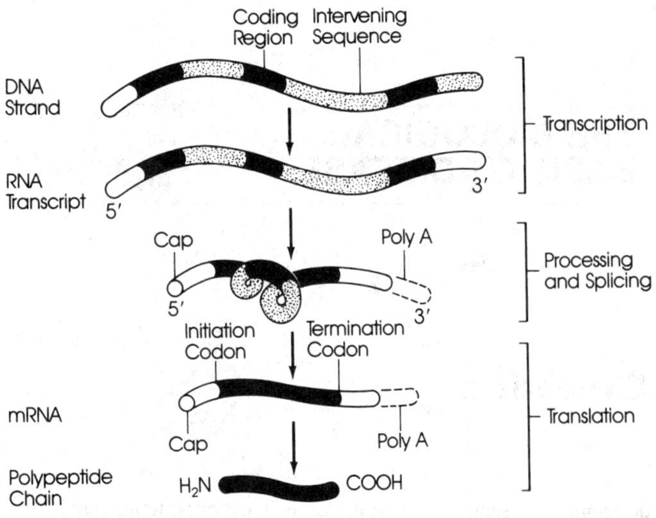

FIGURE 5-2 A schematic diagram of the genetic control of protein synthesis, illustrating the flow of genetic information from the base sequence of DNA to the RNA transcript (transcription) to mRNA (processing) to the polypeptide chain of a protein molecule (translation). Although DNA exists in a double-stranded form, only one of the two strands is used as a template for transcribing the RNA transcript. Solid sections represent coding regions in DNA, RNA transcript, mRNA, and amino acid sequence in polypeptide chain; dotted sections represent intervening sequences in DNA and RNA transcript.

contains altering coding and intervening sequences. The RNA transcript is edited in the nucleus before it passes into the cytoplasm. In the editing process, the intervening sequences are excised, and the coding regions are spliced together to form one continuous gene (Fig. 5-2).

After processing, the edited RNA, which is called *messenger RNA* (mRNA), leaves the nucleus and enters the cytoplasm where it becomes associated with *ribosomes* and thereby serves as a template for the ribosomal synthesis of proteins. Each of the 20 amino acids is attached in the cell cytoplasm to a specific molecule called *transfer RNA* (tRNA). Each tRNA contains a triplet sequence of purine and pyrimidine bases that is "complementary" to a specific codon in the mRNA. These tRNA molecules with their attached amino acids line up along the mRNA molecule in the precise order dictated by the genetic code. Under the action of cytoplasmic enzymes (initiation factors, elongation factors, and termination factors), peptide bonds are formed between the various amino acids, and the completed protein is released from the ribosome. For a more detailed account of the molecular basis of gene expression, see Chap. 6.

MAINTENANCE OF GENETIC DIVERSITY THROUGH TRANSMISSION AND SEGREGATION OF GENES The amount of DNA in the nucleus of each human cell is sufficient to code for more than 50,000 genes and hence to specify more than 50,000 polypeptide chains. The genes are arranged in a linear sequence of DNA that together with certain histone proteins form rod-shaped bodies called *chromosomes*. Each somatic cell contains 46 chromosomes, arranged in 23 pairs, one of each pair derived from each parent. Thus, each individual inherits two copies of each chromosome and hence two copies of each gene. The chromosomal location of the two copies of each gene is termed the *genetic locus*. When a gene occupying a genetic locus exists in two or more different forms, these alternate forms of the gene are referred to as *alleles*.

In humans, a given gene always resides at a specified genetic locus on one particular chromosome. For example, the genetic locus for the Rh blood group is on the short arm of chromosome 1; at this site there are two Rh genes, one on chromosome 1 derived from the mother and the other on chromosome 1 derived from the father. When two genes at the same genetic locus are identical, the individual is a *homozygote*. When the two genes differ (i.e., two different alleles are present at the locus), the individual is a *heterozygote*. Each normal human is heterozygous at approximately 20 percent of genetic loci and homozygous at 80 percent. Figure 5-3 shows a map of human chromosome 1, illustrating the location of a representative sample of genes that have been assigned loci on this chromosome.

The genetic information carried on chromosomes is transmitted to daughter cells under two different sets of circumstances. One of these occurs whenever a somatic cell (i.e., a nongerm cell) divides. This process, called *mitosis*, transmits identical copies of each gene to each daughter cell, thus maintaining a uniform genetic makeup in all cells of a single individual. The other set of circumstances prevails when genetic information must be transmitted from one individual to an offspring. This process, called *meiosis*, produces germ cells (i.e., ova or spermatozoa) that possess only one copy of each parental chromosome, thus allowing for new combinations of chromosomes to occur when ovum and sperm cell fuse during fertilization.

During meiosis, the 46 chromosomes of an immature germ cell arrange themselves in 23 pairs at the center of the nucleus, each pair being composed of one chromosome derived from the mother and its homologous chromosome derived from the father. At a specified point in the meiotic process, the two partner chromosomes separate, only one of each pair going into each daughter cell, or gamete. Thus, meiosis produces gametes with a reduction in the number of chromosomes from 46 to 23, each gamete having received one chromosome from each of the 23 pairs. The assortment of the chromosomes within each pair is random so that each germ cell receives a different combination of maternal and paternal chromosomes. During the process of fertilization, the fusion of ovum and sperm cell, each of which has 23 chromosomes, produces an individual with 46 chromosomes.

The independent assortment of chromosomes into gametes during meiosis produces an enormous diversity among the possible genotypes

FIGURE 5-3 Gene map of human chromosome 1, illustrating a representative sample of the genes that have been localized to this chromosome. The black bands represent those genetic regions of the chromosome that stain brightly by a fluorescent dye such as quinacrine; the white bands are the negatively staining regions; the hatched area is a variable region that stains differently (i.e., either brightly or negatively) in the chromosomes of different individuals. Each gene is listed opposite its genetic locus on the right. (*Data provided by VA McKusick.*)

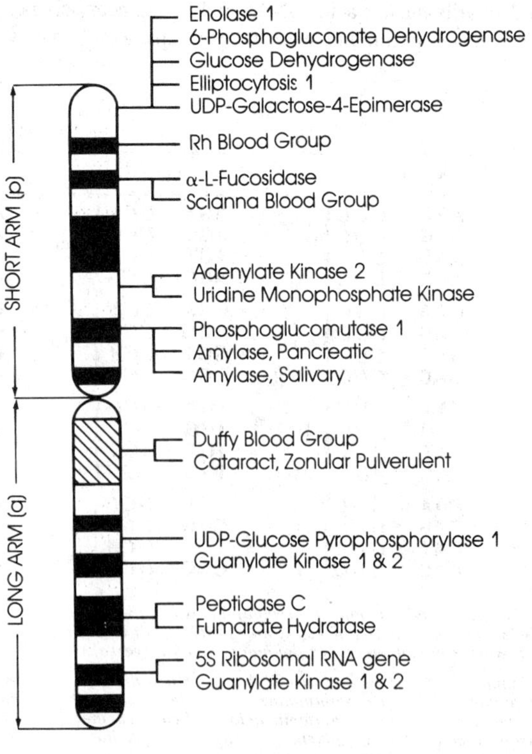

of the progeny. For each 23 pairs of chromosomes, there are 2^{23} different combinations of chromosomes that could occur in a gamete, and the likelihood that one set of parents will produce two offspring with the identical complement of chromosomes is one in 2^{23} or one in 8.4 million (assuming no monozygotic or identical twins).

RECOMBINATION Adding to the genetic diversity in humans is the phenomenon of *genetic recombination*. During meiosis, when homologous chromosomes are paired, bridges frequently form between corresponding regions of the chromosome pair. These bridges, or *chiasmata*, are regions in which the two chromosomes break at identical points along their length and subsequently rejoin, the distal segments having been switched from one homologous chromosome to another. This process is designated *crossing over*. Although no net change in the amount of genetic material occurs during crossing over, a recombination of genes does occur. For example, consider a chromosome with two loci, A and B, located at opposite ends of the same chromosome. On this particular chromosome, the A locus has a rare allele *x*, and the B locus also has a rare allele *y*. Without the phenomenon of recombination every offspring that inherited the *x* allele at the A locus would also inherit the *y* allele at the B locus. However, if recombination occurs, the A locus with the *x* allele would then be on the opposite chromosome from the B locus with the *y* allele. In this case any offspring that inherited the *x* allele at the A locus could not inherit the *y* allele at the B locus.

Crossing over occurs with great frequency in every meiosis in humans, and the resultant recombination of genes may occur at any point on a chromosome. The farther apart two genes are on the same chromosome, the greater is the likelihood that a crossing over will occur in the space between them. When two genes are on the opposite ends of a long chromosome, the probability of recombination is so great that their respective alleles are transmitted to offspring almost independently of one another, just as if the two gene loci were on different chromosomes. On the other hand, gene loci that are close together on the same chromosome are said to be *linked* so that there is a great likelihood that offspring will inherit the same combination of alleles that are present on the parental chromosome.

Several examples of *gene linkage* can be seen from the map of human chromosome 1 (Fig. 5-3). For example, the locus for the gene specifying the Rh blood group factor and the locus for the gene producing one form of the dominant trait hereditary elliptocytosis occur in close proximity on this chromosome. Thus, if a subject with hereditary elliptocytosis transmits the disease to an offspring, the offspring will usually inherit the allele that is present at the Rh locus on this chromosome. If the Rh allele happens to be a rare one in the population (such as *r'*), one can assume that whichever offspring inherits the *r'* allele at the Rh locus will also inherit the abnormal allele at the elliptocytosis locus. On the other hand, if an offspring does not exhibit the *r'* allele, he or she will not usually have elliptocytosis. The concept of linkage does not imply an association between any particular set of Rh alleles and the disease state elliptocytosis, rather between the two genetic loci. Thus, in different families the abnormal elliptocytosis allele may be linked to the R^1, R^0, r_2, or any other allele at the Rh locus, depending on the allele that happened to be at that locus when the elliptocytosis mutation occurred. Stated another way, the elliptocytosis locus is linked to the Rh locus in every family, but the particular Rh allele with which it is associated differs from family to family.

MUTATION Broadly defined, a *mutation* is a stable, heritable alteration in DNA. Although the causes of mutation in humans are largely unknown, a variety of environmental agents, such as radiation, viruses, and chemicals, are among the factors that are implicated.

Mutations can involve a visible alteration in the structure of a chromosome, such as a deletion or translocation of a portion of a chromosome, or they can involve a minute change in one of the purine or pyrimidine bases of a single gene. Most commonly, such "point" mutations consist of the substitution of one base for another, changing the meaning of the codon containing that base, hence their designation as *missense mutations*. For example, in the gene coding for the β chain of hemoglobin, the sixth position normally contains the nucleotide triplet CTC, which codes for the amino acid glutamic acid (Fig. 5-1). The mutation that gives rise to hemoglobin C produces a change of the first base of this triplet from cytosine to thymine, changing the triplet to TTC, which codes for lysine. On the other hand, the mutation that gives rise to hemoglobin S produces a change in the second base of the same triplet (from thymine to adenine), producing CAC, which codes for valine. Thus, in the sixth position of the β chain of hemoglobin, the normally occurring glutamic acid may be replaced with either lysine (producing hemoglobin C) or valine (producing hemoglobin S). More than 90 such single-base mutations in the hemoglobin β chain have been identified, and many of these mutations produce distinct clinical syndromes. Of all the mutations so far elucidated in humans, most involve such single-base changes.

Besides producing an amino acid substitution, a single-base substitution can also cause another abnormality in protein synthesis—premature chain termination. Three mRNA code words (UAA, UAG, and UGA) normally do not specify an amino acid but constitute the signal that the message has ended and that the protein chain should be released from the ribosome (Fig. 5-1). If a change occurs in DNA that produces one of these mRNA code words [for example, a switch in an mRNA triplet from UAU (tyrosine) to UAA (termination)], the polypeptide chain would be terminated prematurely when translation had reached that point. Such mutations, called *non-sense mutations*, produce short fragments of proteins that have reduced function.

CELLULAR MECHANISM BY WHICH MUTANT GENES PRODUCE DISEASES Critical to the understanding of heredity is the concept that the only information transmitted from generation to generation is the sequence of bases in DNA and that these sequences in turn specify only the primary structure of RNA and protein molecules. All other chemical reactions—such as the synthesis of complex lipids and carbohydrates, the formation of membranes and other cellular organelles, and the accumulation and partitioning of inorganic ions—occur as a secondary consequence of the action of specific proteins. Many of these proteins are enzymes that catalyze the biochemical conversion of one molecule into another. Others are structural proteins such as collagen and elastin, and still others are regulatory proteins that dictate how much of each enzyme and each structural protein is made.

Since proteins are the cellular molecules whose structures are encoded by genes, mutations in genes exert their deleterious effects by altering the structure of enzymes, structural proteins, or regulatory proteins. For example, in a disease such as glycogen storage disease, type I (von Gierke's disease), massive accumulation of glycogen in the liver is due not to a primary structural abnormality in the polysaccharide glycogen but to a structural abnormality in a protein, glucose-6-phosphatase, an enzyme that is required to liberate glucose so as to permit glycogen breakdown. Other examples of the biochemical mechanisms by which mutant genes alter cellular metabolism are discussed below under "Simply Inherited Disorders."

GENETIC HETEROGENEITY When two or more mutations can produce a similar clinical syndrome, genetic heterogeneity is said to exist. Hemophilia is one example of a genetically heterogeneous syndrome. A clinically similar bleeding disorder can be caused by mutations at either of two loci on the X chromosome, one leading to a deficiency of factor VIII (classic hemophilia) and the other causing a deficiency of factor IX (Christmas disease). Most, if not all, hereditary diseases, when carefully analyzed, will probably prove to be genetically heterogeneous.

Genetic heterogeneity may result from the existence of a series of different mutations at a single genetic locus (allelic mutations) or from mutations at different genetic loci (nonallelic mutations). For example, drug-induced hemolysis of red blood cells can occur in patients with several different types of allelic mutations at the glucose-6-phosphate dehydrogenase locus. On the other hand, hemophilia is an example of a syndrome in which nonallelic mutations can produce a similar clinical picture (see above).

In some cases of heterogeneity, both the genetic locus and the mode of inheritance differ. Diseases such as spastic paraplegia, Charcot-Marie-Tooth peroneal muscular atrophy, and retinitis pigmentosa are inherited as autosomal dominant traits in some families, as autosomal recessives in others, and as X-linked recessives in still others. The identification of such genetic heterogeneity in these disorders is of obvious importance for correct genetic counseling.

TAKING THE FAMILY HISTORY

The investigation of a patient with a possible genetic disorder begins with the *family history*. The first step is to obtain certain information on the *proband* or *index case* (i.e., the clinically affected person who has brought the family to attention) and on each of the *first-degree relatives* (i.e., the parents, siblings, and offspring of the proband). This information includes the given name, surname, maiden name, birth date or current age, age at death, cause of death, and name or description of any disease or defect.

The second step is to ask questions designed to survey the family for the presence of disease or defect. (1) Has any relative an identical or similar trait? (2) Has any relative a trait that is absent in the proband but is known to occur in some patients with the same disease? This question requires that the physician have some knowledge about the manifestations of the disease in question. For example, when obtaining the family history from a proband with dissecting aneurysm caused possibly by Marfan's syndrome, one should ask about the occurrence of eye abnormalities, cardiac abnormalities, and skeletal abnormalities in the relatives. (3) Has any relative a trait that is recognized to be genetically determined? The purpose of this question is to ascertain the occurrence of hereditary disease in the family even though the particular patient may not be involved. (4) Has any relative an unusual disease, or has any relative died of a rare condition? The purpose of this question is to identify a condition that might be genetically determined though not recognized as such by the informant. In addition, this question may help to identify conditions in relatives that might be etiologically related to the patient's problem. For example, a patient with pheochromocytoma should be suspected of having von Recklinghausen's disease if he or she has a brother with scoliosis and mental retardation, both of which can be manifestations of the neurofibromatosis (von Recklinghausen's) gene. (5) Is there any consanguinity in the family? This inquiry should be made directly. In addition, one should ask whether common last names appear in the families of husband-wife pairs. Consanguineous marriage may be the source of a rare autosomal recessive syndrome, and sometimes its presence in the family may not be known by the proband. (6) What is the ethnic origin of the family? Persons of various ethnic origins, such as blacks, Jews, and Greeks, have increased chances of specific genetic diseases. Table 5-1 lists examples of simply inherited disorders that are found with increased frequency in various ethnic groups.

TABLE 5-1 Examples of simply inherited disorders that occur with increased frequency in specific ethnic groups

Ethnic group	Simply inherited disorder
African blacks	Hemoglobinopathies, especially Hb S, Hb C, persistent Hb F, α and β thalassemias Glucose-6-phosphate dehydrogenase deficiency
Armenians	Familial Mediterranean fever
Ashkenazi Jews	Abetalipoproteinemia Bloom's syndrome Dystonia musculorum deformans (recessive form) Factor XI (PTA) deficiency Familial dysautonomia (Riley-Day syndrome) Gaucher's disease (adult form) Neimann-Pick disease Pentosuria Tay-Sachs disease
Chinese	α-Thalassemia Glucose-6-phosphate dehydrogenase deficiency Adult lactase deficiency
Eskimos	Pseudocholinesterase deficiency Adrenogenital syndrome
Finns	Congenital nephrosis Mulibrey nanism
French Canadians	Tyrosinemia
Japanese	Acatalasemia
Lebanese	Homozygous familial hypercholesterolemia
Mediterranean peoples (Italians, Greeks, Sephardic Jews)	β-Thalassemia Glucose-6-phosphate dehydrogenase deficiency Familial Mediterranean fever Glycogen storage disease, type III
Northern Europeans	Cystic fibrosis
Scandinavians	Alpha$_1$-antitrypsin deficiency LCAT (lecithin:cholesterol acyltransferase) deficiency
South African whites	Porphyria variegata Homozygous familial hypercholesterolemia

CATEGORIES OF GENETIC DISORDERS

Genetic diseases generally fall into one of three categories: (1) *Chromosomal disorders* involve the lack, excess, or abnormal arrangement of one or more chromosomes, producing excessive or deficient genetic material. (2) *Mendelian or simply inherited disorders* are determined primarily by a single mutant gene. These disorders display inheritance patterns which can be classified into autosomal dominant, autosomal recessive, or X-linked types. (3) *Mulifactorial disorders* are caused by an interaction of multiple genes and multiple exogenous or environmental factors. Although many of these multifactorial disorders, such as essential hypertension and cleft lip and palate, are said to run in families, the inheritance pattern is complex and the risk to relatives is less than in the single-gene (mendelian) disorders. Each of these categories presents different problems with respect to causation, prevention, diagnosis, genetic counseling, and treatment.

CHROMOSOMAL DISORDERS The karyotype of an individual (i.e., the number and structure of the chromosomes) can be ascertained from readily accessible body tissues, such as peripheral blood lymphocytes or skin, by growing them in tissue culture until active cell proliferation occurs and then preparing single cells for examination of chromosomes by microscopy. Each individual chromosome can be identified by special staining of DNA sequences, for example, by the affinity of fluorescent dyes (such as quinacrine hydrochloride) for certain chromosomal segments that can be visualized by fluorescence microscopy or by treatment with special dyes (Giemsa) and proteolytic enzymes (trypsin). These techniques produce characteristic *banding patterns* for each chromosome (Fig. 5-4).

The number of chromosomes in normal individuals is 46, of which 44 are the 22 pairs of *autosomes* and the other two are the *sex chromosomes*. Women have two X chromosomes (XX), and men have one X chromosome and one Y chromosome (XY). Each of the 22 pairs of autosomes and the two sex chromosomes can be distinguished on the basis of size, location of the centromere (which divides the chromosome into arms of equal or unequal length), and the unique banding pattern (Fig. 5-4). The relative length of the arms and the position of the centromere are used as further criteria to divide the human chromosomes into seven groups (designated A to G) (Fig. 5-4).

For a complete discussion of the etiology and clinical features of chromosomal abnormalities affecting humans, the reader is referred to Chap. 7.

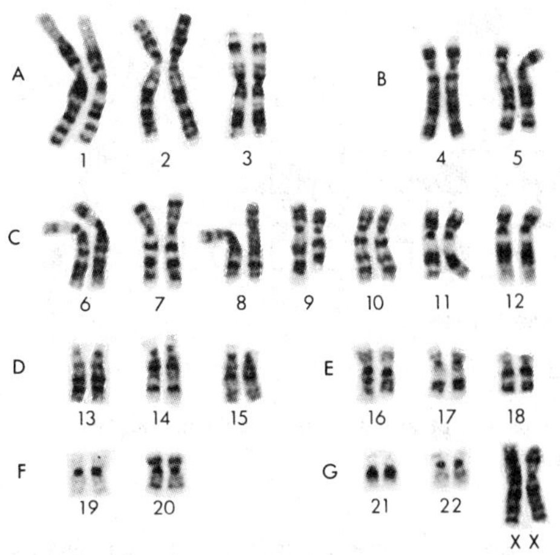

FIGURE 5-4 The karyotype of a normal female showing the chromosomes of a single somatic cell in the metaphase stage of cell division. The photographic images of the chromosomes have been cut out and arranged according to descending length and varying arm ratio. The chromosomes have been stained by the Giemsa technique, which allows each chromosome pair to be identified by its unique banding pattern. Chromosomes 1 to 22 are the autosomes. The sex chromosomes in this normal female are both X. The normal male has an identical karyotype except for the absence of one X chromosome and the presence instead of one Y chromosome. (*Courtesy of David H. Ledbetter.*)

SIMPLY INHERITED DISORDERS Disorders caused by the transmission of a single mutant gene show one of three simple (or mendelian) patterns of inheritance: (1) autosomal dominant, (2) autosomal recessive, or (3) X-linked. The distinction between "dominant" and "recessive" is one of convenience in pedigree analysis and does not imply a fundamental difference in genetic mechanism. The term *dominant* implies that a mutation is clinically manifest when an individual has a single dose of this mutation (or is *heterozygous* for it), while *recessive* implies that a double dose (or *homozygosity*) is required for clinical detection. Genes are never dominant or recessive; their effects, however, produce clinical patterns that are classified as dominant or recessive. Despite their overall clinical "normality," individuals who are heterozygous for "recessive" genes often have biochemical abnormalities that are demonstrable in the laboratory; on the other hand, those who are homozygous for "dominant" genes are usually more severely affected than are the heterozygotes.

With few exceptions, each of the approximately 1200 mendelian diseases is rare. However, as a group these disorders constitute an important cause of morbidity and death, accounting directly for more than 5 percent of all hospital admissions.

The genes for more than 200 simply inherited diseases have been assigned to specific chromosomes. Disease-producing genes assigned to the X chromosome outnumber those so far assigned to any single autosome. This is because assignment to the X chromosome requires only pedigree studies showing X-linked inheritance (see below). Assignment to an autosome is more complicated, requiring sophisticated techniques of somatic cell hybridization or pedigree studies showing linkage between a disease-producing gene and a "marker" gene that is known to be on a certain chromosome. Table 5-2 shows a partial list of those human genetic diseases that have been mapped to specific chromosomes.

The demonstration that a particular disease or syndrome shows one of the three mendelian patterns of inheritance implies that its pathogenesis, no matter how complex, is due to an abnormality in a single protein molecule. For example, in sickle cell anemia, the entire clinical syndrome, including such seemingly unrelated disturbances as anemia, pain crises, nephropathy, and predisposition to pneumococcal infections, are all the physiologic consequences of having thymine instead of adenine at a specific site in the gene that codes for the β chain of hemoglobin, producing a substitution of a valine for a glutamic acid in the sixth amino acid position in the protein sequence.

In many mendelian disorders, especially in those with dominant inheritance, it is not possible to demonstrate directly the protein that is primarily altered by the mutation. In such cases (e.g., adult polycystic kidney disease and tuberous sclerosis) only the distal physiologic effects of the mutation are recognizable. Nevertheless, it is safe to assume that a single primary defect exists whenever a disease is transmitted by a single-gene mechanism and that the various manifestations of the disease all can be related to the mutational event by a more or less complicated "pedigree of causes."

TABLE 5-2 Partial list of human genetic diseases that have been mapped to specific chromosomes

Chromosome	Disease
1	Elliptocytosis
	RH erythroblastosis
	Porphyria cutanea tarda
2	Protein C deficiency
3	Protein S deficiency
	Orotic aciduria
4	Huntington's disease
5	Gardner syndrome
	Familial polyposis coli
6	Hemochromatosis
	Congenital adrenal hyperplasia (21-hydroxylase deficiency)
7	Cystic fibrosis
	Ehlers-Danlos syndrome (one form)
	Osteogenesis imperfecta (one form)
9	Galactosemia
	Nail-patella syndrome
10	Multiple endocrine neoplasia, type 2
11	Syndrome of Wilms' tumor, aniridia, gonadoblastoma, retardation
	β-Thalassemia
	Sickle cell anemia
	Acute intermittent porphyria
12	Phenylketonuria
	von Willebrand's disease
13	Retinoblastoma
	Wilson's disease
14	Nucleoside phosphorylase deficiency (immunodeficiency)
	Alpha$_1$-antitrypsin deficiency
15	Prader-Willi syndrome
	Tay Sachs disease
16	α-Thalassemia
	Gout due to adenine phosphoribosyltransferase deficiency
	LCAT deficiency
17	Growth hormone deficiency (type 1A)
	von Recklinghausen neurofibromatosis
19	Familial hypercholesterolemia
	Familial type 3 hyperlipoproteinemia
	Myotonic dystrophy
	Complement C3 deficiency
20	Adenosine deaminase deficiency (immunodeficiency)
21	Alzheimer's disease
	Homocystinuria
22	Metachromatic leukodystrophy
	Hurler syndrome (mucopolysaccharidoses I)
	Scheie's syndrome (mucopolysaccharidoses V)
X	X-linked ichthyosis due to placental steroid sulfatase deficiency
	Ocular albinism
	Chronic granulomatous disease
	Duchenne muscular dystrophy
	Testicular feminization syndrome
	Phosphoglycerate kinase deficiency (hemolytic anemia)
	Fabry's disease
	Lesch-Nyhan syndrome
	Fragile site associated with X-linked mental retardation
	Color blindness
	Hemophilia A
	Glucose-6-phosphate dehydrogenase (G6PD) deficiency

SOURCE: McKusick.

TABLE 5-3 Some relatively frequent mendelian disorders affecting adults

AUTOSOMAL DOMINANT DISORDERS
Familial hypercholesterolemia
Hereditary hemorrhagic telangiectasia
Marfan's syndrome
Hereditary spherocytosis
Adult polycystic kidney disease
Huntington's chorea
Acute intermittent porphyria
Osteogenesis imperfecta tarda
von Willebrand's disease
Myotonic dystrophy
Idiopathic hypertrophic subaortic stenosis (IHSS)
Noonan's syndrome
Neurofibromatosis
Tuberous sclerosis
AUTOSOMAL RECESSIVE DISORDERS
Deafness
Albinism
Wilson's disease
Hemochromatosis
Sickle cell anemia
β-Thalassemia
Cystic fibrosis
Hereditary emphysema (alpha$_1$-antitrypsin deficiency)
Homocystinuria
Familial Mediterranean fever
Friedreich's ataxia
Phenylketonuria
X-LINKED DISORDERS
Hemophilia A
Glucose-6-phosphate dehydrogenase deficiency
Fabry's disease
Ocular albinism
Testicular feminization
Chronic granulomatous disease
Hypophosphatemic rickets
Color blindness

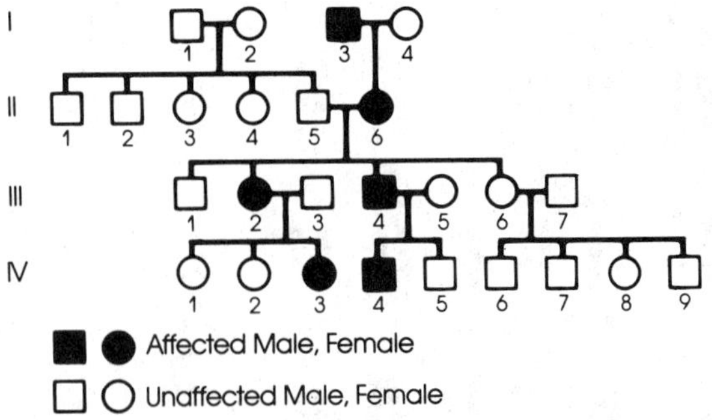

FIGURE 5-5 Pedigree pattern of an autosomal dominant trait. Note the *vertical* pattern of inheritance.

Table 5-3 lists the most commonly encountered mendelian disorders affecting adults.

Autosomal dominant disorders Dominant diseases are those manifest in the heterozygous state, that is, when only one abnormal gene (*mutant allele*) is present and the corresponding partner allele on the homologous chromosome is normal. The gene responsible for an autosomal dominant disorder is located on one of the 22 autosomes, and both males and females can be affected. Since alleles segregate independently at meiosis, there is a 1 in 2 chance that the offspring of an affected heterozygote will inherit the mutant allele and, similarly, a 1 in 2 chance of the offspring inheriting the normal allele.

Figure 5-5 shows a typical pedigree involving an autosomal dominant trait. The following features are characteristic: (1) Each affected individual has an affected parent (unless the condition arose by a new mutation or is mildly expressed in the affected parent); (2) an affected individual will bear, on the average, both normal and affected offspring in equal proportions; (3) normal children of an affected individual will have only normal offspring; (4) males and females are affected in equal proportions; (5) each sex is equally likely to transmit the condition to male and female offspring, with male-to-male transmission occurring; and (6) vertical transmission of the condition through successive generations occurs, especially when the trait does not impair reproductive capacity.

While half of the offspring of an individual with an autosomal dominant condition will inherit the disease, it is not necessarily true that each affected person must have an affected parent. In every autosomal dominant disease a certain proportion of affected persons owe their disorder to a new mutation rather than to an inherited mutation. Since the estimated frequency of mutation is 5×10^{-6} mutations per gene per generation and since a dominant trait, by definition, requires a mutation in only one of a pair of alleles, one would expect that about 1 in 100,000 newborn persons would possess a new mutation at any given genetic locus. Many of these mutations either do not impair the function of the gene product or involve a recessive function so that the mutation is clinically silent. Others, however, cause a defective gene product that gives rise to a dominant trait. The parent in whose germ cells the mutation arose is clinically normal. Likewise, the siblings of the affected individual are normal since the mutation affects only a single germ cell. However, the affected individual transmits the disease to half of his or her children.

The proportion of patients with dominant disorders who represent new mutations is inversely proportional to the effect of the disease in question on biologic fitness. The term *biologic fitness* refers to the ability of an affected individual to produce children who survive to adult life and reproduce. In the extreme case, if a dominant mutation produced absolute infertility, then all observed cases would of necessity represent new mutations, and it would be impossible to prove the genetic transmission of the trait. In less severe disorders, as in tuberous sclerosis, the severe mental retardation reduces biologic fitness to about 20 percent of normal, and the proportion of cases due to new mutations is about 80 percent. Other examples of the relation between biologic fitness and the proportion of new mutations in dominant disorders are shown in Table 5-4.

Many new mutations appear to occur in the germ cells of fathers who are of relatively advanced age. Such a "paternal age effect" is seen, for example, in Marfan's syndrome in which the average age of fathers of sporadic or "new mutation" cases (37 years) is in excess of the mean age of fathers generally (30 years) and also in excess of the age of fathers who transmit Marfan's disease due to an inherited mutation (30 years).

Before one concludes that a dominant disorder in a given patient with unaffected parents is the result of a new mutation, it is important to consider two other possibilities: (1) that the gene may be carried by one parent in whom the disease is of low expressivity (discussed below), and (2) that extramarital paternity may have occurred. The

TABLE 5-4 Approximate percentage of patients affected by new mutations in some autosomal dominant disorders

Disorder	Percentage
Achondroplasia	80
Tuberous sclerosis	80
Neurofibromatosis	40
Marfan's syndrome	30
Myotonic dystrophy	25
Huntington's chorea	4
Adult polycystic kidney disease	1
Familial hypercholesterolemia	Very low

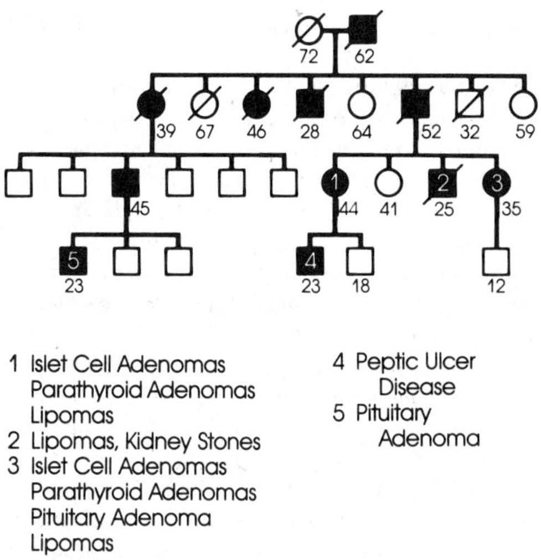

FIGURE 5-6 Pedigree of a family affected with the multiple endocrine adenoma–peptic ulcer syndrome, a disorder inherited as an autosomal dominant trait. Circles denote females; squares, males. Open circles and squares denote unaffected relatives; closed circles and squares denote affected relatives. Deceased relatives are indicated by the oblique line. The age of each relative is indicated below his or her symbol. Note the marked variation in clinical expression among living affected heterozygotes.

latter is found in about 3 to 5 percent of randomly studied children in the United States.

Most autosomal dominant disorders show two characteristic features that are not usually seen in recessive syndromes: (1) *delayed age of onset* and (2) *variability in clinical expression.* Delayed age of onset is seen in disorders such as Huntington's chorea and adult polycystic kidney disease. These disorders do not manifest clinically until adult life, even though the mutant gene is present from the time of conception. Variability in clinical expression is illustrated dramatically by the multiple endocrine adenoma–peptic ulcer syndrome. Patients in the same family inheriting the same abnormal gene may have hyperplasia or neoplasia of one or more endocrine glands (including the pancreas, parathyroid glands, and pituitary gland), as well as of adipose tissue. The resulting clinical manifestations are diverse; different members of the same family may develop peptic ulcers, hypoglycemia, kidney stones, multiple lipomas of the skin, or bitemporal hemianopsia. The recognition that each family member suffers from the same genetic abnormality can be difficult, as illustrated by the family pedigree in Fig. 5-6.

Dominant mutations involve a type of gene product that produces clinical symptoms when only 50 percent of the gene product is defective. The defective genes usually do not encode enzymes, since a 50 percent deficiency of most enzymes produces no symptoms (see "Recessive Disorders" below). Rather, dominant diseases are likely to involve abnormalities in two classes of proteins: (1) those that regulate complex metabolic pathways, such as membrane receptors and rate-limiting enzymes in pathways under feedback control, and (2) key structural proteins, such as hemoglobin or collagen.

The basic biochemical defects have been identified in only a handful of the approximately 600 autosomal dominant disorders. These include familial hypercholesterolemia (abnormal cell surface receptor that binds plasma low-density lipoprotein and thereby regulates cholesterol metabolism); osteogenesis imperfecta (abnormal collagen molecule); hereditary methemoglobinemia and several hemolytic anemias due to unstable forms of hemoglobin (abnormal hemoglobin molecule); hereditary angioneurotic edema (abnormal protein inhibitor of an enzyme involved in the serum complement system); acute intermittent porphyria (abnormal enzyme that catalyzes a rate-limiting step in the heme biosynthetic pathway); and pseudohypoparathyroidism, type 1 (abnormal guanine nucleotide-binding regulatory component or G-protein of the adenylate cyclase system).

Autosomal recessive disorders Autosomal recessive conditions are clinically apparent only in the homozygous state, that is, when both alleles at a particular genetic locus are mutant. By definition, the gene responsible for an autosomal recessive disorder must be on one of the 22 autosomes; thus, both males and females can be affected.

Figure 5-7 shows a pedigree in which an autosomal recessive trait is present in the family. The following features are characteristic: (1) the parents are clinically normal; (2) only siblings are affected, and vertical transmission does not occur; and (3) males and females are affected in equal proportions.

The relative infrequency of recessive genes in the population and the requirement for two abnormal genes for clinical expression combine to create special conditions for autosomal recessive inheritance: (1) the more infrequent the mutant gene in the population, the stronger the likelihood that affected individuals are the product of consanguineous matings (see below); (2) if a husband and a wife are both carriers for the same autosomal recessive gene, 25 percent of the children will be normal, 50 percent will be heterozygous carriers, and 25 percent will be homozygous and affected with the disease; (3) if an affected individual marries a heterozygote (as may occur with consanguineous marriage), half the children will be affected, and a pedigree simulating dominant inheritance will result; and (4) if two individuals with the same recessive disease marry, all their children will be affected.

The clinical picture in autosomal recessive disorders tends to be more uniform than that of dominant diseases, and the age of onset is often early in life. As a general rule, recessive disorders are more commonly diagnosed in children, while dominant diseases are more frequently encountered in adults.

Since with recessive inheritance only one of four children in a sibship is expected to be affected, multiple cases in a family may not occur. This is especially true in a society in which small families are common. Consider, for example, 16 families in which both parents are heterozygous for the same recessive disorder. If each family has two children, 9 of the families will have no affected children, 6 will have one affected and one normal child, and only 1 of the 16 families will have two affected children. In the United States physicians usually see sporadic or isolated cases of a recessive disorder without an affected sibling to alert them to the possibility of a genetic disorder. Fortunately, because of the relatively uniform clinical picture of recessive disorders and because most can be diagnosed directly by biochemical tests, the correct diagnosis can usually be made even when no other members of a family are clinically affected.

The basic biochemical lesions underlying many autosomal recessive disorders have been identified. Of the three types of proteins in which mutations could occur (i.e., enzymes, structural proteins, and regulatory proteins), the enzymes have been the easiest to study. A mutation that destroys the catalytic activity of an enzyme generally does not impair the health of a heterozygote (i.e., an individual who has one mutant allele specifying a functionless enzyme and one

FIGURE 5-7 Pedigree pattern of an autosomal recessive trait. Note the *horizontal* pattern of inheritance.

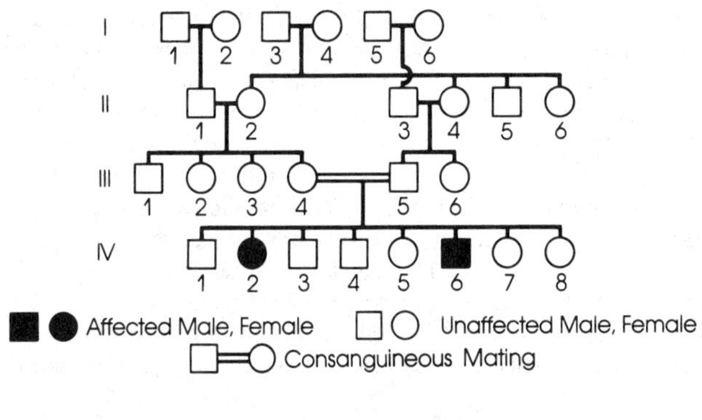

normal allele on the partner chromosome specifying a normal enzyme). In this situation each cell in the body usually produces about 50 percent of the normal number of active enzyme molecules. However, normal regulatory mechanisms function to avert any clinical consequences of this 50 percent deficiency, and so heterozygotes usually are clinically normal. On the other hand, when an individual inherits functionless alleles at both loci specifying an enzyme, the reduction in enzyme activity is too great for a compensatory mechanism to overcome, and a disease results. For example, heterozygotes for phenylketonuria have half the normal activity of phenylalanine hydroxylase, but they are clinically asymptomatic because the body compensates for the half-normal level of the enzyme by raising the substrate concentration approximately twofold. Under these conditions a normal amount of phenylalanine can be metabolized with no symptoms. On the other hand, the homozygote for phenylketonuria has such a severe reduction in phenylalanine hydroxylase activity that enormous levels of phenylalanine and its derivatives accumulate, causing detrimental brain development. As in the case of phenylketonuria, the majority of enzyme deficiency states produce *simultaneously* both a simple accumulation of one or more metabolites preceding the enzymatic block and a deficient production of other metabolites distal to the block in the metabolic pathway.

Most of the genetic enzyme deficiencies that have been elucidated are not only inherited as recessive traits but also tend to involve enzymes that participate in catabolic pathways. Frequently these enzymes degrade organic molecules that are ingested in the diet, such as galactose (galactosemia), phenylalanine (phenylketonuria), and phytanic acid (Refsum's syndrome). A special class of such catabolic diseases is that in which the deficiency affects an acid hydrolase that occurs within lysosomes. In these *lysosomal storage disorders* the substrate, usually a complex lipid or polysaccharide, accumulates within swollen lysosomes in specific organs, giving the cells a foamy appearance. Examples of such lysosomal diseases include the mucopolysaccharidoses such as Hurler's syndrome (α-iduronidase deficiency) and the lipid storage diseases such as Gaucher's disease (glucocerebrosidase deficiency).

In general, recessive diseases are rare because the reduced biologic fitness of homozygotes acts to remove the mutant gene from the population. However, a few recessive disorders, such as cystic fibrosis and sickle cell anemia, are common. To explain this paradox, it has been postulated that the biologic fitness of heterozygotes is greater than that of noncarriers for these genes. In such a case the frequency of the gene in the population depends on the balance between the increased fitness of the relatively numerous heterozygotes and the reduced fitness of the less common homozygotes. A small selective advantage of the heterozygote over the normal results in a high gene frequency and hence a high birth frequency of homozygotes even when the disease is lethal. Thus, about 1 in 22 Caucasians is a heterozygous carrier for the genetically lethal disease cystic fibrosis, and the disease occurs in about 1 in 2000 Caucasian births. To maintain such a high gene frequency, heterozygotes for cystic fibrosis must have a definite reproductive advantage over noncarriers, but the nature of this advantage is unknown. In sickle cell anemia, another recessive disorder with high frequency among certain populations, heterozygotes appear to have increased resistance to malaria.

Inasmuch as recessive diseases require the inheritance of a mutation at the same genetic locus from each parent, when the genes are rare, the likelihood of any two parents being carriers for the same defect becomes small. However, if the parents have a common ancestor and if that ancestor was a carrier for the recessive gene, then the likelihood that two of the descendants have inherited the gene becomes relatively great. The rarer the recessive gene, the stronger the likelihood that an affected individual will have resulted from such a consanguineous mating. On the other hand, certain recessive genes are so common in the population that the likelihood of two random parents being carriers is great enough to eliminate the need for consanguinity. For common traits such as sickle cell anemia, phenylketonuria, cystic fibrosis, and Tay-Sachs disease, all of which have a high carrier frequency in certain populations, consanguinity in the parents is unusual.

In general, consanguinity is infrequent in families with recessive diseases in the United States. This is because the rate of consanguinity in the general population is low. In most of the United States (as opposed to areas with relative geographic isolation such as northern Norway and Switzerland), a disorder must indeed be rare before it is associated with an important frequency of consanguinity. For example, consanguinity is expected in a large proportion of families having children with very rare disorders such as the Laurence-Moon-Biedl syndrome and abetalipoproteinemia.

Genetic compounds represent a special type of recessively inherited disorder in which the affected individual's two mutant genes, although located at the same genetic locus, are not identical. The mutations in the paternal and maternal alleles presumably involve different alterations in the DNA of the same gene. SC hemoglobinopathy is an example of such a *heteroallelic* compound state in which individuals have a gene for sickle cell hemoglobin on one chromosome and a gene for hemoglobin C on the homologous chromosome.

X-linked disorders The genes responsible for X-linked disorders are located on the X chromosome; therefore, the clinical risk and severity of the disease are different for the two sexes. Since a female has two X chromosomes, she may be either heterozygous or homozygous for a mutant gene, and the trait may therefore demonstrate either recessive or dominant expression. Males, on the other hand, have only one X chromosome, so they can be expected to display the full syndrome whenever they inherit the gene regardless of whether the gene behaves as a recessive or as a dominant trait in the female. Thus, the terms *X-linked dominant* or *X-linked recessive* refer only to the expression of the gene in women.

An important feature of all X-linked inheritance is the absence of male-to-male (i.e., father-to-son) transmission of the trait. This follows because a male must always contribute his Y chromosome to his sons; hence, he can never contribute his X chromosome. On the other hand, a male contributes his one X chromosome to all his daughters.

The pedigree in Fig. 5-8 illustrates the characteristic features of X-linked recessive inheritance. (1) In contrast to the vertical transmission in dominant traits (parents and children affected) and the horizontal transmission in autosomal recessive traits (siblings affected), the pedigree pattern in X-linked recessive traits tends to be oblique because of the occurrence of the trait in the sons of normal carrier sisters of affected males (uncles and nephews affected) (Fig. 5-8*A*); (2) male offspring of carrier women have a 50 percent chance of being affected; (3) all female offspring of affected males are carriers, and affected males do not transmit the disease to their sons (Fig. 5-8*C*); (4) unaffected males do not transmit the trait to any offspring; and (5) affected homozygous females occur only when an affected male fathers the child of a carrier female (Fig. 5-8*B*).

Examples of X-linked recessive disorders in humans include hemophilia A, nephrogenic diabetes insipidus, the Lesch-Nyhan syndrome, Duchenne form of muscular dystrophy, glucose-6-phosphate dehydrogenase deficiency, testicular feminization, and Fabry's disease. Color blindness is also inherited as an X-linked recessive trait, but it is sufficiently frequent (occurring in about 8 percent of white males) that the occurrence of homozygous color-blind females is no rarity.

X-linked dominant inheritance is illustrated by the pedigree in Fig. 5-9. Its characteristic features are as follows: (1) Females are affected about twice as often as males; (2) an affected female transmits the disorder to half of her sons and half of her daughters; (3) an affected male transmits the disorder to all his daughters and to none of his sons; and (4) the syndrome is more variable and less severe in heterozygous affected females than in hemizygous affected males. One common trait, the Xg(a+) blood group, is inherited as an X-linked dominant trait, as is vitamin D–resistant rickets (hypophosphatemic rickets).

Some rare conditions may be inherited as X-linked dominant traits

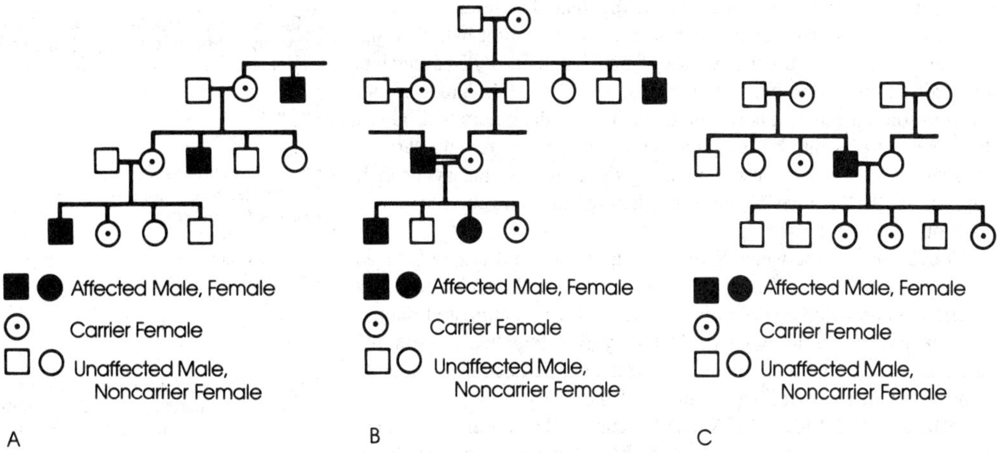

FIGURE 5-8 Pedigree patterns of an X-linked recessive trait. *A*. Note the oblique pattern of inheritance. *B*. An affected female can result from the mating of an affected male and a carrier female, as in the consanguineous marriage shown here. *C*. An affected male mating with a normal noncarrier female has all normal sons and all carrier daughters.

in which there is lethality in the hemizygous male. The characteristics of this form of inheritance are illustrated by the pedigree in Fig. 5-10: (1) The disorder occurs only in females who are heterozygous for the mutant gene; (2) an affected mother transmits the trait to half of her daughters; (3) an increased frequency of abortions occurs in affected women, the abortions representing affected male fetuses. Conditions that appear to be transmitted by this mode of inheritance include incontinentia pigmenti, focal dermal hypoplasia, orofaciodigital syndrome, and hyperammonemia due to ornithine transcarbamylase deficiency.

Expression of X-linked traits in females tends to be variable because of the phenomenon of X-chromosome inactivation. Early in embryonic development one of the two X chromosomes in each somatic cell of a female is inactivated. The inactivation process is random, so that for each cell there is an equal probability that the paternally or maternally derived X chromosome will be inactivated. The inactivated X chromosome is rendered permanently nonfunctional, so that all progeny of the initial cell inherit the same active and inactive X chromosomes. Thus, each female is a mosaic; on the average, half of her cells express the X chromosome of the father, and half express the X chromosome of the mother. If a mutation in a gene is carried on one of her X chromosomes, about one-half of the cells in each tissue will be normal and the other half will manifest the mutant phenotype. However, chance or selection of one or the other set of clones of cells may disturb these proportions in any given individual. Depending on the proportions of mutant and normal X chromosomes in each tissue, a genetically heterozygous female may either be clinically normal or have mild or severe manifestations of the disease. To illustrate, mothers of boys with the X-linked recessive Duchenne form of muscular dystrophy may occasionally show mild manifestations of the disease, such as limb girdle weakness or hypertrophied calves.

In each female cell the nonfunctional X chromosome can be visualized by several techniques. By ordinary staining, the inactivated X chromosome in metaphase appears heteropyknotic (condensed in appearance), and it replicates late in the mitotic cycle (''late-labeling'' with tritiated thymidine). In nondividing cells the inactivated X chromosome can be observed as a clump of chromatin at the periphery of the nucleus—the so-called X chromatin or Barr body. In abnormal states with more than two X chromosomes such as 47, XXX, all but one of the X chromosomes are inactivated, so female cells may have multiple X chromatin bodies (see Chap. 7).

Since a single mutant allele is sufficient for the expression of X-linked recessive disorders, consanguinity does not increase the likelihood of expression in males, unlike the case in the rare autosomal recessive disorders. On the other hand, just as in the dominantly inherited disorders, new mutations can be a factor. In general, if an X-linked recessive condition reduces biologic fitness to zero, one-third of affected males will be a result of new mutations, and an additional one-third will be born to mothers who themselves are carriers as a result of a new mutation. Thus, only one-third will come from a classic pedigree manifesting oblique transmission. An example of such a disease is the Duchenne form of muscular dystrophy in which affected hemizygous males are so severely disabled that they never reproduce. In hemophilia A, in which the biologic fitness is greater than zero, about 20 percent of affected males represent new mutations.

In families in which only one male is affected with an X-linked recessive disease and there is no other family history of the trait, it

FIGURE 5-9 Pedigree pattern of an X-linked dominant trait.

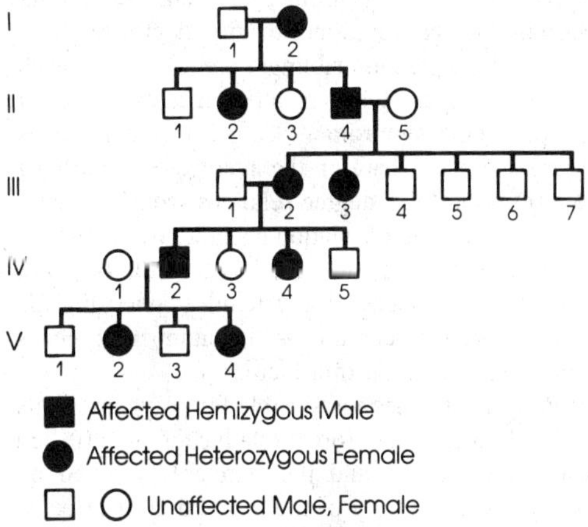

FIGURE 5-10 Pedigree pattern of an X-linked dominant trait lethal in the hemizygous male.

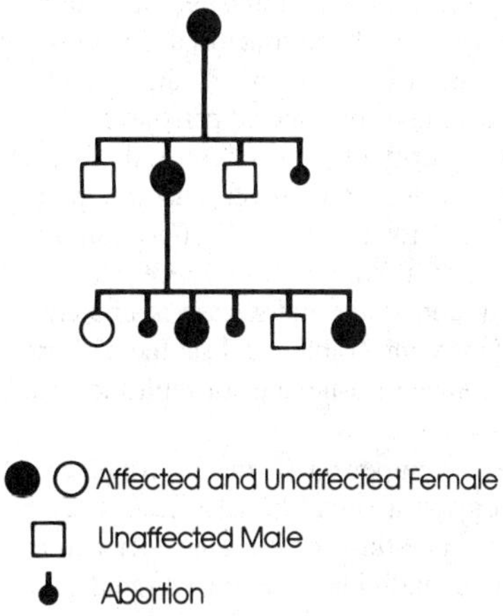

is essential for proper genetic counseling that the mother undergo biochemical tests or other relevant studies to determine whether she is a carrier. If she is a carrier, half of her daughters will be carriers and half of her sons will be affected. On the other hand, if her affected son represents a new mutation, only his daughters will inherit the gene. At present, biochemical tests can identify female carriers for several X-linked diseases including the Lesch-Nyhan syndrome, Fabry's disease, Hunter's syndrome, hemophilia, and the Duchenne form of muscular dystrophy.

The distinction between X-linked inheritance and *sex-influenced autosomal dominant inheritance* is important. Baldness is probably inherited as an autosomal dominant trait, yet it is manifested mainly in men and rarely in women. Heterozygous females express the baldness gene only when a source of testosterone becomes available as occurs with a masculinizing tumor of the ovary.

MULTIFACTORIAL GENETIC DISEASES The common chronic diseases of adults (such as essential hypertension, coronary heart disease, diabetes mellitus, peptic ulcer disease, and schizophrenia) as well as the common birth defects (such as cleft lip and palate, spina bifida, and congenital heart disease) have been long known to "run in families." They fit best into the category of *multifactorial genetic diseases*. The genetic element in these disorders rarely manifests itself in an all-or-none fashion as it does in the simply inherited (mendelian) disorders and in chromosomal aberrations. Instead, it is the interaction of multiple genes with multiple environmental factors that produces the familial aggregation.

In the multifactorial genetic diseases, there is a *polygenic component* consisting of a series of genes that interact in a cumulative fashion. An individual who inherits the right combination of these genes passes beyond a "threshold of risk," at which point an *environmental component* determines whether and to what extent that person is clinically affected. In order for another individual in the same family to express the same syndrome, the same or similar combination of genes must be inherited. Since the first-degree relatives of an affected individual (i.e., parents, siblings, and offspring) each share half of that person's genes, they are all at increased risk of exhibiting the same polygenic syndrome. Second-degree relatives (uncles, aunts, and grandparents) share on the average one-fourth of an individual's genes $(\frac{1}{2})^2$, and third-degree relatives (cousins) share one-eighth $(\frac{1}{2})^3$. Thus, as the degree of relation becomes more distant, the likelihood of a relative inheriting the same combination of genes becomes less. Moreover, the chances of any relative inheriting the right combination of risk genes decrease as the number of genes required for the expression of a given trait increases.

Since the precise number of genes responsible for polygenic traits is unknown, the risk of inheritance for a relative of an affected individual is difficult to calculate, and the standard is based on empiric risk figures (i.e., a direct tally of the proportion of affected relatives in previously reported families). In contrast to the simply inherited disorders in which 25 or 50 percent of the first-degree relatives of an affected proband are at genetic risk, multifactorial genetic disorders are generally observed empirically to affect no more than 5 to 10 percent of first-degree relatives. Moreover, in contrast to mendelian traits, the recurrence risk of multifactorial conditions varies from family to family, and its estimation is significantly influenced by two factors: (1) the number of affected persons already present in the family, and (2) the severity of the disorder in the index case. The greater the number of affected relatives and the more severe their disease, the higher the risk to other relatives. For example, the risk of cleft lip in the siblings of a child with unilateral cleft lip is about 2.5 percent, but if the lesion in the index case is bilateral, the risk in the siblings rises to 6 percent. Table 5-5 lists the empiric risk figures for the familial recurrence of a number of multifactorial genetic diseases.

The hypothesis of a polygenic component in the inheritance of multifactorial diseases has been given a sound basis in recent years by the demonstration that at least one-third of all gene loci harbor polymorphic alleles that vary among individuals. Such a large degree of variation in normal genes undoubtedly provides the substrate for variations in genetic predisposition with which environmental factors can interact. So far, the genetic loci most strikingly associated with predisposition to specific diseases are those that constitute the HLA system (also called the *major histocompatibility gene complex*) (see Chap. 14). The HLA gene complex is located on the short arm of chromosome 6. It consists of four closely linked but distinct loci (A, B, C, and D). The products of these genes are proteins that are found on the surface of body cells and that enable an individual's immune system to distinguish its own cells from those of someone else. Each HLA locus in the population consists of multiple alleles, each of which produces an immunologically distinct protein. For example, an individual may inherit any 2 of 20 alleles at the HLA-B locus.

An important observation of recent years has been the finding that certain alleles at the HLA loci predispose individuals to certain specific diseases. For example, if the B27 allele at the HLA-B locus is inherited by an individual, that person has a 121-fold greater chance of developing ankylosing spondylitis than an individual who lacks this allele (Table 5-6). Ankylosing spondylitis remains a multifactorial disease, however, because its development clearly requires one or more other factors in addition to the B27 allele. Thus, less than 15 percent of people who inherit this allele develop this disease. Table 5-6 lists some of the diseases associated with alleles at the HLA loci. Several of them are suspected to be of viral etiology, suggesting that the HLA loci may dictate the mode of expression of certain viral diseases. A more detailed discussion of the HLA system is presented in Chap. 14.

Multifactorial disorders are heterogeneous in the sense that the relative contribution of the polygenic factors ("risk genes") and environmental factors to the etiology vary greatly from patient to patient. However, it is important to remember that among common

TABLE 5-5 Empiric risks for some common multifactorial genetic diseases affecting adults

Disorder in index case	Estimated absolute risk for first-degree relatives, %
Cleft lip and/or palate	3
Congenital heart disease	4
Coronary heart disease	8 for male relatives 3 for female relatives
Diabetes mellitus	5–10
Epilepsy	5–10
Hypertension	10
Manic-depressive psychosis	10–15
Psoriasis	10–15
Schizophrenia	15
Thyroid disease (autoimmune disorders including hyperthyroidism, thyroiditis, primary myxedema, simple goiter)	10

TABLE 5-6 Alleles at the HLA loci associated with multifactorial genetic diseases

Disease	HLA locus	Specific allele	Relative risk*
Ankylosing spondylitis	B	B27	121
Reiter's syndrome	B	B27	40
Psoriasis with arthritis	B	B27	5
Celiac disease	B	B8	10
Chronic active hepatitis	B	B8	4
Myasthenia gravis	B	B8	4
Diabetes mellitus (insulin-dependent)	DR	DR3/DR4	33
Hyperthyroidism	DR	DR3	4
Addison's disease	B	B8	7
	DR	DR4	10
Multiple sclerosis	DR	DR2	7

* *Relative risk* is the probability of the disease developing in an individual with the specific allele, divided by the probability of its development in an individual who does not possess this specific allele.

TABLE 5-7 Examples of inherited disorders involving an abnormal response to drugs

Disorder	Molecular abnormality	Mode of inheritance	Frequency	Clinical effect	Drugs producing abnormal response
Slow inactivation of isoniazid	Isoniazid acetylase in liver	Autosomal recessive	~50% of U.S. population	Polyneuritis	Isoniazid, sulfamethazine, sulfamaprine, phenelzine, dapsone, hydralazine
Suxamethonium sensitivity	Pseudocholinesterase in plasma	Autosomal recessive	Several mutant alleles; most common affects 1 in 2500	Apnea	Suxamethonium, succinylcholine
Warfarin insensitivity	? Altered receptor or enzyme in liver with increased affinity for vitamin K	Autosomal dominant	Rare	Inability to achieve anticoagulation with usual doses of drug	Warfarin
Glaucoma	Unknown	? Autosomal dominant	Common	Increased intraocular pressure	Glucocorticoids
Malignant hyperthermia	Unknown	Autosomal dominant	~1 in 20,000 anesthetized patients	Severe hyperpyrexia, muscle rigidity, death	Such anesthetics as halothane, succinylcholine, methoxyfluorane, ether, cyclopropane
Unstable hemoglobins:					
Hemoglobin Zurich	Arginine substitution for histidine at sixty-third position of β chain of hemoglobin	Autosomal dominant	Rare	Hemolysis	Sulfonamides
Hemoglobin H	Hemoglobin composed of four β chains	Autosomal dominant	Rare	Hemolysis	Sulfisoxazole
Glucose-6-phosphate dehydrogenase deficiency	Glucose-6-phosphate dehydrogenase in erythrocytes	X-linked recessive	~ 1×10^8 affected persons in world; common in persons of African, Mediterranean, Asiatic origin; multiple mutant alleles	Hemolysis	Analgesics, sulfonamides, antimalarials, nitrofurantoin, other drugs

SOURCE: ES Vesell, N Engl J Med 287:904, 1972.

phenotypes which are largely multifactorial, often a small proportion will be created by major mutant genes. For example, although coronary heart disease is usually of multifactorial etiology, about 5 percent of subjects with premature myocardial infarctions are heterozygotes for familial hypercholesterolemia, a single-gene disorder that produces atherosclerosis in the absence of any other predisposing factor. Similarly, in a small proportion of patients with other common diseases such as peptic ulcer disease or "essential" hypertension, the condition is not multifactorial but determined by a single gene, as in the multiple endocrine adenoma–peptic ulcer syndrome or the medullary thyroid carcinoma–pheochromocytoma syndrome, respectively.

INTERACTION BETWEEN SINGLE GENETIC AND ENVIRONMENTAL FACTORS

Many diseases result from an interaction between a specific genotype and a specific environmental factor. In particular, inherited single-gene mutations may produce clinically significant and often life-threatening idiosyncratic responses to certain drugs.

Table 5-7 lists the most important of these *pharmacogenetic disorders,* which encompass all the mendelian modes of inheritance. Perhaps the most common is glucose-6-phosphate dehydrogenase deficiency, an X-linked recessive trait in which a variety of drugs may precipitate a hemolytic anemia. Plasma pseudocholinesterase deficiency and hepatic transacetylase deficiency are examples of autosomal recessive traits which alter drug catabolism so that when the muscle relaxant suxamethonium or the antituberculous drug isoniazid is administered, apnea or peripheral neuropathy, respectively, may ensue. Malignant hyperthermia is an autosomal dominant trait in which acute hyperpyrexia, muscle rigidity, and hyperkalemic cardiac arrest may be induced by administration of any one of several anesthetic agents. Acute intermittent porphyria is another example of a genetic disorder that is exacerbated by drugs, such as barbiturates.

Misinterpretation of adverse drug reactions may result in serious harm to patients. In general, all unusual idiosyncratic reactions should be considered to be genetically determined until proved otherwise. Fortunately, the pharmacogenetic disorders are a group of diseases for which therapy is straightforward: avoidance of the noxious drug by patient and relatives.

In addition to drugs, other factors in the environment may aggravate specific genetic traits. Cigarette smoke may have deleterious effects on persons homozygous and possibly heterozygous for alpha$_1$-antitrypsin deficiency, who are predisposed to the development of emphysema. Patients with xeroderma pigmentosa and anhydrotic ectodermal dysplasia are unusually sensitive to sunlight and high temperatures, respectively. Avoidance of milk at an early age prevents many of the complications ordinarily seen in persons with galactosemia.

Genetic-environmental interactions are particularly important in pregnancy. Women who are affected with phenylketonuria may develop high plasma phenylalanine levels during pregnancy, and thus their offspring may suffer from a variety of phenylalanine-induced birth defects even though the offspring may not themselves have phenylketonuria. Other examples of diseases resulting from an adverse genetic relation between the mother and fetus include erythroblastosis caused by Rh incompatibility and diabetic embryopathy, a term that refers to a series of major birth defects occurring in about 5 percent of the offspring of women who are clinically diabetic during pregnancy.

REFERENCES

EMERY AEH, RIMOIN DL: *Principles and Practice of Medical Genetics,* Vols. 1 and 2. Edinburgh, Churchill Livingstone, 1983

LEWIN B: *Genes,* 3d ed. New York, Wiley, 1987

MCKUSICK VA: *Mendelian Inheritance in Man: Catalogs of Autosomal Dominant, Autosomal Recessive and X-Linked Phenotypes,* 8th ed. Baltimore, Johns Hopkins, 1988

SCRIVER CR et al: *The Metabolic Basis of Inherited Disease*, 6th ed. New York, McGraw-Hill, 1989
THOMPSON JS, THOMPSON MW: *Genetics in Medicine*, 4th ed. Philadelphia, Saunders, 1986
VOGEL F, MOTULSKY AG: *Human Genetics: Problems and Approaches*, 2d ed. Berlin, Springer-Verlag, 1986

6 MOLECULAR GENETICS AND MEDICINE

ARTHUR L. BEAUDET

The haploid human genome contains about 3×10^9 (3 billion) base pairs of DNA and is estimated to encode 30,000 to 100,000 gene products. The length of DNA frequently is quantitated in thousands of bases (kilobases, kb), e.g., the human genome is 3 million kb in length. Each individual inherits two copies of this genome, and the DNA is packaged as 23 pairs of chromosomes. Each chromosome contains a single linear duplex DNA molecule. Most of the DNA sequences that encode proteins occur as unique (single copy) sequences in the genome. Many gene products show similarities in amino acid sequence and can be viewed as members of large gene families, e.g., the globin gene family or the immunoglobulin superfamily. A large amount of DNA in the genome *appears* not to be functional. Hundreds, if not thousands, of repetitive DNA sequences of uncertain function are present in the genome; some are dispersed, and some are clustered.

If one were to print *one copy* of *one strand* of the human genome, it would fill a text 170 times the size of *Harrison's*. The analogy of the human genome to a large book can be carried further. The book can be envisioned as being bound into 46 separate volumes, each the equivalent of one chromosome. Individuals would inherit one paternal set of 23 volumes and one maternal set of 23 volumes. Sickle cell anemia would be the equivalent of changing a single letter on one page of one volume from each of the sets, while deletion of the alpha-globin gene cluster in α-thalassemia might represent the equivalent of the loss of one or two pages of text in each set. Digestion of genomic DNA with restriction enzymes, which recognize specific short DNA sequences and cut DNA at these sites, would be the equivalent of cutting the line of text each time a specific word occurred.

The human genome is extraordinarily polymorphic, but the DNA differences have a broad range of biologic significance. Beginning at the single nucleotide level, the DNA sequence for the human genome can be variable or relatively constant at a given position. As an example, a DNA base would be highly variable if 60 percent of genes in the population had an A (adenine) nucleotide at the position, 40 percent of genes had a G (guanine) nucleotide, and none had a C (cytosine) or T (thymine) nucleotide. Nucleotide positions where more than 1 percent of genes show a nonmajority sequence are designated *polymorphic sites*. Only 1 in 200 to 1 in 500 nucleotide positions qualify as polymorphic. Most nucleotide positions are relatively invariant, the vast majority having the same sequence. The remaining positions have intermediate frequencies of variation. Nucleotide sequence variation is greater in nonfunctional parts of the genome, less in regions of the genome that encode protein sequence or have other important functions. The consequence is that each copy of the human genome varies from every other copy in millions of sequence-specific ways. The nucleotide variations might be envisioned as a multimillion digit serial number embedded within each copy of the human genome. The variability in primary sequence goes beyond single-base changes to include presence or absence of whole segments of DNA. Indeed, considerable length variations occur in the human genome. Inversions of DNA sequence also occur, and translocations between chromosomes also cause DNA variation.

The second type of genetic variation involves phenotypic effect. The alteration of a single nucleotide or single gene may have a dramatic effect. Indeed, certain DNA sequence alterations may be lethal at the stage of the gamete, fertilized egg, or preimplantation embryo. These instances in which a single alteration has a large effect on the phenotype are single-gene disorders; such disorders have been the focus of most efforts to understand human genetic disease up to the present. However, most of the nucleotide differences between human genomes do not cause any significant phenotypic effect. A continuum exists whereby variations in DNA sequence have phenotypic effects ranging from none to minuscule, to small, to moderate, to large, or to overwhelming. In many instances, multiple genetic loci may interact with each other and/or with environmental factors to produce a phenotypic effect. For example, genetic variations in lipoprotein genes, lipoprotein receptor genes, genes that influence intermediary metabolism, and other genes probably interact with diet, smoking, and additional environmental factors to determine susceptibility to atherosclerosis. Together, variations in DNA sequence and in the biologic effect caused by these differences create individuality. Individuals differ as much in DNA, biochemistry, pharmacokinetics, and susceptibility to disease as in facial appearance, fingerprints, and personality.

ANALYSIS OF THE HUMAN GENOME

Molecular analyses of medical relevance rely heavily on four strategic features: (1) the ability to clone and characterize nucleic acid sequences, (2) the specificity of nucleic acid hybridization, (3) the specificity of restriction endonucleases, and (4) the power of DNA amplification using the polymerase chain reaction (PCR). Various combinations of these capabilities are used to accomplish diverse diagnostic procedures.

MOLECULAR CLONING AND SEQUENCING The size, the complexity, and the variability of the human genome constitute barriers to the analysis of individual traits and genes. The feasibility for such analysis was greatly enhanced by the development of recombinant DNA technology. This technology allows for the analysis of one DNA fragment at a time and has provided an "index" for the human genome and made it possible to locate and isolate individual genes, segments of genes, or nucleotide sequences from the vast DNA library. One of the most powerful of these techniques, so-called cloning of DNA, makes it possible to isolate individual genes or portions of genes, to make an unlimited number of copies of such DNA fragments, to determine the nucleotide sequence of the DNA, and to transcribe and translate the genes so isolated. The various genes and gene products can then be utilized for diverse studies of gene structure and function in normal and disease states. Other recombinant DNA techniques make it possible to analyze genetic variation in individuals directly using clinical samples. Using DNA-hybridization techniques, restriction enzyme digestion, and DNA amplification, to be described below, disease traits can be analyzed both directly and by genetic linkage to polymorphic sites.

The cloning of DNA involves isolation of DNA fragments and insertion of a sequence into the nucleic acid from another biologic source (vector) for manipulation and propagation. The most widely used vectors are based on bacterial plasmids or bacteriophage such as phage λ or M13, some variations of which can accommodate DNA fragments up to 45 kb in size. In addition, vectors designed to function as yeast artificial chromosomes (YAC vectors) can be utilized for cloning DNA fragments up to hundreds of kilobases in size. Space does not allow presentation of the various methods for DNA cloning, but these are well described in Watson et al. and in Sambrook et al. For purposes of this discussion, it is adequate to point out that cDNA (DNA complementary to mRNA) clones have been isolated for hundreds of human genes. Most of these cDNAs have been cloned after characterization of the gene product to obtain amino acid sequence data or specific antibodies. Genomic DNA clones are also

*Hae*III	5′-G-G | C-C-3′ 3′-C-C ↓ G-G-5′		*Hind*III	5′-A | A-G-C-T-T-3′ 3′-T-T-C-G-A ↓ A-5′		*Mst*II	5′-C-C | T-N-A-G-G-3′ 3′-G-G-A-N-T ↓ C-C-5′

FIGURE 6-1 DNA sequence specificity and nuclease activity for three restriction endonucleases. *Hae*III leaves a blunt end while the other enzymes leave single-stranded ends.

available for hundreds of human genes. In addition, many hundreds of *anonymous* genomic DNA clones are in widespread use. These anonymous DNA clones are generally of interest because they detect polymorphisms that map to a particular location in the human genome, as will be discussed below. Human genomic DNA libraries have been prepared containing most or all of the human genome in fragments of 15 to 45 kb. Radioactive, biotinylated, or otherwise modified copies of DNA can be prepared from any cloned fragment and can serve as a specific molecular *probe*. Biotinylated probes can be detected using avidin and secondary detection methods. Cloned DNA can be sequenced using manual or semiautomated methods, and the sequence of millions of base pairs of human DNA is already known, although only about 0.1 percent of the human genome was sequenced as of early 1989. If a gene or a genomic segment has been cloned, it is relatively straightforward to clone the same region from individual patients and determine the sequence for any mutation. The availability of sequence data allows for the use of the polymerase chain reaction for DNA amplification. Thus, some of the fruits of molecular cloning are the availability of probes for analytical procedures, the determination of disease mutations, and the availability of sequence data to allow for DNA amplification. Cloned DNA can also be used for production of proteins, for detection of sequences of infectious organisms, and for research activities.

NUCLEIC ACID HYBRIDIZATION Many of the steps in recombinant DNA analysis take advantage of the fact that the complementary nature of nucleic acid interaction is the result of base pairing during the synthesis of DNA and RNA (see Chap. 5). Linear pieces of double-stranded (native) DNA can be treated with heat or alkali to dissociate the two strands to yield single-stranded (denatured) DNA. The denatured DNA can be incubated under conditions that allow for nucleic acid hybridization, i.e., the recognition of two complementary strands and re-formation of double-stranded molecules by base pairing. Nucleic acid hybridization is so sensitive that a single-stranded DNA molecule can be hybridized specifically to a complementary strand of RNA or DNA present at about 1 part in 10,000. Many recombinant DNA studies involve the preparation of one radioactive or biotinylated strand of nucleic acid which is then used as a "probe" in the analysis. It is possible to identify and distinguish both fully homologous sequences and partially homologous sequences. The specificity of nucleic acid hybridization, often in combination with fractionation or amplification procedures, allows detection of a single gene among tens of thousands or of a viral sequence in the midst of other nucleic acid sequences.

A variation on nucleic acid hybridization involves the use of allele-specific oligonucleotides (ASO): The DNA probe is a synthetic, single-stranded oligonucleotide, usually 15 to 20 bases in length. The oligonucleotides are synthesized to be complementary to each of two or more sequences that represent polymorphisms or mutations in the genome. The variable nucleotide is in the midportion of the oligonucleotide. Hybridization conditions are adjusted so that the oligonucleotide detects a perfectly matched sequence but fails to hybridize if there is a single base mismatch. Allele-specific oligonucleotides can be used in combination with Southern blotting but are now more widely used in combination with DNA amplification, as described below. The majority of hybridization probes have been prepared in radioactive form, but the use of nonradioactive detection methods is likely to increase.

RESTRICTION ENDONUCLEASES The discovery in microorganisms of restriction endonucleases, commonly known as restriction enzymes, facilitated recombinant DNA manipulations. The enzymes recognize a specific oligonucleotide sequence in double-stranded DNA and cleave the DNA at this site. Many enzymes are known, each recognizing a unique DNA sequence (Fig. 6-1). Some enzymes recognize sequences only four base pairs in length. For example, the enzyme *Hae*III cleaves the sequence 5′-GGCC-3′. By convention, only one strand of DNA is printed as the recognition site, but the enzymes recognize double-stranded DNA. Other enzymes recognize sequences six base pairs in length. The enzyme *Hind*III cleaves the sequence 5′-AAGCTT-3′. Other enzymes, such as *Mst*II, recognize a seven-base-pair sequence but tolerate any base pair in the middle position. The sequence specificity of restriction enzymes is a powerful tool in dissection of large genomes. When human DNA is digested with a particular restriction enzyme, hundreds of thousands of DNA fragments are generated with remarkable reproducibility. Such fragments can vary from a few base pairs to several thousand base pairs in length, depending on the enzyme used. Restriction enzymes that recognize a sequence only four base pairs long cleave the DNA into smaller fragments than enzymes that recognize a six-base-pair sequence. With the use of multiple restriction enzymes to analyze a particular segment of DNA, it is possible to define a detailed map of restriction endonuclease cleavage sites for the region. Such a map can span a region of from several hundred to tens of thousands of base pairs of DNA. As described below, variations in the sequences of those cleavage sites can be analyzed as polymorphisms or mutations in the human genome.

SOUTHERN BLOTTING Many analyses of the human genome involve a specific application of DNA-DNA hybridization, the blotting procedure developed by E.M. Southern. For clinical analysis, *Southern blotting* (Fig. 6-2) begins with the isolation of genomic DNA from cells such as peripheral leukocytes or fetal cells. The high-molecular-weight genomic DNA is digested with a restriction enzyme to yield a series of reproducible fragments. These DNA fragments are separated by electrophoresis in agarose gels. After electrophoresis, the DNA is transferred from the gel to a membrane that binds the DNA. The membrane is treated to denature the DNA and is soaked in a solution containing a radioactive single-stranded nucleic acid probe. The probe will form a double-stranded nucleic acid complex at sites on the membrane where homologous DNA is present. The membrane is washed to remove unbound radioactivity, and regions on the membrane where homologous DNA sequences were bound are detected using x-ray film. The sensitivity of Southern blotting is achieved by splitting the DNA into small segments, fractionating the fragments, and applying a sensitive detection method to pick out specific fragments (nucleic acid hybridization). Overall, this method can detect genomic DNA fragments that represent a single gene or about 1 part in 1 million in the genome. The clinical power of Southern blotting resides in the ability it gives to analyze a tiny portion of the primary structure of human genomic DNA taken from an individual.

An analogous procedure starting with RNA for analysis has been termed *northern* (in contrast to Southern) *blotting*. In this procedure, the presence or absence of a particular mRNA as well as its approximate size can be determined. The term *immunoblotting* or *western blotting* describes a derivative procedure designed to analyze protein antigens. Proteins are separated by electrophoresis and transferred to a solid membrane through a blotting procedure. The membrane is analyzed by incubation with antibodies followed by a second step for enzymatic or radioactive detection of bound antibody. Thus, Southern blotting, northern blotting and immunoblotting or western blotting each combines a fractionation and a detection method to provide a sensitive technique for the analysis of DNA, RNA, and protein, respectively (Table 6-1).

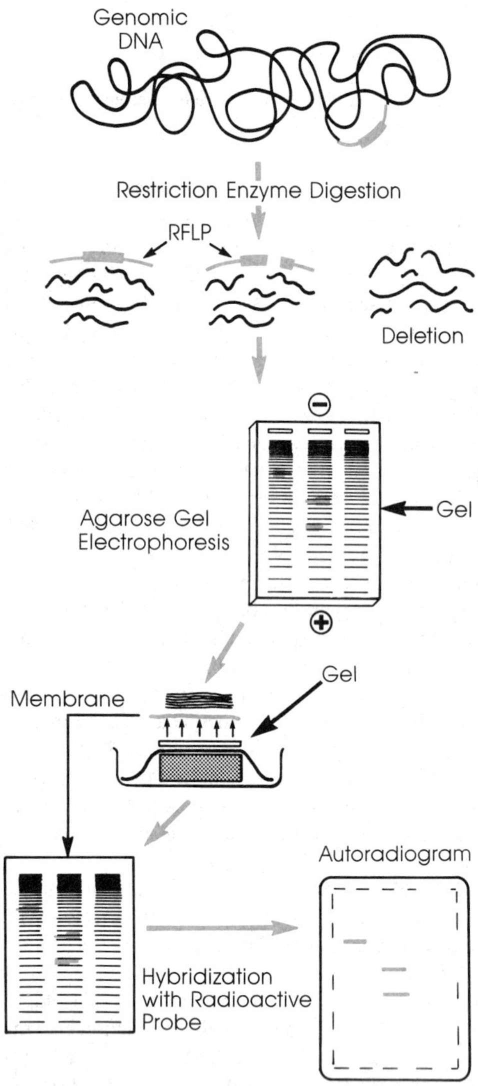

FIGURE 6-2 Southern blotting analysis of genomic DNA.

POLYMERASE CHAIN REACTION (PCR) FOR DNA AMPLIFICATION The technique of PCR for DNA amplification is a powerful method that has had a revolutionary impact on molecular diagnosis. The method was pioneered and patented by workers at the Cetus Corporation. The technique is based on knowing the nucleic acid sequence for a region which, for a diagnostic application, is to be analyzed repeatedly. Oligonucleotide primers are prepared that are complementary to opposite strands of the DNA and are separated by up to a few hundred base pairs (Fig. 6-3). The oligonucleotide primers are incubated with the target DNA to be amplified and with a DNA polymerase that synthesizes a complementary strand in a 5′-to-3′ direction. Considerable specificity is provided by the requirement that primers must lead to convergent synthesis for amplification to be effective. The reaction is subjected to a series of temperature variations including a denaturing temperature where double-stranded DNA is dissociated to single-stranded DNA, an annealing temperature where oligonucleotide primers hybridize to target DNA, and a polymerization temperature for the synthetic step. The reaction is usually carried out using heat-resistant *Taq* (from *Thermus aquaticus*) polymerase such that the polymerase remains active during the

TABLE 6-1 Analytical blotting procedures

Blot method	Material analyzed	Fractionation	Detection
Southern	DNA	Electrophoresis	Nucleic acid hybridization
Northern	RNA	Electrophoresis	Nucleic acid hybridization
Western or immunoblot	Protein	Electrophoresis	Immunologic

FIGURE 6-3 Polymerase chain reaction for amplification of DNA. The target DNA is shown as a solid line in cycle 1. Newly synthesized DNA is indicated by dotted lines in each cycle. Primer oligonucleotides are indicated by solid rectangles. Each DNA strand is marked with an arrow indicating 5′-to-3′ orientation. The polymerase chain reaction is patented by Cetus Corporation.

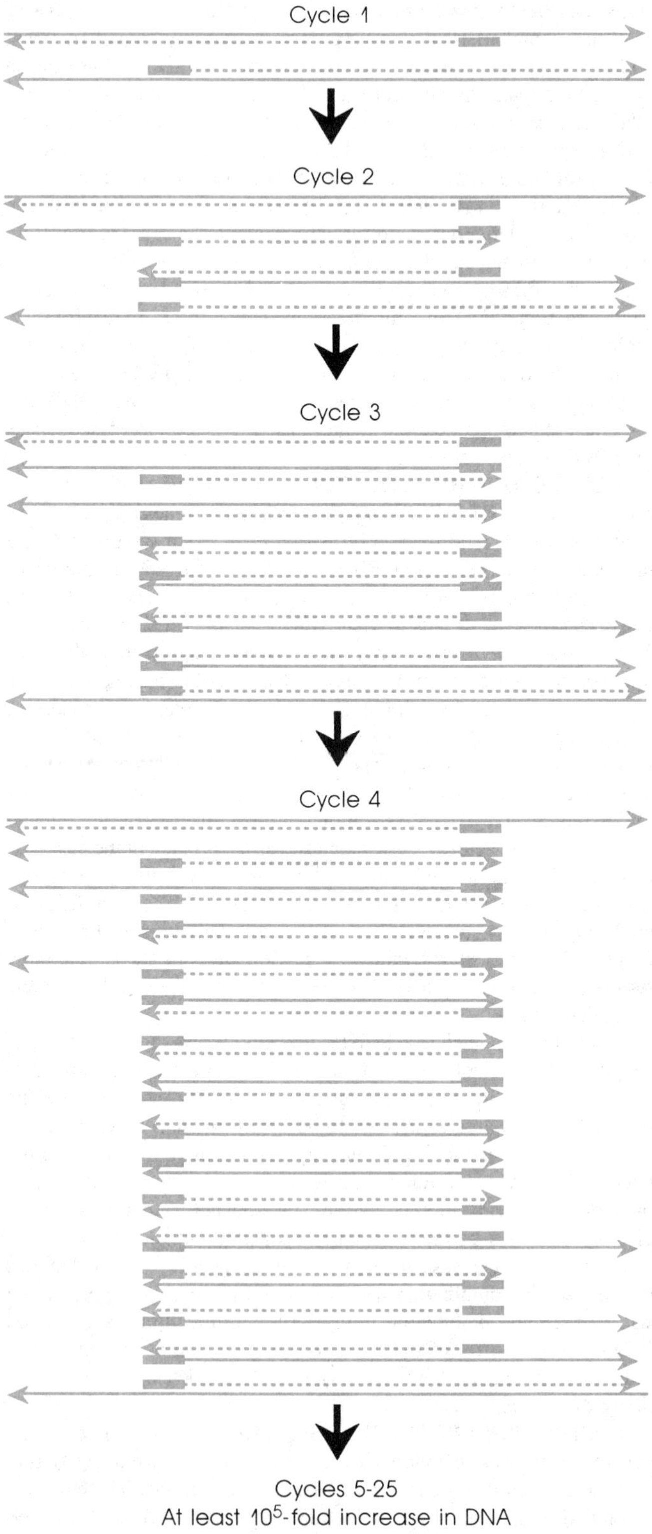

temperature cycles (usually ranging from 50 to 95°C). After a number of such cycles, typically 20 to 30 or more, hundreds of thousands of copies of the original target sequence are synthesized as depicted in Fig. 6-3. The bulk of the product is a double-stranded DNA fragment of specific length. The technique has been used to amplify and analyze DNA from a single human sperm which contains one duplex target DNA molecule. Molecular diagnosis with PCR depends on determining the presence or the absence of an amplified product, digesting the amplified product with a restriction enzyme, hybridizing the PCR product with allele-specific oligonucleotides, and direct sequencing of the PCR product, or on other methods of analysis. Many variations and modifications have been devised to take advantage of the PCR concept. These include synthesis of cDNA with reverse transcriptase followed by amplification of the cDNA. Single-stranded DNA can be synthesized by altering the ratio of the oligonucleotide primers. Research applications include preparation of recombinant DNA constructs, mutagenesis of cloned DNA, detection of rare nucleotide sequences, and detection of nucleotide sequences of infectious agents. The PCR method offers extremely rapid analysis (single day), ease of automation, relative economy, and extraordinary specificity.

A LINKAGE MAP OF THE HUMAN GENOME Linkage analysis has been used for decades to study the genetics of *Escherichia coli, Drosophila,* mouse, and other organisms. Although some clinically relevant linkage relationships were identified by techniques of classic genetics (e.g., that between ABO blood group and nail-patella syndrome), linkage analysis in human beings was enhanced by the advent of recombinant DNA techniques. The feasibility of human linkage analysis was revolutionized in 1978 when Kan and Dozy demonstrated genetic variation in the size of fragments generated after digestion of normal human DNA with restriction endonucleases. These restriction fragment length polymorphisms (RFLPs) are the consequence of the DNA sequence polymorphisms discussed above and are inherited according to Mendelian principles. Restriction enzyme digestion and Southern blotting made it possible to identify these polymorphisms and utilize them as genetic markers for sites within the genome. If one of the base pairs in the recognition sequence for a restriction enzyme is variable between individual copies of the genome or if there is a length variation in the DNA, there will be variation in the size of DNA fragments generated by the restriction enzyme digestion. The inheritance of a RFLP is depicted in Fig. 6-4.

A particularly informative subset of RFLPs occurs at variable number tandem repeat (VNTR) sites. These are sites of length variation in the genome where a short DNA sequence is tandemly repeated a different number of times on different chromosomes. The result is that there are many different sizes of DNA fragments, which can be regarded as different alleles at a VNTR site. Inheritance of a VNTR is depicted in Fig. 6-5. These polymorphic VNTR sites are informative for genetic testing and are valuable for identity testing, as in forensic or paternity analyses. In fact, PCR can be combined with ASO to detect single-base polymorphisms without relying on the fortuitous concurrence of restriction enzyme sites and polymorphisms (see below, Fig. 6-11).

Genetic linkage can be assessed between any group of markers, one of which may represent a disease mutation. The general concepts of genetic recombination and linkage are discussed in Chap. 5. For autosomal genes, each new individual inherits one copy of each chromosome from each parent. Each chromosome is a unique mosaic of polymorphic DNA sequences derived by crossing-over between grandparent chromosomes through the process of meiotic recombination (Fig. 6-6). Genes on different chromosomes are inherited

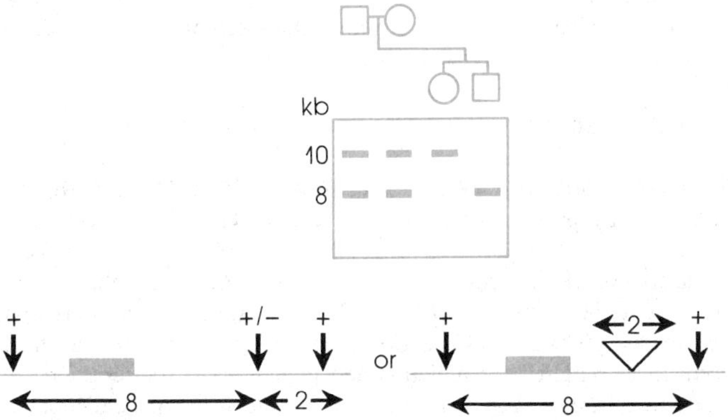

FIGURE 6-4 Example of restriction fragment length polymorphism (RFLP) in human DNA using Southern blotting. The solid blocks indicate segments of DNA used as probe. Parents are heterozygous and children are homozygous for the RFLP. Symbols above the arrows indicate cutting (+) or noncutting (−) by the restriction endonuclease. Numbers indicate DNA length in kilobases.

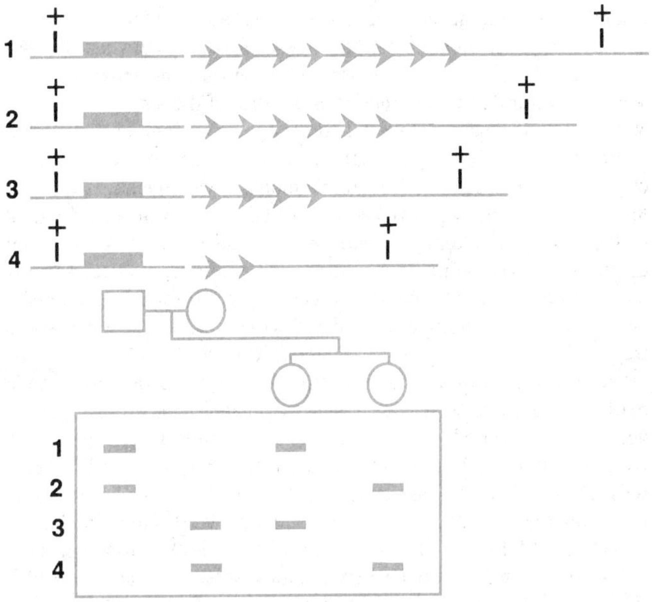

FIGURE 6-5 Example of a variable number tandem repeat (VNTR) polymorphism. Four possible alleles are indicated in the upper portion with the variable number of repeat units indicated by horizontal arrows in the DNA strand. The location of restriction enzyme sites and the DNA probe are indicated as in Fig. 6-4. Inheritance of the alleles within a family as detected by Southern blot is shown below.

FIGURE 6-6 Depiction of two chromosomes (one in solid lines and one in dotted lines) from an individual before (*above*) and after (*below*) meiotic crossing over. The individual is heterozygous for a disease locus with a normal allele (filled square) and a disease allele (open square) and for three RFLPs with alleles *A*/*B*, *M*/*N*, and *Y*/*Z*. See discussion in text.

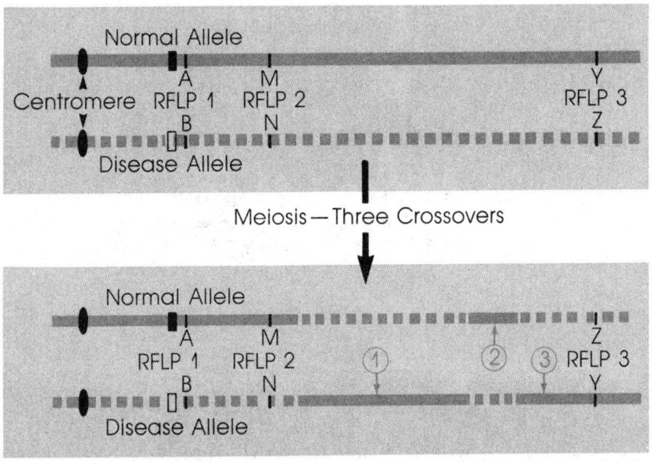

independently, but genes close together on the same chromosome are inherited together unless a meiotic crossover occurs between the two genes. Genes far apart on the same chromosome are inherited as if they were on different chromosomes because of the strong likelihood of meiotic crossovers between two distant loci. Genetic distance is expressed in centimorgans (cM) and is a measure of the likelihood of crossover between two loci. A common clinical concern is whether the disease gene or the normal gene was transmitted from an individual to the next generation. Linkage analysis can be used for prenatal diagnosis, presymptomatic diagnosis, and heterozygote detection. If the mutation in a gene can be detected directly by DNA analysis, genetic linkage need not be considered. However, diagnostic analysis frequently relies on a genetic variation near the disease locus. This often means utilization of an RFLP or VNTR as the nearby genetic marker. If the cloned disease gene is available as a probe, there is negligible likelihood of a crossover between the disease gene and RFLPs within and immediately adjacent to the gene (RFLP 1, Fig. 6-6). If the cloned disease gene is not available, it may be possible to use another cloned DNA fragment a moderate distance (perhaps a few hundred kilobases) from the disease gene. In this instance, there will be occasional crossovers between the disease locus and the RFLP (RFLP 2, Fig. 6-6). Other RFLPs may be so far from the disease locus that no linkage is demonstrable (RFLP 3, Fig. 6-6). There are on average 30 to 35 crossovers during meiosis in males and perhaps twice as many during meiosis in females. The frequency of meiotic crossing-over is not uniform along the length of the chromosomes.

With the availability of an unlimited number of DNA markers, an effort is underway to develop a detailed linkage map for the human genome. Hundreds of polymorphisms detected with specific genes and with anonymous DNA probes are being analyzed. Over 500 individuals from 40 large families are being genotyped in a collaborative effort developed by the CEPH (Centre d'Étude du Polymorphisme Humain). Detailed physical maps of the human genome are also being developed using techniques to map restriction enzyme sites over hundreds of kilobases of DNA. Major international commitments are being made to obtain a detailed map of the human genome, with the ultimate goal of determining its sequence. A short-term product of this effort is the precise mapping of many of the loci causing the more common human single-gene disorders.

REVERSE GENETICS Most genes have been cloned by first identifying the gene product. *Reverse genetics* is a term that has been used to imply various strategies, but in this context it refers to the cloning of a gene prior to knowing the gene product. The first step in cloning a disease gene by a reverse genetic strategy is to identify a DNA polymorphism that is linked to the disease locus. Figure 6-7 depicts analysis for linkage to an autosomal dominant disorder using two randomly selected DNA markers, one of which has *A* and *B* alleles and resides near the disease gene on the same chromosome, and one of which has *Y* and *Z* alleles and is on a different chromosome. Inspection of the family data suggests linkage of the marker with *A* and *B* alleles to the disease locus, and analysis of sufficient pedigree data can provide conclusive evidence that a polymorphic DNA marker is near a disease gene. Analogous efforts can be applied to autosomal recessive diseases. The frequency of crossovers can be used to estimate the genetic distance between the DNA marker and the disease locus. Any DNA clone can be mapped to a chromosome. In 1983 this strategy was used to identify an anonymous (random) DNA segment linked to the Huntington's chorea locus at a distance of 3 to 5 cM on the short arm of chromosome 4. Subsequently, polyposis of the colon, cystic fibrosis, Friedreich's ataxia, adult polycystic kidney disease, neurofibromatosis, and a rare form of Alzheimer's disease have been mapped to human chromosomes 5, 7, 9, 16, 17, and 21, respectively.

With an increasingly detailed genetic map of DNA markers, it is usually possible to identify DNA markers within 1 to 2 cM of a disease gene once the gene is mapped to a chromosome. On average, a genetic distance of 1 cM is equivalent to approximately 1 megabase (1000 kb). Intensive efforts are being applied to clone disease genes once a close linkage is established. These efforts rely on long-range restriction mapping, chromosome walking by isolation of overlapping genomic clones, and chromosome hopping, which involves isolation of the ends of a genomic DNA fragment after deletion of a large intervening region. Having narrowed down the region of genomic DNA that must contain the disease gene, RNA transcripts from this region must be identified and evaluated as candidate gene products. Proof that the disease gene has been located depends on genetic and functional criteria.

FIGURE 6-7 Example of a search for linkage of DNA markers to an autosomal dominant disease. *A* and *B* are DNA marker alleles at one site, and *Y* and *Z* are alleles at another site. Two pairs of chromosomes are depicted for each parent. The B haplotype and the disease allele are inherited together from the father except for the last-born child in whom a crossover occurred, and the A haplotype was inherited with the disease allele.

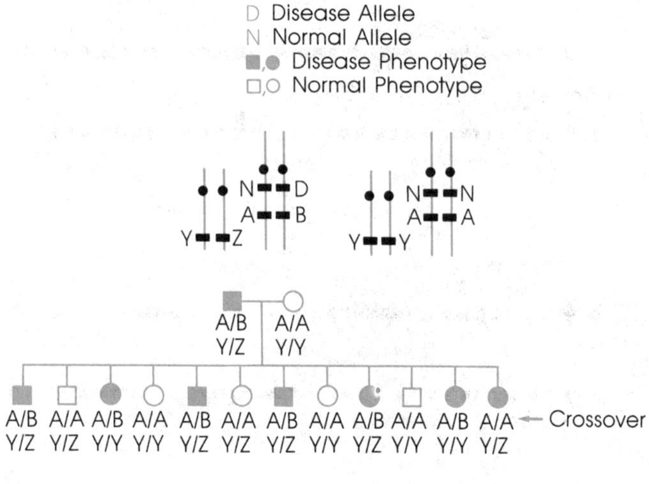

TABLE 6-2 Methods for molecular genetic diagnosis

Strategy	Southern	PCR
Direct detection of mutations		
Large DNA defects	+	+
Altered restriction site	+	+
Any mutation with allele-specific oligonucleotides	+/−*	+
Direct DNA sequencing	−	+
Linkage analysis		
RFLP or VNTR	+	+
Any sequence polymorphism with allele-specific oligonucleotide	+/−*	+

* Although Southern blotting is feasible, it would not be used in current practice.

STRATEGIES AND PITFALLS Molecular genetic diagnosis can be accomplished using Southern blotting and PCR in several ways (Table 6-2). Although these are powerful techniques, there are many clinical and laboratory pitfalls. An erroneous diagnosis in an index case is a common problem, e.g., confusion of von Willebrand's disease or hemophilia B with hemophilia A. Failure to recognize nonpaternity, mislabeling of samples, and other simple errors occur. Laboratory problems such as incomplete digestion with a restriction enzyme or contamination of genomic DNA samples with cloned or amplified DNA have caused misdiagnoses.

DIAGNOSIS OF GENETIC DISEASE

MUTATIONS IN A TYPICAL GENE AND GENETIC HETEROGENEITY A typical gene produces an mRNA that is translated into a protein (Fig. 6-8); also see Chap. 5. The end of the gene where transcription (RNA synthesis) originates is referred to as the *5' end,* relative to the orientation of the mRNA. The site where transcription begins is referred to as the *Cap site.* At least some of the DNA sequences required for initiation and regulation of transcription are located upstream from this region (opposite from the direction of

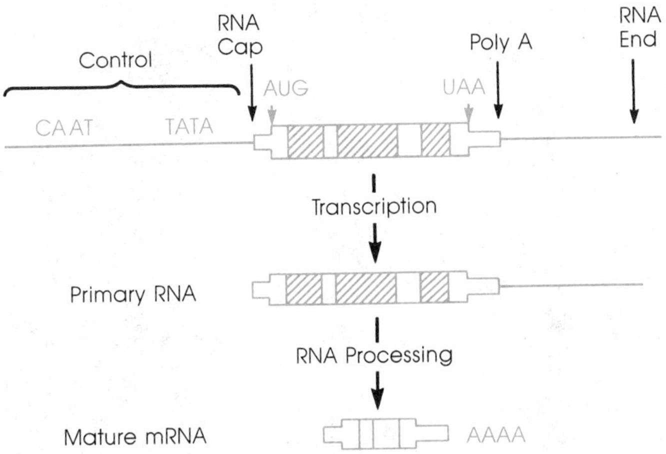

FIGURE 6-8 A typical gene encoding a protein product. Sequences included in mature mRNA (exons) are represented by open blocks with narrower regions for untranslated sequences. Introns (intervening sequences) are shown as hatched blocks.

transcription, to the left in Fig. 6-8). Many upstream regions contain sequences referred to as *TATA boxes* and *CAAT boxes,* which sequences are involved in the initiation and control of transcription. Important sequences for gene regulation may also occur even further upstream and downstream from the Cap site. The segments of DNA sequence that are retained in mature processed mRNA are called *exons.* These exons are separated by segments called *intervening sequences* (IVS) or *introns,* which initially are copied into RNA but which are spliced out in the formation of mature mRNA; i.e., the initial transcript contains an RNA copy of both introns and exons, whereas mature mRNA contains copies only of exons. Untranslated RNA sequences are present in mature mRNA and occur upstream from the protein initiator (AUG) codon and downstream from the terminator (UAA, UAG, or UGA) codon. Transcription proceeds beyond the site where mature mRNA will end. The initial RNA transcript is processed by nuclease cleavage at a poly(A) recognition site and subsequent addition of A (adenine) nucleotides to the 3′ end of the mRNA.

Many types of mutation are known. The gene can be entirely deleted. The gene can be rearranged by partial deletion, insertion, or inversion of significant segments. Single-base changes in the coding region generate missense or nonsense codons that cause amino acid substitution or premature chain termination. Mutations in the initiator or terminator codon also can cause disease. In addition, mutations can cause abnormalities of mRNA splicing, usually by changing conserved sequences near intron-exon boundaries. These abnormalities of splicing usually generate mRNAs that do not produce a functional product. Mutations also can occur in control regions and in the polyadenylation signal. In addition, disease mutations may occur in parts of the genome that do not encode proteins, although there are few examples of such instances. The diversity of mutations means that detection of mutant genes at a DNA level can be quite complex.

The extent of molecular heterogeneity is exemplified by the human globin loci. Many different deletions occur in the alpha-globin and beta-globin clusters. Hundreds of single-base changes are known to cause amino acid substitutions. Molecular heterogeneity underlying β-thalassemia is particularly common, with numerous mutations causing nonsense codons, frameshift, abnormal splicing, abnormal transcription, and impaired RNA cleavage and polyadenylation (Fig. 6-9).

STRATEGIES FOR DIAGNOSIS OF MENDELIAN DISORDERS Approaches for diagnosis of human single-gene disorders can be categorized as follows: (1) direct detection of mutations, (2) linkage analysis with negligible recombination, and (3) linkage analysis with measurable recombination. Linkage disequilibrium is of lesser importance.

Direct detection of mutations Initially, large deletions and genomic DNA rearrangements were the easiest to detect directly using Southern blotting. It is now possible to detect any mutation that occurs widely in the population if the defect is first characterized by DNA sequencing. Southern blotting is rapidly being replaced by PCR, which can be used to determine the presence or absence of a genomic DNA region, to analyze RFLPs or VNTRs, and to prepare material for analysis with ASO or direct DNA sequencing. These techniques have been widely used for human globin gene analysis. For large deletions of major portions of a globin gene cluster, Southern blotting analysis can demonstrate the presence of a homozygous defect (Fig. 6-10). Gene deletions are common causes of α-thalassemia, and prenatal diagnosis of these defects is straightforward using either cDNA or genomic DNA probes. Identification of heterozygous deletions requires either careful quantitation (dosage analysis) or demonstration of abnormal junction fragments from the deleted site. Large deletions are a less frequent cause of mutations in the beta-globin cluster, but such deletions can be demonstrated in hereditary persistance of fetal hemoglobin (Fig. 6-10) and in some forms of δβ-thalassemia.

A Southern blot of the type depicted in Fig. 6-10 would appear

FIGURE 6-9 Point mutations in β-thalassemia. The beta-globin gene is shown with numbered hatched areas representing the coding regions of exons. Boxed open areas between the exons are introns, and boxed open areas at the 5′ and 3′ ends of the gene are untranslated regions that appear in the messenger RNA. The various types of mutations are depicted by different symbols. *(From AH Kazazian, Jr. CD Boehm, Blood 72:1107, 1988.)*

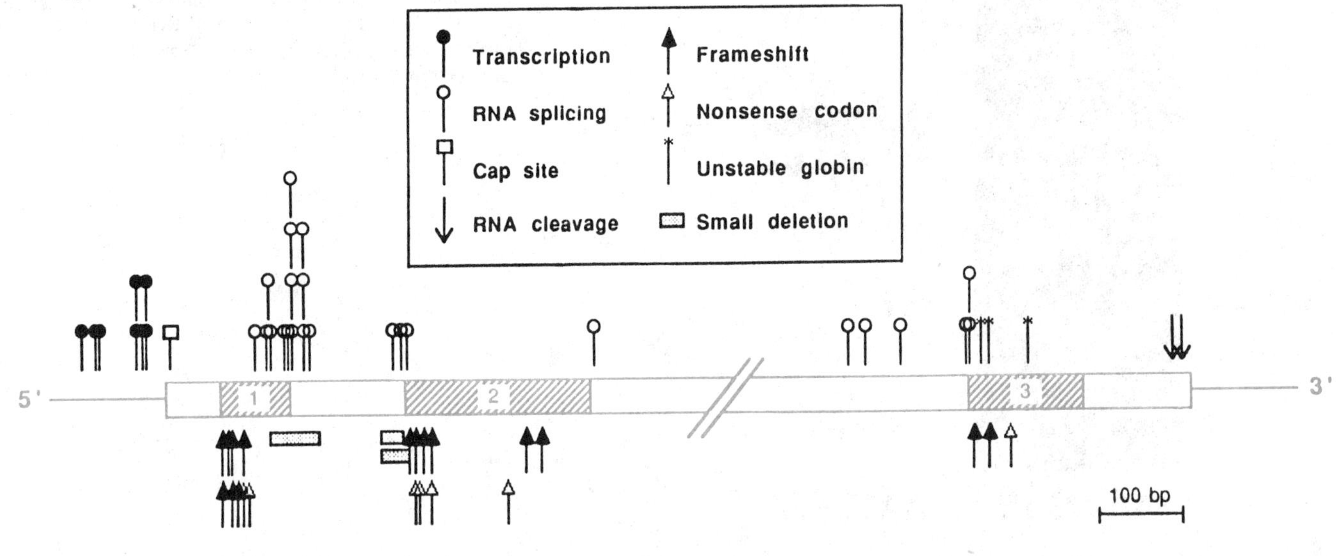

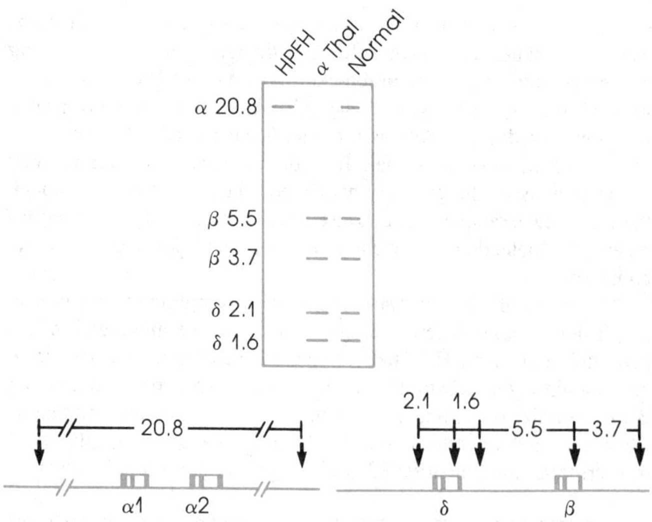

FIGURE 6-10 Depiction of Southern blot analysis of human globin genes. Above, DNA was isolated from a normal individual and from patients with homozygous hereditary persistence of fetal hemoglobin (HPFH) or homozygous α-thalassemia. DNA was digested with the enzyme *Eco*RI. A mixed DNA probe was prepared by reverse transcription of reticulocyte globin mRNA. Below, arrows indicate *Eco*RI cut sites in the alpha- and beta-globin regions, and numbers indicate DNA fragment sizes in kilobases. *(Adapted from YW Kan, AM Dozy, Proc Natl Acad Sci USA 75:5631, 1978.)*

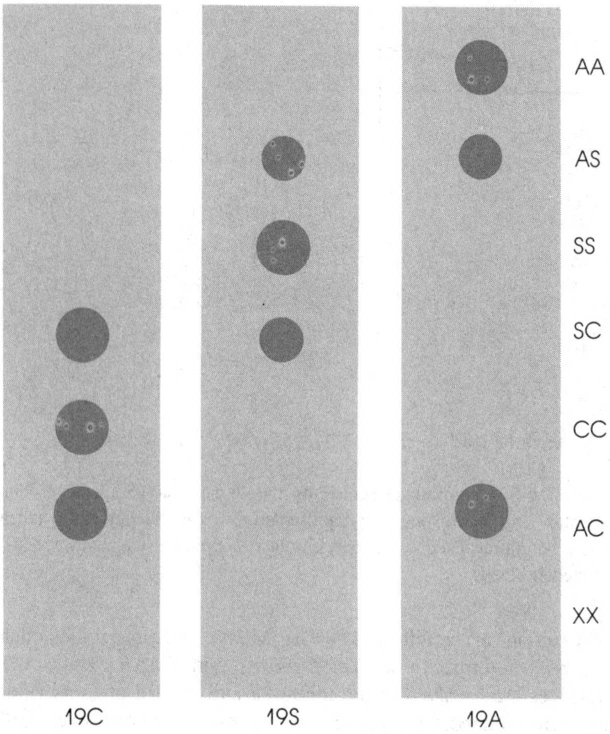

FIGURE 6-11 Genotype analysis of PCR amplified genomic DNA using allele-specific oligonucleotides (ASO) probes. DNA was extracted from the blood of individuals of beta-globin genotypes AA, AS, SS, SC, CC, and AC and homozygous deletion (XX). The DNA was applied to replicate filters for hybridization with ASO as follows: β^A probe (19A), β^S probe (19S), or β^C probe (19C). *(From K Mullis et al, Cold Spring Harbor Symp Quant Biol 51:263, 1986.)*

normal in an individual with sickle cell anemia. However, many options are now available for direct detection of single-base mutations, such as that causing sickle cell anemia. One procedure for direct detection of the sickle mutation utilized a variation on Southern blotting in which the hybridization probe was a synthetic 19-base oligonucleotide that represented a perfect match for either the β^S or the β^A sequence, i.e., an ASO. The ASO technique can be combined with PCR for DNA amplification rather than with Southern blotting. The ASO and PCR techniques can also be combined to detect any single-base variation that must be analyzed repeatedly in the population. The ability to distinguish beta-globin genotypes is depicted in Fig. 6-11.

Another method for direct detection of the sickle cell mutation takes advantage of the fact that a variety of restriction enzymes cut the β^A but not the β^S sequence. A portion of the nucleotide sequence in the β^A gene is 5′-CCTGAGG-3′, and the corresponding sequence in the sickle gene is 5′-CCTG*T*GG-3′. The GAG to GTG change causes the substitution of valine for glutamic acid. The restriction enzyme *Mst*II (or *Oxa*NI) cuts the sequence 5′-CCTNAGG-3′ (N = any nucleotide) and hence will cut the β^A but not the β^S sequence at this site. Initially this strategy was combined with Southern blotting for direct detection of the sickle mutation, but restriction enzyme digestion can now be combined with PCR for rapid direct detection of the sickle mutation as depicted in Fig. 6-12. No complex equipment

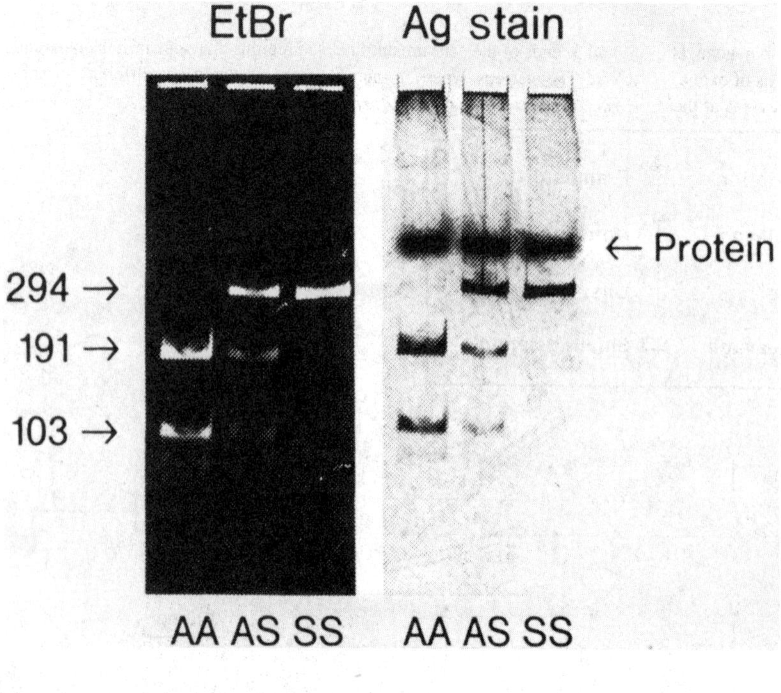

FIGURE 6-12 Diagnosis of sickle cell genotype using PCR and restriction enzyme digestion. Genomic DNA was amplified to yield a 294-base pair fragment. The product was digested with the restriction enzyme *Oxa*NI which cuts the product from the normal gene but does not cut the product from the sickle gene. The DNA fragments can be detected with ethidium bromide (EtBr) or silver (Ag) stain. *(From FF Chehab et al, Nature 329:293, 1987.)*

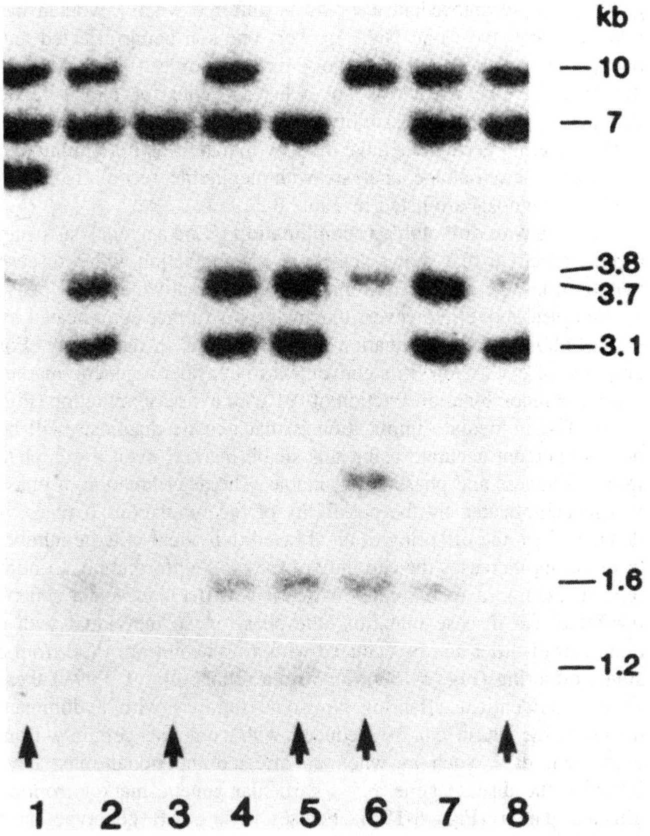

FIGURE 6-13 Detection of deletions in the DNA isolated from Duchenne's muscular dystrophy patients using a dystrophin cDNA probe. Southern blot analysis detects deletions (absence of fragments) in five of eight patients (arrows). A junction fragment is clearly demonstrated in patient 6. *(From M Koenig et al, Cell 50:509, 1987.)*

or radioactivity need be used, and the methods can be applied in underdeveloped areas.

Another example of direct detection of mutations can be drawn from Duchenne's muscular dystrophy. Fragments of the cDNA from this very large gene can be used for Southern blotting to detect deletions in half or more of patients (Fig. 6-13). Heterozygote detection depends on dosage analysis when genomic DNA fragments are absent but is easier and more definitive when junctional DNA fragments are detected (as in patient 6 in Fig. 6-13). Certain portions of the Duchenne locus are particularly prone to deletion, and PCR can be used to demonstrate the absence of selected portions of the gene.

Direct detection of mutations has been accomplished for numerous disorders (Table 6-3 and see Cooper and Schmidtke). A fraction of mutations for most diseases are easily detected either because they cause large DNA defects or because they alter a restriction enzyme site. Certain DNA sequences, particularly those containing methylated cytosine in CpG dinucleotides, have increased mutation rates, often leading to the loss of sites for the restriction enzymes *Msp*I or *Taq*I. Any mutant allele that is widespread in the population can be detected using PCR with ASO.

Linkage with negligible recombination The general concepts for genetic recombination and linkage are discussed earlier in this chapter and in Chap. 5. Genetic diagnosis by linkage is utilized when it is not possible to demonstrate by direct analysis the mutation or the mutant gene product. For clinical linkage analysis, it is essential that some genetic marker near the disease locus (or near the mutation if the locus is very large) be *informative*. The genetic marker is informative if an individual who is heterozygous for the disease locus is also heterozygous for the marker. Linkage analysis is appropriate when an individual carries one mutant gene and one normal gene and the goal is to determine which has been transmitted to the next generation. Most analyses can be made informative since RFLPs are frequent and since it is usually possible to identify useful polymorphisms near genes causing diseases.

A second requirement for linkage analysis is that of *phase* information between the two loci for genetic analysis. If an individual is heterozygous for a RFLP (genotype 1/2) that is tightly linked to a mutation, it must be determined whether allele 1 for the RFLP is on the chromosome with the disease gene or on the chromosome with the normal gene, assuming that allele 2 for the RFLP would be on the chromosome with the alternate gene. When the genetic marker is informative and the phase is known, genetic diagnosis can be carried out in the form of heterozygote detection, presymptomatic diagnosis, detection of lack of penetrance, and prenatal diagnosis. When the DNA probe is a portion of the gene that is mutated, crossing-over between the genetic marker (often a RFLP) and a mutation is usually negligible. Duchenne's muscular dystrophy is an exception with an extremely large gene in which crossing-over within the gene does occur at a detectable frequency.

Examples of molecular diagnosis by linkage, when there is negligible recombination between the loci, are presented in Fig. 6-14. Genetic marker data are presented as letters that might represent simple RFLP alleles or haplotypes of RFLPs. A *haplotype* is a cluster of tightly linked genetic marker information on a chromosome. Phase can usually be determined from a single index case for autosomal recessive disorders (Fig. 6-14*A*). Phase can also be determined for

TABLE 6-3 Examples of the role of molecular analysis for diagnosis of genetic disease

Disease	Detection of mutation*	Linkage with gene probe	Linkage with linked marker	Comments
Sickle cell anemia	+ + + +			PCR with ASO or restriction enzyme
Other globin disorders	+ + +	+		Very heterogeneous
Hemophilia A	+	+ +	+	
Phenylketonuria	+ +	+ +		
α_1-Antitrypsin ZZ	+ + + +			PCR with ASO
Familial hypercholesterolemia	+ +	+ +		Biologic tests valuable
Lesch-Nyhan syndrome	+ +	+ +		Heterozygote detection
Tay-Sachs disease	+ +	+ +		Enzyme valuable
Duchenne's muscular dystrophy	+ +	+ +		Many deletions
Retinoblastoma	+ + +	+		Inherited form
Huntington's disease			+ + +	
Myotonic dystrophy			+ + +	
Adult polycystic kidney disease			+ + +	
Fragile X syndrome			+ + +	
Cystic fibrosis			+ + +	
Neurofibromatosis			+ + +	
Polyposis of colon			+ + +	

* + = relative importance of an approach as of early 1989; the status for disorders could change rapidly. PCR, polymerase chain reactions; ASO, allele specific oligonucleotide

recessive disorders in the absence of an index case if a reliable biologic or biochemical heterozygote test is available, as might occur for β-thalassemia (Fig. 6-14*B*). Fetuses of AA genotype are predicted to be affected in Fig. 6-14*A* and *B*. For autosomal dominant disorders, linkage phase usually cannot be determined from a single affected individual (Fig. 6-14*C*). Exceptions would occur in retinoblastoma or polyposis of the colon, when analysis of tumor DNA may distinguish the allele on the abnormal chromosome (often retained in the tumor) from the allele on the normal chromosome (often lost in the tumor). Linkage phase for autosomal dominant disorders can be determined from two appropriate individuals; it is not essential that both be affected (Fig. 6-14*D* and *E*). Fetuses of AB genotype are predicted to be affected in Fig. 6-14*D* and *E*. For X-linked disorders, phase information is most readily obtained from a single affected male individual (Fig. 6-14*F*). In general, linkage information can be used to determine the genotype of offspring of individuals of known genotype. Linkage information generally cannot be used consistently to determine the genotype of antecedents of individuals of known genotypes because of the possibility of new mutation from one generation to the next. This is exemplified by an X-linked disorder, where linkage information will not clarify whether or not the mother of an isolated affected male is a heterozygote (Fig. 6-14*G*). This represents an important difference between direct detection of a mutation and linkage analysis. Occasionally, linkage analysis can suggest the genotype of an antecedent. Note in Fig. 6-14*G* that the mutation arose on the chromosome from the unaffected maternal grandfather; the maternal grandmother and the maternal aunt of the index case do not carry the mutation, and either the mother or the index case is the recipient of the new mutation. The situation is similar in Fig. 6-14*H* except that the mutation is on the chromosome from the maternal grandmother and the site of the new mutation is unknown and could go back further in the family. Still by linkage analysis, the maternal aunt is not a carrier of the mutation. The genotype of an antecedent also can be inferred when a woman has two sons with the same DNA marker, one son being affected and one son being unaffected with the X-linked disorder (Fig. 6-14*I*). In this instance, the mother is not a heterozygote for the X-linked disorder, although the possibility of gonadal mosaicism (i.e., some of the maternal germ cells have the new mutation) is not eliminated. Diseases where linkage analysis with negligible recombination is used for diagnosis are listed in Table 6-3.

Linkage with detectable recombination Linkage analysis using a genetic marker that shows detectable recombination with a disease mutation has the same requirements for informativeness and phase as discussed above. However, the analysis is further complicated by the possibility of recombination at each meiosis in the family. For purposes of discussion, it is convenient to consider a genetic marker that has a recombination fraction of 0.1 with a disease mutation (Fig. 6-15). The immediate implication is that genetic diagnosis will be only 90 percent accurate using this single marker, even if complete informativeness and phase are available. The determination of phase is also complicated by the possibility of recombination. If phase is deduced from the offspring of an affected individual, a large number of offspring increases the certainty of the phase information. Continuing to assume a recombination fraction of 0.1 between a genetic marker and a disease mutation, the phase in an individual with a dominant disorder can be deduced with a probability of 0.90 from a single offspring (Fig. 6-15*A*) but with a probability of 0.99 if there were two identical offspring. In some families with a dominant disorder, the phase can be deduced with complete certainty from antecedent data, such as when an affected individual must have inherited the disease gene and a particular genetic marker from an affected parent (Fig. 6-15*B*). Fetuses of the AB genotype have probabilities of being affected of approximately 0.81 and 0.90 in Fig. 6-15*A* and *B*, respectively, since crossovers may occur in the meioses leading to conception of the fetus. For autosomal recessive

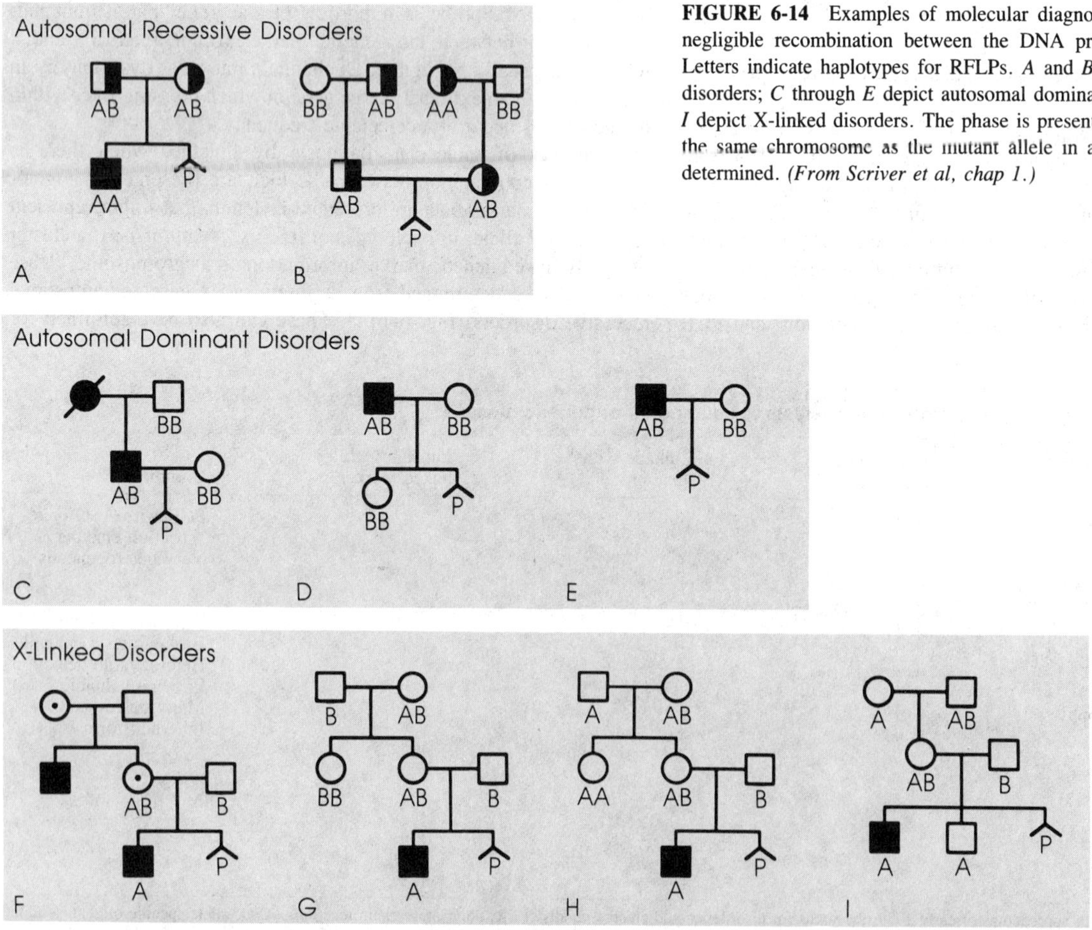

FIGURE 6-14 Examples of molecular diagnosis by genetic linkage with negligible recombination between the DNA probe and the disease locus. Letters indicate haplotypes for RFLPs. *A* and *B* depict autosomal recessive disorders; *C* through *E* depict autosomal dominant disorders; and *F* through *I* depict X-linked disorders. The phase is presented with the A haplotype on the same chromosome as the mutant allele in all cases in which it can be determined. *(From Scriver et al, chap 1.)*

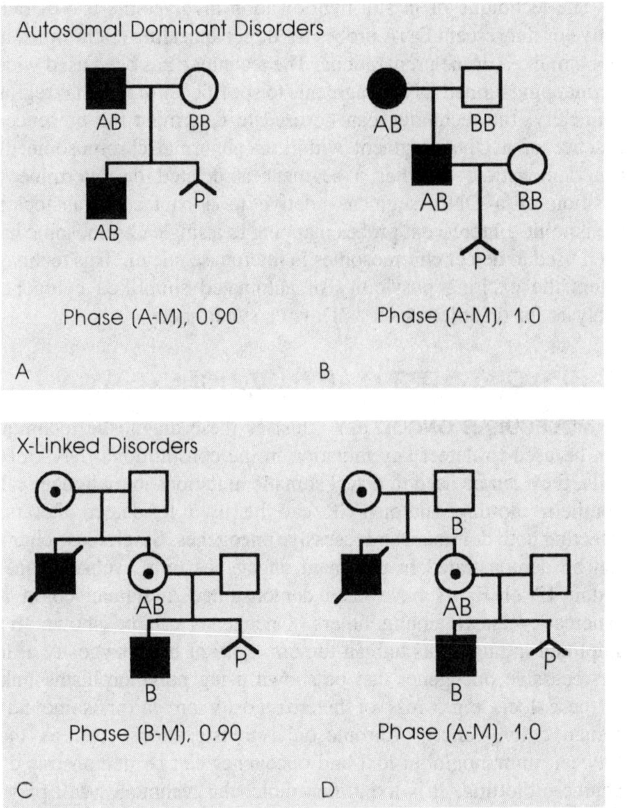

FIGURE 6-15 Examples of molecular diagnosis using genetic linkage with detectable recombination between the DNA probe and the disease locus. Letters indicate haplotypes detected with RFLPs. *A* and *B* depict autosomal dominant disorders; *E* and *F* depict X-linked disorders. The probability of phase at the bottom of each panel indicates the probability that a given haplotype is on the chromosome with mutant allele (M) in the parent of the pregnancy (P). For example, phase (A-M), 0.90, in *A* indicates that the probability is 0.90 that the A haplotype is on the chromosome with a mutant allele in the father of the pregnancy. The recombination fraction is presented as 0.1 for all cases; see text for discussion. *(Modified from Scriver et al, chap 1.)*

disorders, the considerations are analogous. For X-linked disorders, phase can be deduced from offspring of heterozygous females, but more definitive phase information can often be obtained by analysis of the fathers of heterozygous females. In Fig. 6-15*C* and *D*, the same family is depicted with and without data from the maternal grandfather. If an unwise counselor (Fig. 6-15*C*) fails to obtain a sample from the maternal grandfather, the data suggest that the A marker is on the chromosome with the disease gene in the pregnant woman. The phase is known with only 90 percent certainty, and prenatal diagnosis would provide accuracy of approximately 81 percent because of the possibility of crossing-over in either of the meioses leading to the offspring of the heterozygous mother. If a wiser counselor (Fig. 6-15*D*) recognizes the absolute necessity of a sample from the maternal grandfather, the phase in the heterozygous mother becomes known with certainty, and it is evident that the affected son represents a crossover between the genetic marker and the disease mutation. Prenatal diagnosis now becomes 90 percent accurate, but, more important, the prediction of disease or nondisease has been reversed for the presence of a given marker in a male fetus. If phase is to be determined for heterozygous females based on their offspring, the accuracy of phase information increases with increasing numbers of offspring as for the autosomal disorders.

Diseases for which linkage analysis with detectable recombination is used for diagnosis are listed in Table 6-3. An example of the use of PCR to detect a RFLP for diagnosis of cystic fibrosis is shown in Fig. 6-16. An example of linkage analysis using Southern blotting

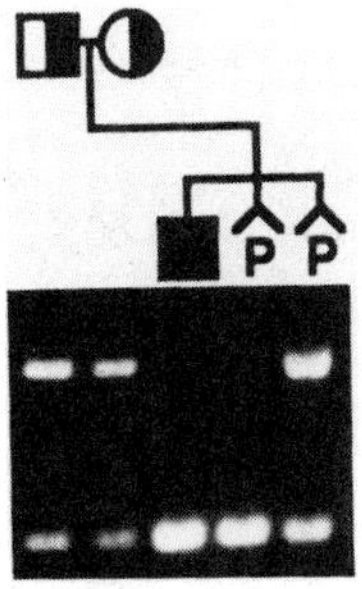

FIGURE 6-16 Use of PCR to detect a RFLP for prenatal diagnosis of cystic fibrosis. A DNA fragment was amplified at the site of an RFLP originally identified by the probe KM-19. The product was digested with the enzyme *Pst*I and the fragments detected with ethidium bromide staining. Both parents are heterozygous for the RFLP. The first fetus was predicted to be affected, and the second fetus was predicted to be a carrier.

to detect a VNTR linked to the locus for adult polycystic kidney disease is shown in Fig. 6-17.

Linkage disequilibrium Linkage disequilibrium refers to the fact that certain alleles at two or more nearby loci may be found together more often than would be predicted from their frequency in the general population. Although linkage disequilibrium occurs routinely between multiple polymorphic sites, for purposes of genetic diagnosis, this is most readily discussed in terms of a genetic marker and a disease mutation. Figure 6-18 depicts the occurrence of a disease susceptibility mutation (*Z*) at a locus where the normal allele is represented as *Y*. The mutation arises on a chromosome carrying the A allele for a nearby DNA polymorphism. With the passage of time, chromosomes carrying the A allele for the DNA haplotype and the *Z* allele for the disease locus grow to represent 10 percent of the chromosomes in the population. *Linkage disequilibrium* is the term used to describe the fact that the disease susceptibility mutation (*Z*) is found preferentially, and in this case exclusively, on chromosomes bearing the *A* form of the DNA polymorphism. Not all chromosomes carrying the *A* form of the polymorphism carry the disease susceptibility allele, but chromosomes carrying the *A* form of the polymorphism are associated with increased risk of disease. This model also implies that it might be possible at a future date to identify and detect directly the *Z* mutation to provide a more accurate prediction of disease susceptibility. For linkage disequilibrium to be present, the two genetic markers must be tightly linked. In addition there must be one or only a few origins for the disease mutations, or the mutations will be found randomly with different alleles for the marker site. Linkage disequilibrium can often be found using a group of close genetic markers to form a haplotype.

Linkage disequilibrium is extensive within the HLA complex, and numerous diseases are found in association with various HLA

FIGURE 6-17 Southern blotting analysis of a family affected with adult polycystic kidney disease. Alleles *C*, *D*, *G*, *J*, and *H* are detected with a linked, highly polymorphic probe. Designations above each lane refer to pedigree positions, and every person with the *C* allele also has polycystic disease. *(From ST Reeders et al, Nature 317:542, 1985; reprinted with permission.)*

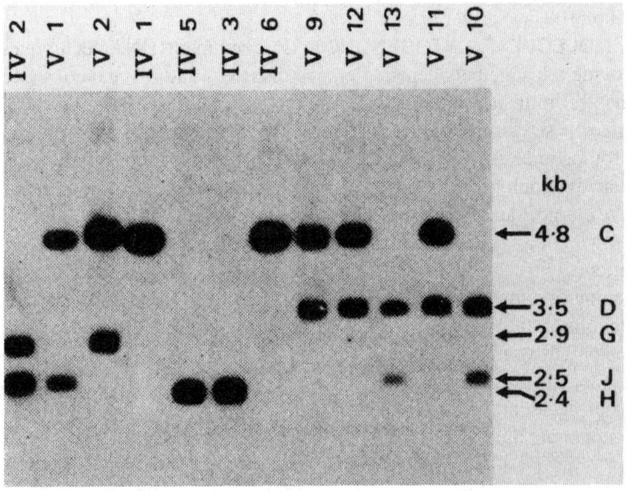

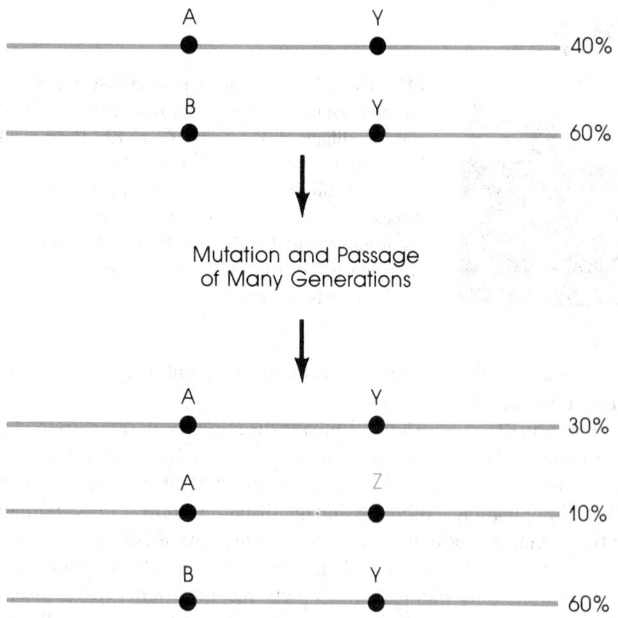

FIGURE 6-18 Depiction of the development of linkage disequilibrium within a population of chromosomes. *A* and *B* indicate alleles for a DNA polymorphism. *Y* represents a normal allele and *Z* a disease susceptibility allele at a locus. See text for discussion.

haplotypes (see Chap. 14 in this text and Chap. 4 in Scriver et al.). For example, insulin-dependent diabetes mellitus is associated with HLA-DR3 and HLA-DR4, and susceptibility to this disease may be attributable to the presence of an aspartic acid residue in position 57 of the HLA-DQβ locus. The genotype at this position can be directly determined using PCR and allele-specific oligonucleotides. By comparison to Fig. 6-18, the HLA-DR data for diabetes could be equivalent to the A/B marker, while the aspartic acid residue could be the equivalent of the Z mutation. By analogy, DNA polymorphisms near any gene might detect linkage disequilibrium with a disease susceptibility. Using this rationale, attempts have been made to determine if certain DNA markers adjacent to the apolipoprotein genes might be associated with increased risk of atherosclerosis. If such associations are proven, they would imply that some genetic variation in the coding or regulatory portions of an apolipoprotein gene itself is responsible for the altered disease susceptibility. Ultimately these genetic variations could be used directly for assessment of disease risks.

RFLPs showing strong linkage disequilibrium with cystic fibrosis have also been identified. The DNA markers are close to the cystic fibrosis locus, and a single mutation accounts for a major proportion of the mutant genes in the population. The linkage disequilibrium information can be used for genetic counseling for cystic fibrosis (see Chap. 108 in Scriver et al.).

MOLECULAR CYTOGENETICS Recombinant DNA techniques provide a bridge between single-gene disorders and cytogenetics (see Chap. 7 in this text and Chap. 9 in Scriver et al.). Genetic alterations range in size from single-base changes to gain or loss of an entire chromosome. As an example, some patients with Duchenne's muscular dystrophy have gross cytogenetic abnormalities, some patients have large deletions of DNA detectable by molecular but not cytogenetic analysis, and presumably others have single-base changes. Patients with detectable cytogenetic abnormalities have facilitated the cloning of numerous X-linked genes, the cloning of the retinoblastoma gene, and the mapping of the locus for polyposis of the colon. Reciprocally, molecular probes have been used to define cytogenetic translocations, deletions, and insertions. DNA probes have been used to detect Y chromosome–specific sequences in 46, XX males and to demonstrate the absence of Y chromosome regions in 46, XY females.

The technique of in situ hybridization involves the use of radioactive or fluorescent DNA probes for direct annealing to chromosomal DNA in fixed tissue preparations. The technique has been used widely for mapping cloned DNA fragments to specific chromosomal regions. Clinically, the technique can be used to determine the presence or absence of a DNA segment within an abnormal chromosome; this can demonstrate whether a segment is deleted or determine the position of a DNA segment relative to a balanced translocation breakpoint. Fluorescent probes mapping to a single chromosome have been used to detect chromosomes in interphase nuclei. This technique offers the exciting possibility of automated simplified cytogenetic analysis for disorders such as Down's syndrome.

OTHER DIAGNOSTIC APPLICATIONS

MOLECULAR ONCOLOGY Just as these diagnostic techniques can be used to detect any mutation in the constitutional DNA of all cells, they can be used to detect somatic mutations in malignant cells. Southern blotting and/or PCR can be used to detect alterations affecting both dominant and recessive oncogenes. Single-base changes can be demonstrated in dominant oncogenes, e.g., substitutions in codon 12 of H-*ras* have been demonstrated in human colon and pancreatic cancer among others. Oncogenes can be shown to be amplified in numerous human tumors. Loss of heterozygosity at loci for recessive oncogenes can be shown using polymorphisms linked to these loci, e.g., loss of heterozygosity on chromosome 5q in human colon cancer. Chromosomal translocations such as those between immunoglobin loci and oncogenes can be demonstrated by Southern blotting. It is likely that molecular techniques will play an increasing role in the analysis of the basic alterations in tumor cells, in the classification and staging of tumors, and in the monitoring of therapeutic strategies.

DIAGNOSTIC VIROLOGY AND MICROBIOLOGY Virtually all microorganisms have DNA or RNA sequences that can be detected by nucleic acid hybridization techiques. As discussed above, nucleic acid hybridization is very sensitive and specific, and it can be combined with PCR to detect an extraordinarily low abundance of foreign nucleic acid sequences. Many other diagnostic procedures such as detection of infectious antigens with monoclonal antibodies and detection of human immune responses with immunoblotting can also provide rapid, sensitive, and specific diagnostic procedures. Each strategy offers special advantages. Some advantages of the detection of foreign nucleic acid sequences are as follows: (1) sequences can be detected without the delay required for the host to mount immune responses, (2) sequences can be detected without regard to passive acquisition of antibody whether by maternal transfer or by transfusion, (3) sequences can be detected even if the host fails to mount an immune response, (4) sequences can be detected even if no foreign proteins are being synthesized, and (5) the extraordinary ability of PCR to detect even a single molecule in a sample may provide the most sensitive technique in many circumstances. These techniques have been used for a broad range of viral diagnoses including cytomegalovirus, rotavirus, Epstein-Barr virus, and others. PCR has been used to detect hepatitis B sequences in serum and to detect HIV-1 sequences in peripheral blood mononuclear cells. In one study using PCR, HIV-1 sequences were detected in 100 percent of specimens from seropositive, virus culture–positive homosexual men and in 64 percent of specimens from seropositive, virus culture–negative homosexual men. DNA amplification required 3 days rather than the 3 to 4 weeks required for virus isolation.

IDENTITY TESTING Analysis with only a few highly polymorphic VNTR probes provides the ability to distinguish the genotype of virtually all individuals except identical twins. This powerful method of identification finds application in paternity testing, in settling immigration disputes, in criminal investigations, and in monitoring bone marrow transplantation. The combination of PCR with VNTR analysis is particularly powerful for forensic analysis,

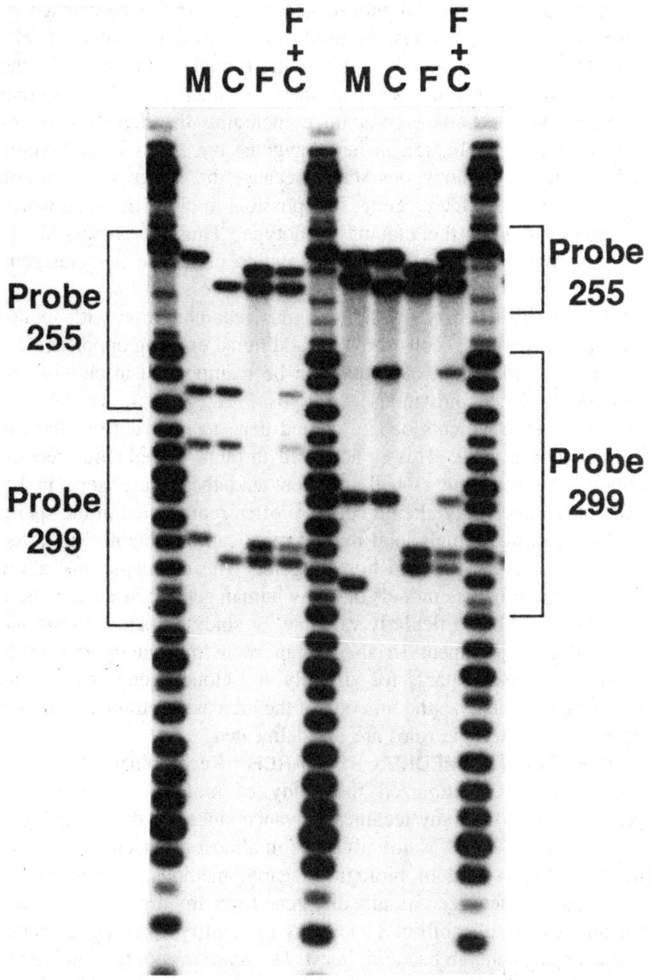

FIGURE 6-19 Paternity analysis in two families using Southern blotting and two highly polymorphic VNTRs. M, mother; C, child; F, putative father; F+C, putative father and child loaded in a single lane. A ladder of marker fragments is loaded in the center and outer lanes. Each individual demonstrates two alleles with each probe. The putative father is not excluded with either probe in the family on the left. In the family on the right, the putative father is not excluded with the probe 255, but is excluded with probe 299. *(Courtesy of R Giles, GeneScreen, Inc, using Lifecodes technology; see Balazs et al.)*

since identification can be made from minuscule samples of semen, blood, hair root, skin, or other tissue. Tissue typing at the HLA loci is also feasible using molecular analysis of polymorphisms. An example of a paternity analysis using highly polymorphic VNTR probes is shown in Fig. 6-19.

THERAPEUTIC APPLICATIONS

PHARMACEUTICALS Cloned DNA sequences can be used for synthesis of proteins and peptides. The major advantages of this strategy are the ability to obtain unlimited amounts of purified products not previously available and the avoidance of contamination by pathogens. Production can be carried out in bacteria, yeast, cultured animal cells, or whole animals. Just as glucocorticoids and their synthetic derivatives have been explored for the treatment of endless numbers of human diseases, so now it will be possible to evaluate the therapeutic potential of innumerable naturally occurring and specially engineered protein products.

Bacteria do not splice eukaryotic messenger RNA properly, so the coding region is usually provided as cDNA clones or as synthetic DNA sequences. The coding region must be linked to bacterial DNA segments that control transcription and initiation of translation. The major difficulties with bacterial synthesis involve the lack of eukaryotic mechanisms for posttranslational processing. Almost all bacterial and eukaryotic proteins undergo proteolytic cleavage at the amino terminus to remove the initiator methionine, and multiple proteolytic cleavages may be involved, as in the production of various hormones from the proopiomelanocortin gene. Other forms of posttranslational modification include removal of leader sequences, carbohydrate addition, phosphorylation, acylation, formation of disulfide bridges, and vitamin K–dependent carboxylation. Improperly or incompletely processed proteins may or may not function normally and may be antigenic. These obstacles have been overcome to produce a number of human proteins that are efficacious and safe. Proteins are also being produced in yeast, and proteins that require extensive posttranslational modification may be produced in cultured animal cells. It is also feasible to create transgenic animals that will secrete large amounts of recombinant proteins into milk. These proteins could then be purified for pharmaceutical use.

Several hormones have been produced by recombinant methods, including human insulin and human growth hormone. Human insulin offers the potential advantage of reduced immunologic response in comparison to animal insulins. Growth hormone represents an instance where the natural product was in extremely short supply. Recombinant clotting factors are being evaluated for clinical use. The fact that many hemophilia patients became infected with HIV-1 again demonstrates the potential advantages of a recombinant product free of human infectious agents. Numerous recombinant cytokines such as tumor necrosis factor, interferons, interleukins, and colony-stimulating factors are being evaluated in the treatment of various diseases, primarily malignancies and AIDS. There is a suggestion that colony-stimulating factor may be efficacious in chronic granulomatous disease. Recombinant α_1-antitrypsin is being evaluated for replacement therapy for that deficiency. Thrombolytic treatment with various forms of recombinant plasminogen activator offers considerable promise in the treatment of acute myocardial infarction. Efforts are under way to engineer novel forms of recombinant plasminogen activator that might be superior to naturally occurring proteins (see Haber et al.). Recombinant erythropoetin produced in bacteria is not biologically active, whereas glycosylated erythropoetin produced in cultured mammalian cells is active. Approximately 96 recombinant proteins in some 23 different therapeutic areas are approved, undergoing clinical trials, or under development (see Copsey and Delnatte).

The value of recombinant DNA products that must function intracellularly is more tenuous. Although recombinant enzyme could be produced for replacement therapy, the problems of intracellular, tissue-specific targeting remain. For example, large amounts of α-galactosidase A and glucocerebrosidase could be produced for therapy of Fabry's disease and Gaucher's disease, respectively, but delivery systems are unproven. Proteins for which there is no mechanism for endocytosis and proteins required in the central nervous system are unlikely candidates for such replacement therapy.

VACCINES Recombinant DNA techniques make it possible to produce recombinant proteins to be used as antigens for vaccination. For example, recombinant hepatitis B surface antigen has been produced in yeast for preparation of a vaccine now in widespread use. There is great interest in the possibility for development of a recombinant vaccine for HIV, but there are significant obstacles such as the hypervariability in the envelope protein of this virus.

Another strategy for recombinant vaccine production involves the use of live recombinant vaccine such as that which might be produced with attenuated vaccinia virus (see Moss et al.). One or more antigens from a virus can be introduced into the vaccinia genome. Live vaccines offer considerable advantages in terms of efficacy, but attenuation must be monitored to reduce the risk of rare complications. Experimental animals have been protected with recombinant vaccinia viruses against diseases caused by hepatitis B, influenza, herpes simplex, rabies, Friend leukemia, Epstein-Barr, and respiratory syncytial viruses.

RESEARCH APPLICATIONS

TRANSGENIC AND MUTANT MICE The germ-line DNA of mice can be manipulated in a variety of powerful ways (Fig. 6-20). The creation of transgenic mice typically involves microinjection of cloned DNA sequences into the male pronucleus of fertilized mouse eggs. The injected DNA becomes integrated into the mouse chromosomal DNA in a fraction of the injected cells. The transgenic DNA can be expressed in the resulting animals and can be present in the germ cells so that a series of transgenic descendant animals can be obtained. Each site of integration of foreign DNA behaves as a single Mendelian trait, and heterozygous and homozygous animals can be obtained.

Up to the present, transgenic animals have been used most widely to evaluate cis-acting regulatory DNA sequences that control tissue-specific and temporal aspects of gene expression. Putative regulatory sequences are linked to a reporter gene, which produces an easily detectable product. Using this strategy, short DNA sequences have been found to provide exquisite tissue specificity for genes such as insulin and elastase while more complex and distant regulatory sequences control the expression of globin genes. Another application of the transgenic method has involved introduction of viral or cellular oncogenes to induce tumors in animals. This opens up a variety of approaches for the study of tumor biology. A tissue-specific regulatory sequence can be linked to the SV40 T antigen to produce tumors in specific cell types. Another transgenic mouse strategy involves linking of regulatory sequences to a toxin which will selectively kill cells that express the sequence. As an example, linking of insulin regulatory sequences to diphtheria toxin can generate mice with selective absence of pancreatic beta cells. In yet another application, larger transgenic animals can be used for production of pharmaceuticals to be harvested from milk or blood.

Since integration of transgenic DNA is relatively random, it results in interruption of normal mouse genes in a certain percentage of cases. Retroviruses can also be used to infect mouse embryonic cells with the goal of relatively random insertional mutagenesis in the mouse. Mutant phenotypes can then be sought in the resulting heterozygous or homozygous mice including the identification of defects which are benign in heterozygotes but result in embryonic lethality in the homozygous state. Because the cloned DNA inserts at the site of the affected gene, it is possible to clone the gene which is associated with the mutant phenotype. Thus, it is possible to identify many new mouse mutants and to clone the relevant gene rather quickly.

The ability to carry out homologous recombination with mouse embryonic stem (ES) cells provides additional exciting opportunities. ES cells are totipotent cells that can be manipulated in culture and then reintroduced into mouse embryos. Strategies are available to use modified fragments of any cloned gene to interrupt or alter the normal mouse gene. This is achieved through homologous recombination between the cloned fragment and the mouse gene in ES cells. The genetically altered cells are often represented in the sperm of the resulting animals, and mutant mice can be obtained and bred to study heterozygotes and homozygotes. The technique will allow for creation of mouse models of many human genetic diseases. These models should be particularly valuable for studying pathogenesis and for conducting therapeutic trials. Perhaps more importantly, the ability to obtain mouse mutants for virtually any cloned gene provides an opportunity to analyze the function of the increasing number of cloned genes whose biologic roles are not delineated.

FIGURE 6-20 Various strategies for producing transgenic and mutant mice. DNA can be injected into the male pronucleus of fertilized mouse eggs followed by implantation in pseudopregnant mothers. Mouse embryos can be infected with retroviruses in vivo or in vitro. Transgenic mice may be mosaic, but the transgene can be recovered in nonmosaic form in the offspring of these mice. These strategies are depicted on the left. On the right, cultured embryonic stem (ES) cells can be modified by homologous or nonhomologous recombination or by retroviral infection. The modified cells can be selected and injected into a mouse blastocyst to produce a chimeric mouse with subsequent recovery of the mutation in the germ line of the offspring of the chimeric mouse.

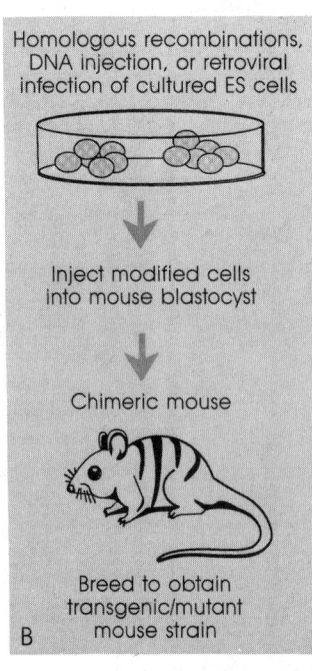

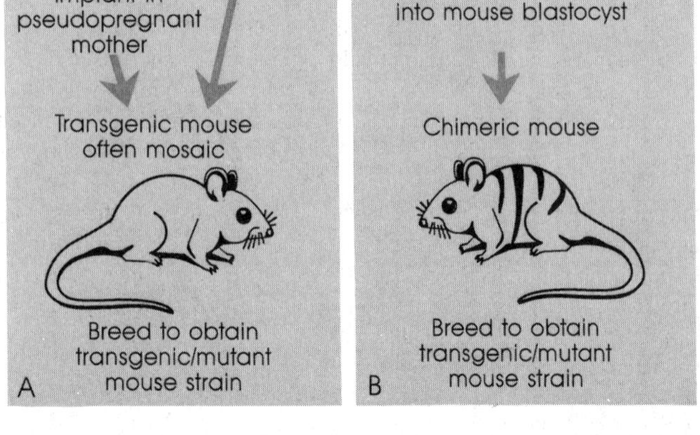

IMPACT ON BIOMEDICAL RESEARCH Recombinant DNA techniques have revolutionized the study of biology and medicine, probably more than any technical advance since the development of the light microscope. Major advances in almost all disciplines utilize these most powerful of biologic research methods. The ability to clone and characterize virtually any gene from any organism provides for universal applicability. The ability to identify homologous genes and gene segments in bacteria, yeast, *Drosophila*, mouse, and human beings brings basic science and medicine closer together. The ability to use organisms other than humans to study genetics and function often allows for deduction of the role of a human gene by analogy. For example, the identification of classes of developmental genes (e.g., homeotic genes in *Drosophila*) has led to the identification of related genes in mouse and human beings. The ability to mutate these genes in mice is likely to clarify their function in humans and lead to the identification of human mutations. These techniques make the study of neurobiology and developmental biology in mammals particularly exciting for research.

THE PROSPECTS OF GENE REPLACEMENT THERAPY For human genetic disorders in which the mutant gene is identified and the cloned normal gene is available, a number of strategies can be considered for gene replacement therapy. Gene replacement therapy has a major theoretical advantage over enzyme or factor replacement, since a single treatment could provide permanent correction. If the disease is caused by simple deficiency of the product, as in the case of most enzyme deficiencies and clotting disorders, any restoration of the synthesis of normal product might be beneficial, and neither normal tissue-specific expression nor precise regulation of gene expression may be an absolute requirement. For other gene products such as globins, an appropriate level of gene expression and tissue-specific expression would be critical. When a mutant gene product has a deleterious effect, elimination of the deleterious gene might be as necessary or more important than provision of a replacement gene. Initially, efforts at gene therapy should be directed at patients with serious life-threatening illness where risk-benefit ratios are acceptable.

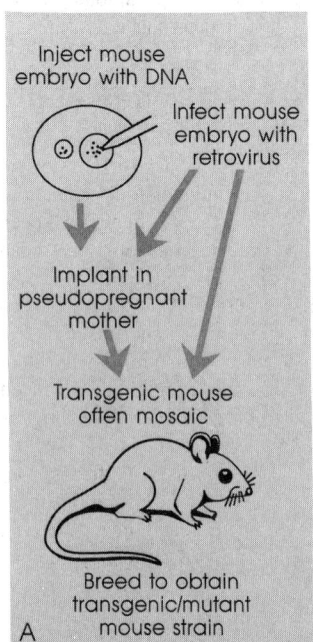

At least three types of DNA replacement can be envisioned. In one instance, a cDNA might be inserted under the control of a foreign promoter so that the product is synthesized without proper regulation. In a second strategy, genomic DNA could include the sequences necessary for proper regulation of the level and tissue specificity of expression. Artificial "minigene" constructions that link genomic regulatory regions with cDNA may provide constructions that are of manageable size and that show proper regulation. These strategies would typically involve random insertion of DNA sequences into the chromosome, although expression of extrachromosomal sequences is also a possibility. A third strategy would utilize site-specific recombination so that the mutant region was replaced by normal DNA sequence. This approach is theoretically optimal and is feasible as the result of the achievement of homologous recombination in cultured mouse embryonic stem cells. One can at least imagine the possibility of culturing human bone marrow stem cells and selecting for clones that are corrected through homologous recombination with cloned normal DNA.

Retroviral vectors are potential agents for gene therapy. Such vectors have the ability to produce viral particles that encode foreign nucleic acid and contain mechanisms for chromosomal integration. One current strategy (Fig. 6-21) involves insertion of cDNA or minigene DNA constructions between two viral long terminal repeats (LTRs) in a plasmid vector. These constructions can be introduced into cultured cell lines that provide the viral proteins necessary to package pseudovirus particles that include the gene sequence of interest. For example, bone marrow cells could be removed from a patient with a specific defect, bone marrow stem cells could be infected with these viral particles, and the patient's bone marrow could be repopulated with his or her altered cells. Delivery to tissues such as liver would be more complex, but can be envisioned.

Alternative strategies might include packaging of DNA in liposomes, development of other viral vectors, and use of vectors that remain in an extrachromosomal state. The risk-benefit ratio for somatic gene replacement therapy must be estimated on an individual basis. Random insertion of DNA sequences into the genome is likely to have some risk for carcinogenesis. However, based on the experience with retroviruses that do not contain oncogenes, this risk might be relatively low if viral progeny are not produced in the recipient. Such risks may be acceptable in patients with life-threatening illness where no reasonable alternative therapy is available. Several human diseases are candidates for early attempts (Table 6-4). Life-threatening, recessive diseases involving bone marrow–derived cells would be excellent choices (e.g., adenosine deaminase deficiency, chronic granulomatous disease, and leukocyte adhesion deficiency), as are disorders in which extracellular products such as hormones or clotting factors might be produced in altered bone marrow cells. Dominant, neurologic disorders such as Huntington's disease appear to be the least approachable. If proper regulation of globin genes could be achieved, sickle cell anemia and thalassemia would constitute important opportunities because of the accessibility of bone marrow for in vitro treatment, because of the frequency of the diseases and because of their serious nature. Human experiments using retroviral vectors to monitor an immunotherapeutic approach to malignancy appear feasible, and this experience may guide attempts at therapy for genetic disease.

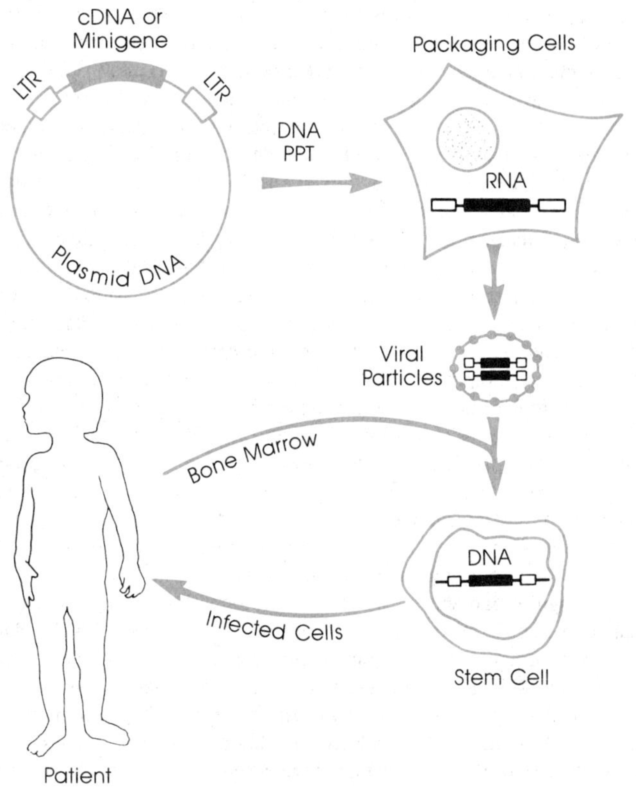

FIGURE 6-21 One strategy for attempting somatic gene replacement therapy.

ETHICAL CONSIDERATIONS Molecular genetic diagnosis provides an increasing capacity for presymptomatic and prenatal diagnosis of disease and disease susceptibility. It is possible to diagnose a newborn infant with familial polyposis of the colon, Huntington's

TABLE 6-4 Human diseases as candidates for gene replacement therapy

Disorder	Burden of disease	Alternative treatment	Disease frequency	Requirement for tissue specificity	Regulation	Relative feasibility*
Hemoglobinopathies	Great	Transfusion, fair to poor	1 in 600 in ethnic groups	Erythroid	Required	+ + +
Lesch-Nyhan syndrome	Great	Poor	Rare	Brain, ?other	?Not essential	+ +
Adenosine deaminase and nucleoside phosphorylase deficiency	Great	Transplant, enzyme replacement, fair to good	Very rare	Bone marrow	?Not essential	+ + +
Leukocyte adhesion deficiency	Great	Transplant, fair to poor	Very rare	Bone marrow	?Not essential	+ + + +
Phenylketonuria	Small to moderate	Diet, good	1 in 11,000	Liver, ?other	?Not essential	+ +
Urea cycle disorders	Moderate to great	Diet, drug, good to poor	1 in 30,000 for all types	Liver, ?other	?Not essential	+ + +
Alpha$_1$ antitrypsin	Moderate	Poor, ?recombinant drug	1 in 3500	Liver, ?other	?Not essential	+ + +
Hemophilia A & B	Moderate to great	Replacement, fair	1 in 10,000 males	?Any organ, f. VIII	?Not essential	+ + + +
Lysosomal storage diseases	Great	Poor	1 in 1500 for all types	Brain for many	?Not essential	+
Familial hypercholesterolemia	Great	Diet, drug, fair	1 in 500 heterozygotes	Liver, ?other	Some importance	+ +
Cystic fibrosis	Great	Supportive, fair/poor	1 in 2500 whites	?	?	?
Duchenne's muscular dystrophy	Great	Poor	1 in 10,000 males	?Muscle	?	?Poor
Huntington's disease	Great	Poor	1 in 20,000	?Brain	?	?Poor

* Attempts to take into account requirements for regulation, accessibility of target organs, alternative treatment, and risk vs benefit.

disease, or dominant polycystic kidney disease decades before the onset of symptoms. What might be the impact of such diagnosis on the psychological development, career opportunities, and insurability of such individuals? Diagnosis of major increased susceptibility to coronary disease, diabetes, colon cancer, breast cancer, and other disorders is also likely to bring both the potential for therapeutic intervention and the risk of anxiety and discrimination. Prenatal diagnosis is now possible for diseases with a wide range of burden, such as alpha$_1$-antitrypsin deficiency, phenylketonuria, sickle cell anemia, muscular dystrophy, and familial hypercholesterolemia. Societies and individuals are divided regarding the suitability of abortion under such circumstances. Development of gene replacement therapy and other means of treating presently untreatable genetic diseases may ultimately result in a reduced utilization of abortion.

Gene replacement therapy raises other ethical considerations. Somatic gene replacement therapy requires conventional risk-benefit analyses for individual patients. So long as there is no modification of the germ-line DNA, few people have serious ethical concerns other than the question of whether such treatment is in the best interest of an individual patient. Experience with cancer chemotherapy suggests that some unintentional low level of damage to germ-line DNA might be an acceptable undesirable risk of such therapy if the patient received great benefit. In the future, it is conceivable that methods for site-specific recombination would allow replacement of mutant DNA in the germ line with normal material. If one could permanently correct the cystic fibrosis mutation, the Huntington's disease mutation, or the sickle cell mutation in the germ line of an individual and if such treatment were safe and effective, would society consider such therapeutic intervention?

REFERENCES

BALAZS I et al: Human population genetic studies of five hypervariable DNA loci. Am J Hum Genet 44:182, 1989

COOPER DN, SCHMIDTKE J: Diagnosis of genetic disease using recombinant DNA. Hum Genet 77(Suppl):66, 1987

COPSEY DN, DELNATTE SYJ (eds): *Genetically Engineered Human Therapeutic Drugs*. New York, Stockton Press, 1988

ERLICH H et al (eds): *Polymerase Chain Reaction*. Cold Spring Harbor, Cold Spring Harbor Laboratory, 1989

HABER E et al: Innovative approaches to plasminogen activator therapy. Science 243:51, 1989

Molecular Biology of Homo sapiens. Cold Spring Harbor Symp Quant Biol 51:1, 1986

MOSS R et al: Roles of vaccinia virus in the development of new vaccines. Vaccine 6:161, 1988

OU CY et al: DNA amplification for direct detection of HIV-1 in DNA of peripheral blood mononuclear cells. Science 239:295, 1988

PALMITER RD, BRINSTER RL: Germ-line transformation of mice. Annu Rev Genet 20:465, 1986

SAMBROOK J et al: *Molecular Cloning, A Laboratory Manual*, 2d ed. Cold Spring Harbor, Cold Spring Harbor Laboratory, 1989

SCRIVER CR et al (eds): *The Metabolic Basis of Inherited Disease*. New York, McGraw-Hill, 1989

WATSON JD et al: *Recombinant DNA, A Short Course*. New York, Scientific American Books, distributed by Freeman, 1983

7 CYTOGENETIC ASPECTS OF HUMAN DISEASE

JAMES GERMAN

The chromosome complement of humans, like that of other species, is guarded carefully against change; most chromosome mutations, either structural or numerical, are deleterious. Only rarely is a balanced structural rearrangement (one that results in neither deficiency nor duplication of significant chromosome segments) introduced into the population and transmitted from generation to generation. As a rule an abnormal number of autosomes results in early death, except for trisomy of the shortest chromosome. In contrast, an abnormal number of sex chromosomes is often tolerated reasonably well, although infertility or subfertility usually is present. Nevertheless, among human embryos abnormalities in chromosome structure and number are common and are, in fact, the major known cause of embryonic and early fetal wastage. However, not every fetus with an abnormal chromosome complement is aborted, and those that survive constitute the material of medical cytogenetics.

Clinical disorders resulting from chromosome imbalance present varying features including abnormal anatomic development, mental deficiency, behavioral disorders, and disturbances in growth and sexual development. Sometimes infertility, repeated abortion, or the birth of malformed children is the presenting complaint of persons with abnormal chromosome complements whose own general development is normal.

The disorders just referred to are due to chromosome imbalance that affects tissues throughout the body. In addition, change can occur in the chromosome complement in a single cell of some somatic tissue. Such a mutant cell may have a proliferative advantage over normal cells, in which case a clone bearing the abnormal chromosome complement can develop among otherwise normal cells. Although such mutant clones are in many cases clinically insignificant, they are also important in the etiology of cancer.

This chapter is addressed to those aspects of normal chromosome structure and function that constitute the basis for an understanding of the chromosome alterations in human disease. In addition, the chromosome alterations important in adult medicine and their consequences are summarized.

CHROMOSOME STRUCTURE AND FUNCTION The human autosomes are numbered 1 through 22, and the sex chromosomes are denoted X and Y. (Figure 7-1 shows the normal human chromosome complement. In the legend of the figure several terms used in human cytogenetics are defined.) Each is recognizable microscopically by morphologic features such as relative length and position of the centromere and by staining characteristics (banding pattern). A mammalian chromosome consists of one double-stranded helix of DNA that extends from one end through the centromere to the other end.

Cell-division cycle Chromosomes must duplicate before cell division can occur. This duplication occurs over a period of several hours prior to the onset of mitosis or meiosis in a phase of the cell cycle termed *S*, for synthesis of DNA (Fig. 7-2). Thus, from the completion of S to the completion of metaphase, each chromosome contains two identical double-stranded helices of DNA, and the nucleus contains four times as much DNA as a spermatozoon or ovum. During mitosis chromosomes are condensed, and the two sister chromatids can be visualized by late prophase or early metaphase (Fig. 7-1). (Metaphase is the stage in the cell-division cycle ordinarily employed for cytogenetic analysis.)

At the onset of anaphase the centromeric regions of each chromosome separate, and the two chromatids move quickly to opposite poles of the mitotic spindle. As soon as each pole receives one full complement of chromatids (now called chromosomes), a nuclear membrane—it had been disassembled late in prophase—is assembled about each cluster to complete formation of the nuclei of the two sister cells that emerge at telophase. The sister cells emerge in what is called the G_1 phase of the cell cycle, in which they remain unreplicated unless another division is to be prepared for, whereupon they enter the S phase. Cells engaged in some differentiated function ordinarily remain unreplicated.

Most normal cells in the human body are diploid; i.e., they have twice the haploid number of chromosomes, the number in a gamete (haploid = 23, diploid = 46). In the germ line, which is devoted to gamete formation, cells destined eventually to differentiate into spermatozoa or ova undergo mitotic cell cycles until they enter the two specialized divisions termed *meiosis*. In meiosis, pairing of homologous chromosomes occurs (the paternally derived chromosome 1 with the maternally derived chromosome 1, and so on), and genetic recombination takes place (see Chap. 5). At the first meiotic division

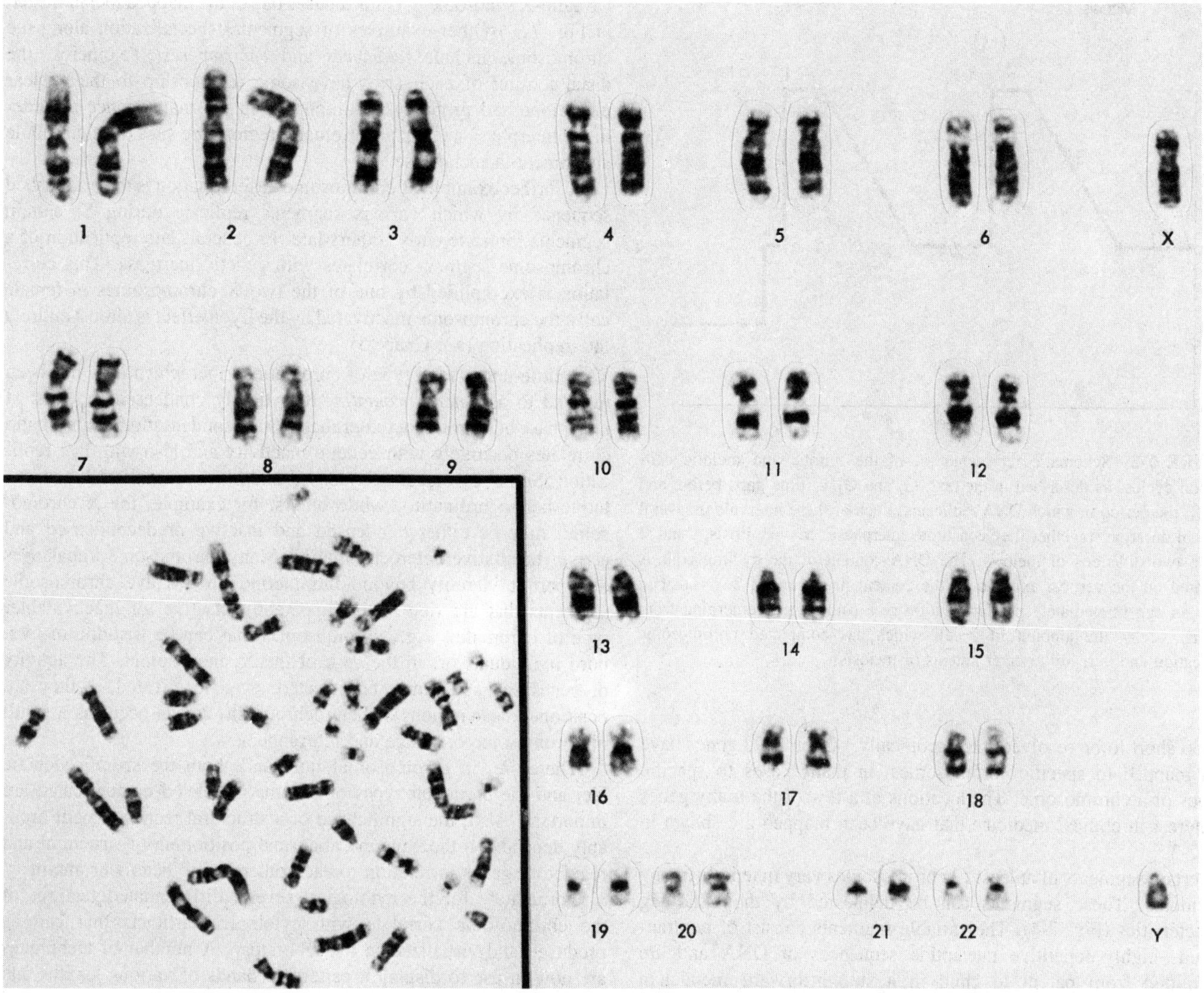

FIGURE 7-1 Normal human lymphocyte chromosomes arrested in metaphase and stained for G bands (G standing for Giemsa). The inset shows the arrangement of chromosomes in an intact cell, and the remainder of the figure shows their ordered arrangement into a karyotype. By the time mitosis begins, each chromosome consists of two identical parts called sister chromatids and is identified by its relative length, the location of its centromere, and a distinctive sequence of bands of varying lengths and depth of staining. The number of bands visible microscopically varies from cell to cell, depending on the degree of chromosome condensation. The 300 to 400 bands seen in this particular cell can be increased to several times that number if cells with longer chromosomes are chosen for analysis, i.e., many of the bands seen here will resolve into subbands. Normally, the G-band patterns of the two chromosomes of a pair are alike, with the exception of certain polymorphic regions, examples of which are shown in Fig. 7-4.

The centromere of a chromosome divides it into a short arm (p) and a long arm (q). Numbers 13 to 15, 21, 22, and Y are called acrocentric because of the nearly terminal positions of their centromeres; the minute p of each acrocentric autosome bears a nucleolus-organizing region which often causes a secondary constriction in the metaphase chromosome (the constriction at the centromere being the primary constriction).

By standard nomenclature, this karyotype is described as 46,XY, indicating that its chromosome number is 46, its sex chromosomes are an X and a Y, and the autosomes (those besides the X and Y) number 44. The following examples show the general use of this nomenclature: A normal female karyotype is described as 46,XX. A female cell with an extra chromosome 18 (trisomic for 18) would be described as 47,XX, + 18. A cell with only one sex chromosome, an X, and with deletion in the short arm of chromosome 5 would be described as 45,X,5p −. A male cell with a translocation between chromosomes 2 and 3, with breakpoints in band 13 of 2p and band 22 of 3p, would be described as t(2;3) (9q13;p22). (See also Table 7-2 footnote.)

homologous chromosomes are segregated, and the diploid chromosome number is reduced to the haploid; i.e., each cell then contains one of each of the 22 (duplicated) autosomes plus one (duplicated) sex chromosome. No S phase takes place between the first and second meiotic divisions (depicted in Fig. 7-2, right), so that at the second division, in which sister chromatids separate, emerging cells maintain the haploid number of chromosomes but are reduced in their content of DNA to half the amount of diploid G_1 cells of somatic tissues. With fertilization of an ovum by a spermatozoon, both the chromosome constitution and the DNA content of the zygote are restored to that of a G_1 somatic cell. An S period in the zygote then permits reinstitution of regular cell-division cycles characteristic of the somatic cells.

Chromosome differentiation A chromosome is differentiated along its length, and some aspects of this differentiation are resolvable, by either light or electron microscopy. The DNA is complexed with a number of proteins in a highly specific way. The DNA-protein complex together with some associated RNA is referred to as *chromatin*. The fine structure, the manner in which the DNA is compacted and interacted with proteins, and the organization of chromatin in the interphase nucleus are thought to pertain to the control of RNA production and DNA replication and perhaps to cellular differentiation as well.

The sequences of nucleotide bases in DNA that constitute the genes and that can be transcribed into messenger RNA are distributed throughout the length of the various chromosomes. (These sequences

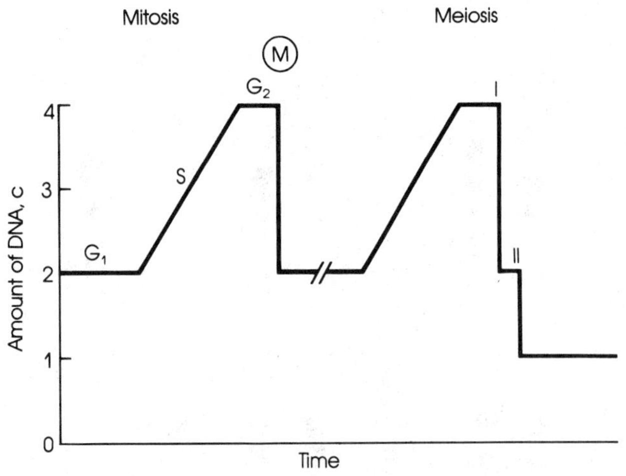

FIGURE 7-2 Schematic representation of the mitotic and meiotic cell-division cycles, as described in the text. G_1 and G_2 = time gaps before and after S, the period in which DNA replicates. Each of these intervals is several hours in duration; together they constitute interphase. M = mitosis; I and II = the two divisions of meiosis. The DNA content of the cycling cells is indicated on the vertical axis: 1c = the content in a gamete; 2c = that in either an egg immediately postfertilization or a somatic cell emerging from mitosis; 4c = the amount in a cell which has completed chromosome duplication and is ready to enter mitosis or meiosis.

are too short to be resolved microscopically.) Over 1000 genes have been mapped to specific chromosomes, in many cases to specific regions of a chromosome. The locations of a few of the many genes of interest in clinical medicine that have been mapped are shown in Fig. 7-3.

Certain segments of at least 12 chromosomes vary in length among individuals. These segments can be delineated by their staining characteristics (Fig. 7-4). The variable segments consist of nontranscribed, highly repetitive nucleotide sequences of DNA and are transmitted from parent to child in a straightforward mendelian fashion. Techniques of molecular genetics, which are useful as an extension of the microscopic observation of human chromosomes, permit the identification and molecular definition of an even greater number of variable segments of DNA, segments that are submicroscopic. These are referred to as *restriction fragment length polymorphisms* (RFLPs). Variations in both microscopically visible and invisible segments are unassociated with detectable phenotypic effect. However, they can serve as useful cell markers in prenatal diagnosis when they lie close to or within disease-associated loci (e.g., in Duchenne's muscular dystrophy) and in determination of zygosity of twins, paternity, and survival of transplants.

Other microscopically recognizable segments in the short arms of the acrocentric autosomes are devoted to the production of ribosomal RNA and nucleoli. As mitosis progresses, these nucleolus-organizer regions tend to remain relatively uncondensed later than other regions. Consequently, at metaphase they appear understained and thereby demarcate condensed segments of chromatin distal to them on the chromosome arms—*satellites*. (Satellites are examples of the polymorphic segments just mentioned.) Several other regions that remain relatively uncondensed at metaphase and that are seen more often than the remainder of the chromatin to undergo outright disruption ("breakage") are recognizable in a low percentage of cells from some normal individuals and sometimes are called *fragile sites*. In a few cases studied the tendency for such fragile sites to be visible at metaphase is a dominantly transmitted trait. The only such region known to be of significance in relation to a human trait is one located near the distal end (the end away from the centromere) of the long arm of the X chromosome; it segregates in certain families as an X-linked trait in association with a syndrome that features mental defectiveness, a characteristic facies, and macroorchia—the "fragile-X syndrome." (This locus is one of the mapped loci indicated in Fig. 7-3.) Other examples of segmental specialization along the chromosome include *telomeres* and *centromeres*. Telomeres, the distal termini of each arm, have some relationship to the nuclear membrane and probably are important in the maintenance of order in the interphase nucleus; centromeric regions are sites of microtubule attachment at metaphase.

A further example of chromosome differentiation is the established sequence by which various segments replicate during S; certain segments replicate early, others late. In general, late replication of a chromosome segment correlates with genetic inertness. This correlation is exemplified by one of the two X chromosomes in female cells; the chromosome inactivated by the Lyon effect is almost entirely late-replicating (see Chap. 5).

A little-understood type of chromatin is that which long has been referred to as *heterochromatin*. It is tightly condensed, not just at metaphase but throughout interphase. Such condensation of chromatin correlates positively with genetic inactivity and also with late replication. Some regions are condensed and inactive in all cells (constitutive heterochromatin), while others, for example, the X chromosome, may be either condensed and inactive or decondensed and active (facultative heterochromatin). Many chromosome imbalances that permit viability beyond intrauterine life involve chromosome segments that are rich in this apparently inactive, or inactivatable, type of chromatin, e.g., chromosomes that can be trisomic in liveborn individuals or, in the case of the X, monosomic. The activity of genes can sometimes be affected, even inactivated, if they are positioned near regions of heterochromatin, as can occur as a result of chromosome breakage and rearrangement.

Therefore, in chromosomal imbalance both the specific genetic loci and the particular types of chromatin deleted or duplicated are important. Also, the significance of a structural rearrangement probably depends on the new and abnormal positioning of structural and regulatory genes in relation to each other and to heterochromatin.

Fortunately for the cytologist, several differentiated features of the chromosome correlate with cytological artifacts that can be produced and visualized in the laboratory. A number of techniques are now in use to display a pattern of bands of various lengths and staining characteristics (Figs. 7-1 and 7-4). These patterns are identical in each chromosome 1, each chromosome 2, etc., varying only in the inert polymorphic regions mentioned above, so that they can be used in clinical cytogenetics to identify chromosomes and to detect and define structural rearrangements.

Sources of error A large number of genetic loci must be active to produce the numerous enzymes and structural proteins required to initiate and complete a cycle. Remarkable precision and accuracy are demanded over and over in matters such as the passage of a cell from G_1 into S, orderly progression of replication, assembly of the mitotic spindle, and spindle function in segregating chromatids during mitosis. Additional loci are activated to permit a cell of the germ line to pass successfully through the complicated stages of meiotic prophase, including pairing of homologous chromosomes, genetic recombination, and then disjoining of chromosomes. Probably all these mechanisms and processes are subject to errors, some spontaneous, others promoted by some unfavorable environmental influence (e.g., Fig. 7-5) or by the presence of deleterious mutations involving one of the many steps just mentioned. Furthermore, the genetic material itself is subject to damage, and certain types of unrepaired or erroneously repaired lesions in DNA theoretically may predispose to chromosome rearrangement. Errors at many of these steps lie behind chromosome imbalance. Errors that occur in germ cells, during fertilization, and in early postfertilization divisions are important in relation to embryonic maldevelopment and infertility; errors in somatic cells are important in relation to neoplasia.

CHROMOSOME ABNORMALITIES Mutations of a single base in a gene and deletions and duplications of chromosome segments involving even hundreds of base pairs are not visible to the cytogeneticist. In fact, for the normal chromosome banding pattern to be

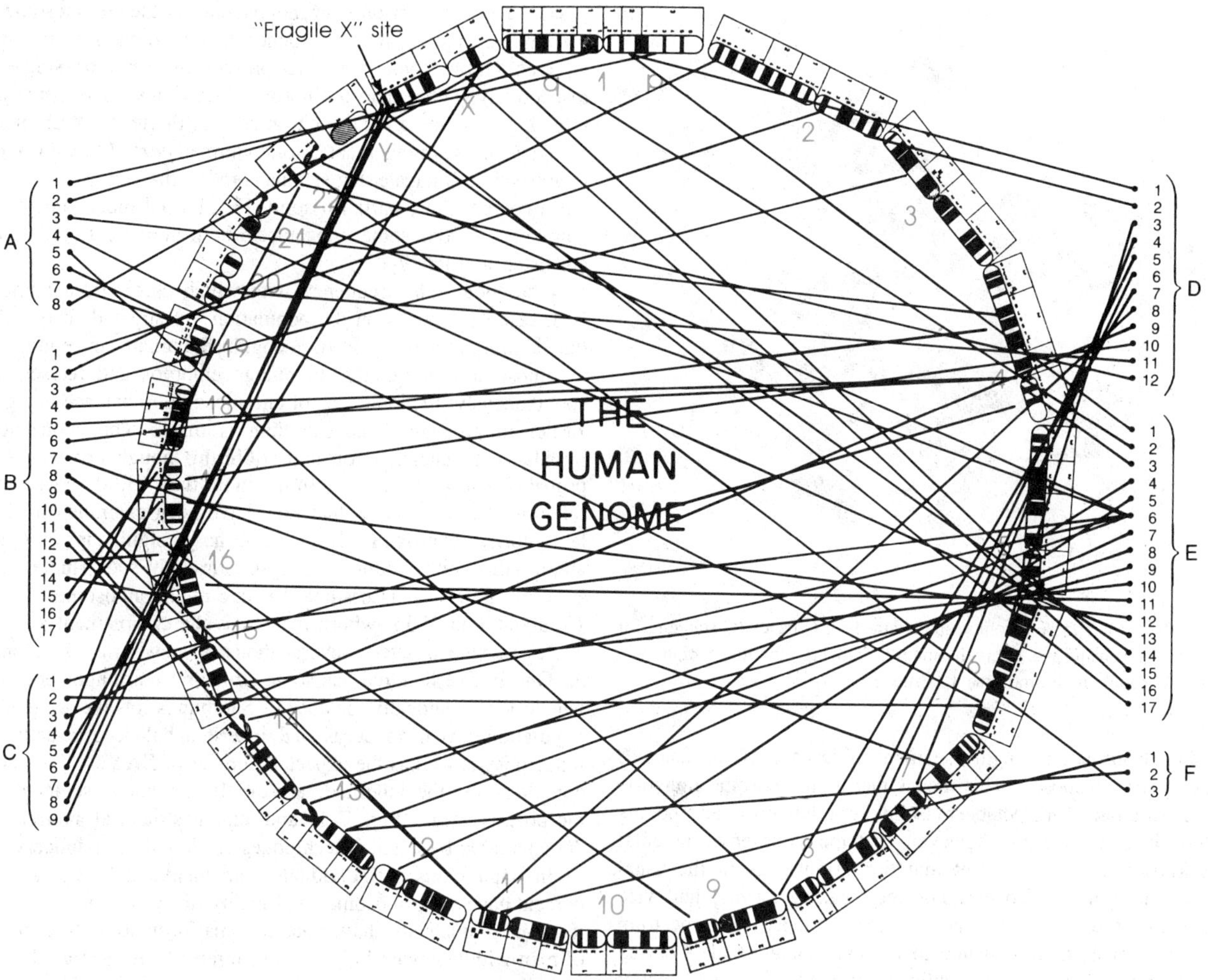

A: CELL SURFACE ANTIGENS
1 = Rhesus
2 = Duffy
3 = MNSs
4 = MHC
5 = ABO
6 = Lewis
7 = Lutheran
8 = Xg

B: DIFFERENTIATED CELL PRODUCTS
1 = Immunoglobulin kappa-light chain
2 = Glucagon
3 = Transferrin
4 = Albumin
5 = Alpha-fetoprotein
6 = Fibrinogen
7 = Collagen I
8 = Interferon (leukocyte)
9 = Insulin
10 = Hemoglobin-beta
11 = Immunoglobulin heavy chain
12 = Beta-2-microglobulin
13 = Hemoglobin-alpha
14 = Haptoglobin
15 = Myosin heavy chain
16 = Growth hormone
17 = Immunoglobulin lambda-light chain

C: GENES FOR DISEASE
1 = Huntington's chorea
2 = Congenital adrenal hyperplasia
3 = Prader-Willi syndrome
4 = Familial hypercholesterolemia (LDL receptor)
5 = Duchenne's muscular dystrophy
6 = Hunter's syndrome
7 = Hemophilia B
8 = Hemophilia A
9 = X-linked mental deficiency

D: CELLULAR ONCOGENES
1 = *N-ras*
2 = *N-myc*
3 = *myb*
4 = *erb B*
5 = *mos*
6 = *myc*
7 = *abl*
8 = *H-ras*
9 = *fes*
10 = *erb A*
11 = *src*
12 = *sis*

E: MISCELLANEOUS
1 = Phosphoglucomutase
2 = 5S ribosomal RNA
3 = Phosphoglucomutase-2
4 = Dihydrofolate reductase
5 = Lactate dehydrogenase A
6 = Ribosomal RNA
7 = Lactate dehydrogenase B
8 = Esterase D
9 = DNA segment D14S1
10 = Hexosaminidase-A
11 = Metallothionein
12 = Thymidine kinase
13 = Superoxide dismutase-1
14 = Testis-determining factor
15 = Steroid sulfatase
16 = DNA segment DXS7
17 = G-6-PD

F: "CANCER GENES"
1 = Wilms's tumor
2 = Retinoblastoma
3 = Meningioma

FIGURE 7-3 The 24 human chromosomes arrayed in a circle. The distinctive bands demonstrable by cytogenetic techniques are shown, with the numerical designations that were agreed upon by a series of international conferences. From the many genes that have been mapped to specific chromosome regions, a few of interest in medicine have been selected and their diverse locations indicated. In addition to the many hundreds of genes that code for enzymes and structural proteins that have been located, the map of the human genome has been blanketed with noncoding marker segments of DNA (RFLPs) for which molecular probes are available. (For a current listing of all known human gene localizations, see *Human Gene Mapping 9*.)

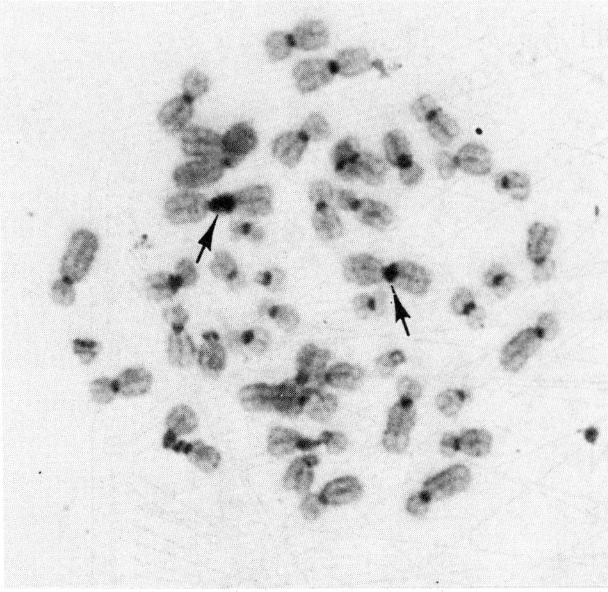

FIGURE 7-4 Metaphase chromosomes stained for C bands (C standing for centromeric or constitutive heterochromatin), showing inherited variation in lengths of C bands in chromosome 1 (arrows).

detectably disturbed, a lengthy segment of DNA must be deleted, duplicated, or transposed. This means that a chromosome mutation that is microscopically detectable must involve relatively huge amounts of DNA. It is noteworthy, however, that the same environmental agents known to produce point mutations (mutagens in the usual sense) are in general also chromosome-breaking agents, and vice versa. Thus, it seems safe to assume the existence of a spectrum extending from mutations visible to the cytogeneticist all the way down to those that must be defined by nucleotide sequencing. Mutations visible to the cytogeneticist ordinarily exert a more widespread effect on development than do point mutations; ordinary genes—often many of them—as well as other specialized types of chromatin whose function usually is unknown are involved in cytologically visible mutations.

If an entire chromosome is affected in an imbalance, the genome is said to be either trisomic or monosomic for the chromosome (thus, trisomy 13, monosomy X). Genes and chromatin carried on the affected chromosome then are present in triple or single dose, respectively, rather than the normal double dose. Abnormal dosage affecting less than an entire chromosome, the result of chromosome breakage and rearrangement, is often termed *partial trisomy* or *partial monosomy,* to indicate that segments rather than entire chromosomes are involved (thus, partial trisomy 13q, partial monosomy 4p). The commoner chromosome imbalances, both numerical and structural, are listed in Table 7-1.

FIGURE 7-5 Breaks and rearrangements (arrows) in metaphase chromosomes of a blood lymphocyte that received ionizing irradiation before being stimulated by phytohemagglutinin to enter S and divide.

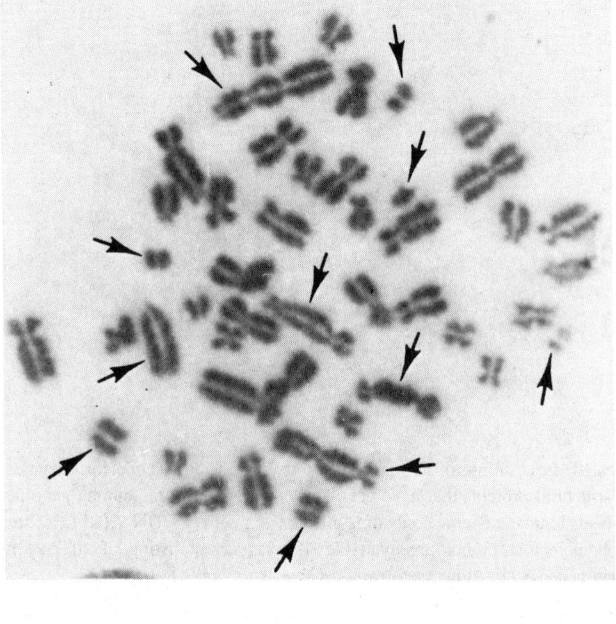

Incidence The frequency with which chromosomal imbalance is detectable depends on the population investigated. It is estimated that a minimum of 1 in 10 recognized human conceptions has a chromosome abnormality. In human embryos and fetuses aborted spontaneously, the incidence of chromosome imbalance is higher the earlier in pregnancy the sampling is made. The contribution of imbalance to late abortion and stillbirth, though not well studied, probably also is significant. In the more than 65,000 consecutive or random live-born babies that now have been examined in different laboratories, approximately 1 in 200 has a significant chromosome abnormality, either numerical or structural. In such studies, at least 1 in 700 newborns is trisomic for one of the autosomes 21, 18, or 13; about 1 in 350 newborn males has the complement 47,XXY or 47,XYY. One in every several thousand newborns has monosomy X. One in five hundred has some structural rearrangement, most of which are genetically balanced. Samplings of the general adult population reveal an occasional inherited balanced structural rearrangement as well as the expected number of XXY, XYY, and XXX complements; the inherited, apparently innocuous segmental polymorphisms (e.g., Fig. 7-4) and minor structural rearrangements demonstrable by banding techniques are found in abundance.

In populations of individuals with mental deficiency, 10 to 15 percent have a chromosome abnormality, the proportion being greater if the individuals also have anatomic malformations. In some groups of men with behavioral disorders or infertility an increased incidence of individuals with an extra X or Y chromosome is found. Infertile women also include many individuals with extra or missing sex chromosomes and an appreciable number with structural chromosome rearrangement; approximately one-fourth of women with primary amenorrhea have some abnormality of the X chromosome. Among infertile men and women, individuals with genes that interfere with meiosis, so-called meiotic mutants, are also found occasionally.

Numerical abnormalities Trisomy (47 chromosomes) is the most common chromosome imbalance in early spontaneous abortuses, followed by monosomy (45 chromosomes) and triploidy (69 chromosomes). The extra or missing chromosomes can be either paternal or maternal in origin, and the error in segregation of chromosomes can occur in the germ line, fertilized egg (zygote), or early embryo. Trisomy of every chromosome except the no. 1 has been observed in spontaneous abortions, trisomy 16 most frequently.

Sex chromosomal trisomy (XXY, XYY, and XXX) is compatible with intrauterine survival; in contrast, autosomal trisomy rarely permits survival to term. However, a small proportion of autosomal trisomics are live-born. For practical purposes these are only trisomy 21, 18, and 13, in decreasing frequency. Trisomies 18 and 13 cause death during infancy. Therefore trisomies of significance in adults are trisomy 21, XXY, XXX, and XYY. A few other autosomal trisomies, such as trisomy 8, have occasionally been reported, usually in mosaicism with a normal cellular component. (Mosaicism is the coexistence of multiple, genetically different populations of cells, all derived originally, however, from a single zygote.)

Autosomal monosomy is rare even among abortion material. In contrast, monosomy X (45,X) occurs in approximately 1.5 percent of recognized conceptions. It is common among spontaneously aborted human embryos (approximately 10 percent) and is present in one in every several thousand live-born babies. The reason for the death of 45,X embryos and fetuses is unknown, although developmental abnormalities doubtless contribute; cardiovascular and renal anomalies

TABLE 7-1 Common chromosome imbalances that recur in the human population and result in clinically recognizable syndromes*

Imbalance	Chromosomes affected	Karyotypes†	Clinical features‡
Monosomy	X	45,X	Turner's syndrome
Segmental deficiency—"partial monosomy"	X	46,XX,p−; 46,XX,q−; 46,X,r(X); 46,X,iso(Xp); 46,X,iso(Xq);	Turner's syndrome or some features of it
	Y	46,XY,p−; 46,XY,q−; 46,X,r(Y); 46,X,iso(Yp); 46,X,iso(Yq)	Turner's syndrome, or some features of it, sometimes with "mixed gonadal dysgenesis" when a 45,X cell line coexists
	4	46,XY,4p−	Gr, Cf, Mi, Ey, Sk, Ge, Ht, Co, Me
	5	46,XY,5p−	Cri-du-chat syndrome: Cr, Mi, Cf, Me
	8	46,XY,8q−	Langer-Gildion syndrome
	11	46,XY,11p−	WT, Ge, Me
	13	46,XY,13q−	RB, Cf, Me
	15	46,XY,15q−	Prader-Willi syndrome
	17	46,XY,17p−	Miller-Dieker syndrome
	18	46,XY,18p−	Gr, Cf, Ea, Te, Po, Sk, Ht, Me
	18	46,XY,18q−	Cf, Hy, Sk, Ey
	21	46,XY,r(21)	Cf, Hp, Ea, Me
Trisomy	X	47,XXX	Se, Me (mild), Ps
	X	47,XXY	Klinefelter's syndrome
	Y	47,XYY	Ta, Ac, Su, B; but often normal
	8	46,XY/47,XY,+8	Cf, Sk, Me (moderate)
	13	47,XY,+13	Trisomy 13 syndrome: Cp, Ey, Pd, Po, Ht, D, V, Sc, F, Ar, Me
	18	47,XY,+18	Trisomy 18 syndrome: Cf, Ea, V, F, Gr, D, He, Me
	21	47,XY,+21	Trisomy 21 syndrome (Down's syndrome)
Segmental duplication—"partial trisomy"	Y	46,X,t(X;Y)§	XX male
	9	9p+†	Cf
	22	22q+¶	Gr, Cf, Ea, Cp, Hy, Co
Chimerism	Entire complement	46,XY/46,XX	Pseudo- or true hermaphroditism; dimorphism of blood-cell-surface antigens
Triploidy	Entire complement	69,XXY	Hc, Me, Sy, Ht, Ge, D

* For complete listing, consult DeGrouchy and Turleau.
† The sex chromosome constitution might be either XY or XX, but in the example karyotypes given, XY arbitrarily is used.
‡ The clinical features given include only some of the more constant ones. Deficiency of one segment often is accompanied by duplication of another, and the phenotypic effect is the consequence of the combined imbalance. Abbreviations are defined below.
§ Translocation onto an X of a segment of the Y bearing the locus Y responsible for testicular differentiation. Random inactivation of either the normal X or the one bearing Y material determines the gonadal phenotype(s)—testis or ovary, respectively.
¶ Brought about through any of several rearrangements.
Abbreviations: Ac, acne; Ar, arrhinencephaly; B, behavior disorder; Cr, characteristically abnormal cry; Cf, characteristic craniofacial dysmorphism; Co, convulsions; Cp, cleft lip–palate; D, early death; Ea, characteristically abnormal ears; Ey, eye anomaly; F, characteristically flared, overlapping fingers; Ge, abnormality of external genitalia; Gr, severe growth deficiency; Hc, hydrocephaly; Hp, hypertonia; Ht, cardiac malformation; Hy, infantile hypotonia; Me, intellectual deficit; Mi, microcephaly; Om, omphalocele; Po, characteristically abnormal posture; Pd, polydactyly; Ps, psychotic predisposition; RB, retinoblastoma; Sc, scalp defect; Se, secondary amenorrhea; Sk, skeletal anomalies; Su, subfertility; Sy, syndactyly; Ta, tallness; Te, characteristically abnormal teeth; V, visceral anomalies; WT, Wilms's tumor with aniridia.

are common in the few that survive. In monosomy X, the missing sex chromosome can be either a Y or an X and is either paternal or maternal in origin. Often the second sex chromosome is not completely absent but is replaced by a structurally rearranged Y or X. Mosaicism is common in live-borns with monosomy X; here, tissues are populated not only by cells with a 45,X complement but by other cells, perhaps with a normal complement, either 46,XY or 46,XX, or with a complement in which the second sex chromosome is rearranged in some way.

Triploidy is rare in live-born babies and usually leads to early death, even when in a mosaicism with normal cells: 46,XY/69,XXY. The phenotypic effects of the autosomal trisomies, of 47,XXY, and of monosomy X (45,X) are characteristic and well defined so that their diagnosis usually is not difficult (see Chap. 324). The effects of the 47,XYY and 47,XXX constitutions are less striking, and therefore these complements are underdiagnosed. Mosaicism with coexistence of abnormal and normal populations of cells can cause an abnormal phenotype to approach the normal.

The mechanisms responsible for the numerical abnormalities are undefined and may be multiple. In trisomy 21 the extra chromosome is of maternal origin in 80 percent and of paternal in 20 percent of cases. A striking but unexplained maternal age effect exists in trisomies 21, 18, 13, XXY, and XXX. Over a third of babies with trisomy 21 are born to women over 35, whereas only something over a tenth of all births occur in this group. The frequency of trisomy 21 rises from 0.5 to 0.7 per 1000 live births between ages 21 and 23 to 3.1 per 1000 at age 35, 10.5 per 1000 at age 40, and 33.6 per 1000 at age 45. After a child with trisomy 21 is born, the risk to the parents of recurrence in future pregnancies is increased to approximately 1 percent. As to the cause of monosomy X, the frequent association of the 45,X complement in mosaicism with normal complements and with structural rearrangements of the X and Y suggests that the zygote or the preimplantation embryo is often the target of a chromosome-breaking event.

Structural abnormalities Some structural chromosome rearrangements are inherited, and others represent new mutations. The cause of the new rearrangements is unknown, although they are assumed to be partly spontaneous and partly the effect of environmental agents such as mutagenic chemicals or ionizing radiation (Fig. 7-5) acting on the germ line, zygote, or early embryo. The majority of de novo rearrangements are paternal in origin.

Many of the known chromosome rearrangements have been

detected only once or a few times. Others are detected repeatedly, the same one occurring in unrelated individuals and families. For example, the commonest translocation, one that can occur either as a result of de novo mutation or by inheritance, affects one chromosome 13 and one 14 at or near their centromeres. In this translocation, only inert chromatin or functional chromatin represented elsewhere in the genome—the nucleolus-organizing regions referred to earlier—is lost from the tiny short arms. Also common is a similar translocation affecting chromosomes 14 and 21.

Chromosome complements bearing rearrangements can be genetically balanced or effectively so, thus imparting no unfavorable phenotypic effect to their bearers; about two-thirds of rearrangements detected during surveys of consecutive live-born babies are balanced. Or, the complement can be unbalanced and affect development adversely, the usual case when rearrangements are detected during surveys of spontaneous abortuses or of individuals with multiple anomalies and mental deficiency.

Some balanced rearrangements are transmitted from generation to generation without producing clinical effects. In other cases, however, they are profoundly important to members of the kindred transmitting them, by being responsible for the conception of embryos with unbalanced genomes. For example, inherited translocations involving chromosome 21 predispose to the trisomy 21 syndrome. Approximately 5 percent of live-borns with that syndrome have a translocation, and in about a fifth of those it is detectable in one of the parents. Because most babies with the trisomy 21 syndrome due to translocation are born to women under 30, a search for a translocation is important when a child with this clinical syndrome is born to young parents.

Different translocations bestow on their carriers different risks of having offspring with unbalanced rearrangements. These risks cannot be predicted on the theoretical basis. Useful empirical risk figures have been accumulated for common translocations; e.g., the 14;21 translocation bestows a 2 percent risk on a balanced male carrier and more than a 10 percent risk on a female carrier of having a child with the trisomy 21 syndrome. In contrast, the balanced carrier of a 21;21 translocation can expect only unbalanced offspring. Information of this type is indispensable to those undertaking genetic counseling in relation to chromosome disorders.

DISEASE ASSOCIATIONS Various combinations of abnormalities in malformed and defective individuals have been correlated with variations in the chromosome complement. In this way, clinical syndromes due to specific chromosome imbalances have been defined. (Many of the pediatric conditions are of little significance in adult medicine because of their lethality in infancy or early childhood.)

Autosome imbalance Of the three autosomal trisomies found in live-born babies, only trisomy 21 is compatible with survival past infancy. The phenotype produced by the presence of an extra chromosome 21, formerly known as *mongolism* but now termed the *Down syndrome* or the *trisomy 21 syndrome*, is characteristic and easily diagnosed from birth: mental deficiency, short stature, muscular hypotonia, brachycephaly, short neck, typical facies (oblique orbital fissures, flat nasal bridge, small simple or folded ears, nystagmus, mouth hanging open), narrow palate, short broad hands with incurving fifth fingers, gaps between the first and second toes, and characteristic dermatoglyphics. Additional findings may include congenital heart disease, blepharitis and conjunctivitis, Brushfield's spots of the iris, straight pubic hair, abnormal teeth, a protruding furrowed tongue, a high-arched palate, loose skin of the neck, transverse palmar creases, and hyperflexibility of the joints. Cardiac malformations lead to death in infancy in a third of individuals with trisomy 21, and other malformations and infections may also cause early death. However, subjects who survive infancy often reach adulthood, and some even old age, at which time features of Alzheimer's disease become common. The proneness to develop leukemia in affected infants is not maintained in later life. Females occasionally become pregnant, and, as expected, approximately half their children have trisomy 21.

Mosaicism of trisomy 21 with normal cells (46/47, +21) may occur in individuals with modified features of the trisomy 21 syndrome, and it is probable that many individuals with this mosaicism go undiagnosed. The risk of such persons having trisomic children is increased, but unfortunately their mosaicism is usually detected only after they have had an affected child.

Partial trisomy, partial monosomy, or a combination of the two explains many of the instances in both children and adults of multiple developmental defects combined with mental deficiency. Sometimes a balanced autosomal translocation is detected in normally developed adults who have repeated spontaneous abortion or subnormal fertility, with or without abnormal live-born children.

Although the phenotypic effects of many of the different segmental chromosome imbalances which can occur are varied and nonspecific, the resulting anomalies sometimes compose recognizable clinical syndromes. Two examples are the following: (1) If a rearrangement causes partial trisomy of just the distal band of the long arm of 21, the clinical features composing the full syndrome associated with an extra chromosome 21 develop. (A triple dose of other segments of the long arm of chromosome 21 also produces adverse effects but not the trisomy 21 syndrome.) (2) Partial monosomy of a short segment within the short arm of chromosome 5 causes mental deficiency, a characteristic facies, and a characteristic cry during infancy. This group of signs is known as the *5p−* (five-p-minus) or *cri-du-chat syndrome*.

Additional specific syndromes produced by imbalance of many different chromosome segments now are known (Table 7-1), e.g., the 4p−, 9p partial trisomy, 13q−, and 18q− syndromes, to name a few. Furthermore, the application of high-resolution banding techniques makes possible identification of the exact band(s) deficient or duplicated. Rearrangements not previously described, partly because they were not visible without high-resolution banding or molecular cytogenetics techniques, and their corresponding clinical syndromes still are being recognized. Any of these syndromes may appear as the result either of de novo chromosome rearrangement or through formation of a genetically unbalanced gamete in a person carrying in balanced state a rearrangement affecting the segment involved.

In most individuals with chromosome imbalance, regardless of which segments are affected, a degree of phenotypic similarity is present. These recurring and nonspecific features include mental deficiency, growth deficiency, dysmorphic ears, nose, and mouth, cardiac malformations of standard types, abnormalities of dermal ridges and creases, and dysmorphic digits. (As a rule, autosomal imbalance need not be considered in the etiology of anatomic defects unaccompanied by mental deficiency.) Why similar abnormalities occur with so many different segmental imbalances is unknown, but when several such features are observed in a single individual, they can be a valuable clinical indication for cytogenetic analysis. Imbalance affecting certain segments also causes specific phenotypic changes, examples being the anomalous cry in the 5p− syndrome mentioned above, retinoblastoma, in relation to one particular band of chromosome 13, and the Prader-Willi syndrome which is often associated with a disturbance of a band near the centromere of chromosome 15. Whereas the nonspecific changes serve to call the clinician's attention to the possibility of some chromosome imbalance, the specific features can suggest the exact segment of the genome affected.

Sex chromosome imbalance (See also Chap. 324) In contrast to autosome imbalance, sex chromosome imbalance has relatively mild phenotypic effects. This is because X chromosomes beyond one in the complement of somatic cells are usually almost totally inactivated and because the Y chromosome bears relatively few genes. X-linked loci (in contrast to autosomal loci) function normally in single dose: the female is functionally hemizygous for most loci on the X through the Lyon effect; the male, with only one X chromosome, is hemizygous for X-linked genes with the exception of loci clustered in a segment at the end of Yp that is homologous to a comparable so-called pseudoautosomal segment at the end of Xp. The addition of an extra sex chromosome to the normal male or female complement has a phenotypic effect but insufficient to interfere with intrauterine survival. Since major anatomic defects are usually absent, individuals with the complements 47,XXY and 47,XYY, both of whom are males, and 47,XXX, who are females, ordinarily go unrecognized till adolescence or later, often never to be diagnosed at all.

The *Klinefelter syndrome* (Chap. 324), which in classic form consists of small testes, infertility, gynecomastia, and variable degrees of underandrogenization, sometimes with mild mental deficiency, antisocial behavior, or both, is the consequence of the addition of an extra X to the male complement: 47,XXY. The extra X interferes in some way with the survival of germ cells, and atrophy of the spermatogenic tubules and azoospermia are the consequence. Sometimes the phenotypic effects are surprisingly mild, the testicular atrophy being the only noteworthy feature in otherwise healthy and socially well-adjusted men. The mosaicism 46,XY/47,XXY sometimes occurs and may ameliorate the phenotypic effect of the extra X. More extreme phenotypic effects and mental deficiency result when more than one extra sex chromosome is added to the normal male complement: 48,XXXY or 49,XXXXY.

The phenotypic effect of 47,XYY is less well defined; although increased height, behavioral difficulties, and infertility are common, the extra Y is sometimes found in otherwise normal men. The rare complement 48,XXYY results in infertility, probably because of the extra X, as in the 47,XXY Klinefelter syndrome. The phenotype associated with 47,XXX is also poorly defined; although women with mild mental deficiency, psychosis, and menstrual abnormalities sometimes are found to have this complement, it is also sometimes detected in normal, healthy women. Further clarification is needed concerning the effects on personality and behavior of all three of the complements 47,XXY, 47,XYY, and 47,XXX.

Loss of the Y or of the second X has drastic effects on development. If it does not cause abortion, it may or may not be recognizable at birth. Loose nuchal skin folds and edema of the hands and feet in a newborn girl, with or without renal or cardiovascular anomalies, may point to the diagnosis of the 45,X complement. The *Turner syndrome* is the manifestation in subsequent life (Chap. 324): short stature, infantilism of otherwise normal female external and internal genitalia, germ-cell-free gonads referred to as gonadal streaks, and variable renal, cardiovascular, skeletal, and ectodermal anomalies. Without estrogen administration breast development remains infantile and menstruation does not occur. Although mental deficiency is not a feature, a poorly defined emotional immaturity is common.

The Turner syndrome may be the developmental consequence of several chromosome constitutions besides 45,X. Mosaicism as well as structural abnormalities affecting certain segments of a second sex chromosome, either a Y or an X, cause a spectrum of disorders at both the clinical and cytogenetic levels. A normal male or normal female cellular component may be present along with the 45,X cellular component, or one component may bear a structurally abnormal chromosome. Common abnormalities of the Y and X are isochromosome formation (one arm deleted and the other duplicated) or deletion of part or all of one arm. In some affected individuals, all cells have 46 chromosomes, with one normal X plus an abnormal Y or X, for example, 46,XXp−, deletion of a segment of the short arm of one of the X chromosomes. In others, a second or third cellular component may be present as well, for example, 45,X/46,XX/46,XXp−. Clinically pure Turner syndrome may be found in association with various combinations of these karyotypes if one of them is either monosomic or partially monosomic for X. However, when Y-bearing cells coexist with the 45,X cells, for example, 45,X/46,XY, genital ambiguity often develops, and gonads may vary from streaks to functional testes (the syndrome of *mixed gonadal dysgenesis*); here the risk of gonadal neoplasia is significant. When 46,XX cells coexist with 45,X, varying degrees of ovarian function may be maintained, including ovulation. Although the phenotype may approach a normal male or female pattern when normal and abnormal cells coexist, the effects of mosaicism are unpredictable. Thus, the clinical syndrome associated with monosomy X and structurally abnormal Ys or Xs ranges from a predominantly male phenotype, through Turner syndrome, to an almost normal female phenotype.

Two other rare conditions deserve mention—*true hermaphroditism* and the *46,XX male* (see also Chap. 324). First, true hermaphroditism is present when testicular and ova- and follicle-containing ovarian tissue coexist in the same individual. In most cases 46,XX is the chromosome complement, and it appears normal by banding. Exceptionally, true hermaphrodites have the complement 46,XY, or chimerism 46,XY/46,XX, each of the two cellular components having been derived from a different zygote. Second, males occasionally have the complement 46,XX. As in 47,XXY men, the second X interferes with meiosis, and azoospermia results. In both the 46,XX true hermaphrodite and the 46,XX male, the rule that a Y is required for testicular differentiation appears to break down. The explanation for some XX males is that the testis-determining locus has been translocated from Yp to Xp, demonstrable not by microscopy but by molecular cytogenetics. True hermaphroditism probably is on the basis of mutation affecting the same lcous.

X-linked mental deficiency In the general population more males than females are mentally deficient, and mental deficiency when familial affects males preferentially. In some such kindreds, mental deficiency segregates as an X-linked trait, and several X-linked mental deficiency syndromes are now recognized.

Although chromosome imbalance is not responsible, one cause of X-linked mental deficiency can be diagnosed by cytogenetic techniques. In a significant proportion of families in which mental deficiency is segregating, the X in the affected males and that same X in their mothers is, or can be made, recognizable cytogenetically by technical manipulations. In a variable but usually small proportion of metaphases from affected persons this phenotypically unusual X chromosome exhibits a fragile site, denoting the fragile-X syndrome. This syndrome is the most common form of X-linked mental deficiency and accounts for almost half of all cases.

Chromosome change in cancer The theory that an alteration in the chromosomal complement may cause cancer was advanced many years ago. Nevertheless, only with improved cytogenetic techniques during the past three decades and with the advent of recombinant DNA technology has firm evidence supporting the theory became available. Chromosome changes are plentiful in cancer, but this very fact—too many changes—was a major reason many rejected them as having etiologic significance. Support for the idea that chromosome alteration is involved in the etiology of human cancer comes from three sets of observations: (1) the known environmental "causes" of human cancer—carcinogenic chemicals and ionizing radiation—are also chromosome-breaking agents (Fig. 7-5); (2) several recessively inherited disorders feature increased chromosome breakage and rearrangement (Bloom's syndrome is the prototype of these disorders), and in each the risk of cancer is increased; and (3) a specific chromosome rearrangement is found in one of the major human leukemias: the so-called Philadelphia chromosome in chronic granulocytic leukemia. Thus, the known environmental and genetic causes of increased chromosome mutation all predispose to cancer, and at least one example of specificity of a chromosome mutation in a human neoplasm is available.

Now it is clear that most human cancers have chromosome complements that are altered in a microscopically detectable way. Table 7-2 lists some of those found with regularity. In the leukemias, lymphomas, and certain myeloproliferative disorders the alterations are less extensive than in solid tumors and, therefore, easier to define. As examples, in certain lymphomas chromosome 14 is often found to have undergone structural rearrangement, with the breakpoint near or in a specific region, namely, the immunoglobulin heavy chain locus; the rearrangement translocates the *myc* locus from its normal position on chromosome 8 to chromosome 14. Also, in over 95 percent of cases of chronic granulocytic leukemia (CGL) a translocation affecting chromosomes 9 and 22 is readily detected, resulting in the Philadelphia, or Ph^1 (p-h-one), chromosome, an abnormally short no. 22. If the leukemia progresses into a "blastic" phase, the

TABLE 7-2 Some of the recurring chromosome abnormalities encountered in human neoplasms

Neoplasm	Aberration	Chromosome regions affected
Leukemia		
Chronic granulocytic	Translocation	9q34 and 22q11
Acute nonlymphocytic		
M1	Translocation	9q34 and 22q11
M2	Translocation	8q22 and 21q22
M3	Translocation	15q22 and 17q11
Chronic lymphocytic	Trisomy	12
Acute lymphocytic		
L1–L2	Translocation	9q34 and 22q11
L3	Translocation	4q21 and 11q23
	Translocation	8q24 and 14q32
Lymphoma		
Burkitt's	Translocation	8q24 and 14q32
Follicular	Translocation	14q32 and 18q21
Solid tumors		
Benign		
Meningioma	Deletion or monosomy	22q
Parotid, mixed	Translocation	3p25 and 8q21
Malignant		
Ewing's sarcoma	Translocation	Bands 11q24 and 22q12
Germ cell tumors, testis	Deletion	12p
	Duplication	12q
Lung, small cell	Deletion	Bands 3p14 to 3p23
Neuroblastoma	Deletion	Bands 1p31 to 3p36
Ovary, cystadenocarcinoma	Translocation	6q21 and 14q24
Retinoblastoma	Deletion	Band 13q14
Wilms's tumor	Deletion	Band 11p13

NOTE: The FAB (French-American-British) classification of leukemias is employed above. The chromosome breakpoint and band nomenclature is that of the Paris Conference (Birth Defects: Original Articles Series VIII (7):1–46, 1971). The chromosome and chromosome-arm designation (e.g., 9q means the long arm of chromosome no. 9) appears first and is followed by the chromosome region and band on that arm (e.g., 9q34 means the fourth band in the third region of the long arm of chromosome no. 9).

already mutated karyotype evolves; certain new chromosome changes are added stepwise in a nonrandom sequence. In CGL and certain other leukemias, the chromosome changes, demonstrable either microscopically or by microscopy supplemented by molecular probes (molecular cytogenetics), may have diagnostic utility as well as considerable value in prognosis and choice of therapy.

The microscopically visible chromosome mutations that are found with regularity in human neoplasms often affect loci that play growth regulatory roles in normal cells, and in some cases the chromosome breakpoints affect known cellular oncogenes. In the examples just given, *myc* in its new position on chromosome 13 is abnormally regulated. In the Ph^1 chromosome, *abl* is translocated from its normal position on chromosome 9 into a specific region called *bcr* on chromosome 22, thereby creating a new genetic determinant; in myeloid cells, this mutant locus is transcribed, and the mRNA is translated into a novel protein that presumably plays a causative role in the autonomous growth of the neoplastic cell lineage.

Another chromosome mechanism known to be important in human neoplasia is somatic crossing-over. (Somatic crossing-over contrasts with germ line crossing-over, where recombination is legitimate.) Through crossing-over, a recessive mutation at a genetic locus concerned with growth regulation—a mutation that preexisted in a cell but remained occult because of the presence of a normal locus on the homologous chromosome—can become homozygous. The consequence of homozygosity at the mutant locus is loss of normal growth control. Such mutations were first recognized in the rare neoplasms retinoblastoma and Wilms's tumor; the loci affected were on chromosomes 13 and 11, respectively. In some cases the original (recessive) mutation consisted of outright deletion of the locus. Transmission through the germ line of such occult recessive mutations explains familial instances of those neoplasms.

Thus, chromosome mutations of at least three types constitute crucial steps in the initiation and progression of malignant neoplasia: (1) translocations that disturb the regulation of loci concerned with growth; (2) deletion-mutation of recessive loci that play a presently obscure role in oncogenesis (e.g., the retinoblastoma locus just referred to), mutations that can either be inherited through the germ line or that occur de novo in a somatic cell; and (3) recombination yielding homozygosity for preexisting mutations affecting this last-mentioned type of locus. These mutations and their oncogenic consequences are now the subject of considerable investigation, both basic and clinical. In turn, the breakpoints in neoplasms of various types are helping identify hitherto unrecognized genetic determinants that together orchestrate normal cellular proliferation and tissue growth; thus the cytogenetics of human cancer is contributing to the understanding of normal cell biology.

Solid tumors, which generally are studied later in their natural course than neoplasms of the bone marrow, show extensive karyotypic changes, both structural and numerical. Different cells from a single tumor have similar numerical changes and structural rearrangements, but in the same direction. This apparent lack of specificity is partly due to the complexity of the karyotypic changes, however, and some chromosome alterations are specific for solid tumors (Table 7-2). The cytogenetic findings in both leukemias and solid tumors demonstrate the clonal nature of human cancer.

TECHNICAL CONSIDERATIONS Human metaphase chromosomes can be examined with light microscopy in any tissue in which sufficient cells are cycling. Preparations can therefore be made directly from almost any embryonic tissue and from adult bone marrow, lymphoid tissue, and selected malignant tissues. In searches for mosaicism, the study of multiple tissues is often required. Some tissues unlikely to contain cells in metaphase can be placed in culture, and chromosome preparations can be made from cells that reach mitosis in vitro. Blood T lymphocytes stimulated to enter cell-division cycles by phytohemagglutinin are the standard material for diagnosing constitutional chromosome imbalance in live-born individuals. Fetal tissue from aborted material can also be examined. In some myeloproliferative disorders and leukemias, unstimulated circulating blood cells divide spontaneously after a few hours in culture. Long-term cultures of fibroblasts can be derived from minute skin biopsies or from fragments of many other types of tissue, although more elaborate laboratory facilities and a longer period of time are required before cytogenetic preparations can be made. Amniotic fluid is among the sources of cells suitable for culture, and the cells, which are fetal in origin, are widely used in the prenatal diagnosis of chromosome imbalance, particularly in pregnancy in women of advanced age or who already have borne a child with a chromosome imbalance. Metaphase preparations also can be made from chorionic villi biopsied in the first trimester of pregnancy.

Meiotic chromosome preparations from testicular biopsies are sometimes useful in obscure cases of infertility. Translocations and genetically determined disturbances in meiotic pairing may be identified.

Recombinant DNA technology has been employed in conjunction with conventional cytogenetic techniques to define chromosome abnormalities in finer detail. Now that a vast number of probes for specific loci or chromosome segments have become available, molecular cytogenetics makes it possible to identify segments of chromosomes involved in rearrangements in which banding techniques had lacked the required resolution, by using molecular hybridization either to Southern blots or directly onto metaphase chromosome fixed to a slide. In prenatal diagnosis, probes for RFLPs sometimes are used to identify which chromosome has been inherited by the conceptus. This can be useful in pregnancies at risk of X-linked disease, determining in males whether the single X chromosome is the one that bears a particular undesirable locus that one of the parents is known to carry. Recombinant technology also can be useful in conditions that follow a dominant pattern of inheritance, such as Huntington's chorea, to determine whether the undesired mutant gene is present in the complement of the conceptus by discovering whether an RFLP closely linked to the mutant gene is or is not present. In a few instances, probes for undesirable mutant genes themselves or for RFLPs within the genes, are already available. Probes specific for the Y chromosome can define the sex of an embryo or fetus if a few cells can be obtained by amniocentesis or chorionic villus biopsy. They also can be of diagnostic value in obscure cases of intersex in which a Y chromosome, or a segment of the Y, is being sought. In relation to neoplasia, the use of molecular probes can identify rearrangements that affect specific chromosome regions. With the polymerase chain reaction even a small population of cells bearing some specific translocation, e.g., the Ph^1 chromosome breakpoint, can be identified.

Sometimes, metaphase, or anaphase chromosomes are analyzed to determine whether damage to the genetic material has been induced by some environmental agent (radiation, chemical, virus), or whether constitutional genomic instability is present. Cells that have proliferated in vivo and then been incubated only briefly in vitro may be used in search of evidence of damage to the genetic material of a given person or of a population (e.g., Fig. 7-5). The number of chromatid gaps, breaks, and rearrangements can be estimated directly in cells reaching their first mitosis in vitro. Another approach is to estimate the amount of in vivo damage by counting the number of exchanges that occur between sister chromatids during growth for two cell-division cycles in 5-bromodeoxyuridine. A test system less laborious than metaphase chromosome analysis, but one capable of showing that excessive chromosome breakage has occurred either in vivo or in vitro, is the determination of the proportion of nondividing cells having micronuclei. A micronucleus is produced when a chromosome fragment lacking a centromere lags at anaphase (as it will be obliged to do) and is encompassed in a separate nuclear membrane at telophase. The micronucleus assay is useful in the survey of populations for clastogen exposure, which is equivalent to mutagen and carcinogen exposure.

REFERENCES

De Grouchy J, Turleau C: *Clinical Atlas of Human Chromosomes*, 2d ed. New York, Wiley, 1984

German JL: Studying human chromosomes today. Am Sci 58:182, 1970

———: Gonadal dimorphism explained as a dosage effect of a locus on the sex chromosome, the gonad-differentiation locus (*GDL*). Am J Hum Genet 42:414, 1988

Heim S, Mitelman R: *Cancer Genetics*. New York, Alan R Liss, 1987

Human Gene Mapping 9. Ninth International Workshop on Human Gene Mapping. Cytogenet Cell Genet 46:1, 1987

McKusick VA: The human gene map. Clin Genet 27:207, 1985

Rooney DE, Czepulkowski BH (eds): *Human Cytogenetics: A Practical Approach*. Oxford and Washington, IRL Press, 1986

Schwarzacher HG: *Methods in Human Cytogenetics*. New York, Springer-Verlag, 1974

Simpson JL: *Disorders of Sexual Differentiation*. New York, Academic, 1976

8 TREATMENT AND PREVENTION OF GENETIC DISORDERS

DAVID VALLE

The complex processes of normal development and physiologic homeostasis depend on the coordinated interactions of the products of many genes working together in developmental and metabolic systems. These systems are adaptable within limits, allowing normal development and physiologic homeostasis to occur over a range of environmental conditions. For instance, the products of some 30 to 40 genes participate in blood glucose homeostasis; the result is maintenance of a relatively constant blood glucose concentration despite intermittant and highly variable ingestion of glucose precursors. Moreover, developmental and homeostatic interactions of 10,000 or so gene products are believed to be necessary for normal development and function of the central nervous system. Mutations that reduce the adaptive capacity of these systems result in maldevelopment and/or dyshomeostasis that we recognize as genetic disease. The mutant gene may so compromise a particular developmental or homeostatic system that the system functions poorly or not at all in any environmental circumstance, thereby producing a monogenic disorder. Alternatively, the mutant gene may have modest effects under ordinary conditions but in certain environments cause maldevelopment or dyshomeostasis that we recognize as a multifactorial disorder. Thus, the role of the genes in health and disease is both central and complex. Consequently, treatment of genetic disease is both difficult and frequently less than completely effective.

TREATMENT

Effective treatment of genetic disorders requires accurate diagnosis, early intervention prior to development of irreversible tissue damage, and an understanding of the abnormal biochemistry or metabolic pathophysiology. The rapid progress in delineating the molecular basis of genetic disease has improved our capability for rapid and accurate diagnosis of monogenic disorders. Understanding of the metabolic pathophysiology is increasing at a slower rate mainly because progress in this area often requires elucidation of integrative physiology by study of the intact organism. The development of noninvasive metabolic monitoring techniques such as positron emission tomography and topical magnetic resonance spectrometry as well as new genetic technologies for the production of specific animal models of human genetic disease offers promise for progress in this area.

Approaches to treatment of genetic disease can be organized biologically proceeding from the clinical phenotype through the levels of the abnormal metabolites and dysfunctional protein to the level of the defective gene (Table 8-1).

TREATMENT OF THE CLINICAL PHENOTYPE Treatment at the level of the clinical phenotype includes a variety of conventional medical practices such as patient education, pharmacologic interventions, and surgical procedures. It depends on a thorough understanding of the natural history of the particular disorder so that potential complications can be avoided or addressed early in the course to minimize the consequences. Although therapy at this level is not aimed at correcting the primary defect, it can markedly improve the patient's quality of life. Examples include instruction to patients with albinism or xeroderma to limit sun exposure or to patients with glucose-6-phosphate dehydrogenase deficiency to avoid the offending drugs; administration of β-blockers to Marfan syndrome patients to prevent or slow dilatation of the aortic root, anticonvulsants to patients with neurogenic disorders, or antihypertensive agents to patients with secondary hypertension; and a host of surgical interventions for patients with genetic malformations, skeletal dysplasias, and malignancies.

TREATMENT OF THE METABOLIC PHENOTYPE Treatment at the metabolite level involves nutritional or pharmacologic approaches and is dependent on understanding the biochemical pathophysiology (Fig. 8-1). Deficient function of a mutant protein may result in a disease phenotype because a substrate accumulates to toxic levels (precursor toxicity); because the product of an alternative pathway is produced in excessive amounts (alternative pathway overflow); because of reduced formation of the reaction product or some downstream metabolite (product deficiency); or some combination of these possibilities. Although this paradigm is most easily visualized for enzymes in a metabolic pathway, it holds for virtually all proteins. The pathophysiology may involve *local* effects within the cell or tissue normally expressing the mutant protein, or it may involve *distant* biochemical effects as a consequence of pertubations of metabolite concentrations in the extracellular fluid. For example, the neurologic phenotype of Tay Sachs disease results from destruction of neurons caused by deficiency of resident hexosaminidase A whereas the mental retardation characteristic of untreated phenylketonuria due to defi-

TABLE 8-1 Some treatments for monogenic disorders

Level of treatment and method	Disorder(s)
CLINICAL PHENOTYPE	
Patient education	
Avoidance of aggravating agents (high carbohydrate diet, exposure to cold)	Periodic paralysis syndromes
Avoidance of certain drugs	Pharmacogenetic disorders, acute intermittent porphyria
Avoidance of sun exposure	Xeroderma pigmentosa, albinism
Avoidance of certain physical activity	Chondrodystrophies
Notify physician for rapid increase in size of mass or tinnitus	Neurofibromatosis
Pharmacologic	
β-Blockers	Marfan's syndrome
Anticonvulsants	Neurodegenerative disorders
Surgical	
Orthopedic reconstruction	Chondrodystrophies
Colectomy	Familial polyposis coli
Plastic reconstruction of facial malformations	Treacher-Collins syndrome, several monogenic cleft lip and/or palate syndromes
METABOLIC PHENOTYPE	
Metabolite alteration	
Substrate restriction	
Phenylalanine	Phenylketonuria
Branch chain amino acids	Maple syrup urine disease
Galactose	Galactosemia
Fructose	Hereditary fructose intolerance
Lactose	Lactase deficiency
Phytanic acid	Refsum's disease
Alternate pathway utilization	
Benzoate and phenylacetate	Urea cycle disorders
Glycine	Isovaleric acidemia
Carnitine	Organic acidosis
Cysteamine	Cystinosis
Penicillamine	Wilson's disease
Metabolic inhibition	
Allopurinol	Gout
Mevinolin	Familial hypercholesterolemia
Replacement of deficient products	
Glucose polymers (cornstarch)	Glycogen storage disease I, III
Uridine	Hereditary orotic aciduria
Glucocorticoids	Congenital adrenal hyperplasia
Thyroxine	Familial goiter
Biotin	Biotinidase deficiency
Protein alteration	
Activation of the mutant protein	
Pyridoxine (vitamin B_6)	Homocystinuria
Thiamine	Maple syrup urine disease
Hydroxycobalamin (vitamin B_{12})	Some forms of methylmalonic acidemia
Replacement of the mutant protein	
Growth hormone	Growth hormone deficiency
Factor VIII	Classic hemophilia
Alpha$_1$-antitrypsin	Alpha$_1$-antitrypsin deficiency
Polyethylene glycol-adenosine deaminase	Adenosine deaminase deficiency
Organ transplantation	
As a source for a specific protein	
Allogeneic bone marrow	Lysosomal storage diseases, β-thalassemia
Liver	Glycogen storage disease, type I, familial hypercholesterolemia, ornithine transcarbamylase deficiency
As a protein source and replacement of damaged organ	
Liver	Alpha$_1$-antitrypsin deficiency, hepatorenal tyrosinemia
Kidney	Cystinosis

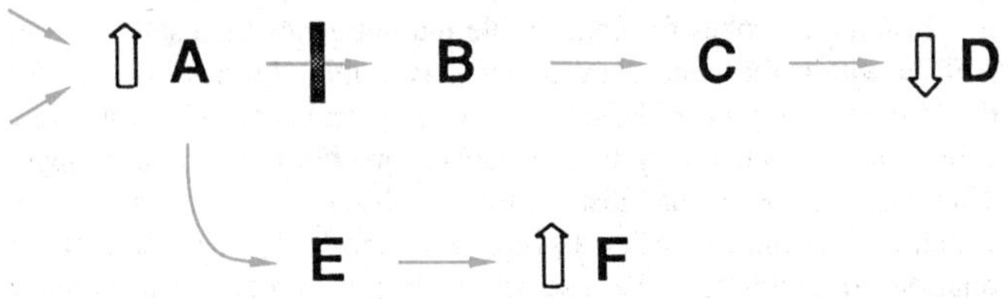

FIGURE 8-1 Pathophysiological consequences of a genetic defect in a metabolic pathway. Substrate A is converted via a series of intermediates to a final product, D. The enzymes catalyzing these reactions are indicated by the horizontal arrows. A also is converted to F in an alternative pathway. Genetic deficiency of the enzyme converting A to B (indicated by the hatched rectangle) may have pathophysiological consequences related to accumulation of A (precursor toxicity), overflow to F (alternative pathway overflow), reduced formation of D (product deficiency), or some combination of these possibilities.

ciency of hepatic phenylalanine hydroxylase is mediated by the systemic accumulation of phenylalanine.

Precursor toxicity Correction of precursor toxicity frequently involves dietary restriction of a particular substrate whose major source is nutritional. Inborn errors of amino acid and carbohydrate metabolism provide good examples of this approach. A diet restricted in the branch chain amino acids (leucine, isoleucine, valine) is effective in preventing the mental retardation associated with maple syrup urine disease caused by deficiency of branch chain ketoacid decarboxylase (see Chap. 334). Such diets should be started soon after birth, continued for life, and monitored in such a way that intake of these essential amino acids is just sufficient for normal growth. Illnesses that cause protein catabolism (e.g., those associated with intercurrent infections or trauma) periodically complicate this therapy by releasing large amounts of the offending amino acids from the breakdown of endogenous protein. These episodes may require hospitalization for administration of intravenous fluids and even dialysis. Similarly, lifetime restriction of dietary galactose in patients with galactosemia due to deficiency of galactose-1-phosphate uridyl transferase corrects growth failure, prevents cataracts, and improves intellectual outcome (see Chap. 337).

Alternate pathway utilization For some disorders alternative metabolic pathways may be utilized to remove toxic metabolites. The effectiveness of this approach is limited by the capacity of the alternate pathway and often must be combined with dietary restriction of the offending substrate. Administration of benzoate and phenylacetate to patients with inborn errors of urea metabolism is a good example of this approach. These compounds are conjugated with endogenous glycine and glutamine, forming hippurate and phenylacetylglutamine, respectively. When used in conjunction with restriction of dietary protein, this therapy reduces the accumulation of ammonia in patients with inborn errors of the urea cycle and organic acid metabolism. Similar approaches include the administration of carnitine, which conjugates with a variety of accumulated CoA esters in patients with defects of organic acid metabolism; cysteamine, which helps to eliminate excess cyctine in cystinosis; and penicillamine to reduce excessive stores of copper in Wilson's disease and iron in hemochromatosis.

Inhibition of an overactive pathway For other disorders, particularly those in which alternative pathway overflow produces a toxic level of a particular metabolite, it may be possible to prevent the accumulation by inhibiting an enzyme in the affected pathway. This approach may lead to accumulation of upstream substrates that must be well tolerated if the treatment is to be successful. For instance, in gout and other disorders in which excessive purine degradation leads to uric acid accumulation, inhibition of xanthine oxidase by allopurinol reduces uric acid production and lowers the incidence of uric acid nephropathy and gouty arthritis. Xanthine, which accumulates as a consequence, has greater aqueous solubility than uric acid and usually is well tolerated. In a similar fashion, hypercholesterolemic patients heterozygous for mutations at the low density lipoprotein receptor locus exhibit significant reductions in plasma cholesterol when treated with lovastatin, a potent inhibitor of hydroxymethylglutaryl coenzyme A reductase that catalyzes an important early and rate-limiting step in the synthesis of cholesterol.

Product deficit For disorders in which the pathophysiology involves product deficit, nutritional or pharmacologic approaches to replenishing the product can be effective if the administered material reaches the appropriate physiologic compartment. For example, many of the inborn errors in hormone biosynthesis such as the various forms of congenital adrenal hyperplasia and hereditary defects in thyroid hormone biosynthesis respond well to pharmacologic replacement of the deficient hormones. By contrast, the administration of melanin to albinos would not correct the pigment deficit in melanocytes.

TREATMENT DIRECTED TO THE PROTEIN PHENOTYPE Therapy at the level of dysfunctional protein involves either activation of the mutant protein or replenishment of the missing protein.

Activation of the mutant protein Activation may be possible if the protein requires a vitamin cofactor and the vitamin is one that is well tolerated in pharmacologic doses. Obviously, not all mutations of a gene encoding a vitamin-dependent protein will respond. Those that do are likely to be missense mutations that either decrease the affinity of the enzyme for its cofactor or destabilize the protein in a way that can be partially overcome by substantial increments in cofactor concentration. About one-third of the cases of homocystinuria due to deficiency of the pyridoxal phosphate-requiring enzyme, cystathione-β-synthase, exhibit a significant increment in the activity when treated with pharmacologic doses (50 to 500 mg/d) of pyridoxine (vitamin B_6). The actual increase in enzyme activity may be small but suffices to improve metabolic flux in the impaired pathway. Since activation of residual activity both reduces precursor accumulation and increases product formation, knowledge of the pathophysiologic mechanism is less critical for this form of treatment.

Protein replacement therapies An alternative therapeutic approach involves replacement with an exogenous supply of the protein. To be successful, the protein must be administered directly into or eventually reach the appropriate physiologic compartment. Thus, blood proteins or proteins that traverse the vascular compartment (e.g., peptide hormones) are candidates for this approach. Other considerations include the availability, stability, and immunogenicity of the administered protein. Recombinant DNA technology can sometimes be utilized to supply sufficient amounts of the pure protein (e.g., human growth hormone and alpha$_1$ antitrypsin). Other proteins (e.g., clotting factor VIII) are available from natural sources but may eventually be produced by recombinant technology. This advance ensures an adequate supply and avoids the risk of transmission of pathologic viruses contaminating the protein purified from natural sources.

ORGAN TRANSPLANTATION Organ transplantation is on the borderline between therapy at the level of the dysfunctional protein and gene therapy. On the one hand a transplanted organ supplies a deficient protein; on the other, the transplant tissue also brings new genetic information which, in contrast to standard models of gene therapy, is not integrated into the recipient's genome. Kidney, liver, and bone marrow transplantation are utilized for a variety of genetic diseases. The development of more effective and specific immunosuppressants (particularly cyclosporin) and the inadequacy of many less invasive therapies account, in part, for the increased utilization of this form of treatment. In some instances, the goal of transplantation is to supply the recipient with a tissue that can replace a mutant protein (e.g., liver transplant for deficiency of low density lipoprotein receptor or one of the urea cycle enzymes). For other disorders (e.g., alpha$_1$ antitrypsin deficiency or hepatorenal tyrosinemia) the transplant both provides the protein and replaces a severely damaged organ. The pathophysiologic mechanism of the disease is relevant; the physician must consider if the newly supplied protein will only be used locally or, if not, will gain access to the involved tissue(s). The long-term efficacy and consequences of organ transplantation as treatment for genetic disorders remain to be determined.

PROSPECTS FOR GENE THERAPY Several methods are now available to introduce new, functional genetic material into mammalian cells. These methods allow consideration of a more direct approach to treatment of genetic disease, namely gene therapy or introduction of a functional gene to replace or supplement the activity of a resident defective gene. Typically, two general strategies have been considered, germline and somatic cell gene therapy, which differ in the nature of the recipient cells. In the germline model foreign DNA is introduced into the zygote or early embryo with a significant probability that the newly introduced material will contribute to the germline, i.e., be passed on to the next generation. By contrast, in somatic gene therapy models, the new genetic material is introduced only into somatic cells and is not transmitted to the germ cells. A third approach to gene therapy involves activation of endogenous genes to augment or circumvent a defective gene.

Much of the technology for germline gene therapy has been developed in work on transgenic mice. Fertilized mouse eggs are harvested from a superovulated female, microinjected with DNA molecules, and reimplanted in a pseudopregnant female. Several murine genetic diseases, including deficiency of growth hormone, myelin basic protein, and β-globin have been "treated" in this fashion with the general result that the disease phenotype is markedly ameliorated. These experiments have provided considerable information on the regulation of gene expression and the pathogenesis of genetic disease. However, the process is inefficient: only 15 to 20 percent of injected eggs produce transgenic animals, and of these only 20 to 30 percent actually express the introduced gene. Furthermore, there are appreciable risks including damage to a resident gene by the random insertion of the foreign DNA (insertional mutagenesis). In practice, availability of the molecular reagents for this approach makes prenatal diagnosis possible. The certainty of having an unaffected child as established by prenatal diagnosis is preferable to the uncertainty and risks of the transgenic approach. Thus, germline gene therapy is not applicable to human genetic disease.

Conversely, somatic gene therapy experiments will be tried for human genetic disease (Fig. 8-2). The methods for introducing the genetic material and the recipient cells will vary depending, in part, on the disease to be treated. Currently, modified retroviral vectors that allow high efficiency introduction of foreign DNA into dividing cells are favored. Bone marrow stem cells, hepatocytes, and fibroblasts are candidate recipient cells, and favorable results have been obtained in tissue culture systems. Difficulties with long-term, high-level expression of the introduced gene and with reintroduction of the recipient cells into the organism are obstacles to progress in this area. Developments in directing the introduced gene to its normal location in the genome (homologous recombination) offer promise for achieving normal regulation of the introduced gene and elimination of detrimental effects of the endogenous mutant gene. The lessons learned from more conventional therapies will apply to somatic gene therapy. The importance of early intervention, consideration of pathophysiologic mechanism(s), and the need for regulated interactions of the product of the introduced gene with other members of the involved homeostatic system are all relevant. Each disorder will have its own therapeutic requirements and problems. These considerations suggest that somatic gene therapy eventually will be useful for certain genetic diseases but is unlikely to be broadly effective.

By contrast to the first two models, activation of the expression of endogenous genes is a form of gene therapy that is already being attempted for human genetic disease. Interferon γ, a potent transcriptional regulator of several genes including those involved in X-linked chronic granulomatous disease (X-CGD), improves neutrophil function in that subset of X-CGD patients with mutations that impair a cytochrome involved in superoxide metabolism (see Chap. 81). Likewise, hydroxyurea increases the expression of the gamma globin gene in some patients with sickle cell disease, providing an alternative, nonsickling hemoglobin. The long-term efficacy of these approaches and the possible detrimental effects of administering agents that markedly affect the expression of many genes are unknown.

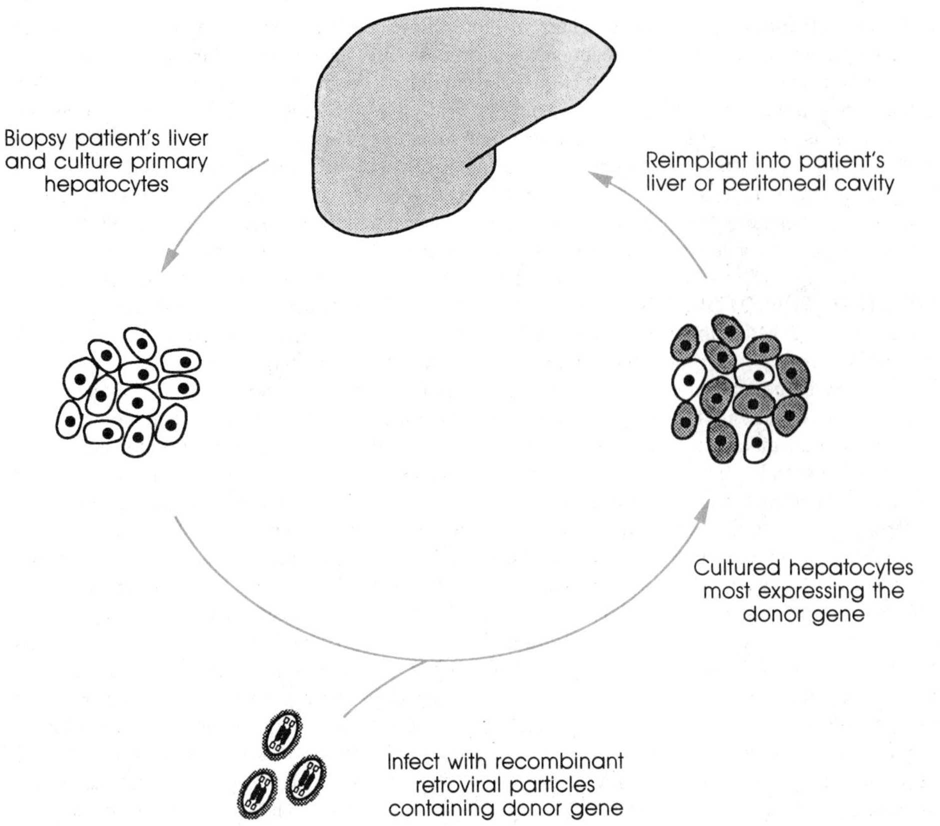
Biopsy patient's liver
and culture primary
hepatocytes
Reimplant into patient's
liver or peritoneal cavity
Cultured hepatocytes
most expressing the
donor gene
Infect with recombinant
retroviral particles
containing donor gene

FIGURE 8-2 One model for somatic gene therapy involving retroviral-mediated gene transfer into hepatocytes.

EVALUATION OF THERAPY FOR GENETIC DISEASE

Two general questions should be posed in an evaluation of therapy for a genetic disease. First, does the treatment provide therapeutic benefit? Second, does the treatment restore the patient to full physiologic normality as if he or she did not have the disease? These questions can be asked of any disease treatment but have special significance for genetic disorders that are predictable and preventable. Studies by Costa, Scriver, and Childs evaluated the effectiveness of therapy of 351 representative monogenic disorders on three basic variables, life span, reproductive capability, and social adaptation; in their study available therapies returned life span to normal in only 15 percent, allowed reproductive capability in only 11 percent, and improved social adaptation in only 6 percent of the disorders. Only slightly better outcomes were found with a subset of 65 diseases in which the basic defect is known. Because more severe diseases are more quickly recognized, this sample may be skewed toward diseases most difficult to treat. Nevertheless, the results of therapy are worse than expected, emphasize the difficulty in developing effective therapies for genetic diseases, and highlight the need for continued work in this area. The results also underscore the value of preventive measures as therapy for genetic disease.

PREVENTION OF GENETIC DISEASE

Recognition of the limitation of therapy in genetic disease plus the predictability of the pattern of transmission of genes from one generation to the next has focused attention on prevention as the most reliable and effective means of dealing with hereditary disorders. The preventive approach includes genetic screening, counseling, and prenatal diagnosis.

GENETIC SCREENING There are two types of genetic screening programs for autosomal recessive disorders: homozygote screening programs search for individuals who have the disorder; by contrast, heterozygote screening programs search for individuals who are carriers of a mutant gene and thus are at increased risk of having offspring with a particular disorder. Successful homozygote screening programs require an inexpensive and reliable test, the recognition of some benefit (treatment, counseling) of early diagnosis, and education of the individuals and/or families screened so that they understand the significance of the results. The best example of such programs are the newborn screening programs. The diseases screened for vary from state to state but often include phenylketonuria, homocystinuria, maple syrup urine disease, galactosemia, cystic fibrosis, hypothyroidism, and sickle cell disease. In each instance the screening test allows early detection and the opportunity to initiate appropriate therapy prior to the onset of irreversible damage. Also, the parents of an affected individual are made aware of the risk to future offspring and have the option of prenatal diagnosis. Heterozygote screening programs are best exemplified by the program to detect carriers of Tay Sachs disease, a fatal, autosomal recessive lysosomal storage disease for which there is no effective treatment. Heterozygote screening of defined subpopulations with an increased carrier frequency (e.g., Ashkenazi Jews where the carrier frequency is approximately 1/25 as compared to approximately 1/300 in Anglo Saxons) identifies couples at risk in which both potential parents are carriers with a 25 percent chance of having an affected child. Prenatal diagnosis is possible, and the procedure provides a means for the couple to have unaffected children.

GENETIC COUNSELING Prospective parents who seek information regarding the risk of genetic disease in their offspring may come to the physician for genetic counseling. Thus, all physicians should become familiar with the principles of medical genetics and use this knowledge to understand and counsel patients. The couples may be identified as having an increased risk for having a child with a genetic disease because of a previously affected child or other near relative. Alternatively, one or both parents may belong to a known high risk group (e.g., identified as a carrier in a heterozygote screening test), or advanced maternal age ($>$ 35 years at the time of delivery) may be associated with increased risk of having a baby with an autosomal trisomy.

One aspect of genetic counseling involves determination of the risk for having an affected child and transmission of this information to the prospective parents so that they can make informed reproductive decisions. The first step is to determine the reliability of the diagnosis. This usually requires critical examination of existing medical data and/or additional evaluation of affected family member(s). The information is then assembled in the format of the family pedigree to determine the pattern of transmission within the particular family and to compare it with that expected for the diagnosed condition. Depending on the type of disease (monogenic, multifactorial, or chromosomal) and reliability of the diagnosis, the risk to subsequent offspring may be predicted with a degree of certainty ranging from a rough estimate to nearly perfect. The reliability of the diagnosis will be influenced by the existence of multiple etiologies for a particular phenotype and the availability of specific diagnostic tests. Molecular tests that directly and unambiguously determine the parental genotype are becoming increasingly available and allow precise prediction of the risk of recurrence and prenatal diagnosis for some monogenic disorders (see Chap. 7). For autosomal recessive and X-linked disorders in which a primary biochemical defect is known, reliable diagnosis is possible by a functional test of the gene product (e.g., assay of enzyme activity). For most autosomal dominant disorders the primary biochemical defect is not known and, thus, identification of parental genotype is subject to error resulting from heterogeneity of etiology. Availability of linked molecular markers, e.g., RFLPs, and identification of the involved genes will greatly improve the realiability and precision of counseling for some of these conditions.

Counseling for many common multifactorial disorders (e.g., diabetes, hypertension, atherosclerotic cardiovascular disease, congenital malformations, and psychiatric disorders) is imperfect and will be so until we have a better understanding of the interactions of the various genes and environmental factors that produce these diseases. In some families the etiology may involve a major contribution of a single gene, and in others a mix of multiple genes and environmental factors is the cause. In the former the risk may be predicted by a monogenic model while in the latter no simple model suffices. In these instances, the physician must resort to empiric risk estimates derived from retrospectively assembled data based on the average reproductive outcome in many different families.

Other information in addition to determining risk should be obtained prior to counseling. The prognosis and treatment of the disorder should be reviewed and the availability of prenatal diagnosis and carrier testing should be determined. Finally, the counselor must be sensitive to the emotional impact this information may have on those counseled.

During the counseling session, effective communication of the information depends on clearly expressing the essentials in language understandable to the subjects. Written notes and diagrams frequently are helpful and can be given to them at the end of the session. Finally, review at subsequent visits helps correct misconceptions and increase retention of the information. In this regard, the physician who has an established relationship with the family may have advantage over a trained counselor who meets with the subjects on only one or two occasions.

PRENATAL DIAGNOSIS Following genetic counseling, the couple at risk for having a child with a genetic disease has several options depending, in part, on the type of disorder. They may be reassured and proceed despite the risk without any subsequent monitoring. Or, they may view the risks as too high and choose to have no additional children or to adopt. Alternatively, when both parents are heterozygous for an autosomal recessive disorder, they may choose to reduce the risk by utilizing artificial insemination by donor. The magnitude of the decrease in the risk provided by this option will depend on the carrier frequency for the particular disorder in the general population. For a couple with a 1 in 4 or 25 percent chance of having a child with phenylketonuria, the risk with donor insemination will drop to 1 in 130 ($\frac{1}{2} \times \frac{1}{65}$) or less than 1 percent because the carrier frequency in the general population is 1 in 65. In the instance that mutant alleles for the gene in question are preferentially associated with particular linked markers (linkage dysequilibrium), it may be possible to reduce the risk further by avoiding donors with the mutant-associated markers.

Finally, if the disorder can be detected antenatally, the couple may decide to proceed with reproduction and utilize prenatal diagnosis with elective abortion of affected fetuses. Because the risk of having an affected fetus ranges from a maximum of 50 percent for heterozygotes with autosomal dominant disorders to < 10 percent for nearly all chromosomal and multifactorial disorders, the great majority of pregnancies monitored by prenatal diagnosis have an unaffected fetus. This relatively low frequency of affected fetuses, together with an increase in reproductive activity which often results from the reassurance provided by the availability of prenatal diagnosis, leads to significant increases in the family size of at risk couples. Thus, in contrast to some public misconceptions, availability of prenatal diagnosis actually results in increased numbers of offspring. The indications for prenatal diagnosis are developed from a comparison of the risk of the procedures with the risk of having an affected child (Table 8-2).

Several methods for prenatal diagnosis are available (Table 8-3). Choice of a method depends on the disorder in question and on family preferences. Measurement of alpha fetoprotein (AFP) and other fetal proteins in maternal serum is noninvasive and can be used to screen for pregnancies at risk for neural tube defects (increased maternal serum AFP) and for fetal aneuploidies (decreased maternal serum AFP). It is possible by ultrasonography to visualize many fetal malformations and growth abnormalities and to monitor more invasive fetal sampling techniques with attendant reductions in the risks of the procedures. Although second trimester (15 to 16 weeks of gestation) fetal sampling by amniocentesis is the most widely used method for obtaining fetal cells, the techniques of transcervical and transabdominal chorionic villus sampling (CVS) can also be performed at 9 to 12 weeks of gestation. CVS has the advantage of allowing the diagnosis to be made earlier, and if an abortion is chosen, it will take place at a stage of pregnancy when maternal-fetal bonding is

TABLE 8-2 Major indications for prenatal diagnosis

Indication	Risk for affected fetus, %	Method of detection
Chromosomal disorders		
Advanced maternal age (>35 y)	1–10 depending on maternal age	
Parent with a balanced translocation	3–20 depending on the transloca-tion	Chromosomal analysis of cells obtained by CVS* or amniocentesis
Previous child with chromosomal abnormality	~1	
Monogenic disorders		
Couple at risk for having a child with an inborn error of metabolism	25	Biochemical and/or molecular analysis of cells obtained by CVS or amniocentesis
Couple at risk for having a child with a monogenic disorder for which molecular markers are available	25–50	Molecular analysis of DNA obtained from cells obtained by CVS or by amniocentesis
Couple at risk for having a child with a monogenic malformation syndrome without biochemical or molecular markers	25–50	Fetal imaging by ultrasound
Malformation disorders		
Couples at risk for having a child with a neural tube defect (anencephaly or meningomyelocele) or other multifactorial malformation syndrome	1–10	Fetal imaging by ultrasound and, for neural tube defects, measurement of alpha fetoprotein and other fetal markers in amniotic fluid obtained by amniocentesis

* CVS, chorionic villus sampling

TABLE 8-3 Methods of prenatal diagnosis

Method	Stage of gestation, weeks	Sample	Fetal disorders	Risks
Maternal serum sampling	15–18	Alpha fetoprotein and other fetal proteins	Neural tube defects, aneuploidies	Negligible
Fetal ultrasonography	6–40	Image	Fetal dating, morphologic abnormalities, skeletal dysplasis	Negligible
Fetal sampling				
Chorionic villus sampling	9–12	Fetal trophoblastic tissue	Cytogenetic, biochemical, molecular	1–2% fetal loss
Amniocentesis	15–18	Amniotic fluid and cells	Cytogenetic, biochemical, molecular, neural tube defects	0.2–0.5% fetal loss
Fetal biopsy	18–20	Fetal skin	Dermatologic	~2% fetal loss
		Fetal liver	Liver-specific, enzyme deficiencies	2–5% fetal loss
		Umbilical cord, blood	Blood disorders	~2% fetal loss

less. Finally, elective abortion at 12 weeks of gestation is a 2- to 3-h outpatient procedure whereas a second trimester elective abortion requires a 1- to 3-day hospitalization. The risks of CVS are still being assessed but, in experienced hands, appear to compare well with those of amniocentesis. The tissue obtained at CVS is fetal trophoblastic tissue, expresses nearly all enzymes found in amniocytes, and provides an excellent source of fetal DNA.

REFERENCES

Scriver CR et al (eds): *The Metabolic Basis of Inherited Disease*, 6th ed. New York, McGraw Hill, 1989

Filkins K, Russo JF (eds): New York, Marcel Dekker, 1985

Friedmann T: Progress toward human gene therapy. Science 244:1275, 1989

Costa T, Scriver CR, Childs B: The effect of mendelian disease on human health: A measurement. Am J Med Genet 21:231, 1985

section 2 Cell growth and regulation

9 GROWTH FACTORS

LEWIS T. WILLIAMS

Many diseases involve abnormalities in the rate of proliferation of cells (Table 9-1). The most obvious of these, cancer, is associated with uncontrolled cell division. A more subtle form of abnormal cell proliferation is found in atherosclerosis, a disease in which vascular smooth-muscle cells proliferate excessively, but not in a malignant fashion, and eventually obstruct blood flow. Diseases that involve nonmalignant proliferation of cells include fibroproliferative processes such as pulmonary interstitial fibrosis, and some forms of glomerulonephritis, cirrhosis, and myelofibrosis. In these processes normal tissue is replaced by fibroblasts and their extracellular products. Several of the disease syndromes are caused by inappropriately low levels of cell proliferation. Thus, in the anemia of renal disease there may be a sluggish proliferation and maturation of erythroid precursors in the bone marrow caused by the inadequate production of erythropoietin by the kidney.

One of the most important findings in the study of cell proliferation has been the recognition that both normal and abnormal proliferation of cells are under control of polypeptide growth factors that serve as intercellular messengers. In general growth factors can act in one of three ways. First, some growth factors are released into the circulation and act at a distance, essentially in the same manner as hormones. This mode of *endocrine* action is typified by erythropoietin and insulin-like growth factor 1. Second, a cell may release a factor into its local environment, perhaps into the extracellular matrix, where the factor acts on adjacent cells. This mode of action, termed *paracrine*, may be the most common way in which growth factors regulate tissue repair and embryonic development. Third, growth factors may act by *autocrine* mechanisms, in which a cell responds to a factor that the cell produces.

Growth factors were originally discovered by measuring their ability to regulate the proliferation of specific target cells in vitro. There have been three general sources for the identification and purification of most factors: serum, tissue extracts, and media "conditioned" by cultured cells. Most of the factors described in this chapter have been purified from these sources, and amino acid sequences of small peptide fragments have been determined directly. Based on these sequences DNA probes were designed and used to isolate full-length cDNA coding sequences by hybridization screening. A similar method has been used to clone the cDNA for several growth factor receptors. An alternative approach has been to express a pool of cDNAs in cells and identify clones by measuring the activity or immunoreactivity of the expressed factor or receptor ("expression cloning"). With these methods it has been possible to express many of these molecules in large quantities. The result has been an explosion of information about the biology of growth factors and a recognition of their potential roles in diseases and therapy. The following sections include discussions of the individual factors that regulate proliferation of mesenchymal, epithelial, endothelial, and neuronal cells (Table 9-2) followed by discussions of the hematopoietic growth factors and the lymphokines.

PLATELET-DERIVED GROWTH FACTOR Platelet-derived growth factor (PDGF) was discovered by the convergence of two lines of investigation. First, for over 50 years tissue culture workers recognized the importance of serum factors in stimulating the growth of animal cells. In retrospect, much of the growth-promoting effect of serum on fibroblasts could be attributed to the PDGF released from activated platelets. A second line of work involved factors that stimulate the proliferation of smooth-muscle cells in atherosclerotic plaques. This

TABLE 9-1 Some diseases that involve abnormal cell proliferation

Cancer	Polycystic kidney
Atherosclerosis	Scleroderma
Pulmonary fibrosis	Rheumatoid arthritis
Primary pulmonary hypertension	Ankylosing spondylitis
Neurofibromatosis	Myelodysplasia
Acoustic neuroma	Some anemias
Tuberous sclerosis	Cirrhosis
Psoriasis	Esophageal stricture
Keloid	Sclerosing cholangitis
Fibrocystic breast	Retroperitoneal fibrosis
Polycystic ovary	

TABLE 9-2 Growth factors for mesenchymal, epithelial, endothelial, and neuronal cells

Platelet-derived growth factor (PDGF AA, PDGF BB, PDGF AB)	Vascular smooth muscle, fibroblasts, glial cells, skeletal myoblasts
Epidermal growth factor family (EGF, TGF-α, vaccinia virus factor)	Epithelial cells, fibroblasts, glial cells
Transforming growth factor	Most cells
Nerve growth factor (NGF)	Sensory and sympathetic neuronal cells, some melanocytes, Schwann cells, capillary endothelial cells
Fibroblast growth factor family (basic FGF, acidic FGF, *int*-2 gene product, *Hst*/Kaposi FGF)	Endothelial cells, fibroblasts, FGF vascular smooth-muscle cells, skeletal myoblasts, neuronal cells
Keratinocyte fibroblast growth factor	Keratinocytes
Tumor necrosis factor (TNF-α, TNF-β)	Some fibroblasts, endothelial cells, T cells
Interleukin 1 (IL-1α, IL-1β)	Fibroblasts, smooth-muscle cells, T cells

work culminated in the purification of PDGF from serum and from human platelets, although other sources of this factor may be important in vivo. For example, endothelial cells are an abundant source of PDGF in blood vessels. The production and release of PDGF from these cells is closely regulated by molecules that accumulate at the site of tissue injury. PDGF is also produced by activated macrophages, mesangial cells, smooth-muscle–like cells in blood vessels, a number of embryonic cells, and several types of tumor cells.

It is likely that the main physiological roles of PDGF are in the earliest stages of embryonic development and in wound healing. In adult tissues, only a limited number of cells respond to PDGF; these include vascular smooth-muscle cells, glial cells, and fibroblasts. The ability of PDGF to stimulate the migration and proliferation of mesenchymal cells, as well as to enhance the production of extracellular matrix proteins, has suggested a role for PDGF in a number of fibroproliferative pathologic processes including atherosclerosis and restenosis following vascular angioplasty. The evidence includes the finding of a high level of expression of PDGF in atherosclerotic vessels and an unusually high number of PDGF receptors in proliferative atherosclerotic lesions biopsied during carotid endarterectomy. Further research should determine whether PDGF is involved in other nonmalignant fibroproliferative processes including glomerulonephritis, pulmonary fibrosis, myelofibrosis, keloid formation, and rheumatoid arthritis.

The possibility that PDGF plays a role in cancer was first recognized in studies of the simian sarcoma virus (SSV) that was isolated from a spontaneously occurring monkey fibrosarcoma. This virus reproducibly causes tumors when inoculated into monkeys and will also transform cells in vitro by the expression of the viral oncogene v-*sis*. Introduction and expression of the v-*sis* oncogene into appropriate fibroblast cell lines transforms the cells into tumor cells that will form solid tumors when implanted in nude mice. The discovery that the v-*sis* oncogene encodes a form of PDGF was revolutionary in the field of growth factors. The v-*sis*-encoded form of PDGF appears to activate PDGF receptors in intracellular compartments before the receptors have a chance to be fully processed and expressed at the cell surface. This autocrine activation of receptors is prevented in most normal cells by the mutually exclusive expression of either PDGF or PDGF receptors. But some human tumor cell lines express both PDGF and its receptor and therefore may utilize similar autocrine pathways. It is possible that the autocrine activation of PDGF receptors is one of several steps required to transform cells in vivo and may be a critical event in initiation of some tumors.

Future studies of the role of PDGF in disease will be based on a better understanding of the structure of the factor and its receptor. PDGF was initially purified from human platelets as a 32-kDa molecule consisting of two polypeptide chains, termed A and B, that form an AB heterodimer. Several other tissues including endothelial cells and glial progenitor cells produce homodimeric AA or BB forms of PDGF. The biological differences between these forms are not yet clearly understood. There are at least two types of structurally related receptors for PDGF, each with a distinctive specificity pattern for binding the multiple forms of the factor. Current attempts to develop antagonists of PDGF for use in treating fibroproliferative diseases are based on molecular analysis of the structural domains that mediate the binding of PDGF to its receptors and on specific cellular reactions that are stimulated by the receptor.

EPIDERMAL GROWTH FACTOR Epidermal growth factor (EGF) was discovered by the remarkable observation that injection of extracts of mouse salivary gland into newborn mice caused precocious opening of eyelids and eruption of incisors. Using these responses as an assay, Stanley Cohen purified and characterized the polypeptide. Eyelid opening could be ascribed to epidermal growth and keratinization stimulated by EGF. Later it was shown that EGF stimulated the proliferation of epithelial cells and fibroblasts in vitro.

The biological effects of EGF are mediated by a single type of membrane receptor that is found predominantly on epithelial cells and fibroblasts. This receptor also binds and responds to at least two additional EGF-like growth factors. These include transforming growth factor alpha (TGF-α), a polypeptide first isolated from media conditioned by tumor cells, and the vaccinia virus growth factor that is encoded by a vaccinia virus gene. These three ligands are only approximately 20 percent identical in amino acid sequence. They appear to act as mitogens in vitro and differ only subtly in their ability to bind to the EGF receptor.

A major surprise in the growth factor field was the discovery that the cytoplasmic domain sequence of the EGF receptor is closely related to the sequence of a transforming gene (oncogene) of the avian erythroblastosis virus, v-*erb*B gene. The precise molecular mechanism by which the differences convert the normal EGF receptor into a transforming protein is not known. Acknowledging the relationship of the EGF receptor to the v-*erb*B oncogene, the normal cellular gene of the EGF receptor has been designated c-*erb*B. Another virus, the avian leukosis virus, utilizes the EGF receptor to transform cells by a different mechanism, in which expression of the EGF receptor is increased by insertion of viral sequences into the flanking regions of the receptor gene. The altered expression of this gene causes erythroblastosis.

A close relative of the EGF receptor gene is the *neu* proto-oncogene, which also has been designated HER-2/*neu*. The HER-2/*neu* gene is 50 percent identical to the EGF receptor gene in its coding sequence and is located on human chromosome 17. The structure of protein encoded by HER-2/*neu* predicts that it is a growth factor receptor, although its ligand has yet to be identified. One of the most provocative findings from studies of this gene is that the critical difference between the *neu* oncogene and the normal HER-2/*neu* gene is a single amino acid replacement in the transmembrane domain. This finding supports the hypothesis that *well-defined mutations in normal growth regulatory molecules may be involved in carcinogenesis* (see Chap. 10).

Other studies have suggested that there is an increased expression of the EGF receptor or the HER-2/*neu* gene in human cancer. For example, the HER-2/*neu* proto-oncogene is amplified in 25 to 30 percent of human primary breast cancers, and this alteration is predictive of disease outcome. A similar association has been reported in ovarian cancer. The concept that alterations in HER-2/*neu* gene expression are important in tumorigenesis has been strengthened by the observations that (1) overexpression of the normal HER-2/*neu* proto-oncogene can induce transformation in mouse cells in vitro and (2) that the mutated rat *neu* gene expressed in transgenic mice causes development of breast adenocarcinomas. Such studies may lead to improved diagnosis and therapeutic strategies for breast and ovarian cancer as well as for other tumors of epithelial cell origin.

TRANSFORMING GROWTH FACTORS A number of growth factors have been isolated from media conditioned by tumor cells. Two of these were purified on the basis of their synergistic actions in stimulating the growth of fibroblasts in soft agar, an assay often used as an index of cell "transformation." Since cancer cells grow in soft agar, the growth factors were first thought to be mitogens involved in tumorigenesis and were called *tumor growth factors*. However their main role appears to be in embryonic development and in tissue repair.

Transforming growth factor alpha (TGF-α) is a mitogen for epithelial cells and appears to mimic EGF in its ability to bind and activate EGF receptors. The major difference between TGF-α and EGF appears to be in their respective patterns of expression, especially during embryogenesis. Both of these factors have the unusual property of being synthesized as precursor proteins that have transmembrane sequences and are probably localized to the cell surface. The precursor may activate EGF receptors on adjacent cells through direct cell-cell interactions that do not involve soluble factors. This type of interaction may be especially important in organogenesis.

Transforming growth factor-beta (TGF-β) has been historically linked to TGF-α, but the functional differences between them are more apparent than their similarities. The biological activities of the TGF-β family span a confusing spectrum of celllular responses including proliferation of some cells (especially connective tissue cells), inhibition of proliferation of other cells (e.g., lymphocytes or epithelial cells), enhanced collagen and extracellular matrix production, and expression of cell adhesion molecules. Given this set of in vitro reactions, it is not surprising that when experimental animals are injected with TGF-β an exuberant granulation and fibrotic response can be seen at the site of injection within an hour. TGF-β factor may play a role in the fibrosis seen in pulmonary fibrosis, keloid formation, cirrhosis, scleroderma, rheumatoid arthritis, or proliferative vitreoretinopathy. An even more compelling case has been made for the role of TGF-β in embryonic formation of bone and cartilage. It may be possible to use TGF-β to stimulate formation of bone matrix and perhaps accelerate fracture healing. The recent finding of large amounts of TGF-β in cardiac myocytes and its increased expression during experimental myocardial infarction has suggested a role for this factor in repair of myocardial injury. There has also been considerable attention focused on the growth inhibitory effect of TGF-β. It is possible that a loss of this negative control of cell proliferation contributes to tumorigenesis.

FIBROBLAST GROWTH FACTORS The fibroblast growth factors (FGFs) constitute a group of structurally homologous polypeptides that stimulate the proliferation of endothelial cells, fibroblasts, vascular smooth muscle cells, skeletal muscle myoblasts, and some forms of epithelial cells. They are also trophic factors for neurons. The FGFs have the unusual ability to elicit the formation of new blood vessels, a process termed angiogenesis, by stimulating endothelial cells to migrate through the vessel wall and to proliferate as capillary sprouts. While angiogenesis may be beneficial in some contexts, such as in embryonic development or in ischemic myocardium, it may have deleterious effects in a number of pathologic conditions such as diabetic retinopathy or the formation of new blood vessels required for tumors to grow beyond a certain size (tumor angiogenesis). In a sense, FGF-induced angiogenesis recapitulates the normal embryonic development of new blood vessels. In fact, FGFs are expressed at the earliest stages of vertebrate embryogenesis, suggesting that these factors have other roles in development.

The FGF family includes at least seven distinct but structurally related molecules, each encoded by a different gene. The first two FGFs (acidic and basic) were purified from tissues known to release mitogenic and angiogenic factors. Several additional FGFs (e.g., FGF-5, Kaposi sarcoma FGF, and the *int*-2 gene product) were identified by their ability to transform cells that coexpress FGF receptors. It has been shown that there are not only multiple FGFs, but also multiple forms of the FGF receptor, each with a distinctive ligand-binding domain. The therapeutic challenge is to learn how to specifically block the deleterious effects of FGFs, such as in tumor angiogenesis, or to enhance the beneficial effects, for example, in nerve regeneration or angiogenesis in ischemic tissue.

GROWTH HORMONE AND INSULIN-LIKE GROWTH FACTOR 1 Growth hormone (see Chaps. 313 and 314) produced by the pituitary gland was one of the first known growth regulatory molecules. Its important role in bone elongation in vivo was recognized by its ability to restore normal growth rates in children and in experimental animals with growth hormone deficiency. Many of the effects of growth hormone can be attributed to the stimulation of systemic release of insulin-like growth factor 1 (IGF-1) from liver. IGF-1 acts as a direct mitogen on cells containing the IGF-1 receptor, a member of the tyrosine kinase family of signal transducing molecules. Whether growth hormone has direct effects other than those mediated by the action of IGF-1 has been the subject of intense investigation. The growth hormone receptor is a molecule that is found either as a membrane receptor that lacks tyrosine kinase sequences or in a truncated soluble form without a transmembrane region that functions as a circulating growth hormone binding protein.

Interestingly there are several abnormal patterns of growth in humans that involve the growth hormone or IGF-1 systems. In Laron dwarfism there is a total absence of high-affinity growth hormone binding proteins (presumably the truncated soluble form of the receptor) in plasma and a virtual absence of hepatic growth hormone receptors. African pygmies appear to have a less severe defect in growth hormone binding protein levels. A rare syndrome of IGF-1 resistance and dwarfism involves a like reduction of IGF-1 receptors.

NERVE GROWTH FACTOR In 1952, Rita Levi-Montalcini showed that transplants of mouse sarcoma tissue onto the chorioallantoic membrane of embryos resulted in a marked increase in the size and number of chicken sensory and sympathetic neurons. This finding could be attributed to enhanced survival of neurons which would normally degenerate during ontogenesis. The factor responsible for this process was purified and designated *nerve growth factor* (NGF) but was considered to be primarily a "survival" or "maintenance" factor rather than a mitogenic compound. Subsequently, many experiments have documented a role for NGF in neuron survival and in the targeting of sensory neurons to specific tissues. It has recently been shown that NGF has effects in the central nervous system as well as in other tissues and may be involved in a number of nonneuronal processes. Thus, NGF receptors are found on capillary endothelium cells, myoepithelium cells, perivascular cells, and mast cells.

Nerve growth factor has been isolated as a complex of noncovalently associated alpha, beta, and gamma subunits. The beta subunit is responsible for the biologic responses of NGF and binds as a dimer to the NGF receptor. Although the primary amino acid sequence of the receptor is known, little is understood about its mechanism of action since, unlike the receptors for PDGF, EGF, insulin, and IGF-1, the NGF receptor is not a tyrosine kinase. The major clinical interest in NGF has centered on the proposal that it might be useful therapeutically in promoting nerve regeneration. It is also possible that a deficiency of NGF or related factors may play a role in degenerative diseases.

GROWTH FACTORS FOR BLOOD CELLS The control of proliferation and differentiation of blood cells are vital processes for the maintenance of adequate levels of circulating cells and for the responses of the immune system to foreign substances. This control is achieved in large part by paracrine mechanisms in which one type of cell, sensing environmental cues, releases factors that act, often at short distances, to regulate proliferation or differentiation of a second type of cell. The complex system of cell-cell interactions is maintained by the highly specific control of expression not only of the growth factors but also of their receptors in the responding cells. This is the basis of a complex network of interactions among numerous cell types in tissues such as bone marrow and lymph nodes or at sites of inflammation. While the molecular and cellular analysis of these processes has led to understanding of the general principles by which the growth and differentiation of hematopoietic cells are regulated, the terminology used in this field is confusing. Classification of these factors into hematopoietic factors and lymphokines is helpful in understanding their biological roles (see Chaps. 13 and 285).

Hematopoietic factors The first insight into the role of hematopoietic growth factors came from attempts to grow myeloid cells in culture. The culture of these cells could only be achieved in the presence of "feeder" cells that produced factors required for the growth of bone marrow-derived progenitors of each type of myeloid cell. The term *colony stimulating factor* was used to refer to the peptides that stimulated growth and maturation of granulocyte or monocyte lineages in soft agar. These assays permitted purification and characterization of the factors. Some factors, e.g., macrophage colony stimulating factor (CSF-1) appeared to be specific for one lineage whereas others, e.g., granulocyte-macrophage colony stimulating factor (GM-CSF), appeared to act on more than one lineage (Table 9-3). However, it has become apparent that initial classification of these factors by responsive cell type may be an oversimplification. For example G-CSF, which was originally thought to act exclusively on granulocytic lineages, appears to act on multiple lineages at several different stages of differentiation.

The study of myeloid cell growth factors has suggested novel approaches for the treatment of a number of diseases. The most obvious of these is the exogenous administration of growth factors to patients with cytopenia. G-CSF and GM-CSF are capable of raising blood granulocyte levels in patients with mild bone marrow suppression caused by cytotoxic drugs or who have disorders such as chronic neutropenia, myelodysplasia, aplastic anemia, AIDS, hairy cell leukemia, or cyclic hematopoiesis. The efficacy of G-CSF and GM-CSF in these syndromes does not necessarily imply that the diseases are caused by factor deficiency, but may reflect a clinically beneficial, stimulation of stem cell proliferation and differentiation in response to the exogenous factors. It is noteworthy that GM-CSF not only leads to an elevation of circulating neutrophils, eosinophils, and monocytes but also causes an increase in lymphocytes, platelets and reticulocytes, indicating the complexity of the effects of GM-CSF.

A more controversial potential use of hemopoietic growth factors is in the treatment of myeloid leukemias. This application is based on the observation that, in addition to their proliferative effects, these factors have the ability to induce differentiation of some populations of myeloid precursors. GM-CSF and G-CSF are known to induce differentiation of leukemic cells in vitro. However the obvious concern that such treatment might accelerate the progress of the disease in patients with leukemia has led to reluctance to use these factors in this setting even for treatment of cytopenias.

Erythropoietin, a factor that was studied for over 50 years before it was fully characterized, is produced primarily by the kidney but also by the liver and bone marrow macrophages. It differs from many of the hematopoietic factors and lymphokines in that it acts in vivo more as a hormone (i.e., at "long" distances) than as a local "paracrine" growth factor. When administered to patients with end-stage renal failure, it can stimulate an increase in red cell mass with relatively mild side effects of transient dyspnea, arthralgia, myalgia, flushing sensation, bone pain, or an increase in diastolic blood pressure. Erythropoietin is likely to be useful in other conditions such as anemia of chronic disease and marrow suppression induced by chemotherapy.

TABLE 9-3 Hematopoietic growth factors

Factor	Other nomenclature	Responsive lineage
CSF-1	MCSF, MAI-1m	Macrophage
G-CSF	MGI-1G, pluripoietin, differentiation factor	Granulocyte
GM-CSF	MGI-1GM, CSF-α, CSF-2, pluripoietin-α	Macrophage and granulocyte
IL-3	Multi-CSF-α, stem cell activating factor, hematopoietic growth factor, hematopoietin 2, burst promoting activity, mast cell growth factor	Macrophage, granulocyte, eosinophil, megakaryocyte, mast cell
Erythropoietin		Erythroid cells
Thrombopoeitin		Megakaryocyte

NOTE: CSF, colony stimulating factor; MGI, macrophage growth inducer; IL, interleukin.

One of the most specific of the hemopoietic factors is the macrophage colony stimulating factor (CSF-1). This factor acts on specific monocyte receptors that are closely related structurally and, to some extent, mechanistically to the receptors for PDGF. The CSF-1 receptor appears to play a role in monocytes analogous to the role of PDGF receptors in vascular smooth muscle cells. The CSF-1 receptor also has an oncogenic form, the v-*fms* gene product, which has been found in some feline tumors. Thus the CSF-1 receptor is also known as the "c-*fms* proto-oncogene."

Lymphokines (cytokines) The search for factors that support the growth of normal lymphocytes in vitro led to the identification of a group of molecules, termed *lymphokines* or *interleukins*, that were initially believed to be specific extracellular signals between different populations of cells in the immune system (see Table 13-4). However it has become evident that neither the production nor the response to lymphokines is restricted to immunocompetent cells. Therefore the more general term *cytokine* has been used for the group of proteins. The growth and maturation of lymphocytes depends on a highly regulated pattern of expression of these factors and on their receptors in different cell populations. Activation of immune responses depends on an equally complex pattern of regulation (see Chap. 13).

Interleukin 1 (IL-1) is made by many cell types and has a diverse group of actions including a number of reactions involved in the acute phase response. It has mitogenic effects on both T-cells and vascular smooth muscle cells especially when it acts in conjunction with other growth factors. The tumor necrosis factors share many of the actions of IL-1. IL-2 plays an important role in T-cell proliferation and maturation and also enhances the cytolytic activity of a population of killer cells that may destroy tumor cells. Thus its potential use for tumor therapy is under investigation. IL-3 stimulates growth and differentiation of hematopoietic precursors of multiple cell lineages and is also a growth factor for mast cells. IL-3, IL-4, and IL-5 appear to play important roles in allergic and antiparasitic inflammatory responses.

The lymphokines are now more noted for the diversity of responses elicited by each factor than for their restricted specificity. There is much overlap in their actions, and many of them act indirectly by inducing the expression and release of other lymphokines. Most act locally as paracrine factors but some of them act as autocrine factors. For this reason the potential use of lymphokines as therapeutic agents may be complicated by numerous side effects. However understanding these important factors should provide insight into a number of diseases of the immune system.

MECHANISM OF GROWTH FACTOR ACTION The mechanism by which growth factors stimulate cells to leave a stage of quiescence, designated "G_0" in cell cycle terminology, and enter the G_1 phase that culminates in DNA synthesis (S phase) involves interactions among several cytoplasmic molecules. Although there are differences among growth factor receptors in their mechanisms of action, there are some common features. First, transcription of a group of specialized growth regulatory genes appears to be required (Fig. 9-1). Second, most growth factor receptors activate cellular kinases and the hydrolysis of phosphatidylinositol. The receptors for many growth factors, including PDGF, EGF, FGF, and IGF-1, are tyrosine kinases. The mechanism of action of this family of receptors is understood best. Upon binding ligand, the receptor phosphorylates several specific substrates on tyrosine residues. These substrates include serine/threonine kinases, phospholipase C, and phosphatidylinositol kinase. The serine/threonine kinases are thought to increase transcription of growth regulatory genes perhaps by regulating the phosphorylation state of cytoplasmic transcription factors. The enzymes phospholipase C and phosphatidylinositol kinase act on membrane phosphatidylinositol to generate diacylglycerol, which activates protein kinase C, a known regulator of gene transcription. In addition, cytoplasmic inositol phosphate second messengers are released, but their precise role in growth regulation has not been defined.

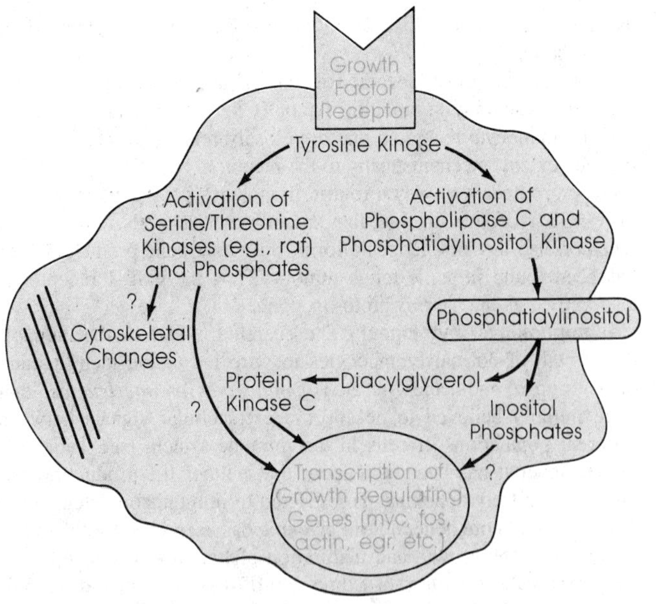

FIGURE 9-1 Scheme depicting the action of a tyrosine kinase growth factor receptor.

Membrane receptors other than the tyrosine kinase family of growth factor receptors may impact on some but not all of these pathways. For example, an alpha$_1$-adrenergic receptor, serotonin receptor, or angiotensin receptor, that can activate phospholipase C through guanylyl nucleotide binding proteins (see Chap. 11) may stimulate the diacylglycerol-mediated events but fail to initiate some of the other reactions that depend on tyrosine kinase. Thus under some circumstances, catecholamines, serotonin, or angiotensin might function as growth factors.

Several of the tyrosine kinase growth factor receptors as well as other cellular tyrosine kinases can be expressed as oncogenic (cancer-causing) proteins. The oncogenic forms of the nonreceptor kinases (*src, yes, fes, fps,* etc.) and of tyrosine kinase receptors (v-*erb*B, v-*fms*, and v-*kit*) stimulate growth regulatory pathways in an unregulated manner (see Chap. 10). Other oncogenes encode activated forms of the *raf* serine/threonine kinase, the *myc* and *fos* proteins, and other cellular proteins that regulate the pathways shown in Fig. 9-1. The net result of expression of an oncogene protein is that a normal growth regulatory pathway is usurped by a constitutively high activity that is independent of the presence of a growth factor.

The mechanism by which a growth factor binds to its receptor and activates the receptor is pivotal to the actions of all growth factors. The structures of the ligand binding domains of the factors and receptors are currently being studied and should yield information that would permit the design of novel growth factor agonists and antagonists. The effects of ligand binding on the receptor molecule vary among receptors. In some cases the ligand may induce receptor dimerization and formation of a cytoplasmic dimeric domain that has enhanced activity. In the case of tyrosine kinases, intermolecular receptor "autophosphorylation" may occur when the receptor dimerizes. Alternatively the ligand may cause the receptor to interact directly with other cellular molecules, perhaps through a conformational change induced in a cytoplasmic transmembrane domain. An understanding of these processes should lead to new approaches by which growth factor-stimulated events can be mimicked or antagonized.

REFERENCES

CARPENTER G: Receptors for epidermal growth factor and other polypeptide mitogens. Ann Rev Biochem 56:881, 1987

PAUL WE: Pleiotropy and redundancy: T cell-derived lymphokines in the immune response. Cell 57:521, 1989

SLAMON DJ et al: Studies of the HER-2/neu proto-oncogene in human breast and ovarian cancer. Science:244:707, 1989

STEWARD WP, SCARFIE JH: Clinical trials with hemopoietic growth factors. Progr Growth Factor Research 1:1, 1989

WILLIAMS LT: Signal transduction by the platelet-derived growth factor receptor. Science 243:1564, 1989

10 ONCOGENES AND NEOPLASTIC DISEASE

PAUL NEIMAN

Upon dividing, cancer cells transmit the neoplastic phenotype to daughter cells. For that reason, it has been generally assumed that the inheritance of the neoplastic phenotype is determined by specific genes. This assumption explains the great appeal of oncogenic viruses for cancer researchers. In spite of their relative genetic simplicity, these agents are capable of inducing all of the pathologic and clinical changes associated with neoplastic disease. In some cases a virus introduces into a normal cell a single gene (oncogene) whose product can initiate and maintain the neoplastic state. In the case of retroviruses, these viral oncogenes represent altered forms of cellular proto-oncogenes, which have important cellular functions in the normal state. Human homologues of some of these oncogenes appear to play a role in human cancer. This situation prompts a number of questions about the nature of oncogenes, the control of their expression, the biochemical nature of their gene products, and the mechanism of interaction with the metabolism of the host cell.

RETROVIRAL ONCOGENES Interaction of retroviruses with host cells The discovery of oncogenes was a result of study of the molecular biology of oncogenic retroviruses. Retroviruses are widespread in nature, and infection with some of them induces neoplastic disease in animals. The retroviral genome is an RNA molecule of between 8000 and 10,000 nucleotides. The distinctive feature in the life cycle of these agents is that after receptor-mediated entry of the virus into the cell the genomic RNA molecule is copied into DNA (reverse transcription) and integrated into the chromosomal DNA of the host cell (hence the name *retroviruses*) (Fig. 10-1). This integrated DNA is termed a *provirus*. The structure of typical proviruses is shown schematically in Fig. 10-2. Long terminal repeats (LTRs) containing sequences copied from both ends of viral genomic RNA are located at each end of the DNA provirus and linked directly to host DNA. These LTRs contain regulatory sequences for the expression of the genes required for viral replication: *gag*, coding for the internal structural protein; *pol*, coding for reverse transcriptase; and *env*, coding for the viral envelope glycoprotein. The regulatory sequences include signals for the initiation and termination of transcription. They usually also include powerful enhancer sequences that amplify the rate of transcription of viral genes so that proviral RNA transcripts may comprise as much as 0.1 to 1 percent of total cellular messenger RNA. The transcriptional promoter-enhancer sequences of some retroviruses function only when introduced into particular cell types, accounting for tissue-specific expression of viral genes. In other cases the activity of these enhancer sequences is regulated by steroid hormones. In contrast to many other viruses, retroviruses usually do not kill the host cell when the replicative process is completed; instead their life cycle results in the introduction and expression of exogenous genes and thus in alteration of the phenotype of the host cells.

Acute transforming retroviruses and their oncogenes Infection of animals with retroviruses encoding only the *gag, pol,* and *env* genes results in neoplastic disease after a long latent period. In contrast, acute transforming retroviruses can induce neoplastic disease in vivo in days to weeks and can transform cultured cells in vitro. The prototype of this class of viruses is the Rous sarcoma virus.

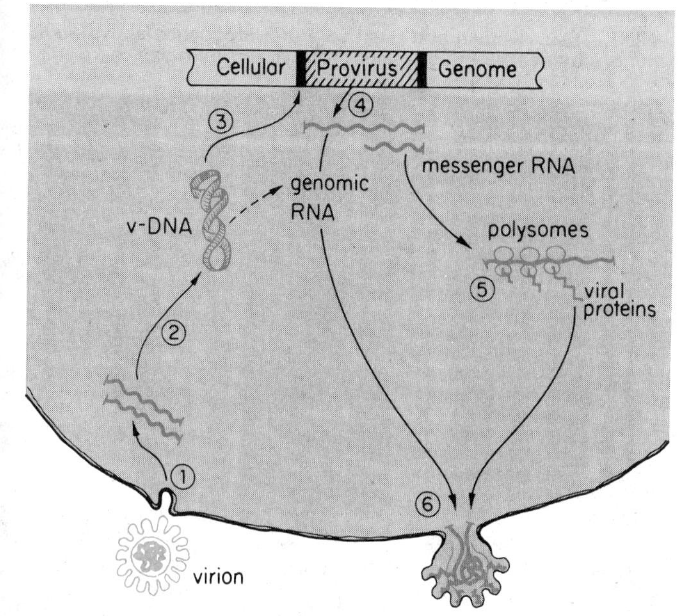

FIGURE 10-1 Replication of retroviruses. (1) Envelope glycoprotein on the surface of viral particles (virions) recognizes receptors that mediate entry into the cell and release of viral genomic RNA. (2) There are two viral RNA molecules per virion which are copied by reverse transcriptase into viral DNA molecules. (3) Some of the viral DNA molecules integrate into host chromosomal DNA at a precise point on the viral DNA molecule and a random, or near random, site on host chromosomes. (4) The integrated viral DNA copy, or provirus, is transcribed into both messenger RNA, which is translated into viral proteins on cellular polysomes (5), and full-length genomic viral RNA, which contains specific sequences serving as packaging signals for virus assembly. (6) Viral RNA and proteins are assembled into particles which bud from the cell surface. The whole process can occur without cytopathic effect on host cells.

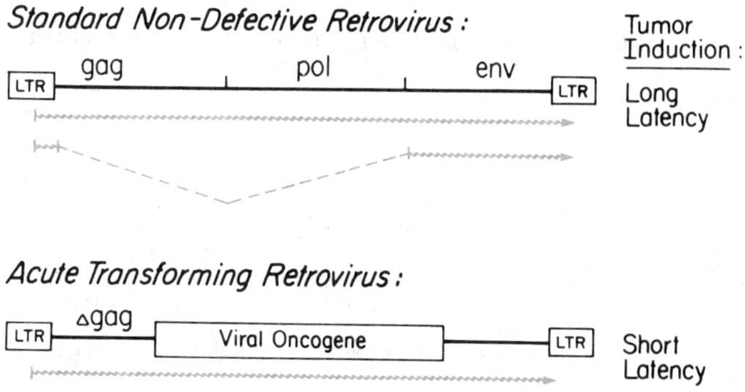

FIGURE 10-2 Comparative structure of the proviruses of standard nondefective replication retroviruses and acute transforming retroviruses. In both cases the provirus is bounded by direct long terminal repeat sequences (LTRs), which contain essential regulatory elements including transcriptional promoters and enhancers, signals for the termination of viral RNA transcripts (poly A addition signals), and signals for integration into the host DNA. Between tne LTRs of standard retroviruses are three genes: *gag* (internal structural proteins), *pol* (reverse transcriptase), and *env* (envelope glycoprotein), which are required for infection and replication. In the acute transforming viruses, all or part of the replicative genes have been replaced by a transforming oncogene, which mediates the oncogenic properties of the virus. The most common structure is a fusion of the 5′ portion of the *gag* gene with the oncogene. The standard provirus is transcribed into full-length genomic viral RNA and spliced messenger RNAs for viral proteins. The acute transforming provirus often expresses only one size RNA transcript and requires coinfection with a standard retroviral "helper" in order to replicate. The Δ*gag* symbol indicates that part of the *gag* sequence is missing because it has been deleted.

The structure of proviruses from these two classes of oncogenic agents is illustrated in Fig. 10-2. Most known acute transforming retroviruses are defective; that is, they have lost part of the genes required for replication and hence require coinfection with a standard helper retrovirus for propagation. Such defects result from the replacement of replicative genes of the virus by an oncogene that mediates the direct transforming properties of the virus. Although there is variability as to which segment of the viral genome is replaced by the oncogene, a common configuration for acute transforming retroviruses is as depicted in Fig. 10-2. In this case, the oncogene is fused to a 5′ portion of the viral *gag* gene, resulting in the synthesis of a transforming protein that contains *gag* peptides at its amino terminus.

Table 10-1 lists some viral oncogenes (designated by their acronyms), the natural host species, and the types of tumors they induce. In the case of the Rous sarcoma virus, the role of the *src* gene in neoplastic transformation was established by genetic and biochemical means. Mutations that cause reversible inactivation of the *src* gene product at elevated temperature (temperature-sensitive mutations) bring about a reversal of the transformed phenotype to the normal state when infected cells are exposed to elevated temperatures. When the temperature is lowered, the cells again revert to the transformed state. Likewise, deletions of the *src* gene destroy the ability of this virus to induce acute neoplasms. Similar but less complete data exist for other viruses listed in Table 10-1. A small number of acute transforming viruses contain a second oncogene which enhances the transforming activity of the principal viral oncogene. Two important examples are *erb*A, which cooperates with *erb*B in avian erythroblastosis virus, and *ets,* which accompanies *myb* in the E-26 strain of avian myeloblastosis virus.

Almost all the acute transforming viruses can be detected in vitro by their ability to induce transformation of cultured cells. The standard assay is the formation by infected fibroblasts (or fibroblast-like cell lines) of morphologically altered cells. Some of the leukemia-inducing viruses can transform macrophages and/or hematopoietic cells in vitro.

PROTO-ONCOGENES The oncogenes of retroviruses are closely related to normal cellular genes. This relationship was deduced from the discovery of nucleotide sequence homology between the transforming oncogene of Rous sarcoma virus, v-*src* (viral-*src*), and a normal chicken gene, c-*src* (cellular *src*). Apparently, Rous sarcoma virus originated from a recombination event between c-*src* and an ancestral standard avian retrovirus. This mechanism, recombination between a viral gene and a gene of host origin, is the apparent explanation for the formation of the transforming viruses listed in Table 10-1. The function of the normal genes and their role in nonviral tumor formation is, therefore, a subject of intense interest and investigation.

The normal forms of the oncogenes are highly conserved in nature. There are human homologues of each, and homologues of some are present in all eukaryotic organisms, including invertebrate species and yeasts. This conservation implies that these genes have vital functions in normal cells and suggests that the oncogenic potential of the genes is acquired only after functionally significant alteration (such as occurs from recombination with a retrovirus). Such genes are referred to as *proto-oncogenes.*

The nucleotide sequences of the protein coding regions of viral oncogenes differ from those of the proto-oncogenes. There are also major differences in the regulation of expression of the viral and cellular genes. For example, the normal cellular form of an oncogene can be expressed without transforming the cell, although usually at a lower level and/or in a more strictly regulated fashion than are viral oncogenes expressed from proviruses. The contributions of overexpression, altered regulation, and structural mutation to the transforming activity of viral oncogenes may all be important to degrees that vary with the individual oncogene and target cell type.

Infection with retroviruses that lack oncogenes can induce neoplastic disease in some animals after a long latent period. A common

TABLE 10-1 Viral oncogenes that cause acute transformation

Name	Virus	Tumors in vivo
AVIAN		
src	Rous sarcoma virus (RSV)	Sarcomas
yes	Y73 sarcoma virus	Sarcomas
fps/fes	Fujinami sarcoma virus	Sarcomas
ros	UR11 avian sarcoma virus	Sarcomas
*erb*B, *erb*A	Avian erythroblastosis virus (AEV)	Erythroid leukemia
myb	Avian myeloblastosis virus (AMV)	Myeloid leukemia
myc	Avian myelocytomatosis virus (MC-29)	Leukemia, endothelioma
ski	Avian SKV770 virus	Unknown
jun	Avian sarcoma virus 17	Sarcomas
crk	Avian sarcoma virus CT10	Sarcomas
sea	Avian sarcoma virus S-13	Erythroid leukemia
rel	Reticuloendotheliosis virus (REV)	Lymphomas
MOUSE		
abl	Abelson leukemia virus	B lymphomas
mos	Moloney murine sarcoma virus (MoMSV)	Sarcomas
fos	FBJ osteosarcoma virus	Osteosarcoma
raf	3611 murine sarcoma virus	Sarcomas
RAT		
Ha-*ras*[1]	Harvey murine sarcoma virus (HaMSV)	Sarcomas, erythroid leukemia
Ki-*ras*[2]	Kirsten murine sarcoma virus (KiMSV)	Sarcomas, erythroid leukemia
CAT		
fes/fps	Snyder Thielen feline sarcoma virus (ST-FeSV)	Sarcomas
fms	McDonough feline sarcoma virus (SM-FeSV)	Sarcomas
fgr	Gardner-Rasheed feline sarcoma virus (GR-FeSV)	Sarcomas
kit	HZ4 feline sarcoma virus (HZ4-FeSV)	Sarcomas
MONKEY		
sis	Simian sarcoma virus (SSV)	Sarcomas

TABLE 10-2 Known and putative proto-oncogenes activated in tumors by nearby integration of retroviral proviruses

Target gene or locus	Virus	Tumor
c-*myc*	Avian leukosis virus	B-cell lymphomas (chicken)
c-*myc*	Feline leukemia virus	Lymphomas (cat)
c-*myb*	Murine leukemia virus	Myeloid leukemia (mouse)
c-*myb*	Avian leukemia	B-cell lymphoma (chicken)
c-*erb*B	Avian leukosis virus	Erythroid leukemia (chicken)
Pim-1, *Mis*-1, c-*myc*	AKR-murine leukemia virus	T-cell lymphoma (mouse)
Mlvi-1, *Mlvi*-2, *Mlvi*-3	Moloney murine leukemia virus	T-cell lymphoma (rat)
Int-1, *Int*-2, *Int*-3	Mouse mammary tumor virus	Mammary adenocarcinoma (mouse)
Evi-1, *fim*-3	Friend murine leukemia virus	Myeloid leukemia (mouse)

mechanism for the oncogenic activity is the activation of cellular proto-oncogenes, as illustrated by the induction of lymphomas in the bursa of Fabricius of chickens by avian leukosis virus (ALV). In these neoplasms, a proto-oncogene called c-*myc* is expressed at high levels as a result of the integration of the promoter-enhancer of the ALV genome near c-*myc*. Table 10-2 lists cellular proto-oncogenes that are known to be activated in retrovirus-induced neoplasms of long latency. Some (*myc*, *myb*, and *erb*B) are homologues of known viral oncogenes. Others (*Int*-1, *Int*-2, *Int*-3, *Pim*-1, *Mis*-1, *Mlvi*-1, *Mlvi*-2, *Mlvi*-3, *fim*-3, and *Evi*-1) have not been identified as a part of the genomes of acute-transforming viruses. Their oncogenic potential, originally inferred by analogy, has been demonstrated recently in some cases by cloning and expression in experimental test systems.

HUMAN ONCOGENIC VIRUSES Human T-cell leukemia viruses (HTLV) are retroviruses that replicate preferentially in human lymphocytes. Infection with HTLV type I is associated with the development of a specific type of adult T-cell leukemia that occurs with increased frequency in southern Japan and the Caribbean basin. In vitro infection of human T cells by HTLV-I in culture confers a capacity for growth that is independent of exogenous T-cell growth factors (immortalization). The HTLVs do not appear to contain a host cell–related oncogene. Instead, unique transacting viral regulatory genes have been shown to have oncogenic potential in animals and may alter host cell behavior in humans. Infection with a different group of retroviruses, human immunodeficiency viruses (HIV), causes the acquired immunodeficiency syndrome. Normal human DNA contains sequences that appear to be proviruses and that are genetically transmitted in the germ line. Their pathologic significance is unknown.

A number of types of DNA viruses induce abnormal host cell growth through the action of viral genes that, in contrast to retroviral oncogenes, are not closely related to host cellular genes. Two important examples in humans are Epstein-Barr virus (EBV), which is implicated in both endemic African Burkitt's lymphoma and nasopharyngeal carcinoma, and certain strains of human papillomavirus (HPV) which appear to be etiologic factors in anogenital cancer. In addition, hepatitis B virus (HBV) infection is associated with hepatocellular carcinoma, and herpes simplex viruses (HSV) have been implicated by some investigators in cervical carcinoma. The mechanism of these possible oncogenic effects is at present not known.

ACTIVATION OF CELLULAR ONCOGENES IN HUMAN NEOPLASMS DETECTED BY TRANSFECTION **The transfection assay for oncogenes** Certain established cell lines have the property of incorporating exogenous DNA into chromosomal DNA with an efficiency that makes experimental gene transfer practical in tissue culture. The transfection technique commonly involves precipitating the DNA onto the surface of the target cells with calcium phosphate. The uptake of the DNA into cells by pinocytosis follows. Some of the ingested DNA molecules are transported to the cell nucleus where they are integrated into chromosomal DNA. If the transfected DNA contains a gene that can be expressed as a dominant, selectable marker in the recipient cells, transfected cells expressing this trait can be recovered. Many of the viral oncogenes in Table 10-1 can induce transformation in this type of assay. Such transformation can be achieved either with cloned oncogene DNA or with total chromosomal DNA from cells transformed by retroviruses.

Activated cellular oncogenes can also be detected by this technique in the DNA of tumors not known to be induced by viruses. For example, DNA from chemically transformed animal cells and DNA from a variety of naturally occurring animal and human tumor cells contain transforming genes. Normal high-molecular-weight human DNA does not transform cells, while DNA from neoplastic cells in some instances may induce transformation in tissue culture and/or by outgrowth of tumors in animals receiving transfected cells.

The *ras* family of cellular oncogenes Some of the transforming genes detected by transfection of cells with DNA from human tumor cells have been identified (Table 10-3). The most common oncogenes belong to a family of genes called *ras*. The first to be identified was the human homologue of the oncogene of Harvey murine sarcoma virus (Table 10-1) called c-*ras*^{H}, which codes for a protein of molecular weight 21,000 called p21 and is activated in a human cell line derived from bladder carcinoma. In cells transformed by Harvey sarcoma virus, p21 is expressed at high levels, and high-level expression of c-*ras*^{H} by experimental linkage of the cellular gene to viral regulatory elements is sufficient to induce cellular transformation. Nevertheless, c-*ras*^{H} is not expressed at high levels in those human tumor cell lines in which it is detectable. Instead, the ability of c-*ras* gene to transform cells is conferred by point mutations that cause amino acid changes either at amino acid positions 12, 13, or 61 of the p21 protein.

These activating mutations can be detected by techniques employing synthetic oligonucleotide probes which are convenient for screening large numbers of human tumor samples. By this approach it was found that a second member of the *ras* family is more frequently activated in human tumors, e.g., the human homologue of the transforming gene of the Kirsten murine sarcoma virus called c-*ras*^{K}. For example, about one-third of human colorectal cancers and most carcinomas of the exocrine pancreas contain mutations predominantly at codon 12. Activation of c-*ras*^{K} is also described in a variety of other human neoplasms. The protein encoded by c-*ras*^{K} is also a p21 molecule, and this activating mutation in p21 is not present in normal tissues of individuals with carcinomas containing an activated c-*ras*^{K} gene, suggesting that activation is a somatic event that occurs during tumor formation. Finally, in transfection experiments and mutational analysis of some tumors activation of a third member of this family, called *ras*^{N}, was detected. For example, mutation of *ras*^{N} occurs in 10 to 20 percent of human acute myeloid leukemias.

Fibroblast growth factor (FGF)–related oncogenes A second group of related oncogenes, called K-*fgf*, *hst*, and FGF-3, has recently been detected in some human tumor DNAs. These are highly conserved genes with extensive homology both to the known mitogens' acid and basic FGF and to the *Int*-2 proto-oncogene activated in mouse adenocarcinomas by mouse mammary tumor virus (Table 10-2). The transforming activity of these genes can be activated by overexpression. The clinical associations of abnormal expression of the FGF family are still being defined.

TABLE 10-3 Oncogenes implicated in human neoplasia

Oncogene	Tumor
By tumor DNA transfection assay:	
c-*ras*^{H}	Rare occurrence, bladder, lung, mammary carcinosarcoma
c-*ras*^{K}	About 10–20% of many types of neoplasms and most pancreatic carcinomas
c-*ras*^{N}	About 10–20% of acute myeloid leukemia, occasionally other tumors
hst-1, (K-*fgf*, FGF-3)	Stomach, colon, and liver carcinoma, Kaposi's sarcoma*
abl, *met*, *trk*, *mos*	Various individual observations†
By chromosomal translocation:	
c-*myc*	Burkitt's lymphoma (>90%), T-cell lymphoma (occasionally)
c-*abl*	Chronic myelogenous leukemia (>90%), acute lymphocytic leukemia (10–20%)
bcl-2	Follicular lymphoma (90%), diffuse lymphoma (20%)
By DNA amplification or other overexpression:	
c-*erb*B	Gliomas
*erb*B-2 (*neu*, HER-2)	Breast cancer†
hst-1, *bcl*-1, *Int*-2	Breast cancer†
N-*myc*, C-*ras*^{N}	Neuroblastoma†
N-*myc*, L-*myc*, c-*myc*	Small cell carcinoma of the lung†
By loss of heterozygosity (recessive oncogene):	
Rb-1	Retinoblastoma, breast cancer*

* Association with specific tumors and/or incidence yet to be established.
† Putative marker of poor prognosis and/or advanced disease.

ONCOGENES IMPLICATED IN HUMAN TUMOR FORMATION A major line of evidence for the activation of oncogenes during tumor formation is derived from the analysis of cytogenetic changes in human neoplasms. Most human tumors are clonal or oligoclonal, that is, composed of cell populations dominated by the progeny of single cells. The dominant cell clones of certain neoplasms are marked by consistent chromosomal abnormalities, such as reciprocal translocations between chromosomes 9 and 22 in chronic myelogenous leukemia (producing the Philadelphia chromosome, Ph^1) or between chromosomes 8 and 14 in Burkitt's lymphoma. Indeed, characteristic nonrandom chromosomal changes have been identified in many neoplasms. Genes at or near the site of the DNA rearrangements underlying these cytogenetic changes are thought to play a role in the development of the tumors. Advances in in situ hybridization and other techniques of somatic cell genetics along with molecular cloning have made it possible to locate the cytogenetic positions of a number of proto-oncogenes on human chromosomes and to demonstrate that some of these genes are located near or at the breakpoints of chromosomes that are translocated in particular tumors.

Rearrangement of the c-*myc* locus in Burkitt's lymphoma The human c-*myc* gene is located on chromosome 8. This chromosome is invariably involved in a translocation in Burkitt's lymphoma. At the DNA level the translocation involves recombination between the c-*myc* locus on chromosome 8 and an immunoglobulin gene locus, usually near a heavy chain gene on chromosome 14, less often near a light chain gene on chromosomes 2 or 22. The specific region of the breakpoint at c-*myc* on chromosome 8 differs between the sporadic, EBV-negative, American and European Burkitt's lymphoma and the endemic, EBV-positive, African form of the disease. In both types this translocation does not appear to affect the structure of the protein-coding portion of the c-*myc* locus but instead affects the regulation of its expression.

Alteration of c-*abl* by chromosomal translocation in chronic myelogenous leukemia and acute lymphoblastic leukemia The Ph^1 chromosome is present both in leukemic cells and in normal marrow cell lineages from 90 to 95 percent of patients with chronic myelogenous leukemia (CML). In this disease, the marrow and peripheral blood are thought to be populated by the progeny of a hematopoietic stem cell that retains its ability to differentiate into red cells, megakaryocytes, and granulocytes. The proliferation of granulocytes, however, is abnormal and excessive, producing the clinical manifestations of CML. Genes whose expression is altered as a consequence of the formation of the Ph^1 chromosome are strong candidates for involvement in the development of CML. The human homologue of the proto-oncogene c-*abl* (Table 10-1) is located near the breakpoint on chromosome 9 for the 9-22 translocation and is transferred to chromosome 22 in the exchange. The additional Ph^1 chromosomes that sometimes appear in blastic crisis of CML result from duplication of the original Ph^1 chromosome. Amplification of the translocation region can also occur within the Ph^1 chromosome. The protein gene product of the c-*abl* locus in CML cells is a distinct fusion product of the c-*abl* gene and a gene called *bcr* (breakpoint cluster region) at the breakpoint on chromosome 22 of the recombinant Ph^1 chromosome. This hybrid *bcr*/*abl* gene product is a tyrosine protein kinase of 210,000 mol wt.

The Ph^1 chromosome also appears in 5 to 20 percent of acute lymphoblastic leukemias. The 9-22 recombination event in about half of these cases is located differently than is seen in CML, and produces a distinct *bcr*/*abl* fusion gene associated with a high level of expression of an *abl*-derived tyrosine protein kinase of 185,000 mol wt.

Translocations in non-Hodgkin's lymphoma The most consistent cytogenetic abnormality in this group of lymphoproliferative diseases is a 14-18 translocation which joins the immunoglobulin heavy chain locus on chromosome 14 to a gene of unknown function called *bcl*-2 on chromosome 18. This event occurs in nearly 90 percent of low-grade follicular lymphomas in the United States and a smaller fraction, about 20 percent, of diffuse large cell lymphomas. Other translocations, including an 11-14 translocation at a locus called *bcl*-1 in B-cell neoplasms and 8-14 translocation in T-cell lymphomas, have been described. The latter event joins the c-*myc* locus on chromosome 8 to a T-cell receptor gene on chromosome 14.

Overexpression of proto-oncogenes in human tumors An increase in gene copy number per cell (gene amplification) can sometimes be manifested at the cytogenetic level by the formation of small chromosome-like structures called *double minute chromosomes* or by the appearance of homogeneous staining regions (HSRs) on regular chromosomes. HSRs are the result of amplification of segments of DNA within the chromosome to the extent that they are identifiable cytogenetically. As a consequence, the structure contains multiple copies of the gene(s) encoded by the DNA segment. Gene amplification in nontransformed cells can sometimes be induced by growing cells under special conditions. For example, cells containing an amplification of the dihydrofolate reductase gene, which is required for DNA replication, can be selected when cells are grown in the presence of low levels of methotrexate, an inhibitor of dihydrofolate reductase. This increase in gene copy number enhances the amount of enzyme in the cell and overcomes the effects of the inhibitor. Double minute chromosomes and HSRs are present in a variety of tumor cells, suggesting that genes critical to the growth of neoplastic cells may amplify during tumor formation.

The first amplified oncogene recognized in a human tumor cell was the c-*myc* gene, which was expressed at a high level in one case of promyelocytic leukemia, both in fresh tumor cells and in a derived cell line. Amplification of c-*myc* appears to be a rare event in this neoplasm and has not been observed in other promyelocytic leukemias. However, double minute chromosomes, amplification of c-*myc* genes, and elevated levels of c-*myc* RNA have been reported in some gastric cancers and small cell carcinomas of the lung. Human neuroblastomas are characterized by a high frequency of double minute chromosomes and HSRs. A gene called N-*myc* which is related to the c-*myc* gene is amplified and/or expressed at a high level in most neuroblastomas. This overexpression correlates with more advanced stages of the disease. Similarly amplification of N-*myc* and a third family member, L-*myc*, in small cell carcinoma of the lung correlates strongly with disease progression. A distinct relative of the *erb*B oncogene (Table 10-2) called c-*erb*B-2 (or *neu* or HER-2), originally detected as an activated transforming gene in chemically induced rat neuroglioblastoma, is amplified in 10 to about 30 percent of human breast cancers. Amplification of c-*erb*B-2 in breast cancer is reported to correlate with poor prognosis. Several oncogenes located on chromosome 11 at band q13, including *int*-2, *hst*-1, and *bcl*-1, have also been reported to be amplified in poor-prognosis breast cancer and a variety of metastatic tumors. The c-*erb*B gene is closely related to or identical with the gene for the receptor for epidermal growth factor (EGF). Amplification and rearrangement of the EGF receptor gene has also been implicated in the formation of human primary gliomas.

RECESSIVE ONCOGENES IN HUMAN NEOPLASIA Dominant oncogenes are not the only mechanism by which tumors arise. The activation of dominant oncogenes is usually a late event associated with widespread disease and metastasis, suggesting that other events may initiate malignant growth. A clue that there might be another class of oncogenes comes from epidemiologic studies of families with inherited forms of cancer. Within these families tumors that usually occur sporadically in the general population are clustered in affected family members. In the early 1970's Knudson and Comings postulated that if *both* copies of a given gene had to be altered before tumor formation occurred, these families might be at such high risk because affected members had inherited *one* altered copy in all cells. Only one further alteration in the hundreds of million cells present in a susceptible tissue would be required to initiate abnormal proliferation. Since dominant oncogenes are inappropriately activated growth stimulatory genes (that are not influenced by the remaining normal copies of the original growth stimulatory genes) it is not surprising that dominant oncogenes have never been linked to the familial cancer syndromes. It was necessary instead to infer the

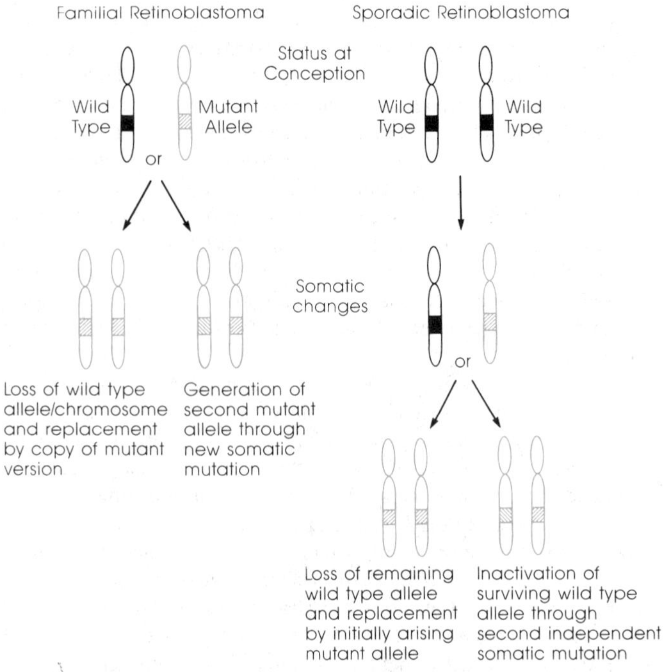

FIGURE 10-3 Mechanisms of loss of the *Rb* gene function. Patients with familial retinoblastoma have one mutant *Rb* allele at conception and therefore all cells have only one wild type *Rb* gene. One single further event in the target cell, either loss of the wild type allele or generation of a second mutant, results in there being no functional *Rb* protein. Patients with sporadic retinoblastoma must undergo at least two mutational events to inactivate the two normal *Rb* alleles. (*Adapted from Friend et al 1988, N Engl J Med.*)

presence of another class of oncogenes termed "recessive oncogenes' or "antioncogenes." Unlike the dominant oncogenes that are a normal part of growth stimulatory pathways, recessive oncogenes must function normally to limit the growth of cells. When both copies are inactivated, tumors are able to occur. Additional evidence suggesting the presence of such genes came from experiments showing that fusion of normal cells with tumor cells generally leads to loss of the malignant phenotype. This would not occur if dominant oncogenes determined the transformed phenotype. However, reversion would be expected if the fusion reintroduced a normal growth-limiting gene into a tumor cell containing inactivated growth-limiting genes.

The first recessive oncogene to be isolated was the retinoblastoma gene *Rb*. It is so named because families with affected members carrying one inactivated copy of the Rb gene almost invariably present with a malignant retinoblastoma of the eye before age 3. A model of the difference between the sporadic and inherited forms of retinoblastoma is shown in Fig. 10-3. The *Rb* gene is located on a subregion of the long arm of chromosome 13 and encodes a 928-amino acid, 205-kDa nuclear phoshoprotein that binds DNA nonspecifically. Tumor formation is a result of a wide range of alterations of the gene, including deletions, point mutations, and insertions that differ for each tumor. Because of this diversity no one probe can be used to detect the alteration as is done, for example, in the detection of sickle cell disease. Nevertheless, the *Rb* gene is altered in all retinoblastoma samples that have been studied at the protein level, and it is likely that inactivation of the *Rb* gene is necessary and sufficient to induce abnormal retinal cell proliferation. Proof that the gene isolated is in fact the *Rb* gene was obtained by demonstrating that the *Rb* gene can act as a tumor suppressor and stop the growth of tumor cells that lack the normal allele.

The *Rb* gene is frequently altered in other tumors as well. Soft tissue sarcomas and osteosarcomas occur at higher frequencies in families with hereditary retinoblastoma, and these tumors frequently exhibit inactivation of the *Rb* gene. The majority of small cell lung carcinomas and bladder carcinomas also have changes at the *Rb*

TABLE 10-4 Location of potential recessive oncogenes and their association with specific tumors

Chromosome location	Associated tumors
2	Uveal melanoma
3p	Renal cell carcinoma, small cell carcinoma lung, von-Hippel Lindau
5q	Colon, leukemia
10	Gliomas, MEN type 2A
11p	Ductal breast carcinoma, Wilms' tumor, rhabdomyosarcoma
11	
13q14	Retinoblastoma, osteosarcoma, soft tissue sarcomas, small cell carcinoma lung, bladder carcinoma, ductal breast carcinoma
17p	Colon, osteosarcoma, astrocytoma
18q	Colon
22	Bilateral acoustic neurofibromatosis, meningioma

locus. However, these tumors do not occur at higher frequencies in families with hereditary retinoblastoma.

Inactivation of the *Rb* gene is due to structural alterations at the DNA level. The DNA tumor virus transforming proteins use a different mechanism and inactivate the *Rb* gene at a functional level. DNA tumor viruses (such as SV40, adenovirus, and the papilloma virus) have proteins that allow these viruses to transform cells. Mutations that prevent binding of these transforming proteins to specific cellular genes destroy their ability to carry out transformation. The Rb gene product p105 is one of the cellular proteins that bind these transforming proteins, and therefore it is believed that these DNA tumor viruses inactivate recessive oncogenes, including the *Rb* gene, as a mechanism of transformation. Thus, inactivation of recessive oncogenes is probably the way in which the human papilloma viruses potentiate cervical carcinomas.

Nine other putative recessive oncogenes have been detected. Table 10-4 shows their chromosomal location and the tumors with which they are associated. In each case their presence has been suggested in one of two ways. The strongest indications have come from linkage studies among the familial forms of these tumors. In these families there are specific chromosomal subregions that can be directly linked with a predisposition to the respective tumors. The other indications have come from comparing normal and tumor DNA for loss of specific DNA markers in the transition to the malignant phenotype. Both criteria have been met for some tumors such as bilateral acoustic neurofibromatosis. There are tumors for which it is virtually certain that recessive oncogenes play a role. Beyond the *Rb* gene, *p53* is the only other recessive oncogene that has been isolated. It is located on chromosome 17, encodes a nuclear phosphoprotein, and is inactivated in sarcomas, brain tumors, and colon cancer.

Whereas retinal cells are transformed by the inactivation of a single recessive oncogene, this simple model will probably not apply to most other tumors. Bladder cancer, small cell carcinoma of the lung, and colon cancer undergo multiple changes, apparently including both inactivation of several recessive oncogenes and activation of dominant oncogenes within the cells. Such complexity hampers the ability to link the inactivation of specific recessive oncogenes with determinants of diagnosis and prognosis. Eventually, the recessive oncogenes are likely to define growth stimulatory pathways of the dominant oncogenes.

FUNCTIONS OF ONCOGENES Studies of the proteins encoded by the viral oncogenes and their normal cellular homologues have provided insight into the functions of these genes. The protein product of the v-*src* gene of Rous sarcoma virus acts as a tyrosine protein kinase, and the oncogenic properties of v-*src* depend upon this enzymatic activity. The viral oncogene proteins of *yes* and *fgr* (Table 10-1) and a series of cellular genes (*fyn, lyn, lck, hck*) are structurally related to the *src* protein and form a subfamily of tyrosine protein kinases. The *abl* gene product is the prototype of a second subfamily of tyrosine protein kinases which includes those encoded by *fes/fps* viral oncogenes and a human cellular gene, ARG. In addition *raf, mos,* and *pim*-1 viral and cellular oncogenes encode serine-threonine protein kinases. The problem has been to identify the cellular proteins that are modified by these cytoplasmic kinases and that are critical for transformation. For example, in cells transformed by Rous sarcoma virus, a number of cellular proteins are modified by the addition of phosphate groups to tyrosine residues, but a specific role for such changes in oncogenesis has not been established.

Growth factors and receptors (See also Chap. 9) An important conceptual advance has come from separate lines of research on oncogene function and growth factor function (Fig. 10-4). The proliferation and differentiation of normal cells are regulated by signals derived from the binding of growth factors to receptors on the cell surface. Three of the better characterized growth factors are platelet-derived growth factor (PDGF), which promotes the growth of connective tissue and smooth muscle cells; epidermal growth factor (EGF), which is required for optimal growth of epithelial cells in vitro; and fibroblast growth factors (acid and basic FGF), which can act as fibroblast mitogens. The receptors for PDGF and EGF are transmembrane proteins that possess a tyrosine protein kinase activity within their cytoplasmic domain that is activated by binding of PDGF or EGF (see Fig. 9-1). More recently hematopoietic and lymphoid

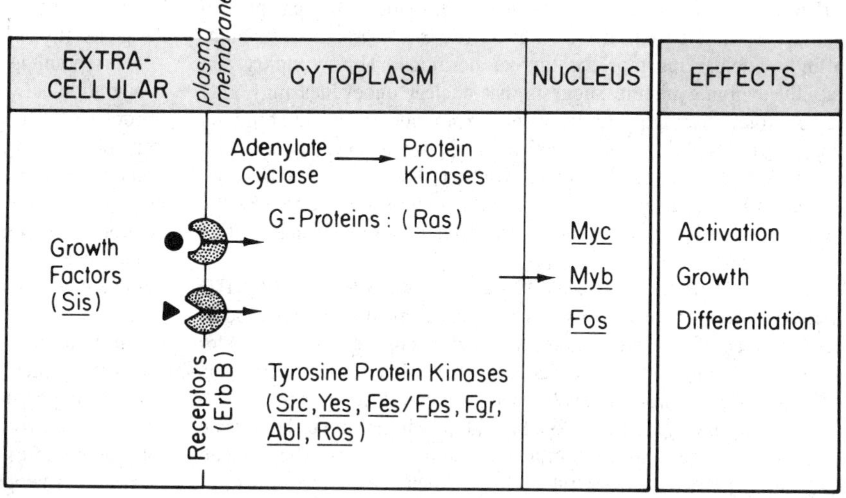

FIGURE 10-4 Relationships between the molecular biology of growth factors and the functions of oncogenes. Growth factors are small molecules that signal cell activation, replication, and differentiation by binding to specific receptors on the surface of target cells. As shown, a number of the proteins made by oncogenes fit into the general pathway for growth factor activity. Oncogenes may transform cells by transmitting a constitutive, unregulated signal for cell growth from their particular position in the pathway. For details see text.

growth factor genes have been isolated including those for several colony-stimulating factors and interleukins.

In addition to the FGF-related oncogenes mentioned before, a protein encoded by the viral oncogene of simian sarcoma virus, *sis,* is closely related to PDGF. In addition, the *fms* oncogene of a strain of feline sarcoma virus is an altered form of the receptor of a macrophage growth factor called colony-stimulating factors (CSF-1). As mentioned before, the *erb*B oncogene is an altered form of the receptor for EGF which can produce a transforming growth signal without normal binding to the growth factor. The cellular oncogenes c-*erb*B-2 (*neu,* HER-2), *trk, met,* and *ret* all have growth factor receptor–like properties. These observations have led to the postulate that the unregulated growth signal involved in neoplastic transformation might result from changes in growth factors, their receptors, or other elements in the pathway. An elaboration of this concept derives from the observation that transformed cells sometimes secrete novel growth factors as a secondary change. Examples are tumor cell growth factors alpha and beta (TGF-α and -β), which can induce transformed morphology and growth of normal cells that are reversible with removal of the growth factor. Thus, autocrine and paracrine stimulation of growth by such factors may contribute to tumorigenesis.

***Ras* oncogene proteins** The proteins encoded by *ras* oncogenes are associated with the inner surface of the cell membrane. They share a functional activity, the binding of guanosine triphosphate (GTP), with a family of GTP-binding or G proteins on the inner surface of the cell membrane that participate in the transmission of signals from the cell surface (see Chap. 68). Mutations that activate the transforming potential of *ras* gene alter the interaction of *ras* proteins with guanine nucleotide substrates. Thus, transforming *ras* proteins are a class of G proteins that transmit a constitutive growth signal.

Oncogene proteins in the cell nucleus The proteins encoded by six of the oncogenes in Table 10-1, *myb, myc, ski, jun, erb*A, and *fos,* act in the cell nucleus. The normal homologue of *myb* is expressed at low levels and is cell cycle–regulated in many cell types, but is expressed at high levels independent of cell cycles in early T-cell, B-cell, and hematopoietic progenitors. Expression of *myc* family genes is elevated in many developing tissues during embryogenesis, but only c-*myc* itself is expressed in most or all lineages in postnatal life. Expression of c-*myc* and c-*fos* can be closely tied to the growth factor pathways. When growth-arrested fibroblasts are exposed to PDGF, a specific set of genes is expressed, including the proto-oncogenes c-*fos* and c-*myc,* and cellular messenger RNA and protein levels for these genes increase. Expression of c-*myc* is also enhanced in resting B and T lymphocytes after exposure to appropriate mitogens. Once cells enter the growth cycle, the expression of c-*myc* remains constant. When cells lose the ability to divide, for example, in postmitotic differentiated cells, c-*myc* expression decreases or ceases. The protein of the cellular *jun*A gene is a DNA-binding protein closely related or identical to a transcription factor for many genes called AP-1, and the c-*fos* protein has been found in nuclear protein complexes in association with AP-1. The *erb*A protein is a high-affinity nuclear receptor for thyroid hormone. This complex and rapidly evolving picture suggests that nuclear oncogenes may play pivotal roles in setting patterns of gene expression. They may function normally as regulators of cell "activation," growth, and differentiation and may be nuclear targets for growth factor–derived signals. When altered or deregulated, they may provide a constitutive drive for the uncontrolled cell growth and abnormal differentiation that characterize the neoplastic state.

EXPERIMENTAL INTRODUCTION OF ACTIVE ONCOGENES INTO CELLS One approach to establishing experimental animal models for analysis of human tumor-associated oncogenes is to transfer activated oncogenes into normal cells in vivo and to observe the effects of these genes on development. Several different genes, such as those specifying immunoglobulin and growth hormone, have been introduced by microinjection into fertilized mouse eggs. The injected "transgenes" become integrated into the genome of progeny mice and, in some cases, are expressed in appropriate cell types (for example, immunoglobulin transgenes are expressed predominantly in B lymphocytes).

The introduction by this technique of a T-antigen gene from the DNA tumor virus SV40 into the germ line of mice resulted in the formation of choroid plexus papillomas. Likewise, the introduction of activated *neu* (*erb*B-2, HER-2) transgenes with promoter-enhancer sequences derived from mouse mammary tumor virus into the germ line of mice uniformly caused the development of polyclonal mammary adenocarcinomas involving the entire mammary epithelium. In contrast, an analogous c-*myc* transgene acted as a predisposing factor to the development of mammary adenocarcinoma in some mice. A *myc* transgene fused to immunoglobulin-regulating elements caused pre-B-cell proliferation preceding the development of B-cell lymphomas. Transgenic mice carrying a human c-*ras*^{H} gene with an activating mutation fused to an elastase gene regulatory element develop adenocarcinoma of the exocrine pancreas shortly after pancreatic differentiation.

Introduction into transplantable stem cells of bone marrow and lymphoid organs is done by infecting stem cells ex vivo with retrovirus-derived vectors containing the genes and then transplanting the cells into appropriately prepared hosts. The introduction of the v-*myc* gene by this technique into the stem cells of the chicken bursa induced preneoplastic proliferative lesions that precede the development of B-cell lymphomas. Introduction of hematopoietic growth factor genes, e.g., for interleukins and granulocyte-macrophage colony-stimulating factor (GM-CSF), using viral vectors into mouse marrow stem cells produces characteristic myeloproliferative changes.

ONCOGENES AND MULTISTAGED TUMORIGENESIS Human cancer and chemically induced neoplasia in animals usually develop by a multistep process in which an abnormal preneoplastic cell type evolves into a cell population successively dominated by clones with increasingly malignant characteristics. This evolution of tumor development is thought to be preceded by a latent period, and the whole process may take a significant fraction of the life span of the affected individual. In contrast, acute transforming viruses carrying activated forms of oncogenes that are implicated in nonviral cancer appear to induce neoplasms within days or weeks, i.e., with kinetics that suggest a single-step process. This difference may be due to several factors. First, many of the viral oncogenes encode kinases with multiple cellular targets and may induce abrupt changes that would require several different mutations in more slowly evolving neoplasms. Second, expression of the viral oncogenes is driven by powerful regulatory elements (promoters and enhancers in the proviral LTRs). The transforming potential of the cellular homologues of these same genes can be activated by mechanisms that do not involve such high-level expression, for example, the point mutations at amino acids 12 or 61 of the proteins encoded by the human *ras* tumor-associated oncogenes. In these situations the concerted activity of several genes may be required to induce the same transformed phenotype that can be induced by very high level, unregulated expression of just one of the genes (as occurs with acute transforming retroviruses).

This point is illustrated by transfection experiments suggesting cooperation between oncogenes in inducing transformation of cultured fibroblasts. The activated *ras* genes from human tumor cells can transform immortalized cell lines but cannot induce full morphologic transformation of primary cell cultures. The combination of activated *myc* and *ras* gene clones, however, produces the fully transformed phenotype in primary cell cultures. Thus, in this system *myc* (and other oncogenes that do not alter these cells by themselves) can complement the transforming activation of human *ras* oncogenes. However, when powerful transcriptional enhancer sequences are engineered into the activated *ras* oncogene, this gene can itself transform primary fibroblast cultures, presumably because of a higher level of expression of the oncogene. The requirement for multiple genes in transformation may be conditioned, in part, by the level of oncogene expression, and more than one cellular oncogene may be activated in neoplasms in vivo.

IMPLICATIONS FOR CLINICAL ONCOLOGY

The clinical impact of the identification and analysis of human oncogenes and their products may be extensive, indeed, revolutionary. For example, efforts to identify and control environmental and nutritional factors that may cause or prevent cancer depend heavily on epidemiologic techniques, animal studies, and clinical trials where disease incidence and mortality are endpoints for measurement. Knowledge of the specific proto-oncogenes that are the targets of environmental carcinogens and of the nature of the changes induced may provide better methods for assessing the actual role of candidate carcinogens and for devising preventive approaches. Delineation of the molecular anatomy of neoplastic change in specific cell lineages will add new dimensions to diagnosis. Classification of disease on the basis of specific molecular changes (e.g., in CML, ALL, and non-Hodgkin's lymphomas) and detection of molecular changes associated with poor prognosis (e.g., in breast cancer) appear to hold promise for the immediate future. As the complex picture of the molecular mechanisms employed by oncogenes to transform cells is progressively revealed, it is reasonable to expect that this new knowledge will improve treatment by providing more precise and more specific means for targeting pharmacologic intervention.

REFERENCES

ALT TW et al (eds): Nuclear oncogenes, in *Current Communications in Molecular Biology*. Cold Spring Harbor Laboratory, New York, 1987

BISHOP JM: The molecular genetics of cancer. Science 235:305, 1987

DREAZEN O et al: The molecular biology of chronic myelogenous leukemia. Semin Hematol 25:35, 1988

FRIEND SH et al: Oncogenes and tumor-suppressing genes. N Engl J Med 318:618, 1988

KNUDSON AG: Hereditary cancer, oncogenes and anti-oncogenes. Cancer Res 45:1437, 1985

WEINBERG RA: The action of oncogenes in the cytoplasm and nucleus. Science 230:770, 1985

———: Finding the anti-oncogene. Sci Am 259:44, 1988

11 TRANSMEMBRANE SIGNALING BY RECEPTORS

CHARLES F. STEVENS

Our cells live in a watery world, and their life depends absolutely on the integrity of the barrier to water soluble molecules that defines the cell's boundaries, the cell membrane. Because this membrane is constructed of a phospholipid bilayer, it forms a virtually impregnable shield against the entry and exit of all hydrophilic molecules dissolved in the extracellular and intracellular aqueous environments. Although the surface membrane is necessary for the cell's existence, its very impregnability poses problems for the functioning of the cell: certain essential metabolites must, in a regulated way, be able to cross the membrane, and information about the outside environment must be communicated to the cell's interior. The first of these problems is solved by a variety of transport systems, and the second by a class of molecules, termed *receptors,* that are the subject of this chapter.

The term *receptor* is generally defined in two distinct ways. The *operational definition* identifies receptors by their binding characteristics; any cell surface molecule that binds tightly a specific molecular species is called a receptor for what is bound. "Receptors" identified in this way include a rather wide variety of functional types of molecules including such entities as cell adhesion molecules used to attach cells together and uptake proteins that transport molecules like glutamate across the surface membrane. In this chapter, the *functional definition* of receptors is used: a class of proteins residing in the cell's surface membrane that transmit information across the membrane about the presence of specific molecules outside the cell. Receptors, by this definition, are signaling molecules that inform the inside of the cell about the external environment.

TABLE 11-1 The three receptor families

Receptor family	Typical receptor ligands	Primary signal	Typical signal results
Channel	Acetylcholine, glycine, GABA, glutamate	Ionic current	Voltage change in neuron
G protein coupled	Acetylcholine, GABA, norepinephrine, cholecystokinin, substance P	Activated G protein	Increased cyclic AMP levels and activation of A kinase
Tyrosine kinase	Insulin, platelet-derived growth factor	Phosphotyrosine residue	Enzyme activation leading to mitogenesis

Receptors fall into three categories according to their mechanism of signaling: channels, G protein–coupled receptors, and tyrosine kinases (Table 11-1). Doubtless additional categories will be added as more is learned about the relevant gene families responsible for encoding receptors. These three classes of receptors are considered in turn.

RECEPTORS INCORPORATING ION CHANNELS Four receptor channel types are now recognized, although others very likely exist. The four current classes, named by their ligand, are acetylcholine, glycine, gamma-aminobutyric acid (GABA), and glutamate receptor channels. The first three proteins have known sequences deduced from molecular genetic analysis of complementary DNA (cDNA) clones; molecular structures are not yet available for glutamate receptor channels. Within each class, a number of subclasses—perhaps half a dozen—are known.

Receptor channels are membrane-spanning proteins defined by their signaling mechanism: ligand binding induces a conformational change that opens a transmembrane aqueous pore in the receptor and permits ions to cross the membrane's lipid bilayer. The signal, then, is a voltage change produced by the ion flux; however, in one case, a type of glutamate receptor channel, a calcium ion influx and the resultant concentration change within the target cell constitute an important aspect of the signal. Which ions flow, and what voltage change occurs, depends on the channel type. Acetylcholine and glutamate receptor channels permit sodium and potassium ions to cross the membrane, and cause positive voltage changes (depolarization of the cell). One type of glutamate receptor channel, the one noted above, additionally permits a calcium ion influx. The GABA and glycine receptor channels let chloride ions permeate and, in the usual situation, produce negative voltages changes (hyperpolarization). Thus, acetylcholine and glutamate are excitatory, and GABA and glycine are inhibitory.

Receptor channels of one sort or other are universally present on neurons, where they subserve synaptic transmission. The ligand, a neurotransmitter such as acetylcholine, is released by presynaptic nerve impulses, and the receptor channels located in the postsynaptic membrane respond to the neurotransmitter to signal the arrival of the nerve impulses. Receptors of this type are found, in addition, on many other cell types such as muscle (where they function in neuromuscular transmission), secretory cells (where they are involved in excitation-secretion coupling), and lymphocytes (where they participate in the response to mitogens).

The nicotinic acetylcholine receptor channel is the best-studied example of this class. This receptor is a pentameric protein composed of four distinct subunits, each with a molecular mass on the order of 50 kDa, encoded by four different genes (Fig. 11-1). The subunits are all highly homologous and fit together like the staves of a barrel to form a membrane-spanning structure with a central pore that can be opened and closed by ligand binding–induced conformation change. Each of the subunits has an extracellular domain (where the ligand

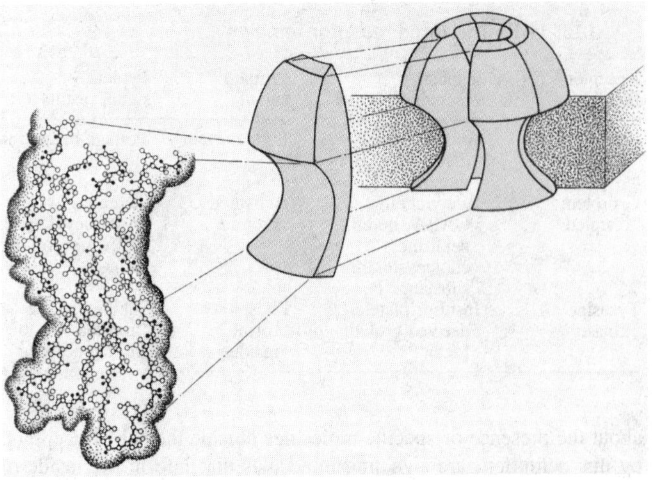

FIGURE 11-1 Exploded view of an acetylcholine receptor channel. The subunits are thought to be arranged, as shown at the right, somewhat like staves of a barrel around a central pore through which the ion traffic flows. Each subunit is shaped much like the others even though they are encoded by separate genes. The far left part of the figure represents the four membrane-spanning peptide chains that constitute the portion of the subunit embedded in the membrane. Compare this structure with that of the G protein–coupled receptor illustrated in Fig. 68-1.

binds on one special subunit), four membrane-spanning regions, and a smaller, intracellular domain. The GABA and glycine receptor channels are proteins encoded by other membranes of the same gene superfamily and are believed to have the same general structure as the acetylcholine receptor.

A number of drugs act by disrupting channel function. For example, curare competes with acetylcholine for its binding site, strychnine similarly blocks glycine receptor channels, phencyclidine (angel dust) inhibits, by a different mechanism, the function of a subtype of glutamate receptor channel, and benzodiazepines enhance the effect of GABA on its receptor (see Chap. 346).

RECEPTORS COUPLED TO G PROTEINS Very many receptors, dozens and possibly hundreds, are G protein coupled, with a signaling mechanism described below. These receptors, generally named according to a ligand they bind tightly, include ones that recognize peptides (e.g., β-endorphins, atrial natriuretic peptide, and cholecystokinin), acetylcholine (muscarinic), biogenic amines (e.g., dopamine and serotonin), amino acids (e.g., GABA and glutamate), and purines (e.g., adenosine). It should be emphasized that some of the same ligands, GABA and acetylcholine, for example, can activate both the receptor channels described above and the G protein–coupled receptors considered here. This situation can lead to terminologic confusion where two different entities have the same name. In many of these cases some further distinction is made. Thus, one speaks of $GABA_A$ and nicotinic acetylcholine receptors (channels) and also of $GABA_B$ and muscarinic acetylcholine receptors (G protein–coupled).

G protein–coupled receptors all work in basically the same way, but some variations on the general theme result finally in a very complex range of actions (see Chap. 68). In every case, ligand binding to the receptor produces a conformational change that causes an entity called a *G protein* to be converted from an inactive to an active form. The "G" in this name refers to guanosine di- or triphosphate (GDP, GTP) because activation of the G protein involves dissociating GDP and binding GTP at a special site. The active G protein then binds to a target and this leads to a final result, as described in more detail below. Much amplification of the original signal (ligand binding) occurs because a single receptor can activate many copies of a G protein, and each activated G protein can be used multiple times on its targets. A G protein remains active so long as it retains GTP in its binding site, and the active state is terminated by an enzymatic activity of the G protein itself that converts the bound GTP into GDP (see also Chap. 68).

The complexity in action of G protein–coupled receptors arises from the fact that many distinct types of receptors can specifically activate different types of G proteins, of which about a dozen are presently recognized. These various G protein species can bind specifically to perhaps a dozen different intracellular targets. Further, different types of G proteins can exhibit antagonistic effects on their targets, thus one G protein species can stimulate whereas another can inhibit some target action. In addition, G protein targets, which are often enzymes, act on a wide range of secondary targets, and these targets can have still other sites of action so that a rather complex regulatory cascade results.

This general regulatory scheme is best understood in terms of a specific example: Norepinephrine causes the heart to beat more forcefully through the action of a G protein–coupled receptor, the beta-adrenergic receptor. An agonist binding to this receptor activates a G protein that in turn enables adenylate cyclase to convert ATP to cyclic AMP. The cyclic AMP produced by the adenylate cyclase then activates yet another enzyme, called *A kinase*, and this enzyme phosphorylates a particular membrane protein, a *calcium channel* (note that this channel is a member of a different superfamily than the receptor channels discussed above), responsible for letting calcium ions into the cardiac myocyte. The intracellular calcium ions act on the heart muscle contractile proteins to result in muscular contraction. The phosphorylated calcium channel permits more calcium ions to enter the myocyte each time the channel is turned on, and the larger influx of calcium ions produces a greater calcium concentration. This greater concentration results, by the law of mass action, in an increased activation of contractile proteins, that is, a more forceful heart beat.

In this example, the regulatory cascade has four levels. The primary target of the activated G protein is the enzyme adenylate cyclase, and this enzyme, through the cyclic AMP it produces, acts on a secondary target, the A kinase. The A kinase then phosphorylates the tertiary target, a calcium channel. This channel lets calcium ions enter in greater quantities when it is phosphorylated, and produces, by the calcium ion action on contractile proteins, the quaternary target, a stronger heart beat. Each G protein–coupled receptor acts through a regulatory cascade of this same general type. G protein actions are often hard to define, and difficult to keep straight, because the intracellular cascades have many levels, each with its own complexities.

Several generalizations can be made about the action of G protein–coupled receptors. First, the various G proteins themselves can be classified. For immediate purposes, the best classification is perhaps the simplest: Many G proteins are either stimulatory (G_s) or inhibitory (G_i) so that they constitute the accelerator and brake characteristic of all biologic regulatory systems. Second, the G proteins act, as far as is now known, on three distinct second-messenger systems: ion channels (membrane proteins responsible for electric excitability of cells), the cyclic AMP system, and the phosphoinositol (PI) turnover system. Some G proteins bind directly to certain channels to alter their function. G proteins also bind to adenylate cyclases (to make the second messenger, cyclic AMP) and to phospholipases, which break phospholipids into inositol-3-phosphate (IP3) and diacylglycerol (DAG), molecules that function as second messengers. Finally, IP3 and cyclic AMP activate kinases (designated C and A, respectively) that in turn phosphorylate various targets to alter their functions. These kinases act on a wide range of substrates and can affect cell electric excitability, activity of various enzyme systems, and expression of specific genes.

G protein–coupled receptors occur on all cell types and are especially common in the brain and gut. As might be expected, the nervous system expresses many different types of G protein–coupled receptors. The ligands for these receptors are contained in presynaptic vesicles and released by nerve activity. Although formerly ligands for all classes of receptors in the brain were called *neurotransmitters*, this term now is reserved generally for those ligands that bind to receptor channels. The ligands that bind to G protein–coupled receptors are termed *neuromodulators* to recognize that they operate through a mechanism different from that of neurotransmitters. Because the same chemical entity can bind to both receptor types, some ligands—acetylcholine, for example—are simultaneously neurotransmitters and neuromodulators.

Over a dozen G protein–coupled receptors, all members of the same gene family, have been cloned and sequenced, and more are on the way. The structures that have been determined include several adrenergic receptors, muscarinic acetylcholine receptors, serotonin receptors, peptide receptors (substance K, atrial natriuretic peptide, and angiotensin), a dopamine receptor, and rhodopsin (a photoreceptor molecule included because it is G protein–coupled and in the same gene family). In all cases, the receptors are monomeric proteins with an extracellular domain that binds ligand, an intracellular G protein–binding domain, and seven transmembrane helices. Because of the seven membrane-spanning helices, these receptors are known as members of the "Magnificent Seven" family. The precise nature of the conformational change that permits the G proteins to be activated has not been determined (see Chap. 68).

Many of the drugs that affect the brain—opiates and antipsychotics, for example—act on G protein–coupled receptors either as agonists or antagonists. Some G protein–coupled receptors are cellular homologues of oncogenes. (The angiotensin receptor was discovered through its homology to the *mas* oncogene and *ras* is a type of G protein.) The precise role of these signaling systems in cancer is, however, still not fully understood (see Chap. 10).

RECEPTORS WITH TYROSINE KINASE ACTIVITY Receptors in the third category phosphorylate tyrosine residues in themselves and in certain other proteins. This receptor family is usually considered to bind growth factors primarily, but some members constitute a link in the chain subserving the actions of hormones, such as insulin. Further, cell-cell interactions during development also make use of these receptors, but the mechanisms involved have not yet been extensively studied. Three main subfamilies of tyrosine kinase receptors have been identified: those related to the insulin receptor, to the epidermal growth factor (EDGF) receptor, and to the platelet-derived growth factor (PDGF) receptor (see Chap. 9).

Receptors in this family all work through tyrosine kinase activity that is enabled by ligand binding. Even now little is known about the targets for this kinase activity, nor is it understood just what these targets do. One clear target, however, is the receptor itself; these receptors autophosphorylate and thereby increase their own activity. Receptor activation often results in cell division and growth. The activated receptors affect various enzyme systems that facilitate mitogenesis and they also participate in the regulation of gene expression. The insulin receptor, of course, plays a role in normal cell function throughout life, but other related receptors are involved in determining cell fate during development.

All cells possess receptors in this class. The brain, as could be anticipated, is particularly richly endowed.

All receptors with tyrosine kinase activity have extracellular, transmembrane, and cytoplasmic domains, and all are rather large proteins with about a thousand amino acids. The extracellular domain binds agonist, characteristically quite tightly (n*M* dissociation constant), and the intracellular domain is the location of kinase activity. Unlike the receptors of the other classes described above, the tyrosine kinases appear to possess only a single membrane-spanning region. Members of the insulin receptor subfamily are composed of two distinct subunits, one of which contains the transmembrane segment and the tyrosine kinase activity, and the second of which is purely extracellular with the agonist binding site. Members of both the EDGF and PDGF families have ligand binding and tyrosine kinase activity within a single large polypeptide chain.

Although understanding of the mechanisms by which receptors of this type act is still quite limited, these molecules have attracted great interest because they are often the cellular homologues of oncogenes, and their activity promotes the expression of additional cytoplasmic oncogene homologues such as *myc* and *fos*. For example, the EDGF receptor is the cellular homologue of *v-Erb*B, and all of these receptor types belong to the same superfamily as do the *Src* and *Abl* families of oncogenes. Because of these connections, many workers believe that with increased understanding of the mechanisms through which this receptor category operates, insight into the pathogenesis of certain cancers will follow (see Chap. 10).

REFERENCES

HANKS SK et al: The protein kinase family: Conserved features and deduced phylogeny of the catalytic domains. Science 241:42, 1988

NEER EJ, CLAPHAM DE: Roles of G protein subunits in transmembrane signalling. Nature 333:129, 1988

UNWIN N et al: Arrangement of the acetylcholine receptor subunits in the resting and desensitized states, determined by cryoelectron microscopy of crystallized torpedo postsynaptic membranes. J Cell Biol 107:1123, 1988

12 BIOLOGY OF AGING

ITAMAR B. ABRASS

Over a third of patients seen by a primary-care physician are now older adults; this number will exceed 50 percent in the next century. The numbers of older adults (age 65 and older) in the United States have grown in absolute and relative terms both because of an increase in the mean life span and a decrease in birth rates. Growth in the group over age 75 is even more rapid. The result is a greater demand on the health care system (see also Chap. 4).

The gain in survival includes both active and dependent years. As mean life span has increased and maximum life span has remained unchanged, it has been widely assumed that the time of dependency will decrease as life expectancy increases. The available data do not support such an outcome. If anything, the mean prevalence of disability seems to be getting worse with time. These observations are in conflict with the widespread impression that older persons are now healthier and more active. In fact, there may be a bimodal distribution with some individuals getting healthier and others becoming more disabled as the result of survival with a problem that was previously fatal. It is important to define the factors that lead to "successful" aging. Delivering the needed health care and decreasing the time of disability present a challenge to both clinician and scientist.

With aging two phenomena occur: a physiologic decline and an increase in disease. Although these processes influence each other, physiologic decline occurs independently of disease.

In healthy older adults many physiologic functions are maintained in the basal resting state, but decrements in function occur in most organ systems and homeostatic mechanisms when the system is challenged or stressed. Furthermore, chronic disease of multifactorial etiology becomes more common with age. Mortality curves are exponential after the age of 30, with cardiovascular and neoplastic diseases being the commonest causes of death. However, even in the oldest, despite the prevalence of disease, the interaction of disease and physiological control mechanisms remains important. In such individuals the pathologist may identify many lesions without defining the cause of death. In fact, the cause of death may have been a relatively minor perturbation of homeostatic mechanisms.

MOLECULAR AND CELLULAR MECHANISMS OF AGING Theories of aging fall into two general categories: accumulation of damage to molecules or the regulation of specific genes.

DNA undergoes continuous change both in response to exogenous agents and intrinsic processes. Stability is maintained by the double strandedness of DNA that makes possible repair of change by specific repair enzymes. It has been proposed that biological aging is due to somatic mutagenesis, either due to greater susceptivility to mutagenesis or deficits in repair mechanisms. In fact, the longevity of different species correlates with DNA repair enzymes. However, in humans the spontaneous rate of mutagenesis is not adequate to account for the number of changes that take place, and there is no evidence that failure in repair functions causes aging.

A related theory, the error catastrophe theory, proposes that errors occur in DNA, RNA, and protein synthesis, each augmenting the other and finally culminating in an error catastrophe. Protein synthesis is considered the most likely source for age-dependent errors, since it is the final common pathway. However, increased translational errors have not been found in aging either in vivo or in vitro. Amino acid substitutions do not increase with age, although some enzyme activities may be altered by changes in posttranslational modification of proteins, such as glycosylation.

The major by-products of oxidative metabolism include superoxide radicals that can react with DNA, RNA, proteins, and lipids and lead to cellular damage and aging. Several scavenging enzymes and some small molecules, such as vitamin C and vitamin E, protect the cell from oxidative damage. There is no significant loss of scavenging enzymes in aging, and treatment with vitamins C and E does not increase longevity in experimental animals.

The most widely accepted concept of aging is that it is regulated by specific genes. Support for this hypothesis has been mostly gained from in vitro models of aging. In adulthood, cells can be divided into three categories based on their replicative capacity: continuously replicating, replicating in response to a challenge, and nonreplicating. Epidermal, gastrointestinal, and hematopoietic cells are continuously renewed; liver can regenerate in response to injury; and neurons and cardiac muscle and skeletal muscle do not regenerate.

In vitro replication is closely related to in vivo proliferation. Neurons and cardiac myocytes from adults can be maintained in culture but do not divide, whereas marrow cells, endothelial cells, and fibroblasts replicate in vitro. Since they are easily obtained from skin, fibroblasts have been the most extensively studied cell type. Although some cells replicate continuously in intact organisms, they have a finite replicative life. For fibroblasts in vitro, this is about 50 doublings. Replicative life in vitro also correlates with the age of the donor, so that the older the donor the fewer doublings. With time, doubling time increases, and ultimately cell division ceases.

When fibroblasts from younger donors are fused with nonreplicating senescent cells, DNA synthesis is inhibited in both old and young nuclei. Transient inhibition of protein synthesis immediately following fusion leads to increased DNA synthesis in both nuclei, suggesting that a protein factor in senescent cells may be involved in the inhibition of replication. When senescent cytoplasts (cells without nuclei) are fused with young, dividing cells, DNA synthesis is also depressed, suggesting that the inhibitory factor(s) is present in cytoplasm. Growth arrest both in vivo and in vitro is associated with the appearance of a specific protein that may be involved in DNA replication, and this protein is a candidate molecule for the inhibition in DNA synthesis associated with senescence.

These experiments help define the finite life span of cells in vitro but do not themselves explain aging in intact organisms, since organisms do not suddenly die because all cells stop replicating. However, factors associated with finite cell replication may indirectly influence in vivo aging. Fibroblasts aged in vitro or obtained from older adult donors are less sensitive to many growth factors at both the receptor and postreceptor levels. A decrease in these growth factors, a change in sensitivity to growth factors, and/or a slowing of the cell cycle may slow wound healing and perhaps place the older individual at greater risk for infection.

For tissues with nonreplicating cells, cell loss may lead to a permanent deficit. With aging, dopaminergic neurons are lost, impairing gait and balance and enhancing susceptibility to the side-effects of drugs. With further decrements such as ischemia or viral infection, Parkinson's disease may develop. Similar cell loss and/or functional deficits in other neurotransmitter systems may lead to autonomic dysfunction, alteration in mental function, and impairment of neuroendocrine control.

The immune system demonstrates similar phenomena with aging. Lymphocytes from older adults have a diminished proliferative response to mitogens. This diminished response may be due to a decrease in lymphokines and a decreased response to extracellular signals. As the thymus involutes postpuberty, thymic hormone (thymosins) levels decrease. With age basal and stimulated interleukin 2 (IL-2) production and responsiveness also diminish. The latter appears to be due, at least in part, to a decreased expression of IL-2 receptors. Some immune functions can be restored by the addition of these hormones to lymphocytes in vitro by their administration to intact, aged animals. The proliferative defect can also be reversed in vitro by calcium ionophores and activators of protein kinase C, suggesting that the T-cell defect may be in transduction of extracellular signals to intracellular function.

In vivo, molecular mechanisms such as those described above are believed to contribute to physiologic deficits and altered homeostatic mechanisms that predispose older individuals to dysfunction in the face of stress and disease.

PHYSIOLOGIC AGING In assessing studies on physiologic function with age, several factors need to be considered: (1) In healthy older adults, decreases in function are usually demonstrable only under stress; (2) data generally represent means, and with aging there is usually a wide intragroup variability; and (3) most data are cross-sectional rather than longitudinal. It is also important to assess how health status was defined.

Cardiovascular Early data suggested that cardiac output at rest declines progressively from about age 20 to age 90. However, such subjects were not screened for occult coronary artery disease. The findings are quite different when the population under scrutiny is screened for coronary artery disease with stress thallium images. In such a population, resting cardiac output in normals is unaffected by age from the 3rd to the 8th decades. Cardiac output during graded exercise is also unchanged with age. However, heart rate is decreased, and end-diastolic and end-systolic volumes increase with age. Thus, in the older subjects, cardiac output during exercise is maintained by utilization of the Frank-Starling mechanism. These individuals use reserve mechanisms to maintain cardiac output and may, therefore, be more vulnerable to decompensation when disease is superimposed.

These findings are also consistent with the concept that myocardial beta-adrenergic responsiveness decreases with age. Such changes occur in both humans and animals. Heart rate response to isoproterenol infusion decreases with age, and in animals, myocardial contractility also decreases. This deficit is related to beta-adrenergic mechanisms and not to intrinsic contractile capacity. Basal and stimulated norepinephrine levels increase with age. Whether the defect in beta-adrenergic responsiveness is due to desensitization by endogenous catecholamines or other age related phenomena is not known.

Older individuals also have decreased baroreceptor reflex sensitivity, i.e., cardiovascular responses to changes in intravascular volume are altered. Such changes may put the older patient at greater risk during rapid volume expansion and may contribute to the higher prevalence of orthostatic hypotension in older adults.

Pulmonary Except for increases in residual volume, most pulmonary volumes are unaltered in healthy nonsmoking older adults. However, compliance increases and small airways tend to collapse as the elastic structures decrease. These changes in small airways lead to an increase in closing volumes such that by the mean age of 65 years not all the airways are opened during regular breathing in the sitting position. In the recumbent position, this phenomenon occurs by age 45. As a consequence, older individuals are more prone to develop atelectasis and pneumonia particularly when lying in bed for prolonged periods of time.

Endocrine Aging is associated with the development of glucose intolerance. The primary defect appears to be insulin resistance, since most studies demonstrate increased insulin levels. However, abnormal regulation of insulin secretion may also be a factor, because the insulin levels may not be appropriate for the degree of hyperglycemia. The cause of this impairment in carbohydrate metabolism has not been fully defined. Body weight, activity, and dietary composition influence carbohydrate metabolism, but they are not the sole factors in the carbohydrate intolerance of aging. At the tissue level, the insulin resistance of aging appears to be at some undefined post-receptor defect since insulin receptor numbers and affinities in monocytes and adipose tissue are unaltered with age.

Although the glucose intolerance of aging is not diabetes mellitus, it may have important consequences. Even within the normal range of an oral glucose tolerance test, those at the upper range have an increased risk of coronary artery disease compared to those with the lowest levels. In healthy older adults fasting blood sugars remain in the normal range, but glycosylated hemoglobin levels rise. Similar glycosylation may occur in other structural proteins and enzymes to modify their function. Furthermore, hyperinsulinemia is an independent risk factor for atherosclerosis and may contribute to the prevalance of vascular disease in older adults.

The metabolic clearance rate of thyroid hormone decreases with age. With an intact hypothalamic-pituitary-thyroid axis, normal thyroxine levels are maintained. However, with thyroid disease, when exogenous thyroxine is administered, the replacement dose must be adjusted downward to compensate for the change in clearance.

The most marked endocrine change with aging is decrease in estrogen at the time of the menopause. Decreased estrogen causes changes in reproductive tissues, and marked alteration in bone metabolism that leads to the development of osteoporosis in those with other risk factors. It has also been hypothesized that the difference in longevity between men and women is the result of differences in atherogenesis, that this in turn is mediated by difference in lipoprotein metabolism, which in turn is determined by gender-specific sex hormone levels. At adolescence, low density lipoprotein (LDL) levels rise and high density lipoprotein (HDL) levels decline more in boys than in girls. At the menopause, LDL levels increase in women, exceeding those in men throughout the postmenopausal period. If the LDL/HDL ratio is utilized as an index of atherogenic risk, the sex differential in this ratio can account for a substantial proportion of the sex differential in atherosclerosis and, thus, for a major fraction of the sex differential in human longevity. The high male to female ratio of coronary heart disease mortality decreases after the menopause. Some studies have reported a reduction in the incidence of coronary heart disease and in mortality from all causes in women using postmenopausal estrogens. These benefits may be mediated by the effects of estrogen on lipoprotein metabolism. Although suggestive, these studies do not directly confirm the hypothesis related to the influence of endogenous steroids on the sex differential in longevity.

Sex hormones do not decline acutely in men as in women at the menopause. However, some studies have demonstrated a progressive decline in testosterone levels with age in men. In most individuals these levels do not reach the hypogonadal range. Although sexual activity decreases with age, it does not appear to be related directly to testosterone levels. The effects of decreasing testosterone levels on other metabolic activities have not been well defined. Muscle mass and strength decline with age, but whether testosterone contributes to this change is unclear.

Fluid and electrolytes Under normal circumstances there is no change in sodium, potassium, hydrogen ion concentration, or extracellular fluid volume with age. However, adaptive mechanisms are impaired, and acute illness is often complicated by derangements in fluid and electrolyte balance.

The response to sodium restriction is blunted. Older individuals are able to decrease sodium excretion with restriction, but the response is sluggish and the sodium deficit incurred before the decline in sodium excretion becomes maximal is greater than in younger individuals. This salt-losing tendency is contributed to by several factors: (1) nephron loss with age and a consequent increased osmotic load per nephron; (2) decrease in renin, both in the basal and stimulated state with age; and (3) diminished aldosterone levels consequent to the changes in renin.

With or without preexisting myocardial disease, older adults are at increased risk for volume expansion. They are less able to excrete an acute salt load and require a longer time to reestablish balance. These changes relate to a decrease in glomerular filtration rate and decreased baroreceptor reflex sensitivity.

Potassium handling is also altered with age, and older individuals are at increased risk for developing hyperkalemia. With a decreased glomerular filtration rate and decreased aldosterone secretion, renal potassium excretion is altered. Insulin and catecholamines modulate potassium transport into cells. With decreased insulin and beta-adrenergic responsiveness, these adaptive mechanisms are blunted.

Dehydration is a particular problem in older adults when fluid intake is limited and/or insensible loss is increased. Water conservation and urine concentrating ability are impaired. Thirst mechanisms are also impaired, compromising the adaptive response to dehydration. Combined with the salt losing tendency, hypertonic volume depletion is a common presentation.

Possibly the most serious and least-well recognized fluid and electrolyte problem in older adults is water intoxication. Basal vasopressin levels are unaltered in normal aging. However, infusion of hypertonic saline leads to a greater increase in plasma vasopressin than in younger individuals. Conversely, infusion of alcohol leads to a lesser suppression of vasopressin in older individuals. These data suggest increased osmoreceptor sensitivity in older adults with a higher "set-point" for vasopressin secretion. As a result, certain drugs as well as pulmonary and central nervous system disorders are more likely to precipitate the syndrome of inappropriate antidiuretic hormone secretion (SIADH) in older patients.

Renal In cross-sectional studies, renal blood flow, glomerular filtration rate, and creatinine clearance decrease with age. However, creatinine generation also decreases with age, and serum creatinine may not directly reflect creatinine clearance. These changes are important because it is necessary to adjust the dosage of drugs that are excreted primarily by the kidney. Longitudinal studies suggest that renal function does not deterioriate with age in all individuals; in some it remains relatively unchanged, in some it deteriorates only slightly, and in some more markedly. This is in keeping with the variability of aging, but the possibility of decrease in renal function still needs to be considered, particularly in those who are ill

Vision and hearing Age associated changes in vision and hearing may contribute to significant functional impairment in older adults. Visual acuity may decrease due to changes in the retina or neural elements, and changes in refractive power may lead either to increased hyperopia or myopia. Loss of accommodation leads to hyperopia, and nuclear sclerosis leads to cataracts and myopia. Diminished tear secretion in older individuals, especially in postmenopausal women, may lead to dryness of the eyes, which can cause irritation and discomfort and endanger the intactness of the corneal surface.

Hearing changes occur both in the peripheral auditory system and at the level of the cerebral cortex. Loss for hearing of pure tones, particularly for higher frequencies in men, can interfere with both hearing and understanding speech. Brainstem changes may lead to problems in localizing sounds and hearing in noisy environments. Cortical changes may cause difficulty with speech and language. In summary changes in auditory function are more complex than just pure tone loss.

PROGNOSIS With changes in the environment mean life span has increased and is approaching that predicted by "ideal" survival curves. Maximum lifespan, about 120 years for humans, appears not to be changing. Newer techniques of cell and molecular biology will almost certainly define the genetic factors that determine maximum life span, but at present prospects for prolonging it are not realistic.

The molecular and cellular events that limit species longevity lead in vivo to decrements in homeostatic mechanisms and increasing vulnerability of the organism to the environment. Understanding these molecular and cellular changes and the influence of the environment on them should ultimately lead to interventions that increase mean life span and more importantly decrease disability.

REFERENCES

ARNETZ BB et al: The influence of aging on hemoglobin A_c (HbA_{1c}). J Gerontol 37:648, 1982

DAVIDSON MG: The effect of aging on carbohydrate metabolism. A review of the English literature and a practical approach to the diagnosis of diabetes mellitus in the elderly. Metabolism 28:688, 1979

FINCH CE: The regulation of physiological changes during mammalian aging. Quart Rev Biol 51:49, 1976

———, SCHNEIDER EL (eds): *Handbook of the Biology of Aging*. New York, Van Nostrand Reinhold, 1985

FINK RI et al: Mechanisms of insulin resistance in aging. J Clin Invest 71:1523, 1983

FRIEDMAN JR et al: Correlation of estimated renal function parameters versus 24-hour creatinine clearance in ambulatory elderly. J Am Geriatr Soc 37:145, 1989

GOLDSTEIN S et al: Some aspects of cellular aging. J Chron Dis 36:103, 1983

HARMAN SM et al: Pituitary-thyroid hormone economy in healthy aging men: basal indices of thyroid function and thyrotropin responses to constant infusions of thyrotropin releasing hormone. J Clin Endocrinol Metab 58:320, 1984

HAYFLICK L: Biology of aging. N Engl J Med 295:1302, 1976

HAZZARD WR: The sex differential in longevity, in *Principles of Geriatric Medicine*, 2d ed, WR Hazzard et al (eds). New York, McGraw-Hill, 1990, pp 37–47

HELDERMAN JH et al: The response of arginine vasopressin to intravenous ethanol and hypertonic saline in man: The impact of aging. J Gerontol 33:39, 1978

KANE RL et al: *Essentials of Clinical Geriatrics*, 2d ed. New York, McGraw-Hill, 1989

LEBLANC P et al: Effects of age and body position on "airway closure" in man. J Appl Physiol 28:448, 1970

LINDEMAN RD et al: Longitudinal studies on the rate of decline in renal function with age. J Am Geriatr Soc 33:278, 1985

MADER S. Hearing impairment in elderly persons. J Am Geriatr Soc 32:548, 1984

RODEHEFFER RJ et al: Exercise cardiac output is maintained with advancing age in healthy human subjects: Cardiac dilation and increased stroke volume compensate for a diminished heart rate. Circulation 69:203, 1984

ROWE JW et al: Age-related failure of volume-pressure-mediated vasopressin release. J Clin Endocrinol Metab 54:661, 1982

——— et al: Characterization of the insulin resistance of aging. J Clin Invest 71:1581, 1983

WABBA WM: Influence of aging on lung function—clinical significance of changes from age twenty. Anesth Analg 62:764, 1983

section 3 Immunology

13 THE IMMUNE SYSTEM

BARTON F. HAYNES / ANTHONY S. FAUCI

Basic research in immunology has resulted in advances in many clinical areas, ranging from allergy and rheumatology to neurology and cardiology. Monoclonal antibody technology has revolutionized the study of cell surface antigens of effector and regulatory immune cells and provided specific reagents for essentially any target molecules. The isolation, cloning, and sequencing of genes for antigen receptors on B cells, T cells, and products of the major histocompatibility locus has yielded the probes necessary to begin to understand immune effector function. These probes are being used to explain diversification of the T- and B-cell antigen repertoire, induction of self-tolerance (self-antigen nonreactivity), and regulation of immune cell growth and differentiation. Molecular biology techniques have likewise enabled production of large quantities of secreted molecules that regulate immune cell function, e.g., lymphokines from lymphocytes and monokines from monocytes.

Finally, of great significance has been the discovery of the human T-cell lymphotropic virus (HTLV) family of retroviruses (see Chap. 134) that causes forms of leukemia (HTLV type I, adult T cell leukemia) and immunodeficiency [human immunodeficiency virus (HIV), acquired immunodeficiency syndrome (AIDS)]. Analysis of the genetic mechanisms of retrovirus alteration of normal T cell growth has led to a deeper understanding of normal and abnormal immune cell growth. This understanding should bring about new and specific modes of therapy for diseases of disordered immunoregulation such as autoimmune diseases, immunodeficiency diseases, and malignant diseases of the immune system. The aim of this chapter is to provide the essentials of immunology with particular emphasis on those principles relevant to understanding at a basic level the protean clinical and laboratory manifestations of disordered immunity.

PHENOTYPE AND FUNCTION OF IMMUNE CELLS

The dual limbs of the immune system are the thymus-derived (T) lymphocyte and the bone marrow-derived or bursa-equivalent (B) lymphocyte, both of which derive from a common stem cell. Other cell types such as the monocyte-macrophage play major roles in the inductive, regulatory, and effector phases of the immune response. The principal effector and regulator cells of the immune system are T, B, and large granular lymphocytes, and monocyte-macrophages. Nonlymphoid cells such as neutrophils, eosinophils, basophils, and tissue mast cells play roles in the inflammatory response that results from certain immune-mediated reactions and as such must be considered in the scheme of immune cell function. With the advent of monoclonal antibody technology has come the discovery of numerous functional immune cell surface molecules, which have recently been given standardized names based on the reactivity of monoclonal antibodies that bind to them (Table 13-1).

The proportion and distribution of immunocompetent cells in various tissues reflect cell traffic, homing patterns, and functional

TABLE 13-1 Surface molecules of human immune and inflammatory cells

CD group	Other names	Distribution and/or cellular function mediated by surface molecules
T LYMPHOCYTES		
CD1	T6	HLA-related molecules on cortical thymocytes and Langerhan's cells; function unknown.
CD2	T11, sheep erythrocyte receptor	T-cell adhesion and activation
CD3	T3	T-cell-receptor–associated molecules (CD3γ, δ, ϵ, ζ, η) involved in T-cell triggering.
CD4	T4	Marker of inducer-helper T cells and a subset of cytotoxic T cells; also expressed on monocytes. By binding to HLA class II antigen, facilitates antigen recognition by CD4+ cells. CD4 is the surface recognition molecule by which HIV infects CD4+ cells.
CD5	Ly1, T1	T-cell activation; present on T cells and subset of autoantibody-producing B cells.
CD7	3A1	T-cell activation; earliest marker of T lineage.
CD8	T8	Marker of suppressor and cytotoxic T cells. By binding to HLA class I molecule, facilitates CD8+ T-cell recognition of antigen.
T-cell receptor for antigen	TCRαβ or TCRγδ	T-cell activation by antigens.

TABLE 13-1 Surface molecules of human immune and inflammatory cells *(continued)*

CD group	Other names	Distribution and/or cellular function mediated by surface molecules
B LYMPHOCYTES		
CD5	Ly1, T1	Present on autoreactive B cells.
CD9	p24	On B cells, platelets, and activated T cells; function unknown.
CD10	Common acute lymphoblastic leukemia antigen (CALLA) J-5	CD10 is the enzyme-neutral endopeptidase involved in peptide hormone inactivation; present on normal and malignant pre-B cells.
CD19	B4	On most normal and malignant B cells. B-cell activation.
CD20	B1	B-cell activation.
CD21	B2	EBV receptor on B cells; receptor for C3d component of complement.
CD23	Blast-2	Activation antigen of B cells; Fc receptor for IgE.
B cell receptor for antigen	IgM, IgD, IgA, IgG, or IgE	B-cell activation by antigen
MYELOID LINEAGES		
CD11b	MO-1, MAC-1	C3bi receptor (CR3) on monocytes, neutrophils, and dendritic cells.
CD16		Low-affinity Fc receptor for IgG on neutrophils, large granular lymphocytes, and macrophages.
CD32	p40	Fc receptor for IgG.
CD34	My10	Present on myeloid progenitor cells.
CD35		C3b receptor (CR1) present on monocytes, granulocytes, erythrocytes, B cells, dendritic cells, and renal glomerular cells.
OTHER HEMATOPOIETIC MOLECULES		
CD18	LFA-1 β chain	Adhesion molecule present on hematopoietic cells.
CD44	p80, Hermes	Homing receptor on lymphocytes; adhesion molecule on other cell types.
CD45	Leukocyte common antigen, T200	Present on most hematopoietic cell types, function unknown.
CD58	LFA-3	Endogenous ligand for T-cell CD2 molecules on erythrocytes, thymic epithelial cells, and monocytes; general adhesion molecule involved in T-cell activation.
CD54	Intracellular adhesion molecule 1 (ICAM-1)	Adhesion molecule present on multiple cell types; ligand for LFA-1 molecule; cellular receptor for rhinoviruses.

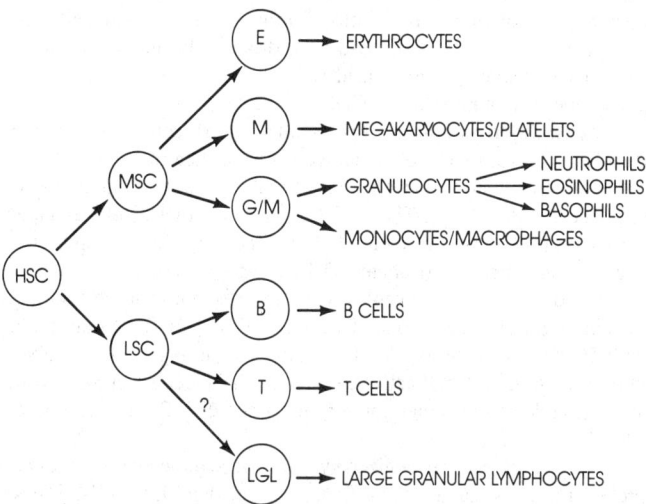

capabilities. Bone marrow is the major site of maturation of B cells, monocyte-macrophages, and granulocytes and contains pluripotent stem cells which, under the influence of various colony stimulating factors (CSF), are capable of giving rise to all hematopoietic cell types (Fig. 13-1). G-CSF stimulates the production of neutrophils; GM-CSF stimulates neutrophil, monocyte, eosinophil, erythroid and megakaryocytoid cell growth; M-CSF drives monocyte differentiation, while IL-3 (multi-CSF) drives neutrophil, monocyte, eosinophil, basophil, erythroid, and megakaryocytoid differentiation. T-cell precursors also arise from hematopoietic stem cells but leave the yolk sac, fetal liver, or bone marrow while immature and home to the thymus for completion of maturation. Mature T lymphocytes, B lymphocytes, and monocytes enter the circulation and home to peripheral lymphoid organs (lymph nodes, spleen) and the gut associated lymphoid tissue (tonsil, Peyer's patches, and appendix) and await activation by foreign antigens. Mature myeloid effector cells (neutrophils, eosinophils, basophils) leave the bone marrow and circulate in peripheral blood as well as home to tissues to perform effector functions associated with the response to foreign antigens (Fig. 13-1).

T CELLS T lymphocytes arise from yolk sac, fetal liver, and bone marrow precursor cells that migrate to the thymus during fetal and early postnatal life. T lymphocytes differ from other immune effector cell types in that the pool of effector T cells is established in the thymus early in life and is maintained throughout life by antigen-driven expansion of long-lived T cells that reside primarily in peripheral lymph organs and recirculate in blood and lymph. Mature T lymphocytes contribute 70 percent to 80 percent of normal peripheral blood lymphocytes, 90 percent of thoracic duct lymphocytes, 30 percent to 40 percent of lymph node cells, and 20 percent to 30 percent of spleen lymphoid cells. In lymph nodes T cells occupy deep paracortical areas around B cell germinal centers and in spleen are in periarteriolar areas of white pulp (see Chap. 63). T cells are the primary effectors of cell-mediated immunity with subsets of T cells maturing into cytotoxic cells capable of lysis of virus-infected or foreign cells. T cells are also the primary regulator cells of T and B lymphocyte and monocyte function by the production of lymphokines and by direct cell contact; in addition, T cells regulate erythroid cell maturation in bone marrow.

Human T cells express cell surface proteins that mark stages of intrathymic T-cell maturation; many of these molecules mediate or augment specific T-cell functions (Table 13-1; Fig. 13-2).

T-cell maturation The earliest identifiable cells of T lineage are CD7+ pro-T cells (i.e., cells in which T-cell receptor genes are neither rearranged nor expressed); they are found in fetal liver, yolk sac, and postnatal bone marrow. In the thymus, CD7+ T-cell precursors first express the T-cell adhesion molecule CD2 and begin cytoplasmic (c) synthesis of components of the CD3 complex of T-cell-receptor–associated molecules (Fig. 13-2). Within CD7+, CD2+, and cCD3+ T-cell precursors, T-cell receptor (TCR) gene rearrangement begins; it eventuates in two T-cell lineages, expressing either TCRαβ chains or TCRγδ chains. T cells expressing the TCRαβ chains comprise the majority of peripheral T cells in blood, lymph

FIGURE 13-1 Model of hematopoietic stem cell differentiation. Multipotential hematopoietic stem cells (HSC) may give rise to more restricted progenitor cells with self-renewal capacity. Thus, lymphocyte-committed stem cells (LSC) give rise to T and B cells. Another group of hematopoietic cells, for which the immediate progenitor is a more differentiated myeloid stem cell (MSC), includes erythrocytes, megakaryocytes, and platelets as well as the granulocyte, monocyte-macrophage series; the origin of large granular lymphocytes in this schema is hypothetical. *(Adapted from MD Cooper et al.)*

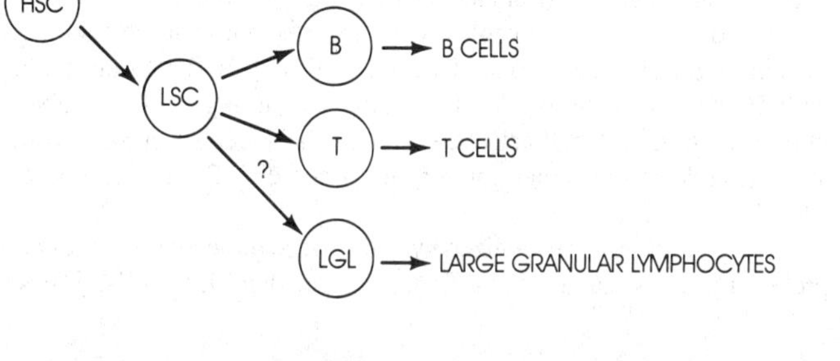

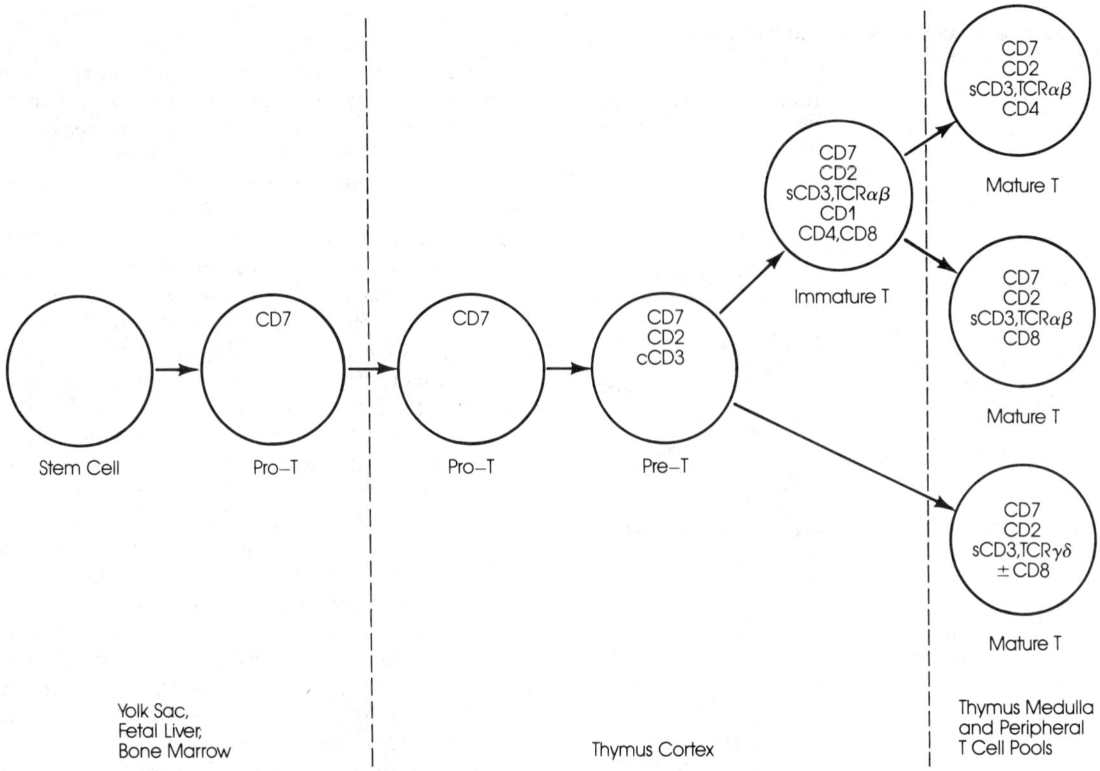

FIGURE 13-2 Model of human T-cell maturation. CD7 pro-T cells migrate to the thymus and stimulate expression of CD2 molecules and the cytoplasmic (c) expression of components of the CD3 complex. CD7+/CD2+/cCD3+ pre-T cells then develop into either surface (s) CD3 TCRαβ+ cells or sCD3 TCRγδ+ cells.

node, and spleen and terminally differentiate into either CD4 or CD8 cells. Cells expressing TCRγδ chains circulate as a minor population in blood; their functions, although not fully known, have been postulated as immune surveillance at epithelial surfaces. CD1 is expressed on immature cortical thymocytes, but with functional maturity, T-cell expression of CD1 ceases and subset antigens CD4 and CD8 are reciprocally expressed. Mature CD4+ TCRαβ+ cells induce B-cell differentiation, induce CD8+ cytotoxic T-cell proliferation, produce various lymphokines, and regulate certain stages of erythropoiesis. A subset of CD4+ cells may also function as cytotoxic effector cells, recognizing foreign antigen of HLA class II. CD8+ TCRαβ+ cells function as suppressors of B-cell antibody synthesis and as cytotoxic effectors, recognizing foreign antigen of HLA class I (see Chap. 14).

T-cell maturation stages are clinically relevant in that T-cell malignancies are derived from one or another of these stages. T-cell acute lymphoblastic leukemia and lymphomas share phenotypic similarities with pro-T, pre-T, or immature T cells and thus are malignancies of immature T cells. Forms of cutaneous T-cell lymphoma (mycosis fungoides, Sézary syndrome) and the syndrome of adult T-cell leukemia (associated with HTLV-I infection) share the phenotype of mature (usually CD4+) T cells.

T-cell antigen receptors The T-cell antigen receptor is a complex of molecules consisting of an antigen-binding heterodimer of either αβ or γδ chains noncovalently linked with five CD3 subunits (γ, δ, ϵ, ζ, and η) (Fig. 13-3). The CD3 ζ chains are either disulfide-linked homodimers (CD3-ζ_2) or disulfide-linked heterodimers composed of one ζ chain and one η chain. TCRαβ or -γδ molecules must be associated with CD3 molecules to be inserted into the cell surface membrane, TCRα being paired with TCRβ and TCRγ being paired with TCRδ. Molecules of the CD3 complex are thought to be involved in transduction of T-cell activation signals via T-cell receptors, while TCRαβ and -γδ molecules combine to form the TCR antigen-binding site.

Foreign antigen is recognized by cell surface molecules on antigen-presenting cells such as macrophages or dendritic cells. These molecules are encoded by HLA-complex genes. Antigen-presenting cells "process" the foreign antigen and display its peptide fragments on their surfaces, where the fragments bind to TCRαβ or -γδ chains of T reactive cells. CD4 molecules act as adhesives and, by direct binding to HLA class II (DR, DQ, or DP) molecules, stabilize the interaction of TCR with the antigen. Similarly CD8 molecules stabilize the TCR-antigen interaction by direct binding to HLA class I (A, B, or C) molecules.

The α, β, γ, and δ T-cell antigen receptor molecules have amino acid sequence homology and structural similarities to immunoglobulin heavy and light chains, and like many functionally relevant molecules of immune cells (e.g., HLA, CD2, CD4, CD8) they are therefore

FIGURE 13-3 Molecules of the T-cell antigen receptor–CD3 complex. T-cell receptor (TCR) heterodimers are composed of either αβ or γδ chains. CD3 molecules are γ, δ, and ϵ chains and a disulfide-linked dimer of either two ζ chains or a ζη heterodimer.

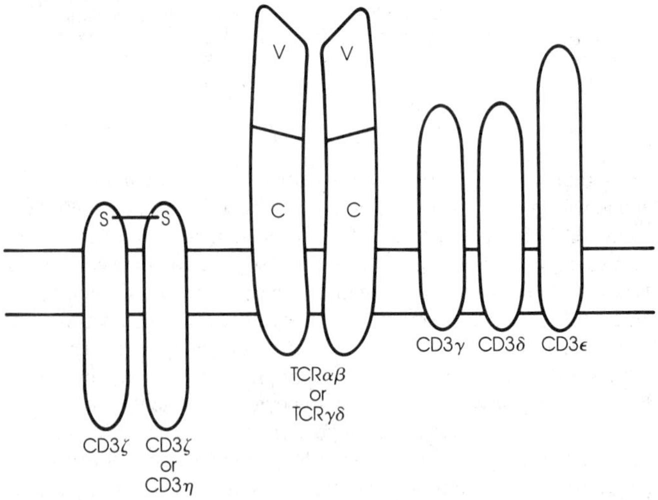

members of the *immunoglobulin gene superfamily*. The TCRβ and -δ chains contains four separately encoded regions, namely the V (variable), D (diversity), J (joining) and C (constant) regions, and the TCRα and -γ chains consist of V, J, and C regions. Thus, molecules of the T-cell antigen receptor have constant and variable regions, and the genes encoding the α, β, γ, and δ chains of these molecules undergo rearrangement during T-cell maturation, culminating in synthesis of the completed molecule.

The variable region elements of α, β, γ, and δ genes, which are separate in the germline, are brought together by DNA rearrangement and deletion during differentiation of the T lymphocyte. Thus, TCR diversity is due to the large numbers of V-J combinations formed during TCR gene rearrangement.

The specificity of mature T cells is largely determined within the thymus. For example, elimination of T cells capable of reacting against autologous (self) antigens (*self tolerance*), thus preventing autoimmune reactivity, may occur there, as may positive selection for T cells that can respond to foreign antigen, i.e., immunocompetent T cells. As mentioned, T cells recognize foreign antigens in association with cell surface molecules encoded for by the major histocompatibility or HLA complex on antigen-presenting cells. Specifically, cytotoxic CD8+ T cells recognize antigens in association with autologous HLA class I (A, B, and C) molecules, and CD4+ helper and CD4+ cytotoxic T cells recognize and respond to foreign antigens bound to autologous HLA class II molecules. This ability to corecognize foreign antigen with autologous class I and II HLA molecules on antigen-presenting cells is referred to as *HLA or MHC restriction* of immune cell interactions.

Nonlymphoid cells of the thymic microenvironment play major roles in the differentiation of T cells. Thymic macrophages and dendritic cells impart to developing thymocytes HLA restriction for immune cell interactions. Thymic epithelial cells produce a variety of cytokines and thymic hormones important in T-cell activation, participate in induction of T-cell tolerance to self antigens, and drive pro-T cells (Fig. 13-2) to proliferate and differentiate.

B CELLS Mature B cells comprise 10 percent to 15 percent of human peripheral blood lymphocytes, 50 percent of splenic lymphocytes, and approximately 10 percent of bone marrow lymphocytes. B cells express on their surface intramembrane immunoglobulin molecules that function as B-cell antigen receptors. B cells also express surface receptors for the Fc region of IgG molecules as well as receptors for activated complement components (C3d, C3b). The primary function of B cells is to produce antibodies. Mature B cells are derived from bone marrow precursor cells that arise continuously throughout life (Fig. 13-1). Like myeloid and erythroid cells, B cells are constantly replaced every few days through cell division from marrow precursor cells. However, the maturation of B lymphocytes differs from myeloid and erythroid cell lines in that B lymphocytes have antigen-dependent and antigen-independent phases of maturation (Fig. 13-4). Pre-B cells arise from precursor cells in bone marrow and are identified by the presence of cytoplasmic immunoglobulin M (cIgM) (initially IgM heavy chain followed by cytoplasmic light chain synthesis). Pre-B cells mature to immature B cells that no longer express cIgM but rather surface IgM (sIgM) molecules. Immature B cells migrate to the periphery and continue antigen-independent maturation, expressing surface IgD, diversifying the B-cell antigen repertoire, and switching the B-cell surface immunoglobulin isotype such that either surface IgM, IgG, IgA, or IgE is expressed alone with IgD. Only one Ig heavy and light chain variable region and thus only one antigen specificity is expressed by each B cell. In lymphoid organs, B cells are the principal cells in lymph node cortical germinal centers and medullary cords and in primary and secondary germinal centers in the white pulp of spleen (see Chap. 63). On contact with antigen, mature B cells in peripheral lymph nodes and spleen either terminally differentiate into antibody-secreting plasma cells or proliferate to form populations of long-lived memory B cells that are capable of interaction when rechallenged with the same antigen (Fig. 13-4).

LARGE GRANULAR LYMPHOCYTES Large granular lymphocytes (LGL) (previously called "null cells") constitute approximately 5 percent to 10 percent of peripheral blood lymphocytes, and are nonadherent, nonphagocytic cells with large azurophilic cytoplasmic granules. LGL express surface receptors for the Fc portion of IgG, and many LGL express some T-lineage markers and proliferate in response to interleukin 2 (T-cell growth factor). Functionally, LGL share features with both monocyte-macrophages and neutrophils in that subsets of LGL mediate antibody dependent cellular cytotoxicity (ADCC) and natural killer (NK) activity. ADCC is the binding of an opsonized (antibody-coated) target cell to an Fc-receptor–bearing effector cell via the Fc region of antibody resulting in lysis of the target by the effector cell. Natural killer cell activity is the nonimmune (i.e., effector cell never having had previous contact with the target), non-antibody-mediated killing of target cells, which are usually malignant cell types. Thus, LGL that mediate NK activity may play an important role in immune surveillance and destruction of cells that spontaneously undergo malignant transformation in vivo. Lymphokine-activated killer, or LAK, cells are lymphocytes that proliferate in vitro to high levels of IL-2 and develop the ability to efficiently

FIGURE 13-4 Model of B-cell differentiation. B cells undergo antigen-independent and antigen-dependent maturation stages that culminate in terminal differentiation into either antibody-secreting plasma cells or memory B cells.

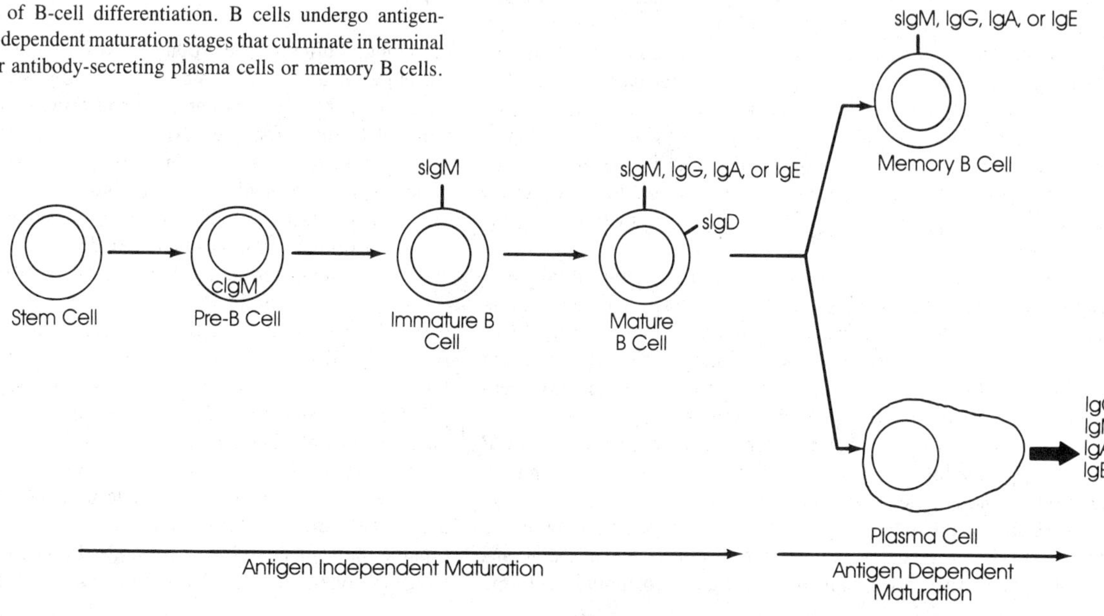

kill tumor cells. LAK cells generated with IL-2 in vitro from patients with solid tumors such as renal cell carcinomas have shown promising antitumor activity in vivo when infused back into patients.

MONOCYTE-MACROPHAGES Monocytes arise from precursor cells within bone marrow (Fig. 13-1) and circulate with a half-life ranging from 1 to 3 days. Monocytes leave the peripheral circulation by marginating in capillaries and then migrating into a vast extravascular pool. Tissue macrophages arise by migration of monocytes from the circulation and by proliferation of macrophage precursors in tissue. Common locations of tissue macrophages (and some of their specialized names) are lymph node; spleen; bone marrow; perivascular connective tissue; serous cavities such as peritoneum, pleura, and synovium; skin connective tissue; lung (alveolar macrophage); liver (Kupffer cell); bone (osteoclast); and central nervous system (microglia). In addition, two types of bone-marrow–derived cells of the myeloid lineage that specialize as antigen-presenting cells are present in many tissues and are called dendritic cells (in lymph nodes, spleen, and thymus) and Langerhan's cells (in skin and thymus) (see Chap. 63).

The monocyte-macrophage system plays a major role in the expression of immune reactivity by mediation of functions such as the presentation of antigen to lymphocytes and the secretion of factors such as interleukin 1 that are central to activation of T lymphocytes. Under certain circumstances monocytes can also mediate immunoregulatory functions such as suppressor cell activity. In addition, monocyte-macrophages mediate effector functions such as destruction of antibody-coated bacteria, tumor cells, or even normal hematopoietic cells in certain types of autoimmune cytopenias. Activated macrophages can also mediate NK-like activity and eliminate cell types such as tumor cells in the absence of antibody. Monocyte-macrophages express surface receptors for a number of molecules, including the Fc region of IgG, activated complement components, and various lymphokines (macrophage inhibitory and activating factors) (Table 13-1). In addition, monocyte-macrophages express cell surface HLA class II (Ia-like) antigens and specific cell surface differentiation antigens. Finally, macrophage secretory products are more diverse than those known for any other cell of the immune system. These secretory products allow the macrophage to exert both pro- and anti-inflammatory effects and to regulate other cell types. Among monocyte-macrophage secreted products are hydrolytic enzymes, products of oxidative metabolism, tumor necrosis factor, and interleukin 1 (IL-1), also called *leukocytic pyrogen* and *lymphocyte activating factor*, which affects lymphocytes, hepatocytes, fibroblasts, synoviocytes, and cells within the hypothalamus.

NEUTROPHILS, EOSINOPHILS, AND BASOPHILS Granulocytes are present in nearly all forms of inflammation and are nonspecific amplifiers and effectors of specific responses. Unchecked accumulation and activation of granulocytes can lead to host tissue damage as seen in neutrophil- and eosinophil-mediated necrotizing vasculitis. Granulocytes are derived from stem cells in bone marrow (Fig. 13-1). Each type of granulocyte (neutrophil, eosinophil, basophil) is derived from a different subclass of progenitor cell which is stimulated to proliferate by colony-stimulating factors. During terminal maturation of granulocytes, class-specific nuclear morphology and cytoplasmic granules appear that allow for histologic identification of granulocyte type.

Neutrophils express Fc receptors for IgG and activated complement components (C3b, C3d) (Table 13-1). Upon interaction of neutrophils with immune complexes, azurophilic granules (containing myeloperoxidase, lysozyme, elastase, and other enzymes) and specific granules (containing lactoferrin, lysozyme, collagenase, and other enzymes) are released, and microbicidal superoxide radicals (O_2^-) are generated at the neutrophil surface. The generation of superoxide is thought to lead to inflammation by direct injury to tissue and cells and by alteration of macromolecules such as collagen and DNA.

Eosinophils express Fc receptors for IgG and are potent cytotoxic effector cells for various parasitic targets. Intracytoplasmic contents of eosinophils, such as major basic protein, eosinophil cationic protein, and eosinophil-derived neurotoxin, are capable of directly damaging tissues and may be responsible in part for the organ system dysfunction in the hypereosinophilic syndromes (see Chap. 64). Since the eosinophil granule contains anti-inflammatory types of enzymes (histaminase, arylsulfatase, phospholipase D) eosinophils may down-regulate or terminate ongoing inflammatory responses in normal homeostasis.

TABLE 13-2 Mediators released from human mast cells and basophils

Mediator	Actions
Histamine	Smooth muscle contraction, increased vascular permeability
Slow reacting substance of anaphylaxis (SRSA) (leukotriene C4, D4, E4)	Smooth muscle contraction
Eosinophil chemotactic factor of anaphylaxis (ECF-A)	Chemotactic attraction of eosinophils
Platelet activating factor	Activates platelets to secrete serotonin and other mediators; smooth muscle contraction; induce vascular permeability
Neutrophil chemotactic factor (NCF)	Chemotactic attraction of neutrophils
Leukotactic activity (leukotriene B4)	Chemotactic attraction of neutrophils
Heparin	Anticoagulant
Basophil kallikrein of anaphylaxis (BK-A)	Cleaves kininogen to form bradykinin

The normal functions of basophils and tissue mast cells are not completely understood; the capacity of basophil mediators to increase local delivery of antibodies and complement by increasing vascular permeability is hypothetical. Thus, the basophil is identified principally with allergic reactions and some delayed cutaneous hypersensitivity states. Certainly the promotion of increased vascular permeability by basophils is important in the genesis of inflammatory lesions in some vasculitis syndromes (see Chap. 276). Basophils express surface receptors for IgE, and upon cross linking of basophil-bound IgE by antigen, release histamine, eosinophil chemotactic factor of anaphylaxis, and neutral protease—all mediators of components of immediate (anaphylaxis) hypersensitivity responses (Table 13-2). In addition basophils express surface receptors for activated complement components (C3a, C5a), through which mediator release can be directly effected (see Chap. 267 for a discussion of tissue mast cells).

HUMORAL MEDIATORS OF IMMUNITY: IMMUNOGLOBULINS

Immunoglobulins are the products of differentiated B cells and mediate the humoral arm of the immune response. Their primary functions are to bind specifically to antigen and bring about the inactivation or removal of the offending toxin, microbe, parasite, or other foreign substance from the body. The structural basis of immunoglobulin molecule function and immunoglobulin gene organization has provided insight into the role of antibody in normal protective immunity and in unwanted immune-mediated damage by immune complexes and autoantibody formation against host determinants.

All immunoglobulins have the basic structure of two heavy and two light chains (Fig. 13-5). Immunoglobulin isotype (i.e., G, M, A, D, E) is determined by the type of heavy and light chain present. IgG and IgA isotypes can further be divided into subclasses (G1, G2, G3, G4, and A1, A2) based on specific antigenic determinants on heavy chains. The characteristics of human immunoglobulins are outlined in Table 13-3. The four chains are covalently linked by disulfide bonds. Each chain is made up of a variable (V) region and constant (C) regions (also called domains), themselves made up of homologous units of 110 amino acids. Light chains have one variable (VL) and one constant (CL) region; heavy chains have one variable

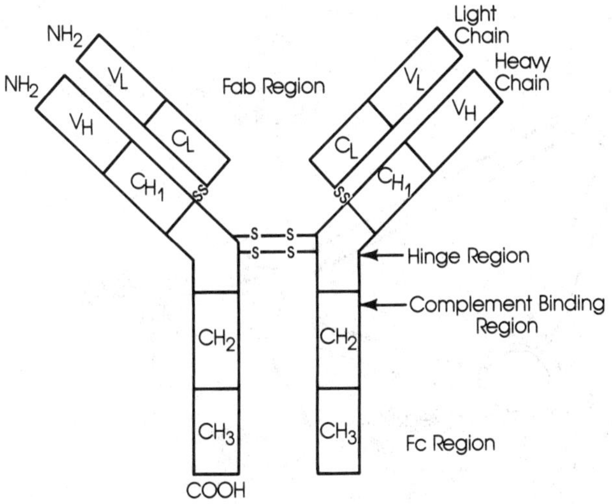

FIGURE 13-5 Schematic structure of the immunoglobulin G (IgG) molecule.

region (VH) and 3 or 4 constant (CH) regions, depending on isotype. As the name suggests, constant regions are made up of homologous sequences and share the same primary structure as all other chains of the same isotype and subclass. Constant regions are involved in biological functions of immunoglobulin molecules. The CH_2 domain of IgG and the CH_4 domain of IgM are involved with binding of the C1q portion of C1. The CH region at the carboxyterminus end of the IgG molecule, the Fc region (Fig. 13-5) binds to surface Fc receptors of macrophages, large granular lymphocytes, B cells, neutrophils, and eosinophils.

Variable regions (VL and VH) constitute the antibody-binding (Fab) region of the molecule. Within the VL and VH regions are hypervariable regions of extreme sequence variability that constitute the antigen-binding site unique to each immunoglobulin molecule. The *idiotype* is the specific region of the Fab portion of the immunoglobulin molecule to which antigen binds. Antibodies against the idiotype portion of an antibody molecule are called *anti-idiotype antibodies*. The formation of anti-idiotype antibodies in vivo during a normal B-cell antibody response may generate a negative (or "off") signal to B cells to terminate antibody production (see "Autoimmune Disease," below).

IgG comprises approximately 75 percent of the total serum immunoglobulin. The four IgG subclasses are numbered in order of their level in serum, IgG1 being found in greatest amounts and IgG4 the least. IgG subclasses have clinical relevance in their varying ability to bind macrophage and neutrophil Fc receptors and to activate complement (Table 13-3). IgG antibodies are frequently the antibody made after rechallenge of the host with antigen (secondary antibody response). Of the immunoglobulin isotypes only IgG crosses the placenta.

IgM antibodies normally circulate as a 950,000-Da pentamer with 160,000-Da monomers joined by a molecule called the J chain, a 15,000-Da nonimmunoglobulin molecule that also effects polymerization of IgA molecules. IgM is the first immunoglobulin to appear in the immune response (primary antibody response) and is the initial type of antibody made by neonates. Membrane IgM in the monomeric form also functions as a major antigen receptor on the surface of the mature B cell. IgM is an important component of immune complexes in autoimmune diseases. For instance, IgM antibodies against IgG molecules (*rheumatoid factors*) are present in high titers in rheumatoid arthritis, other collagen diseases, and some infectious diseases (subacute bacterial endocarditis). IgM antibody binds the C1 component of complement via the CH_4 domain and thus is a potent activator of complement.

IgA comprises only 10 to 15 percent of total serum immunoglobulin but is the predominant class of immunoglobulin in secretions. IgA in secretions (tears, saliva, nasal secretions, GI tract fluid, and human milk) is in the form of secretory IgA (sIgA), a polymer consisting of two IgA monomers, a joining molecule called the J chain, and a glycoprotein called the secretory piece. Of the two IgA subclasses, IgA1 is primarily found in serum, whereas IgA2 is more prevalent in secretions. IgA fixes complement via the alternative pathway and has potent antiviral activity in man by prevention of virus binding to respiratory and gastrointestinal epithelial cells.

IgD is found in minute quantities in serum (Table 13-3) and along with IgM is a major receptor for antigen on the B-cell surface.

Present in serum in very low concentrations (Table 13-3), IgE is

TABLE 13-3 Characteristics of human immunoglobulins

						Complement activation			
Isotype	Molecular weight	Heavy chain	Light chain	Adult average serum level (mg/dL)	Half-life (days)	Classical pathway	Alternative pathway	Binding to cells via Fc	Other biologic properties
IgG	150,000	γ_1, γ_2, γ_3, γ_4	κ or λ	1250±300	23.0	IgG1, IgG2, IgG3, yes; IgG4 no	IgG1, IgG2, IgG3, no; IgG4 yes	Macrophages, neutrophils, eosinophils large granular lymphocytes	Placental transfer
IgM	190,000 (950,000)*	μ	κ or λ	125±50	5.1	Yes	No	Lymphocytes	Primary antibody response, rheumatoid factor
IgA	160,000 (385,000)†	α_1, α_2	κ or λ	210±50	5.8	No	Yes	Lymphocytes	Antibody in mucous secretions
IgD	175,000	δ	κ or λ	4	2.8	No	Yes	None	Primary lymphocyte surface molecule
IgE	190,000	ε	κ or λ	0.03	2.5	No	Yes	Mast cells, basophils, B cells	Mediates anaphylaxis, allergy

* IgM circulates as a pentameric molecule.
† Secretory IgA is a dimer.
SOURCE: Adapted with permission from DJ Jeske, JD Capra, Immunoglobulin: Structure and Function, in *Fundamental Immunology*, WE Paul (ed), New York, Raven, 1984.

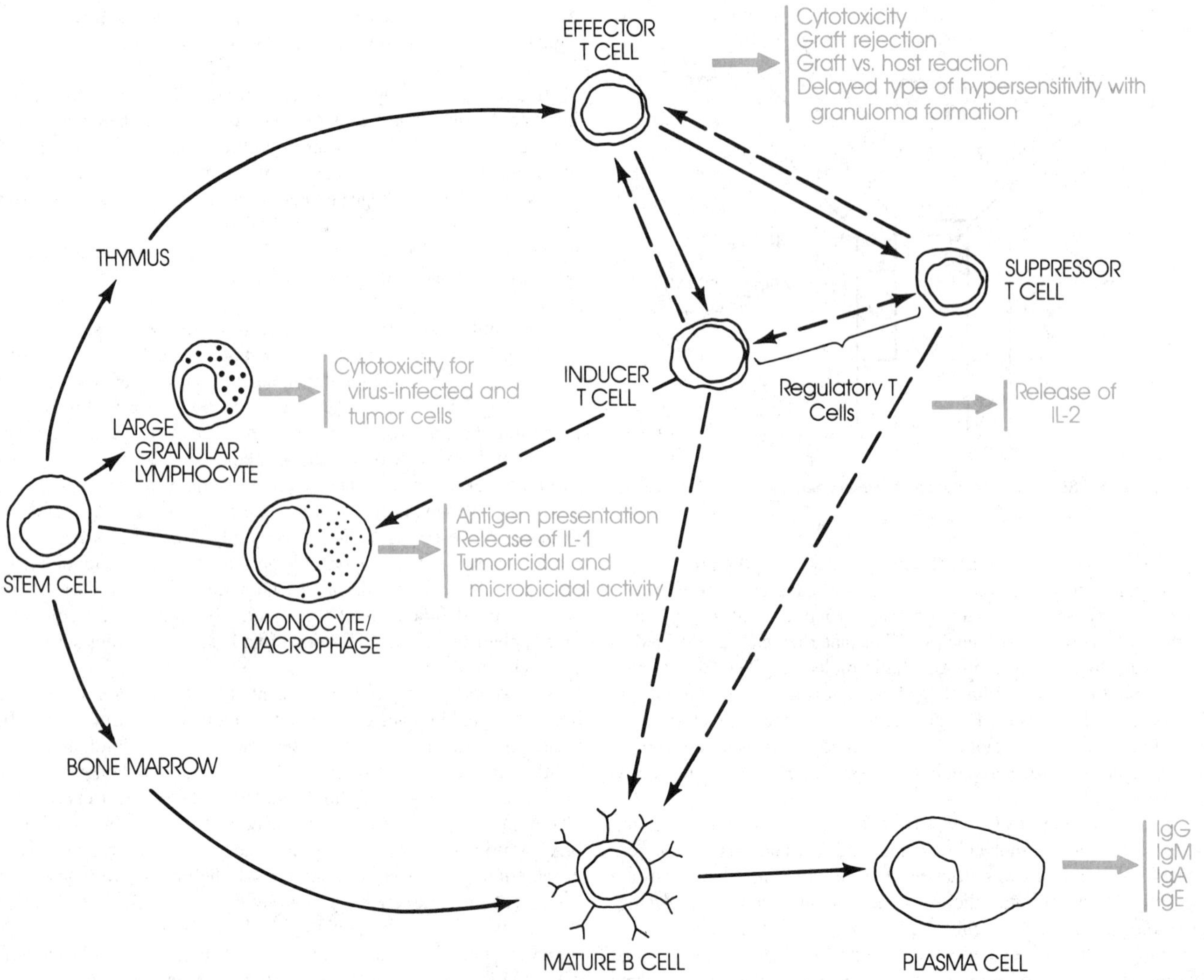

FIGURE 13-6 Schematic representation of cellular interactions involved in the generation of cell-mediated and humoral immunity. *[Adapted with permission from AS Fauci, in WN Kelly et al (eds).]*

the major class of immunoglobulin involved in arming mast cells and basophils by binding to these cells via the Fc region. Antigen crosslinking of IgE molecules on basophil and mast cell surfaces results in release of mediators of the immediate hypersensitivity response.

Similar to the genes for the T-cell antigen receptor, the heavy and light chains of immunoglobulin are each encoded by multiple genetic elements physically separated in germline DNA but brought together to create a single active gene in B cells.

The variable regions of light chains (e.g., kappa light chains) are constructed from two genes called VK and JK. These genes, though on the same chromosome, are far apart in the germline but during B lymphocyte maturation are brought close together with excision of intervening DNA sequences (gene rearrangement). There are approximately 300 VK genes and 5 JK genes resulting in the pairing of VK and JK genes to create 1500 different light chain combinations. The number of distinct kappa light chains that can be generated is increased by somatic mutations within the VK and JK genes, thus creating a large number of specificities from a limited amount of germline genetic information.

In heavy chain immunoglobulin gene rearrangement the VH domain is created by the joining of three types of germline genes called *VH, DH,* and *JH,* thus allowing for even greater diversity in the variable region of heavy chains than for light chains. (See Chap. 263 for more on generation of clonal diversity of B cells.)

CELLULAR INTERACTIONS IN REGULATION OF THE NORMAL IMMUNE RESPONSE

The net result of activation of the humoral (B-cell) and cellular (T-cell) arms of the immune system by foreign antigen is the elimination of antigen directly by effector cells or in concert with specific antibody. In addition, a series of regulatory cells are activated which modulate T-effector-cell activation and B-cell antibody production. Figure 13-6 is a simplified schematic diagram of the immune system outlining some of these cellular interactions.

MONOCYTE–T CELL INTERACTIONS Many of the activation and regulatory effects of lymphocytes and monocytes occur via soluble mediators (Table 13-4). Monocyte-macrophages are required for optimal activation of T cells by antigens or by mitogens (nonspecific activators of lymphocytes). A soluble macrophage product, IL-1, can substitute in some cases for intact macrophages. Upon contact with antigens or mitogens, macrophages secrete IL-1, two effects of which are (1) the induction of receptors for T-cell growth factor or interleukin 2 (IL-2) on T cells and (2) the induction of IL-2 secretion. IL-2 in turn activates T cells, resulting in expansion of effector and regulatory T cells that have also been induced to express IL-2 receptors. Effector T cells mediate a variety of functions including the killing of virus-infected cells, graft rejection, graft-versus-host reaction, delayed-type hypersensitivity, and the release of lymphokines (Table 13-4).

TABLE 13-4 Selected soluble mediators of cellular and humoral immune responses

Factor	Source	Target cells	Effects
IL-1	Monocyte-macrophages, dendritic cells, large granular lymphocytes, B- and T-cell lines, endothelial cells, epidermal cells, thymic epithelial cells, fibroblasts, astrocytes	B cells, T cells, fibroblasts, synovial cells, neutrophils, macrophages, lymphocytes, large granular lymphocytes, hypothalamus	Induces fever; induces T and B cell activation; induces fibroblast, synovial cell, and endothelial cell growth; induces tissue catabolism; enhances natural killer cell activity; chemoattractant for neutrophils, macrophages, lymphocytes
IL-2	T cells	T and B cells	Induces growth of T and B cells, induces cytotoxic T cell activity, induces natural killer and lymphokine-activated killer cell activity
IL-3	T cells	Hematopoietic stem cells, erythroid and myeloid progenitor cells	Drives differentiation of erythroid, myeloid, and multipotent progenitor cells
IL-4	Activated T cells	T and B cells	Induces proliferation of B and T cells; increases IgE secretion by B cells
IL-5	T cells	B cells, eosinophils	Induces differentiation of B cells and eosinophils
IL-6	Monocytes, fibroblasts, various malignant cell lines	B cells, fibroblasts, hepatocytes	Induces B cell growth, induces HLA antigen on fibroblasts, induces production of acute-phase proteins by hepatocytes
IL-7	Bone marrow stromal cells	B-cell and T cell precursors	Promotes growth of B- and T-cell precursors
Interferon γ	T cells, large granular lymphocytes	B cells, monocytes-macrophages, large granular lymphocytes, endothelial cells, fibroblasts, epithelial cells	Augments B-cell proliferation, augments antimicrobial and tumoricidal activity of monocyte-macrophages, induces IgG Fc receptor expression on monocytes and HLA class II expression on many cell types, augments natural killer cell activity

SOURCE: Adapted with permission from O'Garra et al, Immunol Today 9:45, 1988.

T CELL–T CELL AND T CELL–B CELL INTERACTIONS The expression of immune cell function is the result of a complex series of events occurring in phases. Both T and B lymphocytes mediate immune functions, and each of these cell types, when given appropriate signals, passes through stages, from activation and induction through proliferation, differentiation, and ultimately effector functions. The effector function expressed may be at the end point of a response, such as secretion of antibody by a differentiated plasma cell, or it might serve a regulatory function that modulates other functions such as is seen with inducer or suppressor T lymphocytes, which modulate both differentiation of B cells and activation of cytotoxic T cells. As shown schematically in Fig. 13-6, upon activation by IL-1 and IL-2, regulatory T-cell subsets are generated that exert positive and negative forces on effector cells. Thus, for B cells and cytotoxic (CD4+ or CD8+) T cells, there are CD4+ inducer and CD8+ suppressor cells that either facilitate or down-regulate effector cell function. For B cells, trophic effects are mediated by a variety of cytokines, particularly T-cell–derived B-cell growth factor (BCGF or IL-4) and B-cell differentiating factor (BCDF or IL-6), which act at sequential stages of B-cell maturation, resulting in B-cell proliferation, differentiation, and ultimately antibody secretion (Table 13-4). For T cells, trophic factors include inducer T-cell secretion of IL-2. In addition, B cells themselves are capable of processing and presenting antigens to T cells.

These complex cellular and humoral interactions involve a delicate balance among positive and negative influences and ultimately result in expression of an appropriate immune response. The slightest imbalance in these immunoregulatory circuits may result in aberrant immune function leading to clinically apparent immune-mediated disease.

THE COMPLEMENT SYSTEM

The complement system is a cascading series of plasma enzymes, regulatory proteins, and proteins capable of cell lysis whose principal site of synthesis is the liver. There are two arms of the complement system (Fig. 13-7). Activation of the classical complement pathway via C1, C4, and C2 and activation of the alternative complement pathway via factor D, C3, and factor B both lead to cleavage and activation of C3. C3 is a protein whose activation fragments, when bound to target surfaces such as bacteria and other foreign antigens, are critical for opsonization (coating by antibody and complement) in preparation for phagocytosis.

The protein fragment C3b, split from C3, is necessary for activation of the terminal complement components, C5–9. These form the so-

FIGURE 13-7 Components of the complement system. *[Adapted with permission from WE Paul, in WE Paul (ed).]*

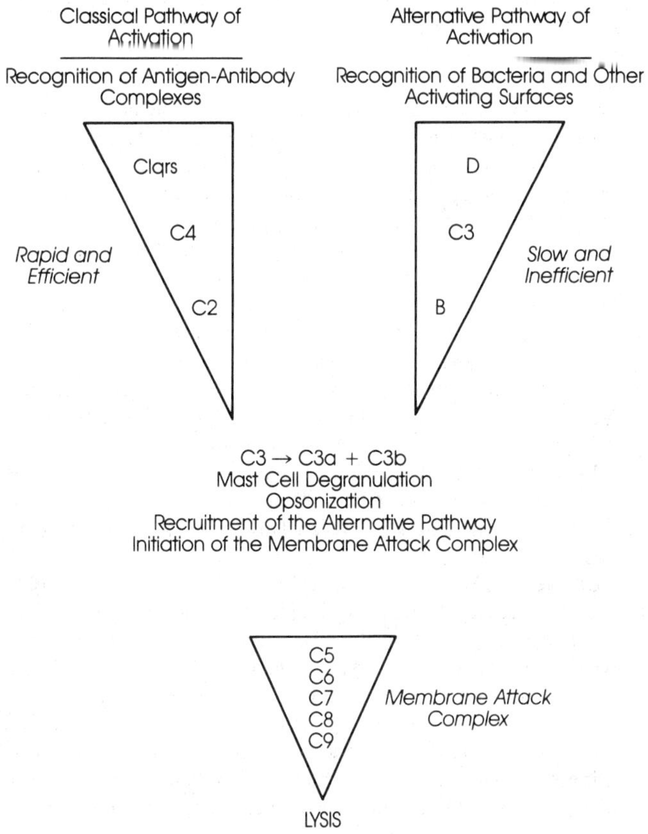

called membrane attack complex which, when inserted into cell membranes brings about osmotic lysis of the cell.

C3b also joins with a cleavage product of factor B (called Bb) to form C3bBb, also known as the *alternative pathway C3 convertase*. Activation of the classical complement pathway results in cleavage of C4 and C2 with a resulting complex of fragments, C4b2a, also called the *classical pathway C3 convertase*. Both the classical C3 convertase (C4b2a) and the alternative pathway C3 convertase (C3bBb) function to cleave C3 to form active C3b, thus driving activation of the C5–9 membrane attack complex. The fact that C3b can combine with Bb to form the alternative C3 convertase gives rise to a potent positive feedback loop for production of C3b and thus continued activation of terminal complement components.

Activation of the classical complement pathway is by interaction of antigen and antibody to form immune complexes that bind C1q, a subunit of C1. Immunoglobulin isotypes that bind C1q and activate the classical pathway are IgM, IgG1, IgG2, and IgG3. In contrast, IgA1, IgA2, and IgD activate complement via the alternative pathway. Activation of the complement cascade via the classical pathway by IgG- or IgM-containing immune complexes is a rapid and efficient, pathway to activation of terminal components. In contrast, activation of the alternative pathway via IgA-containing immune complexes or by bacterial endotoxin is a slower and less efficient pathway to terminal component activation. Thus, the immunoglobulin isotype composition of immune complexes is a critical factor in determining complement activation and, therefore, the efficiency of clearance of immune complexes by C3-receptor-bearing cells.

In addition to the role of complement in opsonization and cell lysis, several complement component fragments are potent mediators of cell activation. C3a and C5a bind to receptors on mast cells and basophils, resulting in release of histamine and other mediators of anaphylaxis. C5a is also a potent chemoattractant for neutrophils and monocyte-macrophages (Table 13-5).

TABLE 13-5 Biologic activities of some complement components

Component	Activity
C4a weak anaphylatoxin	Evokes histamine release from basophils and mast cells.
C3a	Anaphylatoxin; evokes histamine release from basophils and mast cells.
C5a	Anaphylatoxin; evokes histamine release from basophils and mast cells; potent chemoattractant for monocytes and neutrophils.
C3b, C3bi	Enhancement of phagocytosis by neutrophils and monocytes. Promotes immune complex binding to cells within monocyte-macrophage system, as well as neutrophils. C3b with Bb forms alternative pathway C3 convertase and amplifies alternative pathway. Promotes solubilization of immune complexes.
C5–9	Membrane attack complex; forms transmembrane channels leading to cell destruction.

SOURCE: Adapted with permission from Ruddy S: Plasma protein effectors of inflammation: Complement, in WN Kelley et al (eds).

MECHANISMS OF IMMUNE DAMAGE

Several responses by the host to foreign antigen culminate in the rapid and efficient elimination of nonself substances (Table 13-6). In these scenarios the classic weapons of the immune system (T cells, B cell, macrophages) interface with cells and soluble products that are mediators of inflammatory responses (neutrophils, eosinophils, basophils, kinin and coagulation systems, and complement cascade).

There are three general phases of host defense: (1) specific and nonspecific recognition of foreign antigens mediated by T and B lymphocytes, macrophages, and the alternative complement pathway, (2) amplification of the inflammatory response with recruitment of specific and nonspecific effector cells by complement components, lymphokines and monokines, kinins, arachidonic acid metabolites, and mast cell–basophil products, and (3) macrophage, neutrophil, and lymphocyte participation in antigen destruction with ultimate removal by phagocytosis of antigen particles (by macrophages or neutrophils) or by direct cytotoxic mechanisms (involving macrophages, neutrophils, and lymphocytes). Under normal circumstances, orderly progression of host defenses through these phases results in a well-controlled immune and inflammatory response that protects the host from the offending antigen. However, regulatory dysfunction of any of the host defense systems can damage host tissue and produce clinically apparent disease.

IMMUNE COMPLEX FORMATION (TYPE III REACTION) Clearance of antigen by immune complex formation between antigen and antibody is a highly effective mechanism of host defense. However, depending on the level of immune complexes formed and their physicochemical properties, immune complexes may or may not result in host and foreign cell damage. After antigen exposure, certain types of soluble antigen-antibody complexes freely circulate and, if not cleared by the reticuloendothelial system, can be deposited in blood vessel walls and in other tissues such as renal glomeruli. The precise mechanisms whereby immune complexes damage tissues, particularly blood vessels, are discussed in Chaps. 268 and 276.

IgE MEDIATED ALLERGIC REACTIONS–ANAPHYLAXIS (TYPE I) Mast cells and basophils have receptors for the Fc portion of IgE, and cell-bound IgE effectively "arms" basophils and mast cells. Mediator release is triggered by antigen interaction with Fc-receptor–bound IgE; the mediators released are responsible for the pathophysiologic changes of allergic disease (Table 13-2). Mediators released from mast cells and basophils can be divided into three broad categories of action. Those which: (1) increase vascular permeability and contract smooth muscle (histamine, platelet activating factor, SRS-A, BK-A); (2) are chemotactic for or activate other inflammatory cells (ECF-A, NCF, leukotriene B4); and (3) modulate the release of other mediators (BK-A, platelet activating factor).

CYTOTOXIC REACTIONS OF ANTIBODY (TYPE II) In this type of immunologic injury, complement-fixing (C1 binding) antibodies against normal or foreign cells or tissues (IgM, IgG1, IgG2, IgG3) bind complement via the classical pathway and initiate a sequence of events similar to that initiated by immune complex deposition, resulting in cell lysis or tissue injury. Examples of type II antibody-mediated cytotoxic reactions include red cell lysis in transfusion reactions, Goodpasture's syndrome with antiglomerular basement

TABLE 13-6 Mechanisms of immunologically mediated inflammation

Mechanism type	Characteristics of inflammatory response	Clinical disease type
I Allergic (IgE-mediated)	Basophil and mast cell products leading to immediate flare-and-wheal.	Atopy, anaphylaxis
II Cytotoxic or tissue-specific antibody (IgM- or IgG-mediated)	Acute inflammation via phagocytic cells and deposition of complement in tissues, lysis or phagocytosis of target cells.	Goodpasture's syndrome, autoimmune cytopenias, anti-red cell antibodies in transfusion reactions
III Immune complex (IgG-, IgM-, IgA-mediated)	Accumulation of neutrophils, macrophages, complement components.	Systemic necrotizing vasculitis, systemic lupus erythematosus, serum sickness syndromes
IV Delayed hypersensitivity	T cell–induced mononuclear cell accumulation of regulatory and effector T cells and macrophages. Lymphokines and monokines released. Often granuloma formation.	Tuberculosis, sarcoidosis, Wegener's granulomatosis and other forms of granulomatous vasculitis

membrane antibody formation, and possibly juvenile onset diabetes mellitus with anti-islet cell antibody production.

CLASSICAL DELAYED-TYPE HYPERSENSITIVITY REACTIONS (TYPE IV) Inflammatory reactions initiated by mononuclear leukocytes and not by antibody alone have been termed delayed-type hypersensitivity reactions. The term "delayed" has been used to contrast a secondary cellular response which appears 48 to 72 h after antigen exposure to an "immediate" hypersensitivity response generally seen within 12 h of antigen challenge and initiated by basophil mediator release or preformed antibody. For example, in an individual previously infected with mycobacterium tuberculosis (TB) organisms, intradermal placement of TB purified protein derivative (PPD) as a skin test challenge results in an indurated area of skin a 48 to 72 h, indicating previous exposure to TB.

The cellular events that result in classical delayed-type hypersensitivity responses are centered around T cells, their soluble products and macrophages. In the general scheme outlined in Fig. 13-6, antigen is processed by macrophages and presented to T cells expressing a cell surface receptor specific for the antigen. Macrophage-secreted IL-1 amplifies the clonal expansion of antigen-specific T cells, and lymphokines are secreted to recruit other T cells and macrophages nonspecifically to participate in the inflammatory response. Once recruited, macrophages frequently undergo epithelioid cell transformation and form giant cells. This type of mononuclear cell infiltrate is termed *granulomatous inflammation*. Examples of diseases in which delayed-type hypersensitivity plays a major role are fungal infections (*histoplasmosis*), mycobacterial infections, chlamydial infections (*Lymphogranuloma venereum*), helminth infections (*schistosomiasis*), reactions to toxins (*berylliosis*), and hypersensitivity reactions to organic dusts (*hypersensitivity pneumonitis*). In addition, delayed-type hypersensitivity responses may play a role in *rheumatoid arthritis* and *Wegener's granulomatosis* (see Chaps. 270 and 276).

AUTOIMMUNE DISEASE Autoimmune disease is characterized by production of either antibodies that react with host tissue or immune effector T cells that are autoreactive. Since B-cell responses in man generally require inducer T cells, a B-cell autoantibody response directly implies disordered T-cell immunoregulatory control. In some instances, autoantibodies may arise by a normal T- and B-cell response activated by foreign organisms or substances that contain antigens, particularly polysaccharides, that cross react with similar polysaccharides in body tissues. Examples of clinically relevant autoantibodies are antibodies against acetylcholine receptors in myasthenia gravis; and anti-DNA, antierythrocyte, and antiplatelet antibodies in systemic lupus erythematosus.

The clonal selection theory was put forth by Burnet in 1949 to explain autoimmunity. Burnet proposed that the contact of antibody-forming cells with their respective antigens during fetal or early postnatal life lead to their elimination. Thus, in this theory self-reactive clones are avoided unless they arise in later life by somatic mutation of lymphocytes. The progeny of such mutant cells would give rise to self-reacting antibodies. As the study of autoimmunity has progressed, it has become clear that the genesis of autoimmune B and T cells is far more complex than originally thought. Certain drugs (procainamide, phenytoin) and infectious agents (Epstein-Barr virus, *Mycoplasma pneumoniae*) can elicit the production of autoantibodies to a wide array of host antigens in otherwise normal persons. Moreover, normal mice produce autoantibodies when given injections of nonspecific activators of lymphocytes (mitogens). In all of these circumstances, the autoantibodies combine with ubiquitous antigens: DNA, IgG (as the target of an IgM rheumatoid factor), phospholipids (cardiolipins), erythrocytes, lymphocytes, or cytoskeletal components (vimentin, keratins). Thus, production of autoantibodies is an inherent property of the normal immune system. The immune system controls the tendency to produce autoantibodies by a feedback network of T and B cells. It is thought that B cells normally are inhibited from terminal differentiation by suppressor T cells, a lack of inducer T cells, or both. In autoimmunity an imbalance between the two types of T cells can perturb the immunoregulatory network; this may bring about activation of autoreactive B cells.

As mentioned above in the description of immunoglobulins, the unique portion of the variable region of the immunoglobulin molecule where antigen binds is called the *idiotype*, and an antibody that reacts specifically with that region is called an *anti-idiotype antibody*. The specificity of antibody molecules and the regulation of antibody production have been probed by making rabbit antihuman idiotypic antibodies. There are also autologous anti-idiotypes (auto-anti-idiotypes) that arise during the course of the normal immune response. For example, auto-anti-idiotypes against antitetanus antibodies develop during normal immunization of humans to tetanus toxoid and may serve to deliver "off" signals to B cells secreting antitetanus antibodies. Idiotypes and auto-anti-idiotype antibodies may be an important component of the immunoregulatory network. Anti-idiotype antibodies may also be relevant to two types of autoimmunity: (1) dysfunction of the idiotype–anti-idiotype antibody system could lead to B-cell hyperreactivity by failure to generate "off" signals for B-cell differentiation, and (2) some antireceptor antibodies produced in autoimmune diseases (antiacetylcholine receptor antibodies in myasthenia gravis, anti-insulin receptor antibodies in forms of Type I diabetes mellitus, and antithyrotropin receptor antibodies in thyrotoxicosis) may be anti-idiotype antibodies made against the antibody combining site (idiotype) of an autoantibody.

Finally, genetic factors likely play a role in the genesis of autoimmune disease, either by selecting for inherent B-cell hyperreactivity and tendency toward autoantibody formation or via other unknown factors. Linkage of autoimmune diseases with known genetic loci such as the major histocompatibility complex has provoked great interest. Myasthenia gravis, thyrotoxicosis and pernicious anemia are all associated with HLB B8 (Class I) and DR3 (Class II) alloantigen expression (see Chap. 14) and are also associated with certain immunoglobulin heavy chain allotypic markers. Genetic marker systems such as HLA types and immunoglobulin heavy chain allotypic antigens may be associated with autoimmunity by making the host susceptible in some way to antiself immune cell activation. Thus, multiple genes and/or events are operative in the ultimate generation of the clinical autoimmune state.

CLINICAL EVALUATION OF IMMUNE FUNCTION Clinical assessment of immunity requires investigation of the four major components of the immune system that participate in host defense and in pathogenesis of autoimmune diseases: (1) humoral immunity (B cells), (2) cell-mediated immunity (T cells, monocytes), (3) phagocytic cells of the reticuloendothelial system (macrophages), as well as polymorphonuclear leukocytes, and (4) complement. Clinical problems that require an evaluation of immunity include chronic infections, recurrent infection, unusual infecting agents, and certain autoimmune syndromes. The type of clinical syndrome under evaluation can provide information regarding possible immune defects. Defects in cellular immunity generally result in viral, mycobacterial, and fungal infections. An extreme example of deficiency in cellular immunity is the acquired immunodeficiency syndrome (see Chap. 264). Antibody deficiencies result in recurrent bacterial infections, frequently with organisms such as *Streptococcus pneumoniae* and *Haemophilus influenzae* (see Chap. 263). Disorders of phagocyte function frequently are manifested by recurrent skin infections, often due to *Staphylococcus aureus* (see Chap. 81). Finally, deficiencies of early and late complement components are associated with autoimmune phenomena and recurrent *Neisseria* infections (Table 13-7). Table 13-8 summarizes useful initial screening tests of immune function. For evaluation of antibody-mediated immunity, measurement of total serum immunoglobulin levels, measurement of specific antibody titers to commonly adminstered antigens (such as tetanus toxoid), and determination of isohemagglutinin titers yield information necessary for institution of appropriate therapy. In certain cases of hypogammaglobulinemia, quantitation of B-cell markers and in vitro B-cell functional assays are of use.

For assessment of cell-mediated immunity, the total lymphocyte

TABLE 13-7 Complement deficiencies and associated diseases

Component	Associated diseases
Classical pathway	
C1q, C1r, C1s, C4	Immune complex syndromes*, pyogenic infections
C2	Immune complex syndromes*, few with pyogenic infections
C1 inhibitor	Rare immune complex disease; few with pyogenic infections
C3 and alternative pathway	
C3	Immune complex syndromes*; pyogenic infections
D	Pyogenic infections
Properdin	*Neisseria* infections
I	Pyogenic infections
H	Hemolytic uremic syndrome
Membrane attack complex	
C5	Recurrent *Neisseria* infections; immune complex disease
C6	Recurrent *Neisseria* infections; immune complex disease
C7	Recurrent *Neisseria* infections; immune complex disease
C8	Recurrent *Neisseria* infections; immune complex disease
C9	Rare *Neisseria* infections

* Immune complex syndromes include SLE and SLE-like syndromes, glomerulonephritis, and vasculitis syndromes.

SOURCE: Adapted with permission from PJ Lachmann and MJ Walport, Genetic deficiency diseases of the complement system, in GD Ross (ed), *The Immunobiology of the Complement System*. Orlando, Academic, 1986; and from JA Schifferli and DK Peters, Lancet 88, 957, 1983.

count coupled with an appropriately placed battery of intradermal skin tests provides a useful index of T-cell and macrophage response to antigens in vivo.

Anergy is the absence of an appropriate delayed-type hypersensitivity reaction and may be either general, with lack of T-cell responses to many types of antigens, or specific, with lack of T-cell responses to one antigen type. Anergy is determined by absence of reactivity in delayed-type hypersensitivity skin testing to antigens against which the patient is sensitized. For example, a battery of skin tests including *Candida*, histoplasmin, trichophytin, and mycobacterium tuberculosis antigens are placed intradermally. Most normal adult subjects should react to one of these four antigens. If there is no response on two separate occasions, the subject is said to be anergic. The causes of anergy vary in different diseases. Generalized anergy occurs in chronic fungal and TB infections and in sarcoidosis. An example of specific anergy is lack of T-cell responses to *Candida* antigen in mucocutaneous candidiasis.

Quantitation of total T cells and CD4 and CD8 T-cell subsets can be clinically useful. However, changes in the CD4/CD8 (T4/T8) ratio

TABLE 13-8 Initial screening tests of immune function

Humoral immunity	
	Quantitative immunoglobulin levels, IgG, IgM, IgA, IgE
	Tests of specific antibody formation (antitetanus toxoid)
	Isohemagglutinin titer (anti-A, anti-B): measures IgM response
Cell-mediated immunity	
	White blood cell count with differential: measures total lymphocyte level
	Delayed hypersensitivity skin tests: measures specific T-cell and macrophage response to antigens
Phagocytosis	
	White blood cell count with differential: measures total neutrophils
	Nitroblue tetrazolium test (NBT), superoxide production: measures metabolic function
	Chemotaxis: measures cell motility
	Quantitative measurement of intracellular bacterial killing
Complement	
	Total hemolytic complement (CH_{50}): quantitates complement activity
	Assay of individual complement components: defines complement component deficiencies

SOURCE: Adapted with permission from AJ Ammann, in DP Stites et al (eds).

occur in many clinical conditions and are not specific. In certain situations, such as evaluation of a transplant recipient for response to donor antigens, it is useful to measure lymphocyte activation by determination of the amount of tritiated thymidine incorporated into lymphocyte DNA in response to donor antigens and mitogens.

The evaluation of patients with recurrent cutaneous skin infections, such as Job's syndrome and chronic granulomatous disease, requires quantitation of neutrophil numbers and tests of neutrophil function. Functional neutrophil tests include NBT test, superoxide generation, chemotaxis, and quantitation of the ability of neutrophils to kill bacteria (see Chap. 81).

The total hemolytic complement (CH_{50}) determination measures the ability of a test sample of serum to lyse 50 percent of a standard suspension of sheep erythrocytes coated with rabbit antisheep erythrocyte antibody. This reaction requires the entire classical complement reaction sequence. For the classical activation pathway (C1, C4, C2) or the terminal sequence (C5–C9) the CH_{50} determination is a reliable screen for homozygous deficiencies. A normal CH_{50}, however, does not exclude heterozygous partial deficiencies of classical complement components. When the CH_{50} level is subnormal, individual complement measurements are required to determine specific component deficiency states.

REFERENCES

BUTCHER E, WEISSMAN IL: Lymphoid tissues and organs, in *Fundamental Immunology*, WE Paul (ed). New York, Raven, pp 109–127, 1984

CLARK SC, KAMEN R: The human hematopoietic colony-stimulating factors. Science 236:1229, 1987

COOPER MD, et al: Lymphocytes, in *Fundamental Immunology*, WE Paul (ed). New York, Raven, 1984

DAVIS MM: Molecular genetics of T cell antigen receptors. Hosp Practice 23:157, 1988

DENNING SM, HAYNES BF: Differentiation of human T cells. Clin Lab Med 8:1, 1988

FAUCI AS, LANE HC, VOLKMAN DJ: Activation and regulation of human immune responses. Implications in Normal and Disease States. Ann Int Med 99:61, 1983

KELLEY WN et al (eds): *Textbook of Rheumatology*, 2d ed. Philadelphia, Saunders, 1985, Chaps 2, 7, 9, and 10

MARRACK P, KAPPLER J: The T cell receptor. Science 238:1073, 1987

O'GARRA A et al: "B cell factors" are pleotropic. Immunol Today 9:45, 1988

PAUL WE: Introduction to the immune system, in *Fundamental Immunology*, WE Paul (ed). New York Raven, 1984

PLAUT, M LICHTENSTEIN LM: Cellular and chemical basis of the allergic inflammatory response in Allergy, in *Allergy Principles and Practice*, E Middleton, CE Reed, EF Ellis (eds). St. Louis, Mosby, 1978, pp 115–138

ROMAIN PL, SCHLOSSMAN SF: Human T cell subsets. Functional heterogeneity and surface recognition structures. J Clin Invest 74:1559, 1984

SHOENFELD Y, SCHWARTZ RS: Immunologic and genetic factors in autoimmune disease. New Engl J Med 312:1100, 1985

STITES DP et al (eds): *Basic and Clinical Immunology*, 5th ed. Los Gatos CA, Lange Medical Publishers, 1984

14 THE MAJOR HISTOCOMPATIBILITY GENE COMPLEX

CHARLES B. CARPENTER

Antigenic differences between members of a species are called *alloantigens*, and when these play a determining role in the rejection of allogeneic tissue grafts they are called *histocompatibility antigens*. Evolution has conserved a single closely linked region of histocompatibility genes, the products of which are prominently displayed on cell surfaces and provide a strong barrier to allotransplantation. The terms *major histocompatibility antigens* and *major histocompatibility gene complex* (MHC) refer to the gene products and genes of this chromosomal region. Many minor histocompatibility antigens, in contrast, are encoded throughout the genome. They represent weaker allotypic differences on molecules that serve a variety of functions. Structures bearing MHC antigens play a major role in immunity and in self-recognition in the differentiation of cells and tissues. Much of the evidence for MHC control of the immune response comes from work in animal models in which immune-response genes have been mapped within the mouse (H-2), rat (RT1), and guinea pig (GPLA) MHC. In humans the MHC is called *HLA*. The individual letters of HLA have various meanings, and by international agreement HLA is the logo for the human MHC.

Several generalizations can be made about the MHCs. *First,* three classes of gene products are encoded within the small [<2 cM (centimorgans)] region of the MHC. Class I molecules, expressed on virtually all cell surfaces, consist of one heavy and one light polypeptide chain and are the products of three reduplicated loci: HLA-A, HLA-B, and HLA-C. Class II molecules, restricted in expression to B lymphocytes, some monocytes, and activated T lymphocytes, consist of two polypeptide chains (α and β) of unequal length and are the products of several closely linked genes, collectively termed the HLA-D region. Class III molecules are the C4, C2, and Bf components of complement. *Second,* class I and class II molecules form complexes with immunogenic peptides (e.g., from bacteria or viruses), and they are conjointly recognized by T lymphocytes having appropriate antigen receptors. Self versus nonself discrimination in the initiation and effector phase of the immune response is thereby intimately directed by class I and II molecules. *Third,* restricted cell-to-cell interactions involving suppressor T lymphocytes are not clearly defined in humans, but HLA genes are important for some suppressor activities. *Fourth,* genes for enzyme systems having no apparent relationship to immunity are located in the region of the MHC, as are genes of importance in skeletal growth and development. *Fifth,* genes for tumor necrosis factors TNFα and TNFβ lie also within the MHC. The known loci of the HLA region on the short arm of chromosome 6 are shown in Fig. 14-1.

LOCI OF THE HLA SYSTEM Class I antigens HLA antigens of the class I type are defined serologically by human sera, principally from multiparous females, and to a limited extent by monoclonal antibodies. They are present in varying densities in most body tissues,

FIGURE 14-1 Schematic representation of human chromosome 6, showing the location of the HLA region in the 21 region of the short arm. The HLA-A, HLA-B, and HLA-C loci encode class I heavy chains (44,000 Da), while the beta$_2$-microglobulin light chain (11,500 Da) of the class I molecule is encoded by genes of chromosome 15. HLA-D region (class II) is centromeric to the A, B, C loci, with genes for closely linked complement components C4A, C4B, Bf, and C2 in the B-D region. Two genes for tumor necrosis factor (TNFα,β) also lie between HLA-B and the complement genes (not shown). The order of the complement genes is uncertain. Each D region class II molecule is made up of an α and a β chain. They appear on the cell surface in distinct sets, DP, DQ, and DR. The numbers preceding α or β indicate that there are different genes for the chains of a given set; e.g., for DR, there are three β-chain genes. The expressed molecule may be 1βα or 3βα. The 2β gene is not expressed (pseudogene). The antigens DRw52 and DRw53 are on the 3β chain, while the other DR antigens are on 1β. DRα is not polymorphic, while molecules bearing the DQ antigens have polymorphism in both α and β chains (1α1β). The other DQ set (2α2β) appears to be pseudogenes. Polymorphism in DP is confined to the 1β chain. The overall length of the HLA region is about 3 cM.

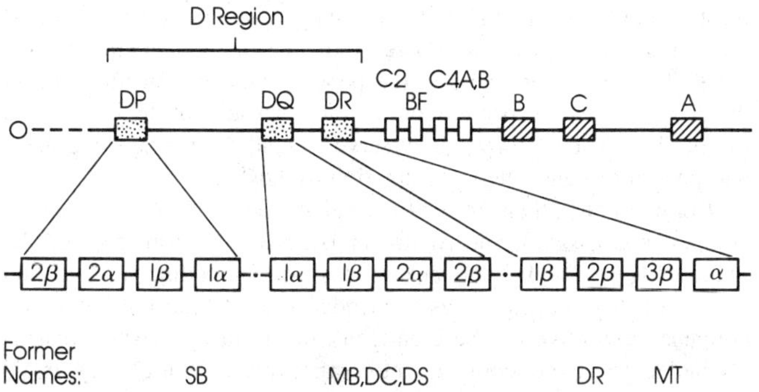

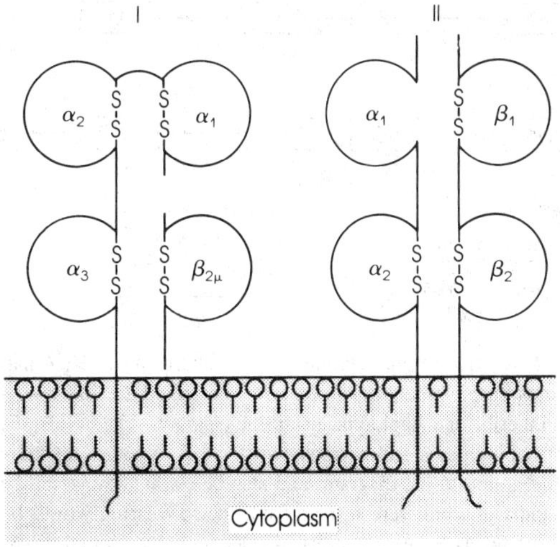

FIGURE 14-2 Schematic representation of class I and class II molecules on the cell surface. Class I molecules are composed of two polypeptide chains. The 44,000-Da heavy chain passes through the plasma membrane. Its external portion consists of three domains (α_1, α_2, α_3) formed by disulfide bonding. The beta$_2$-microglobulin ($\beta_{2\mu}$) light chain (11,500 Da) encoded by chromosome 15 is noncovalently bound to the heavy chain. Amino acid sequence homology among class I molecules is 80 to 85 percent, falling to 50 percent or less in portions of α_1 and α_2 which represent the sites of alloantigenic polymorphism. Class II molecules consist of two noncovalently associated polypeptide chains, a 34,000-Da α and a 29,000-Da β. Each chain has two domains formed by disulfide bridging (the α_1 domain lacks a sulfide bridge). (*From Carpenter and Strom.*)

including B cells, T cells, and platelets, but not in mature red blood cells. The number of serologically defined specificities is large, and the HLA system is the most polymorphic genetic system known in humans. Three clearly defined loci are recognized within the HLA complex for class I, serologically defined (SD) HLA antigens. Each class I antigen consists of an 11,500-Da beta$_2$-microglobulin subunit and a 44,000-Da heavy chain that carries the antigenic specificities (Fig. 14-2). There are over 60 clearly defined A and B specificities, and 11 C-locus specificities are known. Antigens of the major complex are prefixed by HLA, but this may be omitted when the context is clear. Antigens tentatively accepted by the World Health Organization have a *w* after the locus designation. The number following the locus designation is the name of the antigen. The HLA antigens of African, Asian, and Oceanic peoples are less well defined at present, although they include some of the antigens commonly found in people of western European ancestry. The distribution of HLA antigens is distinctive for certain racial groups and can serve as anthropologic markers in the study of migration patterns and diseases.

Since chromosomes are paired, each individual has six serologically defined HLA-A, HLA-B, and HLA-C antigens, three from each parent. Each of these chromosomal sets is termed a *haplotype,* and by simple Mendelian inheritance one-fourth of siblings have identical haplotypes, one-half share a haplotype, and the remaining one-fourth are completely incompatible (Fig. 14-3). Evidence that this gene complex plays the major role in the transplantation response comes from the fact that haplotype-matched sibling donor-recipient combinations show excellent results in kidney transplantation, in the vicinity of 85 to 90 percent long-term survival (see Chap. 225).

Class II antigens The HLA-D region is adjacent to the class I loci on the short arm of chromosome 6 (Fig. 14-1). This region encodes a series of class II molecules, each consisting of a 29,000-Da β chain and a 34,000-Da α chain (Fig. 14-2). Incompatibility for this region, particularly concerning the DR antigens, determines the in vitro proliferative response of lymphocytes to mismatched haplotypes. This mixed lymphocyte response (MLR) is assessed by the degree of proliferation of a *mixed lymphocyte culture* (MLC) and is

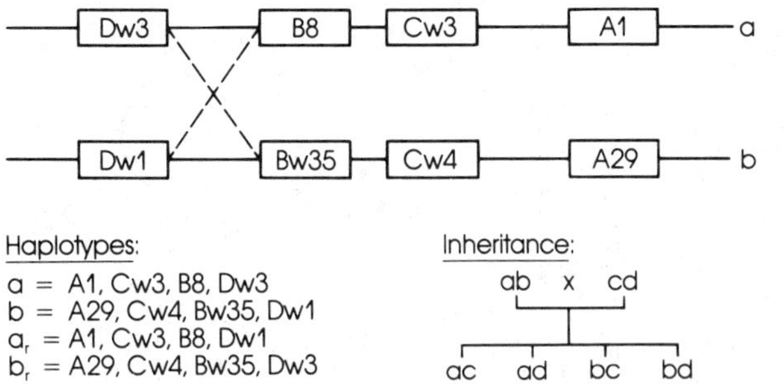

FIGURE 14-3 HLA region, chromosome 6: inheritance of HLA haplotypes. Each chromosomal segment of linked genes is termed a haplotype, and each individual inherits one haplotype from each parent. The A, B, C, and D antigens of haplotypes a and b are shown for this hypothetical individual in chromosomal order on the diagram, and also below as they would be written in text. If individual ab were to marry cd, their offspring would be of four types only, as far as HLA is concerned. Occasionally (dotted cross) recombination occurs in the germ line (meiosis) of a parent, resulting in an altered haplotype. The frequency of recombinant children is a measure of the map distance (1 percent recombination frequency = 1 cM; see Fig. 14-1). (*From CB Carpenter, Kidney International, 14:283, 1978.*)

positive even when HLA-A, HLA-B, and HLA-C antigens are identical (Fig. 14-3). When parental recombination has occurred between HLA-B and -DR, for example, a new haplotype appears in the child, who will be identical for class I but different for class II (a versus a_r in Fig. 14-3). HLA-D antigens are defined by reference-stimulating lymphocytes that are homozygous for HLA-D and are inactivated by x-irradiation or mitomycin C to make the reaction unidirectional. There are 24 such antigens recognized by homozygous typing cells.

Attempts to define HLA-D by serology first established a series of D-related (DR) antigens expressed on class II molecules of B lymphocytes, monocytes, and activated T lymphocytes. Macrophages, dendritic cells, and skin Langerhans cells are also class II–positive. Other closely related antigen systems were soon discovered and given various local names (MB, MT, DC, SB), which have been replaced by subregion names DR, DQ, and DP. The separate identity of these sets of class II molecules is now established, and the genes for their respective α and β chains have been isolated and sequenced. The class II gene map shown in Fig. 14-1 describes a minimal number of genes and molecular sets. Although a class II molecule may be composed of a DRα from one parental haplotype and a DRβ from the other parent (transcomplementation), α and β combinations outside of each DP, DQ, DR set rarely, if ever, occur. DR, and to some extent DQ, molecules provide the stimuli for the primary mixed lymphocyte response. The secondary MLR is called the *primed lymphocyte test* (PLT) and occurs rapidly over 24 to 36 h instead of 6 to 7 days. DP alloantigens were discovered from their ability to provide PLT stimulation, although they do not produce a primary MLR. DQ and DP molecules can also be identified serologically. While B lymphocytes and activated T lymphocytes express all three sets of class II molecules, DQ antigens are not expressed on 60 to 90 percent of monocytes, which are virtually all DP- and DR-positive.

Molecular genetics Each polypeptide chain of class I and class II molecules bears several polymorphic sites in addition to the "private" antigen defined by alloantisera. In the *cell-mediated lympholysis* (CML) test the specificity of killer T cells (T_c), which arise during the proliferative events in MLR, is determined by testing upon target cells from donors other than those providing the MLR stimulus. Antigen systems defined by this method show a close but imperfect correlation with class I private antigens. Cloning of cytotoxic cells has revealed the presence of a variety of polymorphic target determinants on HLA molecules, some of which are identifiable by alloantisera or monoclonal antibodies derived from immunization of mice with human cells. Some of these reagents can be used to identify private determinants of HLA, while others are directed to more "public" (sometimes called supertypic) determinants. One such system of public HLA-B antigens has two alleles, Bw4 and Bw6. Most HLA-B private antigens are associated with either Bw4 or Bw6. Other systems are restricted to subsets of HLA antigen groups. For example, HLA-B-bearing heavy chains carry additional sites that are common to B7, B27, Bw22, and B40 or to B5, B15, B18, and Bw35. Other types of shared antigenic determinants exist, as exemplified by a monoclonal antibody which reacts with a site shared between HLA-A and HLA-B heavy chains.

The amino acid sequence and peptide maps of several HLA molecules show that the class I hypervariable regions are clustered in the outer α_1 domain (Fig. 14-2) and the adjacent portion of α_2. Variability in the sequences of class II molecules differs from locus to locus. Remarkably, the class I α_3 domain, the class II α_2 and β_2 domains, and the portions of the CD8 (T8, Leu 2) cell surface molecule that function in T-cell interactions (see Chap. 13) all show significant amino acid sequence homologies with immunoglobulin constant regions. These findings suggest evolutionary elaboration within a family of gene products that have immune recognition functions. When genomic DNA for HLA is examined, typical exon-intron sequences of DNA have been found for class I and class II, exons having been identified for signal peptides (5′), each of the domains, a transmembrane hydrophobic segment, and a cytoplasmic segment (3′). cDNA probes are available for most of the HLA chains, and enzymatic digests have been used to study patterns of *restriction fragment length polymorphisms* (RFLP), many of which correlate with class II serologic and MLR patterns. There are 20 to 30 class I genes, however, making assessment of polymorphism by RFLP difficult. Many of these genes are not expressed (pseudogenes), while some could represent additional class I loci that are expressed only on activated T cells, and are of uncertain function. The detection of variable nucleotide sequences (tissue types) by means of the polymerase chain reaction technique is under study. This technique seeks to amplify specific segments of DNA, as defined by oligonucleotide primers, from genomic DNA. Such an approach offers the possibility of rapid HLA typing by hybridization with specific oligonucleotide probes.

Three-dimensional structure of HLA X-ray diffraction studies of the HLA-A2 molecule show a groove on the surface facing away from the cell membrane with dimensions sufficient to bind a peptide fragment 8- to 20-amino acids long, depending upon the degree of helix formation. The margins of the groove are formed by α helices, and the base is floored by a series of β strands, with the α_1 and α_2 domains contributing more or less equally to each side of the structure (Fig. 14-4). It is remarkable that the HLA variable regions and sites for alloantibody binding or cytotoxic T-cell recognition lie along the α helices that form the margins of the groove. Although class II molecules have yet to be studied to the same resolution, preliminary results suggest a similar groove formed by the α_1 and β_1 domains, and the known sequence polymorphisms would also lie along the presumed location of the groove. In brief, it appears that the site of antigen presentation by MHC molecules has been visualized. The known processing of protein antigens into smaller fragments by macrophages can now be related to the binding of certain of these fragments to class II molecules for recognition by the T-cell receptor. The phenomenon of MHC restriction, which indicates that the T cell must recognize both self-MHC and antigen, can now be viewed as the function of a single T-cell receptor that binds to both α-helical sides of the HLA groove and the peptide lying within it. Some of the polymorphism, especially on the inner surfaces of the helices and on the floor of the groove, may serve to bind the peptide fragments and possibly to alter their presentation to the T-cell receptor.

Complement (class III) Structural genes for three complement components, C4, C2, and Bf (factor B), are present in the HLA-B-D region (Fig. 14-1). There are two loci for C4, coding for C4A and C4B, formerly recognized as the Rodgers and Chido red blood cell antigens, respectively. These antigens are, in fact, adsorbed plasma C4 molecules. Other complement components are not closely linked

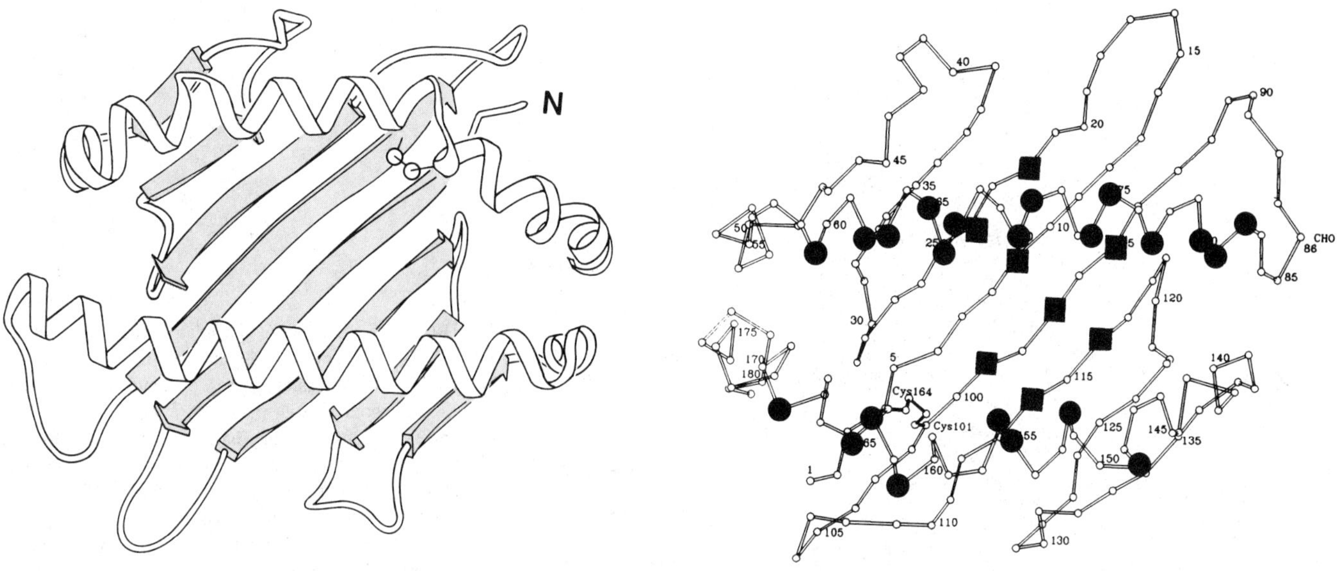

FIGURE 14-4 Structure of the HLA class I molecule as determined by x-ray crystallography. *A*. Shown is the face of the HLA-A2 molecule that points away from the cell surface. This ribbon diagram shows the groove that is formed by two α helices, and is supported by a floor of eight β strands. N is the amino terminal of the α_1 domain; the two small circles represent a disulfide bond. (*From PA Bjorkman et al.*) *B*. Composite display of polymorphic sites from several human and mouse class I alleles, using the HLA-A2 structure as the model. The symbols show a composite of the polymorphisms along the groove. Localization of variable amino acids and/or sites for alloantibody and/or cytotoxic T-cell recognition is shown to be along the α helices (circles). Polymorphic sites exist also in the β strands (squares). The numbers indicate the amino acid sequence. (*After PA Bjorkman et al.*)

to HLA. No crossovers have been found between the C2, Bf, and C4 loci. They are all encoded within a 100-kilobase segment between HLA-B and HLA-DR. There are two alleles of C2, four of Bf, seven of C4A, and three of C4B, plus blanks (null genes) for each locus (QO). The extensive polymorphism of complement types (complotypes) makes them useful for genetic studies. The four most common extended haplotypes found in people of western European ancestry are shown in Table 14-1. MLRs between unrelated individuals who are matched for these extended haplotypes are nonreactive, whereas reactivity is common if unrelated individuals are matched for only HLA-DR and -DQ. Such identical extended haplotypes may be conserved from a common ancestor.

Other sixth-chromosome genes Deficiency of steroid 21-hydroxylase, an autosomal recessive trait, results in the syndrome of congenital adrenal hyperplasia (Chaps. 317 and 324). The gene for the enzyme is localized in the HLA-B-D region. The 21-hydroxylase gene adjacent to C4A is deleted in affected individuals along with C4A (C4AQO), and the HLA-B locus gene may have been altered to convert B13 to the rare Bw47 found only in affected haplotypes. A late-onset variant of 21-hydroxylase deficiency is also linked to HLA. Congenital adrenal hyperplasia due to 11β-hydroxylase deficiency is not HLA-linked. Idiopathic hemochromatosis, an autosomal recessive disorder, is linked to HLA, as has been shown in several family studies (see Chap. 327). Although the pathogenesis of this disease is unknown, the gene that modulates gastrointestinal iron absorption is near HLA-A (Table 14-2).

Immune response genes HLA-D is analogous to the mouse H-2I region as established by studies of in vitro responses to synthetic polypeptide antigens, keyhole limpet hemocyanin, collagen, and tetanus toxoid. Presentation of antigenic fragments on the surfaces of macrophages or other cells bearing class II molecules requires conjoint recognition of a class II + antigen complex by T lymphocytes bearing the appropriate receptor(s) (see also Chap. 13). The crux of this "self + X" or "altered self" hypothesis is that in the T-dependent immune response, help from the T helper-inducer cell (T_H) occurs only if the appropriate class II determinant can be synthesized. The genes for the latter are Ir (immune response) genes. Since allogeneic class II determinants are perceived as already altered, the allogeneic mixed lymphocyte response represents a model for the immune system in which additional nominal antigen does not need to be added (Fig. 14-5). Effector phases of immunity require recognition of nominal antigen together with a self structure. The latter in humans, as in mice, is the molecule bearing class I histocompatibility antigens. Human cell lines infected with influenza virus are lysed by immune cytotoxic T lymphocytes (T_c) only if an HLA-A- or HLA-B-locus antigen is shared between the attacking and target cells. Again, the allogeneic MLR provides a model for development of class I restricted cytotoxic T lymphocytes (Fig. 14-5). When primed cells are propagated and cloned, an array of restrictions to different class I and II molecules and epitopes can be discerned. At the level of the antigen presenting cell, for example, a given T_H clone recognizes an antigenic fragment conjointly with a specific site on a class II molecule via its receptor (T_i). The restriction elements for some microbial antigens are DR or Dw alleles. The association of CD4-positive T cells with responses to class II antigens and of CD8-positive T cells with responses to class I antigens appears to be the result of direct interaction of CD4 and CD8 with class II

TABLE 14-1 Common extended HLA haplotypes

HLA-B	HLA-DR	Bf	C2	C4A	C4B
8	3	S	C	QO	1
7	2	S	C	3	1
57	7	S	C	6	1
44	7	F	C	3	1

TABLE 14-2 Linkage of genetic defects to HLA

	Gene location	Common haplotype found
C2 deficiency	HLA-B-D	Aw25, B18, BfS, DR2
21-OH deficiency	HLA-B-D	A3, Bw47, BfF, DR7
21-OH deficiency (late onset)	HLA-B-D,	B14, BfS, DR1
Idiopathic hemochromatosis	HLA-A	A3, B14
Paget's disease	HLA-A-D	
Spinocerebellar ataxia	HLA-A-D	
Hodgkin's disease	HLA-A-D	

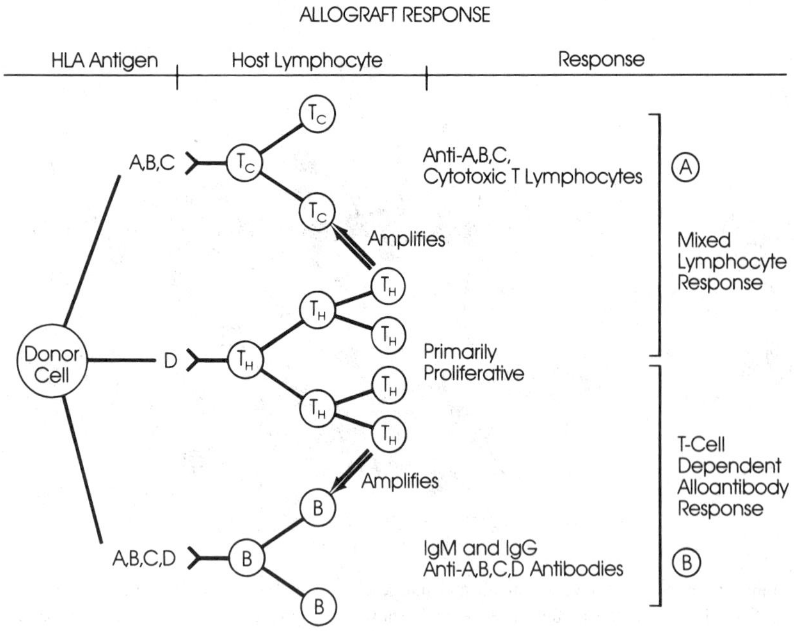

FIGURE 14-5 Schema of the relative roles of HLA-A, HLA-B, HLA-C, and HLA-D antigens in initiation of the alloimmune response and in the development of effector cells and antibodies. Two main classes of T lymphocytes recognize antigens: T_c, the precursors to the cytotoxic "killer" cells, and T_H, the helper cells for amplification of the cytotoxic response. T_H also provide help to B lymphocytes for production of a fully mature IgG response. Note that T_c generally recognize class I antigens, while the T_H signal is provided by antigens of the HLA-D region (class II). *(From CB Carpenter, Kidney International, 14:283, 1978.)*

and class I antigen-presenting molecules, respectively. Suppression of immune responses (i.e., low responder status) to cedar pollen, streptococcal antigen, and schistosomal antigen is linked to HLA-DQ as a dominant trait, suggesting the existence of immune suppressor (Is) genes. Specific allele associations with immune response (e.g., ragweed Ra5 antigen with DR2 and collagen with DR4) have also been demonstrated.

DISEASE ASSOCIATIONS If the major histocompatibility complex serves a critical natural biologic function, what might that be? One hypothesis is that it plays a role in immune surveillance against neoplastic cells that develop in the course of an individual's lifetime. The system could also play an important role in pregnancy because of the histoincompatibility that always exists between the mother and the fetus. The high degree of polymorphism may also ensure survival of the species in relation to the large numbers of microbiologic agents present in the environment. Self-tolerance which happens to cross-react with microbiologic agents would produce a high degree of susceptibility, resulting in lethal infection, whereas the polymorphism in the HLA system ensures that segments of the population recognize offending agents as foreign and initiate the appropriate response. All these hypotheses relate to the survival value of the system under selective evolutionary pressures, and there is some evidence for each of them.

Circumstantial evidence for the role of the HLA complex in immunobiology comes from the finding that a number of disease processes are positively associated with certain HLA antigens within the population. The search for such associations has been stimulated by the discovery of immune response genes linked to the H-2 complex in the mouse. Table 14-3 summarizes the most significant HLA and disease associations.

Most striking is the increased frequency of HLA-B27 in certain rheumatic diseases, particularly ankylosing spondylitis, a condition with a strong familial tendency. B27 is present in about 7 percent of people of western European ancestry, while it appears in 80 to 90 percent of patients with ankylosing spondylitis. Expressed as a relative risk, the antigen B27 confers a susceptibility to the development of ankylosing spondylitis that is 87 times that in the general population. Similarly, acute anterior uveitis, Reiter's syndrome, and reactive arthritis to at least three bacterial infections (yersinia, salmonella, and gonococcus) show a high degree of association with B27. Although the ordinary form of juvenile rheumatoid arthritis (JRA) also shows a similar association with B27, the pauciarticular form of JRA with iritis is DR5-associated. The increased incidence of B27 in psoriatic arthritis is also significant for the central type (axial skeleton) of the disorder, while Bw38 is associated with both the central and peripheral types. Psoriasis is associated with Cw6. Patients with degenerative arthritis or gout show no alteration in antigen frequencies.

Most other disease associations are with HLA-D region antigens. Narcolepsy is virtually 100 percent associated with DR2 in both Japanese and whites. Affected individuals need inherit only a single gene dose of DR2. Although there is no apparent autoimmune component to this condition, there is speculation that an abnormality in a neurotransmitter or its receptor may be influenced by the DR2 gene or another closely linked gene. Gluten-sensitive enteropathy (celiac disease, nontropical sprue) in children and adults is associated with DR3 (relative risk = 21). The actual percentage of such patients having this antigen ranges from 63 to 96 percent compared to 22 to 27 percent of controls. The same antigen is also present in increased frequency in patients with chronic active hepatitis and in patients with dermatitis herpetiformis who also have gluten-sensitive enteropathy. Juvenile-onset insulin-dependent diabetes mellitus (type I) is associated with DR4 and DR3 and is negatively associated with DR2. Resistance to type I diabetes is strongly associated with the inheritance of aspartate at position 57 of the β chain of HLA-DQ, in linkage disequilibrium with HLA-DR2. Other amino acids at position 57, especially when HLA-DR3 or -DR4 are on the same haplotype, are associated with an increased risk of disease. Maturity-onset diabetes is not HLA-associated. A rare allele of Bf (F1) is also found in 17 to 25 percent of cases of type I diabetes. Hyperthyroidism in the United States is associated with B8, Dw3, while in Japanese populations the association is with Bw35. More extensive studies of healthy and diseased members of various races will help in clarification of which HLA markers are universal. For example, B27 is rare in healthy Japanese but is common in subjects with ankylosing spondylitis. Also, DR4 seems to be the common marker for type I diabetes in all races. Sometimes an HLA marker is clearly associated only with a subgroup within a syndrome. For example, myasthenia gravis without thymoma is more strongly B8, DR3-associated, and the association of DR2 with multiple sclerosis is strong in patients with rapidly progressive deterioration. Goodpasture's syndrome due to autoimmunity to glomerular basement membrane, idiopathic membranous glomerulonephritis, which may be an autoimmune process involving antibodies to an antigen of the glomerulus, and gold-induced membranous nephritis are strongly HLA-DR-associated.

LINKAGE DISEQUILIBRIUM Although the distribution of HLA alleles varies in racial and ethnic populations, the most salient feature

TABLE 14-3 HLA antigens and disease, showing the most highly associated antigens

Disease	Antigen	Relative risk*
RHEUMATIC		
Ankylosing spondylitis	B27	69.1
Reiter's syndrome	B27	37.0
Acute anterior uveitis	B27	8.2
Reactive arthritis (yersinia, salmonella, gonococcus)	B27	18.0
Psoriatic arthritis, central	B27	10.7
	Bw38	9.1
Psoriatic arthritis, peripheral	B27	2.0
	Bw38	6.5
Juvenile rheumatoid arthritis	B27	3.9
	DRw8	3.6
Juvenile arthritis, pauciarticular	DR5	3.3
Rheumatoid arthritis	Dw4/DR4	3.8
Sjögren's syndrome	Dw3	5.7
Systemic lupus erythematosus	DR3	2.6
Systemic lupus erythematosus (hydralazine)	DR4	5.6
GASTROINTESTINAL		
Gluten-sensitive enteropathy	DR3	11.6
Chronic active hepatitis	DR3	6.8
Ulcerative colitis	B5	3.8
HEMATOLOGIC		
Idiopathic hemochromatosis	A3	6.7
	B14	26.7
	A3, B14	90.0
Pernicious anemia	DR5	5.4
SKIN		
Dermatitis herpetiformis	Dw3	17.3
Psoriasis vulgaris	Cw6	7.5
Psoriasis vulgaris (Japanese)	Cw6	8.5
Pemphigus vulgaris (Jews)	DR4	14.6
	A10	4.8
Behçet's disease	B5	3.8
ENDOCRINE		
Type 1 diabetes mellitus	DR4	3.6
	DR3	4.8
	DR2	0.2
	BfF1	15.0
Hyperthyroidism	B8	2.5
	Dw3	3.7
Hyperthyroidism (Japanese)	Bw35	4.4
Adrenal insufficiency	Dw3	10.5
Subacute thyroiditis (de Quervain)	Bw35	13.7
Hashimoto's thyroiditis	DR5	3.2
Congenitial adrenal hyperplasia	Bw47	15.4
NEUROLOGIC		
Myasthenia gravis	B8	2.7
	DR3	2.5
Multiple sclerosis	DR2	2.7
Manic-depressive disorder	Bw16	2.3
Narcolepsy	DR2	130.0
Schizophrenia	A28	2.3
RENAL		
Idiopathic membranous glomerulonephritis	DR3	5.7
Goodpasture's syndrome (anti-GBM)	DR2	15.9
Minimal change disease (steroid response)	B12	4.2
Polycystic kidney disease	B5	2.6
IgA nephropathy	DR4	3.1
Gold nephropathy	DR3	14.0
	DR4	0.3
INFECTIOUS		
Tuberculoid leprosy (Asians)	B8	6.8
Paralytic polio	Bw16	4.3
Low vs. high response to vaccinia virus	Cw3	12.7
IMMUNODEFICIENCY		
IgA deficiency (blood donors)	DR3	13.0

* Relative risk $= \dfrac{(\%\ \text{antigen-positive patients})(\%\ \text{antigen-negative controls})}{(\%\ \text{antigen-negative patients})(\%\ \text{antigen-positive controls})}$.

of population genetics of HLA antigens is the presence of linkage disequilibria among certain antigens of the A and B, B and C, and B, D, and complement loci. Linkage disequilibrium means that antigens of closely linked loci appear together more frequently than predicted by random association. The classic example is the linkage disequilibrium present between the A-locus antigen HLA-A1 and the B-locus antigen HLA-B8 in people of western European ancestry. The coincidence of A1 and B8 should be the product of their individual gene frequencies ($0.17 \times 0.11 \cong 0.02$). The observed frequency of A1 and B8 is 0.08, four times that expected, an increase of 0.06. The latter value is termed Δ (delta), and is a measure of the disequilibrium. Other A- and B-locus haplotype disequilibria have been recognized and include (A3, B7), (A2, B12), (A29, B12), and (A11, Bw35). Furthermore, some D-region determinants are in linkage disequilibrium with B-locus antigens (for example, DR3 and B8), as are some B-locus and C-locus antigens. Serologically defined HLA antigens can serve as markers for the genes of an entire haplotype within a family and as markers for specific genes within a population but only where a linkage disequilibrium exists.

Linkage disequilibrium is of importance because such gene associations may have some bearing on their function. For example, selective pressures during the course of evolution may have been the major factor in the survival of certain gene combinations in a haplotype. Such a theory suggests, for example, that A1 and B8, along with certain D-region and other determinants, conferred a selective advantage in the face of epidemics such as the plague or smallpox. It would also follow that the descendants of the survivors may display susceptibility to certain diseases because their unique gene complex happens to confer an abnormal response to other environmental agents. The major difficulty with this hypothesis is the assumption that selection must work on several genes simultaneously to account for the observed Δ's; however, the need for complex interactions among the products of the several loci of the major histocompatibility complex is only beginning to be appreciated, and selection might force multiple linkage disequilibria. The conservation of certain extended haplotypes, mentioned above, supports this view.

On the other hand, the selection hypothesis is not necessary to explain linkage disequilibrium. When a population lacking certain antigens is crossed with one in which a high frequency of antigens is in equilibrium, a Δ can develop within a few generations. For example, the increasing Δ value for A1,B8 found in populations from east to west, from India to western Europe, can be explained on the basis of migration and fusion. In smaller groups, consanguinity, founder effects, and gene drift may account for disequilibria. Finally, certain linkage disequilibria could occur as a result of nonrandom crossing over during gametic meiosis, because of chromosomal segments which are either more or less likely to break. Unless there are selective pressures or restrictions in crossing over, linkage disequilibria disappear over a period of several generations. A large number of nonrandom associations occur throughout the HLA gene complex, and elucidation of the reasons for their existence may provide insight into the mechanism underlying certain disease susceptibilities.

LINKAGE AND ASSOCIATION The diseases listed in Table 14-2 are examples of HLA linkage wherein the inherited conditions are marked within families by the relevant HLA haplotypes. For C2 deficiency, 21-hydroxylase deficiency, and idiopathic hemochromatosis the mode of inheritance is recessive, with heterozygotes showing partial deficiencies. These genetic defects are also HLA-associated, with an excess of certain HLA alleles in affected unrelated individuals. Also, C2 deficiency is commonly linked to the HLA-Aw25, B18, Bfs, D/DR2 haplotype, and idiopathic hemochromatosis exhibits both linkage and strong association with HLA-A3 and -B14. The high degree of linkage disequilibria in these HLA-linked diseases may result from mutations in a single founder, and a sufficient period of time may not have passed to bring the gene pool back into equilibrium. In this view, the HLA antigens are simple markers for the linked gene. Alternatively, expression of the defect may require interaction with specific HLA alleles. This latter hypothesis would require a higher mutation rate, with defective gene expression occurring only when linked with certain HLA genes.

Paget's disease and spinocerebellar ataxia are HLA-linked autosomal dominant traits in families having multiple affected members, and Hodgkin's disease shows an HLA-linked recessive pattern of inheritance. No HLA associations have been discerned for these disorders, suggesting that there were multiple founders with mutations in linkage with different HLA alleles.

HLA linkage is readily recognized when recessive or dominant inheritance patterns are clear-cut, i.e., when expressivity is high and the process is mostly, if not entirely, determined by a single gene defect. In most of the associations HLA markers represent risk factors involving the operation and modulation of the immune response under the influence of multiple genes. An example of a polygenic immunologic disease is atopic allergy, in which the association to HLA may be evident only in individuals whose genetically controlled (non-HLA) levels of IgE production are low. Another is IgA deficiency (Table 14-3), which is HLA-DR3-associated.

CLINICAL APPLICATIONS The clinical value of HLA typing for diagnosis of disease is limited to B27 and ankylosing spondylitis, where nevertheless there are 10 percent false-positive and false-negative rates. HLA studies are also of value in genetic counseling and early recognition of disease in families with idiopathic hemochromatosis or congenital adrenal hyperplasia due to steroid 21-hydroxylase deficiency, particularly as HLA typing can be performed upon cells obtained by amniocentesis. The high degree of polymorphism of the HLA system also makes it a powerful tool for paternity testing and other medicolegal applications. The implications for diseases such as type I diabetes mellitus and the other diseases showing HLA associations require further study of the components of the HLA system and their role in the pathogenesis of disease. Matching for HLA antigens in allogeneic transplantation is reviewed in Chap. 225.

REFERENCES

BIDWELL J: DNA-RFLP analysis and genotyping of HLA-DR and DQ antigens. Immunol Today 9:18, 1988

BJORKMAN PA et al: Structure of the human class I histocompatibility antigen, HLA-A2. Nature 329:506, 1987

——— et al: The foreign antigen binding site and T cell recognition regions of class I histocompatibility antigens. Nature 329:512, 1987

CARPENTER CB, STROM TB: Immunobiology of renal transplantation, in *Renal Transplantation*, EL Milford et al (eds), *Contemporary Issues in Nephrology*, vol 19. New York, Churchill Livingstone, 1989

DEGOS L, DAUSSET J: Human migrations and linkage disequilibrium of HLA system. Immunogenetics 3:195, 1974

DUQUESNOY RJ, TRUCCO M: Genetic basis of cell surface polymorphism encoded by the major histocompatibility complex in humans. CRC Crit Rev Immunol 8:103, 1988

MARSH DG et al: Epidemiology and genetics of atopic allergy. N Eng J Med 305:1551, 1981

MATSUSHITA S et al: HLA linked nonresponsiveness to *Cryptomeria japonica* pollen antigen: I. Nonresponsiveness is mediated by antigen-specific suppressor T cells. J Immunol 138:109, 1987

Nomenclature for factors of the HLA system, 1987. Tissue Antigens 32:177, 1988

SASAZUKI T et al: HLA-linked gene controlling immune response and disease susceptibility. Immunol Rev 70:51, 1983

TIWARI JL, TERASAKI PI: *HLA and Disease Associations*. New York, Springer Verlag, 1985

TODD JA et al: HLA-DQ beta gene contributes to susceptibility and resistance to insulin-dependent diabetes mellitus. Nature 329:599, 1987

WHITE PC et al: HLA-linked congenital adrenal hyperplasia results from a defective gene encoding a cytochrome P-450 specific for steroid 21-hydroxylation. Proc Natl Acad Sci USA 81:7505, 1984

PART TWO CARDINAL MANIFESTATIONS OF DISEASE

section 1 Pain

15 PAIN: PATHOPHYSIOLOGY AND MANAGEMENT

RAYMOND MACIEWICZ / JOSEPH B. MARTIN

Pain is the most common symptom of disease. Although the nature, location, and etiology of pain differ in each case, approximately half of all patients who visit a physician have a primary complaint of pain. For most, the correct treatment of a self-evident, limited disease process (such as a broken bone) alleviates pain. However, in some patients uncontrolled pain continues to be a major problem. In these cases, the symptom of pain requires careful assessment and evaluation to interpret its significance and to establish an approach for its effective treatment.

The evaluation of the patient with pain is frequently complex, partially because pain is a perception rather than a sensation. A person's physical state, past experience, and anticipation all influence the way pain is interpreted. For example, soldiers and athletes may deny pain despite an acute injury, while certain patients with chronic pain may continue to suffer despite the lack of an obvious source of disease. Our knowledge of pain and most of our treatments for it focus on decreasing the nociceptive sensory input; however, a patient's interpretation of a sensation, emotional response, and associated behavior are equally important factors that deserve the physician's careful attention.

ORGANIZATION OF PAIN PATHWAYS **Nociceptive afferents** Sensory stimuli of potentially tissue-damaging intensity activate free nerve endings in skin, underlying tissue, and viscera. Nociceptive signals are conveyed to the spinal cord by unmyelinated and small myelinated sensory axons. In humans, stimulation of individual small sensory axons can evoke the report of pain in the area of skin supplied by that fiber, clearly demonstrating that under certain conditions even single axons can transmit activity that is interpreted as "pain" by the brain.

Many unmyelinated nociceptive afferents exhibit "polymodal" responses. Such fibers can be activated by intense mechanical stimulation, potentially tissue-damaging thermal stimulation, and chemical stimulation by substances injected into skin. Any intense stimulus applied to normal skin can produce a "triple response" that consists of a red flush at the site of stimulation, a surrounding red flare due to arterial dilatation, and local edema caused by increased vascular permeability. Many substances likely play an important role in this response. Some of these agents are released by damaged tissue (potassium, histamine, serotonin, prostaglandins), while others enter from the circulation (bradykinin) or come from local nerve endings themselves (substance P). Certain of these substances also activate free nerve endings, and their long-lasting effects may partially explain the hypersensitivity of the skin that often follows a noxious stimulus.

Dorsal horn Sensory fibers extend distally and proximally from cells located in the segmental dorsal root ganglia. Nociceptive afferents enter the spinal cord through the dorsal root to terminate on dorsal horn neurons (Fig. 15-1*A*). Many of the fine afferents ending in these regions contain neuropeptides, including substance P, cholecystokinin, and somatostatin. There is increasing evidence that these peptides play an important role in normal sensory transmission. Chemical destruction of substance P fibers in animals produces analgesia in certain tests for pain, and there is also a marked decrease in substance P terminal staining in the dorsal horn in patients with congenital neuropathies that are associated with decreased sensitivity to pain.

The spinal dorsal horn can be divided into a series of layers based on cell morphology and arrangement. Neurons that process nociceptive information are found in several of these layers. Unmyelinated afferents terminate principally in layer II (the *substantia gelatinosa*), while myelinated nociceptive afferents end in layers I and V. The output neurons that project to brainstem and thalamus are found principally in layers I and V. The axons of these dorsal horn neurons form a crossed pathway that ascends in the ventrolateral quadrant of the spinal cord, the spinothalamic tract.

Spinothalamic system The axons of nociceptive dorsal horn neurons that form the spinothalamic tracts terminate in several brainstem and thalamic nuclei. The spinothalamic tract can be divided conceptually into two systems based on these connections: a direct spinothalamic system that carries sensory discriminative information about pain to thalamic levels, and a phylogenetically older spinoreticulothalamic system that terminates more diffusely in brainstem reticular nuclei.

The direct spinothalamic system that ends in the thalamus may be important for the conscious perception of nociceptive sensations. This system terminates in an orderly fashion within the *nucleus ventralis posterolateralis* (VPL). The terminal field of the spinothalamic tract in VPL overlaps the dorsal column–medial lemniscal input that relays light touch and joint sensation. The organized pattern of terminations and the convergence of light touch and pain information within VPL may be important for perception of the sensory discriminative aspects of pain, including the location, nature, and intensity of a noxious input. Consistent with this view, cells in VPL project principally to the primary somatosensory cortex.

The more diffuse spinoreticulothalamic system may mediate the autonomic and affective components of pain. Ascending spinoreticular fibers terminate at several levels of the brainstem reticular formation, forming part of a polysynaptic system that terminates in the medial thalamic nuclei (*nucleus centralis lateralis* and *nucleus parafascicularis*). Cells throughout the spinoreticulothalamic system often have large, bilateral sensory receptive fields that can include the entire body surface. These cells often respond best to noxious sensory input. Such cells are probably not involved in sensory discrimination or localization; more likely, they are important for arousal or orientation to a painful stimulus.

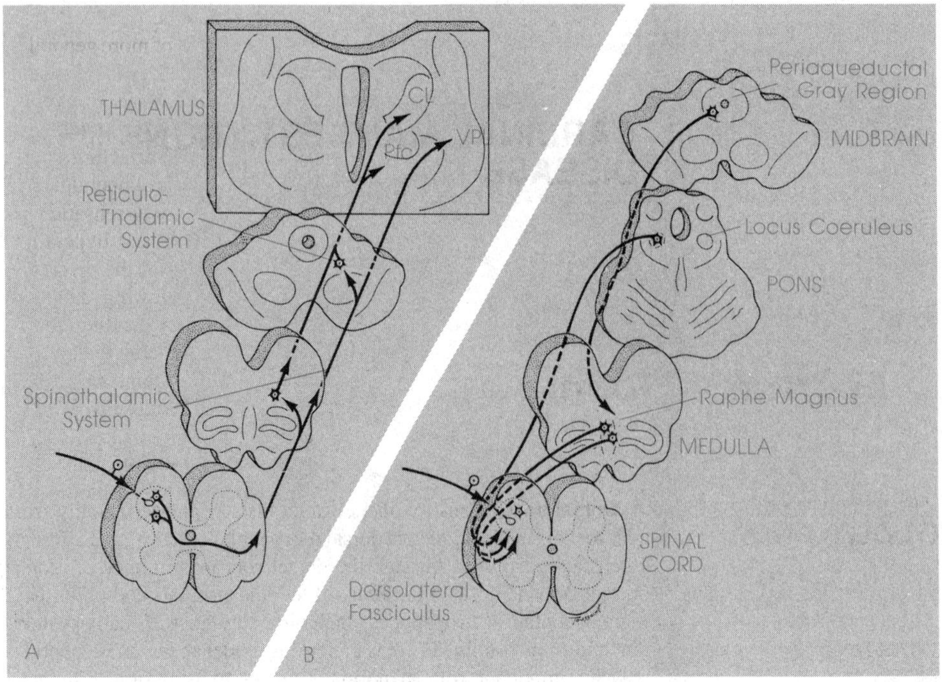

FIGURE 15-1 *A*. Ascending nociceptive pathways. The direct spinothalamic tract terminates in the nucleus ventroposterolateralis (VPL). The indirect, spinoreticulothalamic pathway relays through the brainstem reticular formation and ends in nuclei of the medial and intralaminar thalamus [nuclei parafascicularis (Pfc) and centralis lateralis (CL)]. *B*. Descending analgesia pathways. Periaqueductal gray neurons project to nucleus raphe magnus. A descending projection from raphe magnus inhibits the nociceptive responses of dorsal horn neurons. A separate inhibitory pathway from the nucleus locus coeruleus also directly ends in the dorsal horn.

Descending analgesic pathways In addition to the major ascending pain pathways outlined above, the brain contains powerful descending circuits that suppress nociceptive inputs (Fig. 15-1*B*). In animals, electrical stimulation of the midbrain periaqueductal gray region can produce generalized analgesia without other obvious sensory or motor responses. A similar system may exist in humans, as stimulation of the nearby periventricular gray is reported to relieve clinical pain. This effect appears to be at least partly mediated at the spinal level, since it can be blocked in animals by cutting pathways that carry descending projections from brainstem to dorsal horn. However, few periaqueductal gray cells project directly to the spinal cord. Instead, the descending pathway important for analgesia appears to first synapse in the midline raphe nuclei of the medulla (principally *nucleus raphe magnus*). Raphe neurons in turn project to the spinal cord, where they inhibit the nociceptive responses of dorsal horn neurons. This descending system can potentially gate the flow of nociceptive information from the level of the first synapse in the dorsal horn.

The periaqueductal gray region, the medullary raphe, and the dorsal horn all contain a high density of endogenous opiate peptides and opiate receptors. Systemic narcotic analgesics may, in part, work by activating the descending analgesia system at these sites. High densities of opiate receptors are also found in the medial thalamus and limbic forebrain; these structures may play an additional, important role in the analgesic response to and the addictive potential of systemically administered narcotics.

Biogenic amines represent another class of neurotransmitters found in the descending pathways that modulate nociception. Serotonin is contained in many of the raphe neurons that end in dorsal horn, and some serotonergic axon terminals end directly on spinothalamic tract neurons. A major descending inhibitory pathway containing norepinephrine also arises in the nucleus locus coeruleus of the pons; this system appears to inhibit the nociceptive responses of dorsal horn neurons by an alpha-adrenergic mechanism. Drugs that potentiate the central effects of biogenic amines, such as the tricyclic antidepressants, may therefore be effective analgesic adjuvants that work by enhancing the effects of these descending pathways.

EVALUATION OF THE PATIENT WITH PAIN **Somatic pain** Pain usually occurs when a potentially tissue-damaging stimulus excites peripheral nociceptive afferents. When a noxious stimulus activates receptors in skin, muscle, or joint, the somatic pain that results is usually well-localized and easily described by the patient (Table 15-1). In contrast, pain of visceral origin is often poorly localized and may be referred to an area of skin supplied by the same sensory roots that innervate the diseased visceral organ. For example, myocardial pain activates visceral afferents terminating in the upper four thoracic segments of the spinal cord. This nociceptive information converges on the same neurons that receive cutaneous input from the upper thoracic dermatomes, and the reported pain is therefore frequently referred to the left shoulder and arm. In a similar fashion, the sensory innervation of cranial blood vessels terminates on brainstem trigeminal neurons that also have a cutaneous input. This convergence likely explains the referral of vascular headache pain to the ipsilateral forehead and eye.

Convergence also occurs between muscle, joint, and cutaneous nociceptive afferents. Chronic activation of these pathways can evoke referred pain, local sympathetic effects, segmental muscular contraction, and generalized postural muscle changes. This constellation of features may, with time, result in sustained changes that contribute to the development of certain chronic, painful disorders. For example, following injury or disease, many patients develop a condition of fibromyositis, with pain evoked by movement of specific muscle groups. On examination, such patients often have limitation of movement and tender muscular "trigger points" that reproduce their pain, which is often referred. Myofascial pain of this sort is often prominent in temporomandibular joint disorders, chronic cervical pain, or low back disorders. Untreated myofascial pain can frequently lead to progressive disability, loss of range of motion, and increased pain.

Both cutaneous and visceral pain are common experiences and do not always signal a disease process. The somatic pain resulting from

TABLE 15-1 Evaluation of pain

Somatic pain	Neuropathic pain
1 Nociceptive stimulus usually evident.	*1* No obvious nociceptive stimulus.
2 Pain is usually well-localized; visceral pain may be referred.	*2* Pain is often poorly localized.
3 Pain is similar to other somatic pains in the patient's experience.	*3* Pain is unusual, dissimilar from somatic pain.
4 Pain is relieved by anti-inflammatory or narcotic analgesics.	*4* Pain is only partially relieved by narcotic analgesics.

a new injury or illness is therefore generally familiar to the patient and described in the context of prior similar pains. Somatic pain due to activation of normal nociceptive mechanisms is usually effectively relieved by a brief course of an appropriate analgesic.

Neuropathic pain Pain can also result from injury to, or chronic changes in, peripheral or central somatosensory pathways. This may be due to an abnormal or disordered pattern of afferent neuronal activity that reaches the dorsal horn and more central structures. Damage to sensory pathways may also decrease the inhibitory controls that are normally activated by a peripheral input. Neuropathic pain that follows damage to sensory pathways can develop and persist without an obvious noxious input. The patient often uses unusual terms to describe the pain, emphasizing the distinction between perception of normal somatic pains and neuropathic sensations.

The sensory symptoms in neuropathic pain can be either focal or more generalized. Trauma or irritation to a peripheral nerve may result in a *neuralgia*, which is defined as pain in the distribution of a single nerve; the pain is often (but not always) accompanied by signs of nerve dysfunction, such as sensory loss or weakness of muscles innervated by the nerve. Frequently the pain consists of a background spontaneous burning or aching sensation (*dysesthesia*) that can be associated with paroxysmal jabs of sharp pain within the affected region. Despite an elevated sensory detection threshold, patients will often have an exaggerated response to a noxious stimulus (*hyperalgesia*) or to touch (*hyperesthesia*) or perceive a nonnociceptive stimulus as painful (*allodynia*). These terms for altered hypersensitivity to sensory stimuli are commonly grouped under the less specific term *hyperpathia* (see also Chap. 28).

In some forms of neuralgia (such as trigeminal neuralgia) paroxysmal, lancinating pain predominates without other signs of nerve dysfunction. In contrast, *causalgia* following nerve injury is characterized by a continuous, severe burning pain, allodynia, and evident sympathetic dysfunction. Pain can also be a feature of more generalized neuropathies associated with degeneration of small-caliber axons. In such cases there can be multiple locations for the pain as well as a variety of types of pain. In diffuse sensory or sensorimotor neuropathies, the pain is usually symmetric and distal, affecting the feet and, with progression, the hands. As with more focal neuralgias, the pain often consists of a spontaneous aching or burning sensation with superimposed paroxysmal jabs of pain. Allodynia and hyperalgesia are common features during acute, painful phases of the disease.

Pain may also be a debilitating symptom following damage to central somatosensory pathways. Lesions of the ascending somatosensory pathways at the level of the cord, brainstem, thalamus, or cortex can result in a syndrome of continuous spontaneous pain that is referred to the periphery, often with superimposed sensory abnormalities as discussed above.

MANAGEMENT OF PATIENTS WITH PAIN **Moderate pain** Many acute somatic pains can be treated effectively with oral, nonnarcotic analgesics such as aspirin 650 mg or acetaminophen 650 mg orally every 4 h (Table 15-2). These drugs have few side effects, do not cause sedation, and are not associated with tolerance or dependence. Other nonsteroidal anti-inflammatory drugs (NSAIDs), such as naproxen, indomethacin, ibuprofen, or trisalicylate, are also often effective for minor or moderately severe somatic pain; however, there is little evidence that these agents are clearly better than aspirin, and aspirin is much less expensive. Acetaminophen has little anti-inflammatory action compared to aspirin and indomethacin; pain associated with inflammatory disease is therefore better managed with the latter drugs. However, the side effects of NSAIDs and aspirin, particularly dyspepsia, gastrointestinal bleeding, and inhibition of platelet aggregation can limit their usefulness in certain

TABLE 15-2 Drugs for relief of pain

NONNARCOTIC ANALGESICS: USUAL DOSES AND INTERVALS

Generic name	PO dose, mg	Interval	Comments
Acetylsalicylic acid	650	q 4 h	Enteric-coated preparations available
Acetaminophen	650	q 4 h	Side effects uncommon
Ibuprofen	400	q 4–6 h	Available without prescription
Naproxen	250–500	q 12 h	Delayed effects may be due to long half-life
Suprofen	200	q 6 h	Little anti-inflammatory effect
Trisalicylate	1000–1500	q 12 h	Fewer gastrointestinal or platelet effects
Indomethacin	25–50	q 8 h	Gastrointestinal side effects common

NARCOTIC ANALGESICS: USUAL DOSES AND INTERVALS

Generic name	Parenteral dose, mg	PO dose, mg	Comments
Codeine	30–60 q 4 h	30–60 q 4 h	Nausea common
Oxycodone	—	5–10 q 4–6 h	Usually available with acetominophen or aspirin
Morphine	10 q 4 h	60 q 4 h	
Morphine sustained release	90 q 12 h	Oral slow release preparation	
Hydromorphone	1–2 q 4 h	2–4 q 4 h	Shorter acting than morphine sulfate
Levorphanol	2 q 6–8 h	4 q 6–8 h	Longer acting than morphine sulfate; absorbed well PO
Methadone	10 q 6–8 h	20 q 6–8 h	Delayed sedation due to long half-life
Meperidine	75–100 q 3–4 h	300 q 4 h	Poorly absorbed PO; normeperidine a toxic metabolite

ANTICONVULSANTS

Generic name	PO dose, mg	Interval
Phenytoin	100	q 6–8 h
Carbamazepine	200–300	q 6 h
Clonazepam	1	q 6 h

TRICYCLIC ANTIDEPRESSANTS

Generic name	Uptake blockade 5HT	NE	Sedative potency	Anticholinergic potency	Orthostatic hypotension	Cardiac arrhythmia	Average dose, mg/day	Range, mg/day
Doxepin	+ +	+	High	Moderate	Moderate	Less	200	75–400
Amitriptyline	+ + + +	+ +	High	Highest	Moderate	Yes	150	75–300
Imipramine	+ + + +	+ +	Moderate	Moderate	High	Yes	200	75–400
Nortriptyline	+ + +	+ +	Moderate	Moderate	Low	Yes	100	40–150
Desipramine	+ + +	+ + + +	Low	Low	Low	Yes	150	75–300

patients; these side effects may be less common with trisalicylate and are not observed with acetaminophen.

Severe pain Narcotic analgesics are usually required for relief of severe pain. In general, patients should be treated with only one narcotic agent at a time, and therapy should be begun with an intermediate-strength narcotic such as codeine 30 mg every 4 to 6 h or oxycodone 5 mg every 4 to 6 h. In oral doses, codeine is relatively safe, potent, and well-tolerated. Aspirin or acetaminophen potentiates the analgesic effect of codeine, and so the two drugs can be used together. Oxycodone 5 mg is commonly available only in tablet form combined with aspirin or acetaminophen. Low-strength narcotic analgesics such as propoxyphene (dextropropoxyphene) or mixed agonist/antagonist drugs such as pentazocine have few indications. The analgesic effectiveness of these drugs is often little better than aspirin, and the frequency of side effects is much greater. Mixed agonist/antagonist drugs can also precipitate withdrawal in patients habituated to stronger narcotics.

If codeine 60 mg (or oxycodone 10 mg) orally every 4 h fails to provide relief, it should be discontinued, as larger doses of codeine increase the frequency of side effects without clearly adding to its analgesic effectiveness. In these situations codeine should be stopped and a higher-potency narcotic used, such as intramuscular morphine 10 mg every 4 h or oral hydromorphone 4 mg every 3 to 4 h. There is substantial variation in the effective analgesic dose and the duration of action of narcotics in individual patients. Dosages should therefore be individualized according to the patient's needs.

A variety of drugs, including antihistamines, amphetamines, and antidepressants, may enhance the analgesic effects of narcotics and can be useful in certain situations. Oral hydroxyzine 25 mg four times daily can potentiate narcotic analgesia without adding to the sedative effects. In patients who are excessively sedated by narcotics, oral dextroamphetamine 5 mg twice daily can make the patient more alert while enhancing analgesia. Benzodiazepines and phenothiazines have numerous side effects and often do not enhance analgesia; they should be used for their specific indications and not routinely.

The pharmacokinetics of narcotics are greatly influenced by disease. Hepatic cirrhosis or renal failure can enhance the bioavailability and decrease the elimination of narcotics. This is a particular problem with meperidine (pethidine). In debilitated patients receiving high doses of meperidine, the active metabolite normeperidine can accumulate, resulting in symptoms of tremor, confusion, and seizures. Morphine may be a superior drug to use when chronic, large doses of narcotics are required in debilitated patients, since the pharmacokinetics of morphine do not appear to be altered in cirrhosis.

Although side effects can result from the use of excess or inappropriate narcotics, a far more common problem is underutilization of analgesics. Hospitalized patients, including postoperative and cancer cases, frequently receive inadequate doses of narcotic analgesics. The reasons that underlie inadequate narcotic use in patients with evident painful disease are unclear. Concerns about inducing dependence and addiction in a medically ill population are largely unfounded. Similarly, concerns over respiratory depression and delayed recovery in patients on narcotics are often overstated; more often, *inadequate* analgesia in postoperative patients produces a reduction in tidal volume due to splinting and delays patient mobilization. When indicated, therefore, narcotic analgesics should be given frequently enough and in high enough doses to alleviate pain. A single narcotic medication should be offered the patient on a routine rather than on an "as needed" basis, with the understanding that the patient can refuse the drug if the level of analgesia is sufficient. Changes in analgesic doses and the need to taper narcotics as the acute phase of pain passes should be understood by the patient.

Chronic diseases usually cause recurrent bouts of acute pain rather than continuous discomfort. The management of acute painful exacerbations should be the same as the treatment of any new, acute pain. Analgesics should be available to the patient when pain is present, with the understanding between patient and physician that the drugs will be discontinued as the acute episode subsides.

Pain in advanced illness Patients with terminal diseases such as metastatic cancer often suffer from continuous or recurrent acute pain. For such patients, pain management is often the single most important treatment a physician can provide.

In outpatients with somatic pain due to cancer, oral codeine 30 mg or oxycodone 5 mg and acetaminophen 325 mg every 4 h may provide acceptable pain control. Patients with bony metastases often benefit from the addition of an NSAID, such as oral trisalicylate 1000 mg or naproxen 500 mg twice daily. If a total daily dose of 30 to 40 mg of oxycodone does not adequately relieve pain, the patient should be switched to a stronger narcotic such as oral hydromorphone 4 mg or levorphanol 2 mg as needed; however, there is little evidence that these drugs are more effective than oral morphine. Slow-release oral morphine preparations have little potential for abuse and can be administered every 12 h, with supplemental doses of regular oral morphine given as needed. The 12-h dosing schedule for slow-release morphine results in more continuous analgesia and often allows patients to sleep through the night without pain. Methadone also has a very long half-life and may therefore be useful in individual patients; however, the cumulative effects of methadone over many days requires careful follow-up monitoring of patients.

Essentially all patients on narcotics develop constipation. In cancer patients this can be significant, and should be anticipated.

In cancer patients an increase in pain often signals recurrence or extension of their disease. However, in some patients tolerance to medications can become an important factor. Although the underlying disease process remains essentially unchanged, increasing doses of narcotic analgesics may be necessary in such patients to maintain satisfactory analgesia. The rate at which patients clinically develop tolerance to narcotics is variable; some patients require a doubling of their dose as often as every 1 to 2 weeks. There is no absolute tolerance barrier, however, and patients tolerant to even very high doses of narcotics can still achieve analgesia by doubling or tripling their medication dosage. Although tolerance is an important issue, it should also be emphasized that most cancer patients develop tolerance only gradually, and remain responsive to relatively low doses of narcotics throughout the course of their disease.

As narcotic doses are increased, the frequency of side effects, including sedation and dysphoric reactions, may also increase. When these side effects limit the use of analgesics or require the use of continuous intravenous narcotics, surgical approaches to pain relief are worth considering. An anterolateral cordotomy can provide effective relief in patients with pain that is isolated to a single leg or hip. Touch sensation, motor power, and bladder control are all usually spared by the procedure. Cordotomy is less effective in patients with pain involving the upper extremity or involving both sides of the trunk. In evaluating patients for this procedure, the extent of disease may be as important as the location of pain. A patient with unilateral pain but evidence of bilateral or midline disease (such as extensive vertebral metastases) is not likely to get substantial relief from a cordotomy.

Spinal morphine therapy is worth considering in certain cancer patients. Morphine injections through spinal epidural or intrathecal catheters can provide substantial analgesia, potentially minimizing some of the side effects of large systemic doses of narcotic. Several systems are now available that allow patients to continue administering their own spinal morphine injections at home. The clinical indications for the use of such systems remain controversial.

For most cancer patients, however, surgical pain-relieving procedures are unnecessary. Usually a change in drug, dose, or the addition of an adjuvant analgesic can improve pain relief while minimizing adverse reactions.

Management of neuropathic pain Neuropathic pain is often a chronic disabling condition that can involve pathophysiologic changes at many levels of the nervous system. The medical management of neuropathic pain is disappointing; patients rarely achieve substantial, lasting improvement with any single therapy. For patients with neuropathic pain, conventional analgesics are only rarely effective.

The search for improved forms of treatment in such patients has resulted in a number of approaches.

ANTICONVULSANTS In patients with neuropathic pain with little or no evidence of sympathetic dysfunction, anticonvulsants and antidepressant drugs are frequently prescribed, although there is only limited evidence that such medications are effective.

Phenytoin, carbamazepine, or clonazepam may be helpful in certain patients with painful neuropathies or neuralgias. Anticonvulsants are particularly effective in treating the sharp, lancinating pains associated with focal neuralgias such as trigeminal neuralgia. They are less effective for the more constant dull, burning sensations that are a major component of conditions such as postherpetic neuralgia or diabetic neuropathy.

ANTISYMPATHETIC AGENTS In some patients, traumatic neuralgias can present with spontaneous burning pain and a disturbance in the sympathetic innervation of the affected limb. Some patients with sympathetically maintained pain (''reflex sympathetic dystrophy'') may achieve substantial pain relief with a series of temporary sympathetic blocks or a surgical sympathectomy. When pain relief follows a sympathetic block, treatment with intravenous regional or systemic antisympathetic drugs such as guanethidine also may provide sustained relief in some patients.

TRICYCLIC ANTIDEPRESSANTS Antidepressant drugs are frequently used to treat pain following peripheral nerve injury. Tricyclic iminodibenzyl derivatives are the most commonly used drugs. Their pharmacologic effects include facilitation of monoamine transmission by inhibition of transmitter reuptake at the synapse and changes in pre- and postsynaptic adrenergic receptor sensitivity. The important site of action of tricyclic antidepressants for pain relief is not clear. However, they may act to potentiate the brainstem inhibition of nociceptive transmission at the level of the dorsal horn. Tricyclic antidepressants also have major effects on ascending monoaminergic systems that project into the forebrain. It seems probable that these ascending systems are also important in pain perception, although how antidepressant drugs influence sensory pathways at the level of the thalamus and cortex remains speculative.

TRANSCUTANEOUS ELECTRICAL NERVE STIMULATION (TENS) Electrical stimulation with a TENS unit applied to the painful region or over the proximal nerve may provide substantial pain relief in patients with painful nerve injuries. However, the duration of the effect is usually limited to the period of stimulation. After a period of days to months, in many patients the analgesic response to TENS habituates, and electrical stimulation may actually worsen the pain.

Management of chronic pain Unrelieved pain that has continued to be a major, disabling condition for a minimum of 6 months is usually referred to as ''chronic'' pain. Patients with chronic pain often present special problems in evaluation and management.

In certain pain patients, particularly those with chronic pain, there is often little correlation between the severity of active disease and the amount of pain behavior. Although restricted activity and analgesic medications are important components of the treatment of most patients with acute pain, these forms of therapy may be counterproductive in patients with chronic pain. After an extended period of inactivity due to pain, patients often become physically deconditioned. Fibromyositis is a common problem, with a loss of strength and range of motion associated with tenderness over postural muscles. Patients can become fatigued with minor efforts, and simple chores quickly exacerbate their pain. They learn to avoid activities that may be associated with pain, and become socially withdrawn. Within the family, pain often becomes a focus of attention, argument, and subtle secondary gain. In this setting, the continued use of sedating analgesic medications reinforces the sick role and often simply adds to the patient's degree of disability and progressive loss of function.

PSYCHOLOGICAL ASPECTS Several categories of psychological diagnoses can be associated with chronic pain syndromes. The two most common presentations are patients with depression and patients with somatoform disorders.

DEPRESSION Depressive symptoms are common in patients with chronic pain, and depressive illness is found in approximately 30 percent. Many pain patients deny depression and do not show a depressed affect. In such patients vegetative signs of insomnia, diminished libido, and lack of energy may be present.

The relationship between pain and depression is complex. The pain threshold is lowered in clinically depressed patients, and pain is a common complaint among patients with primary depression. Patients with pain associated with chronic somatic disease also frequently develop depressive symptoms. However, the incidence of depression defined by strict clinical criteria is not clearly different in chronic pain patients when compared to medically ill patients without pain.

In an effort to more clearly delineate the relationship between pain and depression, a subgroup of chronic pain patients with a ''pain-prone'' disorder has been described. Such patients tend to have a hypochondriacal preoccupation with their pain. The pain is often continuous in nature and obscure in origin. Associated with the pain complaint, the patient may have depressive symptoms of insomnia, fatigue, and despair. Pain-prone individuals have developmental histories characterized by stress and unmet dependency needs. There may be a family history of depression, alcoholism, or physical abuse. Before the onset of their pain, however, such individuals have an idealized view of themselves and their family relations, denying conflicts. They may also have compulsive work records and hold several jobs. Chronic pain in this group of individuals may be associated in part with unresolved personal or interpersonal conflicts.

Consistent with the association of pain and depression, antidepressant drugs can stabilize the sleep pattern and improve the dysphoric symptoms of patients with chronic pain. There is often a reduction in the intensity of reported pain that may be associated with a decrease in the requirement for analgesics. Antidepressants may therefore have an important role in the management of chronic pain, although it is still uncertain whether these drugs act primarily to potentiate analgesics or to relieve subclinical depression.

SOMATOFORM DISORDERS Patients with somatoform disorders have symptoms that suggest an organic disease but have no evidence of a physical disorder that might explain these symptoms. The heading ''somatoform disorders'' includes patients with somatization disorders, conversion disorders, hypochondriasis, or psychogenic pain disorders. Although symptoms of chronic pain are often part of the presentation of a somatoform disorder, patients with this diagnosis do not have depressive symptoms and do not usually respond to antidepressants. However, such patients seek out doctors and undergo repetitive tests to evaluate vague complaints. Anxiolytics and muscle relaxants are usually prescribed, with little or no benefit. Surgical procedures are often performed for pain relief without success.

Patients with somatoform disorders need frequent reassurance that their pain is not associated with serious illness; the management of these conditions is therefore primarily supportive. These patients should have careful follow-up from a small number of care-givers to minimize unnecessary tests and reduce the amount of medication prescribed. In this group of patients diagnosing new pains that signal true organic pathology can be a clinical challenge.

When patients with long-standing chronic pain are seen for a new evaluation, they often have unrealistic expectations of the physician. Frequently they state that none of their prior physicians was competent and that this is their last hope for relief from their suffering. A detailed medical history will often reveal poor compliance with previous treatment recommendations made by other physicians.

To avoid another treatment failure, the chronic pain patient should be evaluated by a multidisciplinary group of specialists skilled in managing chronic pain complaints. The specialists composing this group may vary, depending on the nature of the pain complaint and the resources available at an institution. At a minimum, however, a patient should receive a medical, psychological, neurologic, and physical therapy evaluation. A group approach avoids potential confrontation between patient and physician that may stall progress; it also enhances the credibility of the treatment group, increasing the likelihood of patient compliance. The goal of this evaluation is to establish a treatment plan with specific objectives. Each objective should be accomplished according to a timetable mutually agreed on by the patient and the treatment team.

In general, three main goals should be emphasized. First, drug treatment should be simplified and minimized. In many chronic pain patients, common analgesics and muscle relaxants are only minimally effective. The patient therefore tends to increase the dosage in the hope of enhancing pain relief. With the patient's understanding, the number of medications should be reduced by eliminating redundant or ineffective drugs. The dosages of the remaining medications should then be decreased systematically to a point where the patient is taking only drugs that have a definite beneficial effect with minimal side effects.

The second goal of therapy is to help the patient develop a better understanding of the pain and the factors that exacerbate it. Stress management and relaxation training may provide patients with skills to control factors that contribute to their pain. The psychological significance of the pain and its relationship to developmental or interpersonal factors may be worth exploring with individual patients. Antidepressant medications may also have a role in the management of affective symptoms in certain chronic pain patients.

The third goal of therapy should be increased mobilization and functional ability. Under the direction of a specialist in rehabilitation medicine, a program of physical treatments for pain relief (TENS, massage, etc.) should be coupled with an exercise program to increase range of motion and endurance. In some patients, vocational rehabilitation can form an important part of this program. For all patients, realistic timetables should be set for a return to self-care and independent function consistent with the patient's level of objective physical disability.

Social and interpersonal factors may perseverate pain; certain chronic pain patients are therefore refractory to treatment on an outpatient basis. Admission to an inpatient multidisciplinary pain treatment facility can provide an opportunity for an intensive program of evaluation and treatment of such patients. Standards for such inpatient units have been established by the Committee on Accreditation of Rehabilitation Facilities and the American Pain Society. Studies of the effectiveness of pain treatment units demonstrate decreased reports of pain, decreased drug use, and increased functional ability in the majority of patients completing this type of program. However, the ultimate success of such programs depends on maintained functional improvement in patients over long periods following discharge. Careful follow-up and reevaluation of patients with chronic pain is therefore an essential part of successful management.

REFERENCES

Asbury A, Fields HL: Pain due to peripheral nerve damage: An hypothesis. Neurology 34:1587, 1984

Basbaum AI, Fields HL: Endogenous pain control systems: Brainstem spinal pathways and endorphin circuitry. Ann Rev Neurosci 7:309, 1984

Blumer D, Heilbronn M: Chronic pain as a variant of depressive disease. J Nerv Ment Dis 170:381, 1982

Fields HL: *Pain*. New York, McGraw-Hill, 1987

Foley KM, Intruissi CE (eds): *Opioid Analgesics in the Management of Clinical Pain. Advances in Pain Research and Therapy*, vol 8. New York, Raven Press, 1986

———, Payne RM (eds): *Current Therapy of Pain*. Toronto, Decker, 1989

Hackett TP: The pain patient: Evaluation and treatment, in *Massachusetts General Hospital Handbook of General Hospital Psychiatry*, TP Hackett (ed.) Boston, Massachusetts General Hospital, 1978, p 41

Hannington-Kiff JG: Antisympathetic drugs in limbs, in *Textbook of Pain*, PD Wall, R Melzack (eds). New York, Churchill Livingstone, 1984

Maciewicz R, Fields HL: Pain pathways, in *Diseases of the Nervous System*, A Asbury, G McKann (eds). London, Saunders, 1985

Melzack R (ed): *Pain Measurement and Assessment*. New York, Raven Press, 1983

Sweet WH, Poletti CE: Causalgia, in *Evaluation and Treatment of Chronic Pain*, G Aronoff (ed). Baltimore, Urban and Schwarzenberg, 1985

Tasker RR: Deafferentation, in *Textbook of Pain*, PD Wall, R Melzack (eds). New York, Churchill Livingstone, 1984, p 119

Taub A, Collins WF: Observations on the treatment of denervation dysesthesia with psychotropic drugs: Postherpetic neuralgia, anesthesia dolorosa, peripheral neuropathy, in *Advances in Neurology*, JJ Bonica (ed). New York, Raven Press, 1974, p 309

White JC, Sweet WH: *Pain and the Neurosurgeon—A Forty Years' Experience*. Springfield, Ill., Charles C. Thomas, 1969

Yaksh TL, Hammond DL: Peripheral and central substrates involved in the rostrad transmission of nociceptive information. Pain 13:1, 1982

16 CHEST DISCOMFORT AND PALPITATION

LEE GOLDMAN / EUGENE BRAUNWALD

CHEST DISCOMFORT

Chest discomfort is one of the most frequent complaints for which patients seek medical attention; the potential benefit (or harm) resulting from the proper (or improper) assessment and management of the patient with this complaint is enormous. Failure to recognize a serious disorder, such as ischemic heart disease, may result in the dangerous delay of much-needed treatment, while an incorrect diagnosis of a potentially hazardous condition such as angina pectoris is likely to have harmful psychological and economic consequences and may lead to unnecessary cardiac catheterization. There is little relation between the severity of chest discomfort and the gravity of its cause. Therefore, a frequent problem in patients who complain of chest discomfort or pain is distinguishing trivial complaints from coronary artery disease and other serious disorders (Table 16-1).

PATHOPHYSIOLOGY **Discomfort due to myocardial ischemia** Discomfort due to myocardial ischemia occurs when the oxygen supply to the heart is deficient in relation to the oxygen need. Oxygen consumption is closely related to the physiologic effort made during contraction, and coronary venous blood is normally much more desaturated than that draining other areas of the body. As a consequence, the removal of more oxygen from each unit of blood, which

TABLE 16-1 Some causes of chest discomfort

I Cardiac
- *A* Coronary artery disease
- *B* Aortic stenosis
- *C* Hypertropic cardiomyopathy
- *D* Pericarditis

II Vascular
- *A* Aortic dissection
- *B* Pulmonary embolism
- *C* Pulmonary hypertension
- *D* Right ventricular strain

III Pulmonary
- *A* Pleuritis or pneumonia
- *B* Tracheobronchitis
- *C* Pneumothorax
- *D* Tumor
- *E* Mediastinitis or mediastinal emphysema

IV Gastrointestinal
- *A* Esophogeal reflux
- *B* Esophogeal spasm
- *C* Mallory-Weiss tear
- *D* Peptic ulcer disease
- *E* Biliary disease
- *F* Pancreatitis

V Musculoskeletal
- *A* Cervical disk disease
- *B* Arthritis of the shoulder or spine
- *C* Costochondritis
- *D* Intercostal muscle cramps
- *E* Interscalene or hyperabduction syndromes
- *F* Subacromial bursitis

VI Other
- *A* Disorders of the breast
- *B* Chest wall tumors
- *C* Herpes zoster

is one of the adjustments commonly utilized by exercising skeletal muscle, is already employed in the heart in the basal state. Therefore, the heart must rely primarily on an increase in the coronary blood flow for obtaining additional oxygen.

The blood flow through the coronary arteries is directly proportional to the pressure gradient between the aorta and the ventricular myocardium during systole and the ventricular cavity during diastole, but is also proportional to the fourth power of the radius of the coronary arteries. A relatively slight alteration in coronary luminal diameter below a critical level can produce a large decrement in coronary flow, provided that other factors remain constant. Coronary blood flow occurs primarily during diastole, when it is unopposed by systolic myocardial compression of the coronary vessels.

When the epicardial coronary arteries are narrowed critically (>70 percent stenosis of the luminal diameter), the intramyocardial coronary arterioles dilate in an effort to maintain total flow at a level that will avert myocardial ischemia at rest. Further dilatation, which normally occurs during exercise, is therefore not possible. Hence, any condition in which increased heart rate, arterial pressure, or myocardial contractility occurs in the presence of coronary obstruction tends to precipitate anginal attacks by increasing myocardial oxygen needs in the face of a fixed oxygen supply.

By far the most frequent underlying cause of myocardial ischemia is organic narrowing of the coronary arteries secondary to coronary atherosclerosis (see also Chap. 190). A *dynamic* component of increased coronary vascular resistance, secondary to spasm of the major epicardial vessels (often near an atherosclerotic plaque) or more frequently to constriction of smaller coronary arterioles, is present in many, perhaps the majority, of patients with chronic angina pectoris. There is no evidence that systemic arterial constriction or increased cardiac contractile activity (rise in heart rate or blood pressure, or increase in contractility due to liberation of catecholamines or adrenergic activity) due to emotion can precipitate angina unless there is also organic or dynamic narrowing of the coronary vessels. Acute thrombosis superimposed on an atherosclerotic plaque is frequently the cause of unstable angina and acute myocardial infarction.

Aside from conditions which narrow the lumen of the coronary arteries, the only other frequent causes of myocardial ischemia are disorders such as valvular aortic stenosis (Chap. 188) or hypertrophic cardiomyopathy (Chap. 192), which cause a marked disproportion between the perfusion pressure and the heart's oxygen requirements. Under such conditions, the rise in left ventricular systolic pressure is not, as in hypertensive states, balanced by a corresponding elevation of aortic perfusion pressure. Recent epidemiologic studies indicate that chest pain is no more common in patients with mitral valve prolapse than in those without it.

An increase in heart rate is especially harmful in patients with coronary atherosclerosis and with aortic stenosis, because it both increases myocardial oxygen needs and shortens diastole relatively more than systole, thereby decreasing the total available perfusion time per minute. Tachycardia, a decline in arterial pressure, thyrotoxicosis, or diminution in arterial oxygen content (such as occurs in anemia or arterial hypoxia) are precipitating and aggravating factors rather than underlying causes of angina.

Discomfort due to pericarditis The visceral surface of the pericardium ordinarily is insensitive to pain, as is the parietal surface, except in its lower portion, which has a relatively small number of pain fibers carried in the phrenic nerves. The pain associated with pericarditis is believed to be due to inflammation of the adjacent parietal pleura. These observations explain why noninfectious pericarditis (e.g., that associated with uremia and with myocardial infarction) and cardiac tamponade with relatively mild inflammation are usually painless or accompanied by only mild pain, whereas infectious pericarditis, being nearly always more intense and spreading to the neighboring pleura, is usually associated with pain (Chap. 193).

Vascular causes of chest pain *Aortic dissection* develops as a result of a subintimal hematoma, which may start either because a tear has developed in the intima of the aorta or because of bleeding into the vasa vasorum. Antegrade movement of this hematoma can compromise major branches off the aorta, just as retrograde spread can occlude a coronary artery, disrupt the aortic valve annulus, or rupture into the pericardial space.

Pulmonary emboli These commonly originate from thrombi in the venous circulation, especially in the lower extremities. Venous thrombosis is usually related to stasis or slowing of blood flow because of inactivity or impedance to venous return, to damage in the vessel wall, or to alterations in the coagulation system. When thrombi from any source embolize to the pulmonary arterial circulation, they can cause not only mechanical obstruction but also vasoconstriction and elevated pulmonary vascular resistance related to the release of humoral factors, such as histamine, serotonin, and prostaglandins. As a result, hypoxemia and, occasionally, right heart failure can ensue, and an acute fall in cardiac output can lead to sudden death. The acute pain from massive pulmonary emboli is thought to be related to pulmonary hypertension and to distention of the pulmonary artery. Infarction of a segment of the lung that is adjacent to the pleura commonly irritates the pleural surface and causes chest discomfort hours or even days later (see Chap. 213).

Other pulmonary causes of chest discomfort A variety of diseases of the lung can cause chest discomfort. Pleural pain, which is usually brief, sharp pain that is precipitated by inspiration, is very common and generally results from stretching of an inflamed parietal pleura.

Gastrointestinal causes of chest discomfort Esophageal pain includes *esophageal reflux* and *esophageal spasm.* Esophageal discomfort usually results from chemical (acid) irritation of the esophageal mucosa because of acid reflux or spasm of the esophageal muscle. Rupture of the esophagus, such as in a Mallory-Weiss tear that is caused by severe vomiting, causes severe acute chest pain (Chap. 237)

Occasionally, other gastrointestinal diseases including *peptic ulcer disease, biliary disease,* and *pancreatitis* may present with chest discomfort as well as abdominal discomfort.

Neuromusculoskeletal causes of chest discomfort Neuromusculoskeletal chest discomfort can be caused by *cervical disk disease,* because of compression of nerve roots, by *arthritis of the shoulder or spine,* or by *costochondritis,* which is an inflammation of the costochondral junctions. Inflammation of the subacromial bursa or, less commonly, the supraspinatus or deltoid tendon may cause pain that radiates to the chest. *Intercostal muscle cramps* may occur throughout the chest. Anterior scalene and hyperabduction syndromes can also cause chest discomfort.

Other causes of chest discomfort A variety of *disorders of the breast,* including inflammatory breast disease, benign and malignant tumors, and mastodynia, can cause chest discomfort, usually in association with local abnormalities of the breast. *Chest wall tumors,* including metastases from other organs or malignant disease in the ribs, can also present as chest discomfort. The pain of *herpes zoster* may antedate the typical rash by a day or more, making early diagnosis difficult (Chap. 136).

DIFFERENTIAL DIAGNOSIS The key issue in the evaluation of the patient with chest discomfort is to distinguish potentially life-threatening conditions such as coronary artery disease, aortic dissection, and pulmonary embolism from other causes of chest discomfort. Even patients who have brief episodes of pain and are otherwise in apparently excellent health may have intermittent myocardial ischemia or even recurrent pulmonary emboli.

The radiation of pain arising in the thoracic viscera can usually be explained by known neuroanatomic relationships (Chap. 15). Pain impulses which enter one cord segment may spill over and excite nearby cord segments.

The chest discomfort of myocardial ischemia, most commonly from coronary artery disease but also occasionally from the other causes of ischemia noted above, is angina pectoris. Myocardial ischemia from coronary atherosclerosis is more common in patients who have hypercholesterolemia, diabetes mellitus, hypertension, or obesity or who smoke cigarettes (Chap. 195). Toxins, including cocaine ingestion or withdrawal of chronic exposure to nitroglycerin, can cause sufficient coronary vasoconstriction to result in myocardial ischemia, and cocaine can also cause myocardial infarction.

Angina pectoris is usually described as a heaviness, pressure, or squeezing, or as a sensation of strangling or constriction in the chest, but may also be described as aching, burning, or even as indigestion. Some patients steadfastly deny pain but will admit to a discomfort or unusual feeling or may complain of difficulty in breathing.

Typically angina pectoris develops gradually during exertion, after heavy meals, and with anger, excitement, frustration, and other emotional states; it is not precipitated by coughing, respiratory movements, or other motion. When angina is induced by walking, it often forces the patient to stop or to reduce speed. Angina occurs most typically in the substernal region, anteriorly across the midthorax; it may radiate to or rarely occur alone in the interscapular region, in the arms, shoulders, teeth, and abdomen. It rarely radiates to below the umbilicus, to the back of the neck or the occiput. The more severe the attack, the greater the radiation from the substernal areas to the left arm, especially its ulnar aspect. Although the radiation of chest discomfort to the left arm increases the likelihood that myocardial ischemia or infarction is present, impulses from the skin and from visceral structures, such as the esophagus and heart, converge on a common pool of neurons in the posterior horn of the spinal cord. Their origin may be confused by the cerebral cortex; hence almost any condition capable of causing chest discomfort may induce radiation to the left arm. Also, stimulation of one of the thoracic nerves that also innervates the heart by, for example, protrusion of an intervertebral disk, may be misinterpreted as pain originating from the heart.

When the history is atypical, as is often the case, the correct diagnosis of angina pectoris may be aided by noting that the pain disappears more rapidly (usually within 5 min) and more completely when sublingual nitroglycerin is used. The demonstration that the time required for a given exercise to produce pain is consistently and considerably longer when it is undertaken within a few minutes after a sublingual nitroglycerin pill than after a placebo may, in some instances, represent powerful clinical evidence for the diagnosis of angina pectoris. Angina is rarely relieved within a few seconds of lying down, nor is it precipitated by stooping forward.

Myocardial infarction is usually associated with a discomfort similar in quality and distribution to that of angina but of longer duration (usually 30 min) and usually of greater intensity. In contrast to angina, the pain of myocardial infarction is not rapidly relieved by rest or by coronary dilator drugs and may require large doses of narcotics. It may be accompanied by diaphoresis, nausea, and hypotension (Chap. 189).

The physical examination in patients with myocardial ischemia frequently is totally normal. However, myocardial ischemia can cause a third or fourth heart sound because of an impairment of myocardial contraction or relaxation. Ischemic papillary muscle dysfunction can cause transient mitral regurgitation and its associated murmur. Myocardial infarction, and less commonly severe and generalized ischemia, can cause congestive heart failure.

The chest discomfort from myocardial ischemia that is caused by aortic stenosis, hypertrophic cardiomyopathy, and non-atherosclerotic causes of coronary artery disease is generally similar to that of angina pectoris from coronary atherosclerosis. However, the physical examination will usually reveal classic findings of an aortic systolic murmur in patients with aortic stenosis (Chap. 188) and will reveal dynamic outflow obstruction in many patients with hypertrophic cardiomyopathy (Chap. 192).

Pericarditis can cause pain in several locations (Chap. 193). Since the central part of the diaphragm receives its sensory supply from the phrenic nerve (which arises from the third to fifth cervical segments of the spinal cord), pain arising from the lower parietal pericardium and central tendon of the diaphragm is felt characteristically at the tip of the shoulder, the adjoining trapezius ridge, and the neck. Involvement of the more lateral part of the diaphragmatic pleura, supplied by branches from the sixth to ninth intercostal nerves, causes pain not only in the anterior part of the chest but also in the upper part of the abdomen or corresponding region of the back, sometimes simulating the pain of acute cholecystitis or pancreatitis.

Pericardial pain commonly has a pleuritic component, i.e., it is related to respiratory movements and aggravated by cough and/or deep inspiration, because of pleural irritation. It is sometimes brought on by swallowing, because the esophagus lies just behind the posterior portion of the heart, and is often altered by a change of bodily position, becoming sharper and more left-sided in the supine position and reduced when the patient sits upright, leaning forward. It is frequently referred to the neck and lasts longer than the pain of angina pectoris.

In some patients, however, pericardial pain may be described as a steady substernal discomfort that can mimic the pain of acute myocardial infarction. The mechanism of this steady substernal pain is not certain, but it may arise from marked inflammation of the relatively insensitive inner parietal surface of the pericardium, or from irritated afferent cardiac nerve fibers lying in the periadventitial layers of the superficial coronary arteries. Occasionally, both pleuritic and steady pain may be present simultaneously.

Patients with marked *right ventricular hypertension* may have exertional pain which is quite similar to that of angina. This discomfort probably results from relative ischemia of the right ventricle brought about by the increased oxygen needs and by the elevated intramural resistance, with reduction of the normally large systolic pressure gradient which perfuses this chamber.

The pain due to *acute dissection of the aorta* (Chap. 197) or to an expanding aortic aneurysm results from stimulation of nerve endings in the adventitia. The pain usually begins abruptly, reaches an extremely severe peak rapidly, is felt in the center of the chest and radiates to the back, lasts for hours, and requires unusually large amounts of analgesics for relief. Patients commonly describe a true pain rather that the vague discomfort that is sometimes described with myocardial ischemia. The pain is not aggravated by changes in position or respiration.

The pain resulting from *pulmonary embolism* (Chap. 213) may resemble that of acute myocardial infarction, and in massive embolism it is located substernally. In patients with smaller emboli the pain is located more laterally, is pleuritic in nature, and may be associated with hemoptysis.

Pleural pain from fibrinous pleurisy or any pneumonic process is very common. It generally results from stretching of inflamed parietal pleura and is similar in character to the pleural pain of pericarditis (see above). Pneumothorax and tumors involving the pleural space may also irritate the parietal pleura and cause pleural pain; the latter is sharp, knifelike, superficial in quality, and its aggravation by each breath and by coughing distinguishes it from the deep, dull, relatively steady pain of myocardial ischemia. Substernal discomfort also frequently occurs in the presence of *tracheobronchitis;* it is commonly described as a burning sensation accentuated by coughing.

The pain of *mediastinal emphysema* (Chap. 216) may be intense and sharp and may radiate from the substernal region to the shoulders; often a distinct crepitus is heard. The pain associated with *mediastinitis* and *mediastinal tumors* usually resembles that of pleuritis but is more likely to be maximal in the substernal region, and the associated feeling of constriction or oppression may cause confusion with myocardial infarction.

The several *abdominal disorders* which may at times mimic anginal pain may usually be suspected from the history. Esophageal pain commonly presents as a deep thoracic burning discomfort, which is the hallmark of acid-induced pain. Substernal discomfort usually suggests a hiatus hernia. Intake of aspirin, alcohol, or certain foods typically exacerbates this burning discomfort, and the discomfort may be relieved promptly by antacids or even by one or two swallows of food or water. Patients may have accompanying dysphagia, regurgitation of undigested food, or weight loss. The symptoms of a hiatus hernia tend to be exacerbated by lying down, and all forms of acid-peptic disease may be worse in the early morning when acidic secretions are not neutralized by food. Esophageal spasm, which may be induced by reflux of gastric acid into an esophagus in which the mucosa has been previously irritated, can cause a squeezing pain that may be indistinguishable from myocardial ischemia and that may even have a similar pattern of radiation. Pain resulting from gastric or duodenal ulcer (Chap. 238) is epigastric or substernal, usually commences about 1 to $1\frac{1}{2}$ h after meals, and is usually relieved in several minutes by antacids or milk.

The discomfort caused by acute cholecystitis is more commonly described as an ache, which may be epigastric or substernal. It most commonly tends to occur an hour or so after meals and not in relation to exertion.

The presence of an abdominal disorder, such as a hiatus hernia or a duodenal ulcer, does not constitute proof that the patient's chest pain is related to it. Such disorders are frequently asymptomatic and are not at all uncommon in patients who also have angina pectoris.

Musculoskeletal pain The *costochondral and chondrosternal articulations* are the commonest sites of anterior chest pain. Objective signs in the form of swelling (Tietze's syndrome), redness, and heat are rare, but sharply localized tenderness is common. The pain may be darting and last for only a few seconds, or may be a dull ache enduring for hours or days. An associated feeling of tightness due to muscle spasm (see below) is frequent. *Pressure on the chondrosternal and costochondral junctions and on the pectoralis muscles is an essential part of the examination of every patient with chest pain* and will reproduce the pain arising from these tissues. A large percentage of patients with costochondral pain, especially those who also have minor and innocent T-wave alterations, are erroneously labeled as having coronary disease.

Pain secondary to *subacromial bursitis, biceps tendonitis,* and *arthritis of the shoulder and spine* may be precipitated by motion but not by general exertion. Pain arising in the chest wall or upper extremity may develop as a result of muscle or ligament strains brought on by unaccustomed exercise and felt in the costochondral or chondrosternal junctions or in the chest wall muscles. Other causes are *osteoarthritis* of the dorsal or thoracic spine and *ruptured cervical disk disease.* Pain in the left upper extremity and precordium may be due to compression of portions of the brachial plexus by a cervical rib or by spasm and shortening of the scalenus anticus muscle secondary to high fixation of the ribs and sternum. Deep breathing, turning or twisting of the chest, and movements of the shoulder girdle and arm may elicit and duplicate the pain of which the patient complains. The pain may be very brief, lasting only a few seconds, or aching and persist for hours. The duration is, therefore, likely to be either longer or shorter than untreated angina pectoris, which usually lasts for only a few minutes.

Emotional disorders are also common causes of chest pain. Usually, the discomfort is experienced as a sense of "tightness," sometimes called "aching," and occasionally it may be sufficiently severe as to be designated a pain of considerable magnitude. Since the discomfort has almost always the additional quality of tightness or constriction and is often localized at least in part beneath the sternum, it is not surprising that this type of discomfort is frequently confused with that of myocardial ischemia. Ordinarily, it lasts for a half hour or more, unrelated to exertion, and with slow fluctuation of intensity. The association with fatigue or emotional strain is usually clear, although this may not be volunteered by the patient. Associated hyperventilation can cause innocent changes in the T waves and ST segments, which can be confused with coronary disease.

APPROACH TO THE PATIENT WITH CHEST DISCOMFORT A detailed and *meticulous history* of the behavior of the pain is the cornerstone of the evaluation. The location, radiation, quality, intensity, and duration of the episodes are important. Even more so is the story of the aggravating and alleviating factors. A history of intense aggravation by breathing, coughing, or other respiratory movements will usually point toward the pleura and pericardium or mediastinum as the site, although chest wall pain is likewise affected by respiratory motion. Similarly, a pain which regularly appears on rapid walking, or with other exertion such as sexual activity, and vanishes within a few minutes upon standing still suggests the diagnosis of angina pectoris, although a similar story will occasionally be obtained from patients with skeletal disorders.

While data from the history are of cardinal importance in the assessment of chest discomfort, physicians should not be misled into overreliance on any single feature. For example, acute myocardial infarction sometimes presents with pain that may be described as burning or even as sharp and may not be principally located in the substernal area.

A thorough *physical examination* can provide important clues to the cause of chest discomfort. Blood pressure should be checked in both arms if aortic dissection is being considered. Examination of the skin may reveal cyanosis, which suggests hypoxemia either from diminished cardiac output or impaired respiratory function, or xanthelasthma, which would suggest hyperlipidemia and associated coronary disease. The finding of lymphadenopathy suggests a tumor. The examination of the chest wall should include both inspection and palpation to search for costochondritis and other musculoskeletal abnormalities. Lung examination may reveal a pleural rub, signs of pneumonic consolidation, or evidence of congestive heart failure. The physical examination may be totally normal in persons with severe myocardial ischemia, but it may also demonstrate abnormalities of vital signs, a third or fourth heart sound, or mitral regurgitation from papillary muscle dysfunction. Aortic stenosis will be accompanied by its typical murmur (Chap. 188). The cardiac examination should also search for an increased pulmonic second sound that may indicate elevated pulmonary artery pressure, such as is found in pulmonary embolism, and the pericardial friction rub that strongly suggests pericarditis. A careful upper abdominal examination may be the first clue to peptic ulcer disease or cholecystitis.

Critical information can often be obtained by attempts to produce or alleviate the pain, such as with nitroglycerin. Careful palpation of the chest wall, subacromial bursa, deltoid tendon, abdomen, and other structures may be very helpful if it reproduces the chest discomfort. Shoulder and arm motion commonly reproduces pain related to these structures. However, the finding that such maneuvers can cause chest discomfort does not mean that such musculoskeletal diseases are the cause of the presenting complaint unless one can be sure that the patient's syndrome is reproduced precisely. Alternatively, the demonstration that a localized pain can be completely relieved by infiltration of a local anesthetic will be conclusive in convincing both the patient and the physician. Evaluation of the patient at the time of a spontaneous episode, such as with an electrocardiogram during pain, is also extremely helpful.

APPLICATION OF THE PRINCIPLES OF CLINICAL REASONING The assessment of the probability of the various causes of chest pain requires the integration of multiple pieces of data, because no single clinical feature can be considered decisive. Each of the conditions that can cause chest discomfort can have varied presentations, and the diagnostic tests upon which physicians often rely can also have false-positive or false-negative results. Thus, the principles of clinical reasoning (Chap. 2) should be applied to the evaluation of the patient with chest discomfort.

History and physical examination The information obtained from a careful medical history and physical examination can be used to develop a differential diagnosis of the causes of chest discomfort in an individual patient, to rank these diagnostic possibilities, and often to assign approximate percent probabilities to them. Although the various causes of chest discomfort have typical characteristics, these characteristics must be interpreted in light of the prior probability that a person with a given age and sex, and with a particular past medical history, would have such a cause of chest discomfort. For example, the possibility of angina pectoris as a cause of precordial or substernal discomfort must be seriously considered in a middle-aged man with coronary risk factors such as hypercholesterolemia and smoking, even if the description of the discomfort is not perfectly typical for angina pectoris. Conversely, when a 20-year old woman describes the onset of new discomfort in a way that is seemingly classic for angina pectoris, such a diagnosis is relatively unlikely because the prior probability of ischemic heart disease, given her age and sex, is so low.

Although it is not always possible to assign numerical probabilities to the various causes of chest discomfort in an individual patient, experienced clinicians either implicitly or explicitly assess the relative likelihoods of various potential explanations for any chest discomfort syndrome to help guide their future diagnostic evaluations and therapy. For example, a middle-aged or elderly man with typical characteristics for angina pectoris has about an 80 to 85 percent probability of having hemodynamically significant coronary artery disease. By comparison, the same man with a history of chest discomfort that has some characteristics that are typical for angina pectoris but other characteristics that are atypical will have a probability of important coronary disease ranging from about 30 to 60 percent. Even persons with chest pain that is decidedly unlikely to represent coronary disease still have some finite possibility of coronary disease, which may range from exceedingly unlikely in a young woman to the 10 percent range in a middle-aged man with many coronary risk factors.

Diagnostic tests Although myocardial ischemia commonly is associated with electrocardiographic changes (Chap. 190), many patients have normal tracings between attacks, and some may even be normal during an episode of pain. However, depression of the ST segments, caused by myocardial ischemia, typically occurs during exertion and is accompanied by anginal discomfort; moreover, electrocardiographic evidence of myocardial ischemia may occur at rest and with or without accompanying chest discomfort. The finding of flat or down-sloping ST-segment depressions of 0.1 mV or greater during an attack of pain substantially increases the likelihood that the pain is anginal in origin. Exercise electrocardiography will show ischemic changes in about 50 to 80 percent of persons with symptomatic coronary disease, but also in about 10 to 15 percent of patients who do not have coronary disease. The accuracy of ambulatory ischemia monitoring in the general population is less clear. Exercise thallium scintigraphy (Chap. 177) will demonstrate a perfusion defect in about 75 to 85 percent of patients with angina pectoris and will be falsely positive in about 10 percent of patients who have chest discomfort from noncoronary causes.

The evaluation of patients with suspected pulmonary embolism should usually focus on the documentation of deep venous thrombosis (Chap. 213) and the evaluation of pulmonary perfusion with a lung scintigram and/or pulmonary arteriography (Chap. 203). Aortic dissection is often suggested by the routine chest radiograph, and the diagnosis may be established by echocardiography, computed tomography, or magnetic resonance imaging. Aortography is the definitive test, but because of its invasiveness it is usually reserved for situations in which the suspicion of dissection is moderate or high and definitive anatomic documentation or localization is needed, often because of the need to consider a surgical repair.

Esophageal or peptic-ulcer diseases can often be diagnosed by an upper gastrointestinal roentgenogram. Esophageal manometry and measurement of lower esophageal sphincter pressure are useful in identifying esophageal spasm. The Bernstein acid perfusion test, in which an attempt is made to reproduce the pain by infusing hydrochloric acid into the esophagus, can help establish acid reflux as the cause of pain (Chap. 237).

Integration of clinical data and test results It is often useful to subdivide patients into those with an *acute* onset of a new or worsened chest pain syndrome versus those with more *chronic* pain. Acute chest pain, with a duration of minutes to hours prior to the patient's presentation to a physician, could be caused by many of the entities described in this chapter and would be especially suspicious for acute myocardial infarction, aortic dissection, pulmonary embolism, biliary colic, or acute musculoskeletal trauma. In many situations, the patient may have had prior pain that was similar to but less severe than the current discomfort; this prior pain may be an important clue to recurrent problems such as biliary colic or esophageal spasm. Some, but certainly not all, patients with acute myocardial infarctions will have had a prior history of angina pectoris.

Accumulated data from large numbers of patients who have presented to emergency departments with acute chest pain can aid the assessment of the probability that an individual is having an acute myocardial infarction. By integrating information from the history, physical examination, and electrocardiogram, such empirically derived algorithms have been able to predict which patients are having acute myocardial infarctions more accurately than are the physicians who actually saw the patients in the emergency department. For example, a person without a history of known coronary disease is unlikely to be having an acute myocardial infarction if the electrocardiogram is normal and the chest pain does not radiate to the neck or left shoulder or arm. Although no algorithm can be considered a perfect predictor that can be used in a vacuum, physicians have the opportunity to improve patient management by incorporating such information into their decision-making.

In patients with chronic or recurrent chest pain, the prior pain pattern is usually very helpful in establishing the current diagnosis. For patients with recurrent myocardial ischemia, a worsening of a stable pain pattern may herald unstable angina pectoris (Chap. 190). Unlike acute chest pain, where decision-making revolves around the need for immediate hospitalization and electrocardiographic monitoring to avoid sudden death, chronic chest pain, unless indicative of unstable angina pectoris, may be clarified by outpatient diagnostic testing, such as exercise electrocardiography and exercise thallium scintigraphy.

Although exercise electrocardiography and exercise thallium scintigraphy are of value in distinguishing between cardiac and noncardiac causes of chest discomfort, the results must be interpreted in light of the prior probability of coronary artery disease, which is the probability that the patient has coronary disease based on the presenting clinical characteristics, age, and sex (see Fig. 2-2, p. 9). Since exercise thallium scintigraphy appears to provide information that is correlated with the standard exercise electrocardiogram no more than would be expected by chance, it can provide additional independent information (Chap. 2) and further change the probability of coronary artery disease (Fig. 16-1). If absolute diagnostic knowledge is required, cardiac catheterization with coronary angiography serves as the gold standard, i.e., the test that is considered definitive regarding the presence or absence of coronary disease, even though the presence of anatomic disease does not guarantee that the coronary stenoses are causing the chest discomfort.

A sequence of consistently negative cardiologic test results reduces the probability of coronary artery disease to below 10 percent in patients with atypical chest discomfort. However, even after a normal exercise electrocardiogram and exercise thallium scintigram, the probability of coronary disease will still be about 30 percent in a patient with a typical history of angina pectoris (Fig. 16-2). By recognizing the potential change in probabilities that can be obtained with positive and negative results of the diagnostic tests that are planned, the physician can decide whether these potential changes in probability are sufficient to warrant the test. For example, the physician should commonly decide that a patient with typical angina pectoris and a positive exercise electrocardiogram does not require an exercise thallium scintigram to *diagnose* coronary disease, although under some circumstances it might aid in the estimation of the patient's subsequent prognosis.

A useful test result is commonly one that moves the likelihood of a diagnostic possibility across a threshold, so that the test result would lead to a change in management, either by influencing the decision to order additional tests or by causing a change in treatment. In the case of chest discomfort, the decisions cannot be based on a 50 percent threshold: Probabilities of coronary artery disease, pulmonary embolism, or aortic dissection that are well below 50 percent may still demand further evaluation because of the dire consequences

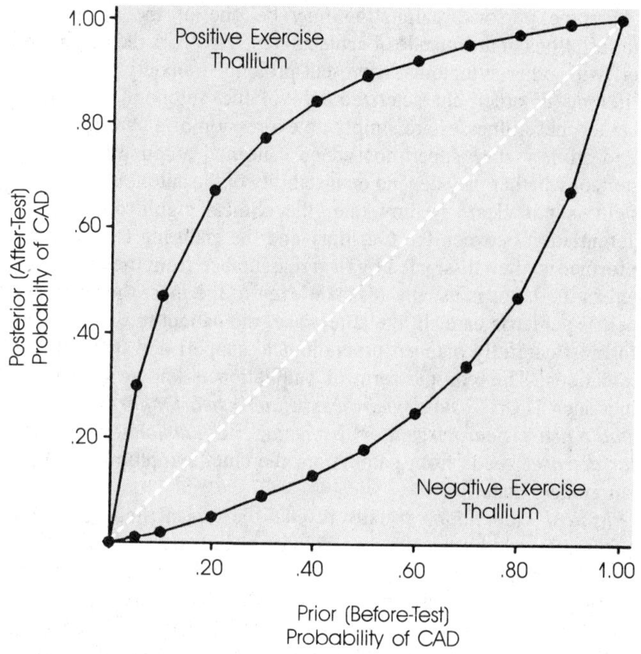

FIGURE 16-1 The curves show the posterior (after-test) probability as a function of the prior (before-test) probability for positive versus negative exercise thallium scintiscans, defined as a perfusion defect that is produced by exercise and resolves with rest. The before-test probability could be estimated from the clinical presentation or could be a postexercise electrocardiogram probability derived from Fig. 2-2 (p. 9). [*From L Goldman, in W Branch, Jr (ed): The Office Practice of Medicine, 2d ed, Philadelphia, Saunders, 1987.*]

of missing one of these important diagnoses. The physician must be prepared to embark on an appropriate evaluation when the history and physical examination do not exclude these diagnoses with a reasonable degree of certainty. The degree of certainty must be determined for the individual condition and patient at hand, typically after an appropriately full and frank discussion between the patient and the physician.

PALPITATION

Palpitation is a common, disagreeable symptom which may be defined as an awareness of the beating of the heart, an awareness most commonly brought about by a change in the heart's rhythm or rate or by an augmentation of its contractility. Palpitation is not pathognomonic of any particular group of disorders; indeed, often it signifies not a primary physical disorder but rather a psychological disturbance. Even when it occurs as a more or less prominent complaint, the diagnosis of the underlying disease is made largely on the basis of other associated symptoms and data. Nevertheless, palpitation is frequently of considerable importance in the minds of patients, who fear that it may indicate heart disease. Concern is all the more pronounced in patients who have been told that they *may* have heart disease; to them palpitation may seem to be an omen of impending disaster. Since the resulting anxiety may be associated with increased activity of the autonomic nervous system, with consequent increases of the cardiac rate and rhythm and the vigor of contraction, the patient's awareness of these changes may then lead to a vicious cycle, which may ultimately be responsible for incapacitation.

Palpitation may be described by the patient in various terms, such as "pounding," "fluttering," "flopping," and "skipping," and in most cases it will be obvious that the complaint is of a sensation of disturbed heartbeat. The sensitivity to alterations in cardiac activity among different individuals varies widely. Some patients seem to be unaware of the most serious and chaotic dysrhythmias; others are seriously troubled by an occasional extrasystole. Patients with anxiety states often exhibit a lowered threshold at which disorders of rate and rhythm result in palpitation. The awareness of the heartbeat also tends to be more common at night and during introspective moments, but is less marked during activity. Patients with organic heart disease and chronic disorders of cardiac rate, rhythm, or stroke volume tend to accommodate to these abnormalities and are often less sensitive than normal persons to such events. Persistent tachycardia and/or atrial fibrillation may not be accompanied by continuous palpitation, in contrast to a sudden, brief alteration in cardiac rate or rhythm which often causes considerable subjective discomfort. Palpitation is particularly prominent when the precipitating cause for increased heart rate or contractility or arrhythmia is recent, transient, and episodic. Conversely, in emotionally well-adjusted individuals palpitation commonly becomes progressively less disconcerting as it becomes more chronic.

PATHOGENESIS OF PALPITATION Under ordinary circumstances the rhythmic heartbeat is imperceptible to the healthy individual of placid or even average temperament. Palpitation may be experienced by normal persons who have engaged in strenuous physical effort or have been aroused emotionally or sexually. This type of palpitation is physiologic and represents the normal awareness of an overactive heart—i.e., a heart that is beating at a rapid rate and with an increased contractility. Palpitation due to overactivity of the heart may also occur in certain pathologic states, e.g., fever, acute or severe anemia, or thyrotoxicosis.

When palpitation is heavy and regular, it is usually caused by an augmented stroke volume. Pathologic states, such as aortic regurgitation or a variety of hyperkinetic circulatory states (anemia, arteriovenous fistula, and thyrotoxicosis) should be considered, as well as the benign so-called idiopathic hyperkinetic heart syndrome. Palpi-

FIGURE 16-2 Approximate probability of coronary artery disease before and after noninvasive testing of a patient with typical (*A*) and atypical (*B*) angina pectoris. The percentages demonstrate how the sequential use of an exercise electrocardiogram and an exercise thallium test may affect the probability of coronary artery disease. [*From L Goldman, in W Branch, Jr (ed): The Office Practice of Medicine, 2d ed, Philadelphia, Saunders, 1987.*]

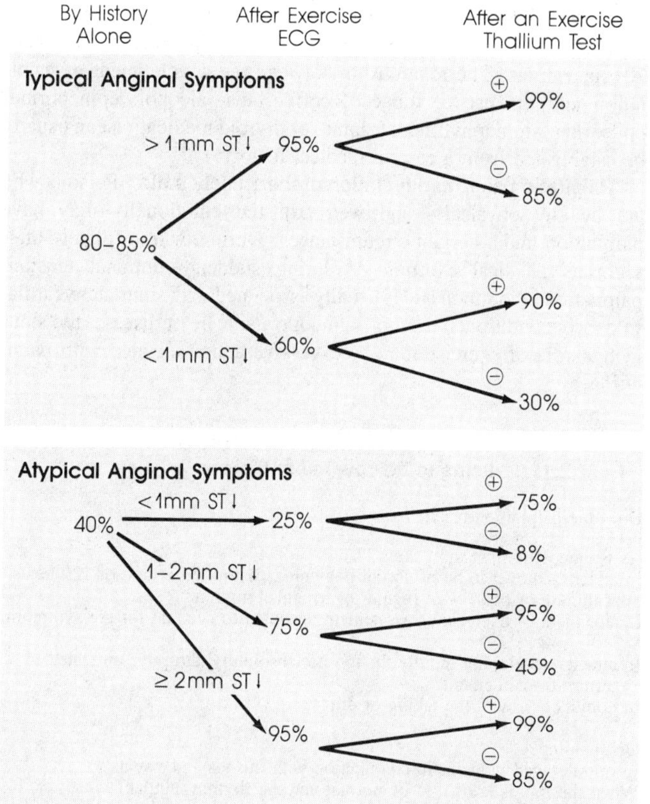

tation may also occur immediately after the onset of cardiac slowing, as with the sudden development of complete atrioventricular block, or upon the conversion from atrial fibrillation to sinus rhythm. Unusual movements of the heart within the thorax are also frequently the mechanism of palpitation. Thus, the ectopic beat and/or the compensatory pause may be appreciated, since both are associated with alterations in cardiac motion.

IMPORTANT CAUSES OF PALPITATION (See also Chap. 185)

Extrasystoles In most cases the diagnosis will be suggested by the patient's story. The premature contraction and postpremature beat are often described as a "flopping," or the patient may say that it feels as if "the heart were turning over." The pause following the premature contraction may be felt as an actual cessation of the heartbeat. The first ventricular contraction succeeding the pause may be felt as an unusually vigorous beat and will be described as "pounding" or "thudding."

When extrasystoles are numerous, clinical differentiation from atrial fibrillation can be made by any procedure that will bring about a definite increase in the ventricular rate. In persons without serious underlying heart disease, the extrasystoles usually diminish in frequency and then disappear at increasingly rapid heart rates, whereas the ventricular irregularity of atrial fibrillation increases.

Tachycardias These conditions, which are considered in detail in Chap. 185, are common and medically important causes of palpitation. Ventricular tachycardia, one of the most serious arrhythmias, rarely is manifested as palpitation; this may be related to the abnormal sequence, and hence impaired coordination and vigor, of ventricular contraction. If the patient is seen between attacks, the diagnosis of ectopic tachycardia and its type will have to depend on the history, but the precise diagnosis can be made only when an electrocardiogram and observations on the effect of carotid sinus pressure are made during the episode. The mode of onset and offset gives the most important lead in distinguishing sinus from one of the various forms of ectopic tachycardias. Ectopic rhythms characteristically begin instantaneously, while sinus tachycardia has a more gradual onset and ending over seconds or minutes. Continuous ambulatory (Holter) electrocardiography and asking the patient to record the time of onset and cessation of the palpitations in a diary are extremely helpful in determining the cause of this symptom.

Other causes These include thyrotoxicosis (Chap. 316), hypoglycemia (Chap. 320), pheochromocytoma (Chap. 318), fever (Chap. 20), and drugs. The relationship between the development of palpitation and the use of tobacco, coffee, tea, alcohol, epinephrine, ephedrine, aminophylline, atropine, or thyroid medication can usually be established from a careful medical history.

Palpitation as a manifestation of the anxiety state Persons who are healthy physically and well adjusted emotionally may have palpitation under certain circumstances. During or immediately after vigorous physical exertion or during sudden emotional tension, palpitation is common and is usually associated with sinus tachycardia. In poorly conditioned persons without organic heart disease, the sinus tachycardia of exercise may be excessive and associated with palpitation.

In some persons, palpitation may be one of the outstanding manifestations of an episode of acute anxiety. In others the palpitation may, with other symptoms, represent prolonged anxiety neurosis or a lifelong disorder characterized by volatile autonomic function. Whether these illnesses are simply an expression of a chronic, deep-seated anxiety state superimposed on a normal autonomic nervous system or whether they depend on instability of the autonomic nervous system is not clear. At any rate, the clinical significance of the differentiation between the transitory and the enduring forms is that the former is often dissipated by firm reassurance from the physician, whereas the latter is usually resistant even to the most thorough and expert psychiatric care. In the latter case, the patient must be treated with most carefully planned psychological support and tranquilizing medications. This chronic form of palpitation is known by various names such as *Da Costa's syndrome, soldier's heart, effort syndrome, irritable heart, neurocirculatory asthenia,* and *functional cardiovascular disease.* Aside from palpitation, the chief symptoms are those of an anxiety state.

Physical examination usually reveals the typical findings of the hyperkinetic syndrome. These include a left parasternal lift, a precordial or apical systolic murmur, a wide pulse pressure, rapidly rising pulse, and excessive perspiration. The electrocardiogram may display minor depressions of the ST junction and inversion of T waves and so occasionally lead to a mistaken diagnosis of coronary disease; this is particularly likely to occur when these findings are associated with complaints by the patients of an aching feeling of substernal tightness, commonly present in emotional stress. The presence of any kind of organic disease is one of the commonest causes of the underlying anxiety which frequently precipitates this functional syndrome. Thus, even when a patient presents undoubted objective evidence of organic cardiac disease, the possibility that a superimposed anxiety state may be responsible for the symptoms described above should be considered. Palpitation associated with organic cardiac disease is nearly always accompanied by arrhythmia or tachycardia, whereas the symptom may exist with regular rhythm and with a heart rate of 80 beats per minute or less in patients with the anxiety state. An anxiety state, in contrast to heart disease, causes a sighing type of dyspnea. Also pain localized to the apex, either brief and lancinating in character or lasting for hours or days and accompanied by hyperesthesia, is due usually to an anxiety state, not to structural cardiac disease. Giddiness due to this syndrome can usually be reproduced by hyperventilation or by change from the recumbent to the erect posture.

The *treatment* of the anxiety state with palpitation is difficult and depends on removal of the cause. In many instances a thorough examination of the heart and a statement that it is normal will suffice. Instructions to take more rather than less physical exercise will reinforce these statements. When the anxiety state is a manifestation of chronic anxiety neurosis or related emotional disorder, the symptoms are more likely to persist.

Table 16-2 summarizes the main points of information to be ascertained in the history in elucidating the significance of palpitation. The recording of an ambulatory electrocardiogram and the precise

TABLE 16-2 Items to be covered in history

Does the palpitation occur:	If so, suspect:
As isolated "jumps" or "skips"?	Extrasystoles
In attacks, known to be of abrupt beginning, with a heart rate of 120 beats per minute or over, with regular or irregular rhythm?	Paroxysmal rapid heart action
Independent of exercise or excitement adequate to account for the symptom?	Atrial fibrillation, atrial flutter, thyrotoxicosis, anemia, febrile states, hypoglycemia, anxiety state
In attacks developing rapidly though not absolutely abruptly, unrelated to exertion or excitement?	Hemorrhage, hypoglycemia, tumor of the adrenal medulla
In conjunction with the taking of drugs?	Tobacco, coffee, tea, alcohol, epinephrine, ephedrine, aminophylline, atropine, thyroid extract, monoamine oxidase inhibitors
On standing?	Postural hypotension
In middle-aged women, in conjunction with flushes and sweats?	Menopausal syndrome
When the rate is known to be normal and the rhythm regular?	Anxiety state

temporal correlation of the cardiac rate and rhythm with the presence of palpitation are extremely useful in the identification or exclusion of an arrhythmia if the symptom does not occur when the patient is under direct observation. The effectiveness of antiarrhythmia treatment can also be assessed objectively in this manner, without the necessity of relying only on the patient's subjective symptoms. Beta-adrenergic blockade with propranolol, beginning with 40 mg/d in divided doses, and ranging as high as 400 mg/d, or with equivalent doses of newer beta-adrenergic antagonists can be extremely effective in patients with palpitation and sinus rhythm or sinus tachycardia.

One point merits special emphasis. *As a rule palpitation produces anxiety and fear out of all proportion to its seriousness.* When the cause has been accurately determined and its significance explained to patients, their concern is often ameliorated and may disappear entirely.

REFERENCES

CONSTANT J: The clinical diagnosis of nonanginal chest pain: The differentiation of angina from nonanginal chest pain by history. Clin Cardiol 6:11, 1983

DIAMOND GA et al: Computer-assisted diagnosis in the noninvasive evaluation of patients with suspected coronary artery disease. J Am Coll Cardiol 1:444, 1983

GOLDMAN L: Atypical chest pain, in *Difficult Diagnosis*, RB Taylor (ed). Philadelphia, Saunders, 1985, p 71

GOLDMAN L et al: A computer protocol to predict myocardial infarction in emergency department patients with chest pain. N Engl J Med 318:797, 1988

GOLDSCHLAGER N: Use of the treadmill test in the diagnosis of coronary artery disease in patients with chest pain. Ann Intern Med 97:383, 1982

POZEN MW et al: A predictive instrument to improve coronary care unit admission practices in acute ischemic heart disease: A prospective multicenter clinical trial. N Engl J Med 310:1273, 1984

RIFKIN RD, HOOD WB: Bayesian analysis of electrocardiographic exercise stress testing. N Engl J Med 297:681, 1977

RUSTGI AK, CHOPRA S: Chest pain of esophageal origin. J Gen Intern Med 4:151, 1989

RUTHERFORD JD et al: Chronic ischemic heart disease, in *Heart Disease*, 3d ed, E Braunwald (ed). Philadelphia, Saunders, 1988, chap 39, p 1314

WOLF MA: Palpitations and disturbances of cardiac rhythm, in *Office Practice of Medicine*, 2d ed, WT Branch Jr (ed). Philadelphia, Saunders, 1987, chap 2, p 19

17 ABDOMINAL PAIN

WILLIAM SILEN

The correct interpretation of acute abdominal pain is one of the most challenging demands made of any physician. Since proper therapy often requires urgent action, the luxury of the leisurely approach suitable for the study of other conditions is frequently denied. Few other clinical situations demand greater experience and judgment, because the most catastrophic of events may be forecast by the subtlest of symptoms and signs. Nowhere in medicine is a meticulously executed, detailed history and physical examination of greater importance. The etiologic classification in Table 17-1, although not complete, forms a useful frame of reference for the evaluation of patients with abdominal pain.

The diagnosis of "acute or surgical abdomen" so often heard in emergency wards is not an acceptable one because of its often misleading and erroneous connotation. The most obvious of "acute abdomens" may not require operative intervention, and the mildest of abdominal pains may herald the onset of an urgently correctable lesion. Any patient with abdominal pain of recent onset requires early and thorough evaluation with specific attempts at accurate diagnosis.

SOME MECHANISMS OF PAIN ORIGINATING IN THE ABDOMEN

Inflammation of the parietal peritoneum The pain of parietal peritoneal inflammation is steady and aching in character and is located directly over the inflamed area, its exact reference being possible because it is transmitted by overlapping somatic nerves supplying the parietal peritoneum. The intensity of the pain is dependent upon the type and amount of foreign substance to which the peritoneal surfaces are exposed in a given period of time. For example, the sudden release into the peritoneal cavity of a small quantity of *sterile* acid gastric juice causes much more pain than the same amount of grossly contaminated neutral fecal material. Enzymatically active pancreatic juice incites more pain and inflammation than does the same amount of sterile bile containing no potent enzymes. Blood and urine are often so bland as to go undetected if exposure of the peritoneum has not been sudden and massive. In the case of bacterial contamination, such as in pelvic inflammatory disease, the pain is frequently of low intensity early in the illness until bacterial multiplication has caused the elaboration of irritating substances.

TABLE 17-1 Some important causes of abdominal pain

- *I* Pain originating in the abdomen
  - *A* Parietal peritoneal inflammation
    - *1* Bacterial contamination, e.g., perforated appendix, pelvic inflammatory disease
    - *2* Chemical irritation, e.g., perforated ulcer, pancreatitis, mittelschmerz
  - *B* Mechanical obstruction of hollow viscera
    - *1* Obstruction of the small or large intestine
    - *2* Obstruction of the biliary tree
    - *3* Obstruction of the ureter
  - *C* Vascular disturbances
    - *1* Embolism or thrombosis
    - *2* Vascular rupture
    - *3* Pressure or torsional occlusion
    - *4* Sickle cell anemia
  - *D* Abdominal wall
    - *1* Distortion or traction of mesentery
    - *2* Trauma or infection of muscles
  - *E* Distention of visceral surfaces, e.g., hepatic or renal capsules
- *II* Pain referred from extraabdominal sources
  - *A* Thorax, e.g., pneumonia, referred pain from coronary occlusion
  - *B* Spine, e.g., radiculitis from arthritis
  - *C* Genitalia, e.g., torsion of the testicle
- *III* Metabolic causes
  - *A* Exogenous
    - *1* Black widow spider bite
    - *2* Lead poisoning and others
  - *B* Endogenous
    - *1* Uremia
    - *2* Diabetic ketoacidosis
    - *3* Porphyria
    - *4* Allergic factors (C'1 esterase inhibitor deficiency)
- *IV* Neurogenic causes
  - *A* Organic
    - *1* Tabes dorsalis
    - *2* Herpes zoster
    - *3* Causalgia and others
  - *B* Functional

So important is the rate at which the irritating material is applied to the peritoneum that cases of perforated peptic ulcer may be associated with entirely different clinical pictures dependent only upon the rapidity with which the gastric juice enters the peritoneal cavity.

The pain of peritoneal inflammation is invariably accentuated by pressure or changes in tension of the peritoneum, whether produced by palpation or by movement, as in coughing or sneezing. Consequently, the patient with peritonitis lies quietly in bed, preferring to avoid motion, in contrast to the patient with colic, who may writhe incessantly.

Another of the characteristic features of peritoneal irritation is tonic reflex spasm of the abdominal musculature, localized to the involved body segment. The intensity of the tonic muscle spasm accompanying peritoneal inflammation is dependent upon the location of the inflammatory process, the rate at which it develops, and the integrity of the nervous system. Spasm over a perforated retrocecal appendix or perforated ulcer into the lesser peritoneal sac may be minimal or absent because of the protective effect of overlying viscera. As in pain of peritoneal inflammation, a slowly developing process often greatly attenuates the degree of muscle spasm. Catastrophic abdominal emergencies such as a perforated ulcer have been repeatedly associated with minimal or occasionally no detectable pain or muscle spasm in obtunded, seriously ill, debilitated elderly patients or in psychotic patients.

Obstruction of hollow viscera The pain of obstruction of hollow abdominal viscera is classically described as intermittent, or colicky. Yet the lack of a truly cramping character should not be misleading, because distention of a hollow viscus may produce steady pain with only very occasional exacerbations. Although not nearly as well localized as the pain of parietal peritoneal inflammation, some useful generalities can be made concerning its distribution.

The colicky pain of obstruction of small intestine is usually periumbilical or supraumbilical and is poorly localized. As the intestine becomes progressively dilated with loss of muscular tone, the colicky nature of the pain may become less apparent. With superimposed strangulating obstruction, pain may spread in the lower lumbar region if there is traction on the root of the mesentery. The colicky pain of colonic obstruction is of lesser intensity than that of the small intestine and is often located in the infraumbilical area. Lumbar radiation of pain is common in colonic obstruction.

Sudden distention of the biliary tree produces a steady rather than colicky type of pain; hence the term *biliary colic* is misleading. Acute distention of the gallbladder usually causes pain in the right upper quadrant with radiation to the right posterior region of the thorax or to the tip of the right scapula, and distention of the common bile duct is often associated with pain in the epigastrium radiating to the upper part of the lumbar region. Considerable variation is common, however, so that differentiation between these may be impossible. The typical subscapular pain or lumbar radiation is frequently absent. Gradual dilatation of the biliary tree as in carcinoma of the head of the pancreas may cause no pain or only a mild aching sensation in the epigastrium or right upper quadrant. The pain of distention of the pancreatic ducts is similar to that described for distention of the common bile duct but in addition is very frequently accentuated by recumbency and relieved by the upright position.

Obstruction of the urinary bladder results in dull suprapubic pain, usually low in intensity. Restlessness without specific complaint of pain may be the only sign of a distended bladder in an obtunded patient. In contrast, acute obstruction of the intravesicular portion of the ureter is characterized by severe suprapubic and flank pain which radiates to the penis, scrotum, or inner aspect of the upper region of the thigh. Obstruction of the ureteropelvic junction is felt as pain in the costovertebral angle, whereas obstruction of the remainder of the ureter is associated with flank pain, which often extends into the corresponding side of the abdomen.

Vascular disturbances A frequent misconception, despite abundant experience to the contrary, is that pain associated with intraabdominal vascular disturbances is sudden and catastrophic in nature. The pain of embolism or thrombosis of the superior mesenteric artery or that of impending rupture of an abdominal aortic aneurysm certainly may be severe and diffuse. Yet just as frequently, the patient with occlusion of the superior mesenteric artery has only mild continuous diffuse pain for 2 or 3 days before vascular collapse or findings of peritoneal inflammation appear. The early, seemingly insignificant discomfort is caused by hyperperistalsis rather than peritoneal inflammation. Indeed, absence of tenderness and rigidity in the presence of continuous, diffuse pain in a patient likely to have vascular disease is quite characteristic of occlusion of the superior mesenteric artery. Abdominal pain with radiation to the sacral region, flank, or genitalia should always signal the possible presence of a rupturing abdominal aortic aneurysm. This pain may persist over a period of several days before rupture and collapse occur.

Abdominal wall Pain arising from the abdominal wall is usually constant and aching. Movement and pressure accentuate the discomfort and muscle spasm. In the case of hematoma of the rectus sheath, now most frequently encountered in association with anticoagulant therapy, a mass may be present in the lower quadrants of the abdomen. Simultaneous involvement of muscles in other parts of the body usually serves to differentiate myositis of the abdominal wall from an intraabdominal process which might cause pain in the same region.

REFERRED PAIN IN ABDOMINAL DISEASES Pain referred to the abdomen from the thorax, spine, or genitalia may prove a vexing problem in differential diagnosis, because diseases of the upper part of the abdominal cavity such as acute cholecystitis, perforated ulcer, or subphrenic abscesses are frequently associated with intrathoracic complications. A most important, yet often forgotten, dictum is that the possibility of intrathoracic disease must be considered in every patient with abdominal pain, especially if the pain is in the upper part of the abdomen. Systematic questioning and examination directed toward detecting the presence or absence of myocardial or pulmonary infarction, pneumonia, pericarditis, or esophageal disease (the intrathoracic diseases which most often masquerade as abdominal emergencies) will often provide sufficient clues to establish the proper diagnosis. Diaphragmatic pleuritis resulting from pneumonia or pulmonary infarction may cause pain in the right upper quadrant and pain in the supraclavicular area, the latter radiation to be sharply distinguished from the referred subscapular pain caused by acute distention of the extrahepatic biliary tree. The ultimate decision as to the origin of abdominal pain may require deliberate and planned observation over a period of several hours, during which time repeated questioning and examination will provide the proper explanation.

Referred pain of thoracic origin is often accompanied by splinting of the involved hemithorax with respiratory lag and decrease in excursion more marked than that seen in the presence of intraabdominal disease. In addition, apparent abdominal muscle spasm caused by referred pain will diminish during the inspiratory phase of respiration, whereas it is persistent throughout both respiratory phases if it is of abdominal origin. Palpation over the area of referred pain in the abdomen also does not usually accentuate the pain and in many instances actually seems to relieve it. The frequent coexistence of thoracic and abdominal disease may be misleading and confusing, so that differentiation might be difficult or impossible. For example, the patient with known biliary tract disease often has epigastric pain during myocardial infarction, or biliary colic may be referred to the precordium or left shoulder in a patient who has suffered previously from angina pectoris. For the explanation of the radiation of pain to a previously diseased area, see Chap. 15.

Referred pain from the spine, which usually involves compression or irritation of nerve roots, is characteristically intensified by certain motions such as cough, sneeze, or strain and is associated with hyperesthesia over the involved dermatomes. Pain referred to the abdomen from the testicles or seminal vesicles is generally accentuated by the slightest pressure on either of these organs. The abdominal discomfort is of dull aching character and is poorly localized.

METABOLIC ABDOMINAL CRISES Pain of metabolic origin may simulate almost any other type of intraabdominal disease. Here several mechanisms may be at work. In certain instances, such as hyperlipemia, the metabolic disease itself may be accompanied by an intraabdominal process such as pancreatitis, which can lead to unnecessary laparotomy unless recognized. C'1 esterase deficiency associated with angioneurotic edema is also often associated with episodes of severe abdominal pain. Whenever the cause of abdominal pain is obscure, a metabolic origin must always be considered. Abdominal pain is also the hallmark of familial Mediterranean fever (Chap. 278).

The problem of differential diagnosis is often not readily resolved. The pain of porphyria and of lead colic usually is difficult to distinguish from that of intestinal obstruction, because severe hyperperistalsis is a prominent feature of both. The pain of uremia or diabetes is nonspecific, and the pain and tenderness frequently shift in location and intensity. Diabetic acidosis may be precipitated by acute appendicitis or intestinal obstruction, so that if prompt resolution of the abdominal pain does not result from correction of the metabolic abnormalities, an underlying organic problem should be suspected. Black widow spider bites produce intense pain and rigidity of the abdominal muscles and of the back, an area infrequently involved in disease of intraabdominal origin.

NEUROGENIC CAUSES Causalgic pain may occur in diseases that injure nerves of sensory type. It has a burning character and is usually limited to the distribution of a given peripheral nerve. Normal stimuli such as touch or change in temperature may be transformed into this type of pain, which is also frequently present in a patient at rest. A helpful finding is the demonstration that cutaneous pain spots are now irregularly spaced, and this may be the only indication of an old nerve lesion underlying causalgic pain. Even though the pain may be precipitated by gentle palpation, rigidity of the abdominal muscles is absent, and the respirations are not disturbed. Distention of the abdomen is uncommon, and the pain has no relationship to the intake of food.

Pain arising from spinal nerves or roots comes and goes suddenly and is of a lancinating type (see Chap. 19). It may be caused by herpes zoster, impingement by arthritis, tumors, herniated nucleus pulposus, diabetes, or syphilis. Again, it is not associated with food intake, abdominal distention, or changes in respiration. Severe muscle spasm, as in the gastric crises of tabes dorsalis, is common but is either relieved or is not accentuated by abdominal palpation. The pain is made worse by movement of the spine and is usually confined to a few dermatome segments. Hyperesthesia is very common.

Psychogenic pain conforms to none of the aforementioned patterns of disease. Here the mechanism is hard to define. The most common problem is the hysterical adolescent or young woman who develops abdominal pain; she frequently loses an appendix and other organs because of it. Ovulation or some other natural event that causes brief mild abdominal discomfort may sometimes be experienced as an abdominal catastrophe.

Psychogenic pain varies enormously in type and location but usually has no relation to meals. It is often at its onset markedly accentuated during the night. Nausea and vomiting are rarely observed, although occasionally the patient reports these symptoms. Spasm is seldom induced in the abdominal musculature and if present does not persist, especially if the attention of the patient can be distracted. Persistent localized tenderness is rare, and if found, the muscle spasm in the area is inconsistent and often absent. Restriction of the depth of respiration is the most common respiratory abnormality, but this is in the nature of a smothering or choking sensation and is part of an anxiety state (see Chap. 29). It occurs in the absence of thoracic splinting or change in the respiratory rate.

APPROACH TO THE PATIENT WITH ABDOMINAL PAIN There are few abdominal conditions that require such urgent operative intervention that an orderly approach need be abandoned, no matter how ill the patient. Only those patients with exsanguinating hemorrhage must be rushed to the operating room immediately, but in such instances only a few minutes are required to assess the critical nature of the problem. Under these circumstances, all obstacles must be swept aside, adequate access for intravenous fluid replacement obtained, and the operation begun. Many patients of this type have died in the radiology department or the emergency room while awaiting such unnecessary examinations as electrocardiograms or films of the abdomen. *There are no contraindications to operation when massive hemorrhage is present.* Although exceedingly important, this situation fortunately is relatively rare.

Nothing will supplant an orderly, painstakingly *detailed history*, which is far more valuable than any laboratory or roentgenologic examination. This kind of history is laborious and time-consuming, making it not especially popular even though a reasonably accurate diagnosis can be made on the basis of the history alone in the majority of cases. In cases of *acute* abdominal pain, a diagnosis is readily established in most instances, whereas success is not so frequently achieved in patients with *chronic* pain. Since the irritable bowel syndrome is one of the most common causes of abdominal pain, the possibility of this diagnosis must always be kept in mind (see Chap. 242). The *chronological sequence of events* in the patient's history is often more important than emphasis on the location of pain. If the examiner is sufficiently open-minded and unhurried, asks the proper questions, and listens, the patient will often provide the diagnosis. Careful attention should be paid to the extraabdominal regions which may be responsible for abdominal pain. An accurate menstrual history in a female patient is essential. Narcotics or analgesics should be withheld until a definitive diagnosis or a definitive plan has been formulated, because these agents often make it more difficult to secure and to interpret the history and physical findings.

In the examination, simple critical inspection of the patient, e.g., of facies, position in bed, and respiratory activity, may provide valuable clues. The amount of information to be gleaned is directly proportional to the *gentleness* and thoroughness of the examiner. Once a patient with peritoneal inflammation has been examined in a brusque manner, accurate assessment by the next examiner becomes almost impossible. For example, eliciting rebound tenderness by sudden release of a deeply palpating hand in a patient with suspected peritonitis is cruel and unnecessary. The same information can be obtained by gentle percussion of the abdomen (rebound tenderness on a miniature scale), a maneuver which can be far more precise and localizing. Asking the patient to cough will elicit true rebound tenderness without the need for placing a hand on the abdomen. Furthermore, the brusque demonstration of rebound tenderness will startle and induce protective spasm in a nervous or worried patient in whom true rebound tenderness is not present. A palpable gallbladder will be missed if palpation is so brusque that voluntary muscle spasm becomes superimposed upon involuntary muscular rigidity.

As in history taking, there is no substitute for sufficient time spent in the examination. It is important to remember that abdominal signs may be minimal but nevertheless, if accompanied by consistent symptoms, may be exceptionally meaningful when carefully assessed. Signs may be virtually or actually totally absent in cases of pelvic peritonitis, so that careful *pelvic and rectal examinations are mandatory in every patient with abdominal pain.* The presence of tenderness on pelvic or rectal examination in the absence of other abdominal signs must not lead the examiner to exclude such important operative indications as perforated appendicitis, diverticulitis, twisted ovarian cyst, and many others.

Much attention has been paid to the presence or absence of peristaltic sounds, their quality, and their frequency. Auscultation of the abdomen is probably one of the least rewarding aspects of the physical examination of a patient with abdominal pain. Severe catastrophes such as strangulating small-intestinal obstruction or perforated appendicitis, may occur in the presence of normal peristalsis. Conversely, when the proximal part of the intestine above an obstruction becomes markedly distended and edematous, peristaltic sounds may lose the characteristics of borborygmi and become weak or absent even when peritonitis is not present. It is usually the severe chemical peritonitis of sudden onset which is associated with the truly silent abdomen. Assessment of the patient's state of hydration is important. The hematocrit and urinalysis permit an accurate estimate of the severity of dehydration, so that adequate replacement can be carried out.

Laboratory examinations may be of enormous value in the assessment of the patient with abdominal pain, yet with but a few exceptions they rarely establish a diagnosis. Leukocytosis should never be the single deciding factor as to whether or not operation is indicated. A white blood cell count greater than 20,000 per cubic millimeter may be observed with perforation of a viscus, but pancreatitis, acute cholecystitis, pelvic inflammatory disease, and intestinal infarction may be associated with marked leukocytosis. A normal white blood cell count is by no means rare in cases of perforation of abdominal viscera. The diagnosis of anemia may be more helpful than the white blood cell count, especially when combined with the history.

The urinalysis is also of great value in indicating to some degree the state of hydration or to rule out severe renal disease, diabetes, or urinary infection. Determination of the blood urea nitrogen, blood sugar, and serum bilirubin levels may also be helpful. The serum amylase determination is overrated, since in carefully controlled series of patients with proven pancreatitis where the determination has been done within the first 72 h, amylase was less than 200 Somogyi units in one-third of the cases, between 200 and 500 in another one-third of the cases, and greater than 500 in one-third. Since many diseases other than pancreatitis, e.g., perforated ulcer, strangulating intestinal obstruction, and acute cholecystitis, may be associated with very marked increase in the serum amylase, great care must be exercised in denying an operation to a patient solely on the basis of an elevated serum amylase level. The determination of the serum lipase may have a somewhat greater accuracy than the serum amylase.

Peritoneal lavage is a safe and effective diagnostic maneuver in patients with acute abdominal pain. It is of special value in patients with blunt trauma to the abdomen in whom evaluation of the abdomen may be difficult because of other multiple injuries to the spine, pelvis, or ribs and in whom blood in the peritoneal cavity produces only a very mild peritoneal reaction. The gallbladder is the only organ which may continue to seep fluid following accidental perforation, so that the region of this organ must be assiduously avoided. Determination of the pH of the aspirated fluid to ascertain the site of a perforation is misleading, because even highly acid gastric juice is rapidly buffered by peritoneal exudate.

Plain and upright or lateral decubitus roentgenograms of the abdomen may be of the greatest value. They are usually unnecessary in patients with acute appendicitis or strangulated external hernias. However, in cases of intestinal obstruction, perforated ulcer, and a variety of other conditions, films may be diagnostic. During a search for free air, the patient should be kept in the decubitus or upright position for at least 10 min before the appropriate film is taken lest a small pneumoperitoneum be missed. In rare instances, barium or water-soluble medium examination of the upper part of the gastrointestinal tract may demonstrate partial intestinal obstruction which may elude diagnosis by other means. If there is any question of obstruction of the colon, oral administration of barium sulfate should be avoided. On the other hand, barium enema is of inestimable value in cases of colonic obstruction and should be used with greater frequency where the possibility of perforation does not exist. Ultrasound recently has proved to be useful in detecting an enlarged gallbladder or pancreas, the presence of gallstones, an enlarged ovary, a tubal pregnancy, or a localized collection of fluid or pus. Radioisotopic scans (HIDA) may help differentiate acute cholecystitis from acute pancreatitis. A computed tomography scan may demonstrate an enlarged pancreas or a ruptured spleen, but it should be used only for *specific* questions such as these.

Sometimes, even under the best of circumstances with all available auxiliary aids and with the greatest of clinical skill, a definitive diagnosis cannot be established at the time of the initial examination. Nevertheless, despite lack of a clear anatomic diagnosis it may be abundantly clear to an experienced and thoughtful physician and surgeon that on clinical grounds alone operation is indicated. Should that decision be questionable, watchful waiting with repeated questioning and examination will often elucidate the true nature of the illness and indicate the proper course of action.

REFERENCES

De Dombal FT: Acute abdominal pain. Scand J Gastroenterol (Suppl) 14:29, 1979

Lee PWR: The plain x-ray in the acute abdomen: A surgeon's evaluation. Br J Surg 63:763, 1976

Leek BF: Abdominal and pelvic visceral receptors. Br Med Bull 33:163, 1977

Silen W: *Cope's Early Diagnosis of the Acute Abdomen*, 17th ed. London, Oxford Press, 1987

Staniland JR et al: Clinical presentation of acute abdomen: Study of 600 patients. Br Med J 2:393, 1972

Valman HB: Acute abdominal pain. Br Med J 282:1858, 1981

18 HEADACHE

JOSEPH B. MARTIN*

Although the term *headache* should encompass all pains located in the head, in common parlance its application is restricted to unpleasant sensations in the cranial vault. Facial, pharyngeal, laryngeal, and cervical pain, which usually signify other disorders, are described in Chaps. 19 and 360. (See also Table 18-1.)

Headache is one of the most frequent human discomforts. Its significance is often abstruse, for it may signal serious disease or represent only tension, fatigue, or a migrainous disorder. Fortunately, in most instances it reflects one of the latter, and only exceptionally does it warn of a serious intracranial abnormality. It is this dual significance, however, the benign and the potentially malignant, that requires the astute attention of the physician. A systematic approach to the headache problem necessitates a broad knowledge of the medical and surgical diseases of which it is a symptom and a clinical methodology that leaves none of the common and treatable causes unexplored.

GENERAL CONSIDERATIONS The quality, location, duration, and time course of the headache and conditions that produce, exacerbate, or relieve it should be carefully reviewed. Unfortunately, except in special circumstances such as temporal arteritis, physical examination of the head itself is seldom useful.

The patient is rarely helpful in describing the *quality* of cephalic pain. In fact, persistent questioning on that point occasions surprise, for the patient usually assumes that the word *headache* conveys adequate information about the nature of the discomfort. Most headaches are dull, deeply located, and of aching character. Occasionally superficial burning or stinging pain localized to the skin is reported. The patient may describe tightness, pressure, or a bursting feeling, terms that may give clues to anxiety or depression.

Queries about *intensity* of pain are seldom useful, since they reflect more the patient's attitude toward the condition than the true severity. The stoical person tends to minimize discomfort, whereas the neurotic or depressed patient dramatizes it. Degree of incapacity is a better index. A severe migraine attack seldom allows performance of the day's work. The pain which awakens the patient from sleep at night, or prevents sleep, is also more likely to have a demonstrable organic basis. As a rule, the most intense cranial pains are those that accompany subarachnoid hemorrhage and meningitis, which have grave implications, or migraine and paroxysmal nocturnal *cluster* headaches, which are benign.

Data regarding *location* of the headache are often informative. If the source is in extracranial structures, as is often the case, the correspondence with the site of the pain is fairly precise. Inflammation of an extracranial artery causes pain localized to the site of the vessel. Lesions of paranasal sinuses, teeth, eyes, and upper cervical vertebrae induce a less sharply localized pain, but one that is still referred in a regional distribution that is fairly constant. Intracranial lesions in the posterior fossa cause pain in the occipital-nuchal region; it is homolateral if the lesion is one-sided. Supratentorial lesions induce frontotemporal pains, again homolateral to the lesion if it is on one side. But localization can also be uninformative or misleading. Ear pain, for example, although it may mean disease in the ear, more often is referred from other regions such as the neck, and eye pain may be referred to the occiput or cervical spine.

Duration and *time-intensity curve* of headaches both during the attack itself and in their life profile are most useful. The headache of bacterial meningitis or subarachnoid hemorrhage occurs usually in single attacks over a period of days. Single, brief, momentary (1 to 2 s) pains in the cranium (icepick-like headaches) are common but

* Revision of chapter by Raymond D. Adams and Joseph B. Martin published in the eleventh edition.

rarely indicate serious underlying disease. Classic migraine has its onset in the early morning hours or daytime, reaches a peak of severity in a half hour or so, lasts, unless treated, for several hours up to 1 to 2 days, is often accompanied by nausea or vomiting, and is terminated by sleep. A frequency of more than a single attack every few weeks is uncommon. A migraine patient having several attacks per week usually proves to have a combination of migraine and tension headaches. In contrast to this is the nightly occurrence (2 to 3 h after onset of sleep) over a period of several weeks to months of the rapidly peaking, nonthrobbing orbital, supraorbital, or temporal pain of cluster headache, which tends to dissipate within an hour. The headache of intracranial tumor can occur at any time of day or night, can interrupt sleep, varies in intensity, and lasts a few minutes to hours. The natural history is one of increasing frequency and intensity over a period of months. Tension headache, once commenced, may persist continuously for weeks or months, often waxing and waning from hour to hour or day to day.

Headache that bears a more or less constant relationship to certain biologic events and also to physical environmental changes may prove to be informative. Premenstrual headaches, most typically of migrainous or tension type, may occur as part of the premenstrual syndrome; they usually dissipate after the first day of vaginal bleeding. The headaches of cervical arthritis are most typically intense after a period of inactivity, and the first movements in the morning are both difficult and painful. Hypertensive headaches are uncommon, but like those of cerebral tumor, tend to occur on waking in the morning; excitement and tension may provoke them. Headache from infection of nasal sinuses may appear, with clocklike regularity, upon awakening and in midmorning, and is characteristically worsened by stooping and jarring of the head. Eyestrain headaches may follow prolonged use of the eyes. Anger, excitement, or irritation may initiate common migraine in certain disposed persons; this is more typical of common migraine than of classic type. Change of position, stooping, straining, cough, and sexual intercourse are each known to produce a special type of headache, described below. Exertional headaches, another well-known type, are usually benign (only 1 in 10 will have an intracranial lesion) and disappear within weeks to months.

PAIN-SENSITIVE STRUCTURES OF THE HEAD Understanding of headache has been greatly augmented by observations made during surgery of pain-sensitive structures. The following are sensitive to mechanical stimulation: (1) skin, subcutaneous tissue, muscles, arteries, and periosteum of skull; (2) tissues of the eye, ear, and nasal and sinus cavities; (3) intracranial venous sinuses and their tributary veins; (4) parts of the dura at the base of the brain and the arteries within the dura mater and pia-arachnoid; and (5) the trigeminal, glossopharyngeal, vagus, and first three cervical nerves. Interestingly, pain is practically the only sensation produced by stimulation of these structures. The bony skull, much of the pia-arachnoid and dura, and the parenchyma of the brain lack sensitivity.

Sensory stimuli from the head are conveyed to the central nervous system via the trigeminal nerves for structures above the tentorium in the anterior and middle fossae of the skull and via the first three cervical nerves for those in the posterior fossa and infradural structures. The ninth and tenth cranial nerves supply part of the posterior fossa and refer the pain to the ear and throat. The pain of intracranial disease is commonly referred to a part of the cranium lying within the areas supplied by these nerves. There may be associated local tenderness of the scalp at the site of reference. Dental or jaw pain may also have cranial reference. The pain of disease in other parts of the body is not referred to the head, although it may initiate headache by other means.

Headache can occur as a result of (1) distention, traction, or dilatation of intracranial or extracranial arteries, (2) traction or displacement of large intracranial veins or of their dural envelope, (3) compression, traction, or inflammation of cranial and spinal nerves, (4) voluntary or involuntary spasm, inflammation, and trauma to cranial and cervical muscles, and (5) meningeal irritation and raised intracranial pressure. More specifically, intracranial mass lesions cause headache only if they deform, displace, or exert traction on vessels, dural structures, or cranial nerves at the base of the brain, and this may happen long before intracranial pressure rises. Raised intracranial pressure causes headache in a bioccipital or bifrontal distribution which is rapidly relieved by lumbar puncture and lowering of the cerebrospinal fluid (CSF) pressure.

Dilatation of the extracranial, temporal, and intracranial *arteries* with stretching of surrounding sensitive structures is believed to be the mechanism of most of the pain of migraine. Extracranial, temporal, and occipital arteries, when involved in giant cell arteritis (cranial or "temporal" arteritis), a disease which usually afflicts individuals over 50 years of age, give rise to headache of dull aching and throbbing type, at first localized and then more diffuse. Characteristically it is severe and persistent over a period of weeks or months. The offending artery, strangely, is not always tender to pressure, yet section of it, as in biopsy, may relieve the pain (Chap. 276). Evolving atherosclerotic thrombosis of internal carotid, anterior, and middle cerebral arteries is sometimes accompanied by pain in the forehead or temple; with vertebral artery thrombosis the pain is postauricular, and basilar artery thrombosis causes referred pain in the occiput and sometimes the forehead.

In *infection or blockage of paranasal sinuses,* pain is usually felt over the antrum or in the forehead; with the *ethmoid* and *sphenoid sinuses,* the pain localizes around the eyes on one or both sides or in the vertex. Usually it is associated with tenderness of the skin in the same distribution. The pain may have two remarkable properties: (1) When throbbing, it may be abolished by compressing the carotid artery on the same side. (2) It tends to recur and subside at the same hours, i.e., it occurs on awakening, gradually disappears when the person is upright, and comes again in the late morning hours. The time relations are believed to yield information concerning the mechanism; morning pain is ascribed to the sinuses filling at night and its relief on arising to emptying after the erect posture has been assumed. Stooping, blowing the nose, and jarring the head intensify the pain; and inhalant sympathomimetic drugs such as phenylephrine, which reduce swelling and congestion, tend to relieve the pain. Sinus pain may persist after all purulent secretions have disappeared, probably because of persistent blockage of the draining orifices eliciting a vacuum or suction effect on the sinus wall (*vacuum sinus headaches*). The condition is relieved when aeration is restored. During air flights both earache and sinus headache tend to occur on descent, when the relative pressure in the blocked viscus falls.

Headache of ocular origin is usually located in the orbit, forehead, or temple, and has a steady, aching quality which may follow prolonged use of the eyes in close work. Ocular muscle imbalance, hyperopia, astigmatism, and impaired convergence and accommodation may give rise to sustained contraction of extraocular as well as frontal, temporal, and even occipital muscles. Raised intraocular pressure in acute glaucoma or iridocyclitis causes steady, aching pain felt in the eye. When intense, it may radiate throughout the distribution of the ophthalmic division of the trigeminal nerve. The pain of diabetic third nerve palsy, intracranial aneurysm, pituitary tumor, cavernous sinus thrombosis, and Raeder's paratrigeminal syndrome is often referred to the eye.

The *headaches accompanying disease of ligaments, muscles, and apophyseal joints* in the upper part of the spine, which are referred to occipital and upper cervical regions, are difficult to separate from the more common muscular contraction (tension) headaches. Such referred pains are especially frequent in middle and late adult life in patients with rheumatoid arthritis and cervical spondylosis and tend also to occur after whiplash injuries to the neck. If the pain is articular or synovial in origin, the first movements after being still for some hours are both stiff and painful. In fact, evocation of pain by active and passive motion of the spine should indicate traumatic or other disease of movable parts. The pain of *myofibrositis,* evidenced by tender nodules near the cranial insertion of cervical and other muscles, is more obscure (see Chap. 15). There are no pathologic data as to the nature of these vaguely palpable lesions, and it is uncertain

TABLE 18-1 Common types of headache

Type	Site	Age and sex	Clinical characteristics	Diurnal pattern	Life profile
Common migraine	Frontotemporal Uni- or bilateral	Children, young to middle-aged adults, both sexes, female > male	Throbbing and/or dull ache; worse behind one eye or ear, nausea or vomiting Headache becomes generalized	Upon awakening or later in day Duration: hours to 1–2 days	Irregular interval, weeks to months Tends to disappear in middle age and during pregnancy
Classic migraine	Same as above	Same as above	Same as above; visual prodrome common	Same as above	Same as above
Cluster, histamine headache, or migrainous neuralgia	Orbital or temporal Unilateral	Adolescent and adult males (80–90%)	Intense, nonthrobbing pain	Usually nocturnal; occurs one or more hours after falling asleep Rarely diurnal	Nightly for several weeks to months (cluster) Recurrence: years later
Tension headaches	Generalized	Children, adolescents, and adults, both sexes	Pressure (nonthrobbing); tightness Aching	Continuous, variable intensity	Recurrent episodes lasting hours to days
Meningeal irritation (meningitis, subarachnoid hemorrhage)	Generalized	Any age, both sexes	Intense, steady deep pain, may be worse in neck	Duration: days to a week or more	Single episode
Brain tumor	(See text)	Any age, both sexes	Variable in intensity May awaken patient Steady pain	Lasts minutes to hours; increasing severity	Once in a lifetime: weeks to months
Temporal arteritis	Unilateral, temporal, or occipital	Over 50 years, either sex	Persistent burning, aching	Continuous or intermittent	Persists for weeks to a few months

SOURCE: After J Patten, Neurological Differential Diagnosis, London, Harold Starke, Springer-Verlag, 1977.

whether the pain actually arises in them. They may represent only the deep tenderness felt in the region of referred pain or the involuntary secondary protective spasm of muscles. Characteristically, the pain is steady (nonthrobbing) and spreads from one to both sides of the head. Exposure to cold or draft may precipitate it. Though severe at times, it seldom prevents sleep. Massage of muscles and heat have unpredictable effects but relieve the pain in some cases.

The *headache of meningeal irritation* (infection or hemorrhage) is acute in onset, severe, generalized, deep-seated, constant, especially intense at the base of the skull, and associated with stiffness of the neck on bending forward. Dilatation and congestion of inflamed meningeal vessels are probably the main cause of the pain.

Lumbar puncture headache is characterized by a steady occipital-nuchal or bifrontal pain that comes on a few minutes after arising from a recumbent position and is relieved within a few minutes by lying down. Its cause is persistent leakage of CSF into the lumbar tissues through the needle site. The CSF pressure is low. The headache is usually increased by compression of the jugular veins and is unaffected by digital obliteration of one carotid artery. It is probable that in the upright position a low intraspinal and negative intracranial pressure exerts traction on dural attachments and dural sinuses by caudal displacement of the brain. Understandably, then, headache following cisternal puncture is rare. As soon as the leakage of CSF stops and CSF pressure is gradually restored (usually from a few days up to a week or so), the headache disappears. "Spontaneous" low-pressure headache may also follow a sneeze or strain, presumably because of rupture of the spinal arachnoid space along a nerve root.

The mechanism of the *throbbing or steady headache that accompanies febrile illnesses,* located in frontal or occipital regions or generalized, is probably vascular. It is much like histamine headache in that it is relieved on one side by carotid artery compression and on both sides by jugular vein compression or the subarachnoid injection of saline solution. It is increased by shaking the head. It seems probable that the meningeal vessels pulsate unduly and stretch pain-sensitive structures around the base of the brain. In certain cases, however, the pain may be lessened by compression of temporal arteries, and in these cases a component of the headache seems to be derived from the walls of extracranial arteries, as in migraine.

The pain felt in *tension headaches* of patients with anxiety or depression has been alleged to be due to spasm of cranial and cervical muscles. There is, however, no direct evidence to support such a mechanism. Combinations of tension and vascular headaches give rise to "mixed headaches," which are one of the most common types of headache.

PRINCIPAL CLINICAL VARIETIES OF HEADACHE Usually there is no difficulty in diagnosing the headache of glaucoma, purulent sinusitis, bacterial meningitis, and brain tumor, and a fuller account of these special headaches will be found where these diseases are described in other sections of the book. It is when headache is chronic, recurrent, and unattended by other important signs of disease that the physician faces one of the most difficult medical problems.

The types of headache subsequently described should then be considered.

Migraine The term *migraine* refers to periodic, hemicranial, throbbing headaches often accompanied by nausea and vomiting which usually begin in childhood, adolescence, or early adult life and recur in diminishing number and intensity during advancing years. Migraine is frequent, with a prevalence of 20 to 30 percent in the population. Women are affected three times as often as men. There is a tendency for the headaches to occur during the period of

TABLE 18-1 Common types of headache *(continued)*

Provoking factors	Associated features	Treatment
Bright light, noise, tension, alcohol Dark room and sleep relieve Scalp sensitive Pressure helps	Nausea in some cases	Ergot preparation at onset Propranolol, calcium channel blockers, methysergide for prevention
Same as above	Blindness and scintillating lights Unilateral numbness Disturbed speech Vertigo Confusion	Same as above
Alcohol in some	Lacrimation, congested eye	Ergot preparation at bedtime Amitriptyline and lithium carbonate for prevention
Fatigue and nervous strain	Depression, nervousness, anxiety, insomnia	Antianxiety and antidepressant drugs
None	Neck stiff on forward bending Kernig and Brudzinski signs	For meningitis or bleeding (see text)
None Sometimes position	Papilledema Vomiting Slow mentation	Glucocorticoids Mannitol Glycerol Treatment of tumor
Scalp sensitive Tender arteries	Intermittent or permanent loss of sight Rheumatic myalgia Fever	Glucocorticoid therapy

premenstrual tension and fluid retention and to decrease during pregnancy. The immediate family history is positive for migraine in over 60 percent of cases. Migraine or vascular headaches present in one of four clinical patterns: (1) classic migraine, (2) common migraine, (3) complicated migraine, and (4) cluster headache.

Classic migraine begins with a prodrome of prominent neurologic symptoms such as visual scintillations, dazzling zigzag lines (fortification spectra), photophobia and spreading scotomas, or dizziness and tinnitus. Classic migraine may be heralded hours before the attack by premonitory symptoms, most commonly a feeling of elation, excessive energy, thirst, a craving for sweet foods, or drowsiness. At other times, there may be a slowing of mentation or a feeling of impending doom or of depression, or there may be no warning whatsoever. The disturbance of vision that commences the attack may be followed by homonymous hemianopic field defects; sometimes they are bilateral, and even total blindness may rarely occur.

In *common migraine* there is an unheralded onset of headache, often with nausea and sometimes vomiting, following the same temporal pattern but without the antecedent neurologic symptoms. Both classic and common migraine respond to ergot preparations, if administered early in the attack.

Complicated migraine refers to headaches accompanied by neurologic symptoms that may either precede or accompany the headache. Numbness and tingling of the lips, face, hand, and leg on one side may occur, sometimes in combination with an aphasic disorder. The arm and leg may become weak or paralyzed on one side, mimicking a stroke. The numbness or weakness spreads from one part of the body to another slowly over a period of minutes. Full recovery usually occurs after a period of minutes or hours. However, permanent deficits consisting of hemianopsia (lesion in distribution of the posterior cerebral artery), hemiplegia or hemianesthesia (lesion in territory of middle cerebral artery), or ophthalmoplegia (usually third nerve lesion) may occur.

Several other neurologic syndromes have been delineated in association with complicated migraine. Bickerstaff first called attention to *basilar migraine,* in which the visual disorder and paresthesias are bilateral and are accompanied by confusion, stupor, rarely coma, aggressive outbursts, vertigo, diplopia, and dysarthria. While the full syndrome is infrequent, partial basilar syndromes are found in some 30 percent of children with migraine. Alternating hemiplegias in children have also been attributed to basilar migraine but could be due as well to alternating involvement of the middle cerebral arteries.

It is also recognized that neurologic syndromes may occur due to migraine which are not followed by headache. In children, abdominal pain and vomiting, sometimes cyclical, may occur without headache as the sole expression of migraine; the same is true of some cases of paroxysmal vertigo in children. Such *migraine equivalents* may be manifest as pain localized in the thorax, pelvis, or extremities; bouts of fever; paroxysmal vertigo; transient disturbances in mood (*psychic equivalents*). The first neurologic syndrome due to migraine may occur in late adult life in a person not previously known to have migraine. Fisher refers to these as *transient migrainous accompaniments* to distinguish them from transient cerebral ischemic attacks (TIAs).

Cluster headache, also called paroxysmal nocturnal cephalalgia, migrainous neuralgia, histamine headache, and Horton's syndrome, has a fourfold higher incidence in men than in women. It is characterized by constant, unilateral orbital pain, with onset usually within 2 or 3 h after falling asleep. It tends to occur during the phase of rapid eye movement (REM) sleep. The pain is intense and steady (nonthrobbing) with lacrimation, blocked nostril, then rhinorrhea, and sometimes miosis, ptosis, flush, and edema of cheek, all lasting approximately an hour or two. It tends to recur nightly for several weeks or a few months (hence the term *cluster*), followed by complete freedom for months or even years. The pain of a given attack may leave as rapidly as it began. Clusters may recur over the years, being possibly more likely in times of stress, prolonged strain, overwork, and with upsetting emotional experiences. Episodes of cluster headache lasting 2 to 3 weeks may recur several times over a lifetime. Often the pain involves the same orbit in each cluster. Occasionally alcohol, nitroglycerin, or tyramine-containing foods precipitate an attack. Rarely, the condition may occur in daytime and may not cluster but continue for years. The picture is so characteristic that its presentation is diagnostic, though to those unfamiliar with it the possibility of a carotid aneurysm, hemangioma, brain tumor, or sinusitis may be suggested.

The relationship of the cluster headache to migraine remains conjectural. A portion of the cases have a background of migraine, which led to the earlier designation of migrainous neuralgia, but the majority do not.

MECHANISM AND PATHOPHYSIOLOGY A satisfactory theory of the pathophysiology of migraine has eluded clinical investigators. Certain facts appear indisputable; the symptoms of migraine are associated with changes in cerebral blood flow, presumably secondary to changes in vessel caliber; the prodromal phase with neurologic symptoms is accompanied by arteriolar constriction and decreased cerebral blood flow beginning most often in the posterior part of the brain; the decrease in cerebral blood flow in migraine proceeds at a rate of about 2 mm/min, resembling the spreading depression originally described by Leão, which is characterized by a transient self-propagating perturbation of brain electrical activity followed by hypoperfusion. The earlier assumption that the headache that follows is due to vascular dilatation has not been supported by direct measurements of cerebral blood flow during the headache phase. Regional cerebral blood flow, measured by xenon 133, shows oligemic regions of cortex during the entire migraine attack with diminished vascular reactivity to carbon dioxide, suggesting an abnormality of vascular responsivity. Between attacks of migraine, patients show normal regulation of brain circulation.

The factors that elicit these changes in cerebral blood flow are unknown. Two general hypotheses about the cause of migraine have emerged. The first is that it is due to a central nervous system neurovascular disorder that triggers alterations in vasomotor regulation. The premonitory symptoms of changes in mood, appetite, and thirst have led some to consider a central hypothalamic or brainstem disorder affecting biogenic amine regulation (norepinephrine or serotonin). The second considers migraine to be a systemic metabolic disregulation with attacks elicited secondary to intravascular events associated with changes in serotonin metabolism. Changes in platelet serotonin levels, shown to fall during the attack, accompanied by increased urinary excretion of serotonin and of 5-hydroxyindoleacetic acid support the contention that migraine is a systemic disorder. Further support for a role of serotonin comes from observations that reserpine, which triggers serotonin release, causes migraine in some patients and that antiserotonin drugs, like methysergide, show greatest success in its treatment. However, there is difficulty in understanding how changes in intravascular serotonin, which has little direct effect on vessel contraction, can induce the changes of migraine, and it is now conceded that these changes are likely secondary to a central disregulation. Lance considers the mechanism of migraine to involve changes in biogenic amine or neuropeptide neurotransmitters in the central nervous system, associated with or followed by platelet release reactions. Recent work has focused on the neurotransmitters found in nerve fibers that innervate cerebral blood vessels. Moskowitz has demonstrated that cerebral vessels are innervated by nerves that contain substance P, a peptide important for pain transmission (see Chap. 15) and also thought to be capable of eliciting local tissue reactions resembling inflammation. Other neuropeptides found in cerebral blood vessels and known to affect vascular tone include vasoactive intestinal polypeptide, neurotensin, and neuropeptide Y.

There is persistent debate concerning factors that trigger the migraine attacks. Dietary factors are important in some patients. Sensitivity to milk and wheat products is found in some patients with severe refractory migraine. Many patients learn to avoid alcohol (particularly red wine), chocolate, coffee, tea, or other agents with pharmacologically active ingredients. How these substances elicit the attacks is unknown. Some patients describe exposure to sunlight, exercise, tension, or the use of oral contraceptives as increasing the frequency and severity of migraine.

DIFFERENTIAL DIAGNOSIS Classic migraine usually causes no difficulty in diagnosis. Difficulties arise from two sources: (1) ignorance of the fact that a progressively unfolding neurologic syndrome may be migrainous in origin, and (2) lack of appreciation that the neurologic disorder may occur without headache.

The neurologic symptoms of the migraine syndrome may resemble focal epilepsy, the clinical picture of a vascular malformation such as an angioma or aneurysm, or some other vascular disease such as a thrombotic or embolic stroke. The pace of the neurologic symptoms of migraine, rather than their character, reliably distinguishes them from epilepsy. The clinical profile of the aura of epilepsy is measured in seconds, for it depends on spreading neural excitation, in contrast to the slow progression of migraine, which is based on spreading depression of nervous tissue. Nevertheless, there are instances where episodes of coma with electroencephalogram (EEG) abnormality may be either migraine or epilepsy. Furthermore, a seizure is often followed by a generalized headache.

Ophthalmoplegic migraine always suggests a carotid aneurysm, and carotid arteriography may be necessary to exclude it. Despite many claims that vascular malformations may cause hemicranial pain occurring invariably on the same side of the head (unlike migraine), larger series of cases have shown this only rarely to be the case. Focal epilepsy, protracted headache, stiff neck and bloody CSF, a persistent neurologic deficit, and cranial bruit are indicative of a vascular type of headache associated with angioma or aneurysm. Only in the earlier stages, when periodic throbbing headache is the sole symptom, are these conditions confused with true migraine.

Tension headache The tension headache is usually bilateral, often with diffuse extension over the top of the cranium. Occipital-nuchal or bifrontal localization is common. Although the sensation may be described as pain, close questioning may uncover other sensations, viz., fullness, tightness, or pressure (as if the head is surrounded by a band or in a vise), on which waves of aching pain are superimposed. The onset of a given attack is more gradual than in migraine, and not infrequently a throbbing "vascular" type of headache is described. Tension headache may occur acutely under conditions of emotional duress or intense worry and lasts for hours or a day or two. More often it persists unremittingly for weeks or months. In fact, this is the only type of headache that exhibits the peculiarity of being absolutely continuous day and night for long periods of time. Although sleep may be possible, whenever the patient awakens, the headache is present; a common feature is the finding that analgesic remedies have relatively little effect in alleviating the pain. In contrast to migraine, in which pain is periodic and lifelong, with tendency to lessen in late adult years, tension headache occurs more often in middle age and may persist for many years.

It is unlikely that the origin of the pain is sustained muscle activity, since electromyographic (EMG) investigations show no changes in forehead or neck muscles. On the other hand, elicitation of headache after administration of amyl nitrite, a vasodilator, in about 50 percent of patients suggests a vascular contribution to the pain. Histamine can also cause headaches in these patients.

It is a common experience for both tension headache and common migraine to coexist in the same patient. The management of such patients may require therapy of both types of headache.

Psychological studies of groups of patients with tension headaches have revealed prominent symptoms of depression, anxiety, and, in some, hypochrondriasis. Kudrow records that 65 percent of depressed patients have this type of headache and that over 60 percent of his patients with tension headaches were depressed.

Headache of angioma and aneurysm The temporal profile of any given attack shows the onset to be sudden or very acute, with the pain reaching a peak within minutes. Neurologic disturbances such as defects in vision, unilateral numbness, weakness, or aphasia may precede or occur after the onset of headache and outlast it. Should hemorrhage occur, the headache is often extremely severe and localizes in the occiput and neck, lasting many days in association with stiff neck. A cranial or cervical bruit and the presence of blood in the CSF establish the diagnosis. The claim that vascular malformations may give rise to migraine is probably untenable. Statistical data show migraine to be no more frequent in this group of patients than in the general population. Vascular lesions may exist for long periods of time without headache, or headache may develop many years after other manifestations such as epilepsy and hemiplegia (see Chap. 351).

Traumatic headaches Severe, chronic, continuous, or intermittent headaches often associated with giddiness, vertigo, or tinnitus appear as the cardinal symptoms of the posttraumatic syndrome. The cause of the headache is unknown, but it is a clear-cut disorder unrelated in most instances to medicolegal issues of compensation. *Posttraumatic dysautonomic cephalalgia* is a term given by Vijayan and Dreyfus to severe, episodic, throbbing, unilateral headaches accompanied by ipsilateral mydriasis and excessive facial sweating. The condition follows injury to the neck in the region of the carotid sheath. It was postulated that the sympathetic nervous supply of the cranium had been disinhibited, and there was clinical and pharmacologic evidence of sympathetic dysfunction.

Headache and dizziness of fluctuating severity, followed by drowsiness, stupor, coma, and hemiparesis, are the usual manifestations of *chronic subdural hematoma*. The head injury may have been minor and forgotten by patient and family. The headaches are deep-seated, steady, unilateral or generalized, and respond to the usual analgesic drugs. The typical attack profile of the headache and other symptoms is one of increasing frequency and severity over several weeks or months. Diagnosis is established by computed tomography (CT), magnetic resonance imaging (MRI), or angiography (see Chap. 352).

Headaches of brain tumor Headache is the outstanding symptom of cerebral tumor. Unfortunately, the quality of the pain has no specific feature. It tends to be deep-seated, nonthrobbing (or throbbing), and aching or bursting. Attacks last a few minutes to an hour or more and occur once or many times during the day. Activity and, frequently, change in the position of the head may provoke pain, while rest in bed diminishes its frequency. Nocturnal awakening because of pain, although typical, is by no means diagnostic. Unexpected forceful (projectile) vomiting may punctuate the illness in its later stages. As the tumor grows, the pain becomes more frequent and severe; it sometimes is nearly continuous terminally. If unilateral, the headache is homolateral to the tumor in 9 out of 10 patients. Supratentorial tumors are felt anterior to the interauricular circumference of the skull; posterior fossa tumors behind this line. Bifrontal and bioccipital headache, coming on after unilateral headache, signifies the development of increased intracranial pressure.

Headaches related to medical disorders Experienced physicians are aware of many conditions in which headache figures as a dominant symptom. These include fevers of any cause, carbon monoxide exposure, chronic lung disease with hypercapnia (headaches often nocturnal), hypothyroidism, Cushing's syndrome, withdrawal of corticosteroid medication, chronic nitrite or ergot exposure, occasionally Addison's disease, aldosterone-producing adrenal tumors, use of contraceptive medications, acute rises in blood pressure, e.g., from pheochromocytoma, and acute anemia with hemoglobin below 10 g. Hypertension per se is an uncommon cause of headache.

Unusual types of headache Sharp, jabbing pains in the head (icepick-like pains) last a second or two, and have no clinical significance. They are reported in up to 3 percent of the normal population and in 46 percent of migrainous patients. The pain is usually felt in the temporal or orbital region.

Cough and exertional headache or headache brought on by stooping follows the initiating action by a few seconds and lasts a minute or two. Usually no explanation is apparent, but exceptionally it occurs in patients with arteriovenous malformations, Paget's disease of the skull, Arnold-Chiari malformation, or an intracranial tumor. In a series of 103 patients followed for 3 years or longer by Rooke, only 10 developed neurologic signs. The mechanism of this headache may be venous distention, for jugular compression induces it in some patients.

Coital headaches are generalized, often severe headaches that begin suddenly during coitus or immediately after orgasm. They are uncommon, occur more often in men than in women, and usually do not signify a serious underlying pathology. They may last minutes or hours. In the latter circumstance they must be differentiated from a subarachnoid hemorrhage due to a ruptured aneurysm.

Erythrocyanotic headache is a rare form of generalized throbbing headache which occurs in conjunction with flushing of the face and hands and numbness of the fingers (erythromelalgia). The condition has been reported in association with (1) mastocytosis (infiltration of tissues with mast cells, which elaborate histamine, heparin, and serotonin); (2) carcinoid tumors; (3) some tumors of pancreatic islets; (4) pheochromocytoma.

HEADACHE AND FACIAL PAIN The facial neuralgias are discussed in Chap. 360 (see Table 18-2).

APPROACH TO THE PATIENT WITH HEADACHE Obviously very different possibilities are raised by a patient who presents for the first time with severe headache and a patient who has had recurrent headache over a period of years. The chances of uncovering the cause in the first instance are much greater than in the second and in the former the underlying conditions (meningitis, subarachnoid hemorrhage, epidural or subdural hematoma, glaucoma, and purulent sinusitis) often are more serious. In general, severe, persistent headache with stiff neck and fever means meningitis, and the same combination without fever, subarachnoid hemorrhage. A lumbar puncture is mandatory. Acute persistent headache over a period of hours or days may occur in systemic infections such as influenza (febrile) or as a manifestation of an acute tension state. If there is a diagnosable febrile disease and no stiffness of the neck, lumbar puncture may be deferred. The first attack of migraine may also present in this way, but of course there is no fever.

In searching for the cause of recurrent headache one should investigate the status of cardiovascular and renal systems by blood pressure and urine examination, eyes by funduscopy, intraocular pressure, and refraction, the sinuses by transillumination and x-rays, the cranial arteries by palpation (and biopsy?), the cervical spine by the effect of passive movement of the head and x-rays, the nervous system by neurologic and psychological evaluation.

Hypertension, although frequent in the general population, is not often a cause of recurrent headaches. Severe hypertension with diastolic blood pressures of over 110 mmHg may be associated with headache. If headache is severe and frequent, the possibilities of underlying anxiety or tension state or a common migraine syndrome should be considered.

The adolescent with daily frontal headaches represents a special type of problem. Often the relationship of the headaches to eyestrain is unclear, and refraction of the eyes and new eyeglasses do not relieve the condition. Anxiety or tension is probably a factor in such cases, but it is difficult to be certain of a causal relationship. Some of the most persistent and inexplicable headaches, which have led to a survey by a battery of diagnostic procedures for tumor, have proved in the end to be associated with endogenous depression.

Equally puzzling is the somber, tense adult whose primary complaint is headache, or the migrainous person who in late life or at menopause begins to have daily headaches. Here it becomes important to assess mental status along the lines suggested in Chaps. 29 and 30, looking for evidence of anxiety, depression, and hypochondriasis. The quality and persistence of the headache are suggestive of the possibility of psychiatric illness. Sometimes asking the patient what is the matter may reveal suspicion and fear of brain tumor. Antidepressant drugs given as an empirical test may relieve the headache, thus clarifying the diagnosis.

The most worrisome type of patient is the one who has headache of increasing frequency and severity over a period of months or a year or so. Since an intracranial mass lesion (tumor, abscess, subdural hematoma) is a leading possibility, a complete neurologic survey, including careful inspection of optic discs, CT or MRI, and electroencephalogram, should be performed.

Every person over 50 to 55 years with severe headache of some few days' or weeks' duration should be considered as possibly having cranial arteritis (see Chap. 276). The overall incidence in patients over 50 years is 1 in 750; that of polymyalgia rheumatica in the same age group is 1 in 200. Women are more often affected than men (4:1), and there is an associated polymyalgia in 25 percent of cases. Conversely, in 50 percent of polymyalgia rheumatica patients there is a cranial arteritis. Increased sedimentation rate, fever, and anemia may occur. The findings of a thickened, tender temporal artery and claudication of jaw muscles from involvement of facial arteries are important. The disease may cause blindness and/or ophthalmoplegia but rarely involves intracranial arteries. Arterial biopsy and response to glucocorticoids establish the diagnosis.

TREATMENT The most important steps in the treatment of headache are those measures which uncover and remove the underlying disease or functional disturbance.

For the *common everyday headache* due to fatigue, acute stress, or excessive use of alcohol and tobacco, the physician advises avoidance of the offending activity or agent, and symptomatic therapy in the form of aspirin, 0.6 g, or acetaminophen, 0.6 g, given every 4 to 6 h. Chronic headaches falling into the common migraine or

TABLE 18-2 Types of facial pain

Types	Site	Clinical characteristics	Aggravating-relieving factors	Diseases	Treatment
Trigeminal neuralgia (tic douloureux)	Second or third division of trigeminal nerve, unilateral	Men : women = 1:3 Over 50 years Paroxysms (10–30 s) of stabbing, burning pain Trigger points, intermittent ache No sensory or motor paralysis	Touching face, chewing, smiling, talking, blowing nose	Idiopathic If in young adults unilateral or bilateral, multiple sclerosis Vascular anomaly Tumor of fifth cranial nerve	Carbamazepine Phenytoin Radiofrequency lesion of ganglion
Atypical facial neuralgia	Unilateral or bilateral	Predominantly female 30–50 years Continuous intolerable pain Mainly maxillary areas	None	Depressive and anxiety states Hysteria Idiopathic	Antidepressant and antianxiety medication
Supraorbital ciliary, infraorbital, sphenopalatine neuralgias	Unilateral in eye, cheek, ear, neck	Persistent, aching pain	Occasional nasal obstruction	Idiopathic Paranasal sinus disease	Decongestant nasal medication ?Nerve section and injection
Postzoster neuralgia	Unilateral Any one of trigeminal divisions	History of zoster Aching, burning pain; jabs of pain Paresthesia, slight sensory loss Dermal scars	Contact, movement	Herpes zoster	Carbamazepine, phenytoin, and antidepressants
Costen's syndrome	Unilateral, near temporomandibular joints	Elderly females Severe aching pain, intensified by chewing Tenderness over joints Malocclusion	Chewing, pressure over temporomandibular joint	Loss of teeth, rheumatoid arthritis	Bite correction and surgery
Tolosa-Hunt syndrome	Unilateral, mainly orbital	Intense sharp, aching pain; associated ophthalmoplegias of varying degree Pupil inequality, sensory loss	None	?Arteritis and granulomatous lesions	Glucocorticoids
Raeder's paratrigeminal syndrome	Unilateral, frontotemporal and maxilla	Intense sharp, aching pain Pupil inequality, sensory loss	None	Tumors, granulomatous lesions, injuries	Depends on type of lesion

SOURCE: After J Patten, Neurological Differential Diagnosis, London, Harold Starke, Springer-Verlag, 1977.

tension category are much more difficult to manage. Analgesics may alleviate the pain, but rarely abolish it. Patients commonly self-administer four to eight tablets daily of aspirin or acetaminophen for years despite acknowledging minimal benefit. Such headaches often respond to amitriptyline given in gradually increased doses to 100 to 150 mg, preferably administered as a single bedtime dose. *Premenstrual headache,* if troublesome, can often be helped by the use of a diuretic for the week preceding the menstrual period and a mixture of mild analgesic and sedative medications (aspirin or acetaminophen, 0.6 g, and barbiturate). If the headaches are severe and incapacitating, they should be treated as common migraine.

Migraine may require no treatment at all, other than an explanation of its nature to the patient and a reassurance that it will do no harm. Some patients know, or allege to know, that certain factors induce attacks, and these should be avoided. In some patients alcoholic drinks, particularly red wine, are invariably followed by a migraine. Others claim reduction of attacks of headache by an elimination diet, correction of refractive error, or by psychotherapy. Biofeedback can reduce the number of migraine attacks in some patients, and practiced relaxation is beneficial in others.

Drugs used for treatment of migraine can be separated into agents used for the acute attack and those administered for prophylaxis. Patients who experience more than three or four severe attacks each month should be considered for preventive treatment. Treatment of the neurologic aura of migraine is rarely required or possible because of its brevity. Some patients find relief with ergot preparations given orally, 1 to 3 mg held under the tongue until dissolved, or ergotamine tartrate, 0.25 mg by intravenous injection. These treatments if given early will abort a classic migraine attack in 80 to 90 percent of patients. Sometimes the combination of caffeine, 100 mg with 1 mg ergotamine, is preferred (Cafergot or equivalent). It may be taken in the form of tablets (two at the onset of headache and a third in half an hour) or as rectal suppositories (2 mg ergotamine and 100 mg caffeine) if vomiting prevents oral administration.The acute migraine attack is managed best with an ergotamine-caffeine combination. Some patients find relief with ergotamine given orally in a dose of 1 to 3 mg. If oral administration is not tolerated because of nausea, or is ineffective, rectal administration of ergotamine is indicated. One-half suppository given at the onset of the attack followed by another half in 10 to 15 min and a whole suppository in 20 to 30 min, if necessary, is often effective. Medication should be limited to no more than two suppositories per day or four per week because of the danger of vasospasm. Ergotamine inhalation is more acceptable to some patients; one inhalation is given at the start of the attack, another in 5 min, and a third at 10 min. Inhalations should be limited to three per day or six per week. In patients who have vascular disease or are pregnant, ergot preparations must be used cautiously, if at all, because of the danger of prolonged vascular spasm.

Once the headache has become intense (after 30 min), ergot is of little help, and one must resort to codeine sulfate, 30 mg, or meperidine, 50 mg, as the only means of terminating the pain. If sleep customarily terminates the headache, 50 mg of promethazine or an equivalent drug orally is helpful; it also relieves vomiting.

In individuals with frequent migrainous attacks (more than four per month), efforts at prevention are worthwhile. Some success has been obtained with preparations of ergot, 0.5 mg, atropine, 0.3 mg, and phenobarbital, 15 mg, two or three times a day for a few weeks. Propranolol, 20 to 40 mg three times a day, has been effective in reducing the frequency and intensity of attacks in approximately one-half of cases. For the most severe forms of the disorder, methysergide in a dose of 6 to 8 mg per day given for several weeks or months has proved effective in reducing the frequency of or abolishing attacks. The main adverse effect has been retroperitoneal and pulmonary fibrosis; this complication has been reported in several dozen cases when the patient has been treated continuously for more than 6 months. Discontinuing treatment for 1 month out of every 6 has greatly reduced the incidence of this complication. Some patients benefit from tricyclic antidepressants such as doxepin or amitriptyline, which should be started in doses of 25 to 75 mg at bedtime and increased gradually every third or fourth night to 100 to 150 mg. Calcium channel blockers such as nifedipine 10 to 40 mg per day in divided doses or verapamil 80 mg given three times daily may be beneficial. Some patients experience an initial exacerbation of migraine attacks on first taking calcium channel blocking drugs, and then obtain relief. Severe attacks of common migraine lasting for several days or even weeks have been treated successfully with chlorpromazine in doses of 50 to 100 mg daily administered for 7 to 10 days. Prednisone in divided doses of 20 mg three or four times a day is also effective in some severe cases. Newer drugs with antiserotonergic effects are currently nearing approval for clinical use in migraine.

All experienced physicians appreciate the importance of helping patients rearrange their schedules so as to control the tensions and hard-driving ways of living so often a feature of migrainous patients. There is no one way of accomplishing this, but, in general, long and costly psychotherapy has not been helpful, or at least one can say there are no substantial data as to its value.

Cluster headaches have proved to be most resistant to treatment. The acute attack can be terminated with oxygen or ergotamine inhalation. However, the most effective treatment is the administration of drugs to prevent headache episodes until the cluster is over. Success has been obtained in individual cases with amitriptyline, 100 to 150 mg daily, methysergide, 6 to 8 mg per day, prednisone, 40 mg daily for 5 days then reduced to an amount necessary to control headaches, lithium carbonate in an initial dose of 250 mg three times a day, and calcium channel blockers. Histamine desensitization, originally proposed by Horton, has been little used in recent years because of inconvenience and inconsistent results. Persistent cluster headaches have also been treated effectively with indomethacin.

Hypertensive headaches respond to agents that lower blood pressure and relieve muscle tension.

Muscle tension headaches respond best to massage, relaxation, and a combination of drugs which relieve depression (e.g., amitriptyline or imipramine) and anxiety (e.g., diazepam and alprazolam). Pain-relieving medicine of non-habit-forming type (e.g., aspirin and propoxyphene hydrochloride) should be added when throbbing headache is present. Stronger analgesic medication (codeine or meperidine hydrochloride) should be avoided. Psychotherapy may be helpful in this group of patients.

The headache of the *posttraumatic syndrome* requires supportive psychotherapy in the form of reassurance and frequent explanation of its benign and transient nature, a program of increasing physical activity, and drugs which allay anxiety and depression. However, the tricyclic antidepressants are generally less effective than in the mixed tension and throbbing headaches of anxious depressions. Tender scars from scalp laceration may be novocainized repeatedly (subcutaneous injection of 5 mL of 1% procaine) with some degree of success. Settlement of litigation as soon as possible works to the patient's advantage.

Heat, massage, salicylates, and indomethacin or phenylbutazone usually effect some improvement in those arthritic diseases of the cervical spine that are associated with cervicocranial pain (see Chaps. 270 and 281). A soft collar and traction may be beneficial.

Glucocorticoid therapy is indicated in *cranial arteritis* to prevent disastrous blindness by occlusion of the ophthalmic arteries, which occurs in 50 percent of untreated patients. Prednisone should be given in full doses (40 to 60 mg per day) for at least a month and continued until all symptoms and laboratory abnormalities have disappeared. The headaches of brain tumor often respond promptly to large doses of glucocorticoids.

REFERENCES

Appenzeller O: Migraine and cluster headache, in *Current Therapy in Neurologic Disease*, RT Johnson (ed). Philadelphia, Decker, 1987, vol 2, p 59

Bickerstaff ER: Basilar artery migraine. Lancet 1:15, 1961

Bogduk N, Lance JW: Pain and pain syndrome including headache, in *Current Neurology*, SF Appel (ed). New York, Wiley, 1981, vol 3, chap 14

Caviness VS, O'Brien P: Headache. N Engl J Med 302:446, 1980

Couch JR, Hassaneim RS: Platelet aggregability in migraine. Neurology 27:843, 1977

Critchley M et al (eds): *Advances in Neurology*, vol 33: *Headache: Physiopathological and Clinical Aspects*. New York, Raven Press, 1982

Diamond S: Prolonged benign exertional headache. Headache 22:96, 1982

Ehyai A, Fenichel GM: Natural history of acute confusional migraine. Arch Neurol 35:368, 1978

Fisher CM: Late-life migraine accompaniment—further experience. Stroke 17:1033, 1986

Gelmers HJ: Nimodipine, a new calcium antagonist, in the prophylactic treatment of migraine. *Headache* 23:106, 1983

Greenberg DA: Calcium channel antagonists and the treatment of migraine. Clin Neuropharmacol 9:311, 1986

Hockaday JM: Basilar migraine in children. Dev Med Child Neurol 21:455, 1979

Johns D: Benign sexual headache within a family. Arch Neurol 43:1158, 1986

Kayan A, Hood JD: Neuro-otological manifestations of migraine. Brain 107:1123, 1984

Lake A et al: Biofeedback and rational-emotive therapy in the management of migraine headache. Appl Behav Anal 12:127, 1979

Lance JW: Headache. Ann Neurol 10:1, 1981

———: Headaches related to sexual activity. J Neurol Neurosurg Psychiat 39:1226, 1976

Lauritzen M, Hansen AJ: Spreading depression of Leão. Possible relation to migraine pathophysiology, in *Basic Mechanisms of Headache*, vol 2: *Pain Research and Clinical Management*, J Olesen, L Edvinsson (eds). Amsterdam, Elsevier, 1988, p 439

———, Olesen J: Regional cerebral blood flow during migraine attacks by xenon-133 inhalation and emission tomography. Brain 107:447, 1984

Meyer JS, Hardenberg J: Clinical effectiveness of calcium entry blockers in prophylactic treatment of migraine and cluster headaches. Headache 23:266, 1983

Moskowitz M: Neurobiology of vascular head pain. Ann Neurol 16:157, 1984

Olesen J: Pathophysiological implications of migraine and symptomatology, in *Basic Mechanisms of Headache*, vol 2: *Pain Research and Clinical Management*, J Olesen, L Edvinsson (eds). Amsterdam, Elsevier, 1988, p 353

———, Edvinsson L (eds): *Basic Mechanisms of Headache*, vol 2: *Pain Research and Clinical Management*. Amsterdam, Elsevier, 1988

Peroutka J: The pharmacology of calcium channel antagonists: Novel class of anti-migraine agents? Headache 23:278, 1983

Raskin NH: Migraine, in *Diseases of the Nervous System*, AK Asbury, GM McKhann, WI McDonald (eds). Philadelphia, Saunders, 1986, p 961

Spierings EL: Clinical and experimental evidence for a role of calcium entry blockers in the treatment of migraine. Ann NY Acad Sci 522:676, 1988

Vijayan N, Dreyfus PM: Posttraumatic dysautonomic cephalalgia: Clinical observations and treatment. Arch Neurol 32:649, 1976

Vinken PJ, Bruyn GW (eds): *Handbook of Clinical Neurology*, vol 5: *Headache and Cranial Neuralgias*. Amsterdam, North-Holland, 1968

19 BACK AND NECK PAIN

HENRY J. MANKIN*

ANATOMY AND PHYSIOLOGY OF THE LOWER PART OF THE BACK

The bony spine is a complex structure, anatomically divisible into two parts. The anterior part consists of a series of cylindrical vertebral bodies connected to one another by the intervertebral disks and held together by the anterior and posterior longitudinal ligaments. The posterior part consists of more delicate elements that extend from the vertebral body as pedicles and broaden posteriorly to form laminae, which together with ligamentous structures form the vertebral canal. The posterior elements are joined to adjacent vertebrae by two small facetal synovial joints which allow a modest degree of motion between any two segments, but in aggregate produce a rather extensive range (Fig. 19-1). Stout transverse and spinous bony processes project laterally and posteriorly and serve as the attachments of muscles which move, support, and protect the vertebral column. The stability of the spine depends on two types of support: that provided by the bony articulations (principally by the diskal joints and the synovial articulations of the posterior elements) and a second type provided by the ligamentous (passive) and muscular (active) supporting structures. The ligamentous structures are quite strong, but because neither they nor the vertebral body–disk complexes have sufficient integral strength to resist the enormous forces acting on the column during even simple movements, voluntary and reflex contractions of the sacrospinalis, abdominal, gluteal, psoas, and hamstring muscles afford much of the stability.

The vertebral and paravertebral structures derive their innervation from the recurrent branches of the spinal nerves. Pain endings and fibers have been demonstrated in the ligaments, muscles, periosteum of bone, outer layers of annulus fibrosus, and synovium of the articular facets. The sensory fibers from these structures and the sacroiliac and lumbosacral joints join to form the sinovertebral nerves which pass via the recurrent branches of the spinal nerves of the first sacral and the fifth to first lumbar vertebrae into the gray matter of the corresponding segments of the spinal cord. Efferent fibers emerge from these segments and extend to the muscles through the same nerves.

The parts of the back that possess the greatest freedom of movement, and hence are most frequently subject to injury, are the lumbar and cervical regions. In addition to the voluntary motions required for bending, twisting, and other movements, many actions of the spine are reflex in nature and are the basis of posture.

GENERAL CLINICAL CONSIDERATIONS

TYPES OF LOW BACK PAIN Four types of pain may be differentiated: local, referred, radicular, and that arising from secondary (protective) muscular spasm.

Local pain is caused by any pathologic process that impinges upon or irritates sensory endings. Involvement of structures which contain no sensory endings is painless. The central, medullary portion of the vertebral body may be destroyed by tumor, for example, without evocation of pain, whereas cortical fractures, or tears and distortions of the periosteum, synovial membranes, muscles, annulus fibrosus, and ligaments are often exquisitely painful. The latter structures are innervated by afferent fibers of the posterior primary rami. Although painful states are often accompanied by swelling of the affected tissues, this may not be apparent if a deep structure of the back is the site of disease. Local pain is often described as steady but may be intermittent, varying considerably with position or activity. The pain may be sharp or dull and although often diffuse is always felt in or near the affected part of the spine. Reflex splinting of the spine segments by paravertebral muscles is frequently noted, and certain movements or postures that alter the position of the injured tissues aggravate the pain. Firm pressure or percussion upon superficial structures in the region involved usually evokes tenderness, which is of aid in identifying the site of the abnormality.

Referred pain is of two types: that projected from the spine into regions lying within the area of the lumbar and upper sacral dermatomes and that projected from the pelvic and abdominal viscera to the spine. Pain due to diseases of the upper part of the lumbar spine is usually referred to the anterior aspects of the thighs and legs; that from the lower lumbar and sacral segments is referred to the gluteal regions, posterior thighs, calves, and sometimes feet. Pain of this type, although of deep, aching quality and rather diffuse, tends at times to be superficially projected. In general the referred pain parallels in intensity the local pain in the back. In other words, maneuvers that alter local pain have a similar effect on referred pain, though not with such precision and immediacy as in radicular, or "root," pain. Referred pain may be confused with pain from visceral disease, but the latter is usually described as "deep" and tends to radiate from the abdomen through to the back. Also, visceral pain is usually unaffected by movement of the spine, does not improve with recumbency, and may be modified by the activity of the involved viscus.

Radicular, or "root," *pain* has some of the characteristics of referred pain but differs in its greater intensity, distal radiation, circumscription to the territory of a root, and the factors which excite it. The mechanisms are principally distortion, stretching, irritation, and compression of a spinal root, most often central to the intervertebral foramen. In addition, it has been suggested that in patients with spinal stenosis the "lumbar claudication" pattern may be due to a relative ischemia associated with compression. Although the pain itself is often dull or aching, various maneuvers which increase the irritation of the root or stretch it may greatly intensify the pain, eliciting a lancinating quality. Nearly always the radiation of pain is from a central position near the spine to some part of the lower extremity. Cough, sneeze, and strain are characteristically evocative maneuvers; but since they may also jar or move the spine, they may aggravate local pain as well. Forward bending with the knees extended or "straight-leg raising" in disease of the lower part of the lumbar spine excites radicular pain on the basis of stretch; jugular vein compression, which raises intraspinal pressure and may cause a shift in the position of or pressure on the root, may have a similar effect. Irritation of the fourth and fifth lumbar and first sacral roots, which form the sciatic nerve, causes pain that extends mainly down the posterior aspects of the thigh, the postero- and anterolateral aspects of the leg, and into the foot—termed sciatica. Tingling, paresthesias,

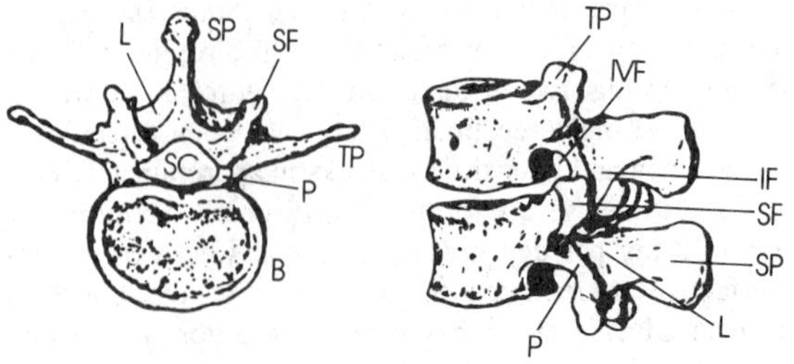

FIGURE 19-1 *Left:* Superior view of a stripped lumbar vertebra. *Right:* Lateral view of two articulated lumbar vertebrae. B = body; SC = spinal canal; IVF = intervertebral foramen; IF = inferior articular facet; SF = superior articular facet; P = pedicle; TP = transverse process; SP = spinous process; L = lamina. *(Adapted from DB Levine, in Arthritis and Allied Conditions: A Textbook of Rheumatology, 10th ed, DJ McCarty (ed), Philadelphia, Lea & Febiger, 1985.)*

* The author wishes to acknowledge the contribution of Raymond D. Adams to this chapter, which is a revision of their joint chapter in the eleventh edition.

and numbness or sensory impairment of the skin, soreness of the skin, and tenderness along the nerve usually accompany classic sciatic pain, and on physical examination, reflex loss, weakness, atrophy, fascicular twitching, and occasionally stasis edema may occur if the motor fibers of the anterior root are involved.

Pain resulting from muscular spasm is usually mentioned in relation to local pain, but the anatomic or physiologic basis is more obscure. Muscle spasm associated with many disorders of the spine can produce significant distortions of the normal posture; as a result, chronic tension in muscles may give rise to a dull and sometimes cramping ache. In this instance one can feel the tautness of the sacrospinalis and gluteal muscles and demonstrate by palpation that the pain is localized to these structures.

Other pains often of undetermined origin are sometimes described by patients with chronic disease of the lower part of the back. Unilateral symptoms of drawing, pulling, cramping sensations (without involuntary muscle spasm), tearing, throbbing, or jabbing pains, or feelings of burning or coldness are difficult to interpret but, like paresthesias and numbness, should always suggest the possibility of nerve or root disease.

In addition to assessing the character and location of the pain, one should determine the factors that aggravate and relieve it, its constancy, and its relationship to recumbency and such stereotypical movements and maneuvers as forward bending, cough, sneeze, and strain. Frequently the most important lead comes from the knowledge of the mode of onset and circumstances that initiated the pain. Inasmuch as many painful afflictions of the back are the result of injury incurred during work or in an accident, the possibility of exaggeration or prolongation of pain for purposes of compensation or other personal reasons, or because of hysteria or malingering, must always be kept in mind.

EXAMINATION OF THE LOWER PART OF THE BACK

Inspection of the normal spine shows a dorsal kyphosis and lumbar lordosis in the sagittal plane, which in some individuals may be exaggerated (swayback). In patients with spinal disorders, one should seek excessive curvature, flattening of the normal lumbar arch, presence of a gibbus (a short, sharp, kyphotic angulation usually indicative of a fracture or congenital abnormality), lateral curvature and/or rotation (scoliosis), pelvic tilt or obliquity, or asymmetry of the paravertebral or gluteal musculature. In severe sciatica, one may observe that the affected limb is held with the hip and knee flexed, presumably to reduce tension on the irritated part.

The spine, hips, and legs should be observed during certain motions, but no advantage accrues from trying to find out how much pain the patient can endure. It is more important to assess when and under what conditions the pain commences. Normally, the motion of forward bending produces flattening and reversal of the lumbar lordotic curve and exaggeration of the dorsal curve. With ruptured lumbar disks or lesions that involve the posterior ligaments, articular facets, or sacrospinalis muscle, protective reflexes prevent stretching of these structures; as a consequence, the sacrospinalis muscles remain taut and limit motion in the lumbar part of the spine, causing forward bending to occur at the hips and at the lumbar-thoracic junction. With disease principally affecting the spinal roots or the lumbosacral joints, forward bending occurs in such a way as to avoid tensing the hamstring muscles, which puts undue leverage upon the pelvis. In unilateral "sciatica," with its increased curvature toward the side of the lesion, the lumbar and lumbosacral motions are splinted, and bending is mainly at the hips; at a certain point the knee on the affected side is flexed to relieve hamstring spasm, and tilting of the pelvis occurs to slacken the lumbosacral roots and sciatic nerve.

With lumbosacral lesions and sciatica, passive lumbar flexion in the supine position causes little pain and is not limited as long as the hamstrings are relaxed and the sciatic nerve is not stretched. With lumbosacral and lumbar spine disease (e.g., arthritis), passive flexion of the hips is free, whereas flexion of the lumbar spine may be impeded and painful. Passive straight-leg raising (possible in most normal individuals up to 80 to 90° except in those who have unusually tight hamstrings), like forward bending with the knees extended in the standing posture, places the sciatic nerve and its roots under tension, thereby producing pain. It may also cause an anterior rotation of the pelvis around a transverse axis, increasing stress on the lumbosacral joint, and thus causing pain if this segment is arthritic or otherwise impaired. Consequently, in diseases of the lumbosacral joints and lumbosacral roots, this movement is limited on the affected side and to a lesser extent on the opposite side. Evocation of such a response (pain and limitation of movement during flexion of the hip when the knee is extended) is known as Lasègue's sign and is considered to be a useful test of this condition. A positive contralateral straight-leg raising sign is believed by some to be a sign of a more extensive lesion, such as an extruded disk fragment, rather than a simple prolapse or protrusion. It is important to remember, however, that the evoked pain is always referred to the diseased side, no matter which leg is flexed.

Hyperextension is best evaluated with the patient standing or lying prone. If the condition causing back pain is acute, it may be difficult to extend the spine in the standing position. A patient with lumbosacral strain or disk disease can usually extend or hyperextend the spine without aggravation of pain. If the lesion is in the upper lumbar segments or if an active inflammatory process, fracture of the vertebral body, or a very tight canal (vertebral stenosis) is present, hyperextension may be markedly limited.

Palpation and percussion of the spine are the last steps in the examination. It is preferable to palpate first those regions which are the least likely to evoke pain. At all times the examiner should know what structures are being palpated (see Fig. 19-2). Localized tenderness is seldom pronounced in disease of the spine because the involved structures are so deep that they rarely give rise to surface tenderness.

FIGURE 19-2 (1) Costovertebral angle. (2) Spinous process and interspinous ligament. (3) Region of the articular fifth lumbar to the first sacral facet. (4) Dorsum of sacrum. (5) Region of iliac crest. (6) Iliolumbar angle. (7) Spinous processes of fifth lumbar to first sacral vertebrae (tenderness = faulty posture or occasionally spina bifida occulta). (8) Region between posterior superior and posterior inferior spines. Sacroiliac ligaments (tenderness = sacroiliac sprain, often tender with fifth lumbar to first sacral disk). (9) Sacrococcygeal junction (tenderness = sacrococcygeal injury, i.e., sprain or fracture). (10) Region of sacrosciatic notch (tenderness = fourth to fifth lumbar disk rupture and sacroiliac sprain). (11) Sciatic nerve trunk (tenderness = ruptured lumbar disk or sciatic nerve lesion).

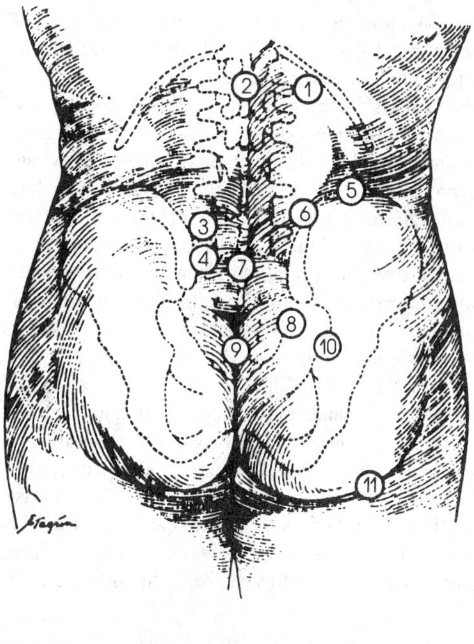

Mild superficial and poorly localized tenderness signifies only a disease process within the affected segment of the body, i.e., dermatome.

Tenderness over the costovertebral angle often indicates renal disease, adrenal disease, or an injury to the transverse processes of the first or second lumbar vertebra. Hypersensitivity on palpation of the transverse processes of the other lumbar vertebrae as well as the overlying sacrospinalis muscles may signify fracture of the transverse process or a strain of muscle attachments. Tenderness of a spinous process or aggravation of pain by the jarring of gentle percussion may be nonspecific but frequently indicates the presence of a disk lesion at the site deep to it, inflammation (as in disk space infection), or fracture. Tenderness in the region of the articular facets between the fifth lumbar and first sacral vertebrae is consistent with disease of a lumbosacral disk [Fig. 19-2 (3)]. It is also frequent in rheumatoid arthritis.

In palpation of the spinous processes, it is important to note any deviation in the lateral plane (this may be indicative of fracture or arthritis) or in the anteroposterior plane. A ''step-off'' forward displacement of the spinous process may be an important clue to the presence of a spondylolisthesis one segment below the displaced level.

Abdominal, rectal, and pelvic examination and assessment of the status of the peripheral vascular system are important parts of the examination of the patient with complaints in the lower back and should not be omitted. They may provide evidence for vascular, visceral, neoplastic, or inflammatory disorders which may extend to the spine or cause pain to be referred to this region. Finally, a careful neurologic examination should be performed, with special attention given to motor, reflex, and sensory changes, particularly in the lower extremities (see ''Protrusion of Lumbar Intervertebral Disks,'' below).

SPECIAL LABORATORY PROCEDURES Useful laboratory tests, depending on the nature of the problem and the circumstances, include a complete blood count, erythrocyte sedimentation rate (especially helpful in screening for infection or myeloma), measurement of serum calcium, phosphorus, alkaline phosphatase, acid phosphatase (the last mentioned is of importance if one suspects metastatic carcinoma from the prostate), immunoglobulin electrophoresis, and tests for rheumatoid factor. Roentgenograms of the lumbar part of the spine in the anteroposterior, lateral, and oblique planes should be obtained in every patient with low back pain and sciatica. Special spot views or stereoscopic or laminographic films may provide further information in certain cases. Bone scans are of particular aid in revealing some fractures and neoplastic and inflammatory lesions.

Examination of the spinal canal with a contrast medium is often of value, especially if a spinal cord tumor is suspected or if a patient is thought to have a disk herniation and fails to improve on a conservative regimen. Myelography can be combined with tests of dynamics of the cerebrospinal fluid, and a sample of the fluid should always be removed for cytologic and chemical examination prior to the instillation of the contrast medium (Pantopaque, Myodil, or a water-soluble contrast medium). Injection and removal of Pantopaque require special skill and should not be attempted without previous experience with the procedure. If done properly, the procedure has a very low incidence of significant complications. Injection of contrast medium directly into the intervertebral disk (diskograms) has waxed and waned in popularity over the years and remains controversial. The technique of this procedure is more complicated than that of myelographic examination, and the risk of damage to the disk or nerve roots and the possibility of introduction of infection is not inconsiderable.

Computed tomography (CT) and, more recently, magnetic resonance imaging (MRI) have become extremely valuable instruments for the study of the spinal canal, bony segments, and adjacent soft tissues. CT, if combined with instillation of water-soluble contrast media, provides excellent definition of a narrow canal, destructive lesions of the vertebral bodies and posterior elements, or the presence of a paravertebral soft tissue mass, and by appropriate computerized reconstruction techniques can also identify disk herniations, sometimes with greater accuracy than the myelogram. The MRI has in recent years virtually replaced CT for the study of the degenerate disk and its relationship to the adjacent roots. The definition of soft tissue alterations and even edema surrounding the roots is remarkable, especially with sagittal projections. The use of gadolinium to enhance regions of inflammation with MRI provides even better resolution of the defects (see Chap. 348).

Confirmation of proximal motor and sensory nerve and root disease can be obtained by nerve conduction studies, H and F responses, and electromyography (see Chap. 362).

PRINCIPAL CONDITIONS THAT GIVE RISE TO DISABLING PAIN IN THE LOWER PART OF THE BACK

CONGENITAL ANOMALIES OF THE LUMBAR SPINE One of the most common disorders is a failure of fusion of the laminae of the neural arch (spina bifida) of one or several of the lumbar vertebrae or of the sacrum. Hypertrichosis or hyperpigmentation in the sacral area may betray the condition, but in most patients the spine defect remains entirely occult until disclosed by x-ray. The anomaly has greater potentiality for pain if accompanied by malformation of vertebral joints, and usually the pain is induced by injury. Other congenital anomalies that affect the lower lumbar vertebrae, such as asymmetric facetal joints, abnormalities of the transverse processes, sacralization of the fifth lumbar vertebra (in which L5 is firmly fixed to the sacrum), or lumbarization of the first sacral vertebra (in which the first sacral segment resembles a sixth lumbar), are rarely the cause of specific symptomatology.

Spondylolysis consists of a bony defect probably caused by trauma to a congenitally abnormal segment in the pars interarticularis (a segment near the junction of the pedicle with the lamina) of the lower lumbar area. The defect is best visualized on oblique projections or with CT. In some individuals the defect is bilateral. In the circumstance of either a single injury or repeated minor injuries, the vertebral body, pedicles, and superior articular facets slip anteriorly, leaving the posterior elements behind. This latter abnormality, known as *spondylolisthesis*, usually results in symptoms, often proportional to the degree of forward slip. The patient may complain of pain in the low back radiating into the thighs, and a limitation of motion may be noted. Often tenderness is elicited near the segment which has ''slipped'' forward (most often L5 on S1 or occasionally L4 on L5), and one can feel a ''step'' on deep palpation of the posterior elements of the segment above the spondylolisthetic joint. In moderately severe displacements the pelvis is sometimes rotated and hip flexion limited by hamstring spasm. A variety of usually minor neurologic deficits indicative of radiculopathy may be present. In exceptionally severe degrees of spondylolisthesis the trunk may be shortened and the abdomen protuberant, both the result of the extreme forward displacement of L5 on S1.

TRAUMATIC AFFLICTIONS OF THE LOWER PART OF THE BACK Trauma constitutes the most frequent cause of acute low back pain, and such injured patients should be very carefully evaluated. In severe acute injuries which involve fracture or dislocation of the vertebral segments, the examining physician must be careful to avoid further damage. Tests of mobility and forceful manipulations should be avoided until a diagnosis has been made and adequate measures have been instituted for the proper care of the patient. A patient complaining of back pain and inability to move the legs may have a fractured spine. The neck should not be flexed, nor should the patient be allowed to sit up. (See Chap. 361 for further discussion of spinal cord injury.)

Sprains, strains, and derangements The terms lumbosacral *sprain* and *strain* are often used loosely by physicians, and do not clearly relate to a known anatomic lesion. The author prefers the term *low back derangement* or *strain* for minor, self-limited injuries usually associated with lifting a heavy object, a fall, or a sudden deceleration as may occur in an automobile accident. Occasionally, these syndromes are more chronic in nature, suggesting that diskal or arthritic factors may play a role. The patients with low back derangement are often acutely discomfited and may assume unusual postures related to spasm of the sacrospinalis muscles. The pain is usually confined to the lower back and is usually relieved by rest and analgesic medication within a few days. More extensive or longer lasting problems, formerly classified as sacroiliac strain or sprain, are now known to be due in most instances to disk disease (see below).

Vertebral fractures Most fractures of the lumbar vertebral body result from flexion injuries and consist of anterior wedging or compression. With more severe trauma the patient may sustain a fracture dislocation, "bursting" fracture, or asymmetric fracture involving not only the body but the posterior elements. The initiating trauma which causes fractures of the vertebrae is usually a fall from a height (in which case the calcanei may also be fractured), sudden deceleration in an automobile accident, or other major violence. When fractures occur with minimal trauma (or even spontaneously), the bone is presumed to have been previously weakened by some pathologic process. Most of the time, particularly in older individuals, the cause of such an event is senile or postmenopausal osteoporosis (see Chap. 341), but there may be other underlying systemic disorders such as osteomalacia, hyperparathyroidism, hyperthyroidism, multiple myeloma, metastatic carcinoma, and a large number of local conditions that may play a role in weakening the vertebral body. Spasm of the lumbar muscles, limitation of motion of the lumbar segments, and the roentgenographic appearance of the damaged vertebra (with or without neurologic abnormalities) are the basis for the clinical diagnosis. The pain is usually immediate, though occasionally it may be delayed in onset for a few days, and the patient may develop a mild paralytic ileus or urinary retention during the acute period.

Fractures of the transverse processes are almost always associated with severe injury to the paravertebral muscles, principally the psoas. A significant retroperitoneal hemorrhage may be present (identified on CT or MRI) which can result in a marked depression in the hematocrit and, in extensive fractures, hypovolemic shock. Such injuries may be diagnosed by the finding of deep tenderness at the site of the injury, local muscle spasm on one side, and limitation of all movements which stretch the lumbar muscles. Radiologic evidence (especially CT or MRI) provides the final confirmation. Fractures of multiple transverse processes, although seemingly trivial, should be the object of considerable concern, and the patient should be carefully watched for internal hemorrhage.

Protrusion of lumbar intervertebral disks This condition is the major cause of severe chronic or recurrent low back and leg pain. It is most likely to occur between the fifth lumbar and first sacral vertebrae, and, with lessening frequency, between the fourth and fifth lumbar, the third and fourth lumbar, the second and third lumbar, and, rarely, between the first and second lumbar vertebrae. Rare in the thoracic portion of the spine, it is next most frequent between the sixth and seventh and fifth and sixth cervical vertebrae. The cause is usually a flexion injury, but in many cases no trauma is recalled. Degeneration of the posterior longitudinal ligaments and the annulus fibrosus, which occurs in most adults of middle and advanced years, may have taken place silently or have been manifested by mild, recurrent lumbar ache. A sneeze, lurch, or other trivial movement may then cause the nucleus pulposus to prolapse, pushing the frayed and weakened annulus posteriorly. In more severe cases of disk disease, the nucleus may protrude through the annulus or become extruded to lie as a free fragment in the vertebral canal.

The fully developed syndrome of ruptured lumbar intervertebral disk consists of backache, abnormal posture, and limitation of motion of the spine (particularly flexion). Nerve root involvement is indicated by radicular pain, sensory disturbances (paresthesias, hyper- and hyposensitivity in dermatome pattern), coarse twitching and fasciculation, muscle spasms, and impairment of a tendon reflex. Motor abnormalities (weakness and muscle atrophy) may also occur but are usually less prominent than the pain and sensory disorder. Since herniation of the intervertebral lumbar disks most often occurs between the fourth and fifth lumbar vertebrae and the fifth lumbar and first sacral vertebrae with irritation and compression of the fifth lumbar and first sacral roots, respectively, it is important to recognize the clinical characteristics of lesions of these two roots. *Lesions of the fifth lumbar root* produce pain in the region of the hip, groin, posterolateral thigh, lateral calf to the external malleolus, dorsal surface of the foot, and the first or second and third toes. Paresthesias may be in the entire territory or only in the distal parts of these territories. The tenderness is in the lateral gluteal region and near the head of the fibula. Weakness, if present, involves the extensor of the great toe and less often of the foot. The knee and ankle reflexes are seldom altered, although occasionally the ankle jerk is moderately depressed. Walking on the heels may be more difficult, because of weakness of dorsiflexion of the foot, and more uncomfortable than walking on the toes. In *lesions of the first sacral root* the pain is felt in the midgluteal region, posterior part of the thigh, posterior region of the calf to the heel, and the plantar surface of the foot and fourth and fifth toes. Tenderness is most pronounced over the midgluteal region (sacroiliac joint), posterior thigh area, and calf. Rarely it may be referred to the rectum, testicles, or labia. Paresthesias and sensory loss are mainly in the lower leg and outer toes, and weakness, if present, involves the flexor muscles of the foot and toes, abductors of the toes, and hamstring muscles. The ankle reflex is diminished or absent in the majority of cases. Walking on the toes is more difficult, because of weakness of plantar flexors, and more uncomfortable than walking on the heel. With lesions of either root there may be limitation of straight-leg raising during the acute, painful stages.

Degeneration of the intervertebral disk without frank extrusion of a fragment of disk tissue may give rise to low back pain, or the disk may herniate into the adjacent vertebral body, giving rise to a Schmorl's node, usually visualized by x-ray. Such cases often show no signs of nerve root involvement though the back pain may be referred to the thigh and leg.

The rarer *lesions of the fourth and third lumbar roots* give rise to pain in the anterior part of the thigh and knee, with corresponding sensory loss. The knee jerk is diminished or abolished. An inverted Lasègue sign (pain with hyperextension of the limb in relation to the trunk, best elicited with the patient in the prone position) is often positive when the third lumbar root is affected.

The lumbar disk syndromes are usually unilateral. Occasionally with massive derangements of the disk or with the extrusion of a large, free fragment into the canal the symptoms and signs are bilateral. Often one side is affected more than the other and the pain, motor, and sensory changes may be associated with paralysis of the sphincters. The pain of lumbar disk disease is variable and may be mild or severe. There may be back pain with little or no leg pain, and occasionally the patient experiences leg pain with little or no discomfort in the back. Some patients present with evidence of multiple disk ruptures affecting both cervical and lumbar segments, suggesting a diffuse disorder of the connective tissue of the disks, possibly including both the annulus fibrosus and the nucleus pulposus.

When all components of the syndrome are present, the diagnosis is easy; when only one part is present (particularly backache), it may be difficult, especially if there has not been a clearly remembered initiating traumatic event. Since similar symptoms may occur without demonstrable disk rupture, other diagnostic procedures are required. Plain roentgenograms usually show no abnormality or at most a narrowing of the intervertebral space, sometimes more on the side of the rupture. Traction spurs, which are indicative of disk degeneration, may be present; in extreme cases, there may be a "vacuum" disk sign, in which a gas-density shadow is present in the intervertebral space, usually on lateral roentgenogram. CT transverse images with or without contrast sometimes show the herniated disk very clearly, and at times the MRI will demonstrate a remarkably sharp image of cauda equina or nerve root compression by a bulging or extruded disk fragment. Less frequently than in the past do clinicians resort to Pantopaque or soluble contrast myelography (both of which have potential complications) to demonstrate the disk herniation. The myelogram remains the most reliable of the studies, and many surgeons are loathe to consider laminectomy without such a study. Occasionally, the electromyogram is helpful in showing denervation of paravertebral and leg muscles (see Chap. 362).

It should be noted in evaluating patients with herniated disks that epidural or intradural tumors of the spinal canal may produce a syndrome similar to that of ruptured disk. These lesions may present with unremitting pain even with bed rest and predominant sphincter disturbances even early in the course (see Chap. 361).

OTHER CAUSES OF LOW BACK PAIN AND SCIATICA In a sizable number of patients disk rupture types of symptoms occur, but the problem has a different cause. Often these patients have had multiple operations for diskogenic disease with or without arthrodesis of the lumbar vertebrae, but the pain and disability have not remitted. The indications for the original surgery may have been questionable, with only a disk bulge noted on CT, MRI, or myelogram and no definite neurologic signs. To explain these chronic pain states a number of pathologic entities have been introduced, some of uncertain status. Entrapment of one or more nerve roots may be the consequence not only of a disk rupture but also as a result of spondylotic spurs with variable stenosis of the lateral recess and intervertebral canal, hypertrophy of apophyseal facets, or a more nebulous cause.

The syndrome that is caused by spondylotic spurs and stenosis of the lateral recess and intervertebral foramen has not been clearly distinguished from that of ruptured disk. Known variously as vertebral stenosis, lumbar claudication, degenerative spinal stenosis, and narrow canal, the cause appears to be related principally to an encroachment on roots of the cauda equina by bony excrescences usually attributed to osteoarthritis but possibly related to spondylolisthesis, old trauma, Paget's disease, or a congenital abnormality of the shape or size of the canal. Many of these patients are elderly, and the pattern must be clearly distinguished from peripheral vascular claudication. The pain, often bilateral along the sciatic distribution, becomes increasingly severe with standing and walking and is relieved by a short period of rest. Although some of the patients have no physical findings, motor, reflex, and sensory changes may be present.

The *facet syndrome* is closely related to the above but tends to be unilateral. Reynolds et al. have reported 22 cases in which a lumbar monoradiculopathy had simulated a ruptured disk: 16 had an L5 radiculopathy, 3 an S1 radiculopathy, and 3 an L4 radiculopathy. Coexisting back pain was present in 15 of the cases. No disk rupture was found by myelography. At operation the spinal root was compressed against the floor or roof of the intervertebral canal by an enlarged superior or inferior facet. Foraminotomy and facetectomy relieved the symptoms in 12 of the 15 operated cases.

Lumbar adhesive arachnoiditis with radiculopathy has waxed and waned over the years as an entity employed to explain low back pain persisting after treatment. Most often it is considered in patients who have had multiple lumbar operations and myelograms and are left with backache and leg pain in combination with mild to moderate motor, sensory, and reflex changes. On surgical exploration, the arachnoidal membrane is thickened and opaque, adherent to dura, and tightly bound to pia and roots. The contrast medium during myelography does not fill the root sheaths and tends to be irregularly loculated. Disk rupture, multiple Pantopaque myelograms, operative procedures, infection, and subarachnoid hemorrhage, in various combinations, are factors that favor its development. Treatment is unsatisfactory; lysis of adhesions and intrathecal steroid therapy have been of only limited value.

In patients with persistent chronic low back pain and sciatica after failed disk surgery or due to spondylitic spurs, spondylolysis, facetal joint degeneration, or arachnoiditis, some surgeons have attributed the disability in part, at least, to "instability" of the lumbar segments, and the perpetuation of the pain to excessive or abnormal movements of the lumbar vertebral segments. For such patients spinal fusion is occasionally advocated and can in certain circumstances provide a measure of relief. A posterior arthrodesis of the fourth and fifth lumbar segments to the sacrum may reduce motion at these parts and decrease pressure on the nerve roots associated with abnormal movements. More often than not, however, the patient continues to have pain (although often reduced in degree), and the procedure should not be regarded as a panacea. The author rarely advocates such an operative intervention, unless clear anatomic evidence exists for a mechanical problem that could be alleviated by stabilization of the spine.

ARTHRITIS Arthritis of the spine is a major cause of backache, cervical pain, and occipital headache.

Osteoarthritis (See also Chap. 281) This more frequent type of osteoarthritic spinal disease occurs usually in later life and may involve any part of the spine. It is most prevalent in the cervical and lumbar regions, however, and the exact location determines the localization of the symptoms. Patients often complain of pain centered in the spine that is increased by motion and is almost invariably associated with complaints of stiffness and limitation of motion. There is a notable absence of systemic symptoms such as fatigue, malaise, and fever, and the pain usually can be relieved by rest. The severity of the symptoms often bears little relation to the radiologic findings; pain may be present when there are minimal findings on an x-ray, and, conversely, marked osteophytic overgrowth with spur formation, ridging, and bridging of vertebrae can be seen in asymptomatic patients in middle and later life. Osteoarthropathic changes in the cervical spine and to a lesser extent in the lumbar spine may by their location compress roots or even the cauda equina or spinal cord, giving rise to the spondylitic form of radiculopathy or myelopathy (see Chap. 361).

Rheumatoid arthritis and ankylosing spondylitis (See also Chaps. 270 and 274) Arthritic disease of the spine takes two distinct forms, ankylosing spondylitis (the more common) and rheumatoid arthritis.

Patients with *ankylosing spondylitis* (also called Marie-Strümpell arthritis) are usually young men who complain of mild to moderate pain which early in the course of the disease is centered in the back and on occasion radiates to the back of the thighs. The symptoms may be vague at first and the diagnosis may be overlooked for a considerable period. Although the pain is often intermittent, the finding of limitation of movement is constant and progressive and over a period of time tends to dominate the picture. Early in the course, this finding is described as "morning stiffness" or increasing stiffness after periods of inactivity, and may be present long before radiologic changes are manifest. Limitation of chest expansion, tenderness over the sternum, and decreased motion and flexion contractures of the hips may also be present early in the course. The radiologic hallmarks of the disease are periarticular destructive changes and subsequent obliteration of the sacroiliac joints, development of syndesmophytes on the margins of the vertebral bodies, followed by bridging by bone to produce the characteristic "bamboo spine." The entire spine becomes immobilized, often in a flexed position, and usually the pain then subsides. Patterns of restricted movement, indistinguishable from those of ankylosing spondylitis, may accompany Reiter's syndrome, psoriatic arthritis, and chronic inflammatory bowel diseases. Patients with these disorders rarely show the joint manifestations of peripheral rheumatoid arthritis, and seldom do they display involvement of the hips or knees. The rheumatoid factor is usually absent, but the sedimentation rate is often rapid, and many of the patients are found to have an HLA-B27 antigen.

Occasionally ankylosing spondylitis is complicated by progressively destructive vertebral lesions. This complication should be suspected whenever the pain returns, after a period of quiescence, or becomes localized. The etiology of these lesions is not known, but they may represent an exaggerated healing response to fracture or excessive production of fibrous inflammatory tissues. Rarely they may result in collapse of a segment of the spine and compression of the spinal cord. Another complication of severe ankylosing spondylitis is bilateral ankylosis of the ribs to the spine, which, coupled with a decrease in the height of axial thoracic structures, causes marked impairment of respiratory function.

Spinal rheumatoid arthritis tends to be localized to the cervical apophyseal joints and atlantoaxial articulation; the pain, stiffness, and limitation of motion are then in the neck and back of the head. Unlike ankylosing spondylitis, rheumatoid arthritis is rarely confined to the spine, and it does not lead to significant degrees of intervertebral bridging. Because of major affection of other joints, the diagnosis is relatively easy to make, but significant involvement of the neck may be overlooked. In the advanced stages of the disease, one or several of the vertebrae may be displaced anteriorly, or a synovitis of the atlantoaxial joint may damage the transverse ligament of the atlas, resulting in forward displacement of the atlas on the axis, i.e., atlantoaxial subluxation. In either instance, serious and even life-threatening compression of the spinal cord may occur gradually or suddenly (see Chaps. 270 and 361). Lateral roentgenograms in flexion and extension, performed cautiously, are sometimes necessary to visualize dislocation or subluxation.

OTHER DESTRUCTIVE DISEASES **Neoplastic, infectious, and metabolic diseases** Metastatic carcinoma (breast, lung, prostate, thyroid, kidney, gastrointestinal tract), multiple myeloma, and non-Hodgkin's and Hodgkin's lymphomas are the malignant tumors which most frequently involve the spine. Since the primary site may be overlooked or asymptomatic, the presenting complaint in such patients may be pain in the back. The pain tends to be constant and dull, and is often unrelieved by rest. Indeed, it may be worse at night. Radiographic changes may be absent early in the disease, but when they appear, usually are manifest as destructive lesions in one or several vertebral bodies with little or limited involvement of the disk space, even in the face of a compression fracture. A ^{99m}Tc diphosphonate bone scan is helpful in demonstrating "hot spots," indicating areas of increased blood flow and reactive bone formation associated with destructive, inflammatory, or arthritic lesions. It should be noted, however, that myeloma and sometimes metastatic thyroid carcinoma may fail to show increased activity on a bone scan.

Infection of the vertebral column is usually the result of pyogenic organisms (staphylococci or coliform bacilli) or, less commonly today, the tubercle bacilli. Patients complain of pain in the back of subacute or chronic nature that is exacerbated by motion but not materially relieved by rest. There is limitation of motion, tenderness over the spine of the involved segments, and pain with jarring of the spine, such as occurs with walking on the heels. Usually, these patients are afebrile and often do not have a leukocytosis although the erythrocyte sedimentation rate is almost invariably elevated. Radiographs may demonstrate narrowing of a disk space with erosion and destruction of the two adjacent vertebrae. A paravertebral soft tissue mass evident on contrast CT or MRI may be present, indicating an abscess, which may in the case of tuberculosis drain spontaneously at sites quite remote from the vertebral column. In addition to a bone scan, a gallium scan is sometimes helpful in identifying a soft tissue inflammatory or infectious lesion even when overt bone destruction is not visible in x-rays.

Special mention should be made of the spinal *epidural abscess* (usually staphylococcal), which necessitates urgent surgical treatment. The symptoms are a localized pain, occurring spontaneously, aggravated by percussion and palpation. The patient is febrile and usually has severe radicular complaints, often bilateral, progressing rapidly to a flaccid paraplegia (see Chap. 348). Chronic drug abusers are particularly prone to this problem. Patients with AIDS have also been noted to have increased incidence of epidural abscess and of pyogenic and granulomatous osteomyelitis.

In metabolic bone diseases (hyperparathyroidism, osteoporosis, or osteomalacia) a considerable degree of loss of bone substance may occur without any symptoms whatsoever. Many patients with such conditions do, however, complain of aching in the lumbar or thoracic area. This is most likely to occur following an injury, sometimes trivial in nature, which leads to collapse or wedging of a vertebra. Certain movements greatly enhance the pain, while certain positions relieve it. One or more spinal roots may be involved. Paget's disease of the spine is readily identifiable on x-ray and is often painless. The disease may, however, lead to compression of the spinal cord or roots because of encroachment on the canal or foramina by the pagetoid bone. The recognition of these bone disorders is discussed in some detail elsewhere (Chaps. 341 and 344).

In general, patients thought to have neoplastic, infectious, or metabolic disease of the spine should be thoroughly evaluated by means of radiographs, bone scans, CT or MRI scans, and appropriate laboratory studies (see above).

REFERRED PAIN FROM VISCERAL DISEASE The pain of disease of the pelvic, abdominal, or thoracic viscera is often felt in the region of the spine; i.e., it is referred to the posterior parts of the spinal segment that innervates the diseased organ. Occasionally back pain may be the first and only sign. The general rule is that pelvic diseases are referred to the sacral region, lower abdominal diseases to the lumbar region (centering around the second to fourth lumbar vertebrae), and upper abdominal diseases to the lower thoracic spine (eighth thoracic to the first and second lumbar vertebrae). Characteristically local signs or stiffness of the back are not elicited, and motion may be of full range without augmentation of the pain. However, some positions, e.g., flexion of the lumbar area of the spine in the lateral recumbent position, may be more comfortable than others.

Low thoracic and upper lumbar pain in abdominal disease Peptic ulceration or tumor of the wall of the stomach and of the duodenum most typically induces pain in the epigastrium (see Chaps. 238 and 261); but if the posterior wall is involved, and particularly if there is retroperitoneal extension, the pain may be felt in the region of the spine. The pain may be central in location or more intense on one side, or it may be felt in both locations. If very intense, it may seem to encircle the body. It tends to retain the characteristics of pain from the affected organ; e.g., if due to peptic ulceration, it appears about 2 h after a meal and is relieved by food and antacids.

Diseases of the pancreas (peptic ulceration with extension to the pancreas, cholecystitis with pancreatitis, cyst, or tumor) are apt to cause pain in the back, being more to the right of the spine if the head of the pancreas is involved and to the left if the body and tail are implicated.

Diseases of retroperitoneal structures, e.g., lymphomas, sarcomas, and carcinomas, may evoke pain in the adjacent part of the spine with some tendency toward radiation to the lower part of the abdomen, groin, and anterior thighs. A secondary tumor of the iliopsoas region on one side often produces a unilateral lumbar ache with radiation toward the groin, labia, or testicle; there may also be signs of involvement of the upper lumbar spinal roots. An aneurysm of the abdominal aorta may induce pain which is localized to this region of the spine but may be felt higher or lower, depending on the location of the lesion.

The sudden appearance of obscure lumbar pain in a patient receiving anticoagulants should arouse the suspicion of retroperitoneal bleeding.

Lumbar pain with lower abdominal diseases Inflammatory diseases of segments of the colon (colitis, diverticulitis) or tumor of the colon cause pain which may be felt in the lower part of the abdomen between the umbilicus and pubis, in the midlumbar region, or in both places. If very intense, the pain may have a beltlike distribution around the body. A lesion in the transverse colon or first part of the descending colon may be central or left-sided, and its level of reference to the back is to the second to third lumbar vertebrae. If the sigmoid colon is implicated, the pain is lower, in the upper sacral region and anteriorly in the midline suprapubic region or left lower quadrant of the abdomen.

Sacral pain in pelvic (urologic and gynecologic) diseases The pelvis is seldom the site of a disease which causes obscure low back pain although gynecologic disorders may manifest themselves in this manner. Of painful pelvic lesions less than a third are due to inflammatory disease; other more hypothetical entities, such as relaxation of uterine supporting structures, retroversion of uterus, pelvic varicosities, and adnexal edema, have been largely discredited. Recently, CT, MRI, or diagnostic laparoscopy has been recommended as a valuable supplement to rectal and pelvic examinations, sigmoidoscopy, and intravenous pyelography for patients with obscure pelvic pain. The importance of psychiatric illness in the majority of undiagnosed cases has been stressed.

Menstrual pain itself may be felt in the sacral region. It is rather poorly localized, tends to radiate down the legs, and is often described as cramplike. The most important source of chronic back pain from the pelvic organs, however, is thought to be the uterosacral ligaments. Endometriosis or carcinoma of the uterus (body or cervix) may invade these structures, while malposition of the uterus may cause traction on them. The pain is localized centrally in the sacrum below the lumbosacral joint but may be more on one side than the other. In endometriosis the pain begins during the premenstrual phase and often continues until it merges with menstrual pain. Malposition of the uterus (retroversion, descensus, and prolapse) is thought by some to lead to sacral pain, especially after the patient has been standing for several hours. One may observe the effect of postural influences here as when a fibroma of the uterus pulls on the uterosacral ligaments. Carcinomatous pain due to involvement of nerve plexuses is continuous and becomes progressively more severe; it tends to be more intense at night. The primary lesion may be inconspicuous, being overlooked upon pelvic examination. Papanicolaou smears, pyelogram, and CT scan are the most useful diagnostic procedures. X-ray therapy of these tumors may produce sacral pain consequent to necrosis of tissue and injury to nerve roots. Low back pain with radiation into one or both thighs is a common phenomenon during the last weeks of pregnancy.

Chronic prostatitis, evidenced by prostatic discharge, burning and frequency of urination, and sometimes a reduction in sexual potency, may be attended by a nagging sacral ache; it may be mainly on one side, with radiation into one leg if the seminal vesicle is involved on that side. Carcinoma of the prostate with metastases to the lower part of the spine is another more common cause of sacral or lumbar pain. It may be present without urinary frequency or burning. Spinal nerves may be infiltrated by tumor cells, or the spinal cord itself may be compressed if the epidural space is invaded. The diagnosis is established by rectal examination, imaging studies and bone scans of the spine, and measurement of acid phosphatase (particularly the prostatic phosphatase fraction). Lesions of the bladder and testes are usually not accompanied by back pain. When the kidney is the site of disease, the pain is ipsilateral, being felt in the flank or lumbar region.

Visceral derangements of whatever type may intensify the pain of arthritis, and the presence of arthritis may alter the distribution of visceral pain. With disease of the spine in the lumbosacral region, for example, distention of the ampulla of the sigmoid by feces or a bout of colitis may aggravate the arthritic pain. In patients with arthritis of the cervical or thoracic spine the pain of myocardial ischemia may radiate to the back.

OBSCURE TYPES OF LOW BACK PAIN AND THE QUESTION OF PSYCHIATRIC DISEASE The practitioner is frequently consulted by persons who complain of low back pain of obscure origin. Usually the disorder is benign in nature and results from some minor derangement, muscular strain, or diskal prolapse. This is particularly true for those lesions which are of acute onset, aggravated by motion, and relieved by rest. Considerably more difficult are patients with chronic pain, especially those who have had prior back surgery or chronic visceral disease, or those who have severe and progressive pain in which neoplasia or infection is considered.

Even when exhaustive studies have been performed, there remains a group of patients in whom no anatomic or pathologic lesion can be found. These patients generally fall into two categories: those with what might be termed "postural back pain" and those with psychiatric illness.

"Postural" back pain Some slender asthenic young individuals complain of a vague pain in the back, diffuse in nature and most frequently noted with prolonged sitting or standing. Similarly, some obese middle-aged patients describe a discomfort in the back, either thoracic or lumbar in location. The physical examination in these patients is negative except for slack musculature and what may be best termed "poor posture." Imaging studies and laboratory evaluation usually show no abnormalities, and characteristically the pain is relieved by bed rest. Exercises to strengthen the paraspinal and abdominal muscles are sometimes therapeutic.

Psychiatric illness Low back pain may be encountered in compensation hysteria and malingering, in chronic anxiety states or depression, and in many individuals whose symptoms and complaints do not fall within any category of psychiatric illness. It is important to be certain that pain in the back in such patients does not signify disease of the spine and adjacent structures, and all such patients should be carefully studied. However, even when organic factors are found, the pain may be exaggerated, prolonged, or woven into a pattern of invalidism or disability because of coexistent psychological factors. This is especially true when there is the possibility of secondary gain (notably compensation for a work-related injury) (see Chap. 15).

PAIN IN THE NECK AND SHOULDER

It is useful to distinguish three major categories of painful disease—of the spine, brachial plexus (thoracic outlet), and shoulder. Although pain in these three regions of the body may overlap, the patient can usually indicate the site of origin.

Cervical spine Pain arising from the cervical spine is felt in the neck and back of the head (though it may often be projected to the shoulder, arm, and even forearm and hand), is evoked or enhanced by certain movements or positions of the neck, and is accompanied by tenderness and limitation of motions of the neck.

Osteoarthritis of the cervical spine may cause pains which radiate into the back of the head, shoulders, and arms on one or both sides of the thorax. Coincident involvement of nerve roots is manifested by paresthesias, sensory loss, weakness, or deep tendon reflex change. Should bony ridges form in the spinal canal (spondylosis) the spinal cord may be compressed (see Chap. 361). A myelogram, CT, or MRI may reveal the degree of encroachment on the spinal canal (narrowing of the canal to less than 11 mm in the anteroposterior diameter) at the level at which the spinal cord is affected. Difficulty may be experienced in distinguishing the syndrome associated with spondylosis with or without disk rupture and spinal cord compression from primary neurologic diseases (syringomyelia, amyotrophic lateral sclerosis, or tumor) with an unrelated osteoarthritis of the cervical portion of the spine, particularly at the fifth to sixth and sixth to seventh cervical vertebrae, where the disk spaces are often narrowed in the adult. The newer imaging studies such as CT or MRI are helpful in this regard. A painful injury to ligaments and muscles after an accident in which the neck is forcibly extended and flexed (e.g., "whiplash" injury to spine) may be a difficult diagnostic problem, particularly if the patient has some ostensible spurring and especially if in the course of the injury a cerebral concussion has occurred. If the pain is persistent and limited to the neck, imaging studies will sometimes prove that the problem is due to disruption of a disk, but it is often complicated by psychological factors.

Thoracic outlet Pain resulting from abnormalities of the thoracic outlet is experienced in and around the shoulder in the supraclavicular region, or between the shoulders; is induced by the performance of certain tasks and by certain positions; and is associated with tenderness of structures above the clavicle. There may be a palpable abnormality above the clavicle (aneurysms of the subclavian artery, tumor, cervical rib). The combination of circulatory symptoms and signs referable to the lower part of the brachial plexus, manifested in the hand by obliteration of pulse when the patient holds a full breath with the head tilted back or turned (Adson's test), unilateral Raynaud's phenomenon, trophic changes in the fingers, and sensory loss over the ulnar side of the hand with or without interosseous atrophy complete the clinical picture. Roentgenograms and other imaging studies showing a cervical rib, deformed thoracic outlet, or superior sulcus tumor of the lung (Pancoast's syndrome) corroborate disease in this location. Electromyography and conduction studies along the plexus from points stimulated above and below the clavicle, and studies of arterial and venous circulation (venograms, noninvasive Doppler techniques) are especially helpful in evaluating this problem.

Shoulder Pain localized to the shoulder region is often worse at night and may be associated with local tenderness over the shoulder. The pain is characteristically aggravated by abduction, internal rotation, and extension. Most often shoulder lesions are in the form of a tendonitis or bursitis (sometimes calcific) usually affecting the supraspinatus tendon, the adjacent subdeltoid bursa, or the biceps tendon; occasionally the lesion is more extensive and consists of a rupture of the rotator cuff, in which case the patient may have weakness on abduction and forward flexion. In some such patients there is an adhesive capsulitis, leading to profound limitation of motion, designated as a "frozen shoulder." Partial cuff tears, impingement of the cuff under the acromion, and slight subluxations produce a variety of symptoms about the shoulder particularly with exercise or maintaining the arm in abduction for long periods of time. The pain of shoulder disease may at times radiate into the arm or hand, but the sensory, motor, and reflex changes which indicate disease of nerve roots, plexus, or peripheral nerves are absent.

RUPTURED CERVICAL DISKS One of the commonest causes of neck, shoulder, and arm pain is disk herniation in the lower cervical region. As with rupture of the lumbar disks, the complete syndrome includes the disorder of spinal function and evidence of neural involvement. It may develop after trauma either major or minor (sudden hyperextension of the neck, diving injuries, forceful manipulations, etc.). Virtually every patient exhibits a diminution in range of motion of the neck (often accompanied by intensification of pain). Hyperextension is the movement that most consistently aggravates the pain, although one occasionally sees patients whose principal limitation is in flexion. Rotation and lateral movements are often moderately restricted by pain. With laterally situated disk lesions between the fifth and sixth cervical vertebrae, the symptoms and signs are referred to the sixth cervical roots. The full syndrome is characterized by pain felt at the trapezius ridge, tip of the shoulder, anterior upper part of the arm, radial forearm, and often in the thumb; paresthesias and sensory impairment or hypersensitivity in the same regions; tenderness in the area above the spine of the scapula and in the supraclavicular and biceps regions; weakness in flexion of the forearm; and diminished to absent biceps and supinator reflexes (triceps retained or exaggerated). When the protruded disk lies between the sixth and seventh cervical vertebrae, the seventh cervical root is involved. Under these circumstances, in the patient with the complete syndrome, the pain is in the region of the shoulder blade, pectoral region and medial axilla, posterolateral upper arm, elbow and dorsal forearm, index and middle fingers, or all the fingers; tenderness is most pronounced over the medial aspect of the shoulder blade opposite the third to fourth thoracic spinous processes, in the supraclavicular area and triceps region; paresthesias and sensory loss are most pronounced in the second and third fingers or tips of all the fingers; weakness is seen in extension of the forearm, in the extension of the wrist, and in the hand grip; the triceps reflex is diminished to absent, and the biceps and supinator reflexes are preserved. Either of these syndromes may be incomplete in that only one of several of the typical findings (e.g., pain) is present. Usually the patient states that cough, sneeze, and downward pressure on the head in the hyperextension position exacerbate pain and that traction (even manual) tends to relieve it.

Unlike lumbar disks, the cervical ones, if large and centrally situated, may result in compression of the spinal cord (central disk, all the cord; paracentral disk, part of the cord). The central disk is often nearly painless, and the cord syndrome may simulate a degenerative disease (amyotrophic lateral sclerosis, combined system disease). A common error is to fail to think of a ruptured disk in the cervical region in patients with obscure symptoms in the legs. The diagnosis of ruptured cervical disk should be confirmed by the same laboratory procedures that were mentioned under "Spondylosis," above.

OTHER CONDITIONS Metastases to the cervical spine are fortunately less common than to other parts of the vertebral column. They are frequently painful and the cause of disordered root function. Compression fractures or extension of the tumor posteriorly may lead to rapid development of quadriplegia.

Shoulder injuries (rotator cuff), subacromial or subdeltoid bursitis, the frozen shoulder (periarthritis or capsulitis), tendonitis, and arthritis may develop in patients who are otherwise well, but these conditions are also frequent in hemiplegics or in individuals suffering from coronary heart disease. The pain is often severe and extends toward the neck and down the arm into the hand. The dorsum of the latter may tingle without other signs of nerve involvement. Vasomotor and arthropathic changes also may occur in the hand (shoulder-hand syndrome, reflex dystrophy), and after a time, osteoporosis and atrophy of cutaneous and subcutaneous structures occur (Sudeck's atrophy or Sudeck-Leriche syndrome). These conditions fall more within the province of orthopaedics than of medicine and are not discussed here in detail. The physician, however, must know that they can often be prevented by proper exercises.

The *carpal tunnel syndrome,* with paresthesias and numbness in palmar distribution of the median nerve and aching pain which extends up into the forearm, may be mistaken for disease of the shoulder or neck. Similarly, other less common forms of nerve entrapment may involve the ulnar, radial, or median nerves and lead to a mistaken diagnosis of brachial plexus lesion or cervical syndrome. Electromyography and conduction studies are especially helpful in such conditions (Chap. 362).

MANAGEMENT OF BACK AND NECK PAIN

Without doubt the preventive aspects of back pain are important. There would be far fewer back problems if adults kept their trunk muscles in optimal condition by regular exercise such as swimming, bicycle riding, walking briskly, running, or calisthenic programs. A weight reduction diet and a regular exercise program to strengthen abdominal and paraspinal muscles is frequently very beneficial for patients with chronic low back discomfort. Morning is the ideal time since the back of the older adult tends to stiffen during the night because of inactivity. This happens regardless of whether a bed board or a stiff mattress is used. Sleeping with back hyperextended and sitting for long times in an overstuffed chair or a badly designed auto seat commonly cause difficulties for the patient with low back problems. It is estimated that pressures between disks are increased 200 percent by changing from a recumbent to a standing position and by 400 percent by sitting slumped in an easy chair. Correct sitting posture lessens this. Long trips in a car or plane without change in position put maximal strain on disk and ligamentous structures in the spine. Lifting from a position of flexed trunk, as in removing a suitcase from the trunk of a car, is dangerous (always lift with the object close to the body). Sudden strenuous activity without conditioning and warm-up also is likely to cause trouble to disks and their ligamentous envelopes (the commonest sources of back pain).

Muscular and ligamentous strains and minor disk prolapses are usually self-limited, responding to simple measures in a relatively short period of time. The basic principle of therapy is rest in a recumbent position for several days to weeks. When weight bearing is resumed, a light lumbosacral support is occasionally helpful in continuing the immobilization until the patient is restored to full health. Physical measures such as heat, cold, diathermy, or massage are of limited value; of considerably greater importance are active exercises to both reduce the spasm and improve muscle tone. Analgesic medication should be given liberally during the first few days: codeine, 30 mg, and aspirin, 0.6 g, or pentazocine, 50 mg, propoxyphene, 65 mg, or meperidine, 50 mg. Muscle relaxants are often a valuable adjunct, particularly in that such drugs as diazepam, 8 to 40 mg in divided doses, may make bed rest more tolerable. If an inflammatory component is suspected, indomethacin, 75 mg per day (in divided doses), ibuprofen, 600 mg three or four times daily, or naproxen, 375 to 500 mg once or twice daily, may be helpful.

In the treatment of a clearly diagnosed acute or chronic rupture of a lumbar or cervical disk, complete bed rest is essential, at least initially, and analgesic medication may be required. Traction is of little value in lumbar disk disease, and it is best to permit the patient to find the most comfortable position. Cervical traction with a halter may be of considerable benefit to patients with cervical disk syndrome. It can be administered with the patient in recumbency, or after sufficient improvement to allow ambulation, can be performed intermittently in the erect, slightly forward flexed position using special equipment. During the recumbent phase of treatment of lumbar disk disease, exercises to reduce spasm, muscle relaxants, and anti-inflammatory agents as described above may be of considerable value. After 2 to 3 weeks in bed, the patient can be allowed to slowly resume activities, usually with the protection of a brace or light spinal support. Exercise programs designed to increase the strength of the abdominal and paraspinal muscles are helpful at this point. The patient may suffer some minor recurrence of the pain but be able to carry on his or her usual activities, and eventually most individuals will recover. If the pain and neurologic findings do not disappear on prolonged, conservative management, or if the patient suffers frequently recurring acute episodes, surgical management may be indicated. This should always be preceded by a CT, MRI, or myelogram to localize the lesion (and rule out the presence of intra- or extradural tumors). The surgical procedure most often indicated is a hemilaminectomy with excision of the disk involved. Arthrodesis of the involved segments is indicated only in cases in which there is extraordinary instability usually related to an anatomic abnormality (such as spondylolysis) or in the cervical region when an extensive laminectomy has rendered the spine unstable. The result of conservative management of patients with diskal disease and sciatica is that approximately 80 percent improve at the end of 4 weeks regardless of whether traction, exercises, manipulation, or corset, or some combination thereof, is used. Therefore, only a small number of patients should be considered to require surgery.

Spondylosis of the cervical spine, if painful, is helped by bed rest and traction; if signs of spinal cord involvement are present, a collar to limit movement may lead to improvement. Decompressive laminectomy or anterior fusion is reserved for severe instances of the disease with advancing neurologic symptoms. The shoulder-hand syndrome may benefit from stellate ganglion blocks or ganglionectomy, but the basic treatment is physiotherapy, with or without medication, and surgical procedures are used only as measures of last resort.

The management of patients with thoracic outlet syndrome is complex and requires first a careful study to be certain that the cause of the lesion is really a mechanical encroachment of the brachial plexus in the interspace between the clavicle and first rib. Exercises to reduce the tension in this region are mainly designed to strengthen the clavicular musculature and improve posture, thus opening the outlet. Many patients benefit from change of work circumstances, and for women with pendulous breasts, a better designed brassiere is sometimes helpful. Nonsteroidal anti-inflammatory agents are sometimes beneficial, as are muscle relaxants such as diazepam. In the event that the patient's difficulties are intractable or the root compression causes neurologic deficits, exploration of the anterior scalene triangle with resection of the first rib is advocated with usually excellent results.

REFERENCES

Bell GR, Parkman RH: The conservative treatment of sciatica. Spine 9:54, 1984

Bogduk N: The innervation of the lumbar spine. Spine 8:286, 1983

Brady LP et al: An evaluation of the electromyogram in the diagnosis of lumbar disk lesion. J Bone Joint Surg 51A:539, 1969

Buchanan JR et al: A comparison of the risk of vertebral fracture in menopausal osteopenia and other metabolic disturbances. J Bone Joint Surg 70:704, 1988

Bundschuh CV et al: Epidural fibrosis and recurrent disk herniation in the lumbar spine: MR imaging assessment. AJR 150:923, 1988

Collier B: Treatment for lumbar sciatic pain in posterior articular lumbar joint syndrome. Anesthesia 34:202, 1979

Deyo RA, Diehl AK: Measuring physical and psychosocial function in patients with low back pain. Spine 8:635, 1983

Friedenberg AB, Miller WT: Degenerative disk disease of the cervical spine. J Bone Joint Surg 45A:1171, 1963

Frymoyer JW: Back pain and sciatica. N Engl J Med 318:291, 1988

Grabias SL: The treatment of spinal stenosis. J Bone Joint Surg 62A:308, 1988

———, Mankin HJ: Pain in lower back. Bull Rheum Dis 30:1040, 1980

Masaryk TJ et al: High-resolution MR imaging of sequestered lumbar intervertebral disks. AJR 150:1155, 1988

Mikhael MH et al: Neurologic evaluation of lateral recess syndrome. Radiology 140:97, 1981

Modic MT et al: Imaging of degenerative disk disease. Radiology 168:177, 1988

Murphy RW: Nerve roots and spinal nerves in degenerative disk disease. Clin Orthop 129:46, 1977

Naylor A: The changes in the human intervertebral disk in degeneration and nuclear prolapse. Orthop Clin North Am 2:343, 1971

Pleatman CW, Lukin RR: Lumbar spinal stenosis. Semin Roentgenol 23:106, 1988

Raskin SP: Computerized tomographic findings in lumbar disk disease. Orthopedics 5:419, 1981

Reynolds AV et al: Lumbar monoradiculopathy due to unilateral facet hypertrophy. Neurosurgery 10:480, 1982

Rothman RC, Simeone F: *Lumbar Disc Disease*. Philadelphia, Saunders, 1975, pp 443–458

Williams AL et al: Computed tomography in the diagnosis of herniated nucleus pulposus. Radiology 135:95, 1980

Wilson ES, Brill RF: Spinal stenosis: The narrow lumbar canal syndrome. Clin Orthop 122:244, 1977

section 2 Alterations in body temperature

20 CHILLS AND FEVER

RICHARD K. ROOT / ROBERT G. PETERSDORF

Body temperature is normally regulated between 35.8 and 37.2°C (96.5 and 99°F) in healthy persons, with a diurnal variation (see Chap. 377). When heat production exceeds the capacity of heat loss, as during vigorous exercise, the core body temperature may exceed 39°C (103.2°F) for variable time periods until heat is dissipated by sweating, hyperventilation, and cutaneous vasodilation. These transient physiologic elevations in core temperature must be distinguished from sustained elevations found in a number of disease states and termed *fever*. At the onset of fever an abrupt increase in core temperature can occur by means of violent muscle contractions (*rigors*) coupled with cutaneous vasoconstriction and piloerection ("goose flesh"), a symptom complex defined as chills.

PATHOGENESIS OF FEVER Pyrogens Fever may be produced by many stimuli including bacteria and their endotoxins, viruses, yeasts, spirochetes, protozoa, immune reactions, progestational hormones, and drugs and synthetic polynucleotides. These substances, which have been termed collectively *exogenous pyrogens*, are both diverse and complex. Substantial evidence supports a key intermediary role in fever production for cytokines, termed *endogenous pyrogens*, which are produced by cells interacting with exogenous pyrogens. These endogenous pyrogens act centrally on thermosensitive neurons in the preoptic hypothalamus to trigger increased heat production and to decrease heat loss. The core body temperature rises until a higher stable point is reached. The temperature of the blood bathing the hypothalamus is equivalent to the new "set point," and the patient is usually flushed and warm. Defervescence occurs through activation of heat loss mechanisms, in particular sweating, until the core body temperature reaches its baseline and a new equilibrium is established. Hyperthermia from other causes is not accompanied by a resetting of the central thermostat.

The major endogenous pyrogens identified in experimental animals and humans are interleukin 1α and 1β (IL-1), and cachectin, also known as tumor necrosis factor-α (TNF). Similar in size (17-kDa glycoproteins), many actions, and highly conserved in nature, the IL-1 and TNF molecules are structurally discrete. IL-1β is the predominant species in humans (see Chap. 13). Recently, the interferons α, β, and γ (IFN-α, -β, -γ) have been shown to have pyrogenic action, although the mechanisms remain to be defined. Monocytes, macrophages, and macrophage-derived cells are major sources of IL-1 and TNF. Endothelial cells, keratinocytes, and brain astrocytes can also produce IL-1. During phagocytosis or stimulation by bacterial endotoxins, up to 5 percent of the total protein produced by macrophages consists of IL-1 and TNF. Administration of endotoxin to humans is followed by the appearance of fever and free TNF in the plasma; during severe bacterial sepsis both IL-1 and TNF may be found.

A positive feedback mechanism for IL-1 production by macrophages and endothelial cells has been demonstrated, triggered by both IL-1 and TNF. Activation of macrophages by IFN-γ can augment IL-1 and TNF production in response to other stimuli. Production of both IL-1 and TNF involves the synthesis of new specific mRNA as well as the IL-1 and TNF molecules themselves, which are then secreted by the stimulated cells. Glucocorticoids can block both the elaboration of specific mRNA and its eventual translation into synthesis of IL-1 and TNF; release of preformed IL-1 or TNF is not affected. Prostaglandins of the E series also exert an inhibitory effect on IL-1 and TNF production. Both glucocorticoids and prostaglandin E_2 (PGE_2) appear to be important regulatory molecules for IL-1 and TNF production and action. In addition other negative regulatory molecules for IL-1 have been described, and IL-1 may downregulate its own receptors on target cells.

Once released from stimulated cells TNF and IL-1 can have actions on target cells in the immediate locale or in distal sites to which they are transported in the plasma. IL-1 that remains bound to the plasma membranes of stimulated cells also has potent biologic activity. The ability of target cells to respond to their actions is a function of specific receptors for IL-1 and TNF. Despite similarities in molecular weight, production, and in a wide variety of actions the cellular receptors for IL-1 and TNF differ, suggesting that they trigger common intracellular pathways in responding cells and tissues.

In support of this thesis, multiple actions of both compounds are mediated through the induction of arachidonate metabolism. Within the hypothalamus, IL-1 and TNF act by promoting the synthesis of prostaglandins of the E series using arachidonate released from target cell membranes. PGE_2 activates heat generating and conserving mechanisms; synthesis of cyclic adenyl monophosphate (AMP) is involved. The precise molecular mechanisms linking PGE_2 and cyclic AMP actions to "resetting" the central thermostat remain to be elucidated as do the central actions of the IFNs. Aspirin and nonsteroidal anti-inflammatory drugs (NSAIDs) are antipyretic by inhibiting cyclooxygenase activity and the synthesis of PGE_2, not by inhibiting TNF or IL-1 production. Glucocorticoids may be antipyretic through dual mechanisms involving production of IL-1 and TNF as well as inhibition of arachidonate release centrally.

GENERAL ACTIONS OF IL-1 AND TNF Besides fever, a wide variety of actions characteristic of the acute inflammatory response can be triggered jointly by IL-1 and TNF. Many of these actions also involve arachidonate intermediates. These include myelopoiesis, release of neutrophils, and augmentation of some neutrophil functions; vasodilation and induction of cell adhesion proteins, platelet activating factor (PAF) production, and thrombomodulin expression by endothelial cells; proteolysis and glycogenolysis in muscles; mobilization of lipids from adipocytes; induction of acute phase protein synthesis and glycogenolysis in the liver; induction of fibroblast proliferation, osteoclast activation, and release of collagenase from chondrocytes; induction of slow-wave sleep activity in the brain; a variety of endocrine responses including release of ACTH, β-endorphins, growth hormone, and vasopressin from the pituitary; and the release of insulin from pancreatic cells and of cortisol and catecholamine from the adrenals. TNF and, to a lesser extent, IL-1 may contribute to the wasting (cachexia) characteristic of chronic infections and other inflammatory or neoplastic diseases by these mechanisms as well as by inhibiting appetite. In all of these actions, as well as in the production of fever, IL-1 and TNF can act synergistically or additively.

In contrast to TNF, IL-1 has major actions in triggering and amplifying the specific immune response through activating T cells and elaboration of interleukin 2 (IL-2). IL-1 also promotes B-cell proliferation (see Chap. 13). Interestingly, in vitro T-cell activation and mitogenesis as well as responses to IL-2 are enhanced at febrile body temperature, reaching an optimum at 39.5°C (103.1°F). By this means fever, as part of the inflammatory response, may exert a positive feedback on the specific immune response to infecting organisms.

Both fever and specific events mediated by IL-1 and TNF have a broad and highly integrated role in the characteristic responses to infection and/or acute inflammation. The interferons, in particular IFN-γ, may augment these responses (see Chap. 13). Some of these responses may be viewed as protective, whereas others contribute to deleterious symptoms and signs. In fact, when these responses are exaggerated or unchecked the syndrome of septicemia or septic shock (see Chap. 89) may develop. Given this complexity, it is not surprising that conflict still surrounds the need to treat fever with antipyretics and other means. While symptoms might be relieved, the cost could be interference with normally protective mechanisms, including the specific immune response and the mobilization of nutrients and cellular protective and proliferative responses necessary to promote a successful recovery.

DISEASES ACCOMPANIED BY FEVER Omitting disorders that may involve cerebral thermoregulatory centers directly, such as brain tumors, intracranial hemorrhage or thrombosis, or heat stroke, the following disease states may be accompanied by fever:

1 All *infections* whether caused by bacteria, rickettsias, chlamydiae, viruses, or parasites (in particular protozoa) may cause fever.
2 Diseases due to *immune mechanisms* often are associated with fever. These include the connective tissue disorders, drug reactions, disorders due to other immunologic abnormalities (including immune-mediated hemolysis), and the acquired immunodeficiency syndrome (AIDS). In the latter, particular care must be taken to exclude complicating infection.
3 Diseases characterized by *vascular inflammation or thrombosis*, tissue *infarction*, or *trauma* are often accompanied by fever. These include phlebitis; the giant-cell arteridites; myocardial, pulmonary, and cerebral infarctions; crushing mechanical trauma; and rhabdomyolysis. In all cases, complicating infection must be excluded.
4 *Granulomatous disorders* such as sarcoid and granulomatous hepatitis often have fever as a major manifestation.
5 *Inflammatory bowel disease* (ulcerative colitis and Crohn's disease) as well as other intraabdominal inflammatory processes (acute pancreatitis and hepatitis) may have fever associated with them.
6 *Neoplastic disorders*, in particular those arising from the lymphoreticular or hematopoietic systems, may have fever as a prominent manifestation at the beginning or later in the course. Rarely other solid tumors (hypernephroma; carcinoma of the pancreas, lung, and bone; or hepatoma) present with fever. Fever complicating most solid tumors is usually related to widespread metastases with tumor necrosis or obstruction and infection of drainage ducts.
7 Certain *acute metabolic disorders* such as gout, porphyria, Fabry's disease, Addisonian or thyroid crises, and, rarely, pheochromocytoma are sometimes associated with fever. The pathogenesis varies from activation of the inflammatory response (e.g., gout) to alterations in thermogenesis and heat regulation (e.g., hyperthyroidism and pheochromocytoma).

ACCOMPANIMENTS OF FEVER **Systemic symptoms** The perception of fever by patients varies enormously. Some persons can tell with considerable accuracy when their body temperatures are elevated; others with chronic febrile illnesses (e.g., patients with tuberculosis) may be wholly unaware of body temperature as high as 39.9°C (103°F). Often patients may pay no attention to fever because of other unpleasant symptoms such as headache or pleuritic pain. Pain in the back, generalized myalgias, and arthralgias without arthritis are commonly associated with fever. To what extent these symptoms can be ascribed to specific infectious agents as opposed to the actions of IL-1 and TNF (e.g., muscle proteolysis) is not clear, but whatever the mechanism, many of these symptoms may be reduced or abolished with aspirin or NSAID administration.

Chills Abrupt onset of fever with a *chill* or *rigor* is characteristic of some diseases and, in the absence of antipyretic drugs, rare in others. Although repeated rigors are typical of pyogenic infection with bacteremia, a similar pattern of fever may occur in noninfectious diseases such as vasculitis or lymphoma. A true chill, which is usually accompanied by teeth chattering and bed shaking, must be differentiated from the chilly sensations which occur in almost all fevers, particularly those in viral infections. Rarely, a true rigor occurs in viremia. Chills may be evoked or perpetuated by the intermittent administration of aspirin or other antipyretics when their action wears off or if there is an exaggerated hypothermic response. These unpleasant side effects may be minimized by administering antipyretics at 2 to 3 h intervals around the clock, rather than prescribing them only for elevations of temperature above a certain level.

Sweats When the stimulus to fever production is removed or inhibited, for example, by the action of antipyretics, defervescence is achieved by activation of heat loss mechanisms. Diffuse sweating, sometimes soaking clothing or bedsheets, allows rapid dissipation of heat by evaporation and may add to patient discomfort. In some patients, this may be the most prominent manifestation of repetitive fevers followed by defervescence (e.g., tuberculosis).

Changes in mental status Febrile episodes may be accompanied by obtundation, irritability, or frank delirium in some patients without evidence for central nervous system involvement by the primary disease process. This is most striking in the very old and in the very young, and in patients with other disorders such as alcoholism, cardiovascular disease, or senility. The soporific actions of TNF and IL-1 as well as release of β-endorphins may contribute to these events. The sensorium usually clears with defervescence in the absence of underlying disease of the central nervous system.

Convulsions Infants and young children (less than age 5) may sometimes develop seizures when the temperature is elevated. A family history of epilepsy may be present, but usually febrile convulsions do not signal serious cerebral disease. When they occur, however, a primary disorder affecting the central nervous system must be excluded, as is also mandatory for patients with marked alteration in mental status.

Herpes labialis Elevations of body temperature can activate latent herpes simplex virus (HSV) infection (''fever blisters''). For unclear reasons this is more common in acute pyogenic bacterial infections (pneumococcal, streptococcal, meningococcal), malaria, and the rickettsioses than in other infections or noninfectious causes of fever. Activation of latent HSV infection is also a manifestation of suppressed cellular immunity.

CLINICAL IMPORTANCE OF FEVER Properly measured, the temperature is a simple, objective, and accurate indicator of a physiologic state and is much less subject to external and psychogenic stimuli than the other vital signs, such as pulse, respiratory rate, and blood pressure. For these reasons, determination of the body temperature assists in estimating the severity of an illness, its course and duration, and the effect of therapy, or even in deciding which person has an organic illness. In general, determination of rectal temperature is easily performed and most accurately reflects core body temperatures. In seriously ill patients or those in whom oral temperatures are unreliable (e.g., failure to cooperate, hyperventilation) *rectal temperature monitoring is mandatory*.

Benefit of fever Beyond drawing attention to its cause, it has been difficult to relate more rapid resolution or decreased complications of a disease state to the presence and degree of fever. Fever therapy was used in the past to diminish the manifestations of neurosyphilis or some forms of chronic arthritis. To what extent beneficial effects could be ascribed to high core body temperature as opposed to the action of mediators of the febrile process is unclear. In vitro IL-1–mediated activation of the specific immune response is accelerated at febrile body temperatures. Similarly, minor increases of chemotactic, phagocytic, and bactericidal activity of human polymorphonuclear leukocytes have been observed. In cold-blooded animals a warm environment has been demonstrated to augment the inflammatory response.

Detrimental aspects of fever Many of the alleged detrimental effects of fever may be due to the concurrent actions of IL-1, TNF, and other mediators at a variety of sites and may be independent of temperature elevation per se. Muscle wasting with myalgias, adipose tissue loss, other metabolic changes, and perhaps CNS alterations in febrile disorders are examples of such effects. Nevertheless, in febrile patients basal metabolism rates are increased as are cardiac output and work. Sweating may aggravate loss of salt and water. There may be general discomfort due to malaise, myalgias, headache, photophobia, or an unpleasant sensation of warmth. Fever may precipitate seizures in epileptic patients. The rigors and profuse sweats of hectic fevers are particularly unpleasant for many patients. In elderly patients, particularly those with cardiac or cerebrovascular disease, fever and its associated manifestations may be deleterious.

MANAGEMENT OF FEVER The most important aspects of fever management should be directed at its cause. Since fever ordinarily does little harm, imposes no great discomfort, and may benefit host defense mechanisms, antipyretic drugs are rarely essential to patient welfare and may obfuscate the effect of a specific therapeutic agent or of the natural course of the disease. There are situations, however, in which lowering of the body temperature is of vital importance, e.g., heat stroke and malignant hyperthermia (see Chap. 377), epileptic seizures, or when cardiac or CNS function is impaired. Under these circumstances lowering the temperature is indicated. Cooling blankets set at hypothermic temperatures can be a highly effective means for external cooling. However, their effects may be negated if they induce further cutaneous vasoconstriction and shivering. Sponging the body surface with cool saline or water or applying cool compresses to the skin and forehead may be helpful. There is no advantage to sponging with alcohol, which, because of its pungent odor, may add to patient discomfort. When high internal temperature is combined with cutaneous vasoconstriction, as in heat stroke or malignant hyperthermia, external cooling should be combined with massage of the skin in order to promote surface vasodilation. Immediate immersion in a tub of ice water or packing with ice should be considered as a measure of last resort and can be lifesaving in patients with heat stroke if the internal body temperature is in excess of 42.2°C (108°F). In most instances cooling blankets, if available, are safer and more comfortable.

Antipyretic drugs, such as aspirin (0.650 g every 4 h) or acetaminophen (0.650 to 1.0 g every 4 h) are often employed in lowering temperature and relieving other manifestations of febrile illness. Acetaminophen is generally preferred because of its lack of adverse effects on gastric mucosa, platelet function, or the subsequent development of Reye's syndrome in some children with viral illnesses given aspirin (see Chap. 256). Candidates for antipyretic therapy include patients who are uncomfortable or those in whom fever poses a high risk, as in patients with ischemic heart disease, heart failure, febrile seizures (usually children), head injury, mental disorders, or pregnancy. Antipyretics are sometimes associated with unpleasant diaphoresis, an alarming fall in blood pressure, and the subsequent return of fever accompanied by a chill; these can be mitigated by enforcing a liberal fluid intake and by administering the drugs regularly and frequently at 2- to 3-h intervals. NSAIDs such as ibuprofen (200 mg every 6 h), indomethacin (50 mg every 6 to 8 h), or naproxen (250 mg bid) also have potent antipyretic effects and have been useful in controlling chronic fevers in patients with malignancy. Although glucocorticoids are effective antipyretics, they must be used with caution because of their tendency to precipitate abrupt falls in temperature accompanied by hypotension. The capacity of these drugs to mask other manifestations of infection and inflammation as well as potential adverse side effects constitute a relative contraindication to their use.

The discomfort of a rigor can be alleviated in many patients by the intravenous injection of calcium salts. This procedure will stop the shivering and chilliness, but has no influence on the ultimate height of the fever. Severe rigors can also be abolished with morphine sulfate (10 to 15 mg subcutaneously) or with parenteral chlorpromazine (10 to 25 mg). When this approach is employed, the patient must be carefully monitored for hypotension.

DIAGNOSTIC CONSIDERATIONS IN FEVER In many illnesses fever is the most prominent and often the only manifestation of disease. While certain fever patterns may suggest a particular type of disease, fever per se is only an indication of a reaction to injury comparable with an elevated leukocyte count or rapid erythrocyte sedimentation rate.

Fever patterns Fever may be intermittent, remittent, sustained, or relapsing. In *intermittent fever* the temperature falls to normal each day in an exaggeration of the circadian rhythmn. When the variation between the peak and the nadir is very large, the fever is called *hectic* or *septic*. Intermittent fevers are characteristic but not diagnostic of pyogenic infections, particularly abscesses, lymphomas, and miliary tuberculosis. In *remittent fever* the temperature falls each day, usually by morning, but does not return to normal. Most fevers are remittent and this type of febrile response is not characteristic of any disease. A *sustained fever* is characterized by persistent temperature elevation without significant diurnal variation. It is exemplified by the fever of untreated typhoid, typhus, or infectious endocarditis. With *relapsing fever* short febrile periods occur between one or several days of normal temperature. Examples of relapsing fever are the following:

Malaria (see Chap. 159), in particular that caused by infection with *Plasmodium vivax*, produces relapsing fevers at 2- to 3-day intervals. Relapsing fever caused by infection with *Borrelia* species is discussed in Chap. 131; typically 7- to 10-day febrile episodes are interspersed with 5- to 7-day afebrile periods. *Rat-bite fever* can be caused by either *Spirillum minus* or *Streptobacillus moniliformis*, both transmitted by the bite of a rat (see Chap. 98). The periodic exacerbations of fever usually follow a 7- to 10-day pattern, following a history of rat bite 1 to 10 weeks prior to the onset of symptoms. The diagnosis is made by cultures of blood, joints, or other inflamed sites or by serology.

Localized *pyogenic infections* may in rare instances produce periodic bouts of fever. The so-called Charcot's intermittent biliary fever, i.e., cholangitis with episodic biliary obstruction due to stones, is an example. Similarly, periodic ureteral obstruction due to small stones or inspissated pus may cause a relapsing fever pattern in the presence of urinary infection.

Pel-Ebstein fever—bouts of fever lasting 3 to 10 days, separated by a febrile and asymptomatic period of 3 to 10 days—is the eponym for relapsing fever occurring as a manifestation of Hodgkin's disease or other lymphomas. In some patients these cycles may be repeated for months until other manifestations of the illness become apparent. Although the pattern may suggest the nature of the underlying disease, most patients with Pel-Ebstein relapsing fever have causes other than Hodgkin's disease.

Epidemiology of fever The diagnosis of febrile illness must take into account the epidemiologic setting. For example an acute febrile illness in southeast Asia or Africa is probably due to malaria (see Chap. 159) or one of the arboviruses (see Chap. 148); in a college student in the United States it may result from infectious mononucleosis or some other viral infection; and in a hospitalized octogenarian following prostatectomy it is probably an indication of urinary tract infection, wound infection, phlebitis from an intravenous catheter, aspiration pneumonia, or pulmonary infarction. In children, prolonged fevers are more likely to be due to infections than in adults. Travelers returning from trips to foreign countries must be evaluated for diseases indigenous to the countries visited, but they are more likely to have febrile diseases that are more common at home. Patients whose host defenses are altered by malignancy, cytotoxic or steroid therapy, or congenital or acquired immunodeficiency are more likely to have infections caused by unusual opportunistic organisms than are normal hosts.

Rare versus common diseases Unless host defense mechanisms have been severely altered by disease or immunosuppressive therapy, fever is much more likely to be a manifestation of a common than a rare disease. On the other hand, patients with abnormal host defenses are no less prone to infections with common agents than are normal hosts. For example, while pneumococcal pneumonia is a leading cause of pulmonary infiltrates and fever in the elderly, it also is an important cause of illness in patients with AIDS, although not as frequent as *Pneumocystis carinii* (see Chap. 264).

Febrile illnesses of short duration Acute febrile illnesses of less than 2 weeks' duration are common in medical practice. In most cases they run their course, progressing to complete recovery, and a precise diagnosis is not, nor need be, made. It is likely that the vast majority of such illnesses are infectious although short febrile episodes may be characteristic of thromboembolic disease, gout, or drug allergies in which the drug is discontinued.

Symptomatic infections with respiratory viruses are usually short-lived and self-limited. The presence of cough, coryza, and pharyngitis associated with fever supports this diagnosis (see Chap. 140). Similarly during summer months short-lived fever and malaise ("grippe") are characteristic of many enteroviral infections (see Chap. 144). It is neither practical nor cost-effective to carry out detailed diagnostic studies for these agents. In bacterial infections, however, laboratory diagnosis is simpler and can be indispensible to proper therapy.

The following characteristics, though not restricted solely to acute infections, are highly suggestive that infection is present:

1 Abrupt onset
2 High fever, i.e., 38.9 to 40.6°C (102 to 105°F) with or without chills
3 Respiratory symptoms—sore throat, cough, coryza
4 Severe malaise, with muscle or joint pain, photophobia, pain on movement of the eyes, headache
5 Nausea, vomiting, or diarrhea
6 Acute tender enlargement of the lymph nodes or spleen
7 Meningeal signs with or without spinal fluid pleocytosis
8 Dysuria, urinary frequency, and flank pain

None of the symptoms and signs listed is encountered solely in infections. Acute leukemias or vasculitis may have similar features on presentation. Nevertheless, in a given instance of acute febrile illness with some or all of the manifestations listed, the probabilities strongly favor infection.

It is desirable, of course, to establish an accurate diagnosis, and whatever steps are practicable in the circumstances to establish the cause should be taken. Cultures of the blood, urine, and other suspected sites of infection should be obtained before institution of antibacterial chemotherapy (see Chap. 80). Skin and/or serologic tests should also be carried out when indicated.

There is a tendency to rely immediately and excessively on the laboratory in ascertaining the cause of fever. In many instances, a thorough history and a complete and, if necessary, repeated physical examination along with a complete blood count (CBC) and urinalysis will provide the answer. Measurement of the erythrocyte sedimentation rate can help differentiate fevers caused by infection or inflammation from other causes. Often a little patience, in the form of watchful waiting before embarking on an expensive and extensive laboratory workup, will lead to the diagnosis.

Prolonged febrile illness Some of the knottiest problems in medicine are posed by cases of prolonged fever in which the diagnosis remains obscure for weeks or even months. Eventually, however, the true nature of the illness usually reveals itself, since a disease which causes injury sufficient to evoke temperature elevations to 38.3°C (101°F) or higher for several weeks does not often subside without leaving some clue as to its nature. The evaluation of problems of this sort calls for skillful application of all diagnostic methods—careful history, thorough physical examination, and the carefully considered and staged use of laboratory examinations and imaging techniques.

FEVER OF UNKNOWN ORIGIN In some, fever becomes the dominant sign or symptom in a patient's illness, and when its cause escapes detection, it is defined as a fever of unknown origin (FUO). This term should be reserved for patients who have elevations in temperature greater than 38.3°C (101°F) for a prolonged period (at least 2, and preferably, 3 weeks) and in whom the diagnosis cannot be made during at least 1 week of intensive study. These rigid criteria eliminate from this diagnostic category patients with common viral or bacterial infections, those in whom the diagnosis is obvious by simple physical and/or laboratory examination, and those whose fever is due to a sequential occurrence of etiologically unrelated diseases. An example is a patient febrile after a myocardial infarction, who then develops thrombophlebitis followed by multiple pulmonary emboli, each accompanied by recurrence of fever. Much of the confusion in the literature concerning causes of FUO is due to failure to define the criteria employed in classifying patients.

DISEASES CAUSING PROLONGED FEVERS Table 20-1 lists some of the diseases responsible for prolonged fever.

Infections Infections that are relatively resistant to rapid eradication by host defenses (e.g., localized pyogenic infections or intracellular infections) often pursue a chronic or subacute course. As a cause for FUO, infections account for about 30 percent, a figure that appears to be decreasing due to the common practice of administering antibiotics to any patient in whom fever persists for more than a few days. Consequently many infections may be eradicated by more or less "blind" therapy without accurate determination of their nature or location.

ABSCESSES (See also Chap. 91) Abscesses are the most common form of bacterial infection presenting as FUO and are important because they can be cured with early diagnosis and treatment. Failure to make a diagnosis may result in a fatal or permanently disabling outcome. Intraabdominal abscesses arising in the liver or spleen, in the subphrenic space, related to a ruptured diverticulum or appendix, or in the pelvis may be associated with more fever than pain. Ultrasonography, computed tomographic (CT) scanning, or magnetic resonance imaging (MRI) have simplified the detection and localization of abscesses. In many cases percutaneous needle aspiration under imaging guidance can be employed for both diagnosis and treatment, without the need to resort to laparotomy.

RENAL INFECTION Fever in uncomplicated pyelonephritis is usually limited to 5 to 7 days (see Chap. 95). Prolongation of fever beyond this time should suggest intra- or extrarenal obstruction or abscess. Prostate abscesses should be considered in males; sometimes there is no associated rectal pain or dysuria. Occasionally focal pyelonephritis may cause prolonged fever. Ultrasonography coupled with CT scanning will detect obstruction and abscesses with a high degree of reliability.

INTRAVASCULAR INFECTIONS Because of a high index of suspicion, the ubiquitous use of blood cultures, and widespread application of antibiotics, which must cure some patients, bacterial endocarditis has become a rare cause of FUO. Antibiotic use or infection by highly fastidious organisms including fungi and rickettsias are important factors in "culture-negative" endocarditis (see Chap. 90). Organisms that give rise to chronic or intermittent bacteremia without prominent localizing findings include *Salmonella (S. typhosa, S. choleraesuis), Neisseria* (both gonococci and meningococci), and *Brucella*. Consideration of the epidemiologic setting, using appropriate serologic testing, and informing laboratories of the need to look for fastidious organisms in blood cultures are useful in establishing the diagnosis.

OTHER BACTERIAL INFECTIONS These include sinusitis or mastoiditis, exacerbations of chronic or subacute osteomyelitis (in particular vertebral osteomyelitis), and retroperitoneal infection such as an aortic aneurysm filled with secondarily infected organizing clot. Enteric pathogens (including *Escherichia coli, Bacteroides,* and *Salmonella*) have been frequent isolates from patients with such infections. Blood cultures may be intermittently positive. For screening of bone infections, bone scan can demonstrate foci of increased uptake; however, the changes must be differentiated from those caused by fractures, neoplasm, or other causes of osteoblastic activity. Imaging techniques including ultrasonography, CT scan, and, if necessary, MRI can assist in establishing the diagnosis of retroperitoneal, sinus, and bone infections. Surgery is necessary for both diagnosis and therapy of infected aneurysms. In addition some patients with dissecting aneurysms have fever without infection.

TABLE 20-1 Disease entities in the United States causing prolonged fever

- *I* Infections
  - *A* Pyogenic infections
    - *1* Upper abdominal infections
      - *a* Cholecystitis (stone), empyema of gallbladder
      - *b* Cholangitis
      - *c* Liver abscess
      - *d* Lesser sac abscess
      - *e* Subphrenic abscess
      - *f* Splenic abscess
    - *2* Lower abdominal infections
      - *a* Diverticulitis (abscess)
      - *b* Appendicitis
    - *3* Pelvic inflammatory disease
      - *a* Pelvic abscess
    - *4* Urinary tract infections
      - *a* Pyelonephritis (rare)
      - *b* Intrarenal abscess
      - *c* Perinephric abscess
      - *d* Ureteral obstruction
      - *e* Prostatic abscess
    - *5* Sinusitis
    - *6* Osteomyelitis
    - *7* Cat-scratch fever
  - *B* Intravascular infections
    - *1* Bacterial endocarditis (acute and subacute)
    - *2* Intravascular catheter infections
  - *C* Bacteremias without overt primary focus
    - *1* Meningococcemia
    - *2* Gonococcemia
    - *3* Typhoid
    - *4* Vibriosis
    - *5* Listeriosis
    - *6* Brucellosis
    - *7* Coliform bacteremia in patients with cirrhosis
  - *D* Granulomatous infections
    - *1* Tuberculosis
    - *2* Deep-seated fungus infections
    - *3* Atypical mycobacterial infections
  - *E* Viral, rickettsial, and chlamydial infections
    - *1* Infectious mononucleosis
    - *2* Cytomegalovirus
    - *3* Hepatitis
    - *4* Group B coxsackievirus diseases
    - *5* Mucocutaneous lymph node syndrome (children)
    - *6* Human immunodeficiency virus infection (ARC, AIDS)
    - *7* Q fever (including endocarditis)
    - *8* Psittacosis
  - *F* Parasitic diseases
    - *1* Amebiasis
    - *2* Malaria
    - *3* Toxoplasmosis
    - *4* *Pneumocystis carinii* pneumonia
    - *5* Trichinosis
  - *G* Spirochetal infections
    - *1* Leptospirosis
    - *2* Relapsing fever
    - *3* Lyme Disease
- *II* Neoplasms
  - *A* Solid (localized)
    - *1* Kidney
    - *2* Lung
    - *3* Pancreas
    - *4* Liver
    - *5* Large Bowel
    - *6* Atrial myxoma
  - *B* Metastatic
    - *1* From gastrointestinal tract
    - *2* From lung, kidneys, bone, cervix, ovary
    - *3* Melanoma
    - *4* Sarcoma
  - *C* Tumors of the reticuloendothelial system
    - *1* Hodgkin's disease
    - *2* Non-Hodgkin's lymphoma
    - *3* Malignant histiocytosis
    - *4* Immunoblastic lymphadenopathy
    - *5* Lymphomatoid granulomatosis
- *III* Connective tissue disease
  - *A* Rheumatic fever
  - *B* Systemic lupus erythematosus
  - *C* Rheumatoid arthritis (particularly Still's disease)
  - *D* Giant cell arteritis (polymyalgia rheumatica)
  - *E* Hypersensitivity vasculitis
  - *F* Periarteritis nodosa
  - *G* Wegener's granulomatosis
  - *H* Panaortitis
- *IV* Granulomatous diseases
  - *A* Sarcoidosis
  - *B* Granulomatous hepatitis
  - *C* Crohn's disease (regional enteritis)
  - *D* Erythema nodosum
- *V* Miscellaneous
  - *A* Drug fever
  - *B* Pulmonary emboli
  - *C* Thyroiditis
  - *D* Hemolytic states
  - *E* Cryptic trauma with bleeding into enclosed spaces (hematomas)
  - *F* Dissecting aneurysm
  - *G* Whipple's disease
  - *H* Weber-Christian Disease
- *VI* Metabolic and inherited diseases
  - *A* Familial Mediterranean fever
  - *B* Hypertriglyceridemia and hypercholesterolemia with pancreatitis
  - *C* Fabry's disease
  - *D* Cyclic neutropenia
- *VII* Thermoregulatory disorders
  - *A* Central
    - *1* Brain tumor
    - *2* Cerebrovascular accident
    - *3* Encephalitis
  - *B* Peripheral
    - *1* Hyperthyroidism
    - *2* Pheochromocytoma
- *VIII* Psychogenic fevers
  - *A* Factitious fever
  - *B* Habitual hyperthermia
- *IX* Undiagnosed
  - *A* Resolved
    - *1* Without treatment
    - *2* With antibiotics
    - *3* With anti-inflammatory drugs
  - *B* Recurrent
    - *1* Suppressed with steroids

Cat-scratch fever (see Chap. 98) may run a prolonged course with multiple systems involved. Diagnosis is made by lymph node biopsy.

IATROGENIC INFECTIONS These include infections of catheters, arteriovenous fistulas, ventricular-peritoneal shunts, and other foreign bodies. Usually their cure requires removal of the infected material as well as antimicrobial therapy. Intravascular graft infection may give rise to prolonged bacteremia and poses a particularly difficult management problem.

GRANULOMATOUS INFECTIONS Formation of granulomas is characteristic of chronic infection with mycobacteria and of the primary deep mycoses, particularly histoplasmosis and coccidioidomycosis (see Chap. 151). Tuberculosis (see Chap. 125) and atypical mycobacterial infections (see Chap. 127) continue to cause FUO. Reservoirs of tuberculosis exist in patients with a previous contact with an active case, and the prevalence is higher among blacks, native Americans, southeast Asians, and natives of other countries where tuberculosis is still endemic. Symptomatic progressive disseminated infection due to *Mycobacterium avium-intracellulare* (MAI) is a common complication of AIDS (see Chap. 264) and is seen in other patients on immunosuppressive treatment, particularly in association with high-dose glucocorticoids. Most of these infections are extrapulmonary and may involve the bones, lymph nodes, genital or urinary organs, or the liver. Many of these patients are debilitated and have overwhelming mycobacterial disease. The diagnosis can be established by stain and culture of biopsy material from bone marrow, liver, lymph nodes, or other involved tissues. Granuloma formation does not occur in AIDS patients, and the number of organisms is so high that blood cultures are usually positive. Even with far-advanced disease, patients with tuberculosis may respond well to treatment with bactericidal drugs, in particular isoniazid and rifampin, making the establishment of this diagnosis imperative. In contrast, no effective treatment for progressive MAI infection is available.

VIRAL, RICKETTSIAL, AND CHLAMYDIAL INFECTIONS Older patients with Epstein-Barr virus (EBV) or cytomegalovirus infection may have prolonged febrile illness without prominent localizing findings (see Chap. 137). Lymphadenopathy, splenomegaly, and evanescent skin rashes are variable findings. Usually atypical lymphocytosis and abnormalities of liver function tests are present. The diagnosis can be made by serology or culture. Patients with HIV infection often have periods of prolonged fever, either as a manifestation of primary infection or later as full-blown AIDS develops (see Chap. 264). While opportunistic infections are usually present in febrile AIDS patients, fever and lymphadenopathy can be manifestations of HIV infection alone.

Mucocutaneous lymph node (Kawasaki) syndrome (see Chaps. 56 or 59) affects children with a prolonged infectious mononucleosis-like illness, including aseptic meningitis and cardiac disease; a viral etiology appears likely. Psittacosis may look much like typhoid fever, and Q-fever endocarditis has been a particularly puzzling and lethal illness that must be treated both with antibiotics and valve replacement. Both infections may be diagnosed serologically, and contacts with birds, sheep, or cattle are important epidemiologic clues.

PARASITIC DISEASES Amebiasis can present as an FUO either in the form of diffuse hepatitis or, more commonly, as liver abscesses. The diagnosis of malaria is simple when the importance of exposure to endemic areas is considered. Generalized toxoplasmosis may present with prolonged fever and lymphadenopathy. In AIDS patients or those on glucocorticoids, *carinii* pneumonia may cause prolonged fever before cough, dyspnea, hypoxemia, and chest x-ray findings appear (see Chap. 163).

SPIROCHETAL INFECTIONS Besides relapsing fever caused by *Borrelia*, leptospirosis (see Chap. 130), secondary syphilis (see Chap. 128), and Lyme disease (see Chap. 132) can all have prolonged and occasionally relapsing fever as one of their major manifestations. Clinical suspicion of a characteristic syndrome and serologic methods are central to establishing the diagnosis in the latter three illnesses.

Neoplasms HODGKIN'S DISEASE Fever may be the principal symptom and only objective finding early in the course of Hodgkin's disease (see Chap. 302), especially as patients with this disease who present with FUO may have only intraabdominal or retroperitoneal disease or involvement of the bone marrow. The diagnosis is usually made by biopsy or staging laparotomy. It is important to arrive at the diagnosis early because, with proper chemotherapy, prolonged remissions and even cure may be achieved.

NON-HODGKIN'S LYMPHOMA These diseases usually present with fever, nonspecific symptoms, and lymphadenopathy which the patient recognizes. Hepatosplenomegaly, bone pain, and tenderness may be present. Primary lymphomas of the small intestine present with fever and malabsorption. The laboratory findings usually consist of anemia, leukocytosis, and sometimes atypical lymphocytosis leading to confusion with EBV infection. The diagnosis is usually made by lymph node biopsy, but biopsies can be mistaken for reactive hyperplasia or atypical lymphocytic infiltrates. Prolonged remissions can occasionally be achieved with newer chemotherapy regimens (see Chap. 302).

LYMPHOMA-LIKE SYNDROMES Several disease entities with features similar to Hodgkin's disease have been recognized but may have a better prognosis or respond differently to steroids or antitumor agents. All may present as FUOs and they include immunoblastic lymphadenopathy, lymphomatoid granulomatosis, and acute megakaryocytic myelosis. Rarely, disseminated Kaposi's sarcoma presents with fever as a prominent manifestation. These disorders are discussed more fully in Chaps. 302 and 264.

LEUKEMIAS It is not uncommon for acute leukemia to be mistaken for acute infection at the onset. High fever [40.6°C (105°F)] and the absence of blast cells in the peripheral blood may delay the diagnosis. Either neutropenia or neutrophilic leukocytosis may be present, and most patients are anemic. Bone marrow aspiration and biopsy usually reveal the diagnosis (see Chap. 296), although rarely only myeloid dysplasia, a preleukemic syndrome, may be the only finding. In patients with chronic lymphatic or granulocytic leukemia, fever is most often a manifestation of concomitant infection. Similarly, before it is assumed that fever in any patient with leukemia is due to the blood dyscrasia, infection must be ruled out by appropriate tests and cultures, and attempts to treat the "most likely" pathogen must be made, particularly if the patient has neutropenia.

SOLID TUMORS Fever is not a common occurrence in the vast majority of solid tumors, unless drainage ducts are obstructed and infection has set in or metastases with tumor necrosis have developed. Imaging techniques (ultrasound, CT, MRI) are the most useful in detecting tumor masses, which may be biopsied percutaneously or at laparotomy. Occasionally disseminated carcinomatosis with bone marrow invasion causes leukemoid reactions. Nucleated erythrocytes present in the peripheral blood smear indicate marrow injury; bone marrow biopsy makes the diagnosis. Patients are usually older and the sites of the primary tumor vary widely and include the kidney, pancreas, bowel, liver, lung, and, rarely, the uterus, ovaries, breast, or prostate.

ATRIAL MYXOMA Patients with fever, changing heart murmurs, peripheral embolic pneumonia, and joint pains are usually suspected of having bacterial endocarditis, rheumatic fever, or occasionally some other connective tissue disease. Most intracardiac tumors are readily detected by two-dimensional echocardiography and the diagnosis should be suspected upon the finding of a pedunculated intraatrial (rarely intraventricular) mass, the occasional presence of calcification associated with negative blood cultures, or serologic tests. MRI and angiography may be needed to confirm the suspicion before surgical removal.

Connective tissue disease RHEUMATIC FEVER Episodic outbreaks of rheumatic fever still occur in the United States and worldwide. Most victims are young and there will not be a definite history of antecedent sore throat in all patients. Similarly, serologic evidence for recent streptococcal infection may be lacking in 5 to 10 percent of patients. The diagnosis is made on clinical grounds and requires the exclusion of other connective tissue disorders or infectious diseases (see Chap. 101).

SYSTEMIC LUPUS ERYTHEMATOSUS (SLE) The widespread availability of a variety of serologic tests has simplified the diagnosis of SLE and its variant syndromes (see Chap. 269). These disorders no longer comprise as large a part of FUO series as they once did. Fever can be either a manifestation of active lupus or due to complicating infection, particularly if steroid or cytotoxic immunosuppressive treatment is given. In the face of negative cultures or histologic evidence of infection, high titers of anti double-stranded DNA antibodies, and low serum hemolytic complement, C4 or C3 levels support a diagnosis of active SLE.

RHEUMATOID ARTHRITIS In its classic form this disease is not difficult to recognize and high titers of serum rheumatoid factor will support the diagnosis. Some patients, usually children or young adults, may present with a seronegative version (Still's disease) in which high fever, hepatosplenomegaly, lymphadenopathy, evanescent rashes, anemia, and leukocytosis are variably present. Joint changes may not appear until late in the disease. The diagnosis is made only after prolonged observation and the exclusion of other diseases. The prognosis is generally good and patients respond well to aspirin, NSAIDs, or steroids. Other arthritis syndromes in which fever may be prominent include ankylosing spondylitis (see Chap. 274), psoriatic arthritis (see Chap. 283), and Lyme disease (see Chap. 132).

OTHER CONNECTIVE TISSUE DISEASES These include classic periarteritis nodosa and other vasculitic syndromes that involve small and medium-sized arteries as well as the aorta and its main branches. Serologic evidence of infection with hepatitis B virus may be present in some patients but other serologic parameters of autoimmune disease are usually absent (see Chap. 276). Angiography and biopsy can be useful in establishing this diagnosis. Fever in Wegener's granulomatosis is usually due to complicating sinusitis, otitis media, or pulmonary infection. Most patients respond to treatment with steroids and cytotoxic agents.

GIANT CELL ARTERITIS (POLYMYALGIA RHEUMATICA) This is a disease of elderly persons who complain of fever, headache, and pain in the muscles and joints, particularly those of the shoulder girdle. Overt arthritis is rare. At times fever is the only symptom and there are no abnormal physical findings. The sedimentation rate is characteristically very rapid and anemia of chronic disease is present. Dramatic improvement may occur in patients with polymyalgia rheumatica (PMR) with low doses of steroids, which can be used as a therapeutic trial once other disorders are excluded. Patients with classic temporal arteritis may have a PMR syndrome as a prodrome. They may present with additional complaints of visual disturbances or jaw claudication (see Chap. 276). Swelling and tenderness of the cranial arteries are variably present, and temporal artery biopsy in the untreated state usually discloses a granulomatous vasculitis. In contrast to PMR, longer-term treatment with high doses of steroids is indicated in temporal arteritis to induce remission and prevent catastrophic complications such as blindness.

Granulomatous diseases SARCOIDOSIS Ordinarily fever is not characteristic of sarcoidosis but may be prominent in patients with arthritis, hilar lymphadenopathy, and cutaneous lesions of erythema nodosum, or in those with extensive hepatic involvement. The diagnosis is suggested by the youthful age and black race of most patients, mediastinal lymphoid enlargement with interstitial pulmonary infiltrates, and, in rare patients, infiltration of the parotid or lacrimal glands with or without uveitis or a lymphocytic meningitis. Serum angiotensin-converting enzyme activity is often increased (see Chap. 277). Noncaseating granulomas are found on biopsy of the skin, submaximal salivary glands, lymph nodes, or liver. There may be symptomatic improvement with steroid therapy although the natural history appears not to be affected.

GRANULOMATOUS HEPATITIS Patients present with fever, weight loss, variable hepatomegaly, anemia of chronic disease, and elevated alkaline phosphatase, but with relatively normal bilirubin, transaminases, and prothrombin time. Liver biopsy shows noncaseating granulomas, and specific diseases which cause this reaction must be excluded. These include tuberculosis, Hodgkin's disease, histoplasmosis, sarcoidosis, primary biliary cirrhosis, drug reactions, schistosomiasis, and berylliosis, to name only some. The fever generally subsides over a period of weeks to months and can be mitigated with glucocorticoids. In the majority of patients and certainly in all with a positive tuberculin reaction, concomitant treatment with antituberculosis medications should be given until the diagnosis of tuberculosis can be excluded.

ERYTHEMA NODOSUM These tender subcutaneous nodules (see Chap. 58) can appear with fever over extensor surfaces of the extremities as a complication of sarcoidosis, tuberculosis, histoplasmosis, coccidioidomycosis, drug reactions, inflammatory bowel disease, or rarely without precipitating cause.

Miscellaneous causes of fever DRUG FEVER This is an important cause of cryptic fever; a careful history of drug intake should be taken in every patient with unexplained fever. Fever due to allergy to an antibiotic may become superimposed on the fever of the infection for which the drug was given, resulting in a very confusing picture. Common drugs which can cause fever include sulfonamides, penicillins and cephalosporins, barbiturates, antituberculous medications, nitrofurantoin, phenytoin, procainamide, quinidine, phenolphthalein—including laxatives, allopurinol, and thioureas. Fever due to drug allergy must be distinguished from that which is a predictable part of a drug response such as amphotericin-induced fever. Fever in drug allergy may be accompanied by other manifestations of hypersensitivity, including rash, neutropenia, hemolytic anemia, eosinophilia, or thrombocytopenia or it may be the sole manifestation. Any question of drug fever can usually be resolved within several days by discontinuing all medications. If essential, the diagnosis can be further substantiated by giving a test dose of the drug after fever has subsided, but this may result in a very unpleasant or even dangerous reaction in some patients.

MULTIPLE PULMONARY EMBOLI Symptomless thrombosis of deep calf or pelvic veins may cause prolonged febrile illness either because of thrombophlebitis or as a result of repeated pulmonary emboli. These emboli may not be manifested by pleuritic pain or hemoptysis, but cough, dyspnea, and vague thoracic discomfort are likely to be present. Lung scans, venography, and, if necessary, pulmonary angiography should reveal the diagnosis. Some patients may have nephrotic syndrome due to renal vein thrombosis. Pelvic thrombophlebitis with or without pulmonary emboli is an important cause of FUO in postpartum patients.

HEMOLYTIC EPISODES Most episodes of acute or subacute hemolysis are characterized by bouts of fever and sometimes in acute hemolytic crises by shaking chills and marked temperature elevation. The hemolysis may be due to genetic disorders such as a crisis in sickle cell disease and its variants or to immune mechanisms. Chronic hemolytic disorders, such as spherocytosis or the thalassemias, are not usually associated with fever unless there is complicating infection. Since infection is an important precipitating cause of sickle cell crisis, it must be searched for diligently and if necessary treated presumptively. Besides the appearance of sickled or fragmented erythrocytes on blood smear, the presence of hemolysis will be suggested by the rapid development of anemia without apparent bleeding, reticulocytosis, and indirect hyperbilirubinemia. Evaluation for hemoglobinopathies, glucose-6-phosphate dehydrogenase deficiency, or antibody and/or complement bound to erythrocytes will reveal the diagnosis (see Chap. 61).

CRYPTIC HEMATOMAS Accumulation of old blood in closed spaces, for instance, at sites of remote trauma, particularly in the perisplenic area, the pericardium, or retroperitoneal area, may give rise to prolonged fever. This diagnosis should be thought of in any patient receiving anticoagulants. Evacuation of the clot is usually curative. Fever commonly accompanies intraluminal dissection of the aorta.

FAMILIAL MEDITERRANEAN FEVER (See Chap. 278) This diagnosis should be suspected in patients of Armenian or Mediterranean ancestry who have short-lived episodes of fever accompanied by abdominal or pleuritic chest pain, but without evidence for infection or connective tissue disorder.

THERMOREGULATORY DISORDERS These rare disorders include central disturbances of temperature control in patients with CNS dysfunction caused by encephalitis, stroke, or hemorrhage or with unusual congenital defects affecting the hypothalamus. Such patients may have exaggerated responses in temperature during the course of other fever-producing diseases. The diagnosis is made by exclusion; some patients respond to chlorpromazine. Patients with hyperthyroidism, particularly thyroid storm or pheochromocytoma, may have episodic or sustained temperature elevations due to their hypermetabolic state. Patients taking medications that impair parasympathetic function (phenothiazines, tricyclic antidepressants, anti-Parkinsonian drugs) may develop elevated body temperatures in a warm environment; this may predispose to heat stroke (see Chap. 377).

Psychogenic fever FACTITIOUS FEVER Occasionally patients will produce either false elevations in recorded body temperature or self-administer pyrogenic substances. Typical patient groupings range from children wishing to avoid school, medically sophisticated persons (most often women), with more serious psychopathology, or malingerers with drug-seeking behavior. Clues to false elevations are a dissociation between pulse and temperature, fevers greater than 41.1°C (106°F) in adults, and the absence of chills, sweats, or tachycardia. Repeating the temperature measurement under observation or finding rectal temperatures which are substantially lower than oral will usually reveal the nature of the problem. Pyrogenic substances which may be injected include fecal material, milk or other liquids, and bacterial cultures; an inflammatory response will occur at the injection sites.

Psychopathology ranges from "borderline syndromes" to patients with serious self-mutilating behavior; the prognosis is guarded. Others, mostly young girls, falsify their temperatures as a means of asking for psychiatric help and do well with psychotherapy.

HABITUAL HYPERTHERMIA Some patients may have a body temperature range which is slightly above normal limits without apparent associated physical illness. However, if the patient is past middle age, such elevations should be viewed as indicative of organic disease unless proven otherwise. A special problem termed "habitual hyperthermia" is encountered in young females. The patient may have temperatures ranging from 37.2 to 38.0°C (99.0 to 100.5°F) regularly or intermittently for years and also a variety of complaints characteristic of psychoneurosis such as fatigability, insomnia, asthenia, vague aches, and bowel distress. Some of these individuals may have a variation of the "chronic fatigue syndrome" attributed to EBV infection (see Chap. 137). Prolonged study and observation usually fail to reveal evidence of an organic disease. Unfortunately many of these patients go from physician to physician and are subject to a variety of unpleasant, expensive, and even harmful tests, treatments, and operations. The diagnosis of this syndrome can be made with reasonable certainty after a suitable period of observation and study; if the patient can be convinced of its validity a real service will have been rendered.

Patients with FUO who remain undiagnosed These patients divide themselves into several groups. Some have a self-limited, prolonged viral infection that resembles infectious mononucleosis, cytomegalovirus, or hepatitis, but in which the causative agents are not isolated and the serologic findings are not definitive. They recover spontaneously and completely. Others appear to have responded to antibiotics and can be presumed to have had a cryptic bacterial infection. A third group has a steroid-responsive fever which resembles, but is not diagnostic of, immunologically mediated diseases. Some of these patients eventually no longer require steroids for suppression of fever, but some do not stay free of fever or other inflammatory symptoms without steroids. An occasional elderly patient may display a superannuated form of juvenile rheumatoid arthritis (Still's disease).

DIAGNOSTIC PROCEDURES IN FEVER OF UNKNOWN ORIGIN

With so large a number of diagnostic possibilities, it is obvious that no single plan can be outlined for the systematic study of every problem in unexplained fever. In any given patient the history, physical examination, and, most importantly, epidemiologic setting must determine the diagnostic approach. If the features suggest infectious disease, the main dependence will be upon microbiologic methods, while in a person in the "cancer age group" with an obscure febrile disorder, the best chance of an early diagnosis may lie in x-ray studies, scans, and biopsy. Since most infectious diseases are treatable or self-limited these must be excluded first.

History Careful attention to the patient's past history and the chronologic development of symptoms may provide important leads. Places of recent residence, travel, diet, contact with domestic or wild animals and birds, preceding acute infectious diseases such as diarrheal illness or boils, and contact with persons with tuberculosis at any point in life may provide clues to infection. Localizing symptoms may provide a lead to the affected organ system. It is important to query the patient repeatedly. All too often facts of historical importance do not come to light until several interviews have been held.

Physical examination A careful search should be made for skin lesions and for petechial hemorrhages in the ocular fundi, conjunctivae, nail beds, and skin. The lymph nodes should be carefully palpated, with special attention given to the supraclavicular, axillary, and epitrochlear areas. The finding of a heart murmur may be important, particularly if it occurs in diastole. Detection of an abdominal mass may be the first lead to the diagnosis of neoplastic disease. Palpable enlargement of the spleen suggests infection, leukemia, or lymphoma and points away from a diagnosis of solid tumors. Enlargement of the liver and spleen suggests lymphoma, leukemia, chronic infection, or cirrhosis. A large liver without a palpable spleen may point to liver abscess or metastatic cancer. The rectum and the female pelvic organs may reveal masses or abscesses; the testicles may reveal tumor or tuberculosis.

Laboratory tests Patients with FUO are subjected to a large number of laboratory tests, often repeatedly and to excess. The following may be useful guidelines in the use of these tests.

HEMATOLOGY These tests are often abnormal, showing anemia, leukopenia, thrombocytopenia or thrombocytosis, and elevation in the sedimentation rate. They are rarely specific. Blood smears for morphology show many abnormalities but, by virtue of the type of patient who presents with FUO, are rarely diagnostic.

CHEMISTRY Unless specific organ dysfunction is defined, these tests are rarely useful. Tests of liver function can reveal evidence of inflammatory, obstructive, or infiltrative disease, even in the absence of specific symptoms, and are usually indicated.

IMMUNOLOGIC TESTS These are most helpful in the diagnosis of fevers caused by connective tissue disorders or, occasionally, because of secondary immune complex disease or infectious endocarditis.

MICROBIOLOGY In the initial evaluation of prolonged fever, blood cultures are indicated. However, in no instance should more than six blood cultures (which are expensive) be performed on any one patient. Smears and cultures of pus are useful but in sick patients should not delay institution of therapy. Anaerobic cultures of all abscesses should be performed. Mycobacterial cultures continue to be the mainstay in the diagnosis of acid-fast disease. Cultures and special stains or biopsies of suspected tissues are often required to diagnose disseminated fungal infections.

SEROLOGY Serologic testing is useful in Epstein-Barr virus, hepatitis A and B infection, syphilis, Lyme disease, Q fever, and occasionally cytomegalovirus infections and in amebiasis or coccidioidomycosis. Routine febrile agglutinins are rarely helpful but may reveal brucellosis.

SKIN TESTS These are rarely helpful, due to anergy or nonspecificity for acute infection. Many patients with far-advanced neoplasia are anergic. Not all patients with disseminated tuberculosis have positive tuberculin tests. Patients with disseminated histoplasmosis or coccidioidomycosis are usually skin test–negative.

Imaging techniques ROENTGENOGRAMS Chest x-rays and flat abdominal films are the most valuable films in the diagnosis of FUO. Review of earlier films, including those performed at other institutions, often turns up important clues when viewed by a fresh observer. Conversely, there is nothing to be gained by repeating earlier films that are technically satisfactory, provided such films were obtained within a reasonable period of time. Sinus and bone films are often useful. In contrast, gastrointestinal x-rays; intravenous pyelograms; oral intravenous, transhepatic, or retrograde endoscopic cholangiograms; aortograms; and lymphangiograms are helpful only if there are clues that clearly indicate the likelihood of an abnormality in the organ or organ system to be imaged. In many cases, imaging of abdominal and thoracic organs and vessels with CT scan or MRI is preferable to standard radiography.

ULTRASONOGRAPHY This technique is simple and useful to screen for abdominal, renal, retroperitoneal, or pelvic mass lesions. It is probably the method of choice for imaging the gallbladder and bilary tree and can rapidly detect renal obstruction, cardiac valve vegetations, or intracardiac masses.

COMPUTED TOMOGRAPHY SCANS CT scans are very useful in the detection of subphrenic, abdominal, and pelvic abscesses and are the most effective method for imaging the retroperitoneum, which is often the site of the cause of FUO in the form of retroperitoneal lymph nodes, tumors, abscesses, or hematomas. CT scanning is excellent for detecting space-occupying lesions in the liver and is the procedure of choice for suspected intracranial masses. MRI provides the best resolution of tissue planes of differing density and is supplanting CT scanning of the bones, spinal cord, brain, pelvis, and thoracic large vessels or where metal (e.g., surgical clips) creates obscuring artifacts.

RADIONUCLIDE SCANS Ventilation/perfusion lung scans are indicated in suspected pulmonary emboli. Bone scans may detect osseous metastases or osteomyelitis more readily than x-rays. The technetium sulfocolloid liver-spleen scan, while useful in detecting space-occupying lesions of the liver, has been largely replaced by the CT scan. Gallium scanning is subject to many false-positive and false-negative tests and has been overrated. Indium-111 leukocyte scanning may be more reliable in the diagnosis of intraabdominal abscesses, but has also produced false-positive activity in some patients with FUO.

Biopsies Often the best means of definitive diagnosis is a biopsy.

Bone marrow biopsy may be helpful not only in clarifying the histologic nature of the marrow but also for occasional demonstration of other disease processes such as metastatic carcinoma or granulomas and for culture. Bone marrow is one location where blind sampling is productive.

Needle biopsy of the liver, while often abnormal, has a low diagnostic yield. It may be particularly helpful in granulomatous diseases. It rarely yields the diagnosis if there are no abnormalities in liver function tests, ultrasonography, or CT scan.

Biopsies of other tissues that appear abnormal on physical examination or by noninvasive imaging tests are more likely to be helpful in the diagnosis than of tissues that are biopsied blindly. These include biopsies of the lung, muscle, skin, gastrointestinal mucosa, bone, and arteries. The technique of fine-needle aspiration biopsy has made percutaneous approaches safer. Occasionally, "blind biopsies" of muscle or temporal artery will yield abnormalities, but even here tenderness of the affected part makes finding an abnormality much more likely.

Lymph node biopsy is helpful in the diagnosis of many diseases, including the lymphomas, metastatic cancer, tuberculosis, cat-scratch fever, toxoplasmosis, and mycotic infections. Inguinal nodes are notoriously unsatisfactory for biopsy and are too frequently chosen because of their easy accessibility. Axillary, cervical, and supraclavicular nodes are much more likely to yield helpful information, and the node aspirated or excised need not necessarily be large.

Exploratory laparotomy In the past exploratory laparotomy has been advocated as the most definitive diagnostic maneuver in FUO but is valuable only when other investigations, including history, physical examination, noninvasive imaging techniques, and laboratory data point to the abdomen as a possible source of disease. Laparotomies are most helpful in patients with solid tumors, intraabdominal abscesses not amendable to percutaneous biopsy or aspiration, or, rarely, for granulomatous disease or vasculitis. The clues to intraabdominal disease are often subtle, but they are present nonetheless. Blind exploration of the abdomen simply because the diagnosis is obscure is not good practice, and should be discouraged.

Therapeutic trials It is common to give a trial of antibiotics to patients with unidentified febrile disorders. Occasionally, this kind of therapeutic marksmanship is sound, but in general, blind therapy does more harm than good. Undesirable features include drug toxicity, superinfection due to resistant pathogenic bacteria, and interference with accurate diagnosis by cultural methods. Furthermore, a coincidental fall in temperature not due to therapy is likely to be interpreted as response to treatment, with the conclusion that an infectious disease is present. If therapeutic trials are instituted, they should be as specific as possible. Examples are *isoniazid* and *ethambutol* or *rifampin* for tuberculosis; *metronidazole* for hepatic amebiasis; or *aspirin* for rheumatic fever. Relatively few trials with antibiotics will be successful; those with aspirin, NSAIDs, and steroids are more likely to be effective in reducing symptoms, but these drugs should be used with caution and only in patients in whom the likelihood of connective tissue disease is high and in whom granulomas, infection, and cancer have been ruled out as definitively as possible.

Prognosis in FUO The intelligent application of appropriate diagnostic maneuvers should provide the answer in approximately 90 percent of patients with prolonged obscure febrile illness. The mortality rate in patients with FUO is high among elderly patients, particularly since cancer is the most likely cause of the fever in this age group. Fortunately, most of the remaining patients respond to medical or surgical treatment or recover spontaneously. Of those who do come to autopsy (about 10 percent), fewer than half have had potentially curable disease.

A brief philosophy about patients with FUO Many patients are placed in the FUO category because attending physicians overlook, disregard, or reject an obvious clue. This statement implies no malice; it simply means that physicians, being human, are far from perfect. No algorithms or computers are likely to reverse this trend; moreover, even the new technology is not sufficiently sophisticated to sort out the causes of fever in these patients who often present in very atypical fashion.

In order to mitigate these human errors, clinicians have to work harder. This requires repeated histories and physical examinations, frequent chart reviews to look for the "clue" that is there but has not been appreciated, extensive discussion of the problem with colleagues, and last but not least, time spent in quiet contemplation of the clinical enigma. It does not mean yet another barrage of tests, some of which might be painful and all of which are likely to be expensive, or dousing the patient with more drugs, or, in the absence of corroborating data and as a last resort, subjecting the patient to exploratory surgery. Physicians who care for patients with FUO need to observe them, to talk to them, and to think about them. There are no substitutes for these simple clinical principles.

REFERENCES

Pathogenesis of fever

BEUTLER B, CERAMI A: Cachectin: More than a tumor necrosis factor. N Engl J Med 316:379, 1987

DINARELLO CA: Biology of interleukin-1. FASEB J 2:108, 1988

——— et al: New concepts in the pathogenesis of fever. Rev Infect Dis 10:168, 1988

GIRARDIN E et al: Tumor necrosis factor and interleukin-1 in the serum of children with severe infectious purpura. N Engl J Med 319:397, 1988

MICHIE HR et al: Detection of circulating tumor necrosis factor after endotoxin administration. N Engl J Med 318:1481, 1988

Fever of unknown origin

ADUAN RP et al: Factitious fever and self-induced infection: A report of 32 cases and review of the literature. Ann Intern Med 90:230, 1979

DATZ FL, THORNE DA: Gastrointestinal tract radionuclide activity on In-111 labeled leukocyte imaging: Clinical significance in patients with fever of unknown origin. Radiology 160:635, 1986

HALL S et al: The therapeutic impact of temporal artery biopsy. Lancet ii:1217, 1983

——— et al: Takayasu arteritis: A study of 32 North American patients. Medicine 64:89, 1985

LARSON EB: Adult Still's disease. Evolution of a clinical syndrome and diagnosis, treatment and follow-up of 17 patients. Medicine 63:82, 1984

——— et al: Fever of undetermined origin: Diagnosis and follow-up of 105 cases. 1970–1980. Medicine 61:269, 1982

MACKOWICK PA, LEMAISTRE CF: Drug fever: A critical appraisal of conventional concepts. Ann Intern Med 106:728, 1987

MARGILETH D et al: Systemic cat-scratch disease: Report of 23 patients with prolonged or recurrent severe bacterial infection. J Infect Dis 155:390, 1987

MODIE MT et al: Vertebral osteomyelitis: Assessment using MR. Radiology 157:157, 1985

SIMON HB, WOLFF SM: Granulomatous hepatitis and prolonged fever of unknown origin: A study of 13 patients. Medicine 52:1, 1973

WOLFF SM et al: Unusual etiologies of fever and their evaluation. Ann Rev Med 26:277, 1975

Fever: Treatment

CHANG JC, GROSS HM: Utility of naproxen in the differential diagnosis of fever of undetermined origin in patients with cancer. Am J Med 76:597, 1984

section 3 Nervous system dysfunction

21 FAINTNESS, SYNCOPE, AND SEIZURES

JOSEPH B. MARTIN / JERRY RUSKIN[1]

Episodic faintness, light-headedness, and reduced alertness are frequently difficult to distinguish, tending to shade into one another. The difference between faintness and frank syncope is often only quantitative. Types of episodic weakness, such as myasthenia gravis, cataplexy, and familial periodic paralysis, which cause striking reduction of muscular strength but no impairment of consciousness, should be set apart (see Chaps. 366 and 367). Seizures, an important cause of altered consciousness, usually differ from syncope, but in some instances distinguishing the two may be difficult. The features that distinguish seizures from syncope are discussed at the end of this chapter and in Chap. 350.

SYNCOPE AND FAINTNESS

Syncope comprises a generalized weakness of muscles, with loss of postural tone, inability to stand upright, and a loss of consciousness. The term *faintness,* in contrast, refers to lack of strength, with sensation of impending loss of consciousness (*presyncope*). At the beginning of a syncopal attack the patient is nearly always in the upright position, either sitting or standing [the Stokes-Adams attack (see Chap. 184) is exceptional in this respect]. Usually the patient is warned of the impending faint by a sense of "feeling bad." A sense of giddiness and movement or swaying of the floor or surrounding objects ensues. The senses become confused; the patient yawns or gapes, there are spots before the eyes, vision may dim, and the ears may ring. Nausea and sometimes vomiting accompany these symptoms. There is a striking pallor or ashen gray color of the face, and very often the face and body are bathed in cold perspiration. In some patients, a deliberate onset may allow time for protection against injury; in others the occurrence of syncope is sudden and without warning.

The depth and duration of unconsciousness vary. Sometimes the patient is not completely oblivious of the surroundings, or there may be profound coma with complete lack of awareness and of capacity to respond. The patient may remain in this state for seconds to minutes or even as long as half an hour. Usually the patient lies motionless with skeletal muscles relaxed, but a few clonic jerks of the limbs and face may occur shortly after the beginning of the unconsciousness. Sphincter control is usually maintained. The pulse is feeble or cannot be felt; the blood pressure may be low to undetectable; and breathing may be almost imperceptible. Once the patient is in a horizontal position, gravitation no longer hinders the flow of blood to the brain. The strength of the pulse may then improve, color begins to return to the face, breathing becomes quicker and deeper, and consciousness is regained. There is usually an immediate recovery of consciousness. Some patients may, however, be keenly aware of physical weakness, and rising too soon may precipitate another faint. In other patients, particularly those with transient tachyarrhythmias, there may be no residual symptoms following the initial syncope. Headache and drowsiness, which, with mental confusion, are the usual sequelae of a convulsion, do not follow a syncopal attack.

ETIOLOGY The list of causes in Table 21-1 is based on established or assumed physiologic mechanisms. The commoner types of faint are reducible to a few simple mechanisms. Syncope results from a sudden impairment of brain metabolism usually brought about by hypotension with reduction of cerebral blood flow.

Several mechanisms subserve circulatory adjustments to the upright posture. Approximately three-fourths of the systemic blood volume is contained in the venous bed, and any interference with venous return may lead to a reduction in cardiac output. Cerebral blood flow may still be maintained, as long as systemic arterial vasoconstriction

TABLE 21-1 Causes of recurrent weakness, faintness, and disturbances of consciousness

I Circulatory (reduced cerebral blood flow)
- *A* Inadequate vasoconstrictor mechanisms
  - *1* Vasovagal (vasodepressor)
  - *2* Postural hypotension
  - *3* Primary autonomic insufficiency
  - *4* Sympathectomy (pharmacologic, due to antihypertensive medications such as methyldopa and hydralazine, or surgical)
  - *5* Diseases of central and peripheral nervous systems, including autonomic nerves (Chap. 363)
  - *6* Carotid sinus syncope (see also "Bradyarrhythmias," below)
  - *7* Hyperbradykininemia
- *B* Hypovolemia
  - *1* Blood loss—gastrointestinal hemorrhage
  - *2* Addison's disease
- *C* Mechanical reduction of venous return
  - *1* Valsalva maneuver
  - *2* Cough
  - *3* Micturition
  - *4* Atrial myxoma, ball valve thrombus
- *D* Reduced cardiac output
  - *1* Obstruction to left ventricular outflow: aortic stenosis, hypertrophic subaortic stenosis
  - *2* Obstruction to pulmonary flow: pulmonic stenosis, primary pulmonary hypertension, pulmonary embolism
  - *3* Myocardial: massive myocardial infarction with pump failure
  - *4* Pericardial: cardiac tamponade
- *E* Arrhythmias (Chaps. 184 and 185)
  - *1* Bradyarrhythmias
    - *a* Atrioventricular (AV) block (second- and third-degree), with Stokes-Adams attacks
    - *b* Ventricular asystole
    - *c* Sinus bradycardia, sinoatrial block, sinus arrest, sick-sinus syndrome
    - *d* Carotid sinus syncope (see also inadequate vasoconstrictor mechanisms, above)
    - *e* Glossopharyngeal neuralgia (and other painful states)
  - *2* Tachyarrhythmias
    - *a* Episodic ventricular tachycardia with or without associated bradyarrhythmias
    - *b* Supraventricular tachycardia without AV block

II Other causes of weakness and episodic disturbances of consciousness
- *A* Altered state of blood to the brain
  - *1* Hypoxia
  - *2* Anemia
  - *3* Diminished carbon dioxide due to hyperventilation (faintness common, syncope seldom occurs)
  - *4* Hypoglycemia (episodic weakness common, faintness occasional, syncope rare)
- *B* Cerebral
  - *1* Cerebrovascular disturbances (cerebral ischemic attacks, see Chap. 351)
    - *a* Extracranial vascular insufficiency (vertebral-basilar, carotid)
    - *b* Diffuse spasm of cerebral arterioles (hypertensive encephalopathy)
  - *2* Emotional disturbances, anxiety attacks, and hysterical seizures (see Chap. 29)

[1] A revision of the chapter by Raymond D. Adams and Joseph B. Martin in the eleventh edition.

occurs; but when this adjustment fails, serious hypotension with resultant cerebral underperfusion to less than half of normal results in syncope. Normally, the pooling of blood in the lower parts of the body is prevented by (1) pressor reflexes which induce constriction of peripheral arterioles and venules, (2) reflex acceleration of the heart by means of aortic and carotid reflexes, and (3) improvement of venous return to the heart by activity of the muscles of the limbs. Placing a normal person on a tilt table to relax the muscles and tilting upright slightly diminishes cardiac output and allows the blood to accumulate in the legs to a slight degree. This may then be followed by a slight transitory fall in systolic arterial pressure and, in patients with defective vasomotor reflexes, may be a means of producing faints.

TYPES OF SYNCOPE Vasovagal (vasodepressor) syncope This syncope is the common faint that may be experienced by normal persons; it is frequently recurrent and tends to take place during emotional stress (especially in a warm, crowded room), after an injurious, shocking accident, and during pain. Mild blood loss, poor physical condition, prolonged bed rest, anemia, fever, organic heart disease, and fasting are other factors which increase the possibility of fainting in susceptible individuals. A short premonitory phase is characterized by nausea, perspiration, yawning, epigastric distress, hyperpnea, tachypnea, weakness, confusion, tachycardia, and pupillary dilatation. Physiologically, there is first a marked fall in arterial pressure and systemic vascular resistance which is most notable in the skeletal muscular beds. Cardiac output may be within normal limits but fails to exhibit the expected increase which normally occurs with hypotension. Output declines when vagal activity leads to marked bradycardia, replacing tachycardia, resulting in further lowering of arterial pressure and reduction of cerebral perfusion. Assumption of the supine posture with elevation of the legs and removal of the offending stimulus will rapidly restore consciousness. While both components of the abnormal reflex (vasodilatation and bradycardia) are active in most patients, in some individuals one component may predominate, accounting for the range of clinical presentations of this syndrome.

Postural hypotension with syncope This type of syncope affects persons who have a chronic defect in, or variable instability of, vasomotor reflexes. The fall in blood pressure on assumption of upright posture is due to a loss of vasoconstriction reflexes in resistance and capacitance vessels of the lower extremities. Though the character of the syncopal attack differs little from that of the vasovagal or vasodepressor type, the effect of posture is its cardinal feature; sudden arising from a recumbent position or standing still are precipitating circumstances.

Postural syncope tends to occur under the following conditions:

1 In otherwise normal persons who for some unknown reason have defective postural reflexes (this may be familial). In such individuals fainting may occur when they are tilted on a table. Under such circumstances it has been found that the blood pressure at first diminishes slightly and then stabilizes at a lower level. Shortly thereafter, the compensatory reflexes suddenly fail and the arterial pressure falls precipitously.

2 In *primary autonomic insufficiency* and in the *dysautonomias*. At least three syndromes have been delineated:

ACUTE OR SUBACUTE DYSAUTONOMIA. In this disease an otherwise healthy adult or child develops over a period of a few days or weeks a partial or complete paralysis of the parasympathetic and sympathetic nervous systems. Pupillary reflexes are lost, as are lacrimation, salivation, and sweating, and there is impotence, paresis of bladder and bowel musculature, and orthostatic hypotension. The CSF protein is increased. Sensory and motor nerve fibers are demonstrably intact, but nonmedullated autonomic ones have degenerated. Recovery occurs within a few months, possibly hastened by prednisone therapy. The disease is believed to represent a variant of acute idiopathic polyneuritis, akin to Guillain-Barré syndrome.

CHRONIC POSTGANGLIONIC AUTONOMIC INSUFFICIENCY. This is a disease of middle-aged and elderly individuals who gradually develop chronic orthostatic hypotension, sometimes in conjunction with impotence and sphincter disturbances. Upon standing for 5 to 10 min, the blood pressure decreases at least 35 mmHg and the pulse pressure narrows, both without increase in pulse rate, pallor, or nausea. Men are more often affected than women. The condition is relatively benign and seemingly irreversible.

CHRONIC PREGANGLIONIC AUTONOMIC INSUFFICIENCY. In this condition orthostatic hypotension with variable anhidrosis, impotence, and sphincter disturbances is combined with a disorder of the central nervous system. The disorders include (1) tremor, extrapyramidal rigidity, and akinesia (Shy-Drager syndrome); (2) progressive cerebellar degeneration, some instances of which are familial; and (3) a more variable extrapyramidal and cerebellar disorder (striatonigral degeneration). These syndromes lead to disability and often death within a few years. (See Chap. 359.)

The differentiation of the chronic peripheral postganglionic and central preganglionic insufficiency is based on pathologic and pharmacologic evidence. In the postganglionic type, neurons of the sympathetic ganglia degenerate, whereas in the central type, the lateral horn cells of the thoracic spinal cord degenerate. In the postganglionic peripheral type, the resting levels of norepinephrine are subnormal because of failure to release norepinephrine from postganglionic endings, and there is hypersensitivity to injected norepinephrine. In the central type, resting levels of norepinephrine are normal. On standing, unlike the reaction in the normal individual, there is little if any rise in norepinephrine levels in either type. And in both types, the levels of plasma dopamine β-hydroxylase (the enzyme that converts dopamine to norepinephrine) are subnormal.

The distinction between the various types of orthostatic hypotension has therapeutic significance. In the peripheral postganglionic type, the most effective treatment is 9α-fluorohydrocortisone (oral dose 0.1 to 0.2 mg/d) and salt loading to increase blood volume, supplemented by mechanical devices to prevent pooling of blood in the legs and lower trunk (g suit). However, salt together with mineralocorticoids may induce serious supine hypertension, and the dose of the drug must be adjusted for this. For the central preganglionic type, there has been greater success with use of a sympathomimetic amine such as tyramine (which releases norepinephrine from intact postganglionic endings) supplemented by a monoamine oxidase inhibitor (to prevent destruction of the amine), and possibly propranolol. Levodopa has been effective in some cases. In the postganglionic type, judicious use of phenylephrine or ephedrine may be beneficial. Initial reports of the effectiveness of indomethacin in chronic orthostatic hypotension have not been substantiated.

OTHER CAUSES OF POSTURAL SYNCOPE (1) After physical deconditioning, e.g., after prolonged illness with recumbency, especially in elderly individuals with reduced muscle tone. (2) After a sympathectomy that has abolished vasopressor reflexes. (3) In diabetic, alcoholic, and other neuropathies; syringomyelia; and diseases of the nervous system which cause muscular atrophy and paralysis of vasopressor reflexes. The most common form of neurogenic orthostatic hypotension is that which accompanies diseases of the peripheral nervous system. Diabetic polyneuropathy, beriberi, amyloid polyneuropathy, and the Adie syndrome are examples. Usually the orthostatic hypotension is associated with disturbances in sweating, impotence, and sphincter difficulties. Presumably the lesion involves postganglionic, nonmedullated fibers in peripheral nerves. (4) In patients receiving antihypertensive and vasodilator drugs as well as those who may be hypovolemic because of diuretics, excessive sweating, or adrenal insufficiency.

Micturition syncope, a condition usually seen in the elderly during or after urination, particularly after arising from the recumbent position, is probably a special type of postural syncope. It has been suggested that release of intravesicular pressure causes sudden vasodilatation, augmented by standing, and that vagally mediated bradycardia is a contributory factor.

Hyperbradykininemia Deficient kinin-inactivating enzymes with apparently normal sympathetic function may result in symptoms of faintness or syncope on assumption of upright posture. Hyperbradykininemia causes arteriolar and venular dilatation giving rise to postural hypotension and syncope with tachycardia. The pathophysiology of this condition remains uncertain. Treatment with beta-receptor antagonists has been beneficial.

Syncope of cardiac origin (cardiac syncope) Cardiac syncope results from a sudden reduction in cardiac output, caused most commonly by a cardiac arrhythmia. In normal individuals slow ventricular rates, but above 35 to 40 beats per minute, and fast ones not exceeding 180 beats per minute do not reduce cerebral blood flow, especially if the person is in the supine position. However, changes in pulse rate outside these limits may impair cerebral circulation and function. Upright posture, cerebrovascular disease, anemia, and coronary, myocardial, or valvular disease all reduce the tolerance to alterations in rate.

High-degree atrioventricular block is one of the commonest arrhythmias that leads to fainting, and syncopal episodes associated with this arrhythmia are known as the Stokes-Adams-Morgagni syndrome. The etiology of disturbances in atrioventricular conduction is considered elsewhere (Chap. 184), but in patients with these attacks the block may be persistent or intermittent and is often preceded or followed by disturbed conduction in one or more of the three fascicles through which the ventricles are normally activated. When the block is high-grade or complete and the pacemaker below the block fails to function, syncope occurs. Stokes-Adams attacks occur usually without more than a momentary sense of weakness, the patient suddenly losing consciousness. After cardiac standstill of more than several seconds, the patient turns pale, falls unconscious, and, as in other types of fainting, may exhibit a few clonic jerks. With longer periods of asystole, the ashen gray pallor gives way to cyanosis, stertorous breathing, fixed pupils, incontinence, and bilateral Babinski signs. While recovery following a Stokes-Adams attack is usually prompt and complete, prolonged confusion and neurologic signs due to cerebral ischemia may occur in some patients, and permanent impairment of mental function may occasionally result, although focal neurologic signs are rare. Cardiac faints of this type may recur several times a day. Commonly the heart block is transitory, and the electrocardiogram taken later may not show any arrhythmia. In some patients, ventricular tachycardia or fibrillation may follow a period of asystole, resulting in syncope or sudden death.

Disorders of sinus node automaticity or sinoatrial conduction may also result in asystole or bradycardia of sufficient severity to cause presyncope or syncope. This disorder is most frequently detected with ambulatory electrocardiographic monitoring. Findings consistent with a diagnosis of sinus node dysfunction include symptomatic sinus pauses (>3 s) resulting from sinus arrest or sinoatrial block and severe unexplained sinus bradycardia (<40 beats per minute). The *bradycardia-tachycardia syndrome* is a common form of sinus node dysfunction in which syncope generally occurs as a result of marked sinus pauses following termination of paroxysmal supraventricular tachycardia. In occasional patients with syncope and suspected sinus node dysfunction in whom the diagnosis is not established by ambulatory ECG recording, electrophysiologic testing may be helpful in unmasking diagnostic abnormalities.

Recurrent paroxysmal tachyarrhythmias may also cause presyncope and syncope as a result of a sudden reduction in cardiac output. The magnitude of tachycardia-induced hypotension is dependent upon the interaction of several variables including the rate and mechanism of the tachycardia, the type and severity of underlying cardiac disease, the patient's posture and activity level at the onset of the tachycardia, sensitivity of the tachycardia to catecholamines, and the integrity of compensatory autonomic reflexes. Supraventricular tachyarrhythmias are not commonly associated with syncope. However, even in the absence of structural heart disease, the combination of extremely high heart rates and loss of atrial transport may impair cardiac filling and output sufficiently to cause loss of consciousness. These tachycardias result most commonly from the occurrence of paroxysmal atrial flutter, atrial fibrillation, or reentry involving the atrioventricular node or accessory pathways which bypass part or all of the atrioventricular conduction system. Patients with the Wolff-Parkinson-White syndrome are susceptible to several forms of supraventricular tachycardia, the most dangerous of which is atrial fibrillation with rapid antegrade conduction to the ventricles over an accessory atrioventricular connection which may result in syncope and, in rare instances, sudden death. When supraventricular tachycardia is suspected as a cause of syncope, electrophysiologic testing is indicated to define the mechanism and pathway of the tachycardia and to facilitate the selection of an effective antiarrhythmic intervention (see also Chap. 184).

Paroxysmal ventricular tachycardia is a relatively common cause of syncope, particularly in patients with structural heart disease. Typically, the tachycardias are rapid and associated with abrupt loss of consciousness without premonitory symptoms. More often than not, the patient is unaware of palpitations, and recovery following an episode is usually prompt and complete without residual neurologic or cardiac sequelae. The occurrence of unexplained syncope in a patient with structural heart disease is a potentially ominous finding and merits careful evaluation. The presence of pathologic Q waves on the electrocardiogram indicative of a prior transmural myocardial infarction is strongly associated with ventricular tachycardia as a cause of syncope in patients with ischemic heart disease. Other forms of heart disease such as hypertrophic and dilated cardiomyopathy, right ventricular dysplasia, and the long-QT-interval syndromes are also frequently associated with paroxysmal ventricular tachycardia and syncope.

In another form of cardiac syncope the heart block is reflexive and is due to irritation of the vagus nerves. Examples of this phenomenon have been observed in patients with esophageal diverticula, mediastinal tumors, gallbladder disease, carotid sinus disease, glossopharyngeal neuralgia, and pleural and pulmonary irritation. However, in these conditions reflex bradycardia is more commonly of the sinoatrial than the atrioventricular type.

Cardiac syncope may also result from *acute massive myocardial infarction*, particularly when associated with cardiogenic shock. *Aortic stenosis* often sets the stage for exertional syncope, most commonly by limiting cardiac output in the face of peripheral vasodilatation, but sometimes during exertion, with resultant myocardial and cerebral ischemia and occasionally arrhythmias. *Idiopathic hypertrophic subaortic stenosis* may also lead to exertional syncope, because of intensified obstruction and/or ventricular arrhythmias (Chap. 192). In *primary pulmonary hypertension* a relatively fixed cardiac output and bouts of acute right ventricular failure may be associated with syncope (Chap. 191). However, vagal reflexes may be involved in this condition as well as in the syncope that occurs with *pulmonary embolism*. Ball valve thrombus in the left atrium, left atrial myxoma, or thrombosis or malfunction of a prosthetic valve may produce sudden mechanical obstruction of the circulation and syncope. *Tetralogy of Fallot* is the congenital cardiac malformation most commonly responsible for syncope. In this condition systemic vasodilatation, perhaps associated with infundibular spasm, greatly increases the right-to-left shunt and produces arterial hypoxia, which leads to syncope (Chap. 186).

Carotid sinus syncope The carotid sinus is normally sensitive to stretch and gives rise to sensory impulses carried via the nerve of Hering, a branch of the glossopharyngeal nerve, to the medulla oblongata. Massage of one or both of the carotid sinuses, particularly in elderly persons, causes (1) a reflex cardiac slowing (sinus bradycardia, sinus arrest, or even atrioventricular block), the so-called vagal type of response, and (2) a fall of arterial pressure without cardiac slowing, the so-called depressor type of response. Both types of carotid sinus response may coexist.

Syncope due to carotid sinus sensitivity may be initiated by turning of the head to one side, by a tight collar, or, as in a few reported cases, by shaving over the region of the sinus. Spontaneous attacks may also occur. The attack nearly always begins when the patient is in an upright position, usually when standing. The period of unconsciousness seldom lasts longer than a few minutes. Full consciousness is regained immediately. Most reported cases have been in men. In a patient displaying faintness on compression of one carotid sinus, it is important to distinguish between the benign disorder (hypersensitivity of one carotid sinus) and a much more serious condition—atheromatous narrowing of the opposite carotid or of the basilar artery (see Chap. 351).

Other forms of vasovagal syncope have been described. Exceptionally intense pain of visceral origin may inhibit cardiac action through vagal stimulation, e.g., cardiac standstill during an attack of gallbladder colic, a lesion of the esophagus or mediastinum, bronchoscopy, pleural or peritoneal taps, intense vertigo from labyrinthine or vestibular disease, and needling of body cavities. Occasionally, a patient with a severe migraine attack will sustain a syncopal episode.

Vagal and glossopharyngeal neuralgia Occasionally this induces a reflex type of fainting. Again the sequence is always pain, then syncope; in this instance the pain is localized to the base of the tongue, pharynx or larynx, tonsillar area, and ear. It may be triggered by pressure at these sites. Section of the appropriate branches of the ninth or tenth cranial nerve relieves the condition. The cardiovascular effects are attributable to excitation of the dorsal motor nucleus of the vagus via collateral fibers from the nucleus of the tractus solitarius.

Tussive syncope (laryngeal vertigo) This is a rare condition that results from a paroxysm of coughing, usually in men with chronic bronchitis. After hard coughing the patient suddenly becomes weak and loses consciousness momentarily. The intrathoracic pressure becomes elevated and interferes with the venous return to the heart, as does the Valsalva maneuver (exhaling against a closed glottis).

Syncope associated with cerebrovascular disease This is usually caused by partial or complete occlusion of the large arteries in the neck. Physical activity may then critically reduce blood flow to the upper part of the brainstem, causing abrupt loss of consciousness (see Chap. 351).

PATHOPHYSIOLOGY OF SYNCOPE The loss of consciousness in each type of syncope is caused by reduction of oxygenation to those parts of the brain which subserve consciousness. There are demonstrable reductions in cerebral blood flow, cerebral oxygen utilization, and cerebrovascular resistance. If the ischemia lasts only a few minutes, there are no lasting effects on the brain. Prolonged ischemia may result in necrosis of brain tissue in the border zones of perfusion between the vascular territories of the major cerebral arteries.

In a patient with faintness or syncope attended by bradycardia, one has to distinguish that due to failure of neurogenic reflexes from that due to a cardiogenic (Stokes-Adams) attack. The electrocardiogram is decisive, but even without it, the Stokes-Adams attacks can be recognized clinically by their longer duration, by the greater constancy of the slow heart rate, by the presence of audible sounds synchronous with atrial contractions, by atrial contraction (A) waves in the jugular venous pulse, and by marked variation in intensity of the first sound, despite the regular rhythm (Chap. 184).

DIFFERENTIAL DIAGNOSIS OF CONDITIONS INVOLVING EPISODIC WEAKNESS AND FAINTNESS BUT NOT SYNCOPE

Anxiety attacks and the hyperventilation syndrome These symptoms are discussed in Chaps. 29 and 368. The giddiness of anxiety is frequently interpreted as a feeling of faintness without actual loss of consciousness. Such symptoms are not accompanied by facial pallor and are not relieved by recumbency. The diagnosis is made on the basis of the associated symptoms, and part of the attack can be reproduced by hyperventilation. Two of the mechanisms known to be involved in the attacks are reduction in carbon dioxide as the result of hyperventilation and the release of epinephrine. Hyperventilation results in hypocapnia, alkalosis, increased cerebrovascular resistance, and decreased cerebral blood flow.

Hypoglycemia When severe, hypoglycemia is usually traceable to a serious disease, such as a tumor of the islets of Langerhans or advanced adrenal, pituitary, or hepatic disease, or to excessive administration of insulin. The clinical picture is one of confusion or even a loss of consciousness. When mild, as is usually the case, hypoglycemia is often of the reactive type (Chap. 320), occurring 2 to 5 h after eating, and is not usually associated with a disturbance of consciousness. The diagnosis depends on the history and the documentation of reduced blood sugar during an attack.

Acute hemorrhage Acute hemorrhage, usually within the gastrointestinal tract, is an occasional cause of syncope. In the absence of pain and hematemesis the cause of the weakness, faintness, or even unconsciousness may remain obscure until the passage of a black stool.

Cerebral transient ischemic attacks Such attacks occur in some patients with arteriosclerotic narrowings or occlusion of the major arteries of the brain. The main symptoms vary from patient to patient and include dim vision, hemiparesis or sudden drop attacks, numbness of one side of the body, dizziness, and thick speech. In any one patient all attacks are of identical type and indicate a temporary deficit of function in a certain region of the brain due to inadequate circulation (see Chap. 351).

Hysterical fainting Fainting usually occurs under dramatic circumstances. The attack is unattended by any outward display of anxiety. The evident lack of change in pulse and blood pressure or color of the skin and mucous membranes distinguishes it from the vasodepressor faint. The diagnosis is based on the bizarre nature of the attack in a person who exhibits the general personality and behavioral characteristics of the hysteric.

Type of onset When the attack begins over the period of a few seconds, carotid sinus syncope, postural hypotension, sudden atrioventricular block, asystole, or ventricular tachycardia is likely. When the symptoms develop gradually during a period of several minutes, hyperventilation or hypoglycemia should be considered. Onset of syncope during or immediately after exertion suggests aortic stenosis, idiopathic hypertrophic subaortic stenosis or excessive bradycardia, and, in elderly subjects, postural hypotension. Exertional syncope is seen occasionally in persons with aortic insufficiency and with severe occlusive disease of cerebral arteries. In patients with ventricular standstill or ventricular fibrillation, loss of consciousness occurs several seconds later, followed rapidly by cessation of electroencephalographic activity and then often by brief clonic muscle contractions.

Position at onset of attack Epilepsy and syncopal attacks due to hypoglycemia, hyperventilation, or heart block are likely to be independent of posture. Faintness associated with a decline in blood pressure (including carotid sinus attacks) and with ectopic tachycardia usually occurs only in the sitting or standing position, whereas faintness resulting from orthostatic hypotension is apt to set in shortly after change from the recumbent to the standing position.

Associated symptoms Symptoms such as palpitation may be present when the attack is due to anxiety or hyperventilation, to ectopic tachycardia, or to hypoglycemia. Numbness and tingling in the hands and face are frequent accompaniments of hyperventilation. Genuine convulsions during the attack may occasionally occur with heart block, asystole, or ventricular tachycardia. When *duration of attack* is very brief, i.e., a few seconds to a few minutes, carotid sinus syncope or one of the several forms of postural hypotension is most likely. A duration of more than a few minutes but less than an hour suggests hypoglycemia or hyperventilation.

SPECIAL METHODS OF EXAMINATION In many patients who complain of recurrent weakness or syncope but who do not have a spontaneous attack while under observation, an attempt to reproduce attacks is of great assistance in diagnosis.

When hyperventilation is accompanied by faintness, the pattern of symptoms can be reproduced readily by having the subject breathe rapidly and deeply for 2 to 3 min. This test is often of therapeutic value also, because the underlying anxiety tends to be lessened when the patient learns that the symptoms can be produced and alleviated at will simply by controlling breathing.

Among other conditions in which the diagnosis is commonly clarified by reproducing the attacks are carotid sinus hypersensitivity (massage of one or the other carotid sinus), orthostatic hypotension and orthostatic tachycardia (observations of pulse rate, blood pressure, and symptoms in the recumbent and standing positions), and tussive syncope (by inducing the Valsalva maneuver). In all these instances the crucial point is not whether symptoms are produced (the procedures mentioned frequently induce symptoms in healthy persons) but whether the exact pattern of symptoms that occurs in the spontaneous attacks is reproduced in the artificial ones. Continuous ambulatory electrocardiographic monitoring may be extremely useful in identifying an arrhythmia responsible for the syncopal episode, particularly in patients with frequently recurring symptoms. Monitoring is most helpful if it shows that the syncopal episode is characterized by a bout of asystole, extreme bradycardia, or tachyarrhythmia.

In cases of recurrent syncope of unknown cause in which ambulatory ECG monitoring is unrevealing, the use of intracardiac electrophysiologic techniques with programmed stimulation can be helpful in detecting cardiac rhythm abnormalities and in establishing effective treatment. During stimulation, up to two-thirds of such patients can be shown to have rapid ventricular tachycardia, His bundle conduction delays, atrial flutter, sick-sinus syndrome, or hypervagotonia. The technique is particularly useful in patients with ischemic heart disease and prior myocardial infarction, a common clinical setting for recurrent ventricular tachycardia. The diagnostic yield of electrophysiologic testing is lower with patients with non-ischemic heart disease and patients with structurally normal hearts than with patients with ischemic heart disease. Recently the signal-averaged surface electrocardiogram has proved to be useful in identifying patients with unexplained syncope who are likely to have ventricular tachycardia induced by electrophysiologic study.

Head-up tilt testing is a useful provocative technique for the diagnosis of vasodepressor syncope. Upright tilt to a maximum of 60 to 70° usually precipitates symptomatic hypotension or syncope within 10 to 30 min in patients with this syndrome. In normal subjects, passive tilting to 60° causes a small decrease in systolic blood pressure and an increase in diastolic blood pressure and heart rate. Recently, tilt testing has been used in conjunction with electrophysiologic testing to assess the efficacy of prophylactic pacing in selected patients with vasodepressor syncope and to evaluate the impact of posture on the hemodynamic consequences of some tachyarrhythmias.

The electroencephalogram may be helpful in differentiating syncope from seizures. In the interval between epileptic seizures it may show some degree of abnormality in 40 to 80 percent of cases. In the interval between syncopal attacks it should be normal.

TREATMENT In most instances fainting is relatively benign. In dealing with patients who have fainted, the physician should think first of those causes of fainting that constitute a therapeutic emergency. Among them are massive internal hemorrhage and myocardial infarction, which may be painless, and cardiac arrhythmias. In elderly persons a sudden faint, without obvious cause, should arouse the suspicion of complete heart block or a tachyarrhythmia, even though all findings are negative when the patient is seen.

Patients seen during the preliminary stages of fainting or after they have lost consciousness should be placed in a position which permits maximal cerebral blood flow, i.e., with head lowered between the knees, if sitting, or in the supine position. All tight clothing and other constrictions should be loosened and the head turned so that the tongue does not fall back into the throat, blocking the airway. Peripheral irritation, such as sprinkling or dashing cold water on the face and neck or the application of cold moist towels, is helpful. If the temperature is subnormal, the body should be covered with a warm blanket. Since emesis is frequent, aspiration should be prevented. The head should be turned to the side and nothing given by mouth until the patient has regained consciousness. Patients should not be permitted to rise until the sense of physical weakness has passed and should be watched carefully for a few minutes after rising.

The *prevention* of fainting depends on the mechanisms involved. In the usual vasovagal faint of adolescents, which tends to occur in periods of emotional excitement, fatigue, hunger, etc., it is enough to advise the patient to avoid such circumstances. In postural hypotension, patients should be cautioned against arising suddenly from bed. Instead, they should first exercise their legs for a few seconds, then sit on the edge of the bed and make sure they are not light-headed or dizzy before starting to walk. Sleeping with the headposts of the bed elevated on wooden blocks 8 to 12 in high and wearing a snug elastic abdominal binder and elastic stockings are often helpful. Drugs of the ephedrine group may be useful if they do not cause insomnia. If there are no contraindications, a high intake of sodium chloride, which expands the extracellular fluid volume, may be beneficial.

In the syndrome of chronic orthostatic hypotension, special mineralocorticoid preparations (fludrocortisone acetate tablets, 0.1 to 0.2 mg/d in divided doses) have given relief in some cases. Binding of the legs (g suit) and sleeping with head and shoulders elevated are helpful.

The treatment of carotid sinus syncope involves first of all instructing the patient in measures that minimize the hazards of a fall (see below). Loose collars should be worn, and the patient should learn to turn the whole body, rather than the head alone, when looking to one side. Atropine or the ephedrine group of drugs should be used, respectively, in patients with pronounced bradycardia or hypotension during attacks. If atropine is not successful, a demand pacemaker should be inserted into the right ventricle. Radiation or surgical denervation of the carotid sinus has apparently yielded favorable results in some patients, but it is rarely necessary. Once it has been concluded that the attacks are due to a narrowing of major cerebral arteries, some of the surgical measures discussed in Chap. 351 must be considered.

The treatment of the various cardiac arrhythmias which may induce syncope is discussed in Chap. 184. The treatment of hypoglycemia is found in Chap. 320.

The chief hazard of a faint in most elderly persons is not the underlying disease but fracture or other trauma due to the fall. Therefore, patients subject to recurrent syncope should cover the bathroom floor and bathtub with rubber mats and should have as much of their home carpeted as is feasible. Especially important is the floor space between the bed and the bathroom, because faints are common in elderly persons when walking from bed to toilet. Outdoor walking should be on soft ground rather than hard surfaces, and the patient should avoid standing still, which is more likely than walking to induce an attack.

SEIZURES

A brain seizure or convulsion is defined as an abrupt alteration in cortical electrical activity manifested clinically by a change in consciousness or by a motor, sensory, or behavioral symptom. Seizures, which may be due to a variety of causes, become important in the differential diagnosis of syncope when the episode occurs with minimal or no warning and results in only a brief loss of consciousness. *Epilepsy* (discussed in Chap. 350) is the term used to describe recurrent seizures present over months or years, often with a stereotyped clinical pattern.

CLINICAL CHARACTERISTICS OF SEIZURES A detailed account of the types of seizures, of their pathophysiology, and of their treatment is found in Chap. 350. The purpose here is to recount briefly the varieties of seizures that occur (Table 21-2), and to outline their clinical presentation, particularly with respect to their distinction from syncope. A single seizure may occur during the course of many medical illnesses; its importance derives from the fact that it signifies involvement of the central nervous system by the disease process.

Partial seizures (focal seizures) The appearance of focal motor or sensory manifestations provides clinical documentation of the localization of the cerebral lesion. Deviation of the eyes and head to

TABLE 21-2 Classification of seizures

I Partial or focal seizures
- *A* Simple partial seizures (with motor, sensory, autonomic, or psychic signs)
- *B* Complex partial seizures (psychomotor or temporal lobe seizures)
- *C* Secondary generalized partial seizures

II Primary generalized seizures
- *A* Tonic clonic (grand mal)
- *B* Absence (petit mal)
- *C* Myoclonic
- *D* Atonic or akinetic

one side (aversive seizure) usually points to an irritative focus in the opposite prefrontal region. A Jacksonian seizure begins as a clonic movement in one portion of the body, often the thumb, the corner of the mouth, or the great toe, and spreads to adjacent muscular groups over a few seconds or minutes. The seizure may progress to involve the entire side or become generalized with attendant loss of consciousness. Jacksonian seizures almost always are accompanied by an abnormal interictal EEG.

Complex partial seizures (temporal lobe or psychomotor seizures) These differ from generalized motor seizures by (1) the frequent occurrence of an aura that arises from discharges in the autonomic, visceral, and olfactory portions of the temporal lobe and limbic system; and (2) the loss of awareness or contact with the environment, often associated with behavioral or complex motor movements for which the patient is amnesic after the attack. Subjective experiences of the aura include hallucinations (olfactory, gustatory, visual, or auditory), illusions (spatial distortions, shrinkage, or angulation), aberrations in cognition (déjà vu, a sense of familiarity; jamais vu, a sense of unfamiliarity; or recurrent memory), and affective changes (anxiety, fear, and, very rarely, rage). The seizure may terminate with only the subjective component or may progress to the motor phase which is often evident by repetitive motor acts like smacking the lips, swallowing, undressing, and incoherent or dysphasic speech.

The abrupt onset of complex partial seizures often indicates a disorder of the temporal lobe and its connection to the limbic system. Complete investigation in search of the cause is indicated.

Tonic-clonic (grand mal) seizure The abrupt presentation, without warning, of a generalized motor seizure is one of the commonest indications of involvement of the cerebral cortex by a disease process. Grand mal seizures usually begin with opening of the eyes and mouth, flexion and abduction of the arms, and extension of the legs. The *tonic* phase of the seizure is often heralded by contraction of the respiratory muscles resulting in a vocalization. These motor signs are followed by closure of the jaw, often with laceration of the tongue, respiratory arrest with plethora and cyanosis, and urinary, or less commonly, fecal incontinence. The tonic phase of the seizure, which usually persists for only 15 to 30 s, is followed immediately by the *clonic* phase, characterized by violent rhythmic muscular contractions affecting the whole body including the muscles of respiration. Eye movements, facial grimacing, and persistence of respiratory apnea are evident. The clonic movements subside in amplitude and frequency, and the seizure terminates, usually within 1 to 2 min. Normal respiration resumes and the patient falls asleep; arousal may occur in a few minutes but lethargy, fatigue, and postseizure (postictal) confusion are common and may persist for several hours. Postictal headache is also common.

The generalized seizure occurring in the course of a major medical illness signifies involvement of the central nervous system by the disorder and requires careful assessment and investigation. Such a seizure may accompany high fever, hyponatremia, metabolic acidosis, alcohol or drug withdrawal, and renal or liver failure, indicating the presence of a *metabolic encephalopathy*, without requiring the postulation of another separate neurologic illness. The determination that a metabolic encephalopathy may be responsible is dependent upon documentation of the systemic illness and careful attention to the exclusion of an additional infectious, vascular, or neoplastic lesion in the nervous system. Central nervous system evaluation should include a careful history, a detailed neurologic examination searching for focal neurologic deficit, and, in many cases, electroencephalography and computed tomography (CT) scan. If infection is suspected, an examination of the cerebrospinal fluid is mandatory. Recurrent seizures (status epilepticus) indicate a serious compromise of cerebral cortical function and require vigorous treatment to prevent hypoxic damage to the brain and, following termination of the seizures, a thorough investigation of the cause.

An isolated generalized seizure occurring in an otherwise healthy, asymptomatic patient when observed by family or other bystanders is not difficult to distinguish from syncope. More difficult to assess is the circumstance of sudden loss of consciousness occurring without warning and unwitnessed by an observer or an akinetic "drop-seizure" (atypical petit mal). The latter may be indistinguishable from syncope. Postictal confusion or drowsiness, injury such as laceration of the tongue, urinary or fecal incontinence, or muscle soreness suggests that a convulsion has occurred. One common clinical presentation is the sudden occurrence of a brief clonic seizure during a minor surgical or dental procedure. The patient is usually in a seated position and the episode is considered to be due to cerebral ischemia associated with systemic hypotension and bradycardia accompanying vasovagal syncope. There are usually only two or three clonic movements, without a prior tonic phase, and recovery is rapid without postictal symptoms. Such patients should have a neurologic examination and an EEG and, if these are normal, be treated with reassurance and not given anticonvulsants. There is no evidence to indicate an underlying cerebral lesion in such patients.

Generalized seizures may be preceded by a specific warning or *aura*, and attention to these symptoms may be important in aiding in the localization of the seizure focus and can assist in distinguishing the episode from syncope. Tingling or numbness points to involvement of the parietal lobe, and visual or auditory sensations suggest occipitotemporal localization. More complex psychological and cognitive sensations may accompany temporal lobe seizures and also transient cerebral ischemic attacks (see Chap. 351), but in the latter symptoms usually persist for many minutes or hours.

Absence (petit mal) seizures Absence seizures, in contrast to grand mal, are noted for their brevity and for the degree of loss of awareness accompanied by minimal motor manifestations. They are abrupt in onset and are often evident only by a stare or cessation of ongoing behavior; they may be accompanied by fluttering of the eyelids or by a few facial twitches. Full recovery occurs in 5 to 10 s, and the episode may go unnoticed by the patient, the family, or the teacher. Loss of postural tone (atonic or akinetic seizure) with falling is uncommon but when present requires distinction from syncope. The EEG is diagnostic in such cases, consisting of three-per-second spike and wave discharges. This condition, which indicates a specific generalized disorder of cerebral electrical activity, is responsive to specific drug treatments (see Chap. 350).

DIFFERENTIAL DIAGNOSIS OF SEIZURES AND SYNCOPE Syncope must be distinguished from disturbances of cerebral function, caused by a seizure. A seizure may occur day or night, regardless of the position of the patient; syncope rarely appears when the patient is recumbent, the only common exception being the Stokes-Adams attack. The patient's color may not change in seizures, though there may be cyanosis; pallor is an early and invariable finding in all types of syncope, except chronic orthostatic hypotension and hysteria, and it precedes unconsciousness. Seizures are often heralded by an aura, which is caused by a focal seizure discharge and hence has brain localizing significance. It is usually followed by rapid return to normal or by loss of consciousness. The onset of syncope is usually more deliberate and without aura. Injury from falling is frequent in a seizure and rare in syncope, for the reason that only in seizures are protective reflexes abolished instantaneously. Tonic-convulsive movements with upturning eyes are a feature of seizures and usually do not occur with syncope, although, as stated above, brief tonic clonic seizure-like activity can accompany fainting episodes. The period of unconsciousness tends to be longer in seizures than in syncope. Urinary incontinence is frequent in seizures and rare in syncope. The return of consciousness is prompt in syncope, slow after a seizure. Mental confusion, headache, and drowsiness are common sequelae of seizures; physical weakness with a clear sensorium characterizes the postsyncopal state. Repeated spells of unconsciousness in a young person at a rate of several per day or month are more suggestive of epilepsy than of syncope. No one of these points will absolutely differentiate a seizure from syncope, but taken as a group and supplemented by electroencephalograms, they provide a means of distinguishing the two conditions.

REFERENCES

ALMQUIST A et al: Provocation of bradycardia and hypotension by isoproterenol and upright posture in patients with unexplained syncope. N Engl J Med 320:346, 1989

CHEN MY et al: Cardiac electrophysiologic and hemodynamic correlates of neurally mediated syncope. Am J Cardiol 63:66, 1989

DAY SC: et al: Evaluation and outcome of emergency room patients with transient loss of consciousness. Am J Med 73:15, 1982

DELGADO-ESCUETA AV et al: The treatable epilepsies (2 parts). N Engl J Med 308:1508 and 1576, 1983

DIMARCO JP et al: Approach to the patient with syncope of unknown cause. Mod Concepts Cardiovasc Dis 52:11, 1983

EAGLE KA et al: Evaluation of prognostic classifications for patients with syncope. Am J Med 79:455, 1985

ECTOR H et al: Bradycardia, ventricular pauses, syncope, and sports. Lancet 1:591, 1984

EWING DJ et al: The natural history of diabetic autonomic neuropathy. Q J Med 49:95, 1980

HICKLER R: Fainting, in *Signs and Symptoms,* 6th ed, RS Blacklow (ed). Philadelphia, Lippincott, 1977, chap 33

JOHNSON RH, SPAULDING JMK: *Disorders of the Autonomic Nervous System.* Philadelphia, Davis, 1974

KAPOOR WN et al: Diagnostic and prognostic implications of recurrences in patients with syncope. Am J Med 83:700, 1987

——— et al: A prospective evaluation and follow-up of patients with syncope. N Engl J Med 309:197, 1983

KENNY RA et al: Head-up tilt: A useful test for investigating unexplained syncope. Lancet II:1352, 1986

LEE JE et al: Episodic unconsciousness, in *Diagnostic Approaches to Presenting Syndromes,* JA Barondess (ed). Baltimore, Williams & Wilkins, 1971, pp 133–167

MCLEOD JG, TUCK RR: Disorders of the autonomic nervous system. 1. Pathophysiology and clinical features. Ann Neurol 21:419, 1987

———, ———: Disorders of the autonomic nervous system. 2. Investigation and treatment. Ann Neurol 21:519, 1987

POLINSKY RJ et al: Pharmacologic distinction of different orthostatic hypotension syndromes. Neurology 31:1, 1981

RICHARDS AM et al: Syncope in aortic valvular stenosis. Lancet 1:1113, 1984

SILVERSTEIN MD et al: Patients with syncope admitted to medical intensive care units. JAMA 248:1185, 1982

STREETER DHP et al: Hyperbradykininism: A new orthostatic syndrome. Lancet 2:1048, 1972

SUTHERLAND JM, EADIE MJ: *The Epilepsies,* 3d ed. Edinburgh, Churchill Livingstone, 1980

WEISSLER AM, WARREN, JV: Syncope and shock, in *The Heart,* 4th ed, JW Hurst et al (eds). New York, McGraw-Hill, 1978, p 705

WINTERS SL et al: Signal averaging of the surface QRS complex predicts inducibility of ventricular tachycardia in patients with syncope of unknown origin: A prospective study. J Am Coll Cardiol 10:775, 1987

WRIGHT KE JR, MCINTOSH MD: Syncope: Review of pathophysiological mechanisms. Prog Cardiovasc Dis 13:580, 1971

YOUNG RR et al: Pure pandysautonomia with recovery. Description and discussion of diagnostic criteria. Brain 98:613, 1975

22 DIZZINESS AND VERTIGO

ROBERT B. DAROFF

Dizziness is a common and often vexing symptom. Patients use the term to encompass a variety of sensations including those that seem semantically appropriate (e.g., lightheadedness, fainting, spinning, giddiness, etc.) and those that are seemingly inappropriate, such as confusion, blurred vision, headache, tingling, "walking on cotton," etc. Moreover, some patients with gait disturbances, and no abnormal cephalic sensations, will describe their problem as "dizziness." A careful history is necessary to determine exactly what a patient who states, "Doctor, I'm dizzy," is experiencing.

After eliminating misleading symptoms such as confusion, "dizziness" usually means either *faintness* (analogous to the feelings that precede syncope) or *vertigo* (an illusory or hallucinatory sense of environmental or self-movement). In other instances, neither of these terms accurately describes a patient's symptoms, and the explanation may only become apparent when the neurologic examination reveals spasticity, parkinsonism, or other ambulation disturbances as the cause of the complaint. Operationally, dizziness is classified into four categories: (1) faintness, (2) vertigo, (3) miscellaneous head sensations, and (4) gait disturbances.

FAINTNESS Fainting (syncope) is a loss of consciousness secondary to cerebral ischemia, more specifically ischemia to the brainstem (see Chap. 21). Prior to the actual faint, there are often prodromal symptoms (*faintness*) reflecting ischemia to a degree insufficient to impair consciousness. The sequence of symptoms is reasonably stereotyped and includes increasing lightheadedness, visual blurring proceeding to blindness, and heaviness in the lower limbs progressing to postural sway. The symptoms increase in severity until consciousness is lost or the ischemia is corrected, often by assumption of the recumbent position. True vertigo almost never occurs during the presyncopal state.

The causes of faintness are described in Chap. 21 and include the multiple etiologies of decreased cardiac output, postural (orthostatic) hypotension, and mimics such as vertebrobasilar insufficiency and seizures.

VERTIGO Vertigo is a hallucination of self- or environmental movement, most commonly a feeling of spinning, usually due to a disturbance in the vestibular system. The end organs of this system, situated in the bony labyrinths of the inner ears, consist of the three semicircular canals and the otolithic apparatus (utricle and saccule) on each side. The canals transduce angular acceleration while the otoliths transduce linear acceleration and static gravitational forces, the latter providing a sense of head position in space. The neural output of the end organs is conveyed to the vestibular nuclei in the brainstem via the eighth cranial nerves. The principal projections from the vestibular nuclei are to the nuclei of cranial nerves III, IV, and VI, the spinal cord, cerebral cortex, and cerebellum. The vestibuloocular reflex (VOR) serves to maintain visual stability during head movement and depends upon direct projections from the vestibular nuclei to the sixth cranial nerve (abducens) nuclei in the pons and, via the medial longitudinal fasciculus, to the third (oculomotor) and fourth (trochlear) cranial nerve nuclei in the midbrain. These connections account for the nystagmus (to-and-fro oscillation of the eyes) which is an almost invariable accompaniment of vestibular dysfunction. The vestibulospinal pathways assist in the maintenance of postural stability. Projections to the cerebral cortex, via the thalamus, provide conscious awareness of head position and movement. The vestibular nerves and nuclei project to areas of the cerebellum (primarily the flocculus and nodulus) which modulate the VOR.

The vestibular system is one of three sensory systems subserving spatial orientation and posture; the other two are the visual system (retina to occipital cortex) and the somatosensory system that conveys peripheral information from skin, joint, and muscle receptors. The three stabilizing systems overlap sufficiently to compensate (partially or completely) for each other's deficiencies. Vertigo may represent either physiologic stimulation or pathologic dysfunction in any of the three systems.

Physiologic vertigo This occurs when (1) the brain is confronted with a mismatch among the three stabilizing sensory systems or (2) the vestibular system is subjected to unfamiliar head movements to which it has never adapted, such as in seasickness. Intersensory mismatch explains carsickness, height vertigo, and the visual vertigo most commonly experienced during motion picture chase scenes; in the latter the visual sensation of environmental movement is unaccompanied by concomitant vestibular and somatosensory movement cues. *Space sickness*, a frequent transient effect of active head movement in the weightless zero-gravity environment, is another example of physiologic vertigo.

Pathologic vertigo This results from lesions of the visual, somatosensory, or vestibular systems. Visual vertigo is caused by new or incorrect spectacles or by the sudden onset of an extraocular muscle paresis with diplopia; in either instance, central nervous system compensation rapidly counteracts the vertigo. Somatosensory vertigo, rare in isolation, is usually due to a peripheral neuropathy which reduces the sensory input necessary for central compensation when there is dysfunction of the vestibular or visual systems.

The most common cause of pathologic vertigo is vestibular dysfunction. The vertigo is frequently accompanied by nausea, jerk nystagmus, postural unsteadiness, and gait ataxia.

LABYRINTHINE DYSFUNCTION This causes severe rotational or linear vertigo with the hallucination of movement, whether of environment or self, directed away from the side of the lesion. The fast phases of nystagmus beat away from the lesion side, and the tendency to fall is toward the side of the lesion.

When the head is straight and immobile, the vestibular end organs generate a tonic resting firing frequency which is equal from the two sides. With any rotational acceleration, the anatomic positions of the semicircular canals on each side necessitate an increased firing rate from one and a commensurate decrease from the other. This change in neural activity is ultimately projected to the cerebral cortex where it is summed with inputs from the visual and somatosensory systems to produce the appropriate conscious sense of rotational movement. The end organs' response to deceleration continues for some time after cessation of prolonged rotation. The side with the initially increased firing rate decreases that rate below the steady state level and the other side increases it. A sense of rotation in the opposite direction is experienced; since there is no actual head movement, this hallucinatory sensation is *vertigo*. Any disease state that changes the firing frequency of an end organ, producing unequal neural input to the brainstem and ultimately the cerebral cortex, causes vertigo. The symptom can be conceptualized as the cortex inappropriately interpreting the abnormal neural input from the brainstem as indicating actual head rotation. Transient deficits produce short-lived symptoms. With a fixed unilateral deficit, central compensatory mechanisms ultimately diminish the vertigo. Since compensation depends upon the plasticity of connections between the vestibular nuclei and cerebellum, patients with brainstem or cerebellar disease have diminished adaptive capacity and symptoms may persist indefinitely. Compensation is always inadequate for severe fixed bilateral lesions despite normal cerebellar connections; these patients are symptomatic indefinitely.

Acute unilateral labyrinthine dysfunction is caused by infection, trauma, ischemia, and toxins (usually drugs or alcohol). Often, no specific etiology is uncovered and the nonspecific term *acute labyrinthitis* or, preferably, *acute peripheral vestibulopathy* is used to describe the event. It is impossible to determine whether a patient recovering from the first bout of vertigo will have recurrent episodes.

Schwannomas involving the eighth cranial nerve (*acoustic neuroma*) grow slowly and produce such a gradual reduction of labyrinthine output that central compensatory mechanisms usually prevent or minimize the vertigo; auditory symptoms of hearing loss and tinnitus are the most common manifestations. While lesions of the brainstem or cerebellum can cause acute vertigo, associated signs and symptoms permit distinction from a labyrinthine etiology (Table 22-1). Rarely, an acute lesion of the vestibulocerebellum may present with monosymptomatic vertigo indistinguishable from a labyrinthopathy.

Recurrent unilateral labyrinthine dysfunction, in association with signs and symptoms of cochlear disease (progressive hearing loss and tinnitus), is usually due to Ménière's disease. When auditory manifestations are absent, the term *vestibular neuronitis* denotes recurrent monosymptomatic vertigo. Transient ischemic attacks of the posterior cerebral circulation (vertebrobasilar insufficiency) almost never cause recurrent vertigo without concomitant motor, sensory, cranial nerve, or cerebellar signs.

TABLE 22-1 Differentiation of peripheral and central vertigo

Sign or symptom	Peripheral (labyrinth)	Central (brainstem or cerebellum)
Direction of associated nystagmus	Unidirectional; fast phase opposite lesion*	Bidirectional or unidirectional
Purely horizontal nystagmus without torsional component	Uncommon	Common
Vertical or purely torsional nystagmus	Never present	May be present
Visual fixation	Inhibits nystagmus and vertigo	No inhibition
Severity of vertigo	Marked	Often mild
Direction of spin	Toward fast phase	Variable
Direction of fall	Toward slow phase	Variable
Duration of symptoms	Finite (minutes, days, weeks) but recurrent	May be chronic
Tinnitus and/or deafness	Often present	Usually absent
Associated central abnormalities	None	Extremely common
Common causes	Infection (labyrinthitis), Ménière's, neuronitis, ischemia, trauma, toxin	Vascular or demyelinating disease, neoplasm, trauma

* In Ménière's disease, the fast phase is variable in direction.

Positional vertigo is precipitated by a recumbent head position, either to the right or to the left. Benign paroxysmal positional vertigo (BPPV) is particularly common. Although the condition may be due to head trauma, usually no precipitating factors are identified. It generally abates spontaneously after weeks or months. The vertigo and accompanying nystagmus have a distinct pattern of latency, fatigability, and habituation that differs from the less common central positional vertigo (Table 22-2) due to lesions in and around the fourth ventricle. Moreover, the pattern of nystagmus in BPPV is often distinctive. The lower eye displays a large-amplitude torsional nystagmus, and the upper eye has a lesser degree of torsion combined with upbeating nystagmus. If the eyes are directed to the upper ear, the vertical nystagmus in the upper eye increases in amplitude.

Position*al* must be distinguished from position*ing* vertigo. The latter is provoked by head movement rather than head position and is an invariable feature of *all* vestibulopathies, central or peripheral. Since vertigo increases with quick head movements, patients tend to hold their heads still.

Vestibular epilepsy, vertigo secondary to temporal lobe epileptic activity, is rare, and almost always intermixed with other epileptic manifestations.

Psychogenic vertigo, usually a concomitant of agoraphobia (fear

TABLE 22-2 Benign paroxysmal positional (BPPV) and central positional vertigo

Features	BPPV	Central
Latency*	3–40 s	None: immediate vertigo and nystagmus
Fatigability†	Yes	No
Habituation‡	Yes	No
Intensity of vertigo	Severe	Mild
Reproducibility§	Variable	Good

* Time between attaining head position and onset of symptoms.
† Disappearance of symptoms with maintenance of offending position.
‡ Lessening of symptoms with repeated trials.
§ Likelihood of symptom production during any examination session.

of large open spaces, crowds, or leaving the safety of home), should be suspected in patients so "incapacitated" by their symptoms that they adopt a prolonged housebound status. Despite their discomfort, most patients with organic vertigo attempt to function. Vertigo should be accompanied by nystagmus; a psychogenic etiology is almost certain when nystagmus is absent during a vertiginous episode.

EVALUATION OF PATIENTS WITH PATHOLOGIC VESTIBULAR VERTIGO The evaluation depends upon whether a central etiology is suspected (Table 22-1). If so, computed tomography, with emphasis upon the posterior fossa, or a magnetic resonance imaging (MRI) scan of the head, is mandatory. Such an examination is rarely helpful in cases of recurrent monosymptomatic vertigo with a normal neurologic examination. Typical BPPV requires no investigation after the diagnosis is made (Table 22-2).

Vestibular function tests serve to (1) demonstrate an abnormality when the distinction between organic and psychogenic is uncertain, (2) establish the side of the abnormality, and (3) distinguish between peripheral and central etiologies. The standard test is electronystagmography (ENG) where warm and cold water (or air) is applied, in a prescribed fashion, to the tympanic membranes, and the slow phase velocities of the resultant nystagmus from the right and left ears are compared. A velocity decrease from one side indicates hypofunction ("canal paresis"). An inability to induce nystagmus with ice water denotes a "dead labyrinth." Some institutions have the capability of quantitatively determining various aspects of the vestibuloocular reflex using computer-driven rotational chairs and precise oculographic recording of eye movements.

Treatment of acute vertigo consists of bed rest and vestibular suppressant drugs such as antihistaminics (meclizine, dimenhydrinate, promethazine), centrally acting anticholinergics (scopolamine), or a tranquilizer with GABA-ergic effects (diazepam). If the vertigo persists beyond a few days, most authorities advise ambulation in an attempt to induce central compensatory mechanisms, despite the short-term discomfiture to the patient. Chronic vertigo of labyrinthine origin may be treated with a systematized exercise program to facilitate compensation.

Prophylactic measures to prevent recurrent vertigo are variably effective. Antihistamines are commonly utilized. Ménière's disease may respond to a very low salt diet (1 g per day). The unusual examples of persisting (beyond 4 to 6 weeks) BPPV respond dramatically, within 7 to 10 days, to a specific exercise program.

There are a variety of surgical procedures for all forms of refractory chronic or recurrent vertigo, but these are only rarely necessary.

MISCELLANEOUS HEAD SENSATIONS This designation is used, primarily for purposes of initial classification, to describe dizziness which is neither faintness nor vertigo. However, cephalic ischemia or vestibular dysfunction may be of such low intensity that the usual symptomatology is not clearly identified. For example, a small decrease in blood pressure or a slight vestibular imbalance may cause sensations different than distinct faintness or vertigo but which may be identified properly during provocative testing techniques. Other causes of dizziness in this category are hyperventilation syndrome, hypoglycemia, and the somatic symptoms of a clinical depression. All these patients should have normal neurologic examinations and vestibular function tests.

GAIT DISTURBANCES Some individuals with gait disorders complain of dizziness despite the absence of vertigo or other abnormal cephalic sensations. The causes include peripheral neuropathy, myelopathy, spasticity, parkinsonian rigidity, and cerebellar ataxia. In this context, the term dizziness is being used to describe disturbed mobility. There may be mild associated lightheadedness, particularly with impaired sensation from the feet or poor vision; this is known as *multiple sensory defect dizziness* and occurs in elderly individuals who complain of dizziness only during ambulation. Decreased position sense (secondary to neuropathy or myelopathy) and poor vision (from cataracts or retinal degeneration) create an overreliance on the aging vestibular apparatus. A less precise, but sometimes comforting, designation is *benign dysequilibrium of aging*.

EVALUATION OF THE DIZZY PATIENT The most important diagnostic tool is a careful history focused upon the meaning of "dizziness" to the patient. Is it faintness? Is there a sensation of spinning? If either of these is affirmed and the neurologic examination is normal, appropriate investigations for the multiple etiologies of cephalic ischemia or vestibular dysfunction are undertaken.

When the source of the dizziness is uncertain, provocative tests may be helpful. These office procedures simulate either cephalic ischemia or vestibular dysfunction. The former becomes obvious if the dizziness is duplicated during orthostatic hypotension. Further provocation involves the Valsalva maneuver, which decreases cerebral blood flow and should reproduce ischemic symptoms.

The simplest provocative test for vestibular dysfunction is rapid rotation and abrupt cessation of movement in a swivel chair. This always induces vertigo which the patients can compare to their symptomatic dizziness. The intense induced vertigo may be unlike the spontaneous symptoms, but shortly thereafter, when the vertigo has all but subsided, a lightheadedness supervenes which may be identified as "my dizziness." When this occurs, the dizzy patient, originally classified as suffering from "miscellaneous head sensations," is now properly diagnosed as having mild vertigo secondary to a vestibulopathy.

Patients with symptoms of positional vertigo should be appropriately tested (Table 22-2); positional testing is more sensitive with special spectacles that preclude visual fixation (Frenzel lenses).

A final provocative test, requiring the use of Frenzel lenses, is vigorous head shaking in the horizontal plane for about 10 s. If nystagmus develops after the shaking stops, even in the absence of vertigo, vestibular dysfunction is demonstrated. The maneuver can then be repeated in the vertical plane. If the provocative tests establish the dizziness as a vestibular symptom, the previously described evaluation of vestibular vertigo is undertaken.

Hyperventilation is the cause of dizziness in many anxious individuals; tingling of the hands and face may be absent. Two minutes of forced hyperventilation is indicated for patients with enigmatic dizziness and normal neurologic examinations. Similarly, depressive symptoms (which patients usually insist are "secondary" to the dizziness) must alert the examiner to a clinical depression as the *cause*, rather than the effect, of the dizziness.

Central nervous system disease can produce dizzy sensations of all types. Consequently, a neurologic examination is always required even if the history or provocative tests suggest a cardiac, peripheral vestibular, or psychogenic etiology. Any abnormality on the neurologic examination should prompt appropriate neurodiagnostic studies.

REFERENCES

Baloh RH et al: Benign postional vertigo: Clinical and oculographic features in 240 cases. Neurology 37:371, 1987

Barber HO, Sharpe JA: *Vestibular Disorders*. Chicago, Year Book Medical, 1988, chaps 5, 9, 14, and 17

Dell'Osso LF et al: Nystagmus and saccadic intrusions and oscillations, in *Clinical Ophthalmology*, TD Duane, EA Jaeger (eds). Philadelphia, Lippincott, 1988, chap 11, p 11–12, 19–20

Leigh RJ, Zee DS: *The Neurology of Eye Movements*. Philadelphia, Davis, 1984, chaps 2 and 9

Zee DS: Perspectives on the pharmacotherapy of vertigo. Arch Otolarnygol 3:609, 1985

23 DISTURBANCES OF VISION AND OCULAR MOVEMENTS

SHIRLEY H. WRAY / THOMAS L. SLAMOVITS / RONALD M. BURDE

THE HUMAN VISUAL SYSTEM

The visual system functions to form color images instantly over a wide range of background illumination. In addition, the image is placed simultaneously on the foveas of both eyes producing a three-dimensional construct of the image (stereopsis).

Light entering the eye is focused first by the cornea, which has a fixed refractile power throughout adult life, and then by the lens, which can change focal length to form a sharp image on the retina. The variation in lens shape allows objects to be seen clearly at both near and far distances. Focusing an image on the retina is called *refraction*, and optical aberrations can be corrected by spectacles or contact lenses.

The lens is fully pliable at birth. It becomes more spherical when the zonules arising from the ciliary body relax, allowing an increase in its refractive power and a clear near image. With age the lens becomes less malleable, its protein changes and by the fifth decade it can no longer focus near objects. This accommodative loss (presbyopia) leads to the need for reading glasses. Progressive change in lenticular protein with age can also cause opacification and impaired vision (cataract).

The retina is a multilayered structure lining the posterior wall of the globe. Light reaches the retina after passing through the cornea, aqueous humor, lens, and vitreous humor. Light must also pass through all layers of the retina to reach the photoreceptor cells. Photoreceptors are specialized neurons whose most distal segment consists of a stack of membranes containing wavelength-specific photopigments (vitamin A congeners) connected to a neuron-specific protein. The particular photopigment and the structural anatomy of the cell (whether rod or cone) determine its function. Since each photoreceptor connects with multiple ganglion cells, the photoreceptor cell participates in more than one function.

The retina is divided into a system of rods, dealing with light detection and motion, and a system of cones, dealing with higher visual function (acuity and color perception). Rods contain one photopigment (rhodopsin) and are achromatic; cones contain one of three photopigments (red, blue, yellow) which respond to chromatic stimuli producing color vision. Incoming light is perceived by the photoreceptors as present or absent. The signals are then integrated by a network of neurons, including horizontal, bipolar, and amacrine cells, before reaching the ganglion cells. In the periphery of the retina (containing mostly rods) there is considerable convergence of information; hundreds of thousands of rods influence the response of one ganglion cell. In the foveamacular area, which subserves central vision, there is much less convergence, and for some bipolar cells there is a one-to-one relationship: one photoreceptor is connected to one bipolar cell to one ganglion cell.

Ganglion cells are of several types, each with specialized functions. Ganglion cell axons project to the brain through the optic nerve, optic chiasm, and optic tracts. The majority of axons project to the lateral geniculate body. Axon collaterals, which form proximal to the lateral geniculate body, project to pupillomotor centers in the pretectum and to ocular, sensory, and motor centers in the superior colliculus. Second-order neurons in the lateral geniculate nucleus project to the occipital cortex via the optic radiations.

The image formed by the retina is inverted and reversed. The temporal retina images the nasal visual field while the nasal retina images the temporal field. Similarly, the superior retina perceives the inferior visual field and the inferior retina the superior field.

The fovea-macula projection (papillomacular bundle) is the major ocular-cortical outflow. The central 5° of retina is subserved by 25 to 27 percent of the axons, and the central 20° by 90 percent of the axons. The temporal field axons (nasal retina), which account for 52 percent of axons in the optic nerve, cross in the chiasm to project to the contralateral lateral geniculate nucleus, where they synapse and project to the striate cortex in the occipital lobe.

CLINICAL ASSESSMENT OF DISTURBANCES OF VISION

ACUITY Acuity is a perceptual response of a subject to a stimulus of minimal magnitude. There are many different types of visual acuity in addition to that determined by the standard Snellen chart, such as resolution, orientation, motion, color, contrast sensitivity, and stereopsis. Visual disturbances are characterized by subnormal visual acuity (less than 20/20 Snellen acuity; see below) and by abnormalities of visual field, color vision, contrast sensitivity, and depth perception. A corrected visual acuity of less than 6/60 metric (20/200 conventional) bilaterally constitutes legal blindness. Refractive errors (myopia, hyperopia, astigmatism) commonly cause subnormal visual acuity and must be assessed for by measuring *best corrected* (i.e., best refracted) visual acuity. A pinhole can be used for a reasonable approximation of best corrected visual acuity. Visual acuity at distance is measured with a Snellen chart [normal 6/6 meters (20/20 feet)]. In the fractional denotation—e.g., 6/60 metric (20/200 conventional), the numerator 6 (or 20) stands for the testing distance (in meters or feet) and the denominator 60 (or 200) for the test letter's size normally seen at that denominator distance. Near acuity is measured with a near card (Jaeger chart). Bifocals or near spectacles must be worn by presbyopes (who have difficulties with accommodation) when testing near vision.

COLOR VISION Acquired color vision abnormalities in red/green perception usually imply optic neuropathy. Bedside testing may consist of gross recognition or comparison of prime colors, or the use of a series of color charts (Ishihara pseudoisochromatic or American Optical Hardy-Rand-Rittler plates). Color desaturation tests rely on a comparison of the subjective perception of a colored target (e.g., red bottle top) in the right and left eyes or in the nasal and temporal half-fields of a single eye. The test detects unilateral or hemianopic abnormalities.

CONTRAST SENSITIVITY Testing of this acuity requires manipulation of both contrast and spatial frequency by measuring the minimum contrast necessary to see patterns of various sizes. Contrast sensitivity plates (Arden or American Optical) can be used at the bedside.

STEREOPSIS There is a linear relationship between stereoacuity and Snellen visual acuity. Individuals with normal 6/6 (20/20) vision in each eye and binocular fixation (no manifest strabismus) have an average stereopsis of 40 seconds of arc. Stereoacuity is reduced with decreasing acuity down to 6/60 (20/200) at which level monocular and binocular responses become identical. The Titmus stereoacuity test is used in children and adults who have been corrected for presbyopia and is suitable for bedside use. This linearity may not exist in the presence of optic nerve damage even if visual acuity returns to normal.

VISUAL FIELDS It is possible to perform a visual field test using any perceptual stimulus. The bedside exam is performed by confrontation. Two types of "formal" field testing are in common use:

1. On *kinetic perimetry* (Goldmann, tangent screen), the patient is instructed to look at a central fixation target while test objects of varying brightness and size (white or chromatic) are moved from the periphery toward the fixation point until the patient signals that the test object is visualized. The normal field using white objects is approximately 90° temporally, 50° nasally, 50° superiorly, and 65° inferiorly. Concentric contraction of the visual field binocularly to less than 10° constitutes legal blindness.

2. On *automated static perimetry* (Humphrey, Octopus), the patient fixes on a central target in a hemisphere with a homogeneous white background, while a nonmoving light of fixed size and brightness is presented at various points in the hemisphere. Brightness is increased until the patient recognizes the presence of the stimulus above background. Thus, static perimetry measures brightness sensitivity of various retinal points.

Visual field defects are localizable on the basis of the anatomy of the visual pathway. Retinal and optic nerve lesions affect one of three types of nerve fiber bundles, leading to blind spots (scotomas) termed: (1) central/cecocentral, (2) arcuate, or (3) radial. Loss of nerve fibers between the optic nerve and macula (maculopapillary bundle) leads to central or cecocentral scotomas, i.e., involving the center of the visual field or extending between the center and the physiologic blind spot (cecum) (Fig. 23-1*D* and *E*). Temporal retinal lesions above and below the maculopapillary bundle or those involving the superotemporal or inferotemporal optic nerve affect the *arcuate* bundles and cause inferonasal or superonasal visual field defects, respectively. Because such field defects abut the horizontal midline, they are at times referred to as *altitudinal* (Fig. 23-1*B*). Lesions involving the nasal retinal or optic nerve fibers (radial nerve fiber bundle defects) lead to inferotemporal and superotemporal visual field defects that extend toward the physiologic blind spot (Fig. 23-1*A*).

FIGURE 23-1 Types of monocular visual field loss in left eye. *A*. Superior arcuate scotoma (inferior nerve fiber bundle defect). *B*. Inferior altitudinal field defect respecting the horizontal meridian (superior nerve fiber bundle defect). *C*. Enlargement of the blind spot in the left eye. *D*. Central scotoma, normal blind spot. *E*. Centrocecal scotoma. *F*. Temporal hemianopsia respecting the vertical meridian but with involvement of central vision. *G*. Generalized constriction of the visual field to 2 isopters. *H*. Nonorganic "corkscrew" field defect to 1 isopter. *(From Wray, 1985; by permission.)*

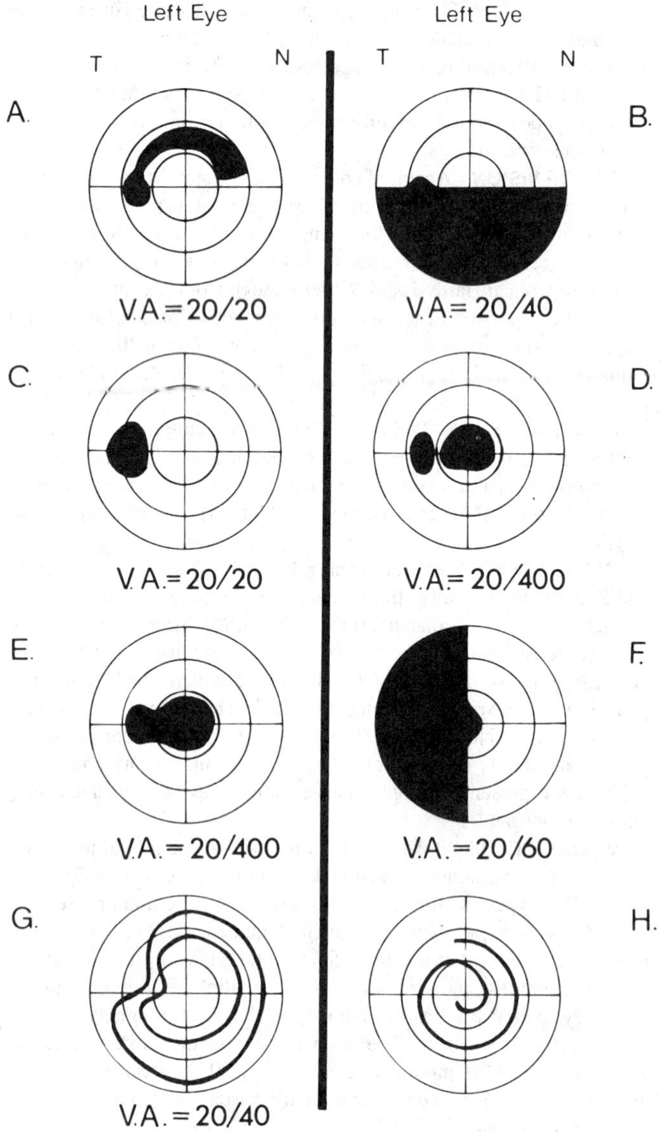

Retinal field defects frequently correspond to lesions seen with the ophthalmoscope, i.e., areas of infarction, inflammation, or degenerative change. Macular lesions produce central scotomas. Retinitis pigmentosa usually produces constricted fields and equatorial ring scotomas.

Discrete lesions, frequently ischemic, primarily in the anterior optic nerve may produce *arcuate field defects*. Such lesions include anterior ischemic optic neuropathy, glaucoma, and optic atrophy secondary to papilledema. The central/cecocentral scotoma is a specific and common sign of optic nerve disease. It occurs in a variety of conditions both intrinsic (demyelinating, infiltrative, metabolic-toxic) and compressive in nature.

At the chiasm, the visual afferents become divided into a right and left half so that the right brain sees left visual space and the left brain sees right visual space. A discrete vertical midline is the hallmark of all visual pathway disorders at or posterior to the chiasm. A chiasmal lesion most often causes bitemporal hemianopsia (Fig. 23-2*B*), but several different patterns can occur: junctional scotoma, superior or inferior bitemporal quadrantanopsia, or monocular temporal hemianopsia. Each type can occur with chiasmal compression due to a pituitary tumor, craniopharyngioma, or aneurysm. Pseudochiasmal or ocular syndromes that can mimic chiasmal lesions include tilted optic discs, drug toxicity (chloroquine), sector retinitis pigmentosa, and bilateral retinal detachments. A mass in the retrochiasmatic region impinging upon or displacing the optic tract results in homonymous hemianopsia of two types: an incongruous homonymous hemianopsia or a complete homonymous hemianopsia.

Homonymous field defects due to lesions of the anterior optic radiation tend to be incongruous. Those due to damage to the radiations close to the visual cortex are congruous. (Congruity is said to be present when the edge of the field defect in each eye is identical in shape.) Depending on its site, the lesion may involve only the upper or lower fibers of the radiation and thus cause a lower or upper quadrant defect in the opposite half-field; e.g., temporal lobe radiation lesion causes "pie in the sky" (Fig. 23-2*E*) whereas a parietal lobe radiation lesion causes "pie on the floor" (Fig. 23-2*G*). A complete hemianopic defect to bilateral simultaneous visual stimulation (attention defect) may, however, be the only detectable sign of visual dysfunction in lesions of the parietal area. Left temporoparietal lesions are associated with defective recognition of visual symbols, alexia, and agraphia; lesions of the right temporoparietal area are manifested by impaired judgment of spatial relationships, as in topographic agnosia and constructional apraxia (see Chap. 32).

Destruction of the visual cortex of one occipital lobe produces a contralateral congruous homonymous hemianopsia. This is the commonest type of cortical field defect and is frequently the result of embolic occlusion of the posterior cerebral artery. Other patterns of visual loss permit precise localization of the deficit. These defects are congruous homonymous hemianopic scotoma, congruous homonymous hemianopsia sparing the temporal crescent, or, rarely, a monocular field defect due to loss of the temporal crescent, bilateral homonymous hemianopsia, bilateral altitudinal scotoma, cortical blindness, and tunnel or keyhole vision.

PUPILLARY EXAMINATION Normal pupillary responses consist of prompt, symmetric constriction (miosis) on exposure to light or on attempted near convergence. Diminished response to a direct light stimulus, combined with a normal consensual pupillary response following stimulation of the contralateral eye, is termed a relative afferent pupillary defect (RAPD). The RAPD is an important objective sign of ipsilateral optic neuropathy. The best way to elicit the RAPD is to perform a swinging flashlight test (Fig. 23-3). Anisocoria (unequal pupil size) and abnormal pupillary reflexes are two clinically

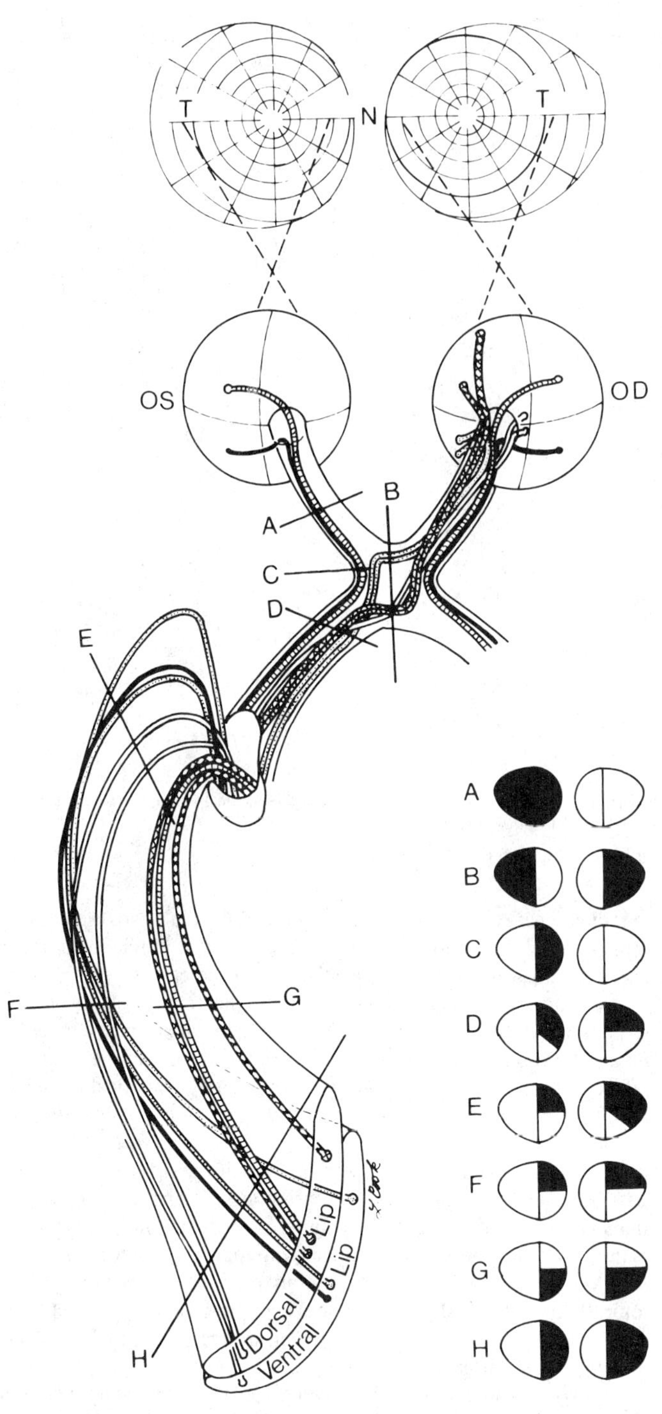

FIGURE 23-2 Nerve fiber anatomy of the visual pathways from retina to occipital cortex. The effect of the fields of vision produced by lesions at various points along the optic pathway is shown on the right. *A*. complete blindness in left eye. *B*. Bitemporal hemianopsia. *C*. Nasal hemianopsia of left eye. *D* and *E*. Right incongruous homonymous hemianopsia. *F* and *G*. Right upper and lower homonymous quadrantanopia. *H*. complete right homonymous hemianopsia. *Courtesy of DD Donaldson. (From Wray, 1985; by permission.)*

important pupillary abnormalities. Comparing pupil size in the dark and in room light and observing direct light responses help to determine whether the smaller or larger pupil is the abnormal one. With parasympathetic anisocoria, the difference in pupil size will be accentuated in room light since the affected (large) pupil constricts subnormally. With oculosympathetic paresis, the anisocoria is more marked in dim light because the affected (small) pupil dilates subnormally.

Isolated chronic pupillary dilation (mydriasis) is almost never caused by a lesion in the oculomotor nerve; it may be constitutional (physiologic, "benign"), pharmacologic (induced by local instillation of mydriatics), traumatic, or a result of a parasympathetic lesion at or distal to the ciliary ganglion (tonic pupil, Adie's pupil). The diagnostic workup utilizes changes in pupil size in response to topical agents (Table 23-1).

Unilateral mydriasis with impaired direct-light and near response, ipsilateral ptosis, and extraocular muscle paresis of the superior, medial, and inferior rectus and inferior oblique muscles constitutes an oculomotor nerve palsy. Unilateral miosis with normal direct-light response and mild ipsilateral ptosis constitutes an oculosympathetic lesion or Horner syndrome. The diagnosis of the Horner pupil can be confirmed by pharmacologic testing (Table 23-1).

Light-near dissociation (LND) of the pupillary response is bilateral and characterized by an impaired response to light with an intact response to near vision. When LND is bilateral and symmetric it occurs with dorsal midbrain lesions (hydrocephalus, pineal region

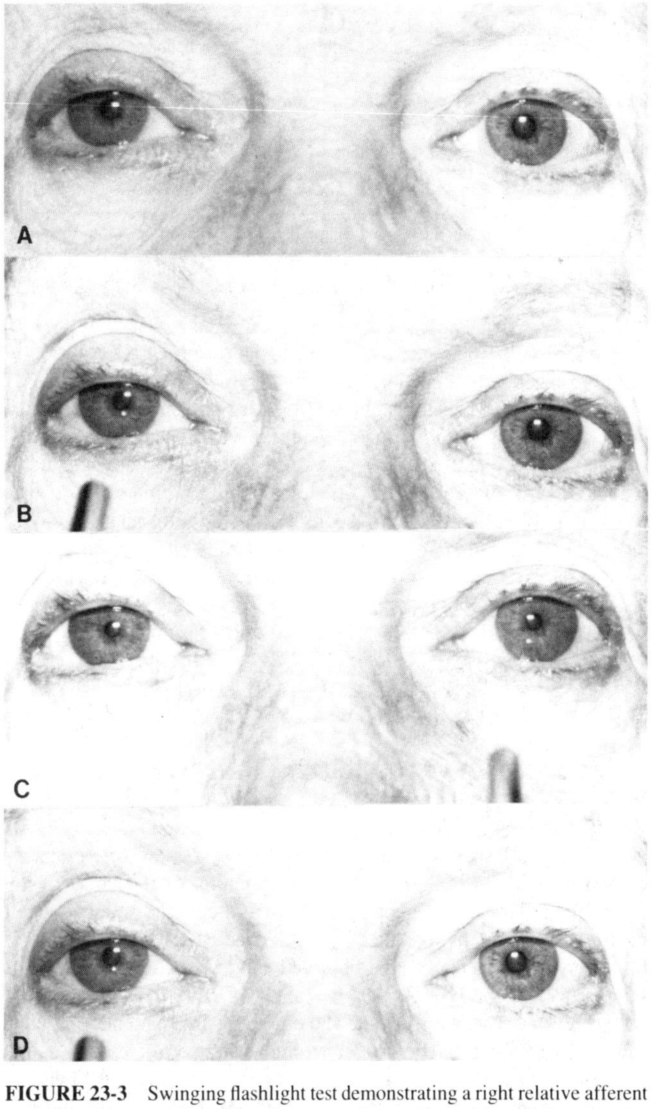

FIGURE 23-3 Swinging flashlight test demonstrating a right relative afferent pupillary defect (RAPD) in a patient with giant cell arteritis and right anterior ischemic optic neuropathy. The patient is fixating on a distant target to avoid near effort and related accommodative miosis. *A*. Pupils in a dimly lit room. *B*. Flashlight illuminates right eye, leading to minimal direct constriction of right pupil and minimal consensual constriction of left pupil. *C*. Flashlight is swung to the left eye, causing obvious pupillary constriction directly on left and consensually on right. *D*. Flashlight is again swung to right eye, leading to bilateral pupillary dilation—a result of the right optic nerve conduction deficit.

TABLE 23-1 Characteristics of pupils encountered in neuroophthalmology

	General characteristics	Responses to light and near stimuli	Room condition in which anisocoria is greater	Response to mydriatics	Response to miotics	Response to pharmacologic agents
Essential anisocoria	Round, regular	Both brisk	No change	Dilates	Constricts	Normal and rarely needed
Horner's syndrome	Small, round, unilateral	Both brisk	Darkness	Dilates	Constricts	Cocaine 4%, poor dilation; Paredrine 1%, no dilation if third-order neuron damage
Tonic pupil syndrome (Holmes-Adie syndrome)	Usually larger* in bright light; sector pupil palsy, vermiform movement Unilateral or, less often, bilateral	Absent to light, tonic to near; tonic redilation	Light	Dilates	Constricts	Pilocarpine 0.1% or 0.125% constricts; Mecholyl 2.5% constricts
Argyll Robertson pupils	Small, irregular, bilateral	Poor to light, better to near	No change	Poor	Constricts	
Midbrain pupils	Mid-dilated; may be oval; bilateral	Poor to light, better to near (or fixed to both)	No change	Dilates	Constricts	
Pharmacologically dilated pupils	Very large†, round, unilateral	Fixed‡	Light		No‡	Pilocarpine 1% will not constrict
Oculomotor palsy (nonvascular)	Mid-dilated (6–7 mm), unilateral (rarely bilateral)	Fixed	Light	Dilates	Constricts	

* Tonic pupil may appear smaller following prolonged near-effort or in dim illumination; affected pupil is initially large, but with passing time gradually becomes smaller.
† Atropinized pupils have diameters of 8 to 9 mm. No tonic, midbrain, or oculomotor palsy pupil ever is this large.
‡ Pupils may be weakly reactive, depending on interim after instillation.
SOURCE: TL Slamovits and JS Glaser in *Clinical Ophthalmology*, T Duane (ed) Vol 2, Philadelphia, Lippincott, 1988

tumors). Argyll-Robertson pupil is a special form of LND caused by syphilis; the pupils are miotic and usually irregular in shape. LND can also occur in diabetes mellitus. LND accompanied by bilaterally poor vision is generally due to anterior visual pathway disease. Unilateral LND is most commonly seen in patients with ipsilateral retinal or optic nerve disease. Bilateral pupillary enlargement with subnormal direct and near responses occurs with pharmacologic blockade, botulism, or diphtheria. Bilaterally miotic pupils are produced by the use of parasympathomimetics for glaucoma; a pontine lesion (pinpoint pontine pupils) or narcotic (heroin) overdose should be considered in a comatose patient with bilateral miosis.

OCULAR DISEASES

THE CONJUNCTIVE AND CORNEA Diseases of the conjunctiva and cornea can produce loss of visual acuity, pain, and discharge. Examination should first be directed to the lids and lid margins as well as to the lashes. Chronic infectious processes are often characterized by scaling around the lashes or pointing of the ducts of the meibomian glands. It is to be noted that basal cell and squamous cell carcinomas often involve the lids. Evidence of discharge from the conjunctiva can frequently be observed as crusting, either nasally or temporally, on the lids.

The eyes are ordinarily white and quiet. When a patient complains of discomfort or discharge the upper and lower fornix as well as the palpebral conjunctiva should be inspected, by pulling the lower lid out and down or everting the upper lid on the tarsus. Discharge, foreign bodies, and Kaposi's sarcoma may go undetected without such an examination.

The presence of perilimbal injection is indicative of anterior uveal inflammation and such patients should be referred for ophthalmologic evaluation.

Diseases of the conjunctiva and cornea may occur as a result of direct trauma, drying associated with disorders of tearing, exposure to radiant energy (ultraviolet light, sun, and welding guns), allergens (pollen, mold), infectious agents (bacteria, viruses, fungi, and ameba) and inflammatory, metabolic, and neoplastic processes.

Neonatal infection of the cornea or conjunctiva is usually due to staphylococci or gonococci, or in some geographic areas to chlamydiae. Prophylactic silver nitrate treatment in the newborn is effective against gonococci but may itself cause a chemical conjunctivitis. Tetracycline or erythromycin ointment is equally effective for gonococcal prophylaxis. Congenital syphilis can produce interstitial keratitis late in the last decade of life, resulting in bilateral corneal vascularization, photophobia, and visual loss. Herpes simplex infections cause dendritic keratitis. Failure to recognize herpetic keratopathy and its inappropriate treatment with topical glucocorticoids can lead to corneal "melting" and perforation. Treatment with acyclovir topically or systemically can suppress herpetic keratopathy (see Chap. 135). Herpesvirus can become latent in the trigeminal ganglia, allowing recurrent keratitis to occur in some patients.

Adenovirus infection is the leading cause of keratoconjunctivitis in adults; it is usually self-limiting and benign. In sexually active young adults, inclusion conjunctivitis is common (see Chap. 155). In developing countries, trachoma and onchocerciasis are leading causes of corneal scarring and blindness.

Chronic indolent amebic ulcers of the cornea can occur in soft–contact lens wearers who have a break in the corneal epithelium; such ulcers are difficult to treat. However, this complication is rare in those who remove and clean contact lenses daily. Debilitated patients can develop keratitis due to gram-negative bacteria (*Klebsiella, Pseudomonas*) or fungi. Malnutrition and avitaminosis A can lead to conjunctival and corneal scarring with keratinization (xerosis) and severe visual loss.

Keratoconjunctivitis can also occur in patients with Stevens-Johnson syndrome (Chap. 272), Wegener's granulomatosis (Chap. 276), rheumatoid arthritis (Chap. 270), atopic dermatitis (Chap. 56), and cicatricial pemphigoid (Chap. 58). These processes are often associated with corneal ulceration. Band keratopathy is caused by corneal deposition of calcium salts, especially within the palpebral fissure (Fig. A4-10). It occurs as a result of chronic inflammation (keratouveitis) or of systemic hypercalcemia (see Chap. 340).

Corneal clouding is prominent in G_{M1} gangliosidosis (Chap. 331), in certain of the mucopolysaccharidoses (Chap. 331), and in aminoaciduria [cystinosis (Chap. 335)]. In Wilson's disease (Chap. 330) and in chronic biliary cirrhosis, copper deposits form a golden-brown ring (Kayser-Fleischer ring) (Fig. A4-16) in the cornea at the level of Descemet's membrane. Corneal drug deposition may occur following systemic use of chloroquine, phenothiazine, gold, silver, or amiodarone.

THE LENS AND CATARACTS Opacification of the normally clear and transparent crystalline lens is termed a cataract. Visual symptoms are blurred vision, glare, altered color perception, and monocular diplopia. *Congenital* cataracts occur as a complication of intrauterine rubella, herpes simplex, herpes zoster, syphilis, and cytomegalic inclusion disease. The majority are idiopathic or inherited. Acquired cataracts result from trauma, radiation, drugs, metabolic disorders, ocular inflammatory disorders, or aging (senile cataract). Cataracts develop earlier in patients with diabetes mellitus (type I and type II) and in some patients with a strong family history of cataract formation. Metabolic disorders complicated by cataract include galactosemia (Chap. 337), chronic hypercalcemic states (Chap. 340), Fabry's disease, Wilson's disease (Chap. 330), and Lowe's syndrome (Chap. 231). More than one-third of patients with myotonic dystrophy have multicolored crystalline opacities scattered throughout the lens. Cataracts may also be associated with chromosomal disorders; with the Alport, cri-du-chat, Conradi, Crouzon, and Down syndromes; and with gonadal dysgenesis. Inflammatory ocular diseases, drugs and toxic substances such as haloperidol, glucocorticoids, and iron can also cause cataracts. Cataract extraction is performed by removing the lens nucleus and cortex from within the lens capsule. In most adults, a plastic lens is then implanted within the capsule.

The zonules holding the lens may be broken in one region, allowing the lens to move eccentrically, often leaving its edge in the pupillary axis (subluxation) or totally broken, allowing the lens to move into the anterior chamber or into the vitreous cavity (luxation). The most common cause of subluxation or luxation is trauma. Others include homocystinuria (Chap. 334), Marfan's syndrome, spherophakia, and sulfite oxidase insufficiency.

UVEAL DISEASES The uvea consists of the iris and ciliary body anteriorly and the choroid posteriorly. Anatomically, the choroid has three layers of vessels and a cellular matrix including pigmented cells. Common diseases of the uvea are inflammatory or neoplastic. Inflammation can involve the iris (iritis), ciliary body (cyclitis), or choroid (choroiditis) or any combination of the three (uveitis). Uveitis causes photophobia, ocular discomfort and visual blurring. Chronic uveitis can cause cystoid macular edema with decreased central acuity, cataract formation, and secondary glaucoma. The commonest form of uveitis is idiopathic. Systemic diseases causing uveitis include pauciarticular juvenile rheumatoid arthritis (rheumatoid factor negative), juvenile nevoxanthogranuloma, rheumatoid arthritis, sarcoidosis, Lyme disease, and relapsing polychondritis. Treatment of uveitis (dependent on severity) includes cycloplegic drops and glucocorticoids (topically or systemically), and sometimes immunosuppressive drugs (chlorambucil, azathioprine, cyclophosphamide, and cyclosporin A).

Ocular malignant melanoma is a primary neoplastic disease of the choroid. Choroidal involvement also occurs as a result of metastases (lung, breast, prostate) and in association with lymphoma of the central nervous system (reticulum cell sarcoma)—conditions that are sometimes responsive to low-dose radiation.

RETINAL DISEASES Retinal abnormalities are best seen by performing a dilated fundus examination. Retinal diseases involving the macula cause distortion of straight lines (metamorphopsia), loss of central acuity, and visual field abnormalities. Nonmacular retinal disorders cause scotomata involving the peripheral or paracentral visual field, correlating with the site of retinal pathology. Retinopathies can be due to diseases of the retinal vessels, neurosensory retina, or the retinal pigment epithelium.

Retinal vasculopathies occur in many systemic conditions. In hypertensive retinopathy, the severity of retinal changes correlates closely with the level of systemic hypertension (see Chap. 196). Grade I consists of arteriolar narrowing; Grade II includes arteriovenous nicking, minimal exudation, and splinter hemorrhages; Grade III includes retinal edema, hemorrhages, and cotton-wool spots (focal ischemia in the nerve fiber layer); Grade IV includes Grade III changes plus papilledema, often with a macular star produced by deposition of cellular debris (hard exudates). Hypertensive retinopathy can be seen with all forms of hypertension—essential and secondary. Cotton-wool spots, a common feature of malignant hypertension, may also occur in anemia, leukemia, collagen vascular disease, dysproteinemia, infective endocarditis, and diabetes mellitus. They are the most common ophthalmic lesions in acquired immunodeficiency syndrome (AIDS) (see Chap. 264). Other ocular manifestations of AIDS include cytomegalovirus (CMV) retinitis (Fig. A4-14) and toxoplasmic and fungal retinal infections. Nonretinal ocular manifestations of AIDS include optic neuropathy, Kaposi's sarcoma of the conjunctiva, and orbital lymphoma.

Diabetic retinopathy is classified into two groups: (1) background retinopathy (Fig. A4-12) characterized by microaneurysms, dot-blot hemorrhages, cotton-wool spots, hard exudates, intraretinal microvascular shunt vessels, and venous beading, sometimes with related macular edema; and (2) proliferative retinopathy (Fig. A4-13) characterized by neovascularization, proliferation of fibrous tissue into the vitreous cavity, and eventually traction retinal detachments with visual loss (see Chap. 319). Panretinal photocoagulation is beneficial in maintaining vision in early proliferative retinopathy. The progression of diabetic retinopathy correlates best with the concentration of hemoglobin A_{1c}, reflecting the long-term metabolic control. The lower the hemoglobin A_{1c} concentration the slower the progression. The acute induction of so-called tight control is often associated with a short-term aggravation of the retinopathic process (e.g., insulin infusion pump or multiple injection regime).

Somewhat similar retinal vascular changes ("sea fan" proliferation) occur in sickle cell diseases (S-S, S-C, S-Thal) and in the retinopathy of prematurity. In sickle cell disease focal photocoagulation is helpful. Focal cryotherapy may be of benefit in the acute retinopathy of prematurity.

Permanent blindness occurs with *infarction* of the inner retina due to occlusion of the central retinal artery (CRA). Funduscopic examination shows rectangular "box-car" segmentation of venous blood flow and an opaque white retina due to axoplasmic stasis in ganglion cell axons. A central cherry-red spot is due to visualization of the choroid in the macular area devoid of axons (Fig. A4-2). CRA occlusion may be embolic (ipsilateral internal carotid artery, aorta, or heart) or thrombotic due to giant cell arteritis, arteriosclerosis, collagen vascular disease, or hyperviscosity states. CRA occlusion is an ophthalmic emergency. Treatment may include ballotement of the globe, retrobulbar anesthetic block, and paracentesis of aqueous humor in an attempt to move embolic material into peripheral arterioles.

Monocular transient blurring of vision (amaurosis fugax) lasting seconds to minutes may herald CRA occlusion but, more importantly, may be a precursor of a stroke. These patients require evaluation of the aortic arch and carotid circulation as well as the heart (see Chap. 351).

Central (Fig. A4-3) and branch retinal vein occlusion may occur spontaneously or in association with hypertension or elevated intraocular pressure. Venous stasis retinopathy mimics early vein occlusion with venous dilatation, hemorrhages, and cotton-wool spots; it is due to impaired retinal perfusion produced by carotid occlusive disease and Takayasu's disease. Systemic coagulopathies such as thrombocytopenia, erythematosus disseminated intravascular coagulopathy, and systemic lupus erythematosus with circulating anticoagulants (cardiolipin), may cause retinal hemorrhages, clotting in the submacular choriocapillaris, choroidal hemorrhages, and detachment of the retina. Perivenous sheathing occurs in primary retinal vasculitis (Eales disease), leukemia, and optic nerve demyelination. Fundus changes may be the mark of an abused child presenting with multiple retinal hemorrhages (subhyaloid lakes, blot and flame hemorrhages) and cotton-wool spots. This retinopathy is caused by severe shaking or choking of the child.

Retinal vascular anomalies are rare and among them are to be found retinal telangiectasia (Coat's disease), retinal angiomatosis [von Hippel-Lindau syndrome (Chap. 358)], direct arteriovenous connections [Wyburn-Mason syndrome (A4-15)], miliary aneurysms, cavernous retinal hemangiomas.

Nonvascular diseases of the retina include infections such as congenital and acquired toxoplasmosis, herpes retinitis, and *Monilia* and nematode infestations. Inflammatory diseases of the outer retina and choroid include the presumed ocular histoplasmosis syndrome, acute multifocal placoid pigment epitheliopathy, serpiginous retinopathy, "bird-shot" chorioretinopathy, multiple evanescent white dot syndrome, and neoplastic diseases such as retinoblastoma.

Retinal degenerative disease may involve the retinovitreal interface with focal capillary sclerosis and hole formation (lattice degeneration) or may appear as isolated areas of retinovitreal adhesion and vitreous liquefaction (syneresis) leading to retinal traction, retinal horseshoe-shaped tears, and detachment. Lightning-like flashes and/or an acute vitreous hemorrhage producing a spiderweb-like shadow and blurred vision may herald detachment. These patients must be examined by an ophthalmologist utilizing an indirect ophthalmoscope. Emergency surgery (laser, cryotherapy) is required to seal the tears. Degeneration of the outer retina and pigment epithelium is characteristic of retinitis pigmentosa (Fig. A4-9) which occurs in sporadic, X-linked, autosomal recessive, and autosomal dominant forms. Symptoms are loss of night vision, progressive concentric contraction of the visual field, and eventually, loss of central vision.

Multisystem disorders that cause retinal degeneration are abetalipoproteinemia (Bassen-Kornzweig syndrome, Chap. 326), neuronal ceroid lipofuscinosis (Batten-Mayou disease), Refsum's disease (Chap. 363), certain mucopolysaccharidoses, and the Kearns-Sayre syndrome (Chap. 365).

Certain lysosomal storage diseases including G_{M1} and G_{M2} gangliosidosis and the sphingolipidoses affect ganglion cell function, leading to blindness; cherry-red spots are invariably present (Chap. 331). Toxic retinopathy may follow the use of phenothiazine derivatives, especially thioridazine (Mellaril), chloroquine, and hydroxychloroquine. Long-term therapy with these agents should be monitored at regular intervals with static perimetry or kinetic perimetry with red and white targets.

DISEASES OF BRUCH'S MEMBRANE Bruch's membrane is a multilayered structure formed by the choriocapillaris and the pigment epithelium of the retina. With aging, the pigment epithelium may accumulate intracellular material, leading to age-related macular degeneration. Visual loss is slowly progressive, associated with metamorphopsia, and rarely causes less than 6/120 (20/400) Snellen acuity. A second type of age-related macular degeneration can occur in the paramacular foveal area and cause visual loss. It results from degeneration of Bruch's membrane with the formation of large or small breaks in its integrity and subretinal neovascularization. Subsequent exudation and hemorrhage causes a further elevation of the sensory or pigment epithelium of the retina. Visual loss is often acute and catastrophic in nature, decreasing acuity to less than 6/120 (20/400) with a large central scotoma that is defined by the anatomic detachment. Laser ablation of the neovascular net may delay blindness. Angioid streaks are large breaks in Bruch's membrane (Fig. A4-8). They are associated with Paget's disease, acromegaly, pseudoxanthoma elasticum, sickle cell disease and severe myopia.

DISEASES OF THE OPTIC NERVE

The optic disc is the exit site of all retinal ganglion cell axons. The axons leave the globe in the optic nerve by passing through the lamina cribrosa. Just posterior to the lamina, the nerve fibers become myelinated. The blood supply of the nerve head is primarily derived from choroidal and posterior ciliary branches of the ophthalmic artery.

GLAUCOMA Glaucoma is characterized by progressive field loss due to nerve damage from elevated intraocular pressure. It is an important cause of blindness worldwide and in the United States occurs in 1 to 2 percent of patients above age 60. The disease may be asymptomatic with painless, slow loss of peripheral and paracentral visual fields. Early detection depends upon a routine eye examination with intraocular pressure measurement (tonometry), funduscopy with attention to optic disc appearance, and visual field testing. In the normal eye the optic cups are symmetric and the neural rim is pink (Fig. A4-1). In glaucoma, either localized notching or generalized enlargement of the optic cup can be seen (Fig. A4-11). The rim, although thinned, remains pink until late. The central optic cup diameter can be compared to the diameter of the disc and a ratio of the horizontal and vertical dimensions can be recorded. The normal cup-disc ratio is less than 0.2 to 0.3. Vertical disparity in one or both eyes is an early sign of glaucoma. Glaucoma is often asymmetric and the finding of asymmetry of the cup-disc ratio implies glaucoma. Early visual field loss includes nonspecific constriction and small paracentral scotomas. Eventually, arcuate nerve fiber bundle defects develop with a characteristic *nasal step* (e.g., arcuate bundle defect extending to the nasal horizontal raphe forms a steplike configuration on kinetic visual field testing). The papillomacular bundle and acuity are spared until late in the disease. Intraocular pressure reflects the balance between the production and outflow of aqueous humor, and the normal range is 2.09 ± 0.33 kPa (15.8 ± 2.5 mmHg) measured by applanation tonometry. (Schiotz tonometers measure intraocular pressure by indentation of the cornea, whereas most tonometers measure by planating the corneal surface, hence applanation.)

Glaucoma is an appellation for many disease states. It results from decreased outflow of aqueous humor through the pupil, trabecular meshwork, and Schlemm's canal, leading to elevated intraocular pressure. Chronic or *primary open-angle glaucoma,* the most common of adult glaucomas, is asymptomatic and detected only by routine eye examination. It is associated with a relative obstruction to aqueous outflow through the trabecular meshwork and is of unknown cause. Treatment includes the use of topical agents including cholinergic (pilocarpine, carbachol, echothiophate) or adrenergic agonists (epinephrine, dipivefrin), or antagonists, i.e., beta-adrenergic blockers (timolol, levobunalol, betaxolol). If topical agents do not reduce the intraocular pressure satisfactorily, systemic carbonic anhydrase inhibitors (acetazolamide or methazolamide) are added. Laser trabeculoplasty or filtration surgery, to improve aqueous outflow, is indicated when medical therapy fails.

Secondary open-angle glaucoma may develop in patients with ocular inflammatory or neoplastic disease, with mature cataracts or elevated episcleral venous pressure, or during a course of long-term glucocorticoid therapy, either topical or systemic.

Angle-closure glaucoma occurs when the iris blocks egress of aqueous humor through the trabecular meshwork. In the primary form, an anatomic abnormality of the eye leads to pupillary block and obstruction of the trabecular meshwork. An acute rise in intraocular pressure occurs with dilation of the pupil causing severe eye and face pain, nausea, vomiting, colored halos around lights and loss of visual acuity. Conjunctival hyperemia, corneal edema, and a fixed mid-dilated pupil are common signs. Urgent reduction of the intraocular pressure is best accomplished by the use of hyperosmotic agents including oral glycerine and sorbitol or intravenous mannitol. Laser or surgical iridotomy is curative in most cases.

Secondary angle-closure glaucoma can occur when the lens or ciliary body becomes swollen, pushing the iris against the trabecular meshwork or sealing the iris to the trabecular meshwork as a result of the formation of a neovascular network. This process occurs in patients with diabetic retinopathy, advanced ocular ischemic syndrome due to severe occlusive carotid disease, or inflammatory adhesions (synechiae).

OPTIC NEUROPATHIES Diseases of the optic nerve cause acuity loss, subjective color and brightness desaturation, changes in contrast sensitivity, and visual field loss. There is almost always a relative afferent pupillary defect (RAPD) (Fig. 23-3). Papilledema (optic disc edema secondary to elevated intracranial pressure) and infiltration of the optic nerve sheath cause visual dysfunction late in the course of the disease. In acute optic neuropathy the optic disc may be normal or swollen. In chronic optic neuropathy the disc is swollen or pale (atrophy).

Optic neuritis most commonly afflicts patients in their twenties or thirties, women more than men, and can either be a primary demyelinating disease of unknown etiology or associated with past, present, or future manifestations of multiple sclerosis (see Chap. 356). There is acute, typically central visual loss, retrobulbar pain with eye movement, and RAPD. In the acute phase the nerve is normal (retrobulbar optic neuritis) or swollen (anterior optic neuritis or papillitis). Acute optic neuritis is generally unilateral. Bilateral recurrent bouts in the same or contralateral eye can occur, especially with multiple sclerosis.

Anterior ischemic optic neuropathy (AION) occurs most often in patients over 40 years of age. Typically sudden visual loss and altitudinal field loss occurs, i.e., a superior or inferior visual field defect with one border along the horizontal midline, associated with disc swelling due to infarction of the nerve head (Fig. A4-6). It occurs in two forms: (1) nonarteritic (median age 56 years) in which the risk factors are diabetes mellitus in younger patients and hypertension in older patients; (2) an arteritic (giant cell arteritis) variety (median age 74 years). Symptoms of giant cell arteritis (anorexia, malaise, proximal arthralgia, myalgia, headache, and jaw claudication) and an elevated erythrocyte sedimentation rate are indications for prompt systemic glucocorticoid therapy and a temporal artery biopsy. Untreated, arteritic ischemic optic neuropathy may affect the contralateral eye and cause blindness in 40 percent of cases.

Compression (intrinsic or extrinsic) of the optic nerve causes insidious progressive acuity and field loss. The disc may be normal, swollen, or atrophic (Fig. A4-7). Intrinsic tumors include optic nerve sheath meningioma and glioma. In Graves' ophthalmopathy, the optic neuropathy is due to compression of the nerve in the orbital apex by the enlarged extraocular muscles. Benign or malignant orbital tumors, metastatic lesions, tumors arising from the adjacent paranasal sinuses and middle cranial fossa, and giant pituitary adenomas can each lead to compressive optic neuropathy.

Infiltrative and toxic optic neuropathies are rare. Progressive disc swelling and visual loss characterize infiltration by inflammatory disease (sarcoidosis), infection (cryptococcosis), or neoplasia (leukemia, lymphoma, metastatic carcinoma). Toxic agents (methanol, ethambutol) cause a more acute visual loss with normal or swollen discs, whereas nutritional amblyopias are associated with a more insidious course.

Leber optic neuropathy This condition, which affects males primarily, is transmitted via female carriers through cytoplasmic DNA in the ovum (mitochondrial). It is characterized by rapid loss of central vision occurring during early adult life. Both eyes are affected either simultaneously or sequentially. The visual fields contain scotomas that are initially central and rapidly become cecocentral in location. In acute Leber optic neuropathy the ophthalmoscopic findings are (1) circumpapillary telangiectatic microangiopathy; (2) swelling of the nerve fiber layer around the disc; and (3) absence of leakage from the disc or papillary region on fluorescein angiography with arteriovenous shunting present in the area of the telangiectatic vessels. In chronic Leber optic neuropathy the optic disc is atrophic. About 15 percent of patients recover useful vision in one or both eyes many years after the ictus.

Papilledema Optic disc swelling resulting from elevated intracranial pressure (Fig. A4-4) is typically bilateral, often asymmetric, and is associated with transient visual loss lasting seconds (visual obscurations) and horizontal diplopia. Optic atrophy, impaired vision, and field loss may ensue if papilledema becomes chronic. Increased intracranial pressure may be caused by mass lesions, inflammatory disease, or idiopathic pseudotumor cerebri (benign intracranial hypertension), but the immediate obligation is to exclude an intracranial mass lesion with appropriate neuroimaging tests (see Chap. 353).

Pseudopapilledema Pseudopapilledema is usually due to congenital disc anomalies, giving rise to apparent rather than true disc swelling. Small or absent optic cups, abnormal branching of the major retinal vessels, and calcific excrescences [optic disc drusen (Fig. A4-5)] may be seen.

DISORDERS OF EYE MOVEMENT

Disorders of eye movement in the adult usually present with diplopia. The diagnostic approach to determine the cause is based on a series of specific questions and a step-by-step analysis of the eye movements to establish first whether the double vision is monocular or binocular. If diplopia is present with one eye covered, the patient has monocular diplopia. Monocular diplopia almost never signals a neurologic disorder but is most often due to an optical problem (refractive error, keratoconus, or cataract). It may be psychogenic or functional. Binocular diplopia resolves with occlusion of vision to either eye and is due to ocular misalignment, whether caused by disorders of the ocular motor nerves, of the myoneural junction (myasthenia gravis, see Chap. 366) or of the extraocular muscles themselves. Myasthenia gravis can usually be diagnosed with the edrophonium or prostigmine test. Restriction of extraocular muscle function can result from inflammation (orbital myositis), infiltration (thyroid ophthalmopathy or metastatic disease), or entrapment (blow-out fracture of the orbital floor). Restriction of movement of the globe can be confirmed with a positive forced duction test. Topical proparacaine is used to anesthetize the eye, especially over the insertion of the rectus muscles to be manipulated. While the patient looks in the direction of gaze limitation, the physician, using a cotton-tipped applicator or toothed forceps, attempts to move the globe in the direction of gaze deficit. The inability to overcome the eye movement limitation signifies the presence of a restrictive process.

Once restrictive disease and myasthenia gravis are excluded, the major cause of binocular diplopia is a cranial nerve lesion. The type of binocular diplopia—horizontal, vertical, or oblique—provides clues in determining which muscle is affected. A red glass test allows a more exact documentation of the type of diplopia.

ISOLATED OCULAR MOTOR NERVE PALSIES Oculomotor nerve (third cranial nerve) The oculomotor (third nerve) nuclear complex is a compact midline structure in the rostral midbrain, containing somatic motor and visceral nuclei. Motoneurons project ipsilaterally to the medial rectus, inferior rectus, and inferior oblique muscles and contralaterally to the superior rectus muscle. One central caudal nucleus innervates the levator palpebrae superioris bilaterally. Axons from the visceral nuclei project ipsilaterally, as the preganglionic, parasympathetic outflow to the ciliary ganglion, controlling pupillary sphincter function and accommodation.

The fascicular portion of the third nerve courses through the red nucleus and ventral mesencephalon to emerge in the interpeduncular fossa. It then runs forward beneath the posterior cerebral artery and lateral to the posterior communicating artery, pierces the dura, and enters the cavernous sinus. The pupillary fibers travel superficially in the dorsomedial portion of the nerve. At the superior orbital fissure, where the nerve enters the orbit, it divides into a superior (levator, superior rectus) and inferior division (medial and inferior rectus, inferior oblique, pupillomotor fibers).

A complete third nerve lesion causes ptosis and inability to turn the eye upward, downward, or inward. At rest, the eye is deviated down and temporally. Whether the iris sphincter is involved or spared, as determined by pupillary size and reactivity, is critical in determining the appropriate workup of the patient over age 50 years.

An acute, total, isolated painful third nerve palsy with a dilated nonreactive pupil suggests aneurysm of the posterior communicating artery compressing the third nerve. Pupillary sparing (normal size and reflex response) is the hallmark of a third nerve palsy due to microinfarction as occurs in diabetes mellitus. Initial pupillary sparing can be found in 8 to 15 percent of aneurysms, but pupillary involvement usually occurs within 5 to 7 days. Prompt consideration of cerebral angiography and surgery is indicated in all third nerve palsies with pupil involvement at all ages. Patients over age 50 with an isolated oculomotor palsy in which there is pupillary sparing and without signs of subarachnoid hemorrhage can be followed expectantly.

Recovery within three to four months is common in cases of microinfarction. In compressive or traumatic oculomotor palsies, regeneration is often aberrant, consisting of activation of inappropriate muscle groups on eye movements, e.g., producing lid retraction on down gaze or pupillary constriction with adduction.

The common causes of third nerve palsies in adults are aneurysms and vascular disease (hypertension, atherosclerosis, diabetes mellitus, temporal arteritis). Trauma and tumor (pituitary tumor, cavernous sinus meningioma or metastasis) each account for 10 to 15 percent of cases. Parasellar mass lesions can cause acute onset of a third nerve palsy after only minor trauma. (A similar relation holds for fourth and sixth nerve palsies as well.) Aberrant regeneration without a history of an antecedent oculomotor palsy indicates an indolent mass lesion in the cavernous sinus.

Trochlear nerve (fourth cranial nerve) The neurons of the fourth nerve nucleus lie dorsally in the rostral brainstem at the level of the inferior colliculi, contiguous to the caudal end of the oculomotor complex. The axons run dorsally and decussate in the anterior medullary velum (the roof of the fourth ventricle) where they are vulnerable to head trauma. The nerve exits the brainstem dorsally, crosses the superior cerebellar artery, runs forward in the cavernous sinus, and enters the orbit through the superior orbital fissure to innervate the superior oblique muscle.

A superior oblique palsy causes vertical diplopia with hypertropia and excylotorsion of the eye. Many patients compensate for this by adapting a head tilt toward the uninvolved side (i.e., a patient with a right superior oblique palsy will often have a left head tilt). Some patients who have a congenital fourth nerve palsy may be asymptomatic until later in life when the ability to fuse is lost. Such patients generally have a head tilt documented on childhood and adult photographs.

Trauma is the commonest cause of fourth nerve palsies. Vascular diseases (hypertension, atherosclerosis, diabetes mellitus) account for approximately 20 percent of cases. Miscellaneous causes include aneurysm (cavernous internal carotid artery or basilar artery), hydrocephalus, or sequelae to intracranial surgery. Management is usually conservative using vertical prism glasses or unilateral patching to alleviate symptoms. A variety of surgical procedures on the superior oblique or inferior oblique muscle can be performed if conservative treatment is unsatisfactory.

Abducens nerve (sixth nerve) The abducens nucleus is located beneath the floor of the fourth ventricle and lateral to the midline of the pons at the junction of the pons and medulla. The genu of the facial nerve curves over the dorsal and lateral surface. The medial longitudinal fasciculus lies adjacent and medial to it. The abducens nucleus contains motor neurons that innervate the ipsilateral lateral rectus muscle and a pool of interneurons whose axons cross the midline and ascend in the medial longitudinal fasciculus to reach the contralateral oculomotor subnucleus innervating the medial rectus muscle of the opposite eye. The abducens nucleus thus participates in the control of horizontal gaze.

The fascicular portion of the sixth nerve passes ventrally, laterally, and caudally through the pons, medial to the olivary nucleus, to exit the brainstem in a groove between the pons and the medulla. The proximity of the sixth nerve nucleus and its fascicular portion to the motor nucleus of the facial nerve, facial nerve fascicle, the vestibular nucleus, and descending sympathetic fibers within the brainstem explains the association of sixth nerve deficits with a multitude of disease states.

After emerging from the brainstem, the nerve runs along the face of the bony clivus to penetrate the dura below the crest of the petrous bone to enter the cavernous sinus. The sixth nerve is not situated within the sinus wall, like the third and fourth cranial nerves, but instead lies within the body of the sinus itself. It enters the orbit through the superior orbital fissure within the annulus of Zinn to innervate the lateral rectus muscle. A sixth nerve palsy causes an inward deviation of the eye and paresis of abduction. Causes of sixth nerve palsy include infarction, aneurysm, tumor, trauma, leptomeningitis, and multiple sclerosis, However, in spite of improved diagnostic techniques, many cases of monocranial nerve palsy remain unexplained (idiopathic).

MULTIPLE OCULAR MOTOR NERVE PALSIES The localization of lesions that cause combinations of third, fourth, or sixth nerve palsies depends upon the accurate assessment of the various combinations of associated neurologic deficits.

Lesions producing ophthalmoplegia involving the functions of more than one ocular motor nerve and associated with pain or hypesthesia in the distribution of the trigeminal nerve (fifth nerve) can be localized depending upon the extent of fifth nerve involvement. The lesion is at the superior orbital fissure or anterior cavernous sinus region, if only the first division of nerve V is involved; is at the middle to posterior cavernous sinus region, if the first (V1) and second (V2) divisions are involved; and is in the parasellar region, if all three divisions are involved. If the ipsilateral optic nerve is affected, the lesion must be in the orbital apex. Causes of these syndromes include nasopharyngeal carcinoma, granulomatous inflammatory processes (pseudotumor of the orbit or ''Tolosa Hunt'' syndrome), and lymphoma. Pituitary tumors, menigiomas, chordomas, and other rarer tumors can produce cavernous sinus–orbital apex syndromes. The diagnosis is aided by neuroimaging of the suspected area, including the nasopharynx.

SUPRANUCLEAR DISORDERS The neurologic signs The bedside diagnosis of brainstem disorders is aided by the understanding of the neuroanatomy of ocular motor control.

There are two classes of eye movements, rapid or *saccadic* movements and slow or *pursuit* movements. Both systems alter the direction of gaze (eye position in space). Rapid eye movements are used to bring new images onto the fovea. Pursuit eye movements are used to hold the object's image stationary on the moving retina.

Saccadic eye movements are tested by observation of eye movements on command, refixation saccades between two targets, and quick phases of optokinetic nystagmus and/or vestibular stimulation. Saccades and quick phases share the same immediate premotor neural circuitry within the brainstem. The descending pathways transmitting saccadic signals for gaze control are part of a corticobulbar pathway with connections between visual, frontal, and brainstem structures. All decussate in the midbrain to terminate in the contralateral pontine paramedian reticular formation (PPRF) in the brainstem, just rostral to the sixth nerve nucleus. Pursuit eye movements are tested by observation of the eyes tracking a target horizontally and vertically. Three visual cortical areas in the temporal-occipital junction are concerned with control of pursuit eye movements. They are the middle temporal and medial superior temporal cortex and the fundus of the superior temporal cortex. Pursuit pathways descend ipsilaterally to the dorsal lateral pontine nuclei, the Purkinje cells in the cerebellar flocculus, to the vestibular nuclei, and onward to the final common brainstem pathway, the PPRF.

Direct vertical gaze requires bilateral cortical activation. The rostral PPRF acts as the first brainstem center from which fibers project to the pretectal rostral interstitial nucleus of the median longitudinal fasciculus, which is the final vertical gaze center. Paralysis of horizontal and vertical gaze can be produced by lesions affecting cortical, mesencephalic, and pontine centers of their projections. Destruction of the ocular motor nuclei, fascicles, or nerves as well as myasthenia gravis can mimic a gaze palsy. Isolated upward gaze paralysis (Parinaud's syndrome) and isolated downward gaze or complete vertical gaze paralysis are produced by lesions involving the mesencephalon and pretectum. Tumors in the region of the pineal gland produce Parinaud's syndrome or the sylvian aqueduct syndrome; ocular signs include a supranuclear paralysis of upward gaze, light-near dissociation of the pupils, convergence paresis, skew deviation, and convergence retraction nystagmus. Brainstem infarction is possibly the only cause of selective paralysis of downward gaze, due to occlusion of a single perforating vessel, the posterior thalamosubthalamic paramedian artery.

Degenerative diseases e.g., progressive supranuclear palsy (see Chap. 359) may selectively or primarily involve the supranuclear structures of the brainstem. Vertical saccades are affected first, being slow and then small. Eventually there is complete loss of voluntary vertical refixations. With chronicity, the horizontal eye movements become similarly affected. Convergence may be impaired. The disease may progress to total ophthalmoplegia. Other degenerative diseases—Huntington's chorea, abetalipoproteinema, amyotrophic lateral sclerosis, and olivopontocerebellar degeneration—may be associated with a supranuclear disorder of vertical as well as horizontal gaze. Supranuclear vertical gaze disorders also occur in multiple sclerosis, Whipple's disease, syphilis, brucellosis, tetanus, encephalitis, neurofibromatosis, and tuberculoma as well as brainstem trauma, including neurosurgical procedures.

Opsoclonus is a striking disorder of saccadic eye movements reflecting the presence of unwanted saccades. It consists of involuntary, arrhythmic, multidirectional, high-amplitude, conjugate back-to-back saccades. The eye movements are usually continuous and persist during sleep. Opsoclonus can occur with encephalitis, trauma, intracranial tumors, hydrocephalus, thalamic hemorrhage, and toxic and metabolic encephalopathies. It occurs as a paraneoplastic or remote effect of neuroblastoma in children and, less commonly, of other carcinomas (ovary, lung, breast) in adults (Chap. 310).

INTERNUCLEAR OPHTHALMOPLEGIA Clinically, internuclear ophthalmoplegia (INO) is characterized by (1) paresis or paralysis of adduction of the ipsilateral eye on attempted horizontal gaze to the contralateral side, and (2) horizontal jerk nystagmus in the contralateral abducting eye. Typically convergence is intact if the lesion does not extend to the mesencephalon; gaze-evoked vertical nystagmus on upward gaze is frequent. Unilateral INO is due to the interruption of the ipsilateral medial longitudinal fasciculus (MLF), after fibers have crossed from the interneurons of the contralateral abducens nucleus projecting to the ipsilateral medial rectus subnucleus. Unilateral internuclear ophthalmoplegia is most commonly due to multiple sclerosis in young adults and to vascular infarction in the elderly. Prognosis for full recovery is good.

Bilateral INO is usually due to brainstem glioma in children and to multiple sclerosis in adults. Myasthenia gravis can mimic both unilateral and bilateral INO.

NYSTAGMUS AND OTHER ENTITIES THAT MIMIC NYSTAGMUS (See also Chap. 22) Nystagmus is a repetitive, to-and-fro movement of the eyes. *Pendular nystagmus* consists of smooth sinusoidal oscillations, and *jerk nystagmus* consists of slow drift alternating with corrective quick phases. Normal subjects develop nystagmus in response to vestibular and optokinetic stimuli.

Normally, the vestibular, optokinetic, and pursuit systems each act to hold images steady on the retina, and a neural integrator allows maintenance of eccentric positions of gaze. Disorders of these systems create nystagmus. Identification of the cause of nystagmus requires historical information—especially of drug use or alcohol abuse—and a complete ocular motor evaluation. The most important clinical types of nystagmus are discussed below and in Chap. 22.

Congenital nystagmus Congenital nystagmus is a pendular or jerk nystagmus that remains horizontal in all positions of gaze, is dampened by convergence, and is associated with better vision at near rather than far distances. Patients with congenital nystagmus often have afferent visual system dysfunction.

Labyrinthine-vestibular nystagmus Disease of the vestibular system causes constant velocity slow-phase drifts with corrective quick phases that create a "saw-tooth" jerk nystagmus. By convention, the side of the nystagmus is designated by the direction of the quick corrective saccade (fast phase). Vestibular nystagmus may be due to a peripheral or central lesion. In peripheral vestibular disease, the nystagmus is usually of mixed type. For example, in benign positional nystagmus, a mixed vertical-torsional nystagmus is common. In unilateral labyrinthine destruction, a mixed horizontal-torsional nystagmus occurs. Peripheral vestibular nystagmus is suppressed by fixation and exacerbated by changes in head position. Peripheral nystagmus if often associated with severe vertigo, nausea, vomiting, and oscillopsia. Disturbances of central vestibular connections are associated with a central imbalance between semicircular canal inputs and disruption of ascending vestibular or cerebellovestibular connections. Mixed nystagmus can be caused by peripheral labyrinthine or central vestibular disease. Purely bilateral vertical (upbeat, downbeat), torsional, or horizontal nystagmus can only occur with central vestibular disease. Central vestibular nystagmus is poorly suppressed by fixation but exacerbated or induced by changes in head position (Chap. 22).

Four forms of primary position vestibular nystagmus have anatomic localizing value: downbeat, upbeat, horizontal, and torsional nystagmus. Downbeat nystagmus in the primary position and accentuated on lateral gaze occurs with cervicomedullary junction disorders, such as Arnold-Chiari malformation and basilar invagination, and in multiple sclerosis, brainstem infarction, cerebellar atrophy, hydrocephalus, metabolic disorders, familiar periodic ataxia, or as a toxic side effect of anticonvulsant drugs. Lesions associated with primary position upbeat nystagmus are in the tegmentum of the rostral medulla and caudal pons; causes include infarction, demyelination, myelinolysis, and diffuse infiltration with glioma. Horizontal primary position nystagmus is rare and is usually due to peripheral vestibular disease.

Primary position torsional nystagmus is common in the lateral medullary syndrome. With this lesion the nystagmus may be horizontal or mixed with both torsional and vertical components. Typically the horizontal nystagmus beats away from the side of the medullary infarction with the eyes in a primary position but beats ipsilaterally when gaze is directed toward the lesion. Vertical nystagmus, if present, is usually upbeating.

Gaze-evoked nystagmus Gaze-evoked nystagmus implies a weakness in holding the eyes in an eccentric position due to a defect in the integrator in the brainstem. It is commonly caused by drugs such as sedatives or anticonvulsants. Asymmetric but conjugate horizontal gaze-evoked nystagmus occurs with unilateral cerebellar disease and cerebellopontine-angle tumors such as acoustic neuroma or meningioma.

REFERENCES

AMERICAN ACADEMY OF OPHTHALMOLOGY: *Basic and Clinical Science Course*, Sections I and II. San Francisco, 1988–1989

BURDE RM et al: *Clinical Decision in Neurophthalmology*. St. Louis, Mosby, 1985

DUANE T (ED): *Clinical Ophthalmology*. Philadelphia, Lippincott, 1988

GLASER JS: *Neuroophthalmology*. Philadelphia, Lippincott 1989

LEIGH RJ, ZEE DS: *The Neurology of Eye Movements*. Philadelphia, Davis, 1983

MILLER NR: *Walsh and Hoyt's Clinical Neuroophthalmology*, 4th ed. Baltimore, Williams & Wilkins, 1982

24 DISTURBANCES OF SMELL, TASTE, AND HEARING

JAMES B. SNOW, JR. / JOSEPH B. MARTIN

SMELL The sense of smell determines the flavor and palatability of food and drink. It serves along with the trigeminal system as a monitor of inhaled chemicals including dangerous substances such as natural gas, smoke, and air pollutants. Although qualitative sensations of smell are subserved by the olfactory neuroepithelium, many substances are capable of producing somatic sensations of coolness, warmth, and irritation through the trigeminal, glossopharyngeal, and vagal afferents in the nose, oral cavity, tongue, pharynx, and larynx. The sense of smell should be considered as one of several chemosensory systems since most chemical substances initiate olfactory, trigeminal, and taste perceptions.

The *olfactory neuroepithelium* is located in the superior part of the nasal cavities. It contains an orderly arrangement of bipolar olfactory receptor cells, microvillar cells, sustentacular cells, and basal cells. The dendritic process of the bipolar cell has a bulb-shaped knob or vesicle that projects into the mucous layer and bears six to eight cilia. The receptor sites for odorant molecules are located on the cilia. The microvillar cells are located adjacent to the receptor cells on the surface of the neuroepithelium. The sustentacular cells, unlike their counterparts in the respiratory epithelium, are not specialized to secrete mucus. Their function is unknown. The basal cells are progenitors of other cell types in the olfactory neuroepithelium including the bipolar receptor cells. There is a regular turnover of the bipolar receptor cells, which function as the primary sensory neurons. In addition with injury to the cell body or its axon, the receptor cell is replaced by a basal cell which reestablishes a central neural connection. *Hence, these primary sensory neurons are unique among sensory systems in that they are regularly replaced and regenerate after injury.*

The unmyelinated axons of the receptor cells form the fila of the olfactory nerve, pass through the cribriform plate, and terminate within spherical masses of neuropil, termed glomeruli, in the olfactory bulb. The glomeruli are a focus of a high degree of convergence of information, since many more fibers enter than leave them. The main second-order neurons are the mitral cells. The primary dendrite of each mitral cell extends into a single glomerulus. Axons of the mitral cells project along with the axons of adjacent tufted cells to the limbic system, including the anterior olfactory nucleus, the prepiriform cortex, the periamygdaloid cortex, the olfactory tubercle, the nucleus of the lateral olfactory tract, and the corticomedial nucleus of the amygdala. Cognitive awareness of smell requires stimulation of the prepiriform cortex or the amygdaloid nuclei.

Odorants are absorbed into the mucus overlying the olfactory neuroepithelium, diffuse to the cilia, and reversibly bind to membrane receptor sites. The process causes conformational changes in the receptor proteins which induce a chain of biochemical events that results in generation of action potentials in the primary neurons. Intensity appears to be coded by the amount of firing in the afferent neurons. Indeed, a clear relationship exists in humans between psychophysical measures of intensity and the magnitude of the evoked potential from the olfactory neuroepithelium. Little is known about quality coding. Individual receptor cells are responsive to a wide range of stimuli. It is thought that more than one type of receptor site is present on each cell.

Disturbances of the sense of smell Disturbances of the sense of smell are caused by conditions that interfere with the access of the odorant to the olfactory neuroepithelium (transport loss), injure the receptor region (sensory loss), or damage central olfactory pathways (neural loss).

Transport olfactory loss can result from swollen nasal mucous membrane in acute viral upper respiratory infections, herpes simplex, viral hepatitis, bacterial rhinitis, sinusitis, and allergic rhinitis and with structural changes in the nasal cavity such as deviations of the nasal septum, polyps, and neoplasms. Nasopharyngeal tumor or lymphoma can interfere with smell perception. It is also likely that abnormalities of mucous secretion in which the olfactory cilia are immersed could result in a loss of olfactory sensitivity. Currently little is known about alterations in the mucus environment of the olfactory neuroepithelium.

Sensory olfactory losses are caused by destruction of the olfactory neuroepithelium by viral infections, neoplasms, the inhalation of toxic chemicals, drugs that affect cell turnover, and radiation therapy to the head. *Neural olfactory losses* occur in head trauma, with or without fracture of the base of the anterior cranial fossa or cribriform plate area; Parkinson's disease, Alzheimer's disease, Korsakoff's psychosis, and vitamin B_{12} deficiency; neoplasms of the anterior cranial fossa; neurosurgical procedures; administration of neurotoxic drugs (e.g., ethanol, amphetamines, topical cocaine, aminoglycosides, tetracycline, cigarette smoke); and in some congenital disorders such as Kallmann's syndrome. Other endocrine disorders, including Cushing's syndrome, hypothyroidism, and diabetes mellitus, can affect smell perception.

From the psychophysical point of view, disturbances of the sense of smell may be categorized by either the patient's complaint or the objective sensory measurements as *total anosmia* (general anosmia)—inability to detect any qualitative olfactory sensations; *partial anosmia*—ability to detect some, but not all, qualitative olfactory sensations; *specific anosmia*—loss of ability to appreciate only one or a very limited number of odorants; *total hyposmia* (general hyposmia)—decreased sensitivity to all odorants; *partial hyposmia*—decreased sensitivity to some odorants; dysosmia (cacosmia or paraosmia)—distortion in the perception of an odor, that is, the perception of an unpleasant odor when a pleasant odorant is being presented or the perception of an odor when there is no odorant in the environment; *total hyperosmia* (general hyperosmia)—increased sensitivity to all odorants; *partial hyperosmia*—increased sensitivity to some odorants; and *agnosia*—inability to classify, contrast, or identify odor sensations verbally, even though the ability to distinguish between odorants or to recognize them may be normal.

CLINICAL EVALUATION The history of the onset and development of the disturbance of the sense of smell may be of paramount importance in making an etiologic diagnosis. Unilateral anosmia is rarely a complaint. Only by separate testing of smell in each nasal cavity can it be recognized. Bilateral anosmia, on the other hand, does bring patients to medical attention. Anosmic patients usually complain of a loss of the sense of taste even though their taste thresholds may be within normal limits. In actuality, they are complaining of a loss of flavor detection, which is mainly an olfactory function. Flavor appreciation depends on the olfactory detection of volatile substances in food and beverages as well as the sense of taste. The physical examination should include a complete examination of the ears, upper respiratory tract, and head and neck. A neurologic examination emphasizing the cranial nerves is essential. Computed tomography scans of the head with enhancement is required to rule out neoplasms of the anterior cranial fossa, unsuspected fractures of the anterior cranial fossa, paranasal sinusitis, and neoplasms of the nasal cavity and paranasal sinuses.

The sensory evaluation of olfactory function is necessary for corroboration of the patient's complaint, evaluation of the efficacy of treatment, and determination of the degree of permanent impairment. The first step in the sensory evaluation is to determine the degree to which qualitative sensations are present. For this assessment, a smell identification test is used that consists of a 40-item, forced choice, microencapsulated odor, scratch-and-sniff paradigm. For example, one of the items reads, "This odor smells most like (a) chocolate, (b) banana, (c) onion, or (d) fruit punch," and the patient is instructed to answer one of the alternatives. The test is highly reliable (short-term test-retest reliability $r = 0.95$) and is sensitive to age and sex differences (Fig. 24-1). It is an accurate quantitative

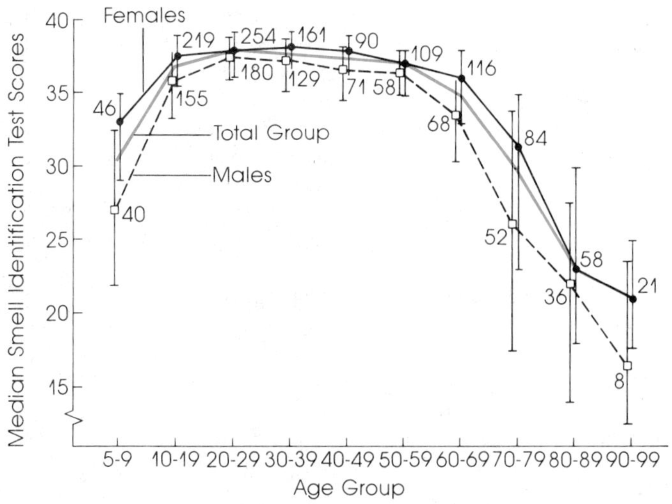

FIGURE 24-1 Smell identification test. Scores for a group of male and female subjects 5 to 99 years in age are shown. *(Reprinted with permission from RL Doty et al. Copyright 1984 by the AAAS.)*

determination of the relative degree of olfactory deficit. Persons with a total loss of smell function score in the range of 7 to 19 out of 40. The average score for total anosmics is slightly higher than that expected on the basis of chance because of the inclusion of some odorants which act by trigeminal stimulation.

The second step is to establish a detection threshold for the odorant phenyl ethyl alcohol, using a graduated stimulus. Although the detection threshold usually agrees with the results of the smell identification test, in some instances patients who fail the smell identification test perform well on the threshold test. However, the reverse is much less common. Since the threshold test can be influenced by trigeminal and nonolfactory nerve clues, the results of the smell identification test are relied upon more heavily in the sensory evaluation. Sensitivity for each side of the nose is determined with a detection threshold for phenyl ethyl methyl ethyl carbinol. Nasal resistance is measured with anterior rhinomanometry for each side of the nose.

Techniques have been developed to biopsy the olfactory neuroepithelium, but in view of the widespread degeneration of the olfactory neuroepithelium and intercalation of respiratory epithelium in the olfactory area of adults with no apparent olfactory dysfunction, biopsy material must be interpreted cautiously.

DIFFERENTIAL DIAGNOSIS At the present time there are no psychophysical methods to differentiate sensory from neural olfactory losses. Fortunately, the history of the disease provides important clues to the cause. The leading causes of olfactory disorders are head trauma and viral infections. Head trauma is a more frequent cause of anosmia in children and young adults, and viral infections are more important causes of anosmia in older adults.

Cranial trauma is followed by uni- or bilateral impairment of smell in 5 to 10 percent of cases. Frontal injuries and fractures disrupt the cribriform plate and olfactory axons which perforate it. Sometimes there is an associated cerebrospinal fluid (CSF) rhinorrhea resulting from a tearing of the dura overlying the cribriform plate and paranasal sinuses. If the anosmia is unilateral, it is usually on the side of the CSF leak, and this fact aids in localization of the fistula. Anosmia may also follow blows to the occiput. Once traumatic anosmia develops, it is usually permanent; only about 10 percent of patients ever improve or recover. Perversion of the sense of smell may occur as a phase in the recovery process.

The occurrence of a permanent hyposmia or anosmia may follow viral infections and is called *postviral anosmia*. In this instance the sensory epithelium of the olfactory zone is destroyed by the virus and replaced by respiratory epithelial and goblet cells and scar tissue. The congenital anosmias, one type of which is associated with a hypothalamic defect [Kallmann's syndrome, or congenital anosmia with hypogonadotropic hypogonadism (see Chap. 313)], are rare but important causes of anosmia or hyposmia. Anosmia can also occur in albinos. The receptor cells are present but hypoplastic, lack cilia, and do not project above the surrounding supporting cells.

Meningioma of the inferior frontal region is the most frequent neoplastic cause of anosmia; rarely anosmia can occur with glioma of the frontal lobe. Occasionally pituitary adenomas, craniopharyngiomas, suprasellar meningiomas, and aneurysms of the anterior part of the circle of Willis extend forward and damage olfactory structures. These tumors and hamartomas may also induce seizures with olfactory hallucinations, indicating involvement of the uncus of the temporal lobe.

Paraosmia and dysosmia, subjective distortions of olfactory perception, may occur with intranasal disease that partially impairs smell, or may represent a phase in the recovery from a neurogenic anosmia. Most paraosmic disturbances consist of disagreeable or foul odors, and they may be accompanied by distortions of taste. Dysosmia may also be a symptom in elderly patients with depression. Every article of food has an extremely unpleasant odor (cacosmia). Sensations of disagreeable taste are often noted (cacogeusia).

Olfactory hallucinations are descriptions of smelling an odor that no one else can smell. They occur in alcohol withdrawal, in which olfactory hallucinations are occasionally associated with other types of hallucinations, and in uncal seizures, which are brief and clearly related to a derangement of consciousness and other epileptic components. In other settings, olfactory hallucinations usually signify a psychiatric disease. A huge range of odors may be reported, most of them foul. Some patients perceive the smell as emanating from themselves (intrinsic); others perceive the source to be external (extrinsic). Most are associated with schizophrenia and depressive illnesses.

TREATMENT Therapy for patients with transport olfactory losses due to allergic rhinitis, bacterial rhinitis and sinusitis, polyps, neoplasms, and structural abnormalities of the nasal cavities can be undertaken rationally and with a high chance of improvement. Allergy management, antibiotic therapy, topical and systemic glucocorticoid therapy, and operations for nasal polyps, deviation of the nasal septum, and chronic hyperplastic sinusitis are frequently effective in restoring the sense of smell.

There is no treatment with demonstrated efficacy for sensorineural olfactory losses. Fortunately spontaneous recovery often occurs. Zinc and vitamin therapy are advocated by some. Profound zinc deficiency can undoubtedly result in losses and distortion of the sense of smell, but it is not a clinical problem except in very limited geographic areas. Vitamin therapy has mainly been in the form of vitamin A. The epithelial degeneration associated with vitamin A deficiency can cause anosmia, but vitamin A deficiency is not a common clinical problem in the United States. Unfortunately at the present time there are no effective therapeutic strategies for the sensorineural disorders of the sense of smell.

TASTE Many patients with a loss of olfactory sensitivity also complain of a loss of the sense of taste. On psychophysical testing, most of these patients have normal detection thresholds for taste. Disturbances of the sense of taste are far less frequent than disturbances of the sense of smell.

The taste receptor cells are located in the taste buds, spherical groups of cells arranged like the segments of a citrus fruit. At the surface, the taste bud has a pore into which microvilli of the receptor cells project. Taste buds have a similar appearance wherever they are located. Unlike the olfactory system the receptor cell is not the primary neuron. Instead, gustatory afferent nerve fibers contact individual taste receptor cells.

The sense of taste is mediated through the facial, glossopharyngeal, and vagal nerves. The gustatory system consists of at least five receptor populations. Taste buds are located in the foliate papillae along the lateral margin of the tongue, in the fungiform papillae throughout the dorsum of the tongue, in the circumvallate papillae at the junction of the dorsum and the base of the tongue, and in the palate, epiglottis, larynx, and esophagus. The chorda tympani branch of the facial nerve subserves taste from the anterior two-thirds of the tongue. The posterior one-third of the tongue is supplied by the lingual branch of the glossopharyngeal nerve. Afferents from the palate travel with the greater superficial petrosal nerve to the geniculate ganglion and thence via the facial nerve to the brainstem. The internal branch of the superior laryngeal nerve of the vagus nerve contains the taste afferents from the larynx including the epiglottis and esophagus.

The central connections of the nerves terminate in the brainstem in the nucleus of the tractus solitarius. The fibers of the chorda tympani and greater superficial petrosal nerves go to the cephalic portion of the nucleus. The glossopharyngeal gustatory fibers go to the middle, and the superior laryngeal nerve fibers to the caudal portion of the nucleus. The central pathway from the nucleus of the tractus solitarius projects to the ipsilateral parabrachial nuclei of the pons. Two divergent pathways project from the parabrachial nuclei. One ascends to the gustatory relay in the dorsal thalamus, synapses, and continues to the cortex of the insula. There is also evidence for a direct pathway from the parabrachial nuclei to the cortex. (Olfaction and taste appear to be unique among sensory systems in that at least some fibers bypass the thalamus.) The other pathway from the parabrachial nuclei goes to the ventral forebrain including the lateral hypothalamus, substantia innominata, central nucleus of the amygdala, and the stria terminalis.

Tastants gain access to the receptor cells through the taste pore. Four classes of taste are recognized: sweet, salt, sour, and bitter. Individual gustatory afferent fibers almost always respond to a number of different chemicals. Response patterns of gustatory afferent axons can be grouped into classes based on the stimulus chemical that produces the largest response. For example, for sucrose-best response neurons, the second-best stimulus is almost always sodium chloride. The fact that individual gustatory afferent fibers respond to a large number of different chemicals led to the *across-fiber-pattern* theory of gustatory coding, while the best-stimulus analysis led to the concept of *labeled* afferents. It appears that labeled fibers are important for establishing gross quality, but the across-fiber-pattern within a best-stimulus category, and perhaps among categories, is needed for discriminating chemicals within qualities. For example, sweetness may be carried by sucrose-best neurons, but the differentiation of sucrose and fructose may require a comparison of the relative activity among sucrose-best, salt-best, and quinine-best neurons. As with olfaction and other sensory systems, intensity appears to be encoded by the quantity of neural activity.

Disturbances of the sense of taste Disturbances of the sense of taste are caused by conditions that interfere with the access of the tastant to the receptor cells in the taste bud (transport loss), injure receptor cells (sensory loss), or damage gustatory afferent nerves and central gustatory pathways (neural loss).

Transport gustatory losses result from xerostomia due to many causes including Sjögren's syndrome, heavy metal intoxication, and bacterial colonization of the taste pore. The salivary milieu of the receptors may prove to be important to diverse causes of gustatory loss.

Sensory gustatory losses are caused by inflammatory and degenerative diseases in the oral cavity, a vast number of drugs, particularly those that interfere with cell turnover such as antithyroid and antineoplastic agents, radiation therapy to the oral cavity and pharynx, viral infections, endocrine disorders, neoplasms, and aging.

Neural olfactory losses occur with neoplasms, trauma, and operations in which the gustatory afferents are injured. Taste buds degenerate when their gustatory afferents are transected but remain when their somatosensory afferents are severed.

CLINICAL MANIFESTATIONS From the psychophysical point of view disturbances of the sense of taste may be categorized by either the patient's complaint or the objective sensory measurements as *total ageusia*—inability to detect the qualities of sweet, salt, bitter, or sour; *partial ageusia*—ability to detect some but not all of the qualitative gustatory sensations; *specific ageusia*—inability to detect the taste quality of certain substances; *total hypoguesia*—decreased sensitivity to all tastants; *partial hypogeusia*—decreased sensitivity to some tastants; *dysgeusia*—distortion in the perception of a tastant, that is, the perception of the wrong quality when a tastant is presented or the perception of a taste when there has been no tastant ingested. Confusions of sour and bitter are common and, at times, may be semantic misunderstandings. Frequently, however, they have physiologic or pathophysiologic bases.

It may be possible to differentiate between the loss of flavor recognition in patients with olfactory losses who complain of a loss of taste as well as smell by asking if they are able to taste sweetness in sodas, saltiness in potato chips, etc.

Patients who complain of loss of taste should be evaluated psychophysically for gustatory function in addition to being evaluated for olfactory function. The first step is to perform suprathreshold whole-mouth taste testing for quality, intensity, and pleasantness perception with sucrose, citric acid, caffeine, and sodium chloride. In the quantification of the sense of taste, detection thresholds are obtained by applying graduated dilutions to the tongue quadrants or by whole-mouth sips. Finally, suprathreshold magnitude estimation may be used to shed further light on the patient's complaint. Electric taste testing (electrogustometry) is used clinically to identify taste deficits in specific quadrants of the tongue.

Biopsy of the foliate or fungiform papillae for histopathologic study of taste buds remains experimental but holds promise of shedding light on the categorization of taste disorders.

DIFFERENTIAL DIAGNOSIS As with olfaction, psychophysical methods for differentiating transport, sensory, and neural gustatory losses are not available. Once there is objective evidence of a disorder of taste, it is important to establish, as is done in other neurologic deficits, an anatomic diagnosis before proceeding to an etiologic diagnosis. The history of the disease often provides important clues to the cause. For example, absence of taste on the anterior two-thirds of the tongue associated with a facial paralysis indicates that the lesion is proximal to the point of junction of the chorda tympani branch with the facial nerve in the mastoid.

TREATMENT Therapy for gustatory losses remains limited. Artificial saliva benefits some patients with a disturbed salivary milieu. Treatment for bacterial and fungal infections of the oral cavity are appropriate and may be helpful. Withdrawal of drugs affecting cell turnover are usually helpful if the patient's general condition permits. Zinc and vitamin therapy for gustatory losses are advocated by some, but lack demonstrated efficacy. No therapeutic strategies exist for the sensorineural disorders of taste.

HEARING Hearing occurs by air conduction and bone conduction. In air conduction, sound waves reach the ear by propagation in air, enter the external auditory canal, and set the tympanic membrane in motion, which in turn moves the malleus, incus, and stapes. Movement of the footplate of the stapes causes pressure changes in the fluid-filled inner ear eliciting a traveling wave in the basilar membrane of the cochlea. The traveling wave moves from the base to the apex of the cochlea. Hairs of the hair cells of the organ of Corti, which rests on the basilar membrane, are imbedded in the tectorial membrane and are deformed by the traveling wave. A point of maximal displacement of the basilar membrane determined by the frequency of the stimulating tone occurs with each traveling wave. High-frequency tones cause maximal displacement of the basilar membrane near the base of the cochlea. As the frequency of the stimulating tone decreases, the point of maximal displacement moves toward the apex of the cochlea. Hearing by bone conduction occurs when the sounding source, in contact with the head, results in vibration of the bones of the skull including the temporal bone, producing a traveling wave in the basilar membrane.

The deformation of the hairs of the hair cells produces several bioelectric phenomena. The cochlear microphonic, an alternating current response that faithfully represents the frequency and intensity of the stimulating tone, occurs about 0.5 ms prior to the eighth nerve action potential. This latency is taken as evidence for release of an as yet unidentified neurotransmitter at the hair cell and cochlear nerve dendrite interface. Each of the cochlear nerve neurons can be activated at a frequency and intensity specific for that cell. This phenomenon of the characteristic or best frequency occurs at each point of the central auditory pathway: dorsal and ventral cochlear nuclei, trapezoid body, superior olivary complex, lateral lemniscus, inferior colliculus, medial geniculate body, and auditory cortex. At low frequencies, individual auditory nerve fibers can respond more or less synchronously with the stimulating tone. At higher frequencies, phase-locking occurs so that neurons take turns in responding to particular phases of the cycle of the sound wave. Intensity is encoded by the amount of neural activity in individual neurons, the number of neurons that are active, and the specific neurons that are activated.

Disturbances of the sense of hearing A loss of hearing can result from lesions in the external auditory canal, middle ear, inner ear, or central auditory pathways. Lesions in the external auditory canal or the middle ear cause conductive hearing losses while lesions in the inner ear or eighth nerve cause sensorineural hearing losses.

Conductive hearing losses result from obstruction of the external auditory canal by cerumen, debris and foreign bodies, swelling of the lining of the canal, and stenosis and neoplasms of the canal. Perforations of the tympanic membrane, as in chronic otitis media, disruption of the ossicular chain, as occurs with necrosis of the long process of the incus in trauma or infection, fixation of the ossicles as in otosclerosis, and fluid, scarring, or neoplasms in the middle ear also result in conductive hearing losses. *Sensory hearing losses* are due principally to damage to the hair cells of the organ of Corti caused by intense noise, viral infections, ototoxic drugs, fractures of the temporal bone, meningitis, cochlear otosclerosis, Ménière's disease, and aging. Neural hearing losses are due mainly to cerebellar angle tumors such as acoustic neuromas, but may also result from any neoplastic, vascular, demyelinating, infectious, or degenerative disease or trauma affecting the central auditory pathways.

CLINICAL EVALUATION OF HEARING The physical examination should evaluate the external ear canal and tympanic membrane. Careful inspection of the nose, nasopharynx, and the upper respiratory tract is indicated. The other cranial nerves should be carefully evaluated. Conductive and sensorineural hearing losses can be differentiated by comparing the threshold of hearing by air conduction with that elicited by bone conduction. Testing the hearing by air conduction is accomplished by presenting the stimulus in air. Hearing by air conduction is affected by the patency of the external auditory canal, the efficiency of the middle ear, and the integrity of the inner ear, eighth nerve, and the central auditory pathways. Testing the hearing by bone conduction is accomplished by placing an oscillator or the stem of a vibrating tuning fork in contact with the head. Hearing by bone conduction bypasses the external auditory canal and middle ear and tests the integrity of the inner ear, eighth nerve, and central auditory pathways. If air conduction thresholds are elevated and bone conduction thresholds are in the normal range, the lesion causing hearing loss is in the external auditory canal or middle ear. If both air conduction and bone conduction thresholds are elevated, the lesion is in the inner ear, eighth nerve, or central auditory pathways. Of course, conductive and sensorineural hearing losses can coexist, in which case both the air conduction and bone conduction thresholds are elevated, but in this case, air conduction thresholds are elevated more than bone conduction thresholds.

The Weber and Rinne tuning fork tests are used to differentiate conductive from sensorineural hearing losses. The Weber tuning fork test may be performed with a 256- or 512-Hz fork. The Rinne tuning fork test is most sensitive in detecting mild conductive hearing losses if a 256-Hz fork is used. Weber's test is performed by placing the stem of a vibrating tuning fork on the head in the midline and asking the patient whether the tone is heard in both ears or better in one ear than in the other. With a unilateral conductive hearing loss, the tone is perceived in the affected ear. With a unilateral sensorineural hearing loss, the tone is perceived in the unaffected ear. Rinne's test compares the ability to hear by air conduction with the ability to hear by bone conduction. The tines of a vibrating tuning fork are held near the opening of the external auditory canal and then the stem is placed on the mastoid process. The patient is asked to indicate whether the tone is louder by air conduction or bone conduction. Normally a tone is heard louder by air conduction than by bone conduction. With a conductive hearing loss, the bone conduction stimulus is perceived as louder than the air conduction stimulus. With sensorineural hearing losses, both air and bone conduction perceptions are reduced, but the air conduction stimulus is perceived as louder, as it is in normal hearing. The combined information from the Weber and Rinne tests permits a tentative conclusion as to whether a conductive or sensorineural hearing loss is present.

Measurement of hearing Quantification of hearing loss is obtained with an audiometer, an electronic device that allows the presentation of specific frequencies at specific intensities to each ear by either air or bone conduction. The testing is done in a sound-attenuated chamber, and masking, usually with broad-spectrum noise, is presented to the nontest ear so that responses are based on perception from the ear under test. Frequencies from 250 to 8000 Hz are used in clinical testing. The responses are measured in decibels. A decibel (dB) is equal to 10 times the logarithm of the ratio of the acoustic power required to achieve threshold in the patient to the acoustic power required to achieve threshold in a normal hearing person. An audiogram is a plot of intensity in decibels versus frequency.

The audiometric pattern of hearing loss is often of diagnostic value. Conductive hearing losses usually have a fairly equal threshold elevation for each frequency. Conductive hearing losses with a large mass component, as is often seen in middle ear effusions, have a greater elevation of thresholds in the higher frequencies. Conductive hearing losses with a large stiffness component, as in fixation of the footplate of the stapes in early otosclerosis, have a greater elevation of thresholds in the lower frequencies. In general, sensorineural hearing losses tend to have a greater threshold elevation at each higher frequency. Interesting exceptions to this generalization are noise-induced hearing loss, in which the loss at 4000 Hz is greater than it is at higher frequencies, and in Ménière's disease, particularly in the early stages of the disease, where thresholds are elevated more in lower than in higher frequencies.

Speech audiometry provides essential additional information. The *spondee threshold* is defined as the intensity at which speech is recognized as a meaningful symbol and is obtained by presenting through an audiometer two-syllable words with an equal accent on each syllable. The intensity at which the patient can repeat 50 percent of the words correctly is the spondee threshold and usually approximates the average threshold at the speech frequencies (500, 1000, and 2000 Hz). Once the spondee threshold is determined, the discrimination ability is tested by presenting one-syllable words at 25 to 40 dB above the spondee threshold. An individual with normal hearing can repeat 90 to 100 percent of the words correctly. Likewise, individuals with a conductive hearing loss do well in discrimination testing. On the other hand, patients with a sensorineural hearing loss have a loss of discrimination attributable to the loss of peripheral analysis of sound in the inner ear or eighth nerve. With a lesion in the inner ear, the discrimination is moderately affected, usually in the 50 to 80 percent range, while with neural lesions the discrimination is severely affected, often in the 0 to 50 percent range.

The discrimination testing may then be done at higher intensities than 25 to 40 dB above the spondee threshold to determine the performance-intensity function. A deterioration in discrimination ability at higher intensities suggests a lesion in the eighth nerve or central auditory pathways.

Tympanometry measures the impedance of the middle ear to sound. A sounding source and microphone are introduced into the ear canal with an airtight seal. The amount of sound that is absorbed through the middle ear or reflected from the middle ear is measured at the microphone. In conductive hearing losses, more sound is reflected than in the normal middle ear. The pressure in the ear canal can be increased or decreased from atmospheric pressure. Normally the middle ear is most compliant at atmospheric pressure. With a negative pressure in the middle ear, as with eustachian tube obstruction, the point of maximal compliance occurs with negative pressure in the ear canal. With discontinuity of the ossicular chain, no point of maximal compliance can be obtained. Tympanometry is particularly useful in the identification and diagnosis of middle ear effusions in children.

During tympanometry, an intense tone (80 dB above the hearing threshold) elicits contraction of the stapedius muscle. The change in compliance of the middle ear with contraction of the stapedius muscle can be detected. The presence or absence of this *acoustic reflex* is important in the anatomic localization of facial nerve paralysis. The presence or absence of *acoustic reflex decay* helps differentiate sensory from neural hearing losses. In neural hearing loss, the reflex adapts or decays with time.

In order to evaluate a patient with a loss of hearing the minimum audiologic assessment should include the measurement of pure tone air and bone conduction thresholds, spondee threshold, discrimination score, performance-intensity function, tympanometry, acoustic reflexes, and acoustic reflex decay. This information provides a comprehensive screening evaluation of the whole auditory system and allows one to determine whether further differentiation of a sensory (cochlear) from a neural (retrocochlear) hearing loss is indicated.

In addition to these tests, testing for recruitment, the short increment sensitivity index, tone decay, Békésy audiometry, and auditory brainstem evoked responses (ABR) help differentiate sensory from neural hearing losses. Of these, ABR is the most powerful means of differentiating the site of sensorineural hearing loss (see Chap. 349). In response to sound, five distinct waves can be recorded with computer averaging from scalp surface electrodes. Poor or absent waveforms, abnormal latency of waves, and abnormal interwave latency are evidence of lesions in the eighth nerve and brainstem. In addition, ABR is valuable in situations in which patients cannot or will not give reliable voluntary thresholds. It is also used to measure auditory function in neonates and young children and to monitor the integrity of the auditory nerve and brainstem in various clinical situations, including intraoperatively and in determination of brain death.

CLINICAL ASSESSMENT OF A COMPLAINT OF HEARING LOSS In evaluating patients who complain of loss of hearing, associated symptoms of tinnitus, vertigo, difficulty with balance, earache, otorrhea, and aural fullness should be sought along with a careful reconstruction of the history of evolution of the hearing deficit. A sudden onset of unilateral hearing loss, with or without tinnitus, may represent a viral infection in the inner ear. Gradual progression in a hearing deficit is common with otosclerosis, noise-induced hearing loss, acoustic neuroma, or Ménière's disease. In the latter case, intermittent tinnitus and vertigo are usual. Hearing loss can occur with demyelinative lesions in the brainstem. Hearing loss is a hallmark of several genetic diseases, some with onset at birth, others occurring in children or adults (see Konigsmark for review).

Tinnitus is defined as the perception of a sound when there is no sound in the environment. It may have a buzzing, roaring, or ringing quality and may be pulsatile (synchronous with the heartbeat). Tinnitus is usually associated with a conductive or sensorineural loss of hearing. The pathophysiology of tinnitus is not well understood. The cause of the tinnitus can usually be determined by finding the cause of the associated hearing loss. Tinnitus may be the first symptom of a serious condition such as an acoustic schwannoma. Pulsatile tinnitus requires evaluation of the vascular system of the head to exclude vascular tumors such as glomus jugulare tumors, aneurysms, and stenotic lesions.

DIFFERENTIAL DIAGNOSIS Many patients with sensorineural hearing losses should have the vestibular system evaluated with electronystagmography and caloric testing (see Chap. 22). Most patients with conductive hearing losses should have computed tomography of the temporal tones. Patients with unilateral or asymmetric sensorineural hearing losses should have magnetic resonance imaging of the head with Gadolinium enhancement.

PREVENTION Conductive hearing losses may be prevented by prompt and appropriate antibiotic therapy of adequate duration for acute otitis media and by reventilation of the middle ear with tympanostomy tubes in middle ear infusions lasting 6 weeks or longer. Loss of vestibular function and deafness due to aminoglycoside antibiotics can largely be prevented by careful monitoring of serum peak and trough levels. Noise-induced hearing loss can be prevented by avoidance of exposure to loud noise or by regular use of ear plugs or glycerine-filled muffs to attenuate intense sound.

TREATMENT Most patients with conductive hearing losses can have the middle ear reconstructed using procedures such as tympanoplasty after chronic otitis media and trauma and stapedectomy for otosclerosis. Tympanostomy tubes allow the prompt return of hearing to normal in children and adults with middle ear effusions. Hearing aids are effective and well-tolerated for patients with conductive hearing losses. Patients with mild, moderate, and severe sensorineural hearing losses are regularly rehabilitated with hearing aids of varying configuration and strength. The profoundly deaf benefit from cochlear implants.

The treatment of tinnitus is particularly problematic. The frequency range and intensity of tinnitus can often be matched with the use of an audiometer. Relief of the tinnitus may be obtained by masking it with background music. Hearing aids also are helpful in tinnitus suppression, as are tinnitus maskers, devices that present a sound to the affected ear which is more pleasant to listen to than the tinnitus. The use of a tinnitus masker is often followed by several hours of inhibition of the tinnitus.

REFERENCES

ALBERTI PW, RUBEN RJ (eds): *Otologic Medicine and Surgery*. New York, Churchill Livingstone, 1988

COLE P: Upper respiratory airflow, in *The Nose: Upper Airway Physiology and the Atmospheric Environment*, DF Proctor, IB Anderson (eds). Amsterdam, Elsevier, 1982, pp 163–189

DALLOS P: *The Auditory Periphery: Biophysics and Physiology*. New York, Academic Press, 1973

DOTY RL: A review of olfactory dysfunctions in man. Am J Otolaryngol 1:57, 1979

——— et al: Smell identification ability: Changes with age. Science 226:1441, 1984

———: Presence of both odor identification and detection deficits in Alzheimer's disease. Brain Res Bull 18:597, 1987

———: Olfactory dysfunction in Parkinsonism: A general deficit unrelated to neurological signs, disease stage or disease duration. Neurology 38:1237, 1988

JERGER JR: *Modern Developments in Audiology*, 2d ed. New York, Academic Press, 1973

KONIGSMARK BW: Hereditary diseases of the nervous system with hearing loss, in *Handbook of Clinical Neurology*, PJ Vinken, GW Bruyn (eds). Elsevier, Amsterdam, 1975, vol 22, chap 23, pp 499–526

LEVINE SB, SNOW JB: Pulsatile tinnitus. Laryngoscope 97:401, 1987

LOWELL MA et al: Biopsy of human olfactory mucosa: An instrument and a technique. Arch Otolaryngol 108:247, 1982

NAKASHIMA T et al: Structure of human fetal and adult olfactory neuroepithelium. Arch Otolaryngol 110:641, 1984

NORGREN R: The gustatory system in mammals. Am J Otolaryngol 4:234, 1983

RINTELMAN WF: *Hearing Assessment*. Baltimore, Baltimore University, 1979

SNOW JB: Sudden deafness, in *Otolaryngology*, 2d ed, MM Paprella, DA Shumrick (eds). Philadelphia, Saunders, 1980, pp 1751–1767

——— et al: Central auditory imperception. Laryngoscope 87:1450, 1977

———: Clinical problems in chemosensory distrubances. Am J Otolaryngol 4:224 1983

TALAMO BR et al: Pathological changes in olfactory neurons in patients with Alzheimer's disease. Nature 337:736, 1989

25 PARALYSIS AND MOVEMENT DISORDERS

JOHN H. GROWDON / J. STEPHEN FINK[1]

Impairments of motor function may be subdivided into (1) paralysis due to lesions of corticospinal, corticobulbar, or brainstem descending (subcorticospinal) neurons, (2) abnormalities of movement and posture due to disease of the extrapyramidal motor system, (3) apraxic or nonparalytic disturbances of purposive movement due to involvement of the cerebrum, (4) abnormalities of coordination (ataxia) due to lesions in the cerebellar system, including its inputs and outputs, and (5) paralysis due to disorders of the motor unit including bulbar or spinal motor neurons, neuromuscular junction, and muscle. This chapter reviews signs and symptoms that result from lesions of lower motor neurons, descending corticospinal and other tracts, and the extrapyramidal system. It also includes consideration of apraxic disorders. The cerebellar system is discussed in Chap. 26. Signs and symptoms that result from lesions of the neuromuscular junction and muscle are discussed in Chaps. 365 and 366.

FUNCTIONAL ANATOMY OF PRINCIPAL MOTOR TRACTS AND THE MOTOR UNIT

PYRAMIDAL SYSTEM The chief element, the corticospinal tract, is the only direct connection between the cerebrum and the spinal cord. At the level of the medulla the tract contains approximately 1 million axons, far exceeding in number the 30,000 giant Betz cells of the motor cortex (area 4 of Brodmann). Thus, smaller Betz cells of area 4, cells of the adjacent precentral cortex (area 6), and those of the secondary motor cortex in the superior frontal convolution and postcentral cortex (areas 1, 2, 3, 5, and 7) all contribute to the pyramidal system. It is now known that the cells of origin of the corticospinal tract reside in cortical layer V; only 30 percent of the corticospinal and corticobulbar axons originate in area 4.

[1] The authors acknowledge the contribution to this discussion of Robert R. Young, coauthor in the 11th edition.

At the level of the internal capsule corticospinal fibers are intermingled with many others—some destined to end in the striatum, globus pallidus, substantia nigra, red nucleus, and reticular substance; others ascending from the thalamus. Fibers to the cranial nerve nuclei become separated at about the level of the midbrain, where they cross the midline to the contralateral cranial nerve nuclei. These fibers form the corticomesencephalic, corticopontine, and corticobulbar tracts and are included in the pyramidal system of motor neurons because they have functions similar to those of the corticospinal tract. The decussation of the corticospinal tract at the lower end of the medulla is variable. Most of the crossing fibers come to occupy a position in the posterolateral part of the lateral funiculus; a few cross to form an anterior funiculus. A small number of fibers, 10 to 20 percent, do not cross but descend ipsilaterally as the uncrossed corticospinal tract in the anterior funiculus of the spinal cord. Exceptionally, all of the corticospinal fibers cross; rarely, they remain uncrossed. Axons that travel in the lateral corticospinal tract terminate upon (1) neurons of the dorsal horn, (2) interneurons in the intermediate zone of spinal gray matter, and (3) motor neurons located dorsolaterally in the anterior horn. Not more than 25 percent of pyramidal tract neurons establish direct synaptic connection with anterior horn cells (Fig. 25-1). The corticospinal tract in the anterior funiculus terminates bilaterally upon motor neurons located in the ventromedial anterior horn; these neurons innervate axial muscles.

The motor area of the cerebral cortex includes that part of the precentral convolution which contains Betz cells (area 4), but it also extends anteriorly into area 6 and the secondary motor area of the superior frontal convolution and posteriorly into the anterior parietal lobe, where it overlaps the sensory areas. Physiologically the motor cortex is defined as the region of electrically excitable cortex from which isolated movements can be evoked by stimuli of minimal intensity. The muscle groups of contralateral face, arm, trunk, and leg are represented in the motor cortex, those of the face being at the lower end of the precentral convolution and those of the leg in the paracentral lobule on the medial surface of the cerebral hemisphere. The parts of the body capable of the most delicate movements have, in general, the largest cortical representation. One of the functions of the motor cortex is to synthesize simple movements into an infinite variety of finely graded, highly differentiated patterns.

VENTROMEDIAL BULBOSPINAL SYSTEM In addition to the pyramidal (corticospinal and corticobulbar) tract, the spinal gray

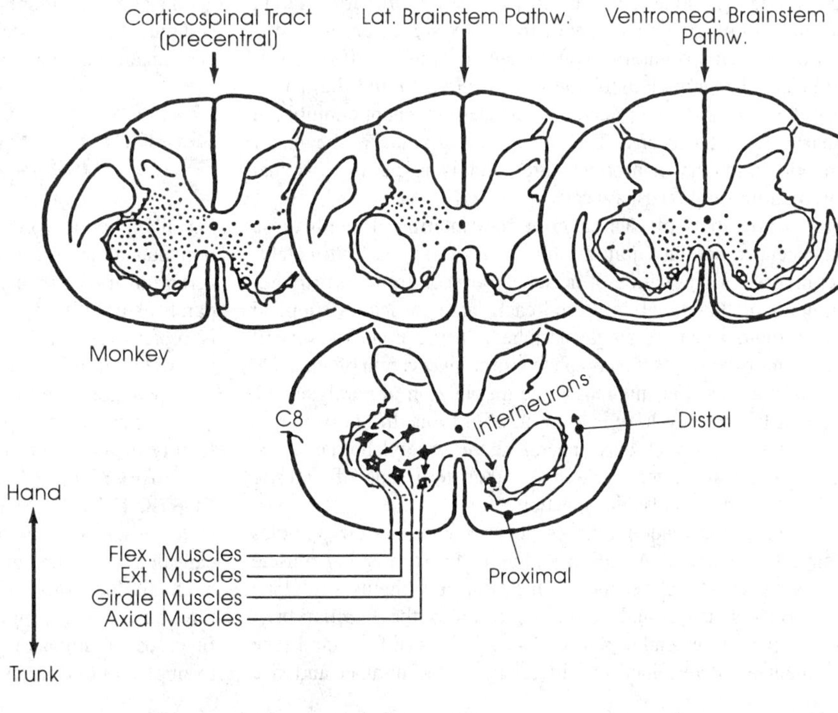

FIGURE 25-1 The distribution of terminations of cortical and brainstem descending pathways (dots) in the spinal intermediate zone and motor neuronal cell groups in rhesus monkey. Note that lateral brainstem pathways (arising from the magnocellular red nucleus and the ventrolateral pontine tegmentum) end on interneurons concerned principally with hand muscles. Ventromedial brainstem pathways (from the superior colliculus, interstitial nucleus of Cajal, pontine, medullary and mesencephalic medial reticular formation, and vestibular nuclei) end on interneurons concerned with trunkal and limb girdle muscles. [*From HGJM Kuypers, in JE Desmedt (ed). New Developments in Electromyography and Clinical Neurophysiology, Basel, Karger, 1973, vol. 3.*]

matter receives axons from two groups of descending pathways from the brainstem. Major contributions to the *ventromedial system* come from the lateral and medial vestibulospinal tracts originating in the lateral and medial vestibular nuclei, the reticulospinal tract originating in the reticular formation of the medulla and pons, and the tectospinal tract originating in the superior colliculus of the midbrain. Neurons originating in the raphe nuclei of the medulla (containing serotonin, substance P, and TRH), in the region of the locus coeruleus in the dorsal brainstem (containing norepinephrine), and in the interstitial nucleus of Cajal also contribute axons to the ventromedial brainstem descending system. These descending ventromedial axons terminate largely upon motor neurons located in the ventromedial anterior horn that innervate axial and proximal muscles; this pool of motor neurons is important in the maintenance of posture and balance. The ventromedial system is also richly collateralized in the upper and lower spinal cord.

DORSOLATERAL BULBOSPINAL SYSTEM Neurons in the red nucleus of the midbrain contribute axons to the rubrospinal tract, which is the major component of the *dorsolateral system* of brainstem descending pathways. Like the corticospinal tract in the lateral funiculus, the dorsolateral system terminates in the lateral portion of the intermediate zone and on motor neurons located dorsolaterally in the anterior horn; these motor neurons innervate distal muscles.

FUNCTIONAL ANATOMY OF THE MOTOR UNIT Each motor nerve cell, through extensive arborization of the terminal part of its fiber, comes into contact with hundreds of muscle fibers; together they constitute the "motor unit." Motor neurons in the spinal cord gray matter are organized topographically (Fig. 25-1). Motor neurons innervating a single muscle are distributed longitudinally through two to four spinal segments. Within the anterior horn, groups of motor neurons located medially project to axial muscles, such as neck and back, whereas neurons located laterally in the anterior horn innervate the distal muscles of the limbs. There is an additional topographic representation of flexor and extensor muscles in the anterior horn; motor neurons that are located more dorsally terminate on flexor muscles, and extensor muscles are innervated by motor neurons located more ventrally. Motor neuron excitability is modulated by segmental afferent and suprasegmental descending pathways. Descending corticospinal axons are believed to release aspartic acid and glutamic acid as neurotransmitters. Afferent modulation of motor unit activity is provided, in part, by axons of dorsal root ganglia cells which innervate most lamina of the dorsal horn, the intermediate zone, and some motor neurons directly. Substance P and the excitatory neurotransmitter glutamic acid are released by the primary afferent neurons and can modulate the gain of the reflex arc. Aspartic acid is believed to mediate excitatory impulses among spinal cord interneurons. Release of gamma-aminobutyric acid (GABA) and the neuropeptide enkephalin from interneurons increases presynaptic inhibition of primary afferent neurons. The amino acid glycine is the major postsynaptic inhibitory neurotransmitter and is released by spinal cord interneurons and Renshaw cells.

Motor nerve fibers of each anterior root intermingle with those from adjacent roots and join to form plexuses and, ultimately, peripheral nerves. Innervation of muscles proceeds from corresponding segments of the spinal cord, and each large muscle is supplied by two or more roots. A single peripheral nerve contains several roots and usually provides the complete motor innervation of a muscle or group of muscles. For this reason the distribution of paralysis due to disease of the anterior horn cells or anterior roots differs from that which follows a lesion of a peripheral nerve. Acetylcholine is the excitatory neurotransmitter released by axon terminals of anterior horn cells at the neuromuscular junction.

Muscle tone and tendon reflexes depend upon muscle spindles and their afferent fibers. A tap on a tendon, by stimulating muscle spindles, activates stretch receptors which transmit impulses to alpha motor neurons in the spinal cord. The result is the familiar brief muscle contraction or tendon reflex. All variations in force and type of movement are determined by differences in the number and size of motor units called into activity, the frequency of their firing rates, and the patterns of activity in different muscles. Feeble movements recruit few units; the number and size of motor units increase in a stereotyped fashion with stronger movements. Motor units involved in tonic contractions have muscle fibers known as type I that are rich in oxidative enzymes and mitochondria; those controlling phasic contractions innervate muscle fibers that have anaerobic metabolism (type II fibers) (see also Chap. 362). When a motor neuron becomes diseased, as in progressive muscular atrophy, its axon may manifest increased irritability and all the muscle fibers that it controls may discharge sporadically, in isolation from other units. The result of the contraction of one or several such units is a muscular twitch, or *fasciculation,* which can be observed visibly and recorded in the electromyogram (EMG). If the motor neuron or its axon is destroyed, all of the muscle fibers to which it is attached undergo profound denervation atrophy. As a result, individual muscle fibers become hypersensitive to acetylcholine and contract spontaneously, although they are unresponsive to nerve impulses. Isolated activity of individual muscle fibers is called *fibrillation;* it is so fine that it cannot be seen through the intact skin and can be recorded only as a short-duration spike potential in the EMG (see Chap. 362).

All motor activity, even of the most elementary reflex type, requires the cooperation of several muscles. Analysis of a relatively simple movement, such as clenching the fist, affords some idea of the complexity of the underlying neural arrangements. In this act the primary movement is a contraction of the flexor muscles of the fingers, the flexor digitorum sublimis and profundus, the flexor pollicis longus and brevis, and the adductor pollicis brevis. These muscles act as *agonists,* or *prime movers,* in this act. In order for flexion to be smooth and forceful, finger extensor muscles act as *antagonists* and must relax at the same rate at which the flexors contract. The muscles which flex the fingers also tend to flex the wrist; and since that weakens the grip, muscles which extend the wrist must be brought into play to prevent its flexion. The action of the wrist extensors is *synergic,* and these muscles are called synergists in this particular act. The elbow and shoulder must be stabilized by appropriate flexor and extensor muscles, which serve as *fixators.* The coordination of agonists, antagonists, synergists, and fixators involves reciprocal innervation and is managed entirely by segmental spinal mechanisms with guidance from proprioceptive input. Only the agonist movement in a voluntary act is believed to be initiated at a cortical level. There are many other basic motor activities, such as the maintenance of certain postures and stepping movements, where agonists and antagonists contract simultaneously (see Chap. 26). In general, the more delicate the movement, the more precise the coordination between agonist and antagonist muscles.

CLINICAL MANIFESTATIONS OF MOTOR SYSTEM DISEASES

When applied to voluntary muscles, *paralysis* means loss of contraction due to interruption of one or more motor pathways from the cerebrum to the muscle fiber. In everyday medical parlance, motor paralysis usually means either partial or complete loss of strength; it is preferable to use *paresis* for slight and *paralysis* or *plegia* for severe loss of motor strength. Motor paralysis may result from lesions of upper motor neurons (corticospinal, corticobulbar, or subcorticospinal neurons) or of the motor unit. In addition to weakness, impaired facility of movement is an important functional deficit.

PARALYSIS DUE TO DISEASES OF PYRAMIDAL AND SUBCORTICOSPINAL NEURONS Corticospinal paralysis may be due to lesions in the cerebral cortex, subcortical white matter, internal capsule, brainstem, or spinal cord. Lesions confined to one of these anatomic locations without damaging adjacent parts of the brain are rare, but afford an opportunity to assess pure pyramidal tract function. In cases of unilateral pyramidal tract damage in the medulla, for example, initial paralysis may be striking but there is a remarkable degree of recovery of motor function in the affected contralateral arm and leg, leaving only slight spasticity, an increase in phasic myotatic or tendon reflexes, and an extensor plantar reflex (Babinski's sign). The extent of recovery is surprising, and may be due to preservation of a few fibers in the pyramid or to preservation of lateral brainstem pathways. This picture of pure pyramidal tract damage is much different from the extensive deficits that generally accompany most spastic hemiplegic syndromes. In clinical practice, most lesions of the upper motor neurons interrupt descending fibers from the cerebral cortex (corticospinal, corticorubral, corticostriatal, corticopallidal, corticopontine, and corticoreticular) and from the brainstem (reticulospinal, vestibulospinal, and rubrospinal). Damage to the nonpyramidal fibers increases the degree of paralysis and accounts for dysfunction in segmental motor neurons subserving reflex, postural, and locomotor functions. In most cases, it is therefore inaccurate to refer to spastic hemiplegia as the "pyramidal syndrome."

With corticospinal lesions in humans the distribution of the paralysis varies with the lesion site, but there are certain common features. Paralysis due to a lesion of upper motor neurons always involves a group of muscles, never individual muscles. In general, hand, arm, and leg muscles are most affected after a corticospinal lesion; of the cranial musculature, only the lower face and tongue are involved to any significant degree. Whatever volitional movement remains, the maximum effort is attained more slowly than in the normal limb, fewer motor units are recruited, and the frequency of their discharge is reduced. Corticospinal paralysis never involves all the muscles on one side of the body, even with a complete hemiplegia. Movements that are invariably bilateral, such as those of the eyes, jaw, pharynx, larynx, neck, thorax, and abdomen, are usually unaffected. The cortical control of all movements is to some extent bilateral. Examples that prove this point are hemiplegias that worsen when the contralateral motor system is interrupted by disease. Corticospinal paralysis is rarely complete for long; in this respect it differs from the total and absolute paralysis due to a complete destruction of anterior horn cells and their axons. The paralyzed arm may suddenly move during yawning and stretching, and various spinal reflexes can be elicited at all times.

Acute lesions of the corticospinal and subcorticospinal motor system at lower levels, such as the cervical cord, produce a distinctive picture of total paralysis and areflexia known as *spinal shock*. After a few days to weeks flaccidity subsides, muscular tone reappears, and the affected limbs become spastic; paralysis persists unchanged. *Spasticity* is a feature of all lesions of the motor system at cerebral, capsular, midbrain, and pontine levels. Spasticity is defined as a motor disorder characterized by a velocity-dependent increase in tonic stretch reflexes ("muscle tone") with exaggerated tendon jerks, resulting from hyperexcitability of the stretch reflex; it is one component of the "upper motor neuron" syndrome. Spasticity is related to excessive activity of motor neurons that are released from inhibition consequent to lesions of the corticospinal or descending brainstem pathways. The postures of the arm and leg inform us that certain spinal neurons are more active than others. With supraspinal lesions, the arm is maintained in a pronated, flexed position and the leg in an adducted, extended position. Attempts to extend the arm or flex the leg passively will elicit increasing resistance which abruptly subsides (*clasp-knife phenomenon*). When the limb is left in the new position, the resistance reappears (*lengthening and shortening reactions*). With combined lesions of corticospinal and other suprasegmental tracts, sustained resistance to movement (*hypertonus*) is more common than the clasp-knife type of spasticity. Upper motor neuron lesions also release the nocifensive spinal flexion reflexes, including Babinski's sign, and diminish or abolish the cutaneomuscular abdominal and cremasteric reflexes. Other signs of corticospinal or upper motor neuron lesions include exaggerated stretch and cutaneous reflexes in cranial as well as in limb and trunk muscles. If the corticospinal lesions are bilateral, there is *pseudobulbar paralysis* (dysarthria, dysphonia, and dysphagia with bifacial paralysis) accompanied by forced crying and laughing. Prolonged flexor and extensor spasms occur with lesions of the spinal cord; they are due to a release of cutaneous reflexes.

Spasticity is present with paresis as well as paralysis and can add to disturbances of voluntary movements. In general, all attempts by the patient to move the hemiparetic extremities appear to be hampered. Discrete movements of individual fingers and finely coordinated movements of the hand are lost, but voluntary control over proximal muscles is generally maintained. Synergies of movements eventually appear. For example, in the upper extremity a flexion synergy consisting of finger flexion, wrist flexion and pronation, elbow flexion, and shoulder elevation and abduction is produced in a slow, massive, stereotyped fashion upon attempted grasp of an object. Attempts to push with the hand result in a weak pronation of the hand, extension or flexion of the fingers, extension of the wrist and elbow, adduction of the upper arm, and lowering of the shoulder. In the lower extremity the extensor synergy (thigh adduction, thigh and knee extension, and plantar flexion of the toes and foot) is more powerful than the flexor synergy of hip abduction, hip and knee flexion, and dorsiflexion and inversion of toes and foot. A bias toward extensor synergy facilitates weight-bearing and walking, which are eventually achieved by nearly all hemiplegic patients. These synergies indicate that there is a diminution in voluntary anterior horn cell activation (the negative effect of a motor lesion) and excessive reflex and synergistic discharges in the same motor neuron pools (the positive effects of the lesion). Strong-willed effort to move the paretic limb may also evoke symmetric associated (mirror) movements in the normal limb.

In spasticity, where the neurons responsible for excitation of the extensor muscles of the leg and flexors of the arm are overactive, it is not known whether there is a functional excess of excitatory neurotransmitters or a deficiency of inhibitory transmitters or both. Current evidence indicates that drugs that decrease spasticity act at the spinal cord level to alter neurotransmitter function. Baclofen slows conduction in the spinal cord reflex arc, perhaps by interfering with the release of excitatory neurotransmitters, including substance P, from primary afferent neurons. Diazepam facilitates GABA-mediated presynaptic inhibition of primary afferent excitatory transmitter release.

PARALYSIS DUE TO DISEASES OF THE MOTOR UNIT Damage to the lower motor neurons can produce paresis or paralysis as a direct result of physiologic block or destruction of anterior horn cells or their axons in anterior roots and nerves. The signs and symptoms of the lower motor neuron syndrome vary according to the location of the lesion: the most important question for clinical purposes is whether sensory changes coexist with muscular weakness. The combination of flaccid areflexic paralysis and sensory loss usually indicates involvement of mixed motor and sensory nerves or damage to both anterior and posterior roots. If sensory changes are absent, the lesion must be situated in the gray matter of the spinal cord, in the anterior roots, in a purely motor branch of a peripheral nerve, or in motor axons alone. The distinction between nuclear (spinal) and anterior root (radicular) lesions may at times be impossible to make.

If all or practically all peripheral motor nerves supplying a muscle are destroyed, voluntary, postural, and reflex movements are abolished. The muscle becomes soft and yields excessively to passive stretching, a condition known as *flaccidity*. Muscle tone—the slight resistance that normal relaxed muscle offers to passive movement—is reduced (*hypotonia* or *atonia*). The denervated muscles undergo extreme atrophy, and lose 70 to 80 percent of their original bulk within 4 months. The reflex reaction of the muscle to sudden stretch, as by tapping its tendon, is lost. If only a few motor units in the muscles are affected, partial paralysis will ensue. With partial denervation, EMG evidence of fibrillations may also be obtained. Clinical features that distinguish lower motor and upper motor neuron lesions are summarized in Table 25-1.

APRAXIC OR NONPARALYTIC DISORDERS OF MOTOR FUNCTION Loss of learned movements can simulate paresis of a limb, even though the pyramidal tract and spinal cord motor units are intact. This condition is called *apraxia* and is defined as a disorder

TABLE 25-1 Differences between paralysis due to lesions of upper versus lower motor neurons

Upper motor neuron paralysis	Lower motor neuron paralysis
Muscle groups affected diffusely, never individual muscles	Individual muscles may be affected
Atrophy slight	Atrophy pronounced, 70 to 80% of total bulk
Spasticity with hyperactivity of the tendon reflexes	Flaccidity and hypotonia of affected muscles with loss of tendon reflexes
Extensor plantar reflex, Babinski's sign	Plantar reflex, if present, is of normal flexor type
Fascicular twitches not produced	Fasciculations may be present
	Electromyogram reveals reduced numbers of motor units and fibrillations

of learned movement that is not due to weakness, incoordination, sensory loss, or failure to comprehend commands. A failure to execute a designated action while retaining the ability to carry out the individual movements upon which such an act depends is the main feature of apraxia. A clinical test of motor deficits of this type is to observe a series of self-initiated actions such as using a comb, a razor, a toothbrush, or a common tool, or gesturing, e.g., waving goodbye, saluting, shaking the fist as though angry, or blowing a kiss. These actions can be normally elicited by a command or a request to imitate the examiner. Of course, failure to follow a spoken or written request may be due to an aphasia that prevents understanding of what is asked or to an agnosia that prevents recognition of the tool or object to be used. But when these difficulties are excluded, there remains a peculiar motor deficit in which the patient appears to understand but has lost the memory of how to perform a given act, especially if it is called for in an unnatural setting. The patient may have the idea of what to do but cannot translate the idea of the sequence of movements into a precise, well-executed act. An apraxic deficit may be evident both after a spoken command and in requests to imitate the gestures of the examiner. Sometimes these two conditions may be dissociated; the patient, while not aphasic, cannot execute a spoken command but can still imitate the act if it is called forth by gesture. Also, if merely given the tool, the patient may use it properly in an automatic fashion.

To understand the anatomic basis of apraxia, it is necessary to appreciate that the production of complex motor behavior results from association among several cortical brain areas. The motor response of right-handed (and most left-handed) persons to a command requires the integrity of the left parietal and temporal lobes, especially the region around the left supramarginal gyrus, and their connection with the left premotor regions for control of the right hand. Information flows through the corpus callosum from the left to the right motor cortex for control of the left side of the body. Disconnection of the supramarginal area from motor areas of the right hemisphere (most commonly by lesions of the midcallosum, dominant frontal association cortex, or posterior parietal lobe) results in apraxia of left limbs when tested by response to verbal commands. Traditionally, abnormalities in the execution of single gestures resulting from lesions of these brain areas have been referred to as *ideomotor apraxia*. The anatomic basis of *ideational apraxia*, in which the execution of a multistep activity is faulty although the constituent movements can be performed, has not been clearly delineated. Because pure disorders of these subtypes of apraxia are uncommon, and precise anatomic correlates are lacking, clinical distinctions between ideomotor and ideational apraxia are difficult to make.

EXAMINATION SCHEME FOR MOTOR PARALYSIS AND APRAXIA The first step in examination is to inspect the paralyzed limb, taking note of its posture and whether there are signs of muscular hypertrophy, atrophy, or fascicular twitchings. Slight atrophy may be due to disuse from any cause, i.e., pain, fixation as the result of a cast, or any type of paralysis. Pronounced atrophy usually occurs only with denervation of several weeks' or months' standing. The patient is then called upon to move each muscle group, and the power and facility of movement are graded and recorded. The examiner then determines the range of passive movement and the degree of resistance encountered moving all the joints. This provides information concerning alterations of muscle tone, i.e., hypotonia, spasticity, and rigidity. Dislocations, diseased joints, and ankyloses may also be revealed by these same maneuvers. The tendon reflexes are then tested. The usual routine is to try to elicit the jaw jerk (increased in pseudobulbar palsy) and the biceps, triceps, quadriceps, and Achilles tendon reflexes. Two cutaneous reflexes are then tested, the abdominal and plantar reflexes.

If there is no evidence of upper or lower motor neuron disease, but motor acts are nonetheless imperfectly performed, one should look for a disorder of postural control associated with cerebellar incoordination, or consider that rigidity with abnormalities of posture and movement may be due to disease of the basal ganglia. In the absence of these disorders, the possibility of an apraxic disorder may be investigated by watching the patient's own movements and those called forth by specific command and gesture.

DIFFERENTIAL DIAGNOSIS OF PARALYSIS The diagnostic consideration of paralysis may be simplified by the following subdivisions, which relate to the location and distribution of weakness. Paralysis may result from dysfunction of upper motor neurons (corticospinal, corticobulbar, and subcorticospinal neurons) or of the motor unit (bulbar and spinal motor neurons, neuromuscular junction, and muscle). In general, the presence or absence of atrophy of muscles in a monoplegic limb can assist the clinician to arrive at an anatomic and clinical diagnosis.

Monoplegia It is necessary to determine carefully the distribution of muscle weakness. For example, patients who complain of weakness of one extremity often have unnoticed weakness in another limb, and the condition is actually hemiplegia or paraplegia. A comprehensive physical examination should be conducted in order to determine whether there is weakness of all the muscles in a limb or only isolated muscle groups. The examination should also exclude nonparalytic conditions such as ataxia, sensory disturbances, mechanical limitation resulting from arthritis, the rigidity of parkinsonism, or pain in an extremity; such conditions are often interpreted by the patient as weakness.

PARALYSIS WITH LITTLE OR NO ATROPHY The most frequent cause of monoplegia without muscular wasting is a lesion of the cerebral cortex; diseases that interrupt the corticospinal tract at the level of the internal capsule, brainstem, or spinal cord rarely cause monoplegia because corticospinal fibers to arm and leg are intermingled at subcortical levels. A cortical vascular lesion (thrombosis or embolus) is the commonest cause of monoplegia, but a discrete traumatic lesion, tumor, or abscess may have the same effect. Multiple sclerosis and spinal cord tumor, early in their course, may cause isolated weakness of one extremity, usually the leg. Weakness due to damage of the corticospinal and subcorticospinal system is usually accompanied by spasticity, increased reflexes, and an extensor plantar reflex (Babinski's sign). Acute traumatic or inflammatory lesions that destroy the motor tracts in the spinal cord are exceptions to this rule because immediately after damage the tendon reflexes are reduced or absent and muscle tone is flaccid (spinal shock). This does not occur in partial or slowly evolving lesions and occurs only to minimal degree, if at all, in lesions of brainstem and cerebrum. In acute diseases affecting the lower motor neurons, such as poliomyelitis, the tendon reflexes are always reduced or abolished, but atrophy may not appear for several weeks. Hence one must take into account the mode of onset and the duration of the disease in evaluating the tendon reflexes, muscle tone, and degree of atrophy before reaching an anatomic diagnosis.

PARALYSIS WITH MUSCULAR ATROPHY Atrophy of muscles in a paralyzed limb usually indicates a lesion of some portion of the motor unit (spinal cord, spinal roots, peripheral nerve, or muscle). Disease of the neuromuscular junction is not associated with muscular atrophy.

In addition to the paralysis, reduced or abolished tendon reflexes, and decreased tone, there may be visible fasciculations. The EMG shows decreased numbers of motor units (often of large size), fasciculations at rest, and fibrillations. The location of the lesion can usually be decided by the distribution of the palsied muscles (whether the pattern is one of muscles, nerve, spinal root, or spinal cord involvement), by the associated neurologic symptoms and signs, and by special tests (cerebrospinal fluid examination, CT or magnetic resonance imaging scans of the spine, myelogram, serum muscle enzymes, EMG, and biopsy). A clinical approach to the signs and symptoms that assist the clinician in arriving at an anatomic diagnosis of diseases of the motor unit (spinal cord, spinal motor nerves, neuromuscular junction, or muscle) are described in more detail in Chaps. 362 and 363.

The anatomic pattern of paralysis with atrophy may suggest the clinical diagnosis. Atrophic monoplegia affecting the arm should suggest brachial plexus trauma in an infant; poliomyelitis in a child; and poliomyelitis, syringomyelia, amyotrophic lateral sclerosis, or neuritis of the brachial plexus in an adult. Crural monoplegia (affecting the leg) is more frequent than brachial monoplegia and may be caused by any lesion of thoracic or lumber cord, including trauma, tumor, myelitis, or multiple sclerosis. Multiple sclerosis almost never causes atrophy, and ruptured intervertebral disk and the many varieties of neuritis rarely paralyze all or most of the muscles of a limb. Muscular dystrophy may begin in one limb, but by the time the patient is seen the typical pattern of symmetric proximal limb and trunk involvement is usually evident. A unilateral retroperitoneal tumor may paralyze the leg by implicating the lumbosacral plexus. Prolonged disuse of a limb may lead to atrophy, but this is usually not so marked as in diseases that denervate muscles. In disuse atrophy the tendon reflexes are normal, and the responses of the muscles to electric stimulation and on EMG are unaltered.

Hemiplegia Loss of strength in the arm, leg, and sometimes face on one side of the body is the most frequent distribution of paralysis in humans. With rare exceptions (a few unusual cases of poliomyelitis or motor system disease) this pattern of paralysis is due to involvement of the descending motor tracts. The site or level of the lesion that produced hemiplegia can usually be deduced from the associated neurologic findings. Diseases localized in the cerebral cortex, cerebral white matter (corona radiata), and internal capsule usually evoke weakness or paralysis of the face, arm, and leg in the side of the body contralateral to the brain lesion. The occurrence of convulsive seizures or the presence of a defect in speech (aphasia), a cortical type of sensory loss (astereognosis and loss of two-point discrimination), anosognosia, or defects in the visual fields suggest a cortical or subcortical rather than a capsular location. A pure, isolated motor hemiplegia affecting simultaneously the face, arm, and leg indicates a small discrete lesion in the posterior limb of the internal capsule, cerebral peduncle, or medullary pyramids.

Damage to the corticospinal and corticobulbar tracts in the upper portion of the brainstem will cause paralysis of the face, arm, and leg in the side opposite the lesion, plus deficits in cranial nerve function on the same side as the lesion. Some of the classic brainstem syndromes permit precise localization of the lesion, which is usually vascular. Paralysis of the oculomotor nerve on the same side as the lesion with contralateral limb paresis is known as Weber's syndrome. With low pontine lesions, an ipsilateral abducens or facial palsy combined with a contralateral weakness or paralysis of the arm and leg is the Millard-Gubler syndrome. Lesions of the lowermost part of the brainstem, i.e., in the medulla, affect the tongue and sometimes the pharynx and larynx on one side and arm and leg on the other side. Ataxic hemiplegia with or without dysarthria indicates a lesion in the contralateral basis pons. These "crossed paralyses" that are so characteristic of brainstem diseases are described in Chap. 351.

Hemiplegia that spares cranial musculature may be caused by a lesion in the lateral column of the cervical spinal cord. At this level, however, the pathologic process often induces bilateral signs, with resulting quadriparesis or quadriplegia. Homolateral paralysis, if combined with a loss of vibratory and position sense on the same side and contralateral loss of pain and temperature (Brown-Séquard syndrome), signifies disease of the spinal cord (Chap. 361).

Muscle atrophy of minor degree is often associated with hemiplegia but never reaches the proportions seen in diseases of the lower motor neurons. Atrophy secondary to upper motor neuron damage is largely due to disuse. There is an important exception to this rule: When the motor cortex and adjacent parts of the parietal lobe are damaged in infancy or childhood, the normal development of the muscles and the skeletal system in the affected limbs is retarded, and the palsied limbs and even the trunk on one side are small. Developmental atrophy does not occur, however, if the paralysis begins after puberty when the greater part of skeletal growth has been attained. In hemiplegia due to spinal cord injury, muscles at the level of the lesion may undergo atrophy if there is associated damage to anterior horn cells or ventral roots.

Vascular diseases of the cerebrum and brainstem are the most common causes of hemiplegia. Trauma (brain contusion, epidural and subdural hemorrhage) ranks second, followed by other diseases such as brain tumor, demyelinative disease, brain abcess, and encephalitis. Complications of meningitis, tuberculosis, and syphilis were common causes of hemiplegia in the past but are much less evident in current practice.

Paraplegia Paraplegia denotes a condition of weakness or paralysis of both lower extremities with sparing of the upper extremities. Paraplegia most commonly occurs in diseases of the spinal cord, spinal roots, or peripheral nerves. Among cerebral causes, parasagittal tumors and hydrocephalus cause leg weakness. If the onset is acute, it may be difficult to distinguish spinal from neural paralysis, because sudden damage to either may result in flaccidity and abolition of reflexes. As a rule, in acute spinal cord diseases the paralysis affects all muscles below a given level; often, if the white matter is extensively damaged, sensory loss below a particular level (loss of pain and temperature sense from lateral spinothalamic tracts involvement and loss of vibratory and position sense from posterior columns damage) is conjoined. Also, in bilateral disease of the spinal cord the bladder and bowel sphincters are paralyzed. Alterations of cerebrospinal fluid (dynamic block and increases in protein or cells) are frequent. In peripheral nerve diseases both sensory loss and motor loss tend to involve the distal muscles of the legs more than the proximal ones (an exception is acute idiopathic polyneuritis), and the sphincters are spared or only briefly deranged in function. Sensory loss, if present, is more likely to consist of distal impairment of touch, vibration, and position sense, with pain and temperature sense spared in many instances. The cerebrospinal fluid protein level may be normal or elevated. Studies of nerve conduction through spinal roots (F waves) are always abnormal.

Acute paraplegia most commonly occurs after trauma or in association with metastatic neoplasia. Uncommon causes of acute paraplegia include a medial pontine lesion affecting the leg fibers which are near the midline (as in pontine infarction or central pontine myelinolysis); spontaneous hematomyelia with bleeding from a vascular malformation (angioma, telangiectasis); thrombosis of a spinal artery with infarction (myelomalacia); and dissecting aortic aneurysm or atherosclerotic occlusion of nutrient spinal arteries arising from the aorta with resulting infarction (myelomalacia). Postinfectious or postvaccinal myelitis, acute demyelinative myelitis (Devic's disease if the optic nerves are affected), necrotizing myelitis, and epidural abscess or hemorrhage with spinal cord compression tend to develop somewhat more slowly over a period of hours or days, but they may have an acute onset. Poliomyelitis, in those countries where immunization is incomplete, presents as a purely motor disorder with meningitis, and must be distinguished from the other acute myelopathies.

Subacute or chronic paraplegia in adults results from such common diseases as cervical spondylosis and multiple sclerosis. Other causes are subacute combined degeneration, spinal cord tumor, ruptured cervical disk, syphilitic meningomyelitis, chronic epidural infections (fungus and other granulomatous diseases), motor system disease, and syringomyelia. Familial spastic paraparesis is a rare cause of paraplegia in which there is symmetric demyelination of the dorsolateral corticospinal tract. (See Chap. 361 for discussion of these spinal cord diseases.) The several varieties of polyneuritis, including Guillain-Barré syndrome and polymyositis, must be considered in the differential diagnosis, for they, too, may cause paraparesis. Friedreich's ataxia and familial spastic paraplegia, progressive muscular dystrophy, and the chronic varieties of polyneuritis tend to appear during late childhood and adolescence and are slowly progressive.

Paraplegia (or paraparesis) may be due to a lesion of the leg areas of the motor cortex. Arterial (anterior cerebral arteries) or venous (superior sagittal sinus and tributary cerebral veins) distribution cerebral infarction are causes of acute paraplegia; parasagittal meningioma is a cause of asymmetric chronic paraplegia. Usually other signs such as confusion, stupor, or seizures indicate the cerebral localization, and differential diagnosis is not a problem.

Quadriplegia All that has been written about the common causes of paraplegia applies to quadriplegia except that the lesion is in the cervical rather than the thoracic or lumbar segments of the spinal cord. If it is situated in the low cervical segments and involves the anterior half of the spinal cord, as in occlusion of the anterior spinal artery, the arm paralysis may be flaccid and areflexic and the leg paralysis spastic (anterior spinal syndrome). There are only a few points of difference between the common paraplegic and quadriplegic syndromes. One of the most common causes of subacute quadriplegia is the Guillain-Barré syndrome due to inflammatory demyelination of motor neuron axons in the anterior roots. Repeated cerebral vascular accidents may lead to bilateral hemiplegia, usually accompanied by pseudobulbar palsy. An unusual cause of quadriplegia is bilateral infarctions of the medullary pyramids.

Isolated paralysis Paralysis of isolated muscle groups usually indicates a lesion of one or more peripheral nerves. The basis for diagnosing a lesion of an individual peripheral nerve is the presence of weakness or paralysis of the muscle or group of muscles and impairment or loss of sensation in the distribution of the nerve in question (Chap. 363). Complete transection or severe injury to a peripheral nerve is usually followed by atrophy of the muscles it innervates and by loss of their tendon reflexes. Trophic changes in the skin, nails, and subcutaneous tissue may also occur. It is of considerable importance to decide whether the lesion is only a temporary one (conduction block), or whether there has been a dissolution of axonal continuity, requiring nerve regeneration for recovery.

THE BASAL GANGLIA

The basal ganglia subserve motor functions that are distinct from those attributed to the pyramidal (corticospinal) tract. The term *extrapyramidal* underscores this distinction and calls attention to a set of neurologic illnesses caused by lesions that affect the basal ganglia. In addition to motor impairments, diseases of the basal ganglia are often associated with disturbances of affect and cognition. Familiar examples of extrapyramidal disorders include Parkinson's disease, Huntington's disease, and Wilson's disease. This section reviews aspects of the anatomy, biochemistry, and physiology of the basal ganglia and describes the clinical symptoms and signs that arise from their dysfunction.

ANATOMIC CONNECTIONS AND NEURONAL TRANSMITTERS IN THE BASAL GANGLIA The basal ganglia are paired subcortical masses of gray matter that form anatomically distinct nuclear groups. The major nuclei are the caudate and the putamen (which together are called the striatum), the internal and external segments of the globus pallidus, the subthalamic nucleus, and the substantia nigra (Fig. 25-2). The striatum receives afferent inputs from many sources, including the cerebral cortex, thalamic nuclei, brainstem raphe nuclei, and the substantia nigra. There are two anatomically and functionally distinct subdivisions of the striatum: the striosomes and the matrix. Afferents to the striosomal region originate in the frontal cortex, insula, amygdala, and midline thalamus; afferents to the matrix arise from neurons in the sensory and motor cortex, parietal-temporal-occipital association cortex, and intralaminar thalamic nuclei. Cortical neurons that project to the striatum release the excitatory amino acid glutamate. Neurons that project to the striatum from the raphe nuclei synthesize and release serotonin (5-HT). Neurons in the pars compacta of the substantia nigra synthesize and release dopamine (DA), which acts as an inhibitory neurotransmitter on striatal neurons. DA neurons in the substantia nigra pars compacta project to striosomes, whereas DA neurons in the ventral tegmental area project to the matrix. Transmitters released by thalamic projections are unknown. The striatum contains two distinct classes of cells: local circuit neurons, whose axons do not project beyond the confines of the nucleus, and other neurons whose axons project to the globus pallidus and substantia nigra. Local circuit neurons synthesize and release acetylcholine (ACh), GABA, and neuropeptides, including somatostatin and vasoactive intestinal polypeptide. Neurons in the striosomes project to the medial part of the pars compacta of the substantia nigra; the main output of the extrastriosomal matrix goes to the pallidum and pars reticulata of the substantia nigra. Striatal neurons that inhibit the pars reticulata of the substantia nigra release GABA, whereas those that

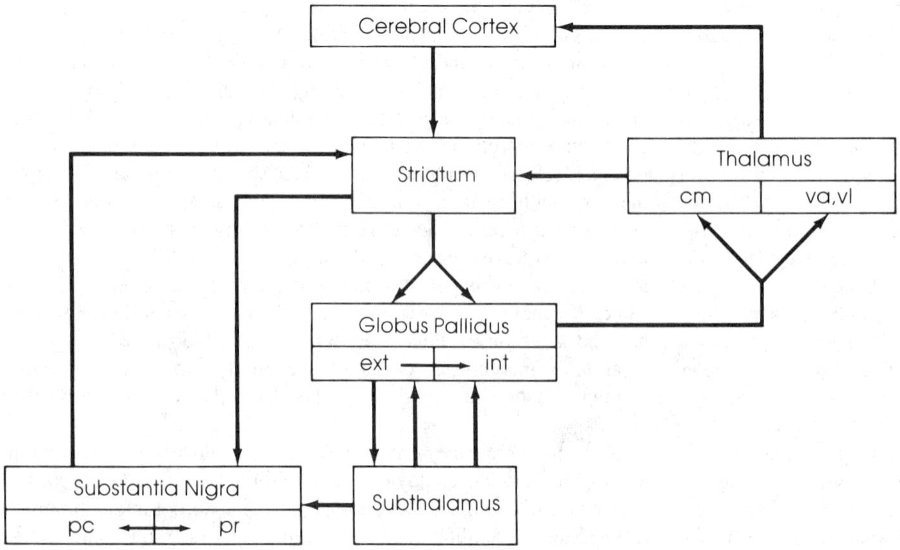

FIGURE 25-2 Simplified schematic diagram of the major neuronal connections between the basal ganglia, thalamus, and cerebral cortex. The projection from the internal segment of the globus pallidus constitutes the principal efferent pathway from the basal ganglia. Abbreviations: ext = external, int = internal, pc = pars compacta, pr = pars reticulata, cm = centromedian, va = ventroanterior, vl = ventrolateral.

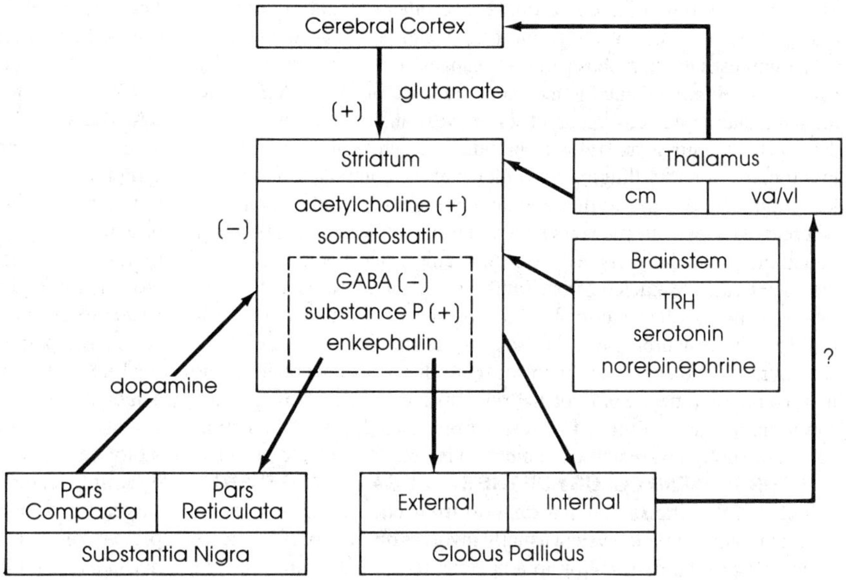

FIGURE 25-3 Schematic diagram of the excitatory and inhibitory effects of neuroregulators released by neurons in the basal ganglia pathways. The area (enclosed by dashed lines) in the striatum indicates neurons with efferent projection systems. The other striatal transmitters are present in intrinsic neurons. Plus sign (+) indicates an excitatory postsynaptic effect. Minus sign (−) indicates an inhibitory effect. Abbreviations: cm = centromedian nucleus, GABA = gamma-aminobutyric acid, TRH = thyrotropin releasing hormone, va/vl = ventroanterior and ventrolateral.

excite the pars compacta release substance P (Fig. 25-3). Transmitters released in the striatal projections to the globus pallidus include GABA, the enkephalins, and substance P.

Axons that originate in the internal segment of the globus pallidus form the main efferent projection from the basal ganglia. There is a massive projection around and through the internal capsule (the ansa and fasciculus lenticularis that pass through the fields of Forel) to the ventral anterior and ventral lateral thalamus as well as to intralaminar thalamic nuclei, including the centromedian nucleus. Chemical transmitters released by this pathway are unknown. Other efferent projections from the basal ganglia include direct dopaminergic connections from the ventral tegmental area to regions of limbic and frontal cerebral cortex; the pars reticulata of the substantia nigra also sends a projection to thalamic nuclei and to the superior colliculus.

Recent anatomic studies have clarified the cortical distribution of ascending thalamic fibers. Ventral thalamic neurons project to premotor and motor cerebral cortices; medial thalamic nuclei project primarily to prefrontal cortex. The supplementary motor cortex receives a prominent input from the basal ganglia, including a dopaminergic projection from the substantia nigra, whereas the primary motor and premotor cortex receives a major input from the cerebellum. Thus there are a series of parallel loops reciprocally linking specific basal ganglionic structures and cerebral cortical regions. Although the exact mechanism whereby these various inputs are translated into coordinated volitional acts remains uncertain, it is clear that most of the basal ganglionic and cerebellar influences on the motor system are funneled through this ventral plane of thalamic nuclei. The major cerebellar output, which exits the cerebellum through the superior cerebellar peduncle, terminates with the pallidal-thalamic fibers in the ventroanterior and ventrolateral thalamic nuclei. This region of the thalamus forms an essential link in the ascending fiber systems from both the basal ganglia and the cerebellum to the motor cortex. Despite the apparently crucial nature of these structures, lesions placed stereotactically in the ventral thalamus can abolish essential-familial tremor or the rigidity and tremor in Parkinson's disease without producing functional deficits. Ascending thalamocortical fibers pass through the internal capsule and cerebral white matter, so lesions in these parts or in the cortex may simultaneously affect both corticospinal and extrapyramidal systems.

Axons from some cortical neurons form the internal capsule (the corticobulbar and corticospinal tracts); these and others also project to the striatum. This forms a complete loop—from cerebral cortex to striatum, to globus pallidus, to thalamus, to cerebral cortex. Axons that originate in the centromedian nucleus of the thalamus project back to the striatum, thus completing a subcortical loop from striatum to globus pallidus, to centromedian nucleus, to striatum. There is another subcortical loop between the striatum and the substantia nigra: Dopaminergic neurons in the pars compacta of substantia nigra project to the striatum, and separate striatal neurons that release GABA and substance P send projections to the pars reticulata of the substantia nigra. There are reciprocal connections between the pars reticulata and pars compacta of the substantia nigra; the pars reticulata sends projections to ventral thalamus, superior colliculus, and brainstem reticular formation structures as well. The subthalamic nucleus receives fibers from the neocortex and from the external segment of the globus pallidus; neurons within the subthalamic nucleus form reciprocal connections with the external segment of the globus pallidus and also send axons to the internal segment of the globus pallidus and pars reticulata of the substantia nigra. The neurochemicals involved in these pathways remain unknown, although GABA has been implicated.

PHYSIOLOGY OF THE BASAL GANGLIA Recordings from neurons in the globus pallidus and substantia nigra in awake, performing primates confirm the main motor function of the basal ganglia. Cells within these regions clearly participate in the initiation of movement, because they increase their firing rates before movement is observed clinically or detected by EMG. Discharges in the basal ganglia are related principally to contralateral rather than ipsilateral limb movements. Many neurons increase their firing rates during slow (ramp) movements, but some others discharge during more rapid (ballistic) movements. There is somatotopic localization of leg, arm, and face within the internal segment of the globus pallidus and pars reticulata of the substantia nigra. This observation provides a possible explanation for the occurrence of restricted dyskinesias: Focal dystonia and buccal-lingual-masticatory tardive dyskinesia may result from localized pallidal or nigral biochemical lesions that affect only regions with hand or face representation.

Although the basal ganglia are motor nuclei, it is not possible to identify a specific type of basal ganglia movement. Hypotheses about the function of the basal ganglia in human beings derive from correlations between clinical signs and sites of pathologic lesions in patients with extrapyramidal diseases. The basal ganglia are a constellation of nuclei centered around the globus pallidus, through which impulses are channeled to the thalamus and onward to the cerebral cortex (Fig. 25-2). Neurons in each satellite nucleus contribute excitatory and inhibitory impulses, and the sum of these influences on the main pathway from basal ganglia to thalamus and cerebral cortex, modified by the cerebellum, determines smooth motor function as expressed through the corticospinal and other descending cortical tracts. If one or more of the supporting nuclei is damaged, the sum of the impulses to the globus pallidus changes and disordered mobility can occur. Hemiballismus is the most dramatic of these; damage to the subthalamic nucleus apparently removes inhibitory influences on the substantia nigra and globus pallidus, which results in violent, involuntary, rotatory flinging movements of the contralateral arm and leg. Similarly, damage to the caudate nucleus often results in chorea, whereas the opposite phenomenon, akinesia, typically occurs when dopamine-producing cells in the substantia nigra degenerate, releasing the intact caudate nucleus from inhibition. Lesions restricted to the globus pallidus often cause flexion dystonia and impaired postural reflexes. The neurologic substrates of cognitive impairments in extrapyramidal diseases are more obscure than those accounting for motor abnormalities. Some of the cognitive impairments in Parkinson's disease are postulated to result from frontal lobe dysfunction due to disruption of reciprocal connections with the caudate nucleus.

NEUROPHARMACOLOGY OF THE BASAL GANGLIA: GENERAL PRINCIPLES Transfer of information from one cell to another in the mammalian nervous system usually involves one or more chemicals released from the first neuron to a specific receptor site on a second neuron, thereby altering the biochemical and physical properties of the second neuron. These chemicals taken together are called neuroregulators. There are three distinct classes of neuroregulators: neurotransmitters, neuromodulators, and neurohormones. Neurotransmitters, such as the catecholamines, ACh, and amino acids such as glutamate and GABA, are the best known and clinically most important class of neuroregulators. They cause short-latency, brief postsynaptic effects (e.g., depolarization) close to their point of release. Neuromodulators, such as the endorphins, somatostatin, substance P, and other neuropeptides, also exert effects close to the point of release; they can enhance or diminish effects of the classic neurotransmitters. Many neurons that contain classic neurotransmitters also contain neuromodulator peptides. Substance P coexists within raphe neurons that synthesize 5-HT, for example, and vasoactive intestinal polypeptide coexists with ACh in many cortical cholinergic neurons. Neurohormones, such as vasopressin and angiotensin II, differ from other regulators because they are released into the bloodstream and are transported to remote receptors. Their effects are slow in onset and have a long duration of action. The distinction between the various classes of neuroregulators is not absolute. DA, for example, acts as a neurotransmitter in the caudate nucleus but is believed to act as a neurohormone in the hypothalamus.

Neuroregulators of the neurotransmitter class are the best-studied transmitters in the basal ganglia and the ones on which most drugs exert their effects. Neurotransmitters are synthesized in the presynaptic terminals of neurons and are stored in vesicles. Following the arrival of an electric impulse, neurotransmitters are released from the presynaptic terminal into the synaptic cleft, diffuse across the synaptic gap, and combine with specific receptor sites on the postsynaptic cell. This initiates a series of biochemical and biophysical changes; the sum of all postsynaptic excitatory and inhibitory influences determines the likelihood that a given neuron will discharge. The biogenic amines DA, norepinephrine (NE), and 5-HT are inactivated by enzymatic degradation (monamine oxidase and catechol-*O*-methyltransferase) and by uptake into the presynaptic terminals; ACh is inactivated by intrasynaptic hydrolysis. There are also receptor sites on the presynaptic terminal, called autoreceptors, and their stimulation generally causes a decrease in synthesis and release of the transmitter. The affinity of an autoreceptor for its neurotransmitter is often much greater than that of the postsynaptic receptor. Drugs that stimulate DA autoreceptors can be expected to decrease dopaminergic transmission and possibly be useful in the treatment of hyperkinetic movement disorders such as Huntington's disease and tardive dyskinesia. Receptors may be further subdivided based on response to pharmacologic agents. There are at least two separate populations of DA receptors, for example: Stimulation of D-1 sites activates adenylate cyclase, whereas D-2 receptor stimulation inhibits adenyl cyclase. The ergot alkaloid bromocriptine, used in the treatment of Parkinson's disease, stimulates D-2 but blocks D-1 receptors; most neuroleptics block D-2 receptors.

CLINICAL MANIFESTATIONS OF LESIONS OF THE BASAL GANGLIA Akinesia When extrapyramidal diseases are analyzed along classic neurologic lines into primary functional deficits (negative symptoms due to loss of connectivity) and secondary release effects (positive symptoms of excessive activity), akinesia stands as a principal negative or deficit symptom. *Akinesia* refers to the inability to initiate changes in activity and to perform ordinary volitional movements rapidly and easily. The terms *bradykinesia* and *hypokinesia* are employed to describe lesser degrees of impairment. In contrast to paralysis, which is the negative symptom of corticospinal tract lesions, strength is preserved although there is a delay in achieving peak power. Akinesia is also distinct from *apraxia*, in which the command to perform a particular action never reaches the motor centers that direct the desired movement. Akinesia is the most disabling feature of Parkinson's disease. Akinetic patients display severe immobility and underactivity. They sit motionless for long periods of time without shifting postures and take double the time normally required to eat, dress, and bathe. Poverty of movement reveals itself in the loss of automatic associated motions, such as eye blinks and freely swinging arms when walking. Akinesia probably accounts for such common symptoms in Parkinson's disease as facial immobility, vocal hypophonia, micrographia, and difficulty in arising from a chair and beginning to walk. Akinesia can affect the mind as well; slowed speed of thought is called bradyphrenia. Although pathophysiologic details remain uncertain, clinical analysis of akinesia supports the hypothesis that the basal ganglia are mainly responsible for initiation and automatic execution of learned motor plans. Neuropharmacologic evidence suggests that akinesia itself results from DA deficiency.

Rigidity *Muscle tone* is defined as the amount of resistance encountered when a relaxed limb is moved passively. In rigidity, the muscles are in continuous contraction and resistance to passive movement is constant. Rigidity secondary to extrapyramidal disorders may superficially resemble spasticity due to corticospinal tract lesions in that both produce increases in muscular tone. A few clinical guidelines provide help in distinguishing these conditions at the bedside. The distribution of increased tone often differs in rigidity and spasticity. Although rigidity is present in both flexor and extensor muscle groups, it tends to be more prominent in those that maintain a flexed posture. Rigidity is easy to detect in large muscle groups, but smaller muscles of the face, tongue, and larynx are also often affected. In contrast to rigidity, spasticity usually produces increased tone in the extensor muscles of the legs and the flexor musculature of the arms. The quality of hypertonus can also be used to distinguish the two conditions. Resistance to passive movements is constant in rigidity, accounting for terms such as "lead pipe" and "plastic" resistance. In spasticity, there may be a free interval followed classically by the clasp-knife phenomenon; muscles do not contract until they are stretched a bit, and later during stretch the augmentation in muscle tone quickly subsides. Deep tendon reflexes are normal in rigidity but increased in spastic states. Spasticity results from hyperactivity of the stretch reflex arc due to central changes but without increased sensitivity of the muscle spindle; spasticity can be abolished by sectioning posterior spinal roots. Rigidity has less relationship with hyperactivity of segmental reflex arcs and depends more upon heightened discharge of alpha motor neurons. A special type of rigidity is the cogwheel phenomenon, which is especially common in Parkinson's disease. When the hypertonic muscle is passively stretched, the resistance may be rhythmically jerky, as though the resistance of the limb were controlled by a ratchet.

Chorea Derived from the Greek word meaning "dance," chorea refers to widespread arrhythmic movements of a forcible, rapid, jerky, restless type. Choreic movements are noted for their irregularity and variability; they are generally continuous, may be simple or quite elaborate, and affect any part of the body. They may resemble voluntary movement in complexity, but they are never combined into a coordinated act unless the patient incorporates them into a deliberate movement in order to make them less noticeable. Normal volitional movements are possible because there is no paralysis, but they may be excessively quick, poorly sustained, and deformed by choreic movements. Chorea may be generalized or limited to one side of the body. Generalized chorea is the predominant involuntary movement in Huntington's disease and in rheumatic (Sydenham's) chorea, and usually involves the face, trunk, and limbs; it is often seen with levodopa toxicity in patients with Parkinson's disease. Another common choreiform disorder, tardive dyskinesia, occurs in association with chronic neuroleptic administration. Choreic movements in this disorder are generally restricted to the buccal, lingual, and mandibular musculature, although trunk and limbs may be involved in severe cases. Sedatives such as phenobarbital or a benzodiazepine are used in treating Sydenham's chorea; neuroleptics are commonly used to suppress chorea in Huntington's disease. Drugs that increase cholinergic neurotransmission, such as phosphatidylcholine and physostigmine, have been used to suppress chorea in about 30 percent of patients with tardive dyskinesia.

A special type of paroxysmal chorea, sometimes with athetosis or dystonic features, occurs sporadically, or as an autosomal dominant disorder. These disorders usually appear during childhood or adolescence and continue throughout life; patients have paroxysms that last minutes to hours. In one special subtype, the chorea is kinesogenic, which means that it may be initiated by a sudden voluntary movement. Alcohol, hypernatremia, and phenytoin may precipitate paroxysmal chorea, especially in patients who have had Sydenham's chorea in childhood. In some cases, anticonvulsant drugs, including phenobarbital and clonazepam, and in other instances levodopa have prevented attacks.

Athetosis This term is from a Greek word meaning "unfixed" or "changeable." Athetosis is characterized by an inability to sustain the muscles of the fingers, toes, tongue or any other group of muscles in one position. The maintained posture is interrupted by continuous slow, purposeless movements. These are most pronounced in the digits and hands and consist of extension, pronation, flexion, and supination of the arm with alternating flexion and extension of the fingers. Athetotic movements are slower than those associated with chorea, but gradations are commonly seen and termed *choreoathetosis* when it is impossible to distinguish between the two. Generalized athetosis may be seen in children with static encephalopathy (cerebral palsy); it can also occur in Wilson's disease, in torsion dystonia, and following cerebral anoxia. Posthemiplegic athetosis is unilateral and occurs especially in children who have suffered a stroke. Patients whose athetosis is due to cerebral palsy or cerebral anoxia have variable degrees of additional motor deficit due to associated corticospinal tract disease. Discrete individual movements of the tongue, lips, and hands are often impossible, and attempts to perform such voluntary movements result in contraction of all the muscles in the limb and other parts of the body. Variable degrees of rigidity are generally associated with all forms of athetosis and may account for the slower quality of movement in this disorder in contrast to chorea. Treatment of athetosis is generally unsatisfactory, although some patients improve with the drugs used to suppress chorea and dystonia.

The dystonias Dystonia refers to abnormally increased muscular tone that causes fixed abnormal postures. Some patients with dystonia also have shifting postures resulting from irregular, forceful twisting movements that affect trunk and extremities and produce bizarre, grotesque movements and positions of the body. The mobile spasms of dystonia are similar to those of athetosis but are generally slower and involve axial (trunk) rather than appendicular (extremity) muscles. Dystonic movements increase during volitional motor activity, nervousness, and emotional stress; they diminish during relaxation and, like most extrapyramidal movement disorders, disappear completely during sleep. *Primary torsion dystonia,* formerly known as dystonia musculorum deformans, is frequently inherited as an autosomal dominant characteristic; families of Ashkenazic Jews with an autosomal recessive pattern of inheritance have been described. Spontaneous cases without family histories of dystonia are also common. Manifestations of dystonia usually begin in the first two decades of life, but adult forms are recognized. Generalized torsion spasms can also occur in children with kernicterus and after cerebral hypoxia.

The term dystonia is also used in another sense, to describe any fixed posture which may be the end result of a motor system disease. For example, dystonia secondary to a stroke (flexed arm and extended leg) is often called hemiplegic dystonia, and that associated with parkinsonism called flexion dystonia. In contrast to these permanent dystonic states, drugs such as the neuroleptics, and levodopa in patients with parkinsonism, can induce dystonic postures and spasms that subside once the offending medication is discontinued.

Secondary or *focal dystonias* are more common than torsion dystonia and include such disorders as spasmodic torticollis, writer's cramp, blepharospasm, spastic dysphonia, and Meige's syndrome. In the focal dystonias as a group, symptoms tend to be highly localized; they remain stable, and rarely spread to involve other body parts. Focal dystonias occur more frequently in adults and most often arise spontaneously without known genetic transmission or antecedent illness. Spasmodic torticollis is the most common focal dystonia. There are intermittent or continuous spasms of the sternocleidomastoid, trapezius, and other neck muscles, usually more prominent on one side than the other, that cause turning or tipping of the head. Torticollis is involuntary and cannot be inhibited, and thereby differs from habit spasm or tic. Torticollis is worse when the patient sits, stands, or walks; placing a finger to the chin or side of the jaw often alleviates the muscle imbalance. Women are affected twice as often as men; the average age of onset is 40.

Torsion dystonia is classified as an extrapyramidal disease even though no pathologic lesions have been observed in the basal ganglia or elsewhere in the brain. Development of rational therapy is further impaired by the lack of information regarding possible neurotransmitter abnormalities. Symptomatic relief is sometimes achieved with sedatives such as the benzodiazepines and high doses of anticholinergic drugs; levodopa has been helpful in some instances. Biofeedback therapy has sometimes been beneficial but psychiatric treatment is ineffectual. Blepharospasm has been successfully treated by injecting a dilute solution of botulinum toxin into periocular muscles. The toxin produces a mild neuromuscular blockade; its effect is transient and treatment must be repeated every 2 or 3 months. Preliminary reports indicate that injection of toxin into the appropriate muscle is effective treatment for torticollis, spastic dysphonia, and occupational finger dystonias. When spasmodic torticollis is severe, surgical denervation of the affected muscles (C1 to C3 bilaterally and C4 on one side) has given favorable results in most patients.

Myoclonus This is a descriptive term for very brief, involuntary, random muscular contractions. Myoclonus can occur spontaneously at rest, in response to sensory stimuli, or with voluntary movements. Myoclonus may involve a single motor unit and simulate a fasciculation, or it may simultaneously involve groups of muscles that displace the limb or distort its voluntary movement. Myoclonus is a symptom that occurs in a wide variety of generalized metabolic and neurologic disorders collectively called the myoclonias. Posthypoxic intention myoclonus is a special myoclonic syndrome that occurs as a sequel to transient cerebral anoxia such as might occur, for example, during a brief cardiorespiratory arrest. Cognitive abilities are usually preserved; however, there are signs of cerebellar dysfunction and voluntary movements are marred by action myoclonus involving the extremities, facial muscles, and even the voice. Action myoclonus deforms all movements and severely limits the patient's ability to eat, talk, write, or even walk. Myoclonus may also result from lipid storage disease, encephalitis, Creutzfeldt-Jakob disease, or metabolic encephalopathies due to respiratory failure, chronic renal failure, hepatic failure, or electrolyte imbalance. Posthypoxic intention myoclonus and idiopathic myoclonus may be treated with the 5-HT precursor 5-hydroxytryptophan (Fig. 25-4); alternative therapies include baclofen, clonazepam, and valproic acid.

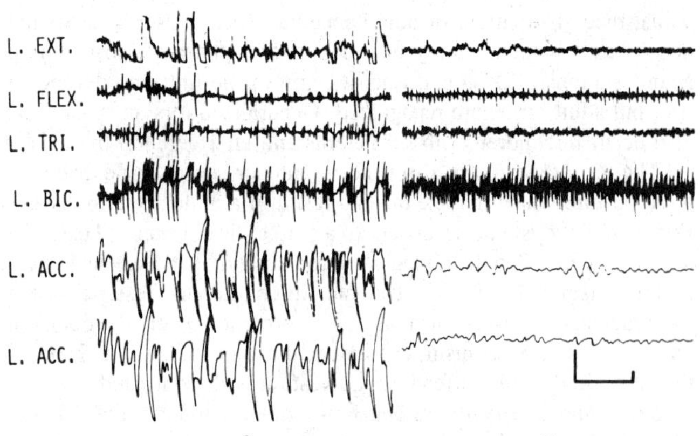

FIGURE 25-4 Recordings from the left arm of a patient with posthypoxic intention myoclonus (*A*) before and (*B*) during treatment with 5-hydroxytryptophan. In both, the arm was held out horizontally from the shoulder. The upper four traces are EMGs from wrist extensors, wrist flexors, triceps, and biceps. The lower two traces are from accelerometers at right angles to one another on the hand. The horizontal calibration is 1 s. *A*. The continuous, large, jerky movements during voluntary activity are produced by arrhythmic bursts of EMG activity interspersed with irregular periods of EMG silence. The former positive and latter negative abnormalities occurred synchronously in antagonistic muscle groups. *B*. Only a little irregular tremor remains, and the EMG is much more continuous. (*From JH Growdon et al, Neurology 26:1135, 1976.*)

Asterixis Quick arrhythmic movements that occur due to brief interruptions in background tonic muscular contractions are called asterixis; in a sense, asterixis may be considered as negative myoclonus. Asterixis may be observed in any voluntary muscle during contraction but is usually demonstrated clinically as a brief lapse of posture with prompt restoration during voluntary extension of the limb with dorsiflexion of the wrist or ankle. Asterixis is characterized by 50- to 200-ms silent periods in ongoing EMG activity in all muscle groups in one limb (Fig. 25-5). This results in a downward movement of the wrist or ankle due to gravity before muscular activity resumes and restores the limb to its original position. Asterixis is commonly observed bilaterally in metabolic encephalopathies, and its description in hepatic failure accounted for the original term "liver flap." Asterixis may be caused by drugs, including all anticonvulsants and the radiographic contrast agent metrizamide. Unilateral asterixis can occur after brain lesions in the distributions of the anterior or posterior cerebral arteries. The smallest brain lesion that can cause unilateral asterixis involves structures that are destroyed during stereotactic ventrolateral thalamotomy.

Hemiballismus Hemiballismus is a hyperkinetic movement disorder characterized by violent flinging motions in the arm contralateral to a lesion (usually vascular) in or near the subthalamic nucleus. The movements in ballism also have a rotary component at the shoulder and hip; there may be concomitant flexion and extension movements in the hand and foot as well. The involuntary motions persist throughout the day but generally attenuate during sleep. Strength and muscle tone may be slightly decreased in the affected extremities and accurate movements are impaired, but patients with hemiballismus are not paralyzed. Both experimental and clinical observations indicate that the subthalamic nucleus probably exerts a controlling influence on the globus pallidus. Damage to the subthalamic nucleus destroys this restraining influence and results in hemiballismus. The exact biochemical consequences of these lesions remain unclear, but indirect evidence suggests that there is an increase in dopaminergic tone in the remaining basal ganglia structures. Medical treatment with neuroleptic drugs given to block DA receptors are generally effective in suppressing ballismus. Surgery is reserved for refractory cases; a stereotactic lesion placed in the ipsilateral globus pallidus, thalamic fasciculus, or ventrolateral thalamus can also abolish hemiballismus and restore normal function. Although recovery can be complete, many patients are left with variable amounts of hemichorea involving the hand and foot.

Tremor This common symptom consists of a rhythmic oscillation of a part of the body around a fixed point. Tremors usually involve the distal parts of limbs; the head, tongue, or jaw; and rarely the trunk. There are several different types of tremor, and each has its own clinical setting, pathophysiology, and therapeutic requirements. Often several different tremors exist in the same patient and must be treated individually. In a general hospital, most patients who appear tremulous actually have asterixis as a manifestation of one or another metabolic encephalopathy. Tremors may be subdivided clinically according to their distribution, amplitude, and relationship to volitional movement.

Tremor at rest is a coarse tremor with an average rate of four to five beats per second. It is most often localized in one or both hands and, occasionally, in the jaw or tongue. It is frequently a feature of Parkinson's disease. It characteristically occurs with postural (tonic) contraction of axial and limb girdle musculature when the limb is in an attitude of repose; willed movement temporarily suppresses it (Fig. 25-6). If the proximal muscles are completely relaxed, the tremor usually disappears, but the average patient rarely achieves this state. In some cases the tremor is constant; in others it varies from time to time and may extend from one group of muscles to another as the disease progresses. In some patients with Parkinson's disease there is no tremor; in others the tremor tends to be rather gentle and more or less limited to the distal muscles, whereas in a minority of parkinsonian patients and in patients with Wilson's disease (hepatolenticular degeneration), it often has a wider range and involves proximal muscles. In many cases there is a variable degree of rigidity of a plastic type in the tremulous limb or elsewhere. Although it is

FIGURE 25-5 Asterixis recorded from the outstretched left arm of a patient with metrizamide-induced encephalopathy. The upper four EMG traces are identical to those in Fig. 25-4. The bottom trace is from an accelerometer on the dorsum of the hand. Calibration is 1 s. Note the continuous voluntary EMG interrupted at the arrow by a brief involuntary silent period in all four muscles. This silent period is followed by a lapse of posture and its jerky restitution, which is recorded by the accelerometer.

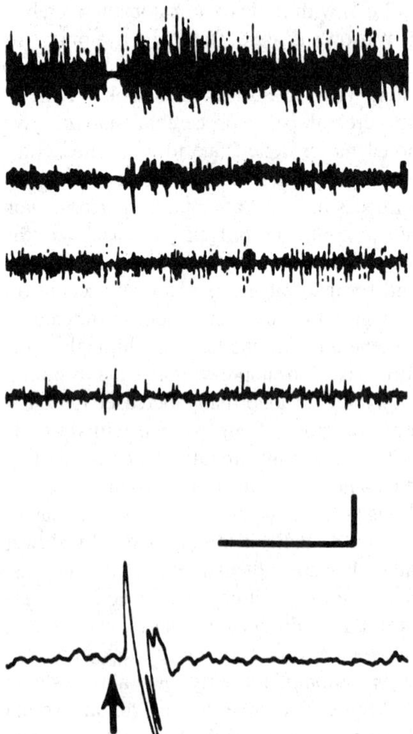

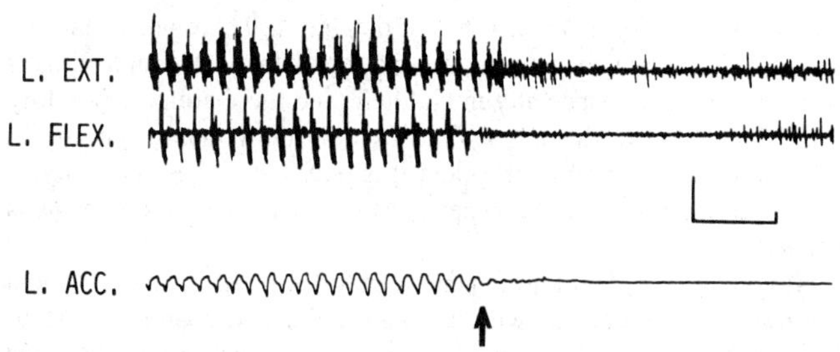

FIGURE 25-6 Tremor at rest in a patient with Parkinson's disease. The upper two traces are surface EMG recordings from extensors and flexors of the left wrist; the lower trace is from an accelerometer attached to the left hand. The horizontal calibration denotes 1 s. Note the tremor at rest results from alternating contractions of antagonistic muscles at approximately 5 Hz. At the arrow, the patient is asked to dorsiflex the left wrist, and the tremor at rest disappears.

a source of great embarrassment and often is deemed responsible for all of a patient's motor difficulties, this type of tremor interferes with voluntary movements surprisingly little: It is not uncommon to see a patient who has been trembling violently raise a full glass of water to the lips and drain the contents without spilling a drop. It is the combination of tremor at rest, slowness of movement, rigidity, flexed postures without true paralysis, and postural instability that constitutes Parkinson's syndrome. Often patients with Parkinson's disease also suffer from the tremor of stage fright (one of the enhanced physiologic tremors—see below) or from essential-familial tremor. Both may be exaggerated by increased levels of catecholamines in the bloodstream and may be suppressed by drugs, such as propranolol, that block beta-adrenergic receptors.

The exact pathologic anatomy of *tremor at rest* is unknown. In Parkinson's disease, the visible lesions are predominantly in the substantia nigra. In Wilson's disease, in which tremor is mixed with cerebellar ataxia, the lesions are diffuse. Elderly persons may develop resting tremor without rigidity, slowness of movement, flexed postures, or masked facies. Unlike patients with parkinsonism, individuals with this syndrome do not progress to motor disability; their tremor does not respond to anti-parkinsonian drugs. In any given case it is not predictable whether a tremor is the initial sign of Parkinson's disease. Patients with titubation and a proximal tremor at rest (rubral tremor) as a symptom of cerebellar system dysfunction can be differentiated by the presence of ataxia and dysmetria from those with Parkinson's disease.

Action tremor refers to tremors present when the limbs are active, either when maintained in a certain position, as when outstretched, or throughout voluntary movement. Tremor amplitude may increase slightly as the action of the limbs becomes more precise, but it never approaches the degree of augmentation seen with cerebellar ataxia/dysmetria. In contrast to tremor at rest, action tremors disappear when the limbs are relaxed. Some of the action tremors are an exaggeration of normal *physiologic tremor;* such enhanced physiologic tremors are extremely common. They are experienced occasionally by all normal persons as well as by patients with essential-familial tremor or Parkinson's disease. They involve the outstretched hand as well as head, lips, and tongue. In general, they are due to a hyperadrenergic state and sometimes are iatrogenic (Table 25-2). Activation of $beta_2$ receptors in muscle alters the mechanical properties of muscle, eliciting action tremor. These alterations are reflected in discharges of muscle spindle afferents which modify the timing of activity around the stretch reflex arc and serve to augment the amplitude of preexisting physiologic tremor. Only patients without functional stretch reflex arcs are immune to these tremors. Peripherally active drugs that block $beta_2$-adrenergic receptors diminish enhanced physiologic tremors. This type of tremor is seen in numerous medical, neurologic, and psychiatric diseases and is therefore more difficult to interpret than tremor at rest.

Essential-familial tremor (Fig. 25-7) is a somewhat slower action tremor which may occur as the only neurologic abnormality either sporadically or in several members of a family. It may begin in childhood but usually comes on later and persists throughout adult life. It becomes a source of embarrassment because it suggests to the onlooker that the patient is nervous. A curious fact about this tremor is that one or two drinks of an alcoholic beverage may abolish it but it will become worse after the effects of the alcohol have worn off. Essential-familial tremors are suppressed by primidone or CNS-active beta-adrenergic blocking agents such as propranolol.

Intention tremor is an ambiguous term: The abnormal movements are certainly not intentional, and the abnormality is best described as an oscillatory ataxia generated proximally rather than as tremor. True tremors tend to affect distal musculature and the movements are more rhythmic and tend to be in one plane. Cerebellar ataxia, in which the direction of abnormal movement varies from second to second, requires for its full expression the performance of an exacting, precise, willed movement. Ataxia is absent when the limbs are inactive and during the first part of a voluntary movement, but develops as the action continues and greater precision is demanded (e.g., in touching a target such as the patient's nose or the examiner's finger). Ataxia is a jerky, arrhythmic interruption of forward progression in a voluntary motion, often with side-to-side oscillations. Ataxia continues for a fraction of a second or so after the act is completed, and may seriously interfere with the patient's performance of skilled acts. Sometimes the head is involved (titubation). This movement disorder invariably indicates disease of the cerebellar system including its connections. When the disease is very severe, every movement, even lifting a limb, causes a wide-ranging oscillation of such violence that the patient is thrown off balance. This state is occasionally seen in multiple sclerosis, Wilson's disease, and vascular, traumatic, and

TABLE 25-2 Conditions that enhance physiologic tremors

HYPERADRENERGIC STATES
Anxiety
Bronchodilators and other beta agonists
Excitement
Hypoglycemia
Hyperthyroidism
Pheochromocytoma
Peripheral metabolites of levodopa
Stage fright
POSSIBLE HYPERADRENERGIC STATES
Amphetamines
Antidepressants
Withdrawal from alcohol or opiates
Xanthines in tea and coffee
STATES OF UNCERTAIN ETIOLOGY
Glucocorticoid therapy
Exercise
Fatigue
Lithium therapy

FIGURE 25-7 Action tremor in a patient with essential-familial tremor. Recordings from the right upper extremity are with the hand actively dorsiflexed; otherwise, traces are similar to Fig. 25-4. The horizontal calibration denotes 500 ms. Note that during this action tremor, bursts of EMG activity at approximately 8 Hz occur synchronously in antagonistic muscles.

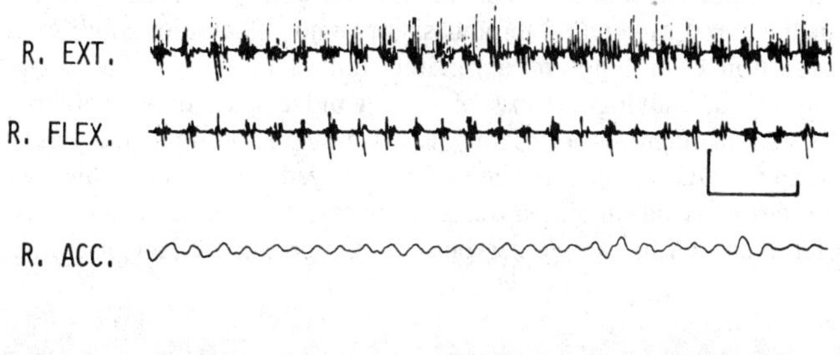

other lesions of the tegmentum of the midbrain and subthalamus but not of the cerebellum.

Habit spasms and tics Many individuals develop habitual movements that persist unchanged throughout life. Common examples include sniffing, clearing the throat, protruding the chin, and pulling on the collar. These are called habit spasms. Affected individuals admit that the movements are voluntary, but that they feel compelled to make them in order to relieve tension. Habit spasms can be inhibited for a time by a willful effort but reappear when attention is diverted. In certain cases, they become so ingrained that the person is unaware of them and unable to control them. Children between 5 and 10 years of age are especially likely to have habit spasms.

Tics are characterized by stereotyped, purposeless, and irregularly repetitive movements. Gilles de la Tourette syndrome is the most common and severe form of multiple tic disorder. This syndrome is a neuropsychiatric disorder with motor and behavior abnormalities; it usually begins in the first two decades of life and affects boys four times more frequently than girls. Motor symptoms include multiple brief muscular spasms, known as convulsive tics, in the face, neck, and shoulders. Vocal tics, including grunts and barking sounds, are also common. Behavioral abnormalities include coprolalia (swearing and repeating other vile utterances) and repeating the words of others (echolalia). The cause of Tourette's syndrome is unknown, and its pathophysiology remains obscure. Treatments with neuroleptic drugs will decrease the severity and frequency of tics in 75 to 90 percent of patients with Tourette's syndrome, regardless of disease severity. The noradrenergic agonist clonidine has also been reported to suppress symptoms.

EXAMINATION AND DIFFERENTIAL DIAGNOSIS OF EXTRAPYRAMIDAL SYNDROMES In broad terms, all of the extrapyramidal disorders should be viewed in terms of primary deficit (negative symptoms) and of the new phenomena (abnormal postures and involuntary movements) that have appeared. The positive symptoms are ascribed to release from inhibition or disequilibrium of undamaged motor parts of the nervous system. The physician must cultivate the habit of accurately observing and describing abnormalities of movement and must not be content merely to give the condition a name or to force it into some superficial category. The fully developed extrapyramidal motor syndromes can be recognized without difficulty once the physician has become familiar with the typical pictures. A mental picture of Parkinson's disease, with its slowness of movement, poverty of facial expression, tremor at rest, and muscular rigidity, should be fixed in mind. Similarly, the gross distortions of posture found in dystonia, whether widespread in trunk muscles or involving only neck muscles as in spasmodic torticollis, should be easily recognized. Athetosis, with its instability of postures, ceaseless movements of finger and hands, and intention spasm; chorea, with its rapid and complicated movements; and myoclonus, with its abrupt movements that flit over the body, are other standard syndromes. There tends to be a mild defect in the voluntary use of the affected parts in all extrapyramidal syndromes.

Early or mild forms of these conditions, like all medical diseases, may offer special difficulties in diagnosis. Cases of Parkinson's disease, seen before the appearance of tremor, are often overlooked. Uncertainty of balance and short gait (*marche à petit pas*) in the elderly is often incorrectly attributed to loss of confidence and fear of falling. Patients may complain of being nervous and restless and describe a stiffness and aching in parts of the body. Because there is no weakness or change in reflexes, the disorder may then be considered rheumatic or even psychogenic. Parkinson's disease often begins in a hemiplegic distribution, and for this reason, the illness may be misdiagnosed as cerebral thrombosis or tumor. Facial immobility, a suggestion of a limp, mild rigidity, failure of an arm to swing naturally in walking, or loss of certain movements of cooperation will help in diagnosis at this time. Every case presenting with atypical extrapyramidal symptoms should be surveyed for Wilson's disease in order to avoid missing a treatable illness. Mild or early chorea is often mistaken for simple nervousness. Observing the patient at rest as well as in action is critical to the diagnosis. There are instances, nonetheless, in which it is impossible to distinguish simple fidgets from early chorea, especially in children, and there are no laboratory tests to aid in the diagnosis. The first postural manifestations of dystonia may suggest hysteria, and it is only later when the fixity of the postural abnormality becomes apparent that accurate diagnosis is reached.

Motor disorders seldom appear in pure form, and extrapyramidal syndromes often coexist with lesions in the corticospinal tract or cerebellar systems. For example, syndromes such as progressive supranuclear palsy, olivopontocerebellar atrophy, or the Shy-Drager syndrome have many elements of Parkinson's disease but also have paralysis of voluntary eye movements, ataxia, apraxia, postural hypotension, or spasticity with bilateral Babinski signs. Wilson's disease usually displays tremor at rest, rigidity, slowness of movement, and flexion dystonia of the trunk, but exceptionally there are athetosis, dystonia, and intention tremor. Emotional or cognitive abnormalities may be the presenting signs in Wilson's disease. Hallervorden-Spatz disease may take the form of universal rigidity and flexion dystonia, but choreoathetosis is sometimes observed. In some forms of Huntington's disease, particularly with juvenile onset, rigidity replaces choreoathetosis. Corticospinal and various extrapyramidal disorders may be associated in patients with cerebral diplegia. Some of the neurodegenerative diseases in which corticospinal tract and basal ganglia lesions coexist are described in Chap. 359.

Anatomic and neuropathologic studies of the basal ganglia, coupled with biochemical analyses of neurotransmitter content and behavioral responses to neuropharmacologic agents, provide the basis for understanding disorders involving the basal ganglia and for guiding their treatment. Results of studies in Parkinson's disease and Huntington's disease clearly illustrate these principles. In Parkinson's disease, the DA content of the striatum is depleted owing to a loss of neurons in the substantia nigra and degeneration of their axonal projection to the striatum. As a result of decreased DA release, neurons within the striatum that synthesize ACh are released from inhibition. This results in the preponderance of cholinergic neurotransmission relative to dopaminergic transmission that accounts for most of the symptoms in Parkinson's disease. Recognition of this imbalance provides the basis for rational pharmacologic treatments. According to this formulation, drugs that increase dopaminergic neurotransmission, such as levodopa or bromocriptine, would be expected to rectify the imbalance between cholinergic and dopaminergic tone. These drugs, often prescribed in combination with anticholinergic drugs, are now standard therapy in Parkinson's disease. Excess levodopa or bromocriptine in patients with Parkinson's disease may induce a wide variety of abnormal movements that result from excessive stimulation of DA receptors in the striatum. The most frequent of these is craniofacial choreoathetosis, but more generalized choreoathetosis, facial and cervical spasms, dystonic postures, and myoclonic jerks may also occur. On the other hand, administration of drugs that block DA receptors (such as the neuroleptics) or deplete DA storage (such as reserpine or tetrabenazine) may produce a parkinsonian syndrome in an otherwise normal individual.

Huntington's disease is in many ways the clinical and pharmacologic opposite of Parkinson's disease. In Huntington's disease, characterized by personality change and dementia, gait abnormality, and chorea, there is a loss of neurons within the caudate and putamen, with resultant depletion of GABA and ACh but preserved DA content. The symptoms of chorea are believed to result from relative excess of DA compared with other transmitters in the striatum; drugs that block DA receptors, such as the neuroleptics, generally suppress chorea, whereas levodopa administration increases it. Similarly, physostigmine, given to increase cholinergic neurotransmission, may suppress chorea, whereas anticholinergic drugs enhance it.

These examples of clinical pharmacology further confirm the existence of delicate balances between excitatory and inhibitory impulses in the basal ganglia. In any one patient, the variable clinical manifestations seen during therapy are due to alterations in the neurochemical environment; the anatomic lesions remain unchanged. These examples illustrate the power of neuropharmacologic therapy in basal ganglia disease and provide the basis for optimism regarding the future ability of drugs to benefit patients with extrapyramidal movement disorders.

REFERENCES

ALEXANDER GE et al: Parallel organization of functionally segregated circuits linking basal ganglia and cortex. Ann Rev Neurosci 9:357, 1986

FAHN S et al: Classification and investigation of dystonia, in *Movement Disorders 2*. CD Marsden, S Fahn (eds). London, Butterworths, 1987, pp 332–358

GESCHWIND N: The apraxias: Neural mechanisms of disorders of learned movement. Am Sci 63:188, 1975

GRAYBIEL AM: Neuropeptides in the basal ganglia, in *Neuropeptides in Neurologic and Psychiatric Disease*, JB Martin, JD Barchas (eds). New York, Raven Press, 1986, pp 135–161

GROWDON JH, SCHEIFE RT: Medical treatment of extrapyramidal diseases, in *Update III: Harrison's Principles of Internal Medicine*. KJ Isselbacher et al (eds). New York, McGraw-Hill, 1982, pp 185–208

JAGIELLA WM, SUNG JH: Bilateral infarction of the medullary pyramids in humans. Neurology 39:21, 1989

JANKOVIC J, ORMAN J: Botulinum A toxin for cranial-cervical dystonia: A double-blind, placebo-controlled study. Neurology 37:616, 1987

KUYPERS HGJM: Anatomy of the descending pathways, in *Handbook of Physiology*, Section 1, *The Nervous System*, vol II: *Motor Control*, Part I, VB Brooks (ed). Bethesda, American Physiological Society, 1981, pp 597–666

MARSDEN CD: The mysterious motor function of the basal ganglia. Neurology 32:514, 1982

MARTIN JB: Huntington's disease: New approaches to an old problem. Neurology 34:1059, 1984

PENN RD et al: Intrathecal baclofen for severe spinal spasticity. N Engl J Med 320:1517, 1989

YOUNG RR: Treatment of spastic paresis. N Engl J Med 320:1553, 1989

26 ATAXIA AND DISORDERS OF BALANCE AND GAIT

SID GILMAN

In the assessment of patients with neurologic disorders, it is important when taking the history to inquire about posture and gait and to examine these functions routinely as part of the neurologic examination. Abnormalities of posture and gait can result from disorders affecting several levels of the nervous system, and the type of abnormality observed clinically often indicates the site affected.

NEURAL STRUCTURES REQUIRED FOR STANDING AND WALKING The structures in the central nervous system that control standing and walking are the basal ganglia, a "locomotor region" in the mesencephalon, the cerebellum, and the spinal cord. The cerebral cortex doubtless is important in many aspects of standing and walking, but in experimental animals, complete removal of the cerebral cortex during the neonatal period, preserving the basal ganglia, thalamus, and lower structures, leaves stance and locomotion essentially normal. If the cerebral cortex, basal ganglia, and thalamus are removed, leaving the mesencephalon and lower brainstem intact, standing and walking are still possible. Electrical stimulation in a region of the mesencephalon termed the "locomotor region" evokes walking motions, and the speed and form of locomotion can be modified from a slow walk to a trot or gallop with changes in stimulation strength. This region receives projections from the basal ganglia, including the subthalamic and endopeduncular nuclei and the substantia nigra.

The spinal cord contains neural circuitry that coordinates the muscles for locomotion. After experimental transection of the spinal cord in the midthoracic region, the hindlimbs maintain the capacity to perform coordinated walking movements when placed on a moving treadmill. With increased treadmill speed, walking movements can switch to simultaneous movements of the hindlimbs, as in a gallop. After a high spinal transection, both the forelimbs and the hindlimbs can generate alternating movements and the sets of limbs remain coordinated. Thus, neural circuitry in the spinal cord can coordinate movements among all four limbs. The cerebellum controls many of the movements required for walking. Ablation of the cerebellum results in severe disorders of standing and walking.

In summary, walking is the result of integrated activity of the basal ganglia, mesencephalon, cerebellum, and spinal cord. Sensory inputs from movements of joints and muscle afferents provide important components for the control of walking. Without appropriate sensory feedback information, the pattern of walking is severely disrupted.

THE CEREBELLUM The cerebellum functions in concert with the motor cortex, basal ganglia, and many brainstem structures in executing a variety of movements. The cerebellum is needed to maintain proper posture and balance for walking and running; to perform fine voluntary movements such as those needed for writing, dressing, and eating; to carry out rapidly alternating and repetitive movements as in playing a musical instrument or working with a computer; and to coordinate smooth tracking movements of the eyes. The cerebellum controls certain properties of movements, including trajectory, velocity, and acceleration. Voluntary movements can be performed in the absence of cerebellar function, but the movements are clumsy and disorganized. The disturbances of movement from cerebellar dysfunction are termed *dyssynergia* (also *asynergia* or *ataxia*).

The cerebellum consists of a midline vermal region and two hemispheres, which are attached to the medulla, pons, and midbrain by three peduncles on each side. A layer of gray matter, the cerebellar cortex, covers the cerebellar surface and encloses an internal core of white matter. Three pairs of deep cerebellar nuclei are buried within the cerebellum. From medial to lateral these consist of the fastigial, interposed (globose and emboliform), and dentate nuclei.

The cerebellum consists of three lobes. The *flocculonodular lobe*, which is the oldest part of the cerebellum phylogenetically (archicerebellum), consists of the paired flocculi and the nodulus. This lobe receives input principally from the vestibular nuclei. The *anterior lobe*, the second oldest part (paleocerebellum), consists of vermal and paravermal structures in the anterior superior portion of the cerebellum. The anterior lobe receives input chiefly from the spinal cord. The *posterior lobe* is the largest and phylogenetically newest part of the cerebellum (neocerebellum) and is located between the other two lobes. The posterior lobe receives projections from the cerebral hemispheres via the pontine nuclei.

The cerebellar cortex contains three layers: an outermost *molecular layer*, a middle *Purkinje cell layer*, and an inner *granular layer*. The afferent fibers reaching the cerebellar cortex send collateral projections to the deep cerebellar nuclei and terminate either in the granule cell layer as *mossy fibers* or upon the dendrites of Purkinje cells as *climbing fibers*. Mossy fiber afferents are derived from the spinal cord, pontine nuclei, vestibular receptors and nuclei, trigeminal nuclei, reticular nuclei, and deep cerebellar nuclei. Climbing fiber afferents are derived exclusively from the inferior olive. Both mossy fiber and climbing fiber inputs are excitatory to the deep cerebellar nuclei and the cortex. Purkinje cells provide the only route for all information exiting from the cerebellar cortex and are inhibitory to the deep cerebellar and vestibular nuclei.

Projections to the cerebellum also originate in the locus coeruleus and the raphe nuclei of the brainstem. The afferents to the cerebellum from the locus coeruleus are noradrenergic; those from the raphe nuclei are serotonergic; and both sets of afferents are inhibitory. Several amino acids have been identified as putative neurotransmitters in the cerebellum. These include glutamate, which is used by mossy fibers and the axons of granule cells (parallel fibers); aspartate, which is used by climbing fibers; and γ-aminobutyric acid, which is used by the axons of Purkinje cells, Golgi cells, and basket cells.

The *inferior cerebellar peduncle* (*restiform body*) consists chiefly of afferent fibers. The peduncle contains a single efferent tract, the fastigiobulbar tract, which projects to the vestibular nuclei and

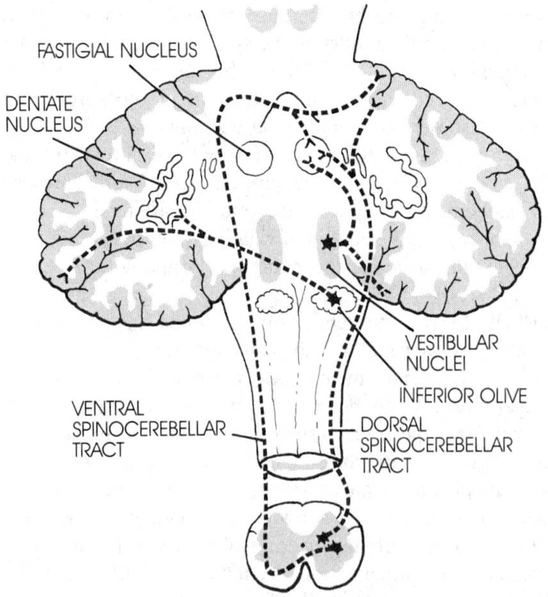

FIGURE 26-1 The central nervous system connections of the dorsal and ventral spinocerebellar tracts, the fastigial nuclei, and the vestibular nuclei. *(Adapted from S Gilman and S Winans Newman, in Manter & Gatz's Essentials of Clinical Neuroanatomy and Neurophysiology, 7th ed, Philadelphia, Davis, 1987.)*

completes a vestibular circuit through the cerebellum. Afferent fibers enter the inferior cerebellar peduncle from at least six sources (Fig. 26-1): (1) fibers from the vestibular nerve and nuclei; (2) olivocerebellar fibers from the inferior olivary nuclei; (3) the dorsal spinocerebellar tract; (4) some of the fibers from the ventral spinocerebellar tract; (5) the cuneocerebellar tract from the accessory cuneate nuclei in the medulla; and (6) reticulocerebellar fibers. *The middle cerebellar peduncle* (*brachium pontis*) consists almost entirely of crossed afferent fibers from the pontine nuclei in the gray substance of the basal part of the pons (pontocerebellar or transverse pontine fibers) (Fig. 26-2). The major projections to the pontine nuclei originate within the cerebral cortex. The *superior cerebellar peduncle* (*brachium conjunctivum*) consists principally of efferent projections from the cerebellum. Fibers arising in the dentate and interposed nuclei project to the reticular formation, red nucleus, and thalamus. Some of the fastigiobulbar tract fibers also run with the superior peduncle for a short distance before they enter the inferior cerebellar peduncle. The superior cerebellar peduncle contains afferent projections from the ventral spinocerebellar tract, a portion of the rostral spinocerebellar tract, and trigeminocerebellar projections.

FIGURE 26-2 The central nervous system connections of the dentate nucleus and interposed (emboliform and globose) nuclei. *(Adapted from S Gilman and S Winans Newman, in Manter & Gatz's Essentials of Clinical Neuroanatomy and Neurophysiology, 7th ed, Philadelphia, Davis, 1987.)*

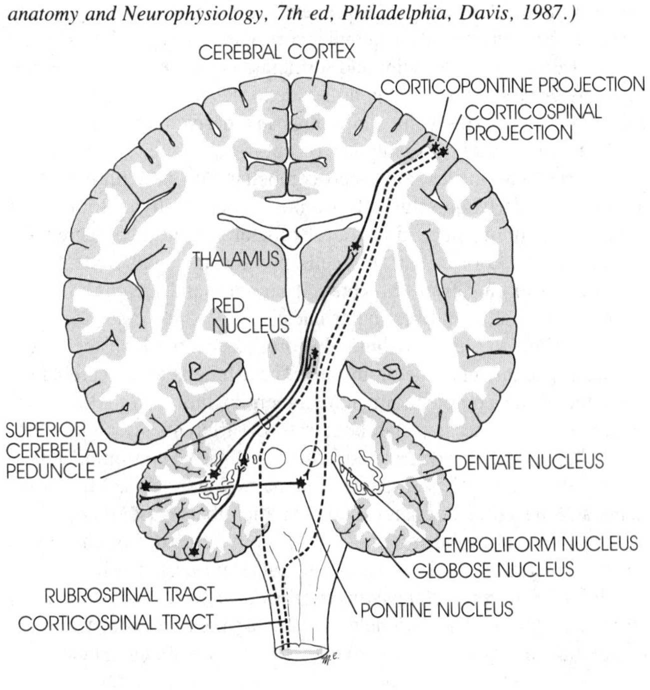

Except for direct projections of Purkinje cells onto vestibular nuclei, the efferent pathways of the cerebellum begin with the deep nuclei. The fastigial nucleus sends fibers to the reticular and vestibular nuclei of the brainstem. These nuclei project into the spinal cord and are concerned with posture and balance. The interposed nuclei of each side of the cerebellum project axons through the superior cerebellar peduncle to the red nucleus of the contralateral side. The red nucleus sends fibers into the rubrospinal tract (Fig. 26-2), and this tract crosses the midline before descending into the spinal cord. The origin of this pathway in the interposed nuclei and the terminal portion in the spinal cord are on the same side of the body. Both the dentate and the interposed nuclei send fibers through the superior cerebellar peduncle to the contralateral ventrolateral nucleus of the thalamus. The ventrolateral nucleus relays fibers to the motor regions of the ipsilateral frontal lobe. The thalamic endings in the cerebral cortex make connection with corticospinal neurons whose efferent fibers pass through the pyramidal tract and cross to the contralateral side of the spinal cord. Thus, the origin of the cerebellothalamocortical pathway in the dentate and interposed nuclei and its termination in the spinal cord are on the same side of the body (Fig. 26-2).

For clinical purposes, a useful method of describing the cerebellum is based upon the existence of longitudinal sagittal zones. Each half of the cerebellum is subdivided into three longitudinal strips arranged from medial to lateral, including the cerebellar cortex, underlying white matter, and deep cerebellar nuclei: (1) a midline zone consisting of the vermal region with the fastigial nucleus; (2) an intermediate zone, the paravermal region, with the interposed nuclei; and (3) a lateral zone consisting of the cerebellar hemisphere with the dentate nucleus. Lesions of the midline zone cause disorders of stance and gait, truncal ataxia and titubation, and rotated or tilted postures of the head. Lesions of the lateral zone lead to disturbances in coordinated limb movement (ataxia), dysarthria, hypotonia, nystagmus, and kinetic tremor. Lesions of the intermediate zone cause symptoms characteristic of involvement of both the midline and lateral zones.

Ataxia is the result of dysmetria and decomposition of movement. *Dysmetria* is a disturbance of the trajectory or placement of a limb during active movement in which the limb falls short of its target (*hypometria*) or extends beyond its target (*hypermetria*). *Decomposition of movement* refers to errors in the sequence and speed of the component parts of a movement. The result is a lack of speed and skill in acts requiring the smoothly coordinated activity of several muscles. Movements previously fluid and accurate become halting and imprecise. *Ataxia* appears clinically as a disturbance in the rate and extent of an individual movement and commonly occurs from lesions of the cerebellum or of the sensory systems. Ataxia of gait consists of irregularities in the rate, length, and consistency of walking movements, with veering to one side or the other.

PHYSIOLOGIC RESPONSES IMPORTANT IN STANDING AND WALKING Maintenance of the upright posture results from the actions of a number of postural reflex responses: (1) local static reactions acting on individual limbs; (2) segmental static reactions linking the extremities together; and (3) general static reactions resulting from the position of the head in space. *Local static reactions* include the stretch reflex and the positive supporting reaction. The simplest *stretch reflex* is illustrated by the muscle stretch response (deep tendon reflex), a brief muscle twitch evoked by rapid stretch of the muscle's tendon. Maintenance of muscle extension results in sustained contraction of that muscle through the stretch reflex. The *positive supporting reaction*, as elucidated in animal studies, results from a light cutaneous contact of the skin of the foot and also by proprioceptive stimulation owing to stretch of the interosseous muscles. The result of these stimuli is an extensor thrust by the limb.

The *segmental static reactions* include the crossed extension reflex and interlimb coordination. In the crossed extension reflex, application of noxious stimulation to an extremity results in flexion of that limb and simultaneous extension of the contralateral limb. With stronger stimulation, the crossed extension reflex triggered from a hindlimb can induce flexion in the contralateral forelimb and extension in the ipsilateral forelimb. Thus, the whole body moves along a diagonal path through the extended contralateral hindlimb and ipsilateral forelimb, thereby removing the stimulated limb from the source of noxious stimulation. This diagonal pattern of interlimb coordination also provides postural adjustments in various situations.

The *general static reactions* consist of two general types. The first, the *tonic neck* and *labyrinthine reflexes*, function together to adjust body posture when the head moves relative to the trunk in space. The second, the *righting reflex*, is triggered by labyrinthine, neck, and visual stimuli and helps the animal to regain an upright position after a fall. The *grasp reflex* is a component of the righting reflex. Other forms of general static reactions include the placing and hopping reactions as well as adjustment of body postures during limb movements.

CLINICAL APPROACH TO DISORDERS OF EQUILIBRIUM AND GAIT When evaluating a disorder of gait, the physician should inquire whether the disturbance occurs more in the dark than in the light; whether vertigo, giddiness, or lightheadedness accompanies the disorder; and whether there is pain, numbness, tingling, or other type of paresthesias of the limbs. Inquiry should search for weakness, bowel and bladder dysfunction, and limb stiffness or rigidity. The physician should ask whether there is difficulty in the initiation or termination of walking.

Examination of stance and gait is performed best in a setting in which the physician can observe the patient walk from the front, back, and sides. The patient should rise quickly from a chair, walk normally at a slow pace, then more rapidly, and then turn around. The patient should walk on the heels, on the toes, and in tandem, placing the heel of one foot directly in front of the toes of the opposite foot, attempting to progress in a straight line. The patient should stand erect with the feet together and the head straight, first with the eyes open and then with the eyes closed to determine whether balance can be maintained (Romberg's sign). It is often helpful to observe the gait initially as the patient comes into the examining room when the patient is unaware that gait and stance are being examined.

With normal walking the body should be held erect, the head should be straight and the arms should hang loosely at the sides, each moving in rhythm with movement of the opposite leg. The shoulders and hips should be level and the arms should swing equally. The steps should be straight and equal in length. The head should not be tilted, and there should be no appreciable scoliosis or lordosis. With each step the hip and knee should flex smoothly, the ankle should dorsiflex, and the foot should clear the ground easily. The heel should strike the ground first, and the weight of the body should be transferred successively onto the sole of the foot and then onto the toes. The head and body should rotate slightly with each step without lurching or falling movements. Each person walks in a characteristic fashion that is often familial. Some people walk with the toes turned inward, others with the toes turned outward. Some people stride with large steps and others shuffle, making small steps. A person's gait is often a reflection of personality traits and can reflect shyness and timidity or aggressiveness and self-confidence.

Hemiparesis The patient with weakness of the limbs on one side of the body from a lesion of the corticospinal tract usually develops a characteristic gait disorder. The severity of the disorder depends upon the degree of weakness and stiffness of the affected limbs. The severely hemiparetic subject will stand and walk with the affected arm adducted at the shoulder and flexed at the elbow, wrist, and fingers and the affected leg stiffly extended at the hip, knee, and ankle. There is difficulty in flexing the hip and knee and dorsiflexing the ankle. Thus, the paretic leg swings outward at the hip so that the foot does not scrape the floor. The leg is held stiffly and rotates in a semicircle, first away from and then toward the trunk in a circumduction movement. Often the upper body tilts slightly to the opposite side during the leg movement. The arm on the hemiparetic side usually swings little during walking. The loss of arm swing can be an early sign of a progressive hemiparesis. A person with a mild hemiparesis may show a gait disorder similar to that of the severely hemiparetic individual, but with a lesser degree of abnormality. In this case, a decrease in arm swing may be associated with subtle circumduction of the leg, without clear stiffness or weakness of the affected limbs.

Paraparesis Diseases of the spinal cord that affect leg function produce a characteristic gait resulting from a combination of spasticity and weakness of the lower extremities. Walking requires considerable effort and consists of slow, stiff movements at the hips and knees. The legs are usually maintained extended or slightly flexed at the hips and knees and adducted at the hips. In some people with paraparesis the legs may cross with each step, producing a scissoring motion. The steps usually are regular and short, and the patient may move the trunk from side to side, attempting to compensate for the stiff movements of the legs. The legs circumduct at the hips, and the feet scrape along the floor so that the soles of the shoes become worn at the toes.

Parkinsonism Parkinson's disease produces a characteristic posture and gait. The severely affected individual stands in a posture of flexion, with the thoracic spine bent forward, the head bent downward, the arms moderately flexed at the elbows and the legs slightly flexed at the hips and knees. The patient sits or stands with striking immobility, showing a fixed facial expression with infrequent blinking and making few automatic movements of the limbs. The patient seldom crosses the legs or adjusts body posture when seated in a chair. Although the arms are held immobile, often a tremor involves the fingers and wrists at four to five cycles per second. In some people the tremor also occurs at the elbows and even at the shoulders. In advanced cases there may be drooling and a rhythmic tremor of the jaw. The patient usually gets up slowly to walk and, with walking, the trunk bends even farther forward and the arms remain immobile at the sides of the body or become further flexed and carried a bit ahead of the body. The arms fail to swing. As forward progression begins, the legs remain bent at the hips, knees, and ankles. Characteristically, the steps are short so that the feet barely clear the ground and the soles of the feet shuffle and scrape the floor. With forward locomotion the steps become successively more rapid, and the patient may fall unless assisted (*festination*). If the patient is pushed forward or backward, compensatory flexion or extension movements of the trunk fail to occur, and the patient is forced to make a series of propulsive or retropulsive steps.

Patients with Parkinson's disease often have great difficulty in rising from a chair or walking after standing still. The individual may initiate walking with several small steps before taking longer strides. Walking may stop involuntarily with attempts to pass through a doorway or into an elevator. Parkinsonian patients at times can walk with surprising speed and dexterity for brief intervals. In times of acute emergency, as in a fire, a person previously immobile can walk rapidly or even run briefly.

Cerebellar disease Disease of the cerebellum causes difficulty in standing without support and in walking. The disorder may result from lesions intrinsic to the cerebellum or from lesions in the connecting pathways to and from the cerebellum. The difficulty is worsened by attempts to walk with a narrow base. The affected person usually stands with the legs apart, and standing may provoke *titubation*, a coarse forward and backward tremor of the trunk. Attempting to stand with the feet together provokes swaying or falling. The instability is the same whether the eyes are open or closed. The patient walks cautiously, taking steps of varying lengths, and lurches from side to side. The patient complains of difficulty with balance, is fearful of walking without support, and may insist upon holding onto objects such as a bed or chair, moving cautiously between these objects. Frequently the individual does not need to be supported; simply touching a wall or an object in the room makes it possible to walk with a greater sense of security. When a mild gait disorder is present, walking may deteriorate with attempts to walk in tandem in a straight line. This causes the patient to lose balance and, in response, to place one foot to the side to avoid falling. With unilateral lesions of the cerebellum, balance is lost toward the side of the lesion.

When disease is restricted to the midline (vermal) portions of the cerebellum, as occurs in alcoholic cerebellar degeneration, disorders of stance and gait may develop without other signs of cerebellar dysfunction such as limb ataxia or nystagmus. In contrast, disease of the cerebellar hemispheres, either unilaterally or bilaterally, often causes marked limb ataxia and nystagmus in association with a gait disorder. With a lesion confined to one cerebellar hemisphere, ipsilateral disturbances of posture and movement commonly accompany the gait disorder. The patient usually stands with the shoulder on the side of the lesion lower than the other, and there may be an accompanying scoliosis. The limbs on the side of the cerebellar lesion show diminished resistance to passive manipulation (hypotonia). On walking the patient staggers and deviates toward the affected side. This can be demonstrated by asking the patient to walk around a chair. Rotation toward the affected side results in a fall into the chair, and rotation toward the normal side causes movement away from the chair in a spiral. The affected arm and leg show marked ataxia in tests of coordinated movement such as successively touching the patient's nose and then the examiner's finger or running the heel of the affected leg down the shin of the opposite leg.

Sensory ataxia A characteristic gait disorder results from loss of sensation in the lower extremities due to disease processes in the peripheral nerves, dorsal roots, dorsal columns of the spinal cord, or medial lemnisci. The most disabling component of the sensory disorder is the loss of joint position sense, but loss of input from muscle spindle receptors, vibration detectors, and cutaneous receptors also contributes to the disability. People with sensory ataxia are unaware of the position of the lower extremities and consequently have difficulty in both standing and walking. The patient usually stands with the legs spread widely apart. The patient remains stable if asked to stand with the feet together and the eyes open, but sways and often falls (positive Romberg's sign) when the eyes are closed. The test for Romberg's sign cannot be performed if the subject is unsteady when standing with the feet together and the eyes open, as may occur with cerebellar disease.

The patient with sensory ataxia walks with the legs spread widely apart, watching the ground carefully. The legs are lifted higher than necessary at the hips and are flung forward and outward in abrupt motions. The steps vary in length, and the feet make characteristic slapping sounds as they contact the floor. The patient usually holds the body somewhat flexed at the hips, often using a cane for support. If vision is impaired or the patient attempts to walk in the dark, the gait disturbance worsens. The patient becomes unsteady and often falls when attempting to wash the face because of the temporary loss of visual compensation occurring with closure of the eyes.

Cerebral palsy This term encompasses a number of different motor abnormalities, most of them resulting from hypoxic-ischemic injury to the central nervous system in the perinatal period. The severity of the gait disturbance varies with the nature and extent of the lesion. Mild limited lesions can lead to increased deep tendon reflexes and extensor plantar responses with a slight degree of talipes equinovarus, without a clear gait disorder. More severe and extensive lesions commonly lead to bilateral hemiparesis. The patient stands and walks with a paraparetic posture and gait. The arms are adducted at the shoulders and flexed at the elbows and wrists.

Movement disorders commonly alter the gait in people with cerebral palsy. Athetosis occurs frequently and consists of slow or moderately rapid serpentine movements of the arms and legs, with postures alternating between the extremes of flexion with supination and extension with pronation. On walking, people with athetotic cerebral palsy show involuntary limb movements that are accompanied by rotary movements of the neck and frequent facial grimacing. The arms are usually flexed and the legs are extended, but asymmetric limb postures can occur with ambulation. For example, one arm may flex and supinate, and the other may extend and pronate. Asymmetric limb postures commonly occur as the head rotates from side to side. Usually when the chin turns to one side, the arm on that side extends and the opposite arm flexes.

Chorea Individuals with choreic movements often develop a characteristic gait disorder. Chorea occurs most frequently in children with Sydenham's chorea, in adults with Huntington's disease, and occasionally in adults with Parkinson's disease treated with excessive amounts of dopamine agonist medications. Choreic movements consist of intermittent rapid movements of the face, trunk, neck, and limbs. Flexion, extension, and rotary movements of the neck occur along with grimacing movements of the face, twisting movements of the trunk and limbs, and rapid piano-playing movements of the digits. Frequently, in early chorea, flexion and extension movements of the hips occur so that the individual constantly seems to be crossing and uncrossing the legs. The patient may scowl, frown, and smile involuntarily. Walking usually accentuates the choreic movements. Sudden forward or sideward thrusting movements of the pelvis and rapid twisting movements of the trunk and limbs result in a gait that resembles a series of dance steps. The steps are usually irregular in size, and the patient has difficulty walking in a straight line. The rate of progression varies from slow to rapid owing to variability in the rate and amplitude of each step.

Dystonia This is an involuntary postural and movement disorder affecting children (dystonia musculorum deformans or torsion dystonia) and adults (dystonia of adult onset). The condition may occur sporadically without known cause, as a genetic disorder, or as part of another process such as Wilson's disease. In dystonia musculorum deformans, which commonly begins in children, the first symptom often consists of an abnormal gait. Characteristically the patient will walk with one foot inverted at the ankle, placing weight on the lateral side of the foot; as the disease progresses, this problem worsens and other postural abnormalities develop. These include elevation of one shoulder, elevation of a hip, twisted postures of the trunk, and excessive flexion of the wrist and fingers of one upper limb. Intermittent spasms of the trunk and limbs may interfere with walking. Eventually torticollis, tortipelvis, lordosis, and scoliosis may supervene. In extreme cases, the patient becomes unable to walk. Adult-onset dystonia often results in a similar progression of movement disorders.

Muscular dystrophy Marked weakness of the muscles of the trunk and proximal portions of the legs causes a characteristic stance and gait. In attempting to rise from a seated position, the affected person bends forward, flexing the trunk at the hips, places the hands on the knees, and pushes the trunk upward by working the hands up the thighs. Standing occurs with exaggerated lumbar lordosis and a protuberant abdomen owing to weakness of the abdominal and paravertebral muscles. The patient walks with the legs spread widely apart and develops a waddling motion of the pelvis because of weakness of the gluteal muscles. The shoulders often slope forward, and winging of the scapulae may be seen with walking.

Frontal lobe disease Bilateral frontal lobe disease causes a characteristic gait disorder that is usually associated with dementia and frontal lobe release signs including grasp, suck, and snout reflexes. The patient characteristically stands with the feet spread widely apart and takes a first step only after a long delay. This hesitancy is followed by very small shuffling steps and then by a few steps of moderate amplitude after which time the patient freezes, unable to continue walking. The cycle then is repeated. Affected individuals usually do not show muscular weakness, abnormalities of the deep tendon reflexes, sensory changes, or extensor plantar reflex responses. Usually the patient can perform the individual limb movements required for walking if asked to mimic walking movements while lying supine. The gait disorder with frontal lobe disease is a form of apraxia, i.e., a disturbance in the performance of a motor function in the absence of weakness of the muscles required for the function.

Normal-pressure hydrocephalus Normal-pressure hydrocephalus (NPH) is a disorder characterized by dementia, gait apraxia, and urinary incontinence. Computed tomography reveals large cerebral ventricles, widening of the callosal angle, and lack of filling with cerebrospinal fluid of the subarachnoid space over the cerebral hemispheres. Injection of radioactive isotope into the lumbar subarachnoid space demonstrates pathologic reflux of the isotope into the ventricular system and inadequate penetration into the cortical subarachnoid spaces.

The gait in NPH resembles that seen in apraxia from frontal lobe disease, consisting of a series of small, shuffling steps making it appear that the feet are glued to the floor. Initiation of walking is impaired, and slow and small angular displacements of the hip, knee, and ankle joints occur along with low clearance of the foot from the floor so that the patient appears to be sliding the feet along the floor. There is continuous contraction of the antigravity muscles of the legs but low muscle activity in the calf muscles. The gait disorder in NPH is thought to result from impaired function of the frontal lobes. In about half the patients with NPH the gait is improved by surgical shunting of cerebrospinal fluid from the cerebral ventricles into the venous system.

Aging Changes in gait and difficulties with balance occur with aging. Elderly men develop forward flexion of the upper portion of the trunk with flexion of the arms and knees, decreased arm swing, and shortening of step length. Elderly women develop a waddling gait with shortening of step length. Abnormalities of gait and balance predispose the elderly to falls. About half the falls in the aged result from environmental factors, including poor illumination, stairs, and uneven or slippery surfaces. Other causes of falls include drop attacks, orthostatic hypotension, turning movements of the head, and vertigo.

Lower motor neuron disorders Diseases of the lower motor neurons or peripheral nerves characteristically cause distal limb weakness. Foot drop is a common manifestation. In the case of lower motor neuron disease, the limb weakness occurs in association with fasciculations and muscle atrophy. The patient usually cannot dorsiflex the foot and compensates by raising the knees higher than usual, thereby walking with a "steppage gait." If proximal muscles are affected, the gait also can take on a waddling quality.

Hysterical gait disorders Hysterical disorders of gait commonly appear in association with hysterical paralysis of one or more limbs. Usually the gait is bizarre, easily recognized as hysterical, and unlike any disorder of gait evoked by organic disease. In other instances, however, hysterical gait disorders may resemble organic gait disorders and can be difficult to identify. Hysterical gait disorders can occur in men or women and can appear in youth, young adulthood, and middle age.

In hysterical hemiplegia, the patient drags the affected leg along the ground behind the body and does not circumduct the leg or use it effectively to support the body weight. At times the hemiplegic leg may be pushed ahead of the patient and used mainly for support. The arm on the affected side often remains limp, hanging uselessly beside the body and does not develop the flexed posture commonly seen in hemiplegia from organic causes. The patient with hysterical hemiplegia usually shows "give way" weakness. This is tested by asking the patient to make a maximum contraction of a set of muscles in an affected limb. Initially a strong contraction may occur, but as the examiner attempts to oppose the contracting muscles, the contraction suddenly gives way. Hysterical patients also commonly contract their muscles very slowly upon request, displaying great concentration and effort to evoke the contraction. Objective signs of neurologic disease are absent; the affected limbs show normal resistance to passive manipulation, the deep tendon reflexes are equal on the two sides of the body, and the plantar responses are downgoing.

In hysterical paraplegia, the patient usually walks with one or two crutches or lies in bed with the legs maintained either completely limp or stiffly extended. The term *astasia-abasia* refers to patients who cannot stand or walk but who can carry out natural movements of the limbs when lying in bed. Some patients with hysterical paraparesis walk with seeming difficulty but show normal power and coordination when lying in bed. On walking, the hysterical person clings to the bed or the furnishings of the room. If asked to walk without support the patient may lurch forward dramatically, veering from side to side at regular intervals. The patient can manage feats of extraordinary balance to avoid falling and may assume a variety of postures, walking with the legs in stiff extension, as if the legs are granite pillars, or walking with the legs in flexion and teetering from side to side. The hysterical patient may fall with walking, but only when a nearby physician or family member can catch the patient or when soft objects are available to cushion the fall. The gait disturbance is usually dramatic when an audience is present, and the patient can display remarkable agility in the rapid postural adjustments that occur.

REFERENCES

DIETZ V et al: Afferent control of human stance and gait: Evidence for blocking of group I afferents during gait. Exp Brain Res 61:153, 1985

GILMAN S: Cerebellar deficit, in *Diseases of the Nervous System,* AK Asbury et al (eds). Philadelphia, Saunders, 1986, pp 401–422

——— et al: *Disorders of the Cerebellum.* Philadelphia, Davis, 1981

GRILLNER S: Neurobiological bases of rhythmic motor acts in vertebrates. Science 228: 143, 1985

HORAK FB, NASHNER LM: Central programming of postural movements: Adaptation to altered support-surface configurations. J Neurophysiol 55:1369, 1986

KNUTSSON E, LYING-TUNELL U: Gait apraxia in normal-pressure hydrocephalus: Patterns of movement and muscle activation. Neurology 35:155, 1985

SMITH JC et al: Neural mechanisms generating locomotion studied in mammalian brainstem–spinal cord in vitro. FASEB J 2:2283, 1988

27 PAIN, SPASM, AND CRAMPS OF MUSCLE

ROBERT C. GRIGGS

Spontaneous or exercise-related discomfort from muscles or joints is usually benign and does not signal neuromuscular disease. Such symptoms may, however, provide clues to disabling disorders that too often evade diagnosis. The terms *pain*, *spasm*, and *cramp* are often used interchangeably by patients to describe symptoms referable to muscles. Other terms, including *aching*, *heaviness*, *stiffness*, and *rheumatism*, are also used, and usually connote less certainty about the source or localization of the discomfort. In clinical terminology, *spasm* refers to a brief, unsustained contraction of a single or multiple muscles. *Cramp* is a paroxysmal, spontaneous, prolonged, and painful contraction of one or more muscles.

SPASMS Abnormal movements of muscle may arise from abnormal electrical activity of the central nervous system mediated via the motor neuron, or occur within the muscle fiber itself. It may be difficult on clinical grounds alone to determine the precise site of origin of the abnormal motor activity. In general, movements originating in the central nervous system affect the entire side of the body, an entire limb, or a group of muscles. Central disorders may be rhythmic or intermittent; those arising in the periphery are usually random. The electroencephalogram may provide evidence for altered cortical activity in some conditions with a central nervous system etiology. The electromyogram (EMG) is less helpful because it reflects motor activity from any cause. EMG evidence of an underlying nerve disease may, however, be helpful in diagnosis (see Chap. 362), and certain abnormal muscle contractions have characteristic EMG features.

Intermittent, nonrhythmic movements of an entire limb, of the trunk, or of a portion of the face may result from cerebral seizure activity (Chap. 349) or from myoclonus (Chap. 25). Flexor and extensor spasms of an entire side or of the lower limbs result from a loss of motor inhibition within the central nervous system (Chap. 25). *Segmental myoclonus* results from focal disease within the brainstem or spinal cord that causes an abnormal discharge of groups of motor neurons. Localized vascular disease, tumor, or another lesion may be implicated.

Abnormal facial movements *Hemifacial spasm* results from paroxysmal facial nerve activity, sometimes triggered by pressure from a tortuous blood vessel adjacent to the facial nerve as it leaves the brainstem. Hemifacial spasm commonly occurs in muscles about the eye, but may also involve or spread to the entire side of the face. Symptoms are often intermittent and intensified when patients are using facial muscles in activities such as speaking. Hemifacial spasm is painless but embarrassing, especially to individuals dealing with the public. Since it is often intensified and more severe when the patient is in stressful situations, an erroneous diagnosis of tic (habit spasm) is often made. Cerebellopontine angle lesions can occasionally produce a similar disorder. Neuroradiologic investigation is indicated in patients with hemifacial spasm. Anticonvulsant medications occasionally alleviate the spasms, but surgical exploration and shielding of the facial nerve from the adjacent vessel is curative (Chap. 360).

Facial *tics* (habit spasms) are stereotyped movements of the face such as eye blinking, head turning, or grimacing that are under voluntary control but may be suppressed only by effort and anxiety on the part of the subject (see Chap. 25). Some tics are so frequently encountered as to be considered mannerisms, analogous to excessive clearing of the throat. The repetitious elevation of the eyebrows by frontalis muscle contraction is an example. Certain hereditary movement disorders such as Gilles de la Tourette syndrome are characterized by multiple tics (Chap. 25).

Synkinesias of the face result from aberrant regeneration of the facial nerve following facial paralysis from Bell's palsy or other facial nerve lesions. Nearly 50 percent of patients who recover from Bell's palsy display such movements; an example is *jaw winking*, where voluntary movements of the lower face elicit contraction of the orbicularis oculi muscle with eye closure (Chap. 360).

Trigeminal neuralgia (tic douloureux) is characterized by brief, paroxysmal, lancinating pain in one side of the face (see Chap. 360). Although the portion of the nerve involved is almost exclusively sensory, the severity of the pain causes involuntary contraction of facial muscles; hence the name tic. Abnormal movements do not occur in the absence of pain.

Facial myokymia refers to a nearly continuous, fine or coarse rippling and fascicular twitching of facial muscles. Although often benign, it may result from lesions of the pons such as a neoplasm or multiple sclerosis. Similar movements occur in motor neuron diseases such as amyotrophic lateral sclerosis or occasionally as an isolated, hereditary condition.

Abnormal limb movements No movement should be visible in totally relaxed muscles. Diseases of motor neurons or their proximal axons are often associated with *fasciculations*, the spontaneous firing of an entire motor unit. Fasciculations are visible on inspection of muscle or perceived by the patient as a pulsation or quivering within muscle. Fasciculations occur at times in most normal individuals, and unless weakness is present, are seldom of any significance. Fasciculations are normal if observed in incompletely relaxed muscles. *Myokymia*, consisting of numerous, repetitive fasciculations, may also occur in limb muscles, giving a writhing appearance. Myokymia disappears with neuromuscular blockade, proving that the activity originates in anterior horn cells or in peripheral nerve. In patients with long-standing muscle denervation and reinnervation, motor unit size enlarges and fasciculations may be so large as to produce movement of the limbs, particularly of the fingers, a condition termed *minipolymyoclonus*. Similarly, the enlarged motor units of chronic denervation may be associated with a tremor of the fingers on extension.

Certain conditions are characterized by a compulsion to move the extremities. *Akathisia*, or motor restlessness, occurs in Parkinson's disease and other disorders of the basal ganglia including drug-induced movement disorders. The *restless legs syndrome* describes an uncomfortable sensation in muscles, usually in the legs and thighs, which occurs most commonly in middle-aged women. Patients feel they need to move their legs to relieve the abnormal sensation. The restless leg syndrome is frequent in uremia and may occur in other neuropathies, suggesting that the sensation is caused by an underlying neuropathy. It may also be familial, and detailed study of such patients has failed to demonstrate any evidence of neuropathy. The restless sensation may be accompanied by myoclonic jerks of muscle often occurring during sleep. These myoclonic jerks are similar to the myoclonus observed in normal individuals entering REM sleep (see Chap. 34).

These forms of muscle spasm and myoclonus are somewhat similar to a group of unusual and unexplained *startle* syndromes or *hyperexplexias* characterized by sudden jerking of limbs or occasionally of trunk muscles. Sudden noise or touch may cause a patient to jump or to fling an extremity. The cause is unknown.

SUSTAINED MUSCLE CONTRACTIONS Distinguishing central from peripheral causes of sustained muscle contraction is often difficult. Abnormal muscle contractions with increased muscle tone usually result from central nervous system disease. Thus, loss or disturbance of central nervous system inhibition may lead to abnormal muscle contraction characteristic of spasticity, rigidity, or "paratonic" rigidity. In most instances there is other evidence of central nervous system disorder (Chap. 25). Diseases of the basal ganglia, presumably resulting from altered neurotransmitter release, may lead to dystonia (Chaps. 25 and 26).

Abnormal muscle contractions may also arise from repetitive depolarization of the component portions of the motor unit: the motor neuron; the peripheral axon of the neuron; the neuromuscular junction; or muscle fibers. Electrically inactive contractions may arise from disorders of the muscle contractile system.

Motor neuron disorders *Cramp* is a term often used by patients to refer to a painful, involuntary contraction of a single muscle or a muscle group. Muscle cramps can arise from spontaneous firing of groups of anterior horn cells followed by contraction of many motor units. EMG recordings indicate that motor units fire at a rate of up to 300 per second, much higher than occurs with voluntary contraction. Cramps occur frequently in the legs in elderly patients and when severe are followed by residual tenderness and evidence of muscle fiber necrosis including elevation of serum creatine kinase. Cramps in the calf muscles are so common as to be considered normal, but more generalized cramps may be a sign of chronic disease of the motor neuron such as amyotrophic lateral sclerosis. They may be particularly troublesome during pregnancy, in patients with electrolyte disturbances (hyponatremia), and in patients on hemodialysis. When recurrent and localized to one muscle group they suggest nerve root disease. In many instances, however, it is impossible to determine the cause of cramps. Benign cramps, occurring commonly at night, may be relieved by quinine sulfate. Other causes of contractions arising from the motor neuron include *tetanus* (Chap. 105) and the *stiff-man syndrome*. In both disorders a loss of inhibitory neuronal input to anterior horn cells may result in repeated firing of motor neurons, producing severe, painful muscle contraction. A similar clinical picture may occur acutely with *strychnine poisoning*. Diazepam improves these spasms but may cause respiratory depression in doses sufficient to alleviate muscle contraction.

Peripheral nerve *Tetany* is characterized by contractions of predominantly distal muscles, particularly in the hand (carpal spasm) and feet (pedal spasm). Laryngospasm may also occur. Tetany results from increased excitability of peripheral nerves. The muscle contractions are initially painless, but if sustained may cause muscle damage with pain. Severe tetany may involve spine musculature to produce opisthotonus. Tetany is usually caused by hypocalcemia, but may occur with hypomagnesemia or severe respiratory alkalosis (see Chap. 340). Idiopathic normocalcemic tetany, *spasmophilia*, occurs in both hereditary and sporadic forms.

Muscle MYOTONIA Repetitive depolarization of muscle cells can cause muscle contraction resulting in muscle stiffness and impaired relaxation. Myotonia is usually painless, but may disable patients by interfering with fine hand movements or by slowing ambulation. Myotonic dystrophy is the commonest disorder associated with myotonia although other manifestations of the disease such as cataracts and muscle weakness are usually more symptomatic (see Chap. 365). Myotonia congenita and paramyotonia congenita are less common, but more troublesome in terms of severity of myotonia. Myotonia is often worsened by cold and characteristically is attenuated by repeated muscle activity. *Paradoxical myotonia* worsens with repeated activity and is characteristic of paramyotonia congenita; these patients also suffer from episodic and cold-induced weakness (Chap. 367). Impaired muscle relaxation that is electrically inactive is characteristic of the delayed relaxation of myxedema. This delay produces the characteristic "hung-up" ankle reflexes but is essentially asymptomatic.

CONTRACTURE Muscle contracture is a painful shortening of a muscle unassociated with muscle membrane depolarization. It occurs in disorders where a metabolic defect such as myophosphorylase deficiency limits the production of high-energy phosphates. Contractures are precipitated by exercise and are usually intensely painful. This use of the term *contracture* is confusing since the same word is used to describe the unrelated limitation of joint movement by shortening of muscle tendons seen in rheumatologic disorders, cerebral palsy, or chronic myopathies. Muscle rigidity from metabolic contracture can occur in the malignant hyperthermia syndrome, usually associated with general anesthesia (Chap. 20). In the neuroleptic malignant syndrome, muscle rigidity arises from central nervous system overactivity, and intense electrical activity is present in muscle (Chap. 20).

MUSCLE PAIN, ACHING, AND TENDERNESS Painful muscles do not always imply muscle disease. Joint and bone disease frequently produce complaints of muscle pain and may further confuse the anatomic localization of symptoms by resulting in disuse atrophy and moderate muscle weakness. Pain from disease of overlying subcutaneous tissue or fascia and of tendons may also be referred to muscle. Additionally, disease of major peripheral nerves or of their small intramuscular branches may produce both muscle pain and weakness. Muscle pain may be a major symptom in inflammatory, metabolic, endocrine, and toxic myopathies (Chaps. 364 and 365).

Muscle trauma Vigorous activity, even in conditioned athletes, may be associated with muscle and tendon tears which lead to temporary acute muscle pain, swelling, and tenderness. Rupture of muscle tendons such as the biceps or gastrocnemius muscle may produce visible muscle shortening.

The almost-pleasurable ache and fatigue of muscles after strenuous activity is separable only by degree from more severe, but still normal pain following severe, unaccustomed activity. Such symptoms are often associated with laboratory evidence of profound muscle damage including a rise in serum enzymes (creatine kinase) and widespread muscle necrosis on biopsy. Myoglobinemia and myoglobinuria may occur. Particularly likely to produce muscle pain and necrosis are certain types of exercise: brief periods of contracting a muscle while it is lengthening (eccentric contractions); and prolonged exercise such as marathon running. The point at which such symptoms become abnormal is not clear. Many patients have pain with moderate activity. Such exertional muscle pain is also characteristic of metabolic disorders of muscle including carnitine palmityl transferase deficiency and myoadenylate deaminase deficiency; deficiencies of enzymes of glycolysis are more commonly associated with contractures (see Chap. 365). The majority of patients with exertional and postexertional muscle pain do not have a definable abnormality.

Diffuse myalgias Muscle pain in the absence of muscle weakness can occur in acute infections caused by influenza and Coxsackie viruses. Fibrositis, fibromyalgia, and fibromyositis are synonyms for a disorder associated with pain and tenderness of muscle and adjacent connective tissue. Focal "trigger points" of tenderness can be identified, and systemic symptoms such as fatigue, insomnia, and depression are frequently present (see Chap. 364). Although patients often identify painful swellings, histologic evaluation discloses no abnormality of muscle or connective tissue. Symptoms may respond partially to nonsteroidal anti-inflammatory agents, but the disorder tends to be chronic and unrelenting. Patients whose symptoms persist for months or years are often considered to have a psychiatric disorder, but its nature has not been defined.

Polymyalgia rheumatica occurs in patients over age 50 and is characterized by stiffness and pain in shoulder and hip musculature. Despite symptoms of pain localized to muscles, there is convincing evidence that the disease includes a proximal, inflammatory arthritis; joint effusions are often present in knees and other peripheral joints as well. Patients often develop profound disuse atrophy of muscles and complain of weakness, giving rise to a suspicion of polymyositis. However, creatine kinase levels are usually normal, and muscle biopsy shows atrophy without evidence of muscle necrosis or inflammation. The erythrocyte sedimentation rate is elevated in most patients, and temporal arteritis may be present (see Chap. 276). Treatment with nonsteroidal anti-inflammatory agents is advocated except in patients with temporal arteritis, for whom prednisone (40 to 60 mg daily) is recommended. Patients with polymyalgia rheumatica who fail to respond to nonsteroidal anti-inflammatory agents may require low-dose prednisone (10 to 20 mg daily). Myalgias are also frequent in other rheumatologic disorders including rheumatoid arthritis, systemic lupus erythematosus, polyarteritis nodosa, scleroderma, and the mixed connective tissue syndrome. When muscle pain occurs as an early symptom, it may erroneously suggest a primary muscle disease, and the myalgia may be due to inflammatory muscle involvement that can occur in each of these conditions (see Chap. 364). Patients with polymyositis and dermatomyositis may have myalgias, although in the majority, muscle pain is lacking or minimal (Chap. 364).

EPISODIC WEAKNESS The term *weakness* is often used by a patient to describe a loss of stamina or decreased "energy." Even careful efforts at eliciting a history of true as opposed to subjective weakness may fail to distinguish the two conditions. The most helpful strategy is to ask the patient to identify whether a discrete loss of function has occurred and to elicit the circumstances in which symptoms are noted.

Weakness whether true or perceived may be due to disorders of the central or peripheral nervous system. Weakness from central nervous system disorders such as transient cerebral ischemia is usually associated with a change in level of consciousness or cognition, with increased muscle tone and muscle stretch reflexes, and often with alterations of sensation. Most neuromuscular causes of intermittent weakness are associated with normal mental function but diminished muscle tone and muscle stretch reflexes. The major causes of intermittent weakness are listed in Table 27-1. Central causes are considered in Chap. 351.

EPISODIC ASTHENIA Patients who describe intermittent "weakness" as *fatigue* and loss of *stamina* suffer from asthenia, which can be separated from true weakness by the fact that patients do not lack the ability to do a task but rather the ability to perform it repetitively. Asthenia is a major problem in many patients with serious renal, hepatic, cardiac, or pulmonary disease. Examination of such patients usually confirms their ability to do all functional activities at least once, such as rising from a knee bend, climbing stairs, or rising from a chair. Fatigue is also characteristic of relatively selective damage to central nervous system descending motor tracts, in which signs of neurologic abnormality may be minimal.

Intermittent weakness due to peripheral neuromuscular disease may result from abrupt changes in peripheral nerve function; inter-

TABLE 27-1 Causes of episodic generalized weakness

Electrolyte disturbances
- Hypokalemia: Primary aldosteronism (Conn's syndrome); barium poisoning; renal tubular acidosis; juxtaglomerular apparatus hyperplasia (Bartter's syndrome); villous adenoma of colon; alcoholism; diuretics; licorice; para-aminosalicylic acid; glucocorticoids
- Hyperkalemia: Addison's disease; chronic renal failure; hyporeninemic hypoaldosteronism; recurrent rhabdomyolysis
- Hypercalcemia
- Hypocalcemic tetany
- Hyponatremia
- Hypophosphatemia
- Hypermagnesemia

Neuromuscular junction disorders
- Myasthenia gravis
- Lambert-Eaton syndrome

Central nervous system causes
- Cataplexy and sleep paralysis associated with narcolepsy
- Multiple sclerosis
- Transient ischemic attacks

Disorders with only subjective weakness: hyperventilation, hypoglycemia

mittent destruction of muscle; alterations of electrophysiologic properties of muscle from abnormalities of blood electrolytes; and intermittent failure of neuromuscular transmission.

FAILURE OF PERIPHERAL NERVE CONDUCTION A number of uncommon peripheral neuropathies are associated with recurrent weakness. *Hereditary liability to pressure palsies*, often termed *tomaculous* neuropathy because of the sausage-like appearance of myelin on nerve biopsy, is an autosomal dominant disorder characterized by abrupt paralysis following compression of a peripheral nerve. The paralysis is usually self-limited, lasting days to weeks. Other types of peripheral neuropathy may also predispose to the development of reversible, compressive neuropathies (see Chap. 363).

DISORDERED NEUROMUSCULAR JUNCTION TRANSMISSION *Myasthenia gravis*, particularly in its initial manifestations, is characterized by transient weakness. Cranial muscles are usually affected first, causing double vision, ptosis, dysphagia, and dysarthria. Rarely, limb weakness may herald the onset of myasthenia gravis and in the absence of cranial muscle dysfunction may escape diagnosis for months. Diurnal variation in strength is typical, and reflexes are preserved. Other, less-common defects of the neuromuscular junction such as the Lambert-Eaton syndrome may also present with intermittent weakness (see Chap. 366).

INTERMITTENT ALTERATIONS IN ELECTROLYTES Transient shifts in serum potassium are associated with profound alterations in muscle strength. Although the primary periodic paralyses (hypo- and hyperkalemic periodic paralysis) spring to mind in a patient with weakness and an abnormality in serum potassium, other causes of abnormal serum potassium are more frequently the cause of episodic weakness (see Chap. 367). Familial periodic paralysis seldom presents after age 30; other causes are usually present in older patients. Hypokalemic periodic paralysis may occur in patients with hyperthyroidism. Episodic weakness due to hypokalemia may occur with renal or gastrointestinal potassium loss; major causes include renal tubular acidosis, diuretic- or laxative-induced hypokalemia, primary aldosteronism, Bartter's syndrome, and villous adenoma of the colon.

Hyperkalemic weakness occurs in chronic renal or adrenal insufficiency, with hyporeninemic hypoaldosteronism, and on an iatrogenic basis from injudicious administration of oral potassium preparations alone or in combination with potassium-sparing diuretics such as triamterene, amiloride, and spironolactone. The use of potassium salts as a substitute for table salt may cause hyperkalemia in patients with impaired potassium excretion.

Other electrolyte disturbances may occasionally produce intermittent weakness as the initial clinical manifestation of a severe metabolic abnormality. These include elevation or depression of serum sodium, calcium, or magnesium as well as hypophosphatemia.

METABOLIC MUSCLE DISEASE (See Chap. 355) A number of uncommon defects in glycogen and lipid utilization are associated with impaired energy production by muscle and cause intermittent weakness, usually accompanied by muscle pain. Carnitine palmityl transferase deficiency is one such condition. Other metabolic defects of muscle such as mitochondrial disorders and the purine nucleotide cycle defect known as myoadenylate deaminase deficiency may also cause episodic weakness. This latter disorder occurs in approximately 1 percent of the population, but inexplicably causes symptoms in a small proportion of subjects deficient in the enzyme.

Recurrent attacks of a feeling of "weakness" often occur in patients with the *hyperventilation syndrome;* such patients are, however, of normal strength when tested. Similarly, *recurrent hypoglycemic episodes* are associated with subjective weakness though hypoglycemia is uncommon as the cause of this symptom. Central nervous system disorders may cause generalized weakness without an associated alteration of consciousness. *Drop attacks* resulting from impaired blood supply to the motor pathways of the brainstem cause sudden paraparesis or quadriparesis, usually lasting only a few seconds. Patients with narcolepsy may have sudden loss of muscle strength and tone during episodes of *cataplexy*. A disorder of the reticular activating system is responsible for these episodes as well as for *sleep paralysis* that occurs as narcoleptic patients are falling asleep or awakening (see Chap. 34).

REFERENCES

Barchi RL: The myotonic syndromes. Neurol Clin 6:473, 1988

Clark S et al: Clinical characteristics of fibrositis. II. A "blinded," controlled study using standard psychological tests. Arthritis Rheum 28:132, 1985

Jankovic J, Tolosa E (ed): Facial dyskinesias, in *Advances in Neurology*. New York, Raven Press, 1988, vol 49

Layzer RB: Muscle pain, cramps and fatigue, in AG Engel, BQ Banker (eds), *Myology*. New York, McGraw-Hill, 1986

Riggs JE: The periodic paralyses. Neurol Clin 6:485, 1988

28 NUMBNESS, TINGLING, AND SENSORY LOSS

ARTHUR K. ASBURY

Normal somatic sensation is a continuous process that commands considerable moment-to-moment nervous system activity. Little of the activity intrudes upon consciousness or exacts notice. In contrast, disordered sensation, particularly pains and paresthesias, may be highly intrusive, alarming, and tenacious and may dominate attention. Abnormalities of sensation tend to bring patients quickly to medical attention. When abnormal sensations are perceived as painful, medical advice is even more quickly sought. For a consideration of pain, see Chap. 15. The physician must have a framework of knowledge in order to assess abnormal sensations, estimate their likely site of origin, and recognize their implications.

POSITIVE AND NEGATIVE PHENOMENA It is useful to divide all abnormal sensory phenomena into two great categories, positive and negative. Positive phenomena include tingling, pins-and-needles, pricking, bandlike sensations, lightning-like shooting feelings (lancinations), aching, and knifelike, twisting, drawing, pulling, tightening, burning, searing, electrical, and raw sensations. These descriptors are frequently the actual words used by patients. Such sensations may or may not be experienced as painful. It is thought that the pathophysiologic basis of positive phenomena resides in the ectopic generation of volleys of impulses at some site of lowered neural threshold along the sensory pathways, either in peripheral or central sensory fibers. Such trains of ectopically generated afferent impulses arising from sites other than normal peripheral nerve receptors determine the quality of the abnormal sensation experienced, depending upon the number, rate, and distribution of impulses and the type and function of nerve fibers in which they arise.

Positive phenomena represent heightened activity in sensory pathways; therefore they are not necessarily associated with any demonstrable sensory deficit upon examination, an important point for the examiner to bear in mind.

Negative phenomena result from loss of sensory function and are characterized by numbness, or diminution or absence of feeling in a particular distribution. Negative phenomena, in contrast to positive phenomena, are accompanied by abnormal findings on sensory examination. In disorders affecting peripheral sensation, it is estimated that at least one-half of afferent fibers innervating a given site must be lost or functionless in order for sensory deficit to be demonstrated. This estimate probably varies according to how rapidly sensory fibers have lost function. If the rate of loss is slow and chronic, lack of cutaneous feeling may be unnoticed by the patient and difficult to demonstrate on examination, even though few sensory fibers are functioning. Rapidly evolving sensory abnormality usually evokes positive phenomena of some type and is more readily recognized by patients than insidious deafferentation. Subclinical degrees of sensory dysfunction not demonstrable on clinical sensory examination may be revealed by sensory nerve conduction studies or somatosensory cerebral evoked potentials (see Chaps. 349 and 362).

Terminology Two general types of medical terms are used to characterize abnormal sensation, those referring to symptoms of which patients complain (both positive and negative phenomena) and those describing abnormalities found on examination (only negative phenomena). *Paresthesia* and *dysesthesia* are terms used to denote positive phenomena. Paresthesia carries the implication that the abnormal sensation is perceived without an apparent stimulus; whereas dysesthesia is a more general term used to describe all types of positive sensations whether stimulus-generated or not. Abnormalities on examination are denoted by *hypesthesia* or *hypoesthesia* (reduction of cutaneous sensation to a specific type of testing such as pressure, light touch, and warm or cold stimuli), *anesthesia* (complete absence of skin sensation to the same stimuli plus pinprick), and *hypalgesia* (referring to loss of pain perception, i.e., nociception, such as the pricking quality elicited by a pin). *Hyperesthesia* connotes exaggerated perception of sensations in response to mild stimuli (light touch or stroking of the skin). Similarly *allodynia* describes the situation in which an ordinarily nonpainful stimulus, once perceived, is experienced as painful, even excruciating. An example is elicitation of a painful sensation by application of a vibrating tuning fork. *Hyperalgesia* denotes an exaggerated response to a noxious stimulus, and *hyperpathia,* a broad term, encompasses the phenomena implied by hyperesthesia, allodynia, and hyperalgesia.

Disorders of deep sensation, arising from muscle spindles, tendons, and joints, deserve special comment. Normally these afferents subserve proprioception (position sense) and the moment-to-moment sense of the state of muscle contraction. If a significant number of these special nerve endings become denervated, the resulting manifestations include imbalance, particularly with eyes closed or in the dark, clumsiness of precision movements, and unsteadiness of gait, all of which is referred to as *sensory ataxia* (see Chap. 26). Other findings on examination are reduced or absent joint position and vibratory sensibility and absent deep tendon reflexes in the affected limbs. Romberg's sign is positive, which means that the patient sways or topples when asked to stand with feet close together and eyes closed.

In severe states of deafferentation involving deep sensation, the patient cannot walk or stand unaided, or even sit unsupported. Continuous, sometimes wormlike involuntary movements, called *pseudoathetosis,* of the hands and arms occur, particularly with eyes closed. Such patients are severely disabled.

Normal sensation Cutaneous afferent innervation is subserved by a rich variety of receptors, both naked endings (nociceptors and thermoreceptors) and encapsulated terminals (mechanoreceptors). Each has its own set of sensitivities to specific stimuli (see Table 28-1), size and distinctness of receptive fields, and adaptational qualities. Much of the knowledge about these receptors has come from the development of techniques to study single intact nerve fibers intraneurally in alert unanesthetized human subjects. It is possible not only to record from single nerve fibers, large or small, but also to stimulate single fibers in isolation. A single impulse, whether elicited by a natural stimulus or evoked by electrical microstimulation, in a large myelinated afferent fiber may be both perceived and localized.

Afferent fibers in peripheral nerve trunks sort themselves into topographically coherent patterns as they approach the dorsal roots and enter the dorsal horn of the spinal cord. From there, the polysynaptic projections of the smaller fibers (unmyelinated and small myelinated), which in general subserve nociception and temperature sensibility, cross and ascend in the contralateral spinothalamic tract through spinal cord, through brainstem, to the ventral posterolateral nucleus (VPL) of the thalamus, and ultimately project to the postcentral gyrus of the parietal cortex (see Chap. 15). This is the spinothalamic pathway. The larger fibers which subserve tactile and position sense and kinesthesia project rostrally in the ipsilateral posterior column of the spinal cord and finally make their first synapse in the gracile or cuneate nuclei of the lower medulla (see Fig. 28-1). The second-order neuron decussates and ascends in the medial lemniscus located medially in the medulla and in the tegmentum of the pons and midbrain, and synapses in VPL. The third-order neuron projects to parietal cortex; this system is referred to as *lemniscal.*

Although the fiber types and functions which make up the spinothalamic and lemniscal systems are relatively well known, it has been found that many other fibers, particularly those associated with touch, pressure, and position sense, ascend in a diffusely

TABLE 28-1 Human cutaneous sensory receptors*

Receptor type	Location	Activating stimulus	Afferent nerve fiber	Sensation evoked	Central pathway
Meissner's corpuscle	S	Light pressure, once or repetitive	LM	Tapping, fluttering	Lemniscal
Merkel's disk	S	Sustained pressure	LM	Sense of pressure	Lemniscal
Pacinian corpuscle	D	Light touch, once or repetitive	LM	Sense of vibration	Lemniscal
Ruffini's ending	D	Sustained, angulated pressure	LM	None, thought to be proprioceptive	Lemniscal
Naked ending	S	Noxious	SM	Sharp pain	Spinothalamic
Naked ending	S	Noxious	UM	Dull pain, itch	Spinothalamic
Naked ending	S	Thermal, 34–50°C	UM	Warmth	Spinothalamic
Naked ending	S	Thermal, range uncertain	SM	Coldness	Spinothalamic

* LM = large myelinated fiber; SM = small myelinated fiber; UM = unmyelinated fiber; D = deep; S = superficial.
SOURCE: After Lindblom and Ochoa, 1986.

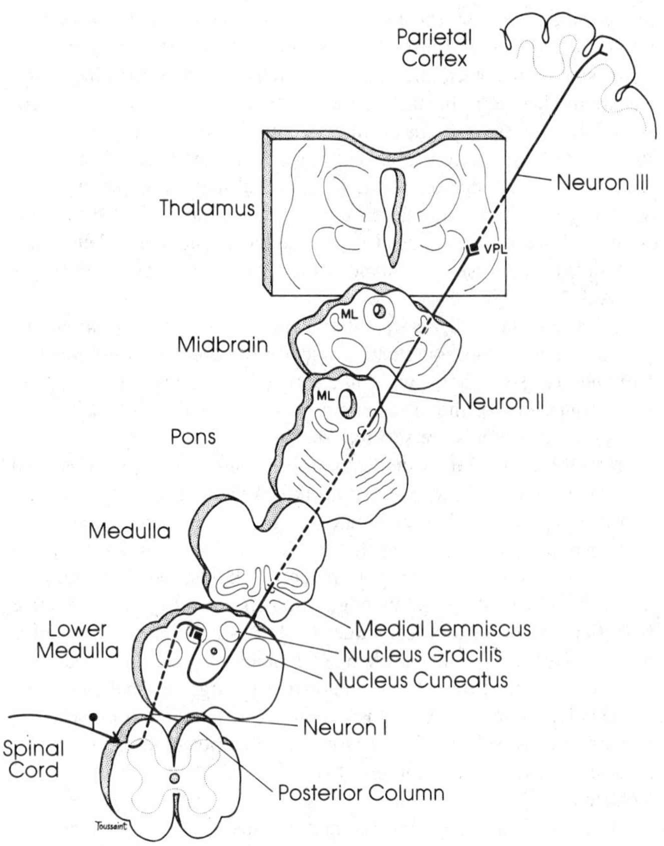

FIGURE 28-1 Schematic diagram of lemniscal system which subserves proprioception and discriminative touch.

distributed pattern both ipsilaterally and contralaterally in the anterolateral quadrants of the spinal cord. These anatomic facts explain why an individual with a known complete lesion of the posterior columns of the spinal cord may have little sensory deficit on examination.

EXAMINATION OF SENSATION The initial step in examination of the somatosensory system is to do the tests of primary sensation, which by convention include the sense of pain, touch, vibration, joint position, and thermal sensation, both hot and cold. These tests have gradually become codified through tradition, but they do appear to assess, if crudely, the major afferent functions and pathways (see Table 28-2). Testing of both primary sensation and cortical sensory function can be carried out in the office or at the bedside with a minimum of special equipment.

Some general principles pertain to the sensory examination. First, it should be remembered that the examiner is depending upon subjective patient response; therefore, discriminating responses depend upon the level of alertness, motivation, and intelligence of the patient and also upon the skill with which the examiner has made the task clear. In a stupefied or obtunded patient, the examiner is reduced to observing the briskness of withdrawal and the complexity of defensive movements of the patient in response to a pinch or other noxious stimulus. In the alert but uncooperative patient, it is often possible to get some idea of proprioceptive function by noting the patient's best performance in casually observed movements requiring balance and precision, but cutaneous sensation may be unexaminable.

Second, sensory examination should not be pressed if the patient is fatigued. An abbreviated survey will suffice until a more extensive examination can be carried out when the patient has rested. Third, sensory examination in a patient who has no neurologic complaints should be quite abbreviated and may consist of pin, touch, and vibration testing in the hands and feet plus evaluation of station and gait including Romberg's maneuver, which also tests the integrity of motor and cerebellar systems. Fourth, patients should be tested with their eyes closed or covered during both primary sensation and cortical sensory function examination.

Primary sensation (see Table 28-2) The sense of pain is usually tested with a pin, asking the patient to focus on the pricking or unpleasant quality of the stimulus and not just the pressure or touch sensation elicited. Areas of hypalgesia should be mapped by proceeding from the most hypalgesic zones to less affected ones (see Figs. 28-2 and 28-3).

Temperature sensation, both to hot and to cold, is probably best tested by touching the skin for a couple of seconds with a water flask filled with water of the desired temperature, using a thermometer to verify the temperature. For most purposes, it is satisfactory if a patient can identify as warm the flask that is 35 or 36°C and as cool the one that is 28 to 32°C. Between 28 and 32°C, most individuals can distinguish temperature differences in 1°C steps. Both cold and warm should be tested because different receptors respond to each.

Touch is usually tested with a wisp of cotton or a fine camel's hair brush. In general, it is better to avoid testing touch on hairy skin because of the profusion of sensory endings which surround each hair follicle. The patients, whose eyes are covered, should be asked to say "now" each time they feel the stimulus. They may also be asked to point to the site where the stimulus was felt, although this tests not only the sense of touch but also touch localization (see cortical sensory testing below).

Joint position testing is a measure of proprioception, one of the most important functions of the sensory system. Joint position is usually tested first in the great toe and in the fingers. Patients are asked to keep their eyes closed and to relax completely the part to be examined. In the case of the great toe, one starts with the toe in

TABLE 28-2 Testing primary sensation

Sense	Test device	Endings activated	Fiber size mediating	Central pathway*
Pain	Pinprick	Cutaneous nociceptors	Small	SpTh, also D
Temperature, heat	Flask with warm water	Cutaneous thermoreceptors for hot	Small	SpTh
Temperature, cold	Flask with cold water	Cutaneous thermoreceptors for cold	Small	SpTh
Touch	Cotton wisp, fine brush	Cutaneous mechanoreceptors, also naked endings	Large and small	Lem, also D and SpTh
Vibration	Tuning fork, 128 Hz	Mechanoreceptors, especially pacinian corpuscles	Large	Lem, also D
Joint position	Passive movement of specific joints	Joint capsule and tendon endings, muscle spindles	Large	Lem, also D

* D = diffuse ascending projections in ipsilateral and contralateral anteriolateral columns; SpTh = spinothalamic projection, contralateral; Lem = posterior column and lemniscal projection, ipsilateral.

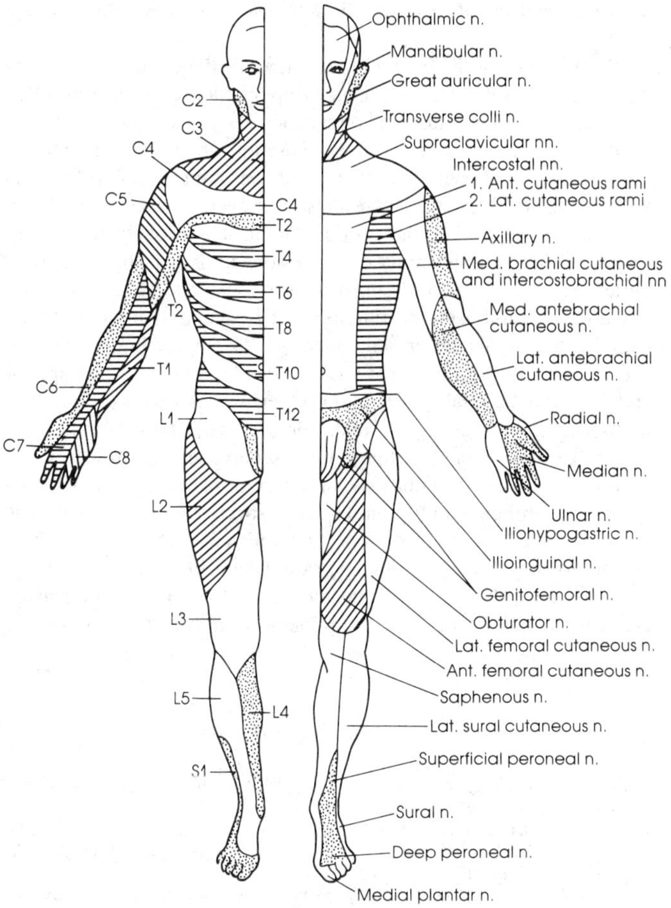

FIGURE 28-2 Anterior view of dermatomes (left) and cutaneous areas supplied by individual peripheral nerves (right). *(Modified from MB Carpenter and J Sutin, in Human Neuroanatomy, 8th ed, Baltimore, Williams & Wilkins, 1983.)*

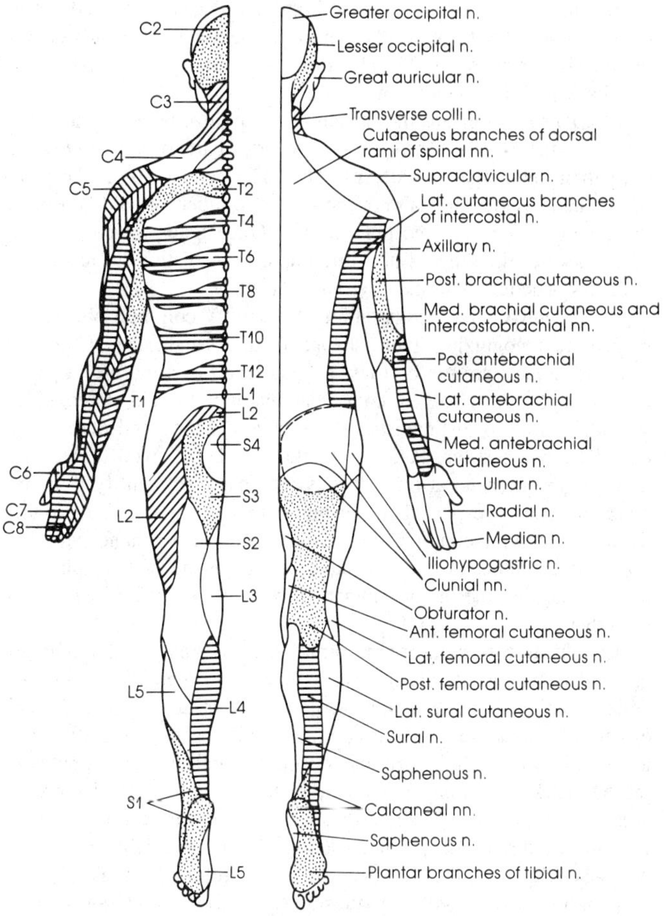

FIGURE 28-3 Posterior view of dermatomes (left) and cutaneous areas supplied by individual peripheral nerves (right). *(Modified from MB Carpenter and J Sutin, in Human Neuroanatomy, 8th ed, Baltimore, Williams & Wilkins, 1983.)*

a neutral position and grasps it lightly between the thumb and the forefinger on either side of the toe (not top and bottom) and then the toe is moved a few degrees either in a dorsal or a plantar direction, and the patient is asked to say whether the movement was up or down. One must make sure that the patient understands that it is the direction of movement which is being tested and not the direction the toe is pointing when it stops. A patient with absence of position sense in the part being tested will have a 50 percent error rate because only two choices are available. Answers which are consistently greater than 50 percent in error should be viewed with skepticism. If errors are made in recognizing the direction of passive movements of the toe, then passive movements of the ankle or even of the knee should be undertaken in the same way. Similarly, position sense at the proximal interphalangeal joint of the index finger may be tested, and if abnormal, other finger joints and the wrist and elbow joints should also be tested. A test of proximal joint position sense, primarily at the shoulder, can be carried out by asking the patient to bring the two index fingers together with the arms extended and the eyes closed. Normal individuals should be able to do this quite accurately with errors of a centimeter or less.

The sense of vibration is tested with a tuning fork, preferably a large one which vibrates at 128 Hz. The decay of vibration using this fork is slow enough to be of quantitative use because it requires between 15 and 20 s to decay below the threshold of perceptibility. Vibration is usually tested at bony prominences, specifically the malleoli at the ankles, the patella, the anterior iliac spine, the spinous processes of the vertebral bodies, the metacarpal-phalangeal joints (knuckles), the styloid process of the ulna, the elbow, and the acromion of the shoulder. Control sites at which to test vibration are the sternum and on the forehead. The examiner can compare the threshold at a given site for both patient and self. A crude approximation of degree of vibratory sense loss can be made by counting the seconds that the examiner can feel the sense of vibration longer than the patient. It must be clear to the patient that it is the sense of vibration and not just the pressure of the end of the tuning fork to which attention is directed.

Cortical sensation Cortical sensory testing includes two-point discrimination, touch localization, stereognosis, graphesthesia, and bilateral simultaneous stimulation, to name the most commonly used methods. Abnormalities of these sensory tests, in the presence of normal primary sensation and an alert cooperative patient, signify a lesion of the parietal cortex or thalamocortical projections to the parietal lobe. If primary sensation is altered, it is not possible to test for these cortical discriminative functions.

Two-point discrimination is tested by special calipers whose points may be set from 2 mm to several centimeters apart and then applied simultaneously to the site to be tested. The pulp of the fingertips is a common site to test; a normal individual can distinguish about 3-mm separation of points there. One can distinguish more closely set points on the tongue and lips, but the threshold for discriminating two points may be centimeters at other sites on the body. Comparisons should always be made between analogous sites on the two sides of the body, since the deficit, with a specific parietal lesion, is likely to be hemilateral. This point holds true for all cortical sensory testing.

Touch localization is usually carried out by light pressure with the examiner's fingertip, asking the patient, whose eyes are closed, to identify the site of touch. It is usual to ask the patient to touch the same site with a fingertip. Bilateral simultaneous stimulation at analogous sites (e.g., the dorsa of both hands) can be carried out to determine whether the perception of touch is extinguished consistently on one side or the other. The phenomenon is referred to as extinction on bilateral simultaneous stimulation.

Graphesthesia means the capacity to recognize letters or numbers drawn by the examiner's fingertip on various parts of the body while the patient maintains closed eyes. The usual comparison is the palm of one hand versus the palm of the other. Numbers should be drawn large enough to occupy most of the palm. Once again, the comparison of one side to the other is of prime importance. Failure to recognize numbers or letters is termed *agraphesthesia*.

Stereognosis refers to the ability to identify common objects by palpation, recognizing their shape, texture, and size. Common standard objects are the best test objects, such as a marble, a paper clip, a small rubber ball, or coins. Patients with normal stereognosis should be able to distinguish a dime from a penny and certainly a nickel from a quarter. Patients should only be allowed to feel the object with one hand at time. If they are unable to identify it in one hand, it should be placed in the other for comparison. Individuals unable to identify common objects and coins in one hand who can do so in the other are said to have *astereognosis* of the abnormal hand. Note that the major comparison is one side of the body with the other.

Localization of sensory abnormalities Peripheral neuropathies are generally graded, distal, and symmetric in their distribution of deficit. Although most peripheral neuropathies are pansensory and affect all modalities of sensation, selective sensory dysfunction according to nerve fiber size may occur. In small fiber neuropathies, the hallmark is burning, painful dysesthesias with reduced pinprick and thermal sensation but with sparing of proprioception, motor function, and even deep tendon jerks. Touch is variably involved, but when spared, the sensory pattern is referred to as sensory dissociation (see below). In contrast to small fiber neuropathies, large fiber neuropathies are characterized by position sense deficit, imbalance, absent tendon jerks, variable motor dysfunction, but preservation of most cutaneous sensation and few or no dysesthesias.

Paresthesias and dysesthesias may be of either peripheral nerve or spinal cord origin, and probably can arise in the brainstem, but in every instance are thought to represent abnormal showers of impulses generated from an ectopic focus or foci. By themselves, paresthesias may not be localizable, but when accompanied by other signs of neuropathy or of myelopathy, the correct site of origin may be deduced.

Dissociated sensory deficit patterns, in which pinprick and thermal sensation are lost but touch is spared, are usually a sign of spinothalamic tract involvement in the spinal cord, especially if the deficit is unilateral and has an upper level on the torso. Bilateral spinothalamic tract involvement occurs with lesions affecting the center of the spinal cord, such as happens with expansion of the central canal in hydromyelia or syringomyelia. Sensory dissociation may also occur in peripheral neuropathies in which afferent cutaneous nerve fibers of small diameter are preferentially affected. Neuropathies in which sensory dissociation may occur include leprous neuritis, hereditary sensory neuropathy, and certain cases of amyloid and diabetic polyneuropathy (see Chap. 363).

Hemisensory disturbance with tingling numbness from head to foot is usually thalamic in origin. If abrupt in onset, the thalamic lesion is likely to be due to a small stroke (lacunar infarction). Occasionally, with lesions affecting the posterolateral thalamus (VPL) or adjacent white matter, a syndrome of thalamic pain, also called Déjerine-Roussy syndrome, may ensue. This is a persistent unrelenting hemipainful state often described in dramatic terms such as "like the flesh is being torn from my limbs" or "as though that side is bathed in acid" (see Chap. 15). Harlequin patterns of sensory disturbance, in which one side of the face and the opposite side of the body are affected, localize to the lateral medulla where a small lesion may damage both the ipsilateral descending trigeminal tract and ascending spinothalamic fibers (lateral lemniscus) subserving the opposite arm, leg, and hemitorso (see "Lateral Medulla Syndrome," Chap. 351).

With lesions of the parietal lobe, either of the cortex or subjacent white matter, the most prominent symptoms are contralateral hemineglect, hemi-inattention, and a tendency not to use the contralateral hand and arm. Tests of primary sensation are usually normal or minimally altered, but tests of cortical sensation are often severely abnormal (see Chap. 32). Dysesthesias or even a sense of numbness are unusual except in the special circumstance of focal sensory seizures. These are generally due to lesions in or near the postcentral gyrus. Symptoms of focal somatosensory seizures are usually combinations of numbness and tingling, but frequently additional, more complex sensations are present, such as a rushing feeling, a sense of warmth, a sense of movement without visible motion, or an unpleasantly dysesthetic quality. Duration of seizures is variable; they may be transient, lasting only seconds, or may persist for hours. Focal motor features (clonic jerking) may supervene, and seizures can become generalized with loss of consciousness. Likely sites of symptoms are unilaterally in the lips, face, digits, or foot, and symptoms may spread as in a Jacksonian march. On occasion, symptoms may occur in a symmetric bilateral fashion, for instance, in both hands; this results from involvement of the second sensory area (unilaterally) located in the rolandic area at and just above the Sylvian fissure.

REFERENCES

Culp W, Ochoa JL (eds): *Abnormal Nerves and Muscles as Impulse Generators*. Oxford University, New York, 1982

Dyck PJ et al: Detection thresholds of cutaneous sensation in humans, in PJ Dyck, PK Thomas, EH Lambert, RP Bunge (eds), *Peripheral Neuropathy*, 2d ed. Philadelphia, Saunders, 1984, pp 1103–1138

Lindblom U, Ochoa JL: Somatosensory function and dysfunction, in AK Asbury, GM McKhann, WI McDonald (eds), *Diseases of the Nervous System*. Philadelphia, Saunders, 1986, pp 283–298

Mackel R: Single unit analysis of regenerated cutaneous afferents in man. Ann Neurol 18:165, 1985

Vallbo AB et al: Somatosensory, proprioceptive, and sympathetic activity in human peripheral nerve. Physiol Rev 59:919, 1979

29 BEHAVIORAL AND EMOTIONAL DISTURBANCES

EDWIN H. CASSEM

Patients often seek medical attention with complaints that are difficult to ascribe to a specific clinical disorder: fatigue, tension, nervousness, listlessness, anxiety, depression. Other patients have somatic complaints—dizziness, shortness of breath, unsteadiness, or persistent pain (headache, backache, cramps)—but the intensity of the complaint is out of proportion to the physical findings, if any. The clinical challenge in such patients is to discern the contributions of emotional or psychiatric problems to the physical complaints. Some patients disclose their psychiatric disorder immediately by their complaint, as when one complains that his thoughts are being broadcast through the local television station, or another that she has lost all interest in living since shortly after the birth of her last child. Even when the patient has no complaint, clues to psychiatric disorders may be obvious, such as profuse sweating, virtual absence of eye contact, use of a handkerchief to open the door, or repeated demands for analgesic prescriptions.

When are mental and emotional disturbances "abnormal"? No person escapes stress of some sort in daily life. Anxiety or despondency may be a normal response to a threat, disappointment, or loss. When symptoms are vague and unexplained by the physical examination or laboratory assessment, and when the patient denies any psychological cause, discovery of a diagnosis that explains them may be difficult. Many of these complaints are caused by common and treatable psychiatric disorders like the anxiety and affective disorders. Another common difficulty arises when the patient has an obvious disorder, such as Parkinson's disease, appropriate treatment is prescribed that leads to significant improvement in the core symptoms of rigidity and bradykinesia, yet the patient continues to complain of exhaustion, insomnia, and inability to concentrate. In this case the patient may suffer from both Parkinson's disease and major depression and requires treatment for both conditions.

This chapter formulates an approach to the diagnosis of mental, emotional, and behavioral complaints and abnormalities. The classification of such symptoms, as defined in the *Diagnostic and Statistical Manual of Mental Disorders* (DSM III-R), is organized to ascertain whether the patient's complaints and findings meet diagnostic criteria for psychiatric disorders.

PSYCHIATRIC METHOD OF CLINICAL EVALUATION Occasionally the psychiatrist is able to approach a chief complaint with a beginning question almost the same as that asked by the neurologist, i.e., where is the lesion? That is, one can ask if the primary difficulty is in the realm of thought, of mood and feeling, or of behavior. Although not anatomic, these three areas cover the major psychiatric disorders. The delusion of the patient who complained that his thoughts were being broadcast on television, for example, is readily identifiable as a disturbance of thought, and a history and examination might swiftly confirm that his most likely diagnosis was schizophrenia. Likewise the postpartum mother might meet all the diagnostic criteria for major depression.

At present one cannot confirm either diagnosis by a laboratory test that is more reliable than the clinical diagnosis itself. In a sense, then, the psychiatrist makes a diagnosis similar to an internist's diagnostic evaluation of a systemic illness. The postpartum mother must meet five or more of the nine DSM III-R diagnostic criteria for major depression, just as a patient with bilateral, symmetric, inflammatory polyarthritis must meet seven of eleven criteria for a definite diagnosis of rheumatoid arthritis. Of the eleven criteria for rheumatoid arthritis, two are historical, four demonstrable on physical examination, and five provided by laboratory examination. Even though major mood disorders have characteristic biologic manifestations, these have yet to generate laboratory tests sufficiently useful for routine diagnostic use (see Chap. 368). Psychiatric diagnosis, therefore, remains largely a clinical effort.

Furthermore, in psychiatric diagnosis shortcuts are seldom available. A medical patient's history of cough and fever may justify a chest x-ray that confirms a diagnosis of pneumonia. Sputum can be cultured promptly, antibiotics prescribed and, on the basis of culture results, changed to more specific agents at a later time. For psychiatric disorders no x-rays or cultures can be ordered that will make the history unnecessary or indicate the psychotropic drug specific to the disorder. Hence the history and the clinical examination for a psychiatric disorder must have each step specifically addressed if the physician wishes to avoid a misdiagnosis. The steps of the psychiatric examination are outlined below.

THE PSYCHIATRIC HISTORY The salient components of the psychiatric history are summarized in Table 29-1.

PSYCHIATRIC EXAMINATION After the history has been completed, a systematic mental status examination should assess: (1) appearance and behavior; (2) flow, rate, quantity, and content of speech; (3) mood; (4) thought and perception (hallucinations, delusions, obsessions, derealization, and depersonalization); (5) orientation; (6) attention; (7) memory; and (8) judgment and insight. This examination is summarized conveniently in the Mini-Mental Status Examination (see Table 29-2). This simple examination provides a numerical score that gives both an estimate of the severity of impairment and a reference point for later comparison, as when a delirious patient begins to recover. Further elaboration on the details of the psychiatric history and examination can be found in Chap. 368.

TABLE 29-1 The psychiatric history

Chief complaint
Source of and reason for referral: why now?
History of present illness
Past psychiatric history
Family psychiatric history
Personal history: delivery, developmental milestones, school and occupational history, peer relations, psychosexual/menstrual history, service/war history, religious history, marital history
Past medical history: febrile seizures, head trauma, prolonged illness, surgery, accidents, disabilities (vision, hearing), sexually transmitted diseases
Habits: drugs, alcohol, tobacco
Current medications

FORMULATION OF THE DIAGNOSIS Proceeding in a manner similar to that for nonpsychiatric symptoms, the physician considers the medical history, the examination, and the laboratory findings and then formulates a differential diagnosis. The differential diagnosis for psychiatric symptoms has two components: (1) exclusion of organic disease and (2) the psychiatric diagnosis.

Exclusion of organic disease The physician begins the differential diagnosis by considering those medical illnesses that might give rise to the symptoms and signs elicited during examination. Dramatically disordered cognition, emotion, and behavior can occur in hypoglycemia, hypertensive encephalopathy, Wernicke's encephalopathy, hypoxemia from pulmonary failure, hepatic encephalopathy, subarachnoid hemorrhage, or drug overdose (see Chap. 30). A hypoglycemic diabetic may be mistaken initially for an inebriated alcoholic because of clouded consciousness, slurred speech, and agitated behavior.

Symptoms of depression, fatigue, insomnia, and poor concentration can be caused by drugs and medical diseases. Alcohol, antihypertensive medications (reserpine, alphamethyldopa, and beta-adrenergic blocking agents), and glucocorticoids are frequently implicated in causing depression. Cimetidine, although more often a cause of confusion, can also produce depression. Cocaine, barbiturates, and amphetamine abuse are often associated with a depressive syndrome. Hypothyroidism, hyperparathyroidism, Cushing's disease, and subcortical dementias like Huntington's and Parkinson's diseases are often heralded by depression. Anemia, hypo- and hyperglycemia, hyponatremia, hypercalcemia, hypokalemia, encephalitis, and an occult malignancy may produce symptoms of weakness and fatigue that are mistakenly ascribed to depression.

Symptoms of anxiety are defined by somatic symptoms: "butterflies" or a "knot" in the stomach, sweating, tremulousness, palpitations, flushing, breathlessness, numbness, muscular tension, dry mouth, urinary frequency. Caffeine can induce acute and chronic anxiety. Withdrawal from alcohol, barbiturates, meprobamate, and benzodiazepines can produce dramatic anxiety, occasionally progressing to a life-threatening medical emergency. Symptoms similar to anxiety can occur in hyperthyroidism, paroxysmal atrial tachycardia, mitral valve prolapse, pheochromocytoma, insulinoma, myocardial infarction, or hypoglycemia. Excess thyroid medication, sympathomimetic amines, and bronchodilators such as theophylline can produce tachycardia and anxiety. Pulmonary conditions such as asthma, obstructive pulmonary disease, and pulmonary embolism can cause breathlessness and make the patient anxious. Pulmonary edema and congestive heart failure do the same. These conditions are not often mistaken for an emotional disorder unless they are subtle—as occult, intermittent showers of pulmonary emboli may be.

Fear is a common emotion that may be produced by a complex partial seizure. Carcinoid tumor, the commonest endocrine neoplasm of the digestive tract, is of special interest because its clinical episodes of flushing and tachycardia may be triggered by intense emotion. In such a case a patient may relate that anger caused the feeling of being "on fire." Patients who receive neuroleptic medications occasionally develop akathisia, a side effect characterized by extreme restlessness, inability to remain seated (which gives the condition its name), and

TABLE 29-2 Mini-mental status examination

EXAMINATION

Patient ____________
Examiner ____________
Date ____________

Maximum score	Score	Orientation
5	( )	What is the (year)(season)(date)(day)(month)?
5	( )	Where are we? (state)(county)(town)(hospital)(floor)
		Registration
3	( )	Name 3 objects: 1 s to say each. Then ask the patient all 3 after you have said them. Give 1 point for each correct answer. Then repeat them until he learns all 3. Count trials, and record: Trials ____________
		Attention and calculation
5	( )	Serial 7s. 1 point for each correct. Stop after 5 answers. Alternative: Spell "world" backwards.
		Recall
3	( )	Ask for the 3 objects repeated above. Give 1 point for each correct.
		Language
9	( )	Name a pencil and wristwatch (2 points) Repeat the following: "No ifs, ands, or buts." (1 point) Follow a 3-stage command: "Take a paper in your right hand, fold it in half, and put it on the floor." (3 points) Read and obey the following: Close your eyes (1 point)
		Write a sentence (1 point)
		Copy design (1 point)
		Total score ________
		Assess level of consciousness along a continuum ____________ Alert Drowsy Stupor Coma

INSTRUCTIONS FOR ADMINISTRATION

Orientation
Ask for the date. Then ask specifically for parts omitted, e.g., "Can you also tell me what season it is?" One point for each correct.
Ask in turn "Can you tell me the name of this hospital?" (town, country, etc.). One point for each correct.

Registration
Ask the patient if you may test his memory. Then say the names of 3 unrelated objects, clearly and slowly, about 1 s for each. After you have said all 3, ask him to repeat them. This first repetition determines his score (0–3), but keep saying them until he can repeat all 3, up to 6 trials. If he does not eventually learn all 3, recall cannot be meaningfully tested.

Attention and calculation
Ask the patient to begin with 100 and count backwards by 7. Stop after 5 subtractions (93, 86, 79, 72, 65). Score the total number of correct answers. If the patient cannot or will not perform this task, ask him to spell the word "world" backwards. The score is the number of letters in correct order: e.g., dlrow = 5, dlorw = 3.

Recall
Ask the patient if he can recall the 3 words you previously asked him to remember. Score 0–3.

Language
Naming: Show the patient a wristwatch and ask him what it is. Repeat for pencil. Score 0–2.
Repetition: Ask the patient to repeat the sentence after you. Allow only one trial. Score 0–1.
3-Stage command: Give the patient a piece of plain blank paper and repeat the command. Score 1 point for each part correctly executed.
Reading: On a blank piece of paper print the sentence "Close your eyes," in letters large enough for the patient to see clearly. Ask him to read it and do what it says. Score 1 point only if he actually closes his eyes.
Writing: Give the patient a blank piece of paper and ask him to write a sentence for you. Do not dictate a sentence, it is to be written spontaneously. It must contain a subject and verb and be sensible. Correct grammar and punctuation are not necessary.
Copying: On a clean piece of paper, draw intersecting pentagons, each side about 1 in, and ask him to copy it exactly as it is. All 10 angles must be present and 2 must intersect to score 1 point. Tremor and rotation are ignored.

Estimate the patient's level of sensorium along a continuum, from alert on the left to coma on the right.

SOURCE: Reproduced with permission from Folstein et al.

a state difficult to distinguish from anxious agitation. Failure to recognize this side effect may cause the physician to increase the dose of the neuroleptic, which only worsens the akathisia. Paradoxically, even though depression and anxiety are classified as two separate categories of psychiatric disorder, anxiety is one of the most common and most severe features of major depression. Treatment of the depression often alleviates the anxiety.

Delusions and hallucinations are the hallmark of a psychosis (see Chap. 368). Somatic delusions (that one's body is giving off a foul odor, for example), grandiose and paranoid delusions, and hallucinations (auditory, visual, olfactory, tactile), while characteristic of the major psychoses, can also occur in patients with confusional states due to medical illness or drug effects. Amphetamine and cocaine abuse may produce paranoid states. Levodopa, administered to patients with Parkinson's disease, may produce paranoid, manic, or confusional states. Lysergic acid (LSD), mescaline, phencyclidine (PCP), and other psychotomimetic agents may produce isolated hallucinations or delusions or both; PCP is particularly associated with severe confusional states marked by agitation and violence (see Chap. 372). Characteristic organic delusions are described with neurologic disorders, such as denial of blindness after bilateral occipital lobe lesions (Anton's syndrome) or the denial of hemiparesis after a parietal lobe injury. This latter lesion may be associated with the delusion that the involved side of the body has multiple limbs. Ideas of reference, e.g., a sudden intense belief that the television news commentator is referring to oneself, may be the result of a complex partial seizure. Degenerative brain disease (such as Alzheimer's disease) or toxic/metabolic disorders may be associated with psychotic manifestations, and it may be the psychotic manifestation that first leads to a consultation with the physician (see Chap. 30).

Hallucinations are often associated with organic conditions. Visual hallucinations should be considered as due to an organic etiology until proven otherwise. Alcoholic hallucinosis, as distinguished from delirium tremens, is unique in usually being *auditory*, with a paranoid theme (accusatory voices). The sensorium is clear, there is often no tremor, and it occurs during drinking, not withdrawal (see Chap. 370). It usually occurs after many years of drinking. Formed visual hallucinations have also been reported with alcohol withdrawal, digoxin and pentazocine, in viral encephalitis and Creutzfeldt-Jakob disease, and with sensory deprivation. Macropsia, micropsia (the illusion of objects expanding or shrinking in size), formed visual hallucinations, olfactory hallucinations, déjà vu or jamais vu, and amnesic episodes are symptoms common to focal epilepsy of the temporal lobe or subcortical limbic structures (see Chap. 350). Confusional states are discussed in Chap. 30.

Patients who appear "hyper"—expansive, elated, hypertalkative, egotistical, distractable, and boundlessly energetic with a decreased need for sleep—may be manifesting a lifelong personality style or be either manic or hypomanic; or they may be medically ill. If ill, the cause is either drug ingestion or brain disease. The drugs most commonly associated with manic-like symptoms are glucocorticoids and adrenocorticotropic hormone (ACTH); stimulants like cocaine, amphetamines, sympathomimetics; and excessive thyroid medication, antidepressants, and antiparkinsonian agents.

Rarely brain tumor, ACTH-producing tumors, viral encephalitis (including human immunodeficiency virus infection), temporal lobe seizures, neurosyphilis, multiple sclerosis, Huntington's disease, uremia, hyperthyroidism, vitamin B_{12} deficiency, carcinoid syndrome, and dialysis dementia syndrome can cause mania. Whenever manic symptoms appear in a patient over 50 years of age who has no prior history of either mania or depression, the abnormal state is almost always *secondary* to one of the conditions listed above and not a *primary* psychiatric disorder.

Psychiatric differential diagnosis The internist cannot be expected to become an expert in psychiatric disorders. Some disorders, however, are so common that generalists not only see them frequently but see more of them than do psychiatrists. This is most often the case, for example, with major depression. Estimates suggest that up to 60 percent of depressed patients are seen by general physicians and internists and 20 percent by psychiatrists or other mental health professionals, while 20 percent consult no professional for help with their disorder. The generalist who includes depression in the differential diagnosis is in an excellent position to recognize this disorder when it appears and to treat it appropriately.

The term *neurotic*, or *psychoneurotic*, while descriptive of certain conflicts that patients carried with them from early life, is no longer a psychiatric diagnosis. Certain other terms, like *neurasthenia, psychasthenia, neurocirculatory asthenia,* and *soldier's heart* have also been eliminated from lists of psychiatric diagnoses because more precise diagnostic categories have replaced them (see DSM III-R for current usage).

Like all physicians, the psychiatrist's basic activities are diagnosis and treatment. Intuition develops with clinical experience, but even the most gifted clinician must continue to cover the basic components of the psychiatric history and examination.

REFERENCES

American Psychiatric Association: *Diagnostic and Statistical Manual of Mental Disorders* (DSM III-R). Washington, DC, 1987

Folstein MF et al: "Mini-mental state," a practical method for grading the cognitive state of patients for the clinician. J Psychiatr Res 12:189, 1975

Hackett TP, Cassem NH (eds): *Massachusetts General Hospital Handbook of General Hospital Psychiatry*, 2d ed. Littleton, MA, PSG Publishing, 1987

Kaplan HI, Sadock BJ (eds): *Comprehensive Textbook of Psychiatry/V*. Baltimore, Williams & Wilkins, 1989

Nicholi AM Jr (ed): *The New Harvard Guide to Psychiatry*. Cambridge, MA, Harvard, 1988

30 ACUTE CONFUSIONAL STATES, AMNESIA, AND DEMENTIA

MARTIN M. BROWN / VLADIMIR C. HACHINSKI

The brain functions with marvelous complexity when it reasons, formulates language, or calculates. Because of this complexity and the vulnerability of neuronal function to biochemical and physiologic alterations, cognitive function is easily disturbed. The resulting syndromes are common and may result from a wide variety of conditions. Many systemic illnesses and brain diseases come to notice because of disruption of cognitive function, often without other neurologic symptoms or signs. It is important to recognize the pattern of the resulting organic neurobehavioral syndromes to avoid mistaken psychiatric diagnoses and begin appropriate management early. The examination of cognitive function is an important bedside clinical skill for the student and physician to acquire and practice so that minor degrees of confusion are not overlooked and more confused patients can be approached with confidence. Careful testing of individual components of cognitive function allows identification of specific areas of abnormality and is an essential prerequisite to establishing the diagnosis of a neurobehavioral syndrome.

SYNDROME DEFINITION

This chapter discusses the examination of cognitive function in three related syndromes—confusion, amnesia, and dementia—in which an intellectual disorder is the major presenting feature.

CONFUSION Any disorder of cognitive function may cause confusion, which can be defined as a lack of clarity and coherence of thought, perception, understanding, or action. Confusion is often the first feature of cognitive impairment noticed by relatives or the examiner. The confusion in acute confusional states and dementia reflects global or multifocal impairment of cognition and in amnesia reflects impairment of memory. Confusion may also appear to be the presenting complaint in isolated focal disorders of cognitive function such as aphasia or visuospatial agnosia (see Chap. 32), but careful examination will show that the confusion is related to a single deficit.

ACUTE CONFUSIONAL STATE The acute confusional state is a common neurobehavioral syndrome in which acute and global impairment of cognitive function is accompanied by impairment of attention and consciousness. The impairments of cognition usually include disorientation, abnormal perception, disordered reasoning, and poor memory. A wide variety of causes may be responsible.

DELIRIUM Some authors (e.g., Lipowski) use the term *delirium* as synonymous with the acute confusional state, but delirium is best reserved to describe a clinically distinct variety of acute confusional

TABLE 30-1 Clinical features of the acute confusional state and dementia compared

	Acute confusional state	Dementia
Onset	Acute	Usually insidious
Duration	Transient (hours to weeks)	Persistent (months to years)
Course	Fluctuating over hours; diurnal variation common	Stable over days
Sleep-wake cycle	Disrupted	Normal
Conscious level	Depressed	Normal
Attention	Impaired	Normal
Orientation	Impaired	Impaired
Language	Incoherent	Aphasia common
Memory		
Digit span	Shortened	Normal
Long-term memory	Impaired	Impaired
Perception	Impaired (illusions, delusions, hallucinations)	Normal early, agnosia later
Mood	Agitation or fear common	Apathy or disinhibition common
Autonomic changes	Common	Unusual
Psychomotor changes (depressed motor activity or restlessness)	Common	Uncommon
Involuntary movements	Common	Uncommon
EEG	Diffuse slow-wave activity	Mild slowing

state characterized by periods of agitation, heightened mental activity, increased wakefulness, marked readiness to respond to certain stimuli (such as sudden noises), intrusive visual hallucinations, motor hyperactivity, and autonomic stimulation. The features essential to the acute confusional state of impairment of consciousness and attention are present despite the apparent arousal (see "Consciousness," below). The agitation of delirium characteristically fluctuates and may alternate with or progress to a subdued confusional state. The clinical picture is exemplified by the excited hallucinatory state of *delirium tremens* which follows alcohol withdrawal. However, delirium may be seen in acute confusional states from any cause.

DEMENTIA This is also a common syndrome of acquired global or multifocal impairment of cognitive function, involving decline in intellect, memory, and personality in the presence of normal consciousness. Normal alertness and attention distinguish dementia from the acute confusional state, although there are other differences (see Table 30-1). The decline in intellect usually involves all intellectual functions, but in early or limited disease, the diagnosis may be established by impairment of any three of the following spheres: language, memory, visuospatial skills, emotion, personality, or cognition. Loss of a single intellectual function such as speech or memory, however devastating, is not sufficient. Dementia is not necessarily progressive, and in some instances can be reversed or halted by appropriate treatment. It is therefore important to recognize dementia as a syndrome with many causes.

AMNESIA This term describes an isolated disorder of memory characterized by inability to remember past events and to learn new information despite normal consciousness and attention. Like the other syndromes discussed in this chapter, amnesia has a variety of possible causes.

OBSERVABLE COMPONENTS OF COGNITION

Despite the complexity of mental activity, certain aspects can be assessed reliably at the bedside as part of the neurologic examination. A sequence of cognitive functions proceeding from the initial sensory input (the examiner's question) to motor or verbal output (the patient's response) can be distinguished, as well as a number of influences on the sequence (see Fig. 30-1).

CONSCIOUSNESS Consciousness is the state of awareness of self and the environment and has various facets (see also Chap. 31). The *content* of consciousness represents the sum of cognitive and affective mental functions and can be assessed only by inference. *Arousal* is closely allied to the appearance of wakefulness and *alertness,* i.e., the readiness to respond to stimulation. *Attention* includes the capacity to attend selectively to relevant stimuli and to manipulate abstract ideas. Consciousness also includes the concepts of *insight* and recognition of self. *Clouding of consciousness* is an essential feature of acute confusional states and describes the mildest impairment of consciousness on the continuum from full consciousness to deep coma. In most instances clouding of consciousness involves all facets of consciousness but does not necessarily imply reduced wakefulness. In delirium the patient may appear awake or excited, but the content of consciousness, awareness of the surroundings and self, and the capacity to attend selectively to relevant stimuli are all impaired.

PERCEPTION Perception involves conscious awareness and selection and identification of a stimulus from the environment. Even under normal conditions the perception of a stimulus depends on numerous factors, both physiologic (such as lighting) and psychological (such as mood and expectation). With clouding of consciousness attention falters, and perception becomes more subject to these influences. For example, poor vision or deafness may make the elderly more prone to misperception, and the sensory deprivation of confinement to bed or the advent of darkness often contributes to delirium. Coherent perception requires intact visuospatial or language function. Disturbances of perception are frequent in acute confusional states and include *illusions* (misperceptions of actual sensory stimuli) and *hallucinations* (perceptions experienced without apparent sensory

FIGURE 30-1 Observable components of cognition. Cognition from sensory input to verbal or motor output involves a sequence of separate but interrelated functions. The arrows indicate the influence at every stage of the level of consciousness and degree of attention, as well as the effect of mood and memory. These functions should be individually assessed at the bedside.

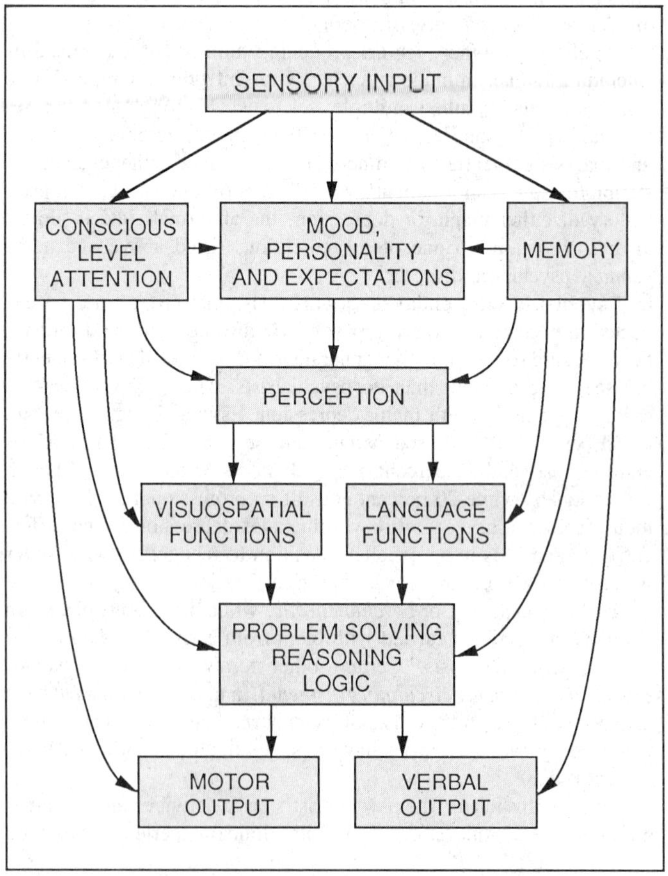

stimulation). In dementia misperception more commonly results from focal impairments of visuospatial or language function such as agnosia or aphasia.

MEMORY Three classes of memory can be distinguished at the bedside depending on the length of recall. This distinction is important in the differentiation of acute confusional states, dementia, and amnesic syndromes. The *immediate memory* system holds information close to consciousness for a few seconds while it is used for mental activity. It can be tested by the reproduction of a string of numerals and has a finite capacity for information at around seven digits, which are retained within the span of attention for only seconds or minutes unless the information is rehearsed by internal repetition. Normal attention is therefore required for immediate memory function, and impairment of immediate memory and a shortened digit span are diagnostic features of the acute confusional syndrome. Immediate memory is relatively normal in dementia and amnesic syndromes. Immediate memory appears to be mediated by a separate system that does not necessarily lead to longer-term storage. Recall of information after a delay of a few minutes requires a process of consolidation or learning and is mediated by the *long-term* or *secondary memory* system, with almost limitless capacity and durability. In contrast to immediate memory, recall of information from long-term memory is often selected by its relevance to the individual and usually incorporates the meaning of the information rather than exact words or pictures. Clinically, *recent memory,* the recall of information presented within minutes, hours, or days, is distinguished from *remote memory,* the recall of events months or years earlier. Recent and remote memory probably both involve the same long-term memory system, but access to remote memories is less sensitive to interference (e.g., from the effect of head injury) than recent memory. Impaired recent memory is usual in dementia and acute confusional states, and is the defining feature of amnesic syndromes.

MOOD AND PERSONALITY *Mood* refers to the prevailing emotional state, while *affect* is the emotional experience evoked by a particular stimulus. Individual reactions to any situation are closely related to underlying personality, previous experience, expectations, and degree of insight. These need to be taken into account when assessing cognitive function. The prevailing mood may have a profound affect on all aspects of cognition, especially at the extremes of the continuum of mood. Hypomania may be accompanied by illusions, flight of ideas, and extreme motor and verbal output sometimes mimicking delirium. In contrast, depression may exhibit slowing of thought, speech, and activity (psychomotor retardation) which, if severe, may be mistaken for dementia. Extreme anxiety may also interfere with the organization and coherence of thought and speech. Many diseases of the brain alter mood and affect. Frontal lobe lesions, in particular, may cause either lack of drive and initiative (abulia) with indifference to outcome or sometimes fatuous euphoria with social and sexual disinhibitions, which may interfere with cognitive function.

PROBLEM SOLVING Thought is intangible and elusive. However, the processes of reasoning, logic, and the ability to solve problems using language or mathematics can be assessed more easily using tests of words or numbers. Disorder of these processes is an essential feature of the acute confusional states and dementia, but in contrast reasoning is intact in the amnesic syndrome, except when recent memory is required. One manifestation of defective reasoning seen in acute confusional states and sometimes in dementia is the occurrence of delusions (false beliefs maintained in spite of convincing contradictory evidence). Delusions are also seen in psychiatric illnesses such as schizophrenia but tend to be more organized and persistent than in acute confusional states.

APPROACH TO THE PATIENT WITH DISORDERS OF COGNITION

HISTORY A careful history taken from close relatives or friends is essential to establish the first appearance of intellectual impairment and the subsequent tempo of the disease. Was the onset over hours or days, suggesting an acute confusional state, or over months or years, making dementia a more likely diagnosis? Was there an organic precipitating event such as a head injury, or did the confusion follow an emotional crisis, suggesting a psychiatric cause or deliberate drug overdose? Questioning should include inquiries about impairment of memory, personality and mood change, and how the patient copes with work, driving, and the activities of daily life. The history should include questioning about symptoms which suggest focal pathology such as those of raised intracranial pressure (headaches, nausea, vomiting, and ataxia), strokelike events, or seizures. Attention to past medical and family history, drugs, alcohol, and toxic exposure is important (see also Chap. 347). The handedness of the patient should be determined to assess the likelihood that the left hemisphere is dominant for speech.

EXAMINATION OF COGNITIVE FUNCTION The main focus is to establish the level of consciousness and to determine whether one or more areas of intellectual function are impaired. It is important as an initial step to determine the patient's premorbid level of intellect. A rough indicator can be obtained from the patient's profession or occupation and the amount of schooling completed. The physician is sometimes surprised to discover that a patient never learned to read or write, sometimes because of developmental dyslexia.

Examination of cognitive function needs to be adjusted according to the previous and current intellectual state, but it is useful to have a sequence of questions that the examiner has applied regularly to intellectually intact patients so as to have a good understanding of the normal range of replies. The patient's answers to questioning should be carefully recorded so that deterioration or improvement can be easily confirmed at a later evaluation. A number of pitfalls may cause the patient's intellectual function to be underestimated. Perseveration, usually a sign of frontal lobe disease, may cause the patient to repeat replies and have difficulty switching attention to a new task. Aphasia, with difficulty understanding commands or expressing the correct answer in response to questions, may cloud interpretation of the examination. The incoherence or mutism resulting from isolated expressive aphasia is commonly misinterpreted as a confusional state or dementia.

Orientation Orientation to person, place, and time (including date, time of day, month, and year) should be tested first as a guide to the degree of amnesia and confusion. In most cases, the more severe the impairment of memory the more inaccurate the date. If the patient cannot name the place accurately, some assessment of reasoning powers can be gauged by asking the patient to identify the type of place (e.g., hospital or home).

Consciousness Detecting clouding of consciousness requires careful observation. The normally alert individual engages in conversation or some other diversional activity, while the patient with impairment of consciousness remains quiet or engages in purposeless repetitive activities. More obtunded patients may drift into sleep when undisturbed but awaken promptly during the stimulation of questioning or physical examination. The demented patient may also lack spontaneous activity or conversation but shows normal alertness and responsiveness to questioning.

Attention Attention is assessed during history taking. Does the patient pay attention to questions, or is the patient easily distracted, giving equal notice to relevant and irrelevant stimuli? The capacity for sustained attention and concentration can be tested by asking for sequential subtraction of 7 from 100 down to zero, but the response should be interpreted with caution, as immediate memory and mathematical ability are also required. Forward and reverse digit span are also specific tests of attention as well as of immediate memory (see below).

Abnormalities of perception Abnormalities of perception should be sought by specific questioning about perception of the environment. The presence of hallucinations may be betrayed by the patient brushing or picking nonexistent objects off the bed covers or turning to answer an imaginary question.

Language Aphasia resulting in nonfluency of speech, hesitation, circumlocution, neologisms, or jargon is usually appreciated during routine conversation and history taking (see Chap. 33). It is also useful to ask the patient to name common and uncommon objects to assess for nominal aphasia, and to give a complex two- or three-stage conditional command to test for minor degrees of receptive dysphasia. (For example, "If I take my pen out of my pocket, please touch your left ear with your right index finger.") Agraphia should be sought by asking the patient to write his or her name and a short spontaneous sentence. Reading should be assessed using a standard text or newspaper article including an explanation of its meaning by the patient. Simple sums are given to assess mathematical skills.

Visuospatial function The most useful test of visuospatial function is to ask the patient to copy a drawing, starting with a simple object such as a five-pointed star and progressing to a more difficult object such as a three-dimensional box. Constructional apraxia, or visuospatial agnosia, results in difficulty in drawing the lines required in the correct spatial orientation or position. Other deficits of cortical function such as perseveration or visual neglect may also be revealed by this test. The visual recognition of common objects will have been tested when examining for nominal aphasia, but bedside testing for difficulty in recognition of faces (prosopagnosia) requires a newspaper or magazine containing photographs of famous people, unless individuals who should be well known to the patient can be presented without other clues such as voice to aid recognition.

Memory *Immediate memory* and attention are tested by determining *digit span.* The patient is asked to repeat a string of numerals after the examiner starting with a short string and working up to the normal digit span of six or seven consecutive numbers presented at about half-second intervals. A shorter string of numerals or a short word can be given to repeat or spell backwards. This test requires sustained attention as well as immediate memory. *Recent memory* should be assessed by asking the patient to learn the names of three common objects or a simple address. After confirming that the patient has registered the information, recall is tested after 2 and 5 min, depending on the degree of anticipated amnesia. If the patient fails to recall the information, then the severity of the amnesia can be gauged by giving the patient a clue, and if this fails, recognition can be tested by asking the patient to identify the correct answer from a choice. Recent memory for events over the last few days or weeks is assessed by asking for a description of events of personal or world importance. A relative or friend may need to corroborate the appropriateness of the description. *Remote long-term memory* can be tested by asking for items of common general knowledge such as the dates of important past events, names of important political figures, or location of major cities.

Mood and personality Judgments about personality, mood, affect, and insight should be made during history taking and examination. The appearance of the patient, content of conversation, and speed of movement provide the most useful clues to mood. Affect is signaled by language, facial expression, gestures, and posture, all of which should be studied closely. The presence of euphoria, disinhibition, or abulia should be noted.

Thought and problem solving Incoherence of reasoning and logical thought will usually have been detected during history taking or testing of language skills and mathematics. More subtle disorder of thought is sometimes revealed by asking the patient to explain the meaning of well-known proverbs or sayings.

Cognitive scales A number of scales [e.g., Blessed Dementia Scale; Mini-Mental State Examination (see Chap. 29)] have been developed to make an approximate assessment of cognitive function. These are not true psychometric tests but questionnaires that can be completed fairly quickly by untrained staff to provide a score that roughly reflects the degree of intellectual and behavioral impairment. Another scale, the Ischemic Score, helps to distinguish multi-infarct from degenerative dementia. On the whole, these scales are less useful in diagnosis than a careful cognitive examination conducted in the manner described above.

ACUTE CONFUSIONAL STATES AND DELIRIUM

Acute confusional states occur in about 10 percent of all hospitalized patients and in 30 to 50 percent of hospitalized geriatric patients; patients with dementia are particularly vulnerable.

PATHOPHYSIOLOGY *Neurologic diseases* cause confusional states in a variety of ways, including depression of consciousness level. Consciousness is normally maintained by the ascending reticular activating system in the brainstem and thalamic regions. Focal diseases (such as a brain tumor or subdural hematoma) may depress consciousness by compression of the brainstem or thalamus or by producing hydrocephalus. Many other neurologic diseases present with confusion as a result of diffuse impairment of neuronal function (e.g., concussion or encephalitis). Multifocal disease (e.g., multiple metastases or multiple infarcts) may also present with confusion if the loci of disease cause several separate deficits of cognitive function with impaired attention. Usually lesions in both hemispheres are necessary, but occasionally a single right nondominant hemispheric lesion (usually a parietal infarct) presents with an acute confusional state because of impairment of attention, which appears to be a predominant right hemisphere function.

Systemic diseases mostly result in confusion from diffuse impairment of neuronal function. This may be due to inadequate supply of oxygen (hypoxia), glucose (hypoglycemia), or other factors required for metabolism, including vitamins and hormones. In metabolic encephalopathy the mechanisms include acid-base disturbance, electrolyte imbalance, and circulating toxins (e.g., ammonia in liver failure). In systemic infections there are several possible factors, including high fever, hypoxia, dehydration, and circulating bacterial toxins. Most drug-induced confusional states result from direct interference with synaptic transmission. In delirium following drug withdrawal the excited state may result from the sudden overactivity of a previously depressed transmitter system that has developed the equivalent of denervation hypersensitivity.

In many cases of acute confusion multiple mechanisms can be identified, particularly in the elderly. Preexisting disease of the brain, blindness or deafness, age-related changes in the metabolism, and pharmacology of drugs, mild organ failure, and an unfamiliar environment may all contribute. At any age, the brain may be made more vulnerable by preexisting brain damage, sleep and sensory deprivation, or an unfamiliar environment.

CLINICAL FEATURES Because most causes of the acute confusional state affect neuronal function diffusely, all aspects of intellectual function are impaired to a lesser or greater degree (Table 30-1). The cardinal feature is *clouding of consciousness*, manifested by impaired alertness, awareness, and attention. This impairment is usually mild but can advance to coma if untreated. Depression of consciousness is distinguished from natural drowsiness by observing that the patient cannot easily be aroused. Reduced attentiveness can range from mild apathy and a failure to grasp complex details to reduced interaction with the examiner, lack of normal spontaneous comment or questions, and neglect of bodily needs. In delirium, arousal is evidenced by a readiness to respond to certain stimuli, insomnia, and excessive reactions to noise or bright lights. This is accompanied by a reduced ability to focus attention, distractibility, and inability to concentrate.

Variability in the level of arousal is a common feature of the acute confusional state. Reduced responsiveness may be interspersed with outbursts of delirium. Sleep-wake cycles are frequently disrupted or reversed, and confusion is often more marked during the night. The early symptoms of delirium often include insomnia and vivid unpleasant dreams before a frank confusional state supervenes.

Impairment of memory with reduced digit span, poor recent memory, and defective recall for distant events is an important feature. One of the earliest signs of this impairment is disorientation for time, and later, disorientation for place. Knowledge of personal identity is usually retained if the patient can understand the question. The memory deficit is characteristically patchy so that distortions of memory (para-amnesia) and partially correct information may be incorporated into confabulatory answers or delusions. When the patient recovers, partial or total amnesia for the period of confusion is usual, although isolated events, especially vivid hallucinations, may be remembered in detail.

Impairment of cognitive function leads to difficulty performing tasks requiring logic, mathematics, or spatial organization. Thought processes are slowed, although the agitated delirious patient may have flight of ideas. In all cases, thinking is disorganized and disjointed. Speech is incoherent, rambling, and often inappropriate. Comprehension of complex material is impaired, and errors in the naming of objects or in writing may be elicited.

Impaired perception may compound confusion. The patient often misperceives surroundings and attendants as those more familiar to the patient. More concrete illusions and hallucinations are common, especially following drug withdrawal and in alcoholic delirium tremens. Hallucinations are most frequently visual, but may involve any sensory modality.

Disturbances of emotion may include blunting of affect or emotional lability. Mood disturbances include dysphoria, depression, agitation, or fear, and these may be accompanied by appropriate autonomic responses. *Autonomic hyperactivity* including tachycardia, diaphoresis, and anxiety are particularly prominent with drug and alcohol withdrawal.

Psychomotor changes are common. In most patients, spontaneous motor activity is depressed, but hyperactivity and restlessness characterize delirium. Repetitive stereotyped motor behavior, such as plucking at the bed clothes or tossing from side to side, is frequent. *Involuntary movements,* including irregular tremor, asterixis, and myoclonus, are usually seen in drug withdrawal or metabolic encephalopathy. Rarely, patients show catatonic behavior.

DIFFERENTIAL DIAGNOSIS The first essential distinction to be made is whether the confusional state results from primary neurologic disease or as a complication of systemic illness. This distinction can normally be made on examination and is then supported by investigation (see Table 30-2).

Neurologic causes These can usually be recognized by the presence of focal neurologic signs in addition to disordered intellectual function. Examples include hemiparesis in *cerebral infarction,* neck stiffness in *meningitis* or *subarachnoid hemorrhage,* and gait disturbance in *hydrocephalus.* However, diffuse neurologic diseases such as *encephalitis, epileptic confusion,* or *small-vessel vasculitis* may cause no focal neurologic signs apart from the disorder of cognition. *Neoplasias* of the nervous system usually cause headache and focal signs, but midline tumors may present with a gradually evolving confusional state. Acute onset may be caused by brainstem compression or acute hydrocephalus.

Impairment of consciousness is uncommon following nonhemorrhagic *stroke* unless the stroke is large enough to cause midline mass effects. However, impairment of consciousness and confusion may occur when a cerebral ischemic event is superimposed on preexisting cerebral infarcts. *Subarachnoid hemorrhage* may present with a confusional state secondary to widespread vasospasm, and the typical history of headache may not be obtained. *Postictal confusion* after a minor seizure lasts only a few seconds and after a major seizure usually resolves within an hour unless complicated by head injury, hypoxia, or status epilepticus. However, a persistent confusional state may occur with continuous or serial minor seizures (*minor epileptic status*) (see Chap. 350). Acute confusional states may accompany *encephalitis* or *brain abscess* without systemic signs of infarction always being present.

Systemic causes Systemic causes are usually characterized by absence of focal neurologic signs apart from cognitive disorders, although minor signs such as reflex asymmetry or extensor plantar responses may be seen. An exception to this rule is occasionally seen in hypoglycemia, which may be accompanied in the elderly by hemiparesis. In *metabolic encephalopathy,* acidotic hyperventilation, tremor, asterixis, or myoclonus may suggest the diagnosis. *Wernicke's encephalopathy* (see Chap. 370) should be considered in patients with a history of alcoholism or malnutrition. *Drugs* often cause confusion, especially in the elderly and those on multiple medications. *Endocrine dysfunction* (see Chap. 313 and 316) rarely causes acute

TABLE 30-2 Differential diagnosis of the acute confusional state

NEUROLOGIC (focal neurologic signs are uncommon)

- Trauma
  - Concussion
  - Intracranial hematoma
  - Subdural hematoma
- Vascular disorders
  - Multiple infarcts
  - Right hemisphere or posterior circulation infarcts
  - Hypertensive encephalopathy
  - Vasculitis (e.g., systemic lupus erythematosus, polyarteritis nodosa, giant cell arteritis)
  - Air and fat embolism
  - Subarachnoid hemorrhage
- Neoplasia
  - Multiple parenchymal metastases
  - Meningeal carcinomatosis
  - Midline brain tumors
  - Brain tumors elsewhere with brainstem compression, edema, or hydrocephalus
  - Paraneoplastic syndromes (limbic encephalitis)
- Infections
  - Meningitis and encephalitis (viral, bacterial, fungal, protozoal)
  - Multiple abscesses
  - Progressive multifocal leukoencephalopathy
- Inflammations
  - Acute disseminated encephalomyelitis
  - Postinfectious encephalitis
- Epilepsy
  - Postictal state
  - Minor epileptic status (temporal lobe)

SYSTEMIC (focal neurologic signs are uncommon)

- Substrate depletion
  - Hypoglycemia
  - Diffuse hypoxia
    - Pulmonary
    - Cardiac
    - Carbon monoxide poisoning
- Metabolic encephalopathy
  - Diabetic ketoacidosis
  - Renal failure
  - Liver failure
  - Electrolyte, fluid, and acid-base imbalance (especially Na^+, Ca^{2+}, Mg^{2+})
  - Hereditary metabolic disease, e.g., porphyria, metachromatic leukodystrophy, mitochondrial cytopathy
- Vitamin deficiency
  - Thiamine (Wernicke's encephalopathy)
  - Nicotinic acid (pellagra)
  - B_{12} deficiency
- Endocrine; over- or underactivity
  - Thyroid
  - Parathyroid
  - Adrenal
- Infection
  - Septicemia
  - Malaria
  - Subacute bacterial endocarditis
  - Focal infection, e.g., pneumonia
- Thermal injuries
  - hypothermia
  - heat stroke
- Hematologic disorders
  - Hyperviscosity syndrome
  - Severe anemia
- Toxic causes
  - Drug and alcohol intoxication (therapeutic, social, or illegal)
  - Drug withdrawal, e.g., alcohol, barbiturates, narcotics
  - Chemical toxins, e.g., heavy metals, organic toxins

PSYCHIATRIC

- Acute mania
- Depression or extreme anxiety
- Schizophrenia
- Hysterical fugue states

confusional state but should always be considered, particularly if there is hyponatremia. *Systemic infections*, especially *septicemia* and *subacute bacterial endocarditis* can cause acute confusional states, particularly in the elderly in whom fever may not always be evident, as can meningitis or brain abscess complicating the systemic infection.

Psychiatric causes In *anxiety*, extreme *grief*, or *depression*, orientation for person and place is usually preserved, and with encouragement the patient can concentrate and improve cognitive performance. Hyperactivity, diminished need for sleep, pressure of speech, delusions, short attention span, and distractibility in *acute mania* may be confused with the hyperexcitability of delirium. Mania is characterized by a sustained elevation of mood and preservation of orientation. Hyperactivity persists throughout the manic episode in contrast to delirium, in which hyperactivity may be interspersed with somnolence. *Disassociative or hysterical disorders*, for example, psychogenic amnesia and fugue states, are usually distinguished from organic confusional states by the focal nature of the amnesia. *Acute schizophrenia* may simulate the acute confusional state, but consciousness, normal sleep-wake cycles, orientation, and attention are usually preserved (see Chap. 368).

INVESTIGATION Investigation is an urgent procedure. A *biochemical profile*, including blood sugar level, readily diagnoses the common metabolic disorders. A *blood count* detects hematologic disorders, and a neutrophilia suggests infection. If in doubt, a raised *erythrocyte sedimentation rate* supports the diagnosis of an organic disorder. *Arterial blood gas analysis* is a useful screen for hypoxia, respiratory failure, and acidosis. *Chest x-ray* and *blood and urine cultures* should be performed even if there is no fever. A complete infectious disease screen is indicated if there is a stronger suspicion of infection. *Endocrine tests* and *vitamin* B_{12} measurement may be indicated in individual patients. *Drug and toxicologic screen* are indicated for suspicion of drug overdose or toxic exposure. *Cerebrospinal fluid* (*CSF*) *examination* is mandatory in all patients with fever or neck stiffness so long as raised intracranial pressure or intracranial mass is not suspected and is also helpful in distinguishing metabolic from neurologic disease. The CSF white cell count is usually normal in metabolic disease, whereas leukocytosis implies neurologic disease, especially a central nervous system (CNS) infection. The *electroencephalogram* (EEG) is useful if the presence of encephalopathy is uncertain; it is almost always abnormal in organic causes, but does not necessarily distinguish between neurologic and systemic causes. Certain patterns may suggest metabolic disorders (particularly liver failure), encephalitis (especially herpes simplex), or epileptic status; and focal abnormalities may point to a stroke, abscess, or tumor. A *magnetic resonance imaging* (*MRI*) *or computed tomography* (*CT*) *scan* is not an emergency procedure unless examination or the EEG suggests a focal lesion, but should be considered if no systemic cause is found after initial investigation.

MANAGEMENT The patient with acute confusion state is often agitated, and before the appropriate examination and investigations can be completed, the cooperation of the patient is required. Patients can frequently be calmed by a sympathetic and friendly physician. A relative or friend can often help and should be encouraged to stay with the patient. Nursing care should be given in a well-lit, relatively quiet environment with facilities for frequent observation. Sedation is seldom required with these measures. However, in some agitated, violent, or paranoid patients parenteral medication may prevent harm to the patient or others and allow completion of the examination, investigation, or treatment. A long-acting oral or intramuscular major tranquilizer such as chlorpromazine or haloperidol is usually suitable, but for short-term sedation, such as during a CT scan, an intravenous benzodiazapine may be appropriate. The possibility that psychopharmaceutical agents may exacerbate an abnormal mental state or disguise the neurologic signs of deterioration should be borne in mind.

Management begins with identification and correction of hypoxia, hypoglycemia, hyperthermia, or dehydration. Parenteral thiamine should be given to all patients suspected of Wernicke's encephalopathy. Subsequent treatment depends on the underlying cause. If the confusional state does not quickly resolve, attention to the hydration and nutrition of the patient is required to prevent perpetuation of the confusional state.

AMNESIA

PATHOPHYSIOLOGY The anatomic basis of memory is only partly understood, but clearly involves the temporal lobes. Most lesions cause long-term memory loss without affecting immediate memory or attention. As a rule, significant amnesia occurs only after bilateral lesions of the medial temporal lobes. Unilateral lesions of the speech dominant temporal lobe cause deficits of verbal memory, and unilateral lesions of the nondominant temporal lobe result in deficits in visual or nonverbal recall, but these deficits are rarely significant in the absence of preexisting contralateral temporal lobe pathology. The minimum lesion required to produce amnesia has not been established, but involvement of limbic structures appears crucial. Cholinergic neurons may play an important role. For example, anticholinergic drugs disrupt memory storage, and cholinergic drugs may on occasion improve memory.

CLINICAL FEATURES The classic example of amnesia is *Korsakoff's syndrome*, secondary to chronic alcoholism (see Chap. 357 and Chap. 370). The cardinal feature is an inability to recall new information despite a normal level of consciousness. Immediate memory, digit span, and attention are normal. Memory of knowledge acquired before the onset of illness is relatively intact, but memory for new events is severely impaired. Patients are disoriented in place and time and incapable of recalling information for more than the duration of immediate memory. They are thus condemned to be brief visitors to the present; their inner world consists only of memories of their remote past. On first encounter, they may seem relatively normal, taking part in ward routine and engaging in conversation. Because of intact immediate memory they retain information briefly but forget as soon as they are distracted. In the pure syndrome, tests of intelligence not requiring long-term memory may be normal. Compensation is by confabulation, giving more or less plausible answers incorporating some relevant information and sometimes fantastic elaboration. Although characteristic, confabulation is not universal in Korsakoff's syndrome and may be seen in amnesia of all causes and in acute confusional states. Amnesic subjects can slowly and laboriously learn some tasks, such as tactile or visual mazes, tunes on the piano, and the use of a computer. Despite evidence that the subjects acquire and retain new skills, they do not recall learning and deny the new skills, demonstrating dramatically a disassociation between recollection and retention of information.

DIFFERENTIAL DIAGNOSIS The diagnosis of *Korsakoff's syndrome* is usually clear from its association with chronic alcoholism. It often follows an episode of Wernicke's encephalopathy, and the amnesic deficit becomes evident with recovery from the acute confusional state. Nonalcoholic causes of *thiamine deficiency* (see Chap. 357) may cause Korsakoff's syndrome. Similar clinical syndromes may occur after bilateral temporal lobe lesions resulting from *medial temporal lobectomy, head injury, herpes simplex encephalitis, strokes*, or *brain tumors*. *Alzheimer's disease* (see below) may also cause isolated amnesia before generalized dementia becomes evident.

Temporary amnesia is a common feature of *head injury* (see Chap. 352). The memory disturbance occurs both for events before (*retrograde amnesia*) and after (*posttraumatic amnesia*) the time of injury. *Anterograde amnesia* refers to impairment in learning new material, which accompanies posttraumatic amnesia. Almost invariably, retrograde amnesia causes permanent inability to recall the few minutes prior to the head injury, implying disruption of the immediate memory system and failure to register long-term memory. In severe head injuries retrograde amnesia may extend back for hours or weeks. With recovery, the duration of retrograde amnesia shrinks and may resolve. During retrograde amnesia, remote memory is usually accessible. The length of posttraumatic amnesia generally corresponds to the length of postconcussive confusion and may be present despite normal immediate memory and digit span. The duration of posttraumatic amnesia is an indicator of the severity of head injury, the ability to learn new material often being the last cognitive deficit to recover.

Transient global amnesia is a syndrome in which a previously well person suddenly becomes confused and amnesic. The attacks are usually spontaneous but occasionally follow immersion in cold or hot water, emotional stimuli, physical exertion, sexual intercourse, or travel in a motor vehicle. The patient appears bewildered and repeatedly asks questions about present and recent events. Orientation for person and sometimes place is preserved, but recent memory is impaired and the patient cannot recall new information after a few minutes delay. Behavior is otherwise normal and appropriate. Examination during an attack shows intact immediate memory but severe impairment of recall of recent and sometimes more distant events. General intellectual function is normal. By definition, no other neurologic signs are present. The attacks usually last 2 to 12 h. Headache, nausea, and vomiting may occur. Recovery is complete, and recurrence is unusual. The cause of transient global amnesia is a mystery. Associations with migraine-like phenomena, temporal lobe ischemia, and epilepsy have been described. The disorder is usually benign; rarely, the attack is due to an underlying temporal lobe tumor.

Brief "blanks" in memory may cause difficulties in diagnosis. Occasionally *complex partial seizures* may occur without the patient being conscious of any associated signs or loss of awareness, apart from the disruption of memory during the seizure. Amnesia may also rarely accompany *classical migraine*. A number of *drugs*, including alcohol and short-acting benzodiazepines, may impair memory and cause amnesia for events during the period of their use. *Electroconvulsive therapy* (ECT) causes temporary retrograde and anterograde amnesia.

Psychogenic amnesia for personally important memories is common, although whether this results from deliberate avoidance of unpleasant memories or from unconscious repression may be impossible to establish. This *event-specific amnesia* is particularly common after violent crimes such as homicide of a close relative but uncommon in nonviolent crimes. This type of amnesia is also associated with severe drug or alcohol intoxication and sometimes with schizophrenia. More prolonged psychogenic amnesia occurs in *fugue states* that also commonly follow severe emotional stress. The patient with a fugue state suffers from a sudden loss of personal identity and may be found wandering far from home. In contrast to organic amnesia, fugue states are associated with amnesia for personal identity and events closely associated with the personal past. At the same time, memory for other recent events and the ability to learn and use new information are preserved. The episodes usually last hours or days and occasionally weeks or months while the patient takes on a new identity. On recovery there is a residual amnesic gap for the period of the fugue.

MANAGEMENT The cause of temporary amnesia is usually evident from the history. In patients with transient global amnesia investigations to exclude an underlying structural cause (MRI or CT), epilepsy (EEG), and vascular risk factors are appropriate. Unless the investigations are positive, reassurance is the only further measure required. The management of persistent amnesia is more demanding. Although Wernicke's encephalopathy responds to thiamine, established Korsakoff's syndrome does not, and the amnesia is usually permanent. Nevertheless, a course of thiamine should be given in newly diagnosed cases to prevent further deterioration.

DEMENTIA

Dementia is common, affecting about 4 million people in the United States alone, and is the major cause of long-term disability in old age. The prevalence of dementia increases rapidly with age, afflicting about 2 percent of the population between ages 65 and 70 and 20 percent of people above 80. With increasing longevity of the population and decreasing birth rates, the prevalence will continue to rise.

PATHOPHYSIOLOGY Some authorities separate dementia occurring before the age of 65 (presenile dementia) from that occurring after (senile dementia). This distinction was based on the assumption that the causes were different: rare degenerations in the young and vascular disease or senescence in the elderly. Although the expression of diseases may differ at different ages, the major findings in demented patients of all ages are similar, and the distinction arbitrary.

Most diseases causing dementia are either widespread neuronal degenerations or multifocal disorders. The initial symptoms depend on where the dementing process starts, but the location and numbers of neurons lost that are required to cause dementia is difficult to establish. Aging results in a gradual loss of neurons and of brain mass, but this is not accompanied by significant intellectual decline in the absence of disease. Indeed, brain mass is a poor guide to intellectual function. Patients with a degenerative dementia in the sixth decade may have a greater brain mass than intellectually normal patients in their eighth decade. Consequently, documentation of generalized atrophy by CT scan is not a clear indication of dementia.

Dementia may result from cortical disease (e.g., Alzheimer's disease) or from disease of subcortical structures such as the basal ganglia, thalamus, and deep white matter (e.g., Huntington's disease). Cortical dementia is characterized by loss of cognitive functions such as language, perception, calculation; in contrast, subcortical dementia exhibits slowing of cognition and information processing ("bradyphrenia"), flattening of the affect, and disturbances of motivation, mood, and arousal. Memory is impaired in both types. The features of subcortical dementia also occur in cortical processes affecting the frontal lobes and probably reflect damaged projections to and from the frontal lobes.

In Alzheimer's disease, which is the commonest cause of dementia, the dementia results from loss of cortical tissue especially in the temporal and frontal lobes. This is accompanied in most cases by increased space between the gyri and enlargement of the ventricles. The histologic hallmark is the presence of numerous neurofibrillary tangles and senile plaques (see Chap. 359). Plaques and tangles are found in normal elderly brains but are increased in number in Alzheimer's disease, especially in the hippocampus and temporal lobes. The hippocampal involvement probably accounts for the memory disorder, which may be partially mediated by a reduction in cholinergic activity. The activities of other neurotransmitters including norepinephrine, serotonin, dopamine, glutamate, and somatostatin are also reduced. These changes are accompanied by reductions in cerebral blood flow and decreased metabolism of oxygen and glucose.

DIFFERENTIAL DIAGNOSIS The causes of dementia are numerous (Table 30-3). However, a small number of diseases account for most cases. In most of the western world, Alzheimer's disease is responsible for 50 to 90 percent and vascular disease for 5 to 10 percent of cases of dementia referred to hospital. In Japan and parts of Scandinavia, vascular disease appears to be more prevalent than Alzheimer's disease, at least in hospitalized patients. Cerebral infarction contributes to intellectual loss in a further 15 percent of patients with Alzheimer's disease documented at autopsy (*mixed dementia*). Dementia attributed to ethanol abuse may account for 5 to 10 percent of cases. Metabolic disturbances, cerebral neoplasms, subdural hematoma, and normal-pressure hydrocephalus account for around 10 percent of cases, and Huntington's chorea for about 2 percent. The remainder of causes, including Creutzfeldt-Jakob disease, are rare, accounting for less than 1 percent of cases. In human immunodeficiency virus (HIV) infection, dementia is present in 30 to 40 percent of patients.

An important aim of diagnosis is to identify treatable causes of dementia. The differential diagnosis depends primarily on a careful history and examination, supported by investigation. Illnesses that cause dementia can be divided into those in which dementia is the

TABLE 30-3 Differential diagnosis of dementia

- Primary dementia with no other signs
  - Alzheimer's disease
  - Pick's disease
  - Frontal lobe degeneration
- Dementia with signs of vascular disease
  - Multi-infarct dementia*
  - Thalamic infarction
  - "Binswanger's disease"* and lacunar state*
  - Vasculitis,* e.g., systemic lupus erythematosus, polyarteritis nodosa, granulomatous angiitis of the central nervous system, Behçet's disease
- Dementia with evidence of chronic infection†
  - Human immunodeficiency virus
  - Syphilis*
  - Papovavirus (progressive multifocal leukoencephalopathy)
  - Subacute sclerosing panencephalitis
  - Creutzfeldt-Jakob disease (subacute spongiform encephalopathy)
  - Tuberculosis,* fungal* and protozoal infections*
  - Sarcoidosis*
  - Whipple's disease*
- Secondary dementia with signs of the underlying neurologic condition
  - Neoplasia and mass lesions
    - Primary and secondary tumors*
    - Carcinomatous meningitis
    - Paraneoplastic encephalitis
    - Chronic subdural hematoma*
    - Hydrocephalus*
  - Movement disorders
    - Parkinson's disease
    - Lewy body dementia
    - Huntington's chorea
    - Progressive supranuclear palsy (Steele-Richardson syndrome)
    - Multisystem degeneration (Shy-Drager syndrome)
    - Hereditary ataxias
  - Motor neuron disease (amyotrophic lateral sclerosis)
  - Multiple sclerosis
- Dementia following diffuse brain damage‡
  - Acute head injury
  - Pugilistic dementia
  - Anoxia
  - Encephalitis
- Endocrine disorders and vitamin deficiency
  - Hypothyroidism*
  - B_{12} deficiency*
  - Thiamine deficiency*
  - Nicotinic acid deficiency* (pellagra)
  - Adrenal insufficiency* and Cushing's syndrome*
  - Hypo-* and hyperparathyroidism*
  - Chronic hypoglycemia*
- Toxic disorders
  - Drug and narcotic poisoning*
  - Alcoholic dementia*
  - Heavy metal intoxication*
  - Organic toxins*
  - Dialysis dementia*
- Psychiatric
  - Chronic schizophrenia
  - Pseudodementia*
- Additional conditions to consider in adolescents or young adults
  - Movement disorders
    - Wilson's disease*
    - Hallervorden-Spatz disease
  - Tuberous sclerosis
  - Progressive myoclonic epilepsy*
  - Metabolic diseases, e.g., leukodystrophies, mitochondrial cytopathy, storage diseases, Leigh's disease, homocystinuria

*Condition in which treatment may reverse or prevent progression of dementia.
†Systemic, hematologic or CSF findings suggest infection except in Creutzfeldt-Jakob disease.
‡History of acute injury with depression of consciousness usual, except in pugilistic dementia.

primary manifestation of the disease (other neurologic signs are absent); those in which dementia is secondary to other neurologic disorders (additional neurologic findings are usually present); and systemic diseases in which dementia is usually associated with signs outside the central nervous system.

In the elderly, dementia must be distinguished from the minor degree of forgetfulness that accompanies aging (*benign senescent forgetfulness*); the latter is often accompanied by slowing of physical and mental agility, inability to change course, and rigidity of thinking. This is by no means universal with aging and may reflect an unidentified disease process. Benign senescent forgetfulness is not disabling in the activities of daily life and does not progress to more severe disability. The early symptoms and signs of the degenerative dementias are often indistinguishable from those of benign senescence, and it is only the young age of the patient or progression of the symptoms that allows the diagnosis of dementia to be confirmed.

Primary dementia The diagnosis of *Alzheimer's disease* is only certain at autopsy but is usually reliably suggested by the characteristic history and signs, supported by negative investigations excluding other causes of dementia. Series of well-investigated patients with dementia attributed to Alzheimer's disease always include cases with an alternative diagnosis established at autopsy. The term *dementia of Alzheimer type* is sometimes used for patients with the characteristic clinical picture and negative investigations in whom pathologic confirmation has not been obtained.

The mean duration from the onset of symptoms to death is 8 years, with a range of 2 to 15 years. The course may be more rapid in younger patients. The early features vary according to the initial brain site involved. The onset is insidious and subtle, and can rarely be pinpointed. In most cases, insight is lost early, and the patient attributes failures to old age or oversight. Some have no spontaneous complaints but become disturbed when unable to answer simple questions. The history is almost invariably given by a relative. Early loss of spontaneity and initiative is frequent. The patient may give up hobbies and lose interest in social contacts or conversation. Lapses of memory, difficulty learning new information, and failure to remember names and appointments are noticed. At this stage, the memory deficit is more likely to involve recent events. In the early stages, social graces are usually preserved, and routine behavior and simple conversation are normal, so that friends and relatives may be unaware that anything is wrong, unless the patient is tested by an unfamiliar situation or by a formal examination of cognitive function. As the disease progresses, inexplicable mistakes are made in the activities of everyday life, and dress, appearance, and personal hygiene are neglected. Spatial disorientation may become evident, especially in unfamiliar surroundings. The patient may oscillate between apathy and unprovoked irritability or aggression.

Examination in the early stage usually shows impairment of memory for recent events with varying degrees of cognitive deficit. The patient often appears puzzled in response to questioning. Primitive reflexes such as palmomental response or suck reflex may be present.

As the disease advances, the impairments of memory, speech, and behavior become so marked that patients are unable to care for themselves, repeat questions over and over again, and fail to recognize friends and relatives. Restlessness is common especially at night, and patients become lost if allowed to wander. Delusions, paranoia, and hallucinations may occur. On examination at this stage, the patient remains alert but is disoriented to time and place and has poor memory for recent and distant events. Digit span is usually preserved. Speech lacks spontaneity and fluency and exhibits minor aphasic errors, and there is difficulty understanding complex commands. Nonfluent aphasia, especially in younger patients, may be striking. Motor and constructional apraxia and agnosia may be present. Extrapyramidal signs, including stooped posture, slow shuffling gait, generalized bradykinesia, and rigidity, are common. The tendon reflexes may be brisk, but extensor plantar responses are rare. Grasp reflexes may be elicited. In the last stage the patient is immobile, mute, and incontinent. The patient no longer recognizes relatives, and testing of cognitive function is not possible. Seizures and myoclonus may become prominent. Weight loss and a shrunken appearance may precede death, often from intercurrent infection.

Pick's disease is characterized by circumscribed cortical atrophy, usually confined to the frontal and temporal lobes, associated with a characteristic histologic appearance of degenerative neurons in the cortex, basal ganglia, and brainstem (Pick's bodies) (see Chap. 359). The age at onset and course are similar to Alzheimer's disease. Patients with Pick's disease suffer slowly progressive dementia and in the early stages may show frontal-temporal lobe features uncommon in Alzheimer's disease, including personality and emotional changes, disinhibition, lack of restraint, poor social and sexual conduct, and lack of foresight. Later, patients may appear euphoric or retreat into increasing apathy and abulia in association with nonfluent aphasia, which progresses to mutism. Comprehension of speech and spatial functions are relatively spared. Some cases of Pick's disease are indistinguishable clinically from Alzheimer's disease, and some cases of Alzheimer's disease show a frontal predominance so that the distinction may only be made at autopsy. A similar picture of *frontal lobe dementia* may occur in association with primary neuronal degeneration in the frontal and anterior temporal lobes without the neuropathologic findings of either Alzheimer's or Pick's disease.

Vascular dementia In most instances vascular dementia results from multiple areas of discrete infarction and not from chronic diffuse ischemia. The term *multi-infarct dementia* emphasizes this distinction. The diagnosis of vascular dementia is strongly suggested by an abrupt onset, especially if there is a history of previous stroke. The course characteristically fluctuates with periods of improvement and stepwise deterioration, in contrast to the steady progression of Alzheimer's disease. Hypertension is usual in vascular dementia but rare in Alzheimer's disease. Nocturnal confusion, relative preservation of personality, emotional lability, somatic complaints, and depression are more common in vascular dementia but not diagnostic. Focal neurologic signs (other than those of the cognitive deficits) including pseudobulbar palsy, visual field deficits, hemiparesis, or extensor plantar responses may suggest vascular dementia but may also be symptomatic of other neurologic causes such as a tumor.

Multi-infarct dementia can result from all types of cerebral vascular disease but is most likely to result from recurrent bilateral cerebral embolism from the heart or carotid arteries. It can also occur following a single episode such as severe hypotension or cardiac arrest if the degree of bilateral brain damage is sufficient. Multi-infarct dementia may also result from widespread involvement of small vessels by vasculitis, from a few strategically placed large cortical infarcts, or from multiple small infarcts in subcortical structures, such as occurs in the *lacunar state* secondary to hypertensive small-vessel disease (see Chap. 351). Hypertensive or atherosclerotic disease with thickening of the perforating deep vessels and capillaries supplying the subcortical white matter may also cause *Binswanger's disease* (*subcortical arteriosclerotic encephalopathy*) in which dementia is associated with diffuse loss of subcortical white matter and enlargement of the underlying ventricle. In contrast to multi-infarct dementia, major stroke is unusual in Binswanger's disease, and examination shows features of subcortical dementia (see above), a characteristic small-stepped, wide-based gait (marche à petit pas), pseudobulbar palsy, and corticospinal signs.

Chronic infections Chronic infections are important to consider, as the dementia may be treatable. Infections of the CNS are usually associated with systemic manifestations, meningeal involvement, abnormal CSF, and abnormalities on MRI or CT scan. Cerebral *syphilis* was a major cause and should still be excluded in all patients (see Chap. 128). *Human immunodeficiency virus* infection, also sexually transmitted, is an important cause of dementia in young people (see Chap. 134) but should also be considered in all patients at risk. The dementia usually occurs as a part of acquired immunodeficiency syndrome (AIDS) but may be the first manifestation. Dementia may also arise from "slow" virus infections. *Subacute sclerosing panencephalitis* causes dementia in children and occasionally in adolescents due to persistent replication of the measles virus in the brain many years after initial infection (see Chap. 355). *Creutzfeldt-Jacob disease* (*subacute spongiform encephalopathy*), a rare dementia, has been transmitted by an unknown agent to animals and to humans by corneal transplantation, neurosurgical instrumentation, or injections of growth hormone extracted from human pituitaries. In most cases the route of infection is unknown. After incubating for several years, the illness occurs in middle or late life and progresses to death within months. The dementia is often combined with ataxia, corticospinal signs, abnormal movements, cortical blindness, and myoclonus (see Chap. 355). Bizarre behavior and hallucinations are sometimes striking. In contrast to most other infections of the nervous system, signs of intracranial inflammation are absent and the CSF is normal.

Neoplasia and mass lesions *Primary or secondary brain tumors* may present with dementia, particularly slowly growing, deep, midline tumors of the corpus callosum or frontal lobe. Frontal meningiomas are the most important to consider in all patients as they are benign and the dementia potentially curable. Other curable mass lesions include *chronic subdural hematoma*. The head trauma in such cases may have been remote, trivial, or forgotten, particularly in the elderly. Diffuse primary tumors and multiple secondary tumors may also cause dementia. Features of raised intracranial pressures (such as headaches or papilledema) and focal signs apart from the cognitive disorders may be absent, although minor signs such as a grasp reflex or extensor plantar response are often present. Most causes of dementia due to mass lesions or raised intracranial pressure are easily diagnosed from the MRI or CT scan.

Malignancy arising outside the nervous system may also cause dementia through *metastatic carcinomatous meningitis* or from a *nonmetastatic paraneoplastic encephalitis* (see Chap. 353). The latter condition usually begins insidiously and progresses slowly. Depression of consciousness is absent in the early stages, and psychiatric disturbances may be striking. The CSF is usually abnormal in these conditions.

Obstructive or communicating hydrocephalus in adults characteristically presents with subacute progressive dementia and is an important treatable cause. A history of headache may be obtained, and ataxia and gait disturbance are usual. Signs of raised intracranial pressure may be absent. The diagnosis is hampered in the elderly by the difficulty of distinguishing the scan appearances of hydrocephalus due to abnormal CSF dynamics from hydrocephalus "ex vacuo" secondary to atrophy. However, the combination of dementia, urinary incontinence, and gait disorder suggests the syndrome of *normal- or low-pressure hydrocephalus*. In this condition, routine measurements of CSF pressure at lumbar puncture or ventriculography are normal, but intermittent waves of increased CSF pressure may be detected if patients are monitored for several days. Such cases may respond to ventricular drainage.

Movement disorders A number of degenerative neurologic diseases other than the primary dementias may also cause dementia, usually as a late manifestation. Movement disorders provide the largest group, of which the most common is *idiopathic Parkinson's disease*, where dementia develops in the late stages of the disease in 15 to 30 percent (see Chap. 359). Another important cause is Huntington's chorea, partly because the diagnosis has genetic implications (see Chap. 359). In these conditions, the cause of the dementia is usually evident from the history or clinical signs of the underlying neurologic disease, but very occasionally the dementia may be the only feature.

Diffuse brain damage In dementia secondary to *head injury, anoxia, hypoglycemia,* or *encephalitis* the cause is usually obvious from the history. The initial insult almost invariably causes loss of consciousness, and the dementia becomes evident when consciousness is regained after prolonged coma. If the patient recovers but then declines intellectually, the possibility of a secondary cause of dementia such as hydrocephalus should be considered. Repeated, less severe head trauma, such as occurs in boxers, may also lead to dementia later in life (*dementia pugilistica,* or the "punch drunk" syndrome), associated with extrapyramidal signs, dysarthria, and ataxia.

Endocrine disorders and vitamin deficiency Imbalances sufficient to affect neuronal function usually cause an acute confusional state with disturbance of attention and consciousness, but on occasion the presentation may be more chronic and mimic dementia. These conditions are treatable and cause reversible dementia, and they must be excluded in all patients. *Hypothyroidism* is the most common endocrine condition to present with dementia.

Toxic disorders Intoxications usually present with acute confusional state, often fluctuating according to the exposure. However, chronic intoxication may result in a reversible dementia. *Drugs* are an important cause, especially in the elderly, and the medication history should be carefully reviewed. The list of potential agents is large and includes drugs of abuse, psychotherapeutic agents (including barbiturates, sleeping tablets, tranquilizers, and antidepressants), drugs used in Parkinson's disease (levodopa and anticholinergics), and anticonvulsants. *Alcohol* is the most prevalent intoxicant implicated in dementia. Chronic inebriation results in reversible intellectual impairment but may also lead to a persistent deficit. In some cases, this is pure amnesia due to Korsakoff's psychosis, but in others it is a global dementia, associated with cerebral atrophy. Factors accounting for dementia in alcoholics include vitamin deficiency, repeated head injury, anoxia or hypoglycemia during alcoholic stupor, chronic liver failure, or the rare complication of *Marchiafava-Bignami disease,* which causes widespread demyelination in the cerebral hemispheres.

Dementia in adolescents and young adults This requires consideration of a further group of conditions in addition to those already mentioned (Table 30-3). Late presentation of *Wilson's disease* is another important example of a treatable dementia and should be excluded in all patients under the age of 40. Metabolic diseases are the largest group. There is usually evidence of a systemic disorder such as a peripheral neuropathy, myopathy, retinopathy, or hepatosplenomegaly. Specific diagnosis relies on special investigation.

Pseudodementias Nonorganic causes of apparent intellectual decline are not rare, although it is probably more frequent for organic dementia to be misdiagnosed initially as a psychiatric illness. A mistaken diagnosis is particularly common in the elderly, in whom the behavioral changes of dementia may be attributed to depression. Conversely, the severely depressed patient may appear disoriented and perform poorly in all aspects of intellectual function. These deficits are caused by the psychomotor retardation, apathy, and loss of interest that accompanies depression. Such intellectual impairments may be due to reversible neurochemical changes that mimic the irreversible changes of degenerative dementias. The distinction may be difficult, but the correct diagnosis of depression is often suggested by a history of sudden onset, marked sleep disturbance, a previous history of psychiatric illness, or precipitation by an emotional event. In addition, depressed patients often complain to a greater extent about difficulties with mentation that seems justified from their performance on tests of intellectual function. In contrast, the patient with true dementia rarely complains appropriately about deficits that are obvious on examination. Dementia due to depression may also be suggested by inconsistency during the history; for example, patients may give a clear account of some topic of interest to them or recount the history and details of their personal lives reasonably well but then show inconsistent difficulties with specific questions, often failing even to attempt an answer. Variability in performance during testing, particularly improvement with encouragement, is characteristic. Negative neurologic investigation supports the diagnosis of pseudodementia but may also be found in organic dementia. The only way to confirm the diagnosis is to demonstrate improvement in intellectual functioning with appropriate psychiatric treatment (see Chap. 368).

Pseudodementias may also occur as a *hysterical phenomenon,* when amnesia is often striking. In one variety of pseudodementia (Ganser syndrome) the answers to simple questions are often inaccurate but the patient may retain a sense of the purpose of the question ("approximate" answers) indicating that, despite the absurdity of the answer, the question is understood and the correct answer is known to the patient. In hysterical pseudodementia and the Ganser syndrome the apparent severe disturbance of intellect is not reflected in the patient's behavior. Frank simulation of dementia is rare, although the distinction between hysteria and malingering is not always clear. Intellectual impairment is a feature of *mania* and *schizophrenia;* the diagnosis is made from the accompanying thought disorder (see Chap. 368).

INVESTIGATION The age, history, and clinical findings will dictate the selection of screening tests (Table 30-4). Investigations essential in all patients are aimed at excluding reversible causes of dementia. Ideally, every patient with dementia should have an *MRI* or *CT scan* to exclude treatable intracranial pathology, especially in the presence of focal clinical signs, a history of subacute illness, or a younger age of patient. Scanning is less likely to influence management if the patient is elderly and has a long history of degenerative dementia. In Alzheimer's disease the scan may show progressive cortical atrophy and ventricular dilatation, but this is not invariable and can also be found in normal aging. The CT or MRI may show areas of low attenuation or abnormal signal in the deep white matter, particularly in the periventricular regions and centrum semiovale, referred to by the descriptive term *leuko-araiosis.* These findings are characteristic of Binswanger's disease but are not specific and can also be seen in Alzheimer's disease, in patients with cerebrovascular disease who are not demented, and in apparently normal subjects. The *electroencephalogram* may show features that support the diagnosis of Alzheimer's disease, subacute sclerosing panencephalitis, or Creutzfeldt-Jakob disease. *CSF examination* is normal in the primary degenerative dementias but may be useful if there is doubt about the diagnosis and is essential if there is a suspicion of intracranial infection. *Regional cerebral blood flow studies* (e.g., single-photon emission computed tomography) may sometimes be useful in distinguishing between frontal lobe dementias and Alzheimer's disease or in demonstrating multifocal deficits in vascular dementia. *Cerebral angiography* is rarely helpful except for the further investigation of suspected vascular dementia, vasculitis, or intracranial masses. *Neuropsychologic testing* (such as the Wechsler Adult Intelligence Scale) may help document intellectual decline or identify pseudodementia. *Meningeal and brain biopsy* may occasionally be justified when infection, vasculitis, or treatable tumor is suspected and occasionally in younger patients when etiology remains in doubt.

MANAGEMENT The initial management includes treatment of any reversible cause of dementia or superimposed confusional state. Approximately 10 percent of patients with dementia have a treatable neurologic or systemic illness, and another 10 percent have pseudodementia due to treatable psychiatric illnesses. A modifiable contributory cause such as alcoholism or hypertension is present in a further

TABLE 30-4 Investigation of dementia

In all cases:
- Blood count and erythrocyte sedimentation rate
- Blood sugar
- Serum electrolytes and calcium
- Liver function tests
- Thyroid function tests
- Serum B_{12} and folate
- Serology for syphilis
- Chest x-ray
- Electroencephalogram
- CT or MRI scan

In selected cases:
- CSF examination
- Neuropsychologic testing
- Human immunodeficiency virus antibodies
- Infectious diseases screen
- Autoantibody screen and immunoglobulins
- Serum copper and ceruloplasmin
- Drug and toxin screen
- Arterial blood gases
- Cerebral angiography
- Cerebral blood flow studies

In very selected cases:
- Brain biopsy

In suspected metabolic diseases:
- White cell enzyme screen
- Urinary and plasma amino acids
- Plasma pyruvate and lactate
- Urinary and fecal porphyrins
- Bone marrow, liver, nerve, muscle, or rectal biopsy

10 percent. Unfortunately, the remainder have irreversible dementia so that management aims to support the patient and the family.

The mildly demented patient may continue relatively normal activities at home but rarely at work. As the dementia progresses, more supervision is required, but the patient may still be capable of simple tasks. As the disorder deepens, the patient requires increasing help with the activities of daily life. The supervision required depends on the individual. Some fairly severely impaired patients can live alone if they have support from the community, including daily visits from family or friends, regular visits by a community nurse, the provision of meals, and help from neighbors. Many mildly demented individuals become disoriented and confused when removed to unfamiliar surroundings such as a hospital but may manage adequately in their homes.

In the early stages the patient may be helped by treatment of associated depression, anxiety, agitation, psychotic symptoms, or insomnia with appropriate psychotropic medication. However, psychotropic drugs may make demented patients more confused, requiring reduction or withdrawal of the medication. The demands on relatives caring for a severely demented patient are high, especially if the patient is restless at night and requires constant supervision to prevent wandering or personal harm. The fact that individuals may live for many years in such a state increases the burden. The situation often becomes intolerable when incontinence develops. Sleep deprivation and physical exhaustion aggravate the stress of caring for a demented relative, who may appear ungrateful, cantankerous, aggressive, or disinhibited. Sympathetic attention to the relatives of the demented is therefore important. It may help to obtain a "baby sitter" to allow the caregiver regular time off. If the caregiver can do so without undue feelings of guilt, an annual holiday while the patient is placed in a nursing home temporarily is invaluable.

Eventually, many demented patients require full-time nursing care in a residential home or hospital. Relatives should be encouraged to plan for this and should be counseled not to regard this outcome as a personal failure. In the later stages management aims at preserving the patient's dignity and comfort.

REFERENCES

ANTHONY JC et al: Limits of the "Mini-Mental State" as a screening test for dementia and delirium among hospital patients. Psychol Med 12:397, 1982

BLESSED G et al: The association between quantitative measures of dementia and of senile change in the cerebral grey matter of elderly subjects, appendix. Br J Psychiatry 114:797, 1968

BROWN MM, HACHINSKI VC: Vascular dementia. Curr Opinion Neurol Neurosurg 2:78, 1989

CUMMINGS JL: Subcortical dementia: Neuropsychology, neuropsychiatry, and pathophysiology. Br J Psychiatry 149:682, 1989

——— et al: Reversible dementia: Illustrative cases, definition, and review. JAMA 243:2434, 1980

GESCHWIND N: Disorders of attention: A frontier in neuropsychology. Phil Trans R Soc Lond 198:173, 1982

GUBERMAN A, STUSS D: The syndrome of bilateral paramedian thalamic infarction. Neurol 33:540, 1983

GUSTAFSON L: Frontal lobe degeneration of non-Alzheimer type. Clinical picture and differential diagnosis. Arch Geront Geriat 6:209, 1987

HACHINSKI VC et al: Cerebral blood flow in dementia. Arch Neurol 32:632, 1975

KOPELMAN MD: Amnesia: Organic and psychogenic. Br J Psychiatry 150:428, 1987

LIPOWSKI ZJ: Delirium (acute confusional state), in *Handbook of Clinical Neurology*. Amsterdam, Elsevier, 1985, vol 46, pp 523–559

LISHMAN WA: Organic Psychiatry: The Psychological Consequences of Cerebral Disorder, 2d ed. Oxford, Blackwell, 1987

MESULAM M et al: Acute confusional states with right middle cerebral artery infarctions. J Neurol Neursurg Psychiatry 39:84, 1976

MILLER JW et al: Transient global amnesia: Clinical characteristics and prognosis. Neurol 37:733, 1987

ROMAN GC: Senile dementia of the Binswanger type: A vascular form of dementia in the elderly. JAMA 258:1782, 1987

ROTH M, IVERSEN LL (eds): Alzheimer's disease and related disorders. Br Med Bull 42:1, 1986

SCHOLTZ CL: Dementia in middle and late life. Curr Top Pathol 76:105, 1988

WADE JPH, HACHINSKI VC: Multi-infarct dementia, in *Dementia (Medicine in Old Age)*, BM Pitt (ed). London, Churchill Livingstone, 1987, pp 209–228

31 COMA AND OTHER DISORDERS OF CONSCIOUSNESS

ALLAN H. ROPPER / JOSEPH B. MARTIN

Coma is a common problem in general medicine; it is estimated that up to 3 percent of admissions to the emergency ward of large municipal hospitals are due to diseases that cause a disorder of consciousness. The importance of this class of neurologic disorders points to the necessity of acquiring a systematic approach to their diagnosis and management.

The increased availability of computed tomography (CT) and magnetic resonance imaging (MRI) has resulted in an artificial focus on lesions that are radiologically detectable (e.g., hemorrhages, tumors, or hydrocephalus) in the diagnosis of coma. This approach, although at times expedient, is often imprudent because most coma is metabolic or toxic in origin. The physician confronted with an unresponsive patient should formulate a differential diagnosis based on the history and the clinical signs before leaving the bedside. Certain signs observed during general and neurologic examination allow the physician to decide which of several generic diseases is responsible for coma, thus limiting the diagnostic possibilities. A rational approach to the precise diagnosis and subsequent management can then be planned and clinical changes anticipated. The clinical approach must be coupled with knowledge of the pathologic entities that cause coma. This chapter describes a practical approach to coma based on the anatomy and physiology of consciousness, the general and neurologic examination, and CT and MRI.

Coma is epitomized by unresponsiveness and as such is easily recognized. The interesting and sometimes subtle distinctions made between coma, stupor, and drowsiness are at times clinically useful to transmit information concisely, but are largely semantic, because there is no anatomic or physiologic basis for distinguishing them except as relative degrees of unresponsiveness. A narrative description of the clinical state of the patient and of responses evoked by various stimuli, precisely as they are observed at the bedside, remains the optimal way to characterize coma and related disturbances of consciousness. Such a description is preferable to summary terms such as *semicoma* or *obtundation,* which are often ambiguous and commonly differ between observers. *Stupor,* as currently used, implies a state from which the patient can be aroused by vigorous stimuli but verbal responses are slow or absent and the patient makes some effort to avoid uncomfortable stimuli; *coma* suggests a state from which the patient cannot be aroused by stimulation, and no purposeful attempt is made to avoid painful stimuli.

Although the definition of consciousness is a psychological and philosophical matter, the distinction between *level* of consciousness, or wakefulness, and *content* of consciousness, or awareness, has physiologic significance. Wakefulness or alertness is maintained by a diffuse system of upper brainstem and thalamic neurons, the reticular activating system (RAS), and its connections to the cerebral hemispheres as a whole. Therefore, depression of either hemispheral or RAS activity may cause reduced wakefulness. Awareness is dependent on integrated and organized material thoughts, subjective experience, emotions, and mental processes, each of which resides to some extent in anatomically defined regions of the brain. The inability to maintain a coherent sequence of thoughts and actions is called *confusion* and is a disorder of content of consciousness. Reduced wakefulness often precludes evaluation of content of consciousness (for example, most stuporous patients can be said to be confused), but content of consciousness can be severely impaired, as in confusion, without affecting arousal. Confusion is used to describe a state of inattention and lack of clarity in thinking (see Chap. 30). In special cases it is accompanied by illusions (misperceptions of environmental sight, sound, or touch) or hallucinations (spontaneous endogenous perceptions). Psychiatrists often use the term *delirium* for any confusion, but delirium is usually reserved as a description for an agitated, hypersympathotonic, frequently hallucinatory state most often due to specific causes such as alcohol or drug withdrawal. Usually, the confused patient is subdued, not inclined to speak, and less active physically than usual. Many processes that ultimately lead to coma begin with confusion, and diagnostic considerations should address the primary problem as an alteration in the level of consciousness. Confusion alone generally indicates a metabolic derangement, although focal cerebral lesions that cause deficits in language, orientation, or memory may make the patient appear to be confused.

ANATOMIC CORRELATES OF CONSCIOUSNESS A normal level of consciousness (wakefulness) depends upon activation of the cerebral hemispheres by groups of neurons located in the brainstem RAS. Both of the cerebral hemispheres, the RAS, and the connections between them must be preserved for normal consciousness. The principal causes of coma are, therefore, (1) bilateral hemispheral damage or suppression by drugs or toxins and (2) a brainstem lesion or metabolic derangement that damages or suppresses the RAS. There is some evidence that large, purely unilateral hemispheral lesions particularly on the left may cause drowsiness (though not coma) even in the absence of damage to the opposite hemisphere or RAS.

Reticular activating system The RAS is best defined as a physiologic system, not an anatomic one. It is contained within the reticular formation, which consists of loosely grouped neurons located bilaterally in the medial tegmental gray matter of the brainstem extending from the medulla to the posterior diencephalon. These neurons have been shown in neuroanatomic studies to span long rostrocaudal distances within the reticular formation. Animal experiments and human clinical-neuropathologic observations have established that the *neurons located in the region extending from the rostral pons to the caudal diencephalon are of primary importance for maintaining wakefulness.* Lesions here that produce coma also commonly affect adjacent brainstem structures concerned with control of pupillary constriction and mechanisms for eye movements (Fig. 31-1). Abnormalities in these systems on physical examination provide signposts of brainstem damage. Lesions confined to the cerebral hemispheres do not directly affect the brainstem RAS, though secondary dysfunction of the upper brainstem may result from compression by a mass in a cerebral hemisphere.

Brainstem RAS neurons project rostrally to the cortex, primarily via "nonspecific" thalamic relay nuclei which exert a tonic influence on the activity of the cerebral cortex. Experimental work in primates suggests that the brainstem RAS indirectly affects the level of consciousness by suppressing the activity of the nonspecific nuclei. Electrical stimulation of the pontine and midbrain RAS desynchronizes the electroencephalogram (EEG), a pattern associated with behavioral arousal. Stimulation of the thalamic relay nuclei opposes this activity, resulting in synchronization and slowing of the EEG. The basis of behavioral arousal by environmental stimuli (somesthetic, auditory, and visual) depends on the rich innervation of the RAS by each sensory system.

The relay between the RAS and thalamic and cortical areas is accomplished by neurotransmitters. Of these, the influences of acetylcholine and norepinephrine on arousals have been studied most extensively. Cholinergic fibers connect the midbrain to other areas of the upper brainstem, thalamus, and cortex. These pathways are thought to mediate the clinical and EEG arousal observed after administration of cholinergic drugs such as physostigmine. Serotonin and norepinephrine also subserve important functions in the regulation of the sleep-wake cycle (see Chap. 34). Their roles in arousal and coma have not been clearly established, although the alerting effects of amphetamines are likely to be mediated by catecholamine release.

Cerebral hemispheres and consciousness The specialized functions of the cerebral cortex in language, control of movement, and perception are regionalized (see Chaps. 30, 32, and 33). In contrast, wakefulness is related in a semiquantitative way to the total mass of functioning cortex (and RAS connections) and is not focally represented in any region of the hemispheres. Hemispheral lesions may cause coma in one of three ways: (1) most commonly, bilateral, generalized hemispheral lesions or metabolic derangements such as occur in encephalitis, generalized epilepsy, drug ingestion, global brain ischemia, and hypoglycemia interfere with awareness in a graded fashion as more cortical territory is damaged or rendered functionally inactive; (2) rarely, enlarging masses or secondary brain swelling initially confined to one side of the brain may compress the contralateral hemisphere, effectively creating bilateral hemispheral lesions; and (3) large lesions in one or both hemispheres may compress the brainstem and diencephalic RAS causing coma indirectly. *The degree of decrease in alertness is often related to the acuteness of onset of the cortical dysfunction.*

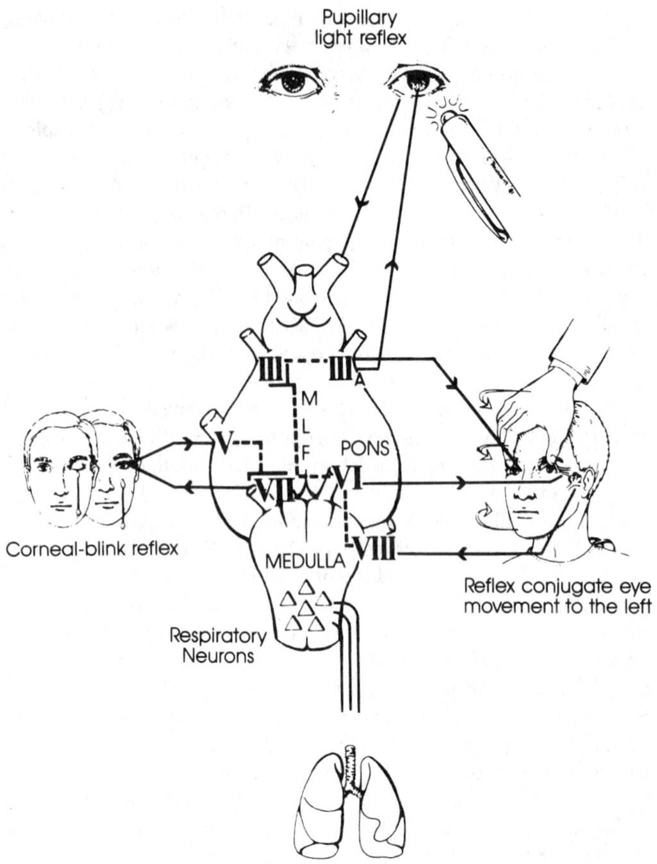

FIGURE 31-1 Brainstem reflexes in the coma examination. Midbrain and third nerve function are tested by pupillary reaction to light, pontine function by spontaneous and reflex eye movements and corneal responses, and medullary function by respiratory and pharyngeal responses.

Reflex conjugate, horizontal eye movements are dependent upon the medial longitudinal fasciculus (MLF) interconnecting the sixth and contralateral third nerve nuclei. Eye movements are elicited by head rotation (oculocephalic reflex) or caloric stimulation of the labyrinths (oculovestibular reflex). These reflex movements are suppressed in the awake patient by the cerebral hemispheres via their connections to the brainstem.

The concept of *transtentorial herniation* with progressive brainstem compression has been used to explain neurologic signs in coma caused by supratentorial mass lesions. Herniation refers to displacement of brain tissue away from a mass, past a less mobile structure such as dura, and into a space that it normally does not occupy. Herniation suggests a degree of irreversibility because the tissue is trapped in its new location. The common herniations seen at postmortem are transfalcial (under the falx in the anterior midline), transtentorial (into the tentorial opening), and cerebellar tonsillar (into the foramen magnum). Uncal transtentorial herniation, or impaction of the uncal gyrus into the cistern between the free edge of the tentorium and lateral edge of the midbrain, causes compression of the third nerve with pupillary dilation and subsequent coma due to midbrain compression. Central transtentorial herniation denotes downward movement of the diencephalon (thalamic region) through the tentorial opening in the midline and is heralded by miotic pupils and drowsiness. In both cases, an orderly progression of rostral to caudal compression of first the midbrain, then the pons, and finally the medulla leads to the sequential appearance of neurologic signs corresponding to the level damaged, and to progressively diminished alertness. However, many patients with supratentorial masses do not follow these stereotypic patterns; an orderly progression of signs from midbrain to medulla is rarely seen in catastrophic lesions where all brainstem functions are lost almost simultaneously. Furthermore, drowsiness and stupor typically occur with moderate lateral shifts at the level of the diencephalon (3 to 8 mm) when there is only 1- to 3-mm vertical displacement of structures near the tentorial opening, and before actual downward herniation is evident on a CT or MRI scan.

PATHOPHYSIOLOGY OF COMA The pathophysiologic basis of coma is either mechanical destruction of crucial areas of the brainstem or cerebral cortex (anatomic coma) or global disruption of brain metabolic processes (metabolic coma). Coma of metabolic origin may be produced by interruption of energy substrate delivery (hypoxia, ischemia, hypoglycemia) or by alteration of the neurophysiologic responses of neuronal membranes (drug or alcohol intoxication, epilepsy, or acute head injury).

The brain is markedly dependent on continuous blood flow and delivery of oxygen and glucose, which are consumed at rates of 3.5 mL per 100 g/min and 5 mg per 100 g/min, respectively. Brain stores of glucose provide energy for approximately 2 min after blood flow is interrupted, although consciousness is lost within 8 to 10 s. When hypoxia occurs simultaneously with ischemia, available glucose is exhausted more rapidly. Normal resting cerebral blood flow (CBF) is approximately 75 mL per 100 g/min in gray matter and 30 mL per 100 g/min in white matter (mean = 55 mL per 100 g/min). This provides for adequate metabolic supplies with a modest safety factor to accommodate most physiologic changes. When mean CBF diminishes to 25 mL per 100 g/min, the EEG becomes diffusely slowed (typical of metabolic encephalopathies), and at 15 mL per 100 g/min brain electrical activity ceases. If all other conditions such as temperature and arterial oxygenation remain normal, CBF less than 10 mL per 100 g/min causes irreversible brain damage.

Coma due to hyponatremia, hyperosmolarity, hypercapnia, and the encephalopathies of hepatic and renal failure are associated with a variety of metabolic derangements of neurons and astrocytes. The toxic effects of these conditions on the brain are not well understood, but may be multifactorial, producing impaired energy supplies, changes in resting membrane potentials, neurotransmitter abnormalities, and in some instances morphologic changes. For example, the high brain ammonia concentration associated with hepatic coma has been theorized to interfere with cerebral energy metabolism and the Na^+,K^+-ATPase pump, increase the number and size of astrocytes, result in increased concentrations of potentially toxic products of ammonia metabolism, and result in abnormalities of neurotransmitters, including possible "false" neurotransmitters, which may act competitively at monoaminergic receptor sites.

The exact cause of the encephalopathy of renal failure is also poorly understood. Unlike ammonia, urea itself does not produce nervous system toxicity. A multifactorial cause is likely, including increased permeability of the blood-brain barrier to toxic substances such as organic acids and an increase in brain calcium or cerebrospinal fluid (CSF) phosphate content.

Abnormalities of osmolarity are involved in the coma and seizures caused by several medical disorders including diabetic ketoacidosis, the nonketotic hyperosmolar state, and hyponatremia. In hyperosmolarity, brain volume is reduced while hypoosmolarity leads to brain swelling. Brain water volume correlates best with level of consciousness in hyponatremic-hypoosmolar states but other factors probably also play a role. Sodium levels below 115 mmol/L are associated with coma and convulsions, depending to some extent on the rapidity with which the hyponatremia develops. Serum osmolarity is generally above 350 mosmol/L in hyperosmolar coma.

Hypercapnia produces a diminished level of consciousness proportional to the P_{CO_2} tension in the blood and to acuteness of onset. A relationship between CSF acidosis and severity of symptoms has been established. The pathophysiology of other metabolic encephalopathies such as hypercalcemia, hypothyroidism, vitamin B_{12} deficiency, and hypothermia are incompletely understood but probably reflect multifaceted derangements of cerebral biochemistry.

Central nervous system (CNS) depressant drugs and some endogenous toxins probably produce coma by suppression of metabolic and membrane electrical activities in both the RAS and cerebral cortex. For this reason combinations of cortical and brainstem signs occur in drug overdose and other metabolic comas which may lead to a specious diagnosis of structural brainstem damage. Certain anesthetic agents also have a predilection for affecting the brainstem RAS neurons out of proportion to the cortex.

Although all metabolic derangements alter neuronal electrophysiology, the disturbance of brain electrical activity most commonly encountered in clinical practice is epilepsy. Continuous, generalized electrical discharges of the cortex may be associated with coma even in the absence of epileptic motor activity. Coma following seizures (postictal state) may be due to exhaustion of energy metabolites or be secondary to locally toxic molecules produced during the seizures. Recovery from postictal unresponsiveness occurs when neuronal metabolic balance is restored. The postictal state produces a pattern of continuous, generalized slowing of the background EEG activity similar to that of metabolic encephalopathy.

Endogenous "excitatoxins" such as glutamate released after injury have been found to cause secondary neuronal damage in experimental models of ischemia. These endogenous "neurotoxins" act to allow calcium influx into cells, a mechanism thought to lead to neuronal death. This mechanism may play a role in the genesis of coma, or at least in its neuropathologic changes, after global ischemia.

PRACTICAL APPROACH TO THE COMATOSE PATIENT The diagnosis and acute management of coma depend on understanding the pitfalls of examining the comatose patient, an interpretation of brainstem reflexes, and the wise use of diagnostic tests. Acute respiratory and cardiovascular problems should generally be attended to prior to neurologic diagnosis. The complete medical evaluation, except for the vital signs, fundoscopy, and examination for nuchal rigidity, may be deferred until the neurologic evaluation has established the severity and nature of coma.

History In many cases the cause of coma is immediately evident (e.g., trauma, cardiac arrest, and known drug ingestion). However, in the remainder, historical information about the onset of coma is often sparse. The most useful historical points, when obtainable, are (1) the circumstances and temporal profile of the onset of neurologic symptoms, (2) the precise details of preceding neurologic symptoms (weakness, headaches, seizures, dizziness, diplopia, or vomiting), (3) the use of drugs or alcohol, and (4) history of liver, kidney, lung, heart, or other medical disease. Telephone calls to family and observers on the scene are an important part of the initial evaluation.

Physical examination and general observations The temperature, pulse, respiratory rate and pattern, and blood pressure should be measured. Fever suggests systemic infection, bacterial meningitis, or a brain lesion that has disturbed the temperature-regulating centers. High body temperature, 42 to 44°C, associated with dry skin should arouse the suspicion of heat stroke or anticholinergic drug intoxication. Hypothermia is observed with bodily exposure; alcoholic, barbiturate, or phenothiazine intoxication; hypoglycemia; peripheral circulatory failure; or myxedema. Hypothermia causes coma directly only when the temperature is below 31°C. Aberrant respiratory patterns that may reflect brainstem disorders are discussed below. A change of pulse rate combined with hyperventilation and hypertension may signal an increase in intracranial pressure. Marked hypertension occurs in patients with hypertensive encephalopathy, cerebral hemorrhage, and other causes of acutely increased intracranial pressure. Hypotension occurs in the coma of alcohol or barbiturate intoxication, internal hemorrhage, myocardial infarction, gram-negative bacillary septicemia, and Addisonian crisis. The funduscopic examination is useful in detecting subarachnoid hemorrhage (subhyaloid hemorrhages), hypertensive encephalopathy (exudates, hemorrhages, vessel-crossing changes), and increased intracranial pressure (papilledema). Generalized cutaneous petechiae suggest thrombotic thrombocytopenic purpura or a bleeding diathesis associated with intracerebral hemorrhage.

General neurologic assessment An exact description of spontaneous and elicited movements in coma is of great value in establishing the level of neurologic dysfunction. The patient's state is observed first without examiner intervention. The nature of respirations, similarity to sleep, and spontaneous movements are observed. Patients who toss about, reach up toward the face, cross the midline with an arm, cross their legs, yawn, swallow, cough, or moan are closest to being awake. Adventitious movements or postures may be subtle and must be specifically sought. For example, the only sign of seizures may be small excursion twitching of a foot, finger, or facial muscle. An outturned leg at rest or lack of restless movements on one side suggests a hemiparesis.

The terms *decorticate* and *decerebrate rigidity* or "posturing" have been adapted from animal experiments to describe stereotyped tonic flexor and extensor arm movements, respectively, with extension of the legs. Spontaneous flexion of the elbows and wrists and arm supination (decortication) suggest severe bilateral damage in the hemispheres above the midbrain, while extension of the elbows and wrists with pronation (decerebration) suggests damage in the midbrain or diencephalon. Arm extension with weak leg flexion or flaccid legs has been associated with lesions in the low pons. Acute lesions, however, frequently cause limb extension regardless of location, and almost all extensor posturing becomes flexor in nature as time passes, so posturing alone cannot be depended upon to make an accurate anatomic localization. Metabolic coma, especially after acute hypoxia, may also produce vigorous spontaneous extensor (decerebrate) rigidity. Posturing may alternate or coexist with purposeful limb movements, usually reflecting subtotal damage to the motor system. Multifocal myoclonus is almost always an indication of metabolic disorder, particularly azotemia, or drug ingestion. In an awake, confused patient, asterixis is a certain sign of metabolic encephalopathy or ingestion of a drug, particularly phenytoin.

Elicited movements and level of arousal A sequence of increasingly intense stimuli is used to determine the patient's best level of arousal and the optimal motor response of each limb. If the patient is not aroused by conversational voice, shouting should be tried. Shaking the patient is attempted next, then painful pressure on the limbs. Nasal tickle with a cotton wisp is a strong arousal stimulus. Deep pressure on the knuckles or bony prominences is the preferred and humane form of noxious stimulus. Pinching the skin over the face or chest may cause unsightly ecchymoses and is rarely necessary.

Responses to noxious stimuli should be appraised critically. Abduction avoidance movement of a limb is a purposeful, cortically derived action and denotes an intact corticospinal system to that limb. If abduction is present in all limbs, it is a reliable sign of only minimal motor dysfunction. Stereotyped posturing following stimulation of a limb indicates severe dysfunction of the corticospinal system. Adduction and flexion of the stimulated limbs may occur as reflex movements and do not imply an intact corticospinal system. Brief clonic or twitching limb movements frequently occur at the end of extensor posturing excursions and should not be mistaken for seizures.

Brainstem reflexes Brainstem signs are a key to the localization of the causative lesion in coma (Fig. 31-1). As a rule, coma associated with normal brainstem function indicates widespread and bilateral hemispheral disease or dysfunction. The brainstem contains several intrinsic reflexes that are convenient to examine. Normal pupillary symmetry, size, shape, and reaction to light indicate intact functioning of the upper midbrain and efferent parasympathetic fibers of the third cranial nerve responsible for pupillary constriction. (The afferent component of the light reflex utilizes the optic nerve.) Pupillary reaction should be examined with a bright diffuse light and, if absent, confirmed with a magnifying lens. Light reaction in pupils smaller than 2 mm is often difficult to appreciate. Excessive room lighting mutes pupillary reactivity. Equal and reactive round pupils (2.5 to 5 mm in diameter) usually exclude midbrain damage as the cause of coma. An enlarged (greater than 5 mm) and unreactive or poorly reactive pupil can result either from an intrinsic midbrain lesion (on the same side) or, far more commonly, can be secondary to compression of the midbrain and/or third nerve as occurs in transtentorial herniation. Unilateral pupillary enlargement usually denotes an ipsilateral mass but rarely can occur contralaterally by compression of the midbrain against the opposite tentorial margin. Oval and slightly eccentric pupils (corectopia) often accompany early midbrain–third nerve compression. Bilaterally dilated and unreactive pupils indicate severe midbrain damage, usually from secondary compression by transtentorial herniation or metabolically by ingestion of drugs with anticholinergic activity. The use of mydriatic eye drops by a previous examiner, self-administration by the patient, or direct ocular trauma may cause misleading pupillary enlargement. Reactive and bilaterally small but not pinpoint pupils (1 to 2.5 mm) are most commonly seen in metabolic encephalopathy or after deep bilateral hemispheral lesions such as hydrocephalus or thalamic hemorrhage. This has been attributed to dysfunction of sympathetic nervous system efferents emerging from the posterior hypothalamus. Profound barbiturate-induced coma may produce similar-sized pupils. Very small but reactive pupils (less than 1 mm) denote narcotic overdose but may also occur with acute, extensive bilateral pontine damage, usually from hemorrhage. The response to naloxone and the presence of reflex eye movements (see below) distinguishes these. The unilaterally small pupil of a Horner's syndrome is rare in coma but may occur ipsilateral to a large cerebral hemorrhage.

Eye movements are the foundation of physical diagnosis in coma because their examination permits exploration of a large portion of the rostrocaudal extent of the brainstem. The eyes are first observed by elevating the lids and noting the resting position and spontaneous movements of the globes. Horizontal divergence of the eyes at rest is normally observed in drowsiness. As patients either awaken or slip deeper into coma, the ocular axes become parallel again. An adducted eye at rest indicates lateral rectus paresis (weakness) due to a sixth nerve lesion and may indicate damage to the pons. However, sixth nerve paresis, often bilateral, occurs with increased intracranial pressure and is then a falsely localizing sign. An abducted eye at rest, often accompanied by ipsilateral pupillary enlargement, indicates medial rectus paresis due to third nerve paresis. With few exceptions, vertical separation of the ocular axes, or *skew deviation,* results from pontine or cerebellar lesions. In hydrocephalus with dilatation of the third ventricle, the eye globes frequently rest below the horizontal meridian. Conjugate ocular deviation at rest is discussed below.

When spontaneous eye movements are present in coma, they generally take the form of conjugate horizontal roving. This motion exonerates the midbrain and pons and has the same meaning as normal reflex eye movements (see below). Cyclic vertical downward movements are seen in specific circumstances. "Ocular bobbing" describes a brisk conjugate downward and slow upward movement of the globes in situations in which horizontal eye movement mechanisms have been disrupted and is diagnostic of bilateral pontine damage. "Ocular dipping" is a slow downward movement followed by a faster upward movement in patients with normal reflex horizontal gaze. Dipping occurs particularly in patients with diffuse anoxic damage to the cerebral cortex and may be preceded by sustained up or down gaze. The eyes may turn down and inward in thalamic and upper midbrain lesions.

Doll's-eye, or *oculocephalic,* movements are tested by moving the head from side to side or vertically, first slowly then briskly. Reflex eye movements are evoked in the opposite direction to head movement (Fig. 31-1). These responses are mediated by brainstem mechanisms originating in the labyrinths, vestibular nuclei, and cervical proprioceptors. They are normally suppressed by visual fixation mediated by the cerebral hemispheres in awake patients. The neuronal pathways for reflex horizontal eye movements require integrity of the region surrounding the sixth nerve nucleus and are yoked to the contralateral third nerve via the medial longitudinal fasciculus (MLF) (Fig. 31-1). Two disparate pieces of information can be obtained from the reflex eye movements. *First,* in coma resulting from bihemispheral disease or early metabolic or drug depression, the eyes move easily or "loosely" from side to side in a direction opposite to the direction of head turning. The ease with which the globes move toward the opposite side is a reflection of disinhibition of brainstem reflexes by damaged cerebral hemispheres. In drowsy patients, the first two or three head rotations cause opposite conjugate eye movements following which the maneuver itself usually causes arousal and the reflex movements stop. *Second,* full conjugate oculocephalic movements demonstrate the integrity of brainstem pathways extending from the high cervical spinal cord and medulla, where vestibular and proprioceptive input from head turning originates, to the midbrain, where the third nerve originates. Thus, the oculocephalic maneuver is a convenient way to demonstrate the functional integrity of a large segment of brainstem pathways and to exclude a lesion in the brainstem as the cause of coma. Lack of complete adduction indicates an ipsilateral midbrain (third nerve) lesion or, alternatively, damage to the pathways mediating reflex eye movements in the MLF (i.e., internuclear ophthalmoplegia). Third nerve damage is usually associated with an enlarged pupil and horizontal ocular divergence at rest, whereas MLF destruction shows neither. Adduction of the globes is by nature more difficult to obtain with head turning than abduction, and subtle symmetric abnormalities in the doll's-eye maneuver should be interpreted with caution.

Caloric stimulation of the vestibular apparatus (*oculovestibular* or *vestibuloocular response*) is a useful adjunct to the oculocephalic test and acts as a stronger stimulus to reflex eye movements. Irrigation of the external auditory canal with cold water causes convection currents in the endolymph of the labyrinths of the inner ear. With the head at approximately 30° elevation from the supine position, endolymph movement is induced primarily in the horizontal semicircular canals. An intact brainstem response is indicated with variable latency, by tonic deviation of both eyes (lasting 30 to 120 s) to the side of cold-water irrigation. Bilateral conjugate eye movements have the same significance as full oculocephalic responses. If the cerebral hemispheres are intact, a rapid corrective conjugate movement is generated away from the side of tonic deviation. The absence of this saccadic, nystagmus-like quick phase signifies damage to the cerebral hemispheres.

Conjugate ocular deviation at rest or incomplete conjugate eye movements with head turning indicates damage in the pons on the side of the gaze paresis or frontal lobe damage on the opposite side. This phenomenon may be summarized by the phrase "the eyes look toward a hemispheral lesion and away from a brainstem lesion." It is usually possible to overcome the ocular deviation associated with frontal lobe damage by brisk head turning. Seizures may also cause aversive (opposite) eye deviation with rhythmic, jerky movements to the side of gaze. On rare occasions, the eyes may turn paradoxically away from the side of a deep hemispheral lesion ("wrong-way eyes").

A major pitfall in coma diagnosis may occur when reflex eye movements are suppressed by drugs. The eyes often move with the head as it is turned as if locked in place, thus spuriously suggesting anatomic brainstem damage. Overdoses of phenytoin, tricyclic antidepressants, and barbiturates are commonly implicated as well as, on occasion, alcohol, phenothiazines, diazepam, and neuromuscular blockers such as pancuronium. The presence of normal pupillary size and light reaction will distinguish most drug-induced coma from brainstem damage (except for pontine infarction or hemorrhage in which the pupils remain small). Small to midposition, 1- to 3-mm, nonreactive pupils may also occur with very high serum levels of barbiturates or secondary to hydrocephalus (see below).

Although the *corneal reflexes* are rarely useful alone, they may corroborate eye movement abnormalities because they also depend on the integrity of pontine pathways. By touching the cornea with a wisp of cotton, a response consisting of brief bilateral lid closure may be observed. The corneal response may be lost when the afferent fifth nerve, the efferent seventh nerve, or their reflex connections within the pons are damaged. The normal efferent response is bilateral, with closure of both eyelids. Nervous system depressant drugs diminish or eliminate the corneal responses soon after the reflex eye movements become paralyzed but before the pupils become unreactive to light.

Respiration Respiratory patterns have received much attention in coma diagnosis but are of inconsistent localizing value. Shallow, slow, but well-timed regular breathing suggests metabolic or drug depression. Rapid, deep (Kussmaul) breathing usually implies metabolic acidosis but may also occur with pontomesencephalic lesions. Cheyne-Stokes respiration in its classic cyclic form, ending with a brief apneic period, signifies mild bihemispheral damage or metabolic suppression and commonly accompanies light coma. Agonal gasps reflect bilateral lower brainstem damage and are well known as the terminal respiratory pattern of severe brain damage. In brain-dead patients, shallow respiratory-like movements with irregular, nonrepetitive back arching may be produced by hypoxia and are probably generated by the surviving cervical spinal cord and lower medulla. Other cyclic breathing variations are not usually diagnostic of specific local lesions.

COMA-LIKE SYNDROMES AND RELATED STATES The simple observation of inability to arouse a patient characterizes most comatose states. Several syndromes, however, render patients unresponsive or insensate but are considered separately because of their unusual features. The *vegetative state,* an unfortunate term, occurs in patients who were earlier comatose but whose eyelids have subsequently opened giving the appearance of being awake. There may be yawning, grunting, and random limb and head movements. These are associated with signs of extensive damage to both cerebral hemispheres, i.e., Babinski signs, decerebrate or decorticate posturing, absence of response to visual stimuli, and absent corrective nystagmus on oculovestibular testing. Autonomic nervous system functions such as cardiovascular and thermoregulatory and neuroendocrine control are preserved and may be subject to periods of overactivity. The syndrome is best viewed as a severe dementia resulting from global damage to the cerebral cortex and differs somewhat from akinetic mutism because of a complete inability to respond to commands or communicate. *Akinetic mutism* refers to a partially or fully awake patient who is immobile and silent. The state may result from hydrocephalus, from masses in the region of the third ventricle, or with lesions in the cingulate gyrus or other portions of both frontal lobes. *Abulia* is a mild form of akinetic mutism in which the patient is hypokinetic and slow to respond but generally gives correct answers. Lesions in the periaqueductal or low diencephalic regions may cause a similar state in which hypophonia is prominent. The *locked-in syndrome* (pseudocoma) describes patients who are awake but selectively deefferented, i.e., have no means of producing speech or limb, face, or pharyngeal movements. This results from infarction or hemorrhage of the ventral pons, which transects all descending corticospinal and corticobulbar pathways but spares the RAS arousal system. Vertical eye movements and lid elevation are partially preserved because these midbrain functions are outside the field of infarction in some cases of basilar artery thrombosis. Such movements can be used by the patient to signal to the examiner. A similar awake state simulating unresponsiveness may occur in severe cases of acute polyneuritis or myasthenia gravis as a result of total paralysis of limb, ocular, or bulbar musculature. Unlike basilar artery stroke, vertical eye movements are not selectively spared in these nerve and muscle diseases.

Certain psychiatric states mimic coma because they produce apparent unresponsiveness. *Catatonia* is a term for peculiar motor activities associated with major psychosis. In the typical hypomobile form catatonic patients appear awake with eyes open but make no voluntary or responsive movements, though they blink spontaneously and may not appear distressed. There may be associated "waxy flexibility" in which limbs maintain their posture when lifted by the examiner. Upon recovery, such patients have full memory of events that occurred during their catatonic stupor. Patients with *pseudocoma conversion* states (trance) have signs which indicate voluntary attempts to appear comatose. They may resist eyelid elevation, blink to threat when the lids are held open, and move the eyes concomitantly with head rotation, all signs belying brain damage.

LABORATORY EXAMINATION IN COMA Four laboratory tests are used most frequently in the diagnosis of coma: chemical-toxicologic analysis of blood and urine, CT or MRI, EEG, and cerebral spinal fluid examination.

Chemical blood determinations are routinely made to investigate metabolic, toxic, or drug-induced encephalopathies. The major metabolic aberrations encountered in clinical practice are those of electrolytes, calcium, blood urea nitrogen (BUN), glucose, and hepatic dysfunction. Toxicologic analysis is of great value in any case of coma where the diagnosis is not immediately clear. However, the presence of exogenous drugs or toxins, especially alcohol, does not ensure that other factors, particularly head trauma, may not also contribute to the clinical state.

The notion that a normal CT scan excludes anatomic lesions as the cause of coma is erroneous. Early bilateral hemisphere infarction, small brainstem lesions, encephalitis, mechanical shearing of axons as a result of closed head trauma, absent cerebral perfusion associated with brain death, sagittal sinus thrombosis, and subdural hematomas that are isodense to adjacent brain are some of the lesions that may be overlooked by CT. Nevertheless, in coma of unknown etiology, a CT scan should be obtained early in the evaluation. In those cases in which the etiology is clinically apparent, the CT provides verification and defines the extent of the lesion. For technical reasons MRI is difficult to perform in comatose patients. It also has the disadvantage of not demonstrating hemorrhages as well as CT (see Chap. 348).

The EEG is rarely diagnostic in coma, with the occasional exceptions of coma due to ongoing clinically unrecognized seizures, herpes virus encephalitis, and Creutzfeldt-Jakob disease. The EEG, however, may suggest metabolic encephalopathy and provide important information about the general electrophysiologic state of the cortex. The amount of background slowing of the EEG is useful for gauging and following the severity of any diffuse encephalopathy. The EEG pattern of "alpha coma" is defined by widespread, invariant 8- to 12-Hz activity superficially resembling the normal alpha rhythm of waking, but which is unresponsive to environmental stimuli. Alpha coma results from either high pontine or diffuse cortical damage and is associated with a poor prognosis. Coma due to persistent epileptic discharges that are not clinically manifested may be revealed by EEG recordings. Normal alpha activity on the EEG may also alert the clinician to the "locked-in" syndrome. Evoked potential recordings (auditory and somatosensory) are currently under investigation as additional methods of coma diagnosis and monitoring.

Lumbar puncture is now used more judiciously than previously because the CT scan excludes intracerebral hemorrhages and most subarachnoid hemorrhages. The use of lumbar puncture in coma is limited to diagnosis of meningitis-encephalitis, occasional cases of subarachnoid hemorrhage, and cases with normal CT in which the origin of coma is obscure. If the CT is normal or unavailable and suspicion of meningeal infection or subarachnoid hemorrhage remains, then the CSF should be examined for white cells, microorganisms, and blood. Xanthochromia is documented by spinning the CSF in a large tube and comparing the supernatant to water. Yellow coloration indicates preexisting blood in the CSF and permits exclusion of a traumatic puncture. In addition, initial and final tubes should be inspected for a decrement in the number of erythrocytes, indicating traumatic puncture.

DIFFERENTIAL DIAGNOSIS OF COMA In most instances, coma is part of an obvious medical problem such as known drug ingestion, hypoxia, stroke, trauma, or liver or kidney failure. Attention is appropriately focused on the primary illness. A complete listing of all diseases which cause coma would serve little purpose since it would not aid diagnosis. Some general rules, however, are helpful. Illnesses which cause sudden or acute coma are due to drug ingestion or to one of the catastrophic brain lesions—hemorrhage, trauma, hypoxia, or, rarely, acute basilar artery occlusion. Coma which appears subacutely is usually related to preceding medical or neurologic problems, including the secondary brain swelling which surrounds a preexisting lesion. Coma diagnosis, therefore, requires familiarity with the common intracerebral catastrophies. These are described in more detail in Chap. 351, but may be summarized as follows: (1) basal ganglia and thalamic hemorrhage (acute but not instantaneous onset, vomiting, headache, hemiplegia, and characteristic eye signs); (2) subarachnoid hemorrhage (instantaneous onset, severe headache, neck stiffness, vomiting, third or sixth nerve lesions, transient loss of consciousness, or sudden coma with vigorous extensor posturing); (3) pontine hemorrhage (sudden onset, pinpoint pupils, loss of reflex eye movements and corneal responses, ocular bobbing, posturing, hyperventilation, and sweating); (4) cerebellar hemorrhage (occipital headache, vomiting, gaze paresis, and inability to stand); (5) basilar artery thrombosis (neurologic prodrome or warning spells, diplopia, dysarthria, vomiting, eye movement and corneal response abnormalities, and asymmetric limb paresis). The commonest stroke, namely, infarction in the territory of the middle cerebral artery, does not cause coma acutely. The syndrome of acute hydrocephalus causing coma may accompany many intracranial catastrophes, particularly subarachnoid hemorrhage. Acute symmetric enlargement of both lateral ventricles causes headache and vomiting. Further ventricular enlargement leads to drowsiness that may progress quickly to coma, with extensor posturing of the limbs, bilateral Babinski signs, often small (1 mm diameter) nonreactive pupils, and impaired vertical oculocephalic movements.

If the history and examination are not typical for any neurologic diagnosis and metabolic or drug causes are excluded, then information obtained from CT may be used as outlined in Table 31-1. The neurologic examination remains preeminent because it allows localization of lesions to one or both hemispheres or to the brainstem (with the exceptions noted above). The CT scan is useful to focus the differential diagnosis, and because of its accuracy and general availability, the diagnoses which it facilitates are listed in the table. The majority of medical causes of coma are established without a CT or with the study being normal.

COMA AFTER HEAD TRAUMA Concussion is a common form of transient coma which probably results from torsion of the hemispheres about the midbrain-diencephalic junction with brief interruption of RAS function. Persistent coma after head trauma presents a more complex and serious problem (Chap. 352).

EMERGENCY TREATMENT OF THE COMATOSE PATIENT The immediate goal in acute coma is prevention of further nervous system damage. Hypotension, hypoglycemia, hypoxia, hypercapnia, and hyperthermia should be rapidly and assiduously corrected. An oropharyngeal airway is adequate to keep the pharynx open in drowsy patients who are breathing normally. Tracheal intubation is indicated if there is obvious apnea, hypoventilation, or emesis, or if the patient is liable to aspirate. Mechanical ventilation is required if the patient is apneic or hypoventilating or if there is an intracranial mass and hypocapnia is therapeutically necessary. An intravenous access is established and naloxone and dextrose administered if narcotic overdose or hypoglycemia are even remote possibilities. Thiamine is generally administered with glucose in order to prevent an exacerbation of Wernicke's encephalopathy. The veins of intravenous drug abusers may be difficult to cannulate; in such cases, naloxone can be injected sublingually through a small-gauge needle. In cases of suspected basilar thrombosis with brainstem ischemia, intravenous heparin is administered after obtaining a CT scan, keeping in mind that cerebellar and pontine hemorrhages resemble the syndrome of basilar artery occlusion. Physostigmine, when used by experienced physicians with careful monitoring, may awaken patients with anticholinergic-type

TABLE 31-1 Approach to the differential diagnosis of coma

I Normal brainstem reflexes, no lateralizing signs
- *A* Anatomic lesions of hemisphere found
  - *1* Hydrocephalus
  - *2* Bilateral subdural hematomas
  - *3* Bilateral contusions, edema, or axonal shearing of hemispheres due to closed head trauma, subarachnoid hemorrhage
- *B* Bilateral hemispheral dysfunction without mass lesion (CT normal)
  - *1* Drug-toxin ingestion (toxicologic analysis)
  - *2* Endogenous metabolic encephalopathy (glucose, ammonia, calcium, osmolarity, P_{O_2}, P_{CO_2}, urea, sodium)
  - *3* Shock, hypertensive encephalopathy
  - *4* Meningitis (CSF analysis)
  - *5* Nonherpetic viral encephalitis (CSF analysis)
  - *6* Epilepsy (EEG)
  - *7* Reye's syndrome (ammonia, increased intracranial pressure)
  - *8* Fat embolism
  - *9* Subarachnoid hemorrhage with normal CT (CSF analysis)
  - *10* Acute disseminated encephalomyelitis (CSF analysis)
  - *11* Acute hemorrhagic leukoencephalitis
  - *12* Advanced Alzheimer's and Creutzfeldt-Jakob disease

II Normal brainstem reflexes (with or without unilateral compressive third nerve palsy), lateralizing motor signs (CT abnormal)
- *A* Unilateral mass lesion found
  - *1* Cerebral hemorrhage (basal ganglia, thalamus)
  - *2* Large infarction with surrounding brain edema
  - *3* Herpes virus encephalitis (temporal lobe lesion)
  - *4* Subdural or epidural hematoma
  - *5* Tumor with edema
  - *6* Brain abscess with edema
  - *7* Vasculitis with multiple infarctions
  - *8* Metabolic encephalopathy superimposed on preexisting focal lesions (i.e., stroke)
  - *9* Pituitary apoplexy
- *B* Asymmetric signs accompanied by diffuse hemispheral dysfunction
  - *1* Metabolic encephalopathies with asymmetric signs (blood chemical determinations)
  - *2* Isodense subdural hematoma (brain scan, angiogram)
  - *3* Thrombotic thrombocytopenic purpura (blood smear, platelet count)
  - *4* Epilepsy with focal seizures or postictal state (EEG)

III Multiple brainstem reflex abnormalities
- *A* Anatomic lesions in brainstem found
  - *1* Pontine, midbrain hemorrhage
  - *2* Cerebellar hemorrhage, tumor, abscess
  - *3* Cerebellar infarction with brainstem compression
  - *4* Mass in hemisphere causing advanced bilateral brainstem compression
  - *5* Brainstem tumor or demyelination
  - *6* Traumatic brainstem contusion-hemorrhage (clinical signs, auditory-evoked potentials)
- *B* Brainstem dysfunction without mass lesion
  - *1* Basilar artery thrombosis causing brainstem stroke (clinical signs, angiogram)
  - *2* Severe drug overdose (toxicologic analysis)
  - *3* Brainstem encephalitis
  - *4* Basilar artery migraine
  - *5* Brain death

drug overdose, but many physicians believe that this is justified only to treat associated cardiac arrhythmias. Intravenous fluid should be carefully monitored in any serious acute nervous system illness because of the potential for exacerbating brain swelling by excess water administration. Neck injuries must not be overlooked, particularly prior to attempting the oculocephalic maneuver. Headache accompanied by fever and meningismus indicates a need for examination of the CSF to diagnose meningitis, and *lumbar puncture should not be delayed while awaiting a CT scan.*

Enlargement of one pupil usually indicates secondary midbrain compression by a hemispheral mass and demands immediate reduction of intracranial pressure. Normal saline or lactated Ringer's solution are safest because they are iso- or hyperosmolar. Therapeutic hyperventilation may be used to achieve an arterial P_{CO_2} of 3.7 to 4.2 kPa (28 to 32 mmHg). This acts rapidly to reduce intracranial pressure, but the beneficial effect rarely lasts more than 1 to 2 h. Hyperosmolar therapy with mannitol may be used simultaneously with hyperventilation in critical cases, but its effects are not apparent for several minutes. It is generally best to administer mannitol before attempting to intubate a patient with suspected impending herniation. A ventricular puncture may be necessary to decompress hydrocephalus if medical measures fail. Virtually all patients who survive to arrive in an emergency room can be protected from further brain damage by these means until definitive therapy is possible. The use of high-dose barbiturates soon after cardiac arrest has not been shown in clinical studies to be beneficial, although they may still be useful in lowering intracranial pressure in other circumstances.

BRAIN DEATH Brain death results from total cessation of cerebral blood flow and global infarction of the brain at a time when cardiovascular and respiratory functions are preserved with artificial support. It is the only type of irrevocable loss of brain function currently recognized by law as death. Many sets of roughly equivalent criteria have been advanced for the diagnosis of brain death, and it is essential to adhere to those approved locally and recognized as standard practice. Ideal criteria are ones that are simple, conducted at the bedside, and which allow no chance of diagnostic error. Widespread cortical destruction is usually shown by unresponsiveness to the environment, midbrain damage by absent pupillary light reaction, pontine damage by absent oculovestibular and corneal reflexes, and medullary dysfunction by apnea. Some period of observation, usually 6 to 24 h, is desirable during which this state is shown to be sustained. The pupils need not be fully dilated but should not be constricted. The absence of spinal reflexes is not required since the spinal cord remains functional in many cases. Most centers use an isoelectric EEG as a confirmatory test for cortical death. The possibility of profound drug-induced or hypothermic nervous system depression should always be excluded. It is often advisable to delay clinical testing for up to 24 h if a cardiac arrest has caused brain death.

The demonstration of apnea generally requires that the P_{CO_2} be high enough to stimulate respiration. This can be safely accomplished in most patients by removal of the respirator and use of diffusion oxygenation sustained by a tracheal cannula connected to an oxygen supply. In brain-dead patients, CO_2 tension increases approximately 0.3 to 0.4 kPa/min (2 to 3 mmHg/min) during apnea. At the end of an appropriate interval, arterial P_{CO_2} should be at least above 6.6 to 8.0 kPa (50 to 60 mmHg) for the test to be valid. Large posterior fossa lesions that compress the brainstem, nervous system–depressant drugs, and profound hypothermia can simulate brain death, but adherence to recognized protocols for diagnosis will prevent these errors. Radionuclide brain scanning, cerebral angiography or transcranial Doppler measurements may be used to demonstrate the absence of cerebral blood flow in brain death. These techniques have the virtue of rapidity but are often cumbersome and have not been extensively correlated with pathologic material.

There is no implicit pressure to make the diagnosis of brain death except when organ transplantation or difficult resource allocation (intensive care) issues are involved. Although it is commonly accepted that the respirator can be disconnected from a brain-dead patient after proper explanations to the family, there is no obligation to do so, and some physicians prefer to await the inevitable cardiovascular failure that follows brain death if full medical support is omitted, usually within a week.

PROGNOSIS OF COMA Interest in predicting the outcome of coma is oriented toward allocating medical resources and limiting the support of hopeless cases. To date, no collection of clinical signs except those of brain death assuredly predicts outcome of coma. Children and young adults may have ominous early clinical findings such as abnormal brainstem reflexes and yet recover. All schemes for prognosis should, therefore, be taken as only approximate indicators, and medical judgments must be conservatively tempered by other factors such as age, underlying disease, general medical condition, and the previously expressed wishes of the patient. In an attempt to collect prognostic information from large numbers of patients with head injury, a "coma scale" scoring system has been devised which empirically has predictive value in cases of brain trauma (see Chap. 352). Major points include a 95 percent death rate in patients whose pupillary reaction or reflex eye movements were absent 6 h after onset of coma, and a 91 percent death rate if the pupils were unreactive at 24 h (though 4 percent made a good recovery).

Prognostication of nontraumatic coma is more difficult because of the heterogeneity of contributing diseases. Unfavorable signs in the first hours after admission have been reported to be the absence of any two of pupillary reaction, corneal reflex, or the oculovestibular response. One day after the onset of coma, the above signs, in addition to absence of eye opening and muscle tone, predicted death or severe disability and the same signs at 3 days strengthened the prediction of a poor outcome. In many patients precise combinations of predictive signs do not occur and coma scales lose their value. The use of evoked potentials has recently been shown to aid prognostication in head-injured and postcardiac arrest patients. Bilateral absence of cortical somatosensory evoked potentials is associated with death or a vegetative state in most cases. It may be wisest to fully support all but those patients whose extreme signs convincingly suggest a poor outcome. Medical practitioners are becoming less reluctant to withdraw support from brain-dead patients as predictions become more reliable and resources more limited.

REFERENCES

Choi D: Glutamate neurotoxicity and diseases of the nervous system. Neuron 1:623, 1988

Finklestein S, Ropper A: The diagnosis of coma: Its pitfalls and limitations. Heart Lung 8:1059, 1979

Fisher CM: The neurological examination of the comatose patient. Acta Neurol Scand 45 (Suppl 6):1, 1969

Ivan L, Bruce D: *Coma*. Springfield, Ill, Charles C Thomas, 1982

Jennet B et al: Prognosis of patients with severe head injury. Neurosurgery 4:283, 1979

Levy D et al: Prognosis in non-traumatic coma. Ann Intern Med 94:229, 1981

Plum F, Posner J: *The Diagnosis of Stupor and Coma*, 3d ed. Philadelphia, Davis, 1980

Ropper AH: Coma and acutely raised intracranial pressure, in *Diseases of the Nervous System*, A Asbury, G McKhann, I McDonald (eds). Philadelphia, Saunders, 1986

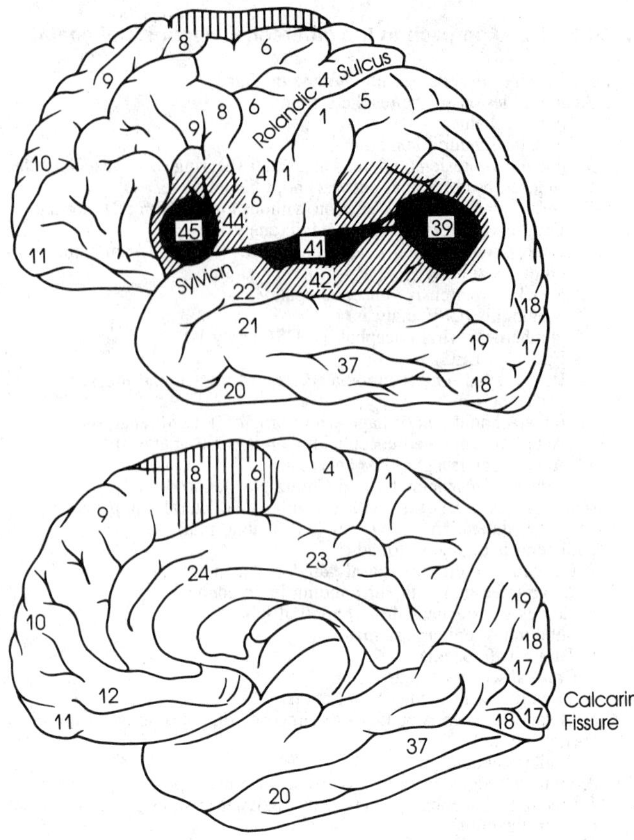

FIGURE 32-1 Diagram to show cortical areas, numbered according to the scheme of Brodmann. The speech areas are in black, the three main ones of which are 39, 41, and 45. The zone marked by vertical stripes in the superior frontal convolution is the secondary motor area which, like Broca's area 45, if stimulated causes vocal arrest. *(After Handbuch der Inneren Medizin, Berlin, Springer-Verlag, 1939.)*

32 SYNDROMES DUE TO FOCAL CEREBRAL LESIONS

RAYMOND D. ADAMS / MAURICE VICTOR

In addition to the general syndromes described in Chap. 30, there are many others that relate to lesions of particular parts of the cerebrum. Recognition of these constitutes irrefutable evidence that all parts of the cerebrum are not functionally equivalent. Some of the symptoms and signs that make up these syndromes have the same diagnostic value as a hemiplegia and, once identified, require the same type of clinical analysis as to cause and pathophysiologic mechanism.

These focal syndromes will be described in terms of the conventional anatomic divisions of the cerebrum, but it will be obvious that most diseases do not respect these boundaries. Hence the syndromes may overlap or occur in a number of combinations.

FRONTAL LOBES In Fig. 32-1, it is seen that the frontal lobes lie anterior to the central (rolandic) sulcus and superior to the Sylvian fissure. They consist of several functionally different parts, which are conventionally designated in the neurologic literature by numbers (according to the scheme devised by Brodmann) or by letters (according to the scheme of von Economo and Koskinas).

The posterior parts, areas 4 and 6 of Brodmann, are specifically related to motor function. There is also a supplementary motor area, located in the posterior part of the superior frontal convolution. Voluntary movement in humans depends on the integrity of these areas, and lesions in them produce a spastic paralysis of the contralateral face, arm, and leg. This is discussed in Chap. 25. A lesion limited more or less to the premotor area (area 6 and the supplementary motor area) is accompanied by less paralysis and more spasticity, as well as by a contralateral grasp reflex, and bilateral lesions of these parts are accompanied by a suck reflex. A lesion in area 8 of Brodmann interferes with the mechanism for turning the head and eyes contralaterally. In addition, a lesion of the left supplementary motor area can result in mutism at its onset; in time the condition resolves to a state of transcortical motor aphasia, with reduced language output and preserved repetition and naming. Ideomotor apraxia is another manifestation of area 6 lesions observed in some patients. A lesion in area 44 (Broca's area) of the dominant cerebral hemisphere, usually the left one, results in at least a temporary loss of verbal expression. A phonetic-articulatory defect (cortical dysarthria) and agrammatism, with retention of "content words," are characteristic. More extensive lesions, including adjacent insular and motor cortex, result in a more severe and persistent motor speech disorder, agraphia, and apraxia of the face, lips, and tongue (see Chap. 33). Lesions of the anterior cingulate gyrus, in the acute stages, may cause a speechless, aphonic state; with recovery, speech returns through whispering and hoarseness rather than dysarthria and aphasia, according to Brown. Lesions in the medial limbic or piriform cortex (areas 23 and 24), where the mechanisms controlling respiration, circulation, and micturition are organized bilaterally, have relatively unclear clinical effects.

The remaining parts of the frontal lobes (areas 9 to 12 of Brodmann), sometimes called the *prefrontal areas*, have less specific and measurable functions. In contrast to the motor areas of the frontal lobes and other areas of the brain, electrical stimulation of the prefrontal areas in humans has yielded a paucity of findings. Many patients with gunshot wounds of these areas have shown only mild and inconsistent abnormalities of behavior. Nevertheless, the following groups of symptoms have been observed in patients with large lesions of one or both of the frontal lobes and of the central white matter and the anterior part of the corpus callosum by which they are joined:

1 Lack of initiative and spontaneity in conjunction with diminished speech and with motor inactivity (apathetic, akinetic, or abulic state). Necessary daily activities are neglected. Interpersonal social reactions are reduced and shallow.
2 Change of personality, usually expressed as lack of concern over the consequences of any action and social disinhibition. Sometimes it may take the form of a childish excitement, an inappropriate joking and punning, a thoughtless impulsivity, an instability and superficiality of emotion, or irritability. The capacity for worry, anxiety, and depression (tortured self-concern) is reduced. These are especially prominent in orbital frontal lesions.
3 Slight impairment of intelligence, usually described as a lack of concentration, vacillation of attention, inability to carry out planned activity, difficulty in changing from one activity to another, or perseveration. These cognitive impairments are more prominent in dorsolateral frontal lesions. Goldstein reduced the difficulty to a loss of the capacity for abstract thinking, but the authors believe this tendency to concrete thinking to be another manifestation of abulia and perseveration. According to Luria, who views the frontal lobe as a regulating mechanism of the organism's activities, planned action is deficient with respect to steady control and goal orientation. With left frontal lesions, intelligence is reduced more (10 points on the IQ scale) than with right frontal lesions, probably because of reduced verbal skills. There is also a memory impairment, usually slight, probably because the mental strategies needed for memorization and recall are impaired.
4 A decomposition of gait and upright stance, consisting of a wide-based gait, flexed posture, and small shuffling steps, and culminating in an inability to stand (Bruns' frontal lobe ataxia or gait apraxia) accompanied by abnormal postures, reflex grasping or sucking, and incontinence of sphincters.

Some differences have been noted between the dominant (left) and right prefrontal lobes. In psychological tests, left-sided lesions impair verbal fluency and cause a greater degree of perseveration, and right-sided ones impair the learning of visual spatial patterns and cause impersistence (see Hecaen and Albert, and Luria for details).

From all the foregoing comments it should be evident that the frontal lobes do not have a unitary function, but comprise a number of interconnected functional components, each subserving a different aspect of motor function, speech, and behavior.

TEMPORAL LOBES The boundaries of the temporal lobes are illustrated in Fig. 32-1. The Sylvian fissure separates the superior surface of each temporal lobe from the frontal lobe and anterior part of the parietal lobe. Posteriorly there is no definite anatomic boundary between the temporal and the occipital and parietal lobe. The temporal lobe includes the superior, middle, and inferior temporal, fusiform, and hippocampal convolutions and the transverse convolutions of Heschl, which are the auditory receptive area on the superior surface, within the Sylvian fissure. The hippocampal convolution was once believed to be related to olfactory function, but now it is known that lesions here do not cause anosmia. Only the medial and anterior parts of the temporal lobes (uncal regions) are related to smell. The lower fibers of the geniculocalcarine pathway (from the inferior retina) swing in a wide arc over the temporal horn of the ventricle into the white matter of the temporal lobe en route to the occipital lobes, and lesions that interrupt them characteristically produce a contralateral upper homonymous quadrantanopsia. Hearing, localized in the superior surfaces of the temporal lobes (Heschl's gyri), is bilaterally represented, which accounts for the fact that both temporal lobes need to be affected to cause deafness. Loss of equilibrium has not been observed with temporal lobe lesions, although electrical stimulation (or a seizure discharge) of the superior surface of the temporal lobe, posterior to the auditory cortex, evokes vertigo. Disease in the superior convolution of the left temporal lobe and adjacent inferior parietal lobule in right-handed individuals results in a Wernicke's aphasia. This syndrome, discussed in Chap. 33, consists of paraphasic speech or jargon aphasia and inability to read, write, repeat, or understand the meaning of spoken words.

Between the auditory and olfactory projection areas there is a large expanse of temporal lobe, subserving three specific functional systems. In the inferolateral parts (areas 20, 21, and 37) are located some of the visual-associated projections from the striate and peristriate cortex of the occipital lobes. In the superior-lateral parts (areas 22, 41, and 42) are the primary and secondary areas for acoustic perception. In the mediobasal parts are the limbic structures (amygdaloid nuclei and hippocampi) where the neural organizations for emotional and memory processes lie. Bilateral lesions of the geniculocalcarine pathways result in cortical blindness; lesions of the visual cortex of the dominant temporal lobe result in a variety of agnosias, apparently based on a loss of visual memories: recognition of written words (alexia), visual naming (anomia), loss of pattern discrimination, and possibly color recognition (achromatopsia) and object agnosia. Bilateral hippocampal/parahippocampal lesions produce a deficit in which the patient is unable to record events and information, i.e., has a loss of memory, in both its general and specific aspects (see Chap. 30). Also, the temporal lobes include a large part of the limbic system, which subserves the emotional and motivational aspects of behavior and vegetative functions ("visceral brain"). Lesions involving both the visual and limbic areas contribute to the Klüver-Bucy syndrome. This syndrome, first produced in monkeys by removal of both temporal lobes, has been observed only rarely in human beings, usually after an attack of herpes simplex encephalitis. It consists of apathy, impaired recognition of objects and persons, uncontrollable oral exploration, hypersexuality, amnesia, and bulimia. Usually the syndrome is incomplete.

Apart from aphasia, psychological studies have shown a difference between the effects of dominant and nondominant temporal lobe lesions. With dominant lesions there is impairment in learning auditorially presented verbal material; with nondominant lesions there is a failure in learning visually presented nonverbal material. In addition, about 20 percent of patients with either a right or left lobectomy have shown an alteration of personality similar to that described after lesions in the prefrontal parts of the brain (see above).

The study of patients with uncinate seizures, with the characteristic dreamy state, olfactory or gustatory hallucinations, and masticatory movements, suggests that all these functions are organized through the temporal lobes. Stimulation of the posterior parts of the temporal lobes of fully conscious epileptic patients during surgical procedures has brought to light the interesting fact that complex memories and visual and auditory images, some with strong emotional content, can be aroused. Studies of the effects of stimulation of the amygdaloid nucleus, which is in the anterior and medial part of the temporal lobe, have shed additional light on this subject. Some symptoms like those of schizophrenia and mania may be evoked. Complex emotional experiences that had occurred previously may be revived. There are also remarkable autonomic effects: the blood pressure rises, pulse increases, respirations increase in frequency and depth, and the patient looks frightened. In temporal lobe epilepsy, there may be an intensification of the patient's emotional reactions, vague preoccupation with moral and religious issues, a tendency to write excessively, and sometimes aggressiveness. Ablation of the amygdaloid nuclei has eliminated uncontrollable rage reactions in psychotic patients. Hippocampal and adjacent convolutions have been excised bilaterally, with a disastrous loss of ability to learn or to establish new memories (Korsakoff's psychosis).

The abnormalities consequent upon lesions of the temporal lobes may be summarized as follows:

1 Effects of unilateral disease of the dominant temporal lobe
  a Upper homonymous quadrantanopsia
  b Wernicke's aphasia

- *c* Impairment in tests of verbal material presented through the auditory sense
- *d* Dysnomia or amnesic aphasia
- *e* Amusia (inability to name musical scores and to read and write music)

2 Effects of unilateral disease of nondominant temporal lobe
- *a* Upper homonymous quadrantanopsia
- *b* Inability to judge spatial relationships in rare cases
- *c* Impairment in tests of nonverbal visually presented material
- *d* Inability to recognize melodies and other nonlexical qualities of music

3 Effects of disease of either temporal lobe
- *a* Auditory illusions and hallucinations
- *b* Psychotic behavior (aggressivity)
- *c* Upper homonymous quadrantanopsia

4 Effects of bilateral disease
- *a* Korsakoff's amnesic defect
- *b* Apathy and placidity } Klüver-Bucy syndrome
- *c* Increased sexual activity } Klüver-Bucy syndrome
- *d* Sham rage } Klüver-Bucy syndrome
- *e* Cortical deafness
- *f* Loss of other unilateral functions

PARIETAL LOBES The postcentral convolution is the terminus of somatic sensory pathways from the opposite half of the body. However, destructive lesions here do not abolish cutaneous sensation but cause mainly a defect in sensory discrimination with variable impairment of primary sensation. In other words, the perception of painful, tactile, thermal, and vibratory stimuli is affected little or not at all, whereas stereognosis (ability to recognize the size, shape, and texture of objects by touch), sense of position, distinction between single and double contacts (two-point threshold), and the localization of sensory stimuli are impaired or lost (atopognosia). There is also the phenomenon of extinction, i.e., if a stimulus (tactile, painful, visual) is delivered simultaneously to corresponding parts of the body or visual fields, only the stimulus on the normal side is perceived. This type of sensory disturbance, sometimes called *cortical sensory defect,* is really a disturbance of somatic sensory perception, and is discussed in Chap. 28. Extensive lesions deep in the white matter of the parietal lobes produce an impairment of all forms of sensation contralaterally, and if these lesions encroach upon the uppermost part of the temporal lobe, there may be a contralateral homonymous hemianopsia, often incongruous and tending to be greater in the inferior quadrants. Lesions of the angular gyrus of the dominant hemisphere result in an inability to read (alexia).

Recent interest has centered more on the function of the parietal lobes in the perception of one's position in space, the interrelationships of objects in space, and the relationship of the various parts of the body to one another. Since the time of Babinski it has been known that patients with large lesions of the minor parietal lobe are often unaware of their hemiplegia and hemianesthesia. Babinski called this condition *anosognosia.* Related psychological disorders are lack of recognition of the left arm and leg, neglect of the left side of the body (as in dressing) and of external space on the left side, and constructional apraxia (an inability to perceive and construct simple figures). While all of these disorders may occur with left-sided lesions as well, they are observed less frequently, in part because the aphasia that occurs with lesions of the left hemisphere precludes adequate testing of other parietal lobe functions.

Another frequent constellation of symptoms, usually referred to as *Gerstmann's syndrome,* occurs only with lesions of the dominant parietal lobe. This consists of inability to write (agraphia), calculate (acalculia), distinguish right from left, and identify fingers (finger agnosia) and other parts of the body. This syndrome is a true *agnosia,* since it represents a defect in the formulation and use of symbolic concepts (including the significance of numbers and letters and the names of parts of the body), in which a unilateral (dominant) lesion evokes the defect bilaterally. An ideomotor apraxia may or may not be associated. *Apraxia* and *agnosia* are discussed in Chaps. 25 and 28.

The effects of disease of the parietal lobes may be summarized as follows:

1 Effects of unilateral disease of the parietal lobe, right or left
- *a* Cortical sensory syndrome and sensory extinction (or total hemianesthesia with large acute lesions of white matter)
- *b* In children, mild contralateral hemiparesis and hemiatrophy
- *c* Visual inattention and sometimes anosognosia, constructional and dressing apraxias, and neglect of the opposite one-half of the body and extrapersonal space (all of these defects are observed far more frequently with right than with left parietal lesions)
- *d* Abolition of optokinetic nystagmus to one side

2 Effects of unilateral disease of the dominant parietal lobe (left hemisphere in right-handed patients), additional phenomena
- *a* Disorders of language (especially alexia)
- *b* Gerstmann's syndrome
- *c* Bimanual astereognosis (tactile agnosia)
- *d* Bilateral ideational or ideomotor apraxia

In all parietal lesions, if sufficiently extensive, there may be a bland mood, indifference to illness or neurologic defects, reduction in the capacity to think clearly, inattentiveness, and impaired memory.

OCCIPITAL LOBES The occipital lobes are the termini of the geniculocalcarine pathways and are essential for visual sensation and perception. Destructive lesions in one occipital lobe result in a contralateral homonymous hemianopsia, i.e., a loss of vision in part or all of the homonymous fields. Occasionally patients complain of changes in the form and contour of visually perceived objects (metamorphopsia), as well as illusory displacement of images from one side of the visual field to another (visual allesthesia), or of abnormal persistence of the visual image after the object has been removed (palinopsia). Visual illusions and elementary (unformed) hallucinations may also occur. Bilateral lesions cause "cortical" blindness, a state of blindness without change in the optic fundi or pupillary reflexes.

Lesions in Brodmann's areas 18 and 19 of the dominant hemisphere (Fig. 32-1) cause a loss of recognition of objects presented visually, despite the ability to see, at least to some degree—a state termed *visual object agnosia.* In the classic form of this disorder, individuals with intact mental powers are unable to recognize objects visually, even though by tests of visual acuity and perimetry they appear to see sufficiently well to do so; they are able to recognize objects by tactile or other nonvisual senses. In these terms, *alexia,* or inability to read, represents a visual verbal agnosia or "word blindness." Patients can see letters and words but do not know their meaning, although they can still recognize them through tactile or auditory senses. Several other types of agnosia are observed with bilateral occipital lesions: disorders of *spatial or topographic localization,* in which the patient cannot describe or find his or her way in familiar surroundings (usually due to bilateral occipitoparietal lesions); failure to identify a familiar face (*prosopagnosia*), often with achromatopsia (inferomesial occipitotemporal lesions); an inability to scan the peripheral field and to grasp an object under visual guidance, coupled with visual inattention (*Balint's syndrome,* due usually to bilateral occipitoparietal lesions); and a failure to perceive simultaneously all the elements of a scene (*simultanagnosia*). In actuality these agnosias represent the effects not of purely occipital lesions but of either occipitotemporal or occipitoparietal disconnections.

The details of these syndromes of the different lobes of the cerebrum can be found in the textbook of Adams and Victor and the monographs by Walsh and Mesulam.

CORPUS CALLOSUM AND THE DISCONNECTION SYNDROMES Considerable attention has been devoted to the study of each of the two cerebral hemispheres in isolation. This is possible only when the corpus callosum, which forms a bridge between the two hemispheres, is surgically sectioned (for epilepsy) or destroyed by infarction or tumors. From these studies emerges the well-known fact that the left hemisphere is dominant in all language functions and auditory perception and the right hemisphere is superior in spatial and visual perception. Partial lesions of the corpus callosum or of the long tracts in the cerebral white matter are found to be associated with a number of interesting syndromes (commissural and intrahemispheric) described below.

When the corpus callosum is sectioned by a surgical procedure or destroyed by an anterior cerebral artery occlusion (anterior four-fifths), the language and perceptual areas of the left hemisphere are isolated from the sensory and motor areas of the right hemisphere. These patients, if blindfolded, are then unable to match an object held in one hand with an identical object in the other hand. Further, they cannot match an object seen in the right half of the visual field with one in the left half. If given verbal commands, they perform correctly with the right hand but not with the left. Without vision, objects placed in the right hand are named correctly, but not those in the left. In lesions confined to the posterior fifth of the corpus callosum (splenium), only the visual part of the disconnection syndrome occurs. Occlusion of the left posterior cerebral artery provides the best examples of this. Infarction of the left occipital lobe causes a right homonymous hemianopsia, as a consequence of which all visual information needed for activating the speech areas of the left hemisphere must come from the right occipital lobe, across the splenium of the corpus callosum. If there is a lesion in the corpus callosum (or in other portions of the crossing fibers), the patient cannot read or name colors because the visual information cannot reach the left angular gyrus. There is no difficulty in copying words, though the patient cannot read what he or she has written (alexia without agraphia); matching colors without naming them is done without error. Apparently the visual information for activating the left motor area crosses the corpus callosum more anteriorly. A lesion that is limited to the anterior third of the corpus callosum does not result in a left-sided apraxia (a failure of the left hand to obey commands, the right one performing perfectly). A section of the entire corpus callosum does result in such an apraxia, indicating that the fiber systems connecting the left to the right motor areas cross posterior to the genu (but anterior to the splenium).

There are also intrahemispheric disconnections, of which the most important are the following:

1 *Conduction aphasia* (also called *central* aphasia). The patient has fluent but paraphasic speech and writing with nearly perfect comprehension of spoken or written language. Repetition of what is heard or read is, however, severely impaired. The lesion is presumably in the arcuate fasciculus, which connects Wernicke's area with Broca's area.

2 *Pure word deafness*. Although the patient is able to hear and identify nonverbal sounds, there is a loss of ability to comprehend spoken language. The patient's speech remains normal. The defect has been attributed to a subcortical lesion, undercutting Wernicke's area.

DIAGNOSIS AND MANAGEMENT OF PATIENTS WITH FOCAL CEREBRAL LESIONS These involve the same principles described in Chap. 30. Special tests, mostly of the psychological type, are available for each of the focal cerebral syndromes. The investigation and care of individual patients will also be governed by the underlying disease, of course.

REFERENCES

Adams RD, Victor M: *Principles of Neurology*, 4th ed. New York, McGraw-Hill, 1989

Brodal A: *Neurological Anatomy in Relation to Clinical Medicine*, 3d ed. New York, Oxford University Press, 1981

Brown JW: Frontal lobe syndromes, in *Handbook of Clinical Neurology*, JAM Frederiks (ed). Amsterdam, Elsevier Science, 1985, vol 45, chap 3

Dimond SJ: The disconnection syndromes, in *Modern Trends in Neurology*, D. Williams (ed). London, Butterworth, 1975

Geschwind N: Disconnection syndromes in animals and man. Brain 88:237, 585, 1965

Hecaen H, Albert ML: Disorders of mental functioning related to the frontal lobes, in *Modern Trends in Neurology*, D Williams (ed). London, Butterworth, 1975

Heilman KM, Valenstein E: *Clinical Neuropsychology*, 2d ed. Oxford, Oxford University Press, 1985

Luria AR: *The Working Brain: An Introduction to Neuropsychology*. New York, Basic Books (translation Penguin Books Ltd), 1973

Marlowe WH et al: Complete Klüver-Bucy syndrome in man. Cortex 11:53, 1975

Mesulam M-M (ed): *Principles of Behavioral Neurology*. Philadelphia, Davis, 1985

Walsh KW: *Neuropsychology: A Clinical Approach*. London, Churchill Livingstone, 1978

33 DISORDERS OF SPEECH AND LANGUAGE

JAY P. MOHR

Language and speech are fundamental both to social intercourse and to intellectual life. When disordered as a consequence of disease of the brain, the loss exceeds blindness, deafness, or paralysis in gravity.

TERMS The terms *speech* and *language* are separated here to emphasize that the two are not synonymous. A given brain lesion may affect them in different ways and degrees of severity.

The term *speech* is usually taken to mean the execution of acquired motor skills for the pronunciation of words, putting the expected emphasis on given syllables; the intonation of strings of words to make questions or statements; the grouping of words into phrases; and production of the speech "melody" that is distinctive for given languages and regional dialects. The skillful use of speech is often essential to communication. For example, the meaning of what is a sincere expression in written words may be radically altered when it is spoken in a sarcastic manner. While necessary for the communication of language, speech skills are mainly a modality by which language is conveyed from one person to another and are not themselves sufficient to produce communication. Even when speech is poorly executed (as for example in *dysarthria*), it may nonetheless permit communication.

Language has a wider connotation and refers to the selection and serial ordering of words according to rules that permit a person using one or more of the modalities of speech to modify the behavior of another, and to express that poorly understood cerebral activity termed *thinking*. Disturbances of language usage or comprehension, apart from disorders in the modalities of speech by which the words are discriminated or produced, are known broadly as *aphasia*. Since the disorder clinically encountered is rarely complete, some insist the state is better described by the term indicating a partial disturbance, namely, *dysphasia*. Because of its more common use, aphasia will be used in this chapter.

CEREBRAL DOMINANCE: RELATION TO SPEECH AND HANDEDNESS The side dominant for language is inferred from which eye, hand, or foot is chosen preferentially for intricate, complex acts. Such preference is more complete in some persons than in others. Hereditary, anatomic and developmental factors play a role. Over 90 percent of people are right-handed. Left-handedness may be hereditary or may result from disease of the left cerebral hemisphere in early life. Left hemisphere dominance for language occurs in 95 percent of right-handed people and in 50 percent of those who are left-handed.

Anatomic differences exist between the dominant and the nondominant cerebral hemispheres. The planum temporale, a part of Wernicke's language zone, is larger in the left hemisphere in right-handed individuals. Formerly, many children were shifted at an early age from left to right (shifted sinistrals) because it is a handicap to be left-handed in a right-handed world. A disturbance in language is produced in almost all right-handers by unilateral brain damage that affects the left hemisphere. Positron emission tomography has shown the left hemisphere to be activated more for verbal tasks, the right for spatial motor tasks.

LANGUAGE DISORDERS IN MEDICAL PRACTICE

Language disorders may be divided into four categories:

1 *Aphasia* is defined as a state in which there is a loss more or less exclusively of the production and/or comprehension of speech and language from an acquired cerebral lesion.
2 *Dysarthria* is a defect in articulation usually related to poor pronunciation of consonants. These defects are pure motor disorders of the muscles of articulation in the presence of intact mental functions and may be due to flaccid or spastic paralysis, rigidity, repetitive spasms (stuttering), or ataxia.
3 *Aphonia or dysphonia* is the loss of voice due to a disease of the larynx or its innervation, causing inability to produce the basic vowel sounds.
4 *Disturbances of language* occur with diseases that produce delirium and dementia (see Chap. 30). Speech is seldom lost, and language is deranged as part of a general impairment of cerebral functions.

APHASIA As a general orientation, most lesions that lead to aphasia occur in the perisylvian regions (frontal, temporal, and parietal) of the dominant cerebral hemisphere, i.e., the left side in right-handed individuals. The anatomic site of the lesion can usually be demonstrated by computed tomography (CT scan) or magnetic resonance imaging (MRI).

Anteriorly placed sylvian lesions mainly disturb the acts of speaking. These range from mutism through impaired articulation, to disordered transitions from syllable to syllable, to abnormalities in phrasing, intonation, and melody. Lesions more posterior produce malpositioning of the tongue, lips, and other structures in the oropharynx with anticipatory errors from some syllables occurring out of sequence. Lesions grouped around the posterior sylvian fissure including the superior temporal lobe and its auditory gyri are manifested by disordered understanding of spoken words, resulting in poor repetition of speech sounds.

The language deficits that are superimposed on the speech disturbances are less well correlated with anatomic pathology. Language disturbances can be separated by pathoanatomic considerations into two large groups. Large anterior lesions involving the bulk of the frontal operculum (that region which lies above the insula) and the insula itself result in agrammatism, featuring sharply contracted sentence structure, absence of most small words, and a preservation of words serving mainly a predicative, interjectional, or substantive function. The patient may only be able to say "hi," "no," and "hello" or to use simple nouns, i.e., "ball," "top," "key." Large posterior sylvian lesions show almost the opposite, with simple speech elements missing or replaced by substitutions in which the desired response is only approximated (*paraphasias*). These latter may consist of faulty pronunciations (*literal paraphasias*) or faulty word selections (*verbal paraphasias*). Verbal paraphasias may approximate the desired word with a similarity of sound or of spelling (*formal verbal paraphasias*), such as "stock" for "stop" or by similarity of meaning (*semantic verbal paraphasias*) such as "slow" for "stop." Disturbances in understanding language, both auditory and visual speech, occur in both types of major paraphasias.

Diseases of the cerebral surface gray matter produce a more significant deficit than those confined to the white matter: tumors, located largely in the white matter, usually reach a large size before causing a speech or language deficit. Infarcts or traumatic lesions of one or more centimeters in diameter are usually associated with an evanescent deficit that fades to functional insignificance within weeks or months.

Deficits due to acute lesions are most easily demonstrated in the acute phase. Improvements over weeks to months occur in all but the largest vascular lesions, but those due to tumors show progression. The site is more significant than the size of the lesion: the former determines the qualitative features of the deficit, while size determines the severity of the syndrome. Furthermore, deficits in speech function predominate in smaller lesions, while major disturbances in language are superimposed on the speech disturbance in the larger lesions.

Lesions well away from the sylvian region either cause no disturbance of human communicative skills or alter them only secondarily. An example of the latter is the lesion of the anterior frontal lobes, especially the medial and orbital parts, that impairs all motor activities and often results in lack of attention and responsiveness (abulia), verging on the akinetic mute state (see Chap. 32). The speech is laconic with long pauses between utterances, and there is an inability to sustain monologue and narrative. Extensive occipital lesions impair reading and reduce the utilization of all visual, lexical stimuli. Thalamic and deep cerebral lesions impair alertness and cause fluctuating states of inattention and disorientation, thereby inducing fragmentation of words (neologisms) and phrases, and protracted, uncontrollable talking (logorrhea). Strong stimulation to increase momentarily the level of awareness and alertness usually will show that such patients have intact language mechanisms.

The nondominant hemisphere provides the substratum for several types of behavior: motor responses of mimicry, social anticipation (smiling, handshaking, modesty reactions), and self-care (washing and feeding); avoidance behavior to noxious stimuli; and the capability of cross matching visually when presented simple words with pictures. It follows that tests which elicit these behaviors are no guide to functions of the hemisphere dominant for language.

Lesions of the frontal (motor) regions are generally believed to produce syndromes independent from those of the posterior (sensory) regions; the dysphasias can be classified as motor (Broca's) or sensory (Wernicke's) and can be further specified as subcortical, cortical, or transcortical in location. Subcortical lesions are believed to interfere with the main efferent or afferent projections of the cerebrum; lesions of the surface involve the "centers" themselves; transcortical lesions isolate these centers from one another or from other regions of the brain related to speech. Although an oversimplification, these basic concepts provide a rough guide for the classification of the aphasias, but they are not reliable to predict the lesion's site and size. Positron emission studies have challenged formerly popular concepts of functional connections between the major language areas.

TYPES OF APHASIA Disturbances of speech and language can result from several abnormalities. Classifications have been based upon the predominant form, the presumed physiologic or psychological bases, and the anatomy of the underlying diseases. The classification utilized here has been formulated on the basis of the anatomic localization and the clinical presentation (see Table 33-1). The prognoses are helpful in management, particularly in the choice of corrective measures in therapy. Aphasias have also been classified according to the severity of impediment to speech production and flow. *Fluent aphasias* are characterized by runs of well-articulated speech, of basically normal rhythm and flow, although lacking in language meaning. The defect is usually a lesion in the dominant parietal or temporal lobe. *Nonfluent aphasias* are characterized by slow, incorrectly articulated words and sentences. The lesion usually lies in the dominant frontal lobe.

Total (global) aphasia In total, or global, aphasia the causative lesion destroys a large part of the speech and language areas of the major cerebral hemisphere, producing a severe aphasic deficit which has the poorest prognosis for improvement of any aphasic syndrome.

Most patients with total aphasia say but a few words; they do not read or write, and they understand only a few words of the speech of others. Related signs include right hemiplegia, hemianesthesia, and homonymous hemianopsia. The alert patient may participate in common gestures of greeting, may show modesty and avoidance reactions, and is able to engage in self-help activities. The early appearance of clearly vocalized stereotyped words, such as "hi" and "yes," are often falsely encouraging signs; they may reflect the uninhibited function of the right hemisphere. After weeks or months

TABLE 33-1 Classification of aphasic disorders

	Clinical manifestations	Anatomic location	Etiology	Associated clinical symptoms
MAJOR SYNDROMES				
Global aphasia	Minimal speech; nonfluent aphasia; comprehension poor for spoken and written language	Large lesion of dominant frontal, parietal, and superior temporal lobe	Infarction in distribution of internal carotid or middle cerebral artery; trauma; tumor	Contralateral hemiplegia; hemisensory loss; hemianopsia
Broca's aphasia	Nonfluent aphasia; agrammatic sentences; poor articulation; dysprosody; may be mute	Cortical and subcortical lesion of prefrontal and frontal regions	Infarction in distribution of superior frontal branch middle cerebral artery; hemorrhage; tumor	Contralateral hemiparesis; minor or no sensory loss; no visual field disturbance; oral dyspraxia; cortical dysarthria; severe impairment in writing
Wernicke's aphasia (central or sensory aphasia)	Fluent speech; total incomprehension of spoken speech; inability to read or to repeat sounds or words; alexia, agraphia, paraphasia common	Posterior perisylvian structures of the parietal and temporal lobe	Infarction in distribution of lower division of middle cerebral artery; tumor; herpes simplex encephalitis	Parietal lobe sensory deficits; hemianopsia; no motor disturbance
MINOR CENTRAL APHASIA SYNDROMES				
Conduction aphasia	Paraphasia; difficulty in repetition of speech and in reading aloud; aware of deficit; adequate comprehension of written and spoken words	Upper bank of sylvian fissure; inferior parietal lobule	Embolic occlusion of posterior branches of middle cerebral artery	Contralateral hemihypesthesia or homonymous hemianopsia; abnormal optokinetic nystagmus
Mainly auditory (pure word deafness)	Impaired auditory comprehension; inability to repeat a sentence or write a dictation	Lesion in superior temporal gyrus	Infarction; tumor; abscess	Rarely deafness
Mainly visual (dyslexia with dysgraphia)	Visual language compromised more than auditory; cannot read or write	Parietooccipital lesion	Infarction; tumor, lobar hemorrhage	Hemianopsia
OTHER SYNDROMES				
Pure word blindness	Normal spoken language and writing, with inability to read	Left occipitostriate cortex, adjacent association cortex, and posterior corpus callosum (splenium)	Infarction in distribution of posterior cerebral artery; tumor, lobar hemorrhage	Hemianopsia
Isolation of speech areas	Parrot-like speech; echolalia	Ischemic infarction in border (watershed) zones between anterior, middle, and posterior cerebral artery distributions	Systemic hypotension or hypoxia; cardiac arrest	Decreased alertness and responsiveness; bilateral leg weakness
Amnesic-dysnomic aphasia	Inability to recall names of objects or parts of objects; difficulty with recent memory	Deep temporal lobe lesions, parahippocampal, hippocampal gyrus	Tumor; Alzheimer's disease; infarction in distribution posterior cerebral artery; herpes simplex encephalitis	Apraxia; dementia; no motor or sensory abnormalities; upper quadrantic visual field defect

the understanding of spoken speech improves slightly and a few words may be uttered.

Infarction from occlusion of the left internal carotid or the middle cerebral artery, a large hemorrhage, major tumor, or penetrating trauma is most often responsible. In the rare instances of rapid improvement, the main cause is postconvulsive paralysis, posttraumatic edema, or transitory ischemia from a fragmenting embolus. Rarely, hyperthermia, infection, or hyponatremia may transiently cause a temporary relapse of aphasia due to an old lesion.

Broca's aphasia (major motor aphasia) This term designates a complex syndrome with severely disturbed speech and writing, accompanied by simplified grammar skills (agrammatism) in speaking and writing and a less obvious impairment in language comprehension. The syndrome results from a large lesion involving cortical and subcortical structures along the insula and superior sylvian fissure, not simply Broca's area, a circumscribed lesion in the inferior frontal convolution. CT scan may underestimate the lesion because the angle of the imaged lesion may seem to merge with the sylvian fissure.

The lesions are smaller than those causing complete aphasia and usually involve the sensorimotor rolandic region, producing an accompanying persisting hemiparesis and hemisensory syndrome. Initially, a transient ipsilateral deviation of the eyes is observed due to the frontal infarction.

In the acute phase, the entire language mechanism appears to be inactivated, and the helplessly mute, noncommunicative, and uncomprehending patient presents the syndrome of complete or global aphasia. Within weeks to years, the disorder of comprehension abates somewhat, and this improvement exceeds that found in speaking and writing, leaving the motor speech deficits that gave the syndrome its original name.

For a time an apraxia of the lingual and oropharyngeal apparatus retards efforts to make purposeful movements. Imitation may be better performed than execution of acts on command. Certain stereotyped and simple phrases, such as "hi," "good morning," or curses are uttered more easily, and words of popular songs may be sung surprisingly well. The patient's efforts to speak and facial expressions suggest an awareness of his or her ineptitudes and mistakes, and an accompanying exasperation and despair are common.

As improvement occurs, words are enunciated slowly and laboriously, with greatly impaired melody of speech (prosody). Speech is sparse and consists mainly of nouns, transitive verbs, and important adjectives; many of the small words (articles, prepositions, conjunctions) are omitted, giving the speech an agrammatic and telegraphic character. The preservation of substantive words allows the patients to communicate despite the gross mechanical and agrammatic language difficulties. This hesitant, laconic speech has been termed nonfluent aphasia.

Most patients with Broca's aphasia have a correspondingly severe impairment in communication by writing with either hand. However, communication by writing is superior to that by speaking, suggesting a certain independence between these two acts as vehicles of language.

The syndrome is most often due to embolic occlusions of the

upper division of the left middle cerebral artery; major putaminal hypertensive hemorrhage, huge frontal lobe tumor or abscess, metastatic lesions, subdural hematoma, and encephalitis are less common causes.

Minor motor aphasia More circumscribed focal lesions along the anterior and superior sylvian operculum and insula produce remarkably discrete effects on the speech skills which may resemble major motor aphasia except for the satisfactory understanding of spoken and written words. The prognosis for nearly full recovery is excellent. Indeed, *none of these focal lesions produces significant or lasting deficits in language usage.*

Broca's area infarction affects the lower premotor cortex adjacent to the motor cortex controlling the oropharynx, larynx, and respiratory apparatus. The infarct interrupts skilled movements of these muscle groups, and the resultant dyspraxia in speech features impaired transitions between syllables in words and disruption of the melodic intonation of phrases (dysprosody). Involvement of this region alone is insufficient to produce the major syndrome referred to as Broca's aphasia. *Rolandic infarction* involves the sensorimotor cortex itself; either the syndrome of dysprosody occurs, or speech has poor articulation and lowered volume and pitch, while a nasal quality to the voice reveals the paresis of the nasopharyngeal musculature. *Postcentral, anterior parietal infarction* is associated with errors in the positioning of the oral cavity for individual sounds, syllables, and whole words; the acoustic features of the utterance are often distorted by these malpositions of the oral cavity and strike the ear as literal paraphasias.

Lesions in the more anterior parts of the dominant frontal lobe, sparing Broca's area, may also cause an aphasic disorder. Usually speech output is reduced and nonfluent, and auditory comprehension is intact. Repetition of words spoken by the examiner is preserved. This condition has been called *transcortical motor aphasia* but may be part of the broader frontal lobe syndromes in which spontaneous speech is lacking (mutism) and all motor activity is reduced (akinesia).

Most such focal lesions are due to emboli to the sequential branches of the upper division of the middle cerebral artery. Deeper, larger lesions or larger emboli involving the stem of the upper division can cause several types of deficit in a single patient, making these individual distinctions less clear and blending with the major syndrome of Broca's aphasia. Facial, lingual, and sometimes brachial paresis and ideomotor dyspraxia of the face and left, nondominant limbs commonly accompany the speech disorder. Most of these syndromes recede within weeks or months.

Wernicke's aphasia (major central or sensory aphasia) This term encompasses a range of syndromes that arise from lesions of the posterior perisylvian structures or the posterior temporal, parietal, and occipital regions supplied by the lower division of the middle cerebral artery. There is disruption of the whole array of language behavior. When restricted to the temporal lobe, the main disturbance is most evident in language tasks involving words heard; and when more parietal and occipital, in words seen.

Spoken and written efforts in communication as well as in auditory and visual comprehension are affected, a combination that justifies the term *central aphasia*. The term *sensory aphasia* was formerly used to accentuate the contrast with motor (Broca's) aphasia. Instead of the difficult articulation, faulty transitions, dysmelodic speaking, and disproportionate condensation of grammatical forms that characterize Broca's aphasia, the speech of Wernicke's aphasia is fluent, hence the name *fluent aphasia*.

In severe cases, the patient utters a series of incomprehensible syllables, makes illegible marks on a page in attempts at writing, cannot be made to repeat aloud or copy correctly at sight, and treats the examiner's attempts at written and verbal communication as if they were in a wholly unfamiliar foreign language. In less severe cases, the patient can repeat aloud and copy, but echoes the words heard with faulty pronunciation or copies the words in a slavish manner, imitating even the examiner's handwriting style, as though the test words were unfamiliar. The disturbance in language does not simply reflect a disturbance in hearing or in vision. In the mildest cases, the deficits are manifested in errors in word comprehension and usage. The patient may choose words that show approximation to the desired response, the words often belonging to the same functional class [i.e., *cow* for *pig*, but not *cow* for *yellow* (such errors are labeled *semantic verbal paraphasias*)]; or the words may be similar in sound or shape (*formal verbal paraphasias*) such as "flee" for "tree"; there may be errors in word structure, with improper tenses, prefixes, suffixes (i.e., *beautifuling*), or other errors that resemble those of normal people unfamiliar with the language in question. Some such patients pass for normal in brief or casual conversation. In its milder form or later in the course of the illness, the speech resembles that of a person tired or distracted, and the abnormality is detected only on tests of complex language function.

CT scanning and MRI are the best methods to delineate the topography of the lesion. Arteriographic findings are an unreliable basis of correlation because the vascular occlusions, most often due to cerebral embolism, frequently fail to show the embolus because it has disintegrated or drifted distally into one or more smaller branches. Radionuclide brain scanning is useful only for the largest lesions.

Minor central aphasia syndromes In time, Wernicke's aphasia improves, and a number of lesser syndromes appear. These latter, however, may be present in comparatively pure form from the beginning, when only a small, restricted lesion involves some part of the territory of the lower division of the middle cerebral artery.

The posterior sylvian region, comprising posterosuperior temporal, opercular, supramarginal, and posterior insular gyri, appears to encompass a variety of language functions. Seemingly minor changes in size and locale of the lesion are associated with important variations in the elements of Wernicke's aphasia. Depending on the location of the lesion, language behavior dependent on auditory function (hearing spoken words, echoing sounds and speech, relating the spoken to the written word, and finally repeating and writing it) may be deranged partially or completely. The same is true of language behavior dependent upon visual function, when the left posterior parietal lobe is involved. These partial syndromes are termed *conduction aphasia*, *pure word deafness*, *dyslexia with dysgraphia*, and *pure word blindness*.

CONDUCTION APHASIA: SEPARATION OF WERNICKE'S AND BROCA'S LANGUAGE AREAS The principal abnormality resembles Wernicke's aphasia. There is the same degree of paraphasia in self-initiated speech, in repeating what is heard, and in reading aloud. However, little or no difficulty is encountered in comprehending words that are heard or seen. Because the motor regions are unaffected, no element of dysarthria or dysprosody occurs. The patient is alert and unaware of the deficit. The mistakes take the form of literal paraphasia; i.e., errors in oropharyngeal positioning produce detectably different sounds from those intended. The disorder in repeating from dictation becomes more apparent when the rate of presentation of auditory material is increased, the uttered words are polysyllabic, or the words are unfamiliar, e.g., sets of nonsense syllables. Since nouns are usually the longest words in sentences, one may gain an impression that they are specifically affected.

The lesion at autopsy is located in the cortex and subcortical white matter in the upper bank of the sylvian fissure, involving the supramarginal gyrus of the inferior parietal lobule. The posterior part of the superior temporal region is occasionally affected. The usual cause is an embolus in the ascending parietal or posterior temporal branch of the middle cerebral artery. Deeper, larger lesions that interrupt the arcuate fasciculus connecting the temporal and frontal lobes may produce the syndrome, but usually they involve other pathways as well, giving rise to a more extensive speech deficit (Wernicke's aphasia or amnesic aphasia). However, these latter types of aphasia, as they regress, may resolve into conduction aphasia. More anterior insular lesions usually include some degree of Broca's aphasia.

PURE WORD DEAFNESS Instead of a disturbance confined to auditory comprehension, this syndrome is considered to be the auditory form of Wernicke's aphasia. The most obvious findings are an impaired auditory comprehension and inability to repeat what is said or to write to dictation. Spoken language is less impaired but rarely normal, and occasionally the paraphasic speech leads to an initial diagnosis of Wernicke's aphasia. By audiometric testing little defect in hearing is found. The patient frequently learns to use visual cues well enough to overcome much of the difficulty. Comprehension of visually presented material such as printed matter, although not normal, is better than auditory comprehension. When there is full preservation of reading skill, the traditional term *pure word deafness* can be applied.

In most autopsy studies the lesion is embolic, bilateral in the superior temporal gyrus, in position to damage the primary auditory cortex in the transverse gyrus of Heschl and to impair its relation to the associated areas of the superior, posterior part of the temporal lobe. The occasional unilateral lesions are localized in this part of the major (dominant) temporal lobe and encroach on those regions whose involvement precipitates the larger syndrome of Wernicke's aphasia.

DYSLEXIA WITH DYSGRAPHIA This language disturbance is often a late sequela of the larger syndrome of Wernicke's aphasia, most evident in reading and writing. The syndrome is the visual form of Wernicke's aphasia. Errors occur in response to lexical stimuli. Auditory comprehension, while not normal, is less impaired than visual comprehension. Since conversational testing is frequently the only type of clinical evaluation in such patients, satisfactory auditory comprehension, ability to repeat aloud, and mild paraphasic errors in spontaneous speech frequently lead to a misdiagnosis of mild Wernicke's aphasia. Detailed testing of reading aloud and reading for comprehension and tests of spontaneous writing and of writing in response to dictated and visually presented material reveal a greater disturbance in these tasks.

The parietal and occipital region is usually affected. Although a discrete embolism is unusual, a small clot may pass through the more proximal territory and lodge distally. Tumors, abscess, and lobar hemorrhages usually disrupt other structures as well, and this syndrome is often a less conspicuous part of a larger clinical picture. Systemic hypotension and hypoxia may leave dyslexia with dysgraphia as a residual impairment, but more often they produce a more severe defect, described below under "Isolation of speech areas."

PURE WORD BLINDNESS In the fully developed syndrome, the victims lose the ability to read and usually to name colors. The patient is unable to name or point to a letter or word on command. However, understanding spoken language, repetition of what is heard, writing to dictation, conversation and writing, are all intact. The condition is also sometimes termed *dyslexia without dysgraphia*. Because the victim may be unaware the deficit exists, the examiner is often required to test for its presence, rather than simply assume the complaint will be volunteered. The errors may be minimal and the defect obscured if other visual cues are available, such as the bottle on which the words Coca-Cola appear. The naming of common colors presented singly and of objects is also impaired. When the syndrome is less severe, reading is impaired mainly in the affected visual field, producing a dyslexia for the letters on the affected side of the longer words (so-called hemidyslexia).

Right homonymous hemianopsia, an amnesic defect, and a hemisensory defect on the right reflect the involvement of the left occipital lobe and its callosal decussation, the left fornix, and the left thalamus, respectively, a combination that nearly always signifies thrombosis or embolism of the left posterior cerebral artery, placing the origin of this syndrome rather remote from the main language zone supplied by the middle cerebral artery.

Autopsy usually demonstrates a lesion that destroys the left visual striate cortex (area 17) and visual association areas (18 and 19), as well as the connections of the right visual cortex and association areas with the temporoparietal region. This latter "disconnection" usually is due to interruption of the fibers passing through the posterior part (splenium) of the corpus callosum, which connect the visual association areas of the two hemispheres. Rarely, a lesion deep in the left parietooccipital region prevents visual information from either occipital lobe from reaching the left language region. Right homonymous hemianopsia may be absent. Aside from infarction, the syndrome may occur from a primary or secondary tumor, multifocal leukoencephalopathy, or even from multiple sclerosis.

Isolation of speech areas Following prolonged hypoxia, widespread cerebral ischemia can affect the vascular border zones linking the major cerebral arteries and their distal branches on the cerebral surfaces and spread centripetally into their adjacent territories. The central fields of supply of these arteries may be spared. In the middle cerebral artery territory, this sparing leaves largely intact the sylvian region and its speech areas. With much of the rest of the brain out of action in patients who survive such episodes, the speech mechanism can be activated by spoken words. There is parrotlike repetition of words and sounds (echolalia) and similar findings which indicate that the auditory-vocal loop is functional. Scant evidence of comprehension or self-initiated conversation is present, reflecting the widespread injury outside the speech regions. The syndrome is common following cardiac arrest.

Amnesic-dysnomic aphasia This may be a relatively early or an isolated syndrome in patients with CNS disease. The patient has difficulty recalling names on demand, not only nouns but also adjectives and other descriptive parts of speech. There are usually pauses in speech, groping for words, and substitution of another word or phrase that conveys the meaning (circumlocution). The function of an object may be described, but its name forgotten. The difficulty applies not only to common objects seen but also to the names of things heard or felt. By contrast, other verbal tasks, including recall of the names of the letters and digits, reading, writing, spelling, etc., are far better performed.

The causative lesion is usually deep in the temporal lobe, presumably interrupting connections of sensory speech areas with the hippocampal-parahippocampal regions concerned with learning and memory (see Chap. 32). Masses such as a tumor or abscess are the most frequent causes; as they enlarge, an upper contralateral quadrantic visual field defect or Wernicke's aphasia is added. Dysnomia may be part of the syndromes produced by occlusion of the temporal branches of the posterior cerebral artery. Alzheimer's disease may begin with a dysnomic or amnesic type of aphasia; by the time the patient's difficulty is fully recognized, other disorders of speech and indifference, apathy, and abulia are conjoined. Dysnomia may also be present in confusional states caused by metabolic, infectious, intoxicative, or other acute medical illnesses, but then it has no certain localizing value.

The combination of dysnomia and major impairment of auditory comprehension with a remarkable retention of the ability to repeat what is heard is called *transcortical sensory aphasia*. The causative lesion spares the auditory cortex and Wernicke area and involves the inferior temporal cortices, particularly area 37.

DISORDERS OF ARTICULATION AND PHONATION The highly coordinated act of speaking involves the larynx, pharynx, palate, tongue, lips, and respiratory musculature, which are innervated by the hypoglossal, vagal, facial, and phrenic nerves. Their nuclei are controlled through the corticobulbar tracts by both motor cortices and by extrapyramidal influences from the cerebellum and basal ganglia. The current of air is produced by expiration and is finely regulated by the activity of the various muscles engaged in speech. *Phonation*, or the production of vocal sounds, is a function of the larynx. Changes in the size and shape of the glottis and in the length and tension of the vocal cords are controlled by the laryngeal muscles, which transmit their vibrations to the column of air passing over the vocal cords. Sounds thus formed are modified as they pass through the nasopharynx and mouth, which act as resonators. *Articulation* consists of contractions of the tongue, lips, pharynx, and palate, which interrupt or alter the vocal sounds. Vowels are of laryngeal origin, as are some consonants, but the latter are formed for the most part during articulation. For instance, the consonants *m, b,* and *p* are labial; *l* and *t* are lingual; and *nk* and *ng* are nasoguttural.

Disorders of phonation prompt examination of the vocal cords, tongue, palate, and pharynx. Defects in articulation can be subdivided into paretic dysarthria; spastic and rigid dysarthria; and choreic, myoclonic, and ataxic dysarthria.

Aphonia Some speech disorders involve disturbances of voice. Paresis of the respiratory movements, as in poliomyelitis and acute infectious polyneuritis, or incoordination as part of extrapyramidal disease may affect the voice because insufficient air is provided for phonation and speech. Reduced volume of speech due to limited excursion of the breathing muscles is common; the patient is unable to speak above a whisper or to shout. Whispering speech is also a feature of stupor, but strong stimulation may make the voice audible.

Paresis of both vocal cords causes complete aphonia. There is no voice, and the patient can speak only in whispers. Since the vocal cords normally separate during inspiration, their failure to do so when paralyzed may result in an inspiratory stridor. If one vocal cord is paralyzed, the voice becomes hoarse, low-pitched, and rasping. Involvement of one of the tenth cranial nerves by tumor, for example, may also cause a nasal voice because the posterior nares do not close during phonation. Consonants such as *b, p, n,* and *k* are followed by escape of air into the nasal passages. The abnormality may be less pronounced in recumbency and may increase when the head is thrown forward. Hoarseness may also be due to structural changes in the vocal cords caused by cigarette smoking, chronic inflammation, polyps, etc.

Spastic dysphonia is a poorly understood neurologic disorder similar to dystonia. Many patients, middle-aged or elderly, otherwise healthy, gradually lose the ability to speak quietly and fluently. Any effort to speak results in contraction of the speech musculature so that the voice is strained and phonation is labored. The patients are not neurotic, and psychotherapy and speech therapy are ineffective. The condition differs from the stridor caused by spasm of the laryngeal muscles in tetany. It is nonprogressive but may be combined with restricted extrapyramidal disorders such as blepharospasm and spasmodic torticollis. Surgical section of the superior laryngeal nerve on one side has been found to at least partially diminish the rigidity.

Paretic dysarthria This disorder of articulation is due to a neural or bulbar (medullary) weakness or paralysis of the articulatory muscles (lower motor neuron paralysis). There is a special difficulty in the correct utterance of vibratives, such as *r;* the voice develops a nasal quality due to palatal weakness; as the paralysis becomes more complete, lingual and labial consonants are not pronounced. In the advanced stages, the shriveled tongue lies inert on the floor of the mouth, and the lips are relaxed and tremulous. Saliva collects in the mouth because of dysphagia and spills over the lips causing drooling. Bulbar palsy, peripheral neuropathies, and muscle diseases, including myasthenia gravis, are common causes.

Spastic and rigid dysarthria This disorder is a supranuclear weakness of articulation. Diseases that involve the corticobulbar or subcortical tracts cause pseudobulbar palsy. In the past, the patient may have had a minor stroke affecting the corticobulbar fibers on one side; but since the bulbar muscles are probably represented in both motor cortices, there is no impairment in speech or swallowing from a unilateral lesion. Should another stroke then occur, involving the other corticobulbar tract and possibly the corticospinal tract at the pontine, midbrain, or capsular level, the patient becomes anarthric or dysarthric and dysphagic. Often the muscles of facial expression on both sides are weakened as well. Unlike bulbar paralysis due to lower neuron involvement, this condition entails no atrophy or fasciculation of the paralyzed muscles; the jaw jerk and other facial reflexes are exaggerated; the palatal reflexes are retained; emotional control is poor (pathologic laughter and crying); and sometimes breathing is periodic (Cheyne-Stokes). When the frontal operculum alone is involved, the speech deficit may be a pure dysarthria but usually without the impairment in emotional control. In the beginning, the patient may be totally anarthric and aphonic, but when improvement occurs or when the patient has a milder version of the same condition, speech is notably slow, thick, and indistinct, much like that of partial bulbar paralysis.

An extrapyramidal disturbance of articulation occurs in Parkinson's syndrome. The patient speaks hastily and articulates poorly, slurring over many syllables and trailing the ends of sentences. The voice is low-pitched, monotonous, and lacking in inflection; voice volume diminishes. In advanced cases speech is almost unintelligible; only whispering is possible.

In many cases of capsular hemiplegia or partially recovered Broca's aphasia, residual dysarthria may be difficult to distinguish from a pure articulatory defect.

Choreic and myoclonic dysarthria In chorea and myoclonus, speech may also be characteristic. Unlike the defect of pseudobulbar palsy or parkinsonism, chorea and myoclonus abruptly interrupt the pronunciation of words by the abnormal movements. Grimacing and other characteristic motor signs suggest the diagnosis.

Ataxic dysarthria This is characteristic of acute and chronic cerebellar lesions and may be observed in multiple sclerosis, Friedreich's ataxia, cerebellar atrophy, and heat stroke. The principal speech abnormality is slowness; imprecise enunciation, monotony, and unnatural, irregular separation of the syllables of words (scanning) are additional features. Coordination of speech and respiration are poor. There may not be enough breath to utter certain words, and others may be ejaculated explosively. Myoclonic jerks involving the speech musculature may be superimposed on cerebellar ataxia in a number of diseases.

CLINICAL APPROACH TO LANGUAGE DISORDERS

DIAGNOSIS **Aphasia** Conversational testing permits quick assessment of the motor aspects of speech (praxis and prosody), apparent language formulation, and auditory comprehension. Disabilities in the purely motor aspects of speech suggest a motor aphasia, and this possibility can be pursued by tests of repeating from dictation and by tests of praxis of the oropharyngeal and respiratory apparatus. Disabilities in language formulation such as literal paraphasias with impaired comprehension are indicative of Wernicke's aphasia. Disorders confined to naming, generally without paraphasias, when other language functions (reading, writing, spelling, etc.) are adequate, are diagnostic of amnesic dysnomia.

Dyspraxia of limbs and speech musculature in response to spoken commands or to visual mimicry is generally associated with Broca's aphasia and sometimes with Wernicke's aphasia. Bilateral or unilateral homonymous hemianopsia without motor weakness is often linked with pure word blindness (alexia or dyslexia) or to amnesic-dysnomic aphasia. Bilateral hemiplegias due to extensive frontal lesions are accompanied not infrequently by pure word muteness.

When conversation shows virtually no disabilities, other tests may be revealing. Reading aloud single letters, words, and text may reveal pure word blindness, while tests of writing in this syndrome are normal. Literal and verbal paraphasic errors may appear in milder cases of Wernicke's aphasia as the patient reads aloud from text or from words in the examiner's handwriting. Similar errors occur more frequently when the patient is asked to explain the text, read aloud, or give explanations in writing. Adequacy of response channels is determined by presenting tasks that permit a response physically identical with the test stimulus, such as copying visual stimuli and repeating aloud from auditory stimuli. Inadequacy of receptive or response channels precludes further analysis of the deficit involving that channel in more complex types of tests, except in the unlikely instance that the more complex test is better performed. If reception and response channels are adequate in these initial tests, they may then be used in tests requiring all types of language function, such as writing from dictation, vocal naming of visual stimuli, matching physically dissimilar stimuli having a name in common (e.g., the word *cow* and a picture of a cow). By using the same test material as in the earlier tests, direct comparison of performances in spoken naming, written naming, and matching can be made from visual, auditory, and palpated stimuli. A performance profile can be constructed separately for each type of stimulus material tested (objects, pictures, words, letters, numbers, colors, etc.). The resultant profile can then be used to determine whether the main deficits fall across one or more input or response channels. These data provide a baseline against which later changes may be compared.

Articulatory-phonation disorders Disturbances of articulation point to involvement of a different set of neural structures, such as the motor cortices; the corticobulbar pathways; the seventh, ninth, and tenth nuclei; the brainstem; and extrapyramidal nuclei and tracts. It may be necessary to use other neurologic findings to decide which of these are implicated. It is particularly important to distinguish between the pseudobulbar or supranuclear palsies and the bulbar palsies. The information obtained by separating these two types of dysarthria is particularly helpful in differential diagnosis.

Dysphonia should lead to an investigation of laryngeal disease, either primary or secondary to an abnormality of innervation. Inspection of the vocal cords is necessary.

TREATMENT Except for almost pure motor defects, most patients show remarkably little concern over the sudden loss of speech. The very lesion that deprives them of speech also appears to cause a partial loss of insight into the disability. Nonetheless, as improvement occurs, many patients become discouraged. Reassurance and a positive program of speech rehabilitation are the best ways of helping the patient at this stage.

As a rule, speech therapy is not advisable in the first few days of an aphasic illness, because one does not know how lasting it will be. Also, if a global aphasia is present, the speech therapist is helpless. Under such circumstances, it is preferable to wait until some of the language function has begun to return. In milder aphasic disorders speech therapy can be begun as soon as the illness is stabilized. Although speech therapy has not been proved, in controlled studies, to be of benefit to recovery, its value in terms of support for the patient and the family needs to be emphasized.

There is no special treatment for the dysarthric disturbance of speech.

PROGNOSIS The outcome depends on the underlying disease and the magnitude of the lesion within the speech areas. Global aphasias lasting more than a week or two usually have a bad outcome. Seldom is there enough recovery of communicative speech to permit resumption of occupation or profession. Partial aphasias frequently improve, sometimes to a gratifying degree, if of vascular or encephalitic origin. Aphasias due to embolism, whether global or restricted, may disappear in hours to days or may persist.

Most aphasias are due to vascular disease of the brain, and some degree of spontaneous improvement usually occurs over days to months after the stroke. Sometimes recovery is complete within hours or days; at times not more than a few words are regained after a year or two of assiduous speech training. Nevertheless, many experts in the field believe that speech training is worthwhile.

REFERENCES

Albert ML et al: *Clinical Aspects of Dysphasia.* New York, Springer-Verlag, 1981

Chase TN et al: Wechsler adult intelligence scale performance. Cortical localization by fluorodeoxyglucose F18-positron emission tomography. Arch Neurol 41:1244, 1984

Damasio AR, Geschwind N: The neural basis of language. Ann Rev Neurosci 7:127, 1984

Kempler D et al: A metabolic investigation of a disconnection syndrome: Conduction aphasia. Ann Neurol 22:134, 1987

Ludlow CL et al: Brain lesions associated with nonfluent aphasia fifteen years following penetrating head injury. Brain 109:55, 1986

Metter EJ et al: A study of Broca's aphasia by 18F-fluorodeoxyglucose positron emission tomography. Ann Neurol 22:134, 1987

Mohr JP, Sidman M: Aphasia: Behavioral aspects, in *American Handbook of Psychiatry,* vol 4, M Reiser (ed). New York, Basic Books, 1975, pp 279–298

Petersen SE et al: Positron emission tomography studies of the cortical anatomy of single-word processing. Nature 331:585, 1988

Posner MI et al: Localization of cognitive operations in the human brain. Science 240:1627, 1988

34 DISORDERS OF SLEEP AND CIRCADIAN RHYTHMS

CHARLES A. CZEISLER / GARY S. RICHARDSON / JOSEPH B. MARTIN

Disturbed sleep is among the most frequent health complaints physicians encounter. One-third of adults in the United States experience occasional or persistent sleep disturbances. Sleep deprivation or disruption of the circadian timing system can lead to serious impairment of daytime functioning. Sleep disorders may either contribute to or result from related medical or psychiatric conditions. Twenty years ago, many such complaints were treated with hypnotic medications without further diagnostic evaluation. A distinct class of sleep and arousal disorders has now been identified, and the field of sleep disorders is now an established clinical discipline. Two principal neurobiologic systems govern the sleep-wake cycle: one that actively generates sleep and sleep-related processes and another that times sleep within the 24-h day. Either intrinsic abnormalities in these systems or extrinsic disturbances (environmental, drug- or illness-related) can lead to sleep or circadian rhythm disorders.

PHYSIOLOGY OF SLEEP AND WAKEFULNESS

Most adults sleep 7 to 8 h per night, although the timing, duration, and internal structure of sleep vary among apparently healthy individuals and as a function of age. At the extremes, infants and the elderly have frequent interruptions of sleep. In the United States, individuals of intermediate age tend to have one consolidated sleep episode per day, although in some cultures sleep may be divided into a midafternoon nap and a shortened night sleep. Infants sleep more than half the day, and the elderly sleep less than half that amount. While there is a wide range of normal sleep lengths, adults with habitual sleep durations of fewer than 4 h or greater than 9 have increased mortality rates as compared to those who sleep 7 to 8 h per night.

STATES AND STAGES OF SLEEP States and stages of human sleep are defined on the basis of characteristic patterns in three electrophysiologic parameters, the electroencephalogram (EEG), the electrooculogram (EOG—a measure of eye-movement activity), and the electromyogram (EMG). In routine sleep recordings, the EEG is recorded from a single central derivation (C3 or C4 in the 10 to 20 standard EEG nomenclature), and sleep states are defined on the basis of the EEG pattern. The EOG is recorded from electrodes placed on the outer canthus of each eye, and the EMG is recorded from the submentalis muscle of the chin. The continuous recording of this array of electrophysiologic parameters to define sleep and wakefulness is termed *polysomnography* (see Table 34-1).

Polysomnograpahic profiles define two states of sleep: (1) rapid-eye-movement (REM) sleep (also known as dreaming, paradoxical, desynchronized, or "D" sleep) and (2) non-rapid-eye-movement (NREM) sleep. NREM sleep is in turn subdivided into four stages. NREM stage 1 is the transition from wakefulness and is characterized by disappearance of the regular alpha pattern and emergence of a low-amplitude, mixed-frequency pattern, predominantly in the theta range (2 to 7 Hz) (Fig. 34-1) and slow "rolling" eye movements. The amplitude of the EMG attenuates and its variability is reduced. NREM stage 2 is defined by the occurrence of K complexes and sleep spindles superimposed upon a background activity similar to that of stage 1. K complexes are slow, high-amplitude, negative (upward) discharges followed immediately by a positive (downward) deflection. Sleep spindles are high-frequency (12 to 14 Hz) discharges lasting 0.5 to 2.0 s with a characteristic waxing-waning amplitude. Eye-movement activity is absent, and the EMG is similar to stage 1. NREM stage 3 is sleep with at least 20 percent but less than 50

TABLE 34-1 Electrophysiologic correlates of human sleep states and stages

	Electroencephalogram	Electrooculogram	Electromyogram
Wake (eyes open)	Low amplitude, mixed, (high) frequency	Rapid	High, variable
Wake (eyes closed)	Low amplitude, alpha (8–13 Hz) dominates, particularly over occipital region	Absent, but slow "rolling" eye movements	Reduced
NREM stage 1	Low amplitude, mixed frequency (alpha absent)	Slow "rolling" eye movements	Reduced
NREM stage 2	Low amplitude with addition of characteristic EEG patterns (K complexes and sleep spindles)	Absent	Reduced
NREM stage 3	Increased amplitude, decreased frequency 20–50% of record dominated by delta (0.5–2.0 Hz)	Absent	Reduced
NREM stage 4	>50% of record dominated by delta EEG activity	Absent	Reduced
REM	Low amplitude, mixed frequency	Rapid, conjugate	Absent

SOURCE: Modified from: Rechtschaffen A, Kales A (eds): *A Manual of Standardized Terminology, Technique and Scoring System for Sleep Stages of Human Subjects.* Los Angeles, UCLA Brain Information Service/Brain Research Institute, 1968.

percent high-amplitude delta (0.5 to 2 Hz) activity. Sleep spindles may persist, eye-movement activity is absent, and EMG activity persists at a reduced level. In NREM stage 4, the high-voltage, slow EEG pattern of stage 3 comprises at least 50 percent of the record. NREM stages 3 and 4 are referred to, collectively, as "slow-wave," "delta," or "deep" sleep.

FIGURE 34-1 Electroencephalogram of human sleep stages. The first trace illustrates alpha activity seen in quiet wakefulness (eyes closed) and the beta activity of an alert subject. Stage 1 theta activity is seen in the second trace; stage 2 sleep (with associated sleep spindle and K complex) in the third. The fourth and fifth traces show slow-wave (stages 3 and 4) sleep, with prominent delta activity. This synchronous activity is absent in REM sleep (sixth trace), which resembles stage 1 EEG. However, REM sleep is accompanied by rapid eye movements and muscle paralysis. (*Reproduced from Horne.*)

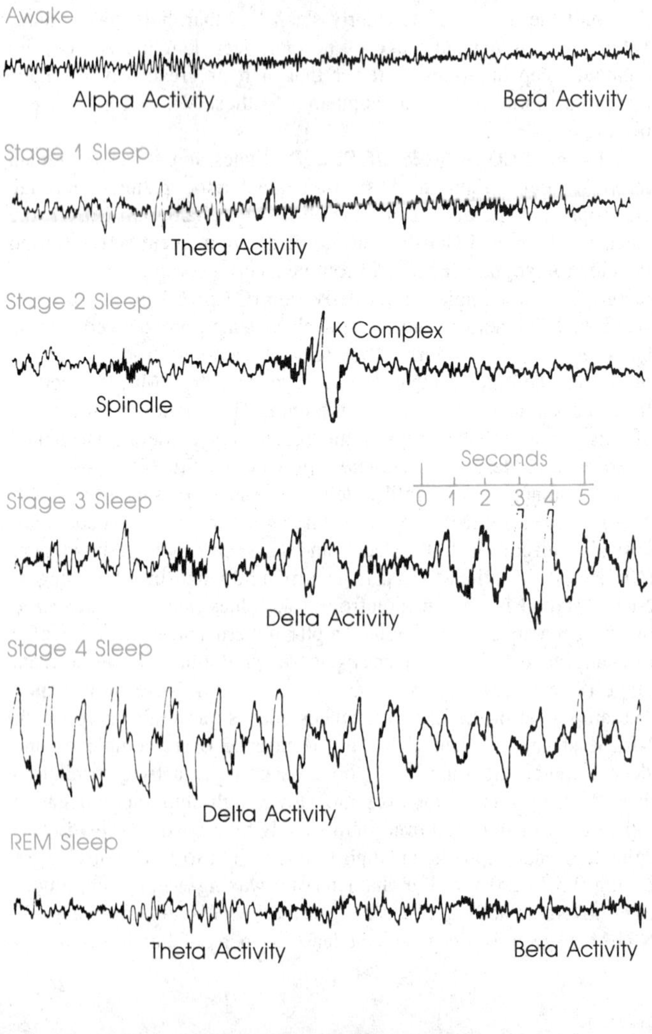

The second state of human sleep, REM, is characterized by a low-amplitude, mixed-frequency EEG similar to that of NREM stage 1. Superimposed are bursts of 3- to 5-Hz activity with sharp negative deflections (Fig. 34-1). The EOG shows REM indistinguishable from that seen during eyes-open wakefulness. EMG activity is absent, reflecting the characteristic descending motor paralysis of the state.

ORGANIZATION OF HUMAN SLEEP Normal nocturnal sleep in adults displays a consistent organization from night to night (Fig. 34-2). After sleep onset, sleep usually progresses through NREM stages 1 to 4 within 45 to 60 min. Slow-wave sleep (NREM stages 3 and 4) predominates in the first third of the night and comprises 15 to 25 percent of total nocturnal sleep time in young adults. The percentage of slow-wave sleep is influenced by several factors, most notably age (see below). In addition, prior sleep deprivation increases both the rapidity with which slow-wave sleep begins and its percentage of total sleep.

After the first slow-wave sleep episode, the progression of NREM stages reverses; the first REM sleep occurs, usually not less than 80 min after sleep begins. More rapid onset of REM sleep (particularly less than 30 min) suggests pathology such as endogenous depression, narcolepsy, or circadian rhythm disorders. NREM and REM alternate through the night with an average cycle of 90 to 110 min (the "ultradian" cycle). In time the portion of each cycle composed of slow-wave sleep decreases and that of REM sleep increases. Overall, REM sleep is 20 to 25 percent of total sleep, NREM stages (1 and 2) are 50 to 60 percent (increasing in elderly subjects).

BEHAVIORAL CORRELATES OF SLEEP STATES AND STAGES Age has a large impact on sleep state organization (Fig. 34-2). Slow-wave sleep is most prominent during childhood, decreasing sharply at puberty and across the second and third decades of life. After age 30, there is a progressive, almost linear decline in the amount of slow-wave sleep, and the amplitude of delta EEG activity comprising slow-wave sleep is reduced. In the otherwise healthy elderly, slow-wave sleep may be completely absent.

A different age profile exists for REM sleep. In infancy, REM sleep may comprise 50 percent of total sleep time, and the percentage is inversely proportional to developmental age. The amount of REM sleep falls off sharply over the first postnatal year as a mature REM-NREM cycle develops. During the rest of life into extreme old age, REM occupies a remarkably constant percentage of total sleep time.

Polysomnographic staging of sleep correlates with behavioral changes during specific states and stages. Sleep onset is associated with marked decrements in perception of both auditory and visual stimuli and lapses of consciousness. At stage 1 subjects may respond to faint auditory or visual signals without "awakening." Furthermore, although memory incorporation appears to be inhibited at the onset of NREM stage 1, subjects aroused from that stage frequently deny having been asleep. In contrast, subjective and objective assessments of sleep agree more closely for subjects awakened from NREM stage 2. This has led some investigators to define sleep onset as the

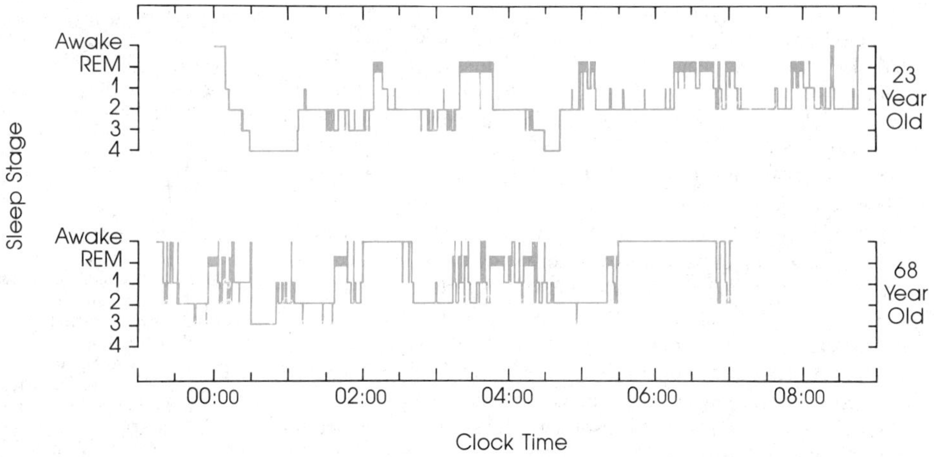

FIGURE 34-2 Plots of the stages of REM sleep (solid bars) and the four stages of NREM sleep over the course of the entire night for representative young (upper panel, age 23) and elderly (lower panel, age 68) adult men. The recording in the elderly subject illustrates the reduction of delta sleep, frequent spontaneous awakenings, early sleep onset, and early morning awakening that are characteristic features of sleep in the aged, even in the absence of specific medical or psychiatric pathology. (*From the Center for Circadian and Sleep Disorders Medicine, Brigham and Women's Hospital.*)

occurrence of the first K complex or sleep spindle suggestive of NREM stage 2 and to define NREM stage 1 as a "transitional stage." The progression of subsequent NREM stages corresponds with increasing depth of sleep as measured by threshold for arousal with a variety of auditory stimuli.

Awakenings from REM sleep are associated with recall of vivid dream imagery more than 80 percent of the time. The reliability of dream recall increases with REM periods occurring later in the night. Imagery may also be reported after NREM sleep interruptions, though these typically lack the detail and vividness of REM dreams. The incidence of NREM dream recall can be increased by selective REM sleep deprivation, suggesting that REM sleep and dreaming per se are not inexorably linked.

PHYSIOLOGIC CORRELATES OF SLEEP STATES AND STAGES All major physiologic systems are influenced by sleep. In some cases, concomitant behavior changes such as supine posture or inactivity are the proximal causes of altered physiologic function, but in most cases the sleep state itself appears to be responsible. Changes in cardiovascular function include a decrease in blood pressure and heart rate during NREM and particularly during slow-wave sleep. During REM sleep, phasic activity (bursts of eye movements) is associated with variability in both blood pressure and heart rate mediated principally by the vagus. Cardiac dysrhythmias may occur selectively during REM sleep. Respiratory function also changes (see Chap. 217). Respiratory rate and minute ventilation decrease during NREM sleep and become variable during phasic REM sleep. The ventilatory response to carbon dioxide attenuates during NREM sleep, resulting in a higher P_{CO_2}. During REM sleep the ventilatory response to both hypercapnia and hypoxia shows marked variability. Respiratory musculature, including that responsible for upper airway patency, is hypotonic throughout sleep and more so during REM sleep, resulting in an increase in airway resistance. In addition, the cough reflex is attenuated or absent during sleep. These changes in respiratory function may be relevant to the pathogenesis of obstructive sleep apnea (OSA) and sudden infant death syndrome (SIDS) (see Chap. 217).

Endocrine function also varies with sleep. The most prominent changes are apparent in neuroendocrine parameters. Slow-wave sleep is associated with secretion of growth hormone in humans, while sleep in general is associated with augmented secretion of prolactin. Sleep has a complex effect on the secretion of luteinizing hormone (LH); during puberty sleep is associated with increased LH secretion while sleep in the mature female inhibits LH secretion in the early follicular phase of the menstrual cycle. Sleep onset (and probably slow-wave sleep) is associated with inhibition of thyroid-stimulating hormone (TSH) and of the adrenocorticotropic hormone (ACTH)–cortisol axis, an effect that is independent of the circadian rhythms in the two systems (see Fig. 34-3).

Sleep is also associated with alterations of thermoregulatory function. NREM sleep is associated with an attenuation of thermoregulatory responses to either heat or cold stress, and animal studies of thermosensitive neurons in the hypothalamus document a NREM-dependent reduction of the thermoregulatory set-point. REM sleep is associated with complete absence of thermoregulatory responsivity resulting in effective poikilothermy. However, the potential adverse impact of this failure of thermoregulation is blunted by inhibition of REM sleep by extreme ambient temperatures.

Neuroanatomy of sleep Lesion studies in animals and neurologic diseases in humans have suggested distinct neuroanatomic sites in the generation of normal sleep and wakefulness. The studies of von Economo of patients with encephalitis lethargica suggested that the anterior hypothalamus contained a "sleep center" while the posterior hypothalamus contained a "wake center." Experimental studies in animals have variously implicated the medullary reticular formation, the thalamus, and the basal forebrain in the generation of sleep, while the brainstem reticular formation, the midbrain, the subthalamus, the thalamus, and the basal forebrain have all been suggested to play a role in the generation of wakefulness or EEG arousal (see also Chap. 31).

Despite many studies, there is little evidence for either a single, discrete "sleep center" or a single, discrete "wake center." Current hypotheses suggest that the capacity for sleep and wake generation is distributed along an axial "core" of neurons extending from the brainstem rostrally to the basal forebrain. Complex comingling of neuronal groups occurs at many points along this basal forebrain axis.

However, the neuroanatomic correlates of REM sleep appear to be more discretely localized. Specific regions in the pons are associated with each of the neurophysiologic correlates of REM sleep. Small lesions in the dorsal pons produce REM sleep without the descending muscle inhibition normally associated with that state; microinjections of carbachol into the same area produce atonia without other features of REM sleep. These experimental manipulations are mimicked by pathologic conditions in humans and animals. In narcolepsy, for example, abrupt, complete or partial paralysis (cataplexy) occurs in response to a variety of stimuli. In dogs with this condition, physostigmine, a central cholinesterase inhibitor, increases the frequency of cataplectic attacks while atropine decreases their frequency. Conversely, in REM sleep behavior disorder (see below), patients suffer from incomplete motor inhibition during REM sleep resulting in involuntary, occasionally violent movement during REM sleep.

Neurochemistry of sleep Early experimental studies that focused on the raphe nuclei of the brainstem appeared to implicate serotonin as the primary sleep-promoting neurotransmitter, while catecholamines were considered to be responsible for wakefulness. Subsequent work has demonstrated that the raphe-serotonin system may facilitate sleep but is not necessary to its expression. The extensive pharmacology of sleep and wakefulness suggests roles for other neurotransmitters as well. The alerting influence of caffeine implicates adenosine while the hypnotic effect of benzodiazepines and barbiturates suggests a role for endogenous ligands of the GABA-receptor complex.

A variety of sleep-promoting substances have been identified.

These are principally peptides, and the hypnotic effect is commonly limited to NREM or slow-wave sleep, although peptides that increase REM sleep have also been reported. Many of these "sleep factors," including interleukin 1 and prostaglandin E_2, are immunologically active as well, suggesting a link between immune function and sleep-wake states.

PHYSIOLOGY OF CIRCADIAN RHYTHMICITY The sleep-wake cycle is the most evident of the many 24-h rhythms in humans. Prominent daily variations also occur in endocrine, thermoregulatory, cardiac, pulmonary, renal, gastrointestinal, and cognitive functions. However, in evaluating a daily variation, it is important to distinguish between those rhythmic components passively evoked by periodic environmental or behavioral changes (e.g., the increase in blood pressure and heart rate upon assumption of the upright posture), and those actively driven by an endogenous oscillatory process (e.g., the circadian variation in plasma cortisol that persists under a variety of environmental and behavioral conditions).

The suprachiasmatic nuclei (SCN) of the hypothalamus act as the central neural pacemakers of the circadian timing system in mammals. The persistence of some rhythmicity after SCN lesions suggests that they synchronize subsidiary rhythms rather than serving as the sole source of rhythmicity. The period and phase of the endogenous neural oscillator are normally synchronized to the 24-h period of the environmental light-dark cycle. Entrainment of mammalian circadian rhythms by the light-dark cycle is mediated via the retinohypothalamic tract, a monosynaptic pathway that links the retina to the SCN.

The principal properties characterizing an endogenous circadian pacemaker are its *intrinsic period, phase, amplitude,* and *resetting capacity*. In human subjects living in controlled laboratory environments free of time cues (*free-running*), the duration of the behavioral rest-activity cycle averages 25 h. However, the rest-activity cycle often oscillates with a period that is different from that of other physiologic measures (such as body temperature, plasma cortisol, and urinary potassium). This state of "internal desynchronization" implies that the endogenous circadian pacemaker actually has a shorter period, averaging about 24.6 h. Therefore, synchronization of the endogenous circadian pacemaker to the 24-h day requires that the pacemaker be reset by about 0.6 h each day, which is normally achieved by exposure to the environmental light-dark cycle.

Exposure to light can shift the phase of the endogenous circadian pacemaker, but both the magnitude and direction of the phase shifts induced by light depend on the timing and intensity of the light. Properly timed exposure to light of sufficient intensity can, within 2 to 3 days, reset the human circadian pacemaker (presumably the SCN).

The timing and internal architecture of sleep are directly coupled to the output of the endogenous pacemaker. Spontaneous sleep duration, sleepiness, REM sleep propensity, and both the ability and the tendency to sleep vary with the circadian phase as marked by the endogenous circadian temperature cycle in humans. Sleep tendency, sleepiness, and REM sleep propensity all peak just after the nadir of the endogenous circadian temperature cycle (approximately 3 h before awakening). In addition, 85 percent of all spontaneous awakenings of subjects living in constant environmental conditions occur on the rising slope of the temperature cycle. Furthermore, there are certain times (wake maintenance zones) when it is very difficult to fall asleep, even in subjects who are sleep deprived. Misalignment of the output of the endogenous circadian pacemaker with the desired sleep-wake cycle is thought to be responsible for certain types of insomnia, as well as for the decrements of alertness and performance in night-shift workers and after jet lag.

DISORDERS OF SLEEP AND WAKEFULNESS

An international classification of sleep disorders (Table 34-2) divides these conditions into three major groups: dyssomnias, parasomnias, and medical psychiatric sleep disorders. A detailed description of each of these disorders may be found in the publication of the American Sleep Disorders Association.

TABLE 34-2 International classification of sleep disorders

- *I* Dyssomnias
  - *A* Intrinsic sleep disorders
    - *1* Psychophysiologic insomnia
    - *2* Idiopathic insomnia
    - *3* Narcolepsy
    - *4* Recurrent or idiopathic hypersomnia
    - *5* Posttraumatic hypersomnia
    - *6* Sleep apnea syndromes
    - *7* Periodic limb movement disorder
    - *8* Restless legs syndrome
  - *B* Extrinsic sleep disorders
    - *1* Inadequate sleep hygiene
    - *2* Environmental sleep disorder
    - *3* Altitude insomnia
    - *4* Adjustment sleep disorder
    - *5* Sleep-onset association disorder
    - *6* Food allergy insomnia
    - *7* Nocturnal eating (drinking) syndrome
    - *8* Drug- or alcohol-dependent sleep disorders
  - *C* Circadian rhythm sleep disorders
    - *1* Time-zone change (jet-lag) syndrome
    - *2* Shift-work sleep disorder
    - *3* Delayed sleep phase syndrome
    - *4* Advanced sleep phase syndrome
    - *5* Non-24-h sleep-wake disorder
- *II* Parasomnias
  - *A* Arousal disorders
    - *1* Confusional arousals
    - *2* Sleepwalking
    - *3* Sleep terrors
  - *B* Sleep-wake transition disorders
    - *1* Rhythmic movement disorder
    - *2* Sleep talking
    - *3* Nocturnal leg cramps
  - *C* Parasomnias usually associated with REM sleep
    - *1* Nightmares
    - *2* Sleep paralysis
    - *3* Impaired sleep-related penile erections
    - *4* Sleep-related painful erections
    - *5* REM sleep-related cardiac arrhythmias
    - *6* REM sleep behavior disorder
  - *D* Other parasomnias
    - *1* Sleep bruxism
    - *2* Sleep enuresis
    - *3* Nocturnal paroxysmal dystonia
- *III* Sleep disorders associated with medical/psychiatric disorders
  - *A* Associated with mental disorders
  - *B* Associated with neurologic disorders
    - *1* Cerebral degenerative disorders
    - *2* Parkinsonism
    - *3* Fatal familial insomnia
    - *4* Sleep-related epilepsy
    - *5* Sleep-related headaches
  - *C* Associated with other medical disorders
    - *1* Sleeping sickness
    - *2* Nocturnal cardiac ischemia
    - *3* Chronic obstructive pulmonary disease
    - *4* Sleep-related asthma
    - *5* Sleep-related gastroesophageal reflux
    - *6* Peptic ulcer disease
    - *7* Fibrositis syndrome

SOURCE: Modified from *International Classification of Sleep Disorders,* prepared by the Diagnostic Classification Committee, Thorpy MJ, Chairman. American Sleep Disorders Association, in press, 1990.

APPROACH TO THE PATIENT WITH A SLEEP COMPLAINT Several general principles are useful to the physician with a patient who complains of sleep disruption. The first is recognition that the severity of the reported chronic sleep disruption (i.e., the complaint of chronic insomnia) is often exaggerated relative to objective measurement. In addition, nocturnal sleep and daytime alertness are linked in a predictable way. With the advent of objective measurements of sleep tendency (see below), quantification of the impairment of daytime alertness is a valuable adjunct in the assessment of sleep problems. As a rule, the clinical approach to a patient with disrupted sleep but without impaired daytime alertness should be conservative. Chronic treatment of isolated insomnia with hypnotic medications is rarely justified.

Laboratory investigation In addition to the three electrophysiologic variables used to define sleep states and stages (see above), the standard clinical polysomnogram includes measures of respiration (respiratory effort, air flow, and oxygen saturation), lower extremity EMG, and ECG. Assessment of daytime functioning as an index of the adequacy of sleep can be made with the multiple sleep latency test (MSLT), which involves repeated measurement of sleep latency (time to onset of sleep) at 2-h intervals under standardized conditions during a day following quantified nocturnal sleep. The average latency across five to seven tests (administered every 2 h across the waking day) is taken as an objective measure of daytime sleep tendency. Disorders of sleep that result in pathologic, daytime somnolence can be reliably distinguished with the MSLT. In addition, the multiple measurements of sleep onset identify direct transitions from wakefulness to REM sleep that are indicative of specific pathologic conditions (e.g., narcolepsy). Finally, evaluation of penile tumescence during sleep can be used to determine whether the etiology of erectile dysfunction in a patient is psychogenic or organic (see Chap. 52).

INSOMNIA Insomnia is a common complaint that increases in prevalence with advancing age. As many as half of people between 65 and 79 years of age complain of disturbed sleep. This may account for the fact that 40 percent of all sleeping pills are consumed by the elderly who represent only 11 percent of the general population. To reduce the number of patients dependent on hypnotics, it is important for physicians to make an effort to determine the underlying cause of insomnia before initiating treatment. Insomnia is usually subdivided into *sleep onset, sleep maintenance,* or *premature awakening* type. Transient insomnia can last up to 3 to 4 weeks; after that, it is considered chronic. It is important to note that patients often cannot estimate actual sleep time. Objective polysomnographic recording can indicate that a patient slept 6 to 7 h, even though that same patient reports having been "up all night."

Psychophysiologic insomnia Persistent psychophysiologic insomnia is a behavioral disorder in which patients are preoccupied with a perceived inability to sleep at night. The sleep disturbance is often triggered by an emotionally stressful event; however, the poor sleep habits acquired during the stressful period persist long after the initial incident. Such patients become hyperaroused by their own persistent efforts to sleep, and the insomnia is a conditioned or learned response. Patients with psychophysiologic insomnia fall asleep more easily at unscheduled times (when not trying) or outside the home environment. In these cases, polysomnographic recording reveals an objective sleep disturbance, often with an abnormally long sleep latency, frequent nocturnal awakenings, and an increased amount of stage 1 transitional sleep. Behavioral therapy is often beneficial; relaxation training can improve the sleep of patients in whom anxiety is prominent. Limited use of hypnotic medications, which can serve as a catalyst for successful behavioral therapy, may be appropriate. Extrinsic factors may contribute to this condition (see below). Rigorous attention should be paid to sleep hygiene (see below) and correction of counterproductive, arousing behaviors before bedtime.

Extrinsic insomnia A number of sleep disorders are the result of extrinsic factors that interfere with sleep. *Adjustment sleep disorder,* also called *transient situational insomnia,* can occur after a change in the sleeping environment (e.g., in an unfamiliar hotel or hospital bed) or before or after a significant life event, such as a change of occupation, loss of a loved one, illness, or anxiety over a deadline or examination. Increased sleep latency, frequent awakenings from sleep, and early morning awakening can all occur. Recovery generally occurs rapidly, certainly within 2 to 3 weeks. *Inadequate sleep hygiene* is characterized by a behavior pattern prior to sleep and/or a bedroom environment that is not conducive to sleep. On taking a careful history, physicians may learn that some insomniac patients are attempting to sleep with the television on throughout the night or are attempting to sleep just after coming home from work at midnight. Noise and/or light in the bedroom can interfere with sleep, as can a bed partner with periodic limb movements during sleep or one who snores loudly. Luminous clocks can arouse the patient, heightening anxiety about the time it has taken to fall asleep. Large meals, extensive exercise, or hot showers just before sleep may interfere with sleep onset. Patients should be counseled to develop a soporific bedtime ritual and to prepare and reserve the bedroom environment for sleeping.

Altitude insomnia Sleep disturbance is a common consequence of exposure to high altitude. Periodic breathing of the Cheyne-Stokes type occurs during NREM sleep about half the time at altitude, with restoration of a regular breathing pattern during REM sleep. Central rather than obstructive sleep apnea appears to be responsible, and the regularity of the respiratory pauses distinguishes this breathing pattern from central sleep apnea seen at sea level. Both hypoxia and hypocapnia are thought to be involved in the development of periodic breathing. Frequent awakenings and poor quality sleep characterize altitude insomnia, which is generally worst on the first few nights at high altitude but may persist. The duration of sleep is unchanged, but there are more arousals after sleep onset and less time in slow-wave (stages 3 and 4) sleep. Pretreatment with acetazolamide can decrease time spent in periodic breathing and substantially reduce hypoxia during sleep. Medroxyprogesterone acetate (MPA) also reduces periodic breathing but does not significantly reduce hypoxia during sleep at altitude.

Drug- or alcohol-dependent sleep disorders Disturbed sleep can result from ingestion of a wide variety of agents. Caffeine is perhaps the most common pharmacologic cause of insomnia in sensitive patients. It produces increased latency to sleep onset, more frequent arousals during sleep, and a reduction in total sleep time for up to 8 to 14 h after ingestion. Some patients are surprised to learn that their insomnia may be related to coffee consumption; a careful history will reveal that such patients may drink 15 to 20 cups per day. As few as 3 to 5 cups of coffee can significantly disturb sleep in some patients; therefore, a 1- to 2-month caffeine withdrawal period should be attempted in patients with these symptoms. Similarly, alcohol and nicotine can interfere with sleep, although many patients use them to relax and promote sleep. Although alcohol can increase drowsiness and shorten sleep latency, even moderate amounts of alcohol increase awakenings after sleep onset by interfering with the ability of the brain to maintain sleep. In addition, alcohol ingestion prior to sleep is contraindicated in patients with sleep apnea because of the inhibitory effects of alcohol on respiration. Acutely, amphetamines and cocaine suppress REM sleep, which returns to normal with chronic use. Withdrawal leads to a REM sleep rebound. Finally, rebound insomnia associated with the acute withdrawal of hypnotics can be severe, especially following the use of benzodiazepines with a short half-life. For this reason, hypnotics should rarely be prescribed for habitual use; doses should be low to moderate, the total duration of hypnotic therapy should be limited to 2 to 3 weeks, and drug dosage should be reduced prior to withdrawal.

NARCOLEPSY Excessive daytime sleepiness with involuntary daytime sleep episodes, disturbed nocturnal sleep, and cataplexy (sudden weakness or loss of muscle tone, often elicited by emotion) are the most common symptoms of narcolepsy. Some patients also experience muscular paralysis and/or hallucinations at sleep onset or upon awakening. The severity varies. Patients may have two to three cataplectic attacks per day or per decade, and the extent and duration of an attack may vary from a transient sagging of the jaw to flaccid paralysis of the entire voluntary musculature for 20 to 30 min.

Narcolepsy affects over 100,000 people in the United States and appears to have a genetic basis. Experiments in some canine models of narcolepsy suggest an autosomal recessive pattern of inheritance. First-degree relatives of narcoleptic patients commonly exhibit excessive daytime somnolence and have at least a hundredfold higher incidence of narcolepsy than the general population. In addition, nearly all narcoleptics are positive for the human leukocyte antigen DR2 (see Chap. 14).

Symptoms typically begin in the second decade, although the onset ranges from ages 5 to 50. An identifiable stress (e.g., sleep-wake cycle disruption, divorce, loss of a loved one) may precede symptom onset.

Diagnosis Classically, the diagnosis of narcolepsy required the presence of the "narcolepsy tetrad," consisting of (1) excessive daytime somnolence, (2) cataplexy, (3) hypnogogic hallucinations (the occurrence of vivid hallucinatory dream imagery at sleep onset), and (4) sleep paralysis (an awareness that voluntary musculature is paralyzed coincident with the onset of sleep). The last three symptoms of the tetrad are all manifestations of the abnormal REM sleep regulation inherent in the syndrome. All patients with narcolepsy have objectively verifiable daytime somnolence, but the other three symptoms are variably present. Eighty percent have cataplexy of some degree and smaller percentages report hyponogogic hallucinations and/or sleep paralysis. Other associated symptoms are useful but not specific. A history of "automatic behavior" during wakefulness (a trancelike state during which simple motor behaviors persist) serves principally to corroborate the presence of daytime somnolence but is not specific for mechanism. Patients with narcolepsy also commonly report severe disruption of nocturnal sleep, a feature that may distinguish narcolepsy from other causes of daytime somnolence.

A family history is important in the evaluation of the patient with excessive daytime somnolence. Careful observation of the children and siblings of known narcoleptics, particularly at the typical age of onset (second decade), can lead to early diagnosis. The diagnosis of narcolepsy in a patient with a suggestive history depends upon (1) objective verification of excessive daytime somnolence, typically using the MSLT after nocturnal sleep recording, and (2) documentation of abnormal REM sleep regulation as evidenced by direct wake-to-REM sleep transitions either during the nocturnal recording or on one or more of the MSLT determinations.

Treatment The treatment of narcolepsy is symptomatic. Somnolence is treated with stimulants. Amphetamine use is limited due to side effects, tolerance, and drug dependence. Methylphenidate is considered the drug of choice by most, but pemoline has a longer half-life and is associated with fewer side effects.

Treatment of cataplexy, hypnogogic hallucinations, and sleep paralysis requires the tricyclic antidepressants, which are effective, in part, because of potent REM-suppressive effects; within this class of compounds, protriptyline is most commonly used in the United States. Efficacy is limited largely by anticholinergic side effects. New compounds including viloxazine hydrochloride and fluoxetine are under evaluation.

Gamma-hydroxy-butyrate (GHB), a drug available in Europe and Canada but still under evaluation in the United States, appears to be particularly useful to reverse nocturnal sleep disruption and, perhaps as a consequence of this mechanism, may also substantially improve daytime somnolence and cataplexy. Lastly, behavioral modifications, particularly nocturnal sleep restriction and structured daytime napping, may help the narcoleptic deal with excessive daytime somnolence but are not usually a substitute for pharmacologic therapy.

SLEEP APNEA SYNDROMES Respiratory dysfunction during sleep is a common, serious cause of excessive daytime somnolence, as well as of disturbed nocturnal sleep. An estimated 2 to 5 million people in the United States stop breathing for 15 to 150 s, from a dozen to several hundred times every night during sleep. These cessations of breathing may be due to either an occlusion of the airway (*obstructive sleep apnea*), absence of respiratory effort (*central sleep apnea*), or a combination of these factors (*mixed sleep apnea*). Failure to recognize and appropriately treat these conditions may lead to serious cardiovascular complications and increased mortality. This problem is particularly prevalent in the elderly. Occult sleep-related breathing disorders may result in significant impairment of daytime alertness and functioning in otherwise healthy elderly persons. Readers are referred to Chap. 217 for a comprehensive review of the diagnosis and treatment of patients with these conditions.

DYSSOMNIA ASSOCIATED WITH LIMB MOVEMENTS **Restless legs syndrome** Patients with dyssomnia associated with the restless legs syndrome report an irresistible urge to move their legs when awake and inactive, especially when lying in bed just prior to sleep. This interferes with the ability to fall asleep. They report a creeping or crawling sensation deep within their calves that is only relieved by movement, particularly walking. In contrast, paresthesia secondary to peripheral neuropathy persists with activity. The severity of this chronic, idiopathic disorder may wax and wane with time and can be exacerbated by caffeine. Nearly all patients with restless legs also experience periodic limb movement disorder during sleep, although the reverse is not the case. Together, these conditions constitute the principal diagnosis in one-eighth of patients with insomnia.

Periodic limb movement disorder Periodic limb movement disorder, also known as *nocturnal myoclonus,* is the principal objective polysomnographic finding in 17 percent of patients with insomnia and 11 percent of those with excessive daytime somnolence. Stereotyped, rhythmic, 0.5- to 5.0-s extensions of the great toe and dorsiflexion of the foot recur every 20 to 40 s during NREM stages 1 and 2 sleep, in episodes lasting from minutes to hours. Most such episodes occur during the first half of the night. The disorder occurs in a wide variety of sleep disorders (including narcolepsy, sleep apnea, and various forms of insomnia) and is associated with frequent arousals and an increased number of sleep-stage transitions. However, it has not been demonstrated that these sleep disturbances lead to insomnia. In fact, periodic limb movement may be secondary to chronic sleep-wake disturbance rather than the cause of it. The incidence increases with age; 44 percent of healthy subjects over age 65 without a sleep complaint and all patients with the restless legs syndrome have periodic limb movements (see below). The pathophysiology is not well understood. Polysomnography with bilateral EMG recording of the anterior tibialis, triceps, and biceps is used to establish the diagnosis. Treatment options are limited; some patients may respond to clonazepam.

PARASOMNIAS The term *parasomnia* refers to behavioral disorders during sleep that are associated with brief or partial arousals but not with marked sleep disruption or impaired daytime alertness. The presenting complaint is usually related to the behavior itself. They are more common in children but may persist into adulthood when their occurrence may have more pathologic significance.

Sleepwalking (somnambulism) Patients affected by this disorder carry out automatic motor activities that range from minor to complex. Individuals may leave the bed, walk, urinate inappropriately, or exit from the house while remaining unconscious or uncommunicative. Arousal is difficult, and untoward or even fatal activities can occur. Sleepwalking occurs in stage 3 or 4 NREM sleep. It is most common in children and adolescents. Episodes are usually isolated but may be recurrent in 1 to 6 percent of patients. The cause is unknown, and no effective treatments have been developed.

Sleep terrors This disorder, also called *pavor nocturnus,* occurs primarily in young children during the first several hours after sleep onset, in stages 3 and 4 of NREM sleep. The child suddenly screams, exhibiting autonomic arousal with sweating, tachycardia, and hyperventilation. The individual may be difficult to arouse and rarely recalls the episode on awakening in the morning. Recurrent attacks are rare, and treatment is usually by way of reassurance of parents. Both sleep terrors and sleepwalking represent abnormalities of arousal. In contrast, *nightmares* (dream anxiety attacks) occur during REM sleep and cause full arousal, with memory for the dream-associated unpleasant episode.

REM sleep behavior disorder This disorder is a parasomnia arising from REM sleep instead of slow-wave sleep, as is characteristic of the other common parasomnias. It primarily afflicts men of middle age or older, many of whom have a history of prior neurologic disease (e.g., Guillain-Barré syndrome, dementia, subarachnoid hemorrhage). Presenting symptoms are of violent behavior during sleep, reported by a bed partner. In contrast to typical somnambulism, injury to patient or bystander is common, and, upon awakening, the patient reports vivid, often unpleasant dream imagery. The principal differential diagnosis is that of nocturnal seizures, which can be excluded with polysomnography. In REM sleep behavior disorder, seizure activity is absent, and the EEG/EOG REM sleep pattern exhibits a high-amplitude EMG. Complex, purposeful motor behavior occurs during REM sleep episodes. The pathogenesis is unclear, but the preexisting neurologic disease may have involved brainstem areas responsible for descending motor inhibition during REM sleep. In support of this hypothesis are the remarkable similarities between the REM sleep behavior disorder and the sleep of animals with bilateral lesions of the pontine tegmentum in areas controlling REM sleep motor inhibition. Treatment with clonazepam or tricyclic antidepressants has been successful in early trials.

Sleep bruxism Bruxism is an involuntary, forceful grinding of teeth during sleep. The patient is usually unaware of the problem, and data on this parasomnia come from roommates and bed partners, alarmed by the loud grinding noise, and from dentists who see evidence of destruction of tooth enamel and dentum. The prevalence of bruxism has been estimated at 10 to 20 percent of the general population. The typical age of onset is 17 to 20 years and spontaneous remission usually occurs by age 40. Sex distribution appears to be equal.

Hypotheses about the pathophysiology suggest contributory roles for dental abnormalities, e.g., malocclusion, and for central neural mechanisms. Psychological factors may also play a role in that stress exacerbates the disorder. Treatment is dictated by the risk of dental injury. In many cases, the diagnosis is made during dental examination, damage is minor, and no treatment is indicated. In more severe cases, treatment with a rubber tooth guard is necessary to prevent permanent and disfiguring tooth injury. Psychotherapy can be useful when bruxism is a manifestation of severe stress. Useful pharmacologic therapy has not been described.

Sleep enuresis Bedwetting, like sleepwalking and night terrors, is another parasomnia occurring during slow-wave sleep in the young. Before age 5 or 6, nocturnal enuresis should probably be considered a normal feature of development. The condition usually spontaneously improves at puberty, has a prevalence in late adolescence of 1 to 3 percent, and is rare in adulthood. The age threshold for initiation of treatment depends on parental and patient concern about the problem. Persistence of enuresis into adolescence or adulthood may reflect a variety of underlying conditions. In older patients with enuresis a distinction must be made between primary and secondary enuresis, the latter being defined as bedwetting in patients who have been fully continent for 6 to 12 months. Treatment of primary enuresis is reserved for patients of appropriate age (older than 5 or 6 years) and consists of bladder training exercises and behavioral therapy. Important causes of secondary enuresis include emotional disturbances, urinary tract infections, cauda equina lesions, epilepsy, sleep apnea, and urinary tract malformations. In the patient with secondary enuresis, underlying causes need to be eliminated. In the patient for whom enuresis may be a source of significant stress, symptomatic pharmacotherapy may be appropriate while attention is also paid to underlying causes. This is usually accomplished with oxybutynin chloride or imipramine. Intranasal desmopressin has been used in some patients.

Miscellaneous parasomnias Other clinical entities fulfill the definition of a parasomnia in that they occur selectively during sleep and are associated with some degree of sleep disruption. Examples include *jactatio capitis nocturna* (nocturnal headbanging), sleep talking, nightmares, and nocturnal leg cramps.

SLEEP DISORDERS ASSOCIATED WITH MEDICAL/PSYCHIATRIC DISORDERS **Sleep disorders associated with mental disorders** Although some differences are present in sleep architecture and physiology in *schizophrenia* (such as a decreased amount of stage 4 sleep and a lack of augmentation of REM sleep following REM sleep deprivation), chronic schizophrenics usually sleep well. In contrast, patients with other psychiatric disorders (anxiety disorders, affective illness, obsessive-compulsive disorders, and chronic alcoholism) often sleep poorly. There is considerable heterogeneity, however, in the nature of the sleep disturbance both between conditions and among patients with the same condition.

Depression can be associated with sleep onset insomnia, sleep maintenance insomnia, and/or early morning wakefulness. However, hypersomnia occurs in some depressed patients, especially adolescents and those with seasonal (fall/winter) depression (see also Chap. 368). Indeed, sleep disturbance is an important vegetative sign of depression, and may commence before any mood changes are perceived by the patient and then return to normal at the beginning of remission. Consistent polysomnographic findings in depression include decreased REM sleep latency, lengthened first REM sleep episode, and shortened first NREM sleep episode; however, the extent of these changes varies with age and symptomatology.

In *mania* and *hypomania,* sleep latency is increased, and total sleep time can be reduced. Patients with *obsessive-compulsive disorders* have sleep disturbances similar to those of endogenously depressed patients. Finally, *chronic alcoholics* lack slow-wave sleep, have decreased amounts of REM sleep, and have frequent arousals throughout the night. This is associated with impaired daytime alertness. The sleep of chronic alcoholics remains disturbed for years after discontinuance of alcohol usage.

Sleep disorders associated with neurologic disorders A variety of neurologic diseases result in sleep disruption through both indirect, nonspecific mechanisms (e.g., pain in cervical spondylosis or low back pain) or by impairment of central neural structures involved in the generation and control of sleep itself. Headache syndromes may show sleep-associated exacerbations (*migraine* or *cluster headache*) (see also Chap. 18). The mechanism of association between sleep and headache is unknown.

Epilepsy may also present as a sleep complaint (see also Chap. 350). Often the history is of abnormal, occasionally violent activity during sleep, and the differential diagnosis includes REM sleep behavior disorder, sleep apnea syndrome, and periodic movements of sleep (see above). Diagnosis requires nocturnal EEG recording. Other neurologic diseases associated with abnormal movements, such as *Parkinson's disease, hemiballismus, Huntington's chorea,* and *Gilles de la Tourette syndrome*, are also associated with disrupted sleep, presumably through secondary mechanisms.

Fatal familial insomnia is a rare hereditary disorder that causes bilateral degeneration of anterior and dorsomedial nuclei of the thalamus. Insomnia is a prominent early symptom. Progressively, the syndrome produces autonomic dysfunction, dysarthria, myoclonus, coma, and death. The pathogenesis of the thalamic destruction is unknown.

Sleep disorders associated with other medical disorders A number of medical conditions are associated with disruptions of sleep. The association may be nonspecific, for example, that between sleep disruption and chronic pain from rheumatologic disorders. Attention to this association is important in that many such patients present with only sleep-associated symptoms.

Among the most prominent associations is that between sleep disruption and *asthma.* In many asthmatics there is a prominent daily variation in airway resistance, probably related to daily rhythms in catecholamine and histamine levels, which results in marked increases in asthmatic symptoms at night. In addition, treatment of asthma with theophylline-based compounds, adrenergic agonists, or glucocorticoids can independently disrupt sleep. When sleep disruption is a prominent side effect of asthma treatment, inhaled steroids (e.g., beclomethasone) that do not disrupt sleep may provide a useful alternative.

Cardiac ischemia may also be associated with sleep disruption. Variability in autonomic nervous system function during REM sleep may account for the association of sleep and angina, although this remains unproven. Patients may present with complaints of nightmares or vivid disturbing dreams, with or without awareness of the more classical symptoms of angina. *Paroxysmal nocturnal dyspnea* can also occur as a consequence of sleep-associated cardiac ischemia that causes pulmonary congestion exacerbated by recumbent posture.

Chronic obstructive pulmonary disease is also associated with sleep disruption, the pathogenesis of which is presumed to be sleep-

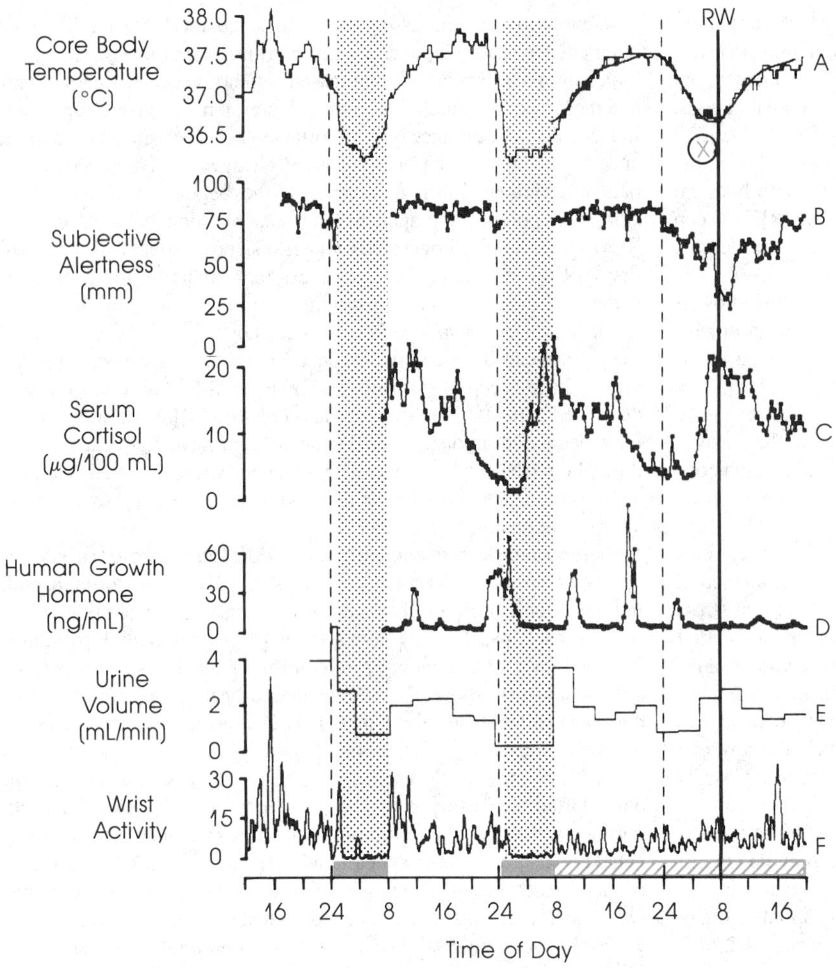

FIGURE 34-3 Circadian rhythms recorded during both the baseline and the constant routine in a single normal subject (age 21). The solid horizontal bar indicates lights out, and the cross-hatched bar indicates the 40-h constant routine. The solid vertical line (RW) indicates the subject's customary waketime. A harmonic regression model fitted to the temperature data is superimposed on the raw data during the constant routine, and an encircled X marks the time of the fitted minimum of the endogenous component of the temperature cycle. Note that all variables except wrist activity and growth hormone continue to show a circadian variation during the constant routine.

related exacerbation of hypoxia and hypercapnia secondary to alveolar hypoventilation. In addition, recumbent posture results in suboptimal ventilation-perfusion ratios. Other conditions associated with sleep disruption include *cystic fibrosis, menopause, hyperthyroidism, gastroesophageal reflux, chronic renal failure,* and *liver failure.*

CIRCADIAN RHYTHM SLEEP DISORDERS

A subset of patients presenting with either insomnia or hypersomnia may have a disorder of sleep *timing* rather than sleep *generation.* Disorders of sleep timing can either be organic (i.e., due to an intrinsic defect in the circadian pacemaker or its responsiveness to entraining stimuli) or environmental (i.e., due to a disruption of exposure to entraining stimuli from the environment). Regardless of etiology, the symptoms reflect the influence of the underlying circadian pacemaker on sleep-wake function. Thus, effective therapeutic approaches should aim to entrain the oscillator at an appropriate phase.

ENDOGENOUS CIRCADIAN PHASE ASSESSMENT Abnormal synchronization of the circadian pacemaker to the 24-h day can be assessed clinically by studying patients under standardized behavioral and environmental conditions. Exogenous factors (such as variations in light exposure, room temperature, activity level, posture, nutritional intake), which can evoke physiologic responses, must be held constant to assess the phase and amplitude of endogenous circadian rhythms. Patients are studied for 30 to 50 h of enforced semirecumbent wakefulness in constant indoor room light, with their daily nutritional and fluid intake equally divided into hourly snacks. During such a constant routine, the body temperature cycle serves as a reliable marker of the output of the endogenous circadian pacemaker (Fig. 34-3). In normal young men, the endogenous component of the body temperature cycle under such conditions reaches its nadir about 3 h before the habitual waketime. The technique can be used to determine whether there is an organic basis consistent with a diagnosis of delayed sleep phase syndrome, non-24-h sleep-wake schedule, or advanced sleep phase syndrome.

RAPID TIME-ZONE CHANGE (JET LAG) SYNDROME More than 60 million people experience transmeridian air travel annually, which is often associated with excessive daytime sleepiness, sleep onset insomnia, and frequent arousals from sleep, particularly in the latter half of the night. Gastrointestinal discomfort is common. The syndrome is transient, typically lasting 2 to 14 days depending on the number of time zones crossed, the direction of travel, and the traveler's age and phase-shifting capacity. Travelers who spend more time outdoors reportedly adapt more quickly than those who remain in hotel rooms, presumably due to bright (outdoor) light exposure.

SHIFT-WORK SLEEP DISORDER About 7 million workers in the United States regularly work at night, either on a permanent or rotating schedule. Studies of shift workers indicate that the circadian timing system of the average night-shift worker fails to adapt successfully to such work schedules. This leads to a misalignment between the desired work-rest schedule and the output of the pacemaker and in disturbed daytime sleep. Consequent sleep deprivation and misalignment of circadian phase produce decreased alertness and performance and cause increased safety hazards among night-shift workers. In addition, shift workers are believed to have higher rates of cardiac, gastrointestinal, and reproductive disorders.

Treatment must be aimed at minimizing both circadian disruption and sleep deprivation. The work schedule should: (1) favor a phase delay (clockwise) direction of shift rotation; (2) minimize the frequency of shift rotation so that shifts do not rotate more than once every 2 to 3 weeks; and (3) reduce the number of consecutive days worked at night from 7 (which is typical) to 4 or 5. These steps can lead to marked improvements in employee health and performance and to reduced accident rates among shift workers.

DELAYED SLEEP PHASE SYNDROME Delayed sleep phase syndrome is characterized by: (1) reported sleep onset and wake times intractably later than desired; (2) actual sleep times at nearly the same clock hours daily; and (3) essentially normal all-night polysomnography except for delayed sleep onset. Patients exhibit an abnormally delayed endogenous circadian phase, with the temperature minimum during the constant routine occurring later than normal. This delayed phase could be due to: (1) an abnormally long intrinsic period of endogenous circadian pacemaker; (2) an abnormally reduced phase-advancing capacity of the pacemaker; or (3) an irregular prior sleep-wake schedule, characterized by frequent nights when the patient chooses to remain awake well past midnight (for social, school, or work reasons). In most cases, it is difficult to distinguish among these factors, since patients with an abnormally long intrinsic period are more likely to "choose" such late-night activities because they are unable to sleep at that time. Patients tend to be young adults. This self-perpetuating condition can persist for years and does not usually respond to attempts to reestablish normal bedtime hours.

Patients respond to a rescheduling regimen in which bedtimes are successively delayed by about 3 h per day until the desired (and earlier) bedtime is achieved. Treatment methods involving bright-light phototherapy also show promise in these patients.

ADVANCED SLEEP PHASE SYNDROME Advanced sleep phase syndrome is the converse of the delayed sleep phase syndrome and tends to occur in the elderly. Patients with this condition report excessive daytime sleepiness during the evening hours, when they have great difficulty remaining awake, even in social settings. The patients awaken from 3 to 5 A.M. each day, often several hours before their desired wake times. Although such patients have not been studied extensively, some of these patients may benefit from bright-light phototherapy designed to reset the circadian pacemaker to a later hour.

NON-24-H SLEEP-WAKE DISORDER This condition occurs when the maximal phase-advancing capacity of the circadian pacemaker is not adequate to accommodate the difference between the 24-h geophysical day and the intrinsic period of the pacemaker in the patient. Patients affected are not able to maintain a stable phase relationship between the output of the pacemaker and the 24-h day. Such patients typically present with an incremental pattern of successive delays in sleep onsets and wake times, progressing in and out of phase with local time. When the patient's endogenous rhythms are out of phase with the local environment, insomnia coexists with excessive daytime sleepiness. Conversely, when the endogenous rhythms are in phase with the local environment, symptoms remit. The intervals of alternation between symptomatic vs. asymptomatic intervals may last several weeks to several months. Blind subjects unable to perceive light are particularly susceptible to this disorder.

MEDICAL IMPLICATIONS OF CIRCADIAN RHYTHMICITY Understanding the role of circadian rhythmicity in the pathophysiology of illness may lead to improvements in diagnosis and treatment. For example, prominent circadian variations have been reported in the incidence of *acute myocardial infarction, sudden cardiac death,* and *stroke,* the leading causes of death in the United States. Platelet aggregability is increased after arising in the early morning hours, coincident with the peak incidence of these cardiovascular events. A better understanding of the possible role of circadian rhythmicity in the acute destabilization of a chronic condition such as atherosclerotic disease could improve the understanding of the pathophysiology.

Diagnostic procedures may also be affected by the time of day at which data are collected. Examples include blood pressure, body temperature, the dexamethasone suppression test, and plasma cortisol levels. Few physicians realize the extent to which routine measures are affected by the time (or sleep/wake state) when the measurement is made.

In addition, both the toxicity and effectiveness of drugs can vary during the day. For example, more than a fivefold difference has been observed in mortality rates following administration of toxic agents to experimental animals at different times of day. Anesthetic agents are particularly sensitive to time-of-day effects.

REFERENCES

ANCH AM et al: *Sleep: A Scientific Perspective.* Englewood Cliffs, NJ, Prentice Hall, 1988

COLEMAN RM et al: Sleep-wake disorders based on a polysomnographic diagnosis: A national cooperative study. JAMA 247:997, 1982

CZEISLER CA et al: Bright light induction of strong (Type O) resetting of the human circadian pacemaker. Science 244:1328, 1989

DIAGNOSTIC CLASSIFICATION COMMITTEE, Thorpy MJ (chairman): *International Classification of Sleep Disorders.* American Sleep Disorders Association, 1990

DINGES DF, BROUGHTON RJ (eds): *Sleep and Alertness.* New York, Raven Press, 1989

FAIRBANKS DN et al (eds): *Snoring and Obstructive Sleep Apnea.* New York, Raven Press, 1987

GUILLEMINAULT C (ed): *Sleeping and Waking Disorders: Indications and Techniques.* Menlo Park, Calif, Addison-Wesley, 1982

HORNE J: *Why We Sleep: The Functions of Sleep in Humans and Other Mammals.* Oxford, Oxford University Press, 1988

KRYGER MH et al (eds): *Principles and Practice of Sleep Medicine.* Philadelphia, Saunders, 1989

LUGARESI E et al: Fatal familial insomnia and dysautonomia with selective degeneration of thalamic nuclei. N Engl J Med 315:997, 1986

LYDIC R, BIEBUYCK JF (eds): *Clinical Physiology of Sleep.* Bethesda, MD, American Physiological Society, 1988

MENDELSON WB: *Human Sleep: Research and Clinical Care.* New York, Plenum, 1987

PARKES JD: *Sleep and Its Disorders.* Philadelphia, Saunders, 1985

ROTH B: *Narcolepsy and Hypersomnia.* Basel, Karger, 1980

SCHENCK CH et al: Rapid eye movement sleep behavior disorder: A treatable parasomnia affecting older adults. JAMA 257:1786, 1987

WILLIAMS RL et al (eds): *Sleep Disorders: Diagnosis and Treatment,* 2d ed. New York, Wiley, 1988

section 4 Alterations in circulatory and respiratory function

35 COUGH AND HEMOPTYSIS

EUGENE BRAUNWALD[1]

COUGH

Cough, one of the most frequent cardiorespiratory symptoms, is an explosive expiration which provides a means of clearing the tracheobronchial tree of secretions and foreign bodies.

MECHANISM Coughing may be initiated either voluntarily or reflexively. As a defensive reflex it has both afferent and efferent pathways. The *afferent limb* includes receptors within the sensory distribution of the trigeminal, glossopharyngeal, superior laryngeal, and vagus nerves. The *efferent limb* includes the recurrent laryngeal nerve (which causes glottic closure) and the spinal nerves (which cause contraction of the thoracic and abdominal musculature). The *sequence of a cough* includes an appropriate stimulus which initiates a deep inspiration. This is followed by glottic closure, relaxation of

[1] The late Gennaro M. Tisi was the senior author of this chapter in the 11th edition, and this chapter represents a revision of that work.

the diaphragm, and muscle contraction against a closed glottis so as to produce maximally positive intrathoracic and intraairway pressures. These positive intrathoracic pressures result in a narrowing of the trachea, produced by an infolding of its more compliant posterior membrane. Once the glottis opens, the combination of a large pressure differential between the airways and the atmosphere coupled with this tracheal narrowing produces flow rates through the trachea close to the speed of sound. The shearing forces which are developed aid in the elimination of mucus and foreign materials. A tracheostomy short-circuits and an endotracheal tube prevents glottic closure. Therefore, both decrease the effectiveness of the cough mechanism.

ETIOLOGY Cough is produced by inflammatory, mechanical, chemical, and thermal stimulation of the cough receptors. *Inflammatory* stimuli are initiated by edema and hyperemia of the respiratory mucous membranes, and by irritation from exudative processes, such as postnasal drip and gastric reflux with aspiration. Such stimuli may arise either in the airways (as in laryngitis, tracheitis, bronchitis, and bronchiolitis) or in the alveoli (as in pneumonitis and lung abscess). *Mechanical* stimuli are produced by inhalation of particulate matter, such as dust particles, and by compression of the air passages and pressure or tension upon these structures. Lesions associated with airway compression may be either extramural or intramural in type. The former include aortic aneurysms, granulomas, pulmonary neoplasms, and mediastinal tumors; intramural lesions include bronchogenic carcinoma, bronchial adenoma, foreign bodies, granulomatous endobronchial involvement, and contraction of airway smooth muscle (bronchial asthma). Pressure or tension upon the air passages is usually produced by lesions associated with a decrease in pulmonary compliance. Examples of specific causes include acute and chronic interstitial fibrosis (Chap. 211), pulmonary edema, and atelectasis. *Chemical* stimuli may result from inhalation of irritant gases, including cigarette smoke and chemical fumes. Finally, *thermal* stimuli may be produced by inhalation of either very hot or cold air.

Cough is commonly associated with episodic wheezing secondary to bronchoconstriction in symptomatic patients with bronchial asthma (Chap. 204). Chronic, persistent cough may be the *sole* presenting manifestation of bronchial asthma (''cough asthma''). Such patients are characterized by (1) absence of a history of episodic wheezing and (2) no evidence of expiratory airflow obstruction by spirometry, but (3) hyperreactive airways (characteristic of asthma) when challenged with a cholinergic agent, methacholine.

DIAGNOSTIC EVALUATION The history is the most important aspect of the evaluation. It should address the following issues:

1 Is the cough acute or chronic?
2 Is it associated with fever?
3 Is it associated with sputum? If so, what is its character?
4 Is it seasonal?
5 Does the patient have important risk factors for disease? (e.g., homosexuality, cigarette smoking, intravenous drugs, immobilization, environmental exposures?)
6 What is the past medical history?

The physical examination, chest roentgenogram, sputum examination, and screening pulmonary function studies (static lung volumes and dynamic flow rates) may then indicate a specific cause. The *history* may indicate specific diagnoses. Acute episodes of cough may be associated with such viral infections as acute tracheobronchitis or pneumonitis or with bacterial bronchopneumonia. Cough associated with an acute febrile episode and associated with hoarseness is usually produced by viral laryngotracheobronchitis. Postnasal drip is also a common cause of chronic cough.

The character of the cough may suggest the anatomic site of involvement: the patient with a ''barking'' type of cough may have epiglottal involvement (i.e., ''whooping cough'' due to *Haemophilus pertussis* infection in young children), while the cough associated with tracheal or major airway involvement is often loud and ''brassy.'' Cough associated with generalized wheezing may be produced by acute bronchospasm. The time of occurrence of a cough may indicate a specific cause: a cough which occurs selectively at night suggests congestive heart failure; one related to meals suggests a tracheoesophageal fistula, a hiatal hernia, or an esophageal diverticulum; a cough precipitated by a change in position suggests a lung abscess or a localized area of bronchiectasis. The description of sputum or secretions produced in conjunction with the cough should include color, consistency, odor, and volume: purulent and/or large amounts of sputum suggests lung abscess and bronchiectasis; bloody sputum, bleeding (see ''Hemoptysis,'' below); frothy and pink-tinged sputum, pulmonary edema; mucoid and massive sputum, alveolar cell carcinoma.

The general *physical examination* may point to a nonpulmonary cause of cough, such as heart failure, primary nonpulmonary neoplasm, acquired immunodeficiency disease, etc. The character of the auscultatory findings may suggest the site of disease: inspiratory stridor and wheezing may be present in laryngeal disease, inspiratory and expiratory rhonchi favor tracheal and major airway involvement, coarse subcrepitant inspiratory rales may indicate interstitial fibrosis and/or edema, fine crepitant rales may indicate a process such as pneumonitis or pulmonary edema, which fills the alveoli with fluid. The *chest roentgenogram* may reveal the cause of the cough; it may show an intrapulmonary mass lesion which may be either central or peripheral (Chap. 215), an alveolar filling process which may be pneumonic or nonpneumonic, an area of honeycombing and cyst formation which may indicate an area of localized bronchiectasis, or bilateral hilar adenopathy which may indicate sarcoidosis or a lymphoma.

A careful *sputum examination* may be more enlightening than a patient's description of the character of the sputum. Examination shows whether the sputum is thin or viscid, purulent, foul-smelling, blood-tinged, or scant or copious. In pneumococcal pneumonia the sputum has a ''rusty'' color, while in *Klebsiella* pneumonia it may look like ''currant jelly.'' Gram stain and culture of deep-cough specimens may reveal a specific bacterial, fungal, or mycoplasmal causation, while sputum cytology may result in a positive diagnosis of a pulmonary neoplasm.

Bronchoscopy may reveal the cause of otherwise unexplained chronic cough. *Pulmonary function* studies (Chap. 201) may also be helpful. Significant expiratory obstruction to airflow (as determined from a forced expiratory flow maneuver), coupled with a history of cough and significant sputum production, suggests that irrespective of other lesions the patient has significant bronchitis. Decreased lung volume (as determined from the static lung volumes) suggests that a restrictive type of lung disease (Chap. 211) is present. Perhaps more important than providing a specific diagnosis, pulmonary function studies are useful in quantifying the severity of disease, its progression over time, and in assessing the efficacy of an intervention.

Two features of cough should be highlighted: (1) A cough is often so common in the cigarette smoker as to be ignored or minimized. *Any change in the nature or character of a chronic cigarette cough should initiate immediate diagnostic evaluation, with particular attention directed to detection of bronchogenic carcinoma.* (2) Female patients are inclined to swallow sputum and not to expectorate as male patients do. This tendency may lead to the incorrect conclusion that a cough in a female patient is irritative and nonproductive.

COMPLICATIONS Three complications may be produced by the coughing mechanism: paroxysms of coughing may precipitate syncope (cough syncope, Chap. 21), and strenuous coughing may produce rupture of an emphysematous bleb, rib fractures, and costochondritis. A potential mechanism for cough syncope includes the development of markedly positive intrathoracic and alveolar pressures which decrease venous return, producing a decrease in cardiac output and resultant syncope. Although cough fractures of the ribs may occur in otherwise normal patients, their occurrence should at least raise the possibility of pathologic fractures, which are seen in multiple myeloma, osteoporosis, and osteolytic metastases.

THERAPY Definitive treatment of cough depends on determining its precise cause and then initiating specific therapy for the underlying cause. Symptomatic therapy should be considered when the cause of the cough is idiopathic and the cough performs no useful function or represents a potential hazard to the patient. An irritative, nonproductive cough may be suppressed by an antitussive agent, such as codeine or dextromethorphan, 15 mg qid. These drugs are useful symptomatic therapy by interrupting prolonged, self-perpetuating paroxysms. However, a cough productive of significant quantities of sputum should not be suppressed, since retention of sputum in the tracheobronchial tree may interfere with the distribution of ventilation, alveolar aeration, and the ability of the lung to resist infection. When secretions are tenacious and thick, adequate hydration, expectorants, and humidification of the air with an ultrasonic nebulizer may be helpful. Ipratropium (a class of bronchodilator with antimuscarinic actions) may prove especially useful in patients with cough asthma.

HEMOPTYSIS

For purposes of definition hemoptysis includes both blood-streaked sputum and gross hemoptysis. Any patient with gross hemoptysis should be given appropriate diagnostic tests so that a specific cause may be found. The patient with blood-streaked sputum should also be studied unless one can be certain that this type of hemoptysis is due to a benign condition. Recurrent episodes of hemoptysis should not be automatically ascribed to a previously established diagnosis, such as chronic bronchiectasis or bronchitis. Such an approach may result in missing a serious but potentially treatable lesion.

ETIOLOGY AND INCIDENCE Prior to embarking upon an extensive diagnostic workup of hemoptysis, it is essential to determine that the blood is in fact coming from the respiratory tract, not from the nasopharynx or gastrointestinal tract. Distinguishing hemoptysis from hematemesis is difficult at times. In hemoptysis, the prodrome is usually a tingling in the throat or a desire to cough, the blood is coughed up, and it is usually bright-red and *frothy*; in hematemesis, the prodrome includes nausea and abdominal discomfort, the blood is vomited, and it is usually *dark red* in color. Once this point is established, the diagnostic tests for hemoptysis may proceed. Although there are numerous single case reports of diseases which have been associated with hemoptysis, Table 35-1 presents the more common disorders.

The incidence of the diagnoses listed in Table 35-1 depends upon the nature of the series reported and whether one includes both gross bleeding and blood streaking of the sputum. If both types of bleeding are included, then the major causes (approximately 60 to 70 percent) are chronic bronchitis and bronchiectasis. If the definition is restricted to gross bleeding (greater than several tablespoons) then the incidence depends upon the type of series reported. Surgical series favor the incidence of mass lesions and operable lesions (carcinoma, 20 percent; localized, segmental, or lobar bronchiectasis, 30 percent). Those from centers with a large tuberculosis population favor this condition (incidence varying between 2 and 40 percent). Combined medical-surgical series include a wider representation of those lesions which present with hemoptysis (carcinoma, 20 percent; bronchiectasis, 30 percent; bronchitis, 15 percent; other inflammatory lesions including tuberculosis, 10 to 20 percent; other lesions including the vascular, traumatic, and hemorrhagic etiologies listed in Table 35-1, 10 percent). Despite the most extensive of evaluations, 5 to 15 percent of cases entailing gross hemoptysis remain undiagnosed.

TABLE 35-1 Causes of hemoptysis

1 Inflammatory
- *a* Bronchitis
- *b* Bronchiectasis
- *c* Tuberculosis
- *d* Lung abscess
- *e* Pneumonia, particularly *Klebsiella*

2 Neoplastic
- *a* Lung cancer: squamous cell, adenocarcinoma, oat cell
- *b* Bronchial adenoma

3 Other
- *a* Pulmonary thromboembolism
- *b* Left ventricular failure
- *c* Mitral stenosis
- *d* Traumatic, including foreign body and lung contusion
- *e* Primary pulmonary hypertension; arteriovenous malformation; Eisenmenger's syndrome; pulmonary vasculitis including Wegener's granulomatosis and Goodpasture's syndrome; idiopathic pulmonary hemosiderosis; and amyloid
- *f* Hemorrhagic diathesis including anticoagulant therapy

Two points should be highlighted with reference to diseases associated with hemoptysis: (1) hemoptysis is rare in metastatic carcinoma to the lung; (2) although hemoptysis may occur at some time during the course of a viral or pneumococcal pneumonia, it is usually scanty and its occurrence should always raise the question of a more serious underlying process.

DIAGNOSIS As is the case for cough, *history* is of enormous value. Recurrent, chronic hemoptysis in a young, otherwise asymptomatic female favors the diagnosis of a bronchial adenoma; recurrent hemoptysis with chronic, marked sputum production associated with ring shadows, tram lines (abnormal air bronchograms), and cyst formation on the roentgenogram suggests a diagnosis of bronchiectasis; putrid sputum production suggests a lung abscess; weight loss and anorexia in a male smoker over the age of 40 raise the possibility of a bronchogenic carcinoma; a recent history of blunt trauma to the chest suggests a lung contusion; and acute pleuritic chest pain raises the possibility of pulmonary embolism with infarction or some other pleurally based lesion (lung abscess, coccidioidomycosis cavity, and vasculitis). Several findings on the *physical examination* may also suggest a specific diagnosis: a pleural friction rub suggests those diagnoses just mentioned in connection with pleuritic pain; the findings of pulmonary hypertension raise the diagnostic possibilities of primary pulmonary hypertension, mitral stenosis, recurrent or chronic thromboembolism, and Eisenmenger's syndrome; a localized wheeze over a major lobar airway suggests an intramural lesion such as a bronchogenic carcinoma or a foreign body; systemic arteriovenous communications or the presence of a murmur over the lung fields suggest the diagnosis of Osler-Rendu-Weber disease with pulmonary arteriovenous malformation; evidence of significant expiratory obstruction to airflow coupled with sputum production suggests that whatever other lesion may be present, the patient has significant bronchitis. The *chest roentgenogram* is critical to diagnosis. The presence of ring shadows favors a diagnosis of bronchiectasis; an air-fluid level, the diagnosis of a lung abscess; and a mass lesion, the diagnosis of a central or peripheral pulmonary neoplasm. A mass lesion which may cause hemoptysis should be distinguished from an area of blood pneumonitis caused by aspiration of blood into contiguous areas.

One of the most demanding diagnostic problems is the identification of the site of bleeding in a patient with normal findings on physical examination and a normal roentgenogram of the chest. A patient with hemoptysis tends to keep the bleeding side dependent. Otherwise, gravitational drainage would cause aspiration into the noninvolved dependent lung. The patient may also be able to give a history of a burning or deep pain which may localize the side of bleeding; bronchoscopy may then be useful. This procedure generally is most helpful when the bleeding is scant, and of least help when the bleeding is massive, since blood may be aspirated into contiguous airways. Such aspiration may produce alveolar filling (i.e., a "blood pneumonitis") that may obscure the etiology of the hemoptysis on the initial chest roentgenogram. Blood pneumonitis usually clears within a week, and once clearing has occurred, a repeat chest roentgenogram may disclose the origin of the hemoptysis.

Following the history and physical examination, the diagnostic approach to a patient with hemoptysis includes whatever specialized studies and procedures are required to make a specific diagnosis. The first step is to obtain a roentgenogram. Usually computed tomography is the procedure employed next, followed by bronchoscopy. Rigid bronchoscopy permits visualization of the more central airways. It is of particular value when the source of bleeding is in this portion of the airway system, the degree of hemoptysis is massive, and selective endobronchial intubation is being considered. Fiberoptic bronchoscopy (Chap. 203) includes within the range of visualization airways as small as several millimeters in diameter. This endoscopic technique may provide definitive visual, biopsy, or cytologic information. Since direct visualization of more peripheral portions of the airway system is now possible, the indications for bronchography in the evaluation of hemoptysis are being modified. The principal indications for bronchography in such patients are (1) to establish the presence of localized bronchiectasis (including a sequestered lobe) and (2) to rule out the presence of more generalized bronchiectasis in a patient with localized disease who is regarded as a surgical candidate because of either repetitive hemoptysis or recurrent infections. The majority of patients with bronchiectasis have a normal chest roentgenogram, but the diagnosis can usually be established by computed tomography (Chaps. 202 and 203). A PPD and, if sputum is present, examination for acid-fast bacilli should be obtained. The laboratory evaluation should also rule out a bleeding disorder (Chap. 288).

THERAPY Since hemoptysis is such an alarming symptom, there is a tendency to overtreat the patient. Usually hemoptysis is scant and will stop spontaneously without specific therapy. If the hemoptysis is substantial, the mainstays of therapy include keeping the patient calm, instituting complete bed rest, excluding unnecessary diagnostic procedures until the hemoptysis has begun to subside, and suppressing cough if it is present and an aggravating feature of the hemoptysis. The emergency care of such a patient demands that intubation and suctioning equipment be at the bedside. In patients in danger of asphyxiation by flooding of the lung contralateral to the site of hemorrhage, intubation by a technique which isolates the hemorrhaging lung and prevents contralateral aspiration of blood should be carried out. This can be accomplished by strategic location of a balloon catheter whose introduction into the bronchus in question is facilitated by direct visualization through a fiberoptic bronchoscope.

The management of potentially lethal massive hemoptysis remains controversial. The choice between a medical approach and surgical intervention hinges on the words *potentially lethal*. Massive hemoptysis, usually defined as greater than 600 to 800 mL in 24 h, is an alarming clinical situation in which asphyxiation due to aspiration of blood represents the principal threat to life. The choice between surgical and medical management relates most often to the anatomic basis for the massive hemoptysis. In patients with cavitary tuberculosis, anaerobic lung abscess, and lung cancer, the risk of mortality is far greater than when the cause of the hemoptysis is bronchitis or bronchiectasis. Operation may occasionally be necessary in the former, but virtually never in the latter group. In either case the initial management should include the conservative measures suggested above. With such management, spontaneous cessation of bleeding usually occurs. Surgical intervention should be considered in that small group of patients with a definable lesion on chest roentgenogram (i.e., cavitary disease, lung abscess, lung cancer) who have evidence of uncontrollable respiratory or hemodynamic compromise. If a patient is a surgical candidate, bronchoscopy should be performed to identify the specific site of bleeding. Otherwise bronchoscopy should be deferred for several days because of the tendency of this procedure to aggravate cough and thereby perpetuate the hemoptysis. Bronchial arterial catheterization and embolization are currently under evaluation for the nonsurgical control of massive hemoptysis, especially in patients with nonresectable lung cancer. Laser (neodymium YAG—yttrium aluminum garnet) therapy should also be considered as a palliative modality for massive hemoptysis in such patients.

REFERENCES

ADELMAN M et al: Cryptogenic hemoptysis: Clinical features, bronchoscopic findings, and natural history in 67 patients. Ann Intern Med 102:829, 1985

BOUSHEY HA et al: Medical staff conference: Evaluating and treating intractable cough. West J Med 143:223, 1985

CONLAN AA: Massive hemoptysis: Diagnostic and therapeutic implications. Surg Ann 17:337, 1985

CORRAO WMC et al: Chronic cough as the sole presenting manifestation of bronchial asthma. N Engl J Med 300:633, 1979

GROSS NJ et al: Anticholinergic, antimuscarinic bronchodilators. Am Rev Resp Dis 129:856, 1984

LEITH DE: The development of cough. Am Rev Respir Dis 131:S39, 1985

SACKNER MA: Cough, in *Textbook of Respiratory Practice*, JF Murray, JA Nadel (eds). Philadelphia, Saunders, 1988, pp 397–408

WILLIAMS MH: Management of massive hemoptysis. Pulmonary Perspectives, a publication of the American College of Chest Physicians 1:3, 1984

36 DYSPNEA AND PULMONARY EDEMA

ROLAND H. INGRAM, JR. / EUGENE BRAUNWALD

DYSPNEA

The breathing pattern is controlled by a series of higher central and peripheral mechanisms which can increase ventilation in excess of metabolic demands in conditions such as anxiety and fear, and can increase ventilation appropriate to increased metabolic demands during physical activity. A normal resting person is unaware of the act of breathing, and while he or she may become conscious of breathing during mild to moderate exertion, no discomfort is experienced. However, during and following exhausting exertion an individual may become unpleasantly aware of breathing, yet feel reasonably assured that the sensation will be transitory and is appropriate to the level of exercise. Therefore, as a cardinal symptom of diseases affecting the cardiorespiratory system, dyspnea is defined as an *abnormally uncomfortable awareness of breathing*.

Although dyspnea is not painful in the usual sense of the word, it is, like pain, involved with both the perception of a sensation and the reaction to that perception. Patients experience a number of uncomfortable sensations related to breathing and use an even larger number of verbal expressions to describe these sensations, such as "cannot get enough air," "air does not go all the way down," "smothering feeling in the chest," "tightness in the chest," "fatigue in the chest," and a "choking sensation." It may be necessary, therefore, to review meticulously the patient's history in order to ascertain whether the more abstruse descriptions do, in fact, represent dyspnea. Once it is established that a patient does have dyspnea, it is of paramount importance to define the circumstances in which it occurs and to assess associated symptoms. There are situations in which breathing appears labored but in which dyspnea does not occur. For example, the hyperventilation in association with metabolic acidemia is rarely accompanied by dyspnea. On the other hand, patients with apparently normal breathing patterns may complain of shortness of breath.

QUANTITATION OF DYSPNEA The gradation of dyspnea may usefully be based upon the amount of physical exertion required to produce the sensation. In actual practice the major functional classifications of patients with heart or lung disease are based largely on dyspnea in relation to degree of exertion. However, in assessing the severity of dyspnea, it is important to obtain a clear understanding of the patient's general physical condition, work history, and recreational habits. For example, the development of dyspnea in a trained runner upon running 2 mi may signify a more serious disturbance than a similar degree of breathlessness in a sedentary person upon running a fraction of this distance. Another variable to consider in assessing the degree of dyspnea as an index of the severity of underlying heart or lung disease is the interindividual variation in perception. Some patients with extremely severe disease may complain of only mild dyspnea; others with mild disease may experience more severe shortness of breath. Thus, rather like variations in pain thresholds, patients have different degrees of subjective tolerance to cardiopulmonary dysfunction. There is some evidence that persons with relatively blunted ventilatory drives tolerate their disease with less dyspnea than those who have a heightened level of ventilatory responsiveness. Some patients with lung or heart disease may have such reduced capabilities due to other disease (e.g., peripheral vascular insufficiency or severe osteoarthritis of the hips or knees) that exertional dyspnea is precluded despite serious impairment of pulmonary or cardiac function.

Some patterns of dyspnea are not directly related to physical exertion. Sudden and unexpected dyspneic episodes at rest can be associated with pulmonary emboli, spontaneous pneumothorax, or anxiety. Nocturnal episodes of severe paroxysmal dyspnea are characteristic of left ventricular failure. Dyspnea upon assuming the supine posture, *orthopnea* (see below), thought to be mainly characteristic of congestive heart failure, may also occur in some patients with asthma and chronic obstruction of the airways and is a regular finding in the rare occurrence of bilateral diaphragmatic paralysis. *Trepopnea* is used to describe the unusual circumstance in which dyspnea occurs only in the left or right lateral decubitus position, most often in patients with heart disease, while *platypnea* is dyspnea which occurs only in the upright position. Both of these patterns remain to be fully explained but may be related to positional alterations in ventilation-perfusion relations (Chap. 201).

MECHANISMS OF DYSPNEA Physicians usually relate the symptom of dyspnea to a process such as obstruction of the airways or congestive heart failure and generally proceed with further diagnostic and/or therapeutic attempts, having satisfied themselves that they understand the mechanism of the dyspnea. In fact, elucidation of the *actual* mechanism(s) of dyspnea has eluded clinical investigators.

Dyspnea occurs whenever the work of breathing is excessive. Increased force generation is required of the respiratory muscles to produce a given volume change if the chest wall or lungs are less compliant or if resistance to airflow is increased. Increased work of breathing also occurs when the ventilation is excessive for the level of activity. Although an individual is more apt to become dyspneic when the work of breathing is increased, the work theory does not account for the perceptual difference between a deep breath with a normal mechanical load and a normal-sized breath with an increased mechanical load. The work might be the same with both breaths, but the normal one with the increased load will be associated with discomfort. In fact, with respiratory loading, such as adding a resistance at the mouth, there is an increase in respiratory center output, as gauged by newer indexes, that is disproportionate to the increase in work of breathing. It has been postulated that whenever the force that muscles actually generate during breathing approach some fraction of their maximal force-generating ability, which may vary among individuals, dyspnea ensues due to transduction of mechanical to neural stimuli. Such a theory would still not explain why patients who are completely paralyzed, either by cord transections or neuromuscular blockade, experience dyspnea although aided by a mechanical ventilator. It is probable, in these circumstances, that signals from the lungs and/or airways travel via the vagus nerve to the central nervous system to account for the sensation.

In all likelihood several different mechanisms operate to different degrees in the various clinical situations in which dyspnea occurs. Perhaps, in some circumstances, dyspnea is evoked by stimulation of receptors in the upper respiratory tract; in others it may originate from receptors in the lungs, airways, respiratory muscles, or some combination of those structures. In any event, dyspnea is characterized by an excessive or abnormal activation of the respiratory centers in the brainstem. This activation comes about from stimuli transmitted from or through a variety of structures and pathways including (1) intrathoracic receptors via the vagi; (2) afferent somatic nerves, particularly from the respiratory muscles and chest wall, but also from other skeletal muscles and joints; (3) chemoreceptors in the brain, aortic and carotid bodies, and elsewhere in the circulation; (4) higher (cortical) centers; and perhaps (5) afferent fibers in the phrenic nerves. In general, despite the interindividual variations described above, there is a reasonable correlation between the severity of dyspnea and the magnitude of disturbances of pulmonary or cardiac function which are responsible.

DIFFERENTIAL DIAGNOSIS Obstructive disease of airways (See also Chaps. 204 and 210) Obstruction to airflow can be present anywhere from the extrathoracic airways out to the small airways in the periphery of the lung. Large extrathoracic airway obstruction can occur acutely, as with aspiration of food or a foreign body or with angioedema of the glottis. Circumstantial evidence or testimony from witnesses should cause the physician to suspect aspiration, and an allergic history together with a few scattered hives should raise the possibility of glottic edema. The acute form of upper airway obstruction is a medical emergency. More chronic forms can occur with tumors or with fibrotic stenosis following tracheostomy or prolonged endotracheal intubation. Whether acute or chronic, the cardinal symptom is dyspnea, and the characteristic signs are stridor and retraction of the supraclavicular fossae with inspiration.

Obstruction of intrathoracic airways can occur acutely and intermittently or can be present chronically with worsening during respiratory infections. Acute intermittent obstruction with wheezing is typical of *asthma*. Chronic cough with expectoration is typical of *chronic bronchitis* and *bronchiectasis*. Most often there is a prolongation of expiration and coarse rhonchi which are generalized in chronic bronchitis and may be localized in the case of bronchiectasis. Intercurrent infection results in worsening of the cough, increased expectoration of purulent sputum, and more severe dyspnea. During such episodes the patient may complain of nocturnal paroxysms of dyspnea with wheezing relieved by cough and expectoration of sputum.

Many years of exertional dyspnea progressing to dyspnea at rest characterize the patient with predominant *emphysema* (Chap. 210). Although a parenchymal disease by definition, emphysema is invariably accompanied by obstruction of airways.

Diffuse parenchymal lung diseases (See also Chap. 211) This category includes a large number of diseases ranging from acute pneumonia to chronic disorders such as sarcoidosis and the various forms of *pneumoconiosis*. History, physical findings, and radiographic abnormalities often provide clues to the diagnosis. The patients are often tachypneic with arterial P_{CO_2} and P_{O_2} values below normal. Exertion often further reduces the arterial P_{O_2}. Lung volumes are decreased and the lungs are stiffer, i.e., less compliant than normal.

Pulmonary vascular occlusive diseases (See also Chap. 213) Repeated episodes of dyspnea at rest often occur with recurrent pulmonary emboli. A source for emboli, such as phlebitis of a lower extremity or the pelvis, is quite helpful in leading the physician to suspect the diagnosis. Arterial blood gases are almost invariably abnormal, but lung volumes are frequently normal or only minimally abnormal.

Diseases of the chest wall or respiratory muscles (See also Chap. 217) The physical examination establishes the presence of a chest wall disease such as severe kyphoscoliosis, pectus excavatum, or spondylitis. Although all three of these deformities may be associated with dyspnea, only severe kyphoscoliosis regularly interferes with ventilation sufficiently to produce chronic cor pulmonale and respiratory failure. Even though vital capacity, lung volumes, and airflow rates are normal with pectus excavatum, there is some evidence that cardiac compression from the posteriorly displaced sternum interferes with diastolic filling of the ventricle during the increased demands of exercise. Hence a cardiogenic component to the dyspnea may be present in this condition.

Both weakness and paralysis of respiratory muscles can lead to respiratory failure and dyspnea (Chap. 217), but most often the signs and symptoms of the neurologic or muscular disorder are more prominently manifested in other systems.

Heart disease In patients with cardiac disease exertional dyspnea occurs most commonly as a consequence of an elevated pulmonary capillary pressure; aside from uncommon causes such as obstructive disease of the pulmonary veins (Chap. 186), pulmonary capillary hypertension is a consequence of left atrial hypertension, which in turn may be due to left ventricular dysfunction (Chaps. 181 and 182), reduced left ventricular compliance, and mitral stenosis. The elevation of hydrostatic pressure in the pulmonary vascular bed tends to upset the Starling equilibrium (see "Pulmonary Edema," below) with resulting transudation of liquid into the interstitial space, reducing the compliance of the lungs and stimulating J (juxtacapillary) receptors in the alveolar interstitial space. When prolonged, pulmonary venous hypertension results in thickening of pulmonary vessels and an increase in perivascular cells and fibrous tissue, causing a further reduction in compliance. The competition for space between vessels, airways, and increased liquid within the interstitial space compromises the lumina of small airways, increasing the airways' resistance. Diminution in compliance and an increase in airways' resistance increase the work of breathing which, to some degree, is minimized by a reduction in tidal volume which is compensated for by an increase in frequency of respiration. In severe heart disease, usually involving elevation of both pulmonary and systemic venous pressures, hydrothorax may develop, further interfering with pulmonary function and intensifying dyspnea. In patients with heart failure and a severely diminished cardiac output, dyspnea may also be related to fatigue of the respiratory muscles as a consequence of their reduced perfusion. The metabolic acidosis characteristic of severe heart failure may play a contributory role. Dyspnea may also be associated with severe systemic and cerebral hypoxia, as occurs during exertion in patients with congenital heart disease and right-to-left shunts.

Cardiac dyspnea usually begins as breathlessness on strenuous exertion and, over the course of months or years, progresses until the patient is dyspneic at rest. Occasionally, a nonproductive cough developing in the recumbent position, particularly at night, may be the first complaint.

Orthopnea, i.e., dyspnea in the recumbent position, and *paroxysmal nocturnal dyspnea*, i.e., attacks of shortness of breath which usually occur at night and awaken the patient from sleep, are characteristic of more advanced forms of heart failure associated with elevations of pulmonary venous and capillary pressures and are discussed in Chap. 182. Orthopnea is the result of the alteration of gravitational forces when the recumbent position is assumed. This augmentation of intrathoracic blood volume elevates pulmonary venous and capillary pressures which increases the pulmonary closing volume (Chap. 201) and reduces the vital capacity. An additional factor associated with recumbency is the elevation of the diaphragm, which results in a lower end-expiratory lung volume. This combination of lower end-expiratory lung volume and increase in closing volume results in a significant alteration of alveolar-capillary gas exchange.

PAROXYSMAL (NOCTURNAL) DYSPNEA Also known as *cardiac asthma*, this condition is characterized by attacks of severe shortness of breath which generally occur at night and usually awaken the patient from sleep. The attack is precipitated by stimuli which aggravate the previously existing pulmonary congestion; frequently the total blood volume is augmented at night because of the reabsorption of edema from dependent portions of the body during recumbency; the redistribution of blood volume which takes place results in an increase in intrathoracic blood volume and therefore produces pulmonary congestion. A sleeping patient can tolerate relatively severe pulmonary engorgement and may awaken only when actual pulmonary edema and bronchospasm have developed, with the feeling of suffocation and with wheezing respirations.

CHEYNE-STOKES RESPIRATION See Chap. 182.

DIAGNOSIS The diagnosis of cardiac dyspnea depends on the recognition of heart disease on the basis of the history and physical examination. There may be a history of antecedent myocardial infarction, third and fourth heart sounds may be audible, and/or there may be evidence of left ventricular enlargement, jugular neck vein distention, and/or peripheral edema. Often there are radiographic signs of heart failure, with evidence of interstitial edema, pulmonary vascular redistribution, and accumulation of liquid in the septal planes and pleural cavity. Cardiomegaly is often present, but the overall heart size may be normal, particularly in patients with dyspnea due to acute myocardial infarction or mitral stenosis; an enlarged left atrium is usually evident in the latter condition. The electrocardiogram (Chap. 176) is rarely specific for heart disease and cannot specifically indicate whether a patient's dyspnea is caused by heart disease; however, it is rarely normal in patients with cardiac dyspnea.

Differentiation between cardiac and pulmonary dyspnea In most patients with dyspnea there is obvious clinical evidence of disease of either heart or lungs. The dyspnea of chronic obstructive lung disease tends to develop more gradually than that of heart diseases; exceptions, of course, occur in patients with obstructive lung disease who develop an episode of infectious bronchitis, pneumonia, or pneumothorax, or an exacerbation of asthma. Like patients with cardiac dyspnea, patients with chronic obstructive lung disease may also waken at night with dyspnea, but this is usually associated with sputum production; the dyspnea is relieved after these patients rid themselves of secretions.

The difficulty in the distinction between cardiac and pulmonary dyspnea may be compounded by the coexistence of diseases involving both organ systems. Patients with a history of chronic bronchitis or asthma who develop left ventricular failure tend to develop recurrences of bronchoconstriction and wheezing in association with bouts of paroxysmal nocturnal dyspnea and pulmonary edema. This condition, i.e., cardiac asthma, usually occurs in patients with overt clinical evidence of heart disease. Acute cardiac asthma is further differentiated from acute attacks of bronchial asthma by the presence of diaphoresis, more bubbly airway sounds, and the more common occurrence of cyanosis.

It is desirable to carry out pulmonary function testing in patients in whom the etiology of dyspnea is not clear, for these tests should be helpful in determining whether dyspnea is produced by heart disease, lung disease, abnormalities of the chest wall, or anxiety. In addition to the usual means of assessing patients for heart disease (Chap. 174), determination of the ejection fraction at rest and during exercise by radionuclide ventriculography (Chap. 178) is helpful in the differential diagnosis of dyspnea; the left ventricular ejection fraction is depressed in left ventricular failure while the right ventricular ejection fraction may be low at rest or may decline during exercise in patients with severe lung disease; both ejection fractions are normal at rest and during exercise in dyspnea due to anxiety or malingering. Careful observation during the performance of an exercise treadmill test will often help in the identification of the patient who is malingering or whose dyspnea is secondary to anxiety. Under these circumstances the patient usually complains of severe shortness of breath but appears to be breathing either effortlessly or totally irregularly. In less than obvious cases, measurements of P_{O_2}, pH, and P_{CO_2} in arterial blood and CO_2 and O_2 levels in mixed expired gas may be helpful in establishing either that gas exchange is normal or that a significant abnormality that is not detectable at rest exists during exercise.

Anxiety neurosis Dyspnea experienced by someone with an anxiety neurosis is a difficult symptom to evaluate. The signs and symptoms of acute and chronic hyperventilation do not serve to distinguish between anxiety neurosis and other processes, such as recurrent pulmonary emboli. Another potentially confusing situation is seen when chest pain and electrocardiographic changes accompany the hyperventilation syndrome. When present and attributable to this condition, often referred to as *neurocirculatory asthenia* (Chap. 16), the chest pain is often sharp, fleeting, and in various loci, and the electrocardiographic changes are most often seen during repolarization; yet occasional ventricular ectopic activity can be seen as well. A rather extensive series of pulmonary and cardiac function tests, carried out both at rest and during exercise, may be needed to be certain that anxiety is, in fact, the cause of the dyspnea. Certain clues are helpful in leading one to suspect a psychogenic origin. Frequent sighing respirations and a bizarre, irregular breathing pattern are helpful. Often the breathing pattern returns to normal during sleep.

PULMONARY EDEMA

CARDIOGENIC PULMONARY EDEMA An increase in pulmonary venous pressure, which results initially in the engorgement of the pulmonary vasculature, is common in most instances of dyspnea in association with congestive heart failure. The lungs become less compliant, the resistance of small airways increases, and there is an increase in lymphatic flow which apparently serves to maintain a constant pulmonary extravascular liquid volume. At this early stage there is usually mild tachypnea, and if arterial blood gases are measured, the arterial P_{O_2} and P_{CO_2} are both lowered with an increase in the alveolar-to-arterial oxygen difference. Tachypnea itself, which might result from stimulation of receptors in the pulmonary interstitium, apparently increases lymphatic flow by augmenting ventilatory pumping of lymphatic vessels. The changes described are seen well in advance of auscultatory findings or radiographic signs pointing to congestive heart failure. If sufficient both in magnitude and duration, the increase in intravascular pressure results in a net gain of liquid in the extravascular space despite further increases in lymphatic flow. It is at this point that symptoms worsen, tachypnea increases, gas exchange deteriorates further, and radiographic changes, such as Kerley B lines and loss of distinct vascular margins, are seen. Even at this intermediate stage, the capillary endothelial intercellular junctions have been shown to widen and allow passage of macromolecules into the interstices. Up to and including this stage, the edema is purely *interstitial*. Sufficient further elevations in intravascular pressure result in disruption of the tighter junctions between alveolar lining cells, and alveolar edema ensues with outpouring of liquid, which contains both red blood cells and macromolecules. At this point *alveolar edema* is present. Although at one time considered an early and subtle radiographic sign of interstitial edema, current evidence suggests that an antigravity redistribution of pulmonary blood flow occurs only after the onset of alveolar edema. With yet more severe disruption of the alveolar-capillary membrane, edematous liquid floods the alveoli and airways. At this point, full-blown clinical pulmonary edema with bilateral wet rales and rhonchi will occur, and the chest radiograph may show diffuse haziness of the lung fields with greater density in the more proximal hilar regions. Typically, the patient is anxious and perspires freely, and the sputum is frothy and blood-tinged. Gas exchange is more severely compromised with worsening hypoxia and possibly hypercapnia. Without effective treatment (Chap. 182), progressive acidemia, hypoxia, and respiratory arrest ensue.

The earlier sequence of liquid accumulation described above follows the Starling law of capillary–interstitial fluid exchange:

$$\text{Liquid accumulation} = K[(P_c - P_{IF}) - \sigma(\pi_{pl} - \pi_{IF})] - Q_{lymph}$$

where K = permeability coefficient
P_c = mean intracapillary pressure
π_{IF} = oncotic pressure of interstitial liquid
σ = reflection coefficient of macromolecules
P_{IF} = mean interstitial liquid pressure
π_{pl} = oncotic pressure of the plasma
Q_{lymph} = lymphatic flow

The pressures tending to move liquid out of the vessel are P_c and π_{IF}, which are normally more than offset by pressures tending to move liquid back into the vasculature, i.e., the algebraic sum of P_{IF} and π_{pl}. Implicit in the above equation is that lymphatic flow can increase in the case of imbalance of forces and result in no net accumulation of interstitial liquid. However, in later sequences, with opening of first the endothelial and then the alveolar intercellular junctions, the permeability and reflection coefficients change strikingly. Thus, the initial process of hemodynamic pulmonary edema is one of liquid filtration and clearance. With further increasing pressures, disruption of both the structure and the function of the alveolar-capillary membrane occurs.

NONCARDIOGENIC PULMONARY EDEMA There are several clinical conditions which are associated with pulmonary edema based upon an imbalance of Starling forces other than through primary elevations of pulmonary capillary pressure. Although diminished plasma oncotic pressure in hypoalbuminemic states (e.g., severe liver disease, nephrotic syndrome, protein-losing enteropathy) might be expected to lead to pulmonary edema, the balance of forces normally so strongly favors resorption that even under these conditions some elevation of capillary pressure is necessary before interstitial edema develops. Increased negativity of interstitial pressure has been implicated in the genesis of unilateral pulmonary edema following rapid evacuation of a large pneumothorax. In this situation the findings may be apparent only by radiography, but occasionally the patient experiences dyspnea with physical findings localized to the edematous lung. It has been recently proposed that large negative intrapleural pressures during acute severe asthma may be associated with the development of interstitial edema. If this proposal can be supported by sufficient clinical data, then asthma would represent an additional example of edema due to increased negativity of interstitial pressure. Lymphatic blockade secondary to fibrotic and inflammatory diseases or lymphangitic carcinomatosis may lead to interstitial edema. In such instances both clinical and radiographic manifestations are dominated by the underlying disease process.

There are other conditions characterized by increases in the interstitial liquid content of the lungs which begin neither with an imbalance between intravascular and interstitial forces nor with alterations in lymphatics, but rather appear to be associated primarily with disruption of the alveolar-capillary membranes. Any number of spontaneously occurring or environmental toxic insults, including diffuse pulmonary infections, aspiration, shock (particularly due to gram-negative septicemia and hemorrhagic pancreatitis, and following cardiopulmonary bypass), are associated with diffuse pulmonary edema which clearly does not have a hemodynamic origin. These conditions, which may lead to the adult respiratory distress syndrome, are discussed in Chap. 218.

Other forms of pulmonary edema There are three forms of pulmonary edema which have not been clearly related to increased permeability, inadequate lymphatic flow, or an imbalance of Starling forces; hence their precise mechanism remains unexplained. *Narcotic overdose* is a well-recognized antecedent to pulmonary edema. Although illicit use of parenteral heroin has been the most frequent cause, parenteral and oral overdoses of legitimate preparations of morphine, methadone, and dextropropoxyphene have also been associated with pulmonary edema. Thus the earlier idea that injected impurities lead to the disorder is untenable. Available evidence suggests that there are alterations in the permeability of alveolar and capillary membranes rather than elevation of pulmonary capillary pressure.

Exposure to high altitude in association with severe physical exertion is a well-recognized setting for pulmonary edema in unacclimatized, yet otherwise healthy, persons. Recent data show that acclimatized high-altitude natives also develop this syndrome upon return to high altitude after a relatively brief sojourn at low altitudes. The syndrome is far more common in persons under the age of 25 years. The mechanism for high-altitude pulmonary edema remains obscure, and studies have been conflicting, some suggesting pulmonary venous constriction and others indicating pulmonary arteriolar constriction as the prime mechanisms. A role for hypoxia at altitude is suggested by the fact that patients respond to the administration of oxygen and/or return to lower altitudes. Hypoxia per se does not alter permeability of the alveolar-capillary membrane. Hence, increased cardiac output and pulmonary arterial pressures with exercise combined with hypoxic pulmonary arteriolar constriction, which is more prominent in young persons, may combine to make this an example of prearteriolar, high-pressure pulmonary edema.

Neurogenic pulmonary edema has been suspected in patients with central nervous system disorders and without apparent preexisting left ventricular dysfunction. Although most experimental equivalents have implicated sympathetic nervous system activity, the mechanism whereby sympathetic efferent activity leads to pulmonary edema is a matter of speculation. It is known that a massive adrenergic discharge leads to peripheral vasoconstriction with elevation of blood pressure and shifts of blood to the central circulation. In addition, it is probable that a decrease in left ventricular compliance also occurs, and both factors serve to increase left atrial pressures sufficiently to induce pulmonary edema on a hemodynamic basis. Some experimental evidence suggests that stimulation of adrenergic receptors increases capillary permeability directly, but this effect is relatively minor as compared to the imbalance of Starling forces.

TREATMENT OF PULMONARY EDEMA See Chap. 182.

REFERENCES

CHERNIACK NS, ALTOSE MD: Mechanisms of dyspnea. Clin Chest Med 8:207, 1987

INGRAM RH JR, BRAUNWALD E: Pulmonary edema: Cardiogenic and noncardiogenic, in *Heart Disease*, E. Braunwald (ed). Philadelphia, Saunders, 1988, p 544

MALIK AB: Mechanisms of neurogenic pulmonary edema. Circ Res 57:1, 1985

MCFADDEN ER, INGRAM RH JR: Relationship between diseases of the heart and lungs, in *Heart Disease*, E Braunwald (ed). Philadelphia, Saunders, 1988, p 1870

RASANEN J et al: Continuous positive airway pressure by face mask in acute cardiogenic pulmonary edema. Am J Cardiol 55:296, 1985

ROUSSOS C, MACKLEM PT: Disorders of the respiratory muscle function, in *Update III: Harrison's Principles of Internal Medicine*, KJ Isselbacher et al (eds). New York, McGraw-Hill, 1982, p 83

SCHOENE RB et al: High altitude pulmonary edema: Characteristics of lung lavage fluid. JAMA 256:63, 1986

SPRUNG CL et al: The spectrum of pulmonary edema: Differentiation of cardiogenic, intermediate, and noncardiogenic forms of pulmonary edema. Am Rev Resp Dis 124:718, 1981

WASSERMAN K, CASABURI R: Dyspnea: Physiological and pathophysiological mechanisms. Ann Rev Med 39:503, 1988

37 HYPOXIA, POLYCYTHEMIA, AND CYANOSIS

EUGENE BRAUNWALD

HYPOXIA

The fundamental purpose of the cardiorespiratory system is to deliver oxygen (and substrates) to the cells and to remove carbon dioxide (and other metabolic products) from them. Proper maintenance of this function depends on intact cardiovascular and respiratory systems and a supply of inspired gas containing adequate oxygen. Changes in oxygen and in carbon dioxide tension as well as changes in the intraerythrocytic concentration of certain *organic phosphate compounds*, especially 2,3-diphosphoglyceric acid (2,3-DPG), cause shifts in the oxygen dissociation curve. These are discussed in detail in Chap. 290 and are illustrated in Fig. 290-4. When hypoxia results as a consequence of respiratory failure, Pa_{CO_2} usually rises (Chap. 210), and the oxygen dissociation curve tends to be displaced to the right. Under these conditions the percentage saturation of the hemoglobin in the arterial blood at a given level of alveolar oxygen (Pa_{O_2}) tension declines. Thus arterial hypoxia and cyanosis are likely to be more marked in proportion to the degree of depression of Pa_{O_2} when such depression results from pulmonary disease than when the depression occurs as the result of a decline in the partial pressure of oxygen in the inspired air, in which case Pa_{CO_2} falls and the oxygen dissociation curve is displaced to the left.

DIFFERENTIAL DIAGNOSIS **Anemic hypoxia** Any decrease in hemoglobin concentration is attended by a corresponding decline in the oxygen-carrying capacity. The Pa_{O_2} remains normal, but the absolute amount of oxygen transported per unit volume of blood is diminished. As the anemic blood passes through the capillaries, and the usual amount of oxygen is removed from it, the P_{O_2} in the venous blood declines to a greater degree than would normally be the case.

Circulatory hypoxia As in anemic hypoxia, Pa_{O_2} is normal, but venous and tissue P_{O_2} are reduced as a consequence of reduced tissue perfusion in the face of normal tissue oxygen consumption. For this reason the term *stagnant hypoxia* may be used for this condition. Generalized circulatory hypoxia occurs in heart failure (Chap. 182) and in most forms of shock (Chap. 39).

Specific organ hypoxia Decreased circulation to a specific organ resulting in localized stagnant hypoxia may be due to organic arterial or venous obstruction or may occur as a consequence of vasoconstriction. The latter may occur in the upper extremities in Raynaud's phenomenon. Reduced circulation may occur in all limbs in patients with heart failure or hypovolemic shock in an attempt to maintain adequate perfusion to more vital organs. Ischemic hypoxia with accompanying pallor occurs in organic arterial obliterative disease. Localized hypoxia may also result from venous obstruction and the resultant congestion. Edema, which increases the distance through which oxygen diffuses before it reaches the cells, can also cause localized hypoxia.

Increased oxygen requirements Even if oxygen diffusion into blood perfusing the pulmonary capillary bed is unhampered and the hemoglobin is qualitatively and quantitatively normal, the P_{O_2} in venous blood (hence, capillary and tissue P_{O_2}) may be reduced if the oxygen consumption of the tissues is elevated without a corresponding increase in volume flow per unit of time. Such a situation may be encountered when fever or thyrotoxicosis occurs in patients in whom the cardiac output cannot rise normally. Under such conditions the circulation may be considered deficient relative to the metabolic requirements.

Ordinarily, the clinical picture of patients with hypoxia due to an elevated basal metabolic rate is quite different from that in other types of hypoxia; the skin is warm and flushed, owing to increased cutaneous blood flow which dissipates the excessive heat produced, and cyanosis is usually absent.

Exercise is a classic example of increased tissue oxygen requirements. The increased demands are normally met by several mechanisms: (1) increasing the cardiac output and ventilation and thus oxygen delivery to the tissues; (2) preferentially directing the blood to the exercising muscles and away from resting muscles and skin (by changing vascular resistances in various circulatory beds, directly and/or reflexly); (3) increasing oxygen extraction from the delivered blood and widening the arteriovenous oxygen differences; (4) reducing the pH of the tissues and capillary blood, thereby unloading more oxygen from hemoglobin. If the capacity of these mechanisms is exceeded, then hypoxia, especially of the exercising muscles, will result.

Carbon monoxide intoxication (Chap. 374) This condition is analogous to anemic hypoxia in that the hemoglobin which is combined with the carbon monoxide (carboxyhemoglobin) is unavailable for oxygen transport. In addition, the presence of carboxyhemoglobin shifts the dissociation curve of hemoglobin to the left, so that the oxygen can be unloaded only at lower tensions. By such formation of carboxyhemoglobin a given degree of reduction in oxygen-carrying power produces a far greater degree of tissue hypoxia than the equivalent reduction in hemoglobin due to simple anemia.

Improper oxygen utilization Cyanide (Chap. 374) and several other similarly acting poisons cause a paradoxic state in which the tissues are unable to utilize oxygen and as a consequence the venous blood tends to have a high oxygen tension. This condition has been termed *histotoxic hypoxia*. Cyanide produces cellular hypoxia by paralyzing the electron-transfer function of cytochrome oxidase so that it cannot pass electrons to oxygen, whereas diphtheria toxin is believed to inhibit the synthesis of one of the cytochromes and thus interfere with oxygen consumption and energy production by the cells involved.

EFFECTS OF HYPOXIA Changes in the central nervous system, particularly the higher centers, are especially important. Acute hypoxia produces impaired judgment, motor incoordination, and a clinical picture closely resembling that of acute alcoholism. When hypoxia is long-standing, fatigue, drowsiness, apathy, inattentiveness, delayed reaction time, and reduced work capacity occur. As hypoxia becomes more severe, the centers of the brainstem are affected, and death usually results from respiratory failure. With reduction of Pa_{O_2}, cerebrovascular resistance decreases and cerebral blood flow increases, which tends to reduce the cerebral hypoxia. On the other hand when the reduction of Pa_{O_2} is accompanied by hyperventilation and diminution of Pa_{CO_2}, cerebrovascular resistance rises, blood flow falls, and hypoxia is enhanced. Compared with the brain, the phylogenetically older spinal cord and peripheral nerves are relatively insensitive to hypoxia. Hypoxia also causes pulmonary arterial constriction, which serves the useful function of shunting blood away from poorly ventilated areas toward better-ventilated portions of the lung. However, it has the disadvantage of causing increased pulmonary vascular resistance and increased right ventricular afterload.

A complex disturbance of cellular functions results from the metabolic effects of severe acute hypoxia. In liver and muscles the breakdown of the primary foodstuff, carbohydrate, normally proceeds anaerobically (i.e., without oxidation) to the stage of formation of pyruvic acid. The breakdown of pyruvate requires oxygen, and when this is deficient, increasing proportions of pyruvate are reduced to lactic acid, which cannot be broken down further (Chap. 51). Hence, there is an increase in the blood lactate, with decrease in bicarbonate and a corresponding metabolic acidosis. Under these circumstances the total energy obtained from foodstuff breakdown is greatly reduced, and the amount of energy available for continuing resynthesis of energy-rich phosphate compounds becomes inadequate, leading to a complex disturbance of cellular function.

Most of the useful respiratory response to hypoxia originates in special chemosensitive cells in the carotid and aortic bodies, although the respiratory center is also stimulated directly by oxygen lack. The resultant increase in ventilation, with loss of carbon dioxide, leads to respiratory alkalosis. On the other hand, the diffusion of additional quantities of lactic acid from the tissues into the blood tends to produce metabolic acidosis. In either case the total amount of bicarbonate, and hence the carbon dioxide–combining power, tends to be diminished.

Diminished oxygen tension in any tissue results in local vasodilatation, and the diffuse vasodilatation which occurs in generalized hypoxia causes an elevation of total cardiac output (Fig. 290-5). In patients with preexisting heart disease, particularly coronary artery disease, the combination of hypoxia and the requirements of the peripheral tissues for an increase of cardiac output may precipitate congestive heart failure. Prolonged or severe hypoxia may also impair hepatic and renal function.

One of the important mechanisms of compensation for prolonged hypoxia is an increase in the quantity of hemoglobin in the blood (Fig. 290-5). This is due not to direct stimulation of the bone marrow but to the effect of erythropoietin, which originates primarily in the kidneys (Chap. 290). Assayable levels of erythropoietin are increased by hypoxia, and its production has been found to be regulated by the balance between tissue oxygen supply and demand.

POLYCYTHEMIA (See also Chap. 297)

The term *polycythemia* signifies an increase above the normal in the number of red blood cells in the circulating blood. This elevation is usually, though not always, accompanied by a corresponding increase in the quantity of hemoglobin and in the hematocrit. The increase may or may not be associated with an elevation in the total quantity of red blood cells in the body. It is important to distinguish between *absolute* polycythemia (an increase in the total red cell mass) and *relative* polycythemia, which occurs when, through loss of blood plasma, the *concentration* of the red cells becomes greater than normal in the circulating blood. This may be the consequence of abnormally lowered fluid intake, of the loss of plasma into the interstitial fluid, or of the marked loss of body fluids, such as occurs in persistent vomiting, severe diarrhea, copious sweating, or acidosis.

Because the term polycythemia is used loosely to refer to all varieties of increase in the number of red corpuscles, the terms *erythrocytosis* and *erythremia* are preferred in referring to two forms of *absolute* polycythemia. Erythrocytosis denotes absolute polycythemia which occurs in response to some known stimulus (secondary polycythemia); erythremia (polycythemia vera) refers to the disease of unknown etiology (Chap. 297). An approach to the differential diagnosis of erythrocytosis should begin with a consideration of its mechanisms (Table 37-1). Erythrocytosis develops as a consequence of a variety of factors and represents a physiologic response to conditions of hypoxia.

Sojourn at high altitudes leads to defective saturation of arterial blood with oxygen and stimulates the production of more red cells. The oxygen saturation, rather than oxygen tension, appears to be the more important determinant of the erythropoietic response to chronic hypoxia (Fig. 37-1). A disorder may set in insidiously after several years of continued residence at high altitudes, leading to the development of a condition known as *chronic mountain sickness* or *seroche* (Monge's disease), which appears to be caused by the development of alveolar hypoventilation superimposed on a lowered inspired O_2 concentration. Prominent manifestations are a florid color which turns to cyanosis on mild exertion, mental torpor, fatigue, and headache. Those affected are usually in the fourth to sixth decades. Return to sea level promptly relieves the symptoms. Living at high altitudes also evokes a number of compensatory reactions which act to increase oxygen delivery to the tissues. These include hyperventilation, which reduces the oxygen gradient between inspired and alveolar air, an augmentation of pulmonary capillary blood volume, an increase of diffusing capacity, and an increase in cardiac output.

Any pulmonary disease which produces chronic hypoxia may lead to erythrocytosis. The increased blood viscosity secondary to the polycythemia elevates pulmonary arterial pressure and, combined with the elevation of pulmonary vascular resistance resulting from

TABLE 37-1 Differential diagnosis of erythrocytosis

ABSOLUTE (↑ RED CELL MASS)

I Autonomous erythroid proliferation (↓ EP*); polycythemia vera
II Secondary erythroid proliferation
- *A* Autonomous or inappropriate increase in EP
  - *1* Neoplasm
  - *2* Renal lesions
  - *3* Familial erythrocytosis (autosomal recessive inheritance)
- *B* Secondary increase in EP
  - *1* Hypoxia (↓ arterial P_{O_2})
    - *a* High altitude
    - *b* Alveolar hypoventilation
    - *c* Pulmonary disease
    - *d* Cardiac right-to-left shunt
  - *2* Abnormal hemoglobin function (normal arterial P_{O_2})
    - *a* High-affinity variants (autosomal dominant inheritance)
    - *b* Congenital methemoglobinemia
    - *c* Carboxyhemoglobin (smokers')
- *C* Hormonal stimulus to erythropoiesis
  - *1* Cushing's syndrome
  - *2* Androgen or corticosteroid administration

RELATIVE (REDUCED PLASMA VOLUME, NORMAL RED CELL MASS)

I Dehydration
II Stress erythrocytosis

* Erythropoietin.
SOURCE: Adapted from HF Bunn et al, *Human Hemoglobins*, Philadelphia, Saunders, 1988.

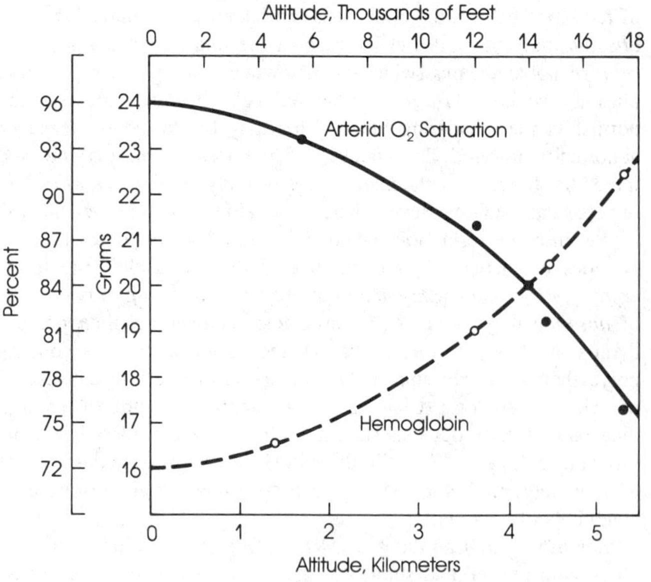

FIGURE 37-1 Relationship between mean arterial oxygen saturation (percent) and the mean hemoglobin content (grams per deciliter) in healthy male residents at various altitudes. *(From Hurtado, by permission of Annals of Internal Medicine.)*

hypoxia, further elevates right ventricular pressure, contributing to the development or intensification of cor pulmonale (Chap. 191). The *abnormal ventilatory conditions* present in very obese individuals may cause alveolar hypoventilation and result in arterial unsaturation, erythrocytosis, hypercapnia, and somnolence (the Pickwickian syndrome, Chap. 217). This syndrome is observed less commonly in nonobese persons (sleep-apnea syndrome) in whom decreased sensitivity of the respiratory center to CO_2 may play a role (Chap. 217).

The partial shunting of blood from the pulmonary circuit, such as occurs in *congenital heart disease,* causes the most striking erythrocytosis resulting from abnormalities in the heart or lungs (Chap. 186). Erythrocyte counts as high as 13 million per microliter, which are possible only when the red corpuscles are smaller than normal, have been observed in such patients, with volumes of packed red blood cells as high as 860 mL/L (86 mL/dL) of blood. As the polycythemia develops, there is a progressive elevation of blood viscosity, which begins to rise logarithmically when the volume of packed red blood cells exceeds 55 percent. The commonest defects producing such polycythemia in the adult are tetralogy of Fallot and Eisenmenger's complex. Other conditions include transposition of the great arteries, tricuspid atresia, and persistent truncus arteriosus. The polycythemia of cyanotic congenital heart disease may lead to spontaneous thrombosis at any site, including the central nervous system. The increase in hematocrit and the sharp increase in viscosity which occur when these patients become dehydrated are particularly hazardous. This condition may also be accompanied by a variety of blood coagulation defects, including reduced fibrinogen and prothrombin concentrations, as well as thrombocytopenia. Reduction in red blood cell volume (phlebotomy with reinfusion of the plasma) is sometimes performed in severely symptomatic patients with extremely high hematocrit levels, but it must be carried out slowly and with caution. It results in a reduction of the elevated blood viscosity which improves blood flow.

The excessive use of coal-tar derivatives and other forms of chronic poisoning, by producing abnormal hemoglobin pigments such as *methemoglobin* and *sulfhemoglobin* (Chap. 295), also may cause erythrocytosis. Patients with abnormal hemoglobins which displace the oxygen dissociation curve to the left and interfere with oxygen unloading in the tissues stimulate the production of erythropoietin and a secondary erythrocytosis *unassociated* with leukocytosis or thrombocytosis (Chap. 295).

Mild erythrocytosis is sometimes found in *Cushing's syndrome* and can be produced by the administration of large amounts of adrenocortical steroids. Androgens also exert an erythropoietic effect and when administered to normal individuals can produce erythrocytosis. Especially intriguing are the instances of erythrocytosis observed in association with various *tumors* which produce erythropoietin or an erythropoietin-like substance. These have been chiefly of two varieties, *infratentorial* and *renal.* The tumors in the posterior fossa have usually been vascular (hemangioblastomas). The renal tumors have included renal cell carcinoma, adenoma, and sarcoma. Other tumors that have been associated with erythrocytosis include uterine myoma, hepatic carcinoma, and pheochromocytoma. Erythrocytosis also has been reported in association with solitary and polycystic disease of the kidneys, with hydronephrosis, and with renal artery stenosis. However, only a small proportion of the renal disorders mentioned above have been associated with polycythemia. Plasma erythropoietin levels have been found to be elevated in a number of these patients. Erythropoietin-like activity has been demonstrated in tumor extracts and in renal cyst fluid, and erythrocytosis has disappeared after the associated tumor was removed.

The term *stress erythrocytosis* has been applied to the polycythemia seen occasionally in very active, hard-working, middle-aged white males who are typically hypertensive and overweight and in a state of anxiety, who appear florid but who have none of the other characteristic signs of polycythemia vera—no splenomegaly or leukocytosis with immature cells in the blood. In such persons the total red blood cell mass is normal, and the plasma volume is below normal. Thus, they have an elevated hematocrit and *relative* polycythemia. *Smokers' polycythemia* is a closely related condition, but the high carboxyhemoglobin concentration may cause a small absolute increase in red cell mass which is often associated with a reduced plasma volume.

The *clinical features* of polycythemia include, in addition to the symptoms of the underlying condition (in the secondary forms), a characteristic ''ruddy'' cyanosis, dizziness, headache, epistaxes, and an increased incidence of thrombotic complications.

The *differential diagnosis* of absolute polycythemia is discussed in Chap. 297. In polycythemia vera, erythropoietin levels are usually absent, leukocyte alkaline phosphatase and vitamin B_{12} levels and platelet and total white blood cells are usually elevated, and splenomegaly is common; the bone marrow shows hyperplasia of all elements. In secondary polycythemia with hypoxia, Pa_{CO_2} is reduced, erythropoietin levels are elevated, while levels of leukocyte alkaline phosphatase, serum vitamin B_{12}, platelet, total white blood cell, and differential counts are all normal, and the liver and spleen are not enlarged; the bone marrow shows only erythroid hyperplasia. In the absence of features of either polycythemia vera or polycythemia secondary to hypoxia or to a tumor, a hemoglobin with a high affinity for oxygen should be sought for.

CYANOSIS

Cyanosis refers to a bluish color of the skin and mucous membranes resulting from an increased amount of reduced hemoglobin, or of hemoglobin derivatives, in the small blood vessels of those areas. It is usually most marked in the lips, nail beds, ears, and malar eminences. The ''red cyanosis'' of polycythemia vera (Chap. 297) must be distinguished from the true cyanosis discussed here. A cherry-colored flush, rather than cyanosis, is caused by carboxyhemoglobin (Chap. 374). The degree of cyanosis is modified by the quality of cutaneous pigment, the color of the blood plasma, and the thickness of the skin, as well as by the state of the cutaneous capillaries. The accurate clinical detection of the presence and degree of cyanosis is difficult, as proved by oximetric studies. In some instances central cyanosis can be reliably detected when the arterial saturation has fallen to 85 percent; in others, particularly dark-skinned persons, it may not be detected until the saturation has declined to 75 percent.

The increase in the quantity of reduced hemoglobin in the cutaneous vessels which produces cyanosis may be brought about either by an increase in the quantity of venous blood in the skin as the result of dilatation of the venules and venous ends of the capillaries, or by a reduction in the oxygen saturation in the capillary blood. In general, cyanosis becomes apparent when the mean capillary concentration of reduced hemoglobin exceeds 50 g/L (5 g/dL). It is the *absolute* rather than the *relative* quantity of reduced hemoglobin which is important in producing cyanosis. Thus, in a patient with severe anemia the relative amount of reduced hemoglobin in the venous blood may be very large when considered in relation to the total amount of hemoglobin. However, since the concentration of the latter is markedly reduced, the *absolute* quantity of reduced hemoglobin may still be small, and therefore patients with severe anemia and even *marked* arterial desaturation do not display cyanosis. Conversely, the higher the total hemoglobin content, the greater the tendency toward cyanosis; thus, patients with marked polycythemia tend to be cyanotic at higher levels of arterial oxygen saturation than patients with normal hematocrit values. Likewise, local passive congestion, which causes an increase in the total amount of reduced hemoglobin in the vessels in a given area, may cause cyanosis. Cyanosis also is observed when nonfunctional hemoglobin such as methemoglobin or sulfhemoglobin (Chap. 295) is present in blood.

Cyanosis may be subdivided into *central* and *peripheral* types. In the *central* type, there is arterial blood unsaturation or an abnormal hemoglobin derivative, and the mucous membranes and skin are both affected. *Peripheral* cyanosis is due to a slowing of blood flow to an area and abnormally great extraction of oxygen from normally saturated arterial blood. It results from vasoconstriction and diminished peripheral blood flow, such as occurs in cold exposure, shock, congestive failure, and peripheral vascular disease. Often, in these conditions the mucous membranes of the oral cavity or those beneath the tongue may be spared. Clinical differentiation between central and peripheral cyanosis may not always be simple, and in conditions such as cardiogenic shock with pulmonary edema there may be a mixture of both types.

DIFFERENTIAL DIAGNOSIS (See Table 37-2) **Central cyanosis** Decreased arterial oxygen saturation results from a marked reduction in the oxygen tension in the arterial blood. This may be brought about by a decline in the tension of oxygen in the inspired air without sufficient compensatory alveolar hyperventilation to maintain alveolar oxygen tension. Cyanosis does not occur in a significant degree in an ascent to an altitude of 2500 m (8000 ft) but is marked in a further ascent to 5000 m (16,000 ft). The reason for this becomes clear on studying the *S* shape of the oxygen dissociation curve (Fig. 290-4). At 2500 m (8000 ft) the tension of oxygen in the inspired air is about 120 mmHg, the alveolar tension is approximately 80 mmHg, and the hemoglobin is nearly completely saturated. However, at 5000 m (16,000 ft) the oxygen tensions in atmospheric air and alveolar air are about 85 and 50 mmHg, respectively, and the oxygen dissociation curve shows that the arterial blood is only about 75 percent saturated. This leaves 25 percent of the hemoglobin in the reduced form, an amount likely to be associated with cyanosis in the absence of anemia. Similarly, a mutant hemoglobin with a low affinity for oxygen (Hb Kansas) causes lowered arterial oxygen saturation and resultant central cyanosis (Chap. 295).

TABLE 37-2 Causes of cyanosis

I Central cyanosis
- *A* Decreased arterial oxygen saturation
  - *1* Decreased atmospheric pressure—high altitude
  - *2* Impaired pulmonary function
    - *a* Alveolar hypoventilation
    - *b* Uneven relationships between pulmonary ventilation and perfusion (perfusion of hypoventilated alveoli)
    - *c* Impaired oxygen diffusion
  - *3* Anatomic shunts
    - *a* Certain types of congenital heart disease
    - *b* Pulmonary arteriovenous fistulas
    - *c* Multiple small intrapulmonary shunts
  - *4* Hemoglobin with low affinity for oxygen
- *B* Hemoglobin abnormalities
  - *1* Methemoglobinemia—hereditary, acquired
  - *2* Sulfhemoglobinema—acquired
  - *3* Carboxyhemoglobinemia (not true cyanosis)

II Peripheral cyanosis
- *A* Reduced cardiac output
- *B* Cold exposure
- *C* Redistribution of blood flow from extremities
- *D* Arterial obstruction
- *E* Venous obstruction

Seriously *impaired pulmonary function,* through alveolar hypoventilation or perfusion of unventilated or poorly ventilated areas of the lung, is a common cause of central cyanosis (Chap. 201). This may occur acutely, as in extensive pneumonia or pulmonary edema, or with chronic pulmonary diseases (e.g., emphysema). In the last situation polycythemia is generally present and clubbing of the fingers may occur. However, in many types of chronic pulmonary disease with fibrosis and obliteration of the capillary vascular bed, cyanosis does not occur because there is relatively little perfusion of underventilated areas.

Another cause of decreased arterial oxygen saturation is *shunting of systemic venous blood into the arterial circuit.* Certain forms of congenital heart disease are associated with cyanosis (Chap. 186). Since blood normally flows from a higher pressure to a lower pressure region, in order for a cardiac defect to result in a right-to-left shunt, it must ordinarily be combined with an obstructive lesion distal to the defect or with elevated pulmonary vascular resistance. The commonest congenital cardiac lesion associated with cyanosis in the adult is the combination of ventricular septal defect and pulmonary outflow tract obstruction (tetralogy of Fallot). The more severe the obstruction, the greater the degree of right-to-left shunting and resultant cyanosis. The mechanisms for the elevated pulmonary vascular resistance which may produce cyanosis in the presence of intra- and extracardiac communications without pulmonic stenosis are discussed elsewhere (Chap. 186). In patients with patent ductus arteriosus, pulmonary hypertension, and right-to-left shunt, *differential cyanosis* results; i.e., cyanosis occurs in the lower extremities but not in the upper extremities.

Pulmonary arteriovenous fistulas may be congenital or acquired, solitary or multiple, microscopic or massive. The degree of cyanosis produced by these fistulas depends upon their size and number. They occur with some frequency in hereditary hemorrhagic telangiectasia (Chap. 288). Arterial oxygen unsaturation also occurs in some patients with cirrhosis, presumably as a consequence of pulmonary arteriovenous fistulas or portal vein–pulmonary vein anastomoses.

In patients with cardiac or pulmonary right-to-left shunts, the presence and severity of cyanosis depend on the size of the shunt relative to the systemic flow as well as on the oxyhemoglobin saturation of the venous blood. In patients with central cyanosis due to arterial oxygen unsaturation, the severity of cyanosis increases with exercise. With increased extraction of oxygen from the blood by the exercising muscles, the venous blood returning to the right side of the heart is more unsaturated than at rest, and shunting of this blood or its passage through lungs incapable of normal oxygenation intensifies the cyanosis. Also, since the systemic vascular resistance normally decreases with exercise, the right-to-left shunt is augmented by exercise in patients with congenital heart disease and communications between the two sides of the heart. Secondary polycythemia occurs frequently in patients with arterial unsaturation and contributes to the cyanosis.

Cyanosis can be caused by small amounts of circulating methemoglobin and by even smaller amounts of sulfhemoglobin (Chap. 295). Although they are uncommon causes of cyanosis, these abnormal hemoglobin pigments should be sought by spectroscopy when cyanosis is not readily explained by malfunction of the circulatory or respiratory systems. Generally, clubbing does not occur with them. The diagnosis of methemoglobinemia can be suspected, if, on mixing the patient's blood in a test tube and exposing it to air, it remains brown.

Peripheral cyanosis Probably the most common cause of peripheral cyanosis is generalized vasoconstriction resulting from exposure to cold air or water. This is a normal response. When cardiac output is low, as in severe congestive heart failure or shock, cutaneous vasoconstriction occurs as a compensatory mechanism, so that blood is diverted from the skin to more vital areas such as the central nervous system and heart (Chap. 182), and intense cyanosis associated with cool extremities may result. Even though the arterial blood is normally saturated, the reduced volume flow through the skin and the reduced oxygen tension at the venous end of the capillary result in cyanosis.

Arterial obstruction to an extremity, as with an embolus, or arteriolar constriction, as in cold-induced vasospasm (Raynaud's phenomenon, Chap. 198), generally results in pallor and coldness, but there may be associated cyanosis. If there is venous obstruction and the extremity is congested and with stagnation of blood flow, cyanosis is also present. Venous hypertension, which may be local (as in thrombophlebitis) or generalized (as in tricuspid valve disease or constrictive pericarditis), dilates the subpapillary venous plexuses and thereby intensifies cyanosis.

APPROACH TO THE PATIENT WITH CYANOSIS Certain features are important in arriving at the proper cause of cyanosis:

1 The history, particularly the duration (cyanosis present since birth is usually due to congenital heart disease); possible exposure to drugs or chemicals which may produce abnormal types of hemoglobin.
2 Clinical differentiation of central as opposed to peripheral cyanosis. Objective evidence by physical or radiographic examination of disorders of the respiratory or cardiovascular systems. Massage or gentle warming of a cyanotic extremity will increase peripheral blood flow and abolish peripheral but not central cyanosis.
3 The presence or absence of clubbing of the fingers. Clubbing without cyanosis is frequent in patients with infective endocarditis and in association with ulcerative colitis, it may occasionally occur in healthy persons, and in some instances it may be occupational, e.g., in jackhammer operators. Slight cyanosis of the lips and cheeks, without clubbing of the fingers, is common in patients with mitral stenosis and is probably due to minimal arterial hypoxia resulting from fibrotic changes in the lungs secondary to long-standing congestion combined with reduction of cardiac output (Chap. 188). The combination of cyanosis and clubbing is frequent in many patients with certain types of congenital cardiac disease and is seen occasionally in persons with pulmonary disease such as lung abscess or pulmonary arteriovenous shunts. On the other hand, peripheral cyanosis or acutely developing central cyanosis is not associated with clubbed fingers.
4 Determination of arterial blood oxygen tension or oxygen saturation, spectroscopic and other examinations of the blood for abnormal types of hemoglobin.

CLUBBING The selective bullous enlargement of the distal segment of a digit due to an increase in soft tissue is termed *clubbing*. It may be hereditary or idiopathic, or acquired and associated with a variety of disorders, including cyanotic heart disease, infective endocarditis, and a variety of pulmonary conditions (among them, primary and metastatic lung cancer, bronchiectasis, lung abscess, and mesothelioma), as well as with some gastrointestinal diseases (including regional enteritis, chronic ulcerative colitis, and hepatic cirrhosis). Primary lung cancer, mesothelioma, neurogenic diaphragmatic tumors, and rarely cyanotic congenital heart disease may be associated with hypertrophic osteoarthropathy, the subperiosteal formation of new bone in the distal diaphyses of the long bones of the extremities. Although the mechanism of clubbing is unclear, it appears to be secondary to a (presumably humoral) substance which causes dilation of the vessels of the fingertip.

REFERENCES

Doll DC, Greenberg BR: Cerebral thrombosis in smokers' polycythemia. Ann Intern Med 102:786, 1985

Erslev AJ: Erythrocytosis (sec 17, Chaps 73–75), in *Hematology*, 4th ed, WJ Williams et al (eds). New York, McGraw-Hill, 1990, p 705

Hurtado A: Some clinical aspects of life at high altitudes. Ann Intern Med 53:247, 1960

Lupinetti FM et al: Pathophysiology of chronic cyanosis in a canine model. Functional and metabolic response to global ischemia. J Thorac Cardiovasc Surg 90:291, 1985

Rosenthal A, Tyler DC: Effect of red cell volume reduction or pulmonary blood flow in polycythemia of cyanotic congenital heart disease. Am J Cardiol 33:410, 1974

Schoene RB, Hornbein TF: High altitude adaptation, in *Textbook of Respiratory Medicine*, JF Murray, JA Nadel (eds). Philadelphia, Saunders, 1988

Smith JR, Landaw SA: Smokers' polycythemia. N Engl J Med 298:6, 1978

Szidon JP, Fishman AP: Cyanosis and clubbing, in *Pulmonary Diseases and Disorders*, 2d ed, A Fishman (ed). Philadelphia, Saunders, 1988, 351

38 EDEMA

EUGENE BRAUNWALD

Edema is defined as an increase in the extravascular (interstitial) component of the extracellular fluid volume, which may expand by several liters before the abnormality is recognized. Therefore, a weight gain of several kilograms usually precedes overt manifestations of edema, and a similar weight loss from diuresis can be induced in a slightly edematous patient before "dry weight" is achieved. *Ascites* (Chap. 48) and *hydrothorax* refer to accumulation of excess fluid in the peritoneal and pleural cavities, respectively, and are considered to be special forms of edema. *Anasarca* refers to gross, generalized edema. Depending on its etiology and mechanism, edema may be localized or have a generalized distribution; it is recognized in its generalized form by puffiness of the face, which is most readily apparent in the periorbital areas, and by the persistence of an indentation of the skin following pressure; this is known as "pitting" edema. In its more subtle form, it may be detected by the fact that after the stethoscope is removed, the rim of the bell leaves an indentation on chest skin for a few minutes. An early symptom a patient may note is the ring on a finger fitting more snugly than in the past, or difficulty in putting on shoes, particularly in the evening.

PATHOGENESIS (See also Chap. 50) About one-third of the total-body water is confined to the extracellular space. This compartment, in turn, is composed of the plasma volume and the interstitial space. Under ordinary circumstances the plasma volume represents about 25 percent of the extracellular space, and the remainder is interstitial fluid. The forces that regulate the disposition of fluid between these two components of the extracellular compartment are frequently referred to as the Starling forces (see p. 223). In general terms, the hydrostatic pressure within the vascular system and the colloid oncotic pressure in the interstitial fluid tend to promote movement of fluid from the vascular to the extravascular space. In contrast, the colloid oncotic pressure contributed by the plasma proteins and the hydrostatic pressure within the interstitial fluid, referred to as the *tissue tension,* promote the movement of fluid into the vascular compartment. As a consequence of these forces there is a movement of water and diffusible solutes from the vascular space at the arteriolar end of the capillaries. Fluid is returned from the interstitial space into the vascular system at the venous end of the capillary and by way of the lymphatics, and unless these channels are obstructed, lymph flow tends to increase if there is net movement of fluid from the vascular compartment to the interstitium. These forces are usually balanced so that a steady state exists in the size of the intravascular and interstitial compartments, and yet a large exchange between them is permitted. However, should any one of these forces be altered significantly, a net movement of fluid from one component of the extracellular space to the other will occur.

An increase in capillary pressure as a cause of edema may result from an increase in venous pressure due to local obstruction in venous drainage, to congestive heart failure, or rarely to the simple expansion of the vascular volume by the administration of large volumes of fluid at a rate in excess of the ability of the kidneys to excrete them. The colloid oncotic pressure of the plasma may be reduced, owing to any factor that may induce severe hypoalbuminemia, such as malnutrition, liver disease, loss of protein into the urine or into the gastrointestinal tract, or a severe catabolic state.

Edema may also result from damage to the capillary endothelium, which increases its permeability and permits the transfer to the interstitial compartment of fluid containing more protein than usual. Injury to the capillary wall can result from chemical, bacterial, thermal, or mechanical agents. Increased capillary permeability may also be a consequence of a hypersensitivity reaction and is characteristic of immune injury. Damage to the capillary endothelium is presumably responsible for inflammatory edema, which is usually nonpitting, localized, and accompanied by other signs of inflammation—redness, heat, and tenderness.

To formulate a hypothesis about the pathophysiology of an edematous state, it is important to discriminate between the *primary* events, such as venous or lymphatic obstruction, reduction of cardiac output, hypoalbuminemia, trapping of fluid in spaces such as the peritoneal cavity, or an increase in capillary permeability, and the predictable *secondary* consequences, which include the renal retention of salt and water in an attempt to restore the plasma volume. There are also instances in which an abnormal positive balance of salt and water may, in fact, be the primary disturbance. In these circumstances the edema is a secondary manifestation of the generalized increase in extracellular fluid volume. These special instances are usually related to conditions characterized by a reduction in renal function (either acute, as in acute tubular necrosis or acute glomerulonephritis, or chronic, as in chronic renal failure). Vasodilators such as minoxidil can also induce primary renal sodium retention.

The pathogenesis of edema depends on one or more alterations in the Starling forces so that there is a net movement of fluid from the vascular system into the interstitium or into a "third space" or from the arterial compartment of the vascular space into the chambers of the heart or into the venous circulation itself. The *effective arterial blood volume,* an as yet poorly defined parameter of the filling of the arterial tree, is reduced, and as a consequence a series of physiologic responses designed to restore it to normal are set into motion. A key element of these responses is the retention of an increment of salt and therefore of water, and in many instances this repairs the deficit of the effective arterial blood volume; often this occurs without the development of overt edema. If, however, the retention of salt and water is insufficient to restore and maintain the effective arterial blood volume, the stimuli are not dissipated, the retention of salt and water continues, and edema develops. This sequence of events is operative in dehydration and hemorrhage. Although in these conditions there is a reduction of effective arterial blood volume and activation of the entire sequence shown in the center of Fig. 38-1, including the diminished excretion of salt and water, edema does not occur because the net sodium and water balance is negative. In most conditions that lead to edema the mechanisms responsible for maintaining a normal effective osmolality in the body fluids operate efficiently so that sodium retention promotes thirst and secretion of the antidiuretic hormone, which, in turn, lead to the ingestion and retention of approximately 1 L of water for each 140 mmol sodium retained. In edematous states, isotonic expansion of the extracellular fluid space may be massive, while the intracellular fluid volume is changed little or not at all.

Reduced cardiac output A reduction of cardiac output, whatever the cause, is associated with a reduction of the effective arterial blood volume as well as of renal blood flow and an elevation of the filtration fraction, i.e., the ratio of glomerular filtration rate to renal plasma

FIGURE 38-1 Sequence of events leading to the formation and retention of salt and water and the development of edema. ANP, atrial natriuretic peptide; RPF, renal plasma flow. Inhibitory influences are shown by dashed lines.

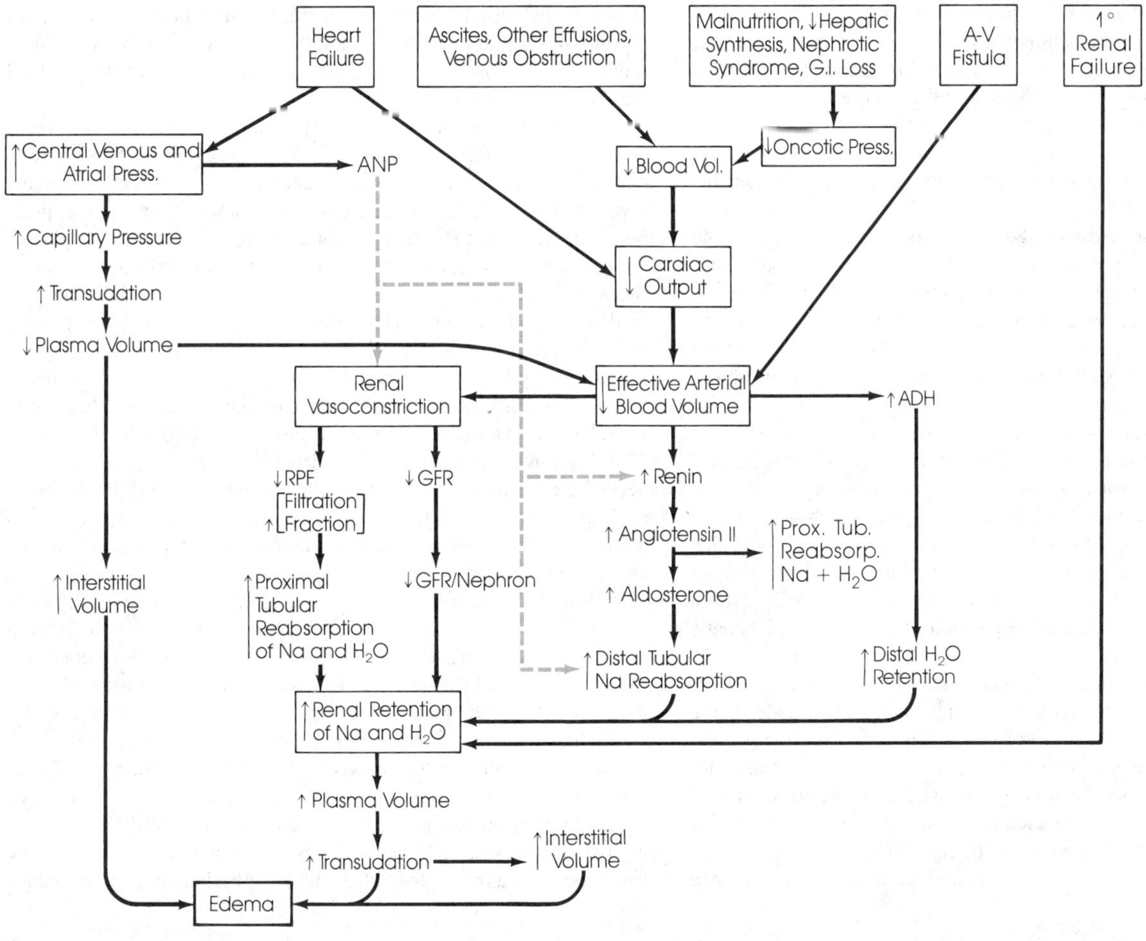

flow. In severe heart failure the blood flow to the outer renal cortex, in particular, is reduced with less depression in the more central regions of the kidney, and there is a reduction in the glomerular filtration rate. This constriction of renal cortical vessels plays an important role in the retention of salt and water and in the formation of edema in heart failure. At different stages of heart failure, activation of the sympathetic nervous system or of the renin-angiotensin systems is responsible for renal vasoconstriction. Activation of the former can be counteracted by the administration of alpha-adrenergic blocking agents, a finding which indicates that the elevated renal vascular resistance in heart failure is mediated, at least in part, by sympathetic stimuli. The augmented renal blood flow and diuresis induced by treatment with angiotensin-converting enzyme inhibitors point to the involvement of the renin-angiotensin system in the retention of salt and water in heart failure.

Renal factors An increase in the tubular reabsorption of glomerular filtrate plays a principal role in the salt and water retention of heart failure. Although there is evidence for both proximal and distal increases in sodium reabsorption in heart failure, the precise role of each tubule segment, including the thick ascending limb of Henle and the collecting duct, requires further elucidation. Alterations in intrarenal hemodynamics appear to play a significant role. Heart failure, by augmenting renal arteriolar constriction, reduces the hydrostatic pressure and raises the colloid osmotic pressure in the peritubular capillaries, thus enhancing salt and water reabsorption in the proximal tubule. The reduction of renal perfusion pressure may be responsible for augmentation of sodium reabsorption in the ascending limb of the loop of Henle.

In addition, the diminished renal blood flow characteristic of states in which the effective arterial blood volume is reduced is translated by the renal juxtaglomerular cells into a signal for increased renin release (Chap. 317). The specific nature of the signal is complex. One factor involves a baroreceptor mechanism, in which reduced renal perfusion results in incomplete filling of the renal arterioles and diminished stretch of the juxtaglomerular cells, a signal that provides for the elaboration or release, or both, of renin. A second mechanism involves the macula densa; as a result of reduced glomerular filtration the sodium chloride load reaching the distal renal tubules is reduced. This is sensed by the macula densa, which in an undefined manner signals the neighboring juxtaglomerular cells to secrete renin. A third mechanism involves the sympathetic nervous system and circulating catecholamines. Activation of the beta-adrenergic receptors in the juxtaglomerular cells stimulates renin release. These three mechanisms generally act in concert.

The renin-angiotensin-aldosterone system Renin, an enzyme with a molecular weight of about 40,000, acts on its substrate, angiotensinogen, an alpha$_2$ globulin synthesized by the liver, to release angiotensin I, a decapeptide, which is broken down to angiotensin II, an octapeptide. This has vasoconstrictor properties and independently increases Na reabsorption in the proximal tubule. The intrarenal production of angiotensin II may also contribute to renal vasoconstriction and to the salt and water retention in heart failure. Angiotensin II also enters the circulation and stimulates the production of aldosterone by the zona glomerulosa of the adrenal cortex. In patients with heart failure, not only is aldosterone secretion elevated, but the biologic half-life of aldosterone is prolonged, which further increases the plasma level of the hormone. A depression of hepatic blood flow, particularly during exercise, secondary to a reduction in cardiac output, is responsible for the reduced hepatic catabolism of aldosterone.

Although increased quantities of aldosterone are secreted in heart failure and in other edematous states and although blockade of the action of aldosterone by spironolactone often induces a moderate diuresis in edematous states, persistent augmented levels of aldosterone (or other mineralocorticoids) do not always promote accumulation of edema, as witnessed by the lack of striking fluid retention in most instances of primary aldosteronism (Chap. 317). Furthermore, although normal subjects retain some salt and water under the influence of a potent mineralocorticoid, such as deoxycorticosterone acetate or fludrocortisone, the accumulation is self-limiting, despite continued exposure to the steroid and to salt and water (mineralocorticoid escape). The failure of normal subjects to accumulate large quantities of fluid is probably a consequence of an increase in glomerular filtration rate, other hemodynamic influences, and most importantly the increase in volume which promotes an increased excretion of salt that is independent of the filtered load of sodium, i.e., through the action of natriuretic substance(s) or of pressure natriuresis. The role of aldosterone in the accumulation of fluid in edematous states may be more important because these patients are unable to repair the deficit in effective arterial blood volume.

Atrial natriuretic peptide Atrial distention and/or a sodium load cause release into the circulation of atrial natriuretic peptide (ANP), a polypeptide (Chap. 173); a high-molecular-weight precursor of ANP is stored in secretory granules within atrial myocytes. Release of ANP causes (1) excretion of sodium and water by augmenting glomerular filtration rate, inhibiting sodium reabsorption in the papillary collecting duct, and inhibiting release of renin and aldosterone; and (2) arteriolar and venous dilatation. Thus, ANP has the capacity to oppose sodium retention and arterial pressure elevation in states characterized by hypervolemia. There is also some evidence for the existence of a distinctly different natriuretic factor, a low-molecular-weight substance that is activated or released as a result of the expansion of the extracellular fluid and causes natriuresis by inhibiting renal sodium reabsorption through inhibiting ouabain-sensitive Na^+,K^+-ATPase. The role of this factor and of ANP in normal and pathophysiologic conditions requires clarification. For example, it is not yet clear why patients with heart failure and hepatic cirrhosis have low rates of sodium excretion despite often having high circulating levels of ANP.

Obstruction of venous (and lymphatic) drainage of a limb In this condition the hydrostatic pressure in the capillary bed upstream to the obstruction increases so that more fluid than normal is transferred from the vascular to the interstitial space; since the alternate route (i.e., the lymphatic channels) may also be obstructed, this event causes an increased volume of interstitial fluid in the limb, i.e., a trapping of fluid in the extremity, at the expense of the blood volume in the remainder of the body, thereby reducing effective arterial blood volume and leading to the consequences shown in Fig. 38-1.

As fluid accumulates in the interstitium of the limb in which venous and lymphatic drainage are obstructed, tissue tension rises until it counterbalances the primary alterations in the Starling forces, at which time no further fluid accumulates in that limb. At this point the additional accumulation of fluid repairs the deficit in plasma volume, and the stimuli to retain more salt and water are dissipated. The net effect is an increase in the volume of interstitial fluid in a local area, and the secondary responses repair the plasma volume deficit incurred by the primary event. This same sequence occurs in ascites and hydrothorax in which fluid is trapped or accumulates in the cavitary space, depleting the intravascular volume and leading to secondary salt and fluid retention as already described.

Congestive heart failure (See also Chap. 182) In this disorder the defective systolic emptying of the chambers of the heart and/or the impairment of ventricular relaxation promotes an accumulation of blood in the heart and venous circulation at the expense of the arterial volume, and the aforementioned sequence of events (Fig. 38-1) is initiated. In some instances of mild heart failure, a small increment of total blood volume may repair the deficit of arterial volume and establish a new steady state because, through the operation of Starling's law of the heart, up to a point, an increase in the volume of blood within the chambers of the heart promotes a more forceful contraction and may thereby increase the cardiac output (Fig. 182-1). However, if the cardiac disorder is more severe, retention of fluid cannot repair the deficit in effective arterial blood volume. The increment accumulates in the venous circulation, and the increase in hydrostatic pressure therein promotes the formation of edema. The formation of edema in the lungs (Chap. 36) impairs gas exchange and may induce hypoxia, which embarrasses cardiac function still further.

Incomplete ventricular emptying and/or inadequate ventricular relaxation leads to an elevation of ventricular diastolic pressure. If the impairment of cardiac function involves the right ventricle, pressures in the systemic veins and capillaries may rise, thereby augmenting transudation of fluid into the interstitial space and enhancing the likelihood of peripheral edema. The elevated systemic venous pressure is transmitted to the thoracic duct with consequent reduction of lymph drainage, further increasing the accumulation of edema.

If the impairment of cardiac function (incomplete ventricular emptying and/or inadequate relaxation) involves the left ventricle, then pulmonary venous and capillary pressures rise [leading in some instances to pulmonary edema (Chap. 36)], as does pulmonary artery pressure; this in turn interferes with the systolic emptying of the right ventricle, leading to an elevation of right ventricular diastolic and central and systemic venous pressures, enhancing the likelihood of formation of peripheral edema.

Nephrotic syndrome and other hypoalbuminic states (See also Chap. 227) The traditional view holds that the primary alteration in this disorder is a diminished colloid oncotic pressure due to massive losses of protein into the urine. This promotes a net movement of fluid into the interstitium, causes hypovolemia, and initiates the sequence of events described above, including activation of the renin-angiotensin-aldosterone system. As long as the hypoalbuminemia is severe, the salt and water retained cannot be restrained within the vascular compartment, and hence the stimuli to retain salt and water are not abated. A similar sequence of events occurs in other conditions which lead to *severe* hypoalbuminemia, including severe nutritional deficiency states, protein-losing enteropathy, congenital hypoalbuminemia, and severe, chronic liver disease. However, in the nephrotic syndrome, particularly when the serum albumin exceeds approximately 2 g/dL, edema is probably more related to primary renal sodium retention.

Cirrhosis (See also Chaps. 48 and 254) The *total* blood volume in cirrhosis of the liver is commonly increased when the disorder is accompanied by a system of dilated venous radicles and multiple small arteriovenous fistulas. On the other hand, effective systemic perfusion, the effective arterial blood volume, and the intrathoracic blood volume appear to be diminished, probably as a consequence of the passage of blood through these fistulas, as well as from the portal venous hypertension and the obstruction of the lymphatic drainage of the liver. These alterations are frequently complicated by reduced serum albumin, which reduces the effective arterial blood volume even further, leading to activation of the renin-angiotensin-aldosterone system and other salt- and water-retaining mechanisms. Initially, the excess interstitial fluid is localized preferentially behind the congested portal venous system and obstructed hepatic lymphatics, i.e., in the peritoneal cavity. In late stages of the disease, particularly when there is severe hypoalbuminemia, peripheral edema may also be noted.

Idiopathic edema This syndrome, which occurs almost exclusively in women, often with psychosocial difficulties, is characterized by periodic episodes of edema, frequently accompanied by abdominal distention. Fairly large, diurnal alterations in weight occur, so that the patient may weigh several pounds more after having been in the upright posture for several hours. Such large diurnal weight changes suggest an increase in capillary permeability which appears to fluctuate in severity and is aggravated by hot weather. The fact that it occurs most commonly in women, appears to be most prominent during the premenstrual period, and may be improved by progesterone administration suggests that there may be a hormonal effect on the permeability of the vessels that permits the loss of plasma volume into the interstitial space in the upright position and that leads in turn to a contraction in plasma volume and the subsequent retention of salt and water. There are also some cases in which the edema appears to be ''diuretic-induced.'' It has been postulated that in these patients, chronic diuretic administration leads to mild blood volume depletion which causes chronic hyperreninemia and juxtaglomerular hyperplasia. *Acute* withdrawal of diuretics can then leave the sodium-retaining forces unopposed, leading to fluid retention and edema.

The treatment of idiopathic cyclic edema includes a reduction in salt intake, rest in the supine position for several hours each day, the wearing of elastic stockings which are put on before arising in the morning, and an attempt to understand any underlying emotional problems. A variety of pharmacologic agents including angiotensin-converting enzyme inhibitors, progesterone, the dopamine receptor agonist bromocriptine, and the sympathomimetic amine dextroamphetamine have all been reported to be useful when administered to patients who do not respond to simpler measures. Diuretics are initially useful but may lose their effectiveness with continuous administration; accordingly, they should be employed sparingly, if at all. Persistent discontinuation of diuretics paradoxically leads to diuresis in ''diuretic-induced'' edema, described above.

DIFFERENTIAL DIAGNOSIS As a rule, localized edema can be readily differentiated from generalized edema. The great majority of patients with generalized edema of significant degree suffer from advanced cardiac, renal, hepatic, or nutritional disorders. Consequently, the differential diagnosis of generalized edema should be directed toward identifying or excluding these several conditions.

Localized edema Edema originating from inflammation or hypersensitivity is usually readily identified. Localized edema due to venous or lymphatic obstruction may be caused by thrombophlebitis, chronic lymphangitis, resection of regional lymph nodes, filariasis, etc. Lymphedema is particularly intractable because restriction of lymphatic flow results in increased protein concentration in the interstitial fluid, a circumstance which aggravates retention of fluid.

Edema of heart failure Evidence of heart disease, as manifested by cardiac enlargement and gallop rhythm together with evidence of cardiac failure, such as dyspnea, basilar rales, venous distention, and hepatomegaly, usually provides an indication on clinical examination that edema results from heart failure. Noninvasive tests such as echocardiography and radionuclide angiography may be helpful in establishing the diagnosis of heart failure (see also Chaps. 177 and 182).

Edema of the nephrotic syndrome Massive proteinuria (> 3.5 g/d), severe hypoalbuminemia, and in some instances hypercholesterolemia are present. This syndrome may occur during the course of a variety of kidney diseases, which include glomerulonephritis, diabetic glomerulosclerosis, and hypersensitivity reactions. A history of previous renal disease may or may not be elicited (see also Chap. 227).

Edema of acute glomerulonephritis and other forms of renal failure The edema occurring during the acute phases of glomerulonephritis is characteristically associated with hematuria, proteinuria, and hypertension. Although some evidence supports the view that the fluid retention is due to increased capillary permeability, in most instances the edema in this disease results from primary retention of sodium and water by the kidneys owing to renal insufficiency. This state differs from congestive heart failure in that it is characterized by a normal or increased cardiac output and a normal arterial–mixed venous oxygen difference. Patients commonly have evidence of pulmonary congestion on chest roentgenograms before cardiac enlargement is significant and do not usually develop orthopnea. Patients with chronic impairment of renal function (including some patients with the nephrotic syndrome *without* severe hypoalbuminemia) may also develop edema due to primary renal retention of sodium and water.

Edema of cirrhosis Ascites and evidence of hepatic disease (collateral venous channels, jaundice, and spider angiomas) characterize edema of hepatic origin. The ascites is frequently refractory to treatment because it collects as a result of a combination of obstruction of hepatic lymphatic drainage, portal hypertension, and hypoalbuminemia. Edema may also occur in other parts of the body in these patients as a result of hypoalbuminemia. Furthermore, the sizable accumulation of ascitic fluid may increase intraabdominal pressure and impede venous return from the lower extremities; hence, it tends to promote accumulation of edema in this region as well (see also Chap. 254).

Edema of nutritional origin A grossly deficient diet over a prolonged period may produce hypoproteinemia and edema, which may be intensified by beriberi heart disease, in which multiple peripheral arteriovenous fistulas result in reduced effective systemic perfusion and effective arterial blood volume, thereby enhancing edema formation (Chap. 194). Edema may actually become intensified when these famished subjects are first provided with an adequate diet. The ingestion of more food may increase the quantity of salt ingested, which is then retained along with water. Refeeding edema may also be linked to increased release of insulin, which directly increases tubular sodium reabsorption. In addition to hypoalbuminemia, hypokalemia and caloric deficits may be involved in the edema of starvation.

Other causes of edema These include hypothyroidism, in which myxedema may be located typically in the pretibial region and which may also be associated with periorbital puffiness. Exogenous hyperadrenocortism, pregnancy, and administration of estrogens and vasodilators, particularly the calcium antagonist nifedipine, may also all cause edema.

Distribution The distribution of edema is an important guide to the cause. Thus, edema of one leg or of one or both arms is usually the result of venous and/or lymphatic obstruction. Edema resulting from hypoproteinemia characteristically is generalized, but it is especially evident in the very soft tissues of the eyelids and face and tends to be most pronounced in the morning because of the recumbent posture assumed during the night. Edema associated with heart failure, on the other hand, tends to be more extensive in the legs and to be accentuated in the evening, a feature also determined largely by posture. When patients with heart failure have been confined to bed, edema may be most prominent in the presacral region. In the rare types of cardiac disease, such as tricuspid stenosis and constrictive pericarditis, in which orthopnea is absent and the patient actually prefers the recumbent posture, the factor of gravity may be equalized and facial edema observed. Less common causes of facial edema include trichinosis, allergic reactions, and myxedema. Unilateral edema occasionally results from lesions in the central nervous system affecting the vasomotor fibers on one side of the body; paralysis also reduces lymphatic and venous drainage on the affected side.

Additional factors in diagnosis The color, thickness, and sensitivity of the skin are significant. Local tenderness and increase in temperature suggest inflammation. Local cyanosis may signify a venous obstruction. In individuals who have had repeated episodes of prolonged edema, the skin over the involved areas may be thickened, indurated, and often red.

Measurement of the venous pressure is of importance in evaluating edema. Elevation in an isolated part of the body usually reflects localized venous obstruction. Generalized elevation of systemic venous pressure usually suggests the presence of congestive heart failure, although it may occur with the hypervolemia that accompanies acute renal insufficiency. Ordinarily, significant increase in venous pressure can be recognized by the level at which cervical veins collapse; in doubtful cases and for accurate recording, the central venous pressure should be measured manometrically. In patients with obstruction of the superior vena cava, edema is confined to the face, neck, and upper extremities, where the venous pressure is elevated compared with that in the lower extremities. Measurement of venous pressure in the upper extremities is also useful in patients with massive edema of the lower extremities and ascites; it is elevated when the edema is on a cardiac basis (e.g., constrictive pericarditis or tricuspid stenosis) but is normal when it is secondary to cirrhosis. Severe heart failure may cause ascites that may be distinguished from the ascites caused by hepatic cirrhosis by the jugular venous pressure, which is elevated in heart failure and low-normal in cirrhosis.

Determination of the concentration of serum albumin aids importantly in identifying those patients in whom edema is due, at least in part, to diminished intravascular colloid oncotic pressure. The presence of proteinuria affords useful clues. The total absence of protein in the urine is evidence against renal disease as a cause of edema. Slight to moderate proteinuria is the rule in patients with heart failure, whereas persistent massive proteinuria is usually due to the nephrotic syndrome.

APPROACH TO THE PATIENT WITH EDEMA A significant question to ask is whether the edema is localized or generalized. If it is localized, those phenomena that may be responsible should be concentrated upon. In this context, *localized* edema may include hydrothorax, ascites, or both, in the absence of congestive heart failure or hypoalbuminemia. Either of these collections may be a consequence of local venous or lymphatic obstruction, as in inflammatory disease or carcinoma.

If the edema is generalized, it should be determined, first, if there is hypoalbuminemia of significant degree, e.g., serum albumin concentration less than 2.5 g/dL. If there is, the history, physical examination, urinalysis, and other laboratory data will help evaluate the question of cirrhosis, severe malnutrition, protein-losing gastroenteropathy, or the nephrotic syndrome as the underlying disorder. If hypoalbuminemia is not present, it should be determined if there is evidence of congestive heart failure of a severity to promote generalized edema. Finally, it should be ascertained whether the patient has an adequate urine output, or if there is significant oliguria or even anuria. These abnormalities are discussed in Chaps. 49, 223, and 224. The major differential diagnosis in patients with generalized edema and normal serum albumin is between primary renal retention of salt and water and congestive heart failure.

REFERENCES

BERNARD DB: Extrarenal complications of the nephrotic syndrome. Kidney Int 33:1184, 1988

GOLDEN MHN: Protein deficiency, energy deficiency, and the oedema of malnutrition. Lancet 1:1261, 1982

ROSE BD: Edematous states, in *Clinical Physiology of Acid-Base and Electrolyte Disorders*. New York, McGraw-Hill, 1989, pp 416–463

SEIFTER JL et al: Control of extracellular fluid volume and pathophysiology of edema formation, in *The Kidney*, 3d ed, BM Brenner, FC Rector (eds). Philadelphia, Saunders, 1986, p 343

STAUB NB, TAYLOR AE (eds): *Edema*. New York, Raven Press, 1984

STREETEN DHP: Idiopathic edema: Pathogenesis, clinical features, and treatment. Metabolism 27:353, 1978

SUZUKI H et al: Effect of the angiotensin converting enzyme inhibitor, captopril (SQ14, 225), on orthostatic sodium and water retention in patients with idiopathic edema. Nephron 39:244, 1985

39 SHOCK

JOSEPH E. PARRILLO

Shock may be defined as the state in which profound and widespread reduction of tissue perfusion leads first to reversible, and then, if prolonged, to irreversible, cellular injury. Since reduction of tissue perfusion is central to this definition, it is useful to consider the factors that control this vital function.

CONTROL OF ARTERIAL BLOOD PRESSURE Maintenance of adequate perfusion of vital organs is critical for survival. Organ perfusion is dependent on an appropriate perfusion pressure, which, in turn, is determined by two variables, the cardiac output and the systemic vascular resistance. The latter is proportional to the vessel length and the viscosity of blood and inversely proportional to the fourth power of the vessel radius. Therefore, the cross-sectional area of a vessel is the overriding determinant of the resistance to blood flow. Since vascular smooth-muscle tone regulates the cross-sectional area of the arteriolar bed (the major site of systemic resistance in the vascular tree), any variable that affects vascular smooth-muscle tone has a profound effect on vascular resistance and, in turn, on perfusion pressure.

The second critical determinant of arterial pressure is the cardiac output, which itself is the product of stroke volume and heart rate. The stroke volume is a function of three major variables, as discussed in detail in Chap. 181: (1) preload, generally reflected in the ventricular end-diastolic volume; (2) impedance to blood flow (afterload), which is related to the systemic vascular resistance; and (3) myocardial contractility.

Physiologic mechanisms can affect the arterial pressure by acting on one or more of the variables mentioned above. These mechanisms include the local release of vasodilator metabolites such as adenosine; the activity of the autonomic (sympathetic and parasympathetic) nervous system and the modulation of this activity by baroreceptor reflexes and the vasomotor center in the brainstem, which, in turn, is acted on by higher centers in the nervous system; the release into the bloodstream of the catecholamines epinephrine or norepinephrine by the adrenal medulla and sympathetic nerve endings (Chap. 67); the activity of the renin-angiotensin system (Chap. 317); the release of vasopressin (Chap. 315); the release of vasodilators, including the kinins and prostaglandins; and alterations in intravascular volume via control of fluid and electrolyte balance (Chap. 38). All of these can affect the arterial pressure by altering the vascular resistance and/or cardiac output. Through the integrated operation of these several mechanisms the mean arterial pressure (the average pressure throughout the cardiac cycle) in young, healthy adults is maintained within a relatively narrow range of 90 to 100 mmHg.

CLASSIFICATION OF SHOCK A classification of shock based on etiology is shown in Table 39-1.

Oligemic or hypovolemic shock Hemorrhage or a large loss of fluid secondary to vomiting, diarrhea, burns, or dehydration leads to inadequate ventricular filling, i.e., to severely decreased preload, reflected in decreased left and right ventricular end-diastolic volumes and pressures. These changes lead to shock by causing an inadequate stroke volume and inadequate cardiac output. This is probably the most frequent cause of shock and also the best studied, because all gradations of oligemic shock can be produced in animal models.

Cardiogenic shock (See Chap. 189) This is due to a severe depression of systolic cardiac performance. Systolic arterial pressure is <80 mmHg. The cardiac index is reduced below 1.8 $(L/min)/m^2$, and the left ventricular filling pressure is elevated, generally above 18 mmHg; pulmonary edema may or may not be evident. The patient is frequently obtunded, the urine output is less than 20 mL/h, and the extremities are cold and cyanotic. The most frequent cause is infarction involving 40 percent or more of the left ventricular myocardium, leading to a severe reduction in left ventricular contractility and failure of the left ventricular pump. Other causes include acute myocarditis and the depression of myocardial contractility following cardiac arrest and prolonged cardiac surgery.

Another form of cardiogenic shock is caused by mechanical abnormalities of the ventricle. Acute mitral or aortic regurgitation or acutely acquired ventricular septal defect or ventricular aneurysm, usually caused by acute myocardial infarction, can cause a severe reduction in *forward* cardiac output (blood flow through the aortic valve into the systemic arterial circulation) and thereby result in cardiogenic shock.

Extracardiac obstructive shock This form of shock is best exemplified by pericardial tamponade (Chap. 193). Physiologically, the major abnormality is the inability of the ventricle to fill during diastole, markedly limiting the stroke volume and ultimately the cardiac output. Another common cause of extracardiac obstructive shock is massive pulmonary embolism (Chap. 213). Although the mechanism responsible for the reduced cardiac output in extracardiac obstructive shock differs from that in cardiogenic shock, the actual cause of shock, i.e., the severe reduction in tissue perfusion, is similar.

Distributive shock Examples of this form of shock are septic shock (Chap. 89), neurogenic shock, and anaphylactic shock (Chap. 267), all of which usually cause a profound *decrease* in peripheral vascular resistance; the first is now the most common cause of death in intensive care units in the United States. The pathogenesis of septic shock probably involves abnormalities of both the peripheral vascular system and the heart. It is considered in detail below.

Patients may suffer from more than one form of shock simultaneously. Thus, septic and oligemic shock sometimes coexist. These two forms of shock may produce dissimilar, even opposing cardiovascular effects, and treatment of one form may unmask the presence of the other.

PATHOGENESIS Some characteristics of the pathogenesis of shock are the same regardless of the underlying cause. The final pathway of shock is cell death. Once large numbers of cells from vital organs have reached this stage, shock becomes irreversible, and death occurs despite correction of the underlying cause. This concept of irreversibility is useful because it emphasizes the need to prevent the progression of shock.

The pathogenetic mechanism leading to cell death is incompletely understood. One of the common denominators of the first three forms of shock listed in Table 39-1 is a low cardiac output (see Fig. 39-1). Patients with oligemic shock, cardiogenic shock, extracardiac obstructive shock, and a minority of patients with distributive shock develop a severe decrease in cardiac output and, hence, in perfusion of vital organs. Initially, compensatory mechanisms such as vasoconstriction may maintain arterial pressure at a near-normal level. However, if the process causing shock continues, these compensatory mechanisms ultimately fail, leading to the clinical manifestations of the shock syndrome. If shock persists, cell death will ensue and result in irreversible shock.

Of the forms of shock with low cardiac output, *oligemic shock* has been studied the most carefully, both in humans and in animal models, and it provides lessons applicable to other forms of low-output shock. A healthy adult can compensate for the loss of 10 percent of total blood volume using the mechanisms described previously, principally sympathetically mediated vasoconstriction. However, if 20 to 25 percent of the blood volume is lost, the compensatory mechanisms usually begin to fail, and the clinical shock syndrome ensues. The cardiac output declines, and there is hypotension despite generalized vasoconstriction. Regulation of local blood flow maintains perfusion of the heart and brain until late in the course, when these mechanisms also fail. Vasoconstriction, which

TABLE 39-1 Classification of forms of shock

- Cardiogenic shock
  - Myopathic (reduced systolic function)
    - Acute myocardial infarction
    - Dilated cardiomyopathy
    - Myocardial depression in septic shock
  - Mechanical
    - Mitral regurgitation
    - Ventricular septal defect
    - Ventricular aneurysm
    - LV outflow obstruction (aortic stenosis, idiopathic hypertrophic subaortic stenosis)
  - Arrhythmic
- Extracardiac obstructive shock
  - Pericardial tamponade
  - Constrictive pericarditis
  - Pulmonary embolism (massive)
  - Severe pulmonary hypertension (primary or Eisenmenger)
  - Coarctation of the aorta
- Oligemic shock
  - Hemorrhage
  - Fluid depletion
- Distributive shock
  - Septic shock
  - Toxic products, e.g., overdose
  - Anaphylaxis
  - Neurogenic shock
  - Endocrinologic shock

SOURCE: Adapted with permission from Parker and Parrillo.

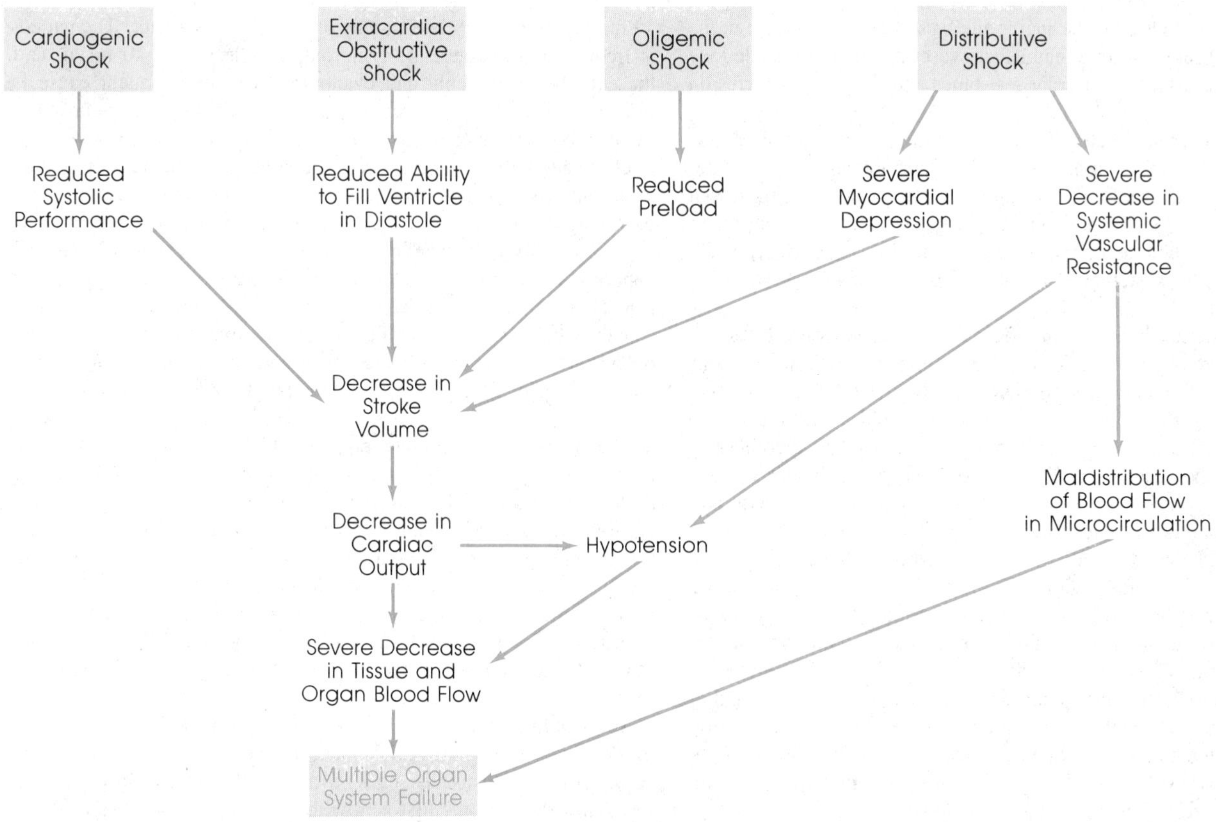

FIGURE 39-1 Pathogenesis of shock in humans. This schematic diagram depicts our present understanding of the pathogenetic relationships among the different types of shock and the cardiovascular abnormalities they usually produce.

begins as a compensatory mechanism in shock, may become excessive in some tissues and cause destructive lesions such as ischemic necrosis of the intestines or digits. A myocardial depressant factor has been characterized in the dog with hemorrhagic shock, but this factor has not been clearly related to clinical myocardial dysfunction. Ultimately, if shock continues, end organ damage occurs, precipitating the adult respiratory distress syndrome (Chap. 218), acute renal failure (Chap. 223), disseminated intravascular coagulation (Chap. 288), and multiorgan failure leading to death.

Distributive shock has a different and more complicated pathogenesis. Septic shock (Chap. 89) is characterized, at least initially, by a low systemic vascular resistance and an elevated cardiac output. As shown in Fig. 39-2, septic shock usually begins with a nidus of infection that releases microbes and/or one or more mediators into the bloodstream. Many mediators [e.g., histamine, kinins, most prostaglandins, lipid A (the toxic component of endotoxin), endorphins, tumor necrosis factor, interleukin 1, and interleukin 2] produce vascular dilatation, while others (some prostaglandins and leukotrienes) produce vasoconstriction. The peripheral vasodilatation results in a reduced systemic vascular resistance and a high cardiac output; the latter occurs in virtually all patients with septic shock, who are *volume-loaded.* The maldistribution of blood flow, evidenced by lactic acidemia despite a high cardiac output, probably results from circulating mediators with either dilating or constricting properties, causing inappropriate dilatation in some vascular beds and constriction in others.

It has been argued that the high cardiac output in humans with septic shock suggests good ventricular function. However, left and right ventricular ejection fractions are reduced and the ventricles dilate during the initial phase of septic shock. Both ventricles are usually dilated; the increase in preload maintains a normal stroke volume despite the depression of myocardial contractility. The normal stroke volume, combined with tachycardia, results in an elevated cardiac output. However, expansion of blood volume in such patients demonstrates depressed ventricular function curves (Chap. 181), i.e., the response of stroke work as a function of filling pressure is subnormal. The reduced ejection fraction, ventricular dilatation, and decreased ventricular stroke work response to volume infusion all demonstrate that myocardial depression occurs frequently in human septic shock. A similar pattern of cardiac dysfunction has been reported with anaphylactic shock. The mechanism of this depressed ventricular performance is unknown; a circulating myocardial depressant substance probably plays a role.

If septic shock persists, the combined peripheral vascular abnormalities and the myocardial depression result in a mortality of approximately 50 percent (Fig. 39-2). Death results from unrelenting hypotension and/or organ system failure. The hypotension is usually associated with a severe and irreversible reduction in systemic vascular resistance, though occasionally (in 10 to 20 percent of nonsurvivors) myocardial depression progresses and results in a low cardiac output that worsens the hypotension. Death from multiple organ failure usually results from insufficiency of kidney, liver, brain, or lung function.

Other pathogenetic mechanisms in septic shock appear to relate to neutrophil aggregation, which produces microthrombi and endothelial cell injury that contribute to alterations in microvascular perfusion. These are discussed in Chap. 89.

CLINICAL MANIFESTATIONS Some symptoms and signs are the same for all types of shock. This condition is almost always characterized by hypotension, which in adults generally refers to a mean arterial pressure of less than 60 mmHg. However, in interpreting any given level of arterial pressure the *chronic* level of pressure must be considered. Thus, patients with severe, chronic hypertension may be hypotensive when their mean arterial pressure declines by 40 mmHg, even if it still exceeds 60 mmHg. Conversely, patients with chronic hypotension may not exhibit acute relative hypotension until mean pressures decline below 50 mmHg. Other common manifestations of shock are tachycardia, oliguria, a clouded sensorium, and cool, mottled extremities indicative of reduced blood flow to the skin (the latter sign usually is not characteristic of distributive shock).

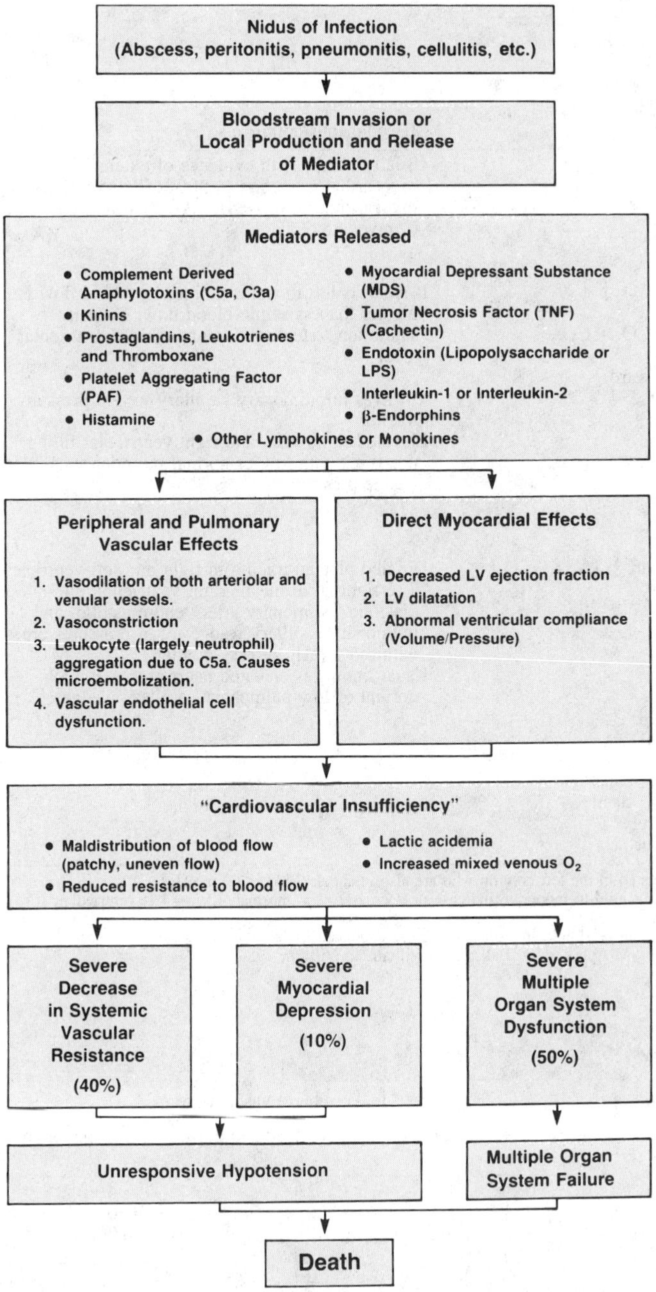

FIGURE 39-2 Pathogenesis of human septic shock. This schematic diagram represents our present understanding of the interrelationships in the pathogenesis of septic shock in humans. *(Adapted from JE Parrillo, in Major Issues in Critical Care Medicine, JE Parrillo, SM Ayres, eds, Baltimore, Williams & Wilkins, 1984.)*

Metabolic acidosis, often due to elevated blood lactic acid levels (Chap. 51), reflects prolonged inadequate blood flow to multiple tissues.

Other clinical manifestations are specific to the type of shock. Patients with cardiogenic shock usually have symptoms and signs of heart disease, including elevated filling pressures, a gallop rhythm, and other evidence of acute heart failure. Mechanical causes of cardiogenic shock frequently cause heart murmurs, such as those of acute mitral regurgitation or ventricular septal defect. Patients with pericardial tamponade may demonstrate evidence of pericardial effusion, e.g., pulsus paradoxus, distant heart sounds. Patients with oligemic shock frequently have a history of gastrointestinal bleeding or hemorrhage from another site or clear evidence of large volume losses via diarrhea and/or vomiting. In patients with distributive shock due to sepsis in the absence of severe neutropenia there may be evidence of a localized infection (pneumonitis, pyelonephritis, or abdominal abscess) as well as fever and chills. Patients with septic shock and severe neutropenia are less likely to have a clinically evident nidus of infection and may be septic from their own skin or bowel flora.

CLINICAL EVALUATION OF THE SHOCK PATIENT Shock is usually an emergency. Optimal management requires a balance of the need to institute therapy before shock causes irreversible damage to vital organs against the need to complete the clinical assessment required to ensure a comprehensive understanding of the cause. A practical approach is to make a rapid evaluation initially, based on a limited history, physical examination, and specific diagnostic procedures directed to determining the cause and severity of shock. Initial laboratory tests may include a chest x-ray, electrocardiogram, arterial blood P_{O_2}, P_{CO_2}, and pH; a right heart catheterization with a balloon-tipped flow-directed (Swan-Ganz) catheter; and other x-rays or tests directed at specific questions raised by the initial examination. Once this brief evaluation is completed and if the shock is severe or progressive, therapy should be initiated. After the condition has stabilized, a more comprehensive conventional diagnostic evaluation should be undertaken, and the response to the initial therapeutic interventions should be assessed.

Use of right heart catheterization to evaluate shock The different categories of shock (Table 39-1) have different cardiovascular profiles (Table 39-2). Patients with mild hypovolemic shock may be treated successfully with fluid replacement, the nature of the fluid depending upon the cause of the shock. However, in patients with moderate or severe shock, the flow-directed balloon-tipped pulmonary artery (Swan-Ganz) catheter is often useful for providing hemodynamic assessment and following the response to therapy, because clinical evaluation is frequently incorrect in estimating filling pressure and cardiac output.

Table 39-2 summarizes the usual hemodynamic profiles of patients with the different forms of shock. When these profiles are combined with clinical findings and the calculation of systemic vascular resistance, the etiology of most bouts of shock can be categorized, allowing the physician to concentrate attention on management.

MANAGEMENT Whenever possible, patients should be treated in an intensive care unit and should receive continuous electrocardiographic monitoring and an arterial line to provide a beat-to-beat measure of systolic, diastolic, and mean arterial pressures. In most cases of shock that cannot be rapidly reversed, serial measurement of left and right ventricular filling pressures and cardiac output should be performed. Frequent determinations of arterial blood gases (P_{O_2}, P_{CO_2}, and pH), electrolytes, complete blood count, and clotting parameters should be made. Serum calcium and phosphorus values should be followed, because substantial reductions in these ions can be associated with myocardial depression. The frequency of measurements should depend on the clinical course and the perceived need to assess the response to therapy.

In general, the goals of treating shock are threefold: (1) Maintain blood flow to those organs most frequently damaged by shock, i.e., kidney, liver, central nervous system, and lungs. It is useful to follow urine flow hourly as a rough guide to renal perfusion. (2) Maintain mean arterial pressure above 60 mmHg (in a normal adult) to ensure adequate perfusion of vital organs. (3) Maintain arterial blood lactate below 22 mmol/L. (Since lactate measurements are not usually available "on line," the last goal must often be assessed retrospectively.)

Specific forms of shock require therapy directed at the underlying process.

Oligemic shock usually presents with clinical evidence of blood or fluid loss and low pulmonary artery wedge and right atrial pressures. Rapid infusion of blood plasma or plasma expanders is the correct therapy while the source of blood or fluid loss is identified and corrected.

In *cardiogenic shock* (Chap. 189) therapy should be directed toward reducing ischemia and salvaging severely ischemic but re-

TABLE 39-2 Use of right heart catheterization to diagnose the etiology of shock*

Diagnosis	Pulmonary capillary wedge pressure†	Cardiac output (CO)	Miscellaneous comments
Cardiogenic shock	↑ ↑	↓ ↓	
Cardiogenic shock due to myocardial dysfunction			Usually occurs with evidence of extensive myocardial infarction (>40% of left ventricular myocardium destroyed), severe cardiomyopathy, or myocarditis
Cardiogenic shock due to a mechanical defect			
Acute ventricular septal defect	↑ or nl	LVCO ↓ ↓ and RVCO > CO	If shunt is left to right, pulmonary blood flow is greater than systemic blood flow: oxygen saturation "step-up" occurs at right ventricular level
Acute mitral regurgitation	↑ ↑	Forward CO ↓ ↓	V waves in pulmonary capillary wedge pressure tracing
Right ventricular infarction	nl or ↓	↓ ↓	Elevated right atrial and right ventricular filling pressures with low or normal pulmonary capillary wedge pressures
Extracardiac obstructive forms of shock			
Pericardial tamponade	↑ ↑	↓ or ↓ ↓	Dip and plateau tracing in right and left ventricles. The right atrial mean, right ventricular end-diastolic, pulmonary artery end-diastolic, and pulmonary capillary wedge mean pressures are within 5 mmHg of one another
Massive pulmonary emboli	nl or ↓	↓ ↓	Usual finding is elevated heart pressures with normal or low pulmonary capillary wedge
Oligemic shock (hypovolemia)	↓ ↓	↓ ↓	
Distributive forms of shock			
Septic shock	↓ or nl	↑ ↑ or nl, rarely ↓	
Anaphylactic shock	↓ or nl	↑ or nl	

* The hemodynamic profiles summarized in this table refer to patients with the diagnosis listed in the left column who are also in shock (MAP <60 mmHg).
† ↑ ↑ or ↓ ↓ designates a moderate-to-severe increase or decrease; ↑ or ↓ designates a mild-to-moderate increase or decrease; nl = normal; LV = left ventricular; RV = right ventricular.
NOTE: Systemic vascular resistance is increased, initially, in all forms of shock except distributive shock, in which it is usually reduced.
SOURCE: Modified from JE Parrillo, in *Major Issues in Critical Care Medicine,* JE Parrillo, SM Ayres (eds), Baltimore, William & Wilkins, 1984.

TABLE 39-3 Commonly used vasopressor agents (relative potency*)

		Cardiac		Peripheral vasculature		
Agent	Dose	Heart rate	Contractility	Vasoconstriction	Vasodilatation	Dopaminergic
Dopamine	1–4 (μg/kg)/min	2+	2+	0	2+	4+
	4–20 (μg/kg)/min	2+	2+	2–3+	0	0
Levarterenol (norepinephrine)	2–8 μg/min	2+	2+	4+	0	0
Dobutamine	1–10 (μg/kg)/min	1+	4+	1+	2+	0
Isoproterenol	1–4 μg/min	4+	4+	0	4+	0
Epinephrine	1–8 μg/min	4+	4+	4+	3+	0
Phenylephrine	20–200 μg/min	0	0	4+	0	0

* The 1 to 4+ scoring system represents an arbitrary quantitative scoring system to allow a judgment of comparative potency among these vasopressor agents.
SOURCE: Adapted from JE Parrillo, *Major Issues in Critical Care Medicine,* JE Parrillo, SM Ayres (eds), Baltimore, Williams & Wilkins, 1984.

versibly damaged myocardium at the infarct border. This may be accomplished by administration of oxygen and nitrates, institution of intraaortic balloon pumping to unload mechanically the ventricle and augment coronary perfusion, and, perhaps most importantly, by attempting to restore myocardial perfusion to salvage nonirreversibly damaged myocardium. Depending on the specific situation, the latter may include the administration of thrombolytic agents, cardiac catheterization and coronary arteriography to define coronary anatomy, and early coronary angioplasty or coronary bypass surgery in patients with appropriate anatomy. This aggressive approach may reduce the mortality of cardiogenic shock from approximately 90 to approximately 60 percent. Prospective, randomized studies are needed to document the true efficacy of this approach. Cardiogenic shock also occurs after a prolonged period of induced cardiac arrest, often during reparative cardiac surgery. The impaired (stunned) myocardium may require hours or days to recover sufficiently to support the circulation. Treatment consists of the combination of intraaortic balloon counterpulsation and sympathomimetic amines such as dopamine or dobutamine (Table 39-3). In cardiogenic shock due to mechanical abnormalities, such as acute mitral regurgitation or ventricular septal defect, surgical correction is usually necessary.

Pericardial tamponade, the prototype of *extracardiac obstructive shock,* may be recognized by clinical manifestations (hypotension, pulsus paradoxus, distended neck veins) and characteristic findings on electrocardiography (Chap. 193) or by echocardiography (Chap. 177). Although expansion of intravascular volume and the administration of inotropic agents, particularly sympathomimetic amines such as norepinephrine and/or dopamine, may temporarily improve hemodynamics and act as a "holding maneuver," pericardiocentesis or surgical pericardial drainage is the only effective treatment.

The management of *septic shock* is discussed in Chap. 89.

REFERENCES

BONE RC et al and the Methylprednisolone Severe Sepsis Study Group: A controlled clinical trial of high-dose methylprednisolone in the treatment of severe sepsis and septic shock. N Engl J Med 317:653, 1987
CONNORS AF et al: Evaluation of right-heart catheterization in the critically ill patient without acute myocardial infarction. N Engl J Med 308:263, 1983
ELLRODT AG et al: Left ventricular performance in septic shock: Reversible segmental and global abnormalities. Am Heart J 110:402, 1985
GUYTON AC: Local control of blood flow by the tissues; and nervous and humoral regulation, in *Human Physiology and Mechanisms of Disease*, 3d ed. Philadelphia, Saunders, 1982, pp 161–169
———: Cardiac output and circulatory shock, in *Human Physiology and Mechanisms of Disease*, 3d ed. Philadelphia, Saunders, 1982, pp 187–200
NATANSON C et al: Gram negative bacteremia produces both severe systolic and diastolic cardiac dysfunction in a canine model that simulates human septic shock. J Clin Invest 77:259, 1986
OGNIBENE FP et al: Neutrophil aggregation activity and septic shock in humans: Neutrophil aggregation by a C5a-like material occurs more frequently than complement component depletion and correlates with depression of systemic vascular resistance. J Crit Care 3:103, 1988
——— et al: Depressed left ventricular performance in response to volume infusion in patients with sepsis and septic shock. Chest 93:903, 1988
PARKER MM, PARRILLO JE: Septic shock and other forms of distributive shock, in *Current Therapy in Critical Care Medicine*. Toronto, B.C. Decker, 1987, pp 44–55
PARRILLO JE: Septic shock in humans: Clinical evaluation, pathogenesis, and therapeutic approach, in *Textbook of Critical Care*, 2d ed, W.C. Shoemaker et al (eds). Philadelphia, Saunders, 1989, pp 1006–1023
——— et al: A circulating myocardial depressant substance in humans with septic shock: Septic shock patients with a reduced ejection fraction have a circulating factor that depresses *in vitro* myocardial cell performance. J Clin Invest 76:1539, 1985
ROCK P et al: Efficacy and safety of naloxone in septic shock. Crit Care Med 13:28, 1985
SCHAER GL et al: Norepinephrine alone versus norepinephrine plus low-dose dopamine: Enhanced renal blood flow with combination pressor therapy. Crit Care Med 13:492, 1985
ZIEGLER EJ et al: Treatment of gram-negative bacteremia and shock with human antiserum to a mutant *Escherichia coli*. N Engl J Med 307:1225, 1982

40 CARDIOVASCULAR COLLAPSE, CARDIAC ARREST, AND SUDDEN DEATH

ROBERT J. MYERBURG / AGUSTIN CASTELLANOS

OVERVIEW AND DEFINITIONS

Cardiac disorders account for the vast majority of natural sudden deaths. The magnitude of the problem of *cardiac* causes is highlighted by estimates that more than 300,000 sudden cardiac deaths (SCD) occur each year in the United States, and that as many as 50 percent of all cardiac deaths are sudden and unexpected. Since techniques and systems are now available to save patients who have out-of-hospital cardiac arrest, which was uniformly fatal in the past, understanding the SCD problem has practical importance.

SCD must be defined carefully. In the context of time, "sudden" was previously defined as death within 24 h of the onset of the clinical event which led to a fatal cardiac arrest; this was subsequently shortened for most clinical and epidemiologic purposes to 1 h or less between the onset of the terminal illness and death. However, because of community-based interventions, victims may remain biologically alive for days or weeks after a cardiac arrest that has resulted in irreversible central nervous system damage. Confusion in terms can be avoided by adhering strictly to definitions of death, cardiac arrest, and cardiovascular collapse, as outlined in Table 40-1. Death is biologically, legally, and literally an absolute and irreversible event. Death may be delayed in a survivor of cardiac arrest, but "survival after sudden death" is contradictory. Currently, the accepted definition of SCD is *natural death* due to *cardiac* causes, heralded by abrupt loss of consciousness within *1 h* of the onset of acute symptoms, in an individual who may have known *preexisting* heart disease, but in whom the *time* and *mode* of death are *unexpected*. When biologic death of the cardiac arrest victim is delayed because of interventions, the relevant pathophysiologic event remains the sudden and unexpected cardiac arrest which leads ultimately to death, even though delayed by artificial methods. Thus, the terminology used should reflect the fact that the index event was a cardiac arrest, and that death was due to its delayed consequences.

TABLE 40-1 Distinction between death, cardiac arrest, and cardiovascular collapse

Term	Definition	Qualifiers or exceptions
Death	Irreversible cessation of all biologic functions	None
Cardiac arrest	Abrupt cessation of cardiac pump function which may be reversible by a prompt intervention but will lead to death in its absence	Rare spontaneous reversions; likelihood of successful intervention relates to mechanism of arrest and clinical setting
Cardiovascular collapse	A sudden loss of effective blood flow due to cardiac and/or peripheral vascular factors which may reverse spontaneously (e.g., vasodepressor syncope) or only with interventions (e.g., cardiac arrest)	Nonspecific term which includes cardiac arrest and its consequences and also events which characteristically revert spontaneously

SOURCE: Myerburg and Castellanos, with permission.

CAUSES, CONTRIBUTING FACTORS, AND CLINICAL EPIDEMIOLOGY

Extensive epidemiologic studies have identified populations at high risk for SCD. In addition, a large body of pathologic data provide information on the underlying *structural abnormalities* in victims of SCD, and clinical/physiologic studies highlight the *contributing functional factors* which may convert a long-standing underlying structural abnormality from a stable to an unstable state (Table 40-2). This mass of information is developing into an understanding of the causes and mechanisms of SCD.

Cardiac disorders constitute the most common causes of sudden *natural* death. After an initial peak incidence of sudden death between birth and 6 months of age (the sudden infant death syndrome), the incidence of sudden death falls abruptly and then increases to a second peak in the age range of 45 to 75 years. Moreover, increasing age is a powerful risk factor for sudden *cardiac* death. It follows that the *proportion* of *cardiac* causes among all sudden *natural* deaths increases dramatically with advancing years. From 1 to 13 years of age, only one of five sudden natural deaths is due to cardiac causes. Between 14 and 21 years of age, the proportion increases to 30 percent, and then to 88 percent in the middle aged and elderly.

Men and women have very different susceptibilities to SCD, which tend to decrease with advancing age. The overall male/female ratio is approximately 4:1, but in the 55- to 64-year-old age group, the male SCD excess is nearly 7:1. It falls to approximately 2:1 in the 65- to 74-year-old age group. The difference in risk for SCD parallels the risks for other manifestations of coronary heart disease in men and women. As the gap for other manifestations of coronary heart disease closes in the seventh and eighth decades of life, the excess risk of SCD narrows. Despite the lower incidence in women, the classic coronary risk factors still operate in the proportionately smaller subgroup of women—cigarette smoking, diabetes, hyperlipidemia, hypertension.

Hereditary factors contribute to the risk of SCD, but largely in a nonspecific manner, merely as one expression of the hereditary predisposition to coronary heart disease. Except for a few very

TABLE 40-2 Cardiac arrest and sudden cardiac death

I Structural causes

- *A* Coronary heart disease
  - *1* Coronary atherosclerosis
    - *a* Chronic obstructive lesions
    - *b* Acute lesion (plaque fissuring, platelet aggregation, acute thrombosis)
  - *2* Myocardial infarction
    - *a* Healed
    - *b* Acute
- *B* Myocardial hypertrophy
  - *1* Secondary
  - *2* Hypertrophic cardiomyopathy
    - *a* Obstructive
    - *b* Nonobstructive
- *C* Cardiomyopathy, dilated
- *D* Myocarditis
- *E* Valvular heart disease
- *F* Electrophysiologic abnormalities, structural
  - *1* Anomalous pathways
  - *2* Conducting system disease

II Functional contributing factors

- *A* Transient ischemia and reperfusion
  - *1* Loss of substrates
  - *2* Generation of injurious substances
  - *3* Disturbed membrane electrical properties
- *B* Low cardiac output states
  - *1* Heart failure
    - *a* Chronic
    - *b* Acute decompensation
  - *2* Shock
- *C* Systemic metabolic abnormalities
  - *1* Electrolyte imbalance
  - *2* Hypoxemia, acidosis
- *D* Neurophysiologic disturbances
  - *1* Autonomic fluctuations
    - *a* Central, neural, humoral
  - *2* Receptor function
  - *3* Long QT syndrome, congenital
- *E* Toxic responses
  - *1* Proarrhythmic drug effects
  - *2* Cardiac toxins

infrequent syndromes, such as the genetic hyperlipoproteinemias (Chap. 326), there are no *specific* hereditary risk factors for SCD. Higher levels of life stress, lower levels of education, social isolation, changes in lifestyle after myocardial infarction, cigarette use, alcohol consumption, obesity, absence of regular exercise, and type A–personality features, all have been *suggested* as contributors to risk of SCD. Among women, those who are unmarried, and those who have fewer children or have greater educational disparity with their spouses, appear to be at higher risk.

The major categories of structural causes of, and functional factors contributing to, the SCD syndrome are listed in Table 40-2. Worldwide, and especially in western cultures, coronary atherosclerotic heart disease is the most common structural abnormality associated with SCD. Up to 80 percent of all SCDs in the United States are due to the consequences of coronary atherosclerosis. The cardiomyopathies (dilated and hypertrophic, collectively, Chap. 192) account for another 10 to 15 percent of SCDs, and all of the remaining diverse etiologies cause only 5 to 10 percent of these events. The relative role of various factors contributing to the initiation of cardiac arrest has not been quantitated as well as the structural basis. Transient ischemia in the previously scarred or hypertrophied heart, electrolyte disturbances, fluctuations in autonomic nervous system activity, and transient changes in the electrophysiologic properties of the diseased heart have all been implicated as mechanisms responsible for transition from electrophysiologic stability to instability.

PATHOLOGY Data from necropsies of SCD victims parallel the clinical observations on the prevalence of coronary heart disease as the major structural etiologic factor. More than 80 percent of SCD victims have pathologic findings of coronary heart disease which are commonly accompanied by ruptured atherosclerotic plaques and/or coronary thrombi. The most consistent *coronary artery* abnormality is extensive coronary atherosclerosis. Seventy-five percent of the victims have two or more major vessels with $\geq$75 percent stenosis. In one study, atherosclerotic plaque fissuring, platelet aggregates, and/or acute thrombosis were observed in 95 of 100 individuals who had pathologic studies after SCD. The majority of these acute changes were superimposed on preexisting chronic lesions. However, only 44 percent of the SCD victims had more than 50 percent luminal narrowing by recent coronary thrombi, raising issues about interactions between breakdown of preexisting noncritical lesions, local thrombus formation and spontaneous lysis, and acute coronary spasm with ischemia in the initiation of the terminal event.

The pathology of the *myocardium* in SCD also reflects the extensive coronary heart disease which usually precedes the fatal event. As many as 70 to 75 percent of males who die suddenly have prior myocardial infarctions (MIs), and 20 to 30 percent have recent acute MIs. A high incidence of left ventricular (LV) hypertrophy coexists with prior MIs. Clinical and epidemiologic data suggest that LV hypertrophy itself predisposes to SCD, and it is likely that coexistence with prior MI adds a dimension of risk.

CLINICAL DEFINITION OF FORMS OF CARDIOVASCULAR COLLAPSE The definitions of the terms listed in Table 40-1 have important clinical applications. Cardiovascular collapse is a general term connoting loss of effective blood flow due to acute dysfunction of the heart and/or peripheral vasculature. Cardiovascular collapse may be caused by vasodepressor syncope (vasovagal syncope, postural hypotension with syncope—see Chap. 21), a transient severe bradycardia, or by cardiac arrest. The latter is distinguished from the transient forms of cardiovascular collapse in that it requires an intervention to achieve resuscitation. In contrast, vasodepressor syncope and many primary bradyarrhythmic syncopal events are transient, and the patient will regain consciousness spontaneously.

The most common electrical mechanism for true cardiac arrest is ventricular fibrillation (VF), which is responsible for 65 to 80 percent of cardiac arrests. Severe persistent bradyarrhythmias and asystole cause another 20 to 30 percent. Sustained ventricular tachycardia (VT) with hypotension is a less common cause, as is electromechanical dissociation in which organized electrical activity is present but no mechanical response. Acute low cardiac output states, having precipitous onset, may also present clinically as a cardiac arrest. The causes include massive acute pulmonary emboli, internal blood loss from ruptured aortic aneurysm, intense anaphylaxis, cardiac rupture after myocardial infarction, and unexpected fatal arrhythmia due to electrolyte disturbances.

CLINICAL CHARACTERISTICS OF CARDIAC ARREST

PRODROME, ONSET, ARREST, DEATH Long-term studies in both unselected and high-risk populations suggest that SCD may be presaged by days, weeks, or months of increasing angina, dyspnea, palpitations, easy fatigability, and other nonspecific complaints. However, these *prodromal complaints* are generally predictive of any major cardiac event; they are not specific for predicting SCD. In one study, nearly 50 percent of SCD victims saw a physician within the month prior to death, but the complaints generally appeared to be unrelated to the heart. Among survivors of out-of-hospital cardiac arrest, 28 percent retrospectively reported new onset of worsening angina pectoris or dyspnea prior to cardiac arrest. Prodromes are useful for identifying patients at risk for cardiovascular events, but not for identifying the subgroup of SCD victims.

The *onset of the terminal event*, leading to cardiac arrest, may be abrupt and instantaneous or may be heralded by up to 1 h of symptoms reflecting an acute change in cardiovascular status. Continuous ECG recordings, fortuitously obtained prior to a cardiac arrest, demonstrate changes in cardiac electrical activity in the minutes or hours before the event. There is a tendency for the heart rate to increase and for advanced grades of premature ventricular contractions to evolve. Most cardiac arrests that occur by the mechanism of VF begin with a run of sustained or nonsustained VT which then degenerates into VF.

In the clinical classification proposed by Hinkle and Thaler, sudden unexpected loss of effective circulation was separated into ''arrhythmic events'' and ''circulatory failure.'' Arrhythmic events are characterized by a high incidence of patients being awake and actively moving immediately prior to the event, are dominated by VF as the electrical mechanism, and have a short duration of terminal illness (<1 h). In contrast, circulatory failure deaths occur in patients who are inactive or comatose, have a higher incidence of asystole than VF, have a tendency to a longer duration of terminal illness, and are dominated by noncardiac events preceding the terminal illness.

The onset of cardiac arrest may be characterized by typical symptoms of an acute cardiac event, such as prolonged angina or the pain of myocardial infarction, acute dyspnea or orthopnea, or the sudden onset of palpitations, sustained tachycardia, or light-headedness. However, in many patients, the onset is precipitous, without forewarning.

Cardiac arrest is, by definition, abrupt. Mentation may be impaired in patients with sustained VT during the onset of the terminal event. However, complete loss of consciousness is a *sine qua non* in cardiac arrest. Although rare spontaneous reversions occur, it is generally accepted that cardiac arrest progresses to death within minutes (i.e., SCD has occurred) if active interventions are not undertaken promptly.

The ability to resuscitate the victim of cardiac arrest is related to the setting in which the event occurs, the mechanism (VF, VT, electromechanical dissociation, asystole), and the clinical status of the patient prior to the cardiac arrest. Those settings in which it is possible to institute prompt cardiopulmonary resuscitation (CPR) provide a better chance of a successful outcome. However, the outcome in intensive care units and other in-hospital environments is heavily influenced by the patient's preceding clinical status. The immediate outcome is good for cardiac arrest occurring in the intensive care unit in the presence of an acute cardiac event or transient metabolic disturbance, but the outcome for patients with advanced noncardiac disease (e.g., renal failure, pneumonia, sepsis, diabetes, cancer) is no more successful in hospital than in the out-of-hospital environment.

The success rate for initial resuscitation and ultimate survival from an out-of-hospital cardiac arrest depends in part upon the mechanism of the event. When the mechanism is VT, the outcome is best (67 percent); VF is the next most successful (30 percent), and asystole and electromechanical dissociation have dismal outcome statistics (Fig. 40-1). Age also influences the chances of successful resuscitation, with statistics for the elderly being poor.

Progression to biologic death is a function of the mechanism of cardiac arrest and the length of the delay before interventions. VF or asystole, without CPR within the first 4 to 6 min, has a poor outcome, and there are few survivors among patients who have had no life support activities for 8 min. Outcome statistics are dramatically improved by lay bystander intervention (basic life support—see below) prior to definitive interventions (advanced life support—defibrillation). The most common causes of death during hospitalization after resuscitated cardiac arrests are related to the severity of injury to the central nervous system. Anoxic encephalopathy and infections subsequent to prolonged respirator-dependence account for 60 percent of the deaths. Another 30 percent occur as a consequence of low cardiac output states which fail to respond to interventions. Paradoxically, recurrent arrhythmias are the least common cause of death, accounting for only 10 percent of in-hospital deaths.

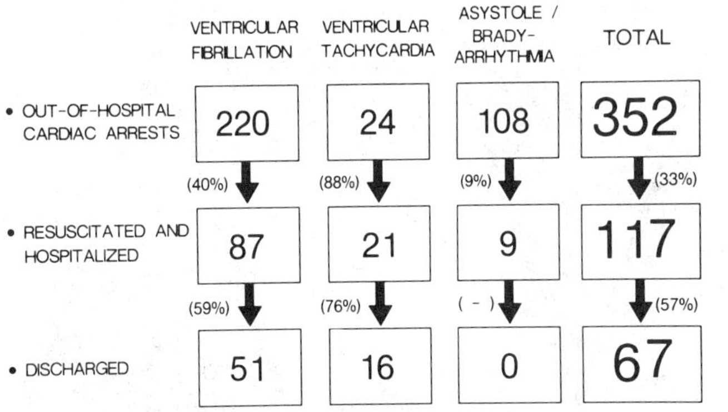

FIGURE 40-1 Initial electrophysiologic mechanisms recorded during out-of-hospital cardiac arrest. The figures highlighted by the boxes indicate the number of patients in each of three mechanism categories (ventricular fibrillation, ventricular tachycardia, and bradyarrhythmia/asystole), plus totals. In each category, the data indicate the number of prehospital cardiac arrests (*top*), the number of patients successfully resuscitated in the field and transferred to the hospital alive (*middle*), and the number of patients who survived to be discharged from hospital (*bottom*). The percentages in parentheses indicate survivals between each level of care for each category. *(Modified from Myerburg RJ et al: Clinical, electrophysiologic, and hemodynamic profile of patients resuscitated from prehospital cardiac arrest. Am J Med 68: 568, 1980, with permission).*

Outcome during hospitalization, particularly in patients with acute MI, is very different for patients with primary and secondary cardiac arrests. *Primary* cardiac arrests refer to those which occur in the absence of hemodynamic instability, and *secondary* cardiac arrests are those which occur in patients in whom abnormal hemodynamics dominate the clinical picture before cardiac arrest. The success rate for immediate resuscitation in primary cardiac arrest during acute MI should approach 100 percent. In contrast, as many as 70 percent of patients with secondary cardiac arrest succumb immediately or during the same hospitalization.

IDENTIFICATION OF PATIENTS AT RISK FOR SUDDEN CARDIAC DEATH Primary prevention of cardiac arrest depends upon the ability to identify individual patients at high risk. One must view the problem in the context of the total number of events and the population pools from which they are derived. In Fig. 40-2, the inverted triangle demonstrates that the annual incidence of SCD among an unselected adult population is 1 to 2 per 1000 population, largely reflecting the prevalence of those coronary heart disease patients among whom SCD is the first clinical manifestation (20 to 25 percent of first coronary events). The incidence (percent per year) increases progressively with addition of coronary risk factors to populations free of prior coronary events. The most powerful factors are age, elevated blood pressure, cigarette smoking, elevated serum cholesterol level, obesity, and nonspecific electrocardiographic abnormalities. These coronary risk factors are not specific for SCD, but rather represent increasing risk for all coronary deaths. The proportion of coronary deaths that are sudden remains at approximately 50 percent in all risk categories. Despite the marked *relative* increase of risk of SCD with addition of multiple risk factors (from 1 to 2 per 1000 population per year in an unselected population to as much as 50 to 60 per 1000 in the highest risk subgroups), the *absolute* incidence remains relatively low when viewed in terms of the relationship between the number of individuals to have a preventive intervention versus the number of events which can be prevented. Specifically, a 50 percent reduction in annual SCD risk would be a huge *relative* decrease, but would require an intervention in up to 200 unselected individuals to prevent one sudden death. These figures highlight the importance of primary prevention of coronary heart disease. Control of coronary risk factors may be the only practical method to prevent SCD in major segments of the population, since the majority of events occur in the large unselected subgroups rather

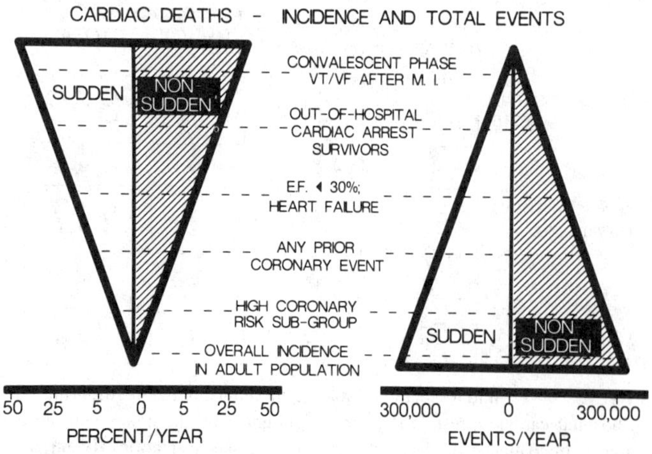

FIGURE 40-2 Incidence of sudden and nonsudden cardiac deaths in population subgroups, and the relation of total number of events per year to incidence figures. Approximations of subgroup incidence figures, and the related population pool from which they are derived, are presented. Approximately 50 percent of all cardiac deaths are sudden and unexpected. The incidence triangle on the left (''Percent/Year'') indicates the approximate percentage of sudden and nonsudden deaths in each of the population subgroups indicated, ranging from the lowest percentage in unselected adult populations (0.1 to 2 percent/year), to the highest percentage in patients with VT or VF during convalescence after an MI (approximately 50 percent/year). The triangle on the right indicates the total number of events per year in each of these groups, to reflect incidence in context with the size of the population subgroups. The highest risk categories identify the smallest number of total annual events, and the lowest incidence category accounts for the largest number of events per year. (EF = ejection fraction; VT = ventricular tachycardia; VF = ventricular fibrillation; MI = myocardial infarction.)

than the specific high-risk subgroups (contrast ''Events/Year'' to ''Percent/Year'' in Fig. 40-2).

For patients with acute or prior clinical manifestations of coronary heart disease, high-risk subgroups having a much higher ratio of SCD risk to population base can be identified. The acute, convalescent, and chronic phases of MI provide large population subsets with more highly focused risk (Chap. 189). The potential risk of cardiac arrest from the onset through the first 72 h after acute MI (the acute phase) may be as high as 15 to 20 percent. The highest risk of SCD in relation to MI is found in the subgroup who have VT or VF during the convalescent phase (3 days to 8 weeks) after MI. A 50 to 80 percent mortality in 6 to 12 months has been observed among these patients, when managed with conventional therapy, and at least 50 percent of the deaths are sudden. Aggressive interventions appear to reduce the incidence dramatically to 15 to 20 percent in 18 months, or better.

Chronic premature ventricular complexes (PVCs) after the acute phase of MI identify a long-term risk for total cardiac mortality and SCD. Increasing *frequency* of PVCs, with a plateau above the range of 10 to 30 PVCs per h on 24-h ambulatory monitor recordings, indicates increased risk; but advanced *forms* (salvos, nonsustained VT) are probably the more powerful predictor. PVCs interact strongly with the size of MI, as reflected by decreased left ventricular ejection fraction (EF). The combination of frequent PVCs, salvos or nonsustained VT, and an EF ≤ 30 percent identifies patients who have an annual risk of 20 percent. The risk falls off sharply with decreasing PVC frequency and the absence of advanced forms, and with higher EF. Whether suppression of PVCs alters risk has not yet been determined.

Beyond the specific problem of coronary heart disease, the general factors of extent of underlying disease due to any cause and a prior clinical expression of risk of SCD (i.e., survival after out-of-hospital cardiac arrest, not associated with acute MI) identify very high risk patients. Survival after out-of-hospital cardiac arrest predicts a 30 percent 1-year recurrent cardiac arrest rate in the absence of specific interventions (see below) in this group of patients.

A general rule is that the risk of SCD is approximately one-half of the total cardiovascular mortality rate. Thus, the SCD risk is approximately 20 percent per year for patients with advanced coronary heart disease or dilated cardiomyopathy severe enough to result in a 40 percent 1-year total mortality rate. Figure 40-2 demonstrates a much more focused population fraction (''Percent/Year'') for identifying high-risk patients for interventions in the high-risk subgroups, but the overall impact on the population, indicated by the absolute number of preventable events (''Events/Year''), is considerably smaller.

MANAGEMENT OF CARDIAC ARREST

The individual who collapses suddenly is managed in five stages: (1) the initial response; (2) basic life support; (3) advanced life support; (4) postresuscitation care; and (5) long-term management. The initial response and basic life support can be carried out by physicians, nurses, paramedical personnel, and trained lay persons. There is a requirement for increasing skills as the patient moves through the stages of advanced life support, postresuscitation care, and long-term management.

INITIAL RESPONSE The initial response will confirm whether a sudden collapse is indeed due to a cardiac arrest. Observations for respiratory movements, skin color, and the presence or absence of pulses in the carotid or femoral arteries will immediately determine whether a life-threatening cardiac arrest has occurred. Agonal respiratory movements may persist for a short time after cardiac arrest, but it is important to observe for severe stridor with a persistent pulse as a clue to aspiration of a foreign body or food. If this is suspected, a prompt Heimlich maneuver (see below) may dislodge the obstructing body. A precordial blow, or ''thump,'' delivered firmly to the junction of the middle and lower third of the sternum may occasionally revert VT or VF, but there is concern about converting VT *to* VF. Therefore, it has been recommended to use precordial thumps only in monitored patients; this recommendation remains controversial. The third action during the initial response is to clear the airway. The head is tilted back and chin lifted so that the oropharynx can be explored to clear the airway. Dentures or foreign bodies are removed, and the Heimlich maneuver is performed if there is reason to suspect that a foreign body is lodged in the oropharynx. If respiratory arrest precipitating cardiac arrest is suspected, a second precordial thump is delivered after the airway is cleared.

BASIC LIFE SUPPORT More popularly known as cardiopulmonary resuscitation (CPR), basic life support is intended to maintain organ perfusion until definitive interventions can be accomplished. The elements of CPR are the establishment and maintenance of ventilation of the lungs and compression of the chest. Mouth-to-mouth respiration may be used if no specific rescue equipment is immediately available (e.g., plastic oropharyngeal airways, esophageal obturators, masked Ambu bag). Conventional ventilation techniques during CPR require the lungs to be inflated once every 5 s when two persons are performing the resuscitation, and twice in succession every 15 s when one person is carrying out both ventilation and chest wall compression. Chest compression is based on the assumption that cardiac compression allows the heart to maintain a pump function by sequential filling and emptying of its chambers, with competent valves maintaining forward direction of flow. The technique is illustrated in Fig. 40-3. The palm of one hand is placed over the lower sternum, with the heel of the other resting on the dorsum of the lower hand. The sternum is depressed, with the arms remaining straight, at a rate of approximately 80/min. Sufficient force is applied to depress the sternum 3 to 5 cm, and relaxation is abrupt. This conventional technique for CPR is currently being compared to a new technique based on simultaneous compression and ventilation. While measurable carotid artery flow can be achieved with conventional CPR, experimental data and theoretical considerations suggest

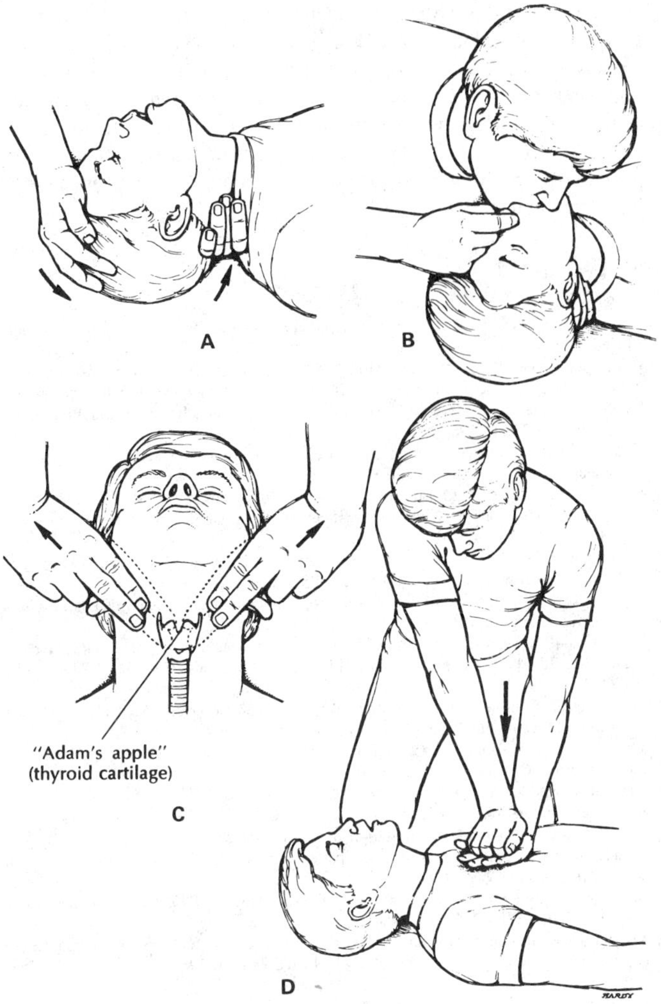

FIGURE 40-3 Major steps in cardiopulmonary resuscitation. *A*. Make certain the victim has an open airway. *B*. Start respiratory resuscitation immediately. *C*. Feel for the carotid pulse in the groove alongside the "Adam's apple" or thyroid cartilage. *D*. If pulse is absent, begin cardiac massage. Use 60 compressions a minute with one lung inflation after each group of 5 chest compressions. *(From J Henderson, Emergency Medical Guide, 4th ed, New York, McGraw-Hill, 1978.)*

that flow may be optimized by a pumping action produced by pressure changes in the entire thoracic cavity, as is achieved by simultaneous compression and ventilation. However, it is not yet clear whether this technique causes an unacceptable impedance of coronary blood flow, and whether the increased *carotid flow* produces equivalent increases in *cerebral perfusion*. Until these issues are clarified, conventional CPR remains the generally accepted technique.

ADVANCED LIFE SUPPORT Advanced life support is intended to achieve adequate ventilation, control cardiac arrhythmias, stabilize the hemodynamic status (blood pressure and cardiac output), and to restore organ perfusion. The activities carried out to achieve these goals include: (1) intubation with an endotracheal tube; (2) defibrillation/cardioversion and/or pacing; and (3) insertion of an intravenous line. Ventilation with O_2 (room air if O_2 is not immediately available) may promptly reverse hypoxemia and acidosis. The speed with which defibrillation/cardioversion is carried out is an important element for successful resuscitation. When possible, immediate defibrillation should precede intubation and insertion of an intravenous line; CPR should be carried out while the defibrillator is being charged. As soon as a diagnosis of VT or VF is obtained a 200-J shock should be delivered. Additional shocks at higher energies, up to a maximum of 360 J, are tried if the initial shock does not successfully abolish VT or VF. If the patient is less than fully conscious upon reversion, or if two or three attempts fail, prompt intubation, ventilation, and arterial blood gas analysis should be carried out. Intravenous $NaHCO_3$, which was formerly used in large quantities, is no longer considered routinely necessary and may be dangerous in larger quantities. However, the patient who is persistently acidotic after successful defibrillation and intubation should be given 1 mmol/kg of $NaHCO_3$ initially, and a 50 percent addition of the dose repeated every 10 to 15 min.

After initial defibrillation attempts, whether successful or not, a bolus of 1 mg/kg of lidocaine is given intravenously (Chap. 189) and the dose repeated in 2 min in those patients who have persistent ventricular arrhythmias or remain in VF. This is followed by a continuous infusion at a rate of 1 to 4 mg/min. If lidocaine fails to provide control, intravenous procainamide (loading infusion of 100 mg/5 min to a total dose of 500 to 800 mg, followed by continuous infusion at 2 to 5 mg/min) or bretylium tosylate (loading dose 5 to 10 mg/kg in 5 min; maintenance dose 0.5 to 2 mg/min) may be tried. For persistent VF, epinephrine (0.5 to 1.0 mg) may be given intravenously every 5 min during resuscitation with attempts to defibrillate between each dose. The drug may be given by an intracardiac route if intravenous access is not available. Intravenous calcium gluconate is no longer considered safe or necessary for routine administration. It is used only in patients in whom acute hyperkalemia is known to be the triggering event for resistant VF, in the presence of known hypocalcemia, or in patients who have received toxic doses of calcium channel antagonists.

Cardiac arrest secondary to bradyarrhythmias or asystole are managed differently. Once it is known that this type of rhythm is present, there is no role for external shock. The patient is promptly intubated, CPR is continued, and an attempt is made to control hypoxemia and acidosis. Epinephrine and/or atropine are given intravenously or by an intracardiac route. External pacing devices are now available to attempt to establish a regular rhythm, but the prognosis is generally very poor in this form of cardiac arrest. The one exception is bradyarrhythmic/asystolic cardiac arrest secondary to airway obstruction. This form of cardiac arrest may respond promptly to removal of foreign bodies by the Heimlich maneuver; or, more commonly in hospitalized patients, by intubation and suctioning of obstructing secretions in the airway.

POSTRESUSCITATION This phase of care is determined by the clinical setting of the cardiac arrest. *Primary VF in acute MI* (Chap. 189) is generally very responsive to life support techniques and easily controlled after the initial event. Patients are maintained on a lidocaine infusion at the rate of 2 to 4 mg/min for 24 to 72 h after the event. In the in-hospital setting, respirator support is usually not necessary or needed for only a short time, and hemodynamics stabilize promptly after defibrillation or cardioversion. In *secondary VF in acute MI* (those events in which hemodynamic abnormalities predispose to an arrhythmic event), resuscitative efforts are less often successful; and in those patients who are successfully resuscitated, the recurrence rate is high. The clinical picture is dominated by hemodynamic instability. In fact, the outcome is determined more by the ability to control hemodynamic dysfunction than electrophysiologic abnormalities. Bradyarrhythmias, asystole, and electromechanical dissociation are commonly secondary events in hemodynamically unstable patients, and are less responsive to interventions.

The outcome after in-hospital cardiac arrest associated with *noncardiac* diseases is poor; and in the few successfully resuscitated patients, the postresuscitation course is dominated by the nature of the underlying disease. Patients with cancer, renal failure, acute central nervous system disease, and uncontrolled infections, as a group, have a survival rate of less than 10 percent after in-hospital cardiac arrest. Some major exceptions to the poor outcome of cardiac arrest due to noncardiac causes are patients with transient airway obstruction, electrolyte disturbances, proarrhythmic effects of drugs, and severe metabolic abnormalities, most of whom may have an excellent chance of survival if they can be promptly resuscitated and maintained while the transient abnormalities are being corrected.

POST-CARDIAC ARREST CARE AFTER SURVIVAL FROM OUT-OF-HOSPITAL CARDIAC ARREST This form of care has evolved into a major area of specialized clinical activities since the development of community-based emergency rescue systems. Patients who do not suffer irreversible injury of the central nervous system and who become hemodynamically stable should have extensive diagnostic and therapeutic testing to guide long-term management. This aggressive approach is driven by the fact that early statistics indicated survival after out-of-hospital cardiac arrest was followed by a 30 percent recurrent cardiac arrest rate at 1 year, 45 percent at 2 years, and a total mortality rate of almost 60 percent at 2 years. Historical comparisons suggests that these dismal statistics may be significantly improved by newer interventions.

Among those patients in whom a transmural, acute MI is the cause of out-of-hospital cardiac arrest, the management is the same as any other patient who suffers cardiac arrest during the acute phase of a documented MI (see Chap. 189). For almost all other categories of patients, however, extensive diagnostic studies are carried out to determine etiology, functional impairment, and electrophysiologic instability as guides to future management. In general, patients who have out-of-hospital cardiac arrest due to chronic ischemic heart disease, without an acute MI, are evaluated to determine whether transient ischemia or chronic electrophysiologic instability was the more likely cause of the event. If there is reason to suspect an ischemic mechanism, anti-ischemic surgery or medical interventions (angioplasty, drugs) are used to reduce the ischemic burden. Electrophysiologic instability is best identified by the use of programmed electrical stimulation to determine whether the patient is inducible into a sustained VT or VF (Chap. 184). If so, this information can be used as a baseline against which to evaluate drug efficacy for prevention of inducibility, which is considered a satisfactory endpoint for long-term management. Using this technique for patients with ejection fractions of 30 percent or more, the recurrent cardiac arrest rate is less than 10 percent during the first year of follow-up. The outcome is not as good for patients with ejection fractions under 30 percent, but is still better than the apparent natural history of survival after cardiac arrest. For patients for whom successful drug therapy cannot be identified by this technique, insertion of an automatic implantable cardioverter/defibrillator or antiarrhythmic surgery (coronary bypass surgery, aneurysmectomy, cryoablation), should be considered (Chap. 184). The array of interventions available for these patients, properly applied, is providing continuing improvement in long-term outcome.

REFERENCES

BEDELL SE et al: Survival after cardiopulmonary resuscitation in the hospital. N Engl J Med 309:569, 1983

BIGGER JT, FLEISS JL, KLEIGER R, MILLER JP, ROLNITZKY LM, AND THE MULTICENTER POST-INFARCTION RESEARCH GROUP: The relationships among ventricular arrhythmias, left ventricular dysfunction, and mortality in the two years after myocardial infarction. Circulation 69:250, 1984

COBB LA, HALLSTROM AP: Community-based cardiopulmonary resuscitation: What have we learned? Ann NY Acad Sci 382:330, 1982

HEIMLICH HJ: A life-saving maneuver to prevent food-choking. JAMA 234:398, 1975

HINKLE LA, THALER HT: Clinical classification of cardiac deaths. Circulation 65:457, 1982

KANNEL WB, SCHATZKIN A: Sudden death: Lessions from subsets in population studies. J Am Coll Cardiol 5 (Suppl 6): 141B, 1985

KULLER L et al: An epidemiological study of sudden and unexpected deaths in adults. Medicine 46:341, 1967

MYERBURG RJ, CASTELLANOS A: Cardiac arrest and sudden cardiac death, in *Heart Disease*, 3d ed, E Braunwald (ed). Philadelphia, Saunders, 1988, chap 24, pp 742–777

——— et al: Long-term survival after prehospital cardiac arrest: Analysis of outcome during an 8-year study. Circulation 70:538, 1984

——— et al: A biological approach to sudden cardiac death: Structure, function, and cause. Am J Cardiol, 63:1512, 1989

PACKER M: Sudden unexpected death in patients with congestive heart failure: A second frontier. Circulation 72:681, 1985

ROBERTS WC, JONES AA: Quantitation of coronary arterial narrowing at necropsy in sudden cardiac death. Analysis of 31 patients and comparison with 25 controls. Am J Cardiol 44:39, 1979

Standard and guidelines for cardiopulmonary resuscitation (CPR) and emergency cardiac care (ECC). JAMA 255:290, 1986

WILBER DJ et al: Out-of-hospital cardiac arrest: Use of electrophysiologic testing in the prediction of long-term outcome. N Engl J Med 318:19, 1988

section 5 Alterations in gastrointestinal function

41 ORAL MANIFESTATIONS OF DISEASE

JOHN S. GREENSPAN / PAUL GOLDHABER

A thorough oral examination, to include the oral and pharyngeal soft tissues as well as the teeth, is an important part of the physical examination. The common oral diseases are due to infection by bacteria, fungi, and viruses. The complex development of the orofacial structures leads to close interposition of a wide range of tissues, most of which are prone to developmental anomalies, growth disturbances, and neoplasia.

DISEASES OF THE TEETH

DENTAL CARIES, PULPAL AND PERIAPICAL DISEASE, AND COMPLICATIONS Dental caries is a destructive disease of the hard tissues of the teeth due to infection with *Streptococcus mutans* and other bacteria. Formerly one of the commonest human diseases, caries has shown marked changes in recent years. In the United States fewer than half of those 17 years and younger now have carious lesions, although in many segments of the population and in the third world this decrease has not occurred. Much of the decline is due to artificial fluoridation of drinking water to a level of 1 part per million, with additional effects due to fluoride-containing toothpastes and topical fluoride administration. Conversely, retention of teeth and the aging of the population have led to an increase in root caries. Increasing numbers of patients surviving with the consequences of cancer therapy and other special populations (diabetics and those with xerostomia due to Sjögren's syndrome or to medications) may experience severe caries unless appropriate topical fluoride prophylaxis is used. Treatment of caries involves removal of the softened and infected hard tissues, sealing of the exposed dentine, and restoration of the lost tooth structure with silver amalgam, composite plastic, gold, or porcelain.

If the carious lesion progresses, infection of the dental pulp may occur, causing *acute pulpitis*. The tooth may become sensitive to hot or cold and then severe continuous throbbing pain ensues. At this stage, pulp damage is irreversible and it becomes necessary to remove the contents of the pulp chamber and root canals, followed by thorough cleaning, antisepsis, and filling with an inert material (root canal therapy). Alternatively, extraction of the tooth may be indicated.

If the pulpitis is not successfully treated, infection may spread beyond the tooth apex into the periodontal ligament. If the infection causes acute inflammation, pain on chewing or percussion is present and a *periapical abscess* may form, while chronic inflammation can produce a *periapical granuloma* within the alveolar bone. This may cause slight pain and tenderness or may be asymptomatic. Proliferation of epithelial cell rests may convert the granuloma into a *periapical cyst*. Both the granuloma and the cyst produce periapical radiolucencies, whereas the periapical abscess does not do so unless it forms as a complication of one of the other two lesions. The pus in the periapical abscess may track through the alveolar bone into soft tissues, causing cellulitis and bacteremia, or may discharge into the oral cavity (*parulis* or *gumboil*), into the maxillary sinus, or through the skin of the face or submandibular area. A severe form of cellulitis, *Ludwig's angina*, originates from an infected mandibular molar, involves the submandibular space, and extends throughout the floor of the mouth, with elevation of the tongue, dysphagia, and difficulty in breathing. Glottal edema may occur, necessitating emergency tracheotomy.

EFFECT OF SYSTEMIC FACTORS ON TEETH Systemic factors, occurring in utero or in infancy during the stages of crown formation, may influence the development and structure of the teeth. Enamel hypoplasia of the primary and/or permanent teeth, manifested by alterations ranging from white spots to gross defects in the surface structure of the crowns, may be caused by disturbances of calcium and phosphate metabolism such as are found in vitamin D–resistant rickets, hypoparathyroidism, gastroenteritis, and celiac disease. Premature birth or high fevers may also give rise to enamel hypoplasia. Tetracycline, given during the second half of pregnancy, in infancy, and in childhood up to 8 years of age, causes both a permanent discoloration of the teeth and enamel hypoplasia. Daily ingestion of more than 1.5 mg fluoride can result in enamel discoloration (*mottling*). Prenatal factors appear to influence crown size. Larger teeth are associated with maternal diabetes, maternal hypothyroidism, and large birth size. Tooth size is reduced in Down's syndrome. Premature loss of the deciduous dentition is frequently the first symptom in juvenile hypophosphatasia. Systemic disease may give rise to pain that simulates pulpal disease. Maxillary sinusitis is frequently manifested as pain in the maxillary teeth, including sensitivity to thermal changes and percussion. Cardiac disease with angina pectoris may result in pain referred to the lower jaw, probably through the vagus nerve.

PERIODONTAL DISEASES

In adults, chronic destructive periodontal disease becomes responsible for more loss of teeth than caries, particularly in the aged. However, the prevalence and incidence of periodontal disease also appears to be declining in the United States. The commonest form of periodontal disease starts as inflammation of the marginal gingiva (*gingivitis*) which is painless, although the gingiva may bleed on brushing. The disease spreads to involve the periodontal ligament and alveolar bone. As the latter is slowly resorbed, there is loss of periodontal ligament attachment between tooth and bone. The soft tissue separates from the tooth surface, causing ''pocket'' formation with bleeding on probing and during chewing. Acute inflammation may become superimposed on this chronic process, with the production of pus and the formation of a *periodontal abscess*. Ultimately, extreme bone loss, tooth mobility, and recurrent abscess formation leads to tooth exfoliation or may mandate tooth extraction.

Gingivitis and periodontitis are infections associated with the accumulation of *bacterial plaque* which may become mineralized (*calculus*) and which can be prevented by appropriate *oral hygiene* measures including tooth brushing, flossing, antibacterial mouth rinses, and the removal of impacted food debris. Poorly fabricated or deteriorated restorations may contribute through overextended or inadequate margins, while the role of occlusal trauma is unclear. Therapy is directed at the causative microflora and consists of removal of plaque and calculus, debridement of the pocket lining and superficial infected cementum, combined with elimination of other contributing factors.

Periodontal disease appears to be a group of conditions, including *adult periodontitis*, associated with *Bacteroides gingivalis*, *B. intermedius*, and other gram-negative organisms. *Localized juvenile periodontitis* (LJP) causes rapid, severe pocketing and bone loss and is associated with *Actinobacillus actinomycetemcomitans* (*A.a*), *Capnocytophaga*, *Eikenella corrodens*, and other anaerobes. *Acute necrotizing ulcerative gingivitis* (ANUG) involves sudden inflammation of the gingivae with necrosis, tissue loss, pain, bleeding, and halitosis and is associated with *B. intermedius* and spirochetes. ANUG and an aggressive and rapid form of periodontitis (HIV-P) are seen in association with human immunodeficiency virus (HIV) infection. Some of these cases progress to a destructive gangrenelike lesion of oral soft tissues and bone (*necrotizing stomatitis*) resembling the *noma* formerly seen in severely malnourished populations. Therapy involves local antibacterial measures, debridement and, in severe cases, systemic antibiotics effective against gram-negative anaerobes.

Host factors may be involved in the pathogenesis of periodontal disease in other populations also. Thus, familial defects in neutrophil chemotaxis are found in LJP and these may predispose to tissue destruction caused by the toxins of *A.a.* including leucotoxin, collagenase, endotoxin, and a factor further inhibiting neutrophil chemotaxis. Patients with IgA deficiency and agammaglobulinemia probably have less periodontal disease than matched healthy individuals, whereas in *Down's syndrome* and *diabetes mellitus* severe periodontal disease may occur. During pregnancy there may be severe gingivitis and the formation of localized *pyogenic granulomas*. Certain drugs, notably the anticonvulsant *phenytoin* and the antiangina calcium channel blocker *nifedipine*, cause *fibrous hyperplasia* of the gingiva which may cover the teeth, interfere with eating, and be unsightly. Similar clinical appearances can be due to *idiopathic familial gingival fibromatosis*. Surgical management is used for both conditions, although a change in medication may be appropriate for the drug-induced form.

Periapical and periodontal bacterial infections can cause transient bacteremia after tooth extraction and even routine dental prophylaxis. These can lead to bacterial endocarditis in patients with a history of rheumatic fever, other valvular disease, valvular graft, or heart or joint prostheses. Antibiotic coverage is appropriate in such cases.

DISEASES OF THE ORAL MUCOSA

INFECTIONS Most oral mucosal diseases involve microorganisms (see Table 41-1).

PIGMENTED LESIONS (See Table 41-2)

DERMATOLOGIC DISEASES (See Tables 41-1, -2, and -3 and Chaps. 55 to 60)

DISEASES OF THE TONGUE (See Table 41-4)

HALITOSIS (See Table 41-5)

HIV DISEASE AND AIDS (See Table 41-6 and Chaps. 134 and 264) Immunosuppression induced by HIV infection predisposes to numerous oral infections, neoplasms, and autoimmune and idiopathic lesions. Some of these, such as *oral candidiasis* and *hairy leukoplakia* (a benign epithelial hyperplasia associated with Epstein-Barr virus, or EBV), are common features of HIV disease and often precede or accompany full-blown AIDS. Some, such as oral Kaposi's sarcoma and lymphoma, are diagnostic of AIDS. While most oral lesions of HIV disease are also found in the general population, both hairy leukoplakia and HIV-P are strongly associated with HIV infection and are seen only very rarely in other circumstances. Only small and variable amounts of HIV can be found in saliva but blood, tissue fluid, and gingival crevicular exudate, found in the mouth as a result of lesions or of clinical manipulation, are certainly sources of other

TABLE 41-1 Vesicular, bullous, or ulcerative lesions of the oral mucosa

Condition	Usual location	Clinical features	Course
VIRAL DISEASES			
Primary acute herpetic gingivostomatitis (herpes simplex virus type 1, rarely type 2)	Lip and oral mucosa	Labial vesicles which rupture and crust, and intraoral vesicles which quickly ulcerate; extremely painful; acute gingivitis, fever, malaise, foul odor, and cervical lymphadenopathy; occurs primarily in infants, children, and young adults	Heals spontaneously in 10–14 days unless secondarily infected
Recurrent herpes labialis	Mucocutaneous junction of lip perioral skin	Eruption of groups of vesicles which may coalesce, then rupture and crust; painful to pressure or spicy foods	Lasts about 1 week, but condition may be prolonged if secondary infection occurs
Recurrent intraoral herpes simplex	Palate and gingiva	Small vesicles which rupture and coalesce; painful	Heal spontaneously in about 1 week
Chickenpox (varicella-zoster virus)	Gingiva and oral mucosa	Skin lesions may be accompanied by small vesicles on oral mucosa that rupture to form shallow ulcers; may coalesce to form large bullous lesions that ulcerate; mucosa may have generalized erythema	Lesions heal spontaneously within 2 weeks
Herpes zoster (reactivation of varicella-zoster virus)	Cheek, tongue, gingiva, or palate	Unilateral vesicular eruption and ulceration in linear pattern following sensory distribution of trigeminal nerve or one of its branches	Gradual healing without scarring; postherpetic neuralgia is common
Infectious mononucleosis (Epstein-Barr virus)	Oral mucosa	Fatigue, sore throat, malaise, low-grade fever, and enlarged cervical lymph nodes; numerous small ulcers usually appear several days before lymphadenopathy; gingival bleeding and multiple petechiae at junction of hard and soft palates	Oral lesions disappear during convalescence
Warts (papillomavirus)	Any place on skin and oral mucosa	Single or multiple papillary lesions, with thick, white keratinized surfaces containing many pointed projections; cauliflower lesions covered with normal colored mucosa or multiple pink or pale bumps (focal epithelial hyperplasia)	Lesions grow rapidly and spread
Herpangina (coxsackievirus A; also possibly coxsackievirus B and echovirus)	Oral mucosa, pharynx, tongue	Sudden onset of fever, sore throat, and oropharyngeal vesicles, usually in children under 4 years, during summer months; diffuse pharyngeal injection and vesicles (1–2 mm), grayish white surrounded by red areola; vesicles enlarge and ulcerate	Incubation period 2–9 days; fever for 1–4 days; recovery uneventful
Hand, foot, and mouth disease (type A coxsackieviruses)	Oral mucosa, pharynx, palms, and soles	Fever, malaise, headache with oropharyngeal vesicles which become painful, shallow ulcers	Incubation period 2–18 days; lesions heal spontaneously in 2–4 weeks
Primary HIV infection	Gingiva, palate, and pharynx	Acute gingivitis and oropharyngeal ulceration, associated with febrile illness resembling mononucleosis and including lymphadenopathy	Followed by HIV seroconversion; asymptomatic HIV infection and usually ultimately by HIV disease
BACTERIAL OR FUNGAL DISEASES			
Acute necrotizing ulcerative gingivitis ("trench mouth", Vincent's infection)	Gingiva	Painful, bleeding gingiva characterized by necrosis and ulceration of gingival papillae and margins plus lymphadenopathy and foul odor	Continued destruction of tissue followed by remission, but may recur
Prenatal (congenital) syphilis	Palate, jaws, tongue, and teeth	Gummatous involvement of palate, jaws, and facial bones; Hutchinson's incisors, mulberry molars, glossitis, mucous patches, and fissures of corners of mouth	Tooth deformities in permanent dentition irreversible
Primary syphilis (chancre)	Lesion appears where organism enters body; may occur on lips, tongue, or tonsillar area	Small papule developing rapidly into a large, painless ulcer with indurated border; unilateral lymphadenopathy; chancre and lymph nodes containing spirochetes; serologic tests positive by third to fourth weeks	Healing of chancre in 1–2 months, followed by secondary syphilis in 6–8 weeks
Secondary syphilis	Oral mucosa frequently involved with mucous patches, primarily on palate, also at commissures of mouth	Maculopapular lesions of oral mucosa, 5–10 mm in diameter with central ulceration covered by grayish membrane; eruptions occurring on various mucosal surfaces and skin accompanied by fever, malaise, and sore throat	Lesions may persist from several weeks to a year
Tertiary syphilis	Palate and tongue	Gummatous infiltration of palate or tongue followed by ulceration and fibrosis; atrophy of tongue papillae produce characteristic bald tongue and glossitis	Gumma may destroy palate, causing complete perforation

(*continued*)

TABLE 41-1 Vesicular, bullous, or ulcerative lesions of the oral mucosa *(continued)*

Condition	Usual location	Clinical features	Course
BACTERIAL OR FUNGAL DISEASES			
Gonorrhea	Lesions may occur in mouth at site of inoculation or secondarily by hematogenous spread from a primary focus elsewhere	Earliest symptoms are burning or itching sensation, dryness, or heat in mouth followed by acute pain on eating or speaking; tonsils and oropharynx most frequently involved; oral tissues may be diffusely inflamed or ulcerated; saliva develops increased viscosity and fetid odor; submaxillary lymphadenopathy with fever in severe cases	Lesions may resolve with appropriate antibiotic therapy
Tuberculosis	Tongue, tonsillar area, soft palate	A solitary, irregular ulcer covered by a persistent exudate; ulcer has an undermined, firm border	Lesions may persist
Cervicofacial actinomycosis	Swellings in region of face, neck, and floor of mouth	Infection may be associated with an extraction, jaw fracture, or eruption of molar tooth; in acute form resembles an acute pyogenic abscess, but contains yellow "sulfur granules" (gram-positive mycelia and their hyphae)	Acute form may last a few weeks; chronic form lasts months or years; prognosis excellent; actinomycetes respond to antibiotics (tetracyclines or penicillin) but not to antifungal drugs
Histoplasmosis	Any area in mouth, particularly tongue, gingiva, or palate	Numerous small nodules which may ulcerate; hoarseness and dysphagia may occur because of lesions in larynx, usually associated with fever and malaise	May be fatal
Candidiasis	Any area of oral mucosa	Pseudomembranous form with white patches which are easily wiped off leaving red, bleeding, sore surface; erythematous form is flat and red while rarely candida leukoplakia appears as white patch in tongue which does not rub off; angular cheilitis due to *Candida* involves sore cracks and redness at angle of mouth; *Candida* seen on KOH preparation in all forms	Responds to antifungals
DERMATOLOGIC DISEASES			
Mucous membrane pemphigoid	Primarily mucous membranes of the oral cavity, but may also involve the eyes, urethra vagina, and rectum	Painful, grayish white collapsed vesicles or bullae with peripheral erythematous zone; gingival lesions desquamate, leaving ulcerated area	Protracted course with remissions and exacerbations; involvement of different sites occurs slowly; glucocorticoids may temporarily reduce symptoms but do not control the disease
Erythema multiforme (Stevens-Johnson syndrome)	Primarily the oral mucosa and skin of hands and feet	Intraoral ruptured bullae surrounded by an inflammatory area; lips may show hemorrhagic crusts; the "iris," or "target" lesion, on the skin is pathognomonic; patient may have severe signs of toxicity	Onset very rapid; condition may last 1–2 weeks; may be fatal; acute episodes respond to steroids
Pemphigus vulgaris	Oral mucosa and skin	Ruptured bullae and ulcerated oral areas; mostly in older adults	With repeated recurrence of bullae, toxicity may lead to cachexia, infection, and death within 2 years; often controllable with steroids
Lichen planus	Oral mucosa and skin	White striae in mouth; purplish nodules on skin at sites of friction; occasionally causes oral mucosal ulcers and erosive gingivitis	Protracted course, may respond to topical steroids
NEOPLASTIC DISEASES			
Squamous cell carcinoma	Any areas in mouth, most commonly on lower lip, tongue, and floor of mouth	Ulcer with elevated, indurated border; failure to heal, pain not prominent; lesions tend to arise in areas of leukoplakia or in smooth or atrophic tongue	Invades and destroys underlying tissues and may metastasize to regional lymph nodes
Acute leukemia	Gingiva	Gingival swelling and superficial ulcerations followed by hyperplasia of gingiva with extensive necrosis and hemorrhage; deep ulcers may occur elsewhere on the mucosa complicated by secondary infection	Fatal if untreated
Lymphoma	Gingiva, palate, tongue, and tonsillar area	Elevated, ulcerated area which may proliferate rapidly, giving the appearance of a traumatic inflammatory lesion; swelling of regional lymph nodes	Fatal if untreated
Metastatic tumors	Deep in jaw bone, usually in premolar-molar area of mandible	May arise from carcinoma of distant organ such as breast, lung, or kidney; advanced lesion may expand and destroy bone, loosen and spread teeth, involve inferior alveolar nerve, cause pain and numbness of lower lip	Usually fatal

(continued)

TABLE 41-1 Vesicular, bullous, or ulcerative lesions of the oral mucosa *(continued)*

Condition	Usual location	Clinical features	Course
OTHER CONDITIONS			
Recurrent aphthous ulcers	Any place on nonkeratinized oral mucosa (lips, tongue, buccal mucosa, floor of mouth, soft palate, oropharynx)	Single or clusters of painful ulcers with surrounding erythematous border; lesions may be 1–2 mm in diameter in crops (herpetiform), 1–5 mm (minor), or 5–15 mm (major)	Lesions heal in 1–2 weeks but may recur monthly or several times a year; topical steroids give symptomatic relief; systemic glucocorticoids may be needed in severe cases; a tetracycline oral suspension may decrease severity of herpetiform ulcers
Behçet's syndrome	Oral mucosa, eyes, genitalia, gut, and CNS	Multiple aphthous ulcers in mouth; inflammatory ocular changes, ulcerative lesions on genitalia; inflammatory bowel disease and CNS disease	Ulcers may persist for several weeks and heal without scarring
Traumatic ulcers	Any place on oral mucosa; dentures frequently responsible for ulcers in vestibule	Localized, discrete ulcerated lesion with red border; produced by accidental biting of mucosa, penetration by a foreign object, or chronic irritation by a denture	Lesions usually heal in 7–10 days when irritant is removed, unless secondarily infected

viruses, such as herpes simplex virus (HSV) and EBV, and the same may be true for HIV.

HEMATOLOGIC AND NUTRITIONAL DISEASE Gingival bleeding, necrotic ulcers, and enlargement due to malignant infiltrates are seen in all forms of leukemia, particularly *monocytic leukemia*. In agranulocytosis severe oral mucosal ulcers are seen, while in *thrombocytopenia* oral petechiae, ecchymoses, and gingival bleeding occur. In *Plummer-Vinson syndrome* (see Chaps. 290 and 291), atrophy of oral mucosa, particularly the tongue papillae, causes redness and soreness as well as dysphagia. This is associated with increased susceptibility to oral cancer. A smooth tongue can also be seen in *pernicious anemia* (Chap. 292). Severe oral mucositis with ulcers, candidiasis, bacterial infections, and xerostomia complicate local radiotherapy for head and neck malignancies as well as chemotherapy for both local and other malignancies. Although now rarely seen in the United States, oral features of vitamin deficiency include oral mucositis and ulcers, glossitis, and burning sensations in the tongue (*B group vitamins*) and petechiae, gingival swelling, bleeding, and ulceration as well as loosening of teeth (*scurvy* of vitamin C deficiency).

ORAL CANCER

Oral *squamous cell carcinoma* accounts for 2 to 4 percent of malignancies in the United States (excluding skin carcinomas) and

TABLE 41-2 Pigmented lesions of the oral mucosa

Condition	Usual location	Clinical features	Course
Oral melanotic macule	Any area of the mouth	Discrete or diffuse localized, brown to black macule	Remains indefinitely
Diffuse melanin pigmentation	Any area of the mouth	Diffuse pale to dark-brown pigmentation; may be physiologic (''racial'') or due to smoking	Remains indefinitely
Nevi	Any area of the mouth	Discrete, localized, brown to black pigmentation	
Malignant melanoma	Any area of the mouth	Can be flat and diffuse, painless, brown to black, or can be raised and nodular	Expands and invades early; metastasis leads to death
Addison's disease	Any area in mouth but mostly on buccal mucosa	Blotches or spots of bluish-black to dark-brown pigmentation occurring early in the disease, accompanied by diffuse pigmentation of skin; other symptoms of adrenal insufficiency	Condition controlled by steroid therapy
Peutz-Jeghers syndrome	Any area in mouth	Dark-brown spots on lips, buccal mucosa, with characteristic distribution of pigment around lips, nose, eyes, and on hands; concomitant intestinal polyposis	Pigmented lesions remain indefinitely; polyps may become malignant
Drug ingestion (tranquilizers, oral contraceptives, antimalarials)	Any area in mouth	Brown, black, or gray areas of pigmentation	Disappears following cessation of drug
Amalgam tattoo	Gingiva and mucobuccal fold	Small blue-black pigmented areas associated with embedded amalgam particles in soft tissues; these may show up on radiographs as radiopaque particles in some cases	Remains indefinitely
Heavy metal pigmentation (bismuth, mercury, lead)	Gingival margin	Thin blue-black pigmented line along gingival margin; due to prior treatment for syphilis with bismuth or mercury or from accidental absorption of lead	Long-lasting
Black hairy tongue	Dorsum of tongue	Elongation of filiform papillae of tongue, which take on a brown to black coloration	Long-lasting but may disappear spontaneously
Fordyce's ''disease''	Buccal and labial mucosa	Aggregation of numerous small yellowish spots just beneath mucosal surface; no symptoms; due to hyperplasia of sebaceous glands	Remains without apparent change indefinitely

TABLE 41-3 White lesions of oral mucosa

Condition	Usual location	Clinical features	Course
Lichen planus	Buccal mucosa, tongue, gingiva, and lips; skin	Striae, white plaques, red areas, ulcers in mouth; purplish papules on skin; may be asymptomatic, sore, or painful; lichenoid drug reactions may look similar	Protracted; responds to topical steroids
White sponge nevus	Oral mucosa, vagina, anal mucosa	Painless white thickening of epithelium; adolescent/early adult onset; familial	Benign and permanent
Smokers leukoplakia and smokeless tobacco lesions	Any area of oral mucosa, sometimes related to location	White patch that may become firm, rough, or red fissured and ulcerated; may become sore and painful but usually painless	Occasionally premalignant; may or may not resolve on cessation of habit
Nicotinic stomatitis	Palate in pipe smokers	White nodular elevations on hard palate with central red areas	Benign; usually resolves on cessation of pipe smoking
Frictional keratosis	Any area in mouth	Elevated white lesion due to hyperkeratosis and thickening of the oral epithelium secondary to chronic irritation	Removal of irritant leads to healing in 2–3 weeks
Candidiasis (''candidosis,'' ''moniliasis'')	Any area in mouth	*Pseudomembranous type* (''thrush''): creamy white curdlike patches that reveal a raw, bleeding surface when scraped; found in sick infants, debilitated elderly patients receiving high doses of glucocorticoids or broad spectrum antibiotics, or in patients with AIDS	Responds favorably to antifungal therapy and correction of predisposing causes where possible
		Erythematous type: flat, red, sometimes sore areas, same groups of patients	
		Candidal leukoplakia: nonremovable white thickening of epithelium due to *Candida*	Responds to prolonged antifungals
		Angular cheilitis: sore fissures at corner of mouth	Responds to topical antifungals
Hairy leukoplakia	Usually lateral tongue, rarely elsewhere on oral mucosa	White areas ranging from small and flat to extensive and ''hairy''; found in HIV carriers in all risk groups for AIDS; rarely causes discomfort	Due to EBV; many patients develop AIDS; responds to high dose acyclovir but recurs
Chemical burns	Any area in mouth	White slough due to necrosis of epithelium and underlying connective tissue caused by contact with agents (e.g., aspirin) applied locally or the use of undiluted sodium perborate or hydrogen peroxide as a mouthwash; removal of slough leaves a raw, painful surface	Lesion heals in several weeks if not secondarily infected

in most western countries, but represents up to 50 percent of malignancies in India. Globally, oral cancer is fourth in incidence for men and sixth for women. The disease is age related, occurring in those over 40 years of age and increasing in incidence with age. The male/female ratio is 3:1 but the incidence of lip and mouth cancer is decreasing in white males and increasing in black males and in females. However, both the overall incidence and death rate are fairly static. *Lip cancer* has shown significant decreases in incidence in recent years, probably because of changes in pipe-smoking habits, while *tongue cancer* has become commoner. Lip cancer is still the commonest oral site followed by tongue, floor of mouth, and other intraoral locations. The etiology involves *tobacco* smoked in pipes, cigars,and cigarettes and chewed or ''dipped.'' The role of pipe smoking in lip cancer may also include the effects of

TABLE 41-4 Alterations of the tongue

Type of change	Clinical features
SIZE OR MORPHOLOGY CHANGES	
Macroglossia	Enlarged tongue that may be part of a syndrome found in developmental conditions such as Down's syndrome; may be due to tumor (hemangioma or lymphangioma), metabolic disease (such as primary amyloidosis), or endocrine disturbance (such as acromegaly or cretinism)
Fissured (''scrotal'') tongue	Dorsal surface and sides of tongue covered by painless shallow or deep fissures that may collect debris and become irritated
Median rhomboid glossitis	Congenital abnormality of tongue with ovoid, denuded area in median posterior portion of the tongue; may be associated with candidiasis and may respond to antifungals
COLOR CHANGES	
''Geographic'' tongue (benign migratory glossitis)	Asymptomatic inflammatory condition of the tongue, with rapid loss and regrowth of filiform papillae, leading to appearance of denuded red patches ''wandering'' across the surface of the tongue
Hairy tongue	Elongation of filiform papillae of the medial dorsal surface area due to failure of keratin layer of the papillae to desquamate normally; brownish-black coloration may be due to staining by tobacco, food, or chromogenic organisms
''Strawberry'' and ''raspberry'' tongue	Appearance of tongue during scarlet fever due to the hypertrophy of fungiform papillae plus changes in the filiform papillae
''Bald'' tongue	Atrophy may be associated with xerostomia, pernicious anemia, iron-deficiency anemia, pellagra, or syphilis; may be accompanied by painful burning sensation; may be an expression of erythmematous candidiasis and respond to antifungals

TABLE 41-5 Causes of halitosis

I Upper respiratory infection
  A Bronchiectasis
  B Lung abscess
II Oral infection
  A Acute primary herpetic gingivostomatitis
  B Acute necrotizing ulcerative gingivitis
  C Periodontal disease
  D Caries
III Smoking
IV Hepatic failure (fishy odor)
V Azotemia (ammoniacal or urinary odor)
VI Diabetic ketoacidosis (sweet, fruity odor)

heat and other irritants. Other factors include *alcohol*, iron deficiency (Plummer-Vinson syndrome), and deficiencies of vitamins. Evidence linking oral *syphilitic* lesions and oral *candidiasis* with oral cancer is circumstantial, but a growing body of data indicates roles for *herpes simplex virus* and *human papillomavirus*. There are no data supporting the idea that irritation from sharp teeth or dental appliances cause oral cancer.

The most common precancerous lesion in the oral cavity presents as *leukoplakia*, a white patch on the mucosa that cannot be rubbed off. Histologically such lesions show hyperkeratosis, acanthosis, and *atypia* (*dysplasia*). Leukoplakias include homogeneous and nonhomogeneous types. The nonhomogeneous nodular leukoplakias (white nodules on a red background), have a much higher potential for malignant transformation than homogeneous leukoplakia. Recent evidence suggests that the asymptomatic, red velvety lesion (*erythroplasia*) of the floor of the mouth, ventrolateral aspect of the tongue, or soft palate–anterior pillar complex is more likely to be carcinoma in situ or invasive carcinoma than is the white lesion. All chronic ulcerative lesions that fail to heal within 1 to 2 weeks should be considered potentially malignant and must be biopsied in order to make a definitive diagnosis. It is noteworthy that in their early stages intraoral squamous cell carcinomas are rarely painful, in contrast to similar-appearing inflammatory lesions.

The prognosis for patients with carcinoma of the lip is usually good, since these malignant tumors are noted sooner and apparently metastasize later. Patients with carincoma of the tongue have a poorer prognosis, particularly if the tumor occurs more posteriorly on the tongue. Intraoral carcinomas may spread by direct invasion to the underlying bone. Depending on the site of origin of the intraoral carcinoma, metastases usually spread to the submaxillary or cervical lymph nodes. Death may result from recurrent or uncontrollable disease above the clavicles, metastatic disease beyond the neck, treatment complications, or a second primary cancer, usually in the oral cavity or the upper parts of the gastrointestinal or respiratory tract. Metastatic tumors to the jaw may occur from carcinomas of the lung, breast, kidney, or gastrointestinal tract.

TABLE 41-6 Oral lesions of HIV disease and AIDS

I Fungal
  A Candidiasis
    1 Pseudomembranous
    2 Erythematous
    3 Candidal leukoplakia
    4 Angular cheilitis
  B Histoplasmosis
  C Cryptococcosis
II Bacterial
  A Acute necrotizing ulcerative gingivitis
  B HIV-gingivitis
  C HIV-periodontitis
  D Necrotizing stomatitis
  E Mycobacterium avium intracellulare complex and tuberculosis
  F Stomatitis due to enteric organisms
III Viral
  A Herpes simplex
  B Herpes zoster
  C Hairy leukoplakia
  D Warts
IV Neoplastic
  A Kaposi's sarcoma
  B Lymphoma
V Other
  A Recurrent aphthous ulcers
  B Immune thrombocytopenic purpura
  C Xerostomia
  D Salivary gland enlargement

DISEASES OF THE SALIVARY GLANDS

The major and minor salivary glands can be involved in mumps, sarcoidosis, tuberculosis, lymphoma, and Sjögren's syndrome (Chap. 273). The latter may cause dry eyes and dry mouth (*xerostomia*) and be associated with features of connective tissue diseases, including rheumatoid arthritis or systemic lupus erythematosus. Xerostomia may also be due to medications such as diuretics, antihistamines, or tricylic antidepressants as well as therapeutic irradiation for head and neck cancer. It may cause *cervical or incisal caries* and oral candidiasis. Management includes fluoride mouth rinses and topical applications, saliva substitutes, salivary stimulation with sugarless candies, and the avoidance of sugar-containing drinks or food. Candidiasis is treated with nystatin or other antifungals. Salivary stones (*sialolithiasis*), usually in the duct of a major salivary gland, cause *sialoadenitis* with pain and swelling, often on eating. Recurrent parotitis without apparent cause is seen in children.

The commonest neoplasm of the salivary glands is the *pleomorphic adenoma* which is benign but will recur unless fully enucleated; malignant tumors include *mucoepidermoid carcinoma*, *adenoid cystic carcinoma*, and *adenocarcinoma*. The pleomorphic adenoma causes a firm, slowly growing mass in the parotid, palate, or cheek while malignant tumors grow faster and can cause ulceration and invade nerves, producing numbness or facial paralysis.

NEUROLOGIC DISTURBANCES AND OROFACIAL PAIN

The mouth and face may be the site of pain from a number of vascular, neurologic, muscle/connective tissue, or joint conditions. Interdisciplinary diagnosis and management programs involving neurologists, restorative dentists, oral surgeons, otorhinolaryngologists, and other specialists, together with new imaging techniques to diagnose or exclude organic lesions, have begun to clarify this complex field. *Temporal arteritis* causes pain in the face, jaws, and tongue and may mimic temporomandibular joint disease. Glucocorticoids may provide relief. *Myofascial pain* is a dull, constant ache with local tenderness in the muscles of the jaws and difficulty in opening the mouth. This may be related to clenching and grinding habits (*bruxism*). *Arthralgia* of the temporomandibular joint causes local pain which may extend to the face and head. Both myofascial pain and arthralgia can be relieved with heat, rest, and anti-inflammatory agents. Displacement of the meniscus or condyle may cause pain, clenching, or locking of the mandible in the open position. The joint may become involved in *osteoarthritis* with minimal symptoms, while *rheumatoid arthritis* causes pain and swelling in the joint, limitation of movement and, in the *juvenile* form, severe malocclusion in children. *Ankylosis* may occur, necessitating condylectomy (see Chap. 270).

Trigeminal neuralgia (tic douloureux) causes sudden, severe, unilateral lancinating pain initiated by touching a "trigger zone" or occurring spontaneously. Confusion with pulpal or periapical pain is common, leading to inappropriate endodontic or surgical therapy. Many cases respond to carbamazepine and phenytoin although, for a few, surgical intervention to decompress the trigeminal nerve is indicated. Similar symptoms in the distribution of the ninth cranial nerve (tongue, pharynx, soft palate) are due to *glossopharyngeal neuralgia*, which may be triggered by swallowing and may produce referred pain in the temporomandibular joint. *Postherpetic neuralgia* may follow trigeminal herpes zoster (see Chap. 360) and cause burning, aching, and long-lasting pain. *Facial palsy* is usually unilateral and may be due to trauma, surgical intervention, tumor, or infection of the seventh cranial nerve. *Bell's palsy* is a form with acute onset and unknown cause, possibly viral infection such as herpes zoster. The corner of the mouth droops, there may be difficulty in speech, eating, and in closing the eye. The symptoms usually disappear spontaneously but residual facial immobility and lip drooping may persist. Abnormal or reduced *taste sensation* may be due to xerostomia, disturbances of the facial and glossopharyngeal nerves or their central connections, aging, or the wearing of dentures. Disease involving the hypoglossal nerve may cause atrophy of the tongue muscles with protrusion, if bilateral, or deviation towards the affected side, if unilateral.

REFERENCES

GENCO R et al: *Contemporary Periodontics*. St. Louis, Mosby, 1989

GREENSPAN D et al: *AIDS and the Dental Team*. Chicago, Yearbook, 1987

LYNCH MA et al: *Burket's Oral Medicine, Diagnosis and Treatment*, 8th ed. Philadelphia, Lippincott, 1984

NEWBRUN E: *Cariology*, 3d ed. Chicago, Quintessence, 1989

WRIGHT BA et al: *Oral Cancer: Clinical and Pathological Considerations*. Boca Raton, Fla. CRC Press, 1988

42 DYSPHAGIA

RAJ K. GOYAL

Dysphagia is defined as a sensation of "sticking" or obstruction of the passage of food through the mouth, pharynx, or the esophagus.

Dysphagia should be distinguished from other symptoms related to swallowing. *Aphagia* signifies complete esophageal obstruction, which is usually due to bolus impaction and represents a medical emergency. *Difficulty in initiating a swallow* occurs in disorders of the voluntary phase of swallowing. Once initiated, however, swallowing is completed normally. *Odynophagia* means painful swallowing. Frequently, odynophagia and dysphagia occur together. *Globus hystericus* is the sensation of a lump lodged in the throat. No difficulty, however, is encountered when actual swallowing is performed. *Phagophobia,* meaning fear of swallowing, and *refusal to swallow* may occur in hysteria, rabies, tetanus, and pharyngeal paralysis due to fear of aspiration. Painful inflammatory lesions that cause odynophagia may also cause refusal to swallow. Some patients may feel the food as it goes down the esophagus. This esophageal sensitivity is not associated with sticking of the food or obstruction, however. Similarly, the *feeling of fullness in the epigastrium* that occurs after a meal or after swallowing air should not be confused with dysphagia.

PHYSIOLOGY OF SWALLOWING The process of swallowing begins with a voluntary (oral) phase during which a bolus of food is pushed backward into the pharynx. The bolus activates oropharyngeal sensory receptors which initiate the involuntary (pharyngeal and esophageal) phase, or deglutition reflex. The deglutition reflex is a complex series of events which serves both to propel food through the pharynx and the esophagus and to prevent its entry into the airway. At the same time as the bolus is propelled backward by the tongue, the larynx moves forward and the upper esophageal sphincter opens. As the bolus moves into the pharynx, contraction of the superior pharyngeal constrictor against the contracted soft palate initiates a peristaltic contraction that proceeds rapidly downward to move the bolus through the pharynx and the esophagus. The lower esophageal sphincter opens as the food enters the esophagus and remains open until the peristaltic contraction has swept the bolus into the stomach. Peristaltic contraction in response to a swallow involves inhibition followed by sequential contraction of muscles along the entire swallowing passage and is called *primary peristalsis.* The inhibition that precedes the peristaltic contraction is called *deglutitive inhibition*. Local distention of the esophagus due to food activates intramural reflexes in the smooth muscle and results in *secondary peristalsis,* limited to the thoracic esophagus. *Tertiary contractions* are nonperistaltic as they occur simultaneously over a long segment of the esophagus. Tertiary contractions may occur in response to a swallow or esophageal distention, or they may occur spontaneously.

PATHOPHYSIOLOGY OF DYSPHAGIA The normal transport of an ingested bolus through the swallowing passage depends on (1) the size of the ingested bolus, (2) the luminal diameter of the swallowing passage, (3) the peristaltic contraction, and (4) deglutitive inhibition, including normal relaxation of upper and lower esophageal sphincters during swallowing. Dysphagia caused by a large bolus or luminal narrowing is called *mechanical dysphagia,* while dysphagia due to incoordination or weakness of peristaltic contractions or to impaired deglutitive inhibition is called *motor dysphagia*.

Mechanical dysphagia Mechanical dysphagia could be caused by a very large food bolus, intrinsic narrowing, or extrinsic compression of the lumen. In an adult, the esophageal lumen can distend up to a diameter of 4 cm because of the elasticity of the esophageal wall. When the esophagus cannot dilate beyond 2.5 cm in diameter, dysphagia can occur, but it is always present when it cannot distend beyond 1.3 cm. Circumferential lesions produce dysphagia more consistently than do lesions that involve only a portion of circumferences of the esophageal wall, as uninvolved segments retain their distensibility. The causes of mechanical dysphagia are listed in Table 42-1. Common causes include: (1) carcinoma, (2) peptic and other benign strictures, and (3) lower esophageal ring.

Motor dysphagia Motor dysphagia may result from difficulty in initiating a swallow or abnormalities in peristalsis and deglutitive inhibition due to diseases of the esophageal striated or smooth muscle.

Diseases of the striated muscle involve the pharynx, upper esophageal sphincter, and the upper part of the esophagus. The striated muscle is innervated by a somatic component of the vagus with cell bodies of the lower motor neurons located in the nucleus ambiguus. These neurons are cholinergic and excitatory and are the sole determinant of the muscle activity. Peristalsis in the striated muscle segment is due to sequential central activation of neurons innervating muscles at different levels along the esophagus. Motor dysphagia of the pharynx results from neuromuscular disorders causing muscle paralysis, simultaneous nonperistaltic contraction, or loss of opening of the upper esophageal sphincter. Loss of opening of the upper sphincter is caused by paralysis of geniohyoid and other suprahyoid muscles or loss of deglutitive inhibition of the cricopharyngeus muscle. Because each side of the pharynx is innervated by ipsilateral nerves, a lesion of motor neurons occurring only on one side leads to unilateral pharyngeal paralysis. Although lesions of striated muscle also involve the cervical part of the esophagus, the clinical manifestations of pharyngeal dysfunction usually overshadow the manifestations due to esophageal involvement.

Diseases of the smooth muscle segment involve the thoracic part of the esophagus and the lower esophageal sphincter. The smooth muscle is innervated by the parasympathetic component of the vagal preganglionic fibers and postganglionic neurons in the myenteric ganglia. These nerves exert a predominantly inhibitory influence on the lower esophageal sphincter and cause inhibition followed by contraction in the esophageal body. Peristalsis in this segment is due to neuromuscular mechanisms in the wall of the esophagus itself. Dysphagia results when the peristaltic contractions are weak or nonperistaltic or when the lower sphincter fails to open normally. Loss of contractile power occurs due to muscle weakness, as in scleroderma, or to loss of myenteric neurons, as in achalasia. The cause of nonperistaltic contractions, typically seen in diffuse esoph-

TABLE 42-1 Causes of dysphagia

Mechanical dysphagia	Motor (neuromuscular) dysphagia
I Luminal	*I* Difficulty in initiating swallowing reflex
A Large bolus	*A* Oral lesions and paralysis of tongue
B Foreign body	*B* Oropharyngeal anesthesia
II Intrinsic narrowing	*C* Lack of saliva (e.g., Sjögren's syndrome)
A Inflammatory condition causing edema and swelling	*D* Lesions of sensory components of vagus and glossopharyngeal nerves
1 Stomatitis	*E* Lesions of swallowing center
2 Pharyngitis, epiglottitis	*II* Disorders of pharyngeal and esophageal striated muscle
3 Esophagitis	*A* Muscle weakness
a Viral (herpes simplex, varicella-zoster, cytomegalovirus)	*1* Lower motor neuron lesion (bulbar paralysis)
b Bacterial	*a* Cerebrovascular accident
c Fungal (candidal)	*b* Motor neuron disease
d Mucocutaneous bullous diseases	*c* Poliomyelitis
B Webs and rings	*d* Polyneuritis
1 Pharyngeal (Plummer-Vinson syndrome)	*e* Amyotrophic lateral sclerosis
2 Esophageal (congenital, inflammatory)	*f* Familial dysautonomia
3 Lower esophageal mucosal ring (Schatzki ring)	*2* Neuromuscular
C Benign strictures	*a* Myasthenia gravis
1 Peptic	*3* Muscle disorders
2 Caustic and pill-induced	*a* Polymyositis
3 Inflammatory (Crohn's disease, candidal, mucocutaneous lesions)	*b* Dermatomyositis
4 Ischemic	*c* Myopathies (myotonic dystrophy, oculopharyngeal myopathy)
5 Postoperative, postirradiation	*B* Simultaneous onset contractions or impaired deglutitive inhibition
6 Congenital	*1* Pharynx and upper esophagus
D Malignant tumors	*a* Rabies
1 Primary carcinoma	*b* Tetanus
a Squamous cell carcinoma	*c* Extrapyramidal tract disease
b Adenocarcinoma	*d* Upper motor neuron lesions (pseudobulbar paralysis)
c Carcinosarcoma	*2* Upper esophageal sphincter (UES)
d Pseudosarcoma	*a* Paralysis of suprahyoid muscles (causes same as paralysis of pharyngeal musculature)
e Lymphoma	*b* Cricopharyngeal achalasia
f Melanoma	*III* Disorders of esophageal smooth muscle
g Kaposi's sarcoma	*A* Paralysis of esophageal body causing weak contractions
2 Metastatic carcinoma	*1* Scleroderma and related collagen vascular diseases
E Benign tumors	*2* Hollow visceral myopathy
1 Leiomyoma	*3* Myotonic dystrophy
2 Lipoma	*4* Metabolic neuromyopathy (amyloid, alcohol?, diabetes?)
3 Angioma	*5* Achalasia (classical)
4 Inflammatory fibroid polyp	*B* Simultaneous-onset contractions or impaired deglutitive inhibition
5 Epithelial papilloma	*1* Esophageal body
III Extrinsic compression	*a* Diffuse esophageal spasm
A Cervical spondylitis	*b* Achalasia (vigorous)
B Vertebral osteophytes	*c* Variants of diffuse esophageal spasm
C Retropharyngeal abscess and masses	*2* Lower esophageal sphincter
D Enlarged thyroid gland	*a* Disorders of achalasia
E Zenker's diverticulum	*(1)* Primary
F Vascular compression	*(2)* Secondary
1 Aberrant right subclavian artery	*(a)* Chagas' disease
2 Right-sided aorta	*(b)* Carcinoma
3 Left atrial enlargement	*(c)* Lymphoma
4 Aortic aneurysm	*(d)* Neuropathic intestinal pseudoobstruction syndrome
G Posterior mediastinal masses	*(e)* Toxins and drugs
H Pancreatic tumor, pancreatitis	*b* Lower esophageal muscular (contractile) ring
I Postvagotomy hematoma and fibrosis	

ageal spasm, is not understood. Impairment of deglutitive inhibition of the lower esophageal sphincter is associated with a defect in inhibitory nerves to the sphincter and is the major cause of dysphagia in achalasia.

The causes of motor dysphagia are listed in Table 42-1. The important causes are pharyngeal paralysis, cricopharyngeal achalasia, scleroderma of the esophagus, achalasia, diffuse esophageal spasm and related motor disorders.

APPROACH TO THE PATIENT WITH DYSPHAGIA **History** The history can provide a correct presumptive diagnosis in over 80 percent of patients. The type of food causing dysphagia provides useful information. Difficulty only with solids implies mechanical dysphagia with a lumen that is not severely narrowed. The impacted bolus may be forced through the narrowed area by drinking liquids. In advanced obstruction dysphagia occurs with liquids as well as solids. In contrast, motor dysphagia due to achalasia and diffuse esophageal spasm is equally affected by solids and liquids from the very onset. Patients with scleroderma have dysphagia to solids that is unrelated to posture and to liquids in the recumbent but not in the upright posture. When peptic stricture develops in these patients dysphagia becomes more persistent.

The duration and course of dysphagia are helpful in diagnosis. Transient dysphagia of short duration may be due to an inflammatory process. Progressive dysphagia of a few weeks' to a few months' duration is suggestive of carcinoma of the esophagus. Episodic dysphagia to solids of several years' duration indicates a benign disease and is characteristic of a lower esophageal ring.

The localization of dysphagia is helpful when it is described in the chest, where the site of dysphagia generally correlates with the site of esophageal obstruction. However, localization of dysphagia to the neck is of no diagnostic value because lesions of even the lower esophagus may cause dysphagia to be perceived in the neck.

Associated symptoms provide important diagnostic clues. Nasal regurgitation and tracheobronchial aspiration with swallowing are hallmarks of pharyngeal paralysis or a tracheoesophageal fistula. Tracheobronchial aspiration unrelated to swallowing may be secondary to achalasia, a Zenker's diverticulum, or gastroesophageal reflux. Severe weight loss out of proportion to the degree of dysphagia is highly suggestive of carcinoma. When hoarseness precedes dysphagia, the primary lesion is usually in the larynx. Hoarseness following dysphagia may suggest involvement of the recurrent laryngeal nerve by extension of esophageal carcinoma beyond the walls of the esophagus. Sometimes hoarseness may be due to laryngitis secondary to gastroesophageal reflux. Association of laryngeal symptoms and dysphagia also occurs in various neuromuscular disorders. Hiccups suggest a lesion in the distal portion of the esophagus. Unilateral wheezing with dysphagia indicates a mediastinal mass involving the esophagus and a large bronchus. Chest pain with dysphagia occurs in diffuse esophageal spasm and in related motor disorders. Chest pain resembling diffuse esophageal spasms also may occur in acute aphagia due to a large bolus. A prolonged history of heartburn and reflux preceding dysphagia indicates peptic stricture. Similarly, a history of prolonged nasogastric intubation, ingestion of caustic agents, ingestion of pills without water, previous radiation therapy, or associated mucocutaneous diseases may provide the cause of esophageal stricture. If odynophagia is present, candidal or herpes esophagitis should be suspected. In patients with AIDS or other immunodeficiency states, esophagitis due to opportunistic infections such as *candida*, herpes simplex virus, cytomegalovirus, and tumors such as Kaposi's sarcoma and lymphoma should be suspected.

Physical examination Physical examination is important in motor dysphagia due to skeletal muscle, neurologic, and oropharyngeal diseases. Signs of bulbar or pseudobulbar palsy, including dysarthria, dysphonia, ptosis, tongue atrophy, and hyperactive jaw jerk, in addition to evidence of generalized neuromuscular disease, should be carefully searched for. The neck should be examined for thyromegaly or a spinal abnormality. A careful inspection of the mouth and pharynx should disclose lesions that may cause interference with passage of food from the mouth or esophagus because of pain or obstruction. Changes in the skin and extremities may suggest a diagnosis of scleroderma and other collagen vascular diseases, or mucocutaneous diseases such as pemphigoid or epidermolysis bullosa which may involve the esophagus. Metastatic diseases to lymph nodes and liver may be evident. Pulmonary complications of acute aspiration pneumonia or chronic aspiration may be present.

Diagnostic procedures Dysphagia is one of the major symptoms of esophageal disease, and a cause for this symptom can invariably be determined. Therefore, all patients with dysphagia must be thoroughly investigated until a specific cause is determined. This is particularly important because the treatment depends upon the underlying cause of dysphagia. Barium swallow with cineradiography, esophagogastroscopy with biopsy and exfoliative cytology, and esophageal motility study are the main diagnostic procedures (see Chap. 237). The treatment is dependent upon the cause of dysphagia.

REFERENCES

CASTELL DO, JOHNSON LF (eds): *Esophageal Function in Health and Disease*. New York, Elsevier Biomedical, 1983

DURANCEAU A et al: Oropharyngeal dysphagia and operations on the upper esophageal sphincter. Surg Annu 19:317, 1987

ENTERLINE H, THOMPSON, J: *Pathology of the Esophagus*. New York, Springer-Verlag, 1984

FRIEDMAN SL, OWEN RL: Gastrointestinal manifestations of AIDS and other sexually transmitted diseases, in *Gastrointestinal Diseases*, MH Sleisenger, JS Fordtran (eds). Philadelphia, Saunders, 1989, pp 1250–1251

GIDDA JS, GOYAL RK: Regional gradient of initial inhibition and refractoriness in esophageal smooth muscle. Gastroenterology 89:843, 1985

GOYAL RK, PATERSON WG: Esophageal motility, in *Handbook of Physiology: Gastrointestinal System I. American Physiological Society 1989, pp 865–908*

OTT DJ: Radiologic evaluation of esophageal dysphagia. Curr Probl Diag Radiol 17:1, 1975

SCHULZE-DELNIEU K, CHRISTENSEN J: The esophagus, in *The Gastroenterology Annual*, F Kern, A Blum (eds). New York, Elsevier Science, 1984, pp 1–28

43 ANOREXIA, NAUSEA, VOMITING, AND INDIGESTION

LAWRENCE S. FRIEDMAN / KURT J. ISSELBACHER

ANOREXIA

Anorexia is a loss of appetite or lack of desire to eat. It must be differentiated from specific food intolerances and early satiety, a sense of fullness after the ingestion of a small amount of food. Anorexia is a prominent symptom in a wide variety of intestinal and extraintestinal disorders but as an isolated symptom is of little specific diagnostic value.

The mechanisms whereby hunger and appetite are modified in various disease states are poorly understood. Food intake is regulated by two hypothalamic centers—a lateral "feeding center" and a ventromedial "satiety center." The latter inhibits the feeding center following a meal, leading to the sensation of satiety. The brain-gut peptide cholecystokinin (CCK) appears to have a satiety effect and may be involved in the regulation of feeding behavior.

Anorexia is commonly seen in *diseases of the gastrointestinal tract and liver*. For example, it may precede the appearance of jaundice in acute hepatitis, or it may be a prominent symptom in gastric carcinoma. In the setting of intestinal disease, anorexia should be clearly differentiated from *sitophobia* (fear of eating because of subsequent abdominal discomfort). In such circumstances, appetite may persist, but the ingestion of food is curtailed nonetheless. Sitophobia may occur, for example, in regional enteritis (especially with partial obstruction) or in chronic mesenteric vascular insufficiency ("abdominal angina").

Anorexia may also be a prominent feature of *extraintestinal diseases*. Chronic pain from any source may lead to loss of appetite. Anorexia may be profound in severe congestive heart failure and may be a major symptom in patients with uremia, respiratory failure, and various endocrinopathies (e.g., hyperparathyroidism, Addison's disease, and panhypopituitarism). In patients with cancer, anorexia may result from anxiety, depression, pain, a decreased sense of taste and smell, the effect of the tumor on the gastrointestinal tract (e.g., partial intestinal obstruction) or liver (metastases), chemotherapeutic agents, and, possibly, the release of an anorectic substance by the tumor (possibly tumor necrosis factor). Medications such as antihypertensives, diuretics, digitalis, and narcotic analgesics may cause anorexia. Finally, anorexia often accompanies psychogenic disturbances such as depression and may result from emotional upset, boredom, or exposure to unpleasant sights, odors, or thoughts. For a discussion of anorexia nervosa, see Chap. 73.

NAUSEA AND VOMITING

Nausea and vomiting may occur independently of each other but generally are closely allied and are presumed to be mediated by the same neural pathways, so that they may be considered together. *Nausea* denotes the feeling of an imminent desire to vomit, usually referred to the throat or epigastrium. *Vomiting* (or emesis) refers to the forceful oral expulsion of gastric contents. *Retching* denotes the labored rhythmic contraction of respiratory and abdominal musculature that frequently precedes or accompanies vomiting.

Nausea often precedes or accompanies vomiting. It is usually associated with diminished functional activity of the stomach (e.g., hypotonicity, hypoperistalsis, and hyposecretion) and altered small-intestinal motility (e.g., hypertonicity and reversed peristalsis of the duodenum). Often accompanying severe nausea is evidence of altered autonomic (especially parasympathetic) activity, such as skin pallor, increased perspiration, hypersalivation, defecation, and, occasionally, hypotension and bradycardia (vasovagal syndrome); anorexia is also usually present.

Nausea, retching, and hypersalivation frequently precede the act of vomiting, which is a highly integrated sequence of involuntary visceral and somatic motor events. The stomach plays a relatively passive role in the vomiting process, the major ejection force being provided by the abdominal musculature. With relaxation of the gastric fundus and gastroesophageal sphincter, a sharp increase in intraabdominal pressure is brought about by forceful contraction of the diaphragm and abdominal wall muscles. This, together with concomitant annular contraction of the gastric pylorus, results in the expulsion of gastric contents into the esophagus. Increased intrathoracic pressure results in the further movement of esophageal contents into the mouth. Reversal of the normal direction of esophageal peristalsis may play a role in this process. Reflex elevation of the soft palate during the vomiting act prevents the entry of the expelled material into the nasopharynx, whereas reflex closure of the glottis and inhibition of respiration help to prevent pulmonary aspiration.

Repeated emesis may have deleterious effects in a number of ways. The process of vomiting, if forceful, may lead to pressure rupture of the esophagus (Boerhaave's syndrome) or to linear mucosal (Mallory-Weiss) tears in the region of the cardioesophageal junction with resulting hematemesis. Prolonged vomiting may lead to dehydration, the loss of gastric secretions (especially hydrochloric acid) resulting in metabolic alkalosis with hypokalemia, malnutrition with various deficiency states, and dental caries. In states of central nervous system depression (e.g., coma), gastric contents may be aspirated into the lungs, with a resulting aspiration pneumonitis.

VOMITING MECHANISM The act of vomiting is under the control of two functionally distinct medullary centers: the *vomiting center* in the dorsal portion of the lateral reticular formation and the *chemoreceptor trigger zone* in the area postrema of the floor of the fourth ventricle. The vomiting center controls and integrates the actual act of emesis. It receives afferent stimuli from the gastrointestinal tract and other parts of the body, from higher brainstem and cortical centers, especially the labyrinthine apparatus, and from the chemoreceptor trigger zone. Persons vary considerably in the threshold of their vomiting centers to different stimuli. The important efferent pathways in vomiting are the phrenic nerves (to the diaphragm), the spinal nerves (to the intercostal and abdominal musculature), and visceral efferent fibers in the vagus nerve (to the larynx, pharynx, esophagus, and stomach). The vomiting center is located near other medullary centers regulating respiratory, vasomotor, and autonomic functions that may be involved in the act of vomiting.

The chemoreceptor trigger zone by itself is incapable of mediating the act of vomiting; rather activation of this zone results in efferent impulses to the medullary vomiting center, which in turn initiates emesis. The chemoreceptor trigger zone is an emetic chemoreceptor that can be activated by a variety of stimuli or drugs, including apomorphine and other opiates, levodopa (after decarboxylation to dopamine), digitalis, bacterial toxins, radiation, and metabolic abnormalities as occur with uremia and hypoxia.

CLINICAL CLASSIFICATION Nausea and vomiting are common manifestations of many organic and functional disorders. The precise mechanisms triggering vomiting in various clinical conditions are not well understood, making classification of mechanisms difficult.

Many *acute abdominal emergencies* which lead to the "surgical abdomen" are associated with nausea and vomiting. Vomiting may be seen with inflammation of a viscus, as in acute appendicitis or acute cholecystitis, intestinal obstruction, or acute peritonitis (see Chap. 246).

Other *disorders of the alimentary tract,* including those associated with chronic indigestion (see below), are frequently accompanied by nausea and vomiting. In peptic ulcer, emesis may be either spontaneous or self-induced and may lead to relief of symptoms, particularly if antral or pyloric edema has resulted in gastric outlet obstruction. Nausea and vomiting are also prominent in patients with disordered gastrointestinal motility, including postvagotomy, diabetic, or idiopathic gastroparesis (gastric atony), other gastric "dysrhythmias" resulting from abnormal myoelectric activity, and intestinal pseudo-obstruction due to abnormal intestinal myogenic or neurogenic function. Gastroparesis may be demonstrated by gastric scanning after a radiolabeled meal or by radiography after ingestion of indigestible radiopaque solid markers. Experimentally, some patients with otherwise unexplained nausea and vomiting have been demonstrated to have accelerated ("tachygastria") or irregular ("gastric tachyarrhythmia") gastric electrical activity as measured by electrodes implanted surgically on the serosa of the stomach or placed on the abdominal surface ("electrogastrogram"). Typically intestinal obstruction of any cause (e.g., adhesions, malignancy, hernia, volvulus) leads to vomiting, as do other disorders of the liver, pancreas, and biliary tract. Nausea and vomiting may accompany the distention and pain seen in the aerophagic syndromes (see below).

Viral, bacterial, and parasitic *infections of the intestinal tract* are typically associated with severe nausea and vomiting, often with diarrhea. *Acute systemic infections* with fever, especially in young children, are also frequently accompanied by vomiting and often by severe diarrhea. The mechanism whereby infections remote from the gastrointestinal tract produce these manifestations may relate to stimulation of the medullary chemoreceptor trigger zone by toxins or abnormal metabolites.

Central nervous system disorders which lead to increased intracranial pressure (e.g., neoplasms, encephalitis, hydrocephalus) may be accompanied by vomiting, which is often *projectile* (intensely forceful). Vertigo due to disorders of the labyrinthine apparatus, such as acute labyrinthitis and Ménière's disease, may be accompanied by vomiting with nausea and retching. Similarly, motion sickness is typically associated with anorexia, nausea, and vomiting as well as apathy, increased salivation, cold sweating, and headache. Additionally, migraine headaches, tabetic crises, acute meningitis, and the reactive phase of hypotension with syncope may be associated with nausea and vomiting.

Nausea and vomiting may be present in *acute myocardial infarction*, especially when posterior in location or transmural in extent, and in *congestive heart failure*, perhaps in relation to congestion of the liver. The possibility that these symptoms may also be due to drugs (e.g., opiates or digitalis) should always be borne in mind in patients with cardiac disease. Nausea and vomiting are common in cancer patients, especially those who are terminally ill.

Nausea and vomiting commonly accompany several *metabolic and endocrinologic disorders,* including uremia, diabetic ketoacidosis, hypo- and hyperparathyroidism, hyperthyroid crisis, and adrenal insufficiency, especially adrenal crisis. The morning sickness of early pregnancy is another instance of nausea and vomiting possibly related to hormonal changes; the term *hyperemesis gravidarum* is applied when fluid and electrolyte disturbances or nutritional deficiency results.

The *side effects of many drugs and chemicals* include nausea and vomiting. In some cases drugs have central emetic effects, as with digitalis, morphine, histamine, and some chemotherapeutic agents. In other cases drug-induced gastric irritation leads to stimulation of the medullary vomiting center, as with salicylates, aminophylline, and ipecac. The ingestion of a toxin (e.g., food poisoning) may also cause acute vomiting.

Psychogenic vomiting refers to chronic or recurrent vomiting which may result from an emotional or psychological disturbance. Often patients with emotional disorders and chronic vomiting maintain a relatively normal state of nutrition because only a relatively small amount of the ingested food is vomited. In some cases regurgitation rather than vomiting may predominate, and the degree of weight loss may be out of proportion to the patient's description of the frequency and severity of vomiting. As discussed in Chap. 73, anorexia nervosa and bulimia are emotional disturbances which may be associated with vomiting and weight loss.

DIFFERENTIAL DIAGNOSIS Vomiting should be distinguished from *regurgitation,* which refers to the expulsion of food in the absence of nausea and without the abdominal diaphragmatic muscular contraction associated with vomiting. Regurgitation of esophageal contents may occur with esophageal strictures or diverticula. Regurgitation of gastric contents is generally seen with gastroesophageal sphincter incompetence, especially with hiatus hernia and gastroesophageal reflux, with pyloric spasm or obstruction due to peptic ulcer, or with gastroparesis. *Rumination* is the regurgitation, rechewing, and reswallowing of food from the stomach, one mouthful at a time; psychological factors are thought to play a role.

The temporal relationship of vomiting to eating may be of help diagnostically. Vomiting that occurs predominantly in the morning is often seen early in pregnancy and in uremia. Alcoholic gastritis is also commonly accompanied by early-morning retching and emesis, the so-called dry heaves. Vomiting that occurs during or shortly after eating may suggest psychogenic vomiting or peptic ulcer with pylorospasm. Vomiting that occurs 4 to 6 h or longer after eating and involves the elimination of large quantities of undigested food often indicates gastric retention (e.g., pyloric obstruction, gastroparesis) or certain esophageal disorders (achalasia, Zenker's diverticulum). Vomiting that is projectile or without antecedent nausea suggests the possibility of a central nervous system lesion.

Associated symptoms may also provide diagnostic clues. For example, vertigo and tinnitus indicate the possibility of Ménière's disease. A long history of vomiting with little or no weight loss suggests psychogenic vomiting. Relief of abdominal pain with vomiting is typical of peptic ulcer. Early satiety is typical of gastroparesis.

The character of the vomitus also offers clues to the diagnosis. If the vomitus contains large amounts of free hydrochloric acid, gastric outlet obstruction due to an ulcer or a hypersecretory state such as Zollinger-Ellison syndrome should be considered. Absence of free hydrochloric acid is more compatible with gastric malignancy. A feculent or putrid odor reflects the results of bacterial action on the intestinal contents and may occur with distal intestinal obstruction, peritonitis, or gastrocolic fistula. Bile is commonly present in gastric contents whenever vomiting is prolonged; it has no significance unless constantly present in large quantities, when it may signify an obstructing lesion below the ampulla of Vater. The presence of blood in the gastric contents usually denotes bleeding from the esophagus, stomach, or duodenum.

TREATMENT Effective therapy of nausea and vomiting usually depends on correction of the underlying cause. *Antiemetic agents* vary in their usefulness depending on the cause of the symptoms, responsiveness of the patient, and occurrence of side effects. *Antihistamines* such as dimenhydrinate and promethazine hydrochloride are effective for the control of nausea and vomiting due to inner ear dysfunction; they do not act on the chemoreceptor trigger zone and are of little value in other causes of vomiting. *Anticholinergics* such as scopolamine are also effective in motion sickness. *Phenothiazine* derivatives such as prochlorperazine and the structurally related butyrophenone haloperidol inhibit cerebral dopamine receptors and act principally at the chemoreceptor trigger zone. They are often ineffective for severe nausea and vomiting and have the potential for causing sedation, hypotension, and Parkinson-like effects. *Metoclopramide* is the prototype of selective dopamine antagonists called *substituted benzamides*. In contrast to the phenothiazines, which have anticholinergic effects, metoclopramide has powerful peripheral cholinergic effects that enhance gastric emptying. Metoclopramide may be superior to phenothiazines in the treatment of severe nausea and vomiting and is particularly useful in the treatment of gastroparesis. The usual oral dosage is 5 to 20 mg four times daily, but intravenous doses up to 1 to 3 mg/kg may be effective as prophylaxis prior to potent chemotherapeutic agents (e.g., cisplatin). Unfortunately, neurologic side effects are frequent, including muscle spasm, tremor, parkinsonism, and confusion. Experimental agents (not yet licensed for use in the United States) such as *domperidone* and *cisapride* exert peripheral antiemetic effects without the central nervous system side effects of metoclopramide. *Tetrahydrocannabinol*, the active ingredient of marijuana, is marketed as dronabinal for the prevention of nausea and vomiting after cancer chemotherapy; the mechanism of action is unknown.

INDIGESTION

Indigestion is a term frequently used by patients to describe a variety of symptoms generally appreciated as distress associated with the intake of food. The term is nonspecific and may not have the same meaning for the patient and physician. Thus, in approaching the patient with indigestion, it is important for the physician first to elicit a precise description of this complaint. To some patients indigestion refers to actual abdominal pain, pressure, or heartburn. Others may use the term to describe either a vague feeling that digestion has not proceeded naturally or intolerances to specific foods. Still others may use it to describe belching, a feeling of excessive gas, or flatulence. The term *dyspepsia* has often been used interchangeably with indigestion but is increasingly used to refer specifically to upper abdominal pain or discomfort typical of (but not necessarily due to) peptic ulcer.

After having ascertained the patient's definition of indigestion, it is important to determine (1) the location and duration of the discomfort, (2) the temporal relation of the symptoms to the ingestion of food, and (3) the possible relation of the symptoms to the ingestion of specific types of food (e.g., milk, fatty foods) or drugs.

Indigestion may occur in association with diseases of the gastrointestinal tract or pathologic states in other organ systems. As a result of a systematic clinical and laboratory investigation, a definable pathophysiologic process sometimes can be shown to be responsible for the symptoms in a given case of indigestion. Frequently, however, a clear etiologic explanation for the patient's complaint of indigestion cannot be established. If the symptoms are typical of peptic ulcer, but an ulcer is not found, the designation *nonulcer dyspepsia* may be applied. Other cases may be designated as "functional indigestion," with the implication that psychosomatic factors underlie the complaint. Although it is evident that psychological factors may lead to symptoms of indigestion, the designation of "functional indigestion" is rarely a satisfactory explanation, serving only to rephrase the patient's description of the symptoms. Moreover, on the basis of electrophysiologic studies, some cases of functional indigestion, including some cases of nonulcer dyspepsia, appear to result from subtle disturbances of gastrointestinal motility. Indeed, some patients with functional indigestion also have features of the irritable bowel syndrome, suggesting a diffuse intestinal motility disturbance (see Chap. 242).

SYNDROMES COMMONLY DESCRIBED AS INDIGESTION

Pain A careful elucidation of the pattern of pain may provide important diagnostic information. Visceral abdominal pain is mediated by visceral afferent nerves which accompany the abdominal sympathetic pathways (see Chap. 17). Visceral pain is described as dull and aching in nature, with a diffuse midline localization, or as fullness or pressure. The location of the discomfort generally corresponds to the segmental level of neural innervation of the affected organ. Abdominal visceral pain can be produced experimentally by artificially increasing pressure in a hollow viscus and results from distention or exaggerated muscular contraction of the viscus. Inflammation generally lowers the threshold for pain from such stimuli.

The visceral pain of indigestion should be distinguished from the sharp, localized pain patterns of many acute abdominal processes involving the peritoneum. In contrast to visceral pain, this somatic pain is mediated by cerebrospinal afferent nerves.

In view of the diffuse nature of visceral abdominal pain, the main clue to the cause comes from the *location* of the pain and the corresponding segmental level of neural innervation; however, in any given segmental region there is no way of determining which of several viscera is the source of the pain (Table 43-1). The following rules, already described in Chap. 17, are useful: *Substernal pain* of gastrointestinal origin usually arises from disorders of the esophagus

TABLE 43-1 Distribution of visceral pain and examples of disorders frequently involving the specific organ

Organ	Location of pain	Examples of disorders
Esophagus	Substernum, epigastrium	Peptic esophagitis, stricture, esophageal spasm, carcinoma
Stomach	Epigastrium	Gastritis, gastric ulcer, carcinoma
Duodenum (first and second portions)	Epigastrium	Duodenal ulcer
Small intestine (excluding first and second portions of duodenum)	Periumbilical region	Infectious gastroenteritis, regional enteritis, lymphoma, intestinal obstruction
Gallbladder	Epigastrium, right upper quadrant, right upper back	Cholelithiasis, cholecystitis
Pancreas	Epigastrium, left upper quadrant, left side of back	Pancreatitis, pancreatic carcinoma
Liver	Right upper quadrant	Hepatitis, cirrhosis, passive congestion
Colon	Below umbilicus	Infectious colitis, ulcerative colitis, carcinoma, partial obstruction

or cardia of the stomach. Because pain in this area can emanate from the heart, cardiac disease must be carefully considered and excluded. *Epigastric pain* is generally of gastric, duodenal, biliary, or pancreatic origin. (The epigastrium is also a frequent location for "functional" pain.) As pathologic processes in the biliary tract or pancreas become more intense, pain may lateralize and localize, e.g., biliary pain to the right upper quadrant and tip of the scapula and pancreatic pain to the left upper quadrant and back. *Periumbilical pain* is generally associated with disease involving the small intestine. *Pain below the umbilicus* is often of appendiceal, colonic, or pelvic origin.

The unraveling of the *temporal relationships* of the patient's symptoms often provides additional diagnostic clues. It is important to ascertain whether the symptoms are *constant* (continually present over extended periods of time), as may occur with an infiltrating gastric carcinoma, or *intermittent,* as in acute gastritis or biliary colic. The symptoms may have a *diurnal* pattern, as in reflux esophagitis in which pain often occurs nocturnally and with recumbency. Pain that awakens the patient from a sound sleep may occur with duodenal ulcer. Occasionally symptoms are *seasonal,* as in peptic ulcer disease, in which some patients experience more discomfort in the spring and autumn than at other times.

Another helpful diagnostic feature is the relation of pain to *food ingestion.* Early postprandial symptoms may reflect esophageal disease, acute gastritis, or gastric carcinoma. Late postprandial indigestion, i.e., occurring several hours after eating, may reflect failure of the stomach to empty adequately, as in gastric outlet obstruction, gastroparesis and other disorders of gastric motility, or duodenal ulcer, in which case pain results from exposure of ulcerated mucosa to acid secreted by the stomach and unbuffered by food. Conversely, the relief of pain following ingestion of food or antacids is characteristic of duodenal ulcer and is presumably due to the neutralization of acid. Late postprandial indigestion also may result from impaired digestive and absorptive processes, as in pancreatic insufficiency.

It is important to recognize that the pain patterns and relationships to the intake of food described above are generalizations, and many cases do not conform to classic "textbook" descriptions. For example, although pain limited to the right upper quadrant is often caused by gallbladder disease, about half of patients with this condition experience only epigastric pain. Similarly, there are some patients with peptic ulcer whose pain is not relieved by food or antacids; there are other patients with functional indigestion and even gastric carcinoma whose pain improves with food or antacids.

Nonulcer dyspepsia Nonulcer dyspepsia (also referred to as *idiopathic* or *essential dyspepsia*) refers to symptoms that suggest a diagnosis of peptic ulcer despite the absence of an ulcer by endoscopy or barium x-ray studies and the absence of any other demonstrable organic disorder (e.g., biliary tract disease) or evidence of the irritable bowel syndrome to account for the symptoms. Nonulcer dyspepsia is twice as common as peptic ulcer and may affect up to 20 to 30 percent of the population. The pathogenesis is poorly understood; most patients with nonulcer dyspepsia have normal gastric acid secretion, and a relation between nonulcer dyspepsia and duodenitis or duodenal ulcer has not been demonstrated. Similarly, the role of *Helicobacter pylori* and associated chronic gastritis in causing dyspeptic symptoms in persons without peptic ulcer is uncertain (see Chap. 238). A role for disordered gastroduodenal and small-intestinal motility in nonulcer dyspepsia has been suggested but requires further investigation. In contrast to peptic ulcer, nonulcer dyspepsia improves inconsistently following antacids and other standard ulcer therapy.

Heartburn Heartburn, or pyrosis, is a sensation of warmth or burning located substernally or high in the epigastrium with radiation into the neck and occasionally to the arms. Occasional heartburn is common in normal persons, but frequent and severe heartburn is generally a manifestation of esophageal dysfunction. Heartburn may result from abnormal motor activity or distention of the esophagus, reflux of acid or bile into the esophagus, or direct esophageal mucosal irritation (esophagitis).

Heartburn is most often associated with gastroesophageal reflux (see Chap. 237). In this setting, heartburn typically occurs after a large meal, with stooping or bending, or when the patient is supine. It may be accompanied by the spontaneous appearance in the mouth of fluid which may be salty ("water brash"), sour (gastric contents), or bitter and green or yellow (bile). Heartburn may arise following the ingestion of certain foods (e.g., citrus fruit juices) or drugs (e.g., alcohol and aspirin). Characteristically heartburn is alleviated promptly, even if only temporarily, by antacids.

Heartburn may also occur in the absence of a demonstrable anatomic or physiologic condition. In this setting, it is frequently accompanied by aerophagia, which may represent an attempt by the patient to relieve discomfort, and is often attributed to psychological factors for lack of other explanations.

Food intolerance In some persons specific foods or types of foods appear to be related to indigestion. Careful documentation of this relationship is sometimes of great help in arriving at an etiologic diagnosis.

Some foods may be poorly tolerated because of their consistency. Patients with esophageal stricture or carcinoma may tolerate liquids well but may experience discomfort, especially substernal distress, after ingesting solids (see Chaps. 42 and 237). Citrus fruits, with their relatively low pH, often provoke symptoms in patients with peptic ulcer disease or peptic esophagitis. Certain foods may be tolerated poorly because of impaired intestinal digestion or absorption, as with the ingestion of fatty foods in patients with pancreatic or biliary tract disease.

Patients may have a congenital or acquired *deficiency of a specific enzyme* required for intestinal absorption of a certain nutrient. One example is the deficiency of lactase, the intestinal mucosal enzyme which catalyzes the hydrolysis of lactose. In persons who are lactase-deficient, the ingestion of milk (which contains lactose) results in abdominal cramps, distention, diarrhea, and flatulence (Chap. 240). Certain nutrients may lead to profound systemic effects because of *biochemical defects* in the patient that render the substances particularly hazardous, as in galactose intolerance in persons with galactosemia (see Chap. 337).

Some foods may initiate *allergic reactions,* which should be suspected when symptoms occur immediately after ingestion of the food, recur on challenge testing, and are associated with other features of an allergic reaction, such as lip swelling, urticaria, angioedema, asthma, or, rarely, anaphylactic shock. Other foods may exert *toxic effects* on the intestine in susceptible persons (e.g., gluten in patients with celiac sprue).

In many instances we do not understand the mechanism by which indigestion is associated with the ingestion of specific foods. Thus, a history of fatty food intolerance or distress after eating spicy foods is commonly obtained from patients with indigestion; however, the mechanisms leading to these symptoms in these circumstances are often unclear.

Aerophagia Patients with a complaint of *chronic, repetitive eructation* (belching) can usually be observed to precede each belch with a swallow of air, most of which passes only partway down the esophagus and is then regurgitated. Thus, excessive eructation results from *aerophagia,* or air swallowing, not from excessive gas production in the stomach or the intestine. A degree of aerophagia occurs in normal persons, but some individuals gulp air excessively because of chronic anxiety, rapid eating, drinking carbonated beverages, gum chewing, postnasal drip, poorly fitting dentures, or esophageal speech. Because eructation which follows aerophagia may provide a temporary sense of relief to the patient, a vicious cycle of aerophagia and eructation may ensue.

About 20 to 60 percent of intestinal gas represents swallowed air. Because nitrogen and oxygen are the only gases present in the atmosphere in appreciable concentrations and because they are not produced in the gastrointestinal tract, their detection on chromatographic analysis of intestinal gas indicates that swallowed air is the source. Swallowed air that is not eructated passes into the stomach and intestine. Accumulation of swallowed air in the stomach may lead to postprandial fullness and pressure and the finding by x-ray of a large amount of air in the gastric fundus. This symptom complex, referred to as the *magenblase* (i.e., gastric bubble) *syndrome,* may occur when a patient lies supine after a large meal, thereby permitting gastric air to be "trapped" below the gastroesophageal junction by overlying fluid and unable to be eructated. Inability to eructate is also thought to underlie the "gas-bloat" syndrome observed after surgical repair of a hiatal hernia. Acute gastric distention by swallowed air can sometimes produce sharp pains which may mimic angina pectoris. Swallowed air which successfully passes the stomach may either produce diffuse abdominal distention or become trapped in the splenic flexure of the colon. The latter condition, or *splenic flexure syndrome,* is characterized by a sensation of left upper quadrant fullness and pressure with radiation to the left side of the chest. Relief of pain often follows defecation or the expulsion of flatus. The diagnosis is suggested by the finding of increased tympany in the extreme left lateral portion of the upper abdomen on physical examination or of large amounts of air in the splenic flexure of the colon on a plain abdominal radiograph.

Gaseousness, bloating, and flatulence Despite the widely held belief that feelings of *diffuse abdominal pain and bloating* are often caused by excessive quantities of intestinal gas, studies employing an intestinal gas wash-out technique suggest that patients complaining of excessive gas have normal volumes of intestinal gas. The primary abnormality causing functional bloating and pain in such persons appears to be a motility disturbance that causes the patient to perceive pain with an intestinal gas volume that is well tolerated by normal subjects. Alternatively, intestinal motility may be normal in such persons, but they may be excessively responsive to normal impulses arising from the intestinal tract.

A major source of intestinal gas is the fermentative action of intestinal bacteria on carbohydrates and proteins within the lumen. Normally such bacteria are limited to the colon, and the principal gases produced are carbon dioxide and hydrogen (in addition to minute quantities of odoriferous gases—indole, skatols, and sulfur-containing compounds—which give flatus its characteristic odor). In the upper small bowel carbon dioxide is also produced when hydrochloric acid from the stomach or ingested fatty acids are neutralized by bicarbonate. (This may explain, in part, indigestion associated with fatty foods.) About one-third of adults produce appreciable quantities of methane in the colon; this appears to be a familial trait and unrelated to food ingestion.

An increase in intraluminal gas production resulting in *abdominal distention, bloating, and flatulence* occurs following the ingestion of certain foods, such as legumes and some grains, which contain significant quantities of nonabsorbable carbohydrates that pass into the colon where they supply gas-forming substrates for colonic bacteria. The best-studied example of this is beans, which contain oligosaccharides (stachyose and raffinose) that cannot be split by intestinal mucosal enzymes but are metabolized by colonic bacteria. Increased intraluminal gas production may also result from abnormal bacterial colonization of the small intestine (bacterial overgrowth syndrome) or infection with *Giardia lamblia.*

Indigestion due to extraintestinal disease A number of extraintestinal diseases may lead to indigestion. Thus, indigestion may be prominent in congestive heart failure, pulmonary tuberculosis, neoplastic disease, and uremia. Also, a variety of drugs such as aspirin, nonsteroidal anti-inflammatory agents, and glucocorticoids may cause indigestion because of their ulcerogenic properties.

DIAGNOSTIC APPROACH TO THE PATIENT WITH INDIGESTION Indigestion represents a challenging and difficult diagnostic problem because of its nonspecific nature. It is essential to obtain a clear and detailed description of the specific symptoms, particularly the patient's definition of the term indigestion. The nature of the distress, its frequency and time of occurrence, its relationship to meals, and the special circumstances which lead to its exacerbation or relief should be elicited. Associated intestinal symptoms such as nausea and vomiting, abnormal bowel habits, diarrhea, steatorrhea, and melena should be sought, and an assessment of nutritional status, appetite, and changes in weight should be made. A careful history should also include an assessment of the patient's general health, including the possible presence of extraintestinal disorders which may produce indigestion. A careful evaluation of psychological factors is crucial, because they often play an etiologic or contributory role; of particular importance are anxiety, depressive symptoms, and hysteria.

Physical examination rarely establishes the specific diagnosis but may be useful in detecting diseases in other organ systems which can affect intestinal function (e.g., congestive heart failure). Stools should be examined for appearance and occult blood.

Whether further diagnostic studies are indicated depends on the specific nature of the patient's complaints and the patient's age (concern about the possibility of gastrointestinal malignancy being greater in older patients). Abdominal pain may be evaluated with radiologic and imaging studies of the esophagus, stomach, small intestine, colon, pancreas, and biliary tract. Esophagogastroscopy, endoscopic cholangiopancreatography, sigmoidoscopy, or colonoscopy may also be helpful or necessary. On the other hand, in patients under age 40 with epigastric pain typical of peptic ulcer, routine diagnostic studies are unlikely to disclose serious diseases (such as gastric carcinoma) and are often in fact negative; thus, an empiric trial of antacids, H-2-receptor-blocking drugs, or sucralfate may be appropriate. Esophagogastroscopy may be reserved for patients with symptoms that persist despite therapy or that recur soon after therapy is discontinued. In patients with *C. pylori* on endoscopic antral biopsy, a trial of bismuth subsalicylate or an oral antibiotic active against *C. pylori* (or both) may be considered. In individuals complaining of excessive eructation, a simple demonstration that aerophagia reproduces the symptoms may suffice to confirm the diagnosis and hopefully break the habit. Patients complaining of excessive gas, bloating, distention, and flatulence must be questioned carefully about dietary preferences and the relation of symptoms to ingestion of specific foods. In some cases elimination of certain foods (e.g., milk, legumes) from the diet followed by rechallenge may be confirmatory. In other cases a more detailed assessment, including stool examination for fat and muscle fibers and for parasites such as *G. lamblia,* breath tests to detect carbohydrate malabsorption, and gastrointestinal motility studies, may be desirable. The therapeutic value of activated charcoal in reducing gaseousness associated with carbohydrate malabsorption is uncertain.

In many cases of indigestion no clear explanation is obtained, even after careful diagnostic studies and therapeutic trials. Some cases represent nonulcer dyspepsia or intestinal motility disturbances, perhaps due to subtle physiologic derangements not detectable by currently available methods. In some such instances, an empiric trial of dopamine antagonists (e.g., metoclopramide) which augment gastrointestinal motility may be beneficial. Other cases represent early stages of actual disease processes which may only be diagnosed by conventional methods at a later date. Still others are psychogenic and may respond to appropriate psychiatric measures. The ultimate evaluation of indigestion requires, therefore, the utmost in sensitivity, diligence, and concern on the part of the examining physician.

REFERENCES

FELDMAN M: Nausea and vomiting, in *Gastrointestinal Disease*, 4th ed, MH Sleisenger, JS Fordtran (eds). Philadelphia, Saunders, 1989, pp 222–238

HANSON JS, MCCALLUM RW: The diagnosis and management of nausea and vomiting. Am J Gastroenterol 80:210, 1985

HEALTH AND PUBLIC POLICY COMMITTEE, AMERICAN COLLEGE OF PHYSICIANS: Endoscopy in the evaluation of dyspepsia. Ann Intern Med 102:266, 1985

HEATLEY RV, RATHBONE BJ: Dyspepsia: A dilemma for doctors? Lancet ii:779, 1987

LEVITT MD, BOND JH: Intestinal gas, in *Gastrointestinal Disease*, 4th ed, MH Sleisenger, JS Fordtran (eds). Philadelphia, Saunders, 1989, pp 257–263

MALAGELADA J-R, CAMILLERI M: Unexplained vomiting: A diagnostic challenge. Ann Intern Med 101:211, 1984

TALLEY NJ, PHILLIPS SF: Non-ulcer dyspepsia: Potential causes and pathophysiology. Ann Intern Med 108:865, 1988

VANTRAPPEN G et al: Gastrointestinal motility disorders. Dig Dis Sci 31:5S, 1986

44 CONSTIPATION AND DIARRHEA

STEPHEN E. GOLDFINGER

NORMAL COLONIC FUNCTION Each day approximately 9 L of fluid enters the digestive tract; 2 L represents ingested fluids and the remainder comes from salivary, gastric, biliary, pancreatic, and intestinal secretions that are needed to provide an appropriate milieu for food digestion. Most of this fluid is absorbed in the upper bowel. Approximately 1 L containing undigested dietary residue and cellular debris passes across the ileocecal valve to the colon. Little of nutritional value remains following the extensive digestive processing and absorption that occurs in the small intestine. The colon's principal function is to convert this liquid ileal effluent to solid feces before it is advanced to the rectum and evacuated. Several important physiologic processes underlie normal colonic function; among these are *absorption* of fluid and electrolytes; *peristaltic contractions* that facilitate mixing, desiccation, and passage of feces to the rectum; and, finally, *defecation*.

Absorption of fluid and electrolytes (See also Chap. 240) In western societies where dietary fiber content is relatively low, the average daily stool weight is less than 200 g, of which 60 to 80 percent is water. Thus, the colon normally absorbs approximately 80 to 90 percent of the fluid it receives, and this occurs well within its absorptive capacity of 6 L water and 800 mmol sodium per day. Fluid and electrolyte absorption occurs primarily in the ascending and transverse colon. Water absorption occurs passively, osmotically following the active transport of sodium and chloride ions. In addition, bicarbonate is secreted in exchange for chloride. The secreted bicarbonate is converted, in part, to carbon dioxide by reacting with acids produced by colonic bacteria.

The term *diarrhea* generally connotes *frequent* or *loose* stools. Based on physiologic events described above, diarrhea may be defined more quantitatively as a fecal output exceeding 200 g per day when dietary fiber content is low. Diarrhea can be further classified on the basis of underlying mechanisms (see Table 44-1). In *secretory diarrhea*, fecal fluid rich in sodium and potassium is lost as a consequence of impaired absorption and/or excessive secretion of electrolytes by the bowel. In *osmotic diarrhea,* absorption of water is decreased by the osmotic effect of nonabsorbable, intraluminal molecules. *Exudative diarrhea* is caused by an outpouring of necrotic mucosa, colloid, fluid, and electrolytes from an inflamed colon which, in addition, is less able to carry out its normal absorptive function. Increased amounts of arachidonic acid metabolites present in inflamed mucosa may also promote increased ion secretion. *Anatomic derangements* of the bowel and *motility disorders* cause diarrhea by reducing the surface area or the contact time necessary for adequate absorption to occur.

Colonic innervation and motility The colon and rectum are innervated by fibers that release norepinephrine, acetylcholine, and a variety of other neurotransmitters. Signals transmitted by autonomic nervous system fibers originating centrally, local reflex arcs confined to the autonomous "enteric nervous system," and intrinsic contractile responses of smooth muscle all play a part in the coordination of colonic motility. Parasympathetic nerves, which stimulate peristaltic contraction as well as electrolyte secretion, dominate the neurogenic regulation of colonic motor activity; adrenergic tone inhibits cholinergic stimulation and also increases electrolyte absorption. The precise integration of all neural and nonneural mediators of colonic motility and ion transport remains poorly understood.

The basal motor activity of the colon corresponds to the function of its various segments. In the ascending colon, where most fluid absorption occurs, rhythmic, retrograde contractions occur to prolong fecal contact time. In the midcolon, segmental contractions continue the process of absorption while feces are gradually advanced to the left colon. The most distal portion of the colon, which is under the greatest neurogenic control, propels feces caudally in preparation for defecation. In addition, massive peristalsis occurs several times per day.

Since colonic motility plays an important role in both absorption and movement of contents to the rectum, alterations of bowel tone occurring as a result of disease, stress, or various drugs tend to have an important influence on bowel movements. In view of the number of pharmacologic agents that may influence smooth muscle contractility, it is essential to take a careful drug history when evaluating patients with constipation or diarrhea of recent onset.

TABLE 44-1 Classification of diarrhea

Type	Mechanism	Stool characteristics	Examples
Secretory	↑ Secretion of electrolytes ↓ Absorption of electrolytes	Clear Negative osmotic gap* No polymorphs	Cholera Diarrheogenic islet cell tumors Bile salt enteropathy
Exudative	Impaired colonic absorption; outpouring of cells and colloid	Purulent Polymorphs present Gross or occult blood	Ulcerative colitis Shigellosis Amebiasis
Decreased absorption			
Osmotic	Nonabsorbable intraluminal molecules	Clear High osmotic gap* No polymorphs	Lactase deficiency Mg^{2+}-containing cathartics
Anatomic derangement	Decreased absorption surface	Variable	Subtotal colectomy Gastrocolic fistula
Motility disorder	Decreased contact time	Variable	Hyperthyroidism Irritable bowel syndrome

* See Shiau et al.

Defecation The defecatory reflex is initiated by acute distention of the rectum. When it is allowed to progress by supraspinal centers, sigmoidal and rectal contractions heighten the pressure within the rectum and also obliterate the rectosigmoidal angle. Concomitant relaxation of the internal and external anal sphincters then permits the evacuation of feces. This can be augmented by an increase in intraabdominal pressure created by the Valsalva maneuver. Conversely, defecation may be consciously prevented by the voluntary contraction of the striated muscles of the pelvic diaphragm and external anal sphincter. The functional value of voluntary control of defecation requires little elaboration, but the opportunity for individuals to resist the defecatory urge, when abused, may lead to chronic rectal distention, reduced afferent signals, lax tone, and chronic constipation.

DIARRHEA AND CONSTIPATION The bowel habits of apparently healthy persons vary widely. For this reason, the complaint of *diarrhea* and *constipation* should be evaluated in terms of the degree of change from an individual's customary pattern. Reasonably detailed information is important in either abnormality. When patients complain of diarrhea, it is important to obtain an estimate of the volume as well as frequency of fecal output and, whenever possible, to examine directly a stool sample for consistency, blood, oiliness, and malodor. For example, the repeated elimination of small quantities of solid material admixed with gas, so typical in the irritable bowel syndrome, has a far different connotation than the same number of movements of liquid, blood-tinged feces. It is also useful to learn if fecal incontinence is present. Involuntary loss of feces may be an embarrassing symptom for a patient to verbalize, but such information may point to a potentially correctable anal sphincter abnormality. The term *constipation* may be used by the patient to refer to a variety of changes including reduction in frequency of defecation, a constant sensation of rectal fullness with incomplete evacuation of feces, and sometimes painful defecation due to hard stools or perianal pathology. Excessively hard stools are usually due to increased absorption of fluid as a result of prolonged contact of the luminal contents with the colonic mucosa consequent to delayed transit. In an assessment of complaints of diarrhea or constipation, it is important to consider the patient's emotional state since in many instances the recent onset of psychological stress is the major reason for altered bowel habits. However, it can be hazardous to assume this to be the case, even when the relationship seems convincing. For this reason, the judicious use of laboratory, proctoscopic, and radiologic procedures is recommended to make certain that organic disease will not be overlooked.

Acute diarrhea Diarrhea of abrupt onset occurring in otherwise healthy persons is usually due to an infectious cause. A variety of accompanying symptoms are often observed, including fever, headache, anorexia, vomiting, malaise, and myalgia, but they cannot be used to distinguish with certainty among viral, bacterial, and protozoal causes. When bacterial and protozoal pathogens are not recovered from the feces, so-called nonspecific diarrhea is usually considered to be of viral etiology. However, enterotoxin-producing strains of *Escherichia coli*, which are not distinguishable from "normal flora" on routine culture, may account for a number of cases that are usually ascribed to viral infection.

Acute diarrhea presumed to be of viral etiology typically lasts for a period of 1 to 3 days; death is extremely rare except in previously debilitated individuals who become severely dehydrated. When human volunteers have been infected with the Norwalk virus, which is believed to account for approximately one-third of epidemics of acute viral diarrhea in American adults, transient malabsorption of fat and xylose has been described. Changes in the small intestine include abnormalities of intestinal cell morphology such as villous shortening, an increase in the number of crypt cells, and increased cellularity of the lamina propria. The colonic mucosa is unaffected in viral diarrhea; this is consistent with the absence of polymorphonuclear leukocytes when fresh stool is examined microscopically after preparation with Loeffler's methylene blue.

Bacterial diarrhea is likely if there is a history of a similar and simultaneous illness in individuals who have shared contaminated food with the patient. Diarrhea developing within 12 h of the meal is most likely due to ingestion of a preformed toxin (e.g., staphylococcal exotoxin). A lag period of up to 3 days after consumption of contaminated food can occur with salmonellosis. The pathogenesis of bacterial diarrhea is due to two mechanisms, direct mucosal invasion by bacteria and the elaboration of toxins; the latter may cause direct tissue damage (cytotoxin) or promote intestinal secretion without causing any morphologic change (enterotoxin). Invasive bacteria (shigella, salmonella, *Campylobacter, Vibrio parahaemolyticus*) and cytotoxin-producing bacteria (*Clostridium difficile, Escherichia coli* 0157:H7) typically cause edema, leukocytic infiltration, and frank ulceration of colonic mucosa. Lower abdominal cramps and tenderness are prominent, as are tenesmus and rectal urgency. In severe cases the stool is grossly bloody. Microscopic examination of the stool will often reveal neutrophils along with erythrocytes. The prototypical example of enterotoxin-mediated bacterial diarrhea is *cholera*, in which the organism *Vibrio cholerae* adheres to, but does not invade, the surface epithelial cells and releases an enterotoxin which stimulates massive secretion of fluid and electrolytes by the small intestine. This may be produced experimentally in animals by placing the enterotoxin, free of the organism itself, into isolated intestinal loops. Hypersecretion reaches a peak at 4 to 6 h and is mediated by the stimulation of mucosal adenylate cyclase by the toxin. Because mucosal morphology is essentially normal and intestinal absorptive capacity is preserved, cholera is effectively treated by oral rehydration therapy with solutions containing simple sugars and sodium chloride, the former stimulating absorption of the latter. Other species of bacteria that produce enterotoxins include *E. coli, Clostridium, Staphylococcus aureus*, and *Aeromonas*.

Protozoal infections may also be responsible for acute diarrhea. *Entamoeba histolytica*, prevalent in some areas of the United States and in the homosexual male population, produces an inflammatory colitis which can closely mimic idiopathic ulcerative colitis. Giardiasis is a cause of nonexudative diarrhea that may last for weeks or even months; it is acquired by drinking contaminated water. *Cryptosporidial* infection, initially described as occurring in immunocompromised patients, has also been linked to diarrheal illness in otherwise normal persons. Careful microscopic examination of fresh stools by experienced personnel is required for the diagnosis of protozoal infection.

Travelers' diarrhea may result from any one or several of the pathogens described above. When no specific agent is identified, the etiology is usually assumed to be due to enterotoxin-producing coliform organisms or viruses; both Norwalk virus and rotavirus have been implicated. Prolonged bowel irregularity often occurs following the acute illness.

Ulcerative colitis and *Crohn's disease* may begin as acute diarrhea (Chap. 241). Bloody stools, abdominal cramping, tenderness, and fever are often observed. When Crohn's disease is limited to the small bowel (regional enteritis), the diarrhea tends to be milder, is often nonbloody, and is associated with right lower quadrant pain and tenderness. Diarrhea may be caused by a variety of *drugs*, including cholinergic agents, magnesium-containing antacids, antimetabolites used in cancer chemotherapy, and many antibiotics. A necrolytic toxin produced by *Clostridium difficile* is the cause of pseudomembranous colitis occurring during or after antibiotic use. Diarrhea due to *diverticulitis* is usually accompanied by fever, tenesmus, and rectal urgency, together with cramps and tenderness in the left lower quadrant (Chap. 243). When there is no evidence of acute inflammation, diarrhea in the presence of colonic diverticula is probably due to a spastic (irritable) colon, a disorder which may set the stage for the development of diverticula. In elderly and debilitated individuals with *fecal impaction*, the presenting symptom may be the frequent expulsion of small amounts of liquid stool overflowing from colonic distention behind the impaction. This is sometimes termed *paradoxical diarrhea*. Fecal incontinence due to anal sphincter impairment is a problem that may be encountered in certain neurologic disorders or following local surgical procedures (e.g., hemorrhoidectomy, episiotomy). Acute *psychological stress* can cause diarrhea at any age.

DIAGNOSTIC APPROACH The appropriate tempo and approach in the evaluation of acute diarrhea depend so heavily on the clinical setting in which it occurs that only very general guidelines can be offered. It is entirely reasonable to withhold studies in mild, self-limited cases such as are seen as part of an epidemic viral illness. When dealing with sporadic severe diarrhea or when a suggestive epidemiologic history is obtained, bacterial cultures and microscopic examination of the stool for parasites and inflammatory cells are appropriate. Proctoscopy is generally reserved for patients with bloody diarrhea or those who show no improvement within 10 days. Likewise, radiologic studies should usually be deferred until the initial course of the illness has been observed. In cases of massive fluid loss, measurement of serum electrolytes is useful to aid in determining replacement therapy.

TREATMENT General and nonspecific treatment of acute diarrhea includes rest and encouragement of fluid intake. Intravenous fluid and electrolyte replacement may be necessary in infants and the elderly. The use of opiate-containing drugs to control diarrhea is potentially dangerous if an enteroinvasive organism is suspected, but is a reasonable comfort measure in cases of mild, undifferentiated diarrhea. As a result of success achieved with cholera patients, the use of oral sugar-electrolyte solutions is being extended to the treatment of patients with acute diarrhea considered to be due to other enterotoxin-producing bacteria. The relative pros and cons of antimicrobial treatment of specific enteric infections are reviewed in their respective sections of this textbook. Biofeedback therapy has proved helpful for some patients who suffer from fecal incontinence due to anal sphincter impairment.

Chronic diarrhea Diarrhea persisting for weeks or months, whether constant or intermittent, may be a functional symptom or a manifestation of serious illness. For this reason, it is incumbent upon the physician to search carefully for evidence of organic disease, such as fever, weight loss, malnutrition, or anemia. Abdominal tenderness and fever suggest the presence of inflammation. When there is involvement of the large bowel, the major diseases to be considered include ulcerative colitis, Crohn's disease of the colon, amebiasis, and diverticulitis. Crohn's disease of the small intestine may involve one or more of its segments. The ileum is most frequently affected. Other diarrheal conditions that may resemble Crohn's disease radiographically include tuberculous and fungal enteritis, lymphoma, amyloidosis, and argentaffin (carcinoid) tumors of the small bowel.

Prolonged diarrhea without evidence of inflammation may reflect a primary malabsorptive disorder. Selective derangements of absorption, such as those due to *bile salt enteropathy* and *lactase deficiency,* are usually not accompanied by weight loss or malnutrition. *Mucosal disorders,* best exemplified by sprue, are frequently associated with weight loss, malodorous stools, abdominal distention, and anemia, and, when more severe, with osteomalacia, bleeding due to hypoprothrombinemia, avitaminotic neuropathies, and tetany. Both osmotic and secretory mechanisms contribute to the diarrhea of sprue. *Pancreatic insufficiency* resulting from chronic pancreatitis, carcinoma, resection, or cystic fibrosis produces steatorrhea and weight loss of varying severity. A number of factors may be responsible for *postgastrectomy diarrhea* (see Chap. 238). These include the dumping syndrome, postvagotomy motility derangements, inadequate stimulation of pancreatic digestive enzymes, and incomplete mixing of these enzymes with food. On rare occasions severe postgastrectomy diarrhea and malnutrition are due to the inadvertent creation by the surgeon of a gastroileostomy instead of a gastrojejunostomy. *Bacterial overgrowth* in the small intestine, as may occur with extensive diverticulosis and prolonged bowel stasis secondary to disorders of peristalsis (e.g., scleroderma, diabetic visceral neuropathy), can also lead to chronic diarrhea and weight loss. This has been attributed to the secretory action of deconjugated bile salts and hydroxylated fatty acids that are produced by bacterial enzymes, to consumption of nutrients by the microorganisms, and to mucosal abnormalities believed to be caused by bacteria or their metabolites (see Chap. 240). At times, diarrhea may accompany stasis in the absence of bacterial overgrowth.

Endocrine disorders that may be accompanied by chronic diarrhea include thyrotoxicosis, diabetes mellitus, adrenal insufficiency, and hypoparathyroidism. The release of potent secretagogues from neoplastic tissue in the Zollinger-Ellison syndrome (gastrin), medullary carcinoma of the thyroid (calcitonin, prostaglandins), the pancreatic cholera syndrome (vasoactive intestinal peptide), and the carcinoid syndrome (serotonin) makes diarrhea a prominent feature of these disorders. *Rectal villous adenomas* may secrete large quantities of fluid and electrolytes, which are promptly evacuated as a clear, odorless liquid. When marked fluid loss occurs, hypokalemia and dehydration may result.

Habitual *cathartic abuse* must be suspected when the cause of prolonged diarrhea remains perplexing. Even if this is denied by the patient, a stool sample should be alkalinized with sodium hydroxide; this will produce a lavender color if phenolphthalein-containing laxatives have been surreptitiously ingested. The observation of melanosis coli by sigmoidoscopy indicates chronic usage of anthraquinone laxatives.

Constipation Constipation is a common complaint often resulting from the inordinate expectation of "regularity" in bowel-conscious individuals. Stools are described as infrequent, incomplete, or unduly hard; unusual straining may be required to achieve defecation. A review of the patient's habits often reveals contributory and correctable causes, such as insufficient dietary roughage, lack of exercise, suppression of defecatory urges arising at inconvenient moments, inadequate allotment of time for full defecation, and prolonged travel. Appropriate adjustments of these patterns and reassurance are preferable to the prescription of laxatives and may be all that is required for improvement. When the patient also has symptoms such as fatigue, malaise, headaches, or anorexia, the possibility should be considered that such symptoms reflect an underlying depression of which constipation is but one component. Decreased colonic motility is responsible for the constipation associated with the use of parasympatholytic drugs, spinal cord injury, scleroderma, and Hirschsprung's disease. A variety of derangements have been described in patients with severe idiopathic constipation. These include: histopathologic abnormalities of the myenteric plexi; functional outlet obstruction during defecation due to incomplete relaxation of the internal anal sphincter; excessive contraction of the external sphincter (anismus); a reduced anorectal angle as detected by defecatory radiography; and absence of rectosigmoid myoelectric and pressure responses to feeding. It is uncertain whether these abnormalities represent primary or secondary events and whether any of them will be responsive to specific therapeutic interventions.

Hemorrhoids, anal fissures, perineal abscesses, and rectal strictures often prevent easy and adequate stool evacuation. When constipation and tenesmus of recent onset are reported, the possibility of carcinoma of the rectum or sigmoid colon must be seriously considered. In such instances sigmoidoscopic and barium enema examinations should be obtained early and are virtually obligatory if fecal blood has been observed or if occult blood is detected on any of three successive stool specimens. Stools of abnormally thin caliber occur in patients with rectal or sigmoid colon carcinoma but are more commonly due to a spastic colon. Other mechanical causes of constipation include volvulus of the sigmoid colon, diverticulitis, intussusception, and hernias. A variety of metabolic abnormalities, such as hypothyroidism, hypercalcemia, hypokalemia, porphyria, lead poisoning, and dehydration are often associated with constipation. Prolonged fecal retention, leading to impaction, may occur in certain neurologic disorders (e.g., spinal cord injury, multiple sclerosis, cerebral palsy, senility), and in these instances, when autonomous regulation of evacuation is unachievable, vigorous and sustained enema programs are often necessary.

IRRITABLE BOWEL The irritable bowel syndrome (also referred to as *spastic colon* and *mucous colitis*) is one of the most frequent gastrointestinal disorders (see Chap. 243). This condition is characterized by periodic or chronic bowel symptoms which include diarrhea, constipation, a sense of incomplete evacuation, and abdominal pain. These symptoms flare during periods of psychological stress, but the anxiety produced by the bowel disturbance is sometimes regarded by the patient as the fundamental cause of the emotional upset. During periods of discomfort, stools are apt to become thin, fragmented, or pelletlike, and are accompanied by excessive mucus and gas. It is estimated that 17 percent of adults have irritable bowel syndrome, but most do not seek medical evaluation; those who do are apt to have greater concern about personal health and fear of illness. Efforts to ameliorate symptoms with mild cathartics or various drugs may yield adverse and exaggerated responses. A number of therapeutic approaches, including the avoidance of foods which tend to upset the patient, addition of bulk-forming agents, judicious use of antispasmodics and tranquilizers, and psychotherapy may provide some degree of relief. If the patient's life goals can be shifted away from the quixotic search for the perfect stool, much can be accomplished. At the same time, it must be remembered that such individuals are not exempt from developing bowel cancer, and any worrisome deviation from their general pattern of derangement must be seriously evaluated.

FLATULENCE A significant amount of flatus is passed each day by normal persons, and the complaint of flatulence often reflects a heightened and embarrassing awareness of this natural occurrence. Excessive quantities of flatus may be caused by aerophagia or the formation of increased amounts of gas by intestinal bacteria. The latter process can be associated with malabsorption syndromes but is more frequently a consequence of eating foods such as beans, broccoli, and cabbage which have a high content of nondigestible polysaccharides. The oligosaccharides stachyose and raffinose, isolated from beans, are particularly effective substrates for fermentation to carbon dioxide, hydrogen, and methane by colonic flora. Chromatographic analysis of a sample of flatus will show these gases to predominate, in contrast to the high nitrogen levels that occur when excessive flatus is caused by aerophagia. The treatment of flatulence is generally undertaken to reduce embarrassment and consists of measures to decrease aerophagia along with avoidance of foods that cause excessive gas.

REFERENCES

Antony MA et al: Infectious diarrhea in patients with AIDS. Dig Dis Sci 33:1141, 1988

Blacklow NR, Cukor GC: Viral gastroenteritis. N Engl J Med 304:397, 1981

Christensen J: Motility of the colon, in *Physiology of the Gastrointestinal Tract*, LR Johnson et al (eds). New York, Raven Press, 1981, vol 1, chap 14

Drossman DA et al: Psychosocial factors in the irritable bowel syndrome. Gastroenterology 95:701, 1988

Field M et al (eds): *Secretory Diarrhea*, Clinical Physiology Series. Bethesda, Md, American Physiological Society, 1980

Gershon MD, Erde SM: The nervous system of the gut. Gastroenterology 80:1571, 1981

Krejs GT, Fordtran JS: Diarrhea, in *Gastrointestinal Disease*, MH Sleisenger, JS Fordtran (eds). Philadelphia, Saunders, 1983, chap 16

Lieberman DA: Common anorectal disorders. Ann Intern Med 101:837, 1984

Read NW et al: Chronic diarrhea of unknown origin. Gastroenterology 78:2644, 1980

Reynolds JC et al: Chronic severe constipation. Gastroenterology 92:414, 1987

Schultz SG: Ion transport by mammalian large intestine, in *Physiology of the Gastrointestinal Tract*, LR Johnson et al (eds). New York, Raven Press, 1981, vol 2, chap 38

Shiau YF et al: Stool electrolyte and osmolality measures in the evaluation of diarrheal disorders. Ann Intern Med 102:773, 1985

Shouler P, Keighley MRB: Changes in colorectal function in severe idiopathic chronic constipation. Gastroenterology 90:414, 1986

Snooks SJ et al: Damage to the innervation of the pelvic floor musculature in chronic constipation. Gastroenterology 89:977, 1985

Waldron D et al: Colonic and anorectal motility in young women with severe idiopathic constipation. Gastroenterology 95:1388, 1985

45 GAIN AND LOSS IN WEIGHT

DANIEL W. FOSTER

GENERAL PRINCIPLES In normal persons weight is stable because food intake is matched to energy expenditure by the coordinated activity of "feeding" and "satiety" centers in the hypothalamus. The signals that regulate the interactions of these centers are probably multifactorial, and both short- and long-term controls are thought to be operative. Whatever the mechanisms, the system is normally efficient over periods of months to years.

Gain or loss in tissue mass is determined by the net balance between food intake and energy expenditure. Food intake is determined by availability and attractiveness of food and by emotional and physical factors. The bulk of energy expenditure is due to basal metabolism and physical activity. The former is defined as the requirement when the body is in the supine position, motionless except for quiet respiration; it is the energy required to maintain structural and functional integrity of the body in the absence of physical activity. About half the total daily intake is normally consumed by basal processes. Nonsedentary persons spend about 40 percent of energy in physical activity; athletes may utilize 50 percent or more of ingested energy in exercise. Persons sedentary because of habit, illness, or obesity expend far less in activity. In nonobese, nonsedentary subjects 10 percent of ingested food is released as heat associated with the absorption of food, a process called *dietary thermogenesis*. This fraction, previously designated *specific dynamic action*, is usually considered a separate component of energy costs. Heat generated during and after exercise and heat released for maintenance of body temperature (*regulatory thermogenesis*) are included in the energy costs of physical activity and basal metabolism, respectively.

Change in body weight as a consequence of voluntary alteration in diet or exercise is never worrisome; change in weight that is not deliberately sought, on the other hand, is a frequent reason for consultation with the physician and often indicates the presence of disease. Changes in weight may reflect alteration in either tissue mass or body fluid content. Even when tissue mass is changing, fluid loss or gain plays a major role in the measured change in weight, particularly over the short run. This point is illustrated in Table 45-1, where the composition of weight loss was estimated during a 24-day period of semistarvation in 13 normal men [daily intake, 4200 kJ (1010 kcal)]. During the first 3 days 70 percent of the decrease in weight was due to water loss, while in subsequent stages a diminution of protein and fat accounted for essentially all the weight loss. This varying contribution of fluid explains why a fixed formula cannot be used for predicting weight loss or gain. It is frequently stated that a net change of 32,000 kJ (7700 kcal) will be accompanied by a 1-kg change in body mass. While this estimate is reasonable for long-term changes in food intake, the apparent cost per kilogram of weight lost or gained varies with the accompanying fluid shifts. In the experiment

TABLE 45-1 Percentage composition of mean daily weight loss in 13 young men during food restriction for 24 days

Days	Mean weight loss, kg/day	Water, %	Fat, %	Protein, %	Food equiv. of weight loss, kJ/kg (kcal/kg)
1–3	0.80	70	25	5	10,900 (2600)
11–13	0.23	19	69	12	29,500 (7000)
22–24	0.17	0	85	15	36,400 (8700)

SOURCE: After Brožek et al.

summarized in Table 45-1, for example, a negative balance of only 10,900 kJ (2600 kcal) resulted in the loss of 1 kg of weight between days 1 and 3, while between days 22 and 24, loss of 1 kg of weight required a deficit of 36,400 kJ (8700 kcal). In general if weight loss or gain has occurred over a period of weeks or months, it is safe to assume that change in tissue mass has occurred; weight loss or gain limited to a several-day period may be due to fluid shifts alone. Occasionally true loss of tissue mass is obscured by fluid retention as in the case of the patient with cirrhosis of the liver who develops ascites or the patient with anorexia nervosa who has significant edema.

WEIGHT GAIN

While obesity is a major public health concern (see Chap. 72), its diagnosis is usually uncomplicated. Obese subjects often deny overeating, but the true situation can be assessed either by tabulating actual food intake and determining its caloric content from standard tables, by interviewing the patient's family and friends, or by estimating metabolic rates from indirect calorimetry.

Regardless of history, excess caloric intake is the cause of obesity in the majority of cases. Pathologic causes are rare. In the adult, Cushing's syndrome can result in acquired obesity, but usually the diagnosis is suggested by the pattern of fat distribution and the clinical picture. Other endocrine diseases such as hypothyroidism, hypogonadism, and insulin-secreting tumors are frequently listed in the differential diagnosis of obesity but do not represent significant diagnostic problems. Congenital diseases that cause obesity such as the Prader-Willi, Laurence-Moon-Biedl, and Alström syndromes are readily recognizable and appear early in life. Rarely, a disease involving the hypothalamus, such as craniopharyngioma, may cause acquired obesity. Extensive workup of the central nervous system is not indicated in obesity, however, in the absence of suspicious symptoms (headache, visual difficulties, vomiting, or endocrine changes).

WEIGHT LOSS

Weight loss in the absence of deliberate dieting is a more serious problem than weight gain, because there is a high chance that organic disease is present. Mechanisms include decreased food intake, accelerated metabolism, and loss of calories in urine or stool, acting singly or in combination. Almost any serious illness can cause weight loss either through direct effects or by inducing malaise and depression. The signals that cause decreased appetite and accelerated tissue loss are not known. The negative nitrogen balance that occurs following trauma, surgery, or stressful illness is likely mediated at least partially by glucagon and other catabolic hormones. Additional candidate molecules for disease-induced weight loss are cytokines such as tumor necrosis factor (cachectin) and adipsin, but proof of their involvement is lacking.

The general categories of disease that need to be considered when weight loss is a prominent complaint are discussed next.

DIABETES MELLITUS Initial weight loss with the onset of diabetes is largely fluid and is due to the osmotic diuresis induced by hyperglycemia. Subsequently, loss of tissue mass occurs in the insulin-dependent form of the disease as a result of caloric wastage (the consequence of glycosuria) and of the hormonal abnormalities that characterize the illness. Insulin deficiency and glucagon excess result in impaired synthesis of protein and fat and simultaneously cause accelerated proteolysis and lipolysis such that the net energy state is catabolic. Weight loss in diabetes is frequently associated with increased food intake.

ENDOCRINE DISEASE Thyrotoxicosis is the most common endocrine disease producing weight loss. Increased appetite and food intake are the rule, and patients often consume a high-carbohydrate diet. Energy expenditure is enormous, primarily because of an increased metabolic rate, but increased motor activity also plays a role. The molecular mechanism whereby thyrotoxicosis causes weight loss is not settled. In rodents thyroid hormone increases Na-K adenosine triphosphatase (ATPase) activity in many tissues resulting in a futile cycle of ATP synthesis and breakdown with energy lost as heat. This abnormality does not appear to operate in humans. Whatever the mechanism, metabolism is ''uncoupled'' in thyrotoxicosis, accounting for excess generation of heat and caloric wastage.

In ''apathetic'' hyperthyroidism weight loss and weakness may predominate with little evidence of nervousness or other symptoms. Another cause of weight loss due to hypermetabolism is pheochromocytoma, the inducing agent being catecholamine release. Panhypopituitarism and adrenal insufficiency are often associated with weight loss, largely as a consequence of diminished appetite secondary to cortisol deficiency.

GASTROINTESTINAL DISEASE Overt or occult steatorrhea due to sprue, chronic pancreatitis, or cystic fibrosis may produce wasting despite major increases in food intake. A variety of other diseases of the gastrointestinal tract cause weight loss: inflammatory bowel disease, parasites, esophageal strictures, obstruction secondary to chronic peptic ulcer, pernicious anemia, and cirrhosis of the liver. Mechanisms of weight loss include anorexia, obstruction with vomiting, malabsorption, and the effects of inflammation. Intraabdominal masses (e.g., massive splenomegaly) act by compressing the stomach, while weight loss in heart failure is due to visceral congestion.

INFECTION Hidden infection must always be sought in patients with unexplained weight loss. Tuberculosis, fungal disease, amebic abscess, and subacute bacterial endocarditis should be high on the list of suspects. Infection with human immunodeficiency virus must be considered, especially in high-risk groups (male homosexuals, intravenous drug users, recipients of multiple transfusions). Weight loss with infection is probably due to inflammatory cytokines.

MALIGNANCY Occult malignancy is probably the most common cause of weight loss in the absence of major signs and symptoms. In the search for malignancy particular emphasis must be placed on the gastrointestinal tract, pancreas, and liver. Lymphoma and leukemia should also be considered. While silent (except for weight loss) malignancy can occur in any organ, the gastrointestinal tract is the most common site. Mechanisms of weight loss in cancer vary, and more than one factor is often operative. Anorexia is usually present, but increased metabolism may also play a role, particularly in lymphomas and leukemias. Thus far, no increase in weight-loss-inducing cytokines has been documented.

PSYCHIATRIC DISEASE The classic psychiatric illness associated with profound weight loss is anorexia nervosa (Chap. 73). Conversion disorders, schizophrenia, and depression may also cause weight loss due to decreased food intake. While organic disease causing both anorexia and depression has to be ruled out, ordinarily the psychiatric nature of the problem will be clear.

RENAL DISEASE One of the earliest manifestations of uremia is anorexia. As a consequence all patients with unexplained weight loss should be given screening renal function tests.

SUMMARY

Weight loss is more often a diagnostic problem than weight gain and more often a sign of serious organic illness. If the weight loss is associated with increased food intake, the diagnosis is likely diabetes, thyrotoxicosis, or malabsorption; less frequently, leukemias or lymphomas cause weight loss in the presence of increased food intake. If food intake is normal or decreased, malignancy, infection, renal disease, psychiatric syndromes, or endocrine deficiency is more common.

REFERENCES

BEUTLER B, CERAMI A: Cachectin: More than a tumor necrosis factor. N Engl J Med 316:379, 1987

BROŽEK J et al: Changes in body weight and body dimensions in men performing work on a low calorie carbohydrate diet. J Appl Physiol 10:412, 1957
FLIER JS et al: Severely impaired adipsin expression in genetic and acquired obesity. Science 237:405, 1987
FOSTER DW: Eating disorders: Obesity and anorexia nervosa, in *Williams Textbook of Endocrinology*, 7th ed, JD Wilson, DW Foster (eds). Philadelphia, Saunders, 1985, p 1081
GARFINKEL PE et al: Differential diagnosis of emotional disorders that cause weight loss. Can Med Assoc J 129:939, 1983
MARTON KI et al: Involuntary weight loss: Diagnostic and prognostic significance. Ann Intern Med 95:568, 1981
MORLEY JE: Neuropeptide regulation of appetite and weight. Endocrine Rev 8:256, 1987
SOCHER SH et al: Tumor necrosis factor not detectable in patients with clinical cancer cachexia. J Natl Cancer Inst 80:595, 1988

46 GASTROINTESTINAL BLEEDING

JAMES M. RICHTER / KURT J. ISSELBACHER

Hematemesis is defined as the vomiting of blood, and *melena* as the passage of stools rendered black and tarry by the presence of altered blood. These symptoms of gastrointestinal hemorrhage should bring the patient to medical attention and suggest the anatomic site of bleeding. The color of vomited blood will vary depending on the concentration of hydrochloric acid in the stomach and its mixture with the blood. Thus, if vomiting occurs shortly after the onset of bleeding, the vomitus appears red; and later the appearance will be dark red, brown, or black. Precipitated blood clots in the vomitus will produce a characteristic "coffee grounds" appearance. Hematemesis usually indicates bleeding proximal to the ligament of Treitz, since blood entering the gastrointestinal tract below the duodenum rarely enters the stomach.

While bleeding sufficient to produce hematemesis usually results in melena, less than half of patients with melena have hematemesis. *Melena* usually denotes bleeding from the esophagus, stomach, or duodenum, but lesions in the jejunum, ileum, and even ascending colon may cause melena provided the gastrointestinal transit time is sufficiently prolonged. Approximately 60 mL of blood is required to produce a single black stool; acute blood loss greater than this may produce melena for up to 3 days. After the stool color returns to normal, tests for occult blood may remain positive for up to a week or longer. The black color of stools secondary to intestinal bleeding results from contact of the blood with hydrochloric acid to produce hematin. Characteristically, such stools are tarry ("sticky"). This tarry consistency is in contrast to black or dark stools occurring after the ingestion of iron, bismuth, or licorice. Similarly, red stools may result from the ingestion of beets or intravenous administration of sulfobromophthalein. Gastrointestinal bleeding, even if detected only by positive tests for occult blood, indicates potentially serious disease and must be further investigated.

Hematochezia, the passage of red blood per rectum, generally signifies bleeding from a source distal to the ligament of Treitz. However, since blood must remain in the gut for approximately 8 h to produce melena, rapid hemorrhage into the esophagus, stomach, or duodenum may also result in hematochezia.

The clinical manifestations of gastrointestinal bleeding depend upon the extent and rate of hemorrhage and the presence of coincidental diseases. Blood loss of less than 500 mL is rarely associated with systemic signs; exceptions include bleeding in the elderly or in the anemic patient in whom smaller amounts of blood loss may produce hemodynamic alterations. Rapid hemorrhage of greater volume results in decreased venous return to the heart, decreased cardiac output, and increased peripheral resistance due to reflex vasoconstriction. Orthostatic hypotension greater than 10 mmHg usually indicates a 20 percent or greater reduction in blood volume. Concomitant symptoms include syncope, lightheadedness, nausea, sweating, and thirst. When blood loss approaches 40 percent of blood volume, shock frequently ensues with pronounced tachycardia and hypotension. Pallor is prominent, and the skin is cool.

In the setting of rapid hemorrhage the hematocrit may not accurately reflect magnitude of blood loss, since equilibration with extravascular fluid and hemodilution require several hours. Common laboratory findings include mild leukocytosis and thrombocytosis which develop within 6 h after the onset of bleeding. The blood urea nitrogen may be mildly elevated, particularly in upper gastrointestinal bleeding, due to breakdown of blood proteins to urea by intestinal bacteria as well as from a mild reduction in the glomerular filtration rate.

Occult bleeding, detected by the physician or patient with a simple card test for hemoglobin peroxidase, has been recognized as an important means of finding colorectal neoplasia at early stages, when it is more amenable to cure. Testing is advocated for patients over age 40 as a part of the periodic checkup, and test kits are available for purchase by patients. The interpretation of the test is complicated by the need for examining multiple stools (usually two samples from three stools) and multiple examinations for positive tests. A positive result can be due to physiologic blood loss, dietary peroxidases, vitamin C, or any cause of upper or lower gastrointestinal bleeding. In order to limit the confounding variables, patients should be tested on a high-fiber and low-meat diet with no ingestion of nonsteroidal anti-inflammatory agents or vitamin C.

ETIOLOGY OF UPPER GASTROINTESTINAL BLEEDING A careful history and physical examination of the oropharynx and nasal cavity should serve to exclude swallowed blood as a source of hematemesis or melena.

The four most common causes of upper gastrointestinal hemorrhage are (1) peptic ulceration, (2) erosive gastritis, (3) varices, and (4) esophagogastric mucosal tear. These entities account for up to 90 percent of all cases of upper gastrointestinal hemorrhage in which a definite lesion can be found.

Peptic ulcer Peptic ulcer is the most common cause of upper gastrointestinal bleeding; the majority of such ulcers are found in the duodenum. Because hemorrhage may be the initial manifestation of a peptic ulcer, this lesion should be seriously considered even when a history characteristic of ulcer disease is not obtained.

Gastritis Gastritis may be associated with recent alcohol ingestion, portal hypertension, or the use of anti-inflammatory drugs, such as aspirin or ibuprofen. Gastric erosions also frequently develop in patients with major trauma, surgery, and severe systemic disease, particularly burn victims and patients with increased intracranial pressure. Because there are no characteristic physical findings, the diagnosis of gastritis must be suspected when the appropriate clinical setting is encountered. When a specific diagnosis is required, endoscopy is usually needed to confirm the diagnosis since radiologic examination generally lacks sufficient sensitivity.

Varices Variceal bleeding is characteristically abrupt and massive; chronic gastrointestinal blood loss is unusual. Bleeding from esophageal or gastric varices is usually the result of portal hypertension, secondary to cirrhosis. Although alcoholic cirrhosis is the most prevalent cause of esophageal varices in the United States, any condition producing portal hypertension, even in the absence of hepatic disease (i.e., portal vein thrombosis or idiopathic portal hypertension), may result in variceal bleeding. Further, while the presence of varices usually connotes long-standing portal hypertension, acute hepatitis or severe fatty infiltration of the liver may occasionally produce varices which disappear once the hepatic abnormality resolves. Although upper gastrointestinal bleeding in a patient with cirrhosis suggests a variceal source, approximately half those patients will be bleeding from other lesions (e.g., gastritis, ulcers). Consequently, it is essential to exclude nonvariceal causes of bleeding so that the appropriate treatment can be instituted.

Esophagogastric mucosal tear (Mallory-Weiss syndrome) With the advent of esophagogastroduodenoscopy, the Mallory-Weiss syndrome has been demonstrated with increasing frequency as a cause of acute upper gastrointestinal hemorrhage (see also Chap. 43). Mucosal laceration occurs in the region of the esophagogastric junction and is often characterized historically by retching or nonbloody vomiting followed by hematemesis.

Other lesions Less common bleeding esophageal lesions include esophagitis and carcinoma; these generally cause chronic blood loss and rarely produce massive bleeding.

Gastric carcinoma may result in chronic gastrointestinal bleeding. Lymphoma, polyps, and other tumors of the stomach and small bowel are uncommon and are infrequent causes of hemorrhage. Leiomyoma and leiomyosarcoma are likewise rare, but they can lead to massive hemorrhage. Bleeding from duodenal and jejunal diverticula is relatively unusual. Vascular insufficiency of the mesenteric vessels, including occlusive and nonocclusive disease, may lead to bloody diarrhea.

Arteriosclerotic aortic aneurysms may rupture into the small intestine; such an event is almost always fatal. Rupture usually occurs following arterial reconstructive surgery with fistula formation between synthetic graft and bowel lumen. A small or herald bleed may precede a sudden massive hemorrhage from an aortoenteric fistula. Sudden bleeding may also occur after trauma resulting in hepatic laceration; this may result in blood loss into the bile ducts (i.e., hemobilia).

Primary blood dyscrasias, vasculitis, and connective tissue disorders may result in significant gastrointestinal bleeding. Uremia may produce gastrointestinal blood loss; the most common presentation is chronic, occult bleeding from diffuse involvement of the mucosa of the stomach and small bowel.

ETIOLOGY OF LOWER GASTROINTESTINAL BLEEDING **Anal and rectal lesions** Small amounts of bright red blood on the surface of the stool and toilet tissue are often caused by hemorrhoids; such bleeding is generally precipitated by the strained passage of a hard stool. Anal fissures and fistulas may present in a similar fashion. Proctitis is another source of rectal bleeding. It is often an idiopathic, limited variant of ulcerative colitis. In others, particularly male homosexuals, proctitis may be due to gonorrheal or mycoplasma infections. Rectal trauma is a cause of hematochezia, and the placement of foreign objects in the rectal vault may precipitate perforation as well as acute rectal hemorrhage. It must be emphasized that anal pathology does not preclude other sources of blood loss, and these must be sought and excluded.

Colonic lesions Carcinoma of the colon, as well as colonic polyps, may produce chronic blood loss. Angiodysplasia, a mucosal telangiectasia usually involving the ascending colon, is a major source of acute or chronic bleeding in elderly patients. Frankly bloody diarrhea is common and may be the presenting symptom in patients with ulcerative colitis; it is less frequent in granulomatous colitis, but occult blood may be present in the stool. Bleeding may also accompany diarrhea due to infections such as shigellosis, amebiasis, campylobacterosis, and rarely, salmonellosis. In the elderly patient, ischemic colitis may be a cause of bloody diarrhea; this lesion may also be seen in younger women who use oral contraceptive agents.

Diverticula Colonic diverticula are most often located in the sigmoid colon; however, diverticular bleeding may originate anywhere in the colon. Bleeding from colonic diverticula is a cause of massive lower gastrointestinal hemorrhage. The usual presentation of a diverticular hemorrhage is that of painless passage of a maroon-colored stool. Meckel's diverticulum, a congenital anomaly of the distal ileum, is present in about 2 percent of the population and is an important cause of acute hemorrhage in children and young adults. Although only about 15 percent of these diverticula contain gastric mucosa, half of the lesions which cause acute bleeding contain gastric mucosa.

APPROACH TO THE PATIENT WITH GASTROINTESTINAL BLEEDING The approach to the bleeding patient depends upon the site, extent, and rate of bleeding. Patients with hematemesis have usually bled greater amounts (often greater than 1000 mL) than those who have melena alone (usually 500 mL or less), and mortality with the former is about twice that of the latter. When first seen, the patient may be in shock. Prior to taking a history and performing a thorough physical examination, vital signs should be noted, blood sent for typing and cross-matching, and a large-bore intravenous line placed for infusion of saline or other plasma expanders. The primary consideration in the care of the bleeding patient is maintaining adequate intravascular volume and hemodynamic stability.

History A history or symptoms suggestive of ulcer disease may provide a useful clue. Similarly, recent heavy use of alcohol or anti-inflammatory drugs should make erosive gastritis suspect. If such alcohol use has been long-standing, esophageal varices may be a more likely source of hemorrhage. Aspirin use may also cause gastroduodenitis, peptic ulceration, and bleeding. Prior history of gastrointestinal bleeding may be helpful, as may a family history of intestinal disease or hemorrhagic diathesis. Recent retching followed by hematemesis should suggest the possibility of the Mallory-Weiss syndrome. The acute onset of bloody diarrhea may indicate the presence of inflammatory bowel disease or an infectious colitis. Associated systemic illnesses, burns, or recent trauma may lead to erosive gastritis.

Physical examination Following evaluation for orthostatic changes in pulse and blood pressure and institution of volume repletion, the patient should be examined for clues to the underlying illness. A nonintestinal bleeding source should be excluded by careful examination of the oral cavity and nasopharynx. Dermatologic examination may disclose the characteristic telangiectasia of Osler-Weber-Rendu disease (although these will not be visible if severe anemia is present), the perioral pigmentation of Peutz-Jeghers syndrome, the dermal fibromas of neurofibromatosis, the sebaceous cysts and bony tumors of Gardner's syndrome, the palpable purpura frequently seen with vasculitis, or the diffuse pigmentation seen in hemochromatosis. Stigmata of chronic liver disease such as spider angiomata, gynecomastia, testicular atrophy, jaundice, ascites, and hepatosplenomegaly suggest portal hypertension resulting in bleeding from esophageal or gastric varices. Significant lymph node enlargement or abdominal masses may reflect underlying intraabdominal malignancy. Careful rectal examination is important to exclude local pathology as well as to observe the color of the stool.

Laboratory studies Initial studies should include the hematocrit, hemoglobin, careful assessment of red blood cell morphologic features (hypochromic, microcytic red blood cells suggest that blood loss is chronic), white blood cell count, differential, and platelet count. Prothrombin time, partial thromboplastin time, and other coagulation studies are needed to exclude primary or secondary clotting defects. Radiography of the abdomen is rarely helpful in establishing a diagnosis unless a perforated or ischemic viscus is suspected. Though the initial studies are valuable and essential, repeated evaluation of the laboratory data is important as one follows the clinical course of the bleeding.

Diagnostic and therapeutic approach The diagnostic approach to the patient with gastrointestinal hemorrhage must be individualized. The management of gastrointestinal bleeding is often under the direction of the internist, but it is prudent to consult a surgeon in the event that surgery is required.

When there is a history of melena or hematemesis or the suspicion of bleeding from the upper part of the gastrointestinal tract, the patient should have a nasogastric tube passed to empty the stomach and to determine whether the bleeding is in the esophagus, stomach, or duodenum. If the initial nasogastric aspirate is clear, the tube should be left in place for several hours, since active duodenal bleeding may occur with an initially clear nasogastric aspirate. If the aspirate is negative for blood during a period of active bleeding, it is reasonable to conclude that active bleeding is not occurring in the gastroduodenal region, and the nasogastric tube can be removed. However, if there is no evidence of active bleeding at the time the nasogastric tube is placed, one cannot assume bleeding did not come from the stomach or duodenum and endoscopy may be required.

If red blood or "coffee grounds" material is aspirated from the nasogastric tube, saline irrigation of the stomach should be initiated. Irrigation serves two purposes: it provides the clinician with an assessment of the rapidity of the bleeding, and it clears the stomach of old blood prior to possible endoscopy. Subsequent diagnostic maneuvers will depend on whether bleeding continues; this can be assessed by vital signs, transfusion requirements, and the number and consistency of stools.

If the bleeding has stopped and the patient is stable, one may proceed with either esophagogastroduodenoscopy or upper gastrointestinal barium studies. Although *endoscopy* provides a higher diagnostic yield, it has not been proved conclusively that survival is increased by early endoscopy. *Barium examination* may identify a potential source of hemorrhage, but there are important limitations to such x-rays. First, lesions such as erosive gastritis and Mallory-Weiss lacerations are not visualized by x-ray. Second, if the patient rebleeds following a barium exam, the retained contrast material will make endoscopy difficult and angiography impossible. Clearly the approach in this setting must be individualized. The decision to employ esophagogastroduodenoscopy or barium studies will depend on several variables, including the availability of an experienced endoscopist and the condition of the patient. Although studies have shown that emergency endoscopy and a vigorous diagnostic approach do not generally decrease patient morbidity or mortality, emergency endoscopy may be important in planning therapy in certain patients with cirrhosis or previous gastric surgery. By identifying other patients with visible vessels and thus a high risk for recurrent bleeding, possible complications can be anticipated.

Persistent upper gastrointestinal hemorrhage must be viewed differently, and most clinicians would proceed immediately to esophagogastroduodenoscopy (Fig. 46-1). Determination of the site and cause of bleeding is essential to plan for appropriate therapy, particularly if varices are suspected. Thus, anticipation of surgery, angiography, or the suspicion of bleeding varices are strong indications for esophagogastroduodenoscopy in the evaluation of the patient with persistent upper gastrointestinal bleeding. Bleeding from an arteriole in a peptic ulcer may be controlled by endoscopic coagulation using Nd:YAG laser, heater probe, or electrocautery. However, esophagogastroduodenoscopy is more difficult in the evaluation of *massive* hemorrhage, since large amounts of blood obscure visualization of mucosal pathology, and angiography may be required in addition to endoscopy.

Should bleeding continue and endoscopy fail to reveal the bleeding source, the site of hemorrhage may be beyond the ligament of Treitz. In this situation angiography is frequently valuable in establishing a diagnosis. Angiographic demonstration of the bleeding site requires blood loss at a rate of at least 0.5 mL/min. Clinical correlates reflecting this degree of blood loss include postural hypotension and the necessity for blood transfusion to maintain stable vital signs. Emergency angiography may localize the site of bleeding; however, the cause of the bleeding may not be determined unless varices, vascular malformations, or aneurysms are present.

Therapeutic angiography is a helpful approach to the control of persistent hemorrhage. Continuous intraarterial infusion of vasoconstrictor agents, such as vasopressin, is often successful in controlling hemorrhage due to gastric ulcer or Mallory-Weiss tear. Additionally, embolic material may be injected directly into the artery perfusing the bleeding site. However, intravenous infusions of vasopressin and endoscopic sclerosis for control of variceal bleeding are more valuable than angiographic techniques.

If bleeding esophageal varices are identified on upper endoscopy, peripheral infusions of vasopressin may control the bleeding. The response to such therapy depends upon the general condition of the patient as assessed by clinical and laboratory parameters. It has been shown that intraarterial vasopressin is no more effective than intravenous administration in the control of variceal bleeding. Endoscopic sclerosis of varices has emerged as an effective therapy for bleeding esophageal varices and when available should be attempted prior to surgery. Periodic endoscopic sclerotherapy also appears to limit further bleeding in patients who have bled from varices. Varices may also be controlled by balloon tamponade with a Sengstaken-Blakemore tube. Unlike vasopressin, this technique is generally used as a preoperative stabilizing measure which should be followed by definitive therapy within 48 h whenever possible.

In the evaluation of *lower gastrointestinal bleeding* the most important procedures are the digital examination, anoscopy, and sigmoidoscopy. The last of these may identify a bleeding site or document bleeding coming from above the range of the instrument. Colonoscopy is a valuable technique for the evaluation of patients with small to moderate lower gastrointestinal bleeds. Preparation of the colon with saline lavage solutions permits a colonoscopic evaluation of the bowel within hours. Many colonic abnormalities can be detected and treated with polypectomy or electrocoagulation. If bleeding is brisk, arteriography may serve to localize the bleeding site and allow local infusion of vasoconstrictor agents to control bleeding. Because arteriography detects actively bleeding lesions only when blood loss exceeds 0.5 mL/min and gastrointestinal bleeding tends to be intermittent, arteriography is often nondiagnostic. Radiolabeled erythrocyte scanning is more sensitive than arteriography in detecting blood loss of 0.1 mL/min and may be used to investigate less severe bleeding. However, bleeding scans are less specific than arteriography, generally localizing the lesion and seldom making a discrete diagnosis. Bleeding scans are most helpful in detecting active, low-grade, or intermittent bleeding in order to better time arteriography and obtain the maximal diagnostic yield. Finally, a barium enema has a limited role in the evaluation of acute rectal bleeding. Although it may localize potential bleeding sources, it will not define the

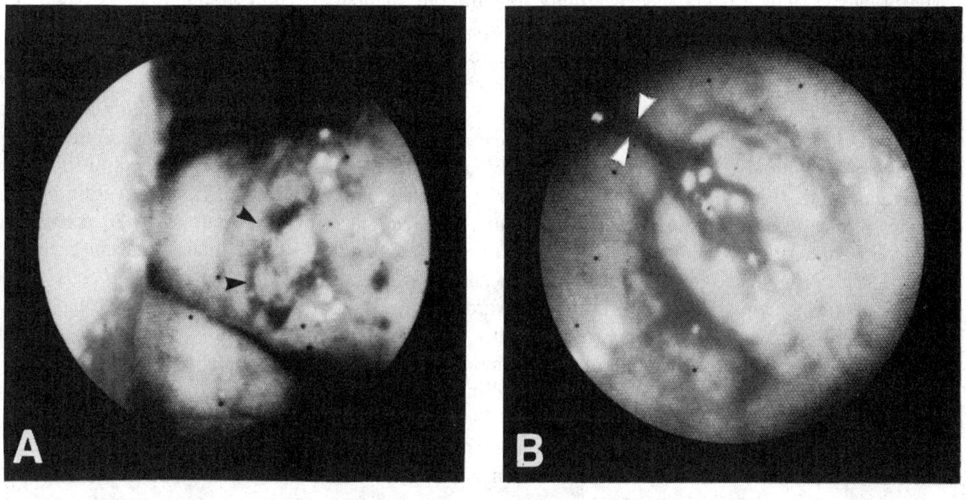

FIGURE 46-1 Endoscopic photographs from a patient with hematemesis. *A*. A gastric ulcer along the lesser curvature of the stomach is identified (*arrows*). *B*. The same ulcer is bleeding actively from a spurting artery (*arrows*).

bleeding site. Furthermore, if brisk bleeding recurs, subsequent colonoscopy or angiography will be difficult to interpret due to retained contrast material. Therefore, it is advisable to withhold barium studies of both the upper and lower bowel for at least 48 h after the cessation of active bleeding.

Patients with occult bleeding are evaluated principally to exclude colorectal neoplasia. Any symptoms or history of disease should be investigated as well. If there are no symptoms, evaluation should focus on the colon with either a barium enema and sigmoidoscopy or colonoscopy. If there is no symptom or anemia, evaluation of the colon is sufficient. Patients with anemia are unlikely to have a physiologic or trivial basis for their test result, and the evaluation should be pursued until a full explanation is obtained.

REFERENCES

CELLO JP et al: Endoscopic sclerotherapy versus portacaval shunt in patients with severe cirrhosis and acute variceal hemorrhage; Long-term follow-up. N Engl J Med 316:11, 1987

CHOJKIER M et al: A controlled comparison of continuous intra-arterial and intravenous infusions of vasopressin in hemorrhage from esophageal varices. Gastroenterology 77:540, 1979

LAINE L: Multipolar electrocoagulation in the treatment of active upper gastrointestinal tract hemorrhage. N Engl J Med 316:1613, 1987

LEVY M: et al: Major upper gastrointestinal tract bleeding; Relation to the use of aspirin and other nonnarcotic analgesics. Arch Intern Med 148:281, 1988

LICHTENSTEIN JL: Accuracy and reliability of endoscopy and x-ray in upper gastrointestinal bleeding. Dig Dis Sci 26:70s, 1981

PETERSON WL et al: Routine early endoscopy in upper gastrointestinal tract bleeding: A randomized, controlled trial. N Engl J Med 304:925, 1981

PRIEBE HJ et al: Antacid versus cimetidine in preventing acute gastrointestinal bleeding. A randomized trial in 75 critically ill patients. N Engl J Med 302:426, 1980

RICHTER JM et al: Angiodysplasia: Clinical presentation and colonoscopic diagnosis. Dig Dis Sci 29:481, 1984

STEER ML, SILEN W: Diagnostic procedures in gastrointestinal hemorrhage. N Engl J Med 309:646, 1983

47 JAUNDICE AND HEPATOMEGALY

KURT J. ISSELBACHER

JAUNDICE

Jaundice, or *icterus,* refers to the yellow pigmentation of the skin or scleras by bilirubin. This in turn is a result of elevated levels of bilirubin in the bloodstream. Jaundice may be brought to clinical attention by a darkening of the urine or a yellow discoloration of the skin or sclera; the latter often is the site where clinical icterus may first be detected. Scleral pigmentation is attributed to richness of this tissue in elastin, which has a special affinity for bilirubin. Jaundice must be distinguished from other causes of yellow pigmentation such as carotenemia (see Chap. 76), which is due to carotenoid pigments in the bloodstream and is associated with a yellowish discoloration of the skin but not of the sclera.

Normal serum bilirubin concentrations range from 5 to 17 μmol/L (or 0.3 to 1.0 mg/dL), and normally most of this is unconjugated (see Fig. 47-1). The precise level at which jaundice becomes clinically evident varies, but it can usually be recognized when the total serum bilirubin exceeds 34 to 43 μmol/L (2 to 2.5 mg/dL). With pronounced jaundice the skin may take on a greenish hue because of the conversion of bilirubin to biliverdin, an oxidation product of bilirubin. Oxidation occurs more readily with conjugated bilirubin, and hence a greenish hue is seen more frequently in conditions with pronounced conjugated hyperbilirubinemia. When bilirubin is exposed to visible blue light (430 to 470 nm), metastable isomers of bilirubin are produced. These photoisomers are polar (because they permit no intramolecular hydrogen bonding) and can

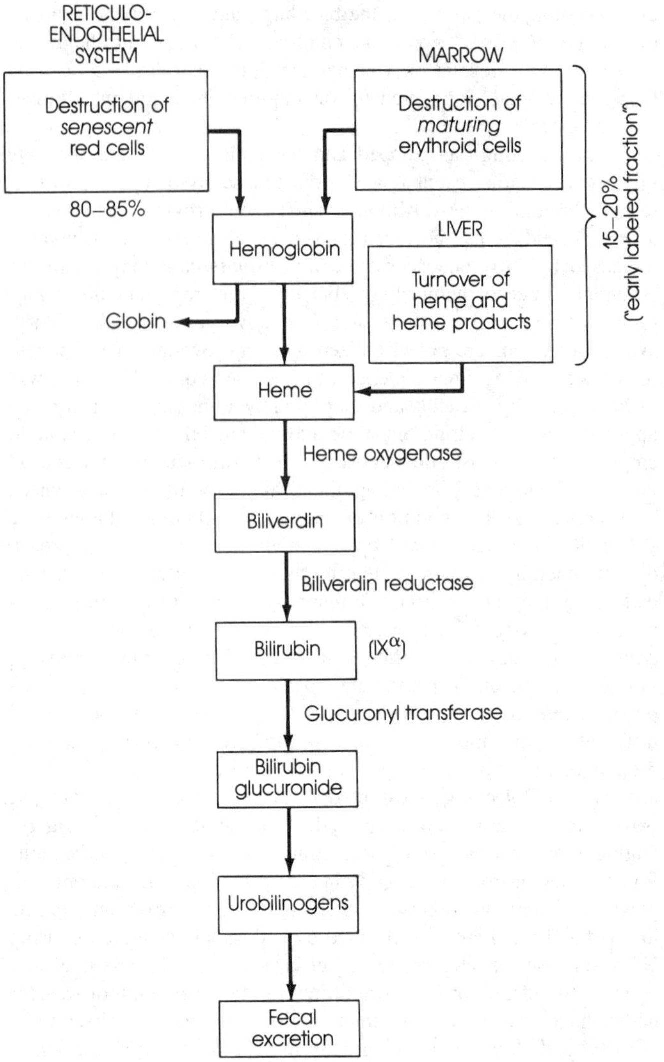

FIGURE 47-1 The sources and precursors of bilirubin and steps in its subsequent metabolism and excretion.

be excreted by the liver into bile without having to be conjugated (see below and Fig. 47-2).

PRODUCTION AND METABOLISM OF BILIRUBIN Normal sources of bilirubin (Fig. 47-2) Most bilirubin is derived from the catabolism of hemoglobin present in senescent red blood cells. This normally accounts for about 80 to 85 percent of the daily bilirubin production. When a circulating red blood cell reaches the end of its normal life span of approximately 120 days, it is destroyed in the reticuloendothelial system. In the catabolism of hemoglobin, globin is first dissociated from heme, after which the heme moiety (ferro-protoporphyrin IX) is oxidatively cleaved and converted to biliverdin by a microsomal heme oxygenase (which is inhibited by protoporphyrins; see below). This enzyme system requires oxygen and a cofactor, reduced nicotinamide adenine dinucleotide phosphate (NADPH). Bilirubin (in the chemical form of bilirubin IXα) is then formed from biliverdin by biliverdin reductase.

About 15 to 20 percent of the bilirubin is derived from sources other than senescent erythrocytes. One source is the *destruction of maturing erythroid cells in the bone marrow,* or so-called ineffective erythropoiesis (see Chap. 294). The other is *nonerythroid components,* especially in the liver, and involves the turnover of heme and heme proteins (such as cytochrome, myoglobin, and heme-containing enzymes). These two sources of bilirubin are collectively referred to as the *early labeled fraction,* a term derived from experiments with labeled glycine and Δ-aminolevulinic acid (ALA). Thus when labeled glycine is administered to a normal subject, approximately 15 percent

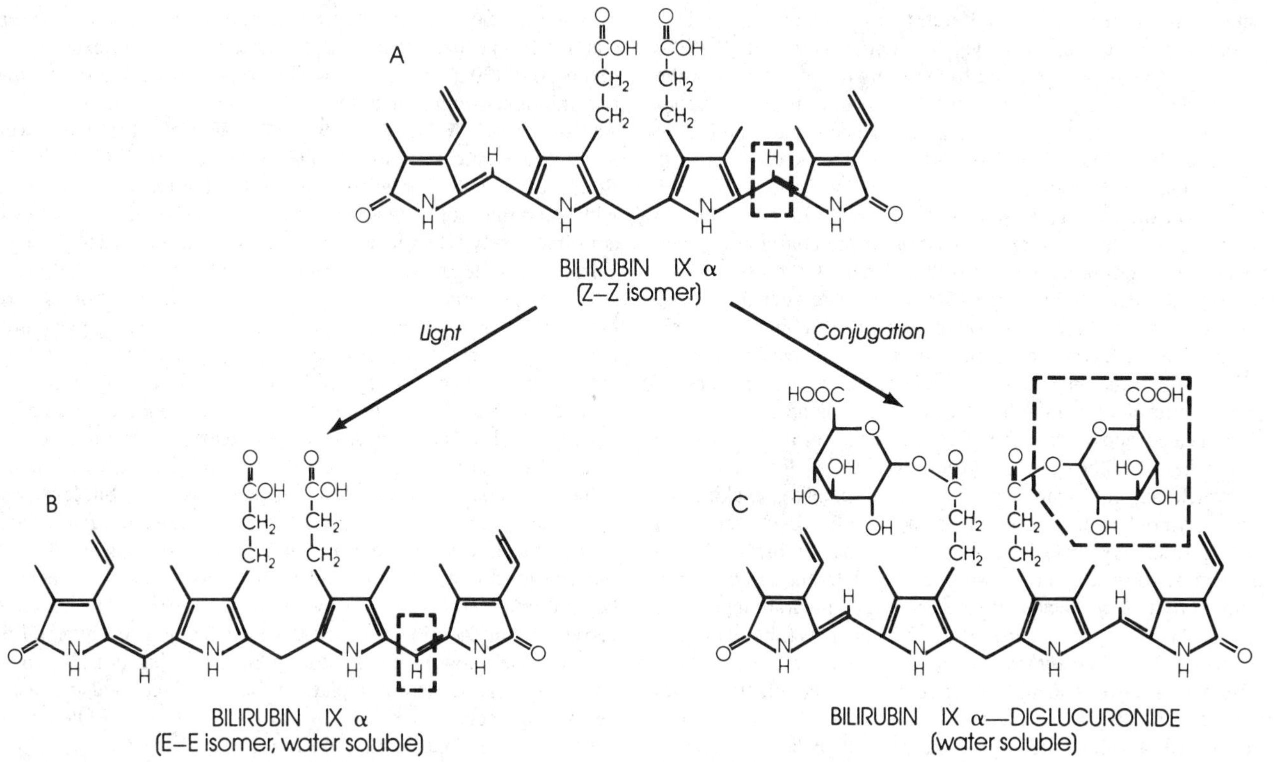

FIGURE 47-2 Scheme showing the conversion of bilirubin IXα to water-soluble derivatives by photoisomerization or conjugation. In *A* the normal, unconjugated pigment Z-Z isomer is shown; the dashed line shows the upright position of the hydrogen at the methene bridges linking the pyrrole molecules. *B* shows the effect of light leading to the formation of the water-soluble E-E isomer; the dashed-line box serves to emphasize the inversion of the hydrogens at the methene bridges between the pyrrole molecules. *C* shows the formation of water-soluble bilirubin diglucuronide formation; the dashed-line box encloses one of the two glucuronic acid moieties.

of the label appears in stool urobilinogens in the first 3 to 5 days; 85 percent of the label appears over a broad range with the peak at about 120 days and reflects bilirubin produced from the normal destruction of senescent red blood cells.

Transport of bilirubin Following liberation of unconjugated bilirubin into the plasma, virtually all the pigment is tightly *bound to albumin.* The maximum binding capacity is 2 mol bilirubin per mole of albumin in a reversible, noncovalent manner. Certain organic anions, such as sulfonamides and salicylates, compete with bilirubin for common binding sites on albumin and may displace bilirubin from albumin, permitting it to enter tissues such as the central nervous system. Most of the evidence for albumin binding has been obtained from studies using unconjugated bilirubin. Conjugated bilirubin is also bound to albumin, but in both a reversible and an irreversible manner. The reversible binding is similar to the noncovalent binding of unconjugated bilirubin, but the binding is much weaker. The second type involves a very tight, irreversible albumin-bilirubin complex that appears in the serum when hepatic excretion of bilirubin is impaired (i.e., with cholestasis). Due to the nature of the binding, the complex does *not* appear in urine. Also this bilirubin-albumin conjugate may remain detectable in the serum for several weeks after the relief of the obstruction or during recovery from hepatocellular jaundice.

Bilirubin is found in body fluids (cerebrospinal fluid, joint effusions, cysts, etc.) in proportion to the albumin content of the fluids and is absent from true secretions such as tears, saliva, and pancreatic juice. The appearance of jaundice is also influenced by blood flow and edema. Paralyzed extremities and edematous areas tend to remain uncolored, and "unilateral" jaundice in patients with hemiplegia and edema may be seen if jaundice develops.

Hepatic metabolism of bilirubin (Fig. 47-3) The liver occupies a central role in the metabolism of the bile pigments. Three distinct phases are recognized: (1) *hepatic uptake,* (2) *conjugation,* and (3) *excretion* into bile. Of these three steps, excretion appears to be the rate-limiting step and the one most susceptible to impairment when the liver cell is damaged.

UPTAKE Unconjugated bilirubin bound to albumin is presented to the liver cell, and upon entry the pigment and albumin become dissociated. The uptake phase and subsequent hepatocyte storage of bilirubin involves binding of bilirubin to certain cytoplasmic anionic binding proteins, especially ligandin. This binding may prevent efflux of bilirubin back into the plasma.

CONJUGATION Unconjugated bilirubin is water-insoluble and must be converted to a *water-soluble derivative* in order to be excreted by the liver cell into bile. This is accomplished by conjugation whereby bilirubin is predominantly converted to bilirubin glucuronide. The reaction occurs in the endoplasmic reticulum of the hepatocytes

FIGURE 47-3 Scheme of bilirubin uptake, conjugation, and excretion by the liver cell. Although the conversion of BMG to BDG appears to be catalyzed by glucuronyl transferase, some have also postulated its formation by a plasma membrane transglucuronidase. B = bilirubin; BMG = bilirubin monoglucuronide; BDG = bilirubin diglucuronide; UDP = uridine diphosphate.

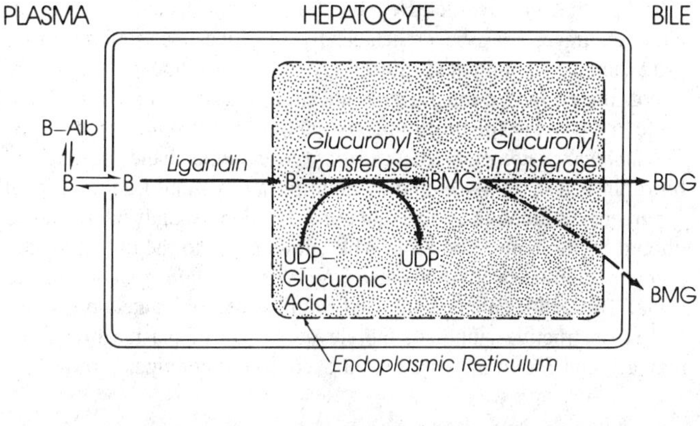

by action of bilirubin glucuronyl transferase. As shown in Fig. 47-3, this appears to be a two-step reaction, resulting first in the formation of the monoglucuronide followed by the production of the diglucuronide. Normally, bile contains 85 percent of bilirubin diconjugates and 15 percent monoconjugates. Unconjugated bilirubin usually is *not* excreted by the liver into the bile (except following photooxidation, see below).

EXCRETION OR SECRETION INTO BILE Normally, for bilirubin to be excreted into bile, *the pigment must be in the conjugated form.* Although the overall process is not well understood, the excretion of conjugated bilirubin into bile appears to be an energy-dependent and *rate-limiting* step in the hepatic metabolism of bilirubin. When this step is compromised, two consequences occur: (1) decreased excretion of bilirubin into the bile and (2) "regurgitation," or reentry of conjugated bilirubin from the liver cells into the bloodstream.

As indicated above, bilirubin IXα can exist as four geometric isomers. The naturally occurring isomer is the Z-Z form (see Fig. 47-2), which permits intramolecular hydrogen bonding, making the molecule hydrophobic. The other isomers (Z-E, E-Z, and E-E, depending on the position of the hydrogens at the two bridge double bonds) can be formed upon exposure to blue light and are unstable. They are *water-soluble* because their geometric configuration prevents intramolecular hydrogen bonding. Thus, these isomers (photoisomers) can be *excreted* into bile *without having to be conjugated.* The natural Z-Z isomer is also rendered water-soluble by conjugation with glucuronic acid. Bilirubin glucuronide formation prevents intramolecular hydrogen bonding, makes the molecule polar, and permits excretion of the pigment into bile (Fig. 47-2).

Intestinal phase of bilirubin metabolism After its appearance in the intestinal lumen, bilirubin glucuronide may be excreted in the stool or metabolized to urobilinogen and related products. Because of its polarity, *conjugated bilirubin is not reabsorbed* by the intestinal mucosa, a mechanism which may serve to rid the body of this pigment. The formation of urobilinogen from conjugated bilirubin requires the action of bacteria and occurs in the lower part of the small intestine and colon.

In contrast to conjugated bilirubin, *urobilinogen is reabsorbed* from the small intestine into the portal blood and is thus subject to the enterohepatic circulation. Some urobilinogen is reexcreted by the liver into the bile; the rest is excreted in the urine in an amount usually not exceeding 4 mg daily. When the hepatic excretory mechanism is impaired (e.g., in hepatocellular disease) or the production of bilirubin is greatly increased (e.g., in hemolytic anemia), the urinary urobilinogen may increase significantly.

The normal output of fecal urobilinogen ranges from 50 to 280 mg per day. Under conditions of decreased excretion of conjugated bilirubin into the intestine (e.g., liver disease, bile duct obstruction) or suppression of intestinal flora by antibiotics, fecal output will be diminished. In hemolytic anemia, urinary and fecal urobilinogen excretion is greatly increased.

In a normal person with a blood volume of 5 L and a hemoglobin concentration of 150 g/L (15 g/dL), the total circulating hemoglobin is 750 g. Because approximately 0.8 percent of the red blood cells are destroyed daily, 6.3 g hemoglobin is released for catabolism.

Renal excretion of bilirubin Normally the urine contains no bilirubin that can be detected by the methods usually employed, although traces may be detectable by sensitive spectrophotometric procedures. Unconjugated bilirubin, being tightly bound to albumin, is not filtered by the renal glomeruli, and because there is no tubular secretory process for bilirubin, *unconjugated bilirubin (as the IXα, Z-Z isomer) is not excreted in urine.* On the other hand, conjugated bilirubin is less tightly bound to albumin, and a small fraction (about 5 percent) is unbound. The unbound fraction is dialyzable and is filtered by the renal glomeruli. Thus, in contrast to the unconjugated pigment, a fraction of plasma *conjugated bilirubin appears in the urine.* Bile salts enhance the dialyzability of conjugated bilirubin, and in obstructive jaundice, the elevated level of plasma bile acids may account for an increased renal excretion of conjugated bilirubin. This may also explain why in biliary tract obstruction, serum conjugated bilirubin levels tend to plateau and not to exceed 510 to 680 μmol/L (30 to 40 mg/dL), while with severe hepatocellular injury bilirubin levels higher than this may occur.

CHEMICAL TESTS FOR BILE PIGMENTS The most widely employed chemical test for the bile pigments in serum is the van den Bergh reaction. In this reaction the bilirubin pigments are diazotized with sulfanilic acid, and the chromogenic products are measured colorimetrically. The van den Bergh reaction can be used to distinguish between unconjugated and conjugated bilirubin because of the different solubility properties of the pigments. When the reaction is carried out in an *aqueous* medium, the water-soluble conjugated bilirubin reacts to give the so-called direct van den Bergh reaction. When the reaction is carried out in *methanol,* the intramolecular hydrogen bonds of unconjugated bilirubin are broken; thus, both conjugated and unconjugated pigments react, giving a measure of the *total* bilirubin level. The total minus the direct-reacting bilirubin give the *indirect* value, which is a measure of the unconjugated bilirubin level.

In the direct van den Bergh reaction, the most accurate measurements are those carried out at 1 min. If the reaction is allowed to proceed longer, a small amount of the unconjugated pigment may begin to react in the aqueous medium. As a result, if the reaction is carried out at 30 min in a patient with unconjugated hyperbilirubinemia, falsely low values for the indirect-reacting bilirubin may be obtained. This serves to emphasize that the direct and indirect van den Bergh reactions represent *approximations* (not absolute measurements) of the conjugated and unconjugated pigments.

The most accurate method for measuring bilirubin in biologic fluids involves the formation of bilirubin methyl esters (by alkaline methanolysis) and measuring the products by high-performance liquid chromatography (HPLC). Studies with this procedure show that *normal serum contains mostly unconjugated bilirubin* with less than 4 percent of the total bilirubin being conjugated. This confirms the long-held suspicion that the small amount of "direct-reacting" bilirubin measured by the van den Bergh method (2 to 5 μmol/L or 0.1 to 0.3 mg/dL) is not correct and is an overestimate of the amount of conjugated bilirubin actually present in normal serum. The HPLC method also shows that in patients with liver disease and conjugated hyperbilirubinemia, the serum contains significant amounts of *monoconjugates as well as diconjugates.* A summary of the key differences in the properties and reactions of the bilirubin pigments is presented in Table 47-1.

The qualitative measurement of bilirubin in the urine may be carried out with Ictotest tablets or the dipstick method. The foam test is also a simple and qualitatively valid procedure. When normal urine is vigorously shaken in a test tube, the foam is absolutely white. In urine containing bilirubin, the foam will be yellow. This difference may be subtle and may become evident only by comparing a normal urine specimen and one containing bilirubin side by side.

Except for concentrated urine, the most common cause of a deep-yellow-brown or dark urine is bilirubinuria. However, other mechanisms and diseases associated with a dark urine need to be considered. These include yellow urine due to drugs (e.g., sulfasalazine); red

TABLE 47-1 Comparison of the major differences between conjugated and unconjugated bilirubin

Properties and reactions	Unconjugated*	Conjugated
Water solubility	0	+
Affinity for lipids	+	0
Renal excretion	0	+
van den Bergh reaction	Indirect (total minus direct)	Direct
Binding to serum albumin (reversible)	+ + +	+
Formation of bilirubin-albumin complex (irreversible)	0	+†

* These properties apply to the naturally occurring bilirubin IXα. Other geometric and photoisomers behave like conjugated bilirubin. See text for details.
† Detectable in plasma under conditions of cholestasis (see text).

urine due to porphyria, hemoglobinuria, myoglobinuria, or drugs (e.g., pyridium); and dark-brown or black urine due to homogentisic acid (in ochronosis) or melanin (with melanoma).

APPROACH TO THE PATIENT WITH JAUNDICE Once jaundice is recognized clinically or chemically, it is important to determine whether it is predominantly due to unconjugated or to conjugated hyperbilirubinemia. *A simple clue in this regard is to determine whether bilirubin is present in the urine.* Its absence in the urine suggests unconjugated hyperbilirubinemia (since this pigment is not filtered by the glomerulus); its presence indicates conjugated hyperbilirubinemia. One can then proceed to the chemical measurement of the bilirubin pigments in the serum. In predominantly unconjugated hyperbilirubinemia, 80 to 85 percent of the total serum bilirubin is measured as unconjugated by the van den Bergh reaction, but more than 96 percent by the more accurate HPLC method. The patient is considered to have predominantly conjugated hyperbilirubinemia when more than 50 percent of the serum bilirubin is of the conjugated type. The serum of such patients will contain both mono- and diglucuronide conjugates.

An approach to the classification of jaundice based on this important distinction is presented in Table 47-2. Derangements of bilirubin metabolism may occur through any of four mechanisms: (1) overproduction, (2) decreased hepatic uptake, (3) decreased hepatic conjugation, and (4) decreased excretion of bilirubin into bile (due to both intrahepatic and extrahepatic factors). Jaundice may also be described on the basis of the pathogenetic mechanisms or disease processes leading to increased bilirubin levels. Thus, the terms *hemolytic jaundice, hepatocellular jaundice,* and *obstructive* (or *cholestatic*) *jaundice* are often used. Though these classifications and terms are helpful, in any one patient more than a single derangement or more than one "type" of jaundice may be present. For example, a patient with cirrhosis may have not only impaired liver cell function (and hence hepatocellular jaundice) but also hemolysis. Furthermore, obstructive jaundice may be due to either *mechanical* obstruction of the biliary radicles or *functional* factors causing impaired hepatic excretion of bilirubin into bile.

In the present chapter a brief description of the major types of jaundice is given. A more detailed discussion of the individual disease entities is found in Chap. 251.

TABLE 47-2 Classification of jaundice based on underlying derangement of bilirubin metabolism

I Predominantly *unconjugated* hyperbilirubinemia
- *A* Overproduction
  - *1* Hemolysis (intra- and extravascular)
  - *2* Ineffective erythropoiesis
- *B* Decreased hepatic uptake
  - *1* Drugs (e.g., flavaspidic acid)
  - *2* Prolonged fasting [< 1255 kJ/d (< 300 kcal/d)]
  - *3* Sepsis
- *C* Decreased bilirubin conjugation (decreased glucuronyl transferase activity)
  - *1* Gilbert's syndrome (*mild* decrease in transferase)
  - *2* Crigler-Najjar type II (*moderate* decrease in transferase)
  - *3* Crigler-Najjar type I (*absent* transferase)
  - *4* Neonatal jaundice
  - *5* Acquired transferase deficiency
    - *a* Drug inhibition (e.g., pregnanediol, chloramphenicol)
    - *b* Hepatocellular disease (hepatitis, cirrhosis)*
  - *6* Sepsis

II Predominantly *conjugated* hyperbilirubinemia
- *A* Impaired hepatic excretion (intrahepatic defects)
  - *1* Familial or hereditary disorders
    - *a* Dubin-Johnson syndrome; Rotor syndrome
    - *b* Recurrent (benign) intrahepatic cholestasis
    - *c* Cholestatic jaundice of pregnancy
  - *2* Acquired disorders
    - *a* Hepatocellular disease* (e.g., viral or drug-induced hepatitis)
    - *b* Drug-induced cholestasis (e.g., oral contraceptives, methyltestosterone)
    - *c* Sepsis
- *B* Extrahepatic biliary obstruction (mechanical obstruction, e.g., stones, stricture, tumor of bile duct)

* In hepatocellular disease (hepatitis and cirrhosis) there is usually interference in the three major steps of bilirubin metabolism—uptake, conjugation, and excretion. However, excretion is the rate-limiting step and is usually impaired to the greatest extent. As a result, conjugated hyperbilirubinemia predominates.

Jaundice with predominantly unconjugated bilirubin in the serum OVERPRODUCTION OF BILIRUBIN When an increased amount of hemoglobin is released from red blood cells into either the bloodstream or tissues, increased bilirubin production occurs. This is reflected by an increase in unconjugated bilirubin levels in the serum, but with levels rarely exceeding 51 to 68 μmol/L (3 to 4 mg/dL). There may also be a slight increase in conjugated bilirubin, but on a percentage basis the amount is comparable to what is found in normal serum, i.e., 4 percent or less of total bilirubin. For a detailed description of the causes of increased bilirubin production, see Chap. 251.

IMPAIRED HEPATIC UPTAKE OF BILIRUBIN As indicated previously, the uptake of bilirubin by the liver cell involves dissociation of the pigment from albumin, and then binding to ligandin. In some cases of drug-induced jaundice (e.g., due to flavaspidic acid) and possibly in some patients with Gilbert's syndrome, there may be a derangement in this phase of bilirubin metabolism (see Chap. 251).

IMPAIRED GLUCURONIDE CONJUGATION Both acquired and genetic derangements in hepatic glucuronyl transferase occur. In the fetus and at birth, glucuronyl transferase activity is low and appears to account in part for the *neonatal jaundice* normally found between the second and the fifth days of life. *Mild* decreases in glucuronyl transferases occur in Gilbert's syndrome, *moderate* decreases are found in Crigler-Najjar syndrome type II, and the enzyme is totally *absent* in the rare Crigler-Najjar syndrome type I (see Chap. 251).

Acquired defects in bilirubin glucuronyl transferase activity may be produced by drugs (i.e., enzyme inhibition) or intrinsic liver disease. However, with liver cell damage, the excretory capacity of the liver is impaired to a greater extent than is the conjugating capacity. Therefore in most hepatocellular diseases, the hyperbilirubinemia is predominantly of the conjugated type (see Chap. 251).

Jaundice with predominantly conjugated bilirubin in the serum IMPAIRED EXCRETION OF BILIRUBIN BY THE LIVER The impaired excretion of bilirubin into the biliary canaliculi, whether due to functional or mechanical factors, results in predominantly conjugated hyperbilirubinemia and bilirubinuria. The presence of *bilirubin in the urine is evidence of conjugated hyperbilirubinemia* and is a most important point in the differential diagnosis of jaundice. Such findings are identical to those occurring in complete obstruction of the bile duct, emphasizing that *jaundice due to hepatocellular disease can seldom be differentiated from that due to extrahepatic obstruction solely on the basis of changes in bile pigment metabolism.* Indeed there are often instances when the two conditions are not distinguishable by any biochemical criteria, and liver biopsy or other diagnostic procedures (e.g., ultrasound) are needed for the definitive diagnosis.

When there is interference in the excretion of conjugated bilirubin into bile, by what mechanism does this pigment enter the systemic circulation? Several postulates have been proposed for this "reentry": (1) rupture of the bile canaliculi secondary to the necrosis of the hepatic cells that constitute their walls; (2) occlusion of the canaliculi by inspissated bile or their compression by swollen hepatic cells; (3) obstruction of the terminal intrahepatic bile ducts (cholangioles) by inflammatory cells; (4) altered hepatic cell permeability; and (5) impaired excretion, resulting in accumulation of conjugated bilirubin in the hepatocytes, and secondary diffusion into the plasma. Although some of these postulates are speculative, it is likely that several of these mechanisms occur. For example, occasionally in histologic sections, escape of bile through rents in the walls of canaliculi in areas of necrosis is apparent. Also, microscopic studies of the liver of rats injected with fluorescent dyes have shown reflux of bile from canaliculi into sinusoids. However, no anatomic damage needs to be invoked, because when unconjugated bilirubin is infused into normal subjects at high rates, conjugated hyperbilirubinemia occurs; this is explained most logically by passive diffusion.

EXTRAHEPATIC BILIARY OBSTRUCTION Complete obstruction of the extrahepatic bile ducts leads to jaundice with predominantly conjugated hyperbilirubinemia, bilirubinuria, and clay-colored stools. Failure of bile to reach the intestine results in virtual disappearance of urobilinogen from the stool and urine. The concentration of bilirubin rises progressively but then usually plateaus at a level of 510 to 680 μmol/L (30 to 40 mg/dL). To some extent this plateau may be explained by a balance between renal excretion and diversion of bilirubin to other metabolites. In hepatocellular jaundice, such a plateau tends not to occur, and bilirubin levels in excess of 855 μmol/L (50 mg/dL) may be found, in part due to concomitant hemolysis and renal insufficiency.

Partial obstruction of the extrahepatic bile ducts can also give rise to jaundice but only if the intrabiliary pressure is increased, because the excretion of bilirubin does not diminish until the intraductile pressure approaches the maximal secretory pressure of approximately 250 mmHg bile. Jaundice may occur at much lower pressures if the obstruction is complicated by infection of the ducts or hepatocellular injury. Therefore, jaundice, bilirubinuria, and clay-colored stools are inconstant findings in partial biliary obstruction, and the amount of urobilinogen in urine and stool varies with the degree of occlusion.

The functional reserve of the liver is so great that *occlusion of the intrahepatic bile ducts* does not give rise to jaundice unless the drainage of bile from a large segment of the parenchyma is interrupted. Either of the two major hepatic ducts or a large number of secondary radicles may be occluded without production of jaundice. In experimental animals the ducts draining at least 75 percent of the parenchyma must be occluded before jaundice appears.

Additional points of terminology In clinical practice, a patient may be described as having *obstructive,* or *cholestatic,* jaundice. By this is meant that clinically, and especially biochemically, there is little to suggest hepatocellular damage and that the main features point to interference with, or obstruction in, the flow of bile. Typically one would expect such a patient to show (1) predominantly conjugated hyperbilirubinemia, (2) minimal biochemical changes of parenchymal liver damage, and (3) a moderate to a marked increase in the serum alkaline phosphatase level [usually three or four times normal (or greater than 250 IU/L)]. As emphasized in Chaps. 248 and 250, an *elevated alkaline phosphatase level* in a patient with jaundice or liver disease, in the absence of other disorders such as bone disease, is most suggestive of interference with bile secretion or an infiltrative process in the liver. However, *laboratory tests alone may not permit differentiation of intrahepatic from extrahepatic cholestasis.*

Some clinicians reserve the term *obstructive jaundice* for those cases in which anatomic obstruction can be demonstrated and use the term *cholestatic jaundice* for cases of parenchymal liver disease in which the obstructive phase is on a functional basis. Nevertheless, because these two entities frequently are indistinguishable by clinical and biochemical criteria, the terms obstructive jaundice and cholestatic jaundice are often used interchangeably.

Hepatocellular disorders in which jaundice associated with an obstructive, or cholestatic, phase occurs include (1) occasional cases of viral hepatitis, (2) drug reactions, especially those due to chlorpromazine and methyltestosterone, (3) some cases of alcoholic hepatitis or alcohol-induced fatty liver, (4) jaundice in the last trimester of pregnancy, (5) most cases of Dubin-Johnson or Rotor syndrome, (6) benign recurrent intrahepatic cholestasis, and (7) certain types of postoperative jaundice. These and other conditions are discussed in Chaps. 251 and 252.

In summary, all forms of conjugated hyperbilirubinemia have by definition an impairment in the excretion of bilirubin into bile. In most cases of parenchymal liver disease, a broad derangement is shown by the biochemical tests of liver function. However, when the major detectable alterations of liver function tests include (1) conjugated hyperbilirubinemia and (2) moderate to marked elevation of the serum alkaline phosphatase level, the terms obstructive or cholestatic jaundice may be appropriate. Additional procedures, including operation, are often needed to determine the cause of the cholestasis (see Chaps. 247 to 249).

HEPATOMEGALY

In the supine position, the major part of the liver lies beneath the right rib cage. In some normal persons the liver edge may be palpable 1 to 2 cm below the right costal margin, and a palpable liver edge by itself does not necessarily indicate hepatomegaly. In evaluating liver size by physical examination, two factors other than ability to palpate the liver edge need to be considered, namely, (1) the location of the upper border of liver dullness by percussion and (2) the body habitus.

Normally, the upper edge of liver dullness on the right side in the midclavicular line is at the level of the fifth rib, but in asthenic habitus it may be lower. The liver edge normally descends 1 to 3 cm with deep inspiration. In hypersthenic subjects, the liver may extend over to the left side of the abdominal wall, with the lower edge high and not palpable; in hyposthenic subjects with a very acute costal angle, the liver may lie in the right half of the abdomen, the edge being palpable by as much as 6 to 8 cm below the right costal margin lateral to the right rectus abdominis muscle. Thus, palpability does not necessarily imply hepatomegaly.

In determining liver enlargement by palpation, one should be certain that the liver is being palpated rather than other right upper quadrant masses such as gallbladder, colonic neoplasm, or fecal material in the colon. Liver enlargement is often confirmed by radiologic studies, including hepatic scintiscans, computed tomography, and ultrasonography.

In many cases of generalized liver enlargement, the left lobe will be felt in the epigastrium between the xiphoid and umbilicus. The liver should be carefully palpated during deep inspiration to determine whether the edge is tender, regular or irregular, firm or soft, rounded and thickened, or sharp. The edge is tender and often rounded with hepatic inflammation, as in hepatitis, or when the liver is acutely congested, as in cardiac decompensation. Pulsation of the liver may be found with tricuspid valvular incompetence. A carcinomatous liver may be rocklike in hardness; the cirrhotic liver is very firm in consistency. The largest livers are often found with carcinoma (primary or metastatic), marked fatty infiltration, congestive cardiac decompensation, Hodgkin's disease, and amyloidosis. Rapid decrease in liver size may occur with improvement of congestive failure, mobilization of fat from the liver, or massive hepatic necrosis.

In a patient with hepatomegaly, auscultation is sometimes helpful.

TABLE 47-3 Causes of a palpable liver and hepatomegaly

I Palpable liver without hepatomegaly
- *A* Right diaphragm displaced downward (e.g., emphysema, asthma)
- *B* Subdiaphragmatic lesion (e.g., abscess)
- *C* Aberrant lobe of liver (Riedel's lobe)
- *D* Extremely thin or relaxed abdominal muscles
- *E* Occasionally present in normal persons

II Hepatomegaly
- *A* Vascular congestion (e.g., congestive heart failure, hepatic vein thrombosis)
- *B* Bile duct obstruction (e.g., lesion in common duct leading to hepatomegaly and subsequently to biliary cirrhosis)
- *C* Infiltrative disorders
  - *1* Bone marrow and reticuloendothelial cells
    - *a* Extramedullary hematopoiesis
    - *b* Leukemia
    - *c* Lymphoma
  - *2* Fat
    - *a* Fatty liver (e.g., secondary to alcohol, diabetes, or toxins)
    - *b* Gaucher's disease and some other lipidoses
  - *3* Glycogen (e.g., diabetes, especially after insulin excess)
  - *4* Amyloid
  - *5* Iron (hemochromatosis and hemosiderosis)
  - *6* Granuloma (tuberculosis, sarcoid)
- *D* Inflammatory disorders
  - *1* Hepatitis—due to drugs or infectious agents
  - *2* Cirrhosis—except in late stages when prolonged scarring may lead to a *small,* shrunken liver
- *E* Tumors—primary or metastatic
- *F* Cysts—polycystic disease, congenital hepatic fibrosis

A friction rub may be audible (and palpable) in the right upper quadrant; it is usually due to a recent biopsy, tumor, or perihepatitis. In portal hypertension a venous hum may be audible between the umbilicus and the xiphoid. An arterial murmur or bruit over the liver may indicate tumor, usually hepatocellular carcinoma.

Some of the causes of a palpable liver and hepatomegaly are given in Table 47-3.

REFERENCES

BERLIN N, BERK P: Quantitative aspects of bilirubin metabolism for hematologists. Blood 57:983, 1981

BLANKAERT N, SCHMID R: Physiology and pathophysiology of bilirubin metabolism, in *Hepatology: A Textbook of Liver Disease*, D Zakim, T Boyer (eds). Philadelphia, Saunders, 1982, pp 246–296

CHOWDHURY JR et al: Hereditary jaundice and disorders of bilirubin metabolism, in *The Metabolic Basis of Inherited Disease*, 6th ed, CR Scriver et al (eds). New York, McGraw-Hill, 1989, pp 1367–1408

KAPPAS A et al: Sn-Protoporphyrin use in the management of hyperbilirubinemia in term newborns with direct Coombs-positive ABO incompatibility. Pediatrics 81:485, 1988

McDONAGH AF et al: Blue light and bilirubin excretion. Science 208:145, 1980

MURACA M et al: Relationship between serum bilirubins and production and conjugation of bilirubin. Studies in Gilbert's syndrome, Crigler-Najjar disease, hemolytic disorders and rat models. Gastroenterology 92:309, 1987

VAN HOOTEGEM P et al: Serum bilirubins in hepatobiliary disease: Comparison with other liver function tests. Hepatology 5:112, 1985

WEISS JS et al: The clinical importance of a protein-bound fraction of serum bilirubin in patients with hyperbilirubinemia. N Engl J Med 309:147, 1983

48 ABDOMINAL SWELLING AND ASCITES

ROBERT M. GLICKMAN / KURT J. ISSELBACHER

ABDOMINAL SWELLING Abdominal swelling or distention is a common problem in clinical medicine and may be the initial manifestation of a systemic disease or of otherwise unsuspected abdominal disease. *Subjective* abdominal enlargement, often described as a sensation of fullness or bloating, is usually transient and is often related to a functional gastrointestinal disorder when it is not accompanied by objective physical findings of increased abdominal girth or local swelling. *Obesity* and lumbar lordosis, which may be associated with prominence of the abdomen, may usually be distinguished from true increases in the volume of the peritoneal cavity by history and careful physical examination.

Clinical history Abdominal swelling may first be noticed by the patient because of a progressive increase in belt or clothing size, the appearance of abdominal or inguinal hernias, or the development of a localized swelling. Often, considerable abdominal enlargement has gone unnoticed for weeks or months, either because of coexistent obesity or because the ascites formation has been insidious, without pain or localizing symptoms. Progressive abdominal distention may be associated with a sensation of "pulling" or "stretching" of the flanks or groins and vague low back pain. Localized *pain* usually results from involvement of an abdominal organ (e.g., a passively congested liver, large spleen, or colonic tumor). Pain is uncommon in cirrhosis with ascites and when it is present, pancreatitis, hepatoma, or peritonitis should be considered. Tense ascites or abdominal tumors may produce increased intraabdominal pressure, resulting in *indigestion* and *heartburn* due to gastroesophageal reflux or *dyspnea, orthopnea,* and *tachypnea* from elevation of the diaphragm. A coexistent pleural effusion, more commonly on the right, presumably due to leakage of ascitic fluid through lymphatic channels in the diaphragm, may also contribute to respiratory embarrassment. The patient with diffuse abdominal swelling should be questioned about increased alcoholic intake, a prior episode of jaundice or hematuria, a change in bowel habits, or a past history of rheumatic heart disease. Such historical information may provide the clues that will lead one to suspect an occult cirrhosis, a colonic tumor with peritoneal seeding, congestive heart failure, or nephrosis.

Physical examination A carefully executed *general physical examination* can yield valuable clues concerning the etiology of abdominal swelling. Thus palmar erythema and spider angiomas suggest an underlying cirrhosis, while supraclavicular adenopathy (Virchow's node) should raise the question of an underlying gastrointestinal malignancy. *Inspection* of the abdomen is an important but often cursorily performed aspect of the abdominal examination. By noting the abdominal contour, one may be able to distinguish localized from generalized swelling. The tensely distended abdomen with tightly stretched skin, bulging flanks, and everted umbilicus is characteristic of ascites. A prominent abdominal venous pattern with the direction of flow away from the umbilicus often is a reflection of portal hypertension; venous collaterals with flow from the lower part of the abdomen toward the umbilicus suggest obstruction of the inferior vena cava; flow downward toward the umbilicus suggests superior vena cava obstruction. "Doming" of the abdomen with visible ridges from underlying intestinal loops is usually due to intestinal obstruction or distention. An epigastric mass, with evident peristalsis proceeding from left to right, usually indicates underlying pyloric obstruction. A liver with metastatic deposits may be visible as a nodular right upper quadrant mass moving with respiration.

Auscultation may reveal the high-pitched, rushing sounds of early intestinal obstruction or a succussion sound due to increased fluid and gas in a dilated hollow viscus. Careful auscultation over an enlarged liver occasionally reveals the harsh bruit of a vascular tumor, especially a hepatoma, or the leathery friction rub of a surface nodule. A venous hum at the umbilicus may signify portal hypertension and an increased collateral blood flow around the liver. A fluid wave and flank dullness which shifts with change in position of the patient are important signs that indicate the presence of peritoneal fluid. In obese patients, small amounts of fluid may be difficult to demonstrate; on occasion the fluid may be detected by abdominal percussion with patients on their hands and knees. Doubt about the presence of peritoneal fluid may be resolved by careful paracentesis with a small-gauge (no. 19 or 20) needle. Careful percussion should serve to distinguish generalized abdominal enlargement from localized swelling due to an enlarged uterus, ovarian cyst, or distended bladder. Percussion can also outline an abnormally small or large liver. Loss of normal liver dullness may result from massive hepatic necrosis; it may also be a clue to free gas in the peritoneal cavity, as from perforation of a hollow viscus.

Palpation is often difficult with massive ascites, and ballottement of overlying fluid may be the only method of palpating the liver or spleen. A slightly enlarged spleen in association with ascites may be the only evidence of an occult cirrhosis. When there is evidence of portal hypertension, a soft liver suggests that obstruction to portal flow is extrahepatic; a firm liver suggests cirrhosis as the likely cause of the portal hypertension. A very hard or nodular liver is a clue that the liver is infiltrated with tumor, and when accompanied by ascites, it suggests that the latter is due to peritoneal seeding. The presence of a hard periumbilical lymph node (Sister Marie Joseph's nodule) suggests metastatic disease from a pelvic or gastrointestinal primary tumor. A pulsatile liver and ascites may be found in tricuspid insufficiency.

An attempt should be made to determine whether a mass is solid or cystic, smooth or irregular, and whether it moves with respiration. The liver, spleen, and gallbladder should descend with respiration unless they are fixed by adhesions or extension of tumor beyond the organ. A fixed mass not descending with respiration may indicate that it is retroperitoneal. Tenderness, especially if localized, may indicate an inflammatory process such as an abscess; it may also be due to stretching of the visceral peritoneum or tumor necrosis. Rectal and pelvic examinations are mandatory; they may reveal otherwise undetected masses due to tumor or infection.

Radiographic and laboratory examinations are essential for confirming or extending the impressions gained on physical examination. Upright and recumbent films of the abdomen may demonstrate the dilated loops of intestine with fluid levels characteristic of intestinal obstruction or the diffuse abdominal haziness and loss of psoas margins suggestive of ascites. Ultrasonography is often of value in detecting ascites, determining the presence of a mass, or evaluating the size of the liver and spleen. CT scanning provides similar information. A plain film of the abdomen may reveal the distended colon of otherwise unsuspected ulcerative colitis and give valuable information as to the size of the liver and spleen. An irregular and elevated right side of the diaphragm may be a clue to a liver abscess or hepatoma. Studies of the gastrointestinal tract with barium or other contrast media are usually necessary in the search for a primary tumor.

ASCITES The evaluation of a patient with ascites requires that the *cause* of the ascites be established. In most cases ascites will appear as a part of a well-recognized illness, i.e., cirrhosis, congestive heart failure, nephrosis, or disseminated carcinomatosis. In these situations, the physician should determine that the development of ascites is indeed a consequence of the basic underlying disease and not due to the presence of a separate or related disease process. This distinction is necessary even when the cause of ascites seems obvious. For example, when the patient with compensated cirrhosis and minimal ascites develops progressive ascites that is increasingly difficult to control with sodium restriction or diuretics, the obvious temptation is to attribute the worsening of the clinical picture to progressive liver disease. However, an occult hepatoma, portal vein thrombosis, spontaneous bacterial peritonitis, or even tuberculosis may be responsible for the decompensation. The disappointingly low success in diagnosing tuberculous peritonitis or hepatoma in the patient with cirrhosis and ascites reflects the too-low index of suspicion for the development of such superimposed conditions. Similarly, the patient with congestive heart failure may develop ascites from a disseminated carcinoma with peritoneal seeding. The thorough evaluation of each patient with ascites, even in the presence of an "obvious" cause, will help avoid these errors.

Diagnostic paracentesis (50 to 100 mL) should be part of the routine evaluation of the patient with ascites. The fluid should be examined for its gross appearance; and protein content, cell count, and differential cell count should be determined, and Gram's and acid-fast stains and culture performed. Cytologic and cell-block examination may disclose an otherwise unsuspected carcinoma. Table 48-1 presents some of the features of ascitic fluid typically found in various disease states. In some disorders, such as cirrhosis, the fluid has the characteristics of a transudate (less than 25 g protein per liter and a specific gravity less than 1.016); in others, such as peritonitis, the features are those of an exudate. Although there is variability of the ascitic fluid in any given disease state, some features are sufficiently characteristic to suggest certain diagnostic possibilities. For example, blood-stained fluid with more than 25 g protein per liter is unusual in uncomplicated cirrhosis but is consistent with tuberculous peritonitis or neoplasm. Cloudy fluid with a predominance of polymorphonuclear cells and a positive Gram stain are characteristic of bacterial peritonitis; if most cells are lymphocytes, tuberculosis should be suspected. The complete examination of each fluid is most important, for occasionally only *one* finding may be abnormal. For example, if the fluid is a typical transudate but contains more than 250 white blood cells per microliter, the finding should be recognized as atypical for cirrhosis, nephrosis, or congestive heart failure and should warrant a search for tumor or infection. This is especially true in the evaluation of cirrhotic ascites where occult peritoneal infection may be present with only minor elevations in the white blood cell count of the peritoneal fluid (300 to 500 cells per microliter). Since Gram's stain of the fluid may be negative in a high proportion of such cases, careful culture of the peritoneal fluid is mandatory. Direct visualization of the peritoneum (laparoscopy) may disclose peritoneal deposits of tumor, tuberculosis, or metastatic disease of the liver. Biopsies are taken under direct vision often adding to the diagnostic accuracy of the procedure.

Chylous ascites refers to a turbid, milky, or creamy peritoneal fluid due to the presence of thoracic or intestinal lymph. Such a fluid shows Sudan-staining fat globules microscopically and an increased triglyceride content by chemical examination. A turbid fluid due to leukocytes or tumor cells may be confused with chylous fluid (pseudochylous), and it is often helpful to carry out alkalinization and ether extraction of the specimen. Alkali will tend to dissolve cellular proteins and thereby reduce turbidity; ether extraction will lead to clearing if the turbidity of the fluid is due to lipid. Chylous

TABLE 48-1 Ascitic fluid characteristics in various disease states

				Cell count		
Condition	Gross appearance	Specific gravity	Protein, g/dL	Red blood cells, >10,000/µL	White blood cells, per µL	Other tests
Cirrhosis	Straw-colored or bile-stained	<1.016 (95%)*	<25 (95%)	1%	<250 (90%);* predominantly mesothelial	
Neoplasm	Straw-colored, hemorrhagic, mucinous, or chylous	Variable, >1.016 (45%)	>25 (75%)	20%	>1000 (50%); variable cell types	Cytology, cell block, peritoneal biopsy
Tuberculous peritonitis	Clear, turbid, hemorrhagic, chylous	Variable, >1.016 (50%)	>25 (50%)	7%	>1000 (70%); usually >70% lymphocytes	Peritoneal biopsy, stain and culture for acid-fast bacilli
Pyogenic peritonitis	Turbid or purulent	If purulent, >1.016	If purulent, >2.5	Unusual	Predominantly polymorphonuclear leukocytes	+Gram's stain, culture
Congestive heart failure	Straw-colored	Variable, <1.016 (60%)	Variable, 15–53	10%	<1000 (90%); usually mesothelial, mononuclear	
Nephrosis	Straw-colored or chylous	<1.016	<25(100%)	Unusual	<250; mesothelial, mononuclear	If chylous, ether extraction, Sudan staining
Pancreatic ascites (pancreatitis, pseudocyst)	Turbid, hemorrhagic, or chylous	Variable, often >1.016	Variable, often >25	Variable, may be blood-stained	Variable	Increased amylase in ascitic fluid and serum

* Since the conditions of examining fluid and selecting patients were not identical in each series, the percentage figures (in the parentheses) should be taken as an indication of the order of magnitude rather than as the precise incidence of any abnormal finding.

ascites is most often the result of lymphatic obstruction from trauma, tumor, tuberculosis, filariasis (see Chap. 169), or congenital abnormalities. It may also be seen in the nephrotic syndrome.

Rarely, ascitic fluid may be *mucinous* in character, suggesting either pseudomyxoma peritonei (Chap. 246) or rarely a colloid carcinoma of the stomach or colon with peritoneal implants.

On occasion, ascites may develop as a seemingly isolated finding in the absence of a clinically evident underlying disease. It is then that a careful analysis of ascitic fluid may indicate the direction the evaluation should take. A useful framework for the workup starts with an analysis of whether the fluid is an exudate or transudate. *Transudative ascites* of unclear etiology is most often due to occult cirrhosis, right-sided venous hypertension raising hepatic sinusoidal pressure, or hypoalbuminemic states such as nephrosis or protein-losing enteropathy. Cirrhosis with well-preserved liver function (normal albumin) resulting in ascites invariably is associated with significant portal hypertension (see Chap. 254). Evaluation should include liver function tests, liver spleen scan or other hepatic imaging procedure (i.e., CT or ultrasound) to detect nodular changes in the liver, or a colloid shift of isotope to suggest portal hypertension. On occasion a wedged hepatic venous pressure can be useful to document portal hypertension. Finally, if clinically indicated, a liver biopsy will confirm the diagnosis of cirrhosis and perhaps suggest its etiology. Other etiologies may result in hepatic venous congestion and resultant ascites. Right-sided cardiac valvular disease and particularly constrictive pericarditis should raise a high index of suspicion and may require cardiac imaging and cardiac catheterization for definitive diagnosis. Hepatic vein thrombosis is evaluated by visualizing the hepatic veins using imaging techniques (angiography, CT scans, magnetic resonance imaging) to demonstrate obliteration, thrombosis, or obstruction by tumor. Uncommonly, transudative ascites may be associated with benign tumors of the ovary, particularly fibroma (Meigs's syndrome) with ascites and hydrothorax.

Exudative ascites should initiate an evaluation for primary peritoneal processes, most importantly infection and tumor. Routine bacteriologic culture of ascitic fluid often will yield a specific organism causing infectious peritonitis. Tuberculous peritonitis (Table 48-1) is best diagnosed by peritoneal biopsy, either percutaneously or via laparoscopy. Histologic examination invariably shows granulomata that may contain acid-fast bacilli. Since cultures of peritoneal fluid and biopsies for tuberculosis may require 6 weeks, characteristic histology with appropriate stains allows antituberculosis therapy to be started promptly. Similarly the diagnosis of peritoneal seeding by tumor can be made by cytologic analysis of peritoneal fluid or by peritoneal biopsy. Appropriate diagnostic studies can then be undertaken to determine the nature and site of the primary tumor. Pancreatic ascites (Table 48-1) is invariably associated with an extravasation of pancreatic fluid from the pancreatic ductal system, most commonly from a leaking pseudocyst. Ultrasound or CT examination of the pancreas followed by visualization of the pancreatic duct by direct cannulation (viz., endoscopic retrograde cholangiopancreatography, ERCP) will usually disclose the site of leakage and permit resective surgery to be carried out.

An analysis of the physiologic and metabolic factors involved in the production of ascites (see Chap. 254 for details), coupled with a complete evaluation of the nature of the ascitic fluid, will invariably disclose the etiology of the ascites and permit appropriate therapy to be instituted.

REFERENCES

CATTAN EL JR et al: The accuracy of the physical examination in the diagnosis of suspected ascites. JAMA 247:1146, 1982

EPSTEIN M: Treatment of refractory ascites. N Engl J Med 321:1675, 1989

GARCIA-TSAO G et al: The diagnosis of bacterial peritonitis. Hepatology 5:91, 1985

PINTO PC et al: Large volume paracentesis in nonedematous patients with tense ascites: Its effect on intravascular volume. Hepatology 8:207, 1988

RECTOR WG JR, REYNOLDS TB: Superiority of the serum: Ascites albumin difference over the ascites total protein concentration in separation of "transudative" and "exudative" ascites. Am J Med 77:83, 1984

RUNTON BA: Patients with deficient ascitic fluid opsonic activity are predisposed to spontaneous bacterial peritonitis. Hepatology 8:632, 1988

section 6 Alterations in urinary function and electrolytes

49 ALTERATIONS IN URINARY FUNCTION

FREDRIC L. COE

AZOTEMIA, OLIGURIA, AND ANURIA

AZOTEMIA Measurements of urea and creatinine concentrations in serum are often obtained to assess the glomerular filtration rate (GFR). Both substances are produced at a reasonably constant rate, by the liver and muscles, respectively. As discussed in Chap. 222, they undergo complete glomerular filtration and are not reabsorbed extensively by the renal tubules; hence their clearances tend to reflect the GFR. An increase in their serum concentrations, termed *azotemia* (*azo*, "containing nitrogen"), occurs as the GFR falls. Creatinine is a more reliable index of GFR than urea because of the latter's lower back diffusion from tubule lumen to peritubular blood. The GFR may be reduced by a fall in the filtration rates of individual functioning nephrons or by a reduction in the total number of functioning nephrons. (See Table 49-1.)

Reduced single-nephron GFR TUBULAR FUNCTION NORMAL An important response of the normal kidney to a severe sodium-conserving stimulus, such as extracellular fluid volume depletion, is reduction of the single-nephron glomerular filtration rate (SNGFR) and subsequent reabsorption of an increased fraction of the reduced amounts of NaCl and water that enter the tubules. The resulting azotemia is called *prerenal azotemia*, in which urinary Na concentration falls below 20 (often below 1) mmol/L (see Table 49-1). The fractional excretion of Na can be calculated (see Chap. 223) and used as an additional index of prerenal azotemia. Secretion of vasopressin is stimulated by depletion of extracellular fluid volume, and as a consequence, the distal tubules and collecting ducts become fully permeable to water. The concentrating mechanisms in the inner medulla (Chap. 222) are very efficient when flow rates through the loops of Henle and the collecting ducts are low. As a result, the filtrate that escapes reabsorption in the proximal tubule undergoes maximal osmotic concentration, the urine volume becomes small, and it has a high osmolality, above 500 mosmol per kilogram of water. Most of the filtered creatinine escapes tubular reabsorption,

TABLE 49-1 Pathophysiologic mechanisms of azotemia

Mechanism of reduced GFR	Clinical examples	Laboratory findings: Oliguria	Urine osm, mosmol/kg	Urine [Na^+], mmol/L	$\left(\frac{U}{P}\right)_{creat}$	$\left(\frac{U}{P}\right)_{urea}$	$\frac{BUN}{Serum\ creat}$
REDUCED SNGFR							
Tubules normal (prerenal azotemia)	Severe dehydration, edema-forming states, diuretic agents, systemic hypotension, acute glomerular disease,* acute urinary obstruction, incomplete renal vascular obstruction	Nearly always present	>500	<20	>40	>8	>10
Tubules damaged (acute renal failure)	Acute tubular necrosis, nephrotoxic agents, glomerulonephritis with tubule injury	Common	<350	>40	<20	>2	10
REDUCED NEPHRON NUMBER							
Elevated SNGFR	Chronic tubulointerstitial-renal disease Surgical loss of renal tissue	Rare†	[290	>40	3–10	3–10]	10
Normal SNGFR	Diffuse chronic glomerulonephritis Diabetic nephropathy	Rare†	[100–350‡	10–100‡	>10	>3]	>10
Reduced SNGFR	Any of the factors that can reduce SNGFR (listed above) may lower SNGFR in a patient who has a reduced number of functioning nephrons	Common	290	>20	>10	<3	>10

* Acute obstruction causing reduced SNGFR is called postrenal azotemia.
† Occurs only when total GFR is below 5% normal; urine chemistry values are helpful only when oliguria is present and are therefore enclosed in brackets.
‡ Varies with diet and with the level of GFR. When GFR is below 20% normal, osmotic concentration of the urine is usually impossible.
NOTE: osm = osmolality; creat = creatinine concentration; U = urine; P = plasma.

and consequently the ratio of the urine-to-plasma (U/P) creatinine concentrations is very high, 40 or more. Because urea can back-diffuse more completely than creatinine, the blood urea nitrogen (BUN) level rises more than the serum creatinine concentration. Normally, the ratio of BUN to serum creatinine concentration is 10:1; with depletion of the extracellular fluid volume this ratio rises. An elevated ratio can also be produced by unrelated factors such as tetracycline administration, adrenocortical steroid therapy, the presence of blood in the gastrointestinal tract, and increased protein turnover due to trauma or burn.

Prerenal azotemia can occur in any edema-forming condition during the phase in which NaCl and water accumulate. Typical examples include the nephrotic syndrome and hepatic cirrhosis with ascites (Chaps. 38 and 227). When a diuretic is being administered to inhibit the tubular reabsorption of NaCl, urine volume and Na concentration may be normal or elevated, even though SNGFR falls in response to the combination of the underlying edema-forming stimulus and further extracellular fluid volume depletion from the drug. Oliguria may appear upon withdrawal of the drug as the renal tubules resume intense reabsorption of NaCl and water. Prerenal azotemia may also be seen when renal blood flow is reduced by systemic hypotension, incomplete renal arterial or venous occlusion, or other cause (Chap. 132). Acute incomplete obstruction of the ureter and acute glomerular injury may also reduce SNGFR and leave tubule function relatively intact; postrenal azotemia is a term often applied when acute obstruction lowers SNGFR and causes azotemia. Whenever chronic obstruction of any portion of the urinary tract or glomerulonephritis damages nephrons extensively, the high urinary osmolality, U/P ratios for creatinine or urea, and low urinary Na concentrations disappear, and the kidneys behave as they do when nephron number is reduced.

TUBULE FUNCTION IMPAIRED Certain acute renal diseases which produce azotemia lower SNGFR and at the same time damage the tubules sufficiently to reduce or even abolish their reabsorptive function, producing *acute renal failure*. Acute tubular necrosis, nephrotoxic agents, and all forms of acute tubulointerstitial disease are excellent examples. Azotemia and oliguria appear, but the urinary Na concentration exceeds 20 mmol and usually 40 mmol/L; the U/P ratios for urea and creatinine are below 2 and 20, respectively; and urine osmolality is below 350 mosmol per kilogram of water. The ratio of BUN to serum creatinine is not elevated (see Chap. 223).

Reduced nephron number INCREASED SNGFR If one kidney is removed, the other grows larger, its nephrons enlarge, and the SNGFR increases until the total GFR becomes nearly normal for two kidneys. The tubules are overperfused with filtrate, but they appear to cope well with their increased reabsorptive burdens, perhaps in part because they are longer and wider and possess more cells. If more kidney tissue is removed, the remnant nephrons enlarge further, and their SNGFR rises. Extreme overperfusion of the tubules interferes with Na conservation. At the same time, total GFR comes to depend more and more upon expansion of the extracellular fluid volume largely because the increase in SNGFR is due not only to anatomic growth of the glomeruli but also to a relatively high rate of blood flow per glomerulus. Nephron adaptations to reduced nephron number are detailed in Chap. 222.

Azotemia occurs because the total GFR, i.e., the product of the elevated SNGFR and the markedly reduced nephron number, is low. Tubular conservation of filtered H_2O and Na conservation are poor, so fluid and salt intake must be liberal. Clinical states that produce this picture include surgical loss of renal substance secondary to trauma, neoplasm, stone, and destruction of kidneys by bacterial infection or tuberculosis, polycystic and medullary cystic renal diseases, and all the chronic tubulointerstitial nephropathies (Chaps. 229 and 231). In each of these disorders, the nephrons that remain viable are either fully intact or behave as though the SNGFR is better preserved than tubule function.

SNGFR NORMAL The SNGFR does not appear to increase despite a reduction of nephron number in diseases such as glomerulonephritis and diabetic glomerulosclerosis, where the glomerulus is the primary site of damage. In these diseases total GFR falls directly with nephron number and is not supported by elevated SNGFR. Since the tubules are not confronted with an excessive reabsorptive burden, sodium conservation is adequate. In these disorders, superimposed conditions that lower SNGFR, such as depletion of extracellular fluid volume, can cause oliguria with low urine sodium concentration and U/P ratios for creatinine and urea above 20 and 3, respectively. The serum urea to creatinine ratio will rise distinctly.

SNGFR REDUCED In patients with chronic renal disease in whom total GFR has been sufficient to support life only because of a very high SNGFR, inadvertent dehydration or any other factor (Table 49-1 and Chaps. 222 and 223) that lowers the SNGFR can provoke oliguria and severe azotemia. Under these circumstances, urine Na concentration falls, but not below 20 mmol/L, as in the normal person, because SNGFR, though reduced from a previously elevated level, may still be above normal. The U/P ratios for creatinine and urea will be low, usually below 10 and 3, respectively, despite oliguria, and urine osmolality will not rise above the plasma level. The serum urea to creatinine ratio may rise, but not above 20. In less extreme situations, reduction of SNGFR will worsen azotemia and alter urine chemistry in the same directions but to a lesser extent.

OLIGURIA AND ANURIA *Oliguria* refers to a urine volume insufficient to sustain life, usually less than 400 mL per day in an adult of average size. Daily urine volume is difficult to measure when flow rate is low, because small absolute errors of volume measurement, in the range of 50 to 100 mL of urine each day, or of timing of collection, may represent large percentage errors.

Anuria, which is the absence of urine flow, is caused mainly by urinary obstruction, which must be excluded as a first step (Chap. 233). Total renal arterial and venous occlusion is another important cause. Severe renal diseases such as cortical necrosis and rapidly progressive glomerulonephritis produce anuria in the adult, but so rarely that anuria should never be ascribed to a primary renal disease until patency of the urinary tract and major renal blood vessels has been established.

Approach to the patient with azotemia or oliguria A critical issue is whether azotemia has been stable and long-standing (chronic renal failure, Chap. 221) or is recent and increasing (acute renal failure, Chap. 223; pre- and postrenal azotemia). If azotemia is recent, and oliguria present, the most discriminating additional measurements include serum urea and creatinine concentrations, and the Na, urea, and creatinine concentrations and osmolality of a concurrent urine sample. Reduction of SNGFR with well-preserved tubule function is usually present when urine osmolality exceeds 500 mosmol per kilogram of water, Na $<$ 20 mmol/L, the U/P ratios for urea and creatinine $>$ 8 and 40, respectively, the urinalysis is normal, and the BUN is more than 10 times the serum creatinine concentration. The prognosis for recovery of adequate GFR is good, if the cause of reduced SNGFR can be reversed. When urine osmolality is below 350 mosmol per kilogram of water, Na $>$ 40 mmol, the U/P values for urea and creatinine $<$ 2 and 20, respectively, and the BUN exceeds the serum creatinine by only tenfold, tubule function has been lost, and some form of acute or chronic renal failure usually is present.

ABNORMAL URINARY CONSTITUENTS

PROTEINURIA Normal adults may excrete up to 150 mg protein daily. Of this, only 10 to 15 mg is albumin; the rest is composed of over 30 different plasma proteins and of glycoproteins that derive from the renal cells. Tamm-Horsfall mucoprotein, the most prevalent of the urine proteins that do not arise from plasma, is produced by the cells of the ascending limb of the loop of Henle and is excreted at the rate of 25 mg per day. Daily excretion of more than 150 mg protein is properly termed *pathologic proteinuria,* but in common usage the word *proteinuria* suffices. Protein excretion above 3.5 g per 24 h is termed *massive* proteinuria and usually occurs when glomeruli have been damaged enough to allow plasma proteins, especially albumin, to enter the urine. Urinary albumin loss lowers serum albumin concentration, and the consequent fall in intracapillary oncotic pressure fosters the accumulation of tissue edema (Chap. 38); serum lipids rise, for reasons detailed in Chap. 227. The combination of *massive proteinuria, hypoalbuminemia, edema,* and *hyperlipidemia* is often called the *nephrotic syndrome;* but this term is becoming synonymous with massive urinary protein loss alone. Hypoalbuminemia, elevated blood lipids, and edema are pathophysiologic consequences of massive proteinuria and occur only when hepatic albumin synthesis, though normal or even increased, fails to compensate for urine albumin losses; these features are not a direct result of renal disease.

Detection of proteinuria Proteinuria is usually detected by urine "dipsticks" that register a trace result in response to as little as 50 mg protein per liter, and a distinct color change of the 1+ level at about 300 mg protein per liter. Since proteinuria can be missed if the urine is very dilute, fasting morning samples that tend to be concentrated are usually studied. Dipsticks respond best to albumin, so that a negative result can occur when large amounts of other protein, or protein fragments such as light chains, are being excreted. Dipstick proteinuria requires additional evaluation by the measurement of 24-h excretion rate. If total protein excretion is abnormal, it is helpful to characterize the proportions of albumin and globulins in the urine by cellulose acetate electrophoresis or other methods. Immunoelectrophoresis is required to identify immunoglobulin fragments, kappa or lambda light chains, when their presence is suggested by a monoclonal peak on routine urine electrophoresis.

Mechanisms of proteinuria TUBULAR PROTEINURIA Normal low-molecular-weight ($<$40,000) serum proteins, such as beta$_2$ microglobulin (11,600 mol wt), lysozyme (14,000 mol wt), or light chains (22,000 mol wt) are readily filtered by the glomeruli but are reabsorbed so efficiently that only trace amounts enter the urine. Diseases that selectively damage the tubules more than glomeruli (Chap. 229) cause excessive excretion of these small proteins with little or no increase in albumin excretion. The resulting proteinuria is usually between 1 and 3 g per 24 h, and edema and lipid disorders do not occur because albumin losses are small. Bence Jones protein, which is probably a dimer of two light chains, light chains themselves, and myoglobin are examples of proteins whose plasma concentrations may increase as a consequence of disease. If their filtered load rises enough to exceed tubular reabsorptive capacity, "overflow" proteinuria may occur.

GLOMERULAR PROTEINURIA Normal glomeruli filter very little albumin or globulin. Glomerular capillary endothelial cells form a barrier penetrated by pores of about 100 nm diameter that holds back cells and other particles but offers no impediment to most proteins. The glomerular basement membrane traps molecules about 5 nm in effective radius, above 100,000 daltons molecular mass. The *foot processes (podocytes)* of the visceral epithelial cells (Fig. 49-1) cover the urinary aspect of the glomerular basement membrane and produce a series of narrow channels through which molecules that traverse the basement membrane must pass. Anionic molecules, like albumin, are filtered less freely than are neutral or positively charged molecules of the same size, so little albumin enters the filtrate. This charge selectively appears to be due to anionic glycoproteins that cover the surfaces of the foot processes and contribute to the matrix structure of the basement membrane (Chap. 222). The glycoproteins are anionic because they contain the dicarboxylic amino acids, glutamic and aspartic acid, and sialic acid. At the pH of blood (7.4) or urine (4.5 to 7.5) carboxylic and sialic acid residues are dissociated and, therefore, have a negative charge; albumin also carries an overall negative charge. The negatively charged portions of the glycoproteins repel those of albumin and retard filtration.

Glomerular disease can disrupt any of these filtration barriers. Injury limited to the polyanion glycoproteins would tend to produce selective losses of anionic proteins, such as albumin, that would be filtered more completely by the normal glomerulus but for their charge. Extensive injury that involves the entire basement membrane, not only its polyanion components, may increase losses of very large proteins as well as albumin.

The selectivity of proteinuria varies with the extent of glomerular injury. However, the clinical value of measuring selectivity has not been fully defined. The basis of such measurements is to express the

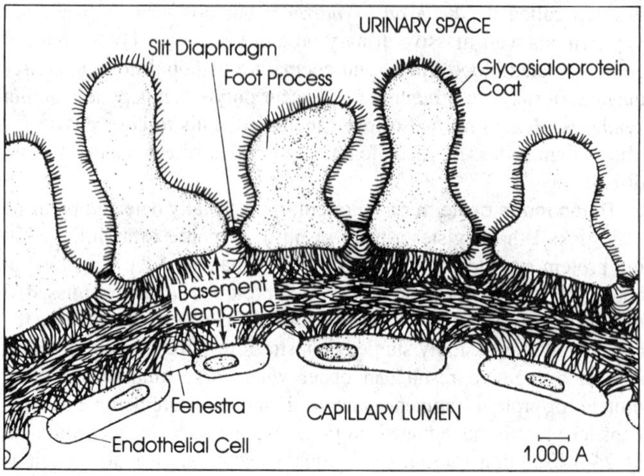

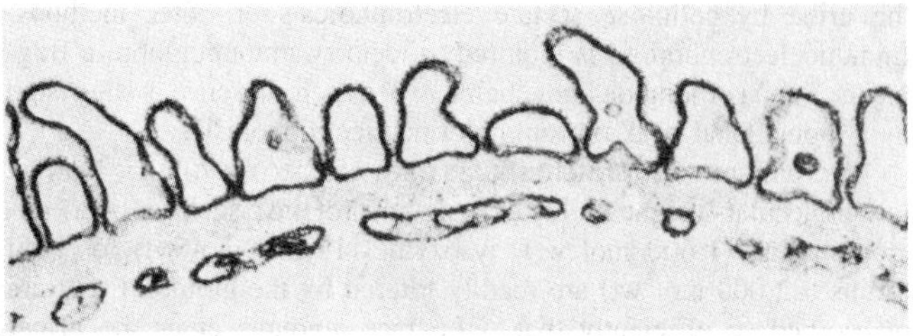

FIGURE 49-1 Top. Diagram showing normal structures separating the capillary lumen and urinary space in the glomerulus. In the process of glomerular filtration, an ultrafiltrate of plasma traverses the glomerular capillary wall through endothelial fenestrae, basement membrane, and slit diaphragms. Macromolecules in the plasma are believed to be restricted from entry into glomerular urine by each of these wall structures. In addition, circulating polyanions (e.g., albumin) are thought to be retarded by negatively charged glycosialoproteins, which, as shown by the shaded area in the upper panel, are distributed throughout the glomerular wall. Bottom. A corresponding electron micrograph of the same structures. *(Drawing by NL Gahan from BM Brenner, R Beeuwkes, Hosp Prac, vol 13, no 7, 1978. Reproduced with permission.)*

excretion rate of a protein as a fraction of its theoretical maximal filtered load, which is the product of its serum concentration and the GFR. This fraction must reflect the relative filtration efficiency of the protein to that of a completely filtered GFR marker, usually inulin or creatinine, provided that tubular reabsorption and renal production or catabolism are negligible. The slope of a plot of such a clearance ratio against the molecular weight for a variety of serum proteins is one index of filtration selectivity. A more practical version of this test is based upon the ratio of the clearance fractions of two proteins of different molecular weight, such as IgG and transferrin (Chap. 227).

Approach to the patient with proteinuria Given dipstick proteinuria of the 1+ level or more, 24-h urine protein excretion should be measured. If it is above 150 mg, electrophoresis should be carried out to determine the proportions of albumin and other proteins. Excretion mainly of albumin signifies a glomerular lesion. When the total daily protein excretion exceeds 3.5 g, by definition the nephrotic syndrome is considered to be present; milder albuminuria is called an *asymptomatic urinary abnormality*. The initial steps in evaluating proteinuria are outlined in Chap. 221. Subsequent details of differential diagnosis are in Chaps. 227 and 228. Tubular proteinuria usually reflects a hereditary or acquired tubular disorder (Chap. 231) or tubulointerstitial nephropathy (Chap. 229). The presence of large amounts of Bence Jones protein suggests that multiple myeloma may be present (Chap. 265).

HEMATURIA AND CASTS **Isolated hematuria** Bleeding in the urinary tract from the urethra to the renal pelvis produces isolated hematuria, without significant proteinuria, cells, or urinary casts. Total hematuria, which occurs evenly throughout voiding, means that blood has had the opportunity to mix fully with the bladder urine. When bleeding occurs mainly at the beginning or end of micturition, a prostatic or urethral origin is more likely.

Common causes of *isolated* hematuria are urinary tract stones, benign and malignant neoplasms of the urinary tract, tuberculosis, trauma, and prostatitis; few primary renal diseases cause it. As discussed in Chaps. 221 and 227, *focal glomerulitis,* in the syndrome of benign recurrent hematuria or in Berger's disease, i.e., IgA nephropathy, is usually associated with red blood cell casts. Analgesic nephropathy and sickling states cause isolated hematuria, but modest proteinuria; papillary necrosis or azotemia often is present and suggests a renal origin. Hemoglobin electrophoresis is appropriate whenever a sickling disorder is suspected.

Examination of the prostate and external urethra is the basic first step in the evaluation of isolated hematuria. Intravenous pyelography and renal ultrasonography are the next. If no lesion is found and no obvious cause of bleeding such as renal stone passage is present, cystoscopy and retrograde pyelography may become necessary. At cystoscopy, blood may be found to issue from only one ureter, a helpful clue which indicates a localized lesion rather than a primary renal disease. Disorders of coagulation, and thrombocytopenia, as well as urinary infection, must be excluded. Because infection with tuberculosis and fungi may be difficult to detect, multiple urine samples must be cultured and examined by microscopy. Computed tomography of the kidney and sometimes renal arteriography may be needed to disclose anatomic lesions such as cysts or tumors. Urine cytology may give a clue to malignant neoplasms of the kidneys or urinary tract that otherwise escape detection.

Hematuria associated with urinary tract infection Bacterial infection of the lower urinary tract or of the kidneys frequently causes hematuria. The presence of associated pyuria suggests the diagnosis of infection, and the demonstration of pathogenic bacteria in concentrations above 10^5 colonies per milliliter of urine establishes it. Acute cystitis or urethritis in women is an especially common cause of gross hematuria; in such symptomatic patients infection is documented by colony counts above 10^2 colonies per milliliter. Urinary tuberculosis can produce isolated hematuria, but pyuria often is present as well.

Hematuria with evidence of renal disease NEPHRONAL HEMATURIA Blood that enters the tubular fluid anywhere along the nephron can be trapped in a cylindrical mold of gelled Tamm-Horsfall protein to produce red blood cell casts. Tamm-Horsfall protein gels when concentrated at a low pH, as occurs during dehydration, or when exposed to myoglobin, hemoglobin, albumin, Bence Jones protein, and pyelographic contrast media. Degenerated red blood cells and clumps of hemoglobin can produce deeply pigmented casts that have the same significance—nephronal hematuria—as red blood cell casts.

Nephronal hematuria always connotes significant renal disease such as glomerulonephritis, tubulointerstitial injury, or a vasculitis that has damaged the circulation of the nephron. Glomerular or tubular proteinuria often accompanies renal bleeding, as a consequence of nephron injury. In general, nephronal hematuria, or proteinuria alone, arise from primary renal diseases that have a better prognosis than those in which proteinuria and hematuria occur in combination (Chap. 221).

Hematuria with proteinuria or casts Frequently, hematuria is accompanied by proteinuria, but red blood cell and deeply pigmented granular casts are absent. The presumption then is that bleeding is of nephronal origin, but a coincident independent lesion of the urinary tract must always be considered, because common renal diseases, such as diabetic glomerulosclerosis and arteriolar nephrosclerosis associated with hypertension, produce mainly proteinuria.

TYPES OF CASTS Heavy albuminuria or dehydration can cause showers of transparent, refractile "hyaline" casts. During heavy proteinuria, tubule cells fill with cholesterol-rich lipid droplets that display a Maltese-cross appearance in polarized light. Casts that incorporate these cells are called *fatty casts* because the lipid droplets are prominent. The same lipid-rich cells free in urine are called *oval fat bodies*.

White blood cell and *epithelial cell casts* can occur in any inflammatory state that involves the nephrons. White blood cell casts are particularly common in pyelonephritis, in nephritis associated with systemic lupus erythematosus, and during transplant rejection. When white blood or epithelial cells degenerate, they form granular nonpigmented casts that contain cellular debris and aggregated proteins. So-called *waxy* casts, with few granules and very distinct margins, arise when cell debris has broken down to a fine dispersion so that granules are no longer visible and are most common in chronic and progressive renal diseases.

Broad casts, of unusual width, are thought to arise in the dilated tubules of enlarged nephrons that have undergone compensatory hypertrophy in response to a reduction of functioning renal mass. A urine sample that contains a combination of broad and waxy casts as well as cellular or granular casts or red blood cells indicates a chronic smoldering process and has been termed a *telescoped* urine. This abnormality, first described in polyarteritis nodosa and systemic lupus erythematosus, can also be found in many chronic forms of glomerulonephritis with active glomerulitis.

Approach to the patient with hematuria Many urinalyses should be performed to determine whether the hematuria is isolated or associated with other features of primary renal disease, i.e., cells, casts, or proteinuria. The magnitude and type of associated proteinuria should be determined. As a general rule intravenous pyelography should be performed, if it can be done safely, even when the hematuria is of definite nephronal origin. Not only lesions of the urinary tract, but renal tumors or cysts, discrete areas of papillary necrosis, or signs of renal venous obstruction may be present. The source of isolated hematuria must always be ascertained, and this means a detailed examination of the urinary tract by cystoscopy, retrograde pyelography, and arteriography to disclose tumor, stone, cysts, or other cause. Renal ultrasonography and computed tomography are particularly helpful in detecting and evaluating renal cysts and tumors and should precede cystoscopy and arteriography. If all the studies disclose normal structures, a nephronal origin of hematuria is likely even if no red blood cell casts are present. The role of renal biopsy in such cases is detailed in Chaps. 227, 228, and 229. Hematuria with infection or overt renal disease usually requires no steps beyond intravenous pyelography. Evaluation of hematuria is detailed further in Chap. 215.

POLYURIA AND NOCTURIA

POLYURIA A reasonable definition of polyuria is a urine volume above 3 liters per day, but this should be qualified to exclude normal individuals who desire a large fluid intake and therefore form large volumes of urine. Patients cannot always distinguish polyuria from urinary frequency, the frequent voiding of small volumes. Since voiding volumes may not be clear from the history, polyuria must be substantiated by 24-h urine collection before one begins an investigation of causes.

Causes Polyuria can arise from inadequate secretion of vasopressin, failure of the renal tubules to respond to vasopressin, solute diuresis, or natriuresis (Table 49-2). It may also occur as a physiologic adaptation to deliberate excessive water drinking. The normal physiology of urine formation and mechanisms responsible for renal water conservation are discussed in Chap. 222.

DIABETES INSIPIDUS (See also Chap. 315) The term *diabetes insipidus* is applied to situations in which inadequate renal water conservation causes polyuria and secondary thirst. Either vasopressin insufficiency (central diabetes insipidus) or renal unresponsiveness to vasopressin (nephrogenic diabetes insipidus) may be responsible. In both, water reabsorption is reduced all along the distal nephron, because passive water movement from tubules into the hypertonic outer and inner medullary interstitium is slow. But even though the rate of water movement out of the collecting ducts is low for a given osmotic difference between the tubule lumen and interstitial fluid, the fluid that enters the collecting ducts is so abnormally dilute and copious in volume that more water enters the inner medulla than under normal circumstances and medullary solutes are washed out into the vasa recta. Wash-out is incomplete and vasopressin administration can lead to formation of an osmotically concentrated urine, but the maximal urine osmolality that can be attained is below normal.

TABLE 49-2 Causes of polyuria

I Inadequate renal water conservation
- *A* Diabetes insipidus
  - *1* Vasopressin-sensitive (posthypophysectomy; posttrauma; postpituitary ablation; idiopathic, supra- or intrasellar tumors or cysts; histiocystosis or granuloma; encroachment by aneurysm; Sheehan's syndrome, meningoencephalitis; Guillain-Barré syndrome; fat embolus; empty sella)
  - *2* Nephrogenic
    - *a* Acquired tubulointerstitial renal disease (pyelonephritis, analgesic nephropathy, multiple myeloma, amyloidosis, obstructive uropathy, sarcoidosis, hypercalcemic or hypokalemic nephropathy, Sjögren's syndrome, sickle cell anemia, renal transplantation)
    - *b* Drugs or toxins (lithium, demeclocycline, methoxyflurane, ethanol, diphenylhydantoin, propoxyphene, amphotericin)
    - *c* Congenital (hereditary nephrogenic diabetes insipidus, polycystic or medullary cystic disease)
- *B* Solute diuresis (glucosuria, high-protein tube feedings, urea or mannitol infusion, radiographic contrast media, chronic renal failure)
- *C* Natriuretic syndromes (salt-losing nephritis, diuretic phase of acute tubular necrosis, diuretic agents)

II Primary polydipsia
- *A* Psychogenic
- *B* Hypothalamic disease
- *C* Drugs (thioridazine, chlorpromazine, anticholinergic agents)

Vasopressin-sensitive (central) diabetes insipidus may be idiopathic or secondary to hypophysectomy or trauma or to neoplastic, inflammatory, vascular, or infectious causes (Table 49-2). Idiopathic diabetes insipidus can be inherited as an autosomal dominant trait; but more commonly it is sporadic and appears in childhood. In both forms there is selective destruction of the neurons that produce vasopressin in the supraoptic nucleus.

Rarely, nephrogenic diabetes insipidus is familial and congenital; but usually it is acquired from renal disease (Table 49-2). Hypercalcemia and hypokalemic nephropathy are important reversible causes of nephrogenic diabetes insipidus. Lithium carbonate, methoxyflurane anesthesia, and demeclocycline can also produce nephrogenic diabetes insipidus.

SOLUTE DIURESIS Excessive filtration of a poorly resorbed solute such as glucose, mannitol, or urea can depress reabsorption of NaCl and water in the proximal tubule and cause their loss in the urine, producing polyuria. Urine Na concentration is below that of blood, so that more water than salt is lost from the body and serum hypertonicity can be produced. Glucosuria in diabetes mellitus is a common cause of solute diuresis. Iatrogenic solute diuresis may arise from mannitol infusion, angiographic contrast media, and high-protein gavage feedings, which produce an excessive excretion of urea. Any degree of solute diuresis can cause polyuria, so further evaluation of renal concentrating ability should be postponed until the solute diuresis is corrected.

NATRIURETIC SYNDROMES Excessive chronic Na loss may occur during the course of tubulointerstitial or cystic renal diseases. Polyuria and polydipsia are accompanied by an unusually large daily Na requirement. Examples of this phenomenon include medullary cystic disease, Bartter's syndrome, and the diuretic phase of acute tubular necrosis, in which Na and water losses are very large.

PRIMARY POLYDIPSIA Whether because of habit, predilection, psychiatric disorder, a specific lesion in the brain, or medication (Table 49-2), some people drink enough water every day to produce polyuria. The body and the kidneys rarely if ever are injured by chronic polydipsia, but the condition can be confused with diabetes insipidus, which it resembles closely. During deliberate polydipsia, extracellular fluid volume is normal or high, and vasopressin secretion is reduced to a basal level because serum osmolality tends to be near the lower limits of normal. Reabsorption of water from the end distal convoluted tubule and collecting ducts is reduced so that all the surplus water can be excreted into the urine. The inner medulla loses its urea and NaCl gradients because of wash-out, as in diabetes insipidus. Wash-out may be more severe than in diabetes insipidus because primary polydipsia tends to cause expansion of the extracellular fluid volume, whereas primary renal water loss does the opposite. Volume expansion raises total delivery of NaCl and water to the thick ascending limb of Henle's loop and therefore to the inner medulla, all things being equal. It also raises renal blood flow, and increased flow through the vasa recta reduces their ability to trap solutes in the medulla.

Approach to the patient with polyuria Solute diuresis and natriuretic syndromes usually are apparent from the history, physical examination, urinalysis (glucosuria), clinical setting, blood count, blood glucose, and serum creatinine or the BUN. Diagnostic problems occur mainly when stable, chronic polyuria and polydipsia of uncertain origin are present. Here, one must try to distinguish between vasopressin-sensitive diabetes insipidus, nephrogenic diabetes insipidus, and primary polydipsia; the best-established way to do this is by measuring the response of urine osmolality to water deprivation and the administration of vasopressin.

The patient should have free access to water and receive a normal diet that provides approximately 100 mmol NaCl per day for 3 days; then a total fast is instituted. During the fast, pulse and blood pressure should be measured every 30 min and body weight every hour, using an accurate balance. When 3 percent of the initial body weight has been lost or 14 h have elapsed, urine and serum osmolality are measured. The normal subject will lower urine volume below 0.5 mL/min and raise urine osmolality to above 700 mosmol per kilogram of water. In complete diabetes insipidus, nephrogenic or vasopressin-sensitive, the urine osmolality will remain below 200 mosmol/kg water and urine flow above 0.5 mL/min, but some rise in osmolality and fall in flow will occur in incomplete diabetes insipidus. If urine osmolality is below 700 mosmol/kg water, by the end of the fasting period, 5 mU/min of aqueous vasopressin is administered by intravenous drip. Patients with complete or partial vasopressin-sensitive diabetes insipidus will raise their urine osmolality above the level achieved by fasting alone by more than 9 percent (see Chap. 315). No increase will occur given complete nephrogenic diabetes insipidus, although incomplete forms of nephrogenic diabetes insipidus will permit some response to vasopressin. Infusion of hypertonic saline (Chap. 315) is useful in defining defects of osmoregulator function.

The response of patients with primary polydipsia is quite different. During fluid restriction the secretion of vasopressin increases, and at the completion of the test the flow rate and osmolality of the urine will reflect a physiologic level of vasopressin acting upon normal tubules that traverse a medullary interstitium whose urea and NaCl concentrations have been reduced by chronic wash-out. In other words, the wash-out will set the upper limit on urine osmolality, and patients with primary polydipsia thus demonstrate a submaximal concentrating ability in spite of intact vasopressin secretion. Exogenous vasopressin can increase urine osmolality very little, < 9 percent, because medullary wash-out, not vasopressin insufficiency or insensitivity, is the main limiting factor. Usually the urine osmolality will be above 400 mosmol/kg water by the end of the fluid deprivation test, in contrast to the lower values of approximately 200 mosmol/kg water encountered in patients with diabetes insipidus; but it may be impossible to distinguish incomplete diabetes insipidus from primary polydipsia, in some cases, by using the fluid deprivation test alone. However, measurement of serum antidiuretic hormone levels by radioimmunoassay may increase diagnostic accuracy.

NOCTURIA Whether an individual sleeps through the night without urinating depends upon a diurnal rhythm in which the volume of urine formed during sleep does not exceed bladder capacity, because of reduced renal osmotic concentration, high sodium excretion, solute diuresis, or low bladder capacity.

All the polyuric states may cause nocturia. Urinary concentrating ability falls in most renal diseases (Chap. 222), often at an early stage. Even though overt polyuria may be absent, overnight urine volume frequently exceeds bladder capacity. Nocturia also occurs in edema-forming states. In congestive heart failure, nephrotic syndrome, and hepatic cirrhosis with ascites, fluid accumulates preferentially in dependent portions of the body during the day. At night, with recumbency, tissue capillary forces change and some edema fluid is mobilized, producing the effect of an intravenous saline infusion. Venous insufficiency may produce dependent edema of the legs that is often also mobilized at night, causing nocturia.

Reduced bladder capacity also causes nocturia. Infection, tumor, or stone can cause inflammation and increased irritability. Chronic partial bladder-outflow obstruction, from prostatic hypertrophy, urethral stricture, or benign or malignant neoplasm or stone, causes a frequent stimulus to void and also a thickening of the muscular wall that reduces its compliance. Frequent small voidings may be a clue to this lower urinary tract cause of nocturia, but in its earlier phases chronic obstruction may lead to only one nocturnal voiding of reasonable volume.

DYSURIA, FREQUENCY AND URGENCY, INCONTINENCE, AND ENURESIS

DYSURIA, FREQUENCY, AND URGENCY *Dysuria* refers to pain or a burning sensation during urination. *Urinary frequency* means voiding at abnormally brief intervals, due to a sense of bladder fullness that is due not to a full bladder but to a bladder that is irritable and feels full even when it is not. *Urgency* is an exaggerated sense of needing to urinate, due to an irritable or inflamed bladder.

Mechanisms of dysuria REDUCED BLADDER COMPLIANCE When the bladder has a decreased ability to expand, frequency, nocturia, and urgency usually result. When decreased expansion is due to inflammation of the mucosa (cystitis) from infection, radiation, chemicals, or foreign bodies (catheters, stones), a burning sensation usually is more prominent than when it is due to infiltration of the muscle by tumors of the bladder or from adjacent organs (prostate, rectum, uterus).

INFECTION Acute bacterial cystitis, which occurs more frequently in women, usually causes great frequency day and night, a burning sensation on urination, and, not infrequently, gross hematuria. Prostatitis or prostatocystitis in men can cause a picture similar to acute cystitis in women. When only the prostate is involved, milder symptoms such as vague pain or discomfort in the lower abdomen, groin, perineum, rectum, testes, or penis occur. The symptoms may be associated with urination but more frequently are noticed at times other than during micturition or ejaculation.

PSYCHOSOMATIC CYSTITIS The functional bladder syndrome and chronic glandular urethrotrigonitis are synonyms for a very common but poorly understood affliction of middle-aged and older women, in which pain is usually vague, aching in nature, and in the lower abdomen or vagina. There is daytime frequency without nocturia; pyuria is absent. A complete urologic evaluation usually becomes necessary because symptoms are chronic and hard to eradicate. The functional bladder syndrome must be distinguished from the effects of a cystocele, which can be repaired surgically.

Approach to the patient with dysuria The medical history should focus on past as well as present urinary problems. A pelvic examination in women and prostatic examination in men are necessary components of the physical examination. Microscopic examination of a two-glass urinary sediment in all patients and of the prostatic fluid in men, obtained by prostatic massage, is also necessary. The first 20 mL of a voiding, if collected separately, may contain a higher concentration of leukocytes and bacteria than the remainder of the voided urine, when the urethra is the principal site of inflammation or infection. Normal prostatic fluid, not subjected to centrifugation, contains less than 10 leukocytes per high-power field; excessive leukocytes in the prostatic fluid are an important clue to prostatitis and may, when prostatitis is chronic, be the only detectable abnormality. Further diagnostic studies will depend upon such positive findings as a history of chronic or recurrent episodes or associated fever, which are rare in lower urinary tract infections except in acute prostatitis, or an abnormality on physical examination such as a pelvic or rectal mass or tenderness, hematuria or pyuria, or excessive leukocytes and macrophages in the prostatic fluid. Serum acid phosphatase may be elevated when carcinoma of the prostate has extended beyond the boundary of the prostatic capsule.

Additional evaluation of dysuria, when the cause is not evident from clinical examination, may include cultures of urine and prostatic fluid for aerobic and anaerobic bacteria, tubercle bacilli, and mycoplasmas; excretory urography; and voiding cystourethrography. If these examinations do not reveal the diagnosis, but symptoms are troublesome, urologic evaluations, including cystoscopy and urethroscopy with endoscopic biopsies of visualized abnormalities, and dynamic urinary tract studies may be useful.

INCONTINENCE *Incontinence* refers to the inability to retain urine in the bladder. It results from neurologic or mechanical disorders of the complicated system that controls normal micturition.

Normal bladder function The detrusor muscle, which provides the propulsive force for emptying the bladder, consists of interlacing fibers of smooth muscle that are under parasympathetic autonomic control through the pelvic nerves from sacral spinal cord segments S2, S3, and S4. The smooth muscle of the trigonal portion of the bladder, between the ureteral orifices and the posterior area of the bladder outlet, is innervated by motor fibers from thoracolumbar segments (T11 to L2) of the sympathetic nervous system, in which alpha receptor sites predominate. This layer of muscle extends into the posterior urethra and acts as an involuntary internal sphincter that helps maintain urinary continence even in the absence of voluntary control. The external urethral sphincter and perineal muscles are under voluntary control via the pudendal nerves.

Sensory tracts of pain, temperature, and distention pass from the bladder via the pelvic nerves to sacral spinal levels S2, S3, and S4, creating a simple spinal voiding reflex between the bladder and the sacral spinal cord. The sensory tracts from the bladder further ascend through sacrobulbar pathways to the medulla of the brain and ultimately to cortical centers, from which impulses arise, pass back down the lateral and ventral reticulospinal tracts, and normally suppress the sacral spinal reflex arc controlling bladder emptying.

The normal adult bladder can accommodate as much as approximately 400 mL fluid without a significant increase in intravesical pressure (< 20 cmH_2O). Above this point, sensations of fullness are transmitted to the sacral cord. If not suppressed by cortical control, the sacral cord reflexly discharges motor impulses that cause powerful sustained detrusor contraction. Urination can be prevented by cortical suppression of the reflex arc or by voluntary contraction of the external sphincter and perineal muscles. Infants, and adults with spinal cord damage above S2, urinate spontaneously when the bladder fills sufficiently.

Normal urination is initiated by voluntary suppression of cortical inhibition of the reflex arc and by relaxation of the muscles of the pelvic floor and the external sphincter. The base of the bladder falls; then the trigone contracts, an action that occludes the ureters as they pass through the bladder wall and helps to prevent vesicoureteral reflux of urine during voiding. Finally, the detrusor contracts and voiding occurs.

Causes of incontinence DETRUSOR INSTABILITY In this condition, the bladder becomes prone to uncontrollable contractions—that cause incontinence—because inhibitory neural pathways are damaged. Among the elderly, detrusor instability causes as much as 70 percent of urinary incontinence, and arises from diseases of the central nervous system such as cerebrovascular accidents, Alzheimer's dementia, neoplasm, and, possibly, normal pressure hydrocephalus. Any lesion that disrupts the lateral and ventral reticulospinal tracts can reduce or abolish descending inhibiting impulses to the sacral spinal reflex and can result in detrusor instability. If the descending tracts are completely destroyed, the bladder will empty automatically. Bladder or pelvic infection or tumor, fecal impaction, uterine prolapse, and prostatic hypertrophy are other causes. Whatever the cause, the usual clinical picture is of unpredictable, involuntary voiding, usually >160 mL each time. Imipramine, 25 mg at bedtime, or calcium channel blockers (such as nifedipine) reduce detrusor contractions, and improve continence. Local infection, tumors, or fecal impaction are treated conventionally.

STRESS INCONTINENCE This condition is common in postmenopausal parous women. The structures of the female urethra atrophy when deprived of estrogen, and many become unable to resist the passage of urine under the stress of increased intraabdominal pressure during coughing, sneezing, climbing stairs, and other physical activity, so small amounts of urine escape. Parturition may damage the pelvic support of the bladder so that the bladder and urethra can slip downward from their normal position above the pelvic diaphragm. As they do, the urethra shortens, and the normal urethrovesical angle, important in closing the urethral sphincter, is lost. In men, stress incontinence usually is secondary to prostatic surgery for benign prostatic hypertrophy or prostatic carcinoma. If the external sphincter has also been damaged during operation, total incontinence may result. Surgical elevation of the urethrovesical angle is helpful in women. Estrogen replacement therapy may prevent atrophy of the urethral mucosa.

MECHANICAL INCONTINENCE Some congenital anomalies, extrophy of the bladder, patent urachus, and ectopic ureteral openings distal to the vesical neck cause mechanical incontinence. They are correctable only by surgery. Mechanical incontinence can follow transurethral resection of the prostate that damages both the internal and external sphincter mechanisms. Pelvic surgery or irradiation of the uterus or rectum may cause incontinence because of vesicovaginal, ureterovaginal, vesicoperineal, or ureteroperineal fistulas.

OVERFLOW OR PARADOXICAL INCONTINENCE This form of incontinence arises from large residual volumes of urine secondary to obstruction at the bladder neck or along the urethra (urethral stricture) or from neurologic damage. Benign prostatic hypertrophy afflicts upward of 75 percent of older men. It is manifested by nocturia, reduced size and force of the urinary stream, straining to urinate, and terminal dribbling, all due to outflow obstruction. Functional outflow obstruction can occur because of spinal cord disease; the detrusor and external sphincter contract dyssynergistically, i.e., at the same time. Hypotonic neurogenic bladders may occur in diseases which produce autonomic peripheral neuropathy, such as diabetes mellitus, uremia, hypothyroidism, chronic alcoholism, Guillain-Barré syndrome, collagen vascular diseases, and toxic neuropathies associated with some carcinomas (especially lung and kidney). It also may occur because of prolonged overdistention of the bladder. Hydronephrosis and impaired renal function can occur in patients with chronic overflow incontinence. All causes produce a dilated, palpable bladder. Especially in diabetes, patients can control micturition but lose their sensory awareness of bladder filling. Their incontinence can be avoided by scheduled reminders. Outlet obstruction is treated surgically. If the bladder has become adynamic because of prolonged overfilling, bethanechol chloride, 50 to 100 mg per day, may improve emptying.

PSYCHOGENIC AND FUNCTIONAL INCONTINENCE Children, and even some young adults, draw attention to themselves by feigning incontinence and thereby derive some secondary emotional satisfaction. A complete diagnostic evaluation usually is necessary to rule out organic disease even when psychogenic incontinence is strongly suspected. In elderly people, especially those who have a limited ability to walk or who are confused because of central nervous system disease or drugs, incontinence may be *functional,* i.e., due simply to an inability to reach a toilet in time. Treatment depends upon correcting the individual problem in each case.

ENURESIS *Enuresis* refers to the involuntary passage of urine at night or during sleep—hence, the synonym bed-wetting. Some clinicians reserve the term enuresis for those bed wetters who have no gross urologic abnormalities, but it should be used for bed-wetting in general.

The sacral spinal reflex arc alone controls urination in the infant; therefore, enuretic incontinence is normal under the age of 2 years. As the nervous system matures, cortical control over the spinal reflex arc results in the voluntary control over urination and defecation by the age of 2½ years. Even so, enuresis beyond the age of 3 years occurs to some degree in approximately 10 percent of all otherwise normal children and probably is due to a delay in maturation of bladder control, which may be familial.

Although the majority of bed wetters will be dry by the age of puberty, organic diseases, especially infections of the urinary tract, obstructive lesions with overflow incontinence, neurovesical dysfunction, and polyuric conditions that overload the bladder must be suspected in any child who is enuretic beyond the age of 3 years. Patients with organic disease usually, but not always, are incontinent during the day as well as at night. For the majority, who have no overt lesions, imipramine (75 mg at bedtime) may be useful.

REFERENCES

Azotemia, oliguria, and anuria

Abuelo JG: Proteinuria: Diagnostic principles and procedures. Ann Intern Med 98:186, 1983

Brenner BM et al: Molecular basis of proteinuria of glomerular origin. N Engl J Med 298:826, 1978

Bridges CR et al: Glomerular charge alterations in human minimal charge nephropathy. Kidney Int 22:677, 1982

Glassock RJ et al: Primary glomerular diseases, in *The Kidney*, 3d ed, BM Brenner, FC Rector Jr (eds). Philadelphia, Saunders, 1986, p 929

Kurtzman NA (ed): *Seminars in Nephrology: Acute Renal Failure*, JP Knochel (guest ed). New York, Grune & Stratton, 1981

——— (ed): *Seminars in Nephrology: Chronic Renal Failure*, G Eknoyan (guest ed). New York, Grune & Stratton, 1981

Levey AS et al: Idiopathic nephrotic syndrome. Ann Intern Med 107:697, 1987

Oken DE: On the differential diagnosis of acute renal failure. Am J Med 71:916, 1981

Pardo V et al: Benign primary hematuria: Clinicopathologic study of 65 patients. Am J Med 67:817, 1979

Polyuria and nocturia

Berl T (ed): Disorders of water metabolism, in *Seminars in Nephrology*, vol 4. New York, Grune & Stratton, 1984, p 285

Robertson GL, Berl W: Pathophysiology of water metabolism, in *The Kidney*, 3d ed, BM Brenner, FC Rector Jr (eds). Philadelphia, Saunders, 1986, p 385

Schrier RW, Bichet DG: Osmotic and nonosmotic control of vasopressin release and the pathogenesis of impaired water excretion in adrenal, thyroid, and edematous disorders. J Lab Clin Med 98:1, 1981

Zerbe RL, Robertson GL: A comparison of plasma vasopressin measurements with a standard indirect test in the differential diagnosis of polyuria. N Engl J Med 305:1539, 1981

Dysuria, frequency and urgency, incontinence, and enuresis

Bradley WE: Diagnosis of urinary bladder dysfunction in diabetes mellitus. Ann Intern Med 92:323, 1980

———, Scott FB: Physiology of the urinary bladder, in *Urology*, 4th ed, JH Harrison et al (eds). Philadelphia, Saunders, 1978, vol 1, p 87

DeGroat WC, Booth AM: Physiology of the urinary bladder and urethra. Ann Intern Med 92:312, 1980

Hindmarsh HR, Byrne PO: Adult enuresis: A symptomatic and urodynamic assessment. Br J Urol 52:88, 1980

Kellogg JA et al: Clinical relevance of culture versus screens for the detection of microbial pathogens in urine specimens. Am J Med 83:739, 1987

Meares EM Jr: Prostatitis syndromes: New perspectives about old woes. J Urol 123:141, 1980

Mikkelsen EJ, Rapoport JL: Enuresis: Psychopathology, sleep stage, and drug response. Urol Clin North Am 7:361, 1980

Platt R: Quantitative definition of bacteriuria. Infectious Diseases Symposium, July 28, 1983, p 44, Supplement to Am J Med

Turner-Warwick R, Whiteside CG (eds): *Symposium on Clinical Urodynamics: The Urologic Clinics of North America*, vol 6. Philadelphia, Saunders, 1979

Williams ME, Pannell FC: Urinary incontinence in the elderly. Ann Intern Med 97:895, 1982

50 FLUIDS AND ELECTROLYTES

NORMAN G. LEVINSKY

SODIUM AND WATER

PHYSIOLOGIC CONSIDERATIONS (See also Chap. 222) Both physiologically and clinically, sodium and water metabolism are closely interrelated. The sodium content of the body depends on the balance between dietary intake and renal excretion of sodium. In health, extrarenal losses of sodium are negligible. Renal sodium excretion is closely regulated to match dietary content. Within 2 to 4 days after sodium intake stops, urinary excretion decreases to 5 mmol/d or less. If dietary sodium is abruptly increased, sodium excretion promptly rises and equals intake within a few days. Thus, in normal persons the sodium content of the body remains quite constant despite wide variations in sodium intake; over the range of 0 to 400 mmol/d, total body sodium varies only by about 10 percent.

Renal sodium excretion This is regulated by the interplay of multiple control mechanisms. Sodium loads or deficits tend to produce corresponding changes in the central blood volume. Receptors, apparently located in the atria and central arteries, respond to changes in local pressure or flow which signal the volume/capacity relation of the central circulation (*effective blood volume*). If the effective volume is depleted, salt retention is induced, while expansion triggers multiple factors that favor natriuresis. With volume (salt) depletion, renal blood flow falls, due to decreased cardiac output, increased renal sympathetic nerve activity, and activation of the renin-angiotensin system. Glomerular filtration also tends to fall, which reduces filtered sodium. Tubular reabsorption of sodium is enhanced. Proximal reabsorption is stimulated by changes in Starling forces (e.g., increased plasma protein concentration) in the peritubular circulation and by sympathetic nerves which innervate proximal segments directly. Distal tubular reabsorption is enhanced by aldosterone, which is secreted at an increased rate in response to stimulation of the adrenal gland by angiotensin. Volume expansion leads to the opposite changes in renal hemodynamics and in these various regulators of tubular transport. Moreover, one or more natriuretic hormones are released in response to increased extracellular volume. A natriuretic peptide secreted by the atria augments sodium excretion both by increasing glomerular filtration and by inhibiting tubular sodium reabsorption. Another natriuretic hormone may decrease tubular salt transport by inhibiting Na^+, K^+ adenosine triphosphatase (ATPase). Prostaglandins and kinins secreted within the kidney reduce sodium reabsorption in distal nephron segments. The exact role of these natriuretic factors in the regulation of sodium excretion is uncertain.

Undoubtedly, other regulatory mechanisms remain to be defined. The multiplicity of control mechanisms prevents abnormalities of any single mechanism from grossly distorting the regulation of sodium excretion. For example, increased aldosterone secretion leads only to limited and transient sodium retention, because the initial accumulation of sodium stimulates opposing natriuretic factors such as increased glomerular filtration and decreased proximal tubular sodium reabsorption.

Distribution of sodium All but 2 to 5 percent of the sodium in the body is located in the extracellular fluids. (Approximately 40 percent of total body sodium is in bone, but this fraction does not participate significantly in most physiologic processes and will not be considered further.) Except for minor differences in concentration due to the Gibbs-Donnan effect of plasma proteins, the electrolyte compositions of plasma and interstitial fluid are essentially equal. Consequently, plasma composition can be considered representative of the entire extracellular compartment. Total extracellular volume approximates 20 percent of body weight. Of this, 5 percent represents plasma volume and 15 percent the volume of interstitial fluids. Thus, in a 70-kg individual with plasma sodium concentration of 140 mmol/

L, extracellular sodium content will approximate 2000 mmol. The volume of intracellular fluid is approximately twice as great as that of extracellular fluid, i.e., about 40 percent of body weight. However, since intracellular sodium concentration is less than 5 mmol/L, total intracellular sodium content is only about 100 to 150 mmol. The asymmetric distribution of sodium across cell membranes is maintained by expenditure of a large fraction of the energy derived from cell metabolism, which is required constantly to pump sodium out of cells against its electrochemical gradient. All the principal electrolytes are asymmetrically distributed across cell membranes. The principal electrolytes of the extracellular fluids are sodium, chloride, and bicarbonate. The major electrolytes of the intracellular fluids are potassium, magnesium, calcium, and organic anions, including proteins.

Since sodium salts account for more than 90 percent of the total osmolality of the extracellular fluid, variations in plasma sodium concentration are almost always reflected in equivalent changes in plasma osmolality. Exceptions due to accumulation of other solutes in plasma are discussed later. Although the electrolyte compositions of intracellular and extracellular fluids differ markedly, they are always in osmotic equilibrium, since water moves rapidly across cellular membranes to dissipate osmotic gradients. Therefore, although sodium is largely confined to extracellular fluids, plasma sodium concentration is an index of not only the relative proportions of sodium and water in those fluids but also the relation between total body solute and total body water. An example is the effect of shift of sodium from extracellular to intracellular fluid without a change in total body solute. Movement of sodium into cells would not cause hyponatremia, since water would shift into cells with the sodium. On the other hand, a primary decrease in the concentration of osmotically active solute within cells would decrease total body solute; although there would be no change in total body sodium or water, hyponatremia would result from the shift of intracellular water into the extracellular compartment.

Role of antidiuretic hormone A very effective mechanism involving the *hypothalamus,* the *neurohypophysis,* and the kidney regulates plasma osmolality. Changes of 2 percent or less in plasma osmolality can be detected by osmoreceptors in the hypothalamus. Small increases in osmolality stimulate the secretion of vasopressin (the antidiuretic hormone, ADH) from the neurohypophysis, while small decreases suppress secretion of the hormone. Normal plasma osmolality is approximately 280 to 300 mosmol per kilogram of water; the exact level is determined by the "set" of the hypothalamic osmoreceptors in a given individual. When ADH secretion is maximal, urine volume will be about 500 mL/d, and urine osmolality will be 800 to 1400 mosmol/kg. In the absence of ADH, minimal urine osmolality is 40 to 80 mosmol/kg, and maximum water diuresis can reach 15 to 20 L/d or more. The capacity of this receptor-effector system is sufficient to maintain plasma osmolality within narrow limits despite large variations in the volume and concentration of dietary fluids. ADH secretion is also regulated by changes in extracellular volume. A reduction of 10 percent or more may trigger ADH release even in the absence of changes in plasma osmolality. If volume contraction is sufficiently severe, volume-mediated stimulation of ADH may override osmotic signals and cause water retention despite progressive dilution of body fluids. Conversely, extracellular volume expansion tends to suppress ADH release even if the body fluids are hypertonic.

The total sodium *content* of the body is determined by the renal sodium regulatory mechanisms described earlier. However, the principal determinant of plasma sodium *concentration* is water metabolism rather than total body sodium content. If excess sodium were to be ingested and retained, hypernatremia would be only transient. Water intake would increase because of thirst, and the fluid ingested would be retained because hypernatremia (hyperosmolality) would stimulate ADH secretion. Expanded extracellular volume, not hypernatremia, would be the end result. Conversely, if the osmoregulatory system is functioning normally, loss of moderate amounts of sodium without water would not result in permanent reduction of plasma sodium concentration. The initial reduction would shut off secretion of ADH, and a water diuresis would ensue. The final outcome would be contraction of extracellular volume, while plasma sodium concentration would be restored to normal. It follows that changes in total sodium content tend to cause changes in extracellular volume. In this sense, the sodium content of the extracellular fluid determines extracellular volume. On the other hand, changes in plasma sodium concentration reflect altered regulation of water excretion, not changes in total body sodium content alone. Clinically, plasma sodium concentration per se gives no information about the amount of sodium present in the body. Total body sodium content is determined by the volume of extracellular fluids as well as by the concentration of sodium in these fluids. Extracellular volume is usually the dominant factor since changes in volume tend to be proportionately greater than changes in sodium concentration. Plasma sodium concentration reflects the relative proportions of sodium and water (or, more exactly, of total body solute and water), not the absolute amount of sodium in the body. Either hyponatremia or hypernatremia may occur when total body sodium content is decreased, normal, or increased.

CLINICAL DISORDERS Deficits and excesses of sodium and water occur in a great variety of clinical circumstances. The manifestations of the underlying illness may overshadow the clinical features of the fluid and electrolyte disorder. Theoretically, disturbances of sodium and water metabolism can be classified into four categories, reflecting a primary excess or deficit of water or sodium. Practically, such isolated disturbances are uncommon. A primary excess of sodium leads to edema; it is not ordinarily considered as an electrolyte disorder but as a feature of underlying disease, such as congestive heart failure, hepatic cirrhosis, or nephrotic syndrome. Primary sodium deficits are nearly always accompanied by water depletion, leading to the clinical syndrome of extracellular volume depletion. Pure or disproportionate water excess leads to hyponatremia, relative or absolute water depletion to hypernatremia. A practical clinical classification of the principal disorders of sodium and water metabolism is given in Table 50-1.

VOLUME DEPLETION Combined sodium and water deficits are far more frequent than isolated deficits of either constituent. Although the term *dehydration* is often used for combined deficits, this usage is confusing. Dehydration should be used to describe relatively pure water depletion leading to hypernatremia; *volume depletion* or some similar term should be used for combined deficits.

Pathogenesis As noted earlier, elimination of sodium from the diet will not by itself lead to sodium depletion in the presence of normal renal function, since urinary sodium excretion will quickly fall to very low levels. Therefore, sodium depletion is always due either to extrarenal losses or to abnormal renal losses.

GASTROINTESTINAL The most common cause of volume depletion is loss of a significant fraction of the 8 to 10 L of gastrointestinal fluids secreted daily. As the sodium concentration of these fluids is high, their loss causes combined sodium and water deficits. Since the principal secretions contain potassium and hydrogen ion or bicarbonate in large amounts, volume depletion due to such losses is often combined with potassium depletion and acidosis or alkalosis.

Significant volume depletion may be caused by sequestration of secretions within an obstructed gastrointestinal tract or within the peritoneal cavity in peritonitis. Rapid reaccumulation of ascites after paracentesis may reduce the effective circulating blood volume.

SKIN The sodium concentration of sweat varies from 5 to 50 mmol/L; sodium concentration increases with higher rates of sweating and in adrenal insufficiency. Because sweat is always a hypotonic solution, sweating leads to water deficits out of proportion to sodium losses. In burns, capillary damage may lead to sequestration of large amounts of sodium and water in the injured skin.

RENAL Abnormal losses of sodium and water in the urine may occur in both acute and chronic renal diseases. Early in the recovery (diuretic) phase of *acute renal failure,* urinary sodium concentration tends to be high (50 to 100 mmol/L), and substantial deficits of both

TABLE 50-1 Disorders of sodium and water metabolism*

I Combined sodium and water depletion (volume depletion)
- *A* Extrarenal losses
  - *1* Gastrointestinal (vomiting, diarrhea, gastrointestinal suction, fistulas)
  - *2* Abdominal sequestration (peritonitis, rapid reaccumulation of ascites)
  - *3* Skin (sweating, burns)
- *B* Renal losses
  - *1* Renal disease (diuretic phase of acute renal failure, postobstructive diuresis, chronic renal failure, salt-wasting tubular disease)
  - *2* Diuretic excess
  - *3* Osmotic diuresis (diabetic glycosuria)
  - *4* Mineralocorticoid deficiency (Addison's disease, hypoaldosteronism)

II Hyponatremia
- *A* Associated with extracellular volume depletion (see list of causes above)
- *B* Associated with extracellular volume excess and edema
- *C* Associated with normal or modestly expanded extracellular volume (no edema)
  - *1* Acute and chronic renal failure
  - *2* Temporary impairment of water diuresis (pain, drugs, emotion)
  - *3* Syndrome of inappropriate secretion of antidiuretic hormone (SIADH)
  - *4* Endocrine (glucocorticoid deficiency, hypothyroidism)
  - *5* Severe polydipsia
  - *6* Essential (''sick cell syndrome'')
- *D* Without plasma hypoosmolality
  - *1* Osmotic (hyperglycemia, mannitol)
  - *2* Artifactual (hyperlipemia, hyperproteinemia, laboratory error)

III Hypernatremia
- *A* Due solely to water loss
  - *1* Extrarenal
    - *a* Skin (insensible losses)
    - *b* Lungs
  - *2* Renal
    - *a* Diabetes insipidus (central, nephrogenic)
  - *3* Hypothalamic dysfunction
- *B* Due to water loss associated with sodium loss
  - *1* Extrarenal
    - *a* Sweat
  - *2* Renal
    - *a* Osmotic diuresis (glycosuria, urea)
- *C* Due to sodium gain
  - *a* Excessive sodium administration
  - *b* Adrenal hyperfunction (hyperaldosteronism, Cushing's syndrome)

* For differential diagnosis, see Fig. 50-1, p. 283.

sodium and water may ensue. With rare exceptions, severe sodium and water wasting does not persist beyond the first few days. It is important to discriminate between increased excretion, which represents elimination of excess retained during the oliguric period, and true tubular sodium and water wasting, which depletes normal extracellular volume. Only the latter requires replacement. Acute salt and water wasting due to tubular damage may also occur immediately after relief of prolonged *obstruction* of the urinary tract. Although such a postobstructive diuresis may be severe, it rarely persists for more than several days as a clinically important phenomenon.

Patients with *chronic renal failure* have limited ability to decrease sodium and water excretion in response to decreased intake. They will become progressively volume-depleted if their intake is restricted by the anorexia, nausea, and vomiting characteristic of uremia or because of their physician's instructions. Large deficits may develop insidiously over many days or weeks. A ''self-perpetuating cycle'' may result, in that volume depletion will tend further to compromise renal function. Severe sodium-wasting renal disease, i.e., negative sodium balance when dietary sodium is normal, is rare. It occurs in occasional patients with tubulointerstitial diseases of the kidney, especially medullary cystic disease.

Renal sodium wasting in the presence of normal intrinsic renal function occurs in three clinical circumstances. Perhaps the most common is sodium depletion due to continued administration of potent *diuretics* to patients after edema has been relieved or to patients whose edema is sequestered and cannot be mobilized. For example, attempted treatment of cirrhotics with ascites may result in depletion of extracellular volume rather than mobilization of ascitic fluid. An obligatory *osmotic diuresis* may also cause renal sodium and water wasting despite normal renal function. Marked glycosuria in uncontrolled diabetes mellitus is the most frequent clinical example. Volume depletion in patients receiving high-protein enteral or parenteral alimentation may be due to an osmotic diuresis of urea formed by protein metabolism. Administration of solutes such as mannitol, which act as osmotic diuretics, may cause volume depletion. Finally, renal sodium wasting despite normal intrinsic function occurs in Addison's disease and hypoaldosteronism due to a *deficiency* of *mineralocorticoids*.

Clinical features and diagnosis The cause of volume depletion can usually be suspected from a history of inadequate salt and water intake together with vomiting, diarrhea, or excessive sweating; the symptoms of poorly controlled diabetes mellitus or of renal or adrenal disease may be elicited. The key findings on physical examination are those of interstitial and plasma volume depletion. Decreased interstitial volume may be recognized from reduced skin turgor, which is usually present in patients with significant volume contraction but may be difficult to evaluate in the elderly. It can be estimated clinically by noting the slow rate of return of skin to its original position when it is raised between the examiner's fingers. An area of skin normally free of wrinkles and not subject to wide variations in the thickness of subcutaneous tissue, such as that over the sternum, should be selected for this maneuver. Oral mucous membranes may be dry and axillary sweating decreased; these are less reliable diagnostic features than decreased skin turgor. Plasma volume depletion is indicated by changes in blood pressure. With moderate volume depletion, blood pressure is usually normal when the patient is recumbent, although resting tachycardia may be present. Postural hypotension, i.e., a drop of at least 5 to 10 mmHg in the sitting or standing position, is often present. With greater degrees of volume depletion, even recumbent blood pressure is reduced, and frank shock may occur. The patient with moderate or severe degrees of volume contraction is often lethargic, weak, confused, or obtunded. Such patients are usually oliguric, even when recumbent blood pressure is normal. However, an osmotic diuresis, as occurs in hyperglycemia, tends to prevent oliguria despite volume contraction.

LABORATORY FINDINGS The hematocrit and plasma protein concentration are increased, but increases within the normal range are interpretable only if prior values are known. Plasma sodium concentration may be decreased, normal, or increased, depending upon the proportion between deficits of sodium and of water. Plasma creatinine and urea nitrogen are usually increased, since the glomerular filtration rate is decreased (''prerenal azotemia''). Blood urea nitrogen (BUN) tends to rise proportionately more than plasma creatinine. Urinary sodium concentration may be of value in differentiating extrarenal and renal sources of sodium loss if the probable cause is not clear from the history. With extrarenal losses, urinary sodium concentration is less than 10 mmol/L; the concentration will usually exceed 20 mmol/L if renal or adrenal disorders are at fault. However, urinary sodium may ultimately fall below this level even in patients with renal salt wasting if sodium depletion becomes severe.

Treatment The principal clinical manifestations of extracellular volume depletion are due to reduction of plasma and interstitial fluid volume. Since there is no convenient clinical method for quantifying these volumes, the effect of treatment must be determined by following the changes in clinical features such as blood pressure, urine output, and skin turgor. Modest deficits of sodium and water can often be corrected by increased oral intake in patients not suffering from gastrointestinal disorders. Severe depletion requires therapy with intravenous solutions. Isotonic saline (0.85%) is the infusion of choice in patients whose serum sodium concentration is approximately normal. The amount to be infused can be estimated from the history of prior losses and from the severity of the physical findings of extracellular volume contraction. Patients with moderate volume contraction usually require replacement with 2 to 3 L of saline, while patients with severe depletion may require much larger volumes. The need for correction of other concurrent electrolyte abnormalities may alter the composition of the required infusion; e.g., some of the sodium may be given as bicarbonate to patients with volume contraction and metabolic acidosis, or potassium may be added in patients with concurrent potassium depletion. In estimating the total amount to be infused, allowance for ongoing losses must be included. Since the amount to be infused cannot be calculated precisely, patients should be monitored carefully to avoid fluid overload and congestive failure.

HYPONATREMIA Pathophysiology Hyponatremia indicates that the body fluids are diluted by an excess of water relative to total solute. Hyponatremia is not equivalent to sodium depletion, which is only one of the clinical states in which it may occur (see Table 50-1). Most types of hyponatremia result from defective urinary dilution. The normal response to dilution of body fluids is a water diuresis, which corrects the hypoosmotic state. Normal water diuresis requires three factors: (1) Secretion of ADH must be suppressed. (2) Sufficient sodium and water must reach the diluting sites of the nephron, in the ascending limb of Henle's loop and the distal convoluted tubule. (3) These nephron segments must function normally, reabsorbing sodium while remaining impermeable to water.

Correspondingly, three mechanisms may cause defective water diuresis in patients with hyponatremia. (1) Secretion of ADH may continue "inappropriately" despite hypotonicity of extracellular fluid, which normally shuts off secretion of the hormone. This may be due to unregulated release of ADH by neoplasms or to nonosmotic stimuli to ADH secretion. The latter include volume depletion, neural factors such as pain and emotion, and certain drugs. (2) Insufficient sodium may reach the diluting segments to permit the formation of an adequate amount of dilute urine. Inadequate delivery of tubular fluid to distal sites may be due to reduced glomerular filtration and/or enhanced proximal tubular reabsorption. Even in the absence of ADH, distal tubular segments are not absolutely impermeable to water; small amounts of water continue to leak from the hypotonic tubular fluid into the isotonic cortical and slightly hypertonic medullary interstitial fluid. The amount of water leaking back in this manner becomes an increasingly larger fraction of the volume of dilute urine formed, as the diluting process is progressively limited by decreasing delivery. Hence, urine osmolality rises progressively. In some instances, this mechanism may even result in excretion of a urine hypertonic to plasma, despite the absence of ADH. (3) Sodium transport in the diluting segments may be defective, or water permeability may be excessive at these sites even in the absence of ADH. One of these three factors can account for most types of hyponatremia, as described below.

Types of hyponatremia (Table 50-1) In patients with extracellular *volume depletion,* delivery of sodium and water to the diluting segments of the nephron is reduced because of decreased glomerular filtration, increased proximal tubular reabsorption, or both. ADH secretion is stimulated by the volume contraction. These changes in renal function and hormone secretion limit water diuresis during extracelluar volume depletion. Hyponatremia per se is usually of little clinical significance in sodium (volume) depletion. The major features are those of extracellular volume contraction, described above. Reduction of plasma sodium concentration by more than 10 to 15 mmol/L is rare in the absence of obvious decreases in skin turgor, postural or recumbent hypotension, and some degree of azotemia. Treatment is directed to correction of the volume deficits. In the occasional symptomatic patient with sodium depletion whose plasma sodium concentration is less than 125 mmol/L, some of the intravenous sodium replacement fluids should be administered as hypertonic saline.

Multiple factors contribute to hyponatremia caused by *diuretics.* Salt loss may cause volume depletion, which limits water diuresis by mechanisms already described. Furosemide, ethacrynic acid, and thiazides inhibit salt reabsorption in the diluting segments of the nephron and thereby directly limit water diuresis. Thiazides appear to be the diuretics most commonly associated with hyponatremia, probably because they interfere with elaboration of a hypotonic urine by inhibiting sodium reabsorption in the distal convoluted tubule but, unlike loop diuretics, do not limit urine concentration and water retention by interfering with salt transport in the loop of Henle. In addition, potassium depletion caused by many diuretics contributes to hyponatremia through uncertain mechanisms. Hyponatremia due to diuretic therapy is frequent but usually minor in severity. However, moderate or severe hyponatremia may occur in patients who receive diuretics and who drink large quantities of water or other hypotonic fluids. Progressive hyponatremia is an important complication of diuretic therapy in edematous patients, in whom the underlying disease tends to cause hyponatremia (see below) and to whom large doses of diuretics may be given. The treatment of hyponatremia due to diuretics is water restriction and repletion of potassium deficits.

In *edematous states* such as congestive heart failure, cirrhosis, and the nephrotic syndrome, hyponatremia paradoxically appears to result from mechanisms similar to those that cause hyponatremia in patients with volume depletion. Although total extracellular volume is increased in edematous patients, it is believed that the "effective" volume is reduced by decreased cardiac output or sequestration of fluid outside the central circulation. The decrease in "effective" volume results in diminished delivery of sodium and water to nephron diluting segments, because of reduced glomerular filtration, increased proximal tubular reabsorption, or both. Volume-mediated secretion of ADH is also triggered in these conditions. In some edematous patients essential hyponatremia may be an additional mechanism (see below). In edematous states, the severity and frequency of hyponatremia correlate to some extent with the magnitude of the edema and the seriousness of the underlying condition. Hyponatremia is usually present in patients with advanced disease unless water intake is restricted. The hyponatremia itself is often of little clinical significance. The principal features are those of the underlying disease. However, symptomatic hyponatremia may occur, most often in connection with vigorous diuretic therapy or excessive oral or parenteral intake of dilute fluids.

Hyponatremia associated with edema responds to effective treatment of the underlying disease. Moderate nonprogressive hyponatremia in edematous patients usually does not cause symptoms. Attempts to correct such hyponatremia by restriction of fluid intake induce thirst and discomfort without improving the clinical picture or longevity. Patients with severe or progressive hyponatremia may require some restriction of water intake, especially during vigorous treatment with diuretics. However, moderate limitation to the range of 1 to 1.5 L/d will often suffice to avoid symptoms of progressive hyponatremia. More severe restriction should be instituted only if specific clinical or laboratory observations warrant. Since edematous subjects have excess total extracellular sodium, hypertonic saline should not be administered except in rare instances in which clinical manifestations of extreme hyponatremia, such as coma or convulsions, justify emergency measures. Furosemide should be given concurrently in such cases to avoid further expansion of the extracellular space. Dialysis can also be used to correct severe hyponatremia without increasing volume in edematous patients.

Hyponatremia may result from *impaired water excretion* not associated with a substantial deficit or excess of salt. In this case, extracellular volume is only modestly expanded. Since excess water is distributed throughout both intracellular and extracellular fluids in proportion to their volumes, only one-third of a water excess will be retained in the extracellular compartment. *Oliguric* patients develop dilutional hyponatremia if the volume of oral and intravenous fluids is not restricted appropriately. The ability to excrete a normal volume of dilute urine is progressively limited in advancing *chronic renal failure*. Regulation of water intake by thirst usually prevents dilutional hyponatremia. However, hyponatremia may be precipitated by increased fluid intake (for example, if the patient is instructed to force fluids). Since the ability to regulate salt excretion is also limited in chronic renal failure, in many patients hyponatremia is associated with edema or salt depletion. In patients with normal renal function, *water diuresis* may be *limited temporarily* by ADH secretion induced by various neural stimuli such as pain and narcotics. In the postoperative state, these factors, together with administration of large volumes of hypotonic fluids, may cause hyponatremia. The etiology of hyponatremia due to impaired water excretion is usually evident from the clinical setting and a careful review of fluid intake and output. This type of hyponatremia is treated by water restriction. Only if severe symptoms occur is hypertonic saline infusion required.

In the *syndrome* of *inappropriate antidiuretic hormone* (SIADH) secretion (see also Chap. 315), ADH is released "inappropriately" despite dilution of body fluids and increased extracellular volume. Hyponatremia in patients with SIADH is principally due to water retention, but urinary losses of sodium may also contribute to a mild negative sodium balance. Renal sodium wasting is due to water retention and consequent modest volume expansion, which increases sodium excretion by mechanisms discussed above. Clinically, SIADH is characterized by a number of features: (1) Urine osmolality is not maximally dilute even when marked hyponatremia is induced by water loading. In most cases, urine osmolality exceeds plasma osmolality. (2) Plasma creatinine and urea are normal or low, indicating that the glomerular filtration rate is normal or increased. (The elaboration of hypertonic urine is presumptive evidence of ADH secretion if the glomerular filtration rate is normal.) (3) During fluid loading (even if the fluid is saline), hyponatremia increases due to water retention and urinary sodium wasting. It should be noted that sodium wasting during volume expansion may be minimal or even absent in patients with extreme degrees of hyponatremia. (4) Since hyponatremia and salt wasting are not direct effects of vasopressin but are due to retention of ingested water, they are corrected by restriction of fluid intake. This response is helpful in occasional patients in whom it may be difficult to distinguish SIADH from mild volume depletion as the cause of hyponatremia. The plasma uric acid also may be of value in making this distinction. Since uric acid excretion tends to vary with "effective" extracellular volume, hyperuricemia is common in volume depletion while hypouricemia is usual in SIADH.

SIADH occurs commonly in patients with oat cell carcinoma of the lung but has also been described in patients with a variety of other *neoplasms*. In some of these patients the tumor secretes ADH or a substance with analogous biologic activity (see also Chap. 315). The syndrome has also been reported in patients with various disorders of the *central nervous system*, including meningitis, encephalitis, tumors, trauma, stroke, and in acute *porphyria*. It is assumed that ADH in these patients is secreted in response to direct stimulation of the hypothalamic osmoreceptors. *Pulmonary* diseases associated with SIADH, in addition to tumors, include a wide variety of infections, asthma, and chronic obstructive lung disease.

Pharmacologic agents that induce SIADH include (1) the oral hypoglycemic agents chlorpropamide and tolbutamide; (2) the antineoplastic and immunosuppressive agents vincristine and cyclophosphamide; (3) psychoactive drugs such as haloperidol, thioridazine, carbamazepine, and amitriptyline; and (4) clofibrate. These agents exert their antidiuretic effect either by potentiating the tubular action of small amounts of ADH or by stimulating inappropriate secretion of ADH.

Hyponatremia due to SIADH can be treated by limiting fluid intake; restriction to the range of 1 to 1.2 L/d is ordinarily adequate. Occasional patients who are symptomatic despite water restriction may be treated by enhancing water excretion. This can be accomplished either by increasing solute excretion (by taking a high-salt, high-protein diet or ingesting urea) or by antagonizing ADH with demeclocycline or lithium. Initial therapy with hypertonic saline infusions may be required in a few patients with marked hyponatremia. Concurrent administration of furosemide may facilitate correction of hyponatremia in those patients who do not respond promptly to hypertonic saline alone.

Hyponatremia may occur in certain *endocrine* disorders, notably adrenal insufficiency and hypothyroidism. Multiple factors appear to play a role in limiting water diuresis in patients with *adrenal insufficiency*. Deficient secretion of mineralocorticoid hormones may lead to sodium depletion, with consequent reduction of glomerular filtration and enhancement of proximal tubular sodium reabsorption. Moreover, glucocorticoid deficiency directly reduces filtration. Therefore, adrenal insufficiency will tend to decrease delivery of sodium to diluting sites. In addition, glucocorticoid deficiency prevents the maintenance of normal water impermeability in distal diluting segments of the nephron. This appears to be due to inappropriate secretion of ADH, although glucocorticoid deficiency may have a direct effect on water permeability of distal tubular epithelium. Since patients with adrenal insufficiency may have the combination of defective dilution of the urine and sodium wasting, hyponatremia due to Addison's disease can occasionally be confused with SIADH. Usually, other clinical features of adrenal insufficiency such as hyperkalemia, pigmentation, and hypoglycemia suggest the correct diagnosis. However, specific tests of adrenal function are indicated whenever the diagnosis is in doubt. Hyponatremia due to adrenal insufficiency is corrected by appropriate hormonal therapy.

Hyponatremia may develop in moderate or severe *hypothyroidism*. Decreased delivery of tubular fluid to diluting segments and persistent release of ADH both limit water excretion in this condition. The diagnosis of this type of hyponatremia is made by recognizing the clinical features of hypothyroidism and from the response to treatment with thyroid hormone.

The normal kidney can excrete 15 to 20 L of dilute urine per day. Normal water intake, regulated by thirst and habit, is a small fraction of this maximum excretory capacity. Rarely, *psychogenic polydipsia* may be so severe that the rapid ingestion of huge quantities of fluids may overwhelm normal excretory capacity and produce symptomatic dilutional hyponatremia despite normal renal diluting mechanisms. Hyponatremia of this type is diagnosed from the history of massive fluid intake, most often in patients with other evidence of psychiatric illness. Since water excretory capacity is normal, the urine is maximally dilute in this condition. Hyponatremia due to psychogenic polydipsia responds to water restriction. Rare patients who are symptomatic due to extreme degrees of hyponatremia may require intravenous infusion of hypertonic saline.

Some patients may be hyponatremic in the absence of a defect in water diuresis. The terms *essential hyponatremia* and *sick cell syndrome* have been applied to this category. Osmoreceptor cells in the hypothalamus are thought to be "reset" to maintain a decreased level of body fluid osmolality as though it were normal. Urine becomes dilute or concentrated, respectively, if plasma sodium falls or increases slightly from the new "normal" level for the particular patient. The genesis of such a syndrome is speculative. Changes in cellular metabolism may lead to a primary reduction in cellular osmolality. Another possibility is that essential hyponatremia is a variant of SIADH in which there is a nonosmotic stimulus to ADH secretion. When plasma osmolality is reduced sufficiently, osmotic suppression of ADH secretion overcomes the nonosmotic stimulus.

Essential hyponatremia may occur in a variety of chronic illnesses, such as pulmonary tuberculosis, congestive heart failure, and hepatic cirrhosis. This type of hyponatremia is asymptomatic; skin turgor, blood pressure, and renal function are normal, unless altered by the primary disease. Definitive diagnosis of essential hyponatremia requires the demonstration of normal urinary dilution in response to water loading, normal urinary concentration during dehydration, and normal renal sodium excretory responses to sodium loading and restriction. This type of hyponatremia does not require treatment.

Hyponatremia due to *accumulation* of *osmotically active solutes* in the plasma is the sole exception to the rule that hyponatremia means decreased plasma osmolality. In this type of hyponatremia, plasma osmolality is increased. Plasma sodium is diluted by movement of water out of cells along the osmotic gradient created by the addition of a solute such as glucose or mannitol. (High plasma urea levels in patients with renal failure do not cause hyponatremia because urea concentration is equal across cell membranes.) The diagnosis of hyponatremia due to increased plasma concentrations of osmotically active solutes is usually apparent from the history and clinical features of uncontrolled diabetes. Plasma sodium concentration will decrease by about 1.6 mmol/L with every elevation of 1 g/L in plasma glucose above normal. This type of hyponatremia should also be considered whenever there is a history of recent administration of mannitol, especially to oliguric patients unable to excrete it promptly. Since plasma osmolality is increased, clinical manifestations of hypotonicity are absent in this type of hyponatremia.

In patients with severe hyperlipemia or, very rarely, with extreme hyperproteinemia, *artifactual* hyponatremia may be reported by the laboratory. In severe hyperlipemia part of any unit volume of plasma taken for analysis will be lipid, which is sodium-free. This type of hyponatremia rarely occurs unless the plasma is grossly milky. In patients with extreme hyperproteinemia, proteins occupy more than the normal 7 percent of plasma volume, thereby reducing the proportion of aqueous sodium-containing fluid per unit of plasma taken for analysis. In both cases, hyponatremia will be reported by the laboratory because the sodium concentration will be low in millimoles per liter of plasma. However, sodium concentration per liter of plasma water and plasma osmolality are normal; hence, this type of hyponatremia has no clinical significance. Laboratories increasingly have adopted the sodium-selective electrode as the method for measuring plasma sodium. This technique eliminates artifactual hyponatremia because it gives accurate values regardless of plasma lipid or protein concentration.

Differential diagnosis Although the type of hyponatremia can be defined easily in most patients, precise diagnosis may be difficult in some. Figure 50-1 is a flow chart that outlines the major steps in determining the cause of hyponatremia. First, assess extracellular fluid (ECF) volume. The history and physical examination are usually sufficient to determine whether the hyponatremia is associated with a decreased, increased, or normal extracellular volume. In occasional patients, moderate volume depletion may not readily be separable from normovolemia by clinical examination. In that event, measurement of BUN and plasma creatinine may be helpful. The plasma creatinine, and especially the BUN, tend to be increased when hyponatremia is associated with volume depletion and normal or decreased when it is associated with a normal or expanded extracellular volume, as in SIADH. The various types of normovolemic hyponatremia can frequently be recognized by a careful review of specific features of the history, such as associated diseases, drug therapy, and fluid intake. However, laboratory tests, such as measurement of serum cortisol, may be needed to confirm a diagnosis.

Measurements of urinary sodium concentration and osmolality are common in the workup. *Urinary sodium concentration* is low (under 10 mmol/L) if hyponatremia is associated with edema or with volume depletion due to extrarenal causes. Urine sodium concentration usually exceeds 20 mmol/L if hyponatremia is due to renal salt losses or to renal failure with water retention. In SIADH, urine sodium concentration usually exceeds 20 mmol/L unless fluid intake has been restricted. Since impaired water diuresis is the mechanism of most types of hyponatremia, measurement of *urinary osmolality* is not usually of value. A maximally dilute urine would be expected only in hyponatremia due to extreme polydipsia or during water loading in essential hyponatremia. With other causes, urinary osmolality exceeds 150 mosmol per kilogram of water; usually the urine is hypertonic to plasma.

Clinical manifestations Neurologic dysfunction is the principal clinical manifestation of hyponatremia. It is due to intracellular movement of water, leading to swelling of brain cells. The severity of symptoms is related both to the degree of hyponatremia and to the rapidity with which it develops. In chronic hyponatremia, the degree of brain swelling caused by any given reduction in body fluid osmolality is reduced because solute, largely potassium and sodium chloride, is lost from the cells. Patients may be lethargic, confused, stuporous, or comatose. If hyponatremia develops rapidly, signs of hyperexcitability such as muscular twitches, irritability, and convulsions may occur. Hyponatremia rarely causes clinical symptoms when plasma sodium is above 125 mmol/L, although symptoms may occur at higher levels if the decrease in concentration has been rapid.

Treatment Appropriate therapy for the various types of hyponatremia has been outlined. Hyponatremia itself is often of little significance and requires no specific treatment. If severe, symptomatic hyponatremia requires intravenous treatment; the amount of sodium given should be calculated by multiplying the deficit in plasma sodium concentration (millimoles per liter) by the total body water (approximately 50 to 60 percent of body weight). Although the administered sodium will remain in the extracellular compartment, the osmotic

FIGURE 50-1 Flow chart for differential diagnosis of causes of hyponatremia. Categories (A, B, C, D) and types (C1–6) are keyed to Table 50-1. Abbreviations: Nl = normal; ECF = extracellular fluid; creat = creatinine; CHF = congestive heart failure; BP = blood pressure; Uosm = urinary osmolality; U_{Na} = urinary Na, mmol/L; ↓ = decreased, ↑ = increased; Hx = history, PE = physical examination.

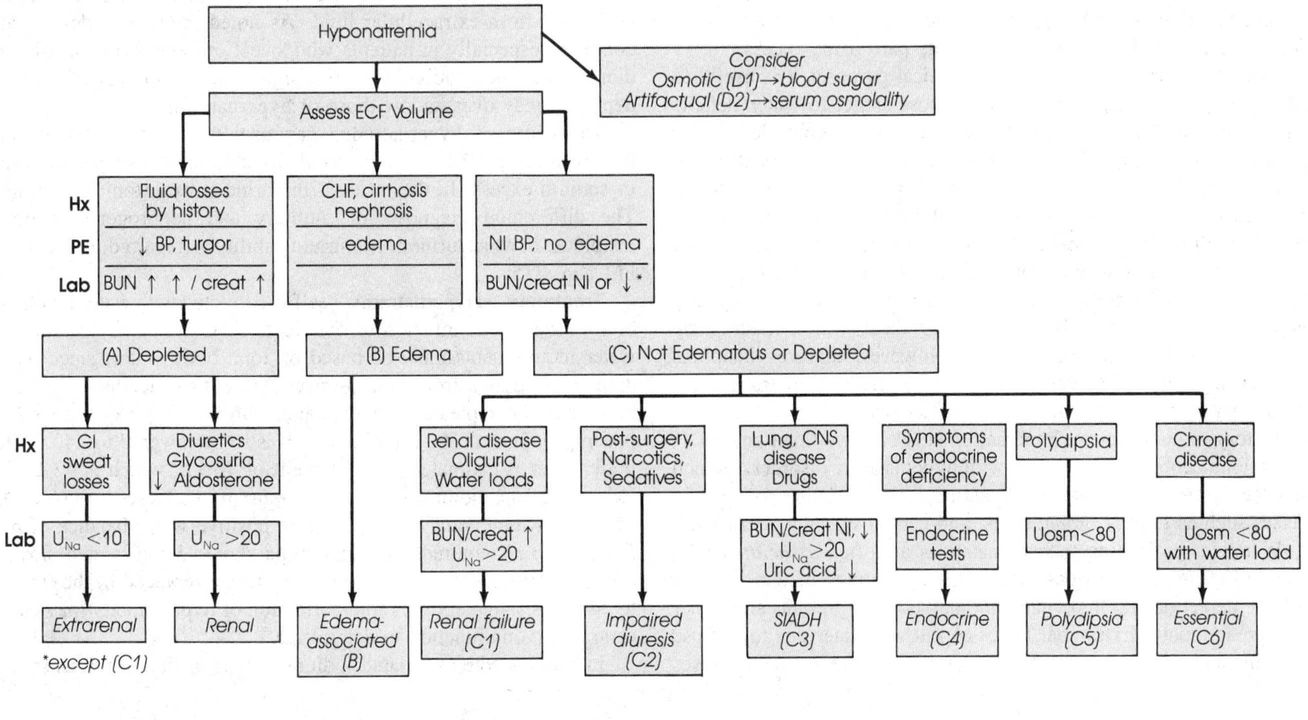

effect of hypertonic saline will cause water to shift out of cells. The appropriate rate and extent of initial correction of hyponatremia is controversial. Severe hyponatremia itself is potentially hazardous; on the other hand, some studies suggest that rapid correction of hyponatremia may cause neurologic damage (central pontine myelinolysis). Although the issue has not yet been resolved, the following regimen seems reasonable. The amount of hypertonic (5%) saline needed to raise plasma sodium to 125 mmol/L should be calculated and infused at a rate estimated to increase plasma sodium by 1 to 2 mmol/h. The symptoms and clinical status, especially with respect to circulatory congestion, should be carefully assessed throughout the infusion. Furosemide may be given if fluid overload is present initially or develops during the infusion. Complete correction of hyponatremia, if indicated, is usually best carried out more slowly by water restriction or oral sodium supplementation if possible.

HYPERNATREMIA Pathophysiology Hypernatremia is due to a deficit of body water relative to total body solute or sodium content. Without exception, hypernatremia indicates that the body fluids are hypertonic. Normally, minimal increases in tonicity stimulate both thirst and release of ADH. Although renal water retention induced by ADH helps to correct hypernatremia, thirst appears to be the principal defense mechanism. Hypernatremia is usually modest in patients with diabetes insipidus, who lack ADH and may excrete 15 L or more of urine per day. Thirst stimulates water intake enough to balance even such large water losses. Severe persistent hypernatremia occurs only in patients who cannot respond to thirst by voluntary ingestion of fluid, e.g., infants or mentally obtunded patients, or in rare patients with disorders of thirst mechanisms. In such individuals, loss of dilute body fluids progressively elevates body fluid osmolality. Initial losses of water are from the extracellular compartment, but water deficits are rapidly equilibrated throughout total body water. The rise in extracellular fluid tonicity causes intracellular water to shift into the extracellular compartment. In effect, approximately two-thirds of pure water deficits are derived from intracellular fluid. Hence, extracellular volume depletion is clinically significant in patients with relatively pure deficits of water only when such deficits are large. The principal clinical features are attributable to decreased intracellular volume, especially dehydration of cells in the central nervous system. Brain cells appear to adapt to chronic hyperosmolality by accumulating increased intracellular solute. When hyperosmolality is rapidly corrected, the increase in total intracellular solute may promote brain swelling even at normal or slightly elevated plasma osmolality. These mechanisms may account for the fact that rapid correction of hypertonicity sometimes causes deterioration of central nervous function. The identity of the excess brain solute is uncertain; electrolyte accumulation accounts for only part of the excess.

Pathogenesis (Table 50-1) For clinical purposes it is useful to classify hypernatremia as due to water loss alone; to water deficits associated with, but proportionately in excess of, sodium deficits; or to retention of sodium. *Pure water deficits* may be due to extrarenal or renal water losses that are not replaced. Insensible losses of water from the skin or lungs may reach several liters per day, especially in patients with fever, increased respirations, or extensive burns. Renal losses may lead to hypernatremia in diabetes insipidus. Alert patients with diabetes insipidus ordinarily maintain normal or only slightly hypertonic body fluids despite massive renal water wasting by increasing fluid intake appropriately. However, diabetes insipidus may develop acutely after cerebral trauma or neurosurgical procedures. In such patients, careful attention to replacement of urinary losses is mandatory to avoid severe hypernatremia. Defective thirst and ADH regulation occurs in rare patients with hypothalamic disorders, which may be idiopathic (''essential hypernatremia'') or due to specific causes such as tumors, granulomas, and cerebrovascular accidents.

Water losses leading to hypernatremia are often *associated with sodium deficits*. In such cases, the clinical features of extracellular volume depletion and hypernatremia may both be present, and either may predominate. Extrarenal losses of salt and water due to profuse sweating and renal losses due to osmotic diuresis are the major causes of hypernatremia in this category. Since sweat is hypotonic, hypernatremia will develop if profusely sweating patients cannot drink. In an osmotic diuresis, urinary sodium concentration is less than plasma concentration; therefore, hypernatremia tends to occur. Hypernatremia due to urea diuresis may develop when patients unable to complain of thirst are placed on high-protein feeding. Examples include patients with severe cerebrovascular accidents who are unable to swallow and postoperative neurosurgical patients. In the syndrome of hyperosmolar nonketotic diabetic coma, severe hyperosmolality of the body fluids is due to a combination of hyperglycemia and relative or absolute hypernatremia. The hypernatremia is a consequence of an intense glucose osmotic diuresis in patients who are unable to ingest fluids. Since hyperglycemia itself causes hyponatremia by inducing a shift of water from cells, the presence of hypernatremia in the face of extreme hyperglycemia indicates that total body water is severely depleted.

Infrequently, hypernatremia may result from an absolute *excess of sodium* rather than from water depletion. Examples are hypernatremia caused by accidental substitution of salt for sugar in infant feeding formulas and administration of excessive amounts of hypertonic sodium chloride or bicarbonate infusions to comatose adults unable to drink. The cause of the common mild hypernatremia in patients with adrenal hyperfunction is uncertain. Presumably, stimulation of renal tubular sodium reabsorption by adrenal steroids initiates the hypernatremia, and the hypervolemia that results resets upward the threshold for ADH release. It is not known why the thirst mechanism fails to maintain normal body fluid osmolality.

Clinical features and diagnosis The principal manifestations of hypernatremia are observed in the central nervous system. Confusion and other evidence of altered mental state; increased neuromuscular irritability, such as twitching and seizures; and obtundation, stupor, or coma may all occur. The magnitude of symptoms depends on the severity of the hyperosmolality. The symptoms are similar whether hyperosmolality is due to hypernatremia or extreme hyperglycemia. The neurologic symptoms appear to be due to dehydration of brain cells. The clinical manifestations of acute hypernatremia are more marked than those of slowly developing hypernatremia. Severe hyperosmolality may cause irreversible neurologic sequelae, apparently due to vascular consequences such as venous sinus thrombosis and hemorrhage from vessels that rupture when the brain shrinks. High mortality rates are associated with extreme hyperosmolality, especially in children and in the elderly.

In patients with pure water deficits, manifestations of extracellular volume depletion are minimal because only one-third of the deficit is derived from extracellular fluid. As noted, combined deficits are common, especially in patients who sweat or experience an osmotic diuresis; in such individuals, the signs and symptoms of volume depletion may overshadow those of hypernatremia.

The cause of hypernatremia can usually be inferred from the history when it is due to extrarenal water loss, an osmotic diuresis, or sodium excess. In these cases, the urine is hypertonic to plasma. The differential diagnosis of pituitary and nephrogenic diabetes insipidus, in which urine concentrating ability is impaired, is discussed in Chap. 315.

Treatment Hypernatremia itself is corrected with water by mouth or by intravenous infusion of 5% dextrose in water. Calculation of water requirements must be based on total body water, since water deficits are drawn from both intracellular and extracellular fluid and both must be repleted. For example, suppose a 70-kg man has a plasma sodium of 160 mmol/L which is to be lowered to 140. Total body water is estimated as 60 percent of 70 kg, which is 42 L. To reduce plasma sodium, this volume must be increased to $(160/140) \times 42$ L, which equals 48 L. Thus, a positive water balance of 6 L $(48 - 42)$ is required. Hypernatremia should be corrected slowly; no more than half the water deficit should be replaced in the first 12 to 24 h. As stated above, rapid correction of hypertonicity may cause central nervous function to deteriorate.

In patients with associated sodium deficits, saline solutions should be infused. If the predominant clinical feature is extracellular volume depletion with circulatory insufficiency, treatment should begin with 0.9% saline to replete extracellular volume promptly. If the neurologic effects of hypertonicity predominate, therapy can start with 0.45% saline. In patients with hyperosmolar diabetic coma, sodium deficits are usually large, due to prior glucose osmotic diuresis. Plasma hypertonicity is due to both hyperglycemia and hypernatremia. Treatment consists of isotonic saline (0.9%) to replete extracellular volume and insulin to lower plasma glucose and thereby partly correct hypertonicity. Later, hypotonic saline (0.45%) can replace the remaining water and salt deficits and return plasma sodium to normal.

POTASSIUM

PHYSIOLOGIC CONSIDERATIONS Potassium is the principal intracellular cation. Active transport mediated by Na^+,K^+–stimulated ATPase in cell membranes maintains a cellular concentration of approximately 160 mmol/L, 40 times that in extracellular fluid. All but 2 percent of the 2500 to 3000 mmol potassium in the body is within cells. Since potassium is a large fraction of total cellular solute, it is a major determinant of the volume of the cell and the osmolality of the body fluids. Moreover, potassium is an important cofactor in a number of metabolic processes. Extracellular potassium, while a small fraction of the total, greatly influences neuromuscular function. The ratio of intracellular to extracellular potassium concentration is the principal determinant of membrane potential in excitable tissues. Since extracellular potassium concentration is low, small deviations in concentration produce large variations in this ratio; conversely, only large changes in intracellular potassium influence the ratio significantly. These relationships have practical consequences. For example, toxic effects of hyperkalemia can be mitigated by inducing movement of potassium from extracellular fluid into cells.

With the exception of changes in acid-base balance (see below), in most circumstances extracellular and intracellular potassium change in the same direction. Hence, alterations in plasma potassium are a useful index of alterations in total body potassium. During potassium depletion, plasma potassium initially decreases about 1 mmol/L for each 100 to 200 mmol lost. However, plasma potassium falls more slowly after it reaches 2 mmol/L. Thus, a plasma potassium in the range of 2 to 3.5 mmol/L is a reasonably accurate guide to the magnitude of depletion, but plasma potassium concentrations less than 2 mmol/L may reflect a wide range of deficits, from moderate to severe. Plasma concentration increases about 1 mmol/L after acute administration of 100 to 200 mmol potassium. Assuming an extracellular volume of 15 L, 150 mmol would be expected to raise plasma potassium by about 10 mmol/L. Thus, the largest fraction of administered potassium rapidly enters cells. Renal excretion also increases promptly. Chronic exposure to high-potassium diets enhances both tissue uptake and renal excretion of the ion; the mechanism of these adaptations is uncertain. Sustained hyperkalemia rarely is caused by excess intake, because these mechanisms normally function so efficiently. Impaired renal excretion and cellular transfer are the usual causes of hyperkalemia.

The relation between plasma and cellular potassium is influenced by acid-base balance and by hormones. Acidosis tends to shift potassium out of cells, and alkalosis favors movement from extracellular fluid into cells. The relation between blood pH and plasma potassium is complex and is influenced by several factors, including the type of acidosis, the duration of the altered acid-base state, and the change in plasma bicarbonate per se. In general, plasma potassium changes less with respiratory acidosis than with metabolic acidosis and less with alkalosis than with acidosis. While the magnitude of the change in plasma potassium cannot be predicted from changes in blood pH alone, a patient with normal total body potassium tends to be hyperkalemic if acidotic and hypokalemic if alkalotic. Hormones appear to be important parts of the mechanism for moving potassium loads out of plasma. Insulin and beta-adrenergic catecholamines promote movement of potassium into cells. Conversely, alpha-adrenergic agonists impair potassium uptake into cells.

Of the usual potassium intake of 50 to 150 mmol/d, most is excreted in the urine. Normally, stool and sweat contain only about 5 mmol/d. As noted, the kidneys respond to acute and chronic changes in potassium intake by corresponding changes in excretion. Excess potassium is excreted promptly; about half of an acute load appears in the urine within 12 h. The renal response to potassium depletion is more sluggish. Excretion does not fall to minimal levels for 7 to 14 days. During this period, a deficit of 200 mmol or more may develop in an individual on a potassium-deficient diet. Renal excretory mechanisms for potassium are complex. Potassium in the urine is derived almost entirely from potassium secreted in the distal convoluted tubule and collecting duct; filtered potassium is nearly quantitatively reabsorbed in more proximal segments. Potassium secretion appears to be determined by the potassium concentration of tubular cells and by an electrochemical gradient favoring diffusion of the ion into tubular fluid. Among the key influences on potassium secretion are aldosterone, distal tubular fluid flow rate, acid-base balance, and factors that alter distal tubular electronegativity. Aldosterone stimulates potassium secretion. Thus, hyperkalemia increases potassium excretion by two mechanisms: it stimulates adrenal secretion of aldosterone, and it directly enhances renal secretion, presumably via increased tubular cell potassium. Potassium secretion in the distal tubule is flow-dependent; increased distal delivery of tubular fluid favors potassium excretion. For example, loop diuretics, which enhance distal volume delivery, increase potassium excretion, especially in patients with edema and secondary aldosteronism. Alkalosis enhances and acidosis depresses renal potassium secretion, probably by inducing corresponding changes in tubular cell potassium. If delivery to distal segments of sodium salts of unreabsorbable anions such as excess bicarbonate or carbenicillin is augmented, tubular electronegative potential will increase as sodium is reabsorbed. The enhanced electrical gradient will promote potassium excretion.

POTASSIUM DEPLETION AND HYPOKALEMIA Pathogenesis The principal causes of potassium depletion are listed in Table 50-2. As noted above, renal excretion of potassium falls slowly in persons on potassium-deficient diets. During the 10 to 14 days before balance is achieved, significant deficits may occur. Thus, in contrast to sodium, moderate potassium depletion may result from *poor intake* alone. Potassium deficiency is frequent in *gastrointestinal disorders* in which vomiting, diarrhea, or loss of gastrointestinal secretions is prominent. Diarrhea may cause large potassium deficits, since the potassium concentration of liquid stool is 40 to 60 mmol/L. *Loss of*

TABLE 50-2 Causes of potassium depletion and hypokalemia

I Gastrointestinal
- *A* Deficient dietary intake
- *B* Gastrointestinal disorders (vomiting, diarrhea, villous adenoma, fistulas, ureterosigmoidostomy)

II Renal
- *A* Metabolic alkalosis
- *B* Diuretics, osmotic diuresis
- *C* Excessive mineralocorticoid effects
  - *1* Primary aldosteronism
  - *2* Secondary aldosteronism (including malignant hypertension, Bartter's syndrome, juxtaglomerular cell tumor)
  - *3* Licorice ingestion
  - *4* Glucocorticoid excess (Cushing's syndrome, exogenous steroids, ectopic ACTH production)
- *D* Renal tubular diseases
  - *1* Renal tubular acidosis
  - *2* Leukemia
  - *3* Liddle's syndrome
  - *4* Antibiotics
- *E* Magnesium depletion

III Hypokalemia due to shift into cells (no depletion)
- *A* Hypokalemic periodic paralysis
- *B* Insulin effect
- *C* Alkalosis

gastric secretions through vomiting or nasogastric suction is also a common cause of potassium depletion. The potassium concentration of gastric fluid is only 5 to 10 mmol/L; direct losses contribute modestly to negative potassium balance. The potassium deficit is primarily due to increased renal excretion. Potassium excretion appears to be stimulated by three mechanisms. Loss of gastric acid leads to *metabolic alkalosis,* which increases tubular cell potassium concentration. The elevated plasma bicarbonate concentration also increases delivery of bicarbonate and fluid to the distal nephron. At that site, as noted above, excess bicarbonate acts as a nonreabsorbable anion to augment potassium excretion. Finally, secondary hyperaldosteronism due to associated extracellular volume contraction may play a role in maintaining potassium excretion at high levels despite potassium depletion.

Diuretics are among the most frequent causes of hypokalemia and potassium depletion. Thiazides, loop diuretics, and carbonic anhydrase inhibitors all increase potassium excretion. These agents augment sodium and fluid delivery to the distal potassium secretory site by inhibiting reabsorption in more proximal nephron segments. Carbonic anhydrase inhibitors such as acetazolamide, which inhibit proximal bicarbonate reabsorption, also enhance potassium excretion by increasing distal delivery of nonreabsorbable bicarbonate. Hypokalemia and potassium depletion are frequent when diuretics are used to treat edematous patients, in whom secondary aldosteronism is the rule. Although hypokalemia also occurs in patients receiving diuretics for treatment of hypertension, potassium depletion is modest if dietary potassium is normal. Surreptitious abuse of diuretics should be considered when hypokalemic patients have renal potassium wasting of uncertain cause.

Potassium excretion is increased during an *osmotic diuresis.* This mechanism leads to potassium depletion in patients with diabetic ketoacidosis, in whom the osmotic diuresis is due to glycosuria and to increased excretion of keto acid anions. However, plasma potassium may be normal or even high due to the shift of potassium out of tissues caused by the diabetic acidosis and insulin deficiency. Failure to recognize potassium depletion may lead to serious cardiotoxicity from sudden hypokalemia when the acidosis is corrected with insulin or alkali. A normal plasma potassium concentration in an acidotic patient strongly suggests potassium depletion.

Urinary potassium loss is often due to *excessive mineralocorticoid activity.* Hypokalemia is characteristic of *primary aldosteronism* (Chap. 317). It may be minimal in patients with restricted sodium intake because potassium excretion is limited by decreased distal salt and fluid delivery. *Secondary aldosteronism* causes renal potassium wasting and hypokalemia in patients with malignant hypertension, Bartter's syndrome, and renin-secreting renal tumors. However, patients with congestive heart failure, hepatic cirrhosis, and nephrotic syndrome usually are not hypokalemic despite secondary aldosteronism. The decrease in effective blood volume in such patients reduces distal delivery of salt and fluid, thereby limiting potassium excretion. As noted above, treatment with diuretics, which increase distal delivery, will often provoke hypokalemia in these patients. Some forms of *licorice* contain a compound with mineralocorticoid activity; patients who consume huge amounts may become hypokalemic. Excessive levels of *glucocorticoids* stimulate secretion of renal potassium (and hydrogen), leading to hypokalemia and alkalosis in patients with *Cushing's syndrome* (Chap. 317) and some receiving *therapeutic steroids.*

Renal tubular potassium wasting is a feature of *renal tubular acidosis* (Chap. 231). Some patients with monocytic or myelomonocytic *leukemia* develop hypokalemia. The mechanism is uncertain. Renal potassium wasting in some patients appears to correlate with lysozymuria, and the enzyme may interfere with tubular function. In *Liddle's syndrome,* a rare familial disorder (Chap. 231), renal potassium wasting is an intrinsic tubular abnormality. Certain *antibiotics* may cause hypokalemia by increasing potassium excretion. Carbenicillin in large amounts promotes distal tubular secretion by acting as an unreabsorbed anion; amphotericin B alters distal tubular permeability. Gentamicin has also been reported to cause hypokalemia by unknown mechanisms.

Magnesium depletion can cause potassium depletion, apparently due to increased renal and possibly gastrointestinal losses. Increased aldosterone secretion may play a role in stimulating potassium excretion. Hypokalemia in this condition is associated with hypocalcemia.

Clinical features and diagnosis The most prominent features of hypokalemia and potassium depletion are neuromuscular. Moderate degrees of depletion may be asymptomatic, especially if they develop slowly. Some patients, however, complain of muscle weakness, especially in the lower extremities. With more severe or acute degrees of hypokalemia and potassium deficiency, marked and generalized weakness of skeletal muscles is prominent. Very severe or abrupt development of hypokalemia may lead to virtually total paralysis, including the respiratory muscles. Rhabdomyolysis may occur. On physical examination, in addition to decreased motor power, the patient may demonstrate decreased or absent tendon reflexes. The smooth muscle of the gastrointestinal tract may be affected, resulting in paralytic ileus.

Abnormalities in the electrocardiogram are common (Chap. 176). The characteristic changes include flattening and inversion of the T wave, increased prominence of the U wave, and sagging of the ST segment. These alterations are not well correlated with the severity of the disturbance in potassium metabolism and cannot be relied on as indexes of the clinical significance of a potassium deficit. Although moderate potassium depletion rarely affects cardiac action, severe or rapid reduction in serum potassium may cause cardiac arrest. Potassium deficiency enhances the cardiac toxicity of digitalis preparations. A variety of atrial and ventricular arrhythmias may occur in hypokalemia, especially in patients receiving digitalis.

Renal tubular function is markedly impaired by potassium depletion (Chap. 229). The most prominent abnormality is decreased concentrating ability, which may cause polyuria and polydipsia. Glomerular filtration rate is normal or slightly reduced; moderate reductions may occur with chronic potassium depletion nephropathy. Renal regulation of potassium excretion remains normal. The urinalysis is benign: protein excretion is normal or minimally increased, and the urinary sediment is normal or demonstrates only a slight increase in hyaline or granular casts.

DIAGNOSIS The cause of hypokalemia and potassium depletion is usually evident from the history. However, patients whose potassium deficiency is caused by chronic abuse of laxatives; psychogenic, self-induced vomiting; or surreptitious use of diuretics rarely volunteer an accurate history. Patients with villous adenomas of the rectum sometimes report that their feces are formed; careful questioning will reveal the elimination of the characteristic mucous secretion of the tumor.

Figure 50-2 is a flow chart that outlines the steps in differential diagnosis of hypokalemia when the cause is not evident from the history. The presence of *hypertension,* which suggests hyperaldosteronism (except Bartter's syndrome) or glucocorticoid excess, may be a clue to diagnosis. Blood pressure is normal in patients whose potassium depletion is due to the other causes listed in Table 50-2. Evaluation of *urinary potassium excretion* may be helpful in determining the origin of the potassium deficit. If gastrointestinal losses have occurred, urinary excretion is usually less than 20 to 25 mmol/L or per day. Although renal conservation of potassium is slow, excretion falls to these levels by the time that clinically significant deficits of potassium have accumulated. On the other hand, when renal potassium wasting is the cause, urinary excretion usually exceeds 20 to 25 mmol/L or per day. However, lower concentrations and lower excretion rates may be found in severe depletion, in those patients with excessive mineralocorticoid activity while on low sodium intake, and in patients whose diuretics have been stopped at the time of examination. Evaluation of blood *acid-base status* may help in differential diagnosis. Hypokalemia is associated with metabolic acidosis in renal tubular acidosis, diarrhea, and diabetic ketoacidosis,

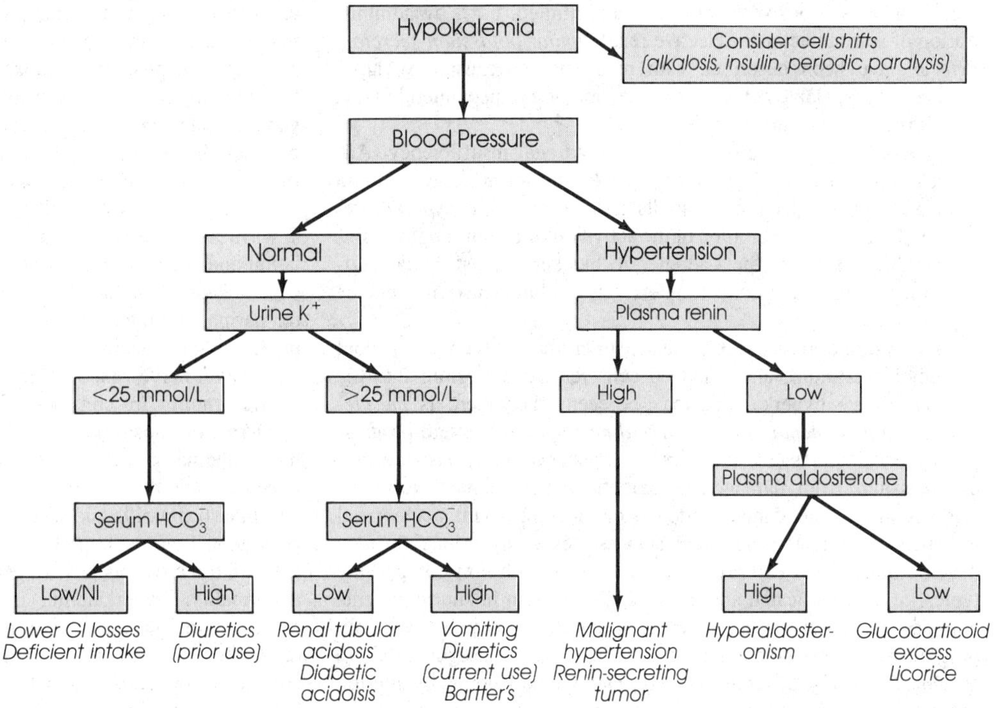

FIGURE 50-2 Flow chart for differential diagnosis of principal causes of hypokalemia. Nl = Normal.

and in patients treated with carbonic anhydrase inhibitors. With other causes of hypokalemia, blood bicarbonate is normal, or elevated due to associated metabolic alkalosis.

Treatment When possible, potassium depletion should be corrected by increased dietary intake or supplementation with potassium salts. Potassium chloride is the salt of choice, especially in alkalotic patients. It may be given in the form of an elixir or in tablets in which potassium chloride crystals are imbedded in a wax. Enteric-coated potassium chloride tablets have been responsible for ulceration of the small bowel, due to release of high concentrations of potassium salts, and should be avoided. Organic salts such as gluconate or citrate are adequate in patients who are not severely alkalotic and often are used to treat hypokalemia due to renal tubular acidosis. In edematous patients treated with diuretics that cause hypokalemia, potassium deficits should be prevented or treated by increased dietary potassium intake, supplementation with potassium chloride, or addition of "potassium-sparing" diuretics such as spironolactone. More controversial is the need for routine dietary supplements in patients receiving diuretics for treatment of hypertension. Patients with adequate dietary potassium intake usually do not develop significant hypokalemia and probably do not require routine supplements to prevent potassium depletion. However, those who do develop hypokalemia despite adequate diets should probably receive potassium salts, since hypokalemia may be associated with an increased frequency of arrhythmias.

Intravenous treatment is required for patients with gastrointestinal disorders or when the potassium deficiency is severe. It must be emphasized that the potassium *concentration* in commonly available intravenous solutions of potassium chloride is 2000 mmol/L. Concentrations in intravenous infusions should not exceed 40 or at the most 60 mmol/L. The rate of infusion should not exceed 20 mmol/h or approximately 200 to 250 mmol/d, unless the need for more rapid infusion has been demonstrated in the individual patient by evidence of continuing losses large enough to justify more intensive therapy. The results of treatment are best monitored by repeated determinations of plasma potassium and evaluation of clinical symptoms such as muscular weakness or paralysis. Disappearance of electrocardiographic abnormalities correlates only roughly with improvement in total body potassium content. However, during rapid intravenous administration of potassium, the electrocardiogram should be monitored to avoid cardiac toxicity from inadvertent hyperkalemia.

Hypokalemia and hypocalcemia may occur together, for example, in patients with malabsorption syndrome. The neuromuscular effect of each electrolyte abnormality is masked by the other. Treatment of either disorder alone may precipitate symptoms. Thus, treatment of hypokalemia alone may precipitate tetany, and conversely, treatment of hypocalcemia without correcting the hypokalemia may exacerbate the manifestations of potassium deficiency.

HYPERKALEMIA **Pathogenesis** The causes of hyperkalemia are shown in Table 50-3. *Inadequate renal excretion* is the most frequent cause (see also Chaps. 223 and 224). When oliguria or anuria is present, as in acute renal failure, progressive hyperkalemia is the rule. Plasma potassium rises by about 0.5 mmol/L per day if there are no abnormal loads. Chronic renal failure does not cause severe or progressive hyperkalemia unless oliguria supervenes. Adaptive changes of unknown etiology increase potassium excretion per residual nephron as chronic renal failure progresses. However, patients with chronic renal failure function at the limits of their excretory capacity. Hence, hyperkalemia may develop rapidly if the potassium

TABLE 50-3 Causes of hyperkalemia

I Inadequate excretion
- *A* Renal failure
  - *1* Acute renal failure
  - *2* Severe chronic renal failure
  - *3* Tubular disorders
- *B* Adrenal insufficiency
  - *1* Hypoaldosteronism
  - *2* Addison's disease
- *C* Diuretics which inhibit potassium secretion (spironolactone, triamterene, amiloride)

II Shift of potassium from tissues
- *A* Tissue damage (muscle crush, hemolysis, internal bleeding)
- *B* Drugs: succinylcholine, arginine, digitalis poisoning, beta-adrenergic antagonists
- *C* Acidosis
- *D* Hyperosmolality
- *E* Insulin deficiency
- *F* Hyperkalemic periodic paralysis

III Excessive intake

IV Pseudohyperkalemia
- *A* Thrombocytosis
- *B* Leukocytosis
- *C* Poor venipuncture technique
- *D* In vitro hemolysis

load is increased or excretory capacity is limited, e.g., by administration of spironolactone. Selective renal *tubular potassium secretory defects* have been described with renal disease caused by lupus erythematosus, sickle cell disease, rejection of a transplanted kidney, or obstructive uropathy.

Hyperkalemia is a cardinal feature of adrenal insufficiency (Addison's disease) and of selective *hypoaldosteronism*. The common form of the latter disorder in adults is *hyporeninemic hypoaldosteronism* (Chap. 317). Inhibition of the activity of the renin-angiotensin-aldosterone system by beta-adrenergic blockers, nonsteroidal anti-inflammatory drugs, or converting enzyme inhibitors also may induce hyperkalemia.

A kilogram of tissue such as muscle or erythrocytes contains about 80 mmol potassium, and damaged cells release potassium into the plasma. Hence hyperkalemia may be seen when there is *muscle-crushing injury, hemolysis,* or *internal hemorrhage*. Severe progressive hyperkalemia is not ordinarily a consequence of increased release of potassium from damaged or acidotic tissues alone. However, acidosis and tissue damage often occur together with acute renal insufficiency; under these circumstances, severe hyperkalemia may develop quickly. In contrast to the increase of 0.5 mmol/L per day typical of uncomplicated anuria, plasma potassium in anuric patients with tissue damage may increase 2 to 4 mmol/L per day. Such rapidly progressive hyperkalemia may be an important cause of death in military casualties. Several *drugs* may cause hyperkalemia by altering tissue uptake of potassium. In patients with trauma, burns, or neuromuscular diseases such as paraplegia and multiple sclerosis, the muscle relaxant succinylcholine may cause dangerous hyperkalemia. This agent apparently releases potassium from muscle by depolarizing cell membranes. Arginine hydrochloride, used to treat metabolic alkalosis, drives potassium out of cells. If potassium excretion is impaired, clinically significant hyperkalemia may occur during arginine infusions. Extreme digitalis poisoning may cause severe hyperkalemia; potassium leaks out of cells because Na^+,K^+-ATPase is inhibited by the drug. Beta-adrenergic blockers may induce hyperkalemia by interfering with the action of endogenous beta-catecholamines to enhance movement of potassium into tissues. *Metabolic acidosis* causes hyperkalemia by shifting potassium out of cells. Respiratory acidosis has less striking effects. *Hyperosmolality* also enhances potassium movement from cells. *Insulin deficiency* is conducive to hyperkalemia because the action of insulin to promote potassium movement into cells is diminished. Hyperosmolality or metabolic acidosis may be additional mechanisms of hyperkalemia in insulin-deficient patients. In *hyperkalemic periodic paralysis,* the hyperkalemia is associated with repeated attacks of muscular paralysis. The mechanism of this syndrome is not understood. Ingestion of increased amounts of potassium may precipitate attacks.

The severity of hyperkalemia caused by large oral or intravenous *potassium loads* is influenced by factors that modulate tissue uptake and renal excretion of potassium. For example, insulin deficiency and treatment with beta-adrenergic blockers tend to augment hyperkalemia by limiting tissue uptake. Volume depletion enhances hyperkalemia by limiting the rate at which the kidney excretes such loads.

Patients with extreme thrombocytosis or, more rarely, extreme leukocytosis in leukemia may demonstrate the phenomenon of pseudohyperkalemia. Platelets or white blood cells release potassium during blood clotting in vitro. While serum potassium may be grossly abnormal, plasma potassium is not increased. Artifactual elevation of plasma potassium may occur if blood is drawn after repeated fist clenching to make veins more prominent during application of a tourniquet, due to leakage of potassium from exercising muscle. Improper technique during collection or processing of blood samples may cause hemolysis and hence hyperkalemia in vitro. Artifactual hyperkalemia may be suspected when electrocardiographic abnormalities are absent despite elevation of measured potassium levels.

Clinical features and diagnosis The most important toxic effects of hyperkalemia are cardiac arrhythmias. The characteristic sequence of electrocardiographic changes is shown in Fig. 176-15. The earliest manifestation is the development of high-peaked T waves, especially prominent in precordial leads. Hyperkalemia does not prolong the QT interval, unlike other disorders which induce peaking of the T waves. Later changes include prolongation of the PR interval, complete heart block, and atrial asystole. As plasma potassium rises further, ventricular complexes may deteriorate. The QRS complex becomes progressively prolonged and finally tends to merge with the T wave in a sine wave configuration. Terminally, ventricular fibrillation and standstill may occur.

Occasionally moderate or severe hyperkalemia has striking effects on peripheral muscles. Ascending muscular weakness can occur, progressing to flaccid quadriplegia and respiratory paralysis. Cerebral and cranial nerve function are normal, as is sensation.

Treatment In considering therapy, it is helpful to classify hyperkalemia according to degree of severity. The seriousness of hyperkalemia is best estimated by considering both the plasma potassium and the electrocardiogram. When the plasma potassium is less than 6 mmol/L and electrocardiographic changes are limited to peaking of T waves, hyperkalemia is mild. When the plasma potassium is 6 to 8 mmol/L and T-wave peaking is the only electrocardiographic abnormality, hyperkalemia is moderate. Severe hyperkalemia is present if the plasma potassium exceeds 8 mmol/L or if electrocardiographic abnormalities include absent P waves, widened QRS complexes, or ventricular arrhythmias. Mild hyperkalemia can usually be treated by elimination of a cause, such as potassium-sparing diuretics, or by treatment of accompanying acidosis.

More severe or progressive hyperkalemia requires vigorous therapy. Severe cardiac toxicity responds most rapidly to infusion of calcium; 10 to 30 mL of 10% calcium gluconate may be infused intravenously within a period of 1 to 5 min under constant electrocardiographic monitoring. While calcium infusions do not alter plasma potassium, they counteract the adverse effects of potassium on neuromuscular membranes. The effect of calcium infusions, while almost immediate, is transient if the hyperkalemia is not treated directly.

In moderate or severe hyperkalemia, infusion of hypertonic glucose solutions decreases toxicity by provoking insulin release and shifting potassium into cells. In the first 30 min, 200 to 500 mL of 10% glucose may be given. An additional 500 to 1000 mL may be infused over the next several hours. Ten units of regular insulin are given intravenously or subcutaneously, although this is probably necessary only in insulin-deficient diabetic patients. This treatment may reduce serum potassium by 1 to 2 mmol/L, and effects persist for a number of hours. The infusion of sodium bicarbonate also helps lower serum potassium rapidly by causing potassium to shift into cells; 50 to 150 mmol alkali (two to three ampuls) may be added to a liter of glucose. Although this agent is most valuable in acidotic patients, it also is effective in individuals with normal acid-base status. The effect occurs within 1 h and persists for a number of hours. The infusion of hypertonic sodium solutions may also be effective in reversing cardiac toxicity, especially in hyponatremic or volume-depleted patients. In part, the effect depends simply on dilution of plasma potassium, but there may be a direct effect of elevated plasma sodium to antagonize hyperkalemic neuromuscular toxicity as well. Glucose, bicarbonate, and sodium may be combined in a "therapeutic cocktail," formulated by adding an ampul or two of sodium bicarbonate to a liter of 5% dextrose in 0.9% saline.

None of the measures just described removes potassium from the body. Cation exchange resins such as sodium polystyrene sulfonate are useful to remove potassium in the treatment of moderate or severe hyperkalemia. Fifty grams of the resin is mixed with 50 mL of 70% sorbitol and 100 mL of tap water and given by retention enema. Enough potassium may be removed by a single enema to reduce potassium by 0.5 to 2 mmol/L within an hour, and repeated enemas can be given. These resins can also be given repeatedly by mouth to maintain low plasma potassium concentration. Twenty grams is given three or four times a day together with 20 mL of a 70% sorbitol solution, as required to ensure the passage of several loose stools daily. In patients with renal failure, hemodialysis and peritoneal dialysis effectively control hyperkalemia. However, they are relatively slow techniques, and patients with severe hyperkalemia should be treated first with one of the methods previously discussed.

REFERENCES

Sodium and water

AYUS JC et al: Treatment of symptomatic hyponatremia and its relation to brain damage. N Engl J Med 317:1190, 1987

NARINS RG et al: Diagnostic strategies in disorders of fluid, electrolyte and acid-base homeostasis. Am J Med 72:496, 1982

ROBERTSON GL: Thirst and vasopressin function in normal and disordered states of water balance. J Lab Clin Med 101:351, 1983

STERNS RH et al: Osmotic demyelination syndrome following correction of hyponatremia. N Engl J Med 314:1535, 1986

WEINER M, EPSTEIN FH: Signs and symptoms of electrolyte disorders. Yale J Biol Med 43:76, 1970

WEISBERG LS et al: Pseudohyponatremia: A reappraisal. Am J Med 86:315, 1989

ZERBE R et al: Vasopressin function in the syndrome of inappropriate diuresis. Ann Rev Med 31:315, 1980

Potassium

BIA MJ, DEFRONZO RA: Extrarenal potassium homeostasis. Am J Physiol 240:F257, 1981

HOLLENBERG NK, BROWN RS (eds): Electrolytes and cardiovascular disease. Am J Med 77(5A):1, 1984

KNOCHEL JP: The syndrome of hyporeninemic hypoaldosteronism. Ann Rev Med 30:145, 1979

———: Neuromuscular manifestations of electrolyte disorders. Am J Med 72:521, 1982

———: Hypokalemia. Adv Int Med 30:317, 1984

PONCE SP et al: Drug-induced hyperkalemia. Medicine 64:357, 1985

RICHARDSON RMA, KUNAU RT JR: Renal regulation of potassium: Abnormal, in *The Kidney: Physiology and Pathophysiology,* 2d ed, DW Seldin, G Giebisch (eds). New York, Raven, 1985, p 1251

SELDIN DW, GIEBISCH G (eds): *The Regulation of Sodium and Chloride Balance.* New York, Raven, 1989, 350 pp

STERNS RH et al: Internal potassium balance and the control of the plasma potassium concentration. Medicine 60:339, 1981

STOKES JB: Potassium intoxication: Pathogenesis and Treatment, in *The Regulation of Potassium Balance*, DW Seldin, G Giebisch (eds). New York, Raven, 1989, p 269

TANNER RL: Diuretic-induced hypokalemia. Kidney Int 28:988, 1985

51 ACIDOSIS AND ALKALOSIS

NORMAN G. LEVINSKY

PHYSIOLOGIC CONSIDERATIONS Acids are produced continuously during normal metabolism. Despite the addition of some 20,000 mmol of carbonic acid and 80 mmol of nonvolatile acids to body fluids daily, the free hydrogen ion concentration of these fluids is fixed within a narrow range. The pH of extracellular fluid is normally between 7.35 and 7.45 (hydrogen ion, 45 to 35 nmol/L). The pH of intracellular fluids cannot be determined with precision, but most methods suggest a mean intracellular pH in the range of 6.9. Intracellular hydrogen ion concentration is not uniform; it varies among intracellular organelles within individual cells. Although the free hydrogen ion concentration of body fluids is low, protons are so reactive that even minute changes in concentration influence enzymatic reactions and physiologic processes. Immediate defense against untoward changes in pH is provided by buffers that can take up or release protons instantaneously in response to changes in acidity of body fluids. Regulation of pH ultimately depends on the lungs and the kidneys.

Role of the lungs The principal acid product of metabolism is carbon dioxide, equivalent to potential carbonic acid. The normal concentration of carbon dioxide in body fluids is fixed around 1.2 mmol/L [P_{CO_2} = 5.3 kPa (40 mmHg)] by the lungs; at this concentration, pulmonary excretion equals metabolic production. Although carbon dioxide reacts with water and body buffers during transport from cells to pulmonary alveoli, no net change in body fluid composition results, since the CO_2 excreted by the lungs is equal to the CO_2 produced by cells.

Nonvolatile acids When a nonvolatile acid is produced by metabolism, the protons are removed instantaneously from body fluids by reaction with buffers. In extracellular fluid, bicarbonate is converted to water and carbon dioxide, which is excreted by the lungs. Although this mechanism minimizes changes in acidity, it destroys bicarbonate and uses up cell buffer capacity. The total buffer capacity of the body fluids is about 15 mmol per kilogram of body weight. Thus, the normal rate of production of nonvolatile acids would be sufficient to deplete the body buffers completely in 10 to 20 days, were it not for the ability of the kidney to eliminate protons from the body by secretion into the urine, thereby regenerating bicarbonate and cell buffer capacity.

The principal source of nonvolatile acid is metabolism of methionine and cystine in dietary proteins, which produces sulfuric acid. Additional sources include the incomplete combustion of carbohydrates and fats, which produces organic acids; the metabolism of nucleoproteins, which produces uric acid; and the metabolism of organic phosphorus compounds, which releases protons and inorganic phosphates. The diet does not normally contain significant amounts of preformed acid or alkali, but significant amounts of potential acid (e.g., an excess of cationic acids, such as lysine) or alkali (e.g., citrate) may be present.

Role of the kidneys The principal functions of the kidney in acid-base metabolism can be viewed as retention of existing bicarbonate and generation of new bicarbonate to replace that used to buffer nonvolatile acids. Bicarbonate is reabsorbed in both proximal and distal segments by secretion of protons into tubular fluid. New bicarbonate is generated by secretion of protons onto urinary buffers. Normally, one-third is titrated onto phosphate, converting HPO_4^{2-} to $H_2PO_4^-$, and the remainder onto ammonia. The amount of free acid which can be excreted in the urine is negligible, even at the minimum urine pH of 4.8. However, acidification of the urine is essential for titration of protons onto phosphate and ammonia. Changes in the pH of body fluids lead to regulatory responses by the kidney. Acidosis stimulates renal hydrogen ion secretion. Ammonia production increases, and more protons can be excreted as ammonium. In extreme acidosis, ammonia production may increase tenfold or more above the normal rate of 40 to 50 mmol/d. The bicarbonate concentration of extracellular fluid is, in effect, set by the renal rate of proton secretion (bicarbonate reabsorption and generation). If plasma bicarbonate rises without an increase in renal reabsorptive capacity, bicarbonate is excreted rapidly and normal plasma bicarbonate is restored promptly. For example, chronic ingestion of even large amounts of sodium bicarbonate normally produces only minimal sustained elevation of plasma bicarbonate.

The rate of proton secretion is influenced by a number of factors, important among them carbon dioxide tension of body fluids, extracellular volume, aldosterone, and body potassium stores. Bicarbonate reabsorption is directly related to carbon dioxide concentration; hypercapnia tends to stimulate, and hypocapnia tends to inhibit, renal bicarbonate retention. Contraction of extracellular volume enhances tubular bicarbonate reabsorption, while volume expansion has the opposite effect. Aldosterone stimulates renal proton secretion; by this effect, hyperaldosteronism promotes metabolic alkalosis, while hypoaldosteronism causes acidosis. In experimental animals, renal bicarbonate reabsorption is inversely related to body potassium stores. In humans, the relation is less clear, but severe potassium depletion has been associated with increased bicarbonate reabsorption and metabolic alkalosis.

The respiratory response to changes in blood pH is almost instantaneous. Acidosis stimulates and alkalosis depresses ventilation. The respiratory center in the medulla appears to respond to a pH intermediate between those of blood and cerebrospinal fluid.

EVALUATION OF ACID-BASE BALANCE In practice, classification of acid-base disorders is based on measurements of changes in the bicarbonate–carbonic acid system, the principal buffer of extracellular fluid. Because intracellular and extracellular buffers are functionally linked, measurement of the plasma bicarbonate system provides useful information about total body buffers. The relationship among the elements of the bicarbonate system is usually described in terms of the Henderson-Hasselbalch equation:

$$pH = pK + \log \frac{[HCO_3^-]}{[H_2CO_3]}$$

Acidosis is defined as a disturbance which tends to add acid or remove alkali from body fluids, while *alkalosis* is any disturbance which tends to remove acid or add base. Since compensatory processes may minimize or prevent a change in the hydrogen ion concentration of the plasma, some authors prefer to use the terms *acidemia* and *alkalemia* to indicate those situations in which the pH of the plasma is measurably altered. *Metabolic* disorders are those in which the primary disturbance is in the concentration of bicarbonate. Since bicarbonate appears in the numerator of the buffer salt/acid ratio in the Henderson-Hasselbalch equation, increased bicarbonate concentration causes increased pH (alkalemia) while a decrease in bicarbonate causes decreased pH (acidemia). *Respiratory* disorders are those in which the primary change is in the concentration of carbon dioxide (carbonic acid). As can be seen from the Henderson-Hasselbalch equation, a fall in carbon dioxide concentration causes alkalemia, while an increase in carbon dioxide concentration causes acidemia.

A major problem in the assessment of acid-base disorders results from the compensatory responses of the lungs and the kidney. A primary change in carbon dioxide concentration induces a compensatory renal response which alters plasma bicarbonate in the same direction. Conversely, a primary alteration of plasma bicarbonate induces a compensatory respiratory response, which changes plasma carbon dioxide in the same direction. Consider a patient with chronic respiratory insufficiency who has the following set of acid-base parameters: P_{CO_2} = 9.3 kPa (70 mmHg), $[HCO_3^-]$ = 31 mmol/L, pH = 7.25. The clinician needs to know whether the elevation of plasma bicarbonate is merely the appropriate renal response to the primary hypercapnia or a metabolic acid-base disorder is superimposed. No calculations or a priori reasoning will provide the answer to this key question. Such information can be derived only from in vivo observations in which the usual compensatory response to a given degree of chronic hypercapnia is determined.

Clinical and experimental observations in humans (and animals) have been made in all common primary acid-base disturbances. They are most readily visualized and used for analysis of clinical acid-base disorders by the "confidence band" technique, as shown in Fig. 51-1. Each band represents the mean ±2 SD, that is, 95 percent of observations, for the compensatory response to each primary disturbance. In the example under discussion, inspection of the confidence band marked *chronic respiratory acidosis* indicates that 95 percent of individuals with chronic elevation of P_{CO_2} to 9.3 kPa (70 mmHg) would have $[HCO_3^-]$ between 34 and 44 mmol/L, due to renal compensation. Thus, the $[HCO_3^-]$ of 31 mmol/L in the example cannot be interpreted as the sole result of an appropriate compensatory response to chronic hypercapnia. A second acid-base disorder, presumably metabolic acidosis, must be superimposed to account for the fact that plasma bicarbonate, although increased in response to hypercapnia, is not as high as usually observed when P_{CO_2} is 9.3 kPa (70 mmHg). Obviously, the use of this figure is no panacea, nor does it obviate the need for commonsense clinical evaluation of alternative possibilities. For example, if the patient under discussion had only recently developed hypercapnia, the $[HCO_3^-]$ of 31 mmol/L would be too high for a purely compensatory response to acute respiratory acidosis and would be interpreted as superimposed metabolic alkalosis. The difference between these two interpretations depends entirely on the clinical recognition of the chronicity of the primary respiratory disorder. The use of Fig. 51-1 in each type of acid-base disturbance is described in the appropriate sections of this chapter.[1]

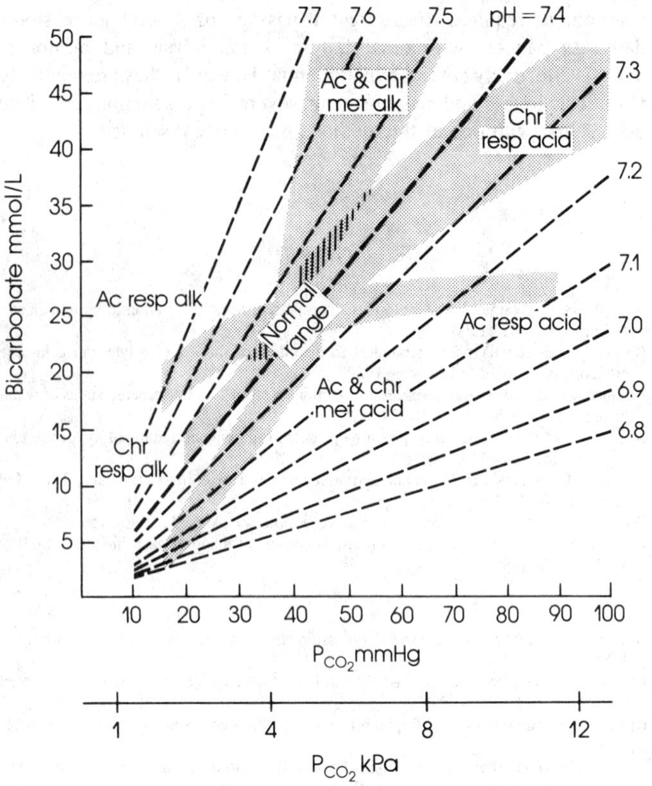

FIGURE 51-1 Nomogram, showing bands for uncomplicated respiratory or metabolic acid-base disturbances in intact subjects. Each "confidence" band represents the mean ±2 SD for the compensatory response of normal subjects or patients to a given primary disorder. Ac = acute; chr = chronic, resp = respiratory; met = metabolic; acid = acidosis; alk = alkalosis. (*Modified from Arbus.*)

METABOLIC ACIDOSIS

PATHOPHYSIOLOGY Metabolic acidosis is caused by one of three mechanisms (see Table 51-1): (1) increased production of nonvolatile acids, (2) decreased acid excretion by the kidney, (3) loss of alkali. In intracellular fluid excess protons replace potassium, which shifts out of cells, tending to elevate plasma levels. Extracellular bicarbonate is reduced by reaction with hydrogen ions or, in patients wasting alkali, by loss of bicarbonate in urine or stool. The decrease in pH stimulates respiration, and P_{CO_2} is lowered. Inspection of the confidence band for metabolic acidosis (Fig. 51-1) indicates that a decrease in P_{CO_2} of about 0.16 kPa (1.2 mmHg) can be expected for each decrement of 1 mmol/L in plasma bicarbonate. Complete respiratory compensation for primary metabolic acidosis does not occur. Respiratory compensation for acute acidosis tends to be somewhat greater than for chronic metabolic acidosis. The minimum level of P_{CO_2} that can be attained is approximately 1.3 kPa (10 mmHg); levels below 2 to 2.7 kPa (15 to 20 mmHg) are rarely maintained in chronic metabolic acidosis. When kidney function is normal, net acid excretion increases promptly in response to metabolic acidosis. Most of the initial rise is due to increased titration of urinary phosphate as urine pH falls below 5.2. Over several days, ammonia

[1] Although the confidence band method does not permit automatic identification of simple or complicated acid-base disorders, it is preferable to techniques such as "buffer base" or "base excess-deficit" for reasons discussed in detail by Schwartz and Relman, N Engl J Med 268:1382, 1963. These terms are not used in this chapter.

TABLE 51-1 Causes of metabolic acidosis

Increased anion gap
- *I* Increased acid production
  - *A* Ketoacidosis
    - *1* Diabetic
    - *2* Alcoholic
    - *3* Starvation
  - *B* Lactic acidosis
    - *1* Secondary to circulatory or respiratory failure
    - *2* Associated with various disorders (see text)
    - *3* Drugs and toxins
    - *4* Enzyme defects
  - *C* Poisoning (salicylates, ethylene glycol, methanol)
- *II* Renal failure

Normal anion gap (hyperchloremic)
- *III* Renal tubular dysfunction
  - *A* Renal tubular acidosis
  - *B* Hypoaldosteronism
  - *C* "Potassium-sparing" diuretics
- *IV* Loss of alkali
  - *A* Diarrhea
  - *B* Ureterosigmoidostomy
  - *C* Carbonic anhydrase inhibitors
- *V* Ammonium chloride, cationic amino acids (excess intake)

production by the kidney increases and becomes the most important mechanism for excreting excess protons. Net acid excretion may increase 5 to 10 times above normal, reaching a maximum of several hundred millimoles per day.

The most common cause of *acute* metabolic acidosis is increased production of nonvolatile acids. In *diabetic ketoacidosis,* acetoacetic and β-hydroxybutyric acids are produced more rapidly than they can be metabolized (Chap. 319). Severe ketoacidosis may occur in *association* with *acute* and *chronic alcoholism.* Typically patients give a history of prolonged abstention from food, protracted vomiting, and appreciable alcohol intake just before development of the ketoacidosis. β-Hydroxybutyrate, acetoacetate, and lactate accumulate in the plasma. The ketosis may be overlooked because the ratio of β-hydroxybutyrate to acetoacetate tends to be high; the nitroprusside test used for clinical detection of plasma ketones responds only to the latter. Blood sugar is usually normal or mildly elevated in these patients. The mechanism of the syndrome is uncertain. *Starvation* may cause mild ketoacidosis because of increased fat catabolism.

Lactic acidosis This is one of the most common types of metabolic acidosis. Metabolic production and consumption of lactate are normally in balance. Under basal conditions the liver and kidney consume lactate produced by tissues such as erythrocytes, skin, intestine, and muscle. However, if oxygen delivery is inadequate to meet energy requirements, any tissue will generate lactate. Deficient oxygen impairs electron flow through the cytochrome transport chain; ATP formation is decreased and cell redox pairs, such as NADH/NAD, are shifted toward the reduced state. Decrease in ATP and reciprocal increases in ADP and AMP concentrations activate phosphofructokinase, the key enzyme regulating glycolysis. Accelerated glycolysis leads to increased production of pyruvate and the increase in NADH/NAD ratio decreases its oxidation. Pyruvate and lactate are in a near-equilibrium reaction catalyzed by lactic dehydrogenase, as follows:

$$\text{Pyruvate} + \text{NADH} + H^+ \rightleftharpoons \text{lactate} + \text{NAD}$$

Thus lactate will tend to increase when pyruvate concentration increases and when the ratio of NADH to NAD rises. Since both conditions occur when tissues are oxygen-deprived, lactate formation is increased. Lactate will accumulate because it can be consumed only by conversion back to pyruvate, which is blocked so long as pyruvate concentration and the NADH/NAD ratio are elevated. Since the overall process of glycolysis generates one H^+ for each lactate produced, acid production increases proportionately with lactate production.

These mechanisms, probably compounded by decreased uptake or, even, production of lactate by the liver, account for the development of lactic acidosis in patients with *shock* due to any cause (e.g., sepsis, myocardial infarction, hemorrhage) or with respiratory arrest. Since severe acidosis depresses myocardial and arteriolar contractility, lactic acidosis may compound the underlying cause of shock. Less commonly, lactic acidosis may be caused by *pulmonary diseases* leading to extreme hypoxia or by diminished blood oxygen–carrying capacity in severe *anemia* and *carbon monoxide* poisoning. The mortality rate is high in patients with lactic acidosis secondary to shock and tissue hypoxia. During vigorous *exercise* or convulsions, local disproportion between oxygen supply and demand in contracting muscle may lead to transient, clinically benign lactic acidosis.

Lactic acidosis also is *associated* with disorders in which tissue hypoxia does not appear to be present. It has been reported in patients with leukemia, lymphoma, and solid tumors; with poorly controlled diabetes mellitus; and with severe hepatic failure. Mechanisms causing lactic acidosis in these disorders are poorly understood. Overproduction of lactate by neoplastic tissue probably is a factor in lactic acidosis associated with tumors. Insulin deficiency, which inhibits pyruvate oxidation, presumably is an important factor in patients with poorly controlled diabetes. Decreased hepatic lactate metabolism seems a likely mechanism in severe liver disease.

A variety of *drugs* and *toxins* have been associated with lactic acidosis. *Drugs* include fructose used in parenteral alimentation; sodium nitroprusside; epinephrine and norepinephrine infusions; and, before the drug was removed from general use, the biguanide hypoglycemic agent, phenformin. Lactic acidosis may contribute to the severe acidosis in *poisoning* by salicylates, ethylene glycol, or methanol. Ethanol elevates serum lactate but clinically significant lactic acidosis does not occur in alcohol intoxication unless there are associated disorders such as hepatic or circulatory failure.

In infants and children a number of congenital defects in enzymes of carbohydrate metabolism cause lactic acidosis. These include defects of glucose-6-phosphatase, fructose-1,6-biphosphatase, pyruvate carboxylase, and pyruvate dehydrogenase. *Primary* lactic acidosis in patients without an underlying disease has been reported, but the existence of such a spontaneous disorder is uncertain.

Acute metabolic acidosis *Poisoning* and drug toxicity are causes of acute metabolic acidosis. Among the more common agents are salicylates, ethylene glycol, and methyl alcohol (Chap. 374). Salicylates create a metabolic block, which leads to production of a mixture of endogenous organic acids. Methanol and ethylene glycol are converted to acid metabolites, methanol to formic acid and ethylene glycol to glyoxylic and oxalic acids. In addition, these intoxicants create metabolic blocks, which may lead to increased production of endogenous organic acids. Salicylates have the additional effect of stimulating the respiratory center directly. Respiratory alkalosis is the earliest derangement in salicylate intoxication and may be the only acid-base disorder in some patients.

Chronic metabolic acidosis Renal disease is the most common cause of *chronic* metabolic acidosis. In *chronic renal failure* (Chap. 224), the principal defect is decreased ability to excrete ammonium, but some patients also waste bicarbonate, especially at plasma levels of 18 mmol/L or above. Acidification of the urine and formation of titratable acidity are usually normal. Plasma bicarbonate tends to fall progressively as renal insufficiency becomes increasingly severe, but plasma bicarbonate usually stabilizes at levels of 12 to 18 mmol/L; it rarely falls below 10 mmol/L, even in advanced uremia. The mechanisms of stabilization are thought to be (1) stimulation of acid excretion by advancing acidosis, which occurs to some extent even in the diseased kidney; and (2) buffering of the daily metabolic acid load by carbonate and phosphate in bone. In *acute renal failure* (Chap. 223), plasma bicarbonate decreases by about 1 to 2 mmol/L per day if reduced renal acid excretion is the only cause of metabolic acidosis. Greater rates of fall suggest the presence, in addition, of some cause of increased acid production.

Chronic metabolic acidosis is the hallmark of *renal tubular acidosis* (Chap. 231), which may be an isolated disorder of tubular acid excretion; part of a Fanconi syndrome, in which other tubular functions are also abnormal; or associated with nonrenal primary disorders (Chap. 335). The acidosis is due to defective renal tubular acidification mechanisms, which limit renal conservation and regeneration of bicarbonate.

Aldosterone stimulates distal tubular acid and potassium secretion. In *hypoaldosteronism,* loss of this effect leads to metabolic acidosis and hyperkalemia. The acidosis is due not only to loss of the direct effect of aldosterone on acid excretion but also to the hyperkalemia, which decreases renal ammonia production. The same factors account for metabolic acidosis caused by the diuretic spironolactone, which blocks the action of aldosterone, and other "potassium-sparing" diuretics such as triamterene and amiloride, which directly inhibit distal tubular secretion of acid and potassium.

Loss of alkali may cause acute or chronic metabolic acidosis. Severe *diarrhea* or intestinal malabsorption usually causes mild to moderate acidosis due to the loss of bicarbonate in liquid stool, in which concentrations of 40 to 60 mmol/L may be present. Ureterosigmoidostomy, i.e., transplantation of the ureters into the sigmoid colon, leads to metabolic acidosis both because of exchange of chloride for bicarbonate by intestinal epithelium and because renal disease (obstructive uropathy and pyelonephritis) often develops. However, acidosis is not a problem with the more modern technique for urinary diversion, in which a bladder is formed from a small isolated loop of ileum. Carbonic anhydrase inhibitors, such as acetazolamide, cause mild to moderate acidosis by increasing bicarbonate loss in the urine.

Acidosis can be caused by administration of ammonium chloride and lysine or arginine hydrochloride, which form HCl during metabolism. This type of acidosis also may occur during parenteral alimentation with amino acid infusates that contain an excess of the cationic amino acids arginine, lysine, and histidine.

CLINICAL FEATURES AND DIAGNOSIS There are few specific symptoms or signs of metabolic acidosis; diagnosis depends on recognition of the clinical setting and appropriate laboratory studies. In acute metabolic acidosis, hyperventilation is usual and may be intense (Kussmaul respiration). However, it is ordinarily impossible to detect increased respiration by physical examination in patients with chronic metabolic acidosis, despite substantial reduction of P_{CO_2}. Acute, severe acidosis produces a variety of nonspecific symptoms ranging from fatigue through confusion, stupor, and coma. Cardiovascular effects include decreased cardiac contractility and vasodilatation, which may lead to heart failure or hypotension. Chronic metabolic acidosis may produce no symptoms or may be associated with fatigue and anorexia, although it is usually difficult to determine whether these symptoms reflect the acidosis per se or are related to the underlying disease.

The characteristic laboratory features are reduction of plasma bicarbonate and blood pH, together with a compensatory reduction in P_{CO_2} (see Fig. 51-1). Hyperkalemia is often present, due to shift of potassium out of cells. This phenomenon may mask significant potassium depletion (see Chap. 50). Hypokalemia is a clue to conditions in which concomitant potassium depletion is severe, for example, diarrhea or diabetic ketoacidosis, or in which renal potassium-regulating mechanisms are affected, such as renal tubular acidosis or administration of carbonic anhydrase inhibitors.

When the cause of metabolic acidosis is not evident from the history or clinical setting, calculation of unmeasured anions (anion gap) may help in differential diagnosis. Unmeasured anions are calculated by subtracting the sum of plasma bicarbonate and chloride from plasma sodium concentration; the normal value is 8 to 16 mmol/L. The negative charges on plasma proteins, principally albumin, make up most of the anion gap. Phosphate, sulfate, and organic acid anions normally contribute to unmeasured anions to a lesser degree. When metabolic acidosis is due to increased acid production or renal insufficiency (categories I and II, Table 51-1), the anion gap is usually increased. In acidosis resulting from increased acid production, the increased anion gap is due to accumulation in plasma of the anions of the various acids such as acetoacetate or lactate, which are produced faster than they can be metabolized or excreted. In renal failure, the anion gap increases because sulfate, phosphate, and organic acid anions are not excreted efficiently.

The cause of acidosis with an increased anion gap usually is easily determined from the clinical setting and simple laboratory tests. *Ketoacidosis* should be considered when acidosis occurs in patients with uncontrolled diabetes mellitus (Chap. 319), alcoholism, or starvation. Ketonemia can be detected by testing serum dilutions with nitroprusside (Acetest) reagent. In occasional patients this test, which reacts to acetoacetate but not β-hydroxybutyrate, may be misleading. If the clinical diagnosis is uncertain, a specific assay for β-hydroxybutyrate is available. The diagnosis of *lactic acidosis* is suspected in patients with severe circulatory insufficiency when other causes of acidosis can be ruled out. A specific assay for plasma lactate is available if the diagnosis is uncertain. Plasma salicylate concentration in the toxic range [>2.9 mmol/L (>40 mg/dL)] will confirm suspected *salicylate intoxication* (Chap. 374). Acidosis due to *poisoning* with ethylene glycol or methanol (Chap. 374) may be suspected if measured plasma osmolality exceeds calculated plasma osmolality [(2 × plasma Na) + glucose/18 + BUN/2.8 (with plasma Na in mmol/L, glucose and BUN in mg/dL)]. This "osmolal gap" reflects the plasma level of methanol or ethylene glycol, small molecules that at toxic concentrations add significantly to plasma osmolality. (Since ethanol has a similar effect, it must be measured if alcohol intoxication is suspected.) Detection of an "osmolal gap" in a patient with severe acidosis may permit prompt treatment to be instituted while awaiting confirmation of the diagnosis with specific tests for the toxins.

In all other types of metabolic acidosis (categories III, IV, V, Table 51-1), the anion gap is normal since there is neither increased production nor decreased excretion of organic acids, sulfate, and phosphate. Plasma chloride concentration is increased approximately as much as plasma bicarbonate is decreased (hyperchloremic acidosis). In diabetic ketoacidosis a variety of plasma acid-base patterns may develop, depending on the balance between production and renal excretion of ketoacid anions. In most patients there is renal dysfunction, and the anions are retained, leading to an anion-gap acidosis in which the elevation in plasma unmeasured anion is about equal to the reduction in bicarbonate concentration. Patients whose renal function is not impaired may present with a component of hyperchloremic acidosis due to renal excretion of ketone anions and retention of chloride. After therapy that repairs volume depletion and hence renal dysfunction, most patients develop some degree of hyperchloremia, due to the same mechanisms.

TREATMENT The treatment of metabolic acidosis depends on its cause and severity. In *chronic renal failure,* mild or moderate metabolic acidosis does not require treatment. When plasma bicarbonate falls below 15 mmol/L, it is reasonable to treat patients with oral alkali, such as sodium bicarbonate or sodium citrate. The dose is gradually increased until plasma bicarbonate concentration rises to about 18 to 20 mmol/L. Some patients appear to benefit symptomatically from elevation of bicarbonate to this level, and fatigue, anorexia, and malaise tend to be alleviated. Caution must be exerted to avoid excessively rapid alkalination of the plasma, which may precipitate tetany; excess sodium given with alkali may aggravate hypertension or edema. Acidosis should be corrected as completely as possible in patients with type 1 (distal) *renal tubular acidosis;* this will avoid hypercalciuria, osteomalacia, nephrocalcinosis, and lithiasis. In type 2 (proximal) renal tubular acidosis, therapy is usually not required (see Chap. 231). Patients with *acute renal failure* also do not ordinarily require specific therapy for acidosis. Dialysis instituted for management of the renal failure should maintain an adequate plasma bicarbonate.

Diabetic *ketoacidosis* responds to insulin, and most patients do not require treatment with alkali (see Chap. 319). However, when acidosis is extreme (pH less than 7.1 or [HCO_3^-] less than 6 to 8 mmol/L), intravenous bicarbonate therapy is justified. The ketoacidosis associated with alcoholism responds rapidly to infusions of glucose and saline. Insulin is not required, nor should alkali be given unless acidosis is extreme. The ketoacidosis of starvation is mild and requires no specific treatment.

In *lactic acidosis,* if the underlying disorder can be reversed, the acidosis will be corrected by metabolism of lactate, which generates bicarbonate. Since lactic acidosis is usually associated with severe circulatory or respiratory failure, the mortality rate is high. Because production of lactate and H^+ in lactic acidosis can be very rapid, it is usually resistant to treatment with alkali. Large amounts of bicarbonate may be required to raise or even to stabilize plasma bicarbonate. Some studies have suggested that alkali therapy in lactic acidosis may be counterproductive because correction of acidosis appears to increase lactate production. However, extreme acidosis may contribute to circulatory collapse (see above), thereby perpetuating the underlying cause of the lactic acidosis. Hence, it seems reasonable to treat lactic acidosis with intravenous bicarbonate at a rate at least sufficient to maintain plasma bicarbonate at 8 to 10 mmol/L and pH above 7.10. If vigorous administration of sodium bicarbonate leads to circulatory overloading, diuretics should be given or dialysis with a bicarbonate-buffered fluid may be instituted. Dichloroacetate, an investigational agent that enhances pyruvate dehydrogenase activity, has shown promise for treating lactic acidosis in experimental and clinical studies.

The acidosis due to *diarrhea* or loss of alkaline upper intestinal secretions is usually associated with volume depletion and potassium deficiency. Treatment of such electrolyte disorders with intravenous infusions appropriate for the patient's specific abnormalities may be required.

Some general points about therapy with alkali are worth emphasis. Oral treatment with sodium bicarbonate should usually begin with 1 g three times daily and be increased to maintain the desired plasma bicarbonate level. Some patients find that sodium bicarbonate leads to upper gastrointestinal discomfort; a 10% sodium citrate solution may be more palatable. In the intravenous treatment of acute metabolic acidosis, sodium bicarbonate is the agent of choice. The amount of bicarbonate to be given depends upon the severity of the acidosis and any associated disorders of serum sodium concentration. Typically, concentrations of bicarbonate between 50 and 150 mmol/L are achieved by adding one to three vials of sodium bicarbonate to a liter of dextrose in water. The concentration of bicarbonate in these vials is 1000 mmol/L (50 mmol in 50 mL); these bicarbonate solutions should never be given undiluted in the treatment of acidosis, since rapid infusion may induce serious or even fatal cardiac arrhythmias, especially if given as a bolus through a central venous catheter.

The total amount of alkali needed to raise plasma bicarbonate can be estimated from the effects of administration of acid loads. Approximately equal amounts of acid appear to be buffered by extracellular bicarbonate and by intracellular buffers. (In severe acidosis, a greater fraction of the acid load may be buffered within cells.) Therefore, it is appropriate to calculate the amount of alkali needed by assuming that approximately half will accept protons from intracellular buffers and be destroyed; the other half will elevate plasma bicarbonate concentration. Thus, the calculation would be: millimoles of bicarbonate required equals desired increment in plasma concentration (millimoles per liter) times 40 percent of body weight. The 40 percent figure represents twice the extracellular volume. It is rarely desirable to infuse enough alkali to elevate plasma bicarbonate to normal. Possible untoward effects include hypokalemic cardiac toxicity in patients who are substantially potassium-depleted, tetany in patients with renal failure or hypocalcemia, and congestive failure due to excess sodium. Moreover, alkalosis may supervene. Cerebrospinal fluid bicarbonate does not equilibrate rapidly with plasma. Hence the respiratory center, which responds to acidity both of blood and cerebrospinal fluid, maintains some degree of hyperventilation as plasma bicarbonate is increasing. This type of respiratory alkalosis may sometimes persist for several days after correction of metabolic acidosis. In acute acidosis due to overproduction of metabolic acids, successful treatment of the primary disorder will cause rapid metabolic conversion of lactate and ketone bodies to bicarbonate. Thus, excessive administration of bicarbonate early in therapy also may lead to metabolic alkalosis at a later stage of treatment, when endogenous bicarbonate has been reconstituted by improvement in metabolism.

METABOLIC ALKALOSIS

PATHOPHYSIOLOGY Metabolic alkalosis is usually initiated by increased loss of acid from the stomach or the kidney. However, excretion of bicarbonate at high plasma concentrations is normally so rapid that alkalosis will not be sustained unless bicarbonate reabsorption is enhanced or alkali is continuously generated at a great rate. Clinically, maintenance of metabolic alkalosis is most often due to stimulation of bicarbonate reabsorption by a volume (chloride) deficit. During volume depletion, renal conservation of sodium takes precedence over other homeostatic mechanisms, such as correction of alkalosis. Since in alkalosis a large fraction of plasma sodium is paired with bicarbonate, complete reabsorption of filtered sodium requires reabsorption of bicarbonate as well. Alkalosis is sustained until volume depletion is corrected by administration of sodium chloride. This diminishes tubular avidity for sodium and provides chloride as an alternative anion for reabsorption with sodium; excess bicarbonate can then be excreted with sodium.

The other major mechanism which can maintain metabolic alkalosis is hypermineralocorticoidism. Mineralocorticoids stimulate renal hydrogen ion secretion. In patients with excess mineralocorticoid activity, elevation of plasma bicarbonate is initiated by increased urinary loss of protons as ammonium and titratable acidity. Stimulation of tubular acid secretion also enhances bicarbonate reabsorption, thereby sustaining the metabolic alkalosis. Patients with excess mineralocorticoid activity are not volume- or chloride-deficient. Hence, this type of metabolic alkalosis does not respond to sodium chloride administration.

The relation between metabolic alkalosis and potassium is incompletely understood. Alkalosis and hypokalemia often occur together. Alkalosis may cause hypokalemia and potassium depletion through mechanisms discussed in Chap. 50. Conversely, potassium depletion may help to sustain metabolic alkalosis because tubular acid secretion, and hence bicarbonate reabsorption, is stimulated. Whether potassium depletion alone can generate metabolic alkalosis is uncertain; if so, severe potassium depletion is required.

Respiratory compensation for metabolic alkalosis is limited. Alveolar ventilation decreases, and P_{CO_2} is elevated. However, since this response is limited by hypoxia, P_{CO_2} rarely rises above 7.3 to 8 kPa (55 to 60 mmHg).

PATHOGENESIS The principal causes of metabolic alkalosis are outlined in Table 51-2. *Vomiting* and *gastric drainage* usually induce only minimal or moderate alkalosis, but occasional patients, especially those with increased gastric acid secretion, e.g., with acid-peptic disease or the Zollinger-Ellison syndrome, may develop very severe alkalosis. Loss of hydrochloric acid in the gastric fluid initiates the alkalosis. Water and sodium chloride are lost in the vomitus or gastric aspirate. Initially, sodium is lost in the urine as well, coupled

TABLE 51-2 Causes of metabolic alkalosis

I Associated with volume (chloride) depletion
- *A* Vomiting or gastric drainage
- *B* Diuretic therapy
- *C* Posthypercapnic alkalosis

II Associated with hyperadrenocorticism
- *A* Cushing's syndrome
- *B* Primary aldosteronism
- *C* Bartter's syndrome

III Severe potassium depletion

IV Excessive alkali intake
- *A* Acute
- *B* Milk-alkali syndrome

to increased bicarbonate excretion (which results from elevation of plasma bicarbonate above the tubular reabsorptive threshold). These losses cause a volume (chloride) deficit, which stimulates tubular reabsorption of bicarbonate and thus maintains the elevated plasma bicarbonate generated by gastric losses of hydrochloric acid.

Alkalosis may be present in patients treated with "loop" *diuretics* (furosemide, ethacrynic acid, bumetanide) or with thiazides. The diuretics cause extracellular volume contraction and inhibit sodium chloride reabsorption in the loop of Henle or distal convoluted tubule, which increases delivery of tubular fluid to more distal nephron segments. The volume deficit and consequent hyperaldosteronism stimulate proton secretion in these segments, generating and maintaining the alkalosis. Alkalosis due to treatment with oral diuretics is usually mild. Acute administration of potent intravenous diuretics such as furosemide or ethacrynic acid to patients on low-sodium diets may induce more severe alkalosis due to rapid loss of sodium chloride in the urine. Sudden contraction of extracellular volume elevates plasma bicarbonate; renal excretion of excess bicarbonate is prevented by the mechanism discussed above. Diuretics that specifically inhibit bicarbonate reabsorption, such as acetazolamide, or inhibit distal cation secretion, such as spironolactone, amiloride, and triamterene, cause acidosis rather than alkalosis (see above).

Patients with chronic hypercapnia due to respiratory insufficiency maintain high plasma bicarbonate concentrations (see "Respiratory Acidosis," below). If respiration improves, P_{CO_2} falls promptly. However, urinary excretion of excess bicarbonate previously generated by renal compensatory mechanisms takes a number of days. In patients on low-salt diets or diuretics who have a volume (chloride) deficiency, *posthypercapnic* alkalosis of this type may persist indefinitely unless sodium or potassium chloride is added to the diet. The mechanism in this condition is the same as that which causes persistent alkalosis in vomiting, described earlier.

Alkalosis is variable in patients with excess mineralocorticoid activity. Minimal or moderate alkalosis is usually present in patients with *Cushing's syndrome* or *primary aldosteronism*. More marked alkalosis may be seen in patients with extreme adrenal hyperfunction associated with ACTH-secreting tumors, such as bronchogenic carcinoma. Moderate alkalosis is typical of patients with *Bartter's syndrome*.

Although alkalosis and *potassium depletion* are often associated, mild or moderate potassium depletion does not cause sustained metabolic alkalosis. However, extreme degrees of potassium depletion (serum potassium usually 2 mmol/L or less) may cause metabolic alkalosis. This type of alkalosis is not corrected by administration of sodium chloride but does respond to administration of potassium.

For reasons noted earlier, alkalosis due to administration of alkali cannot be sustained unless large amounts are given. When renal function is compromised, alkalosis may be sustained by small exogenous loads. This is apparently the mechanism of alkalosis in the milk-alkali syndrome, in which hypercalcemic nephropathy and alkalosis develop in response to excessive intake of absorbable alkali. The nephropathy limits bicarbonate excretion, thus maintaining the alkalosis.

CLINICAL FEATURES AND DIAGNOSIS There are no specific clinical signs or symptoms. Severe alkalosis may cause apathy, confusion, and stupor. If serum calcium is borderline or low, rapid development of alkalosis may lead to tetany. The diagnosis of metabolic alkalosis depends on recognition of the clinical setting and appropriate laboratory studies. Plasma bicarbonate is increased. P_{CO_2} increases by about 0.01 kPa (0.6 mmHg) for each mmol/L increase in bicarbonate. Elevation of P_{CO_2} is insufficient to prevent alkalemia (see Fig. 51-1). Plasma potassium concentration is often reduced, and the electrocardiogram may reveal changes in T and U waves typical of hypokalemia (Chap. 176). These changes may be due to alkalosis itself or to associated alterations in potassium metabolism. Despite elevation of plasma bicarbonate, the urine pH is usually less than 7 in patients with sustained metabolic alkalosis. This "paradoxical aciduria" reflects the fact that bicarbonate reabsorption must be increased if metabolic alkalosis is to be sustained.

Differential diagnosis is usually made from clinical features, such as a history of vomiting or the manifestations of Cushing's syndrome. The urinary chloride concentration may be a helpful clue if the diagnosis is not evident. When the alkalosis is associated with volume contraction (category I, Table 51-2), urinary chloride is low, usually less than 10 mmol/L. When the alkalosis is caused by hyperadrenocorticism or severe potassium depletion (categories II and III), urinary chloride is higher, usually 20 mmol/L or more.

TREATMENT Mild or moderate metabolic alkalosis rarely requires specific treatment. In patients with gastric alkalosis, infusion of saline solutions is usually sufficient to enhance renal bicarbonate excretion and to correct alkalosis by mechanisms discussed above. Administration of potassium chloride is also helpful in treating or preventing alkalosis in these patients and those with diuretic-induced alkalosis. In patients with adrenal hyperfunction, alkalosis is corrected by specific treatment of the underlying disease. In Bartter's syndrome hypokalemia, potassium wasting, and alkalosis may be partly corrected by treatment with prostaglandin synthetase inhibitors such as indomethacin. Whenever alkalosis and potassium depletion occur together, potassium depletion should be treated with potassium chloride, not with an organic salt of potassium.

Rarely, with prolonged gastric metabolic alkalosis losses may be severe enough to require intravenous therapy with acidifying agents. Dilute hydrochloric acid or acidifying salts such as ammonium chloride or arginine hydrochloride may be given slowly under such circumstances. In most patients the use of acidifying agents can be avoided by appropriate treatment with saline and potassium chloride. In patients who are volume-expanded or in whom volume loading is inadvisable, therapy with acetazolamide, which enhances renal bicarbonate excretion, may be helpful.

RESPIRATORY ACIDOSIS

PATHOPHYSIOLOGY Failure of ventilation promptly increases P_{CO_2} (carbonic acid) because metabolic production of carbon dioxide is so rapid. Acute respiratory acidosis is modulated to a limited degree by tissue buffers. As can be seen from the curve labeled *acute respiratory acidosis* in Fig. 51-1, immediate tissue buffering elevates plasma bicarbonate only slightly, by about 1 mmol/L for each increase of 1.3 kPa (10 mmHg) in P_{CO_2}. If hypercapnia is sustained, renal acid excretion is enhanced, and bicarbonate reabsorption is stimulated. Over a period of several days, plasma bicarbonate rises approximately 3 mmol/L for each increase of 1.3 kPa (10 mmHg) in P_{CO_2}, thereby minimizing the degree of acidemia. The increment in plasma bicarbonate attributable to renal activity is represented by the difference between the curves marked *chronic respiratory acidosis* and *acute respiratory acidosis*.

PATHOGENESIS (See also Table 217-1) *Acute* respiratory acidosis occurs whenever there is a sudden failure of ventilation. Common causes include depression of the respiratory center by cerebral disease or drugs, neuromuscular disorders, and cardiopulmonary arrest. *Chronic* respiratory acidosis occurs in pulmonary diseases such as chronic emphysema and bronchitis, in which ventilation and perfusion are mismatched and effective alveolar ventilation is decreased. Chronic hypercapnia may also result from primary alveolar hypoventilation or from alveolar hypoventilation related to extreme obesity (Pickwickian syndrome). Acute and chronic diseases characterized principally by interference with alveolar gas exchange, such as chronic pulmonary fibrosis, pneumonia, and pulmonary edema, usually cause hypocapnia rather than hypercapnia. In these conditions, hypoxia stimulates increased ventilation; since carbon dioxide is much more diffusible than oxygen, excretion of carbon dioxide is enhanced despite the barrier to gas exchange. Hypercapnia occurs only with respiratory fatigue or extremely severe disease.

CLINICAL FEATURES AND DIAGNOSIS It is often difficult to separate the manifestations of respiratory acidosis from those of associated hypoxia. Moderate hypercapnia, especially if it develops slowly, probably has no specific clinical features. When P_{CO_2} exceeds 9.3 kPa (70 mmHg), patients become progressively confused and obtunded. Asterixis may be present. Papilledema may occur, apparently because intracranial pressure is increased by the cerebral vasodilation characteristic of hypercapnia. Dilatation of conjunctival and superficial facial blood vessels may be noted.

The diagnosis of acute respiratory acidosis is usually evident from the clinical situation, especially if respiration is obviously depressed. Proof requires laboratory confirmation that P_{CO_2} is elevated. Acidemia is always present in patients with *acute* hypercapnia. Acidosis in acute cardiopulmonary arrest is usually a combination of a metabolic lactic acidosis and acute respiratory acidosis. Patients with *chronic* hypercapnia are usually acidemic. However, some individuals with minimal or moderate chronic hypercapnia may have normal or even slightly elevated plasma pH, as may be seen from Fig. 51-1. The mechanism of full compensation or of ''overcompensation'' in such instances is unknown. However, significant elevation of pH in patients with chronic hypercapnia is almost always due to complicating metabolic alkalosis. Diuretics, low-sodium diets, and posthypercapnic alkalosis are frequent causes of this type of superimposed acid-base disorder.

Because of the differences between plasma bicarbonate in acute hypercapnia and in chronic hypercapnia, proper interpretation of acid-base parameters in respiratory acidosis depends on clinical information.

TREATMENT The only worthwhile approach to treatment of respiratory acidosis is correction of the underlying disorder. Rapid infusion of alkali is justified in cardiopulmonary arrest. In other circumstances, infusions of alkali have no role in practical management of respiratory acidosis.

RESPIRATORY ALKALOSIS

PATHOPHYSIOLOGY Acute reduction in carbon dioxide concentration releases hydrogen ion from tissue buffers, which minimize alkalemia by reducing plasma bicarbonate. Acute alkalosis also enhances glycolysis; increased production of lactic and pyruvic acids lowers serum bicarbonate and raises plasma concentrations of the corresponding anions by a millimole or two. In chronic hypocapnia, plasma bicarbonate is further reduced because the decreased P_{CO_2} inhibits tubular reabsorption and generation of bicarbonate. As in respiratory acidosis, compensation for the chronic state is much more complete than for the acute (Fig. 51-1). In acute hypocapnia, plasma bicarbonate falls only about 2 mmol/L for each 1.3-kPa (10-mmHg) reduction in P_{CO_2}. In chronic hypocapnia, plasma bicarbonate is reduced by 4 to 5 mmol/L for each 1.3-kPa (10-mmHg) decrease in P_{CO_2}. The decrement in plasma bicarbonate attributable to renal compensatory activity is shown by the difference between the curves labeled acute and chronic respiratory alkalosis in Fig. 51-1.

PATHOGENESIS Respiratory alkalosis is due to acute or chronic hyperventilation, which lowers P_{CO_2}. The causes of respiratory alkalosis are shown in Table 51-3.

TABLE 51-3 Causes of respiratory alkalosis

I Hypoxia
  A Acute (e.g., pneumonia, asthma, pulmonary edema)
  B Chronic (e.g., pulmonary fibrosis, cyanotic heart disease, high altitudes)
II Respiratory center stimulation
  A Anxiety
  B Fever
  C Salicylate intoxication
  D Cerebral disease (tumor, encephalitis, etc.)
III Exercise
IV Gram-negative sepsis
V Hepatic cirrhosis
VI Pregnancy
VII Excessive mechanical ventilation

CLINICAL FEATURES AND DIAGNOSIS Depending on its severity and acuteness, hyperventilation may or may not be clinically apparent. In acute respiratory alkalosis, the clinical picture is rather characteristic: patients complain of paresthesias, numbness, and tingling; of light-headedness; and, if alkalosis is sufficiently severe, of manifestations of tetany. Alkalosis directly enhances neuromuscular excitability; this effect, rather than the modest decrease in ionized plasma calcium induced by alkalosis, is probably the major cause of tetany. Severe respiratory alkalosis may cause confusion or loss of consciousness, perhaps due to cerebral vasospasm induced by hypocapnia.

The diagnosis may be suspected from the clinical setting but must be confirmed by analysis of the plasma bicarbonate system. Hypocapnia together with a variable degree of alkalemia is found; plasma bicarbonate is decreased but is rarely below 15 mmol/L.

TREATMENT The only successful treatment for respiratory alkalosis is elimination of the underlying disorder. In the acute hyperventilation syndrome, sedation, reassurance, and, if symptoms are sufficiently severe, rebreathing into a bag will usually terminate the attack.

REFERENCES

ADROGUE HJ et al: Plasma acid-base patterns in diabetic ketoacidosis. N Engl J Med 307:1603, 1982
ARBUS GS: An in vivo acid-base nomogram for clinical use. Can Med Assoc J 109:291, 1973
BATTLE DC, KURTZMAN NA: Renal regulation of acid-base homeostasis: Integrated response, in *The Kidney: Physiology and Pathophysiology,* 2d ed, DW Seldin, G Giebisch (eds). New York, Raven, 1986, p 1539
EMMETT M, NARINS RG: Clinical use of the anion gap. Medicine 56:38, 1977
HARRINGTON JT: Metabolic alkalosis. Kidney Int 26:88, 1984
KASSIRER JP, MADIAS NE: Respiratory acid-base disorders. Hosp Practice 15:57, 1980
LEVY LH et al: Ketoacidosis associated with alcoholism in non-diabetic subjects. Ann Intern Med 78:213, 1973
MADIAS NE: Lactic acidosis. Kidney Int 29:752, 1986
NARINS RG, EMMETT M: Simple and mixed acid-base disorders: A practical approach. Medicine 59:161, 1980
ROCHER LL, TANNEN RL: The clinical spectrum of renal tubular acidosis. Ann Rev Med 37:319, 1986
SCHWARTZ WB, RELMAN AS: A critique of the parameters used in the evaluation of acid-base disorders. N Engl J Med 268:1382, 1963
SELDIN DW, GIEBISCH G (eds): *Regulation of Acid-Base Balance.* New York, Raven, 1989, 616 pp
STACPOOLE PW et al: Dichloroacetate in the treatment of lactic acidosis. Ann Int Med 108:58, 1988

section 7 Alterations in reproductive and sexual function

52 IMPOTENCE

JOHN D. MCCONNELL / JEAN D. WILSON

A variety of endocrine, vascular, neurologic, and psychiatric diseases disrupt normal sexual and reproductive function in men. Furthermore, sexual dysfunction may be the presenting symptom of systemic disease.

NORMAL SEXUAL FUNCTION

Penile erection is initiated by neuropsychologic stimuli that ultimately produce vasodilation of the sinusoidal spaces and arteries within the paired corpora cavernosa. Erection is normally preceded by sexual desire (or libido), which is regulated in part by androgen-dependent psychic factors. Although nocturnal and diurnal spontaneous erections are suppressed in men with androgen deficiency, erections in response to erotic stimuli may continue. Thus, continuing action of testicular androgens appears to be required for normal libido but not for the erectile mechanism itself.

The penis receives innervation from sympathetic, parasympathetic, and somatic fibers. Somatic fibers in the dorsal nerve of the penis form the afferent limb of the erectile reflex by transmitting sensory impulses from the penile skin and glans to the S2-S4 dorsal root ganglia via the pudendal nerve. Unlike the corpuscular-type endings in the penile shaft skin, the majority of afferent terminations in the glans are free nerve endings. The efferent limb begins with parasympathetic preganglionic fibers from S2-S4 which pass in the pelvic nerves to the pelvic plexus. Sympathetic fibers emerging from the intermediolateral gray areas of T11-L2 travel through the paravertebral sympathetic chain ganglia, superior hypogastric plexus, and hypogastric nerves to enter the pelvic plexus along with parasympathetic fibers. Somatic efferent fibers from S3-S4 traveling in the pudendal nerve to the ischiocavernosus and bulbocavernosus muscles—as well as postganglionic sympathetic fibers innervating the smooth muscle of the epididymis, vas deferens, seminal vesicle, and internal sphincter of the bladder—mediate rhythmic contraction of these structures at the time of ejaculation.

Autonomic nerve impulses, integrated in the pelvic plexus, project to the penis through the cavernous nerves which course along the posterolateral aspect of the prostate before penetrating the pelvic floor muscles immediately lateral to the urethra. Distal to the membranous urethra, some fibers enter the corpus spongiosum, while the remainder enter the corpora cavernosa along with the terminal branches of the pudendal artery and exiting cavernous veins. If disruption of the cavernous nerves occurs following pelvic trauma or surgery, erectile impotence may ensue.

The brain exerts an important modulatory influence over spinal reflex pathways that control penile function. A variety of visual, auditory, olfactory, and imaginative stimuli elicit erectile responses that involve cortical, thalamic, rhinencephalic, and limbic input to the medial preoptic–anterior hypothalamic area, which is an important integrating center. Other areas of the brain, such as the amygdaloid complex, may inhibit sexual function.

Although the parasympathetic nervous system is the primary effector of erection, the transformation of the penis to an erect organ is a vascular phenomenon. In the flaccid state the arteries, arterioles, and sinusoidal spaces within the corpora cavernosa are constricted due to active contraction of smooth muscle in the walls of these structures. The venules between the sinusoids and the dense tunica albuginea surrounding the cavernosa open freely to the emissary veins. Erection begins when relaxation of the smooth muscles leads to dilatation of the sinusoids and a decrease in peripheral resistance, causing a rapid increase in arterial blood flow through internal pudendal and cavernosal arteries. Blood is trapped in the expanding sinusoidal system, which compresses the venules against the tunica albuginea, resulting in venous occlusion. The increase in intracorporeal pressure leads to tumescence and rigidity. Full rigidity, however, may in addition require stimulation of somatic fibers in the pudendal nerve and contraction of the ischiocavernosus muscle.

The neurotransmitter responsible for vasodilation in the penis has not been identified. Although the corpora cavernosa have cholinergic terminals, acetylcholine is unlikely to be the transmitter directly responsible for erection. Indeed, acetylcholine may produce vasodilation indirectly, either by acting on vascular endothelium to release a vasodilator substance, *endothelium-derived relaxing factor*, which then acts on the smooth muscle, or by decreasing adrenergic-induced tone. A variety of neuropeptides in corporal tissues, including vasoactive intestinal peptide (VIP) and substance P, produce tumescence when injected into the penis but have uncertain physiologic roles. Furthermore, high tissue levels of norepinephrine and the rich concentration of adrenergic receptors (predominantly alpha) suggest an important role of adrenergic mechanisms in both tumescence and detumescence, perhaps via synaptic "cross talk" with cholinergic nerves.

Seminal emission and ejaculation are under control of the sympathetic nervous system. Emission results from alpha-adrenergic-mediated contraction of the epididymis, vas deferens, seminal vesicles, and prostate, which causes seminal fluid to enter the prostatic urethra. Concomitant closure of the bladder neck prevents retrograde flow of semen into the bladder. Antegrade ejaculation results from contraction of the muscles of the pelvic floor, including the bulbocavernosus and ischiocavernosus muscles.

Orgasm is a psychosensory phenomenon in which the rhythmic contraction of the pelvic muscles is perceived as pleasurable. Orgasm can occur without either erection or ejaculation and in the presence of retrograde ejaculation.

Detumescence after orgasm and ejaculation is incompletely understood. Presumably, active tone in the vessels of the sinusoidal spaces is restored by active (probably adrenergic-mediated) contraction of smooth muscles, which decreases the inflow of blood to the penis and promotes emptying of the erectile tissue. Following orgasm, there is an refractory period that varies with age, physical condition, and psychic factors during which erection and ejaculation are inhibited.

IMPOTENCE

Simply defined, impotence is the failure to achieve erection, ejaculation, or both. Men with sexual dysfunction present with a variety of complaints, either singly, or in combination: loss of libido, inability to initiate or maintain an erection, ejaculatory failure, premature ejaculation, or inability to achieve orgasm. Sexual dysfunction can be secondary to systemic disease processes or their treatment, to specific disorders of the urogenital or endocrine systems, or to psychological disturbance. Previously, it was felt that the majority of men with erectile impotency had a psychogenic etiology for their dysfunction. It is now believed that the majority of impotent men have a component of underlying organic disease. Since the selection and success of subsequent therapy depends upon the specific etiology, it is essential to evaluate all aspects of the erectile mechanism.

LOSS OF DESIRE A decrease in sexual desire, or libido, may be due to androgen deficiency (arising from either pituitary or testicular disease), psychological disturbance, or to some types of prescribed or habitually abused drugs. The possibility of androgen deficiency can be tested by measurement of plasma testosterone and gonadotropins. The level of testosterone required for normal erectile function remains unknown. Hypogonadism may also result in the absence of emission, secondary to decreased secretion of ejaculate by the seminal vesicles and prostate.

FAILURE OF ERECTION The organic causes of erectile impotence can be grouped into endocrine, drug, local, neurologic, and vascular causes (Table 52-1).

Decreased plasma testosterone secondary to testicular failure is an uncommon but easily recognized and treated disorder. However, hyperprolactinemia may cause impotence in some men with pituitary tumors and may not be obvious on physical examination; hyperprolactinemia suppresses luteinizing hormone–releasing hormone (LHRH) production, resulting in plasma gonadotropins and testosterone values in the low normal range. Bromocriptine, a dopamine agonist, may lower prolactin levels and reverse impotence in such patients.

TABLE 52-1 Some organic causes of erectile impotence in men

I Endocrine causes
- *A* Testicular failure (primary or secondary)
- *B* Hyperprolactinemia

II Drugs
- *A* Antiandrogens
  - *1* H-2 blockers (e.g., cimetidine)
  - *2* Spironolactone
  - *3* Ketoconazole
- *B* Antihypertensives
  - *1* Central-acting sympatholytics (e.g., clonidine and methyldopa)
  - *2* Peripheral acting sympatholytics (e.g., guanadrel)
  - *3* Beta blockers
  - *4* Thiazides
- *C* Anticholinergics
- *D* Antidepressants
  - *1* Monoamine oxidase inhibitors
  - *2* Tricyclic antidepressants
- *E* Antipsychotics
- *F* Central nervous system depressants
  - *1* Sedatives (e.g., barbiturates)
  - *2* Antianxiety drugs (e.g., diazepam)
- *G* Drugs of habituation or addiction
  - *1* Alcohol
  - *2* Methadone
  - *3* Heroin

III Penile diseases
- *A* Peyronie's disease
- *B* Previous priapism
- *C* Penile trauma

IV Neurologic diseases
- *A* Anterior temporal lobe lesions
- *B* Diseases of the spinal cord
- *C* Loss of sensory input
  - *1* Tabes dorsalis
  - *2* Disease of dorsal root ganglia
- *D* Disease of nervi erigentes
  - *1* Radical prostatectomy and cystectomy
  - *2* Rectosigmoid operations
- *E* Diabetic autonomic neuropathy and various polyneuropathies

V Vascular disease
- *A* Aortic occlusion (Leriche syndrome)
- *B* Atherosclerotic occlusion or stenosis of the pudendal and/or cavernosal arteries
- *C* Venous leak
- *D* Disease of the sinusoidal spaces

Although many drugs are associated with impotence, antihypertensive agents, cimetidine, and monoamine oxidase (MAO) inhibitors are more likely to lead to erectile dysfunction. Antihypertensive drugs with peripheral and central sympatholytic action or beta-adrenergic-receptor blocking activity are the most frequently implicated. Angiotensin-converting enzyme inhibitors, calcium channel blockers, and peripheral vasodilators do not cause a significant incidence of sexual dysfunction. Histamine (H-2)-receptor antagonists, such as cimetidine, have antiandrogenic properties in addition to increasing prolactin secretion. MAO inhibitors, antipsychotic drugs, and tricyclic antidepressants may impair sexual function via anticholinergic and sympatholytic action.

Penile diseases including previous priapism, penile trauma, and Peyronie's disease can cause impotence due to fibrosis of the sinusoidal spaces of the corpora cavernosa, corporeal artery occlusion, or neurogenic mechanism. Peyronie's disease is not rare; patients present with a painful plaque on the dorsum of the penis and may progress to development of penile curvature and decreased rigidity.

Many types of neurologic disorders cause impotence, including lesions in the anterior temporal lobe, spinal cord disorders, insufficiency of sensory input such as can occur in tabes dorsalis, or damage to parasympathetic nerves, for example, following surgical procedures such as radical (total) prostatectomy or cystectomy. In contrast, transurethral prostatectomy does not cause organic impotence. Furthermore, the nerve supply to the penis (the nervi erigentes) runs on the posterolateral surface of the prostate, and if the nerves are preserved during radical prostate and bladder surgery, potency can be preserved in many men. If spinal cord injury is above the thoracolumbar region, reflex erections may occur, whereas diffuse injury of the spinal cord results in total impotence. As many as half of men with diabetes mellitus develop impotence within 6 years of the onset of diabetes, and impotency may be the first clinical manifestation of diabetic neuropathy. Several factors contribute to neuropathic impotence, including abnormalities in afferent sensory pathways, motor neuropathy in the cavernosal nerves (which carry the efferent pathways for vasodilation in the penis), and decreased level of cavernosal neurotransmitters. Although the autonomic pathways in the penis cannot be tested directly, most patients demonstrate other manifestations of autonomic neuropathy on careful examination. Many of the other polyneuropathies associated with impotence have similar effects.

Men with vasculogenic impotence may present with total erectile impotence, decreased penile rigidity, or loss of erection during intercourse. Vascular insufficiency may be due to aortic occlusion (Leriche syndrome) or to more distal atherosclerotic disease in the hypogastric, pudendal, and cavernosal arteries. Significant disease in the pudendal and cavernosal arteries can occur in the absence of other clinical manifestations of peripheral vascular disease. Together with neuropathy, vascular insufficiency contributes to the impotence in many men with diabetes mellitus.

PREMATURE EJACULATION This disorder seldom has an organic cause. It is usually related to anxiety in the sexual situation, unreasonable expectations about performance, or emotional disorder. A variety of successful therapeutic modalities have been described by Levine.

ABSENCE OF EMISSION This symptom may be produced by (1) retrograde ejaculation, (2) sympathetic denervation, (3) androgen deficiency, or (4) drugs. Retrograde ejaculation may occur following surgery on the bladder neck or develop spontaneously in diabetic men. Demonstration of sperm in a postcoital urine specimen establishes the diagnosis. Following sympathectomy or occasionally after extensive retroperitoneal surgery, the autonomic innervation of the prostate and seminal vesicles is lost, resulting in absence of smooth-muscle contraction at the time of ejaculation. Androgen deficiency results in a decrease in secretions of the prostate and seminal vesicles and in a diminution of the volume of ejaculate. Finally, drugs such as guanethidine, phenoxybenzamine, and phentolamine primarily impair ejaculation rather than erection or libido.

ABSENCE OF ORGASM If libido and erectile function are normal, the absence of orgasm is almost always due to a psychiatric disorder.

FAILURE OF DETUMESCENCE

Priapism is a persistent painful erection, often unrelated to sexual activity. Priapism can be distinguished from a normal erection by the absence of tumescence of the glans penis. Priapism may be idiopathic but can be associated with sickle cell anemia, chronic granulocytic leukemia, spinal cord injury, or injection of vasodilator agents (such as papaverine) into the penis. The disorder may be secondary to clotting of blood within the sinusoidal spaces of the penis or to abnormalities of the adrenergic-mediated mechanism for detumescence. Failure to treat priapism promptly usually results in fibrosis and subsequent loss of erectile function. In early phases, detumescence can sometimes be achieved by aspiration, irrigation of the corpora cavernosa, and injection of dilute vasoconstrictors. If this fails, surgical relief by shunting procedures may be necessary. In patients with priapism secondary to sickle cell anemia, conservation measures such as transfusion, oxygenation, and irrigation are generally preferred to shunting procedures.

EVALUATION OF IMPOTENCE

The relative frequency of organic as opposed to psychogenic causes of erectile impotence is still debated. Nevertheless, anxiety and depressive states are common causes of impotence (see Chap. 29). Other psychological factors such as disinterest in the sexual partner, fear of sexual incompetence, marital discord, guilt about deviant sexual attitudes, worry, fatigue, and ill health often operate in various combinations to reduce sexual impulse. The central issue in the evaluation of impotence is to separate those instances due to psychological factors from those due to organic causes (Table 52-1). Often, the separation can be made on the basis of history. With the exception of those with severe depression, men with psychogenic impotence usually have normal nocturnal and early morning erections. From early childhood through the eighth decade, erections occur during normal sleep. This phenomenon, termed *nocturnal penile tumescence* (NPT), occurs during rapid eye movement sleep, and the total time of NPT averages 100 min per night. Consequently, if the impotent man gives a history of rigid erections under any circumstances (often when awakening in the morning), the efferent neurologic and circulatory systems that mediate erection are intact, and dysfunction is probably due to a psychiatric disorder. In these patients the workup should be limited. (Occasional patients with early sensory neuropathy may have nocturnal erections.)

If the history of nocturnal erections is questionable, measurements of NPT can be made with the use of a strain gauge attached to a recorder or by snap gauge. Although false-negative and false-positive results are possible, this procedure helps to differentiate psychogenic and organic impotence. Patients with vasculogenic impotence may have some degree of penile tumescence without the development of adequate rigidity, which may result in a false-positive NPT test. Other features in favor of organic impotence include a similar degree of erectile dysfunction under all circumstances, onset not associated with any particular psychiatric symptomatology, a previous uninterrupted period of normal erectile function, and persistent sexual desire.

Having deduced an organic cause, the fundamental problem is the differential diagnosis of the etiology (Table 52-1). The history should be probed for diabetes mellitus, manifestations of peripheral neuropathy or bladder dysfunction, symptoms referable to the vascular system such as intermittent claudication, and symptoms of penile disease such as a history of priapism or penile curvature (Peyronie's). A thorough drug history should be obtained, and inquiry made concerning past surgery that may have produced neurologic damage.

Physical examination should include a detailed genital examination to identify abnormalities of the penis, especially Peyronie's disease which is usually easily felt as a fibrotic plaque on the dorsum of the penis. The testes should be palpated for size, symmetry, and abnormal masses; if the length is less than 3.5 cm, hypogonadism should be considered. Evidence of feminization such as gynecomastia and abnormal body hair distribution should be sought. All pulses should be palpated, and the presence of bruits should be sought. Often, the pulse in the dorsal penile artery can be felt. If there is an indication from either history or physical examination of a vascular etiology, direct measurement of penile blood flow may be indicated.

Pudendal arteriography provides the most accurate assessment of penile arterial disease, but it is expensive and invasive. Moreover, distal arterial lesions may not be identified unless the procedure is performed under conditions of chemical erection (papaverine injection). The penile/brachial index can be used to estimate penile blood flow, by dividing the penile systolic blood pressure, as determined by Doppler technique, by the simultaneously determined supine brachial systolic pressure. An index of less than 0.6 is suggestive of vasculogenic impotence. However, the test only evaluates flow through the dorsal penile artery, which is not directly involved in the erectile process. Significant disease may be present in the cavernosal arteries despite normal flow through the dorsal artery. Pulsed Doppler analysis and high-resolution ultrasonography can be used in conjunction with intracorporeal papaverine to assess blood flow in the cavernosal arteries. Abnormalities in the venous occlusive mechanism of the penis can cause impotence due to venous leak and can be diagnosed with the use of papaverine-induced erection in combination with ultrasonography. The incidence of venous leakage in men with normal erectile function is unknown. Moreover, venous leak may be secondary to arterial inflow and sinusoidal disease. Nevertheless, in carefully selected patients, surgical ligation or clinical obliteration of the incompetent veins can improve erectile function.

The neurologic examination should measure anal sphincter tone, perineal sensation, and the bulbocavernosus reflex. This reflex is elicited by squeezing the glans penis and noting the degree of anal sphincter constriction. An examination for peripheral neuropathy, including assessment of distal muscle function, the tendon reflexes in the legs, and vibratory, position, tactile, and pain sensation, should also be performed. In the presence of peripheral neuropathy, tests to evaluate penile neuropathy are seldom necessary. In cases with an uncertain neurogenic component, electromyographic sacral signal tracing of the bulbocavernosus reflex may be helpful. A specific test to document abnormalities in the penile autonomic efferent pathways is not available.

In the absence of hypogonadism or feminization, the serum testosterone is usually normal. Hyperprolactinemia, however, may not be suspected on the basis of history and physical examination. Although endocrine causes of erectile dysfunction are uncommon, measurement of serum prolactin and pooled serum testosterone and LH (see Chap. 321) is appropriate since abnormalities of these parameters are treatable.

TREATMENT OF IMPOTENCE

Medical therapy with androgens offers little more than placebo benefit except in hypogonadal men, and empirical therapy may actually delay identification of organic etiologies. If a prolactin-secreting pituitary tumor is present, however, either surgical removal or treatment with bromocriptine usually results in return of potency. Surgical therapy may be useful in the treatment of decreased potency related to aortic obstruction; however, potency can be lost rather than improved after aortic surgery if the autonomic nerve supply to the penis is damaged. The efficacy of penile revascularization and balloon embolization therapy for vasculogenic impotency remains uncertain. Men with primary venous leak impotency, without associated arterial or sinusoidal disease, may benefit from venous ligation.

A variety of vasoactive substances produce erection when injected into the corpora cavernosa. Self-injection with papaverine, with or without phentolamine, produces erection in patients with psychogenic, neurogenic, and mild vasculognic impotency. Lack of FDA approval, pain on injection, and the possible complications of priapism and penile fibrosis limited the use of this therapy. Commercially available mechanical devices that utilize a vacuum to produce an erection and a rubber band to restrict venous return at the base of the penis, provide a successful nonsurgical alternative in many patients, including some with diabetes mellitus.

Penile prostheses are the most common therapeutic alternative in impotent patients refractory to other forms of therapy. Malleable silastic rode implanted into the penis provide the simplest system and the lowest complication rates; however, the cosmetic and functional performance of the device is not uniformly satisfactory. Multicomponent, hydraulically operated prostheses offer the advantage of more physiologic erection and greater increase in penile diameter. However, these devices are subject to mechanical failure.

Even in patients with organic impotence, psychotherapy is often beneficial in alleviating concomitant psychogenic factors that limit the success of medical and surgical therapy.

REFERENCES

ABRAMOWICZ M et al: Drugs that cause sexual dysfunction. Med Lett 29:65, 1987

DEGROAT WC, STEERS WD: Neuroanatomy and neurophysiology of penile erection, in *Contemporary Management of Impotence and Infertility*, EA Tanagho et al (eds). Baltimore, Williams & Wilkins, 1988, pp 3–27

FISHMAN JF et al: Experience with inflatable penile prosthesis. Urol 23:86, 1984

GOLDSTEIN I: Electromyography: Evoked-response evaluations, in *Controversies in Neuro-Urology*, DM Barret, AJ Wein (eds). New York, Churchill Livingstone, 1984

KAISER FE, KORENMAN SG: Impotence in diabetic men. Am J Med 85(Suppl 5A):147, 1988

KWAN M et al: The nature of androgen action on male sexuality: A combined laboratory–self-report study on hypogonadal men. J Clin Endocrinol Metab 57:557, 1983

LEVINE SB: Marital sexual dsyfunction: Ejaculation distubances. Ann Intern Med 84:575, 1976

LEWIS RW, PUYAU FA: Procedures for decreasing venous drainage. Semin Urol 4:263, 1986

LUE TF, TANAGHO EA: Functional anatomy and mechanism of penile erection, in *Contemporary Management of Impotency and Infertility*, EA Tanagho et al (eds). Baltimore, Williams & Wilkins, 1988, pp 39–50

——— et al: Functional evaluation of penile veins by cavernosography in papaverine-induced erection. J Urol 135:479, 1986

MEYER J: Disorders of sexual function, in *Textbook of Endocrinology*, JD Wilson, DM Foster (eds). Philadelphia, Saunders, 1985, vol 7, pp 476–491

NATH RL et al: The multidisciplinary approach to vasculogenic impotence. Surgery 89:124, 1981

SAYPOL DC et al: Impotence. Are the newer diagnostic methods a necessity? J Urol 130:260, 1983

WABEK AJ: Bulbocavernosus reflex testing in 100 consecutive cases of erectile dysfunction. Urology 25:495, 1985

WALSH PC et al: Impotency following radical prostatectomy: Insight into etiology and prevention. J Urol 128:492, 1982

WINTER CC: Priapism. Urol Surv 28:163, 1978

WITHERINGTON R: Vacuum constriction device for management of erectile impotence. J Urol 141:320, 1989

ZORGNIOTTI AW: Auto-injection of the corpus cavernosum with a vasoactive drug combination for vasculogenic impotence. J Urol 133:39, 1985

53 DISTURBANCES OF MENSTRUATION AND SEXUAL FUNCTION IN WOMEN

BRUCE R. CARR / JEAN D. WILSON

Complaints related to the female reproductive tract can usually be categorized as disturbances of menstruation, pelvic pain, disturbances in sexual function, or infertility. However, a single disorder, for example, leiomyoma of the uterus, can present with symptoms referable to any one or more of these categories. Furthermore, sexual dysfunction can interdigitate with other complaints in several ways. On the one hand, in women who present with complaints related to other reproductive tract functions, the underlying problem may actually be severe sexual dysfunction or marital conflict. Alternatively, women with severe organic disorders of the pelvis, for example, pelvic inflammatory disease, may present with sexual dysfunction such as dyspareunia which in fact is only a minor manifestation of the underlying disease.

Since normal reproductive function depends on the integrated action of the central nervous system, the endocrine glands, and the reproductive organs, menstrual cycle abnormalities, sexual dysfunction, and infertility may be the result of a variety of systemic and psychological disorders as well as of primary defects in the endocrine and reproductive organs. The endocrine and physiologic control—normal and abnormal—of puberty, reproductive life, and menopause are discussed in Chap. 322. The focus of this chapter is on the initial evaluation of women with disturbances of the reproductive tract.

DISTURBANCES IN MENSTRUATION Disorders of menstruation can be divided into abnormal uterine bleeding and amenorrhea.

Abnormal uterine bleeding The menstrual cycle is defined as the interval between the onset of one bleeding episode and the onset of the next. In normal women the cycle averages 28 ± 3 days, the mean duration of menstrual flow is 4 ± 2 days, and the average blood loss is 40 to 100 mL. Between menarche and the menopause most women experience one or more episodes of abnormal uterine bleeding, here defined as any bleeding pattern outside the normal ranges of frequency, duration, and/or amount of blood loss described above. The decision to evaluate a patient with an abnormal bleeding pattern depends on the severity and frequency of the abnormal bleeding episodes.

When uterine bleeding is suspected, it is essential to establish first that the blood observed by the patient is derived from the uterine endometrium. Rectal, bladder, cervical, and vaginal sources of bleeding must be excluded. Once the bleeding is documented to be uterine in origin, a pregnancy-related disorder (such as threatened or incomplete abortion or ectopic pregnancy) must be excluded by physical examination and appropriate laboratory tests. Abnormal uterine bleeding may also be the initial or principal manifestation of a generalized bleeding diathesis. The remaining causes of abnormal uterine bleeding can be divided into those associated with ovulatory cycles and those associated with anovulatory cycles.

OVULATORY CYCLES Menstrual bleeding with ovulatory cycles is spontaneous, regular in onset, predictable in duration and amount of flow, and frequently associated with discomfort. Uterine bleeding with ovulatory cycles is due to progesterone withdrawal at the end of the luteal (postovulatory) phase and requires prior estrogen priming of the endometrium during the follicular (preovulatory) phase of the cycle. When deviations from an established pattern of menstrual flow occur but the cycles are still regular, the usual cause is organic disease of the outflow tract. For example, regular, prolonged, excessive bleeding episodes unassociated with a bleeding diathesis are usually due to abnormalities of the uterus such as submucous leiomyomas, adenomyosis, or endometrial polyps. On the other hand, cyclic, predictable menstruation characterized by spotting or light bleeding is often due to obstruction of the outflow tract as with uterine synechiae or scarring of the cervix. Intermittent bleeding between cyclic ovulatory menses is often due to cervical or endometrial lesions.

ANOVULATORY CYCLES Uterine bleeding that is irregular in occurrence, unpredictable as to amount and duration of flow, and usually painless is called dysfunctional uterine bleeding. This type of bleeding is the result of a failure of normal follicular maturation with consequent anovulation and may be either transient or chronic. Transient disruption of the synchronous hypothalamic-pituitary-ovarian hormonal control necessary for ovulatory cycles occurs most often in the early menarcheal years, during the perimenopausal period, or as the secondary consequence of a variety of stresses and intercurrent illnesses. Persistent dysfunctional uterine bleeding during the reproductive years can occur in several organic diseases that affect ovarian function and is most often due to estrogen breakthrough bleeding. Estrogen breakthrough bleeding occurs when prolonged continuous estrogen stimulation of the endometrium is not interrupted by cyclic progesterone withdrawal. For example, chronic acyclic estrogen production not associated with ovulation can occur in polycystic ovarian disease.

Amenorrhea Amenorrhea is defined as failure of menarche by age 16, regardless of the presence or absence of secondary sexual characteristics, or the absence of menstruation for 6 months in a woman with previous periodic menses. Amenorrhea in a woman who has never menstruated is termed primary; cessation of menses is termed secondary amenorrhea. Because some disorders can cause both primary and secondary amenorrhea, we prefer a functional classification based upon the nature of the underlying defect, namely anatomic defects of the outflow tract (uterus, cervix, or vagina), ovarian failure, and chronic anovulation.

Anatomic defects of the outflow tract include congenital defects of the vagina, imperforate hymen, transverse vaginal septa, cervical stenosis, intrauterine adhesions (synechiae), absence of the vagina or uterus, and uterine maldevelopment. The diagnosis of an anatomic defect is usually made by physical examination and confirmed by demonstrating failure of bleeding following administration of estrogen plus a progestogen for 21 days or by a hysterosalpingogram or hysteroscopy.

Causes of *ovarian failure* include gonadal dysgenesis, deficiency of 17α-hydroxylase or 17,20-desmolase, resistant ovary syndrome, and premature ovarian failure. Ovarian failure encompasses those disorders in which the ovary is deficient in germ cells and those in which the germ cells are resistant to FSH (follicle-stimulating hormone). The diagnosis of ovarian failure as the cause of amenorrhea is confirmed by a plasma FSH greater than 40 IU/L.

Women with *chronic anovulation* fail to ovulate spontaneously but have the capability of ovulating with appropriate therapy. In some women with chronic anovulation estrogen production is adequate, but estrogen is not secreted in a cyclic fashion. In others estrogen production is deficient.

Women who have adequate estrogen production and demonstrate withdrawal bleeding after progesterone challenge usually have polycystic ovarian disease (see Fig. 322-7). Unusual causes include hormone-secreting ovarian and adrenal tumors. Women with deficient or absent estrogen production, and therefore with absence of withdrawal bleeding after progestogen administration, usually have hypogonadotropic hypogonadism due either to organic or functional disorders of the pituitary or central nervous system such as brain tumors, pituitary tumors (especially prolactin-secreting adenomas), primary hypopituitarism, or Sheehan's syndrome.

PELVIC PAIN Pelvic pain may originate in the pelvis or be referred from another region of the body. A pelvic source for such pain is often suggested by the history (for example, dysmenorrhea and dyspareunia) and physical findings, but a high index of suspicion must be entertained for extrapelvic disorders that refer to the pelvis, such as appendicitis, cholecystitis, intestinal obstruction, and urinary tract infections (see Chap. 17).

"Physiologic" pelvic pain PAIN ASSOCIATED WITH OVULATION ("MITTELSCHMERZ") Many women experience low abdominal discomfort with ovulation, typically a dull aching pain at midcycle in one lower quadrant lasting from a few minutes to hours. It is rarely severe or incapacitating. The relationship of the pain to the mechanisms of ovulation is unknown. It may result from peritoneal irritation by follicular fluid released into the peritoneal cavity at the time of ovulation. The onset at midcycle and a short duration of pain are often diagnostic.

PREMENSTRUAL OR MENSTRUAL PAIN In normal ovulatory women somatic symptoms during the few days prior to menses may be insignificant or disabling. Such symptoms include edema, breast engorgement, and abdominal bloating or discomfort. A symptom complex of cyclic irritability, depression, and lethargy is known as the *premenstrual syndrome* (PMS). The cause of PMS is unknown, and there is no consensus about therapy.

Severe or incapacitating uterine cramping in women with ovulatory menses but no demonstrable disorders of the pelvis is termed *primary dysmenorrhea*. Primary dysmenorrhea is caused by prostaglandin-induced uterine ischemia and is treated with prostaglandin synthetase inhibitors or oral contraceptive agents.

Pelvic pain due to organic causes Severe dysmenorrhea associated with disease of the pelvis is termed *secondary dysmenorrhea*. Organic causes of pelvic pain can be classified as (1) uterine, (2) adnexal, (3) vulvar or vaginal, and (4) pregnancy-associated.

UTERINE PAIN Pain of uterine etiology is often chronic and continuous and increases in intensity during menstruation and intercourse. Causes include leiomyomas of the uterus (particularly submucous and degenerating leiomyomas), adenomyosis, and cervical stenosis. Infections of the uterus associated with intrauterine manipulation following dilatation and curettage or with intrauterine devices can also cause significant pelvic pain (see Chap. 322). Pelvic pain due to endometrial or cervical cancer is usually a late manifestation of disseminated disease (see Chap. 322).

ADNEXAL PAIN The most common cause of pain in the adnexae (fallopian tubes and ovaries) is infection (see Chap. 94). Acute salpingo-oophoritis presents as low abdominal pain, fever, and chills, begins a few days after a menstrual period, and is usually due to chlamydia or gonococcal disease with or without a superimposed pyogenic infection. Chronic pelvic inflammatory disease results from either a single episode or multiple episodes of infection and may present as infertility associated with chronic pelvic pain that increases in intensity with menses and intercourse. On physical examination the adnexae are tender, and adnexal thickening with or without masses may be present. Pelvic inflammatory disease may become a surgical emergency if peritonitis results from rupture of a tuboovarian abscess. Ovarian cysts or neoplasms may cause pelvic pain that becomes more severe with torsion or rupture of the mass, and ectopic pregnancy must be considered in the differential diagnosis (see below). Endometriosis involving fallopian tubes, ovaries, or peritoneum may cause both chronic low abdominal pain and infertility; the magnitude of tissue involvement does not always correlate with the severity of symptoms. Endometriosis pain typically increases with menstruation and, if the posterior ligaments of the uterus are involved, with intercourse.

VULVAR OR VAGINAL PAIN Pain in these areas is most often due to infectious vaginitis caused by organisms such as *Monilia, Trichomonas,* or *Gardnerella* and is characteristically associated with vaginal discharge and pruritus. Herpetic vulvitis, condyloma acuminatum, and cysts or abscesses of Bartholin's glands may also cause vulvar pain.

PREGNANCY-ASSOCIATED DISORDERS Pregnancy must be considered in the differential diagnosis of pelvic pain during the reproductive years. Threatened abortion or incomplete abortion often presents with uterine cramping, bleeding, or passage of tissue following a period of amenorrhea. Ectopic pregnancy may be insidious in presentation and result in severe intraperitoneal hemorrhage and maternal death.

Evaluation of pelvic pain The evaluation of pelvic pain includes a careful history and pelvic examination. This often leads to the correct diagnosis and institution of appropriate treatment. If the pain is severe and the diagnosis is unclear, the workup should follow that outlined for the acute abdomen (Chap. 17). A culdocentesis is indicated if a ruptured ectopic pregnancy is suspected. If there is a question of an adnexal mass or if the patient is so obese as to preclude a thorough pelvic examination, sonography may be useful. Serial human chorionic gonadotropin (hCG) measurements may be helpful in establishing a diagnosis of tubal pregnancy. Finally, diagnostic laparoscopy and laparotomy may be indicated with severe or prolonged pain of undetermined etiology.

SEXUAL DYSFUNCTION Some women with sexual dysfunction describe minor complaints related to the reproductive tract as a means of bringing sexual problems to the attention of the physician. Alternatively, sexual dysfunction may be thought to be the cause of low abdominal discomfort or dyspareunia when the actual etiology is organic. However, more and more women seek medical advice because of sexual problems that interface in provenance between medicine and sociology.

The normal sexual response begins with sexual arousal which causes genital vasocongestion that results in vaginal lubrication in preparation for intromission. The lubrication is due to the formation of a transudate in the vagina and in conjunction with genital congestion produces the so-called orgasmic platform prior to orgasm. Sexual stimuli (visual, tactile, auditory, and olfactory) as well as healthy vaginal tissue are prerequisites for genital vasocongestion and vaginal lubrication. During the second stage of the sexual response involuntary contractions of the muscles of the pelvis result in a pleasurable cortical sensory phenomenon known as orgasm. Direct or indirect stimulation of the clitoris is important in the production of the female orgasm. In simple terms, sexual dysfunction can be due to interference with the arousal or orgasmic phases of the sexual response. Either disorder can be due to an organic or functional cause or both.

Illnesses that impair neurologic function such as diabetes mellitus or multiple sclerosis may prevent normal sexual arousal. Local pelvic diseases such as vaginitis, endometriosis, and salpingo-oophoritis may preclude normal sexual response because of resulting dyspareunia. Debilitating systemic diseases such as cancer and cardiovascular diseases may impair normal sexual response indirectly.

More commonly, failure of a normal sexual response is due to psychological factors that impair sexual arousal. Such problems include misinformation, for example, the perception of sexual satisfaction as bad, or feelings of guilt about previous psychologically traumatic events such as incest, rape, or unwanted pregnancy. In addition, women who have had previous hysterectomy or mastectomy may perceive themselves as "incomplete." Stresses such as anxiety, depression, fatigue, and marital or interpersonal conflicts may lead to failure of the vasocongestive response and prevent normal vaginal lubrication. Women with such experiences may be unable to achieve normal sexual response unless they receive professional counseling by a family physician, psychiatrist, or sex therapist. Such problems are approached by attempting to identify and reduce the causative stresses.

Failure to achieve orgasm is a specific form of sexual dysfunction. In the absence of orgasm many women enjoy sexual encounters to variable degrees because of the pleasure derived from closeness in a cherished relationship, particularly with a loving partner. However, for other women sexual relations with rare or absent orgasms are frustrating and unsatisfying. In many instances, failure of orgasm is due to insufficient clitoral stimulation and may be rectified by appropriate counseling and patient education.

A specific entity, "vaginismus," painful, involuntary contractions of the musculature surrounding the entrance to the vagina, is a rare cause of dyspareunia. It is a conditioned response to a previous real or imagined frightening or traumatic sexual experience. Treatment is directed to elimination of the conditioned response by progressive vaginal dilation by the patient in conjunction with marital therapy.

REPRODUCTION Problems of infertility are discussed in detail in Chap. 322. The approach to infertile couples always involves evaluation of both the man and woman. The initial evaluation includes a thorough history and physical examination. The history should elicit information as to the frequency of intercourse, the sexual responses of both, the use of contraceptives or lubricants, previous or past medical illnesses, and all medications taken.

Male-associated factors account for a third of infertility problems. Therefore, one of the first procedures in the workup of infertile couples should be a semen analysis (see Chap. 321). The initial evaluation of the female includes documentation of normal ovulatory cycles. A history of regular, cyclic, predictable, spontaneous menses usually indicates ovulatory cycles, which may be confirmed by basal body temperature graphs, properly timed endometrial biopsies, or plasma progesterone measurements during the luteal phase of the cycle. Also, the diagnosis of luteal-phase dysfunction (low progesterone secretion during the luteal phase) can be established by these methods. If the woman is anovulatory, attempts to induce ovulation can be undertaken by a variety of methods including clomiphene, human menopausal gonadotropins, bromocriptine, luteinizing hormone–releasing hormone (LHRH) agonists, or wedge resection of the ovaries (Chap. 322).

The most common cause of infertility in women is tubal disease, usually due to infection (pelvic inflammatory disease) or endometriosis. Tubal disease can be evaluated by obtaining a hysterosalpingogram or by diagnostic laparoscopy. The treatment of tubal causes of infertility is primarily surgical.

A cervical factor as a cause of infertility is identified by a properly timed postcoital examination. During this examination the sperm motility in cervical mucus is observed. Also, immunologic etiologies for infertility can be tested for by a variety of laboratory tests. The cause of infertility is unknown in 10 percent of couples. In many instances of infertility reproductive technology now makes possible the successful use of in vitro fertilization and embryo transfer, gamete intrafallopian tube transfer, transfer of cryopreserved ova and embryos, and intrauterine insemination.

The desire for fertility control or contraception is also a frequent cause for women to seek medical treatment or evaluation. The most widely used methods for fertility control include (1) rhythm and withdrawal techniques, (2) barrier methods, (3) intrauterine devices, (4) oral steroid contraceptives, (5) sterilization, and (6) abortion. A discussion of these methods and the possible complications of each is found in Chap. 322.

REFERENCES

Cunningham FG et al: *Williams Obstetrics*, 18th ed. Norwalk, Appleton-Century-Crofts, 1989

Droegemuller W et al: *Comprehensive Gynecology*. St. Louis, Mosby, 1987

Fordney DS: Dyspareunia and vaginismus. Clin Obstet Gynecol 21:205, 1978

Hatcher RA et al: *Contraceptive Technology 1986–1987*. New York, Irvington, 1986

Masters W, Johnson V: *Human Sexual Response*. Boston, Little, Brown, 1966

———, ———: *Human Sexual Inadequacy*. Boston, Little, Brown, 1970

Speroff L et al: *Clinical Gynecologic Endocrinology and Infertility*, 4th ed. Baltimore, Williams & Wilkins, 1988

54 HIRSUTISM AND VIRILIZATION

WILLIAM J. KOVACS / JEAN D. WILSON

Hirsutism, male pattern hair growth in women, is a common and perplexing problem. The distribution and growth of hair in normal persons is under complex genetic and endocrine control so that there is considerable variability in hair growth in normal men and women. As a consequence, abnormal hair growth is sometimes difficult to define: Some patients may seek medical attention because of what the physician may consider an insignificant cosmetic defect. Others, because of personal or cultural differences, may be undisturbed by surprising degrees of hirsutism. The central issue in dealing with such patients is the separation of those infrequent instances in which hirsutism is a manifestation of a serious and remediable underlying disorder from the vast majority of hirsute women in whom excess hair is fundamentally a cosmetic problem.

CONTROL OF NORMAL HAIR GROWTH AND DISTRIBUTION

Endocrine control Androgens are the major determinants of hair distribution in both sexes. There are three principal circulating androgens in women—dehydroepiandrosterone, derived from the adrenal; androstenedione, which is derived equally from adrenal and ovary; and testosterone, which is both secreted by the ovary and adrenal and formed in peripheral tissue from circulating dehydroepiandrosterone and androstenedione. The production of adrenal androgen is regulated primarily by ACTH, while ovarian androgen secretion is regulated by luteinizing hormone (LH). These various androgens must be converted to testosterone (or dihydrotestosterone) before they can bind to the androgen receptor of target cells and induce an androgenic response. Thus, adrenal androgens virilize only in so far as they serve as precursors for testosterone and dihydrotestosterone.

Several types of relationships can be defined between hair growth and androgens in normal individuals. Eyebrows, eyelashes, and lanugo (fine, downy hair) are not dependent on androgens, while axillary and lower pubic hair are sensitive to the small amounts of androgen secreted by the adrenal. Hair in these regions therefore grows to an approximately equal extent in men and women. Hair growth in areas typical of males appears to require the greater androgen levels normally produced by the testes; such areas include the face, upper pubic triangle, chest, and ears. Finally, scalp hair exhibits androgen-mediated regression. The reason different body regions respond differently to the same or similar androgen is unknown. Theoretically, the metabolism of androgens might differ in the various sites, or hormone receptors might vary. The hair follicle, like some other androgen targets, requires conversion of testosterone to dihydrotestosterone for expression of androgen action, and hair follicles from all regions of the body perform this conversion equally well. Moreover, the same receptor that is essential for androgen action in other cells (Chap. 321) mediates the effects of dihydrotestosterone in the hair follicle. Genetic disorders with normal testosterone production but absent androgen receptor have deficient or absent axillary, pubic, facial, truncal, and limb hair (Chap. 324). Regional differences in androgen responsiveness of hair in normal individuals may be the consequence of regional differences in the amount of androgen receptor in hair follicles.

Genetic factors Despite similar hormone levels, there is considerable diversity in the distribution of hair between individuals and among different racial groups in regard to facial, truncal, and pubic hair. Dark-haired, darkly pigmented whites of either sex tend to be more hirsute than blond or fair-skinned persons. Orientals, American Indians, and blacks on average are less hirsute than whites. Orientals rarely have facial or body hair except in the pubic and axillary regions, and American Indians, in addition, rarely develop baldness in either sex. Heterogeneity of hair patterns also exists within families. The inheritance of hair patterns is complex and probably polygenic in nature.

Other factors Aging is a prerequisite for the expression of some types of hair development. For example, in men hair on the trunk and extremities frequently increases for several years after maximal levels of plasma androgens have been reached. Conversely, loss of androgen may not result in diminution of normal hair growth in men or complete reversal of hirsutism in women. The appearance of pubic hair is frequently the heralding event of puberty in females. Women in the first trimester of pregnancy commonly observe increased hairiness of the face, extremities, and breasts. Menopause is often associated with the loss of hair in the pubic area, axillae, and extremities, whereas growth of hair on the face increases in postmenopausal women. The physiologic basis for these changes is unclear and cannot be explained entirely by changes in androgen levels.

PATHOLOGIC HAIR GROWTH AND DISTRIBUTION A central consideration in the evaluation of women with hirsutism is whether evidence of virilization or defeminization is also present (Table 54-1) since such signs suggest a more significant degree of androgen excess. In patients with overproduction of androgen, defeminizing signs, such as disturbances of menstruation, are more frequently observed than are the signs of virilization. However, the presence or absence of overt virilization should be interpreted with caution for at least two reasons. First, signs of virilization (clitoromegaly, balding, coarsening of the hair, hirsutism) indicate androgen excess at some time in the patient's life but do not necessarily mean that active disease is present at the time of evaluation. It is necessary to measure plasma androgen levels and/or production rates to determine if androgen excess is ongoing. Second, severe overandrogenization may exist in the absence of marked virilization; i.e., at the same level of androgen production clitoromegaly may be present in one patient and not another.

TABLE 54-1 Clinical signs of defeminization and virilization

Signs of defeminization	Signs of virilization
Amenorrhea	Frontal balding
Decrease in breast size	Increase in size of shoulder girdle muscles
Loss of female body contours	Clitoromegaly
	Coarsening of the voice
	Acne

After Karp L, Herrmann WL: Diagnosis and treatment of hirsutism in women. Obstet Gynecol 41:283, 1973.

Diagnostic considerations DRUGS Excessive hair growth can be caused by drugs that do not produce signs of defeminization or virilization. Such drugs include phenytoin, minoxidil, diazoxide, cyclosporin, and hexachlorobenzene. Androgens produce hirsutism as well as virilization. Some synthetic progestogens have androgenic activity.

TUMORS The rapid onset of hair growth with or without accompanying signs of frank virilization suggests a neoplastic source of androgen. Such tumors include androgen-secreting adenomas and carcinomas of the adrenal and ovarian tumors such as arrhenoblastoma, which secrete androgens directly, and Krukenberg tumors of the ovary, which stimulate the surrounding ovarian stromal tissue to produce excess androgen.

POLYCYSTIC OVARIAN DISEASE The most common cause of ovarian hyperandrogenism is polycystic ovarian disease. This disorder has a broad clinical spectrum that ranges from mild hirsutism to complete amenorrhea and virilization. The salient feature for the diagnosis is the pubertal onset of chronic anovulation and hirsutism; enlarged cystic ovaries, obesity, and amenorrhea (i.e., the Stein-Leventhal syndrome) are present in only half or fewer of women with this disorder and need not be present for the diagnosis (see Chap. 322). The fundamental abnormality in polycystic ovarian disease is not fully understood. Elevation of plasma LH concentration causes enhanced androgen secretion by stromal and thecal cells of the ovary.

ATTENUATED FORMS OF ADRENAL HYPERPLASIA The adrenal can also be the source of excess androgen in the absence of tumor. Heritable defects in adrenal steroidogenesis (congenital adrenal hyperplasia) such as 21-hydroxylase deficiency, 11β-hydroxylase deficiency, and 3β-hydroxysteroid dehydrogenase deficiency can produce virilization, and each of these enzyme deficiencies can occur in a "late-onset" form in which hirsutism or virilization and menstrual irregularities appear at the time of expected puberty or in adulthood (see Chap. 324). The clinical presentation in these cases is usually indistinguishable from polycystic ovarian disease. Late-onset 21-hydroxylase deficiency is the most common of these attenuation forms of congenital adrenal hyperplasia and has been most extensively studied; its incidence in the general population of hirsute, oligomenorrheic women is probably on the order of a few percent. The presence of elevated plasma levels of adrenal androgens (such as dehydroepiandrosterone sulfate) or of dexamethasone-suppressible hyperandrogenism does not necessarily imply that the overandrogenization is due to a specific adrenal steroidogenic defect, but these findings may be useful as a guide to therapy.

IDIOPATHIC HIRSUTISM In many women with hirsutism a specific diagnosis cannot be made. The term *idiopathic hirsutism* applies to those women with evidence of androgen excess but with normal menses, normal-sized ovaries, no evidence of tumors of the adrenal or ovary, and normal adrenal function. Slight elevations of plasma androstenedione and testosterone are commonly present in such women, and testosterone production rates are increased above normal, although to a lesser degree than in patients with polycystic ovarian disease.

Experience outside the United States with the antiandrogen cyproterone acetate indicates that this form of hirsutism is androgen-mediated, since therapy results in improvement. Women with idiopathic hirsutism could constitute the extreme end of a normal continuum of androgen production or represent a true pathologic subset. Some women with the tentative diagnosis of idiopathic hirsutism actually have mild or early polycystic ovarian disease, but in most, hirsutism is not accompanied by or followed by signs of ovarian dysfunction. If such women are merely extremes of the normal range of androgen production, then their hirsutism is fundamentally a cosmetic defect.

DIAGNOSTIC EVALUATION The decision as to when to undertake a complex diagnostic evaluation depends on several factors. Such evaluation is appropriate in all women with hirsutism and virilization; whether it should be performed in women with isolated hirsutism depends upon the severity, distribution, and rate of hair growth. An approach to the diagnostic evaluation of hirsute patients is shown in Fig. 54-1. The clinical history is taken with particular attention to drug ingestion and to the details of pubertal development and menstrual history and their relation to the onset of excessive hair growth. The physical examination is directed to the assessment of sites of growth of androgen-dependent hair (pubic, axillary, facial, truncal, and extremity) and evaluation for signs of virilization, which correlate with higher levels of androgen overproduction and raise the concern of androgen-producing neoplasms. Such signs include laryngeal enlargement (deepening of the voice), temporal balding, clitoromegaly, and increased muscle mass in the limb girdles. Signs of cortisol excess (plethora, centripetal obesity, striae, and dorsocervical and supraclavicular fat pads) should also be sought. Pelvic examination should include a search for palpable ovarian masses. Appropriate laboratory tests include measurement of serum androgens and, when appropriate, radiologic imaging of ovaries and adrenal glands. Basal measurements of dehydroepiandrosterone sulfate greater than 22 nmol/L (8000 ng/mL) or of serum testosterone over 7 nmol/L (2ng/mL) suggest neoplastic sources of androgen excess; plasma testosterone levels in the normal range are more difficult to interpret because total levels in women do not necessarily reflect the free or unbound levels of hormone under conditions when testosterone-binding globulin levels are either increased or decreased. Suspected Cushing's syndrome should be evaluated with standard dexamethasone suppression testing if a screening test (such as urinary free cortisol excretion or overnight dexamethasone suppression test) is abnormal. The diagnosis of polycystic ovarian disease is made from the history and clinical features in a woman with chronic anovulation. Women with severe hirsutism associated with cystic acne may be screened for delayed-onset adrenal hyperplasia by the short cosyntropin stimulation test and measurement of plasma 17-hydroxyprogesterone (see Chap. 317).

MANAGEMENT In the case of drug-induced hirsutism and neoplastic disease of the ovary or adrenals treatment is straightforward; administration of the drugs should be stopped, or the tumor should be removed. Adrenal steroidogenic defects are treated with glucocorticoids to suppress excess ACTH and hence inhibit adrenal androgen secretion. In most instances (polycystic ovarian disease as well as idiopathic hirsutism) both cosmetic treatment and suppression of androgen production or antagonism of its action at the receptor level need to be employed.

Cosmetic therapy is directed at the concealment or removal of hair from exposed skin areas. Small amounts of hair can be bleached with hydrogen peroxide. Methods for removal of hair are classified as depilatory (removal of hair from the surface of the skin) or epilatory (removal of the intact hair with the root). Depilatory techniques include shaving and chemical methods. Shaving does not have an adverse effect on hair growth rate or coarseness (although the blunt ends may feel coarse), but shaving of areas other than axillae or legs is unacceptable to most women. Chemical depilatories are effective for limited areas of hair removal and are generally safe if used properly. Most available depilatories are substituted mercaptans, such as thioglycollic acid, which reduce the disulfide bonds in the peptide chains of keratin. The hair fiber swells and softens to a consistency that can be washed from the skin. Care must be taken to avoid skin irritation because of the alkalinity of these preparations. Temporary epilation can be achieved by plucking (useful only for isolated hairs) or wax treatment. The waxes are melted and applied to the skin. When the wax cools and sets, it is stripped off, removing hair with it. The procedure is uncomfortable, and best results can be obtained by salon treatments. Permanent epilation can be achieved only by electrolysis. The treatments are expensive and time-consuming, and success depends on the skill of the electrologist.

While cosmetic treatment is undertaken, attempts to suppress androgen overproduction may also be appropriate. Treatment with combination oral contraceptives suppresses ovarian androgen secretion when restoration of fertility is not an objective. To minimize side effects the lowest effective dosage of estrogen should be used. Women over 35 years of age, smokers, and those with hypertension, a history

FIGURE 54-1 Diagnostic approach to the hirsute patient. T = testosterone; DHEA-S = dehydroepiandrosterone sulfate.

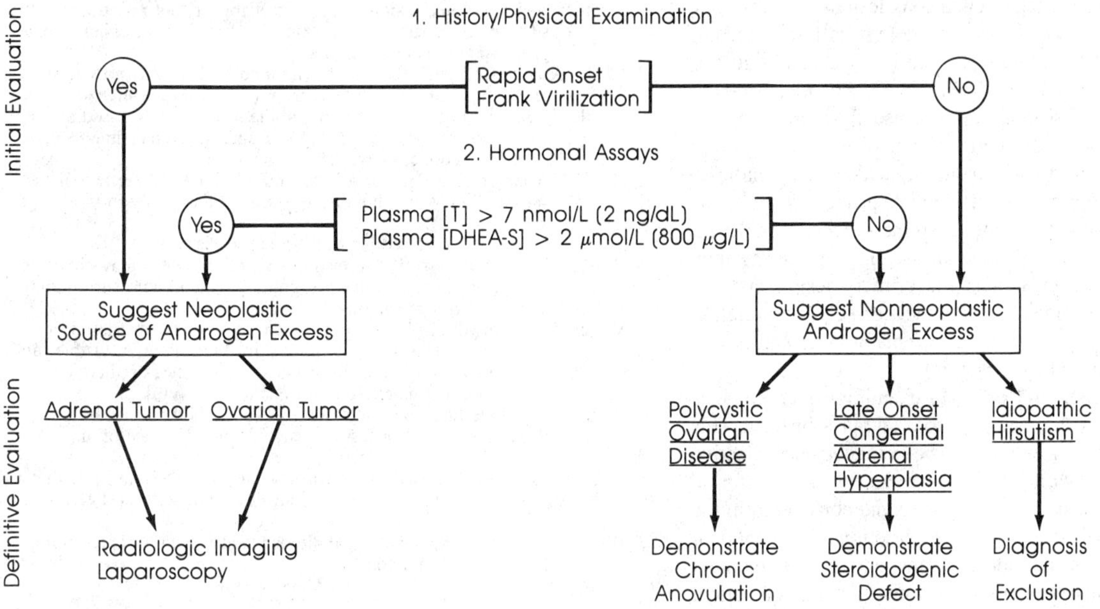

of thromboembolic disease, impaired liver function, or suspected estrogen-dependent neoplasm should not be treated with oral contraceptives. Suppression of adrenal androgen overproduction can be achieved with small doses of dexamethasone and is useful in the treatment of women with late-onset 21-hydroxylase deficiency.

Antagonism of the effects of androgens at the hair follicle is the basis for the other main treatment modality, the antiandrogens. Cyproterone acetate has been used with success but is unavailable in the United States. Spironolactone has a dual action of blocking the androgen receptor and of inhibiting androgen production and is a useful alternative therapy. Cimetidine also binds to the androgen receptor and acts as an androgen antagonist, but it is not of general benefit in the treatment of hirsutism.

If pharmacologic therapy is undertaken, the patient should be prepared to make a commitment of 6 months for an adequate trial of efficacy. Even when treatment is long-term, dramatic reversal of established hair growth is unlikely to be achieved by interference with androgen synthesis or action. Such hormonal manipulations can arrest or slow the rate of hair growth, but established hair must be dealt with by use of cosmetic treatment.

REFERENCES

Brodie BL, Wentz AC: Late onset congenital adrenal hyperplasia—a gynecologist's perspective. Fertil Steril 48:175, 1987

Leshin M: Hirsutism. Am J Med Sci 294:369, 1987

Lucky AW et al: Plasma androgens in women with acne vulgaris. J Invest Dermatol 81:70, 1983

Raj SG et al: Normalization of testosterone levels using a low-estrogen-containing oral contraceptive in women with polycystic ovary syndrome. Obstet Gynecol 60:15, 1982

Richards RN et al: Electroepilation (electrolysis) in hirsutism: 35,000 hours experience on the face and neck. J Am Acad Dermatol 15:693, 1986

Rittmaster RS, Loriaux DL: Hirsutism. Ann Intern Med 106:95, 1987

Rubens R: Androgen levels during cyproterone acetate and ethinyl estradiol treatment of hirsutism. Clin Endocrinol 20:313, 1984

Tremblay RR: Treatment of hirsutism with spironoclactone. Clin Endocrinol Metab 15:363, 1986

section 8 Alterations in the skin

55 EXAMINATION OF THE SKIN

THOMAS J. LAWLEY / KIM B. YANCEY

The challenge of examining the skin lies in distinguishing normal from abnormal and significant findings from trivial ones and in integrating pertinent signs and symptoms into an appropriate differential diagnosis. The fact that the largest organ in the body is visible is both an advantage and a disadvantage to those who examine it. It is advantageous because no special instrumentation, other than a magnifying glass, is necessary and because the skin can be biopsied with little morbidity. However, the casual observer can be overwhelmed by a variety of stimuli and overlook important, subtle signs of skin or systemic disease. For instance, the sometimes minor differences in color and shape that distinguish a malignant melanoma from a benign pigmented nevus can be difficult to recognize. To aid in the interpretation of skin lesions, a variety of descriptive terms have been developed to characterize cutaneous lesions (Tables 55-1 and 55-2; Fig. 55-1). Mastery of this terminology is important not only for categorizing the skin lesions of a particular case but also in formulating a differential diagnosis (Table 55-3). For instance, the finding of large numbers of scaling papules, usually indicative of a primary skin disease, places the patient in a different diagnostic category than would hemorrhagic papules, which may indicate vasculitis or sepsis. It is important to differentiate primary skin lesions from secondary skin changes. If the examiner focuses on linear erosions overlying an area of erythema and scaling, he or she may incorrectly assume that the erosion is the primary lesion and the redness and scale are secondary, while the correct interpretation would be that the patient has a pruritic eczematous dermatitis and the erosions have been caused by scratching.

AN APPROACH TO THE PATIENT In examining the skin it is usually advisable to assess the patient before taking a history. This way, the entire cutaneous surface is sure to be evaluated and objective findings can be integrated with relevant historical data. Four basic features of any cutaneous lesion must be noted and considered in the examination of skin: the distribution of the eruption, the type(s) of primary lesion, the shape of individual lesions, and the arrangement of the lesions. In the initial examination it is important that the patient be disrobed as completely as possible. This will minimize chances of missing important individual skin lesions and make it possible to assess accurately the distribution of the eruption. The patient should first be viewed from a distance of about 1.5 to 2 m (4 to 6 ft), so that the general character of the skin and the distribution of lesions can be evaluated. Indeed, distribution of lesions often correlates highly with diagnosis (Fig. 55-2). For example, a hospitalized patient with a generalized erythematous exanthem is more likely to have a drug eruption than is a patient with a similar rash limited to the sun-exposed portions of the face. The presence or absence of lesions on mucosal surfaces should also be determined. Once the distribution of the lesions has been established, the nature of the primary lesion must be determined. Thus, when lesions are distributed on elbows, knees, and scalp, the most likely possibilities based solely on distribution are psoriasis or dermatitis herpetiformis. The primary

TABLE 55-1 Descriptions of primary skin lesions

1 Macule:	A flat, colored lesion, <2 cm in diameter, not raised above the surface of the surrounding skin. A "freckle," or ephelid, is a prototype pigmented macule.
2 Patch:	A large (>2 cm), flat lesion with a color different from the surrounding skin. This differs from a macule only in size.
3 Papule:	A small, solid lesion, <1 cm in diameter, that is raised above the surface of the surrounding skin and hence palpable (e.g., a closed comedone, or whitehead, in acne).
4 Nodule:	A larger (1–5 cm), firm lesion raised above the surface of the surrounding skin. This differs from a papule only in size (e.g., dermal nevus).
5 Tumor:	A firm, solid, raised growth >5 cm in diameter.
6 Plaque:	A large (>1 cm) flat-topped raised lesion; edges may either be distinct (e.g., in psoriasis) or gradually blend with surrounding skin (e.g., in eczematous dermatitis).
7 Vesicle:	A small, fluid-filled lesion <1 cm in diameter that is raised above the plane of surrounding skin. Fluid is often visible, and the lesions are often translucent [e.g., vesicles in allergic contact dermatitis caused by *Rhus* (poison ivy)].
8 Pustule:	A vesicle filled with leukocytes. Note: The presence of pustules does not necessarily signify the existence of an infection.
9 Bulla:	A fluid-filled, raised, often translucent lesion >1 cm in diameter.
10 Cyst:	A soft, raised, encapsulated lesion filled with semisolid or liquid contents.
11 Wheal:	A raised, erythematous papule or plaque, usually representing short-lived dermal edema.
12 Telangiectasia:	Dilated, superficial blood vessels.

TABLE 55-2 Common dermatologic terms

1 Lichenification: A distinctive thickening of the skin that is characterized by accentuated skin-fold markings and that feels thick and firm on palpation.
2 Crust: Dried exudate of body fluids that may be either yellow (serous exudate) or red (hemorrhagic exudate).
3 Milia: Small, firm, white papules that are filled with keratin (and may in part resemble pustules).
4 Erosion: Epithelial deficit resulting in a superficial disruption of skin integrity.
5 Ulcer: Epithelial deficit resulting in a deep surface disruption.
6 Excoriations: Linear, angular erosions that may be covered by crust and are caused by scratching.
7 Atrophy: An acquired loss of substance. In the skin, this may appear as a depression with intact epidermis (i.e., loss of dermal or subcutaneous tissue) or as sites of shiny, delicate, wrinkled lesions (i.e., epidermal atrophy).
8 Scar: A change in the skin secondary to trauma or inflammation. Sites may be erythematous, hypopigmented, or hypertrophic, depending on their age or character. Sites on hair-bearing areas may be characterized by destruction of hair follicles.

lesion in psoriasis is a scaly papule that soon forms erythematous plaques covered with a white scale, while that of dermatitis herpetiformis is an urticarial papule that quickly becomes a small vesicle. In this manner, identification of the primary lesion directs the examiner toward the proper diagnosis. Secondary changes in skin can also be

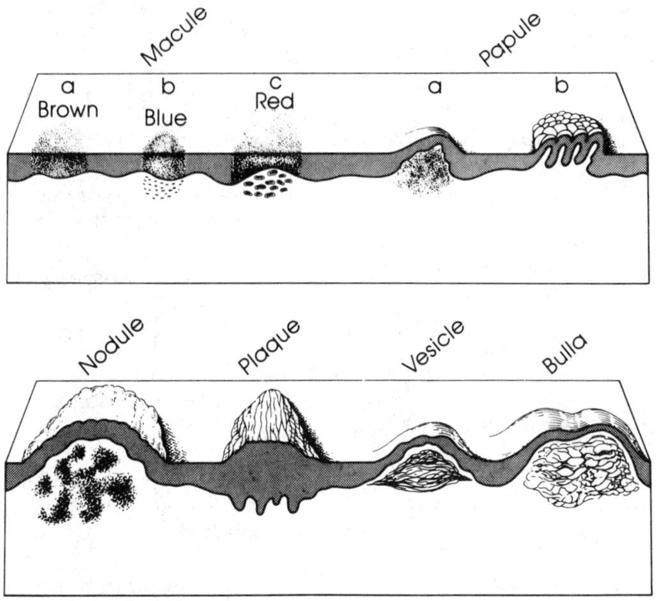

FIGURE 55-1 A schematic representation of several common primary skin lesions (see Table 55-1).

TABLE 55-3 Selected common dermatologic conditions

Diagnosis	Common distribution	Usual morphology
Acne vulgaris	Face, upper back	Open and closed comedones, erythematous papules, pustules, cysts
Rosacea	Blush area of cheeks, nose, forehead, chin	Erythema, telangiectasias, papules, pustules
Seborrheic dermatitis	Scalp, eyebrows, perinasal	Erythema with greasy yellow-brown scale
Atopic dermatitis	Antecubital and popliteal fossae; may be widespread	Patches and plaques of erythema, scaling, and lichenification
Stasis dermatitis	Ankles, lower legs	Patches of erythema and scaling on background of hyperpigmentation associated with signs of venous insufficiency
Dyshidrotic eczema	Palms, soles, sides of fingers and toes	Deep vesicles
Plant dermatitis (poison ivy)	Anywhere	Linear patches of erythema and vesicles
Allergic contact dermatitis	Anywhere	Localized erythema, vesicles, and scale, e.g., fingers, earlobes—nickel; dorsal aspect of foot—shoe dermatitis, etc.
Psoriasis	Elbows, knees, scalp, lower back, fingernails (may be generalized)	Papules and plaques covered with silvery scale; nails have pits
Lichen planus	Wrists, ankles, mouth (may be widespread)	Violaceous flat-topped papules and plaques
Keratosis pilaris	Extensor surfaces of arms and thighs, buttocks	Keratotic follicular papules with surrounding erythema
Melasma	Forehead, cheeks, temples, upper lip	Tan to brown patches
Vitiligo	Periorificial, trunk, extensor surfaces of extremities, flexor wrists, axillae	Chalk-white macules
Actinic keratosis	Sun-exposed areas	Skin-colored or red-brown macule or papule with dry adherent scale
Basal cell carcinoma	Face	Papule with pearly border on sun-damaged skin
Seborrheic keratosis	Trunk, face	Brown plaques with adherent greasy scale; ''stuck on'' appearance
Folliculitis	Any hair-bearing area	Perifollicular pustules
Impetigo	Anywhere	Papules, vesicles, pustules often with honey-colored crusts
Herpes simplex	Lips, genitalia	Grouped vesicles progressing to crusted erosions
Herpes zoster	Dermatomal, usually trunk but may be anywhere	Vesicles limited to a dermatome (often painful)
Varicella	Face, trunk, relative sparing of extremities	Lesions arise in crops and quickly progress from erythematous macules to papules to vesicles to pustules to crusts
Pityriasis rosea	Trunk (Christmas tree pattern) herald patch followed by multiple smaller lesions	Symmetric erythematous patches with a collarette of trailing scale
Tinea versicolor	Chest, back, abdomen, proximal extremities	Scaly hyper- or hypopigmented macules
Candidiasis	Groin, beneath breasts, vagina, oral cavity	Erythematous macerated areas with satellite pustules; white, friable patches on mucous membranes
Dermatophytosis	Feet, groin, beard, or scalp	Varies with site, e.g., tinea corporis—scaly annular patch
Scabies	Groin, axillae, between fingers and toes, beneath breasts	Excoriated papules, burrows
Insect bites	Anywhere	Erythematous papules with central puncta
Cherry angioma	Trunk	Red, blood-filled papules
Keloid	Anywhere (site of previous injury)	Firm tumor; pink, purple, or brown
Dermatofibroma	Anywhere	Firm red to brown nodule that shows dimpling of overlying skin with lateral compression
Acrochordons (skin tags)	Groin, axilla, neck	Fleshy papules
Urticaria	Anywhere	Wheals, sometimes with surrounding flare
Transient acantholytic dermatosis	Trunk, especially anterior chest	Erythematous papules
Xerosis	Extensor extremities, especially legs	Dry, erythematous, scaling patches

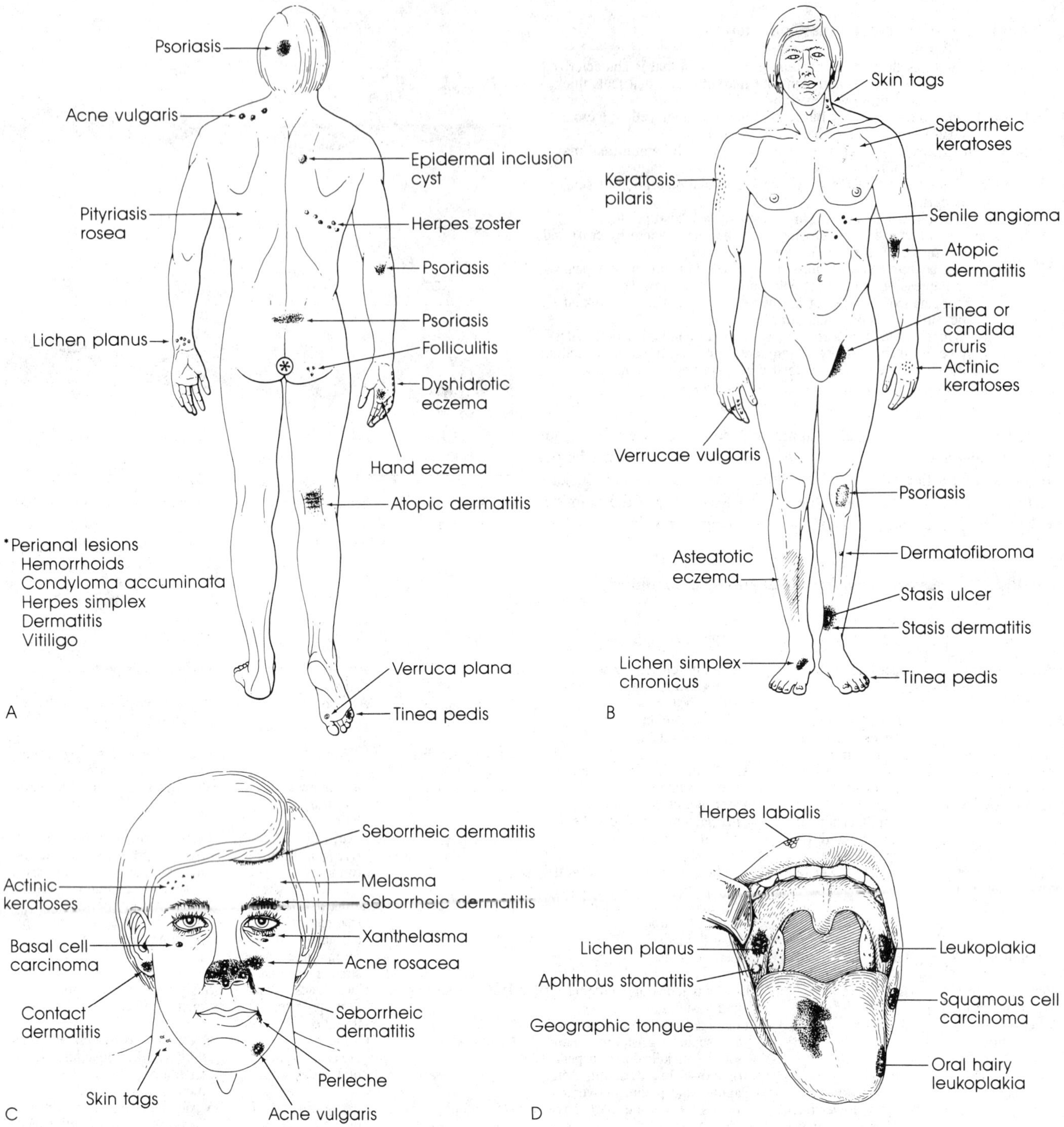

FIGURE 55-2*A–D*. The distribution of some common dermatologic diseases and lesions.

quite helpful. For example, scale represents excessive epidermis, while crust is the result of an inadequate or inconsistent epithelial cell layer. Palpation of skin lesions can also yield insight into the character of an eruption. Thus, red papules on the lower extremities that blanch with pressure can be a manifestation of many different diseases, but red papules that do not blanch with pressure indicate palpable purpura characteristic of necrotizing vasculitis.

The shape of lesions is also an important feature. Flat, round, erythematous macules are common in many cutaneous diseases. However, target-shaped lesions that consist in part of erythematous macules are specific for erythema multiforme. In the same way, the arrangement of individual lesions is important. Erythematous papules and vesicles can occur in many conditions, but their arrangement in a specific linear array suggests an external etiology such as allergic contact or primary irritant dermatitis. In contrast, lesions with an annular or arciform arrangement are common and suggest a systemic etiology.

As in other branches of medicine, a complete history should be obtained to emphasize the following features:

1 Evolution of lesions
   a Site of onset
   b Manner in which eruption progressed or spread
   c Duration
   d Periods of resolution or improvement in chronic eruptions
2 Symptoms associated with eruption
   a Itching, burning, pain, numbness
   b What, if anything, has relieved symptoms
   c Time of day when symptoms are most severe
3 Current or recent medications (prescribed, as well as over-the-counter)

4 Associated systemic symptoms (e.g., malaise, fever, arthralgias)
5 Ongoing or previous illnesses
6 History of allergies
7 Presence of photosensitivity
8 Review of systems

DIAGNOSTIC TECHNIQUES Many skin diseases can be diagnosed on gross clinical appearance, but sometimes relatively simple diagnostic procedures can yield valuable information. In most instances, they can be performed at the bedside with a minimum of equipment.

Skin biopsy A skin biopsy is a straightforward minor surgical procedure; however, it is important to biopsy the anatomic site most likely to yield diagnostic findings. This decision may require expertise in skin diseases and knowledge of superficial anatomic structures in selected areas of the body. In this procedure a small area of skin is anesthetized with 1% xylocaine with or without epinephrine. The skin lesion in question can be excised with a scalpel or removed by punch biopsy. In the latter technique, a punch is pressed against the surface of the skin and rotated with downward pressure until it penetrates to the subcutaneous tissue. The circular biopsy is then lifted with forceps, and the bottom is cut with iris scissors. Biopsy sites may or may not need suture closure, depending on size and location.

KOH preparation A potassium hydroxide (KOH) preparation is performed on scaling skin lesions when a fungal etiology is suspected. The edge of such a lesion is scraped gently with a scalpel blade, and the removed scale is collected on a glass microscope slide and treated with 1 to 2 drops of a solution of 10 to 20% KOH. KOH dissolves keratin and allows easier visualization of fungal elements. Brief heating of the slide accelerates dissolution of keratin. When the preparation is viewed under the microscope, the refractile hyphae will be seen more easily when the light intensity is reduced. This technique can be utilized to identify hyphae in dermatophyte infections, pseudohyphae and budding yeast in *Candida* infections, and fragmented hyphae and spores in tinea versicolor. The same sampling technique can be used to obtain scale for culture of selected pathogenic organisms.

Tzanck smear A Tzanck smear, named after Arnault Tzanck, is a cytologic technique most often used in the diagnosis of herpesvirus infections (simplex or varicella-zoster). An early vesicle, not a pustule or crusted lesion, is unroofed, and the base of the lesion is scraped gently with a scalpel blade. The material is then placed on a glass slide, air-dried, and stained with Giemsa or Wright's stain. Multinucleated giant cells suggest the presence of herpes, but culture must be performed to identify the specific virus.

Diascopy Diascopy is designed to assess whether a skin lesion will blanch with pressure as, for example, in determining whether a red lesion is hemorrhagic or simply blood-filled. For instance, a hemangioma will blanch with pressure, while a purpuric lesion caused by necrotizing vasculitis will not. Diascopy is performed by pressing a microscope slide or magnifying lens against a specified lesion and noting the amount of blanching which occurs. Granulomas often have an ''apple jelly'' appearance on diascopy.

Wood's light A Wood's lamp generates 360 nm ultraviolet (or ''black'') light and causes erythrasma to show a characteristic coral-red color and *Pseudomonas,* a pale blue. Tinea capitis caused by certain dermatophytes such as *Microsporum canis* or *M. audouini* exhibits a yellow fluorescence. Pigmented lesions of the epidermis such as freckles are accentuated, while dermal pigment such as postinflammatory hyperpigmentation fades under a Wood's light. Vitiligo appears totally white under a Wood's lamp, and previously unsuspected areas of involvement often become apparent. A Wood's lamp may also aid in the demonstration of tinea versicolor and in recognition of ash leaf spots in patients with tuberous sclerosis.

Patch tests Patch testing is designed to document sensitivity to a specific antigen. In this procedure a battery of suspected allergens is applied to the patient's back under occlusive dressings and allowed to remain in contact with the skin for 48 h. The dressings are then removed, and the area is examined for evidence of delayed hypersensitivity reactions. This test is best performed by physicians with special expertise in patch testing and is often helpful in the evaluation of patients with chronic dermatitis.

REFERENCES

Fitzpatrick TB et al (eds): *Dermatology in General Medicine,* 3d ed. New York, McGraw-Hill, 1987

Lookingbill DP, Marks JG: *Principles of Dermatology.* Philadelphia, Saunders, 1986

Rook A et al (eds): *Textbook of Dermatology,* 4th ed. Oxford, Blackwell Scientific, 1986

56 ECZEMA, PSORIASIS, CUTANEOUS INFECTIONS, ACNE, AND OTHER COMMON SKIN DISORDERS

THOMAS J. LAWLEY / ROBERT A. SWERLICK

COMMON SKIN DISORDERS

ECZEMA Eczema, or dermatitis, is a reaction pattern manifested by variable clinical and histologic findings. Eczema is the final common expression for atopic dermatitis, allergic contact and irritant contact dermatitis, dyshidrotic eczema, nummular eczema, lichen simplex chronicus, asteatotic eczema, and seborrheic dermatitis. Primary lesions may include papules, erythematous macules, and vesicles, which can coalesce to form patches and plaques. In severe eczema, secondary lesions such as weeping and crusting may predominate. Long-standing dermatitis is often dry and is characterized by thickened, scaling skin (lichenification). The histologic changes correlate with the clinical findings. The histologic features of dermatitis have been divided into three patterns: acute, subacute, and chronic. Acute dermatitis shows a mixture of epidermal and dermal edema, epidermal vesiculation, and a mononuclear cell infiltrate. Chronic dermatitis demonstrates epidermal acanthosis, hyperkeratosis, upper dermal fibrosis, and a predominantly perivascular mononuclear cell infiltrate. Mixtures of these two histologic reaction patterns occur in subacute dermatitis. Any of these patterns may be associated with the various clinical forms of dermatitis, and the histopathologic findings are rarely diagnostic.

ATOPIC DERMATITIS Atopic dermatitis is the cutaneous expression of the atopic state, and up to 70 percent of patients have a family history of asthma, hay fever, or dermatitis. Atopic individuals often have dry, itchy skin, abnormal cutaneous vascular responses, and, in some instances, elevations in serum IgE. The clinical presentation falls into three patterns related to age: the infantile form (ages 2 months to 2 years), the childhood form (ages 4 to 10 years), and the adolescent and adult form. In severe cases, the infantile or childhood forms of the disease may persist into adult life.

The infantile form is characterized by inflammatory patches and weeping, crusted plaques on the face, neck, extensor surfaces, and groin. Pruritus is prominent, and many of the cutaneous findings are secondary to rubbing and scratching. Dermatitis of flexural areas is characteristic of the childhood form, particularly in the antecubital and popliteal fossae. Lesions on the wrists, neck, and face are common. Other cutaneous stigmata that may become apparent at this stage are perioral pallor, an extra fold of skin beneath the lower eyelid (Dennie's line), and increased palmar markings. Cutaneous infections, particularly with *Staphylococcus aureus,* occur frequently.

The adult form is usually more localized than the infantile or childhood forms of the disease. Atopic dermatitis often resolves spontaneously as children enter adulthood, but the persistent variant tends to localize to the hands (see ''Hand Dermatitis''), neck, face, genitalia, or legs and may resemble nummular eczema or lichen simplex chronicus (see below).

Diagnosis is based upon a family history of atopy, presence of other forms of allergy (asthma or allergic rhinitis), history of infantile or childhood eczema, and the pattern of eruption. In severe disease, serum IgE should be measured to rule out the possibility of hyper-IgE syndrome (see Chap. 81). Patients who do not respond to conventional therapies should be considered for patch testing to exclude allergic contact dermatitis.

Therapy of atopic dermatitis should be based upon avoidance of cutaneous irritants, adequate cutaneous hydration, judicious use of low- or midpotency topical glucocorticoids (Table 56-1), and treatment of infected skin lesions. The most common irritants are soaps and hot water. Patients should bathe using warm, but not hot, water and should limit their use of soap, particularly on extremities. Immediately after bathing, the skin should be lubricated with a low- or midpotency topical glucocorticoid in a cream or ointment base. Crusted and weeping lesions should be treated with systemic antibiotics with activity against *S. aureus* and *Streptococcus pyogenes*, since secondary infection often exacerbates eczema. Antihistamines are useful to control the pruritus that accompanies eczema, but sedation may limit their usefulness.

The role of dietary allergens in atopic dermatitis is controversial, but there is little evidence that it plays any role except in infancy. A significant number of children under age 3 who do not respond to conventional therapy have food sensitivities. Unfortunately, parental histories of food intake do not correlate with actual food allergens, and identification of the offending agents is best done with double-blind food challenges.

Treatment with systemic glucocorticoids should be limited to severe exacerbations unresponsive to topical therapy. In the patient with chronic atopic eczema, therapy with systemic glucocorticoids will generally clear the skin only briefly, but cessation of the systemic therapy will invariably be accompanied by return, if not worsening, of the dermatitis. The side effects of daily doses of systemic glucocorticoids preclude chronic use in virtually all patients with atopic dermatitis, and the efficacy of alternate-day regimens in this disease is limited.

ALLERGIC CONTACT DERMATITIS The most commonly recognized form of allergic contact dermatitis (ACD) is phytodermatitis or plant dermatitis. Members of the *Rhus* family, including poison ivy, poison oak, and poison sumac, cause an allergic reaction marked by erythema, vesiculation, and severe pruritus. The eruption is often linear, corresponding to areas where plants have touched the skin. Other allergens are much more difficult to identify, especially if the exposure is chronic and the skin becomes thickened and scaly.

If ACD is suspected and an offending agent is identified and removed, the eruption resolves. Usually, treatment with high-potency fluorinated topical glucocorticoids is enough to relieve symptoms while the ACD runs its course. Patients with particularly widespread disease, or disease involving the face or genitalia, may require treatment with oral glucocorticoids. Since the natural course of ACD is 2 to 3 weeks, therapy should be continued for that length of time. Treatment of ACD with short, rapidly tapered courses of oral glucocorticoids is usually followed by recurrence of skin lesions.

Identification of a contact allergen can be a difficult and time-consuming task. Patients with a dermatitis unresponsive to conventional therapy or with an unusual and patterned distribution should be suspected of having ACD. They should be questioned carefully regarding occupational exposures, topical medications, and oral medications. Common sensitizers include preservatives in topical preparations, nickel sulfate, potassium dichromate, neomycin sulfate, fragrances, formaldehyde, and rubber curing agents. Standard patch test trays are helpful in identifying these agents, but should not be used in patients with widespread active dermatitis or in those on systemic glucocorticoids.

HAND ECZEMA Hand eczema, a common chronic skin disorder, may be associated with other cutaneous disorders such as atopic dermatitis or psoriasis or may occur by itself. Like other forms of dermatitis, both exogenous and endogenous factors play important roles in the expression of hand dermatitis. Chronic, excessive exposure to water and detergents may initiate or aggravate this disorder. It may present with dryness and cracking of the skin of the hands, as well as with variable amounts of erythema and edema. Often, the dermatitis begins under rings, where water and irritants are trapped. A variant of hand dermatitis, dyshidrotic eczema, presents with multiple, intensely pruritic, small papules and vesicles on the thenar and hypothenar eminences and the sides of the fingers. Lesions tend to occur in crops, slowly crust over, and are followed by another outbreak.

Therapy of hand dermatitis is directed toward avoidance of irritants, identification of possible contact allergens, treatment of coexistent infection, and application of topical glucocorticoids. The most common hand irritants are soap and water. Health care professionals, housewives, and food handlers are prone to hand eczema. Use of mild soap, avoidance of hot water, and compulsive use of emollients can alleviate some symptoms. Whenever possible, the hands should be protected by gloves, preferably vinyl gloves, since many patients with hand eczema may become sensitive to curing agents in rubber gloves. Predominant involvement of the dorsal surface of the hands with sparing of the palmar surface should suggest a possible contact dermatitis. Most patients can be treated by application of cool, moist compresses (dressings) to dry and debride acute inflammatory lesions and to decrease swelling, followed by a midpotency topical glucocorticoid in a cream or ointment base. If allergic contact dermatitis is suspected, ointments are preferable. Chronic use of very high potency topical glucocorticoids can lead to cutaneous atrophy and is often accompanied by loss of effectiveness. As with atopic dermatitis, treatment of secondary infection with *Staphylococcus* or *Streptococcus* is essential. All patients with hand dermatitis should be examined for dermatophyte infection by KOH preparation and culture (see "Dermatophyte Infections").

NUMMULAR ECZEMA Nummular eczema is characterized by circular or oval "coinlike" lesions. Initially, this eruption consists of small edematous papules that become crusted and scaly. The most common locations are on the trunk or the extensor surfaces of the extremities, particularly on the pretibial areas or dorsum of the hands. It occurs most frequently in middle-aged men. The etiology is unknown but appears to be related to dryness of the skin and exogenous irritants. Unlike other forms of dermatitis, nummular eczema does not respond well to hydration, topical glucocorticoids,

TABLE 56-1 Selected topical glucocorticoid preparations*

Group†	Generic name	Brand name
1	Clobetasol propionate	Temovate cream 0.05%
	Clobetasol propionate	Temovate ointment 0.05%
	Betamethasone dipropionate	Diprolene cream 0.05%
	Betamethasone dipropionate	Diprolene ointment 0.05%
	Diflorasone diacetate	Psorcon ointment 0.05%
2	Flucinonide	Lidex cream 0.05%
	Flucinonide	Lidex ointment 0.05%
	Betamethasone dipropionate	Diprosone ointment 0.05%
	Halcinonide	Halog cream 0.1%
3	Betamethasone dipropionate	Diprosone cream 0.05%
	Betamethasone valerate	Valisone ointment 0.1%
	Diflorasone diacetate	Maxiflor cream 0.05%
4	Triamcinolone acetonide	Kenalog ointment 0.1%
	Triamcinolone acetonide	Aristocort ointment 0.1%
	Flurandrenolide	Cordran ointment 0.05%
5	Triamcinolone acetonide	Kenalog cream 0.1%
	Fluocinolone acetonide	Synalar cream 0.025%
	Hydrocortisone valerate	Westcort cream 0.2%
6	Desonide	Tridesilon cream 0.05%
	Desonide	DesOwen cream 0.05%
	Alclometasone dipropionate	Alcovate cream 0.05%
7	Hydrocortisone	Many

* List not meant to be comprehensive.
† Preparations grouped according to potency: group 1 is most potent; group 7 is least potent.

or antihistamines. Overt infection should be treated appropriately with antibiotics; however, even in instances where infection is not apparent, treatment with oral antibiotics, such as tetracycline or erythromycin, may be useful.

LICHEN SIMPLEX CHRONICUS Lichen simplex chronicus may represent the end stage of a variety of eczematous disorders. It consists of a well-circumscribed plaque or plaques with lichenified or thickened skin due to chronic scratching or rubbing. Common areas involved include the posterior nuchal region, dorsum of the feet, or ankles. Treatment of lichen simplex chronicus centers around breaking the cycle of chronic itching and scratching. High-potency topical glucocorticoids may be helpful in alleviating pruritus, but in recalcitrant cases application of topical glucocorticoids under occlusion or intralesional injection of glucocorticoids may be required.

ASTEATOTIC ECZEMA Asteatotic eczema, also known as xerotic eczema or "winter itch," is a mildly inflammatory variant of eczematous dermatitis that develops most commonly on the lower legs of elderly individuals during dry times of year. Fine cracks, with or without erythema, resembling cracks seen in china or porcelain characteristically develop on the anterior surface of the lower extremities. Pruritus is variable. Asteatotic eczema responds well to avoidance of excessive dryness, rehydration of the skin, and application of topical emollients, particularly those containing urea or α-hydroxy acids (lactic acid or glycolic acid).

STASIS DERMATITIS AND STASIS ULCERATION Stasis dermatitis develops on the lower extremities secondary to chronic edema and venous incompetence. The disorder usually begins as mild erythema and scaling associated with pruritus over the medial aspect of the ankle, often over a varicose vein. The dermatitis progresses to become pigmented as the result of extravasation of blood and hemosiderin deposition. Stasis dermatitis may become acutely inflamed, with crusting and exudation. Chronic stasis dermatitis is often associated with dermal fibrosis which results in brawny edema and may be complicated by the development of stasis ulcers.

Elevation of the legs, compression stockings, and topical emollients are the cornerstone of therapy. Patients should be instructed to elevate the affected extremity when sitting. Support stockings are a useful adjunct, particularly in individuals who stand for long periods of time. A graded compression stocking is more desirable than an antiembolism hose, which is designed for individuals confined to bed. The dermatitic component can be treated with cool dressings and the application of midpotency topical glucocorticoids. Glucocorticoids should not be applied to ulcerations, since they may retard healing. Secondarily infected lesions should be treated with appropriate oral antibiotics.

Stasis ulcerations are difficult to treat, and resolution of these lesions is slow even under the best of circumstances. The affected limb should be elevated as much as possible. External compression dressings such as an Unna boot are also helpful in aiding healing. The ulcer should be kept clear of necrotic material, and debridement may be facilitated by frequent soaks. The use of semipermeable and hydrocolloid dressings may be helpful. Some ulcerations may take months to heal and require skin grafting. Healed areas are prone to recurrent ulceration.

SEBORRHEIC DERMATITIS Seborrheic dermatitis is a common, chronic disorder usually affecting the central face and scalp, and on occasion the groin, axilla, submammary folds, and gluteal clefts. Rarely, it may cause a widespread generalized dermatitis. Patients commonly complain of itching or burning. It is characterized by greasy scales overlying erythematous patches or plaques. In the scalp it may be recognized as severe dandruff. On the face it affects the eyebrows, eyelids, glabella, nasolabial fold, or ears. Scaling within the external ear is often mistaken for a chronic fungal infection (otomycosis), and postauricular dermatitis often becomes macerated and tender.

Seborrheic dermatitis may be evident in infancy in the scalp ("cradle cap"), face, or groin. It is not seen in children beyond infancy but becomes evident again during adult life. Although it is frequently seen in patients with Parkinson's disease, in those who have had cerebrovascular accidents, and in those with human immunodeficiency virus (HIV-1) infection, the overwhelming majority of individuals with seborrheic dermatitis have no underlying disorder.

Treatment with low- to midpotency topical glucocorticoids in conjunction with shampoos containing coal tar and/or salicylic acid is generally sufficient to control activity of this disorder. Selenium sulfide shampoos may also be effective. Fluorinated topical glucocorticoids should not be used on the face.

PAPULOSQUAMOUS DISORDERS

PSORIASIS Psoriasis is one of the most common dermatologic diseases, affecting 1 to 2 percent of people. It is a chronic inflammatory skin disorder characterized by erythematous, sharply demarcated papules and rounded plaques, covered by silvery micaceous scale. The lesions are variably pruritic. The most common areas of involvement are the elbows, knees, gluteal cleft, and the scalp. Lesions tend to be symmetric. Traumatized areas are often involved (Koebner or isomorphic phenomenon). Most patients will have stable, slowly growing infiltrated plaques, which remain unchanged for long periods. Eruptive psoriasis in children and young adults is notable for the development of many small lesions after upper respiratory tract infection with beta-hemolytic streptococci.

About half of patients have fingernail involvement, appearing as a punctate pitting, nail thickening, or subungual hyperkeratosis. About 5 to 10 percent of psoriatics have joint complaints, often when there is fingernail involvement. Although some have typical rheumatoid arthritis (see Chap. 270), many have joint disease specifically associated with psoriasis: (1) disease limited to a single or a few small joints (70 percent of cases); (2) a seronegative rheumatoid arthritis–like disease; (3) involvement of the distal interphalangeal joints; (4) severe destructive arthritis with the development of "arthritis mutilans"; and (5) disease limited to the spine (see Chap. 283).

The histologic picture can be variable but is usually diagnostic in early lesions or at the advancing edge of a well-established plaque. The epidermis demonstrates elongation of the rete ridges, suprapapillary thinning, loss of the granular layer, parakeratotic keratin, and intraepidermal collections of neutrophils. Dilated capillaries and mononuclear cell infiltrates are common in the dermal papillae.

Treatment depends on the type, location, and extent of disease. All patients should be instructed to avoid excess drying or irritation of the skin and to maintain adequate cutaneous hydration. Most patients with localized plaque-type psoriasis can be managed with midpotency topical glucocorticoids, although their long-term use is often accompanied by loss of effectiveness. The effectiveness of topical glucocorticoids may be increased if used in conjunction with a keratolytic agent, such as salicylic acid, which removes surface scale and allows greater penetration. Crude coal tar (1 to 5% in an ointment base) is an old but useful method of treatment in conjunction with ultraviolet light therapy.

Ultraviolet light is useful for widespread psoriasis. The ultraviolet B (UV-B) spectrum is effective alone or may be combined with coal tar (Goeckerman regimen) or anthralin (Ingram regimen). Natural sunlight or an artificial light source can be used. The combination of the ultraviolet A (UV-A) spectrum and either oral or topical psoralens is also extremely effective for the treatment of psoriasis, but the photosensitizing potential of psoralens and unknown long-term toxicity may limit the use of this therapy.

Other agents can be used for widespread disease. Methotrexate is useful in patients with associated psoriatic arthritis. Long-term liver toxicity limits its use to patients with widespread disease not responsive to standard agents. The synthetic retinoid etretinate is effective in some patients with severe psoriasis, but it is a potent teratogen with an extremely long tissue half-life, thus precluding its use in women of childbearing age.

LICHEN PLANUS Lichen planus is a papulosquamous disorder in which the primary lesions are pruritic, polygonal, flat-topped, violaceous papules. Close examination of the surface of these papules will often reveal a network of grayish lines (Wickham's striae). The skin lesions have a predilection for the wrists, shins, lower back, and genitalia. Involvement of the scalp may lead to hair loss. Lichen planus commonly involves mucous membranes, particularly the buccal mucosa, where it can present as a netlike, whitish eruption. The etiology is unknown, but cutaneous eruptions clinically resembling lichen planus can occur after administration of numerous drugs, including thiazide diuretics, gold, antimalarials, and phenothiazines, and in patients with skin lesions of chronic graft-versus-host disease. Histologic examination of lesions of lichen planus will demonstrate hyperkeratosis, irregular acanthosis, a bandlike dermal infiltrate of lymphocytes adjacent to the epidermis, and damage to the epidermal basal cells. The course is variable, but most patients have spontaneous remissions 6 months to 2 years after the onset of disease. Topical glucocorticoids are the mainstay of therapy.

PITYRIASIS ROSEA Pityriasis rosea is a papulosquamous eruption of unknown etiology that occurs more commonly in the spring and fall. Its first manifestation is the development of a 2- to 6-cm annular lesion (the herald patch). This is followed in a few days to a few weeks by many smaller annular or papular lesions with a truncal predilection. The lesions are generally oval with their long axis parallel to the skin-fold lines. The individual lesions may be red to brown in color with an erythematous border and trailing scale. Many clinical features resemble the eruption of secondary syphilis, but palm and sole lesions are rare in pityriasis rosea. The eruption tends to be moderately pruritic and lasts 3 to 8 weeks. The histologic picture is often not diagnostic, because it can resemble an acute or subacute dermatitis. Treatment is generally directed at alleviating pruritus and consists of oral antihistamines, midpotency topical glucocorticoids, and, in some cases, the use of ultraviolet B phototherapy.

CUTANEOUS INFECTIONS

IMPETIGO AND ECTHYMA *Impetigo* is a common superficial bacterial infection caused by group A beta-hemolytic streptococci or *S. aureus*. The primary lesion is a superficial pustule that ruptures and forms a characteristic yellow-brown "honey-colored" crust. Lesions caused by *Staphylococcus* may be tense, clear bullae, and this form of the disease is called *bullous impetigo*. Lesions may occur on normal skin or in areas already affected by another skin disease. Ecthyma is a variant of impetigo on the lower extremities and causes punched-out ulcerative lesions. In addition to improving hygiene, treatment of both ecthyma and impetigo involves gentle debridement of adherent crusts, which is facilitated by the use of soaks and topical antibiotics in conjunction with appropriate oral antibiotics.

ERYSIPELAS AND CELLULITIS See Chap. 101.

DERMATOPHYTOSIS Fungi that infect skin, hair, and nails include members of the species *Trichophyton*, *Microsporum*, and *Epidermophyton*. Infection of the foot is most common and is referred to as *tinea pedis* (athlete's foot). Tinea pedis is often chronic and is characterized by variable erythema and edema, scaling, pruritus, and occasionally vesiculation. Involvement may be widespread or localized, but almost invariably the web space between the fourth and fifth toes is affected. Infection of the nails (tinea unguium) is characterized by opacified, thickened nails and subungual debris. The groin is the next most commonly involved area, with men affected predominantly. It presents as a scaling erythematous eruption, which spares the scrotum. Microscopic examination of scale after digestion with potassium hydroxide (KOH preparation) of either untreated tinea pedis or tinea cruris usually demonstrates hyphae. However, even short courses of topical antifungal agents may make demonstration of hyphae difficult.

Dermatophyte infection of the scalp (tinea capitis) is quite common, particularly in inner city clinics. The predominant organism, *Trichophyton tonsurans*, can produce a relatively noninflammatory infection that may present with either well-defined or irregular, diffuse areas of mild scaling and hair loss. Close examination of the scalp may reveal many broken off hairs appearing as small black dots. Unlike infections with *Microsporum* sp., which was previously the most common cause of tinea capitis, lesions caused by *Trichophyton tonsurans* are not fluorescent under a Wood's lamp. Tinea capitis caused by *Microsporum audouini* is characterized by a sharply delineated noninflammatory area in which hairs are broken off close to the surface. Hairs infected with *M. audouini* fluoresce bright bluish green when examined with a Wood's lamp. Tinea corporis, or widespread infection on non-hair-bearing skin, may have a variable appearance, depending on the extent of the associated inflammatory reaction. It may have the typical annular appearance of "ringworm" or appear as deep inflammatory nodules (on the scalp known as *kerions*) or granulomas. KOH examination of scale or hair from patients with tinea capitis or inflammatory tinea corporis often does not reveal hyphae, and diagnosis may require culture.

Both topical and systemic therapies may be used to treat dermatophyte infection. Topical imidazoles and triazoles, including miconazole, ketaconazole, and econazole, may be effective. Haloprogin, undecylic acid, ciclopirox olamine, and tolnaftate are also effective, but nystatin is not active against dermatophytes. Griseofulvin is the drug of choice for dermatophyte infections requiring systemic therapy. While older preparations of griseofulvin required the use of as much as 1 to 2 g of drug daily, newer microsized and ultramicrosized preparations are better absorbed and allow treatment with much lower doses of drug. Generally, a daily dose of 500 mg of microsized or 350 mg of ultramicrosized griseofulvin is adequate. Unresponsive infections may respond to doubling the dose. Griseofulvin is best absorbed if administered with a fatty meal. The most common side effects of griseofulvin are gastrointestinal distress and headache. It is also rarely associated with hematologic and liver function abnormalities, and patients on long-term therapy should be carefully monitored.

The choice of treatment depends on the site involved and the type of infection. For chronic noninflammatory tinea pedis, topical imidazoles or keratolytics are useful to limit pruritus and scaling but are rarely curative. Treatment with oral griseofulvin is effective but may require months of therapy for mycologic cure and, even then, is associated with a high relapse rate, particularly if the nails are involved. The therapy of tinea corporis depends on the extent of disease. Localized infection is best treated with topical imidazoles, but widespread disease, particularly in patients with decreased cellular immunity, requires systemic antifugal therapy.

Dermatophyte infection of hair-bearing areas (such as tinea capitis) requires systemic antifungal therapy, and treatment should be continued for 6 to 8 weeks. The adjunctive use of topical antifungals in addition to systemic therapy may be useful, but topical therapy alone is not adequate. Markedly inflammatory tinea capitis may result in scarring and hair loss, and systemic or topical glucocorticoids may prevent this sequela.

TINEA VERSICOLOR Tinea versicolor is caused by a nondermatophyte dimorphic fungus which is a normal inhabitant of the skin. As the yeast form (*Pityrosporum orbiculare*), it generally does not cause disease (except for folliculitis in certain individuals). However, in some individuals, it converts to the hyphal form and causes characteristic lesions. Infection is promoted by heat and humidity. The typical lesions consist of oval scaly macules, papules, and patches concentrated on the chest, shoulders, and back and rarely on the face or distal extremities. On dark skin they often appear as hypopigmented areas, while on light skin they are slightly hyperpigmented. In some darkly pigmented individuals, they may only appear as scaling patches. A KOH preparation from scaling lesions will demonstrate a confluence of short hyphae and round spores (so-called spaghetti and meatballs). There are many effective topical treatments for tinea versicolor. Solutions containing sulfur, salicylic acid, or selenium sulfide will clear the infection if used daily for a week and then intermittently thereafter. Topical imidazoles are also effective.

CANDIDIASIS Candidiasis is caused by a related group of yeasts, whose manifestations may be localized to the skin or may be systemic and life-threatening. The causative organism is usually *Candida albicans* but may also be *C. tropicalis, C. parapsilosis,* and *C. krusei*. These organisms are normal saprophytic inhabitants of the gastrointestinal tract but can overgrow (usually due to broad-spectrum antibiotic therapy) and cause disease at cutaneous sites. Other predisposing factors include diabetes mellitus, chronic intertrigo, and cellular immune deficiency. The oral cavity is commonly involved. Lesions may occur on the tongue or buccal mucosa (thrush) and appear as white plaques. Microscopic examination of scrapings demonstrates both pseudohyphae and yeast forms. Fissured, macerated lesions at the corners of the mouth (perleche) are often seen in individuals with poorly fitting dentures and may also be associated with candidal infection. Additionally, candidal infections have an affinity for sites that are chronically wet and macerated and may occur around nails (onycholysis and paronychia) and in intertriginous areas. Intertriginous lesions are characteristically edematous, erythematous, and scaly, with scattered "satellite pustules." In men there is often involvement of the penis and scrotum as well as the inner aspect of the thighs, and in women the introitus and vagina may be infected. Diagnosis is based upon the clinical pattern and demonstration of yeast on KOH preparation or on culture. Treatment involves removing any predisposing factors such as antibiotic therapy or chronic wetness, the careful control of diabetes mellitus if present, and the use of appropriate topical or systemic antifungal agents.

WARTS Warts are cutaneous neoplasms caused by papillomaviruses. Over 50 different human papillomaviruses (HPV) have been described. Types 1, 2, 4, and 7 cause typical verrucae vulgaris. These lesions are sessile, dome-shaped, usually about a centimeter in diameter, and have a surface made up of many small filamentous projections. These papillomaviruses also cause typical plantar warts and filiform warts in intertriginous areas. Plantar warts are endophytic and are covered by thick keratin. Paring of the wart will generally demonstrate a central core of keratinized debris and punctuate bleeding points. Filiform warts are most common on the face, neck, and skin folds and present as papillomatous lesions on a narrow base. HPV types 3 and 10 are associated with flat warts or verrucae plana. These lesions are only slightly elevated and have a velvety, nonverrucous surface. They have a propensity for the face, arms, and legs and often are spread by shaving.

HPV types 6, 11, 16, 18, 31–35, 39, 48, and 51–54 cause genital tract lesions. Types 6 and 11 are associated with typical lesions of condyloma acuminata, which generally begin as small papillomas and may grow to form large fungating lesions. In women, they may involve either the labia, perineum, or perianal skin. Additionally, the mucosa of the vagina, urethra, and anus can be involved, as well as the cervical epithelium. In men, the lesions often occur initially in the coronal sulcus, but may be seen on the shaft of the penis, the scrotum, perianal skin, or in the urethra. They initially appear as soft, pink filiform lesions, which may enlarge and coalesce to form large cauliflower-like aggregates. HPV types 6 and 11 can also cause juvenile laryngeal papillomas.

HPV also plays a role in the development of neoplasia of the uterine cervix and external genitalia. A high rate of coexistence of condyloma acuminata with cervical dysplasia or carcinoma was initially reported, and HPV DNA has been found in association both with cervical carcinoma and dyplasia and with cancerous and precancerous lesions of the external genitalia. HPV types 16 and 18 have been most intensely studied; other types are also implicated. In men these lesions may initially appear as small, flat, hyperpigmented papules on the penis or perianal skin. The surface of the lesions is generally smooth and velvety, but may be verrucous. The detection of subtle lesions may be improved by treatment with 5% acetic acid, which makes them appear white. In women, cutaneous lesions are generally multiple and often pigmented. They can be located on the labia majora and minora of the vulva and in the perianal region. Histologic examination of biopsies from affected sites may reveal changes associated with typical warts (hyperkeratosis, papillomatosis, and vacuolated cells) and/or features typical of intraepidermal carcinoma (Bowen's disease). Features in the latter include a disordered maturational sequence of dyskeratotic keratinocytes with hyperchromatic nuclei.

Squamous cell carcinomas are also associated with papilloma virus infections in extragenital skin. This has been seen in patients immunosuppressed after renal transplantation and in patients with the disorder epidermodysplasia verruciformis. Patients in both groups tend to develop multiple cutaneous squamous cell carcinomas on sun-exposed sites associated with several HPV types, including types 5, 8, and 14.

There are many ways to treat warts, but none is universally effective. Perhaps the most useful and convenient method is cryotherapy with liquid nitrogen. Equally effective, but requiring much more patient compliance is the use of keratolytic agents such as salicylic acid plasters or combinations of lactic acid and salicylic acid in flexible collodion. Keratolytic agents are of limited use on mucous membranes and genital lesions. For genital warts, podophyllin solution is moderately effective but may be associated with marked local reactions. Other topical agents used include trichloracetic acid or cantharidin. Electrodesiccation and curettage or carbon dioxide laser are also effective but require local anesthesia. Some caution should be exercised with electrodesiccation or carbon dioxide laser ablation as infectious viral particles may be in the vaporized tissue. Recurrence of warts appears to be common to all these modalities because viral genomic material is present in normal-appearing skin adjacent to the clinical lesions. Treatment should be tempered by recognition that most warts in normal individuals resolve spontaneously within 1 to 2 years. Also, only a fraction of warts are associated with neoplasia, and those are almost exclusively located on the genitalia or perianal skin.

HERPES SIMPLEX See Chap. 135.

HERPES ZOSTER See Chap. 136.

ACNE

ACNE VULGARIS Acne vulgaris is usually a self-limited disorder of teenagers and young adults, although 10 to 20 percent of adults may experience some form of the disorder. The permissive factor for the expression of the disease is the increase in sebum release by sebaceous glands after puberty. Small cysts, called comedones, form in hair follicles due to blockage of the follicular orifice by retention of sebum and keratinous material. The action of lipophilic yeast (*Pityrosporum orbiculare*) and bacteria (*Proprionibacterium acnes*) within the comedones releases free fatty acids from sebum, causes inflammation within the cyst, and results in rupture of the cyst wall. An inflammatory reaction develops as a result of extrusion of oily and keratinous debris from the cyst.

The clinical hallmark of acne vulgaris is the comedo, which may be closed (whitehead) or open (blackhead). Closed comedones appear as 1- to 2-mm pebbly white papules that are accentuated when the skin is stretched. They are the precursors of inflammatory lesions, and the contents are not easily expressed. Open comedones, which rarely result in inflammatory acne lesions, have a large dilated follicular orifice and are filled with easily expressible oxidized, darkened oily debris. Closed comedones are usually accompanied by inflammatory lesions: papules, pustules, or nodules.

The earliest lesions in adolescence are generally mildly inflamed or noninflammatory comedones on the forehead followed by more typical inflammatory lesions on the cheeks, nose, and chin. The most common location for acne is the face, but the chest and back may be involved. Most diseases remain mild and do not lead to scarring; a subset of patients develop large inflammatory cysts and nodules, which may drain, and result in significant scarring.

Exogenous and endogenous factors can alter the expression of acne vulgaris. Friction and trauma may rupture preexisting microcomedones and elicit inflammatory acne. This is commonly seen with headbands or chin straps of athletic helmets. Agents that predispose to comedone formation include topical agents in cosmetics or hair preparations such as lanolin, petrolatum, butylstearate, lauryl alcohol, and oleic acid, and chronic topical exposure to certain industrial compounds that contain insoluble cutting oils (impure paraffin oil mixtures), halogenated hydrocarbons, and coal tar and its derivatives. Glucocorticoids, applied topically or administered systemically, may also elicit acne. Other systemic medications such as isoniazid, halogens, dilantin, and phenobarbital may produce acneiform eruptions or aggravate preexisting acne.

Treatment is directed toward elimination of comedones, decreasing the population of lipophilic bacteria and yeast, and decreasing inflammation. Although areas affected with acne should be kept clean, removal of surface oils does not play an important role in therapy. Indeed, overly vigorous scrubbing may aggravate acne due to mechanical rupture of comedones. Oral tetracycline or erythromycin in doses of 250 to 1000 mg daily will decrease follicular colonization with some lipophilic organisms and may have an anti-inflammatory effect independent of antibacterial effects. Topical agents such as retinoic acid, benzoyl peroxide, or salicylic acid may alter the pattern of epidermal desquamation, prevent the formation of comedones, and aid in the resolution of preexisting cysts. Topical antibacterial agents like benzoyl peroxide, topical erythromycin, clindamycin, or tetracycline are also useful adjuncts to therapy. Severe nodulocystic acne not responsive to oral antibiotics and topical therapy may be treated with the synthetic retinoid isotretinoin at doses of 0.5 to 1.0 mg/kg body weight per day for 15 to 20 weeks. The use of this drug is limited by its teratogenicity, and women must be screened for pregnancy prior to initiating therapy, maintain a fail-safe method of birth control during treatment, and be screened for pregnancy during treatment. Patients receiving this medication develop extremely dry skin and cheilitis and must be followed for development of hypertriglyceridemia. Patients treated with isotretinoin, particularly those on long-term therapy for disorders other than acne, are also at risk to develop calcifications of tendons and bony overgrowths of vertebrae.

ACNE ROSACEA Acne rosacea is an inflammatory disorder predominantly affecting the central face. It rarely affects patients under age 30. Rosacea is more common in women, but those most severely affected are men. It is characterized by erythema, telangiectasias, and superficial pustules and is not associated with comedones. Rosacea rarely involves the chest or back.

There is a relationship between the tendency for pronounced facial flushing and the subsequent development of acne rosacea. Initially, individuals with rosacea demonstrate a pronounced flushing reaction. This may be in response to heat, emotional stimuli, alcohol, hot drinks, or spicy foods. As the disease progresses, the flush persists longer and longer, eventually becoming permanent. Papules, pustules, and telangiectasias then become superimposed on the persistent flush.

Rosacea of long standing may lead to connective tissue overgrowth, particularly of the nose (rhinophyma), and may be complicated by inflammatory disorders of the eye, including keratitis, blepharitis, iritis, and recurrent chalazion. These ocular problems potentially threaten vision and warrant ophthalmologic evaluation.

Acne rosacea can generally be effectively treated with oral tetracycline in doses ranging from 250 to 1500 mg/d. Topical metronidazole is also effective, and low-potency, nonfluorinated topical glucocorticoids, particularly after cool soaks, may alleviate facial erythema. Fluorinated topical glucocorticoids should be avoided since chronic use of these preparations may actually elicit rosacea. Topical therapy is not effective for ocular disease.

REFERENCES

FITZPATRICK TB et al (eds): *Dermatology in General Medicine*, 3d ed. New York, McGraw-Hill, 1987

LEVER WP, LEVER GS: *Histopathology of the Skin*, 6th ed. Philadelphia, Lippincott, 1983

MOSCHELLA SL, HURLEY HH (eds): *Dermatology*, 2d ed. Philadelphia, Saunders, 1985

PETO R, ZUR HAUSEN H: *Viral Etiology of Cervical Cancer: Banbury Report*. Cold Spring Harbor, Cold Spring Harbor Laboratory, 1986

PLEWIG G, KLIGMAN AM: *Acne: Morphogenesis and Treatment*. New York, Springer-Verlag, 1975

57 CUTANEOUS DRUG REACTIONS

BRUCE U. WINTROUB / ROBERT S. STERN

Cutaneous reactions are among the most frequent adverse reactions to drugs. Early in drug-induced illness, prompt therapeutic intervention may limit toxicity. This chapter focuses on adverse cutaneous reactions to drugs other than topical agents and reviews the incidence, patterns, and pathogenesis of cutaneous reactions to drugs and therapeutic agents.

USE OF PRESCRIPTION DRUGS IN THE UNITED STATES As of 1981, about 54,000 drug products, comprising nearly 1900 different active agents, were available in the United States with more than 1000 new chemical entities introduced since 1940. Hospital inpatients alone annually receive about 120 million courses of drug therapy, and half of adult Americans receive prescription drugs on a regular outpatient basis. Approximately 1 in 7 hospital days is devoted to treatment for drug toxicity, at a cost exceeding $12 billion per year.

INCIDENCE OF CUTANEOUS REACTIONS Although adverse drug reactions are common, it is difficult to ascertain their incidence, seriousness, and ultimate health effects. The fact that comprehensive information on these reactions is inadequate in part reflects the difficulty in establishing a system for postmarketing surveillance that is both economically feasible and capable of generating clinically useful data. Available information comes from evaluation of hospitalized patients, epidemiologic surveys, premarketing studies, and voluntary reporting.

In one study about 2 percent of medical inpatients had skin reactions consisting of rash, urticaria, or pruritus during hospitalization, and the overall reaction rate per course of drug therapy was 3:1000. Penicillins, sulfonamides, and blood products accounted for two-thirds of cutaneous reactions. In another study of 491 case records, drug-specific reaction rates were estimated for 42 days. This study showed that most cutaneous reactions occur within 1 week of exposure to the drug; exceptions were semisynthetic penicillins and ampicillin; about half of the reactions to these drugs occurred more than 1 week after initial administration. The risk of allergic reactions was not related to age, diagnosis, or blood level of urea nitrogen on admission. Skin reactions were more frequent among women.

In one study of 464 patients with drug eruptions cared for within hospital dermatology departments over a multiyear period, the most common morphologic patterns were classified as exanthematous (46 percent), urticaria and/or angioedema (23 percent), fixed drug eruption (19 percent), erythema multiforme (5.4 percent), and Stevens-Johnson syndrome (4.0 percent). Four percent of cases had exfoliative dermatitis, 3 percent had photosensitivity reactions, 1.5 percent had anaphylaxis, and 1.5 percent had toxic epidermal necrolysis; two patients died. The eruptions were attributed to more than 50 drugs, the most common being sulfonamide- and penicillin-related antibiotics.

PATHOGENESIS OF DRUG REACTIONS

Untoward cutaneous responses to drugs can arise as the result of immunologic or nonimmunologic mechanisms. Immunologic reactions require activation of host immunologic pathways and are designated *drug allergy*. Drug reactions occurring through nonimmunologic mechanisms may be due to activation of effector pathways, overdosage, cumulative toxicity, side effects, ecologic disturbance, interactions between drugs, metabolic alterations, exacerbation of preexisting dermatologic conditions, or inherited protein or enzyme deficiencies. Nonimmunologic cutaneous reactions to drugs are more common, and immunologic reactions are unpredictable when they do occur. It is often not possible to specify the responsible drug or pathogenic mechanism because the skin responds to a variety of stimuli through a limited number of reaction patterns. The mechanism of many drug reactions is unknown.

IMMUNOLOGIC DRUG REACTIONS Drugs frequently elicit an immune response, but only a small number of individuals experience clinical hypersensitivity reactions. For example, most patients exposed to penicillin develop demonstrable antibodies to penicillin but do not manifest drug reactions when exposed to penicillin. Multiple factors determine the capacity of a drug to elicit an immune response, including the *molecular characteristics* of the drug and *host effects*.

Increases in *molecular* size and complexity are associated with increased immunogenicity, and macromolecular drugs such as protein or peptide hormones are highly antigenic. Most drugs are small organic molecules less than 1000 daltons in size, and the capacity of such small molecules to elicit an immune response depends upon their ability to act as haptens, that is, to form stable, usually covalent, bonds with tissue macromolecules. Fortunately, most drugs have little or no ability to form covalent bonds with tissue components, and clinical sensitization results from minor contaminants or conversion of the drugs themselves to reactive metabolic products.

Route of administration of a drug or simple chemical can influence the nature of the *host* immune response. For example, topical application of antigens tends to induce delayed hypersensitivity, and exposure to antigens via oral or nasal cavities stimulates production of secretory immunoglobins, IgA and IgE, and occasionally IgM. Some agents, such as pentadecacatechol, sensitize readily if applied to the skin but do so poorly if orally ingested or applied to a mucosal surface. Frequency of sensitization through intravenous administration of drugs varies, but anaphylaxis is a more likely clinical consequence with this route of exposure.

The degree of drug exposure and individual variability in absorption and metabolism of a given agent may alter immunogenic load. The variable degree of in vivo acetylation of hydralazine provides a clinical example of this phenomenon. Hydralazine produces a lupus-like syndrome associated with antinuclear antibody formation more frequently in patients who acetylate the drug slowly. Frequent high-dose and interrupted courses of therapy are also important risk factors for development of drug allergy.

Pathogenesis of allergic drug reactions IgE-dependent drug reactions are usually manifest in the skin and gastrointestinal, respiratory, and cardiovascular systems (see Chap. 267). Primary symptoms and signs include pruritus, urticaria, nausea, vomiting, cramps, bronchospasm, and laryngeal edema and, on occasion, anaphylactic shock with hypotension and death. Immediate reactions may occur within minutes of drug exposure, and accelerated reactions occur hours or days after drug administration. Accelerated reactions are usually urticarial and may include laryngeal edema. IgE-dependent reactions are usually due to penicillins, manifestations are caused by release from sensitized tissue mast cells or circulating basophilic leukocytes of chemical mediators such as histamine, adenosine, leukotrienes, prostaglandins, platelet activating factor, enzymes, and proteoglycans. Release is triggered when polyvalent drug protein conjugates cross-link IgE molecules fixed to sensitized cells. The clinical manifestations are determined by interaction of the released chemical mediator with its target organ, i.e., skin, respiratory, gastrointestinal, and/or cardiovascular systems. Certain routes of administration favor different clinical patterns (i.e., oral route: gastrointestinal effects; intravenous route: circulating effects).

Immune-complex-dependent reactions Serum sickness is produced by circulating immune complexes and is characterized by fever, arthritis, nephritis, neuritis, edema, and an urticarial, papular, or pruritic rash (see Chap. 268). The syndrome requires an antigen that remains in the circulation for prolonged periods so that when antibody is synthesized, circulating antigen-antibody complexes are formed. Serum sickness was first described following administration of foreign sera, but drugs are now the usual cause. Drugs that produce serum sickness include the penicillins, sulfonamides, thiouracils, cholecystographic dyes, phenytoin, aminosalicylic acid, streptomycin, and antilymphocyte globulin. Symptoms develop 6 days or more after exposure to a drug, the latent period representing the time needed to synthesize antibody. The antibodies responsible for immune-complex-dependent drug reactions are largely of the IgG or IgM class.

Cytotoxic drug-induced reactions Immunologic reactions to drugs may damage kidneys, heart, lungs, liver, muscle, peripheral nerves, or formed elements of the blood by at least three mechanisms. First, a drug may react with the tissue and introduce haptenic groups on a cell surface that renders the tissue susceptible to antibody- or lymphocyte-mediated cytotoxicity. Second, drug-antibody complexes formed in the fluid phase may bind to the cell surface and damage the cell as an "innocent bystander." Third, drugs may induce immune responses that involve formed blood elements such as platelets and erythrocytes but do not cause cutaneous allergic drug reactions.

Cell-mediated immune responses play a role in contact drug hypersensitivity and are suspected to participate in other allergic drug reactions (i.e., pulmonary infiltration).

NONIMMUNOLOGIC DRUG REACTIONS Nonimmunologic mechanisms are responsible for the majority of drug reactions.

Nonimmunologic activation of effector pathways Drug reactions may result from nonimmunologic activation of effector pathways by three mechanisms: First, drugs may directly release mediators from mast cells and basophils and present as anaphylaxis or as urticaria and/or angioedema. Urticarial anaphylactic reactions induced by opiates, polymyxin B, tubocurarine, radiocontrast media, and dextrans may occur by this mechanism. Second, drugs may activate complement in the absence of antibody. This is an additional mechanism through which radiocontrast media may act. Third, drugs such as aspirin and other nonsteroidal anti-inflammatory agents may alter pathways of arachidonic acid metabolism; such drugs inhibit the cyclooxygenase that catalyzes the generation of prostaglandins from arachidonic acid in vitro.

Overdosage The manifestations of overdosage are predictable for most drugs; symptoms are an exaggeration of the drug's pharmacologic action. Overdosage can, at times, be observed in patients given the usual doses of the drug because of differing rates of absorption, metabolism, or excretion. An example is easy bruisability caused by warfarin overdose.

Phototoxicity Phototoxic reactions may be drug-induced or may occur in metabolic disorders in which an appropriate photosensitizing chemical is overproduced. In each case, the phototoxic reaction occurs when enough chromophore (drug or metabolic product) absorbs sufficient radiation in reactive tissue. Drug-induced phototoxic reactions can occur on first exposure, and the incidence of phototoxicity is a direct function of the concentration of sensitizer and amount of light. At least three distinct photochemical mechanisms have been described: First, the reaction between the excited state of a phototoxic molecule and a biologic target may cause formation of a covalent photoaddition product. Second, the phototoxic molecule may absorb protons to form stable photoproducts that are toxic to biologic substrates. Third, radiation of a phototoxic molecule may result in transfer of energy to oxygen molecules and cause formation of toxic oxygen species, such as singlet oxygen, superoxide anion, or hydroxyl radical. Interaction of these species with biologic targets produces photooxidized molecules. Serum protein-dependent systems and circulating effector cells play a role in acute in vivo phototoxic tissue damage due to exogenous agents; normal numbers of polymorphonuclear leukocytes and an intact complement system are required for the full development of demeclocycline-induced phototoxic lesions.

Cumulative toxicity The cumulative effects of drug deposition in skin may cause disturbance in skin color. In some instances, the drug is deposited in phagocytic cells of skin or mucous membranes, as occurs after prolonged administration of silver, bismuth, mercury, or gold. In other instances, the drug or its metabolic derivatives may bind to a component of the skin (for instance, melanin) as in patients taking high doses of chlorpromazine.

Secondary or side effects Secondary effects occur uniformly as part of the normal pharmacologic action of a drug but are not the primary therapeutic objective. Examples include alopecia, gastrointestinal disturbances, or hematopoietic depression during use of chemotherapeutic agents.

Ecologic disturbances These reactions result from drug-dependent alterations of normal flora of the skin, gut, or mucous membranes, permitting overgrowth of an organism (e.g., anogenital and oral candidiasis during administration of a broad-spectrum antibiotic).

Drug interactions Drugs may interact to cause adverse reactions. First, drugs may compete for the same plasma protein binding sites. For example, warfarin may be displaced from its binding site by phenylbutazone or aspirin and result in hemorrhage. Second, a drug may inhibit or stimulate metabolic enzymes important to its degradation or to that of another agent. Third, one drug may interfere with the excretion of another; for example, probenecid reduces penicillin excretion by the kidney.

Metabolic changes Drugs may sufficiently alter nutritional or metabolic status to induce cutaneous changes. For example, drugs, such as phenytoin, that interfere with folate absorption or metabolism increase the risk of aphthous stomatitis. In addition, drugs that alter lipid metabolism, such as isotretinoin, cause xanthomas by elevation of very low-density lipoproteins.

Exacerbation of preexisting diseases A variety of agents can exacerbate preexisting diseases. For example, lithium can exacerbate acne and psoriasis in a dose-dependent manner. Beta-blocking agents may induce a psoriasiform dermatitis, and withdrawal of glucocorticoids can exacerbate psoriasis or atopic dermatitis. Exacerbations of cutaneous lupus have been noted in association with cimetidine use. Vasodilators may exacerbate rosacea.

Inherited enzyme or protein deficiencies Drug reactions may also occur as the result of inherited enzyme deficiencies. For example, patients may be deficient in an enzyme required for metabolism of the drug or clearance of a toxic drug metabolite. The phenytoin hypersensitivity syndrome occurs in patients deficient in epoxide hydrolase, an enzyme required for metabolism of a toxic epoxide derived from phenytoin. Second, patients may be deficient in an enzyme required for normal function of a biochemical pathway, and further drug-induced lowering of the factor may cause pathologic manifestations. An example is warfarin sodium (Coumadin) necrosis of skin in patients with heterozygote deficiency of protein C, a proenzyme required for normal thrombolytic function.

CHARACTERISTIC FEATURES OF CUTANEOUS DRUG REACTIONS

Cutaneous disorders induced by drugs by known mechanisms include: urticaria, photosensitivity, disturbances of pigmentation, vasculitis, phenytoin hypersensitivity syndrome, and warfarin necrosis of skin. Reactions of uncertain mechanism include: morbilliform reactions, erythema multiforme, fixed drug reactions, erythema nodosum, lichenoid reactions, bullous drug reaction, and toxic epidermal necrolysis.

REACTIONS OF KNOWN CAUSE **Urticaria** Urticaria is a skin reaction characterized by pruritic, red wheals. Lesions may vary from a small point to a large area. Individual lesions rarely last more than 24 h. When deep dermal and subcutaneous tissues are also swollen, this reaction is known as *angioedema*. Angioedema may involve mucous membranes and may be part of a life-threatening anaphylactic reaction. Urticarial lesions, along with pruritus and morbilliform (or maculopapular) eruptions, are among the most frequent types of cutaneous reactions to drugs.

Drug-induced urticaria may be caused by three mechanisms: an IgE-dependent mechanism, circulating immune complexes (serum sickness), and nonimmunologic activation of effector pathways. IgE-dependent urticarial reactions usually occur within 36 h but can occur within minutes. Reactions occurring within minutes to hours of drug exposure are termed *immediate reactions,* while those that occur 12 to 36 h after drug exposure are designated *accelerated reactions.* Immune-complex-induced urticaria associated with serum sickness may occur from 4 to 12 days after challenge. In this syndrome, the urticarial eruption may be accompanied by fever, hematuria, and arthralgias, hepatic dysfunction, and neurologic symptoms.

Certain drugs, such as nonsteroidal anti-inflammatory agents and radiographic dyes, may induce urticarial reactions whose time course resembles that of immediate IgE-dependent reactions. Drug-specific antibody does not play a role in such reactions, and they are thought to be induced by the action of drug on cutaneous mast cells, complement, or arachidonic acid–dependent pathways. Although aspirin, penicillin, and blood products are the most frequent causes of urticarial eruptions, urticaria has been observed in association with nearly all drugs.

Drugs may also cause chronic urticaria, which lasts more than 6 weeks. The mechanisms of chronic urticaria are unclear. Aspirin frequently exacerbates this problem.

Photosensitivity eruptions Photosensitivity eruptions are usually most marked in sun-exposed areas but may extend to sun-protected areas. Phototoxic reactions are more common than photoallergic reactions. Phototoxic reactions usually resemble sunburn, can occur with the first exposure to a drug, and are dose-related. The action spectrum for phototoxicity is similar to the ultraviolet absorption spectrum of the drug. No single test system seems to be a successful predictor of the photosensitivity potential for a given compound.

The mechanism for photoallergy to systemic medications is not well defined. Drug, immune response, and light are required to produce clinical photoallergy, and photoallergic reactions may be delayed hypersensitivity responses. Eruptions range from lichenoid papules to eczematous changes.

Orally administered drugs that cause photoallergic or phototoxic reactions include chlorpromazine, tetracycline, thiazides, nalidixic acid, and two nonsteroidal anti-inflammatory agents, benoxaprofen and piroxicam. Based on test systems, the majority of the common photosensitizers seem to have action spectrums in the long-wave ultraviolet (UV-A) range and are usually phototoxic. This is fortunate since phototoxic reactions will abate with removal of either the drug or ultraviolet radiation, but some photoallergic reactions may persist after the drug is withdrawn.

Drugs may also induce photosensitivity diseases. For example, procainamide may induce systemic lupus erythematosus.

Pigmentation changes Drugs may cause a variety of pigmentary changes in the skin. Some drugs stimulate melanocytic activity and increase pigmentation. Drug deposition can also lead to pigmentation; this phenomenon occurs with heavy metals. Phenothiazines may be deposited in the skin and cause a slate-gray color. Antimalarial drugs may cause a slate-gray or yellow pigmentation. Inorganic arsenic, once used to treat psoriasis, is associated with diffuse macular pigmentation. Other heavy metals that cause pigmentary changes include silver, gold, bismuth, and mercury. Long-term use of phenytoin can produce a chloasma-like pigmentation in women. Certain cytostatic agents can also cause pigmentary changes. Histologic examination is often diagnostic for drug deposition diseases.

Clofazimine, an aminophenazine dye used in the treatment of leprosy, causes a red skin color that is so marked that some patients discontinue therapy. Methysergide produces a red color in the skin and an orange-peel-like texture. Nicotinic acid in large doses may cause brown pigmentation. Oral contraceptives may produce chloasma, and adrenocorticotropin may cause a hypermelanosis similar to that of primary adrenal insufficiency. In addition, amiodarone may cause violaceous hyperpigmentation which is increased in sun-exposed skin. Drugs such as heavy metals, copper, antimalarial and arsenical agents, and ACTH may also discolor oral mucosa.

Vasculitis Cutaneous necrotizing vasculitis often presents as palpable purpuric lesions that may be generalized or limited to the lower extremities or other dependent areas (see Chap. 276). Urticarial lesions, ulcers, or hemorrhagic blisters also occur. Vasculitis may involve other organs, including the liver, kidney, brain, and joints. Drugs are only one cause of vasculitis. Immune-complex-dependent mechanisms are probably responsible for drug-induced vasculitis and/or serum sickness. Propylthiouracil induces a cutaneous vasculitis that is accompanied by leukopenia and splenomegaly. Direct immunofluorescent changes in these lesions suggest immune-complex deposition. Drugs implicated in vasculitic eruptions include allopurinol, thiazides, penicillin, and phenytoin.

Phenytoin hypersensitivity reaction The phenytoin hypersensitivity reaction, one of many phenytoin-induced cutaneous reactions, is an erythematous eruption that eventually becomes purpuric and is accompanied by fever, facial and periorbital edema, tender generalized lymphadenopathy, leukocytosis (often with atypical lymphocytes and eosinophils), hepatitis, and sometimes nephritis. The cutaneous reaction usually begins 1 to 3 weeks after phenytoin is begun and resolves rapidly with drug cessation and treatment with systemic glucocorticoids. The eruption recurs with rechallenge. This syndrome apparently results from an inherited deficiency of epoxide hydrolase, an enzyme required for metabolism of a toxic intermediate arene oxide that is formed during metabolism of phenytoin by the cytochrome P_{450} system.

Warfarin necrosis of the skin This rare reaction occurs usually between the third and tenth days of therapy with warfarin derivatives, usually in women. Lesions are sharply demarcated, erythematous, indurated, and purpuric and may resolve or progress to formation of large, irregular, hemorrhagic bullae with eventual necrosis and slow-healing eschar formation.

Development of the syndrome is unrelated to drug dose or underlying condition. Favored sites are breasts, thighs, and buttocks. The course is not altered by discontinuation of the drug after the onset of the eruption. Similar reactions have been associated with heparin. Warfarin reactions are associated with protein C deficiency. Protein C is a vitamin K–dependent protein with a shorter half-life than other clotting proteins and is in part responsible for control of fibrinolysis. Since warfarin inhibits synthesis of vitamin K–dependent coagulation factors, warfarin anticoagulation in heterozygotes for protein C deficiency causes a precipitous fall in circulating levels of protein C, permitting hypercoagulability and thrombosis in the cutaneous microvasculature, with consequent areas of necrosis.

REACTIONS OF UNCERTAIN CAUSE **Morbilliform reactions** Morbilliform or maculopapular eruptions may be the most common of all drug-induced reactions, often start on the trunk or areas of pressure or trauma, and consist of erythematous macules and papules that are frequently symmetric and may become confluent. Involvement of mucous membranes, palms, and soles is variable; the eruption may be associated with moderate to severe pruritus and fever.

The pathogenesis is unclear. A hypersensitivity mechanism has been suggested, although these reactions do not always recur following drug rechallenge. Diagnosis is rarely assisted by laboratory tests; differentiation from viral exanthem is the principal differential diagnostic consideration. While these reactions usually require discontinuation of drug (dechallenge), eruptions may occasionally decrease or fade with continued use of the responsible drug.

Morbilliform reactions usually develop within 1 week of initiation of therapy and last 1 to 2 weeks; however, reactions to some drugs, especially penicillin, may begin more than 2 weeks after therapy has begun, and last as long as 2 weeks after therapy has ceased. These eruptions are common in patients receiving ampicillin, amoxcillin, or allopurinol; trimethoprim-sulfamethoxazole causes frequent reactions in acquired immunodeficiency syndrome (AIDS) patients.

Erythema multiforme Erythema multiforme is an acute, self-limited inflammatory disorder of skin and mucous membranes characterized by distinctive iris or target lesions, often associated with sore throat and malaise. Many drugs, including sulfonamides, penicillin, phenytoin, and phenylbutazone, can cause erythema multiforme; long-acting sulfonamides are the best-studied. Erythema multiforme resulting from sulfonamides typically begins after 1 to 2 weeks of drug therapy and is accompanied by fever and mucous membrane reaction (Stevens-Johnson syndrome). An immune-complex-induced, lymphocyte-mediated mechanism may be responsible.

Fixed drug reactions These reactions are characterized by one or more sharply demarcated, erythematous lesions in which hyperpigmentation results after resolution of the acute inflammation; with rechallenge, the lesion recurs in the same (i.e., "fixed") location. Lesions often involve the face, genitalia, and oral mucosa and cause burning. Fixed drug eruptions have been associated with phenolphthalein, sulfonamides, tetracycline, phenylbutazone, and barbiturates. Although cross-sensitivity appears to occur between different tetracycline compounds, cross-sensitivity was not elicited when different sulfonamide compounds were administered to patients as part of provocation testing.

Documentation of a characteristic papillary-dermal mononuclear cell infiltrate in close approximation to the dermoepidermal junction may confirm the clinical diagnosis. Extensive basal cell degeneration can lead to formation of bullae and pigment dispersion. Even when lesions are completely healed, melanin-laden macrophages are present in the dermis.

Erythema nodosum Erythema nodosum is a panniculitis characterized by tender, subcutaneous, erythematous nodules, usually on the anterior portion of the legs. Drug hypersensitivity, frequently involving oral contraceptives, is one cause of this reaction. The mechanism is unknown.

Lichenoid drug eruptions A lichenoid cutaneous reaction, clinically and morphologically indistinguishable from lichen planus, is associated with a variety of drugs and chemicals. Eosinophils in lichen planus are more common when the reaction is drug-induced. Gold and antimalarials are most often associated with this eruption. Antihypertensive agents, including beta blockers and captopril, have also been reported to cause a lichenoid reaction.

Bullous eruptions Blisters accompany a wide variety of cutaneous reactions, especially the severe morbilliform eruptions, and may be an integral part of erythema multiforme, toxic epidermal necrolysis, and fixed drug eruptions. Nalidixic acid and furosemide cause blistering eruptions indistinguishable from the primary bullous diseases. Other examples are a pemphigus foliaceus–like eruption seen with penicillamine and cicatricial pemphigoid that has been seen with clonidine.

Toxic epidermal necrolysis Toxic epidermal necrolysis is the most serious cutaneous drug reaction and may be fatal. Drugs are the most frequent cause in adults. Onset is generally acute and is characterized by epidermal necrosis with a minimal dermal inflammatory process. This reaction is often associated with allopurinol and has been reported with measles vaccine, fumigants, phenytoin, sulfonamides, and nonsteroidal anti-inflammatory agents.

DRUGS OF SPECIAL INTEREST

PENICILLIN The incidence of reactions to penicillin is about 1 percent. Not all adverse reactions are immunologic, as illustrated by ampicillin-induced morbilliform eruptions and central nervous system reactions to procaine penicillin.

IgG, IgM, and IgE antibodies can be produced; IgG and IgM anti-penicillin antibodies play a role in the development of hemolytic anemia, whereas anaphylaxis and serum sickness appear to be due to IgE antibodies in serum.

Since penicillin reactions often occur in patients without a prior history of penicillin allergy, the utility of accurate and easily administered tests for sensitization is apparent. Current practice is to perform skin testing with a commercially available penicilloyl determinant preparation (Pre-pen, Kremers-Urban) and with fresh penicillin and if possible with another source of minor (nonpenicilloyl) determinants such as aged or base-treated penicillin. Antibodies to minor determinants are common in patients experiencing anaphylaxis. Testing with major determinants alone detects most patients at risk for anaphylaxis.

Twenty-seven percent (10 to 36 percent) of patients with a positive history of penicillin allergy also have a positive skin test, while 6 percent (3 to 10 percent) with a negative history demonstrate a positive skin response to penicillin. Administering penicillin to those patients with a positive skin test produces reactions in a high proportion (50 to 100 percent); conversely, only a few patients (about 0.5 percent) with negative skin tests react to the drug, and reactions tend to be mild and to occur late. Since a negative skin test may occur during or just after an acute reaction, testing should be performed either prospectively or several months after a suspected reaction. As many as 80 percent of patients lose anaphylactic sensitivity and IgE antibody after several years. Radioallergosorbent test (RAST) and other in vitro tests offer no advantage over properly performed skin testing.

Some cross-reactivity exists between penicillin and nonpenicillin β-lactam antibiotics (e.g., cephalosporins). About half of patients who react to penicillin skin testing also react to cephalosporin skin testing; anaphylaxis from cephalosporins has occurred in patients testing positive to penicillin. The benefit of skin testing with penicillin derivatives and cephalosporins in addition to penicillin is uncertain; in one study none of 120 patients with negative results to penicillin skin tests reacted to semisynthetic penicillinase-resistant agents.

In the face of a positive clinical history of penicillin reaction, another drug should be chosen. If this is not feasible or prudent (e.g., in a pregnant patient with syphilis; with enterococcal endocarditis), skin testing with penicillin is warranted. If skin tests are negative, cautious administration of penicillin is acceptable, although some recommend desensitization of such patients. In those with positive skin tests, desensitization is mandatory if therapeutic use of β-lactam antibiotics is to be undertaken. Various protocols are available, including oral and parenteral approaches. Oral desensitization appears to carry a lesser risk of serious anaphylactic reactions during desensitization. However, desensitization carries the risk of anaphylaxis regardless of how it is performed. After desensitization many patients experience non-life-threatening IgE-mediated untoward reactions to penicillin during their course of therapy. Desensitization is not effective in those with exfoliative dermatitis or morbilliform reactions due to penicillin.

NONSTEROIDAL ANTI-INFLAMMATORY DRUGS Nonsteroidal anti-inflammatory drugs (NSAIDs), including aspirin (but not salicylates in general) and indomethacin (indometacin), cause two broad categories of allergic-like symptoms in susceptible individuals: (1) approximately 1 percent of persons experience urticaria or angioedema; (2) about half as many (0.5 percent) experience rhinosinusitis and asthma; however, about 10 percent of adult asthmatics and one-third of individuals with nasal polyposis and sinusitis may respond adversely to aspirin.

Urticaria/angioedema may be delayed up to 24 h and may occur at any age. The rhinosinusitis-asthma syndrome generally develops within 1 h of drug administration. In young people, the reaction pattern often begins as watery rhinorrhea that can be complicated by nasal and sinus infection, and polyposis, bloody discharge and nasal eosinophilia. In many individuals with this syndrome, asthma eventually ensues that can be life-threatening whenever NSAIDs are subsequently ingested, and symptoms may persist despite avoidance of these drugs. Proof of the association of symptoms and NSAIDs use requires either clear-cut history of symptoms following drug ingestion or an oral challenge. For the latter to be performed with relative safety, (1) asthma must be under good control, (2) the procedure must be conducted in a hospital setting by experienced personnel capable of recognizing and treating acute respiratory responses, and (3) the challenge should begin with very low doses (i.e., <30 mg) of aspirin and increase every 1 to 2 h in doubling doses as tolerated to 650 mg. In a study of 50 consecutive patients with a positive history of aspirin-induced bronchospasm, 84 percent developed pulmonary or nasoocular symptoms with aspirin, but 16 percent did not react; moreover, when subjects who initially tested positive to a challenge were reexposed to aspirin, the clinical reaction pattern was identical in only 60 percent.

While cross-reactivity between NSAIDs is common, it is not immunologic, and patients who are sensitive to NSAIDs cannot be identified by assessment of IgE antibody to aspirin, lymphocyte sensitization, or in vitro immunologic testing. All cross-reacting drugs are cyclooxygenase inhibitors, although salicylates also inhibit cyclooxygenase but (except for aspirin) do not cause the response.

"Desensitization" to the adverse effects of NSAIDs can be accomplished by the challenge procedure above, although repeated challenge at the initial provocation dose may be required. Desensitization works by unknown mechanisms, renders the subject tolerant to all NSAIDs yet studied, persists for at least 24 and up to 96 h, and is probably universal but does not have a positive effect on the underlying disorder.

RADIOCONTRAST MEDIA Large numbers of patients are exposed to radiocontrast agents, and 5 to 10 percent of patients receiving them develop some reaction: urticaria in 1 percent, dyspnea in 0.25 percent, and death in 0.01 percent. Reactions consisting of urticaria and angioedema, asthma, and hypotension mimicking anaphylaxis occur in less than 1 percent of radiocontrast procedures. About one-third of those with mild reactions to previous exposure rereact upon reexposure.

There is no proof of an immunologic mechanism for radiocontrast media reactions. Elevations in plasma histamine occur in those with and without reaction, and may be due to the hypertonicity of these media. In addition, complement activation by both classical and alternative pathways occurs in normal and reactive individuals. In short, the mechanism for these reactions is not understood and no test identifies patients at risk for a radiocontrast medium reaction. Because repeat reactions are common, obtaining a thorough history is the best available technique for identifying those most likely to experience an adverse reaction. Several pretreatment regimens are claimed to decrease repeat reaction rate to about 10 percent. One such regimen consists of 50 mg prednisone at 13, 7, and 1 h before the procedure, and 50 mg diphenhydramine 1 h before the procedure.

HYDANTOINS Phenytoin and other hydantoins cause morbilliform eruptions, erythema multiforme, and toxic epidermal necrolysis, as well as a hypersensitivity reaction (described above) and the pseudolymphoma syndrome. In one study, 5 percent of children treated with phenytoin developed a mild dose-dependent, maculopapular eruption lasting 3 to 5 days and occurring within 2 weeks of starting treatment.

The pseudolymphoma syndrome, consisting of lymphadenopathy and histopathologic lymph node atypia, is a more chronic form of the phenytoin hypersensitivity syndrome, and the cutaneous changes are less marked in this syndrome.

Use of phenytoin is frequently associated with gingival hyperplasia and rarely with a syndrome similar to systemic lupus erythematosus, severe exfoliative dermatitis, and polyarteritis nodosa. Because many hydantoin side effects may be dose-related, drugs that interfere with its elimination (e.g., chloramphenicol) effectively prolong those effects.

Sulfasalazine and allopurinol cause reactions that are indistinguishable from the phenytoin hypersensitivity syndrome. Unlike the hydantoins, an immunologic mechanism seems the most likely explanation for hypersensitivity to these drugs.

THIAZIDES AND SULFONAMIDES Thiazides are among the most common causes of drug-induced urticaria and morbilliform eruptions; they also cause erythema multiforme, drug-induced cutaneous vasculitis, and lichenoid and photosensitivity eruptions. Because they are substituted sulfonamides, antibodies to these diuretics may cross-react with sulfonamide antibiotics and sulfonamide-based hypoglycemic agents. The combination of sulfamethoxazole and trimethoprim causes two distinct cutaneous reactions: (1) an urticarial eruption beginning in the first few days of treatment and (2) a morbilliform eruption often occurring more than 1 week after therapy has begun. The morbilliform reaction is frequent in patients with AIDS and is associated with pancytopenia in some patients. The eruption may have an intensely purpuric characacter, independent of the presence of vasculitis. One patient developed toxic epidermal necrolysis and pancytopenia following administration of sulfamethoxazale-trimethoprim.

AGENTS USED IN CANCER CHEMOTHERAPY Since many agents used in cancer chemotherapy inhibit cell division, rapidly proliferating elements of the skin, including hair, mucous membranes, and appendages, are sensitive to their effects; as a result, stomatitis and alopecia are among the most frequent dose-dependent side effects of chemotherapy. Onychodystrophy (dystrophic changes in nails) is also seen with bleomycin, hydroxyurea (hydroxycarbamide), and 5-fluorouracil. Sterile cellulitis and phlebitis and ulceration of pressure areas occur with many of these agents. Urticaria, angioedema, exfoliative dermatitis, and erythema of the palms and soles have also been seen, as has local and diffuse hyperpigmentation. Diagnosis and treatment of these reactions are especially difficult because of the underlying malignancy.

TETRACYCLINES While urticaria and morbilliform eruptions are unusual, tetracyclines sometimes cause other cutaneous side effects, including a photosensitivity reaction (as a result of drug-induced phototoxicity) and onycholysis (sometimes with no apparent cutaneous photosensitivity). These reactions occur with demeclocycline, doxycycline, minocycline, tetracycline, and oxytetracycline. Tetracyclines also cause fixed drug and lichenoid eruptions. An acnelike, gram-negative folliculitis with long-term use of tetracycline is due to overgrowth of resistant bacteria.

Several pigmentary abnormalities have been noted. If used during pregnancy or early childhood, tetracycline stains the teeth, sometimes permanently. Minocyline can cause hyperpigmentation in sun-exposed areas and in areas of previous inflammation. Histiocytes that contain iron are responsible for the pigmentary changes. Tetracycline has also been associated with a flulike syndrome (accompanied by headaches, malaise, and eosinophilia) that recurred with rechallenge. A serum sickness–like reaction to minocycline has also been reported.

GLUCOCORTICOIDS Both systemic and topical glucocorticoids cause a variety of skin changes, including acneiform eruptions, atrophy, striae, and other stigmata of Cushing's syndrome, and in sufficiently high doses can retard wound healing. Patients using glucocorticoids are at higher risk for bacterial, yeast, and fungal skin infections that may be misinterpreted as drug eruptions but are in fact drug side effects instead.

ANTIMALARIAL AGENTS Antimalarial agents are used as therapy for several skin diseases, including the skin manifestations of lupus and polymorphous light eruption, but they also can induce cutaneous reactions. In patients with asymptomatic porphyria cutanea tarda, chloroquine increases porphyrin levels and may exacerbate the disease.

Pigmentation disturbances, including black pigmentation of the face, mucous membranes, pretibial and subungual areas, occur with antimalarials, and quinacrine (mepacrine) causes generalized, cutaneous yellow discoloration. Antimalarial agents may exacerbate psoriasis, and exfoliative dermatitis, fixed drug eruptions, lichenoid dermatitis, and erythema annulare centrifugum have all been reported with their use.

GOLD Chrysotherapy has been associated with a variety of dose-related dermatologic reactions (including maculopapular eruptions) that can develop as long as 2 years after initiation of therapy and require months to resolve. Erythema nodosum, psoriasiform dermatitis, vaginal pruritus, eruptions similar to pityriasis rosea, hyperpigmentation, and lichenoid eruptions resembling those seen with antimalarial agents have been reported. After a cutaneous reaction, it is sometimes possible to reinstitute gold therapy at lower doses without recurrence of the dermatitis.

DIAGNOSIS OF DRUG REACTIONS

Possible causes of an adverse reaction can be assessed as definite, probable, possible, or unlikely, based on six variables: (1) previous experience with the drug in the general population, (2) alternative etiologic candidates, (3) timing of events, (4) drug levels or evidence of overdose, (5) patient reaction to dechallenge, and (6) patient reaction to rechallenge.

PREVIOUS EXPERIENCE Tables of relative reaction rates are available and are useful to assess the likelihood that a given drug is responsible for a given cutaneous reaction. The specific morphologic pattern of a drug reaction, however, may modify these reaction rates by increasing or decreasing the likelihood that a given drug is responsible for a given reaction. For example, since fixed eruptions due to drug are more often seen with barbiturates than with penicillin, a fixed drug reaction in a patient taking both types of agents is more likely to be due to the barbiturate even though penicillins have a higher overall drug reaction rate.

ALTERNATIVE ETIOLOGIC CANDIDATES A cutaneous eruption may be due to exacerbation of preexisting disease or to development of new disease unrelated to drugs. For example, a patient with psoriasis may have a flare-up of disease coincidental with administration of penicillin for streptococcal infection; in this case infection is a more likely cause for the flare-up than drug reaction.

TIMING OF EVENTS Since most drug reactions of the skin occur within 1 to 2 weeks of initiation of therapy, reactions beginning after 2 weeks are less likely to be due to drugs.

DRUG LEVELS Some cutaneous reactions are dependent on dosage or cumulative toxicity. For example, lichenoid dermatoses due to gold administration appear more often in patients taking high doses.

DECHALLENGE Most adverse cutaneous reactions to drugs remit with dechallenge (removal of the suspected agent). A reaction is unlikely to be drug-related if improvement occurs without dechallenge or if a patient fails to improve after dechallenge and appropriate therapy.

RECHALLENGE Rechallenge provides the most definitive information concerning adverse cutaneous reactions to drugs, since a reaction failing to recur on rechallenge with a drug is unlikely to be due to that agent. Rechallenge is frequently impractical, however, because the need to ensure patient safety and comfort outweighs the value of the possible information derived from rechallenge.

DIAGNOSIS OF DRUG ALLERGY

Tests for IgE responses include in vivo and in vitro methods, but such tests are available only for a limited number of drugs, including penicillins and cephalosporins, some peptide and protein drugs (insulin, xenogeneic sera), and some agents used for general anesthesia. In vivo testing is accomplished by prick puncture and/or by intradermal skin testing. A wheal-and-flare response 2 by 2 mm greater than that seen with a saline control within 20 min is considered indicative of IgE-mediated mast cell degranulation, provided (1) the patient is not dermographic, (2) the drug does not nonspecifically degranulate mast cells, (3) the drug concentration is not high enough to be irritating, and (4) the buffer itself does not cause wheal-and-flare responses.

Skin testing with major and minor determinants of penicillins or cephalosporins has proved useful for identifying patients at risk of anaphylactic reactions to these agents. However, skin tests themselves carry a small risk of anaphylaxis. Negative skin tests do not rule out IgE-mediated reactivity, and the risk of anaphylaxis in response to penicillin administration in patients with negative skin tests is about 1 percent; about two-thirds of patients with a positive skin test and history of a previous adverse reaction to penicillin experience an allergic response on rechallenge. Skin tests may be negative in allergic patients receiving antihistamines or in those whose allergy is to determinants not present in the test reagent. Although less well studied, similar techniques can identify patients who are sensitive to protein drugs and to agents such as gallamine and succinylcholine. Most other drugs are small molecules, and skin testing with them is unreliable.

In vitro testing for IgE may be done by assessing the ability of serum to bind to antigen and then to bind radiolabeled antibody to IgE (RAST test) or by assessing the ability of the drug to cause histamine release from basophils from drug-sensitive individuals. The RAST test is sensitive and specific but is not available for most drugs; even in the case of penicillin it is available for major determinants only. Similarly, basophil histamine release is a research technique that is not generally available.

There are no generally available and reliable tests for sensitivity to NSAIDs, to agents that directly degranulate mast cells, or to drugs that cause manifestations via immune-complex-mediated complement activation. Although it is possible to screen for the absence of IgA antibody, the utility of this maneuver in preventing transfusion-associated anaphylaxis in IgA-deficient individuals has not been documented.

REFERENCES

ARNDT KA, JICK H: Rates of cutaneous reactions to drugs. JAMA 235:918, 1976
GREENBERGER PA: Contrast media reaction. J Allergy Clin Immunol 74:600, 1984
———, PATTERSON R: Management of drug allergy in patients with acquired immunodeficiency syndrome. J Allergy Clin Immunol 79:484, 1989
PARKER CW: Drug allergy. N Engl J Med 292:511, 1975
PASRICHA JS: Drugs causing fixed eruptions. Br J Dermatol 100:183, 1979
PLESKOW W et al: Aspirin desensitization in aspirin sensitive asthmatics: Characterization of the refactory period. J Allergy Clin Immunol 69:11, 1982
REVUZ J et al: Toxic epidermal necrolysis: Clinical findings and prognosis factors in 87 patients. Arch Dermatol 123:160, 1987
SAXON A: Immediate hypersensitivity reactions to beta-lactam antibiotics. Rev Infect Dis 5:5368, 1983
SOGN DD: Penicillin allergy. J Allergy Clin Immunol 74:589, 1984
SPEILBERG SP et al: Predisposition to phenytoin hepatotoxicity assessed *in vitro*. N Engl J Med 307:722, 1981
STANLEY J, FALLON-PELLICCI V: Phenytoin hypersensitivity reaction. Arch Dermatol 14:1350, 1978
STERN RS, BIGBY M: An expanded profile of cutaneous reactions to non-steroidal anti-inflammatory drugs. JAMA 252:1433, 1984

58 IMMUNOLOGICALLY MEDIATED SKIN DISEASES

KIM B. YANCEY / THOMAS J. LAWLEY

A number of immunologically mediated skin diseases and the cutaneous manifestations of immunologically mediated systemic disorders are now recognized as distinct entities with relatively consistent clinical, histologic, and immunopathologic findings. Many of these disorders are due to autoimmune mechanisms. Clinically, they are characterized by morbidity (pain, pruritus, disfigurement) and in some instances by mortality (largely due to loss of epidermal barrier function and/or secondary infection). The major features of the more common immunologically mediated skin diseases are summarized in this chapter. See Table 58-1.

PEMPHIGUS VULGARIS Pemphigus vulgaris (PV) is a blistering skin disease seen predominantly in elderly patients. Jewish patients with PV have an increased incidence of the HLA-DR4 haplotype. This disorder is characterized by the loss of cohesion between epidermal cells (a process termed *acantholysis*) with the resultant formation of intraepidermal blisters. Clinical lesions of PV typically consist of flaccid blisters on either normal-appearing or erythematous skin. These blisters rupture easily, leaving denuded areas that may crust and enlarge peripherally. Substantial portions of the body surface may be denuded in severe cases. Manual pressure to the skin of these patients may elicit the separation of the epidermis from the dermis—Nikolsky's sign. This finding, while characteristic of PV, is not specific to this disorder and is also seen in toxic epidermal necrolysis, Stevens-Johnson syndrome, and a few other skin diseases. The skin lesions in PV typically present on the scalp, face, neck, axilla, trunk, and oral cavity. In half or more patients, lesions begin in the mouth; approximately 90 percent of patients have oromucosal involvement at some time during the course of their disease. Involvement of other mucosal surfaces (e.g., pharyngeal, laryngeal, esophageal, conjunctival, vulval, or rectal) can also occur in severe disease. Extensive denudation may be associated with pain of varying severity. Lesions usually heal without scarring except at sites complicated by secondary infection or mechanically induced dermal wounds. Nonetheless, postinflammatory hyperpigmentation is usually present at sites of healed lesions for some time. Although pemphigus occurs in several autoimmune diseases, its association with thymoma and/or myasthenia gravis is particularly significant. To date, more than 30 cases of thymoma and/or myasthenia gravis have been reported in association with pemphigus, usually with pemphigus foliaceus (see below).

Biopsies of early lesions demonstrate intraepidermal vesicle formation secondary to loss of cohesion between epidermal cells (i.e., acantholytic blisters). Blister cavities contain epidermal acantholytic cells which appear as round homogeneous cells containing hyperchromatic nuclei. Basal keratinocytes remain attached to the epidermal basement membrane so that blister formation is within the suprabasal portion of the epidermis. In addition, lesional skin may contain focal collections of intraepidermal eosinophils and granulocytes within blister cavities; dermal alterations are slight, usually limited to an eosinophil-predominant leukocytic infiltrate. Direct immunofluorescence microscopy of normal-appearing, perilesional skin shows IgG on the surface of keratinocytes; deposits of the third component of complement (C3) may occur in the same distribution. These deposits of IgG are derived from a circulating autoantibody directed against keratinocyte cell surface antigens. Circulating autoantibodies can be demonstrated in 80 to 90 percent of PV patients by indirect immunofluorescence microscopy; monkey esophagus is the optimal substrate for demonstration of these autoantibodies. These autoantibodies are responsible for dysadhesion of epidermal cells probably through the activation of endogenous proteases in keratinocytes. The titer of circulating autoantibody (determined by indirect immunofluorescence microscopy) correlates roughly with disease activity. These immunopathologic findings aid the diagnosis of PV and its differentiation from other blistering skin diseases.

PV can be life-threatening. Prior to the availability of glucocorticoids, the mortality ranged from 60 to 90 percent. The current mortality is approximately 5 to 15 percent. Common causes of morbidity and mortality are infection and complications of treatment with glucocorticoids. Bad prognostic factors include advanced age, widespread involvement, and the requirement for high doses of glucocorticoids (with or without other immunosuppressive agents) for control of disease. The course of PV in individual patients is variable and difficult to predict. Some patients achieve remission after variable periods of treatment (40 percent of patients in some series) but others may require long-term treatment or succumb to complications of their disease or its treatment. The mainstay of treatment is systemic glucocorticoids. Patients with moderate to severe disease are usually started on prednisone 60 to 80 mg/d. If new lesions continue to appear after 1 to 2 weeks of treatment, the dose should be increased. Many regimens have combined an immunosuppressive agent with systemic glucocorticoids for control of PV. The two most frequently used are either azathioprine (1 mg/kg per day) or cyclophosphamide (1 mg/kg per day). It is important to

TABLE 58-1 Immunologically mediated blistering skin diseases

Disease	Clinical	Histology	Immunopathology
Pemphigus vulgaris	Flaccid blisters, denuded skin, oromucosal lesions	Blister formed in suprabasal layer of epidermis	Cell surface deposits of IgG on keratinocytes
Pemphigus foliaceus	Crusts and shallow erosions on scalp, central face, neck, upper chest, and back	Blister formed in superficial layers of epidermis	Cell surface deposits of IgG on keratinocytes
Bullous pemphigoid	Large tense blisters on flexor surfaces, oromucosal lesions	Blister formed in subepidermal region, usually eosinophil-rich	Linear band of IgG or C3 at BMZ*
Dermatitis herpetiformis	Extremely itchy small papules and vesicles on elbows, knees, buttocks, and posterior nuchal area	Subepidermal blister with neutrophils in dermal papillae	Granular deposits of IgA in dermal papillae
Linear IgA dermatosis	Extremely itchy small papules and vesicles on extensor surfaces, occasionally larger arciform blisters	Subepidermal blister with neutrophils in dermal papillae	Linear band of IgA at BMZ
Epidermolysis bullosa acquisita	Blisters and scarring on dorsum of hands, elbows, knees, oromucosal lesions	Blister is subepidermal and can be inflammatory or not	Linear band of IgG or C3 at BMZ

* BMZ = basement membrane zone.

bring severe or progressive disease under control quickly to lessen the severity and/or duration of this disorder.

PEMPHIGUS FOLIACEUS Pemphigus foliaceus (PF) is distinguished from PV by several features. In PF, acantholytic blisters are located high within the epidermis, usually just beneath the stratum corneum. Hence, PF is a more superficial blistering disease than PV. The distribution of lesions in the two disorders is much the same except that in the former, mucous membrane lesions are rare and usually limited to superficial erosions. Patients with PF rarely demonstrate intact blisters but rather exhibit shallow erosions associated with erythema, scale, and crust formation. Mild cases of PF resemble severe seborrheic dermatitis; severe PF may cause extensive exfoliation. Sun exposure (ultraviolet irradiation) may be an aggravating factor. A blistering skin disease endemic to south central Brazil known as fogo selvagem or Brazilian pemphigus is clinically, histologically, and immunopathologically indistinguishable from PF.

Patients with PF have immunopathologic features in common with PV. Specifically, direct immunofluorescence microscopy of apparently normal, perilesional skin demonstrates IgG and C3 on the surface of keratinocytes. As in PV, patients with PF frequently have circulating IgG autoantibodies against keratinocyte cell surface antigens. Guinea pig esophagus is the optimal substrate for indirect immunofluorescence microscopy studies of sera from patients with PF.

PF is generally a far less severe disease than PV and carries a better prognosis. Localized disease can be treated conservatively with topical or intralesional glucocorticoids; more active cases can usually be controlled with systemic glucocorticoids, such as prednisone 20 to 40 mg/d.

BULLOUS PEMPHIGOID Bullous pemphigoid (BP) is a subepidermal blistering skin disease usually seen in the elderly. Lesions typically consist of tense blisters on either normal-appearing or erythematous skin. The lesions are usually distributed over the lower abdomen, groin, and flexor surface of the extremities; oral mucosal lesions are found in 10 to 40 percent of patients. Pruritus may be nonexistent or severe. As lesions evolve, tense blisters tend to rupture and be replaced by flaccid lesions or erosions with or without surmounting crust. Nontraumatized blisters heal without scarring. There is no ethnic or HLA association. Patients with BP do not have an increased incidence of malignancy in comparison with appropriately age- and sex-matched controls.

While biopsies of early lesional skin demonstrate subepidermal blisters, the histologic features depend on the character of the particular lesion. Lesions on normal-appearing skin generally show a sparse perivascular leukocytic infiltrate with some eosinophils. Biopsies of inflammatory lesions typically show an eosinophil-rich, leukocytic infiltrate within the papillary dermis, at sites of vesicle formation, and in perivascular areas. In addition to eosinophils, these cell-rich lesions also contain mononuclear cells and neutrophils. It is not always possible to distinguish BP from other subepidermal blistering skin diseases by routine histologic techniques.

Immunopathologic studies have broadened our understanding of this disease and aided its diagnosis. Direct immunofluorescence microscopy of normal-appearing, perilesional skin shows linear deposits of IgG and/or C3 in the epidermal basement membrane. Other immunoreactants such as factor B or C4 may be found in the same location. The sera of approximately 70 percent of these patients contain circulating IgG autoantibodies that bind the epidermal basement membrane of normal human skin in indirect immunofluorescence microscopy. No correlation exists between the titer of these autoantibodies and disease activity. The autoantibodies recognize a 220,000-dalton glycoprotein constituent of the basement membranes of normal stratified squamous epithelial cells. Autoantibodies are believed to develop against this antigen, deposit in situ, activate complement, elicit the accumulation and activation of leukocytes, and prompt dermal mast cell degranulation. The net consequence is to cause blister formation and tissue damage.

BP is generally benign, but may persist for months to years, with exacerbations or remissions. Although extensive involvement may result in widespread erosions and compromise cutaneous integrity, the mortality rate is low even in the absence of treatment. Nonetheless, deaths may occur in elderly and/or debilitated patients. The mainstay of treatment is systemic glucocorticoids. Patients with local or minimal disease can sometimes be controlled with topical glucocorticoids alone; patients with more extensive lesions generally respond to systemic glucocorticoids either alone or in combination with immunosuppressive agents. Patients will usually respond to prednisone 40 to 60 mg/d. In some instances azathioprine (1 mg/kg per day) or cyclophosphamide (1 mg/kg per day) are necessary adjuncts.

DERMATITIS HERPETIFORMIS Dermatitis herpetiformis (DH) is an intensely pruritic, chronic papulovesicular skin disease. The lesions are usually symmetrically distributed over extensor surfaces, including elbows, knees, buttocks, back, scalp, and posterior neck. The primary lesion in this disorder is a papule, papulovesicle, or urticarial plaque. Because pruritus is prominent, patients may present with excoriations and crusted papules but no observable primary lesions. Patients also sometimes report that their pruritus may have a distinctive burning or stinging component, and the onset of these local symptoms reliably heralds the development of distinct clinical lesions 12 to 24 h later. Granular deposits of IgA (with or without C3) are present in the epidermal basement membrane zone in both normal and lesional skin. Thus, while cutaneous deposits of IgA are thought to be very important in the pathogenesis of DH, they are not sufficient to cause lesions. Exactly what else is necessary to induce clinical lesions is not known. Almost all of these patients have an associated, usually subclinical, gluten-sensitive enteropathy (also see Chap. 240) and more than 90 percent express the HLA-B8/DRw3 and HLA-DQw2 haplotypes. Patients with DH and granular deposits of IgA within their epidermal basement membrane zone are distinguished from those with linear deposits of IgA at this site in their skin (see "Linear IgA Dermatosis"). DH may present at any age, including childhood; onset in the second to fourth decades is most common. The disease is typically chronic.

Biopsy of early lesional skin reveals neutrophil-rich infiltrates within dermal papillae. Neutrophils, fibrin, edema, and microvesicle formation at these sites are characteristic of early disease. Older lesions may demonstrate nonspecific features of a subepidermal bulla or an excoriated papule. Because the clinical and histologic features of this disease can be variable and resemble other subepidermal blistering disorders, the diagnosis can be confirmed by direct immunofluorescence microscopy of normal-appearing, perilesional skin. Such studies demonstrate the previously described granular deposits of IgA in the sublamina densa region of the basement membrane zone. Circulating autoantibodies directed against this site in skin have not been demonstrated. Hence, the importance of studying tissue samples for the presence of immunoreactants in situ for evidence of circulating autoantibodies is apparent. IgA deposits in the skin are unaffected by control of disease with medication; however, these immunoreactants may diminish in intensity or disappear in patients maintained for long periods on a strict gluten-free diet (see below).

Although most DH patients do not report overt gastrointestinal symptoms or laboratory evidence of malabsorption, biopsies of small bowel usually reveal blunting of intestinal villi and a lymphocytic infiltrate in the lamina propria. As is true for patients with celiac disease, this gastrointestinal abnormality can be reversed by a gluten-free diet. Moreover, if maintained for a long enough period of time, this diet alone may control the skin disease, and eventually it may not be possible to demonstrate IgA in the epidermal basement membrane zone. Subsequent gluten exposure in the latter patients alters the morphology of their small bowel, elicits a flare of their skin disease, and is associated with the reappearance of IgA in their epidermal basement membrane zone. Patients with DH also have an increased incidence of thyroid abnormalities, achlorhydria, atrophic gastritis, and antigastric parietal cell antibodies. These associations likely relate to the high frequency of the HLA-B8/DRw3 haplotype in these patients since this phenotype is commonly linked to autoimmune disorders. The mainstay of treatment is dapsone. Patients respond rapidly (24 to 48 h) to dapsone but require careful pretreatment evaluation and close follow-up to ensure that complications are avoided or controlled. All patients on more than 100 mg/d dapsone will have some hemolysis and methemoglobinemia. These are expected pharmacologic side effects of dapsone. It is important to employ the lowest possible maintenance dose of dapsone to control symptoms and lesions. Gluten restriction can control DH and lessen dapsone requirements, but this diet must rigidly exclude gluten to be of benefit. Moreover, many months of dietary restriction may be necessary before a beneficial result is achieved. Good dietary counselling by a trained dietitian is essential.

LINEAR IgA DERMATOSIS Linear IgA dermatosis (or linear IgA disease) was formerly considered a variant form of dermatitis herpetiformis. However, this disorder is actually a separate and distinct entity. Clinically, these patients may resemble typical cases of DH, bullous pemphigoid, or other subepidermal blistering skin diseases. Lesions typically consist of papulovesicles, bullae, and/or urticarial plaques, predominantly on extensor (as seen in "classic" DH), central, or flexural sites. Oral mucosal involvement does occur in selected patients. Severe pruritus resembles that in patients with DH. Patients with linear IgA dermatosis do not have an increased frequency of the HLA-B8/DRw3 haplotype or an associated enteropathy and hence are not candidates for a gluten-free diet.

The histologic alterations in early lesions may be virtually indistinguishable from those in DH. However, direct immunofluorescence microscopy of normal-appearing, perilesional skin reveals linear deposits of IgA (and often C3) in the epidermal basement membrane. Selected patients with linear IgA dermatosis demonstrate circulating IgA autoantibodies against normal epidermal basement membrane. As in classic DH, patients respond promptly to treatment with dapsone, 50 to 200 mg/d.

EPIDERMOLYSIS BULLOSA ACQUISITA Epidermolysis bullosa acquisita (EBA) is a rare, noninherited, polymorphic, subepidermal blistering skin disease. Since lesions generally occur in sites prone to minor trauma (e.g., dorsum of the hands, elbows, knees, etc.), EBA is regarded as a mechanobullous disease. Patients with the classic or noninflammatory form of this disease have blisters on noninflamed skin as well as atrophic scarring, milia, nail dystrophy, and oral lesions. Other patients with EBA have widespread inflammatory, scarring, bullous lesions and oromucosal involvement. Cases of inflammatory EBA resemble severe BP. In fact, many cases of EBA were probably incorrectly classified in the past as some other inflammatory blistering skin disease. Some patients present with an inflammatory bullous skin disease that subsequently evolves into the classic noninflammatory form of this disease. In general, EBA is a chronic disorder. Association with multiple myeloma, amyloidosis, inflammatory bowel disease, and diabetes mellitus has been reported. The HLA-DR2 haplotype is found with increased frequency.

The histology of lesional skin varies depending on the type or character of the lesion being studied. Noninflammatory bullae show subepidermal blisters with a sparse leukocytic infiltrate, and resemble those in lesional skin from patients with porphyria cutanea tarda. Inflammatory vesiculobullous lesions consist of a subepidermal blister with a neutrophil-rich leukocytic infiltrate within the superficial dermis. EBA patients have continuous deposits of IgG (and frequently C3) in a linear pattern within the epidermal basement membrane. These immunoreactants are also found in the sublamina densa region in association with anchoring fibrils. Approximately 25 to 50 percent of patients have circulating autoantibodies against normal epidermal basement membrane. These autoantibodies can be distinguished from those in BP by mapping the pattern of binding in indirect immunofluorescence microscopy. In brief, EBA sera bind to the base of 1-*M* NaCl split-skin substrate, while BP sera bind the roof. The antigen recognized by EBA autoantibodies is the globular carboxyl terminal domain of type VII procollagen.

Treatment of EBA is generally unsatisfactory. Some patients with inflammatory EBA may respond to systemic glucocorticoids, either alone or in combination with immunosuppressive agents. Other patients (especially those with neutrophil-rich inflammatory lesions) may respond to dapsone. The chronic, noninflammatory form of this disease is largely resistant to treatment.

AUTOIMMUNE SYSTEMIC DISEASES WITH PROMINENT CUTANEOUS FEATURES

DERMATOMYOSITIS The cutaneous manifestations of dermatomyositis (see Chap. 364) are often distinctive but at times may resemble those of systemic lupus erythematosus (SLE), scleroderma, or other overlapping connective tissue diseases. The extent and severity of cutaneous disease may or may not correlate with the extent and severity of the myositis. Patients with severe muscle involvement may have relatively minor skin changes, while patients with marked skin involvement may have mild muscle disease. The cutaneous manifestations of dermatomyositis are similar whether the disease appears in childhood or old age, except that calcification of subcutaneous tissue is a common late sequela in childhood dermatomyositis.

The cutaneous signs of dermatomyositis may precede or follow the development of myositis by weeks to years. The most common manifestation is a purple/red discoloration of the upper eyelids, sometimes associated with scaling ("heliotrope" erythema) and with periorbital edema. Erythema on the cheeks and nose in a "butterfly" distribution may resemble the eruption in SLE. Erythematous or violaceous scaling patches are common on the upper, anterior chest and the extensor surfaces of the arms, legs, and hands. Erythema and scaling may be particularly prominent over the elbows, knees, and the dorsal interphalangeal joints. Approximately one-third of patients have violaceous, flat-topped papules over the dorsal interphalangeal joints that are pathognomonic of dermatomyositis (Gottron's sign or Gottron's papules). These lesions can be contrasted with the erythema and scaling on the dorsum of the fingers in some patients with SLE which spares the skin over the interphalangeal joints. Periungual telangiectasia may be prominent, and a lacy or reticulated erythema may be associated with fine scaling on the extensor surfaces of the thighs and upper arms. Other patients, particularly those with long-standing disease, develop areas of hypopigmentation, hyperpigmentation, mild atrophy, and telangiectasia, known as poikiloderma vasculare atrophicans. Poikiloderma is rare in both SLE and scleroderma and thus can serve as a clinical sign that distinguishes dermatomyositis from these two diseases. However, cutaneous changes may be similar in scleroderma and dermatomyositis and may include thickening and binding down of the skin of the hands, sclerodactyly, and Raynaud's phenomenon. However, the presence of severe muscle disease, Gottron's papules, heliotrope erythema, and poikiloderma serve to distinguish these patients as having dermatomyositis. Skin biopsy of erythematous, scaling lesions of dermatomyositis may reveal only mild nonspecific inflammation but sometimes may show changes indistinguishable from those found in SLE including epidermal atrophy, hydropic degeneration of basal keratinocytes, edema of the upper dermis, and a mild mononuclear cell infiltrate. Direct immunofluorescence of lesional skin is usually negative. Treatment should be directed at the systemic disease. In the few instances where adjunctive cutaneous therapy is desirable, topical glucocorticoids are sometimes useful. These patients should avoid exposure to ultraviolet irradiation and use photoprotective measures such as sunscreens.

LUPUS ERYTHEMATOSUS The cutaneous manifestations of lupus erythematosus (LE) (see Chap. 269) can be divided into acute, subacute, and chronic (i.e., discoid LE) types. Acute cutaneous LE is characterized by erythema of the nose and malar eminences in a "butterfly" distribution. The erythema is often sudden in onset, accompanied by edema and fine scale, and correlated with systemic involvement. Patients may have widespread involvement of the face as well as erythema and scaling of the extensor surfaces of the extremities and upper chest. These acute lesions, while sometimes evanescent, usually last for days and are often associated with exacerbations of systemic disease. Skin biopsy of acute lesions may show only a sparse dermal infiltrate of mononuclear cells and dermal edema. In some instances cellular infiltrates around blood vessels and hair follicles are notable, as is hydropic degeneration of basal cells of the epidermis. Direct immunofluorescence of lesional skin frequently reveals deposits of immunoglobulin and complement in the epidermal basement membrane zone. Treatment is aimed at control of systemic disease; photoprotection in this, as well as other forms of LE, is very important.

Subacute cutaneous lupus erythematosus (SCLE) is characterized by a widespread photosensitive, nonscarring eruption that may take two forms. About one-half of these patients have SLE in which severe renal and CNS involvement is uncommon. The two forms of SCLE are a papulosquamous eruption that can resemble psoriasis and an annular form that may resemble erythema multiforme. In the papulosquamous form, discrete erythematous papules arise on the back, chest, shoulders, extensor surfaces of the arms, and the dorsum of the hands but are uncommon on the face, flexor surfaces of the arms, and below the waist. The slightly scaling papules tend to merge into large plaques, some with a reticulate appearance. The annular form involves the same areas and also begins as an erythematous papule but tends to develop oval, circular, or polycyclic lesions. The lesions of SCLE are more widespread but have less tendency for scarring than do lesions of discoid LE. Skin biopsy reveals a dense mononuclear cell infiltrate around hair follicles and blood vessels in the superficial dermis, combined with hydropic degeneration of basal cells in the epidermis. Direct immunofluorescence of lesional skin reveals deposits of immunoglobulin at the epidermal basement membrane zone in about half of cases. Most SCLE patients have anti-Ro antibodies. Local therapy is usually unsuccessful, and most patients require treatment with aminoquinoline antimalarials. Low-dose therapy with oral glucocorticoids is sometimes necessary; photoprotective measures are important.

Discoid lupus erythematosus (DLE) is characterized by discrete lesions, most often on the face, scalp, or external ears. The lesions are erythematous papules or plaques with a thick adherent scale that occludes hair follicles (follicular plugging). When the scale is removed, its underside will show small excrescences that correlate with the opening of hair follicles and is termed a "carpet tack" appearance. This finding is relatively specific for discoid LE. Long-standing lesions develop central atrophy, scarring, and hypopigmentation, but frequently have erythematous, sometimes raised, borders at the periphery. These lesions persist for years and tend to expand slowly. Only 5 to 10 percent of patients with DLE meet the American Rheumatism Association criteria for SLE. However, typical discoid lesions are frequently seen in patients with SLE. Biopsy of discoid LE shows hyperkeratosis, follicular plugging, and atrophy of the epidermis. The dermal-epidermal junction reveals hydropic degeneration of basal keratinocytes, and a mononuclear cell infiltrate surrounds hair follicles and blood vessels. Direct immunofluorescence demonstrates immunoglobulin and complement deposits at the basement membrane zone in about 90 percent of cases. Treatment is focused on control of local cutaneous disease and consists mainly of photoprotection and topical or intralesional glucocorticoids. If local therapy is ineffective, use of aminoquinoline antimalarials may be indicated.

SCLERODERMA AND MORPHEA The skin changes of scleroderma (see Chap. 271) usually begin on the hands, feet, and face, with episodes of recurrent nonpitting edema. Sclerosis of the skin begins distally on the fingers (sclerodactyly) and spreads proximally, usually accompanied by resorption of bone of the fingertips, which may have punched out ulcers, stellate scars, or areas of hemorrhage. The fingers may actually shrink in size and become sausage-shaped, and since the fingernails are usually unaffected the nails may curve over the end of the fingertips. Periungual telangiectasias are usually present, but periungual erythema is rare. In advanced cases, the extremities show contractures and calcinosis cutis. Face involvement includes a smooth, unwrinkled brow, taut skin over the nose, shrinkage of tissue around the mouth, and perioral radial furrowing. Matlike telangiectasias are often present, particularly on the face and hands. Involved skin feels indurated, smooth, and bound to underlying structures; hyperpigmentation and hypopigmentation are often also present. Raynaud's phenomenon, that is, cold-induced blanching, cyanosis, and reactive hyperemia, is present in almost all patients with scleroderma and can precede development of scleroderma by many years. The combination of calcinosis cutis, Raynaud's phenomenon, esophageal dysmotility, sclerodactyly, and telangiectasia has been termed the CREST syndrome. Anticentromere antibodies have been reported in a very high percentage of patients with the CREST syndrome but in only a small minority of patients with scleroderma. Skin biopsy reveals thickening of the dermis and homogenization of collagen bundles. Direct immunofluorescence of lesional skin is usually negative.

Morphea, which has been called localized scleroderma, is characterized by localized thickening and sclerosis of skin, usually affecting young adults or children. Morphea begins as erythematous or flesh-colored plaques that become sclerotic, develop central hypopigmentation, and demonstrate an erythematous border. In most cases, patients have one or a few lesions, and the disease is termed *localized morphea.* In some patients, widespread cutaneous lesions may occur, without systemic involvement. This form is called *generalized morphea.* Most patients with morphea do not have autoantibodies. Skin biopsy of morphea is indistinguishable from that of scleroderma. Linear scleroderma is a limited form of disease which presents in a linear, bandlike distribution and tends to involve deep as well as superficial layers of skin. Scleroderma and morphea are usually quite resistant to therapy with medications. For this reason, physical therapy to prevent joint contractures and to maintain function is employed and is often helpful.

Eosinophilic fasciitis is a clinical entity that can sometimes be confused with scleroderma. There is usually the sudden onset of swelling, induration, and erythema of the extremities frequently following significant physical exertion. The proximal portions of extremities (arms, forearms, thighs, legs) are more often involved than are the hands and feet. While the skin is indurated, it is usually not bound down as in scleroderma. These skin findings are accompanied by peripheral blood eosinophilia, increased erythrocyte sedimentation rate, and sometimes hypergammaglobulinemia. Deep biopsy of affected areas of skin reveals inflammation and thickening of the deep fascia overlying muscle. An inflammatory infiltrate composed of eosinophils and mononuclear cells is usually found. Patients with eosinophilic fasciitis appear to be at increased risk to develop bone marrow failure or other hematologic abnormalities. While the ultimate course of eosinophilic fasciitis is uncertain, many patients respond favorably to treatment with prednisone in doses ranging from 40 to 60 mg/d.

REFERENCES

BRAVERMAN IM: Connective tissue diseases, in *Skin Signs of Systemic Disease*. Philadelphia, Saunders, 1981, pp 255–377

GAMMON WR et al: Epidermolysis bullosa acquisita—a pemphigoid-like disease. J Am Acad Dermatol 11:820, 1984

HALL RP: The pathogenesis of dermatitis herpetiformis: Recent advances. J Am Acad Dermatol 16:1129, 1987

KATZ SI et al: Dermatitis herpetiformis: The skin and the gut. Ann Intern Med 93:857, 1980

KORMAN N: Pemphigus. J Am Acad Dermatol 18:1219, 1988

SHULMAN LE: Diffuse fasciitis with eosinophilia: A new syndrome. Arthritis Rheum 20 (Suppl):205, 1977

STANLEY JR: Bullous pemphigoid, in *Symposium on Blistering Disease, Dermatologic Clinics*, BV Jegasothy, GS Lazarus (eds). Philadelphia, Saunders, 1983, pp 205–216

YANCEY KB, LAWLEY TJ: The immunology of the skin, in *Allergy: Principles and Practice*, 3d ed, E Middleton, CE Reed, EF Ellis (eds). St. Louis, Mosby, 1988, pp 206–223

59 SKIN MANIFESTATIONS OF INTERNAL DISEASE

JEAN BOLOGNIA / IRWIN M. BRAVERMAN

It is now a generally accepted concept in medicine that the skin can show signs of internal disease. Therefore in textbooks of medicine, one finds a chapter describing in detail the major systemic disorders that can be identified by cutaneous signs. The underlying assumption of such a chapter is that the clinician has been able to identify the disorder in the patient and needs only to read about it in the textbook. In reality, concise differential diagnoses and the identification of these disorders is actually difficult for the nondermatologist because he or she is not well versed in the recognition of cutaneous lesions or their spectrum of presentations. Therefore the authors of this chapter have decided to cover this particular topic of cutaneous medicine not by discussing individual disorders but by describing and discussing the various presenting clinical signs and symptoms that indicate the presence of these disorders. Concise differential diagnoses will be generated in which the significant diseases will be briefly discussed and distinguished from the more common disorders that have no significance for internal diseases. The latter disorders are reviewed in table form and always need to be excluded when considering the former. For a detailed description of individual diseases, the reader should consult a dermatologic text. The categories of skin lesions that are discussed include: papulosquamous, erythroderma, alopecia, figurate, acne, telangiectasias, hypopigmentation, hyperpigmentation, vesicles/bullae, exanthems, urticaria, papulonodular, purpura, and ulcers. In an attempt to determine the appropriate category for a particular lesion, it is important to carefully examine its surface qualities, shape, and color in addition to the location and distribution (see Chap. 55).

PAPULOSQUAMOUS SKIN LESIONS (Table 59-1) When an eruption is characterized by elevated lesions, papules (<1 cm), or plaques (>1 cm), in association with scale, it is referred to as papulosquamous. The most common papulosquamous diseases—*psoriasis, tinea, pityriasis rosea,* and *lichen planus*—are primary cutaneous disorders (Table 59-2). When psoriatic lesions are accompanied by arthritis, the possibility of psoriatic arthritis or *Reiter's disease* should be considered. A history of oral ulcers, conjunctivitis, uveitis, and/or urethritis point to the latter diagnosis. In *guttate psoriasis*, there is an acute onset of small, widely scattered, uniform lesions, often in association with a streptococcal infection. Lithium, beta blockers, human immunodeficiency virus (HIV) infection, and a rapid taper of systemic glucocorticoids are also known to exacerbate psoriasis. Epidermal hyperproliferation and incomplete maturation are responsible for the plaque formation and scale that is characteristic of psoriasis.

Whenever the diagnosis of pityriasis rosea or lichen planus is made, it is important to review the patient's medications because the eruption can be treated by simply discontinuing the offending agent. Pityriasis rosea-like drug eruptions are seen most commonly with beta blockers, captopril, clonidine, gold, griseofulvin, isotretinoin, metronidazole, penicillin, and tripelennamine, while the drugs which can produce a lichenoid eruption include gold, antimalarials, thiazides, quinidine, phenothiazines, sulfonylureas, furosemide, methyldopa, griseofulvin, beta blockers, and captopril. Lichen planus-like lesions are also observed in chronic graft-versus-host disease. *Bowen's disease* represents squamous cell carcinoma in situ and it usually presents as a single lesion. The plaque is well demarcated, pink to red in color, and the amount of scale varies. Bowen's disease is found in both sun-exposed and sun-protected areas of the body, and the possibility of arsenic exposure should be explored in these patients, and an examination of the palms and soles for arsenical keratoses should be included.

Parapsoriasis is an intermediate disease, for it can remain solely as a primary cutaneous disease or it can progress to cutaneous T-cell lymphoma (CTCL) after a latency period of as long as 40 years. There are several forms of *parapsoriasis*, including small plaque (0.5 to 5 cm), large plaque (>6 cm), and retiform. The lesions of both small plaque and large plaque parapsoriasis are thin and salmon-pink in color with fine white scale. In small plaque, they are commonly on the trunk, but can be widely scattered. In large plaque, the most common location is the "girdle" area, and fine wrinkling secondary to epidermal atrophy is often seen. Retiform parapsoriasis forms a netlike pattern and the individual papules are red-brown and flat-topped. The latter two forms of parapsoriasis, large plaque and retiform, can progress to CTCL.

TABLE 59-1 Causes of papulosquamous skin lesions

Primary cutaneous disorders
- *A* Psoriasis
- *B* Tinea
- *C* Pityriasis rosea
- *D* Lichen planus
- *E* Parapsoriasis
- *F* Bowen's disease

Drugs

Systemic diseases
- *A* Lupus erythematosus
- *B* Cutaneous T-cell lymphoma
- *C* Secondary syphilis
- *D* Reiter's disease
- *E* Bazex' syndrome

TABLE 59-2 Papulosquamous skin diseases (primary cutaneous disorders)

	Characteristic lesion	Location	Other findings	Diagnostic aids
Psoriasis	Pink-red, silvery scale, sharply demarcated	Elbows, knees, scalp, presacral area	Nail dystrophy: pitting, onycholysis, yellow discoloration Arthritis: primarily small joints (hands and feet)	Skin biopsy
Tinea	Pink-red, central clearing common, active, scaling border	Inner thigh (tinea cruris), palms, soles, any area of body	Invasion of stratum corneum by dermatophytes	KOH and/or fungal culture of scale
Pityriasis rosea	Salmon-pink, oval shape, long axis follows lines of cleavage in the skin, peripheral collarette of scale	Trunk, proximal, extremities	Herald patch: initial lesion and usually the largest in size Spontaneous resolution over 2–3 months	Skin biopsy, VDRL to exclude secondary syphilis
Lichen planus	Violet-colored, polygonal, flat-topped, traversed by thin white lines (Wickham's striae)	Flexor wrists, ankles, presacral area, glans penis	Oral mucosa: lacelike white plaques and/or erosions Pruritus	Skin biopsy

Cutaneous T-cell lymphoma (CTCL), *secondary syphilis, lupus* (see "Papulonodular Skin Lesions," below), and *Bazex' syndrome* are less common papulosquamous disorders that are associated with systemic disease. A clue to the development of *CTCL* within lesions of large plaque or retiform parapsoriasis is an increase in the palpable component of the plaque (increased infiltration). In its early stages, CTCL may be confused with ezcema or psoriasis, but it often fails to respond to the appropriate therapy for those inflammatory diseases. The diagnosis of CTCL is established by skin biopsy in which collections of atypical T lymphocytes are found in the epidermis and dermis. As the disease progresses, cutaneous tumors and lymph node involvement may appear.

In *secondary syphilis,* there are scattered red-brown papules with thin scale. The eruption often involves the palms and soles and it can resemble pityriasis rosea. Associated findings are helpful in making the diagnosis and they include annular plaques on the face, nonscarring alopecia, condyloma lata (broad-based and moist), and mucous patches as well as lymphadenopathy, malaise, fever, headache, and myalgias. The interval between the primary chancre and the secondary stage is usually 4 to 8 weeks and spontaneous resolution without appropriate therapy is seen. When psoriasiform lesions are seen on the nose, ears, fingers, and toes, *Bazex' syndrome* should be considered. It is a distinctive paraneoplastic eruption associated with squamous cell carcinomas of the oropharynx, tracheobronchial tree, and esophagus.

ERYTHRODERMA (Table 59-3) Erythroderma is the term used when the majority of the skin surface is erythematous (red in color). There may be associated scale, erosions, or pustules as well as shedding of the hair and nails. Potential systemic manifestations include fever, chills, hypothermia, reactive lymphadenopathy, peripheral edema, hypoalbuminemia, increased transepidermal water loss and high-output cardiac failure. The major etiologies of erythroderma are: (1) *cutaneous diseases* such as psoriasis and dermatitis (Table 59-4); (2) *drugs;* (3) *systemic diseases,* most commonly CTCL; and (4) *idiopathic.* In the first three groups, the location and description of the initial lesions, prior to the development of the erythroderma, aid in the diagnosis. For example, a history of red scaly plaques on the elbows and knees would point to psoriasis. It is also important to examine the skin carefully for a migration of the erythema and associated secondary changes such as pustules or erosions. Migratory waves of erythema studded with superficial pustules are seen in *pustular psoriasis,* whereas erosive migratory erythema of the face and girdle area is seen in *necrolytic migratory erythema* (glucagonoma syndrome).

TABLE 59-3 Causes of erythroderma

Primary cutaneous disorders
- *A* Psoriasis
- *B* Dermatitis (atopic, stasis, contact, sebhorrheic)
- *C* Pityriasis rubra pilaris

Drugs

Systemic diseases
- *A* Cutaneous T-cell lymphoma
- *B* Lymphoma
- *C* Necrolytic migratory erythema

Idiopathic

An erythroderma secondary to an underlying cutaneous disease is most commonly due to *psoriasis* or one of the various forms of *dermatitis* (eczema). Each type of dermatitis has its own distinguishing features, but they may be limited to the initial lesions. Uncontrolled dermatitis can evolve into an erythroderma through a process known as "autosensitization" (conditioned hyperirritability), where initially uninvolved skin becomes pruritic and eventually dermatitic.

Drug-induced erythroderma (exfoliative dermatitis) may begin as a morbilliform eruption or it may arise as diffuse erythema. Fever and peripheral eosinophilia often accompany the eruption. There are a number of *drugs* that can produce an erythroderma, including penicillins, sulfonamides, barbiturates, phenytoin, gold, allopurinol, captopril, D-penicillamine, sulfonylureas, and furosemide. Reactions to allopurinol may also be accompanied by hepatitis and nephropathy, especially in patients with impaired renal function given full doses of allopurinol plus a diuretic.

The most common malignancy that is associated with erythroderma is *CTCL;* in some series, up to 25 percent of the cases of erythroderma were due to CTCL. The patient may progress from isolated plaques and tumors, or the erythroderma may be the initial manifestation (Sézary syndrome). In the Sézary syndrome, there are circulating atypical T lymphocytes, pruritus, and lymphadenopathy. Additional findings include keratoderma and leonine facies. In cases of erythroderma where there is no apparent cause (idiopathic), longitudinal follow-up is mandatory to monitor the possible development of CTCL. Other types of *lymphoma* can be associated with erythroderma, including Hodgkin's and non-Hodgkin's lymphoma, the former being more common. There have also been isolated case reports of erythroderma secondary to some solid tumors—lung, liver, prostate, thyroid, and colon—but it is usually in a late stage of the disease.

ALOPECIA (Table 59-5) The two major forms of alopecia are scarring and nonscarring. In scarring alopecia, there is associated fibrosis, inflammation, and loss of hair follicles. A smooth scalp with a decreased number of follicular openings is usually observed clinically, but in some cases, the changes are only seen in biopsy specimens from the affected areas. In nonscarring alopecia, the hair shafts are gone, but the hair follicles are preserved, explaining the reversible nature of nonscarring alopecia.

Primary cutaneous disorders are the most common causes of nonscarring alopecia and they include *telogen effluvium, androgenetic alopecia, alopecia areata, tinea capitis,* and *traumatic alopecia* (Table 59-6). In women with androgenetic alopecia, an elevation in circulating levels of androgens may be seen as a result of ovarian or adrenal gland dysfunction. When there are signs of virilization, such

TABLE 59-4 Erythroderma (primary cutaneous disorders)

	Initial lesions	Location of initial lesions	Other findings	Diagnostic aids
Psoriasis	Pink-red, silvery scale, sharply demarcated	Elbows, knees, scalp, presacral area	Nail dystrophy, arthritis, pustules	Skin biopsy
Dermatitis:				
Atopic	Acute: Erythema, fine scale, crust, indistinct borders Chronic: Lichenification (increased skin markings)	Antecubital and popliteal fossae, neck, hands	Pruritus Family history of atopy, including asthma, allergic rhinitis or conjunctivitis, and atopic dermatitis Rule out secondary infection with *S. aureus* Rule out superimposed irritant contact dermatitis	Skin biopsy
Stasis	Erythema, crusting, excoriations	Lower extremities	Pruritus, lower extremity edema History of venous ulcers, thrombophlebitis, and/or cellulitis Rule out cellulitis Rule out superimposed contact dermatitis, e.g., topical neomycin	Skin biopsy
Contact (local)	Erythema, crusting, vesicles and bullae	Depends upon offending agent	Irritant—onset often within hours Allergic—delayed type hypersensitivity; lag time of 48 h	Patch testing
Contact (systemic)	Erythema, fine scale, crust	Generalized	Patient has history of allergic contact dermatitis to topical agent then receives systemic medication that is structurally related, e.g., ethylenediamine (topical) aminophyline (IV)	Patch testing
Seborrheic	Pink-red, greasy scale	Scalp, nasolabial folds, eyebrows, intertriginous zones	Flares with stress HIV infection Associated with Parkinson's disease	None
Pityriasis rubra pilaris	Orange-red, perifollicular, papules	Generalized, but characteristic "skip" areas of normal skin	Wax-like keratoderma Rule out cutaneous T-cell lymphoma	Skin biopsy

TABLE 59-5 Causes of alopecia

Nonscarring alopecia
- *A* Primary cutaneous disorders
  - *1* Telogen effluvium
  - *2* Androgenetic alopecia
  - *3* Alopecia areata
  - *4* Tinea capitis
  - *5* Traumatic alopecia
- *B* Drugs
- *C* Systemic diseases
  - *1* Lupus erythematosus
  - *2* Secondary syphilis
  - *3* Hypothyroidism
  - *4* Hyperthyroidism
  - *5* Deficiencies of protein, iron, biotin, and zinc

Scarring alopecia
- *A* Primary cutaneous disorders
  - *1* Lichen planus
  - *2* Folliculitis decalvans
  - *3* Pseudopelade
  - *4* Linear scleroderma (morphea)
- *B* Systemic diseases
  - *1* Lupus erythematosus
  - *2* Sarcoidosis
  - *3* Cutaneous metastases

as a deepened voice and enlarged clitoris, the possibility of an ovarian or adrenal gland tumor should be considered.

Exposure to various *drugs* can also cause diffuse hair loss, usually by inducing a telogen effluvium. An exception is the anagen effluvium observed with antimitotic agents such as daunorubicin. Alopecia is a side effect of the following drugs: warfarin, heparin, propylthiouracil, carbimazole, vitamin A, isotretinoin, etretinate, lithium, beta blockers, levodopa, amphetamines, and thallium. Fortunately, spontaneous regrowth usually follows the discontinuation of the offending agent.

Less commonly, nonscarring alopecia is associated with *lupus erythematosus* and *secondary syphilis*. In systemic lupus, there are two forms of alopecia—one is scarring secondary to discoid lesions (see below) and the other is nonscarring. The latter form may be diffuse and involve the entire scalp or it may localized to the frontal

TABLE 59-6 Nonscarring alopecia (primary cutaneous disorders)

	Clinical characteristics	Pathogenesis
Telogen effluvium	Diffuse shedding of normal hairs Follows either major stress (high fever, severe infection) or change in hormones (post partum) Reversible without treatment	Stress causes the normally asynchronous growth cycles of individual hairs to become synchronous; therefore, large numbers of growing (anagen) hairs simultaneously enter the dying (telogen) phase
Androgenetic alopecia	Miniaturization of hairs along the midline of the scalp Recession of the anterior scalp line in men and some women	Increased sensitivity of affected hairs to the effects of testosterone Increased levels of circulating androgens (ovarian or adrenal source)
Alopecia areata	Well circumscribed, circular areas of hair loss, 2–5 cm in diameter In extensive cases, coalescence of lesions and/or involvement of other hair-bearing surfaces of the body	The germinative zones of the hair follicles are surrounded by T lymphocytes Occasional associated diseases: hyperthyroidism, hypothyroidism, vitiligo, Down's syndrome
Tinea	Varies from scaling with minimal hair loss, to discrete patches with "black dots" (broken hairs), to boggy plaque with pustules (kerion)	Invasion of hairs by dermatophytes, most commonly *Trichophyton tonsurans*
Traumatic alopecia	Broken hairs Irregular outline	Traction with curlers, rubber bands, braiding Exposure to heat or chemicals Mechanical pulling (trichotillomania)

TABLE 59-7 Causes of figurate skin lesions

Primary cutaneous disorders
A Tinea
B Urticaria
C Erythema annulare centrifugum
D Granuloma annulare
Systemic diseases
A Migratory
1 Erythema chronicum migrans
2 Erythema gyratum repens
3 Erythema marginatum
4 Pustular psoriasis
5 Necrolytic migratory erythema
B Nonmigratory
1 Sarcoidosis
2 Subacute lupus erythematosus
3 Secondary syphilis
4 Cutaneous T-cell lymphoma
5 Elastosis perforans serpiginosa

scalp in the form of multiple short hairs (''lupus hairs''). Scattered, poorly circumscribed patches of alopecia with a ''moth-eaten'' appearance are a manifestation of the secondary stage of syphilis (see ''Papulosquamous Skin Lesions''). Diffuse thinning of the hair is also associated with hypothyroidism, hyperthyroidism, hypopituitarism, and deficiencies of protein, iron, biotin, and zinc.

Scarring alopecia is more frequently the result of a primary cutaneous disorder such as *lichen planus, folliculitis decalvans,* or *linear scleroderma (morphea)* than it is a sign of systemic disease. For example, the scarring lesions of *discoid lupus* are seen in patients with systemic lupus; however, in the majority of cases, the disease process is limited to the skin. Less common causes of scarring alopecia include *sarcoidosis* (see ''Papulonodular Skin Lesions''), cutaneous *metastases,* and *pseudopelade.* The latter disease may be idiopathic and arise de novo or it can represent the inactive end-stage phase of a previous inflammatory process such as lichen planus, sarcoid, or discoid lupus. The irregularly shaped areas of alopecia lack inflammation and often arise at an acute angle from the midline.

In the early phases of discoid lupus, lichen planus, and folliculitis decalvans, there are circumscribed areas of alopecia. Fibrosis and subsequent loss of follicles are observed primarily in the center of the individual lesions while the inflammatory process is most prominent at the periphery. The areas of active inflammation in *discoid lupus* are erythematous with scale. The areas of previous inflammation are often hypopigmented with a rim of hyperpigmentation. In *lichen planus,* the peripheral perifollicular papules are violet-colored and postinflammatory hyperpigmentation is a characteristic finding. Complete examination of the skin and oral mucosa combined with a biopsy and direct immunofluorescence will aid in distinguishing these two entities. The peripheral active lesions in *folliculitis decalvans* are perifollicular pustules which routinely grow *Staphylococcus aureus* or normal flora. These patients often have other forms of acne and folliculitis and can develop a reactive arthritis.

FIGURATE SKIN LESIONS (Table 59-7) In figurate eruptions, the lesions form rings and arcs which are usually erythematous, but can be flesh-colored to brown. Most commonly, they are due to primary cutaneous diseases such as *tinea, urticaria, erythema annulare centrifugum,* and *granuloma annulare* (Table 59-8). An underlying systemic illness is found in a second, less common, group of migratory annular erythemas. It includes *erythema gyratum repens, erythema chronicum migrans* (ECM), and *erythema marginatum.*

In *erythema gyratum repens,* one sees hundreds of mobile concentric arcs and wavefronts which resemble the grain in wood. A search for an underlying malignancy is mandatory in a patient with this eruption. *ECM* is the cutaneous manifestation of Lyme disease, which is caused by the spirochete *Borrelia burgdorferi.* In the initial stage (3 to 30 days after tick bite), a single annular lesion is usually seen, which can expand to $\geq$10 cm in diameter. Within several days, approximately half of the patients develop multiple smaller erythematous lesions at sites distant from the bite. Associated symptoms include fever, headache, myalgias, photophobia, arthralgias, and malar rash. *Erythema marginatum* is seen in patients with rheumatic fever, primarily on the trunk. Lesions are pink-red in color, flat to mildly elevated, and transient. If pustules are noted within a figurate eruption, consider *pustular psoriasis,* and if erosions are seen, consider *necrolytic migratory erythema.*

There are additional cutaneous diseases that present as annular eruptions, but they lack an obvious migratory component. Examples include *CTCL,* annular cutaneous *lupus,* also referred to as subacute lupus (see ''Papulonodular Skin Lesions''), secondary *syphilis,* and *sarcoidosis* (see ''Papulonodular Skin Lesions''). The most common clinical setting for the annular form of secondary lues is the face of black patients; a clue to this diagnosis is the presence of central hyperpigmentation. If keratotic plugs are noted within the annular or arciform lesions, particularly if they are localized to the neck and antecubital fossae, consider *elastosis perforans serpiginosa* (EPS). EPS is seen as a side effect of D-penicillamine and in patients with Down's syndrome and disorders of elastin and collagen. The latter include Ehlers-Danlos type IV and Marfan's syndromes, pseudoxanthoma elasticum, and osteogenesis imperfecta.

ACNE (Table 59-9) *Acne vulgaris* and *acne rosacea* are the two major forms of acne (Table 59-10). Estrogens decrease sebaceous gland activity, whereas androgens enhance sebum production. Therefore, acne vulgaris in an adult, especially if it is of recent onset, may be a reflection of increased levels of circulating *androgens.* Dysfunction of the ovary or adrenal gland, e.g., polycystic ovary disease, Cushing's syndrome or partial deficiency of the enzyme 21-hydroxylase, can lead to the hormonal imbalance. Examination of the patient for signs such as hirsutism, androgenetic alopecia, hypertension, and redistribution of subcutaneous fat will aid in the diagnosis. In patients with acne conglobata, a more severe form of acne characterized by multiple cysts and bridging scars, an associated inflammatory arthritis has been described.

Exposure to chlorinated aromatic hydrocarbons such as dioxin (TCDD) leads to a particular form of acne known as chloracne, which is characterized by open comedones and straw-colored cysts. Patients exposed to dioxin can also develop the signs and symptoms of porphyria cutanea tarda (see ''Vesicles''). Exacerbations of acne

TABLE 59-8 Figurate eruptions (primary cutaneous disorders)

	Clinical characteristics	Pathogenesis
Tinea	Active, scaling erythematous border with central clearing Expands slowly	Invasion of stratum corneum by dermatophytes
Urticaria	Central wheal with erythematous flare Transient and/or migratory Pruritic	Release of histamine from mast cells via immunologic (IgE, type 1 hypersensitivity) or nonimmunologic mechanisms
Erythema annulare centrifugum	Enlarges slowly Erythematous, flat or slightly raised ''Trailing scale''—scale on inner aspect of expending ring Buttock, upper thighs	Not known Usually idiopathic Sometimes associated with tinea pedis, drug hypersensitivity Rarely, paraneoplastic
Granuloma annulare	Border composed of flesh-colored to red-brown papules Extremities	Granulomatous process is limited to the skin Unknown etiology Disseminated form is associated with diabetes mellitus

TABLE 59-9 Causes of acneiform eruptions

Primary cutaneous disorders
- *A* Acne vulgaris
- *B* Acne rosacea

Drugs
Systemic diseases
- *A* Increased androgen production
  - *1* Adrenal origin, e.g., Cushing's disease, 21-hydroxylase deficiency
  - *2* Ovarian origin, e.g., polycystic ovary disease
- *B* Cryptococcosis, disseminated

vulgaris follow the ingestion of several *drugs,* such as iodides, bromides, vitamin B_{12}, glucocorticoids, and lithium, as well as the application of oil-containing compounds. In addition, high dose oral glucocorticoids can cause a widespread eruption of perifollicular pustules (folliculitis) on the trunk, characterized by lesions in the same stage of development. In immunocompromised hosts, disseminated *cryptococcosis* may present as an acneiform eruption.

Patients with the carcinoid syndrome have episodes of flushing of the head, neck, and sometimes the trunk. Resultant skin changes of the face, in particular telangiectasias, mimic the clinical appearance of acne rosacea. Suffusion of the face, as is seen in polycythemia vera, can also be confused with acne rosacea.

TELANGIECTASIAS (Table 59-11) In order to distinguish the various types of telangiectasias, it is important to examine the shape and configuration of the dilated blood vessels. *Linear telangiectasias* are seen on the face of patients with *actinically damaged skin* and *acne rosacea* and are found on the legs of patients with *venous hypertension* and *essential telangiectasia* (Table 59-12). Patients with an unusual form of *mastocytosis* (telangiectasia macularis eruptiva perstans), the *carcinoid* syndrome (see "Acne"), and *ataxia-telangiectasia* also have linear telangiectasias. In ataxia-telangiectasia, linear telangiectasias appear on the bulbar conjunctiva during childhood. Eventually, there is involvement of the ears, eyelids, cheeks, and/or flexural areas such as the antecubital and popliteal fossae. Lastly, linear telangiectasias are found in areas of cutaneous inflammation. For example, lesions of discoid lupus frequently have telangiectasias within them.

Poikiloderma is a term used to describe a patch of skin with (1) reticulated hypo- and hyperpigmentation, (2) wrinkling secondary to epidermal atrophy, and (3) telangiectasias. Poikiloderma does not imply a single disease entity—it is seen in skin damaged by *ionizing radiation,* in the disorders *poikiloderma vasculare atrophicans* (PVA) and *xeroderma pigmentosum,* as well as in patients with connective tissue diseases, primarily *dermatomyositis.* PVA is a precursor lesion of CTCL, and the areas of poikiloderma usually begin in the flexural areas of the axillae and groin.

In *scleroderma,* the dilated blood vessels have a unique configuration and are known as *mat telangiectasias.* The lesions are broad macules that usually measure 2 to 7 mm in diameter; occasionally they are larger in size. Mats have a polygonal or oval shape and their erythematous color may be uniform or the result of delicate telangiectasias. The most common locations for mat telangiectasias are the face, oral mucosa, and hands—peripheral sites that are prone to intermittent ischemia. One theory is that the mats represent a form of neovascularization in these areas. In the CREST variant of scleroderma (see Chap. 271), which is associated with a chronic course and anticentromere antibodies, the *T* stands for telangiectasias. Mat telangiectasias are an important clue to the diagnosis of the CREST syndrome as well as systemic scleroderma, for they may be the only cutaneous finding. A minority of the patients with scleroderma will have telangiectasias indistinguishable from those found in hereditary hemorrhagic telangiectasia (see below).

Periungual telangiectasias are pathognomonic signs of the three major connective tissue diseases—*lupus erythematosus, scleroderma,* and *dermatomyositis* (DM). They are easily visualized by the naked eye and they occur in at least two-thirds of these patients. In both DM and lupus, there is associated nailfold erythema and in DM, the erythema is often accompanied by "ragged" cuticles and fingertip tenderness. Under 10× magnification, the blood vessels in the nailfolds of lupus patients are tortuous and resemble "glomeruli," whereas in scleroderma and DM, there is a loss of capillary loops and those that remain are markedly dilated.

In *hereditary hemorrhagic telangiectasia* (Osler-Rendu-Weber disease), the lesions usually appear during adulthood and are most commonly seen on the mucous membranes, face, and distal extremities, including under the nails. They represent arteriovenous (AV) malformations of the dermal microvasculature, are dark red in color, and are usually slightly elevated. When the skin is stretched over an individual lesion, an eccentric punctum with radiating legs is seen. Although the degree of systemic involvement varies in this autosomal dominant disease, the major symptoms are recurrent epistaxis and gastrointestinal bleeding. The fact that these mucosal telangiectasias are actually AV malformations helps to explain their tendency to bleed. Patients should also be screened for pulmonary AV fistulas because of the associated complications of hypoxia, bleeding, and paradoxic emboli.

HYPOPIGMENTATION (Table 59-13) Disorders of hypopigmentation are classified as either diffuse or localized. The classic example of *diffuse* hypopigmentation is *oculocutaneous albinism* (OCA). The two most common forms are tyrosinase-negative OCA and tyrosinase-positive OCA; the former is characterized by a lack of enzyme activity. At birth, both types of OCA appear similar—white hair, gray-blue eyes, and pink-white skin. The patients with tyrosinase-negative OCA maintain this phenotype, whereas those with tyrosinase-positive OCA will acquire some pigmentation of the eyes, hair, and skin as they age. The degree of pigment formation is a function of their racial background, but a pigmentary dilution is readily apparent when they are compared to their first-degree relatives.

The ocular findings in OCA correlate with the degree of hypopigmentation and they include decreased visual acuity, nystagmus, photophobia, and monocular vision. Patients with OCA, particularly those who reside in the tropics, develop cutaneous squamous cell carcinomas in association with severe actinic damage. The diagnosis of tyrosinase-positive OCA in a patient from Puerto Rico (Arecibo region) or southern Holland raises the possibility of the Hermansky-Pudlak syndrome. In addition to the signs and symptoms of OCA, these patients have a bleeding diathesis secondary to a platelet storage pool defect and restrictive lung disease secondary to deposits of

TABLE 59-10 Acne (primary cutaneous disorders)

	Clinical characteristics	Pathogenesis
Acne vulgaris	Erythematous papules, pustules, open comedones (blackheads), closed comedones (whiteheads), and cysts Areas that contain sebaceous glands: face, neck, upper trunk	Epithelial hyperproliferation within the infundibulum of the hair follicle leads to comedone formation Additional factors: sebum-derived free fatty acids, *Propionibacterium acnes*
Acne rosacea	Papules, pustules; central face Telangiectasias of nose and cheeks Facial erythema Flushing reaction to hot foods and alcohol Ocular involvement: conjunctivitis, blepharitis, keratitis	Unknown No increased reactivity of cutaneous blood vessels to vasodilators Sebum production normal

TABLE 59-11 Causes of telangiectasias

Primary cutaneous disorders	Systemic diseases
A Linear	*A* Linear
1 Acne rosacea	*1* Carcinoid
2 Actinically damaged skin	*2* Ataxia-telangiectasia
3 Venous hypertension	*3* Mastocytosis
4 Essential telangiectasia	*B* Poikiloderma
B Poikiloderma	*1* Dermatomyositis
1 Ionizing radiation	*2* Xeroderma pigmentosa
2 Poikiloderma vasculare atrophicans	*C* Mat
C Spider angioma	*1* Scleroderma
1 Idiopathic	*D* Periungual
2 Pregnancy	*1* Lupus erythematosus
	2 Scleroderma
	3 Dermatomyositis
	E Papular
	1 Hereditary hemorrhagic telangiectasia
	F Spider angioma
	1 Cirrhosis

ceroidlike material. Generalized vitiligo, phenylketonuria, and homocystinuria are other unusual causes of diffuse pigmentary dilution. In generalized vitiligo, melanocytes are not found in affected skin, whereas in OCA they are present but have decreased activity. Appropriate laboratory tests exclude the other disorders of metabolism.

The differential diagnosis of *localized* hypomelanosis includes the following primary cutaneous disorders: *vitiligo, chemical leukoderma, piebaldism, nevus depigmentosus* (see below), *postinflammatory hypomelanosis,* and *tinea versicolor* (Table 59-14). In this group of diseases, the areas of involvement are macules or patches with a decrease or absence of pigmentation, and in the first four disorders, secondary changes such as scale or crust are absent. Patients with vitiligo have an increased incidence of several autoimmune disorders, including hypothyroidism, Graves' disease, pernicious anemia, Addison's disease, uveitis, alopecia areata, chronic mucocutaneous candidiasis, and the polyglandular autoimmune syndromes (types I, II, and III). Diseases of the thyroid gland are the most frequently associated disorders, occurring in up to 30 percent of patients with vitiligo. Circulating autoantibodies are often found and the most common ones are antithyroglobulin and antimicrosomal and antiparietal cell antibodies.

There are three systemic diseases which should be considered in a patient with skin findings suggestive of vitiligo—*Vogt-Koyanagi-Harada syndrome, scleroderma,* and *melanoma-associated leukoderma.* A history of aseptic meningitis, nontraumatic uveitis, tinnitus, hearing loss, and/or dysacusis points to the diagnosis of the Vogt-Koyanagi-Harada syndrome. In these patients, the face and scalp are the most common locations of pigment loss. The vitiligo-like leukoderma seen in patients with scleroderma has a clinical resemblance to idiopathic vitiligo that has begun to repigment as a result of treatment; that is, there are perifollicular macules of normal pigmentation within areas of depigmentation. The basis of this leukoderma is unknown; there is no evidence of inflammation in areas of involvement, but it can resolve if the underlying connective tissue disease becomes inactive. In contrast to idiopathic vitiligo, melanoma-associated leukoderma often begins on the trunk and its appearance should prompt a search for metastatic disease. The possibility exists that the destruction of normal melanocytes is the result of an immune response against malignant melanocytes.

There are two systemic disorders that have the cutaneous findings of piebaldism (partial albinism) (Table 59-14). They are Hirschsprung's disease and Waardenburg's syndrome. A possible explanation for both disorders is an abnormal embryonic migration or survival of two neural crest-derived elements, one of them being melanocytes and the other myenteric ganglion cells (Hirschsprung's disease) or auditory nerve cells (Waardenburg's syndrome). The latter syndrome is characterized by congenital sensorineural hearing loss, dystopia canthorum (lateral displacement of the inner canthi, but normal interpupillary distance), heterochromic irises, and a broad nasal root, in addition to the piebaldism.

In *tuberous sclerosis,* the earliest cutaneous sign is the ash leaf spot. These lesions are often present at birth; however, detection may require Wood's lamp examination, especially in fair-skinned individuals. The pigment within them is reduced but not absent. The average size is 1 to 3 cm and the common shapes are oval, polygonal, and lance-ovate, while the less common shapes are dermatomal and confettilike. The terms lance-ovate and ash leaf are used to describe lesions with a particular shape, that is, tapered at one end and round at the other. Examination of the patient for additional cutaneous signs such as adenoma sebaceum (multiple angiofibromas of the face), ungual and gingival fibromas, fibrous plaques of the forehead, and connective tissue nevi (shagreen patches) is recommended. It is important to remember that an ash leaf spot on the scalp will result in poliosis, which is a circumscribed patch of gray-white hair. Internal manifestations include seizures, mental retardation, central nervous system (CNS) and retinal hamartomas, renal angiomyolipomas, and cardiac rhabdomyomas.

Nevus depigmentosus is a stable, well-circumscribed hypomelanosis that is present at birth. There is usually a single circular or rectangular lesion, but occasionally the nevus has a dermatomal or whorled pattern. It is important to distinguish this lesion from ash leaf spots and hypomelanosis of Ito, for it is rarely associated with CNS findings. *Hypomelanosis of Ito* (incontinentia pigmenti achromians) is an autosomal dominant disorder in which swirls and streaks of hypopigmentation run parallel to one another. The pattern resembles that of a marble cake. Associated abnormalities are found in the musculoskeletal system (asymmetry), the CNS (seizures and mental retardation), and the eyes (strabismus and hypertelorism). Chromosomal mosaicism and diploid/triploid mixoploidy have been reported in these patients; this lends support to the hypothesis that the pattern is the result of the migration of two clones of primordial melanocytes, each with a different pigment potential.

Localized areas of decreased pigmentation are commonly seen as a result of cutaneous inflammation (Table 59-14) and have been observed in the skin overlying active lesions of *sarcoidosis* (see

TABLE 59-12 Telangiectasias (primary cutaneous disorders)

Type	Associated disorder	Clinical characteristics	Pathogenesis
Linear: Simple red or blue line that disappears with diascopy (pressure)	Acne rosacea	Face Associated with flushing, erythema, papulopustules, and rhinophyma	Vasodilatation
	Actinically damaged skin	Face, arms, upper trunk Associated with hypopigmentation, hyperpigmentation, and keratoses	Damage to supportive connective tissue
	Essential telangiectasia	Netlike sheets Begins on lower extremities May be widespread More common in women	Unknown
Spider angioma: Central pulsating punctum with radiating legs	Idiopathic Pregnancy	Upper half of the body Halo of pallor secondary to local steal phenomenon	Proliferation of blood vessels in association with increased circulating estrogens

TABLE 59-13 Causes of hypopigmentation

Primary cutaneous disorders	Systemic diseases
A Diffuse	*A* Diffuse
1 Generalized vitiligo	*1* Oculocutaneous albinism
B Localized	*B* Localized
1 Vitiligo	*1* Vogt-Koyanagi-Harada
2 Chemical leukoderma	*2* Scleroderma
3 Piebaldism	*3* Melanoma-associated leukoderma
4 Nevus depigmentosus	*4* Tuberous sclerosis
5 Postinflammatory	*5* Hypomelanosis of Ito
6 Tinea versicolor	*6* Sarcoidosis
	7 Tuberculoid leprosy
	8 Cutaneous T-cell lymphoma

"Papulonodular Skin Lesions") as well as *CTLC*. Cutaneous infections also present as disorders of hypopigmentation and in *tuberculoid leprosy,* there are a few asymmetric patches of hypomelanosis that have associated anesthesia, anhidrosis, and alopecia. Biopsy specimens of the palpable border show dermal granulomas that lack *Mycobacterium leprae* organisms.

HYPERPIGMENTATION (Table 59-15) Disorders of hyperpigmentation are also divided into two groups—localized and diffuse. The *localized* forms are due to an epidermal alteration, a proliferation of melanocytes, or an increase in pigment production. Both *seborrheic keratoses* and *acanthosis nigricans* belong to the first group (Table 59-16). Seborrheic keratoses are common lesions, but in one clinical setting they are a sign of systemic disease, and that setting is the sudden appearance of multiple lesions, often in association with acrocordons (skin tags) and acanthosis nigricans. This is termed the *sign of Leser-Trélat* and it signifies an internal malignancy. *Acanthosis nigricans* can also be a reflection of an internal malignancy, most commonly of the gastrointestinal tract, and it appears as velvety hyperpigmentation (Table 59-16). In the majority of patients, acanthosis nigricans is associated with obesity, but it may be a reflection of an endocrinopathy such as acromegaly, Cushing's syndrome, Addison's disease, the Stein-Leventhal syndrome, or insulin-resistant diabetes mellitus (type A, type B, and lipoatrophic forms).

A proliferation of melanocytes results in the following pigmented lesions: *lentigo,* nevocellular *nevus,* and *melanoma* (Table 59-16). In an adult, the majority of lentigines are related to sun exposure, which explains their distribution. However, in the Peutz-Jeghers and LEOPARD syndromes, lentigines do serve as a clue to systemic disease. The lentigines in patients with *Peutz-Jeghers* syndrome are located primarily around the nose and mouth, on the hands and feet, and within the oral cavity. While the pigmented macules on the face may fade with age, the oral lesions persist. However, similar intraoral lesions are also seen in Addison's disease and as a normal finding in darkly pigmented individuals. Patients with this autosomal dominant syndrome have multiple benign polyps of the gastrointestinal tract, ovarian tumors, and an approximately 6 percent risk of developing a gastrointestinal malignancy when the polyps arise in the stomach, duodenum, or colon.

In the multiple lentigines or *LEOPARD syndrome,* hundreds of lentigines develop during childhood and are scattered over the entire surface of the body. The syndrome consists of *L,* lentigines; *E,* ECG abnormalities, primarily conduction defects; *O,* ocular hypertelorism;

TABLE 59-14 Hypopigmentation (primary cutaneous disorders, localized)

	Clinical characteristics	Wood's lamp examination (UV-A: peak = 365 nm)	Skin biopsy	Pathogenesis
Vitiligo	Acquired; progressive Symmetric areas of complete pigment loss Periorifical—around mouth, nose, eyes, nipples, umbilicus, anus Other areas—flexor wrists, extensor distal extremities Segmental form is less common—unilateral, dermatomal-like	More apparent Chalk-white	Absence of melanocytes Occasional inflammation	Possible autoimmune phenomenon that results in destruction of melanocytes—humoral and/or cellular Alternative hypothesis is self-destruction of melanocytes and circulating antibodies against melanocytes as a secondary phenomenon
Chemical leukoderma	Similar appearance to vitiligo Often begins on hands Satellite lesions in areas not exposed to chemicals	More apparent Chalk-white	Decreased number or absence of melanocytes	Exposure to chemicals that selectively destroy melanocytes, in particular, phenols and catechols (germicides; rubber products) Release of cellular antigens and activation of circulating lymphocytes may explain satellite phenomenon
Piebaldism	Autosomal dominant Congenital, stable White forelock Areas of hypomelanosis contain normally pigmented and hyperpigmented macules of various sizes Symmetric involvement of central forehead, ventral trunk, and mid regions of upper and lower extremities	Enhancement of leukoderma and hyperpigmented macules	Hypomelanotic areas—few to no melanocytes	Defect in migration of melanoblasts from neural crest to ventral skin or failure of melanoblasts to survive or differentiate in these areas
Post-inflammatory	Hypopigmentation can develop within active lesions, as in subacute lupus, or after the lesion fades, as in dermatitis	Depends upon particular disease Usually less enhancement than in vitiligo	Type of inflammatory infiltrate depends upon specific disease	Block in transfer of melanin from melanocytes to keratinocytes could be secondary to edema or decrease in contact time Destruction of melanocytes if inflammatory cells attack basal layer
Tinea versicolor	Common disorder Upper trunk and neck Shawl-like distribution Young adults Macules have fine white scale when scratched	Golden fluorescence	Hyphae and spores in stratum corneum	Invasion of stratum corneum by the yeast *Pityrosporum* Yeast is lipophilic and produces C_9 and C_{11} dicarboxylic acids which in vitro inhibit tyrosinase

TABLE 59-15 Causes of hyperpigmentation

Primary cutaneous disorders
- *A* Localized
  - *1* Epidermal alteration
    - *a* Seborrheic keratosis
    - *b* Acanthosis nigricans (obesity)
  - *2* Proliferation of melanocytes
    - *a* Lentigo
    - *b* Nevus
    - *c* Melanoma
  - *3* Increased pigment production
    - *a* Ephelides (freckles)
    - *b* Café au lait spots
- *B* Localized and diffuse
  - *1* Drugs

Systemic diseases
- *A* Localized
  - *1* Epidermal alteration
    - *a* Seborrheic keratoses (sign of Leser-Trélat)
    - *b* Acanthosis nigricans (endocrine disorders, paraneoplastic)
  - *2* Proliferation of melanocytes
    - *a* Lentigos (Peutz-Jeghers, LEOPARD syndromes)
    - *b* Nevi (LAMB and NAME syndromes)
  - *3* Increased pigment production
    - *a* Café au lait spots (neurofibromatosis, Albright's syndrome)
  - *4* Dermal pigmentation
    - *a* Incontinentia pigmenti
    - *b* Dyskeratosis congenita
- *B* Diffuse
  - *1* Endocrinopathies
    - *a* Addison's disease
    - *b* Nelson's syndrome
    - *c* Ectopic ACTH syndrome
  - *2* Metabolic
    - *a* Porphyria cutanea tarda
    - *b* Hemochromatosis
    - *c* Vitamin B_{12}, folate deficiency
    - *d* Pellagra
    - *e* Malabsorption, Whipple's disease
  - *3* Melanosis secondary to metastatic melanoma
  - *4* Autoimmune
    - *a* Biliary cirrhosis
    - *b* Scleroderma
    - *c* POEMS syndrome
  - *5* Drugs

P, pulmonary stenosis and subaortic valvular stenosis; *A*, abnormal genitalia (cryptorchidism, hypospadias); *R*, retardation of growth; and *D*, deafness (sensorineural). Lentigines are also seen in association with cardiac myxomas and have been described under the mnemonics *LAMB syndrome* and *NAME syndrome*. The findings in these two syndromes overlap and include *L*, lentigines; *A*, atrial myxomas; *M*, mucocutaneous myxomas; and *B*, blue nevi versus *N*, nevus; *A*, atrial myxoma; *M*, myxoid neurofibroma, and *E*, ephelides (freckles). These patients can also have evidence of endocrine overactivity in the form of Cushing's disease, acromegaly, or sexual precocity.

The third type of localized hyperpigmentation is due to a local increase in pigment production and it includes *ephelides* (Table 59-16) and café au lait spots. The latter are most commonly associated with two disorders—neurofibromatosis and Albright's syndrome. *Café au lait* (CAL) spots are flat, uniformly light brown in color, and can vary in size from 0.5 to 12 cm. Approximately 80 percent of the patients with *neurofibromatosis* will have six or more CAL spots measuring 1.5 cm or greater in diameter. Additional findings are discussed in the section on neurofibromas (see "Papulonodular Skin Lesions"). In comparison to neurofibromatosis, the CAL spots in patients with *Albright's disease* (polyostotic fibrous dysplasia with precocious puberty in females) are usually larger, more irregular in outline, respect the midline, and rarely contain macromelanosomes. CAL spots have also been associated with pulmonary stenosis, temporal dysrhythmia, tuberous sclerosis, the LEOPARD syndrome, and ataxia telangiectasia, but a few such lesions can be found in normal individuals.

In incontinentia pigmenti, dyskeratosis congenita, and bleomycin pigmentation, the areas of localized hyperpigmentation form a pattern—swirled in the first, reticulated in the second, and flagellate in the third. Patients with the X-linked dominant disorder *incontinentia pigmenti* can have linear blisters and verrucous papules during infancy. During childhood, parallel swirls and streaks of hyperpigmentation appear on the trunk, and occasionally streaks of hypopigmentation appear on the extremities. Associated findings include seizures, mental retardation, spastic paraplegia, strabismus, cataracts, and delayed or impaired dentition. Biopsy of the streaks will show pigment within dermal macrophages ("incontinent pigment"). In *dyskeratosis congenita,* atrophic reticulated hyperpigmentation is seen on the neck, thighs, and trunk and it is accompanied by nail dystrophy, pancytopenia, and leukoplakia of the oral and anal mucosa. The latter often develops into squamous cell carcinoma. In addition to the flagellate pigmentation (linear streaks) on the trunk, patients receiving bleomycin often have hyperpigmentation on the elbows, knees and small joints of the hand.

Localized hyperpigmentation is seen as a side effect of several other *systemic medications,* including those that produce fixed-drug reactions (phenolphthalein, tetracyclines, sulfonamides, barbiturates,

TABLE 59-16 Hyperpigmentation (primary cutaneous disorders, localized)

	Clinical characteristics	Histopathology
Seborrheic keratosis	Tan to black papule Warty and/or greasy surface "Stuck on" appearance Trunk	Epidermal hyperplasia
Acanthosis nigricans	Velvety surface Neck, axillae, groin Occasionally on dorsum of the hand, corners of mouth	Epidermal folds
Ephelides (freckles)	2–5-mm macule Tan color Sun-exposed surfaces Darkens following sun exposure	Increased pigment in epidermis
Lentigo	0.3–1.5-cm macule Tan to black Most commonly in sun-exposed areas Face, upper trunk, and extremities	Increased number of melanocytes in epidermis
Nevus		
Junctional	Brown to black macule 2–6 mm	Nests of melanocytes at dermoepidermal junction
Compound	Tan to brown papule 2–6 mm	Nests of melanocytes in epidermis and dermis
Dermal	Flesh-colored Papule	Nests of melanocytes in dermis
Melanoma	Variation in color—brown, black, blue, red, white Irregular outline and surface >5 mm in diameter Asymmetric	Malignant neoplasm of melanocytes

and analgesics) and those that can bind to melanin (antimalarials). Fixed-drug eruptions recur in the same location as circular areas of erythema that can become bullous and then resolve as brown macules. The eruption usually appears within hours of administration of the offending agent and common locations include the genitalia, extremities, and perioral region. Chloroquine, hydroxychloroquine, and quinacrine produce gray-brown to blue-black discoloration of the shins, hard palate, and face, while blue macules are seen on the lower extremities and in sites of inflammation with prolonged minocycline administration. Estrogen in oral contraceptives can induce melasma (chloasma)—symmetric brown patches on the face, especially the cheeks, upper lip, chin, and forehead. Similar changes are seen in pregnancy, in patients receiving hydantoin, and in the adult form of Gaucher's disease. In the latter group, there is also hyperpigmentation of the distal lower extremities.

In the *diffuse* forms of hyperpigmentation, the darkening of the skin may be of equal intensity over the entire body or it may be accentuated in sun-exposed areas. The causes of diffuse hyperpigmentation can be divided into four groups—endocrine, metabolic, autoimmune, and drugs. The endocrinopathies that frequently have associated hyperpigmentation include *Addison's disease, Nelson's syndrome,* and *ectopic ACTH syndrome.* In these diseases, the increased pigmentation is diffuse, but it is accentuated in the palmar and plantar creases, sites of friction, scars, and the oral mucosa. An overproduction of any or all of the pituitary hormones α-MSH (melanocyte stimulating hormone), ACTH, and β-lipotropin can lead to an increase in melanocyte activity. All of these peptides are products of the pro-opiomelanocortin gene and therefore they can exhibit homology, e.g., α-MSH and ACTH share 13 amino acids. A minority of the patients with Cushing's disease or hyperthyroidism have generalized hyperpigmentation.

The metabolic causes of hyperpigmentation include *porphyria cutanea tarda* (PCT), *hemochromatosis, vitamin* B_{12} *deficiency, folic acid deficiency, pellagra, malabsorption,* and *Whipple's disease.* In patients with PCT (see "Vesicles/Bullae"), the skin darkening is seen in sun-exposed areas and is a reflection of the photoreactive properties of porphyrins. The increased level of iron in the skin of patients with hemochromatosis stimulates melanin pigment production and leads to the classic bronze color. Patients with pellagra have a brown discoloration of the skin, especially in sun-exposed areas, as a result of nicotinic acid (niacin) deficiency. In the areas of increased pigmentation, there is a thin varnishlike scale. These changes are also seen in patients who are vitamin B_6 deficient, have functioning carcinoid tumors (increased consumption of niacin), or take isoniazid. Approximately 50 percent of the patients with Whipple's disease have an associated generalized hyperpigmentation in association with diarrhea, weight loss, arthritis, and lymphadenopathy. A diffuse slate-blue color is seen in patients with melanosis secondary to *metastatic melanoma* and melanogenuria. There is a debate as to whether the color is due to single-cell metastases in the dermis or to a widespread deposition of melanin resulting from the high concentration of circulating melanin precursors.

Of the autoimmune diseases associated with diffuse hyperpigmentation, *biliary cirrhosis* and *scleroderma* are the most common and, occasionally, both disorders are seen in the same patient. The skin is dark brown in color, especially in sun-exposed areas. In biliary cirrhosis, the hyperpigmentation is accompanied by pruritus, jaundice, and xanthomas, while in scleroderma, it is accompanied by sclerosis of the extremities, face, and, less commonly, the trunk. Additional clues to the diagnosis of scleroderma are telangiectasias, calcinosis cutis, Raynaud's phenomenon, and distal ulcerations (see "Telangiectasias"). The differential diagnosis of cutaneous sclerosis with hyperpigmentation includes the *POEMS syndrome: P,* polyneuropathy; *O,* organomegaly (liver, spleen, lymph nodes); *E,* endocrinopathies (impotence, gynecomastia); *M,* M-protein; and *S,* skin changes. The skin changes include hyperpigmentation, skin thickening, hypertrichosis, hyperhidrosis, and angiomas.

Diffuse hyperpigmentation that is due to *drugs* or metals can result from one of several mechanisms—induction of melanin pigment formation, complexing of the drug or its metabolites to melanin, and deposits of the drug in the dermis. Busulfan; cyclophosphamide; long-term, high-dose ACTH; and inorganic arsenic induce pigment production. Complexes containing melanin or hemosiderin plus the drug or its metabolites are seen in patients receiving chlorpromazine and minocycline. The sun-exposed skin as well as the conjunctivae of patients on long-term, high-dose chlorpromazine can become blue-gray in color. Patients taking minocycline may develop a diffuse blue-gray, muddy appearance in sun-exposed areas in addition to pigmentation of the mucous membranes, teeth, nails, bones, and thyroid. Administration of amiodorone can result in both a phototoxic eruption (exaggerated sunburn) and/or a brown or blue-gray discoloration of sun-exposed skin. Biopsy specimens of the latter show yellow-brown granules in dermal macrophages, which represent intralysosomal accumulations of lipids, amiodarone, and its metabolites. Actual deposits of a particular drug or metal in the skin are seen with silver (argyria), where the skin appears blue-gray in color; gold (chrysiasis), where the skin has a brown to blue-gray color; and clofazimine, where the skin appears reddish-brown. The associated hyperpigmentation is accentuated in sun-exposed areas, and discoloration of the eye is seen with gold (sclerae) and clofazimine (conjunctivae).

VESICLES/BULLAE (Table 59-17) Depending upon their size, cutaneous blisters are referred to as vesicles (<0.5 cm) or bullae (>0.5 cm). The primary blistering disorders include *pemphigus vulgaris, pemphigus foliaceus, pemphigus erythematosus, bullous pemphigoid, herpes gestationis, cicatricial pemphigoid, epidermolysis bullosa acquisita,* and *dermatitis herpetiformis* (see Chap. 58).

Vesicles and bullae are also seen in *contact dermatitis,* both allergic and irritant forms (see "Erythroderma"). When there is a linear arrangement of vesicular lesions, an exogenous cause should be suspected. Bullous disease secondary to the ingestion of drugs can take one of several forms, including phototoxic eruptions, isolated bullae, toxic epidermal necrolysis, and erythema multiforme. Clinically, phototoxic eruptions resemble an exaggerated sunburn with diffuse erythema and bullae in sun-exposed areas. The most commonly associated drugs are chlorothiazides, tetracyclines, sulfonylureas, sulfonamides, phenothiazines, griseofulvin, and psoralens. The development of a phototoxic eruption is dependent upon the dose of both the drug and the UV-A irradiation.

There are several drugs, including penicillins, sulfonamides, D-penicillamine, phenobarbital, phenytoin, furosemide, and nonsteroidal anti-inflammatory agents, that cause isolated bland bullae to arise on normal skin. The characteristics of these blisters are such that they can not be assigned to a particular cutaneous disease. The most common location for these isolated bullae is the distal extremity. In contrast, *toxic epidermal necrolysis* (TEN) is characterized by bullae

TABLE 59-17 Causes of vesicles/bullae

Primary cutaneous diseases	Systemic diseases
A Primary blistering diseases	*A* Infections
1 Pemphigus	*1* Cutaneous emboli
2 Bullous pemphigoid	*B* Metabolic
3 Herpes gestationis	*1* Diabetic bullae
4 Cicatricial pemphigoid	*2* Porphyria cutanea tarda
5 Dermatitis herpetiformis	*3* Porphyria variegata
6 Epidermolysis bullosa acquisita	*4* Pseudoporphyria
B Secondary blistering diseases	*5* Bullous dermatosis of hemodialysis
1 Contact	
2 Erythema multiforme	
3 Toxic epidermal necrolysis	
C Infections	
1 Varicella/zoster*	
2 Herpes simplex*	
3 Staphylococcal scalded-skin syndrome	
4 Bullous impetigo	

* Also systemic.

that arise on widespread areas of erythema and then slough. This results in large areas of denuded skin. The associated morbidity, such as sepsis, and mortality are relatively high and they are a function of the extent of epidermal necrosis. In addition, these patients may also have involvement of the mucous membranes and the intestinal tract. Drugs are the primary cause of TEN, and the most common offenders are phenytoin, barbiturates, sulfonamides, penicillins, allopurinol, phenolphthalein, and phenylbutazone. Severe acute graft-versus-host disease (grade 4) can also resemble TEN.

In *erythema multiforme* (EM), the primary lesions are pink-red macules and edematous papules, the centers of which may become vesicular. The clue to the diagnosis of EM rather than of a drug-induced morbilliform exanthem is the development of a "dusky" violet color or petechiae in the center of the lesions. Target or iris lesions are also characteristic of EM and they arise as a result of active centers and borders in combination with centrifugal spread. However, iris lesions need not be present to make the diagnosis of EM. Preferred sites of involvement include the hands, extensor forearms, palms, soles, and mucous membranes (oral, nasal, ocular, and genital). Hemorrhagic crusts of the lips are characteristic of EM as well as two other blistering disorders—pemphigus vulgaris and TEN. Fever, malaise, myalgias, sore throat, and cough may precede or accompany the eruption. The lesions of EM usually resolve over 3 to 6 weeks, but they may be recurrent.

Drugs can induce EM, in particular sulfonamides, phenytoin, barbiturates, penicillins, phenolphthalein, and carbamazepine, but they do not cause the majority of cases, especially in young adults. Infections with herpes simplex are a common cause of EM in this age group and the lesions appear 7 to 12 days after the viral eruption. Other infectious agents associated with EM include *Mycoplasma pneumoniae, Histoplasma capsulatum, Coccidioides immitis, Yersinia enterocolitica, Francisella tularensis,* and several viruses (echo, coxsackie, Epstein-Barr, and influenza). EM can also follow vaccinations with BCG, poliomyelitis or vaccinia viruses; radiation therapy; and exposure to environmental toxins; and it has been observed in a few patients with lupus erythematosus, Wegener's granulomatosis, and internal malignancy.

In addition to primary blistering disorders and hypersensitivity reactions, bacterial and viral infections can lead to vesicles and bullae. The most common infectious agents are herpes simplex, herpes varicella-zoster, and staphylococci.

Staphylococcal scalded-skin syndrome (SSSS) and bullous impetigo are two blistering disorders associated with staphylococcal (phage group II) infection. In SSSS, the initial findings are redness and tenderness of the central face, neck, trunk, and intertriginous zones. This is followed by short-lived flaccid bullae and a slough or exfoliation of the superficial epidermis. Crusted areas then develop, characteristically around the mouth. SSSS is distinguished from TEN by the following features: younger age group, more superficial site of blister formation, no oral lesions, shorter course, less morbidity and mortality, and an association with staphylococcal exfoliative toxin ("exfoliatin"), not drugs. A rapid diagnosis of SSSS versus TEN can be made by a frozen section of the blister roof or exfoliative cytology of the blister contents. In SSSS, the site of staphylococcal infection is usually extracutaneous (conjunctivitis, rhinorrhea, otitis media, pharyngitis, tonsillitis), and the lesions are sterile, whereas in *bullous impetigo* the lesions are the site of infection. Impetigo is more localized than SSSS and it usually presents with honey-colored crusts. Occasionally, superficial purulent blisters also form. *Cutaneous emboli* from gram-negative infections may present as isolated bullae, but the base of the lesion is purpuric or necrotic and it may develop into an ulcer (see "Purpura").

There are several metabolic disorders that are associated with blister formation including diabetes mellitus, renal failure, and porphyria. Local hypoxia secondary to decreased cutaneous blood flow can also produce blisters, which explains the presence of bullae over pressure points in comatose patients (coma bullae). In *diabetes mellitus,* tense bullae with clear viscous fluid arise on normal skin.

TABLE 59-18 Causes of exanthems

Morbilliform
- *A* Drugs
- *B* Viral
  - *1* Rubeola
  - *2* Rubella
  - *3* Erythema infectiosum
  - *4* Epstein-Barr, echo, coxsackie, and adenovirus
  - *5* Early HIV
- *C* Bacterial
  - *1* Typhoid fever
  - *2* Early secondary syphilis
  - *3* Early Rickettsia
  - *4* Early meningococcus
- *D* Acute graft-versus-host disease

Scarlatiniform
- *A* Scarlet fever
- *B* Toxic shock syndrome
- *C* Kawasaki's disease

The lesions can be as large as 6 cm in diameter and they are located on the distal extremities. There are several types of porphyria, but the most common form with cutaneous findings is *porphyria cutanea tarda* (PCT). In sun-exposed areas (primarily the face and hands), the skin is very fragile and trauma leads to erosions and tense vesicles. These lesions then heal with scarring and formation of milia; the latter are firm 2 to 3 mm white or yellow papules that represent epidermoid inclusion cysts. Associated findings can include hypertrichosis of the lateral malar region (males) or face (females) and, in sun-exposed areas, hyperpigmentation and firm sclerotic plaques. An elevated level of urinary uroporphyrins confirms the diagnosis and is due to a decrease in uroporphyrinogen decarboxylase activity. Precipitating agents include alcohol, estrogen, iron, and chlorinated hydrocarbons.

The differential diagnosis of PCT includes: (1) *porphyria variegata*—the skin signs of PCT plus the systemic findings of acute intermittent porphyria; it has a diagnostic plasma porphyrin fluorescence emission at 626 nm; (2) *drug-induced bullous photosensitivity* (pseudoporphyria)—the clinical and histologic findings are similar to PCT, but porphyrins are normal; etiologic agents are furosemide, tetracycline, nalidixic acid, dapsone, naproxen, and pyridoxine; (3) *bullous dermatosis of hemodialysis*—the same appearance as PCT, but porphyrins are usually normal or occasionally borderline elevated; patients have chronic renal failure and are on hemodialysis; (4) PCT associated with hepatomas, hepatic carcinomas, and hemodialysis; and (5) *epidermolysis bullosa acquisita* (see Chap. 58).

EXANTHEMS (Table 59-18) Exanthems are characterized by an acute generalized eruption. The two most common presentations are erythematous macules and papules (morbilliform) and confluent blanching erythema (scarlatiniform). *Morbilliform* eruptions are usually due to either *drugs* or viral infections. For example, at least 5 percent of the patients receiving penicillins, sulfonamides, captopril, phenytoin, or gold will develop a maculopapular eruption. Accompanying signs may include pruritus, fever, eosinophilia, and transient lymphadenopathy. Similar maculopapular eruptions are seen in the classic childhood viral exanthems including: (1) *rubeola* (measles)—a prodrome of coryza, cough, conjunctivitis, and Koplik's spots on the buccal mucosa whose onset coincides with a second fever spike; the eruption begins behind the ears, at the hair line, and on the forehead then spreads down the body, often becoming confluent; (2) *rubella*—it begins on the forehead and face, then spreads down the body; it resolves in the same order and is associated with retroauricular and suboccipital lymphadenopathy; and (3) *erythema infectiosum* (fifth disease)—erythema of the cheeks is followed by a reticulated pattern on extremities; it is secondary to a parvovirus infection and in adults, an associated arthritis is seen.

Both measles and rubella are seen in unvaccinated young adults and an atypical form of measles is seen in adults immunized with either killed measles vaccine or killed vaccine followed in time by live vaccine. In contrast to classic measles, the eruption of atypical measles begins on the palms, soles, wrists, and knuckles, and the lesions may become purpuric. The patient with atypical measles can have pulmonary involvement and be quite ill. Rubelliform and roseoliform eruptions are also associated with *Epstein-Barr* (5 to 15 percent of patients), *echo, coxsackie,* and *adenovirus* infections. Detection of specific IgM antibodies allows the proper diagnosis. Occasionally, a maculopapular eruption is the result of a drug-viral interaction. For example, about 95 percent of the patients with infectious mononucleosis who are given ampicillin will develop a rash.

Of note, early in the course of infections with *Rickettsia* and *meningococcus,* prior to the development of purpura, the lesions may be erythematous macules and papules. This is also the case in chickenpox prior to the development of vesicles. Maculopapular eruptions are associated with early *HIV* infection, early secondary *syphilis, typhoid fever,* and *acute graft-versus-host* disease. In the last, lesions frequently begin on the palms and soles; the macular rose spots of typhoid fever involve primarily the anterior trunk.

The prototypic *scarlatiniform* eruption is seen in *scarlet fever* and is due to an erythrotoxin produced by group A beta-hemolytic streptococcal infections, most commonly pharyngitis. There are a diffuse erythema, which begins on the neck and upper trunk, and red perifollicular puncta. Additional findings include a white strawberry tongue (white coating with red papillae) followed by a red strawberry tongue (red tongue and red papillae); petechiae of the palate; a facial flush with circumoral pallor; linear petechiae in the antecubital fossae; and desquamation of the involved skin, palms, and soles 5 to 20 days after the onset of the eruption. A similar desquamation of the palms and soles is seen in toxic shock syndrome, Kawasaki's disease, and after severe febrile illnesses. Certain strains of staphylococci also produce an erythrotoxin that leads to the same clinical findings as in streptococcal scarlet fever, except that the antistreptolysin O titers are not elevated.

In *toxic shock syndrome* (TSS), staphylococcal (phage group I) infections produce an exotoxin, which causes the fever and rash, as well as an enterotoxin. Initially, the majority of cases were reported in menstruating women who were using tampons. However, other sites of infection, including wounds and vaginitis, may produce TSS. The diagnosis of TSS is based upon clinical criteria and three of these involve mucocutaneous sites. The clinical criteria are: (1) fever; (2) diffuse erythema of the skin; (3) desquamation of the palms and soles 1 to 2 weeks after onset of illness; (4) hypotension; and (5) involvement of three or more organ systems, including the gastrointestinal tract, muscles, kidney, liver, CNS, hematologic (thrombocytopenia), and mucous membranes. The latter is characterized as hyperemia of the vagina, oropharynx, or conjunctivae.

Although the cutaneous eruption in *Kawasaki's disease* (mucocutaneous lymph node syndrome) is polymorphous, the two common types are morbilliform and scarlatiniform. The majority of cases are seen in children less than 5 years of age, but adult cases have been reported. The diagnosis is based upon a fever lasting more than 5 days plus four of the five following criteria: (1) bilateral conjunctival injection; (2) exanthem; (3) cervical lymphadenopathy, usually unilateral; (4) erythema and edema of the hands and feet followed by desquamation; and (5) diffuse erythema of the oropharynx, red strawberry tongue, and erosions with crusting on the lips. This clinical picture can resemble TSS and scarlet fever, but clues to the diagnosis of Kawasaki's disease are the cervical lymphadenopathy, lip erosions, and increased platelets. The more serious associated systemic finding in this disease is coronary aneurysms secondary to arteritis. The latter may lead to sudden death, primarily within the first 30 days of the illness. Scarlatiniform eruptions are also seen in the early phase of SSSS (see "Vesicles/Bullae") and as reactions to drugs.

URTICARIA (Table 59-19) *Urticaria* (hives) are transient lesions that are composed of a central wheal surrounded by an erythematous halo. Individual lesions are round, oval, or figurate and they are often pruritic. *Acute* and *chronic* urticaria have a wide variety of allergic etiologies. Less common systemic causes of urticaria are mastocytosis (urticaria pigmentosa), hyperthyroidism, malignancy, and juvenile rheumatoid arthritis (JRA). In JRA, the lesions coincide with the fever spike and they are transient, but not migratory as in erythema marginatum.

TABLE 59-19 Causes of urticaria

Primary cutaneous disorders
- *A* Acute and chronic urticaria
- *B* Physical urticaria
  - *1* Dermatographism
  - *2* Solar urticaria
  - *3* Cold urticaria*
  - *4* Cholinergic urticaria*
- *C* Angioedema (hereditary and acquired)

Systemic diseases
- *A* Urticarial vasculitis
- *B* Hepatitis B infection
- *C* Serum sickness
- *D* Angioedema (acquired)

* Also systemic.

The common *physical urticarias* include *dermatographism, solar urticaria, cold urticaria,* and *cholinergic urticaria.* Patients with dermatographism exhibit linear wheals following minor pressure or scratching of the skin. It is a common disorder, affecting approximately 5 percent of the population. Solar urticaria characteristically occurs within minutes of sun exposure and is a skin sign of one systemic disease—erythropoietic protoporphyria. In addition to the urticaria, these patients have subtle pitted scarring of the nose and hands. Cold urticaria is precipitated by exposure to the cold and therefore exposed areas are usually affected. In some cases, the disease is associated with abnormal circulating proteins—more commonly, cryoglobulins and cold hemolysins, and less commonly, cryofibrinogens and cold agglutinins. Additional systemic symptoms include wheezing and syncope, thus explaining the need for these patients to avoid swimming in cold water. Cholinergic urticaria is precipitated by heat, exercise, or emotion and is characterized by small wheals with relatively large flares. It is occasionally associated with wheezing.

Whereas urticaria is the result of dermal edema, subcutaneous edema leads to the clinical picture of *angioedema.* Sites of involvement include the eyelids, lips, tongue, larynx, and gastrointestinal tract as well as the subcutaneous tissue. Angioedema occurs alone or in combination with urticaria, including urticarial vasculitis and the physical urticarias. Both acquired and hereditary (autosomal dominant) forms of angioedema occur (see Chap. 267), and in the latter, urticaria is rarely seen.

Urticarial vasculitis is an immune complex disease that may be confused with simple urticaria. In contrast to simple urticaria, individual lesions tend to last longer than 24 h and they usually develop central petechiae that can be observed even after the urticarial phase has resolved. The patient may also complain of burning rather than pruritus. On biopsy, there is either a lymphocytic or leukocytoclastic vasculitis of the small blood vessels. Although many cases of urticarial vasculitis are idiopathic in origin, it can be a reflection of an underlying systemic illness such as lupus erythematosus, Sjögren's syndrome, or hereditary complement deficiency. There is a spectrum of urticarial vasculitis which ranges from purely cutaneous to multisystem involvement. The most common systemic signs and symptoms are arthralgias and/or arthritis, nephritis, crampy abdominal pain, asthma, and chronic obstructive lung disease. Hypocomplementemia is seen in one- to two-thirds of patients, even in the idiopathic cases. Similar cutaneous, joint, and renal findings can be seen in the prodrome of *hepatitis B* infection, *serum sickness,* and *serum sickness–like illnesses.*

PAPULONODULAR SKIN LESIONS (Table 59-20) In the papulonodular diseases, the lesions are elevated above the surface of the skin and they may coalesce to form plaques. The location, consistency, and color of the lesions are the keys to their diagnosis. This section is organized on the basis of color and the color groups are white, flesh, pink, yellow, red, red-brown, blue, violaceous, purple, and brown-black.

TABLE 59-20 Papulonodular skin lesions according to color groups

White
- *A* Calcinosis cutis

Flesh
- *A* Rheumatoid nodule
- *B* Neurofibromas (von Recklinghausen's disease)
- *C* Angiofibromas (tuberous sclerosis)
- *D* Neuromas (multiple endocrine neoplasia syndrome, type 2b)
- *E* Adnexal tumors
  - *1* Basal cell epitheliomas (basal cell nevus syndrome)
  - *2* Tricholemmomas (Cowden's disease)
- *F* Primary cutaneous disorders
  - *1* Epidermal inclusion cysts
  - *2* Lipomas

Pink/translucent
- *A* Amyloidosis
- *B* Papular mucinosis

Yellow
- *A* Xanthomas
- *B* Tophi
- *C* Necrobiosis lipoidica
- *D* Pseudoxanthoma elasticum
- *E* Sebaceous adenomas (Torre's syndrome)

Red
- *A* Papules
  - *1* Angiokeratomas (Fabry's disease)
  - *2* Hemangioma-like lesions (disseminated cat-scatch disease in AIDS)
- *B* Papules/plaques
  - *1* Cutaneous lupus
  - *2* Lymphoma cutis
  - *3* Leukemia cutis
- *C* Nodules
  - *1* Panniculitis
  - *2* Cutaneous polyarteritis nodosa
  - *3* Systemic vasculitis
- *D* Primary cutaneous disorders
  - *1* Arthropod bites
  - *2* Cherry hemangiomas
  - *3* Infections, e.g., erysipelas, sporotrichosis
  - *4* Polymorphous light eruption
  - *5* Lymphocytoma cutis (pseudolymphoma)

Red-brown
- *A* Sarcoidosis
- *B* Sweet's syndrome
- *C* Urticaria pigmentosa
- *D* Erythema elevatum diutinum (chronic leukocytoclastic vasculitis)
- *E* Lupus vulgaris

Blue
- *A* Cavernous hemangiomas (blue rubber bleb syndrome)
- *B* Primary cutaneous disorders
  - *1* Venous lake
  - *2* Blue nevus

Violaceous
- *A* Lupus pernio (sarcoidosis)
- *B* Lymphoma cutis
- *C* Cutaneous lupus

Purple
- *A* Kaposi's sarcoma
- *B* Angiosarcoma
- *C* Palpable purpura

Brown-black
- See "Hyperpigmentation"

Any color
- *A* Metastases

White lesions In *calcinosis cutis,* there are firm white to white-yellow papules with an irregular surface. When the contents are discharged, a chalky white material is seen. *Dystrophic* calcification is seen at sites of previous inflammation or damage to the skin. It develops in acne scars as well as on the distal extremities of patients with scleroderma and in areas of muscle necrosis in dermatomyositis. The latter is more extensive and is more commonly seen in children. An elevated calcium phosphate product, as in secondary hyperparathyroidism, can lead to nodules of *metastatic* calcinosis cutis, which tend to be subcutaneous and periarticular. This form is often accompanied by calcification of muscular arteries and subsequent ischemic necrosis.

Flesh-colored lesions There are several types of flesh-colored lesions including epidermoid inclusion cysts, lipomas, rheumatoid nodules, neurofibromas, angiofibromas, neuromas, and adnexal tumors such as tricholemmomas. Both *epidermoid inclusion cysts* and *lipomas* are very common mobile subcutaneous nodules—the former are rubbery and compressible and they drain cheeselike material (sebum and keratin) if incised. Lipomas are firm and somewhat lobulated on palpation. When extensive facial epidermoid inclusion cysts develop in childhood or there is a family history of such lesions, the patient should be examined for other signs of Gardner's syndrome, including desmoid tumors (see Chap. 242). *Rheumatoid nodules* are firm 0.5- to 4-cm nodules that tend to localize around pressure points, especially the elbows. They are seen in approximately 20 percent of patients with rheumatoid arthritis and 6 percent of patients with Still's disease. Biopsies of the nodules show palisading granulomas. Similar lesions that are smaller and shorter-lived are seen in rheumatic fever.

Neurofibromas (benign Schwann cell tumors) are soft papules or nodules that exhibit the "button-hole" sign, that is, they invaginate into the skin with pressure in a manner similar to a hernia. Single lesions are seen in normal individuals, but multiple neurofibromas, usually in combination with six or more café au lait spots measuring >1.5 cm (see "Hyperpigmentation") and multiple Lisch nodules, are seen in von Recklinghausen's disease. Lisch nodules are 1-mm yellow-brown spots within the iris that are best observed with 10× magnification. Additional manifestations include axillary freckling and peripheral and CNS tumors (see Chap. 358). In some patients, the neurofibromas are localized and unilateral while in others, they are limited to the CNS.

Angiofibromas are pink to flesh-colored firm papules that measure from 3 mm to several centimeters in diameter. When they are located on the central cheeks (adenoma sebaceum) or under and around the nails, the patient has tuberous sclerosis. It is an autosomal disorder and the associated findings are discussed in the section on ash leaf spots (see "Hypopigmentation").

Neuromas (benign proliferation of nerve fibers) are also flesh-colored firm papules. They are more commonly found at sites of amputation and as rudimentary supernumerary digits. However, when there are multiple neuromas on the eyelids, lips, distal tongue, and/or oral mucosa, the patient should be investigated for other signs of the multiple endocrine neoplasia syndrome, type 2b. Associated findings include marfanoid habitus, protuberant lips, intestinal ganglioneuromas, and medullary thyroid carcinoma (>75 percent of patients) (see Chap. 325).

Adnexal tumors are derived from pluripotential cells of the epidermis that can differentiate toward hair, sebaceous, apocrine, or eccrine glands or remain undifferentiated. *Basal cell epitheliomas* (BCEs) are examples of adnexal tumors that have little or no evidence of differentiation. Clinically, they are translucent papules with rolled borders, telangiectasias, and central erosion. BCEs commonly arise in sun-damaged skin of the head and neck. When a patient has multiple BCEs, especially prior to age 30, the possibility of the basal cell nevus syndrome should be raised. It is inherited as an autosomal dominant trait and is associated with jaw cysts, palmar and plantar pits, frontal bossing, rib anomalies, spina bifida occulta, and calcification of the falx cerebri and diaphragma sellae. *Tricholemmomas* are also flesh-colored adnexal tumors, but they differentiate towards hair follicles and can have a wartlike appearance. The presence of multiple tricholemmomas on the face and oral mucosa points to the diagnosis of Cowden's disease (multiple hamartoma syndrome). The oral tricholemmomas are found primarily on the tongue and gingiva and give these areas a cobblestone appearance. Internal organ involvement (in decreasing order of frequency) includes fibrocystic disease and carcinoma of the breast, adenomas and carcinomas of the thyroid, and gastrointestinal polyposis. Keratoses of the palms, soles, and dorsa of the hands are also seen.

Pink lesions The cutaneous lesions associated with primary systemic *amyloidosis* are pink in color and translucent. Common locations are the face, especially the periorbital and perioral regions, and intertriginous areas. On biopsy, homogeneous deposits of amyloid are seen in the dermis and in the walls of blood vessels; the latter leads to an increase in vessel wall fragility. As a result, petechiae and purpura develop in clinically normal skin as well as in lesional skin following minor trauma, hence the term "pinch purpura." Amyloid deposits are also seen in the striated muscle of the tongue and this results in macroglossia.

Even though specific mucocutaneous lesions are rarely seen in secondary amyloidosis and are present in only about 30 percent of the patients with primary amyloidosis, a rapid diagnosis of systemic amyloidosis can be made by an examination of abdominal subcutaneous fat. By special staining, deposits are seen around blood vessels or individual fat cells in 40 to 50 percent of patients. There are also three forms of amyloidosis that are limited to the skin and that should not be construed as cutaneous lesions of systemic amyloidosis. They are macular amyloid (upper back), lichenoid amyloidosis (usually lower extremities), and nodular amyloidosis. In macular and lichenoid amyloidosis, the deposits are composed of altered epidermal keratin.

Patients with multicentric reticulohistiocytosis also have pink-colored papules and nodules on the face and mucous membranes as well as on the extensor surface of the hands and forearms. They have a polyarthritis that can mimic rheumatoid arthritis clinically. On histologic examination, the papules have characteristic giant cells which are not seen in biopsies of rheumatoid nodules. Pink to flesh-colored papules that are firm, 2 to 5 mm in diameter, and often in a linear arrangement are seen in patients with *papular mucinosis*. This disease is also referred to as lichen myxedematosus or scleromyxedema. The latter name comes from the brawny induration of the face and extremities that may accompany the papular eruption. Biopsy specimens of the papules show localized mucin deposition, and serum protein electrophoresis demonstrates a monoclonal spike of IgG, usually with a λ light chain.

Yellow lesions Several systemic disorders are characterized by yellow-colored cutaneous papules or plaques—hyperlipidemia (xanthomas), gout (tophi), diabetes (necrobiosis lipoidica), pseudoxanthoma elasticum, and Torre's syndrome (sebaceous tumors). Eruptive xanthomas are the most common form of *xanthomas* and they are associated with hypertriglyceridemia (types I, III, IV, and V). Crops of yellow papules with erythematous halos occur primarily on the extensor surface of the extremities and the buttocks in association with elevations of the circulating triglycerides. They spontaneously involute with a fall in serum lipids. Increased β-lipoproteins (primarily types II and III) result in one or more of the following types of xanthoma: xanthelasma, tendon xanthomas, and plane xanthomas. Xanthelasma are found on the eyelids, while tendon xanthomas are frequently associated with the Achilles and extensor finger tendons; plane xanthoma are flat and favor the palmar creases, face, upper trunk, and scars. Tuberous xanthomas are frequently associated with hypertriglyceridemia, but they are also seen in patients with hypercholesterolemia (type II) and they are found most frequently over the large joints or hand. Biopsy specimens of xanthomas show collections of lipid-containing macrophages (foam cells).

Patients with several disorders, including biliary cirrhosis, can have a secondary form of hyperlipidemia with associated tuberous and planar xanthomas. However, patients with myeloma have *normolipemic* flat xanthomas. This latter form of xanthoma may be ≥12 cm in diameter and is most frequently seen on the upper trunk or side of the neck. It is also important to note that the most common setting for eruptive xanthomas is uncontrolled diabetes mellitus. The least specific sign for hyperlipidemia is xanthelasma because at least 50 percent of the patients with this finding have normal lipid profiles.

In tophaceous gout, there are deposits of monosodium urate in the skin around the joints, particularly those of the hands and feet. Additional sites of *tophi* formation include the helix of the ear and the olecranon and prepatellar bursae. The lesions are firm, yellow in color, and occasionally discharge a chalky material. Their size varies from 1 mm to 7 cm and the diagnosis can be established by polarization of the aspirated contents of a lesion. Lesions of *necrobiosis lipoidica* are found primarily on the shins (90 percent) and the majority of patients have diabetes mellitus or develop it subsequently. Characteristic findings include a central yellow color, atrophy (transparency), telangiectasias, and an erythematous border. Ulcerations can also develop within the plaques. Biopsy specimens show necrobiosis of collagen, granulomatous inflammation, and obliterative endarteritis.

In *pseudoxanthoma elasticum* (PXE), there is an abnormal deposition of calcium upon the elastic fibers of the skin, eye, and blood vessels. In the skin, the flexural areas such as the neck, axillae, antecubital fossae, and inguinal area are the primary sites of involvement. Yellow papules coalesce to form reticulated plaques that have an appearance similar to that of plucked chicken skin. In severely affected skin, hanging, redundant folds develop. Some patients have a more subtle macular form of the disease and careful inspection is required. Biopsy specimens of involved skin show swollen and irregularly clumped elastic fibers with deposits of calcium. In the eye, the calcium deposits in Bruch's membrane lead to angioid streaks and choroiditis; in the arteries of the heart, kidney, gastrointestinal tract and extremities, the deposits lead to angina, hypertension, gastrointestinal bleeding, and claudication, respectively. Four types of PXE have been described—two with autosomal dominant and two with autosomal recessive inheritance. The extent of vessel and skin involvement varies depending upon the type.

Adnexal tumors that have differentiated toward sebaceous glands include sebaceous adenoma, sebaceous epithelioma, sebaceous carcinoma, and sebaceous hyperplasia. Except for sebaceous hyperplasia, which is commonly seen on the face, these tumors are solitary and uncommon. Patients with Torre's syndrome have *sebaceous adenomas,* and, in the majority of cases, there are multiple such tumors. These patients can also have sebaceous carcinomas and sebaceous hyperplasia as well as keratoacanthomas. The internal manifestations of Torre's syndrome include *multiple* carcinomas of the gastrointestinal tract (primarily colon) as well as cancers of the larynx, genitourinary tract, ovary, and endometrium. Some patients have a strong family history of cancer.

Red lesions Cutaneous lesions that are red in color have a wide variety of etiologies and in an attempt to simplify their identification, they will be subdivided into papules, papules/plaques, and subcutaneous nodules. Common red papules include *arthropod bites* and *cherry hemangiomas;* the latter are small, bright-red, dome-shaped papules that represent benign proliferation of capillaries. In patients with AIDS, the development of multiple red hemangioma-like lesions points to disseminated *cat-scratch disease,* and biopsy specimens show collections of gram-negative rods. Multiple *angiokeratomas* are seen in Fabry's disease, an X-linked recessive lysosomal storage disease that is due to a deficiency of alpha galactosidase A. The lesions are red to red-blue in color and can be quite small in size (1 to 3 mm) with the most common location being the lower trunk. Associated findings include chronic renal failure, peripheral neuropathy, and corneal opacities (cornea verticillata). Electron photomicrographs of angiokeratomas and clinically normal skin demonstrate lamellar lipid deposits in fibroblasts, pericytes, and endothelial cells that are diagnostic of this disease. Widespread acute eruptions of erythematous papules are discussed in the section on exanthems.

There are several infectious diseases that present as erythematous papules or nodules in a sporotrichoid pattern, that is, in a linear arrangement along the lymphatic channels. The two most common etiologies are *Sporothrix schenckii* (*sporotrichosis*) and *Mycobacterium marinum* (atypical mycobacteria). The organisms are introduced as a result of trauma, and a primary inoculation site is often seen in addition to the lymphatic nodules. Additional causes include *Nocardia, Leishmania,* and other dimorphic fungi; culture of lesional tissue will aid in the diagnosis.

The diseases that are characterized by erythematous plaques with scale are reviewed in the papulosquamous section and the various forms of dermatitis are discussed in the section on erythroderma. Additional disorders in the differential diagnosis of red papules/plaques include *erysipelas, polymorphous light eruption, lymphocytoma cutis, cutaneous lupus, lymphoma cutis,* and *leukemia cutis.* The first three diseases represent primary cutaneous disorders. Polymorphous light eruption (PMLE) is characterized by erythematous papules and plaques in a primarily sun-exposed distribution—dorsum of the hand, extensor forearm, and face. Lesions follow exposure to both UV-B and UV-A, and in northern latitudes PMLE is most severe in the late spring and early summer. A process referred to as "hardening" occurs with continued UV exposure and the eruption fades, but in temperate climates it will recur in the spring. PMLE must be differentiated from cutaneous lupus and this is accomplished by histologic examination and direct immunofluorescence of the lesions. Lymphocytoma cutis (pseudolymphoma) is a *benign* proliferation of lymphocytes in the skin that presents as infiltrated pink-red to red-purple papules and plaques. It must be distinguished from cutaneous lupus and lymphoma cutis.

Several types of red plaques are seen in patients with systemic *lupus* including: (1) erythematous urticarial plaques across the cheeks and nose in the classic butterfly rash; (2) erythematous discoid lesions with fine or "carpet-tack" scale, telangiectasias, central hypopigmentation, peripheral hyperpigmentation, follicular plugging, and atrophy located on the face, scalp, external ears, arms, and upper trunk; and (3) psoriasiform or annular lesions of subacute lupus with hypopigmented centers located on the face, extensor arms, and upper trunk. Additional cutaneous findings include: (1) a violaceous flush on the face and vee of the neck; (2) urticarial vasculitis (see "Urticaria"); (3) lupus panniculitis (see below); (4) diffuse alopecia; (5) alopecia secondary to discoid lesions; (6) periungual telangiectasias and erythema; (7) erythema multiforme-like lesions which may become bullous; and (8) distal ulcerations secondary to Raynaud's phenomenon, vasculitis, or livedoid vasculitis. Patients with only discoid lesions usually have the form of lupus that is limited to the skin. However, 2 to 10 percent of these patients eventually develop systemic lupus. Direct immunofluorescence of involved skin shows deposits of IgG and C3 in a granular distribution along the dermal-epidermal junction.

In *lymphoma cutis,* there is a proliferation of malignant lymphocytes or histiocytes in the skin and the clinical appearance resembles that of lymphocytoma cutis—infiltrated pink-red to red-purple papules and plaques. Lymphoma cutis can occur anywhere on the surface of the skin, whereas the sites of predilection for lymphocytomas are the malar ridge, tip of the nose, earlobes, forearms, and scrotum. Patients with non-Hodgkin's lymphomas have specific cutaneous lesions more often than those with Hodgkin's disease and occasionally the skin nodules precede the development of extracutaneous non-Hodgkin's lymphoma. Arcuate lesions are sometimes seen in lymphoma and lymphocytoma cutis as well as in CTLC. *Leukemia cutis* has the same appearance as lymphoma cutis and specific lesions are seen more commonly in monocytic leukemias than in lymphocytic or granulocytic leukemias. Cutaneous chloromas (granulocytic sarcomas) may precede the appearance of circulating blasts in acute nonlymphocytic leukemia and as such represent a form of aleukemic leukemia cutis.

Common causes of erythematous subcutaneous nodules include inflamed epidermoid inclusion cysts, acne cysts, and furuncles. *Panniculitis,* an inflammation of the fat, also presents as subcutaneous nodules and is frequently a sign of systemic disease. There are several forms of panniculitis including erythema nodosum, erythema induratum, lupus profundus, Weber-Christian disease, α_1-antitrypsin deficiency, facticial, and fat necrosis secondary to pancreatic disease. In all of these disorders, except for erythema nodosum, the lesions may break down and ulcerate or heal with a scar. The shin is the most common location for the nodules of erythema nodosum while the calf is the most common location for lesions of erythema induratum. In erythema nodosum, the nodules are initially red, but then they develop a blue color as they resolve. Patients with erythema nodosum and no underlying systemic illness can still have fever, malaise, leukocytosis, arthralgias and/or arthritis, and unilateral or bilateral hilar adenopathy. However, the possibility of an underlying illness should be excluded and the most common associations are streptococcal infections, upper respiratory infections, sarcoidosis, and inflammatory bowel disease. The less common associations include tuberculosis, histoplasmosis, coccidioidomycosis, psittacosis, drugs (oral contraceptives, sulfonamides, aspartame, bromides, iodides), cat-scratch fever, and infections with *Yersinia, Salmonella,* and *Chlamydia.*

In most patients, erythema induratum/nodular vasculitis is an idiopathic disease, while in a few it may be a reflection of extracutaneous tuberculosis. The lesions of lupus profundus are found primarily on the face, upper arms, and buttocks (sites of abundant fat) and they are seen in both the cutaneous and systemic forms of lupus. The overlying skin may be normal, erythematous, or have the changes of discoid lupus. The subcutaneous fat necrosis that is associated with pancreatic disease is presumably secondary to circulating lipases and is seen in patients with pancreatic carcinoma as well as with acute and chronic pancreatitis. In this disorder and in Weber-Christian disease, there may be an associated arthritis, fever, and inflammation of visceral fat. Histologic examination of deep incisional biopsy specimens will aid in the diagnosis of the particular type of panniculitis.

Subcutaneous erythematous nodules are also seen in *cutaneous polyarteritis nodosa* (PAN) and as a manifestation of *systemic vasculitis,* e.g., systemic PAN, allergic granulomatosis, or Wegener's granulomatosis. Cutaneous PAN presents with painful subcutaneous nodules and ulcers within a red-purple, netlike pattern of livedo reticularis. The latter is due to slowed blood flow through the superficial horizontal venous plexus. The majority of lesions are found on the lower extremity, and while arthralgias and myalgias may accompany cutaneous PAN, there is no evidence of systemic involvement. In both the cutaneous and systemic forms of vasculitis, skin biopsy specimens of the associated nodules will show the changes characteristic of a vasculitis; the size of the vessel involved will depend upon the particular disease.

Red-brown lesions The cutaneous lesions in *sarcoidosis* are classically red to red-brown in color, and with diascopy (pressure with a glass slide) a yellow-brown residual color is observed that is secondary to the granulomatous infiltrate. The waxy papules and plaques may be found anywhere on the skin, but the face is the most common location. Usually there are no surface changes, but occasionally the lesions will have scale. Biopsy specimens of the papules show "naked" granulomas in the dermis, that is, granulomas surrounded by a minimal number of lymphocytes. Other cutaneous findings in sarcoidosis include annular lesions with an atrophic or scaly center, papules within scars, hypopigmented macules and papules, alopecia, acquired ichthyosis, erythema nodosum, and lupus pernio (see below). Additional physical findings are peripheral lymphadenopathy and parotid and lacrimal gland enlargement. When there is cutaneous involvement of the hands, radiographs will often show lytic leisons in the underlying bone.

The differential diagnosis of sarcoidosis includes foreign body granulomas produced by chemicals such as beryllium and zirconium, late secondary syphilis, and *lupus vulgaris.* Lupus vulgaris is a form of cutaneous tuberculosis that is seen in previously infected and sensitized individuals. There is often underlying active tuberculosis elsewhere, usually in the lungs or lymph nodes. At least 90 percent of the lesions occur in the head and neck area and they are red-brown plaques with a yellow-brown color on diascopy. Secondary scarring and squamous cell carcinomas can develop within the plaques. Cultures of the lesions should be done because it is rare for the acid-fast stain to show bacilli within the dermal granulomas.

Sweet's syndrome is characterized by red-brown plaques and nodules that are frequently painful and occur primarily on the head, neck, and upper extremities. The patients also have fever, neutrophilia, and a dense dermal infiltrate of neutrophils in the lesions. In approximately 10 percent of the patients, there is an associated malignancy, most commonly acute nonlymphocytic leukemia. Lymphoma, chronic leukemia, myeloma, myelodysplastic syndromes, and solid tumors (primarily of the genitourinary tract) have also been reported. Extracutaneous sites of involvement include joints, muscles, eye, kidney (proteinuria, occasionally glomerulonephritis), and lung (neutrophilic infiltrates). The idiopathic form of Sweet's syndrome is seen more often in women, following a respiratory tract infection.

A generalized distribution of red-brown macules and papules is seen in the form of mastocytosis known as *urticaria pigmentosa.* Each lesion represents a collection of mast cells in the dermis with hyperpigmentation of the overlying epidermis. Stimuli such as rubbing and heat cause these mast cells to degranulate and this leads to the formation of localized urticaria (Darier's sign). Additional symptoms can result from mast cell degranulation and these include headache, flushing, diarrhea, and pruritus. Mast cells also infiltrate various organs such as the liver, spleen, and gastrointestinal tract in up to 30 to 50 percent of patients with urticaria pigmentosa, and accumulations of mast cells in the bones may produce either osteosclerotic or osteolytic shadows on radiographs. In the majority of these patients, however, the internal involvement remains fairly static. A subtype of chronic leukocytoclastic vasculitis, *erythema elevatum diutinum* (EED), also presents with papules that are red-brown in color. The papules coalesce into plaques on the extensor surface of knees, elbows, and small joints of the hand. Flares of EED have been associated with streptococcal infections.

Blue lesions Lesions that are blue in color are the result of either vascular ectasias and tumors or melanin pigment in the dermis. *Venous lakes* (ectasias) are compressible dark blue lesions that are found commonly in the head and neck region. *Cavernous hemangiomas* are also compressible blue papules and nodules that can occur anywhere on the body, including the oral mucosa. When they are multiple rather than single congenital lesions, the patient may have the blue rubber bleb syndrome or Mafucci's syndrome. Patients with the blue rubber bleb syndrome also have hemangiomas of the gastrointestinal tract that may bleed, whereas patients with Mafucci's syndrome have associated dyschondroplasia and osteochondromas. In the case of single cavernous hemangiomas that are relatively large in size, there can be associated platelet consumption (Kasabach-Merritt syndrome) or musculoskeletal defects. *Blue nevi* (moles) are seen when there are collections of pigment-producing nevus cells in the dermis. These benign papular lesions are dome-shaped and they occur most commonly on the dorsum of the hand and arm.

Violaceous lesions Violaceous papules and plaques are seen in *lupus pernio, lymphoma cutis,* and *cutaneous lupus*. Lupus pernio is a particular type of sarcoidosis that involves the tip of the nose and the earlobes, with lesions that are violaceous in color rather than red-brown. This form of sarcoidosis is associated with involvement of the upper respiratory tract. The plaques of lymphoma cutis and cutaneous lupus may be red or violaceous in color and are discussed above.

Purple lesions Purple-colored papules and plaques are seen in vascular tumors, such as *Kaposi's sarcoma* (see Chap. 264) and *angiosarcoma,* and when there is extravasation of red blood cells into the skin in association with inflammation, as in *palpable purpura* (see purpura). Patients with congenital or acquired arteriovenous fistulas can develop purple papules on the lower extremities that can resemble Kaposi's sarcoma clinically and histologically, and this condition is referred to as pseudo-Kaposi sarcoma (acral angiodermatitis). *Angiosarcoma* is found most commonly on the scalp and face of elderly patients or within areas of chronic lymphedema and it presents as purple papules and plaques. In the head and neck region, the tumor often extends beyond the clinically defined borders and may be accompanied by facial edema.

Brown and black-colored papules are reviewed in the section on hyperpigmentation.

Cutaneous metastases are discussed last because they can have a wide range of colors. Most commonly they present as either firm flesh-colored subcutaneous nodules or red to red-brown firm papulonodules. The lesions of lymphoma cutis range from pink-red to plum in color while metastatic melanoma can be pink, blue, or black in color. Cutaneous metastases develop from hematogenous or lymphatic spread and are most often due to the following primary carcinomas: in men, lung, colon, melanoma, and oral cavity; and in women, breast, colon, and lung. These metastatic lesions may be the initial presentation of the carcinoma, especially when the primary site is the lung, kidney, or ovary.

PURPURA (Table 59-21) Purpura are seen when there is an extravasation of red blood cells into the dermis and, as a result, the lesions do not blanch with pressure. This is in contrast to those erythematous or violet-colored lesions that are due to localized vasodilatation—they do blanch with pressure. Purpura ($\geq$3 mm) and petechiae ($\leq$2 mm) are divided into two major groups, palpable and nonpalpable. The most frequent causes of *nonpalpable* petechiae and purpura are primary cutaneous disorders such as *trauma, solar purpura,* and *steroid purpura.* Less common causes are *capillaritis* and *livedoid vasculitis* (see "Ulcers"). Solar purpura are seen primarily on the dorsum of the hand and extensor forearm while glucocorticoid purpura, secondary to potent topical steroids, or endogenous or exogenous Cushing's syndrome can be more widespread. In both cases, there is alteration of the supporting connective tissue that surrounds the dermal blood vessels. In contrast, the petechiae that result from capillaritis are found primarily on the lower extremities. In capillaritis, there is an extravasation of erythrocytes as a result of perivascular lymphocytic inflammation. The petechiae are bright red, 1 to 2 mm in size, and scattered within annular or coin-shaped yellow-brown macules. The yellow-brown color is caused by hemosiderin deposits within the dermis.

TABLE 59-21 Causes of purpura

Primary cutaneous disorders
- *A* Nonpalpable
  - *1* Trauma
  - *2* Solar purpura
  - *3* Steroid purpura
  - *4* Capillaritis
  - *5* Livedoid vasculitis

Systemic diseases
- *A* Nonpalpable
  - *1* Clotting disturbances
    - *a* Thrombocytopenia
    - *b* Abnormal platelet function
    - *c* Clotting factor defects
  - *2* Vascular fragility
    - *a* Amyloidosis
    - *b* Ehlers-Danlos syndrome
    - *c* Scurvy
  - *3* Thrombi
    - *a* Disseminated intravascular coagulation
    - *b* Monoclonal cryoglobulinemia
    - *c* Thrombotic thrombocytopenic purpura
    - *d* Warfarin reaction
  - *4* Emboli
    - *a* Cholesterol
    - *b* Fat
  - *5* Possible immune complex
    - *a* Gardner-Diamond syndrome (autoerythrocyte sensitization)
    - *b* Waldenström's hypergammaglobulinemic purpura
- *B* Palpable
  - *1* Vasculitis
    - *a* Leukocytoclastic vasculitis (oval outline)
    - *b* Polyarteritis nodosa (irregular outline)
  - *2* Emboli (irregular outline)
    - *a* Acute meningococcemia
    - *b* Disseminated gonococcal infection
    - *c* Rocky mountain spotted fever
    - *d* Ecthyma gangrenosum

Systemic causes of nonpalpable purpura fall into several categories and those secondary to clotting disturbances and vascular fragility will be discussed first. The former group includes *thrombocytopenia, abnormal platelet function* as is seen in uremia, and *clotting factor defects.* The initial site of presentation for thrombocytopenia-induced petechiae is the distal lower extremity. Capillary fragility leads to nonpalpable purpura in patients with systemic *amyloidosis* (see "Papulonodular Skin Lesions") and disorders of collagen production such as *Ehlers-Danlos syndrome* and *scurvy.* In scurvy, there are flattened corkscrew hairs with surrounding hemorrhage on the lower extremities, in addition to gingivitis. Vitamin C is a cofactor for lysyl hydroxylase, an enzyme involved in the posttranslational modification of procollagen that is necessary for cross-link formation.

In contrast to the previous group of disorders in which either capillary fragility or a clotting abnormality is responsible for the nonpalpable purpura, the purpura seen in the following group of diseases are associated with thrombi formation within vessels. It is important to note that these thrombi are demonstrable in skin biopsy specimens. This group of disorders includes *disseminated intravascular coagulation, monoclonal cryoglobulinemia, thrombotic thrombocytopenic purpura* and *reactions to warfarin.* Disseminated intravascular coagulation (DIC) is triggered by several types of infection (gram-negative, gram-positive, viral, and rickettsial) as well as by tissue injury and neoplasms. Widespread purpura and hemorrhagic infarcts of the distal extremities are seen. Similar lesions are found in purpura fulminans, which is a form of DIC associated with fever and hypotension that occurs more commonly in children following an infectious illness such as varicella, scarlet fever, or an upper respiratory tract infection. In both disorders, hemorrhagic bullae can develop in involved skin.

Monoclonal cryoglobulinemia is associated with multiple myeloma, Waldenström's macroglobulinemia, lymphocytic leukemia, and lymphoma. Purpura, primarily of the lower extremities, and hemorrhagic infarcts of the fingers and toes are seen in these patients. Exacerbations of disease activity can follow cold exposure or an increase in serum viscosity. Biopsy specimens show precipitates of the cryoglobulin within dermal vessels. Similar deposits have been found in the lung, brain, and renal glomeruli. Patients with *thrombotic thrombocytopenic purpura* can also have hemorrhagic infarcts as a result of intravascular thromboses. Additional signs include thrombocytopenic purpura, fever, and microangiopathic hemolytic anemia (see Chap. 294).

Administration of *warfarin* can result in painful areas of erythema that become purpuric then necrotic with an adherent black eschar. This reaction is seen more often in women and in areas with abundant subcutaneous fat—breasts, abdomen, buttocks, thighs, and calves. The erythema and purpura develop between the third and tenth day of therapy, most likely as a result of a transient imbalance in the levels of anticoagulant and procoagulant vitamin K–dependent factors. Continued therapy does not exacerbate preexisting lesions, and patients with an inherited or acquired deficiency of protein C are at increased risk for this particular reaction as well as for purpura fulminans.

Purpura secondary to *cholesterol emboli* are usually seen on the lower extremities of patients with atherosclerotic vascular disease. They often follow anticoagulant therapy or an invasive vascular procedure such as an arteriogram, but they also occur spontaneously from disintegration of atheromatous plaques. Associated findings include livedo reticularis, gangrene, cyanosis, subcutaneous nodules, and ischemic ulcerations. Multiple step sections of the biopsy specimen may be necessary to demonstrate the cholesterol clefts with the vessels. Petechiae are also an important sign of *fat embolism* and they occur primarily on the upper body 2 to 3 days after a major injury. By using special fixatives, the emboli can be demonstrated in biopsy specimens of the petechiae. Emboli of tumor or thrombus are seen in patients with atrial myxomas and marantic endocarditis.

In the *Gardner-Diamond* syndrome (autoerythrocyte sensitivity), female patients develop large ecchymoses within areas of painful, warm erythema. An episode of significant trauma frequently precedes the onset of this syndrome. Intradermal injections of autologous erythrocytes or phosphatidyl serine derived from the red cell membrane can reproduce the lesions in most patients; however, there are instances where a reaction is seen at an injection site of the forearm, but not in the midback region. The latter has led some observers to view Gardner-Diamond syndrome as a cutaneous manifestation of severe emotional stress. *Waldenström's hypergammaglobulinemic purpura* is a chronic disorder characterized by petechiae on the lower extremities. There are circulating complexes of IgG; anti-IgG molecules and exacerbations are associated with prolonged standing or walking.

Palpable purpura are further subdivided into vasculitic and embolic. In the group of vasculitic disorders, *leukocytoclastic vasculitis* (LCV), also known as allergic vasculitis, is the one most commonly associated with palpable purpura (see Chap. 276). *Henoch-Schönlein purpura* is a subtype of acute LCV that is seen primarily in children and adolescents following an upper respiratory infection. The majority of lesions are found on the lower extremities and buttocks. Systemic manifestations include fever, arthralgias (primarily of the knees and ankles), abdominal pain, gastrointestinal bleeding, and nephritis. Direct immunofluorescence examination shows deposits of IgA within dermal blood vessel walls. In *polyarteritis nodosa,* specific cutaneous lesions result from a vasculitis of arterial vessels rather than from postcapillary venules as in LCV. The arteritis leads to ischemia of the skin and this explains the irregular outline of the purpura (see below).

Several types of emboli can give rise to palpable purpura. Infectious embolic lesions are usually *irregular* in outline as opposed to the lesions of leukocytoclastic vasculitis which are *circular* in outline. The irregular outline is indicative of a cutaneous infarct, and the size correponds to the area of skin that received its blood supply from that particular arteriole or artery. The palpable purpura in LCV are circular because the erythrocytes simply diffuse out evenly from the postcapillary venules as a result of inflammation. Infectious emboli are most commonly due to gram-negative cocci (meningococcus, gonococcus), gram-negative rods (Enterobacteriaceae), and gram-positive cocci (staphylococcus). Additional causes include *Rickettsia* and, in immunocompromised patients, *Candida* and *Aspergillus.*

The embolic lesions in *acute meningococcemia* are found primarily on the trunk, lower extremities, and sites of pressure, and a gunmetal-gray color often develops within them. Their size varies from 1 mm to several centimeters, and the organisms can be cultured from the lesions. Associated findings include a preceding upper respiratory tract infection, fever, meningitis, disseminated intravascular coagulation, and, in some patients, a deficiency of the terminal components of complement. In *disseminated gonococcal infection* (arthritis-dermatitis syndrome), a small number of papules and vesicopustules with central purpura or hemorrhagic necrosis are found over the joints of the distal extremities. Additional symptoms include arthralgias, tenosynovitis, and fever. To establish the diagnosis, a Gram stain of these lesions should be performed. *Rocky mountain spotted fever* is a tick-borne disease that is caused by *Rickettsia rickettsii.* A several-day history of fever, chills, severe headache, and photophobia precedes the onset of the cutaneous eruption. The initial lesions are erythematous macules and papules on the wrists, ankles, palms, and soles. With time the lesions spread centripetally and become purpuric.

Lesions of *ecthyma gangrenosum* begin as edematous erythematous papules or plaques and then develop central purpura and necrosis. Bullae-formation also occurs in these lesions, and they are frequently found in the girdle region. The organism that is clasically associated with ecthyma gangrenosum is *Pseudomonas aeruginosa,* but other gram-negative rods such as *Klebsiella, E. coli,* and *Serratia* can produce similar lesions. In immunocompromised hosts, the list of potential pathogens is expanded to include *Candida* and *Aspergillus.*

ULCERS (Table 59-22) As an approach to the patient with a cutaneous ulcer, the etiologies are divided into two major groups: (1) primary cutaneous disorders and (2) underlying systemic diseases. Within the group of primary cutaneous disorders, there are three categories: vascular, tumor-associated, and infectious. The *peripheral vascular* group is the first to be discussed because it contains the most common cause of lower extremity ulcers in adults, *venous insufficiency.* Stasis ulcers are characteristically painless and contain adequate granulation tissue. They are often found on the medial malleoli against a background of varicosities, stasis dermatitis, edema, and hemosiderin deposition (yellow-brown discoloration of the skin).

In contrast, lower extremity ulcers due to *arteriosclerosis obliterans* are often painful and are associated with cool, hairless, atrophic skin and dystrophic nails—all a reflection of a decrease in blood flow. The majority of patients are men and they frequently have evidence of atherosclerosis in other large- and medium-sized arteries. *Thromboangiitis obliterans* (Buerger's disease) and *Mönckeberg's arteriosclerosis* are two less common arterial diseases that can lead to ulcers of the distal upper extremity as well as the lower extremity. The latter is found in patients with primary or secondary hyperparathyroidism, and the calcification of the tunica media of involved muscular arteries is seen radiographically as a diffuse pipe-stem

TABLE 59-22 Causes of cutaneous ulcers

Primary cutaneous disorders
- *A* Peripheral vascular disease
  - *1* Venous
  - *2* Arterial
- *B* Livedoid vasculitis
- *C* Squamous cell carcinoma, e.g., within scars
- *D* Infections, e.g., ecthyma

Systemic diseases
- *A* Legs
  - *1* Leukocytoclastic vasculitis
  - *2* Hemoglobinopathies
  - *3* Cryoglobulinemia
  - *4* Cholesterol emboli
  - *5* Necrobiosis lipoidica
- *B* Hands and feet
  - *1* Raynaud's phenomenon
- *C* Generalized
  - *1* Pyoderma gangrenosum
- *D* Mucosal
  - *1* Behçet's syndrome
  - *2* Erythema multiforme

calcification. Buerger's disease occurs primarily in young men (ages 25 to 40) who smoke or have been smokers.

Livedoid vasculitis (atrophie blanche) represents a combination of a vasculopathy with intravascular thrombosis. Purpuric lesions and livedo reticularis are found in association with painful ulcerations of the lower extremities. These ulcers are often slow to heal, but when they do, irregularly shaped white scars are formed. The majority of cases are idiopathic in origin, but possible underlying illnesses include systemic lupus, the antiphospholipid syndrome, scleroderma, and cryoglobulinemia. Patients with the antiphospholipid syndrome have anticardiolipin antibodies, biologic false-positive tests for syphilis, and prolonged activated partial thromboplastin times; the latter are due to a circulating lupus anticoagulant. These antiphospholipid antibodies are seen most commonly in patients with systemic lupus, but they are also associated with other connective tissue diseases. In addition to the lesions of livedoid vasculitis, patients with the antiphospholipid syndrome have recurrent venous thrombosis, arterial thrombosis (including cerebrovascular accidents), spontaneous abortions, and thrombocytopenia.

Several *carcinomas* can present as cutaneous ulcers, e.g., basal cell carcinoma, squamous cell carcinoma, and, less often, melanoma. When an ulcer on the lower extremity does not heal, despite correction of the presumed cause, it should be biopsied to rule out carcinoma, primarily squamous cell carcinoma. The same holds true for ulcers that develop with scars. Bacterial and viral *infections* also lead to cutaneous ulceration, and one of the more commonly isolated organisms is streptococcus. The term ecthyma is used to describe the often widespread ulcerative lesions that are caused by this bacteria. Ecthyma is a primary cutaneous disorder and should not be confused with ecthyma gangrenosum, which is secondary to blood-borne emboli (see "Purpura"). In Meleney's ulcer, a gradually expanding ulcer begins at a site of trauma or surgery. The clinical appearance is similar to that of pyoderma gangrenosum, but it is due to a synergistic infection that usually includes anaerobic streptococci.

For one group of patients with cutaneous ulcers, the lower extremity is the primary location for those due to an underlying systemic disease. In a young patient, ischemic cutaneous ulcers on the leg should raise the possibility of a *hemoglobinopathy* or *hereditary spherocytosis*. Intravascular thrombosis is the presumed cause of these ulcers as well as for the ulcers seen in patients with *monoclonal cryoglobulinemia* (see "Purpura"). Primary and secondary forms of *LCV* as well as *emboli of cholesterol* can result in cutaneous ulceration, again primarily on the lower extremities (see "Purpura"). For example, lower extremity ulcers in patients with rheumatoid arthritis are often due to vasculitis. In addition, the yellow atrophic plaques of *necrobiosis lipoidica* can break down centrally into an ulcer (see "Papulonodular Skin Lesions").

Vasospasm occurs in patients with *Raynaud's phenomenon* and can lead to ulcerations of the hands as well as the feet. Raynaud's phenomenon is defined as a triphasic reaction of pallor, cyanosis, and hyperemia in response to cold or emotional stress. Vasospasm is also seen in patients who receive systemic noradrenaline, vasopressin, ergot, and bleomycin. The patient with Raynaud's phenomenon and ulcerations on the tips of the digits should be examined carefully for periungual and mat telangiectasias, the subtle signs of scleroderma. Raynaud's phenomenon is also seen in patients with dermatomyositis, systemic lupus, cryoglobulinemia, cervical rib and scalenus anticus syndromes, pneumatic hammer disease, and occupational acroosteolysis (associated with the manufacture of polyvinyl chloride).

In *pyoderma gangrenosum*, the border of the ulcers has a characteristic appearance of an undermined necrotic bluish edge and a peripheral erythematous halo. The ulcers often begin as pustules that then expand rather rapidly to a size as large as 20 cm. Although these lesions are most commonly found on the lower extremities, they can arise anywhere on the surface of the body, including sites of trauma (pathergy). An estimated 30 to 50 percent of cases are idiopathic, and the most common associated disorders are ulcerative colitis and Crohn's disease. Less commonly, it is associated with chronic active hepatitis, seropositive rheumatoid arthritis, acute and chronic granulocytic leukemia, polycythemia vera, and myeloma. Additional findings in these patients, even those with idiopathic disease, are cutaneous anergy and a benign monoclonal gammopathy. Because the histology of pyoderma gangrenosum is nonspecific, the diagnosis is made clinically by excluding less common causes of similar-appearing ulcers such as necrotizing vasculitis, Meleney's ulcer (see above), dimorphic fungi, cutaneous amebiasis, spider bites, and facticial. In the myeloproliferative disorders, the ulcers may be more superficial with a pustulobullous border and these lesions provide a connection between classic pyoderma gangrenosum and acute febrile neutrophilic dermatosis (Sweet's syndrome).

The diagnosis of *Behçet's* disease requires the presence of three major clinical criteria, one of which must be recurrent aphthae. The major criteria include: (1) recurrent aphthous stomatitis; (2) recurrent genital ulcers, primarily of the scrotum and labia; (3) uveitis; (4) vasculitis of either cutaneous or large vessels—the skin lesions may be papules, pustules, or nodules; (5) synovitis; (6) meningoencephalitis; and (7) pathergy, which is defined as reproduction of cutaneous lesions by trauma. A test for pathergy is the injection of sterile saline into the dermis. The oral ulcers are painful and well-defined with an erythematous halo, whereas the genital ulcers tend to be deeper and heal with scarring. Patients can also have ulceration of the gastrointestinal tract, superficial and deep thrombophlebitis, pyoderma, and furunculosis. Disorders that must be excluded include recurrent *erythema multiforme* (see "Vesicles/Bullae"), herpes simplex, inflammatory bowel disease, systemic lupus, and Reiter's disease.

REFERENCES

BORK K: *Cutaneous Side Effects of Drugs*. Philadelphia, Saunders, 1988

BRAVERMAN IM: *Skin Signs of Systemic Disease*, 2d ed. Philadelphia, Saunders, 1981

DEVITA VT JR et al: (eds): *Cancer—Principles and Practice of Oncology*, 2d ed. Philadelphia, Lippincott, 1985

JORRIZZO JL: *Dermatology Clinics*, vol 3: No 1: *Urticaria*. Philadelphia, Saunders, 198 .

LEVER WF, SCHAUMBURG-LEVER G: *Histopathology of the Skin*, 6th ed. Philadelphia, Lippincott, 1983

ROOK A et al (eds): *Textbook of Dermatology*, 4th ed. Oxford, Blackwell Scientific, 1986.

60 PHOTOSENSITIVITY AND OTHER REACTIONS TO LIGHT

DAVID R. BICKERS

SOLAR RADIATION Sunlight is the most visible and obvious source of comfort in the environment, and it is in the nature of humans to love light. This natural proclivity for the sun has the beneficial results of warmth and vitamin D synthesis but also can produce pathologic consequences of cutaneous sun exposure. Few effects due to exposure to the sun beyond those on the skin have been identified, but cutaneous exposure to sunlight can alter immunologic responses at sites distant from the skin.

The sun's energy encompasses a broad range from ultrashort ionizing radiation (10^{-2} μm) to ultralong radiowaves of very low photon energy (10^{7} μm). Thus, the emission spectrum has a range of nine orders of magnitude, but the component that reaches the earth's surface is narrow and includes the components of the ultraviolet, visible light, and portions of the infrared. The cutoff at the short end of the ultraviolet is at approximately 290 nm, because stratospheric ozone is formed by ionizing radiation of wavelengths less than 100 nm and ozone absorbs incident energy between 120 and 310 nm. In effect, stratospheric ozone prevents the penetration to the earth's surface of the shorter, more energetic, potentially more harmful wavelengths of solar radiation. Indeed, concern about the destruction of ozone by chlorofluorocarbons released into the atmosphere has led to international agreements to reduce production of these chemicals.

Measurements of solar flux in various areas indicate that there is a twentyfold variation in the amount of ultraviolet B at 300 nm that reaches the surface of the earth. This variability is in part related to seasonal effects, the path of sunlight transmission through ozone and air, the altitude (4 percent increase for each 300 m of elevation), the latitude (increasing intensity with decreasing latitude), and the amount of cloud cover, fog, and pollution.

The major components of the photobiologic action spectrum include the ultraviolet and visible wavelengths between 290 and 700 nm. In addition, the wavelengths beyond 700 nm in the infrared primarily evoke heat, but warming of the skin may enhance the response to wavelengths in the ultraviolet and visible spectrum.

The ultraviolet (UV) spectrum is arbitrarily divided into three major segments: C, B, and A. This includes the wavelengths between 10 and 400 nm. UV-C consists of wavelengths between 10 and 290 nm and does not reach the earth because of its absorption by stratospheric ozone. These wavelengths are not a cause of photosensitivity except in occupational settings where artificial sources of this energy are employed, for example, for germicidal effects. UV-B consists of wavelengths between 290 and 320 nm. This portion of the photobiologic action spectrum is the most efficient in producing redness or erythema in human skin, and hence it is sometimes known as the sunburn spectrum. UV-A represents those wavelengths between 320 and 400 nm and is approximately a thousandfold less efficient in producing skin hyperemia than is UV-B.

The visible wavelengths between 400 and 700 nm include the familiar white light which when directed through a prism can be shown to consist of various colors including violet, indigo, blue, green, yellow, orange, and red. The energy possessed by photons in the visible spectrum usually is not capable of damaging human skin in the absence of a photosensitizing chemical. Photon energy levels are critical to photosensitivity since the absorption process requires that sufficient energy be present. The absorption of a photon is an all-or-none phenomenon, and when absorbed, the photon ceases to exist. The absorption of energy is critical to the development of photosensitivity. Thus, the *absorption spectrum* of a molecule is defined as the range of wavelengths absorbed by it, whereas the *action spectrum* for an effect of incident radiation is defined as the range of wavelengths that evoke the response.

Photosensitivity occurs when a photon-absorbing chemical (*chromophore*) present in the skin absorbs incident energy, becomes excited, and transfers the absorbed energy to various structures or to oxygen. The absorbed energy must subsequently be dissipated by processes including heat, fluorescence, and phosphorescence. It is important to emphasize that absorption spectra and action spectra need not be superimposable, but there must be overlap at some point to produce photosensitization.

STRUCTURE AND FUNCTION OF SKIN The skin is accessible to incident solar radiation and has a structural heterogeneity that permits the absorption of some wavelengths and the transmission of others. Essentially, human skin is a sandwich of two distinctive compartments, the epidermis and dermis. The outer epidermis is a stratified squamous epithelium comprising the surface stratum corneum (a protein- and lipid-rich compact acellular membrane), the stratum granulosum, stratum Malphigii, and the basal cell layer. The basal cell layer contains a heterogeneous population of dividing cells and resting cells, some of which begin an upward migratory process of terminal differentiation that results in keratinization to form the stratum corneum. The cells of the epidermis include resident keratinocytes and melanocytes and immigrant cells including the immunologically active Langerhans cells, lymphocytes, polymorphonuclear leukocytes, monocytes, and macrophages. The epidermis is a major component of the immune system. Branches of sensory nerve endings also reach into this compartment.

The second major component of skin is the dermis, which is relatively large and less densely populated with cells that include fibroblasts, endothelial cells within dermal vessels, and mast cells. Tissue macrophages and sparsely distributed inflammatory cells are also present. All of these cells exist within an extracellular matrix of collagen, elastin, and glycosaminoglycans. In contrast to the epidermis, rich vascularization of the dermis allows it to play an important role in temperature regulation.

UV RADIATION AND SKIN The epidermis and the dermis contain several chromophores capable of interacting with incident solar energy. These interactions include reflection, refraction, absorption, and transmission. The stratum corneum is a major impediment to the transmission of UV-B, and less than 10 percent of incident wavelengths in this region penetrate the basement membrane. Approximately 3 percent of radiation below 300 nm, 20 percent of radiation below 360 nm, and 33 percent of short visible radiation reaches the basal cell layer in untanned human skin. Proteins and nucleic acids absorb intensely in the short UV-B. In contrast, the UV-A penetrates the epidermis efficiently to reach the dermis, where it likely produces changes in structural and matrix proteins that contribute to the appearance of chronically exposed skin, particularly in individuals of light complexion.

Proteins and nucleic acids in the epidermis are major absorbers of UV-B, and one of the consequences of this absorption process is the production in DNA of pyrimidine, particularly thymine dimers. These structural changes are produced primarily by UV-B, but also by UV-A, and can be repaired by mechanisms that result in their excision and the reestablishment of normal base sequences. The efficient repair of these structural aberrations is crucial since individuals with defective DNA repair are at high risk for the development of cutaneous cancer. For example, patients with xeroderma pigmentosum, an autosomal recessive disorder, are characterized by variably decreased repair of UV-induced pyrimidine dimers and may develop the xerotic appearance of photoaging as well as basal cell and squamous cell carcinomas and melanoma in the first two decades of life.

Cutaneous optics and chromophores Chromophores are endogenous or exogenous chemical components that can absorb physical energy. Endogenous chromophores of skin are of two types: (1) chemicals that are normally present in the biologic structure of the skin, including nucleic acids, proteins, lipids, and cholesterol derivatives such as the precursor of vitamin D, and (2) chemicals, such as porphyrins, synthesized elsewhere in the body that circulate in the bloodstream and diffuse into the skin where they can absorb incident radiation and evoke cutaneous photosensitivity. Normally, only trace amounts of porphyrins are present in the skin, but in the porphyrias increased amounts of porphyrins are released into the circulation and are transported to the skin, where they absorb incident energy both in the Soret band around 400 nm (short visible) and to a lesser extent in the red portion of the visible spectrum (580 to 660 nm). This results in structural damage to the skin that may be manifest as erythema, edema, urticaria, or blister formation (see Chap. 328).

Acute effects of sun exposure The immediate cutaneous consequences of sun exposure include sunburn and vitamin D synthesis.

SUNBURN This very common affliction of human skin is the result of sun exposure. Generally speaking, the ability of an individual to tolerate sunlight is inversely proportional to melanin pigmentation. Melanin is a complex polymer of tyrosine that functions as an efficient neutral-density filter with broad absorbance within the UV portion of the solar spectrum. Melanin is synthesized in specialized epidermal dendritic cells termed *melanocytes* and packaged into *melanosomes* that are transferred via dendritic processes into *keratinocytes,* where they provide photoprotection. A single melanocyte can provide melanin pigment for approximately 36 keratinocytes, and this group of cells is termed the *epidermal-melanin unit.* Tolerance of sun exposure is a function of the efficiency of the epidermal melanin unit and can usually be ascertained by asking an individual two questions: (1) Do you always, sometimes, or never burn after sun exposure on unprotected skin? and (2) Do you never, sometimes, or always tan? By the answers to these questions, it is usually possible to divide the population into six skin types varying from type I (always burn, never tan) to type VI (never burn, always tan) (see Table 60-1).

There are two general theories about the pathogenesis of the sunburn response. First, the lag phase in time between skin exposure and the development of visible redness (usually 4 to 12 h) may be due to an epidermal chromophore that causes a delayed production and/or release of vasoactive mediator(s) that diffuse to the dermal vasculature to evoke vasodilatation. Other evidence suggests that the small amount of incident UV-B radiation (10 percent or less) that penetrates to the dermis can be absorbed by endothelial cells in the vasculature, thereby directly resulting in vasodilatation. The issue remains unresolved.

The action spectrum for sunburn erythema includes the UV-B and the UV-A. Photons in the shorter UV-B are perhaps a thousandfold more efficient than photons in the longer UV-B and the UV-A in evoking the response. However, UV-A may contribute to sunburn erythema at midday when much more UV-A than UV-B is present.

The mechanism of injury remains pooly defined, but the action spectrum for UV-B erythema closely resembles the absorption spectrum for DNA after adjusting for the absorbance of incident energy by the stratum corneum. Damaged keratinocytes (so-called sunburn cells) are visible histologically within an hour and are maximal within 24 h of exposure. UV-A is less effective than UV-B in producing sunburn cells. Mast cells may release inflammatory mediators after exposure to UV-B and UV-A radiation. For example, erythema doses of both UV-B and UV-A increase histamine levels in suction blisters of human skin that return to normal by 24 h (before visible erythema has subsided). Prostaglandin E_2 (PGE_2) increases to approximately 150 percent of control levels by 24 h and then diminishes. Since prostaglandins evoke both pain and redness when injected intradermally, their presence in suction blisters after UV-B radiation suggests a role in UV-B erythema. There may be an age-related decline in the amount of inflammatory mediators detectable in human skin after UV-B irradiation. UV-A erythema results in few epidermal sunburn cells, but vascular endothelial injury is greater than with UV-B. In addition, there are increased levels of arachidonic acid and of prostaglandins D_2, E_2, and I_2 that peak within 5 to 9 h and then subside before peak redness occurs. Despite the evidence for elevated prostaglandins in both UV-B- and UV-A-irradiated skin, administration of nonsteroidal anti-inflammatory drugs is more effective in reducing erythema evoked by UV-B than by UV-A.

VITAMIN D PHOTOCHEMISTRY Cutaneous exposure to UV-B causes photolysis of epidermal provitamin D_3 (7-dehydrocholesterol) to previtamin D_3, which then undergoes a temperature-dependent isomerization to form the stable hormone vitamin D_3. This compound then diffuses to the dermal vasculature and circulates to the liver and kidney, where it is converted to the functional hormone 1,25-dihydroxy vitamin D_3 [$1,25(OH)_2D_3$] (see also Chap. 399). There are age-related differences in the rates of conversion of provitamin D_3 to previtamin D_3. Aging substantially decreases the ability of human skin to produce vitamin D_3. This, coupled with the widespread recommended use of sunscreens that filter out UV-B, has led to concern that vitamin D deficiency may become a significant clinical problem in the elderly. Indeed, studies have shown that the use of a sunscreen with a sun protection factor of 8 can prevent the production of vitamin D_3 in human skin.

TABLE 60-1 Skin type and sunburn sensitivity

Type	Description
I	Always burn, never tan
II	Always burn, sometimes tan
III	Sometimes burn, always tan
IV	Never burn, always tan
V	Darker pigment
VI	Darkest pigment

Chronic effects of sun exposure: nonmalignant The clinical features of photodamaged sun-exposed skin consist of wrinkling, blotchiness, telangiectasia, and a roughened irregular "weatherbeaten" appearance. Whether these changes, which some refer to as "photoaging" or dermatoheliosis, represent accelerated chronologic aging or a separate and distinct process is not clear.

Within chronically sun-exposed epidermis there is thickening (acanthosis) and morphologic heterogeneity within the basal cell layer. Higher but irregular melanosome content may be present in some keratinocytes, indicating prolonged residence of the cells in the basal cell layer. These structural changes may help to explain the leathery texture and the blotchy discoloration of sun-damaged skin.

The dermis is the major site for sun-associated chronic damage, manifest as a massive increase in thickened irregular masses of tangled elastic fibers containing uncharacterized electron-dense material. Collagen fibers are also abnormally clumped in the deeper dermis. Fibroblasts are increased in number and show morphologic signs suggesting enhanced metabolic activity. Degraded mast cells may be present in the dermis, the relevance of which remains unclear.

These morphologic changes, both gross and microscopic, are features of chronically sun-exposed skin. The chromophore(s), the action spectra, and the specific biochemical events that result in these changes are unknown. Although topical retinoids, particularly vitamin A acid, are being used for the treatment of these photoaging changes in human skin, neither the efficacy nor the long-term safety has been verified.

Chronic effects of sun exposure: malignant One of the major known consequences of chronic skin exposure to sunlight is nonmelanoma skin cancer. The two types of skin cancer are basal cell and squamous cell carcinoma (see Chap. 307). There are three major steps for cancer induction: initiation, promotion, and progression. Chronic exposure of animal skin to artificial light sources that mimic solar UV radiation results in *initiation,* a step whereby structural (mutational) changes in DNA evoke an irreversible change in the target cell (keratinocyte) that begins the tumorigenic process. Exposure to a tumor initiator is believed to be a necessary but not sufficient step in the malignant process. Thus, initiated cells that are not exposed to tumor promoters do not generally develop into tumors. The second stage in tumor development is promotion, a multistep process whereby initiated cells are exposed to chemical and physical agents that evoke epigenetic changes that culminate in the clonal expansion of initiated cells and cause the development, over a period of weeks to months, of benign growths known as *papillomas*. UV-B radiation is a complete carcinogen, meaning that it can function as both an initiator and a promoter leading to tumor induction. Incomplete carcinogens can initiate tumorigenesis but require additional skin exposure to tumor promoters to cause the production of tumors. The prototype tumor promoter is the phorbol ester 12-*0*-tetradecanoyl phorbol-13-acetate (TPA). Tumor promotion usually requires multiple exposures over time to evoke a neoplasm.

The first tumors that develop in skin exposed to solar radiation are benign papillomas. The final step in the malignant process is the conversion of the benign papillomas into malignant squamous cell carcinomas, a process thought to require additional genetic alterations in already transformed cells.

Sun exposure is believed to promote the development of both nonmelanoma and melanoma cancers of the skin, although the evidence is far more direct for its role in nonmelanoma (basal cell and squamous cell carcinoma) than in melanoma cancers. Approximately 80 percent of nonmelanoma skin cancers develop on exposed body areas, including the face, the neck, and the hands. The nose and cheeks are the most commonly affected sites. Men of fair complexion who work outdoors are twice as likely as women to develop these types of cancers. Whites of darker complexions (e.g.,

Hispanics) have one-tenth the risk of developing such cancers as do light-skinned individuals. Blacks are at lowest risk for all forms of skin cancer. Between 400,000 and 500,000 individuals in the United States annually develop nonmelanoma skin cancer, and the lifetime risk for a white individual to develop such a neoplasm is estimated at approximately 15 percent. A consensus exists that the incidence of nonmelanoma skin cancer is rising as a result of greater opportunities for sun exposure in the population.

The relationship of sun exposure to melanoma is less clear-cut, but suggestive evidence supports an association. Melanomas may develop by the teenage years, indicating that the latent period for tumor growth is less than that of nonmelanomas. Epidemiologic studies of immigrants of similar ethnic stock indicate that individuals born in one area or who migrated to the same locale before age 10 have higher age-specific melanoma rates than individuals arriving later. It is thus reasonable to conclude that life in a sunny climate from birth or early childhood increases the risk of melanoma. In general, risk does not correlate with cumulative sun exposure but may relate to sequelae of sun exposure in childhood. Thus, a blistering sunburn is associated with a doubling of melanoma risk at the site of the reaction.

Immunologic effects Exposure to solar radiation influences both local and systemic immune responses. UV-B appears to be most efficient in altering immune responses, likely related to the capacity of such energy to affect antigen presentation in skin by interacting with epidermal Langerhans cells. These bone marrow–derived dendritic cells possess surface markers characteristic of monocytes and macrophages. Following skin exposure to erythema doses of UV-B, Langerhans cells undergo both morphologic and functional changes that result in decreased contact allergic responses when haptens are applied to the radiated site. This diminished capacity for sensitization is due to the induction of antigen-specific suppressor T lymphocytes. Indeed, while the immunosuppressive effect of irradiation is limited to haptens applied to the irradiated site, the net result is systemic immune suppression to that antigen because of the induction of suppressor T cells that spread throughout the body.

Higher doses of radiation evoke diminished immunologic responses to antigens introduced either epicutaneously or intracutaneously at sites distant from the irradiated site. These suppressed responses are also associated with the induction of antigen-specific suppressor T lymphocytes and may be mediated by as yet undefined factors that are released from epidermal cells at the irradiated site. The implications of this generalized immune suppression in terms of altered susceptibility to infection remain to be defined.

The photoimmunologic effects of solar radiation may also play a role in carcinogenic responses to UV radiation in the skin. UV-induced-tumors in murine skin are antigenic and are rapidly rejected when transplanted into normal syngeneic animals. If the tumors are transplanted into animals previously exposed to subcarcinogenic doses of UV radiation, they are not rejected and instead grow progressively in the recipients. This failure of irradiated animals to reject the transplanted tumors is due to the development of T suppressor cells that prevent the rejection response. While the mechanism of suppression of tumor rejection is unknown, such a response might be a critical determinant of cancer risk in human skin. Namely, in human subjects cutaneous exposure to erythema doses of UV-B causes changes in T-helper- and -suppressor-cell ratios and diminishes the effectiveness of natural killer cell function.

PHOTOSENSITIVITY DISEASES The diagnosis of photosensitivity requires a careful history to define the duration of the signs and symptoms, the length of time between exposure to sunlight, and the development of subjective complaints and visible changes in the skin. The age of onset can also be a helpful clue; for example, the acute photosensitivity of erythropoietic protoporphyria almost always begins in childhood, whereas the chronic photosensitivity of porphyria cutanea tarda typically begins in the fourth and fifth decades. A history of exposure to topical and systemic drugs and chemicals may provide important information. Many classes of drugs can cause photosensitivity either on the basis of phototoxicity or photoallergy. Fragrances such as musk ambrette contained in numerous cosmetic products are also potent photosensitizers.

Examination of the skin may also offer important clues. Anatomic areas that are naturally protected from direct sunlight such as the hairy scalp, the upper eyelids, the retroauricular areas, the infranasal, and the submental regions may be spared when the exposed areas show characteristic features of the pathologic process. These anatomic localization patterns are often helpful but not infallible in making the diagnosis. For example, airborne contact sensitizers that are blown on to the skin may produce dermatitis that can be difficult to distinguish from photosensitivity, despite the fact that such material may trigger skin reactivity in areas shielded from direct sunlight.

Many dermatologic conditions may be caused or aggravated by light (Table 60-2). The role of light in evoking these responses may be dependent upon genetic abnormalities ranging from the well-described defect in DNA repair that occurs in xeroderma pigmentosum to the inherited abnormalities in heme synthesis that characterize the porphyrias. In certain photosensitivity diseases the chromophore has been identified, whereas in the majority, the energy-absorbing agent is unknown.

Polymorphous light eruption After sunburn, the most common type of photosensitivity disease is polymorphous light eruption, the mechanism of which is unknown. Many affected individuals never seek medical attention because the condition is often transient, becoming manifest each spring with initial sun exposure, but then subsiding spontaneously with continuing exposure, a phenomenon known as "hardening." The major manifestations of polymorphous light eruption include pruritic (often intensely so) erythematous

TABLE 60-2 Classification of photosensitivity diseases

Type	Disease
Genetic	Erythropoietic porphyria
	Erythropoietic protoporphyria
	Albinism
	Xeroderma pigmentosum
	Rothmund-Thompson disease
	Bloom's disease
	Cockayne's disease
	Familial porphyria cutanea tarda
	Phenylketonuria
	Hepatoerythropoietic porphyria
Metabolic	Sporadic porphyria cutanea tarda
	Variegate porphyria
	Hartnup disease
	Kwashiorkor
	Pellagra
	Carcinoid
	Pseudoporphyria
Phototoxic	
Internal	Drugs
External	Drugs, plants, food
Photoallergic	
Immediate	Solar urticaria
Delayed	Drug photoallergy
	Persistent light reaction
Neoplastic and degenerative	Photoaging
	Actinic keratoses
	Basal cell carcinoma
	Squamous cell carcinoma
	Melanoma
	Dysplastic nevus syndrome
	Bowen's disease
Idiopathic	Polymorphous light eruption
	Hydroa aestivale
	Actinic reticuloid
Photoaggravated	Lupus erythematosus
	Systemic
	Subacute cutaneous
	Dermatomyositis
	Pemphigus foliaceus
	Herpes simplex
	Lichen planus actinicus
	Acne vulgaris
	Atopic dermatitis
	Transient acantholytic dermatosis

TABLE 60-3 Phototoxic drugs and chemicals

	Topical	Systemic
Coal tar derivatives		
Acridine	+	
Anthracene	+	
Phenanthrene	+	
Drugs		
Amiodarone		+
Dacarbazine		+
5-Fluorouracil	+	+
Furosemide		+
Nalidixic acid		+
Phenothiazines		+
Psoralens	+	+
Retinoids	+	+
Sulfonamides		+
Sulfonylureas		+
Tetracyclines		+
Thiazides		+
Vinblastine		+
Dyes		
Anthraquinone		+
Eosin		+
Methylene blue		+
Rose bengal		+

TABLE 60-4 Photoallergenic drugs and chemicals

	Topical	Systemic
Antibiotics		
Sulfonamides		+
Antifungals		
Fenticlor	+	
Jadit	+	
Multifungin	+	
Diuretics		
Thiazides		+
Fragrances		
Musk ambrette	+	
6-Methylcoumarin	+	
Plant oleoresins	+	
Halogenated salicylanilides		
Bithionol	+	
Tetrachlorosalicylanilides	+	
Tribromosalicylanilide	+	
Nonsteroidal anti-inflammatory agents		
Piroxicam	+	
Phenothiazines		
Chlorpromazine	+	
Promethazine	+	
Sulfonylureas		+
Sunscreens		
p-Aminobenzoic acid and esters	+	
Whitening agents		
Stilbenes	+	

papules that may coalesce into plaques on exposed areas of the face and arms or other areas as well, making the distribution spotty and uneven.

The diagnosis can be confirmed by skin biopsy and by performing phototest procedures in which skin is exposed to multiple erythema doses of the UV-A and UV-B. The action spectrum for polymorphous light eruption is usually within these portions of the solar spectrum.

Treatment of this disease includes the induction of "hardening" by the cautious administration of light either alone or in combination with photosensitizers such as the psoralens (see below).

Phototoxicity and photoallergy Another photosensitivity disorder is related to the topical or systemic administration of drugs and other chemicals. Photosensitivity reactions are of two broad types, phototoxicity and photoallergy, both of which require the absorption of energy by a drug or chemical resulting in the production of an excited state photosensitizer that can transfer its absorbed energy to a bystander molecule or to molecular oxygen, thereby generating tissue-destructive chemical species.

Phototoxicity is a nonimmunologic reaction caused by drugs and chemicals, a few of which are listed in Table 60-3. The usual clinical manifestations include erythema resembling a sunburn that quickly desquamates or "peels" within several days. In addition, edema, vesicles, and bullae may occur.

Photoallergy is distinct in that the immune system participates in the pathologic process. The excited-state photosensitizer may create highly unstable haptenic free radicals that bind covalently to macromolecules to form a functional antigen capable of evoking a delayed hypersensitivity response. Some of the drugs and chemicals that produce photoallergy are listed in Table 60-4. The clinical manifestations typically differ from those of phototoxicity in that an intensely pruritic eczematous dermatitis tends to be predominant and evolves into lichenified, thickened, "leathery" changes in sun-exposed areas. A small subset (perhaps 5 to 10 percent) of patients with photoallergy may develop a persistent exquisite hypersensitivity to light even when the offending drug or chemical is identified and eliminated. This is known as persistent light reaction and may be incapacitating for many years.

Diagnostic confirmation of phototoxicity and photoallergy can often be obtained using phototest procedures. In patients with suspected phototoxicity, determination of the minimal erythema dose (MED) while the patient is exposed to a suspected agent and then repeating the MED after discontinuation of the agent may provide a clue to the causative drug or chemical. Photopatch testing can be performed to confirm the diagnosis of photoallergy. This is a simple variant of ordinary patch testing in which a series of known photoallergens is applied to the skin in duplicate and one set irradiated with a suberythema dose of UV-A. Development of eczematous change at sites exposed to sensitizer and light is a positive result. The characteristic abnormality in patients with persistent light reaction is a diminished threshhold to erythema evoked by UV-B.

The management of drug photosensitivity is first and foremost to eliminate exposure to the chemical agents responsible for the reaction and to reduce sun exposure to the minimum possible. The acute symptoms of phototoxicity may be ameliorated by cool, moist compresses, topical glucocorticoids, and systemically administered nonsteroidal anti-inflammatory agents. In severely affected individuals, a rapidly tapered course of systemic glucocorticoids may be useful. Judicious use of analgesics may be necessary.

Photoallergic reactions require similar management techniques. Furthermore, individuals suffering from persistent light reactivity must be protected against light exposure. In selected patients in whom chronic systemic high-dose glucocorticoids pose unacceptable risks, it may be necessary to employ cytotoxic agents such as azathioprine or cyclophosphamide.

Porphyria The porphyrias (see Chap. 328) are a group of diseases that have in common various derangements in the synthesis of heme. Heme is a nonchelated tetrapyrrole or porphyrin, and the porphyrins are potent photosensitizers that absorb light intensely in both the short (400 to 410 nm) and the long (580 to 650 nm) portions of the visible spectrum.

Heme cannot be reutilized and must be continuously synthesized, and the two compartments with the largest requirement for its production are the bone marrow and the liver. Accordingly, the porphyrias originate in one or the other of these organs with the end result of excessive endogenous production of potent photosensitizers. The porphyrins circulate in the bloodstream and diffuse into the skin, where they absorb solar energy, become photoexcited, and evoke cutaneous photosensitivity. The mechanism of porphyrin photosensitization is known to be a photodynamic or oxygen-dependent reaction that can be mediated by reactive oxygen species such as superoxide anions.

Two forms of human porphyria, porphyria cutanea tarda and erythropoietic protoporphyria, will be discussed briefly. Porphyria cutanea tarda is the most common type of human porphyria and is associated with decreased activity of the enzyme uroporphyrinogen decarboxylase. There are two basic types of porphyria cutanea tarda: the sporadic or acquired type, generally seen in individuals ingesting ethanol or receiving estrogens and associated with increased hepatic iron stores, and the inherited type, in which there is autosomal dominant transmission of deficient enzyme activity.

In both types of porphyria cutanea tarda, the predominant feature is a chronic photosensitivity characterized by increased fragility of sun-exposed skin, particularly areas subject to repeated trauma such as the dorsa of the hands, the forearms, the face, and the ears. The predominant skin lesions are vesicles and bullae that rupture, producing moist erosions often with a hemorrhagic base that heal slowly with crusting and purplish discoloration of the affected skin. Hypertrichosis, mottled pigmentary change, and scleroderma-like induration are associated features. Biochemical confirmation of the diagnosis can be obtained by measurement of urinary porphyrin excretion and by assay of uroporphyrinogen decarboxylase.

Treatment consists of repeated phlebotomies to diminish the excessive hepatic iron stores and/or intermittent low doses of the antimalarial drugs chloroquine and hydroxychloroquine. Long-term remission of the disease can be achieved if the patient eliminates exposure to porphyrinogenic agents.

Erythropoietic protoporphyria originates in the bone marrow and is due to a decrease in the enzyme ferrochelatase. The major clinical features include an acute photosensitivity characterized by subjective burning and stinging of exposed skin that often develops during or just after exposure. There may be associated skin swelling and, after repeated episodes, a waxlike scarring.

The diagnosis is confirmed by demonstration of elevated measurement of free erythrocyte protoporphyrin. Detection of increased plasma protoporphyrin helps to differentiate lead poisoning and iron-deficiency anemia, in both of which elevated erythrocyte protoporphyrin occurs in the absence of cutaneous photosensitivity and of elevated plasma protoporphyrin.

Treatment consists of reducing sun exposure and the oral administration of the carotenoid β-carotene, which is an effective scavenger of free radicals. Many affected individuals are able to tolerate sun exposure while ingesting this drug, but it has no effect upon the metabolic defect in porphyrin-heme synthesis.

PHOTOPROTECTION Since photosensitivity of the skin results from exposure to sunlight, it follows that avoidance of the sun would eliminate these disorders. Unfortunately, social pressures make this an impractical alternative for most individuals, and this has led to a search for better approaches to photoprotection.

Natural photoprotection is provided by structural proteins in the epidermis, particularly keratin and melanin. The amount of melanin and its distribution in cells is genetically regulated, and individuals of darker complexion (skin types IV to VI) are at decreased risk for the development of cutaneous malignancy.

Other forms of photoprotection include clothing and sunscreens. Clothing constructed of tightly woven fabrics irrespective of color affords substantial protection. Wide-brimmed hats, long sleeves, and pants all reduce direct exposure. Sunscreens are of two major types—chemical and physical. Chemical sunscreening agents are chromophores that absorb energy in the UV-B and/or UV-A, thereby diminishing photon absorption by the skin (Table 60-5). Sunscreens are rated for their photoprotective effect by their *sun protective factor* (SPF). The SPF is simply a ratio of the time required to produce sunburn erythema with and without sunscreen application. SPF ratings of 15 or higher provide effective protection against UV-B and, to a lesser extent, UV-A. The major categories of chemical sunscreens include *p*-aminobenzoic acid and its esters, benzophenones, anthranilates, cinnamates, and salicylates. Physical sunscreens are light-opaque mixtures containing zinc oxide, talc, or titanium oxide that scatter light, thereby reducing absorption by the skin.

In addition to light absorption, a critical determinant of the photoprotective effect of sunscreens is their ability to remain on the skin, a property known as *substantivity*. In general, the PABA esters formulated in moisturizing vehicles provide the greatest substantivity.

Photoprotection can also be achieved by limiting the time of exposure during the day. Since as much as half of an individual's total lifetime sun exposure may occur by the age 18, it is important to educate parents and young children about the hazards of sunlight. Simply eliminating exposure at midday will achieve substantial reduction in UV-B exposure.

TABLE 60-5 Properties of selected sunscreens

Ingredients	Trade names	SPF* (outdoors)	Substantivity†
p-Aminobenzoic acid (PABA) (5% in ethanol)	Pre-Sun-15	10–12	Excellent
p-Aminobenzoic acid esters (3.5% padimate A + 3.0% octyldimethyl PABA)	Original Eclipse	4–6	Fair
p-Aminobenzoic acid ester combinations (7.0% padimate 0 + 2.5% oxybenzone + 5.0% dioxybenzone)	Bain de Soleil	9	Excellent
Non-*p*-aminobenzoic acid (3% 2-hydroxy-4-methoxy benzophenone)	Ti-Screen-15	10–12	Excellent
Physical sunscreens (5% titanium Dioxide + 5% methyl anthranilate)	A-Fil	4–6	Good

*SPF = sun protective factor.
†Substantivity = ability to remain on the skin.

PHOTOTHERAPY AND PHOTOCHEMOTHERAPY While greatest attention has been paid to the damaging effects of sunlight in the skin, this same energy is employed in the management of selected dermatologic diseases. The administration of UV-B alone or in combination with topically applied compounds such as emollient ointments with or without crude coal tar induces remissions in psoriasis, an inflammatory disorder in which excessively rapid epidermal cell turnover is associated with thick scaling and redness of the skin.

Photochemotherapy in which UV-A radiation is administered in combination with topically applied or systemically administered psoralens (PUVA) is also effective in treating psoriasis and in the early stages of cutaneous T-cell lymphoma and vitiligo. Psoralens are tricyclic furocoumarins which when intercalated into DNA and exposed to UV-A produce monofunctional adducts to pyrimidine bases and eventually form DNA cross-links. These structural changes are thought to decrease DNA synthesis and effect the improvement that occurs in psoriasis. The reason that PUVA photochemotherapy is effective in cutaneous T-cell lymphoma is not clear.

In addition to its effects on DNA, PUVA photochemotherapy also stimulates melanin synthesis, and this provides the rationale for its use in the depigmenting disease vitiligo. Oral 8-methoxypsoralen and UV-A appear to be most effective in this regard, but as many as 100 treatments extending over 12 to 18 months may be required to promote satisfactory repigmentation.

The major side effects of phototherapy and PUVA photochemotherapy are due to the cumulative effects of photon absorption and include skin dryness, actinic keratoses, and an increased risk of nonmelanoma skin cancer. Despite these risks, the therapeutic index of these modalities is positive.

REFERENCES

Frain-Bell W: *Cutaneous Photobiology*. Oxford, Oxford University Press, 1985
Harber LC, Bickers DR: *Photosensitivity Diseases*, 2d ed. Toronto, Decker, 1989
Magnus IA: *Dermatological Photobiology*. Oxford, Blackwell, 1976
Pathak MA et al: Preventive treatment of sunburn, dermatoheliosis and skin cancer with sun-protective agents, in *Dermatology in General Medicine*, 3d ed, TB Fitzpatrick et al (eds). New York, McGraw-Hill, 1987
Urbach F, Gange RW: *The Biological Effects of UVA Radiation*. New York, Praeger, 1986

section 9 Hematologic alterations

61 ANEMIA

H. FRANKLIN BUNN

By definition patients with anemia have a significant reduction in red cell mass and a corresponding decrease in the oxygen-carrying capacity of the blood. Normally, blood volume is maintained at a nearly constant level. Therefore, anemia entails a decrease in the concentration of red cells or hemoglobin in peripheral blood.

Under unusual circumstances, the blood values do not accurately reflect alterations in the red cell mass. For example, hemoglobin level and hematocrit are falsely elevated in patients who have sustained an acute reduction in plasma volume owing to hemorrhage, extensive burns, vigorous diuresis, or other types of severe dehydration. In contrast, the blood values may be falsely low in patients who have an expanded blood volume, as in pregnancy or congestive heart failure.

Normal blood values for individuals of various ages are shown in the Appendix. In women in the childbearing age group the blood values are 10 percent lower than in men. At high altitudes, higher values are found, roughly in proportion to the elevation above sea level. Anemia may be defined as a reduction of more than 10 percent below the mean values for the sex. However, since the variations in normal hemoglobin values approach this limit, the documentation of mild anemia may be uncertain.

SIGNS AND SYMPTOMS OF ANEMIA The clinical presentation of the anemic patient depends on the underlying disease as well as on the severity and chronicity of the anemia. The manifestations of anemia per se can be explained by the pathophysiologic principles outlined in this chapter and in Chap. 290. Most of these signs and symptoms represent cardiovascular and ventilatory adjustments which compensate for the decrease in red blood cell mass.

The degree to which symptoms occur in an anemic patient depends on several contributing factors. If the anemia has developed rapidly, there may not be adequate time for compensatory adjustments to take place, and the patient may have more marked symptoms than if an anemia of equivalent severity had developed insidiously. Furthermore, the patient's complaints may depend on the presence of local vascular disease. For example, angina pectoris, intermittent claudication, or transient cerebral ischemia may be unmasked by the development of anemia.

Individuals with mild anemia are often asymptomatic. They may complain of fatigue as well as dyspnea and palpitation, particularly following exercise. Severely anemic patients will often be symptomatic at rest and unable to tolerate significant exertion. When the hemoglobin concentration falls below 75 g/L (7.5 g/dL), resting cardiac output rises significantly with an increase in both heart rate and stroke volume. The patient may be aware of this hyperdynamic state and complain of palpitation or a pounding pulse. Symptoms of cardiac failure may develop if the patient's myocardial reserve is reduced.

The symptoms of severe anemia extend to other organ systems. Patients often complain of dizziness and headache and may experience syncope, tinnitus, or vertigo. Many patients are irritable and have difficulty sleeping or concentrating. Because of decreased blood flow to the skin, patients may become hypersensitive to cold. Gastrointestinal symptoms such as anorexia, indigestion, and even nausea or bowel irregularity are attributable to shunting of blood away from the splanchnic bed. Females commonly develop abnormal menstruation, both amenorrhea and increased bleeding. Males may complain of impotence or loss of libido.

Physical findings *Pallor* is the physical finding most commonly associated with anemia. However, the usefulness of this sign is limited by other factors that affect the color of the skin. The thickness and texture of the skin vary widely among individuals. Furthermore, the blood flow to the skin can undergo wide fluctuations. Normal individuals will appear sallow when blood is shunted away from the skin, whereas anemic patients may appear flushed when overheated or during periods of excitement. The concentration of melanin in the epidermis is another important determinant of skin color. Individuals with a fair complexion may look pale even though they are not anemic. Conversely, pallor is difficult to detect in deeply pigmented individuals. Furthermore, acquired disorders of melanin pigmentation (e.g., Addison's disease, hemochromatosis) or jaundice may interfere with detection of pallor. Nevertheless, even in blacks, the presence of anemia may be suspected by the color of the palms or of noncutaneous tissues such as oral mucous membranes, nail beds, and palpebral conjunctivas. The color of the creases of the palm is a useful sign. When they are as pale as the surrounding skin, the patient usually has a hemoglobin of less than 70 g/L (7 g/dL).

Two factors contribute to the development of pallor in patients with anemia. There is, of course, a decrease in the hemoglobin concentration of blood perfusing the skin and mucous membranes. Also, blood is shunted away from the skin and other peripheral tissues, permitting enhanced blood flow to vital organs. Redistribution of blood flow is an important mode of compensation in anemia.

Other physical findings associated with anemia include tachycardia, wide pulse pressure, and a hyperdynamic precordium. A systolic ejection murmur is often heard over the precordium, particularly at the pulmonic area. In addition, a venous hum may be detected over the neck vessels. These cardiac findings disappear when the anemia is corrected. Patients with hemolytic anemia often have icterus and splenomegaly and occasionally develop superficial skin ulceration over the ankle bones.

APPROACH TO THE PATIENT WITH ANEMIA

In evaluating the anemic patient, the physician should proceed in an orderly fashion so that the correct diagnosis can be established with a minimum of laboratory tests and procedures. As in other clinical disciplines, a comprehensive history and meticulous physical examination are of paramount importance in the initial workup of the anemic patient. For example, a family history which reveals a dominant inheritance pattern provides strong support for the diagnosis of hereditary spherocytosis. The discovery of a heart murmur and splenomegaly raises the possibility that the anemic patient may have subacute bacterial endocarditis.

The evaluation of the anemic patient should be based on a firm understanding of the pathophysiologic principles outlined in Chap. 290. As shown in Table 61-1, the clinician must first ask whether the anemia is due to a decreased production of red cells or to enhanced destruction. Moreover, the possibility of blood loss either as the sole etiology or as a contributing factor must always be considered. The examination of the stool for occult blood is an indispensable part of the evaluation of all anemic patients.

TABLE 61-1 Initial evaluation of anemia

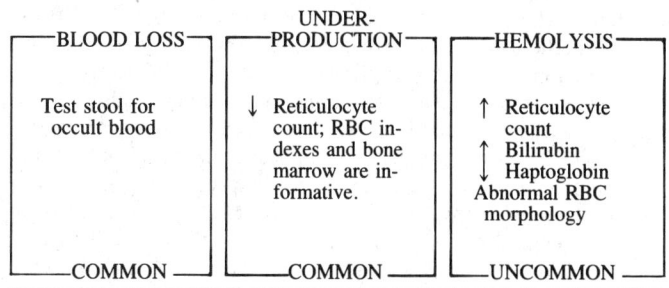

BLOOD LOSS	UNDER-PRODUCTION	HEMOLYSIS
Test stool for occult blood	↓ Reticulocyte count; RBC indexes and bone marrow are informative.	↑ Reticulocyte count ↑ Bilirubin ↓ Haptoglobin Abnormal RBC morphology
COMMON	COMMON	UNCOMMON

RETICULOCYTE COUNT This is the most useful laboratory test for distinguishing underproduction from hemolysis. When an appropriate supravital stain is applied to a sample of peripheral blood, the 1- to 2-day-old red cells exhibit a network of purple strands which are aggregates of ribosomes. Reticulocytosis is a reflection of the release of an increased number of young cells from the bone marrow. The degree of increased erythropoiesis can be assessed more quantitatively by determining the reticulocyte index, which uses the hematocrit or packed cell volume (PCV) and is calculated as follows:

$$\text{Reticulocyte index} = \text{reticulocyte \%} \times \frac{\text{patient's PCV}}{\text{normal PCV}}$$

This measure fails to consider the distribution of reticulocytes between the bone marrow and the peripheral blood. When the marrow is greatly stimulated, marrow reticulocytes enter the circulation prematurely. On a routinely prepared smear, these "shift reticulocytes" appear larger than average and have a lavender hue, so-called polychromatophilia. Since the circulation of "shift reticulocytes" in the peripheral blood is prolonged, the reticulocyte index should be divided by about 2. This factor varies from 1.5 to 3 depending upon the severity of the anemia and the degree of erythropoietin stimulation. This correction should always be made if normoblasts are encountered in the peripheral blood since this finding indicates the premature release of red cell precursors into the circulation.

A failure to produce red cells is reflected in an inappropriately low reticulocyte count. In contrast, a significant elevation of reticulocytes is suggestive of hemolysis. Exceptions include (1) the brisk reticulocyte response that is seen in a patient with hemorrhage, (2) reticulocytosis encountered in patients recovering from impaired erythropoiesis (e.g., an individual with pernicious anemia who received an injection of vitamin B_{12} 1 week earlier), and (3) mild to moderate elevations in reticulocytes (3 to 7 percent) encountered in myelophthisic anemia in which the orderly release of cells is affected by alterations of the marrow stroma owing to tumor, fibrosis, or granulomata. These exceptions are often readily appreciated in the initial evaluation of the patient. Furthermore, a number of ancillary laboratory tests described below are useful in determining to what extent hemolysis is occurring. The measurement of unconjugated bilirubin in the serum is a particularly useful guide to the presence of accelerated red blood cell breakdown. Once this information is obtained, the workup can be directed toward the establishment of a specific etiology.

Three additional baseline studies are of critical importance in the initial workup of the patient with anemia: *measurement of red cell indexes, examination of the peripheral blood smear,* and, in many patients, *bone marrow examination.*

RED CELL INDEXES Red cell indexes can be calculated from determinants of hematocrit, hemoglobin concentration, and red blood cell count. Measuring the hematocrit or PCV is the simplest and one of the most precise ways to ascertain the concentration of red cells in the blood. Generally, a small sample of anticoagulated blood is drawn into a capillary tube which is sealed at one end and centrifuged. The PCV is the ratio of the volume of packed red cells to the total volume. Alternatively, the concentration of hemoglobin can be determined spectrophotometrically from the absorbance of the cyanmethemoglobin form at a specific wavelength. With the advent of automated red blood cell counting technology, very precise measurements of red blood cell indexes are now readily available in nearly all hospitals and clinical laboratories. The electronic counter makes a direct measurement of the red cell count (RBC/μL) and the mean red cell volume (MCV):

$$\text{MCV (fL)} = \frac{\text{PCV (L/L)}}{(\text{RBC}/\mu\text{L}) \times 10^{-9}}$$

This instrument calculates the PCV from the direct measurement of MCV and RBC/L. In addition, hemoglobin concentration is measured directly on a separate channel. The mean corpuscular hemoglobin concentration (MCHC) is then computed as follows:

$$\text{MCHC (g/dL)} = \frac{\text{Hb (g/dL)}}{\text{PCV (L/L)}}$$

A third red blood cell index, the mean corpuscular hemoglobin (MCH), is determined as follows:

$$\text{MCH (pg)} = \frac{\text{Hb (g/dL)}}{(\text{RBC}/\mu\text{L}) \times 10^{-7}}$$

Generally, an automated system provides a printout which includes hemoglobin concentration, red cell count, packed cell volume, and the three red cell indexes (MCV, MCHC, and MCH). The MCHC, when calculated by an electronic counter, is not reliable and is of little use to the clinician.

As Table 61-2 shows, the MCV is particularly useful in classifying the anemias due to decreased red cell production. Microcytic anemias have low MCV values. On microscopic examination, the red cells appear small and often pale. In contrast, in the macrocytic anemias the MCV is elevated and large oval cells (macroovalocytes) are seen on microscopic examination. Unlike the anemias of underproduction, nearly all the hemolytic anemias are normocytic or slightly macrocytic owing to the preponderance of young red cells. Exceptions include the severe forms of thalassemia in which microcytic red cells are accompanied by brisk hemolysis.

TABLE 61-2 Anemias due to decreased red cell production

RBC Indexes	Marrow	Additional lab tests	Diagnosis
Hypochromic, microcytic (↓MCV)	0 Iron	↓ Fe, ↑ TIBC	Iron deficiency
	+ Iron	↑ Hb A_2, ↑ Hb F	β Thalassemia
	Ring sideroblasts	↓ Hb A_2	Sideroblastic anemia
Macrocytic (↑MCV)	Megaloblastic	↓ Serum B_{12}, achlorhydria	Vitamin B_{12} deficiency, pernicious anemia
		↓ Serum folate	Folic acid deficiency
Normochromic, normocytic	Normal	↓ Fe, ↓ TIBC	Anemia of chronic inflammation
		↑ Creatinine	Anemia of uremia
		Abn LFT	Anemia of liver disease
		↓ T_4	Anemia of myxedema
	Aplastic	Pancytopenia	Aplastic anemia
Normoblasts, teardrops	Infiltrated: tumor, lymphoma, etc.		Myelophthisic
	Fibrosis	↑ LAP	Myeloid metaplasia

NOTE: Fe, iron; TIBC, total iron-binding capacity; Hb, hemoglobin; LAP, leukocyte alkaline phosphatase; LFT, liver function tests; Abn, abnormal; MCV, mean corpuscular volume.

EXAMINATION OF THE BLOOD SMEAR In the evaluation of patients with anemia, the physician should take the time to examine a well-stained peripheral blood film. Figures A5-1 to A5-12 show examples of abnormalities in red cell morphology encountered in various types of anemia. Many subtleties escape the attention of the technologist whose primary purpose in examining the slide is to obtain a white cell differential count. Furthermore, the clinician can approach the specimen with a prepared mind and can scrutinize it for specific abnormalities. As suggested above, the examination can confirm the size and color of red cells as estimated by RBC indexes. Furthermore, while these indexes provide mean statistical values, the microscopic examination can reveal variation in red cell size (anisocytosis) or shape (poikilocytosis), changes which are helpful in the diagnosis of specific anemias. Examination of the blood smear is particularly important in evaluating a patient with hemolysis. Most hemolytic anemias have characteristic morphologic abnormalities. Finally, this practice may yield unexpected dividends. The finding of rouleaux suggests the presence of dysproteinemia as occurs in multiple myeloma. The examination may provide the initial clue that the patient has significant thrombocytopenia.

BONE MARROW EXAMINATION A microscopic examination of the bone marrow is generally indicated in the workup of any *unexplained* anemia. Study of the bone marrow is particularly informative in the anemias of underproduction. The more severe the anemia, the more likely that the procedure will be informative. An assessment of the quantity and quality of red cell precursors may determine whether there is a primary defect in cell production. A marrow biopsy is particularly useful in estimating overall cellularity. The normal differential of nucleated cells in the marrow is shown in the Appendix. The ratio of myeloid (M) to erythroid (E) precursors is normally about 2:1 but may be artifactually increased by the inclusion of circulating leukocytes. The ratio is increased in patients with infection, a leukemoid reaction, or neoplastic proliferation of myeloid cells. Rarely, a high M/E ratio is due to selective aplasia of the red cell precursors. A decreased M/E ratio indicates erythroid hyperplasia (seen in hemolysis or hemorrhage) or ineffective erythropoiesis (e.g., megaloblastic and sideroblastic anemias). The morphology of the precursors may reveal a maturation deficit such as megaloblastic anemia. The bone marrow examination is also important in demonstrating the presence of cellular infiltrates such as those found in leukemia, lymphoma, or multiple myeloma. The demonstration of tumor, fibrosis, or granulomata usually requires a biopsy. A portion of the marrow specimen should be stained with Prussian blue. In addition to providing an assessment of iron stores, the iron stain is required for the identification of sideroblasts.

VARIOUS FORMS OF ANEMIA

ANEMIA DUE TO BLOOD LOSS This form of anemia varies considerably in its clinical presentation depending upon the site, severity, and rapidity of the hemorrhage. At opposite extremes are acute fulminant bleeding producing hypovolemic shock and chronic occult blood loss leading to iron-deficiency anemia.

Patients who have sustained an acute hemorrhage generally present with signs and symptoms secondary to hypoxia and hypovolemia. Depending on the severity of the process, the patient will have weakness, fatigue, lightheadedness, stupor, or coma and will often appear pale, diaphoretic, and irritable. Vital signs are a reflection of cardiovascular compensation for the acute blood loss (Chap. 39). The patient will have hypotension and tachycardia in proportion to the degree of hemorrhage. Elicitation of postural signs is useful in the initial evaluation of patients with acute blood loss. If the pulse rises 25 percent or more, or the systolic blood pressure falls 20 mmHg or more upon going from a supine to sitting position, the patient is likely to have significant hypovolemia (blood loss >1000 mL) and requires prompt replacement. Acute blood loss in excess of 1500 mL usually leads to cardiovascular collapse.

If the blood loss has been acute and recent, the peripheral blood may not reveal a significant decrease in packed cell volume or hemoglobin, since the red cell mass and plasma volume are contracted in parallel. There often is a moderate leukocytosis and a "shift to the left" in the white cell differential count. Thrombocytosis may be encountered in both acute and chronic blood loss, particularly when the patient is iron-deficient. During the first few days following an acute hemorrhage there is usually an increase in reticulocytes. Occasionally nucleated red cells may appear in the peripheral blood. Since young red cells are larger than old ones, the patient may develop slightly macrocytic red cell indexes (MCV = 95 to 105 fL). As mentioned above, sustained reticulocytosis will be seen if significant blood loss continues, or until iron stores have been exhausted. Internal bleeding may be accompanied by an increase in unconjugated bilirubin. This abnormality is a reflection of an increase in catabolism of heme from extravasated red cells. Patients with acute gastrointestinal blood loss will often have an elevation of blood urea nitrogen owing to impaired renal blood flow and perhaps to the absorption of digested blood protein.

It is of critical importance to assess these patients promptly and institute treatment without delay. A large-bore intravenous line should be placed. While blood is being typed and cross matched, saline, Ringer's lactate, or, preferably, a colloid such as 5% albumin should be infused to correct hypovolemia. Whole blood is then administered as soon as it is available. Monitoring of vital signs and central venous pressure is useful in determining the appropriate amount of volume replacement. During and following these emergency measures, diagnostic studies may reveal the site or sites of bleeding. If the bleeding is unexplained an emergency coagulation profile should be obtained. Demonstration of bleeding from the gastrointestinal tract may require the insertion of a nasogastric tube. Appropriate radiologic studies may be indicated to determine sites of internal bleeding such as retroperitoneal hemorrhage.

Chronic blood loss is usually due to lesions in the gastrointestinal tract or the uterus. The testing of stool specimens for occult blood is an essential, though frequently overlooked, part of the evaluation of anemia. It may be necessary to examine serial specimens over a prolonged period of time since gastrointestinal bleeding is often intermittent. The hematologic manifestations of chronic blood loss are those of iron-deficiency anemia, discussed in detail in Chap. 291.

ANEMIAS DUE TO DECREASED RBC PRODUCTION As shown in Table 61-2, red cell indexes are useful in classifying the anemias due to underproduction of red cells. They can be conveniently grouped into three major categories: microcytic, macrocytic, and normocytic.

The *microcytic* anemias include iron-deficiency anemia (Chap. 291), sideroblastic anemias (Chap. 291), and the thalassemias (Chap. 295). Collectively, they represent a decrease in the availability or synthesis of one of the three major constituents of the hemoglobin molecule: iron, porphyrin, and globin. Since hemoglobin makes up over 90 percent of the protein within the erythrocyte, it is not surprising that these defects in hemoglobin synthesis result in the formation of small, pale red cells. These disorders involve a variable degree of ineffective erythropoiesis (Chap. 290). In addition, the anemias of chronic inflammation and malignancy may be slightly microcytic (Chap. 293). This phenomenon is due to a defect in the availability of iron. However, these disorders are more often normocytic and have been so classified in Table 61-2. Measurement of serum iron and iron-binding capacity and evaluation of marrow iron stores are particularly useful in distinguishing between these anemias.

The *macrocytic* anemias generally are associated with megaloblastic morphology in the bone marrow. In most cases, a deficiency of either vitamin B_{12} or folic acid results in an impairment of the replication of DNA, particularly in cells having a high turnover rate. Because nuclear maturation lags behind cytoplasmic development, large red cells tend to be produced in the bone marrow. Megaloblastic anemias are discussed in detail in Chap. 292. Like the microcytic anemias, these disorders are maturation defects associated with ineffective erythropoiesis. Macrocytosis, generally of a lesser degree, may also be encountered in patients with liver disease, hypothyroidism, acute blood loss, hemolytic anemia, aplastic anemia, and alcoholism. However, in these conditions, the red cell precursors in the bone marrow do not appear megaloblastic. The macrocytes in liver disease and hypothyroidism may be related to an increased deposition of lipid in the red cell membrane.

The *normocytic* anemias of underproduction comprise a diverse group of disorders. As shown in Table 61-2, this group can be conveniently subdivided into two categories: those secondary to some other underlying disease and those due to intrinsic pathology within the bone marrow.

The primary disorders of the bone marrow are best approached by microscopic examination of a marrow aspirate and biopsy. This group of anemias is often accompanied by leukopenia and thrombocytopenia. Pancytopenia, usually to a lesser degree, can also be seen in hypersplenism and in the megaloblastic anemias. Aplastic anemia and the myelophthisic anemias are discussed in Chap. 298.

The diagnosis of anemia secondary to some underlying disease is usually quite straightforward. Conversely, the presence of an unexplained normocytic anemia should prompt the search for an underlying disorder such as chronic renal failure, infection, or myxedema. If the presence of such an illness is established, the physician is obliged to investigate whether other factors such as blood loss or a nutritional deficiency contribute to the patient's anemia. Generally, the anemias due to liver disease, chronic inflammation, or an endocrinopathy are of only moderate severity. Unlike the other "secondary" anemias, that due to chronic renal failure can be severe. All these anemias are discussed in more detail in Chap. 293.

HEMOLYTIC ANEMIAS Hemolytic anemias (Table 61-3) are encountered much less frequently than the anemias due to decreased red cell production. Although they are a diverse group, the hemolytic anemias have a number of clinical features in common. Signs and symptoms of patients with hemolysis are briefly mentioned above.

A number of laboratory tests are available to establish the presence of accelerated breakdown of red cells. The reticulocyte count is the single most useful test. Patients with hemolysis nearly always have an elevated reticulocyte count. A variety of serum and urine tests are useful in confirming the presence of hemolysis and assessing its magnitude. Serum unconjugated bilirubin and haptoglobin are particularly useful (Table 61-1). Others are described in detail in Chap. 294 and are summarized in Table 294-2.

Classification of hemolytic anemias Once the presence of hemolysis is established, a large battery of laboratory tests is available for determining the specific diagnosis. Some of these tests are listed in Table 61-3. No other area of internal medicine is better suited to detailed and fruitful diagnostic probing. In the interest of time and money, the clinician should use the available tests in an orderly fashion. This complex group of disorders is easier to approach diagnostically if a concise and workable classification is used. The hemolytic anemias can be grouped in several ways: congenital versus acquired, intracorpuscular versus extracorpuscular, or by anatomic site of the erythrocyte defect. The various kinds of hemolytic anemia are discussed in Chap. 294.

TABLE 61-3 Hemolytic anemias

Blood smear	Additional lab tests	Diagnosis
Schistocytes, helmet cells		Traumatic hemolytic anemia
Spherocytes	+Coombs' test	Immunohemolytic anemia
	↑ Osmotic fragility	Hereditary spherocytosis
Spur cells	Abnormal LFT	Spur cell anemia
	+Sucrose lysis	Paroxysmal nocturnal hemoglobinuria
Sickle cells	+Sickle prep	Sickle cell syndromes
Target cells	Abn Hb electrophoresis	Hb C, D, etc.
Heinz bodies	Abn Hb electrophoresis	Congenital Heinz body hemolytic anemia
	↓ G6PD	G6PD deficiency

NOTE: Hb, hemoglobin; G6PD, glucose-6-phosphate dehydrogenase; LFT, liver function tests; Abn, abnormal.

TREATMENT OF ANEMIA

The effective treatment of anemia, like other disorders, is predicated upon a thorough diagnostic evaluation. There is no reason to administer hematinics such as iron, vitamin B_{12}, or folic acid unless a specific deficiency of these substances has been demonstrated or is anticipated. Although the indiscriminate administration of vitamin B_{12} is not deleterious per se, it lulls both the patient and the physician into false security. In contrast, the inappropriate use of iron preparations over a prolonged period of time can be directly harmful, leading to a state of iron overload. Pyridoxine is indicated only in the treatment of sideroblastic anemias.

Many kinds of anemias can be corrected if a precipitating cause can be uncovered and reversed. If a drug or toxin can be incriminated, its withdrawal may allow full recovery. The outcome of the "secondary" anemias is dependent on whether the underlying condition can be corrected. Anemias due to an endocrinopathy or infection should respond favorably to appropriate treatment. Occasionally, the anemia of malignancy is corrected by the removal of the primary tumor. One of the most dramatic sequelae of a successful renal transplant is the prompt correction of the "anemia of uremia." Moreover, the anemia associated with renal failure can be corrected by the administration of recombinant human erythropoietin. This agent may also prove to be effective in the treatment of anemia associated with other chronic disorders such as hepatic cirrhosis, rheumatoid arthritis, or AIDS.

Primary disorders of the bone marrow such as aplastic anemia or myelophthisic anemia are often irreversible and are treated with supportive measures such as transfusions of red cells and platelets. *Androgens* are sometimes employed in this group of anemias, but their efficacy is marginal. The recent availability of recombinant hematopoietic growth factors may provide more specific and effective treatment. Because prognosis is so bleak in these disorders, a radical approach to treatment seems justified. As described in Chaps. 298 and 299, bone marrow transplantation and immunosuppressive therapy are now reasonable therapeutic alternatives in selected cases of severe aplastic anemia and acute leukemia.

Several factors should be weighed in determining whether an anemic patient should be transfused. The risks and complications of the administration of blood products are discussed in Chap. 286. Patients with chronic or long-standing anemias are able to compensate in several ways, discussed earlier in this chapter. A considerable reduction in red cell mass can be surprisingly well tolerated, especially if the patient is young or sedentary. Transfusion is seldom indicated in a patient with a chronic anemia whose hemoglobin is 90 g/L (9 g/dL) or greater. Those who are expected to respond to the administration of a specific agent such as iron, folic acid, or vitamin B_{12} can usually be spared transfusions. If the anemia has precipitated an episode of congestive heart failure or myocardial ischemia, prompt but cautious administration of packed red cells is indicated. In general, whole blood should be given only if the patient is hypovolemic.

Glucocorticoids have only a limited role in the treatment of anemia. These agents are not effective in stimulating erythropoiesis. High doses of a glucocorticoid are indicated in the treatment of immunohemolytic anemia, thrombotic thrombocytopenic purpura, and pure red cell anemia. Otherwise, steroids should be prescribed sparingly unless some coexisting condition dictates their use.

Splenectomy is indicated in the treatment of certain hemolytic anemias. The efficacy of splenectomy correlates with the degree to which the abnormal or defective red cells are sequestered. Splenectomy is virtually curative in hereditary spherocytosis. The operation may be beneficial in selected patients with immunohemolytic anemia, congestive splenomegaly, spur cell anemia, and certain hemoglobinopathies and enzymopathies. The operative morbidity and mortality from elective splenectomy are very low. Occasional patients develop a left subphrenic abscess. Following splenectomy, young children are at risk of developing overwhelming septicemia. This complication is much rarer in adults. Thrombocytosis generally develops promptly following splenectomy. However, in most cases, it is transient. In patients with continued hemolysis or a myeloproliferative disorder (Chap. 297), the thrombocytosis usually persists and may occasionally be associated with thromboembolic phenomena.

REFERENCES

Babior BM, Stossel TP: *Hematology, A Pathophysiological Approach*. New York, Churchill Livingstone, 1984
Beck WS (ed): *Hematology*. 2nd ed. Boston, MIT Press, 1990
Crosby WH: Red cell mass: Its precursors and perturbations. Hosp Prac 15:2, 71, 1980
Erslev AJ, Gabuzda TG: *Pathophysiology of Blood*. Philadelphia, Saunders, 1985
Jandl JH: *Blood, Textbook of Hematology*. Boston, Little, Brown, 1987
Williams WJ et al (eds): *Hematology*. 4th ed. New York: McGraw-Hill, 1990.
Wintrobe MM (ed): *Blood, Pure and Eloquent*. New York, McGraw-Hill, 1980

62 BLEEDING AND THROMBOSIS

ROBERT I. HANDIN

Hemorrhage, intravascular thrombosis, and embolism are common clinical manifestations of many diseases. The normal hemostatic system limits blood loss by precisely regulated interactions between components of the vessel wall, circulating blood platelets, and plasma proteins. However, when disease or trauma damage large arteries and veins, excessive bleeding may occur, despite a normal hemostatic system. Less frequently, hemorrhage is caused by an inherited or acquired disorder of the hemostatic machinery itself. A large number of such bleeding disorders have now been identified.

In addition, unregulated activation of the hemostatic system may cause thrombosis and embolism, which can reduce blood flow to critical organs like the brain and myocardium. Although we understand less about the pathophysiology of thrombosis than of hemostatic failure, certain patient groups have been identified that are particularly prone to thrombosis and embolism. These include patients (1) immobilized after surgery, (2) with chronic congestive heart failure, (3) with atherosclerotic vascular disease, (4) with malignancy, or (5) who are pregnant. Most of these "thrombosis-prone" patients have no identifiable hemostatic disorder. However, there are certain patient groups who have inherited or acquired a "hypercoagulable" or "prethrombotic" state which predisposes them to recurrent thrombosis.

The cardinal manifestations of disordered hemostasis which cause bleeding or thrombosis are discussed below, along with the clinical approach to diagnosis and evaluation of these patients. Certain information in the patient's history, such as the mode of onset and sites of bleeding, a family bleeding tendency, and a record of drug ingestion help establish the correct diagnosis. Physical examination can identify bleeding in the skin or joint deformities due to previous hemarthroses. Ultimately, however, bleeding disorders are diagnosed by laboratory tests. General screening tests are utilized first, to document a systemic disorder, and are then supplemented by specific tests of coagulation protein or platelet function to arrive at an accurate diagnosis.

The hypercoagulable or prethrombotic patient can also be identified by a careful history. There are three important clues to this diagnosis: (1) repeated episodes of thromboembolism without an obvious predisposing condition; (2) a family history of thrombosis; and (3) well-documented thromboembolism in adolescents and young adults. There are, as yet, no clinically useful screening tests for the prethrombotic state. However, several of the prethrombotic disorders can be diagnosed with specific immunologic and functional assays.

NORMAL HEMOSTASIS

Accurate diagnosis and treatment of patients with either bleeding or thrombosis requires some knowledge of the pathophysiology of hemostasis. The process can be divided into primary and secondary components and is initiated when trauma, surgery, or disease disrupt the vascular endothelial lining and blood is exposed to subendothelial connective tissue. *Primary hemostasis* is the name given to the process of platelet plug formation at sites of injury. It occurs within seconds of injury and is of prime importance in stopping blood loss from capillaries, small arterioles, and venules (see Fig. 62-1). *Secondary hemostasis* describes the reactions of the plasma coagulation system which result in fibrin formation. It requires several minutes for completion. The fibrin strands which are produced strengthen the primary hemostatic plug. This reaction is particularly important in larger vessels and prevents recurrent bleeding hours or days after the initial injury. Although presented here as separate events, primary and secondary hemostasis are closely linked. For example, activated platelets accelerate plasma coagulation, and products of the plasma coagulation reaction, such as thrombin, stimulate platelet aggregation.

Effective primary hemostasis requires three critical events—platelet adhesion, granule release, and platelet aggregation. Within a few seconds of injury, platelets adhere to collagen fibrils in vascular subendothelium via a specific platelet collagen receptor made up of glycoprotein Ia and IIa. As shown in Fig. 62-2, this interaction is stabilized by the von Willebrand factor, an adhesive glycoprotein which allows platelets to remain attached to the vessel wall despite the high shear forces generated within the vascular lumen. The von Willebrand factor accomplishes this task by forming a link between a platelet receptor site on glycoprotein Ib and subendothelial collagen fibrils. The adherent platelets then release preformed granule con-

FIGURE 62-1 Schematic presentation of the major events in primary hemostasis. The first event is platelet adhesion, the interaction of platelets with a nonplatelet surface such as vascular subendothelium. This is followed by platelet activation and secretion. Some of the products secreted by platelets are depicted. Abbreviations—ADP, adenosine diphosphate; PDGF, platelet-derived growth factor, vWF, von Willebrand's factor. The final event is the binding of activated platelets to the adherent monolayer in the process of platelet aggregation.

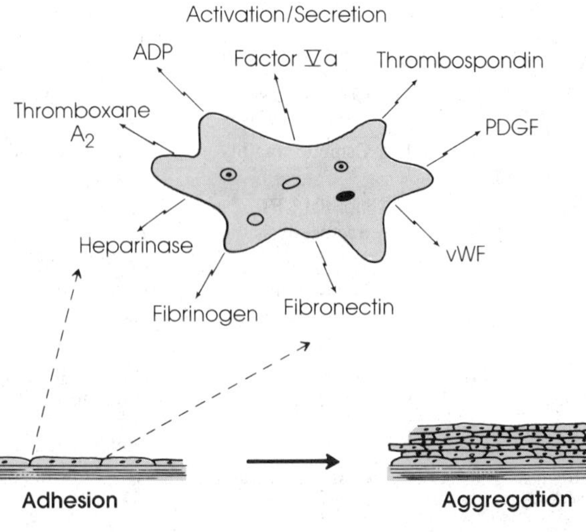

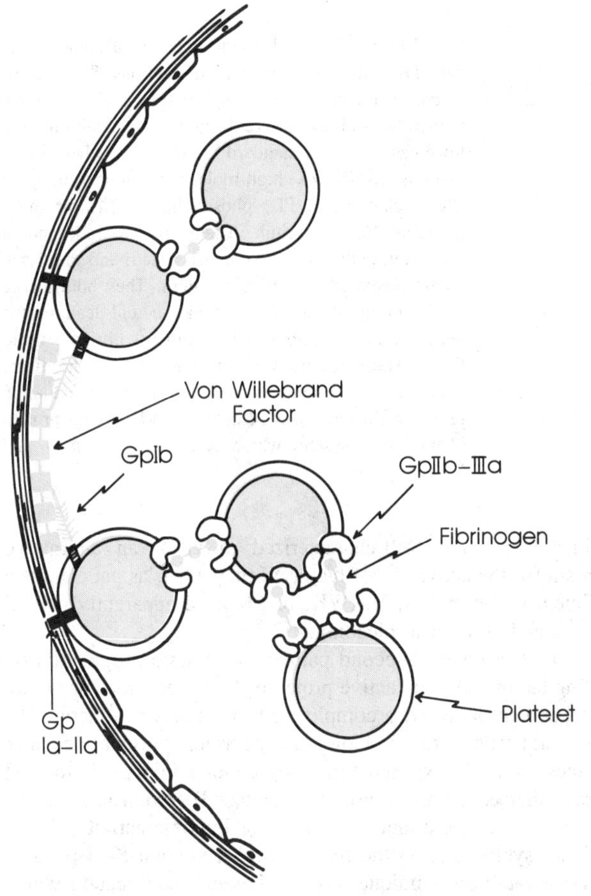

FIGURE 62-2 The molecular basis of platelet adhesion and aggregation. Adhesion of platelets to vascular subendothelium is facilitated by the von Willebrand's factor, which forms a bridge between collagen fibrils in the vessel wall and receptors on platelet glycoprotein Ib (GpIb). In a similar manner, platelet aggregation is mediated by fibrinogen which links adjacent platelets via receptors on the platelet glycoprotein IIb and IIIa complex (GpIIb–IIIa).

stituents and generate de novo mediators like those depicted in Fig. 62-1.

As in other cells, platelet activation and secretion are regulated by changes in the level of cyclic nucleotides, the influx of calcium, hydrolysis of membrane phospholipids, and phosphorylation of critical intracellular proteins. The relevant pathways are depicted in Figs. 62-3 and 62-4. The binding of agonists such as epinephrine, collagen, or thrombin to platelet surface receptors activates two membrane enzymes—phospholipase C and phospholipase A_2. These enzymes catalyze the release of arachidonic acid from two of the major membrane phospholipids, phosphatidylinositol and phosphatidylcholine. Initially, a small quantity of the released arachidonic acid is converted to thromboxane A_2 (TXA_2), which, in turn, can activate phospholipase C. The formation of TXA_2 from arachidonic acid is mediated by the enzyme cyclooxygenase (see Fig. 62-3). This enzyme is inhibited by aspirin and nonsteroidal anti-inflammatory drugs. Inhibition of TXA_2 synthesis is a cause of mild bleeding in some patients, as well as the basis for the action of some antithrombotic drugs.

FIGURE 62-3 Generation of thromboxane A_2 in platelets and prostacyclin (PGI_2) in endothelial cells.

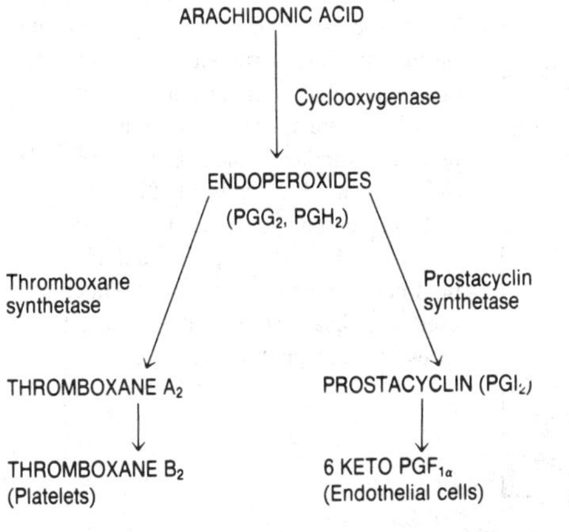

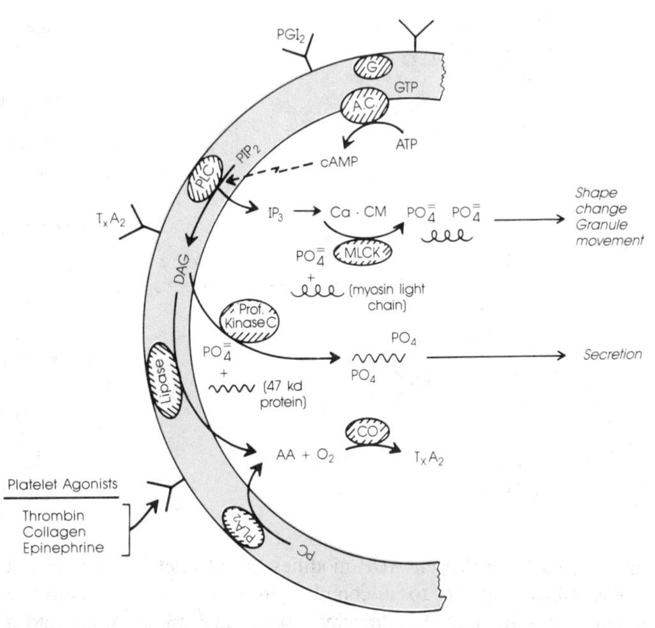

FIGURE 62-4 The biochemical basis of platelet activation and secretion. Binding of agonists such as thrombin, epinephrine, or collagen sets in motion a chain of events which hydrolyzes membrane phospholipids, inhibits adenylate cyclase, mobilizes intracellular calcium, and phosphorylates critical intracellular proteins. The net result is shape change, movement of granules to the canalicular system, generation of mediators like thromboxane A_2, and granule secretion. Abbreviations—A.C., adenylate cyclase; G, guanine nucleotide–binding protein; PIP_2, phosphatidylinositol-4,5-bisphosphate; PLC, phospholipase C; DAG, diacylglycerol; PLA_2, phospholipase A_2; PC, phosphatidylcholine; AA, arachidonic acid; CO, cyclooxygenase; O_2, oxygen; IP_3, inositol triphosphate; cAMP, cyclic AMP; Ca-CM, calcium calmodulin complex; MLCK, myosin light chain kinase.

Hydrolysis of the membrane phospholipid, phosphatidylinositol 4,5-bisphosphate (PIP_2), produces diacylglycerol (DAG) and inositol triphosphate (IP_3), both of which play critical roles in platelet metabolism. IP_3 mediates the movement of calcium into the platelet cytosol and stimulates the phosphorylation of myosin light chains. The latter interact with actin to facilitate granule movement and platelet shape change. DAG activates protein kinase C which, in turn, phosphorylates a 47,000-dalton protein (plekstrin) that may regulate platelet granule secretion.

A finely balanced mechanism controls the rate and extent of platelet activation, which is illustrated in Fig. 62-3. TXA_2, a platelet product of arachidonic acid, increases phospholipase C activity, which stimulates platelet activation and secretion. In contrast, prostacyclin (PGI_2), an endothelial cell product of arachidonic acid, inhibits phospholipase C activity by raising the intraplatelet cyclic AMP levels, which in turn inhibits platelet activation. Similar pathways to regulate activation and secretion occur in other cells.

Following activation, platelets secrete their granule contents into plasma. Endoglycosidases and a heparin-cleaving enzyme are released from lysosomes; calcium, serotonin, and adenosine diphosphate (ADP) are released from the dense granules; and several proteins including the von Willebrand factor, fibronectin, thrombospondin, and a heparin-neutralizing protein (platelet factor 4) are released from

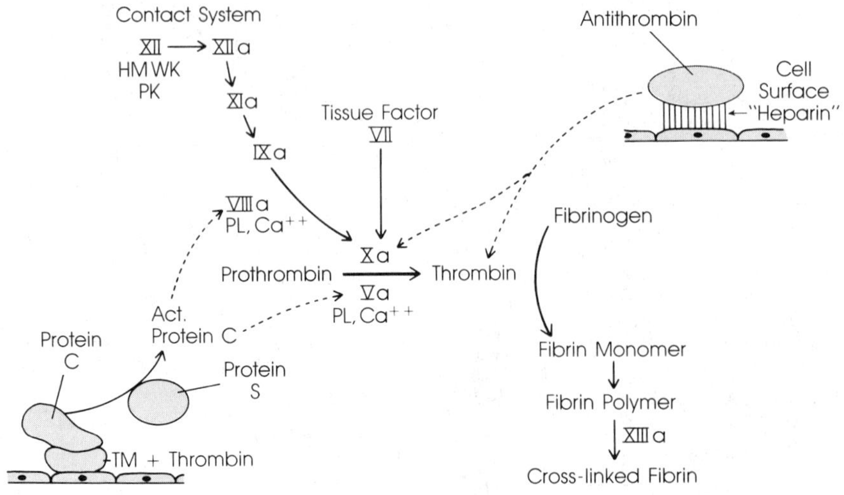

FIGURE 62-5 A schematic diagram of some of the clinically important coagulation reactions. The unactivated or precursor proteins are indicated by roman numerals, and the active form by the addition of a lowercase "a"—a standard convention. Other abbreviations are HMWK, high-molecular-weight kininogen; PK, prekallikrein; PL, phospholipid; TM, thrombomodulin; Ca^{2+}, calcium. There are two independent activation pathways, the contact system and the tissue factor–mediated or extrinsic system. They both merge at the point of factor X activation and lead to the generation of thrombin, which converts fibrinogen into fibrin. These reactions are regulated by antithrombin, which forms complexes with all of the coagulation protein serine proteases except factor VII, and the protein C–protein S system which inactivates factors V and VIII.

alpha granules. Released ADP modifies the platelet surface so that fibrinogen can attach to a complex formed between membrane glycoproteins IIb and IIIa, thereby linking adjacent platelets into a hemostatic plug (Fig. 62-2). Platelet-derived growth factor (PDGF), another alpha granule protein, stimulates the growth and migration of fibroblasts and smooth muscle cells within the vessel wall, which is an important part of the repair process.

As the primary hemostatic plug is being formed, plasma coagulation proteins are activated to initiate secondary hemostasis. An overall picture of the coagulation scheme, including the role of various inhibitors, is shown in Fig. 62-5. The coagulation pathway can be broken down into a series of reactions (outlined in Fig. 62-6) which culminate in the production of sufficient thrombin to convert a small portion of plasma fibrinogen to fibrin. Each of the reactions requires the formation of a surface-bound complex, the conversion of inactive precursor proteins into active proteases by limited proteolysis, and each is regulated by both plasma and cellular cofactors and calcium.

In *reaction 1,* the intrinsic or contact phase of coagulation, three plasma proteins, Hageman factor (factor XII), high-molecular-weight kininogen (HMWK), and prekallikrein (PK) are thought to form a complex on vascular subendothelial collagen. After binding to HMWK, factor XII is slowly converted to an active protease (XIIa), which then converts both PK to kallikrein and factor XI to its active form (XIa). Kallikrein (K) in turn accelerates XII conversion to XIIa, while XIa participates in subsequent coagulation reactions. Although these interactions are well-characterized in vitro, an alternative mechanism for the activation of factor XI may exist, as patients who are deficient in factor XII, HMWK, or PK have apparently normal hemostasis and no clinical bleeding.

Reaction 2 provides a second pathway to initiate coagulation by converting factor VII to an active protease. In this extrinsic or tissue-factor-dependent pathway, a complex is formed between factor VII, calcium, and tissue factor, a ubiquitous lipoprotein present in cellular membranes which is exposed following cellular injury. Factor VII and three other coagulation proteins—factors II (prothrombin), IX, and X—require calcium and vitamin K for biologic activity. These proteins are synthesized in the liver, where a vitamin K–dependent carboxylase catalyzes a unique posttranslational modification which adds a second carboxyl group to certain glutamic acid residues. Pairs of these di-γ-carboxyglutamic acid (Gla) residues bind calcium, which anchors these proteins to negatively charged phospholipid surfaces and confers biological activity. Inhibition of this posttranslational modification by vitamin K antagonists (e.g., warfarin) is the basis of one of the most common forms of anticoagulant therapy.

In *reaction 3,* factor X is activated by the proteases generated in the two previous reactions. In one reaction, a calcium- and lipid dependent complex is formed between factors VIII, IX, and X. Within this complex, factor IX is first converted to IXa by factor XIa that was generated within the intrinsic pathway (reaction 1). Factor X is then activated by factor IXa in concert with factor VIII. Alternatively, both factors IX and X can be activated more directly

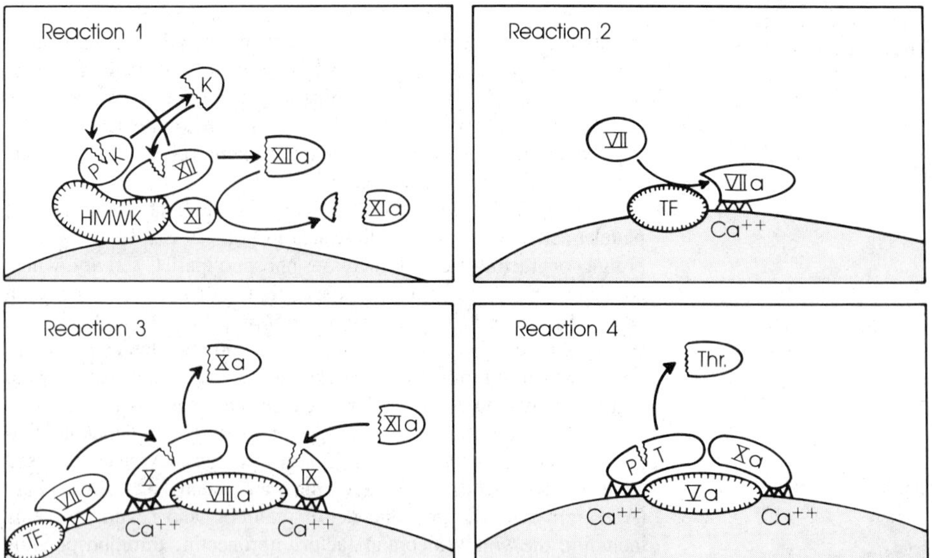

FIGURE 62-6 The major coagulation reactions are subdivided and depicted in schematic form to emphasize their similarity. They all rely on the formation of surface bound enzyme-cofactor complexes. Abbreviations are PK, prekallikrein; K, kallikrein; HMWK, high-molecular-weight kininogen; TF, tissue factor; Ca^{2+}, calcium; PT, prothrombin; Thr, thrombin. By convention other coagulation factors are indicated by roman numerals, with a lowercase "a" appended to indicate their active form. The /\/\/\ is used to indicate the Gla (di-γ-carboxyglutamic acid)–containing domains of factors VII, IX, X, Xa, and PT which bind calcium and phospholipid. Hatching is used to indicate proteins that adhere to surfaces by hydrophobic interaction.

by factor VIIa, which has been generated via the extrinsic pathway (reaction 2). Activation of factors IX and X provides an important link between the intrinsic and extrinsic coagulation pathways (see Fig. 62-5).

Reaction 4, the final step, converts prothrombin to thrombin in the presence of factor V, calcium, and phospholipid. Although prothrombin conversion can take place on various natural and artificial phospholipid-rich surfaces, it accelerates several-thousand-fold on the surface of activated platelets. Thrombin, the product of this reaction, has multiple functions in hemostasis. Although its principal role in hemostasis is the conversion of fibrinogen to fibrin, it also activates factors V, VIII, and XIII and stimulates platelet aggregation and secretion. Following the release of fibrinopeptides A and B from the alpha and beta chains of fibrinogen, the modified molecule, now called fibrin monomer, polymerizes into an insoluble gel. The fibrin polymer is then stabilized by the cross-linking of individual chains by factor XIIIa, a plasma transglutaminase (Fig. 62-5).

Clot lysis and vessel repair begin immediately after the formation of the definitive hemostatic plug. There are three major activators of the fibrinolytic system, Hageman factor fragments, urokinase (UK), and tissue plasminogen activator (t-PA). The principal physiologic activator, t-PA, diffuses from endothelial cells and converts plasminogen, adsorbed to the fibrin clot, into plasmin (see Fig. 62-7). Plasmin then degrades fibrin polymer into small fragments which are cleared by the monocyte-macrophage scavenger system. Although plasmin can also degrade fibrinogen, the reaction remains localized because (1) t-PA activates plasminogen more effectively when it is adsorbed to fibrin clots, and (2) any plasmin that enters the circulation is rapidly bound and neutralized by the alpha$_2$ plasmin inhibitor. The importance of this inhibitor is underscored by the fact that patients who lack it have unchecked fibrinolysis and bleed. In addition endothelial cells release a plasminogen activator inhibitor (PAI) which blocks the action of t-PA.

As noted above, the plasma coagulation system is tightly regulated so that only a small quantity of each coagulation enzyme is converted to its active form. As a consequence, the hemostatic plug does not propagate beyond the site of injury. Precise regulation is important, since there is enough clotting potential in a single milliliter of blood to clot all the fibrinogen in the body in 10 to 15 s. Blood fluidity is maintained by the flow of blood itself, which reduces the concentration of reactants, the adsorption of coagulation factors to surfaces, and the presence of multiple inhibitors in plasma. Antithrombin and proteins C and S are the most important inhibitors which help maintain blood fluidity.

These inhibitors have distinct modes of action. Antithrombin forms complexes with all the serine protease coagulation factors except factor VII (see Fig. 62-5). Rates of complex formation are accelerated by heparin and heparin-like molecules on the surface of the endothelial cells. This ability of heparin to accelerate the activity of antithrombin is the basis for heparin's action as a potent anticoagulant. Protein C is converted to an active protease by thrombin after it is bound to an endothelial cell protein called thrombomodulin. Activated protein C then inactivates the two plasma cofactors V and VIII to slow down two critical coagulation reactions. Protein C may also stimulate the release of tissue plasminogen activator from endothelial cells. The inhibitory function of protein C is enhanced by protein S. As one might predict, reduced levels of antithrombin or proteins C and S, or dysfunctional forms of the molecule, result in a hypercoagulable or prethrombotic state.

The preceding description of blood coagulation implies that the process is uniform throughout the body. In fact, the process is not uniform and composition of the blood clot varies with the site of injury. Hemostatic plugs or thrombi that form in veins where blood flow is slow are richly endowed with fibrin and trapped red blood cells and contain relatively few platelets. They are often called red thrombi due to their appearance in surgical and pathologic specimens. The friable ends of these red thrombi, which often form in leg veins, can break off and embolize to the pulmonary circulation. Conversely, clots that form in arteries under conditions of high flow are predominantly composed of platelets and have little fibrin. These white thrombi may readily dislodge from the arterial wall and embolize to distant sites to cause temporary or permanent ischemia. This is particularly common in the cerebral and retinal circulation and may lead to transient neurologic dysfunction (transient ischemic attacks) including temporary monocular blindness (amaurosis fugax) or strokes. In addition, there is increasing evidence that many episodes of myocardial infarction are due to thrombi which form within atherosclerotic coronary arteries. It is important to remember that there is little difference between hemostatic plugs, which are a physiologic response to injury, and pathologic thrombi. To underscore the similarity, thrombosis is often described as coagulation occurring in the wrong place or at the wrong time.

FIGURE 62-7 A schematic diagram of the fibrinolytic pathway. t-PA (tissue plasminogen activator) is released from endothelial cells, enters the fibrin clot, and activates plasminogen to plasmin. Any free plasmin is complexed with α_2 PI (alpha$_2$ plasmin inhibitor). Fibrin is degraded to low-molecular-weight fragments, abbreviated as FDPs, fibrin degradation products.

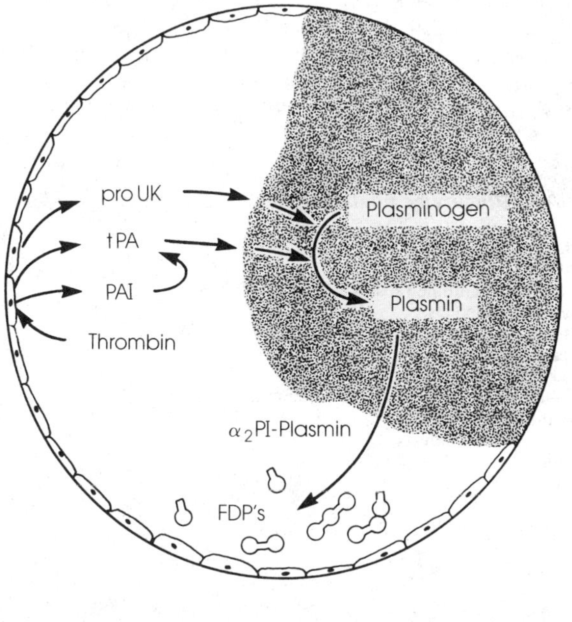

CLINICAL EVALUATION

HISTORY Certain elements of the history are particularly useful in determining whether bleeding is caused by an underlying hemostatic disorder rather than a local anatomic defect. One clue is a history of bleeding following common hemostatic stresses such as dental extraction, childbirth, or minor surgery. Bleeding that is sufficiently severe to require a blood transfusion merits special attention. A family history of bleeding and bleeding from multiple sites that cannot be linked to trauma or surgery also suggest a systemic disorder. Since bleeding can be mild, lack of a family history of bleeding does not exclude an inherited hemostatic disorder.

It may be possible to localize the defect to the platelet or plasma coagulation system (Table 62-1). Bleeding from a platelet disorder is usually localized to superficial sites such as the skin and mucous membranes, comes on immediately after trauma or surgery, and is readily controlled by local measures. In contrast, bleeding from secondary hemostatic or plasma coagulation defects occurs hours or days after injury and is unaffected by local therapy. Such bleeding most often occurs in deep subcutaneous tissues, muscles, joints, or body cavities.

PHYSICAL EXAMINATION In conjunction with a careful history, physical examination can also be of help in evaluating patients with hemostatic disorders. The most common site to observe bleeding is in the skin and mucous membranes. Collections of blood in the skin

TABLE 62-1 Differences in the clinical manifestations of disorders of primary and secondary hemostasis

	Primary hemostasis (platelet defect)	Secondary hemostasis (plasma proteins)
Onset of bleeding after trauma	Immediate	Delayed—hours or days
Sites of bleeding	Superficial—skin; mucous membranes; nose; gastrointestinal, genitourinary tracts	Deep—joints, muscle, retroperitoneum
Physical findings	Petechiae, ecchymoses	Hematomas, hemarthroses
Family history	Autosomal dominant	Autosomal or X-linked recessive
Response to therapy	Immediate; local measures effective	Requires sustained systemic therapy

TABLE 62-2 Causes of thrombocytopenia

I Decreased marrow production of megakaryocytes
- *A* Marrow infiltration with tumor, fibrosis
- *B* Marrow failure—aplastic, hypoplastic anemias

II Splenic sequestration of circulating platelets
- *A* Splenic hypertrophy—tumor, portal hypertension

III Increased destruction of circulating platelets
- *A* Nonimmune destruction
  - *1* Vascular prostheses, cardiac valves
  - *2* Disseminated intravascular coagulation
  - *3* Sepsis
  - *4* Vasculitis
- *B* Immune destruction
  - *1* Autoantibodies to platelet antigens
  - *2* Drug-associated antibodies
  - *3* Circulating immune complexes—systemic lupus erythematosus, viral agents, bacterial sepsis

are called *purpura* and may be subdivided on the basis of the site of bleeding in the skin. Small pinpoint hemorrhages into the dermis due to the leakage of red cells through capillaries are called *petechiae* and are characteristic of platelet disorders—in particular, severe thrombocytopenia. Larger subcutaneous collections of blood due to leakage of blood from small arterioles and venules are *ecchymoses* (common bruises) or, if somewhat deeper and palpable, *hematomas*. They are also common in patients with platelet defects and result from minor trauma. There are other skin and mucous membrane lesions like dilated capillaries or *telangiectasia* that may cause bleeding without any hemostatic defect. In addition, the loss of connective tissue support for capillaries and small veins that accompanies aging increases the fragility of superficial vessels, such as those on the dorsum of the hand, leading to extravasation of blood into subcutaneous tissue—*senile purpura*. Menorrhagia is a serious problem in women with severe thrombocytopenia or platelet dysfunction. In addition, some patients with primary hemostatic defects, especially von Willebrand's disease, may have recurrent gastrointestinal hemorrhage.

As mentioned previously, bleeding into body cavities, retroperitoneum, or joints is a common manifestation of plasma coagulation defects. Repeated joint bleeding may cause synovial thickening, chronic inflammation, and fluid collections and may erode articular cartilage and lead to chronic joint deformity and limited mobility. Such deformities are particularly common in factor VIII and IX deficiency, the two sex-linked coagulation disorders referred to as the hemophilias. For unclear reasons, hemarthroses are much less common in other plasma coagulation defects. Blood collections in various body cavities or soft tissues can cause secondary necrosis of tissues or nerve compression. Retroperitoneal hematomas can cause femoral nerve compression, and large collections of poorly coagulated blood in soft tissues may occasionally mimic malignant growths—the pseudotumor syndrome. Two of the most life-threatening sites of bleeding are in the oropharynx, where bleeding can compromise the airway, and in the central nervous system. Intracerebral hemorrhage is one of the leading causes of death in patients with severe coagulation disorders.

LABORATORY TESTS The most important screening tests of the primary hemostatic system are (1) a *bleeding time* (a sensitive measure of platelet function) and (2) a *platelet count*. The latter is particularly useful as it is readily available and correlates well with the propensity to bleed. The normal platelet count is 150,000 to 450,000 platelets per cubic millimeter of blood. As long as the count is above 100,000 per cubic millimeter, patients are not symptomatic and the bleeding time remains normal. Platelet counts of 50,000 to 100,000 per cubic millimeter cause mild prolongation of the bleeding time and bleeding occurs only after severe trauma or other stress. Patients with platelet counts less than 50,000 per cubic millimeter have easy bruising, which is manifested by skin purpura with minor trauma and bleeding after mucous membrane surgery. Patients with a platelet count below 20,000 per cubic millimeter have an appreciable incidence of spontaneous bleeding, usually have petechiae, and may have intracranial or other spontaneous internal bleeding. The major causes of thrombocytopenia are outlined in Table 62-2.

Patients with qualitative platelet abnormalities have a normal platelet count and a prolonged bleeding time (Table 62-3). The bleeding time is ascertained by making a small, superficial skin incision and timing the duration of blood flow from the wounded area. Although this is a rather crude "bioassay," by careful standardization it has become a reliable and sensitive test of platelet function. The most widely used technique uses a template or an automated scalpel to control the length and depth of the incision (usually 1 mm deep by 9 mm long), and a sphygmomanometer inflated to 40 mmHg to distend the capillary bed of the forearm uniformly. Although any patient with a bleeding time over 10 min has a slightly increased risk of bleeding, the risk does not become great until the bleeding time exceeds 15 or 20 min. When a defect in primary hemostasis is uncovered, specialized testing is needed to determine the cause of the platelet dysfunction (Table 62-3). A precise diagnosis is important since patients with bleeding due to a primary hemostatic disorder may need therapy with platelets, one of several hormones (desmopressin, estrogen, glucocorticoids), or plasma fractions, depending on the nature of the disorder.

Plasma coagulation function is readily assessed with a few simple laboratory tests—the partial thromboplastin time (PTT), prothrombin time (PT), thrombin time (TT), or a quantitative fibrinogen determination (Fig. 62-5, Table 62-4). The PTT screens the intrinsic limb of the coagulation system and tests for the adequacy of factors XII, HMWK, PK, XI, IX, and VIII. The PT screens the extrinsic or tissue factor-dependent pathway. Both tests also evaluate the common coagulation pathway involving all the reactions that occur after the activation of factor X. A specific test for fibrinogen conversion to fibrin is needed when both the PTT and PT are prolonged—either a TT or fibrinogen level can be employed. A test for factor XIII–dependent fibrin cross-linking, such as clot solubility in 5 *M* urea, should be ordered when the PT and PTT are both normal but there

TABLE 62-3 Primary hemostatic (platelet) disorders

Platelet adhesion defects:
- Von Willebrand's disease
- Bernard-Soulier syndrome (absence of platelet GpIb)*

Platelet aggregation defects:
- Glanzmann's thrombasthenia (absence of GpIIb–IIIa)

Platelet release defects:
- Decreased cyclooxygenase activity
  - Drugs—aspirin, nonsteroidal anti-inflammatory agents
  - Congenital
- Granule storage pool defects
  - Congenital
  - Acquired
- Uremia

Platelet coating by drugs (e.g., penicillin or paraproteins)

* Gp = glycoprotein.

TABLE 62-4 Relationship between secondary hemostatic disorders and coagulation test abnormalities

Prolonged partial thromboplastin time (PTT):
- No clinical bleeding—factors XII, HMWK, PK
- Mild or rare bleeding—factor XI
- Frequent, severe bleeding—factors VIII and IX

Prolonged prothrombin time (PT):
- Factor VII deficiency
- Vitamin K deficiency—early
- Warfarin anticoagulant ingestion

Prolonged PTT and PT:
- Factor II, V, or X deficiency
- Vitamin K deficiency—late
- Warfarin anticoagulant ingestion

Prolonged thrombin time (TT):
- Mild or rare bleeding—afibrinogenemia
- Frequent, severe bleeding—dysfibrinogenemia
- Heparin-like inhibitors or heparin administration

Clot solubility in 5 *M* urea:
- Factor XIII deficiency
- Inhibitors or defective cross-linking

Rapid clot lysis
- Alpha$_2$ plasmin inhibitor

NOTE: HMWK = high-molecular-weight kininogen; PK = prekallikrein.

is a strong history of bleeding. The fibrinolytic system can be assessed by measuring the rate of clot lysis with the euglobulin lysis or whole blood clot lysis tests and by measuring the level of alpha$_2$ plasmin inhibitor. When abnormalities are noted in any of the screening tests, more specific coagulation factor assays can be ordered to determine the nature of the defect.

There are no clinical tests to screen patients suspected of having hypercoagulable or prethrombotic disorders, although tests are being developed in research laboratories which measure small peptides or enzyme-inhibitor complexes generated during coagulation. For example, radioimmunoassays have been developed for fibrinopeptides A and B, for the thrombin-antithrombin complex, and for prothrombin cleavage fragments. Elevated levels of these products have been reported in patients with prethrombotic disorders and in patients with thromboembolism. At present, patients suspected of having a hypercoagulable state, on the basis of clinical information, should have specific assays to screen for the small number of known defects. Currently available tests can identify 10 to 20 percent of the cases of familial thrombosis and represent only a small fraction of the many patients who present to physicians with thromboembolism.

Inhibitor syndromes or circulating anticoagulants are usually due to antibodies which impair coagulation factor activity. They are an infrequent cause of bleeding which require specialized diagnostic testing. Inhibitors are likely when screening test abnormalities cannot be reversed by adding normal plasma to patient plasma. Antibodies against specific coagulation factors may develop in (1) postpartum females; (2) patients with autoimmune disorders such as systemic lupus erythematosus; (3) patients taking drugs like penicillin and streptomycin; and (4) otherwise healthy elderly individuals. In addition, between 10 and 20 percent of patients with severe hemophilia who have received multiple plasma infusions develop inhibitor antibodies. Some patients, especially those with systemic lupus erythematosus, may also have a nonspecific form of anticoagulant antibody which interferes with phospholipid binding of coagulation factors and prolongs the PT and PTT but does not cause clinical bleeding. The presence of the lupus anticoagulant may increase the risk of thromboembolism and may cause placental infarction and recurrent midtrimester abortion. Occasionally, patients develop inhibitors that are not antibodies. For example, several patients with circulating mucopolysaccharides that have heparin-like activity have been described with clinical bleeding.

REFERENCES

COLMAN RW et al (eds): *Hemostasis and Thrombosis: Basic Principles and Clinical Practice*, 2d ed. Philadelphia, Lippincott, 1986

HANDIN RI: Physiology of coagulation: The platelet, in *Hematology of Infancy and Childhood*, 3d ed, DG Nathan, FA Oski (eds). Philadelphia, Saunders, 1987, pp 1271–1292

ROSENBERG RD: Physiology of coagulation: The fluid phase, in *Hematology of Infancy and Childhood*, 3d ed, DG Nathan, FA Oski (eds). Philadelphia, Saunders, 1987

WILLIAMS WJ et al (eds): *Hematology*, 4th ed. New York, McGraw-Hill, 1990

63 ENLARGEMENT OF LYMPH NODES AND SPLEEN

BARTON F. HAYNES

Lymph nodes and spleen constitute a major portion of the peripheral immune system, and become enlarged in a wide spectrum of infectious, malignant, autoimmune, and metabolic diseases. Enlargement of lymph nodes (lymphadenopathy) and spleen (splenomegaly) are common clinical findings that can lead to a wide range of diagnostic and therapeutic procedures. The goal of this chapter is to serve as an introduction to these two components of the immune system and to highlight clinical features and diagnostic evaluation of some of the diseases in which lymphadenopathy and splenomegaly occur.

LYMPH NODES

LYMPH NODE STRUCTURE AND FUNCTION Lymph nodes are peripheral lymphoid organs that are connected to the circulation by afferent and efferent lymphatic vessels (Fig. 63-1) and by postcapillary high-endothelial venules. A number of cell types make up the lymph node supportive framework and stroma. Fibroblasts are the predominant cell type in the lymph node capsule and trabeculae. Fibroblast-derived reticular cells are supporting cells found frequently in the follicles and germinal centers, that is, the B-cell areas of lymph nodes. Tissue macrophages derived from circulating monocytes are present throughout the normal node. Within cortical areas are interdigitating reticular cells (also called dendritic cells) and Langerhans cells both of which are specialized nonphagocytic, Ia-bearing cells of bone marrow origin that along with macrophages participate in antigen presentation to thymus-derived (T) and B cells (Chap. 13). The outer lymph node cortex contains lymphoid follicles with germinal centers that are the B-cell areas of lymph node (Fig. 63-1). Primary lymphoid follicles are aggregates of IgM- and IgD-bearing B cells and CD4+ helper/inducer T cells prior to antigenic challenge. Secondary lymphoid follicles are the result of antigen stimulation, and contain an outer or mantle layer of IgM- and IgD-bearing B cells

FIGURE 63-1 Schematic lymph node structure. Lymph flows into nodes via afferent lymphatics (A) and leaves nodes via efferent lymphatics (E). B-cell areas are primary and secondary follicles in lymph node cortex while T cells are concentrated in paracortical areas.

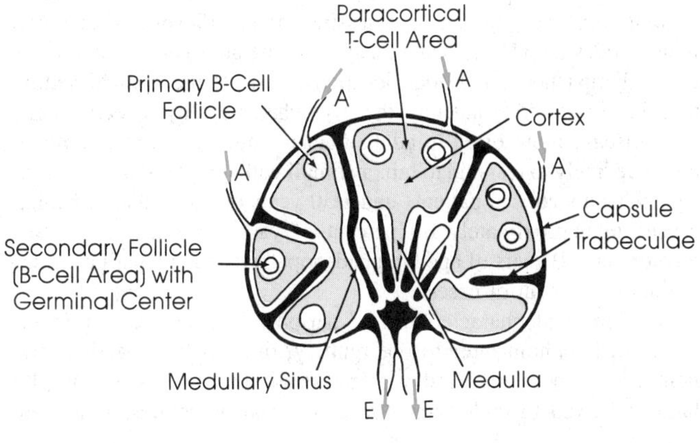

and an inner zone (germinal center) of activated B cells, macrophages, reticular cells, and scattered CD4+ helper T cells. Between primary and secondary follicle areas (interfollicular zones) and inner lymph node medullary regions are T-cell (paracortical) areas. The majority of T cells in lymph nodes are CD4+ helper T cells (approximately 80 percent) while the minority are CD8+ suppressor/cytotoxic T cells (approximately 20 percent).

The two most important factors contributing to the composition and distribution of lymphoid cells within lymph node are (1) generation of memory B and T cells de novo from proliferation of antigen-stimulated percursors within lymph nodes, and (2) selective recirculation to and homing of specific types of lymphoid cells to lymph nodes from the circulation. Traffic through lymph nodes is via two general routes (Fig. 63-1). Afferent lymph, containing lymphocytes, macrophages, and antigens, enters the lymph node via the subcapsular space, and drains through paracortical and medullary areas into medullary sinuses that converge to form efferent lymphatic vessels through which lymph exits. B cells from bone marrow and T cells from the thymus enter lymph nodes from the circulation by binding to specific receptors on cells of postcapillary high-endothelial venules. After activation by antigen and clonal expansion, sensitized T and B cells and antibody-secreting plasma cells leave the node in efferent lymph and rejoin the peripheral blood circulation via the thoracic duct.

Lymph nodes function as sites of macrophage, T-cell, and B-cell contact with antigen, with a specialized structure that gives rise to optimal T cell, B cell, and macrophage interactions.Under normal conditions such interactions result in efficient recognition of antigen, activation of the cellular and humoral arms of the immune response, and ultimate elimination of antigen (see Chap. 13).

Lymph node enlargement can be due to (1) an increase in the number of benign lymphocytes and macrophages during response to antigens, (2) infiltration by inflammatory cells in infections involving lymph nodes (lymphadenitis), (3) in situ proliferation of malignant lymphocytes or macrophages, (4) infiltration of nodes by metastatic malignant cells, or (5) infiltration of lymph nodes by metabolite-laden macrophages in lipid storage diseases.

In normal immune responses, antigen stimulation of macrophages and lymphocytes in lymph nodes exerts profound influences on lymphocyte traffic. One of the earliest effects of antigen is to increase blood flow through the affected node, which during antigen stimulation may reach 10 to 25 times normal levels. Lymphocytes accumulate in antigen-stimulated nodes by increase in traffic through the node, decreased egress of lymphocytes from antigen-stimulated nodes, and proliferation of responding T and B cells. A lymph node may thus reach 15 times its normal size 5 to 10 days after antigenic stimulation.

DISEASES ASSOCIATED WITH LYMPHADENOPATHY Under normal conditions in adults, the inguinal lymph nodes may be palpable, and are generally 0.5 cm to 2 cm in size. Elsewhere in the body, smaller lymph nodes due to past infections may be present normally. Enlargement of lymph nodes requires investigation when there are one or more new nodes present equal to or greater than 1 cm in diameter, and not known to arise from a previously recognized cause. However, this is not a rigid criterion and under certain circumstances new multiple or single smaller lymph nodes may warrant investigation as well. Important factors in assessing the significance of enlarged lymph nodes are (1) the patient's age, (2) the physical characteristics of the lymph node, (3) node locations, and (4) the clinical setting associated with lymphadenopathy. Lymphadenopathy reflects significant disease more often in adults than in children because children are more likely to respond to minor stimuli with lymphoid hyperplasia. Lymphadenopathy in patients under 30 years of age is due to benign causes in approximately 80 percent of cases whereas in patients greater than 50 years of age lymphadenopathy is due to benign causes in only 40 percent of cases.

The physical characteristics of peripheral nodes are important. Nodes of lymphomas tend to be rubbery, firm, matted together, and nontender. Nodes involved with metastatic carcinomas are usually hard and fixed to underlying tissue. In acute infections, nodes are tender, asymmetrically enlarged, matted together, and the overlying skin may be erythematous.

The clinical setting is important in assessing lymphadenopathy. In a young college student with fever and recent onset of lymph node enlargement, infectious mononucleosis syndromes are important to consider. In homosexuals, hemophiliacs, and intravenous drug users with systemic lymphadenopathy, the acquired immunodeficiency syndrome (AIDS) or an AIDS-related complex syndrome should be considered (see Chap. 264).

The location of enlarged lymph nodes may suggest important clues to the diagnosis. Enlarged posterior cervical nodes are frequently present in scalp infections, toxoplasmosis, and rubella, whereas anterior auricular nodes suggest infections of the eyelids and conjunctiva. Lymphomas commonly involve cervical lymph nodes and can occasionally involve posterior auricular and occipital nodes as well. Enlarged suppurative cervical nodes are seen in mycobacterial lymphadenitis (scrofula). Unilateral jugular or mandibular lymph node enlargement suggests lymphoma or nonlymphoid head-and-neck malignancy. Supraclavicular and scalene lymph node enlargement is always significant, and frequently results from metastasis from intrathoracic or gastrointestinal malignancies or from lymphomas. Virchow's node is an enlarged left supraclavicular lymph node infiltrated with metastatic tumor usually from the gastrointestinal tract. Unilateral epitrochlear node enlargement is usually due to hand infections; bilateral epitrochlear node enlargement is seen in sarcoidosis, tularemia, and secondary syphilis.

Unilateral axillary adenopathy can be seen with breast carcinoma, lymphomas, infections of the upper extremities, cat-scratch disease, and brucellosis.

Bilateral inguinal adenopathy can be seen in a variety of venereal infections; however, lymphogranuloma venereum and syphilis are associated with unilateral inguinal adenopathy. Progressive inguinal lymph node enlargement without obvious infection suggests malignant disease. Femoral node involvement has been reported to occur in *Pasteurella pestis* infections and lymphomas.

Symptoms that should raise the suspicion of hilar or mediastinal node enlargement are cough or wheezing due to airway compression, recurrent laryngeal nerve compression with hoarseness, paralysis of the diaphragm, dysphagia with esophageal compression, and swelling of the neck, face, or arms due to superior vena cava or subclavian vein compression. Bilateral mediastinal adenopathy is frequently seen in lymphomas, especially the nodular sclerosing type of Hodgkin's disease. Unilateral hilar adenopathy indicates a high likelihood of metastatic carcinoma (usually lung), while bilateral hilar adenopathy is more often benign and is seen in sarcoidosis, tuberculosis, and systemic fungal infections. Bilateral hilar adenopathy in asymptomatic patients or in association with erythema nodosum or uveitis is almost always due to sarcoidosis (Chap. 277). The association of bilateral hilar adenopathy with an anterior mediastinal mass, pleural effusion, or pulmonary mass suggests neoplastic disease.

Enlarged retroperitoneal and intraabdominal nodes are not usually inflammatory in origin, but are frequently due to lymphomas or other neoplastic diseases. Tuberculosis can cause mesenteric lymphadenitis with large matted and sometimes calcified nodes.

Some of the diseases associated with lymph node enlargement are listed in Table 63-1 and fall into six general categories: infectious diseases, immunologic diseases, malignant diseases, endocrine diseases, lipid storage diseases, and miscellaneous.

The manifestations of infectious diseases are protean and are best considered according to the type of infectious agent. The most common viral infection associated with systemic lymphadenopathy is Epstein-Barr (EB) virus–associated infectious mononucleosis (see Chap. 137). A variety of other viral diseases including viral hepatitis, cytomegalovirus, rubella, and influenza can cause clinical syndromes similar to those induced by the EB virus. AIDS is caused by a retrovirus, human immunodeficiency virus (HIV). In the HIV-associated lymphadenopathy syndrome, cervical, axillary, and occipital nodes are the most commonly involved (see Chap. 264).

TABLE 63-1 Diseases associated with lymph node enlargement

I Infectious diseases
- *A* Viral infections: infectious hepatitis, infectious mononucleosis syndromes (cytomegalovirus, EB virus), AIDS, rubella, varicella–herpes zoster, vaccinia
- *B* Bacterial infections: streptococci, staphylococci, salmonella, brucella, Francisella tularensis, *Listeria monocytogenes, Pasteurella pestis, Haemophilus ducreyi,* cat-scratch disease
- *C* Fungal infections: coccidioidomycosis, histoplasmosis
- *D* Chlamydial infections: Lymphogranuloma venereum, trachoma
- *E* Mycobacterial infections: tuberculosis, leprosy
- *F* Parasitic infections: trypanosomiasis, microfilariasis, toxoplasmosis
- *G* Spirochetal diseases: syphilis, yaws, endemic syphilis (bejel), leptospirosis

II Immunologic diseases
- *A* Rheumatoid arthritis
- *B* Systemic lupus erythematosus
- *C* Dermatomyositis
- *D* Serum sickness
- *E* Drug reactions: phenytoin, hydralazine, allopurinol
- *F* Angioimmunoblastic lymphadenopathy

III Malignant diseases
- *A* Hematologic: Hodgkin's lymphoma, acute and chronic T-, B-, myeloid, and monocytoid cell leukemias and lymphomas, malignant histiocytosis
- *B* Metastatic tumors to lymph nodes: melanoma, Kaposi's sarcoma, neuroblastoma, seminoma, tumors of lung, breast, prostate, kidney, head and neck, gastrointestinal tract

IV Endocrine diseases: hyperthyroidism

V Lipid storage diseases: Gaucher's and Niemann-Pick diseases

VI Miscellaneous diseases and diseases of unknown cause
- *A* Giant follicular lymph node hyperplasia
- *B* Sinus histiocytosis
- *C* Dermatopathic lymphadenitis
- *D* Sarcoidosis
- *E* Amyloidosis
- *F* Mucocutaneous lymph node syndrome
- *G* Lymphomatoid granulomatosis
- *H* Multifocal Langerhans cell (eosinophilic) granulomatosis

Chronic bacterial infections as well as fungal infections may produce considerable lymph node enlargement without signs of local inflammation. Cat-scratch disease is a regional lymphadenitis occurring approximately 2 weeks following a cat scratch or bite. The nodes involved relate to lymph drainage of the wound site with upper extremity adenopathy being the most common, occurring in 50 percent of cases. Fungi associated with primary pulmonary infections (coccidioidomycosis, histoplasmosis) can cause hilar adenopathy. Acute and chronic mycobacterial, parasitic, and spirochetal diseases against which there is a profound cellular and humoral immune response all can result in either systemic or regional enlarged lymph nodes depending on the clinical syndrome in question. Virtually any disease characterized by immune cell activation (systemic lupus erythematosus, rheumatoid arthritis, serum sickness, reactions due to drugs such as diphenylhydantoin, angioimmunoblastic lymphadenopathy) can be associated with regional or systemic adenopathy. Lymph node enlargement associated with malignant disease may be due to direct node involvement by tumor, lymphoid hyperplasia in response to tumor, or both. Generalized lymphoid hyperplasia may occur with hyperthroidism. Patients with lipid storage diseases such as Gaucher's and Niemann-Pick disease can have enlarged lymph nodes, particularly in the abdomen, due to accumulation of lipid-laden macrophages.

A number of diseases of unknown cause are associated with lymphadenopathy and in many of the diseases in this group, lymphadenopathy is a major manifestation of the disease. Sarcoidosis frequently presents with generalized lymph node enlargement, especially in cervical, inguinal, and epitrochlear areas (Chap. 277). Although giant follicular lymph node hyperplasia can occur in extrathoracic lymph nodes, mediastinal or hilar nodes are involved in 70 percent of cases. In sinus histiocytosis, massive cervical lymph node enlargement often associated with generalized lymphadenopathy occurs and is associated with fever and leukocytosis. Patients with exfoliative dermatitis or other dermatologic syndromes can develop enlarged superficial lymph nodes (called dermatopathic lymphadenitis) which usually regress with resolution of the dermatitis. Lymph node involvement occurs in approximately 30 percent of cases of primary and secondary amyloidosis; only rarely is amyloid lymphadenopathy the major or the only organ involvement. The mechanism of node enlargement in amyloidosis is the accumulation of extracellular masses of amyloid fibrils that compress and eventually obliterate normal lymph node architecture (Chap. 266).

Mucocutaneous lymph node syndrome (Kawasaki's disease) is a systemic lymphadenopathy syndrome, the hallmarks of which are fever, conjunctivitis, erythema of the tongue with protrusion of papillae (strawberry tongue), a truncal exanthem with desquamation of palms and soles, and acute nonsuppurative enlargement of cervical lymph nodes (see Chap. 276).

Lymphomatoid granulomatosis is a disease characterized by infiltration of various organs (lungs, skin, central nervous system) with an angiocentric and angioinvasive polymorphic cellular infiltrate consisting of atypical lymphocytes and macrophages. The disease has characteristics of both an inflammatory granulomatous process and a lymphoproliferative disease, with progression to frank lymphoma in up to 50 percent of cases. Lymphadenopathy in the prelymphoma state of lymphomatoid granulomatosis occurs in 40 percent of cases affecting primarily intrathoracic nodes while peripheral adenopathy occurs only rarely (10 percent) (see Chap. 276).

Angioimmunoblastic lymphadenopathy is a disease characterized by fever, generalized lymphadenopathy, hepatosplenomegaly, polyclonal hypergammaglobulinemia, and Coombs-positive hemolytic anemia. Although it is not thought to be a malignant disease, it evolves into B-cell lymphoma in 35 percent of patients (see Chap. 302).

Diseases characterized by benign and malignant proliferation of tissue macrophages (histiocytes) or of specialized bone marrow–derived cells called Langerhans cells have been termed *histiocytoses* or *histiocytosis X*. In the past, these terms encompassed a number of diseases including unifocal and multifocal eosinophilic granuloma, Hand-Schüller-Christian syndrome, Letterer-Siwe disease, and frank neoplasms of undifferentiated histiocytes. Recently, the identification of the Langerhans cell as the predominant cell in forms of eosinophilic granuloma has prompted reevaluation of these syndromes.

One term currently in use for eosinophilic granuloma syndromes is *Langerhans cell (eosinophilic) granulomatosis,* and this term will be used here. The term histiocytosis X is an outmoded term that refers to a spectrum of diseases encompassing both the benign disorder of Langerhans cell (eosinophilic) granulomatosis and malignant lymphomatous disease.

The classic triad of the *Hand-Schüller-Christian syndrome* (exophthalmus, diabetes insipidus, and destructive bone lesions) occurs with 25 percent of cases of multifocal eosinophilic granuloma but also may occur in malignant lymphoma and carcinoma. *Letterer-Siwe disease* is an acute clinical syndrome of unknown etiology in infants that consists of hepatosplenomegaly, lymphadenopathy, hemorrhagic diathesis, anemia, no familial occurrence, and generalized hyperplasia of tissue macrophages in a variety of organs. It is currently felt that Letterer-Siwe disease represents an unusual form of malignant lymphoma, and is distinct from forms of eosinophilic granuloma.

Histologically, Langerhans cell granulomatosis consists of aggregates of mature eosinophils and Langerhans cells. Langerhans cells are bone marrow–derived cells normally found among epidermal cells of skin and rarely in B-cell areas of lymph node and the medulla of thymus. Langerhans cells contain distinct cytoplasmic granules (Birbeck granules) and contain adenosine triphosphatase and alpha naphthyl acetate esterase. Surface markers of Langerhans cells include class II major histocompatibility complex antigens (Ia-like) and the T6 antigen that is also expressed by the cortical (immature) thymocytes (see Chap. 13).

Unifocal Langerhans cell (eosinophilic) granulomatosis is a benign disease of children and young adults, predominantly in males. Occasionally, it occurs as late as 60 to 70 years of age, and presents as a solitary osteolytic lesion in the femur, skull, vertebrae, ribs, or occasionally the pelvis. Since there are no consistent accompanying laboratory abnormalities, the diagnosis of unifocal Langerhans cell granulomatosis requires biopsy of the lytic bone lesion. Treatment of choice of this condition is excision or curettage of the lesion. Rarely, lesions in inaccessible sites such as cervical vertebrae require moderate doses of irradiation [3 to 6 Gy (300 to 600 rad)]. After initial bone scan and radiographic survey to assess extent of disease, follow-up studies should be performed at 6-month intervals for 3 years. If no additional lesions are present 12 months after diagnosis, development of subsequent lesions is unlikely.

Multifocal Langerhans cell (eosinophilic) granulomatosis also usually presents in childhood, and is characterized by the development of multiple bony lesions at virtually any site—though less commonly in the feet and hands.

Transient or permanent diabetes insipidus due to granulomatous involvement of the hypothalamus occurs in one-third of patients; 20 percent develop hepatomegaly, 30 percent splenomegaly, and one-half of the patients have focal or generalized lymph node involvement. Lesions may also involve the skin, vulva, gingiva, lung, and thymus. Laboratory studies are rarely helpful in the diagnosis of multifocal Langerhans cell granulomatosis, necessitating biopsy of lesions. While generally a benign disease, multifocal Langerhans cell granulomatosis is best treated with low to moderate doses of methotrexate, prednisone, or vinblastine, usually with regression of lesions.

EVALUATION OF THE PATIENT WITH LYMPHADENOPATHY Good physical examination techniques for palpation and assessment of lymph nodes are essential for providing useful information on which diagnostic and therapeutic decisions can be based. For serial evaluation of nodes, the documentation of each node with regard to size, location, consistency, and mobility at each examination is critical. For cervical nodes the examiner may stand behind or in front of the seated patient to palpate the neck and to examine in sequence the sites of various groups of nodes. Submental nodes are under the chin in the midline and on either side; submandibular nodes are under the jaw near its angle; jugular nodes are along the anterior border of the sternocleidomastoid muscle; supraclavicular nodes are found behind the mid portion of the clavicle. Suboccipital nodes are found in the apex of the posterior cervical triangle, and pre- and postauricular nodes are found in front of and behind the ear pinnae, respectively. Central axillary nodes occur near the middle of the thoracic wall of the axilla; lateral axillary nodes are located near the upper part of the humerus along the axillary vein and are best felt by having the patient's arm elevated. Subscapular nodes can be felt under the anterior edge of the latissimus dorsi muscle, and pectoral nodes are beneath the lateral edge of the pectoralis major muscle. Infraclavicular nodes can be felt under the distal end of the clavicle. Epitrochlear nodes are located approximately 3 cm proximal to the medial humeral epicondyle. Palpation of epitrochlear nodes is best accomplished by palpation across the epitrochlear node area in an anterior to posterior direction. Enlarged abdominal lymph nodes can be difficult to palpate and may only be felt if the patient has a shallow abdominal cavity. Pelvic nodes are best evaluated with deep palpation of the lower abdomen by rolling the extended fingers over the pelvic brim.

The investigation of lymphadenopathy can be organized according to where nodes occur and the type of clinical symptoms present. Enlarged supraclavicular nodes most often result from lymphoma, gastrointestinal, or intrathoracic tumors and should be biopsied. Acute onset of cervical adenopathy in young adults in the absence of head-and-neck infections suggests the diagnosis of infectious mononucleosis syndromes. If localized cervical node enlargement persists and serologic evaluation for EB virus, cytomegalovirus, and toxoplasmosis infections as well as chest x-ray and intermediate-strength PPD skin test are negative, then lymph node biopsy is indicated to seek lymphoma, sarcoidosis, carcinoma, and other diseases listed in Table 63-1.

Unilateral cervical adenopathy warrants a careful ear, nose, and throat examination for malignancy. In the asymptomatic patient with persistent new axillary and/or inguinal adenopathy, a biopsy specimen should be obtained. If fever and constitutional symptoms are present, the cause of infectious mononucleosis–like syndromes should be sought prior to node biopsy.

Generalized lymph node enlargement can be caused by systemic infections, drug reactions, malignancy, or one of the systemic lymphadenopathy syndromes (Table 63-1). History and physical examination can yield clues regarding the possibility of these diagnoses and direct further evaluation (e.g., complete blood count, blood cultures, chest x-ray, serologies, skin tests). If systemic adenopathy persists without an obvious cause being identified, lymph node biopsy is warranted. Once the decision to perform lymph node biopsy has been made, tissue should be processed for culture of appropriate organisms, frozen in liquid nitrogen for lymphocyte typing or other special diagnostic studies for malignant cell types, and processed for routine pathologic evaluation. One can expect information that will lead to a diagnosis in 50 to 60 percent of lymph node biopsies. About 25 percent of patients with nondiagnostic lymph node biopsies will subsequently develop within a year a disease (usually a lymphoma) related to the indication for biopsy. Therefore there should be little hesitation to repeat a nondiagnostic biopsy, especially if enlarged lymph nodes and symptoms persist.

The term *atypical hyperplasia of lymph nodes* refers to neither a clinical nor a pathologic entity, but designates cases in which the pathologist expresses concern about neoplasia and is unable to unequivocally diagnose lymphoma. Since 30 percent of patients whose lymph node biopsies are read as atypical hyperplasia subsequently develop lymphoma, a repeat biopsy is recommended at a later date if node enlargement persists. Needle aspiration biopsy is a safe technique for initial evaluation of superficial adenopathy. While lymph node aspiration can aid in the diagnosis of metastatic tumor and infections, it is rarely helpful in the diagnosis of lymphomas and other hematologic malignancies.

SPLEEN

SPLEEN STRUCTURE AND FUNCTION The spleen is a lymphoreticular organ that serves at least four major physiologic functions. First, it is an organ of the immune system and a major site of clearance of microorganisms and particulate antigens from the bloodstream and of generation of humoral or cellular responses to foreign antigens. Second, the spleen is instrumental in sequestration and removal of normal and abnormal blood cells. Third, the vasculature of the spleen plays a role in regulation of portal blood flow. Fourth, while hematopoiesis in the normal adult takes place primarily in the bone marrow, under pathologic conditions when the marrow is replaced or overstimulated to respond, the spleen may become a major site of extramedullary hematopoiesis.

The spleen is arranged into units of areas called red and white pulp (Fig. 63-2). Red pulp contains blood-filled sinuses and pulp cords lined by reticuloendothelial cells. White pulp contains centrally located arterioles, surrounded by densely packed small lymphocytes, which are primarily CD4+ helper T lymphocytes. Adjacent to the T-cell periarteriolar lymphocyte sheath is the follicular zone of B lymphocytes which also contains germinal centers made up of B cells and macrophages. The outermost portion of white pulp is another B-cell layer called the marginal zone which blends into red pulp areas.

The blood supply and the route of blood flow are unique in the spleen, and splenic anatomy can best be defined in terms of route of blood flow (Fig. 63-2). Blood enters the spleen by the splenic artery. The splenic artery divides into branches which penetrate into the spleen via connective tissue projections called trabeculae and from the trabeculae branch into smaller arteries called central arteries. From central arteries the bloodstream reaches the arterial capillaries. The periarteriolar lymphoid sheaths of T cells surrounding B-cell follicles persist around the arterial vessels until they become small arterioles. Blood in central arterioles empties partly through arterial capillaries directly into splenic venules and then into splenic veins.

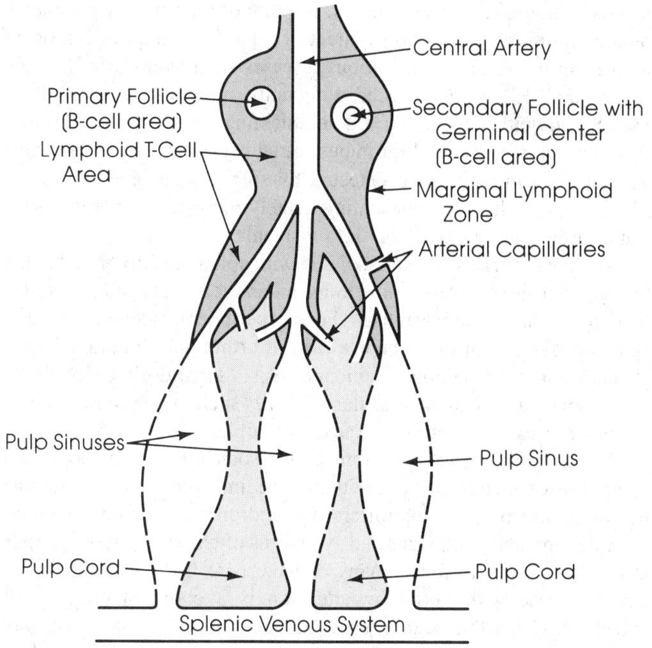

FIGURE 63-2 Schematic spleen structure. The spleen is made up of multiple units of red and white pulp centered around small branches of the splenic artery called central arteries. White pulp areas of spleen are lymphoid areas while red pulp areas include pulp sinuses and pulp cords. In white pulp, B-cell areas are primary and secondary follicles and the marginal lymphoid zone, while T-cell areas are lymphoid cells around follicles and arterial capillaries. (*Redrawn with permission from Videbaek et al.*)

The central arterioles also empty into macrophage-lined sinuses of red pulp and into the fibrous network of reticuloendothelial cells and tissue macrophages called pulp cords. Blood in red pulp sinuses and pulp cords empties directly into the splenic venous system. During red blood cell passage from central arteries to pulp cords, and finally to spleen sinuses, red cells are concentrated in the macrophage-rich pulp cords. Normally circulating red cells accumulate in pulp cords with subsequent passage through critical small openings of sinus endothelium into red pulp sinuses and on to the splenic venous system. Packing of red cells in pulp cords with subsequent passage through small slits into sinuses is termed *erythrocyte conditioning*. Upon senescence, red cells become less deformable and are unable to pass into sinuses; they are retained in pulp cords and phagocytosed by macrophages—a process termed *culling*. Erythrocyte particulate matter such as nuclear material (Howell-Jolly bodies), denatured hemoglobulin (Heinz bodies), or malaria parasites can be pinched off during passage of red cells from pulp cords into sinuses and retained in the spleen while the rest of the red cell passes back into the circulation—a process termed *pitting*.

Many of the mechanisms of spleen enlargement are exaggerated forms of normal spleen function. While there is a wide variety of diseases associated with enlargement of the spleen, there are six basic pathophysiologic mechanisms of splenic enlargement. (1) Splenic enlargement occurs from reticuloendothelial or immune system hyperplasia in infectious diseases such as bacterial endocarditis or in immune diseases such as Felty's syndrome. Reticuloendothelial hyperplasia also occurs in diseases associated with destruction of abnormal red blood cells such as hereditary spherocytosis, thalassemia, or early in the course of sickle cell disease. (2) Splenic enlargement occurs due to altered splenic blood flow in hepatic cirrhosis or splenic, hepatic, or portal vein thrombosis. (3) Malignant neoplasms can involve the spleen either primarily as with lymphomas or angiosarcomas, or secondarily with leukemias or metastatic solid tumors. (4) Splenic enlargement can occur in situations leading to extramedullary hematopoiesis in the spleen such as in myeloid metaplasia or other myelophthisic syndromes. (5) Infiltration of the spleen with abnormal material in amyloidosis and Gaucher's disease can result in splenomegaly. (6) Splenomegaly can also result from space-occupying lesions such as hemangiomas and cysts.

DISEASES ASSOCIATED WITH SPLENIC ENLARGEMENT A wide variety of diseases lead to an increase in cellularity and vascularity of the spleen (Table 63-2). Increase in cellularity in infections is due to lymphocyte and macrophage proliferation in both red and white pulp areas. Splenomegaly is often present in acute systemic bacterial infections. Infectious granulomas due to mycobacterial and fungal infections occur in both red and white pulp. In diseases associated with disordered immunoregulation such as rheumatoid arthritis and systemic lupus erythematosus, splenic enlargement is often due to lymphoid hyperplasia with enlarged lymphoid follicles present in white pulp areas and increased number of plasma cells and macrophages around red pulp arterioles and pulp cords. Splenic enlargement associated with abnormal splenic blood flow is most commonly due to chronic passive congestion from increased portal vein pressure, or from portal vein obstruction. *Banti's syndrome* is *congestive splenomegaly* with hypersplenism associated with cirrhosis and portal hypertension and is manifested histologically by red pulp congestion with accumulation and concentration of erythrocytes in widened pulp cords and sinuses. In congestive splenomegaly, reticuloendothelial hyperplasia occurs with proliferation of cells lining red pulp cords and sinuses. In splenic enlargement in conditions associated with abnormal erythrocytes such as hereditary spherocytosis, there is pooling of abnormal red cells in sinuses and pulp cords because of

TABLE 63-2 Diseases associated with enlargement of the spleen

I Infections
- *A* Infectious mononucleosis
- *B* Bacterial septicemias
- *C* Bacterial endocarditis
- *D* Tuberculosis
- *E* Malaria
- *F* Leishmaniasis
- *G* Trypanosomiasis
- *H* Acquired immunodeficiency syndrome
- *I* Viral hepatitis
- *J* Congenital syphilis
- *K* Splenic abscess
- *L* Disseminated histoplasmosis

II Diseases of disordered immunoregulation
- *A* Rheumatoid arthritis (Felty's syndrome)
- *B* Systemic lupus erythematosus
- *C* Immune hemolytic anemias
- *D* Angioimmunoblastic lymphadenopathy
- *E* Drug reactions with serum sickness syndromes
- *F* Immune thrombocytopenias and neutropenias

III Diseases of disordered splenic blood flow
- *A* Laennec's and postnecrotic cirrhosis
- *B* Hepatic vein obstruction
- *C* Hepatic schistosomiasis
- *D* Portal vein obstruction or cavernous sinus transformation
- *E* Splenic vein obstruction
- *F* Chronic congestive heart failure
- *G* Splenic artery aneurysm

IV Diseases associated with abnormal erythrocytes
- *A* Spherocytosis
- *B* Sickle cell disease
- *C* Ovalocytosis
- *D* Thalassemia

V Infiltrative diseases of the spleen
- *A* *Benign*—amyloidosis, Gaucher's disease, Niemann-Pick disease, Hurler's syndrome, Tangier disease, multifocal Langerhans cell (eosinophilic) granulomatosis, extramedullary hematopoiesis, hamartomas, fibromas, hemangiomas, lymphangiomas, splenic cysts
- *B* *Malignant*—leukemias, lymphomas, Hodgkin's lymphoma, primary splenic tumors, angiosarcomas, metastatic tumors, myeloproliferative syndromes

VI Miscellaneous diseases or diseases of unknown cause
- *A* Idiopathic splenomegaly
- *B* Thyrotoxicosis
- *C* Iron-deficiency anemia
- *D* Sarcoidosis
- *E* Berylliosis

increased red cell rigidity and therefore decreased ability to traverse the red pulp sinusoidal endothelium.

Myelosclerosis with myeloid metaplasia is characterized by splenic intrasinusoidal extramedullary hematopoiesis involving all three myeloid cell lines associated with dilated and distended pulp sinuses. In cases of secondary extramedullary hematopoiesis such as in myelophthisic syndromes, extramedullary hematopoiesis may only involve one or two cell lineages, particularly red cells. Infiltrative malignant disease can cause focal or generalized increases in white pulp lymphoid cells as in the case of Hodgkin's disease and lymphocytic lymphoma, or infiltration of red pulp areas with malignant cells as in chronic granulocytic leukemia, acute leukemia syndromes, systemic mast cell disease, and metastatic carcinoma. Infiltrative diseases of the spleen such as Gaucher's and Niemann-Pick disease produce splenic enlargement by increase in number of splenic red pulp histiocytes. Thyrotoxicosis can be associated with splenomegaly and is due to thyroid hormone–induced lymphoid hyperplasia. Sarcoidosis causes splenic enlargement by the development of areas of granulomatous inflammation in white pulp lymphoid tissue. A splenic artery aneurysm may cause unexplained splenomegaly, cramping, and left upper abdominal pain; a calcified ring in the splenic area may be seen on x-ray.

The degree of splenomegaly varies with the disease entity. Slight or mild enlargement occurs in chronic passive congestion of the liver due to congestive heart failure, acute malaria, typhoid fever, bacterial endocarditis, systemic lupus erythematosus, rheumatoid arthritis, and thalassemia minor. Moderate splenic enlargement occurs in hepatitis, cirrhosis, lymphomas, infectious mononucleosis, hemolytic anemias, splenic abscesses and infarcts, and amyloidosis. Massive enlargement of the spleen occurs in chronic myelocytic leukemia, agnogenic myeloid metaplasia with myelofibrosis, hairy cell leukemia, Gaucher's and Niemann-Pick diseases, sarcoidosis, thalassemia major, chronic malaria, congenital syphilis, leishmaniasis, and in some cases of portal vein obstruction.

DIAGNOSTIC EVALUATION OF THE PATIENT WITH SPLENIC ENLARGEMENT When normal in size and position, the spleen is generally inaccessible to abdominal palpation. A normal-sized spleen is about 12 cm long and 7 cm wide. Because of the oblique orientation of the spleen to the abdominal cavity, its long axis lies behind and parallel to the tenth rib in the midaxillary line, with splenic width located between the ninth and eleventh ribs. Therefore, to percuss for splenic dullness the patient is placed on the right side and the ninth intercostal space is located by finding the tip of the scapula lying in the seventh intercostal space and counting down to the ninth intercostal space. Dullness outside the ninth and eleventh intercostal spaces suggests splenomegaly, although fluid in the stomach and feces in the colon can cause splenic area dullness as well. Palpation of the left upper quadrant is performed with the patient supine or on the right side by the examiner's right hand; the examiner's left hand is placed under the lower thorax grasping the lower ribs posteriorly. Palpation for spleen enlargement is performed with the patient taking deep breaths to permit the examiner to feel the inferior tip of an enlarged spleen. To avoid missing a massively enlarged spleen, palpation of the left upper quadrant should begin in the lower abdominal cavity with gradual movement up to the left upper quadrant.

Demonstration of mild to moderate splenic enlargement by physical examination may be difficult, particularly in obese patients. Other techniques for assessment of spleen size include ^{99}Tc-colloid liver-spleen scan, computed tomography, and ultrasound scanning of the left upper quadrant. These three techniques can be useful in defining splenic defects such as cysts, infarct, or tumors, or in defining accessory splenic tissue that may be due to congenital accessory spleens or residual foci of splenic tissue following splenic rupture (splenosis).

In the evaluation of the patient with splenomegaly, it is helpful to consider splenomegaly with acute or subacute illnesses separately from splenomegaly with chronic illness. Acute left upper quadrant pain with an enlarged tender spleen suggests subcapsular hematoma, splenic rupture, or splenic infarcts. Rupture of the spleen with splenic hematoma most often follows direct or remote trauma but can occur as well in the setting of infectious diseases such as malaria, typhoid fever, and EB virus–induced infectious mononucleosis. Splenic infarcts due either to in situ red cell sickling (in sickle cell disease) or to emboli (from mural thrombus, atrial myxoma, or cardiac valve vegetation) can usually be detected by spleen scan or arteriogram. More unusual disorders presenting acutely are diffuse splenic metastatic disease and hemorrhage into a splenic cyst.

An acute febrile illness associated with splenomegaly may be due to bacterial endocarditis, infectious mononucleosis syndromes, tuberculosis, and histoplasmosis. Fever, peripheral adenopathy, and splenomegaly, with or without a rash or arthralgias should suggest, in addition to infectious mononucleosis, sarcoidosis, Hodgkin's lymphoma, a collagen vascular disease such as systemic lupus erythematosus, or a serum sickness syndrome.

An acute illness with splenomegaly associated with the signs and symptoms of anemia, with or without bleeding, suggests autoimmune hemolytic anemia, myeloproliferative syndromes, or acute leukemia.

Splenomegaly with signs and symptoms of chronic illness suggests a wide range of disorders, many of which are listed in Table 63-2. Liver disease with portal hypertension is a common etiology of splenomegaly in this setting. Patients with congestive splenomegaly from liver disease or portal or splenic vein thrombosis are often asymptomatic. With clinical features of rheumatoid arthritis and leukopenia, Felty's syndrome should be considered. The presence of lymphadenopathy should suggest chronic lymphocytic leukemia or lymphoma. Plethora and an elevated hematocrit suggest polycythemia vera or chronic lung disease, with right heart failure and congestive splenomegaly. Weight loss or other signs of chronic illness suggest leukemia or other myeloproliferative syndromes as well as a variety of hemoglobinopathies. Bone marrow aspiration and biopsy can aid in the diagnosis of leukemia and lymphoma, lipid storage diseases, disseminated fungal or mycobacterial diseases, metastatic malignant diseases, and amyloidosis.

Occasionally laparotomy and splenectomy are indicated in the evaluation of splenomegaly. The decision to perform diagnostic laparotomy in a patient with unexplained splenomegaly is difficult and must take into account the patient's age and clinical signs, symptoms, and laboratory abnormalities present. One study has documented palpable spleens in 3 percent of entering college freshmen and no increased risk of any disease during the ensuing 6 years. In another study of older subjects (average age 49) who had undergone splenectomy for undiagnosed splenomegaly and had signs and symptoms of chronic illness, a diagnosis of an underlying disorder was obtained in the majority of patients by splenectomy.

HYPERSPLENISM The term hypersplenism applies to any clinical situation in which the spleen removes excessive quantities of erythrocytes, granulocytes, or platelets from the circulation. General mechanisms of removal of formed blood elements include increased sequestration of cells due to hemodynamic abnormalities of splenic blood flow, or by production of anti-red cell, granulocyte, or platelet antibodies, making the cells vulnerable to clearance by splenic macrophages. Situations in which passive congestion of the spleen occurs produce abnormal sludging of blood in sinuses and red pulp cords. Under these conditions there is plasma pooling, producing marked intrasplenic hemoconcentration and hypoxia, making blood cells more vulnerable to the phagocytic action of pulp cord macrophages. Criteria for diagnosis of hypersplenism include (1) splenomegaly, (2) splenic destruction of one or more cell lines in the peripheral blood, (3) normal or hyperplastic cellularity of bone marrow with normal representation of the cell line deficient in the circulation, and (4) variably, evidence of increased cell turnover in the cell lines affected, i.e., reticulocytosis, increased band forms of neutrophils, or circulating immature platelet forms.

Therapy for hypersplenism relates in large part to the underlying disease or the underlying pathophysiologic process. If the underlying disorder responsible for hypersplenism cannot be corrected, splenectomy is an option for cases in which a severe deficit is present (see below for indications for splenectomy).

HYPOSPLENISM The terms hyposplenia or asplenia are used to indicate diminished or absent splenic function. The usual causes of hyposplenism are splenectomy, congenital absence of the spleen, sickle cell anemia in patients older than 5 years (with autosplenectomy due to repeated infarcts), and splenic irradiation. In sickle cell anemia, persistence of a palpable spleen after age 5 suggests coexisting α thalassemia. Findings in the peripheral blood that indicate diminished splenic function include the presence of nucleated red cells, erythrocyte Howell-Jolly bodies, erythrocyte Heinz bodies, as well as target and burr forms of red cells.

Splenectomized patients or patients with functional asplenia (such as in sickle cell disease) are prone to bacterial infections, which are frequently overwhelming and life-threatening, particularly with encapsulated organisms such as *Streptococcus pneumoniae, Neisseria meningitidis, Escherichia coli*, and *Haemophilus influenzae*. This is due to a reduction or absence of the filtration function of the spleen for clearance of antibody-coated bacteria as well as to decreased production of IgG and IgM antibodies (opsonins) needed to bind bacteria. Immunization with pneumococcal vaccine is recommended in patients older than 2 years with hyposplenism and prior to elective splenectomy. The presence of peripheral blood manifestations of hyposplenism (Howell-Jolly bodies) in the presence of a normal-sized or enlarged spleen suggests the presence of splenic infiltrative disease such as a primary splenic angiosarcoma.

INDICATIONS FOR SPLENECTOMY Splenic trauma, whether accidental blunt trauma or intraoperative iatrogenic injury, is the most common indication for splenectomy. En bloc removal of the spleen may be indicated either because of tumor involvement or for a splenorectal shunt. Staging laparotomy with splenectomy remains a major diagnostic procedure for many early stage Hodgkin's disease patients being considered for radiation therapy alone. Splenectomy for selected patients with idiopathic splenomegaly is often necessary when other investigations fail to produce a diagnosis; however, the spleen should not be removed simply because it is palpable. Hypersplenism in lymphomas can cause persistent cytopenias and in select cases responds to splenectomy. B-cell hairy cell leukemia frequently presents with hypersplenism, and splenectomy is often beneficial, producing remission in the majority of cases with a 5-year survival of 50 percent.

Felty's syndrome (rheumatoid arthritis and hypersplenism) and Gaucher's disease both require splenectomy when splenomegaly leads to symptomatic neutropenia or other complications of hypersplenism. Immune thrombocytopenic purpura which persists after trials of medical therapy may benefit from splenectomy (see Chap. 287). Of the hemolytic anemias, hereditary spherocytosis, hereditary elliptocytosis, immune hemolytic anemia with warm-reacting IgG antibody, and pyruvate-kinase deficiency have been improved by splenectomy. Splenectomy is usually necessary late in the course of thalassemia major when neutropenia or thrombocytopenia develops, or when transfusion requirements double. Chronic lymphocytic leukemia (CLL), chronic granulocytic leukemia, and agnogenic myeloid metaplasia may be complicated by symptomatic hypersplenism or, in the case of CLL, immune hemolytic anemia and thrombocytopenia, often necessitating splenectomy. (Chaps. 297 and 296.)

REFERENCES

Lymph node enlargement

Butcher E, Weissman I: Lymphoid tissues and organs in *Fundamental Immunology*, WE Paul (ed). New York, Raven, 1984, pp 109–127

Greenfield S, Jordan MC: The clinical investigation of lymphadenopathy, in primary care practice. JAMA 240:1388, 1978

Ioachim HL: *Lymph Node Biopsy*. Philadelphia, Lippincott, 1982

Lennert K, Stein H: The germinal center, in *Morphology, Histochemistry, and Immunohistology in Lymphoproliferative Diseases of Skin*, M Goos, E Christopher (eds). Berlin, Heidelberg, New York, Springer-Verlag, 1982

Lieberman PH et al: A reappraisal of eosinophilic granuloma of bone, Hand-Schüller-Christian syndrome, and Letterer-Siwe syndrome. Medicine 48:375, 1969

Nathwani BN et al: Malignant lymphoma arising in angioimmunoblastic lymphadenopathy. Cancer 41:578, 1978

Poppema S et al: Distribution of T cell subsets in human lymph nodes. J Exp Med 153:30, 1981

Schroer KR, Franssila KO: Atypical hyperplasia of lymph nodes: A follow-up study. Cancer 44:1155, 1979

Sinclair S et al: Biopsy of enlarged, superficial lymph nodes. JAMA 228:602, 1974

Thomas JA et al: Combined immunological and histochemical analysis of skin and lymph node lesions in histiocytosis X. J Clin Pathol 35:327, 1982

Winterbauer RH et al: A clinical interpretation of bilateral hilar adenopathy. Ann Intern Med 78:65, 1973

Yen-Tsu N et al: Lymph node biopsy for diagnosis: A statistical study. J Surg Oncol 14:53, 1980

Splenic enlargement

Butler JJ: Pathology of the spleen in benign and malignant conditions. Histopathology 7:453, 1983

Eichner ER, Whitfield CL: Splenomegaly: An algorithmic approach to diagnosis. JAMA 246:2858, 1981

Enriquez E, Neiman RS (eds): *The Pathology of the Spleen: A Functional Approach*. Chicago, American Society of Clinical Pathologists, 1976

Hermann RE et al: Splenectomy for the diagnosis of splenomegaly. Ann Surg 168:896, 1964

Lewis SM (ed): *Clinics in Haematology*, vol 12: *The Spleen*. London, Saunders, 1983, pp 361–608

McIntyre OR, Ebaugh FG: Palpable spleens in college freshmen. Ann Intern Med 66:301, 1967

Steinberg MH et al: Evidence of hyposplenism in the presence of splenomegaly. Scand J Haematol 31:437, 1983

Videbaek A et al: *The Spleen in Health and Disease*. Chicago, Yearbook, 1982

64 LEUKOCYTOSIS, LEUKOPENIA, AND EOSINOPHILIA

DAVID C. DALE

Alterations of leukocytes occur in many hematologic, infectious, inflammatory, and neoplastic diseases. For this reason, the laboratory evaluation of many patients begins with measurement of leukocyte count and examination of a stained blood smear. Five types of leukocytes usually are seen: neutrophils, lymphocytes, monocytes, eosinophils, and basophils. It is generally accepted that they all derive from a common hematopoietic stem cell. Beyond this common origin, different mechanisms govern their production, distribution, and function. For simplicity, clinical inferences often are made from the total leukocyte count and the differential count expressed as a percentage. It is more precise to express the counts for each type of leukocyte in terms of the concentration or absolute count per microliter. This is determined by multiplying the total count by the percent value or by direct counting on automated systems (Table 64-1).

Several terms are used to describe alteration of leukocyte counts. *Leukocytosis* and *leukopenia* indicate increases or decreases in the total number of leukocytes. *Granulocytosis* and *granulocytopenia* describe increases or decreases of granulocytes, i.e., neutrophils,

TABLE 64-1 Normal values for concentration of blood leukocytes*

Cell type	Mean, cells per microliter	95% Confidence limits, cells per microliter
Neutrophil	3650	1830–7250
Lymphocyte	2500	1500–4000
Monocyte	430	200–950
Eosinophil	150	0–700
Basophil	30	0–150

* Total leukocyte counts from venous blood samples were done in a Coulter counter, and 200 leukocytes were differentiated on Wright-stained blood smears made on coverglass.

eosinophils, and basophils. *Neutrophilia* and *neutropenia, lymphocytosis* and *lymphopenia, monocytosis* and *monocytopenia, eosinophilia* and *eosinopenia* are used for increases or decreases in the absolute counts of neutrophils, lymphocytes, monocytes, and eosinophils, respectively. It is best to use these terms to describe changes to levels above or below the 95 percent confidence limits of normal values (Table 64-1).

LEUKOCYTOSIS

Leukocytosis occurs by several mechanisms. Normally about half of the blood leukocytes are in a *marginal pool,* i.e., loosely adherent to the vascular endothelium or trapped in the microcirculation. With exercise or epinephrine administration, these cells are released into the *circulating pool* and the leukocyte count rises, a process called *demargination.* For neutrophils, but not for other leukocytes, there is a storage pool of mature cells in the marrow, the *marrow neutrophil reserves.* Normally neutrophils are released from the storage pool into the blood in response to stress, with infections, and after corticosteroid administration. With a strong stimulus, e.g., a severe bacterial infection, immature neutrophils, i.e., bands and metamyelocytes, are released, a response sometimes called a *left shift.* Leukocytosis also occurs due to increased cell production. If production is stimulated intensely, the leukocyte counts can rise to 25,000 to 50,000 per microliter, a response called a *leukemoid reaction.* The rates for these processes differ substantially. A shift of cells from the marginal to the circulatory pool can occur within a few minutes, whereas the release of neutrophils from the marrow usually occurs over several hours. Increases in production take several days.

The mechanisms maintaining normal leukocyte production and blood counts are not well understood. It is presumed that under basal conditions, factors made in the marrow, thymus, lymph nodes, and spleen provide local control (see Chaps. 81 and 297). Two groups of factors, the interleukins and colony stimulating factors, may be involved in normal regulation and play important roles in causing leukocytosis. Interleukin 2 (IL-2) and IL-4 are known to expand T- and B-lymphocyte populations, respectively (see Chap. 13). Granulocyte colony stimulating factor (G-CSF), granulocyte-macrophage colony stimulating factor (GM-CSF), macrophage colony stimulating factor (M-CSF), and four interleukins, IL-1, IL-3, IL-5, and IL-6, are involved in neutrophil, monocyte, and eosinophil production (Fig. 64-1).

TABLE 64-2 Causes of neutrophilia

Physiologic:	Exercise, excitement, stress, epinephrine
Infections:	Chiefly bacterial, also fungal, parasitic, and some viral
Inflammation:	Burns, tissue necrosis, as in myocardial and pulmonary infarction, collagen vascular diseases, hypersensitivity states, other inflammatory diseases
Metabolic disorders:	Ketoacidosis, acute renal failure, eclampsia, acute poisoning
Myeloproliferative diseases:	Myelocytic leukemia, myeloid metaplasia, polycythemia vera
Other:	Metastatic carcinoma, acute hemorrhage or hemolysis, glucocorticoids, lithium therapy, idiopathic

Leukocytosis usually is due to neutrophilia (Table 64-2). Leukocytosis due to lymphocytosis occurs in acute and chronic lymphatic leukemia and some infectious diseases, e.g., infectious mononucleosis, infectious hepatitis, infectious lymphocytosis, pertussis, tuberculosis, brucellosis, and syphilis. A moderate increase in the absolute lymphocyte count is seen with thyrotoxicosis and Addison's disease.

Increases in blood monocytes are observed with chronic inflammation, e.g., tuberculosis, bacterial endocarditis, brucellosis, Rocky Mountain spotted fever, malaria and kala azar, sarcoidosis, Crohn's disease, and some collagen vascular diseases. Monocytosis occurs in pre-leukemia. It may be a prominent feature of histiocytic leukemia and the myeloproliferative syndromes.

LEUKOPENIA

NEUTROPENIA Neutropenia is the most frequent cause of leukopenia. It is usually defined as "severe" if the neutrophil count is less than 500 cells per microliter, "moderate" with 500 to 1000 cells per microliter, and "mild" with 1000 to 2000 cells per microliter. Neutropenia is an important risk factor for infections; as the counts decline below about 1000 cells per microliter, the risk of infection increases (see Chap. 82). This risk also relates to the duration of

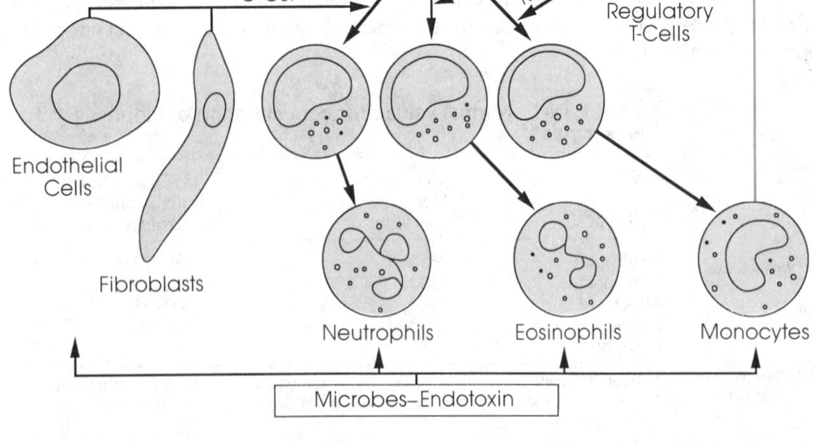

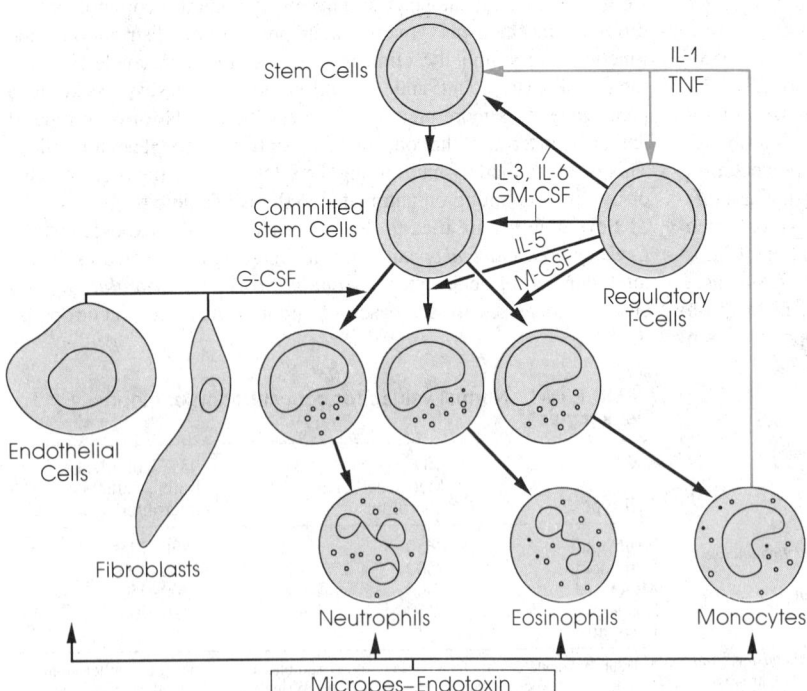

FIGURE 64-1 A simplified schema for the stimulation of neutrophil, eosinophil, and monocyte production by microbial infection or endotoxin. At tissue sites of inflammation, monocytes produce interleukin 1 (IL-1) and tumor necrosis factor (TNF). The IL-1 and TNF directly activate stem cells and stimulate regulatory T lymphocytes to produce additional factors: IL-3, IL-6, and granulocyte-macrophage colony stimulating factor (GM-CSF) from endothelial cells and fibroblasts, and IL-5 and macrophage colony stimulating factor (M-CSF). These factors stimulate production of neutrophils, eosinophils, and monocytes, respectively. All of the colony stimulating factors and interleukins can be produced by other types of cells.

TABLE 64-3 Causes of neutropenia

DECREASED PRODUCTION
Hematologic diseases: Aplastic anemia, leukemia, myelodysplastic syndromes, infantile genetic disorders, cyclic neutropenia, chronic idiopathic neutropenia, neutropenia with clonal expression of T8 cells, Chédiak-Higashi syndrome
Drug-induced: Alkylating agents (nitrogen mustard, busulfan, chlorambucil, cyclophosphamide); antimetabolites (methotrexate, 5-fluorocytosine); noncytotoxic agents [antibiotics (chloramphenicol, penicillins, sulfonamides), phenothiazines, tranquilizers (meprobamate), certain diuretics, anti-inflammatory agents, antithyroid drugs, many others]
Tumor invasion: Myelofibrosis
Nutritional deficiency: Vitamin B_{12}, folate (especially in alcoholics)
Infection: Tuberculosis, typhoid fever, brucellosis, tularemia, measles, infectious mononucleosis, viral hepatitis, malaria, histoplasmosis, leishmaniasis
PERIPHERAL DESTRUCTION
Antineutrophil antibodies and/or splenic trapping
Autoimmune disorders: Felty's syndrome, systemic lupus erythematosus
Drugs: Aminopyrine α-methyldopa, phenylbutazone, mercurial diuretics, some phenothiazines
PERIPHERAL MARGINATION
Overwhelming bacterial infection
Hemodialysis
Cardiopulmonary bypass

neutropenia, the intactness of other host defense mechanisms, and the nature of the primary disease process.

Neutropenia occurs by several mechanisms: reduced or ineffective production, increased margination, accelerated utilization, or a combination of these mechanisms (Table 64-3). Most patients fit into one of the following general categories:

Disorders of production Probably the most frequent cause of severe neutropenia in the United States is marrow suppression from cytotoxic drugs given for cancer or immunosuppressive therapy. Neutropenia is a prominent effect of these drugs because of the high proliferative rate of the neutrophil precursors and the rapid turnover of neutrophils in the blood and tissues. Suppression of neutrophil formation can occur as an idiosyncratic reaction to many other drugs (see below). Neutropenia due to impaired production is a feature of several diseases affecting hematopoietic stem cells, e.g., leukemia and the myelodysplastic syndromes (see Chap. 296) or aplastic anemia (see Chap. 61). With vitamin B_{12} and folic acid deficiency (see Chap. 76), neutropenia is attributed to ineffective production, i.e., defective neutrophils being destroyed in the marrow before they can enter the blood. Most other disorders of production are rare.

GENETIC NEUTROPENIAS *Congenital hypoplastic neutropenia,* Kostmann's syndrome, is a autosomal recessive disease causing severe neutropenia and infections from birth. Some early neutrophil precursors may be present in the marrow, but numbers of more mature cells are severely reduced. With antibiotic therapy and good supportive care, survival to adulthood is not uncommon. Neutropenia with immunodeficiency is a stem cell disorder involving both neutrophils and lymphocytes. It is associated with markedly enhanced susceptibility to infection. Both congenital neutropenia and the immunodeficiency syndromes have been treated successfully with bone marrow transplantation; colony stimulating factors are a promising experimental therapy.

Cyclic neutropenia is an unusual disorder, characterized by fever, malaise, mouth ulcers, cervical adenopathy, and the absence of blood neutrophils, usually at 21-day intervals. Between episodes, the patients are generally well. Cyclic fluctuations of other blood leukocytes, platelets, and reticulocytes also occur. Usually this disease is detected in early childhood, but cases with adult onset are occasionally seen. This disorder is attributed to a regulatory defect of stem cells. It has been shown that G-CSF will stimulate neutrophil production, shorten the duration of neutropenia, and reduce symptoms and infections in these patients.

The Chédiak-Higashi syndrome is discussed in Chap. 81.

NEUTROPENIAS OF UNKNOWN CAUSE In *chronic idiopathic neutropenia,* neutrophils are selectively decreased, and monocytes often are increased. The marrow is normocellular and shows decreased mature neutrophils. In some, but not all cases, antineutrophil antibodies can be detected; but their significance is often unclear. Only individuals with severe neutropenia tend to have recurrent fever and frequent infections.

Spontaneous remissions have occurred, and evolution of idiopathic neutropenia to leukemia has been reported very rarely. Alternate-day glucocorticoids may be helpful. G-CSF recently has been found to elevate the neutrophil counts and reduce infections in severely affected patients.

Syndromes have been described where clonal expansion of T8 cells is associated with neutropenia. T8 cells are granulated T lymphocytes, and patients with T8 cell lymphocytosis have moderate blood and bone marrow lymphocytosis, neutropenia, polyclonal hypergammaglobulinemia, splenomegaly, and absence of lymphadenopathy. They have a chronic and relatively stable course. Recurrent bacterial infections are frequent. It is not clear whether this is a benign or malignant disease. In some patients a spontaneous regression has occurred even after 11 years, suggesting an immunoregulatory defect as the basis for the disorder. It is likely patients with T8 cell lymphocytosis and neutropenia will ultimately be shown to represent a biologically heterogeneous group of patients.

DRUG-INDUCED NEUTROPENIA Idiosyncratic drug reactions are an important cause of neutropenia (see Chap. 66). In most instances, the patient presents acutely ill with fever and a sore throat or perianal ulcerations several weeks or months after beginning a new drug. The total leukocyte count is often 1000 to 2000 per microliter. Mature neutrophils are absent from the blood, and marrow aplasia is rare. If administration of the offending drug is discontinued, recovery is the rule, provided good supportive care is available. The mechanisms responsible for these reactions are poorly understood but probably involve both immunologic and toxic injury to the neutrophils and their precursors. With some drugs, e.g., chloramphenicol, phenothiazines, and propylthiouracil, neutropenia may occur gradually. As a rule, a presumed offending drug should always be discontinued whenever the neutrophil count falls to less than 2000 per microliter.

Neutropenia affecting margination and utilization IMMUNE-MEDIATED NEUTROPENIA Isoimmune neonatal neutropenia is a transient disorder due to the transplacental passage of maternal antibodies directed toward neutrophil specific antigens which were inherited from the patient's father. Ordinarily it resolves spontaneously in the first few months of life and does not recur. Autoimmune neutropenia must be diagnosed by the finding of antineutrophil antibodies in the plasma and on the cells of affected individuals. It is usually a benign condition causing a selective reduction in blood neutrophils. Careful observation and prompt antibiotic therapy for suspected episodes of infection are cornerstones for care of these individuals.

In systemic lupus erythematosus, mild neutropenia is common. Some patients with rheumatoid arthritis have severe neutropenia associated with splenomegaly and very high rheumatoid factor titers, i.e., Felty's syndrome. Usually the marrow is hypercellular. In many patients infections are surprisingly infrequent given the level of the neutrophil counts. Splenectomy usually increases blood neutrophils but should be reserved for patients with well-documented problems with infections. In other autoimmune syndromes, e.g., Sjögren's syndrome and autoimmune hepatitis, autoantibodies and enlargement of the spleen may play a role in the development of neutropenia: splenic trapping of neutrophils may occur.

NEUTROPENIA WITH INFECTIONS Neutropenia can result from bacterial, viral, parasitic, or rickettsial diseases. Depending upon the infection the mechanisms can involve abnormal production, increased margination or utilization, or varying combinations of all. In certain viral infections, e.g., infectious mononucleosis, infectious hepatitis, and human immunodeficiency virus (HIV) infections, severe and protracted neutropenia may be due to infection of the hematopoietic stem cells; neutrophil production is impaired. In addition, antineutrophil antibodies have been described in some HIV-infected patients, and therapy with cytotoxic agents such as azidothymidine may complicate the picture (see Chap. 264). In other infections, neutropenia may be attributed to increased neutrophil adherence to endothelial cells, e.g., measles, influenza, malaria, rickettsial, and *Babesia* infections. With severe bacteremic gram-negative or rarely gram-positive infections, neutropenia is probably due to increased margination and increased utilization at sites of infection. Other bacteremic infections such as typhoid and brucellosis are often associated with a relative but not an absolute neutropenia ($<$ 1500 per microliter) and a left shift with bands seen in the peripheral blood. In tuberculosis, histoplasmosis, and leishmaniasis neutropenia can be associated with marrow invasion by these organisms and decreased myeloid precursors; the mechanism of suppression of myelopoiesis is unknown. With splenomegaly increased trapping of neutrophils may be an additional mechanism for neutropenia.

Miscellaneous causes of neutropenia Conditions which cause splenomegaly (e.g., cirrhosis, sarcoidosis) may have associated neutropenia due to splenic trapping of neutrophils. Neutropenia followed by a neutrophilic leukocytosis is commonly seen in patients undergoing hemodialysis. Increased adhesion of neutrophils to vascular endothelium appears to be responsible for the neutropenia with C5a-mediated increased expression of neutrophil adhesion proteins (see Chap. 87).

LYMPHOCYTOPENIA, MONOCYTOPENIA, EOSINOPENIA Lymphocytopenia, i.e., less than 1500 cells per microliter in adults or less than 3000 cells per microliter in young children, is a feature of the congenital immunodeficiency syndromes; it also occurs acutely following stress, radiation injury, or cytotoxic drug and corticosteroid therapy. Other etiologies include lymphoma, aplastic anemia, renal failure, impaired intestinal lymph drainage, severe right-sided heart failure, and cachexia of any cause. Monocytopenia occurs with acute infections, stress, and following administration of glucocorticoids. Monocytopenia also occurs in aplastic anemia, acute myelogenous leukemia, and as a direct result of myelotoxic and immunosuppressive drugs. Eosinopenia occurs with stress, infections, and after steroid administration.

EOSINOPHILIA

Eosinophilia can be defined as a blood eosinophil count of more than 500 per microliter. The blood eosinophil pool is relatively small compared to the tissue pool; however, significant tissue eosinophilia can occur without an elevated blood count.

TABLE 64-4 Causes of blood eosinophilia

Drug reactions: Iodides, aspirin, sulfonamides, nitrofurantoin, penicillins, cephalosporins

Parasitic infections: Hookworm disease, strongyloidiasis, toxocariasis, trichuriasis, trichinosis, filariasis, schistosomiasis, echinococcosis, cysticercosis

Allergic diseases: Hay fever, asthma, angioedema, serum sickness, allergic vasculitis, eczema, pemphigus

Collagen vascular diseases: Rheumatoid arthritis, dermatomyositis, periarteritis nodosa

Malignancy: Hodgkin's disease, mycosis fungoides, chronic myelogenous leukemia, cancer of lung, stomach, pancreas, ovary, or uterus

Hypereosinophilic syndromes: Loeffler's syndrome, Loeffler's endocarditis, eosinophilic leukemia

There are many causes for eosinophilia (Table 64-4). A useful diagnostic approach is to begin by reexamining the blood smear to be sure the cells are not peculiarly stained neutrophils, i.e., pseudoeosinophilia, and to consider the possibility of chronic myelogenous leukemia, which may present with eosinophilia. Rarely, filarial parasites will be seen on the blood smear. The next step is to review carefully the patient's history with close attention to drugs, diet, and travel. Many drugs can cause eosinophilia (see Chap. 66). The travel and diet history may suggest a specific parasitic infection. The physical examination initially may reveal evidence for a chronic inflammatory disease or a malignancy as the cause of eosinophilia (Table 64-4). Stools should be collected and examined for ova and parasites, in particular looking for evidence of worms (see Chap. 157). If the diagnosis is not obvious, examination of serum for antibodies may reveal infestation with *Dirofilaria immitis* (see Chap. 169) or cysticercosis (see Chap. 171). In most patients, eosinophilia will remit when the primary disease is treated effectively. When other diagnoses are excluded, the *idiopathic hypereosinophilic syndrome* should be considered. This syndrome is characterized by a wasting illness with hepatosplenomegaly, peripheral neuropathy, cardiac murmurs, and congestive heart failure (see Chap. 81).

REFERENCES

CANNISTRA SA, GRIFFIN JD: Regulation of the production and function of granulocyte and monocytes. Semin Hematol 25:173, 1988

DALE DC: "Neutropenia" and "Neutrophilia," in *Hematology*, 4th ed, WJ Williams et al (eds). New York, McGraw-Hill, 1990, pp 807–820

GALLIN JI et al: *Inflammation: Basic Principles and Clinical Correlates*. New York, Raven Press, 1988

GLEICH GJ, LOEGERING DA: Immunobiology of eosinophils. Ann Rev Immunol 2:429, 1984

JOHNSTON RB JR: Monocytes and macrophages. N Engl J Med 318:747, 1988

SHURIN SB: Pathologic states associated with activation of eosinophils and with eosinophilia. Hematol Oncol Clin North Am 2:171, 1988

PART THREE **CLINICAL PHARMACOLOGY**

65 PRINCIPLES OF DRUG THERAPY

JOHN A. OATES / GRANT R. WILKINSON

QUANTITATIVE DETERMINANTS OF DRUG ACTION

Safe and effective therapy with drugs requires their delivery to target tissues in concentrations within the narrow range that yields efficacy without toxicity. Optimal precision in achieving concentrations of drug within this therapeutic "window" can be achieved with regimens that are based on the kinetics of the drug's availability to target sites. This chapter deals with the principles of drug elimination and distribution that form the basis for loading and maintenance regimens for the average patient and considers instances in which elimination of the drug is impaired (e.g., renal failure). The basis for optimal utilization of plasma level data is also discussed.

PLASMA LEVELS AFTER A SINGLE DOSE The levels of lidocaine in plasma following intravenous administration decline in two phases as illustrated in Fig. 65-1; such a biphasic decline is typical for many drugs. Immediately following rapid injection, essentially all of the drug is in the plasma compartment, and the high initial plasma level reflects its confinement to this small volume. Subsequently, the drug is transferred into the extravascular compartment, and the period of time during which this occurs is referred to as the *distribution phase*. For lidocaine the distribution phase is virtually complete within 30 min; then a slower rate of fall ensues, referred to as the *equilibrium phase* or *elimination phase*. During this latter phase, the drug levels in plasma and those in the tissues change in parallel.

Distribution phase Pharmacologic events during the distribution phase depend on whether the level of drug at the receptor site is similar to that in the plasma. If this is the case, the pharmacologic effects, whether favorable or adverse, may be inordinately great during this period because of the high initial levels in plasma. For example, following a small bolus dose (50 mg) of lidocaine, antiarrhythmic effects may be evident during the early distribution phase but disappear as levels fall below those that are minimally effective and even before equilibrium between plasma and tissue is reached. Thus, larger single doses or multiple small doses must be administered to achieve an effect that is sustained into the equilibrium phase. Toxicity resulting from high levels of some drugs during the distribution phase precludes administration of a single intravenous loading dose that will achieve therapeutic levels during the equilibrium phase. For example, the administration of a loading dose of phenytoin as a single intravenous bolus can cause cardiovascular collapse due to the high levels during the distribution phase. If a loading dose of phenytoin is administered intravenously, it must be given in fractions at intervals sufficient to permit substantial distribution of the prior dose before the next is given (for example, 100 mg every 3 to 5 min). For similar reasons, the loading dose of many potent drugs that rapidly equilibrate with their receptors is divided into fractional doses for intravenous administration.

After an oral dose that delivers an equivalent amount of drug into the systemic circulation, plasma levels during the initial period after administration are not as high as after an intravenous bolus dose. Because the drug is not absorbed instantly after oral administration and is delivered into the systemic circulation more slowly, much of the drug is distributed by the time absorption is complete. Thus, procainamide, which is almost totally absorbed after oral administration, can be given as a single 750-mg loading dose with little risk of hypotension; in contrast, loading of the drug by the intravenous route is more safely accomplished by giving the dose in fractions of about 100 mg at 5-min intervals to avoid the hypotension that might ensue during the distribution phase if the entire loading dose were given as a single bolus.

In contrast, other drugs are distributed slowly to their sites of action during the distribution phase. For example, levels of digoxin at the receptor site (and its pharmacologic effect) do not reflect plasma levels during the distribution phase. Digoxin is transported (or bound) to its cardiac receptors more slowly by a process that proceeds throughout distribution. Thus, plasma levels fall during a distribution phase of several hours, while levels at the site of action and pharmacologic effect increase. Only at the end of the distribution phase, when the drug has reached equilibrium with the receptor, does the concentration of digoxin in plasma reflect pharmacologic effect. For this reason, there should be a 6- to 8-h wait after administration before plasma levels of digoxin are obtained for a guide to therapy.

Equilibrium phase After distribution has proceeded to the point where the concentration of drug in plasma is in dynamic equilibrium with that in the tissues outside the vascular compartment, the levels in plasma and tissues fall in parallel as the drug is eliminated from the body. Thus, the *equilibrium phase* is sometimes also referred to as the *elimination phase*. Measurement of drug concentration in plasma provides the best reflection of drug level in tissues during this phase.

Most drugs are eliminated as a first-order process. During the equilibrium phase, a characteristic of the first-order process is that the time required for the level of drug in plasma to fall to one-half the original value (the half-life, $t_{1/2}$) is the same regardless of which point on the plasma level curve is chosen as a starting point for the measurement. Another characteristic of the first-order process is that

FIGURE 65-1 Concentrations of lidocaine in plasma following the administration of 50 mg intravenously. The half-life of 108 min is computed as the time required for levels to fall from any given value during the equilibrium phase (Cp_{initial}) to one-half that level. Cp_0 is the hypothetical concentration of lidocaine in plasma at time zero if equilibrium had been achieved instantly.

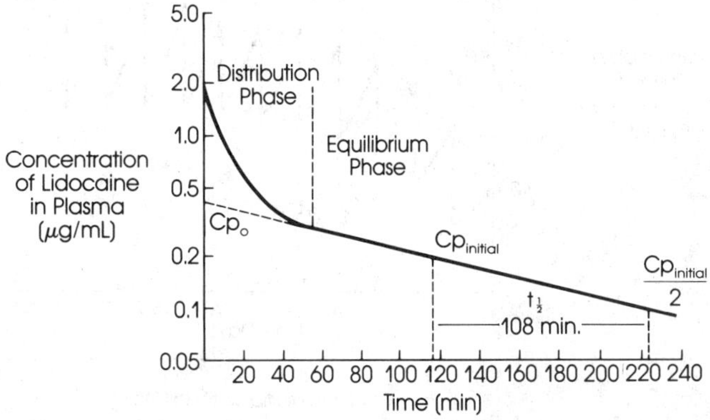

a semilogarithmic plot of the concentrations in plasma versus time during the equilibrium phase is linear. From such a plot (Fig. 65-1) it can be seen that the half-life of lidocaine is 108 min.

One can calculate what amount of the administered dose remains in the body at any multiple of the half-life interval following administration:

Number of half-lives	Amount of dose remaining in the body, %	Amount of dose eliminated, %
1	50	50
2	25	75
3	12.5	87.5
4	6.25	93.75
5	3.125	96.875

In theory, the elimination process never reaches completion. From a clinical standpoint, however, elimination is essentially complete when it has reached 90 percent. Therefore, for practical purposes, *a first-order elimination process reaches completion after 3 to 4 half-lives.*

DRUG ACCUMULATION—LOADING AND MAINTENANCE DOSES With repeated administration of a drug, the amount in the body accumulates if the elimination of the first dose is incomplete when the second dose is given, and both the amount of drug in the body and its pharmacologic effect increase with continuing administration until they reach a plateau. The accumulation of digoxin administered in repeated maintenance doses (without a loading dose) is illustrated in Fig. 65-2. As digoxin's half-life is about 1.6 days in a patient with normal renal function, 65 percent of digoxin remains in the body at the end of 1 day. Thus, the second dose will raise the amount of digoxin in the body (and average plasma level) to 165 percent of that following the first dose. Each subsequent dose will result in greater amounts in the body until a *steady state* is achieved. At this point drug intake per unit of time is the same as the rate of elimination, with the fluctuation between peak and trough plasma levels remaining constant. If the rate of drug delivery is subsequently altered, a different and new steady state will be attained. Continuing infusion of a drug at constant rate will also result in progressive accumulation to a predictable steady state (Fig. 65-3). In this case a constant plasma level (Cp_{ss}) is achieved which is between the peak and trough values attained when the same rate of drug delivery is administered in an intermittent fashion. For *all* drugs with first-order kinetics, the time required to achieve steady state levels can be predicted from the half-life because accumulation also is a first-order process with a half-life identical to that for elimination. Hence, accumulation reaches 90 percent of steady state levels at the end of 3 to 4 half-lives. For digoxin, with a half-life of 1.6 days (with normal renal function), accumulation will be practically complete in 5 days. Continuing

FIGURE 65-2 The time course of digoxin accumulation when a single daily maintenance dose is given without a loading dose. Note that accumulation is more than 90 percent complete by the end of 4 half-lives.

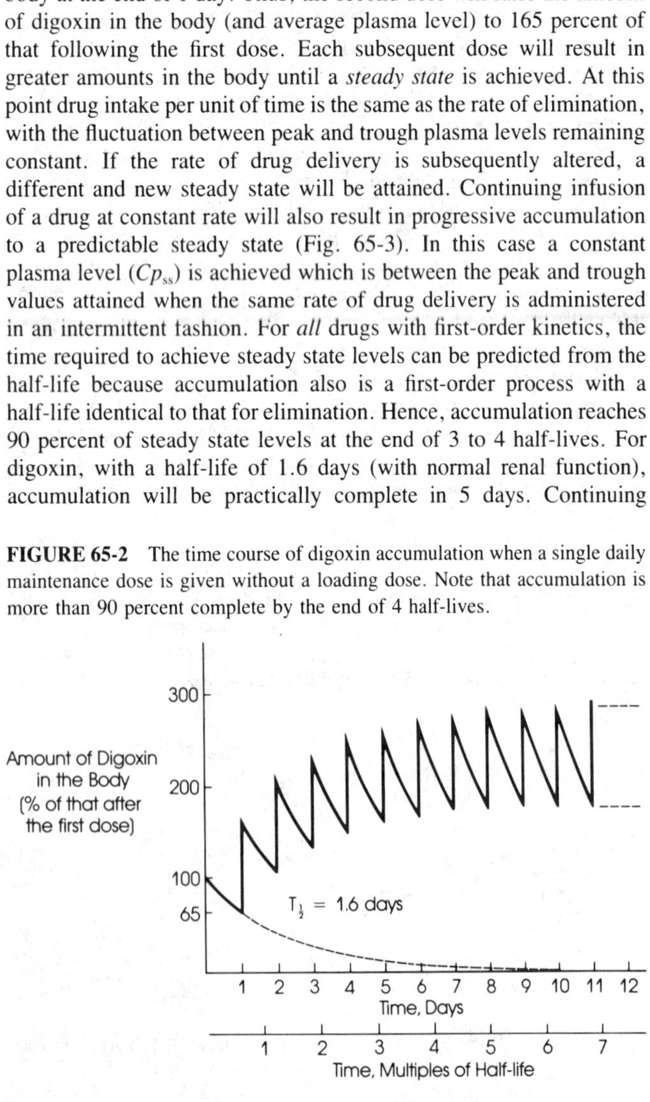

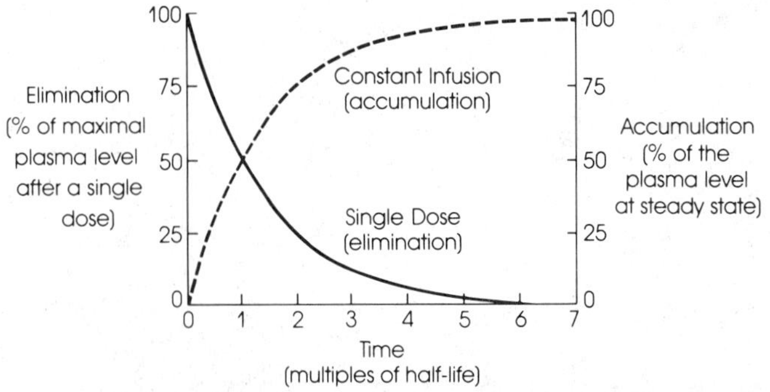

FIGURE 65-3 The time course of plasma levels of a drug following a single intravenous dose (——) compared with those during a constant intravenous infusion (----). This relationship applies to all drugs that rapidly achieve equilibrium between plasma and tissues.

infusion of a drug at a constant rate also will result in progressive accumulation to a steady state with a time course predictable from the elimination curve for that drug (Fig. 65-3).

When the time required to reach steady state levels is longer than one wishes to wait, plasma levels may be achieved more rapidly by the administration of a *loading dose*. Loading entails the administration of an amount that will bring the concentration in plasma (at equilibrium) to the level present during steady state. If the desired plasma level (Cp_{ss}) is known, the loading dose can be estimated with knowledge of the extent of the drug's extravascular distribution at equilibrium; the apparent volume of distribution, or V_d:

$$\text{Loading dose} = \text{desired plasma level at steady state} \times \text{volume of distribution}$$

$$= Cp_{ss} \times V_d$$

Loading may be accomplished by the administration of the loading amount as a single dose, or in the case of drugs for which there is risk of toxicity if all of the drug is introduced into the plasma compartment rapidly, the loading amount is administered in a series of fractions of the total loading amount. As the accumulation of procainamide to 90 percent of steady state by infusion would require approximately 10 h (the $t_{1/2}$ is 3 h), a loading regimen is almost always desirable. The load required to suppress an arrhythmia, however, varies among individuals from 300 to 1000 mg, and rapid intravenous administration of the *average loading dose* causes hypotension during the distribution phase in some patients. Therefore, the intravenous loading dose of procainamide is given in fractions (e.g., 100 mg every 5 min) until the arrhythmia is controlled or adverse effects such as hypotension indicate that no further drug should be given. Dividing the loading dose into fractions is appropriate for most drugs that have a low therapeutic index. (the therapeutic index is the ratio of toxic dose to the therapeutic dose). This permits better individualization of the loading amount and minimizes adverse effects.

The size of the loading dose required to achieve the plasma levels at steady state also can be determined from the fraction of drug eliminated during the dosage interval and the maintenance dose (in the case of intermittent drug administration). For example, if the fraction of digoxin eliminated daily is 35 percent and the planned maintenance dose is to be 0.25 mg daily, then the loading dose to achieve steady state levels should be 100/35 times the maintenance dose, or approximately 0.75 mg. Thus,

$$\text{Loading dose} = \frac{100}{\text{\% of drug eliminated per dosage interval}} \times \text{maintenance dose}$$

The fraction of drug eliminated during any dosage interval can be determined from a semilogarithmic graph, in which the total amount in the body at time zero is set at 100 percent and the fraction remaining at the end of 1 half-life is 50 percent.[1] Conversely, if the loading dose is known, the maintenance dose can be similarly calculated.

To calculate a loading dose designed to achieve the plasma concentration of a known infusion rate at steady state

$$\text{Loading dose} = \frac{\text{infusion rate}}{k}$$

where k is the fractional elimination constant that describes the rate of drug elimination.[1]

Regardless of the size of the loading dose, *after maintenance therapy has been given for 3 to 4 half-lives, the amount of drug in the body is determined by the maintenance dose*. The independence of the plasma levels at steady state from the load is illustrated in Fig. 65-3, which indicates that the elimination of any drug would be practically complete after 3 to 4 half-lives.

DETERMINANTS OF PLASMA LEVELS DURING THE EQUILIBRIUM PHASE An important determinant of the level of drug in plasma during the equilibrium phase after a single dose is the extent to which the drug is distributed outside the plasma compartment. For example, if the distribution of a 3-mg dose of a large macromolecule is confined to a plasma volume of 3 L, then the concentration in plasma will be 1 mg/L. However, if a different drug is distributed so that 90 percent of it leaves the plasma compartment, then only 0.3 mg will remain in the 3-L plasma volume and the concentration in plasma will be only 0.1 mg/L. The *apparent volume of distribution*, or V_d, expresses the relationship between the amount of drug in the body and the plasma concentration at equilibrium:

$$V_d = \frac{\text{amount of drug in body}}{\text{plasma concentration}}$$

The amount of drug in the body is expressed as mass (e.g., milligrams), and the plasma concentration is expressed as mass per volume (e.g., milligrams per liter). Thus V_d is a hypothetical volume into which a quantity of drug would distribute if its concentration in the entire volume were the same as that in plasma. Although it is not a real volume, it is an important concept because it determines the fraction of total drug in the plasma and therefore the fraction available to the organs of elimination. An approximation of V_d in the equilibrium phase can be obtained by estimating the concentration of drug in plasma at time zero (Cp_0) by back-extrapolation of the equilibrium phase plot to zero time as illustrated in Fig. 65-1. Then, after intravenous administration when the amount in the body at time zero is the dose, we have

$$V_d = \frac{\text{dose}}{Cp_0}$$

For the administration of the large macromolecule mentioned above, the measured Cp_0 of 1 mg/L after a 3-mg dose indicates a V_d that is a real volume, the plasma volume. This is the exception, however, for the V_d of most drugs is larger than plasma volume; many drugs are so extensively taken up by cells that cellular levels exceed those in plasma. For such drugs, the hypothetical V_d is large, even greater than the volume of body water. For example, Fig. 65-1 indicates that the Cp_0 obtained by extrapolation after administration of 50 mg lidocaine is 0.42 mg/L, yielding a V_d of 119 L.

As elimination is performed largely by the kidney and liver, it is useful to consider the elimination of drugs according to the *clearance* concept. For example, in the kidney, regardless of the extent to which removal of drug is determined by filtration, secretion, or reabsorption, the net result is a reduction of the concentration of drug in plasma as it passes through the organ. The extent to which the concentration is reduced is expressed as the *extraction ratio*, or E, which is constant as long as first-order elimination occurs.

$$E = \frac{C_a - C_v}{C_a}$$

where C_a = arterial plasma concentration
C_v = venous plasma concentration

If the extraction is complete, $E = 1$. If the total plasma flow to the kidneys is Q (mL/min), the total volume of plasma from which drug is completely removed in a unit time (clearance from the body, Cl) is determined as

$$\text{Cl}_{\text{renal}} = QE$$

If the renal extraction ratio of penicillin is 0.5 and renal plasma flow is 680 mL/min, then penicillin's renal clearance is 340 mL/min. If the extraction ratio is high, as is the case for renal extraction of aminohippurate or hepatic extraction of propranolol, then clearance is a function of organ blood flow.[2]

Clearance from the body is the sum of clearance from all organs of elimination and is the best measure of the efficiency of the elimination processes. If a drug is removed by both the kidney and liver, then

$$\text{Cl} = \text{Cl}_{\text{renal}} + \text{Cl}_{\text{hepatic}}$$

Thus, if penicillin is eliminated by both renal clearance (340 mL/min) and hepatic clearance (36 mL/min) in a normal individual, total clearance is 376 mL/min. If renal clearance is reduced to half, total clearance is 170 + 36 or 206 mL/min. In anuria, total clearance equals hepatic clearance.

Only the drug in the vascular compartment can be cleared during each passage through an organ. To ascertain the effect of a given plasma clearance by one or more organs on the rate of removal of drug from the body, the clearance must be related to the volume of "plasma equivalents" to be cleared, that is, the volume of distribution. If the volume of distribution is 10 L and clearance is 1 L/min, then one-tenth of the drug in the body is eliminated per minute. This fraction, Cl/V_d, is known as a *fractional elimination constant* and is designated as k:

$$k = \frac{\text{Cl}}{V_d}$$

If the fraction k is multiplied by the total amount of drug in the body, the actual rate of elimination at any given time can be determined:

$$\text{Rate of elimination} = k \times \text{amount in body} = \text{Cl}Cp$$

This is the general equation for all first-order processes and expresses the fact that rate is proportional to the declining quantity in a first-order process.

As half-life is a temporal expression of the exponential first-order process, half-life ($t_{1/2}$) can be related to k as follows:

$$t_{1/2} = \frac{0.693}{k}$$

$$\text{Because} \quad k = \frac{\text{Cl}}{V_d}$$

$$\text{then} \quad t_{1/2} = \frac{0.693 V_d}{\text{Cl}}$$

As shown in the section on drug dosage in renal failure, the linear relationship of k to creatinine clearance makes k a useful parameter upon which to estimate changes in drug elimination with reduction in creatinine clearance in renal insufficiency. Half-life is not linearly related to clearance.

[1] Alternatively, the fraction of drug lost from the body during a dosage interval can be determined nongraphically from this equation:

$$\text{Fraction of drug lost from body} = 1 - e^{kt}$$

Values for e^{kt} can be obtained from a table of natural exponential functions or by a calculator, where k (= $0.693/t_{1/2}$) is the fractional elimination constant (described in the next section) and t is the time interval after drug administration.

[2] When drug is present in the formed elements of blood, then calculation of extraction and clearance from blood is more physiologically meaningful than from the plasma.

The important relationship

$$t_{1/2} = \frac{0.693 V_d}{\mathrm{Cl}}$$

indicates clearly the dependency of half-life, a measure of rate of elimination, on the two physiologically independent variables of volume of distribution and clearance, which expresses the efficiency of elimination. Thus, half-life is shortened when phenobarbital induces the enzymes responsible for hepatic clearance of a drug, and half-life is lengthened when a drug's renal clearance is attenuated in renal failure. Also, the half-life of some drugs is shortened when their volume of distribution is reduced. If, as in the case of cardiac failure, the volume of distribution is reduced at the same time that clearance is reduced, there may be little change in drug half-life to reflect the impaired clearance, but steady state plasma levels will be increased, as is the case with lidocaine. In treating patients after an overdose, the effects of hemodialysis on a drug's elimination are dependent on its volume of distribution. When the volume of distribution is large, as with tricyclic antidepressants (V_d of desipramine equals more than 2000 L), the removal of drug, even with a high-clearance dialyzer, proceeds slowly.

The extent to which a drug is bound to plasma protein also determines the fraction extracted by the organ(s) of elimination. Altered binding changes the extraction ratio significantly, however, only when elimination is limited to the unbound (free) drug in plasma. The extent to which binding influences elimination depends on the relative affinity of the plasma binding versus the affinity of the drug for the extraction process. The high affinity of the renal tubular anion transport system for many drugs leads to extraction of bound and unbound drug, and the efficient process by which the liver removes propranolol extracts most of this highly bound drug from blood. However, in the case of drugs with low organ extraction ratios, only unbound drug is available for elimination.

STEADY STATE With a constant infusion of drug, the infusion rate equals elimination rate at steady state. Therefore,

$$\underset{\text{(amt/unit time)}}{\text{Infusion rate}} = \underset{\text{(amt/vol)}}{Cp_{ss}} \times \underset{\text{(vol/unit time)}}{\mathrm{Cl}}$$

when the units for amount, volume, and time are consistent.

Thus, if clearance (Cl) is known, the infusion rate to achieve a given steady state plasma level can be calculated. Estimation of drug clearance is discussed in the section on renal disease.

When the dose is given intermittently instead of by infusion, the above relationship between plasma concentration and the dose administered at each dosage interval can be expressed as

$$\text{Dose} = Cp_{av} \times \mathrm{Cl} \times \text{dosage interval}$$

The average plasma concentration (Cp_{av}) implies, as seen in Fig. 65-2, that levels can be higher and lower than the average during the dosage interval.

When a drug is given orally, the fraction (F) of the administered dose that reaches the systemic circulation is an expression of the drug's *bioavailability*. A reduction in bioavailability may reflect a poorly formulated dosage form that fails to disintegrate or dissolve in the gastrointestinal fluids. Regulatory standards have reduced the extent of this problem. Drug interactions also can impair absorption after oral dosing. Bioavailability may also be reduced due to drug metabolism in the gastrointestinal tract and/or the liver during the absorption process, the *first-pass effect*. This is a particular problem for drugs that are extensively extracted by these organs, and considerable interpatient variability often exists in bioavailability. Lidocaine for the control of arrhythmias is not administered orally because of the first-pass effect. Drugs that are injected intramuscularly may also have low bioavailability, e.g., phenytoin. An unexpected drug response should lead to consideration of bioavailability as a possible factor. Calculation of a dosage regimen should be corrected for bioavailability:

$$\text{Oral dose} = \frac{Cp_{av} \times \mathrm{Cl} \times \text{dosage interval}}{F}$$

DRUG ELIMINATION THAT IS NOT FIRST-ORDER The elimination of some drugs such as phenytoin, salicylate, and theophylline does not follow first-order kinetics when amounts of drug in the body are in the therapeutic range. For these drugs, the clearance changes as levels in the body fall during elimination or after alterations in dose. This pattern of elimination is said to be *dose-dependent*. Accordingly, the time for the concentration to fall to one-half becomes less as plasma levels fall; this halving time is not truly a half-life, because the term *half-life* applies to first-order kinetics and is a constant. The elimination of phenytoin is dose-dependent, and when very high levels are present (in the toxic range), the halving time may be longer than 72 h, whereas as the concentration in plasma declines, the clearance increases and the concentration in plasma will halve in 20 to 30 h. When a drug is eliminated by first-order kinetics, the plasma level at steady state is directly related to the amount of the maintenance dose, and a doubling of the dose should lead to doubling of the steady state plasma level. However, for drugs with dose-dependent kinetics, increases in the dose may be accompanied by disproportionate increases in plasma level. Thus, if the daily dose of phenytoin is increased from 300 to 400 mg, plasma levels rise by more than 33 percent. The extent of increase is not predictable because of the interpatient variability in the extent to which clearance deviates from first order. Salicylates are also eliminated by dose-dependent kinetics at high plasma levels, and in children particular caution must be taken with the administration of high doses. Ethanol metabolism also is dose-dependent, with obvious implications. The mechanisms involved in dose-dependent kinetics may include the saturation of the rate-limiting step in metabolism or a feedback inhibition of the rate-limiting enzyme by a product of the reaction.

INDIVIDUALIZATION OF DRUG THERAPY

Recognition of factors modifying drug action is essential for therapy that provides optimal benefit and minimal risk to each patient.

ALTERATION OF DRUG DOSAGE IN RENAL DISEASE Where urinary excretion is an important route of elimination, renal failure results in decreased drug clearance and therefore slower removal of the drug from the body, so that administration of the usual dosage leads to greater accumulation and an increased likelihood of toxicity. The goal in such cases is to modify the dosage schedule so that a similar drug concentration–time profile is achieved in the plasma of the patient with renal insufficiency and the steady state is reached after a similar time interval as in the patient with normal renal function. This is particularly appropriate for drugs with long half-lives and narrow therapeutic indexes (e.g., digoxin). Since,

$$Cp_{av} = \frac{\text{dose}}{\text{dose interval}} \times \frac{1}{\mathrm{Cl}} = \frac{\text{dose}}{\text{dose interval}} \times \frac{1}{k\,V_d}$$

the Cp_{av} achieved with normal renal function can be obtained in patients with renal impairment, i.e., decreased Cl, by either decreasing the dose while maintaining the normal dosing interval, administering the usual dose but less frequently, or a combination of the two. Moreover, the modification factor for the dosage regimen is dependent on the ratio of the drug's clearance or rate of elimination in renal failure to that in uncompromised patients. Although such pharmacokinetic strategies in renal failure result in the same Cp_{av} during the dosage interval, the peak-to-trough fluctuations differ considerably from those seen in patients with normal renal function. Selection of the most appropriate modifications, therefore, depends on the levels associated with efficacy or toxicity, e.g., peak, Cp_{av}, or trough, and the drug's therapeutic index.

One approach is to calculate the *fraction of the normal dose* that is to be given at the usual dosage interval. This fraction can be determined from either drug clearance (Cl) or the fractional rate constant (k), based on the fact that both renal clearance and k are proportional to creatinine clearance (Cl_{cr}). Creatinine clearance is best determined directly. However, serum creatinine (C_{cr}) may be used to estimate the value by the following equation which is applicable to men:

$$Cl_{cr} = \frac{(140 - \text{age}) \times \text{weight (kg)}}{72 \times C_{cr}\,(\text{mg/dL})}\ (\text{mL/min})$$

For women, the value should be reduced to 85 percent of that estimated by this equation. This approach to estimation of Cl_{cr} is invalid in severe renal insufficiency ($C_{cr} > 5$ mg/dL) or with rapidly changing renal function.

The clearance approach Calculation of drug dosage is most accurately based on the clearance of a drug. From data on the clearance of a drug, the dose in renal insufficiency (Dose_{ri}) may be calculated as follows:

$$\text{Dose}_{ri} = \text{dose} \times \frac{Cl_{ri}}{Cl}$$

where ri = renal insufficiency
Cl = clearance from the whole body with normal renal function
Cl_{ri} = clearance from the whole body with renal insufficiency
Dose = maintenance dose with normal renal function ($Cl_{cr} \sim$ 100 mL/min)

The normal clearance and that in renal impairment can be obtained by employing the data in Table 65-1 in the following equations:

$$Cl = Cl_{renal} + Cl_{nonrenal}$$

$$Cl_{ri} = Cl_{renal} \times \frac{\text{measured } Cl_{cr}}{100\ \text{mL/min}} + Cl_{nonrenal}$$

The Cl_{renal} values in Table 65-1 are those found with $Cl_{cr} = 100$ mL/min, and the renal clearance of drug in renal insufficiency is obtained by multiplying Cl_{renal} by the ratio of measured Cl_{cr} (in milliliters per minute) to 100 mL/min.

For gentamicin, with a normal Cl_{renal} of 78 mL/min and $Cl_{nonrenal}$ of 3 mL/min, Cl = 81 mL/min. Therefore, with a Cl_{cr} of 12 mL/min, $Cl_{ri} = 78 \times (12/100) + 3 = 12.4$ mL/min. If the dose of gentamicin for a given infection should be 1.5 mg/kg per 8 h in the presence of normal renal function, then

$$\text{Dose}_{ri} = \frac{1.5\ \text{mg/kg}}{8\ \text{h}} \times \frac{12.4\ \text{mL/min}}{81\ \text{mL/min}} = \frac{0.23\ \text{mg/kg}}{8\ \text{h}}$$

In the patient with renal insufficiency, this computation provides an average plasma level during a dosage interval that is the same as the average plasma level during the dosage interval with normal renal function; the fluctuations between peaks and troughs, however, will be less pronounced, but the peak value could be below the therapeutic level. Alternatively, the normal (1.5 mg/kg) dose of gentamicin could be administered but the dosage interval prolonged by the modification factor based on the change in clearance

$$8\ \text{h} \times \frac{81\ \text{mL/min}}{12.4\ \text{mL/min}} = 52\ \text{h}$$

TABLE 65-1 Clearance of drugs

Drug	Renal clearance,* mL/min	Nonrenal clearance, mL/min
Ampicillin†	340	12
Carbenicillin	68	10
Digoxin†	110	36
Gentamicin	78	3
Kanamycin	60	0
Penicillin G‡	340	36

* The "normal" renal clearances are those associated with a clearance of creatinine of 100 mL/min.
† The fraction of digoxin absorbed after an oral dose (F) is approximately 0.75, and F for ampicillin is 0.5.
‡ One microgram of penicillin G = 1.6 units.

In this case, the plasma levels may be subtherapeutic for a deleterious length of time during the dosage interval.

In some instances it may be desirable to calculate a dose that will yield a certain plasma level at steady state. This approach is most appropriate for constant intravenous infusions where 100 percent of the dose is delivered to the systemic circulation. When clearance of a drug in a patient with renal insufficiency is calculated as above, then

$$\underset{(\text{amt/unit time})}{\text{Dose}_{ri}} = \underset{(\text{vol/unit time})}{Cl_{ri}} \times \underset{(\text{amt/vol})}{Cp}$$

where the time, amount, and volume terms are uniform.

If a plasma concentration of carbenicillin of 100 μg/mL is the therapeutic objective in a patient with a creatinine clearance of 25 mL/min, the infusion rate is calculated as follows. Carbenicillin clearance is

$$Cl_{ri} = \left(68 \times \frac{25}{100}\right) + 10 = 27\ \text{mL/min}$$

Therefore, carbenicillin should be infused at a rate of 2700 μg/min.

Should the method of calculating dose based on the desired plasma level be applied to intermittent-dose therapy, particular attention should be given to the fact that the calculation is based on an *average* plasma level and that peak plasma levels will be higher. In addition, if an oral drug is not completely absorbed, the computed dose must be divided by the fraction (F) that reaches the systemic circulation (see "Steady State" above).

The fractional rate constant (k) approach For many drugs, clearance data in renal failure are not available. In these cases, the fraction of the normal dose that is required in a patient with renal failure can be approximated from the ratio of the fractional rate constant for elimination from the body in renal failure (k_{ri}) to that with normal renal function (k). This approach requires the assumption that the distribution of the drug (V_d) is not affected by renal disease. The approach is the same as that employed with clearance data:

$$\text{Dose}_{ri} = \text{Dose} \times \frac{k_{ri}}{k}$$

As the ratio k_{ri}/k is the fraction of the usual dose employed in a given degree of renal insufficiency, it is termed the *dose fraction* and may be estimated from the information in Table 65-2 and the nomogram (Fig. 65-4). Table 65-2 gives the fraction of the usual dose of a drug

FIGURE 65-4 Nomogram for estimation of the dose fraction (k_{ri}/k) in patients with renal insufficiency. The application of the nomogram is described in the text.

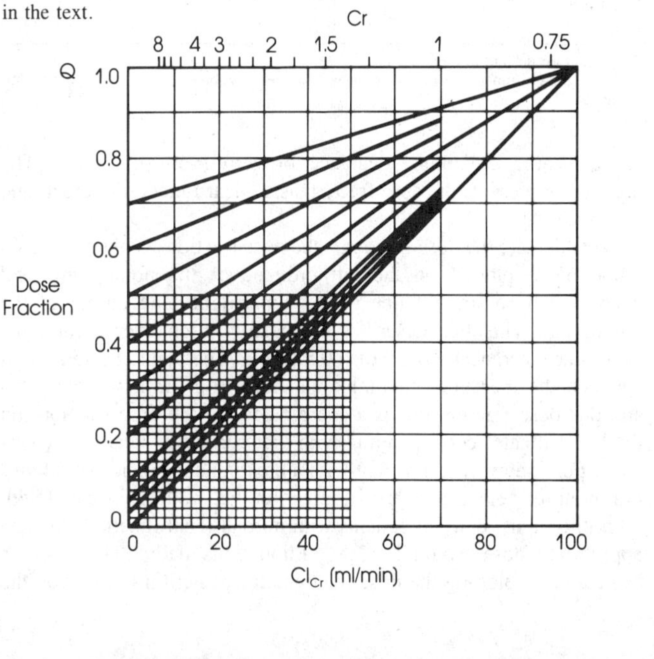

TABLE 65-2 Estimated fraction of usual dose of drug required for a patient with a creatinine clearance of zero (dose fraction$_0$) and average overall fractional elimination rate constant for a patient with normal renal function (k)

Drug	Dose fraction$_0$	k (per hour)
ANTIBIOTICS		
Amikacin	0.05	0.4
Amoxicillin	0.15	0.7
Ampicillin	0.1	0.6
Aztreonam	0.25	0.4
Carbenicillin	0.1	0.6
Cefazolin	0.06	0.35
Cefotaxime*	0.3	0.7
Cefoxitin	0.1	0.8
Ceftazidime	0.1	0.4
Ceftriaxone†	0.5	0.09
Cephalexin	0.04	0.7
Cephalothin	0.02	1.4
Chloramphenicol	0.8	0.3
Ciprofloxacin	0.33	0.2
Clindamycin	0.8	0.2
Cloxacillin	0.25	1.2
Dicloxacillin	0.5	1.2
Doxycycline	0.8	0.03
Erythromycin	0.7	0.5
Gentamicin	0.05	0.3
Imipenim	0.25	0.7
Isoniazid:		
Fast inactivators	0.8	0.5
Slow inactivators	0.5	0.25
Methicillin	0.12	1.4
Minocycline	0.9	0.06
Nafcillin	0.4	1.2
Norfloxacin	0.5	0.2
Oxacillin	0.25	1.4
Penicillin G	0.1	1.4
Piperacillin	0.33	0.5
Rifampin	1.0	0.25
Streptomycin	0.05	0.25
Sulfadiazine	0.45	0.7
Sulfamethoxazole	0.85	0.07
Tetracycline	0.12	0.08
Ticarcillin	0.1	0.6
Tobramycin	0.05	0.35
Trimethoprim	0.45	0.06
Vancomycin	0.03	0.12
MISCELLANEOUS DRUGS		
Chlorpropamide	0.4	0.02
Lidocaine	0.9	0.4
Sulfinpyrazone	0.55	0.3
CARDIAC GLYCOSIDES		
		k (per day)
Digitoxin	0.7	0.1
Digoxin	0.3	0.45

* See text on dosage in renal disease.
† Extrarenal clearance also may be reduced in patients with renal failure who are uremic and/or ill.

required at a creatinine clearance of zero (dose fraction$_0$). The nomogram presents the dose fraction as a linear function of creatinine clearance.

To calculate the dose fraction$_{ri}$, the dose fraction$_0$ is obtained from Table 65-2, plotted on the left ordinate of the nomogram, and connected by a straight line to the upper-right-hand corner of the nomogram. This line describes the dose fraction over a range of creatinine clearances from 0 to 100 mL/min. The point of intersection between the measured creatinine clearance (on the lower abscissa) and this dose fraction line is a coordinate with the dose fraction (on the left ordinate) corresponding with that particular creatinine clearance. For example, if a patient with a creatinine clearance of 20 mL/min requires penicillin G for an infection that would be treated with 10 million units daily in patients with normal renal function, then an appropriate dose would be 2.8 million units daily. This dose is estimated by plotting the dose fraction$_0$ for penicillin G (0.1) on the left-hand ordinate and connecting it to the top right-hand corner of the nomogram (Fig. 65-4). On this dose fraction line for penicillin G, the coordinate for a creatinine clearance of 20 mL/min corresponds on the left ordinate with a dose fraction of 0.28. Hence, the dose is 0.28×10 million units daily.

The loading dose In addition to adjusting the maintenance dose in renal failure, consideration must also be given to the loading dose. Since this dose is designed to bring the plasma concentration, or more particularly the amount of drug in the body, rapidly to the level at steady state, there is no need to modify the usual loading dose, if one is normally used. The elimination of many drugs is sufficiently rapid in patients with normal renal function that the time required to reach steady state is not significant, and no loading dose is usually used. On the other hand, in renal failure where the half-life may be significantly prolonged, this accumulation period may become unacceptably long. In such a case, a loading dose may be indicated; it would be the same amount of drug administered with normal renal function as described in "Drug Accumulation" above.

General considerations for determining dosage in renal insufficiency Because of the differences in volumes of distribution and rates of metabolism, calculations of drug dose in renal failure must be viewed as valuable approximations which prevent the use of doses that are grossly excessive or inadequate for most patients. However, *maintenance dosages are most accurate when plasma level data are employed to enable adjustment of the dose where necessary.*

In all the above calculations, it is assumed that the nonrenal clearance and nonrenal k are constant in renal failure. In fact, when cardiac failure accompanies renal failure, metabolic clearance for many drugs is reduced. Accordingly, when a drug with a narrow therapeutic index, such as digoxin, is used in cardiac failure, an appropriate precaution would be to reduce the value for nonrenal clearance (or k) to about one-half.

Active or toxic metabolites of drugs also may accumulate in renal failure. Meperidine, for example, is cleared largely by metabolism, and its concentration in plasma is little altered by renal insufficiency. However, the plasma concentration of one of its metabolites, normeperidine, is increased when its renal elimination is impaired. As normeperidine has more convulsant activity than meperidine, its accumulation in patients with renal failure probably accounts for the signs of central nervous system excitation such as irritability, twitching, and seizures that result from the administration of multiple doses of meperidine to patients in renal insufficiency.

The metabolite of procainamide, *N*-acetylprocainamide, also has cardiac effects. As *N*-acetylprocainamide is eliminated almost entirely by the kidney, its concentration in plasma is increased by renal failure. Thus, the potential of procainamide to produce toxicity in renal insufficiency cannot be assessed by measuring the plasma concentration of procainamide alone. Cefotaxime is metabolized predominately to desacetylcefotaxime, which also has antimicrobial activity. Desacetylcefotaxime accumulates in renal failure to an even greater degree than does the parent drug, but no adverse effects are known to accrue to the accumulation of this metabolite.

LIVER DISEASE In contrast to the predictable decline in renal clearance of drugs when glomerular filtration is reduced, it is not possible to make a general prediction of the effect of liver disease on hepatic biotransformation of drugs (Chap. 247). Rather, in hepatitis and cirrhosis changes may range from impaired to increased drug clearance. Even in advanced hepatocellular disease, the magnitude of impairment in drug clearance usually is only about two- to fivefold. The extent of such changes, however, cannot be predicted by the common tests of liver function. Consequently, even when it is suspected that drug elimination is altered in liver disease, there is no quantitative base upon which to adjust the dosage regimen other than assessment of clinical response and concentration of drug in plasma.

Portacaval shunting creates a special situation because the effective hepatic blood flow is reduced. This situation has its greatest effect on drugs that normally have a high hepatic extraction ratio so that their clearance is largely a function of blood flow; thus the clearance of such drugs (e.g., propranolol and lidocaine) is remarkably reduced by portacaval shunting. In addition, the fraction of an administered oral dose reaching the systemic circulation is increased, because drug that is shunted around the liver during the absorption process escapes the first-pass metabolism by this organ (e.g., meperidine, pentazocine).

CIRCULATORY INSUFFICIENCY—CARDIAC FAILURE AND SHOCK Under conditions of decreased tissue perfusion, redistribution of the cardiac output occurs to preserve blood flow to the heart and brain at the expense of other tissues (Chap. 39). As a result, the drug is distributed into a smaller volume of distribution, higher drug concentrations are present in the plasma, and the tissues that are best perfused are exposed to these higher concentrations. If either the brain or heart is sensitive to the drug, an alteration in response will occur.

Furthermore, the decreased perfusion of the kidney and liver may impair drug clearance by these organs directly or indirectly. Thus, in severe congestive heart failure, in hemorrhagic shock, and in cardiogenic shock, the response to the usual dose of drug may be excessive, and dosage modification may be necessary. For example, the clearance of lidocaine is reduced by about 50 percent in cardiac failure, and therapeutic plasma levels are achieved at infusion rates of only about half of those usually required. In cardiac failure there also is a significant reduction in lidocaine's volume of distribution which results in the requirement of a smaller loading dose. Similar situations are thought to exist for procainamide, theophylline, and possibly quinidine. Unfortunately, predictors of these types of pharmacokinetic alterations are unavailable. Therefore, loading doses should be conservative, and continued therapy should be monitored closely, following clinical indicators of toxicity and plasma levels.

DISEASE-INDUCED CHANGES IN PLASMA BINDING Many drugs circulate in the plasma partly bound to the plasma proteins. Since only the unbound or free drug can distribute to the site of pharmacologic action, the therapeutic response should be related to the free rather than the total circulating plasma drug concentration. In most cases the degree of binding is fairly constant across the therapeutic concentration range so that significant error is not caused by individualizing therapy on the basis of total drug levels in plasma. However, states such as hypoalbuminemia, liver disease, and renal disease can decrease the extent of drug binding, particularly of acidic and neutral drugs, so that at any total plasma level there is a greater concentration of free drug and a risk of increased response and toxicity. Other conditions, e.g., myocardial infarction, surgery, neoplastic disease, rheumatoid arthritis, and burns, that lead to an increased plasma concentration of the acute-phase reactant alpha$_1$-acid glycoprotein have the opposite effect on the basic drugs that are bound to this macromolecule. The drugs for which changes in binding are important are those that are normally highly bound in the plasma (>90 percent) because a small alteration in the extent of binding produces a large change in the amount of drug in the unbound form.

The consequences of these binding changes, particularly with respect to total drug levels, depend on whether the clearance and distribution are dependent on the unbound or total drug. For many drugs, elimination and distribution are largely restricted to the unbound fraction, and therefore a decrease in binding leads to an increase in the clearance and distribution of the drug. The relative magnitudes of these changes are such that the net effect is to shorten the half-life. The appropriate modification of the dosage regimen in conditions with reduced drug binding, as is the case of phenytoin in renal failure, is simply to administer the usual daily dose of the drug but in divided doses at more frequent intervals. Individualization of therapy can then be based on either the clinical response or the plasma concentration of unbound drug. It is critical that the patient not be titrated into the usual therapeutic range for concentration of *total* drug in plasma since this will lead to excessive response and toxicity.

In the case of drugs bound to alpha$_1$-acid glycoprotein, the disease-induced increase in binding has the opposite effects of reducing the clearance and distribution of total drug. Accordingly, constant rate infusion of lidocaine to control arrhythmias after myocardial infarction leads to an accumulation of total drug. However, the clearance of unbound and pharmacologically active drug remains essentially unchanged. Again, it is critical that the patient not be dosed on the basis of total drug concentrations in the plasma since this will be associated with subtherapeutic levels of unbound drug.

INTERACTIONS BETWEEN DRUGS

The effect of some drugs can be altered markedly by the administration of other agents. Such interactions can sabotage therapeutic intent by producing excessive drug action (with adverse effects) or decreasing the action of a drug, rendering it ineffective. Drug interactions must be considered in the differential diagnosis of unexpected responses to drugs, recognizing that patients often come to the physician with a legacy of drugs acquired during previous medical experiences. A meticulous drug history will minimize the unknown elements in the therapeutic milieu; it should include examination of the patient's medications and calls to the pharmacist to identify prescriptions, if necessary.

There are two principal types of interactions between drugs. *Pharmacokinetic interactions* result from alteration in the delivery of drugs to their sites of action. *Pharmacodynamic interactions* are those in which the responsiveness of the target organ or system is modified by other agents.

An index of the drug interactions discussed in this chapter is provided in Table 65-3. Included are interactions which have verified significance in patients and a few of such potential danger that cognizance should be taken of experimental data or case reports suggesting their likely occurrence.

I PHARMACOKINETIC INTERACTIONS CAUSING DIMINISHED DRUG DELIVERY

***A* Impaired gastrointestinal absorption** Cholestyramine, an ionic exchange resin, binds thyroxine, triiodothyronine, and the cardiac glycosides with sufficiently high affinity to impair their absorption from the gastrointestinal tract. This resin probably also interferes with the absorption of other drugs, and it is safest not to give it within 2 h of their administration. Aluminum ions, present in antacids, form insoluble chelates with the tetracyclines, thereby preventing absorption of these drugs. Ferrous ions similarly block tetracycline absorption. Kaolin-pectin suspensions bind digoxin, and when the drugs are administered together, digoxin absorption is reduced by about one-half. However, when kaolin-pectin is administered 2 h after digoxin, there is no effect on absorption of digoxin.

Ketoconazole is a weak base that dissolves well only at acidic pH. Thus, histamine-2 antagonists such as cimetidine, by neutralizing gastric pH, impair the dissolution and subsequent absorption of ketoconazole. Oral administration of aminosalicylate interferes with the absorption of rifampin by an unknown mechanism.

Impaired absorption results in reduction in the total amount of drug absorbed, with reduced area under the plasma level curve, reduced peak plasma levels, and lower steady state concentrations of the drug involved.

***B* Induction of hepatic drug-metabolizing enzymes** When the elimination of the drug is largely by metabolism, an increase in the rate of metabolism reduces its availability to sites of action. The metabolism of most drugs occurs largely in the liver, because of its mass, high blood flow, and concentration of enzymes that metabolize drugs. The initial step in metabolism of many drugs is executed by a group of mixed-function oxidase isoenzymes in the endoplasmic reticulum. These enzyme systems containing cytochrome P_{450} oxidize the molecule by a variety of reactions including aromatic hydroxylations, *N*-demethylations, *O*-demethylations, and sulfoxidations. The products of these reactions are usually more polar (and more readily excreted by the kidney).

TABLE 65-3 Drug interaction index

Drug	Section of chapter describing interaction
Acetohexamide	IIB
Allopurinol	IIA
p-Aminosalicylate	IA
Amiodarone	IIC
Amphetamine	IC
Antidepressants, tricyclic (desipramine, nortriptyline, imipramine, doxepin, protriptyline, amitriptyline)	IC
Aspirin	IIB, III
Azathioprine	IIA
Barbiturates (class)	IB
Bethanidine	IC
Carbamazepine	IB, IIA
Chlorpromazine	IC
Cholestyramine	IA
Cimetidine	IA, IIA, IIB
Clofibrate	IIA
Clonidine	IC
Cyclosporine	IB, IIA
Dexamethasone	IB
Digitoxin	IA, IB, IIC
Digoxin	IA, IIC
Diuretics	III
Erythromycin	IIA
Ephedrine	IC
Ethanol	IIA
Famotidine	IIA
Guanadrel	IC
Guanethidine	IC
Indomethacin	III
Isoniazid	IIA
Kaolin-pectin	IA
Ketoconazole	IA, IB, IIA
Lidocaine	IIA
6-Mercaptopurine	IIA
Methadone	IB
Methotrexate	IIB
Metronidazole	IB, IIA
Metyrapone	IB
Mexiletine	IB
Nifedipine	IIA
Nonsteroidal anti-inflammatory drugs	III
Oral contraceptive steroids	IB
Phenobarbital	IB
Phenylbutazone	IIA, IIB
Phenytoin (diphenylhydantoin)	IB, IIA
Piroxicam	III
Potassium	III
Prednisone	IB
Probenicid	IIB
Procainamide	IIB
Propranolol	III
Quinidine	IB, IIA, IIC, III
Ranitidine	IA, IIA
Rifampin	IA, IB
Salicylate	IIB
Spironolactone	III
Tetracycline	IA
Theophylline	IIA
Thiazide diuretics	III
Tolbutamide	IIA
Triamterene	III
Triazolam	IIA
Verapamil	IIC
Warfarin	IB, IIA, III

The biosynthesis of some of the mixed-function oxidase isoenzymes is under regulatory control at the transcriptional level, and their content in the liver can be induced by a number of drugs. Phenobarbital is the prototype of these inducers, and all barbiturates in clinical use increase mixed-function oxidase isoenzymes. Induction with phenobarbital can occur with doses of as little as 60 mg daily. Mixed-function oxidases also are induced by rifampin, carbamazepine, phenytoin, and glutethimide, by occupational exposure to chlorinated insecticides such as DDT, and by chronic alcohol ingestion.

Phenobarbital and other inducers lower plasma levels of many drugs, including warfarin, digitoxin, quinidine, mexiletine, ketoconazole, cyclosporine, dexamethasone, prednisolone (the active metabolite of prednisone), oral contraceptive steroids, methadone, metronidazole, and metyrapone. These interactions all have obvious clinical significance. With the coumarin anticoagulants, the patient is placed at major risk when an appropriate level of anticoagulation is achieved while the coumarin drug is coadministered with an inducing agent. Should the inducer then be discontinued, e.g., following discharge from the hospital, plasma levels of the coumarin anticoagulant will rise as the induction effect wears off, leading to excessive anticoagulation. Barbiturates have been shown to lower the plasma levels of phenytoin in some patients, but the clinical effect of reduced phenytoin levels is probably counterbalanced by the anticonvulsant effects of phenobarbital.

There is considerable variation among individuals in the extent to which drug metabolism can be induced. In some patients phenobarbital leads to marked acceleration in the rate of drug metabolism, whereas little induction is seen in others.

In addition to inducing certain of the mixed-function oxidase isoenzymes, phenobarbital has other effects on hepatic function. It increases liver blood flow, bile flow, and the hepatocellular transport of organic anions. The conjugation of drugs and bilirubin may also be enhanced by inducing agents.

C Inhibition of cellular uptake or binding The guanidinium antihypertensives, guanethidine, guanadrel, and bethanidine, are transported to their site of action in adrenergic neurons by an energy-requiring membrane transport system for biogenic monoamines. Although the physiologic function of the transport system is reuptake of the adrenergic neurotransmitter, it also transports a variety of ring-substituted bases, including guanethidine and related guanidiniums, into the adrenergic neuron against a concentration gradient. Inhibitors of norepinephrine uptake prevent the uptake of the guanidinium antihypertensives into adrenergic neurons and thereby block their pharmacologic effects. The tricyclic antidepressants are potent inhibitors of norepinephrine uptake. Consequently, concomitant administration of clinical doses of tricyclic antidepressants including desipramine, protriptyline, nortriptyline, and amitriptyline almost totally abolishes the antihypertensive effects of guanethidine, guanadrel, and bethanidine. Although they are less potent inhibitors of norepinephrine uptake, doxepin and chlorpromazine, when given in doses of greater than 100 mg daily, produce dose-related antagonism of the action of the guanidinium antihypertensives. In patients with severe hypertension, the loss of control of blood pressure from these drug interactions can lead to stroke and malignant hypertension.

Ephedrine, a component of many drug combinations used in asthma, also antagonizes the effect of guanethidine, probably by both inhibition of uptake and displacement from the neuron.

The antihypertensive effect of clonidine is partially antagonized by tricyclic antidepressants. Clonidine lowers arterial pressure by reducing sympathetic outflow from the blood-pressure-regulating centers in the hindbrain (Chap. 196). This central hypotensive action is antagonized by the tricyclic antidepressants.

II PHARMACOKINETIC INTERACTIONS CAUSING INCREASED DRUG DELIVERY

A Inhibition of drug metabolism If the active form of a drug is cleared largely by biotransformation, inhibition of its metabolism leads to a reduced clearance, prolonged half-life, and accumulation of the drug during maintenance therapy. Excessive accumulation due to inhibited metabolism can lead to adverse effects.

Cimetidine is a potent inhibitor of the oxidative metabolism of warfarin, quinidine, nifedipine, lidocaine, theophylline and phenytoin. Adverse reactions, many of them severe, have resulted from the administration of these drugs in conjunction with cimetidine. Cimetidine is a more potent inhibitor of mixed-function oxidases than ranitidine, whereas ranitidine is more potent as a histamine-2 antagonist. Thus, ranitidine, when administered in doses of 150 mg twice daily, does not inhibit the oxidative metabolism of most drugs; where reduced drug elimination has been observed, the effects of ranitidine have been less than those of cimetidine and devoid of appreciable pharmacodynamic consequence. Doses of ranitidine higher than 150 mg, however, may produce greater inhibition of drug oxidation. Famotidine, like ranitidine, is not known to produce clinically appreciable inhibition of drug metabolism.

Erythromycin inhibits the metabolism of several drugs, including cyclosporine, warfarin, carbamazepine, triazolam, and theophylline. Adverse effects, some severe, have been the consequence of these drug interactions. The extent to which disposition of these drugs is impaired by erythromycin is a function of erythromycin concentration in plasma (and its dose) and probably also of the duration of erythromycin administration. Erythromycin is metabolized by an isozyme of cytochrome P_{450} to a nitroso metabolite that binds to and inhibits the P_{450} isozyme.

Other drugs that inhibit biotransformation of pharmacologic compounds include (with examples of drugs that have their metabolism blocked by the inhibitor listed in parenthesis):

Clofibrate (phenytoin, tolbutamide)
Excessive ingestion of ethanol (warfarin)
Isoniazid (phenytoin)
Ketoconazole (cyclosporine)
Metronidazole (warfarin)
Phenylbutazone (warfarin, phenytoin, tolbutamide)

Cyclosporine inhibits the disposition of some other drugs. Cyclosporine lowers the clearance of prednisolone. The administration of lovastatin to cardiac transplant patients receiving cyclosporine has been associated with a high prevalence of rhabdomyolysis that can be severe. As the concentration of lovastatin was noted to be elevated when measured in these patients with rhabdomyolysis, impairment of its clearance by cyclosporine has been inferred but not proved as a cause of this severe drug interaction.

Azathioprine is readily converted in the body to an active metabolite, 6-mercaptopurine, which in turn is oxidized by xanthine oxidase to 6-thiouric acid. When allopurinol, a potent inhibitor of xanthine oxidase, is administered concurrently with standard doses of azathioprine or 6-mercaptopurine, life-threatening toxicity (bone marrow suppression) can result.

***B* Inhibition of renal elimination** A number of drugs are secreted by the renal tubular transport systems for organic anions. Inhibition of this tubular transport system can cause excessive accumulation of a drug. Phenylbutazone, probenecid, and salicylates competitively inhibit this transport system. Salicylate, for example, reduces the renal clearance of methotrexate, an interaction that may lead to methotrexate toxicity. Renal tubular secretion contributes substantially to the elimination of penicillin, which can be inhibited by probenecid.

Inhibition of the tubular cation transport system by cimetidine impedes the renal clearance of procainamide and its active metabolite *N*-acetylprocainamide.

***C* Inhibition of clearance by multiple mechanisms** The concentrations of digoxin and digitoxin in plasma are elevated by quinidine, due largely to inhibition of renal elimination and in part from inhibition of nonrenal clearance as well. An increase in cardiac arrhythmia may occur when quinidine is given in conjunction with a cardiac glycoside.

Amiodarone, cyclosporine, and verapamil also inhibit the clearance of digoxin and increase the concentration of digoxin in plasma.

***III* PHARMACODYNAMIC AND OTHER INTERACTIONS BETWEEN DRUGS** Therapeutically useful interactions occur in which the combined effect of two drugs is greater than that of either drug alone. These favorable drug combinations are described in specific therapeutic sections in this text, and the following is directed toward those interactions that create unwanted effects. Two drugs may act on separate components of a common process and yield effects greater than either alone. For example, small doses of aspirin (less than 1 g daily) do not alter the prothrombin time appreciably in patients who are on warfarin therapy. However, the addition of aspirin to patients anticoagulated with warfarin increases the risk of bleeding because aspirin inhibits platelet aggregation. Thus the combination of impaired functions of platelets and the clotting system increases the potential for hemorrhagic complications in patients receiving warfarin therapy.

Indomethacin, piroxicam, and probably other nonsteroidal anti-inflammatory drugs antagonize the antihypertensive effects of beta-adrenergic receptor blockers, diuretics, converting enzyme inhibitors, and other drugs. The resultant elevation in blood pressure ranges from trivial to severe. Aspirin and sulindac, however, do not elevate the blood pressure in treated hypertensive patients.

Polymorphic ventricular tachycardia (torsades de pointes) during quinidine administration occurs much more frequently in patients receiving diuretics, probably as a consequence of potassium and/or magnesium depletion.

The administration of supplemental potassium leads to more frequent and more severe hyperkalemia when potassium elimination is reduced by concurrent treatment with spironolactone or triamterene.

VARIABLE ACTIONS OF DRUGS CAUSED BY GENETIC DIFFERENCES IN THEIR METABOLISM

ACETYLATION Isoniazid, hydralazine, procainamide, and a number of other drugs are metabolized by acetylation of a hydrazino or amino group. This reaction is catalyzed by *N*-acetyl transferase, an enzyme in the liver cytosol that transfers an acetyl group from acetyl coenzyme A to the drug. Individuals differ markedly in the rate at which drugs are acetylated, and there is a bimodal distribution of the population into "rapid acetylators" and "slow acetylators." The rate of acetylation is under genetic control; slow acetylation is an autosomal recessive trait.

Responses to hydralazine therapy are dependent upon the acetylation phenotype. The hypotensive effect of hydralazine is greater in patients who acetylate the drug slowly, and the lupus erythematosus-like syndrome produced by hydralazine occurs almost exclusively in those with slow acetylation. Thus it may be of value to know the acetylation phenotype as a predictor of which patients with hypertension might benefit from an increase in the dose of hydralazine above the 200 mg daily that can be safely employed in the population at large.

Acetylation phenotype can be determined by measuring the ratio of acetylated to nonacetylated dapsone or sulfamethazine in plasma or urine following administration of a test dose of these acetylation substrates. The ratio of monoacetyldapsone to dapsone in plasma at 6 h after dapsone administration is less than 0.35 for slow acetylators and greater than 0.35 for rapid acetylators. At 6 h following the administration of sulfamethazine, less than 25 percent of the drug in the plasma is in the acetylated form in slow acetylators (rapid acetylators, more than 25 percent); in the urine collected in the 5- to 6-h interval after administration, less than 70 percent of the drug is in the acetylated form in slow acetylators (rapid acetylators, more than 70 percent).

METABOLISM BY MIXED-FUNCTION OXIDASES In healthy individuals taking no other medications, the major determinant of the rate of metabolism of drugs by the hepatic mixed-function oxidases is genetic. Hepatic endoplasmic reticulum contains a family of cytochrome P_{450} isoenzymes with different substrate specificities. Many drugs undergo oxidative metabolism by more than one isoenzyme, and the steady state concentrations of such drugs in the plasma is a function of the sum of the activities of these and other metabolizing enzymes. When a drug is metabolized by multiple pathways, the catalytic activities of the participating enzymes are regulated by a number of genes so that the frequency of clearance rates and steady state concentrations of the drug tend to distribute unimodally within the population. The range of activity may differ markedly (tenfold or more) between different individuals, as is the case for chlorpromazine, and there is no way to make a prior prediction of the rate.

For certain metabolic pathways bimodally distributed activity suggests control by a single gene, and several polymorphisms have been identified. As a result, two phenotypic populations are usually present analogous to the situation with *N*-acetylation (see above). A majority of the population are extensive metabolizers (EM), and a smaller group of individuals of the poor metabolizer phenotype (PM) have an impaired, if not an absent, ability to metabolize the drug. For example, about 8 to 10 percent of whites are unable to form the 4-hydroxy metabolite of the test drug debrisoquin, and this trait is inherited in an autosomal recessive fashion. Importantly, the putatively involved cytochrome P_{450} isoenzyme is also involved in the biotransformation of other drugs whose metabolic fate, therefore, cosegregates with the debrisoquin trait. A similar situation occurs with other oxidative polymorphisms that characterize the metabolism of mephenytoin and possibly tolbutamide. The situation is further complicated by interethnic differences in the frequency of the polymorphisms. For example, impaired hydroxylation of mephenytoin is present in only 3 to 5 percent of whites, but the incidence is about 20 percent in individuals of Japanese descent; likewise, the frequency of the PM phenotype for debrisoquin hydroxylation appears to decrease as one moves from western (8 to 10 percent) to eastern (0 to 1 percent) population groups.

Polymorphisms in drug metabolizing ability may be associated with large differences in the disposition of the drug among individuals, especially when the involved pathway is a major contribution to the overall elimination of the drug. For example, the oral clearance of mephenytoin differs 100- to 200-fold between individuals of the EM and PM phenotypes. As a result, peak plasma concentrations and bioavailability after oral administration may be profoundly increased and the rate of drug elimination decreased in PM individuals. This in turn results in drug accumulation and exaggerated pharmacologic responses, including toxicity, when usual drug dosages are administered to patients with the PM phenotype. Effective individualization of drug therapy is even more critical when using drugs exhibiting polymorphic drug metabolism.

CONCENTRATION OF DRUGS IN PLASMA AS A GUIDE TO THERAPY

Optimal individualization of therapy is assisted by measuring the concentration of certain drugs in plasma. Genetic variation in elimination rates, interactions with other drugs, disease-induced alterations in elimination and distribution, and other factors combine to yield a wide range of plasma levels in patients given the same dose. Furthermore, the problem of noncompliance with prescribed regimens during continuing therapy is an endemic and elusive cause of therapeutic failure (see below). Clinical indicators assist the titration of some drugs into the desired range, and no chemical determination is a substitute for careful observations of the response to treatment. However, the therapeutic and adverse effects are not precisely quantifiable for all drugs, and in complex clinical situations estimates of the action of a drug may be misleading. For example, previously existing neurologic disease may obscure the neurologic consequences of intoxication with phenytoin. Because clearance, half-life, accumulation, and steady state plasma levels are difficult to predict, the measurement of plasma levels is often useful as a guide to the optimal dose. This is particularly so when there is a narrow range between the plasma levels yielding therapeutic and adverse effects. For drugs having such characteristics, e.g., digoxin, theophylline, lidocaine, aminoglycosides, and anticonvulsants, numerous dosing methods have been developed in an attempt to improve the relationship between dosing, plasma drug concentration, and response. Some of these methods are accurate and useful, for example, the Bayesian feedback approach, but others are not accurate or have not been sufficiently validated. Further examination of their cost effectiveness is necessary to establish their place in routine patient care.

The variability among individual responses to given plasma levels must be recognized. This is illustrated by a hypothetical population dose-response curve (Fig. 65-5) and its relationship to the therapeutic range or therapeutic "window" of desired plasma levels. The defined therapeutic window should include the levels at which the majority of patients achieve the intended pharmacologic effect. However, a few people are sensitive to the therapeutic effects of most drugs, responding to lower levels, whereas others are sufficiently refractory as to require levels that impose the likelihood of adverse effects as a price for therapeutic benefit. For example, a few patients with strong seizure foci require plasma levels of phenytoin exceeding 20 μg/mL to control seizures. Dosages to achieve this effect may be appropriate.

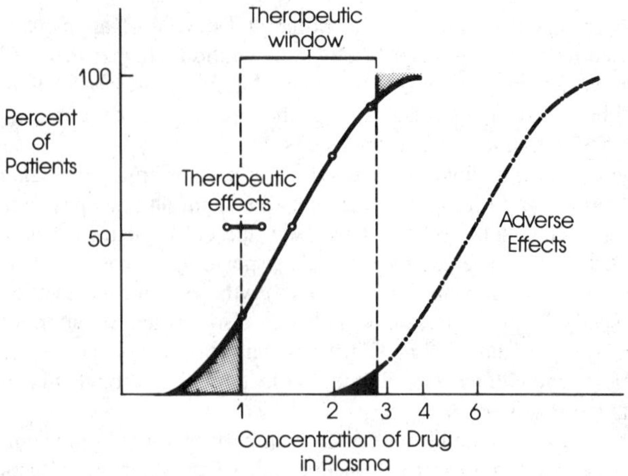

FIGURE 65-5 The cumulative percentage of patients responding to increasing levels of drug in plasma with both therapeutic and adverse effects. The therapeutic "window" defines the range of concentrations of drug that will achieve therapeutic effects in most patients with adverse effects in only a small percentage.

As also illustrated in Fig. 65-5, some patients are prone to adverse effects at levels that are tolerated by most of the population, and therefore elevation of levels to those with a high probability of therapeutic effect may bring on unwanted actions in the exceptional patient. Table 65-4 presents the concentrations of a number of drugs in plasma that are associated with adverse and therapeutic effects in most patients. Its use within the guidelines discussed should permit more effective and safer therapy for those patients who are not "average."

TABLE 65-4 Concentrations of drugs in plasma: Relation to efficacy and adverse effects

Drug	Efficacy*	Adverse effects†
Amikacin (peak)	20 μg/mL	40 μg/mL
Carbenicillin	100 μg/mL‡	300 μg/mL
Carbamazepine	3 μg/mL	10 μg/mL
Digitoxin	12 ng/mL	25–30 ng/mL
Digoxin	0.8 ng/mL	2.0 ng/mL
Ethosuximide	40 μg/mL	100 μg/mL
Gentamicin (peak)	5 μg/mL	10 μg/mL
Gentamicin (predose)		2.5 μg/mL
Lidocaine	1.5 μg/mL	5 μg/mL
Lithium	0.5 meq/liter	1.3 meq/liter
Penicillin G	1–25 μg/mL¶	
Phenytoin (diphenylhydantoin)	10 μg/mL	20 μg/mL
Procainamide	4 μg/mL	10 μg/mL
Quinidine	2.5 μg/mL	6 μg/mL
Theophylline	8 μg/mL	20 μg/mL

* The therapeutic effect is infrequent or slight at levels below these.
† The frequency of adverse effects increases sharply when these levels are exceeded.
‡ Minimal inhibitory concentration (MIC) for most strains of Pseudomonas aeruginosa. MIC for other, more sensitive, organisms is less.
§ Dependent on the MIC. Higher levels may be desired when host defenses are impaired.
¶ There is a wide range of MIC of penicillin for various organisms, and the MIC of all those for which penicillin is used is < 20. "Massive" penicillin therapy with 20 million units daily achieves levels of 20 to 25 μg/mL in patients with clearance of creatinine of 100 mL/min.

EFFECTIVE PARTICIPATION OF THE PATIENT IN THERAPEUTIC PROGRAMS Measurement of the concentration of a drug in plasma is the most effective approach to determining when patients have failed to take the drug. Such "noncompliance" is a frequent problem in the long-term treatment of diseases such as hypertension and epilepsy, occurring in 25 percent or more of patients in therapeutic environments that lack special efforts to involve patients in the responsibility for their own health. Occasionally, noncompliance can be uncovered by sympathetic, nonincriminating questioning, but more often it is recognized only after determining that the concentration of drug in plasma is nil or is recurrently low. Because other factors can cause plasma levels to be lower than expected, comparison with levels obtained during inpatient treatment may be required to confirm that noncompliance did, in fact, occur. Once the physician is certain of noncompliance, a nonaccusatory discussion of the problem with the patient may elucidate a reason for the noncompliance and serve as a basis for more effective participation of the patient in the care subsequently. Many approaches have been tried to enhance the patients' exercise of responsibility for their own treatment, most based on improved communication regarding the nature of the disease and the expectations of treatment success and treatment failure. This communication includes an opportunity for the patient to relate problems associated with treatment, and it may be improved by involving nurses and other paramedical personnel in the process. Minimizing the complexity of the regimen is helpful, both in terms of the number of drugs and the frequency of administration. Educating patients to assume the principal role in their own health care requires a blend of the art and science of medicine.

REFERENCES

BENET LZ, SHEINER LB: Design and optimization of dosage regimens: Pharmacokinetic data, in *Goodman and Gilman's The Pharmacological Basis of Therapeutics*, 7th ed. AG Gilman et al (eds). New York, Macmillan, 1985, p 1663, Appendix II.

BENNETT WM et al: *Drug Prescribing in Renal Failure. Dosing Guidelines for Adults.* Philadelphia, American College of Physicians, 1987

BURTON ME et al: Comparison of drug dosing methods. Clin Pharmacokinet 10:1, 1985

CHENNAVASIN P, BRATER DC: Nomograms for drug use in renal disease. Clin Pharmacokinet 6:193, 1981

ROWLAND M, TOZER TN: *Clinical Pharmacokinetics—Concepts and Applications*, 2d ed. Philadelphia, Lea & Febiger, 1988

SHAND DG et al: Pharmacokinetic drug interactions, in *Handbook of Experimental Pharmacology*, vol 28: *Concepts in Biochemical Pharmacology*, JR Gillette, JR Mitchell (eds). New York, Springer-Verlag, 1975, p 272

SHEINER LB, TOZER TN: Clinical pharmacokinetics: The use of plasma concentrations of drugs, in *Clinical Pharmacology: Basic Principles in Therapeutics*, 2d ed, KL Melmon, HF Morrelli (eds). New York, Macmillan, 1978, p 71

66 ADVERSE REACTIONS TO DRUGS

ALASTAIR J. J. WOOD / JOHN A. OATES

The beneficial effects of drugs are coupled with the inescapable risk of untoward effects. The morbidity and mortality from these untoward effects often present diagnostic problems because they can involve every organ and system of the body.

Major advances in the investigation, development, and regulation of drugs ensure in most instances their uniformity, effectiveness, and relative safety, as well as identify their recognized hazards. However, the large number and variety of drugs available over the counter (OTC) or by prescription make it impossible for patient or physician to obtain or retain the knowledge necessary to use all drugs well. It is understandable, therefore, that many OTC drugs are used unwisely by the public and that restricted drugs may be prescribed incorrectly by physicians.

Most physicians use no more than 50 drug products in their practice, gaining familiarity with their effectiveness and safety. Most patients probably use only a limited number of OTC drugs. Nevertheless, many patients receive care and drug prescriptions from more than one physician, and in any 30-day period patients consume more than three different OTC drug products containing nine or more different chemical agents.

Twenty-five to fifty percent of patients may make errors in self-administration of prescribed medicines, and this can be responsible for adverse drug effects. Elderly patients are most likely to commit such errors. One-third or more of patients also may not take their prescribed medications. Similarly, patients commit errors in taking OTC drugs by not reading or following the directions for use of the medicines on the containers. Physicians must recognize that providing directions with prescriptions does not always guarantee compliance.

Every drug can produce untoward consequences, even when used according to standard or recommended methods of administration. When used incorrectly, the effectiveness may be reduced, and adverse reactions can be expected to occur more frequently. The administration of several drugs during the same period of time also may result in adverse interactions between drugs (see Chap. 65).

In the hospital all drugs a patient is given should be under the control of a physician, and patient compliance is, in general, ensured. Errors may occur nevertheless, in that the wrong drug or dose may be given, or the drug may be given to the wrong patient, although improved drug distribution and administration systems have reduced this problem. On the other hand, there are no means for controlling how ambulatory patients take prescription or OTC drugs.

EPIDEMIOLOGY Epidemiologic studies of adverse drug reactions have been helpful in evaluating the magnitude of the overall problem, in calculating the rate of reactions to individual drugs, and in characterizing some of the determinants of adverse drug effects.

Patients receive on the average 10 different drugs during each hospitalization. The sicker the patient, the more drugs are given, and there is a corresponding increase in the likelihood of adverse drug reactions. When fewer than 6 different drugs are given to hospitalized patients, the probability of an adverse reaction is about 5 percent, but if more than 15 drugs are given, the probability is over 40 percent. Retrospective analyses of ambulatory patients have revealed adverse drug effects in 20 percent.

Thus, the magnitude of drug-induced disease is large. Two to five percent of patients are admitted to the medical and pediatric services of general hospitals because of illnesses attributed to drugs. The case/fatality ratio from drug-induced disease in hospitalized patients varies from 2 to 12 percent. Furthermore, some fetal or neonatal abnormalities are due to medicines taken by the mother during pregnancy or parturition.

A small group of widely used drugs account for a disproportionate number of reactions; aspirin, digoxin, anticoagulants, diuretics, antimicrobials, steroids, and hypoglycemic agents account for 90 percent of reactions.

ETIOLOGY Most adverse reactions can be classified into two groups. The most frequent result from the exaggerated but predicted pharmacologic action of the drug. Other adverse reactions ensue from toxic effects unrelated to the intended pharmacologic actions. These therefore are often unpredictable, are frequently severe, and result from recognized as well as undiscovered mechanisms. Some mechanisms of extrapharmacologic toxicity include direct cytotoxicity, initiation of abnormal immune responses, and perturbation of metabolic processes in individuals with genetic enzymatic defects.

EXAGGERATION OF THE INTENDED PHARMACOLOGIC EFFECT By prior consideration of the known factors that modify drug action, these adverse reactions often are preventable.

Abnormally high drug concentration at the receptor site (site of action) due to the pharmacokinetic variability is the usual cause (see Chap. 65). For example, reduction in the volume of distribution, in the rate of metabolism, or in the rate of excretion all result in higher than expected concentration of drug at the receptor site with consequent increase in pharmacologic effect.

Alteration in the dose-response curve due to increased receptor sensitivity results in an increase in drug effect at the same concentration. An example of this is seen in the excessive response to the anticoagulant warfarin at normal or lower than normal blood levels in the elderly.

The shape of the dose-response curve itself also determines the likelihood of the development of adverse drug reactions. Drugs with a steep dose-response curve are more likely to be associated with dose-related toxicity because of the small increase in dose required to produce a large change in pharmacologic effect. An increase in the dose of drugs which exhibit nonlinear kinetics, such as phenytoin (see previous chapter), may produce a proportionately greater increase in the blood level, resulting in toxicity.

Concomitant drug therapy may affect the pharmacokinetics or pharmacodynamics of other drugs. Pharmacokinetics may be affected by alterations in bioavailability, protein binding, or the rate of metabolism or excretion. Pharmacodynamics may be altered by competition for receptor sites, by prevention of the drug's reaching its site of action, or by antagonism or enhancement of the drug's pharmacologic effect. These subjects are discussed in detail in the previous chapter.

TOXICITY UNRELATED TO A DRUG'S PRIMARY PHARMACOLOGIC ACTIVITY **Cytotoxic reactions** The understanding of so-called idiosyncratic reactions has greatly improved with the recognition that many of these reactions are due to irreversible binding of drug or metabolites to tissue macromolecules by shared electron (covalent) bonds. Some chemical carcinogens such as the alkylating agents combine directly with DNA. Usually, it is only after metabolic activation to reactive metabolites that covalent binding occurs. This activation usually occurs in the microsomal mixed-function oxidase system, the hepatic enzyme system responsible for the metabolism of many drugs (Chap. 65). During the course of drug metabolism, reactive metabolites may covalently bind to tissue macromolecules, causing tissue damage. Because of the reactive nature of these metabolites, covalent binding often occurs close to the site of production, such as the liver, but the mixed-function oxidase system is found in other tissues as well.

An example of this type of adverse drug reaction is the hepatotoxicity associated with isoniazid, which is metabolized principally by acetylation to acetylisoniazid, which is then hydrolyzed to acetylhydrazine. The further metabolism of acetylhydrazine by the mixed-function oxidase system liberates reactive metabolites that covalently bind to hepatic macromolecules, causing hepatic necrosis. The administration of drugs known to increase the activity of the mixed-function oxidase system, such as phenobarbital or rifampin, together with isoniazid, is associated with the production of increased amounts of reactive metabolites, increased covalent binding, and hepatic damage.

The hepatic necrosis produced by overdosage of acetaminophen is also caused by reactive metabolites. Normally these metabolites are detoxified by combining with hepatic glutathione. When glutathione becomes exhausted, the metabolites bind instead to hepatic protein with resultant hepatocyte damage. The hepatic necrosis produced by the ingestion of acetaminophen can be prevented, or at least attenuated, by the administration of substances such as *N*-acetylcysteine, which reduce the binding of electrophilic metabolites to hepatic proteins. The risks of hepatic necrosis are increased in patients receiving drugs such as phenobarbital that increase the rate of drug metabolism and rate of production of toxic metabolite(s).

It is likely, though as yet unproved, that other idiosyncratic reactions are caused by the covalent binding of reactive metabolites to tissue macromolecules, with either direct cytotoxicity or via the initiation of an immunologic response.

Immunologic mechanisms Most pharmacologic agents are poor immunogens since they consist of small molecules with molecular weights less than 2000. Stimulation of antibody synthesis or sensitization of lymphocytes by a drug or one of its metabolites usually requires in vivo activation and covalent linkage to protein, carbohydrate, or nucleic acid.

Drug stimulation of antibody production may mediate tissue injury by one of several mechanisms. The antibody may attack the drug affixed to a cell by covalent linkage and thereby destroy the cell, as occurs in penicillin-induced hemolytic anemia. Complexes of antibody-drug-antigen may be passively adsorbed by a bystander cell which is destroyed by activation of complement; this occurs in quinine- and quinidine-induced thrombocytopenia. Drugs or their reactive metabolites may alter host tissue, rendering it antigenic, and stimulate autoantibodies; for example, hydralazine and procainamide can chemically alter nuclear material, stimulate formation of antinuclear antibodies, and occasionally cause lupus erythematosus. Autoantibodies may be stimulated by drugs which neither interact with the host antigen nor have any chemical similarity to the host tissue; for example, alpha methyldopa frequently stimulates formation of antibodies to host erythrocytes, yet the drug does not itself attach to the erythrocyte or share any chemical similarities with the antigenic determinants on the erythrocyte.

Drug-induced *pure red cell aplasia* (Chap. 298) is due to an immunologic-based drug reaction. Red cell formation in bone marrow cultures can be inhibited by phenytoin and purified IgG obtained from a patient with pure red cell aplasia associated with phenytoin.

Serum sickness (Chap. 267) results from deposition of circulating drug-antibody complexes on endothelial surfaces. Complement activation occurs, chemotactic factors are generated locally, and an inflammatory response appears at the site of complex entrapment. Arthralgias, urticaria, lymphadenopathy, glomerulonephritis, or cerebritis may result. Penicillin is the most common cause of serum sickness today. Many drugs, particularly the antimicrobial agents, induce production of IgE, which affixes to mast cell membranes. Contact with a drug antigen initiates a series of biochemical events within the mast cell and results in the release of mediators that may produce urticaria, wheezing, flushing, rhinorrhea, and occasionally hypotension characteristic of anaphylaxis.

Drugs may also excite cell-mediated immune responses. Topically administered substances may interact with sulfhydryl or amino groups in the skin and react with sensitized lymphocytes to produce the rash characteristic of contact dermatitis. Other types of rashes may also appear from the interaction of serum factors, drugs, and sensitized lymphocytes. The role of drug-activated lymphocytes in the immune mechanisms governing destruction of visceral tissue is unknown.

Toxicity associated with genetically determined enzymatic defects In the porphyrias, drugs that increase the activity of enzymes proximal to the deficient enzyme in the biosynthetic pathway of porphyrins can increase the quantity of porphyrin precursors that accumulate proximal to the deficient enzyme (Chap. 328). These drugs are listed in Table 66-1.

Patients with a deficiency of glucose-6-phosphate dehydrogenase (G6PD) develop hemolytic anemia on primaquine and a number of other drugs (Table 66-1) that do not cause hemolysis in patients with adequate quantities of this enzyme (Chap. 294).

Diagnosis The manifestations of drug-induced diseases frequently resemble those of other diseases and may be produced by different and dissimilar drugs. Recognition of the role of a drug or drugs responsible for illness is dependent upon appreciation of the possible adverse reactions to drugs in any disease, identification of a temporal relationship between drug administration and development of illness, and familiarity with the manifestations most often caused by particular drugs. Although specific reactions have been described as resulting from the use of particular drugs, there is always a "first," and any drug should be suspected of causing an adverse effect if the clinical setting is appropriate.

Illness related to a drug's pharmacologic action may be more easily recognized than illness attributable to immunologic or other mechanisms. For example, side effects such as cardiac arrhythmias in patients receiving digitalis, hypoglycemia in patients given insulin, and bleeding in patients receiving anticoagulants are more easily related to the drug than are symptoms like fever or rash, which may be caused by many drugs or by other factors.

TABLE 66-1 Clinical manifestations of adverse reactions to drugs

I MULTISYSTEM MANIFESTATIONS

Anaphylaxis
- Cephalosporins
- Demeclocycline
- Dextran
- Insulin
- Iodinated drugs or contrast media
- Iron dextran
- Lidocaine
- Penicillins
- Procaine
- Streptomycin
- Sulfobromophthalein

Angioedema
- Captopril
- Enalapril
- Lisinopril

Drug-induced lupus erythematosus
- Acebutolol
- Asparaginase
- Barbiturates
- Bleomycin
- Cephalosporins
- Hydralazine
- Iodides
- Isoniazid
- Methyldopa
- Phenolphthalein
- Phenytoin
- Procainamide
- Quinidine
- Sulfonamides
- Thiouracil

Fever
- Aminosalicylic acid
- Amphotericin B
- Antihistamines
- Novobiocin
- Penicillins

Hyperpyrexia
- Antipsychotics

Serum sickness
- Aspirin
- Penicillins
- Propylthiouracil
- Streptomycin
- Sulfonamides

II ENDOCRINE MANIFESTATIONS

Addisonian-like syndrome
- Busulfan
- Ketoconazole

Galactorrhea (may also cause amenorrhea)
- Methyldopa
- Phenothiazines
- Reserpine
- Tricyclic antidepressants

Gynecomastia
- Calcium channel antagonists
- Digitalis
- Estrogens
- Ethionamide
- Griseofulvin
- Isoniazid
- Methyldopa
- Phenytoin
- Reserpine
- Spironolactone
- Testosterone

Sexual dysfunction

1 Impaired ejaculation:
- Bethanidine
- Debrisoquin
- Guanethidine
- Thioridazine

2 Decreased libido and impotence:
- Beta blockers
- Clonidine
- Diuretics
- Lithium
- Major tranquilizers
- Methyldopa
- Oral contraceptives
- Sedatives

3 Impairment of spermatogenesis or oogenesis:
- Cytotoxics

4 Priapism:
- Trazodone

Thyroid function tests, disorders of
- Acetazolamide
- Amiodarone
- Bromsulfophthalein
- Chlorpropamide
- Clofibrate
- Colestipol and nicotinic acid
- Dimercaprol
- Gold salts
- Iodides
- Lithium
- Oral contraceptives
- Phenindione
- Phenothiazines (long-term)
- Phenylbutazone
- Phenytoin
- Sulfonamides
- Tolbutamide

Vaginal carcinoma
- Diethylstilbestrol (given to mother)

III METABOLIC MANIFESTATIONS

Hyperbilirubinemia
- Novobiocin
- Rifampin

Hypercalcemia
- Antacids with absorbable alkali
- Thiazides
- Vitamin D

Hyperglycemia
- Chlorthalidone
- Diazoxide
- Encainide
- Ethacrynic acid
- Furosemide
- Glucocorticoids
- Growth hormone
- Oral contraceptives
- Thiazides

Hypoglycemia
- Insulin
- Oral hypoglycemics
- Quinine

Hyperkalemia
- Angiotensin converting enzyme inhibitors
- Amiloride
- Cytotoxics
- Digitalis overdose
- Heparin
- Lithium
- Potassium preparations including salt substitute
- Potassium salts of drugs
- Spironolactone
- Succinylcholine
- Triamterene

Hypokalemia
- Alkali-induced alkalosis
- Amphotericin B
- Carbenoxolone
- Corticosteroids
- Diuretics
- Gentamicin
- Insulin
- Laxative abuse
- Mineralocorticoids, some glucocorticoids
- Osmotic diuretics
- Sympathomimetics
- Tetracycline (degraded)
- Theophylline
- Vitamin B_{12}

Hyperuricemia
- Aspirin
- Chlorthalidone
- Cytotoxics
- Ethacrynic acid
- Fructose (IV)
- Furosemide
- Hyperalimentation
- Thiazides

Hyponatremia

1 Dilutional:
- Carbamazepine
- Chlorpropamide
- Cyclophosphamide
- Diuretics
- Octreotide
- Vincristine

2 Salt wasting:
- Diuretics
- Enemas
- Mannitol

Metabolic acidosis
- Acetazolamide
- Paraldehyde (degraded)
- Phenformin
- Salicylates
- Spironolactone

Porphyria exacerbation
- Barbiturates
- Chlordiazepoxide
- Chlorpropamide
- Estrogens
- Glutethimide
- Griseofulvin
- Meprobamate
- Oral contraceptives
- Phenytoin
- Rifampin
- Sulfonamides

(continued)

TABLE 66-1 Clinical manifestations of adverse reactions to drugs *(continued)*

IV DERMATOLOGIC MANIFESTATIONS

- Acne
  - Anabolic and androgenic steroids
  - Bromides
  - Glucocorticoids
  - Iodides
  - Isoniazid
  - Oral contraceptives
  - Troxidone
- Alopecia
  - Cytotoxics
  - Ethionamide
  - Heparin
  - Oral contraceptives (withdrawal)
- Eczema
  - Captopril
  - Cream and lotion preservatives
  - Lanolin
  - Topical antihistamines
  - Topical antimicrobials
  - Topical local anesthetics
- Erythema multiforme or Steven-Johnson syndrome
  - Barbiturates
  - Chlorpropamide
  - Codeine
  - Ethosuximide
  - Penicillins
  - Phenylbutazone
  - Phenytoin
  - Salicylates
  - Sulfonamides
  - Sulfones
  - Tetracyclines
  - Thiazides
- Erythema nodosum
  - Oral contraceptives
  - Penicillins
  - Sulfonamides
- Exfoliative dermatitis
  - Barbiturates
  - Gold salts
  - Penicillins
  - Phenylbutazone
  - Phenytoin
  - Quinidine
  - Sulfonamides
- Fixed drug eruptions
  - Barbiturates
  - Captopril
  - Phenolphthalein
  - Phenylbutazone
  - Quinine
  - Salicylates
  - Sulfonamides
- Hyperpigmentation
  - Bleomycin
  - Busulfan
  - Chloroquine and other antimalarials
  - Corticotropin
  - Cyclophosphamide
  - Gold salts
  - Hypervitaminosis A
  - Oral contraceptives
  - Phenothiazines
- Lichenoid eruptions
  - Aminosalicylic acid
  - Antimalarials
  - Chlorpropamide
  - Gold salts
  - Methyldopa
  - Phenothiazines
- Photodermatitis
  - Captopril
  - Chlordiazepoxide
  - Furosemide
  - Griseofulvin
  - Nalidixic acid
  - Oral contraceptives
  - Phenothiazines
  - Sulfonamides
  - Sulfonylureas
  - Tetracyclines, particularly demeclocycline
  - Thiazides
- Purpura (see also thrombocytopenia)
  - Aspirin
  - Glucocorticoids
- Rashes (nonspecific)
  - Allopurinol
  - Ampicillin
  - Barbiturates
  - Indapamide
  - Methyldopa
  - Phenytoin
- Skin necrosis
  - Warfarin
- Toxic epidermal necrolysis (bullous)
  - Allopurinol
  - Barbiturates
  - Bromides
  - Iodides
  - Nalidixic acid
  - Penicillins
  - Phenolphthalein
  - Phenylbutazone
  - Phenytoin
  - Sulfonamides
- Urticaria
  - Aspirin
  - Barbiturates
  - Captopril
  - Enalapril
  - Penicillins
  - Sulfonamides

V HEMATOLOGIC MANIFESTATIONS

- Agranulocytosis (see also pancytopenia)
  - Aprindine
  - Captopril
  - Carbimazole
  - Chloramphenicol
  - Cotrimoxazole
  - Cytotoxics
  - Gold salts
  - Indomethacin
  - Methimazole
  - Oxyphenbutazone
  - Phenothiazines
  - Phenylbutazone
  - Propylthiouracil
  - Sulfonamides
  - Tolbutamide
  - Tricyclic antidepressants
- Clotting abnormalities/Hypothrombinemia
  - Cefamandole
  - Cefoperazone
  - Moxalactam
- Eosinophilia
  - Aminosalicylic acid
  - Chlorpropamide
  - Erythromycin estolate
  - Imipramine
  - l-Tryptophan
  - Methotrexate
  - Nitrofurantoin
  - Procarbazine
  - Sulfonamides
- Hemolytic anemia
  - Aminosalicylic acid
  - Cephalosporins
  - Chlorpromazine
  - Dapsone
  - Insulin
  - Isoniazid
  - Levodopa
  - Mefenamic acid
  - Melphalan
  - Methyldopa
  - Penicillins
  - Phenacetin
  - Procainamide
  - Quinidine
  - Rifampin
  - Sulfonamides
- Hemolytic anemia (in G6PD deficiency)
  - Aminosalicylic acid
  - Antimalarials, e.g., primaquine
  - Aspirin
  - Chloramphenicol
  - Cotrimoxazole
  - Dapsone
  - Nalidixic acid
  - Nitrofurantoin
  - Phenacetin
  - Probenecid
  - Procainamide
  - Quinidine
  - Sulfonamides
  - Vitamin C
  - Vitamin K
- Leukocytosis
  - Glucocorticoids
  - Lithium
- Lymphadenopathy
  - Phenytoin
  - Primidone
- Megaloblastic anemia
  - Cotrimoxazole
  - Folate antagonists
  - Nitrous oxide (repeated or prolonged exposure)
  - Oral contraceptives
  - Phenobarbital
  - Phenytoin
  - Primidone
  - Triamterene
  - Trimethoprim
- Pancytopenia (aplastic anemia)
  - Carbamazepine
  - Chloramphenicol
  - Cytotoxics
  - Gold salts
  - Mepacrine
  - Mephenytoin
  - Oxyphenbutazone
  - Phenylbutazone
  - Phenytoin
  - Potassium perchlorate
  - Quinacrine
  - Sulfonamides
  - Trimethadione
  - Zidovudine (AZT)
- Pure red cell aplasia
  - Azathioprine
  - Chlorpropamide
  - Isoniazid
  - Phenytoin
- Thrombocytopenia (see also pancytopenia)
  - Acetazolamine
  - Aspirin
  - Carbamazepine
  - Carbenacillin
  - Carbenicillin
  - Chlorpropamide
  - Chlorthalidone
  - Cotrimoxazole
  - Digitoxin
  - Furosemide
  - Gold salts
  - Heparin
  - Indomethacin
  - Isoniazid
  - Methyldopa
  - Moxalactam
  - Novobiocin
  - Oxyphenbutazone
  - Phenylbutazone
  - Phenytoin and other hydantoins
  - Quinidine
  - Quinine
  - Thiazides
  - Ticarcillin

(continued)

Once an adverse reaction is suspected, discontinuance of the suspected drug followed by disappearance of the reaction is presumptive evidence of a drug-induced illness. Reappearance of the reaction upon cautious readministration of the drug may provide confirmatory evidence of the relationship if such confirmation adds useful information to the future management of the patient without entailing undue risk. With concentration-dependent adverse reactions, lowering the dosage may also be followed by disappearance of the reaction, and increasing the dose may cause it to reappear. When the reaction is thought to be allergic, however, readministration

TABLE 66-1 Clinical manifestations of adverse reactions to drugs *(continued)*

VI CARDIOVASCULAR MANIFESTATIONS

- Acute chest pain (nonischemic)
  - Bleomycin
- Angina exacerbation
  - Alpha blockers
  - Ergotamine
  - Excessive thyroxine
  - Hydralazine
  - Methysergide
  - Minoxidil
  - Nifedipine
  - Oxytocin
  - Propranolol withdrawal
  - Vasopressin
- Arrhythmias
  - Adriamycin
  - Antiarrhythmic drugs
  - Atropine
  - Anticholinesterases
  - Beta blockers
  - Daunomycin
  - Digitalis
  - Emetine
  - Guanethidine
  - Lithium
  - Papaverine
  - Phenothiazines, particularly thioridazine
  - Sympathomimetics
  - Thyroid hormone
  - Tricyclic antidepressants
  - Verapamil
- AV block
  - Clonidine
  - Methylclopa
  - Verapamil
- Cardiomyopathy
  - Adriamycin
  - Daunorubicin
  - Emetine
  - Lithium
  - Phenothiazines
  - Sulfonamides
  - Sympathomimetics
- Fluid retention or congestive heart failure
  - Carbenoxolone
  - Diazoxide
  - Estrogens
  - Indomethacin
  - Mannitol
  - Minoxidil
  - Phenylbutazone
  - Propranolol
  - Steroids
  - Verapamil
- Hypotension (see also arrhythmias)
  - Calcium channel blockers, e.g., nifedipine
  - Citrated blood
  - Diuretics
  - Levodopa
  - Morphine
  - Nitroglycerin
  - Phenothiazines
  - Protamine
  - Quinidine
- Hypertension
  - Clonidine withdrawal
  - Corticotropin
  - Cyclosporine
  - Glucocorticoids
  - Monoamine oxidase inhibitors with sympathomimetics
  - NSAIDs (some)
  - Oral contraceptives
  - Sympathomimetics
  - Tricyclic antidepressants with sympathomimetics
- Pericarditis
  - Emetine
  - Hydralazine
  - Methysergide
  - Procainamide
- Thromboembolism
  - Oral contraceptives

VII RESPIRATORY MANIFESTATIONS

- Airway obstruction (bronchospasm, asthma; see also anaphylaxis)
  - Beta blockers
  - Cephalosporins
  - Cholinergic drugs
  - Nonsteroidal anti-inflammatory drugs, e.g., aspirin, indomethacin
  - Penicillins
  - Pentazocine
  - Streptomycin
  - Tartrazine (drugs with yellow dye)
- Cough
  - Angiotensin-converting enzyme inhibitors
- Nasal congestion
  - Decongestant abuse
  - Guanethidine
  - Isoproterenol
  - Oral contraceptives
  - Reserpine
- Pulmonary edema
  - Contrast media
  - Heroin
  - Hydrochlorthiazide
  - Methadone
  - Propoxyphene
- Pulmonary infiltrates
  - Amiodarone
  - Azothioprine
  - Bleomycin
  - Busulfan
  - Carmustine (BCNU)
  - Chlorambucil
  - Cyclophosphamide
  - Melphalan
  - Methotrexate
  - Methysergide
  - Mitomycin C
  - Nitrofurantoin
  - Procarbazine
  - Sulfonamides
- Respiratory depression
  - Aminoglycosides
  - Hypnotics
  - Opiates
  - Polymyxins
  - Sedatives
  - Trimethaphan

(continued)

of the drug may be hazardous, since anaphylactic shock may develop. Readministration is unwise under these conditions unless alternative drugs are not available and treatment is mandatory.

If the patient is receiving many different drugs when an adverse reaction is suspected, the drugs most likely to be incriminated can usually be identified. All drugs may be discontinued at once, or if this is not practical, then drugs should be discontinued one at a time, starting with the drug under greatest suspicion, and the patient observed for signs of improvement. The time taken for the disappearance of a concentration-dependent adverse effect depends on the time for the concentration to fall below the range associated with the adverse effect, and this in turn depends on the initial blood level and on the rate of elimination or metabolism of the drug. Adverse effects of drugs with long half-lives, such as phenobarbital, take a considerable time to disappear.

Drugs recognized as producing a number of reactions are listed in Table 66-1. This table includes well-documented and some less well-documented reactions that are sufficiently devastating as to require consideration. It should be used to suggest the likely causative drug, but the absence of a drug from the table does not mean that it is not responsible for the reaction.

Serum antibody has been demonstrated in some persons with drug allergy involving cellular blood elements, as in agranulocytosis, hemolytic anemia, and thrombocytopenia. For example, both quinine and quinidine can produce platelet agglutination in vitro in the presence of complement and the serum from a patient who has developed thrombocytopenia following this drug.

Eliciting a drug history from patients is important for diagnosis. Attention must be directed to nonprescription, or OTC, as well as to prescription drugs. Each type can be responsible for adverse drug effects, and adverse interactions may occur between OTC drugs and prescribed drugs. In addition, it is common for patients to be cared for by several physicians, and duplicative, additive, counteractive, or synergistic drugs may therefore be taken if the physicians are not aware of the patients' drug histories. Every physician should determine what drugs a patient has been taking, at least during the preceding 30 days, before prescribing any medications. A history of previous adverse drug effects in patients is common. Since these patients have a predisposition to other drug-induced illnesses, eliciting such a history should dictate added caution in prescribing drugs.

Patients with biochemical abnormalities such as erythrocyte G6PD deficiency can be identified; patients with the defect are usually blacks or of Mediterranean descent. Drug-induced hemolytic crisis can be avoided by testing for the enzyme defect before administering these

TABLE 66-1 Clinical manifestations of adverse reactions to drugs *(continued)*

VIII GASTROINTESTINAL MANIFESTATIONS

- Cholestatic jaundice
  - Acetohexamide
  - Anabolic steroids
  - Androgens
  - Chlorpropamide
  - Erythromycin estolate
  - Gold salts
  - Methimazole
  - Nitrofurantoin
  - Oral contraceptives
  - Phenothiazines
- Constipation or ileus
  - Aluminum hydroxide
  - Barium sulfate
  - Calcium carbonate
  - Ferrous sulfate
  - Ganglionic blockers
  - Ion exchange resins
  - Opiates
  - Phenothiazines
  - Tricyclic antidepressants
  - Verapamil
- Diarrhea or colitis
  - Antibiotics (broad-spectrum)
  - Clindamycin
  - Colchicine
  - Digitalis
  - Guanethidine
  - Lactose excipients
  - Lincomycin
  - Magnesium in antacids
  - Methyldopa
  - Purgatives
  - Reserpine
- Diffuse hepatocellular damage
  - Acetaminophen (paracetamol)
  - Allopurinol
  - Aminosalicylic acid
  - Aprindine
  - Dapsone
  - Erythromycin estolate
  - Ethionamide
  - Glyburide
  - Halothane
  - Isoniazid
  - Ketoconazole
  - Methimazole
  - Methotrexate
  - Methoxyflurane
  - Methyldopa
  - Monoamine oxidase inhibitors
  - Niacin
  - Nifedipine
  - Nitrofurantoin
  - Oxyphenisatin
  - Phenytoin and other hydantoins
  - Propoxyphene
  - Propylthiouracil
  - Pyridium
  - Rifampin
  - Salicylates
  - Sodium valproate
  - Sulfonamides
  - Tetracyclines
  - Verapamil
  - Zidovudine (AZT)
- Intestinal ulceration
  - Solid KCl preparations
- Malabsorption
  - Aminosalicylic acid
  - Antibiotics (broad-spectrum)
  - Cholestyramine
  - Colchicine
  - Colestipol
  - Cytotoxics
  - Neomycin
  - Phenobarbital
  - Phenytoin
  - Primidone
- Nausea or vomiting
  - Digitalis
  - Estrogens
  - Ferrous sulfate
  - Levodopa
  - Opiates
  - Potassium chloride
  - Tetracyclines
  - Theophylline
- Oral conditions
  - *1* Dental discoloration:
    - Tetracycline
  - *2* Drymouth:
    - Anticholinergics
    - Clonidine
    - Levodopa
    - Methyldopa
    - Tricyclic antidepressants
  - *3* Gingival hyperplasia:
    - Calcium antagonists
    - Cyclosporine
    - Phenytoin
  - *4* Salivary gland swelling:
    - Bethanidine
    - Bretylium
    - Clonidine
    - Guanethidine
    - Iodides
    - Phenylbutazone
  - *5* Taste disturbances:
    - Biguanides
    - Captopril
    - Griseofulvin
    - Lithium
    - Metronidazole
    - Penicillamine
    - Rifampin
  - *6* Ulceration:
    - Aspirin
    - Cytotoxics
    - Gentian violet
    - Isoproterenol (sublingual)
    - Pancreatin
- Pancreatitis
  - Azathioprine
  - Ethacrynic acid
  - Furosemide
  - Glucocorticoids
  - Opiates
  - Oral contraceptives
  - Sulfonamides
  - Thiazides
- Peptic ulceration or hemorrhage
  - Aspirin
  - Ethacrynic acid
  - Glucocorticoids
  - NSAIDs
  - Reserpine (large doses)

IX RENAL MANIFESTATIONS

- Bladder dysfunction
  - Anticholinergics
  - Disopyramide
  - Monoamine oxidase inhibitors
  - Tricyclic antidepressants
- Calculi
  - Acetazolamide
  - Vitamin D
- Concentrating defect with polyuria (or nephrogenic diabetes insipidus)
  - Demeclocycline
  - Lithium
  - Methoxyflurane
  - Vitamin D
- Hemorrhage cystitis
  - Cyclophosphamide
- Interstitial nephritis
  - Allopurinol
  - Furosemide
  - Penicillins, esp. methicillin
  - Phenindione
  - Sulfonamides
  - Thiazides
- Nephropathies
  - Due to analgesics (e.g., phenacetin)
- Nephrotic syndrome
  - Captopril
  - Gold salts
  - Penicillamine
  - Phenindione
  - Probenecid
- Obstructive uropathy
  - Extrarenal: methysergide
  - Intrarenal: cytotoxics
- Renal dysfunction
  - Cyclosporine
  - NSAIDs
  - Triamterene
- Renal tubular acidosis
  - Acetazolamide
  - Amphotericin B
  - Degraded tetracycline
- Tubular necrosis
  - Aminoglycosides
  - Amphotericin B
  - Cephaloridine
  - Colistin
  - Cyclosporin
  - Methoxyflurane
  - Polymyxins
  - Radioiodinated contrast medium
  - Sulfonamides
  - Tetracyclines

X NEUROLOGIC MANIFESTATIONS

- Exacerbation of myasthenia
  - Aminoglycosides
  - Polymyxins
- Extrapyramidal effects
  - Butyrophenones, e.g., haloperidol
  - Levodopa
  - Methyldopa
  - Metoclopramide
  - Oral contraceptives
  - Phenothiazines
  - Reserpine
  - Tricyclic antidepressants
- Headache
  - Bromides
  - Ergotamine (withdrawal)
  - Glyceryl trinitrate
  - Hydralazine
  - Indomethacin
- Peripheral neuropathy
  - Amiodarone
  - Chloramphenicol
  - Chloroquine
  - Chlorpropamide
  - Clioquinol
  - Clofibrate
  - Demeclocycline
  - Disopyramide
  - Ethambutol
  - Ethionamide
  - Glutethimide
  - Hydralazine
  - Isoniazid
  - Methysergide
  - Metronidazole
  - Mustine
  - Nalidixic acid
  - Nitrofurantoin
- Peripheral neuropathy (*cont.*)
  - Perhexiline
  - Phenelzine
  - Phenytoin
  - Polymyxin, colistin
  - Procarbazine
  - Streptomycin
  - Tolbutamide
  - Tricyclic antidepressants
  - Vincristine
- Pseudotumor cerebri (or intracranial hypertension)
  - Amiodarone
  - Glucocorticoids, mineralocorticoids
  - Hypervitaminosis A
  - Oral contraceptives
  - Tetracyclines
- Seizures
  - Amphetamines
  - Analeptics
  - Imipenem
  - Isoniazid
  - Lidocaine
  - Lithium
  - Nalidixic acid
  - Penicillins
  - Phenothiazines
  - Physostigmine
  - Theophylline
  - Tricyclic antidepressants
  - Vincristine
- Stroke
  - Oral contraceptives

(continued)

TABLE 66-1 Clinical manifestations of adverse reactions to drugs *(continued)*

XI OCULAR MANIFESTATIONS

- Cataracts
  - Busulfan
  - Chlorambucil
  - Glucocorticoids
  - Phenothiazines
- Color vision alteration
  - Barbiturates
  - Digitalis
  - Methaqualone
  - Streptomycin
  - Sulfonamides
  - Thiazides
  - Troxidone
- Corneal edema
  - Oral contraceptives
- Corneal opacities
  - Chloroquine
  - Indomethacin
  - Mepacrine
  - Vitamin D
- Glaucoma
  - Mydriatics
  - Sympathomimetics
- Optic neuritis
  - Aminosalicylic acid
  - Chloramphenicol
  - Clioquinol
  - Ethambutol
  - Isoniazid
  - Penicillamine
  - Phenothiazines
  - Phenylbutazone
  - Quinine
  - Streptomycin
- Retinopathy
  - Chloroquine
  - Phenothiazines

XII EAR MANIFESTATIONS

- Deafness
  - Aminoglycosides
  - Aspirin
  - Bleomycin
  - Chloroquine
  - Erythromycin
  - Ethacrynic acid
  - Furosemide
  - Mustine
  - Nortriptyline
  - Quinine
- Vestibular disorders
  - Aminoglycosides
  - Mustine
  - Quinine

XIII MUSCULOSKELETAL MANIFESTATIONS

- Bone disorders
  - *1* Osteoporosis:
    - Glucocorticoids
    - Heparin
  - *2* Osteomalacia:
    - Aluminum hydroxide
    - Anticonvulsants
    - Glutethimide
- Myopathy or myalgia
  - Amphotericin B
  - Carbenoxolone
  - Chloroquine
  - Clofibrate
  - Glucocorticoids
  - Oral contraceptives
- Myositis
  - Lovastatin

XIV PSYCHIATRIC MANIFESTATIONS

- Delirious or confusional states
  - Amantadine
  - Aminophylline
  - Anticholinergics
  - Antidepressants
  - Bromides
  - Cimetidine
  - Digitalis
  - Glucocorticoids
  - Isoniazid
  - Levodopa
  - Methyldopa
  - Penicillins
  - Phenothiazines
  - Sedatives and hypnotics
- Depression
  - Amphetamine withdrawal
  - Beta blockers
  - Centrally acting antihypertensives (reserpine, methyldopa, clonidine)
  - Glucocorticoids
  - Levodopa
- Drowsiness
  - Antihistamines
  - Anxiolytic drugs
  - Clonidine
  - Major tranquilizers
  - Methyldopa
  - Reserpine
  - Tricyclic antidepressants
- Hallucinatory states
  - Amantadine
  - Beta blockers
  - Levodopa
  - Meperidine
  - Narcotics
  - Pentazocine
  - Tricyclic antidepressants
- Hypomania, mania, or excited reactions
  - Glucocorticoids
  - Levodopa
  - MAO inhibitors
  - Sympathomimetics
  - Tricyclic antidepressants
- Schizophrenic-like or paranoid reactions
  - Amphetamines
  - Bromides
  - Corticosteroids
  - Levodopa
  - Lysergic acid
  - Monoamine oxidase inhibitors
  - Tricyclic antidepressants
- Sleep disturbances
  - Anorexiants
  - Levodopa
  - Monoamine oxidase inhibitors
  - Sympathomimetics

drugs. Similarly, persons with an abnormal serum pseudocholinesterase may have abnormally prolonged apnea when given succinylcholine.

General comments No drug is completely without side effects, and a side effect in one patient may be the desired pharmacologic effect in another. Current drug regulations allow physicians to prescribe drugs with considerable confidence in their purity, bioavailability, and effectiveness. However, physicians have to weigh the potential toxicity against the possible benefits. Thus toxicity that would be acceptable for an effective antineoplastic agent would not be permitted in an oral contraceptive. Because of the necessarily small number of patients treated in premarketing studies, rare adverse reactions cannot be identified, so that the first responsibility for identifying and reporting these effects must rest with the practicing clinician through the use of the various national adverse reaction reporting systems, such as those operated by the Food and Drug Administration in the United States and the Committee on Safety of Medicines in Great Britain. The publication of a newly recognized adverse reaction can in a short time stimulate many similar such reports of reactions that previously had gone unrecognized.

The prevention of adverse drug reactions first involves a high index of suspicion that the development of a new symptom or sign may be drug-related. Reduction of the dose or discontinuation of the suspected agent usually clarifies the position in concentration-dependent toxic reactions. Physicians should be familiar with the common adverse effects of the drugs they use and, if they are in doubt, should consult the literature.

REFERENCES

Davies DM: *Textbook of Adverse Drug Reactions,* 3d ed. New York, Oxford University Press, 1985

Dessypris EN et al: Diphenylhydantoin-induced pure red cell aplasia. Blood 65:789, 1985

Goldstein RA: Drug allergy: Prevention, diagnosis, and treatment. Ann Intern Med 100:302, 1984

Rossi AC, Knatt D: Discovery of new adverse drug reactions. JAMA 252:1030, 1984

Steel K et al: Iatrogenic illness on a general medical service at a university hospital. N Engl J Med 304:398, 1981

Timbrell JA: Drug hepatotoxicity. Br J Clin Pharmacol 15:3, 1983

67 PHYSIOLOGY AND PHARMACOLOGY OF THE AUTONOMIC NERVOUS SYSTEM

LEWIS LANDSBERG / JAMES B. YOUNG

FUNCTIONAL ORGANIZATION OF THE AUTONOMIC NERVOUS SYSTEM

The autonomic nervous system innervates vascular and visceral smooth muscle, exocrine and endocrine glands, and parenchymal cells throughout the various organ systems. Functioning below the conscious level, the autonomic nervous system responds rapidly and continuously to perturbations that threaten the constancy of the internal environment. The many functions governed by this system include the distribution of blood flow and the maintenance of tissue perfusion, the regulation of blood pressure, the regulation of the volume and composition of the extracellular fluid, the expenditure of metabolic energy and supply of substrate, and the control of visceral smooth muscle and glands.

Autonomic responses, like those of the somatic nervous system, are induced promptly and dissipated quickly, in contrast to the slower, more prolonged effects of circulating hormones. The autonomic nervous system, like the endocrine system, regulates the rate of processes that have intrinsic activities of their own, while the somatic nervous system initiates responses de novo. Although certain autonomic responses are discriminating, many are generalized and influence a variety of effectors in different organs. The interface between the autonomic nervous system and the endocrine system is exemplified by the adrenal medulla. This gland, homologous in many respects with the postganglionic sympathetic neuron, secretes a hormone (epinephrine) into the circulation to interact with adrenergic receptors throughout the body.

ANATOMIC ORGANIZATION The autonomic neurons, located in ganglia outside the central nervous system, give rise to the postganglionic autonomic nerves that innervate organs and tissues throughout the body. The activity of autonomic nerves is regulated by central neurons responsive to diverse afferent inputs. After central integration of afferent information, autonomic outflow is adjusted to permit the functioning of the major organ systems in accordance with the needs of the organism as a whole. Connections between the cerebral cortex and the autonomic centers in the brainstem coordinate autonomic outflow with higher mental functions.

The sympathetic and parasympathetic divisions The preganglionic neurons of the parasympathetic nervous system leave the central nervous system in the third, seventh, ninth, and tenth cranial nerves and in the second and third sacral nerves, while the preganglionic neurons of the sympathetic nervous system exit the spinal cord between the first thoracic and the second lumbar segments. Responses to sympathetic and parasympathetic stimulation are frequently antagonistic, as exemplified by their opposing effects on heart rate and gut motility. This antagonism reflects highly coordinated interactions within the central nervous system; the resultant changes in parasympathetic and sympathetic activity, often reciprocal, provide more precise control of autonomic responses than could be achieved by the modulation of a single system.

Neurotransmitters *Acetylcholine* (ACh) is the preganglionic neurotransmitter for both divisions of the autonomic nervous system, as well as the postganglionic neurotransmitter of the parasympathetic neurons. Nerves that release ACh are said to be cholinergic. *Norepinephrine* (NE) is the neurotransmitter of the postganglionic sympathetic neurons; these nerves are said to be adrenergic. Within the sympathetic outflow postganglionic neurons innervating the eccrine sweat glands (and perhaps some blood vessels supplying skeletal muscle) are of the cholinergic type.

THE SYMPATHETIC NERVOUS SYSTEM AND THE ADRENAL MEDULLA

CATECHOLAMINES All three of the naturally occurring catecholamines, NE, *epinephrine* (E), and *dopamine*, function as neurotransmitters within the central nervous system. NE, the neurotransmitter of postganglionic sympathetic nerve endings, exerts its effects locally, in the immediate vicinity of its release. E, the circulating hormone of the adrenal medulla, influences processes throughout the body. A peripheral dopaminergic system also exists but has not been characterized in detail.

Biosynthesis (Fig. 67-1) Catecholamines are synthesized from the amino acid tyrosine, which is sequentially hydroxylated to form dihydroxyphenylalanine (dopa), decarboxylated to form dopamine, and hydroxylated on the beta position of the side chain to form NE. The initial step, the hydroxylation of tyrosine, is rate-limiting and is regulated so that synthesis of dopa is coupled to norepinephrine release. This regulation is achieved by alterations in both the activity and the amount of tyrosine hydroxylase. In the adrenal medulla and in those central neurons utilizing E as neurotransmitter, NE is *N*-methylated to E by the enzyme phenylethanolamine-*N*-methyltransferase (PNMT). A major portion of the blood perfusing the adrenal medulla is enriched with glucocorticoids from the adrenal cortex, and since adrenal PNMT is inducible by glucocorticoids, the capacity of the adrenal medulla to form E may be related to its strategic location within the adrenal cortex.

Catecholamine metabolism (Fig. 67-1) The major metabolic transformations of catecholamines involve *O*-methylation at the meta-hydroxyl group and oxidative deamination. *O*-methylation is catalyzed by the enzyme catechol-*O*-methyltransferase (COMT), and oxidative deamination is promoted by monoamine oxidase (MAO). COMT in liver and kidney is important in the metabolism of circulating catecholamines. MAO, a mitochondrial enzyme present in most tissues including nerve endings, has a lesser role in the metabolism of circulating catecholamines but is important in regulating the catecholamine stores within the peripheral sympathetic nerve endings. The metanephrines and 4-hydroxy-3-methoxymandelic acid (VMA) are the major end products of N and NE metabolism. Homovanillic acid (HVA) is the end product of dopamine metabolism.

STORAGE AND RELEASE OF CATECHOLAMINES Both in the adrenal medulla and sympathetic nerve endings catecholamines are stored in subcellular granules and released by exocytosis. The large stores of catecholamines in these tissues provide an important physiologic reserve that maintains an adequate supply of catecholamines in the face of intense stimulation.

Adrenal medulla The adrenal medullary chromaffin tissue in a pair of normal human adrenal glands weighs about 1 g and contains approximately 6 mg of catecholamines, 85 percent of which is E. Catecholamines are maintained in high concentration within the storage (chromaffin) granule by an active uptake process involving the granule membrane and by an intragranular storage complex that appears to involve ATP, calcium, and a specific granule protein, chromagranin A. The latter, isolated originally from chromaffin granules, has been found to be a common constituent of secretory granules in a number of different endocrine cells, including those of the anterior pituitary, pancreatic islets, and parathyroids. Its role in hormone storage and secretion is still unknown. Catecholamine secretion, stimulated by ACh from the preganglionic sympathetic nerves, occurs after calcium influx triggers fusion of the chromaffin granule membrane and cell membrane; obliteration of the cell membrane at the point of fusion and extrusion of the entire soluble contents of the granule into the extracellular space complete the process of exocytosis (Fig. 67-1). Approximately 2 to 10 percent of the total adrenal medullary catecholamine store is turned over each day.

Peripheral sympathetic nerve endings The peripheral sympathetic nerve endings form a reticulum or ground plexus that brings the terminal fibers into close contact with effector cells. All the NE in peripheral tissues is in the sympathetic nerve endings, and heavily

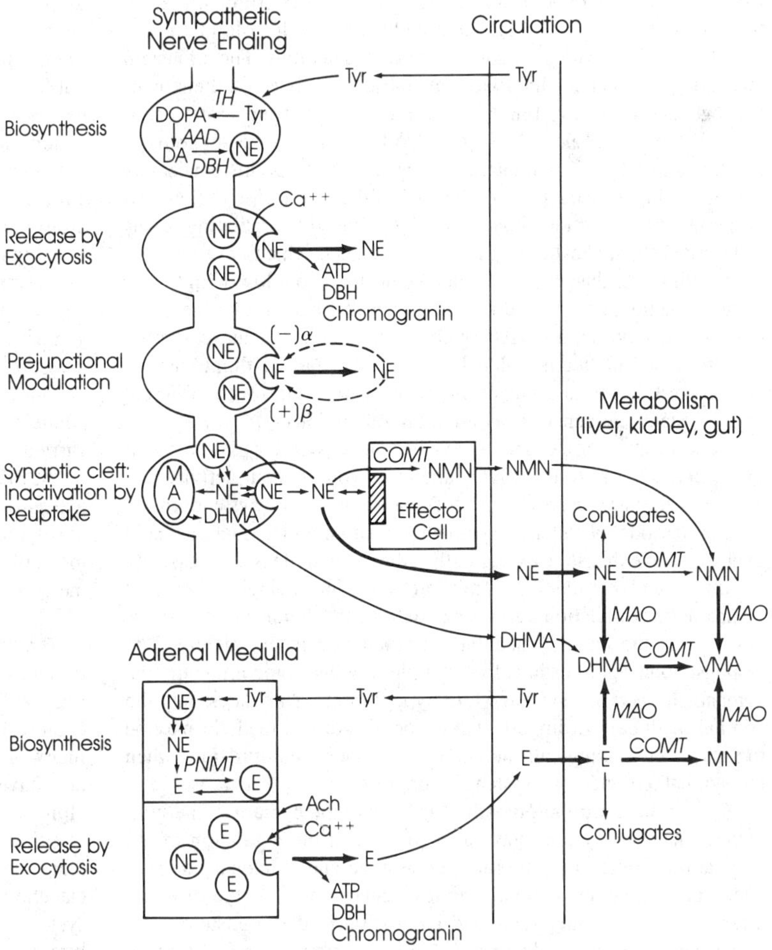

FIGURE 67-1 Catecholamine biosynthesis, release, and metabolism. Schematic representation of a peripheral sympathetic nerve ending is shown at the top; the bulbous areas on the terminal fiber represent varicosities identified by histochemical fluorescence techniques as areas of high neurotransmitter concentration. The processes of biosynthesis, release, modulation, and reuptake are shown sequentially for demonstration purposes only; in vivo they proceed concurrently. Adrenal medullary chromaffin cells are shown at the bottom of the diagram. (TH = tyrosine hydroxylase, AAD = aromatic-L-amino acid decarboxylase, DA = dopamine, DBH = dopamine-β-hydroxylase, NE = norepinephrine, PNMT = phenylethanolamine-*N*-methyltransferase, E = epinephrine, COMT = catechol-*O*-methyltransferase, NMN = normetanephrine, MAO = monoamine oxidase, DHMA = 3,4-dihydroxymandelic acid, VMA = 3-methoxy-4-hydroxymandelic acid.)

innervated tissues contain as much as 1 to 2 μg per gram of tissue. NE stored in the nerve endings is in discrete subcellular particles analogous to the adrenal medullary chromaffin granules. MAO in the mitochondria of the nerve endings plays an important role in regulating the local concentration of NE (Fig. 67-1). Amines in storage vesicles are protected from oxidative deamination; amines within the cytoplasm, however, are deaminated to inactive metabolites. Release from the nerve ending occurs in response to action potentials propagated in terminal sympathetic fibers (Fig. 67-1).

THE PERIPHERAL ADRENERGIC NEUROEFFECTOR JUNCTION **Neuronal uptake** The peripheral sympathetic nerve endings possess an amine transport system that actively takes up amines from the extracellular fluid. A variety of synthetic and naturally occurring amines are substrates for this process. Neuronal uptake or recapture of locally released NE terminates the action of the transmitter and contributes to the constancy of the NE stores (Fig. 67-1).

Prejunctional modulation A variety of factors alter the relationship between neuronal impulse traffic and NE release. Diminished temperature and acidosis, for example, both decrease the amount of NE released in response to sympathetic impulses. Several chemical mediators operate at the peripheral sympathetic nerve ending (referred to as prejunctional or presynaptic sites) to modify sympathetic neurotransmission by influencing the amount of NE released in response to nerve impulses. Prejunctional modulation may be either inhibitory or facilitatory. Certain modulators, such as catecholamines and ACh, may either inhibit or facilitate NE release, antagonistic effects that are mediated by different adrenergic or cholinergic receptors, respectively. Those compounds exerting an *inhibitory* effect on NE release at the prejunctional nerve ending include the following: catecholamines ($alpha_2$ receptor), ACh (muscarinic receptor), dopamine (D-2 receptor), histamine (H-2 receptor), serotonin, adenosine, enkephalins, and prostaglandins. *Facilitatory* prejunctional modulators include catecholamines ($beta_2$ receptor), ACh (nicotinic receptor), and angiotensin II. The overall significance of prejunctional modulation, as well as the relative importance of the various mediators, has yet to be established.

PREJUNCTIONAL ADRENERGIC RECEPTORS Catecholamines reduce NE release via prejunctional alpha receptors in a classic negative feedback system. Feedback regulation is complicated by the fact that beta-receptor activation facilitates NE release. Two hypotheses have been advanced to explain how the antagonistic alpha and beta effects on NE release may be integrated physiologically. One hypothesis is based on the observation that beta-mediated effects occur at lower agonist concentrations than those mediated by the alpha receptor, whereas alpha-mediated responses predominate at higher concentrations of agonist. During low levels of sympathetic stimulation, therefore, when NE concentrations in the synaptic cleft are low, beta-mediated positive feedback may predominate with facilitation of NE release. Conversely, at higher levels of sympathetic stimulation with increased NE concentration in the synaptic cleft, alpha-mediated negative feedback predominates and NE release is inhibited. The other hypothesis is that prejunctional beta receptors ($beta_2$, see below) are more sensitive to E than NE; circulating levels of E, therefore, might stimulate the prejunctional beta receptors, thereby augmenting NE release and enhancing sympathetic neurotransmission.

PREJUNCTIONAL CHOLINERGIC RECEPTORS Though both inhibitory and facilitatory effects of ACh on NE release have been described, the inhibitory effect of ACh, mediated by the muscarinic cholinergic receptor, occurs at lower ACh concentrations and is probably of greater physiologic significance. This peripheral inhibitory effect of ACh on adrenergic neurotransmission may reinforce the reciprocal changes in central parasympathetic and sympathetic outflow that occur in the regulation of numerous physiologic responses.

CENTRAL REGULATION OF SYMPATHOADRENAL OUTFLOW **Brainstem sympathetic centers** Sympathetic outflow is initiated from the reticular formation of the medulla oblongata and pons and from centers in the hypothalamus. Descending fibers originating from these centers synapse in the intermediolateral cell column of the spinal cord with the preganglionic sympathetic neurons. The brainstem sympathetic centers, which have an intrinsic activity of their own, are regulated by many stimuli, including impulses from more rostral areas of the central nervous system (cortex, limbic lobe, hypothalamus); neural afferents that interact at the level of the brainstem centers and at the higher centers; and changes in the physical and chemical properties of the extracellular fluid, including the circulating levels of hormones and substrates. The higher centers, which have connections with the brainstem, coordinate sympathetic outflow with higher mental functions, emotional reactions, and the homeostatic needs of the internal environment. Although the hallmark of intense sympathoadrenal stimulation is a global response (the fight-or-flight reaction of Cannon), discrete changes in sympathetic outflow to different organ systems influence many autonomic functions.

RELATIONSHIP BETWEEN THE SYMPATHETIC NERVOUS SYSTEM AND THE ADRENAL MEDULLA Sympathetic nervous system activity and adrenal medullary secretion are coordinated but not always congruent. During periods of intense sympathetic stimulation, such as cold exposure and exhaustive exercise, the adrenal medulla is progressively recruited, and circulating E reinforces the physiologic effects of sympathetic stimulation. In other situations the sympathetic nervous system and the adrenal medulla are stimulated independently. The response to upright posture, for example, involves predominantly the sympathetic nervous system while hypoglycemia stimulates only the adrenal medulla. An important role for the adrenal medulla may be to provide circulating catecholamines to support vital functions when the sympathetic nervous system is suppressed.

Sympathetic regulation of the cardiovascular system The sympathetic nervous system plays a major role in the regulation of the circulation. Stretch receptors in the systemic and pulmonary arteries and veins continuously monitor intravascular pressures; the resulting afferent impulses, after relay and integration in the brainstem, alter sympathetic activity in defense of blood pressure and blood flow to critical areas (Fig. 67-2).

ARTERIAL BARORECEPTORS An increase in blood pressure stimulates receptors in the carotid sinus and aortic arch. The ensuing afferent impulses, after relay within the nucleus of the solitary tract (NTS) in the brainstem, suppress the brainstem sympathetic centers (Fig. 67-2). This baroreceptor reflex arc forms a negative feedback loop in which a rise in arterial pressure results in the inhibition of central sympathetic outflow. A brainstem noradrenergic pathway interacts with the NTS to participate in suppression of sympathetic outflow. This noradrenergic inhibitory pathway is stimulated by centrally acting alpha-adrenergic agonists and may be involved in the action of certain antihypertensive drugs, such as clonidine, that potentiate the baroreceptor-mediated vasodepressor response (Chap. 196). In the opposite manner, when the blood pressure falls, decreased afferent impulses diminish central inhibition, resulting in an increase in sympathetic outflow and a rise in arterial pressure.

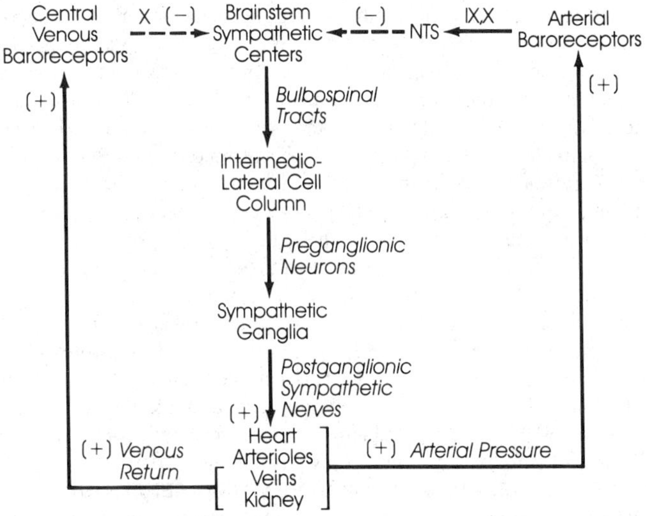

FIGURE 67-2 Sympathetic regulation of the circulation. Receptors in the venous and arterial circulations are stimulated by stretch, caused by an increase in pressure; afferent impulses from these receptors are carried to the central nervous system by the ninth and tenth cranial nerves. The net result of these afferent impulses, after relay in the brainstem, is to inhibit central sympathetic outflow. The arterial baroreceptor reflex involves a relay in the nucleus of the tractus solitarius (NTS). (+ = stimulation; − = inhibition.)

CENTRAL VENOUS PRESSURE Receptors in the walls of the great veins and within the atria are also involved in the regulation of sympathetic outflow. Stimulation of these receptors by high venous pressure suppresses the brainstem sympathetic centers; when central venous pressure is low, sympathetic outflow increases. The central connections are poorly understood, but the afferent impulses are carried in the vagus (Fig. 67-2).

ASSESSMENT OF SYMPATHOADRENAL ACTIVITY The clinical assessment of sympathoadrenal activity involves the measurement of catecholamines in plasma and of catecholamines and catecholamine metabolites in urine. Quantitation of urinary catecholamines and metabolites is useful in the diagnosis of pheochromocytoma (Chap. 318).

Plasma catecholamines Catecholamines in human plasma may be measured by radioenzymatic isotope derivative techniques or by high performance liquid chromatography in conjunction with electrochemical detection. Plasma catecholamine measurements provide an index of sympathetic nervous system and adrenal medullary activity and have been widely used to assess sympathoadrenal activity in clinical investigation in human subjects. The usefulness of plasma catecholamine measurements is, however, compromised by factors that alter the relationship between the plasma concentration of catecholamines and the functional state of the sympathoadrenal system. The clinical usefulness of plasma catecholamine levels is limited to the evaluation of patients with autonomic insufficiency and, on occasion, patients with suspected pheochromocytoma (Chap. 318).

Basal plasma NE concentrations are in the range of 0.09 to 1.8 nmol/L (150 to 350 pg/mL; basal E levels are about 135 to 270 pmol/L (25 to 50 pg/mL). The half-time of disappearance of NE from the circulation is approximately 2 min. The plasma NE level is markedly affected by a variety of factors, including posture; accordingly, the conditions under which blood is obtained for assay must be controlled. By convention, basal plasma NE levels are those obtained through an indwelling intravenous line after the patient has rested supine in a relaxed environment for 30 min.

PLASMA NE RESPONSE TO UPRIGHT POSTURE The predictable increase in circulating NE concentration during upright posture provides a convenient test of sympathetic nervous system function. Five minutes of quiet standing results in a two- to threefold increase in plasma NE level. A normal response requires an intact afferent system, appropriate central nervous system relays, and an intact peripheral sympathetic nervous system; a defect of any of these components reduces the increment in circulating NE.

Plasma E levels are also dependent on the physical and mental state of the subject. Change in plasma E with upright posture is usually small. Hypoglycemia and various types of mental stress, however, can cause large increments in the plasma E level.

PERIPHERAL DOPAMINERGIC SYSTEM

In addition to its role as neurotransmitter in the central nervous system, dopamine functions as an inhibitory transmitter in the carotid body and the sympathetic ganglia. A distinct peripheral dopaminergic system is also believed to exist. Dopamine elicits a variety of responses not attributable to stimulation of classic adrenergic receptors; it relaxes the lower esophageal sphincter, delays gastric emptying, causes vasodilation in the renal and mesenteric arterial circulation, suppresses aldosterone secretion, directly stimulates renal sodium excretion, and suppresses NE release at sympathetic nerve terminals by a presynaptic inhibitory mechanism. The mediation of these dopaminergic effects in vivo is poorly understood. Dopamine does not appear to be a circulating hormone. Unequivocal evidence of peripheral autonomic dopaminergic nerves has not been produced, although such nerves may be present in the kidney. The kidney, furthermore, produces much of the dopamine in the urine since the amount excreted each day (approximately 200 μg per 24 h) cannot be accounted for by clearance of plasma dopamine. Decarboxylation of circulating dopa, which is present in high concentration in the plasma [9 nmol/L (1500 pg/mL)] may contribute to urinary dopamine production. Dopamine generated from the decarboxylation of circulating dopa might also be involved in the mediation of dopaminergic effects in the kidney and other sites. Thus, the nature of the peripheral dopaminergic system is obscure, but the existence of a dopaminergic system in those tissues that respond uniquely to dopamine seems likely.

ADRENERGIC RECEPTORS

Catecholamines influence effector cells by interacting with specific *receptors* on the cell surface. When stimulated by catecholamines, the adrenergic receptor initiates a series of membrane changes followed by a cascade of intracellular events that culminates in a measurable response. Compounds that elicit the response are referred to as *agonists;* those that block the interaction of the agonist with the receptor are referred to as adrenergic *receptor blocking agents* or *antagonists*.

Two major categories of response to catecholamines reflect the activation of two populations of adrenergic receptors, designated *alpha* and *beta*. Selective agonists and antagonists are available, enabling pharmacologic stimulation or blockade of the physiologic effects mediated by one receptor without influencing those mediated by the other. Both alpha and beta receptors have been further divided into subtypes that serve different functions and are susceptible to differential stimulation and blockade.

ALPHA-ADRENERGIC RECEPTORS The alpha-adrenergic receptor mediates vasoconstriction, intestinal relaxation, and pupillary dilatation. E and NE are approximately equipotent as alpha-receptor agonists. Distinct $alpha_1$- and $alpha_2$-receptor subtypes are also recognized. Originally the postsynaptic or postjunctional alpha-adrenergic receptors on effector cells were designated $alpha_1$, while the prejunctional alpha-adrenergic receptors on the sympathetic nerve endings were designated $alpha_2$. Several additional nonneuronal (postsynaptic) processes appear to be mediated by the $alpha_2$ receptor. The $alpha_1$ receptor mediates the classic alpha effects including vasoconstriction; phenylephrine and methoxamine are selective $alpha_1$ agonists, and prazosin is a selective $alpha_1$ antagonist. The $alpha_2$ receptor mediates presynaptic inhibition of NE release from adrenergic nerves and other responses including inhibition of ACh release from cholinergic nerves, inhibition of lipolysis in adipocytes, inhibition of insulin secretion, stimulation of platelet aggregation, and vasoconstriction in some vascular beds. Specific $alpha_2$ agonists include clonidine and α-methylnorepinephrine; these agents, the latter derived from α-methyldopa in vivo, exert an antihypertensive effect by interacting with $alpha_2$ receptors within the brainstem sympathetic centers that regulate blood pressure. Yohimbine is a specific $alpha_2$ antagonist.

BETA-ADRENERGIC RECEPTORS Physiologic events associated with beta-adrenergic receptor responses include stimulation of heart rate and contractility, vasodilation, bronchodilation, and lipolysis. Beta-receptor responses can also be divided into two types. The $beta_1$ receptor responds equally to E and NE and mediates cardiac stimulation and lipolysis. The $beta_2$ receptor is more responsive to E than to NE and mediates responses such as vasodilation and bronchodilation. Isoproterenol stimulates and propranolol blocks both $beta_1$ and $beta_2$ receptors. Other agonists and antagonists that have partial selectivity for the $beta_1$ or $beta_2$ receptors have been used therapeutically where the desired response involves predominantly one of the two subtypes.

DOPAMINERGIC RECEPTORS Specific dopaminergic receptors, distinct from the classic alpha- and beta-adrenergic receptors, are present in the central and peripheral nervous system and in several nonneural tissues. Two types of dopaminergic receptor serve different functions and have different second messengers. Dopamine is a potent agonist of both types of receptor; the action of dopamine is antagonized by phenothiazines and thioxanthenes. The dopamine 1 receptor mediates vasodilation in the renal, mesenteric, coronary, and cerebral vascular beds. Fenoldopam is an investigational agonist selective for the dopamine 1 receptor. The dopamine 2 receptor inhibits transmission in the sympathetic ganglia, inhibits NE release from sympathetic nerve endings by an effect on the presynaptic membrane (Fig. 67-1), inhibits prolactin release from the pituitary, and causes vomiting. Selective agonists of the dopamine 2 receptor include bromocriptine, lergotrile, and apomorphine, while butyrophenones such as haloperidol (active within the central nervous system) and domperidone (does not cross blood-brain barrier readily) and the benzamide sulpiride are relatively selective dopamine 2 antagonists.

STRUCTURE AND FUNCTION OF ADRENERGIC RECEPTORS The utilization of recombinant DNA technology has substantially increased current understanding of the structure and function of adrenergic receptors. cDNAs of the four major adrenergic receptor subtypes have been cloned and their primary amino acid sequences deduced. It is clear from these studies that the adrenergic receptors belong to a family of related membrane proteins that includes the visual protein rhodopsin and the muscarinic acetylcholine receptors. These proteins share significant sequence homologies and, as deduced from the properties of the constituent amino acids, a similar topographic structure in the cell membrane (Chap. 173). The postulated structure of this family of receptor proteins is shown schematically in Fig. 67-3. The characteristic features include seven membrane-spanning hydrophobic domains containing 20 to 28 amino acids each (possibly arranged as alpha helices), a hydrophilic extracellular *N*

FIGURE 67-3 Proposed structure of adrenergic receptors as deduced from primary amino acid sequences. The single protein chain contains a hydrophilic *N* terminus (extracellular) and *C* terminus (intracellular) connected by seven lipophilic membrane-spanning regions (M-I to M-7) which are interconnected by three extracellular loops (E-I to E-III) and three cytoplasmic loops (C-I to C-III). The $beta_1$, $beta_2$, $alpha_1$, and $alpha_2$ adrenergic receptors have appreciable sequence homologies and are believed to fit the general structural model represented. Specificity of agonist binding may be conferred by the tertiary structure of several of the membrane-spanning domains while specificity of intracellular response may be related to the length and tertiary structure of the cytoplasmic loops and *C* terminus. (*Modified from RJ Lefkowitz and MG Caron.*)

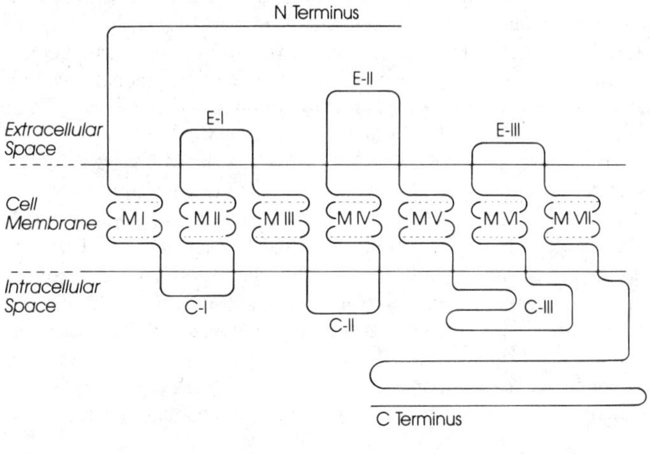

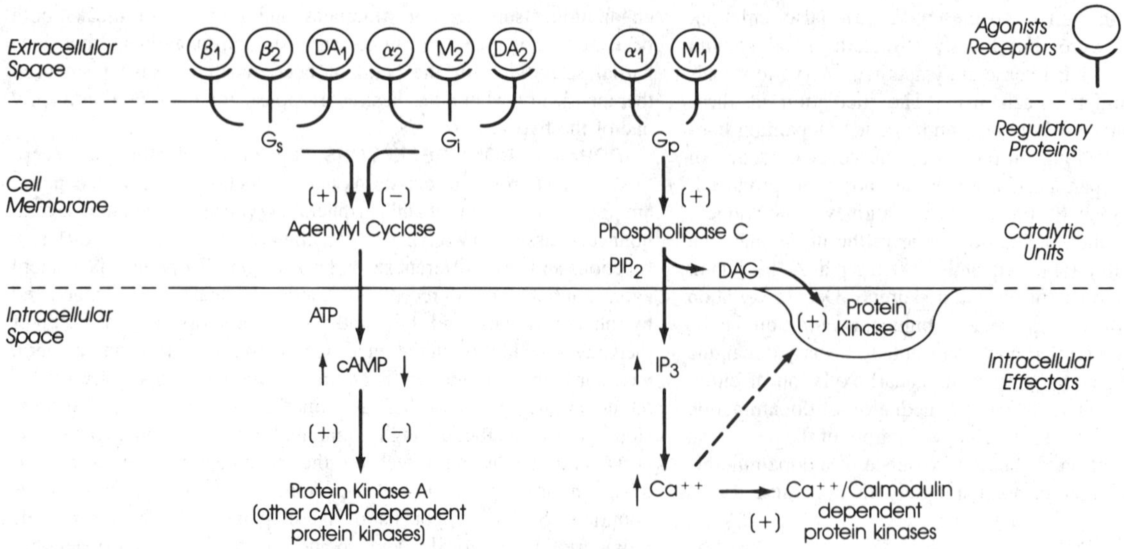

FIGURE 67-4 Interaction of autonomic agonists with membrane-bound regulatory proteins and cellular effectors systems. The designations α and β refer to adrenergic receptors, DA refers to dopaminergic receptors, and M, to muscarinic receptors. G designates the GTP-associated regulatory protein which may have a stimulatory (s) or inhibitory (i) effect on adenylyl cyclase or may stimulate phospholipase C (p). (+) designates stimulation; (−) designates inhibition. PIP_2 = phosphatidylinositol-4,5-bisphosphate; DAG = 1,2-diacylglycerol; IP_3 = inositol-1,4,5-trisphosphate. See text for details.

terminus and three extracellular connecting loops, and a hydrophilic intracellular *C* terminus with three cytoplasmic connecting loops.

Specificity for agonist binding and effector response is apparently conferred by differences in the tertiary structure of the various domains. Beta receptors, for example, have short third cytoplasmic loops (C-III) and long *C*-terminal chains, while the $alpha_2$ receptor has a long C-III and a short *C* terminus. The C-III loop appears to influence binding to the appropriate regulatory protein within the cell membrane (see below). The membrane-spanning domains, particularly M-VII (Fig. 67-3), appear to be important in determining the characteristic agonist binding.

Coupling of receptor occupancy with cellular response The major mediators of adrenergic (as well as many other) cellular responses are a family of regulatory proteins termed G (or N) proteins that, when activated, bind the nucleotide guanosine triphosphate (GTP). The best-characterized G proteins are those that stimulate or inhibit adenylyl cyclase, designated G_s or G_i, respectively (Fig. 67-4) (see Chap 68). The $beta_1$, $beta_2$, and dopamine 1 receptors are coupled to G_s; receptor occupancy is therefore associated with stimulation of adenylyl cyclase and results in an increase in intracellular cyclic adenosine monophosphate (AMP), which in turn results in activation of protein kinase A and other cAMP-dependent protein kinases. The resultant protein phosphorylation alters the activity of enzymes and the function of other proteins, culminating in a cellular response that is characteristic of the tissue being stimulated. The $alpha_2$, M-2 subtype of the muscarinic acetylcholine receptor and the dopamine 2 receptor are coupled to G_i, resulting in diminished adenylyl cyclase activity and a fall in cAMP. The subsequent alterations in enzyme activity and function of other proteins produce an alternate, frequently opposite, series of cellular responses. Not all $alpha_2$ responses can be explained by inhibition of adenylyl cyclase; independent changes in ion fluxes are involved as well.

The $alpha_1$ adrenergic receptor (as well as the M-1 subtype of the acetylcholine receptor) appears to be coupled to a different G protein that activates phospholipase C; this G protein has not been well characterized but is sometimes tentatively designated G_p. Receptor occupancy in this system stimulates phospholipase C, which catalyzes the breakdown of membrane-bound phospholipids, particularly phosphatidylinositol-4,5-bisphosphate (PIP_2) with the production of inositol-1,4,5-trisphosphate (IP_3) and 1,2-diacylglycerol (DAG), both of which act as second messengers (Fig. 67-4). IP_3 rapidly mobilizes calcium from intracellular stores within the endoplasmic reticulum producing an increase in free cytoplasmic calcium which by itself and via calcium-calmodulin–dependent protein kinases influences cellular processes appropriate to the stimulated cell. The transient rise in calcium induced by IP_3 from the intracellular stores is reinforced in the presence of continued agonist stimulation by alterations in membrane calcium flux that result eventually in net calcium uptake from the extracellular fluid by mechanisms that have been incompletely defined.

DAG, the other second messenger produced by the action of phospholipase C on PIP_2 (as well as other membrane phospholipids), remains associated with the cell membrane and activates protein kinase C, which has different substrates than the calcium-calmodulin kinases stimulated by IP_3. Protein phosphorylation stimulated by protein kinase C contributes to the tissue-specific response in ways that remain poorly understood.

REGULATION OF ADRENERGIC RECEPTORS Radiolabeled adrenergic-receptor agonists and antagonists have been utilized as ligands to study adrenergic receptors. In combination with studies of peripheral tissue sensitivity these studies demonstrated that changes in adrenergic receptors occur under a variety of physiologic conditions. Prolonged exposure to alpha- or beta-adrenergic agonists decreases the number of corresponding adrenergic receptors on effector cells. Although the biochemical mechanisms involved are obscure, internalization of the beta-adrenergic receptor within the cell occurs during agonist exposure in some systems, suggesting that internal translocation causes the decrease in receptor number. Alteration in agonist concentration may also affect the affinity of the receptor for the agonist. Adrenergic receptors that utilize adenylate cyclase for the second messenger (beta receptors, $alpha_2$ receptors) exist in high and low affinity states; exposure to agonist diminishes the proportion of receptors in the high affinity state. Such alterations in adrenergic receptors induced by adrenergic agonists are termed *homologous regulation*. Agonist-induced alterations in adrenergic-receptor density and affinity are believed to contribute to the diminished physiologic response that occurs after prolonged exposure of an effector tissue to adrenergic agonist, a phenomenon known as *tachyphylaxis* or *desensitization*. Recent evidence suggests that phosphorylation of the beta receptor by a specific beta-receptor kinase is involved in the desensitization phenomenon.

Adrenergic receptors are also influenced by factors other than adrenergic agonists, so-called heterologous regulation. Enhanced alpha-adrenergic-receptor affinity, for example, may underlie the potentiation of alpha-adrenergic responses that occur in response to lowered environmental temperatures. Thyroid hormones potentiate beta-receptor responses by alterations in beta-receptor number and in the efficiency of coupling receptor occupancy with physiologic response. Estrogen and progesterone alter the sensitivity of the myometrium to catecholamines by effects on alpha-adrenergic receptors. Glucocorticoids may influence adrenergic function by antagonizing agonist-induced decreases in adrenergic receptors, thereby counteracting tachyphylaxis in response to intense adrenergic stimulation. Some forms of heterologous desensitization may involve modifications in the membrane regulatory proteins or in adenylyl cyclase itself.

Alterations in sensitivity to catecholamines also occur as a consequence of postreceptor changes, although the latter remain poorly characterized.

PHYSIOLOGY OF THE SYMPATHOADRENAL SYSTEM

Catecholamines influence all the major organ systems. The effects take place in seconds as compared with the minutes, hours, or days that characterize the actions of the endocrine system and most other control systems that regulate bodily processes. The sympathoadrenal system, moreover, may respond in anticipation of physiologic requirement. An increase in sympathoadrenal activity prior to strenuous exercise, for example, lessens the impact of exercise on the internal environment.

DIRECT EFFECTS OF CATECHOLAMINES Cardiovascular system Catecholamines stimulate vasoconstriction in the subcutaneous, mucosal, splanchnic, and renal vascular beds by an alpha-receptor-mediated mechanism. Since vasoconstriction in the coronary and cerebral circulations is minimal, flow to these areas is maintained. The adaptive significance of this priority given the heart and brain is clear; in both of these organs the metabolic requirements relative to blood flow are high, and continuous perfusion is essential for life. Skeletal muscle vasculature contains beta receptors sensitive to low circulating levels of E so that skeletal muscle blood flow is augmented during adrenal medullary activation.

The effects of catecholamines on the heart are mediated by $beta_1$ receptors and include increase in heart rate, enhancement of cardiac contractility, and increase in conduction velocity. The increase in myocardial contractility is illustrated by a leftward and upward shift of the ventricular function curve (Fig. 181-6) that relates cardiac work to ventricular diastolic fiber length; at any initial fiber length catecholamines increase cardiac work. Catecholamines also enhance cardiac output by stimulating venoconstriction, enhancing venous return, and by increasing the force of atrial contraction, thereby augmenting diastolic volume and hence fiber length. The acceleration of conduction in the junctional tissues results in a more synchronous, and hence more effective, ventricular contraction. Cardiac stimulation increases myocardial oxygen consumption, a major factor in the pathogenesis and treatment of myocardial ischemia.

Metabolism Catecholamines increase metabolic rate. In small mammals mitochondrial respiration in brown adipose tissue is functionally uncoupled by NE. In a reaction unique to brown adipose tissue, NE activates a specific mitochondrial uncoupling protein that dissipates the proton gradient between the inner mitochondrial matrix and the cytoplasm, thereby uncoupling substrate utilization and ATP synthesis. In humans a functional role for brown adipose tissue has not been established with certainty, but increasing evidence suggests a potential role for this tissue in catecholamine-stimulated heat production in human beings.

SUBSTRATE MOBILIZATION In a variety of tissues catecholamines stimulate the breakdown of stored fuel with the production of substrate for local consumption; glycogenolysis in the heart, for example, provides substrate for immediate metabolism by the myocardium. Catecholamines also accelerate fuel mobilization in liver, adipose tissue, and skeletal muscle, liberating substrates (glucose, free fatty acids, lactate) into the circulation for use throughout the body. Activation of enzymes involved in fuel breakdown occurs by a beta-receptor ($beta_1$) mechanism for adipose tissue lipolysis and by alpha- and beta-receptor ($beta_2$) mechanisms for hepatic glycogenolysis and gluconeogenesis. In skeletal muscle catecholamines stimulate glycogenolysis (beta receptor), thereby increasing lactate efflux.

Fluids and electrolytes Catecholamines contribute to the regulation of the volume and composition of extracellular fluid. By a direct action on the renal tubule, NE stimulates sodium reabsorption, thereby defending extracellular fluid volume. Dopamine, in contrast, promotes sodium excretion. NE and E also promote cellular uptake of potassium, thereby defending against the development of hyperkalemia. Effects of catecholamines on calcium, magnesium, and phosphate metabolism are complex and depend on a variety of factors.

Viscera Catecholamines affect visceral function by actions on smooth muscle and glandular epithelium. Urinary bladder and intestinal smooth muscle are relaxed while the corresponding sphincters are stimulated. Gallbladder emptying also involves sympathetic mechanisms. Catecholamine-mediated smooth-muscle contraction in the female aids ovulation and ovum transport along the fallopian tubes, and in the male provides propulsive force for the seminal fluid during ejaculation. Inhibitory $alpha_2$ receptors on cholinergic neurons within the gut contribute to intestinal relaxation. Catecholamines induce bronchodilation by a $beta_2$-receptor mechanism.

INDIRECT EFFECTS OF CATECHOLAMINES The ultimate physiologic response induced by catecholamines involves changes in hormone secretion and in blood flow distribution, both of which support and amplify the direct effects of catecholamines.

Endocrine system Catecholamines influence the secretion of renin, insulin, glucagon, calcitonin, parathormone, thyroxine, gastrin, erythropoietin, progesterone, and, possibly, testosterone. Secretion of each of these hormones is governed by complex feedback loops. With the exception of thyroxine and the gonadal steroids, each is a polypeptide not under the direct control of the pituitary gland. Sympathoadrenal input into the secretion of these hormones provides a mechanism for regulation by the central nervous system and ensures a coordinated hormonal response in accord with the homeostatic needs of the organism.

RENIN The juxtaglomerular apparatus of the kidney is heavily innervated. Sympathetic stimulation increases renin release by a direct beta-receptor effect independent of vascular changes within the kidney. The renin response to volume depletion is sympathetically mediated and is initiated by a fall in central venous pressure. Since renin secretion activates the angiotensin-aldosterone system, angiotensin-induced vasoconstriction supports the direct effects of catecholamines on blood vessels, while aldosterone-mediated sodium reabsorption complements the direct increase in sodium reabsorption induced by sympathetic stimulation. Beta-receptor blocking agents suppress renin secretion.

INSULIN AND GLUCAGON The pancreatic islets also receive an extensive sympathetic innervation. Stimulation of pancreatic sympathetic nerves or an elevation in circulating catecholamines suppresses insulin and increases glucagon release. Inhibition of insulin secretion is mediated by the $alpha_2$ receptor, and stimulation of glucagon is mediated by the beta receptor. This combination of effects supports substrate mobilization, reinforcing the direct effects of catecholamines on hepatic glucose output and lipolysis. Although alpha-receptor-mediated suppression of insulin release usually predominates, a beta-receptor mechanism may augment insulin secretion under some circumstances.

SYMPATHOADRENAL FUNCTION IN SELECTED PHYSIOLOGIC AND PATHOPHYSIOLOGIC STATES Support of the circulation The sympathetic nervous system functions to maintain an adequate circulation. During upright posture and volume depletion, reduction of afferent venous and arterial baroreceptor impulse traffic diminishes an inhibitory input to the vasomotor center, thereby increasing sympathetic activity (Fig. 67-2) and reducing efferent vagal tone. As a result, heart rate is increased, and cardiac output is diverted from the skin, subcutaneous tissues, mucosa, and viscera. Sympathetic stimulation of the kidney increases sodium reabsorption, and sympathetically mediated venoconstriction enhances venous return. With pronounced hypotension, the adrenal medulla is recruited and E reinforces the effects of the sympathetic nervous system. A similar pattern of sympathetic activation occurs in the postprandial state when blood and extracellular fluid are sequestered in the splanchnic circulation and in the lumen of the gut, respectively.

CONGESTIVE HEART FAILURE The sympathetic nervous system also provides circulatory support during congestive heart failure (Chap. 182). Venoconstriction and sympathetic stimulation of the heart increase cardiac output while peripheral vasoconstriction directs blood flow to the heart and brain. The afferent signals are less clear than in simple volume depletion since the venous pressure is usually elevated. In severe heart failure depletion of cardiac NE may impair the effectiveness of sympathetic circulatory support.

TRAUMA AND SHOCK In acute traumatic injury or shock, adrenal catecholamines support the circulation and mobilize substrates. It is presumed, but unproved, that the sympathetic nervous system is activated as well. In the chronic, reparative phase following injury catecholamines contribute to substrate mobilization and to the elevation in metabolic rate.

EXERCISE Sympathetic activation during exercise increases cardiac output, maintains blood flow, and ensures sufficient substrate to meet the increased needs. Central neural factors, such as anticipation, and circulatory factors, such as fall in venous pressure, trigger the sympathetic response. Mild degrees of exercise stimulate the sympathetic nervous system alone; during more severe exertion the adrenal medulla is activated as well. Conditioning is associated with a decrease in sympathetic nervous system activity both at rest and during exercise.

Hypoglycemia Hypoglycemia causes a marked increase in adrenal medullary E secretion. When glucose concentrations fall below overnight fasting levels, regulatory glucose-sensitive neurons in the central nervous system initiate a prompt increase in adrenal medullary secretion. The increase is especially intense when plasma glucose levels drop below 2.8 mmol/L (50 mg/dL) when plasma E levels increase 25 to 50 times above baseline, thereby increasing hepatic glucose output, providing alternative substrate in the form of free fatty acids, suppressing endogenous insulin release, and inhibiting insulin-mediated glucose utilization in muscle. Many clinical manifestations of hypoglycemia, such as tachycardia, palpitations, nervousness, tremor, and widened pulse pressure, are secondary to increased E secretion. These manifestations of epinephrine secretion constitute an ''early warning'' system in insulin-requiring diabetics. In patients with long-standing diabetes mellitus, however, the epinephrine response to hypoglycemia may be diminished or absent, leaving affected patients at greater risk to develop severe hypoglycemia.

Cold exposure The sympathetic nervous system plays a critical role in the maintenance of normal body temperature during exposure to a cold environment. Receptors in the skin and central nervous system respond to a fall in temperature by activating hypothalamic and brainstem centers that increase sympathetic activity. Sympathetic stimulation leads to vasoconstriction in the superficial vascular beds, thereby diminishing heat loss. Heat production is simultaneously increased by shivering, generation of metabolic heat, and substrate mobilization. Acclimatization during chronic cold exposure increases the capacity for metabolic heat production in response to sympathetic stimulation.

Dietary intake Fasting suppresses and overfeeding stimulates the sympathetic nervous system. The reduction in sympathetic activity during fasting or starvation may contribute to the decrease in metabolic rate, bradycardia, and hypotension in these states. Enhanced sympathetic activity during periods of increased caloric intake may contribute to the elevation in metabolic rate associated with a chronic increase in dietary intake.

Hypoxia Chronic hypoxia is associated with stimulation of the sympathoadrenal system, and some of the cardiovascular changes in hypoxia may be dependent upon catecholamines.

THE SYMPATHETIC NERVOUS SYSTEM IN PATHOGENESIS OF SELECTED DISEASE STATES

HYPERTENSION (See also Chap. 196) As shown in Fig. 67-5, regulation of arterial pressure by the sympathetic nervous system involves blood vessels, the heart, and the kidneys. The sympathetic nervous system increases peripheral resistance by direct stimulation of the resistance vessels and by activation of the renin-angiotensin system. Increased cardiac output is the result of enhanced cardiac contractility and augmented venous return, the latter a result of venoconstriction and increased renal sodium reabsorption. Stimulation of sodium retention diminishes the capacity of the kidney to compensate for the increase in blood pressure. Antiadrenergic agents lower blood pressure by interacting at many of the sites shown in Fig. 67-5.

Whether sympathetic overactivity plays a role in the pathogenesis of primary hypertension is uncertain due to the insensitivity of currently available methods of assessing sympathetic activity in humans. It is well established, however, that the sympathetic nervous system plays at least a permissive role in hypertension (Chap. 39). Despite the elevated blood pressure, sympathetic nervous system activity is not suppressed in hypertensive patients, and reflex control of the circulation is retained, due in part to upward resetting of the baroreceptors. In addition, peripheral sensitivity of the vasculature to NE is either normal or enhanced. The maintenance of sympathetic nervous system activity in patients with hypertension accounts for the hypotensive effects of antiadrenergic agents.

During antihypertensive treatment with vasodilators or diuretics, the sympathetic nervous system may be activated in response to decreased pressure in either the venous or arterial circulation (Fig. 67-2). The heightened sympathetic activity that results, in addition to causing tachycardia, may oppose the antihypertensive therapy by activating the various effector systems shown in Fig. 67-5. Antiadrenergic agents, therefore, have a fundamental role in the therapy of most hypertensive patients.

ANGINA PECTORIS (Chap. 190) Sympathetic stimulation of the cardiovascular system increases myocardial oxygen consumption as a consequence of elevated heart rate, enhanced myocardial contractility, and increased myocardial wall tension. Attacks of angina,

FIGURE 67-5 Sympathetic nervous system effects on blood pressure. Sympathetic stimulation (+) increases blood pressure by effects on the heart, the veins, the kidneys, and the arterioles. The net result of sympathetic stimulation is an increase in both cardiac output and peripheral resistance. *[From JB Young, L Landsberg, in P Sleight et al (eds), Scientific Foundations of Cardiology, London, Heinemann, 1981.]*

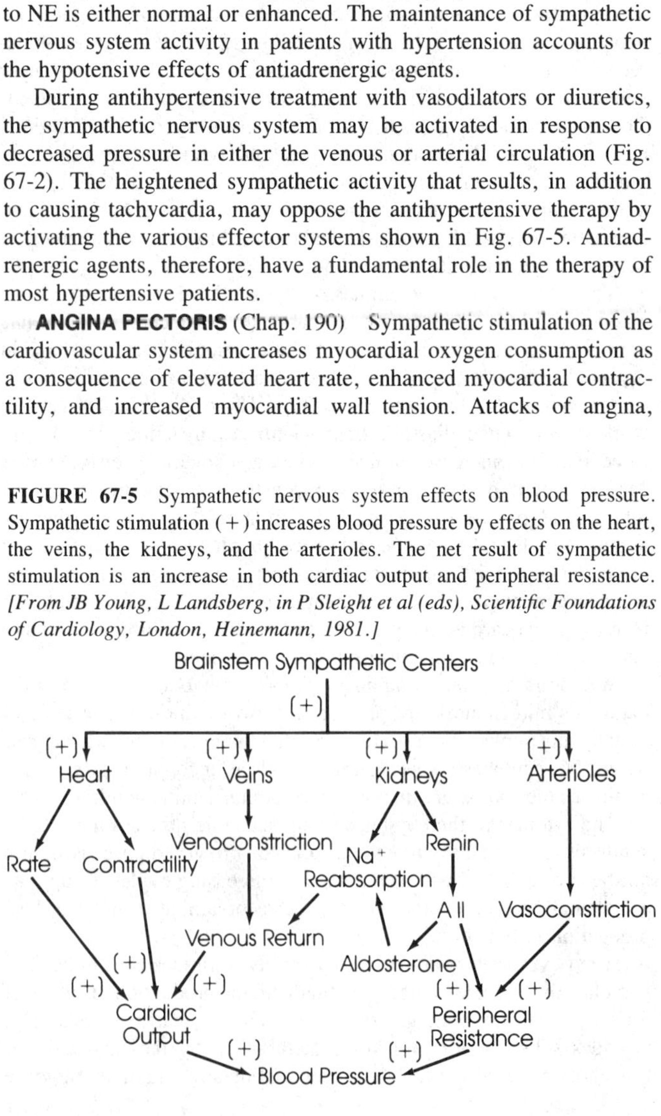

therefore, are often precipitated by situations associated with sympathetic activation such as exercise, eating, and cold exposure. Beta blockade is beneficial in the treatment of angina because of reduction in sympathetic stimulation of the heart. Alpha-adrenergically mediated coronary vasoconstriction may also contribute to coronary spasm.

HYPERTHYROIDISM (Chap. 316) Many of the peripheral manifestations of hyperthyroidism suggest a hyperadrenergic state. Enhancement of beta-receptor responses in hyperthyroidism is due in part to effects on the beta receptor. Thyroid hormone, in some tissues and in some species, increases receptor number; in other tissues, even when beta-receptor number is not increased, coupling of receptor occupancy to the adenylate cyclase cyclic-AMP system is augmented to amplify catecholamine-induced responses. Since thyroid hormone excess does not suppress sympathetic nervous system activity (plasma NE levels are normal in thyrotoxic patients), a "normal" level of sympathetic activity may evoke an exaggerated physiologic response. Many of the adrenergic manifestations of hyperthyroidism are diminished by treatment with beta-receptor blocking agents.

ORTHOSTATIC HYPOTENSION (Chap. 39) The maintenance of arterial pressure during upright posture depends upon an adequate blood volume, an unimpaired venous return, and an intact sympathetic nervous system. Significant postural hypotension, therefore, often reflects extracellular fluid volume depletion or dysfunction of the circulatory reflexes. Diseases of the nervous system, such as tabes dorsalis, syringomyelia, or diabetes mellitus, may disrupt these sympathetic reflexes with resultant orthostatic hypotension. Although any antiadrenergic agent may impair the postural sympathetic response, orthostatic hypotension is most prominent with drugs that block neurotransmission within the ganglia or adrenergic neurons.

The term *idiopathic orthostatic hypotension* refers to a group of degenerative diseases involving either the pre- or postganglionic sympathetic neurons. Involvement of the peripheral sympathetic nervous system is characterized by low basal NE levels, while involvement at the level of the central nervous system or preganglionic sympathetic neurons is associated with normal basal plasma NE levels. In both cases the plasma NE response to upright posture is deficient. Orthostatic hypotension caused by disruption of the preganglionic autonomic neurons within the intermediolateral cell column of the spinal cord often occurs in association with degenerative changes of basal ganglia and other portions of the central nervous system. In the latter situation, known as *multiple systems atrophy*, or the *Shy-Drager* syndrome, orthostatic hypotension occurs along with a variety of neurologic disturbances including Parkinson's disease.

Treatment of orthostatic hypotension is usually unsatisfactory except in the mildest cases. There is no way of reestablishing the normal relationship between fall in venous return and sympathetic neuronal activation. Volume expansion with fludrocortisone and a liberal salt diet in conjunction with fitted stockings to the waist, and elevation of the head of the bed to avoid recumbency, will maintain plasma volume and venous return and frequently provide symptomatic improvement. Rarely a beneficial response may be obtained from treatment with sympathomimetic amines (including clonidine).

PHARMACOLOGY OF THE SYMPATHOADRENAL SYSTEM

A variety of therapeutic agents affect sympathetic nervous system function or interact with adrenergic receptors, making it possible to stimulate or suppress effects mediated by catecholamines with some degree of specificity (Table 67-1).

SYMPATHOMIMETIC AMINES Sympathomimetic amines may directly activate adrenergic receptors (direct acting) or release NE from the sympathetic nerve endings (indirect acting). Many agents have both direct and indirect effects.

Epinephrine and norepinephrine The naturally occurring catecholamines act predominantly by the direct stimulation of adrenergic receptors. NE is employed to support the circulation and elevate the blood pressure in hypotensive states (Chap. 39). Peripheral vasoconstriction is the major effect although cardiac stimulation occurs as well. E, also employed as a pressor, has special usefulness in the treatment of allergic reactions, especially those associated with anaphylaxis. E antagonizes the effects of histamine and other mediators on vascular and visceral smooth muscle and is useful in the treatment of bronchospasm.

Dopamine *Dopamine* is used in treating hypotension, shock (Chap. 39), and certain forms of heart failure (Chap. 182). At low infusion rates it exerts a positive inotropic effect both by a direct action on the cardiac $beta_1$ receptors and by the indirect release of NE from sympathetic nerve endings in the heart. At low doses direct stimulation of dopaminergic receptors in the renal and mesenteric vasculature also results in vasodilation in the gut and kidney and facilitates sodium excretion. At higher infusion rates interaction with alpha-adrenergic receptors results in vasoconstriction, an increase in peripheral resistance, and an elevation of blood pressure.

Beta-receptor agonists *Isoproterenol,* a direct-acting beta-receptor agonist, stimulates the heart, decreases peripheral resistance, and relaxes bronchial smooth muscle. It raises the cardiac output and accelerates atrioventricular conduction while increasing the automaticity of ventricular pacemakers. Isoproterenol is used in the treatment of heart block and bronchoconstriction. *Dobutamine,* a congener of dopamine with relative selectivity for the $beta_1$ receptor and with a greater effect on myocardial contractility than on heart rate, is also used in the treatment of congestive heart failure, often in combination with vasodilators (Chap. 182).

SELECTIVE $BETA_2$-RECEPTOR AGONISTS The cardiac stimulation caused by nonselective beta agonists, such as isoproterenol or epinephrine, is occasionally dangerous when these agents are used in the treatment of bronchoconstriction. Selective $beta_2$ agonists (*metaproterenol, albuterol, terbutaline,* and *isoetharine*) improve the therapeutic ratio by achieving bronchial dilatation with less activation of the cardiovascular system (Chaps. 204 and 210); selectivity is relative, and cardiac stimulation does occur with these agents, particularly at the higher dose levels. *Ritodrine,* another selective $beta_2$ agonist, is used as a tocolytic agent (as is *terbutaline*) to relax the uterus and antagonize premature labor.

Alpha-adrenergic agonists *Phenylephrine* and *methoxamine* are direct-acting alpha agonists that elevate blood pressure by increasing peripheral vasoconstriction. They are used primarily in the treatment of hypotension and paroxysmal supraventricular tachycardia (Chap. 185), in the latter case by increasing cardiac vagal tone through reflex baroreceptor stimulation. Phenylephrine and a related proprietary compound, *phenylpropanolamine,* are common constituents of decongestant medications (often combined with antihistamines) for the treatment of allergic rhinitis and upper respiratory infections.

Miscellaneous sympathomimetic amines with mixed actions *Ephedrine* has both direct beta-receptor agonist properties and an indirect effect on sympathetic nerve endings, from which it releases NE, and is used primarily as a bronchodilator. *Sudephedrine,* a congener of ephedrine, is less potent at dilating bronchi and serves as a nasal decongestant. *Metaraminol* has both direct and indirect effects on sympathetic nerve endings and is employed in the treatment of hypotensive states.

Dopaminergic agonists The dopamine 2–receptor agonist *bromocriptine* is used to suppress prolactin secretion (Chap. 313). *Apomorphine,* another dopamine 2–receptor agonist, is used to induce emesis.

ANTIADRENERGIC OR SYMPATHOLYTIC AGENTS (See also Chap. 196) **Agents inhibiting central sympathetic outflow** The antihypertensive agents *methyldopa, clonidine, guanabenz,* and *guanfacine* diminish central sympathetic outflow by stimulating a central alpha-adrenergic pathway ($alpha_2$ receptor) that diminishes vasomotor outflow. Central nervous system side effects such as sedation are common. When administration of clonidine is stopped abruptly, a withdrawal syndrome characterized by rebound hyperactivity of the

TABLE 67-1 Some commonly used autonomic drugs[a,b,c]

Agent	Indication	Dose and Route	Comment
ADRENERGIC AGONISTS[d]			
Epinephrine	Anaphylaxis	100–500 μg SC or IM (0.1–0.5 mL of 1/1000 solution of hydrochloride salt); 25–50 μg IV (slowly) every 5–15 min; titrate as needed	Nonselective alpha and beta agonist; increases BP, heart rate Bronchodilation
Norepinephrine	Shock Hypotension	2–4 μg of NE base/min IV; titrate as needed	Alpha and beta$_1$ agonist Vasoconstriction predominates Extravasation causes tissue necrosis; infuse through IV cannula
Isoproterenol	Cardiogenic shock Bradyarrhythmias AV block	0.5–5.0 μg/min IV; titrate as needed	Nonselective beta agonist Increases cardiac rate and contractility (beta$_1$) Tachycardia limits usefulness
	Asthma	Inhalation	Dilates bronchi (beta$_2$); cardiac stimulation also occurs
Dobutamine	Refractory CHF Cardiogenic shock	2.5–25 (μg/kg)/min IV	Selective beta$_1$ agonist with greater effect on contractility than heart rate; a congener of dopamine but not a dopaminergic agonist
Phenylephrine	Hypotension	40–180 μg/min IV	Selective alpha$_1$ agonist; useful in antagonizing hypotension of spinal anesthesia
	Supraventricular tachycardia	150–800 μg slow IV push	Pressor effect induces vagotonic response; do not exceed 21 kPa (160 mmHg) systolic BP
Terbutaline	Asthma	2.5–5.0 mg PO tid; 0.25–0.5 mg SC; inhalation every 4–5 h	Selective beta$_2$ agonist; beta$_1$ (cardiac) effects at higher doses
Albuterol	Asthma	2.0–4.0 mg PO tid or qid; inhalation every 4–6 h	Selective beta$_2$ agonist; beta$_1$ effects (cardiac) at higher doses
Isoetharine	Asthma	Inhalation every 2–4 h	Selective beta$_2$ agonist; some beta$_1$ effects
Metaproterenol	Asthma	10–20 mg PO tid or qid; inhalation every 3–4 h	Selective beta$_2$ agonist; some beta$_1$ effects
Ritodrine	Premature labor	100–350 μg/min IV; 10–20 mg every 4–6 h PO	Selective beta$_2$ agonist; hypokalemia. hyperglycemia, hypotension, cardiac stimulation may occur Neonatal hypoglycemia, hypocalcemia reported
DOPAMINERGIC AGONISTS			
Dopamine	Shock	2–5 (μg/kg)/min IV (dopaminergic range) 5–10 (μg/kg)/min IV (dopaminergic and beta range) 10–20 (μg/kg)min IV (beta range) 20–50 (μg/kg)/min IV (alpha range)	Pharmacologic effects are dose dependent: renal and mesenteric vasodilation predominate at lower doses; cardiac stimulation and vasoconstriction develop as the dose is increased
Bromocriptine	Amenorrhea-galactorrhea	2.5 mg PO bid or tid	Selective agonist of dopamine-2 receptor; inhibits prolactin secretion
	Acromegaly	5–15 mg PO tid or qid	Lowers growth hormone in a minority of patients with acromegaly
INHIBITORS OF CENTRAL SYMPATHETIC OUTFLOW			
Clonidine	Hypertension	0.1–0.6 mg PO bid	Selective alpha$_2$ agonist; potentiates central baroreceptor depressor reflex Abrupt discontinuation may result in withdrawal syndrome with rebound hypertension
Methyldopa	Hypertension	250–500 mg PO every 6–8 h	Metabolized by decarboxylation and beta hydroxylation to α-methyl-norepinephrine, a centrally active selective alpha$_2$ agonist
ADRENERGIC NEURON BLOCKING AGENTS			
Guanethidine	Hypertension	10–100 mg PO qd	Concentrated in sympathetic nerve endings; blocks release of NE in response to nerve impulses and depletes NE stores; prominent orthostatic hypotension
Bretylium	Ventricular fibrillation and tachycardia	5 mg/kg IV	In addition to blocking NE release, has direct effect on electrical properties of cardiac muscle
BETA BLOCKING AGENTS[e]			
Propranolol	Hypertension	40–160 mg PO bid (or higher)	Lipophilic, nonselective Dosage highly variable
	Angina	10–40 mg PO tid or qid	
	Myocardial infarction	60–80 mg PO tid	Prolongs survival post MI
	Arrhythmias	10–30 mg PO tid or qid; 1–3 mg IV	
	Hypertrophic cardiomyopathy	20–40 mg PO tid or qid	
	Pheochromocytoma	10–20 mg PO tid or qid; 0.5–2.0 mg IV	After alpha blockade initiated
	Essential tremor	20–80 mg PO tid	
	Migraine	20–80 mg PO bid or tid	
	Hyperthyroidism	10–60 mg PO tid or qid	

TABLE 67-1 Some commonly used autonomic drugs[a,b,c] *(continued)*

Agent	Indication	Dose and Route	Comment
BETA BLOCKING AGENTS[e] *(continued)*			
Metoprolol	Hypertension	50–200 mg PO bid	Selective $beta_1$ (cardiac), lipophilic
	Myocardial infarction	100 mg PO bid	Prolongs survival post MI
Nadolol	Hypertension	80–320 mg PO qd	Hydrophilic, nonselective; lengthen dosage interval with renal failure
	Angina	80–240 mg PO qd	
Timolol	Hypertension	10–30 mg PO bid	Lipophilic, nonselective
	Myocardial infarction	10 mg PO bid	Prolongs survival post MI
Atenolol	Hypertension	50–100 mg PO qd	Selective $beta_1$, hydrophilic; lengthen dosage interval with renal failure
Pindolol	Hypertension	5–30 mg PO bid	Nonselective, lipophilic with partial agonist activity
	Angina	10 mg PO qid	
Acebutolol	Hypertension	200–800 mg qid	Selective $beta_1$, hydrophilic, partial agonist activity
	Arrhythmias	200–600 mg bid	
Esmolol	Supraventricular tachycardia	50–200 (μg/kg)/min after loading dose of 500 (μg/kg)/min for 1 min	Selective $beta_1$, very short duration of action
ALPHA BLOCKING AGENTS			
Phenoxybenzamine	Pheochromocytoma	10–60 mg PO bid; titrate as needed	Noncompetitive, nonselective alpha blockade
Phentolamine	Pheochromocytoma	5 mg IV (after test dose of 0.5 mg)	Competitive, nonselective alpha blockade
Prazosin	Hypertension	1–5 mg PO bid or tid	Competitive, selective $alpha_1$ blockade
	CHF	2–7 mg PO qid	
Terazosin	Hypertension	1–5 mg PO qid	Competitive, selective $alpha_1$ blockade, long duration of action
COMBINED ALPHA-BETA BLOCKING AGENT			
Labetalol	Hypertension	100–1200 mg PO bid; titrate slowly as needed; 20–80 mg IV (by increments up to 300 mg); 2 mg/min by IV infusion	Competitive alpha and beta antagonist with relatively more activity against beta receptors
DOPAMINERGIC ANTAGONIST[f]			
Metoclopramide	Diabetic gastroparesis	10 mg PO qid	Competitive dopaminergic antagonist with prominent cholinergic agonist activity
	Gastroesophageal reflex	10–15 mg PO qid	
	Antiemetic (cancer chemotherapy)	10 mg IV	
GANGLIONIC BLOCKING AGENT			
Trimethaphan	Hypertensive crisis (aortic dissection)	1–3 mg/min IV	Competitive ganglionic blocker; some direct vasodilating effects; inhibits parasympathetic as well as sympathetic nervous system
CHOLINERGIC AGONIST			
Bethanechol	Urinary retention (nonobstructive)	10–100 mg PO tid or qid; 5 mg SC	M-2 receptor agonist
ANTICHOLINESTERASE AGENTS[g]			
Physostigmine	Central cholinergic blockade	1–2 mg IV (slow)	Tertiary amine; penetrates CNS well; may cause seizures; used to reverse central anticholinergic effects produced by overdose of atropine or tricyclic antidepressants
Edrophonium	Paroxysmal supraventricular tachycardia	5 mg IV (after 1.0-mg test dose)	Induces vagotonic response; rapid onset, short duration of action; effects reversed by atropine
CHOLINERGIC BLOCKING AGENTS[h]			
Atropine	Bradycardia and hypotension	0.4–1.0 mg IV every 1–2 h	Competitive inhibition of M-1 and M-2 receptor; blocks hemodynamic changes associated with increased vagal tone

[a] Consult complete prescribing information.
[b] Doses for children are not given.
[c] Only the more common indications and routes of administration are listed.
[d] Dopaminergic agonists are listed separately although dopamine, at high doses, is an adrenergic agonist as well.
[e] Clinical efficacy of most beta blockers appears similar for major indications. Not all beta blockers are FDA approved for all indications listed in the table. When beta blocking agents are discontinued, gradual dosage reduction is recommended.
[f] Neuroleptic and antipsychotic agents are also dopaminergic antagonists; these are not included in the table.
[g] A major use of cholinesterase inhibitors is in the treatment of myasthenia gravis (Chap 368). These agents, quaternary amines that do not penetrate the CNS, are not included in the table.
[h] A wide variety of synthetic atropine derivatives are available for the purpose of (1) diminishing GI tract motility and secretion and (2) increasing urinary bladder capacity. Their usefulness is limited by anticholinergic side effects. Some may be useful as adjuncts in the treatment of peptic ulcer disease.

sympathetic nervous system can produce a syndrome resembling the crises of patients with pheochromocytoma. *Opiates* may also exert a central sympatholytic effect; the sympathetic excitation of morphine withdrawal responds to clonidine and vice versa. *Propranolol* and *reserpine* may exert some sympatholytic effects at the level of the central nervous system.

Ganglionic blocking agents Ganglionic transmission may be antagonized by drugs that block the (nicotinic) cholinergic synapse between the preganglionic and postganglionic autonomic nerves. These agents inhibit the parasympathetic as well as the sympathetic nervous system. Only *trimethaphan* is in general clinical use; its major application is in the treatment of hypertensive crises, particularly aortic dissection, when controlled hypotension and decreased myocardial contractility are desirable (Chap. 197).

Agents acting at the peripheral sympathetic nerve endings Adrenergic neuron-blocking agents depress the function of the peripheral sympathetic nerves by decreasing the amount of neurotransmitter released. *Guanethidine*, the prototype of this class of drugs, is concentrated in the sympathetic nerve endings by the amine-uptake mechanism. Within the terminal it blocks the release of NE in response to nerve impulses and eventually depletes the nerve of NE by displacing it from the intraneuronal storage granules. The drug is occasionally useful in the management of severe hypertension, although orthostatic hypotension is a limiting side effect. *Bretylium*, an agent whose effects are similar to those of guanethidine, is employed in the treatment of ventricular fibrillation (Chap. 185). Both guanethidine and bretylium are antagonized by agents that affect the amine-uptake transport process such as sympathomimetic amines, tricyclic antidepressants, phenoxybenzamine, and phenothiazines. The antihypertensive action of guanethidine may be rapidly reversed by these drugs.

Reserpine depletes catecholamines from the peripheral sympathetic nerve endings, the brain, and the adrenal medulla. Its antihypertensive effect in humans is usually attributed to depletion of peripheral NE stores within sympathetic nerve endings. The sedation and occasionally morbid depression attending its use result from NE depletion within the central nervous system.

Adrenergic-receptor blocking agents Adrenergic blocking agents antagonize the effects of catecholamines at the level of the peripheral tissue.

ALPHA-ADRENERGIC-RECEPTOR BLOCKING AGENTS *Phenoxybenzamine* and *phentolamine* are utilized principally in treating pheochromocytoma (Chap. 318). Phenoxybenzamine produces prolonged, noncompetitive alpha blockade, while phentolamine leads to reversible, competitive blockade. Because of its rapid action and short duration, phentolamine is commonly used in the treatment of acute hypertensive paroxysms secondary to catecholamine excess, such as occur with pheochromocytoma, with pressor reactions in patients receiving monoamine oxidase inhibitors, and in clonidine withdrawal. Both phentolamine and phenoxybenzamine antagonize $alpha_1$ and $alpha_2$ receptors, although phenoxybenzamine is more potent at the $alpha_1$ receptor site. *Prazosin*, an alpha-adrenergic blocking agent with selectivity for the $alpha_1$ receptor, possesses properties that resemble those of primary vasodilators and is used in the treatment of essential hypertension and as an afterload reducing agent in congestive heart failure. Terazosin, a long-acting selective $alpha_1$ blocker, is used in the treatment of essential hypertension. Since none of these agents have much effect on the beta-adrenergic receptor, unopposed beta stimulation may result in tachycardia.

BETA-ADRENERGIC-RECEPTOR BLOCKING AGENTS Beta blocking agents antagonize the cardiovascular effects of catecholamines in angina pectoris, hypertension, and cardiac arrhythmias. The benefit of beta blockade in angina derives from the decrease in myocardial oxygen consumption following reduction in heart rate and myocardial contractility (Chap. 190). The hypotensive effect of beta blockade is not clearly understood (Chap. 196). Diminished cardiac output, decreased NE release at postganglionic sympathetic nerve endings, reduced renin secretion, and suppressed central sympathetic outflow are possible mechanisms. The efficacy of beta blocking agents in the treatment of arrhythmias depends upon reduction of the rate of spontaneous depolarization of pacemaker cells in the sinus node and junctional pacemakers and upon slowing conduction within the atria and atrioventricular node. Beta blockade is also effective in the symptomatic management of hyperthyroidism and the control of tachycardia and arrhythmias in patients with pheochromocytoma. Beta-adrenergic blocking agents are also useful in the treatment of migraine, essential tremor, idiopathic hypertrophic subaortic stenosis, aortic dissection, and possibly in the period following myocardial infarction. Several trials have suggested that beta blocking agents, administered long-term, diminish mortality following acute myocardial infarction. The mechanism may involve antiarrhythmic action, prevention of reinfarction, and reduction in infarct size (Chap. 189).

PHARMACOLOGIC PROPERTIES OF BETA-RECEPTOR BLOCKING AGENTS Eight beta blocking agents (atenolol, acebutolol, esmolol, metoprolol, nadolol, pindolol, propranolol, and timolol) are available for use in the United States. Other agents (alprenolol, bevantolol, oxprenolol, sotalol, etc.) are in use in other countries and investigational within the United States. The utility of these agents is derived predominantly from blockade of beta-adrenergic receptors. In general, the various agents have similar clinical efficacy.

Although much has been written about other pharmacologic properties including cardioselectivity, membrane stabilizing (local anesthetic) effects, intrinsic sympathomimetic (partial-agonist) activity, and lipid solubility, the clinical significance of these additional properties is small. Local anesthetic properties are most prominent with propranolol; however, membrane stabilization probably does not contribute substantially to the clinical utility. The various beta blockers do differ in their water and lipid solubility. The lipophilic agents (propranolol, metoprolol, oxprenolol) are readily absorbed from the gastrointestinal tract, metabolized by the liver, have large volumes of distribution, and penetrate the central nervous system well; the hydrophilic agents (acebutolol, atenolol, nadolol, sotalol) are less readily absorbed, not extensively metabolized, and have relatively long plasma half-lives. As a consequence, the hydrophilic agents may be administered once per day. Hepatic failure may prolong the plasma half-life of the lipophilic agents, and renal failure prolongs the action of the hydrophilic group. The degree of lipid solubility, therefore, may provide a basis for choice of a particular agent in patients with hepatic or renal insufficiency. Although the hydrophilic agents penetrate the central nervous system less well, central nervous system side effects (sedation, depression, hallucinations) probably occur as frequently with the hydrophilic as with the lipophilic agents.

Some beta-adrenergic blocking agents possess beta-agonist activity. This has been referred to as "intrinsic sympathomimetic activity" or "ISA." Agents with partial agonist activity (pindolol, alprenolol, acebutolol, oxprenolol) cause little or no depression of resting heart rate (partial agonist effect) while blocking the increase in heart rate that occurs in response to exercise or the administration of a beta agonist such as isoproterenol. The presence of partial agonist activity may be useful when bradycardia limits treatment in patients with slow resting heart rates. Although intrinsic sympathomimetic activity may also be useful in patients with depressed left ventricular function and reactive airways, no clear advantage of these agents over beta blockers without partial agonist activity has been demonstrated. Pindolol also produces mild vasodilation, perhaps in part related to peripheral $beta_2$ stimulation. On theoretical grounds intrinsic sympathomimetic activity would be undesirable in the treatment of thyrotoxicosis, idiopathic hypertrophic subaortic stenosis, and aortic dissection.

CARDIOSELECTIVE ($BETA_1$)-ADRENERGIC-RECEPTOR BLOCKING AGENTS Propranolol, the prototype of the nonselective beta-adrenergic blocking agent, induces a competitive blockade of both $beta_1$ and $beta_2$ receptors. Other nonselective beta blocking agents include alprenolol, nadolol, oxprenolol, pindolol, sotalol, and timolol. Metoprolol, acebutolol, and atenolol possess relative selectivity for the $beta_1$ receptor. Although $beta_1$ selective agents have the theoretical advantage of producing less bronchoconstriction and less peripheral vasoconstriction, a clear-cut clinical advantage of the cardioselective agents has not been demonstrated, since the $beta_1$ selectivity is only relative. Bronchoconstriction may occur when $beta_1$ selective agents are administered in full therapeutic doses.

ADVERSE EFFECTS OF BETA BLOCKING AGENTS Aside from the effects on the central nervous system, most adverse reactions to beta blocking agents are consequences of beta-adrenergic blockade. These include the precipitation of heart failure in patients in whom cardiac compensation depends upon enhanced sympathetic drive; the aggravation of bronchospasm in patients with asthma; predisposition to the development of hypoglycemia in insulin-requiring diabetics (blockade of catecholamine-mediated counterregulation and antagonism of the adrenergic warning signs of hypoglycemia); the development of hyperkalemia in diabetic or uremic patients with impaired potassium tolerance; and the enhancement of coronary or peripheral arterial vasospasm.

MISCELLANEOUS ADRENERGIC BLOCKING AGENTS *Labetalol*, approved for use in the United States as an antihypertensive agent, is a competitive antagonist of both alpha- and beta-adrenergic receptors. Although labetalol induces relatively more beta- than alpha-receptor blockade, fall in peripheral resistance may be marked following acute administration of the drug. Vasodilation may be mediated in part by a partial agonist effect on the $beta_2$-adrenergic receptor; labetalol does not possess partial agonist activity for the $beta_1$ (cardiac) receptor.

Metoclopramide is a dopaminergic antagonist with cholinergic agonist properties. It enhances gastric emptying, increases the tone of the lower esophageal sphincter, increases prolactin and aldosterone secretion, and antagonizes emesis induced by apomorphine. It is useful clinically in enhancing gastric emptying (in the absence of organic obstruction such as in diabetic gastroparesis), in antagonizing gastroesophageal reflux, and as an antiemetic during cancer chemotherapy.

THE PARASYMPATHETIC NERVOUS SYSTEM

ACETYLCHOLINE Acetylcholine (ACh) serves as the neurotransmitter at all autonomic ganglia, at the postganglionic parasympathetic nerve endings, and at the postganglionic sympathetic nerve endings innervating the eccrine sweat glands. The enzyme choline acetyltransferase catalyzes the synthesis of ACh from acetyl CoA produced within the nerve ending and from choline, actively taken up from the extracellular fluid. Within the cholinergic nerve endings ACh is stored in discrete synaptic vesicles and released in response to nerve impulses that depolarize the nerve terminals and increase calcium influx.

Cholinergic receptors Different receptors for ACh exist on the postganglionic neurons within the autonomic ganglia and at the postjunctional autonomic effector sites. Those within the autonomic ganglia and adrenal medulla are stimulated predominantly by nicotine (*nicotinic receptors*) and those on autonomic effector cells by the alkaloid muscarine (*muscarinic receptors*). Ganglionic blocking agents antagonize the nicotinic receptors while atropine blocks the muscarinic receptors. The muscarinic (M) receptor, furthermore, has been recently subdivided into two types. The M-1 receptor is localized to the central nervous system and perhaps parasympathetic ganglia; the M-2 receptor is the nonneuronal muscarinic receptor on smooth muscle, cardiac muscle, and glandular epithelium. Bethanechol is a selective agonist of the M-2 receptor; pirenzepine, an investigational agent, is a selective antagonist of the M-1 receptor. This agent markedly reduces gastric acid secretion. The M-2 receptor inhibits adenylyl cyclase and utilizes the regulatory G_i protein; the M-1 receptor interacts with G_p and stimulates phospholipase C (Fig. 67-4).

Acetylcholinesterase Hydrolysis of ACh by acetylcholinesterase inactivates the neurotransmitter at cholinergic synapses. This enzyme (also known as specific or true cholinesterase) is present within neurons and is distinct from butyrocholinesterase (serum cholinesterase or pseudocholinesterase). The latter enzyme is present in plasma and nonneuronal tissues and is not primarily involved in the termination of the effects of ACh at autonomic effector sites. The pharmacologic effects of anticholinesterase agents are due to inhibition of neuronal (true) acetylcholinesterase.

PHYSIOLOGY OF THE PARASYMPATHETIC NERVOUS SYSTEM The parasympathetic nervous system participates in the regulation of the cardiovascular system, the gastrointestinal tract, and the genitourinary system. Tissues such as liver, kidney, pancreas, and thyroid also receive parasympathetic innervation, suggesting a role for the parasympathetic nervous system in metabolic regulation as well, although cholinergic effects on metabolism are not well characterized.

Cardiovascular system Parasympathetic effects on the heart are mediated by the vagus nerve. ACh reduces the rate of spontaneous depolarization of the sinoatrial node and decreases heart rate. The heart rate in different physiologic states is the result of coordinated interaction between sympathetic stimulation, parasympathetic inhibition, and the intrinsic activity of the sinoatrial pacemaker. ACh also delays impulse conduction within the atrial musculature while shortening the effective refractory period, a combination of factors which may initiate or perpetuate atrial arrhythmias. At the atrioventricular node ACh reduces conduction velocity, increases the effective refractory period, and thus diminishes the ventricular response during atrial flutter or fibrillation (Chap. 185). The decrease in inotropy induced by ACh is related to a prejunctional inhibitory effect on sympathetic nerve endings as well as to a direct inhibitory effect on the atrial myocardium. The ventricular myocardium is not much affected since innervation by cholinergic fibers is minimal. A direct cholinergic contribution to the regulation of peripheral resistance appears unlikely since parasympathetic innervation of the vasculature is not extensive. The parasympathetic nervous system, however, may influence peripheral resistance indirectly by inhibiting NE release from sympathetic nerves.

Gastrointestinal tract Parasympathetic innervation of the gut is via the vagus nerve and the pelvic sacral nerves. The parasympathetic nervous system increases the tone of gastrointestinal smooth muscle, enhances peristaltic activity, and relaxes the gastrointestinal sphincters. ACh stimulates exocrine secretion from the glandular epithelium and enhances the secretion of gastrin, secretin, and insulin.

Genitourinary and respiratory systems Sacral parasympathetic nerves supply the urinary bladder and genitalia. ACh increases ureteral peristalsis, contracts the urinary detrusor muscle, and relaxes the trigone and sphincter, thereby playing a critical role in the coordination of urination. The respiratory tract is innervated with parasympathetic fibers derived from the vagus nerve. ACh increases tracheobronchial secretions and stimulates bronchial constriction.

PHARMACOLOGY OF THE PARASYMPATHETIC NERVOUS SYSTEM **Cholinergic agonists** ACh itself has no therapeutic role because of its widespread effects and short duration of action. Congeners of ACh are less susceptible to hydrolysis by cholinesterase and have a narrower range of physiologic effects. Bethanechol, the only systemic cholinergic agonist in general use, stimulates gastrointestinal and genitourinary smooth muscle with minimal effect on the cardiovascular system. It is used in the treatment of urinary retention in the absence of outflow tract obstruction and, less commonly, in gastrointestinal disorders such as postvagotomy gastric atony. Pilocarpine and carbachol are topical cholinergic agonists used in the treatment of glaucoma.

Acetylcholinesterase inhibitors Cholinesterase inhibitors enhance the effects of parasympathetic stimulation by diminishing the inactivation of ACh. The therapeutic application of reversible cholinesterase inhibitors depends upon the role of ACh as neurotransmitter at the skeletal muscle neuroeffector junction and within the central nervous system and includes the treatment of myasthenia gravis (Chap. 366), the termination of neuromuscular blockade following general anesthesia, and the reversal of intoxication by agents with a central anticholinergic action. Physostigmine, a tertiary amine, penetrates the central nervous system well, while related quaternary amines (neostigmine, pyridostigmine, ambenonium, and edrophonium) do not. Organophosphorous cholinesterase inhibitors produce irreversible cholinesterase blockade; these agents are used principally as insecticides and are primarily of toxicologic interest. With regard to the autonomic nervous system, cholinesterase inhibitors are of limited use in the treatment of intestinal and bladder smooth-muscle dysfunction such as occurs in paralytic ileus and atonic urinary bladder. Cholinesterase inhibitors induce a vagotonic response in the heart and may be useful in terminating attacks of paroxysmal supraventricular tachycardia (Chap. 185).

Cholinergic-receptor blocking agents *Atropine* blocks muscarinic cholinergic receptors, with little effect on cholinergic transmission at the autonomic ganglia and the neuromuscular junctions. Many of the central nervous system actions of atropine and atropine-like drugs are attributable to blockade of central muscarinic synapses. The related alkaloid, *scopolamine,* is similar to atropine but causes drowsiness, euphoria, and amnesia, effects that make it suitable as a preanesthetic medication.

Atropine increases heart rate and enhances atrioventricular conduction, actions that may be useful in combating the bradycardia or heart block associated with heightened vagal tone. In addition, atropine reverses cholinergically mediated bronchoconstriction and diminishes respiratory tract secretions. These effects contribute to its utility as a preanesthetic medication.

Atropine also decreases gastrointestinal tract motility and secretion. Although various derivatives and congeners of atropine (such as *propantheline, isopropamide,* and *glycopyrrolate*) have been advocated in patients with peptic ulcer or with diarrheal syndromes, the chronic use of such agents is limited by other manifestations of parasympathetic inhibition such as dry mouth and urinary retention. The investigational selective M-1 inhibitor pirenzepine inhibits gastric secretion at doses that have minimal anticholinergic effects at other sites; this agent may be useful in the treatment of peptic ulcer. Atropine and its congener *ipratropium,* when given by inhalation, cause bronchodilation and have been used experimentally in the treatment of asthma.

REFERENCES

BERRIDGE MJ: Inositol trisphosphate and diacylglycerol: Two interacting second messengers. Ann Rev Biochem 56:159, 1987

EXTON JH: Mechanisms of action of calcium-mobilizing agonists: Some variations on a young theme. FASEB J 2:2670, 1988

———: Mechanisms involved in alpha-adrenergic phenomena. Am J Physiol 248:E633, 1985

FRISHMAN WH: Clinical significance of beta$_1$ selectivity and intrinsic sympathomimetic activity in a beta-adrenergic blocking drug. Am J Cardiol 59:33F, 1987

FRISHMAN WH: Beta-adrenoceptor antagonists: New drugs and new indications. N Engl J Med 305:500, 1981

INSEL PA: Identification and regulation of adrenergic receptors in target cells. Am J Physiol 247:E53, 1984

LANDSBERG L, YOUNG JB: Catecholamines and the adrenal medulla, in *Williams Textbook of Endocrinology,* 7th ed, JD Wilson, DW Foster (eds). Philadelphia, Saunders, 1985, p 891

———, ———: The influence of diet on the sympathetic nervous system, in *Neuroendocrine Perspective,* vol 4, EE Muller et al (eds). Amsterdam, Elsevier, 1985, p 191

LEFKOWITZ RJ, CARON MG: Adrenergic receptors: Models for the study of receptors coupled to guanine nucleotide regulatory proteins. J Biol Chem 263:4993, 1988

LIMBIRD LE: Receptors linked to inhibition of adenylate cyclase: Additional signaling mechanisms. FASEB J 2:2686, 1988

WILLIAMSON JR: Role of inositol lipid breakdown in the generation of intracellular signals: State of the art lecture. Hypertension 8(Suppl II):II-140, 1986

68 G PROTEINS AND THE REGULATION OF SECOND MESSENGER SYSTEMS

MICHAEL FREISSMUTH / ALFRED G. GILMAN

For expression of their biological effects, hormones, neurotransmitters, growth factors, and autacoids (local transmitters such as histamine and serotonin) need interaction with specific receptors. These receptors are classified into distinct categories, based on structural homologies and on similarities in their mechanism of action. For example, the receptors for insulin and certain growth factors (e.g., platelet-derived growth factor) are membrane-bound tyrosine protein kinases, and this enzymatic activity is essential for their function (see Chap. 319). The binding site for ANF (atrial natriuretic factor; see Chap. 38) is in the extracellular domain of a guanylate cyclase that spans the plasma membrane; the intracellular portion of this protein synthesizes a second messenger, guanosine-3′,5′-monophosphate (cyclic GMP). Steroid hormones and triiodothyronine form hormone-receptor complexes that act as regulators of gene transcription (see Chap. 311). Yet another class of receptors, exemplified by the nicotinic cholinergic receptor, incorporate ion channels. Lastly, a large family of plasma membrane–bound receptors (the known number approximates 100) activate guanosine triphosphate–binding (GTP-binding) regulatory proteins, or *G proteins,* in the plasma membranes of cells. Each G protein in turn controls the activity of one or more membrane-bound effectors, such as adenylate cyclase, ion channels, and phospholipases (Table 68-1).

G PROTEIN–LINKED RECEPTORS A diverse group of ligands interact with G protein–linked receptors. These include peptide hormones (e.g., glucagon, ACTH), lipids (prostaglandins), nucleosides and nucleotides (adenosine, ATP), and amines (epinephrine, histamine). Nevertheless, all such receptors possess some structural features in common—including the topology of the proteins with respect to the plasma membrane (Fig. 68-1). The amino terminus of each receptor is outside the cell and is attached to *N*-linked oligosaccharides. The carboxyl terminus is intracellular and contains sites that can be phosphorylated and that play a crucial role in desensitization to hormone actions. The central portion of the receptor molecule is believed to fold into seven α helices that span the membrane bilayer and form the hydrophobic core of the receptor. The ligand-binding site lies within this hydrophobic core and is formed by reactive side chains that are contributed by more than one transmembrane helix. Portions of the intracellular loops that connect the individual membrane-spanning α helices form the site of interaction between the ligand-bound receptor and the appropriate G protein.

G PROTEINS AND THEIR EFFECTORS G proteins are composed of three different subunits designated α, β, and γ in order of decreasing mass. A few of the distinctive properties of individual G protein subunits are summarized in Table 68-2.

G Protein α subunit G proteins are classified on the basis of the α subunit. The hormone-sensitive adenylate cyclase system and the retinal cyclic GMP phosphodiesterase that participates in vision have served as models for the elucidation of the mechanisms of G protein–mediated transmembrane signaling. In both cases, the α subunit of the G protein interacts with and regulates the effector. The α subunits bind Mg^{2+} and guanine nucleotide (GTP or GDP) with high affinity and also possess GTPase activity that is essential for deactivation of the pathway. In addition, many G protein α subunits are substrates for bacterial toxins that catalyze the incorporation of an ADP-ribosyl moiety into the polypeptide at specific amino acid residues. G_s (the G protein that activates adenylate cyclase) and G_t (the major retinal G protein that activates the cyclic GMP phosphodiesterase) are substrates for cholera toxin; G_s in intestinal cells is the natural target for the toxin since cholera is an intraluminal infection. The incorporation of ADP-ribose into G_s causes its persistent activation, and

TABLE 68-1 Hormones, neurotransmitters, and autacoids that control G protein–linked second messenger systems

	Adenylate cyclase		Phospholipase C (IP_3, diacylglycerol)	Arachidonic acid release
Agonist	Stimulation	Inhibition	Stimulation	Stimulation
Acetylcholine		+(M_2, M_4)*	+(M_1, M_3, M_5)	+
Adenosine	+(A_2)	+(A_1)		
ADP			+	+
Adrenocorticotropin	+			
Angiotensin		+	+	+
ATP		+(P_2)	+(P_2)	+
Bombesin			+	
Bradykinin			+	
Calcitonin	+			
Chemotactic peptides (e.g., FMLP)			+	+
Cholecystokinin			+	
Dopamine	+(D_1)	+(D_2)		
Enkephalin/endorphin		+(δ, μ?)		
Epinephrine/norepinephrine	+(β_1, β_2)	+(α_2)	+(α_1)	+(α_1)
Follicle stimulating hormone	+			
Glucagon	+(G_2)		+(G_1)	
Histamine	+(H_2)		+(H_1)	+(H_1)
5-Hydroxytryptamine	+($5HT_{1A}$)	+($5HT_{1A}$)	+($5HT_{2, 1B, 1C, 1D}$)	
Leukotrienes			+	+
Luteinizing hormone (LH)	+			
Luteinizing hormone releasing hormone (LHRH)	+		+	
Parathyroid hormone	+			
Platelet activating factor			+	
Prostacyclin	+			
Prostaglandins (e.g., PGE_2)	+	+		
Somatostatin		+		
Tachykinins (substance P,K)			+	
Thromboxane A_2			+	
Thyrotropin releasing hormone (TRH)	+		+	
Vasoactive intestinal peptide (VIP)	+			
Vasopressin	+(V_2)	+(V_1)	+	

*Receptor subtypes, where known, are indicated in parentheses. M = muscarinic; P = purinergic.

this is the crucial reaction in the pathogenesis of cholera. G_o, G_t family, and the G_i's are ADP-ribosylated by pertussis toxin, and this modification blocks the ability of the G protein to interact with receptors. The precise role of ADP-ribosylation in the pathogenesis of whooping cough is not clear.

GS ALPHA SUBUNIT All molecular species of $G_{s\alpha}$ can activate adenylate cyclase and in addition activate Ca^{2+} channels in skeletal and cardiac muscle. The fact that a single G protein α subunit can interact with more than one effector is an important general point. Not only can G proteins integrate the input from several receptors, they also represent a branch point for regulation of multiple effectors in response to a single signal.

GI AND GO ALPHA SUBUNITS G_i mediates hormonal inhibition of adenylate cyclase. The G_i family consists of oligomers with at least

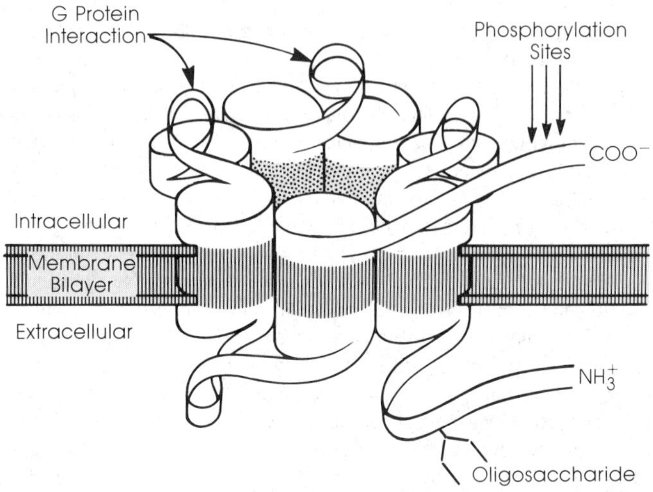

FIGURE 68-1 Schematic representation of the topology of a G protein–coupled receptor. The barrels represent membrane-spanning α helices. The ligand-binding site of the receptor is located within the core formed by these membrane-spanning segments.

three closely related α subunits, designated $G_{i\alpha 1}$, $G_{i\alpha 2}$, and $G_{i\alpha 3}$. $G_{o\alpha}$ is an abundant brain G protein that is structurally similar to the $G_{i\alpha}$ family. While none of the $G_{i\alpha}$ subunits by itself is probably of great relevance in the inhibition of adenylate cyclase (see "Mechanism," below), each of these proteins can activate a K^+ channel in atrial myocardial cells. Stimulation of this pathway by muscarinic cholinergic agonists hyperpolarizes the cell and results in both negative chronotropic and inotropic responses. In the central nervous system, G_o and the G_i family apparently couple a variety of receptors to Ca^{2+} channels; G_o can also modulate K^+ currents in brain cells. The resulting ion fluxes mediate the actions of myriad neurotransmitters. Two or three of the $G_{i\alpha}$ polypeptides and, in some cases, $G_{o\alpha}$ as well control the same effector. The precise role of each α subunit is thus difficult to assess, particularly since single cell types can contain several of these polypeptides. $G_{o\alpha}$- or $G_{i\alpha}$-like polypeptides may also

TABLE 68-2 Properties of G protein subunits

Subunit	$M_r(\times 10^{-3})$	Toxin	Role
α_s (× 4)	44.5–46	Cholera toxin	Activates adenylate cyclase and voltage-sensitive calcium channels
$\alpha_{s,olf}$	44.7	Cholera toxin	Presumed to activate olfactory adenylate cyclase
α_i (× 3)	40.4–40.5	Pertussis toxin	Inhibits adenylate cyclase (weak); stimulates K^+ channels; implicated in pertussis toxin–sensitive activation of phospholipase C
α_o	39.9	Pertussis toxin	Regulates neuronal Ca^{2+} and K^+ channels; implicated in pertussis toxin–sensitive activation of phospholipase C
$\alpha_{t,r}$	40.5	Pertussis toxin, cholera toxin	Activates cyclic GMP phosphodiesterase in retinal rods
$\alpha_{t,c}$	40.9	Pertussis toxin, cholera toxin	Activates cyclic GMP phosphodiesterase in retinal cones
α_z	40.9	Unknown	Pertussis toxin–insensitive events
β (× 2)	37.4	—	βγ required for interaction of α with receptor; deactivates α subunit; direct regulation of effectors(?)
γ (× 3?)	8–10	—	

be involved in the regulation of phospholipase C, since GTP-dependent activation of this enzyme by hormones can be blocked by pertussis toxin in some tissues.

G_T ALPHA SUBUNIT Retinal G protein, G_t or *transducin*, plays a pivotal role in vision. The photon receptor, *rhodopsin*, is localized in membranous disks in the outer segments of retinal rod cells; analogous color receptors are present in the cones. These molecules resemble the other G protein–linked receptors. Upon activation by light, rhodopsin interacts with and activates G_t; G_t in turn activates a cyclic GMP–specific phosphodiesterase. Intracellular concentrations of cyclic GMP fall rapidly, resulting in the closing of Na^+ channels and hyperpolarization of the rod cells. This represents the initial electrical signal that is eventually transmitted to the visual cortex. Retinal rods and cones differ not only in their individual photon receptors; they also have distinct G_t molecules ($G_{t,r}$ and $G_{t,c}$) and distinct cyclic GMP phosphodiesterases.

G_Z ALPHA SUBUNIT G_z is a G protein α subunit that lacks a site for ADP-ribosylation by pertussis toxin and is thus a candidate for regulation of transmembrane signaling pathways that cannot be disrupted by this toxin (e.g., stimulation of phospholipase C in many cells; regulation of certain ion channels).

G protein βγ-subunit complex Two separate genes encode closely related but distinct β subunits (termed β_1 and β_2). Different forms of the γ polypeptide probably exist as well. The functional implication of this heterogeneity is unclear, since the β and γ subunits form a tightly associated complex and have not been resolved in active forms. In addition, the properties of βγ complexes isolated from G_s, G_i, or G_o oligomers are indistinguishable. The βγ complex contributes to the formation of the receptor recognition site on the G protein oligomer and facilitates the attachment of α subunits to the inner face of the plasma membrane. The βγ complex is believed to deactivate the α subunit by formation of the intact G protein. In addition, the free βγ subunit may also regulate effectors, possibly inhibiting adenylate cyclase and activating phospholipase A_2 directly.

MECHANISM OF G PROTEIN–MEDIATED SIGNAL TRANSDUCTION A widely accepted model of the mechanism of G protein–mediated signal transduction is shown schematically in Fig. 68-2. The central thesis is that the G protein α subunit cycles between an inactive, GDP-liganded oligomeric form and an active, GTP-liganded monomeric state. *These two forms of the α subunit represent the "off" and "on" positions of a molecular switch.* The dissociation of GDP from α is the rate-limiting step. That is, the slow rate of spontaneous dissociation of GDP from α holds the switch in the off position. Interaction of the G protein with an agonist-receptor complex (H·R) facilitates dissociation of GDP. Binding of GTP to this ternary complex of hormone, receptor, and G protein has two consequences. First, the affinity of the receptor for the agonist is lowered, resulting in dissociation of the ternary complex. The receptor is thus free to recycle and activate additional G protein molecules, as long as agonist is present. As a result, considerable amplification occurs at this step. Second, the α subunit is activated by its dissociation from the βγ complex. The switch is now on, and the activated α subunit interacts with the appropriate effector and modulates its activity. The G protein switch is programmed to turn itself off automatically, since deactivation results from hydrolysis of bound GTP by the α subunit.

FIGURE 68-2 Model of the regulatory cycles involved in G protein–mediated signal transduction. H = hormone or agonist; R = receptor; E = effector; G = G protein; α and βγ = G protein subunits. Starred complexes are activated species. For further explanation, see text.

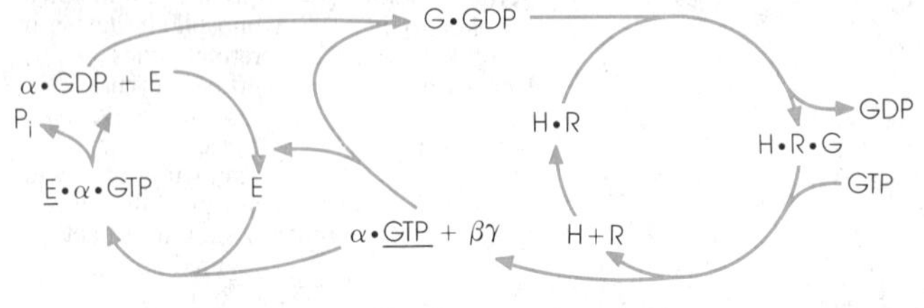

However, the lifetime of the activated α subunit is relatively long (several seconds), since the intrinsic rate of hydrolysis of GTP is slow; this kinetic feature permits additional signal amplification. To complete the cycle, the GDP-bound α subunit associates with βγ, and the system relaxes to its basal state. As mentioned above, the free βγ subunit may itself regulate effectors directly.

Inhibition of adenylate cyclase is attributed at least in part to the capacity of the βγ subunit, released upon activation of G_i, to interact with and deactivate G_s; βγ can thus inhibit adenylate cyclase indirectly. This subunit exchange hypothesis predicts that the activation of one pathway can cause inhibition of effectors that are controlled by other G protein α subunits if the concentration of βγ in the membrane is raised sufficiently.

SECOND MESSENGER SYSTEMS UNDER THE CONTROL OF G PROTEINS (Fig. 68-3) Cyclic AMP The conversion of ATP to cyclic AMP is accomplished by the catalytic subunit of the adenylate cyclase complex. This membrane-bound enzyme is believed to span the plasma membrane several times; the topology of the protein resembles that usually found in transporters and channels.

Cyclic AMP acts as a second messenger for a number of hormones (Table 68-1). The primary mechanism of action of the cyclic nucleotide is to cause dissociation of a dimer of cyclic AMP–binding regulatory subunits from the catalytic subunits of a protein kinase. The free catalytic subunits of the protein kinase are enzymatically active, and they transfer the γ phosphate from ATP to serine and threonine residues in target proteins. Such phosphorylation can either increase the activity (e.g., glycogen phosphorylase kinase, triacylglycerol lipase, protein phosphatase inhibitor 1) or decrease the activity (e.g., glycogen synthase, myosin light chain kinase) of the various substrates.

Termination of cyclic AMP action is accomplished by several mechanisms that are themselves subject to regulation by cyclic AMP and Ca^{2+}-calmodulin, a molecule with related second messenger functions (see below). Cyclic AMP is degraded to 5′-AMP by cyclic nucleotide phosphodiesterases. Some of these isoenzymes are activated by Ca^{2+}-calmodulin; they are inhibited by several drugs, including the methylxanthines (caffeine and theophylline) and milrinone. In addition, most cells possess a mechanism for the facilitated extrusion of cyclic AMP.

The regulatory effects of protein kinases are reversed by phosphoprotein phosphatases, which hydrolytically cleave the phosphate ester bond. These enzymes differ in their substrate specificities and in their regulation. For example, in the presence of elevated concentrations of cyclic AMP, protein phosphatase inhibitor 1 is phosphorylated by the cyclic AMP–dependent protein kinases; in this phosphorylated form, the inhibitor suppresses the activity of protein phosphatase 1. By contrast, protein phosphatase 2B is activated by Ca^{2+}-calmodulin. This network of stimulatory and inhibitory mechanisms integrates input from additional second messenger systems, which is necessary for efficient fine-tuning of cellular activities. All intracellular effects of cyclic AMP were initially believed to result from activation of protein phosphorylation, but ionic (Na^+) channels in olfactory neuroepithelial cells can be regulated (gated) directly by cyclic AMP.

Inositol trisphosphate, diacylglycerol, and calcium Inositol-1,4,5-trisphosphate (IP_3) and diacylglycerol are second messengers generated by activation of a family of phosphoinositidases, commonly termed *phospholipase C*. These enzymes use phosphatidylinositol-4,5-bisphosphate, a phospholipid component of the plasma membrane, as substrate. Inositol trisphosphate can be phosphorylated to inositol-1,3,4,5-tetrakisphosphate, which may also serve as a second messenger. A large number of hormones and related molecules are known to activate phospholipase C (Table 68-1). This pathway is dependent on GTP, and it can be blocked by pertussis toxin in certain cells (e.g., granulocytes and mast cells). By contrast, the toxin has no effect on this response in certain other cells (e.g., cardiac myocytes and hepatocytes). More than one G protein may be involved in the regulation of phospholipase C.

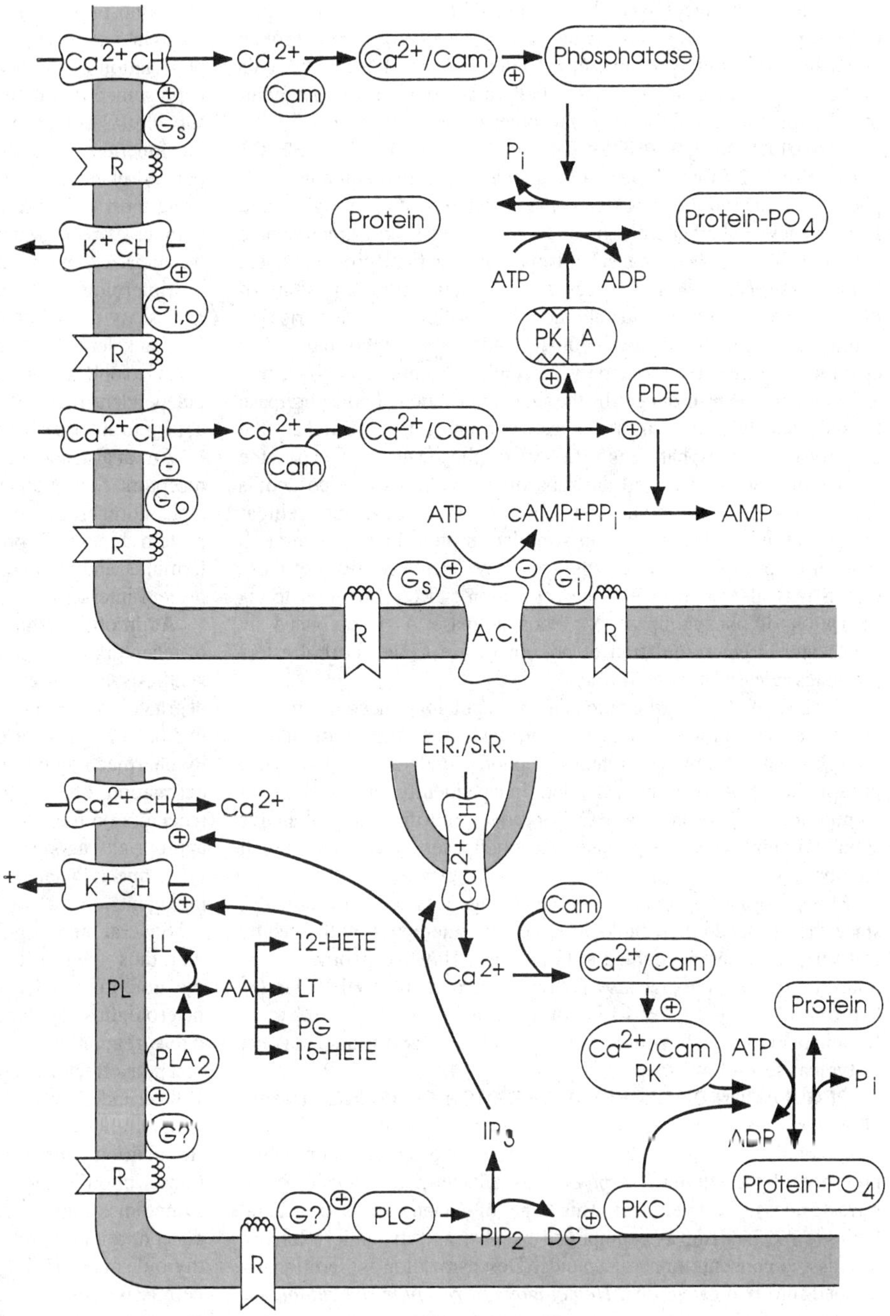

FIGURE 68-3 The role of G proteins in transmembrane signaling. The top panel shows pathways that are regulated by identified G proteins. The bottom panel depicts pathways in which the participation of G proteins is probable, but the specific proteins have not yet been identified.
AA = arachidonic acid
AC = adenylate cyclase
Ca^{2+}/Cam PKC = calcium-calmodulin-dependent protein kinase
Cam = calmodulin
CH = channel
DG = diacylglycerol
E.R./S.R. = endoplasmic/sarcoplasmic reticulum
G = G protein
12-HETE = 12-hydroxyeicosatetraenoic acid
15-HETE = 15-hydroxyeicosatetraenoic acid
IP_3 = inositol trisphosphate
LL = lysophospholipid
LT = leukotriene
PDE = cyclic nucleotide phosphodiesterase
PG = prostaglandin
PIP_2 = phosphatidylinositol trisphosphate
PLC = phospholipase C
PKA = cyclic AMP–dependent protein kinase
PKC = protein kinase C
R = receptor for hormone or agonist

Inositol trisphosphate releases Ca^{2+} from intracellular stores (endoplasmic/sarcoplasmic reticulum) and promotes Ca^{2+} influx from the extracellular fluid. Additional mechanisms for entry of Ca^{2+} into the cytosolic compartment include voltage-gated Ca^{2+} channels and exchange mechanisms activated by other ions. G proteins regulate the activity of some of these channels and exchangers.

Ca^{2+} both regulates the activity of target enzymes directly and, more importantly, exerts its second messenger functions by interactions with Ca^{2+}-binding proteins such as troponin C and calmodulin. Calmodulin is a ubiquitous intracellular protein that binds four molecules of Ca^{2+}. This Ca^{2+}-calmodulin complex regulates several enzymes of the cyclic AMP system, including one type of adenylate cyclase, certain cyclic nucleotide phosphodiesterases, and protein phosphatase 2B (calcineurin). Several protein kinases are also activated by Ca^{2+}-calmodulin; the resulting effect can be either synergistic with (e.g., activation of phosphorylase kinase) or antagonistic to (e.g., activation of myosin light chain kinase) the cyclic AMP–mediated action. The effects of Ca^{2+}-calmodulin on its target enzymes can be blocked by certain phenothiazine drugs. The relationship between this effect and the therapeutic efficacy or toxicity of these drugs is unknown.

Deactivation of the pathway is achieved by active transport of Ca^{2+} into intracellular compartments and extrusion of the ion by plasma membrane–bound, Ca^{2+}-pumping ATPases. Inositol trisphosphate is degraded by sequential dephosphorylation. The phosphatase that catalyzes the removal of phosphate from inositol-1-phosphate is inhibited by Li^+. It is not known whether this effect of Li^+ is related to its efficacy in psychiatric disorders.

The second product of the phospholipase C reaction is diacylglycerol, which acts as a second messenger by activating a family of isoenzymes referred to as *protein kinase C*. Upon binding of diacylglycerol, the requirement of these enzymes for Ca^{2+} decreases into the range of free Ca^{2+} concentrations found in cytosol. Activated protein kinase C phosphorylates many intracellular proteins, including some substrates of cyclic AMP–dependent protein kinase. The phorbol esters, which act as tumor promoters, are structurally related to diacylglycerol and also bind to and activate protein kinase C. This action is believed to explain their carcinogenicity.

The effect of diacylglycerol is terminated by enzymatic recycling to form phosphatidylinositol. Alternatively, diacylglycerol is broken down by a diacylglycerol lipase. Of interest, one of the fatty acids in the diacylglycerol molecule is usually arachidonate, the precursor of prostaglandins, leukotrienes, and other eicosanoids.

STIMULATION OF PHOSPHOLIPASE A_2 AND RELEASE OF ARACHIDONIC ACID Release of arachidonate from membrane phospholipids is the rate-limiting step in the biosynthesis of prostaglandins, leukotrienes, and other eicosanoids (see Chap. 69). Free arachidonate can arise by two distinct mechanisms. First, a family of enzymes, termed *phospholipase A_2*, cleaves the ester bond at the 2 position of the glycerol moiety of membrane phospholipids, giving rise to equimolar amounts of arachidonate and lysophospholipids. The enzymes require Ca^{2+} for activity. Second, as mentioned above, free arachidonate can be produced by the sequential action of phospholipase C and diacylglycerol lipase. Thus, hormones that stimulate the hydrolysis of phosphatidylinositol-4,5-bisphosphate also cause the release of arachidonate and the subsequent synthesis of eicosanoids (Table 68-1). In addition, these hormones increase intracellular concentrations of free Ca^{2+} and stimulate protein kinase C through inositol trisphosphate and diacylglycerol, respectively. Both of these effects may also contribute to the generation of free arachidonate via activation of phospholipase A_2. Phospholipase A_2 is activated by Ca^{2+}, and direct stimulation of protein kinase C by phorbol esters promotes release of arachidonate.

In view of the interdigitation of the regulatory mechanisms that control these pathways, it is not surprising that the regulation of phospholipase A_2 by G proteins is poorly understood. However, phospholipase A_2 can be activated independently of concomitant stimulation of phospholipase C. Moreover, purified G protein $\beta\gamma$ subunit complex may stimulate phospholipase A_2 activity in cell membranes.

Most eicosanoids are not second messengers as defined originally, since they produce their biologic effects by interacting with specific cell surface receptors coupled to G proteins. However, some metabolites of the 12-lipoxygenase pathway, in particular HEPETE (8-hydroxy-11,12-epoxy-5,9,14-icosotrienoic acid), may affect neuronal K^+ channels through a direct intracellular mechanism and thus act as typical second messengers.

REGULATION OF RECEPTOR-EFFECTOR COUPLING Desensitization Prolonged exposure of cells to a hormonal stimulus leads to a gradual attenuation of the biologic response, despite the continuing presence of the stimulus, a process usually termed desensitization, refractoriness, or tolerance. This type of adaptation is a general biologic mechanism, as exemplified by pharmacodynamic tolerance to massive concentrations of opioids. Desensitization is traditionally divided into two categories. *Homologous* or *receptor-specific desensitization* refers to the refractoriness that develops only to agonists that act on the same receptor as the desensitizing stimulus. In addition, stimulation of a particular receptor by an agonist can lead to the subsequent attenuation of the response to multiple hormones that influence the same pathway through distinct receptors. This phenomenon is termed *heterologous desensitization*.

Beta-adrenergic receptor-mediated stimulation of adenylate cyclase has served as a model system for elucidation of the molecular events that underlie desensitization, and both homologous and heterologous desensitization appear to result from phosphorylation of the receptor on its carboxyl-terminal domain.

Homologous desensitization is a multistep process. Initially (within minutes) receptors are uncoupled from G_s, as judged in part by their inability to stimulate adenylate cyclase. This process is reversible upon removal of agonist. However, the continued presence of agonist eventually leads to a decline in the concentration of receptors in the plasma membrane. This "down regulation" occurs over several hours and is not readily reversible, since protein synthesis is required to replenish the receptors on the cell surface. A novel protein kinase termed βARK (beta-adrenergic receptor kinase) specifically phosphorylates the agonist-bound receptor, whereas unliganded or antagonist-bound receptor will not serve as substrate. However, βARK also phosphorylates other agonist-bound receptors that stimulate adenylate cyclase, such as the receptor for prostaglandin E_1. Phosphorylation of the beta-adrenergic receptor uncouples it from G_s and is presumed to initiate sequestration of the receptor into an ill-defined subcellular compartment. The sequestered receptor may recycle to the functionally active pool upon hydrolytic cleavage of the incorporated phosphate by a phosphatase, or it may undergo degradation. Long-term exposure of cells to agonists apparently also reduces the number of receptors by decreasing the steady-state concentration of the mRNA that encodes the protein.

Heterologous desensitization of receptors that stimulate adenylate cyclase is probably mediated predominantly by a classic negative feedback loop. Activation of cyclic AMP–dependent protein kinase leads to phosphorylation of the receptors in a largely agonist-independent manner, and this modification also interferes with their ability to interact with G_s.

An analogous mechanism of desensitization is observed with receptors that mediate stimulation of phospholipase C (e.g., the alpha-adrenergic receptor). As a result of release of diacylglycerol, protein kinase C phosphorylates the receptors near the carboxyl terminus and is thereby presumed to interfere with the receptor–G protein interaction.

Additional forms of regulation The steady-state concentration of receptors in the plasma membrane represents the balance between synthesis and insertion into the bilayer versus internalization and degradation. As mentioned, the continuous presence of agonist tilts this balance in favor of degradation. Conversely, removal of agonist by pharmacologic blockade of the receptor, denervation of tissue, or extirpation of the source of the agonist favors accumulation of receptors on the cell surface and sensitization of target tissues to the appropriate agonist. Such sensitization may underlie the clinical syndrome associated with abrupt withdrawal of beta-adrenergic blocking agents.

Several other regulatory mechanisms influence signal transduction and, thus, the sensitivity of target cells to agonists. Since these events are not promoted by the receptor agonist, they are referred to as heterologous regulation. The most remarkable examples of heterologous regulation at the clinical level are the alterations in adrenergic receptor-effector coupling produced by thyroid and steroid hormones. Both triiodothyronine and glucocorticoids appear to be necessary to maintain normal coupling between beta-adrenergic receptors and G_s. In addition, thyroid hormones and glucocorticoids can increase transcription of mRNA for beta-adrenergic receptors. As one example, symptoms of increased sympathetic activity in the absence of elevated concentrations of plasma catecholamines is characteristic of hyperthyroidism. Similarly, heterologous regulation may underlie the permissive role of glucocorticoids in neurohormonal control of blood pressure.

ROLE OF G PROTEIN SYSTEMS IN DISEASE The pivotal role of G proteins in regulatory biology is understood in considerable detail. Comparatively little is known about the degree to which perturbations of these pathways participate in pathophysiology. However, a link to alterations in a G protein–regulated second messenger system has been established in several entities.

Cholera (See also Chap. 122) Pathogenic strains of *Vibrio cholerae* produce an exotoxin that transfers an ADP-ribosyl moiety to the α subunit of G_s, using intracellular nicotinamide adenine dinucleotide (NAD) as the donor. This reaction can occur in virtually all cells. However, the bacteria remain confined to the intestinal lumen, and the toxin binds to the intestinal epithelium but is not absorbed into the systemic circulation. Cell-surface binding of cholera toxin is dependent on the interaction between the B subunits of the toxin and gangliosides (GM_1) on the cell surface. Following such binding, the catalytically active A subunit of the toxin penetrates the cell. The ensuing modification of $G_{s\alpha}$ leads to its persistent activation, and the resultant high intracellular concentrations of cyclic AMP trigger the secretion of water and electrolytes into the intestinal lumen. The resulting watery diarrhea is the hallmark of cholera. Enteropathogenic strains of *Escherichia coli* produce a heat-labile toxin that is quite similar to cholera toxin and causes diarrhea by an identical mechanism (see Chap. 92). By contrast, other strains of *E. coli* cause diarrhea by elaboration of a low-molecular-weight, heat-stable toxin that activates guanylate cyclase. Enzymes capable of removing mono ADP-ribosyl moieties from cellular proteins have not been detected. Upon removal of the toxin, its effects fade slowly as ADP-ribosylated $G_{s\alpha}$ is gradually replaced by newly synthesized protein. This explains why the symptoms of cholera persist after eradication of the bacteria.

Pertussis (See also Chap. 116) The molecular pathogenesis of whooping cough and cholera are similar. *Bordetella pertussis* remains confined to the bronchi and produces two exotoxins. The first is commonly referred to as pertussis toxin or islet-activating protein. Like cholera toxin, this protein is an enzyme that catalyzes the NAD-dependent ADP-ribosylation of proteins; the targets for pertussis toxin are receptors of the $G_{i\alpha}$ family and $G_{o\alpha}$ (see above). This modification interferes with the ability of these G proteins to interact with receptors; cyclic AMP concentrations are thus elevated. Again, restoration of normal G protein function depends on de novo synthesis of the α subunits, explaining in part why the symptoms of pertussis can persist for weeks after eradication of the microorganisms. In contrast to cholera, the sequence of events that links ADP-ribosylation of G protein α subunits to clinical symptoms is not understood. However, *B. pertussis* also interferes with cellular regulation of cyclic AMP concentrations by another mechanism, since the second exotoxin is itself an invasive calmodulin-dependent adenylate cyclase. Elevated concentrations of cyclic AMP in neutrophils impair their ability to kill ingested bacteria. In addition, ADP-ribosylation of a neutrophil G protein α subunit (presumably $G_{i\alpha 2}$) uncouples the neutrophil chemotactic receptor from the pathway that controls superoxide generation and bactericidal activity. This may contribute to the increased susceptibility to pulmonary infection by other pathogens—a frequent complication of whooping cough.

Anthrax (See also Chap. 104) Cutaneous infection with *Bacillus anthracis* produces a lesion characterized by central necrosis and prominent subcutaneous edema. The edema is due to the presence of a bacterial exotoxin, referred to as *edema factor*. Edema factor is an adenylate cyclase that shares many characteristics with the *B. pertussis* enzyme, including host cell penetration and dependence on calmodulin. Rare patients who ingest *Bacillus* organisms can develop a watery diarrhea indistinguishable from cholera. This syndrome may result from penetration of edema factor into cells of the intestinal mucosa.

Pseudohypoparathyroidism (See also Chap. 340) Pseudohypoparathyroidism type I is an inherited disorder characterized by target organ resistance to parathyroid hormone. In addition, many patients exhibit partial resistance to other hormones that act by stimulation of adenylate cyclase (e.g., thyroid stimulating hormone, vasopressin, glucagon). In one variation of the disorder (termed pseudohypoparathyroidism type Ia), the molecular defect results in reduced cellular concentrations of $G_{s\alpha}$, and this partial deficiency is apparently due to lower cellular levels of the mRNAs that encode the polypeptide. These observations point to a mutation that impairs transcription of the $G_{s\alpha}$ gene or that decreases the stability of the mRNA. Pseudohypoparathyroidism Ib is a similar syndrome in which cellular concentrations of $G_{s\alpha}$ are normal.

Other disorders Alterations of G proteins are postulated to occur in diabetes mellitus and hypertrophic congestive cardiomyopathy. The relationship between these alterations and the pathogenesis of the disease remain to be established.

Certain point mutations within the genes that encode G protein α subunits interfere with the GTPase activity, and in vivo such mutations would be expected to cause constitutive activation of the pathways that they regulate. Analogous mutations also occur in the related guanine nucleotide–binding $p21^{ras}$ proteins of human cancer cells (see Chap. 10). Expression of these mutated $p21^{ras}$ proteins causes transformation of the cells, thus proving a cause-and-effect relationship. Similar mutations in G protein α subunits could also cause human tumors, since the growth rate of some cells (in particular pituitary, adrenal, thyroid, gonads) depends in part on the intracellular concentration of cyclic AMP. Membranes of pituitary adenomas have been reported to contain a constitutively activated $G_{s\alpha}$ subunit. Tumor-promoting phorbol esters are believed to act by persistent activation of protein kinase C, and constitutive activation of this pathway via a mutated G protein α subunit that regulates phospholipase C would conceivably also promote tumor development.

REFERENCES

BERRIDGE MJ: Inositol trisphosphate and diacylglycerol: Two interacting second messengers. Ann Rev Biochem 56:159, 1987

BROWN AM, BIRNBAUMER L: Direct G protein gating of ion channels. Am J Physiol 254:H401, 1988

CARTER A et al: Reduced expression of multiple forms of the α subunit of the stimulatory GTP-binding protein in pseudohypoparathyroidism type Ia. Proc Natl Acad Sci USA 84:7266, 1987

GILMAN AG: G proteins: Transducers of receptor-generated signals. Ann Rev Biochem 56:615, 1987

SIBLEY DR et al: Regulation of transmembrane signaling by receptor phosphorylation. Cell 48:913, 1987

VALLAR L et al: Altered G_s and adenylate cyclase activity in human GH-secreting pituitary adenomas. Nature 330:566, 1987

69 EICOSANOIDS AND HUMAN DISEASE

R. PAUL ROBERTSON

This chapter focuses on the formation and mechanism of action of the physiologically active metabolites of arachidonic acid and on the biologic phenomena in which these compounds may be involved.

FORMATION OF THE EICOSANOIDS Prostaglandins, the first arachidonic acid metabolites to be recognized, were so named because they were originally identified in seminal fluid and thought to be secreted by the prostate. As other active metabolites were characterized, two major pathways—the cyclooxygenase and the lipoxygenase pathways—became apparent. These synthetic pathways are summarized schematically in Fig. 69-1, and structures of representative metabolites are shown in Fig. 69-2. All products of both the cyclooxygenase and the lipoxygenase pathways are called *eicosanoids*. The products of the cyclooxygenase pathway—the prostaglandins and the thromboxanes—are termed *prostanoids*.

The initial synthetic step for both pathways involves the cleavage of arachidonic acid from phospholipid in the plasma membrane of cells. Phospholipase A_2 cleaves arachidonic acid from phospholipid. Free arachidonic acid can also be derived by phospholipase C cleavage of diacylglycerol from phosphoinositides and subsequent cleavage of arachidonic acid from diacylglycerol by diacylglycerol lipase. Free arachidonic acid can then be oxygenated by the cyclooxygenase or lipoxygenase pathway. The first product of the cyclooxygenase pathway is the cyclic endoperoxide prostaglandin G_2 (PGG_2), which is converted to prostaglandin H_2 (PGH_2). PGG_2 and PGH_2 are the key intermediates in the formation of physiologically active prostaglandins (PGD_2, PGE_2, $PGF_{2\alpha}$, and PGI_2) and thromboxane A_2 (TXA_2). The first product of the 5-lipoxygenase pathway is 5-hydroperoxyeicosatetraenoic acid (5-HPETE) which is an intermediate in the formation of 5-hydroxyeicosatetraenoic acid (5-HETE) and the leukotrienes (LTA_4, LTB_4, LTC_4, LTD_4, and LTE_4). Two fatty acids other than arachidonic acid [3,11,14-eicosatrienoic acid (dihomo-γ-linolenic acid) and 5,8,11,14,17-eicosapentaenoic acid] can be converted to metabolites closely related to these eicosanoids. Prostanoid products of the former substrate carry the subscript 1; the leukotriene subscript is 3. Prostanoid products of the latter substrate have the subscript 3 while leukotrienes have the subscript 5. Arachidonic acid forms prostaglandin products with subscripts 2 and leukotrienes with

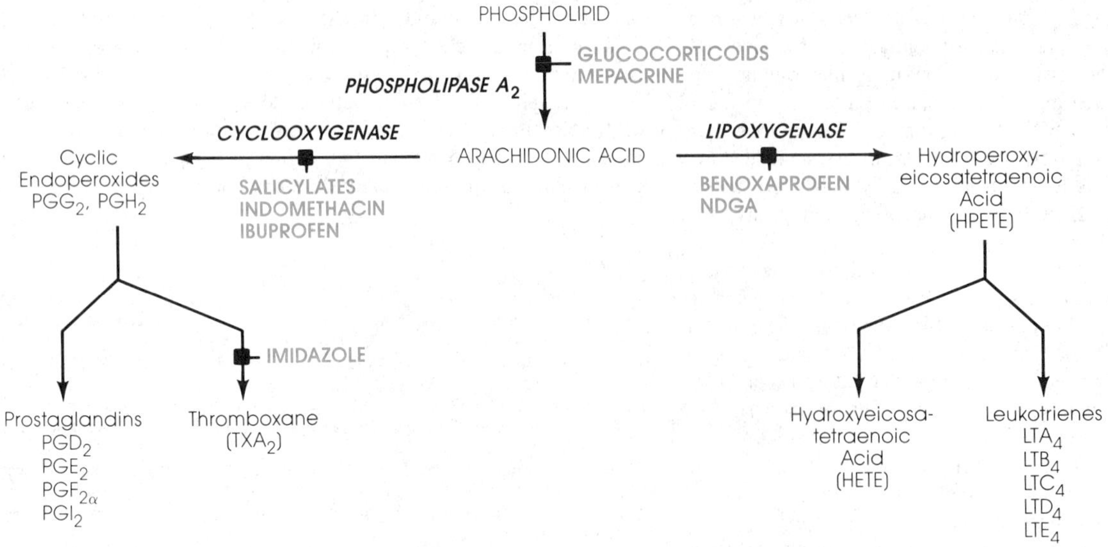

FIGURE 69-1 The overall scheme of arachidonic acid metabolism. The various drugs act at the various enzymatic steps to inhibit the reactions. The major pathways are the cyclooxygenase and the lipoxygenase pathways. Phospholipase A_2 is inhibited by glucocorticoids and mepacrine; cyclooxygenase is inhibited by certain salicylates, indomethacin, and ibuprofen; and lipoxygenase is inhibited by benoxaprofen and nordihydroguaiaretic acid (NDGA). Imidazole prevents TXA_2 synthesis.

the subscript 4. (The subscripts designate the number of double bonds between carbon atoms in the side chains.)

Virtually all cells have the necessary substrates and enzymes to form some of the metabolites of arachidonic acid, but tissues differ in the enzymes they possess and consequently in the products they form. Eicosanoids are synthesized according to immediate need and are not stored in significant amounts for later release.

The cyclooxygenase products Prostaglandins D_2, E_2, $F_{2\alpha}$, and I_2 are formed from the cyclic endoperoxides PGG_2 and PGH_2. Of these, PGE_2 and PGI_2 exert the broadest physiologic effects. PGE_2 has notable effects in, and is synthesized by, many tissues. PGI_2 (also called prostacyclin) is a dominant product of arachidonic acid in the endothelial and smooth muscle cells of vessel walls and in some nonvascular tissues. PGI_2 is a vasodilator and an inhibitor of platelet aggregation. PGD_2 is also believed to play a role in platelet aggregation and brain function. $PGF_{2\alpha}$ plays a role in uterine and ovarian function.

Thromboxane synthetase catalyzes the incorporation of an oxygen atom into the ring of the endoperoxide PGH_2 to form the thromboxanes. TXA_2 is synthesized by platelets and enhances platelet aggregation.

FIGURE 69-2 Structures of representative biologically active eicosanoids.

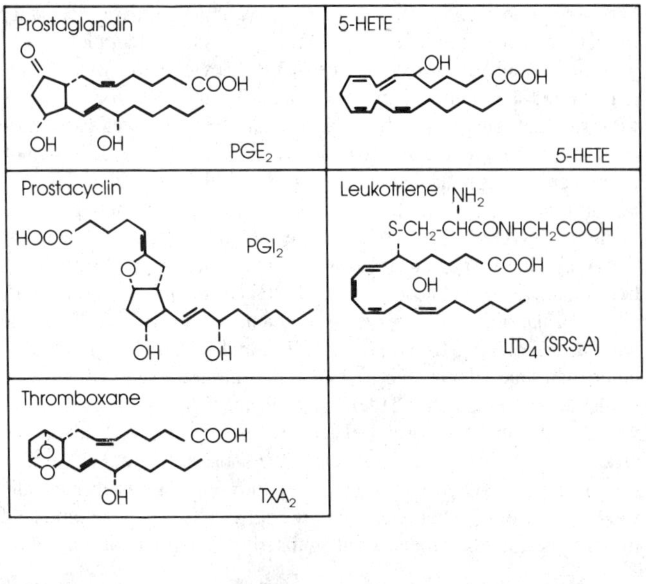

The lipoxygenase products The leukotrienes and HETE are the end products of the lipoxygenase pathway. The leukotrienes have histamine-like actions, including induction of increased vascular permeability and of bronchospasm, and appear to have mediator activities for leukocytes. LTC_4, LTD_4, and LTE_4 together have been identified as slow-reacting substance of anaphylaxis (SRS-A). (The pathophysiology of the leukotrienes is discussed in detail in Chap. 204.)

EFFECTS OF DRUGS ON THE SYNTHESIS OF EICOSANOIDS Many drugs block the synthesis of eicosanoids by inhibiting one or more enzymes in their biosynthetic pathways. Glucocorticoids and antimalarial drugs such as mepacrine interfere with the cleavage of arachidonic acid from phospholipids (Fig. 69-1). Cyclooxygenase is directly inhibited by nonsteroidal anti-inflammatory drugs including salicylates, indomethacin, and ibuprofen. Benoxaprofen, another nonsteroidal anti-inflammatory drug, inhibits the lipoxygenase-mediated conversion of arachidonic acid to HPETE. Tranylcypromine, an antidepressant drug, inhibits the conversion of cyclic endoperoxides to PGI_2, and imidazole inhibits thromboxane synthesis. The fact that a drug inhibits the synthesis of a certain eicosanoid does not mean that a given drug effect is the direct result of a deficiency of that eicosanoid. Most of these drugs inhibit early reactions in the synthetic pathways and therefore block the formation of more than one product. Additionally, some of these drugs have other effects. For example, indomethacin not only inhibits formation of cyclic endoperoxides by cyclooxygenase but may also disrupt calcium flux across membranes, inhibit cyclic adenosine monophosphate (cyclic AMP)–dependent protein kinase and phosphodiesterase, and inhibit one of the enzymes responsible for degradation of PGE_2.

No truly specific synthesis inhibitors nor specific receptor antagonists for individual arachidonic acid metabolites are suitable for human use. The lack of such drugs is a major barrier to elucidating the role of these metabolites in physiologic and pathophysiologic processes.

METABOLISM AND ASSAY OF EICOSANOIDS Arachidonic acid metabolites are catabolized rapidly in vivo. Prostaglandins of the E and F series, although chemically stable, are almost completely degraded during a single passage through the liver or the lung. Thus, essentially all nonmetabolized PGE_2 measurable in urine is derived from renal and seminal vesicle secretion, whereas PGE_2 metabolites in urine represent total-body PGE_2 synthesis. PGI_2 and TXA_2 are both chemically unstable and also rapidly catabolized. Because PGE_2,

PGI_2, and TXA_2 are short-lived in vivo, measurement of their inactive metabolites is commonly used as an index of the rates of their formation. PGE_2 is converted to 15-keto-13,14,-dihydro-PGE_2, PGI_2 is converted to 6-keto-$PGF_{1\alpha}$, and TXA_2 is converted to TXB_2. Five methods are generally available to measure arachidonic acid metabolites in physiologic fluids: bioassay, radioimmunoassay, chromatography, receptor assay, and mass spectrometry. Bioassay provides direct physiologic data but is not very sensitive. Radioimmunoassay is the most convenient and sensitive but, as with bioassay and receptor assay, should be preceded by extraction and chromatography of samples to ensure specificity. Mass spectrometry preceded by chromatography is accurate but laborious. With each method precautions must be taken in handling samples because prostaglandin synthesis may be enhanced during the collection of biologic samples. For example, if blood is allowed to clot or if platelets are not carefully separated from plasma, the generation of large amounts of PGE_2 and TXA_2 during processing can lead to erroneous results. Use of an inhibitor of prostaglandin synthesis in the collection tube minimizes this problem.

PHYSIOLOGY Prostaglandins and leukotrienes have specific receptor sites on the plasma membranes of cells such as liver, corpus luteum, adrenal gland, adipocytes, thymocytes, uterus, pancreatic islets, platelets, and red blood cells. Most of the binding sites exhibit specificity for eicosanoids of a given type. For example, the liver plasma membrane PGE receptor binds PGE_1 and PGE_2 with high affinity but not prostaglandins of the A, F, and I configurations. The postreceptor mechanisms by which the binding of the prostaglandins alters cell function are poorly understood. Some of these mechanisms involve modulation of cyclic AMP production through interactions with two G-proteins, the stimulatory (G_s) and inhibitory (G_i) subunits of adenylate cyclase (see Chap. 68). The normal physiologic actions of eicosanoids are not mediated via the plasma. Instead, eicosanoids act as local, intercellular, and/or intracellular modulators of biochemical activity in the tissues in which they are formed (e.g., a paracrine function). They are autacoids, not hormones. Most are short-lived in the circulation because of chemical instability and/or rapid degradation.

Lipolysis PGE_2 is synthesized by adipocytes, has specific receptors in adipocytes, and is a potent endogenous inhibitor of lipolysis. Since the formation of cyclic AMP is necessary in the action of hormones that stimulate lipolysis, the interactions between PGE and adenylate cyclase have been examined in considerable detail. PGE inhibits lipolysis by decreasing the formation of cyclic AMP in response to epinephrine, adrenocorticotropic hormone (ACTH), glucagon, and thyroid-stimulating hormone (TSH). Thus, PGE may act as an endogenous antilipolytic substance by interfering with the stimulation of cyclic AMP formation by hormones.

Insulin and PGE may act independently during their antilipolytic actions on the adipocyte. For example, insulin but not PGE inhibits the stimulation of lipolysis by exogenous cyclic AMP in isolated adipocytes, but both agents inhibit hormone-stimulated generation of cyclic AMP. This suggests a site of action of insulin distal to the stimulation of adenylate cyclase. In some animals PGE inhibits glucagon-induced lipolysis whereas insulin does not.

Sodium and water balance The renin-angiotensin-aldosterone system is a major regulator of sodium homeostasis, and vasopressin exerts the principal control over water balance. Arachidonic acid metabolites influence both systems. PGE_2 and PGI_2 stimulate renin secretion, and inhibitors of prostaglandin synthesis have the opposite effect. PGI_2 and PGE_2 decrease renal vascular resistance and increase blood flow; this results in redistribution of blood flow from the outer renal cortex to the juxtamedullary region of the kidney. Conversely, inhibitors of prostaglandin synthesis, such as indomethacin and meclofenamate, decrease total renal blood flow and shunt the remaining flow to the outer cortex, which can lead to acute renal venoconstriction and acute renal failure in circumstances such as volume depletion and edematous states. PGE_2 is natriuretic whereas cyclooxygenase inhibitors cause sodium and water retention.

Indomethacin also increases sensitivity to exogenous vasopressin in dogs. Conversely, PGE_2 decreases vasopressin-stimulated water transport. Since this effect of PGE_2 is circumvented by the administration of dibutyryl–cyclic AMP, PGE_2 most likely interferes with the stimulation of adenylate cyclase by vasopressin.

Platelet aggregation Platelets synthesize PGE_2, PGD_2, and TXA_2. Although a physiologic role has not been established for PGE_2 and PGD_2 in platelet function, TXA_2 is a potent stimulator of platelet aggregation; in contrast PGI_2, formed by the endothelial cells of blood vessel walls, is a potent antagonist of platelet aggregation. TXA_2 and PGI_2 may exert their opposing effects by decreasing and increasing, respectively, platelet generation of cyclic AMP.

Inhibitors of endogenous prostaglandin synthesis interfere with platelet aggregation. For example, a single dose of aspirin can suppress normal platelet aggregation for 48 h and longer, presumably by suppressing cyclooxygenase-mediated TXA_2 synthesis. Cyclooxygenase inhibition by a single dose of aspirin is of longer duration in platelets than in other tissues, because the platelet, in contrast to nucleated cells that can synthesize new proteins, does not have the machinery to form new enzyme. Consequently, the effect of aspirin persists until newly formed platelets have been released. Endothelial cells, on the other hand, rapidly recover cyclooxygenase activity following discontinuation of treatment with aspirin, and PGI_2 production is thus restored. This is one reason that patients taking aspirin are not predisposed to excessive formation of platelet thrombi. In addition, the platelet is more sensitive than the endothelial cell to aspirin.

Endothelial damage may lead to platelet aggregation along the blood vessel wall by causing a local decrease in PGI_2 synthesis, thereby allowing unbridled platelet aggregation at the site of vessel wall damage.

Vascular effects The vasoactive properties of arachidonic acid metabolites are among their most impressive actions. PGE_2 and PGI_2 are vasodilators where $PGF_{2\alpha}$, TXA_2, and LTC_4-LTD_4-LTE_4 are vasoconstrictors in most vascular beds. These effects appear to be the result of direct action on the smooth muscle of the vessel wall. Provided that systemic blood pressure is maintained, the vasodilatory arachidonic acid metabolites act to increase blood flow. If blood pressure falls, however, blood flow decreases because with systemic hypotension catecholamine-induced vasoconstriction offsets the vasodilatory effect of the prostaglandins. Thus, significant alterations in systemic blood pressure must be excluded when evaluating the effects of arachidonic acid metabolites on organ blood flow.

Gastrointestinal effects Prostaglandins of the E series influence gastrointestinal function. Infusion of either PGI_2 or PGE_2 into the gastric artery of dogs causes increases in blood flow and inhibition of acid output, and several PGE analogues both inhibit gastric acid output and directly protect the gastrointestinal mucosa when taken orally. In in vitro experiments prostaglandins stimulate gastrointestinal smooth muscle and thereby increase motility, but it is not clear whether these actions are physiologically important.

Neurotransmission PGE inhibits egress of norepinephrine from sympathetic nerve terminals. The effect of PGE on norepinephrine secretion appears to be prejunctional, i.e., at a site on the nerve terminal proximal to the synaptic cleft, and can be reversed by increases in calcium concentration in the perfusing medium. Therefore, PGE_2 may inhibit norepinephrine release by blocking calcium influx. Inhibitors of PGE_2 synthesis can augment norepinephrine release in response to stimulation of adrenergic nerves.

Catecholamines can release PGE_2 from a variety of tissues, probably by an alpha-adrenergic–mediated mechanism. For example, in innervated tissues such as the spleen, nerve stimulation or injection of norepinephrine causes release of PGE_2. This release is blocked after denervation or administration of alpha-adrenergic blockers. Thus, a stimulus that activates the nerve causes release of norepinephrine, which in turn stimulates synthesis and release of PGE_2; PGE_2 then feeds back at the prejunctional level of the nerve terminal to decrease the amount of norepinephrine released.

Pancreatic endocrine function PGE_2 has primarily inhibitory effects on insulin secretion by the pancreatic beta cell in vitro and on insulin response to intravenous glucose. This effect is at least partially mediated by G_i, the inhibitory regulatory subunit of adenylate cyclase, since it is associated with decreased production of cyclic AMP and is preventable by pertussis toxin, an agent that inhibits G_i activity. This inhibitory effect appears to be specific for glucose because the insulin responses to other secretagogues are not influenced by PGE_2. Studies with inhibitors of prostaglandin synthesis support the concept that endogenous PGE_2 acts in vivo to inhibit insulin secretion. In general, such drugs augment insulin secretion and improve carbohydrate tolerance. An exception is indomethacin, which inhibits glucose-induced insulin secretion and can cause hyperglycemia. The discordant results with indomethacin are likely due to some action other than inhibition of cyclooxygenase. The lipoxygenase pathway appears to play a role in potentiating insulin secretion by participating in stimulus-secretion coupling. In this case a likely active arachidonic acid product may be 12-HPETE.

Luteolysis In the sheep hysterectomy during the luteal phase of the ovarian cycle results in maintenance of the corpus luteum, suggesting that the uterus normally produces a luteolytic substance. A candidate for this substance is $PGF_{2\alpha}$ since it can cause luteal regression.

PATHOPHYSIOLOGY Most postulated roles for arachidonic acid metabolites in disease involve excessive production, but a few disorders may be the result of decreased production. The latter could result from dietary deficiency of arachidonic acid (an essential fatty acid), from damage to a tissue required for prostaglandin synthesis, or from therapy with drugs that inhibit enzymes in the synthetic pathway.

Bone resorption: Hypercalcemia of malignancy (Also see Chaps. 309 and 340) Hypercalcemia occurs in association with nonparathyroid malignancies of many different types. Parathyroid hormone excess, as the result either of autonomous production by parathyroid tissue or ectopic formation by the tumor itself, causes a portion of these cases. However, most patients with hypercalcemia of malignancy do not have elevated plasma levels of parathyroid hormone, and the etiology of the hypercalcemia has been the subject of considerable interest.

Prostaglandin E_2 is a potent inducer of bone resorption and of calcium release from bone, and PGE_2 production is elevated in certain hypercalcemic animals with transplantable tumors. Treatment of these animals with inhibitors of PGE_2 synthesis causes reduction of PGE_2 levels and a concomitant decrease in hypercalcemia. Likewise, occasional patients with hypercalcemia and malignancy have excessive amounts of PGE_2 metabolites in urine, whereas equally elevated levels do not occur in normocalcemic patients with otherwise similar malignancies. Drugs that inhibit prostaglandin synthesis decrease circulating calcium levels in some patients with hypercalcemia of malignancy. Thus, a subset of approximately 5 to 10 percent of patients with hypercalcemia and malignancy have elevated PGE production and can be treated with drugs that inhibit prostaglandin synthesis.

The source of the excess PGE_2 in these patients has not been identified. Increased liver and lung degradation of PGE would be expected to compensate if large amounts of PGE were present in the circulation. It is possible, of course, that such large amounts of PGE_2 are released by a tumor into the circulation that liver and lung degradation cannot handle the load. Alternatively, if lung metastases are present, the venous drainage from the tumors could be delivered into the systemic circulation without passing through lung tissue. A third possible mechanism involves metastatic seeding of bone. Tumor cells synthesize PGE in culture, and metastatic tumor cells in bone could synthesize PGE that acts locally to cause bone resorption. Part of this hypothetical mechanism may involve PGE_2 production by circulating white cells which congregate at metastatic sites. Hypercalcemia of malignancy can occur in the absence of demonstrable bone metastases, but the clinical tools for excluding such metastases, such as radioisotope scans, may not be sensitive enough to detect many small lesions.

Bone resorption: Rheumatoid arthritis and dental cysts (See Chap. 270) Overproduction of PGE_2 has been postulated as a cause of the juxtaarticular osteoporosis and bony erosions in some patients with rheumatoid arthritis. Rheumatoid synovia synthesize PGE_2 in tissue culture, and media from these cultures promote bone resorption; moreover, the inclusion of indomethacin in the culture medium blocks this resorptive capacity. Since indomethacin does not prevent bone resorption due to preformed PGE_2, the PGE_2 produced by the synovia is presumed to be responsible for the resorptive activity.

Cells from benign dental cysts also cause bone resorption and synthesize PGE_2 in tissue culture. Again, bone resorption caused by the culture medium from such cells is decreased if indomethacin is added prior to the incubation. A related problem is that of alveolar bone resorption in patients with periodontal disease, a common inflammatory disease of the gums. PGE_2 levels in inflamed gingiva are greater than in healthy gingival tissue. Thus, it is possible that alveolar resorption might be due, in part at least, to local overproduction of these metabolites.

Bartter's syndrome (See Chap. 231) Bartter's syndrome is characterized by elevated levels of plasma renin, aldosterone, and bradykinin; resistance to the pressor effect of angiotensin; hypokalemic alkalosis; and renal potassium wasting in the presence of normal blood pressure. The basis for the postulated role of prostaglandins in the disorder is that PGE_2 and PGI_2 stimulate the release of renin and that the pressor response to infused angiotensin is blunted by the vasodilator effects of PGE_2 and PGI_2. The increase in renin release leads to increased aldosterone secretion, which in turn can increase urinary kallikrein activity.

In keeping with this postulate, elevated levels of PGE_2 and 6-keto-$PGF_{1\alpha}$ are present in urine of patients with the syndrome. Hyperplasia of renal medullary interstitial cells (which synthesize PGE in culture) has also been demonstrated. These findings led to therapeutic trials of inhibitors of prostaglandin synthesis in the disorder. Indomethacin (and other inhibitors) reverse virtually all the abnormalities except hypokalemia. Thus, a prostaglandin, probably PGE_2 and/or PGI_2, probably mediates some of the manifestations of Bartter's syndrome.

Diabetes mellitus (See Chap. 319) Intravenous administration of large amounts of glucose to normal individuals causes a sudden (first-phase) increase in secretion of insulin into plasma followed by a slower, more prolonged response termed second-phase insulin secretion. Patients with type II (non-insulin-dependent, adult-onset) diabetes mellitus have absent first-phase insulin release in response to glucose and a variable decrease in second-phase insulin secretion. Insulin response to other secretagogues, such as arginine, isoproterenol, glucagon, and secretin, is preserved. Thus, diabetics appear to have a specific defect that interferes with normal perception of glucose signals. Since PGE inhibits glucose-induced insulin secretion in normal individuals, inhibitors of endogenous prostaglandin synthesis have been given to patients with type II diabetes mellitus to ascertain whether insulin secretion can be improved. Both sodium salicylate and aspirin elevate basal plasma insulin levels, partially restore the first-phase insulin response, increase second-phase insulin secretion, and improve glucose tolerance. This suggests that the defect in glucose-induced insulin secretion in patients with type II diabetes mellitus may be associated with excessive local production of, or hypersensitivity to, endogenous PGE_2.

Patent ductus arteriosus (See Chap. 186) The ductus arteriosus in sheep is sensitive to the vasodilatory properties of PGE_2, and PGE-like material is present in the ductal wall. Thus, enhanced endogenous PGE_2 might maintain prenatal patency of the ductus. Since inhibitors of prostaglandin synthesis cause constriction of the ductus of fetal lambs, trials with indomethacin were undertaken in premature human infants with isolated patent ductus arteriosus. Such treatment for several days is followed by closure of the vessel in the majority, although some require a second course of therapy, and a minority require surgical ligation. Infants under 35 weeks of gestational age are most likely to respond.

Patients with certain types of congenital heart disease require a patent ductus arteriosus to survive. Ductus-dependent pulmonary blood flow is essential under circumstances in which the ductus is the major channel by which nonoxygenated blood reaches the lungs from the aortic arch, for example, in pulmonary atresia and tricuspid atresia. Since PGE relaxes the smooth muscle in the lamb ductus arteriosus, clinical trials of intravenous PGE were undertaken to attempt to maintain patency of the ductus in such patients as an alternative to emergency surgery. Such PGE infusions for a short time cause a temporary increase in blood flow to the lungs and improve arterial oxygen saturation until the necessary corrective heart surgery can be performed. The large right-to-left shunt in these cardiac malformations allows the intravenously infused PGE_2 to escape pulmonary degradation before arriving at the ductus. In this instance, the disease process itself facilitates delivery of the therapeutic agent.

Peptic ulcer disease (See Chap. 238) Excessive gastric acid secretion in patients with peptic ulcer disease is involved in damaging the mucosa. Various analogues of PGE_2 inhibit gastric acid secretion and are also inherently cytoprotective. These agents are more effective than placebo in relieving pain and decreasing gastric acid secretion in patients with ulcer disease. Moreover, acceleration of the healing of ulcer craters as assessed by endoscopic criteria has been reported in patients receiving PGE analogues as compared with placebo-treated groups.

Dysmenorrhea (See Chap. 322) Dysmenorrhea is usually associated with increased uterine contractions. The fact that some analgesics used to treat this disorder also inhibit prostaglandin synthesis suggests that arachidonic acid metabolites may play a role in the pathogenesis of dysmenorrhea. Prostaglandins of the E and F series are present in human endometrium. Intravenous infusion of either produces uterine contractions, and PGF and PGE levels in menstrual blood are decreased by administration of prostaglandin synthesis inhibitors. Controlled trials comparing prostaglandin synthesis inhibitors with placebo in women with dysmenorrhea suggest that symptomatic improvement is greater following drug therapy.

Asthma (See Chap. 204)

Inflammatory response and immune response (See Chaps. 13 and 267) Drugs such as aspirin have antipyretic, anti-inflammatory, and analgesic effects. Several arguments support a relation between inflammation and the arachidonic acid metabolites: (1) Inflammatory stimuli such as histamine and bradykinin release endogenous prostaglandins in parallel. (2) Leukotriene C_4-D_4-E_4 is more potent than histamine in causing bronchoconstriction. (3) Several arachidonic acid metabolites cause vasodilatation and hyperalgesia. (4) PGE_2 and LTB_4 are present in areas of inflammation. Polymorphonuclear cells release these products during phagocytosis, and they are chemotactic for leukocytes. (5) Some prostaglandins cause increased vascular permeability, a feature of the inflammatory response that gives rise to local edema. (6) Vasodilation induced by PGE is not abolished by atropine, propranolol, methysergide, or antihistamines, known antagonists of other possible mediators of the inflammatory response. Thus, PGE may have a direct inflammatory effect, and some mediators of inflammation may act by influencing PGE release. (7) Some arachidonic acid metabolites can cause pain in animal models and hyperalgesia or an increased sensitivity to pain in humans. (8) PGE can cause fever after injection into the cerebral ventricles or into the hypothalamus of animals. (9) Pyrogens cause increased concentrations of prostaglandins in cerebrospinal fluid, whereas prostaglandin synthesis inhibitors decrease fever and decrease release of prostaglandins into cerebrospinal fluid.

Arachidonic acid metabolites may also play a role in the immune response. Small amounts of PGE_2 can suppress stimulation of human lymphocytes by mitogens such as phytohemagglutinin, and the inflammatory response is associated with the local release of arachidonic acid metabolites; thus, these substances may act as negative modulators of lymphocyte function. The release of PGE by mitogen-stimulated lymphocytes may constitute a portion of a negative feedback control mechanism by which lymphocyte activity is regulated. Sensitivity of lymphocytes to the inhibiting effects of PGE_2 increases with age, and indomethacin augments lymphocyte responsiveness to mitogens to a greater degree in the elderly. Lymphocytes cultured from patients with Hodgkin's disease release more PGE_2 after the addition of phytohemagglutinin, and lymphocyte responsiveness is enhanced by indomethacin. When suppressor T cells are removed from the cultures, the amount of PGE_2 synthesized is diminished, and the responsiveness of the lymphocytes from the Hodgkin's patients and controls is no longer different. Depressed cellular immunity in patients with Hodgkin's disease may be the result of PGE inhibition of lymphocyte function.

REFERENCES

Advances in prostaglandins and gastroenterology. Symposium. Am J Med 83 (1A): 1, 1987

ALESSANDRINI P et al: Thromboxane biosynthesis and platelet function in type I diabetes mellitus. N Engl J Med 319:208, 1988

HEYMAN MA: Prostaglandins and leukotrienes in the perinatal period. Clin Perinatol 14:857, 1987

METZ SA et al: Prostaglandins as mediators of paraneoplastic syndromes: Review and update. Metabolism 30:299, 1981

NEEDLEMAN P et al: Arachidonic acid metabolism. Ann Rev Biochem 55:69, 1986

ROBERTSON RP (ed): Symposium on prostaglandins in health and disease. Med Clin North Am 65:711, 1981

———: Arachidonic acid metabolite regulation of insulin secretion. Diab Metab Rev 2:261, 1986

SCHARSCHMIDT L et al: Glomerular prostaglandins, angiotensin II, and nonsteroidal anti-inflammatory drugs. Am J Med 81(2B):30, 1986

COLOR ATLASES

The skin and mucous membrane may frequently contain a variety of lesions that are rarely a major complaint (see Fig. 47-1). They are, therefore, incidental findings in the general physical examination. The recognition of "bumps and blemishes" is a necessary first step for physicians inasmuch as they will be required to distinguish the trivial from the serious and important skin changes. For example, such a serious lesion as a malignant melanoma may be incidentally discovered during a routine physical examination (see Figs. A1-30 to A1-32 and the discussion in Chap. 302).

The common disorders of the skin that every physician should be able to recognize are presented in this series of color photographs (Figs. A1-1 to A1-23).

A
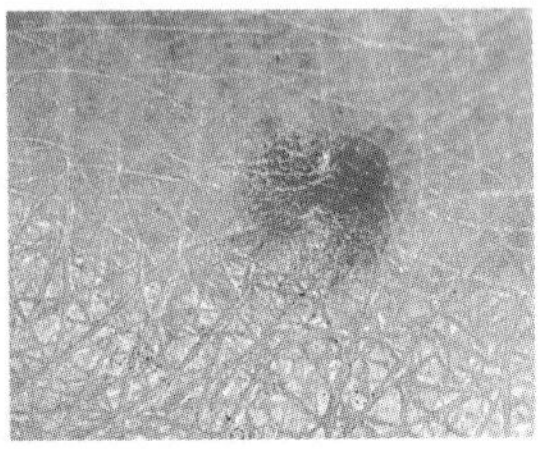
B
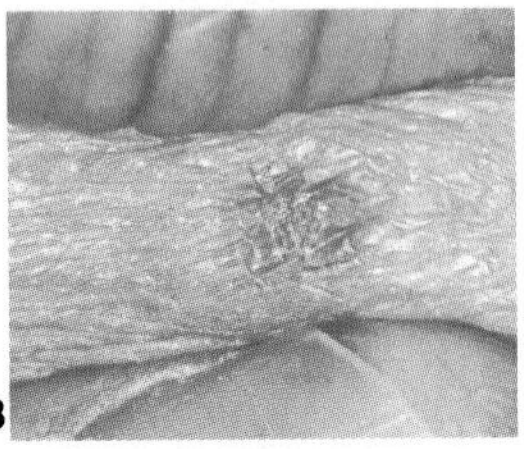

A1-1 **Dermatofibroma** is especially common in middle life and in women. The lesions, when pigmented, are occasionally confused with malignant melanoma. They appear as isolated, slightly elevated, hard, button-like nodules (*A*). In fair-skinned persons, the lesions are not usually skin color, but are pink or dark red, yellowish brown, or gray-black. They are usually less than 1 cm in diameter. A diagnostic sign is that a dermatofibroma dimples or becomes depressed (*B*) when it is laterally compressed; melanocytic nevus and melanoma, however, with which dermatofibroma may be easily confused, become elevated with lateral compression.

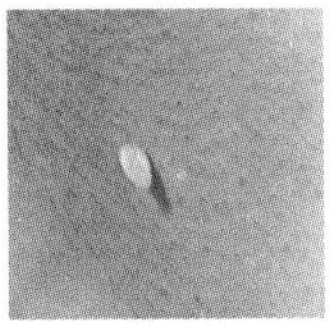

A1-2 **Acrochordon** (skin tag) is very common after middle life and appears on the neck, especially in women, in the axillae, and on the upper part of the trunk. The lesions are small (1 to 5 mm), soft, pedunculated papules, usually of normal skin color.

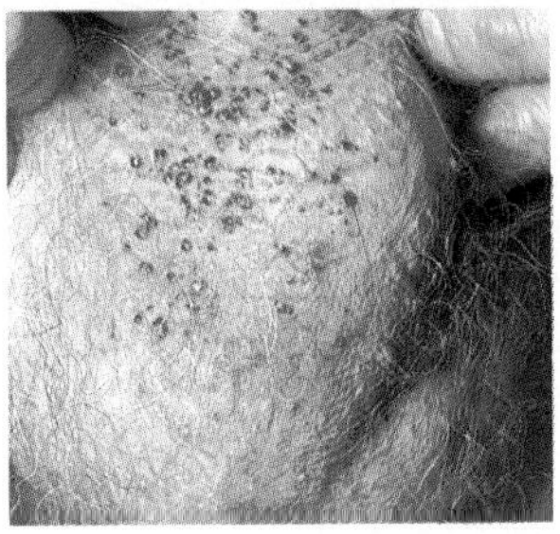

A1-3 **Angiokeratomas** are bizarre vascular dilatations that occur under the tongue and on the scrotum and consist of myriads of 2- to 3-mm purplish red papules. They are of no known significance. When they occur on the trunk and extremities, a biopsy is indicated to rule out glycolipid lipidosis or Fabry's disease

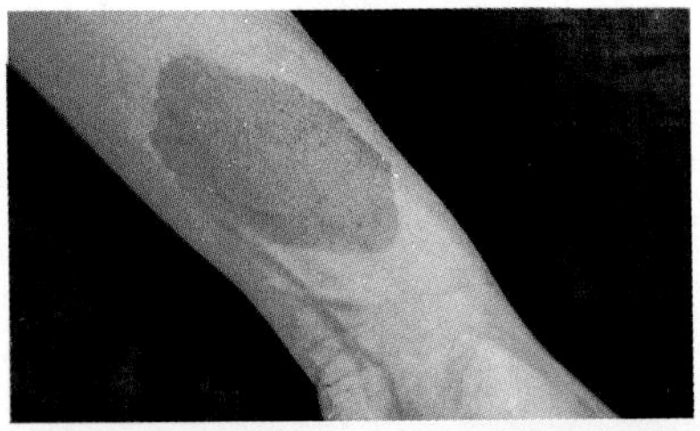

A1-4 **Café au lait macules** are found in about 10 percent of the normal population and, in fair-skinned persons, are light yellowish brown macules, which may also be markers of neurofibromatosis and polyostotic fibrous dysplasia (Albright's syndrome). The presence of six or more café au lait macules with a diameter of 1.5 cm or greater is diagnostic of neurofibromatosis.

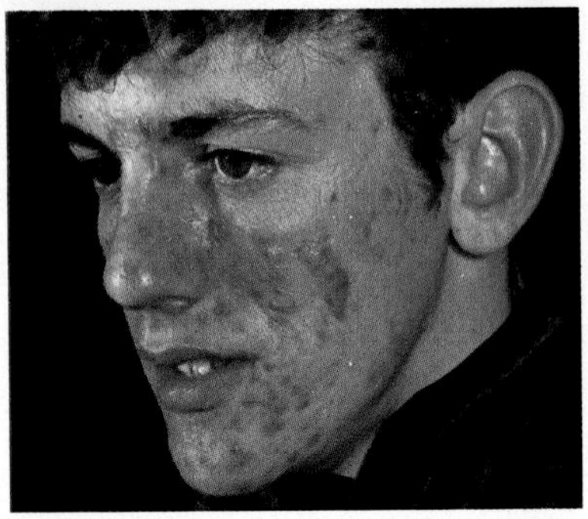

A1-5 **Acne** is a condition in which the most characteristic lesion is the comedo, or "blackhead," that later becomes a conical erythematous papule or pustule. A third type of lesion is the "blind boil," which is a dermal cyst without an orifice. This lesion is often associated with atrophic or hypertrophic scarring. Cystic acne may appear with only a very few comedones; also, comedo-like acne may occur with few cysts or erythematous papules.

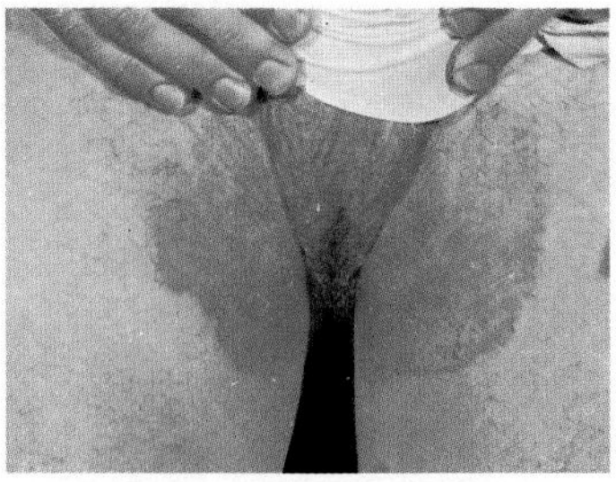

A1-6 **Dermatophytosis** is identified by the striking polycyclic, annular shape of the scaling, especially on the feet and hands, where there is often a scalloped pattern. A positive diagnosis of dermatophytosis is quickly established by direct examination of scales from the advancing border; the mycelia are revealed when the scales are immersed in 10% potassium hydroxide or Swartz stain.

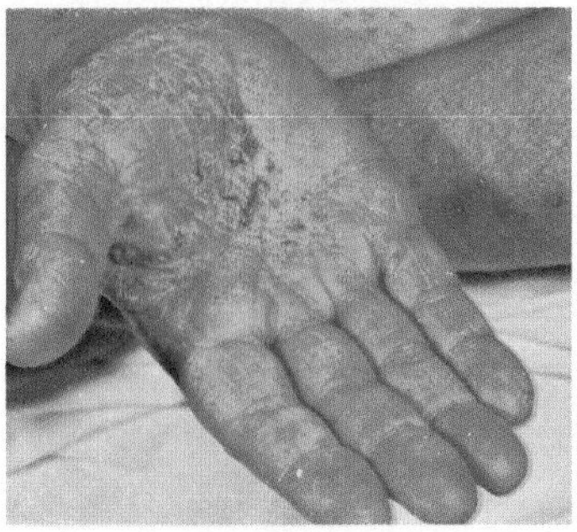

A1-7 **Eczematous dermatitis** is a very common cutaneous reaction that is localized to the hands of housewives, to the legs in patients with chronic venous insufficiency, and behind the ears in patients with seborrheic dermatitis. In subacute eczematous dermatitis, there are mild erythema, dry scales, and often small red papules, many of which are excoriated. In chronic eczematous dermatitis, lichenification is the most prominent feature.

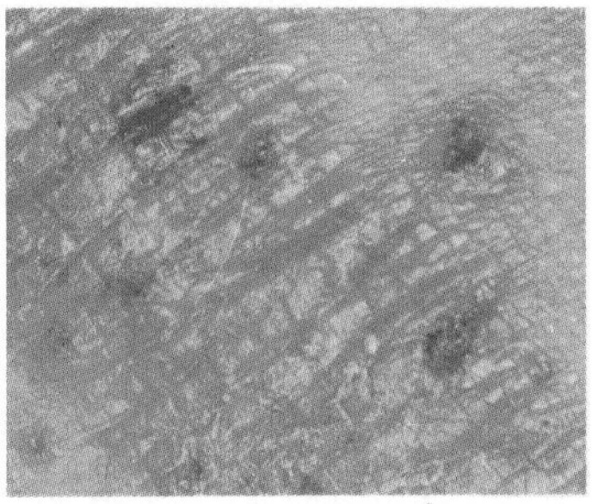

A1-8 **Localized lichenification** results from repeated rubbing of the skin and consists of isolated, circumscribed plaques. These single lesions vary in size from 2 to 10 cm and occur most often on the extensor aspect of the forearm and in the scrotal, nuchal, inguinal, and anogenital areas. The perianal and vulvar areas may become diffusely lichenified. Lichenification is thought to be more frequent in persons with an atopic background.

A1-9 **Melasma (chloasma)** is the so-called "mask" of pregnancy, but it also occurs in men and in women taking progestational agents. The pigmentation is uniform and is limited to the exposed areas of the face. There is no scaling or epidermal change. In fair-skinned persons, the pigment may be any shade from light tan to a very dark brown. It is most often seen on the cheek and upper lip, as here, and on the forehead.

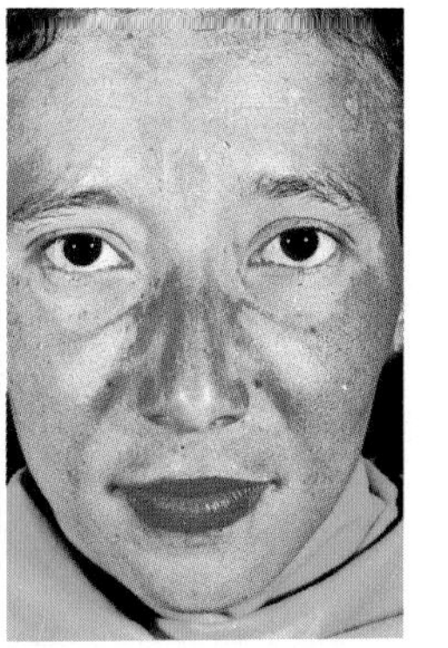

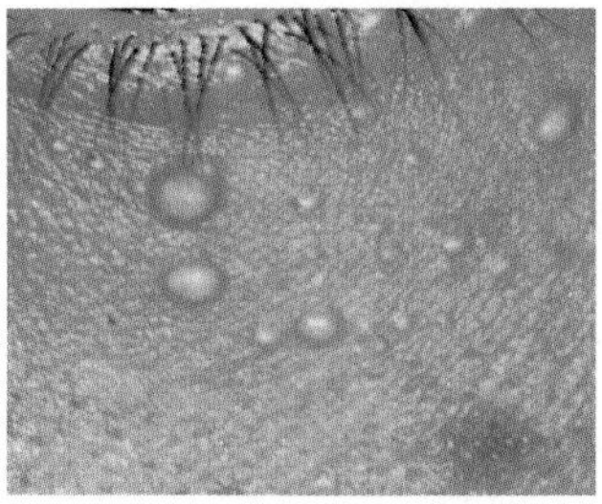

A1-10 **Milia** are a collection of lesions, occurring most commonly on the face, and consist of tiny (1 to 2 mm), white, hard, rounded, superficial papules. There is no orifice, and the keratinous contents are easily expressed by lateral compression after the making of a tiny incision in the dome of the lesion.

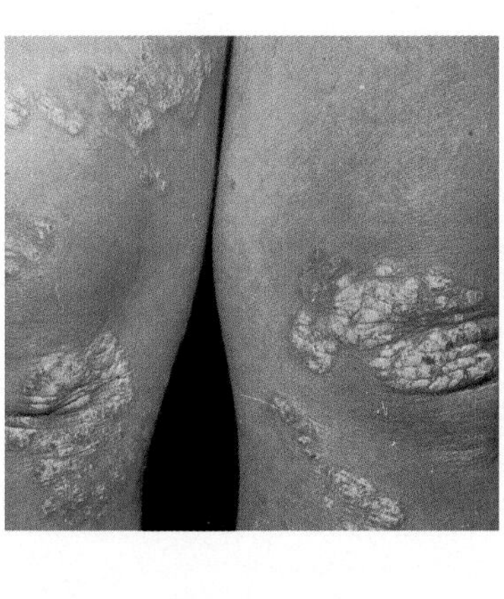

A1-11 **Psoriasis,** affecting more than 2 percent of the population, consists of isolated scaling papules or plaques and is quite commonly observed in the routine physical examination. The lesions occur most frequently on the scalp, elbows, and knees. The color and type of scales are the identifying features of the lesions. The scales are either dense and lamellated with peripherally detached edges or loose and branny. The plaques are pink to deep red, and the borders are distinct.

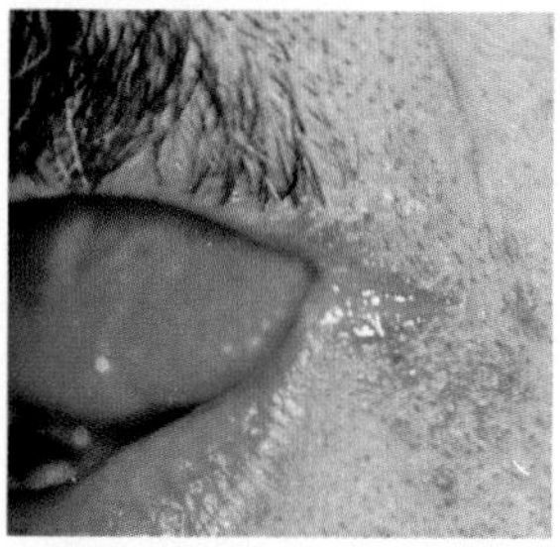

A1-12 **Perlèche** consists of painful small fissures at the angles of the mouth, often covered with yellow crusts. Perlèche most often occurs with poorly fitting dentures and in moniliasis and secondary syphilis.

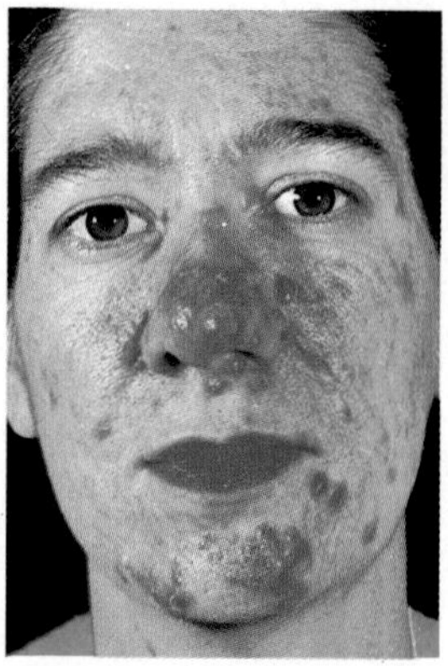

A1-13 **Rosacea,** usually limited to the face, consists of tiny, erythematous papules and pustules 1 to 5 mm in size. The pustules, often tiny and sometimes hardly visible, sit on the dome of the papules. The diffuse redness of the face is due to vasodilatation, as well as to myriad telangiectases. In men, rhinophyma, a disfiguring enlargement of the nose, may occur.

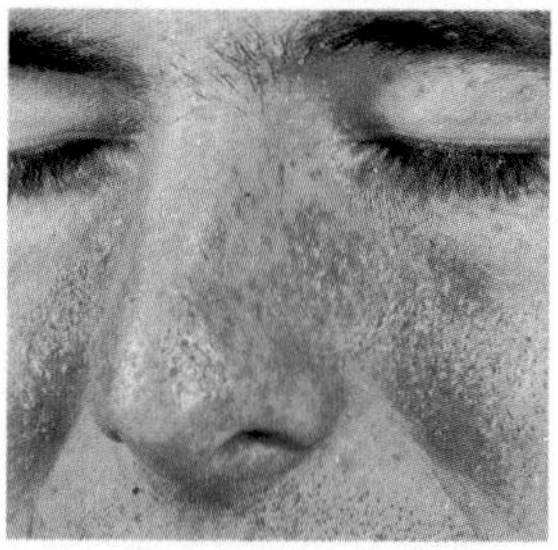

A1-14 **Seborrheic dermatitis,** a common disorder found in all age groups, occurs most frequently on the scalp, eyebrows, and nasolabial folds and behind the ears. Scaling is the prominent feature and is loose and branny; it may be yellow and oily or dry and white. The lesion may become exudative and crusted or eczematous.

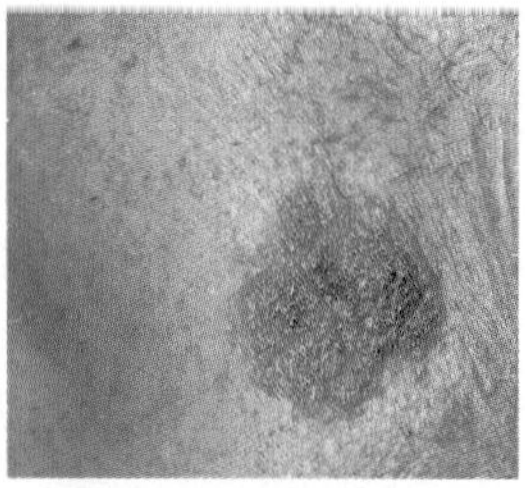

A1-15 **Seborrheic keratosis** appears in middle life and may occur on exposed or unexposed areas but is especially common on the trunk. The lesions are irregularly round or oval flat-topped papules or plaques that seem "stuck" on the skin. The margins are distinct, and the surface is often warty or consists of multiple tiny projections (vegetation). In fair-skinned persons, the lesions are light brown at first but, enlarging, become more heavily pigmented and may be confused with malignant melanoma.

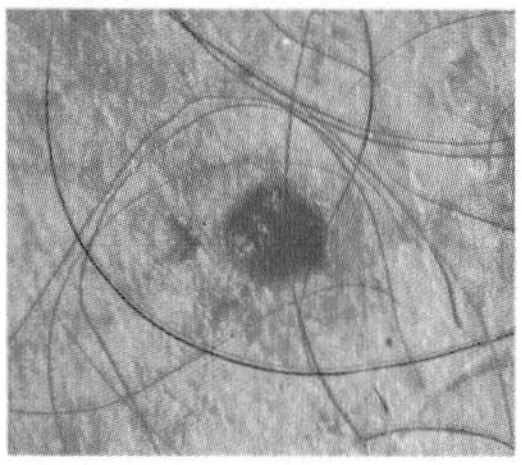

A1-16 **Senile angioma ("cherry red spot")** appears in the third decade. On the lip, the lesion is usually singular and consists of a bluish red round nodule. On the trunk, the lesions are small (2 to 3 mm), bright red, globular papules.

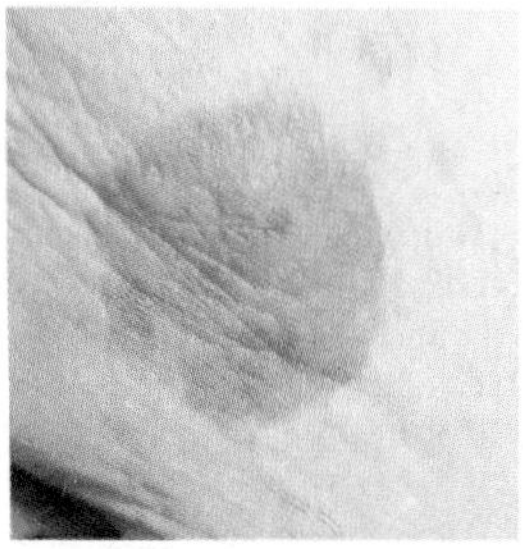

A1-17 **Senile lentigo** occurs as a single macule or as a group of isolated, sharply circumscribed macules on the exposed areas, especially on the dorsal surfaces of the hands and arms and on the forehead and cheeks. The macules are usually light yellowish brown, but may be dark brown; the color is somewhat variegated, rather than uniform as it is in a café au lait macule. Rarely, dark brown *papules* develop in these lesions, and then the condition is called *lentigo maligna,* which may slowly develop, over a period of years, into a melanoma (lentigo maligna melanoma).

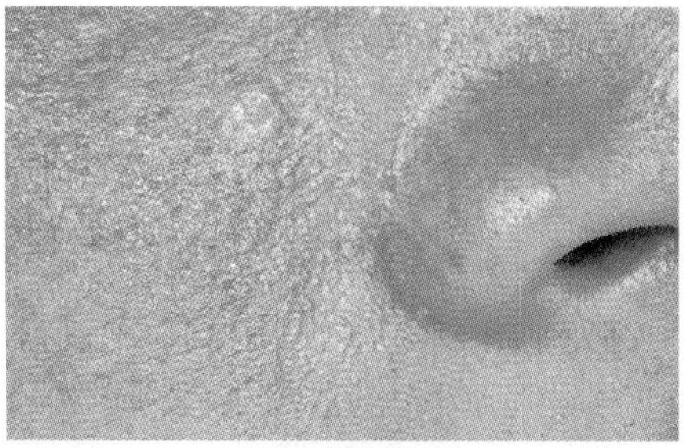

A1-18 **Senile sebaceous adenoma** occurs on the face in patients over 40 and is often diagnosed as basal-cell carcinoma. The lesions are soft, small, flat-topped papules, varying in size from 1 to 8 mm, and are characterized by a minute central depression from which sebaceous material can be exuded by lateral compression.

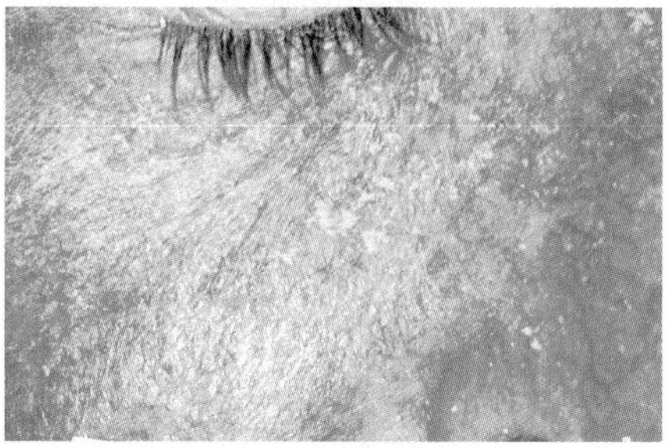

A1-19 **Solar keratosis** (1) occurs usually in persons with light skin prone to sunburn or with darker skin after chronic excessive exposure; (2) is strictly limited to exposed skin, especially on the face and dorsal surfaces of the hands; (3) is more easily felt than seen (gritty and sandpaperish); (4) in fair-skinned persons, consists of skin-colored or light brown macules or slightly raised papules with superficial adherent scales not easily removed; and (5) is associated with marked wrinkling, telangiectasia, and often diffuse, tiny, pale yellow papules indicating solar degeneration of connective tissue ("turkey skin").

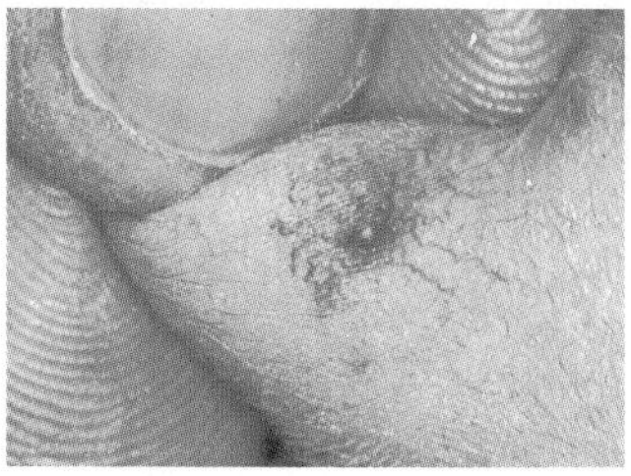

A1-20 **Spider nevus** consists of a central, punctate, bright red macule or papule (the body) from which fine red lines radiate like spider legs. There is often a red flare between the radiating vessels. On diascopy, the central body pulsates.

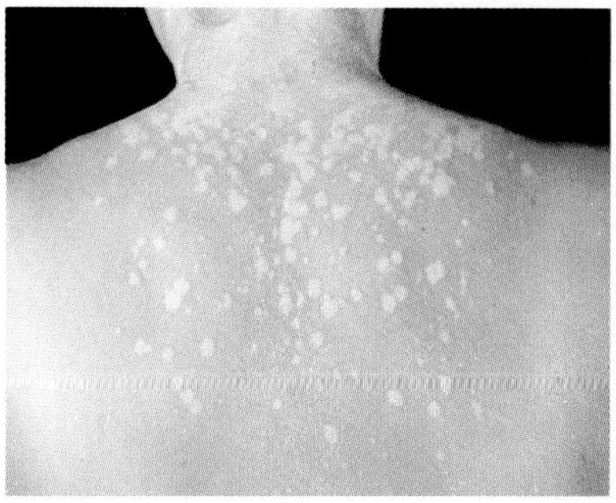

A1-21 **Tinea versicolor** is a relatively common disorder occurring primarily on the trunk and appearing in two forms: as scattered, 3- to 5-mm, very slightly scaling brown macules or as whitish macules that may be confused with vitiligo. The fungal spores and hyphae can be easily demonstrated on direct examination of the scales using Swartz stain.

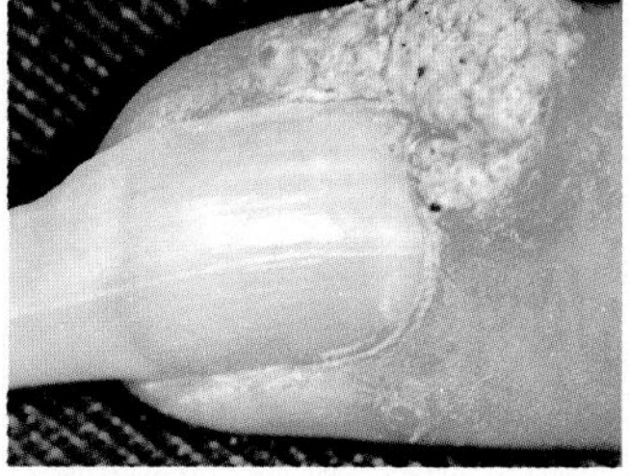

A1-22 **Verruca vulgaris** may occur at any age, but it is most common in children. The lesions, which vary in size from 0.5 to 2.0 cm, are round or oval, firm, skin colored papules with multiple tiny keratotic, rounded or filiform projections covering the surface (vegetation). They occur most frequently on the hands and soles.

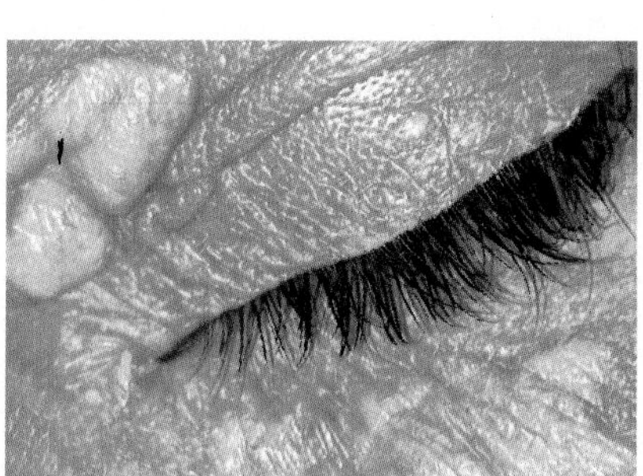

A1-23 **Xanthelasma** consists of one or more bright yellow, sharply marginated plaques with no epidermal change, usually occurring on the eyelids. All patients with xanthelasma should be investigated for evidence of plasma lipid abnormalities.

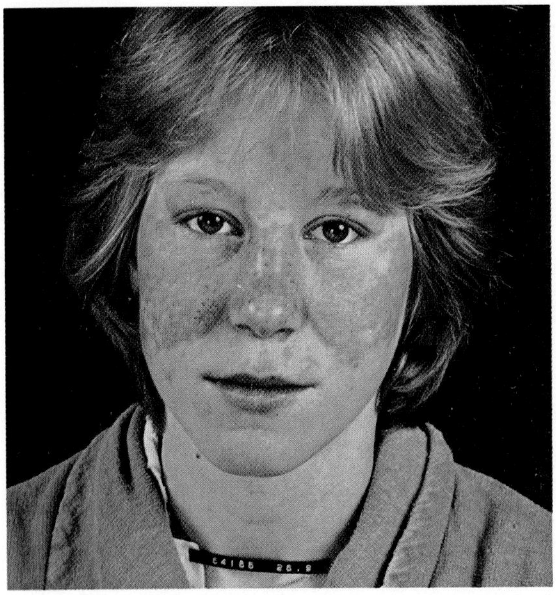

A1-24 **Systemic lupus erythematosus.** Erythematous, confluent, butterfly-like eruption with fine scaling.

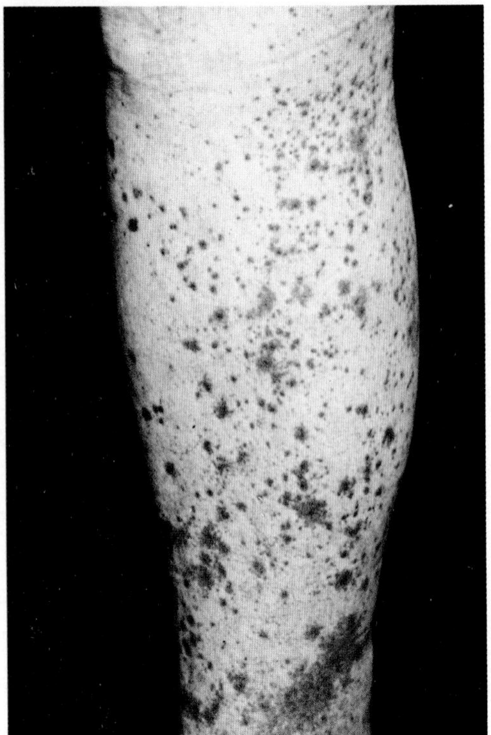

A1-25 **Necrotizing vasculitis syndrome.** Scattered discrete, purpuric eruption on the legs. The purpura is "palpable."

A

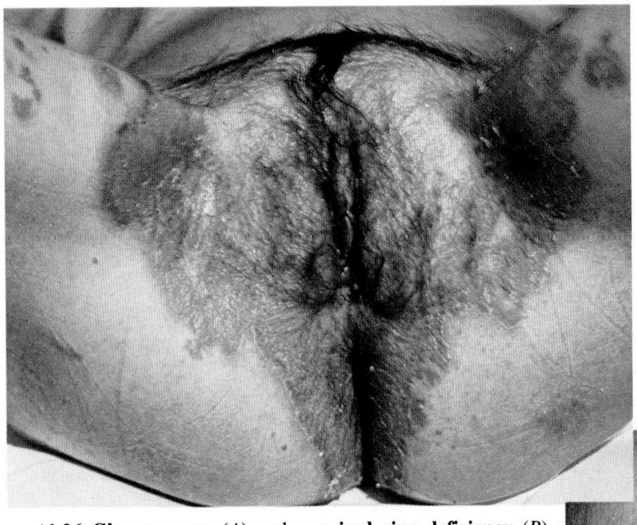

A1-26 **Glucagonoma** (*A*) and **acquired zinc deficiency** (*B*). Circinate and gyrate areas of blistering, erosion, and maceration. The eruption is often mistaken for psoriasis or mucocutaneous moniliasis.

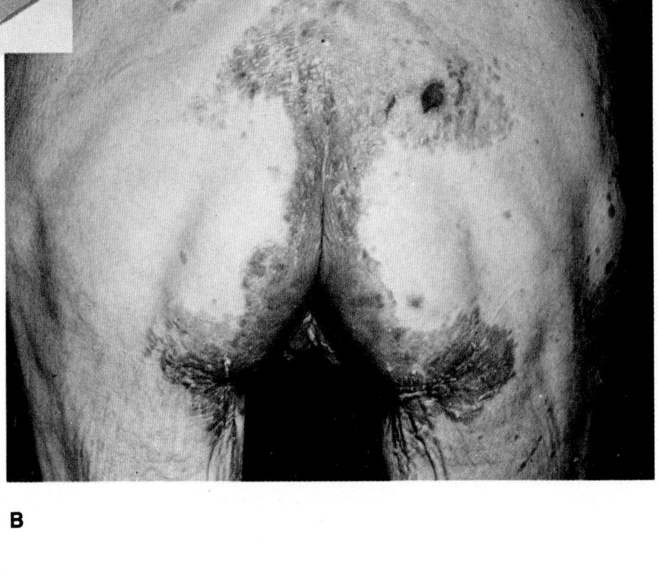

B

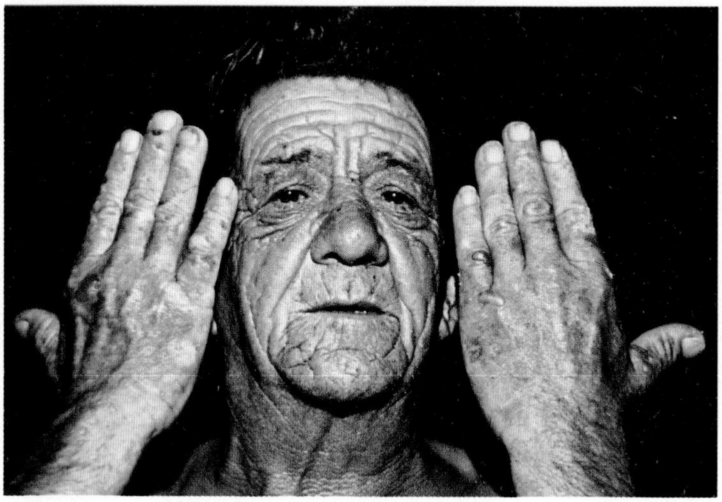

A1-27 **Porphyria cutanea tarda.** Violaceous suffusion in the periorbital skin is evident. There are erosions and pink atrophic scars at sites of previous bullae on the dorsa of the hands.

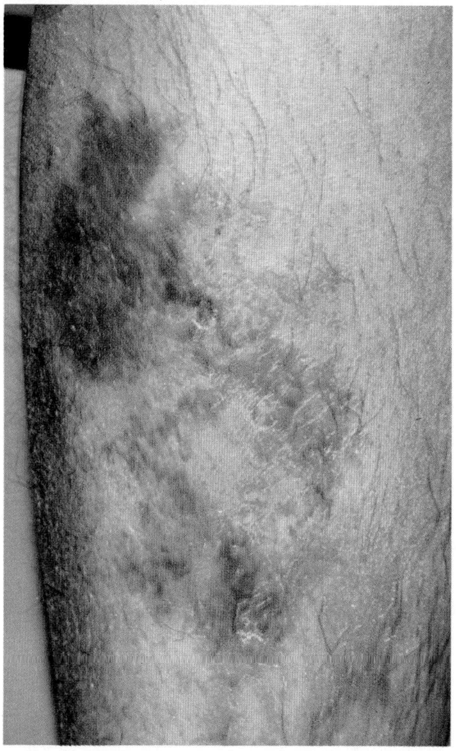

A1-28 **Necrobiosis lipoidica.** The lesion often begins as a small, dusky red, elevated nodule with a sharp border. It slowly enlarges, becomes flattened and eventually depressed as the dermis becomes atrophic. The color becomes brownish yellow except for the border, which may remain reddened. Delicate vessels can be seen through the atrophic epidermis.

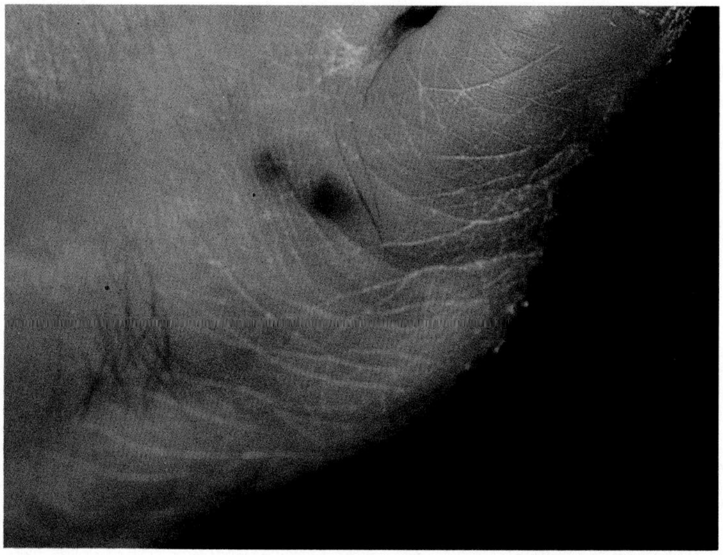

A1-29 Two purplish red nodules of **Kaposi's sarcoma** in a patient with AIDS.

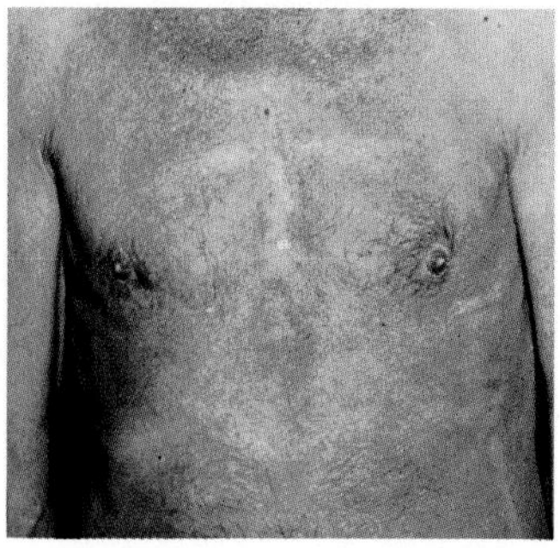

A1-30 **Carcinoid** showing the effect of stroking. In contrast to the flushing that occurs in other disorders, the flush in carcinoid is typically a panorama of colors, ranging from bizarre pinkish orange to bright red to violaceous to blanching white. The flush (which lasts only a few minutes) spreads from the face to the neck, shoulders, chest, and arms.

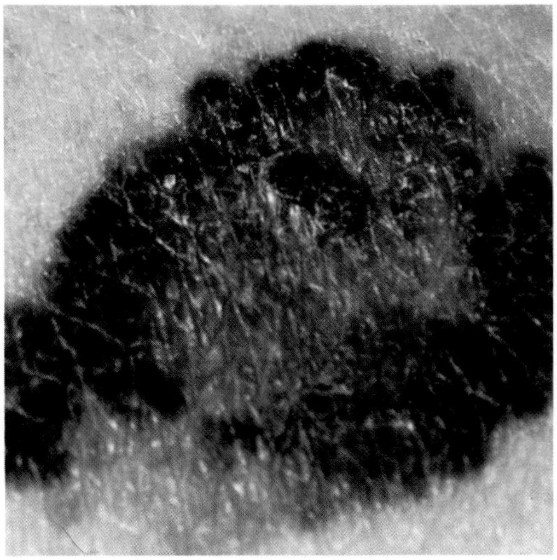

A

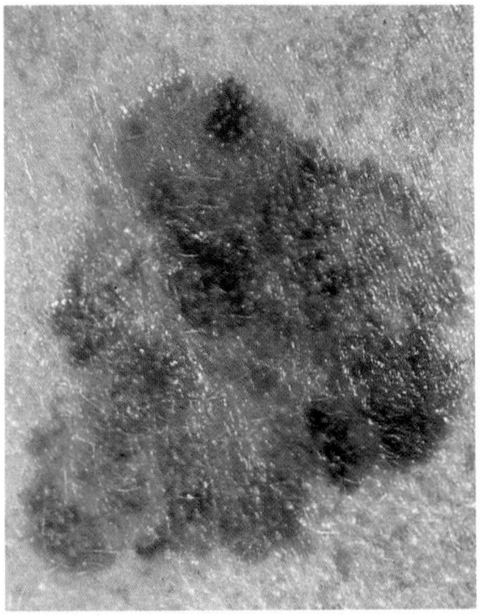

B

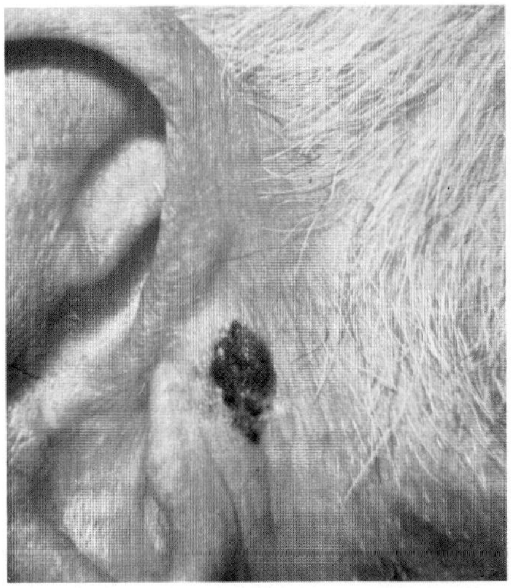

C

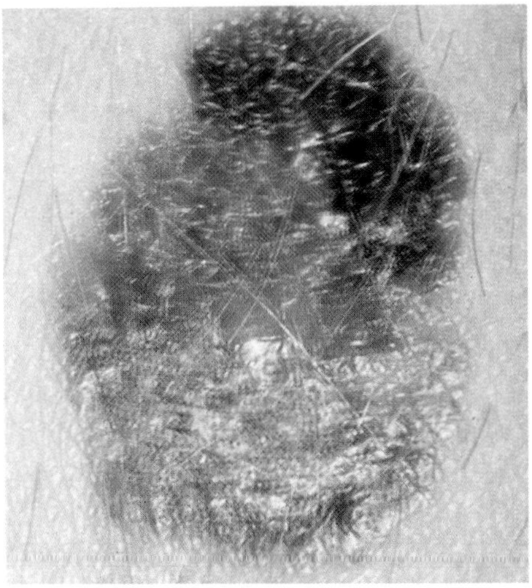

D

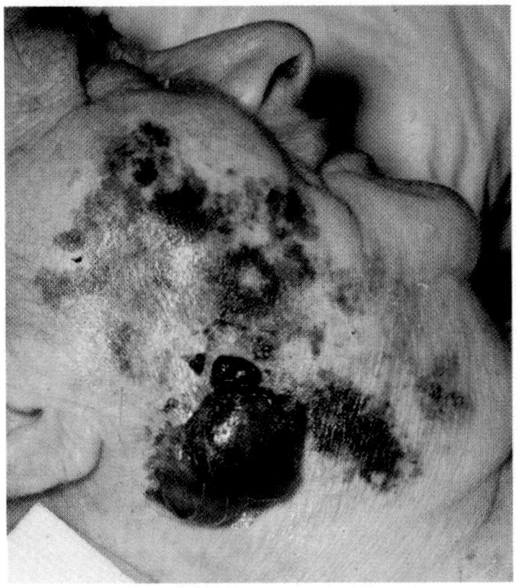

E

A1-31 **Malignant melanoma.** On close inspection melanomas shown are characterized by irregular surface (*A*), irregular border and notching (*B*), and nodularity (*C*). Also shown are a reniform melanoma (*D*), an extensive lentigo maligna on face of patient (*E*) and a regressive melanoma characterized by grayish color infiltrated with pink areas (*F*). (From Hospital Practice, January 1982, with permission.)

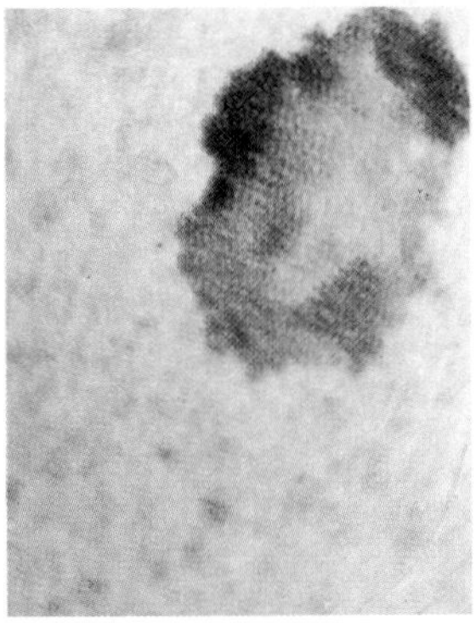

F

A

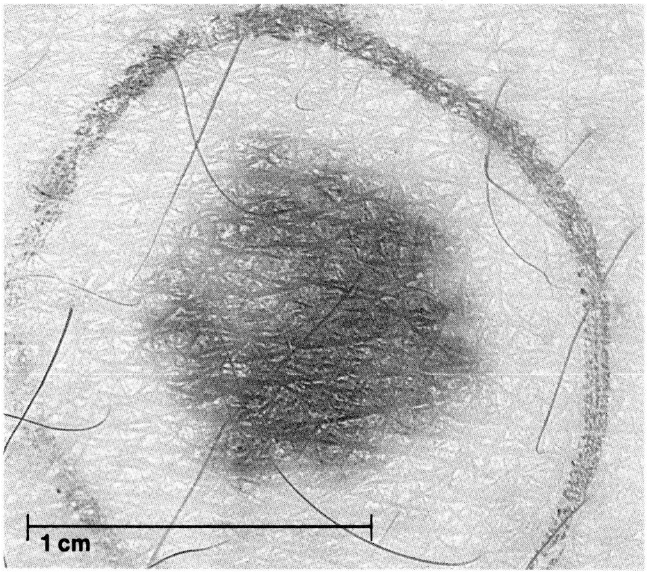

B

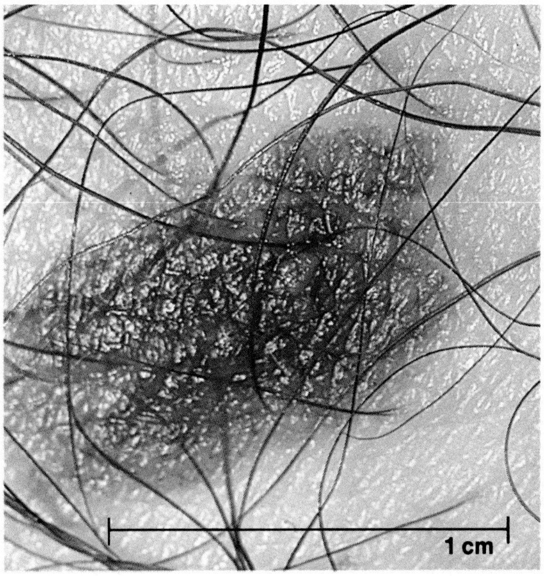

A1-32 **Dysplastic melanocytic nevi.** (*A*) Round, essentially macular lesions in which the slightly elevated area is present at 12:00 o'clock. The elevation is detectable only by oblique lighting. Note striking variegation of color with tan, brown, and pink areas. (*B*) This lesion is more obviously elevated in the central portion. Note "pebbly" surface. Both lesions have indistinct and irregular borders. (From Dermatologic Capsule & Comment 7(4):4, 1985, with permission.)

A1-33 **Malignant melanoma – dysplastic nevus syndrome.** This 28-year-old woman gave a history of a rapidly growing (3 to 6 months), asymptomatic lesion on her right scapular area. Her mother had melanoma and both mother and siblings had many dark "moles." Diagnosis: (1) Superficial spreading melanoma, level IV, 4.75 mm. (2) Regional nodes – of 32 removed, 1 was positive. (3) Dysplastic nevus syndrome with family history of melanoma. Note primary lesion and many dark "moles" on back (*A*) and dysplastic nevi on untanned areas under the bathing suit straps (*B*). (From Dermatologic Capsule & Comment 6(4):3, 1984, with permission.)

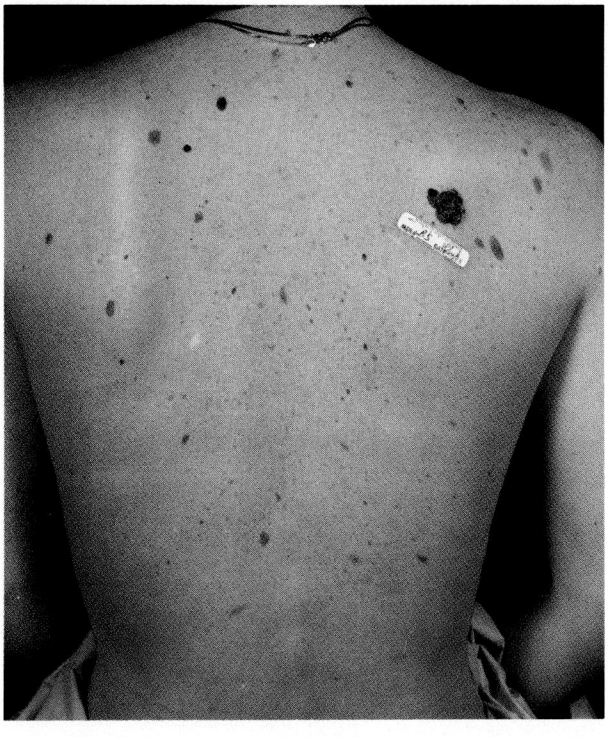

A

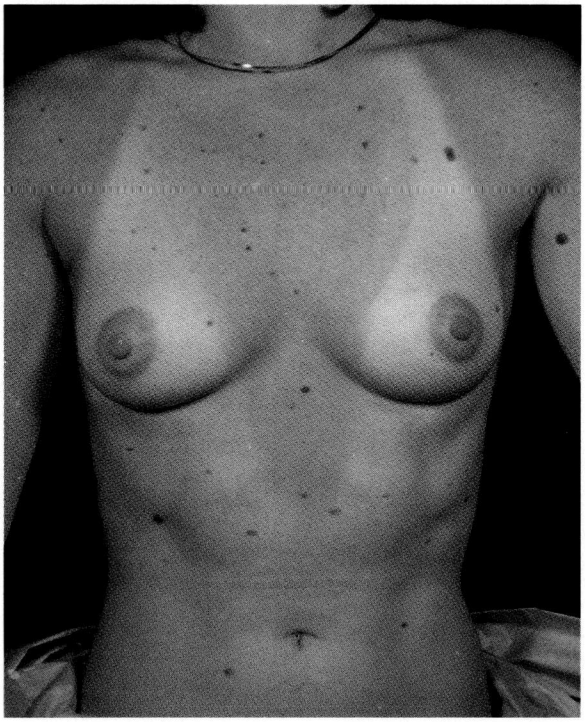

B

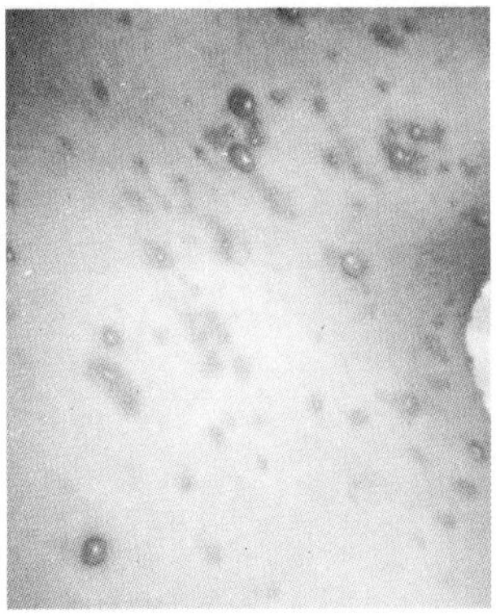

A2-1 **Varicella** (chickenpox).[3]

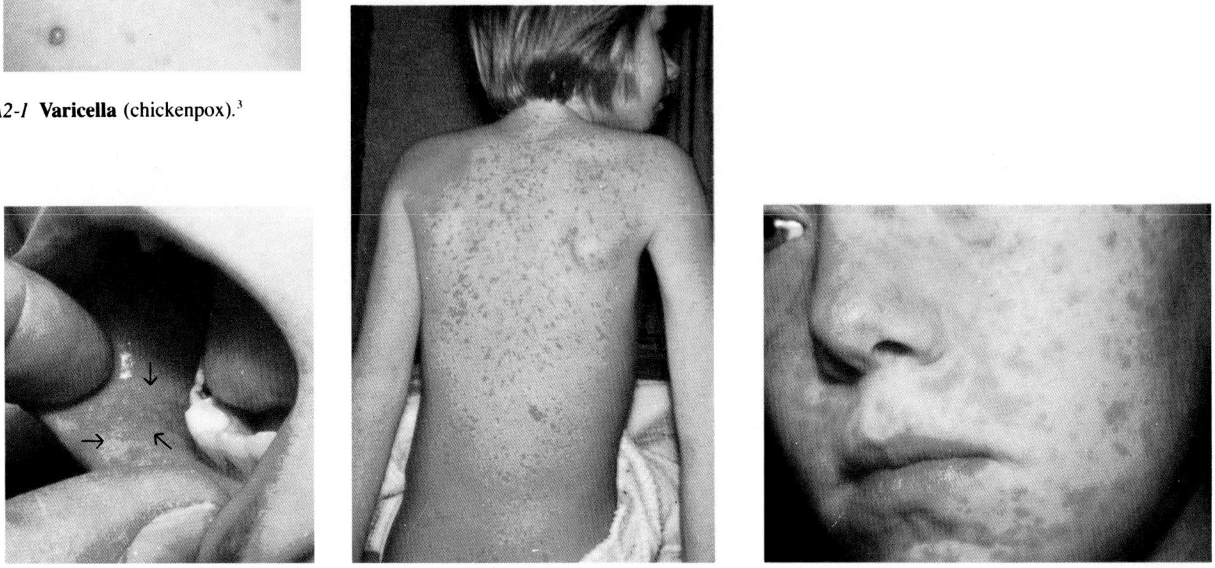

A2-2 **Measles** (rubeola).[3]

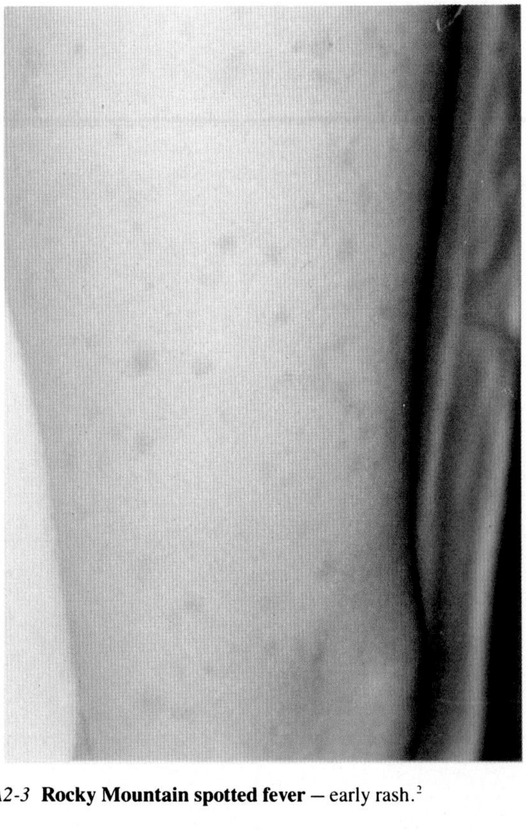

A2-3 **Rocky Mountain spotted fever** – early rash.[2]

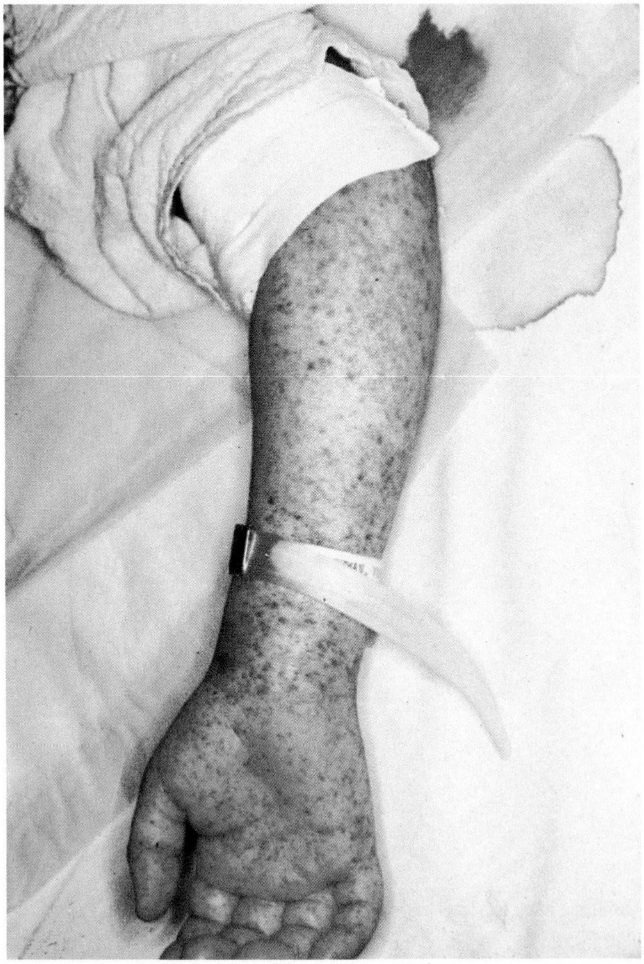

A2-4 **Rocky Mountain spotted fever** – late rash.[2]

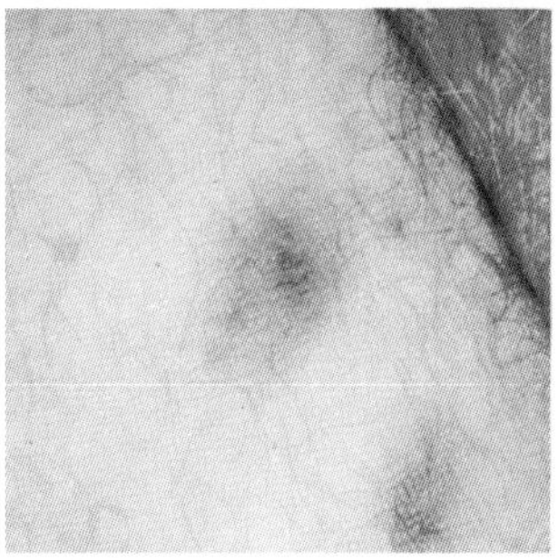

A2-7 **Pseudomonas septicemia**.[3]

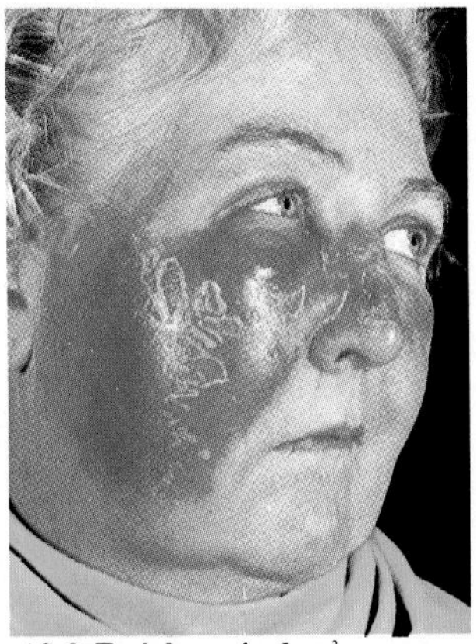

A2-8 **Facial erysipelas**.[3]

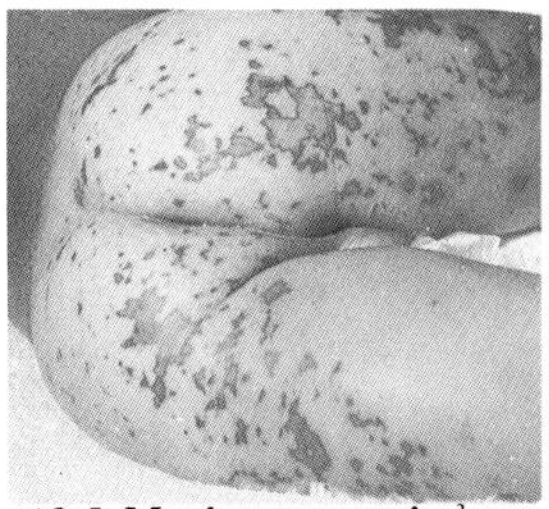

A2-5 **Meningococcemia**.[3]

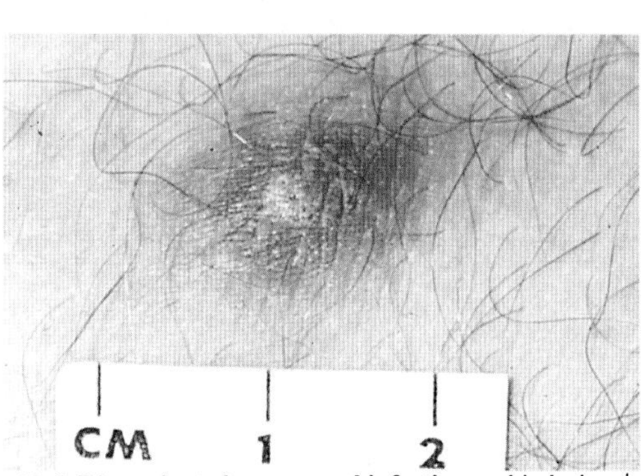

A2-6 **Disseminated gonococcal infection** – skin lesion.[4]

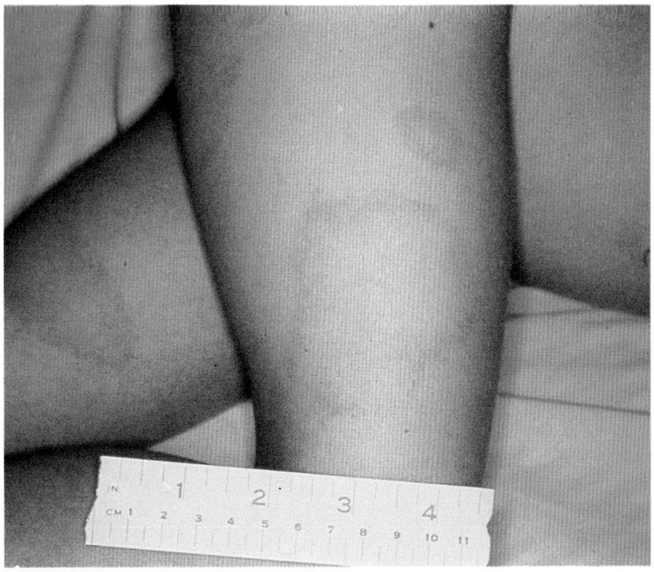

A2-9 **Lyme disease: erythema chronicum migrans** – secondary lesion.[5]

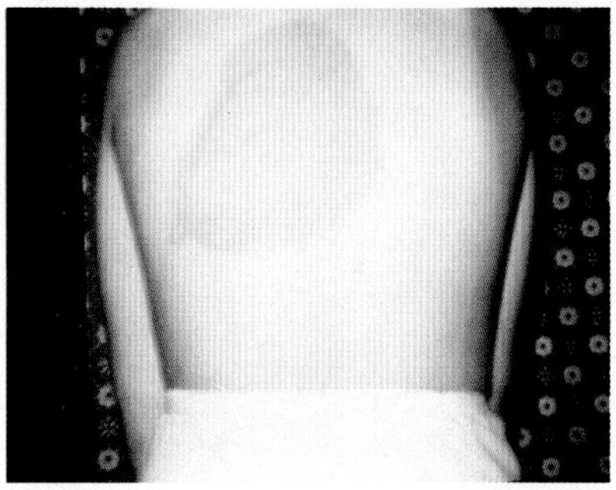

A2-10 **Lyme disease: erythema chronicum migrams** – primary lesion.[5]

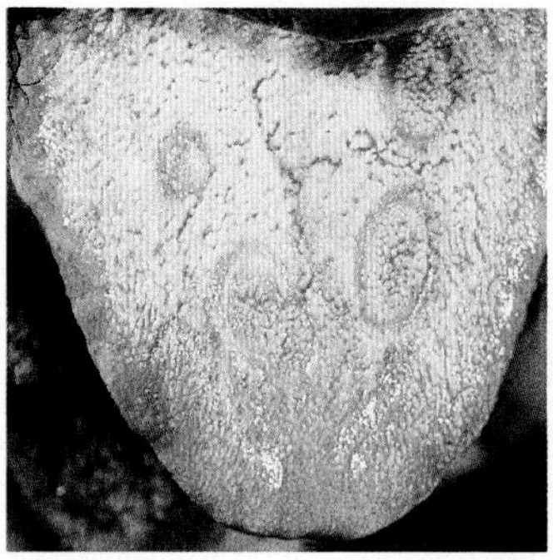

A2-11 Mucous patches involving the tongue in **secondary syphilis**.[4]

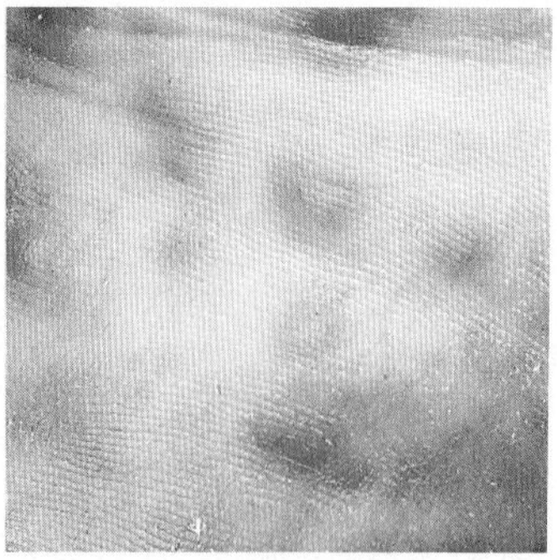

A2-12 **Papulosquamous lesions of secondary syphilis** on the sole of the foot.[4]

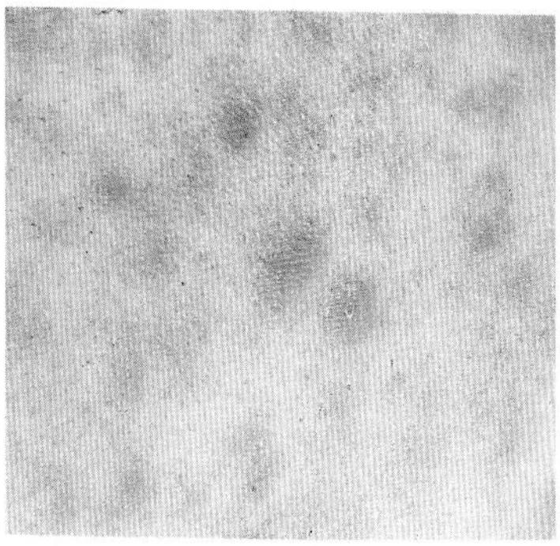

A2-13 **Macular syphilids** in early secondary syphilis.[4]

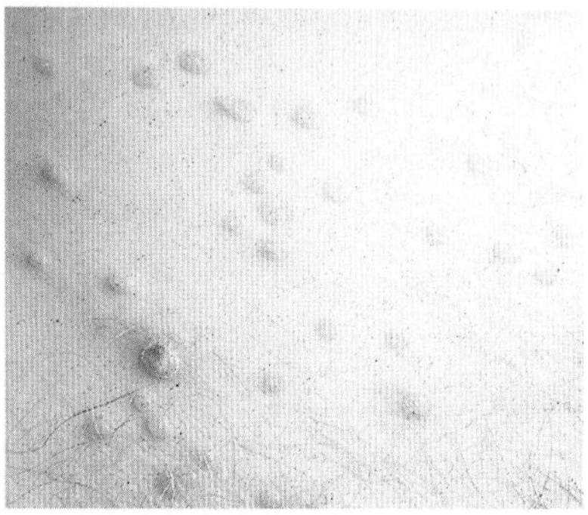

A2-14 **Molluscum contagiosum** of the lower abdomen in a patient with coexisting genital molluscum lesions. Note central umbilication and pale-salmon color.[4]

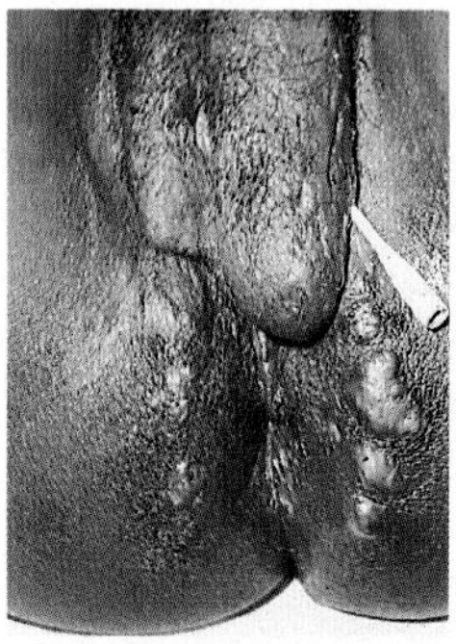

A2-15 **Esthiomene** due to lymphogranuloma venereum.[4]

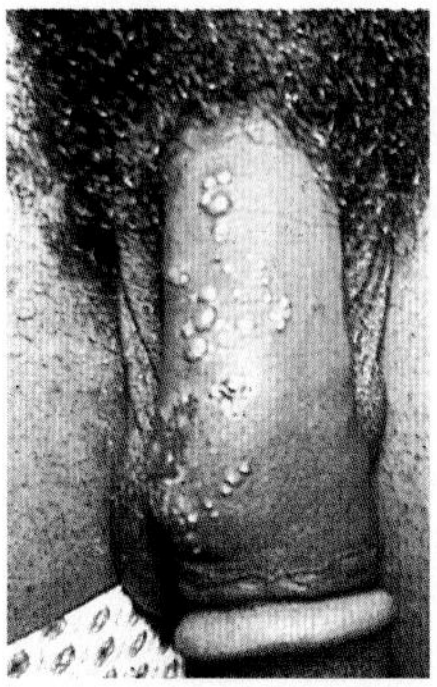

A2-16 **Severe primary HSV* infection** with extensive vesicles, ulcerations, and penile edema.[4]

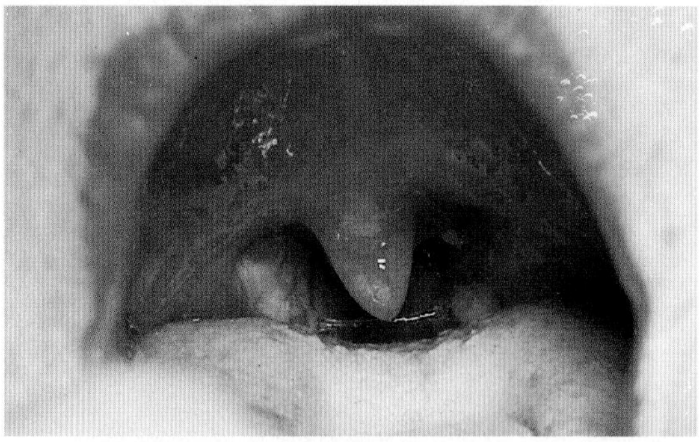

A2-17 **Primary HSV* pharyngitis** showing ulcerative lesions on the uvula and palate together with exudative tonsillitis. HSV-2 was recovered from pharyngeal and genital lesions.[4]

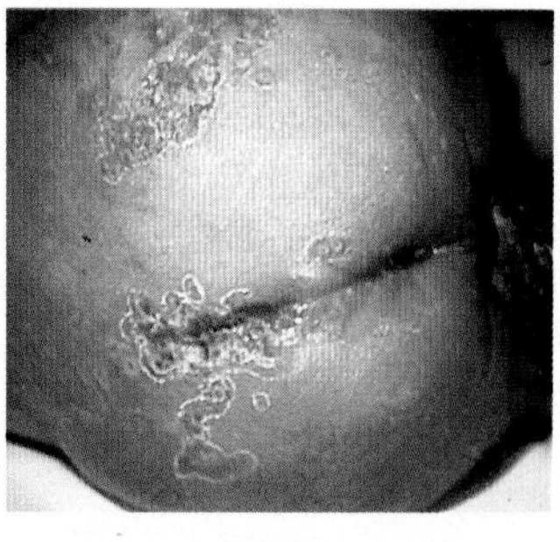

A2-18 **Neonatal HSV* infection.** Ulcers and crusting lesions on the buttocks.[4]

*Herpes Simplex Virus

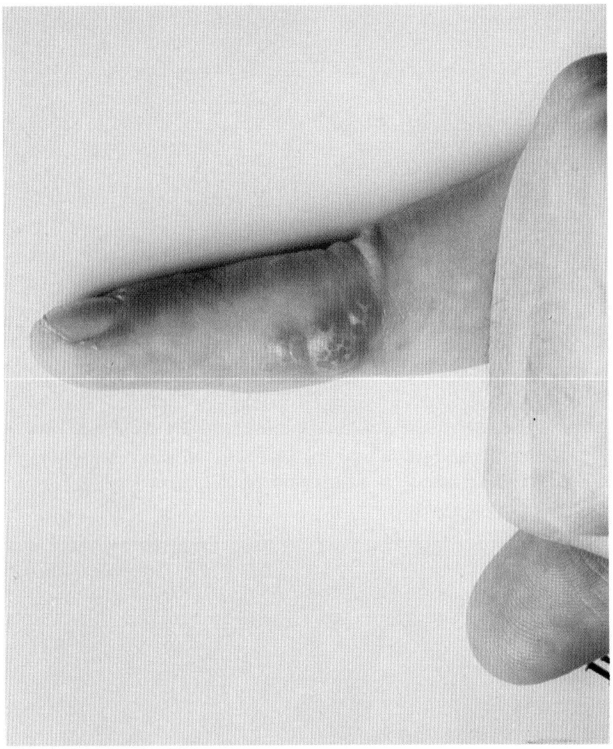

A2-19 **Herpetic whitlow.**[1]

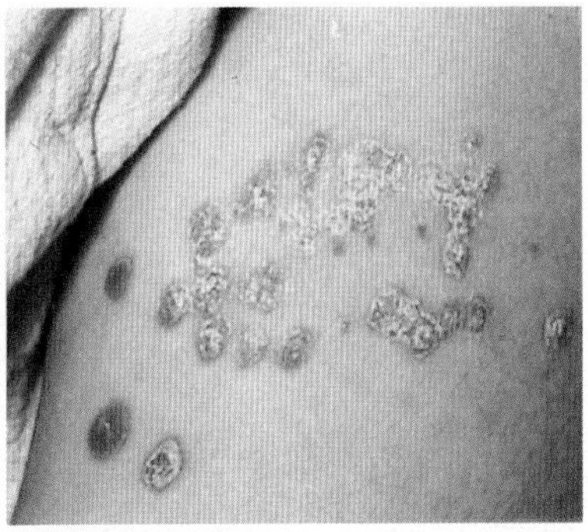

A2-20 **Keratodermia blenorrhagica** in Reiter's syndrome.[4]

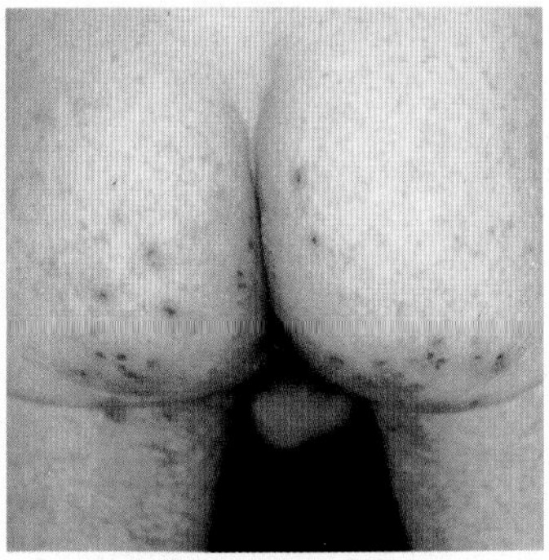

A2-21 Grouped excoriations due to **scabies** on the lower buttocks, simulating dermatitis herpetiformis.[4]

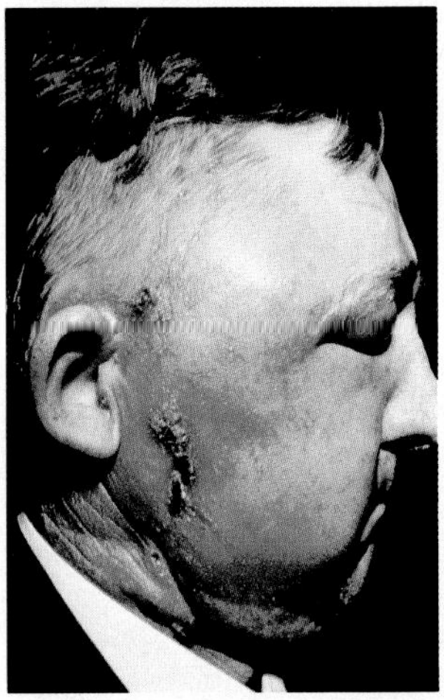

A2-22 **Cervicofacial actinomycosis.**[3]

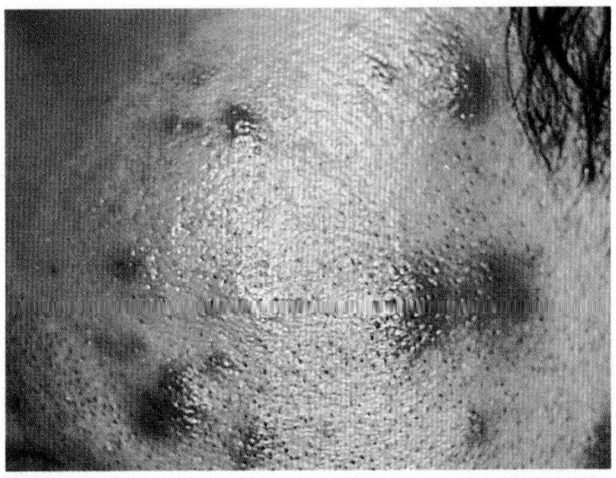

A2-23 Lesions of **Kaposi's sarcoma** on the cheek of a homosexually active man.[4]

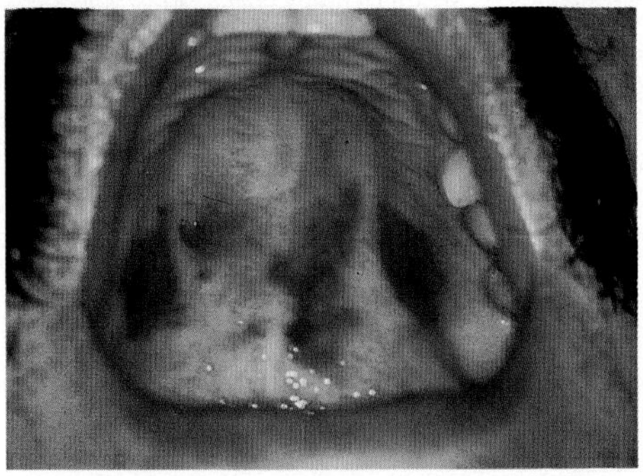

A2-24 **Kaposi's sarcoma** involving the palate of a homosexually active man.[4]

Sources

1 Courtesy of Lawrence Corey, M.D.
2 Courtesy of Theodore E. Woodward, M.D.
3 Fitzpatrick TB et al: *Dermatology in General Medicine*, 2nd ed. New York, McGraw-Hill, 1984
4 Holmes KK et al: *Sexually Transmitted Diseases*. New York, McGraw-Hill, 1984
5 Steere AC et al: Ann Intern Med 86:685, 1977 (reprinted with permission)

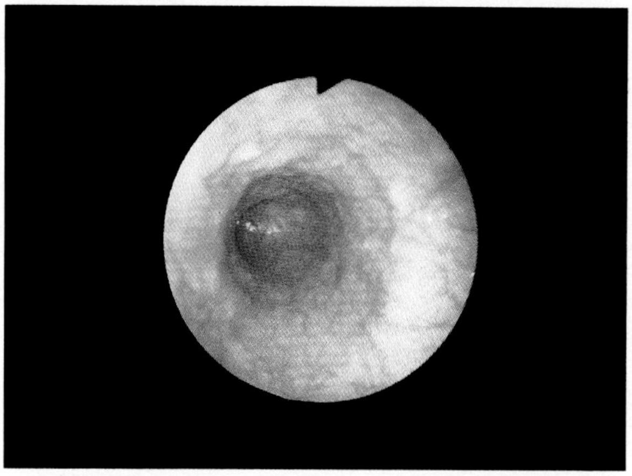

A3-1 **Normal esophagus;** normal fine vasculature can be seen.

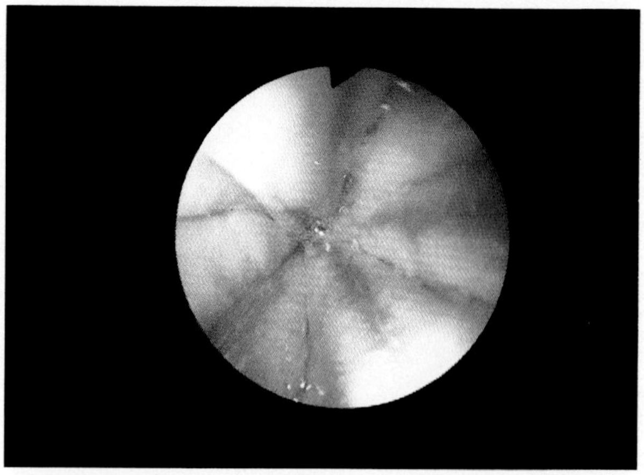

A3-2 **Peptic regurgitant esophagitis;** linear red streaks with a central white streak are noted extending up the esophagus.

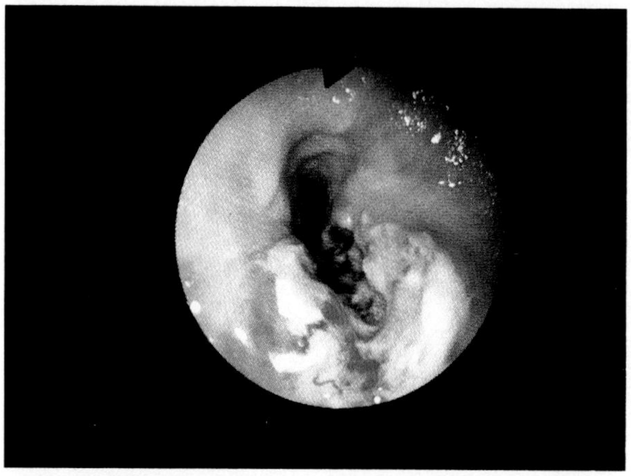

A3-3 **Ulcerated squamous cell carcinoma,** with a depressed center, involving one wall of the esophagus.

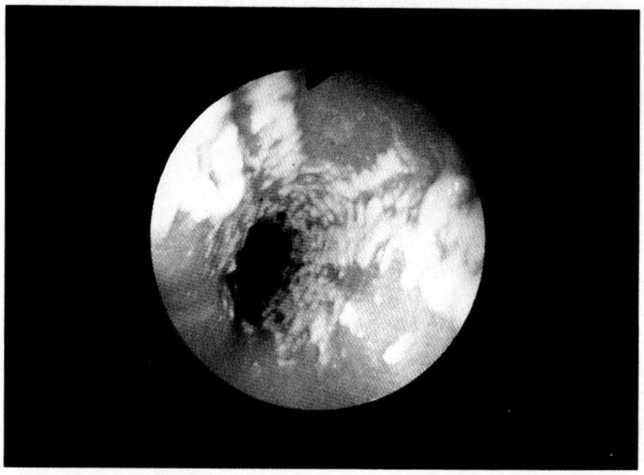

A3-4 **Moniliasis of the esophagus.** A white exudate is seen with underlying erythematous mucosa.

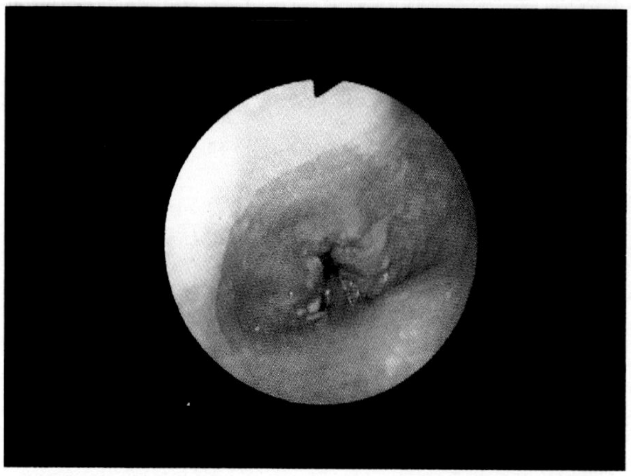

A3-5 **Barrett's metaplasia of the esophagus with an adenocarcinoma.** The squamo-columnar junction is noted in the proximal esophagus. A mucosal irregularity in the center of the photograph was an adenocarcinoma.

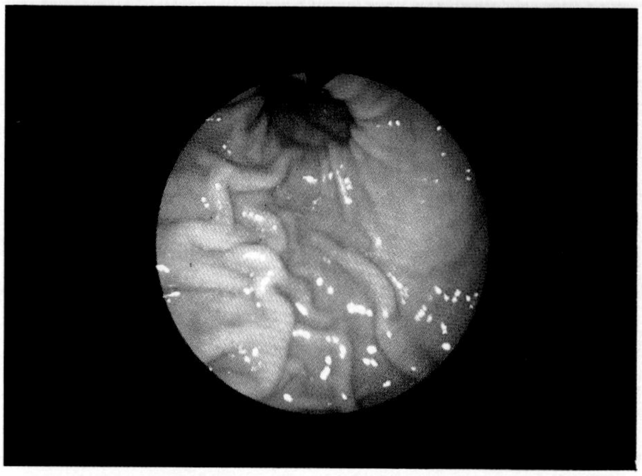

A3-6 **Normal body of the stomach with rugal folds.**

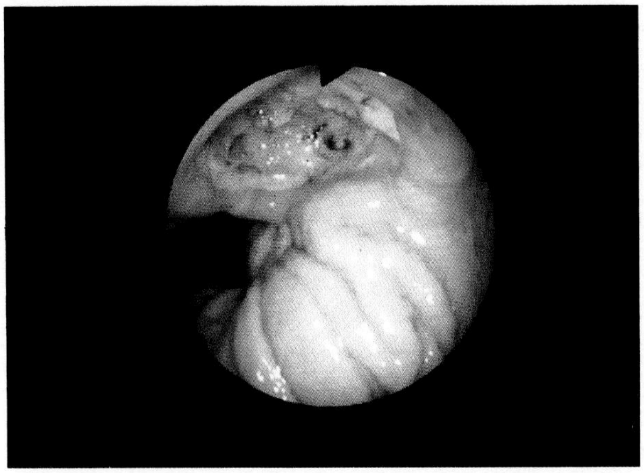

A3-7 **Large, benign, lesser curve, gastric ulcer.** The folds end at the ulcer margin.

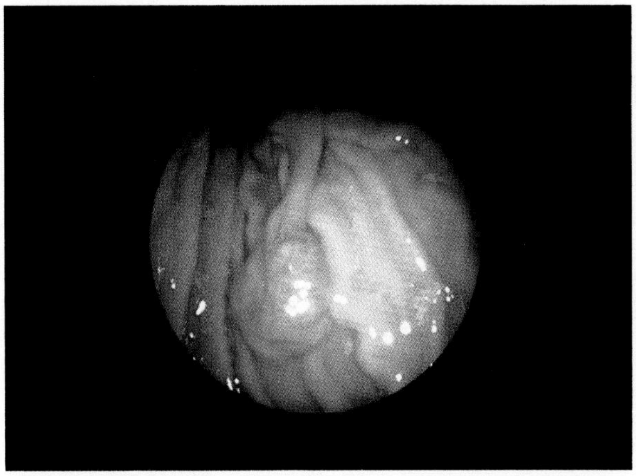

A3-8 **Gastric polyp.** The histologic type must be determined by excision and pathologic examination.

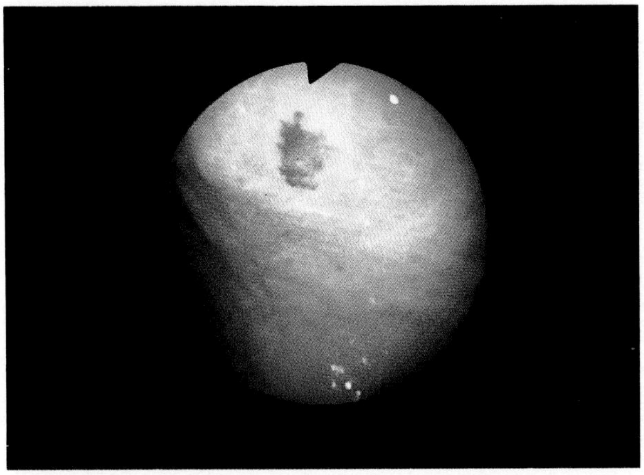

A3-9 **Arteriovenous malformation of the gastric mucosa.**

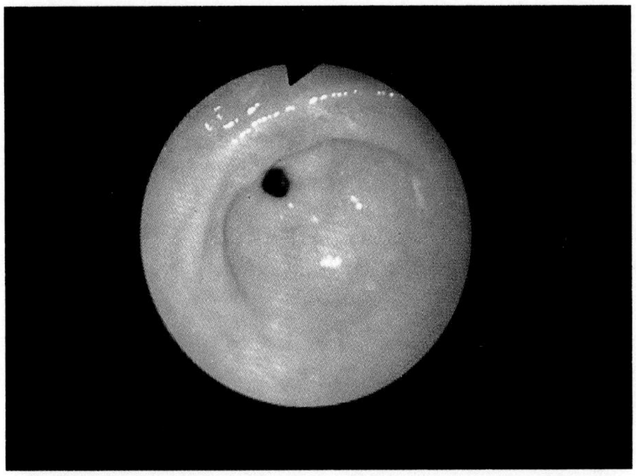

A3-10 **Normal pylorus.** Note the absence of gastric rugal folds in the antrum proximal to the pylorus.

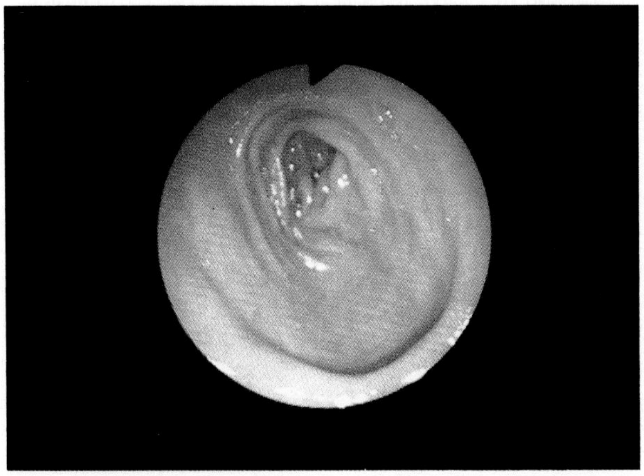

A3-11 **Normal duodenal bulb.**

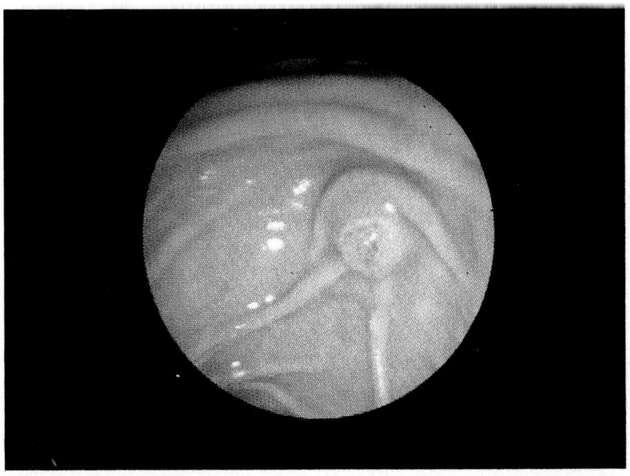

A3-12 **Normal papilla of Vater.** The fold pattern surrounding the papilla is normal; bile is seen adjacent to the papilla.

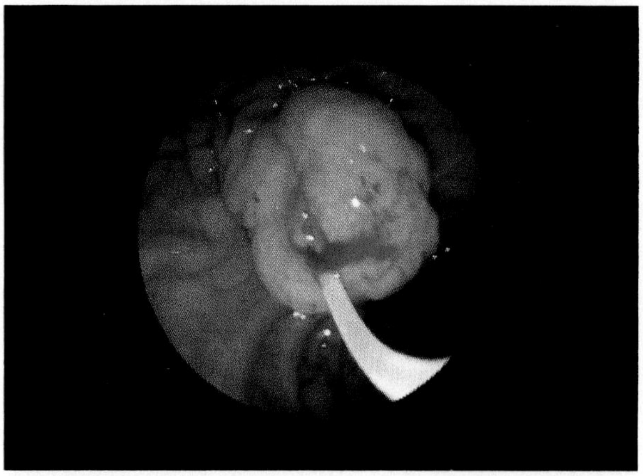

A3-13 **Periampullary carcinoma.** The mass at the papilla of Vater has been catheterized during ERCP.

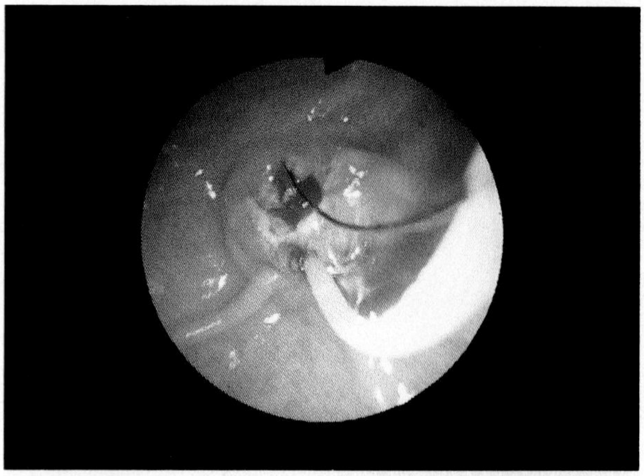

A3-14 **Endoscopic papillotomy.** A papillotome has been passed into the papilla, the wire bowed, and an incision made, with electrosurgical current, in the superior aspect of the papilla.

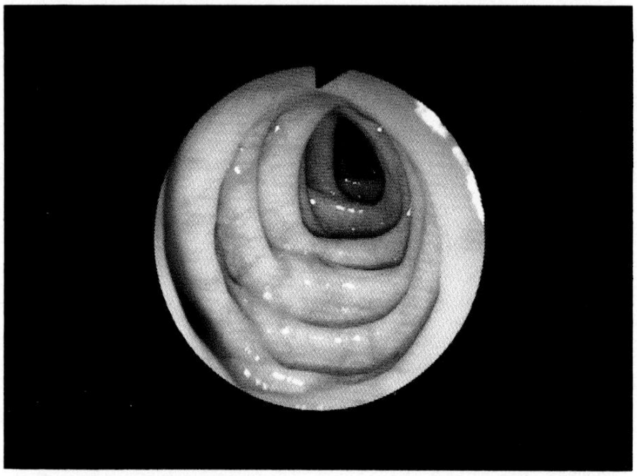

A3-15 **Normal colon;** typical haustral folds and a normal vascular pattern can be seen.

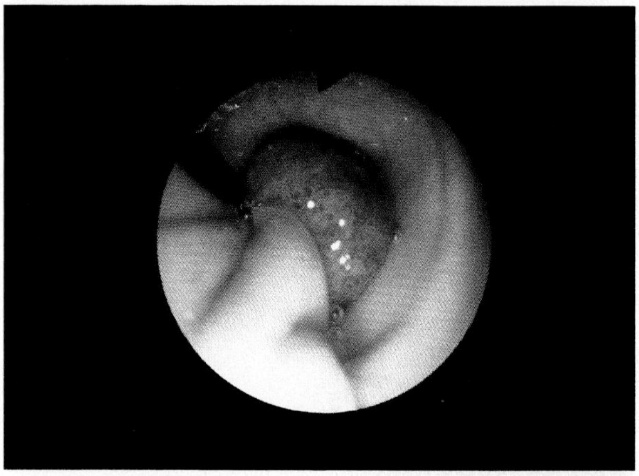

A3-16 **Colonic adenomatous polyp.** The polyp is erythematous; a stalk is seen covered with normal mucosa.

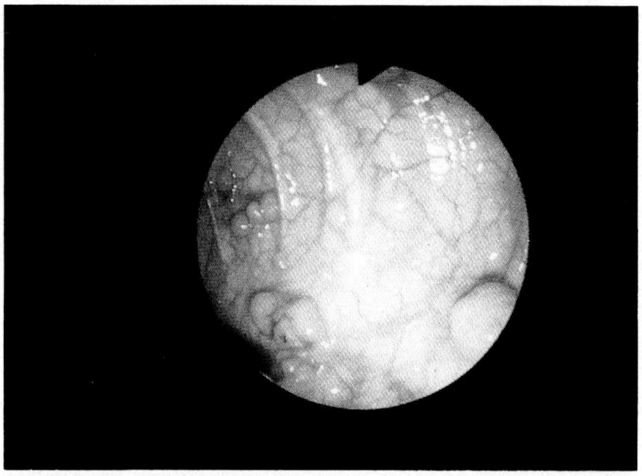

A3-17 **Multiple, small, colonic adenomatous polyps** in a case of familial polyposis coli. This colon must be removed to prevent the development of cancer.

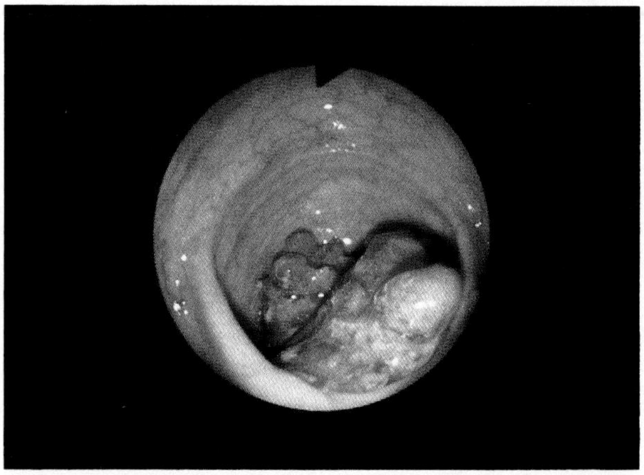

A3-18 **Colon adenocarcinoma.** The cancer is multilobed and growing into the lumen.

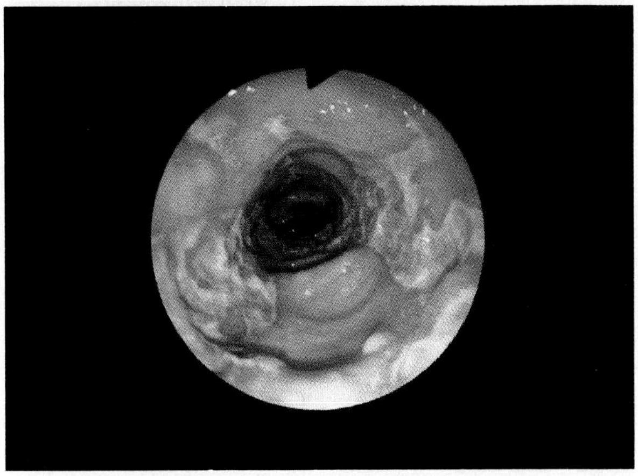

A3-19 **Crohn's colitis** with linear, serpiginous, white-based ulcers surrounded by colonic mucosa which is relatively normal.

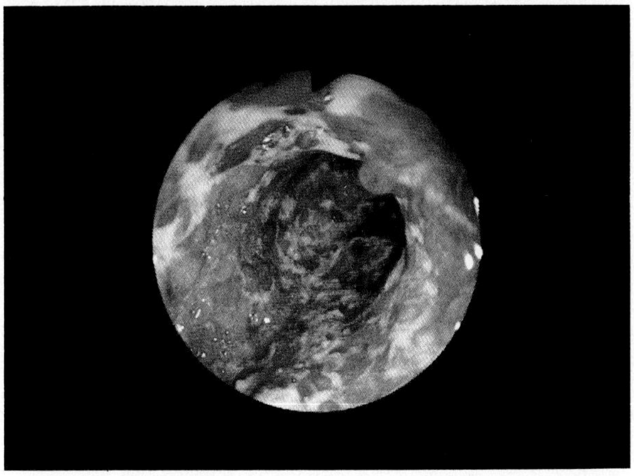

A3-20 **Severe ulcerative colitis** with diffuse ulceration, bleeding, and exudation.

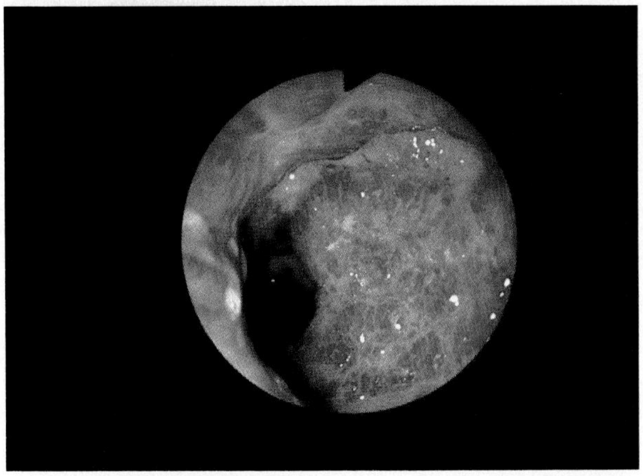

A3-21 **Kaposi's sarcoma involving the colon** in a patient with AIDS. The erythematous lesions involve most of the colonic mucosa in the photograph.

Source: Courtesy of FE Silverstein and GN Tytgat: *Atlas of Gastrointestinal Endoscopy.* Gower Medical Publishing, New York, 1987.

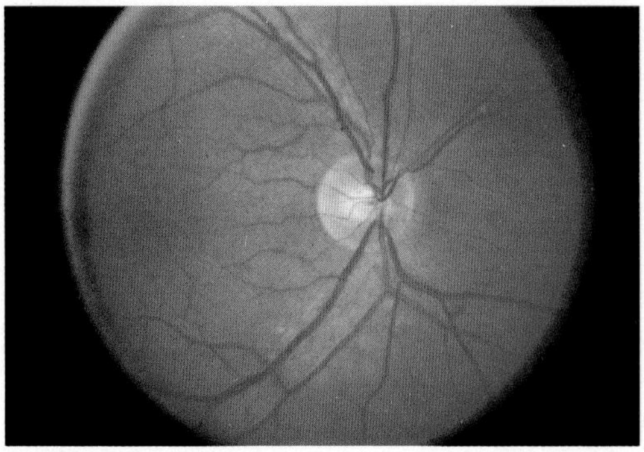

A4-1 **Normal optic nerve and retina.**

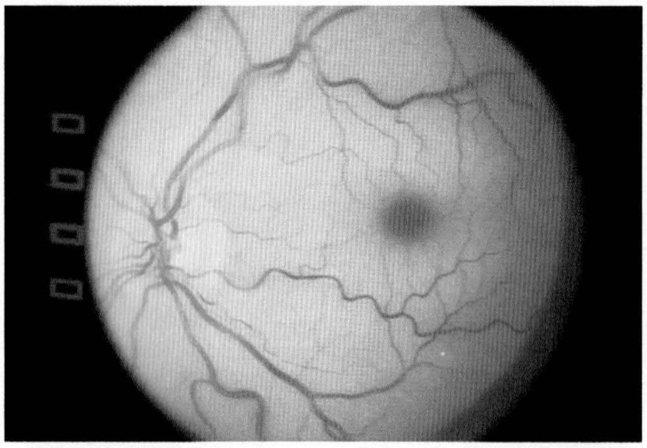

A4-2 **Central retinal artery occlusion.**

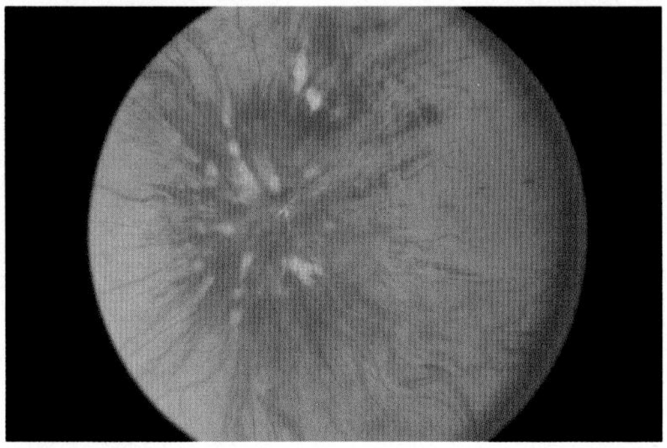

A4-3 **Central retinal vein occlusion.**

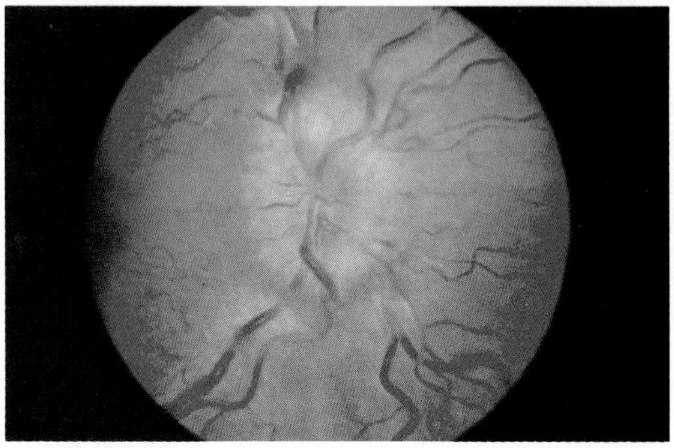

A4-4 **Early papilledema.**

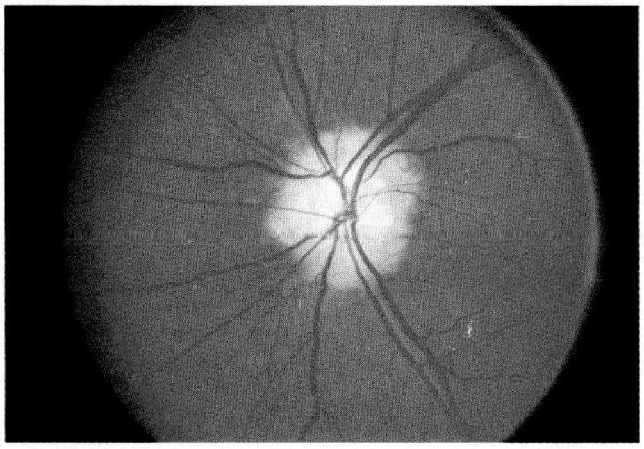

A4-5 **Drusen of the optic nerve head.**

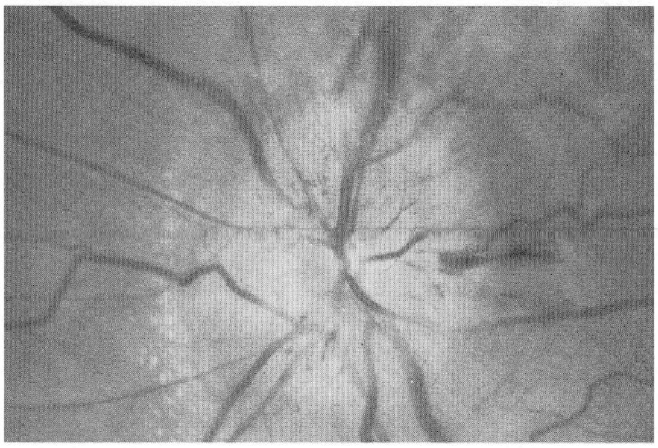

A4-6 **Anterior ischemic optic neuropathy.**

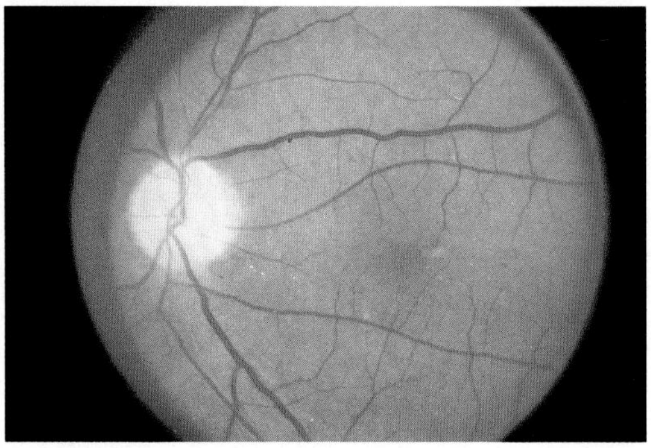

A4-7 **Primary optic atrophy.**

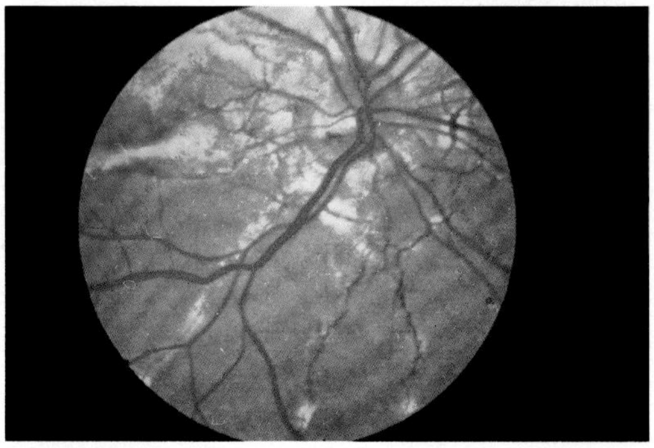

A4-8 **Angioid streaks.**

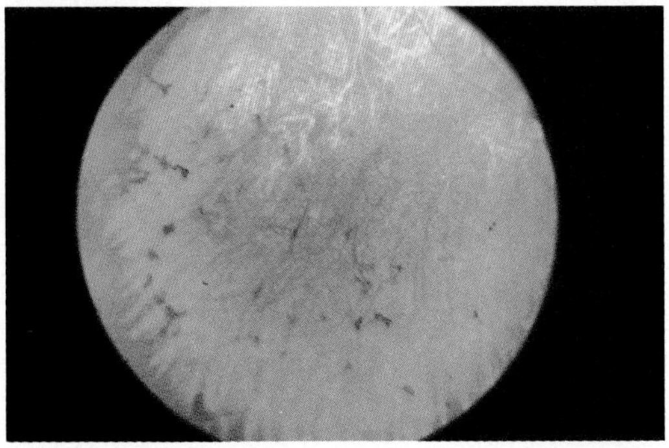

A4-9 **Retinitis pigmentosa.**

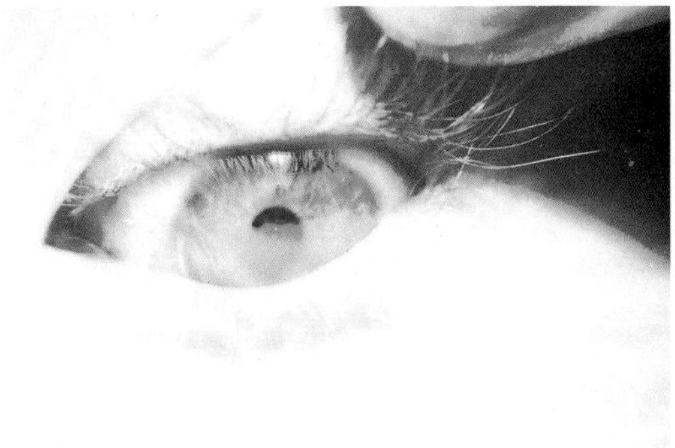

A4-10 **Band keratopathy.**

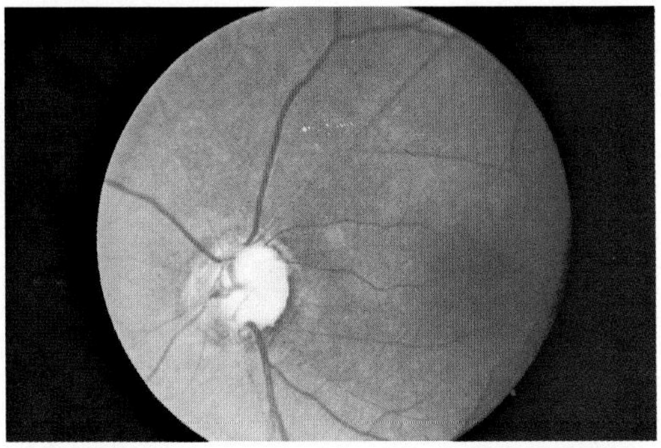

A4-11 **Glaucomatous optic disk with secondary atrophy.**

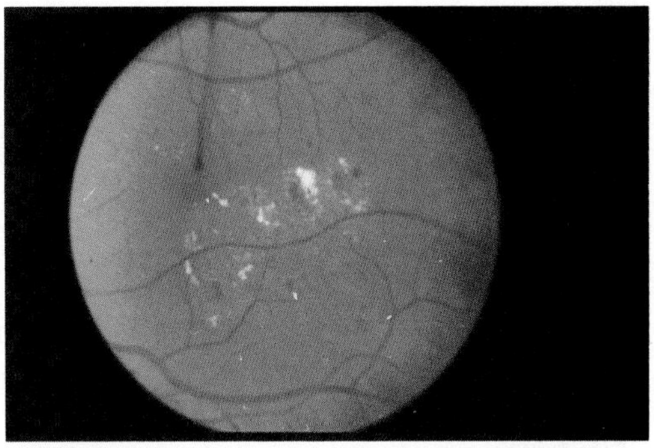

A4-12 **Diabetic retinopathy with microaneurysms.**

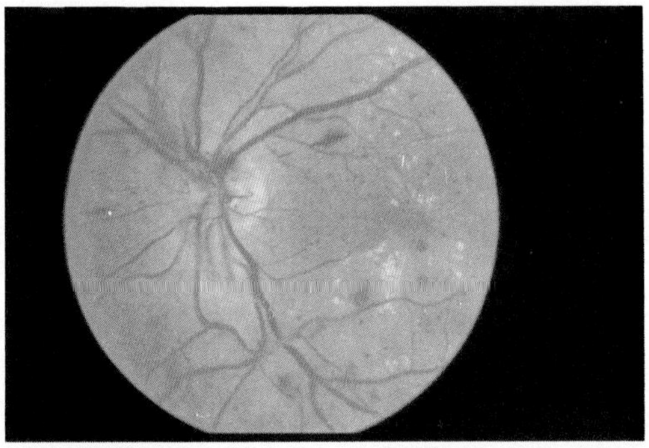

A4-13 **Proliferative diabetic retinopathy.**

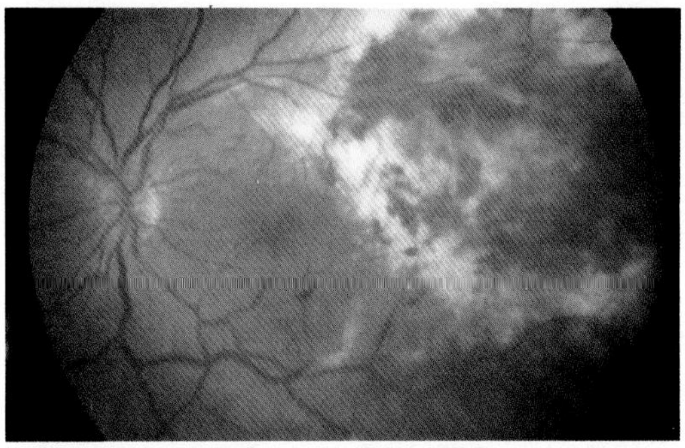

A4-14 **Cytomegalovirus retinitis in AIDS.**
(Courtesy of Donald J. D'Amico, M.D.)

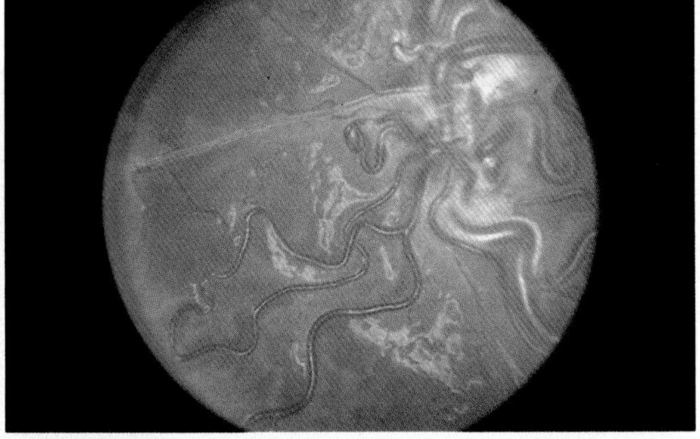

A4-15 **Retinal arteriovenous malformation in the Wyburn-Mason syndrome.**

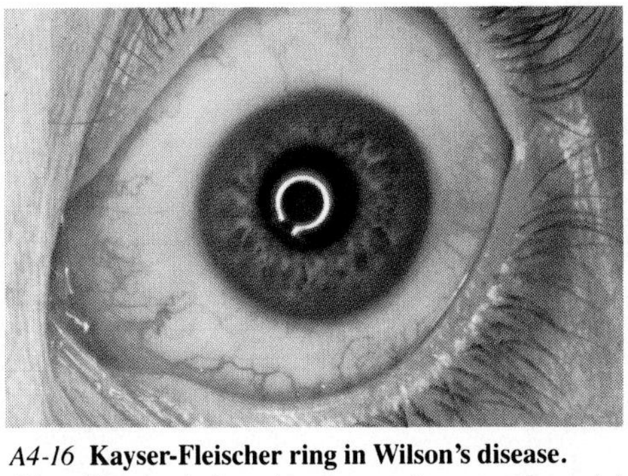

A4-16 **Kayser-Fleischer ring in Wilson's disease.**
(Note: The ring is the golden brown pigment at the periphery of the cornea and is characteristically broader superiorly and inferiorly than it is medially and laterally.)

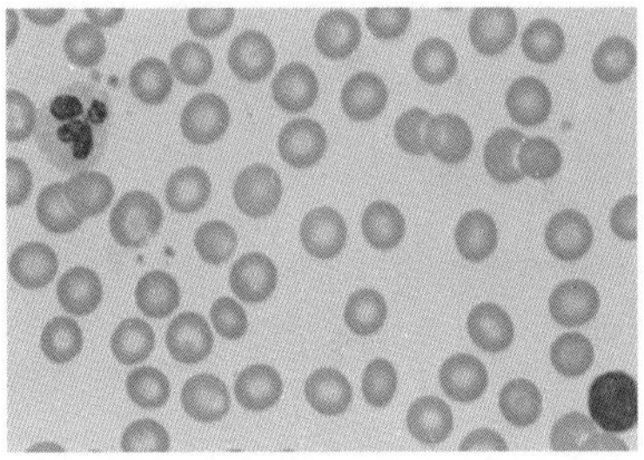

A5-1 **Normal blood smear.** Normal red blood cells are round, possess an area of central pallor, appear slightly smaller than the nucleus of a mature lymphocyte, and vary little in size (anisocytosis) or in shape (poikilocytosis).

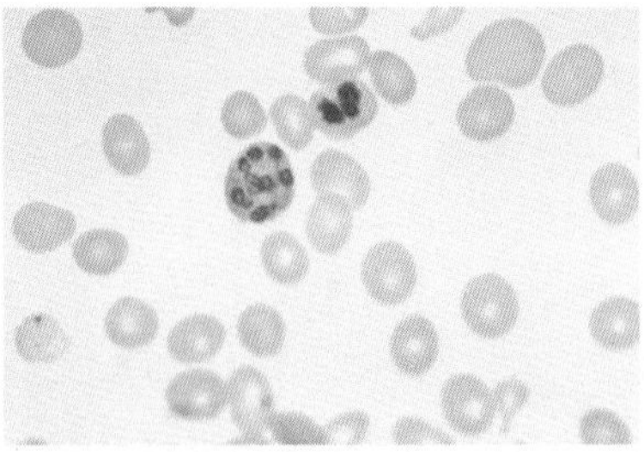

A5-2 **Megaloblastic anemia.** Oval macrocytes, well filled with hemoglobin, are admixed with lesser numbers of small teardrop-shaped red blood cells. Note also hypersegmented granulocyte.

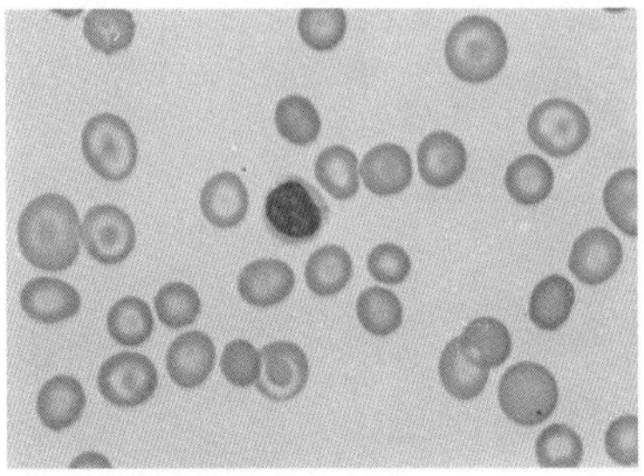

A5-3 **Liver disease.** Round macrocytes of rather uniform size are seen. Many of the macrocytes are also target cells.

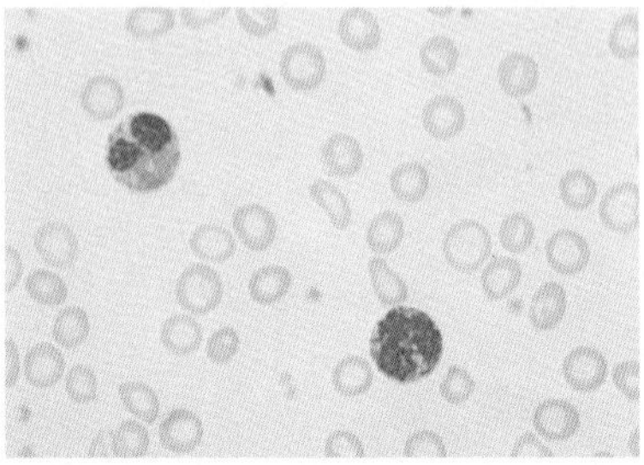

A5-4 **Iron-deficiency anemia.** In severe iron deficiency, the red blood cells are smaller than normal (microcytosis), and their central area of pallor is expanded (hypochromia) so that the cells appear to have only a thin rim of hemoglobin.

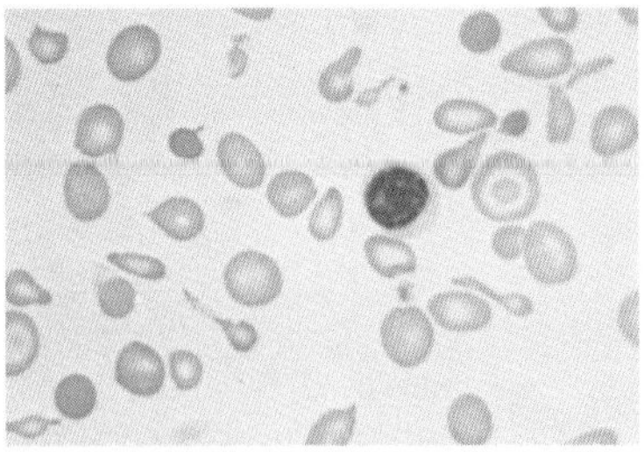

A5-5 **β thalassemia intermedia.** Microcytic and hypochromic red blood cells are seen that resemble the red blood cells of severe iron deficiency anemia shown in Fig. A5-4. Many elliptical and teardrop-shaped red blood cells are noted.

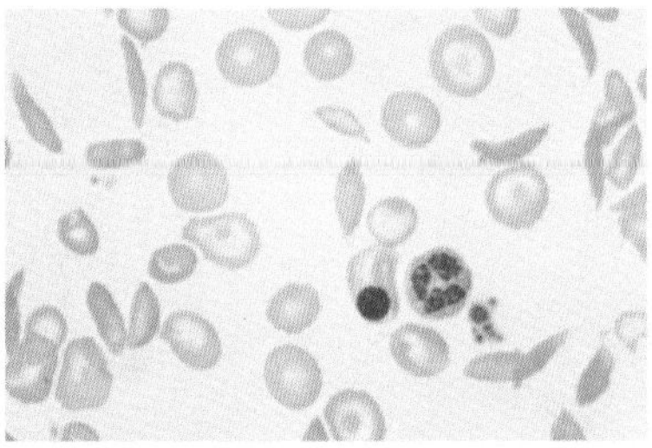

A5-6 **Sickle cell anemia.** The elongated and crescent-shaped red blood cells seen on this smear represent circulating irreversible sickled cells. Target cells and a nucleated red blood cell are also seen.

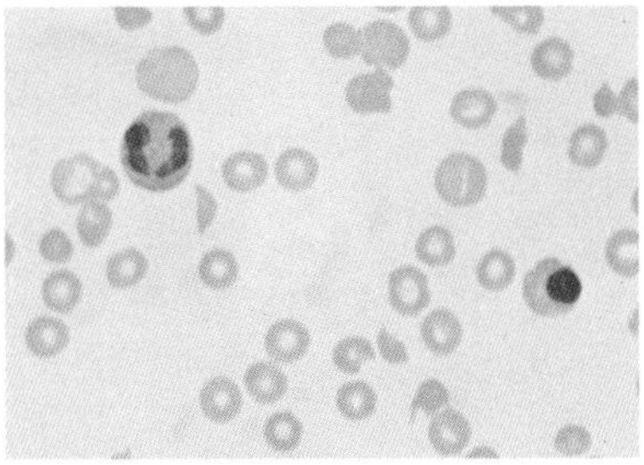

A5-7 **Traumatic hemolysis.** The helmet-shaped red blood cell and the small triangular-shaped red blood cells seen on this smear represent morphologic evidence of mechanical damage to red blood cells within the circulatory tree.

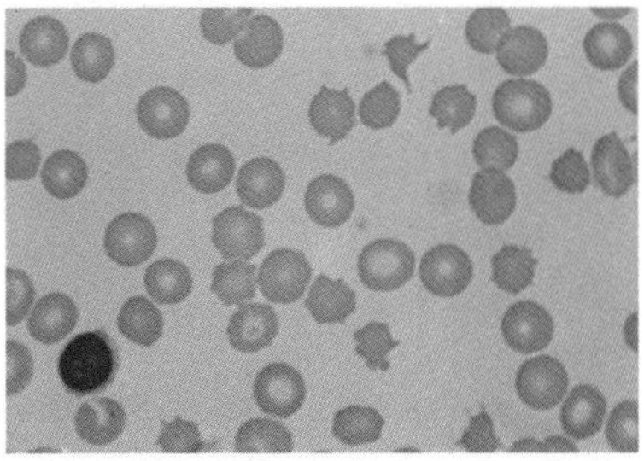

A5-8 **Spur cell anemia.** Spur cells are recognized as distorted red blood cells containing several irregularly distributed thornlike projections. Cells with this morphologic abnormality are also called acanthocytes.

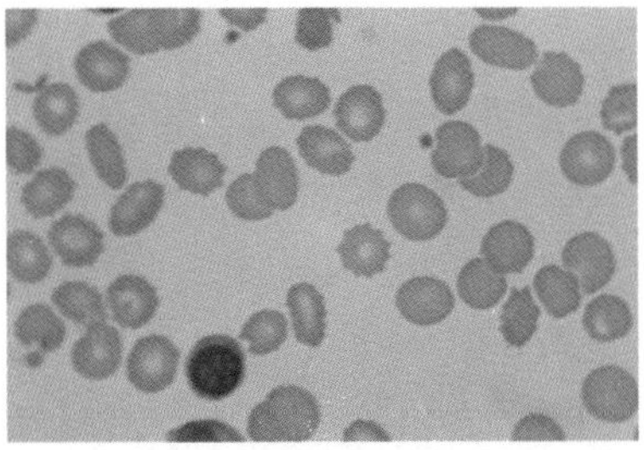

A5-9 **Uremia.** The red blood cells in uremia may acquire numerous, regularly spaced, small spiny projections. Such cells, called burr cells or echinocytes, are readily distinguishable from the irregularly spiculated acanthocytes shown in Fig. A5-8.

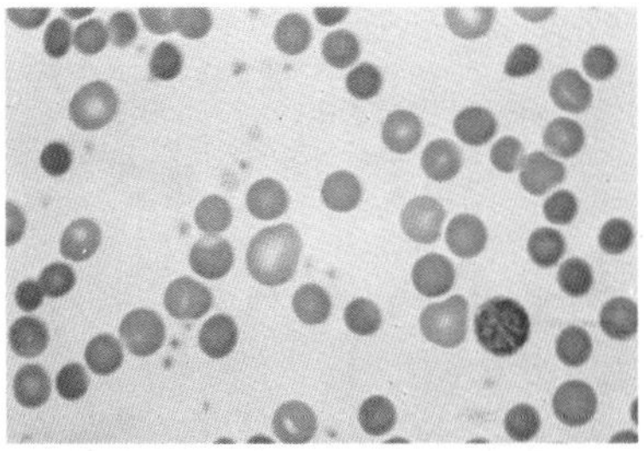

A5-10 **Hereditary spherocytosis.** Small, densely staining red blood cells are seen that have lost their central area of pallor (microspherocytes). Microspherocytes may also be found in other hemolytic disorders (Fig. A5-11).

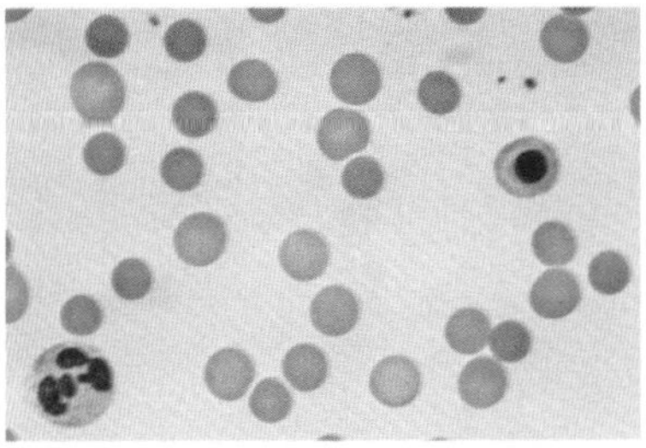

A5-11 **Immunohemolytic anemia.** Microspherocytes are seen on this blood smear along with several macrocytes with a slight purple tinge (polychromasia). The latter represent new red blood cells released early from the bone marrow. The microspherocytes seen in immunohemolytic anemia may be indistinguishable from the microspherocytes seen in hereditary spherocytosis (Fig. A5-10).

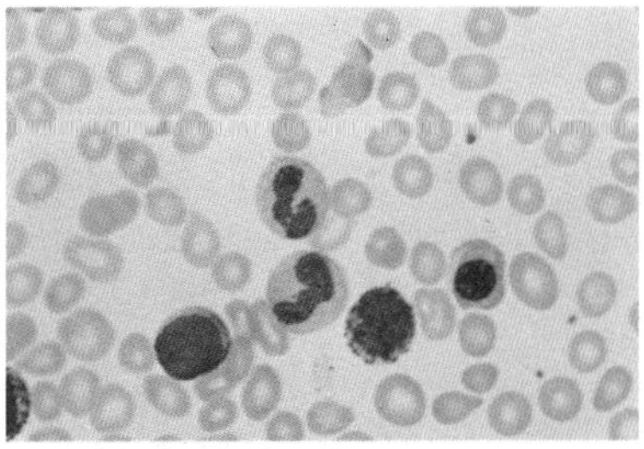

A5-12 **Myeloid metaplasia.** Teardrop-shaped red blood cells, a nucleated red blood cell, and immature myeloid cells are seen on this blood smear.

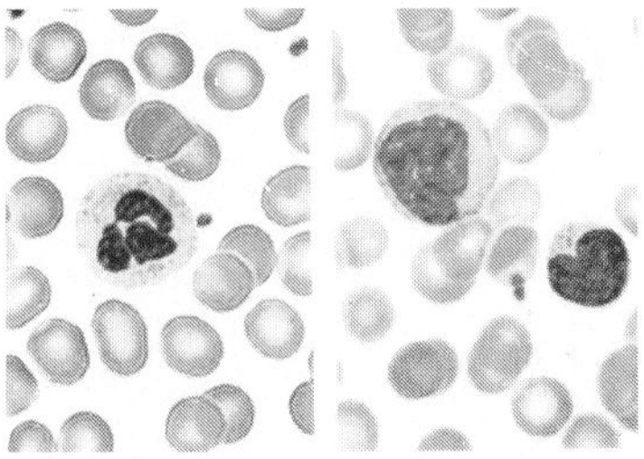

A **B**

A5-13 A. **Normal granulocyte.** The normal granulocyte has a segmented nucleus with heavy, clumped chromatin; fine neutrophilic granules are dispersed throughout its cytoplasm. *B.* **Normal monocyte and lymphocyte.** The normal monocyte is a large cell with an indented or folded nucleus containing loose, strandlike chromatin; the cytoplasm is a blue-gray color and usually contains fine azurophilic granules. The normal lymphocyte is a smaller cell. Its nucleus is usually round but may be indented, as in the cell shown in this plate. The nuclear chromatin has a smudgy appearance; the cytoplasm is a blue color.

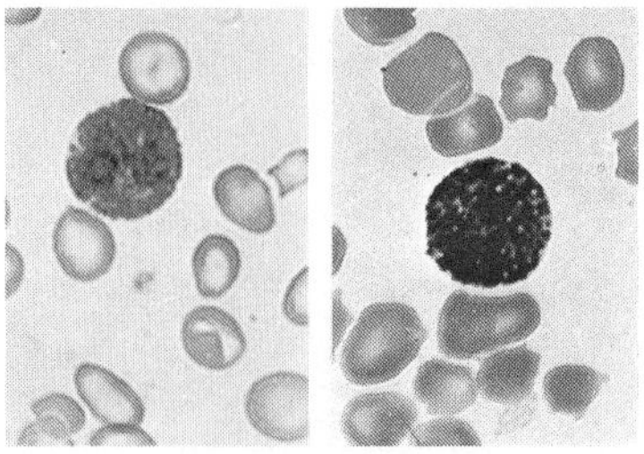

A **B**

A5-14 A. **Normal eosinophil.** The eosinophil contains large, bright-orange granules; the nucleus is bilobed. *B.* **Basophil.** The basophil contains large purple-black granules which fill the cell and obscure the nucleus.

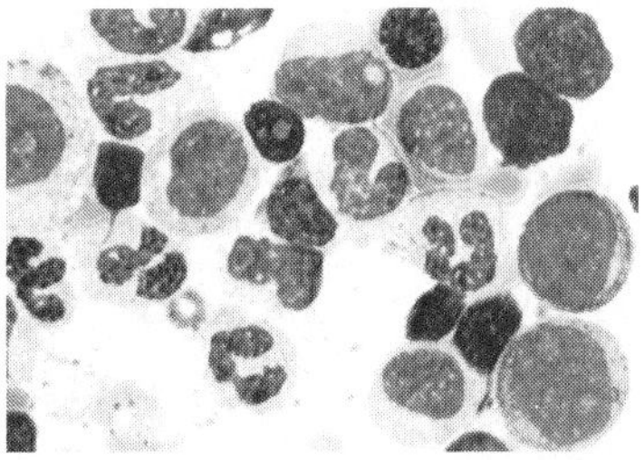

A5-15 **Normal granulocyte precursors in marrow.** The earliest granulocytic precursor (myeloblast) possesses a round nucleus with fine, punctate chromatin and one or more nucleoli; the cytoplasm is blue. As nuclear differentiation proceeds, the nucleoli disappear, the chromatin coarsens, and the nucleus becomes increasingly indented and finally segmented. As cytoplasmic differentiation proceeds, azurophilic granules appear and the cytoplasm changes color from blue to the yellow-pink-gray hue of the mature granulocyte, and as this occurs the azurophilic granules become obscured by fine neutrophilic granules.

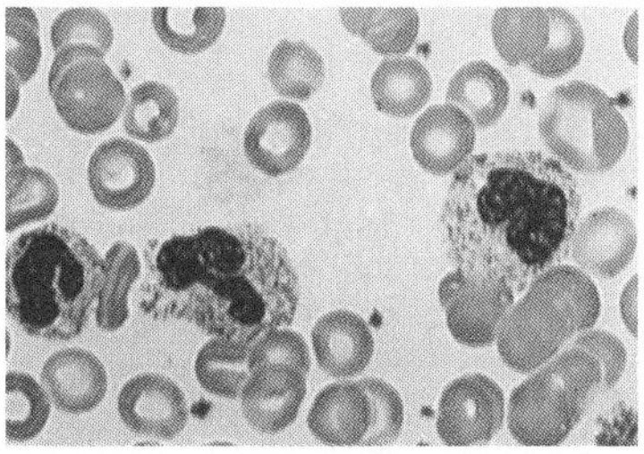

A5-16 **Neutrophils with toxic granulation.** In infection and other toxic states, azurophilic granules may become visible in mature granulocytes as coarse, dark-staining cytoplasmic granules.

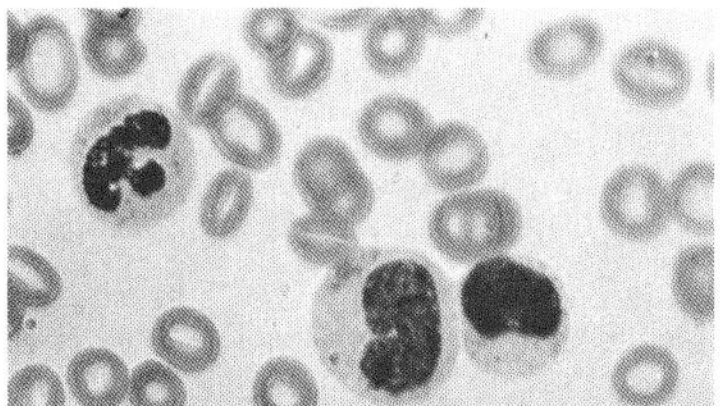

A5-17 **Band with Döhle body** (center). Döhle bodies are discrete, blue-staining, nongranular areas found in the periphery of the cytoplasm of the neutrophil in infections and other toxic states. They represent aggregates of rough endoplasmic reticulum.

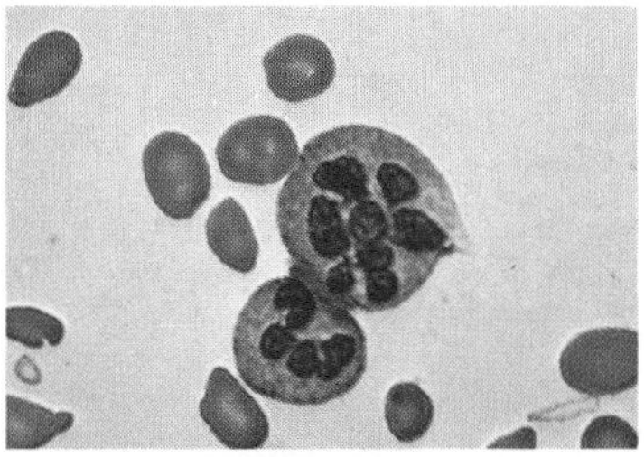

A5-18 **Hypersegmentation.** Frequent five-lobed granulocytes on a blood smear or granulocytes with more than five lobes are evidence of hypersegmentation, an important clue to the diagnosis of megaloblastic anemia.

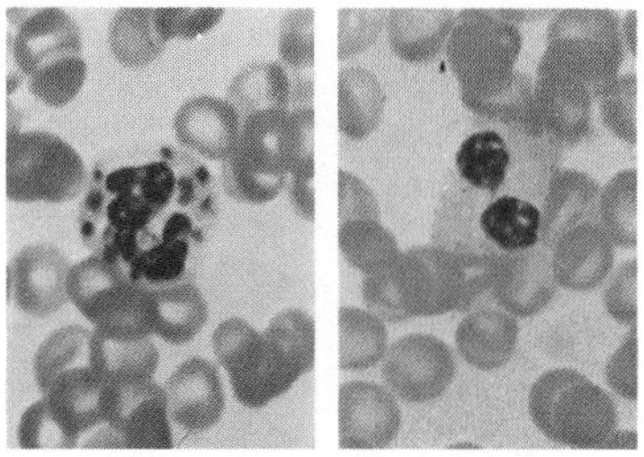

A B

A5-19 A. **Chédiak-Higashi anomaly.** In this ultimately fatal disorder, the granulocytes contain huge cytoplasmic granules, formed from aggregation and fusion of azurophilic and specific granules. Large, abnormal granules are found in other granule-containing cells throughout the body. *B*. **Pelger-Hüet anomaly.** In this benign disorder, the majority of granulocytes are bilobed. The nucleus frequently has a spectacle-like or "pince-nez" configuration.

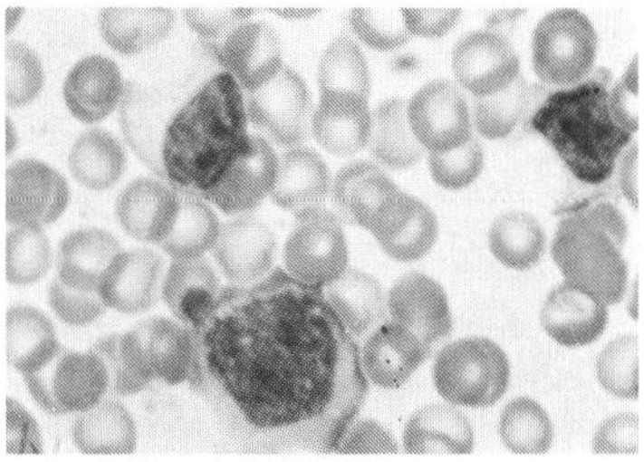

A5-20 **Reactive lymphocytes** (infectious mononucleosis). Reactive lymphocytes are usually large, cytoplasmic lymphocytes. The nucleus may be eccentrically placed and may have irregular borders and indentations (not seen on this plate). The cytoplasm contains areas that stain a darker blue due to their increased content of RNA. The cytoplasm may be indented where it abuts against a red blood cell.

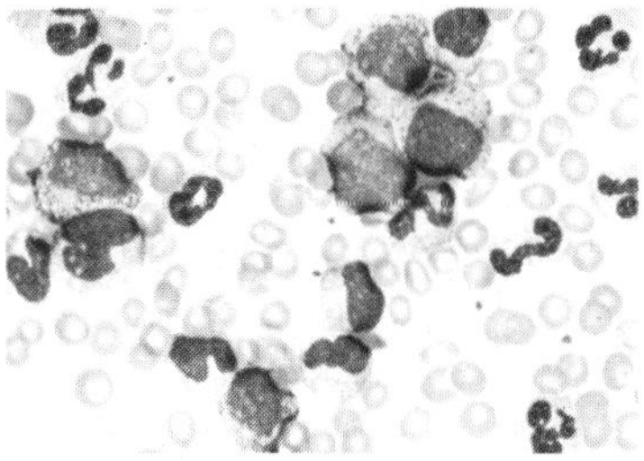

A5-21 **Chronic granulocytic leukemia.** The peripheral blood WBC count is high due to increased numbers of granulocytes and their precursors. The majority of the WBCs are segmented granulocytes or band forms, but as seen on this plate, myelocytes and promyeloblasts (not seen on this plate) may also be found on review of the blood smear.

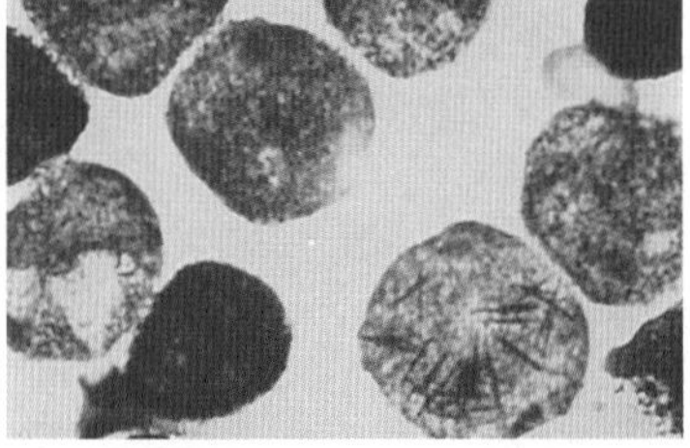

A5-22 **Leukemic cell in acute promyelocytic leukemia.** Note multiple Auer rods.

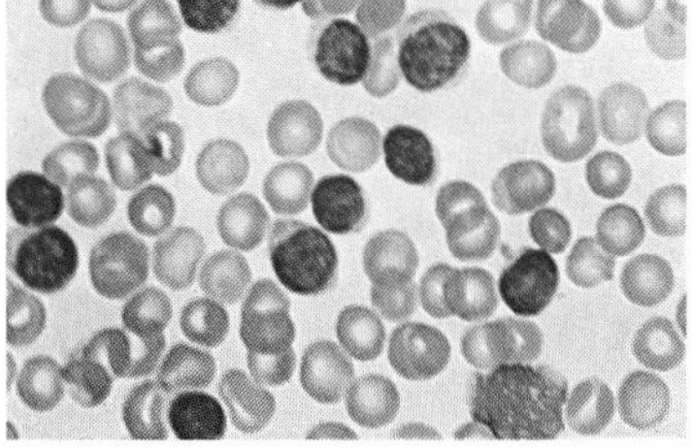

A5-23 **Chronic lymphocytic leukemia.** The peripheral blood WBC count is high due to increased numbers of small, well-differentiated lymphocytes. However, the leukemic lymphocytes are fragile, and substantial numbers of broken, smudged cells are usually also present on the blood smear.

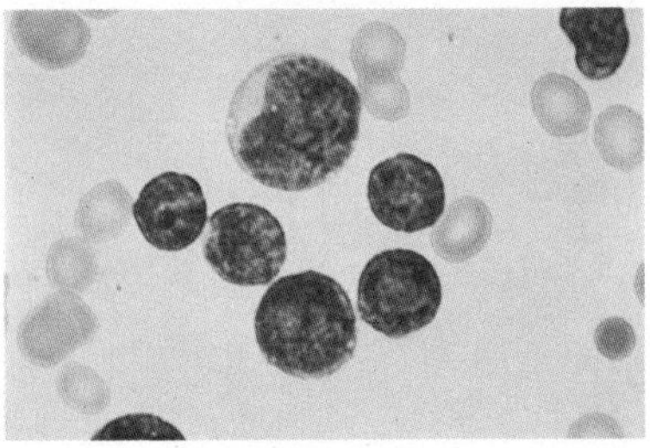

A5-24 **Leukemic cells in acute lymphoblastic leukemia** characterized by round or convoluted nuclei, high nuclear/cytoplasmic ratio and absence of cytoplasmic granules.

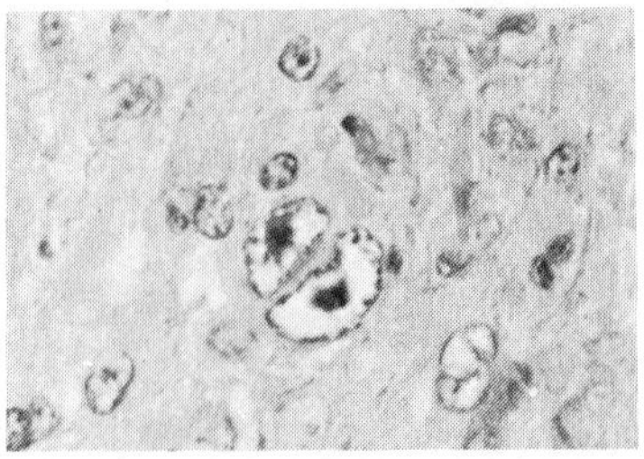

A5-25 **Hodgkin's disease:** Reed-Sternberg cell in marrow (center). The Reed-Sternberg cell is recognized by its bilobed, mirror-image nucleus, which contains in each lobe a giant, inclusion body–like nucleolus. The cytoplasmic borders of the cell cannot be identified on this plate.

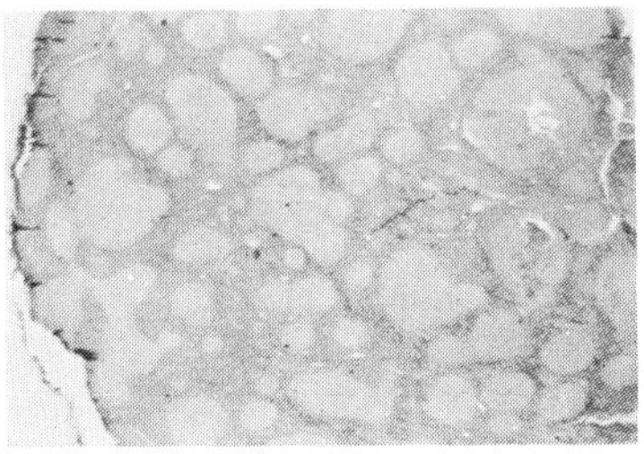

A5-26 **Non-Hodgkin's nodular lymphoma** (lymph node). This low-power view illustrates that a proliferative process has caused the normal architecture of the lymph node to be replaced by multiple nodules of varying size that extend throughout the entire lymph node.

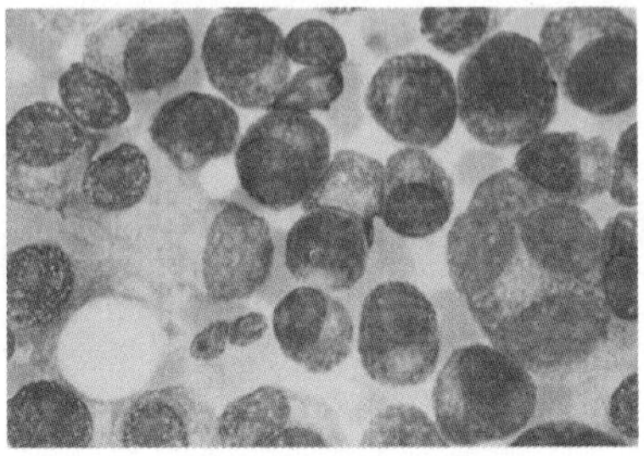

A5-27 **Multiple myeloma** (marrow). The cells bear the characteristic morphologic features of plasma cells, round or oval cells with an eccentric nucleus composed of coarsely clumped chromatin, a densely basophilic cytoplasm, and a perinuclear clear zone (hof) containing the Golgi apparatus. Binucleate and multinucleate malignant plasma cells can also be seen.

PART FOUR NUTRITION

70 NUTRITION AND NUTRITIONAL REQUIREMENTS

IRWIN H. ROSENBERG

Maintenance of good nutrition is essential for both the comprehensive management and the prevention of disease. Many debilitating complications can be prevented or modified by attention to nutritional status and prevention of nutritional deficits. The effective management of the sick patient, therefore, requires detailed evaluation of diet and nutritional status and a projection of the interaction of diet and nutritional status on the clinical course. Only then can proper goals and techniques of nutritional management be selected and nutritional guidance be provided for disease prevention and health promotion.

The purpose of the chapters in this section is to summarize some of the basic considerations for the estimation of nutritional needs and the setting of goals for treatment. Determination of the nutritional needs of the individual patient must take into account both the physiologic responses to normal dietary intake and the nutritional impairments induced by disease.

EATING BEHAVIOR AND NUTRITIONAL NEEDS Eating behavior is by nature intermittent, yet energy needs are continuous. This basic feature of mammalian biology has resulted in the evolution of an elaborate set of metabolic controls that promote the ebb and flow of nutrients after feeding and during the postabsorptive period and, in addition, provide for the maintenance of near-normal function during periods of fasting.

In a nutritional perspective, the mechanisms that control appetite and eating behavior are directed to maintain energy intake adequate for the needs of the healthy adult, for the extra needs of growth in the child, and for the requirements of pregnancy and lactation. Under conditions of disease or trauma, the increased requirements must be met through appropriate modifications in eating behavior or caloric supplementation if energy balance is to be maintained.

The usual remarkable stability of body weight and body composition requires that energy intake and expenditure must be balanced over time. The precise nature of the internal signals that relay the information that caloric intake is appropriate for energy needs during the preceding days is not known. Such signals do not adjust eating behavior on a meal-to-meal time scale. At the time of an individual meal, volume and chemoreceptors in the stomach and small bowel initiate neural and hormonal responses that contribute to satiety. The nutrient density of the food eaten, in terms of the protein or calorie content per unit volume, is not sensitively perceived, and therefore total energy or protein intake can fluctuate substantially over the short run. The neurophysiologic mechanisms that control eating behavior recognize calorie deficiencies on roughly a 24- to 48-h time scale and make compensatory changes in the volume of food eaten over periods of 1 to 2 days. That these controls work remarkably well is attested to by the stability of body weight and general nutritional health of most people who have access to adequate food intake. Aberrations in these control factors can produce serious and even life-threatening imbalance, as evidenced by obesity and syndromes of anorexia and depletion related to manifest disease.

METABOLIC RESPONSES TO CALORIC INTAKE When dietary or energy intake is adequate, several metabolic controls act to maintain essential body functions. One essential function is the maintenance of a steady fuel supply to the brain. Under the usual conditions the brain uses glucose for energy at a rate of about 5 g/h, and such a supply must be available in both the fasted and fed states. The brain is also capable of utilizing ketones as an energy source and will do so in preference to glucose if the ketones are present in sufficiently high concentration. In contrast to tissues such as skeletal muscle, the brain uses energy at a fairly constant rate, whether awake, sleeping, thinking, or dreaming.

During the influx of nutrients into blood after feeding and absorption, the energy and amino acid needs of the body are readily met by the supply entering from the gastrointestinal tract. When this flow of nutrients subsides, however, the body's needs are met by release of energy from stores. In the period immediately after feeding, these stores are generated and maintained under hormonal control, particularly insulin. The excess amino acids, fatty acids, and glucose not required immediately for energy are stored in the form of proteins, triglycerides, and glycogen. This storage process also serves to modulate the large extracellular osmotic shifts that might occur between the fed and the fasting states by depositing excess nutrients in intracellular depots.

NUTRITIONAL REQUIREMENTS To formulate an overall plan for nutritional management, one must consider the nutritional requirements of the patient and the impact of disease on these requirements. Energy balance in simplest terms means energy intake that maintains a steady body weight. Energy insufficiency is reflected in weight loss, and energy overabundance causes weight gain. Conditions that can substantially modify nutritional requirements include infection, trauma (including surgery), alcohol abuse, and malabsorption.

ESTIMATION OF ENERGY REQUIREMENT Malnutrition occurs when nutrient intake is below nutrient needs. Although the disorder can result from excessive nutritional intake, in general the term commonly refers to undernutrition. Undernutrition can be due to inadequate intake or absorption or to increased metabolic requirements imposed by disease, including loss and secretion of nutrients and drug-nutrient antagonisms.

The components of energy requirements in humans are summarized in Table 70-1. Total daily energy requirement consists of basal

TABLE 70-1 Example of estimation of daily energy requirement

The information presented above can be utilized as in the following example: A 45-year-old, 70-kg male office worker presents with rheumatoid arthritis of mild severity. Calorie intake is good, but recent activity has been limited.

Resting energy expenditure (based on weight and sex)	7500 kJ (1800 kcal)
Activity-related expenditure	1700 kJ (400 kcal)
Illness-related expenditure (10 percent of 1800 kcal)	750 kJ (180 kcal)
Diet-induced thermogenesis (10 percent of 2380 kcal)	955 kJ (238 kcal)
Total	10,945 kJ (2618 kcal)

TABLE 70-2 Estimation of resting metabolic rate (RMR)

	Male		Female	
Age (years)	kJ†	kcal†	kJ†	kcal†
3–10	Wt* × 95 + 2110	Wt* × 22.7 + 505	Wt* × 85 + 2033	Wt* × 20.3 + 486
10–18	Wt × 74 + 2754	Wt × 17.7 + 659	Wt × 56 + 2898	Wt × 13.4 + 693
18–30	Wt × 63 + 2896	Wt × 15.1 + 693	Wt × 62 + 2036	Wt × 14.8 + 487
30–60	Wt × 48 + 4653	Wt × 11.5 + 1113	Wt × 34 + 3538	Wt × 8.1 + 846
>60	Wt × 59 + 2459	Wt × 11.7 + 588	Wt × 38 + 2755	Wt × 9.1 + 659

*Body weight in kilograms
†To convert the RMR from kJ to kcal multiply kJ by 0.239.
To convert the RMR from kcal to kJ multiply the kcal by 4.186.
SOURCE: Modified from WN Schofield.

metabolic rate (BMR) plus energy of activity and the thermic effect of food. Basal metabolic rate (BMR) or, more appropriately, resting metabolic rate (RMR) is a measure of the amount of energy expended at rest and without food; energy of activity is a measure of the energy expended to support a variety of physical activities; thermic effect of food (TEF) [also called diet-induced thermogenesis (DIT) and previously called specific dynamic action] is an estimate of the number of calories produced as heat during the digestion, absorption, and metabolism of food. RMR accounts for about two-thirds of the total energy requirements and is affected by body size (height and weight), age, sex, and habitus (Table 70-2). Several clinical methods are available for estimating energy expenditure.

Estimation of resting metabolic rate (RMR) Most methods are based on calorimetry, a measurement of oxygen consumption under carefully controlled conditions, e.g., during fasting, in the morning, and for one hour. A more meaningful metabolic rate would reflect the rate at which energy is consumed in a normal life situation at rest throughout the day, including the period of food assimilation. The usual clinical estimates of RMR discussed below are based on indirect assessments rather than true measurements. Nonetheless, such estimates are frequently very useful.

The method of estimation devised by Harris and Benedict is used most commonly to estimate BMR. The formulas for calculating BMR (in kcal per day) using the four variables of age, height, weight, and sex are as follows:

$$BMR_{women} = 655 + (9.5 \times W) + (1.8 \times H) - (4.7 \times A)$$
$$BMR_{men} = 66 + (13.7 \times W) + (5 \times H) - (6.8 \times A)$$

where W is actual or usual weight (kg), H is height (cm), and A is age (years).

The equations for RMR are simpler than those of Harris and Benedict and are based on more comprehensive data. Because people of the same weight but of different heights have similar RMRs, the formulas are based only on weight, age, and sex (Table 70-2). The values differ from earlier formulas mostly for women, in whom there was an overestimation for weight above 40 kg, reaching an error of nearly 18 percent by a weight of 80 kg. It should be remembered that predicted RMR (or BMR) may over- or underestimate the measured values by 20 or even 30 percent for any individual.

Diet-induced thermogenesis (DIT) The ingestion of nutrients in food causes heat or energy production in excess of basal metabolic rates. A mixed diet causes approximately a 6 to 10 percent increase above basal in calories expended as heat. Thermogenic effect of protein is greatest, that of carbohydrate is next, and fat is least effective. The calorigenic effect of food seems to be closely related to the energy required for ATP formation, in which protein (via amino acid breakdown and urea synthesis) is the oxidative substrate. Most of the effect is generated in the muscle and liver and occurs whether intake is enteral or parenteral. In hypermetabolic patients, diet-induced thermogenesis is less marked because heat production is already elevated. In calculating additional energy requirements for hypermetabolic patients, the DIT should be estimated at no more than 5 percent of total energy requirements.

Estimates of energy for activity The energy expenditure of physical activity accounts for about one-third of total energy expenditures under most conditions and can vary from 6 to 36 kJ (1.5 to 8.5 kcal) per kilogram body weight per hour (Table 70-3). This factor is obviously more important in calculating energy requirements for active, ambulatory patients. Some types of work (e.g., gardening) can fatigue certain muscle groups without using a large number of calories. Usually, any exercise that results in lifting the body from the ground (e.g., running) uses the most calories. Although precise measurements by calorimetry are available for a wide range of activities, it is easiest to use an approximation when estimating energy needs.

Additional energy requirements of illness Heat production increases with fever and inflammation. However, as oxygen consumption increases, DIT decreases, and the energy of activity declines owing to immobility. For these reasons, the daily energy requirement in ill persons is usually only slightly greater than the requirement when well. Indeed, the energy requirement for most patients, even during severe illness, rarely exceeds 12,500 kJ (3000 kcal) per day. (The earlier estimates of massively increased calorie requirements in patients with sepsis have not been substantiated.) Approximately 20 percent should be added to resting energy estimates for a patient confined to bed, and 30 percent should be added for ambulatory patients. Severe illness requires additional caloric supplementation, namely, addition of 10 percent of estimated RMR for mild illness, 25 percent for moderate illness, and 50 percent for severe illness.

Malabsorption is a special cause of increased energy requirement. The most accurate but impractical way to assess calorie loss would be calorimetry of the feces. However, fat excretion in grams per day (as determined in a 72-h fecal fat assay) × 38 kJ (9 kcal) per gram equals the daily energy loss due to fat malabsorption. To estimate total fecal energy loss from all sources, the fecal energy loss from fat (in kJ or kcal) is multiplied by 2.5. This estimate assumes an average dietary composition and equivalent malabsorption of fat, carbohydrate, and protein.

ESTIMATION OF PROTEIN REQUIREMENT Protein balance, like energy balance, is a function of intake relative to utilization and loss. Normally, nitrogen derived from amino acids is excreted in urine and feces and lost from the skin. Unlike the energy stored in triglycerides and glycogen, no proteins (or amino acids) are stored in the body solely for subsequent utilization. Every protein serves either a structural or metabolic function; when excess protein is ingested the amino acids are transaminated, and the nonnitrogenous portion of the molecule serves as a source of calories for storage as glycogen and/or fat.

TABLE 70-3 Estimation of additional energy expenditure by activity

	Calories added to BMR	
Type of work	kJ/d	kcal/d
Sedentary	1670–3350	400–800
Light: office, professional and clerical	3350–5000	800–1200
Moderate: walking, lifting	5000–7500	1200–1800
Heavy: construction, athletic	7500–19,000	1800–4500

SOURCE: Modified from DW Wilmore, *The Metabolic Management of the Critically Ill*. New York, Plenum Press, 1977.

Obligatory nitrogen losses Urea accounts for over 80 percent of urinary nitrogen. The remaining nitrogen is excreted as creatinine, porphyrins, and other nitrogen-containing compounds. Thus, total urine loss of nitrogen = urea nitrogen (mg/dL) × daily volume (dL) ÷ 0.8. Urinary nitrogen is related to the RMR. The larger the body muscle mass, the more transamination of amino acids occurs to fulfill energy needs. Each kilocalorie needed for basal metabolism leads to the excretion of 1 to 1.3 mg of urinary nitrogen. For the same reason, nitrogen excretion increases during exercise and heavy work.

Fecal and skin losses account for a large proportion of nitrogen loss from the body (about 40 percent) in normal circumstances, but the magnitude of these losses varies in disease states. Thus, measurement of urinary nitrogen often provides a useful index of daily nitrogen requirement.

Minimal nitrogen loss (in grams per day) from a 70-kg person on a diet that is nitrogen free but energy adequate approximates 1.9 to 3.1 in urine, 0.7 to 2.5 in stool, and 0.3 from skin for a mean total loss of 4.4 g per day. Equivalent protein loss can be calculated by multiplying nitrogen loss by 6.25 so that total loss by metabolism of protein is 4.4 × 6.25 or 27.5 g/d or about 0.4 g/kg body weight for a 70-kg person. The recommended protein allowance for adults varies from 0.6 to 0.9 g/kg to allow for a margin of safety. Vigorous exercise may increase protein requirements to 1 g/kg body weight or higher.

Protein requirements are highest during the growth spurts of infancy and adolescence. During infancy, total body protein reserve is lowest, and obligatory losses are greatest. Thus, protein deficiency is most common in infancy. Protein requirements decline slightly during childhood and again increase during adolescence. Minimal requirements for these stages of life are about 1.5 g/kg body weight per day. The recommended allowance (2 g/kg body weight per day) exceeds this figure to allow a margin of safety for children who have increased needs or who ingest proteins of low biologic value. Low quality proteins include certain vegetable proteins that do not support growth as well as protein from milk, eggs, or meat. The differences in the nutritional value of protein are largely due to the higher content of essential amino acids in animal proteins and to differences in digestibility. Protein (and energy) requirements also increase during pregnancy and lactation.

CALORIC REQUIREMENTS FOR PROTEIN UTILIZATION Amino acids ingested without other energy sources are not efficiently incorporated into protein partly because of the energy lost during amino acid metabolism. Moreover, incorporation of each amino acid molecule into peptides requires three high-energy phosphate bonds. Consequently, excess of dietary energy over basal needs improves the efficiency of nitrogen utilization. During the period of intense growth in children, about 300 kJ (76 kcal) of nonprotein energy are required for each gram of protein. In ambulatory adults about 200 kJ (50 kcal) from nonprotein sources are needed per gram of protein. This high ratio usually cannot be achieved with parenteral feeding, since energy intake is limited by the volume needed to be infused. Acceptable figures for parenteral nutrition are about 100 to 125 kJ (25 to 30 kcal) from nonprotein sources per gram of protein or 600 to 750 kJ (150 to 180 kcal) per gram of nitrogen.

RECOMMENDED DIETARY ALLOWANCES OF PROTEIN AND MICRONUTRIENTS Guidelines of nutritional requirements in health have been formulated in the reports, updated periodically, of the Food and Nutrition Board of the National Research Council of the United States. These Recommended Dietary Allowances, expressed for age and sex and modified for such conditions as pregnancy and lactation, are designed to cover the requirements of virtually all healthy individuals. With the exception of energy, the allowances are not average requirements but rather a recommended intake sufficient to meet the needs of all healthy individuals.

The recommended dietary allowances for protein (nitrogen), iron, and calcium are based upon experiments in which normal requirement is defined as the intake necessary to achieve zero balance between intake versus output. For most vitamins the recommended allowance is the daily intake required to maintain full function and safe levels of body stores. Most estimates assume normal digestion and absorption and normal metabolism. In some cases, estimates of daily turnover by radioisotope or stable isotope tracer techniques are used to determine the amount of nutrient required to maintain body stores. It follows, therefore, that diseases that influence efficiency of absorption or that change the metabolism or nutritional requirements will change the safe allowance for that individual. It further follows that the recommended dietary allowances are at best a rough guide for requirements for enteral nutrient intake by any individual. Such allowances may be an overestimation of parenteral requirements, particularly in the case of micronutrients, since in that case no allowance need be made for the inefficiency of extraction from food and absorption. A listing of these essential nutrients and an estimation of the ranges of required intake for healthy adults are presented in Table 70-4.

TABLE 70-4 Recommended dietary allowances for healthy adults

	Range of allowance	
	Men	Women
Protein, g	45–63	44–50
Vitamin A, μg retinol equivalents	1000	800
Vitamin D, μg	5–10	5–10
Vitamin E, mg α-tocopherol equivalents	10	8
Vitamin K, μg	45–80	45–65
Vitamin C, mg	50–60	50–60
Thiamine, mg	1.2–1.5	1–1.1
Riboflavin, mg	1.4–1.8	1.2–1.3
Niacin, mg niacin equivalents	15–20	13–15
Vitamin B_6, mg	1.4–2.0	1.4–1.6
Folate, μg	150–200	150–180
Vitamin B_{12}, μg	2.0	2.0
Biotin, μg*	30–100	50–100
Pantothenic Acid, mg*	4–10	4–7
Calcium, mg	800–1200	800–1200
Phosphorus, mg	800–1200	800–1200
Magnesium, mg	270–400	280–300
Iron, mg	10–12	10–15
Zinc, mg	15	12
Iodine, μg	150	150
Selenium, μg	40–70	45–55
Copper, mg*	1.5–3	1.5–3
Manganese, mg*	2–5	2–5
Fluoride, mg*	1.5–4	1.5–4
Chromium, μg*	50–200	50–200
Molybdenum, μg*	75–250	75–250

*Estimated safe and adequate daily dietary intakes. From the National Research Council: *Recommended Dietary Allowances*, 10th ed. Washington, D.C., National Academy of Sciences, 1989.

The recommended dietary allowances make little provision for changes in nutrient requirements for the elderly. Energy requirements decline progressively beyond age 50 or 60 as the lean (muscle) mass declines and resting metabolic energy expenditure decreases. Energy needs for activity also decline as aging often leads to more sedentary lifestyle. There are few studies in the elderly that define specific differences in nutrient requirements. At present, it is prudent to recommend full adult levels of protein, vitamins, and minerals even in the face of declining energy intake. For small elderly people, especially small women, this may require heightened dietary planning and vigilance. Increased physical activity at all ages promotes the retention of lean muscle mass and also increases appetite and food intake.

REFERENCES

ALPERS DH et al: *Manual of Nutritional Therapeutics*. Boston, Little, Brown, 1987, chap 3

HAVEL RJ: Caloric homeostasis and disorders of fuel transport. N Engl J Med 1987:1186, 1972

KISSILEFF HR, VAN ITALLIE TB: Physiology of the control of food intake. Ann Rev Nutr 2:271, 1982

SCHOFIELD WN: Predicting basal metabolic rate, new standards and review of previous work. Human Nutr Clin Nutr 39C(Suppl 1), 1985

THE NATIONAL RESEARCH COUNCIL: *Recommended Dietary Allowances*, 10th ed. Washington, DC, National Academy of Sciences, 1989

71 PROTEIN-ENERGY MALNUTRITION

JOEL B. MASON / IRWIN H. ROSENBERG

Protein-energy malnutrition (PEM), or protein-calorie malnutrition (PCM), is present when there is insufficient energy or protein available to meet metabolic demands. Inadequate dietary intake is only one of several mechanisms by which this may occur: Increased metabolic demands due to disease and increased nutrient losses can also result in PEM. Protein deficiency may also arise in the face of adequate protein intake if the dietary protein is of poor quality (i.e., the content of one or more essential amino acids is inadequate and thus becomes the limiting factor in protein utilization); such is the case when the entire protein intake is derived from a single vegetable source. Protein nutrition is also influenced by the intake of energy relative to the intake of protein because the efficient utilization of dietary protein requires energy from nonprotein calories.

Adaptive responses function over the short term when protein and energy sources are limited. As a consequence, the pathologic consequences of undernutrition require a sustained inadequacy of protein or energy sources. The adaptive mechanisms that respond to protein and calorie deprivation are finite, particularly because protein has no storage form in the body.

The rapidity with which an individual develops PEM and the severity of the resulting syndrome depend on a number of factors, including the nutritional state when the nutritional deprivation begins, the underlying illness, and the developmental stage. Some of these factors are outlined in Table 71-1.

PROTEIN-ENERGY MALNUTRITION AS A GLOBAL PROBLEM Recognition of PEM emerged from studies in the tropics that were focused primarily on the problem in children. Preschool children, particularly infants, are more susceptible to PEM. They are dependent on others for determining the quantity and quality of food intake; protein and energy requirements of children are substantially higher per unit weight; and unhygienic habits and immaturity of the immune system heighten susceptibility to infections. Gastrointestinal infections, in particular, constitute a major precipitant of PEM in infants and children because such illnesses result in altered feeding habits, vomiting, decreased intestinal absorption, increased metabolic needs, and increased metabolic losses. The magnitude of the problem is immense; the World Health Organization estimated in 1983 that 300 million children have growth retardation secondary to malnutrition. Increased mortality and impaired cognitive, social, and economic development are additional features of this condition.

PEM is confined neither to infants and children nor to the less-developed countries. Although the overall prevalence of PEM is low, specific sectors of the U.S. population, such as the institutionalized elderly and children of the poor, have a significant prevalence. For example, the Ten State Survey, which focused on low income areas in the United States, found that 22 to 35 percent of the children aged 2, 4, and 6 were below the 15th percentile for weight. In this survey income level and minority status were predictors of growth retardation among children. Moreover, in large urban teaching hospitals and smaller community hospitals 30 to 70 percent of general medical and surgical patients have anthropometric and/or biochemical evidence of PEM. Similar statistics have been noted in surveys of pediatric inpatients. It is perhaps more disturbing that the nutritional status of the majority of hospitalized patients *declines* during the course of hospitalization. Positive associations between the degree of PEM and the incidence of postoperative infections, impaired healing of surgical wounds, and prolongation of hospitalization indicate that more attention needs to be paid to the maintenance of adequate nutrition in individual patients. There are tangible benefits from such nutritional diligence because aggressive preoperative nutritional restitution of malnourished patients can decrease perioperative morbidity such as infection.

Most modern-day hospital malnutrition is compounded by insufficient attention by medical personnel to nutrition (Table 71-2). Indeed, most factors contributing to the high prevalence of malnutrition in hospitalized patients are reversible or preventable.

PROTEIN-ENERGY METABOLISM DURING STRESS **Physiological adaptation to starvation** During periods of protein and/or energy deficit, compensatory mechanisms serve to lessen the pathologic impact of these deficiencies. To understand how malnutrition develops, it is therefore important to understand the responses to such inadequate intake. During the first 24 h of fasting, circulating glucose, fatty acids, and triglycerides and liver and muscle glycogen are used as fuel sources. However, the sum of these stores in a 70-kg man is only about 5000 kJ (1200 kcal) and provides less fuel than is needed for basal metabolism for a single day. Triglycerides, derived primarily from adipose tissue, can be catabolized to fatty acids and ketone bodies by most tissues. However, over the short run tissues such as the brain can only use glycolytic pathways to obtain energy. Since the conversion of fatty acids to carbohydrate is inefficient in animals, these glycolytic tissues must utilize either glucose or substrates that can be converted to glucose. Amino acids derived primarily from skeletal muscle constitute the major endogenous substrate for glucose production for this purpose. Since there is no storage form of protein in the body, a fasting individual sustains a daily loss of functionally significant protein.

The provision of adequate fuel substrate to critical tissues, particularly the brain, has homeostatic priority during protein/energy deprivation. Brief starvation leads to acute adaptive responses that sustain the supply of glucose to tissues that require it and minimize the amount of protein breakdown to meet this need. To accomplish this end, certain tissues, such as the heart, kidney, and skeletal muscle, change their primary fuel substrate from glucose to fatty acids and ketone bodies. Other tissues, such as the bone marrow, renal medulla, and peripheral nerves, switch from the full oxidation of glucose to anaerobic glycolysis, resulting in the production of

TABLE 71-1 Factors that influence the response to inadequate nutrient intake

I Nutritional factors
- *A* Underlying adequacy of reserves/depot of that nutrient
- *B* Severity and duration of the inadequate intake
- *C* Concurrent deficiencies of other nutrients

II Underlying illnesses
- *A* Fever, infection, trauma, and other conditions associated with increased requirements and catabolic losses
- *B* Malabsorptive and maldigestive states
- *C* Disorders associated with excessive loss of nutrients (e.g., protein-losing enteropathy, nephrotic syndrome, enteric fistulas)
- *D* Conditions associated with altered metabolism of nutrients (e.g., diabetes mellitus, hyperthyroidism)

III Physiologic states in which increased requirements are present
- *A* Pregnancy, lactation
- *B* Growth and development during infancy, childhood, and adolescence

TABLE 71-2 Undesirable practices affecting the nutritional assessment and/or status of hospitalized patients

Failure to record height and weight in the hospital chart
Diffusion of responsibility for patient care
Prolonged use of glucose and saline intravenous feedings
Failure to observe and record dietary intake
Withholding meals because of diagnostic tests
Use of enteral or parenteral feedings of uncertain composition and in inadequate amounts
Ignorance of the composition of nutritional products
Failure to recognize increased nutritional needs due to injury or illness
Lack of communication between physician, nurse, and dietician
Delay of nutritional support until severe depletion has developed
Limited availability of laboratory tests to assess nutritional status; failure to use those that are available
Limited emphasis on nutrition education in medical education

SOURCE: After CE Butterworth, in Nutr Today 9:4, 1974

lactate and pyruvate. These compounds can be converted to glucose in the liver with energy derived from fat oxidation and then released for systemic consumption. This shuttle, the Cori cycle, enables energy stored as fat to be utilized for glucose synthesis and thus conserves protein energy that would otherwise be necessary for the de novo synthesis of glucose.

With more extended starvation other adaptations appear. A decrease in physical exertion decreases energy consumption, and the resting metabolic rate generally declines by about 10 percent. The brain, which ordinarily obtains energy only by glucose oxidation, acquires the ability to use keto acids for its fuel requirements, and this contributes further to protein conservation. Animal studies and, less definitively, human studies suggest that protein that is consumed during relative protein starvation is utilized more efficiently. Moreover, chronic protein deprivation leads to a reduced rate of protein turnover, and amino acids are reutilized more efficiently for the synthesis of new proteins, contributing to savings in both energy and amino acid requirements.

During relative or total caloric starvation, such adaptations allow the body to provide the energy necessary for metabolism and to minimize the obligatory loss of protein, which appears primarily as nitrogen-containing compounds in the urine. After several weeks of starvation, nitrogen loss in the urine may decrease by more than 65 percent. However, these homeostatic mechanisms do not compensate entirely for the imposed deficits, and eventually the negative caloric and/or protein balance lead to pathologic consequences.

Effects of physical stress Infection, trauma, and other physical stress cause inflammatory responses. In such situations, protein and energy metabolism change in ways that increase both energy demands and nitrogen losses and thereby predispose to the development of PEM.

Resting metabolic rate (RMR) increases dramatically during critical illness. Patients with burns over more than 40 percent of the body have a RMR approximately twice normal, and patients with sepsis have a RMR that is about one and a half times normal. Factors that contribute to the increased energy consumption include increases in circulating catecholamines and increase in energy expenditure required for gluconeogenesis.

Nitrogen loss during critical illness is also increased. A healthy adult loses approximately 12 g of nitrogen in urine per day in the fasting state; sepsis and trauma commonly increase that value by 50 to 100 percent. Since 1 g of urinary nitrogen represents approximately 30 g of lean body mass, critical illness induces a daily loss of 0.6 kg of lean body mass. Most of this loss comes from the skeletal muscle, and the efflux of amino acids from skeletal muscle increases two- to sixfold in critically ill patients. Increased efflux from skeletal muscle is probably due to increased protein catabolism rather than decreased protein synthesis.

The amino acids mobilized from skeletal muscle are in part used as fuel and in part taken up by the liver and other visceral organs. The proteolysis of muscle under physical stress thus enables the body to shift protein substrate from the somatic compartment to visceral organs whose function is more critical for immediate survival. Hormonal factors play a significant role in this shift; circulating levels of cortisol, glucagon, epinephrine, and growth hormone are increased in physically stressed individuals. Increased circulating levels of interleukin 1 and tumor necrosis factor in septic and traumatized patients may participate in the sparing of the visceral protein compartment at the expense of the skeletal muscle. Eventually, continued deficits in protein and energy, particularly when superimposed on sustained physical stress, lead to a constriction of the visceral protein compartment and its associated functions.

DIAGNOSIS, ASSESSMENT, AND CLASSIFICATION OF PROTEIN-ENERGY MALNUTRITION Protein-energy malnutrition may be primary, due to an inadequate intake of protein and/or energy source, or secondary, due to illness that impairs intake or utilization of nutrients or that increases nutrient requirements or metabolic losses. Malignancy, intestinal malabsorption, inflammatory bowel disease, acquired immunodeficiency syndrome, and chronic renal failure are a few of the illnesses commonly associated with secondary PEM.

There are no universally accepted criteria for defining the severity of PEM although it is often categorized as mild, moderate, or severe. An effective nutritional assessment requires the synthesis of information provided by a dietary history, physical examination, and anthropometric and biochemical assessment. No single piece of evidence is sufficient to indicate the nutritional status. A corollary is that each parameter used to assess nutritional status can be, and often is, influenced by factors that have little to do with the nutritional state.

In adults, the most commonly used indicator of caloric status is body weight. Standard tables of desirable or ideal body weight are available, but individual variation is such that comparison with the premorbid weight may be most useful in the identification of PEM. An obese individual with ongoing deficits in protein or energy balance, although considerably above ideal body weight, can develop PEM with its pathologic consequences. A decrease of more than 10 percent of the usual body weight, particularly when the rate of loss is greater than 3 to 6 percent per month, is a good predictor of PEM.

Fat stores are the major energy reserve in the body and, as such, can also be used to assess energy status. Reduction in subcutaneous fat together with weight loss constitute the most obvious and constant physical features of PEM in adults. Children with PEM have retarded physical development such as stunted (low height for age) or wasted (low weight for height) body habitus and delayed puberty. Cognitive and psychosocial development is commonly retarded.

Reduction in subcutaneous fat is usually evident by inspection of the extremities or face, although a significant reduction in fat mass can be overlooked unless quantitative criteria are assessed, such as skin-fold measurements or assessment of body composition. The triceps fat fold, when compared to standard values, provides an indication of the adequacy of body fat since more than half of total body fat is subcutaneous (Table 71-3).

Protein nutrition can be assessed in several ways. Separate assessments of the somatic and visceral protein compartments are useful since the two protein depots are handled differently. Decreased muscle mass can frequently be recognized on physical examination, although mild malnutrition is usually underestimated. The somatic compartment (primarily skeletal muscle) can be assessed by comparing the midarm muscle area to normative values (Table 71-4). The creatinine-height index performs a similar function (Table 71-5). The visceral compartment can be assessed by estimation of the total lymphocyte count in peripheral blood and by measuring the delayed cutaneous hypersensitivity response. Levels of serum proteins such as albumin are also useful. However, the validity of serum albumin as a reflection of the status of the visceral protein compartment is poor in the setting of acute or critical illness; the long half-life of albumin (20 days), the fact that it is distributed extensively in the extravascular as well as intravascular compartment, and the fact that its synthesis is influenced by the presence of circulating inflammatory mediators and by liver function all limit its value as a measure of nutrition. Serum proteins with shorter half-lives, such as transferrin, thyroxine-binding prealbumin, and retinol-binding protein, are better than albumin in this regard (Table 71-6).

The reduction in lean body mass in mild to moderate PEM is usually not as great as the reduction in fat mass. Nevertheless, the midarm muscle area or the creatinine-height index may be below the standard values. The decrease in urinary urea nitrogen, in contrast, reflects physiologic adjustments to inadequate intake of protein and/or energy rather than loss in skeletal mass. Functionally, work capacity decreases, particularly in very active individuals. Pregnant women with mild to moderate PEM are at risk of delivering infants with low weight or length for gestational age. The volume and fat and energy content of breast milk in such women are decreased.

More severe forms of PEM cause more marked alterations in body habitus and laboratory parameters. Deficiency states of specific micronutrients (see Chap. 76) may be present although PEM itself

TABLE 71-3 Normative values for triceps skin-fold thickness

Age group, years	Sample size	Estimated population, millions	Mean, mm	Percentile 5	10	25	50	75	90	95
MEN										
18–74	5261	61.18	12.0	4.5	6.0	8.0	11.0	15.0	20.0	23.0
18–24	773	11.78	11.2	4.0	5.0	7.0	9.5	14.0	20.0	23.0
25–34	804	13.00	12.6	4.5	5.5	8.0	12.0	16.0	21.5	24.0
35–44	664	10.68	12.4	5.0	6.0	8.5	12.0	15.5	20.0	23.0
45–54	765	11.15	12.4	5.0	6.0	8.0	11.0	15.0	20.0	25.0
55–64	598	9.07	11.6	5.0	6.0	8.0	11.0	14.0	18.0	21.5
65–74	1657	5.50	11.8	4.5	5.5	8.0	11.0	15.0	19.0	22.0
WOMEN										
18–74	8410	67.84	23.0	11.0	13.0	17.0	22.0	28.0	34.0	37.5
18–24	1523	12.89	19.4	9.4	11.0	14.0	18.0	24.0	30.0	34.0
25–34	1896	13.93	21.9	10.5	12.0	16.0	21.0	26.5	33.5	37.0
35–44	1664	11.59	24.0	12.0	14.0	18.0	23.0	29.5	35.5	39.0
45–54	836	12.16	25.4	13.0	15.0	20.0	25.0	30.0	36.0	40.0
55–65	669	9.98	24.9	11.0	14.0	19.0	25.0	30.5	35.0	39.0
65–74	1822	7.28	23.3	11.5	14.0	18.0	23.0	28.0	33.0	36.0

SOURCE: Heymsfield and Williams.

usually has the most impact on health. There is further loss of subcutaneous fat and worsening of muscle wasting in the extremities; this disorder in children is termed *marasmus*. The decrease in muscle mass can sometimes be recognized in the interosseous muscles in the hand and the temporalis muscles of the head, and confirmation is obtained by determining the midarm muscle area. The loss of subcutaneous fat and muscle mass, in conjunction with a loss of the normal elasticity of the skin, commonly results in loose fitting, wrinkled skin with reduplicated folds. Skin lesions in advanced PEM may be shiny, erythematous, atrophic areas or hyperkeratotic, hyperpigmented regions (''flaky paint'' dermatitis). Decubitus ulcers are also common in severe disease. The hair may become sparse and dry; it loses its usual sheen and can be pulled out with little effort. The color of the hair may change to reddish or dull brown, and alternating periods of nutritional depletion and repletion may give rise to bands of such color changes in the hair.

Lethargy is a common feature. Alterations in gastrointestinal function include constipation and difficulty ingesting normal-sized meals due to early satiety and vomiting. The heart rate, blood pressure, and core body temperature are frequently subnormal. Infections may not be accompanied by fever and appropriate tachycardia.

Severe PEM due to an inadequate intake of both protein and energy (*combined PEM*) is characterized by a diminution in somatic protein out of proportion to the reduction in the visceral protein compartment. Individuals with combined PEM have muscle wasting in the extremities and trunk but maintain a relatively normal visceral compartment. Weakness can be profound. Loss of subcutaneous fat combined with the loss in muscle mass results in a ''skin and bones'' appearance. The fact that edema is absent constitutes the major clinical feature separating combined PEM from pure protein malnutrition.

When inadequate availability of protein outweighs the extent of energy deprivation, the subcutaneous fat and somatic protein compartment tend to be spared in comparison to the reduction in the visceral protein compartment. Interpretation of the anthropometric measurements of the somatic protein and fat compartments may be complicated by the presence of edema, but serum protein levels are consistently low in so-called hypoproteinemic PEM. (In children this disorder is termed *kwashiorkor*.) Pure protein malnutrition is unusual

TABLE 71-4 Normative values for midarm muscle area*

Age group	Arm muscle area percentiles, mm^2: 5	10	25	50	75	90	95
MEN							
16–16.9	3625	4044	4352	4951	5753	6576	6980
17–17.9	3998	4252	4777	5286	5950	6886	7726
18–18.9	4070	4481	5066	5552	6374	7067	8355
19–24.9	4508	4777	5274	5913	6660	7606	8200
25–34.9	4694	4963	5541	6214	7067	7847	8436
35–44.9	4844	5181	5740	6490	7265	8034	8488
45–54.9	4546	4946	5589	6297	7142	7918	8458
55–64.9	4422	4783	5381	6144	6919	7670	8149
65–74.9	3973	4411	5031	5716	6432	7074	7453
WOMEN							
16–16.9	2308	2567	2865	3248	3718	4353	4946
17–17.9	2442	2674	2996	3336	3883	4552	5251
18–18.9	2398	2538	2917	3243	3694	4461	4767
19–24.9	2538	2728	3026	3406	3877	4439	4940
25–34.9	2661	2826	3148	3573	4138	4806	5541
35–44.9	2750	2948	3359	3783	4428	5240	5877
45–54.9	2784	2956	3378	3858	4520	5375	5964
55–64.9	2784	3063	3477	4045	4750	5632	6247
65–74.9	2737	3018	3444	4019	4739	5566	6214

* Estimates based on data from the U.S. Health and Nutrition Examination Survey, 1971–1974 (HANES I).
SOURCE: AJ Frisancho, Am J Clin Nutr 34:2540, 1981.

TABLE 71-5 Normative values for creatinine excretion based on height

Men*: Height, cm	Ideal creatinine, mg	Women†: Height, cm	Ideal creatinine, mg
157.5	1288	147.3	830
160.0	1325	149.9	851
162.6	1359	152.4	875
165.1	1386	154.9	900
167.6	1426	157.5	925
170.2	1467	160.0	949
172.7	1513	162.6	977
175.3	1555	165.1	1006
177.8	1596	167.6	1044
180.3	1642	170.2	1076
182.9	1691	172.7	1109
185.4	1739	175.3	1141
188.0	1785	177.8	1174
190.5	1831	180.3	1206
193.0	1891	182.9	1240

* Creatinine coefficient (men) = 23 mg/kg of ideal body weight.
† Creatinine coefficient (women) = 18 mg/kg of ideal body weight.
SOURCE: GL Blackburn et al., J Parent Ent Nutr 1:11, 1977.

TABLE 71-6 Serum proteins used in nutritional assessment

Serum protein	Approximate molecular mass, Da	Biosynthetic site	Normal value $\bar{X}$ ± SD or (range)*	Half-life, days	Function	Comment†
Albumin	66,000	Hepatocyte	45 (35–50)	14–20	Maintain plasma oncotic pressure; carrier for small molecules	Serum levels are determined by many different processes
Transferrin	77,000	Hepatocyte	2.3 (2.0–3.2)	8–9	Binds Fe^{2+} in plasma and transports to bone	Iron nutriture influences plasma level; increased during pregnancy, estrogen therapy, and acute hepatitis; reduced in protein-losing enteropathy and nephropathy, chronic infections, uremia, and acute catabolic states; often measured indirectly as total iron-binding capacity
Prealbumin	61,000	Hepatocyte	0.30 (0.2–0.5)	2–3	Binds T_3 and to a lesser extent T_4. Carrier for retinol-binding protein	Increased in patients with chronic renal failure on dialysis; reduced in acute catabolic states, after surgery, in hyperthyroidism; serum level determined by overall energy and nitrogen balance
Retinol-binding protein (RBP)	21,000	Hepatocyte	0.0372 ± 0.0073‡	0.5	Transports vitamin A in plasma; binds noncovalently to prealbumin	Catabolized in renal proximal tubular cell; with renal disease RBP increases and $t_{1/2}$ is prolonged; low in vitamin A deficiency, acute catabolic states, after surgery, and in hyperthyroidism

* Units are g/L. Normal range varies between centers; check local values.
† All of the listed proteins are influenced by hydration and the presence of hepatocellular dysfunction.
‡ Normal values are age- and sex-dependent. Table value is for pooled subjects.
SOURCE: Heymsfield and Williams.

in malnourished hospitalized patients, but a mixed form with features of both hypoproteinemic and combined PEM is more common. Such individuals have subnormal fat and somatic protein compartments, as indicated by anthropometric measurements, as well as depressed levels of the serum proteins and accompanying edema. The edema in hypoproteinemic PEM is usually dependent but may be generalized in severe cases. Pure hypoproteinemic PEM is often not recognized because fat and muscle wasting is less marked than that with combined PEM. This does not imply that this type of PEM is associated with less morbidity. Indeed, hospitalized patients with hypoproteinemic PEM may have a worse prognosis and a greater propensity for development of infections than those with combined PEM.

The liver in hypoproteinemic PEM may be enlarged and tender to palpation. Histologic examination reveals fatty infiltration; fat droplets initially appear in the periportal hepatocytes and, with increasing severity, spread to the pericentral regions of the hepatic lobule. The fatty liver is thought to be due to the inadequate movement of lipids out of the hepatic parenchyma caused by the decreased availability of lipoproteins for lipid transport (see Chap. 326). Serum concentrations of very low density lipoproteins (VLDL) and low density lipoproteins (LDL) are subnormal in hypoproteinemic PEM, and the severity of fatty infiltration of the liver correlates with the degree of depression of these lipoproteins.

Several factors influence whether a malnourished child develops a combined, hypoproteinemic, or mixed form of PEM. For example, infection in an undernourished child is more likely to precipitate hypoproteinemic than combined PEM. Individual host responses to the same type of nutritional deprivation may also play a role. Children with combined PEM have a more responsive adrenocortical axis than those with hypoproteinemic PEM, and this difference may maintain the visceral protein compartment at the expense of skeletal muscle.

PHYSIOLOGIC IMPAIRMENTS ASSOCIATED WITH PROTEIN-ENERGY MALNUTRITION **Gastrointestinal tract** The alterations in gastrointestinal structure and function arise partially from undernutrition itself and partially from decreased stimulation of the gut by ingested nutrients. Sustained absence of nutrients in the intestine of a nutritionally-replete, parenterally fed individual causes structural and functional atrophy of the intestine as described below. The changes have been best characterized in malnourished children in the less-developed countries, and similar alterations are presumed to occur in adult PEM. Blunting or absence of the intestinal villi is associated with decreased levels of disaccharidases and aminopeptidases in the mucosa. Gastric and pancreatic secretions are reduced in volume and contain decreased amounts of acid and digestive enzymes. The volume of bile and the concentration of conjugated bile acids in bile are reduced. Substantial populations of facultative and strict anaerobic bacteria in the upper small bowel convert conjugated bile acids to free bile acids. The impairments in pancreatic and biliary function, in conjunction with the structural alterations in the small intestine, result in malabsorption of carbohydrates, vitamins, and fat; the degree of steatorrhea is proportional to the severity of PEM. These alterations in absorption further exacerbate the inability to assimilate nutrients.

Immunologic function PEM impairs both cell-mediated and humoral immune systems. In vitro responses that assess the functional integrity of T lymphocytes, polymorphonuclear leukocytes, and the complement system are uniformly blunted. There is some disagreement as to whether B-lymphocyte function is impaired. A cycle is established in which malnutrition impairs host defenses and thereby enhances the susceptibility to infection, which, in turn, worsens the malnourished state. Additional PEM-associated phenomena, such as impaired epithelial integrity and decreased gastric acid and lysozyme secretion, may accelerate the propensity to infection and promote malnutrition by several mechanisms. These mechanisms include anorexia, which decreases the intake of nutrients; a shift in the balance of protein metabolism, which assumes a catabolic character and thereby promotes the loss of lean body mass; and enhancement of the metabolic rate, which increases about 13 percent for every 1°C elevation of body temperature. The macrophage-derived peptide interleukin 1 (IL-1) may play a role in these secondary effects. Proteolysis-inducing factor (PIF), a cleavage product of IL-1, is present in the blood of infected individuals and causes a marked increase in muscle proteolysis as indicated by increases in the rate of amino acid release from muscle. Cachectin (or tumor necrosis factor) also participates in mediating the effects of infection on host metabolism; it inhibits lipid metabolism and therefore inhibits the utilization of fat stores as an energy source.

Total lymphocyte count and measurements of delayed skin hypersensitivity, as well as some of the nutritional indexes that incorporate these items (see below), serve as reasonable predictors for susceptibility to postoperative infections and, in some cases, to postoperative mortality. Nevertheless, factors other than nutritional status also influence the assessment of lymphocytes (see Chap. 13).

Endocrine function Most hormonal alterations in PEM appear to be the consequence of physiologic adaptations to the undernourished state. Inadequate food intake leads to a decrease in the availability of circulating glucose and amino acids, resulting in low circulating levels of insulin and increased levels of growth hormone and glucagon (see Chap. 320). These alterations, in conjunction with decreased levels of somatomedins and increased levels of glucocorticoids, promote muscle protein catabolism and enhance the incorporation of the liberated amino acids into visceral organs. Urea synthesis is inhibited, decreasing nitrogen loss and enhancing the reutilization of amino acids. Enhancement of lipolysis and gluconeogenesis provides more energy substrate.

The serum levels of triiodothyronine (T_3) and thyroxine (T_4) are commonly decreased in association with increased concentrations of 3,5,5′-triiodothyronine (reverse T_3), resembling the pattern observed in the "euthyroid sick syndrome" (see Chap. 316). The decrease in T_3 levels may play a role in the decrease in metabolic rate and decrease in protein catabolism in PEM. Primary gonadal dysfunction is accompanied by decreased concentrations of circulating testosterone and estrogen and impairment in reproductive potential. Amenorrhea is common. Impaired secretion of luteinizing hormone–releasing hormone (LHRH) may play a role in the hypogonadism. Fertility in women is further reduced by an increased rate of resorption of implanted embryos. In prepubertal children with PEM the basal level of follicle-stimulating hormone and the response of the gonadotropin to LHRH are variously reported to be low or normal. Delay of puberty appears to be related to failure to achieve a critical lean body mass rather than to a decrease in absolute weight.

Cardiovascular system Moderate to severe PEM produces both quantitative and qualitative alterations in the myocardium. Myocardial mass is decreased, although proportionately less than the loss in body weight. Microscopic analysis reveals myofibrillar atrophy, edema, and, less commonly, patchy necrosis and infiltration with chronic inflammatory cells. Involvement of the myocardial conduction system may explain the conduction abnormalities associated with anorexia nervosa and total starvation. The structural changes in the myocardium are also associated with alterations in myocardial performance, most evident under conditions of increased demand as a decrease in cardiac output, stroke volume, and maximal work capacity. The alterations in cardiac structure and function are not irreversible: both left ventricular mass and maximal cardiac output increase after nutritional repletion.

Respiratory system The mass of the diaphragm decreases in proportion to the loss in body weight. This atrophy results in decreases in the maximal inspiratory pressure. Energy deprivation, regardless of nitrogen balance, also blunts the ventilatory drive in response to hypoxia, although the clinical significance of this phenomenon is unclear. In tracheostomy patients, bacterial adherence to tracheal epithelial cells is enhanced. Nutritional repletion leads to reversal of impaired pulmonary function. Repletion associated with weight gain or an improved serum albumin level results in improved respiratory muscle function and a greater likelihood of weaning patients from ventilators.

Wound healing Even mild malnutrition impairs the capacity to deposit collagen in wounds during the early stages of healing, and the provision of adequate nutrition after surgery enhances the deposition of collagen at the wound. Likewise, intestinal anastomoses in well-nourished animals have a higher tensile strength than those in malnourished animals. Nevertheless, those malnourished animals surviving for 8 weeks ultimately develop wounds with equivalent integrity to those of their well-nourished counterparts.

INFLUENCE OF MALNUTRITION ON HOSPITAL COURSE The correlation between those parameters used to assess nutritional status and the outcome of hospitalization is clear-cut. For example, in hospitalized patients a depressed serum albumin or transferrin level, a recent unintentional weight loss of >10 percent of body weight, a decreased total lymphocyte count (<1200/μL) and an anergic skin response to foreign antigens are all predictive of an increased in-hospital incidence of morbid events such as infection. Moreover, some of these parameters are predictors of the duration of postoperative hospitalization as well as of mortality.

Several nutritional indexes, each of which incorporates various combinations of these measurements, have been developed to assess the nutritional status of hospitalized patients, as outlined in Table 71-7. However, every index for the clinical assessment of nutritional status and all indexes that integrate several of them into a single "nutritional score" are also influenced by nonnutritional factors. Consequently, such an index is more properly considered to be an assessment of the severity of illness and of the likelihood of malnutrition rather than to be an indicator of nutritional status alone. It therefore remains unclear whether the ability of these indexes to

TABLE 71-7 Prognostic indices in hospitalized patients

	Incorporated parameters	Correlates with	Reference
Likelihood of malnutrition	Serum folate Serum vitamin C Serum albumin Lymphocyte count Hematocrit Triceps skin fold Arm muscle circumference Weight	Duration of hospitalization	Am J Clin Nutr 32:418, 1979
Prognostic nutritional index	Serum albumin Serum transferrin Delayed hypersensitivity Triceps skin fold	Incidence of postoperative complications and mortality	Cancer 47:2375, 1981
Instant nutritional index	Serum albumin Lymphocyte count	Incidence of postoperative infection	J Parent Ent Nutr 12:195, 1988
Hospital prognostic index	Serum albumin Delayed hypersensitivity Presence of sepsis or cancer	Hospital mortality	Am J Clin Nutr 34:2013, 1981

predict morbidity and mortality is determined solely by nutritional state.

REFERENCES

Arona NS, Rochester DF: Effect of body weight and muscularity on human diaphragm muscle mass, thickness and area. J Appl Physiol 52:64, 1982

Baracos V et al: Stimulation of degradation of muscle proteins during fever. A mechanism for the increased degradation of muscle proteins during fever. N Engl J Med 308:553, 1983

Becker DJ: The endocrine responses to protein calorie malnutrition. Ann Rev Nutr 3:187, 1983

Beutler B, Cerami A: Cachectin: More than a tumor necrosis factor. N Engl J Med 316:379, 1987

Bistrian BR et al: Protein status of general surgical patients. JAMA 230:858, 1974

Bistrian BR et al: Prevalence of malnutrition in general medical patients. JAMA 235:1567, 1976

Cahill GF: Starvation in man. N Engl J Med 282:668, 1970

Dinarello CA: Interleukin 1. Rev Infect Dis 6:51, 1984

Heymsfield SB, Williams PJ: Nutritional assessment by clinical and biochemical methods, in *Modern Nutrition in Health and Disease,* 7th ed, ME Shils, VR Young (eds). Philadelphia, Lea & Febiger, 1988

Heymsfield SB et al: Cardiac abnormalities in cachectic patients before and during nutritional repletion. Am Heart J 95:584, 1978

Keusch GT, Farthing MJG: Nutrition and infection. Ann Rev Nutr 6:131, 1986

Rosenblatt S et al: Exchange of amino acids by muscle and liver in sepsis. Arch Surg 118:167, 1983

Ten-State Nutrition Survey, 1968–70. US Department of Health, Education, and Welfare Publication (HSM) 72, 1972

Weinsier RL et al: A prospective evaluation of general medical patients during the course of hospitalization. Am J Clin Nutr 32:418, 1979

World Health Organization: *Infant and Young Child Nutrition.* Report by the Director General to the World Health Assembly. Document WHA 36/1983/70, March, 1983

72 OBESITY

JERROLD M. OLEFSKY

The ability to store food energy as fat provides survival value when the food supply is scarce or sporadic. Unlike glycogen or protein, triglyceride does not require water or electrolytes for storage purposes and can be retained essentially as pure fat; 1 g adipose tissue yields close to the full theoretical equivalent of 38 kJ (9 kcal). Because of the efficient storage of energy in adipose tissue, an individual of normal weight can survive up to 2 months of total starvation. However, western society is generally not characterized by periodic or insufficient food supply but rather by constant and abundant food. As a consequence, the ability to store fat all too frequently is of negative survival value because of overconsumption and the resulting obesity.

DEFINITION AND INCIDENCE Obesity can most easily be assessed in terms of height and weight. One way is to relate weight to an average range for height and age. This measure of *relative weight* can lead to an underestimation of the incidence of obesity, since in the United States the "average" individual is somewhat obese. Tables of *ideal* and *desirable* weight are based on actuarial estimates of what is consistent with longest life expectancy. Such tables are more useful if adjusted for differences in body build. An alternative method of estimating obesity is the *body mass index* or *BMI* [body weight (in kilograms) divided by height (in meters)^2]. For adults ages 20 to 29, the 85th percentile for BMI is 27.8 for males and 27.3 for females. Although relative weight and BMI correlate with the degree of adiposity, excess poundage can be either lean or fat tissue. For example, heavily muscled individuals would be considered obese using these measurements. Nevertheless, such assessments correlate fairly well with the risk of adverse effects on health and longevity. More precise assessment of obesity can be made with measurements of body density or with isotopic dilution methods, but these are unsuitable for routine use. Alternatively anthropometry can be utilized for assessing the degree of adiposity. Assessment of skin-fold thickness over various areas of the body together with height, weight, and age can be used to assess the degree of adiposity. Triceps and subscapular skin folds are most commonly employed (see Chap. 71). From a health standpoint, certain patterns of obesity may be less desirable than others. Fat deposition about the waist and flank, as evidenced by a high ratio of waist to hip circumference, is associated with a greater health risk than fat deposition at the hips.

The term *obesity* implies an excess of adipose tissue, but the meaning of excess is hard to define. Aesthetic considerations aside, obesity can best be viewed as any degree of excess adiposity that imparts a health risk. This cutoff between normal and obese can only be approximated, and the health risk imparted by obesity is probably a continuum with increasing adiposity. The Framingham Study demonstrated that a 20 percent excess over desirable weight clearly imparted a health risk. A National Institutes of Health consensus panel on obesity agreed with this definition and concluded that a 20 percent increase in relative weight or a BMI above the 85th percentile for young adults constitutes a health risk; by use of these criteria 20 to 30 percent of adult men and 30 to 40 percent of adult women are obese, with the highest rates among the poor and minority groups. Significant health risks at lower levels of obesity can occur in the presence of diabetes, hypertension, heart disease, or other associated risk factors.

The Surgeon General's 1988 Report on obesity notes that even mild obesity increases the risk for premature death, diabetes, hypertension, atherosclerosis, gallbladder disease, and certain types of cancer. In the United States the prevalence of obesity has increased in the past few decades. Because of the high prevalence of obesity and its health consequences, its prevention and treatment should be a high public health priority.

ETIOLOGY When energy intake exceeds expenditure, the excess calories are stored in adipose tissue, and if this net positive balance is prolonged, obesity results, i.e., there are two components to weight balance, and an abnormality on either side (intake or expenditure) can lead to obesity.

The regulation of eating behavior is incompletely understood. To some extent, appetite is controlled by discrete areas in the hypothalamus: a feeding center in the ventrolateral nucleus of the hypothalamus (VLH) and a satiety center in the ventromedial hypothalamus (VMH). The cerebral cortex receives positive signals from the feeding center that stimulate eating (Fig. 72-1), and the satiety center modulates this process by sending inhibitory impulses to the feeding center. In animals destruction of the feeding center results in decreased food intake, and destruction of the satiety center leads to overeating and obesity. Several regulatory processes may influence these hypothalamic centers. The satiety center may be activated by the increases in plasma glucose and/or insulin that follow a meal. It is of interest in this regard that the VMH contains insulin receptors and is insulin-sensitive. Meal-induced gastric distention is another possible inhibitory factor. The total adipose tissue mass may also influence the activity of the hypothalamic centers; i.e., there is a relatively fixed "set point" for body adiposity. An elevated set point may account for the frequent recidivism in obese patients who have lost weight. How the "set point" is established and how the hypothalamus senses total fat stores are unknown. Glycerol release from fat cells, ascending neural impulses, and/or circulation of adipocyte-derived peptides such as adipsin may be signals of adipose tissue size. Additionally, the hypothalamic centers are sensitive to catecholamines, and beta-adrenergic stimulation inhibits eating behavior. This provides at least one rationale for the anorexiant effects of amphetamines.

Ultimately, the cerebral cortex controls eating behavior, and impulses from the feeding center to the cerebral cortex are only one input. Psychological, social, and genetic factors also influence food intake. In many obese subjects these influences are overriding; indeed, obese subjects usually respond to external signals such as time of day, social setting, and smell or taste of food to a greater extent than do persons of normal weight.

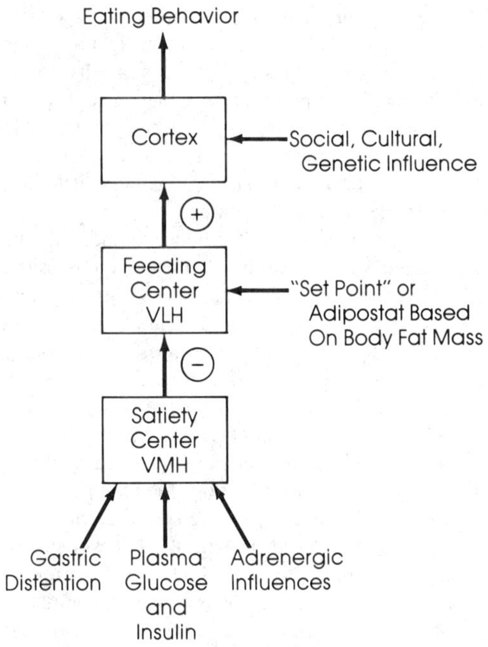

FIGURE 72-1 The regulation of eating. The ventromedial satiety center is considered to be inhibitory, and the ventrolateral feeding center stimulatory. See text for discussion.

Although overeating is the usual cause of obesity, other factors may participate. Daily caloric needs normally range between 110 to 130 kJ (27 to 32 kcal) per kilogram of body weight; this figure is higher in active and lower in sedentary individuals. Physical activity clearly modulates overall caloric balance, and obese individuals tend to be less active. This can be a contributory factor in the maintenance of excess weight, but decreased physical activity is unlikely to be an important cause of major weight gain in most obese subjects. Rather, obesity leads to inactivity. The modest increase in weight that often accompanies the middle years may be related more directly to diminished physical activity. Injury or illness may lead to chronic restricted activity and predispose to weight gain unless caloric intake is appropriately curtailed. Perhaps the greatest factor tending to diminish the output side of the equation is simply a sedentary lifestyle.

Decreased caloric expenditure and a metabolic abnormality associated with overefficient caloric utilization have also been postulated as involved in the pathogenesis of obesity. With rare exceptions major metabolic abnormalities have not been detected in obese individuals, although subtle defects may be undetected. There are three major components to overall energy expenditure: resting metabolic rate, exercise-induced thermogenesis, and the thermic response to food.

The resting metabolic rate accounts for 60 to 75 percent of daily energy expenditure and is measured in a thermoneutral environment while the subject is at rest following an overnight fast and several hours after any significant physical activity. An average resting metabolic rate in a 70-kg man is 6300 kJ (1500 kcal)/d. The resting metabolic rate should be expressed as a function of fat-free body weight (by subtracting the subject's total adipose mass from body weight), since triglyceride mass is metabolically inert in that negligible energy is expended to maintain triglyceride depots. When expressed in this way, the resting metabolic rate is normal in most obese subjects. However, a distinction must be made between static obesity and the actual process of gaining weight. When normal subjects consume hypercaloric diets, less weight is gained than would be predicted on the basis of the excess calories ingested. This effect is most marked when carbohydrate is consumed and disappears when the excess calories consist of fat. Thus, humans can apparently partially adapt to chronic excessive carbohydrate and protein intake, and this protective effect attenuates the weight gain. Part of this adaptive response is related to an increase in thermogenesis manifested as an increase in the resting metabolic rate. The mechanism of adaptive thermogenesis is unknown, but overeating of carbohydrate or mixed nutrients leads to increased plasma levels of triiodothyronine (T_3) and decreased levels of reverse T_3 (rT_3). A converse effect is seen in starvation with decreased T_3 and increased rT_3 levels. The conversion of thyroxine to T_3 occurs largely in the liver; excess food may induce adaptive thermogenesis by increasing the concentration of T_3 relative to that of T_4 and rT_3. Increased central or peripheral sympathetic outflow leading to increased catecholamine-induced caloric utilization and increased heat production may also play a role in the thermogenic response to overnutrition. Adaptive thermogenesis can lead to a 10- to 15-percent increase in resting metabolic rate, and this effect is seen after a 2- to 3-week period of hypercaloric intake. The rate of onset and the degree of adaptive thermogenesis is the same in obese and nonobese individuals when expressed on the basis of fat-free body mass. Specifically, the increase in resting metabolic rate, changes in thyroid hormone metabolism, and thermic responses to infused catecholamines are similar in normal and obese subjects during periods of overnutrition.

Work performance, or energy expenditure per standard physical work load, can be normal or increased in obesity depending on the kind of work performed. The energy expenditure of exercise is increased in obese compared to lean subjects due to the extra effort involved in moving or supporting an increased body mass. When this effect of increased body mass is taken into account, work performance is normal in obesity. Clearly, normal or increased energy expenditure during physical work cannot contribute to the development of obesity. On the other hand, the total daily energy expenditure due to exercise is less in many sedentary obese subjects simply because they engage in less daily physical activity than their lean counterparts.

The third important aspect of caloric balance is the thermic response to food, so-called dietary thermogenesis. This consists of the heat, or energy, expended above the resting metabolic rate for several hours after the ingestion of a meal. About 75 percent of the thermic response to food is due to the energy cost of digestion, absorption, metabolism, and storage of foodstuffs; the remainder is probably due to activation of the sympathetic nervous system. The heat produced following nutrient ingestion is a form of caloric expenditure and is greater for protein and less for carbohydrate and fat. The thermic response to mixed meals can equal 10 to 15 percent of the calories ingested, and decreased thermic responses have been described in some studies of human obesity. This difference may be due to altered flux rates through different pathways of intermediary metabolism, with more energy-efficient pathways being favored in obesity. As an example, the higher the rate of glucose utilization, the greater the thermic response to carbohydrate-containing meals, and small decreases in the thermic response to food may be due to insulin resistance and decreased glucose disposal in obese subjects. It is clear that small differences in caloric utilization maintained over years can lead to a significant net positive caloric balance. However, while it is tempting to postulate that this decreased thermic response may contribute to obesity, most of the published comparisons have been made between normal persons and subjects who are already obese. Thus, the obesity-associated changes in thermic response to food may be secondary to the obese state rather than a primary abnormality. More importantly, differences in the thermic response to meals between the obese and nonobese are at most in the range of 125 to 210 kJ (30 to 50 kcal)/d. Such minor differences can easily be counterbalanced by minor decreases in food intake and/or increases in exercise-induced thermogenesis. Since such compensation does not occur, it seems more probable that obesity is the result of impaired coupling between caloric intake and expenditure.

Another potential regulatory process in the control of adipose tissue mass involves adipose tissue lipoprotein lipase (ATLPL). This enzyme is synthesized within adipocytes, secreted into the extracellular space, and attached to the luminal surface of nearby endothelial cells.

At this location ATLPL hydrolyzes fatty acids from the triglycerides of circulating triglyceride-rich lipoproteins. The released fatty acids are taken up by adipocytes, converted to triglycerides, and stored. Thus, ATLPL participates in the storage of excess fat calories in adipose tissue. The *lipoprotein lipase hypothesis* holds that in some obese states excessive levels of this enzyme induce obesity by causing preferential deposition of fat calories in adipose tissue. In support of this hypothesis, ATLPL levels are increased in obese rodents and humans. More importantly, levels of this enzyme do not return to normal following weight reduction. This latter finding is of particular interest since it is one of the few characteristics of the obese state that is not corrected by weight reduction and could explain the propensity of obese patients to regain lost weight.

Environmental, cultural, and genetic influences all contribute to obesity, and in population studies it is impossible to quantitate the separate impact of these factors. Nevertheless, the importance of genetics has been demonstrated in studies of twins and adopted siblings. The BMI of adopted individuals correlates better with that of the biologic rather than the adoptive parents. Among biologic and adoptive siblings, the amount and distribution of fat is associated with a genetic relationship, and similarities are not as close among adopted siblings. Most likely, both nature and nurture contribute to the etiology of obesity.

SECONDARY OBESITY **Hypothyroidism** Obesity can result from hypothyroidism because of decreased caloric needs. However, only a minority of hypothyroid patients are truly obese, and an even smaller proportion of obese patients are hypothyroid. Indiscriminate use of thyroid hormone in the treatment of obesity is to be deplored and should never be instituted in the absence of documentation of decreased thyroid function.

Cushing's disease Cushing's disease is a rare cause of obesity. Hyperadrenocorticism elicits a typical pattern of obesity with predominantly centripetal fat stores, characteristic rounded or moon facies, and cervical or supraclavicular fat deposits.

Insulinoma Hyperinsulinemia, secondary to an insulinoma, can occasionally cause obesity, presumably because of increased caloric intake secondary to recurrent hypoglycemia. Most patients with islet cell tumors and hypoglycemia are not obese.

Hypothalamic disorders Froehlich's syndrome in boys is characterized by obesity and hypogonadotrophic hypogonadism with other variable features such as diabetes insipidus, visual impairment, and mental retardation. The anterior pituitary is usually normal, and the syndrome is thought to be the result of hypothalamic dysfunction. This syndrome likely includes a number of overlapping disorders having in common a hypothalamic lesion that leads to overeating and to hypogonadotrophism. Occasionally pituitary tumors are present (as in Froehlich's original case) that may physically impair the hypothalamus.

Other rare causes of obesity include the Laurence-Moon-Biedl syndrome, characterized by retinitis pigmentosa, mental retardation, skull deformities, polydactyly and syndactyly, and the Prader-Willi syndrome, which is associated with hypotonia, mental retardation, and a predilection for diabetes mellitus. Both of these disorders also feature obesity and hypogonadism that are thought to be hypothalamic in origin.

PATHOLOGIC SEQUELAE Increased adipose tissue stores are deposited subcutaneously, around all internal organs, throughout the omentum, and in the intramuscular spaces. Obese individuals also have an expansion of lean body mass as evidenced by increased size of the kidneys, heart, liver, and skeletal muscle mass. Fatty livers are common in extreme obesity.

Adipocyte size and number Attempts have been made to classify obese individuals on the basis of the relative degree of adipocyte hypertrophy versus hyperplasia. This classification scheme was generated as the result of experimental data indicating that in several rodent species and in humans the capacity to increase adipocyte number exists for only a limited period in early life and perhaps at the time of puberty. Thus, prior to reaching adulthood the ability to increase the number of adipocytes declines, and after this time expansion of adipose tissue mass is accompanied primarily by an increase in fat-cell size. Individuals with severe obesity have both increased adipocyte size and number, and those with the greatest degree of adipocyte hyperplasia have a strong tendency toward onset of obesity early in life. Patients having mild to moderate obesity show predominantly adipocyte hypertrophy, and the onset is usually during adult life. Weight reduction leads to a decrease in adipocyte size with no change in cell number. The above observations led to the concept of the existence of a "critical period" in early life when final adipocyte number is determined and after which cell number cannot be changed. This formulation implies that alterations in adipocyte number can only be induced during this critical period. However, the concept of a strictly defined critical period for hyperplasia of the adipocytes is only partially correct. When severe obesity is induced in adult rats, both adipocyte number and cell size increase. Adipocyte hypercellularity also occurs in some patients with adult-onset obesity.

Thus while substantial overnutrition at any stage of life can lead to hypertrophy of individual existing adipocytes, there are periods during childhood and adolescence when overnutrition has an enhanced ability to induce the development of new adipocytes. Furthermore, even in adult life, if the degree of overnutrition is sufficient to induce existing adipocytes to enlarge to some limiting size, then new adipocytes will form. Whether this latter population of cells represents new cell formation or simply the filling with lipid of previously undetectable preadipocytes formed earlier in life is not known. Regardless of the cause or time of development of increased adiposity (adipocyte hypertrophy with or without hyperplasia), subsequent weight reduction only leads to a decrease in the size of existing adipocytes and not a decrease in adipocyte number. Thus, once a given complement of adipocytes is attained, this number is fixed and cannot be reduced.

METABOLIC SEQUELAE Obesity has a profound impact on diabetes mellitus and on various hyperlipoproteinemic states primarily through its influences on insulin secretion and insulin sensitivity.

Hyperinsulinemia: Insulin resistance Increased insulin secretion is a common feature of obesity. It occurs in the basal state and in response to a wide variety of insulinogenic agents. A correlation exists between the degree of obesity and the magnitude of the hyperinsulinemia—particularly the basal insulin levels. Some obese patients exhibit hyperglycemia or frank diabetes in the face of hyperinsulinemia. The combination of hyper- or euglycemia and hyperinsulinemia indicates an insulin-resistant state, and decreased hypoglycemic responses to insulin are common in obese humans and animals. Insulin resistance could be due to an abnormal beta-cell product, circulating insulin antagonists, or tissue insulin insensitivity. Since abnormal islet secretory products or circulating antagonists have not been identified, it is thought that the insulin resistance of obesity is primarily due to tissue insensitivity. The initial step in the cellular action of insulin involves binding to cell surface receptors in target tissues. Cells from obese animals and humans contain decreased numbers of insulin receptors, and this decrease doubtless plays a role in the insulin resistance. However, other factors participate. The enlarged adipocytes of obese rats have both a decrease in insulin receptors and an even greater defect in the capacity to metabolize glucose, suggesting a major biochemical abnormality distal to the receptor mechanism. A similar postreceptor defect presumably exists in other insulin target tissues such as muscle and liver. In the obese human insulin resistance is due to a combination of receptor and postreceptor defects in insulin action. In those obese patients with the mildest degree of hyperinsulinemia and insulin resistance, the decrease in insulin action is predominantly due to a decreased number of insulin receptors. As the insulin-resistant state worsens, a postreceptor defect emerges, and in obese subjects with the most severe degree of insulin resistance, the postreceptor defect is the predominant abnormality.

Diabetes mellitus (See also Chap. 319) Although only a minority of obese patients are diabetic, the converse is not the case. Non-insulin-dependent, or type II, diabetes comprises about 90 percent of the diabetic population in the United States, and 80 to 90 percent of type II diabetics are obese. Obesity is an important contributory factor to the diabetes in these patients, predominantly through its influences on insulin resistance. Obesity exacerbates the diabetic state, and in many cases diabetes can be ameliorated by weight reduction.

Hyperlipoproteinemia (See also Chap. 326) Most plasma cholesterol circulates in the low-density lipoprotein (LDL) fraction, and, in the fasting state, very low density lipoproteins (VLDL) contain most of the circulating triglyceride. The association between obesity and elevated LDL levels is modest at best, especially when the relationship is corrected for factors such as age. Total-body cholesterol is increased in obesity, but this is mainly accounted for by adipose tissue cholesterol stores. Cholesterol turnover may be increased, leading to increased biliary excretion of cholesterol. This may contribute to the increased incidence of gallstone formation. Obesity has a more pronounced effect on VLDL metabolism. Hypertriglyceridemia is frequent, and the degree of obesity correlates with the level of hypertriglyceridemia. The increased triglyceride levels are due to increased hepatic VLDL production with no defect in the removal of VLDL from plasma. As discussed above, plasma insulin levels are elevated, particularly in the portal venous blood. Hyperinsulinemia can promote increased hepatic VLDL synthesis and secretion. In addition, increased plasma free fatty acid (FFA) turnover exists in obesity, and FFA extraction by the liver provides an important precursor for hepatic triglyceride synthesis. Thus, the hypertriglyceridemia in obesity may be secondary to increased hepatic VLDL secretion due to hyperinsulinemia and augmented FFA availability.

MANIFESTATIONS AND COMPLICATIONS Gross obesity produces mechanical and physical stresses that aggravate or cause a number of disorders including osteoarthritis (especially of the hips) and sciatica. Varicose veins, thromboembolism, ventral and hiatal hernias, and cholelithiasis are also more common.

Hypertension In significantly obese persons, use of the standard size blood pressure cuff leads to erroneously high readings; an oversize cuff should always be used. A strong association between hypertension and obesity is observed even when accurate measurements are obtained. The mechanism by which obesity causes hypertension is uncertain, but peripheral vascular resistance is usually normal while blood volume is increased. Weight loss leads to reductions in systemic blood pressure independent of changes in sodium balance.

Hypoventilation syndrome (Pickwickian syndrome) The obesity-hypoventilation syndrome is a heterogeneous group of disorders with differing clinical manifestations. The hypersomnolence that can occur in obesity is a manifestation of nighttime sleep apnea. In these individuals, once sleep begins, upper airway obstruction leads to hypoxemia and hypercapnia, causing arousal with return of normal respiration. Many such episodes occur each night, leading to chronic sleep deprivation and daytime somnolence. The combination of the obese habitus plus sleep-induced relaxation of the pharyngeal musculature is believed to be the cause of the intermittent upper airway obstruction. Occasionally such episodes are life-threatening (causing serious cardiac arrhythmias) and require long-term tracheostomy therapy. Chronic daytime hypoventilation is usually not as severe as that occurring during sleep and may be due to abnormalities of the respiratory control centers. Patients with hypoventilation display blunted ventilatory responses to hypercapnia and hypoxia and often develop hypercapnia and hypoxemia due to decreased basal ventilation; in addition, ventilation-perfusion mismatch may result from mechanical factors. In severe cases polycythemia, pulmonary hypertension, and cor pulmonale can result. Weight reduction will reverse these abnormalities if instituted before permanent cardiac damage develops. Some obese patients with sleep apnea and hypersomnolence do not have daytime hypoventilation and have normal ventilatory responses to hypoxia and hypercapnia. Progestational agents have been used therapeutically in the obesity-hypoventilation syndrome since they stimulate the ventilatory response to hypercapnia and hypoxia in normal subjects. Medroxyprogesterone increases ventilation and improves heart failure and erythrocytosis in these patients, although obstructive sleep apnea continues.

Adrenal function Although Cushing's disease can usually be distinguished from simple obesity on clinical grounds, laboratory testing is occasionally necessary. This can lead to confusion since 24-h urinary 17-hydroxycorticoid excretion is often elevated in obesity. Less commonly, plasma cortisol levels are also increased. Corticosteroid levels are usually suppressible with dexamethasone in obesity, but occasionally suppression is incomplete, rendering the diagnosis difficult (also see Chap. 317).

Growth hormone Secretory responses of growth hormone to a variety of stimuli such as hypoglycemia, exercise, and arginine infusion are reduced, and the starvation-induced rise in plasma growth hormone levels is attenuated.

Atherosclerosis Obesity is a risk factor for the development of coronary artery disease and stroke. Most of the risk is mediated through the associated hypertension, hyperlipoproteinemia, and diabetes. Nevertheless, even when these abnormalities are factored out, an additional, smaller risk can be ascribed to obesity per se.

TREATMENT Amelioration of hyperinsulinemia, insulin resistance, diabetes, hypertension, and hyperlipidemia can occur following weight loss. These changes are significant and enduring provided the weight loss is maintained. During weight loss all adipose tissue depots diminish proportionately. Sometimes generalized loss does not produce the attractive cosmetic effects desired. Many techniques have been proposed to effect selective adipose tissue reduction over particular regions of the body, but none is effective.

Methods of weight reduction In instances where obesity is secondary, the appropriate therapy is to treat the underlying disease. Most of the time the difficult problem of primary weight reduction must be undertaken.

Diet Caloric restriction is the cornerstone of weight reduction. From the standpoint of patient and physician this is a frustrating and demanding undertaking. The basic principles are simple. If food intake is less than energy expenditure, stored calories, predominantly in the form of fat, will be consumed. In general, a deficit of 32,000 kJ (7700 kcal) leads to loss of about 1 kg fat. By estimating the patient's daily caloric needs [approximately 125 to 150 kJ (30 to 35 kcal) per kilogram of body weight], one can calculate the daily deficit necessary to achieve a given rate of weight loss.

Dietary restriction can range from total starvation to mild caloric deprivation, and these approaches will be discussed separately. Dietary recommendations are most effective when they are specific and geared to the patient's life-style. A dietitian or a similarly trained health professional should interview each patient and estimate average daily caloric intake, identify food preferences, and characterize the eating patterns. The amount of calories to be consumed on the restricted diet should be carefully explained in terms of quantities of specific foodstuffs. Frequently, the therapist must balance the degree of restriction against potential noncompliance. The more restrictive the diet, the more rapid the weight loss, but this often leads to a greater rate of nonadherence. It is preferable to design a diet with which the patient is comfortable and that produces a modest but steady weight loss.

Schemes for weight reduction have become a profitable business in the United States, and there are almost as many diets as there are therapists. Each proponent claims that the presence or absence of certain foodstuffs is desirable for more effective weight loss. However, little evidence exists to support the claim that calorie for calorie one hypocaloric diet will lead to a greater weight loss than another. The relationship between the patient and the therapist, plus patient education and encouragement, are more important to success than are the specific dietary constituents. The major virtue of "fad" diets is that patients are usually motivated to try them, at least initially, and patient cooperation is often better. Provided a particular diet is not harmful, probably the best course for the therapist is to maintain flexibility in the treatment program. Nevertheless, diets markedly deficient in any major class of foodstuff are to be avoided. For example, whole-food diets that are exceedingly low in carbohydrate are by nature high in fat and, depending on the type and quantity of fat ingested, may lead to hypercholesterolemia. The major virtue of a low-carbohydrate diet is the attendant ketosis (ketone bodies have a central anorexiant effect). This provided part of the rationale for the widely touted liquid or powdered protein diets that were previously popular. These diets have been dubbed "protein-sparing modified fasts," and claims were made that they allowed drastic long-term caloric restriction without inducing negative nitrogen balance. These claims have not been substantiated, nor has it been shown that the diets lead to a greater degree of fat tissue weight loss than mixed diets of equal caloric value. Basically a calorie is a calorie whether it comes from protein, carbohydrate, or fat. Furthermore, deaths have been reported in otherwise healthy individuals participating in such long-term dietary programs, even under medical supervision. This has been attributed to the fact that some of these diets contain mostly collagen-derived protein of low biologic value. Other very low calorie diets involve formula preparations containing 500 to 800 kcal/d, with 50 to 80 g of high-quality protein. The remaining calories consist of carbohydrate and fat. Vitamin and micronutrient supplements are incorporated in the formula or provided as an added supplement. Such high-quality low-calorie diet formulas lead to relatively rapid weight loss but should not be taken continuously as the sole caloric source for more than 6 weeks. In the absence of coexisting diseases such as gout, renal insufficiency, cardiac arrhythmias, etc., such diets are safe when taken under medical supervision. Such very low calorie diets are contraindicated in pregnant women and growing children.

Prior to therapy it is wise to warn patients that when caloric restriction is started, there is usually a marked initial weight loss, in large part due to fluid loss, but such rapid rates of loss will not persist. Likewise, positive shifts in fluid balance can sometimes mask loss of adipose mass, a fact that can sometimes be demonstrated to the patient's satisfaction by recording skin-fold thickness at periodic intervals.

Total-starvation diets have been advocated for the treatment of obesity; provided gout, renal insufficiency, and ketosis-prone diabetes are not present, short-term (2- to 3-day) fasts are usually well tolerated. Ketonemia and hyperuricemia regularly develop during starvation but rarely lead to acidosis or gout. Because of these potential complications, total fasting should be carried out only under medical supervision. Probably the major usefulness of total fasting is as a motivational aid at the beginning of a dietary program or when weight loss has stopped. Even though much of the weight loss during short-term fasting represents fluid, this weight loss can be encouraging to frustrated patients and motivate them to improve compliance with the long-term weight reduction program.

The major problem in the treatment of obesity is not weight reduction but maintenance of the reduced weight. Provided the therapist works hard and long enough, most motivated patients can eventually lose weight. Unfortunately, only the rare patient maintains the weight loss permanently. Obesity is an eating disorder, and the underlying mechanisms are not reversed by limiting food intake.

Behavior modification In recognition of the problems involved, the techniques of behavior modification have been devised to treat abnormal patterns of eating behavior. Many studies demonstrate that obese individuals respond less well than normal individuals to internal cues that regulate eating behavior such as gastric contractions, fear, and previous food ingestion. Conversely, obese subjects overrespond to external cues such as taste, smell, food attractiveness, food abundance, and the ease of obtaining food. Given the fact that the obese individual is unusually susceptible to external stimuli, food intake may be altered by changing the pattern and nature of these external cues, and this is the major premise underlying the behavior modification approach to weight reduction.

Behavior modification begins with a detailed individual history of the patient's eating patterns with respect to time of day, length of eating period, place of ingestion (restaurant, dining table, standing in front of open refrigerator), simultaneous activities (watching television, reading, idleness), emotional state, companions (relatives, friends, or alone), and finally the kinds and quantities of foods ingested. Once this detailed record is obtained, the therapist and patient can design specific behavioral changes aimed at disrupting or aborting recurring behavior patterns which initiate or prolong abnormal eating activity. As examples: if a patient eats in response to certain emotional states, then other activities can be substituted when the patient perceives such a state; if the patient snacks frequently from readily available food storage areas (refrigerators, cookie jars, etc.), then he or she is encouraged to eat only while sitting down at a table with a fixed place setting; if eating frequently occurs while watching television alone, then efforts to avoid this activity can be initiated. Many other examples of specific and general interventions could be given. Results with behavior modification techniques indicate that many patients can maintain long-term weight reduction providing the new behavior patterns are truly "learned."

Exercise Exercise has a place in any weight reduction program. However, the importance of exercise in terms of caloric balance must be clearly understood. Even moderate daily exercise would not lead to a large enough increase in energy expenditure to alter significantly the initial rate of weight reduction (Table 72-1). This does not mean exercise is unimportant in weight reduction, since even modest increases in caloric expenditure can lead to large long-term differences in caloric balance, provided exercise is performed on a regular basis. For example, a daily increase in caloric expenditure of 1250 kJ (300 kcal) over a period of 4 months could lead to a 4.5-kg weight loss. More importantly, incorporation of regular exercise into the overall weight reduction program improves the chances that the patient will maintain the weight loss.

Drugs Two classes of drugs are frequently used in the treatment of obesity: anorexiants and thyroid hormone supplements. The addition of levothyroxine or triiodothyronine to a weight reduction program is ineffective in promoting adipose tissue loss and, if anything, accentuates lean tissue loss and causes negative nitrogen balance. In susceptible individuals, cardiotoxicity may occur. Thus, unless clear-cut hypothyroidism is present, thyroid supplementation has no role in the treatment of obesity.

The major anorexiants are amphetamine-like agents that presumably exert their effect at the level of the hypothalamus. They probably have a modest effect in promoting short-term weight loss in some individuals. However, they are effective only for short periods, and problems of habituation, addiction, and drug abuse limit their usefulness. Two anorexiants, diethylpropion and fenfluramine, may be less addictive and, therefore, somewhat more useful. However, none of these agents treats the underlying eating disorder, and they are of little use in maintenance of weight reduction.

Injections of human chorionic gonadotropin (hCG) have been tried as an adjunct to weight reduction, but no evidence exists to indicate a beneficial effect. The primary effectiveness of the hCG-diet program is due to the calorically restricted diet, frequent physician contact, and placebo effects. Comparable weight loss is achieved if saline injections are substituted for hCG, suggesting a placebo or physiologic effect of the act of parenteral injection.

Jejunoileal shunt Small-bowel bypass is an effective means of achieving weight reduction in morbidly obese patients. However, it is an experimental procedure and should be attempted only in institutions where a trained team is committed to regular, systematic, and long-term follow-up. Because of accompanying morbidity and mortality most such institutions have abandoned this form of surgery in favor of the more benign and effective gastric plication or bypass approach described below.

The most common operative procedures for the jejunoileal shunt

TABLE 72-1 **Energy equivalents of food calories expressed in minutes of activity**

Food	Energy value, kJ (kcal)	Activity: Walking*	Riding bicycle†	Swimming‡	Running§	Reclining¶
Apple, large	422 (101)	19	12	9	5	78
Bacon, 2 strips	401 (96)	18	12	9	5	74
Beer, 1 glass	477 (114)	22	14	10	6	88
Bread and butter	326 (78)	15	10	7	4	60
Carbonated beverage, 1 glass	444 (106)	20	13	9	5	82
Carrot, raw	176 (42)	8	5	4	2	32
Cheese, cottage, 1 tbsp	113 (27)	5	3	2	1	21
Chicken, fried, ½ breast	971 (232)	45	28	21	12	178
Cookie, chocolate chip	213 (51)	10	6	5	3	39
Egg, fried	460 (110)	21	13	10	6	85
Ham, 2 slices	699 (167)	32	20	15	9	128
Ice cream, ⅙ qt	808 (193)	37	24	17	10	148
Mayonnaise, 1 tbsp	385 (92)	18	11	8	5	71
Milk, skim, 1 glass	339 (81)	16	10	7	4	62
Milk shake	1762 (421)	81	51	38	22	324
Orange, medium	285 (68)	13	8	6	4	52
Pancake with syrup	519 (124)	24	15	11	6	95
Peas, green, ½ cup	234 (56)	11	7	5	3	43
Pizza, cheese, ¼	753 (180)	35	22	16	9	138
Potato chips, 1 serving	462 (108)	21	13	10	6	83
Sandwiches:						
Hamburger	1456 (350)	67	43	31	18	269
Tuna fish salad	1163 (278)	53	34	25	14	214
Sherbet, ⅙ qt	741 (177)	34	22	16	9	136

* Energy cost of walking for 70-kg individual = 22 kJ (5.2 kcal)/min.
† Energy cost of riding bicycle = 34 kJ (8.2 kcal)/min.
‡ Energy cost of swimming = 47 kJ (11.2 kcal)/min.
§ Energy cost of running = 81 kJ (19.4 kcal)/min.
¶ Energy cost of reclining = 5 kJ (1.3 kcal)/min.

involve end-to-end or end-to-side anastomosis of about 38 cm of proximal jejunum to 10 cm of terminal ileum. Weight loss is initially rapid, reaching a plateau at 18 to 24 months. While all patients lose weight, few return to ideal weight. The mean weight loss is about 30 to 50 percent of initial excess weight, leaving patients still about 50 percent overweight once a steady state is reached. Although some degree of malabsorption occurs, the major portion of the weight loss is due to decreased food intake.

Teams still performing this surgery select patients who are at least 50 kg overweight and in whom adequate attempts at medical management have failed repeatedly. Because of postoperative morbidity, older patients (>50 years) and psychologically unstable individuals are usually excluded.

The overall surgical mortality ranges from 0.5 to 7.8 percent with an average of around 4 percent. Mortality is inversely related to the experience of the surgical team. The major postoperative morbidity is related to wound infection and thromboembolism. The common serious medical complications are cirrhosis and hepatic failure, nephrolithiasis, electrolyte imbalances, cholelithiasis, and arthritis (Table 72-2). Severe liver disease probably occurs in 5 percent of patients, and milder degrees of hepatic dysfunction are more common. The long-range implications of mild hepatic abnormalities are unknown. Possible causes of liver damage following small-bowel bypass include (1) protein and particularly essential amino acid deficiency, (2) accumulation of hepatotoxic, secondary bile salts, and (3) release of unknown toxic substances from the excluded bowel. Hypokalemia is most likely secondary to diarrhea. Persistent deficiency of calcium and magnesium can result from malabsorption and must be treated with appropriate replacement. Transient depression of plasma 25-hydroxyvitamin D levels may also contribute to abnormal mineral metabolism. Nephrolithiasis occurs in up to 30 percent of patients and is due to hyperoxaluria secondary to calcium malabsorption. It can be treated by calcium supplements and a low oxalate intake. Migratory polyarthritis occurs in up to 6 percent of patients and may be due to circulating immune complexes. This operation is now rarely performed, in part due to the decision of many insurance companies not to render compensation for this procedure.

Gastric surgery Gastroplasty establishes a small upper gastric remnant connected to a larger lower gastric pouch by a narrow 1- to 1.5-cm channel. Gastric bypass excludes the lower 90 percent of the stomach pouch and maintains intestinal continuity of the upper 10 percent via a retrocolic gastrojejunostomy. Both of these procedures

TABLE 72-2 **Complications of bypass surgery**

Complication	Percentage
EARLY	
Perioperative mortality	2–6
Thromboembolic disease	1–5
Wound infection	2–5
Renal failure	3
Severe nausea, vomiting	3
Wound dehiscence	1–3
LATE	
Urinary calculi	3–10
Severe electrolyte imbalance	5–8
Acute cholecystitis	0–5
Progressive liver disease	2–4
Intestinal obstruction	2
Peptic ulcer	1–2
Osteoporosis	?
Tuberculosis	1
MINOR	
Diarrhea	100
Weakness	80
Hypokalemia	80
Hypoproteinemia	50
Vomiting	50
Thirst	50
Hypocalcemia	30
Arthralgias	15
Incisional hernias	3
Hyperuricemia	<10
Anemias	<10

cause patients to limit food intake by delaying gastric emptying and providing a small gastric reservoir so that fullness is experienced after a small meal. Weight loss with these procedures is comparable with that achieved with small-bowel bypass operations but without the complications related to malabsorption, diarrhea, and hepatic dysfunction. The procedure can be reversed if a decision to restore normal anatomy is made at a later time. For these reasons, gastroplasty is frequently performed for the surgical treatment of morbid obesity in patients who have failed standard weight loss regimens.

SUMMARY For most patients obesity is an eating disorder, and a major hope for effective long-term treatment of this disease lies in understanding the causes of overeating. No single etiology explains all cases, and different causes exist for different individuals. At present a variety of techniques are available to effect initial weight loss. Unfortunately, initial weight loss is not the real therapeutic goal. Rather, the problem is that most obese patients eventually regain their weight. An effective means to sustain weight loss is the major challenge in the treatment of obesity today. The technique of behavioral modification, when professionally and rigorously applied, is the best tool for this task. As information develops concerning the hypothalamic "set point," or *adipostat*, and the factors that regulate it, other therapies may emerge that will effect long-term correction of abnormal eating patterns.

REFERENCES

BRAY GA: Current status of intestinal bypass surgery in the treatment of obesity. Diabetes 26:1072, 1977

———, GRAY IS: Treatment of obesity: Overview. Diabetes/Metabolism Rev 4:653, 1988

FOSTER DW: Eating disorders: Obesity and anorexia nervosa, in *Williams Textbook of Endocrinology*, 7th ed, JD Wilson, DW Foster (eds). Philadelphia, Saunders, 1985, p 1081

HASHIM SA, PORIKOS K: Food intake behavior in man: Implications for treatment of obesity. Clin Endocrinol Metab 5:503, 1976

HENRY RR et al: Metabolic consequences of very low calorie diet therapy in obese non-insulin dependent diabetic and non-diabetic subjects. Diabetes 35:155, 1986

HORTON ES, DANFORTH E JR: Energy metabolism and obesity, in *Diabetes Mellitus and Obesity*, SJ Bleicher, BN Brodoff (eds). Baltimore, Williams & Wilkins, 1981, p 261

KOLTERMAN OG et al: Mechanisms of insulin resistance in human obesity. Evidence for receptor and postreceptor defects. J Clin Invest 65:1272, 1980

MANN GV: The influence of obesity on health. N Engl J Med 291:226, 1974

NATIONAL INSTITUTES OF HEALTH CONSENSUS DEVELOPMENT PANEL ON THE HEALTH IMPLICATIONS OF OBESITY: Health implications of obesity. Ann Intern Med 103:147, 1985

OLEFSKY JM et al: Insulin action and insulin resistance in obesity and non-insulin dependent, type II diabetes mellitus. Am J Physiol 243:E15, 1982

SALANS L: The obesities, in *Endocrinology and Metabolism*, 2d ed, P Felig et al (eds). New York, McGraw-Hill, 1987, chap 21, p 1203

STUNKARD AJ et al: An adoption study of human obesity. N Engl J Med 314:193, 1984

The Surgeon General's Report on Nutrition and Health. US Department of Health and Human Services Public Health Service (DHHS PHS) Publication 88-50210, 1988

WOO R et al: Regulation of energy balance, in *Annual Review of Nutrition*, vol 5. Palo Alto, Annual Reviews Inc, 1985, pp 411–433

73 ANOREXIA NERVOSA AND BULIMIA

DANIEL W. FOSTER

Anorexia nervosa and bulimia are eating disorders in young, previously healthy women who develop a paralyzing fear of becoming fat. The population at risk consists largely of white women from middle- and upper-class backgrounds. The disorders rarely occur in black or oriental women, are unusual in the poor, and are almost never seen in men. The driving force is the pursuit of thinness, all other aspects of life being secondary. In the anorexia nervosa syndrome this aim is achieved primarily by radical restriction of caloric intake, the end result being emaciation. In bulimia massive binge eating is followed by vomiting and excessive use of laxatives. Weight loss in bulimic subjects is not great despite the obsession with food. Some authors consider anorexia nervosa and bulimia to be distinct illnesses, while others classify bulimia as a variant of anorexia nervosa. Overlap syndromes exist since emaciated patients fulfilling the criteria of true anorexia nervosa may exhibit bulimic behavior, while subjects with bulimia often pass through a phase of anorexia. In this chapter it is assumed that the two disorders are different clinical expressions of a primary psychologic obsession with body weight.

PREVALENCE Estimates of prevalence for anorexia nervosa range from 0.4 to 1.5 per 100,000 population. In adolescent white girls from middle- or upper-class families rates as high as 1 per 100 have been reported. Prevalence is believed to be increasing. Subclinical variants may occur in up to 5 percent of the socioeconomic group at highest risk. The incidence of bulimia is less certain. Vomiting after eating may occur in as many as 18 percent of women college students. The frequency of self-induced vomiting is probably 1 to 2 percent, but the full-blown bulimic syndrome is less frequent.

DIAGNOSIS The diagnosis of both anorexia nervosa and bulimia is made on clinical grounds. No specific diagnostic tests exist. For many years the criteria of Feighner et al. (Table 73-1) were the basis for diagnosis in research studies. Less strict requirements were formulated for the American Psychiatric Association's *Diagnostic and Statistical Manual of Mental Disorders* (revised, third edition; DSM-IIIR.)

In the revised criteria the weight loss required for diagnosis was decreased from 25 to 15 percent of expected or ideal weight. Three other requirements were listed: intense fear of gaining weight or becoming fat even when underweight; disturbance in the way body weight, size, or shape is experienced such that the individual "feels fat"; and, in women, either primary amenorrhea or secondary amenorrhea for at least three consecutive periods. The Feighner criteria remain useful, although it seems reasonable to substitute the 15 percent figure for weight loss. In actuality the spectrum of restricted eating ranges from a mild disorder of little consequence to life-threatening starvation. For this reason neither set of criteria is definitive.

The uniqueness of the disturbance in body image in patients with eating disorders has been questioned, and some authorities have recommended its omission on the grounds that many normal young women demonstrate the same perceptual distortion. In practice a presumptive diagnosis of anorexia nervosa is justified if the following elements are elicited: (1) a history of major weight loss; (2) absence of organic disease sufficient to account for weight loss; (3) absence of severe primary psychiatric illness that might account for failure to eat; (4) extreme restriction of food intake with or without intermittent induction of vomiting; (4) ritualized exercise; and (5) denial of hunger, fatigue, or emaciation.

The criteria for the diagnosis of bulimia in DSM-IIIR appear to be less useful. The picture is that of a normal- or near-normal-weight subject whose life is dominated by gorging and regurgitation in the absence of profound weight loss.

ETIOLOGY The cause of anorexia nervosa and bulimia is unknown. Although primary dysfunction of the hypothalamus has been

TABLE 73-1 Criteria for the diagnosis of anorexia nervosa

1 Onset prior to age 25
2 Anorexia with weight loss of at least 25 percent of original body weight
3 Distorted attitude toward eating, food, or weight that overrides hunger, admonitions, reassurances, and threats
4 No known medical illness that could account for the weight loss
5 No other known psychiatric disorder
6 At least two of the following manifestations:
 a Amenorrhea
 b Lanugo hair
 c Bradycardia (persistent resting pulse of 60 beats per minute or less)
 d Periods of overactivity
 e Episodes of bulimia
 f Vomiting (may be self-induced)

SOURCE: After Feighner et al.

postulated, the associated hypothalamic abnormalities revert to normal with weight gain and thus are secondary rather than causal.

Most investigators favor a psychiatric etiology, but there is disagreement about its nature. One view holds that the disorders begin in response to inadequate or destructive interpersonal relationships in upper middle class families that are goal-oriented and highly achieving. Despite an outward appearance of normality, interpersonal communication among family members tends to be inadequate, frequently following a pattern in which the father seeks success in his work while the mother turns to her children for fulfillment and in the process becomes overdirective. It is often stated that the families are "enmeshed," meaning that generational boundaries are blurred and that parents and children are constantly involved in each other's problems. Psychoanalytic interpretation tends to focus on anorexia as a mechanism whereby the patient reestablishes control of her own life in a way that is independent of parental direction. It is not clear how this sequence might cause the intense fear of being fat that is the central feature of both anorexia and bulimia.

Although the absence of psychiatric disease is a common criterion for diagnosis (Table 73-1), it is now widely held that depression plays a significant role in the eating disorders. Abnormalities of neurotransmitter concentrations have been reported in blood and cerebrospinal fluid, but such changes are inconsistent and are likely secondary rather than primary.

Cultural issues are also important in anorexia nervosa. The quest for health and slimness is a powerful force in modern western society and may reinforce the fear of fatness in patients with established anorexia or tip the borderline case into full-blown disease. Occupation may play a role; dancers, for example, have a prevalence of anorexia nervosa 10 times that of the general population. Likewise athletes, particularly runners, often seek to decrease body fat to very low levels (5 to 7 percent).

Whatever the mechanism(s) involved, the behavioral response is obsessive and is difficult to treat.

CLINICAL PICTURE While anorexia nervosa and bulimia may coexist in the same patient, the clinical pictures are ordinarily distinct (Table 73-2).

Anorexia nervosa The anorexia nervosa syndrome usually begins before or shortly after puberty but may appear later (rarely later than the middle twenties). Many patients have been overweight in childhood. Emaciation is equivalent to that seen in the concentration camp victims of World War II. Despite profound weight loss the patients deny hunger, thinness, or fatigue. They are often physically active, and ritualized exercise programs are common. Frenzied calisthenics or running may follow food intake. There is a preoccupation with food, and elaborate meals may be prepared for others. If social circumstances require them to eat more than usual, vomiting is induced as soon as possible, often in a public restroom. As noted, episodic binge eating may occur and is also followed by emesis. Amenorrhea usually accompanies or follows weight loss but in a sixth of patients may appear prior to any physical change. Constipation and cold intolerance are common. The latter is presumably due to a defect in regulatory thermogenesis secondary to hypothalamic dysfunction.

TABLE 73-2 The eating disorders

	Anorexia nervosa	Bulimia
Predominant sex	Female	Female
Method of weight control	Restriction of intake	Vomiting
Binge eating	Uncommon	Invariant
Weight at diagnosis	Markedly decreased	Near normal
Ritualized exercise	Usual	Rare
Amenorrhea	~100%	~50%
Antisocial behavior	Rare	Frequent
Cardiovascular changes (bradycardia, hypotension)	Common	Uncommon
Skin changes (hirsutism, dryness, carotenemia)	Usual	Rare
Hypothermia	Usual	Rare
Edema	+/−	+/−
Medical complications	Hypokalemia, cardiac arrhythmias	Hypokalemia, cardiac arrhythmias, aspiration of gastric contents, esophageal or gastric rupture

NOTE: These features are characteristic of pure anorexia nervosa and pure bulimia. Overlap syndromes occur, and anorexia may evolve to bulimia (the bulimia → anorexia transformation is rare).

In advanced cases bradycardia, hypothermia, and hypotension are present. Body fat is undetectable, and the bones protrude through the skin. Interestingly, breast tissue is often preserved. The skin may be dry and scaly and is often yellow due to carotenemia, (particularly visible in the palms). Body hair is often increased; it is usually of fine, lanugo quality, but frank hirsutism may occur. Parotid glands may be enlarged as in other forms of starvation. Mitral valve prolapse is common and is due to valve-ventricular volume mismatch secondary to starvation-induced decrease in left ventricular volume. Edema in the absence of hypoalbuminemia is thought to be due to failure of extracellular fluid volume to diminish proportionately with body mass during weight loss. Because of edema in the legs and parotid enlargement, which gives a fullness to the face, the true state of emaciation may be masked when the patient is fully dressed.

Laboratory abnormalities include anemia and leukopenia (with hypocellularity of the bone marrow), hypokalemia, and hypoalbuminemia. Serum β-carotene levels tend to be elevated. Prerenal azotemia may occur if vomiting or laxative use are prominent. The blood urea nitrogen may be as high as 21 to 25 mmol/L (60 to 70 mg/dL). Renal concentrating ability is impaired, possibly due to blunted responsiveness to antidiuretic hormone. Release of vasopressin in response to an osmotic stimulus is also abnormal. Plasma cholesterol is occasionally high, but triglyceride levels are not increased despite low activities of hepatic and lipoprotein lipases. Glucose tolerance is abnormal as in other forms of starvation.

Miscellaneous abnormalities include low levels of IgG, IgM, and a variety of proteins in the complement pathways. Despite these findings immune function is generally preserved, and serious infections are rare. Plasma iron and ceruloplasmin are normal, but iron binding capacity is decreased. Serum zinc and copper are decreased, but concentrations of these metals are normal in hair. Serum amylase may be increased in the absence of signs or symptoms of pancreatitis.

A variety of endocrine abnormalities are seen. Basal levels of luteinizing hormone (LH) and follicle-stimulating hormone (FSH) are low when weight loss is severe, and the LH response to luteinizing hormone–releasing hormone (LHRH) is impaired. FSH response to LHRH is normal, although time to peak increase may be delayed. Studies of the 24-h circadian pattern of LH secretion show regression of the maturational stage to the pattern characteristic of prepubertal or early pubertal girls; i.e., episodic LH release is missing or occurs only during sleep. These findings presumably account, at least in part, for the amenorrhea. Menses return with weight gain, although the weight required for reinitiation of menstruation may be somewhat higher (~ 10 percent) than that needed for the original induction of menarche. Ovulatory menses may be induced in subjects with anorexia nervosa by prolonged treatment with LHRH agonists, suggesting that pituitary gonadotropin release is impaired because of hypothalamic dysfunction. Prolactin levels are normal. Plasma estradiol levels are low, but plasma testosterone is in the normal female range. Testosterone levels are low in men with anorexia nervosa.

Growth hormone (GH) in the basal state may be normal or elevated. A rise in GH occurs after injection of thyrotropin-releasing hormone (TRH), as in other states with elevated basal levels of GH such as acromegaly, uremia, and protein-calorie malnutrition. Insulin-like growth factor I (somatomedin C) concentrations are low and may contribute to growth hormone elevation via diminished negative feedback. Plasma cortisol levels are high due to increased secretion of corticotropin-releasing hormone from the hypothalamus. The cortisol negative feedback mechanism in the hypothalamus is believed to be impaired. Dexamethasone suppression tests may be abnormal. Norepinephrine concentrations in plasma are depressed.

Thyroxine (T_4) levels are in the low-normal range; free T_4 is normal. Triiodothyronine (T_3) concentrations are reduced, while reverse T_3 (rT_3) levels are increased. Basal levels of thyroid-stimulating hormone (TSH) are usually normal, and TSH response to TRH is intact. The primary defect in thyroid hormone metabolism is decreased activity of the 5′-deiodinase that converts T_4 to T_3 and rT_3 to diiodothyronine in nonthyroidal tissues. These changes are characteristic of starvation and wasting diseases and are not specific for anorexia nervosa.

Bone density is decreased in women with anorexia nervosa. The mechanism is thought to be estrogen deficiency rather than an abnormality in vitamin D metabolism. Cortisol excess may contribute.

Bulimia Bulimia, which means "ox-hunger," refers to the episodic ingestion of large amounts of food in a compulsive fashion, coupled with awareness that the eating pattern is abnormal, a fear that eating cannot be stopped voluntarily, and feelings of depression at completion of the act. Bulimics have a morbid fear of becoming fat. While binge eating may occur in several types of emotional disorders, a high percentage of patients give a history of overt or cryptic anorexia nervosa, suggesting that bulimia is a variant of anorexia nervosa. Episodes of binge eating are followed by induced vomiting, with or without the subsequent ingestion of laxatives. Initially vomiting is induced by placing a toothbrush or fingers in the throat, but eventually most patients learn to vomit reflexly.

Binge eating generally occurs daily in the active phase; in a series of 40 patients the mean number of episodes per week was 12, ranging from 1 to 46. The duration of the eating period averaged 1.2 h but could last as long as 8 h. The amount of food ingested can be enormous, up to 200,000 kJ (50,000 kcal). High-carbohydrate foods are favored, and more than one food is usually eaten. The order of frequency in one report was: ice cream→bread→candy→doughnuts→soft drinks. The term "dietary chaos" describes the eating pattern. Because of the high sugar content of the diet, dental caries are frequent.

Other behavioral abnormalities are common. Secrecy about the eating-vomiting sequence is characteristic so that family and friends are often unaware. Stealing is common, and food is the item most often taken. There is a high rate of alcohol and drug abuse. Depression tends to be more severe than in anorexia nervosa, making suicide a definite risk. Hysterical behavior may occur. Families of patients with bulimia have a higher incidence of affective disorders, alcoholism, and illicit drug use than is seen in families of patients with anorexia nervosa.

Despite the close relationship with anorexia nervosa, a number of differences are noted. While many patients with bulimia are thin, emaciation is not seen; generally weight is within 15 percent of the normal range as defined by life insurance tables of ideal weight. Fluctuating weight is common, with cyclical gains and losses. Some patients are modestly overweight. In contrast to anorexia nervosa, about half of the patients continue to menstruate, and a number have become pregnant. Persistent menstruation probably reflects the absence of extreme weight loss. Sexual activity is greater in bulimic subjects than in those with anorexia.

The physical findings associated with bulimia are usually minimal, although subjects with more extensive weight loss may manifest some of the changes seen with anorexia nervosa.

The most common laboratory abnormality is hypokalemia with metabolic alkalosis secondary to vomiting and laxative use. Endocrine abnormalities are similar to those in anorexia nervosa. One study suggested that LH response to LHRH is exaggerated in bulimic patients, but this has not been confirmed. Dexamethasone suppression is frequently abnormal. Unlike patients with anorexia nervosa, some women with bulimia have low basal prolactin levels and an exaggerated prolactin response to TRH.

COMPLICATIONS Patients with anorexia nervosa are vulnerable to sudden death from ventricular tachyarrhythmias. Electrocardiograms show prolonged QT intervals. The risk of death becomes high when weight loss reaches 35 percent below ideal, probably because of protein deficiency. (Since there is no reserve store of protein, critical enzymes and cellular structures are affected by starvation-induced decreases in lean body mass; see Chap. 71.) Major complications of bulimia include aspiration, esophageal or gastric rupture, pneumomediastinum, hypokalemia with cardiac arrhythmias, pancreatitis, and ipecac-induced myopathy and/or cardiomyopathy.

PROGNOSIS The course of anorexia nervosa is variable. In long-term follow-up about half of patients achieve normal weight, 20 percent improve but remain underweight, 20 percent continue anorexic, 5 percent become obese, and 6 percent die. Even when weight gain occurs, signs of persistent illness remain since intermittent dieting, binge eating, vomiting, and laxative use persist in up to two-thirds of patients. Death is usually due to starvation (cardiac arrhythmias primarily) or suicide. Poor prognostic signs include older age of onset, longer duration of illness, history of bulimia or vomiting, extreme weight loss, and presence of significant depression. Fewer reports of long-term follow-up are available for bulimia than for anorexia nervosa. Because the psychiatric disturbance tends to be more severe (suicide occurs at higher rates) and because the medical dangers of gorging are greater, prognosis is believed to be even worse in bulimia than in anorexia. One report indicates that 40 percent of treated patients remained bulimic after 18 months of treatment and that relapse occurred in 65 percent after 1 year of recovery.

TREATMENT There is no specific treatment for anorexia nervosa or bulimia. The intense fear of becoming fat coupled with a perceptual disturbance that causes overestimation of body size results in powerful resistance to therapy. The benefits of psychiatric intervention are marginal. The same can be said of behavior modification techniques and for group and family therapy. Supportive care by an understanding physician may accomplish as much as formal psychotherapy. The patient should be seen regularly for a review of weight change, diet, and exercise patterns. It is often useful to establish a mutually agreeable explicit contract; e.g., if the patient weighs 65 pounds and ideal body weight determined from life insurance tables is 115 pounds, a goal of 90 pounds might be set as a first stage. At every visit the patient should be reassured by the physician that "we will not let you get fat." A calm but realistic review of the dangers of starvation, including sudden death, should be given, coupled with statements like "my job is to help you deal with this illness so that you can have a normal life expectancy with reasonable happiness." The physician must be perceived not as an enemy or a parental surrogate but an advisor and partner in the struggle.

A similar approach should also be used with bulimic patients. Even if the gorging-regurgitation cycle cannot be stopped, the lesser goal of limiting the load of food ingested (to minimize the chance of aspiration or gastric rupture) and decreasing the frequency of events may be achieved. Because depression and antisocial behavior are more common in bulimia, psychiatric therapy is usually required. It is now common to use antidepressants in both anorexia nervosa and bulimia. Imipramine and phenelzine may be the best choices. Potassium supplementation may be required for vomiters.

Hospitalization may be a lifesaving measure with severe anorexia nervosa. Sudden death may occur at weights more than 35 percent below ideal, particularly if weight loss has been rapid. Hypokalemia, hypotension, and prerenal azotemia due to volume depletion are other indications for hospitalization. If the patient refuses to eat, a nasogastric tube will be required, but it is better to persuade the patient to eat. Supervision of every meal is initially required, ideally by the same person. During the hospitalization the patient should never be allowed to eat alone. Total parenteral nutrition is rarely indicated. Instruction about nutrition, occupational therapy, group work with the family, and individual psychotherapy should be included in the treatment plan. The "safety" of eating and assurances that obesity will not result should be emphasized repetitively. Some specialists feel that all seriously affected anorexia patients benefit from initial hospitalization, but this is not a universal view. Hospitalization for bulimic subjects is normally only required for medical complications (e.g., aspiration).

Treatment of patients with the anorexia-bulimia syndrome is a long-term proposition, rife with failure, and requires perseverance by the subject, family, and physician.

REFERENCES

FEIGHNER JP et al: Diagnostic criteria for use in psychiatric research. Arch Gen Psychiatry 26:57, 1972

FOSTER DW: Eating disorders: Obesity and anorexia nervosa, in *Williams Textbook of Endocrinology*, 7th ed, JD Wilson, DW Foster (eds). Philadelphia, Saunders, 1985, pp 1081–1107

HERZOG DB, COPELAND PM: Eating disorders. N Engl J Med 313:295, 1985

———, ———: Bulimia nervosa—psyche and satiety. N Engl J Med 319:716, 1988

ISNER JM et al: Anorexia nervosa and sudden death. Ann Intern Med 102:49, 1985

LEVY AB: Neuroendocrine profile in bulimia nervosa. Biol Psychiatry 25:98, 1989

——— et al: How are depression and bulimia related? Am J Psychiatry 146:162, 1989

LUCAS AR et al: Anorexia nervosa in Rochester, Minnesota: A 45-year study. Mayo Clin Proc 63:433, 1988

MITCHELL JE et al: Medical complications and medical management of bulimia. Ann Intern Med 107:71, 1987

NEWMAN MM, HALMI KA: The endocrinology of anorexia nervosa and bulimia nervosa. Endocrin Metab Clin North Am 17:195, 1988

74 DIET THERAPY

JOHANNA T. DWYER / JODI ROY

The primary role of diet therapy is to prevent or treat malnutrition, to control diet-related signs and symptoms of disease, to delay the progression of chronic degenerative diseases, and to provide adjunctive support for other medical or surgical treatments. Diet therapy also plays an important role in rehabilitation and in palliation. For example, it may aid in maintaining or enhancing the quality of life in the terminally ill. Nutrition therapy may involve feeding by parenteral and enteral routes and/or use of special purpose oral supplements. Dietary advice may also be useful for health promotion, disease prevention, nutritional support, and rehabilitation.

There are four essential principles for sound diet therapy. First, a nutrition-related problem must be present for which an accepted dietary therapy exists. Second, the diet therapy should be based on a solid scientific rationale. Evidence on the effectiveness of therapeutic diets in ameliorating symptoms, slowing progression, lessening secondary problems or otherwise positively affecting function must be available from sound clinical trials. Anecdotal evidence of improvement alone is insufficient to warrant diet therapy. Third, the patient must be able to eat and must have a functional gastrointestinal tract. (For patients who require enteral nutrition therapy, see Chap. 75.) Finally, the patient must adhere to the diet. Little motivation may be required for a patient to consume a therapeutic diet in the hospital since no other food choice may be available, but a great deal of motivation is needed to buy, prepare, and eat therapeutic diets after discharge.

PLANNING DIET THERAPY

ASSESSMENT Dietary assessment attempts to discover what is eaten, whereas assessment of nutrition status (Chap. 71) is aimed at measuring the interaction of diet, disease, and requirements. Both types of information are needed to identify nutrition-related problems and plan therapeutic diets. Dietary assessment requires cataloging what an individual usually eats and the nutritional quality and adequacy of that diet; it also helps determine nutritional status, establishes or refines differential diagnoses, and furnishes the background information on food intakes and preferences that are needed for implementing dietary therapy.

There are qualitative and quantitative levels of dietary assessment. Qualitative assessment involves determining (1) if the patient is currently eating, following a specific diet, and/or has had recent weight loss or gain; (2) the number of meals per day, any use of nutritional supplements (e.g., amounts and types of vitamin or mineral supplements), special dietary preferences or dietary practices (e.g., consumption of only one or a few foods); and (3) assessment of the physical state (e.g., chewing problems, dysphagia, diarrhea). If the qualitative assessment suggests that nutritional problems may exist, more quantitation should be obtained. For example, the current dietary intake (e.g., the past day) is catalogued using 24-h recalls. The patient is asked to describe, starting with the meal last eaten, what has been consumed over the past 24 h. The intake is then assessed by calculating intakes of nutrients or by comparing intakes to a food grouping system that assumes dietary adequacy. This method is easy to administer, places little burden on the patient, and provides some estimate of intakes. However, 24 h may not be a long enough period to provide a representative intake, and habitual diet may not be assessed. Dietary intake data must reflect a sufficient period of time (weeks or months) for its effects on nutritional status to be meaningful. If changes in intake have occurred, it may also be helpful to recall previous intakes before illness or other events caused dietary alteration.

The patient's habitual diet is assessed using either semiquantitative food-frequency questionnaires, which permit a standardized dietary history to be taken using a list of foods and portion sizes, or the periodic collection of food records for several days at a time. Semiquantitative food-frequency questionnaires make it possible to estimate habitual diet and can be analyzed on a computer. Food records are better for identifying the intake of unusual foods not included on food-frequency questionnaires, but such records are more difficult to obtain and to analyze. Other methods for dietary assessment include the dietary history, in which the patient provides information on usual intakes in an interview with a dietitian. In skilled hands this can reveal usual dietary patterns quickly and is less burdensome to the patient than keeping food records, but training and time are needed to interview in a reproducible manner.

PRESCRIPTION A diet prescription specifies the dietary modifications needed for nutritional therapy. It is usually brief, stated in terms of further assessment needed, the disease to be treated, and the modifications to deal with the disease. The physician is also responsible for making timely changes in diet orders. Failure to make changes can result in such unfortunate events as keeping patients indefinitely on nutritionally inadequate "clear liquid" diets, with resulting debilitation and/or delayed healing.

The rendering of nutrition care requires knowledge about food composition, dietary assessment, diet planning, and diet-counseling techniques. In acute care and inpatient settings the diet order is translated by dietitians to actual foods, menus, or eating plans acceptable to the patient. In outpatient settings, the physician may counsel patients directly, or they may be referred to dietitians.

CARE PLAN The diet order is the first step in the implementation of nutritional intervention. A nutrition care plan is then formulated for the implementation of the diet. The individual who takes responsibility for diet therapy needs to record the nutritional care plan in the medical record and supervise its implementation. The care plan should include a summary of the needs discovered during patient assessment and an implementation plan describing how nutritional objectives are to be reached in terms of food behaviors and any additional resources needed, such as assistance in purchasing food, counseling, education, and help with eating (if necessary). Plans for review, follow-up, and evaluation of progress should also be specified.

IMPLEMENTING DIET THERAPY

USUAL INTAKE The starting point for planning therapeutic diets is the patient's usual intake. The fewer the changes from usual intake, the greater the likelihood that individual preferences will be met and that the new eating plan will be followed. If the usual intake is not nutritionally adequate, the therapeutic plan includes modifications to ensure nutritional sufficiency.

MODIFICATIONS Therapeutic diets involve up to three basic alterations: modifications in route of feeding (see Chap. 75), in consistency, and in food constituents. The appropriate diet for a given condition depends on the stage or severity of disease, characteristics of the patient (age, sex, educational level, ethnicity), the treatment environment (e.g., inpatient, outpatient), and the social situation. For example, there is no single diabetic diet; there are many diets for diabetics, depending upon individual requirements such as whether the patient is on insulin, whether there is a need for weight reduction, and whether coexisting medical complications (such as hyperlipidemia, hypertension or renal disease) are present. Individual planning may be necessary to meet medical demands while ensuring that the planned diet is palatable.

Additional considerations must be taken into account in planning therapeutic diets. The first is meeting the recommended dietary allowances (RDAs) for nutrients (see Table 70-4), and the second is to deal with relevant medical concerns (such as ease of swallowing in a stroke patient, or the timing of feeding in insulin-dependent diabetes mellitus), patient food preferences, and drug-nutrient interactions. Individual hospital manuals specify the diets available in the institution.

Consistency (See Table 74-1) Variations in consistency usually involve two factors. The first is liquidity; major modifications are *clear liquid, full liquid,* and *soft*. The form in which the food constituents are prepared and the type of ingredients constitute the second factor. Options include common foods that have been chopped and blenderized, commercial nutritional supplements formulated with ingredients not usually available in the home, and ''elemental diets'' using nutrients in simple forms such as protein hydrolysates or amino acids. In general, the commercial products are more appetizing because they use stabilizers and other means to keep particles in suspension and because the mixtures are more palatable.

Nutritional adequacy and palatability must be considered in plans that alter consistency. *Clear liquid* diets are nutritionally inadequate and include only a few foods that most people eat regularly, but they may be all that is tolerated immediately after surgery or during severe medical emergencies. *Full liquid* diets include more foods and may be nutritionally adequate, but they are limited in choice compared to normal diets. *Soft* diets are also limited in terms of palatability and deviation from usual diets. For these reasons, modifications in consistency should only be used when absolutely necessary and for as limited a time as feasible.

Composition (See Table 74-2) Modifications in the composition of diets may include energy level, type and amount of nutrients (e.g., lactose-free; low-fat, low saturated fat), or type and amount of other constituents in the diet (e.g., 30 gm soluble fiber, 300 mg cholesterol; low oxalate). Other therapeutic regimens are described in various standard texts.

Several points need emphasis in planning alterations in dietary composition: First, the supporting evidence and documentation of benefits for therapeutic diets vary in their completeness (Table 74-2). For some diseases, such as the hyperlipidemias, the role of diet modification in decreasing serum cholesterol and risk of coronary artery disease is well-documented. For other diseases, such as diabetes mellitus, diet can control acute and short-term symptoms, but its efficacy in altering the long-term sequelae, such as retinopathy and kidney disease, is not established. Patients need to be informed as to what can be expected from the diet therapy instituted.

Second, changes both in consistency and in constituents may be required. For example, simultaneous modifications in a number of constituents are mandatory in diabetes mellitus and renal failure. Such a patient may require an eating plan that controls energy intake, type and amount of carbohydrate, timing of carbohydrate intake, amount of dietary fiber, and the content of fat, protein, and sodium. In some cases there are so many constraints that priority ranking must be given to the most important alteration. With other modifications, less precision is acceptable. Otherwise, it may be impractical to implement the diet therapy.

Third, additional modifications in nutrient composition may be necessary to meet normal physiologic needs (infancy, puberty, pregnancy, lactation). Factors that may need to be considered include inadequacies in recent intake, the timing of nutrient intake (as in insulin-dependent diabetes mellitus), and the presence of specific food allergies or intolerances (e.g., patients on monoamine oxidase

TABLE 74-1 Modifications in diet consistency

Consistency	Purpose	Use	Nutritional adequacy	Comments
Clear liquid: clear broth, gelatin, popsicles, ices; sugar, honey, hard candy; clear fruit juices; clear coffee, tea, and carbonated beverages (as tolerated); low-residue, high-protein, high-calorie clear oral supplements	Short term (1–2 days preferably): to supply fluid and some energy [~2500 kJ/d (~600 kcal/d)] in a form that requires minimal digestion after surgery, trauma, or in acute illness.	Initial feeding after surgery or IV feeding to relieve thirst and hydrate, while minimizing the need to chew and GI-tract stimulation.	Falls seriously short of nutrient needs in energy, protein, vitamins, and minerals; if this diet is to continue beyond 3–5 days, nutritional support is necessary.	Produces few or no feces; greatly different from usual diets.
Full liquid: clear liquids plus: all milk and milk drinks, yogurt; vegetable and fruit juices; refined cooked cereals; butter, margarine; custard, ice cream, pudding; high-protein, high-calorie oral supplements	Supply fluid and meet energy and other nutrient needs more completely with foods that are liquid at body temperature; usually higher in calories than clear liquid diet.	Transition between clear liquid and solid foods after surgery and in acute illness; in esophageal or stomach disorders with strictures or anatomical irregularity; and for inability to chew or swallow solid foods.	May be inadequate in niacin, folacin, and iron due to lack of meat, whole grain, and vegetable intake; adequacy may be improved using high-protein, high-calorie supplements or the addition of a multivitamin supplement.	More complete diet than clear liquid; beneficial as a transitional feeding for weak patients who cannot adequately chew food; greatly different from usual diets.
Soft	Provide foods that can be swallowed with little or no chewing.	For patients who are alert or acutely ill with difficulty in chewing/swallowing, or who are too ill or weak to tolerate a usual diet; for head and neck surgical patients; those with esophageal strictures or poor dentition.	Can be adequate in all nutrients based on menu selection.	Textures can range from pureed (blenderized, strained or smooth foods) to ground, chopped, or soft solids.

TABLE 74-2 Dietary modifications in various diseases

Therapeutic diet modification	Disease	Known benefit(s)	Possible benefit(s)
ENERGY			
Energy controlled	Diabetes mellitus	Increased glucose tolerance, decreased acute side effects	Decreased long-term complications (large vessel atherosclerosis, nephropathy, hypertension)
Low energy	Obesity	Weight loss	
	Hypertension	Decreased systolic and diastolic blood pressure	
	Non-insulin dependent diabetes mellitus	Increased glucose tolerance, decreased short-term symptoms	Decreased long-term complications
High energy	Anorexia	Increased weight, lean body mass, and fat; promotes normal fat and lean tissue	
	Emaciation		
Small feedings	Gastroesophageal reflux	Decreased gastric volume, decreased likelihood of reflux (small feedings in an upright position)	
ENERGY-YIELDING NUTRIENTS			
Protein			
Low protein	Chronic renal failure (end stage renal disease)	Control of blood urea nitrogen, electrolytes, and phosphorus levels (amino acid supplements are used)	
	Hepatic encephalopathy	Prevention of hepatic encephalopathy	
	Early chronic progressive renal disease		Decreased decline in glomerular filtration rate
	Nephrotic syndrome		Decreased protein wasting
Fat			
Low fat	Steatorrhea	Decreased malabsorption	
	Gastroesophageal reflux	Increased lower esophageal sphincter pressure	
	Acute hepatic, pancreatic, and gall bladder disease	Decreased need for bile salts	
	Crohn's disease	Decreased malabsorption in patients with functional lactase deficiency	
	Postgastrectomy dumping	Decreased malabsorption in patients with functional lactase deficiency	
Minerals			
Low sodium	Hypertension	Decreased blood pressure in salt-sensitive individuals	
	Congestive heart failure	Decreased sodium retention, reducing hypertension	
	Chronic renal failure	Decreased sodium retention, reducing hypertension	
	Ascites	Decreased sodium retention	
Low potassium	Hyperkalemia	Decreased serum potassium	
	Chronic renal failure	Decreased serum potassium	
High potassium	Hypokalemia	Increased serum potassium	
High calcium	Osteoporosis		Risk reduction in premenopausal women
Low phosphorus	Hyperphosphatemia	Decreased serum phosphorus	
	Renal failure	Decreased serum phosphorus	
Oxalate			
Low oxalate	Oxalate kidney stones	Decreased concentration of oxalate in the urine	
	Crohn's disease	Decreased malabsorption in patients with steatorrhea	
	Radiation enteritis	Decreased malabsorption	
	Colon, prostate, and breast cancers		Reduced risks in promotional stage via hormonal actions
Low fat, low saturated fat, low cholesterol	Hyperlipidemia	Reduced serum lipids	
	Coronary heart disease	Reduced serum lipids	Fosters regression of some arterial plaques (if diet is extreme and long-continued)

(continued)

inhibitors). Other problems, such as the inability to feed oneself, vegetarianism, religious beliefs that prohibit certain foods, alcoholism, and specific likes and dislikes also need to be taken into account.

Fourth, elaborate diet prescriptions place a burden on patients. Complicated diets may cause only minor problems in the hospitalized patient but create major compliance problems for outpatients. When the continuation of such diets is necessary, diet counseling prior to discharge should be supplemented by frequent outpatient visits.

Even within a given disease category the role of dietary therapy may vary, and there may be no single "therapeutic diet" for a given disease.

Modifications for hypercholesterolemia The associations between dietary modifications and lowering of serum cholesterol are well-described and, at least in men, predictable, and the association between lowering of serum cholesterol and decreases in the complications of coronary artery disease is clear-cut. Hence, diet therapy is the first step in the treatment of most hyperlipidemic states. Table 74-3 summarizes the current recommendations for diet therapy of

TABLE 74-2 Dietary modifications in various diseases *(continued)*

Therapeutic diet modification	Disease	Known benefit(s)	Possible benefit(s)
OTHER CONSTITUENTS			
Fiber			
High fiber	Atonic constipation	Increased stool bulk and decreased transit time	
	Diverticulosis	Increased stool bulk and decreased colonic pressure, preventing the production of diverticula	
	Irritable bowel syndrome	Decreased constipation	
	Colon cancer		Risk reduction
	Crohn's disease (inactive)		Symptom control
	Diabetes mellitus	Improved glycemic control, reduced insulin requirements	
	Hyperlipidemia		Decreased serum cholesterol (high water-soluble fiber)
Low fiber	Crohn's disease/ulcerative colitis (active phase)	Reduced diarrhea and pain	
	Crohn's disease (inactive phase)		Symptom control
Gluten			
Gluten-free	Celiac disease	Decreased malabsorption and gut damage due to gluten enteropathy	
Lactose			
Lactose-free	Lactose intolerance	Decreased malabsorption	

TABLE 74-3 Recommendations of American Heart Association/National Cholesterol Education Program: step 1 and step 2 diets for hypercholesterolemia

Indications
- LDL cholesterol >4.1 mmol/L (>160 mg/dL)
- LDL cholesterol >3.4 mmol/L (>130 mg/dL) with definite coronary disease or two other risk factors*

Minimal goals
- Without coronary disease or two risk factors: Lower LDL cholesterol below 4.1 mmol/L (160 mg/dL)
- With coronary disease or two risk factors: Lower LDL cholesterol below 3.4 mmol/L (130 mg/dL)

	% of total calories	
Recommended intake	Step 1 diet	Step 2 diet (if serum lipid goal not reached)
Total fat	<30%	<30%
Saturated fatty acids	<10%	< 7%
Polyunsaturated fatty acids	<10%	<10%
Monounsaturated fatty acids	10–15%	10–15%
Carbohydrates	50–60%	50–60%
Protein	10–20%	10–20%
Cholesterol	<300 mg/d	<200 mg/d
Total energy intake	To achieve and maintain desirable weight	To achieve and maintain desirable weight

* Risk factors include male sex, family history of premature coronary distress, cigarette smoking, hypertension, low HDL cholesterol level, diabetes mellitus, history of definite cerebrovascular or occlusive peripheral vascular disease, severe obesity.

NOTE: LDL = low-density lipoprotein; HDL = high-density lipoprotein.

SOURCE: Adapted from National Cholesterol Education Program: Arch Intern Med 148:36, 1988.

TABLE 74-4 Nutritional recommendations for patients with diabetes mellitus

Energy intake: Achieve and maintain a desirable body weight.
Carbohydrate: (1) Up to 55–60% of the total calories; (2) Substitute unrefined complex carbohydrates with fiber for highly refined carbohydrates; (3) Modest amounts of sucrose and other refined sugars acceptable.
Protein: Consistent with the RDA of 0.8 g/kg of ideal body weight.
Total fat and cholesterol: Restrict to <30% total calories from fat, and cholesterol <300 mg/d.
Alternative sweeteners: Nutritive and non-nutritive sweeteners both acceptable in moderation.
Salt intake: <3000 mg/d.
Alcohol: If at all, in moderation.
Vitamins and minerals: Meet the RDA.

SOURCE: Adapted from Franz MJ et al: J Am Diet Assoc 87:28, 1987.

those adults at high risk [(e.g., total serum cholesterol >6.2 mmol/L (<240 mg/dL)] jointly endorsed by the National Cholesterol Education Program (NCEP) and the American Heart Association (AHA) and includes the indications for diet therapy in terms of the individual's serum lipid values (also see Chaps. 195 and 326).

The NCEP recommends a "step-care" approach in dealing with hyperlipidemia. Patients at risk are first placed on the step 1 diet (unless they are at very high risk), which is modified in total fat, saturated fat, cholesterol, and energy intake. After a period of 2 months the serum cholesterol is evaluated. Those who, despite adherence, do not achieve the goals of therapy on the step 1 diet are asked to continue the diet trial and are provided with additional assistance. Patients who still fail to lower their serum cholesterol to acceptable levels with diet are moved to the step 2 diet, which is even lower in saturated fat and cholesterol. If serum cholesterol levels are still not reduced sufficiently, drug therapy is added, and, if dietary efforts fail completely, drug therapy alone may be used.

Hyperlipidemic patients may also have hypertension, diabetes mellitus, chronic renal insufficiency, or other diseases that require additional dietary modifications.

Modifications for diabetes mellitus Table 74-4 outlines the nutritional recommendations for individuals with diabetes mellitus, and Table 74-5 summarizes a widely used tool—the exchange list. Exchange lists describe the serving size of various foods in groups that are similar in nutrient value. Exchange lists vary depending on the disease and the desired dietary modifications. Such lists provide an overall meal plan that allows selection of different foods and menus. However, the type and amount of dietary carbohydrate and fat and the energy intake ingested throughout the day need to be considered in planning the diet, drug schedule, and physical activity patterns. Diet therapy in diabetes is helpful in controlling the acute manifestations (excessive thirst, frequent urination, blurred vision, etc.) of hyperglycemia. Diet may also reduce the risk of accelerated atherosclerosis.

Alterations in dietary fiber Modifications in the type and amount of dietary fiber can sometimes ameliorate functional constipation or diarrhea. Increased dietary fiber intakes, particularly of water-insoluble fibers like wheat bran, also provide symptomatic relief in diverticulosis of the colon. Some water-soluble fibers in large doses may decrease serum cholesterol levels; these include fiber derived from oat bran, beans, and psyllium seeds.

Lactose-free diets Many adults, especially Orientals and blacks, have hereditary intestinal lactase deficiency. Lactose intolerance may

TABLE 74-5 Exchange list for meal planning for diabetics

Exchange list food group	Carbohydrate, grams	Protein, grams	Fat, grams	Energy intake, kilojoules (kilocalories)
Starch/bread ½ cup (120 mL) cereal, grain, or pasta 1 ounce (30 g) of a bread product	15	3	Trace	335 (80)
Meat 1 ounce (30 g) cooked				
Lean	—	7	3	230 (55)
Medium-fat	—	7	5	315 (75)
High-fat	—	7	8	415 (100)
Vegetable ½ cup (120 mL) cooked or juice 1 cup (240 mL) raw	5	2	—	105 (25)
Fruit ½ cup (120 mL) fresh or juice ¼ cup (60 mL) dried	15	—	—	250 (60)
Milk 1 cup (240 mL)				
Skim	12	8	Trace	375 (90)
Low-fat	12	8	5	500 (120)
Whole	12	8	8	625 (150)
Fat 1 tsp. butter, margarine, oil, mayonnaise (5 mL) 1 Tbsp. salad dressing (15 mL)	—	—	5	190 (45)

NOTE: Saturated fat, fiber and sodium intakes are controlled by choices within food groups
SOURCE: American Diabetes Association and the American Dietetic Association: *Exchange Lists for Meal Planning*, 1986.

also be secondary, either acquired or as the result of gastrointestinal disease. Elimination of lactose from the diet reduces the diarrhea due to the osmotic action of unabsorbed lactose in the gut lumen (see Chap. 240).

Gluten-free diets Gluten, a protein found primarily in wheat products, produces a toxic reaction causing villous atrophy in patients with sprue or celiac disease. Elimination of gluten from the diet is essential and requires substitution of foods from sources such as rice or potato (see Chap. 240).

Caffeine Caffeine can cause untoward behavioral effects in large doses (e.g., 1000 mg or more—the equivalent of 10 cups of coffee a day). Some patients with reflux esophagitis, hypermotility syndrome, and peptic ulcer disease may also benefit from reducing or eliminating caffeine from the diet.

Unproven dietary remedies Many legitimate therapeutic diets exist in addition to those mentioned in Table 74-2. However, not all popular dietary remedies are well-documented and useful. For example, there is no evidence that special diets have any role in alleviating or treating premenstrual syndrome, migraine headaches, hyperactivity, fibrocystic disease of the breast, or acne; that a polyunsaturated fat diet is beneficial for multiple sclerosis; or that a macrobiotic diet is useful in patients with cancer.

HOW DIETARY CHANGES ARE ACHIEVED Dietary change is achieved by altering the amounts and the frequency of food con-

TABLE 74-6 Rich food sources of vitamins

Vitamin	Alternative names	Richest sources
Vitamin A (plus carotenoids)	Retinol (vitamin A alcohol)	Liver, egg yolk, chicken meat; whole milk, butter; breakfast cereals; margarines fortified with vitamin A
Carotenoids	β-Carotene (most plentiful)	Dark-green leafy vegetables like spinach, chard; yellow vegetables like carrots, squash; yellow fruits like mango, cantaloupe
Vitamin D	D_3 (cholecalciferol) D_2 (ergocalciferol)	Fatty fish like salmon and fish oils; eggs; butter; liver; milk fortified with vitamin D
Vitamin E	Alpha tocopherol	Oils from soybean, sunflower, corn, and cottonseed; germ of whole grains; fish liver oils; nuts
Thiamin	Vitamin B_1	Whole grains, dried legumes; pork muscle, liver; products made with enriched flour
Riboflavin	Vitamin B_2	Milk and milk products; eggs; whole- and enriched-grain products; lean meat, liver, poultry, fish; dark-green vegetables like spinach, asparagus
Niacin	Nicotinic Acid	Meats, poultry, fish; yeast; whole- and enriched-grain products; legumes; nuts; in addition, some of the tryptophan present in meats, poultry, fish, cheese, legumes, and seeds can be converted in the body to niacin
Vitamin B_6	Pyridoxine Pyridoxal Pyridoxamine	Meat, poultry, fish; bananas; yeast; bran; and nuts
Vitamin B_{12}	Cobalamin	Only in foods of animal origin: liver, muscle meats, fish, eggs, and milk and milk products
Folacin	Folic Acid Folate	Liver; dark-green leafy vegetables like spinach, romaine lettuce; dry beans, peanuts, wheat germ, whole grains; yeast
Vitamin C	Ascorbic Acid	Citrus fruits like oranges, lemons, grapefruit; dark-green leafy vegetables like broccoli, asparagus

SOURCE: National Academy of Sciences Committee on Diet and Health: *Diet and Health Report*, 1989.

sumption. Nutrients are not equally distributed throughout all foods, and Tables 74-6 and 74-7 list food sources rich in selected vitamins and minerals.

Substitutions within food groups can alter diet composition. For example, using skim milk instead of whole milk lowers the amount of fat but does not alter its contribution of other nutrients (protein, calcium, and phosphorus). Lean cuts of meat, skinned chicken, and lean fish contain less fat than fried meats, but have the same content of protein, vitamins, and minerals.

When many simultaneous reductions must be made in nutrient intakes, development of a reasonable eating plan can be time-consuming and difficult. Computerized menu planning systems or use of simplified exchange systems and menu-planning guides may be helpful in some circumstances.

ORAL NUTRITIONAL SUPPLEMENTS WITH SPECIAL CHARACTERISTICS Diets to meet therapeutic needs may utilize readily available foods, but flexibility is enhanced by the inclusion of specially formulated dietary products (Table 74-8). These products can be of great help in planning menus that are palatable and that permit some latitude on the part of the patient. Some of the products are particularly useful for complex therapeutic diets.

SPECIAL PROBLEMS IN DIET THERAPY

TRANSITIONS FROM ONE ROUTE OF FEEDING TO ANOTHER Transitional feeding refers to the return to the usual feeding pattern

TABLE 74-7 Rich food sources of minerals

Mineral	Sources
Calcium	Milk, cheese, broccoli, dark-green leafy vegetables such as collard, turnip, and mustard greens
Phosphorus	Meats, milk products, grains, phosphate, food additives
Magnesium	Green vegetables, nuts, seeds, dried beans, whole grains, and meats
Iron	Liver, red meat, whole-grain and enriched-grain products, beans, nuts, and dark-green leafy vegetables
Zinc	Shellfish, meat, poultry, cheese, whole grains, dry beans, nuts
Copper	Crab meat, fresh vegetables and fruits, nuts, seeds, legumes
Sodium	Salt (sodium chloride); cured meats (ham, bacon, sausage, frankfurters, luncheon meats); cheeses, olives; pickles; condiment sauces; frozen and canned meat and fish entrees and dinners; canned and dried soups; commercial pasta, noodle, and potato dishes; salted snacks; commercial mixes for waffles, muffins, and cakes; canned vegetables with sauces; baking powder; baking soda; certain emulsifiers and other food additives; drinking water; drugs such as some antacids.
Potassium	Milk, fruits (especially oranges, prunes, apples, pears, peaches, bananas, and grapefruit), vegetables (especially fresh broccoli, carrots, tomatoes, and potatoes), fish, shellfish, turkey, chicken, and cooked oatmeal.

SOURCE: National Academy of Sciences Committee on Diet and Health: *Diet and Health Report*, 1989.

TABLE 74-8 Nutrient composition of oral nutritional supplements

				Percent of energy			
	Manufacturer	kJ/mL	kcal/mL	Protein	Fat	Carbohydrate	Comments
CLEAR LIQUID FORMULAS							
Citrotein	Sandoz Nutrition	2.8	0.66	25	2	73	
Ross SLD (surgical liquid diet)	Ross	2.9	0.70	21	1	78	
FULL LIQUID FORMULAS							
Milk-based formulas							
Carnation Instant Breakfast	Carnation Company	4.4	1.06	21	27	52	
Meritene Liquid	Sandoz Nutrition	4.0	0.96	24	30	46	
Meritene Powder	Sandoz Nutrition	4.4	1.06	26	29	45	
Sustacal Nutritional Powder	Mead Johnson	5.4	1.30	23	23	54	
Sustagen	Mead Johnson	7.7	1.85	24	8	68	
Blenderized formulas							
Compleat Modified Formula	Sandoz Nutrition	4.5	1.07	16	31	53	Lactose-free; gluten-free
Compleat Regular Formula	Sandoz Nutrition	4.5	1.07	16	36	48	
Vitaneed	Sherwood Medical	4.2	1.00	16	35	49	Lactose-free
Formulas with fiber							
Enrich	Ross	4.6	1.10	14	29	57	Lactose-free; 14 g fiber per L
Sustacal with Fiber	Mead Johnson	4.4	1.06	17	29	54	Lactose-free; 5 g fiber per L
Jevity	Ross	4.4	1.06	16	30	54	Isotonic,* lactose-free; 14 g fiber per L
Lactose-free formulas							
Ensure	Ross	4.4	1.06	14	31	55	Low-residue*
Resource Plus Liquid	Sandoz Nutrition	6.2	1.50	15	32	53	Gluten-free; low-residue
Sustacal Liquid	Mead Johnson	4.2	1.01	24	20	56	Low-residue
Travasorb MCT Diet	Clinitec Nutrition Co.	6.7	1.60	20	30	50	
Resource Instant Crystals	Sandoz Nutrition	4.4	1.06	14	31	55	Low-residue
Resource Liquid	Sandoz Nutrition	4.4	1.06	14	31	55	Gluten-free; low-residue
Comply	Sherwood Medical	6.2	1.50	16	36	48	
Ensure Plus	Ross	6.2	1.50	15	32	53	Low-residue
Sustacal HC	Mead Johnson	6.4	1.52	16	34	50	Low-residue
Ensure Plus HN	Ross	6.2	1.50	17	30	53	Low-residue
Isocal HCN	Mead Johnson	8.4	2.00	15	45	40	
Magnacal	Sherwood Medical	8.4	2.00	14	36	50	Low-residue
Two Cal HN	Ross	8.4	2.00	17	40	43	
Isotonic formulas*							
Attain	Sherwood Medical	4.2	1.00	16	36	48	Lactose-free; low-residue
Osmolite	Ross	4.4	1.06	14	32	54	Lactose-free; low-residue
Precision Isotonic Diet	Sandoz Nutrition	4.0	0.96	12	28	60	Lactose-free; gluten-free; purine-free

(continued)

TABLE 74-8 Nutrient composition of oral nutritional supplements *(continued)*

	Manufacturer	kJ/mL	kcal/mL	Percent of energy: Protein	Fat	Carbohydrate	Comments
FULL LIQUID FORMULAS *(continued)*							
Isotonic formulas* *(continued)*							
Isocal	Mead Johnson	4.4	1.06	13	37	50	Lactose-free; low-residue
Isosource	Ross	5.2	1.25	14	30	56	Lactose-free; low-residue; gluten-free
Isotein HN	Sandoz Nutrition	5.0	1.20	23	25	52	Lactose-free; low-residue; gluten-free
Isosource HN	Sandoz Nutrition	5.4	1.28	17	30	53	High-nitrogen; isotonic; lactose-free; gluten-free; low-residue
Osmolite HN	Ross	4.4	1.06	17	31	52	Lactose-free; low-residue
Specialized use formulas							
Amin-Aid Instant Drink	Kendall McGraw	8.2	1.96	4	21	75	Requires vitamin, mineral, and electrolyte supplementation
Attain L.S.	Sherwood Medical	4.2	1.00	16	36	48	Lactose-free; low-residue
Pre-Attain	Sherwood Medical	2.1	0.50	16	36	48	Lactose-free
Hepatic Aid II Instant Drink	Kendall McGraw	4.9	1.18	15	28	57	Requires vitamin, mineral, and electrolyte supplementation
Lonalac	Mead Johnson	4.2	1.00	21	49	30	
Portagen	Mead Johnson	4.2	1.01	14	41	45	Lactose-free
Precision High Nitrogen Diet	Sandoz Nutrition	4.4	1.05	17	1	82	Lactose-free; low-residue; gluten-free
Precision LR Diet	Sandoz Nutrition	4.2	1.10	9	1	90	Lactose-free; low-residue; gluten-free
Pulmocare	Ross	6.3	1.50	17	55	28	Lactose-free
Stresstein	Sandoz Nutrition	5.0	1.20	23	21	56	Lactose-free; no residue
Traum-Aid HBC	Kendall McGraw	4.2	1.00	24	6	70	Lactose-free; low-residue
TraumaCal	Mead Johnson	6.3	1.50	22	40	38	Lactose-free
Travasorb Hepatic	Clinitec Nutrition Co.	4.6	1.10	11	12	77	Low aromatic amino acids
Travasorb Renal	Clinitec Nutrition Co.	5.7	1.35	7	12	81	Requires vitamin, mineral, and electrolyte supplementation
Hydrolyzed protein-elemental formulas*							
Carnation Peptamen Liquid, Isotonic, Complete, Elemental Diet	Clinitec Nutrition Co.	4.2	1.00	16	34	50	Lactose-free
Criticare HN	Mead Johnson	4.4	1.06	14	3	83	Lactose-free; low-residue
Pepti 2000	Sherwood Medical	4.2	1.00	16	9	75	Lactose-free; low-residue
Travasorb HN	Clinitec Nutrition Co.	4.2	1.00	18	12	70	Lactose-free; low-residue
Travasorb STD	Clinitec Nutrition Co.	4.2	1.00	12	12	76	Lactose-free; low-residue
Vital High Nitrogen	Ross	4.2	1.00	17	10	73	Lactose-free; low-residue
Vivonex HN	Norwich Eaton	4.2	1.00	18	1	81	Lactose-free; no residue
Vivonex Standard	Norwich Eaton	4.2	1.00	9	1	90	Lactose-free; no residue
Vivonex T.E.N.	Norwich Eaton	4.2	1.00	15	3	82	Lactose-free; low-residue
HIGH CALORIE SOFT SUPPLEMENTS		kJ/g	kcal/g				
Puddings							
Ensure Pudding	Ross	7.5	1.8	11	35	54	Gluten-free
Sustacal Pudding	Mead Johnson	7.5	1.7	11	36	53	
Forta Pudding	Ross	7.5	1.8	14	32	54	Lactose free

(continued)

after total parenteral nutrition, peripheral hyperalimentation, or enteral feeding by gastrostomy, jejunostomy, esophagostomy, or nasogastric tube. After extended periods of disuse, the gut may not function normally, and unless the transition process is carefully monitored, ad libitum oral intakes and/or food absorption may be inadequate.

ADHERENCE TO DIET Compliance with therapeutic dietary recommendations is relatively easy to monitor if the patient is hospitalized. A menu that conforms to the diet orders is offered and choices are made in line with the therapeutic prescription (and if the choices are not appropriate, substitutes are made). However, the

TABLE 74-8 Nutrient composition of oral nutritional supplements *(continued)*

	Manufacturer			Percent of energy: Protein	Fat	Carbohydrate	Comments
MODULAR SYSTEMS (SINGLE NUTRIENT SOURCES)		kJ/g or /mL	kcal/g or /mL				
Protein nodules							
Casec	Mead Johnson	15.5	3.7	96	4	<1	Powder
Nutrisource Amino Acids	Sandoz Nutrition	16.3	3.9	100	0	0	Powder
Nutrisource Amino Acids -High BCAA	Sandoz Nutrition	15.9	3.8	100	0	0	Powder
Nutrisource Protein	Sandoz Nutrition	16.7	4.0	75	19	6	Powder
Pro Mod	Ross	17.6	4.2	72	19	9	Powder
Propac	Sherwood Medical	16.7	4.0	77	18	5	Powder
RDP	Corpak, Inc.	15.1	3.6	84	10	6	Powder
Fat nodules							
High Fat Supplement	Corpak, Inc.	25.5	6.12	3	70	27	Powder
MCT Oil	Mead Johnson	32.3	7.7	0	100	0	Liquid
Nutrisource Lipid-Long-Chain Triglycerides	Sandoz Nutrition	9.2	2.2	0	100	0	Liquid
Nutrisource Lipid-Medium Chain Triglycerides	Sandoz Nutrition	8.4	2.0	0	100	0	Liquid
Microlipid	Sherwood Medical	18.8	4.5	0	100	0	Liquid
Carbohydrate nodules							
Liquid Carbohydrate Supplement	Corpak, Inc.	10.5	2.5	0	0	100	Liquid
Moducal	Mead Johnson	15.9	3.8	0	0	100	Powder
Nutrisource Carbohydrate	Sandoz Nutrition	13.4	3.2	0	0	100	Liquid
Polycose Powder	Ross	15.9	3.8	0	0	100	Powder
Polycose Liquid	Ross	8.4	2.0	0	0	100	Liquid
Pure Carbohydrate Supplement	Corpak, Inc.	16.7	4.0	0	0	100	Powder
Sumacal	Sherwood Medical	15.9	3.8	0	0	100	Powder
LOW-PROTEIN PRODUCTS		kJ/50 g	kcal/50 g				
Low-protein noodles	Aproten	322	77	1	2	97	
Low-protein cookies	Kingsmill	1046	250	<1	41	59	
Low-protein bread	Dietary Specialties	527	126	2	20	78	
FIBER SUPPLEMENTS		kJ/20 g	kcal/20 g				
Fiber Med	Purdue Frederick Co.	243	70	11	26	63	
Fiberall	Ciba-Geigy Corp.	331	79	5	46	49	

* Definitions: Low-residue = producing little or no stool; isotonic = having the tonicity of plasma (308 mosmol/L); hydrolyzed protein-elemental formula = nutrients partially or completely digested.

SOURCE: Modified from the American Dietetic Association: *Manual of Clinical Dietetics,* 1988.

patient may refuse to eat or may miss meals because of diagnostic tests. Therefore, nutritional status and patient adherence should be monitored carefully even in the hospital.

To implement outpatient therapeutic diets, the patient must be motivated and must understand the diet instructions and the changes in what is to be eaten. New habits of food buying, food preparation, cooking, and eating may be required. Selections when dining out are also altered. These changes are difficult to make and even more difficult to sustain.

Psychological support; assistance in learning new food preparation, buying, and management skills; help with eating (in disabilities such as stroke); help in obtaining financial assistance to buy special foods; and general education about the importance of diet are as important as nutritional advice.

ASSURING THE CONTINUITY OF NUTRITIONAL CARE: THE TEAM CONCEPT Nutrition is too important to be the sole responsibility of a single member of the health team. Nutritional counseling can and does change dietary habits, and each health-care provider has a critical role in assuring that nutrition is adequate. However, physicians rarely obtain thorough diet histories, address potential barriers to change in eating habits, or offer special guidance on food selection. The major role of physicians is to expand the content of the nutritional information they provide, to emphasize the health benefits of good nutrition, and to refer those requiring help to specialized providers when available.

REFERENCES

NATIONAL RESEARCH COUNCIL: *Recommended Dietary Allowances,* 10th ed. Washington, DC, National Academy of Sciences, 1989

OLSON RE et al: *Present Knowledge in Nutrition.* Washington, DC, The Nutrition Foundation, 1984

PAIGE DM: *Clinical Nutrition.* St Louis, 1988

SHILS ME, YOUNG VR: *Modern Nutrition in Health and Disease. Philadelphia, Lea & Febiger, 1988*

SLEISENGER MH, FORDTRAN JS: *Gastrointestinal Disease: Pathophysiology, Diagnosis and Management,* 4th ed. Philadelphia, Saunders, 1988, pp 1971–2023

75 PARENTERAL AND ENTERAL NUTRITION THERAPY

LYN J. HOWARD

Parenteral and enteral nutrition provide life-sustaining therapy for patients who cannot take adequate nutrition by mouth and who consequently are at risk for the debilitating complications of malnutrition. These complications include greater susceptibility to infection and to the consequences of hypomotility (aspiration, pulmonary embolism), delayed recovery from illness and surgery, and an increased likelihood of death.

Although the term *enteral* refers to feeding via the gut and hence includes normal eating, in the present context it refers to the infusion of chemically defined formulas via a tube into the upper gastrointestinal tract. *Parenteral,* which means outside the gut, refers to the infusion of nutrient solutions into the bloodstream. While these approaches to nutritional support are technically different, the goals of therapy are by and large the same, and the techniques are best discussed concurrently. Wherever feasible, enteral nutrition is the preferred therapy because it better preserves immunologic defense mechanisms and is less expensive than parenteral nutrition.

Enteral tube feeding initially involved large-bore rubber tubes placed via the nose or through an ostomy into the stomach or jejunum, but these large tubes have been replaced by small-bore pliable tubes that remain soft with continued exposure to digestive juices. Endoscopic techniques have also been developed for placement of gastrostomy feeding tubes without the need for a surgical laparotomy. For many years, long-term tube feeding was used principally in hospitalized patients with chronic swallowing dysfunction or upper intestinal obstruction, but enteral feeding is now also used in the home setting.

Parenteral nutrition therapy has younger roots. After the life raft studies in the 1940s by Gamble demonstrated that small amounts of glucose (100 g/d) spared protein in fasting subjects, hypocaloric intravenous glucose infusions became routine therapy for hospitalized patients unable to eat. In the 1960s Dudrick and his colleagues demonstrated that it is possible to provide energy, amino acids, minerals, and vitamins via long-term infusion into a central vein catheter adequate to produce positive nitrogen balance and promote wound healing in adults and to support growth and development in infants. Subsequently, total parenteral nutrition became practical in hospitalized patients and in outpatients.

Isotonic amino acid solutions are more effective than isotonic glucose in counteracting negative nitrogen balance in fasting subjects, and the development of high-energy, isotonic intravenous fat solutions made it possible to deliver adequate amino acids and calories via a peripheral vein. However, peripheral veins usually do not withstand these nutrient infusions indefinitely, and long-term support usually requires access to a central vein.

INDICATIONS FOR ASSISTED THERAPY

The principles of nutritional assessment are discussed in Chap. 71. Some criteria used to define moderate and severe malnutrition in hospitalized patients are summarized in Table 75-1. Since none of these measurements is entirely specific for malnutrition, a weighted combination of the individual measurements has been developed, the so-called prognostic nutritional index. This index predicts, with reasonable sensitivity (0.88) and specificity (0.45), patients at risk for malnutrition-associated complications. Clinical assessment provides a somewhat better combination of sensitivity (0.82) and specificity (0.72). For this purpose the medical history must address recent weight change and the effects of the primary disease on nutritional and functional status, and the physical examination must assess muscle mass and fat, edema, glossitis, and other signs indicative of micronutrient deficiencies. On the basis of this information, the physician categorizes patients as well-nourished, mildly malnourished, or severely malnourished. The inter-observer agreement is high.

In some clinical situations (e.g., the early phase of the extreme short-bowel syndrome, severe hemorrhagic pancreatitis, pseudomembranous colitis, necrotizing enterocolitis, and clinical conditions causing prolonged ileus) parenteral nutrition and bowel rest improve survival (Table 75-2). In other situations, where the need for total bowel rest may not be essential, enteral nutrition or a combination of enteral and limited parenteral nutrition can be successful and perhaps preferable. Disorders in this category include enterocutaneous fistulas, intractable diarrhea of infancy, and the later stages of the extreme short-bowel syndrome.

It is important to demonstrate that nutrition support leads to improved clinical outcome and not just to better nitrogen balance or increased serum albumin. Valid clinical end points include improved survival, fewer complications, or shorter hospital stays.

PERIOPERATIVE PERIOD Perioperative nutrition has a beneficial effect on complications and survival of surgical patients. Studley pointed out in 1936 that mortality rates after surgery for peptic ulcer are greater in patients with severe preoperative weight loss, and subsequent studies have confirmed the association between poor nutrition and poor surgical outcome. In a review of 18 controlled trials, 14 of which involved patient randomization, perioperative parenteral nutrition reduced the relative risk[1] of a major surgical complication, such as wound dehiscence, abscess, prolonged ileus, and sepsis, by a fifth and the relative risk of death by a third. A major complication of parenteral nutrition, including pneumothorax, central vein thrombosis, or sepsis, occurred in 7 percent of this pooled patient sample. In addition preliminary results of a large cooperative Veterans Administration trial indicate that perioperative nutrition also reduces noninfectious complications that relate both to prolonged immobility (pulmonary embolus) and to delayed wound healing in patients with moderative and severe malnutrition. Unfortunately, perioperative parenteral nutrition increased infectious complications, even infections not directly related to the central line. Because of these iatrogenic complications, perioperative nutrition provides medical benefit only to severely malnourished surgical patients.

CANCER Although early nonrandomized studies suggested that significant benefit ensues from parenteral nutritional support of cancer patients, randomized trials have largely shown no clinical benefit,

[1]Relative risk is the absolute difference in rate of events in the control group and represents the proportionate reduction in events attributable to perioperative parenteral nutrition.

TABLE 75-1 Quantitative values commonly used to stratify nutritional status

Method of assessment	Moderately malnourished	Severely malnourished
Ideal weight, %	60–80	<60
Creatinine-height index: (24-h urine creatinine) $\frac{\text{Actual}}{\text{Ideal for height and sex}} \times 100$ (see Table 71-5)	60–80	<60
Serum albumin, g/L (g/dL)	21–30 (2.1–3.0)	<21 (<2.1)
Serum transferrin, g/L (mg/dL)	1–1.5 (100–150)	<1 (<100)
Total lymphocyte count, 10^6/L (per mm^3)	0.8–1.2 (800–1200)	<0.8 (<800)
Delayed hypersensitivity index*	1	0
Prognostic nutritional index, %†	40–50	>50

* Delayed hypersensitivity index quantitates the amount of induration elicited by skin testing with a common antigen such as *Candida,* trichophyton, or mumps. Induration grade: 0 = <0.5 cm, 1 = 0.5 cm, 2 = 1.0 cm.

† Prognostic nutritional index (PNI) is a weighted combination of four individual measurements: PNI (%) = 158 − 1.66 × albumin (g/L) − 0.78 × triceps skinfold (mm) − 2.0 × transferrin (g/L) − 5.8 × delayed hypersensitivity index (0–2).

TABLE 75-2 Indications for nutritional support

HOSPITALIZED PATIENT	Enteral nutrition (EN)	Parenteral nutrition (PN)
Part of routine care	Protein-energy malnutrition [>10% acute weight loss, serum albumin <35 g/L (<3.5 g/dL)], no intake for >5 days Normal nutritional status but no intake for >10 days Severe dysphagia or anorexia Major full-thickness burns Massive small-bowel resection in combination with PN Low output enterocutaneous fistulas	Massive small bowel resection (>70%) Moderate to severe acute pancreatitis Established or clinically predictable malnutrition when the gastrointestinal tract is not usable for >7 days Necrotizing enterocolitis
Usually helpful	Major trauma Radiation therapy Mild chemotherapy Severe hepatic, renal and chronic pulmonary failure	Severe preoperative malnutrition Major surgery, trauma, including burns, where enteral absorption inadequate High output enterocutaneous fistulas Severe Crohn's disease requiring bowel rest or involving marked growth failure Inflammatory adhesions leading to small-bowel obstruction Hyperemesis gravidarum Intensive chemotherapy resulting in severe diarrhea
Benefit not established	Intensive chemotherapy Immediate postoperative period or poststress period Massive small-bowel resection (>90%) Severe diarrhea Severe bowel hypomotility	Minimal stress and trauma, where well-nourished and gastrointestinal tract expected to recover within 10 days Suspected untreatable disease state
Contraindicated	Complete mechanical or functional bowel obstruction High-output fistulas Severe acute pancreatitis Shock and bowel ischemia Necrotizing enterocolitis Prognosis not warranting nutritional support	Patients who have a functional and usable gastrointestinal tract When dependence on PN is anticipated to be <5 days Urgent operation should not be delayed for PN buildup Proven untreatable disease
HOME PATIENT*		
Usually helpful	Chronic severe dysfunction of swallowing Chronic upper gastrointestinal obstruction Gastrointestinal function insufficient to sustain growth or weight Period of gastrointestinal recovery and adaptation after major resection or severe enteritis	Extreme short-bowel syndrome Severe radiation enteritis Chronic obstruction due to adhesions or dysmotility Severe Crohn's disease Enterocutaneous fistula Congenital bowel dysfunction Hyperemesis gravidarum Disorders of multiple systems including GI tract Neoplasms with bowel obstruction AIDS
Benefit not established	Chronic severe brain damage (vegetative state) Malnutrition of systemic illness such as chronic renal, hepatic, pulmonary disease or AIDS	
Contraindicated	Prognosis not warranting aggressive nutritional support Patient refusing treatment Legal surrogate refusing treatment for an incompetent, terminal patient	Patient without adequate social support to deal with risks of therapy Proven untreatable disease where some meaningful quality of life cannot be sustained

* Includes patients in nursing homes.
SOURCE: Adapted from guidelines published by the American Society for Parenteral Enteral Nutrition, J Parent Enteral Nutr 10:441, 1986, 11:342, 439, 1987.

except in severely malnourished cancer patients undergoing surgery. Parenteral nutrition may enable patients to survive toxic chemotherapy and bone marrow transplantation. In patients undergoing bone marrow transplantation, parenteral and enteral nutrition support are equally effective.

LIVER DISEASE Patients with alcoholic liver disease tend to be chronically malnourished, both because of anorexia and because of the substitution of alcohol for food. Patients with both acute and chronic liver disease also may have decreased branched chain amino acids (BCAA) and elevated aromatic amino acids (AAA) in plasma and brain. In randomized prospective trials in patients with borderline hepatic encephalopathy, BCAA-enriched formulas improve nitrogen balance without precipitating encephalopathy, but only one study was large enough to show improved patient survival. Since the BCAA-enriched formula is expensive, it can only be justified in patients with hepatic failure who cannot tolerate adequate protein from standard enteral or parenteral formulas without developing encephalopathy.

RENAL DISEASE One controlled trial reported improved survival of patients with acute renal failure who received parenteral solutions of essential amino acids and glucose. Subsequent studies have suggested similar benefit from solutions that supply equal amounts of essential and nonessential amino acids.

PULMONARY DISEASE Weight loss in patients with advanced pulmonary disease is usually the consequence of increased work of breathing and of poor food intake. In cystic fibrosis, malnutrition may worsen pulmonary deterioration, and enteral feeding via gastrostomy tubes accelerates growth and stabilizes or improves pulmonary function. The greatest benefit is seen in the younger patients. The criteria for patient selection and the psychological costs of such invasive treatment have not been established. Clinical outcome studies of nutrition support are not available for other types of pulmonary disease.

THE DESIGN OF INDIVIDUAL REGIMENS

FLUID REQUIREMENTS These can be estimated by adding the normal daily requirement (120 mL/kg body weight for infants, 40 mL/kg body weight for adults) to any abnormal loss. If the patient is on parenteral therapy, any enteral intake should be subtracted from

TABLE 75-3 Estimation of daily fluid requirements

NORMAL 70-KG MAN

Intake	Output
Normal: 40 × 70 = 2800 mL/d [derived from oral liquids of 1500 mL, or 7 glasses/cups per day, and solid food providing 1300 mL (1000 mL from water in food, 300 mL from water generated by metabolism of foods)]	Urine: 1900 mL/d Insensible loss: 800 mL/d Stool: 100 mL/d (sweat loss can be up to 2 L/d; for each °C of fever add 200 mL/d)

TUBE ENTERAL PATIENT

55 kg-woman recovering from total gastrectomy for gastric cancer and supported by jejunostomy feedings, taking nothing by mouth or intravenously but experiencing 600 mL of diarrheal losses per day.

Normal requirement, 40 × 55	= 2200 mL/d
Abnormal loss, 600 − 100	= 500 mL/d
Total requirement	= 2700 mL/d

PARENTERAL PATIENT

65 kg-man with a high jejunostomy following massive bowel resection for Crohn's disease with oral intake of 2000 mL/d and jejunostomy loss of 4000 mL/d.

Normal requirement 40 × 65	= 2600 mL/d
Abnormal loss (4000 − 100) minus oral intake (2000)	= 1900 mL/d
Total requirement	= 4500 mL/d

the abnormal loss. For clinical examples see Table 75-3. Since abnormal loss of enteric fluid implies significant mineral losses, extra amounts of these nutrients (Table 75-4) must also be added to any standard parenteral or enteral formula.

ENERGY REQUIREMENTS These may be calculated by indirect calorimetry using a bedside metabolic cart and simultaneously measuring urine urea nitrogen and calculating energy expenditure, the respiratory quotient (RQ), and hence the mixture of fuels the patient is burning (fat, carbohydrate, protein). An RQ of greater than 1 suggests the patient is synthesizing fat and is at risk for hepatic dysfunction due to steatosis. If indirect calorimetry is not available, the patient's basal energy expenditure (BEE) can be calculated using the Harris-Benedict equation.

For women:

$$\text{BEE(kcal/d)} = 655.10 + 9.56 \times \text{wt(kg)} + 1.85 \times \text{ht(cm)} - 4.68 \times \text{age(years)}$$

For men:

$$\text{BEE(kcal/d)} = 66.47 + 13.75 \times \text{wt(kg)} + 5.00 \times \text{ht(cm)} - 6.76 \times \text{age(years)}$$

TABLE 75-4 Enteric fluid volumes and their sodium, potassium, chloride and bicarbonate content*

	L/d†	Na, mmol/L	K‡, mmol/L	Cl, mmol/L	HCO_3§ mmol/L
Oral intake	2–3				
Enteric secretions					
Saliva	1–2	10	30	10	30
Gastric juice	2	60	9	90	0
Bile	2–3	150	10	90	70
Small bowel	1	100	5	100	20
Colon	Variable	40	100	15	60

* Enteric secretions are also rich in divalent cations (Ca, Mg, Zn, Cu) and their loss is increased by steatorrhea, a high bowel fistula, or prolonged suction.

† Of the 9 L/d of oral and enteric fluid presented to the upper small bowel, normally 50% is absorbed in the jejunum, 40% in the ileum, and 10% in the colon. In short-bowel patients, the colon can absorb greater amounts, up to 3 L/d.

‡ Potassium losses are small except in secretions distal to the ileocecal valve. The colon ion exchange is partly controlled by aldosterone, and Na^+ depletion increases K^+ loss in the stool.

§ Bicarbonate losses must be replaced in parenteral solutions as acetate or lactate because of potential precipitation of bicarbonate with ingredients such as calcium.

To the BEE should be added a value of 20 percent of the BEE for patients without significant metabolic stress, 50 percent for patients with marked stress such as sepsis and trauma, and 100 percent for patients with severe stress such as a 40 percent surface burn. A simpler method of estimating energy requirements is to provide 105 kJ/kg (25 kcal/kg) body weight per day for unstressed patients and 126, 146, and 167 kJ/kg (30, 35, and 40 kcal/kg) body weight per day for patients who are mildly, moderately, and severely stressed or malnourished, respectively.

The most desirable balance of carbohydrate to fat in parenteral and enteral solutions is unsettled. There is a relative dependence of wound tissue, white blood cells, and the cerebral and renal cortex on glucose metabolism. The majority of energy is usually supplied as glucose in parenteral solutions and as oligosaccharides and disaccharides in enteral solutions. Parenteral lipid solutions are available as 10% or 20% emulsions of vegetable oils (soybean or safflower oils emulsified into artificial lipoproteins with egg phospholipid and made isotonic with glycerin). Polyunsaturated vegetable oils are used in most enteral formulas since they are better absorbed by the compromised gastrointestinal tract. The fat in parenteral and enteral formulas must supply the essential fatty acid requirement (1 to 2 percent of energy from linoleic and linolenic acid), and the provision of 30 percent of energy as fat may reduce the problems that arise from providing excess carbohydrate (e.g., hepatic steatosis and excess carbon dioxide production). Substitution of ω6 polyunsaturated vegetable fat by ω3 polyunsaturated fish oils may reduce the inflammatory response to burn injury, trauma, and radiation by reducing the synthesis of prostaglandins that may alter the gut mucosal barrier.

PROTEIN OR AMINO ACID REQUIREMENTS The recommended dietary protein allowance of 0.8 g/kg body weight per day is adequate for nonstressed patients (e.g., a patient with a high-grade esophageal stricture or anorexia nervosa). More catabolic patients require 1.2 or 1.5 g/kg body weight per day of protein to induce positive nitrogen balance and reconstitute the normal body mass. In a stable patient the adequacy of protein and energy support can be assessed by a balance study:

$$\text{Protein balance} = \text{protein intake} - \text{protein loss}$$

where protein loss = [24-h urine urea nitrogen (g) + 4] × 6.25, and by documenting healing, restoration of normal body composition, or resumption of longitudinal growth.

In states of disturbed protein utilization, such as renal and hepatic failure, azotemia and abnormal plasma amino acid patterns develop. The use of enteral and parenteral solutions to correct these aberrations is justified only in specific clinical circumstances. (See section on medical effectiveness of nutrition support, above.)

Glutamine is an important fuel for the gastrointestinal tract. The oxidation of one molecule of glutamine produces 30 mmol of ATP, which makes this amino acid almost as rich an energy source as one molecule of glucose. The free amino acid pool of the enterocyte is glutamine rich. Although this amino acid can be synthesized endogenously, it appears to be a relatively essential nutrient in stressed patients. Glutamine is fairly insoluble, and it is present in low concentrations in most enteral solutions. Arginine, carnitine, and certain nucleotides may promote optimal gut repair and function in stressed patients. Enteral nutrition provides the best vehicle for supplying nutrients with special trophic and immune benefit for the gut and also stimulates the secretion of gut hormones such as epidermal growth factor and gastrin.

MINERAL AND VITAMIN REQUIREMENTS (See Table 75-5) The parenteral requirements of some vitamins may be higher than the enteral requirements for several reasons: First, the micronutrients are delivered into the systemic rather than the portal circulation, thereby potentially bypassing the liver and being rapidly excreted by the kidneys. Second, many patients requiring parenteral support have large enteric losses that can result in sodium, potassium, chloride, and bicarbonate wasting (Table 75-4) and also in loss of divalent

TABLE 75-5 Daily enteral (EN) and parenteral (PN) requirements of essential fatty acids, minerals, and vitamins

Nutrient	Daily requirement, adult range	
	EN	PN
Essential fatty acids, % kcal	1–2	±2–4
Calcium, g	0.8–1.2	0.4
Phosphorus, g	0.8–1.2	0.4
Potassium, g	2–5	4
Sodium, g	1–3	1–2
Chloride, g	2–5	2
Magnesium, g	0.3	0.3
Iron, mg	10	1–2
Zinc, mg	15	3–12
Copper, mg	2–3	0.3–0.5
Iodine, mg	0.15	0.15
Manganese, mg	2–5	2–5
Chromium, mg	0.05–0.2	0.015
Molybdenum, mg	0.15–0.3	0.01–0.5
Selenium, mg	0.05–0.2	.05–0.1
Ascorbic acid, mg	60	100
Thiamine, mg	1.4	3.0
Riboflavin, mg	1–6	3.6
Niacin, mg	18	40
Biotin, μg	60	60
Pantothenic acid, mg	5	15
Pyridoxine, mg	2.0	4.0
Folic acid, μg	400	400
Cobalamin, μg	3.0	5
Vitamin A, μg	1000	1300
Vitamin D, μg	10	5
Vitamin E, mg	8–10	10–15
Vitamin K, μg	70–140	200

cations and vitamins that normally have an enterohepatic circulation such as folate, cobalamin, vitamin D, and perhaps other fat-soluble vitamins. The tubing and delivery bags themselves and exposure to oxygen and light can also absorb and destroy vitamins (particularly vitamin A) before they reach the patient.

TABLE 75-6 Central vein parenteral nutrition catheters

I Sites of venous access
- *A* Distal tip of catheter best placed in mid-portion of superior vena cava.
- *B* Enters venous system via:
  - *1* Percutaneous stick into the subclavian, external or internal jugular, or anterior cubital vein.
  - *2* Cutdown site on external jugular (via common facial vein), femoral, axillary, or intercostal vein.
- *C* All catheters can be tunneled superficially to a distal site, which:
  - *1* May provide a barrier to skin organisms infecting the line.
  - *2* Places exit site at convenient place for self care in patients going home.

II Types of catheters
- *A* Externalized
  - *1* Single, double, or triple lumen.
    - *a* 2d and 3d channels used for IV medications or drawing of blood.
    - *b* Higher incidence of infectious complications with multiple-lumen catheters.
  - *2* In home patients, avoids the need to do a nightly needle stick but requires constant aseptic dressing.
  - *3* Repair kits available if a leak or tear develops in the externalized portion.
- *B* Subcutaneous port
  - *1* Involves a small reservoir with an overlying rubber diaphragm that is self-sealing.
  - *2* Port must be entered by a J-shaped needle.
  - *3* Not all patients like the daily needle stick.
  - *4* If line is not in use, the buried port makes taking showers and swimming less hazardous.

III Catheter material
- *A* Polyvinylchloride, polyethylene, polyurethane, or polytetrafluoroethylene
  - *1* Advantage:
    - *a* Inherent stiffness allows easy threading into the vein.
  - *2* Disadvantages:
    - *a* Stiffness allows catheter to be in direct contact with vessel wall, causing thrombosis.
    - *b* Stiffness increases over time, causing kinks or fractures.
- *B* Silicone rubber
  - *1* Advantages:
    - *a* Very pliable; less kinking.
    - *b* Less traumatic to vessel wall.
    - *c* Inert, inducing little reaction or adherence.
  - *2* Disadvantages:
    - *a* Difficult to thread into vein.
    - *b* Falls out more easily owing to nonadherence.
    - *c* Potential for tearing.

PARENTERAL NUTRITION

INFUSION TECHNIQUE AND PATIENT MONITORING Partial and short-term parenteral nutrition can be provided via a peripheral vein if the majority of the energy intake is supplied by isotonic fat solutions, but long-term total parenteral support should be administered via a central vein catheter because hypertonic glucose must be rapidly diluted in a high-flow system. The preferred sites for central vein access and the catheter choices available are summarized in Table 75-6, and typical nutrient contents for a standard daily parenteral formula are given in Table 75-7. The glucose content is increased gradually as the patient demonstrates tolerance of the high glucose load. Appropriate clinical and laboratory monitoring for patients on parenteral nutrition is summarized in Table 75-8.

COMPLICATIONS (See Table 75-9) **Mechanical** The insertion of a central venous catheter should only be done by trained personnel using stringently aseptic techniques. Major mechanical complications include pneumothorax, hemothorax from laceration of the subclavian artery or vein, brachial plexus injury, and malpositioning of the catheter in a cerebral vein, the azygos vein, or in the right ventricle. The correct catheter position must be confirmed by x-ray before the hypertonic nutrient solution is infused. Catheters can subsequently back out of the vein, develop leaks, or become detached from the hub and embolize into the heart or pulmonary artery. Catheter thrombosis may occur, especially if the catheter is used for withdrawing blood samples. Thrombosis of the catheter extending to the central vein is frequently coincident with infection. Thrombosed catheters may be unblocked by urokinase treatment.

Metabolic Early problems, especially in elderly and debilitated patients, include fluid overload producing congestive heart failure and glucose overload leading to osmotic diuresis and, as a result of stimulation of insulin secretion, massive extracellular to intracellular shifts of phosphorus and potassium. Such shifts are most likely in cachectic patients with total body phosphorus and potassium depletion and can result in arrhythmias, cardiopulmonary dysfunction, and neurologic symptoms. To avoid these complications, parenteral nutrition should be begun slowly and monitored carefully. Late metabolic complications include cholestatic liver disease with bile sludging and gallstone formation. The exact cause of the liver disease is not understood but appears to be linked to the lack of enteral stimulation; the disease is less likely if some enteral feeding is maintained. Parenteral nutrition induces hypercalcuria, which can result in negative calcium balance and osteopenia. The hypercalcuria appears to reflect several factors, including the calcuric effect of amino acid infusion and the high fixed acid load. Prior to the advent of synthetic amino acid solutions, many protein hydrolysates were contaminated with aluminum, which blocked bone mineralization. Once patients on long-term parenteral nutrition move from catabolic breakdown to sustained anabolism, deficiencies of micronutrients, such as essential fatty acids, trace minerals, and vitamins, may develop unless they are adequate in the parenteral nutrient solution (see Table 75-5).

Infectious Infection of the access line rarely occurs in the first 72 h, and early fever usually points to some alternative infectious site or other cause of hyperpyrexia. Infection of the access line is likely if the patient defervesces when the infusion rate of the parenteral nutrient is tapered. Positive central line cultures suggest catheter

TABLE 75-7 Standard total parenteral nutrition solution (24 h) for a 70-kg adult

Fluid	3L
Protein (amino acids)	0.2–0.3 g nitrogen per kg
Energy value*	105–165 kJ/kg (25–40 kcal/kg)
Essential fatty acids (lipids)	2% of total energy
Electrolytes	
Sodium	100 mmol
Potassium	100 mmol
Chloride	130 mmol
Acetate/gluconate	90 mmol
Calcium	30 mmol
Magnesium	40 mmol
Phosphorus	300 mg
Trace Elements	
Zinc	5 mg
Copper	1.5 mg
Iodine	120 μg
Selenium	100 μg
Chromium	15 μg
Manganese	2 mg
Vitamins	
Ascorbic acid	100 mg
Thiamine	3 mg
Riboflavin	3.6 mg
Niacin	40 mg
Pantothenic acid	15 mg
Pyridoxine	4 mg
Biotin	60 μg
Folid acid	400 μg
Cobalamin	5 μg
Vitamin A	1300 RE
Vitamin D	10 μg
Vitamin E	15 mg
Vitamin K	200 μg

* Provided principally as dextrose.

TABLE 75-8 Monitoring the patient on total parenteral nutrition

Clinical data checked daily
- Patient's sense of well being, symptoms suggesting fluid overload, high or low blood glucose, electrolyte imbalance, etc.
- Patient's strength as judged by graded activity, getting out of bed, walking, stair climbing.
- Vital signs: temperature, blood pressure, pulse rate, and respiratory rate.
- Fluid balance: weight; fluid input (intravenous +/− enteral) versus fluid output (urine, stool, gastric suction, etc.).
- Delivery equipment for parenteral nutrition: composition of nutrient solution, tubing, pump, filter catheter, dressing (skin checked for local infection at time of dressing change).

Laboratory data	
Urine quantitative glucose	Four times daily
Blood glucose Na^+, K^+, Cl^-, HCO_3^- Blood urea nitrogen	Daily until glucose infusion load and patient stable, then twice weekly
Serum albumin, transferrin Liver function studies Serum creatinine Ca^{2+}, PO_4^{2-}, Mg^{2+} Hb/Ht, WBC	Baseline, then twice weekly
Prothrombin time	Baseline, then weekly
Micronutrient tests as indicated	

sepsis, especially if no other infectious source is identified and if the organism is staphylococcus or a *Candida* species. While removal of the central catheter may allow the patient to clear fungemia spontaneously, antibiotic therapy is usually necessary for bacterial infections. Catheter sepsis is less likely if central vein parenteral nutrition is provided via a single-lumen catheter; triple-lumen catheters, even if frequently replaced over a guidewire, are associated with a two or three times greater incidence of sepsis.

ENTERAL NUTRITION

TUBE PLACEMENT AND PATIENT MONITORING The different types of enteral tubes, the techniques for inserting them, their clinical uses, and potential problems are outlined in Table 75-10. Available enteral formulas and their nutrient compositions are listed in Table 74-8. Patients on enteral feeding are at risk for some of the same metabolic complications as parenterally fed patients and should receive the same clinical and laboratory monitoring (Table 75-8). Since small-bore tubes are easily displaced, tube position should be tested by aspirating and measuring the pH of the gut fluid (<4 in stomach, >6 in jejunum). A generic description of the types of tubes required for different enteral formulas is given in Table 75-11.

COMPLICATIONS Aspiration The debilitated patient with poor gastric emptying and an impaired swallow and cough mechanism is at risk for aspiration. In patients on respirators, effective tracheal suctioning induces coughing and provokes gastric regurgitation, and the cuff on the endotracheal tube or tracheostomy seldom provides adequate protection against aspiration. Under these circumstances, it may be safer to use a large-bore rubber feeding tube, rather than a fine-bore soft collapsible tube, to allow for an accurate check of residual gastric contents and, if necessary, temporary removal of gastric contents prior to tracheal suction.

Although normal gastric motility provides a churning and fragmenting activity with intermittent propulsion of liquid and small food fragments into the duodenum, constant gastric infusion of an enteral formula is better tolerated in sick patients than is intermittent bolus feeding. A continuous infusion is best achieved with an enteral feeding pump, especially when using fine-bore feeding tubes that have a greater potential to clog. If long-term gastric feeding is anticipated, endoscopic, radiologic, or surgical placement of a gastric tube is preferable.

A nasojejunal tube reduces the risk of aspiration, but placement

TABLE 75-9 Complications of total parenteral nutrition (PN)

	First 48 h	First 2 weeks	After 3 months
Mechanical	Complications from catheter insertion: Cephalad displacement Pneumothorax Hemothorax Detachment of line at catheter hub with blood loss or air embolism	Catheter coming out vein more common if Silastic Detachment of line at catheter hub with blood loss or air embolism	Detachment of line at catheter hub with blood loss or air embolism Fractures or tears in catheter
Metabolic	Fluid overload Hyperglycemia Hypophosphatemia Hypokalemia	Cardiopulmonary failure Hyperosmolar nonketotic hyperglycemic coma Acid-base imbalance Electrolyte imbalance	Essential fatty acid deficiency Zinc, copper, chromium, selenium, molybdenum deficiency Iron deficiency Vitamin deficiencies Refeeding edema PN metabolic bone disease PN liver disease
Infectious		Catheter-induced sepsis	Catheter-induced sepsis Tunnel infections

TABLE 75-10 Enteral feeding tubes

Type of tube	Placement technique	Clinical uses	Potential problems
Nasogastric	External measurement: nostril, ear to xiphisternum. Placed by professional or, with instruction, by family member or patient. Tube stiffened by ice water or a stylet. Position tested by injecting air and auscultating air bubble passing through fluid, or by aspirating acid gastric contents.	Short-term clinical situations (a few weeks). Placement can be intermittent. Normal gastric emptying required. Bolus feeds or continuous drip.	Aspiration pneumonia from regurgitated stomach contents. Irritation of nasopharynx or esophagogastric junction with bleeding and/or stricture.
Nasoduodenal or nasojejunal	External measurement: nostril, ear to anterior superior iliac spine in adults; to the medial malleolus in infants. Weighted tube may pass spontaneously through pylorus if patient lies on right side; or tube is placed with stiffening stylet under fluoroscopy. Position tested by aspirating alkaline duodenal contents or checking by x-ray.	Short-term clinical situations. Used if gastric emptying is impaired or to infuse beyond a high bowel fistula such as an esophageal tear or gastric or duodenal fistula.	Passing tube through pylorus. Preventing the spontaneous pulling back into stomach. Continuous drip required and tends to cause diarrhea. Tubes stiffen with time, can lacerate pylorus or gastroesophageal junction if pulled out rapidly.
Pharyngostomy/esophagostomy	Tube placed surgically through side of neck into pharynx.	Long-term access. No nasopharyngeal irritation. Once tract is established, tubes can be replaced.	Aspiration if tube in stomach. Pharyngeal scarring causes distortion of normal anatomy.
Gastrostomy	Tube placed through the abdominal wall into the stomach, either by a percutaneous endoscopic technique using local anesthetic or surgically via an abdominal incision using a spinal or general anesthetic.	Long-term access. Once tract is established, tubes can be replaced. Used when swallowing is impaired because of either mechanical obstruction or neurologic discoordination.	Irritation around tube site. Aspiration of stomach contents. Displacement of tube into peritoneal cavity or, if held in situ by balloon, obstruction of the pylorus.
Jejunostomy	Tube placed surgically through abdominal wall into proximal loop of jejunum and tethered to anterior wall by suture. Fine-bore tube inserted by diagonal tract into bowel lumen or large bore secured with an anchoring suture.	Long-term access. Used for defective gastric emptying. Fine-bore tube recommended as postoperative backup when prolonged gastric atony might occur.	Irritation at tube exit site, especially with large-bore tube. Clogging or displacement of tube. Continuous drip usually required. Diarrhea common.
Combined gastrojejunostomy	Tube placed surgically with jejunal arm threaded beyond the pylorus.	Allows for simultaneous gastric suction and jejunal infusion. Used in patient particularly at risk for aspiration of gastric contents.	Not yet widely available.

TABLE 75-11 Types of enteral feeding formulas

Formula category	Description	Clinical indications	Tube of choice	Comments
Blenderized	Mixture of pureed meat, fruit, vegetables, sometimes added nonfat milk, fiber, vitamins, and minerals; highly viscous	Normal digestion and absorption required; used with pharyngostomy, cervical esophagostomy, or gastrostomy tubes	Large-bore (12–18 French)	Lowest cost; 2 or more liters daily; bolus feed
Polymeric	Mixture of whole proteins, polysaccharides, and triglycerides; contains no fiber; lower viscosity than blenderized formulas	Normal digestion and absorption required; can be fed into esophagus, stomach, duodenum or jejunum	Small-bore (8–10 French)	2 or more liters needed daily; bolus, gravity, or pump feed
Monomeric	Mixture of predigested protein, carbohydrate (CHO), and a small amount of triglyceride; contains no fiber; has lowest viscosity of all formulas	Used for inflammatory bowel disease, chronic pancreatitis, GI fistula, enteritis from radiation or chemotherapy, panmalabsorption, or as a transition feeding from parenteral to enteral therapy	Small-bore (5–6 French)	Higher cost than polymeric formulas; 1.5–3 liters needed daily; pump feed
Disease-related	Devised to meet the nutritional needs of specific disease states; varying amounts of protein, amino acid ratios, CHO, and electrolytes; low viscosity.	Used for renal failure, hepatic encephalopathy, stress, trauma, and respiratory failure	Small-bore (5–6 French)	Highest cost; 2 liters or more needed daily; gravity or pump feed
Modular	Made-to-order feedings of individual constituents; viscosity depends on quantities of protein, CHO, and fat	Used for specific metabolic abnormalities, such as glycogen storage disease	Varies, depending on viscosity	Higher cost than monomeric formula; 1.5 or more liters needed daily; bolus, gravity, or pump feed

of such tubes through the pylorus is time-consuming, and such tubes frequently pull back into the stomach. If a debilitated patient with poor gastric emptying goes to surgery, it is appropriate to ask the surgeon to place a jejunostomy tube for feeding. This can involve a traditional rubber tube (12 to 14 French) or a fine-bore (5 to 8 French) tube inserted through an oblique needle track that seals rapidly when the jejunostomy tube is removed.

Diarrhea Enteral feeding often causes diarrhea, especially if absorption is compromised by bowel disease or drugs such as antibiotics. The diarrhea may be controlled by the use of continuous drip or administration of enteral bulking agents, such as psyllium hydrophilic mucilogs or an anticholinergic medication, in the formula. Diarrhea, stimulated by enteral feeding, does not necessarily imply inadequate absorption. Furthermore, since luminal nutrients induce trophic effects on the gut mucosa and stimulate the enteric immunologic barrier, it may be appropriate to persist despite the diarrhea, even when this necessitates temporary supplemental parenteral support.

OVERALL IMPACT OF NUTRITION SUPPORT

In 1986 about 1.5 million patients in the United States received parenteral and enteral nutrition at a cost of about 5 billion dollars, thus accounting for about 1 percent of health-care costs.

HOSPITAL SETTING Most nutrition support is for hospitalized patients, predominantly for patients whose length of stay is four times the average hospital stay and who are high users of other life-sustaining therapies (ventilators, kidney dialysis, intensive care units, cardiac monitoring). Such patients are typically referred from smaller hospitals to tertiary care centers. Perioperative parenteral nutrition is cost-effective for surgical patients who are severely malnourished preoperatively and for well-nourished patients in whom surgery results in ileus of 10 days duration or more. The costs and complications of parenteral nutrition can be reduced if patient management is supervised by a nutrition support service. In one study, catheter sepsis decreased from 28.6 percent to 4.7 percent after such a service was instituted, and in another study routine consultations with a nutrition support service resulted in a 20 percent reduction in average hospital stay and a 26 percent average reduction in costs per patient receiving parenteral nutrition.

NON-HOSPITAL SETTING In patients with benign causes of extreme short-bowel syndrome, home parenteral nutrition therapy is associated with low morbidity and high rates of good rehabilitation. For example, in patients with Crohn's disease on home parenteral nutrition, complete or partial rehabilitation was achieved in 97 percent, the mortality was only 3 percent per year, and the rehospitalization rate was only 1 percent per year. Home parenteral nutrition costs about half as much as similar treatment in hospital.

ETHICAL ASPECTS OF NUTRITIONAL SUPPORT As with all other forms of therapy, nutrition support is contraindicated if the risks exceed the potential benefit, and the consent of the patient or the legal surrogate is required. Because artificially supplied nutrition can protract the terminal phase of many illnesses, withholding or withdrawing nutrition support can be a major ethical and legal problem, especially in incompetent and institutionalized patients.

REFERENCES

ABEL RM et al: Improved survival from acute renal failure after treatment with intravenous essential L. amino acids and glucose. N Engl J Med 288:695, 1973

ALEXANDER WJ et al: The importance of lipid type in the diet after burn injury. Ann Surg 240:1, 1986

ANDERSON GF, STEINBERG EP: DRG's and specialized nutritional support: The need for reform. J Parent Enteral Nutr 10:3, 1986

BLACKBURN GL et al: Peripheral intravenous feeding with isotonic aminoacid solutions. Am J Surg 125:447, 1973

CERRA FB et al: Disease-specific amino acid infusion (F080) in hepatic encephalopathy. A prospective randomized, double blind controlled trial. J Parent Enteral Nutr 9:288, 1985

DETSKY AS et al: Evaluating the accuracy of nutritional assessment techniques applied to hospitalized patients: Methodology and comparisons. J Parent Enteral Nutr 8:153, 1984

———: A cost-effective analysis of the home parenteral nutrition program at Toronto General: 1970–1982. J Parent Enteral Nutr 10:49, 1986

———: Perioperative parenteral nutrition: A Meta analysis. Ann Intern Med 107:195, 1987

DUDRICK SJ et al: Long-term total parenteral nutrition with growth, development and positive nitrogen balance. Surgery 64:134, 1968

FOX AD et al: Effect of glutamine-supplemented enteral diet on methotrexate-induced enterocolitis. J Parent Enteral Nutr 12:325, 1988

HOWARD L et al: Vitamin A deficiency: A complication of long-term parenteral nutrition. Ann Intern Med 93:576, 1980

ISSELL BF et al: Protection against chemotherapy by IV hyperalimentation. Cancer Treat Rep 62:1139, 1978

OASIS Home Nutrition Support Patient Registry, Annual Report, 1986 Data. Oley Foundation, Albany Medical College, Albany, NY, 1986

SHILS ME et al: Long-term parenteral nutrition through an external arteriovenous shunt. N Engl J Med 283:341, 1970

STUDLEY HO: Percentage of weight loss. JAMA 106:458, 1936

SZELUGA DJ et al: Nutritional support of bone marrow transplant recipients: A prospective randomized clinical trial comparing total parenteral nutrition to an enteral feeding program. Cancer Res 47:3309, 1987

WEINSIER RL et al: Cost containment: A contribution of aggressive nutritional support in burn patients. J Burn Care Rehabil 6:436, 1985

WEISDORF S et al: Influence of prophylactic total parenteral nutrition on long-term outcome of bone marrow transplantation. Transplantation 43:833, 1987

76 VITAMIN DEFICIENCY AND EXCESS[1]

JEAN D. WILSON

Vitamins play several roles in human disease. Deficiencies of single vitamins are now rarely endemic, even in developing nations, and are more likely to occur either as a portion of states of general malnutrition, as a result of food faddism, as a complication of more widespread disease such as malabsorption, as a complication of complex therapy such as hemodialysis or total parenteral nutrition, or as the result of an inborn error of metabolism. Indeed, disorders of vitamin excess may now be more common than vitamin deficiency.

In considering the pathophysiology of vitamins several points are worth emphasis. (1) The fact that organic compounds cannot be synthesized within the body and are required constituents of the diet is the result of mutations, and the provision of vitamins in the diet is a form of therapy for an inborn error of metabolism. In some instances, such as the limited ability to synthesize thiamine, the requirement is common to many if not all animals, and the mutation must have occurred early in evolution; in others, such as the single-gene defect that prevents ascorbic acid synthesis, humans share the defect with only a few other species, such as the guinea pig. (2) The feature that separates vitamins from other necessary organic constituents in the diet is that small amounts of them are required, in contrast to the relatively large amounts of essential amino acids and essential fatty acids. This is a consequence of the fact that vitamins function not as building blocks of tissue mass or as substrates for energy production but rather as prosthetic groups for quantitatively minor tissue constituents or as catalytic cofactors for biologic reactions; like most catalysts they are required only in small amounts. (3) Deficiency of some vitamins has never been described in humans (e.g., pantothenic acid) implying that these vitamins are either so ubiquitous in food sources or are conserved so efficiently by the body that deficiency can become manifest, if at all, only in the context of a mixed nutritional and vitamin deficiency. (4) Alcoholism is the background upon which many vitamin deficiencies develop in the United States. This is the consequence of several interlocking factors including diminished intake, impairment of absorption and storage of vitamins, and, in some cases, predisposing genetic factors. (5) Biochemical means of proving vitamin deficiency, once suspected,

[1] For vitamin D, see Chap. 341 and for the hematologic vitamins, see Chap. 292.

are limited, and the role of vitamin deficiency in disease states is frequently not recognized because nonspecific vitamin therapy is a common part of standard supportive care. As a consequence, recognition of the manifestations of vitamin deficiency and a high index of suspicion in the appropriate clinical setting are essential for considering the diagnosis, and demonstration of a response to replacement therapy may be the most accurate way to confirm a diagnosis. (6) The consumption of excessive amounts of vitamins can occur either as the indirect consequence of dietary practice or, more commonly, as the result of deliberate ingestion. Syndromes of excess for the fat-soluble vitamins A and D are well characterized, whereas the toxicity syndromes produced by the water-soluble vitamins are inconsistent and less well understood.

DEFICIENCY STATES

NIACIN (PELLAGRA) Biochemistry *Niacin* is the generic term for nicotinic acid (3-pyridinecarboxylic acid) and derivatives that exhibit the nutritional activity of nicotinic acid (Fig. 76-1). In one sense niacin is not a vitamin since it can be formed from the essential amino acid tryptophan. In the human an average of about 1 mg of niacin is formed from 60 mg of dietary tryptophan. Accordingly, estimates of the adequacy of dietary intake must take into account the tryptophan content of the diet as well as the content of niacin. Many foodstuffs, especially cereals, contain bound forms of niacin from which the vitamin is not nutritionally available.

The absorption, tissue distribution, and metabolism of the vitamin are poorly understood. Approximately one-fifth of the vitamin is decarboxylated to nicotinuric acid, and the remainder is excreted in the urine as methylated products, largely *N*-methylnicotinamide and *N*-methyl-2-pyridone-5-carboxamide.

Mechanism of action Niacin is an essential component of nicotinamide adenine dinucleotide (NAD) and nicotinamide adenine dinucleotide phosphate (NADP), coenzymes for many oxidation-reduction reactions.

Requirements The requirements and recommended daily allowances for niacin and tryptophan are listed in Table 70-1. In contrast to most vitamins, the requirement for niacin does not appear to be increased during pregnancy. Requirement is primarily determined by the amino acid composition of the diet.

FIGURE 76-1 The structure and principal functions of some of the vitamins associated with human disorders.

Vitamin	Active Derivative or Cofactor Form	Principal Function
Niacin 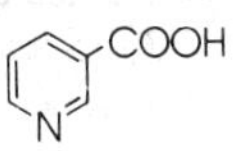	Nicotinamide Adenine Dinucleotide Phosphate (NADP) and Nicotine Adenine Dinucleotide (NAD)	Coenzymes for Oxidations and Reductions
Thiamine 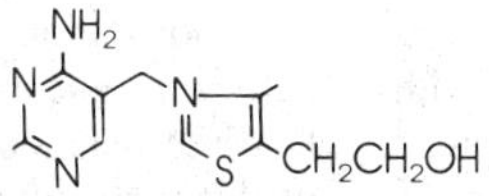	Thiamine Diphosphate	Coenzyme for Cleavage of Carbon-Carbon Bonds
Pyridoxine 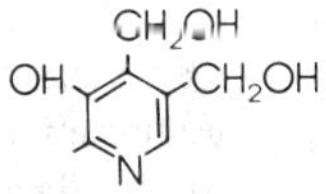	Pyridoxal Phosphate	Cofactor for Enzymes of Amino Acid Metabolism
Riboflavin 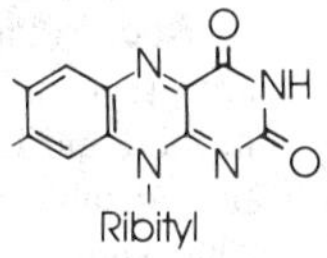	Flavin Mononucleotide (FMN) and Flavin Adenine Dinucleotide (FAD)	Cofactor for Oxidation-Reduction Reactions and Covalently Attached Prosthetic Groups for Some Enzymes
Ascorbic Acid 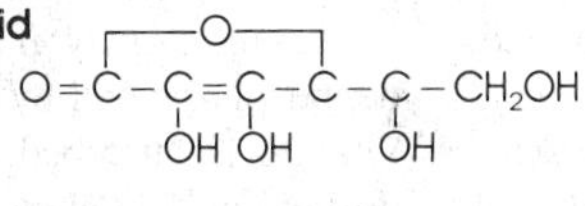	Ascorbic Acid and Dehydroascorbic Acid	Participation as a Redox Ion in Many Biological Oxidation Reactions
Vitamin A 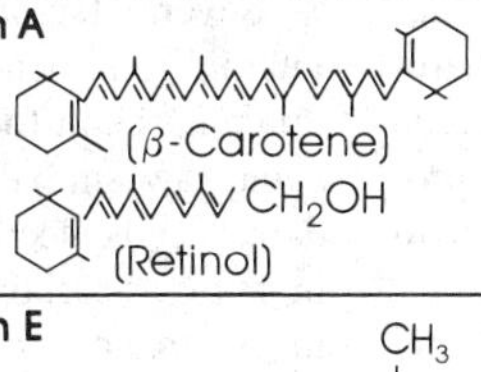	Retinol, Retinal, and Retinoic Acid	Formation of Carotenoid Proteins (Vision) and Glycoproteins (Epithelial Cell Function)
Vitamin E 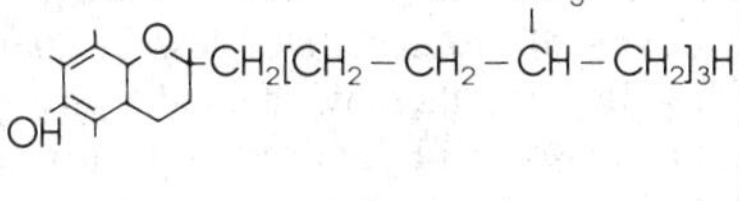	Tocopherol	Antioxidant
Vitamin K 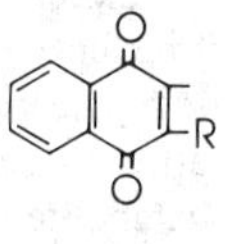	Menaquinone	Cofactor for Post-Translational Carboxylation of Many Proteins Including Essential Clotting Factors

Experimental depletion After the institution of a diet deficient in niacin and tryptophan, the urinary excretion of niacin metabolites reaches minimal values (<1.5 mg/d) after 1 to 2 months and remains constant thereafter. Clinical deficiency develops shortly after excretion becomes stable at a low level and consists of dermatitis, glossitis, stomatitis, diarrhea, proctitis, mental depression, abdominal pain, vaginitis, dysphagia, and amenorrhea, findings similar to those in pellagra.

Clinical deficiency Pellagra was previously an endemic disease in the American south and in many other parts of the world. The endemic disease is usually associated with a high intake of maize (American corn) or of millet (sorghum; jowar) and can be cured by the administration of niacin; nevertheless, the fact that large populations of people exist on a diet in which maize is the major source of protein but nevertheless are free of endemic pellagra implies that the relation between maize intake and the development of the disease is not straightforward. As a consequence, the concept of the pathogenesis of pellagra has evolved from that of a pure vitamin deficiency or a mixed deficiency of tryptophan and available niacin in the diet to a more complicated etiology. The disorder may be due to an imbalance in dietary amino acids or to a complex vitamin deficiency; the niacin equivalent (available niacin and tryptophan) of maize, although low, is no lower than that of some cereals that are unassociated with endemic pellagra. An alternative possibility is that the milling of maize influences the bioavailability of the niacin in the cereal. Treatment of maize with alkali in the preparation of foods in Latin America may serve to hydrolyze bound nicotinic acid and to inactivate toxins that may accumulate in stored grain contaminated with molds. Alternatively, degermination of the cereal during the common milling process in the United States may inhibit the liberation of bound niacin. The effect of these treatments, respectively, would be to prevent or to predispose to the development of pellagra when maize is a major element of the diet.

Whatever the cause, endemic pellagra disappeared coincident with the improvement of nutritional education and with the widespread supplementation of grain cereals with niacin. At present, pellagra is an occasional secondary manifestation of two disorders that profoundly affect tryptophan metabolism, the carcinoid syndrome, in which up to 60 percent of tryptophan is catabolized by what is ordinarily a minor pathway of metabolism (see Chap. 262), and Hartnup disease (see Chap. 335), an inherited disorder in which several amino acids including tryptophan are absorbed poorly from the diet. In both conditions pellagra is due to diminished availability of effective niacin equivalents and can be cured by the administration of large amounts of the vitamin.

Pellagra is a chronic wasting disease typically associated with dermatitis, dementia, and diarrhea. The dermatitis is bilateral, symmetric, and present in sites exposed to sunlight, and is due to photosensitivity. The mental changes are less discrete; fatigue, insomnia, and apathy may precede the development of an encephalopathy characterized by confusion, disorientation, hallucination, loss of memory, and eventually, frank organic psychosis. Paresthesias and polyneuritis may be the result of coexisting deficiencies of other vitamins. Diarrhea, when present, results from widespread inflammation of the mucous surfaces; other mucosal abnormalities include achlorhydria, glossitis, stomatitis, and vaginitis. The course is progressive over a several-year period, and death is usually due to secondary complications.

The relation between the known coenzyme function of NAD and NADP and these various symptoms has not been defined. Levels of NAD and NADP in erythrocytes are lower in patients with pellagra than in normal individuals, but the coenzymes are essential to so many reactions in intermediary metabolism that profound deficiency of the coenzymes is incompatible with life. The mental changes in pellagra may be associated with diminished conversion of tryptophan to serotonin.

No biochemical test is of diagnostic value, and diagnosis must be based upon suspicion and response to replacement therapy. As predicted, excretion in the urine of the metabolites of nicotinic acid and tryptophan is lower than average but not lower than in patients with generalized malnutrition. Plasma tryptophan and erythrocyte NAD and NADP levels are also low. The skin lesions are characterized by hyperkeratosis, hyperpigmentation, and desquamation.

The administration of small amounts of niacin (10 mg/d) in the face of adequate amounts of dietary tryptophan is sufficient to cure endemic pellagra. Large amounts of niacin (40 to 200 mg/d) may be required in Hartnup disease and in the carcinoid syndrome.

THIAMINE (BERIBERI) Biochemistry Thiamine contains pyrimidine and thiazole moieties linked by a methylene bridge (Fig. 76-1). The vitamin is synthesized by a variety of plants and microorganisms but not ordinarily by animals. However, rats and pigeons fed a thiamine-free diet can be protected from deficiency by large quantities of the pyrimidine and thiazole moieties, suggesting a small capacity to couple the subunits together. Small amounts of the vitamin may be synthesized by microorganisms in the gastrointestinal tract. Thiamine is absorbed both by an active-transport process and by passive diffusion. The capacity to absorb the vitamin in the human intestine is about 5 mg/d. Approximately 25 to 30 mg is stored in the body, 80 percent as thiamine diphosphate (pyrophosphate), 10 percent as thiamine triphosphate, and the remainder as thiamine monophosphate. Large amounts are present in skeletal muscles (about one-half of body stores), heart, liver, kidneys, and brain. A number of thiaminase enzymes inactivate thiamine by splitting the vitamin into its two component parts. Several metabolites are excreted in the urine, principally thiamine itself (which is secreted by the renal tubules), an acetylated derivative, and end products of thiamine catabolism, mainly derivatives of thiazole acetate and pyrimidine carboxylate.

Mechanism of action Thiamine diphosphate acts as a coenzyme for several reactions that cleave carbon-carbon bonds—the oxidative decarboxylation of α-keto acids (pyruvate and α-ketoglutarate) and keto analogues of leucine, isoleucine, and valine, and the transketolase reaction in the pentose phosphate pathway. Many features of thiamine deficiency are the result of inhibition of these enzymatic reactions and/or the accumulation of the proximal metabolites. Thiamine may also have a specific role in neurons independent of its coenzymatic function in general metabolism; thiamine and its esters are present in axonal membranes, and electrical stimulation of nerves effects the hydrolysis and release of thiamine diphosphate and triphosphate.

Requirements The recommended daily allowances for thiamine are given in Table 70-1. The vitamin has a widespread distribution in food and is absent only from oils, fats, cassava, and refined sugar. In vegetable products the vitamin is largely in the form of thiamine. The outer layers of cereal grains are especially rich in the vitamin; hence, machine-milled rice is a poor source. In animal tissues thiamine is present largely in the form of phosphate esters. The esters are dephosphorylated by phosphatases in the intestine, and only the free vitamin is absorbed. A substantial loss of the vitamin takes place during cooking above 100°C.

Several factors influence the absorption and metabolism of the vitamin (and hence alter daily requirements). One is the presence of thiaminases in foods such as fresh fish, clams, shrimp, mussels, and some raw animal tissues and in microorganisms in the colon. Two, daily needs decrease when fat forms a large part of the diet and increase as carbohydrate intake increases. Requirements are increased in pregnancy, during lactation, in thyrotoxicosis, and by fever. Accelerated loss of thiamine from the body may occur with diuretic therapy, hemodialysis, peritoneal dialysis, and diarrhea. Defective intestinal absorption can occur in malabsorption states, alcoholism, chronic malnutrition, and folate deficiency.

Experimental depletion Following the institution of a thiamine-free diet in control subjects, thiamine excretion in the urine decreases to 5 percent of the control value after a week and becomes undetectable after 2 weeks. However, the excretion of the pyrimidine and thiazole catabolites of thiamine remains unchanged for as long as a month, indicating that the body pool is slowly utilized during a period of deficient intake.

Within a week after the institution of a deficient diet, subjects develop a resting tachycardia, followed by the onset of weakness, decreased deep tendon reflexes, and (in some) a sensory neuropathy. Subjective symptoms include generalized malaise, headache, nausea, and aching of the muscles. Appearance of these symptoms is paralleled by a fall in red blood cell transketolase activity. Within a week of thiamine repletion (2 mg/d) all abnormal physical findings disappear, and the subjective symptoms clear after 2 weeks. (Experimental depletion in humans has not been carried to the point of development of severe cerebral or cardiovascular symptoms.)

Clinical deficiency In developed nations thiamine deficiency occurs in alcoholics or food faddists or in the context of special clinical situations, such as chronic peritoneal dialysis, hemodialysis, refeeding after starvation, or after the administration of glucose to asymptomatic but thiamine-depleted patients. In developing countries the disorder is commonly due to the consumption of milled rice or foods containing thiaminases or (possibly) other antithiamine factors.

Development of thiamine defeciency in chronic alcoholics is due to low thiamine intake, impaired thiamine absorption and storage, accelerated destruction of thiamine diphosphate, and varying degrees of energy expenditure. However, clinical manifestations develop in only a fraction of alcoholics and other chronically malnourished persons. Genetic factors may be involved in susceptibility.

The two major manifestations of thiamine deficiency involve the cardiovascular (wet beriberi) and nervous systems (dry beriberi and the Wernicke-Korsakoff syndrome). The typical patient has mixed symptoms involving both the cardiovascular and nervous systems, but pure cardiovascular, pure neuropathic, and pure cerebral forms also occur. The factors that determine the relative preponderance of these manifestations are related in part to the duration and severity of the deficiency, the degree of physical exertion, and the caloric intake. Severe physical exertion, high carbohydrate intake, and a moderate degree of chronic deficiency favor wet beriberi with little or no peripheral neuritis, whereas an equal deficiency with caloric restriction and relative inactivity favors the development of dry beriberi.

Beriberi heart disease comprises three major physiologic derangements: (1) peripheral vasodilatation leading to a high-output state, (2) biventricular myocardial failure, and (3) retention of sodium and water leading to edema. In the chronic form peripheral vasodilatation leads to increased arteriovenous shunting of blood, rapid circulation time, tachycardia, increased cardiac output, and a venous congestive state characterized by elevated peripheral venous pressure, elevated right ventricular end-diastolic pressure, decreased arteriovenous extraction of oxygen, sodium retention, and edema. Disordered blood flow (decreased cerebral and renal blood flow and increased flow to muscles) is common. Cardiac output increases so that notwithstanding the lowered peripheral vascular resistance ventricular work, arterial blood pressure, and pulmonary wedge pressure tend to be elevated. Temporary appearance or worsening of hypertension may occur during thiamine repletion, presumably due to closing of arteriovenous shunts and temporary volume overload.

In acute fulminant cardiovascular (shoshin) beriberi, the myocardial lesion is the central feature of a course in which severe dyspnea, restlessness, and anxiety eventuate in acute cardiovascular collapse and death within hours to days. Physical findings include stocking-glove cyanosis, extreme tachycardia, marked cardiomegaly, hepatomegaly, arterial bruits, and neck vein distention. The venous pressure is high, and the circulation time is rapid. Because of the fulminant course edema may be minimal or absent. Administration of thiamine rapidly restores peripheral vascular resistance, but improvement in the myocardial abnormality may be delayed so that low-output failure supervenes during treatment.

Three types of nervous system involvement occur: peripheral neuropathy, Wernicke's encephalopathy (cerebral beriberi), and the Korsakoff syndrome. The neuropathy may or may not be painful and is characterized by a symmetric impairment of sensory, motor, and reflex function that affects the distal segments of limbs more severely than the proximal ones. The histologic lesion is a noninflammatory degeneration of myelin sheaths. No meaningful distinction can be made between this disorder and so-called alcoholic neuropathy on the basis of either clinical or neurologic criteria.

Wernicke's encephalopathy ordinarily develops in an orderly sequence and consists of vomiting, nystagmus (horizontal more commonly than vertical), palsies of the rectus muscles leading to unilateral or bilateral ophthalmoplegia (and decrease in the nystagmus), fever, ataxia, and progressive mental deterioration that eventuates in a global confusional state and may progress to coma and death. Improvement occurs after thiamine replacement, although Korsakoff's syndrome may supervene. Thus, the eye palsies are corrected, the nystagmus improves in one-half, the ataxia improves or disappears in two-thirds, and the global confusional state disappears to be replaced by Korsakoff's syndrome. The latter consists of retrograde amnesia, impaired ability to learn, and (usually) confabulation. The patient is typically alert and responsive and exhibits no serious defect in behavior. Recovery (complete or partial) from Korsakoff's syndrome can be expected only in one-half.

In summary, Wernicke's encephalopathy and the amnesic psychosis of Korsakoff's syndrome are not separate clinical events; instead, the changing ocular and ataxic signs, the transformation of the global confusional state into the amnesic-confabulatory syndrome, and the development of a nonconfabulatory amnesic state are successive stages in the recovery from a single process. The clinical features, differential diagnosis, course, and pathology of cerebral beriberi are discussed in detail in Chap. 357.

Various biochemical tests to detect thiamine deficiency include the measurement of blood thiamine, pyruvate, α-ketoglutarate, lactate, and glyoxylate; measurement of the urinary excretion of thiamine and thiamine metabolites; a thiamine-loading test; and measurement of urinary methylglyoxal. The most reliable is the measurement of whole-blood or erythrocyte transketolase activity. Any enhancement in enzymatic activity resulting from added thiamine diphosphate (TPP) is referred to as the TPP effect (expressed in percent). If the activity of the enzyme is increased more than 15 percent by the added thiamine diphosphate, then a deficiency state is probably present. Due to variability in activity, measurement of isolated transketolase levels is not useful, but demonstration of an increase in activity after treatment coupled with a significant stimulation in vitro by added thiamine diphosphate prior to treatment suggests the presence of thiamine deficiency.

Another criterion for the diagnosis is the assessment of clinical response to thiamine administration. Clinical improvement may be dramatic in cardiovascular beriberi, and an increase in blood pressure and decrease in heart rate may be seen within 12 h after start of therapy. Diuresis and reduction in heart size may be apparent within 1 to 2 days.

Prompt administration of thiamine is indicated when beriberi is diagnosed or suspected. Fifty milligrams per day should be given intramuscularly for several days after which 2.5 to 5 mg/d can be administered by mouth. Larger amounts are usually not absorbed. All patients should also receive other water-soluble vitamins in therapeutic quantities.

Thiamine-responsive inborn errors of metabolism A number of thiamine-responsive inborn errors of metabolism have been described in which patients respond to pharmacologic doses of thiamine. These include thiamine-responsive megaloblastic anemia, for which the mechanism is unknown; thiamine-responsive lactic acidosis, which is due to low activity of pyruvate carboxylase in liver; thiamine-responsive branched-chain ketoaciduria, which is due to low activity of a ketoacid dehydrogenase; and intermittent cerebellar ataxia which may result from an abnormal pyruvate dehydrogenase. In addition, the autosomal recessive disorder subacute necrotizing encephalomyelopathy (Leigh's disease) may be related to a diminished amount of thiamine triphosphate in neural tissue; a factor has been isolated from the urine of such patients that inhibits the enzyme that synthesizes thiamine triphosphate. The clinical response of patients with Leigh's disease to pharmacologic doses of the vitamin appears to be minor, however.

PYRIDOXINE (VITAMIN B_6) Biochemistry The biologic activity of the vitamin B_6 group is displayed by pyridoxine, pyridoxal, and pyridoxamine and their 5-phosphate esters (Fig. 76-1). The coenzyme form is pyridoxal-5-phosphate, and the other compounds owe their activity to conversion to pyridoxal-5-phosphate. The vitamin is widely and uniformly distributed in all foods; muscle meats, liver, vegetables, and whole-grain cereals are among the best sources.

Mechanism of action Pyridoxal phosphate acts as a cofactor for many enzymes involved in amino acid metabolism, including transaminases, synthetases, and hydroxylases. In humans the vitamin is of particular importance in the metabolism of tryptophan, glycine, serine, glutamate, and the sulfur-containing amino acids. Pyridoxal phosphate is also required for the synthesis of the heme precursor δ-aminolevulinic acid. A large portion of body stores of pyridoxine is in muscle phosphorylase, where it functions to stabilize the enzyme rather than as a catalyst. It also plays a poorly understood role in neuronal excitability, possibly as a result of its function in transsulfuration reactions or in γ-aminobutyric acid metabolism.

Requirements The recommended daily allowances are given in Table 70-1. Even more than for most vitamins, the requirement is increased in pregnancy and by the administration of estrogens. In both conditions the pattern of excretion of tryptophan metabolites in urine changes, and this can be prevented by supplementation with pyridoxine. Estrogens appear to inhibit the role of pyridoxal phosphate in tryptophan metabolism. Pyridoxine requirement may also be increased by high protein intake. The ethanol metabolite acetaldehyde displaces pyridoxal phosphate from proteins and thus enhances its degradation.

Experimental depletion The feeding of pyridoxine-deficient diets leads to chemical evidence of deficiency (increased xanthurenic acid and decreased pyridoxine in urine) within a week. Electroencephalographic abnormalities are demonstrable within 3 weeks, and some subjects have grand mal seizures. Deficiency induced with the pyridoxine antagonist deoxypyridoxine causes, in addition, seborrheic dermatitis, cheilosis, glossitis, nausea, vomiting, weakness, and dizziness.

Clinical deficiency The widespread occurrence of the vitamin in food is probably the reason that pure pyridoxine deficiency does not occur except when the pyridoxine content of food is either destroyed or converted to less available protein-bound forms during processing, as has happened in some infant formulas. It is a paradox, therefore, that pyridoxine deficiency is now frequent because many commonly used drugs act as pyridoxine antagonists. Hydrazines such as *isoniazid* combine with pyridoxal and pyridoxal phosphate to form hydrazones. The hydrazones inhibit enzymes such as pyridoxal kinase, induce convulsions directly, and accelerate pyridoxine loss in the urine and thus induce a vitamin deficiency. *Cycloserine* also causes an increase in the excretion of the vitamin in the urine and produces profound neurologic effects, presumably by forming a complex with pyridoxal phosphate that competes with the cofactor for apoenzymes. *Penicillamine* acts as an antagonist by forming a thiazolidine derivative with pyridoxal phosphate. In each of these instances abnormal tryptophan metabolism and convulsions can be prevented by supplementation with the vitamin.

Estimates of vitamin deficiency have been based upon the correction of clinical signs of deficiency following administration of the vitamin, measurement of the excretion of tryptophan metabolites after tryptophan-loading tests, measurement of various amino acid transferase activities in blood, and measurement of the excretion of pyridoxine or its metabolites or of oxalate in urine. The most commonly used index is the measurement of urinary tryptophan metabolites, particularly xanthurenic acid, following tryptophan loading. Alternatively, cystathionine can be assayed after administration of a methionine load. In vitro measurement of red blood cell glutamic pyruvic transaminase in the presence and absence of pyridoxal phosphate may be a better indicator of pyridoxine status than either loading test.

The appropriate management is prevention of deficiency. Supplementation of the diet with 30 mg of pyridoxine returns tryptophan metabolism to normal in pregnancy, in users of oral contraceptives, and in patients taking isoniazid. Doses as high as 100 mg/d may be required in subjects taking penicillamine.

Pyridoxine-responsive diseases Several genetic disorders cause abnormalities in vitamin B_6 metabolism. In one group, infants develop convulsions and brain damage and die if not provided with large daily supplements of pyridoxine; these children have an apoenzyme for glutamic acid decarboxylase that has a decreased binding affinity for pyridoxal phosphate. Consequently they do not form normal amounts of γ-aminobutyric acid, a physiologic inhibitor of neurotransmission. Another group of patients has pyridoxine-responsive chronic anemia; pyridoxine supplementation results in prompt hematologic improvement but does not correct the morphologic abnormality in the erythrocytes.

The synthesis of cystathionine from homocystine and serine and its cleavage to cysteine and homoserine are catalyzed by two pyridoxal phosphate enzymes. The changes that occur in deficiency of these two enzymes and in xanthurenic aciduria due to kynureninase deficiency have been reviewed by Mudd. Some patients with vitamin B_6–responsive xanthurenic aciduria or cystathioninuria have a mutant apoenzyme that interacts abnormally with pyridoxal phosphate, a defect that can be largely corrected by elevated concentrations of the cofactor. In contrast, the vitamin B_6 response in patients with homocystinuria due to cystathionine synthetase deficiency is due to an enhancement of the activity of the residual amount of normal enzyme present rather than a restoration of the affected enzyme levels to normal.

RIBOFLAVIN Riboflavin in the form of the coenzymes flavin mononucleotide (FMN) and flavin adenine dinucleotide (FAD) (Fig. 76-1) participates in a variety of oxidation-reduction reactions. In addition, covalently attached flavins are essential to the structure of such enzymes as succinate dehydrogenase and monoamine oxidase. The vitamin is absorbed from the gastrointestinal tract either as free riboflavin or the 5′-phosphate by a specific transport process. The recommended daily allowance is listed in Table 70-1. Covalently linked vitamin accounts for less than one-tenth of the tissue pool. The vitamin is excreted in urine predominantly in the free form although a small fraction of the daily turnover is the result of catabolism by microorganisms in the gastrointestinal tract.

Riboflavin deficiency can be induced in humans by feeding a riboflavin-deficient diet or by the administration of riboflavin antagonists such as galactoflavin. The deficiency syndrome is characterized by sore throat, hyperemia and edema of the pharyngeal and oral mucous membranes, cheilosis, angular stomatitis, glossitis, seborrheic dermatitis, and normochromic, normocytic anemia due to red cell hypoplasia of the bone marrow. These features can be reversed by riboflavin administration. Thyroid hormones and adrenal steroids enhance FMN and FAD synthesis; certain psychotropic agents (phenothiazines and tricyclic antidepressants) competitively inhibit flavin coenzyme biosynthesis, but these agents alone do not induce deficiency. Instead, riboflavin deficiency almost invariably occurs in combination with other vitamin deficiencies.

VITAMIN C (SCURVY) Biochemistry In most animals ascorbic acid (vitamin C) can be synthesized from glucose. However, humans, other primates, and the guinea pig are unable to synthesize L-ascorbic acid and require vitamin C in the diet. These species can perform the various reactions required for the biosynthesis of the vitamin from D-glucose except for one step, the conversion of L-gluconogammalactone to L-abscorbic acid. The enzyme that catalyzes this reaction (L-gluconolactone oxidase) is missing because of a mutation; thus the need for vitamin C in the diet is the result of an inborn error in carbohydrate metabolism.

Mechanism of action L-Ascorbic acid readily undergoes reversible oxidation and reduction as follows:

$$\text{L-ascorbic acid} \rightleftharpoons \text{dehydro-L-ascorbic acid} + 2H^+ + 2e$$

This property of the vitamin is the key to understanding its role as a redox agent for biologic oxidation. However, ascorbic acid does not act as a conventional cofactor since its requirement can usually be replaced by other compounds with similar redox properties. The best understood function is in the synthesis of collagen; absence of the vitamin leads to impairment of peptidyl hydroxylation of procollagen and a reduction in collagen formation and secretion by connective tissue. Nonhydroxylated collagen is unstable and cannot form the triple helix required for normal tissue structure. Many features of scurvy result from this defect in collagen synthesis, including the capillary fragility that underlies the hemorrhagic features, the poor healing of wounds, and (in part) the bony abnormalities of children. Collagens that normally have the highest content of hydroxyproline are most severely affected, accounting for the early disruption of the adventitia, media, and basal laminae of blood vessels. Ascorbic acid also functions to prevent oxidation of tetrahydrofolate and thus protect the active folic acid pool and to regulate iron distribution and storage, probably by influencing the valence of stored iron and maintaining a normal ratio of ferritin to hemosiderin. Scorbutic patients excrete incompletely oxidized products of tyrosine metabolism, but the significance is not clear.

Requirements The recommended daily allowance for vitamin C is described in Table 70-1. The vitamin is present in milk and some meats (kidney, liver, fish) and is widely distributed in fruits and vegetables. A portion is lost after prolonged storage of unprocessed fruits and vegetables (for example, potatoes), but it is partially preserved (half or greater) by most means of food processing (boiling, steaming, pressure cooking, preserving jams and jellies, freezing, dehydration, and canning). As a consequence the recommended daily allowances can be met with even a modest intake of fruits and vegetables. The utilization of the vitamin is increased during pregnancy and lactation and in thyrotoxicosis, and absorption is decreased in diarrheal states and in achlorhydria.

Experimental depletion The total-body pool of vitamin C varies from 1.5 to 3 g. When a deficient diet is instituted, the pool is depleted at a constant rate that may be as high as 4 percent per day. In monkeys the major catabolic pathway involves oxidation of the alcohol at carbon 6 to an aldehyde and then to an acid. Because of differences in initial pool size and rates of turnover, differences in the completeness of deficiency in various experimental diets, and variation among normal subjects at the cellular or enzymatic level, the time required for development of symptoms ranges from 1 to 3 months in different studies. Manifestations of deficiency correlate better with the total pool size than with plasma or blood levels. The first symptoms (petechial hemorrhages and ecchymoses) develop when the pool size is less than 0.5 g; with further depletion (pool size 0.1 to 0.5 g) manifestations include gum involvement, hyperkeratosis, congested hair follicles, arthralgias, Sjögren's syndrome, coiled hairs, and joint effusions. When depletion is extreme (pool size $<$0.1 g), dyspnea, edema, oliguria, and neuropathy supervene. Progress of the disease may then be rapid.

Symptoms do not improve until the normal pool is repleted, and the larger the therapeutic dose, the more rapid the repletion. However, with doses as small as 6.5 mg/d the body pool eventually returns to normal, and amelioration of symptoms follows.

Clinical deficiency Clinical scurvy now occurs for the most part in areas of urban poverty. An increased incidence occurs at 6 to 12 months of age in infants whose processed milk formulas are unsupplemented with citrus fruit or vegetables as a result of maternal error or neglect. Another peak occurs in middle and old age; edentulous men who live alone and cook for themselves are particularly prone to develop scurvy. Clinical scurvy is more severe than the experimental disease, doubtlessly because affected individuals usually have deficiencies of other dietary constituents as well and because the groups at risk (infants and the elderly) are especially vulnerable.

In adults the features include perifollicular hyperkeratotic papules in which hairs become fragmented and buried; perifollicular hemorrhages; purpura beginning on the backs of the lower extremities coalescing to become ecchymoses (Fig. 76-2); hemorrhage into the muscles of the arms and legs with secondary phlebothromboses; hemorrhages into joints; splinter hemorrhages in the nail beds; gum involvement (only in people with teeth) that includes swelling, friability, bleeding, secondary infection, and loosening of the teeth; poor healing of wounds and breakdown of recently healed wounds; petechial hemorrhages in the viscera; and emotional changes. Symptoms resembling those of Sjögren's syndrome may occur. Terminally, icterus, edema, and fever are common, and convulsions, shock, and death may occur abruptly.

In infancy and childhood hemorrhage into the periosteum of long bones causes painful swellings and may result in epiphyseal separation. The sternum may sink inward, leaving a sharp elevation at the rib margins (scorbutic rosary). Purpura and ecchymoses may develop in the skin, and gum lesions occur if the teeth have erupted. Retrobulbar, subarachnoid, and intracerebral hemorrhages rapidly culminate in death if treatment is delayed.

Severe to moderate anemia is common in children and in adults, is usually normochromic and normocytic, and is due to bleeding into tissues. The anemia may be macrocytic and/or megaloblastic (one-fifth of patients in one series). Many foods that contain vitamin C also contain folate, and diets that cause scurvy may also cause folate deficiency. However, ascorbic acid deficiency also results in an increased oxidation of formyl tetrahydrofolic acid to inactive folate

FIGURE 76-2 Hemorrhages and ecchymoses in a patient with scurvy. *(Photograph courtesy of Leonard L. Madison.)*

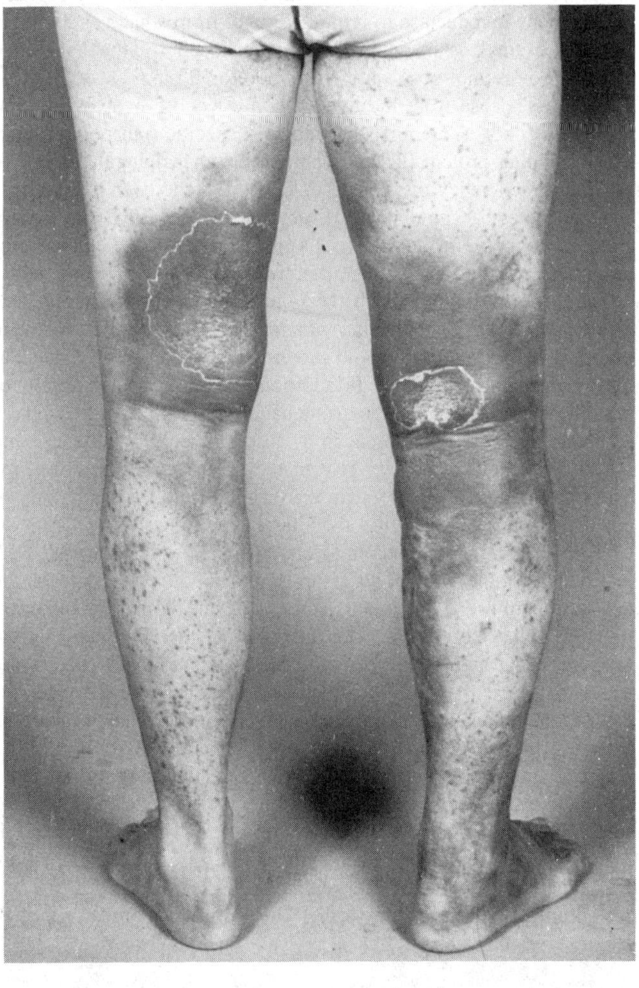

metabolites and may cause a decrease in the active folate pool. Whether changes in iron distribution and storage are involved in the pathogenesis of the anemia is unclear. The anemia is corrected with refeeding and replenishment of vitamin C and the institution of a balanced diet.

In some hospitals platelet ascorbic acid levels are useful in diagnosing scurvy and are usually less than one-fourth of the normal value. Plasma levels of the vitamin correlate less well with the clinical state. In infants x-ray changes of the bones may be diagnostic. Indirect bilirubin is frequently elevated. Capillary fragility is abnormal. The remainder of the laboratory tests are nondiagnostic.

Scurvy is potentially fatal; if the diagnosis is suspected, blood should be obtained, and ascorbic acid therapy should be instituted promptly. The usual dose in adults is 100 mg three to five times a day by mouth until 4 g has been administered, then 100 mg/d. In infants and children administration of 10 to 25 mg three times a day is adequate. A diet rich in vitamin C should be initiated simultaneously. Spontaneous bleeding usually ceases within 24 h, muscle and bone pains subside quickly, and the gums begin to heal within 2 to 3 days. Even large ecchymoses and hematomas resolve in 10 to 12 days, although pigmentary changes in areas of extensive hemorrhage may persist for months. Serum bilirubin becomes normal within 3 to 5 days, and the anemia is ordinarily corrected within 2 to 4 weeks.

VITAMIN A **Biochemistry** Vitamin A (retinol) can either be ingested or synthesized within the body from plant carotenoids (Fig. 76-1). Preformed vitamin A is present in animal tissues, and the best sources are liver, milk, and kidney, where it occurs largely in the form of fatty acid esters. The esters are hydrolyzed during digestion, absorbed in the free form, reesterified with fatty acids within the intestinal mucosa, and enter the circulation in association with lymph chylomicrons. The carotenoid substrates for synthesis of vitamin A, mainly β-carotenes, are widely distributed in plants. β-Carotene can either be absorbed intact or cleaved in the intestinal tract to form two molecules of retinaldehyde. Retinaldehyde is subsequently reduced by an aldehyde reductase to retinol. Retinol from whatever source is stored as retinyl esters in the parenchymal cells of the liver. The normal body retinol pool varies from 300 to 900 mg.

Prior to release from the liver retinyl esters are hydrolyzed, and the free alcohol is mobilized bound to a specific transport protein, retinol-binding protein (RBP), for transport to peripheral tissues. In vitamin A deficiency the release of RBP from the liver is inhibited, and the protein accumulates in liver; with repletion RBP is rapidly released from preformed stores. Approximately equal amounts of retinol are excreted in the bile and urine.

Mechanism of action The best-defined function of vitamin A is its role in vision; in the retina vitamin A constitutes the prosthetic group of a series of carotenoid proteins that provide the molecular basis for visual excitation. In addition, vitamin A is required for growth, reproduction, and the maintenance of life. Retinol-phosphate-mannose glycolipid is present in a variety of cell membranes, and the vitamin plays a primary role in the synthesis of glycoproteins. The importance of glycoprotein to every cell implies that this is an equally important function of the vitamin.

Requirements The recommended daily allowance for vitamin A is listed in Table 70-1. The assumed utilization efficiency for the conversion of β-carotene to vitamin A in the human is one-sixth (0.167). Other carotenoids with provitamin A activity have, on the average, about half the activity of β-carotene. Pregnancy and disease states in which there is impaired absorption or storage, excessive utilization, or increased excretion of vitamin A may lead to increased requirements.

Experimental depletion When experimental subjects are fed a diet deficient in both retinol and carotene, plasma levels fall, and the body pool shrinks to less than half the control value. Deficiency is manifested by follicular hyperkeratosis, impaired dark adaptation, and abnormalities of the electroretinogram. These changes are corrected after supplementation with 150 μg of retinol or 300 μg of β-carotene per day.

Clinical deficiency Endemic deficiency results from inadequate amounts of the vitamin and of the carotene provitamins in the diet and probably always occurs in conjunction with deficiency of other nutrients or complicating diseases. In some developing countries vitamin A deficiency is a major cause of blindness in the young as a consequence of failure to incorporate green leafy vegetables or other sources of the provitamin or vitamin into the diet. Such children appear to be particularly susceptible to the complications of measles. Vitamin A deficiency may also accompany protein-calorie malnutrition, and here the deficiency is due in part to a defective release mechanism from the liver secondary to inadequate retinol-binding protein. In developed nations vitamin A deficiency is usually due either to intestinal malabsorption (as in sprue or after intestinal bypass surgery), abnormal storage (liver disease), or enhanced destruction or excretion of the vitamin (proteinuria). Vitamin A deficiency has also occurred in patients receiving total parenteral nutrition because of loss of vitamin A after prolonged storage of intravenous fluid.

Night blindness is the earliest symptom of deficiency, followed by degenerative changes in the retina. The bulbar conjunctiva becomes dry (xerosis), and small gray plaques with foamy surfaces develop (Bitôt's spots). These early lesions are reversible with vitamin A. The more serious effects of vitamin A deficiency are ulceration and necrosis of the cornea (keratomalacia), leading to perforation, endophthalmitis, and blindness. Such patients may also exhibit dryness and hyperkeratosis of the skin.

Vitamin A levels in plasma are not reliable for the assessment of stores in individual cases. Measurements of dark adaptation, rod scotometry, and electroretinography are useful indicators of vitamin A stores but require trained personnel and expensive equipment; consequently, the diagnosis is usually based upon a high index of suspicion in malnourished children or in patients with known predisposing factors for its development.

Night blindness and the milder conjunctival changes respond well to 30,000 IU of vitamin A daily for a week. Corneal damage constitutes a therapeutic emergency, and the usual treatment is 20,000 IU/kg body weight per day for 5 days. Children who are at risk for vitamin A deficiency and who develop measles should be given 200,000 IU orally each day for 2 days.

VITAMIN E **Biochemistry** Eight naturally occurring tocopherols possess vitamin E activity. The structure of alpha tocopherol, the most widely distributed and most active of the tocopherols, is shown in Fig. 76-1. The vitamin is absorbed from the gastrointestinal tract by a mechanism similar to that for other fat-soluble vitamins and enters the bloodstream via the lymph, associated first with chylomicrons and then with plasma betalipoproteins. Indeed, plasma levels correlate closely with plasma lipid levels. The vitamin is stored in all tissues, and the tissue stores can protect against vitamin deficiency for long periods. Approximately three-fourths of the vitamin is excreted in bile, and the balance is excreted as glucuronides in urine. Metabolites with quinone structures (including one similar to ubiquinone) are present in tissues.

Mechanism of action The vitamin probably acts as an antioxidant rather than as a specific cofactor. In so acting it presumably inhibits oxidation of essential cellular constituents and prevents the formation of toxic oxidation products. Other antioxidants such as selenium, sulfur-containing amino acids, and the ubiquinone group can reverse the symptoms of vitamin E deficiency in animals.

Requirements The recommended daily requirement is 10 to 30 mg/d (Table 70-1). Diets containing large amounts of polyunsaturated fatty acids increase and diets containing antioxidants decrease the requirement. The vitamin is widely distributed in food, so that a primary deficiency state has never been recognized in otherwise healthy children or adults. Newborn infants have plasma concentrations about one-fifth that of maternal levels, implying poor placental transfer, but human milk (in contrast to cow's milk) has sufficient levels to meet the requirements in infants.

Experimental depletion In long-term studies vitamin E concentrations in plasma declined significantly only after months on a deficient diet. No manifestations of the depletion were detected in normal volunteers, making it difficult to establish that tocopherol is a human vitamin.

Clinical deficiency In the appropriate clinical setting vitamin E deficiency is associated with a discrete syndrome. Rarely, deficiency is due to a selective malabsorption of the vitamin. More commonly intestinal fat malabsorption can cause deficiency of all fat-soluble vitamins including vitamin E, and children with chronic cholestatic liver disease appear to be particularly susceptible, due to a combination of malabsorption of vitamin E and trapping of the vitamin in plasma by the associated hyperlipoproteinemia, so that tissue stores may be depleted despite a normal tocopherol level in serum. Indeed, the ratio of serum vitamin E to total serum lipid is the preferred index for assessing vitamin E status. The manifestations of deficiency include areflexia, gait disturbance, decreased proprioceptive and vibratory sensation, and paresis of gaze and are associated with degeneration of the posterior columns of the spinal cord, selective loss of large-caliber, myelinated axons in peripheral nerves, and appearance of spheroids in the gracile and cuneate nuclei of the brain. Treatment (50 to 100 IU/d by mouth) is most effective when initiated early in the course of the disease.

VITAMIN K Vitamin K consists of a quinone ring attached to a side chain (labeled *R* in Fig. 76-1) that varies depending on the source of the vitamin. Vitamin K_1 (phylloquinone) is present in most edible vegetables, particularly in green leaves, and vitamin K_2 is produced by intestinal bacteria. The many compounds with vitamin K activity are structurally related to the simpler compound, 2-methyl-1,4-naphthoquinone (menadione). Menadione is formed in the gut by the removal of the side chain from the vitamin by intestinal bacteria. After absorption, menadione is converted in the body to the active menaquinone. The vitamin is a component of a specialized microsomal enzyme system that effects the posttranslational γ carboxylation of glutamic acid in proteins of the plasma, bone, kidney, and urine, including the precursor proteins for the clotting factors VII, IX, X, and possibly V. Death from hemorrhage in deficiency states ensues before deficiency of the other carboxylated proteins becomes manifest.

Under ordinary circumstances about 80 percent of vitamin K is absorbed from the small bowel into the intestinal lymph. Because the naturally occurring forms of vitamin K are fat-soluble and are poorly stored in the body, deficiency can occur in association with diseases that interfere with fat absorption. In addition, long-term treatment with oral antibiotics may temporarily eliminate intestinal bacteria as a source for vitamin K and promote deficiency when the diet is marginal or deficient. The warfarin anticoagulant drugs induce hypoprothrombinemia by inhibiting the γ carboxylation of the precursor protein.

Newborn infants tend to be deficient in vitamin K and have low plasma levels of several coagulation factors in the prothrombin complex. Such deficiencies result from minimal stores of vitamin K at birth, lack of an established intestinal flora, and a limited dietary intake of the vitamin.

Routine determination of prothrombin should be performed prior to surgical procedures or delivery. Subjects with levels below 70 percent of normal should receive therapy with vitamin K. Vitamin K deficiency can be separated from hypoprothrombinemia of liver disease by measurement of the noncarboxylated prothrombin precursor that accumulates in plasma in the vitamin deficiency.

VITAMIN EXCESS

Fat-soluble vitamins are stored to a variable extent in the body and hence are more likely to cause adverse effects when taken in excess; excess states for vitamins D (see Chap. 341) and A are particularly well characterized. Water-soluble vitamins are readily excreted in the urine and stored only to a limited extent. Consequently, toxicity states for these vitamins only occur when large amounts are taken for prolonged periods.

VITAMIN A AND CAROTENES **Carotenemia** Carotenemia results from excessive intake of vitamin A precursors in foods, principally carrots. Excess carotene is not injurious apart from the cosmetic effect; the fact that carotenemia does not cause hypervitaminosis A indicates that the conversion of carotene to vitamin A must be regulated. Carotenemia is manifested by yellowing of the skin with greatest intensity on the palms and soles and by a corresponding yellowness of serum. The yellowing of the skin can be distinguished from jaundice in that the scleras remain white. Hypothyroid patients are particularly susceptible. The omission of carrots from the diet leads to the rapid disappearance of the pigmentation. Discoloration of the skin can also result from the consumption of excessive amounts of other colored fruits and vegetables.

Vitamin A toxicity Hypervitaminosis A can result from accidental overingestion by hunters or explorers (polar bear liver), as the result of food faddism (usually caused by overly solicitous parents), or as a side effect of inappropriate therapy. Acute toxicity from a single massive dose consists of abdominal pain, nausea, vomiting, headache, dizziness, sluggishness, papilledema, and in infants a bulging fontanel followed within a few days by generalized desquamation of the skin and recovery. Chronic toxicity occurs following ingestion of 25,000 units or more daily for protracted periods and is characterized by bone and joint pain, hyperostoses, hair loss, dryness and fissures of the lips, anorexia, benign intracranial hypertension, low-grade fever, pruritus, weight loss, and hepatosplenomegaly. The only diagnostic laboratory finding is elevation of the vitamin in serum, chiefly in the form of retinyl esters. The concentration of retinol-binding protein is normal, and the excess vitamin A circulates in association with lipoprotein. Relief is prompt on withdrawal of the vitamin from the diet.

VITAMIN E Relatively large doses of vitamin E have been taken by some for extended periods without causing apparent harm. In others, a variety of nonspecific complaints have been reported including malaise, gastrointestinal complaint, headaches, and possibly hypertension. However, true toxicity appears to occur in two situations—in subjects receiving oral anticoagulants and in premature infants. In large amounts, vitamin E can apparently antagonize vitamin K and inhibit prothrombin time; this phenomenon results in a marked potentiation of oral anticoagulants. Premature infants given parenteral vitamin E are reported to have developed ascites associated with hepatosplenomegaly, cholestatic jaundice, azotemia, and thrombocytopenia.

VITAMIN K Large amounts of vitamin K can block the effects of oral anticoagulants and when given to pregnant women can cause jaundice in the newborn.

PYRIDOXINE Most adults can consume up to 10 times the recommended daily allowance of 2 mg pyridoxine per day without adverse effects. However, severe peripheral neuropathies have developed after ingestion of several grams per day for prolonged periods; symptoms include ataxia, perioral numbness, and clumsiness of the hands and feet, and the findings include loss of position and vibration sense without impairment of reflexes or sensory function. Recovery is slow after ingestion ceases. Lower doses (25 mg/d) can antagonize the effects of levodopa in Parkinson's disease and decrease the anticonvulsant effects of phenytoin barbiturates.

VITAMIN C Vitamin C is widely used in megavitamin therapy because of the claim that large amounts of the vitamin (a gram or greater per day) are effective in preventing or minimizing the symptoms of the common cold. However, in controlled studies, no significant differences in occurrence, severity, or duration of colds have been demonstrated in subjects treated with a placebo compared with the vitamin. Use of the vitamin in this way is unwarranted and probably unwise. The long-term use of ascorbic acid in these doses can interfere with the absorption of vitamin B_{12}, enhance blood levels of estrogens in women on exogenous estrogens, cause uricosuria, and predispose to formation of oxalate kidney stones. In addition, large doses enhance the development of metabolizing enzymes in the fetus and may cause rebound scurvy in the offspring of mothers who have ingested large amounts of the vitamin during pregnancy. However, pharmacologic doses (200 mg daily) may correct leukocyte abnormalities in patients with the Chédiak-Higashi syndrome (see Chap. 64).

NIACIN Large doses of niacin are used for treatment of hypercholesterolemia and occasionally for other purposes. The vitamin causes release of histamine, which in turn can cause severe flushing, pruritus, and gastrointestinal disturbances and may aggravate asthma. Acanthosis nigricans may occur. In doses of 3 g/d niacin has been reported to cause elevation of serum uric acid and of fasting glucose. Large doses can also cause hepatic toxicity including cholestatic jaundice.

REFERENCES

General

ELSAS LJ, MCCORMICK DB: Genetic defects in vitamin utilization. Part I: General aspects and fat-soluble vitamins. Vitam Horm 43:103, 1986

GOODHART RS, SHILS ME (eds): *Modern Nutrition in Health and Disease,* 6th ed. Philadelphia, Lea & Febiger, 1980

HOYUMPA AM: Mechanisms of vitamin deficiencies in alcoholism. Alcoholism (NY) 10:573, 1986

MACHLIN LJ (ed): *Handbook of Vitamins. Nutritional, Biochemical, and Clinical Aspects.* New York, Dekker, 1984

MUDD SH: Inborn errors of metabolism. Vitamin-responsive genetic disease. J Clin Pathol 27(Suppl) 8:38, 1974

RUDMAN D, WILLIAMS PJ: Nutrient deficiencies during total parenteral nutrition. Nutr Rev 43:1, 1984

Niacin deficiency

CARPENTER KJ: The relationship of pellagra to corn and the low availability of niacin in cereals. Experientia(Suppl) 44:197, 1983

———, LEWIN WJ: A reexamination of the composition of diets associated with pellagra. J Nutr 115:543, 1985

CASTIELLO RJ, LYNCH PJ: Pellagra and the carcinoid syndrome. Arch Dermatol 105:574, 1972

DE LANGE DJ, JOUBERT CP: Assessment of nicotinic acid status of population groups. Am J Clin Nutr 15:169, 1964

GOLDSMITH GA: Experimental niacin deficiency. J Am Dietetic Assoc 32:312, 1956

HENDERSON LM: Niacin. Ann Rev Nutr 3:289, 1983

LEVY HL: Hartnup disorder, in *The Metabolic Basis of Inherited Disease,* 6th ed, CR Scriver et al (eds). New York, McGraw-Hill, 1989, p 2515

JUKES TH et al: The conquest of pellagra. Fed Proc 40:1519, 1980

Thiamine deficiency

BROWN GM: Biogenesis and metabolism of thiamine, in *Metabolic Pathways,* 3d ed, DM Greenberg (ed). New York, Academic, 1970, p 369

DURAN M, WADMAN SK: Thiamine-responsive inborn errors of metabolism. J Inherited Metab Dis 8(Suppl 1):70, 1985

DYCKNER T et al: Aggravation of thiamine deficiency by magnesium depletion. Acta Med Scand 218:129, 1985

HARPER CG et al: Clinical signs in the Wernicke-Korsakoff complex: A retrospective analysis of 131 cases diagnosed at necropsy. J Neurol Neurosurg Psychiatry 49:341, 1986

HOYUMPA AM: Mechanisms of thiamine deficiency in chronic alcoholism. Am J Clin Nutr 33:2750, 1980

KAWAI C et al: Reappearance of beriberi heart disease in Japan. Am J Med 69:383, 1980

KOZAM RL et al: Cardiovascular beriberi. Am J Cardiol 30:418, 1972

KURIYAMA M et al: Blood vitamin B_1, transketolase, and thiamine pyrophosphate (TPP) effect in beriberi patients. Clin Chim Acta 108:159, 1980

PINCUS JH et al: Thiamine derivatives in subacute necrotizing encephalomyelopathy. Pediatrics 51:716, 1973

VICTOR M et al: *The Wernicke-Korsakoff Syndrome.* Philadelphia, Davis, 1971

ZIPORIN ZZ et al: Excretion of thiamine and its metabolites in the urine of young adult males receiving restricted intakes of the vitamin. J Nutr 85:287, 1965

Pyridoxine deficiency

BHAGAVAN HN, BRIN M: Drug–vitamin B_6 interaction. Curr Concepts Nutr 12:1, 1983

FRIMPTER GW et al: Vitamin B_6–dependency syndromes: New horizons in nutrition. Am J Clin Nutr 22:794, 1969

GERSHOFF SN: Vitamin B_6, in *Nutrition Reviews' Present Knowledge in Nutrition,* 4th ed, DM Hegsted et al (eds). Washington, DC, The Nutrition Foundation, 1976, p 149

HARRIS JW, HORRIGAN DL: Pyridoxine-responsive anemia-prototype and variations on the theme, in *Vitamins and Hormones,* RS Harris et al (eds). New York, Academic, 1964, vol 22, p 721

JAFFE IA: The antivitamin B_6 effect of penicillamine: Clinical and immunological implications, in *Advances in Biochemical Psychopharmacology,* MS Ebodi et al (eds). New York, Raven Press, 1972, vol 4

LUHBY AL et al: Vitamin B_6 metabolism in users of oral contraceptive agents: I. Abnormal urinary xanthurenic acid excretion and its correction by pyridoxine. Am J Clin Nutr 24:684, 1971

MUDD SH: Pyridoxine-responsive genetic disease. Fed Proc 30:970, 1971

SAUBERLICH HE et al: Biochemical assessment of the nutritional status of vitamin B_6 in the human. Am J Clin Nutr 25:629, 1972

Riboflavin deficiency

BATES CJ: Human riboflavin requirements, and metabolic consequences of deficiency in man and animals. World Rev Nutr Diet 50:215, 1987

MERRILL AH JR et al: Formation and mode of action of flavoproteins. Ann Rev Nutr 1:281, 1981

PINTO JT, RIVLIN RS: Drugs that promote renal excretion of riboflavin. Drug Nutr Interact 5:143, 1987

——— et al: Mechanisms underlying the differential effects of ethanol on the bioavailability of riboflavin and flavin adenine dinucleotide. J Clin Invest 79:1343, 1987

Ascorbic acid deficiency

BARNES MJ, KODICEK E: Biological hydroxylations and ascorbic acid, in *Vitamins and Hormones,* P Munson et al (eds). New York, Academic, 1972, vol 30, p 1

BARNESS LA: Nutritional aspects of vegetarianism, health foods, and fad diets. Nutr Rev 59:153, 1977

BOXER LA et al: Correction of leucocyte function in Chédiak-Higashi syndrome by ascorbate. N Engl J Med 295:1041, 1971

BURNS JJ et al: Third conference on vitamin C. Ann NY Acad Sci 498, 1987

ENGLAND S, SEIFTER S: The biochemical functions of ascorbic acid. Ann Rev Nutr 6:365, 1986

HODGES RE et al: Clinical manifestations of ascorbic acid deficiency in man. Am J Clin Nutr 24:432, 1971

LEVINE M: New concepts in the biology and biochemistry of ascorbic acid. N Engl J Med 314:892, 1986

REID GM: Scurvy: Old disease—New insight. Med Hypotheses 12:167, 1983

REULER JB et al: Adult scurvy. JAMA 253:805, 1985

SATO P, UNDENFRIEND S: Studies on ascorbic acid related to the genetic basis of scurvy, in *Vitamins and Hormones,* P Munson et al (eds). New York, Academic, 1978, vol 36, p 33

TOLBERT BM et al: New information on synthesis and metabolism of ascorbic acid. Nutr Rev 35:22, 1977

VILTER RW: Effects of ascorbic acid deficiency in man, in *The Vitamins,* WH Sebrell Jr et al (eds). New York, Academic, 1967, vol 1, p 457

WALLERSTEIN RO, WALLERSTEIN RO JR: Scurvy. Sem Hematol 13:211, 1976

Vitamin A deficiency

BARCLAY AJG et al: Vitamin A supplements and mortality related to measles: A randomised clinical trial. Br Med J 294:294, 1987

DELUCA LM: The direct involvement of vitamin A in glycosyl transfer reactions of mammalian membranes, in *Vitamins and Hormones,* PL Munson et al (eds). New York, Academic, 1977, vol 35, p 1

GOODMAN DS: Vitamin A and retinoids in health and disease. N Engl J Med 310:1023, 1984

HOWARD L et al: Vitamin A deficiency from long-term parenteral nutrition. Ann Intern Med 93:576, 1980

SAUBERLICH HE et al: Vitamin A metabolism and requirements in the human studied with the use of labeled retinol, in *Vitamins and Hormones,* RS Harris et al (eds). New York, Academic, 1974, vol 32

SMITH FR, GOODMAN DS: Vitamin A transport in human vitamin A toxicity. N Engl J Med 294:805, 1976

SOMMER A et al: Clinical characteristics of vitamin A responsive and nonresponsive Bitôt's spots. Am J Ophthalmol 90:160, 1980

TIELSCH JM, SOMMER A: The epidemiology of vitamin A deficiency and xerophthalmia. Ann Rev Nutr 4:183, 1974

VAHLQUIST A: Clinical use of vitamin A and its derivatives—physiological and pharmacological aspects. Clin Exp Dermatol 10:133, 1985

Vitamin A for measles. Lancet 1:1067, 1987

WALD G: Molecular basis of visual excitation. Science 162:230, 1968

Vitamin E deficiency

BIERI JG et al: Medical uses of vitamin E. N Engl J Med 308:1063, 1983

HORWITT MK: Interrelations between vitamin E and polyunsaturated fatty acids in adult men, in *Vitamins and Hormones,* GF Marrian, KV Thimann (eds). New York, Academic, 1962, vol 20, p 541

———: The promotion of vitamin E. J Nutr 116:1371, 1986

PERLMUTTER DH et al: Intramuscular vitamin E repletion in children with chronic cholestasis. Am J Dis Child 141:170, 1987

ROSENBLUM JL et al: A progressive neurologic syndrome in children with chronic liver disease. N Engl J Med 304:503, 1981

SITRIN MD et al: Vitamin E deficiency and neurologic disease in adults with cystic fibrosis. Ann Intern Med 107:51, 1987

SOKOL RJ et al: Vitamin E deficiency with normal serum vitamin E concentrations in children with chronic cholestasis. N Engl J Med 310:1209, 1984

——— et al: Isolated vitamin E deficiency in the absence of fat malabsorption—familial and sporadic cases: Characterization and investigation of causes. J Lab Clin Med 111:548, 1988

TRABER MG et al: Lack of tocopherol in peripheral nerves of vitamin E–deficient patients with peripheral neuropathy. N Engl J Med 317:262, 1987

Vitamin K deficiency

ALLISON PM et al: Effects of a vitamin K-deficient diet and antibiotics in normal human volunteers. J Lab Clin Med 110:180, 1987

BERTINA RM et al: New method for the rapid detection of vitamin K deficiency. Clin Chim Acta 105:93, 1980
DOISY EA JR, MATSCHINER JT: Biochemistry of vitamin K, in *Fat-Soluble Vitamins*, RA Morton (ed). Elmsford, NY, Pergamon, 1970, vol 9, p 293
IBER FL et al: Vitamin K deficiency in chronic alcoholic males. Alcoholism (NY) 10:679, 1986
OLSON RE, SUTTIE JW: Vitamin K and α-carboxyglutamate biosynthesis, in *Vitamins and Hormones*, PL Munson et al (eds). New York, Academic, 1977, vol 35, p 59
SHEARER MJ et al: Studies on the absorption and metabolism of phylloquinone (vitamin K) in man, in *Vitamins and Hormones*, RS Harris et al (eds). New York, Academic, 1974, vol 32, p 513
SUTTIE JW: *Vitamin K Metabolism and Vitamin K-Dependent Proteins*. Baltimore, University Park Press, 1980

Vitamin excess

ALHADEFF L: Toxic effects of water-soluble vitamins. Nutr Rev 42:33, 1984
CHALMERS TC: Effects of ascorbic acid on the common cold. Am J Med 58:532, 1975
CORRIGAN JJ JR: The effect of vitamin E on warfarin-induced vitamin K deficiency. Ann NY Acad Sci 82:361, 1982
HERBERT V: The vitamin craze. Arch Intern Med 140:173, 1980
LEMONS JA, MAISELS MJ: Vitamin E—How much is too much? Pediatrics 76:625, 1985
LOMBAERT A, CARTON H: Benign intracranial hypertension due to A-hypervitaminosis in adults and adolescents. Eur Neurol 14:340, 1976
LORCH V et al: Unusual syndrome with fatalities among premature infants: Association with a new intravenous vitamin E product. Morb Mort Week Rep 33:198, 1984
Megavitamin E supplementation and vitamin K–dependent carboxylation. Nutr Rev 41:268, 1986
SCHAUMBURG H et al: Sensory neuropathy from pyridoxine abuse: A new megavitamin syndrome. N Engl J Med 309:445, 1983
SHIN HB et al: Ascorbic acid–induced uricosuria: A consequence of megavitamin therapy. Ann Intern Med 84:385, 1976
Toxic effects of vitamin overdosage. Med Lett Drugs Ther 26:73, 1984
WOOLLISCROFT JO: Megavitamins: Fact and fancy. Dis-A-Month 24:1, 1983

77 DISTURBANCES IN TRACE ELEMENT METABOLISM

KENNETH H. FALCHUK

CLASSIFICATION AND FUNCTIONS The "trace elements" comprise metals in biologic fluids at concentrations below one microgram per gram of wet weight. Most are essential nutrients for human beings (Table 77-1). Others (As, Ni, Sn, V, Si) are essential for some plants and/or vertebrates including mammals and may be required by humans. The functions of trace elements and of other, more abundant metals (Na, K, Ca, Mg) are determined, in part, by their charges, mobilities, and binding constants to biologic ligands. Elements in one group (Na, K) bind weakly to negatively charged ligands and can cross cellular membranes without major impediment. They are used by living systems as charge carriers to conduct electric impulses along nerves, etc. Those in a second group (Mg, Ca) form moderately stable but not tight complexes with enzymes, nucleic acids, and other ligands. They act as biochemical "triggers," altering and/or controlling the functions of these molecules, e.g., Ca affects muscle contraction and relaxation (Chap. 365). Those in a third group (Fe, Zn, Cu, and others) form strong, static complexes with and become integral functional components of enzymes (Table 77-1).

METAL DEFICIENCY OR TOXICITY Metals can cause disease through deficiency, imbalance, or toxicity. Deficiency usually results when dietary intake is inadequate or when intake is adequate but other conditioning factors come into play. Deficiencies can be caused by metal malabsorption in chronic diarrheal diseases, surgical resection of the small intestine, or formation of metal complexes with dietary components that are not readily absorbed, e.g., between phytates and Zn. Deficiency states can also result from increased losses through urine, pancreatic juice, or other exocrine secretions or from metabolic imbalances produced by antagonistic or synergistic interactions between metals. Large amounts of Ca, for example, decrease the absorption of and induce deficiency of Zn. Similarly, Mo and Cu compete with each other; excessive Mo in cattle leads to Cu deficiency characterized by diarrhea and wasting. Proven manifestations of trace element deficiencies in humans, except for iron, were previously rare but have been recognized more frequently with the use of total parenteral nutrition (TPN) (Chap. 75). Clinical criteria for the recognition of deficiency states include decreases in metal content of whole blood, serum, hair and/or other accessible fluids and tissues, changes in the activities of metalloenzymes, and characteristic signs and symptoms (Table 77-2).

Toxic effects are dependent on the chemical form, the amount ingested, the route of entry into the body, the biologic ligands associated with the metal, the tissue distribution, the concentration

TABLE 77-1 Requirements and functions of trace elements in humans

Element	Requirements, mg/day*	Amount† Total, g per 70 kg body weight	Amount† Serum µmol/L	Amount† Serum µg/dL	Selected biochemical functions	Enzymes Class	Enzymes Example
Fe	10–20	4.0	18	100	Oxygen transport	Oxidoreductases	Cytochrome oxidase
Zn	15–20	3.0	15	100	Nucleic acid and protein synthesis and degradation, alcohol metabolism	Transferases, hydrolases, lyases, isomerases, ligases, oxidoreductases	RNA polymerases, alcohol dehydrogenases, transcription factors
Cu	2–6	0.25	16	100	Hemoglobin synthesis, connective tissue metabolism, bone development	Oxidoreductases	Superoxide dismutase, ferroxidase (ceruloplasmin)
Co	0.0001	1.1	0.0001	0.0007	Methionine metabolism	Transferases	Homocysteine methyltransferase
Mn	2–5	0.02	0.001	0.06	Oxidative phosphorylation; fatty acid, mucopolysaccharide, and cholesterol metabolism	Oxidoreductases, hydrolases, ligases	Diamine oxidase, pyruvate carboxylase
Mo	0.15–0.5	0.07	0.007	0.07	Xanthine metabolism	Oxidoreductases	Xanthine oxidase
Se	0.05–0.2	(−)	1.6	13	Antioxidant	Oxidoreductases, transferases	Glutathione peroxidase
Ni	(−)	(−)	0.02	0.1	?Stabilizing RNA structure	Oxidoreductases, hydrolases	Urease
Cr	0.005–0.2	0.0006	0.004	0.02	?Binding of insulin to cells, glucose metabolism		

* Requirements may differ for different age groups and physiologic states, e.g., pregnancy.
† Reported normal values vary owing to differences in sample preparation, analytical instruments, and small quantities present in biologic materials.
(−), Reported values variable or not available.

TABLE 77-2 Disorders of metal metabolism in humans

Element	Deficiency	Toxicity*
Fe	Anemia	Hepatic failure, diabetes, testicular atrophy, arthritis, cardiomyopathy, peripheral neuropathy, hyperpigmentation
Zn	Growth retardation, alopecia, dermatitis, diarrhea, immunologic dysfunction, failure to thrive, psychological disturbances, gonadal atrophy, impaired spermatogenesis, congenital malformations.	Gastric ulcer, pancreatitis lethargy, anemia, fever, nausea, vomiting, respiratory distress, pulmonary fibrosis
Cu	Anemia, growth retardation, defective keratinization and pigmentation of hair, hypothermia, degenerative changes in aortic elastin, mental deterioration, scurvy-like changes in skeleton	Hepatitis, cirrhosis, tremor, mental deterioration, Kayser-Fleischer rings, hemolytic anemia, renal dysfunction (Fanconi-like syndrome)
Mn	Bleeding disorder (increased prothrombin time)	Encephalitis-like syndrome, Parkinson-like syndrome, psychosis, pneumoconiosis
Co	Anemia (B_{12} deficiency)	Cardiomyopathy, goiter
Mo	? Esophageal cancer	? Hyperuricemia
Cr	? Impairment of glucose tolerance	Renal failure, dermatitis (occupational), pulmonary cancer
Se	Cardiomyopathy, congestive heart failure, striated muscle degeneration	Alopecia, abnormal nails, emotional lability, lassitude, garlic odor to breath
Ni	?	Dermatitis (occupational), lung and nasal carcinomas, liver necrosis, pulmonary inflammation
Si	? Impaired early bone development	Pulmonary inflammation, granuloma, fibrosis
F	? Impaired bone and dental structure	Motted dental enamel, nausea, abdominal pain, vomiting, diarrhea, tetany, cardiovascular collapse

* Symptoms are dependent on route of entry and tissue distribution (see text).

achieved, and the excretion rate. Mechanisms of toxicity include inhibition of enzyme activity by binding to essential amino acid residues, alterations in nucleic acid function and structure, alteration in protein synthesis, effects on membrane permeability, and inhibition of phosphorylation, among others. Metal toxicity in patients undergoing chronic renal dialysis is important because of the frequency and severity of the resulting problems and because of the number of metals involved, e.g., Al, Zn, Cu, Ni, and Sn (Chap. 225). For example, even when it is present only in trace amounts in dialysis fluids, Al is readily absorbed into blood and accumulates in brain, bone, and erythroid tissues, causing disabling neurologic, skeletal, and hematologic disorders. These include malaise, memory loss, asterixis, dementia, twitches, and other manifestations of metabolic encephalopathy including seizures and death. Osteomalacia unresponsive to vitamin D, fractures, muscular pain, weakness, and anemia may occur. Documentation of increase in plasma Al concentration following deferoxamine administration is diagnostic.

DISORDERS OF METABOLISM OF SPECIFIC METALS **Zinc** Absorption of Zn in the small intestine is decreased by fibers, phytate, phosphate, Ca, and Cu. In contrast, amino acids, peptides, iodoquinol and other chelating agents increase Zn absorption. Excretion of Zn occurs principally through secretions of the pancreas and intestine. Nearly 99 percent of total-body Zn is inside cells, the remainder is in plasma and extracellular fluids. Serum Zn, approximately 70 percent of which is loosely bound to albumin and other proteins, is the source of metal for cellular needs. Serum Zn content does not normally vary, but it decreases when intake or absorption is reduced (e.g., in regional enteritis) or when urinary losses are increased (e.g., in nephrotic syndrome; in cirrhosis of the liver or other hypoalbuminemic states; during the administration of penicillamine or other chelating agents; in high catabolic states as after trauma, burns, or surgery; and in hemolytic anemias and sickle cell disease). Plasma Zn also decreases in the acute phase of myocardial infarction, infections, malignancies, hepatitis, and other diseases. The decreases may be due to redistribution from plasma to tissues and are probably mediated by ACTH, cortisol, and/or a leukocyte protein (leukocyte endogenous mediator). Clinical deficiency may follow these decreases in serum content. The Zn requirement of the developing fetus, pregnant woman, and growing child or adolescent is higher than that of adult men or nonpregnant women. Therefore, the former groups are more susceptible to Zn depletion. Zn deficiency in pregnant animals can lead to fetal Zn deficiency, which results in high mortality rates or congenital malformations of nearly all organ systems. Zinc deficiency has not been described in pregnant women, but has been reported in adolescents who eat dirt, in patients who receive TPN without supplemental Zn (see Chap. 75), and in patients with the autosomal recessive defect acrodermatitis enteropathica. In the latter disease, deficiency in plasma Zn may be the consequence of a defect in Zn absorption. The onset of symptoms often occurs when an affected infant is weaned from human to cow's milk. Zn may also play a role in the maintenance of normal taste and in wound healing.

Tissues with a high cellular turnover, including skin, gastrointestinal mucosa, chondrocytes, spermatogonia, and thymocytes are characteristically affected (Table 77-2). The dermatologic abnormalities (hyperkeratosis, parakeratosis, acrodermatitis, and alopecia) call attention to the possibility of Zn deficiency. The usual distribution of the keratotic lesions is in areas that are readily traumatized (elbows, knees), but the lesions can develop in other areas as well. The keratotic lesions can become pustular or crusting, red, scaly plaques. Superinfections are common with either fungi or bacteria.

Toxicity follows inhalation of Zn fumes (by welders), oral ingestion, or intravenous administration. Inhalation of high concentrations of zinc oxide fumes leads to an acute illness called *metal-fume fever* or *brass chills,* manifested by fever, chills, excessive salivation, headaches, cough, and leukocytosis. Dialysis fluids can be contaminated with Zn from the adhesive plaster used on the dialysis coils or from galvanized pipes. The toxic syndrome associated with hemodialysis is characterized by anemia, fever, and central nervous system disturbances (Table 77-2). Toxic amounts of Zn decrease chemotaxis, phagocytosis, pinocytosis, and platelet aggregation.

Copper The liver, kidney, heart, and brain contain the highest amounts of Cu. Over 90 percent of plasma Cu is associated with ceruloplasmin, while 60 percent of that in red blood cells is bound to superoxide dismutase. The major excretory pathway is through the bile. The serum Cu concentration is normally constant. Increases occur in patients with acute myocardial infarction, leukemia, solid tumors, infections, portal and biliary cirrhosis, hemochromatosis, thyrotoxicosis, and connective tissue disorders. The consequences of the increases are unknown. Decreases occur in the nephrotic syndrome, kwashiorkor, the hepatolenticular degeneration of Wilson's disease (see Chap. 330), severe diarrheal diseases with malabsorption, and other conditions associated with increased excretion or decreased synthesis of ceruloplasmin. Premature infants who are fed diets deficient in Cu develop decreased serum ceruloplasmin and Cu levels, anemia, osteopenia, skin and hair depigmentation, and psychomotor retardation. Cu deficiency in subjects receiving TPN causes anemia and neutropenia.

A more complex disorder of Cu metabolism occurs in Menkes' disease, an X-linked recessive disorder (see also Chap. 336). Intestinal Cu uptake is normal, and tissue Cu content varies; that of intestinal, kidney, and skin (fibroblast) cells is normal or high, while that of serum, liver, brain, and (likely) vascular cells is low. Ceruloplasmin content and the activities of some Cu enzymes (e.g., connective tissue amine oxidases) also are decreased. The clinical picture is similar to that of nutritional Cu deficiency in animals except that anemia does not occur (Table 77-2). The patients have kinky hair, and decreased amounts of mature collagen and elastin cause dissecting aneurysms, sudden cardiac rupture, emphysema, and osteoporosis. Death usually occurs in the first 5 years of life.

Excessive oral intake of Cu or hemodialysis with water contaminated with Cu is toxic. The acute symptoms include hemolytic anemia, nausea, vomiting, and diarrhea. The renal and hepatic failure and the central nervous system disorders that eventually develop (Table 77-2) are typical of the Cu toxicity syndrome in hepatolenticular degeneration (Wilson's disease). (See Chap. 330.)

Cobalt Co is a component of vitamin B_{12}, and deficiency syndromes are those associated with deficiency of the vitamin (see Chap. 292). Pharmacologic doses of Co induce erythropoiesis. Chronic administration blocks iodine uptake by the thyroid, resulting in development of goiter.

Cardiomyopathy, congestive heart failure with pericardial effusions, polycythemia, thyroid enlargement, and neurologic abnormalities have been reported as manifestations of Co toxicity in drinkers of beer to which the metal had been added as a foam stabilizer. Co accumulates in the heart, forms a complex with lipoic acid, and interferes with decarboxylation reactions critical to both pyruvate and fatty acid metabolism.

Manganese Mn acts both as an activator of enzymes and as a component of metalloenzymes (Table 77-1). Defects of the skeletal, central nervous, and gonadal systems occur in Mn deficiency in animals. Humans obtain sufficient Mn from normal dietary intake so that a deficiency syndrome is rare. In one reported instance an increase in prothrombin time, unresponsive to Vitamin K, was noted. In serum, Mn is bound to transmanganin. Mn is excreted primarily in bile and pancreatic secretions.

Serum Mn increases following myocardial infarction and decreases for unknown reasons in children with convulsive disorders. Miners who inhale large quantities of Mn dust over long periods of time develop asthenia, anorexia, apathy, headache, impotence, leg cramps, speech disturbances, and occasionally even more severe toxic symptoms (Table 77-2).

Selenium Se is a component of glutathione peroxidase and plays a critical role in the control of oxygen metabolism, particularly in catalyzing the breakdown of H_2O_2. The metal is required for the growth of human fibroblasts and other cells in tissue culture. Furthermore, Se cures or prevents Keshan disease, a syndrome that is endemic to Keshan Province in China where the soil may be deficient in the metal. Keshan disease is characterized by multifocal myocardial necrosis and reduced blood and serum Se content. The clinical severity varies from severe arrhythmias and cardiogenic shock to a mild form with cardiac enlargement as the only significant finding. Peripheral myopathies may develop as a consequence of muscle degeneration (Table 77-2). Children and women of child-bearing age are particularly susceptible. Se protects animals from a number of carcinogenic chemicals and viral agents; a role in human cancer prevention is not established. Se binds Cd, Hg, and other metals and mitigates their toxic effects, even though the measurable levels of the metals remain elevated.

Se toxicity occurs in animals, but humans who have consumed vegetables grown in soil containing high selenium content have not become ill. Se poisoning has been reported due to ingestion of water containing large amounts of the metal.

Other trace elements *Silicon* is present in bone and skin and may play a role in the cross-linkage of collagen. Deficiency in animals results in decreased growth, abnormal early bone development, and decreased hexosamine content of epiphyses and epiphyseal plates. No instance of deficiency in humans has been described. Inhalation of fine particles of SiO_2 causes granuloma formation and chronic fibrosis (silicosis) of the lungs (see Chap. 206).

Fluoride is a constituent of teeth and bone. It prevents dental caries, and its use in patients with osteoporosis has resulted in increased mineralized bone (see Chap. 345). Complications of long-term ingestion by such patients include calcification of bony ligaments and tendons. Chronic intake of fluorides also causes fluorosis, a syndrome characterized by weakness, weight loss, anemia, brittle bones, and mottling of teeth (if taken during stages of enamel formation). Acute ingestion of toxic amounts, as found in some insect poisons, causes severe abdominal pain, nausea, vomiting, diarrhea, and hypocalcemia. Eventually, tetany and cardiorespiratory arrest occur.

A deficiency of any one of *arsenic, nickel, tin,* and *vanadium* causes pathologic manifestations in plants and some vertebrates. Their roles in human health are undefined.

REFERENCES

FALCHUK KH: Effect of acute disease and ACTH on serum zinc proteins. N Engl J Med 296:1129, 1977

KARCIOULU ZA, SARPER RM: *Zinc and Copper in Medicine*. Springfield, Ill., Charles C Thomas, 1980

Metabolic and physiological consequences of trace element deficiency in animals and man. Philos Trans R Soc Lond [Biol] 294:1, 1981

MILLINER DS et al: Use of the deferoxamine infusion test in the diagnosis of aluminum-related osteodystrophy. Ann Intern Med 101:775, 1984

PRASAD AS: *Trace Elements in Human Health and Disease*. New York, Academic, 1976, vol II

REINHOLD JG: Trace elements—A selective survey. Clin Chem 21:476, 1975

TING-KAI L, VALLEE BL: The biochemical and nutritional roles of other trace elements, in *Modern Nutrition in Health and Disease*, 6th ed, RS Goodhart and ME Shils (eds). Philadelphia, Lea and Febiger, 1980

UNDERWOOD EJ: *Trace Elements in Human and Animal Nutrition*, 3d ed. New York, Academic, 1971

WILLIAMS RJP: The Tilden lecture. Q Rev Chem Soc (Lond) 24:331, 1970

PART FIVE INFECTIOUS DISEASES

section 1 Basic considerations in infectious disease

78 INTRODUCTION TO INFECTIOUS DISEASES: PATHOGENIC MECHANISMS AND HOST RESPONSES

FREDERICK P. HEINZEL / RICHARD K. ROOT

THE SCOPE OF INFECTIOUS DISEASES Infectious diseases pervade human existence. Great plagues have shaped our history, literature, plumbing, personal hygiene, and societal mores. Just centuries ago, cities were devastated by bubonic plague, populations scarred by smallpox, and whole armies defeated by vibrio and spirochetes. Fortunately, a century of advance in medicine and public health has markedly attenuated the risk of most infectious diseases. As a result, modern day children no longer fear diphtheria, tetanus, polio, or pertussis. Smallpox has been completely eradicated. Mosquito control has removed malaria and yellow fever as endemic threats in the United States, while improved disposal of human waste has decreased the frequency of bacterial and helminthic enteric infections. Unfortunately, many old enemies are with us still; malaria, typhoid, tuberculosis, and other infections remain prevalent in developing nations, where they continue to impede agricultural and economic development. Sexually transmitted diseases, such as chlamydia and gonorrhea, are rampant in most modern cities. Pneumococcus is still occasionally "the old man's friend."

Some technologic advances have created their own problems; the foremost of these has been the development of antibiotic resistance in microbes. In this regard, hospitals have bred strains of staphylococcus and pseudomonas that are increasingly unresponsive to available antibiotics. Poultry and cattle fed antimicrobials to improve their commercial yield now harbor multiply resistant salmonella that have caused outbreaks of disease among humans. Both falciparum malaria and its mosquito vector have become refractory to formerly effective drugs and insecticides.

Similarly, our advanced medical science has inadvertently provided niches in which less pathogenic microorganisms can produce mischief. Transplant and cancer patients are treated with cytotoxic drugs that attenuate host defenses while receiving antibiotics that remove normal pathogens. These patients become a fertile field for formerly unusual species of pathogenic bacteria and fungus. The use of indwelling metal and plastic prosthetic devices has produced access and microecologies favorable for infection with previously "nonpathogenic" coagulase-negative staphylococci and diphtheroids.

If new tricks learned by old microbes were not trouble enough, novel pathogens have been discovered in the last decade. Most prominent among these is the human immunodeficiency virus (HIV), the cause of acquired immunodeficiency syndrome. The immune devastation produced by this virus has in turn given clinical and research prominence to opportunistic pathogens that were previously mere curiosities. Similarly, the clinical entity of Lyme disease has been described and its causative agent, *Borrelia burgdorferi*, characterized. Human parvovirus and human herpesvirus 6 have been implicated in the etiology of erythema infectiosum and erythema subitum, respectively, both previously idiopathic febrile exanthems of infancy. Even peptic ulcers may prove to be of microbial origin, as evidence accumulates linking *Campylobacter pylori* with that disease.

The need for all health care practitioners to study the pathogenesis, diagnosis, and treatment of infectious diseases has not changed in this century of medical progress. It is still true that the study of medicine is greatly involved with the study of infectious disease. It is also true that to understand infection, we must first know how microbes interact with their human hosts.

MICROBIAL FACTORS Infectious disease occurs when a pathogenic organism causes signs and symptoms of inflammation or organ dysfunction. This may be caused by infection, when the etiologic agent multiplies in the host, or from intoxication of the host by cellular poisons generated by a noninfecting organism. Many infections are subclinical, not producing the usual manifestations of ill health. Whether infection is clinically evident or not, the outcome is (1) eradication of the infecting agent (resolution), (2) chronic infection, (3) prolonged excretion of agent (carrier state), or (4) latency of the agent within host tissues.

A wide variety of viruses, bacteria, protozoa, fungi, helminths, and arthropods have been demonstrated to infect humans. The ability of a specific pathogen to cause disease depends on the interaction between its intrinsic pathogenic potential, or virulence, and the defensive measures used by the host to contain and neutralize the infectious threat (Fig. 78-1). The virulence of a pathogen is a relative term; many organisms with normally low virulence can cause severe disease in hosts with compromised immunity. These are called *opportunistic pathogens.* Virulence factors are characteristics of the organism that allow it to colonize, proliferate, invade, and destroy host tissues. In some cases, tissue damage is caused by mass effect from parasitic accumulations or by exuberant host responses.

A relatively uniform series of events must occur before a particular microbe produces clinical disease in humans. At the most basic level, pathogen and host must meet. All etiologic agents have some normal habitat, or reservoir, where they reside and multiply. The most proximate place that the pathogen exists before transmittal to host is termed the source and may be distinct from the reservoir. An infecting agent can be from endogenous or exogenous sources. Endogenously acquired organisms are typically those residing on mucosal surfaces or resting latent in various tissues. Exogenous pathogens are transmitted from source to host by direct or indirect contact, by common vehicle, by airborne particles, or by arthropod or animal vectors. Transmittal by contact occurs when the host encounters the source directly, as in person-to-person spread, or indirectly through secretions, excretions, or objects contaminated by the source. A common

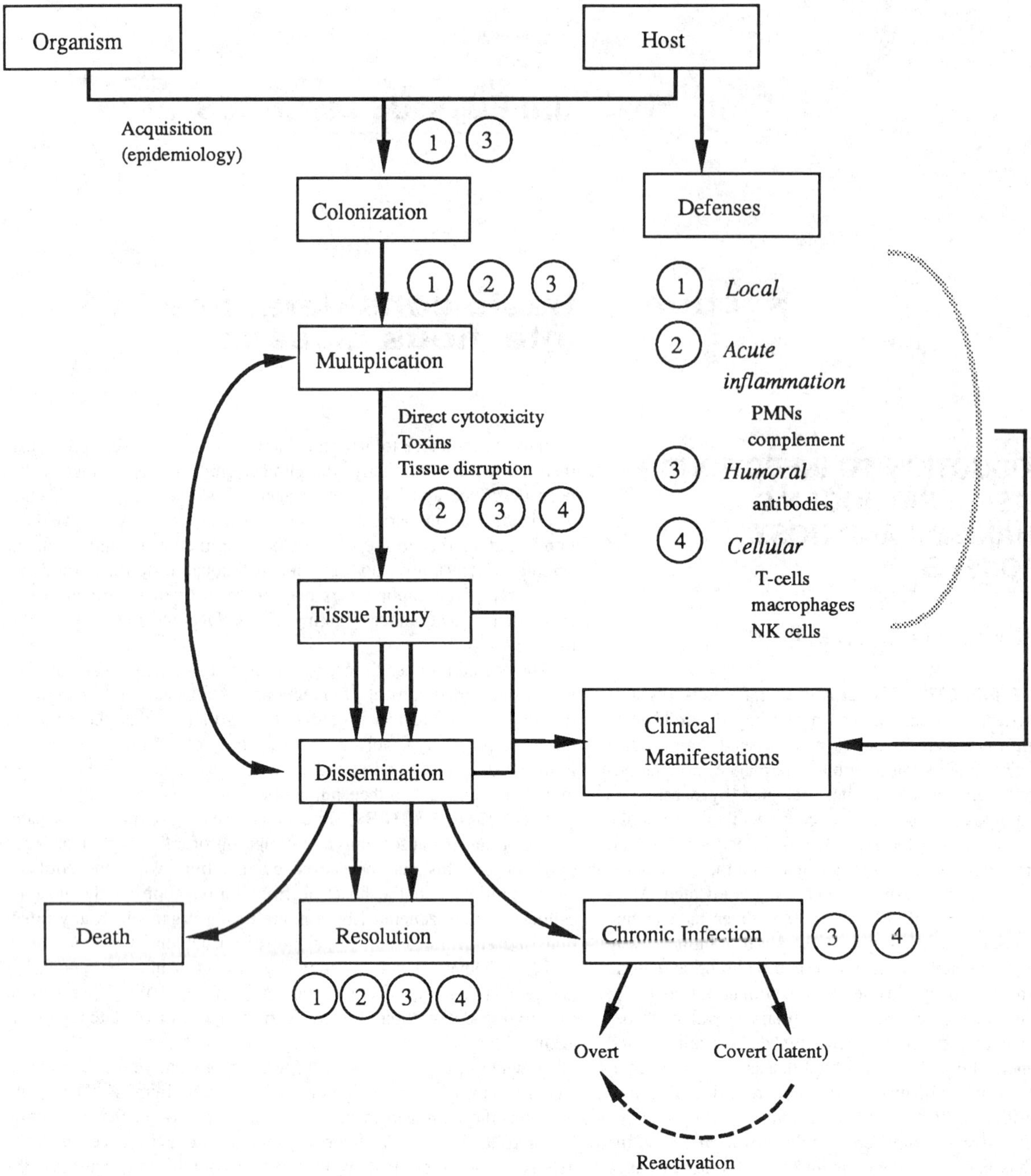

FIGURE 78-1 Schematized interplay between microorganisms and host factors that lead to infection, infectious disease, and resolution. The circled numbers indicate sites at which the designated host responses may interrupt or modify the pathogenesis of disease. *(Modified and used with permission from RK Root, WL Heirholzer, in Clinical Pharmacology: Basic Principles in Therapeutics, 2d ed, KL Melmon, HF Morelli, (eds), Macmillan, New York, 1978.)*

vehicle is a shared item, such as food, water, or blood, that transmits a pathogen to multiple hosts. Airborne transmittal occurs when infectious agents travel through the air on small water or dust particles, often for great distances. Animal or arthropod vectors may transmit disease agents from source to host; in some cases the vector may serve double duty as reservoir and host. Knowledge of the route of transmission of an infectious agent not only will help the physician to understand how disease develops but will provide important diagnostic clues in the case of pet-, travel-, and food-related outbreaks. Additionally, such information is critical to the public health official or hospital epidemiologist who must prevent further illness by disrupting routes of transmission or by removing sources of infection.

Disease does not immediately or inevitably occur once a prospective pathogen is transmitted to its host. Many infections are preceded by colonization of body surfaces, wounds, or hollow viscera with the infecting agent. The agent typically first colonizes at the site to which it is transmitted (the portal of entry). Success there is supported when the infecting dose is sufficiently large and adherence to epithelium or other tissue is possible. Epithelial attachment is promoted by microbial adhesins, molecules that bind to distinct tissue receptors. In bacteria, these molecules are usually located on filamentous structures (pili, fimbriae) and demonstrate affinity for specific epithelial receptors, such as surface glycoproteins and gangliosides. Pili increase the virulence of pathogenic strains of *Escherichia coli* and *Neisseria gonorrheae,* allowing these organisms to attach to uroepithelium, persist against the opposing flow of urine, and thus better cause disease. Surface polysaccharides of other pathogens may serve similar functions. Dextran produced by certain viridans streptococci glues bacteria to tooth surfaces, where they participate in causing gingival disease. Similarly, complex carbohydrate slime secreted by

Staphylococcus epidermidis promotes adherence to prosthetic devices, a common site for infection with that bacterium.

Pathogens that colonize a site in the body may subsequently proliferate there, greatly increasing the opportunity for tissue invasion or toxin production. Growth of the infecting agent at the portal of entry is determined by the prevailing moisture, oxygen content, pH, and availability of nutrients. Additionally, the agent must be able to surmount competition from the normal flora for required nutrients and epithelial attachment sites. When the protective normal flora is diminished by antibiotics or ill health, pathogenic organisms, such as *Clostridium difficile,* may proliferate inappropriately and cause disease. Alternatively, the proliferative phase may not result in invasive disease, but instead continue and cause prolonged excretion of infectious organisms (carrier state).

Infectious disease becomes evident when microbes invade and disseminate in host tissue. Most infections will present as a primary lesion, usually at the site of initial entry, colonization, and proliferation. If proliferation results in spread along mucosal surfaces, lymphatic channels, or fascial planes, lesions may appear at sites distant from the point of entry. Bloodborne infection can result either in symptoms and signs of overwhelming, multisystem sepsis or in distant metastatic infection. Bacteria often localize to specific organs during dissemination, depending on local factors, such as blood flow, oxygen content, and tissue receptors for microbial adherence factors. For instance, the dextran used by viridans streptococci to promote adherence to teeth also may mediate adherence to heart valve lesions, which could explain the propensity of such bacteria to cause infective endocarditis.

Specific virulence factors that allow pathogens to invade tissue in a predictable fashion have been characterized. Entry may be facilitated by digestive enzymes secreted from the invading organism. Schistosomula and hookworm larvae generate proteases that digest a passage as the worm enters through the skin of the host. Similarly, pyogenic bacteria, such as *Staphylococcus aureus, Streptococcus pyogenes, Pseudomonas aeruginosa,* and *Clostridium perfringens,* secrete complex cocktails of collagenases, hyaluronidases, lecithinases, and streptokinases that destroy connective tissue and permit invasion and dissemination of infection.

For viral, bacterial, and protozoan agents which are obligate intracellular pathogens, invasion necessarily precedes proliferation. Most of these organisms possess surface molecules that mediate binding and entry into their cellular targets. Influenza viruses adhere to *N*-acetylneuraminic acid residues on respiratory epithelia via hemagglutinating (H) protein expressed on the viral coat. A viral neuraminidase (N) then allows penetration of the cell membrane and uncoating of the virus. Chlamydia and rickettsia have evolved surface proteins that induce phagocytosis by their normally nonphagocytic host cells. *Leishmania* spp., also obligate intramacrophage parasites, use at least three distinct ligand interactions to ensure that they are efficiently phagocytosed by the cells they infect.

Outside of factors that promote colonization, proliferation, and tissue invasion, important virulence factors include bacterial toxins. These are either secreted proteins (exotoxins) or structural portions of the organism, such as endotoxins. Exotoxins can cause disease without antecedent infection. Toxin preformed in food by *S. aureus* or *Bacillus cereus* will cause food poisoning without any further participation of the bacteria following ingestion. Other exotoxins are produced during local proliferation, causing disease without evidence of invasion. Examples include the diarrhea caused by colonization and proliferation within the intestine of *Vibrio cholerae,* which produces a locally active enterotoxin. Toxins formed during bacterial proliferation at one site may be carried considerable distances in the body to produce dysfunction systemically or in other organ systems, as occurs during staphylococcal toxic shock syndrome, scarlet fever, diphtheria, and tetanus.

In contrast to these protein exotoxins, endotoxins from gram-negative bacteria are highly heterogeneous lipopolysaccharides that are part of the bacterial cell wall. Release of this substance during infection, or during infusion of contaminated parenteral fluids, results in an intense host response. Endotoxin potently activates coagulation, complement, and kallikrein pathways, as well as stimulating production of cytokines that can cause fever, widespread circulatory disturbances, and organ dysfunction. The resulting clinical picture of septic shock is discussed in Chap. 89.

HOST IMMUNE FACTORS Life in such a hostile microbial environment is possible because mammalian hosts possess efficient physical, cellular, and molecular host defenses. The first level of protection is provided by epithelial and epidermal barriers. Would-be pathogens may colonize, but may be unable to penetrate these surfaces. The normally acidic conditions that prevail in the stomach, urine, and vagina additionally limit proliferation of microbes at these sites. Other local secretions contain antimicrobial substances, such as lysozyme and fatty acids, or contain antibodies that block microbial adherence. Surface flow of fluids in the hollow viscera and mucociliary flow of secretions in the respiratory passages further act to prevent internal spread of microbes colonizing the external orifices. Unfortunately, these mechanisms are only as good as their physical integrity, which is often violated by environmental trauma or by the well-meant insertion of urinary and intravenous catheters.

When these external surfaces are penetrated by infectious agents, additional immune mechanisms can be recruited to contain infection (see Chap. 13). The defenses provided by phagocytes, complement, antibodies, and cellular immunity are traditionally described separately, but are in fact tightly interrelated systems that rarely operate in isolation. These responses may occur in either a nonspecific or a specific fashion. Nonspecific responses, although indiscriminate and inefficient, have the advantage of being rapidly available during acute infection and may permit survival of the host until specific responses focus subsequent defenses. Phagocytes and the alternative pathway of complement account for the bulk of nonspecific immune responses, most occurring within hours of the stimulus. In contrast, antibody- and cell-mediated immunities take days to weeks to develop following primary exposure but are often required for complete resolution of disease. Because they have intrinsic memory functions, antibodies and T lymphocytes provide the basis for long-term immunity to reinfection. Their immune specificity is determined by the enormous repertoire of recognition sites available in normal populations of antibodies and T-cell receptors. The importance of these various systems is demonstrated by the markedly increased infectious morbidity and mortality that accompanies genetic or acquired defects of the immune system, which are specifically discussed in Chap. 82.

Polymorphonuclear cells (PMNs) and macrophages are the host's "professional" phagocytes; eosinophils have comparatively minor roles in host defense (see Chap. 64). Polymorphonuclear cells are highly mobile, short-lived blood cells that rapidly enter sites of infection to ingest and destroy microbial invaders. When infection occurs, PMNs can be provided in large numbers from marrow precursors or from preformed pools. Under the guidance of substances diffusing from infection sites, including both microbial products and elicited host factors, PMNs adhere to and cross the endothelium. These same factors then elicit directed migration (chemotaxis) of PMNs to the inflammatory site. Pathogens are bound by PMN surface adhesins, ingested, and subsequently exposed during phagolysosomal fusion to an acidic internal environment rich in hydrolytic enzymes and antibacterial proteins. In addition, the polymorphonuclear cell consumes oxygen during microbial ingestion and generates toxic oxidants such as superoxide anion and hydrogen peroxide. The lysosomal enzyme myeloperoxidase augments the already considerable microbicidal activity of these oxidants by producing hypochlorous acid from chloride ion and hydrogen peroxide. Disorders of phagocytes are discussed in Chap. 81.

In contrast, macrophages circulate transiently and then establish long-lived residency in tissue, particularly the spleen, liver, and lung. They are favorably situated to remove infectious threats in transit through the lungs or bloodstream. Macrophages share many of the phagocytic and microbicidal activities of PMNs. However they can markedly increase these functions when activated by factors, notably γ-interferon, produced by stimulated T lymphocytes. In addition, macrophages have accessory cell functions, such as antigen presentation and interleukin 1 production, that are critical for initiating cellular and humoral immunity.

Complement and antibodies are the major soluble mediators of immunity in serum and provide important specific and nonspecific protection against extracellular and viral pathogens. The complement system is a collection of some 25 proteins that enzymatically generates membrane-associated opsonizing and microbicidal protein complexes. Specific activation of complement, by the classical pathway, is triggered when antibodies bind to microbe. Nonspecific activation (alternative pathway) is stimulated upon exposure to certain types of microbial surface components and does not require the presence of antibody.

Antibodies are complex glycoproteins, produced by B lymphocytes, that bind to microbial antigens and that subsequently activate microbicidal responses. The antigen-binding site of antibody exhibits any of approximately 10^8 variable protein sequences capable of specifically binding to macromolecules, such as microbial antigens, by means of complementary charge and molecular topography. Other portions of the antibody are invariant in structure and are responsible for initiating complement activation, antibody-dependent cellular cytotoxicity (ADCC), or phagocytosis when antibody is bound to a microbial target. Antibodies may, in addition, neutralize viruses, bacteria, and toxins by blocking adhesins or functional sites.

The constant regions of the antibody define the five classes of immunoglobulin: IgM, IgG, IgA, IgD, and IgE. Each class of immunoglobulin has a distinct distribution within host tissues. IgM antibodies are largely found within the intravascular compartment, whereas IgG antibodies are distributed widely throughout the extracellular space. Both may appear on mucosal surfaces during inflammation. Otherwise, mucosal immunity is largely due to IgA secretory antibodies that inhibit colonization, multiplication, and invasion by bacteria and viruses.

Cellular immunity is the host response mediated by macrophages, T lymphocytes, and their soluble products. Whereas PMNs and humoral immunity are most effective against extracellular pathogens, cellular immunity is best suited for the control of intracellular parasites. T lymphocytes are activated by antigen presented in conjunction with major histocompatibility antigen (MHC) on the surfaces of macrophages and B lymphocytes. Following activation, T lymphocytes may assume a variety of functional roles. They may differentiate into T cells that stimulate B-cell growth and synthesis of immunoglobulin. Alternatively, they may secrete proteins that activate the microbicidal or cytotoxic functions of macrophages and cytotoxic T cells. Both macrophages and T lymphocytes secrete other proinflammatory cytokines that cause fever, increase serum levels of acute phase reactants, or stimulate bone marrow production of leukocytes. Other T lymphocytes are capable of lysing host cells infected with virus or that have become neoplastic. Similar cytotoxic functions are provided by large granular lymphocytes that lack T-cell receptors and that do not require MHC for recognition of their target; these lymphocytes are called natural killer (NK) cells.

Each step in the pathogenesis of infectious disease is a complex interplay of microbial action and host reaction. These battle lines are far from static, as many infectious agents have evolved strategies to evade host immunity. Certainly colonizing organisms that elude local host defenses are better able to proliferate and cause eventual disease. Not surprisingly, a wide variety of such stratagems are recognized. One such mechanism is the avoidance of early nonspecific immune responses. For example, antiphagocytic surfaces of encapsulated bacteria protect against ingestion by leukocytes; other bacteria are intrinsically resistant to complement activation when in the bloodstream. Similarly, microbes may evade phagocytes and antibodies by dwelling within host cells, a technique used to great advantage by chlamydia, rickettsia, toxoplasma, and leishmania. Antigenic variation may foil recognition by antibodies and is used by some species of borrelia and trypanosoma, accounting for the chronic, relapsing course of those diseases. Influenza viruses regularly undergo antigenic change; epidemics result when the neoantigen is unrecognized by the human population. Pathogens may generate molecules that inactivate host immune responses. Lumen-dwelling bacteria, such as *N. gonorrhea,* produce IgA proteases that degrade mucosal antibodies, whereas some strains of *S. aureus* and streptococci possess surface proteins that bind immunoglobulin in nonfunctional conformations. Other bacteria, such as clostridia and bordetella, produce toxins that kill or inactivate leukocytes.

The balance of microbial virulence and host immunity determines the outcome of disease. When host responses eradicate the offending agent, resolution occurs—often with complete immunity to reinfection. When host responses are evenly balanced against microbial factors, chronic disease may result. Alternatively, the immune response may simply drive the pathogen into a latent state in some protected site, such as a nerve ganglion cell following infection with herpes simplex or varicella-zoster viruses. Any waning of host surveillance then results in reactivation of infection, as often happens with herpes viruses, toxoplasma, and mycobacteria following immunosuppression. When host defenses eliminate invasive infection but allow continued proliferation of the microbe at mucosal sites, a carrier state may develop.

HOST RESPONSES TO INFECTION Infectious diseases have long been known by the host responses they provoke: fever, chills, local inflammation, leukocytosis, protein catabolism, and the serum acute phase reaction. Fever and chills, often accompanied by increased pulse rate, are the usual herald signs of severe infection. Although the pattern and duration of fever may give useful diagnostic clues, body temperature is better used to assess the course of infection and the response to therapy (see Chap. 20). Signs of inflammation (heat, erythema, pain, and swelling) are the characteristic features of localized infection. Infected viscera become recognizable by tenderness upon palpation, by the inflammatory changes (usually polymorphonuclear leukocytes) present in adjacent body fluids, by their radiographic appearance, or by altered organ function. Like fever, an increased neutrophil count in the peripheral blood gives information about the presence and intensity of infection. However, as the severity of infection increases, neutropenia may develop and is a poor prognostic sign during sepsis or pneumonia. Other blood constituents are affected; thrombocytopenia, anemia, and coagulopathy may accompany subacute or chronic infection.

The profile of serum proteins changes during infection. Collectively referred to as the acute phase reaction, it reflects altered hepatic synthesis of protein. Typically, serum albumin concentration is reduced while serum amyloid A protein, C-reactive protein, and various proteinase inhibitors increase, sometimes up to 1000-fold. Serum levels of zinc and iron decrease in the serum at the same time, probably due to chelation with lactoferrin and similar acute phase products. A catabolic state is further augmented by simultaneous increases in levels of circulating cortisol, glucagon, catecholamines, and other hormones.

Although discrete inflammatory roles have been described for prostanoids, complement products, and monamines, the most dramatic effects are mediated by a few proinflammatory cytokines: interleukin 1, tumor necrosis factor, interleukin 6, and γ-interferon. These factors, singly or in combination, promote fever, stimulate hepatic acute phase responses, produce local inflammatory signs, and trigger catabolic responses. Responding lymphocytes and macrophages similarly elaborate a variety of colony-stimulating factors which promote bone marrow production of leukocytes.

When mild to moderate in intensity, inflammatory responses probably serve important host defense functions. For instance, increased body temperatures accentuate lymphocyte responses and may inhibit viral replication. Inflammatory hyperemia and systemic neutrophilia optimize phagocyte delivery to sites of infection. The decreased availability of iron "starves" certain microbes of a necessary nutrient. However, when these responses become extreme, extensive tissue damage can result, as typified in the extreme by fulminant septic shock (see Chap. 89).

Other infections may be similarly accompanied by deleterious side effects as a result of prolonged or inappropriate immune reactivity. The wasting of body fat and muscle during lengthy infections probably reflects the strong catabolic and anorexic effects of circulating interleukin 1 and tumor necrosis factor. In certain circumstances, antigen and antibody may form immune complexes that will independently initiate inflammatory reactions at sites of deposition, causing vasculitis and glomerulonephritis syndromes. When microbe and host by chance share common immunologic epitopes, autoimmune disease may be triggered. The classic example is provided by rheumatic cardiomyopathy, thought to arise from molecular mimicry of cardiac muscle antigen by streptococcal M protein. Celiac disease, Reiter's syndrome, and juvenile-onset diabetes mellitus may be initiated by similar events.

DIAGNOSIS AND TREATMENT OF INFECTIOUS DISEASES The basic goals of diagnosis in infectious disease are to determine which organ system is affected and which agent is responsible for the disease. This evaluation requires a careful history, complete physical examination, and intelligent use of laboratory tests. The clinician is usually first presented with certain clinical symptoms and signs highly suggestive of infection, including abrupt onset, fever, chills, myalgia, photophobia, pharyngitis, acute lymphadenopathy and splenomegaly, gastrointestinal upset, and leukocytosis or leukopenia. When infectious disease is likely, three important items should be addressed by the history, physical examination, and initial laboratory tests: the organ system involved, the tempo of the illness, and the presence of unusual risk factors. The affected organ system is usually obvious from complaints such as dysuria, productive cough, localized pain, swelling, or erythema. Occasionally symptoms are diffuse and may represent systemic infection. Because certain organs are infected by relatively predictable agents, the classification of the patient's disorder as pneumonia, meningitis, urinary tract infection, septic shock, cellulitis, etc., will help direct diagnostic and therapeutic strategies. This syndromic approach to infectious disease is illustrated in the following chapters. The tempo of onset may incriminate certain types of pathogen as possible causes of infectious disease. For example, viruses and pyogenic bacteria tend to have acute or subacute courses; fungal or mycobacterial infections are indolent and often cause chronic diseases. Relapsing or recurrent symptoms may be critical diagnostic clues during infection with borrelia, plasmodia, or brucella.

Most infectious agents have sharply defined reservoirs and routes of communication, so that unusual exposures should be sought in the patient's history. An extensive review of occupational, travel, sexual, and social information may be required. This is exemplified by the workup for atypical pneumonia, which necessitates a detailed inquiry about travel- and animal-related exposures that might implicate psittacosis, coccidioidomycosis, tularemia, or Q fever. Similarly, sexual histories are essential when genital lesions are present, and information about sexual practices, intravenous drug abuse, or transfusions is required to assess a patient's risk for HIV infection. Many unusual risks are iatrogenic or nosocomially acquired, the most obvious being previous antibiotic use, irradiation, or cytotoxic therapy for neoplasm and organ transplantation (see Chaps. 82 and 83).

Once a list of suspect pathogens has been generated, laboratory tests are used to identify the offender. Direct methods of identification typically include stains and culture of body fluids, secretions, and tissue. The type of stain and culture to use in atypical scenarios is best decided after consultation with the microbiology laboratory (see Chap. 80). Another direct means of microbial diagnosis is to assay for microbial antigen in fluid or tissue using immunofluorescence, ELISA, or RIA techniques. Indirect methods measure the host response to infecting agent by assaying titers of specific antibody or by measuring skin test reactivity. These give less satisfactory diagnostic information because the measured responses often are delayed in onset, persist for years, and may not occur at all in immunocompromised patients. Because no microbiologic or serologic assay is perfect, very few diagnoses are made from these data alone; the clinician must interpret the facts supplied by the laboratory examination in the context of a patient's history and examination.

When infection does occur, numerous therapeutic options are available. Many simple viral infections will, of course, resolve without specific treatment. Minor cutaneous or mucosal infections may respond to topical therapy. With increasing severity of disease, systemic antibiotics become necessary. The choice of agent should be based on the efficacy, toxicity, cost, and ease of administration (see Chaps. 85 to 88). Although sometimes therapy can be initiated on minimal microbiologic data, such as penicillin for streptococcal pharyngitis, nosocomial infections may require a careful review of susceptibility data to uncover acquired antibiotic resistances.

In infectious diseases, prevention is preferable to cure. Immunization has become a cornerstone of modern medicine, and it is essential that it be a part of primary care (see Chap. 84). Most active vaccines contain an immunizing agent that is either inactivated or attenuated and are typically used before infectious exposure can occur. However, administration of vaccine in conjunction with specialized immune globulins may be effective even after exposure to certain infectious agents such as hepatitis B, rabies, and *Clostridium tetani*. Passive immunization alone, such as provided by pooled human serum globulin, is still used to protect travelers against the acquisition of hepatitis A. Other practices to avoid infection have become standard procedure, such as the use of asepsis during surgery and the aggressive debridement and cleaning of traumatic wounds. In appropriate circumstances, antibacterial prophylaxis may additionally decrease the risk of infection inherent in some surgical procedures or from exposure to communicable agents (see Chap. 85).

REFERENCES

BURNET FM, WHITE DO: *Natural History of Infectious Disease*, 4th ed. Cambridge University Press, 1972

MANDELL GL et al (eds): *Principles and Practice of Infectious Diseases*, 3d ed. New York, Wiley, 1990

MIMS CA: *The Pathogenesis of Infectious Disease*, 3d ed. London, Academic, 1987

ROOT RK: Infectious diseases: Pathogenetic mechanisms and host responses, in *Pathophysiology—The Biological Principles of Diseases*, 2d ed, LH Smith Jr, SO Thier (eds). Philadelphia, Saunders, 1985

79 INFECTIOUS DISEASES AND THE NEW BIOLOGY

DON GANEM

Fundamental recent developments in molecular biology have revolutionized our understanding of the basic chemistry of living things. These developments have enormous potential for the study and treatment of human diseases in general and infectious diseases in particular. In this chapter we review selected advances in the study of microbial pathogens that illustrate the nature and scope of progress in this area.

The conceptual cornerstone of molecular biology is the marriage of genetic reasoning and biochemical methodology. In this approach, biochemical phenomena are characterized by the isolation and study of mutant organisms with genetic lesions affecting these phenomena. Initially this was done with simple organisms, most commonly *Escherichia coli* and its bacteriophages. It has since become possible to extend these studies to higher organisms and to the parasites and viruses that infect them. Thus, virtually from its inception, molecular biology has had a disproportionate impact on the study of microorganisms. A major watershed was crossed in the mid-1970s when the technology was developed to clone and characterize segments of DNA from any organism in *E. coli.* (For a discussion of the details of this methodology, see Chap. 6.) This *recombinant DNA* (*rDNA*) technology has further facilitated the study of microbial pathogens and also made possible new approaches to diagnostics and therapeutics. The impact of these developments for our understanding of the origins, pathogenesis, and treatment of human infectious diseases are considered below.

MOLECULAR GENETICS AND PATHOGENESIS

BACTERIAL DISEASES Recent progress in understanding the nature of phase and antigenic variation in gonococci provides a beautiful example of the power of genetic reasoning to understand microbial pathogenesis. Early studies of pathogenic gonococci indicated that piliated strains (i.e., those with the protein *pilin* organized as surface projections called *pili*) are substantially more pathogenic than nonpiliated ones, perhaps because they show increased adherence to mucosal cells or resistance to phagocytosis (see Chap. 110). However, when cultured apart from the host, strains often lose their surface pili; with further passage the same organism can regain surface pili. This is referred to as pilin *phase variation.* It is even more important that the antigenic structure of these pili often changes radically as the organisms grow; such *antigenic variation* is believed to contribute greatly to the organism's ability to evade the host's immune response.

Cloning and characterization of pilin revealed that the gonococcal genome contains many incomplete genes harboring fragmentary coding information for pilin polypeptides in a silent, unexpressed form and only one (or, rarely, two) locus at which pilin genes can be actively expressed as RNA and protein. Variant pilins arise when stretches of coding sequences originating from the silent pilin loci recombine into the expression site. As a result of this genetic exchange, new pilin coding sequences are created. If these sequences are untranslatable, the organism loses its pili altogether (phase variation); if translatable, they often give rise to antigenic variation. These studies indicate that phase and antigenic variation proceed from a single recombinational mechanism and have important potential implications for the design of vaccination strategies.

Another important example of the use of genetics to define virulence pathways has been the study of plasmid-associated virulence factors. For example, both *Yersinia enterocolitica* and *Shigella sonnei* produce an invasive intestinal infection, and both harbor large extrachromosomal DNA molecules (plasmids) that replicate apart from the bacterial genome. In both cases, derivative strains lacking the plasmid have been isolated. When compared with their parental strains, each plasmidless variant was virtually avirulent when inoculated into animal hosts, indicating that important virulence factors are either encoded or regulated by the plasmid sequences. This finding set the stage for the identification of these factors by isolating and characterizing mutants of the plasmid that would not restore virulence upon transfer to plasmidless strains. In this way, multiple plasmid gene products that contribute to virulence have been identified in both organisms. The availability of each of these genes in cloned form now makes possible rigorous study of the biosynthesis and function of their products.

Genetic analysis of bacterial virulence factors is not limited to those mediated by plasmids. In *Yersinia,* for instance, important chromosomal loci exist that mediate additional functions in pathogenesis. It has long been known that *Yersinia* of several species can invade and replicate within eukaryotic host cells, even including cells not overtly specialized for phagocytosis. Two genetic loci governing such invasion have now been identified by cloning *Yersinia* DNA in *E. coli* and screening the recombinant bacteria (carrying cloned sequences) for the ability to invade cells in culture. Two distinct genes of *Yersinia* have emerged from this selection, each of which can mediate entry into host cells, albeit at different efficiencies. At least one of these genes encodes a surface protein involved in cell attachment and invasion. Neither gene, however, allows intracellular growth of *E. coli,* suggesting that additional loci mediate these functions.

This brief survey of genetically identified bacterial virulence factors is intended to be illustrative. Over the years many other equally important virulence determinants have been identified using these approaches. These include enterotoxins (in *Vibrio cholerae* and enterotoxigenic *E. coli*), cytotoxins (in *Pseudomonas aeruginosa, Shigella,* and enterohemorrhagic *E. coli*), adhesins (in uropathogenic and enterotoxigenic *E. coli*), and IgA proteases (in pathogenic *Neisseriae*), to name but a few.

VIRAL REPLICATION Viruses have proven invaluable as tools for the study of gene expression in higher eukaryotic cells. Much of what is currently known about transcription, RNA processing, and translation in mammalian cells was learned through the study of animal viruses. Conversely, in the course of these studies the basics of virus structure and replication were elucidated in great detail, setting the stage for further progress in the understanding of virus-host biology and pathogenesis. In no other area of infectious disease research has the impact of molecular biology been as profound as in virology (see Chap. 133).

The course of research into the acquired immunodeficiency syndrome (AIDS) bears eloquent testimony to this fact (see Chap. 264). In the space of only a few years from the first isolation of human immune virus (HIV), the viral genome was cloned and its complete nucleotide sequence determined. This led to the recognition of a number of new viral genes not previously encountered among standard animal retroviruses, including genes involved in the regulation of viral transcription (*tat*) and RNA processing (*rev*), as well as others affecting viral infectivity and morphogenesis. The molecular basis of the antigenic variation of the viral surface glycoproteins has been determined, and highly conserved sites on this protein involved in receptor binding and membrane fusion identified. Such regions are of obvious importance in the design of potential strategies for immunoprophylaxis. The viral receptor has been identified as the cell surface protein CD4, and the regions of the receptor involved in virus binding have been mapped. Cloning of the receptor itself also has been achieved, and mutant variants of the protein secreted from cultured cells have been shown to block viral infectivity. These recombinant CD4 preparations have been used in clinical trials as candidate antiviral agents.

These advances in the understanding of HIV are particularly striking because they illustrate how rapidly such information can be obtained with contemporary approaches. Most of these technologies were developed through the study of other viruses prior to the advent of the AIDS epidemic. Using these methods, for instance, the receptors for many viruses, including Epstein-Barr virus, poliovirus, and rhinoviruses have been identified and cloned. For some viruses, including poliovirus and influenza, the details of the virion surface structure and receptor-binding site are known at atomic resolution.

Recombinant DNA technology has also made possible the detailed study of many aspects of viral replication and gene expression without the requirement for virus growth in culture. This can be done by transfection of cloned viral genes into cultured cell lines, as well as by the analysis of viral DNA and RNA in infected human or animal tissues. This has allowed characterization of many medically important viruses whose study was impossible by classic virologic means. The hepatitis viruses provide an important case in point. The involvement of reverse transcription in the replication of hepatitis B virus (HBV) was discovered, and its mechanism defined, entirely in the absence of cell culture. The replicative program of the virus of delta hepatitis, a satellite of HBV, was similarly elucidated. More recently a candidate viral genome has been cloned from the serum of a recipient of blood products implicated in the transmission of non-A, non-B hepatitis. Even though this agent (tentatively termed hepatitis C virus) also has not been grown in culture, serodiagnostic tests based on recombinant antigens can now be developed and should have a major positive impact on the safety of the blood supply.

The human papilloma viruses (HPV) also cannot be grown in culture, but analysis of infected tissues with cloned HPV DNA probes has revealed that there is a strong association between cervical and genital carcinoma and infection with specific biotypes of HPV. Tumors arising in the context of infection by these viruses harbor viral DNA sequences integrated into the host genome; analysis of the host DNA invariably reveals the retention of certain regions of the viral genome, while others are typically deleted. These studies have provided powerful clues to the viral genes involved in malignant transformation.

No discussion of contemporary molecular virology would be complete without mention of the use of animal viruses as genetic vectors for the delivery of foreign DNA to somatic cells. Viruses are attractive vehicles for such gene transfer because they have evolved efficient mechanisms for entry into and persistence within host cells. In most strategies for viral vectoring, genes are first removed from the virus genome and replaced with the exogenous DNA of interest. The resulting recombinant genome, once packaged inside the virus particle, is then used to infect the appropriate host cell. Assuming the genes excised from the virus are not required for its replication, the recombinant genome will be capable of replication and spread within the recipient. If the deleted sequences are required for viral growth, the recombinant will be defective (nonviable) and will not spread beyond the original infected cell unless complemented by a helper virus.

Many types of virus has been employed as genetic vectors, including polyomavirus, parvovirus, adenovirus, papillomavirus, retrovirus, poxvirus, and even herpesvirus. As yet only retrovirus, adenovirus, and poxvirus show promise as clinically useful vectors. Defective murine retrovirus is the most likely vector to be used in initial efforts at somatic gene therapy, particularly for disorders involving cells of the blood or bone marrow (e.g., adenosine deaminase deficiency; see Chap. 263). The principal advantages of this virus include its efficient infection of hematopoietic cells and the ability to prepare helper-free stocks of replication-incompetent vectors, which ensures that there will be no spread of the virus in the recipient of the treated marrow.

By contrast, there are situations in which a limited amount of viral replication in the host is desirable—for example, in the design of live-virus vaccines—where this serves to mimic natural infection and provoke both humoral and cell-mediated immunity. For these applications, a nondefective poxvirus (e.g., vaccinia) or adenovirus has found favor. Attenuated live-virus strains with long records of human use as vaccines are available for both virus families; these serve as starting material for recombinant design. Foreign genes encoding antigens of interest are then cloned into nonessential regions of the viral genome and the recombinants isolated in pure culture for use. This practice is most highly developed for vaccinia, where recombinants have been constructed bearing antigens from HBV, HIV, influenza, and even *Plasmodium falciparum*. Like all live-virus vaccines, these recombinant viruses carry with them the risk of disease induction in the immunodeficient host (as well as other potential risks) and will require careful experimental and clinical scrutiny before they can be contemplated for widespread use.

PARASITOLOGY The same features that have allowed molecular biologists to study noncultivatable viruses have also proven useful in the study of difficult-to-grow protozoan and metazoan parasites. Spectacular progress has been made, for example, in the study of the biology of the African trypanosomes, the causative agents of sleeping sickness (see Chap. 161). These organisms undergo a remarkable program of antigenic variation to evade host immune responses during their protracted bloodstream infection. It consists of sequential expression of variants of a major surface glycoprotein, brought about, as in gonococci, by movement of coding information from silent chromosomal reservoirs into active expression sites.

Equally remarkable progress is being made in the study of malarial parasites. Genes governing the production of the major surface protein of the sporozoite have been cloned and extensively characterized, and the protein products of the recombinants have been tested as candidate vaccine components. Similar work is underway to express important antigens from the merozoite (bloodstream) and even the gametocyte stages (see Chaps. 156 and 159). While an effective vaccine has not been developed, there is renewed hope that a combination of such antigens affecting a number of steps in the parasite's complex life cycle may yet prove effective in attenuating disease and preventing transmission.

Perhaps the most surprising and provocative result yet to emerge from the application of molecular biology to parasites concerns the characterization of *Pneumocystis carinii* (see Chap. 163). Examination of the sequence of ribosomal RNA from this organism yields the unexpected finding that this agent, widely classified as a protozoan, is taxonomically closer to yeasts!

DIAGNOSTIC AND THERAPEUTIC APPLICATIONS

Although the aforementioned advances will form the bases of the diagnostic and therapeutic approaches of the future, many more direct applications of rDNA technology are having immediate impact on present-day clinical practice. Some of these are summarized below.

DIAGNOSTICS Once any organism is available in reasonable quantity and purity, molecular clones of its genome can be prepared, irrespective of its ability to be readily grown in culture. These DNA clones can then be used as hybridization probes to detect the organism's genome in clinical specimens. A variety of formats are available for such DNA:DNA hybridization tests, both in solid phase (*filter hybridization*) and in solution. Methods even exist for the detection of microbial genomes or transcripts in histologic specimens (*in situ hybridization*). While detailed consideration of the methodologic aspects of such testing is beyond the scope of this chapter (see Chap. 81), the advantages of these tests can be simply summarized as follows: (1) they can be performed on noncultivatable as well as cultivatable organisms; (2) they can be much more rapid than culture-based tests for organisms that are difficult to grow; and (3) they can display extraordinary specificity. However, such testing is not a diagnostic panacea. Widespread use of these tests has been limited by several features. Optimal sensitivity often requires the use of radiolabeled probes with isotopes with a short half-life; particularly where radiolabeled probes are required, a high level of technical expertise is necessary to maintain quality in the environment of mass testing in clinical laboratories. Finally, like most biochemical tests, the sensitivity of filter hybridization tests is generally less than that of culture, where replication of the organism affords rapid and enormous amplification of the signal. These considerations suggest that such tests will not replace cultures for most conventional bacteria but will be of greatest use in the diagnosis of organisms (e.g., viruses, *Chlamydia*, and parasites) where culture is either impossible, difficult, or inefficient.

An even more powerful DNA-based diagnostic technology has recently been developed that promises to mitigate the problem of sensitivity mentioned above. This is the enzymatic amplification of DNA in vitro also known by its technical name, the polymerase chain reaction (see Chap. 6). Basically, this method uses DNA polymerases to amplify the signal from the microbial genome in the test tube, in a fashion analogous to what authentic replication would do during culture. As a result, each copy of the microbial genome in the specimen undergoes replication many thousandfold in vitro during the brief period (hours) of the reaction. The amplified DNA segment can then be specifically identified by filter hybridization or other means. The method has the advantage of enormous sensitivity, rivaling that of culture for some organisms. Its disadvantages are the expense and high level of technical expertise needed to perform the test. Its exquisite sensitivity may also impose some limits on its clinical utility. False-positive results from degrees of laboratory contamination too trivial to be detected by conventional tests have already occurred.

The other area in which rDNA technology is already having an impact is in the development of improved reagents for serologic testing. The expression of foreign antigens in *E. coli* is now routine and is increasingly being used to generate pure antigens for use in diagnostic serology. This has been particularly valuable for agents that are difficult to grow in quantity or hard to purify. For example, recombinant core and surface antigens of HBV and *gag* and envelope antigens of HIV are now commonly used in commercial testing kits (see Chaps. 252 and 264).

THERAPEUTICS The other major area in which rDNA technology is already affecting clinical practice is in the production of therapeutic agents and vaccines. This area is still in its infancy but will certainly undergo rapid expansion in the future. The development of live virus vaccines based on viral vectors has already been discussed. More conventional vaccines composed of recombinant antigens produced in bacteria, yeast, or cultured cells can be anticipated with certainty. Already one such product has been licensed, recombinant hepatitis B surface antigen (produced in yeast cells). Similar strategies are underway for vaccine development against HIV, herpes simplex, rabies, and other agents.

A wide variety of biologically active polypeptides with therapeutic potential have also been produced using this technology, including a number of growth factors, hormones, and cytokines. Some of these, e.g., hematopoietic growth factors like GM-CSF, may be useful in shortening periods of neutropenia induced by cytotoxic cancer chemotherapy. Other polypeptides with immunoregulatory or antiviral activity, such as interferons or other lymphokines, may also have therapeutic value.

Finally, the expression of microbial products by rDNA technology in large quantities facilitates x-ray crystallographic structure determination. For those proteins (e.g., metabolic enzymes or adhesins) that are good targets for antimicrobial drugs, knowledge of the protein's fine structure may one day make possible the rational design of inhibitors targeted to the relevant active site.

REFERENCES

GANEM D, VARMUS H: The molecular biology of the hepatitis B viruses. Ann Rev Biochem 56:651, 1987

MILLER V, FALKOW S: Evidence for two genetic loci in *Yersinia enterocolitica* that can promote invasion of epithelial cells. Infect Immun 56:1242, 1988

NOTKINS A, OLDSTONE MB (eds): *Concepts in Viral Pathogenesis*. New York, Springer-Verlag, 1984

SCAIFE J et al (eds): *The Genetics of Bacteria*. London, Academic, 1985

SPARLING PF et al: Phase and antigenic variation of pili and outer membrane protein II in *Neisseria gonorrheae*. J Infect Dis 153:196, 1986

TURNER M, ARNOT D (eds): *Molecular Genetics of Parasitic Protozooa*. New York, Cold Spring Harbor Press, 1988

80 THE DIAGNOSIS OF INFECTIOUS DISEASES

JAMES J. PLORDE

The diagnosis of an infectious disease requires the direct or indirect demonstration of a pathogenic microbe on or within the tissues of the afflicted host. The major ways in which this is accomplished are described in this chapter.

DIRECT MICROSCOPIC EXAMINATION

The direct microscopic examination of body fluids, exudates, and tissues is both the simplest and one of the most helpful laboratory procedures available for the diagnosis of infectious diseases. In many situations the examination allows an accurate, highly specific identification of the causative agent. Examples include the recognition of *Borrelia* or *Plasmodium* species in blood smears taken from patients with relapsing fever or malaria. More commonly, only a tentative identification can be made on the basis of microbial morphology. Nevertheless, this is often sufficiently precise to allow the selection of an appropriate chemotherapeutic agent pending the results of more definitive investigations.

WET MOUNTS Dark-field examination of fluid from genital lesions for the spirochete of syphilis is a well-known, but neglected, procedure. More often, wet mounts are used for the diagnosis of fungal and parasitic infections. The examination of hair fragments, skin scrapings, or nail clippings in a drop of 10% KOH or KOH-calcofluor is useful in establishing the presence of superficial mycoses. Occasionally a presumptive diagnosis of a systemic fungus infection can also be established with this procedure. Two examples are cryptococcal meningitis diagnosed by demonstrating the encapsulated organism in an india ink preparation of cerebrospinal fluid, and coccidioidomycosis identified by finding characteristic spherules in expectorated sputum.

Examination of wet mounts of stool or duodenal drainage is also the initial step in establishing the diagnosis of intestinal protozoal infections such as amebiasis, giardiasis, and cryptosporidiosis. Moreover, it is the definitive procedure diagnosing intestinal helminthic infections including ascariasis, trichuriasis, strongyloidiasis, and hookworm. Filariasis and sleeping sickness can be recognized by demonstrating the characteristic motility of microfilariae and trypanosomes in blood or other body fluids.

STAIN-ENHANCED MICROSCOPY Despite many technical advances in the field of microbiology, the Gram stain remains, after 100 years of use, the best single technique available for the rapid diagnosis of bacterial infections. It is of particular value in the examination of exudates, aspirates, and body fluids, including cerebrospinal fluid and urine. Stains are examined first under the lower-power objective to demonstrate the presence of pink-staining inflammatory cells. The paucity of such cells in the presence of many squamous epithelial cells suggests that the specimen was contaminated during the process of collection and may not be representative of the inflammatory process. The smear is then examined for the presence of bacteria using the oil immersion lens; bacteria appear either as dark blue (gram-positive) or pink (gram-negative) bodies. Their color and morphologic appearance often make possible a presumptive identification of the genus and occasionally the species of the organism. The demonstration of pneumococci in the sputum, Enterobacteriaceae in the urine, staphylococci in localized abscesses, gonococci in urethral exudates, clostridia in foul-smelling discharge, and pneumococci, meningococci, or *Haemophilus influenzae* in stained smears of the cerebrospinal fluid permits the initiation of specific chemotherapy with the assurance that the regimen is the proper one.

Mycobacteria have the unique capacity to resist the decolorization by strong mineral acid alcohol solutions once they have been stained with basic carbol-fuchsin (Ziehl-Neelsen, Kinyoun stains) or one of the newer fluorochromes. This allows their immediate recognition in body tissues and fluids. The presence of a large number of acid-fast bacilli in the expectorated sputum establishes the presumptive diagnosis of respiratory tuberculosis and is sufficient evidence for initiating isolation procedures and antituberculosis therapy once additional specimens are collected for culture.

Acid-fast smears can also be used to identify *Cryptosporidium* and *Isospora* spp. in the stool of patients with diarrhea. If mineral acid rather than acid alcohol is used for decolorization, pathogenic strains of *Nocardia* may be visualized in body fluids or exudates.

A number of stains are available for the definitive identification of parasites. *Pneumocystis carinii* can be recognized in induced sputum, bronchial lavage fluid, and transbronchial brush biopsies using a modified Wright's stain, toluidine blue, or methenamine silver. Blood and tissue protozoa such as plasmodia and *Leishmania* can be demonstrated best with Romanowsky-type mixtures containing methylene blue and eosin. These render the nuclei red to violet and the cytoplasm blue. The identification of intestinal protozoa, on the other hand, requires the use of stains such as iron hematoxylin or trichrome to demonstrate the taxonomically important nuclear detail.

IMMUNE MICROSCOPY This method combines the specificity of immunologic procedures with the speed of direct microscopy. In the immunofluorescent technique, smears thought to contain viral, bacterial, fungal, or parasitic organisms are stained with specific antibody preparations labeled with fluorescent compounds and examined with a fluorescent microscope. The most useful application of this technique is the examination of brain tissue for herpes simplex or rabies virus; respiratory specimens for cytomegalovirus, *Legionella* spp., and *P. carinii;* cervical, urethral, conjunctival, and nasopharyngeal specimens for *Chlamydia trachomatis;* and genital lesions for herpes simplex virus. Direct fluorescent antibody staining of nasopharyngeal cells may also be used for the rapid diagnosis of pertussis, influenza, parainfluenza, and respiratory syncytial virus infections.

The accuracy and reliability of immunofluorescent techniques continues to improve as older polyclonal antisera are replaced with more specific monoclonal reagents. The need for expensive fluorescent microscopes and well-trained technologists restricts the routine use of these procedures to larger laboratories.

Enzyme-linked immunosorbent assay (ELISA) tests are similar to the immunofluorescence test except that the antiserum is reacted with an enzyme-labeled antispecies conjugate. After treatment with an appropriate substrate, a color change can be visualized with the ordinary light microscope, obviating expensive equipment.

HYBRIDIZATION MICROSCOPY It has been shown that microbes fixed on glass slides can be hybridized with small, fluorescently labeled, oligonucleotide probes complementary to 16 S ribosomal RNA and visualized by fluorescent microscopy. Identification is accomplished by utilizing probes complementary to group- or species-specific 16 S rRNA sequences. A variety of microbes can be identified on the same microscopic slide with the simultaneous use of multiple probes labeled with different fluors.

DETECTION OF MICROBIAL ANTIGENS, BY-PRODUCTS, AND GENOMES

The relative nonspecificity of many direct microscopic methods and the delay inherent in culture procedures have resulted in the introduction of a variety of techniques aimed at the rapid detection of microbial antigens, by-products, or genomes. Such procedures are particularly useful when prior antibiotic therapy has rendered microscopic and culture tests negative.

PARTICLE AGGLUTINATION Particle (e.g., latex, erythrocytes) agglutination tests are the most commonly employed antigen detection procedures. They are technically simpler and frequently more sensitive than the counterimmunoelectrophoresis (CIE) method which they have supplanted. Agglutination tests have been plagued by false-positive reactions from heat-labile serum and urine components and from rheumatoid factor. Like CIE, latex and coagglutination tests have proved most useful for the rapid detection of pneumococcal, meningococcal, group B streptococcal, or *H. influenzae* antigens in the urine and spinal fluid of children with acute meningitis and cryptococcal antigen in the blood and spinal fluid of patients with chronic meningoencephalitis. Agglutination tests have been introduced for the detection of pneumococci in the sputum, group A streptococci *(Streptococcus pyogenes)* in throat swabs, *Candida* antigen in serum, and rotavirus, as well as a product of *C. difficile,* in stool.

Of these, tests for the detection of *S. pyogenes* in throat swabs have attracted the most clinical attention. Over 30 such assays are commercially available; in each the group A carbohydrate is extracted from the swab with acid or enzyme treatment and then tested in a latex agglutination, coagglutination, or enzyme-linked immunosorbent assay (see below). Results are generally available within minutes. The speed and ease with which these tests can be performed have resulted in their widespread utilization in primary and emergency care settings. Although antigen detection tests have generally demonstrated high specificity (≥90 percent) vis-à-vis culture results, their sensitivities have varied (62 to 100 percent) from study to study. The adequacy of quality control and culture procedures, the skill of the tester, the patient's age, and the number of organisms present on the swab all appear to influence outcome. Of primary concern is the relative insensitivity of these procedures in patients whose simultaneous throat cultures yield fewer than 100 streptococcal colonies. Because a significant proportion of such patients demonstrate fourfold serum streptococcal antibody rises, true infections may be missed by the current generation of antigen tests. While their ultimate role in the diagnosis of streptococcal pharyngitis remains to be determined, they are now widely used as a culture substitute in outpatient settings lacking adequate laboratory services and in patient populations unable or unlikely to return for culture results. In clinical settings where throat cultures are practical, the simultaneous use of both tests may facilitate patient management. Patients with positive antigen test results could then be treated immediately, and therapeutic decisions on the antigen-negative patients postponed pending the availability of culture results.

ENZYME-LINKED IMMUNOSORBENT ASSAYS The method, as described above under "Direct Microscopic Examination," can be adapted for the visual or spectrophotometric detection of microbial antigens. It has largely replaced radioimmunoassay techniques in the diagnosis of hepatitis A and B infections and is extensively utilized to ascertain the presence of rotavirus and enteric adenovirus in the diarrheal stool of infants and immunosuppressed adults. It has been successfully used to detect circulating antigens in candidiasis, aspergillosis, and toxoplasmosis as well as urinary antigens in legionellosis. Enzyme immunoassays are also beginning to play an important role in the diagnosis of *C. trachomatis* and gonococcal cervicitis and urethritis, genital herpes, and viral respiratory tract infections.

URINE SCREENING TESTS A number of nonmicroscopic bacteriuria screening tests are commercially available. Each is designed to decrease the time and cost involved in the diagnosis of urinary tract infections. Bioluminescence, filtration-colorimetry, or chemical procedures are employed to determine the presence or absence ot bacterial and/or leukocytic enzymes in the urine specimen. The tests can be performed reliably by individuals with minimal technical training and require only minutes to complete. Generally, specimens demonstrating a positive screening test are cultured; a negative result is reported as such, and the specimen is discarded. The sensitivity, specificity, and reproducibility of these tests do not differ significantly from those obtained with a microscopic examination of a stained urine smear conducted by a competent microbiologist; all reliably detect specimens containing 10^5 or more colony-forming units (CFU) per milliliter of urine, but are insufficiently sensitive at lower colony counts. The considerably higher cost of the screening tests vis-à-vis microscopic examination is partially offset by their technical simplicity. The ultimate role of these screening tests may be in the selection of specimens requiring culture techniques capable of detecting low colony count bacteriuria.

DNA PROBES The utilization of recombinant DNA techniques has made it possible to isolate, reproduce, and label single-stranded nucleotide sequences from the genome of specific microorganisms that are unique to that particular strain, species, genus, or group. These labeled DNA fragments, or probes, can be added to microbial cultures, body fluids, exudates, or tissues thought to contain the pathogen in question and the mixture treated with heat or chemicals to separate the microbial DNA into single strands. Following treatment, the DNA strands reanneal. This reassociation, or hybridization, is highly specific, occurring only between strands bearing complementary nucleotide sequences. If the specimen contains nucleotide sequences complementary to those of the probe, they will be hybridized and labeled.

The potential advantages of such probes are in their unique

specificity, their capacity to detect a single pathogen among a plethora of others, and the capacity to identify microorganisms that are either difficult or impossible to recover by cultural methods. Their most immediate impact will be on the diagnosis of viral, chlamydial, mycobacterial, enteric bacterial, and parasitic infections. Probes have already been developed for a wide variety of agents, including herpes simplex virus I and II, cytomegalovirus, enteroviruses, Epstein-Barr virus, hepatitis B virus, adenovirus, varicella-zoster virus, rotavirus, human papillomavirus, human immunodeficiency and T-cell leukemia viruses, *Mycoplasma pneumoniae, C. trachomatis,* enterotoxigenic and enteroadherent *Escherichia coli, Yersinia enterocolitica, Salmonella* spp., *Shigella* spp., *Campylobacter* spp., *Legionella* spp., *Mycobacteria* spp., *Leishmania mexicana, L. braziliensis,* and *Plasmodium falciparum.* Only a few of these, including mycoplasmal, mycobacterial, legionella, gonococcal, and human papillomavirus probes, are commercially available.

Ultimately, the utility of DNA probes in clinical medicine will rest on the simplification and commercialization of the hybridization procedure and the development of practical, highly sensitive labels. To date, most probes have utilized radioisotopic markers (usually ^{32}P). These demonstrate a high level of sensitivity but require prolonged processing for autoradiographic detection, have an extremely limited shelf life, and require the storage and disposal of radioactive materials, making them impractical for the clinical laboratory. Colorimetrically detected or fluorescent enzymatic labels have been developed which circumvent these drawbacks; however, all appear to be somewhat less sensitive than the radiometric labels and decidedly less sensitive than most cultural procedures. A gene amplification method known as the polymerase chain reaction (PCR) is capable of synthesizing millions of copies of a single nucleotide sequence within a few hours. Application of the PCR methodology to clinical specimens make it possible, in combination with DNA probes, to detect the presence of microbes present in extremely small numbers (see Chap. 6). This technique has already proved useful in the research laboratory for the detection of human immunodeficiency virus (HIV) in the peripheral blood cells of infected patients. With the anticipated development of more satisfactory, nonradiometric labels, the DNA probe may well alter the diagnosis and management of infectious diseases in a dramatic way. They are unlikely, however, to displace culture methods for infections in which the recovery, characterization, and susceptibility testing of the pathogenic agent is critical to the management of a sick patient.

CULTURE TECHNIQUES

Despite the time and complexity, the isolation of the etiologic agent by cultivation in artificial media, tissue cultures, or animals is generally the most definitive procedure available.

The diagnostic value of a culture specimen, however, depends to a large extent on the likelihood that it has been collected free of contamination with the resident microbial flora and transported to the laboratory in a fashion that ensures survival of fastidious organisms.

SPECIMEN COLLECTION When specimens from deep closed lesions are collected, the site of percutaneous needle aspiration should be cleansed first by using 70% isopropyl or ethyl alcohol and then disinfected with a 2% tincture of iodine or an appropriate iodophor. If the specimen for culture is drawn through an indwelling cannula, the site of withdrawal must be disinfected in the same fashion.

When specimens are to be collected from the uterus or a draining wound or sinus tract, the orifice must be thoroughly cleansed and disinfected as described above, a sterile intravenous catheter or multilumen tube is introduced as deeply as possible through the orifice, and the specimen aspirated into a sterile syringe. Culture from an open lesion may be collected by biopsy, aspiration from the margin, or by swabbing the surface. In the first two situations the wound is prepared as for a deep closed lesion. For swab cultures, the wound surface is cleansed only with sterile saline to remove debris and saprophytic flora.

TRANSPORTATION All specimens submitted for microbial culture should be transported to the laboratory as rapidly as possible, preferably within 1 h. Delay beyond this time may result in death of fastidious organisms, overgrowth of contaminants, and/or change in the number of bacteria unless special procedures are employed to overcome these problems. Respiratory secretions, urine, large pieces of tissue, and large volumes of fluid can be safely transmitted in plastic containers with leakproof lids. Aspirates are conveniently and safely transported in the same syringe used in the collection procedure, providing all air is expressed from the syringe. Alternatively, such fluid may be injected into a sealed gassed-out vial suitable for transport of anaerobic specimens. Small pieces of tissue (less than 1 cm^2) are transported best in sterile rubber-stoppered gassed-out tubes. Swabs should be submitted in one of several commercially available transport media. These prevent both the desiccation of organisms implanted on the swab and the overgrowth of hardy organisms at the expense of more fastidious ones. Although special anaerobic transport materials are available, use of swab specimens for the recovery of such organisms is not encouraged.

UPPER RESPIRATORY TRACT SPECIMENS Because the throat and nasopharynx are normally heavily colonized by both saprophytic and potentially pathogenic bacteria, culture of this area is seldom useful except when a particular bacterial pathogen is being sought, e.g., *S. pyogenes, Bordetella pertussis, Corynebacterium diphtheriae,* meningococci, or gonococci.

When *throat cultures* are submitted to the laboratory without specifying the pathogen being sought, the laboratory will generally report only the presence or absence of *S. pyogenes.* Since a single properly obtained throat swab will detect at least 90 percent of patients with streptococcal pharyngitis, a negative culture is very helpful in excluding the possibility of this disease. Similarly, a heavy or predominant growth of group A beta-hemolytic streptococci in patients presenting with the signs and symptoms of streptococcal pharyngitis is highly predictive of an antibody response to streptococcal antigens and, therefore, presumably disease. It is far more difficult to interpret cultures with a light or nonpredominant growth of *S. pyogenes.* At least half of these patients do not mount an appreciable immunologic response, suggesting that bacterial growth often represents a carrier state.

LOWER RESPIRATORY TRACT SPECIMENS Although culture of expectorated sputum is the most frequently employed technique for the diagnosis of lower respiratory tract infections, both its sensitivity and specificity have been questioned. Studies of patients with bacteremic pneumococcal pneumonia have shown the etiologic agent to be present in the sputum in only 50 to 94 percent of cases. Moreover, expectorated sputum is almost always contaminated with oropharyngeal flora including, in many cases, bacterial species commonly associated with pulmonary infections. Some confusion can be avoided if the specimen is collected appropriately and screened carefully for both gross and microscopic characteristics prior to inoculation of the culture.

Specimens demonstrating a Gram-stain smear with fewer than 10 squamous epithelial cells (SEC) and greater than 25 leukocytes per low-power field are likely to contain lower tract flora. This is particularly true if a single or clearly predominant bacterial type grows, or, in the case of chronic obstructive pulmonary disease, if both pneumococci and *H. influenzae* are isolated. If SEC number more than 10 per low-power field, the specimen can be considered heavily contaminated with oropharyngeal flora and should be discarded. In most cases a second carefully collected expectorated sputum will yield a satisfactory specimen. If the patient is unable to produce sputum, coughing may be stimulated by lowering the head of the patient's bed for a few minutes or exposing the patient to an aerosol of warm hypertonic saline.

Direct endotracheal or endobronchial aspiration may be employed when a satisfactory expectorated or induced sputum cannot be produced. However, such specimens are subject to contamination by oropharyngeal flora which is introduced during the passage of the aspiration instrument. Fiberoptic bronchoscopy, which allows the direct visualization and aspiration of bronchial secretions, may result in a somewhat better specimen. When it is accompanied by a brush biopsy performed through an occluded double-lumen tube, the material obtained is unlikely to be diluted with saliva or topical anesthetics and may be utilized for anaerobic cultures. Alternatively, the specimen may be collected by a technique that totally bypasses the oropharynx. The most widely used is transtracheal aspiration. This method entails a definite risk of hemoptysis, subcutaneous and mediastinal emphysema, vagal discharge, or respiratory embarrassment and is contraindicated in the presence of a bleeding diathesis. It should be used only when results from expectorated sputum are unsatisfactory and the infection is severe enough to merit the attendant risks (see Chap. 207).

Needle aspiration of a pulmonary infiltrate under fluoroscopic control also produces specimens of excellent quality. The percutaneous method gives both a high yield and accurate results but has at least a 5 percent chance of complications, particularly pneumothorax. The morbidity risk is greater than with transtracheal aspiration biopsy, but the diagnostic yield may be superior.

Whatever technique is used to sample the lower respiratory tract, a concomitant blood culture should always be obtained. If a pleural effusion is present, it should also be aspirated and cultured.

In addition to bacterial pathogens, pneumonia can be caused by viruses, *Rickettsia, Chlamydia, M. pneumoniae, Legionella*, and *Pneumocystis* and related agents. Techniques for the recovery of these agents from the sputum are generally not available in a routine clinical microbiology laboratory, and the diagnosis is most frequently made by clinical, immunologic, and/or serologic methods. *P. carinii* and cytomegalovirus can be recovered by bronchoalveolar lavage. *L. pneumophila* can be cultured from expectorated sputum, lung tissue, or empyema fluid. In addition, the organism can be demonstrated by direct fluorescent antibody staining and DNA probing of respiratory specimens, and its antigens may be detected in urine with ELISA procedures. These methods permit early diagnosis and rapid institution of appropriate therapy.

URINE SPECIMENS Voided urine, like expectorated sputum, is usually contaminated with the normal microbial flora, in this case from the urethra and external genitalia. Urine cultures, however, are more reliable than those of expectorated sputum, because the periurethral area can be disinfected and the urethra itself flushed with the first portion of the urine stream before a sample is taken by the clean-voided, midstream collection technique. In addition, quantitation of the bacterial growth is helpful in separating contaminated specimens from true infection. When this procedure is followed conscientiously, a single specimen from a male which yields a colony count in excess of 100,000 organisms per milliliter is highly indicative of bacteriuria. In women, the colony count must exceed 100,000 organisms per milliliter in two consecutive urine specimens before infection can be considered to be present. Because urine is a good culture medium, contaminating organisms will multiply to large numbers if the urine is allowed to stand at room temperature for prolonged periods of time. For this reason, specimens which cannot be dispatched to the laboratory within an hour should be refrigerated. They can be held at 4°C for 4 to 6 h without an appreciable change in the bacterial colony count. In most instances, urinary tract infections are caused by a single bacterial species. The isolation of three or more species in a urine culture usually reflects contamination even when the colony count is high. True polymicrobial bacteriuria does occur but is generally restricted to patients with chronic indwelling urethral catheters. In contrast, colony counts of less than 100,000 organisms per milliliter may represent true bacteriuria. For example, $\geq 10^2$ CFU per milliliter in symptomatic dysuric women and $\geq 10^3$ in symptomatic men are significant counts. In fact, up to one-third of urinary tract infections are associated with counts less than 100,000 organisms per milliliter. Patients receiving antimicrobial therapy and specimens obtained by ureteral or urethral catheterization and by suprapubic aspiration also are likely to contain a low number of organisms.

When an adequate clean-voided urine specimen cannot be obtained, or when anaerobic cultures are desired, suprapubic aspiration may be employed. Specimens obtained in this manner are unlikely to be contaminated, and even slight growth may be significant. When an indwelling catheter is in place, a specimen should be collected directly from the catheter by means of a sterile needle and syringe after careful disinfection of the exterior surface or sampling port. Urine should not be taken from the drainage tube or bag, because these are frequently contaminated.

BLOOD SPECIMENS Cultures should be obtained from all febrile patients who have rigors, are seriously ill, are thought to have endocarditis or intravascular infection, or are immunosuppressed. If viremia, fungemia, brucellosis, tularemia, leptospirosis, or an infection with cell wall–deficient bacteria is suspected, the laboratory should be contacted for special instructions. The sensitivity of most culture techniques is volume-dependent, with yields increasing approximately 2 percent for each milliliter of blood drawn over 5 mL. In general, three blood cultures of 10 to 30 mL taken at intervals of no less than 60 min are adequate to document the presence of bacteremia in an adult. In emergent situations, two cultures taken simultaneously from different anatomic sites will usually suffice. In patients who have received antimicrobial agents within the previous 2 weeks or in whom endocarditis is suspected, a total of six cultures taken over a 2-day period may be useful. If the patient is receiving antimicrobial agents, the cultures should be taken immediately prior to the next dose, and the laboratory should be notified to allow use of an antibiotic removal device, or extensive dilution of the blood specimen. The collection of specimens over and above the number listed above is seldom helpful in detecting occult bacteremia unless the culture procedures, media, or conditions of incubation are altered to allow detection of fastidious organisms.

Specimens are best collected by percutaneous venipuncture. If possible, aspirations from the femoral vein should be avoided since disinfecting the skin of the groin is often difficult and the concentration of organisms in the venous drainage of the lower extremity is generally less than that found in the venous blood of the arms. The increasingly common practice of drawing blood for culture through an indwelling intravascular cannula often results in a higher level of contamination without substantially improving the detection of bacteremia. Similarly there is no evidence that arterial blood cultures possess any advantage over venous cultures. Bone marrow cultures may reveal the etiologic agent when it cannot be obtained by other means in occasional patients with disseminated salmonellosis, tuberculosis, and deep mycoses.

To minimize the chance of contamination with skin flora, the site of aspiration should be carefully disinfected as described above. Following aspiration, the blood should be inoculated into both aerobic and anaerobic broths immediately. The dilution ratio of blood to broth should be at least 1:5 to minimize the normal bactericidal activity of serum and the activity of any antimicrobial agents that may be present. If direct inoculation into broth is not feasible, the blood may be drawn into a sterile Vacutainer tube containing sodium polyethanol sulfanate (SPS). This anticoagulant is anticomplementary and inactivates leukocytes and certain aminoglycoside and polypeptide antibiotics. Nevertheless, it will not delay bacterial death indefinitely, and Vacutainer specimens should be sent to the laboratory for dilution in broth within 30 min of the time the blood is drawn. If fungemia is suspected, the laboratory should be notified since some of the standard techniques described above are less satisfactory for the isolation of fungi.

Approximately two-thirds of blood cultures from bacteremic patients are found to be positive within 24 h and 90 percent within 3 days. Despite strict adherence to disinfectant procedures on the ward and sterile technique in the laboratory, contamination occasionally occurs. The following are characteristics of "false-positive" blood cultures: (1) repeat cultures are seldom positive for the same organism, (2) bacterial growth in broth generally occurs after 2 days of incubation, and (3) the organisms are often identified as diphtheroids, *Bacillus*, or *Staphylococcus epidermidis*. However, any of these species, particularly coagulase-negative staphylococci, can occasionally be responsible for true bacteremia, particularly in immunosuppressed patients.

CEREBROSPINAL FLUID SPECIMENS Bacterial meningitis can be rapidly fatal if treatment is delayed or inadequate, and appropriate therapy often requires specific identification of the etiologic agent. Because of the clinical urgency, CSF specimens should be collected as soon as the diagnosis is considered, and the specimen promptly transported to the laboratory. The laboratory should be notified if the specimen has been collected from an abscess within the central nervous system to ensure that it is cultured both aerobically and anaerobically. If possible, at least 2 mL CSF should be obtained and the specimen sent for glucose, quantitative protein level, and cell count in addition to microbiologic studies. A simultaneous blood sugar also should be drawn for correlation with the CSF glucose level. Fastidious organisms, particularly *Neisseria meningitidis,* may not survive prolonged storage at temperatures below that of the body. If a delay in CSF examination cannot be avoided, specimens should be held at 37°C.

After receipt, the specimen is concentrated by centrifugation or filtration, Gram stained, and cultured. The inflammatory response in the CSF is helpful in distinguishing acute bacterial meningitis from nonbacterial forms of the disease. In bacterial meningitis, polymorphonuclear leukocytes predominate, while in tuberculous, fungal, or protozoal meningitis, the inflammatory cells usually consist of lymphocytes, and the response is less intense. Although polymorphonuclear leukocytes may dominate early in the course of aseptic meningitis, there is usually a clear shift to mononuclear cells within 8 h. Cytologic changes in the CSF may also be seen in patients with brain abscess. However, smears and cultures are generally negative in these cases unless the abscess ruptures into the subarachnoid space or into the ventricles (see Chap. 354). The Gram's stain smear of the CSF should be examined carefully for stainable organisms, particularly meningococci, pneumococci, *Enterobacteriaceae, Listeria,* and staphylococci in patients with atrioventricular shunts. Stainable, but nonviable, organisms occasionally contaminate sterile plastic containers and may result in a "false-positive" Gram's stain. In addition, in cases of partially treated bacterial meningitis there is a tendency for gram-positive organisms to stain gram-negative.

When a large number of organisms are present and specific antiserums are available, the etiologic agent can often be rapidly identified by the particle agglutination tests described above. Moreover, detection of microbial antigens in the CSF is often the only method of identification of an infectious agent from a patient with partially treated meningitis. In the presence of a significant number of mononuclear cells without stainable bacteria cryptococcal antigen can be identified by latex agglutination tests.

Regardless of the results of these studies, the CSF must be cultured and any resulting growth identified to the species level. In patients presenting with an acute mononuclear meningitis, the viral cultures should be submitted simultaneously with bacterial cultures. Coxsackie B, mumps, herpes simplex virus, and HIV may be recovered in appropriate clinical settings. Mycobacterial and fungal cultures should be set up on patients who present with chronic meningitis and a mononuclear inflammatory response in the CSF.

Naegleria fowleri, the cause of amebic meningoencephalitis, can often be recognized by its ameboid movements in wet-mount preparations of cerebrospinal fluid. This organism should be looked for in patients who develop hemorrhagic meningoencephalitis during the summer months (see Chap. 158).

GASTROINTESTINAL TRACT SPECIMENS Cultures of the mouth, periodontal lesions, or saliva usually yield a mixed flora of aerobic and anaerobic organisms including *Actinomyces* spp. and *Candida* spp. The isolation of these organisms is without significance unless the specimen was collected in a way which avoided contamination with indigenous flora. If actinomycosis is suspected, the laboratory should be contacted for special instructions. The diagnosis of oral thrush and Vincent's infection can be made with stained smears from scrapings of the suspected lesion.

Cultures of ileostomy or colostomy stomas, gastrointestinal fistulas, and rectal fissures invariably grow both aerobic and anaerobic intestinal flora. They are seldom helpful, therefore, unless a search is made for specific intestinal pathogens.

Fecal cultures are helpful in determining the etiology of diarrhea and in detecting carrier states. Such specimens are routinely cultured for species of *Salmonella, Shigella,* and *Arizona.* Many laboratories are now also looking for *Vibrio parahaemolyticus, Yersinia enterocolitica, Campylobacter jejuni, E. coli* 0157:H7, and *Clostridium difficile.* Cell culture and particle agglutination techniques can be used for the direct detection of *C. difficile* toxin and other diarrhea-associated products of this organism in the stool of diarrheal patients. There is at present no convenient and reliable cultural method of identifying enterotoxogenic strains of *E. coli* or the Norwalk-like viruses in the clinical laboratory. The laboratory should be alerted as to whether any of these, or any other unusual infection such as candidiasis, clostridial food poisoning, or cholera, is suspected.

Although rectal swabs are adequate for the diagnosis of bacterial diarrhea, they are less satisfactory for the detection of carrier states. If swabs are used, they should show obvious soiling and be sent to the laboratory in appropriate transport media. Whole stool should be collected free of urine, placed in clean, waxed cardboard cartons, and promptly dispatched to the laboratory. If delivery cannot be made within 1 h, the stool should be preserved in phosphate-buffered glycerol to prevent death of fastidious organisms such as *Shigella* spp. It is seldom necessary to submit more than three consecutive daily specimens.

GENITAL TRACT SPECIMENS Genital specimens are submitted primarily for the diagnosis of venereal disease including gonorrhea, syphilis, herpes, chancroid, trichomoniasis, chlamydial, CMV, and HIV infections. Instructions for the collection of specimens should be sought in the sections of the text dealing with these specific diseases. In addition to the venereal pathogens, a number of organisms may infect the endometrium, tuboovarian tissues, and vagina. Endometrial cultures must be collected through a double- or triple-lumen tube inserted through a decontaminated cervical os if contamination with vaginal and cervical flora is to be avoided. The specimens should be delivered to the laboratory in either a gassed-out vial or a sealed syringe to ensure recovery of anaerobic organisms. When a patient presents with vaginitis, a specimen is collected by swabbing the vaginal fornix under direct visualization. Candidiasis and bacterial vaginosis are best diagnosed by examination of a Gram-stained smear.

EXUDATES AND BODY FLUIDS Pus from undrained abscesses as well as pericardial, pleural, peritoneal, and synovial fluids is best collected by syringe and needle aspiration through disinfected skin. Prior rinsing of the syringe with a sterile anticoagulant such as heparin or SPS will help prevent formation of clots. Because anaerobic organisms are commonly involved in infection of these areas, the syringe should be sealed and sent immediately to the microbiology laboratory. Alternatively, the aspirate may be injected into a gassed-out anaerobic transport vial. The use of swabs is not encouraged since the sample size is small and fastidious organisms including anaerobes are unusually susceptible to desiccation and oxidation. Deep suppurative lesions which communicate with the surface of the body through fistulas or sinus tracts present a difficult problem in specimen collection. The communicating pathway is generally colonized by a wide variety of bacterial flora which contaminate drainage being ejected through the fistula opening. The degree of contamination can be lessened in many instances by carefully disinfecting the orifice and aspirating material via a sterile plastic catheter inserted deep into the sinus. Even when these precautions are taken, however, sinus tract cultures often fail to correlate well with pathogens isolated from operative specimens. For this reason, a bacteriologic diagnosis of draining suppurative lesions should be based on a culture of currettings or biopsy rather than sinus drainage. If actinomycosis is suspected, the draining sinus tract may be covered with gauze which is left in place until it is thoroughly saturated. The gauze is then submitted to the laboratory where it is carefully examined for the presence of granules which can be picked out and then identified.

SKIN, SOFT TISSUE, AND SUPERFICIAL WOUNDS Specimens collected from these areas are usually heavily contaminated with the normal flora of their respective sites. Swab cultures should be obtained only if gross pus is present or if there is need to confirm the presence or absence of only a single bacterial pathogen, such as *C. diphtheriae;* in this case, the wound should first be cleansed mechanically with saline to remove as much exudate as possible. Material from bullae and areas of cellulitis is best obtained with a syringe. Successful aspiration of an area of cellulitis may require several thrusts and withdrawals, care being taken to maintain the tip of the needle beneath the surface of the skin and a significant vacuum in the barrel of the syringe. If sterile saline is injected prior to aspiration, this solution should not contain a preservative which may affect the viability of some bacteria. Alternatively, a punch biopsy may be obtained of the area after appropriate disinfection. Similarly, cultures from open lesions may be obtained by biopsy or by aspirating from the margins of these lesions using a syringe and needle. Semiquantitative cultures of burn eschars are useful in identifying patients at risk of bacteremia.

Intravenous and intraarterial catheter segments are best collected by disinfecting the area of the skin penetrated by the catheter, carefully withdrawing the catheter, and aseptically cutting off the 5-cm section that had been located just under the skin into a sterile container. This is then delivered to the microbiology laboratory where semiquantitative cultures are done. In general, catheters which are contaminated during removal will have only a few colonies on agar plates, while infected catheters will show heavy growth.

IMMUNOLOGIC METHODS

These diagnostic methods are intended to supply evidence of past or present infection by demonstrating antibodies in serum or other body fluids, or indicating changed reactivity of the host (hypersensitivity, allergy) to products of the organism.

SEROLOGIC TESTS The finding on a single occasion that a patient's serum contains antibody which reacts with a certain antigen merely indicates that the patient has had previous contact with the antigen or a closely related substance. For this reason, with rare exceptions, the clinical interpretation of serologic tests depends on serial determinations. If the antibody titer is found to *rise or fall significantly,* or, alternatively, if specific IgM antibody is detected, the response likely is a result of recent contact with the antigen. With infections caused by herpes family or other latent viruses, caution must be exercised in interpreting serologic data. Reactivation may occur with or without changes in antibody titer. Cytomegalovirus IgM may persist for months after primary infection in transplant patients. *In any patient with a puzzling illness, a sterile specimen of serum should be preserved in a frozen state so that it can, if necessary, be studied and compared with serum collected at a later date.*

Prior contact with an antigen may be the result of past immunization with vaccines; interpretation of serum agglutinin titers for typhoid bacilli is often made difficult by prior immunization. The so-called anamnestic reaction, a nonspecific stimulation of antibody formation by an acute illness (e.g., a rise in *Brucella* agglutinins in a patient with acute tularemia), occurs only when the two organisms are antigenically related, and rarely presents a serious problem.

Some mention of "nonspecific" serologic changes may serve to emphasize again that clinical laboratory tests have come into use *only because they have been found to correlate reasonably well with clinical findings.* In several diseases it has been found, often accidentally, that serum antibody develops which will react with antigens derived from sources other than the etiologic agent (which may actually be unknown). Common examples are heterophil agglutinins in infectious mononucleosis, cold agglutinins in mycoplasma pneumonia, and the agglutination of certain strains of *Proteus* bacilli by serum of patients with rickettsial diseases. The VDRL test for syphilis and related flocculation tests are performed with antigens derived from sources completely unrelated to *Treponema pallidum.*

The results of serologic tests must be interpreted in the light of other information about the patient, including such factors as previous immunizations and illnesses, the possibility of exposure to chemically but etiologically unrelated antigens, and the importance of a changing titer in serial tests as opposed to a single isolated observation.

VIROLOGIC SPECIMENS

The selection of specimens for the diagnosis of viral illness depends on both the stage of the disease and its clinical presentation. If the patient is seen early in the course of illness, frequently it is possible to demonstrate viral antigen in body tissue or fluids and/or to recover the virus by appropriate culture techniques. If the patient is seen later, during the recovery or convalescent stages, the diagnosis is often best established by serologic means. The type of specimen submitted for culture and the method of specimen transport depend to some extent on the nature of the illness. Throat swabs are helpful in the diagnosis of most viral infections. Because respiratory viruses are extremely labile, the swabs are placed in a buffered, high-protein transport medium containing antibiotic agents. If the specimen is to be transported to another institution, the specimen should be transported on ice (4°C). If delays of more than 24 h are anticipated, specimens should be stored at −60°C and shipped on dry ice.

Cerebrospinal fluid from patients presenting with meningitis or encephalitis can also be submitted for culture. As with throat swabs, these specimens should be stored at low temperatures and shipped on dry ice. Stool should be collected in patients with respiratory illnesses, meningitis, or encephalitis, if either adenoviruses or enteroviruses are thought to be involved. Although these organisms are hardy, the feces should be collected in any sterile screw-top bottle and dispatched promptly to avoid bacterial overgrowth. Urine cultures are helpful in the diagnosis of congenital cytomegalovirus and rubella infections and in the late diagnosis of mumps. Vesicular fluid is a rich source of virus and viral antigen in patients presenting with exanthems. Pericardial fluid may be of help in patients with myocarditis or pericarditis. Viral blood cultures are seldom useful except in the diagnosis of arboviral infections. Isolation techniques for these viruses are highly specialized and are not available in most virus laboratories. Buffy coat cultures for cytomegalovirus and herpesvirus are often helpful in AIDS, transplant, and other immunosuppressed patients. Brain biopsy is the best single method for diagnosing herpes simplex encephalitis (see Chap. 135). The biopsy specimen should be placed in viral transport and dispatched, at 4°C, as quickly as possible.

REFERENCES

CENTOR RM et al: Throat cultures and rapid tests for diagnosis of Group A streptococcal pharyngitis. Ann Intern Med 105:892, 1986

EISENBERG HD et al: Collection, handling and processing of specimens, in *Manual of Clinical Microbiology,* 4th ed, EH Lennette et al (eds). Washington, DC, American Society for Microbiology, 1985

MINNICH LL et al: Cumitech 24, Rapid detection of viruses by immunofluorescence, S Specter (coordinating ed). Washington, DC, American Society for Microbiology, 1988

PEZZLO M: Detection of urinary tract infections by rapid methods. Clin Microbiol Rev 1:268, 1988

SIMOR AE et al: Cumitech 23, Infections of the skin and subcutaneous tissues, JS Smith (coordinating ed). Washington, DC, American Society for Microbiology, 1988

WASHINGTON JA II: Bacterial, fungi and parasites, the clinician and microbiology laboratory, in *Principles and Practice of Infectious Diseases,* 3d ed, GL Mandell et al (eds). New York, Wiley, 1990

81 DISORDERS OF PHAGOCYTIC CELLS

JOHN I. GALLIN

Leukocytes are the major cellular components of inflammatory and immune responses and include neutrophils, lymphocytes, monocytes, eosinophils, and basophils. The blood is the most readily obtainable source of leukocytes and serves as the vehicle for their delivery to the various tissues from the bone marrow, where they are produced. Normal blood leukocyte counts for adults are given in Chap. 64 and those for different ages in the Appendix. The various leukocytes are thought to derive from a common stem cell in the bone marrow. Three-fourths of the nucleated cells of bone marrow are committed to the production of leukocytes. Leukocyte maturation in the marrow is generally thought to be under the regulatory control of a number of different factors, which are incompletely defined (see Chap. 64). Because an alteration in the number and type of leukocytes is a frequent association with disease processes, a total white blood count (WBC) (cells per microliter) and differential counts are obtained frequently. The lymphocytes and basophils are discussed elsewhere. This chapter focuses on the neutrophils, monocytes, and eosinophils.

NEUTROPHILS

MATURATION Important events in the neutrophil life are summarized in Fig. 81-1. In normal humans neutrophils are only produced in the bone marrow. Best estimates indicate that the appropriate number of stem cells necessary to support hematopoiesis is between 400 and 500. There is convincing evidence that human blood monocytes and tissue macrophages produce colony stimulating factors, hormone(s) required for the growth of monocytes and neutrophils in the bone marrow. The hematopoietic system not only produces enough neutrophils (approximately 1.3×10^{11} cells per 80-kg person per day) to carry out physiologic functions but also has a large reserve stored in the marrow which can be mobilized in response to inflammation or infection. An increase in the number of blood neutrophils is called *neutrophilia*, and the presence of immature cells is termed a "shift to the left." A diminution in the number of blood neutrophils is referred to as *neutropenia* (see Chap. 64).

Neutrophils evolve from pluripotent stem cells. The final stages of hematopoiesis are characterized by the appearance of cells with distinct morphologic features. The myeloblast is the first recognizable precursor cell and is followed by the *promyelocyte* (see Fig. A5-15). The promyelocyte evolves when the classic lysosomal granules, called the *primary* or *azurophil granules*, are produced. The primary granules contain hydrolases, elastase, myeloperoxidase, and cationic proteins. The promyelocyte divides to produce the *myelocyte*, a cell responsible for the synthesis of the *specific* or *secondary granules* which contain unique (specific) constituents such as lactoferrin, vitamin B_{12}–binding proteins, and probably cytochrome b, histaminase, and receptors for certain chemoattractants and adherence promoting factors. The secondary granules do not contain acid hydrolases and therefore are not classic lysosomes. They are readily released extracellularly, and their mobilization is probably important in modulating inflammation. During the final stages of maturation there is no cell division and the cell passes through the *metamyelocyte* stage and then to the *band* neutrophil with a sausage-shaped nucleus. As the band cell matures, the nucleus assumes a lobulated configuration.

In settings of severe acute bacterial infection, prominent neutrophil cytoplasmic granules called *toxic granulations* are occasionally seen. Toxic granulations are thought to be immature or abnormally staining azurophil granules. Cytoplasmic inclusions, also called *Doehle bodies*, (see Fig. A5-17) can also be seen during infection and probably represent fragments of endoplasmic reticulum. Large neutrophil vacuoles are often present in acute bacterial infection and probably represent pinocytosed (internalized) membrane.

Neutrophils have long been thought to be a homogeneous population of cells. However, studies of neutrophil function have suggested they are heterogeneous. Recently monoclonal antibodies have been developed that recognize only a subset of mature neutrophils. The meaning of neutrophil heterogeneity is not known.

MARROW RELEASE AND CIRCULATING COMPARTMENTS Specific signals, including interleukin 1, tumor necrosis factor-α, the colony stimulating factors (see Chap. 64), or the complement fragment C3e, mobilize leukocytes from the bone marrow and deliver them to the blood in an unstimulated state. Under normal conditions about 90 percent of the neutrophil pool is in the bone marrow, 2 to 3 percent in the circulation, and the remainder in the tissues. The blood pool exists as two compartments: the marginated pool adherent to endothelial cells and the freely flowing circulating pool. In response to chemotactic stimuli from tissues (e.g., the complement product C5a, the arachidonic acid derivative leukotriene B_4, or the bacterial product *N*-formylmethionylleucylphenylalanine), neutrophil adhesiveness increases and the circulating cells aggregate to each other and adhere to the endothelium. An increased expression of a glycoprotein receptor for C3bi (also called CR3) appears to be intimately involved with the increased adhesion. Receptors for chemoattractants and opsonins are probably also mobilized; the cells orient toward the chemoattractant source in the extravascular space, increase their motile activity (chemokinesis), and migrate with direction (chemotaxis) into tissues. The process of migration into tissues is called *diapedesis* and involves the crawling of neutrophils between postcapillary endothelial cells which open junctions between adjacent cells to permit leukocyte passage. The endothelial responses (increased blood flow secondary to increased vasodilation and permeability) are mediated by anaphylatoxins (e.g., complement products

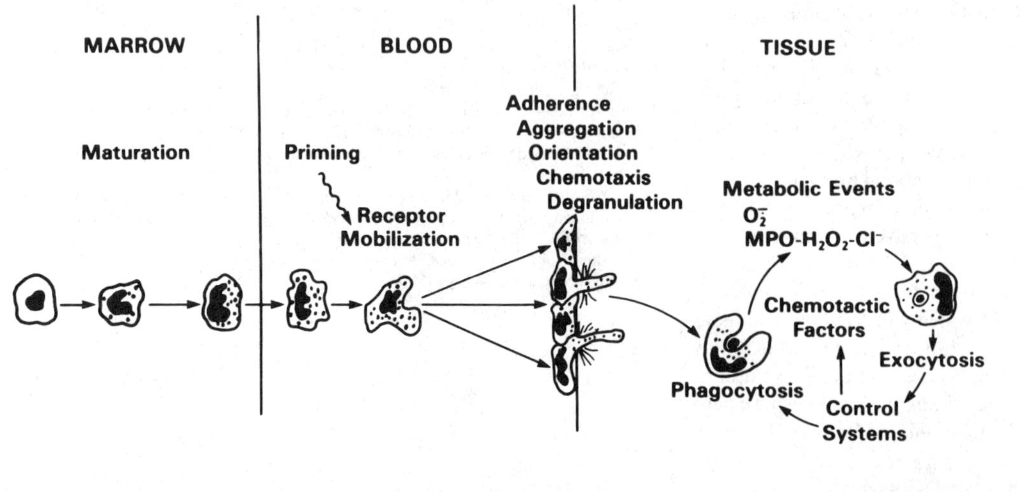

FIGURE 81-1 Schematic diagram of the life cycle of the neutrophil. MPO, myeloperoxidase.

C3a and C5a) as well as vasodilators such as bradykinin and prostaglandins E and I. In the healthy adult most neutrophils leave the body by migration through the mucous membrane of the gastrointestinal tract. Normally neutrophils spend a relatively short time in the circulation with a half-life of 6 to 7 h. Once in the tissues neutrophils release enzymes such as collagenase and elastase, which may help establish abscess cavities. Neutrophils ingest (phagocytose) pathogenic materials that have been properly altered (opsonized) by substances such as immunoglobulin G (IgG) and the complement product C3b. Fibronectin and the tetrapeptide tuftsin facilitate the phagocytic process.

Concomitant with phagocytosis there is a burst of oxygen consumption and activation of the hexose-monophosphate shunt. Nicotinamide-adenine dinucleotide phosphate (NADPH) oxidase is activated, and through a complex enzyme system consisting of membrane and cytosolic components, toxic oxygen products (e.g., hydrogen peroxide and hydroxyl radical) are generated. Hydrogen peroxide + chloride + neutrophil myeloperoxidase provide a particularly toxic system that generates hypochlorous acid, hypochlorite, and chlorine. These products oxidize and halogenate microorganisms and tumor cells and when uncontrolled, can damage host tissue. Strongly cationic proteins and small peptides known as "defensins" also participate in microbial killing. Other enzymes, such as lysozyme and acid proteases, help digest microbial debris. After 1 to 4 days in tissues neutrophils die. Under certain conditions, such as following delayed-type hypersensitivity immunity, a second wave of inflammation, associated with monocyte accumulation, occurs within 6 to 12 h of initiation of inflammation. Neutrophils, monocytes, microorganisms in various states of digestion, and altered local tissue cells make up pus, which derives its characteristic green color from myeloperoxidase. Myeloperoxidase and other factors may be important in turning off the inflammatory process by inactivating chemoattractants and immobilizing phagocytic cells.

NEUTROPHIL DYSFUNCTION A defect anywhere in the neutrophil life cycle summarized in Fig. 81-1 can lead to dysfunction and compromised host defenses. Inflammation is often depressed and the clinical result is often recurrent and severe bacterial and fungal infections creating novel and often difficult management problems. Diagnosis of phagocytic cell disorders is suggested by clinical evaluation. Neutropenia or impaired neutrophil function are frequently associated with depressed inflammation. Aphthous ulcers of mucous membranes (gray ulcers without pus) are common. Gingivitis and periodontal disease are common. Characteristically, patients with phagocyte defects have recurrent and often severe bacterial or fungal infections which often present as difficult management problems. Patients with congenital phagocyte defects can have infections within the first few days of life. Skin, ear, upper and lower respiratory tract, and bone infections are common. Sepsis and meningitis are rare. In some disorders the frequency of infection is variable, and patients can go for months or even years without major infection. Adults over 30 years of age with congenital defects are unusual, suggesting that patients with such defects die at an early age. However, with aggressive management, adults with these diseases are being seen with increasing frequency.

Neutropenia The consequences of absent neutrophils represent a dramatic demonstration of their importance in host defense. When the neutrophil count is below 1000 per microliter, there is an increased risk for infection (Chap. 82); when there are fewer than 200 cells per microliter, the inflammatory process is absent. The causes of neutropenia are multiple and are related to depressed production, peripheral destruction, and peripheral pooling. They are discussed in Chap. 64.

Neutrophilia Neutrophilia results from increased neutrophil production, marrow release, or defective margination. These are discussed in Chap. 64.

ABNORMAL NEUTROPHIL FUNCTION Congenital deficiencies and acquired abnormalities of phagocyte function are described in Table 81-1. The resulting diseases are best considered in terms of the functional defects of adherence, chemotaxis, and microbicidal activity. The distinguishing features of the important congenital lesions are shown in Table 81-2, several of which are discussed below.

Patients with congenitally (autosomal recessive) abnormal phagocyte adherence, *C3bi (CR3) deficiency,* lack the plasma membrane receptor for the fragment of the third complement component called C3bi (CR3 by other terminology). Patients with this syndrome have recurrent bacterial and fungal infections, severe periodontal disease, persistent leukocytosis (15,000 to 20,000 neutrophils per microliter), and usually a history of delayed separation of the umbilical stump. Neutrophils (and monocytes) from these patients have defective adherence, spreading, aggregation, and chemotaxis.

Abnormal neutrophil and monocyte chemotaxis occurs in the *hyperimmunoglobulin E–recurrent infection (Job's) syndrome.* For many years the cold abscesses were thought to be a reflection of impaired chemotaxis with too few phagocytes arriving too late, perhaps secondary to a lymphocyte factor inhibiting chemotaxis. However, it is now clear that the chemotactic defect in these patients is variable and the fundamental basis for the impaired defenses is complex and inadequately delineated.

The most common neutrophil defect is *myeloperoxidase deficiency*, which is inherited as an autosomal recessive trait and may have an incidence as high as about 1 in 2000 persons. Isolated myeloperoxidase

TABLE 81-1 Types of neutrophil dysfunction

Function	Drug-induced	Acquired disease	Congenital disorder
Adherence-aggregation	Aspirin; colchicine; alcohol; glucocorticoids; ibuprofen; piroxicam	Neonates, hemodialysis	C3bi (CR3) receptor deficiency
Deformability		Leukemia, neonates, diabetes mellitus, immature neutrophils	
Chemokinesis-chemotaxis	Glucocorticoids (high-dose); auranofin; colchicine (weak effect); phenylbutazone, naproxen; indomethacin	Thermal injury; malignancy; malnutrition; periodontal disease; neonates; systemic lupus erythematosus; rheumatoid arthritis; diabetes mellitus; sepsis; influenza virus infection; herpes simplex virus infection; acrodermatitis enteropathica; Down's syndrome; α-mannosidase deficiency; severe combined immunodeficiency; Wiskott-Aldrich syndrome	Hyper IgE–recurrent infection (Job's) syndrome; Chédiak-Higashi syndrome; specific granule deficiency
Microbicidal activity	Colchicine; cyclophosphamide; glucocorticoids (high-dose)	Leukemia; aplastic anemia; certain neutropenias; tuftsin deficiency; thermal injury; sepsis; neonates; diabetes mellitus; malnutrition	Chédiak-Higashi syndrome; specific granule deficiency; chronic granulomatous disease

TABLE 81-2 Distinguishing features of congenital phagocyte dysfunction syndromes

Disease/inheritance*	Defect	Clinical manifestations
C3bi (CR3) receptor deficiency/AR	Adherence, aggregation, spreading, chemotaxis, leukemoid reaction	Delayed separation of umbilical stump, depressed inflammation, bacterial infections, gingivitis, periodontal disease
Hyperimmunoglobulin E–recurrent infection (Job's) syndrome/Non X-linked	Variable chemotactic defects, very high IgE with anti-*S. aureus* IgE; low anti-*S. aureus* IgA	"Coarse" facies in most patients, "cold" cutaneous abscesses; recurrent pulmonary, bone, upper airway infections with *S. aureus* or *Haemophilus influenzae;* mild eosinophilia; mucocutaneous candidiasis
Myeloperoxidase deficiency/AR	Absent myeloperoxidase	Minimal unless another defect present, then *Candida albicans* or other fungal infections
Chédiak-Higashi syndrome/AR	Giant lysosomal granules; neutropenia, chemotaxis, degranulation, microbicidal activity, excess O_2 consumption and H_2O_2 production	Recurrent pyogenic infections, especially with *S. aureus;* many patients get lymphomatous-like illness during adolescence; periodontal disease; partial oculocutaneous albinism, nystagmus, progressive peripheral neuropathy
Specific granule deficiency/AR (?)	Absent specific granules; chemotaxis, O_2^- production, bactericidal activity decreased	Recurrent cutaneous, ear, and pulmonary bacterial infections; diminished inflammation
Chronic granulomatous disease/X, AR, AD (rare)	H_2O_2 production absent in neutrophils and monocytes; defective "turn-off" of inflammation	Severe infections of skin, ears, lungs, liver, bone with catalase-positive microorganisms such as *S. aureus, Pseudomonas cepacia, Aspergillus* sp., *Chromobacterium violaceum;* often hard to culture organism; excessive inflammation with granulomas; frequent lymph node suppuration; granulomas can obstruct gastrointestinal or genitourinary tracts; gingivitis, aphthous ulcers

* X = x-linked; AR = autosomal recessive; AD = autosomal dominant.

deficiency is not associated with severely compromised defenses, because other defense systems such as hydrogen peroxide generation are accelerated. However, if another underlying defect in host defense, such as poorly controlled diabetes mellitus, accompanies myeloperoxidase deficiency, then host defenses are likely to be significantly compromised. An acquired form of myeloperoxidase deficiency occurs in myelomonocytic leukemia and acute myeloblastic leukemia (also referred to as myelogenous leukemia).

Chédiak-Higashi syndrome (CHS) is a rare disease with autosomal recessive inheritance. Neutrophils and all cells containing lysosomes from patients with CHS characteristically have large granules (see Fig. A5-19). CHS neutrophils and monocytes have impaired chemotaxis and abnormal rates of microbial killing due to slow rates of fusion of the lysosomal granules with phagosomes.

Chronic granulomatous disease (CGD) represents a group of patients with disorders of neutrophil and monocyte oxidative metabolism. Although CGD is rare, occurring in about 1 in 1 million individuals, it is an important model of defective neutrophil oxidative metabolism. Most often CGD is inherited as an X-linked recessive pattern, although in 35 percent of patients the disease is inherited with an autosomal recessive pattern and an autosomal dominant pattern has been reported in one family. Leukocytes from patients with CGD have severely diminished hydrogen peroxide production. Defects anywhere in the leukocyte's hexose-monophosphate shunt or the NADPH oxidase enzyme system can lead to clinical disease, and specific defects of cell membrane and cytosolic components have been identified. The genes involved in several of the defects have been cloned. Patients with CGD characteristically have increased infection with catalase-positive microorganisms (organisms which destroy their own hydrogen peroxide). When patients with CGD become infected, they often have extensive inflammatory reactions, and lymph node suppuration is common despite the administration of appropriate antibiotics. Aphthous ulcers and chronic inflammation of the nares are usually present. Granulomas are frequent and can obstruct the gastrointestinal or genitourinary tracts. The excessive inflammatory reactions probably reflect abnormal turnoff of inflammation by failure to degrade chemoattractants and antigens which cause persistent neutrophil accumulation. Impaired killing of intracellular microorganisms by macrophages may lead to persistent cell-mediated immunity and granuloma formation.

MONONUCLEAR PHAGOCYTES

The mononuclear phagocyte system is defined as a continuum linking monoblasts, promonocytes, and monocytes with the structurally diverse tissue macrophages which make up what was previously referred to as the reticuloendothelial system. Macrophages are long-lived phagocytic cells capable of many of the functions of neutrophils. In addition, they are important secretory cells that, through their receptors and secretory products, participate in many complex immunologic and inflammatory processes not attributed to neutrophils. Monocytes leave the circulation by diapedesis more slowly than neutrophils and have a half-life in the blood of 12 to 24 h.

After blood monocytes arrive in the tissues, they differentiate into macrophages ("big eaters") with specialized functions suited for specific anatomic locations. Macrophages are particularly abundant in capillary walls of the lung, spleen, liver, and bone marrow, where they function to remove microorganisms and other noxious elements from the blood. Alveolar macrophages, liver Kupffer cells, splenic macrophages, peritoneal macrophages, bone marrow macrophages, lymphatic macrophages, brain microglial cells, and dendritic macrophages all have specialized functions. Macrophage secreted products include lysozyme, neutral proteases, acid hydrolases, arginase, numerous complement components, enzyme inhibitors (plasmin, α_2-macroglobulin), binding proteins (transferrin, fibronectin, transcobalamin II), nucleosides, cachectin, and interleukin 1 (pyrogen). Interleukin 1 (see Chaps. 13 and 20) has many important functions, including stimulating the hypothalamus to initiate fever, mobilizing leukocytes from the bone marrow, as well as activating lymphocytes and neutrophils. Cachectin (also called tumor necrosis factor) is a pyrogen that duplicates many of the actions of interleukin 1 and plays an important role in the pathogenesis of gram-negative shock (see Chap. 89). It can stimulate vigorous production of hydrogen peroxide and related toxic oxygen species by macrophages and neutrophils. In addition, cachectin induces catabolic responses of chronic inflammation which contribute to the profound wasting (cachexia) associated with many chronic diseases.

Other macrophage secreted products include reactive oxygen metabolites, bioactive lipids (arachidonate metabolites and platelet activating factors), a neutrophil chemoattractant, factors regulating synthesis of proteins by other cells, bone marrow colony stimulating factors, factors stimulating fibroblast and microvasculature proliferation, as well as factors inhibiting replication of lymphocytes, tumors, viruses, and certain bacteria (*Listeria monocytogenes*). Macrophages are key effector cells in the elimination of intracellular microorganisms. Their ability to fuse to form giant cells which coalesce into granulomas in response to some inflammatory stimuli is important in the elimination of intracellular microbes and may be under the control of γ-interferon.

Macrophages play an important role in the immune response (see Chap. 13). They process antigen for presentation to lymphocytes, their secreted products modulate lymphocyte function, and macrophages participate in autoimmune phenomena by removing immune complexes and other immunologically active substances from the circulation. Furthermore, they play a role in wound healing, in the disposal of senescent cells, and in the development of atheromas.

DISORDERS OF THE MONONUCLEAR PHAGOCYTE SYSTEM Many disorders of neutrophils extend to mononuclear phagocytes. Thus, drugs which suppress neutrophil production in the bone marrow usually lead to monocytopenia. Transient monocytopenia can also be seen after stress or glucocorticoid administration. Monocytosis is associated with certain infections such as tuberculosis, brucellosis, subacute bacterial endocarditis, Rocky Mountain spotted fever, and malaria. Monocytosis is also seen in kala azar, malignancies, leukemias, myeloproliferative syndromes, hemolytic anemias, chronic idiopathic neutropenias, granulomatous diseases such as sarcoidosis, regional enteritis, and some collagen vascular diseases. Patients with neutrophil C3bi receptor deficiency, the hyperimmunoglobulin E–recurrent infection (Job's) syndrome, Chédiak-Higashi syndrome, and chronic granulomatous diseases all have defects in the mononuclear phagocyte system.

Certain viral infections impair mononuclear phagocyte function. For example, influenza virus infection is associated with abnormal monocyte chemotaxis. Mononuclear phagocytes can be infected by the human immunodeficiency virus (HIV), and abnormal monocyte chemotaxis and abnormal clearance of IgG-coated erythrocytes (discussed below) by macrophages is also seen in the acquired immunodeficiency syndrome (AIDS) (see Chap. 264). It is likely that these defects of the monocyte-macrophage system in AIDS contribute to the disordered immunoregulation and increased susceptibility to opportunistic infection due to intracellular microorganisms such as *Pneumocystis carinii* and *Mycobacterium avium-intracellulare*. T lymphocytes produce γ-interferon, which induces Fc-receptor expression and phagocytosis as well as stimulates hydrogen peroxide production by mononuclear phagocytes. In certain diseases, such as AIDS, γ-interferon production may be deficient, while in other diseases, such as T-cell lymphomas, excessive release of γ-interferon is thought to cause erythrophagocytosis by splenic macrophages.

Specific defects of the mononuclear phagocytes have been described in certain autoimmune diseases. Removal of IgG-coated radiolabeled autologous erythrocytes, presumably via the Fc receptor of splenic macrophages, is profoundly abnormal in patients with active systemic lupus erythematosus. Patients with other autoimmune diseases characterized by tissue deposition of immune complexes, as seen in Sjögren's syndrome, mixed cryoglobulinemia, dermatitis herpetiformis, and chronic progressive multiple sclerosis, also have defects in Fc-receptor function as judged by clearance of IgG-coated erythrocytes (see Chap. 268). Clinically, normal subjects with genetic haplotypes commonly associated with autoimmune disease (i.e., HLA-B8/DRw3) also have an increased incidence of defective Fc receptor–specific functional activity, suggesting that this defect may predispose individuals with this genetic profile to immune-complex disease.

EOSINOPHILS

Eosinophils and neutrophils share similar morphology, many lysosomal constituents, most chemotactic responses, phagocytic capacity, and oxidative metabolism. However, there are major differences between the two cell types, and little is known about the natural function of eosinophils. Eosinophils are much longer lived than neutrophils, and unlike neutrophils, tissue eosinophils can recirculate. During most infections eosinophils do not appear to have any important function. However, in invasive parasite infections, such as hookworm, schistosomiasis, strongyloidiasis, toxocariasis, trichinosis, filariasis, echinococcosis, and cysticercosis, the eosinophil likely plays a central role in host defense. Eosinophils are also associated with bronchial asthma, cutaneous allergic reactions, and other hypersensitivity states.

The characteristic red-staining eosinophil granules (Wright's stain) contain a number of unique constituents. The distinctive feature of the eosinophil granule is its crystalline core consisting of an arginine-rich protein (major basic protein) with histaminase activity, which is probably important in host defense against parasites. Eosinophil granules also contain a unique eosinophil peroxidase which catalyzes the oxidation of many substances by hydrogen peroxide and may facilitate killing of microorganisms.

Eosinophil peroxidase, in the presence of hydrogen peroxide and halide, initiates mast cell secretion in vitro and thereby may contribute to inflammation. Other substances found in eosinophils include cationic proteins, some of which bind to heparin and reduce its anticoagulant activity. Eosinophil cytoplasm contains Charcot-Leyden crystal protein, a hexagonal bipyramidal crystal first described in leukemia and then in sputum from asthma patients, which is lysophospholipase and may function to restrict the toxicity of certain lysophospholipids. Eosinophils also contain a powerful neurotoxin. Because patients with hypereosinophilic syndrome and cerebral spinal fluid eosinophilia exhibit varied neurologic abnormalities, eosinophil-derived neurotoxin may play an important role in central nervous system disease.

Several factors enhance the eosinophil's function in host defense. For example, T-cell-derived eosinophil stimulation promoter enhances the ability of eosinophils to kill parasites. Mast cell–derived eosinophil chemotactic factor of anaphylaxis (ECFa) increases the number of eosinophil complement receptors and enhances eosinophil killing of parasites. In addition, eosinophil colony stimulating factors produced by macrophages may not only increase eosinophil production in the bone marrow but may also activate eosinophils to kill parasites.

EOSINOPHILIA The presence of more than 500 eosinophils per microliter of blood is common in many settings besides parasite infection (see Chap. 64). The most common cause of eosinophilia is probably allergic reactions to drugs such as iodides, aspirin, and sulfonamides. Allergies such as hay fever, asthma, and eczema commonly are associated with eosinophilia. Eosinophilia is also seen in collagen vascular diseases (e.g., rheumatoid arthritis, eosinophilic fasciitis, allergic angiitis, and granulomatosis) and malignancies (e.g., Hodgkin's disease, mycosis fungoides) as well as the hyperimmunoglobulin E–recurrent infection (Job's) syndrome and the chronic granulomatous diseases; the mechanisms for the eosinophilia in these diseases are not known. The most dramatic increases in eosinophils occur in hypereosinophilic syndromes, including Loeffler's syndrome, eosinophilic leukemia, and idiopathic hypereosinophilic syndrome (with counts as high as 50,000 to 100,000 eosinophils per microliter).

The idiopathic hypereosinophilic syndrome represents a heterogeneous group of disorders with the common feature of prolonged eosinophilia of unknown cause and associated organ system dysfunction, including the heart, central nervous system, kidneys, lungs, gastrointestinal tract, and skin. The bone marrow is involved in all subjects, but the most severe complications involve the heart and central nervous system. Eosinophils are found in the involved tissues and are thought to cause tissue damage by local deposition of toxic eosinophil proteins such as eosinophil cationic protein and eosinophil major basic protein. In the heart the pathologic changes lead to thrombosis which may result in endocardial fibrosis and restrictive endomyocardiopathy. Similar pathologic changes are thought to contribute to the damage of tissues in other organ systems. Although the mechanism for the hypereosinophilia is not known, it has been shown that chemotherapy with glucocorticoids usually induces remission. In patients unresponsive to glucocorticoids, a cytotoxic agent such as hydroxyurea has been used successfully to lower the peripheral blood eosinophil counts and to improve markedly the prognosis. Aggressive medical and surgical approaches are also employed when managing patients with cardiovascular complications.

EOSINOPENIA This occurs with stress, such as acute bacterial infection, and following administration of glucocorticoids. The mechanism of eosinopenia of acute bacterial infection is unknown but is independent of endogenous glucocorticoids since it occurs in animals following total adrenalectomy. There is no known adverse effect of eosinopenia.

LABORATORY DIAGNOSIS AND MANAGEMENT OF PHAGOCYTE DYSFUNCTION

Initial studies of white blood count and differential and often a bone marrow examination are followed by assessment of bone marrow reserves (steroid challenge test), marginated circulating pool of cells (epinephrine challenge test), and marginating ability (endotoxin challenge test). In vivo assessment of inflammation is possible with a Rebuck skin window test, in which the ability of leukocytes to accumulate at a superficial abrasion and adhere to a glass coverslip is tested. In vivo clearance of IgG-coated erythrocytes provides a useful way to monitor the mononuclear-phagocytic (reticuloendothelial) system. In vitro tests of phagocyte aggregation, adherence, chemotaxis, phagocytosis, degranulation, and microbicidal activity (for *Staphylococcus aureus*) help pinpoint cellular or humoral lesions which can then be further characterized at the molecular level. Deficiencies of oxidative metabolism are screened with the nitroblue tetrazolium dye (NBT) test, which is based on the ability of products of oxidative metabolism to reduce yellow, soluble NBT to blue-black formazan, an insoluble material which precipitates intracellularly and can be seen microscopically. Further aspects of neutrophil oxidative metabolism are defined by studies of superoxide and hydrogen peroxide production.

The most important aspect of patient management is to appreciate that patients often have delayed inflammatory responses. Therefore, clinical manifestations may be minimal despite overwhelming infection, and unusual infections must always be suspected in some patients. Early signs of infection demand prompt, aggressive use of antibiotics and surgical drainage of abscesses. Prolonged antibiotics are often required, and in life-threatening infections daily white blood cell transfusions (enriched for neutrophils) are probably beneficial, although their use is still controversial. In patients with the chronic granulomatous diseases, prophylactic antibiotics (trimethoprim-sulfamethoxazole) probably diminish the frequency of life-threatening infections. Surgery is required for thorough drainage of abscesses in lung, liver, and bones. Short courses of glucocorticoids have been of benefit in the management of the granulomas of CGD. Recent studies indicate that γ-interferon may correct the biochemical and functional defects in certain patients with CGD. Rigorous oral hygiene reduces but does not eliminate the discomfort of gingivitis, periodontal disease, and aphthous ulcers; tooth brushing with a hydrogen peroxide–sodium bicarbonate paste helps some patients. Ketoconazole has caused dramatic improvement of mucocutaneous candidiasis in patients with the hyperimmunoglobulin E–recurrent infection (Job's) syndrome. Treatment to restore myelopoiesis in patients with neutropenia due to impaired production has included use of androgens, glucocorticoids, lithium, and immunosuppressive therapy. Studies with granulocyte and macrophage colony stimulating factors suggest these agents will be useful in the management of certain forms of neutropenia. Cure of some congenital phagocyte defects is theoretically possible by bone marrow transplantation (see Chap. 299). However, complications of bone marrow transplantation are still great, and with rigorous medical care many patients with phagocytic disorders can go for years without a life-threatening infection. The identification of specific gene defects in certain patients with phagocyte abnormalities makes gene therapy an exciting future possibility.

REFERENCES

ANDERSON DC, SPRINGER TA: Leukocyte adhesion deficiency: An inherited defect in the Mac-1, LFA-1, and p150,95 glycoproteins. Ann Rev Med 38:175, 1987

CLARK RA et al: Genetic variants of chronic granulomatous disease: Prevalence of deficiencies of two discrete cytosolic components of the NADPH oxidase system. N Engl J Med 321:647, 1989

CURNUTTE JT (ed): Phagocyte defects: Abnormalities outside of the respiratory burst. Hematol Clin North Am 2:1988

DONABEDIAN H, BALLIN JI: The hyperimmunoglobulin E–recurrent infection (Job's) syndrome. A review of the NIH experience and the literature. Medicine 62:185, 1983

GALLIN JI: Phagocytic cells: Disorders of function, in: *Inflammation: Basic Principles and Clinical Correlates*, JI Gallin et al (eds). New York, Raven Press, 1988, pp 493–511

———: Neutrophil specific granule deficiency. Ann Rev Med 36:263, 1985

GLEICH GJ, LOEGEUNG DA: Immunobiology of eosinophils. Ann Rev Immunol 2:429, 1984

JOHNSTON RB: Monocytes and macrophages. N Engl J Med 318:747, 1988

LEUNG DYM, GEHA R: Clinical and immunologic aspects of the hyperimmunoglobulin E syndrome. Hematol Oncol Clin North Am 2:81, 1988

LOMAX KJ et al: Recombinant 47-kD cytosol factor restores NADPH oxidase in chronic granulomatous disease. Science 245:409, 1989

——— et al: The molecular biology of selected phagocyte defects. Blood Rev 3:94, 1989

MALECH HL, GALLIN JI: Neutrophils in human disease. N Engl J Med 317:687, 1987

NUNOI H et al: Two forms of autosomal chronic granulomatous disease lack distinct neutrophil cytosol factors. Science 242:1298, 1988

SAMTER M (ed): *Immunological Diseases*, 4th ed. Boston, Little, Brown, 1988

SECHLER JMG et al: Recombinant human interferon-γ reconstitutes defective phagocyte function in patients with chronic granulomatous disease of childhood. Proc Natl Acad Sci USA 85:4874, 1988

SHERRY B, CERAMI A: Cachectin/tumor necrosis factor exerts endocrine, paracrine, and autocrine control of inflammatory responses. J Cell Biol 107:1269, 1988

82 INFECTIONS IN THE COMPROMISED HOST

HENRY MASUR / ANTHONY S. FAUCI

DEFINITION Patients who lack resistance to infection because of a deficiency in any of their multifaceted host defenses are referred to as "compromised hosts." Other terms such as "abnormal host," "immunosuppressed host," or "immunocompromised patient" are often used, but they have different connotations. The latter two refer specifically to a subpopulation of compromised hosts whose major deficiency in antimicrobial activity is related to their defective immune response.

Deficient host defense can be caused by many different factors including inherited disorders, coexisting disease, trauma, alcoholism, malnutrition, or drug therapies. The drugs that most often cause deficient host defense are cytotoxic agents and glucocorticoids, which are administered to treat malignant neoplasms, collagen vascular disorders, and organ transplants. An expanding spectrum of diseases can now be controlled or cured by complex and aggressive surgery, implantation of foreign bodies, or powerful cytotoxic or anti-inflammatory drugs. As noninfectious complications such as hemorrhage or uremia or graft rejection are being managed with increasing success, infection is becoming the major threat to the quality and duration of survival in many different patient populations.

HOST DEFENSE MECHANISMS

Antimicrobial defense mechanisms (Table 82-1) consist of complex, interacting systems that protect the host from endogenous and exogenous microbes (Chap. 78). The degree to which a patient becomes abnormally susceptible to infection by this microbial envi-

TABLE 82-1 Mechanisms of host defense

Physical and chemical barriers
- Morphologic integrity of skin, mucous membranes
- Sphincters
- Epiglottis
- Normal secretory and excretory flow
- Endogenous microbial flora
- Gastric acidity

Inflammatory response
- Circulating phagocytes
- Complement
- Other humoral mediators (bradykinins, fibrinolytic systems, arachidonic acid cascade)

Reticuloendothelial system
- Tissue phagocytes

Immune response
- T lymphocytes and their soluble products
- B lymphocytes and immunoglobulins

ronment depends on the mechanism compromised, the severity of the derangements, and their interactions. For instance, as isolated abnormalities, total absence of serum IgA or complement component C9 would probably have minor, if any, impact on host susceptibility to infection. In contrast, isolated abnormalities such as total absence of circulating neutrophils, serum IgG, or complement component C3 would lead to recurrent and life-threatening infections. Similarly, partial deficiencies in host defense mechanisms can have variable impact on susceptibility to infection depending on the specific mechanism, the degree of deficiency, and the presence of concomitant abnormalities. A modest decrease in circulating neutrophil count to 25 percent of the lower limit of normal or a decrease in serum IgG concentration to 50 percent of the lower limit of normal are usually tolerated with little or no difficulty if either is an isolated and transient abnormality. If such a neutrophil count were present concurrently with a major defect in the skin or mucous membranes for a prolonged period of time, complicating infection is more likely to occur.

Recognition of which specific and nonspecific host defenses are compromised is important in order to develop effective clinical strategies for predicting the probable onset of infection and the most likely causative organisms; for formulating the appropriate diagnostic approach; and for developing the optimal therapeutic and preventive plan. However, based on an understanding of the mechanisms of host defenses, such an approach must be supplemented by clinical experience with specific patient populations. Because there are complexities of various host defense mechanisms that are not fully understood, it cannot be assumed that all patient populations with the same measured deficiency in antimicrobial defense (as assessed by current laboratory techniques) will behave identically. For example, patients with cytomegalovirus infection (Chap. 138) have immunologic profiles that are similar in certain respects to those of patients in the early phases of the acquired immunodeficiency syndrome (AIDS) (Chap. 264). However, the susceptibility of these two populations to life-threatening opportunistic infection is vastly different, with AIDS patients being far more susceptible.

PHYSICAL AND CHEMICAL BARRIERS Physical and chemical barriers (Table 82-1) are part of a complex and interacting system of nonspecific host defense mechanisms that are essential for preventing the introduction and spread of microbial pathogens. These barriers utilize a wide variety of properties to protect the host, including the morphologic and functional integrity of skin or mucous membranes, the epiglottis, or sphincters; chemical processes (e.g., gastric acidity, pancreatic enzymes, cutaneous fatty acids or lysozyme); physical removal of organisms (e.g., peristalsis, sloughing of squamous cells, urine flow); and competition from less virulent flora. Interference with any of these mechanisms can increase the host's susceptibility to infection.

INFLAMMATORY RESPONSES Circulating phagocytes (neutrophils, monocytes, eosinophils, and basophils) arise from the bone marrow and upon appropriate signals enter the peripheral circulation and are distributed to local tissues, where they form the cornerstone of the inflammatory response. Recruitment of phagocytes from the bloodstream is a complicated process which involves the phagocytes' aggregation, adherence to the vascular endothelium, passage through endothelial spaces, and migration to local tissue sites (Chap. 81). An effective inflammatory response depends on the ability of the phagocyte to adhere, deform, have random locomotion, and respond to a chemical signal with directed movement. Humoral mediators influence local structures in ways that affect the phagocyte's ability to reach various loci: an example is the influence the complement cascade (especially C3a and C5a) has on the potential spaces between endothelial cells. Humoral mediators including the complement system, the arachidonic acid cascade, kinin-generating systems, and cellular products such as interleukin 1 and tumor necrosis factor, microbial peptides, or endotoxins also promote directed locomotion of the phagocytes. Once the phagocyte arrives at a focus of infection, it can adhere to the microorganism, ingest it, and digest it, particularly if the organism has been opsonized by antibodies or complement products. A wide variety of bacteria as well as fungi are killed by neutrophils in this manner.

RETICULOENDOTHELIAL SYSTEM Circulating microorganisms are cleared from the bloodstream by tissue phagocytes that are derived from circulating monocytes. These phagocytes include macrophages in the liver (Kupffer cells), spleen, lymph nodes, lung (alveolar macrophages), kidney (mesangial cells), and brain (microglial cells). The antimicrobial activities of these monocytes and macrophages are strongly influenced by opsonins such as IgG or C3b, which enhance the rate of particle ingestion, and by a large variety of soluble mediators produced primarily by mononuclear leukocytes (see Chap. 81). The efficacy of the reticuloendothelial system is also influenced by characteristics of specific organisms which allow the microbes to resist phagocytosis, lysosome-phagosome fusion (toxoplasma), or intraphagosomal inactivation (leishmania).

Immune response The major cellular components of the immune response are T lymphocytes and B lymphocytes (Chap. 13). These cells are distributed throughout the body in the bloodstream and at tissue sites. They interact in a highly complex fashion among themselves and with monocytes, macrophages, immunoglobulins, and the complement cascade. T lymphocytes are major components of the cell-mediated immune system. They secrete a multitude of cytokines which influence the functional status of other T lymphocytes, B lymphocytes, monocytes, and macrophages to eradicate infection, and participate directly in cytotoxic reactions against tumor cells, HLA-incompatible cells, and certain virus-infected host cells. B lymphocytes and plasma cells secrete specific antibodies which have important roles in eradicating certain infections. The ability of the monocytes and macrophages to ingest and kill a wide variety of bacteria, fungi, and protozoa is augmented by lymphokines released by T lymphocytes, in particular, γ-interferon. Production of opsonizing, neutralizing, or microbicidal antibodies can also be profoundly influenced by the regulatory effect of T lymphocytes on B lymphocytes (Chap. 13).

ETIOLOGY AND PATHOGENESIS OF INFECTION

In compromised hosts the development of infections reflects the interaction of impaired immunologic and nonimmunologic host defense mechanisms with the host's endogenous and exogenous microbial environment. Factors which change the microbial flora have an important impact on the organisms that are likely to cause disease. Such factors include antimicrobial therapy, invasive procedures or trauma, ingestion or inhalation of infected material, and hospitalization itself. The type of infections which develop are usually the consequence of specific alterations in host defenses, however. Numerous processes can predispose to serious infection by compromising the anatomic and physical barriers of host defense. For example, the skin and mucous membranes can be breached by tumor invasion, tumor necrosis, or vascular insufficiency induced by arteritis or atherosclerosis; by injury such as burns, pressure, or trauma; by radiation or cytotoxic chemotherapy; by a drug-induced cutaneous slough; and by procedures such as venipuncture or surgery. The respiratory tract can become the site of infection when its anatomic barriers are disrupted: the epiglottis may fail to protect the lower tract when the patient's consciousness is impaired or during intubation or bronchoscopy. The patient's ability to expel organisms may be adversely affected by infection, tumor, or drugs that alter the state of consciousness or prevent coughing; by disruption of mucociliary transport by a congenital disorder of ciliary subunits (such as Kartagener's syndrome) or by smoke or other inhaled toxins, anesthetic agents, or cytotoxic therapy; or by airway obstruction as a result of tumor, a foreign body, or lymph node enlargement. The gastrointestinal tract can become a less effective barrier against entry of organisms if gastric acidity is abolished by a surgical procedure or antacid therapy (infections with *Salmonella* and other gram-negative rods are a particular consequence); or if its mucosa is eroded by tumor or cytotoxic therapy, especially in neutropenic patients. Obstruction of the intestinal or biliary tract by tumor, a stricture, or a stone allows endogenous or introduced flora to gain access to the involved tissues and often the bloodstream. The genitourinary tract can become a portal of entry for infections if its mucosa is eroded by tumor, irradiation, or cytotoxic therapy or there is urinary obstruction. Renal failure associated with oliguria or anuria deprives the genitourinary system of the ability to flush out microorganisms and obviates the antimicrobial effects of urine itself. The insertion of foreign bodies into the urethra during catheterization or cystoscopy allows exogenous organisms to be introduced into the urinary tract. Any locus in the body can become the site of infection if devitalized tissue or foreign bodies are seeded by bacteria or become infected by direct penetration. Hematomas, necrotic tissue, infarcts, calcified heart valves, and prosthetic devices (joints, heart valves, or central nervous system appliances) are particularly prone to bacterial infection.

Defects in inflammatory and immune function may permit infections that would normally be promptly eradicated to progress and cause clinically important disease. These quantitative or qualitative defects may be due to a congenital disorder, an underlying acquired disease, or drug therapy. Several specific types of defects are associated with particularly frequent or severe infectious complications.

LEUKOCYTE DISORDERS The clinical consequences of leukocyte disorders depend on which subpopulations of leukocytes are numerically or functionally affected and the duration of the dysfunction (Table 82-2) (Chap. 81). Neutropenia (less than 1800 neutrophils per

TABLE 82-2 Infections associated with common defects in inflammatory or immunologic response

Host defect	Examples of diseases or therapies associated with defects	Common etiologic agents of infections
INFLAMMATORY RESPONSE		
Neutropenia	Hematologic malignancies, cytotoxic chemotherapy, aplastic anemia	Gram-negative bacilli, *Staphylococcus aureus, Candida* species, *Aspergillus* species
Chemotaxis	Chédiak-Higashi syndrome	*Staphylococcus aureus, Streptococcus pyogenes*
	Job's syndrome Protein-calorie malnutrition	*Staphylococcus aureus, Haemophilus influenzae,* gram-negative bacilli
Phagocytosis (cellular)	Systemic lupus erythematosus, chronic myelogenous leukemia, megaloblastic anemia	*Streptococcus pneumoniae, Haemophilus influenzae*
Splenectomy		*Haemophilus influenzae, Streptococcus pneumoniae,* other streptococci, DF-2, *Babesia microti*
Microbicidal defect	Chronic granulomatous disease	Catalase-positive bacteria and fungi: Staphylococci, *Escherichia coli, Klebsiella* species, *Pseudomonas aeruginosa, Candida* species, *Aspergillus* species, *Nocardia* species
	Chédiak-Higashi syndrome	*Staphylococcus aureus, Streptococcus pyogenes*
COMPLEMENT SYSTEM		
C3	Congenital liver disease	*Staphylococcus aureus, Streptococcus pneumoniae*
	Systemic lupus erythematosus	*Pseudomonas* species, *Proteus* species
C5	Congenital	*Neisseria* species, Gram-negative rods
C6, C7, C8	Congenital, systemic lupus erythematosus	*Neisseria meningitidis, Neisseria gonorrhoeae*
Alternate pathway	Sickle cell disease	*Streptococcus pneumoniae, Salmonella* species
IMMUNE RESPONSE		
T-lymphocyte deficiency/dysfunction	Thymic aplasia, thymic hypoplasia, Hodgkin's disease, sarcoid, lepromatous leprosy	*Listeria monocytogenes, Mycobacterium* species, *Candida* species, *Aspergillus* species, *Cryptococcus neoformans, Herpes simplex, Herpes zoster*
	Acquired immunodeficiency syndrome	*Pneumocystis carinii,* cytomegalovirus, *Herpes simplex, Mycobacterium avium-intracellulare, Cryptococcus neoformans, Candida* species
	Mucocutaneous candidiasis	*Candida* species
	Purine nucleoside phosphorylase deficiency	Fungi, viruses
B-cell deficiency/dysfunction	Bruton's X-linked agammaglobulinemia, agammaglobulinemia, chronic lymphocytic leukemia, multiple myeloma, dysglobulinemia	*Streptococcus pneumoniae,* other streptococci, *Haemophilus influenzae, Neisseria meningitidis, Staphylococcus aureus, Klebsiella pneumoniae, Escherichia coli, Giardia lamblia* *Pneumocystis carinii,* enteroviruses
	Selective IgM deficiency	*Streptococcus pneumoniae, Haemophilus influenzae, Escherichia coli*
	Selective IgA deficiency	*Giardia lamblia,* Viral hepatitis, *Streptococcus pneumoniae, Haemophilus influenzae*
Mixed T- and B-cell deficiency/dysfunction	Common variable hypogammaglobulinemia	*Pneumocystis carinii,* cytomegalovirus, *Streptococcus pneumoniae, Haemophilus influenzae,* various other bacteria
	Ataxia-telangiectasia	*Streptococcus pneumoniae, Haemophilus influenzae, Staphylococcus aureus,* rubella, *Giardia lamblia*
	Severe combined immunodeficiency	*Candida albicans, Pneumocystis carinii,* varicella, rubella, cytomegalovirus
	Wiskott-Aldrich	Infections seen in T- and B-cell abnormalities

microliter) is the most commonly encountered defect in inflammatory host defense mechanisms (Chap. 64). When the neutrophil count falls below 1000 cells per microliter, there is a progressive increase in susceptibility to bacterial and fungal infections and a progressive decrease in the localizing signs and symptoms of inflammation. Susceptibility to infection increases dramatically when the peripheral neutrophil count falls below 500 cells per microliter, particularly when the count falls below 100 cells per microliter. The rate of decline and the duration of neutropenia are also important parameters which influence the development of infection. Neutropenia can occur because of bone marrow failure, peripheral destruction, or pooling or sequestration of cells. The most common causes of neutropenia are cytotoxic chemotherapy, neoplastic invasion of the bone marrow, aplastic anemia, and idiosyncratic drug reactions.

Neutrophil dysfunction can also result in a substantial predisposition to serious infection. Dysfunction may be a manifestation of a congenital disorder such as chronic granulomatous disease or Chédiak-Higashi syndrome (Chap. 81). Glucocorticoids and some multiple drug chemotherapeutic regimens may alter both the number and the function of circulating neutrophils.

Lymphopenia in adults is defined as less than 1000 lymphocytes per microliter. The clinical consequences of lymphopenia depend on which subset(s) is affected. Regardless of the total lymphocyte count, severe infections may occur if profound deficiencies of either B lymphocytes or T lymphocytes are present. Substantial reductions in helper T lymphocytes (<200 per microliter) have particularly important infectious consequences. The most common causes of lymphopenia are hematologic malignancies, glucocorticoid therapy, antilymphocyte globulins, cytotoxic drugs, and infection with certain viruses such as cytomegalovirus (Chap. 138) and HIV (Chap. 264). Congenital lymphopenias can also have severe consequences (Chap. 263).

Lymphocyte dysfunction can predispose to life-threatening infection even if the lymphocyte number is normal. Lymphocyte dysfunction is most often a consequence of therapy with glucocorticoids or cytotoxic drugs.

IMMUNOGLOBULIN DISORDERS Decreased production of functional immunoglobulins, particularly IgG, can cause a marked increase in susceptibility to microbial disease (Chap. 263). Patients with significant reductions in IgG (usually less than 200 to 300 mg/dL) characteristically have recurrent infections due to encapsulated bacteria, particularly *Streptococcus pneumoniae, Haemophilus influenzae,* and *Neisseria meningitidis,* and to certain protozoa (*Pneumocystis carinii* and *Giardia lamblia*). Selective IgA deficiency can lead to respiratory or systemic bacterial infections (particularly when accompanied by IgG_2 deficiency) as well as intestinal giardiasis or severe viral hepatitis. The few documented cases of selective IgM deficiency have also been associated with severe infections, in particular, with gram-negative organisms such as *Neisseria meningitidis*. Clinically important causes of immunoglobulin deficiency or dysfunction include congenital and acquired disorders, such as malignancies (multiple myeloma, chronic lymphocytic leukemia), sickle cell disease, and splenectomy (Table 82-2) (Chap. 263).

COMPLEMENT DISORDERS The consequences of total absence of functional complement proteins depend on which of the specific components are deficient (Table 82-2) (Chap. 13). Deficiencies of C1 or C3 have been associated with pneumococcal infections while deficiencies of C5, C6, C7, or C8 may lead to relapsing *Neisseria meningitidis* or *Neisseria gonorrhoeae* infections. Most severe deficiencies are due to inherited disorders, although there are reports of significant deficiencies in patients with systemic lupus erythematosus, cirrhosis, or splenectomy.

SPLENECTOMY The spleen contains large numbers of B lymphocytes, monocytes, and macrophages and is a major site for T cell–independent immune responses such as the production of antibodies to polysaccharide antigens. The spleen has an important role in the phagocytosis of circulating opsonized organisms. Following splenectomy young children are at high risk for fulminant infections due to *Streptococcus pneumoniae*, *Haemophilus influenzae*, *Neisseria meningitidis,* and the fastidious gram-negative bacterium DF-2. Adults who undergo splenectomy are also at increased risk for these infections, especially during the first 3 years after surgery. Splenectomized patients may develop fulminant infection with intraerythrocytic protozoa such as *Plasmodium malariae* and *Babesia*.

DIAGNOSIS

Clinicians managing compromised patients must recognize that the diagnosis of infectious processes requires special attention, persistence, and expertise. Compromised patients often present initially with manifestations that may be subtle or atypical. All infections can become life-threatening in extremely short time periods in many of these patients, so that the diagnostic evaluation needs to begin promptly when the first signs or symptoms or laboratory abnormalities become apparent. These evaluations should proceed in rapid sequence using tests that have the shortest feasible processing times. A thorough approach is necessary to make certain that the true etiologic agent is being treated and to minimize the likelihood that unnecessary drugs with unneeded toxicities will be employed. The spectrum of potential etiologic agents is usually wide, so that the diagnostic tests must often be broad-gauged as well. Based on knowledge of the factors that render the patient compromised, the organisms associated with particular defects in host defense, and the patient's individual history and presentation, the clinician in concert with the laboratory must consider whether special testing should be done for unusual bacteria, fungi, viruses, helminths, protozoa, or other microorganisms. It is usually desirable to have a standard protocol for evaluating common clinical syndromes (e.g., pneumonia, fevers, meningitis) in compromised patients, with modifications being made in the protocol as warranted by the individual patient's circumstances. For instance, when an HIV-infected patient has a helper-T-lymphocyte (T4-positive or CD4-positive) count below 200 to 300 per microliter, and especially when the count falls below 100 per microliter, mild cough with fever must be evaluated promptly and aggressively since pneumocystis or cytomegalovirus pneumonia are much more likely than in HIV-positive patients with normal T4 counts. Kidney transplant recipients are known to be at very high risk for bacterial wound and urinary tract infections during the first postoperative month, while opportunistic viral, fungal, and protozoan diseases are more common during the second through sixth months. The development of fever during the first postoperative month should prompt an evaluation that focuses initially on the wound and urinary tract, while similar symptoms occurring several months after surgery should direct studies for protozoan, fungal, or viral infections.

Patients with leukemias and lymphomas need particular scrutiny for complicating bacterial or fungal infections when their neutrophil counts fall below 100 cells per microliter (a time that is usually predictable from the pharmacokinetics of the chemotherapeutic regimen).

THERAPY

In compromised patients the therapy of infectious complications should include drainage of localized collections of infected material, specific antimicrobials, and, if possible, reconstitution of deficient antimicrobial defenses. Examples include the infusion of fresh frozen plasma to augment complement components, the administration of immune serum globulin to restore IgG levels, and the tapering of immunosuppressive drugs (such as glucocorticoids or cytotoxic agents) to restore cell-mediated immune mechanisms or neutrophil production. In certain neutropenic patients augmentation or restoration of neutrophils can be achieved temporarily by the use of colony stimulating factors (see Chap. 64) or white blood cell transfusions, or permanently by bone marrow transplantation. Patients must be carefully selected for which of these procedures is likely to be effective.

Empiric antimicrobial therapy is clearly appropriate for some patient populations. For example, newly developing fever in severely neutropenic patients is frequently due to infection with bacteria, and therapy using a broad-spectrum regimen directed against potential major gram-positive and gram-negative pathogens before culture results are available can be lifesaving. The use of antibiotic combinations that are synergistic against infecting bacteria has been more successful in reducing morbidity and mortality from bacterial infection in neutropenic patients than single agents or nonsynergistic combinations. Examples of such combinations are vancomycin, ticarcillin, and amikacin or ceftazidime and amikacin (for dosages see Chap. 85). Empiric use of amphotericin B in the febrile neutropenic patient unresponsive after several days of antibacterial treatment is a common practice and may reduce mortality from fungal superinfection.

PREVENTION OF INFECTION

In compromised patients certain types of infections can be prevented by avoiding damage to physical barriers, bolstering host defenses, reducing acquisition of new potential pathogens, and suppressing colonizing flora. The use of invasive procedures including repeated venipuncture, indwelling peripheral venous catheters, and urinary catheterization should be minimized or avoided completely. Surgical procedures should be chosen only when absolutely essential and performed with meticulous care. Bolstering host defenses can be accomplished directly in some patient groups. For example, immune serum globulin can be given prophylactically to hypogammaglobulinemic patients (see Chap. 263); hyperimmune varicella-zoster immunoglobulin can prevent or reduce the severity of varicella-zoster virus disease after acute exposure; immunization with vaccines against pneumococci, *Haemophilus,* and meningococci may be helpful for patients with conditions of particular susceptibility such as following splenectomy (see Chap. 81).

Maintaining an optimal nutritional status will improve cellular immune mechanisms and aid wound repair. Most other methods to enhance depressed cell-mediated immunity have been clinically ineffective. Colony stimulating factors offer promise in restoring neutrophil numbers and preventing infection in neutropenic subjects but requires further investigation (see Chap. 64). Reducing the acquisition of potential pathogens can be facilitated by simple techniques such as having hospital personnel wash their hands before patient contact and by appropriate isolation from specific potentially contagious organisms such as *Herpes zoster, Mycobacterium tuberculosis,* or multiply antibiotic-resistant gram-negative bacilli (see Chap. 83). More stringent measures such as laminar flow isolation or control of sterility of food and water have not proved to be useful or cost-effective for ultimate survival, although these measures will decrease the rate of infection for patients with prolonged and profound granulocytopenia. Suppression of endogenous bacteria or fungi is an important concept, since they cause more than 80 percent of infections in neutropenic cancer patients. Gut sterilization or prophylactic systemic antibiotics have proved useful as temporary measures in neutropenic patients but cannot be practically sustained for more than a few weeks. Prolonged antimicrobial prophylaxis of certain specific infections that have exceedingly high attack rates in certain defined populations can be quite effective. The impressive protection provided by trimethoprim-sulfamethoxazole or aerosolized pentamidine against *Pneumocystis carinii* pneumonia in patients with AIDS or acute lymphocytic leukemia is a striking example.

REFERENCES

THE EORTC INTERNATIONAL ANTIMICROBIAL THERAPY COOPERATIVE GROUP: Ceftazidime combined with a short or long course of amikacin for empirical therapy of gram-negative bacteremia in cancer patients with granulocytopenia. N Engl J Med 317:1692, 1987

GALLIN JI, FAUCI AS: *Advances in Host Defense Mechanisms,* vol 2, *Lymphoid Cells.* New York, Raven Press, 1983

HUGHES WT et al: Successful chemoprophylaxis for *Pneumocystis carinii* pneumonitis. N Engl J Med 297:1419, 1977

MASUR H et al: CD4 counts as predictors of pneumonias in human immunodeficiency virus infected individuals. Ann Intern Med 111:223, 1989

NOSSAL GJV: Current concepts: Immunology: The basic components of the immune system. N Engl J Med 316:1320, 1987

PIZZO PA, MEYERS J: Infections in the cancer patient, in *Cancer Medicine: Principles and Practice of Oncology,* V DeVita et al (eds). Philadelphia, Lippincott, 1989

——— et al: Fever in the pediatric and young adult patient with cancer: A prospective study of 1001 episodes. Medicine 61:153, 1982

ROSEN FS et al: The primary immunodeficiencies. N Engl J Med 311Z:235, 1984

ROSS SC, DENSEN P: Complement deficiency states and infection. Epidemiology, pathogenesis, and consequences of neisserial and other infections in an immune deficiency. Medicine 63:243, 1984

RUBIN RH, YOUNG LS: *The Clinical Approach to Infection in the Immunocompromised Host,* 2d ed. New York, Plenum, 1988

SANDE MA, VOLBERDING PA: *The Medical Management of AIDS.* Philadelphia, Saunders, 1988

SHENEP JL et al: Vancomycin, ticarcillin, and amikacin compared with ticarcillin-clavulanate and amikacin in the empirical treatment of febrile, neutropenic children with cancer. N Engl J Med 319:1053, 1988

83 HOSPITAL-ACQUIRED INFECTIONS

PIERCE GARDNER / JOSEPH J. KLIMEK

DEFINITIONS Hospital-acquired infections (also called nosocomial infections) are defined as infections occurring in patients after admission to the hospital that were neither present nor incubating at the time of admission. Infections acquired in the hospital but not manifest until after the patient is discharged are also included in this definition. Although many of these infections can be prevented, some cannot, and the term *hospital-acquired infection* should not be equated with *iatrogenic infection,* which indicates an infection caused by a diagnostic or therapeutic intervention such as the insertion of a urethral or intravenous catheter. *Opportunistic infections* occur in patients with impaired host defenses and are commonly caused by infectious agents that do not ordinarily produce disease in healthy individuals. Many opportunistic infections are caused by organisms in the patient's own flora (*autochthonous infections*) and are often unavoidable because they are related to defects in mucosal barriers or other host defenses rather than preventable environmental risks.

ETIOLOGY AND EPIDEMIOLOGY **Incidence and cost** Hospital-acquired infections occur in from 2 to 10 percent (average, 5 percent) of patients admitted to general hospitals. The highest infection rates are reported from municipal hospitals and tertiary-care centers, while the prevalence of these infections is much lower in community hospitals. These differences in rates appear to be due to the greater severity of underlying disease in patients in municipal and tertiary-care hospitals and may also reflect greater utilization of invasive procedures and diagnostic tests in the management of these patients. On the average, hospital-acquired infections have a mortality rate of 1 percent and contribute to the death of at least an additional 3 percent. Therefore the estimated 2 million hospital-acquired infections which occur annually in the United States result in approximately 20,000 deaths and contribute to the mortality of an additional 60,000 patients. Nosocomial infections add over 7.5 million hospital days and over 1 billion dollars to national health care costs.

Causative pathogens Gram-negative bacilli lead the list of nosocomial pathogens. Their statistical importance is due in large part to their role in urinary tract infections, but gram-negative bacilli also are important pathogens at other sites. Many of these organisms, especially pseudomonads and *Klebsiella,* require minimal nutrients and are able to establish reservoirs in the inanimate hospital environment, as well as in patients. In large part, antimicrobial resistance among gram-negative bacilli is due to the acquisition of plasmids called *resistance factors* (R factors). R-factor plasmids consist of extrachromosomal circular DNA, which mediates antibiotic resistance by coding for enzymes that inactivate the drug or by modifying systems involved in antibiotic uptake. Several properties of plasmids are of major public health concern: (1) Resistance to several antibiotics is often linked on the same R factor; (2) R-factor transfer can occur across species and even genera of gram-negative bacilli; (3) small gene fragments encoding for a single antibiotic-inactivating enzyme have been incorporated into diverse plasmids which are spread among many genera of gram-negative bacilli. Certain gram-negative bacilli (most often *Enterobacter, Pseudomonas,* and *Serratia*) have developed an additional chromosomal mechanism of resistance to penicillin and cephalosporin drugs, i.e., the induction of β-lactamase enzymes. Because production of these enzymes is enhanced by exposure to β-lactam antibiotics (especially the newer cephalosporins), widespread use of these antibiotics in hospitals exerts selective pressure for the emergence of these difficult-to-treat gram-negative bacilli.

Among gram-positive cocci, *Staphylococcus aureus,* the scourge of the 1950s and early 1960s, remains the most important pathogen. During the past decade an alarming increase in methicillin-resistant *S. aureus* (MRSA) has been noted, especially in debilitated immunocompromised patients in intensive care units (see Chap. 101). These strains are generally resistant to all β-lactam agents and often to erythromycin, clindamycin, and the aminoglycosides as well. For serious infections caused by these strains, vancomycin is the drug of choice. Other antimicrobials with activity against MRSA include rifampin, ciprofloxacin, and trimethoprim-sulfamethoxazole (see Chap. 85). Bacterial tolerance (organisms are inhibited but not killed by bactericidal drugs) is common among currently isolated strains of *S. aureus* and may dictate the use of bactericidal antibiotic combinations in serious infections, such as endocarditis (see Chap. 90). The enterococcus (group D streptococcus), long recognized as an important pathogen in nosocomial urinary tract infections, is emerging as a significant wound pathogen particularly in patients who have received broad-spectrum cephalosporins (to which enterococci are uniformly resistant).

The spectrum of microorganisms recognized to be important nosocomial pathogens has expanded considerably. Opportunistic infections caused by low-virulence bacteria (*Staphylococcus epidermidis,* JK diphtheroid) and fungi (*Aspergillus, Candida,* and agents causing mucormycosis) have become commonplace. Respiratory viruses, especially respiratory syncytial virus and influenza, have gained increased recognition as causes of significant morbidity when acquired during hospitalization. Other viruses transmissible in blood (hepatitis viruses, human immunodeficiency virus, cytomegalovirus) are of concern to hospital personnel as well as patients.

Transmission of nosocomial pathogens Contact with hospital personnel remains the principal means of transmission of nosocomial pathogens and hand-washing by hospital personnel remains the principal control measure. Other less important modes of transmission include the airborne route, by which infections such as chickenpox and tuberculosis are spread, and contact with environmental sources. The inanimate hospital environment usually is not the source of infecting pathogens. However, environmental reservoirs have proved to be of primary importance in clusters of cases of aspergillosis caused by inhalation of spores from dust or fireproofing material, and in epidemics of Legionnaires' disease.

Host factors The age and underlying disease of patients, the integrity of their mucosal and integumentary surfaces, and the status of their immunologic defenses are among the major determinants of both the incidence and outcome of hospital-acquired infections (see Chap. 82).

COMMON HOSPITAL-ACQUIRED INFECTIONS **Urinary tract infections** Approximately 40 percent of hospital-acquired infections occur in the urinary tract and are usually a consequence of instrumentation of the urethra, bladder, or kidneys. The most common predisposing factor is the insertion of an indwelling urethral catheter which bypasses the normal anatomic barriers to ascending infection. Hospital surveys show that 10 to 15 percent of all adult patients have indwelling urinary catheters, many of which are unnecessary. Because the urinary tract is the most common site of infection resulting in gram-negative bacteremia, steps to prevent catheter-related infections merit special emphasis and include the following:

1 Restrict the use of indwelling catheters except when required for management of bladder outlet obstruction or for close monitoring of urine output.
2 Rigorously adhere to sterile technique during insertion of the catheter.
3 Maintain a system of closed drainage. Good technique can usually keep the urine sterile for 5 to 7 days.
4 Keep the collecting tubing and bag unobstructed and in a dependent position.
5 When urine specimens are required, aspirate the specimen from the sampling port in the collecting tubing by use of a sterile needle and syringe rather than by breaking the closed drainage system.
6 Consider intermittent straight catheterization for patients with anticipated short-term needs for bladder drainage.

Wound infections Most surgical wound infections are caused by organisms introduced directly into the tissues at the time of operative procedures. Most infecting organisms originate from the resident flora of the patient, although personnel in the operating theater may occasionally be the source of infection, especially with group A streptococci or *S. aureus.* The major factors affecting the incidence of wound infection include the type of operation, its duration, the skill of the surgeon, and the basic health of the patient. Operations involving contaminated sites, such as the bowel or vagina, are more likely to be complicated by infection than operations on sites which are sterile prior to surgery. Operations of long duration, or ones in which devitalized tissue, foreign bodies, or hematomas are left behind, are associated with increased rates of wound infection. Adverse host factors include advanced age, poor nutritional status, the presence of distant foci of infection, diabetes mellitus, renal failure, and glucocorticoid therapy.

Most wound infections become apparent from 3 to 7 days following surgery. Early postoperative wound infections (those occurring within 24 to 48 h of surgery) are commonly caused by group A *Streptococcus* or *Clostridium* spp. Staphylococcal wound infections characteristically become evident 4 to 6 days after surgery, and those caused by gram-negative bacilli and anaerobic bacteria may not appear for a week or more. If perioperative antibiotics are used, the manifestations of infection may be delayed. Gram-stained smears of wound exudate, together with culture, often provide valuable early clues to the bacterial cause of wound infections.

In addition to emphasis on maintaining sterility in the operating room and insistence on operative techniques that minimize tissue trauma and blood loss, short prophylactic courses of antibiotics during the perioperative period may be beneficial in certain operations (see Chap. 85). The principles that should govern the use of antibiotics in this situation include (1) beginning the drug during the immediate preoperative period but not earlier, (2) ensuring adequate tissue levels throughout the surgery, giving intraoperative doses of antibiotics if necessary, and (3) discontinuing antibiotic prophylaxis within 24 to 48 h following surgery. These brief courses of antibiotics do not appear to alter the patient's flora or promote colonization with resistant strains. Prolonged pre- and postoperative courses are unnecessary, expensive, and potentially harmful because of the increased risk of drug toxicity and superinfection. Antibiotic prophylaxis administered according to these principles has reduced infectious morbidity in a wide variety of operative procedures that are traditionally associated with major risk of infection including colon surgery and vaginal hysterectomy.

Nonsurgical wounds that are common sites of nosocomial infection include burns, decubitus ulcers, and cutaneous ulcers resulting from venous or arterial occlusive disease. In general, the offending pathogens are similar to those found in surgical wound infections, except that burn wound infections are frequently caused by *Pseudo-*

monas aeruginosa, and ulcers of the pelvis and lower extremities usually contain fecal flora.

Pneumonia Lower respiratory tract infections are the leading cause of mortality among hospital-acquired infections, although they rank third in incidence behind urinary tract infections and wound infections. The major pathogens are the gram-negative bacilli and *S. aureus,* all of which characteristically cause a necrotizing bronchopneumonia. These organisms usually reach the lower respiratory tract by aspiration from the pharynx rather than by hematogenous spread. This is consistent with the observation that the pharyngeal flora of seriously ill patients contains an increased number of gram-negative bacilli. The three settings in which nosocomial pneumonias occur most commonly are in (1) obtunded patients whose gag reflex and cough are ineffective, (2) patients with underlying pulmonary disease or congestive heart failure whose pulmonary clearance mechanisms are impaired, and (3) patients who require respiratory tract instrumentation or ventilatory assistance.

Because antibiotic treatment of nosocomial pneumonia is often ineffective, preventive measures assume special importance. Positioning the patient in a swimmer's or Gatch position is the cornerstone for preventing aspiration in obtunded patients. Treatment of congestive heart failure will improve the effectiveness of the lung's defenses and will reduce lung edema fluid that serves as an excellent culture medium. Emphasis should be placed on sterile technique when performing tracheal toilet, and the breathing circuits on ventilatory assistance equipment must be properly maintained. Nosocomial spread of the tubercle bacillus is uncommon; however, recognition of active cases of pulmonary tuberculosis and prompt institution of respiratory isolation and appropriate chemotherapy are the principal means by which in-hospital spread of the disease can be limited.

Hospital transmission of viral respiratory pathogens is common, but except for influenza and respiratory syncytial virus, rarely results in severe disease. Epidemiologic studies indicate that direct and indirect contact spread of viruses on the hands of personnel is a more important route of transmission than airborne spread. When influenza A is widespread in the community, amantadine prophylaxis should be considered for unimmunized hospital patients identified as being at high risk for complications of influenza. Increasing the immunization levels among hospital personnel is likely to reduce nosocomial transmission of influenza viruses.

Bacteremia Although invasion of the bloodstream can occur in any nosocomial infection, the infected vascular cannula is the most common and also most preventable cause of hospital-acquired primary bacteremia and fungemia. Annually in the United States more than 10 million persons (more than one in four hospitalized patients) receive intravenous therapy, and therefore even a low rate of infection assumes major clinical significance. Infections related to intravenous therapy account for about 5 percent of all nosocomial infections and 10 percent of all positive blood cultures. The most common causative organisms are *S. epidermidis, S. aureus,* gram-negative bacilli, and enterococci; when hyperalimentation fluid is administered through the catheter, *Candida* also is an important pathogen. Although microorganisms can enter a fluid delivery system at any point, contamination most commonly occurs at the site of entry into the skin during cannula insertion or subsequent manipulation and may be followed by migration of organisms along the cannula into the bloodstream. Occasionally hematogenous seeding of the cannula may occur. Intravenous fluids may become contaminated as a result of adding medications, or, rarely, in the process of manufacture. A clue to the possible presence of infusate contamination is unexpected bacteremia caused by one of the few pathogens (*Enterobacter, Klebsiella, Serratia, Pseudomonas cepacia,* or *Citrobacter freundii*) capable of sustained growth in intravenous solutions containing 5% dextrose.

The type of cannula, the choice of insertion site, the adequacy of skin preparation, and the duration of cannula use influence the risk of cannula-related sepsis. Suppurative phlebitis, one of the most feared complications of cannula-related infections, is virtually unknown with steel needles. Arms are better insertion sites than legs owing to lower rates of phlebitis and sepsis. When cannula infection is suspected, semiquantitative microbiologic evaluation of the removed cannula tip by culture or by direct examination of a Gram-stained catheter segment is useful in identifying patients with heavily colonized cannulas who are at high risk of developing bacteremia or fungemia. With meticulous care, central venous catheters used for parenteral hyperalimentation can be maintained free of infection for prolonged periods. However, infectious complications, particularly *Candida* sepsis, are not uncommon in this setting. Intravascular catheters used for pressure monitoring pose many of the same risks as those used for infusion therapy; in addition, the presence of an indwelling pulmonary artery catheter during a period of bacteremia may increase the risk of developing endocarditis.

Transient bacteremia following diagnostic or therapeutic manipulations of the mouth or respiratory, gastrointestinal, or genitourinary tract are usually well-tolerated by the normal host. However, the patient with valvular or congenital heart disease or a prosthetic valve may be at risk of developing endocarditis during such episodes and should receive antibiotic prophylaxis when undergoing procedures associated with significant risk of bacteremia. These procedures include dental manipulations, urinary tract instrumentation, abdominal surgery, and other surgery involving infected tissue. For patients with prosthetic heart valves, these recommendations have been extended. Detailed programs of prophylaxis are given in the chapter on infectious endocarditis (see Chap. 90).

NOSOCOMIAL PATHOGENS OF SPECIAL INTEREST Human immunodeficiency virus (HIV) Nosocomial transmission of HIV has been a major problem for patients with hemophilia and others who have received HIV-infected blood products, but has been reassuringly rare in other health care settings. The incidence of *acquired immunodeficiency syndrome* (AIDS) among health care workers does not exceed the rate in the general public, and the risk of HIV transmission following a needle-stick accident from an infected patient is less than 1 percent. Nevertheless, the recognition of a large reservoir of infected asymptomatic people and the potential risk to health care workers exposed to blood and certain other body fluids (cerebrospinal fluid, pleural fluids, peritoneal fluid, pericardial fluid, and amniotic fluid) has led the Centers for Disease Control to recommend blood and body fluid precautions in the handling of all such specimens. These "universal precautions" might also be expected to reduce health worker risks of nosocomial hepatitis B virus and other bloodborne viruses. Universal precautions represent a significant departure from traditional disease-focused infection control methods. The impact of this approach on HIV and HBV transmission to health care workers and the effects on rates of bacterial nosocomial infections have not been determined (see Chap. 264).

Hepatitis B virus (HBV) The risk of hospital-acquired HBV is significant not only for patients but also for hospital personnel who work with infected patients or handle their blood specimens. Patients at special risk of HBV infection include those who receive blood products or undergo hemodialysis. Screening of blood products for hepatitis B surface antigen (HBsAg) has markedly reduced the incidence of posttransfusion HBV and most posttransfusion hepatitis is now caused by other hepatitis viruses (non-A, non-B hepatitis). However, transmission of HBV remains an endemic problem on many hemodialysis units and oncology services.

Measures to prevent nosocomial HBV infection of health care workers should include: (1) HBV immunization for all hospital personnel whose work places them at risk; (2) meticulous attention to precautions to limit spread of pathogens by needle accidents or body fluid contact (see "Universal Precautions" in Chap. 264); and (3) prompt passive-active immunization with hepatitis B immune globulin and HBV vaccine for susceptible personnel who have been subjected to a specific hepatitis risk (i.e., needle stick from an infectious patient) (see Chap. 252).

Legionnaires' disease Nosocomial Legionnaires' disease usually affects immunocompromised patients. Although contamination of hospital cooling tower water accounts for some cases, sustained epidemic or hyperendemic problems have almost always been traced to heavy contamination of hot tap water by *Legionella* species. Infectious aerosols of tap water can be produced by showers and during operation of some humidifiers and respiratory devices filled with tap water. A causative role of contaminated hospital tap water has been substantiated by the efficacy of hyperchlorination or superheating of hospital tap water in curtailing epidemics.

***Clostridium difficile* colitis** Bacterial superinfection with *C. difficile* is a consequence of alteration of bowel flora by antimicrobial therapy. Patients with *C. difficile* colitis excrete large numbers of organisms and represent a risk to other patients. Therefore, enteric precautions and thorough cleaning of bathroom areas of patients with *C. difficile* disease should be implemented.

CONTROL MEASURES Infection control team The goals of those concerned with infection control are (1) to reduce the risk of patients acquiring infections in the hospital, (2) to provide adequate care for patients with a potentially communicable infection, and (3) to minimize the infectious risks of employees, visitors, and community contacts. The functions of the infection control team include (1) development of enforceable policies necessary for appropriate management of patients with communicable infections; (2) development of a surveillance system which identifies patients with communicable infections, quantitates the incidence and prevalence of hospital-acquired infection, and focuses on problems requiring further investigation; (3) feedback to physicians and other staff regarding identified problems and surveillance findings, including surgical wound infection rates; (4) liaison with personnel from nursing, central supply, housekeeping, maintenance, pharmacy, and other hospital services to ensure that an appropriate infection control environment is maintained; (5) education of employees in appropriate techniques to prevent the spread of infectious agents; (6) communication with employee health services to ensure adequate immunization of hospital employees and to provide care when personnel are exposed to a potentially communicable disease; and (7) monitoring of antibiotic utilization and susceptibility patterns of common nosocomial pathogens. Generally an effective infection control program can reduce nosocomial infection rates by one-third.

Prevention The basic principles of hand-washing between patient contacts, appropriate isolation of patients harboring communicable microorganisms, and application of epidemiologic methods to identify and correct potential sources of infection remain the cornerstones of prevention of nosocomial infections.

EMPLOYEE HEALTH SERVICE Preventive medicine also applies to hospital personnel. The employee health service should maintain an employee surveillance program for communicable diseases such as tuberculosis and routinely offer indicated adult immunizations (see Chap. 84). Personnel of both sexes who are likely to come into contact with pregnant women should be tested for rubella antibodies, and, if susceptible, immunized before being allowed to work in areas where contact with pregnant women is likely. HBV immunization is strongly indicated for all personnel whose work involves frequent handling of blood or direct contact with patients. Annual influenza immunization should be encouraged both to reduce the risk of nosocomial influenza transmission to patients and to minimize winter absenteeism.

Hospital personnel with highly communicable infections should be removed from patient contact during the period of communicability. The dangers of pustular lesions are often underestimated and it is commonly forgotten that susceptible contacts may develop chickenpox following exposure to persons with herpes zoster.

Approximately 1 percent of physicians and dentists are asymptomatic carriers of HBV. Although several instances of transmission from health care workers to patients have been identified, the great majority of HBV-infected personnel do not appear to present a hazard to patients. They should be encouraged to pay particular attention to personal hygiene and hand-washing and should wear gloves during invasive procedures or contact with mucous membranes. If these precautions are observed, their patient-related activities need not be restricted. There is no evidence to suggest that HIV infected health personnel present an infectious risk to patients.

ADMISSION SCREENING A patient scheduled for elective admission who has, or is thought to be incubating, an acute communicable disease should not be admitted until the period of communicability has passed. Screening on admission for communicable infections is particularly important for pediatric patients and for patients being admitted to oncology and transplant services where there may be a concentration of immunocompromised patients. Infections usually considered to be of minor importance, such as chickenpox or measles, can be devastating in such patients.

CONTAINMENT Isolation procedures are time-consuming and expensive and can hinder essential patient care activities if applied too rigidly. They should be used only when necessary and for the shortest period consistent with good medical practice. Several alternative isolation systems are presently in common use: (1) A "category" system of seven unique isolation and precaution practices each designed to protect against one kind of disease transmission such as "respiratory," "enteric," or "wound and skin"; (2) a system listing each disease or pathogen separately along with specific individual isolation practices; (3) a system treating all body substances as potentially infectious (universal precautions).

Differences in patient population and hospital size and function may be important determinants of which system (or combination) is most appropriate for any given institution.

If preventive measures fail and a communicable infection develops in an inpatient, the following principles of containment should be observed:

1 Prevent further transmission of disease by the index case by either isolating the patient or, if the patient's condition allows, arranging for discharge from the hospital.
2 Identify all contacts of the index case and determine their susceptibility and degree of exposure.
3 If prophylactic measures are available, administer them appropriately to exposed susceptible individuals.
4 Design a plan to prevent the spread of the infectious agent from the exposed susceptibles to other patients and personnel. This plan must recognize the epidemiology of the communicable disease in question, the effectiveness and feasibility of various control measures, and the potential consequences of further disease transmission.

Methods commonly employed to limit the tertiary spread of communicable diseases by exposed susceptibles are (1) early discharge of patients when feasible, (2) arranging assignments of exposed personnel to avoid patient contact during the period of communicability, and (3) cohorting exposed susceptible patients and personnel together and treating them as an epidemiologic unit. Although cohorting is cumbersome, it remains a major measure for control of hospital outbreaks of chickenpox and epidemic diarrhea.

PROGNOSIS Most nosocomial infections are diseases of medical progress, and the ever-increasing orientation of modern medicine to technologically sophisticated procedures, both diagnostic and therapeutic, makes it likely that the risk of patients acquiring infections in the hospital will continue to increase. On the other hand, many of the factors that promote infections in the hospital have been identified, and measures for their control have been developed. Influencing hospital personnel to carry out these control measures, such as hand-washing, catheter care, and restraint in the use of antibiotics, remains a major challenge.

REFERENCES

BENNETT JV, BRACHMAN PS (eds): *Hospital Infections*. Boston, Little, Brown, 1985

CENTERS FOR DISEASE CONTROL: Recommendations for prevention of HIV transmission in health care settings. Morb Mort Week Rep Supp 2S, 1987

CHAMBERS HF: Methicillin resistant staphylococci. Clin Microbial Rev 1:173, 1988

MAKI DG et al: Prospective study of replacing administration set for intravenous therapy at 48- vs 72-hour intervals. JAMA 258:1777, 1987

WILLIAMS WW et al: Immunization policies and vaccine coverage among adults. Ann Intern Med 108:616, 1988

YU VL: Nosocomial legionellosis: Current epidemiological issues, in *Current Clinical Topics in Infectious Diseases*, JS Remington, MN Swartz (eds). New York, McGraw-Hill, 1986.

section 2 Prevention and therapy of infectious disease

84 IMMUNIZATION

ADAM FINN / STANLEY A. PLOTKIN

"Prevention is better than cure" is an old and familiar saying that remains valid for the modern physician, nowhere more so than in the field of infectious diseases. Figure 84-1 depicts the three main approaches to the prevention of infection. Of these, removal of the infecting microorganism from the general environment of the host and enhancement of the host immune response to invasion have had by far the greatest impact on disease. Active immunization works through both these strategies. A single vaccine, appropriately administered, can have effects on morbidity and mortality in a population which far outweigh the benefits a single doctor practicing curative medicine could hope to have in an entire lifetime. For example, it has been estimated that during the first 20 years since its licensure, measles vaccine has prevented 52 million cases, 5210 deaths, and 17,370 cases of mental retardation in the United States alone.

PRINCIPLES OF IMMUNIZATION

ACTIVE IMMUNIZATION Active immunization is highly effective because it works through the adaptive immune system, which is specific for an infecting agent and has long-lasting memory (see Chap. 13). Vaccination provides the stimulus to activate this system and arms the vaccinee with protection which may be lifelong. Important factors that affect the development of useful active vaccines include: (1) the number and stability of critical antigens involved in the virulence of microorganisms; (2) the role of local as opposed to systemic immunity in protection against infection by parenteral or orally administered vaccines; (3) the ability of vaccine antigens to stimulate a lasting host response that mimics natural immunity; (4) the safety of the vaccine; and (5) the existence of effective mechanisms

FIGURE 84-1 Ways of preventing infection. Examples of infectious diseases significantly influenced are shown in brackets; i.m.o., infecting microorganism.

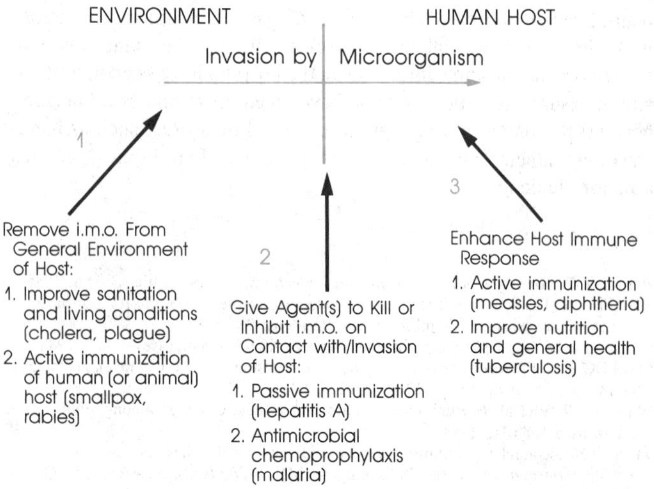

to ensure vaccine delivery and compliance with vaccination strategies in populations at risk.

Antigenic diversity has limited development of effective vaccines against rhinoviruses and is a major problem in the design of a vaccine against the human immunodeficiency virus (HIV). Other factors have limited development of highly effective vaccines against cholera and salmonellae (see Chaps. 107 and 122). Despite the challenges the dramatic successes of active vaccines against smallpox, polio, measles, mumps, rubella, pertussis, diphtheria, tetanus, and, most recently, against hepatitis B virus testify to the value and utility of this approach in the prevention of disease worldwide.

HERD IMMUNITY AND VACCINATION RATES Active immunization has two points of impact on the prevention of disease (see Fig. 84-1). First, it may provide the individual vaccinee with immune protection, and, second, it may reduce the circulation of the infecting agent in the population, thereby protecting unvaccinated individuals as well. This phenomenon is known as *herd immunity* and is of relevance in many immunization programs directed against infections that are transferred from person to person. Once adequate rates of vaccination are achieved, herd immunity will operate and the incidence of the disease will fall rapidly. Highly contagious infections such as measles require higher vaccination rates for effective herd immunity. If vaccination rates fall and the pathogen is still circulating, the incidence of new infections will rise as herd immunity is lost. For example, large outbreaks of pertussis occurred in the mid-1970s in the United Kingdom following a dramatic fall in vaccination rates after reports of possible adverse neurologic effects were publicized in the mass media. The very success of a vaccine mitigates against its continued use because, as the memory of the specific infection fades within the population, so does the will to ensure adequate immunization. All this underlines the need for good education of physicians, other health professionals, and the public about the use and continuing benefits of immunization.

IMMUNIZATION STRATEGIES Vaccine efficacy is determined by its ability to induce a detectable immune response, the documentation of substantially reduced or abolished infection rates under experimental and natural conditions, the production of lasting immunity, proper application of the vaccine to key target populations, and acceptance of vaccination by these populations and their health care providers.

Extensive development and testing must be carried out with documentation of safety and efficacy in well-designed field trials before vaccines are licensed for routine use. When effective vaccines are developed against a particular disease, there are many factors that influence the strategy chosen for subsequent use. A simplified scheme is depicted in Fig. 84-2. The epidemiologic characteristics of the disease will be the primary influence on all the elements of strategy. For example, the severity and widespread endemicity of smallpox, together with its lack of carrier state and lack of nonhuman reservoir, enabled a worldwide strategy to be adopted which led to its complete elimination.

Target population In some cases universal immunization of the population (usually as children) will be appropriate (e.g., for diphtheria-pertussis-tetanus and polio), whereas in others only selected high-risk groups should be vaccinated (e.g., for hepatitis B, influenza). With some vaccines, the target group for vaccination may not be the group which the program is principally designed to protect. Rubella vaccination of all children and females of child-bearing age aims to

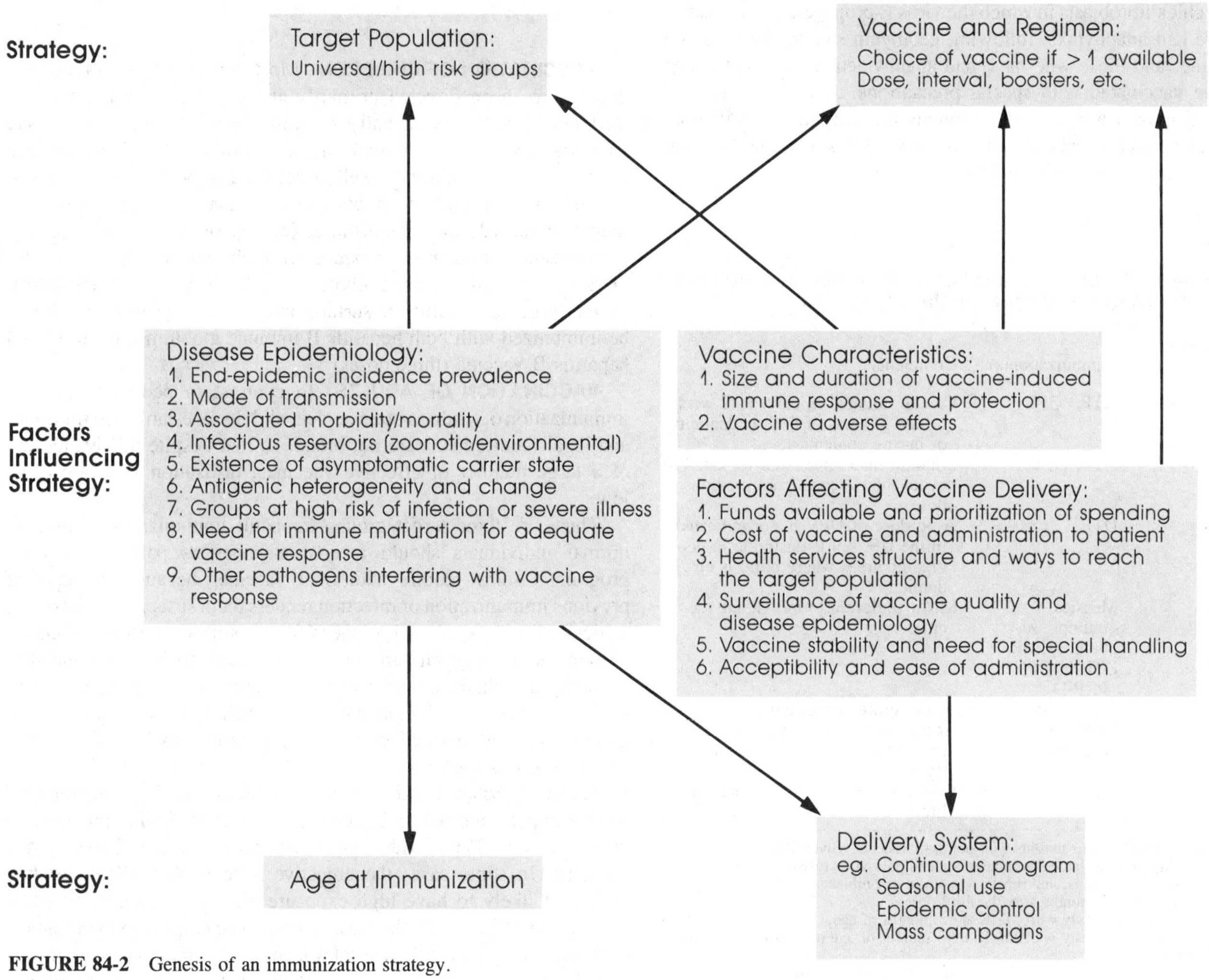

FIGURE 84-2 Genesis of an immunization strategy.

prevent infection of the fetus by reducing the likelihood of primary infection in women during pregnancy.

Vaccine and regimen The choice of vaccine and appropriate dosage regimen can vary with the disease, specific target populations, health systems, and even climates. For example, debate continues concerning the relative efficacies of live and inactivated polio vaccines in both temperate and tropical climates.

Age at immunization Regional differences in infection rates and severity may influence the age at which vaccine is routinely administered. Measles vaccine is administered to children at 15 months of age in the United States; in developing countries it is often given to younger infants, aged 6 to 9 months, since measles infection and mortality rates in infants are high. The aim of this approach is to prevent infection at an earlier age even though seroconversion rates may be somewhat lower because of the persistence of maternal antibody.

Delivery system The delivery system can vary with different diseases, vaccine efficacy, and local practical issues. In countries where health service facilities are not available for a continuing policy of universal vaccination of infants against polio, mass campaigns are often used to vaccinate large numbers in a single day.

SURVEILLANCE AND RECORDS Vaccine programs require continuous and rigorous monitoring. First, the quality and purity of vaccine must be subject to close surveillance in order to avoid the occurrence of mishaps such as the notorious ''Cutter incident'' in 1955 in which 192 vaccinees and their contacts developed paralytic polio as a result of incomplete inactivation of live virus in the Salk-type vaccine. Second, the balance of risks and benefits must be constantly reevaluated in the context of vaccine efficacy and risks of vaccination and the current epidemiology of the disease. In response to data from the United States demonstrating more effective prevention of the congenital rubella syndrome, the strategy of rubella vaccination in the United Kingdom was changed in 1988 from one of selective vaccination of prepubertal females to include universal vaccination of children at 15 months of age. Accurate records of immunizations should be kept by both physicians and vaccinees; such records are often required for travel from one country to another and, in the United States, for entry into school.

LIVE AND "KILLED" VACCINES Live vaccines utilize an attenuated strain of the original pathogen which can replicate and induce an immune response in the host but fails to cause significant illness. These vaccines mimic true infection and tend to induce long-lasting immunity. They may also cause significant illness in a small minority of vaccinees either because of reversion to virulence during replication in the host or because of immune defects in the host. Other intercurrent infection may interfere with live vaccines and prevent an adequate response. ''Killed'' vaccines, really a misnomer as not all of this group are prepared from inactivated organisms, challenge the vaccinee's immune system with antigens common to the original pathogen that do not replicate. In general effective immune responses require relatively large vaccine dosages and protection may be less persistent, but there is no risk of serious vaccine-induced infection. The term ''subunit'' vaccines refers to vaccines that are constructed of key antigenic components of microorganisms essential for infection and/or virulence.

HYPERSENSITIVITY Vaccines occasionally induce allergic reactions ranging from mild to anaphylactic responses that contraindicate further administration of that vaccine. Sometimes these responses are due to materials other than the vaccine itself. For example, measles vaccine contains small quantities of neomycin and traces of protein from the chick fibroblasts in which the virus is propagated. Individuals who have had anaphylaxis following neomycin should not be given the vaccine, and those who have had anaphylactic reactions to eggs should be vaccinated with special precautions. A vague history of allergic symptoms is inadequate grounds for denying an individual the benefit of immunization, and specific recommendations for each vaccine should always be consulted.

TABLE 84-1 Recommended schedule for active immunization of healthy infants and children in the United States

Recommended age	Immunization(s)	Comments
2 Months	DTP,[1] OPV[2]	Can be initiated as early as 2 weeks of age in areas of high endemicity or during epidemics.
4 Months	DTP, OPV	2-month interval desired for OPV to avoid interference from previous dose.
6 Months	DTP	A 3d dose of OPV is not indicated in the US, but is desirable in geographic areas where polio is endemic.
15 Months	Measles, mumps, rubella (MMR)[3]	MMR preferred to individual vaccines.
18 Months	DTP,[4,5] OPV[6] PRP-D[7]	
4–6 Years	DTP,[8] OPV	At or before school entry.
12 Years	MMR or measles	At entrance to middle school. However, may be given instead at entry to kindergarten.
14–16 Years	Td[9]	Repeat every 10 years throughout life.

[1] DTP, diphtheria and tetanus toxoids with pertussis vaccine. Given IM.
[2] OPV, oral poliovirus vaccine containing attenuated poliovirus types 1, 2, and 3.
[3] MMR, live measles, mumps, and rubella viruses in a combined vaccine. Given SC.
[4] Should be given 6 to 12 months after the third dose.
[5] May be given simultaneously with MMR at 15 months of age.
[6] May be given simultaneously with MMR at 15 months of age or at any time between 12 and 24 months of age.
[7] PRP-D, *Haemophilus* b diphtheria toxoid conjugate vaccine. Given IM.
[8] Up to the seventh birthday.
[9] Td, adult tetanus toxoid (full dose) and diphtheria toxoid (reduced dose) for adult use. Given IM.

SOURCE: American Academy of Pediatrics, *Report of the Committee on Infectious Diseases*, 1988.

IMMUNIZATION PROGRAMS

VACCINATION OF CHILDREN Most general immunization programs have been directed primarily at the pediatric population. In the United States, it is currently recommended that all children receive vaccines against eight common diseases (Table 84-1). The practice of vaccination of children is well-established, generally well-accepted by pediatricians and the public, and is reinforced by regulations requiring records of immunization for school entry. Consequently immunization rates in many areas are high. Special indications for extra vaccines are similar to those in adults (Tables 84-3 and 84-4). Infants born to hepatitis B surface-antigen-positive mothers should be immunized with both hepatitis B immune globulin (one dose) and hepatitis B vaccine (three doses).

VACCINATION OF ADULTS In contrast to pediatric practice, immunization of adults is often neglected. It lacks established tradition, and legal requirements are not broad, so that despite the availability of a large number of effective vaccines, utilization rates are often low.

There are three target groups for adult immunization. First, all normal individuals should receive vaccines as part of universal programs. Some require additional vaccines because the lack of previous immunization or infection renders them susceptible. Visitors, students, immigrants, and refugees from countries with poor general immunization programs are particularly likely to be unimmunized, so such individuals should make vaccination a high priority. Table 84-2 lists vaccines documented to be effective in producing an immune response and reducing disease in normal adults and indicates appropriate target groups.

Second, certain conditions or occupations, such as health care work, can place normal adults at significant risk of vaccine-preventable infection and illness. Table 84-3 lists vaccines that fall into this category. In some cases the objective is to prevent illness of key personnel likely to have high exposure rates to influenza, hepatitis B, and rabies. In others, the vaccines are to be employed in outbreaks of disease (e.g., meningococcal vaccine) or immediately upon potential exposure to a lethal infectious agent (e.g., postexposure prophylaxis for rabies). Because of the relatively low frequency of tuberculosis, the lack of proven efficacy in large population studies in the country, and the availability of effective prophylaxis (isoniazid),

TABLE 84-2 Vaccines for active immunization of normal civilian adults in the United States

Vaccine	Schedule and target group	Delivery	Comments
Combined diphtheria and tetanus toxoids (Td)	Each 10 years. All adults (e.g., age 25, 35, 45, etc.). Also, after potentially tetanus-contaminated wound if no immunization in previous 5 years. Primary course: 3 doses at 0, 1–2, 6–12 months.	Primary care offices and clinical emergency rooms.	Td has reduced dose of diphtheria toxin relative to combined vaccine used in primary immunization of children. Td should always be used in preference to tetanus toxoid alone. Previously unimmunized adults seen at time of injury should also receive passive immunization.
Inactivated influenza vaccine for current year	Yearly in autumn. All adults, from age 65 (see also Tables 84-3 and 84-4).	Hospital wards (at discharge). Hospital clinics. Primary care offices and clinics. Residential homes for elderly.	Both this vaccine and 23-valent pneumococcal vaccine can be given simultaneously at separate sites.
23-Valent pneumococcal vaccine	One dose. All adults at age 65 (or over). See also Table 84-4.	See above.	See above.
Live measles vaccine	One dose. All adults (particularly males) without history of previous infection or immunization born after 1956.	College clinics. Primary care offices and clinics.	Serologic testing for immunity is not considered necessary as previous infection or immunization does not contraindicate revaccination. A combined measles-mumps vaccine is available
Live mumps vaccine	One dose. All adults (particularly males) without history of previous infection or immunization.	See above.	See above.
Live rubella vaccine	One dose. All females shown to be seronegative (e.g., on antenatal or hospital employee screening).	Postnatal wards, obstetric and gynecologic clinics. Primary care.	Immunization of the many women of childbearing age who are seronegative is needed so long as rubella continues to circulate in the community.

TABLE 84-3 Vaccines for additional active immunization of normal individuals with high-risk circumstances in the United States

Vaccine	Schedule/target group	Notes
Bacille Calmette-Guérîn (BCG) (against tuberculosis)	One dose. 1. Tuberculin-negative individuals in populations and groups with high frequency of TB transmission and inadequate health provision for normal methods of case detection and isoniazid prophylaxis (e.g., ghettos, alcoholics, and migrants). 2. Tuberculin-negative health care personnel caring for such populations.	BCG should not be given to immunodeficient individuals (e.g., with HIV infection).
Inactivated influenza vaccine for current year	Yearly, in fall. IM (preferred) or SC. 1. Health care personnel caring for high-risk patients (see Table 84-4). 2. Residents of institutions housing patients with chronic medical conditions (see also Tables 84-2 and 84-4).	Acute febrile illness is a contraindication. Most individuals with egg allergy can be immunized with special precautions.
Hepatitis B vaccine	3 Doses at 0, 1, and 6 months. IM in deltoid muscle. Susceptible or probably susceptible individuals in the following groups: 1. Health care personnel (ideally in training) who will be at risk of exposure to blood, blood products, and needles. 2. Household and sexual contacts of known hepatitis B carriers. 3. Clients and staff of institutions for the mentally handicapped. 4. Hemodialysis patients and recipients of clotting factor concentrates. 5. Homosexual men and heterosexual persons with multiple sexual partners. 6. Users of illicit injectable drugs. 7. Prison inmates. 8. Groups with highly endemic disease (e.g., Alaskan Eskimos, Pacific Islanders, immigrants from east Asia and sub-Saharan Africa). 9. Infants born to hepatitis B surface-antigen-positive mothers (see Table 84-5).	Pregnancy is not a contraindication for women at risk of contracting hepatitis B.
Rabies vaccine [human diploid cell vaccine (HDCV) or other licensed vaccine]	1. Preexposure prophylaxis: 3 doses at 0, 7, and 28 days IM (boosters may be necessary). Individuals at high risk of exposure (e.g., veterinarians, laboratory workers). 2. Postexposure prophylaxis: (see Table 84-5).	
Inactivated polio vaccine (enhanced potency)	3 Doses at 0, 1–2, and 6–12 months, SC. Unimmunized adults likely to be exposed to wild poliovirus (health care workers). For immediate risk of exposure [e.g., contact with known polio case, household contact of child receiving oral polio vaccine (OPV)] unimmunized adults should receive OPV 4 doses at 0, 1–2, 3–4, 9–16 months (see also Table 84-4). Previously partially immunized adults should complete course of vaccine.	Routine immunization against polio of adults resident in United States is not recommended.
Meningococcal polysaccharide vaccine	Bivalent (groups A, C) or quadrivalent (gps. A, C, Y, W135) vaccine. One dose, SC. 1. Household contact of patient with type A, C, Y, or W135 meningococcal infection. 2. Local control of outbreak of type A, C, Y, or W135 meningococcal disease (see also Table 84-4).	Type B infection against which there is no vaccine is most common. Contacts are given rifampin also.

BCG (bacille Calmette-Guérin) is not routinely employed in the United States.

Third, because of underlying medical conditions some individuals are likely to develop particularly severe illness from infections which may be prevented by appropriate vaccination. Table 84-4 lists indications for use of influenza, pneumococcal, meningococcal, and polio vaccines in different patient groups in this category.

IMMUNE DEFICIENCY Patients with reduced immunity present a particular problem. On the one hand, they are particularly at risk for severe infections, but on the other, they are often unable to mount a good immune response. Furthermore, live-virus vaccines are as a rule contraindicated, so these patients are usually given less immunogenic toxoids and other inactivated vaccines. When patients will be medically immunosuppressed, for example, as part of cancer chemotherapy or following splenectomy, appropriate vaccination should, whenever possible, be undertaken before initiation of treatment. If this is not feasible, vaccination should be delayed for at least a month after chemotherapy has been completed to allow for immune recovery.

Persons infected with HIV are a group for whom vaccination recommendations are under constant review (see Chap. 264). In the United States it is recommended that symptomatic HIV infection contraindicate the use of some live vaccines [e.g., oral polio vaccine (OPV) and BCG]. Asymptomatic HIV-seropositive individuals with preserved CD4-positive lymphocyte numbers can be given live vaccines except BCG, unless they have household contacts with

TABLE 84-4 Vaccines for additional active immunization of individuals who have an inherently increased risk of severe vaccine-preventable infections

Vaccine	Schedule and target group	Notes
Inactivated influenza vaccine for current year	Yearly, in autumn (children should only be given "split" vaccine). Individuals with chronic cardiovascular, pulmonary, renal, and metabolic (e.g., diabetes mellitus) diseases, severe anemia, and immune deficiency or suppression (including symptomatic HIV infection). See also Tables 84-2 and 84-3.	Acute febrile illness is a contraindication. Most individuals with egg allergy can be immunized with special precautions.
23-Valent pneumococcal vaccine	One dose. Individuals with chronic cardiovascular, pulmonary disease, cirrhosis, renal failure, alcoholism, anatomic or functional asplenia (including sickle cell anemia), Hodgkin's lymphoma, myeloma, cerebrospinal fluid leaks, and immune deficiency or suppression (including symptomatic HIV infection). See Table 84-2.	
Quadrivalent meningococcal vaccine (groups A, C, Y, W135)	One dose. Individuals with anatomic or functional asplenia (including sickle cell anemia). Individuals with terminal complement component defects. See also Table 84-3.	
Inactivated polio vaccine (IPV) (enhanced potency)	3 Doses at 0, 1–2, and 6–12 months. Individuals with immune deficiency or suppression and their household contacts should be given IPV, not oral polio vaccine. See also Table 84-3.	Although immune response may be reduced, some protection may be achieved.

symptomatic HIV infection, in which case inactivated polio vaccine should be used instead of OPV. Measles vaccine, either monovalent or as measles, mumps, and rubella combined vaccine, is advocated for all HIV-infected children because of reports of severe or fatal natural measles in this group and no reports of vaccine complications. Pneumococcal vaccine, preferably administered at a time before depression of CD4-positive lymphocytes occurs, is also recommended.

PREGNANCY In general, the administration of vaccines, like drugs, should be avoided in pregnancy or delayed until the second or third trimester. The theoretical risks include teratogenic effects of vaccines on the fetus and, in the case of live vaccines, of congenital infection. However, diphtheria and tetanus toxoids are considered to be safe, and where there is genuine, substantial, and unavoidable risk of exposure, a nonimmune pregnant woman may be given live oral polio and yellow fever vaccines. Hepatitis B vaccine may also be given to susceptible pregnant women who are at high risk because the risk of infection to the infant outweighs theoretical concerns about the vaccine. Rubella vaccine is of special interest in this context because of the congenital rubella syndrome (CRS). Although the vaccine is contraindicated in pregnancy and transplacental infection of the fetus with the vaccine virus has been observed, CRS has not been reported in infants born to women inadvertently vaccinated in pregnancy. Therefore, such vaccination is not a priori an indication for abortion. In the case of influenza, the risk of severe disease, particularly in the third trimester, is greater than the theoretical risk to the fetus of inactivated vaccine.

PASSIVE IMMUNIZATION Passive immunization involves providing exogenous antibody in an attempt to prevent or to attenuate an anticipated infection. Although this method lacks many of the advantages of active immunization and protection may be short-lived, it has the advantage that the effect is immediate. This is important in the use of antibody preparations in prophylaxis against tetanus and rabies and in the protection of contacts with measles, varicella, and hepatitis A and B (see Table 84-5). Passive immunization is also used to protect travelers against hepatitis A, where no vaccine is yet commercially available. Pooled human serum immune globulins contain a wide variety of IgG antibodies against different agents. The increasing availability of intravenous preparations which can be safely administered in high dosages has broadened the use of this treatment. Individuals with congenital deficiency of immunoglobulins treated with regular infusions of immune globulin have a reduced number of infections due to a wide variety of pathogens (see Chap. 263). There is also limited evidence to suggest that similar therapy reduces the frequency of serious infections in children with symptomatic HIV infection (see Chap. 264). Studies are being conducted to evaluate intravenous gamma globulin treatment in other individuals at high risk for sepsis (e.g., burn and intensive care patients).

Passive immunization may interfere with immune responses to some antigens, as with measles vaccine. However, combined active and passive immunization is used effectively against both rabies and hepatitis B.

IMMUNIZATION OF TRAVELERS The presentation of an individual for immunization advice prior to travel is an opportunity to ensure that routine vaccinations have been performed (Table 84-2). Often the risks of measles and diphtheria will be much greater outside the United States, in underdeveloped countries. The need for supplementary protection will vary not only with the travel destinations but also with the activities planned. For example, immunization against hepatitis B would routinely be undertaken only if the individual were susceptible and expected to have prolonged close contact with the local population in an area of endemic infection (e.g., health care workers). Finally, many countries have regulations governing the immunization status of visitors. Table 84-6 lists some of the immunizations commonly advised for use in travelers. As specific recommendations vary from one area to another and are subject to change, up-to-date information can be obtained in the United States

TABLE 84-5 Preparations currently recommended for passive immunization of exposed or infected patients

Disease	Preparation of choice	Target group and schedule	Comment
POSTEXPOSURE PROPHYLAXIS OF CONTACTS			
Hepatitis A	Immune globulin (human) (IG)	Contacts in day care centers, households, and custodial institutions. 0.02 mL/kg IM.	See Table 84-6 for preexposure prophylaxis for foreign travel.
Hepatitis B	Hepatitis B immune globulin (HBIG)	1. Infants of hepatitis B surface antigen positive mothers. 0.5 mL IM. 2. Possible percutaneous or sexual contact with hepatitis B. 0.06 mL/kg IM.	HBIG is usually given with appropriate doses of hepatitis B vaccine (see Table 84-3).
Varicella	Varicella-zoster immune globulin (VZIG)	1. Exposed infants and children at high risk of severe infection. 2. Exposed susceptible adults. 125 units (1 vial)/10 kg IM (minimum 125, maximum 625).	
Tetanus	Tetanus immune globulin (TIG)	Patients with wounds (other than clean minor wounds) without a clear history of full, up-to-date tetanus immunization 500–3000 units IM, part of dose infiltrated around wound.	Tetanus with diphtheria toxoids (Td) normally given as well.
Rabies	Human rabies immune globulin (HRIG)	Individuals thought to have had significant exposure to a rabid or potentially rabid animal. Patients known to be immune and/or fully immunized against rabies do not require HBIG but only 2 doses of rabies vaccine on days 0 and 3 (see Table 84-3). 20 IU/kg, half infiltrated around wound, half IM.	Give early and follow with a 5-dose course of rabies vaccine on days 0, 3, 7, 14, and 28.
Measles	Immune globulin (human) (IG)	Susceptible household and close contacts, within 6 days of exposure, particularly immunosuppressed individuals (including those with HIV infection) and infants. 0.25 mL/kg IM.	Routine measles vaccination should be postponed until 3 months after IG administration.
Rubella	Immune globulin (human) (IG)	Pregnant women exposed in early pregnancy, where termination is not an option. 0.55 mL/kg IM.	Passive immunization does not ensure protection of the fetus.
TREATMENT OF ESTABLISHED DISEASE			
Botulism	Equine trivalent antitoxin*	Patients with food-borne or wound botulism.	Not used to treat infant botulism.
Diphtheria	Equine diphtheria antitoxin*	Patients with clinical diagnosis of diphtheria.	Probably of no value in cutaneous diphtheria.
Tetanus	Tetanus immune globulin (TIG)	Patients with clinical diagnosis of tetanus.	

* Tests for sensitivity and if necessary desensitization should be undertaken for these products.

TABLE 84-6 Immunizations and chemoprophylaxis commonly required by travelers abroad in addition to routine requirements*

Disease	Schedule	Notes
ACTIVE IMMUNIZATION		
Polio	Where time allows, previously unimmunized adults should receive inactivated polio vaccine (regimen as in Table 84-3). For rapid immunization: killed polio vaccine, 2 doses at least 4 weeks apart. For immediate protection, oral polio vaccine should be given.	If a pregnant woman requires rapid protection against polio, because of significant risk of exposure, oral polio vaccine may be given.
Yellow fever	Single dose of live-virus vaccine must be administered at registered vaccination center, which will issue certificate of vaccination, which may be required for travel in certain areas.	Certificate is valid for 10 years. Vaccination is contraindicated in immune-suppressed persons. Pregnant women and infants less than 6 months old should not be vaccinated unless risk of exposure is unavoidable.
Typhoid	Killed whole-cell vaccine may be used to protect travelers to areas where typhoid is endemic.	These vaccines have relatively high rates of local and systemic adverse effects.
Cholera	Vaccination is not recommended unless it is a requirement for entry into the country of destination.	Infection is more effectively prevented by taking precautions in handling food and drink.
Japanese B encephalitis	Killed-virus vaccine; recommended for travelers to rural areas of the Far East, including China and Korea.	Routinely given to children in endemic areas.
PASSIVE IMMUNIZATION		
Hepatitis A	Up to 0.06 mL/kg immune serum globulin is given by IM injection, affording protection against hepatitis A (HAV) infection for 3–4 months.	Individuals who are seropositive for anti-HAV need not be immunized.
CHEMOPROPHYLAXIS		
Malaria	Chemoprophylaxis should be started prior to departure and continued after return. Regimens change with changing plasmodial resistance.	Chemoprophylaxis does not provide absolute protection.

* Indications and further details should be sought from *Health Information for International Travel.*

from the latest edition of the Centers for Disease Control booklet entitled *Health Information for International Travel.* For recommendations regarding chemoprophylaxis against malaria see Chap. 159.

ASSESSMENT OF IMMUNIZATION PROGRAMS Vaccine efficacy The ultimate test of a vaccine is in its ability to reduce or prevent widespread disease. The dramatic fall in the reported cases of the seven diseases that have been the object of sustained immunization programs in the United States is shown in Table 84-7. Information of this type is much more important than specific measurements of an immune response in vaccinated subjects and testifies to effective application of highly immunogenic vaccines to large populations. The latter involves a well-coordinated and -supported public and private health effort.

Cost-benefit The rising cost of health care in wealthy nations and the limited resources available in many poorer countries mandate the rigorous assessment of cost-benefit for all medical interventions (see Chap. 3). In all analyses to date effective immunization programs have been shown to be less costly than most other preventive health strategies and far less expensive than the cost of treating established disease.

TABLE 84-7 Comparison of maximum and current morbidity of vaccine-preventable diseases

Disease	Maximum cases (year)	1986	% Change
Diphtheria	206,939 (1921)	0	100.00
Measles	894,134 (1941)	6282	99.30
Mumps*	152,209 (1968)	7790	94.88
Pertussis	265,269 (1934)	4195	98.42
Polio (paralytic)	21,269 (1952)	3	99.99
Rubella†	57,686 (1969)	551	99.05
Congenital rubella syndrome	20,000 (1964–5)	14	99.93
Tetanus‡	608 (1948)	64	89.35

* First reportable in 1968.
† First reportable in 1966.
‡ First reportable in 1947.
SOURCE: AR Hinman, in Plotkin and Mortimer.

Legal considerations Successful vaccination programs can militate against their own continued use. This phenomenon is compounded by the growing number of lawsuits filed on behalf of individuals claiming compensation for alleged vaccine-induced damage. Because pediatric vaccination is a legal requirement, persons or the families of persons thought to have been damaged by a vaccine will often consider that they are entitled to compensation, particularly if they were not informed of the inherent risks involved. No vaccines are perfect, although serious adverse effects are extremely rare. Furthermore, it is often impossible to define whether there is a causal connection between a coincidental acute illness and immunization. The costs and uncertainties that accompany such legal proceedings act as disincentives to health professionals to administer vaccines and to pharmaceutical firms to manufacture them. Some programs of immunization, most notably that against pertussis, are under threat as a result, with possibly disastrous consequences. The best solution to this problem may prove to be the institution of an effective no-fault compensation scheme for vaccine-related injury. Several European countries have used such programs successfully, and the United States has recently instituted one.

LICENSED VACCINES IN CURRENT ROUTINE USE

DIPHTHERIA AND TETANUS TOXOIDS These are two of the most successful vaccines ever made. Both are based on the use of an inactivated toxin to produce antitoxin antibodies. The vaccines are protective because the diseases are mediated through the action of extracellular toxins, which are neutralized by the antitoxin.

PERTUSSIS Widespread use of the conventional whole cell pertussis vaccine has greatly reduced the frequency of the infection. Mono- and combined-component acellular pertussis vaccines were developed and used initially in Japan in children over 2 years of age. Field trials of such vaccines in younger infants in Scandinavia and the United States are in progress and suggest that they may be efficacious and have fewer side effects.

POLIO Two types of vaccine are available. One is a live attenuated vaccine administered orally, the other is a formalin-inactivated vaccine administered parenterally. Both are mixtures of the three poliovirus serotypes. While both are effective in individual vaccinees, their relative efficacy in different populations may vary with the local epidemiology of polio. The oral vaccine is preferred for routine use in the United States. The antigenicity of the inactivated vaccine has been enhanced, and this more potent product may eventually receive greater use in the United States.

MEASLES Use of the live attenuated vaccine has brought measles to a low ebb in the United States, but earlier hopes of eradicating the disease have not been borne out. There have been persistent epidemics in unvaccinated infants in poor areas of large cities, and occasional outbreaks in older vaccinated children. Proposed new strategies include strenuous efforts to vaccinate young infants whenever possible, and mass revaccination of students in schools where an outbreak occurs without attempting to confirm old records or to identify seronegative individuals. Live attenuated measles vaccine should be given to previous recipients of the older inactivated vaccine to prevent attacks of atypically presenting measles (see Chap. 141).

MUMPS Epidemic mumps is now virtually gone from the United States through immunization with mumps vaccine, although not every state mandates its use.

RUBELLA Congenital rubella syndrome is now rare, and the high immunity due to vaccination may make eradication of the virus from the United States a possibility.

***HAEMOPHILUS* TYPE B** A particular problem of polysaccharide vaccines, which contain the polymers that constitute the bacterial cell wall, is their poor immunogenicity in children under 2 years. Since much of the most serious illness caused by *Haemophilus influenzae* type b occurs in this age group, a newly licensed vaccine contains the polysaccharide bound to diphtheria toxoid, a protein antigen. This T-cell-dependent antigen enhances immunogenicity and gives added protection to younger children (see Chap. 115).

HEPATITIS B The licensure of recombinant hepatitis B vaccine made in yeast has sharply diminished fears concerning the widespread use of this vaccine for high-risk populations, including medical personnel.

PNEUMOCOCCUS This vaccine has recently been improved to contain 23 capsular serotypes which together cause over 90 percent of bacteremic pneumococcal infections in children and adults. However, this polysaccharide vaccine is poorly immunogenic in infants and some other high-risk groups. Debate persists regarding its efficacy in adult populations at high risk of developing serious pneumococcal infections (e.g., splenectomized and elderly patients). It is generally well-tolerated, and there are few contraindications to its use (see Chap. 99).

INFLUENZA This is a trivalent vaccine, containing two prevalent type A strains with different hemagglutinins, and a type B strain. Each autumn the composition of the vaccine is changed to reflect a prediction of the important strains of the coming winter's epidemic.

NEW DEVELOPMENTS Much work in vaccine development is in progress. Attempts are being made both to improve the quality of vaccines already in use and to develop vaccines against other infectious diseases not hitherto preventable by immunization. In addition, a number of newly developed molecular genetic techniques may enhance vaccine research.

Rabies The main impediment to the use of the highly effective human diploid cell vaccine against rabies in the poorer countries of the world where rabies is common is its high cost. A number of vaccines are becoming available which use animal cell lines to propagate the virus. These may prove to be substantially cheaper.

Adenovirus Live attenuated adenovirus vaccines have been used extensively in military recruits and have been effective in preventing outbreaks of acute respiratory diseases (see Chap. 140). They have not been used in civilians.

Cytomegalovirus (CMV) Congenital CMV infection of the fetus and disseminated CMV infection in transplant recipients are important causes of morbidity and mortality. Both live attenuated and subunit CMV vaccines are under development and may contribute to prevention of these infections (see Chap. 138).

Rotavirus Multiple serotype viruses of this group are a major cause of infantile gastroenteritis throughout the world. A number of live vaccines have been developed from viruses of animal origin. Further work may include genetic manipulation of human rotaviruses to produce a safe and immunogenic multivalent vaccine (see Chap. 145).

Varicella A live attenuated varicella vaccine was developed in Japan in 1974. It has been shown to be safe and immunogenic in several field trials conducted in normal children or children with malignancies. It has been licensed in Japan and Europe, and it may be licensed either for restricted or general use in the United States in the near future (see Chap. 136).

Hepatitis A Several vaccines against hepatitis A are under development. In areas where the disease is prevalent, the induction of lasting immunity by active immunization, perhaps as part of the routine childhood immunization program, would be an important step forward.

Measles The availability of the Edmonston-Zagreb strain of measles virus that is more immunogenic in 7- to 9-month-old children holds promise for future use in areas of the world with high endemic rates in young children.

REFERENCES

American Academy of Pediatrics: Report of the Committee of Infectious Diseases 1986 ("Red Book"), 20th ed., 1986
Bloch AB et al: The health impact of measles vaccination in the United States. Pediatrics 76:524, 1985
Centers for Disease Control: Rubella vaccination during pregnancy-United States 1971–1986. Morb Mort Week Rep 36:457, 1987
———: *Health Information for International Travel.* Atlanta, GA, Centers for Disease Control, United States Department of Health and Human Services, Public Health Service (published annually)
Communicable Disease Statistics 1986: England and Wales. Her Majesty's Stationery Office, ser MB2, no 13, 1986
Fenner F et al: Smallpox and its eradication. Geneva, World Health Organization, 1988
Guide for Adult Immunization. Philadelphia, American College of Physicians, 1985
Herman JJ et al: Allergic reactions to measles (rubeola) vaccine in patients hypersensitive to egg protein. Pediatrics 102:196, 1983
——— et al: Live-inactivated poliovirus vaccine. Pediatr Infect Dis J 6:881, 1987
Plotkin SA, Mortimer EA: *Vaccines.* Philadelphia, Saunders, 1988
Walker D et al: Measles, mumps, and rubella: The need for a change in immunization policy. Br Med J 292:1501, 1986
World Health Organization Expanded Programme on Immunization: Conclusions and recommendations of the Global Advisory Group. Wkly Epidemiol Rec 60:13, 1985

85 THERAPY AND PROPHYLAXIS OF BACTERIAL INFECTIONS

HAROLD C. NEU

INTRODUCTION Changes in the host, the appearance of new pathogens, and the resistance of new and old pathogens to previously available antimicrobial agents explain the large number of antimicrobial agents. Changes in the host include prolonged survival of critically ill patients due to use of cancer chemotherapy, transplantation, and prosthetic devices. The problem of resistance has been severe due to the worldwide dissemination of plasmids that convey resistance to multiple antimicrobial agents. Considerations of efficacy and toxicity have a major impact on the selection of antimicrobial agents, but cost is increasingly important. This chapter deals with general observations on antimicrobial therapy, and a description of most antibacterial agents. Recommendations for therapy of infections are made in the chapters dealing with individual diseases. Tables 85-1 and 85-2 summarize important information concerning the drugs discussed in this chapter.

FACTORS INFLUENCING SELECTION OF ANTIMICROBIALS Several factors bear directly on the selection of an antimicrobial agent. Knowledge of the infecting microorganism may not be available

TABLE 85-1 Serum and body fluid levels after oral administration of various antibiotics

Drug	Unit dose* (oral)	Average peak level, μg/mL: Blood†	Urine‡	Bile§	CSF¶	Half-life, h: C_{cl} >80 mL	C_{cl} <10 mL	Dose adjustment renal failure
Amoxicillin	0.5 g	10	1000	10	NA	1	6	Minor
Ampicillin	0.25 g	1.5	50	5	NA	1	6	Minor
Cefaclor	0.5 g	15	200	5	NA	1	2	No
Cephalexin	0.25 g	8	500	3	NA	1	8–20	Major
Cephradine	0.25 g	8	500	5	NA	1	8	Major
Chloramphenicol	1 g	13	100	3	6	2	5	Minor
Ciprofloxacin	0.75 g	4	300	8	1	3.5	5–10	Major
Clindamycin	0.15 g	2	30	20	NA	2	6–10	Minor
Cloxacillin	0.5 g	8	200	—	NA	1	4	Minor
Dicloxacillin	0.5 g	15	200	—	NA	1	2–4	Minor
Doxycycline	100 mg	2.5	100	15	NA	15–20	15–20	No
Erythromycin estolate	0.25 g	1.4	200	800	NA	1.5–2	4–6	No
Indanyl carbenicillin	1 g	15	600	NA	NA	1–2	15	Major
Metronidazole	0.25 g	5	50	5	2	8	8	Minor
Minocycline	100 mg	2.5	100	15	NA	15	15–25	Minor
Norfloxacin	500 mg	4	200	2	NA	3	8–20	Major
Ofloxacin	400 mg	6	500	5	NA	6	10–20	Major
Penicillin V	0.25 g	2	300	4	NA	1	2	No
Rifampin	8 mg/kg	10	50	100	0.5	1.5–5	1.5–5	No
Sulfadiazine	1.0 g	25	100	25	15	10	12–25	Major
Tetracycline	0.25 g	2.2	100	15	NA	6–8	30–50	Major
TMP/SMX	0.16 g TMP + 0.8 g SMX	1 + 30	10 + 100	3 + 30	0.5 + 15	10	25	Major

* Doses listed are the lowest doses that would normally be employed for adults or children over 32 kg with normal renal function in the treatment of systemic infections.
† Blood levels are at 1–2 h after IM or at the end of 20–30 min IV infusion. In most instances considerably higher serum levels are attainable with higher dosages. For example, 2 g of ampicillin would yield a peak blood level of 70–90 μg/mL, 2 g of cefoxitin a peak blood level of 120–140 μg/mL.
‡ Drug concentrations may be significantly lower if the patient is producing a very dilute urine or if creatinine clearance is below 10 mL/min. Concentration based on mean levels for the first 4 h after drug is administered.
§ Assuming normal liver function.
¶ Meningeal inflammation; in meningitis higher doses than those listed would normally be employed resulting in higher CSF levels.
NOTE: NA = not appropriate therapy for meningitis; — = data not available; TMP/SMX = trimethoprim-sulfamethoxazole.

TABLE 85-2 Serum and body fluid levels after parenteral administration of various antibiotics

Drug	Unit dose[a] (parenteral)	Average peak level, μg/mL: Blood[b]	Urine[c]	Bile[d]	CSF[e]	Half-life, h: C_{cl} >80 mL	C_{cl} <10 mL	Dose adjustment renal failure	Effect of hemodialysis
Amdinocillin	1.0 g IV	70	>1000	20	1–5[f]	1	4	Minor	Yes
Amikacin	5 mg/kg IM or IV	25	200	5	5	2	30	Major	Yes
Ampicillin	1.0 g IV	35	500	10	3[f]	1	4	Minor	Yes
Azlocillin	3.0 g IV	190	>2000	100	16	1	4	Minor	Yes
Aztreonam	1.0 g IV	160	>1000	20	1–5[f]	1.5–2	6	Minor	Yes
Carbenicillin	4.0 g IV	250	>1000	50	20	1	15	Major	Yes
Cefamandole	1.0 g IV	70	1000	100	NA	0.7	8	Minor	Yes
Cefazolin	1.0 g IV	110	>1000	50	NA	2	25	Major	Yes
Cefoperazone	2.0 g IV	250	>1000	>100	1–5	2	2–4	No	No
Cefotaxime	1.0 g IV	80	>1000	15	10[f]	1	4	Minor	Yes
Cefoxitin	1.0 g IV	70	1000	100	1–5	0.8	10	Major	Yes
Ceftazidime	1.0 g IV	80	>1000	5–10	1–20[f]	1.8	1.5	Major	Yes
Ceftizoxime	1.0 g IV	80	>1000	30	1–10[f]	1.6	19	Major	Yes
Ceftriaxone	1.0 g IV	150	>1000	200	1–20[f]	8	16	No	Yes
Cefuroxime	0.75 g IV	40	>1000	10–30	1–20[f]	1.5	20	Major	Yes
Cephalothin	1.0 g IV	70	500	10	0.7	0.5	8	Minor	Yes
Cephapirin	1.0 g IV	70	500	10	NA	0.5	8	Minor	Yes
Chloramphenicol	1.0 g IV	15	100	3	10	1–2	3–5	No	Yes
Ciprofloxacin	300 mg IV	3	100	10	1	3–4	5–10	Yes	Yes
Clindamycin	0.6 g IV	15	30	40	NA	2	6–10	No	No
Erythromycin	1.0 g IV	10	20	80	1	1–2	4–6	No	No
Gentamicin	1.5 mg/kg IM or IV	6	50	2	1	1–2	4–6	Major	Yes
Imipenem	0.5 g IV	30	100	10	1	1	6	Major	Yes
Kanamycin	5.0 mg/kg IM or IV	20	200	5	NA	2	35	Major	Yes
Methicillin	2.0 g IV	80	1000	30	5	0.5	4	Minor	Yes
Metronidazole	8.0 mg/kg IV	25	100	20	10	8	8	Minor	Yes
Mezlocillin	3.0 g IV	190	>2000	100	16	1	4	Minor	Yes
Moxalactam	1.0 g IV	100	>1000	60	1–30[f]	2	19	Major	Yes
Nafcillin	1.0 g IV	70	150	40	2	1	2	Minor	No
Oxacillin	1.0 g IV	70	500	2.5	1	1	2	Minor	No
Penicillin G	3 million units IV	115	300	15	6	1	4	Minor	Yes
Piperacillin	3.0 g IV	190	>2000	50	20	1	4	Minor	Yes
Ticarcillin	3.0 g IV	190	>2000	50	20	1	15	Major	Yes
Tobramycin	1.5 mg/kg IM or IV	6	50	2	1	2	35	Major	Yes
Vancomycin	0.5 g IV	30	100	3	3	6	120	Major	No

[a] Doses listed are the lowest doses that would normally be employed for adults or children over 32 kg with normal renal function in the treatment of systemic infections.
[b] Blood levels are at 1–2 h after IM or at the end of 20–30 min IV infusion. In most instances considerably higher serum levels are attainable with higher dosages. For example, 2 g of ampicillin would yield a peak blood level of 70–90 μg/mL, 2 g of cefoxitin a peak blood level of 120–140 μg/mL.
[c] Drug concentrations may be significantly lower if the patient is producing a very dilute urine or if creatinine clearance is below 10 mL/min. Concentration based on mean levels for the first 4 h after drug is administered.
[d] Assuming no biliary obstruction.
[e] Meningeal inflammation; in meningitis higher doses than those listed would normally be employed resulting in higher CSF levels. For example, 2 g of cefotaxime is usually used.
[f] Value at higher dose.
NOTE: NA = not appropriate therapy for meningitis; — = data not available.

at the time therapy is initiated. Antimicrobial therapy is started empirically in many situations. Empiric selection of an antimicrobial agent should be based on a knowledge of the likely pathogens and their antimicrobial susceptibility. For example, the most common cause of urinary tract infections is *Escherichia coli*. When dealing with outpatient urinary tract infections, therapy should be selected to inhibit this microorganism; therapy for treatment of a nosocomial urinary tract infection might be quite different. Bacteria other than *E. coli* are likely to produce urinary infection, particularly in the presence of an indwelling urethral catheter, and nosocomial pathogens are likely to be resistant to many antibiotics.

The host plays an extremely important role in the selection of an antimicrobial. The antibiotics chosen to treat a febrile, neutropenic patient will be different than those for a healthy individual with a minor infection. Host factors also have an important impact on the route of administration of antimicrobial agents and upon the duration of therapy.

IDENTIFICATION OF THE INFECTING ORGANISMS There are a number of techniques for the rapid identification of the infecting microorganism. A Gram stain is a simple, inexpensive, and rapid method to identify many bacteria and fungi. This technique should be applied to all available body fluids such as urine, wound exudate, synovial fluid, pleural fluid, peritoneal fluid, and cerebrospinal fluid. In situations in which material for diagnosis is not available, knowledge of the most likely pathogens will be beneficial in directing the selection of an antimicrobial agent. For example, following an animal bite an organism such as *Pasteurella multocida* should be suspected. Cellulitis in the foot of a diabetic patient should suggest hemolytic streptococci, *Staphylococcus aureus,* as well as anaerobes.

SUSCEPTIBILITY OF INFECTING MICROORGANISMS There are a number of different methods for determining the susceptibility of bacteria to antimicrobial agents. Susceptibility tests for viruses and fungi are less well developed, and very few laboratories have the ability to determine susceptibility of parasites to antiparasitic drugs.

A commonly used method to determine bacterial susceptibility to antibiotics is a disk diffusion method, which provides data within 24 h. It is semiquantitative, not useful for many slow-growing or fastidious organisms, and has not been adequately standardized for anaerobic bacteria. With the disk method, results are usually given as susceptible, resistant, and intermediate. A *susceptible* zone of inhibition correlates with serum and urine levels that are readily achievable with standard doses of the agent being tested. A *resistant* reading indicates that the zone of inhibition, using regression analysis, is less than that which would correspond to a concentration that could be achieved in blood under normal circumstances. *Intermediate* susceptibility means that the organism falls into a category that is necessary because of the splay in data correlating zone size with minimum inhibitory concentrations (MIC). This is particularly true if the infecting organism is found in a urine specimen in which the concentration of antimicrobial agent would be much higher than in blood or tissues.

Quantitative data on the susceptibility of particular organisms can be determined by micro or macro broth-dilution techniques. These methods detect the lowest concentration of antimicrobial agent that prevents visible growth after an 18- to 24-h incubation period (MIC). To understand MIC values it is essential to understand the pharmacokinetics of an antimicrobial agent. In general, an organism is considered susceptible when the MIC is no more than one-fourth of the readily obtainable peak serum level of the antimicrobial agent. It is also possible to determine the minimal bactericidal concentration (MBC) or minimal lethal concentration (MLC). This is defined as the concentration of drug that reduces the original inoculum by 99.9 percent as judged by subculture on antibiotic-free medium. MBC determinations are necessary in only a few situations that will be discussed below.

The large number of antimicrobial agents has made it difficult to test all antimicrobial agents against an isolate, and a particular compound is used as the class representative for a group of compounds. For example, among the first-generation cephalosporins, cephalothin is the representative drug that, either in a disk or in a broth-dilution system, is used to represent susceptibility to cephapirin, cefazolin, cephalexin, cephradine, and cefaclor. Occasionally, susceptibility tests provide incorrect information. For example, methicillin-resistant *S. aureus* appear susceptible to cephalosporin antibiotics, but are not. Most susceptibility tests do not readily identify a resistant subpopulation.

Some microorganisms have remained susceptible to the same drugs since antibiotics were discovered, and in them development of resistance is exceedingly rare. Examples are group A streptococci which are susceptible to penicillins and cephalosporins. Hence most laboratories do not report susceptibilities of group A streptococci. However, group A streptococci may be resistant to erythromycin, and if the use of this drug is contemplated, susceptibility tests may be necessary. Most strains of *Streptococcus pneumoniae* remain susceptible to penicillin. However, some isolates have intermediate susceptibility; that is, the MICs are between 0.1 and 1.0 μg/mL. Although such a penicillin concentration can readily be achieved in the blood and lung, it may be difficult to achieve cerebrospinal fluid concentrations that are tenfold this level. For this reason, pneumococci isolated from the CSF should be tested for penicillin susceptibility.

CLINICAL PHARMACOLOGY Knowledge of the clinical pharmacology of antimicrobial agents is important in selecting therapeutic programs that are both effective and safe. Antimicrobial agents can be administered by the oral, intramuscular, intravenous, intraperitoneal, or topical routes. After absorption they dissolve in the plasma and are variably bound to plasma proteins. From the plasma they are distributed to various extracellular tissues and fluids in which they may be free or bound. As an antibiotic is distributed into extravascular compartments, there is an initial fall in plasma concentration. Peak concentrations of antimicrobial agents after intravenous infusion occur at the end of the infusion. In contrast, after intramuscular injection, and after oral ingestion, there is an initial slow distribution phase, that is, a combination of absorption and simultaneous excretion or metabolism. Peak serum levels following oral ingestion of antimicrobial agents usually occur in 1 to 2 h. Continued decrease in serum levels of antimicrobial agents is related to renal and biliary excretion and to the hepatic metabolism of some drugs. The amount of drug that reaches the extravascular tissues in which the infection is present depends not only on the concentration gradient from serum to tissue, but also on protein binding in serum and in tissues and the diffusibility of the agent. The diffusibility of antimicrobial agents is a function of their molecular size, dissociation constant, and lipid solubility.

Several pharmacokinetic indexes are useful in adjusting the dosage of antimicrobial agents. The half-life of a drug is the time required for the plasma concentration to fall by one-half as it is being eliminated from the body. Half-life refers to the drug elimination phase after the absorption of the drug has been completed and the drug has been distributed throughout its entire volume of distribution. The assumption is that the fall in plasma concentration parallels the fall in the total amount of drug in the body. Direct extrapolation of the frequency of dosing from half-life considerations is not completely appropriate. The MIC of the infecting organism, site of infection, and host defense mechanisms must be considered in determining dose frequency.

Another pharmacokinetic index that may be useful for guiding therapy is the volume of distribution (V_d). This is the volume in which the total amount of drug in the body would have to be uniformly distributed in order to give the observed plasma concentration. Simplistically it is calculated by the formula $V_d = A/C_p$, where A is amount of drug administered and C_p is plasma concentration. The volume of distribution does not correspond to an actual anatomic or physiologic space. It is useful for determining initial or loading doses and in calculating subsequent or maintenance doses to achieve safe, therapeutic plasma concentrations. When a drug dose is given repetitively at regular intervals, the peak concentration and the minimal concentration eventually reach a constant state if there is no change in the rate of drug elimination. With most antimicrobial agents it is not necessary to use an initial loading dose. However, when agents such as the aminoglycosides are used to treat serious infections such as suspected bacteremia or pneumonia, a loading dose which will provide an initial plasma and tissue concentration well above the MIC of the suspected infecting microorganisms is used.

The half-lives of many antibiotics have been determined in healthy young males. Prolongation of a drug half-life often may result from renal or hepatic dysfunction. Half-life may also be influenced by age and may be shortened in certain disease states. Other drugs administered concomitantly can also either prolong or shorten a drug's half-life.

HOST FACTORS A number of different host factors have a significant influence on the efficacy and toxicity of antimicrobial agents.

Allergic history It is critical to obtain a history of previous adverse reactions to antimicrobial agents since similar reactions may occur to drugs within the same class.

Age Certain antimicrobial agents should not be given to individuals in some age groups. Sulfonamides should not be administered to pregnant females or to newborns because they bind to serum albumin, displacing bilirubin, which may result in kernicterus. Premature and newborn babies produce an inadequate amount of glucuronyltransferase, the enzyme that inactivates chloramphenicol, and some newborns treated with this drug may develop the "gray baby syndrome," which is characterized by progressive pallor, cyanosis, vasomotor collapse, and death. Tetracyclines should not be administered to pregnant females, newborn infants, or to children below 8 years of age because the drugs bind to developing bone and tooth structure, which may cause permanent brownish discoloration of the teeth.

Renal function Many antimicrobial agents are removed from the body by renal excretion. Glomerular and some tubular functions do not develop to adult levels until at least 2 months of age, and drugs administered to premature or newborn infants must be given at different dosage schedules than those used for older children or adults. With advancing age, renal function decreases, and approximately 1 percent of glomerular clearance is lost per year over the age of 30. Antimicrobial agents removed from the body purely by glomerular filtration will accumulate as glomerular filtration declines, resulting in toxicity to other organs or to the kidney itself. Even compounds removed from the body by tubular secretion will accumulate as renal function falls below creatinine clearance of 20 mL/min. Toxic levels of certain penicillins, aminoglycosides, tetracyclines, and quinolones may develop in the presence of markedly reduced renal function. Serum creatinine or blood urea nitrogen may not reflect the true state of renal function in an elderly individual with a small body mass. Hence in calculating the dose of antimicrobial agent it is necessary to consider age, sex, and body weight.

Hepatic function Some antimicrobial agents are metabolized and removed from the body primarily by hepatic mechanisms. These include some of the macrolides, rifamycins, imidazoles, chloramphenicol, quinolones, and linconoid drugs. Reductions in dose may be necessary to avoid toxic concentrations of these agents. Chloramphenicol, clindamycin, and tetracyclines accumulate in patients with severe liver disease. The half-lives of both rifampin and isoniazid are prolonged in patients with extensive hepatic disease. Some drugs which are excreted by biliary mechanisms are excreted by the kidney in the presence of hepatic failure. Conversely, some compounds that are normally excreted by the kidney are excreted in the bile in the presence of renal failure. In the presence of combined biliary and hepatic disease, toxic levels may be reached. Examples are cefoperazone, which is primarily excreted by biliary mechanisms, and carbenicillin and ticarcillin, which are primarily renally excreted but in the presence of combined hepatic and renal failure accumulate in the plasma.

Pregnancy Antimicrobial agents cross the placenta to varying degrees. Most penicillins, cephalosporins, and erythromycins are not teratogenic and are safe in pregnant women. Tetracyclines should not be used in pregnancy not only because of their effect upon fetal dentition but also because they have a propensity to cause fatty necrosis of the liver, pancreatitis, and possible renal damage in pregnant females. If streptomycin is used to treat tuberculosis in pregnancy, it can cause abnormalities of vestibular function and hearing in the child.

Genetic factors A number of different antimicrobial agents will produce hemolysis in patients with glucose-6-phosphate dehydrogenase deficiency. These include sulfonamides, nitrofurantoin, furazoline, chloramphenicol, pyrimethamine, and various sulfones.

The rate at which isoniazid is inactivated by acetylation in the liver is genetically determined. In the United States and North European populations, 50 to 60 percent of individuals are slow inactivators of this drug. Polyneuritis is seen more frequently as a complication of isoniazid therapy in individuals who are slow acetylators.

Site of infection The site of infection is one of the most important factors in determining the choice of a dose and route by which the antimicrobial is administered. Adequate concentrations of a drug must be delivered to the site of the infection. In many situations, if the local concentration of an antimicrobial equals or exceeds the minimum inhibitory concentration of the infecting microorganism, cure will result, but only in those areas of the body in which there are adequate host defenses such as polymorphonuclear cells, complement, and antibody. Where these factors are inadequate or absent, such as in the spinal fluid or on the heart valves, concentrations at least fourfold and preferably five- to tenfold above the MIC, or even MBC, are needed to achieve a cure. Even when concentrations above the MICs are not achieved, there will be an effect on the microorganisms that will aid the host's counterattack. Subinhibitory concentrations of antimicrobial agents alter the adherence properties of microorganisms, thereby decreasing further invasion. Subinhibitory concentrations also alter surface structures, enhancing phagocytosis. Subinhibitory concentrations of antibiotics, by binding to the surface of microorganisms, enhance the intracellular killing of bacteria ingested by phagocytic cells. These factors may explain the unusual circumstances in which antimicrobial agents in seemingly inadequate doses result in clinical cure. Nonetheless, the major goal of therapy should be to achieve concentrations above the MIC in all tissues.

In general, antimicrobial agents are widely distributed and reach adequate concentrations in many infected sites, including pleural, pericardial, and infected joint fluids and infections in muscles or skin structures. An exception are vegetations on the heart valves in endocarditis. Although the valves are exposed to the circulation, the bacteria often are trapped deep within the fibrin vegetation. The organisms are growing less rapidly, making them less susceptible to many antibiotics, and there is inadequate phagocytic function in the focal valvular infection. Because of these factors, therapy of bacterial endocarditis requires bactericidal agents that are administered for long periods of time and that achieve such high concentration in the blood that diffusion of the antibiotic into the vegetation occurs (see Chap. 90).

Meningitis is another disease in which the concentration of antimicrobial agent in the infected site is critical. Many antimicrobial agents cross the blood-brain barrier poorly and do not produce adequate cerebrospinal fluid levels, for example, parenteral aminoglycosides. Lipid-soluble agents can cross the spinal fluid barrier easily, accounting for the utility of chloramphenicol. This agent has proved highly effective in the therapy of meningitis due to *Streptococcus pneumoniae, Haemophilus influenzae,* and *Neisseria meningitidis* because of the bactericidal concentrations it produces in the cerebrospinal fluid. Chloramphenicol is not useful in treating meningitis due to *E. coli* or *Klebsiella pneumoniae,* even if the organisms are susceptible in vitro, because it is not bactericidal for these organisms, and concentrations eightfold above the MBC cannot be achieved within the cerebrospinal fluid. Fortunately, antimicrobials such as cefotaxime, ceftizoxime, ceftriaxone, ceftazidime, and moxalactam all enter the cerebrospinal fluid in concentrations adequate to treat both the common causes of meningitis and the less frequently encountered gram-negative organisms.

An infectious site that may be particularly refractory to treatment involves bones in areas of devitalized tissue, as occurs in diabetics and other patients with inadequate blood supply due to vascular insufficiency. Penetration of the antimicrobial agents to the site of the infection may be only borderline or inadequate. Antimicrobial agents must be administered in high concentrations for prolonged periods to yield adequate concentration within bone. Even with extended therapy, many cases of chronic osteomyelitis are never completely cured since some of the bacteria are in a resting state and do not come into contact with the antimicrobial agent.

In some instances the surgeon's knife is the only mechanism by which an abscess can be cured. Others, like lung abscess, can be treated without surgical intervention in most situations since the abscess can drain via the bronchi, and the antimicrobial agents kill bacteria in the surrounding inflammatory tissue (see Chap. 207). Lung abscesses 8 to 10 cm in diameter frequently do not respond to antimicrobial therapy alone since there is inadequate diffusion of the antimicrobial agent into the cavity and organisms persist. Other abscesses which may respond to antimicrobial therapy alone are those of the ovary, brain, and liver. Ultrasound, computed tomography (CT) scanning, and magnetic resonance imaging (MRI) have demonstrated detectable decreases in abscess size with antimicrobial treatment alone. In general, abscesses in other parts of the abdomen require external drainage, since antimicrobial agents by themselves fail to sterilize the majority of them. Exceptions have been noted with some anaerobic microorganisms; compounds such as metronidazole diffuse into the abscess and destroy the anaerobic organisms.

Local factors within an abscess can have an important impact upon the activity of certain antimicrobial agents. For example, in the case of a mixed aerobic and anaerobic abscess, the anaerobic organisms may produce β-lactamases that will destroy the β-lactam compound that is being used to inhibit the aerobic gram-negative bacilli. Aminoglycoside antibiotics are significantly less active in an anaerobic abscess since they require an aerobic environment for antimicrobial activity. They are less effective at an acid pH than at pH 7.4. Gentamicin or tobramycin might inhibit a *Klebsiella* at 0.1 μg/mL at pH 7.4, but in the infected lung the pH is 6.4 to 6.5. Aminoglycosides are ten- to thirtyfold less active at this pH than they are at pH 7.4. Cellular debris from decaying white cells will complex with aminoglycosides and reduce their activity. In a hyperosmolar environment some β-lactam antimicrobial agents may be less effective because they will not produce death of the microorganism. Agents such as methenamine, nitrofurantoin, and chlortetracycline are more active at an acid pH; the activities of erythromycin, clindamycin, and aminoglycosides are greater in an alkaline milieu.

Foreign bodies have an extremely important effect on the response to antimicrobial agents. Infections of prosthetic heart valves or joint implants usually are not cured by antimicrobial agents even though the organisms infecting the foreign body are highly susceptible to antibiotics. It is thought that a glycocalyx develops that adheres to the foreign material and provides a cover for the microorganisms. Organisms such as *Staphylococcus epidermidis* send projections into small defects in the polypropylene material used in catheters and other foreign devices. The methylmethacrylate used in artificial joints provides a large number of interstices in which microorganisms avoid exposure to antimicrobial agents. Indwelling urethral catheters are another example of a foreign body which makes it virtually impossible to eradicate infecting microorganisms. Unless the catheter is removed, the organisms will not be eradicated. Calculi, whether in the urinary or biliary tracts, provide a haven for microorganisms.

ANTIMICROBIAL COMBINATIONS Although the majority of infections can be treated with a single antimicrobial agent, there are definite situations in which the combination of antimicrobial agents is indicated. However, combination antimicrobial therapy is used much more frequently than necessary and may have deleterious results.

The combination of two or three antimicrobial agents may have one of three different effects. Drugs are *additive* when their activity in combination equals the sum of their separate, independent activities. *Synergistic* activity implies that the activity of two or three antimicrobials is greater than the sum of their independent activities. Drugs are *antagonistic* when the activity of the combination is less than the sum of the independent effects.

Preventing the emergence of resistant organisms is one of the most common indications for combination therapy. For example, the mycobacteria causing tuberculosis consist of a population of organisms of varying susceptibility to antituberculous drugs. The large number of bacilli in a tuberculous lung cavity contain organisms that are intrinsically resistant to the antituberculous agent. Mutants resistant to antituberculosis agents occur at a rate of 1 in 10^{-6} organisms. For this reason, two or three drugs are utilized in the treatment of this disease. The concept of the use of multiple drugs in the treatment of tuberculosis is particularly important for isoniazid-resistant organisms.

Use of rifampin as a single agent to treat staphylococcal infections rapidly results in the emergence of strains resistant to the antibiotic. However, the combination of a β-lactam antibiotic with rifampin reduces the chance for the emergence of such resistant strains. Combination of an aminoglycoside with a cephalosporin has not been shown to prevent the emergence of resistance in *Enterobacter* or *Citrobacter* species.

A second major reason for combination therapy is to treat polymicrobial infections. Intraperitoneal and pelvic infections are usually due to an aerobic and anaerobic flora. Although some antimicrobial agents inhibit both aerobic and anaerobic species, it may not always be feasible to use these drugs clinically. Combination therapy might include an agent effective against the anaerobic organism and an agent effective against the aerobic gram-negative rod. Brain abscesses are frequently caused by *Bacteroides* and anaerobic or microaerophilic streptococci. Metronidazole penetrates extremely well into the abscess and has excellent activity against the *Bacteroides* species. However, it has poor activity against streptococcal species. Penicillin will penetrate into the brain adequately to kill the streptococcal species but cannot be used singly since it would be destroyed in the brain abscess by the β-lactamases frequently elaborated by the *Bacteroides* strains.

A theoretical reason for the use of drug combinations is to lower concentrations of compounds that have toxic potential. However, there is no clinical evidence to substantiate the use of two drugs at lower concentrations than that at which they would normally be utilized.

One of the major indications for combined antimicrobial therapy is to provide a broad spectrum of coverage for the patient who is neutropenic and has significantly compromised host defenses. It has been the practice to use a broad-spectrum antipseudomonas penicillin or cephalosporin combined with an aminoglycoside as initial therapy for the febrile neutropenic patient. The increasing number of infections due to β-lactam-resistant gram-positive species has led to the use of vancomycin in combination with β-lactams.

Although synergism can be demonstrated in the laboratory with many antimicrobial combinations, in only a few clinical settings has combination therapy proved more effective than single agents. The most widely accepted combination therapy is penicillin G or ampicillin with an aminoglycoside, streptomycin or gentamicin, for the treatment of enterococcal endocarditis. The drugs enhance the uptake of each other, and the enterococci are killed. Similar synergism can be demonstrated between semisynthetic penicillinase-resistant penicillins, such as nafcillin or oxacillin, and gentamicin against *S. aureus*. However, clinical data do not show that this combination has advantages over use of a single drug. Combinations of antipseudomonas penicillins with aminoglycosides are synergistic against many strains of *Pseudomonas aeruginosa*. Clinical trials have demonstrated the superiority of these combinations in neutropenic patients.

The combination of trimethoprim with sulfamethoxazole inhibits two critical points in the folic acid cycle, which is part of the production pathway of DNA. In vitro and animal experiments demonstrate that the two drugs are more effective than either drug alone. The major situation in which the combination is necessary is in treatment of *Pneumocystis carinii* infection. In urinary tract infections trimethoprim alone is as effective as the combination.

Examples of drug synergism are combinations of a β-lactam drug with a β-lactamase inhibitor: an amoxicillin and clavulanate (augmentin), ticarcillin and clavulanate (timentin), and sulbactam with ampicillin. Combination of a β-lactamase-susceptible β-lactam with a β-lactamase inhibitor enhances the antibacterial spectrum of a drug that would normally be destroyed by β-lactamase. Amoxicillin-clavulanate and sulbactam-ampicillin inhibit *Haemophilus, Branhamella, E. coli, Salmonella, S. aureus, Fusobacterium, Bacteroides, Neisseria,* and *Klebsiella,* which are resistant to amoxicillin or ampicillin.

Another form of synergy is that shown by amdinocillin, which binds to a specific penicillin-binding protein different from the proteins to which other penicillins and cephalosporins bind. When combined with various β-lactams, amdinocillin synergistically inhibits some gram-negative bacteria.

Disadvantages of antimicrobial combinations There are a few examples of antagonism of antimicrobial agents. In the 1950s it was demonstrated that penicillin alone was more effective than a combination of penicillin and chlortetracycline for the treatment of pneumococcal meningitis.

Combination therapy may result in superinfection with other organisms, particularly fungi, since the combination obliterates the normal protective flora of the oropharynx and the intestine. This problem can be avoided by discontinuing unnecessary empiric combination therapy once the diagnosis has been established. Another adverse effect of combination therapy may be increased drug reactions or other metabolic side effects.

ROUTE OF ADMINISTRATION OF ANTIMICROBIAL AGENTS Having determined the most appropriate agent to treat a given infection, the most appropriate route of administration should be determined. The choice usually lies between the oral and the parenteral route. Oral administration of antimicrobial agents has generally been for infections that are mild and are treated on an outpatient basis. As hospital costs have risen, reevaluation of this concept is necessary. Some serious infections initially may be treated parenterally; then therapy can be completed with an oral antibiotic. Examples would be osteomyelitis, pneumonitis, or severe skin infections that have begun to respond to parenteral therapy. When drugs are administered by the oral route, it is important to be certain that the patient takes the drug in a manner that will result in the best blood and tissue levels. The absorption of many antimicrobial agents is markedly decreased by food. Tetracyclines form a soluble chelate with magnesium, calcium, aluminum, or iron. Quinolone absorption is reduced by aluminum and magnesium but not by calcium. In a number of infections it may be possible to administer an oral antimicrobial agent twice a day rather than four times a day. This may be important for patient compliance.

The parenteral route is used for agents that are not absorbed from the gastrointestinal tract, and for serious infections in which a high concentration of the antimicrobial agent is needed immediately. Examples are suspected bacteremia, meningitis, and gram-negative pneumonia. Intravenous administration of most drugs is preferred since it provides for high serum concentration. There are no definitive data that show whether bolus, 3- to 5-min injection, infusion over 15 to 30 min, or continuous administration of a drug by the intravenous route is more effective in curing bacterial infection. Serum concentrations adequate to treat many infections are achieved after intramuscular administration. With some agents with extremely long half-lives it may be possible to complete therapy of serious infections by administration of the drug intramuscularly once a day. It is rarely necessary to instill antimicrobial agents into infected cavities. Peritonitis in patients receiving peritoneal dialysis may respond better to administration of the antimicrobial agent in the dialysis solution. Meningitis due to *Coccidioides immitis* and some gram-negative species may require intraventricular or intrathecal therapy.

MONITORING PATIENT RESPONSE With some antimicrobial agents it is essential that serum levels of the agent be monitored. For the aminoglycoside antibiotics, peak levels should be obtained to determine that effective concentrations are being achieved and trough levels should be measured to determine that the drugs are not accumulating and producing nephrotoxicity or ototoxicity. Except for renal failure, it is not necessary to monitor serum concentrations of β-lactam antibiotics.

Serum bactericidal titers, defined as the dilution of serum which will kill the infecting pathogen in vitro, have been used extensively to monitor therapy of bacterial endocarditis. There has been wide variation in the performance of serum bactericidal titers, but guidelines for their use have been developed. If a standardized inoculum of organisms is used and standard media and techniques employed, the tests are useful in certain clinical situations. For example, a peak serum bactericidal titer >1:64 correlates with a 98 percent bacteriologic cure of endocarditis. However, clinical cure cannot be predicted since damage to the valve as a result of the endocarditis may result in valvular insufficiency requiring surgery. A peak serum bactericidal titer greater than 1:8 correlates with a successful outcome in osteomyelitis, bacteremia, septic arthritis, and empyema.

PROPHYLAXIS WITH ANTIMICROBIAL AGENTS Antibiotic prophylaxis should be directed at preventing specific bacterial infection. This means that a particular species or several species of microorganisms have been shown to produce the infection, that an effective antibiotic is available, and that the risk of the infection outweighs the hazard of the antibiotic. The antibiotic must achieve adequate concentrations at the site at which infection would occur, and it must prevent colonization or eliminate organisms that could potentially cause infection. In the case of surgical prophylaxis, the antibiotic must be delivered to the site of probable infection in time to inhibit bacteria that would colonize the area and produce subsequent infection, and the agent must be present for 3 to 4 h after the incision. In some situations it is sufficient to decrease the number of pathogens but not eradicate them. The duration of prophylaxis must be short to avoid toxicity and prevent selection of a resistant bacterial flora by eliminating the normal flora.

Prophylaxis can be divided into medical and surgical situations. Medical situations in which it has been successful include meningococcal meningitis, *Haemophilus influenzae* meningitis, recurrence of rheumatic fever, postsplenectomy, pneumococcal or *Haemophilus* infection, cellulitis complicating lymphedema, recurrent cystitis, tuberculosis, and bacterial endocarditis. A special medical problem is the prevention of infection in the neutropenic patient. Many of the bacteremias in neutropenic patients are of gastrointestinal origin, and use of agents that eliminate the aerobic gram-negative flora reduces the incidence of gram-negative sepsis (see Chap. 82).

Numerous surgical situations qualify for prophylaxis—upper gastrointestinal surgery, cholecystectomy, colon surgery, appendectomy, head and neck surgery, cardiac surgery, prosthetic hip and other joint surgery, hysterectomy, and cesarean section. The optimum agent for each clinical situation has not been established.

Prophylaxis can be effective without eradicating all of the bacteria in an area. Topical application of silver sulfadiazine or mafenide to burn eschars will reduce the number of bacteria in the burn eschar to less than 10^5 per gram of tissue. This prevents sepsis in the burn and allows healing.

Antibiotics do not alter an underlying pathophysiologic state. Trimethoprim-sulfamethoxazole (TMP/SMX) will prevent recurrent urinary tract infections in women with recurrent cystitis. However, even if an individual uses TMP/SMX for 6 months, reinfection can recur when the antimicrobial agent is discontinued if the patient's perineal area is recolonized with *E. coli* that have fimbriae with receptors for the urethra and bladder of the patient (see Chap. 95).

SPECIFIC ANTIMICROBIAL AGENTS

β-LACTAM ANTIBIOTICS β-Lactam antibiotics interfere with bacterial cell wall biosynthesis by binding to proteins, referred to as penicillin-binding proteins (PBPs), which by transpeptidation produce crosslinking of peptidoglycan chains that form the bacterial cell wall. The most common form of resistance is that due to β-lactamases. In staphylococci, β-lactamases are plasmid-mediated exoenzymes with affinity primarily for penicillins. In gram-negative aerobic and anaerobic species, β-lactamase synthesis is either plasmid- or chromosomally mediated and the enzymes are in the periplasmic space. β-Lactamases of gram-negatives can have affinity primarily for penicillins or for cephalosporins, or they may be capable of destroying both classes of compounds.

Resistance to β-lactams can be due to failure to bind to PBPs, as occurs with methicillin-resistant staphylococci and penicillin-resistant pneumococci. Resistance can be due to failure of the β-lactam to reach a receptor, i.e., cross the bacterial cell wall. Rarely, resistance of gram-positive bacteria to β-lactams is due to failure to activate autolysins.

PENICILLINS Penicillins can be divided into several classes on the basis of antibacterial activity.

Natural penicillins Penicillin G and penicillin V are the two natural penicillins. Penicillin G is available as an orally, intramuscularly, and intravenously administered compound. Penicillin G is combined with procaine as a 1:1 molar salt which extends the half-life of the drug, and it is combined with benzathine to produce a long-acting repository form. Penicillin V is available only for oral use. The antibacterial activity of penicillin G and penicillin V includes *S. pneumoniae,* beta-hemolytic streptococci, viridans group streptococci, and microaerophilic and anaerobic streptococci. Most *S. aureus* and *S. epidermidis* produce β-lactamases which destroy both penicillin G and V. *Neisseria meningitidis* are susceptible to penicillin G. In many parts of the world penicillinase-producing *N. gonorrhoeae* are a significant problem. Penicillin G has excellent activity against clostridial species and also inhibits many oral *Bacteroides* species and *Fusobacterium* species. Penicillin V does not have good activity against species such as *Haemophilus* or *Branhamella,* which are important pathogens causing sinusitis, otitis, and other upper respiratory infections. Infrequently encountered organisms for which penicillin G remains an excellent drug are *Erysipelothrix, Listeria monocytogenes, Pasteurella multocida, Streptobacillus, Spirillum, Fusospirochetes, Treponema pallidum,* and *Actinomyces israelii,* as well as the *Borrelia* which causes Lyme disease.

Penicillin G is not stable in gastric acid and should not be used as an oral preparation. In contrast, penicillin V is 60 percent absorbed when given orally, and food causes only a minor decrease in absorption. Penicillin V is an effective agent in treatment of streptococcal infections and less serious forms of pneumococcal pneumonia. It should not be used to treat syphilis, gonorrhea, or *Haemophilus* infections. Penicillin G remains the treatment of choice for viridans group streptococcal endocarditis and for most cases of pneumococcal and meningococcal meningitis. Since penicillin G has a short half-life due to rapid tubular secretion, it must be administered on a 4- or 6-hourly basis. Only minor dosage adjustments are necessary until the creatinine clearance falls below 30 mL/min. Even in the presence of renal failure, doses of 4,000,000 to 6,000,000 units per day can be administered safely. Benzathine penicillin, which has a half-life of a week, can be used in the treatment of streptococcal pharyngitis, in the therapy of primary and early syphilis, and in the prevention of recurrences of rheumatic fever when administered once monthly.

Aminopenicillins Aminopenicillins have an amino group on the β-acyl side chain of the penicillin nucleus. A number of different compounds are available. They differ microbiologically to a minor degree. Ampicillin was the first aminopenicillin. Subsequently, amoxicillin was produced, and other agents such as bacampicillin, cyclacillin, epicillin, hetacillin, and pivampicillin have been synthesized. Aminopenicillins retain the in vitro activity of penicillin G. In addition, they inhibit many *H. influenzae* and are more active against *Enterococcus faecalis*. Many *E. coli* are inhibited by aminopenicillins, as are *Proteus mirabilis*. In the United States, many *Salmonella* species and *Shigella* species are inhibited by ampicillin, but in developing countries most strains are resistant to aminopenicillins. Aminopenicillins inhibit most mouth organisms, but do not inhibit *Pseudomonas* species, *Klebsiella, Enterobacter,* and the majority of *Bacteroides fragilis* species. In some parts of the United States, 35 percent of *H. influenzae* contain a β-lactamase, making them resistant to the aminopenicillins.

Amoxicillin and bacampicillin are absorbed approximately twice as well as ampicillin. Bacampicillin is an ester of ampicillin that is converted in the intestinal mucosa and in plasma to free ampicillin. Administered parenterally, ampicillin is well distributed to most body compartments and therapeutic concentrations are achieved in the cerebrospinal, pleural, joint, and peritoneal fluids in the presence of inflammation. Urinary levels are high. Although ampicillin can be administered intramuscularly, orally administered amoxicillin will produce serum levels comparable to those achieved by intramuscular injection of similar amounts of ampicillin. Ampicillin currently is used in the treatment of outpatient urinary tract infections, upper respiratory infections, otitis media, sinusitis, bacterial exacerbations of bronchitis, and community-acquired pneumonia. It is effective therapy for pneumococcal and meningococcal meningitis, and is used in the therapy of enterococcal endocarditis, always in combination with an aminoglycoside. For oral therapy, amoxicillin should replace ampicillin due to its better absorption. The one clinical setting in which amoxicillin is inferior to ampicillin is in the treatment of shigellosis. Amoxicillin and bacampicillin can be administered three times a day and still attain adequate blood, tissue, and urinary levels for treatment of susceptible organisms.

Although allergic reactions of the hypersensitivity type to the aminopenicillins occur with the same frequency as with penicillin G or V, there is an increased risk of skin rash with oral ampicillin. It is estimated that 8 to 10 percent of patients receiving oral ampicillin develop a skin rash. As many as 90 percent of patients with infectious mononucleosis receiving ampicillin develop a maculopapular rash beginning approximately 4 days after therapy is instituted. This rash does not represent true penicillin allergy and does not mean that the patient can never receive a penicillin again.

Penicillinase-resistant penicillins A number of different penicillinase-resistant penicillins were developed for the treatment of staphylococcal infections. These agents inhibit *S. aureus* and coagulase-negative staphylococci, as well as *S. pyogenes* and *S. pneumoniae*. None of them has activity against *E. faecalis* or against aerobic or anaerobic gram-negative bacilli. Methicillin was the first antistaphylococcal β-lactamase-stable penicillin.

S. aureus resistant to all β-lactams are referred to as methicillin-resistant. These isolates have an altered penicillin-binding protein as the basis of their resistance, and hence these *S. aureus* and similar strains of coagulase-negative staphylococci are resistant to all penicillins and to cephalosporins as well. In vitro tests of methicillin-resistant staphylococci against cephalosporins tend to be unreliable, and may show false-positive susceptibility. The drug of choice for methicillin-resistant staphylococci is vancomycin.

Methicillin can only be used parenterally since it is not acid-stable, and it has a short half-life, necessitating intravenous administration every 4 h. Since interstitial nephritis is a relatively common side effect, methicillin is rarely used today.

Nafcillin has more intrinsic activity than methicillin against both staphylococci and streptococci. It is excreted primarily by the liver, and to a lesser extent by the kidney. Nafcillin should not be used orally since absorption by this route is erratic. The usual dosage of nafcillin is 4 to 12 g/d, depending upon the severity of the infection, and 100 to 200 mg/kg per day for children. Intravenous nafcillin may result in more severe phlebitis than other antistaphylococcal penicillins, and in high doses may result in more neutropenia.

The isoxazolyl penicillins consist of oxacillin, which should be used only parenterally due to poor oral absorption, and the oral preparations cloxacillin and dicloxacillin. In many countries, flucloxacillin is also available as an oral drug, and in some countries cloxacillin is available for parenteral use. Although dicloxacillin produces higher blood levels than cloxacillin, it is slightly more protein-bound, 96 vs. 94 percent, than cloxacillin. The active antibiotic levels of the two drugs are quite similar. In general, cloxacillin or dicloxacillin are administered in doses of 0.5 or 0.25 g four times a day, respectively.

Although the primary indication for the use of antistaphylococcal penicillins is infection due to penicillinase-producing staphylococci, they are often administered before the etiologic agent is known. Blood levels with the penicillinase-resistant penicillins are adequate to inhibit *S. pneumoniae,* except in the CSF, and most hemolytic streptococci; therefore, it is not necessary to give both a penicillinase-resistant penicillin and penicillin G simultaneously. However, infections caused by *E. faecalis* and *Neisseria* do not respond to penicillinase-resistant penicillins, and ampicillin should also be used if these organisms are suspected.

Carboxy penicillins Carbenicillin was the first penicillin with activity against *P. aeruginosa* and certain indole-positive *Proteus* species. Ticarcillin is also a carboxy penicillin, but it is fourfold more active than carbenicillin against *P. aeruginosa* and has replaced carbenicillin. These compounds are destroyed by β-lactamases of gram-positive and some gram-negative organisms but are less readily destroyed by the β-lactamases of species such as *Pseudomonas, Enterobacter, Morganella,* and *Proteus-Providencia.* Carbenicillin and ticarcillin are less active than ampicillin against *S. pyogenes, S. pneumoniae,* and *E. faecalis.* They have excellent activity against non-β-lactamase-producing *Haemophilus, N. meningitidis,* and *N. gonorrhoeae.* In general, the antibacterial activity of the carboxy penicillins against *E. coli, Proteus, Salmonella,* and *Shigella* species is similar to ampicillin. They are inactive against *Klebsiella* since they are destroyed by the β-lactamase of these organisms. Ticarcillin has activity against oral and intestinal *Bacteroides* species, although higher concentrations are required than are needed to inhibit the Enterobacteriaceae. Ticarcillin acts synergistically with aminoglycosides to inhibit *P. aeruginosa.* This group of compounds is rarely used intramuscularly since peak serum levels are inadequate for tissue *Pseudomonas* infections, but they provide adequate concentrations in the urine. Ticarcillin is administered in dosage of 200 to 300 mg/kg per day, divided into 4- or 6-hourly doses for 24 h. Ticarcillin is excreted by the renal tubules and accumulates in the presence of renal dysfunction. Since the drug contains 4.7 mmol of sodium, full doses of 12 to 30 g/d may precipitate congestive heart failure. Hypokalemia may also result since the nonreabsorbable portion of the anion is delivered to the distal tubule where it triggers a hydrogen ion exchange, resulting in potassium loss. Ticarcillin and other penicillins bind to ADP receptor sites on platelets and prevent normal platelet aggregation. Bleeding times are prolonged and clinical bleeding may occur in the presence of high serum levels. Ticarcillin cannot be administered in the same solution as aminoglycosides since it complexes with the aminoglycoside, rendering the aminoglycoside inactive. This does not normally occur in the body, except in the presence of renal failure, when very high concentrations of the antipseudomonas penicillins result in complexing with aminoglycosides. Ticarcillin has proved useful in the therapy of aspiration pneumonia in the hospital setting, in the therapy of the febrile neutropenic patient, in treatment of intraabdominal infection, and in treatment of gynecologic infections.

In the United States, there is only one oral antipseudomonas penicillin, indanyl carbenicillin. This is an alpha-carboxy ester of carbenicillin that has no intrinsic activity of its own, but is acid-stable and moderately well absorbed in the gastrointestinal tract, where it is hydrolyzed to yield free carbenicillin. Indanyl carbenicillin does not provide adequate serum or tissue levels for systemic infection and is useful only for the treatment of urinary tract infections or prostatitis. In the presence of decreased renal function, urine levels may be lower and may be inadequate to treat *Pseudomonas* urinary tract infections. This drug should be replaced by the quinolones.

Ureido penicillins Ureido penicillins, azlocillin, mezlocillin, and piperacillin, in contrast to the carboxy penicillins, are derivatives of ampicillin in which the presence of a side chain linked to the amino group on the alpha carbon provides increased binding to penicillin-binding proteins and more rapid passage through porin channels of gram-negative bacteria. Ureido penicillins are destroyed by β-lactamases of *S. aureus, E. coli, Klebsiella,* and *Bacteroides.* Azlocillin is 4 times more active than ticarcillin against *P. aeruginosa* and is less active against indole-positive *Proteus* species. It has the same activity as ampicillin against streptococcal species. It is not absorbed orally and must be given by the intravenous route to provide adequate serum levels to treat *Pseudomonas* infections. Since ureido penicillins show nonlinear pharmacokinetics, these drugs should be used in a larger dose administered at intervals of 6 h, rather than the 4-h interval used for ticarcillin. Azlocillin does not accumulate in the blood in renal failure to the same degree as ticarcillin. Its half-life increases to a maximum of only 4 h, even when renal insufficiency is present, necessitating less adjustment in dosage. Azlocillin enters the cerebrospinal fluid in the presence of meningeal inflammation, but levels are only 10 percent of serum levels. The drug is used primarily to treat *Pseudomonas* infections; the usual dose is 12 to 18 g/d.

Mezlocillin is a ureido penicillin that differs from ticarcillin by being more active against streptococci, particularly enterococci, and it inhibits approximately 60 percent of *Klebsiella pneumoniae* in a concentration of 16 μg/mL; virtually no *Klebsiella* are inhibited by ticarcillin. It is also more active against *B. fragilis* and *H. influenzae.* Mezlocillin has activity against *P. aeruginosa* similar to that of ticarcillin. Mezlocillin can be given at 6-hourly intervals, and the dose needs to be reduced only moderately as renal function declines. It is the least likely of the broad-spectrum penicillins to alter bleeding times, but the clinical significance of this is unknown. The drug has been effective in the treatment of respiratory, urinary, gynecologic, and surgical infections. Usual doses are 12 to 18 g/d for adults.

Piperacillin has excellent activity against streptococcal species, *Neisseria,* and *Haemophilus,* and it is the most active penicillin against *P. aeruginosa.* Like the other acyl ureido penicillins, it is destroyed by β-lactamases. It inhibits some community-acquired *Klebsiella* and *Bacteroides* species but will not inhibit Enterobacteriaceae which contain the plasmid β-lactamase. The human pharmacology of piperacillin is similar to the other ureido penicillins. It should be administered in a dose of 12 to 18 g/d, at 6-hourly intervals.

Other penicillins Amdinocillin is a penicillin active only against gram-negative species since it does not bind to the penicillin-binding proteins of gram-positive organisms. It has poor activity against *Haemophilus* and *Neisseria,* but is extremely active against *E. coli,* many *Klebsiella, Enterobacter,* and *Citrobacter* species. It has variable activity against *Proteus* species and does not inhibit *Pseudomonas* or *Bacteroides fragilis.* Amdinocillin acts synergistically with other penicillins and has been used in this way. Amdinocillin is not acid-stable and cannot be used orally except as the pivolyl ester which is well absorbed and immediately hydrolyzed, yielding the free compound.

Untoward reactions to penicillins The major adverse effects of penicillins are hypersensitivity reactions which range from minor rashes to immediate anaphylaxis. Anaphylactic reactions and accelerated urticarial reactions are due to IgE antibody. Patients who have had such reactions should not receive penicillins. Drug fever is common with all penicillins. Intestinal side effects produced by penicillins are diarrhea or bouts of enterocolitis, some of which are due to overgrowth of *Clostridium difficile.* Neutropenia, platelet dysfunction, and hemolytic anemia have followed the use of all the penicillins. Minor elevations in serum glutamic oxaloacetic transaminase (SGOT) occur most often with oxacillin, nafcillin, or carbenicillin. Neurologic adverse effects in the form of seizures will occur if penicillin G is administered in high doses to patients with decreased renal function. Renal toxicity has varied from allergic angiitis to interstitial nephritis most commonly with methicillin, but this complication can occur with all penicillins.

CEPHALOSPORINS Cephalosporins differ from penicillins by the presence of a dihydrothiazine ring rather than the five-membered thiazolidine ring fused to the four-membered β-lactam ring. Because of their structural configuration, cephalosporins have been modified chemically to produce compounds with different microbiologic and pharmacologic properties. It is useful to divide cephalosporins into so-called generations. In a particular group of cephalosporins, there may be marked differences in microbiologic activity and pharmacologic properties. Like the penicillins, cephalosporins inhibit cell wall biosynthesis and are bactericidal.

First-generation cephalosporins First-generation cephalosporins include some compounds that can be used only parenterally and some that can be used orally. The parenteral agents are cephalothin, cephapirin, cefazolin, and cephradine. Oral compounds are cephalexin, cephradine, cefadroxil, and cefaclor. First-generation cephalosporins inhibit group A, B, C, and G streptococci and most viridans group streptococci. They are active against *S. pneumoniae, S. aureus,* and *S. epidermidis.* Among the Enterobacteriaceae, *E. coli, P. mirabilis,* and *Klebsiella* species are inhibited. None of these first-generation drugs inhibit *Serratia, Enterobacter,* indole-positive *Proteus, P. aeruginosa,* or *B. fragilis* species. Only cefaclor can be considered therapeutically useful against *Haemophilus.* None of these agents is therapeutic for *Neisseria* species, although all of them have some inhibitory activity against these organisms in vitro.

In some hospitals, 20 to 30 percent of *E. coli* and *Klebsiella* are resistant to first-generation cephalosporins. Nonetheless, one of these agents, cefazolin, has continued to be useful. Cefazolin has a half-life of approximately 2 h and can be administered either by the intramuscular or intravenous routes. It accumulates in the body in the presence of decreased renal function, in which event dosage adjustments must be made. It is normally administered in doses of 0.5 to 1 g every 8 h. Cefazolin has proved useful as therapy of respiratory, skin, and urinary tract infections, and as therapy of endocarditis due to viridans streptococci in penicillin-allergic patients. It is also appropriate therapy for osteomyelitis due to staphylococcal species. Cefazolin is useful as a prophylactic antimicrobial agent at the time of orthopedic surgery, prosthetic valve surgery, and upper gastrointestinal operations. Cephalothin and cephapirin have half-lives of 4 h and are converted in the body to less active desacetyl derivatives. These drugs should be administered every 4 h.

Both cephalexin and cephradine are well absorbed after oral ingestion, yielding peak blood levels in the range of 15 to 20 μg/mL after a 0.5-g dose. Although these cephalosporins are less active against *S. aureus* than the parenteral first-generation cephalosporins, serum and tissue concentrations are adequate to treat many minor staphylococcal infections in penicillin-allergic patients. Both drugs have a half-life of approximately 1 h and are usually administered three or four times daily. The drugs are totally excreted in the urine, yielding high concentrations inhibitory to common urinary pathogens.

Cefadroxil is a parahydroxy derivative of cephalexin which has a longer half-life, allowing it to be administered twice daily. Otherwise, its antimicrobial activity is identical to that of cephalexin.

Cefaclor has found utility primarily as a therapeutic agent for respiratory infections in children caused by *H. influenzae* or other susceptible organisms. It is partially β-lactamase-stable, but the concentrations in ear fluid are adequate to eradicate β-lactamase-producing *H. influenzae.* It should not be used for serious infections caused by β-lactamase-producing strains and is ineffective in urinary tract infections due to β-lactamase-producing *E. coli* and *Klebsiella.*

Second-generation cephalosporins Second-generation cephalosporins probably should not be grouped as a class since the compounds within this class have markedly different antibacterial and pharmacologic properties. They are most frequently used by the intravenous route; only cefuroxime axetil can be used orally. Cefamandole has excellent activity against streptococcal and staphylococcal species with the exception of *E. faecalis.* It is more active than first-generation cephalosporins against *E. coli* and *Klebsiella* and has increased activity against *H. influenzae.* It is destroyed by β-lactamases of some gram-negative species, and is not active against *Bacteroides* or *Pseudomonas* species. Cefamandole has a relatively short half-life, 0.7 h, and is administered every 4 to 6 h in doses of 1 to 2 g. The drug does not produce adequate concentrations in the cerebrospinal fluid, and should not be used in patients in whom meningitis is suspected. Because of potential nephrotoxicity, this drug is used rarely and has been replaced by other cephalosporins.

Cefuroxime is a β-lactamase-stable cephalosporin that inhibits most streptococcal and staphylococcal species, *H. influenzae,* penicillinase-producing *N. gonorrhoeae,* and β-lactamase-producing Enterobacteriaceae. It is not active against *E. faecalis, Bacteroides fragilis,* or *P. aeruginosa.* Cefuroxime has a half-life of approximately 1.5 h, permitting administration at 8-hourly intervals. It enters the cerebrospinal fluid in concentrations adequate to treat meningitis due to *H. influenzae, S. pneumoniae,* and *N. meningitidis.* CSF concentrations are inadequate to treat meningitis due to *E. coli* or *Klebsiella* species. Cefuroxime has been used in the therapy of respiratory infections, biliary tract infections, soft tissue infections, osteomyelitis, and urinary tract infections. It can also be used for therapy of meningitis in children and young adults. Cefuroxime axetil is an oral form for use in respiratory infections, particularly those in which β-lactamase-producing *H. influenzae* are suspected, and for cutaneous infections.

Cefonicid is a cephalosporin structurally related to cefamandole. However, substitution of a different moiety at position 3 of the dihydrothiazine ring has provided the compound with a long half-life of approximately 4 to 5 h. Cefonicid activity is similar to that of cefamandole and cefuroxime, with the exception of lower activity against *S. aureus.* Cefonicid has been used in a single daily dose administered either intravenously or intramuscularly to treat respiratory, skin, and urinary tract infections due to susceptible organisms. It should not be used to treat meningeal infections.

Cefoxitin is a cephalosporin which possesses a methoxy group affixed to the β-lactam that provides excellent β-lactamase resistance but decreases activity against gram-positive organisms such as staphylococci. Cefoxitin inhibits most staphylococci at concentrations of 2 to 4 μg/mL, and *S. pneumoniae* are inhibited at similar concentrations. It possesses no activity against *E. faecalis.* Cefoxitin inhibits *E. coli* and *Klebsiella* species resistant to first-generation cephalosporins. It lacks activity against *Enterobacter* and *Citrobacter* species, and does not inhibit *Pseudomonas.* Cefoxitin has good activity against *B. fragilis,* inhibiting 85 percent of clinical isolates at a concentration between 16 to 32 μg/mL, which is readily achieved in humans. Cefoxitin has a half-life of approximately 0.8 h. It does not yield adequate concentrations within the CSF. The drug accumulates in the presence of decreased renal function, so that dose adjustments must be made. Cefoxitin has been widely used as therapy of mixed aerobic and anaerobic intraabdominal infections and in the treatment of gynecologic infections. Cefoxitin combined with doxycycline is effective therapy for pelvic inflammatory disease. Cefoxitin has also been used as a parenteral prophylactic agent for colon surgery, particularly in patients in whom oral prophylactic programs are not feasible.

Third-generation cephalosporins Third-generation cephalosporins can be grouped into several convenient classes. The first of these are the aminothiazolyl iminomethoxy cephalosporins which consist of cefotaxime, ceftizoxime, cefmenoxime, and ceftriaxone. These agents possess excellent activity against hemolytic streptococci and *S. pneumoniae,* inhibiting these species at concentrations <0.1 μg/mL. They do not inhibit *E. faecalis.* The compounds are highly active against *H. influenzae, N. meningitidis,* and *N. gonorrhoeae,* including β-lactamase-producing strains. Because of their high affinity for penicillin-binding proteins, these compounds inhibit the majority of the Enterobacteriaceae at concentrations below 4.0 μg/mL, although some *Enterobacter* and *Citrobacter* are resistant. These four agents do not show adequate activity against *P. aeruginosa* and *Acinetobacter.*

Cefotaxime has a half-life of approximately 1 h, and it is converted to a desacetyl derivative which has a half-life of approximately 1.6 h. Although the desacetyl derivative is less active than the parent compound, it is more active than most second-generation cephalosporins and acts synergistically with the parent compound to inhibit some microorganisms. Cefotaxime produces concentrations in the CSF ranging from 1 to 30 μg/mL, depending upon the degree of inflammation and the dose used. It has proved effective as therapy of meningitis due to group B streptococci, *E. coli, H. influenzae, N. meningitidis, S. pneumoniae,* and *Klebsiella.* Although cefotaxime has a relatively short half-life, its high activity and the presence of an active metabolite indicate that it can be administered 8-hourly in most infections, except in febrile neutropenic patients.

Ceftizoxime has a slightly longer half-life than cefotaxime at 1.6 h, and can be administered every 8 to 12 h in the majority of infections.

Ceftriaxone differs from the aforementioned compounds because it has a half-life of approximately 7 h in normal individuals. Sixty percent of ceftriaxone is cleared by the kidney, and the remainder of the drug is cleared through the biliary system. Although ceftriaxone is 95 percent bound to serum proteins, it produces such high serum levels that adequate free drug is available to inhibit the majority of gram-positive and gram-negative bacteria with the exception of *E. faecalis, Pseudomonas,* and *Bacteroides.* Ceftriaxone enters the CSF and is removed from the CSF extremely slowly. Levels well above the minimum inhibitory concentration for most meningeal pathogens are present 24 h after the administration of a single dose. Ceftriaxone has been administered once and twice daily to treat a variety of infections and offers the possibility of once-daily intramuscular therapy in the home setting to complete treatment initially instituted within the hospital.

Moxalactam is an oxacephalosporin with oxygen replacing the sulfur in the bicyclic ring structure. The drug possesses an *N*-methylthiotetrazole group at position 3 of the bicyclic structure. This structure has been associated with two adverse reactions. The first is a disulfiram reaction when alcohol is ingested. This is caused by interference with alcohol dehydrogenase and the accumulation of acetaldehyde. The second is hypoprothrombinemia which appears related to dimer formation of the *N*-methylthiotetrazole which interferes with the production of vitamin K. Moxalactam administered in doses above 4 g/d also will cause platelet dysfunction due to its effect on ADP receptors on the platelets. Because of these factors, patients receiving moxalactam should receive vitamin K at least twice weekly, and platelet function should be assessed by bleeding times. Concern over bleeding problems associated with moxalactam has limited its use in the United States.

Cefotetan is a 7-alpha-methoxy cephalosporin that has in vitro activity similar to cefoxitin against anaerobic microorganisms and activity slightly less than that of the aminothiazolyl cephalosporins against gram-positive cocci and the Enterobacteriaceae. It does not inhibit *Pseudomonas* species. Cefotetan has a half-life of approximately 4 h, and can be administered twice or three times daily.

Cephalosporins with activity against *Pseudomonas aeruginosa* Cefoperazone inhibits Enterobacteriaceae and the majority of gram-positive microorganisms, and will inhibit most *P. aeruginosa* at concentrations below 32 μg/mL. It is destroyed by some β-lactamase-producing *E. coli, Klebsiella,* and *B. fragilis* strains. Cefoperazone is approximately 85 percent protein bound. Following a 2-g dose, peak blood levels of 250 μg/mL are achieved. The half-life of the drug is approximately 2 h. Only 25 percent of cefoperazone is removed from the body by the kidney; the remainder is removed by biliary mechanisms. Cefoperazone is used in a dose of 2 g twice daily to treat gram-positive and gram-negative infections. Higher doses are usually needed to treat serious *Pseudomonas* infections. Since cefoperazone contains an *N*-methylthiotetrazole group, it can produce disulfiram reactions and prolongation of the prothrombin time. Therefore vitamin K should be administered once a week to patients treated with this agent. It does not alter platelet function.

Ceftazidime is an aminothiazolyl cephalosporin that contains a propyliminocarboxy group which has excellent activity against *P. aeruginosa* and many strains of *P. cepacia* and *Acinetobacter.* It is slightly less active than cefotaxime against streptococcal species and fourfold to eightfold less active against *S. aureus,* but has similar activity against the Enterobacteriaceae. Ceftazidime has no activity against *B. fragilis* and is inactive against many clostridial species. Ceftazidime is cleared primarily by glomerular filtration and has a half-life of approximately 1.8 h. It enters the CSF in concentrations adequate to inhibit the majority of organisms producing meningitis and has been used successfully to treat a number of patients with meningitis caused by *Haemophilus, Neisseria,* and even *P. aeruginosa.* Ceftazidime accumulates in the presence of decreased renal function, and dosage adjustments must be made in patients with markedly decreased renal function. Ceftazidime has proved to be a successful drug in various serious infections, including pneumonia, bacteremia, urosepsis, osteomyelitis, and deep skin structure infections due to Enterobacteriaceae and *P. aeruginosa.* It is widely used to treat suspected infection in the febrile neutropenic patient singly or in combination with vancomycin.

OTHER β-LACTAM ANTIBIOTICS A number of novel compounds belonging to the β-lactam class have been developed. These agents differ widely in their antibacterial and pharmacologic properties.

Imipenem Imipenem is a carbapenem which has excellent in vitro activity against aerobic gram-positive species such as the hemolytic streptococci and *S. pneumoniae;* it inhibits *E. faecalis, S. aureus,* and *S. epidermidis,* including β-lactamase-producing strains, and *Listeria monocytogenes.* The majority of the Enterobacteriaceae are inhibited by concentrations <1 μg/mL, as are *H. influenzae* and *N. gonorrhoeae. P. aeruginosa,* including strains resistant to penicillins and to aminoglycosides, are inhibited by concentrations of 1 to 8 μg/mL. *P. cepacia* and *Acinetobacter* are inhibited, but *P. maltophilia* are resistant. Imipenem inhibits the majority of anaerobic species including *B. fragilis.* Imipenem is not absorbed after oral ingestion due to its instability in gastric acid. It is hydrolyzed in the kidney by a peptidase, dehydropeptidase-1, which is located on the brush border of the proximal renal tubular cells. To overcome the problem of destruction of imipenem, a dehydropeptidase inhibitor, cilastatin, is administered with imipenem.

Imipenem has a relatively short half-life of approximately 1 h; doses of 500 mg to 1 g provide plasma, tissue, and urine concentrations sufficient to inhibit the majority of bacteria. Imipenem has been used to treat bacteremia, respiratory infections, intraabdominal infections, bone and joint infections, endocarditis, and urinary tract infections due to organisms that are susceptible to it and that are resistant to other β-lactams and to aminoglycosides. Nausea occurs in some patients following too rapid infusion. The most important toxic effect is seizures, which occur in less than 5 percent of patients.

Monobactams Aztreonam is a monocyclic β-lactam which inhibits only aerobic gram-negative bacteria and does not inhibit gram-positive or anaerobic organisms. Most Enterobacteriaceae, *Haemophilus,* and *Neisseria* species, including β-lactamase-producing strains, are inhibited by <1 μg/mL. Most *P. aeruginosa* are inhibited by 16 μg/mL. Aztreonam is not absorbed following oral ingestion. It has a half-life between 1.5 and 2 h, and following doses of 1 g, serum and urine concentrations above the MICs of most Enterobacteriaceae and *Pseudomonas* are readily achieved. Aztreonam accumulates in the presence of renal failure with an increase in half-life to 6 h. The drug has been used to treat a variety of serious infections due to aerobic gram-negative species including *E. coli, Klebsiella, Serratia,* and *Pseudomonas.* It has been used in combination with clindamycin, antistaphylococcal penicillins, or vancomycin in mixed infections where it has been utilized as a replacement for the aminoglycosides. Aztreonam enters the CSF, but only a small number of patients with meningitis have been treated. The drug does not cross-react with penicillins and cephalosporins and is safe to administer to patients allergic to these agents.

β-LACTAMASE INHIBITORS Clavulanate is a β-lactamase inhibitor that has minimal antibacterial activity of its own but inhibits the β-lactamases of *S. aureus,* many Enterobacteriaceae, *Bacteroides, Klebsiella,* and *Branhamella* species. Clavulanate is a suicide inhibitor of β-lactamases. Potassium clavulanate is moderately well absorbed from the gastrointestinal tract and peak serum levels occur approximately at the same time as with amoxicillin, with which it is combined. The combination of clavulanate and amoxicillin (augmentin) does not alter the pharmacologic properties of either drug. Augmentin can be administered every 8 h and has been used to treat skin and bite wound infections due to β-lactamase-producing bacteria, otitis due to *H. influenzae,* and urinary tract infections due to β-lactamase-producing *E. coli* and *Klebsiella.* It has also been used in deep cutaneous infections due to anaerobic microorganisms and in upper respiratory infections in which *Branhamella* has been shown to be an important component.

Timentin is a combination of 3 g ticarcillin and 100 or 200 mg of clavulanate. Timentin increases the activity of ticarcillin to include *S. aureus,* β-lactamase-producing *Haemophilus, Branhamella, Bacteroides* species, *Klebsiella,* and many of the β-lactamase-producing *E. coli* strains. Timentin has been used to treat respiratory, cutaneous, gynecologic, and intraabdominal infections, osteomyelitis, and urinary tract infections, and as combination therapy in the febrile neutropenic patient.

Sulbactam is a penicillanic acid sulfone that inhibits the plasmid and chromosomally mediated β-lactamases inhibited by clavulanate. It has been combined with ampicillin, and in the presence of concentrations of 8 μg/mL of sulbactam and 16 μg/mL of ampicillin, most species of staphylococci, *Klebsiella, Haemophilus, Branhamella, E. coli,* and *Bacteroides* are inhibited. Sulbactam has pharmacokinetics in humans similar to ampicillin. It is administered intravenously. The ampicillin-sulbactam combination has been used successfully to treat urinary tract, intraabdominal, skin, gynecologic, and respiratory infections due to β-lactamase-producing microorganisms.

VANCOMYCIN Vancomycin is a glycopeptide that is active only against gram-positive species. It has assumed increasing importance because of the widespread appearance of methicillin-resistant staphylococci and the recognition of antibiotic-associated colitis caused by *C. difficile.* Vancomycin inhibits cell wall synthesis and is bactericidal. It is active against all hemolytic streptococcal species, *viridans* group streptococci, *S. pneumoniae, L. monocytogenes,* and the *Corynebacterium* species resistant to other β-lactam drugs. For most infections vancomycin is administered by the intravenous route. It is eliminated from the body by glomerular filtration and has a half-life of approximately 6 h in individuals with normal renal function. In the presence of anuria, its half-life may be prolonged to between 5 to 9 days, and it may be detected in serum for as long as 21 days after a single 1-g dose. Vancomycin is not absorbed from the gastrointestinal tract. It can be used orally, but not parenterally, to treat enterocolitis, since it is not secreted into the intestine. Following intravenous administration of a 1-g dose, peak levels of 20 to 125 μg/mL are found in serum, and when given orally, concentrations between 100 to 800 μg/mL are found in the stool. Vancomycin enters the CSF poorly. It may be administered once weekly to patients in renal failure as therapy for serious staphylococcal or streptococcal infections. Hemodialysis does not remove vancomycin. Rapid infusion of vancomycin will produce a "red man" syndrome due to histamine release, with fever, chills, and generalized erythema. This reaction can be mitigated by antihistamine drugs, e.g., diphenhydramine. Vancomycin also produces ototoxicity. It is probably minimally nephrotoxic, but when used with an aminoglycoside, nephrotoxicity and ototoxicity may be increased. Vancomycin is the therapy of choice for methicillin-resistant staphylococcal infections and for therapy of *E. faecalis* endocarditis in penicillin-allergic patients. Vancomycin is also useful in the prevention of bacterial endocarditis in patients allergic to penicillin, particularly those who have a prosthetic heart valve (see Chap. 90).

AMINOGLYCOSIDES AND SPECTINOMYCIN Aminoglycoside antibiotics are defined by the presence of amino sugars linked by a glycoside bound to an aminocyclitol ring. All aminoglycosides contain amino groups and hydroxyl groups which are important in the antibacterial activity of the compounds, as well as being the sites of enzymatic inactivation by bacterial enzymes. The drugs' ototoxicity and nephrotoxicity is also determined by their structure. Aminoglycosides are bactericidal since they bind irreversibly to proteins in the ribosomes and cause the interruption of the flow of genetic information. Enzymatic modification of the aminoglycosides by enzymes in plasmid-carrying bacteria results in their inactivation since compounds that have been adenylated, phosphorylated, or acetylated do not bind well to ribosomes and fail to induce a protein which facilitates their uptake by bacteria.

Their antibacterial activity is to inhibit members of the Enterobacteriaceae, that is, *E. coli, Klebsiella, Serratia, Enterobacter,* etc. Gentamicin, tobramycin, amikacin, sisomicin, and netilmicin all inhibit *P. aeruginosa,* but kanamycin does not. None of the agents are active against anaerobic species such as *Clostridium* or *Bacteroides.* They are not active against a number of gram-positive cocci, including *S. pneumoniae* or hemolytic streptococci. Aminoglycosides act synergistically with penicillins to inhibit *E. faecalis* and with antipseudomonas penicillins (aztreonam, imipenem, and ceftazidime) to inhibit *Pseudomonas.* They also act synergistically with nafcillin or oxacillin against *S. aureus.*

Aminoglycosides are highly water soluble and stable over a wide pH range but are markedly less active at acid pH, and their activity is decreased in the presence of divalent cations such as calcium and magnesium. An anaerobic environment decreases their effectiveness against both Enterobacteriaceae and staphylococci. They are inactivated by nucleic acid debris from decaying cells.

Aminoglycosides are not normally absorbed from the intestine. However, the small amounts absorbed can be sufficient to produce toxicity in the patient with markedly decreased renal function. This is particularly true when neomycin is administered orally in large amounts. The drugs can be absorbed when applied to burns or after irrigation of ulcers or wounds if excessive amounts are used, and they will produce oto- and nephrotoxicity following such topical application. Aminoglycosides are well absorbed after intramuscular use. Peak serum levels occur 30 to 90 min after an intramuscular injection, and in normal individuals with creatinine clearances >100 mL, their half-life is approximately 2 h. Aminoglycosides are distributed in the extracellular fluid and enter pleural, peritoneal, and synovial fluids. They do not penetrate the CSF or the eye. Extremely high concentrations are present in renal cortical tissue and persist there for up to several weeks after a course of therapy. All aminoglycosides are removed from the body by glomerular filtration. The drugs are not metabolized, and biliary excretion is minimal. With all the aminoglycosides, there is marked accumulation in the presence of decreased renal function. The half-life of the drugs in the presence of anuria is 35 to 50 h. Urinary concentrations in normal individuals are 25 to 100 times the plasma concentrations. However, in the presence of decreased renal function, only a small amount of drug is present in the urine.

The pharmacokinetics of aminoglycosides in children and the elderly are markedly different than those in young healthy adults. Although the volume of distribution in the elderly is similar to that in young adults, half-lives are considerably longer due to decreased glomerular function. Glomerular function in the elderly may not necessarily be reflected by a higher serum creatinine because of decreased creatinine production in this group. It is therefore important always to use a calculated creatinine clearance in order to estimate the half-life of an aminoglycoside in the elderly. The equation of Cockroft and Gault by which aminoglycoside concentrations may be calculated is

$$C_{cr}(\text{min}) = \frac{(140 - \text{age}) \times \text{wt (kg)}}{\text{Cr (mg/dL)} \times 72}$$

In obese patients, the volume of distribution of aminoglycosides is approximately 75 percent of that in normal patients. In calculating doses, this must be taken into consideration. Conversely, in a markedly protein-malnourished individual, there will be a larger volume of distribution so that the total body weight should be multiplied by 120 percent compared to that of the normal patient.

In initiating therapy with aminoglycosides, a loading dose should be administered in order to achieve a therapeutic serum level as quickly as possible. Reasonable serum levels, 30 to 60 min after the initial dose, are between 5 and 10 μg/mL for gentamicin, tobramycin, netilmicin, and sisomicin, and between 20 and 40 μg/mL for kanamycin and amikacin. A loading dose of 2 mg/kg for gentamicin, tobramycin, and netilmicin and a loading dose of 8 mg/kg for amikacin are satisfactory. The loading dose is the same whether or not elimination is impaired by renal dysfunction. Since loading doses are sizable, they should be given intravenously over 20 to 30 min to avoid the risk of neuromuscular toxicity. In individuals with creatinine clearances >80 mL/min, a dose of 1.5 to 2 mg/kg of gentamicin, tobramycin, or netilmicin every 8 h, or 5 mg/kg of amikacin every 8 h, provides adequate peak and trough levels. The daily dose of aminoglycosides must be reduced in patients whose renal function is impaired. A simple way of calculating the total daily dose is to calculate the patient's creatinine clearance based on age, sex, weight, and serum creatinine. The clearance of aminoglycosides is linearly related to creatinine clearance. Therefore, the ratio of the patient's creatinine clearance to a normal creatinine clearance approximates the aminoglycoside clearance. An individual with a creatinine clearance of 30 mL/min or 30 percent should receive 30 percent of the usual daily dose. Instead of 4.5 to 6 mg/kg per day, the dose should be reduced to 1.5 to 2 mg/kg per day. This dose can be administered either as a reduced dose at the regular time interval of 8 h, or the total dose can be divided and administered at less frequent intervals. Calculated predictions of aminoglycoside levels provide reasonable approximations, but blood levels should be measured, both at the peak and trough, and dose adjustments should be made accordingly.

Toxicity of aminoglycosides All aminoglycosides share similar toxicity. Hypersensitivity is exceedingly rare, but all of these drugs will produce some degree of nephrotoxicity. The initial renal toxicity is nonoliguric renal failure. There is a loss of concentrating ability, proteinuria, casts in the urine, and renal enzymuria. Subsequently, the serum creatinine and blood urea nitrogen (BUN) will rise. Nephrotoxicity involves the proximal tubular cells. Risk factors for development of toxicity are old age, concomitant hypotension at the onset of aminoglycoside therapy, use of other nephrotoxic agents simultaneously, and, perhaps, concomitant liver disease. Aminoglycoside nephrotoxicity is usually mild and reversible. However, it can result in renal failure and may even require dialysis. For this reason, it is critical to follow aminoglycoside blood levels in patients receiving these drugs. Ototoxicity can be aimed at either the cochlea or the vestibular apparatus. The mechanism of the toxicity is the destruction of hair cells within the organ of Corti or those in the ampullar cristae. Once these cells have been damaged, they cannot regenerate. Detectable toxicity occurs in 3 to 5 percent of patients receiving aminoglycosides. Although tinnitus and a feeling of fullness in the ears may precede hearing loss, it is not a useful guide to hearing damage. Since the high tones outside the conversation range are affected first, ototoxicity may not be recognized initially. Less frequent forms of toxicity seen with these drugs are neuromuscular blockade and malabsorption. There is evidence that administration of the total daily dose to nonneutropenic patients as a single dose provides a similar response with less toxicity.

Individual aminoglycosides Streptomycin is used for treatment of selected cases of tuberculosis (for which it is administered twice weekly), tularemia, plague, and brucellosis. It is used in the treatment of endocarditis due to *E. faecalis* or viridans streptococci, provided that the strains are susceptible to less than 2000 μg/mL. Neomycin's sole use today is in bowel preparation for intestinal surgery, combined with erythromycin or metronidazole. Kanamycin has been superseded by other aminoglycosides. Gentamicin remains useful as a first-line agent in the treatment of gram-negative infections, particularly because of its relatively low cost. Tobramycin is more active than gentamicin against *P. aeruginosa* and less active against *Serratia* species. Its clinical efficacy is equivalent to that of gentamicin, but there is some evidence that tobramycin is somewhat less nephrotoxic than gentamicin. Amikacin is less likely to be inactivated by plasmid-mediated resistance enzymes and should be used particularly in those situations in which it is likely that there is aminoglycoside resistance. Netilmicin is a derivative of gentamicin which is less nephrotoxic and ototoxic. It is less active against *Pseudomonas* than is gentamicin or tobramycin, but it inhibits a number of strains of *E. coli, Klebsiella,* and *Serratia* resistant to gentamicin and tobramycin.

Spectinomycin is an amino cyclitol antibiotic that has been used in a single 2-g intramuscular dose to treat gonorrhea due to penicillinase-producing strains. Its use has been superseded by compounds such as ceftriaxone, which can be administered in 125- to 250-mg intramuscular doses to treat penicillinase-producing gonococcal strains.

TETRACYCLINES Tetracyclines are bacteriostatic agents that inhibit protein biosynthesis. By binding to the 30 S ribosome they inhibit binding of aminoacyl tRNA. Resistance to tetracyclines is due to plasmid-mediated synthesis of a protein which results in a drug efflux. Tetracycline-resistant bacteria bind less drug; what does enter is pumped out by an energy-dependent process. They inhibit many gram-positive and gram-negative species and are active against other important organisms, including Rickettsiae, *Chlamydia,* and *Mycoplasma*. They also inhibit *Actinomyces,* but do not inhibit *Nocardia*. Resistance to the tetracyclines has appeared in many species. Some strains of *S. pneumoniae* and *S. pyogenes* are resistant. Many staphylococci are resistant to the tetracyclines as well as many enteric organisms such as *Shigella*. In general, organisms resistant to one tetracycline are resistant to all members of the group. Tetracyclines can be divided into three groups based on pharmacology. The short-acting group consists of tetracycline, chlortetracycline, and oxytetracycline. The intermediate group consists of demeclocycline and methacycline, and the long-acting compounds are doxycycline and minocycline. Tetracyclines are incompletely absorbed from the gastrointestinal tract, and their absorption is increased if they are taken in the fasting state. Their absorption is decreased by milk, milk products, and magnesium-containing antacids and iron. The binding of tetracyclines to plasma proteins varies with the type of drug. They enter the CSF, but concentrations are inadequate for treatment of meningitis. Since the agents cross the placenta, they cannot be given to pregnant women since they will be sequestered into bone and tooth structures causing abnormalities. High concentrations of the drugs are found in the bile, and there is a significant enterohepatic circulation. Minocycline is excreted in saliva and lacrimal secretions producing antibacterial concentrations in the oropharynx; for this reason it has been used as prophylaxis for meningococcal disease. However, since minocycline can cause vestibular toxicity, it has been supplanted by rifampin. With the exception of doxycycline and chlortetracycline, the tetracyclines are eliminated from the body primarily by glomerular filtration. In the presence of renal failure, the half-life of all tetracyclines, except these two drugs, increases markedly.

The tetracyclines may cause skin rashes, particularly with solar exposure. Gastrointestinal effects include nausea, vomiting, and diarrhea. The diarrhea may be either a direct toxic effect, or due to pseudomembranous colitis. Severe hepatotoxicity has occurred during prolonged therapy with high doses, particularly in pregnant women. In some, often debilitated, patients there may be catabolic effects with protein breakdown, weight loss, and nitrogen retention. Tetracycline's effect on the gut flora may cause prolongation of prothrombin time.

Tetracyclines are rarely the drugs of choice in most common bacterial infections because of the large number of other drugs available. There are specific indications for use of these compounds. In rickettsial infections such as Rocky Mountain spotted fever, typhus, or scrub typhus, tetracycline remains the drug of choice. They are drugs of choice in the treatment of sexually transmitted chlamydial infections and are useful in the treatment of *Mycoplasma* infections. Tetracyclines have proved useful in the therapy of Lyme disease in adults, brucellosis, relapsing fever due to *Borrelia*, and, combined with streptomycin, for treatment of complicated plague. They have also proved useful in therapy of infections due to *Actinomyces* and in *Pasteurella multocida* infections in penicillin-allergic patients. Tetracyclines have been used in a number of syndromes such as acne, bacterial exacerbations of bronchitis, malabsorption syndrome, and sinusitis. They are not the drugs of choice for streptococcal or pneumococcal infections or for anaerobic infections in the abdomen.

CHLORAMPHENICOL Chloramphenicol binds to 50 S ribosomes inhibiting peptide bond formation. It is bacteriostatic. Resistance is due to acetylation of the drug by the plasmid-mediated enzyme chloramphenicol transacetylase. Acetylation of the OH of the C-1 carbon prevents binding to ribosomes. Chloramphenicol is extremely active against aerobic and anaerobic bacteria, *Rickettsia, Chlamydia, Mycoplasma,* and *Spirochaeta*. The organisms most commonly causing meningitis in childhood, *H. influenzae, S. pneumoniae,* and *N. meningitidis,* are highly susceptible to this agent and most *Bacteroides* species are inhibited by it.

Chloramphenicol is well-absorbed from the gastrointestinal tract. Blood levels following oral ingestion are superior to those achieved after intravenous injection since the inactive chloramphenicol succinate ester which is used in the intravenous preparation is incompletely hydrolyzed within the body. Chloramphenicol is metabolized in the liver where it is conjugated with glucuronic acid and is excreted in an inactive form by the kidneys. It diffuses well into many tissues and body fluids and produces excellent concentrations in the cerebrospinal fluid and brain tissue. In the presence of renal disease, the half-life of the drug is not significantly increased. In contrast, in patients with hepatic disease, serum levels may increase yielding levels capable of producing bone marrow suppression.

The most important toxic effect of chloramphenicol is on bone marrow. Approximately 1 in 25,000 patients who receive the drug develop aplastic anemia. This is an unpredictable, idiosyncratic response. There is also a dose-related anemia and leukopenia which is predictable when blood levels are above 25 μg/mL. This toxicity is reversible when the antibiotic is discontinued. Chloramphenicol cannot be given to newborns since they are unable to conjugate the drug and develop toxicity due to excessive levels of free compound.

In the United States, chloramphenicol is now rarely used. The new cephalosporins enter the CSF and provide concentrations that are effective against many pathogens. Metronidazole, clindamycin, cefoxitin, and imipenem are available to treat severe *B. fragilis* infections. Many strains of *S. typhi* are resistant to chloramphenicol, and other drugs such as trimethoprim-sulfamethoxazole or ciprofloxacin should be used.

Chloramphenicol undergoes a number of significant drug interactions. It prolongs the half-life of tolbutamide, chlorpropamide, phenytoin, and warfarin by inhibiting hepatic microsomal enzymes.

ERYTHROMYCIN Erythromycin is a macrolide antibiotic that acts primarily in a bacteriostatic fashion by binding to 50 S ribosomes and preventing peptidyl transfer and translocation. Resistance is due to methylation of two adenine nucleotides in the 23 S component of the 50 S RNA. The resistance is normally repressed in nonresistant bacteria and is induced in the presence of a plasmid. The drug inhibits *S. pyogenes, S. pneumoniae,* many strains of *Neisseria,* some strains of *H. influenzae, C. diphtheriae, Clostridium, Listeria, Treponema,* and a number of anaerobic cocci and oral *Bacteroides* species. It is effective against *Mycoplasma pneumoniae* and *Legionella pneumophila*.

Erythromycin is used by either the oral or intravenous route. There are a number of different erythromycin preparations available. Esters and salts of erythromycin are more acid-stable. The erythromycin base and ethyl succinate forms are better absorbed when taken in the fasting state. The stearate form is better absorbed when taken with meals. The estolate salt is associated with more cholestatic hepatitis in adults than are the other forms. The normal half-life of erythromycin is 1.5 h, and appreciable serum levels are maintained for at least 6 h. Therefore, in a number of infections such as streptococcal pharyngitis, the drug can be administered on a twice-daily basis. In anuric patients, reduction in dosage is generally not necessary.

Erythromycin is one of the safest antibiotics, and untoward reactions are extremely uncommon except for cholestatic hepatitis. The main side effect has been epigastric distress and nausea. Hearing loss does occur in association with large doses administered to elderly patients with renal insufficiency. Erythromycin used concomitantly with oral theophylline preparations may cause increased blood levels of theophylline and potential theophylline toxicity. Erythromycin also causes elevation in urinary catecholamines and in 17-hydroxycorticosteroids. The major use of erythromycin is to treat streptococcal pharyngitis in the penicillin-allergic patient, or in the treatment of otitis media in combination with sulfonamides. Erythromycin can also be used during pregnancy to treat skin infections or, in high doses, to treat syphilis in pregnancy. Erythromycin in a dose of 0.5 to 1 g every 6 h is the therapy of choice for *Legionella* pneumonia, and it is the drug of choice for *M. pneumoniae* and some *Ureaplasma* infections.

LINCOMYCIN AND CLINDAMYCIN Lincosamide antibiotics inhibit many of the same organisms as do the erythromycins. Their mechanism of action is inhibition of protein synthesis. Clindamycin is a less effective inducer of the methylating enzyme. The clinical significance becomes evident in the development of resistance of erythromycin-resistant, clindamycin-susceptible *S. aureus* infections. Lincomycin is rarely used today and clindamycin is the primary agent in this class. Clindamycin inhibits *S. pneumoniae, S. pyogenes,* and viridans group streptococci. It lacks activity against *E. faecalis*. Many strains of *S. aureus* and *S. epidermidis* are inhibited by clindamycin, and it has excellent activity against most anaerobic species, including *Clostridium* and *Bacteroides*. It also inhibits *Chlamydia*.

Clindamycin is well-absorbed following oral ingestion and can also be administered intramuscularly or intravenously. The serum half-life is approximately 2.5 h, and the drug is metabolized primarily in the liver. Dosage adjustments are minor except in the presence of hepatic failure. Clindamycin produces high concentrations in bone, and has been found to enter white blood cells. Its most significant toxic effect is diarrhea, which has often been associated with pseudomembranous colitis caused by *C. difficile*. If diarrhea develops during clindamycin therapy, the drug should be discontinued. If diarrhea persists, proctoscopy or assay for *C. difficile* toxin should be performed and therapy with oral vancomycin or metronidazole instituted.

The major therapeutic use of clindamycin is for anaerobic infections or as a combination with an aminoglycoside or aztreonam. Clindamycin provides coverage against streptococcal, staphylococcal, and anaerobic species while the aerobic gram-negative organism is attacked by the other agent. Clindamycin has proved to be an excellent agent for the therapy of anaerobic pulmonary disease, particularly in patients who have failed to respond to penicillin. Topical solutions of clindamycin are useful in the treatment of severe acne. Clindamycin should not be used for serious staphylococcal infections due to erythromycin-resistant bacteria because resistance to clindamycin will develop. Furthermore, its bacteriostatic activity against *S. aureus* makes it a less desirable choice against this organism than active β-lactams or vancomycin.

RIFAMPIN Rifampin is a macrocyclic antibiotic produced by a *Streptomyces*. It inhibits DNA-directed RNA polymerase. Resistance is due to change of one amino acid on the beta subunit of the polymerase altering the binding of rifampin to the enzyme. The degree of resistance is related to the degree that the enzyme is changed. Resistance can develop during therapy due to selection of a subpopulation of microorganisms that contain altered polymerase. Rifampin is available in the United States only for oral use. The drug has been used primarily in the treatment of tuberculosis. However, rifampin inhibits many microorganisms: coagulase-positive and -negative staphylococci, as well as *N. meningitidis, N. gonorrhoeae,* and *H. influenzae*. It is the most active agent known against *L. pneumophila* and is also effective against *L. micdadei* and *L. dumoffei*. It inhibits *C. difficile* at concentrations less than 1 μg/mL and inhibits the majority of streptococci and *S. pneumoniae* at concentrations of less than 0.1 μg/mL. Although rifampin inhibits many of the Enterobacteriaceae and some strains of *Pseudomonas,* resistance develops rapidly. The drug inhibits *Chlamydia,* but *Ureaplasma urealyticum* and *Treponema pallidum* usually are resistant.

Rifampin is well-absorbed from the gastrointestinal tract and, following ingestion of 600 mg in an adult or 10 mg/kg in children, peak serum concentrations of approximately 8 μg/mL are reached. With repeated doses, drug levels decrease slightly because the drug stimulates the hepatic enzymes responsible for its metabolism. The drug is approximately 75 percent protein-bound. Rifampin is both metabolized and excreted by the liver. The desacetyl derivative is not reabsorbed and is excreted via the stool; only 5 to 30 percent of the dose is excreted in the urine. In general, dosage adjustment is unnecessary in renal failure, but a lower dose should be used in patients with severe hepatic dysfunction. Food will interfere with the absorption of rifampin, lowering and delaying peak blood levels. Rifampin penetrates into all body tissues and enters white cells. High concentrations are found in lacrimal and salivary secretions; the drug penetrates well into bone. Cerebrospinal fluid levels as high as 1.3 μg/mL have been observed during treatment of meningitis.

The adverse effects of rifampin are few. On occasion, it will produce a flulike syndrome in individuals who take the drug intermittently. There have also been reports of interstitial nephritis, thrombocytopenia, and hemolytic anemia. Rifampin alters the metabolism of a number of drugs; it decreases the effect of exogenous steroids and interferes with birth control pills. It artificially lowers the serum concentration of thyroxine; tri-iodothyronine remains normal. Patients should be warned that rifampin will cause red discoloration of urine and can cause permanent staining of soft contact lenses. Rifampin crosses the placenta and has produced teratogenic effects in rodents, but such effects have not been observed in humans. However, during pregnancy the drug should be used only for severe tuberculosis. The major use of rifampin is in short-term (6 to 9 months) treatment of tuberculosis, combined with isoniazid (see Chap. 125). It is also used as prophylaxis for contacts of patients with meningococcal meningitis in a dose of 600 mg for 2 days in adults and 20 mg/kg for 2 days in children. It has also been recommended for prophylaxis of children under 4 years of age who have had close contact with a child with *H. influenzae* type B meningitis. Rifampin, combined with cloxacillin, has proved effective in eradicating nasal carriage in individuals with recurrent furunculosis. It may also be used to eradicate methicillin-resistant staphylococci when used in combination with vancomycin or trimethoprim-sulfamethoxazole. Rifampin has been used in the therapy of endocarditis due to tolerant *S. aureus* and for treatment of *Corynebacterium* species endocarditis. It is useful in treating patients with *L. pneumophila* infection who have failed to respond to erythromycin. Rifampin also may be useful combined with nafcillin or vancomycin in the treatment of chronic staphylococcal osteomyelitis.

METRONIDAZOLE Metronidazole is a nitroimidazole which, following reduction of the nitro group of the nitrosohydroxyl amino group, causes breaks in strands of DNA. Plasmids that prevent reduction of imidazoles have been found. The drug kills organisms within a twofold dilution of the inhibitory concentration: 99 percent of *B. fragilis* are inhibited by 8 μg/mL and 100 percent of *Fusobacterium* by 4 μg/mL. Most clostridial species are inhibited by 4 μg/mL. However, anaerobic gram-positive cocci may be less susceptible, as are *Actinomyces* and *Arachnida*. It is highly active against *C. difficile*. *Propionibacterium acnes* are resistant, but *Gardnerella vaginalis, Campylobacter fetus,* and oral *Spirochaeta* are inhibited by metronidazole.

Metronidazole is rapidly and almost completely absorbed when given orally. It can also be absorbed by rectal instillation and is available as an intravenous solution. There is minimal protein binding; the drug has a long half-life of 8 h. Absorption of metronidazole is not affected by food although peak levels are markedly delayed. Metronidazole is metabolized in the liver to a variety of hydroxy and glucuronide derivatives. Both metronidazole and its metabolites are eliminated in the urine and in the feces. Metronidazole dosage does not need to be adjusted in renal failure, but the drug is rapidly removed by hemodialysis. Therefore, additional doses should be given after dialysis. Given its long half-life, dosage of 500 mg every 8 h is adequate.

There are a number of adverse effects related to metronidazole. Rare but important reactions are seizures and encephalopathy, peripheral neuropathy, disulfiram-like reaction with alcohol, potentiation of the effects of warfarin, and, extremely rarely, pseudomembranous colitis. Minor problems that are associated with the drug are development of gastrointestinal disturbance, metallic taste, maculopapular rashes, or vaginal burning. Metronidazole is tumorigenic in rats, but there is no evidence that this occurs in humans. Nevertheless, the drug should probably not be used in pregnancy unless no other drug is feasible.

Metronidazole is effective in treatment of serious anaerobic infections, with some exceptions. It is not useful in actinomycosis, and it has not been very effective in aspiration pneumonia, probably because of the large number of streptococci found in this infection. It is particularly useful in intraabdominal infections since it is able to penetrate abscesses and kill *Bacteroides* within the abscess. It has also been used in other anaerobic infections including bacteremia, endocarditis, osteomyelitis, and head-and-neck infections. Metronidazole can be used in the management of pseudomembranous colitis due to *C. difficile* either orally or parenterally. Metronidazole is useful in the treatment of amebic liver abscess, intestinal amebiasis, and vaginitis due to *Trichomonas*. It may be useful in *Blastocystis hominis* infections. Metronidazole has been used as prophylaxis for elective colonic and gynecologic surgery or at the time of emergency appendectomy. However, it has no activity against gram-positive or gram-negative aerobic organisms.

POLYMYXINS Polymyxins are cyclic basic polypeptides. There are two compounds available, polymyxin B sulfate and polymyxin E, or colistin. Polymyxins are active only against aerobic gram-negative bacteria such as *Pseudomonas* and members of the Enterobacteriaceae. The compounds are not absorbed when given orally and must be administered parenterally. They are rapidly sequestered within the kidney and liver, reducing their clinical value. Both drugs produce very serious neuro- and nephrotoxicity. In view of the large number of other compounds available, there is no reason to use them.

SULFONAMIDES AND TRIMETHOPRIM Sulfonamides are bacteriostatic and act by interfering with folic acid metabolism in bacteria. Resistance is due to the presence of an altered or new dihydropteroic synthetase enzyme that binds para-aminobenzoic acid (PABA) better than sulfonamides. They are generally classified as short-, medium-, or long-acting sulfonamides, sulfonamides limited to the gastrointestinal tract, and topical sulfonamides. Sulfonamides inhibit some gram-positive bacteria and members of the Enterobacteriaceae, including *E. coli, Klebsiella,* and *Proteus*. They are also active against *Haemophilus,* but do not have activity against *P. aeruginosa*. The major problem with sulfonamides is that bacteria have become resistant on the basis of plasmid-mediated production of altered enzymes. Most sulfonamides are administered orally, although sulfamethoxazole is available for intravenous use. Sulfonamides are absorbed rapidly from the small intestine and stomach. The compounds are distributed throughout the body and enter the CSF, synovial, pleural, and peritoneal fluids in concentrations that approximate 80 percent of serum levels. Sulfonamides are metabolized in the liver by acetylation and glucuronidation. They are excreted via glomerular filtration with partial reabsorption and tubular secretion. Sulfonamides differ widely in their protein binding, plasma half-life, metabolism, and solubility.

Sulfonamides produce a number of serious side effects. These include a rash that appears in 3 to 5 percent of individuals (more frequently in AIDS patients), fever, jaundice, serum sickness–like syndrome, and acute hemolysis in the G6PD-deficient patient. They also may cause agranulocytosis, thrombocytopenia, and leukopenia. Sulfonamides cannot be administered during the last month of pregnancy since they cross the placenta and displace bilirubin from albumin and increase the risk of kernicterus. Long-acting sulfonamides have been associated with fatal hypersensitivity reactions; this has been noted particularly with the longer-acting sulfonamides used in malarial preparations. By binding to albumin sites, sulfonamides may displace drugs such as warfarin, methotrexate, and hypoglycemic agents such as chlorpropamide. Sulfonamide concentrations are increased by indomethacin, salicylates, and probenecid. Tubular necrosis due to deposition of sulfa crystals within the kidney rarely occurs today.

Sulfadiazine is the most active sulfonamide attaining the highest blood and cerebrospinal fluid levels. However, it tends more often to produce crystalluria; hence sulfisoxazole and sulfamethoxazole are used more frequently. Mixtures of three sulfonamides are also available and can be used in the treatment of toxoplasmosis. Long-acting sulfonamides should be avoided because of the risk of severe erythema multiforme. Topical sulfonamide preparations such as silver-sulfadiazine or mafenide inhibit Enterobacteriaceae, *P. aeruginosa,* staphylococci, and streptococci and are extremely useful to reduce the number of bacteria in burn eschars.

Trimethoprim is a 2,4-diaminopyrimidine that inhibits dihydrofolate reductase. Resistance is plasmid- and transposon-mediated due to production of altered dihydrofolate reductase enzyme which has markedly reduced affinity for trimethoprim. Trimethoprim is active against most gram-positive cocci and gram-negative rods with the exception of *P. aeruginosa* and *Bacteroides.* It also has relatively poor activity against *Neisseria* species, and against *Chlamydia* and *Nocardia.* Resistance to trimethoprim has been fairly slow to develop. However, in the far east, strains of *Salmonella* and *Shigella* have become resistant, and toxigenic *E. coli* have been isolated in Central America that are resistant to trimethoprim and the combination of trimethoprim and sulfamethoxazole.

Trimethoprim is available as a single agent or a combined agent in a fixed combination of one part trimethoprim to five parts sulfamethoxazole. It is also available as an intravenous combination which contains one part trimethoprim and five parts sulfamethoxazole. Like the sulfonamides, trimethoprim is well-absorbed from the gastrointestinal tract. Most of the drug is excreted in the urine via tubular secretion; it has a serum half-life of 9 to 11 h in normal individuals. Trimethoprim-sulfamethoxazole can usually be given to patients with creatinine clearances greater than 30 mL/min in the usual doses and given in half doses to patients whose creatinine clearances are in the range of 15 to 30 mL/min. Trimethoprim itself may cause fever and rash and depression of white cells and platelets. This problem often can be avoided by the simultaneous administration of folinic acid. Pseudomembranous enterocolitis also can occur following use of trimethoprim-sulfamethoxazole.

Trimethoprim-sulfamethoxazole has been useful in the treatment of urinary tract infections, acute bacterial exacerbations of chronic bronchitis, otitis media, and gastrointestinal infections due to *Salmonella, Shigella,* and toxigenic *E. coli.* Trimethoprim also is useful in the treatment of gonorrhea and chancroid. It can be used to treat *Listeria* meningitis in patients allergic to penicillins. It has had some success in therapy of methicillin-resistant *S. aureus.* Trimethoprim-sulfamethoxazole is used in high-dose oral or intravenous therapy of *Pneumocystis carinii* infections. Trimethoprim-sulfamethoxazole has also proved useful as prophylaxis in neutropenic children and in chronic granulomatous disease of childhood. The combination has been of particular value in the prevention of recurrent bacteriuria in women with recurrent urinary tract infections.

QUINOLONES Quinolones are synthesized chemically. Nalidixic acid which inhibits gram-negative bacteria has been used only for the treatment of urinary tract infections. Quinolones bind to an enzyme, DNA gyrase, which is involved in the production of new DNA molecules. Resistance is due to an altered DNA gyrase A subunit and to failure of uptake of the drugs due to loss of outer membrane proteins.

The compounds can be considered in groups; nalidixic acid, oxolinic acid, and cinoxacin are one group. They inhibit the majority of strains of *E. coli, P. mirabilis, Klebsiella,* and *Enterobacter* at concentrations that can be achieved in urine. *Pseudomonas* species are resistant as are gram-positive organisms, *S. aureus, S. pneumoniae,* and *E. faecalis.* Cross-resistance occurs between all three of the compounds. These agents are given by the oral route and are almost completely absorbed from the gastrointestinal tract. They are metabolized in the liver to biologically active and inactive compounds that are excreted by the kidney. The major difficulty with these agents has been the rapid development of resistance to them; hence they have not proved very effective for urinary tract infections.

The carboxyfluoroquinolones norfloxacin, enoxacin, pefloxacin, ofloxacin, and ciprofloxacin differ from the previously mentioned drugs because they have an extended antibacterial spectrum. All of these agents inhibit virtually all of the Enterobacteriaceae at concentrations below 1 μg/mL. They have varying activity against *Pseudomonas,* depending upon the particular compound. Ciprofloxacin is extremely active against *P. aeruginosa,* inhibiting isolates resistant to β-lactam and aminoglycoside antibiotics at $\leq$ 0.5 μg/mL. The agents also inhibit *Haemophilus, Branhamella,* and methicillin-resistant staphylococci. They tend to have less activity against *S. pneumoniae* and hemolytic streptococci and generally do not inhibit *Bacteroides* and many clostridial species except at high concentrations. Ciprofloxacin inhibits most *S. pneumoniae* and *S. pyogenes* at $\leq$ 2.0 μg/mL.

These agents differ in their oral absorption. Ofloxacin and enoxacin are more readily absorbed than are norfloxacin and ciprofloxacin. Absorption is markedly reduced in the presence of aluminum and magnesium antacids, but not by H-2-blocking agents. The compounds are widely distributed in the body and are metabolized to both active and inactive products within the liver. The majority of excretion products leave the body via the urinary tract or biliary tract. Ciprofloxacin enters the CSF at therapeutic concentrations against *H. influenzae, N. meningitidis,* and Enterobacteriaceae, but not *S. pneumoniae.* High concentrations are achieved in bone. Ciprofloxacin and norfloxacin are available for use in the United States. Ciprofloxacin has been used in the treatment of urinary tract infections, respiratory tract infections, gastrointestinal disease due to *Salmonella* and *Shigella,* and pathogenic *E. coli* and *Campylobacter.* Ciprofloxacin and ofloxacin have been successfully used in the treatment of osteomyelitis and skin infections. Ciprofloxacin has been extremely effective in therapy of *Pseudomonas* infections, including those occurring in cystic fibrosis patients. Norfloxacin has been restricted to use in urinary tract infections.

Toxic and adverse reactions to these agents have been infrequent. Gastrointestinal side effects have included nausea, vomiting, and occasionally diarrhea. Nonspecific rashes and urticaria have occurred. Ophthalmologic side effects are rare. Central nervous system symptoms noted with nalidixic acid include headache, vertigo, seizures, and psychosis, but such reactions are extremely uncommon with ciprofloxacin, norfloxacin, and ofloxacin. Ciprofloxacin prolongs the half-life of theophylline; all the agents increase caffeine's half-life.

ANTITUBERCULOSIS DRUGS See Chap. 125.

ANTIFUNGAL AGENTS See Chap. 87.

ANTIVIRAL AGENTS See Chap. 86.

ANTIPARASITIC AGENTS See Chap. 88.

REASONS FOR FAILURE OF CHEMOTHERAPY

There are few microorganisms with the exception of fungi and viruses that are not susceptible to some antimicrobial agents. Nonetheless, a large number of patients who develop infections continue to die. In these patients, antimicrobial agents appear to have failed. The failure of chemotherapy often is more apparent than real, and may be attributed to a number of different causes.

First, the infection being treated may not be due to a treatable microorganism but to a viral infection that will not respond to the chemotherapeutic agents that are being used. Antibiotics do not prevent bacterial complications of most viral infections.

A second common reason for failure of antimicrobial therapy is that purulent material has not been drained, or that a focus of obstruction or a foreign body has not been removed. Antimicrobial agents do not work well in these situations.

Third, fever may continue, not due to the infection, but as the result of development of hypersensitivity to one of the agents being used to treat the patient. Drug fever is particularly common with antimicrobial agents of the β-lactam and sulfonamide classes.

Occasionally, chemotherapy fails because the incorrect drug has been chosen or the culture results have been misinterpreted. This may be particularly true in respiratory infections. One of the most common errors when such a patient is not responding is to add more antimicrobial agents indiscriminately, when the correct course would be to discontinue therapy and observe the patient.

With many of the new antimicrobial agents, failure to provide an adequate dose of antibiotic is less frequently a problem than it was formerly. However, this still may be true in certain infections in which penetration of the antimicrobial agent to the particular area of the body is inadequate unless large doses are utilized.

More and more, today's patients lack host defenses, and include elderly patients with degenerative and debilitating diseases, or patients who have received multiple antimicrobial agents, antineoplastic or immunosuppressive drugs, or who have undergone major surgical procedures. These individuals will have much more difficulty in responding to antimicrobial therapy than normal uncompromised hosts, most of whom remain free of life-threatening infections.

REFERENCES

ACAR JF, NEU HC (eds): Gram-negative aerobic bacterial infections: A focus on directed therapy, with special reference to aztreonam. Rev Infect Dis 7(Suppl 4):537, 1985

ANDRIOLE VT (ed): *The Quinolones*. London, Academic, 1988

Antimicrobial prophylaxis in surgery. Med Lett Drugs Ther 31:105, 1989

BRUCHAT MA, DAJANI AS (eds): Sulbactam/ampicillin in clinical practice. Drugs 35(Suppl 7):1, 1988

DONOWITZ GR, MANDELL GL: Beta-lactam antibiotics. N Engl J Med 319:419, 1988

DRUSANO GL et al: The acylampicillins: Mezlocillin, piperacillin, and azlocillin. Rev Infect Dis 6:13, 1984

GEDDES AM, STILLE W (eds): Imipenem, the first thienamycin antibiotic. Rev Infect Dis 7(Suppl 3), 1985

LEVY SB et al: Antibiotic use and antibiotic resistance worldwide. Rev Infect Dis 9(Suppl 3):231, 1987

NEU HC (ed): Beta-lactamase inhibition: Therapeutic advances. Am J Med 79(Suppl 5B):1, 1985

——— (ed): Update on antibiotics I. Med Clin North Am 71(6):1051, 1987

——— (ed): Update on antibiotics II. Med Clin North Am 72(3):555, 1988

——— et al (eds): Ciprofloxacin: A major advance in quinolone chemotherapy. Am J Med 82(4A):1, 1987

NORRBY SR et al (eds): Evaluation of new beta-lactam antibiotics. Rev Infect Dis 8(Suppl 3):235, 1986

PLATT R et al: Perioperative antibiotic prophylaxis for herniorrhaphy and breast surgery. N Engl J Med 322:153, 1990

86 ANTIVIRAL CHEMOTHERAPY

RAPHAEL DOLIN

INTRODUCTION The use of antiviral compounds for chemotherapy and chemoprophylaxis of viral diseases is a relatively new development in the field of infectious diseases, particularly when compared to the more than 40 years of experience with antibacterial antibiotics. The principles which underlie the use of antiviral compounds have been modeled after those successfully employed in the treatment of bacterial infections, as outlined in Chap. 85. However, application of these principles to antiviral chemotherapy and chemoprophylaxis presents a number of unique problems.

First, antiviral compounds must possess a high degree of selectivity because of the biologic properties of viruses. Bacteria can replicate extracellularly and have evolved metabolic and structural features which differ considerably from those of mammalian cells. However, viruses must replicate intracellularly and often employ host cell enzymes, macromolecules, and organelles for the synthesis of virus particles. Therefore, safe and effective antiviral compounds must be able to discriminate with a high degree of efficiency between cellular and virus-specific functions. Inhibitors of virus replication which lack this selectivity are likely to be too toxic for clinical use.

Second, because of the nature of virus replication, evaluation of the in vitro sensitivity of virus isolates to antiviral compounds must be carried out in a complex culture system consisting of living cells (e.g., tissue culture). The results from such assay systems vary widely according to the type of tissue culture cells which are employed and the conditions of assay. Furthermore, the precise relationship between the in vitro sensitivity of an isolate and the outcome of antiviral therapy is not well worked out.

Third, information regarding the pharmacokinetics of antiviral compounds, particularly in diverse clinical settings, is limited, particularly when compared to that available for antibacterial antibiotics. For compounds such as acyclovir, considerable detailed pharmacokinetic data are available, while for others such as rimantadine, relatively little information exists. Assays to determine concentrations of antivirals, particularly of active moieties within cells, are not widely available. There are few guidelines with which to adjust dosage levels to maximize antiviral activity and to minimize toxicity. Therefore, clinical use of antiviral compounds must be accompanied by particular vigilance for unanticipated side effects or toxicities.

Fourth, it is clear that highly complex host defense systems play critical roles in the course of viral infections. The presence or absence of preexisting immunity, and the ability to mount humoral and/or cell-mediated immune responses, are especially important determinants in the outcome of viral infections. For example, profound "immunosuppression" may result in infections in which prolonged viral replication is present, and inhibition of such replication by antiviral compounds may be particularly useful. On the other hand, if host defenses are severely depressed, as in bone marrow transplants, antiviral therapy may be relatively ineffective. The state of host defenses and their interactions with antiviral compounds need to be considered when antivirals are utilized or evaluated.

Finally, as with antibacterial antibiotics, the optimal use of antiviral compounds requires that a specific and timely diagnosis be made. For some viral infections, such as herpes zoster, the clinical manifestations are so characteristic that a diagnosis can be made on clinical grounds alone. For other viral infections, such as influenza A, epidemiologic information (i.e., community-wide outbreaks) can be utilized to make a presumptive diagnosis with a high degree of accuracy. However, for most other viral infections, including herpes simplex encephalitis, cytomegalovirus infections, and acute viral gastroenteritis, diagnosis on clinical grounds alone cannot be accomplished with certainty. For such infections, rapid, noninvasive viral diagnostic techniques are sorely needed, and considerable effort is being expended to develop such tests.

Despite the above complexities, the efficacy of several antiviral compounds has been clearly established in rigorously conducted and controlled studies. The compounds which are currently available or likely to be made available in the immediate future for clinical use are discussed below and summarized in Table 86-1.

AMANTADINE AND RIMANTADINE Amantadine (1-adamantanamine hydrochloride) and the closely related compound rimantadine (α-methyl-1-adamantanemethylamine hydrochloride) are primary symmetric amines with antiviral activity limited to influenza A viruses.

TABLE 86-1 Antiviral chemotherapy and chemoprophylaxis

Infection	Antiviral drug	Administration	Dosage	Comment
Influenza A (prophylaxis)	Amantadine	Oral	Adults: 200 mg/d for period at risk Children ≤9 yrs: 4.4–8.8 mg/kg per day not to exceed 150 mg/d	Needs to be administered for the duration of the outbreak. Dosage should be reduced in renal failure and in the elderly. Can be administered along with vaccine.
	or			
	rimantadine	Oral	As above	Not yet licensed by FDA. May be better tolerated than amantadine.
Influenza A (therapy)	Amantadine	Oral	As above for 5–7 days	Both amantadine and rimantadine are effective in uncomplicated influenza. Neither drug has been demonstrated to be effective in complicated influenza (e.g., pneumonia).
	or			
	rimantadine	Oral	As above for 5–7 days	Under study for treatment of complicated influenza in placebo-controlled trials.
Respiratory syncytial virus	Ribavirin	Aerosol	Administered continuously by small-particle aerosol from a reservoir containing 20 mg/mL for 3–6 days	Utilized for treatment of infants and young children hospitalized with RSV pneumonia and bronchiolitis.
Herpes simplex encephalitis	Acyclovir	IV	10 mg/kg every 8 h for 10 days	Acyclovir is the drug of choice for this infection on the basis of comparative trials vs. vidarabine. Optimal results are obtained when therapy is initiated early in illness.
	or			
	vidarabine	IV	15 mg/kg per day as a continous infusion for 12 h for 10 days	
Neonatal herpes simplex	Vidarabine	IV	30 mg/kg per day given as a continuous infusion over 12 h per day for 10 days	Vidarabine reduces mortality, but severe morbidity is frequent. Currently being compared with acyclovir in a clinical trial.
	or			
	acyclovir	IV	10 mg/kg every 8 h for 10 days	
Genital herpes simplex: primary infection	Acyclovir	IV	5 mg/kg every 8 h for 5–10 days	IV route is preferred if infection is of sufficient severity to warrant hospitalization, or if neurologic complications are present.
		Oral	200 mg 5 times per day for 10 days	Preferred route of administration for patients who do not warrant hospitalization. Adequate hydration should be maintained.
		Topical	5% ointment; 4–6 applications per day for 7–10 days	Largely supplanted by oral therapy. May be of use in pregnant women in order to avoid systemic therapy. Systemic symptoms and untreated areas are not affected.
Genital herpes simplex: recurrent infections (therapy)	Acyclovir	Oral	200 mg 5 times per day for 5 days	Clinical effect is modest and is enhanced if therapy is initiated early. No effect on subsequent recurrence rates.
Genital herpes simplex: recurrent infections (suppression)	Acyclovir	Oral	200 mg 3 times per day for up to 6 months	Suppressive therapy is recommended only for patients with frequent recurrences, at least 6 to 10 per year. Occasional "breakthrough" may occur, and asymptomatic shedding of virus occurs.
Mucocutaneous herpes simplex in immunocompromised patients (treatment)	Acyclovir	IV	250 mg/m² every 8 h for 7 days	Choice of intravenous or oral route will depend on severity of infection and whether patient can take oral medication. Oral or IV administration has supplanted topical therapy except for small, easily accessible lesions.
		Oral	200 mg PO 5 times per day for 10 days	
	or	Topical	5% ointment; 4–6 applications per day for 7 days or until healed	
	vidarabine	IV	10 mg/kg per day for 7 days given as a 12-h infusion	Efficacy has been demonstrated in HSV-1 infections and in patients who were older than 40. Appears to be less useful than acyclovir in this setting.
Mucocutaneous herpes simplex in immunocompromised patients (prevention of recurrences during periods of intense immunosuppression)	Acyclovir	Oral	200 mg 4 times per day	Acyclovir is administered during periods when intense immunosuppression is expected, e.g., antitumor chemotherapy, after transplantation. After therapy is discontinued, lesions recur.
		IV	5 mg/kg every 12 h	
Herpes simplex keratitis	Trifluorothymidine	Topical	One drop of 0.1% ophthalmic solution every 2 h while awake (maximum 9 drops per day)	Therapy should be undertaken in consultation with an ophthalmologist.
	or			
	vidarabine	Topical	0.5-in ribbon of 0.5% ophthalmic ointment 5 times per day	As above.
Varicella in immunocompromised patients	Acyclovir	IV	500 mg/m² every 8 h for 7 days	Studies comparing acyclovir with vidarabine in the treatment of varicella have not been performed. Limited placebo-controlled studies suggest the effects of both drugs on varicella are similar.
	or			
	vidarabine	IV	10 mg/kg per day in a 12-h infusion for 5 days	

TABLE 86-1 Antiviral chemotherapy and chemoprophylaxis *(continued)*

Infection	Antiviral drug	Administration	Dosage	Comment
Herpes zoster in immunocompromised patients	Acyclovir	IV	500 mg/m² every 8 h for 7 days	Efficacy of acyclovir and vidarabine are established for localized zoster, particularly when treated early and acyclovir appears to be more effective. Studies of the effect on disseminated zoster of the two drugs are under way. Oral acyclovir (4 g/d) is under study in herpes zoster in immunosuppressed patients and in "normal" hosts.
	or			
	vidarabine	IV	10 mg/kg per day in a 12-h infusion for 5 days	
Herpes zoster ophthalmicus	Acyclovir	Oral	600 mg PO 5 times a day for 10 days	Reduces ocular complications including keratitis and uveitis
Cytomegalovirus infections	Ganciclovir	IV	5 mg/kg twice a day for 14–21 days, then 5 mg/kg per day as maintenance	Investigational drug used to treat CMV infections, particularly in AIDS patients. May be effective in retinitis, colitis, "wasting syndromes" associated with CMV—probably less so in CMV pneumonitis.
Human immunodeficiency virus infection	Zidovudine	Oral	200 mg PO every 4 h	Licensed for treatment of AIDS and ARC patients with CD4 counts less than 200/μL. Beneficial effects on mortality and morbidity wane after 1 year of therapy. Efficacy of lower doses and efficacy in patients with early ARC or with asymptomatic HIV infections are under study.

They inhibit influenza A virus replication at an as yet unspecified step after virus attachment to the cell, possibly through interaction with the influenza A M2 matrix protein. In several experimental systems, rimantadine is two to four times more active than amantadine against isolates of influenza A.

Amantadine and rimantadine have been demonstrated to be effective in the prophylaxis of influenza A in large-scale studies in young adults, and to a lesser extent in children and in elderly subjects. In such studies, efficacy rates of 55 to 80 percent in prevention of influenza-like illness were noted, and even higher rates were reported when virus-specific attack rates were calculated. Amantadine and rimantadine have also been demonstrated to be effective in the treatment of influenza A infection, in studies carried out predominantly in young adults and, to a lesser extent, in children. Administration of these compounds within 24 to 72 h after the onset of illness has resulted in a reduction of duration of signs and symptoms by approximately 50 percent when compared to a placebo-treated group. The effect on signs and symptoms of illness has been demonstrated to be superior to that of commonly used antipyretic-analgesics. Only anecdotal reports are available concerning the efficacy of amantadine or rimantadine in the prevention or treatment of complications of influenza (e.g., pneumonia).

Amantadine and rimantadine are available only in oral formulations and are ordinarily administered in a dose of 200 mg/d for adults, given once or twice daily. Despite their structural similarities, the pharmacokinetics of the two compounds are different. Amantadine is not metabolized and is excreted almost entirely by the kidney, with a half-life of 12 to 17 h and peak plasma concentrations of 0.4 μg/mL. Rimantadine is extensively metabolized to hydroxylated derivatives and has a half-life of 30 h. Only 30 percent of an orally administered dose is recovered in the urine. The peak plasma levels of rimantadine are approximately one-half those of amantadine, but rimantadine is concentrated in respiratory secretions to a greater extent than amantadine. For prophylaxis, the compounds must be administered daily for the period at risk (i.e., the duration of the outbreak). For therapy, amantadine or rimantadine is generally administered for 5 to 7 days.

Although these compounds are generally well tolerated, 5 to 10 percent of amantadine recipients experience mild central nervous system side effects, consisting primarily of dizziness, anxiety, insomnia, and difficulty in concentrating. These side effects are rapidly reversible upon cessation of the drug. In a dose of 200 mg/d, rimantadine is better tolerated than amantadine, and in a large-scale study in young adults, side effects were no more frequent in rimantadine recipients than in placebo recipients. Seizures and worsening of congestive heart failure have also been reported in patients treated with amantadine, although a causal relationship has not been established.

Amantadine is licensed for the prophylaxis and therapy of influenza A in the United States, while rimantadine remains experimental. Because of its effectiveness and lack of toxicity, rimantadine may be particularly advantageous for long-term prophylaxis, or for therapy of influenza in subjects at particular risk for development of CNS toxicity, such as elderly individuals. When amantadine is employed in the latter group, the recommended dose is 100 mg/d.

RIBAVIRIN Ribavirin is a synthetic nucleoside analogue that inhibits a wide range of RNA and DNA viruses. The mechanism of action of ribavirin is not completely defined and may be different for different groups of viruses. Ribavirin-5′-monophosphate blocks the conversion of inosine-5′-monophosphate to xanthosine-5′-monophosphate, and interferes with the synthesis of guanine nucleotides and both RNA and DNA synthesis. Ribavirin-5′-monophosphate also inhibits capping of virus-specific RNA in certain viral systems. In studies demonstrating the effectiveness of ribavirin, the compound has been administered as a small-particle aerosol. It has been utilized to treat respiratory syncytial virus (RSV) infection in infants, and to a lesser extent, parainfluenza infections in children and influenza A and B infection in young adults. In RSV infection in infants, ribavirin administered by continuous aerosol for 3 to 6 days resulted in more rapid resolution of illness, lower respiratory tract signs, and arterial oxygen desaturation when compared to placebo-treated groups. Its use for severe RSV infections in adults has not resulted in any clear benefit. Orally administered ribavirin has not been effective in the treatment of influenza A infections. Ribavirin is under evaluation for adenovirus and arenavirus infections, including Lassa fever, and for patients with acquired immunodeficiency syndrome (AIDS).

Large doses of ribavirin administered orally (800 to 1000 mg/d) have been associated with reversible hematopoietic toxicity, but this has not been observed with aerosolized ribavirin, apparently because little drug is absorbed systemically. Aerosolized administration of ribavirin has been approved for treatment of respiratory syncytial virus infection in infants. Because of the need for aerosolized administration, the drug can only be given for this indication under close supervision. Health care workers exposed to the drug have experienced minor toxicity including eye and respiratory tract irritation.

ACYCLOVIR Acyclovir, 9-[(2-hydroxyethoxy)methyl]guanine, is a highly potent and selective inhibitor of replication of certain herpesviruses, including herpes simplex 1 (HSV-1), herpes simplex 2 (HSV-2), varicella-zoster virus (VZV), and Epstein-Barr virus (EBV). It is relatively ineffective in human cytomegalovirus (CMV) infections.

The high degree of selectivity of acyclovir is related to its mechanism of action, which requires that the compound first be phosphorylated to acyclovir monophosphate. This phosphorylation occurs efficiently in herpesvirus-infected cells by means of a virus-coded thymidine kinase. In uninfected mammalian cells, little phosphorylation of acyclovir occurs, and therefore, the drug is concentrated in herpesvirus-infected cells. Acyclovir monophosphate is subsequently converted by host cell kinases to a triphosphate which is a potent inhibitor of virus-induced DNA polymerase but has relatively little effect on host cell DNA polymerase. Acyclovir triphosphate can also be incorporated into viral DNA, with early chain termination.

Acyclovir is available in intravenous, oral, and topically administered forms. Intravenous acyclovir has been demonstrated to be markedly effective in the therapy of mucocutaneous HSV infections in immunocompromised hosts, reducing time to healing, duration of pain, and virus shedding. When administered prophylactically during periods of intense immunosuppression such as chemotherapy for leukemia or transplantation, but before lesions are present, intravenous acyclovir has also reduced the frequency of HSV-associated disease. After prophylaxis was discontinued, recurrent HSV lesions developed. Intravenous acyclovir has also been demonstrated to be effective in the treatment of HSV encephalitis, and two comparative trials have indicated that acyclovir is more effective than vidarabine for treatment of the latter infection (see below). Varicella-zoster virus is generally less sensitive to acyclovir than is herpes simplex virus, so that higher doses of acyclovir must be used to treat varicella-zoster virus infections. In immunocompromised patients with herpes zoster, intravenous acyclovir reduced the frequency of cutaneous dissemination and visceral complications and was more effective than vidarabine in one comparative trial. Acyclovir administered orally at doses of 800 mg five times a day had a modest beneficial effect on localized herpes zoster lesions in both immunocompromised and immunocompetent patients and is being evaluated in large-scale collaborative trials. Orally administered acyclovir (600 mg five times a day) reduced complications of herpes zoster ophthalmicus in a placebo-controlled trial.

The most widespread use of acyclovir is in the therapy of genital herpes simplex virus infections. Both intravenous and oral formulations have shortened the duration of symptoms, reduced virus shedding, and accelerated healing when employed for the treatment of primary genital HSV infections. Oral acyclovir also had a modest effect in the therapy of recurrent genital HSV infections. However, treatment of either primary or recurrent disease did not reduce the frequency of subsequent recurrences, indicating that acyclovir was ineffective in elimination of latent infection. Chronically administered oral acyclovir for periods ranging from 1 to 6 years has been shown to reduce the frequency of recurrences markedly while on therapy, although once the drug was discontinued, lesions recurred. In AIDS patients chronic administration of acyclovir has been asociated with the development of strains resistant to the action of the drug and with clinical failures.

With the availability of the oral and intravenous forms, there are few indications for topical acyclovir, although treatment with this formulation has shown modest beneficial effects in the therapy of primary genital herpes infections and of mucocutaneous HSV infections in immunocompromised hosts.

Overall, acyclovir is remarkably well tolerated and generally free of toxicity. The most frequently encountered toxicity has been occasional renal dysfunction, particularly after rapid intravenous administration or when patients have been inadequately hydrated. Central nervous system changes, including lethargy and tremors, occasionally have been reported, primarily in immunosuppressed patients. However, whether these changes are related to acyclovir, to concurrent administration of other therapy, or to underlying infection remains unclear. Acyclovir is excreted primarily unmetabolized by the kidney, both by glomerular filtration and tubular secretion. Approximately 15 percent of a dose of acyclovir is metabolized to 9-[(carboxymethoxy)methyl]guanine or other minor metabolites. Reduction in dosage is indicated in patients with creatinine clearances less than 50 mL/min per 1.73 m^2. The half-life of acyclovir is approximately 3 h in normal adults, and peak plasma concentrations after a 1-h infusion employing a 5 mg/kg dose are 9.8 μg/mL. Approximately 22 percent of acyclovir administered orally is absorbed, and peak plasma concentrations of 0.3 to 0.9 μg/mL are attained after administration of a 200-mg dose. Acyclovir penetrates relatively well into the cerebrospinal fluid, with CSF concentrations approaching one-half of those found in plasma.

GANCICLOVIR An analogue of acyclovir, ganciclovir, 9-[(1,3-dihydroxy-2-propoxy)methyl]guanine, has markedly increased activity against CMV. Ganciclovir triphosphate inhibits CMV DNA polymerases and can be incorporated into CMV DNA but, in contrast to acyclovir, does not function as a chain terminator. CMV, unlike HSV, does not code for its own thymidine kinase, and the mechanism by which phosphorylation of ganciclovir takes place in host cells is not defined. Ganciclovir has been utilized most extensively in the treatment of CMV infection in AIDS and otherwise immunosuppressed patients, and the drug has been used in neonatal CMV infections as well. Much of the clinical experience with ganciclovir has been uncontrolled, but available evidence indicates that it is effective in treatment of CMV retinitis for which it is approved by the Federal Drug Administration (FDA). Its efficacy in CMV colitis, CMV-associated "wasting," and, perhaps less so, in CMV pneumonitis remains to be established. It is currently investigational for the latter conditions, and is available only as an intravenous preparation. The most commonly employed dosage for initial therapy is 5 mg/kg twice a day for 14 to 21 days, followed by a maintenance dose of 5 mg/kg per day, possibly for as long as the immunosuppression persists. Administration of ganciclovir has been associated with profound bone marrow suppression, particularly neutropenia, which represents a major limitation of its use in many patients. Bone marrow toxicity is potentiated when other bone marrow suppressants such as zidovudine are used concomitantly. Clinical trials to determine optimal dosage and to evaluate oral formulations of ganciclovir are under way.

Foscarnet is another inhibitor of CMV DNA polymerase which has shown antiviral activity in vitro and in vivo. The major toxicity appears to be renal, with little bone marrow suppression, which makes the drug an attractive alternative in patients who cannot tolerate ganciclovir. It also has activity against human immunodeficiency virus (HIV) in vitro. Clinical trials to determine the efficacy and toxicity of foscarnet are currently being carried out.

ZIDOVUDINE Zidovudine (ZDV), also known as azidothymidine (AZT), inhibits the replication of HIV-1 through a competitive inhibition of HIV reverse transcriptase by AZT triphosphate, and possibly through chain termination of viral DNA synthesis as well. A large-scale placebo-controlled trial carried out in patients with AIDS or with advanced AIDS-related complex (ARC) demonstrated that administration of ZDV was associated with prolonged survival and with a decreased frequency and severity of opportunistic infections. On this basis, ZDV was licensed for treatment of patients with AIDS or patients with ARC who have less than 200 CD4 lymphocytes per microliter in peripheral blood. Median survival for the patients in the study who received ZDV was 85 percent at the end of the first year, but fell markedly during the second year. The reasons for this decline in efficacy are unclear but may be related to the progressive bone marrow toxicity associated with ZDV. Anemia or granulocytopenia sufficient to require blood transfusion and/or interruption or discontinuation of ZDV occurred in 70 percent of subjects during 21 months of study. In addition, relative resistance of HIV-1 to ZDV has been described after more than 6 months of administration of the drug. Trials are underway to define the role of myelopoietic growth factors (G-CSF and GM-CSF) and erythropoietin in reversing ZDV bone marrow toxicity.

The recommended dose of ZDV is 200 mg by mouth every 4 h, but because of drug toxicity, reduced doses, usually to 200 mg by mouth every 8 h, are frequently employed. The efficacy of reduced doses is under study as is the efficacy of ZDV in the prevention of disease progression in patients who are infected with HIV but are asymptomatic or who have early stages of ARC.

Other inhibitors of HIV replication are also being evaluated in laboratory and clinical studies. Among the most promising are dideoxycytidine and dideoxyinosine, which are nucleoside analogues that are active in vitro and have shown anti-HIV-1 activity in phase one studies in humans. Comparative studies of these drugs with ZDV are in progress.

VIDARABINE Vidarabine (9-β-D-arabinofuranosyladenine) is a purine nucleoside analogue with activity against HSV-1, HSV-2, VZV, and EBV. Vidarabine inhibits viral DNA synthesis through its 5′-triphosphorylated metabolite, although the precise molecular mechanisms of action are not completely understood. In the therapy of herpes zoster in immunosuppressed patients, vidarabine, administered in a dose of 10 mg/kg per day for 5 days, resulted in reduction of rates of cutaneous and visceral dissemination, and of postherpetic neuralgia but was less effective than acyclovir in a comparative trial. Beneficial effects have also been observed in the treatment of varicella in immunosuppressed patients. Vidarabine administered in a higher dose (15 mg/kg per day for 10 days) was demonstrated to be effective in the therapy of herpes simplex encephalitis in a placebo-controlled study in which mortality was reduced from 70 to 40 percent in vidarabine recipients at 6 months after therapy. However, comparative studies indicate that acyclovir (30 mg/kg per day) is more effective than vidarabine in the therapy of herpes simplex encephalitis, and acyclovir has supplanted vidarabine as the treatment of choice for that infection. The above studies also indicated that the success of therapy was closely related to administration of the drug early in the illness.

Vidarabine treatment has also reduced the mortality of neonatal herpes simplex infection from 74 percent in placebo recipients to 38 percent, although the majority of survivors have severely impaired central nervous system function. Vidarabine has also been effective in the treatment of HSV mucocutaneous infections in immunosuppressed patients, although the effects observed were limited to patients who had HSV-1 infections and were older than 40. Topically administered vidarabine has been generally ineffective in the treatment of mucocutaneous genital or orofacial HSV infections, but is effective in the treatment of HSV keratitis.

For systemic administration, vidarabine is available only as an intravenous preparation with poor solubility and is administered as a constant 12-h infusion, so that a substantial fluid load can result which may be a significant problem in central nervous system infections. In humans, vidarabine is rapidly deaminated by a serum adenosine deaminase to its hypoxanthine derivative, ara-Hx, which has tenfold less antiviral activity than the parent compound, but is the major antiviral moiety in the plasma.

Large-scale controlled trials of vidarabine at doses of 10 to 15 mg/kg per day have not been attended by significant toxicity. At somewhat higher doses (20 mg/kg per day), vidarabine has been associated with hematopoietic side effects, including anemia, leukopenia, and thrombocytopenia. Neurotoxicity has also been reported, particularly with high dosages, in patients with hepatic or renal insufficiency, and possibly with concurrent interferon or allopurinol administration. The neurotoxic effects have included tremor, alterations in mentation, rarely coma or seizures, and unusual pain syndromes in the extremities, which have lasted up to 6 months after cessation of therapy.

TOPICAL ANTIVIRALS IUdR (5′-iodo-2′-deoxyuridine) is an inhibitor of DNA virus replication, including herpesviruses and poxviruses. It was formerly used systemically to treat herpesvirus infections, including HSV encephalitis, but because of associated toxicity and lack of demonstrated efficacy, its systemic use has largely been abandoned. Topical IUdR has been effective in the treatment of HSV keratitis, particularly in superficial epithelial infections, but has been largely supplanted by topically applied trifluorothymidine or vidarabine.

Trifluorothymidine (TFT) is an analogue of deoxythymidine, which is also effective against herpesvirus infections. Because of bone marrow suppression, its use is restricted to topical application in the eye, where it appears to be somewhat more effective and better tolerated than IUdR, and at least as effective as vidarabine. TFT has also been effective in some patients who had not responded clinically to topical IUdR or vidarabine.

INTERFERONS From its earliest descriptions, considerable interest has existed in the application of interferon to the prophylaxis and/or therapy of viral infections. Early studies with human leukocyte interferon demonstrated an effect in the prophylaxis of experimentally induced rhinovirus infections in humans, and in the treatment of varicella-zoster infections in immunosuppressed patients. DNA recombinant technology has made available highly purified α-, β-, and γ-interferons, which have been evaluated in a variety of viral infections. Results available from such trials have confirmed the effectiveness of intranasally administered interferon in the prophylaxis of rhinovirus infections, although its use has been associated with nasal mucosal irritation. Administration of either intralesional or intramuscular interferons has resulted in beneficial effects on genital warts, and trials of interferon therapy in papilloma virus infection are under way. Interferon therapy is undergoing evaluation in chronic hepatitis B infections, and as an additive treatment to ZDV in therapy of AIDS. α-Interferon has been demonstrated to be effective in reducing the manifestations of Kaposi's sarcoma in AIDS patients.

REFERENCES

DOLIN R: Antiviral chemotherapy and chemoprophylaxis (review). Science 227:1296, 1985

——— et al: A controlled trial of amantadine and rimantadine in the prophylaxis of influenza A infection. N Engl J Med 307:580, 1982

FISCHL M et al. The efficacy of azidothymidine (AZT) in the treatment of patients with AIDS and AIDS-related complex; a double blind placebo-controlled trial. N Engl J Med 317:185, 1987

HALL CB et al: Aerosolized ribavirin treatment of infants with respiratory syncytial viral infection: A randomized double blind study. N Engl J Med 308:1443, 1983

NEYERS JD: Management of cytomegalovirus infection. Am J Med 85(Suppl 2A):102, 1988

REICHMAN RC et al: Treatment of recurrent genital herpes simplex with acyclovir. A controlled trial. JAMA 251:2103, 1984

WHITLEY RJ et al and the NIAID Collaborative Antiviral Study Group: Herpes simplex encephalitis: Adenine arabinoside versus acyclovir therapies. N Engl J Med 314:144, 1986

87 ANTIFUNGAL THERAPY

JOHN E. BENNETT

TOPICAL AGENTS **Imidazoles and triazoles** These synthetic compounds act by inhibiting ergosterol synthesis in the fungal cell wall and when given topically may cause direct damage to the cytoplasmic membrane. Drug resistance rarely arises in the previously sensitive strains. Imidazoles available for cutaneous application include clotrimazole, econazole, and miconazole. Vaginal formulations include three imidazoles: miconazole, clotrimazole, and butoconazole; and one triazole: terconazole. Miconazole lotion is available without prescription. As yet, no substantial difference in efficacy or local intolerance between these agents has appeared. All are effective in treatment of cutaneous candidiasis, tinea versicolor, and mild to moderately severe ringworm of the glabrous skin. Vaginal formulations are effective in vulvovaginal candidiasis. Clotrimazole is poorly absorbed from the gastrointestinal tract, but the oral troche is useful as a topical treatment for oral and esophageal candidiasis.

Polyene macrolide antibiotics These broad-spectrum antifungal agents combine with sterol in the fungal cytoplasmic membrane, increasing membrane permeability. Topically they are not active against ringworm but are effective against candidiasis of the skin and mucous membranes. Nystatin suspension is effective in oral thrush, and vaginal troches are effective in vulvovaginal candidiasis. Both nystatin and amphotericin B are available in topical preparations for cutaneous candidiasis. Natamycin ophthalmic suspension is marketed in some countries (but not in the United States) for mycotic keratitis and conjunctivitis.

Other topical antifungals Ciclopirox olamine, haloprogin, and naftifine have the same clinical spectrum among the cutaneous mycoses as the imidazoles. Tolnaftate and undecylenic acid are effective against ringworm but not candidiasis. Keratolytic agents, such as salicylic acid, are helpful as accessory drugs for some hyperkeratotic skin lesions.

SYSTEMIC ANTIFUNGALS **Griseofulvin** Griseofulvin is a useful drug in treating certain kinds of ringworm; however, it is ineffective in treating candidiasis. The microcrystalline and ultramicrocrystalline preparations differ in dose but not in efficacy. Absorption of both is enhanced when ingested with fat-containing foods. Griseofulvin interacts with phenobarbital and coumarin-type anticoagulants.

Imidazoles and triazoles Ketoconazole is the only systemically absorbed oral drug of this class that is currently available, though similar drugs are undergoing clinical trial. Absorption of ketoconazole is variable between individuals, is not affected by food, and is poor in patients taking cimetidine or other H-2 blocking agents. Simultaneous administration of antacids can also impair absorption. Metabolism is chiefly hepatic, but substantial liver disease has minimal effect on plasma ketoconazole concentrations. Ketoconazole plasma levels are decreased in patients taking rifampin and also in some taking isoniazid. Ketoconazole administration can elevate cyclosporin blood levels and, occasionally, can enhance the anticoagulant effect of warfarin. The drug is contraindicated during pregnancy and, because it appears in breast milk, during breast feeding. Neither renal disease nor hemodialysis affects the metabolism of ketoconazole. The most common toxicity of ketoconazole is dose-related nausea, anorexia and, occasionally, vomiting. Hepatotoxicity is idiosyncratic and usually mild but rarely can be serious and fatal. Several dose-related, temporary endocrine effects have been observed: decreased adrenal cortical reserve; gynecomastia; decreased serum testosterone, libido, and potency in males; and menstrual irregularity in females. Pruritus or rash may also occur. Ketoconazole is effective in blastomycosis, histoplasmosis, paracoccidioidomycosis, chronic mucocutaneous candidiasis, esophageal candidiasis, and some forms of disseminated coccidioidomycosis and pseudallescheriasis. The usual adult dose is 400 mg, taken once daily. Partial improvement may be seen in cutaneous sporotrichosis and chromomycosis. Although vulvovaginal candidiasis, ringworm, and tinea versicolor are responsive to the drug, the toxicity of oral ketoconazole makes topical imidazoles or other drugs preferable for these indications. Miconazole is available as both a topical and an intravenous preparation. The latter is rarely indicated.

Itraconazole and fluconazole are systemic triazoles under clinical investigation. Toxicity and hormonal suppression are less than with ketoconazole. There is preliminary evidence that fluconazole may be useful in cryptococcosis and in coccidioidal meningitis. Itraconazole has compared favorably with ketoconazole for most indications. Therapeutic indications, significant drug interactions, and dosage remain to be defined for both agents.

Amphotericin B A colloidal preparation of this drug is available for intravenous or intrathecal administration. The drug cannot be given intramuscularly and is not absorbed orally. Sodium or potassium salts must not be added to the infusion solutions because the colloidal drug will precipitate out of solution. In-line filters with 0.22-μm pore diameter may trap some of the colloid. Catabolism is extremely slow and is not influenced by renal failure, hepatic failure, or hemodialysis. Penetration into cerebrospinal fluid and vitreous humor is poor; however, concentrations in pleural, peritoneal, and articular exudates are adequate for many mycoses. Histoplasmosis, blastomycosis, paracoccidioidomycosis, candidiasis, and cryptococcosis are the most responsive mycoses. Coccidioidomycosis, extraarticular sporotrichosis, aspergillosis, and mucormycosis are less responsive; chromomycosis, mycetoma, and pseudallescheriasis show little if any response. The usual course is 8 to 10 weeks of 0.4 to 0.6 mg/kg daily. Infusions are generally given in 5% dextrose over 2 to 4 h. Severe febrile reactions to initial doses generally prompt use of an initial test dose with 1 mg, followed by escalating doses based upon the gravity of the patient's infection and tolerance of the drug. Virtually all patients show toxic reactions that are related to the dose and duration of therapy. These side effects include azotemia, anemia, hypokalemia, nausea, anorexia, weight loss, phlebitis and, occasionally, hypomagnesemia. Intrathecal amphotericin B is indicated in coccidioidal meningitis and refractory cryptococcal meningitis, though this therapy is associated with considerable toxicity. Doses of 0.1 to 0.5 mg are given three times per week initially, then with decreasing frequency.

Flucytosine Flucytosine (5-fluorocytosine) is a synthetic oral drug useful in cryptococcosis, candidiasis, and chromomycosis. Within the fungal cell, flucytosine is converted to the antimetabolite 5-fluorouracil. Drug resistance appears rather rapidly when flucytosine is used alone. For this reason the drug is generally used in combination with amphotericin B, permitting a lower dose of the latter. The usual regimen is amphotericin B 0.3 mg/kg daily and flucytosine 37.5 mg/kg every 6 h. Flucytosine is well absorbed from the gastrointestinal tract, even in the presence of food. The drug penetrates well into the cerebrospinal fluid and is excreted unchanged in the urine. Hemodialysis results in significant drug removal. Even modest reductions in renal function may elevate flucytosine blood levels into the toxic range, ≥100 to 125 μg/mL. Elevated levels are associated with a significant incidence of neutropenia and thrombocytopenia. Elevated flucytosine blood levels also seem to predispose to colitis, the other major toxicity of this drug. Hepatotoxicity is idiosyncratic and uncommon. An allergic rash may also occur.

REFERENCES (See Chap. 151)

88 THERAPY OF PARASITIC INFECTIONS

JAMES J. PLORDE

INTRODUCTION Despite some gains, treatment of parasitic diseases remains unsatisfactory. The total number of available agents remains small, and for some infections, including cryptosporidiosis, satisfactory drugs have yet to be developed. Few of the newer chemotherapeutics are at once inexpensive, effective in single oral dose, and safely dispensed with limited medical supervision, essential attributes if they are to be fully useful in developing countries, where the burden of parasitism is greatest. Drug resistance, a phenomenon so common to bacterial pathogens, now threatens the usefulness of several antiparasitic chemicals. This is particularly serious among the antimalarials. Chloroquine-resistant *Plasmodium falciparum,* long present in southeast Asia and Latin America, has spread to most parts of tropical Africa, the area most devastated by this disease. Some Asian strains of this organism have developed resistance to the

TABLE 88-1 Agents available through the parasitic diseases division, CDC*

Infection	Therapeutic agent
Amebiasis	Dehydroemetine
	Diloxanide furoate
Chagas' disease *(Trypanosoma cruzi)*	Nifurtimox
Fascioliasis	Bithionol
Leishmaniasis	Sodium antimony gluconate (stibogluconate sodium)
Malaria	Parenteral quinine dihydrochloride
Onchocerciasis	Ivermectin
	Suramin
Paragonimiasis	Bithionol
Sleeping sickness *(Trypanosoma brucei)*	Melarsoprol
	Suramin

* Parasitic Diseases Division, Centers for Disease Control, Atlanta, Ga 30333. Telephone: (404)639-3670 (day); (404)639-2888 (evenings, weekends, or holidays).

pyrimethamine-sulfadoxine drug combination and to newly introduced agents such as mefloquine, sharply limiting the armamentarium available for the management of this lethal disease. The availability of many antiparasitic drugs is sharply limited, both in the United States and around the world. In fact, many of the drugs recommended in the following chapters have not been approved by the U.S. Food and Drug Administration either for use in this country or for the particular disease indicated. Those available as investigational agents through the Centers for Disease Control are listed in Table 88-1. Others, such as albendazole, DL-α-difluoromethylornithine (DFMO), and ivermectin, must be obtained directly from the manufacturer. When a clinician prescribes such an agent, the patient should be informed of the drug's investigational status and potential side effects.

STRUCTURE AND MODE OF ACTION Characteristically, antiparasitic agents have been synthesized de novo rather than derived from naturally occurring antibiotics. Most are relatively simple, often containing benzene or other ring structures. Nitrocompounds are common, despite studies documenting that chemicals of this class may be teratogenic and carcinogenic in experimental animals. A few of the currently used drugs resemble the original chemotherapeutics in their possession of heavy metal moieties, specifically arsenic or antimony.

It has been difficult to determine the precise mechanisms by which chemotherapeutic agents kill or injure parasites, given the metabolic complexity of these organisms and the difficulties involved in maintaining them in vitro. Nevertheless, there is both direct and indirect evidence that most antiprotozoan agents act by interfering with nucleic acid synthesis. Anthelmintics, in contrast, are thought to compromise glycolytic pathways or interfere with neuromuscular function. As both parasite and host share similar, and in some cases identical, target sites, differential toxicity is achieved by differences in the susceptibility of functionally equivalent sites, metabolic alteration of the drug within the parasite, or preferential uptake by the parasite. The development of parasite resistance usually results from mutation and selection in the face of intensive drug use. The responsible mechanisms most commonly appear to be related to altered uptake of drug.

DRUG CATEGORIES **Heavy metals** Although nearly a century has passed since the introduction of the first organic heavy metal chemotherapeutic agents, a few such agents survive for want of adequate substitutes. Such drugs are thought to inhibit cellular enzyme systems necessary for metabolism by binding to sulfhydryl groups; arsenate ion may block ATP generation through the inhibition of pyruvate kinase. The drugs have their greatest impact on cells that are the most metabolically active, and their differential toxicity for parasites probably results from the intense metabolic activity of these pathogens. Pentavalent compounds, which appear to penetrate mammalian cells less effectively than their trivalent analogues, are generally preferred for human use. They appear, however, to be less effective parasitologic agents than the trivalent compounds and may require intracellular conversion to the trivalent form for full activity. Side chain substitutions of the organic structure alter drug solubility and other pharmacologic properties.

Melarsoprol (Mel B), a trivalent compound capable of penetrating the blood-brain barrier, is the only arsenical still widely used for the treatment of human disease. It is administered for sleeping sickness when less toxic agents have failed or the central nervous system is involved. It must be given intravenously, and tissue extravasation produces an intense inflammatory reaction. Arsenic-induced enteropathy, hepatitis, nephritis, or dermatitis may occur. The most serious side effect is an often fatal encephalopathy, which occurs in up to 20 percent of patients with central nervous system involvement.

Antimonial agents are now restricted to the management of leishmanial infections. In the United States, the pentavalent compound sodium stibogluconate (Pentostam) is the drug of choice. It may be given intravenously, intramuscularly, or, in the case of cutaneous leishmaniasis, by local infiltration. In disseminated disease, prolonged therapy is often required and relapse occurs with some frequency. In localized cutaneous leishmaniasis, cure is usually achieved with a single, relatively brief course. Toxic side effects are similar to that produced by the arsenicals. Anaphylaxis, hemolytic anemia, arthropathies, bradycardia, electrocardiogram abnormalities, and vascular collapse have also been reported.

Antimalarial quinolines Following the isolation of quinine from cinchona bark in 1820, this alkaloid rapidly became the most widely used antimalarial agent in the world. Synthesis of new antimalarials, which share a double-ring quinoline structure with quinine, was stimulated by the interruption of quinine supplies during two world wars and the subsequent development and spread of resistant strains of *P. falciparum*. The synthetic analogues fall into three major groups, the 4-aminoquinolines, 8-aminoquinolines, and 4-quinolinemethanols. The first two appear to block nucleic acid synthesis by intercalation into double-stranded DNA; the failure of the 4-quinolinemethanols to intercalate indicates that other mechanisms, possibly interference with hemoglobin digestion by the malaria parasite, may also be involved. Quinine, 4-aminoquinolines, and 4-quinolinemethanols concentrate in parasitized erythrocytes and rapidly destroy the intracellular schizonts. As these parasite forms are responsible for the clinical manifestations of malaria, blood schizonticides rapidly terminate the acute malarial paroxysm; administered prophylactically, they prevent clinical manifestations should infection occur. As they are not selectively concentrated in tissue cells, hepatic schizonts survive administration of these agents and may later invade the bloodstream and reestablish erythrocytic infection, producing a clinical relapse. The 8-aminoquinolines accumulate in tissue cells and, by damaging parasite mitochondria, destroy hepatic hypnozoites. This prevents subsequent relapse and effects a radical cure. While active against mature gametocytes of all four malaria species, the 8-aminoquinolines are minimally effective against erythrocytic schizonts; accordingly, they are not used in the treatment of acute disease. The discrepancy between the high level of activity demonstrated by these drugs against hepatic hypnozoites and mature gametocytes and their minimal activity against erythrocytic schizonts is not fully understood. As the two former parasitic stages are metabolically dormant, it is possible they lack the capacity for mitochondrial repair, making them more sensitive to the damaging effects of the 8-aminoquinolines.

Quinine is the most toxic of the quinolines. Normal doses produce tinnitus and reversible alterations in auditory and visual acuity (cinchonism). Rapid intravenous administration may induce cardiac arrythmia and/or hypotension. Its use is currently restricted to the treatment of multiresistant strains of *P. falciparum*. Chloroquine phosphate, a 4-aminoquinoline, is the most widely used of the blood schizonticidal drugs. In the doses recommended for long-term malaria prophylaxis, it has proved remarkably free of untoward effects, even in pregnant women. Although irreversible retinopathy has occurred in patients receiving high daily doses over prolonged periods for conditions such as rheumatoid arthritis, this phenomenon has been seen rarely among those taking the lower doses recommended for malaria prophylaxis, even after decades of use. Its use in acute malaria is occasionally accompanied by transient gastrointestinal or visual disturbances. Chloroquine overdose can produce convulsions and cardiorespiratory arrest. The major toxic effect of primaquine phosphate, the 8-aminoquinoline used to eradicate persistent hepatic parasites, relates to its oxidant activity. Methemoglobinemia and hemolytic anemia are particularly frequent in patients with glucose-6-phosphate dehydrogenase deficiency, because they are unable to generate sufficient quantities of NADPH to respond to this oxidant stress. Typically, anemia is severe in patients of Mediterranean and Oriental ancestry and mild in blacks.

Strains of *P. falciparum* resistant to several of the blood schizonticidal agents are spreading rapidly through Asia, Latin America, and Africa. Chloroquine resistance is the most frequent and worrisome because there are few suitable alternatives to this safe and highly effective agent. The mechanism of resistance is not clearly understood. Mefloquine, a newly developed oral 4-quinolinemethanol, displays high level of activity against most chloroquine-resistant parasites. However, its structural similarity to chloroquine, the ready in vitro induction of mefloquine resistance in *P. falciparum,* and reports of mefloquine-resistant falciparum malaria from the field raise the specter that cross-resistance to this new agent may develop quickly.

Folate antagonists In protozoa, as in bacteria, the active form of folic acid is produced in vivo by a simple two-step process. The first, the conversion of para-aminobenzoic acid (PABA) to dihydrofolic acid, is blocked by sulfonamides. The second, the transformation of dihydro- to tetrahydrofolic acid, is suppressed by folic acid analogues (folate antagonists), which competitively inhibit the enzyme dihydrofolate reductase. Used together with sulfonamides, these antagonists are very effective inhibitors of protozoan growth.

The trimethoprim and sulfamethoxazole combination so widely used as an antibacterial agent is also effective in the management of some parasitic diseases, most notably *Pneumocystis carinii* pneumonia. Because of its high affinity for sporozoan dihydrofolate reductase, pyrimethamine has been particularly effective, when used in combination with a sulfonamide, in the management of malaria and toxoplasmosis. Proguanil also demonstrates antimalarial activity. Because this folate antagonist is slow-acting, it is used as a prophylactic rather than a therapeutic agent. Although unavailable in this country, it is used in many endemic areas of Africa and Asia. Acquired protozoan resistance is mutational in origin and generally has been limited to species of plasmodia; the mechanism is presumed to be identical to that described for bacteria. Cross-resistance among drugs of this class is common.

Manifestations of folate deficiency may be seen when these agents are used in individuals with limited folate stores, such as newborns, pregnant women, and the malnourished. It is particularly frequent when large doses are used for a prolonged period of time, as in the treatment of acute toxoplasmosis. When administered with sulfonamides, the entire range of toxicities associated with this class of antimicrobials may be seen. Of particular concern are the serious cutaneous reactions such as erythema multiforme, toxic epidermal necrolysis, and the highly lethal Stevens-Johnson syndrome reported in individuals receiving long-term malaria prophylaxis with the pyrimethamine-sulfadoxine combination. Patients with acquired immunodeficiency syndrome (AIDS) appear to suffer an unusually high incidence of toxic side effects to trimethoprim-sulfamethoxazole given for the treatment of *P. carinii* pneumonia. In approximately half, the reactions are severe enough to require discontinuation of the drugs.

Nitroimidazoles Metronidazole, one of the first of the new generation of antiparasitic agents, was introduced in 1959 for the treatment of trichomoniasis. Subsequently, it was found to be effective in the management of giardiasis and amebiasis as well. In all three of these protozoan agents, generation of energy is dependent upon the presence of low redox potential compounds such as ferredoxin to serve as electron carriers. They reduce the 5-nitro group of the imidazoles to intermediate products responsible for the death of protozoal cells, possibly by alkylation of DNA. Resistance, although uncommon, has been noted in strains of *Trichomonas vaginalis* lacking nitroreductase activity. Since low redox potential compounds are unique to obligate anaerobes, the nitroimidazoles are ineffective against aerobic or facultatively anaerobic pathogens. Metronidazole is rapidly absorbed after oral administration, reaching peak levels in 2 h; it diffuses well into all tissues, including the brain and cerebrospinal fluid. Side effects are uncommon and generally mild, including a metallic taste, epigastric discomfort, urethral and vaginal burning, overgrowth of *Candida,* and reversible neutropenia. Excreted metabolites often impart a reddish-brown color to the urine. Although an Antabuse-like reaction has been reported with metronidazole, this is not common. Rarely, central nervous system toxicity including vertigo, ataxia, sensory neuropathy, and convulsions has been observed. Of greater concern is metronidazole's mutagenicity for a variety of bacteria, an indication of its potential carcinogenicity in mammals. This appears to be mediated by the nitro group's reduction metabolites. Although tumorigenic activity has been demonstrated in chronically dosed rodents, it has not been noted in two retrospective human studies. Longer observation periods will be required before a definitive judgment about human carcinogenicity can be made. Although there is no evidence of teratogenicity in either animals or humans, it is probably unwise to use this agent during the first trimester of pregnancy. Metronidazole is the drug of choice for trichomoniasis and invasive amebiasis. Although not yet approved for treatment of giardiasis, the drug is effective in this infection as well. Tinidazole, a newer nitroimidazole not yet available in the United States, appears to be both more effective and less mutagenic.

Benzimidazoles As the name implies, the basic structure of these broad-spectrum anthelmintic agents consists of linked imidazole and benzene rings. The prototype drug, thiabendazole, acts against both adult and larval nematodes and was shown to be useful in the management of cutaneous larva migrans, trichinosis, and most intestinal nematode infections. It remains the drug of choice of cutanea larva migrans, strongyloidiasis, toxocariasis, and trichinosis. The mechanism by which it exerts its anthelmintic action is uncertain; it is known to inhibit fumarate reductase, an important mitochondrial enzyme of helminths. Thiabendazole is rapidly absorbed from the intestinal tract, reaches peak levels within 1 h of dosing, and, after hydroxylation in the liver, is almost totally eliminated in the urine within 24 h. Most side effects are mild, related to the gastrointestinal tract or liver, and rapidly disappear with the discontinuation of the drug. Occasionally dizziness, paresthesias, and drowsiness are noted. Hypersensitivity reactions, induced either by the drug or by antigens released from the damaged parasite, may occur.

Mebendazole, a carbamate benzimidazole, has a spectrum similar to that of thiabendazole. It also has been found to be effective against a number of cestodes including *Taenia, Hymenolepsis,* and *Echinococcus.* It is the drug of choice for pinworm infections, trichuriasis, ascariasis, and hookworm disease. Although not yet approved for use in tapeworm infections, mebendazole has proved to be useful in the management of the cestode infections mentioned above, particularly as an adjunct to the surgical removal of echinococcal cysts. It irreversibly blocks glucose uptake of both adult and larvae worms resulting in glycogen depletion, cessation of ATP formation, and paralysis or death. It does not appear to affect glucose metabolism in humans and is thought to exert its effect in worms by binding to tubulin and interfering with the assembly of cytoplasmic microtubules, structures essential to glucose uptake. Unlike thiabendazole, the drug is not well absorbed from the gastrointestinal tract, and it may owe part of its effectiveness against intestinal-dwelling adult worms to its high concentrations in the gut. Because of its poor absorption, systemic toxicity is uncommon. Nevertheless teratogenic effects have been observed in experimental animals. Accordingly its use in infants and pregnant women is contraindicated.

Albendazole, a benzimidazole carbamate not yet approved for use in the United States (available from manufacturer), has a spectrum similar to that of its close relative, mebendazole. It may be more effective than mebendazole in the management of echinococciasis, and is effective in the management of many intestinal nematode infections when administered as a single-dose treatment.

Avermectins Avermectins are macrocyclic lactones produced as fermentation products of *Streptomyces avermitilis*. They are effective at extremely low concentrations against a wide variety of nematodes and arthropods, possibly by mimicking the action of the parasites' inhibitory neurotransmitter, γ-aminobutyric acid (GABA), thereby producing neuromuscular paralysis; host immune mechanisms may synergize and prolong drug activity. GABA receptors also are found in the mammalian brain, but because avermectins penetrate the blood-brain barrier poorly, significant untoward effects in humans appear to be uncommon. As might be suspected by their unique mode of action, these antibiotics have not demonstrated cross-resistance with other antiparasitic agents.

Ivermectin, a 22,23-dihydro derivative of avermectin B_1 widely used in veterinary medicine, has become the drug of choice for the treatment of onchocerciasis. Peak blood levels are achieved within 3 h of oral administration, but little is known about subsequent distribution or metabolism of the drug in humans. While pharmacokinetic studies have demonstrated a half-life of only 22 h, microfilaricidal activity appears to persist for months. Dose-dependent, mild to moderate hypotension occurs in approximately 5 percent of drug recipients, but only rarely requires therapy. Rash, tenderness, and lymph node enlargement have also been reported. Ocular reactions are minimal, even in patients with severe corneal involvement. Its usefulness in other nematode infections of humans remains to be established. Not yet approved for use in the United States, the drug may be obtained from the manufacturer for investigational purposes.

Praziquantel As an extremely safe, single-dose oral agent effective against a broad range of cestodes and trematodes, praziquantel more closely approaches the definition of an ideal antiparasitic than any other currently used anthelmintic. This heterocyclic pyrazine-isoquinoline is rapidly absorbed from the gastrointestinal tract and metabolized in the liver; it diffuses well into most tissues, including the central nervous system. Activity appears dependent on the agent's ability to penetrate the helminthic cuticle; the thick outer membrane of the nematodes protects this class of worms from the action of the drug. In the susceptible platyhelminths, praziquantel induces the loss of intracellular calcium with tetanic muscular contraction, paralysis, and tegmental damage. The latter results in the loss of attachment organs and the exposure of surface antigens to the host's immune mechanisms. Differential toxicity appears related to the inability of susceptible worms to metabolize the drug. Aside from the transient, mild gastrointestinal symptoms, the drug is remarkably free of side effects; it is well tolerated by patients with glucose-6-phosphate dehydrogenase deficiency and hemoglobinopathies, and does not appear to be mutagenic or carcinogenic. It is currently the drug of choice for the treatment of schistosomiasis, neurocysticercosis, *Hymenolepsis nana* infections, and all infections produced by hermaphroditic flukes, *Fasciola hepatica* excepted. Good activity has been demonstrated against other common trematode and cestode infections, and it may displace currently used agents for these diseases as well. Its effectiveness as a single dose and its high level of safety make it likely that this agent will play a significant role in worldwide mass therapy campaigns.

Ornithine decarboxylase inhibitors Elfornithine (DL-α-difluoromethylornithine, DFMO) is a potent inhibitor of *Trypanosoma*

TABLE 88-2 Miscellaneous antiparasitic medications

Compound	Drug class	Route	Mechanism of action	Clinical use	Side effects and comments
Bithionol	Phenol	Oral	Uncouples phosphorylation	Paragonimiasis	Rare leukopenia, toxic hepatitis Availability: CDC
Dehydroemetine	Synthetic alkaloid	SQ	Blocks movement of ribosome along messenger RNA	Tissue amebiasis	Occasional GI disturbances, neuropathy, heart failure; use only in severe disease Availability: CDC
Diethylcarbamazine	Piperazine	Oral	Neuromuscular paralysis	Filarial infections	Allergic reactions to filarial antigens Rare loss of vision in onchocerciasis Availability: Lederle
Diloxanide furoate	Acetanilide	Oral	Unknown	Intestinal amebiasis	Flatulence, urticaria Indications: asymptomatic carriers Availability: CDC
Iodoquinol (diiodohydroxyquin)	Halogenated quinoline	Oral	Unknown	Intestinal amebiasis, *Dientamoeba* infections	Rare optic atrophy with prolonged use
Niclosamide	Phenol	Oral	Uncouples phosphorylation	Intestinal tapeworms	Occasional nausea, abdominal pain Does not kill eggs
Nifurtimox	Nitrofuran	Oral	Alkylates DNA	Acute Chagas' disease	Rare convulsions, pulmonary infiltrates Therapy prolonged, effectiveness marginal Availability: CDC
Pentamidine	Diamidine	IV	Binds DNA	Pneumocystosis, leishmaniasis, trypanosomiasis	Extremely toxic
Pyrantel pamoate	Tetrahydropyrimidine	Oral	Neuromuscular blockade Inhibits fumarate reductase	Pinworm infection, hookworm infection, ascariasis	Occasional GI disturbance, fever Single-dose therapy
Suramin	Sulfated naphthylamine	IV	Inhibits a glycerophosphate oxidase and dehydrogenase	African trypanosomiasis, onchocerciasis	Occasional renal toxicity, blood dyscrasia, optic atrophy, shock Not effective in CNS disease

SOURCE: After JJ Plorde.

TABLE 88-3 Fecal egg counts associated with illness

Worm	Approximate egg output per female worm per day	Minimum egg output usually associated with illness
Necator americanus	25,000	>2000/mL
Trichuris trichiura	7500	>3000/g
Schistosoma mansoni	60–300	>200/g

SOURCE: After DP Stevens, Clin Gastroenterol 7:236, 1978.

brucei, the protozoan agent of African trypanosomiasis (sleeping sickness). It acts by specifically and irreversibly inhibiting ornithine decarboxylase (ODC), an enzyme required in the biosynthesis of polyamines such as putrescine, spermidine, and spermine—substances thought to play an important role in cell division and differentiation. In *T. brucei,* DFMO slows nucleic acid synthesis and alters parasite morphology. Its effect appears to be cytostatic; an intact immune system is required for optimal effect. Although ornithine decarboxylase is present in mammalian as well as protozoan cells, *T. brucei* is 100 times more sensitive to the effects of elfornithine than are mammalian cells, possibly related to its high affinity for the trypanosomal enzyme or its active uptake by trypanosomes. Diarrhea, a common side effect, can be controlled with symptomatic therapy and dose reduction. Reversible anemia occurs in one-third of patients. Seizures have occurred in 10 percent of patients with late-stage trypanosomiasis. The drug may be given orally or intravenously and readily penetrates the blood-brain barrier. Early clinical trials in *T.b. gambiense* infections have shown the drug to be highly effective, even in patients failing arsenical therapy. It seems likely that this agent will supplant melarsoprol in the treatment of central nervous system trypanosomal infections. Not yet approved for use in the United States, the drug may be obtained from the manufacturer for investigational purposes.

Miscellaneous agents The names of a number of other important antiparasitic agents, the diseases for which they are used, their mode of action, and other comments are provided in Table 88-2.

THERAPEUTIC GOALS The principles governing the treatment of helminthic infections differ significantly from those employed for the management of prokaryotic or protozoan disease. Unlike the latter pathogens, worms, with few exceptions, do not multiply within the human host. Although they produce prodigious numbers of offspring, these mature to their infectious state outside the body. Subsequent contact of a human with an infectious egg or larva results in the development of a single adult worm within the host's body. Multiple worm infections require the repeated acquisition of infectious stage parasites. Because there is a direct correlation between the total number of worms harbored by the human host and the disability incurred, clinical disease is manifest only in those who have accumulated large worm burdens through repeated infections. Worm burdens do not follow a normal distribution in human populations. Most infected patients harbor fewer than a dozen adult worms; only a small minority harbor the large numbers required to produce clinical illness. In endemic areas, focusing treatment on the clinically ill will alleviate the medical impact of a helminthic disease on a community at a cost dramatically lower than that required for treatment of all who are infected. Short, subcurative doses will often produce sufficient decrease in the worm burden to alleviate clinical symptoms. This approach reduces cost, minimizes the likelihood of drug toxicity, and decreases the transmission of disease by targeting the major reservoir of the helminths. In general, light infections need to be treated only when (1) a small number of worms may be dangerous, as in the case of strongyloidiasis, (2) the chance of reinfection is slight, and/or (3) the anthelmintic agent in question is without serious side effects. The intensity of many infections can be determined by enumerating the eggs found in stool (Table 88-3). Multiplying the total seen on direct smear by 750 provides a rough estimate of the number present per gram of feces. The Stoll dilution and the various modifications of the Kato thick-smear technique provide more precise results.

REFERENCES

CAMPBELL WC, REW RS (eds): *Chemotherapy of Parasitic Diseases.* New York, Plenum, 1986

Drugs for parasitic infections. Med Lett 30:15, 1988

Health Information for International Travel 1988. US Department of Health and Human Services Publication (CDC) 88-8280, 1988

PLORDE JJ: Pathogenesis and chemotherapy of parasitic diseases, in *Medical Microbiology: An Introduction to Infectious Diseases,* 2d ed, JC Sherris (ed). New York, Elsevier–North Holland, 1989

section 3 Clinical syndromes

89 SEPTICEMIA AND SEPTIC SHOCK

RICHARD K. ROOT / RICHARD JACOBS

DEFINITION Septicemia and septic shock are dramatic clinical syndromes which result from acute invasion of the bloodstream by certain microorganisms or their toxic products. Fever, chills, tachycardia, tachypnea, and altered mentation are common acute manifestations of septicemia. When hypotension and signs of inadequate organ perfusion develop, the condition is termed *septic shock.* The circulatory insufficiency is characterized by a lowered systemic vascular resistance, decreased myocardial contractile function, and pooling and altered distribution of blood in the microcirculation. Diffuse cell and tissue injury and, ultimately, widespread organ failure develop. Even with appropriate antimicrobial and supportive care many patients die of septic shock, making strategies for prevention and more effective treatment of critical importance.

ETIOLOGY Manifestations of septicemia can be seen with severe systemic infection with all classes of organisms; however, frank septic shock is most commonly caused by gram-negative bacteria (60 to 70 percent of cases). Staphylococci, pneumococci, streptococci, and other gram-positive organisms are less frequent causes (20 to 40 percent of cases), as are opportunistic fungi (2 to 3 percent), and, rarely, mycobacteria or certain viruses (e.g., dengue–hemorrhagic fever and herpesviruses) or protozoans (e.g., *Falciparum malaria*). In septic shock, *Escherichia coli, Klebsiella-Enterobacter, Proteus, Pseudomonas,* and *Serratia* are the most frequent blood culture isolates, followed by staphylococci and pneumococci. Gram-negative bacteremia is complicated by shock in about 40 percent of patients; shock is seen in 5 to 15 percent of patients with acute bacteremias caused by pneumococci or staphylococci. In the setting of systemic purpura and meningitis, *Neisseria meningitidis* is the most frequent isolate. Patients may develop manifestations of sepsis and frank septic shock with severe localized infection but without detectable organisms on blood culture. The sepsis syndrome and shock are triggered by the interactions of various microbial products in the blood, in particular, gram-negative endotoxins, with host mediator systems.

EPIDEMIOLOGY In the 1970s the incidence of gram-negative rod bacteremia in the United States was estimated at between 100,000 and 300,000 cases per year; the incidence now may approach 300,000 to 500,000 cases per year. About two-thirds of cases are seen in already hospitalized patients, most of whom have underlying diseases or procedures which render their bloodstreams susceptible to invasion. Despite the introduction of new antimicrobial agents, the overall mortality from gram-negative bacteremia has averaged about 25 percent over the past two decades and is highest in patients who have major associated diseases or shock. Predisposing factors include diabetes mellitus; cirrhosis; alcoholism; leukemia; lymphoma or disseminated carcinoma; cytotoxic chemotherapy and immunosuppressive drugs which cause neutropenia; total parenteral nutrition; a variety of surgical procedures; and infections arising from the urinary, biliary, or gastrointestinal tracts. Neonates and elderly patients with urinary tract obstruction or dysfunction are particularly at risk. Gram-positive bacteremias are more often community-acquired except staphylococcal sepsis from indwelling intravenous catheters. In the 1970s gram-positive organisms accounted for less than 10 percent of cases of septic shock in most hospitals, but their relative incidence appears to be increasing and now approximates 30 percent in prospective studies. Opportunistic fungal sepsis is seen most often in immunosuppressed patients with severe neutropenia or in postoperative patients with intravenous catheters and usually follows prolonged antibiotic therapy. The widespread use of antibiotics, glucocorticoids, mechanical ventilation, and urinary and intravenous catheters and drainage tubes in other sites, as well as the increased longevity of patients with chronic diseases, contributes to the changing incidence and profile of this serious clinical problem.

PATHOGENESIS AND PATHOLOGY Most of the bacteria causing gram-negative sepsis are normal commensals in the gastrointestinal tract. From there they may spread to contiguous structures, as in peritonitis after appendiceal perforation, or they may migrate from the perineum into the urethra or bladder. Gram-negative bacteremia follows infection in a primary focus, usually the genitourinary tract, biliary tree, gastrointestinal tract, or lungs and, less commonly, the skin, bones, and joints. In burn patients and in patients with leukemia, the skin or the lungs are often portals of entry. In about 30 percent of cases, notably in patients with debilitating diseases, cirrhosis, and cancer, no primary focus is apparent. Gram-positive bacteremias usually arise from the skin or respiratory tract. Metastatic abscess formation may complicate bacteremia, particularly that caused by gram-positive or anaerobic organisms. More often, however, the autopsy findings in gram-negative sepsis reflect primarily the infection at the primary locus and show involvement of target organs: pulmonary edema, hemorrhage, and hyaline membrane formation in the lungs; tubular or cortical necrosis in the kidney; patchy necrosis in the myocardium; superficial ulceration or even hemorrhagic necrosis in the gastrointestinal tract; and leukocyte-platelet or, less commonly, fibrin thrombi in the capillaries in many tissues.

PATHOPHYSIOLOGY The clinical manifestations of septicemia and septic shock are the result of an interplay between microbial products and host mediator systems. From the standpoint of vascular perfusion and organ function a vicious circle is established that results in altered blood flow in the microcirculation and progressive injury to the capillary endothelium and tissues. Unless this circle is interrupted by control of the infection and correction of the hemodynamic and metabolic alterations, death usually results.

Microbial factors Microbial factors that are most important include gram-negative lipopolysaccharides (LPS), in particular, the lipid A component, peptidoglycans from gram-positive organisms or mannan from fungal cell walls, certain polysaccharides, and extracellular enzymes (e.g., streptokinase) or toxins (e.g., toxic shock enterotoxins of staphylococci) (see Chap. 100). The mechanisms of action of LPS and lipid A have been studied most extensively. LPS can directly activate humoral or cellular systems, which, in turn, promote the development of the septicemic and shock syndromes. Although not as well defined, other microbial products affect the same systems to varying degrees.

Host mediators A variety of host mediators have been implicated in the pathogenesis of septic shock including active metabolites of the complement, kinin, and coagulation systems as well as factors released from stimulated cells, in particular, the cytokines, tumor necrosis factor-α (TNF) and interleukin 1 (IL-1), enzymes and oxidants from polymorphonuclear leukocytes (PMNs), vasoactive peptides (e.g., histamine), and products of the metabolism of arachidonic acid. The precise sequence of events and the critical initiating steps need further clarification. Furthermore, the secretion and action of counterregulatory vasoactive catecholamines, angiotensin, pituitary hormones, insulin, and glucagon all contribute to the clinical and laboratory events in sepsis.

HUMORAL SYSTEMS LPS can directly activate both the *coagulation* and *kinin systems* through its effect on Hageman factor (Fig. 89-1). The intrinsic coagulation cascade is triggered (see Chap. 62); and increased turnover of factors XII, VIII, and V and fibrinogen is measurable in sepsis. Plasmin is also generated by activated Hageman factor. Bradykinin and related kinins are potent vasodilators, increase capillary permeability, and increase gastrointestinal motility. They are produced when activated Hageman factor cleaves prekallikrein to kallikrein. Reduction of these precursors and increases in plasma kinins have both been documented in septic shock.

LPS and other microbial products can activate the *complement system* (see Chap. 13); reduction of C3 levels in septic shock has

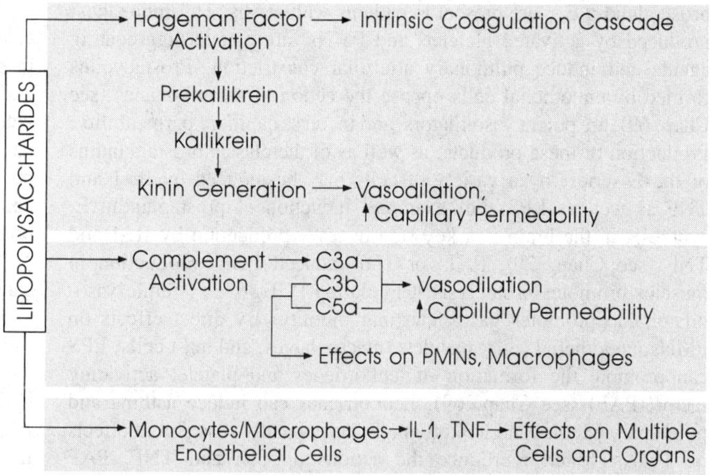

FIGURE 89-1 Schematized interactions between gram-negative lipopolysaccharides (LPS) and host humoral and cellular mediator systems in sepsis. PMNs = polymorphonuclear leukocytes; IL-1 = interleukin 1; TNF = tumor necrosis factor-α.

been correlated with a fatal outcome. Generation of the anaphylatoxins C3a and C5a can contribute to vasodilation and increased capillary permeability; free C5a and C3a have been detected in the plasma of septic patients. Effects on PMNs include aggregation, increased adhesion to endothelial cells, promotion of lysosomal enzyme release, and activation of the superoxide-generating system (see Chap. 81).

CYTOKINES A primary mechanism for the multiple actions of LPS and other microbial products in sepsis appears to reside in their ability to induce formation and release of both IL-1 and TNF (or "cachetin") by macrophages, endothelial cells, and perhaps other cells (see Chap. 20). Cardinal manifestations of sepsis—fever, somnolence, myalgias, and leukocytosis—follow administration of small amounts of recombinant TNF or IL-1 to human beings. Large doses of TNF in experimental animals produce all the systemic and pathologic features of LPS- or bacteria-induced septic shock, including hypotension, pulmonary injury with platelet and leukocyte thrombi, hemorrhagic necrosis of the intestine, acute renal failure, severe metabolic acidosis, and death. Anti-TNF antibodies block the manifestations of experimental LPS- and bacteria-induced sepsis, as does pretreatment with glucocorticoids, which inhibit TNF and IL-1 production, or cyclooxygenase inhibitors, which block their actions.

TNF appears in the plasma of human beings following LPS administration. During naturally occurring sepsis the levels of TNF in some studies correlate with severity and mortality, although more investigation of this is needed. Less precise correlations have been observed with measurements of circulating IL-1; however, it acts synergistically with TNF when administered in vivo to animals. Furthermore, many of the effects of IL-1 may be exerted at a local cellular level by the nonsecreted IL-1α form. The mechanisms by which TNF and IL-1 are produced and act and their relevance to the acute inflammatory responses characteristic of sepsis are discussed in detail in Chap. 20.

In experimental animals TNF and IL-1 can act synergistically to mobilize amino acids from muscles by proteolysis and lipids from adipose tissue, producing hyperlipidemia, and they also promote hepatic glycogenolysis and gluconeogenesis. Albumin synthesis is inhibited and may lead to hypoalbuminemia; formation of acute phase reaction proteins is enhanced. Finally, both TNF and IL-1 can release insulin and glucagon from pancreatic cells, and adrenocorticotropic hormone (ACTH), β-endorphins, growth hormone, and arginine vasopressin (AVP) from the pituitary. These studies suggest that both cytokines contribute to characteristic hormonal and metabolic alterations seen in sepsis in human beings.

Other cytokines found in high levels in the plasma of patients with sepsis include interleukin 6 (IL-6) and interferon γ (IFN-γ). These cytokines may act synergistically with IL-1 and TNF (IL-6) or augment cellular responses to TNF (IFN-γ).

ARACHIDONATE METABOLITES In experimental animals inhibition of cyclooxygenase or thromboxane synthetase has been protective against lethal endotoxin shock. Elevated levels of thromboxane B_2 (TBX_2) and the end product of prostacyclin metabolism, 6-keto-prostaglandin $F_{1\alpha}$, are present in patients with sepsis. Thromboxanes, produced by activated platelets and PMNs, are platelet aggregating agents and induce pulmonary arteriolar constriction. Prostacyclins formed by endothelial cells oppose the action of thromboxanes (see Chap. 69), are potent vasodilators, and increase capillary permeability. Production of these products, as well as of the classic prostaglandins of the E series, by a variety of cells may be induced by IL-1 and TNF as well as LPS. For example, induction of prostaglandin E_2 synthesis in the brain is a key step in fever production by IL-1 and TNF (see Chap. 20); IL-1- or TNF-induced PGE_2 production in muscles promotes proteolysis. Circulating PGE_2 is a systemic vasodilator and promotes gastrointestinal motility. By direct effects on PMNs, endothelial cells, platelets, macrophages, and mast cells, LPS can promote the formation of leukotrienes and platelet activating factor (PAF) (see Chap. 69). Leukotrienes can induce asthma and pulmonary edema, and leukotriene B_4, specifically, has potent effects on PMNs which reproduce the actions of C5a and TNF. PAF aggregates platelets, is a vasodilator, increases capillary permeability, and also has effects on PMNs that duplicate those of the leukotrienes.

Once triggered, the interactions become very complex, with recruitment of a wide array of inflammatory mediators. Endothelial cells and the microcirculation appear to be major targets of this intravascular inflammatory response. There is evidence of cytotoxicity, precapillary shunting, the plugging of postcapillary venules with PMN and platelet thrombi, and fibrin deposition. A generalized capillary leak syndrome manifested in the lungs as pulmonary edema is a common event. Kinins, C3a, C5a, histamine released by mast cells, arachidonate metabolites, proteases, and oxygen products released by activated neutrophils, monocytes, and macrophages can all contribute to the vasomotor alterations characteristic of sepsis and can participate in capillary damage. Widespread tissue hypoxia and eventual cell death result from the disordered microcirculation.

CARDIOPULMONARY MANIFESTATIONS The cardiovascular features of septicemia and septic shock can be distinguished from cardiogenic or hypovolemic shock in that the systemic vascular resistance (SVR) is low and the cardiac output is increased. A maldistribution of blood flow in the microcirculation occurs, presumably through the actions of various vasodilators and constrictors. Leakage of plasma constituents from capillaries contributes to functional hypovolemia. These findings appear to be universal and independent of the type of organism causing the infection. The cardiovascular abnormalities in sepsis with shock are discussed in detail in Chap. 39. In brief, in addition to a low SVR and early functional hypovolemia, which contribute to hypotension, about half the patients exhibit depression of myocardial contractile function. With successful treatment both the SVR and myocardial function return to normal over a several-day period. Death is associated with refractory hypotension and persistently low SVR, progressive lactic acidosis, and evidence of multiple organ failure despite administration of fluids, pressors, and antibiotics.

Hyperventilation is a characteristic early response to sepsis leading to varying degrees of respiratory alkalosis. The precise mechanisms for the initial hyperventilation remain to be defined, but at later stages, increased lung water, decreased compliance, stimulation of lung stretch receptors, and incipient or manifest pulmonary edema all play a role. Hypoxemia and increased blood lactate concentrations also cause hyperventilation through central mechanisms in the brain. Ventilation-perfusion mismatching early in sepsis causes a fall in arterial P_{O_2}. With progression of sepsis a widening alveolar-arterial oxygen gradient often signals lung injury, which becomes fully expressed as the adult respiratory distress syndrome (ARDS).

METABOLIC RESPONSES Blood lactate concentrations rise early in sepsis, and in the late stages marked metabolic acidosis usually predominates. While increased lactate production by poorly perfused tissues may be a factor, reduced removal of lactate by the liver and kidneys appears to play the major role. In the late stages of septic shock generalized hypoperfusion and the use of vasoconstricting pressors also aggravate the acidosis.

Elevations in plasma ACTH, growth hormone, AVP, cortisol, catecholamines, glucagon and insulin, lipids, and amino acids occur in sepsis. Some hormonal responses can exacerbate hyperglycemia in diabetic patients by antagonizing the action of insulin and promoting ketosis (see Chap. 319). Conversely, some patients with sepsis develop hypoglycemia. The mechanisms are not fully understood, but diminished hepatic glycogen stores (in neonates, with starvation, and with preexisting liver disease) and excessive insulin release may both contribute.

COMPLICATIONS **Respiratory failure** Sepsis is the leading cause of ARDS (see Chap. 218). A progressively widening alveolar-arterial oxygen gradient and the appearance of diffuse pulmonary infiltrates on chest x-ray are characteristic features. Histopathologically the lungs show pulmonary edema, hemorrhage, atelectasis, hyaline membrane formation, and platelet-PMN-fibrin capillary thrombi. ARDS develops in 20 to 45 percent of patients with severe sepsis. Infection with gram-negative organisms and the development of clinical shock are the major risk factors. Overly vigorous intravenous fluid administration may also contribute. When ARDS results from sepsis, the mortality rates are 80 to 90 percent in most studies, with complicating secondary pneumonias responsible for many of the deaths which occur late (>48 h) in the course.

Coagulation defects Thrombocytopenia of modest (<150,000 platelets per microliter) to moderate (<50,000 to 100,000 platelets per microliter) degree is seen in up to 70 percent of patients with septicemia. Direct effects of LPS as well as activation of platelet aggregation by multiple mechanisms are responsible. Platelet counts below 50,000 per microliter (in the absence of antecedent marrow failure) are usually associated with evidence of disseminated intravascular coagulation (DIC) (see Chap. 62). Activation of Hageman factor also contributes to this syndrome, as does release of plasminogen activator from macrophages and endothelial cells. The development of overt DIC in septic shock is an ominous prognostic sign.

Renal failure Most patients will have evidence of renal hypoperfusion or renal injury including oliguria, azotemia, variable degrees of proteinuria, and the appearance of tubular and epithelial cells and coarse granular casts in the urine. Late complications include acute tubular necrosis (ATN) (see Chap. 223) or, rarely, renal cortical necrosis as part of a generalized Shwartzman reaction.

Other organs Patchy myocardial necrosis with heart failure, hemorrhagic necrosis of the intestine, and hepatic necrosis may occur terminally in sepsis as in other shock syndromes.

CLINICAL MANIFESTATIONS The abrupt onset of the full-blown picture of sepsis, with fever, chills, tachycardia, tachypnea, mental status changes, and hypotension, is easily recognized. However, during the early stages of sepsis and depending upon various host factors (e.g., age extremes, underlying disease, treatment with glucocorticoids), the clinical manifestations may be subtle and the diagnosis difficult. Fever and chills occur commonly, but up to 13 percent of patients may be hypothermic, with rectal temperature of <36.5°C (97.6°F), at the onset of sepsis, and an additional 5 percent of patients who are not initially hypothermic may fail to mount a febrile response above 37.5°C (99.6°F). The absence of fever is seen primarily in the elderly and in those with underlying diseases such as alcoholism and uremia and has been associated with a poor prognosis. Up to 40 percent of patients who present with hypothermia may have severe infection or bacteremia as the cause, and the mortality rate is higher in those with infection than in those with hypothermia of other causes.

Hyperventilation with respiratory alkalosis and changes in mental status are extremely important signs, because they occur early, often before the onset of fever, chills, and hypotension. In the initial stages of sepsis, alterations in mental status may be subtle, with disorientation or personality change as the only manifestation; later in the disease more obvious changes of obtundation and coma may be present. Focal neurologic signs are absent, and the findings are usually more pronounced in neonates, the elderly, or those with preexisting central nervous system disease, but they may be seen in any patient.

Cutaneous manifestations occur with variable frequency, are diverse in presentation, and are not usually specific for the sepsis syndrome. They are extremely important, however, because a Gram stain of a scraping may confirm the presence of sepsis and indicate a preliminary microbiologic diagnosis. When bacteria or fungi invade the skin, pustules or vesiculopustular lesions are usually seen. In some gram-negative infections, particularly those caused by *Pseudomonas aeruginosa,* necrotizing or bullous skin lesions may occur and have been termed *ecthyma gangrenosum*. Sepsis associated with DIC is often accompanied by acrocyanosis with eventual necrosis of peripheral tissues (tip of the nose, fingertips, toes, and ears).

Gastrointestinal manifestations are seen in approximately one-third of patients. They include nausea, vomiting, diarrhea, or ileus and may obfuscate the diagnosis of septicemia by suggesting the possibility of acute gastroenteritis. Upper gastrointestinal bleeding may occur; on endoscopy small ulcers of the stomach and duodenum are seen. The appearance and prevalence of ulceration is similar to that seen in other conditions of extreme systemic stress (e.g., severe head trauma). Rarely hemorrhagic necrosis of the bowel occurs and may be exacerbated by preexisting atherosclerotic disease. Mild to moderate jaundice may be present, related to a sepsis-induced defect in bile secretion. Less frequently shock-induced hepatic necrosis occurs.

LABORATORY FINDINGS The laboratory data in sepsis are variable and depend primarily upon whether shock with end organ damage and other complications have occurred. There is usually a leukocytosis with a left shift, but normal white blood cell counts and even leukopenia can occur. Toxic granulations, Döhle bodies, and intracytoplasmic vacuolization may been seen within neutrophils. Thrombocytopenia is often present; when severe (<50,000 per microliter), it is usually a manifestation of concomitant DIC and is associated with a prolonged thrombin time, decreased fibrinogen level, and elevated fibrin degradation products. In the absence of DIC with a microangiopathic hemolytic anemia, red blood cell morphology and numbers are usually normal.

Many patients will demonstrate mild abnormalities on urinalysis, such as proteinuria. With shock, acute tubular necrosis (ATN) may develop with oliguria, azotemia, and cellular or granular casts. In patients with normal renal function, the urinary sodium is low (<20 meq/L) in the initial phases of shock but rises in the presence of ATN or with the use of diuretics.

During the early phases of sepsis there is respiratory alkalosis and arterial blood gases reveal an elevated pH and decreased P_{CO_2}. With shock a metabolic acidosis develops with elevated lactate levels. Hypoxemia is present in varying degrees and is most severe when ARDS develops. Abnormalities in the chest x-ray may include an underlying pneumonia as the source of sepsis, congestive heart failure as a result of myocardial depression and volume resuscitation, or the diffuse infiltrates of ARDS. The ECG often shows nonspecific ST-T wave abnormalities; as with any hypotensive patient an initial and follow-up ECGs are indicated to exclude myocardial infarction.

Hypoglycemia is an uncommon manifestation of overwhelming sepsis. Most diabetics will have hyperglycemia, and severe infection is a leading cause of diabetic ketoacidosis which may contribute to the development of shock (see Chap. 314). Abnormalities in serum electrolytes can include an elevated anion gap with reduction of the bicarbonate concentration and metabolic acidosis. Liver function test abnormalities include modest hyperbilirubinemia and elevations of the transaminases that may be more pronounced in severe shock. Hypoalbuminemia, mild at first, may progress as sepsis continues and malnutrition supervenes. Serum lipids are often elevated. Rarely, changes in serum calcium and phosphorus levels are seen.

DIAGNOSIS Because many of the signs and symptoms of sepsis are nonspecific, the bedside diagnosis may be difficult. Once shock with end organ dysfunction has supervened in the febrile patient with a primary focus, the diagnosis is usually obvious. The presence of hyperventilation with a normal chest x-ray and unexplained confusion or disorientation should raise the possibility of sepsis. Other entities often confused with septic shock include myocardial infarction, pulmonary embolus, drug overdose, occult hemorrhage, cardiac tamponade, rupture of an aortic aneurysm, and aortic dissection.

The diagnosis and etiology of sepsis is confirmed by finding pathogenic organisms in the blood or at other sites of infection. Because bacteremia is intermittent and low grade (usually less than 10 organisms per milliliter of blood), obtaining a single small volume of blood (5 to 10 mL) prior to initiating antibiotic therapy may only result in positive cultures 50 to 60 percent of the time. Obtaining a single large volume of blood (30 mL) and dividing it equally into three culture bottles will increase the yield. Blood cultures usually become positive within 3 days of incubation; the failure to do so may be due to the intermittent nature of the bacteremia, prior administration of antibiotics, or the presence of slow-growing, fastidious organisms. In several large prospective studies of septic shock blood cultures were positive in only 50 to 60 percent of patients; the diagnosis was established by documenting infection at a local site. A Gram stain and culture of the primary site of infection or skin lesions, if present, are essential to establish the diagnosis, determine the etiology, and assist in immediate management.

In some patients a rapid diagnosis of bacteremia can be made by doing a Gram stain of the buffy coat. Although results are conflicting, this simple technique has been reported to give positive results in up to 10 to 50 percent of patients with bacteremia. The presence of intracytoplasmic vacuoles in neutrophils may also correlate with the presence of bacteremia.

TREATMENT Reversal of sepsis and septic shock depends upon aggressive treatment of the underlying infection as well as careful monitoring of hemodynamic and respiratory function in order to ensure adequate perfusion and oxygenation of vital organs. In the severely ill patient, clinical assessment of hemodynamic function does not correlate well with values measured more precisely. Even though pulmonary artery catheterization has not been shown to improve survival, its use allows for accurate measurement of volume status, cardiac output, and peripheral resistance, and it is an invaluable aid in monitoring the administration of fluids and pressors. Although not absolutely required, a peripheral arterial line is helpful in monitoring pressure and obtaining arterial samples to assess oxygenation. Management of the patient with sepsis and septic shock requires attention to the following:

Reversal of the underlying disease The outcome of sepsis depends in large part upon the severity of the underlying disease of the patient. Patients who are immunosuppressed by virtue of drugs or a disease will have an improved outcome if the immunosuppressive medication can be decreased or discontinued or if the underlying disease can be effectively treated. In patients with neutropenia or neutrophil dysfunction who have persistent bacteremia despite appropriate antibiotic therapy, granulocyte transfusions should be considered, but their benefit is controversial.

Removal of the source of infection A careful search for the site of origin of a bacteremia is always indicated since, if possible, removal or drainage of the source can turn a potentially fatal disease into an easily treatable one. Intravenous catheters should be removed and replaced. Foley and drainage catheters should be checked for patency and replaced if necessary.

Support of respiration Arterial oxygen should be monitored by pulse oximetry or by direct measurement. Oxygen should be provided nasally or by mask sufficient to maintain arterial oxygen saturations in excess of 95 percent. If respiratory failure develops, intubation with mechanical ventilation should be employed. The use of positive end-expiratory pressure (PEEP) does not prevent ARDS from developing but is useful to improve oxygenation at the lowest possible fraction of inspired oxygen (see Chap. 218).

Hemodynamic support Many patients have a relative depletion of intravascular volume, and the initial response to a falling blood pressure should be the administration of fluid. Whether colloids or crystalloids are superior has not been established. Anemia severe enough to compromise peripheral oxygen delivery (e.g., hematocrit acutely <30 percent) requires red blood cell transfusions. The pulmonary capillary wedge pressure should be maintained between 15 and 20 mmHg or the central venous pressure between 10 and 12 cmH_2O. Adequate fluid usually requires initial administration of 1 to 1.5 L over 1 to 2 h although on occasion much larger volumes are needed. Once volume has been repleted, a diuretic such as furosemide can be given to maintain hourly urine output above 20 mL/h and to prevent the occurrence of pulmonary edema. If the mean arterial pressure is sufficient to maintain adequate mentation and urine output and to prevent chest pain, it is not necessary to raise blood pressure to normal levels. In previously normotensive patients this can usually be accomplished at mean arterial pressures of >60 mmHg. About a third of patients will respond to fluid administration alone with reversal of the hypotension; if volume resuscitation fails to increase blood pressure, pressor drugs should be given. Dopamine is the agent most frequently used. When given in doses of 5 to 10 (μg/kg)/min, it primarily has a $beta_1$ effect, augmenting cardiac output and dilating splanchnic, renal, and cerebral arterioles through stimulation of dopaminergic receptors (see Chap. 39). Higher doses stimulate alpha receptors and can result in peripheral vasoconstriction severe enough to cause ischemia and gangrene. Dobutamine, 2 to 20 (μg/kg)/min, acts primarily on $beta_1$- and $beta_2$-adrenergic receptors and may be particularly useful in the rare patients with low cardiac output states. Because of its $alpha_1$ effect, norepinephrine, 10 to 15 μg/min, should be reserved for situations in which blood pressure cannot be maintained by other means; it can be used in combination with dopamine.

Therapy of acidosis and DIC Acidosis often resolves with therapy of the underlying infection and correction of hypoperfusion. If the pH falls below 7.20, sodium bicarbonate should be given (see Chap. 51).

Treatment of the underlying infection is of critical importance in the management of DIC. Asymptomatic DIC (laboratory abnormalities only) or mild manifestations, such as ecchymoses or oozing at venipuncture sites, do not require specific therapy. If major bleeding is encountered, replacement of clotting factors and platelets is prudent. Use of heparin and fibrinolytic agents is controversial (see Chap. 62).

Antibiotics Antibiotics should be initiated as soon as the diagnosis of sepsis is seriously entertained. Prior to the institution of antibiotics, blood cultures as well as cultures of relevant body fluids and exudates should be obtained, but administration of antibiotics should not be unduly delayed just to obtain cultures. Identification of a portal of entry or localized site of infection can guide initial antibiotic therapy. In the absence of this information, it is important to note that the signs and symptoms of sepsis due to gram-positive and gram-negative organisms are identical and indistinguishable at the bedside. When considering the choice of antibiotics prior to the availability of culture results, an antibiotic or combination of antibiotics should be chosen with activity against both gram-positive and gram-negative organisms. Once the results of culture are known, therapy can be more specific. Drugs should be given intravenously, and, generally, bactericidal drugs are preferred over bacteriostatic agents. The dosage of drug used should be the maximum recommended in order to ensure adequate serum and tissue levels. Knowledge of local bacteriologic patterns is very important in choosing initial therapy. Many nosocomial pathogens may only be susceptible to drugs that may be potentially toxic, such as aminoglycosides. In such cases, even if the patient has renal insufficiency, it is usually necessary to give aminoglycosides to ensure adequate therapy, taking into account that nephrotoxicity from these agents usually requires 3 to 5 days to develop. Ideally, during that period the causative organism will be identified and less toxic drugs can be substituted. In most situations a single agent is adequate to treat sepsis with a known pathogen. Combination therapy is indicated in the following circumstances:

1 As initial therapy to cover all likely pathogens until culture results are available
2 To treat certain pathogens for which antibiotic synergy has been demonstrated, such as *Pseudomonas aeruginosa* and enterococcus
3 For therapy in immunosuppressed patients, particularly those with neutropenia

The following are examples of initial therapy for various infections by site until culture results and antimicrobial susceptibilities are known. The precise antimicrobial dosages are provided in Chap. 85.

Urosepsis is usually caused by gram-negative rods or enterococci, and initial therapy with ampicillin plus gentamicin (vancomycin for the penicillin-allergic patient) is appropriate. If only gram-negative rods are seen in the urine, then gentamicin alone should suffice unless there is reason to suspect resistance to this drug (see Chap. 95).

Intraabdominal infections are usually polymicrobial and caused by anaerobes and enteric gram-negative organisms. They can be treated with metronidazole and gentamicin (ampicillin can be added to cover the possibility of enterococcus). Ticarcillin plus gentamicin or cefoxitin plus gentamicin are equally effective as initial treatment.

Imipenem may be used as a single drug or in combination with an aminoglycoside (see Chap. 108).

Outpatient *pneumonia* in an otherwise healthy adult is usually caused by *Streptococcus pneumoniae,* and penicillin can be used. In alcoholics or smokers, *Klebsiella pneumoniae* and *Haemophilus influenzae* become important pathogens, and a second- or third-generation cephalosporin (e.g., cefuroxime, cefotaxime, or ceftizoxime) can be given (see Chap. 207).

Nosocomial pneumonias frequently are caused by resistant gram-negative rods, and an aminoglycoside (gentamicin or tobramycin), usually in combination with an antipseudomonal penicillin (ticarcillin, mezlocillin, azlocillin, or piperacillin) or ceftazidime, is indicated (see Chap. 207).

Cellulitis is usually caused by streptococci and staphylococci, and a first-generation cephalosporin (e.g., cefazolin) or oxacillin is adequate coverage.

Sepsis from an *intravenous catheter* is usually caused by *Staphylococcus aureus, S. epidermidis,* or gram-negative rods. The catheter should be removed, and therapy with vancomycin and gentamicin is indicated.

Meningitis in adults can be treated with high-dose penicillin to cover *S. pneumoniae* and *Neisseria meningitidis;* if a gram-negative organism is suspected (posttraumatic or nosocomial meningitis) or the Gram stain is negative, a third-generation cephalosporin, such as cefotaxime or ceftriaxone, should be given (see Chap. 354).

In 30 percent of cases no source will be evident, and broad-spectrum coverage for gram-negative and gram-positive bacteria is important. A choice of vancomycin, metronidazole and gentamicin, or cefotaxime and gentamicin is reasonable.

Other agents Studies in animals have suggested that under highly controlled conditions administration of glucocorticoids may reduce mortality in sepsis. The clinical use of these drugs has been controversial due to the lack of well-designed studies evaluating large numbers of septic patients. Two prospective, randomized, placebo-controlled, and blinded studies have assessed the effect of early administration of large doses of glucocorticoids (30 mg/kg methylprednisolone every 6 h for four doses or 30 mg/kg of methylprednisolone followed by a constant infusion of 5 mg/kg per hour for 9 h) on the outcome of patients with severe sepsis and shock. In both studies the addition of glucocorticoids did *not* improve survival, prevent the development of shock, or reverse shock in those who presented with it. Furthermore, superinfection was more likely to occur in patients treated with glucocorticoids, and the mortality rate was higher in steroid-treated patients with azotemia. Based on these data, there is little support for the use of glucocorticoids in the therapy of acute sepsis.

Naloxone, an opiate antagonist, has been demonstrated in animal studies to prevent endotoxin-induced shock. Although uncontrolled studies have suggested that naloxone can reverse septic shock in humans, most controlled studies involving small numbers of patients have not confirmed this finding. Thus, the use of naloxone remains of unproven benefit.

Administration of polyclonal antibodies directed at common core LPS antigens of the J5 mutants of *E. coli* has been shown to decrease mortality in patients with gram-negative bacteremia and septic shock and to prevent the development of shock when given prophylactically to high-risk patients. Immunotherapy for gram-negative sepsis is under investigation using monoclonal antibodies to core components of LPS and to TNF. Results are not yet available, but both techniques hold promise as a possible novel approach to therapy.

PROGNOSIS The outcome of gram-negative sepsis depends more upon host factors than virulence factors of organisms. A major determinant of mortality is the presence of underlying diseases: patients with rapidly fatal diseases (e.g., acute leukemia) have higher mortality rates than do patients with ultimately fatal (likely to be fatal in 5 years) or nonfatal diseases. With the exception of *Pseudomonas aeruginosa,* which has been associated with an increased mortality, the specific organism causing infection is not a major determinant of outcome. The development of complications such as shock, lactic acidosis, DIC, and ARDS all contribute to a poor prognosis. Other less important factors associated with increased mortality include azotemia, failure to mount a febrile response, polymicrobial infections, and high-grade bacteremia (>10 organisms per milliliter of blood). Conversely, early and appropriate antibiotic therapy is associated with improved survival.

The overall mortality in gram-negative sepsis is about 25 percent; most deaths occur in the first 48 h. These early deaths are usually due to acute events such as irreversible shock. Deaths occurring after 48 h are usually due to persistent poorly controlled infection or to other complications of intensive care.

PREVENTION Despite the availability of new broad-spectrum antibiotics with increased activity, the incidence and outcome of sepsis and septic shock have not decreased significantly in the last two decades. This is due in part to the failure of early recognition and therapy of underlying infection, a problem particularly common in the elderly, who may not manifest classic signs of infection. Even more important, though, is the increased longevity of patients with chronic diseases. Up to 75 percent of all episodes of gram-negative sepsis are nosocomial in nature. This fact emphasizes the need to limit invasive procedures, limit the use of intravenous lines, avoid Foley catheterization, and practice good infection control at all times in an attempt to prevent the occurrence of these infections (see Chap. 83). Finally, the use of active and passive immunization against cell wall components of gram-negative organisms holds promise as a preventive measure in the future.

REFERENCES

Ball HA et al: Role of thromboxane, prostaglandins, and leukotrienes in endotoxic and septic shock. Intensive Care Med 12:116, 1986

Beutler B, Cerami A: Cachectin: More than a tumor necrosis factor. N Engl J Med 316:379, 1987

Bone RC et al: A controlled clinical trial of high dose methylprednisolone in the treatment of severe sepsis and septic shock. N Engl J Med 317:653, 1987

DeGroote MA et al: Plasma tumor necrosis factor levels in patients with presumed sepsis. Results in those treated with antilipid A antibody vs. placebo. JAMA 26:2, 1989

Dinarello CA: Interleukin 1. Amino acid sequences, multiple biologic activities, and comparison with tumor necrosis factor. Year Immunol 2:68, 1986

The EORTC International Antimicrobial Therapy Cooperative Group: Ceftazidime combined with a short or long course of amikacin for empirical therapy of gram-negative bacteremia in cancer patients with granulocytopenia. N Engl J Med 317:1692, 1987

Girardin E et al: Tumor necrosis factor and interleukin 1 in the serum of children with severe infectious purpura. N Engl J Med 319:397, 1988

Hack CE et al: Increased plasma levels of interleukin-6 in sepsis. Blood 74:1704, 1989

Harris RL et al: Manifestations of sepsis. Arch Intern Med 147:1895, 1987

Higgins TL, Chenow B: Pharmacotherapy of circulatory shock. Dis-a-Month 33:309, 1987

Jacobs ER, Bone RC: Clinical indicators in sepsis and septic adult respiratory distress syndrome. Medical emergencies I. Med Clin North Am 70:921, 1986

Kreger BE et al: Gram-negative rod bacteremia III: Reassessment of etiology, epidemiology, and ecology in 612 patients. Am J Med 68:332, 1980

——— et al: Gram-negative rod bacteremia IV: Re-evaluation of clinical features and treatment in 612 patients. Am J Med 68:344, 1980

Michie HR et al: Detection of circulating tumor necrosis factor after endotoxin administration. N Engl J Med 318:1481, 1988

Parker MM et al: Profound but reversible myocardial depression in patients with septic shock. Ann Intern Med 100:483, 1984

Roberts DE et al: Effects of prolonged naloxone infusion in septic shock. Lancet 2:699, 1988

Root RK, Sande MS (eds): *Contemporary Issues in Infectious Diseases,* vol 4, *Septic Shock.* New York, Churchill Livingstone, 1985

The Veterans Administration Study Group: Effects of high-dose glucocorticoid therapy in patients with clinical signs of systemic sepsis. N Engl J Med 317:659, 1987

Wilson JJ et al: Infection-induced thrombocytopenia. Semin Thrombos Hemostas 8:217, 1982

Young LS: Gram negative sepsis, in *Principles and Practices of Infectious Diseases,* 3d ed, G Mandell et al (eds). New York, Wiley, 1990, pp 611–635

Ziegler EJ et al: Treatment of gram negative bacteremia and shock with antiserum to a mutant *E. coli.* N Engl J Med 303:1225, 1982

90 INFECTIVE ENDOCARDITIS

DONALD KAYE

DEFINITION Infective endocarditis is an infection which produces vegetations on the endocardium. It is virtually always fatal if untreated. A heart valve is usually involved, but infection may be on a septal defect or mural endocardium. Infection of an arteriovenous shunt or coarctation of the aorta is more properly called endarteritis and produces a similar clinical syndrome. The subsequent discussion of endocarditis also applies to endarteritis.

CLASSIFICATION

Endocarditis can be divided into native valve endocarditis, endocarditis in intravenous drug abusers, and prosthetic valve endocarditis, each with different infecting microorganisms and courses. Endocarditis can also be classified as acute or subacute. Acute endocarditis most frequently is caused by *Staphylococcus aureus,* occurs on a normal heart valve, is rapidly destructive, produces metastatic foci, and untreated, is fatal in less than 6 weeks. Subacute endocarditis usually is caused by viridans streptococci, occurs on damaged valves, does not produce metastatic foci, and untreated, takes more than 6 weeks and even a year to be fatal. Correlations between organism and course are not perfect. Viridans streptococci can be associated with an acute course and *S. aureus* with a subacute course. Most important is classification by infecting organisms (e.g., *S. aureus* endocarditis), because the organism has implications for therapy as well as course.

NATIVE VALVE ENDOCARDITIS Etiology Although almost any bacteria can produce endocarditis, streptococci and staphylococci account for the vast majority of cases.

STREPTOCOCCI Streptococci cause 60 to 80 percent of cases of native valve endocarditis in patients who do not abuse intravenous drugs. Viridans streptococci (most commonly *S. sanguis, S. mutans,* or *S. mitior*) account for over half of these; *S. bovis,* enterococci,[1] and other streptococci cause 25, 15, and 5 percent respectively. Viridans streptococci are normal inhabitants of the oropharynx and generally are highly susceptible to penicillin.

Enterococci and group A beta-hemolytic streptococci attack normal or damaged heart valves and may cause their rapid destruction. Other streptococci are much more likely to infect damaged valves and rarely cause rapid valve destruction. Enterococci and *S. mitior* can cause metastatic abscesses, which are uncommon with other streptococci.

Enterococci are alpha-, beta-, or gamma-hemolytic and are normal inhabitants of the gastrointestinal tract, the anterior urethra, and occasionally the mouth. All enterococci are in Lancefield's group D and may be distinguished from other streptococci by biochemical tests. They are relatively resistant to penicillin G, and an aminoglycoside must be added to achieve a bactericidal effect. Enterococcal endocarditis is most common in males, who develop infection at an average age of 60, while the average age of women with enterococcal endocarditis is under 40. Many patients give a recent history of genitourinary tract manipulation, trauma, or disease (e.g., cystoscopy, urethral catheterization, prostatectomy, abortion, pregnancy, or cesarean section) which occur mainly in older men and younger women.

Two other group D streptococci, *S. bovis* and *S. equinus,* differ from enterococci biochemically and are highly susceptible to penicillin G. Endocarditis caused by these organisms can be treated like viridans streptococcal endocarditis. *S. bovis* endocarditis occurs in elderly individuals (80 percent over 60 years of age), over one-third of whom have a malignant or premalignant gastrointestinal lesion (most often colonic cancer or a villous adenoma or polyp of the colon).

[1] Although enterococci have been classified as a separate genus, in this chapter they are considered with the streptococci.

STAPHYLOCOCCI Staphylococci cause about 25 percent of cases of native valve endocarditis (with *S. aureus* 5 to 10 times more frequent than *S. epidermidis*). *S. aureus* attacks normal or damaged heart valves, often causing rapid destruction. The course is often fulminant, with death from bacteremia within days or heart failure within weeks. Abscesses are common at multiple sites (e.g., kidneys, lungs, and brain). *S. epidermidis* infects abnormal valves without causing rapid destruction.

OTHER BACTERIA Almost all species of bacteria are occasional causes of endocarditis, including *Strep. pneumoniae, Neisseria gonorrhoeae,* enteric gram-negative bacilli, *Pseudomonas, Salmonella, Streptobacillus, Serratia marcescens, Bacteroides, Haemophilus, Brucella, Mycobacterium, N. meningiditis, Listeria, Legionella,* and diphtheroids, and can result in an acute or chronic course.

FUNGI Fungi rarely cause native valve endocarditis in nonintravenous drug abusers. However, *Candida* and *Aspergillus* endocarditis can occur in patients with intravascular catheters who frequently have received glucocorticoids, broad spectrum antimicrobial drugs, or cytotoxic agents. The course is usually subacute. Large friable vegetations are common and give rise to large emboli, often to the lower extremities. The prognosis is grave, partly because of the relatively poor activity of available antifungal agents.

OTHER MICROORGANISMS Spirochetes (e.g., *Spirillum minor*), cell wall–deficient bacteria, rickettsiae (*Coxiella burnetti*), and chlamydiae (*C. psittaci* and *C. trachomatis*) are rare causes of endocarditis.

Epidemiology In native valve endocarditis, the proportion of males is higher than females, and most patients are over age 50. Endocarditis is uncommon in children.

Between 60 and 80 percent of patients have an identifiable predisposing cardiac lesion. *Rheumatic valvular disease* accounts for about 30 percent of cases. The mitral valve is most commonly involved, followed by the aortic. Right-sided endocarditis usually affects the tricuspid valve but is rare on rheumatic valves.

Congenital heart disease other than mitral valve prolapse is the underlying lesion in about 10 to 20 percent of patients with endocarditis. Predisposing lesions include patent ductus arteriosus, ventricular septal defect, tetralogy of Fallot, coarctation of the aorta, pulmonary stenosis, and bicuspid aortic valve but not uncomplicated atrial septal defect. *Mitral valve prolapse* is the underlying lesion in about 10 to 33 percent of cases.

Degenerative heart disease predisposes to endocarditis. *Calcific aortic stenosis* (from degenerative disease or bicuspid valve) is an important lesion in the elderly. Other predisposing but unusual lesions are *asymmetric septal hypertrophy, Marfan's syndrome,* and *syphilitic aortic valve. Arterioarterial* or *arteriovenous fistulas* can also be underlying lesions. In 20 to 40 percent of patients with infective endocarditis, *no underlying heart disease* can be recognized.

ENDOCARDITIS IN INTRAVENOUS DRUG ABUSERS Drug abusers with endocarditis are frequently young males. The skin is the most frequent source of microorganisms responsible for endocarditis; contamination of drugs is less common. *S. aureus* causes over 50 percent of cases, streptococci about 15 percent and fungi (mainly *Candida*) and gram-negative bacilli (usually *Pseudomonas* species) about 10 to 15 percent each. Infection with multiple organisms is common. The onset is usually acute. Only about 20 percent of addicts with their first episode of endocarditis have previously damaged heart valves. The tricuspid valve is infected in over 50 percent of cases, the aortic in 25 percent, and the mitral in about 20 percent. Over 75 percent with *S. aureus* infection and a much lower percent with other organisms have tricuspid valve endocarditis. Pulmonary emboli or pneumonia consequent to septic pulmonary emboli are common in tricuspid valve endocarditis, and murmurs are frequently absent.

PROSTHETIC VALVE ENDOCARDITIS Any intravascular prosthesis predisposes to endocarditis and makes cure difficult. Infections of prosthetic valves now account for 10 to 20 percent of cases of endocarditis. Intravascular sutures, pacemaker wires, and Teflon-Silastic tubes can also be foci of infection. Patients with prosthetic valve endocarditis are mainly males over age 60. Endocarditis occurs in 1 to 2 percent of these patients during the first year after operation and 1 percent per year thereafter. Aortic valve prostheses are much more likely to be involved than mitral valve prostheses. The infection is usually on the suture line.

Early-onset endocarditis (onset of symptoms within 60 days of surgery) is a consequence of valve contamination during the procedure or bacteremia perioperatively. *Late-onset endocarditis* (onset of symptoms after 60 days) may have the same pathogenesis as early endocarditis (especially during the first year) but with a long incubation period, or may result from transient bacteremia.

About half the episodes of early and one-third of late endocarditis are caused by staphylococci, and *S. epidermidis* is more frequent than *S. aureus*. Gram-negative bacilli cause up to 15 percent and fungi (most commonly *Candida*) up to 10 percent of early cases and are less common in late endocarditis. A prosthetic valve may malfunction because of large fungal vegetations. Streptococci are the most frequent single cause of late endocarditis (about 40 percent of cases) but are uncommon in early endocarditis.

Early prosthetic valve endocarditis is often associated with valve dysfunction or dehiscence and a fulminant course. Although late endocarditis may be similarly fulminant, the course is commonly indistinguishable from that of patients without prosthetic valves, especially when the organism is a streptococcus.

PATHOGENESIS AND PATHOLOGY

The characteristic lesions of infective endocarditis are vegetations on valves or elsewhere on endocardium. The disease usually arises secondary to localization of microorganisms on sterile vegetations composed of platelets and fibrin. Sterile vegetations, termed nonbacterial thrombotic endocarditis, form over areas of trauma to the endothelium (e.g., from intracardiac foreign bodies), in areas of turbulence (as on deformed valves), over scars, or in patients with wasting disease, particularly malignancy (marantic endocarditis).

Infection of a sterile vegetation is most likely when bacteremia occurs with bacteria that adhere well to platelets, fibrin, and fibronectin. The vegetation of infective endocarditis then results from deposition of platelets and fibrin over the bacteria, forming a "protected site" into which phagocytic cells penetrate poorly.

Endocarditis tends to occur in high-pressure areas (left side of heart) and downstream from where blood flows through a narrow orifice at a high velocity from a high- to low-pressure chamber (e.g., distal to the constriction in coarctation of the aorta). Endocarditis is unusual in sites with a small pressure gradient, as in atrial septal defects. Endocarditis occurs more frequently in valvular incompetence than pure stenosis and is characteristically on the atrial side of the regurgitant mitral valve and the ventricular surface of the regurgitant aortic valve. A high-velocity stream of blood can produce satellite-infected lesions at distant points of impact.

Microorganisms that possess little pathogenicity in other situations, e.g., viridans streptococci, usually implant only on deformed heart valves with nonbacterial thrombotic endocarditis, but more virulent microorganisms, e.g., *S. aureus* and *Strep. pneumoniae*, can infect apparently normal valves.

Transient bacteremia is common in various infections and during traumatic procedures involving epithelial surfaces that are colonized by a bacterial flora (oropharynx, genitourinary and gastrointestinal tracts, and skin). For example, after trauma to tissues of the mouth, viridans streptococci are the most common bacteria isolated from blood, alone or more often mixed with other bacteria. The frequency and magnitude of bacteremia are related to the severity of periodontal disease and the severity of trauma. The portal of entry for the initiating episode of bacteremia is usually not apparent in viridans streptococcal endocarditis. Dental procedures, the most common apparent portals of entry, precede viridans streptococcal endocarditis in only 15 to 20 percent of cases.

Bacteremia also is common with prostatic surgery, cystoscopy, urethral dilation or catheterization, and procedures on the female reproductive tract. The organisms are usually enterococci and gram-negative bacilli. About 50 percent of patients with enterococcal endocarditis have had a recent operation or instrumentation on the genitourinary or gastrointestinal tracts. About 35 percent with staphylococcal endocarditis have had a preceding staphylococcal infection at a remote site.

The clinical features of endocarditis result from the vegetations and an immune reaction to the infection. Extensive vegetations, especially in fungal endocarditis, may occlude the valve orifice. Rapid destruction with consequent valvular regurgitation may occur, especially with *S. aureus*. Healing may cause scar formation with subsequent valvular stenosis or regurgitation. Infection may extend into the myocardium producing burrowing abscesses. Conduction abnormalities, fistulas (between chambers of the heart and the pericardium or major vessels), or rupture of the chordae, a papillary muscle, or the ventricular septum may result.

Pieces of vegetation break off and embolize to the heart, brain, kidney, spleen, liver, extremities, and lung (in right-sided endocarditis). Infarcts and occasionally abscesses result. Septic embolization to the vasa vasorum or direct bacterial invasion of the arterial wall may result in formation of mycotic aneurysms which may rupture. Mycotic aneurysms most often develop in the cerebral arteries, aorta, sinuses of Valsalva, ligated ductus arteriosus, and the superior mesenteric, splenic, coronary, and pulmonary arteries.

Patients with endocarditis usually have high antibody titers against the infecting microorganism. This contributes to formation of circulating immune complexes that may result in glomerulonephritis (focal, membranoproliferative, or diffuse), arthritis, or various mucocutaneous manifestations of vasculitis.

Myocarditis may be due to small coronary artery emboli, myocardial abscesses, or immune complex vasculitis.

MANIFESTATIONS

Symptoms of endocarditis generally start within two weeks of the precipitating event. The *onset* is usually gradual, with mild fever and malaise, with organisms of low pathogenicity (e.g., viridans streptococci). With organisms of high pathogenicity (e.g., *S. aureus*), the onset is often acute with high fever. *Fever* is present in almost all patients with endocarditis (except occasionally in the elderly or those with renal failure, congestive heart failure, or severe debility). The fever is usually low grade (less than 39.4°C) except with acute disease. Arthralgias are common, and arthritis occurs occasionally.

Cardiac murmurs are almost always present except early in acute endocarditis or in intravenous drug abusers with tricuspid valve infection. True changes in murmurs or the appearance of a new murmur are uncommon except in acute endocarditis where a new murmur (particularly aortic regurgitation) is frequent. Changes in intensities of murmurs are often due to changes in heart rate and/or cardiac output (e.g., from anemia) and not necessarily from progressive valvular damage.

Splenomegaly and *petechiae* each tend to occur in about 30 percent of cases in disease of long duration. Petechiae are most frequently found on the conjunctivae, palate, buccal mucosa, and upper extremities. *Splinter hemorrhages* are subungual, linear, dark-red streaks that may appear in endocarditis but also commonly result from trauma. *Roth spots* (oval, retinal hemorrhages with a clear pale center) are seen in less than 5 percent of patients and may also occur in connective tissue disease and severe anemia. *Osler nodes* (small tender nodules usually on the finger or toe pads which persist for hours to days) occur in 10 to 25 percent of patients but also in other diseases. *Janeway lesions* are small hemorrhages with a slightly nodular character on the palms and soles and are most commonly seen in acute endocarditis. *Clubbing* of the fingers is present in some patients with longstanding disease. *Embolic episodes* are recognized in about one-third of patients and may occur during or after therapy. Emboli to large arteries (e.g., femoral arteries) are often the result of fungal endocarditis with its large friable vegetations. Pulmonary emboli are common in drug abusers with right-sided endocarditis and may be seen in left-sided endocarditis with left-to-right cardiac shunts.

Mycotic aneurysms occur in about 10 percent of patients. Symptoms are usually lacking but may be those of an expanding mass. They can rupture during or even years after therapy. *Neurologic manifestations* are present in about one-third of patients with endocarditis. Major cerebral emboli as well as mycotic aneurysms usually involve the middle cerebral artery system. Brain abscess and purulent meningitis are most common with *S. aureus* endocarditis. *Heart failure* may occur during the course of the disease or long after cure. Contributing factors are valve destruction, myocarditis, coronary artery emboli with infarction, and myocardial abscesses. *Renal disease* is present in most patients with endocarditis and is due to renal emboli or glomerulonephritis. Renal insufficiency may result.

LABORATORY FEATURES

A normocytic normochromic anemia is usual in infective endocarditis. The white blood cell and differential counts are often normal. However, in acute disease, leukocytosis without anemia may be present. Proteinuria and/or microscopic hematuria are found in most patients, and the serum creatinine may be elevated. The erythrocyte sedimentation rate is almost always elevated except when heart failure is present.

About 50 percent of patients with endocarditis for at least six weeks have a positive serum test for rheumatoid factor, and virtually all have circulating immune complexes. These tend to disappear with cure. The serum complement may be decreased, especially with diffuse glomerulonephritis. Large mononuclear cells in the first drop of blood obtained after massage of the ear lobe (''ear lobe histiocytes'') occur in about 25 percent of patients with endocarditis as well as in some with other chronic infections. Serum antibodies to teichoic acid (a cell wall antigen in *S. aureus*) suggest endocarditis or other deep infection in patients with staphylococcal bacteremia. Bacteria can be seen inside leukocytes in buffy coat preparations of blood in about 50 percent of patients with endocarditis.

The critical diagnostic finding in endocarditis is bacteremia or fungemia. Blood cultures are positive in over 95 percent of patients. The bacteremia is continuous; if any cultures are positive, all are likely to be positive. There is no advantage to obtaining cultures at any particular time or body temperature. Arterial blood or bone marrow offers no advantage over antecubital vein blood.

In subacute disease, in the absence of previous therapy, three cultures should be obtained over 3 to 6 h and therapy initiated. With previous therapy, treatment may be expeditiously delayed in an attempt to obtain positive blood cultures. In general, in acute disease, therapy should not be delayed for more than 2 to 3 h while obtaining cultures. Only one culture should be obtained from each venipuncture, using anaerobic as well as aerobic techniques. The yield of positive cultures is increased by observing them over three weeks and making periodic blind Gram stains and subcultures. Addition of pyridoxal hydrochloride to the media will improve the chances of isolating nutritionally deficient variant streptococci.

Blood cultures may be negative in infections with fastidious organisms such as *Haemophilus parainfluenzae*. Fifty percent of patients with *Candida* endocarditis and almost all with *Aspergillus*, *Histoplasma*, and *Coxiella burnetii* endocarditis have negative blood cultures. With fungi, large peripheral emboli are common, necessitating embolectomy. Histologic examination and culture of the embolus may be diagnostic. Serologic tests for *C. burnetii* and *C. psittaci* are positive in endocarditis caused by these organisms.

Although not diagnostic, echocardiograms will demonstrate the vegetation in up to 80 percent of patients with native valve endocarditis. Serial phonocardiography and cineradiography are useful in evaluating infection on prosthetic valves. Disappearance of an opening click or sound produced by a closing valve suggests presence of a vegetation. With dehiscence, cineradiography of the valve will show abnormal motion.

DIAGNOSIS

Endocarditis should be suspected either when a heart murmur and unexplained fever are present for at least 1 week or in febrile intravenous drug abusers even in the absence of a murmur. However, a definitive clinical diagnosis requires positive blood cultures.

Atrial myxoma, nonbacterial thrombotic endocarditis, acute rheumatic fever, lupus erythematosus, and sickle cell disease can duplicate the syndrome of infective endocarditis. Any patient with an existing heart murmur can develop fever related to another occult illness or to drugs. Therefore, in the absence of positive blood cultures, a search must be made for other causes of fever.

Following cardiac surgery, fever may be related to infection at other sites, to the post-cardiotomy syndrome, or to a ''postpump syndrome'' (e.g., cytomegalovirus infection).

TREATMENT

PRINCIPLES OF THERAPY Cure of endocarditis requires eradication of all microorganisms from the vegetation. Therefore, microbicidal drug regimens must be used in high enough concentrations and for a long enough duration to sterilize the vegetation. Regimens including penicillins, cephalosporins, and vancomycin give far better results than when these drugs cannot be used because of resistant organisms or drug reactions.

The minimal inhibitory and bactericidal concentrations (MIC and MBC) should be determined. Evidence suggests that peak serum concentrations of a regimen that are bactericidal at a 1:8 dilution generally indicate adequate therapy. While this determination is not necessary in most cases, it may be useful when infection is caused by organisms other than gram-positive cocci, treatment has failed, or regimens do not include penicillins, cephalosporins, or vancomycin. Except for unusual circumstances, antibiotic administration should be parenteral to guarantee adequate absorption of drugs. The infecting microorganism should be saved for future testing (e.g., serum antibacterial activity, evaluation of different antibiotics, or comparison with a relapse strain).

SPECIFIC ANTIMICROBIAL REGIMENS Therapy before culture results are known The treatment of subacute infective endocarditis on a native valve while awaiting culture results should be for streptococci, and such ''expectant'' therapy should be directed against the most antibiotic-resistant streptococci, enterococci.

With an acute course, therapy should be directed against *S. aureus*. In intravenous drug abusers, therapy should be directed against *S. aureus* and gentamicin should be included for gram-negative bacilli. In many cities, most *S. aureus* isolated from drug abusers are methicillin-resistant and vancomycin must be used. With prosthetic valves, vancomycin plus gentamicin should be used because of the high incidence of methicillin-resistant *S. epidermidis* as well as to cover enterococci.

Once the organism is isolated, the regimen should be altered appropriately. If cultures remain sterile and culture-negative endocarditis is likely, treatment is continued provided that the response is adequate.

Streptococci Most streptococci are inhibited by serum concentrations of 0.1 μg/mL penicillin G. Three regimens including penicillin G (Table 90-1) can be used for these highly penicillin-susceptible strains. Penicillin G alone for 4 weeks (regimen A) gives cure rates of 99 percent. Addition of gentamicin or streptomycin (regimen B) results in a more rapid bactericidal effect and gives equivalent cure rates in 2 weeks. Regimen B should be standard for uncomplicated infection, but regimen A is preferred in patients likely to have side

TABLE 90-1 Therapy of infective endocarditis caused by gram-positive cocci*

STREPTOCOCCI† WITH MIC ≤ 0.1 μg/mL PENICILLIN G	
Regimen A	Penicillin G, 10–20 million units/d IV in divided doses every 4 h × 4 weeks *or*
Regimen B	Penicillin as in regimen A plus streptomycin, 7.5 mg/kg IM every 12 h or gentamicin, 1 mg/kg IV every 8 h, both × 2 weeks *or*
Regimen C	Penicillin plus streptomycin or gentamicin × 2 weeks as in regimen B with penicillin continued 2 weeks longer *or*
Regimen D	Cefazolin 1–2 g IV or IM every 6–8 h × 4 weeks *or*
Regimen E	Vancomycin, 15 mg/kg IV every 12 h × 4 weeks
ENTEROCOCCI OR OTHER STREPTOCOCCI WITH MIC > 0.5 μg/mL PENICILLIN G	
Regimen F	Penicillin G, 20–30 million units/d or ampicillin, 12 g/d IV in divided doses every 4 h plus gentamicin, 1 mg/kg IV every 8 h or streptomycin 7.5 mg/kg IM every 12 h, both × 4–6 weeks *or*
Regimen G	Vancomycin, 15 mg/kg IV every 12 h plus gentamicin or streptomycin as in regimen F, both × 4–6 weeks
STREPTOCOCCI OTHER THAN ENTEROCOCCI WITH MIC > 0.1 BUT < 0.5 μg/mL PENICILLIN G	
Regimen H	Use regimen C *or* regimen E if penicillin allergic
METHICILLIN-SUSCEPTIBLE *S. AUREUS* OR *S. EPIDERMIDIS*	
Regimen I	Nafcillin, 2 g IV every 4 h × 4–6 weeks with or without gentamicin, 1 mg/kg IV every 8 h × the first 3–5 d *or*
Regimen J	Cefazolin, 2 g IV every 6 h × 4–6 weeks with or without gentamicin as in regimen I *or*
Regimen K	Vancomycin 15 mg/kg IV every 12 h × 4–6 weeks with or without gentamicin as in regimen I
METHICILLIN-RESISTANT STAPHYLOCOCCI OR *CORYNEBACTERIUM SP.*	
Regimen L	Vancomycin with or without gentamicin as in regimen K
ENDOCARDITIS ON A PROSTHETIC VALVE	
Regimen C but with 20 million units of penicillin each day and a longer duration of penicillin (a total of 6 weeks)	
Regimen D × 6 weeks with gentamicin or streptomycin × the first 2 weeks	
Regimen E × 6 weeks with gentamicin or streptomycin × the first 2 weeks	
Regimen F or G × 6 weeks	
Regimen H, but continue penicillin × 6 weeks	
Regimen I, J, or K × 6–8 weeks with gentamicin × the first 2 weeks	
Regimen L × 6–8 weeks with gentamicin × the first 2 weeks	
In the presence of *S. epidermidis* also add rifampin, 300 mg orally every 8 h × 6–8 weeks. The use of rifampin with *S. aureus* is controversial.	

* Peak serum concentrations of gentamicin should be about 3 μg/mL. Streptomycin peaks should be about 20 μg/mL. The maximum dose of vancomycin is 1 g every 12 h.
† For Group A streptococci or *S. pneumoniae* use regimen A.
NOTE: MIC = minimal inhibitory concentration.

effects with aminoglycosides (i.e., those with renal insufficiency or eighth nerve disease, or older than 65 years). Penicillin for 4 weeks with an aminoglycoside for the first 2 weeks (regimen C) is used for nutritionally deficient variant strains, a relapse, or complications (e.g., metastatic abscesses or shock). Regimen D can be substituted with a history of a delayed rash to penicillin. Regimen E should be used with a history of anaphylaxis to penicillin.

Penicillin, ampicillin, and vancomycin are not bactericidal for most enterococci. With the addition of an aminoglycoside a synergistic bactericidal effect occurs. Enterococcal endocarditis requires penicillin, ampicillin, or vancomycin plus an aminoglycoside for cure of most patients (regimens F and G, with G used for hypersensitivity to penicillin G). An alternative to regimen G consists of skin testing with major and minor determinants of penicillin, followed by attempts at desensitization to penicillin. This involves a scratch test through a drop of penicillin G (100 units per mL). This is followed in 30 min by graded amounts of penicillin intradermally, begun at 0.01 units in 0.1 mL of saline solution and continued in tenfold increments every 30 min; with increasing amounts, administration is changed to the subcutaneous, intramuscular, and finally intravenous route. Epinephrine and diphenhydramine should be on hand for emergency use during the procedure in case of anaphylaxis, and preferably the procedure should be carried out in an intensive care unit. If a reaction occurs, alternative therapy should be initiated.

Therapy is usually given for 4 weeks but is prolonged to 6 weeks when symptoms have been present for longer than 3 months or the course is complicated. Cephalosporins cannot be used in enterococcal endocarditis because the organisms are highly resistant.

A synergistic bactericidal effect against enterococci occurs with aminoglycosides only when growth is inhibited by 2000 μg/mL. Synergism is most likely with gentamicin. However, enterococci resistant to 2000 μg/mL of gentamicin are more common than in the past. Some of these gentamicin-resistant strains are inhibited by 2000 μg/mL of streptomycin, but most are resistant to 2000 μg/mL of all aminoglycosides. With aminoglycoside-resistant strains, it may be best to exclude aminoglycosides from the regimen and treat for 6 to 8 weeks. However, relapses may occur.

Endocarditis caused by non-enterococcal streptococci with a MIC > 0.1 but < 0.5μg/mL penicillin G is managed with regimen H, a compromise between the regimens for highly susceptible (MIC ≤ 0.1 μg/mL) and relatively resistant (MIC ≥ 0.5 μg/mL) streptococci.

Staphylococci Methicillin-susceptible *S. aureus* and *S. epidermidis* are treated with regimens I or J. Methicillin-resistant staphylococci are resistant to all penicillins and cephalosporins. In these cases, or in patients who cannot tolerate penicillins or cephalosporins, vancomycin as in regimens K and L must be used. Some experts advocate addition of gentamicin for the first 3 to 5 days because of an increase in the rate of bactericidal activity. However, clinical evidence of improved outcome is lacking and routine administration of gentamicin is not recommended. Therapy for 4 weeks is standard, but with metastatic or intracardiac abscess formation or an otherwise complicated course, therapy should be prolonged to 6 weeks or even longer.

As indicated in Table 90-1, in prosthetic valve endocarditis, therapy should be prolonged and combinations containing an aminoglycoside are usually used. When a methicillin-resistant *S. epidermidis* infects a prosthetic valve, results have been improved with addition of rifampin.

Other organisms In endocarditis caused by other organisms, bactericidal antibiotics, preferably a penicillin, cephalosporin, or vancomycin with or without an aminoglycoside, should be given, and therapy continued for 4 to 6 weeks. With gram-negative bacilli, the penicillin or cephalosporin which has the greatest potency against the infecting bacteria in vitro should be administered in large doses intravenously along with an aminoglycoside to which the bacterium is susceptible (e.g., ampicillin, 2 g every 4 h; piperacillin, 3 g every 4 h; cefotaxime, 2 g every 4 to 6 h; or ceftazidime, 2 g every 8 h plus gentamicin 1.7 mg/kg every 8 h). Ciprofloxacin alone, which is bactericidal for gram-negative bacilli, should also be useful.

When the organisms are resistant to penicillins, cephalosporins, ciprofloxacin, and vancomycin, therapy will probably be unsuccessful. Under these circumstances, treatment should be with the bactericidal drug grouping that demonstrates the best activity in vitro. If the response is poor or relapse occurs, antimicrobial therapy plus valve replacement will probably be necessary.

SURGERY IN THE MANAGEMENT OF ENDOCARDITIS When appropriate microbicidal therapy is not available (as in fungal endocarditis) and positive blood cultures persist on therapy or relapse occurs after therapy, the valve should be replaced. Ideally, surgery should be performed after several days of the best available antimicrobial therapy. With organisms that tend to produce metastatic foci, therapy should then be continued long enough to eradicate these foci. Persistence of infection with the same organism following valve replacement has been uncommon. Immediate replacement (even after only hours of therapy) is essential in patients developing heart failure secondary to severe valvular regurgitation. Surgery is necessary to drain myocardial or valve ring abscesses and should be considered with recurrent emboli despite adequate antimicrobial therapy. It should also be considered in patients with aortic valve endocarditis who develop first and second degree atrioventricular block. In some centers, the presence of a large vegetation on echocardiography is also an indication for surgery.

Replacement of a prosthesis is often necessary for infections with organisms other than streptococci, for valve dysfunction or dehiscence, or for myocardial invasion. Myocardial invasion is common with prosthetic valves and is suggested by continued fever after 10 days of therapy, a new regurgitant murmur, and/or atrioventricular conduction disturbance.

COURSE

Defervescence usually occurs after 3 to 7 days of antimicrobial therapy. Blood cultures should be obtained periodically during treatment and generally become negative after several days of therapy. Lack of response of fever and bacteremia may be associated with myocardial or metastatic abscess formation (especially associated with *S. aureus*).

The most common cause of persistent or recurrent fever during therapy is a drug reaction and, less commonly, emboli. If a rash develops, therapy can be continued and antihistamines or even glucocorticoids given to suppress the reaction. If the rash is severe, therapy should be altered.

Weight gain and a rise in hemoglobin may not be seen until weeks after therapy has been completed. Petechiae, Osler nodes, and emboli may occur during and for weeks after successful antimicrobial therapy. Mycotic aneurysms may regress on drug therapy or may rupture weeks to years later. Heart failure may occuring during or after therapy and is the principal cause of death.

Anticoagulants should be used only with a pressing indication (such as certain prosthetic valves, but not including infected emboli) because of increased risk of hemorrhage (especially intracranial). Coumadin is preferable to heparin. Blood cultures 2 and 4 weeks after discontinuation of the therapy detect the vast majority of relapses.

PROGNOSIS

Factors that predispose to a poor prognosis are (1) non-streptococcal disease, (2) development of heart failure, (3) aortic valve involvement, (4) infection on a prosthetic valve, (5) older age, and (6) valve ring or myocardial abscess. The cure rate in streptococcal endocarditis is about 90 percent. Failures are not due to uncontrolled infection but to death from heart failure, embolus, rupture of mycotic aneurysm, or renal failure. The mortality rate in nonaddicts with *S. aureus* endocarditis is at least 40 percent, and most deaths are due to overwhelming infection or heart failure. In drug addicts with *S. aureus* infection on the tricuspid valve, cure rates are over 90 percent and treatment may be shortened in the absence of infected emboli to 2 weeks of nafcillin plus an aminoglycoside. Results are poor in endocarditis caused by fungi and gram-negative bacilli resistant to penicillins and cephalosporins. The presence of large vegetations on echocardiogram may indicate a poorer prognosis than small or absent vegetations. About 10 percent of patients will have additional episodes of endocarditis, months or years later. The prognosis in early prosthetic valve endocarditis is much worse than in late disease, with mortality rates of 40 to 80 percent versus 20 to 40 percent.

ANTIMICROBIAL PROPHYLAXIS OF ENDOCARDITIS

Although the risk of endocarditis is small and there is no proof of efficacy, prophylaxis is recommended for patients with predisposing cardiac lesions undergoing procedures known to cause bacteremia. The conditions for which prophylaxis is recommended are valvular or congenital heart disease (except uncomplicated atrial septal defect), intracardiac prostheses, asymmetric septal hypertrophy, and previous episode of endocarditis. Mitral valve prolapse increases the risk of endocarditis to a low to moderate extent. However, it is so common, that it is neither risk- nor cost-effective to give prophylaxis to all patients with prolapse for all procedures. It is, however, reasonable to use prophylaxis in individuals with mitral valve prolapse who have holosystolic murmurs and who presumably are at greatest risk.

Oral hygiene should be optimal in patients with cardiac lesions that predispose to endocarditis, especially those who are to have prosthetic cardiac valves implanted.

For dental and other procedures in the mouth, nose, or throat likely to cause bleeding or significant trauma, prophylaxis is aimed at viridans streptococci. The regimen recommended by the American Heart Association is penicillin V, 2 g orally, 1 h before the procedure followed by 1 g 6 h later. An effective alternative regimen is a single oral dose of 3 g of amoxicillin 1 h before the procedure. With penicillin allergy, erythromycin is recommended, 1 g orally 1 h before, followed by 0.5 g 6 h later. In high-risk patients (e.g., those with prosthetic valves), the regimen is ampicillin, 2 g intramuscularly or intravenously plus gentamicin, 1.5 mg/kg intramuscularly or intravenously both 30 min before and 1 g penicillin V orally 6 h later or, with penicillin allergy, vancomycin, 1 g intravenously over 1 h starting 1 h before.

For genitourinary and gastrointestinal tract procedures likely to cause significant trauma (e.g., urethral catheterization, prostatic surgery, and colonic or gallbladder surgery), prophylaxis is directed against enterococci. The regimen is ampicillin plus gentamicin as above. With penicillin allergy, the vancomycin regimen above is given, but 1.5 mg/kg gentamicin intravenously or intramuscularly is added 1 h before the procedure. For low-risk patients with minor procedures, amoxicillin may be used, 3g orally 1 h before the procedure followed by 1.5 g 6 h later. Fiberoptic endoscopy without biopsy and barium enema are at such low risk for endocarditis that prophylaxis is difficult to justify. If used, it should be only in high-risk patients.

Prophylaxis for cardiac surgery with placement of intracardiac prostheses, patches, or sutures is directed against staphylococci and has usually consisted of 2 g of cefazolin intravenously plus 1.5 mg/kg gentamicin intravenously starting immediately preoperatively, followed by repeated doses 8 and 16 h later. However, as strains of *S. epidermidis* may be methicillin-resistant, substitution of vancomycin for cefazolin in a dose of 15 mg/kg intravenously over 1 h, starting 1 h before the procedure, 10 mg/kg after completion of by-pass, and then 7.5 mg/kg every 6 h for 3 doses is reasonable. Vancomycin can also be used when patients have hypersensitivity to penicillins and cephalosporins.

Patients with coronary artery bypass grafts or transvenous pacemakers in place do not require prophylaxis for endocarditis nor is it indicated for patients undergoing cardiac catheterization.

REFERENCES

BISNO AL et al: Antimicrobial treatment of infective endocarditis due to viridans streptococci, enterococci and staphylococci. JAMA 261(10):1471, 1989

BUDA AJ et al: Prognostic significance of vegetations detected by two-dimensional echocardiography in infective endocarditis. Am Heart J 112(6):1291, 1986

CHAMBERS HF et al: Right-sided *Staphylococcus aureus* endocarditis in intravenous drug abusers: Two-week combination therapy. Ann Intern Med 109:619, 1988

DURACK D: Prophylaxis of infective endocarditis, in *Principles and Practice of Infectious Diseases*, 3d ed, GL Mandell et al (eds). New York, Churchill Livingstone, 1990

HOFFMAN SA, MOELLERING RC: The enterococcus: "Putting the bug in our ears." Ann Intern Med 106:757, 1987

MACMAHON SW et al: Risk of infective endocarditis in mitral valve prolapse with and without precordial systolic murmurs. Am J Cardiol 59:105, 1987

MCKINSEY DS et al: Underlying cardiac lesions in adults with infective endocarditis. Am J Med 82:681, 1987

Prevention of bacterial endocarditis. Med Lett Drugs Ther 31:112, 1989

SANDE MA et al (eds): *Contemporary Issues in Infectious Diseases*, vol 2: *Endocarditis*. New York, Churchill Livingstone, 1984

SCHELD M, SANDE M: Endocarditis and intravascular infections, in *Principles and Practice of Infectious Diseases*, 3d ed, GL Mandell et al (eds). New York, Churchill Livingstone, 1990

SHULMAN ST et al: Prevention of bacterial endocarditis. Circulation 70:1123A, 1984

SUSSMAN JI et al: Viridans streptococcal endocarditis: Clinical, microbiological and echocardiographic correlations. J Infect Dis 154(4):597, 1986

THRELKELD M, COBBS G: Infections of prosthetic valves and intravascular devices, in *Principles and Practice of Infectious Diseases*, 3d ed, GL Mandell et al (eds). New York, Churchill-Livingstone, 1990

91 LOCALIZED INFECTIONS AND ABSCESSES

JAN V. HIRSCHMANN

GENERAL CONSIDERATIONS

While many pathogens produce a characteristic clinical syndrome, in some infections the location of the process rather than the identity of the responsible organisms determines the clinical manifestations. Examples include abscesses, soft tissue infections, bacterial endocarditis (see Chap. 90), pyogenic infections of the central nervous system (see Chap. 354), urinary tract infections (see Chap. 95), lung abscess (see Chap. 207), mediastinitis (see Chap. 216), appendicitis and appendiceal abscess (see Chap. 245), diverticulitis (see Chap. 243), osteomyelitis (see Chap. 97), and infections of the pericardium (see Chap. 193). Many pathogens can cause infections in these sites; but knowledge of the usual flora causing them should permit appropriate therapy before the results of cultures are available.

ETIOLOGY Localized pyogenic infection can develop in any region or organ of the body, and may be initiated by *trauma* and secondary bacterial contamination, by some *alteration in local conditions* that renders a tissue susceptible to infection with organisms already present as part of the "normal flora" to which it is ordinarily resistant, by *contiguous spread* from a nearby lesion, or by *metastatic implantation* of microorganisms carried in blood or lymph.

Infection in some areas is more likely to be caused by certain organisms, such as staphylococci in the skin and coliform bacteria in the urinary tract, and special features of the tissue reaction produced by some bacterial species make it possible to recognize infection by them with considerable accuracy. The *staphylococci* produce rapid necrosis and early suppuration with large amounts of creamy yellow pus (see Chap. 100). Group A beta-hemolytic streptococcal infections (see Chap. 101) tend to spread rapidly through tissues, causing intense edema and erythema but relatively little necrosis and thin, serumlike exudate; anaerobic bacteria (see Chap. 108) may produce necrosis and profuse, foul-smelling pus.

The identification of infecting organisms is important in the choice of antimicrobial chemotherapy. However, when infection occurs in certain areas, as in paranasal sinuses or cutaneous ulcers, or shows up in sputum, it is unlikely that treatment will render cultured specimens sterile. In these locations, serial cultures during antimicrobial administration are typically unhelpful, and therapy should be guided largely by the clinical response.

PATHOGENESIS Factors predisposing to the initiation and persistence of infection in a tissue include trauma, obstruction of normal drainage (sweat glands, biliary tract, bronchial tree, urinary tract), ischemia (infarction, gangrene), chemical irritation (by gastric contents, bile, or intramuscularly injected drugs), hematoma formation, accumulation of fluid (lymphatic obstruction, cardiac edema), foreign bodies (bullets, splinters, sutures), and others such as the occurrence of stasis or turbulence in the vascular system. When these conditions severely compromise local host defenses almost any common bacteria can initiate an infection, and the organisms responsible are often part of the normal flora of an adjacent cutaneous or mucosal surface.

Infection in soft tissue usually begins as a *cellulitis*, a diffuse acute inflammation with hyperemia, edema, and leukocytic infiltration but little or no necrosis and suppuration. With some organisms, this is followed by necrosis, liquefaction, accumulation of leukocytes and debris, suppuration, loculation of the pus, and formation of one or more *abscesses*.

Infection may spread locally via the path of least resistance along fascial planes or by the lymphatic system, which may lead to lymphangitis or regional lymphadenitis, sometimes with suppuration. Involvement of local venules or large veins may cause infective thrombophlebitis with resulting bacteremia, septic embolization, and systemic dissemination of infection.

Depending upon the infecting organism and the anatomy of the affected region, a small abscess may subside completely; there may be gradual encapsulation of the accumulated pus and persistence of the focus in a quiescent state; or the lesion may "point" and rupture into adjacent tissues or to the outside surface of the body, as usually happens with furuncles. Spontaneous drainage ordinarily leads to resolution of a superficial abscess. However, if it is deeply situated and well encapsulated, persistence of a fistulous tract and the formation of a chronic, draining sinus may occur. *The development of persistent sinuses over an area of suppuration produced by ordinary pyogenic bacteria should always suggest involvement of underlying bone or the presence of a foreign body.* Fistulas that open onto the skin are, of course, soon colonized by microorganisms from the external environment. Routine bacterial cultures of drainage fluid almost invariably show a mixed flora and are unreliable for the etiologic diagnosis of the underlying disease, particularly in disorders that characteristically lead to persistent sinus formation, such as tuberculosis and actinomycosis.

MANIFESTATIONS Infections of the skin and subcutaneous tissues almost invariably produce the classic manifestations: *redness, tenderness, heat,* and *swelling*. Reddish streaks extending proximally and associated with tender enlargement of regional lymph nodes indicate lymphangitis. Systemic symptoms may be absent or mild, or there may be fever, malaise, prostration, and leukocytosis.

Infection and suppuration in deeper tissues or in body cavities often cause pain and tenderness, but locating and determining the exact nature of the lesion may be difficult. Palpating a tender mass is helpful and fluctuation indicates that it contains fluid, usually pus, but muscle spasm and intervening structures often interfere with identifying the site. Auscultation may reveal a friction rub over an abdominal viscus, the pleura, or the pericardium. The rapid development of an effusion in the pericardium, pleura, abdomen, or a joint should suggest infection. Similarly, fluid detected by transillumination of paranasal sinuses or inspection of the tympanic membrane may be the first sign of infection.

An abscess may produce symptoms and signs by encroaching upon adjacent structures. Respiratory obstruction may be the first sign of mediastinal abscess; dysphagia often first calls attention to peritonsillar or retropharyngeal abscesses; and tamponade is sometimes the initial clue to pericardial infection. Localizing signs of dysfunction are especially striking and important with brain and spinal cord abscesses, although brain abscesses may be clinically silent (see Chap. 354). In some patients local pain and tenderness or signs of dysfunction are absent, mild, or equivocal, and fever, prostration, fatigue, and weight loss predominate. The fever may be low-grade but is often hectic, with repeated rigors and drenching night sweats. Fatigue and anemia are frequent, and weight loss may be so rapid that emaciation occurs within a few weeks. A patient with these symptoms and signs may have a chronic intraabdominal abscess without any detectable physical sign to indicate its location.

LABORATORY FINDINGS Peripheral polymorphonuclear leukocytosis is frequent with abscesses, and significant unexplained elevation of the white blood cell count in any patient may indicate localized suppuration. An elevated sedimentation rate is common in infections of all durations, but the "anemia of chronic disease" may occur with a protracted course. Mild albuminuria, occasionally noted in febrile patients, has no diagnostic import.

Pus or fluid obtained by needle aspiration or incision of a suspected lesion should *always* be stained and examined directly in addition to being cultured aerobically and anaerobically. *Failure to examine exudates with Gram's stain is the single greatest deterrent to appropriate antimicrobial therapy.*

Blood cultures are usually positive in intravascular infections such as septic thrombophlebitis and endocarditis and may be positive in localized abscesses, especially when metastatic, as in staphylococcal, streptococcal, and *Salmonella* bacteremias. Moreover, manipulation, including surgical incision, of any localized infection may cause transient bacteremia.

Noninvasive techniques are often helpful in the diagnosis of abscess. Radiographic examinations may indicate localized collections of pus when they show atypical collections of gas, displacement of organs, and tissue densities in abnormal locations. Diagnostic ultrasound is not only useful in localizing abscess but also may provide clues to the size of the abscess and to the presence of multiple abscesses or loculation. Computed tomography (CT) scan is usually the most accurate technique in demonstrating abscesses, especially in the brain and abdominal cavity, including the retroperitoneum. Radionuclide scans using labeled leukocytes may be helpful when other imaging technologies are negative or equivocal, but they also may be misleading. Magnetic resonance imaging (MRI) scans may be preferred when metal causes artifacts or in further defining brain abscesses or those invading soft tissues and contiguous bone (e.g., vertebral body abscesses with spinal cord compression).

THERAPEUTIC CONSIDERATIONS Striking symptomatic improvement usually follows adequate drainage of pus, but incision of infected tissue before the stage of liquefaction is often deleterious, fails to relieve discomfort, and may even at times facilitate spread of infection. For this reason, it is sometimes necessary to wait until an abscess "ripens," i.e., localizes and "comes to a head." The *application of heat* to an area of superficial inflammation may relieve pain and speed the subsidence of cellulitis without suppuration. If necrosis of tissue is already under way, hot applications appear to facilitate localization of the process and accumulation of pus, making incision and drainage feasible at an earlier time. Another procedure that helps reduce swelling and relieve pain is *elevation of the affected part.*

Antimicrobial therapy is used in many types of abscesses. Some agents, notably the penicillins, retain their antibacterial activity in the presence of pus, while others, exemplified by the aminoglycosides, are partially inactivated. The inability of the drug to penetrate into an area of suppuration, however, is rarely the reason for therapeutic failure. Although this possibility exists in some infections, such as osteomyelitis, it is usually overcome by increasing dosage.

An established inflammatory exudate is a relatively poor environment for rapid bacterial multiplication. Because some antibiotics are bactericidal only against multiplying organisms, failure of these agents to eradicate infection in an abscess may be related to the organisms' inactive metabolic state. Because bacteriostatic drugs inhibit, but do not kill, bacteria, the death of organisms in any infection treated with these agents depends on other mechanisms, especially phagocytosis. In fluid-filled cavities, particularly in the metabolically unfavorable milieu of an abscess, phagocytosis may occur, but intracellular killing is reduced. Consequently, despite inhibition of bacterial multiplication, organisms can remain dormant and survive for long periods of time. It is probably a combination of these two circumstances, decreased multiplication of bacteria and decreased phagocytosis, that makes infection in the heart valves, for example, so relatively resistant to antimicrobial therapy. Large doses of bactericidal drugs for long periods are needed to achieve cure.

Antimicrobial drugs may obviate suppuration if given early or prevent spread of an existing abscess, but usually are no substitute for drainage of purulent material. Indeed, their use in the face of a lesion requiring evacuation of pus is one of the most common serious errors in treating pyogenic infections.

In thoracic empyema, suppurative pericarditis, or pyarthrosis, excellent therapeutic results are sometimes achieved by aspiration of pus and systemic antimicrobial therapy. Success, however, depends as fully on the adequacy of drainage as it does upon the administration of the antibiotic, and if loculation occurs or the exudate becomes too viscid to remove, surgical or catheter drainage may be necessary. An exception to the general rule of the essential role of surgical drainage for cure may be seen in the treatment of brain abscesses; if small or inaccessible, good therapeutic responses have been obtained with prolonged (>6 weeks) administration of antimicrobials (see Chap. 354).

In infective thrombophlebitis, surgical interruption of the veins by ligation or, in some cases, by total excision of an infected segment is sometimes indicated to prevent seeding of other organs by infected emboli.

CLINICAL FEATURES OF INFECTIONS IN VARIOUS REGIONS

SUPERFICIAL ABSCESSES Skin and subcutaneous tissues *Impetigo* is a superficial infection caused by group A hemolytic streptococci, sometimes combined with *Staphylococcus aureus.* Primarily a disease of children and common in warm weather, it is characterized by multiple, pruritic, erythematous lesions, which become vesicles and pustules that rupture to form a crust. In adults impetigo is most commonly an infectious complication of a chronic dermatitis. Local spread occurs through scratching and release of infected vesicle fluid. Serious complications are metastatic abscesses and acute glomerulonephritis. Treatment consists of local and general cleansing of the skin, appropriate systemic antibiotics, and therapy of any underlying dermatologic condition.

About one-fourth of cutaneous abscesses, especially on the extremities, are due to *S. aureus.* The rest yield other organisms, usually anaerobes alone or a combination of aerobes and anaerobes. The bacteria isolated are usually part of the normal flora on that region of the skin where the abscess developed. These organisms ordinarily possess little cutaneous virulence, but when inoculated into the dermis or subcutaneous tissue by trauma or other mechanisms, they can produce suppuration. In most patients with normal host defenses the appropriate treatment is incision and drainage of the abscess and packing of the wound. Gram stain, culture, and antibiotic therapy are unnecessary unless the patient is immunocompromised or the lesion is complicated by extensive cellulitis, cutaneous gangrene, or systemic manifestations of infection.

Lymphadenitis with or without suppuration may complicate any pyogenic skin lesion and is often striking with superficial streptococcal infections. Specific diseases characterized by suppurative regional lymphadenitis include lymphogranuloma venereum (see Chap. 155), cat-scratch disease (see Chap. 98), tularemia (see Chap. 120), and bubonic plague (see Chap. 121).

Infections of the hand These are almost invariably secondary to trauma. Because of the rapidity with which infection can spread through the complex fascial spaces of the hand, wrist, and forearm. and produce irreparable functional damage, *any deep infection in this area should receive expert surgical attention immediately.* The availability of antibiotics has in no way lessened the importance of such care.

The ordinary *paronychia,* or "run-around," is a superficial infection of the epithelium lateral to a nail, usually a result of tearing a hangnail and most frequently caused by staphylococcus. Hot applications will lead to subsidence of paronychial cellulitis, but often a superficial blister of pus appears. A small incision or simply separation of the nail fold from the nail will promote adequate drainage. If the infection burrows beneath the nail to form a painful *subungual abscess,* incision and drainage with partial or complete removal of the nail are necessary. Recurrence is common, especially in nail biters, and this seemingly trivial infection can cause painful disability. Chronic paronychial inflammation, usually from *Candida,* occurs in those with prolonged or frequent immersion of hands in water.

What appears to be a small furuncle of the webs of the fingers sometimes produces a *collar-button abscess,* consisting of a superficial and deep compartment connected by a narrow tract. Evacuation of the shallow pocket without emptying the deeper abscess can lead to puzzling persistence of infection. Sometimes a foreign-body granuloma forms in the skin of the digital webs. This is most common in barbers, in whom a hair is the core of the foreign-body granuloma, the "barber's interdigital pilonidal sinus."

Infection of the distal phalanx of a finger, usually acquired by pinprick, thorn prick, burn, or sliver, may lead to the formation of a *felon,* or *whitlow.* This is a suppurative infection in the tightly enclosed fibrous compartments of the finger pulp, that can compromise the distal blood supply by compressing the digital arteries, cause skin necrosis, and produce osteomyelitis of the phalanx. The manifestations are swelling, extreme pain, and tenderness of the palmar surface of the fingertip. The treatment is immediate incision directly over the lesion to drain the locus of purulence.

Suppurative tenosynovitis, usually a complication of a puncture wound, is a very serious hand infection in which early diagnosis and treatment are mandatory to prevent permanent disability from destruction of the tendon or its sheath. The cardinal manifestations of tenosynovitis are (1) generalized swelling of the digit, (2) exquisite tenderness over the flexor tendon sheath, (3) flexion of the fingers, and (4) excruciating pain, most marked at the base of the digit, on extension of the involved finger. *Immediate incision* of the sheath is indicated, to prevent not only tendon damage but also proximal extension of the process into the major fascial spaces of the hand or forearm. Vigorous antibiotic treatment should accompany surgery.

Human bites may lead to hand infections that, if neglected, almost invariably produce a highly destructive, necrotizing lesion contaminated by a mixture of aerobic and anaerobic organisms (see Chap. 98). A deliberately inflicted bite on the hand or elsewhere is usually recognized as dangerously contaminated, but wounds on the knuckles produced by striking an opponent's teeth with the fists may not be recognized as potentially dangerous. In general, bite wounds should be cleaned thoroughly and not sutured. Patients should be given prophylaxis for tetanus and antibiotics, a good choice being amoxicillin-clavulanic acid.

Chronic cutaneous ulcers Chronic cutaneous ulcers from a variety of causes, including vascular disease, burns, bedsores, or neurologic disease, usually become colonized with bacteria, commonly a complex flora of aerobic and anaerobic organisms, often including streptococci, staphylococci, and anaerobic gram-negative bacilli. These organisms ordinarily do not retard healing and tend to persist until the wound becomes covered with epithelium, even in those patients treated with topical or systemic antibiotics. Chronic cutaneous ulcers do not require routine cultures or antimicrobial therapy, which should be reserved for substantial surrounding cellulitis, osteomyelitis, signs of systemic infection, or formation of abscesses, which should be drained.

INFECTIONS OF THE HEAD AND NECK Pustules of the nose and upper lip may be particularly dangerous, because they can extend intracranially through the angular vein to the cavernous sinus. These lesions should be treated conservatively, manipulation or incision should be avoided if possible, and systemic antibiotics should be used if local swelling or redness appears.

Suppurative parotitis Typically, suppurative parotitis occurs in elderly and chronically ill patients who have a dry mouth from decreased oral intake, following general anesthesia and surgery, or from medications with atropine-like effects, such as antihistamines or phenothiazines. In most patients, it is an ascending infection due to *S. aureus,* which can colonize the opening to Stensen's duct. Occasionally, there is an obstructing calculus. Its onset, usually sudden, is heralded by unilateral local pain and swelling, frequently with fever and chills. Frank pus can often be expressed from the duct and may show gram-positive cocci in clumps. The gland itself is firm and tender, often with redness and edema of the overlying skin. Treatment consists of systemic antimicrobial therapy with a penicillinase-resistant penicillin or some other agent effective against *S. aureus,* unless another organism is isolated, combined with improved hydration and oral hygiene. Massage of the gland and sialagogues, like lemon drops, help promote drainage through the duct. Surgery is usually unnecessary and should be reserved for patients failing to improve after several days of medical management.

Miscellaneous infections Antibiotics have reduced the incidence of many suppurative complications of streptococcal pharyngitis. However, as a result of streptococcal sore throat, *Bacteroides* infections of the pharynx, or introduction of infection by trauma to the floor of the mouth or the pharyngeal wall, abscesses of the deep cervical structures still occur. *Suppurative cervical adenitis,* once an all-too-common sequel to streptococcal pharyngitis in children, is now rare. *Peritonsillar abscess* (*quinsy*) is manifested by fever, sore throat, cervical lymphadenopathy, unilateral pain radiating to the ear on swallowing, and enlargement of the tonsil with redness and swelling of the adjacent soft palate. Treatment with penicillin and irrigations of warm saline solution sometimes suffices, but if digital palpation reveals fluctuation, needle aspiration is indicated. Tonsillectomy is usually reserved for patients with recurrent tonsillar infections. Organisms associated with peritonsillar abscess include *Streptococcus pyogenes* and oral anaerobic bacteria.

The course of *deep cervical infections* depends upon the anatomic arrangement of fascial planes. Infection in this area is serious and is attended by fever, prostration, and leukocytosis. It is usually caused by a mixture of aerobes, predominantly streptococci, and anaerobes, particularly *Peptostreptococcus, Fusobacterium,* and *Bacteroides* (mostly *melaninogenicus*) (see Chap. 108).

Infection of the *sublingual* and submandibular spaces, so-called Ludwig's angina, causes brawny induration of the submaxillary region, edema of the floor of the mouth, and elevation of the tongue. It usually originates from apical abscesses of the second and third mandibular molars and causes severe pain, dysphagia, drooling, stiff neck, and, within hours, dyspnea from respiratory obstruction. *Treatment* consists of large doses of penicillin and careful observation. With significant airway obstruction, tracheostomy, tracheal intubation, or cricothyroidotomy is necessary. Since the infection is largely a cellulitis, incision and drainage are reserved for evidence of abscess formation detected by physical or radiographic (especially CT) examination.

The retropharyngeal space lies between the muscles anterior to the cervical vertebrae and the pharyngeal mucosa. *Retropharyngeal abscess,* formerly common in children, is manifested by dysphagia, progressive stridor, pain, and fever. The bulging mass is easily seen and can completely occlude the airway within hours. Incision and drainage are mandatory; spontaneous rupture may lead to death by aspiration. Another complication is extension of infection into the mediastinum, causing posterior mediastinitis, mediastinal abscess that may rupture into the pleura, or pericarditis, frequently with tamponade. Esophageal perforation during endoscopy may result in abscess as a late complication. Tuberculous abscess, secondary to spinal disease, occasionally appears in the retropharyngeal space; it is painless, and relief of obstruction follows surgical incision.

Lateral pharyngeal space infections, occurring in the lateral portion of the neck between the hyoid bone inferiorly and the sphenoid bone superiorly, can develop from infections throughout the neck, including those involving the teeth, lymph nodes, pharynx, and parotids. Patients usually have fever and leukocytosis. When the anterior portion of this space is involved, trismus, indurated edema of the mandibular angle, and medial bulging of the pharyngeal wall are typically present. Infection of the posterior compartment causes fewer signs, and many patients have only fever. A very serious complication of lateral space infections is involvement of the contiguous vessels. Suppurative jugular venous thrombophlebitis can cause bacteremia, septic pulmonary emboli, and thrombosis of the intracranial venous sinuses. Infection adjacent to the carotid artery may result in an aneurysm that may compress nearby structures to produce a Horner's syndrome, or palsies of the ninth to twelfth cranial nerves. These aneurysms may rupture, causing fatal bleeding.

Therapy of head and neck abscesses includes surgical incision and drainage, open treatment of infected wounds, and systemic antibiotics, which should include agents active against anaerobic organisms. Penicillin is usually the drug of choice; clindamycin or chloramphenicol can be used in penicillin-allergic patients.

INTRAABDOMINAL ABSCESSES

A useful classification divides intraabdominal abscesses, according to location, into three major types, each with several subdivisions: (1) intraperitoneal, (2) retroperitoneal, and (3) visceral. The clinical features vary but usually include fever, with no characteristic pattern (ranging from mild to hectic), leukocytosis, and an elevated erythrocyte sedimentation rate. Common, but not universal, are pain near the abscess, anorexia, weight loss, nausea, vomiting, and altered bowel habits. A tender mass may be palpable. Plain abdominal films may suggest an abscess by showing a soft tissue density, displacement of adjacent organs, or extraintestinal gas from a perforated viscus or produced by the infecting organisms within the abscess cavity.

The most useful noninvasive diagnostic techniques are ultrasound and CT examinations. Ultrasound has a diagnostic accuracy of about 80 percent and is most effective in detecting abscesses in the right upper quadrant, retroperitoneum, and pelvis. It shows a sonolucent mass that may have internal echoes when debris and septations are present. The appearance is usually indistinguishable from other fluid-filled masses, but clinical features and, if necessary, needle aspiration of the mass should discriminate among the possible causes. Since gas blocks the beam, ultrasound is not useful when large amounts of gas are present, as occurs in the stomach and splenic flexure, which makes the left upper quadrant a difficult area to examine. Similarly, loops of gas-filled bowel impair evaluation of the midabdomen. Since the transducer must have good skin contact, wounds, fistulas, stomata, and surgical dressings may make ultrasound examination impossible.

These factors do not affect CT scans, which are therefore especially useful in the postoperative patient, when there are no focal signs or symptoms, or when the area of concern is the left upper quadrant, pancreas, or midabdomen. CT scans are positive in over 90 percent of patients with abscesses, characteristically demonstrating fluid collections with well-defined walls that enhance following intravenous administration of contrast material. MRI is preferred to CT scanning if steel clips obscure visualization by artifact; it may also be better for detecting pelvic abscesses. Unless gas lies within the mass, however, these findings do not distinguish abscesses from simple cysts, old hematomas, or mucinous metastases. Clinical features or needle aspiration should determine the correct diagnosis.

Effective treatment must include antimicrobial agents active against the responsible organisms. While the infecting flora varies, it commonly comprises bowel organisms, a complex mixture of aerobic and anaerobic bacteria, including *Bacteroides fragilis.* An appropriate initial therapeutic choice is a combination of an aminoglycoside, such as gentamicin, and an antianaerobic agent such as clindamycin, chloramphenicol, or metronidazole. Cefoxitin, cefotetan, or cefotaxime are effective alternatives, but an aminoglycoside should be added if the infection is hospital-acquired or the patient has received previous antimicrobial therapy.

Antimicrobial therapy alone is often sufficient for some abscesses—appendiceal, renal, and some hepatic—but cure usually also requires drainage of pus, either by surgery or percutaneous catheters, inserted with ultrasonic or CT guidance. Criteria for percutaneous drainage include (1) pus thin enough to be evacuated through the catheter; (2) few abscess cavities or loculations; (3) a drainage route that does not traverse bowel, uncontaminated organs, or sterile pleural or peritoneal spaces. The absence of a safe drainage route prevents catheter drainage in most pelvic and interloop abscesses, and this technique is not very successful in pancreatic abscesses because of its inability to remove thick necrotic debris. When used appropriately, however, its success rate is about 70 percent, with the catheters typically remaining in place for about 10 to 20 days.

INTRAPERITIONEAL ABSCESS These infections usually arise from a generalized peritonitis caused by perforated abdominal viscera, penetrating trauma, or postoperative infections. Some derive from localized peritonitis when infection extends from a contiguous site. With generalized peritonitis, the effects of gravity, intraabdominal pressure, and respiratory movements favor localization to the subphrenic spaces, the pelvis, and paracolic gutters lateral to the ascending and descending colon.

Subphrenic abscess These abscesses occur in the subphrenic space, arbitrarily defined as lying between the diaphragm and the transverse colon and possessing four subdivisions. The *suprahepatic* and *subhepatic* spaces are located on the right side; on the left there is a single *subphrenic* space plus the *lesser sac,* a space posterior to the stomach and anterior to the pancreas. About 55 percent of subphrenic abscesses are right-sided, 25 percent left-sided, and 20 percent multiple. Over 90 percent are complications of abdominal surgery, especially on the biliary tract, stomach, and duodenum. The contamination causing infection can occur during surgery or afterward, especially from anastomotic leaks. Symptoms typically begin 3 to 6 weeks after surgery, but occasionally develop only months later. Fever, nearly universal, is often mild, rather than dramatic. Abdominal pain is usual, but localized tenderness less common, and a palpable mass rare. By causing diaphragmatic irritation, inflammation that spreads to the pleural cavity, and abdominal distention, subphrenic abscesses often produce thoracic symptoms such as cough, dyspnea, and chest pain. Shoulder discomfort, referred pain from an irritated diaphragm, and hiccups sometimes occur. On chest examination there may be dullness to percussion, diminished breath sounds, basilar crackles, and rarely, a pleural friction rub. Chest roentgenograms, usually abnormal, may demonstrate ipsilateral atelectasis, pleural effusion, elevated hemidiaphragm, and basilar pneumonia.

Midabdominal abscess These abscesses include those in the right and left lower quadrants and between loops of bowel (interloop abscesses). *Right lower quadrant abscesses* usually arise as a complication of acute appendicitis, but occasionally from colonic diverticulitis, Crohn's disease, or upper alimentary tract perforations that drain down into the right paracolic gutter. Most commonly, fever, right lower quadrant pain, and a palpable mass occur following symptoms suggesting acute appendicitis. Occasionally, the abscess causes partial or complete small bowel obstruction. Appendiceal abscesses are usually treatable with antibiotics alone. *Left lower quadrant abscesses* complicate left colonic perforations, usually from diverticulitis, carcinoma, or Crohn's disease, and cause fever, left lower quadrant pain, and a palpable mass. *Interloop abscesses* are collections of pus between the folded surfaces of the small and large intestines and their mesenteries, generally arising from anastomotic disruptions, bowel perforations, or Crohn's disease. The clinical features, which are often very subtle, include mild fever, with or without vague abdominal discomfort. Abdominal tenderness, mechanical bowel obstruction, or a palpable mass occasionally occurs. Plain abdominal roentgenograms may show bowel wall edema, separation of bowel loops, localized ileus, and air-fluid levels on upright films.

Pelvic abscess These are complications of acute appendicitis, colonic diverticulitis, or acute salpingitis. The major symptoms are fever and lower abdominal discomfort. Those adjacent to the colon may cause diarrhea; those next to the bladder may cause urinary frequency and urgency. On abdominal examination tenderness is common, but peritoneal signs, guarding, or a palpable mass are unusual. Rectal or vaginal examination may reveal a mass anterior to the rectum or in the cul-de-sac. Pelvic abscesses usually require surgical drainage, but those arising from acute salpingitis typically resolve with antibiotic therapy alone.

RETROPERITONEAL ABSCESS The retroperitoneum is the space between the posterior peritoneum and the transversalis fascia lining the posterior portion of the abdominal cavity. The *anterior retroperitoneal* space, lying between the posterior peritoneum and the anterior renal fascia, contains the extraperitoneal portion of the alimentary tract: the ascending and descending colon, the duodenal loop, and the pancreas. Abscesses in this space usually develop from pancreatitis or perforations in these extraperitoneal parts of the intestines. The major clinical features are fever, abdominal or flank pain and tenderness, and a palpable mass.

The *perinephric* space, situated between the anterior and posterior layers of the renal (Gerota's) fascia on each side of the body, contains the kidney, adrenal, and ureter. Perinephric abscesses usually occur from rupture of a renal parenchymal abscess through the renal capsule. Such an abscess may be staphylococcal following hematogenous dissemination from another site, usually the skin, but more commonly it arises from pyelonephritis, often associated with urinary tract obstruction by stones, malignancies, or other causes. Perinephric abscesses may also follow urologic surgery or, occasionally, suppuration may extend from contiguous infections of the intestinal tract, liver, gallbladder, or bone. The causative organisms, therefore, are usually aerobic gram-negative bacilli or staphylococci; a minority are polymicrobial. The major symptoms are fever, chills, and unilateral flank pain. Dysuria is frequent, and most patients have unilateral flank or abdominal tenderness, often with a palpable mass. Leukocytosis is typical; pyuria, and a positive urine culture occur in about 60 percent. Blood cultures are positive in 20 to 40 percent of patients. Perinephric abscess usually differs clinically from uncomplicated acute pyelonephritis by the longer duration of symptoms before hospitalization (usually more then 5 days) and the failure of patients to become afebrile within 5 days after receiving antimicrobial therapy. Chest roentgenograms often show ipsilateral pneumonia, atelectasis, pleural effusion, or elevated hemidiaphragm. Suggestive findings on excretory urogram occur in about 60 percent of cases and include a nonvisualizing or poorly visualizing kidney, distorted calyces, anterior renal displacement, and unilateral fixation of the kidney, best demonstrated by fluoroscopy or inspiration-expiration films. Ultrasound usually demonstrates the abscess, but is less reliable than CT, which is almost always positive. Treatment includes appropriate systemic antibiotics, drainage of pus by percutaneous catheters or surgery, and relief of any urinary obstruction; occasionally, nephrectomy is necessary.

VISCERAL ABSCESS Hepatic abscess These abscesses are usually amebic (see Chap. 158) or bacterial (pyogenic). Bacterial liver abscesses usually develop by one of five mechanisms: (1) portal vein bacteremia arising from an infected intraabdominal site, such as appendicitis, diverticulitis, or perforated bowel; (2) systemic bacteremia originating from a distant site, causing bacteria to reach the liver via the hepatic artery; (3) ascending cholangitis in a biliary tract completely or partially obstructed by stone, malignancy, or stricture; (4) direct extension from a contiguous focus of infection outside the biliary tract, such as a subphrenic abscess; or (5) trauma, either penetrating, with direct introduction of organisms into the liver, or blunt, causing a hematoma that becomes secondarily infected. In most cases the cause is apparent, but in some the pathogenesis of the abscess is unexplained ("cryptogenic"). Most abscesses are single; multiple abscesses are typically microscopic and are associated with systemic bacteremia or complete biliary tract obstruction. In these cases, the onset is acute, and the clinical features of the predisposing disease usually predominate.

Most other cases of hepatic abscess have a subacute onset, and an illness lasting several weeks is the rule. Fever is nearly always present and is accompanied by such nonspecific symptoms as chills, nausea, vomiting, anorexia, weight loss, and weakness. Right upper quadrant abdominal pain or tenderness is present in about one-half of patients, as is hepatomegaly. Some complain of right pleuritic chest pain. Jaundice is usually evident only when there is biliary tract obstruction.

Laboratory findings in most patients include one or more of the following: anemia, leukocytosis, increased erythrocyte sedimentation rate, increased alkaline phosphatase, decreased serum albumin, and usually mildly increased serum bilirubin. The chest roentgenogram is abnormal in about one-half of patients, showing right-sided basilar atelectasis, pneumonia, pleural effusion, or an elevated hemidiaphragm.

Ultrasound scans are usually positive and can distinguish fluid-filled from solid masses, helping to discriminate between infectious and neoplastic lesions. CT scan is the most accurate method of demonstrating multiple abscesses.

The bacteriology of liver abscesses depends upon the cause. With systemic bacteremia staphylococci or streptococci are common. Abscesses originating from an intraabdominal infection, however, usually contain aerobic gram-negative rods, especially *Escherichia coli* and *Klebsiella-Enterobacter;* anaerobic bacteria, especially anaerobic gram-positive cocci, *F. nucleatum,* and *B. fragilis;* or a mixture of aerobes and anaerobes. Blood cultures are positive in about half of patients but may not grow all the organisms present in the abscess.

Although some patients respond to antibiotic therapy alone, most also require evacuation of pus. Percutaneous catheter drainage, if technically feasible, is generally preferable to surgery, provided that no other indication for laparotomy exists. When the bacteriology is unknown, chloramphenicol or a combination of clindamycin and an aminoglycoside should be effective. Antibiotics are usually continued for several weeks following drainage.

In correctly diagnosed and treated patients, the mortality rate is about 20 to 40 percent and is higher in those with multiple rather than single abscesses.

In patients with clinical and roentgenographic findings suggesting a liver abscess who may have had previous exposure to *Entamoeba histolytica*, it is important to distinguish between a bacterial and an amebic etiology, since the latter rarely requires drainage. Features suggesting an amebic abscess are age under 50; single rather than multiple lesions; an acute presentation (<2 weeks of symptoms); male sex; the presence of *E. histolytica* in the stool; and the absence of a condition predisposing to bacterial liver abscess. The most helpful differential point is that nearly all patients with amebic liver abscesses have a positive serology for *E. histolytica.*

Splenic abscess Most splenic abscesses are multiple, small, and clinically silent lesions found incidentally at autopsy and occurring as a terminal manifestation of uncontrolled infection elsewhere. Clinically important splenic abscesses are generally solitary and arise from (1) systemic bacteremia originating in another site, such as endocarditis or salmonellosis; (2) infection, probably by the hematogenous route, of a spleen damaged by bland infarction (as occurs in hemoglobinopathies, especially sickle cell trait or sickle cell disease), trauma, penetrating or blunt (with superinfection of a subcapsular hematoma), or other diseases (malaria, hydatid cysts); or (3) extension from a contiguous focus of infection, such as a subphrenic abscess. The most common organisms are staphylococci, streptococci, anaerobes, and aerobic gram-negative rods, including *Salmonella*. In neutropenic hosts fungi, predominantly *Candida* species, may cause splenic abscesses.

The onset is typically subacute, and the major features are fever and leukocytosis. Left-sided pain, often pleuritic, may occur in the upper abdomen, lower chest, or flank, sometimes radiating to the left shoulder. Left upper quadrant abdominal tenderness and splenomegaly are common, but an audible splenic friction rub is rare.

Radiographic findings may include (1) a left upper quadrant soft tissue abdominal mass, (2) extraintestinal gas from gas-forming organisms in the abscess, (3) displacement of other organs, including the colon, kidney, and stomach, (4) elevation of the left hemidiaphragm, and (5) left pleural effusion. An ultrasound scan may be positive for macroscopic splenic abscesses, but CT scan is the most reliable diagnostic test.

Treatment consists of appropriate systemic antibiotics and removal of pus by percutaneous catheter, splenotomy, or splenectomy. Splenic abscesses should be considered a possible, although rare, cause of continued bacteremia in acute endocarditis despite appropriate chemotherapy, and splenectomy may be necessary to achieve final eradication of the infection. Successful treatment of fungal splenic abscesses in immunodeficient patients has usually included splenectomy and prolonged administration of amphotericin B, but some patients have been cured with antifungal drugs alone.

Pancreatic abscess These abscesses usually occur in a site of pancreatic necrosis following acute pancreatitis. Typically, the patient improves after the attack of pancreatitis, but about 10 to 21 days later fever, abdominal pain and tenderness, nausea, vomiting, and sometimes persistent ileus occur. Less commonly, the abscess develops shortly after the attack begins. In those cases, persistent fever, leukocytosis, and abdominal findings beyond 7 to 10 days should suggest an abscess. A mass is sometimes palpable. The serum amylase is irregularly elevated, but leukocytosis is usually present. The serum alkaline phosphatase may be increased and the albumin decreased.

Chest roentgenograms often show a left pleural effusion, basilar atelectasis or pneumonia, or a raised hemidiaphragm. Ultrasound is very useful in revealing fluid-filled pancreatic masses but may be unable to distinguish infected from uninfected fluid. CT is the most accurate test for abscesses and may show pancreatic gas, peripancreatic fluid collections, or masses, but only pancreatic gas is diagnostic of infection.

Treatment is appropriate antibiotic therapy and drainage of pus by percutaneous catheters or surgery. Catheter drainage often fails because of inability to remove thick, necrotic debris. Since the usual organisms are coliforms, staphylococci, streptococci, and anaerobes in varying combinations, clindamycin and an aminoglycoside are a reasonable choice until culture results return. Even with appropriate treatment the mortality rate is about 20 to 40 percent, and recurrent abscesses requiring multiple drainage procedures are common.

Renal abscess Single or multiple abscesses of the renal *cortex* may be the result of metastatic implantation of staphylococci from another focus. There is no relationship to previous renal disease; the infection occurs in younger individuals, is usually unilateral, and occurs on the right side oftener than on the left. Many patients give a history of recent skin infection such as furuncle. Medullary abscesses usually develop from acute pyelonephritis when foci of cellular infiltrates in the interstitium coalesce to form single or multiple distinct cavities.

The onset of renal abscess is abrupt, with chills and fever, followed by costovertebral pain and tenderness. If the abscess is cortical, the urine contains *no white blood cells;* medullary abscesses are usually accompanied by pyuria. The stained urinary sediment may show myriads of gram-positive cocci in cortical abscesses and gram-negative organisms in medullary abscesses. Transient gross or microscopic hematuria may occur at the onset. The white blood cell count is usually elevated and may exceed 30,000 cells per cubic millimeter. Physical signs are usually localized to the region of the kidney, but abdominal spasm may lead to confusion with appendicitis, cholecystitis, or pancreatitis. Early in the disease, ureteral calculus or acute hydronephrosis may be considered as possible diagnoses. Sudden onset of *fever, leukocytosis, and renal pain in the absence of pyuria* should suggest the diagnosis of a renal cortical abscess, especially in a patient with infection elsewhere. Obstruction of the ureter by pus or cellular debris may also yield a urine sediment sparse in white blood cells and bacteria. Excretory urograms typically reveal an intrarenal mass, and ultrasound and CT scans usually demonstrate the abscess as a fluid-filled defect. *Treatment* consists of appropriate antibiotics, adequate fluids, and relief of pain. An abscess may suddenly discharge into the renal pelvis, with relief of pain and the passage of cloudy urine containing enormous numbers of leukocytes and bacteria. Recovery is ordinarily prompt, and chronic sequelae are rare. Failure to achieve prompt defervescence following treatment suggests an incorrect diagnosis or the necessity of drainage, by needle aspiration, percutaneous catheter, or surgery.

MISCELLANEOUS ABSCESSES

RETROFASCIAL ABSCESS The retrofascial space, lying between the transversalis and psoas fascias, contains the psoas and quadratus lumborum muscles. Abscesses in this area usually derive from infections in the vertebrae, ilium, and sacroiliac joints. Less frequently, they represent extensions from abscesses in the anterior retroperitoneal space. Sometimes no adjacent source of infection is apparent; these "primary" infections are usually staphylococcal and almost surely have a hematogenous origin. The symptoms of retrofascial abscesses are abdominal pain in the iliac or inguinal region and, particularly with psoas muscle involvement, hip pain and posterior thigh pain and paresthesias. Careful palpation of the lower abdomen or groin often reveals a mass, and rectal or vaginal examination may disclose fullness and tenderness. Pain on hip motion is common, the hip is flexed, and extension or internal rotation of the hip is very painful. Plain abdominal films may demonstrate a mass or loss of the psoas shadow; excretory urograms may show displacement of the kidney or ureter and scoliosis with concavity on the side of infection. Ultrasound usually reveals a soft tissue mass, but CT and MRI scans typically provide more precise information, including evaluation of the adjacent bones. Appropriate antimicrobial therapy alone may sometimes be curative, but drainage by percutaneous catheter or open surgery is often necessary.

PROSTATIC ABSCESS These abscesses, typically occurring in middle age, are complications of acute prostatitis, cystitis, urethritis, or epididymitis. Most patients are *afebrile* and have urinary frequency, retention, or dysuria. Less common features are hematuria, perineal pain, and a purulent urethral discharge. Some patients have persistent or recurrent urinary infections despite apparently adequate antimicrobial therapy. Rectal examination may reveal prostatic tenderness or fluctuance, but sometimes there is only prostatic enlargement or even no abnormality at all. Pyuria and positive urine cultures are usual, but not invariably so. Many of these abscesses are unexpected discoveries at prostatic surgery or endoscopy performed for apparent benign prostatic hypertrophy. Treatment is appropriate antibiotics and surgical drainage by transurethral or perineal incision. The usual pathogens are aerobic gram-negative rods and, less frequently, *S. aureus*.

RECTAL ABSCESS Most of these infections are superficial and involve the perirectal region, and many are associated with fistulas. Infection in the apocrine glands (hidradenitis) or folliculitis in the perianal region, extension of cryptitis or obstructions in the "anal glands'' which open into the crypts of Morgagni, and contamination of submucosal hematomas, sclerosed hemorrhoids, or anal fissures may lead to abscess formation. In most patients, the cause of infection is not apparent. These are usually painful, easily palpable, often visible on inspection. Treatment is incision and drainage, even when no fluctuance is present or the patient is neutropenic. Antibiotics are rarely necessary unless there is extensive perineal cellulitis.

Difficulties in diagnosis are likely to arise with infections higher in the rectum. Most are in the ischiorectal area, but those above the pelvic diaphragm, the so-called supralevator abscess, are particularly elusive. Patients with this type of infection often have fever, malaise, and leukocytosis for several days or even weeks before any symptoms referable to the rectum develop. There is vague pelvic discomfort, relieved by defecation, and constipation punctuated by short episodes of diarrhea is common. In males, the inflammation often involves the base of the bladder, and urinary urgency or retention may occur, falsely centering attention on the urinary tract as the source of fever and malaise. Eventually, the abscess produces severe pain, chills, and fever; palpation and instrumentation will reveal the swelling in the rectal ampulla. Such an abscess may surround the rectum and produce narrowing that is differentiated from neoplasm by the fact that the mucosa remains intact. A useful sign of deep rectal abscess is severe pain with pressure in the region between the anus and the coccyx. The supralevator space is continuous with the ischiorectal space, with both the gluteal and obturator regions, and with the retroperitoneal space. In neglected cases, the abscess may drain through the skin of the perineum, the groin, or the buttock or may extend as high as the perirenal areas. Rectal abscesses often occur in patients with preexisting anorectal disease, diabetes, alcoholism, and neurologic disease; infections in this area are also peculiarly frequent in patients with acute leukemia, especially when neutropenia is present. Because the clinical picture may be that of ''fever of unknown origin'' for a long period, it is important that thorough digital and endoscopic examination of the rectum be carried out in patients with unexplained fever. Identification and localization of the abscess are best achieved by CT or MRI scan. Patients with diabetic ketoacidosis should receive a careful rectal examination because a rectal abscess may be the infection responsible for precipitating the ketoacidosis.

A rectal abscess may be a forerunner of both ulcerative colitis and regional enteritis, and may occur months and even years before other overt manifestations of these diseases. For this reason, proctosigmoidoscopy, colonoscopy, barium enema, and, often, upper gastrointestinal roentgenograms are indicated in nonhealing or recurrent rectal lesions.

Treatment of high rectal abscesses consists of incision and drainage, analgesics, and antibiotics directed at *E. coli*, *Klebsiella-Enterobacter*, *Bacteroides*, and a variety of streptococci, which constitute the polymicrobial flora of these lesions.

REFERENCES

BARNES PF et al: A comparison of amebic and pyogenic abscess of the liver. Medicine 66:472, 1987

BLOMQUIST IK et al: Life-threatening deep fascial space infections of the head and neck. Infect Dis Clin North Am 2:237, 1988

EDELSTEIN H et al: Perinephric abscess. Modern diagnosis and treatment in 47 cases. Medicine 67:118, 1988

GOLIGHER JC: *Surgery of the Anus, Rectum, and Colon*, 5th ed. New York, Macmillan, 1984

GYORFFY EJ et al: Pyogenic liver abscess. Diagnostic and therapeutic strategies. Ann Surg 206:699, 1987

LINSCHEID RL et al: Common and uncommon infections of the hand. Orthop Clin North Am 6:1063, 1975

NELKEN N et al: Changing clinical spectrum of splenic abscess. A multicenter study and review of the literature. Am J Surg 154:27, 1987

PRUETT TL et al: Status of percutaneous catheter drainage of abscesses. Surg Clin North Am 68:89, 1988

STEINER E et al: Complicated pancreatic abscesses: Problems in interventional management. Radiology 167:443, 1988

92 ACUTE INFECTIOUS DIARRHEAL DISEASES AND BACTERIAL FOOD POISONING

CHARLES C. J. CARPENTER

Acute diarrheal illnesses caused by bacterial, viral, or protozoal pathogens vary from slightly annoying bowel dysfunction to fulminant, life-threatening diseases. Largely because of the recognition of enterotoxigenic *Escherichia coli* as a major cause of acute diarrheal disease in adults and the identification of rotavirus as a frequent cause in young children, specific etiologic agents have been isolated from 80 to 85 percent of patients with acute diarrheal illnesses. Those illnesses caused by bacterial pathogens are more often life-threatening, at least among adults, and for that reason they will be addressed first. This chapter is aimed at presenting an overview of these diseases; in most instances, the entities are discussed in more detail in the chapters dealing with the specific etiologic agent.

In considering the bacterial diarrheas, it is useful to divide them into two groups, those caused by invasive and those caused by noninvasive microorganisms. The invasive pathogens, of which *Shigella* (see Chap. 114) may be considered the prototype, generally cause abdominal pain, fever, and other systemic symptoms, often including headache and myalgia. Illness caused by the noninvasive pathogens, of which cholera (see Chap. 122) is the prototype, is generally characterized by the absence of fever and few systemic symptoms (except those directly related to intestinal fluid loss). The invasive pathogens characteristically destroy gut mucosal cells, typically involving the terminal ileum and colon, and both leukocytes and erythrocytes are present, to a variable degree, in the stool. Inflammatory cells are generally absent from the stool in acute diarrheal disease caused by noninvasive bacterial pathogens.

NONINVASIVE BACTERIAL PATHOGENS

ENTEROTOXIGENIC *ESCHERICHIA COLI* **Etiology and epidemiology** Enterotoxin-producing *E. coli* (ETEC), which have the dual capacity to adhere to small-bowel epithelial cells and to produce one or more diarrheagenic toxins, are recognized as a major cause of acute diarrheal disease throughout most of the world and are the most common cause of ''traveler's diarrhea.'' Largely because current techniques for demonstrating toxigenicity remain cumbersome, the epidemiology of ETEC diarrhea is poorly understood. ETEC are responsible for the majority of cases of traveler's diarrhea in visitors to the developing nations in South America, Africa, and Asia. ETEC are also one of the two (with rotavirus) leading causes of acute diarrheal illnesses in children throughout the developing world. ETEC have been implicated as a major cause of fulminant, cholera-like diarrheal disease in adult patients in south and southeast Asia but generally cause milder, self-limited diarrhea in adults in other parts of the developing world. There is no satisfactory explanation for the difference in severity in diarrhea caused by ETEC in different geographic areas. ETEC are occasionally incriminated in episodic diarrheal illness in children and adults in the United States.

Pathogenesis The ability to cause diarrheal disease is not restricted to any one *E. coli* serotype but appears to be dependent upon the presence of both a plasmid-mediated colonization factor, which allows the *E. coli* to adhere to small-bowel mucosal cells, and one or more plasmids which code for the production of one or both of the two distinct classes of diarrheagenic toxins that may be produced by *E. coli*. The kinetics and mode of action of one class, which is heat labile (LT) and of relatively high molecular mass (~83,000 daltons), are similar to those of cholera enterotoxin (see Chap. 122); the diarrheagenic effect results from stimulation of adenylate cyclase in the gut epithelial cells. The other class, which is heat stable (ST) and of a lower molecular mass (<2000 daltons), has a more rapid onset of action and probably exerts its effect through stimulation of guanylate cyclase in the gut mucosal cells. Either or both classes of toxins may be produced by ETEC. Most isolates from patients with severe diarrheal disease in Bangladesh produce both LT and ST, whereas isolates from patients in other developing nations have shown widely varying capacities for the production of LT, ST, or both. The wide clinical spectrum may be, in part, related to the predominant production of either LT or ST by the culpable microorganisms. The nutritional status of the host may also be a factor in determining the clinical response to ETEC.

Manifestations Both clinical observations and volunteer studies indicate that the incubation period is generally between 24 and 72 h. The illness which follows is quite variable, ranging from the fulminant, cholera-like disease often seen on the Indian subcontinent to the much milder Mexican "turista," in which the symptoms of mild, watery diarrhea, abdominal cramps, and occasional low-grade fever are more troublesome than life-threatening. Vomiting occurs in fewer than half the adults with *E. coli* diarrhea and is seldom responsible for major fluid losses.

In fulminant cases, the severe diarrhea seldom lasts longer than 24 to 36 h, and the response to either oral or intravenous electrolyte repletion is predictable and dramatic. With milder disease, the symptoms may subside more gradually, occasionally persisting for a week or longer.

Laboratory findings As with cholera, no erythrocytes and few, if any, polymorphonuclear leukocytes are seen in a stool preparation stained with Loeffler's methylene blue. Because *E. coli* occurs normally among stool flora and its ability to produce enterotoxin is not restricted to any specific serotype, there is no rapid and simple means to make the laboratory diagnosis of enterotoxigenic *E. coli.* Bioassays for LT, based on the ability of *E. coli* isolates to produce fluid in isolated intestinal loops of experimental animals or to stimulate adenylate cyclase in cells in tissue culture, as well as the suckling mouse bioassay for ST, are reliable but of little value in patient management. Newer technology, utilizing DNA probes for rapid identification of the genes responsible for ST and LT production, appears promising and may be adapted for widespread use for epidemiologic purposes in the future.

Treatment The intestinal fluid losses are qualitatively identical to those in cholera. Therefore, in those patients who develop clinically significant saline depletion, the principles of fluid administration are identical to those described for cholera (see Chap. 122). Oral solutions containing electrolytes plus glucose or sucrose are consistently effective in correcting the saline depletion. Antibiotics (tetracycline, 30 mg/kg per day, given orally at 6-h intervals for 48 h; trimethoprim, 200 mg twice daily for 5 days; or trimethoprim, 160 mg, with sulfamethoxazole, 800 mg, twice daily for 5 days) are effective in decreasing the duration of illness but are not essential. One of the quinolone drugs (norfloxacin or ciprofloxacin) is also effective (see Chap. 85). Bismuth subsalicylate, 60 mL hourly for four doses, provides symptomatic relief (less frequent stools, less severe abdominal cramps). Both diphenoxylate and loperamide may provide rapid relief of abdominal cramps, but neither drug has been shown to alter the volume of intestinal fluid loss.

Prognosis Even in the more fulminant cases of disease caused by ETEC, with adequate peroral or intravenous fluid replacement, the prognosis is excellent.

Prevention Careful hygienic practices, with special attention to ingestion of clean water (boiled for 2 min if its source is uncertain) and adequately cooked foods, provide the most certain protection against enterotoxigenic *E. coli.* Doxycycline, 100 mg/d, is 60 to 90 percent effective as a prophylactic agent, the effectiveness varying with the tetracycline sensitivity of the ETEC in the geographic area. Trimethoprim, 160 mg, with sulfamethoxazole, 800 mg, taken once daily, is also effective in prophylaxis against traveler's diarrhea caused by ETEC.

NONTOXIGENIC ENTEROPATHOGENIC *E. COLI* The classically recognized enteropathogenic *E. coli* (EPEC) strains neither invade gut mucosa nor produce an identifiable toxin, yet produce occasional outbreaks of acute, sometimes severe, diarrheal disease in infants and are associated with sporadic cases of mild diarrhea in adults, in both industrialized and developing countries. Most such EPEC strains demonstrate plasmid-encoded adherence to small-gut mucosal cells, which is associated with dissolution of the glycocalyx and effacement of the microvilli. The exact mechanism by which diarrhea is produced is not known. Infants may require oral, or occasionally intravenous, fluid repletion therapy. Since the illness is self-limited, antimicrobial agents are of no demonstrable benefit.

CHOLERA See Chap. 122.

OTHER ENTEROTOXIGENIC ENTEROBACTERIACEAE Noninvasive strains of *Klebsiella* and *Enterobacter* occasionally have been implicated in acute diarrheal disease in developing areas of the world. The clinical illness produced is indistinguishable from the milder cases of diarrhea caused by enterotoxigenic *E. coli,* and treatment is the same.

CLOSTRIDIUM PERFRINGENS (See Chap. 107) This organism remains a significant cause of diarrheal disease and is implicated in many cases of acute food poisoning in the United States. Both the epidemiologic background and the clinical picture of *C. perfringens* diarrhea differ strikingly from those of *E. coli. Clostridium perfringens* diarrhea tends to occur in a microepidemic pattern following ingestion of contaminated meat, poultry products, or legumes. The relatively short incubation period of 6 to 12 h is an important diagnostic clue. Typically, two or more patients who have ingested the same meat dish become ill at roughly the same time. The production of a specific enterotoxin by the actively sporulating microorganisms in the intestinal tract appears to be responsible for all the symptoms. The clinical picture of diarrhea caused by *C. perfringens* is different from that caused by enterotoxigenic *E. coli* in one important respect, because moderately severe cramping abdominal pain, which is usually less prominent with *E. coli,* is a major presenting symptom. Treatment consists of symptomatic therapy to alleviate the cramping abdominal pain and intravenous fluid therapy in the small proportion of patients in whom there is clinical evidence of saline depletion. The illness is self-limited and rarely lasts for more than 24 h. Because of the relatively short natural course of the illness, antimicrobial therapy is of no value. Because *C. perfringens* normally inhabits mammalian and avian intestinal tracts, prevention is dependent upon adequate cooking and handling of meat and poultry products. The practice of allowing cooked meat products to cool slowly toward room temperature over 12 to 24 h permits germination of contaminating clostridial spores and this practice must be avoided.

STAPHYLOCOCCUS AUREUS (See Chap. 100) Acute staphylococcal diarrhea, classic "food poisoning," is due entirely to ingestion of preformed enterotoxin, and the causative organisms are often absent from the stool during the acute illness. This form of diarrhea often occurs in institutional outbreaks and is characterized by a short incubation period (2 to 6 h), relatively short duration (usually less than 10 h), and very high attack rates (often greater than 75 percent of the population at risk). In addition to its distinctive epidemiologic features, acute staphylococcal diarrhea differs from other noninvasive bacterial diarrheas by the prominence of vomiting, which is an almost constant feature and is apparently mediated by a direct effect of the absorbed toxin on the central nervous system. Treatment is directed toward correction of the saline depletion (intravenous fluids are required in 10 to 20 percent of patients) and, when necessary, toward symptomatic relief of vomiting. Because staphylococcal food poisoning is caused by preformed enterotoxin and is not perpetuated by viable microorganisms, antimicrobials are of no value.

A good example of the explosive nature of staphylococcal food poisoning was provided by an outbreak on a jet liner flying from Anchorage to Copenhagen. In this episode, 57 percent of 343 passengers developed an acute illness characterized by vomiting, diarrhea, and cramping abdominal pain. Of the 200 affected individuals, 30 required intravenous fluids, but none had serious sequelae. The food, contaminated by a pustule on the hand of a food handler, had not been adequately refrigerated aboard the plane, allowing abundant growth of the staphylococcus, with production of enterotoxin. Since staphylococci are ubiquitous, the prevention of massive contamination is dependent largely on control of growth conditions, primarily temperature. *Staphylococcus aureus* can multiply at temperatures from 4 to 46°C, and if contaminated food is allowed to remain at ambient temperatures after cooking, these organisms have ample opportunity to multiply, especially in such items as cream pastries, potato salad, and mayonnaise.

BACILLUS CEREUS *Bacillus cereus* is a cause of acute diarrheal disease which, although uncommon, has been identified with increasing frequency in Europe. The illness results from gross contamination of food with this gram-positive rod, which is capable of producing at least two discrete enterotoxins, one having characteristics similar to those of the labile enterotoxin of *E. coli* and the other having effects similar to that of staphylococcal enterotoxin. *Bacillus cereus* may, therefore, cause two distinct clinical syndromes, a diarrheal form resulting from the *E. coli* LT type of enterotoxin and an emetic form caused by the staphylococcal type of enterotoxin. The diarrheal syndrome caused by *B. cereus* is generally similar to that caused by enterotoxin-producing *E. coli,* with the exceptions that abdominal cramps are more common (75 percent of cases) and both the incubation period (6 to 14 h) and median duration of illness (20 h) are shorter. The emetic syndrome is clinically indistinguishable from that caused by staphylococcal enterotoxin, with a short incubation period (median 2 h), short duration (median 9 h), and prominent vomiting (100 percent compared with less than 25 percent in the diarrheal syndrome). Because both syndromes are self-limited and generally mild, no specific therapy is indicated. When *B. cereus* food poisoning is suspected clinically, the diagnosis can be confirmed by demonstration of 10^5 or more *B. cereus* organisms per gram in epidemiologically incriminated food. *Bacillus cereus* grows readily on simple laboratory media, including blood agar, but will not generally be identified as a pathogen unless such identification is specifically requested. Isolation of *B. cereus* from stool alone does not establish it as the etiologic agent because the organism is frequently found in the fecal flora of normal individuals. Since *B. cereus* is ubiquitous in soil, as well as in many raw, dried, and processed foods, proper food handling is the only practical means of preventing this form of food poisoning. The emetic form of *B. cereus* food poisoning almost invariably has been associated with ingestion of contaminated fried rice. *Bacillus cereus* is commonly present in uncooked rice, and its spores survive boiling and germinate, with production of the enterotoxin, when boiled rice is left unrefrigerated. Brief rewarming before serving is not adequate to destroy the relatively heat-stable toxin. Prompt refrigeration of boiled rice will prevent this disease.

INVASIVE AND/OR DESTRUCTIVE ENTERIC PATHOGENS

INTRODUCTION Shigellae characteristically invade the colon and terminal ileum, destroy segments of intestinal mucosa, cause extensive inflammatory changes in the lamina propria, and are the prototype of the invasive and/or destructive enteric bacterial pathogens. Other important invasive bacterial enteric pathogens include *Salmonella, Yersinia enterocolitica, Campylobacter jejuni, Vibrio parahemolyticus,* and enteroinvasive *E. coli* (EIEC). As opposed to the noninvasive pathogens, the invasive enteric organisms frequently cause systemic symptoms, including headache, myalgias, chills, and fever. As a general rule, antiperistaltic agents such as opiates, diphenoxylate, loperamide, and atropine are contraindicated in diarrheal disease caused by invasive enteric pathogens because they clearly worsen the clinical course in shigellosis.

The major therapeutic challenge in invasive bacterial diarrheas is that of distinguishing between (1) shigellosis and yersiniosis, in which antimicrobial therapy decreases the duration and severity of illness and shortens the period of fecal shedding of the pathogen, and (2) infections caused by *Salmonella* in which antimicrobial therapy does not alter the duration of illness and may cause prolonged excretion of the pathogen.

SHIGELLOSIS See Chap. 114.

SALMONELLOSIS See Chap. 113.

YERSINIA ENTEROCOLITICA See Chap. 121.

CAMPYLOBACTER JEJUNI **Etiology and epidemiology** *Campylobacter jejuni* is second only to *Giardia lamblia* among recognized causes of waterborne diarrheal disease outbreaks in the United States. Attack rates have been highest in adolescents and young adults. *C. jejuni* occurs in the intestinal flora of many wild and domestic animals and poultry and can be transmitted to humans by milk and water polluted by such animal carriers. The distribution of *C. jejuni* is worldwide, and *C. jejuni* appears to cause from 5 to 10 percent of acute diarrheal illnesses in adults in both the industrialized and the developing areas of the world. Ingestion of raw milk and of water from contaminated mountain streams has been implicated in *Campylobacter* enteritis in North America; in outbreaks associated with ingestion of raw milk, attack rates have reached 60 percent.

Pathogenesis *C. jejuni* causes patchy destruction of mucosa of both the small intestine, especially the distal ileum, and the colon; the stools, therefore, regularly contain pus cells and occasionally are grossly bloody. *C. jejuni* rarely produces transient bacteremia; when it does, it is likely to occur in an immunocompromised host.

Manifestations An incubation period of 2 to 6 days, longer than that of most bacterial enteric pathogens, is followed by fever, cramping abdominal pain, and diarrhea that is initially watery but later contains blood and mucus. The diarrhea, generally mild but occasionally voluminous, usually ceases within 2 to 5 days without specific antimicrobial therapy; on rare occasions the diarrhea may persist for 3 to 4 weeks. In some cases, the abdominal pain may be more prominent than the diarrhea, and the clinical picture may simulate acute appendicitis or, rarely, pancreatitis. (This may also be true in *Yersinia* enterocolitis; see Chap. 121.) In such cases, laparotomy has revealed acutely inflamed mesenteric lymph nodes as well as patchy inflammation of the small bowel. Acute reactive arthritis, similar to that associated with other invasive bacterial diarrheas (*Shigella, Salmonella, Yersinia*) may follow *C. jejuni* enteritis and is often associated wtih the HLA-B27 antigen.

Laboratory findings Diagnosis depends upon isolating *C. jejuni* from stool. Since this curved, motile bacillus does not compete well with other enteric flora on standard enteric media, it will rarely be isolated from stool unless special techniques are utilized. These include incubation at 42°C in a microaerobic atmosphere on blood agar to which a number of antimicrobials have been added. Serologic diagnosis is rarely helpful, as there are many serotypes of *C. jejuni,* and agglutination tests require use of the homologous organism.

Treatment Since *C. jejuni* usually produces a short, self-limited illness, antimicrobial therapy is not essential to management. Erythromycin, 30 mg/kg per day, does, however, significantly decrease the duration of fecal shedding of *C. jejuni* and may shorten the mean duration of illness. In the occasional patient who develops clinical signs of saline depletion, oral and/or intravenous fluids of the same sort used in cholera are uniformly effective (see Chap. 122).

OTHER *CAMPYLOBACTER* INFECTIONS The observation of small, curved, gram-negative rods with characteristic corkscrew-like motility in many stool specimens from which *C. jejuni* cannot be isolated has led to the identification of several additional species of *Campylobacter* which are associated with human disease. The *Campylobacter* genus causes a broad range of human illness, including gastritis and systemic infection as well as enteritis. All such species, like *C. jejuni,* appear to be epizootic, but precisely which animals are the most common vectors for specific *Campylobacter* species is not known. This discussion will be limited to four species of *Campylobacter,* which represent the spectrum of illness caused by these microorganisms.

Campylobacter coli, although slightly different in biochemical characteristics, is identical to *C. jejuni* in morphology, growth characteristics and epidemiology, as well as in the illness it produces.

Campylobacter fetus is similar to *C. jejuni* in morphology and growth characteristics but has a marked predilection for patients with chronic renal, hepatic, and neoplastic disease, alcoholism, and compromised immune function. Although the intestinal tract of the compromised host is the presumed site of entry, the intestinal infection may be mild or subclinical, and overshadowed by a bacteremic illness, associated with high fever, which often follows a prolonged or relapsing course and may be complicated by endocarditis, infection of preexisting aortic aneurysms, and/or septic phlebitis. Persistent bacteremia may be enhanced by the relative resistance of *C. fetus* to the bactericidal activity of normal serum. Although occasional patients have had self-limited *C. fetus* sepsis, *C. fetus* bacteremia is usually fatal unless treated with antimicrobials. Gentamicin is thought to be the drug of choice, although no controlled observations are available. At least 4 weeks of antimicrobial treatment is recommended because of the tropism of *C. fetus* for intravascular sites.

Campylobacter cinaedi sp. n. has been the most frequently isolated of four *Campylobacter*-like organisms (CLOs) which have been associated with proctitis, proctocolitis, and enteritis in homosexual males. Although morphologically similar to *C. jejuni*, the CLOs grow poorly at 42° (and are therefore missed by the standard technique used to isolate *C. jejuni* and *C. fetus*), and prototype CLO strains show little (< 2 percent) DNA homology with *C. jejuni* and *C. fetus*. The CLO organisms grow slowly in a microaerophilic environment on modified brucella agar supplemented with 10% sheep blood.

A distinct species, *Campylobacter pylori* (formerly *C. pyloridis*), has been strongly associated with antral gastritis and with peptic ulcer disease. *C. pylori* has been isolated from over 50 percent of both adults and children with primary antral gastritis, and from an even higher proportion of patients with demonstrable duodenal ulcers, but rarely from normal gastric mucosa. *C. pylori*–associated antral gastritis has been shown to heal after administration of appropriate antimicrobials. *C. pyloris* is therefore thought to be an etiologic factor in primary antral gastritis and associated peptic ulcer disease. Data are not adequate to determine what proportion of cases of antral gastritis may be associated with *C. pyloris*. *C. pyloris* is readily grown in a microaerobic atmosphere on blood agar to which several antimicrobials have been added; like the CLOs, *C. pyloris* grows well at 37°C but poorly at 42°C.

Despite the differing growth characteristics, the CLOs produce changes which are indistinguishable from those caused by *C. jejuni* on sigmoidoscopic and histologic examination. Although the CLOs are sensitive to erythromycin, no controlled studies of antimicrobial therapy are available.

***VIBRIO PARAHEMOLYTICUS* Etiology and epidemiology** *Vibrio parahemolyticus* is a curved, aerobic, nonmotile, gram-negative bacillus. Although present in coastal waters throughout the temperate zone, it has most commonly been associated with acute diarrheal illness in Japan, presumably in relation to ingestion of raw seafood. It is regarded as the prototype of the halophilic vibrios because it grows more rapidly in 6% NaCl solutions than in the isotonic or hypotonic media used to culture most bacterial pathogens. *V. parahemolyticus* is responsible for a relatively small (<10 percent) proportion of acute diarrheal illnesses in both adults and children in rural Bangladesh, where an association with seafood is less clearly established. It has been implicated in several outbreaks of acute diarrheal disease in the coastal United States, always as a common-source outbreak related to ingestion of inadequately cooked seafood, usually shrimp. Secondary cases caused by person-to-person transmission occur rarely. Several outbreaks of *V. parahemolyticus* infections on cruise ships have occurred.

Pathogenesis Although *V. parahemolyticus* produces a toxin capable of causing intestinal fluid accumulation in experimental animals, the role of this toxin in human disease is not certain. *V. parahemolyticus* causes patchy mucosal damage in both distal ileum and colon; stools usually contain numerous polymorphonuclear leukocytes and are occasionally grossly bloody. The volume of fluid lost with *V. parahemolyticus* infection is relatively small, and intravenous fluids are seldom required. The illness is self-limited, with a median duration of just under 24 h.

Manifestations Within 6 to 48 h after ingestion of raw or inadequately cooked seafood, the patient develops an acute diarrheal illness. The volume of fluid lost is not great, moderately severe abdominal cramps may be a prominent feature, and chills and fever are observed in roughly half the cases. Vomiting is generally not prominent and occurs in no more than one-third of patients. The illness is self-limited, and no deaths have been reported in outbreaks in the United States.

Laboratory findings When a common-source outbreak of acute diarrheal disease occurs in a group exposed to fresh or frozen seafood, the index of suspicion should be high and the diagnosis should be confirmed by plating a rectal swab on thiosulfate–citrate–bile salt–sucrose (TCBS) agar, on which typical colonies of *V. parahemolyticus* appear in 24 h. (This organism grows poorly and is therefore easily overlooked on deoxycholate culture plates.) The stool generally has numerous polymorphonuclear leukocytes and a smaller number of erythrocytes, but these findings are less prominent than in shigellosis.

Treatment No therapy is required for the majority of patients. Antimicrobial therapy shortens neither the course nor the duration of pathogen excretion. Antiperistaltic agents are not of clear-cut benefit. An occasional patient may lose sufficient quantities of intestinal fluid to require oral or intravenous fluid therapy.

Prognosis The outcome is almost always good. Fatal cases, occasionally reported from Japan, have occurred in rare instances in patients with serious underlying disease.

VIBRIO MIMICUS *Vibrio mimicus* has been identified as a pathogen in sporadic cases of acute diarrheal disease, occurring in previously healthy individuals of all age groups who have ingested raw seafood (especially oysters) along the Gulf Coast. The epidemiology of *V. mimicus* infections differs from that caused by *V. parahemolyticus* in that, with the exception of one small outbreak, all isolates have represented single, sporadic cases. Although *V. mimicus*, like *V. cholerae*, is not a halophilic vibrio (it grows more rapidly in 1% NaCl than in higher salt solutions), it does not produce cholera enterotoxin, and it causes an illness in which the presenting features are clinically indistinguishable from those caused by *V. parahemolyticus*.

Fever occurs in at least 40 percent of cases and bloody diarrhea in roughly 15 percent. Since the illness is self-limited, treatment is symptomatic. Antibiotic therapy is of no value.

VIBRIO VULNIFICUS *Vibrio vulnificus*, like *V. parahemolyticus*, is a true halophilic vibrio that is common in shellfish along the Gulf of Mexico and less frequent along the Atlantic and Pacific coasts. It has been recognized as the cause of serious illness in at least 60 individuals in the last decade. *V. vulnificus* produces two clinical syndromes distinct from those caused by other vibrio species. In the compromised host, most frequently in individuals with liver disease, *V. vulnificus* may cause fulminant septicemia, usually associated with the early (within 36 h) development of cutaneous bullae and/or ulcers. In the noncompromised host, after contamination of a superficial wound by seawater, *V. vulnificus* may cause rapid development of intense cellulitis and local ulceration, often associated with bacteremia.

V. vulnificus should be suspected, and therapy with intravenous tetracycline should be initiated immediately in any individual with chronic liver disease who develops signs of septicemia (especially if associated with cutaneous lesions) within 1 to 3 days of ingestion of shellfish.

INVASIVE *ESCHERICHIA COLI* Enteroinvasive *E. coli*, which are far less common pathogens than enterotoxigenic *E. coli*, may cause a clinical syndrome quite similar to shigellosis with the exceptions that vomiting seldom occurs with EIEC and the illness is of shorter duration. Diarrhea caused by EIEC is rare in the United States but has been a significant cause of short-term disability in eastern Europe and southeast Asia. Since the illness is relatively short-lived, antimicrobial therapy has not been shown to be helpful.

ENTEROHEMORRHAGIC *ESCHERICHIA COLI* (EHEC) A small number of *E. coli* strains, most commonly 0157:H7, have been responsible for widely distributed sporadic cases of hemorrhagic colitis in the United States. Undercooked meat, especially hamburger, has been the most frequently identified mode of transmission. All age groups have been affected. The clinical illness is most commonly heralded by crampy abdominal pain and watery diarrhea, followed within 24 h by frankly bloody stools, which may simulate lower gastrointestinal bleeding. Unlike those with other bacteria associated with bloody diarrhea (e.g., *Shigella, Campylobacter*), patients are usually afebrile, and inflammatory cells are seldom present in the stool. Colonoscopy demonstrates inflammation, edema, and hemorrhage, primarily in the ascending and proximal transverse colon. The mean duration of illness has been 8 days.

All isolates tested have been noninvasive (Sereny test negative) but EHEC consistently produce verocytotoxin that is immunologically indistinguishable from the Shiga toxin of *Shigella dysenteriae* type I. Verocytotoxin can be isolated from the stool of virtually all patients with EHEC enteritis. Available data indicate that the hemolytic-uremic syndrome (HUS) is at least as frequent following EHEC colitis as it is following enteritis caused by *S. dysenteriae* type I. Despite the production of a toxin immunologically identical to the Shiga toxin, EHEC are not invasive, appear to cause disease by a direct effect of the verocytotoxin on colonic mucosal cells, and generally cause few systemic symptoms.

With the exception of the individuals who develop HUS, the illness is generally self-limited. HUS may, however, develop in any age group, and the mortality rate has been especially high in elderly individuals who develop this complication. Treatment with appropriate antimicrobials has not been shown to alter the duration or severity of the illness, but the sporadic occurrence of cases has prevented controlled studies of antibiotic therapy.

ACUTE VIRAL DIARRHEAS

Acute viral gastroenteritis is discussed in detail in Chap. 145. These illnesses are both more common and more life-threatening in small children than adults. In the United States, rotaviruses account for a large proportion of diarrheal illnesses during the first 2 years of life and usually occur during the winter. They have seldom been implicated in adult illness. In rural Bangladesh, infection with rotavirus accounts for roughly 60 percent of episodes of diarrhea in children from 6 to 24 months of age and for about 5 percent in the 2- to 5-year-old age group; it seldom occurs in adolescents and adults. The illness usually presents with vomiting followed by watery diarrhea and low-grade fever, with little or no associated abdominal pain. Vomiting is a prominent and almost constant early manifestation of rotavirus enteritis but rarely persists beyond the first 24 h. Diarrhea often persists for 4 to 8 days. Although the illness is generally not life-threatening, many patients require fluid and electrolyte repletion. Since the vomiting is usually short-lived, fluid repletion can generally be achieved by the oral route, using the same fluids that are effective in the treatment of cholera (see Chap. 122).

The diagnosis can be confirmed by a variety of tests including demonstration of the virus in stool by electron microscopy, a rise in complement-fixing antibody titers, and radioimmunoassay. The most useful and reliable test for rapid diagnosis under field conditions consists of direct demonstration of the antigen in stool by the enzyme-linked immunosorbent assay (ELISA).

Norwalk and Norwalk-like viruses, now implicated in roughly a third of episodes of epidemic gastroenteritis involving adults in the United States, usually cause relatively mild, short (<36 h), and self-limited disease, for which neither fluid nor drug therapy is necessary (see Chap. 145).

ACUTE PROTOZOAL DIARRHEAS

Giardia lamblia has emerged as a major cause of acute diarrheal disease (see Chap. 165). Although formerly thought to be a pathogen only in children and later considered to be a significant cause of diarrheal disease only in developing nations, this organism is the pathogen most commonly incriminated in outbreaks of waterborne diarrheal disease in the United States. It occurs most commonly in the Rocky Mountain states and more frequently causes disease in visitors than in the indigenous population. The illness characteristically presents with the sudden onset of watery diarrhea and malabsorption, accompanied by mild to moderate abdominal discomfort, bloating, and flatulence. Symptoms may occasionally persist for weeks unless appropriate antimicrobials are administered. Prolonged disease with malabsorption occurs from time to time in previously normal individuals but is particularly common in patients with IgA deficiency, who tend to have the most severe form of giardiasis.

The attack rate may be quite high (>50 percent) in individuals exposed to contaminated water sources. In North American travelers returning from Leningrad, where the water supply has been heavily contaminated with *Giardia* cysts, up to 60 percent of individuals have developed clinical giardiasis. The usual incubation period is 10 to 20 days. The illness, therefore, frequently develops after a traveler returns home, and the travel history is critical in suspecting the diagnosis. Occasionally the disease occurs endemically in individuals who have not traveled. The diagnosis can be confirmed in approximately half the cases by examining the stool for cysts; if the stool examination is negative in a patient with characteristic clinical features, duodenal aspirates or biopsies will usually yield the characteristic trophozoites. Treatment with quinacrine, 100 mg tid for 5 to 7 days, is generally curative; metronidazole, 250 mg tid for 7 days, is an equally effective alternative.

TRAVELER'S DIARRHEA

Diarrhea is by far the most common health problem of travelers to developing countries. Of more than 16 million travelers annually from industrialized nations to developing countries, approximately one-third will develop diarrhea. The incidence of traveler's diarrhea (TD) varies markedly by destination.

Etiology and epidemiology Virtually all cases of TD are caused by infectious agents, acquired through ingestion of fecally contaminated food and/or water. Especially risky foods include raw vegetables, raw meats, and raw seafood. Foods sold by street vendors are a common source of enteropathogens. Bacterial pathogens account for the great majority of episodes. Overall, the most common etiologic agents in TD are enterotoxigenic *E. coli* (ETEC), which are responsible for 50 to 75 percent of episodes. The culpable ETEC may produce LT, ST, or both enterotoxins, with considerable geographic variation. Other recognized enteropathogens can be isolated from most of the remainder of cases, but with great regional differences in prevalence. For example, *Shigella* causes up to 10 percent of TD in Mexico but is an unusual etiologic agent in North Africa. *Vibrio parahemolyticus* is a relatively common cause of TD in Japanese travelers in Asia but has not been associated with TD in South America. Viruses (rotavirus, Norwalk-like virus) and protozoa (amebas, *Giardia*) are collectively responsible for fewer than 10 percent of cases of TD.

Pathogenesis The pathogenesis varies with the culpable etiologic organism, but most cases of TD, even when caused by *Shigella*, are self-limited and have not been associated with serious sequelae in previously healthy individuals.

Manifestations Episodes of TD usually begin abruptly, with urgent diarrhea, abdominal cramps, nausea, and often low-grade fever. In the great majority of cases, the fluid loss is not voluminous, and symptoms subside within 3 to 5 days.

Treatment For the great majority of patients, fluid losses do not demand specific replacement fluids. Patients want relief from the two specific problems of abdominal cramps and diarrhea. Bismuth subsalicylate, taken as Pepto-Bismol liquid, in a dose of 60 mL qid, can decrease the severity of symptoms. Diphenoxylate and loperamide both provide symptomatic relief, but should not be used in the rare patient with high fever or blood in the stool; the antimotility agents should be discontinued if symptoms persist beyond 48 h. Patients with more severe symptoms (e.g., more than three loose stools within

8 h) may benefit from antimicrobial treatment. Trimethoprim, 160 mg, with sulfamethoxazole, 800 mg, twice daily, or trimethoprim alone, 200 mg twice daily for 3 days, has proved effective in shortening the mean duration of symptoms from 4 to 1.5 days. It is not certain that these antimicrobials will prove equally effective in all parts of the developing world.

Prevention The only sure prevention is to avoid ingestion of contaminated water and food, a goal that is not practical for most travelers. Carefully controlled studies have demonstrated that three antimicrobials, doxycycline, trimethoprim-sulfamethoxazole, and norfloxacin, when taken prophylactically, are consistently effective in reducing the incidence of TD by 50 to 86 percent in various parts of the developing world. Because of the calculable risks of administration of prophylactic antimicrobials to several million travelers annually, balanced against the generally self-limited course of TD, prophylactic antimicrobials are not routinely recommended for prevention of TD. Travelers are advised, however, to obtain therapeutic doses of effective antimicrobial agents prior to travel to high-risk areas, so that the more severe episodes of TD can be treated early, without recourse to potentially dangerous over-the-counter drugs.

REFERENCES

BARKER WH JR et al: *Vibrio parahemolyticus* outbreak in Covington, Louisiana, in August, 1972. Am J Epidemiol 100:316, 1974

BLACKLOW NR, CUKOR G: Viral gastroenteritis. N Engl J Med 304:397, 1981

BLASER MJ et al: *Campylobacter* enteritis in the United States: A multicenter study. Ann Intern Med 98:360, 1983

CARTER AO et al: A severe outbreak of *Escherichia coli* 0157:H7-associated hemorrhagic colitis in a nursing home. N Engl J Med 317:1496, 1987

CLOVER TL, ABER RD: *Yersinia enterocolitica*. N Engl J Med 321:16, 1989

DUPONT HL et al: Pathogenesis of *Escherichia coli* diarrhea. N Engl J Med 285:1, 1971

——— et al: Symptomatic treatment of diarrhea with bismuth subsalicylate among students attending a Mexican university. Gastroenterology 73:715, 1977

——— et al: Treatment of traveler's diarrhea with trimethoprim/sulfamethoxazole and with trimethoprim alone. N Engl J Med 307:841, 1982

GORBACH SL et al: Traveler's diarrhea and toxigenic *Escherichia coli*. N Engl J Med 292:933, 1975

GRIFFIN PM et al: Illnesses associated with *Escherichia coli* 0157:H7 infections. A broad clinical spectrum. Ann Intern Med 109:705, 1988

GUERRANT RL et al: Prospective study of diarrheal illnesses in northeastern Brazil: Patterns of disease, nutritional impact, etiologies and risk factors. J Infect Dis 148:986, 1983

LEVINE MM: *E. coli* that cause diarrhea. J Infect Dis 155:377, 1987

MARSHALL BJ: *Campylobacter pyloridis* and gastritis. J Infect Dis 153:650, 1986

NATIONAL INSTITUTES OF HEALTH: Consensus development conference on traveler's diarrhea. JAMA 253:2700, 1985

NEILL MA et al: Hemorrhagic colitis with *Escherichia coli* 0157:H7 preceding adult hemolytic uremic syndrome. Arch Intern Med 145:2215, 1985

QUINN TC et al: Infections with *Campylobacter jejuni* and Campylobacter-like organisms in homosexual men. Ann Intern Med 101:187, 1984

SACK DA et al: Oral rehydration in rotavirus diarrhea: A double blind comparison of sucrose with glucose electrolyte solution. Lancet 2:280, 1978

TERRANOVA W et al: Current concepts: *Bacillus cereus* food poisoning. N Engl J Med 298:143, 1978

WALKER RI et al: Physiology of *Campylobacter* enteritis. Microbiol Rev 50:81, 1986

93 SEXUALLY TRANSMITTED DISEASES

KING K. HOLMES / H. HUNTER HANDSFIELD

Venereology encompasses not only the five "venerable" venereal diseases (syphilis, gonorrhea, chancroid, lymphogranuloma venereum, and granuloma inguinale) but also a growing number of other diseases which might be considered the "new generation" of sexually transmitted diseases (STDs). The most recently recognized STD, and in certain populations the most important, is infection with human immunodeficiency virus (HIV) (see Chap. 264). Like gonorrhea, many of these newer STDs became epidemic in nearly all countries of the world during the past quarter-century. With increasing interest in these diseases and improved methods for diagnosis has come awareness of the growing consequences of STD to health and society, which extend far beyond the traditional sphere of venereology, encompassing such diverse problems as acquired immunodeficiency syndrome (AIDS), neoplasia, infertility, and serious congenital and perinatal morbidity.

CLASSIFICATION OF SEXUALLY TRANSMITTED DISEASES These diseases can be classified on the basis either of their etiologies or their clinical manifestations. Table 93-1 summarizes the etiologic classification of STD.

APPROACH TO SEXUALLY TRANSMITTED DISEASE No single STD can be regarded as an isolated problem, because multiple coinfections are common and because the presence of an STD denotes the occurrence of high-risk sexual behavior that is often associated with the risk of other, more serious infections. STDs are not endogenous, nor are they transmitted by fomites, food, flies, or casual contact. *At least one infected partner always exists.* The sexual history and management of sexual partners are therefore of paramount importance. Failure to identify and examine or refer the infected partner(s) represents a failure in management, both at the community level (since sources of spread of infection are not identified) and at the patient level (since reinfection is not prevented).

Most persons with genital discharges, lesions, or pain cease sexual activity and seek medical care. Accordingly, those who transmit infection usually are among the minority who are infected but asymptomatic, or who do not understand the implications of their symptoms. Therefore, they do not seek medical attention spontaneously, and physicians must see that they are examined and treated, or referred. In the United States, local health departments will usually identify and treat contacts of some diseases (e.g., syphilis, gonococcal pelvic inflammatory disease), but for most STDs this responsibility is shared by the patient and the physician. With the increasing importance of potentially incurable viral STDs (HIV infection, genital herpes, human papillomaviruses, chronic hepatitis B virus infections), the role of counseling to reduce transmission is growing.

STDs are propagated most efficiently in core populations with high levels of sexual activity and frequent changes of sexual partners. In most of the United States, these core groups consist of predominantly young urbanites of low socioeconomic level, who are disproportionately black and Hispanic. They often reside within circumscribed high-prevalence neighborhoods. The treatable bacterial STDs, such as syphilis, gonorrhea, and chancroid, are heavily concentrated in core populations and increasingly involve prostitutes and their sex partners and others involved in illicit drug use. These individuals are difficult to reach for educational programs and contact tracing and may continue sexual activity despite STD symptoms. Other STDs are more evenly distributed in society, chlamydial infections, for example. For these, available control measures (e.g., widespread screening, contact tracing) have not been widely applied, even in noncore populations. Chlamydial infection and the incurable viral STDs persist, often asymptomatically, and they are propagated widely in populations which do not share the above characteristics of STD core groups. Table 93-2 lists some of the most common clinical syndromes and their complications associated with sexually transmitted pathogens. Strategies for the management of some of the common syndromes are outlined below. AIDS is discussed in Chap. 264.

URETHRITIS IN MEN Urethritis in men is classified as gonococcal or nongonococcal. During the past decade the incidence of gonococcal urethritis has fallen in many western countries, while that of nongonococcal urethritis (NGU) remains at high levels, suggesting that current measures for control of NGU are relatively ineffective. In general, gonorrhea and NGU have similar frequencies among men seen in STD clinics in the United States, whereas NGU is approximately three times as common as gonorrhea among men seen by physicians in private practice and 10 times as common as gonorrhea among college students.

TABLE 93-1 Sexually transmitted pathogens

Bacteria	Virus	Other*
TRANSMITTED IN ADULTS PREDOMINANTLY BY SEXUAL INTERCOURSE		
Neisseria gonorrhoeae	Human immunodeficiency viruses (HIV-1 and -2)	*Trichomonas vaginalis*
Chlamydia trachomatis	Herpes simplex virus, type 2 (HSV-2)	*Phthirus pubis*
Treponema pallidum	Human papilloma virus (genital types HPV 6, 11, 16, 18, 31, 33, 35, 39, 42, 43, 44, 45, 51–56)	*Sarcoptes scabiei*
Calymmatobacterium granulomatis	Cytomegalovirus	
Ureaplasma urealyticum	Molluscum contagiosum virus	
SEXUAL TRANSMISSION REPEATEDLY DESCRIBED BUT NOT WELL DEFINED OR NOT THE PREDOMINANT MODE OF TRANSMISSION		
Mycoplasma hominis	Human T-lymphotrophic virus (HTLV-I)	*Candida albicans*
Gardnerella vaginalis and other vaginal bacteria	(?) Hepatitis C, D viruses	
	Herpes simplex virus type 1 (HSV-1)	
Group B streptococcus	(?) Epstein-Barr virus (EBV)	
TRANSMITTED BY SEXUAL CONTACT INVOLVING ORAL-FECAL EXPOSURE; OF DECLINING IMPORTANCE IN HOMOSEXUAL MEN		
Shigella spp.	Hepatitis A virus†	*Giardia lamblia*
Campylobacter spp.		*Entamoeba histolytica*

* Other includes protozoa, ectoparasites, fungi.
† Among U.S. patients for whom a risk factor can be ascertained, most hepatitis B virus infections are sexually transmitted.

About 40 percent of NGU is caused by *Chlamydia trachomatis*. Herpes simplex virus and, perhaps, *Trichomonas vaginalis* each cause a small additional proportion of NGU cases in the United States, but over half of the cases cannot be attributed to any of these three pathogens. *Ureaplasma urealyticum* has been implicated in case-control studies as a probable cause of many of the *Chlamydia*-negative cases. Two other organisms, *Mycoplasma genitalium* and *Bacteroides urealyticum*, are also under investigation as possible causes of this syndrome. Since facilities for detection of these agents are not widely available and their role is not certain, the diagnosis of male urethritis usually does not include cultures for these organisms. However, diagnostic testing for *C. trachomatis* is now widely available, by isolation of the agent in tissue cell culture or by immunochemical detection of chlamydial antigens. The following steps should be taken in evaluating sexually active men with symptoms of urethral discharge and/or dysuria:

TABLE 93-2 Common STD syndromes and etiologic agents

Syndrome	Primary sexually transmitted (ST) agent
Urethritis: males	*N. gonorrhoeae, C. trachomatis, U. urealyticum,* HSV
Epididymitis	*C. trachomatis, N. gonorrhoeae;* non-ST agent: urinary tract pathogens
Lower genital tract infections: females	
Cystitis/urethritis	*C. trachomatis, N. gonorrhoeae,* HSV; non-ST agent: urinary tract pathogens
Mucopurulent cervicitis	Same as cystitis/urethritis
Vulvovaginitis	*C. albicans, T. vaginalis;* non-ST agent: urinary tract pathogens
Bacterial vaginosis (BV)	BV-associated flora (see text)
Acute pelvic inflammatory disease	*N. gonorrhoeae, C. trachomatis,* BV-associated flora; non-ST agent: coliform bacteria
Ulcerative lesions of the genitalia	HSV-1, HSV-2, *T. pallidum, H. ducreyi, C. trachomatis* (LGV strains), *C. granulomatis;* non-ST agent: pyogenic bacteria (e.g., *S. pyogenes, C. albicans*)
Proctitis	Same as urethritis, cervicitis; *T. pallidum*
Acute arthritis	*N. gonorrhoeae* (e.g., DGI), *C. trachomatis* (e.g., Reiter's syndrome), HBV, HIV
Genital and anal warts	Human papillomavirus (genital types)
AIDS	HIV-1, HIV-2; also many opportunistic pathogens
Glandular fever (acute fever, lymphadenopathy, atypical lymphocytosis)	Cytomegalovirus, HIV; non-ST agent: EBV
Neoplasias	
Squamous cell cancer of the cervix, anus, vulva, or penis	Human papillomavirus (?)
Kaposi's sarcoma	HIV, other (?); non-ST agent: EBV
Lymphoid neoplasia	HIV, HTLV-I
Hepatocellular carcinoma	
Scabies	*S. scabiei*
Pubic lice	*P. pubis*

NOTE: HSV, herpes simplex virus; EBV, Epstein-Barr virus

1 *Establish the presence of urethritis*. Commonly in NGU, and less often in gonorrhea, discharge can be demonstrated only by milking the urethra after the patient has not voided for several hours, preferably overnight. If no overt discharge is demonstrable, urethral inflammation can be documented by inserting a small urethrogenital swab 2 to 3 cm into the urethra and examining the Gram-stained direct smear prepared from this swab for leukocytes. Five or more leukocytes per 1000× field in areas containing cells suggests urethritis. Patients with symptoms who lack objective confirmatory evidence of urethritis on two occasions 1 week apart may have functional problems and generally do not benefit from repeated courses of antibiotics.
2 *Evaluate for complications or alternative diagnoses*. Epididymitis and systemic complications, such as the gonococcal arthritis-dermatitis syndrome and Reiter's syndrome, should be excluded by brief history and examination. Bacterial prostatitis and cystitis should be excluded by appropriate tests in men with dysuria who lack evidence of urethritis or in sexually inactive men with urethritis. Digital examination of the prostate gland is seldom informative in patients with urethritis.
3 *Evaluate for gonococcal and chlamydial infection*. The diagnosis of gonorrhea is confirmed by demonstrating typical gram-negative diplococci within neutrophils. The diagnosis of NGU is warranted if gram-negative diplococci are not found. Isolation of *N. gonorrhoeae* by culture should be attempted to document antimicrobial susceptibility, and also because the predictive value of Gram-stained urethral smears is dependent on the experience of the laboratory. Diagnostic testing for *C. trachomatis* should also be performed if resources are available, regardless of the presence or absence of gonorrhea, since coinfection with *N. gonorrhoeae* and *C. trachomatis* is common in men with urethritis. An approach to the diagnosis of urethritis is illustrated in Fig. 93-1. The treatment of gonorrhea and chlamydial infections is discussed in Chaps. 110 and 155, respectively.

EPIDIDYMITIS Acute epididymitis is almost always unilateral and must be differentiated from testicular torsion, tumor, and trauma. Torsion, a surgical emergency, usually occurs in the second or third

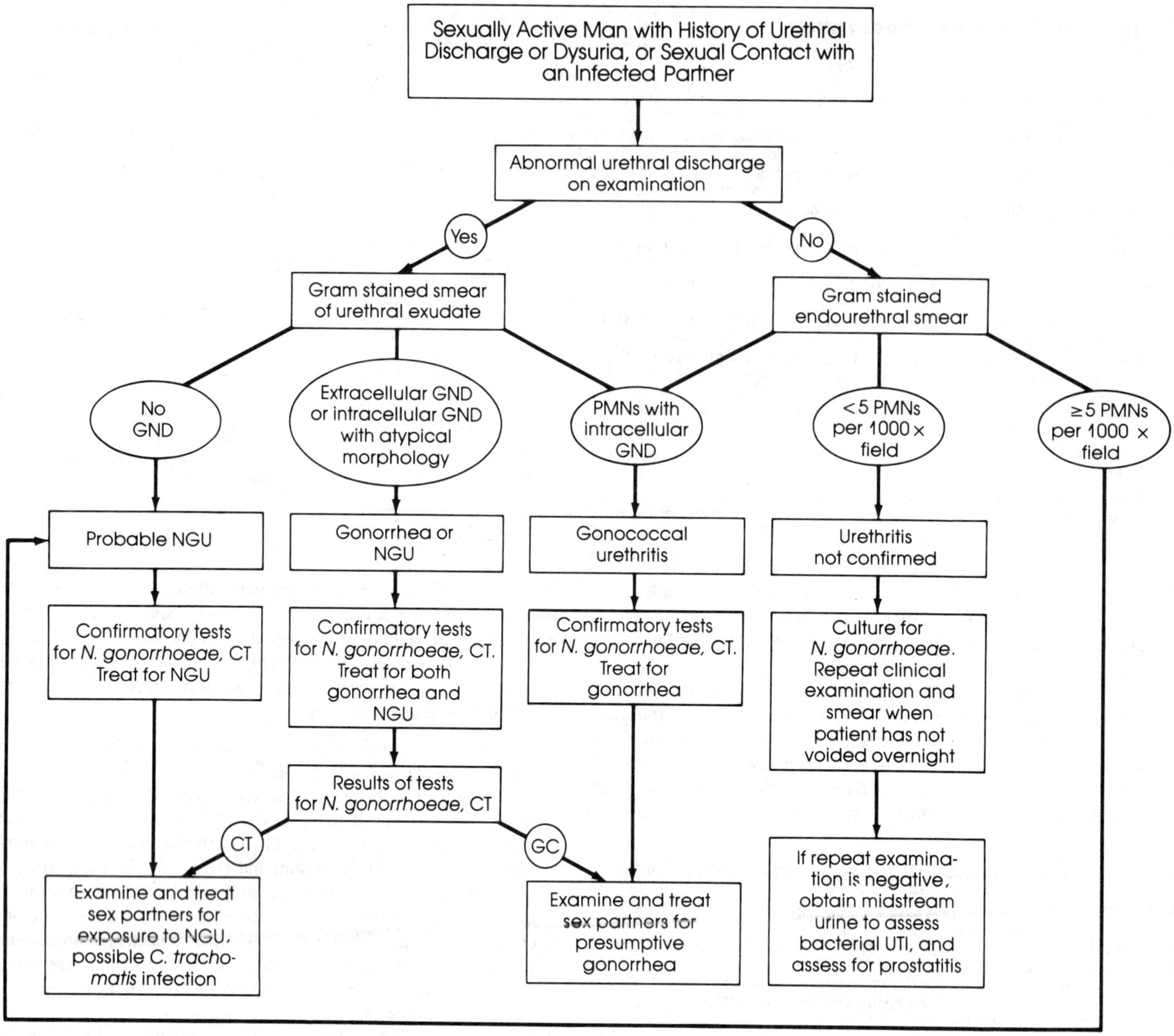

FIGURE 93-1 Evaluation of sexually active men with suspected urethritis. PMN = polymorphonuclear leukocyte; GND = gram-negative diplococci; NGU = nongonococcal urethritis; UTI = urinary tract infection; GC = *Neisseriae gonorrhoeae;* CT = *chlamydia trachomatis.*

decade and is suggested by sudden onset of pain, elevation of the testicle within the scrotal sac, and absence of blood flow on Doppler examination or ^{99}Tc scan. In sexually active men under age 35, acute epididymitis is usually caused by *C. trachomatis,* or less commonly by *Neisseria gonorrhoeae,* and is usually associated with overt or subclinical urethritis. Antimicrobial agents are the mainstay of therapy; optimal treatment for epididymitis due to *C. trachomatis* is doxycycline, 100 mg twice daily for 10 days. For gonococcal epididymitis, the recommended treatment is ceftriaxone, 250 mg intramuscularly, followed by the same doxycycline regimen. Bed rest and scrotal elevation may hasten symptomatic relief.

Acute epididymitis in older men or following urinary tract instrumentation is usually caused by gram-negative bacilli or other urinary pathogens. Urethritis is usually absent, but bacteriuria is present.

LOWER GENITOURINARY TRACT INFECTION IN WOMEN Infections of the female urinary tract, cervix, vulva, and vagina produce dysuria, vulvar irritation, dyspareunia, and increased or altered vaginal discharge. Diagnostic confusion may be attributable not only to the symptomatology, which is nonspecific, but also to the lack of consistent application of available laboratory tests, and to the difficulty in differentiating true inflammatory conditions from functional genitourinary complaints. Two steps are required in the evaluation of lower genitourinary symptoms in women: (1) differentiation among cystitis, urethritis, vaginitis, cervicitis, and cervical ectopy, and (2) exclusion of associated upper tract disease (e.g., pyelonephritis, salpingitis).

Cystitis and urethritis Although dysuria is more common in bacterial urinary tract infection (UTI) than in vaginitis, dysuria is often attributable to vaginitis in young women because vaginitis is substantially more common than UTI. Localization of dysuria as "internal" is suggestive of UTI or urethritis, while "external dysuria" (caused by painful contact of urine with the labia) is associated with vulvovaginitis. Among sexually active young women with internal dysuria, up to 25 percent have fewer than 100 urinary pathogens per milliliter of urine and are considered to have the *urethral syndrome.* About half of these have pyuria, and most of them are infected with *C. trachomatis* or *N. gonorrhoeae.* Sexually active women with urethral syndrome who lack pyuria have no apparent infection, and their symptoms usually resolve spontaneously. In a study of female college students with dysuria, urgency, or frequency without vaginal infection, about half had bacterial cystitis with 10^5 bacteria or more per milliliter of urine, and one-quarter had bacterial cystitis with less than 10^5 bacteria per milliliter (usually between 10^2 and 10^5 per milliliter). About one-quarter had urethral symptoms without bacteriuria. In the latter group, about half had pyuria, and most of these were infected with *C. trachomatis,* while most of those without pyuria had no demonstrable infection and improved with placebo therapy. In populations whose risk of gonorrhea is higher than that of college students, *N. gonorrhoeae* is also a common cause of the urethral syndrome.

DIAGNOSIS AND THERAPY Among women with acute dysuria and frequency, the first step is to exclude evidence of acute pyelonephritis (e.g., costovertebral pain and tenderness, and fever). As outlined in Fig. 93-2, the next step in sexually active women is the differentiation of cystitis or urethritis from vaginal infection. Among women without vaginal infection, bacterial UTI must then be differentiated from the urethral syndrome. The finding of a single conventional urinary pathogen, such as *Escherichia coli* or *Staphylococcus saprophyticus,* in a concentration of $\geq 10^2$ per milliliter in a properly collected midstream urine specimen from a symptomatic woman with pyuria indicates probable bacterial UTI, whereas pyuria with $<10^2$ conventional uropathogens per milliliter of urine (''sterile pyuria'') suggests the diagnosis of acute urethral syndrome due to *C. trachomatis* or *N. gonorrhoeae*. Gonorrhea should be evaluated by Gram stain and culture of the cervix and urethra. Chlamydial infection should be evaluated by culture or specific immunologic tests for chlamydial antigen in urethral and cervical specimens. Treatment with a tetracycline (e.g., doxycycline, 100 mg twice daily for 7 days) has been shown to alleviate dysuria in women with ''sterile'' pyuria, but not in women without pyuria or isolation of a pathogen. The sexual partners of such patients should also be examined and considered for treatment.

VULVOVAGINAL INFECTIONS In self-referred women attending STD clinics, vaginal infection is the most common diagnosis. Bacterial vaginosis is the most common cause of vulvovaginal symptoms, followed by candidiasis and then trichomoniasis. Vaginal infection may be characterized by one or more of the following: increased volume of discharge; abnormal yellow color of discharge caused by increased concentration of polymorphonuclear leukocytes; vulvar itching, irritation, or burning, often with external dysuria; vulvar dyspareunia; and vaginal malodor. An important component of the clinical evaluation of vaginal discharge is ascertaining by speculum examination whether the discharge emanates from the vagina or the cervix, and whether the discharge is, in fact, abnormal. Occasionally, symptoms of increased discharge or other vaginal symptoms are not associated with objective signs of vaginitis or cervicitis. Although psychological testing is normal in most such cases, possible causes of functional symptoms should be explored. The diagnosis and therapy of the three major types of vaginal infection are summarized in Table 93-3.

***Trichomonas vaginalis* vaginitis** (See Chap. 167) Sexual transmission of *T. vaginalis* is well established. Routine culture testing indicates that many women and most men with infection are asymptomatic. However, treatment of asymptomatic as well as symptomatic cases is recommended to reduce the reservoir of infection and the risk of transmission and to prevent the future development of symptoms.

DIAGNOSIS AND THERAPY Trichomoniasis characteristically produces a profuse, yellow, purulent, homogeneous vaginal discharge. The vaginal epithelium is inflamed, and petechial lesions can be seen by colposcopy on the cervix (''strawberry cervix'') in about 50 percent of cases. In women with typical symptoms and signs of trichomoniasis, the diagnosis can usually be confirmed by demonstration of motile trichomonads and polymorphonuclear leukocytes in vaginal secretions mixed with normal saline and promptly examined microscopically. In such patients, wet-mount examination is at least 80 percent as sensitive as culture. However, in women without symptoms or signs, culture is often required to detect the organism. The pH of vaginal secretions is usually ≥ 5.0. The diagnosis of *T. vaginalis* infection in men is more difficult and requires culture of early morning first-voided urine sediment or of a urethral swab specimen obtained before voiding.

Nitroimidazoles are the only consistently effective drugs for treating trichomoniasis. Several studies show that a single 2.0-g oral dose of metronidazole is at least 90 percent as effective as more prolonged dosage schedules. Other nitroimidazoles such as tinidazole and ornidazole have longer half-lives than metronidazole, but have not been clearly shown to give better results in trichomoniasis. Routine treatment of sex partners is recommended to reduce both the risk of reinfection and the reservoir of infection. Metronidazole should not be given to women during the first trimester of pregnancy. Alcohol must be avoided for 24 h after treatment because of a disulfiram-like effect of the drug. The partners of patients with trichomoniasis (and all sexually transmitted infections) should be examined; they should not be treated without examination and counseling.

Bacterial vaginosis Vaginal discharge not associated with *T. vaginalis,* yeast, or cervical infection is usually due to bacterial vaginosis. This syndrome (formerly termed *nonspecific vaginitis* or *Gardnerella-associated vaginal discharge*) is characterized by vaginal malodor and increased white discharge that is homogeneous, low in viscosity, and uniformly coats the vaginal walls. It is unclear whether bacterial vaginosis is a sexually transmitted infection. The syndrome is associated with STD risk factors, such as number of sexual partners and recent intercourse with a new partner, but no single sexually transmitted pathogen has been clearly identified as a cause. Antibiotic treatment of the male sexual partners has not conclusively been shown to influence the recurrence rate in affected women. It is likely that poorly understood factors associated with sexual activity somehow alter the vaginal milieu, resulting in the characteristic alterations of the vaginal flora. Formerly considered a benign condition, bacterial vaginosis has been implicated as a risk factor for acute salpingitis, premature labor, and related neonatal and perinatal complications.

The concentration of *Gardnerella vaginalis* (formerly *Haemophilus vaginalis*), *Mycoplasma hominis, U. urealyticum,* and certain anaerobic bacteria is increased in vaginal washings from women with this syndrome. Two closely related species of curved, motile, gram-negative anaerobic rods (*Mobiluncus curtisii, Mobiluncus mulieris*) are particularly closely associated with this syndrome. The prevalence and concentration of other anaerobic bacteria, such as vaginal *Bacteroides* spp. and *Peptostreptococcus* spp., also are increased and probably contribute to the pathogenesis of bacterial vaginosis. However, many of these are common among women without this syndrome; e.g., *G. vaginalis* has been isolated from the vagina of up to 50 percent of normal women. The aerotolerant *Lactobacillus* species, which constitute most of the normal vaginal flora (e.g., *L. acidophilus, L. jenseni*), are absent or present only in reduced concentration in the vagina in bacterial vaginosis. These species produce lactic acid, hydrogen peroxide, and other factors thought to be important in regulating the vaginal flora.

DIAGNOSIS AND TREATMENT In a patient with symptoms of abnormal vaginal discharge and malodor or objective signs of increased white homogeneous vaginal discharge, the diagnosis of bacterial vaginosis can be made with reasonable certainty by the following:

1. Exclusion of candidal and trichomonal vaginitis and mucopurulent cervicitis, including collection of endocervical specimens to test for *C. trachomatis* and *N. gonorrhoeae.*
2. Microscopic demonstration of ''clue cells'' and characteristic alterations of the vaginal microflora. Clue cells are vaginal epithelial cells coated with coccobacillary organisms. On wet mount, prepared by mixing vaginal secretions 1:1 with normal saline, clue cells have a granular appearance and their borders are obscured (Fig. 93-3). Clue cells also can be detected on a Gram-stained smear, which permits assessment of the vaginal flora; the normally predominant lactobacilli are largely or completely replaced by a profusion of bacterial morphotypes consistent with *G. vaginalis*

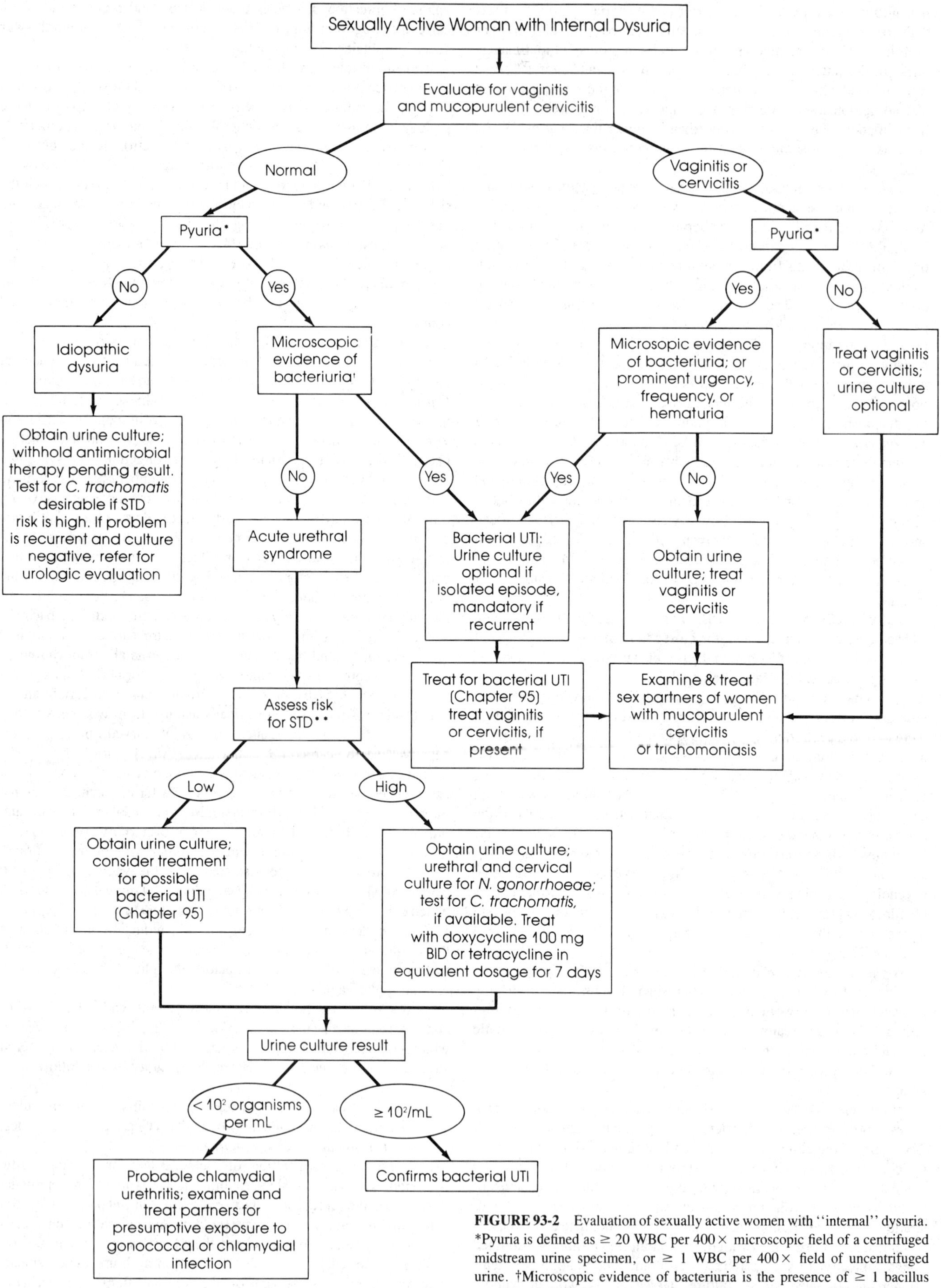

FIGURE 93-2 Evaluation of sexually active women with "internal" dysuria. *Pyuria is defined as ≥ 20 WBC per $400\times$ microscopic field of a centrifuged midstream urine specimen, or ≥ 1 WBC per $400\times$ field of uncentrifuged urine. †Microscopic evidence of bacteriuria is the presence of ≥ 1 bacillus per $400\times$ field of an uncentrifuged midstream specimen of urine. **Evaluation of STD risk is based on number and nature of sexual partner(s), recent change in partner, marital status, past history of STD, etc.

TABLE 93-3 Diagnostic features and management of vaginal infection

	Normal vaginal exam	Yeast vaginitis	Trichomonal vaginitis	Bacterial vaginosis (BV)
Etiology	Uninfected; *Lactobacillus* predominant	*Candida albicans* and yeasts	*Trichomonas vaginalis*	Associated with *G. vaginalis*, various anaerobic bacteria, and mycoplasma
Typical symptoms	None	Vulvar itching and/or irritation, increased discharge	Profuse purulent discharge; vulvar itching	Malodorous, slightly increased discharge
Discharge:				
Amount	Variable; usually scant	Scant to moderate	Profuse	Moderate
Color*	Clear or white	White	Yellow	Usually white or gray
Consistency	Nonhomogeneous, floccular	Clumped; adherent plaques	Homogeneous	Homogeneous, low viscosity; uniformly coating vaginal walls
Inflammation of vulvar or vaginal epithelium	None	Erythema of vaginal epithelium, introitus; vulvar dermatitis common	Erythema of vaginal and vulvar epithelium; colpitis macularis	None
pH of vaginal fluid†	Usually ≤4.5	Usually ≤4.5	Usually ≥5.0	Usually ≥4.7
Amine ("fishy") odor with % KOH	None	None	May be present	Present
Microscopy‡	Normal epithelial cells; lactobacilli predominant	Leukocytes, epithelial cells; yeast, mycelia, or pseudomycelia in up to 80%	Leukocytes; motile trichomonads seen in 80–90% of symptomatic patients, less often in the absence of symptoms	Clue cells; few leukocytes; lactobacilli outnumbered by profuse mixed flora, nearly always including *G. vaginalis* plus anaerobic species on Gram stain
Usual treatment	None	Miconazole or clotrimazole, intravaginally each 100 mg daily for 7 days Nystatin, 100,000 units intravaginally twice daily for 7–14 days	Metronidazole or tinidazole, 2 g orally (single dose) Metronidazole, 500 mg orally twice daily for 7 days	Metronidazole, 500 mg orally twice daily for 7 days
Usual management of sex partner	None	None; topical treatment if candidal dermatitis of penis is present	Examine for STD; treat with metronidazole, 2 g, orally (single dose)	Examine for STD; no treatment if normal

* Color of discharge is determined by examining vaginal discharge against the white background of a swab.
† pH determination is not useful if blood is present.
‡ To detect fungal elements, vaginal fluid is digested with 10% KOH prior to microscopic examination; to examine for other features, fluid is mixed (1:1) with physiologic saline. Gram's stain also is excellent for detecting yeasts and pseudomycelia and for distinguishing normal flora from the mixed flora seen in bacterial vaginosis, but it is less sensitive than the saline preparation for detection of *T. vaginalis*.
SOURCE: From KK Holmes et al.

and anaerobic organisms. The demonstrations of clue cells by wet-mount microscopy and of characteristically altered vaginal flora by Gram stain represent the most sensitive, specific, and objective criteria for the diagnosis of bacterial vaginosis in women with symptoms and/or signs of this condition.

3 Liberation of a distinct fishy odor immediately after mixing vaginal secretions with a 10% solution of KOH. This odor is attributable to volatile amines (e.g., putrescine, cadaverine) present in the vaginal fluid, presumably the result of anaerobic bacterial metabolism.

4 Demonstration of pH of vaginal secretions greater than 4.5. The elevated pH may be partly due to the presence of amines as well as to decreased production of lactate by lactobacilli.

The most consistently effective therapy for bacterial vaginosis is metronidazole, 500 mg twice daily for 7 days, perhaps because of the role of the anaerobes, most of which are highly susceptible to metronidazole in this infection. Amoxicillin, 500 mg three times daily for 7 days, has been effective in about 40 to 50 percent of cases of bacterial vaginosis, and is the primary alternative to metronidazole. Systemic or vaginal therapy with clindamycin is also effective. Sulfonamide-containing vaginal creams are usually ineffective, probably because sulfonamides are inactive against both *G. vaginalis* and many vaginal anaerobes, and there is no rationale for their use. Tetracycline therapy also is ineffective. Treatment of male partners of women with this syndrome is not routinely indicated. However, because bacterial vaginosis is associated with sexual behavioral risks, it is not unreasonable to examine partners for evidence of other STDs.

Vulvovaginal candidiasis The predominant symptom in vulvovaginal candidiasis is vulvar pruritus. There is usually no distinct odor. Vulvar erythema commonly is present. The vaginal discharge typically is white, scanty, and often takes the form of thrush-like plaques or cottage cheese-like curds adhering to the vaginal mucosa. *Candida albicans* accounts for about 80 percent of yeasts isolated from the vagina, while *Torulopsis glabrata* and other less commonly encountered *Candida* species are found in the remainder. Overt vulvovaginitis is more common among women colonized by *C. albicans* than among those colonized with *T. glabrata* or other species. Most cases of vulvovaginal candidiasis probably result from increased growth of yeasts that previously colonized the vagina or the intestinal tract. Some cases of recurrent vulvovaginal candidiasis may be due to sexual transmission from a colonized male.

DIAGNOSIS AND THERAPY The diagnosis of vulvovaginal candidiasis involves demonstration of fungi by microscopic examination of vaginal secretions in saline or 10% KOH, or by Gram's stain. Demonstration of pseudohyphae strengthens the diagnosis of vaginitis due to *C. albicans*. Polymorphonuclear leukocytes usually are present. Microscopic examination is less sensitive than culture, but culture detects asymptomatic carriage in women who may not require therapy. The pH of vaginal secretions is usually less than 4.5, and an amine odor is not produced when vaginal secretions are mixed with 10% KOH. Vulvitis often accompanies vaginitis and may result in superficial erosions that must be differentiated from genital herpes. In most

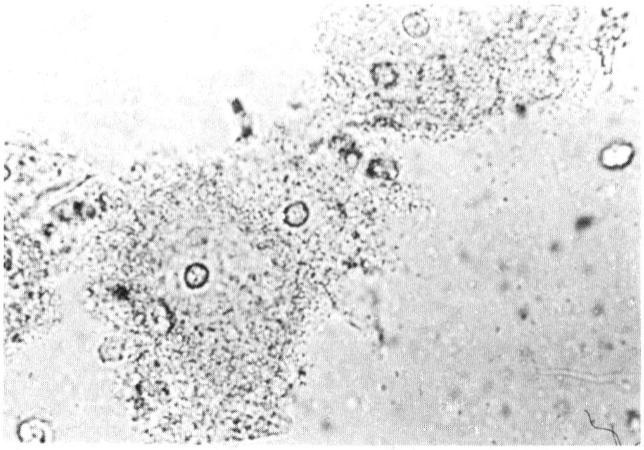

A

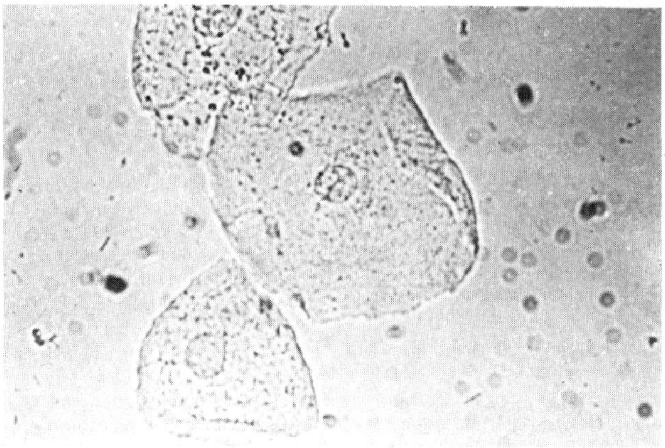

B

FIGURE 93-3 *A*. Vaginal epithelial "clue cells." Note granular appearance due to adherent *G. vaginalis* and indistinct cell margins. 400×. *B*. Normal vaginal epithelial cells. The cell margins are distinct and lack granularity.

circumstances, therapy for candidal vaginal infection is indicated only if the patient is symptomatic, has signs of vulvovaginitis, or if inflammatory cells or pseudohyphae are present. The usual treatment is intravaginal miconazole, clotrimazole, or butoconazole for 3 to 7 days; intravaginal nystatin is less effective. Oral treatment with ketoconazole may be indicated for especially severe or frequently recurrent cases or for cases that do not respond to vaginal therapy. Such patients should be evaluated for HIV infection. Treatment of the sex partner is not routinely indicated, although this has not been studied rigorously.

MUCOPURULENT CERVICITIS Mucopurulent cervicitis refers to inflammation of the columnar epithelium and subepithelium of the endocervix, and of any contiguous columnar epithelium that lies exposed in an ectopic position on the exocervix. Mucopurulent cervicitis in the female can be regarded as the "silent" partner of urethritis in the male, being equally common and caused by the same agents but more difficult to recognize. It is the most common major STD syndrome in women and can lead to pelvic inflammatory disease, and in pregnant women may lead to obstetrical complications. Improved recognition and treatment of this syndrome would greatly improve the control of STD. Mucopurulent cervicitis most commonly is caused by *C. trachomatis* and sometimes by *N. gonorrhoeae*, but about one-third to one-half of cases are associated with neither of these organisms. The syndrome can usually be differentiated clinically from cervicitis caused by primary or recurrent herpes simplex virus infection, which produces lesions on the stratified squamous epithelium of the exocervix, as well as on the columnar epithelium; and from vaginitis caused by *C. albicans* or *T. vaginalis*.

DIAGNOSIS AND THERAPY The diagnosis is made by demonstrating mucopurulent discharge from the cervical os or by demonstrating increased numbers of polymorphonuclear leukocytes in Gram-stained or Papanicolaou smears of endocervical discharge. Cervical ectopy (see below) that is edematous and endocervical bleeding induced by gentle swabbing are common signs of mucopurulent cervicitis due to *C. trachomatis*. The color of cervical mucus on a white swab removed from the endocervix should be noted; a yellow color indicates the presence of mucopus. The cervical mucus should be rolled *thinly* on a slide for Gram staining. An area of the slide should be identified which contains strands of cervical mucus which are not contaminated by vaginal squamous epithelial cells or bacteria. The presence of ≥30 polymorphonuclear cells per 1000× microscopic field within strands of cervical mucus suggests cervicitis. The prevalence of *C. trachomatis* infection or gonorrhea has been significantly greater among women with mucopurulent cervicitis by the above criteria than among women without it. The presence of a characteristic pattern of inflammatory cells on endocervical Papanicolaou smears has been used by cytopathologists to suggest the possibility of chlamydial infection and the need for specific confirmatory testing.

Mucopurulent cervicitis requires antimicrobial therapy. An etiologic diagnosis should always be established to guide management of sexual partners, but therapy should usually be initiated against the most likely causes of this syndrome, while results of diagnostic tests are pending. The diagnosis of gonococcal cervicitis is made by culture of an endocervical specimen. When carefully collected endocervical specimens are examined by experienced personnel, Gram's stain is an insensitive but highly specific test, and observation of intracellular gram-negative diplococci indicates gonococcal infection, even if the culture is negative. The sensitivity of a single endocervical culture for *N. gonorrhoeae* is 80 to 90 percent. Chlamydial infection of the cervix can be confirmed by culture or antigen detection (see Chap. 155).

While diagnostic test results are pending, therapy for mucopurulent cervicitis should be initiated with a single-dose regimen effective for gonorrhea (ceftriaxone, 250 mg intramuscularly), followed by doxycycline, 100 mg twice daily, orally for 1 week. For pregnant women, erythromycin base or stearate, in a dose of 500 mg four times daily for 7 to 14 days, can be substituted for doxycycline. The male sex partners of women with nongonococcal mucopurulent cervicitis should be examined and treated as described for gonococcal and nongonococcal urethritis.

Cervical ectopy Cervicitis must be differentiated from cervical ectopy, which is often mislabeled "cervical erosion." Ectopy represents the presence of the one-cell-thick columnar endocervical epithelium in an exposed visible "ectopic" position on the cervix, where it appears redder than the several-cells-thick stratified squamous vaginal epithelium. When ectopy is present, the cervical os may contain clear or slightly cloudy mucus, but usually not mucopus. Colposcopy shows that the epithelium is intact and not ulcerated. Ectopy is normally present during early adolescence and gradually recedes as squamous metaplasia replaces the ectopic columnar epithelium. Oral contraceptive usage or pregnancy favors persistence or reappearance of ectopy. The use of cauterizing procedures to eliminate simple ectopy is not warranted. The presence of ectopy may make the cervix more susceptible to infection with *N. gonorrhoeae* or *C. trachomatis* by exposing a larger surface area of susceptible columnar epithelium. If mucopurulent cervicitis supervenes, the area of ectopy may become edematous and fragile, with bleeding induced by gentle swabbing. In addition, edema of the cervix may result in eversion of the os, enlarging the apparent area of ectopy.

ULCERATIVE LESIONS OF THE GENITALIA The incidence and etiology of ulcerative lesions of the genitalia vary greatly in different areas of the world. In Asia and Africa, genital ulcers are seen as frequently as gonorrhea in some STD clinics, and chancroid is the commonest cause, while genital herpes is relatively uncommon. In the industrialized western countries, genital ulcers are considerably less common than urethritis, mucopurulent cervicitis, and vaginitis. Genital herpes is the commonest cause, and chancroid is relatively uncommon. Syphilis is the second most common form of genital ulcer in almost all areas of the world and must always be excluded. Lymphogranuloma venereum (LGV) and donovanosis (granuloma inguinale) are very rare in North America and Europe. Other causes include candidiasis and traumatized genital warts, both of which usually are readily recognized; and various nonsexually transmitted dermatoses. Chancroid, syphilis, genital herpes, and probably all causes of genital ulcer enhance the efficiency of sexual transmission and acquisition of HIV. Moreover, genital ulcers, especially chancroid and syphilis, are most common in inner city populations with low socioeconomic status and high rates of prostitution and illicit drug use, independent risk factors for HIV infection. From 1985 through 1988, chancroid and syphilis have been spreading at epidemic rates in such populations.

DIAGNOSIS AND THERAPY In industrialized countries, the differential diagnosis of genital ulceration, when nonsexually transmitted lesions are excluded, usually involves genital herpes simplex virus (HSV) infection, syphilis, and chancroid. The clinical findings are occasionally definitive (e.g., presence of herpetic vesicles), and clinical findings plus epidemiologic considerations usually help to guide initial therapy pending further studies. Nevertheless, most genital ulcerations cannot be diagnosed confidently on clinical grounds. It is axiomatic to exclude syphilis by appropriate serology in all cases. Dark-field examination should also be performed, by experienced technicians when possible, on lesions consistent with primary or secondary syphilis. Direct immunofluorescence using antibodies to *T. pallidum* is at least as sensitive and specific as dark-field microscopy for detection of *T. pallidum* in lesion exudate and can be performed on specimens sent to a central laboratory. This procedure should be used more widely. Selective enrichment media are available for isolation of *Haemophilus ducreyi*.

The following general guidelines are recommended for management of ulcerative genital lesions (Fig. 93-4):

1 *If typical painful herpetic vesicles or pustules are present:* In this case the clinical diagnosis of herpes is warranted, although a serologic test for syphilis should be performed. If desired, the diagnosis can be confirmed by isolation of HSV or by immunochemical detection with specific antibody. Cytologic methods to detect HSV-infected cells (Tzanck preparation or Papanicolaou stain) are insensitive.
2 *If painful nonvesicular ulcer(s) raise the suspicion of herpes or chancroid:* If there are painful lesion(s) or enlarged, tender inguinal lymph nodes or if other features suggest herpes or chancroid, attempts to demonstrate HSV or *H. ducreyi* are indicated. All methods of HSV detection are less sensitive in the ulcerative stage than in the vesicular stage. Syphilis should be excluded by dark-field examination and serologic testing, both of which should be repeated 1 to 2 weeks later if negative initially and if another diagnosis cannot be confirmed.
3 *If painless ulcerative lesions suggest the diagnosis of syphilis:* If lesions are at all suggestive of syphilis, or there are epidemiologic reasons to suspect syphilis, such as recent exposure, then dark-field examination and a rapid serologic test for syphilis should be performed for prompt diagnosis. If these are negative, two more dark-field examinations on successive days are recommended, and the serologic test should be repeated 1, 2, and 6 weeks later. Direct immunofluorescent detection of *T. pallidum* should be used if dark-field examination by experienced examiners is not available.
4 *If genital ulceration is chronic and painless:* In addition to the tests for syphilis and chancroid, biopsy is indicated to exclude donovanosis and carcinoma.

Antibacterial therapy is not indicated for undiagnosed ulcerative genital lesions. Oral acyclovir speeds resolution of systemic and local manifestations of initial episodes of genital and anorectal herpes if started early; therefore, acyclovir should be started promptly if the diagnosis of these forms of herpes seems likely (see Chap. 135). Treatment for syphilis should not be instituted until the diagnosis is established. The value of antimicrobial therapy for idiopathic ulcerative lesions of the genitalia is uncertain, but treatment for presumptive chancroid with ceftriaxone or erythromycin (see Chap. 117) sometimes may be reasonable for lesions of recent onset that persist or progress during several days of observation and that cannot be attributed to herpes or syphilis. Antimicrobial therapy should be given promptly when chancroid is probable, especially if regional lymph node suppuration is present or appears imminent. If patients worsen or do not improve during 1 or 2 weeks of observation and the diagnosis remains obscure, attempts to isolate *H. ducreyi* should be made or repeated, and other noninfectious and infectious etiologies (e.g., donovanosis) should be considered.

PROCTITIS, PROCTOCOLITIS OR ENTEROCOLITIS, AND ENTERITIS Sexually acquired proctitis, or inflammation limited to the rectum, results from direct rectal inoculation of typical STD pathogens. In contrast, inflammation which extends from the rectum to the colon (proctocolitis) and involves the small and large bowel (enterocolitis) or the small bowel alone (enteritis) can result from ingestion of typical intestinal pathogens through sexual contact involving oral-fecal exposure. Anorectal pain and mucopurulent or bloody rectal discharge suggest proctitis or proctocolitis. Proctitis is commonly associated with tenesmus and constipation, whereas proctocolitis and enterocolitis are more often associated with diarrhea. In both, anoscopy usually shows the presence of mucosal inflammation with exudate and easily induced mucosal bleeding (i.e., positive "wipe test"). Petechial or mucosal ulcers also may be observed. Exudate should be sampled for microbiologic studies and Gram stain. Sigmoidoscopy or colonoscopy, performed if possible without an enema, shows inflammation limited to the rectum in proctitis, or disease extending at least into the sigmoid colon in proctocolitis.

Most cases of sexually transmitted intestinal infection have in the past involved homosexual men. During the AIDS era, there has been an extraordinary shift in the clinical and etiologic spectrum of intestinal infections in homosexual men. The number of opportunistic intestinal infections—not described in this chapter—has risen rapidly in homosexual men with AIDS. At the same time, the number of sexually transmitted intestinal infections, described below, has fallen rapidly as high-risk sexual behaviors have become less common in this group.

Most cases of infectious proctitis are due to *N. gonorrhoeae*, HSV, or *C. trachomatis;* these are acquired via receptive rectal intercourse. Primary and secondary syphilis can also produce anal or rectal lesions, with or without symptoms. Gonococcal proctitis and proctitis due to non-LGV strains of *C. trachomatis* typically involve the most distal rectal mucosa and the anal crypts and are clinically mild, without systemic manifestations. In contrast, primary HSV proctitis and LGV proctocolitis usually produce severe anorectal pain and fever. Perianal ulcers and inguinal lymphadenopathy may occur with either, but most commonly are due to herpes. Sacral nerve root radiculopathies, usually with urinary retention, are common in primary herpetic proctitis. Sigmoidoscopy most commonly shows ulcerative proctitis with either herpes or LGV, but may reveal intact vesicopustular lesions with anorectal herpes. In herpes, biopsy of the rectal mucosa shows microulcerations and may show intranuclear inclusions or perivascular lymphocytic cuffing. In LGV, biopsy typically shows crypt abscesses, granulomas, and giant cells, findings that may be indistinguishable from those of Crohn's disease. Syphilis can also produce rectal granulomas, usually associated with infiltration by plasma cells or other mononuclear cells.

The occurrence of diarrhea and abdominal bloating or cramping pain, without anorectal symptoms, in association with normal anoscopy and sigmoidoscopy, is consistent with inflammation of the small intestine or more proximal colon. In homosexual men, without HIV infection, enteritis limited to the small intestine is often attributable to *Giardia lamblia*, while *Campylobacter* spp., *Shigella* spp., and *Entamoeba histolytica* can produce enterocolitis with or without lesions involving the distal colon or rectum. Sexually acquired proctocolitis, enterocolitis, and enteritis due to *Campylobacter* spp., *Shigella* spp., *E. histolytica*, and *G. lamblia* are clinically indistin-

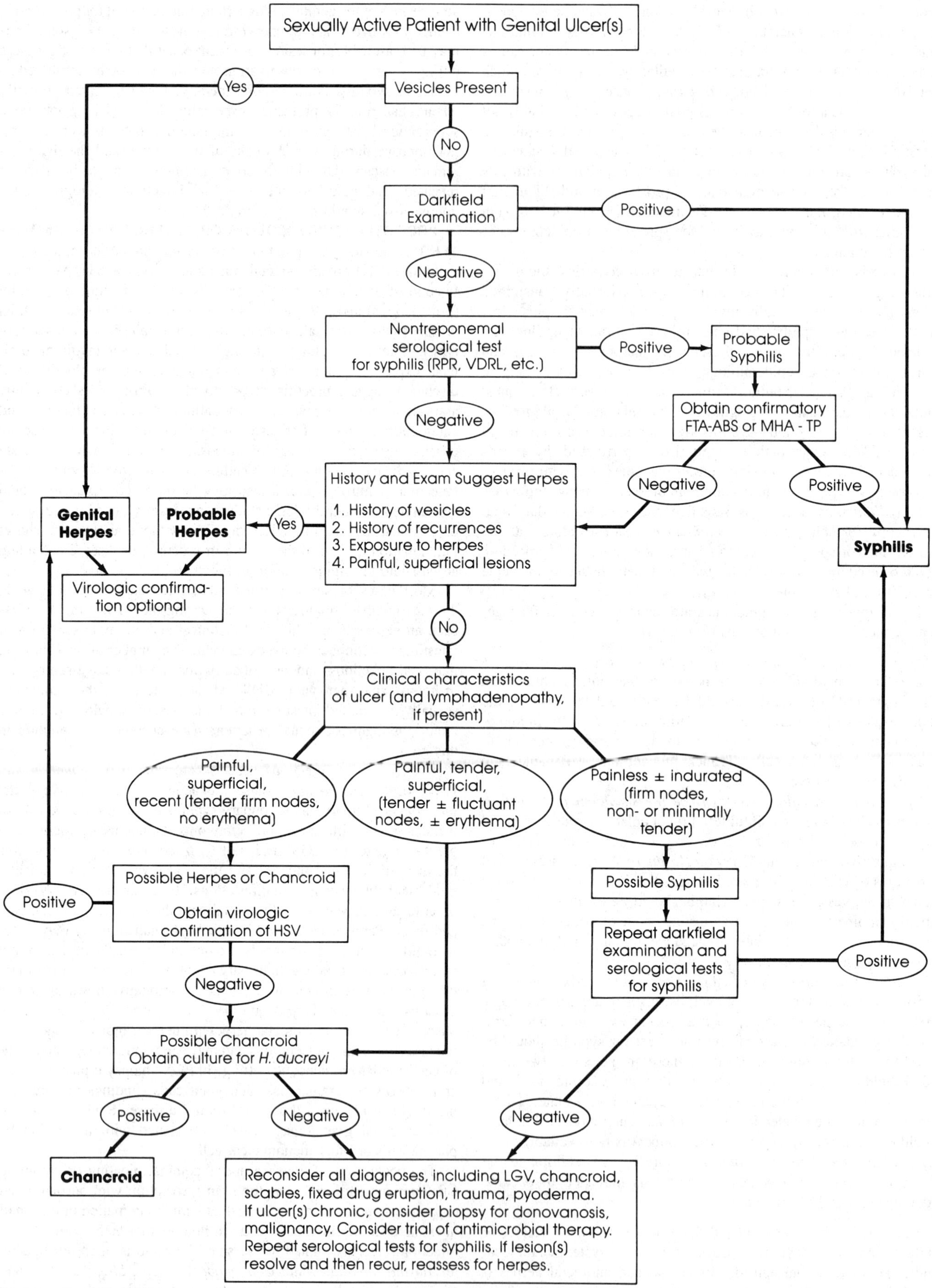

FIGURE 93-4 Evaluation of sexually active persons with genital ulcer-inguinal lymphadenopathy syndromes.

guishable from nonsexually transmitted infections with the same symptoms.

ACUTE ARTHRITIS The gonococcal arthritis-dermatitis syndrome probably is the most common form of acute arthritis in sexually active young adults, and Reiter's syndrome is the second commonest. These must be differentiated from each other and from other forms of infective arthritis, various diseases associated with immune-complex deposition, crystal-induced arthritis, acute rheumatoid arthritis, and other less common rheumatic disorders such as systemic lupus erythematosus. Meningococcemia, *Yersinia* infection, sarcoidosis, and syphilis are other occasional causes of acute arthritis.

Demonstration of *N. gonorrhoeae* by culture or a specific immunochemical method in synovial fluid, blood, skin lesions, or cerebrospinal fluid is diagnostic of DGI. Failing this, gonococcal arthritis is highly probable if *N. gonorrhoeae* is recovered from a mucosal site of infection or from the patient's sex partner, typical pustular or hemorrhagic skin lesions are distributed primarily on the extremities, and a therapeutic antibiotic trial produces prompt improvement. Suspected and confirmed cases of DGI should be treated promptly with an antibiotic effective against antibiotic-sensitive and -resistant gonococci, such as ceftriaxone (see Chap. 110). Some patients with septic gonococcal arthritis may require repeated closed-joint irrigations with saline before improvement occurs.

Reiter's syndrome occurs in a sporadic (apparently sexually transmitted) form and a postdysenteric form, which sometimes occurs in discrete epidemics. It is described in detail in Chap. 274.

VIRAL WARTS See Chap. 150.

PREVENTION AND CONTROL OF SEXUALLY TRANSMITTED DISEASES The control of bacterial STD has traditionally depended on secondary prevention of spread by early diagnosis and treatment. The emergence of the incurable viral STDs has required increasing emphasis on health education and health promotion as primary prevention strategies. Medical students and physicians require training to develop skills in eliciting a sexual history, in determining the extent to which their patients, especially adolescents and young adults, are at risk for STD, and in counseling them appropriately. Public education and personal counseling should begin in early adolescence and should emphasize responsible sexual behavior (abstinence, maintenance of monogamous relationships); the use of condoms for nonmonogamous sexual encounters; avoidance of traumatic sexual practices, such as anal intercourse; the recognition of early symptoms and signs of STD; and early health care for such symptoms and signs. Genital self-examination, analogous to breast self-examination, is a practice to prevent sequelae and improve control of STD.

Maintenance of clinical skills in the recognition, diagnosis, and treatment of STDs is essential for secondary prevention of STD by early treatment. Screening tests for gonorrhea, chlamydial infection, syphilis, and HIV infection should be widely available and used by physicians serving populations at risk. Similarly, health departments should provide high-quality STD clinical services and screening for high-risk populations. Health departments also are responsible for STD surveillance and for coordinating targeted control measures; this requires the cooperation of physicians in reporting cases. Notification of the sexual partners of infected persons is the joint responsibility of the patient and physician. In most communities, the local health department will assist in this effort for cases of syphilis, some cases of gonorrhea, and, increasingly, for cases of HIV infection.

REFERENCES

General

CENTERS FOR DISEASE CONTROL: 1989 sexually transmitted diseases treatment guidelines. Morb Mort Week Rep 38(Suppl 8):1–43, 1989

HANDSFIELD HH (ed): Sexually transmitted diseases. Infect Dis Clin North Am 1:1, 1987

HOLMES KK et al (eds): *Sexually Transmitted Diseases*, 2d ed. New York, McGraw-Hill, 1989

Urethritis in males

BOWIE WR et al: Etiology of nongonococcal urethritis: Evidence for *Chlamydia trachomatis* and *Ureaplasma urealyticum*. J Clin Invest 59:735, 1977

JACOBS NF, KRAUS SF: Gonococcal and nongonococcal urethritis in men: Clinical and laboratory differentiation. Ann Intern Med 82:7, 1975

Epididymitis

BERGER RE et al: Etiology, manifestations, and therapy of acute epididymitis: Prospective study of 50 cases. J Urol 121:750, 1979

Urethral syndrome

STAMM WE et al: Urinary tract infections: From pathogenesis to treatment. J Infect Dis 159:400, 1989

Vaginitis

ESCHENBACH DA et al: Diagnosis and clinical manifestations of bacterial vaginosis. Am J Obstet Gynecol 158:819, 1988

HOLMES KK: Lower genital tract infections in women, in *Sexually Transmitted Diseases*, 2d ed, KK Holmes et al (eds). New York, McGraw-Hill, 1989

SOBEL J: Genital candidiasis, in *Sexually Transmitted Diseases*, 2d ed, KK Holmes et al (eds). New York, McGraw-Hill, 1989

WOLNER-HANSSEN P et al: Clinical manifestations of vaginal trichomoniasis. JAMA 261:571, 1989

Cervicitis

BRUNHAM RC et al: Mucopurulent cervicitis—the ignored counterpart in women of urethritis in men. N Engl J Med 311:1, 1984

Genital ulcers

KROCKTA WP, BARNES RC: Genital ulceration with regional adenopathy. Infect Dis Clin North Am 1:217, 1987

SIMONSEN JN et al: Human immunodeficiency virus infection among men with sexually transmitted diseases. N Engl J Med 319:274, 1988

Proctitis, proctocolitis, enterocolitis, and enteritis

QUINN TC et al: The polymicrobial etiology of intestinal infections in homosexual men. N Engl J Med 309:576, 1983

Arthritis

HANDSFIELD HH, POLLOCK PS: Arthropathies associated with sexually transmitted diseases, in *Sexually Transmitted Diseases*, 2d ed, KK Holmes et al (eds). New York, McGraw-Hill, 1989

94 PELVIC INFLAMMATORY DISEASE

KING K. HOLMES

DEFINITION The term *pelvic inflammatory disease (PID)* usually refers to ascending infection of the uterus, fallopian tubes, and broad ligaments. Intrauterine infection can be primary (spontaneously occurring and usually sexually transmitted) or secondary to invasive intrauterine surgical procedures (e.g., dilatation and curettage, termination of pregnancy, insertion of an intrauterine device, or hysterosalpingography), or to parturition. Endometritis or endomyometritis is particularly common following delivery by cesarean section.

PID is uncommon during pregnancy itself. The uterotubal junction is closed as early as the seventh week of pregnancy, and the chorioamnion becomes approximated to the endocervical os, sealing off the intrauterine cavity, at the twelfth to fifteenth week of gestation. As a consequence, ascending intrauterine infection prior to the twelfth week of gestation may be associated (either as cause or effect) with endometritis and spontaneous abortion, while ascending infection after the twelfth week may be associated with chorioamnionitis. Rarely, infection may extend secondarily to the pelvic organs from adjacent foci of inflammation, such as appendicitis, regional ileitis, or diverticulitis; as a result of hematogenous dissemination, such as tuberculosis; or as a rare complication of certain tropical diseases, such as schistosomiasis.

Spontaneously occurring PID can be divided into chronic and acute types. Chronic PID due to tuberculosis has become uncommon;

other forms of chronic PID, due to chronic infection with *Chlamydia trachomatis* or secondary to IUD usage, have been described but have not been adequately studied.

PID is most often used today to refer to cases of acute spontaneously occurring infection ascending from the cervix or vagina. The clinical diagnosis of PID is imprecise. Use of endometrial biopsy together with laparoscopy provides evidence of a continuum, progressing from cervicitis alone to endometritis, to salpingitis, to pelvic peritonitis, to generalized peritonitis, to perihepatitis, or to pelvic abscess. In this chapter, PID is used to refer to the clinical syndrome which includes each of these conditions, and the term *salpingitis* is restricted to patients with visually or histopathologically confirmed inflammation of the fallopian tubes. The distinction between endometritis and salpingitis may be important, because long-term sequelae are common after salpingitis. These sequelae include infertility due to bilateral tubal occlusion, peritubal adhesions, ectopic pregnancy due to tubal damage without occlusion, chronic pelvic pain, and recurrent PID.

ETIOLOGY The etiology of PID has seemed to vary greatly in several studies for reasons related to patient selection as well as methodology. As is summarized in Table 94-1, the agents most often implicated in acute PID include those which are primary causes of cervicitis (*Neisseria gonorrhoeae* and *C. trachomatis*) and those which can be regarded as abnormal components of the vaginal flora.

In the United States, gonococci were isolated from 44 percent of women with acute PID in a multicity cooperative study during the 1970s. From 1980 through 1989 in Seattle, *N. gonorrhoeae* or *C. trachomatis* have been found in over three-fourths of patients with proven salpingitis and endometritis; about one-fourth had gonorrhea alone, one-fourth had chlamydial infection alone, and one-fourth had both. However, in Scandinavian countries, where gonococcal infection is under much better control, endocervical gonococcal infection has been found in less than one-fourth of women with PID during the past decade, while chlamydial infection has remained common in this group. For example, in Sweden the proportion of women with acute PID who had gonorrhea fell from 50 percent in 1970 to 5 percent in 1985. In general, PID is most often associated with gonorrhea where there is a high incidence of gonorrhea, for example, in developing countries and in indigent, inner city populations in developed countries. In several studies of women with PID, up to two-thirds with positive endocervical cultures for *N. gonorrhoeae* have had positive endometrial, peritoneal, or tubal cultures for this organism. Similarly, studies of women with proven PID have shown that *C. trachomatis* can be demonstrated by culture or immunofluorescent staining in the endometrium or tubes of the majority of those who have endocervical chlamydial infection.

Anaerobic and facultative anaerobic organisms (especially *Bacteroides* species, peptostreptococci, *Escherichia coli*, and groups B and D streptococci) and genital mycoplasmas have been isolated from specimens obtained at laparoscopy from the peritoneal fluid or fallopian tubes in a varying proportion—typically one-fourth to one-third—of women with PID studied in the United States. These vaginal organisms can be found in association with chlamydial or gonococcal infection, as well as in women without them. The importance of vaginal organisms in salpingitis has probably been overestimated in studies based on culture of specimens obtained by culdocentesis or endometrial aspiration, procedures in which contamination of the aspirated specimen by vaginal flora could occur. However, specimens obtained by laparoscopy have also contained anaerobic and facultative species in some patients with PID. It is extremely difficult to determine the exact microbial etiology in the individual patient with PID because of the frequency of mixed infection, the difficulty in sampling the fallopian tube itself, and the complexity of microbiologic techniques required to detect the various fastidious pathogens involved.

TABLE 94-1 Cervical and vaginal organisms most often implicated in acute PID

Cervical pathogens	Vaginal flora
N. gonorrhoeae	Anaerobic bacteria
C. trachomatis	*Bacteroides* spp.
	Peptostreptococci
	Mobiluncus spp.
	Actinomyces spp.
	Facultative bacteria
	Enterobacteriaceae
	H. influenzae
	G. vaginalis
	Streptococcus, groups B, D
	Mycoplasma
	M. hominis
	U. urealyticum

In general, first episodes of acute PID are particularly likely to be caused by *N. gonorrhoeae* and/or *C. trachomatis*. These sexually transmitted pathogens are somewhat less often implicated in recurrent bouts of acute PID, episodes occurring in IUD users, and episodes precipitated by invasive intrauterine diagnostic or therapeutic procedures, which are often associated with ascending infection caused by the more virulent components of the endogenous vaginal flora.

EPIDEMIOLOGY It has been estimated that the annual incidence of PID in the United States during the mid-1970s was about 850,000 cases per year. PID is not a reportable disease in the United States; surveillance of physicians in private practice and of hospital discharges suggests that the incidence of PID increased from the mid-1960s through the mid-1970s and may then have decreased. The incidence of a major sequela of salpingitis, ectopic pregnancy, progressively rose each year from 13,200 cases in 1967 to 78,400 cases in 1985. Similar trends in ectopic pregnancies have been seen in Canada and England. Some of this increase may be due to improved tests for ectopic pregnancy. There is some evidence that involuntary infertility also increased in the United States during the 1970s.

Acute PID is almost exclusively a disease of sexually active women. The risk appears to be greater in sexually active teenagers than among older women. Important risk factors other than young age include a history of gonorrhea or of salpingitis, and use of an intrauterine device, particularly the Dalkon shield. In most studies, the relative risk of PID among IUD users was higher in nulliparous women than in parous women. On the other hand, women using oral contraceptives appear to be at decreased risk of PID. Barrier methods of contraception also prevent PID by reducing the risk of chlamydial and gonococcal infection. Tubal sterilization reduces (but does not completely eliminate) the risk of salpingitis by preventing intraluminal spread of infection into the tubes.

PATHOGENESIS Factors cited as possibly contributing to intracanalicular upward spread of gonococci and *Chlamydia* from the endocervix to the endometrium and endosalpinx include estrogen-dominated (thin) cervical mucus, attachment to sperm which migrate upward into the tubes, use of an intrauterine device, vaginal douching, and menstruation. The onset of symptoms of gonorrhea-associated PID and of *Chlamydia*-associated PID often occurs during or soon after the menstrual period. In fallopian tube organ cultures in vitro, gonococci attach to the surface of the secretory columnar cells (but not the ciliated cells) of the endosalpinx. Gonococcal pili and perhaps other surface proteins are important in this attachment. Gonococci then are taken into the secretory cells by endocytosis. They pass through the cells, and perhaps between cells, and are extruded through the base of the cell into the submucosal connective tissue. Ciliary motion ceases, and then ciliated cells, although not directly invaded by gonococci, are sloughed from the mucosa during this process—a factor which may render the tubes more susceptible to superinfection by other organisms. It is uncertain whether this loss of ciliated cells is irreversible in vivo. Gonococcal endotoxin and peptidoglycan are at least partly responsible for these cytotoxic effects. Gonococci associated with PID have been significantly more resistant to penicillin and less likely to belong to the Arg-Hyx-Ura auxotype than are strains causing uncomplicated gonorrhea.

C. trachomatis also infects the columnar cells of the fallopian tube, but produces little damage in tubal organ cultures, perhaps because the host response is more important in the pathogenesis of chlamydial salpingitis. In chlamydial mucopurulent cervicitis (MPC), cervical biopsies show inclusions containing *Chlamydia* within columnar cells; columnar epithelial infiltration by neutrophils; submucosal and stromal infiltration by plasma cells, lymphocytes, histiocytes, and neutrophils; and lymphoid aggregates containing transformed lymphocytes. Routine endometrial biopsies from consecutive women with chlamydial MPC show endometritis in approximately one-half. Although endometritis detected in this way is sometimes associated with uterine tenderness, abnormal menstrual bleeding, and leukocytosis, symptoms of abdominal pain and fever are usually lacking, underscoring the subclinical nature of many cases of upper genital tract chlamydial infection. It is not known what proportion of those with endometritis also have salpingitis, since laparoscopy has not been performed in the absence of more suggestive symptoms and signs of salpingitis. However, among women with chlamydial MPC who lack such symptoms and signs, the great majority who undergo endometrial biopsy and laparoscopy have both endometritis and salpingitis. Chlamydial inclusions are demonstrable by direct immunofluorescence in columnar epithelial cells of the endometrium and endosalpinx. The endometrial biopsies usually show neutrophils infiltrating the epithelium and plasma cells infiltrating the stroma, findings also seen in gonococcal endometritis, but not in the uninfected endometrium. Other inflammatory changes analogous to those seen in the cervix are also found in the endometrium with chlamydial infection. Experimental inoculation of the fallopian tubes of lower primates produces mild acute salpingitis and ciliary sloughing, which is completely reversible. However, if experimental tubal inoculation is preceded by repeated inoculation of the fallopian tubes or cervix, a more intense salpingitis results and progresses to peritubular scarring. This suggests that in the female genital tract, as in the eye, repeated exposure to *C. trachomatis* leads to the greatest degree of tissue inflammation and damage.

The pathogenesis of PID attributable to mycoplasmas or other vaginal anaerobic or facultative organisms is less well studied. It is possible that other vaginal organisms implicated in PID cause tubal infection in women whose tubes have already been damaged by a primary sexually transmitted pathogen (i.e., *N. gonorrhoeae* or *C. trachomatis*). Since the anaerobic organisms and mycoplasmas implicated in PID are found in the vagina most often and in greatest concentration in bacterial vaginosis (nonspecific vaginitis), it is possible that bacterial vaginosis itself is a predisposing factor for PID (just as poor oral hygiene is a risk factor in aspiration pneumonia).

Certain other iatrogenic factors, such as dilatation and curettage or cesarean section, are known to pose a greater risk of causing PID in women with endocervical gonococcal or chlamydial infection. It remains to be determined whether such procedures are also a greater risk in women with bacterial vaginosis.

CLINICAL MANIFESTATIONS **Tuberculous salpingitis** Unlike nontuberculous salpingitis, genital tuberculosis often occurs in older women, and about half are postmenopausal. In a large review of cases in Sweden, 38 percent had had previously diagnosed tuberculosis. The commonest presenting symptoms were abnormal vaginal bleeding, pain, including dysmenorrhea, and infertility. Most had normal bimanual pelvic examinations, though about one-quarter had adnexal masses. The most common method of diagnosis was endometrial biopsy, showing tuberculous granulomas, often associated with a positive culture.

Nontuberculous salpingitis The evolution of symptoms classically proceeds from a mucopurulent vaginal discharge caused by cervicitis—possibly associated with dysuria and frequency due to urethritis, or with anorectal pain, tenesmus, rectal discharge, and bleeding due to proctitis—to midline abdominal pain and abnormal vaginal bleeding caused by endometritis, followed by bilateral lower abdominal and pelvic pain caused by salpingitis, with nausea and vomiting and increased abdominal tenderness caused by peritonitis. Some patients have diffuse abdominal pain caused by generalized peritonitis, or pleuritic right upper quadrant pain caused by perihepatitis. The pattern in which symptoms evolve varies from patient to patient and is also related to the etiology of the PID.

The onset of IUD-associated PID is typically gradual, and may be preceded by typical malodorous vaginal discharge characteristic of bacterial vaginosis. The onset of gonococcal PID has been more acute than that of chlamydial PID in some, but not all studies, and both are often associated with menses.

The abdominal pain is usually described as dull or aching. In some cases, pain is lacking or is atypical, and active inflammatory changes can be found in the course of an unrelated evaluation or procedure such as a tubal ligation or laparoscopic evaluation for infertility. Abnormal uterine bleeding precedes or coincides with the onset of pain in about 40 percent of women with PID, symptoms of urethritis occur in 20 percent, and symptoms of proctitis in 7 percent of patients.

Speculum examination shows evidence of mucopurulent cervicitis in the majority of women with gonococcal or chlamydial PID. Cervical motion tenderness is produced by stretching of the adnexal attachments on the side toward which the cervix is pushed. Bimanual examination reveals uterine fundal tenderness due to endometritis, and abnormal adnexal tenderness due to salpingitis which is usually, but not necessarily, bilateral. Adnexal swelling is palpable in about one-half of women with acute salpingitis, but evaluation of the adnexae in a patient with marked tenderness is not reliable, even by an experienced examiner. An initial temperature >38°C is found in only about one-third of patients with acute salpingitis, and fever is not required for the diagnosis.

Laboratory findings include elevation of the erythrocyte sedimentation rate (ESR) in 75 percent and elevation of the peripheral white blood cell count in up to 60 percent of patients with acute salpingitis. Microscopic examination of a saline wet-mount preparation of vaginal fluid has revealed more than one polymorphonuclear leukocyte per vaginal epithelial cell in nearly all patients with laparoscopically confirmed salpingitis in Swedish studies. However, exceptions have not been uncommon in U.S. studies of the same population.

Certain clinical manifestations of acute PID have been correlated with etiologic findings. For example, the onset of salpingitis is related to menses in women with gonorrhea or chlamydial infection. Women with gonorrhea or chlamydia-associated salpingitis are significantly younger than women with other forms of salpingitis. Women with chlamydia-associated salpingitis reportedly tend to have an indolent disease with mild symptoms of significantly longer duration and with less fever compared to women who have gonorrhea-associated salpingitis, but paradoxically, those with chlamydia-associated salpingitis have had significantly higher ESR and more severe inflammatory reactions seen at laparoscopy. It is suspected that for all recognized cases of symptomatic *Chlamydia* salpingitis, there is a comparable number of unrecognized cases of indolent subclinical *Chlamydia* salpingitis, and that subclinical chronic or recurrent *Chlamydia* salpingitis may be a major cause of infertility in women.

IUD-associated PID has been much less common since withdrawal of the Dalkon shield from the market. It tends to be indolent and is less often associated with fever, but more often with adnexal masses, than is PID not associated with IUD use.

Perihepatitis and periappendicitis Symptoms of perihepatitis, including pleuritic upper abdominal pain and tenderness, usually localized to the right upper quadrant, occur in 3 to 10 percent of women with acute PID. The onset of symptoms of perihepatitis occurs during or after onset of symptoms of PID and may overshadow the lower abdominal symptoms, leading to a mistaken diagnosis of cholecystitis. In perhaps 5 percent of cases of acute salpingitis, laparoscopy performed early reveals inflammation ranging from edema and erythema of the liver capsule to exudate with fibrinous adhesions between the visceral and parietal peritoneum. When treatment is delayed, and laparoscopy is performed late, dense "violin-string" adhesions are seen over the liver; these cause chronic exertional or positional right upper quadrant pain when traction is placed on the adhesions. Although perihepatitis, also known as the Fitz-Hugh–

Curtis syndrome, was for many years attributed to gonococcal PID, it has been recognized that most cases of perihepatitis have been associated with chlamydial salpingitis. In patients with chlamydial salpingitis, serum microimmunofluorescent antibody titers against *C. trachomatis* are typically much higher when perihepatitis is present than when it is absent, and it has been suggested that repeated chlamydial infections are responsible for perihepatitis.

Physical findings include right upper quadrant tenderness and usually include adnexal tenderness and cervicitis, even in patients whose symptoms are not suggestive of salpingitis.

Liver function tests are nearly always normal, since inflammation is largely limited to the liver capsule, usually sparing the parenchyma. Oral cholecystogram may show nonfunction of the gallbladder, but ultrasonography of the right upper quadrant is normal. The presence of mucopurulent cervicitis and pelvic tenderness in a young woman with subacute pleuritic right upper quadrant pain with normal ultrasonography of the gallbladder points to a diagnosis of perihepatitis.

Periappendicitis (appendiceal serositis without involvement of the intestinal mucosa) has been found in approximately 5 percent of patients undergoing appendectomy for suspected appendicitis, and can occur as a complication of gonococcal or chlamydial salpingitis.

DIAGNOSIS Early diagnosis and initiation of therapy are essential to minimize tubal scarring. Appropriate treatment must not be withheld from patients who have an equivocal diagnosis. Since delay in therapy may lead to progression of tubal scarring, it is better to err on the side of overdiagnosis and overtreatment. On the other hand, it is essential to differentiate between salpingitis and other pelvic pathology, particularly surgical emergencies such as appendicitis and ectopic pregnancy.

No clinical or laboratory finding short of laparoscopy is pathognomonic for salpingitis, and there is reluctance to perform laparoscopy in all cases of suspected salpingitis. Most patients with acute PID have lower abdominal pain of <3 weeks' duration, pelvic tenderness on bimanual pelvic examination, and evidence of lower genital tract infection (e.g., white blood cells outnumber all other cells in the vaginal fluid). Approximately 60 percent of such patients had salpingitis at laparoscopy. Among the patients with these findings, a rectal temperature above 38°C, a palpable adnexal mass, and elevation of the ESR over 15 mm/h also raise the probability of salpingitis, which was found at laparoscopy in 68 percent of patients with one of these additional findings, 90 percent of patients with two or more, and 96 percent of patients with three or more additional findings. However, only 17 percent of all patients with laparoscopy-confirmed salpingitis had three additional findings.

Mucopurulent cervicitis is probably responsible for the presence of neutrophils in vaginal fluid in PID. In a woman with pelvic pain and tenderness, demonstration of an increased number of neutrophils (≥30 per 1000× microscopic field in strands of cervical mucus) increases the predictive value of a clinical diagnosis of acute PID.

Several clinical features other than the presence of cervicitis also favor the diagnosis of acute PID. These include onset with menses, history of recent abnormal menstrual bleeding, presence of an IUD, history of previous salpingitis, and exposure to a male with urethritis. Detection of polymorphonuclear leukocytes in fluid aspirated by culdocentesis supports a diagnosis of suspected salpingitis. Urethritis or proctitis may occur in chlamydial or gonococcal infection but may also represent a urinary tract infection or an intestinal source for the patient's symptoms. Early onset of nausea and vomiting favors appendicitis or other disorders of the gut. A missed menstrual period dictates evaluation for ectopic pregnancy. The more sensitive assays for human beta-chorionic gonadotropin are usually positive. Ultrasonography is sometimes useful to differentiate pelvic abscess from an inflammatory mass involving tubes, ovary, bowel, and omentum, but is not sufficiently sensitive to detect salpingitis.

Laparoscopy is the most specific method for diagnosis of acute salpingitis. Although it may be normal if inflammation is limited to the endosalpinx or endometrium, patients with suspected PID who have normal laparoscopy have a better prognosis, with few if any sequelae, when compared with patients who have abnormal laparoscopic findings. The primary and uncontested value of laparoscopy in women with lower abdominal pain is exclusion of other surgical problems. Table 94-2 clearly shows that the most common and serious problems that may be confused with salpingitis are usually unilateral. Unilateral pain or pelvic mass, though not incompatible with PID, is a strong indication for laparoscopy unless the clinical picture warrants laparotomy instead. Atypical clinical findings such as the absence of lower genital tract infection, a missed menstrual period, or failure to respond to appropriate therapy are other frequent indications for laparoscopy.

TABLE 94-2 Laparoscopic findings in patients with false-positive or false-negative clinical diagnoses of acute PID

False-positive clinical diagnosis		False-negative clinical diagnosis, unexpected PID at laparoscopy	
Laparoscopic diagnosis	Percent	Clinical diagnosis	Percent
Acute appendicitis	24	Ovarian tumor	20
Endometriosis	16	Acute appendicitis	18
Corpus luteum bleeding	12	Ectopic pregnancy	16
Ectopic pregnancy	11	Chronic salpingitis	6
Pelvic adhesions only	7	Acute peritonitis	6
Benign ovarian tumor	7	Endometriosis	5
Chronic salpingitis	6	Uterine myoma	5
Miscellaneous	15	Atypical pelvic pain	6
		Miscellaneous	6

SOURCE: L Jacobsen and L Weström, Am J Obstet Gynecol 105:1088, 1969.

Laparoscopic criteria used for the diagnosis of salpingitis include (1) erythema of the fallopian tube; (2) edema of the fallopian tube; and (3) seropurulent exudate or fresh, easily lysed adhesions at the fimbriated end or on the serosal surface of a fallopian tube. Laparoscopic findings are further scored as mild, where the above manifestations are mild and the tubes are freely movable and patent; moderate, when the above manifestations are more marked, tubes are not freely movable, and patency is uncertain; and severe, when findings consist of an inflammatory mass.

Endometrial biopsy is relatively sensitive and specific for the diagnosis of endometritis when the changes described above are present and are found in at least three-fourths of women with laparoscopically confirmed salpingitis, and absent in women without PID.

The etiologic diagnosis of PID can be further studied by cultures or specimens obtained by endocervical swab, endometrial aspiration, or culdocentesis, or by laparoscopy or laparotomy. Endocervical swab specimens should be examined by Gram stain for neutrophils and gram-negative diplococci and by culture for *N. gonorrhoeae*. The sensitivity of Gram stain is about 60 percent and specificity >95 percent, compared with culture. The endocervical swab specimen should also be tested for *C. trachomatis* by culture, immunofluorescence, or antigen-capture assay. Although isolation of either *N. gonorrhoeae* or *C. trachomatis* from the cervix does not prove that either agent is also present in the upper genital tract, this finding strongly supports the diagnosis of PID. The clinical diagnosis of PID made by expert gynecologists is confirmed by laparoscopy or endometrial biopsy in only about 60 percent of all consecutive patients, but in about 90 percent of those who also have positive cultures for *N. gonorrhoeae* or *C. trachomatis*. There is no evidence that isolation of anaerobes or facultative anaerobes from the cervix or vagina correlates with the presence of these organisms in the upper genital tract in acute PID, but this has not been well studied. The value of culture of culdocentesis and endometrial aspirate specimens is disputed because of the risk of contamination of the specimen with vaginal flora. When laparoscopy is performed, material can be obtained directly from the cul-de-sac or the fimbriated opening of the tube, or by tubal aspiration if pyosalpinx is present. Such specimens should be cultured for anaerobic and facultative pathogens, as well as for *N. gonorrhoeae* and *C. trachomatis*.

TABLE 94-3 Relative activities of the antimicrobial agents most commonly used to treat PID

			Vaginal anaerobes			
	N. gonorrhoeae	*C. trachomatis*	GPC*	GNR†	Facultative GNR	*M. hominis*
Ampicillin/amoxicillin	3+	2+	4+	2+	2+	0
Tetracycline HCl	3+	4+	4+	2+	2+	2+
Doxycycline	3+	4+	4+	3+	2+	2+
Cefoxitin, cefotetan	3+	0	4+	3+	4+	0
Ceftriaxone	4+	0	3+	2+	4+	0
Gentamicin/tobramycin	2+	0	1+	0	4+	2+?
Fluoroquinolones	3 to 4+	Variable	1+	1+	4+	Variable
Clindamycin	1+	2+	4+	4+	0	3+
Metronidazole	0	0	4+	4+	0	0

* GPC = Gram-positive cocci (peptostreptococci).
† GNR = Gram-negative rods (anaerobic GNR include *Bacteroides;* facultative GNR include Enterobacteriaceae, *H. influenzae*).
NOTE: No single antimicrobial agent offers optimal activity against all of these pathogens, but certain combinations (e.g., cefoxitin plus doxycycline, gentamicin plus clindamycin) have complementary activity.

TREATMENT Hospitalization should be considered in all women with PID. Hospitalization is strongly recommended when (1) the diagnosis is uncertain, (2) surgical emergencies such as appendicitis and ectopic pregnancy must be excluded, (3) a pelvic abscess is suspected, (4) severe illness precludes outpatient management, (5) the patient is pregnant, (6) the patient is an adolescent, (7) the patient is assessed as unable to follow or tolerate an outpatient regimen, (8) the patient has failed to respond to outpatient therapy, or (9) clinical follow-up after 48 to 72 h of instituting antibiotic treatment cannot be arranged. The treatment of choice is not established. No single agent is active against the entire spectrum of pathogens (Table 94-3). Several antimicrobial combinations do provide a broad spectrum of activity against the major pathogens in vitro, but many have not been adequately evaluated for clinical efficacy in PID.

Examples of combination regimens with broad activity against major pathogens in PID

1 Doxycycline 100 mg, twice a day, IV, plus cefoxitin 2.0 g, four times a day, IV, or cefotetan 2.0 g, every 12 h, IV. These drugs should be continued IV for at least 48 h after the patient improves. Doxycycline should be continued in a dose of 100 mg by mouth, twice a day, after discharge from the hospital to complete 14 days of therapy. This regimen provides excellent coverage for *N. gonorrhoeae,* including penicillinase-producing *N. gonorrhoeae* (PPNG), and *C. trachomatis.*
2 Clindamycin 900 mg, every 8 h, IV, plus gentamicin 2.0 mg/kg, IV, followed by 1.5 mg/kg, every 8 h, IV, in patients with normal renal function. These drugs should be continued for at least 48 h after the patient improves. After discharge from the hospital doxycycline 100 mg orally, twice a day, should be given to complete 14 days of therapy. This regimen provides good activity against anaerobes and facultative gram-negative rods, and is active against *C. trachomatis* and *N. gonorrhoeae*. Doxycycline provides definitive therapy for chlamydial infection.

Patients who are not hospitalized should also receive a combined regimen with broad activity, such as ceftriaxone 250 mg, IM, followed by doxycycline 100 mg, by mouth, twice a day for 14 days. Cefoxitin, 2.0 g, IM, given concurrently with probenecid 1.0 g, orally, could be used in place of ceftriaxone. Tetracycline could also be used in a dose of 500 mg, four times a day, in place of doxycycline, but requires more frequent dosing which is a major drawback in the treatment of PID.

Management of sexual partners All persons who are sexual partners of patients with PID should be examined for STD and promptly treated with a regimen effective against uncomplicated gonococcal and chlamydial infection.

Follow-up All patients who are treated as outpatients should be clinically reevaluated in 48 to 72 h. Those not responding favorably should be hospitalized. A culture to test whether cure has been achieved should be performed as needed.

Removal of an intrauterine device Although possible benefit of IUD removal on the response of acute salpingitis to antimicrobial therapy and on the risk of recurrent salpingitis has not been proven, removal of the IUD soon after antimicrobial therapy has been initiated seems reasonable. When an IUD is removed, contraceptive counseling is necessary.

Surgery Surgery is necessary only rarely for treatment of salpingitis, except in the face of life-threatening infection such as rupture or threatened rupture of a tuboovarian abscess, or for drainage of an abscess. Ultrasonography is useful for diagnosing and following pelvic abscesses. When surgery is performed, conservative procedures are usually sufficient. Pelvic abscesses can often be drained by posterior colpotomy, and peritoneal lavage can be used if there is generalized peritonitis.

PROGNOSIS In a cooperative trial in the United States, nearly 20 percent of women treated for PID on an ambulatory basis with IM penicillin followed by a 10-day course of ampicillin, or with a 10-day course of tetracycline alone, were judged to be clinical failures.

Among 900 women who underwent long-term follow-up for a mean period of 8 years after successful treatment of the acute episode with various regimens in Sweden, late sequelae included infertility due to bilateral tubal occlusion, ectopic pregnancy due to tubal scarring without occlusion, chronic pelvic pain, and recurrent salpingitis. Chronic pain lasting longer than 6 months was seen in 18 percent of patients and infertility due to tubal occlusion in 17 percent; 4 percent of pregnancies that did occur were ectopic, representing approximately a sixfold increase over the expected rate of ectopic pregnancies. The rate of infertility after salpingitis was found to be related to age of the patient, duration of symptoms when treatment was started, severity of salpingitis by laparoscopy at the time of diagnosis, and number of episodes of salpingitis. The rate of infertility due to tubal occlusion among women exposed to a chance of pregnancy was 14 percent for women 15 to 24 years of age and 26 percent for women 25 to 34 years of age; the risk for women of all ages combined was 11 percent after one episode of salpingitis, 23 percent after two episodes, and 54 percent after three or more episodes. The risk of infertility after gonococcal salpingitis was comparable to the risk after chlamydial salpingitis in one small prospective study.

A striking relationship has also been shown in several countries between infertility due to tubal occlusion and the prevalence and titer of antibody to *C. trachomatis*. Recurrent salpingitis has been seen in approximately 15 to 25 percent of women treated for salpingitis in various studies.

PREVENTION Prevention of PID depends first on the effective control of gonococcal and chlamydial infection. Effective methods include promotion of changes in sexual behavior and use of barrier contraceptives while providing ready access to modern methods of diagnosis and effective treatment, and treatment of sex partners to control further spread. The decline in popularity of the intrauterine device, particularly in nulliparous women, has undoubtedly helped to reduce the incidence of PID. It is also possible, but not proven, that use of oral contraceptives and avoidance of vaginal douching might reduce the risk of PID.

The complications of salpingitis can be minimized by early diagnosis and prompt treatment. It seems logical, but is unproven, that broad-spectrum therapy effective against all of the common causes of PID would offer the best outcome. Similarly, hospitalization to ensure rest and adequate compliance may improve the rather dismal long-term prognosis for tubal function. One placebo-controlled study showed that concurrent anti-inflammatory therapy with prednisolone hastened the reduction of acute inflammatory changes but did not improve the end results as measured by fertility, hysterosalpingographic findings, or chronic pain. However, the potential value of anti-inflammatory therapy remains to be evaluated adequately.

REFERENCES

CATES WJ et al: Worldwide patterns of infertility: Is Africa different? Lancet 2:596, 1985

CENTERS FOR DISEASE CONTROL: 1989 sexually transmitted diseases treatment guidelines. Morb Mort Week Rep 38 (Suppl 8):1, 1989

ESCHENBACH DA et al: Polymicrobial etiology of acute pelvic inflammatory disease. N Engl J Med 293:166, 1975

FALK V et al: Genital tuberculosis in women. Am J Obstet Gynecol 138:974, 1980

HADGU A et al: Predicting acute PID: A multivariate analysis. Am J Obstet Gynecol 155:954, 1986

KIVIAT N et al: Endometrial histopathology in patients with culture-proven upper genital tract infection and laparoscopically diagnosed acute salpingitis. Am J Clin Pathol 1990 (in press)

MÅRDH PA et al: *Chlamydia trachomatis* infection in patients with acute salpingitis. N Engl J Med 296:1377, 1977

MØLLER BR et al: Pelvic infection after elective abortion associated with *Chlamydia trachomatis*. Obstet Gynecol 59:210, 1982

PAAVONEN J et al: Microbiological and histological findings in acute pelvic inflammatory disease. Br J Obstet Gynaecol 94:454, 1987

PLUMMER FA et al: Postpartum upper genital tract infections in Nairobi, Kenya: Epidemiology, etiology, and risk factors. J Infect Dis 156:92, 1987

ST JOHN RK, BROWN ST (eds): International symposium on pelvic inflammatory disease. Am J Obstet Gynecol 138:845, 1980

SVENSSON L et al: Differences in some clinical and laboratory parameters in acute salpingitis related to culture and serologic findings. Am J Obstet Gynecol 138:1017, 1980

——— et al: Infertility after acute salpingitis—with special reference to *Chlamydia trachomatis*-associated infections. Fertil Steril 40:322, 1983

WASSERHEIT JN et al: Microbial causes of proven pelvic inflammatory disease and efficacy of clindamycin with tobramycin. Ann Intern Med 104:187, 1986

WESTRÖM L, MÅRDH PA: Acute pelvic inflammatory disease, in *Sexually Transmitted Diseases*, KK Holmes et al (eds). New York, McGraw-Hill, 1989, pp 593–613

WØLNER-HANSSEN P et al: Outpatient treatment of pelvic inflammatory disease with cefoxitin and doxycycline. Obstet Gynecol 71:595, 1988

——— et al: Atypical pelvic inflammatory disease: Subacute, chronic, or subclinical upper genital tract infections in women, in *Sexually Transmitted Diseases*, KK Holmes et al (eds). New York, McGraw-Hill 1990, pp 615–620

95 URINARY TRACT INFECTIONS AND PYELONEPHRITIS

WALTER E. STAMM / MARVIN TURCK

DEFINITIONS Acute infections of the urinary tract can be subdivided into two general anatomic categories: lower tract infection (urethritis, cystitis, and prostatitis) and upper tract infection (acute pyelonephritis). Infections at these various sites may occur together or independently, and may be asymptomatic or present as the clinical syndromes outlined below.

Microbiologically, urinary tract infection exists when pathogenic microorganisms are detected in the urine, urethra, kidney, or prostate. In most instances, growth of more than 10^5 organisms per milliliter from a properly collected midstream "clean catch" urine sample indicates infection. However, significant bacteriuria may be absent in some circumstances when true urinary infection exists. Especially in symptomatic patients, a smaller number of bacteria (10^2 to 10^4 per milliliter of midstream urine) may accompany infection. In urine specimens obtained by suprapubic aspiration or "in and out" catheterization, or from a patient with an indwelling catheter, colony counts of 10^2 to 10^4 per milliliter generally indicate infection. Conversely, colony counts in excess of 10^5 per milliliter of midstream urine are occasionally due to specimen contamination.

Recurrent infections after antibiotic therapy can be due to the originally infecting strain, as judged by species identification, serotype, and antibiogram, or to reinfection with a new strain. "Same strain" recurrent infections that occur within 2 weeks of cessation of therapy can result from unresolved renal or prostatic infection or from unresolved vaginal colonization that leads to rapid reinfection of the bladder.

Symptoms of dysuria, urgency, and frequency unaccompanied by significant bacteriuria have been termed the acute urethral syndrome. Although widely used, this term lacks anatomic precision because many cases of urethral syndrome are in actuality bladder infections. Moreover, since the causative agent can usually be identified in these patients, the term *syndrome,* implying unknown causation, is inappropriate.

Chronic pyelonephritis refers to chronic interstitial nephritis believed to result from bacterial infection of the kidney (see Chap. 229). Many noninfectious diseases also cause an interstitial nephritis indistinguishable pathologically from chronic pyelonephritis.

ACUTE INFECTIONS OF THE URINARY TRACT: URETHRITIS, CYSTITIS, AND PYELONEPHRITIS

EPIDEMIOLOGY Epidemiologically, urinary tract infections should be subdivided into catheter-associated (or nosocomial) infections and non-catheter-associated (or community-acquired) infections. In either category, infections may be symptomatic or asymptomatic. Acute infections in noncatheterized patients occur very commonly, especially in women, and account for over 6 million office visits annually in the United States. These infections occur in 1 to 3 percent of schoolgirls, and then increase markedly in incidence with the onset of sexual activity in adolescence. The vast majority of acute symptomatic infections occur in young women. Acute symptomatic urinary infections are rare in men under the age of 50. The occurrence of asymptomatic bacteriuria parallels that of symptomatic infection and is rare in men under 50, but is common in women between the ages of 20 and 50. Asymptomatic bacteriuria is most common in elderly men and women.

ETIOLOGY Many different microorganisms can infect the urinary tract, but by far the most common agents are the gram-negative bacilli. *Escherichia coli* causes approximately 80 percent of acute infections in patients without urologic abnormalities or calculi. Other gram-negative rods, especially *Proteus* and *Klebsiella* and occasionally *Enterobacter, Serratia,* and *Pseudomonas,* account for a smaller proportion of uncomplicated infections. These organisms assume increasing importance in recurrent infections and infections associated with urologic manipulation, calculi, or obstruction. They play a major role in nosocomial, catheter-associated infections (see below). *Proteus* species, by virtue of urease production, and *Klebsiella* species, through production of extracellular slime and polysaccharides, predispose to stone formation and are isolated more frequently from patients with calculi.

Gram-positive cocci play a lesser role in urinary tract infections. However, *Staphylococcus saprophyticus,* a novobiocin-resistant, coagulase-negative staphylococcus, accounts for 10 to 15 percent of acute symptomatic urinary tract infections in young females. Enterococci and *Staphylococcus aureus* cause infections in patients with renal stones or previous instrumentation. Isolation of *S. aureus* from the urine should arouse suspicion of bacteremic infection of the kidney.

About one-third of women with dysuria and frequency have either a nonsignificant number of bacteria in midstream urine cultures or completely sterile cultures, and have been previously defined as having the urethral syndrome. About three-quarters of these women have pyuria, while one-quarter have no pyuria and little objective evidence of infection. In the women with pyuria, two groups of pathogens account for the majority of infections. Low quantities (10^2 to 10^4 bacteria per milliliter) of typical bacterial uropathogens such as *E. coli, S. saprophyticus, Klebsiella,* or *Proteus* in midstream urine specimens are found in the majority of these women. They are probably the causative agents in these women because they can usually be isolated from a suprapubic aspirate, are associated with pyuria, and respond to appropriate antimicrobial therapy. In other women with acute urinary symptoms, pyuria, and sterile urine (even on suprapubic aspiration), sexually transmitted urethritis-producing agents such as *Chlamydia trachomatis, Neisseria gonorrhoeae,* and herpes simplex virus are important etiologic agents. These sexually transmitted agents are more frequently found in young, sexually active women with new sexual partners.

Viruses may increase the kidney's susceptibility to infection with gram-negative bacteria. In humans, viruses (cytomegalovirus, for example) are most commonly recovered from the urine without evidence of acute urinary disease, although some adenoviruses cause acute hemorrhagic cystitis. *Candida* and other fungi may colonize the urine of catheterized patients or diabetics, and in some patients cause acute symptomatic infection.

PATHOGENESIS AND SOURCES OF INFECTION The urinary tract should be viewed as a single anatomic unit connected by a continuous column of urine that extends from the urethra to the kidney. In the vast majority of infections, bacteria gain access to the bladder via the urethra. Ascent of bacteria from the bladder may then follow and is probably the usual pathway for most renal parenchymal infections.

The vaginal introitus and distal urethra are normally colonized with diphtheroids, streptococcal species, lactobacilli, and staphylococcal species, but not with the enteric gram-negative bacilli that commonly cause urinary tract infections. In females prone to development of cystitis, however, enteric gram-negative organisms residing in the bowel colonize the introitus, the periurethral skin, and the distal urethra prior to and during episodes of bacteriuria. Factors predisposing to periurethral colonization with gram-negative bacilli remain poorly understood but probably involve alteration of the normal perineal flora by antibiotics or by contraceptives, especially diaphragm and spermicide. Small numbers of periurethral bacteria probably gain entry to the bladder frequently, facilitated in some women by urethral massage during intercourse. Whether bladder infection ensues then depends upon interaction between the pathogenicity of the strain, the inoculum size, and local and systemic host defense mechanisms.

Under normal circumstances, bacteria placed in the bladder are rapidly cleared. This results partly from the flushing and dilutional effects of voiding, but also from direct antibacterial properties of urine and the bladder mucosa. Due mostly to high urea concentration and high osmolarity, the bladder urine of many normal persons inhibits or kills bacteria. Prostatic secretions possess antibacterial properties as well. Polymorphonuclear leukocytes in the bladder wall also appear to play a role in clearing bacteriuria. The role of locally produced antibody remains unclear. Hematogenous pyelonephritis occurs most often in debilitated patients who either have chronic illnesses or who are receiving immunosuppressive therapy. Staphylococcal pyelonephritis may follow bacteremia from distant foci of infection in the bone, skin, endothelium, or elsewhere.

CONDITIONS AFFECTING PATHOGENESIS **Gender and sexual activity** The female urethra appears particularly prone to colonization with colonic gram-negative bacilli, owing to its proximity to the anus, its short length (about 4 cm), and its termination beneath the labia. Urethral massage, as occurs during sexual intercourse, causes introduction of bacteria into the bladder, and appears to be important in the pathogenesis of urinary infections in younger women. (Voiding after intercourse has been shown to reduce the risk of cystitis, probably because it promotes eradication of bacteria introduced during intercourse.) In addition, diaphragm and spermicide use dramatically alter the normal introital bacterial flora and have been associated with a marked increase in vaginal colonization with *E. coli* and risk of urinary infection. In males, prostatitis or urethral obstruction due to prostatic hypertrophy are important factors predisposing to bacteriuria. Homosexuality also predisposes to an increased risk of cystitis, probably associated with rectal intercourse.

Pregnancy Depending on socioeconomic status, urinary infections are detected in 2 to 8 percent of pregnant women. In particular, symptomatic upper tract infections occur more commonly during pregnancy; fully 20 to 30 percent of pregnant women with asymptomatic bacteriuria subsequently develop pyelonephritis. This predisposition to upper tract infection during pregnancy results from the decreased ureteral tone, decreased ureteral peristalsis, and temporary incompetence of the vesicoureteral valves seen in pregnancy. Bladder catheterization during or after delivery causes additional infections. Cystitis and pyelonephritis are no more common in women with toxemia of pregnancy than in other pregnant women. An increased prevalence of prematurity and newborn mortality may result from urinary infections during pregnancy, particularly those involving the upper urinary tract.

Obstruction Any impediment to the free flow of urine—tumor, stricture, stone, or prostatic hypertrophy—results in hydronephrosis and greatly increased frequency of urinary tract infection. Infection superimposed on urinary tract obstruction may lead to rapid destruction of renal tissue. It is of utmost importance, therefore, when infection is present, to repair obstructive lesions. On the other hand, with minor degrees of obstruction that are not progressive or associated with infection, great caution should be exercised in attempting surgical correction. The introduction of infection in such patients may be more damaging than uncorrected minor obstructions that do not significantly impair renal function.

Neurogenic bladder dysfunction Interference with the nerve supply to the bladder, as in spinal cord injury, tabes dorsalis, multiple sclerosis, diabetes, or other diseases, may be associated with urinary tract infection. The infection may be initiated by the use of catheters for bladder drainage and is favored by the prolonged stasis of urine in the bladder. An additional factor often present in these patients is bone demineralization due to immobilization, which causes hypercalciuria, calculus formation, and obstructive uropathy.

Vesicoureteral reflux This condition is defined as reflux of urine from the bladder cavity up into the ureters and sometimes into the renal pelvis. It occurs during voiding or with elevation of pressure in the bladder. In practice, vesicoureteral reflux exists when retrograde movement of radiopaque or radioactive material can be demonstrated. However, since a fluid connection between the bladder and kidney always exists in the patent urinary system, during infections some retrograde movement of bacteria probably occurs normally but is not detected by radiologic techniques. An anatomically impaired vesicoureteral junction facilitates reflux of bacteria.

Vesicoureteral reflux is common in children with anatomic abnormalities of the urinary tract and in children with anatomically normal but infected urinary tracts. In the latter group, reflux disappears with advancing age and probably results from causes other than urinary infection. Follow-up of children with urinary tract infection who were found to have reflux establishes that renal damage correlates with marked reflux, not with infection.

The routine search for reflux would be aided by development of noninvasive tests applicable to young children, where the need is greatest. In the meantime, it appears reasonable to search for reflux in anyone with unexplained failure of renal growth or renal scarring, because urinary tract infection per se is an insufficient explanation for these abnormalities. On the other hand, it is doubtful that all children with recurrent urinary tract infections but normal urinary tracts on pyelography should be subjected to voiding cystoureterography merely to detect the rare patient with marked reflux that did not reveal itself on the intravenous pyelogram.

Bacterial virulence factors Bacterial virulence factors influence the likelihood that a given strain, once introduced into the bladder, will cause urinary tract infection. Not all *E. coli* are equally able to infect the intact urinary tract. The majority of strains that cause symptomatic urinary tract infections in noncatheterized patients belong to a small number of serogroups (O, K, and H), produce hemolysin, and share certain other "uropathogenic" properties. Adherence of bacteria to uroepithelial cells is a critical first step in the initiation of infection. For both *E. coli* and *Proteus,* fimbriae (hairlike surface appendages) mediate bacterial attachment to specific receptors on epithelial cells. Nearly all *E. coli* strains that cause pyelonephritis in patients with anatomically normal urinary tracts possess a particular pilus (the P pilus or gal-gal pilus) that mediates attachment to the digalactoside portion of glycosphingolipids present on uroepithelium. Strains that produce pyelonephritis are also usually hemolysin producers, have aerobactin (a siderophore for scavenging iron), and are resistant to the bactericidal action of human serum. Since most strains that produce acute pyelonephritis in the intact host possess all or nearly all of these virulence factors, the concept has arisen that a small number of uropathogenic clones cause most such cases of infection. In patients with structural or functional abnormalities of the urinary tract, infections are frequently caused by bacterial strains that lack these uropathogenic properties, implying that these properties are not needed for infection of the compromised urinary tract.

Genetic factors Increasing evidence suggests that genetic factors influence susceptibility to urinary infection. The number and type of receptors on uroepithelial cells to which bacteria may attach is at least in part genetically determined. Many of these antigens are found on both erythrocytes and uroepithelial cells. For example, P fimbriae mediate attachment of *E. coli* to P-positive erythrocytes and are present on nearly all strains causing acute uncomplicated pyelonephritis. Conversely, P-negative individuals, who lack these receptors, have a decreased likelihood of pyelonephritis. It has also been demonstrated that nonsecretors of blood group antigens may have an increased risk of recurrent urinary infection.

LOCALIZATION OF INFECTION Infections involving the upper urinary tract usually cause a significant rise in serum antibodies directed against the O antigen of the infecting strain. They also produce a temporary defect in renal concentrating ability in many patients, and may be associated with formation of leukocyte casts. Lower tract infections rarely result in increased antibody titers, concentrating defects, or white cell casts. Unfortunately, these methods of distinguishing renal parenchymal infection from cystitis are neither reliable nor convenient enough for routine clinical use. More sensitive tests for distinguishing pyelonephritis from cystitis (bilateral ureteral catheterization and the bladder wash-out technique originated by Fairley) are inherently invasive and too complex for routine clinical practice. The development of a simpler and clinically applicable test to separate upper and lower tract infections based upon antibody coating of bacteria in the urine has been studied. In this test, urinary bacteria from patients with pyelonephritis demonstrate antibody coating on their surface when they have been exposed to a fluorescein-labeled antihuman globulin and are viewed under a fluorescence microscope. No surface antibodies can be seen on bacteria from patients with cystitis. This antibody response consists mainly of IgG. The antibody-coated bacteria test does not have sufficient sensitivity and specificity to be of value in the routine clinical management of patients. An elevated C-reactive protein often accompanies acute pyelonephritis and rarely is seen in cystitis, but this acute phase reactant is nonspecific and occurs in infections other than pyelonephritis as well.

CLINICAL PRESENTATION Clinical signs and symptoms cannot be relied upon to diagnose urinary tract infection accurately or to localize the site of infection. Many patients with significant bacteriuria (including some with upper tract infection) have no symptoms at all. Of those with significant bacteriuria and symptoms of cystitis, about one-half have lower tract infection and about one-half have clinically silent upper tract infection that is evident only upon performing localization studies. Clinical symptoms and signs of pyelonephritis, though usually suggestive, do not always indicate upper tract infection. Finally, among women presenting with acute dysuria and frequency, only 60 to 70 percent have significant bacteriuria, but the majority of those without significant bacteriuria also have urinary tract or urethral infections.

Enumeration of the number of bacteria in the urine is an extremely important diagnostic procedure. In symptomatic infections of the urinary tract, bacteria are usually demonstrable in the urine in large numbers. Quantitative estimation of the number of bacteria in voided urine specimens as a rule makes it possible to distinguish contaminants from true bacteriuria, and 10^5 or more bacteria per milliliter has been the criterion traditionally used for this purpose. However, in symptomatic women with pyuria, counts of 10^2 to 10^4 *E. coli, Klebsiella, Proteus,* or *S. saprophyticus* per milliliter of midstream urine usually indicate infection, not contamination, and should not be disregarded. In asymptomatic patients, two or three consecutive urine specimens should be examined bacteriologically before instituting therapy, and 10^5 or more per milliliter of a single species should be demonstrable in the repeated specimens. Since the large number of bacteria in the bladder urine is due in part to bacterial multiplication during residence in the bladder cavity, samples of urine from the ureters or renal pelvis may contain fewer than 10^5 bacteria per milliliter and yet indicate infection. Similarly, the presence of bacteriuria of any degree in suprapubic aspirates or of 10^2 or more bacteria per milliliter of urine obtained by catheterization usually indicates infection. In some circumstances (antibiotics, high urea concentration, high osmolarity, low pH), urine will inhibit bacterial multiplication, resulting in a lower number of bacteria in the presence of infection. For this reason, antiseptic solutions should not be used in washing the periurethral area prior to collection of the urine specimen. Water diuresis or recent voiding also reduces the bacterial counts in urine. Rapid methods of detection of bacteriuria have been developed as alternatives to standard culture methods. They detect bacterial growth using photometry, bioluminescence, or other means and provide results rapidly, usually in 1 to 2 h. These methods generally achieve a sensitivity of 95 to 98 percent and >99 percent negative predictive value as compared with urine cultures when bacteriuria is defined as 10^5 cfu/mL. However, the sensitivity of these tests falls to 60 to 80 percent when bacteriuria of 10^2 to 10^4 colony forming units per milliliter is the standard of comparison.

Microscopy of urine from symptomatic patients can be of great diagnostic value. Microscopic bacteriuria, which is best assessed using Gram-stained, uncentrifuged urine, is found in over 90 percent of specimens from patients whose infections have colony counts of 10^5 per milliliter, and is a very specific finding. However, bacteria cannot usually be detected microscopically in lower colony count infections (10^2 to 10^4 per milliliter). The presence of bacteria on urinary microscopy is firm evidence of infection, but its absence does not exclude the diagnosis. When carefully sought using a chamber count microscopy method, pyuria is a highly sensitive indicator of urinary tract infection in symptomatic patients. Its absence should cause the diagnosis to be questioned. The leukocyte esterase "dipstick" method is less sensitive than microscopy in identifying pyuria, but is a useful alternative where microscopy is not available.

Cystitis Patients with dysuria, frequency, urgency, and suprapubic pain usually have cystitis. The urine often becomes grossly cloudy, malodorous, and, in about 30 percent of cases, bloody. White cells and bacteria should be present on examination of the unspun urine in most patients. However, some women with cystitis have only 10^2 to 10^4 bacteria per milliliter of urine, which cannot be seen on Gram's stain of unspun urine. Physical examination generally reveals only a tender urethra or suprapubic tenderness. If a genital lesion or a vaginal discharge is present, especially with fewer than 10^5 bacteria per milliliter on culture, causes of urethritis, vaginitis, or cervicitis such as *C. trachomatis,* gonorrhea, *Trichomonas, Can-*

dida, and *Herpesvirus hominis* should be considered. Prominent systemic manifestations like fever over 38.3°C (101°F), nausea, vomiting, and costovertebral angle tenderness usually indicate concomitant renal infection. However, the absence of these findings does not ensure that infection is limited to the bladder and urethra.

Acute pyelonephritis Symptoms generally develop rapidly over a few hours or a day and include fever which is often 39.4°C (103°F) or greater, shaking chills, nausea, vomiting, and diarrhea. Symptoms of cystitis may or may not be present. Besides fever, tachycardia, and generalized muscle tenderness, physical examination reveals marked tenderness on deep pressure in one or both costovertebral areas or on deep abdominal palpation. In some patients, signs and symptoms of gram-negative sepsis predominate. Most patients have significant leukocytosis, pyuria with leukocyte casts in the urine, and bacteria on a Gram's stain of unspun urine. Hematuria may be present during the acute phase of the disease, but if it persists after acute manifestations of infection have subsided, a stone, tumor, or tuberculosis should be considered.

Except in individuals with papillary necrosis or urinary obstruction, the manifestations of acute pyelonephritis usually subside within a few days, even without specific antibacterial therapy. However, despite the absence of symptoms, bacteriuria or pyuria may persist. With severe pyelonephritis, fever subsides more slowly and may not disappear for several days, even after appropriate antibiotic treatment has been instituted.

Urethritis Approximately 30 percent of women with acute dysuria, frequency, and pyuria have midstream urine cultures that show either no growth or nonsignificant bacterial growth. Clinically, these women cannot be readily distinguished from those with cystitis. In these women distinction should be made between those having sexually transmitted pathogens such as *C. trachomatis, Neisseria gonorrhoeae,* or herpes simplex virus, and those having low-count *E. coli* or staphylococcal infection of the urethra and bladder. Women with a gradual onset of illness, no hematuria, no suprapubic pain, and a history of more than 7 days of symptoms should be suspected of having chlamydial infection. The additional history of a recent sex partner change, especially if the patient's partner has recently had chlamydial or gonococcal urethritis, should heighten the suspicion of a sexually transmitted infection, as would the finding of mucopurulent cervicitis. Gross hematuria, suprapubic pain, abrupt onset of illness, a duration of illness of less than 3 days, and a history of previous urinary tract infections favor *E. coli* or staphylococcal infection.

Catheter-associated urinary tract infections Bacteriuria occurs in at least 10 to 20 percent of hospitalized patients with indwelling urethral catheters. The risk of infection is about 3 to 5 percent per day of catheterization. *Proteus, Pseudomonas, Klebsiella,* and *Serratia,* in addition to *E. coli,* usually cause these infections. Many infecting strains show marked antimicrobial resistance compared with organisms that cause community-acquired urinary infections. Factors associated with an increased risk of infection include female sex, lengthy period of catheterization, severe underlying illness, faulty catheter care, and poorly trained nursing personnel.

Infection occurs when bacteria reach the bladder by one of two routes: by migrating through the column of urine in the catheter lumen (intraluminal route); or by moving up the mucous sheath outside the catheter (periurethral route). Hospital-acquired pathogens reach the patient's catheter or urine-collecting system on the hands of hospital personnel, in contaminated solutions or irrigants, and via contaminated instruments or disinfectants. Entry of bacteria into the catheter system usually occurs at the catheter–collecting tube junction or at the drainage bag portal. Bacteria then ascend intraluminally into the bladder. More often, the patient's own bowel flora migrate to the perineal skin and periurethral area and reach the bladder via the external surface of the catheter. This route is particularly common in women.

Most catheter-associated infections appear to be benign. They cause minimal symptoms, no fever, and often resolve after withdrawal of the catheter. The frequency of upper tract infection associated with catheter-induced bacteriuria is unknown. Gram-negative bacteremia, which follows 1 to 2 percent of cases of catheter-associated bacteriuria, is the most significantly recognized complication of catheter-induced urinary infections. The catheterized urinary tract has repeatedly been demonstrated to be the most common source of gram-negative bacteremia in hospitalized patients. It has also been suggested that bacteriuria in hospitalized catheterized patients is associated with an adjusted increased relative risk of death of approximately threefold compared with similar patients without bacteriuria.

Catheter-associated urinary tract infections can be partially prevented in patients catheterized less than 2 weeks by use of a sterile closed collecting system, attention to aseptic technique during insertion and care of the catheter, use of meatal antiseptic ointments, and by measures to minimize cross infection. Despite these precautions, the majority of patients catheterized longer than 2 weeks develop bacteriuria. The optimal treatment for such patients has not been established. Removal of the catheter and a short course of antibiotics to which the organism is susceptible is probably the best course of action and nearly always eradicates the bacteriuria. If the catheter cannot be removed, antibiotic therapy usually proves to be unsuccessful and may result in infection with a more resistant strain. In this situation, the bacteriuria should be ignored unless the patient develops symptoms or is at high risk of developing bacteremia. In these cases, systemic antibiotics or urinary bladder antiseptics may reduce the degree of bacteriuria and the likelihood of bacteremia. In patients who require long-term catheterization, sterile intermittent in-and-out catheterization performed by a nurse or by the patient results in fewer infections than does continuous indwelling catheterization.

DIAGNOSTIC TESTING Although many authorities have recommended that urine culture and antimicrobial susceptibility testing be performed in any patient with a suspected urinary tract infection, it may be more cost-effective to manage patients who have symptoms and urinalysis findings characteristic of acute uncomplicated cystitis without an initial urine culture. We recommend that patients with symptoms and signs of acute cystitis in whom no complicating factors are present should have urinary microscopy (or alternatively, a leukocyte esterase test or rapid filtration-stain test) performed. If positive for pyuria, hematuria, and/or bacteriuria, these tests provide sufficient documentation of infection that a urine culture and susceptibility testing can be omitted and the patient treated empirically. Urine culture should be obtained, however, in patients in whom symptoms and urine examination findings leave the diagnosis of cystitis in question. Pretherapy cultures and susceptibility testing are also essential in the management of patients with suspected upper tract infections and those in whom complicating factors are present, since in these situations a variety of pathogens may be present and antibiotic therapy is best tailored to the individual organism.

TREATMENT Several therapeutic principles should underlie treatment of urinary tract infections:

1. In most circumstances a quantitative urine culture, a positive Gram stain, or an alternative rapid diagnostic test should be obtained to confirm infection before starting treatment. When cultures are obtained, antimicrobial sensitivity testing should be used to direct therapy.
2. Factors predisposing to infection, such as obstruction, neurogenic bladder, calculi, etc., should be identified and corrected if possible.
3. Relief of clinical symptoms does not always indicate bacteriologic cure.
4. After completion of therapy, each treatment episode should be classified as a failure (bacteriuria not eradicated during therapy or upon the immediate posttreatment culture) or a cure (resolution of symptoms and elimination of bacteriuria). Recurrent infections should be classified as same strain or different strain and early or late.
5. In general, uncomplicated infections confined to the lower urinary tract respond to low doses and short courses of therapy, while upper tract infections require longer periods of treatment. After

therapy, early recurrences with the same strain may result from an unresolved upper tract focus of infection but often (especially after short-course therapy) result from persistent vaginal colonization rather than from recurrent bladder infection. Recurrences that occur more than 2 weeks after the cessation of therapy are nearly always reinfections, even though some may be with the same strain.

6 Community-acquired infections, especially initial infections, are nearly always due to antibiotic-sensitive strains.

7 Patients with repeated infections, instrumentation, or recent hospitalization should be suspected of harboring resistant strains.

The anatomic location of a urinary tract infection greatly influences success or failure of a therapeutic agent. Bladder bacteriuria (cystitis) can usually be eliminated with nearly any antimicrobial to which the infecting strain is sensitive; as little as a single dose of 500-mg intramuscular kanamycin eliminates bladder bacteriuria in most patients. A 7-day course of therapy with oral drugs appears more than adequate. With upper tract infections, however, single-dose therapy fails in the majority of cases and even a 7-day course will be unsuccessful in many patients. Longer periods of treatment (2 to 6 weeks) aimed at eradicating a persistent focus of infection may be necessary in some cases.

In *acute uncomplicated cystitis,* more than 90 percent of infections are due to *E. coli,* and although resistance patterns vary geographically, most strains are sensitive to many antibiotics. Single-dose trimethoprim-sulfamethoxazole (4 to 6 single-strength tablets), trimethoprim (400 mg), and sulfa alone (2.0 g) have been used successfully to treat acute uncomplicated episodes of cystitis. A single 3-g dose of amoxicillin (amoxicilline) appears to result in lower cure rates than the other three agents, especially in women infected with amoxicillin-resistant strains. In most areas, about one-third of *E. coli* strains causing acute cystitis are amoxicillin-resistant. The advantages of single-dose therapy include less expense, ensured compliance, fewer side effects, and perhaps less intense selective pressure for emergence of resistant organisms in the gut or vaginal or perineal flora. However, two studies suggest that more recurrences with the same strain occur shortly after single-dose therapy than after longer treatment and that single-dose therapy does not effectively eradicate vaginal colonization with *E. coli.* Nevertheless, single-dose therapy does appear safe and efficacious for women presenting with *acute uncomplicated cystitis.* Single-dose therapy should be used only in reliable patients, in whom posttreatment follow-up can be ensured, and in patients in whom symptoms have been present for less than 10 days. Three days of therapy may preserve the lower side effects rate of single-dose therapy but may improve efficacy. Single-dose therapy should not be used in women with symptoms or signs of pyelonephritis and in women with urologic abnormalities or stones, or in women with previous infections due to antibiotic-resistant organisms. In these populations, 7 days of therapy with the antimicrobials listed above should be given. Alternatively, broader spectrum agents such as an oral cephalosporin, norfloxacin, or ciprofloxacin can be used. Males with urinary tract infection often have urologic abnormalities or prostatic involvement and positive antibody-coated-bacterial bacteriuria, and hence are not candidates for single-dose or 3-day therapy.

Treatment of the acute urethritis in women depends upon the etiologic agent involved. In chlamydial infection, doxycycline (100 mg orally bid for 7 days) should be used. Women with acute dysuria and frequency, negative urine cultures, and no pyuria do not usually respond to antimicrobial agents.

Acute pyelonephritis without accompanying clinical evidence of calculi or urologic disease is due to *E. coli* in most cases. Although the optimal route and duration of therapy have not been established, a 10- to 14-day course of trimethoprim-sulfamethoxazole, trimethoprim alone, an aminoglycoside, or a cephalosporin usually provides adequate therapy. Ampicillin or amoxicillin should not be used as initial therapy since 20 to 30 percent of *E. coli* are now resistant in vitro. Intravenous antibiotics, at least for the first several days of treatment, should probably be given to most patients, but minimally symptomatic patients can be treated with 2 weeks of oral antibiotics. Some patients relapse following therapy and should be investigated to determine whether unrecognized suppurative foci, calculi, or urologic disease is present. If not, treatment should be extended to 2 to 6 weeks to eliminate a presumed upper tract focus causing recurrent bacteriuria.

When suspected *gram-negative sepsis* complicates acute pyelonephritis, hospitalization, prompt parenteral therapy with an aminoglycoside, and ancillary measures to treat sepsis should be provided (see Chap. 89). When the antibiotic sensitivities of the infecting strain are available, therapy can be changed to a less toxic agent. Similar therapy should be used for infected patients with calculi or urologic abnormalities who have suspected sepsis.

In *pregnancy,* acute cystitis can be managed with 7 days of amoxicillin, nitrofurantoin, or a cephalosporin. After treatment, a culture should be obtained to ensure cure and repeated monthly thereafter. Acute pyelonephritis in pregnancy should be managed by hospitalization and parenteral antibiotics, generally a cephalosporin or an extended-spectrum penicillin. Continuous low-dose prophylaxis with nitrofurantoin should be given to women who have recurrent infections during pregnancy.

Asymptomatic bacteriuria should be documented with at least two positive cultures before treatment is given. Seven days of an oral agent to which the organism is sensitive should be given initially. If bacteriuria persists, it can be followed without further treatment in most patients. In patients who may be at high risk because of neutropenia, compromised host defenses, renal transplant, or previous development of pyelonephritis or bacteremia, further treatment with either 6 weeks of oral therapy or 4 to 6 weeks of combined parenteral and oral therapy should be given.

Optimal treatment regimens for patients with *catheter-associated urinary tract infections* have not been well established. These infections often remit spontaneously or with short-term antibiotic therapy if the catheter can be removed. If the catheter cannot be removed, systemic antibiotics or urinary antiseptics may reduce bacteriuria, but do not usually eliminate it. Asymptomatic bacteriuria in catheterized patients can probably be left untreated in most patients who are not immunosuppressed or who are not at high risk for sepsis because of old age, severe underlying disease, diabetes, or pregnancy.

UROLOGIC EVALUATION Very few women with recurrent urinary tract infections have correctable lesions discovered at cystoscopy or upon intravenous pyelography, and these procedures should not be routinely performed in such patients. In selected women, namely those with relapsing infection, those with a history of childhood infections, those with stones or painless hematuria, and those with recurrent pyelonephritis, urologic evaluation should be performed. All males with urinary infection should be evaluated urologically. Men or women presenting with acute infection and signs or symptoms suggestive of an obstruction or stones should undergo urologic evaluation, generally by means of ultrasound.

PROGNOSIS In patients with uncomplicated cystitis or pyelonephritis, treatment ordinarily results in complete resolution of symptoms. In fact, symptoms usually remit even without specific therapy. Lower tract infections in adult women are of concern mainly because they cause discomfort, minor morbidity, and time lost from work. Cystitis may also result in upper tract infection or in bacteremia (especially during instrumentation), but there is little evidence to suggest that renal impairment follows. When repeated episodes of cystitis occur, they are nearly always reinfections, not relapses. Why a significant subpopulation of adult women develops a predisposition to multiple recurrent infections remains poorly understood. In some cases, residual urine, urethral stenosis, or other anatomic explanations exist, but most women with recurrent infections have no such demonstrable abnormality. Their uroepithelial cells appear highly prone to persistent colonization with *E. coli;* the explanation for this phenomenon is not clear.

Uncomplicated acute pyelonephritis in adults rarely progresses to functional impairment and chronic renal disease. Repeated upper tract infections often indicate relapse rather than reinfection, and a vigorous search for renal calculi or an underlying urologic abnormality should be undertaken. If neither is found, 6 weeks of chemotherapy may be useful in eradicating an unresolved focus of infection.

Repeated symptomatic urinary tract infections in children, and in adults with obstructive uropathy, neurogenic bladder, structural renal disease, or diabetes more often progress to chronic renal disease. Asymptomatic bacteriuria in these groups, as well as in adults without urologic disease or obstruction, predisposes to increased episodes of symptomatic infection but does not result in renal impairment in most instances.

PREVENTION Patients with frequent symptomatic infections may benefit from long-term low-dose antibiotics directed at preventing recurrences. A single dose of trimethoprim-sulfamethoxazole (80 mg trimethoprim and 400 mg sulfamethoxazole daily), trimethoprim alone (100 mg daily), or nitrofurantoin (50 mg daily) have been particularly effective. Prophylaxis should be initiated only after bacteriuria has been eradicated with a full-dose treatment regimen. Women having more than two infections every 6 months should be considered for preventive antibiotics. Low-dose antibiotics (nitrofurantoin 50 to 100 mg) after sexual intercourse may also be of benefit in preventing episodes of symptomatic infections. Other patients for whom prophylaxis appears to have some merit include men with chronic prostatitis; patients undergoing prostatectomy, both during the operation and in the postoperative period; and pregnant women with asymptomatic bacteriuria. All pregnant women should be screened for bacteriuria in the first trimester, and should be treated if bacteriuria is found.

CHRONIC PYELONEPHRITIS

Chronic interstitial nephritis thought to result from bacterial infection of the kidney has been termed *chronic pyelonephritis*. It may occur in patients with predisposing urologic abnormalities (obstruction, vesicoureteral reflux, or neurogenic bladder) or in patients with apparently normal urinary tracts. Unlike acute urinary tract infections, for which simple diagnostic criteria and characteristic clinical syndromes exist, no pathognomonic clinical, laboratory, or pathologic criteria can be used to identify cases of chronic pyelonephritis, and few reliable data on the incidence or prevalence of this condition have been collected. Many patients with renal lesions that fulfill the pathologic criteria for chronic pyelonephritis at autopsy have sterile urine cultures and were not known to have had clinical episodes of bacterial urinary tract infection or urinary obstruction during life. Such cases suggest that other forms of renal injury result in morphologic changes indistinguishable from those produced by bacterial infection. Conversely, relatively few individuals with acute urinary infection develop chronic infection or progressive renal impairment. Most often, this occurs in patients with anatomic obstruction, neurogenic bladder, or vesicoureteral reflux.

Patients with many episodes of urinary tract infection; impaired renal function; pyuria with white cell casts; bacteriuria; an intravenous pyelogram showing an irregularly outlined renal pelvis with caliectasis and cortical scars; and typical pathologic changes can be diagnosed as having chronic pyelonephritis. In less typical patients, the relationship of infection to renal damage is uncertain and the diagnosis often remains unclear.

PAPILLARY NECROSIS

The renal papilla is of major importance in the pathogenesis of chronic interstitial nephritis and, when complicated by bacterial infection, pyelonephritis. It has become evident that a variety of underlying conditions cause primary renal papillary damage, resulting eventually in the renal lesions of chronic interstitial nephritis. When urinary infection does not supervene, the resulting renal disease may progress slowly and silently to the point of renal insufficiency. The pathology of this renal injury may be indistinguishable from that of pyelonephritis. In addition to common diseases such as gout and diabetes mellitus, which cause renal papillary damage, many medications, which achieve enormous concentrations in the urine traversing the renal papilla, may be toxic for that zone of the kidney. The best known of these are phenacetin-containing analgesic mixtures. This problem is much more common than generally recognized, and diagnosis requires a careful history.

It is not known how many other substances may be important in the pathogenesis of primary renal papillary disease. However, in view of the benignity of urinary infection in persons without underlying renal papillary damage, it is reasonable to assume the presence of primary underlying renal papillary damage in any patient with urinary infection who shows the development of or progression to renal damage.

When severe infection of the renal pyramids is present in association with vascular diseases of the kidney or with urinary tract obstruction, renal papillary necrosis is likely to result. Patients with diabetes, sickle cell disease, chronic alcoholism, and vascular disease seem peculiarly susceptible to this complication. Hematuria, pain in the flank or abdomen, and chills and fever are the most common presenting symptoms. Acute renal failure with oliguria or anuria sometimes occurs. Rarely, sloughing of a pyramid may take place without symptoms in a patient with chronic urinary infection, and the diagnosis is made when the necrotic tissue is passed in the urine or identified as a "ring shadow" on pyelography. If renal function deteriorates suddenly in a diabetic or a patient with chronic obstruction, the diagnosis of renal papillary necrosis should be entertained, even in the absence of fever or pain. Although renal papillary necrosis is often bilateral, when it is unilateral, nephrectomy may be lifesaving in the management of overwhelming infection.

RENAL AND PERINEPHRIC ABSCESS

See Chap. 91.

PROSTATITIS

The term *prostatitis* has been used for various inflammatory conditions affecting the prostate, including acute and chronic infections with specific bacteria and, more commonly, instances in which signs and symptoms of prostatic inflammation are present but no specific organisms can be detected. To classify patients with suspected prostatitis correctly, each patient should be evaluated using first-void and midstream urine specimens, a prostatic expressate, and a post-massage urine specimen. All specimens should be quantitatively cultured and evaluated for numbers of leukocytes. Based on the results of these studies, patients can be classified as having acute or chronic bacterial prostatitis, nonbacterial prostatitis, or prostatodynia. Patients with suspected prostatitis usually have low back pain, perineal or testicular discomfort, mild dysuria, and lower urinary obstructive symptoms. Microscopic pyuria may be the only objective manifestation of prostatic disease.

ACUTE BACTERIAL PROSTATITIS This disease generally affects young male adults when it occurs spontaneously, but it may also be associated with an indwelling urethral catheter. It is characterized by fever, chills, dysuria, and a tense or boggy, extremely tender prostate on examination. Although prostatic massage usually produces purulent secretions with a large number of bacteria on culture, bacteremia may result from manipulation of the inflamed gland. For this reason, and because the etiologic agent can usually be identified on urine Gram stain and culture, vigorous prostatic massage should be avoided. In non-catheter-associated cases, the infection is generally due to one of the common gram-negative urinary tract pathogens or *Staphylococcus aureus*. Initially, intravenous trimethoprim-sulfamethoxazole, a cephalosporin, or an aminoglycoside can be utilized if gram-negative rods are seen in the urine Gram stain, and a cephalosporin or nafcillin if gram-positive cocci are seen. Although these drugs do not readily diffuse into the noninflamed prostate gland, the response to antibiotics is usually prompt, perhaps because drugs penetrate more readily into the acutely inflamed prostate. In catheter-associated cases, a broader spectrum of etiologic agents is seen, including hospital-acquired gram-negative rods and enterococci. In such cases, an aminoglycoside or a third-generation cephalosporin should be used for initial therapy until the organism has been isolated and susceptibilities determined. The long-term prognosis is good, although in some instances acute infection may result in abscess formation, epididymoorchitis, seminal vesiculitis, septicemia, and residual chronic bacterial prostatitis. Since the advent of antibiotics, the frequency of acute bacterial prostatitis has diminished markedly. Many so-called cases of acute prostatitis are probably posterior urethritis.

CHRONIC BACTERIAL PROSTATITIS This entity is a major cause of recurrent bacteriuria in males but may be difficult to diagnose. Symptoms are usually absent, the prostate feels normal on palpation, and although many white blood cells may be seen in the urinary sediment, results of conventional bacteriologic studies are often negative. Bacteria may be cultured from the expressed prostatic secretion or postmassage urine. The presence of these bacteria can be determined only by careful quantitative bacteriologic techniques when the bladder urine is sterile. Intermittently, symptoms of frequency, urgency, and dysuria occur when infection spreads to the bladder urine. The pattern of recurrent bladder infection in the male with chronic bacterial prostatitis is clinically not very different from that seen in the recurrent cystourethritis of the female. Antibiotics promptly relieve the symptoms associated with acute exacerbations, but have been less effective in eradicating the focus of chronic infection in the prostate. The relative ineffectiveness of antimicrobials, in terms of long-term cure, in part results from the poor penetration of most antibiotics into the prostate because the low pH which prevails in this organ precludes solubility of most drugs. Macrolides (erythromycin) do enter the prostatic secretions, but these agents are generally ineffective against gram-negative organisms. Sulfonamide-trimethoprim and the fluoroquinolines have been employed successfully in some cases, but they must be given for at least 12 weeks to be effective. Patients with frequent episodes of acute cystitis should be treated with prolonged courses of antimicrobials (usually sulfonamide, trimethoprim, or nitrofurantoin), with a view toward suppressing symptoms and keeping the bladder urine sterile. Total prostatectomy produces cure of chronic prostatitis but is associated with considerable morbidity. Transurethral prostatectomy is safer but cures only one-third of patients.

NONBACTERIAL PROSTATITIS Patients who present with symptoms and signs of prostatitis, increased leukocytes in their expressed prostatic secretions and postmassage urine, and no bacterial growth in cultures are classified as having nonbacterial prostatitis. Prostatic inflammation can be considered present when the expressed prostatic secretion and postmassage urine contain at least tenfold more leukocytes than the first-void and midstream specimens, or when the expressed prostatic secretion contains $\geq$1000 leukocytes per microliter. The presumed infectious etiology of this condition remains unidentified. Evidence for the causative role of both *Ureaplasma urealyticum* and *Chlamydia trachomatis* has been presented, but is not conclusive. Since most cases of nonbacterial prostatitis occur in young, sexually active men, and since many cases arise following an episode of nonspecific urethritis, the causative agent may well be sexually transmitted. The effectiveness of antimicrobial agents in this condition remains uncertain. Some patients benefit from a 4- to 6-week course of erythromycin, doxycycline, or trimethoprim-sulfamethoxazole, but controlled trials are lacking.

PROSTATODYNIA Patients who have symptoms and signs of prostatitis but no evidence of prostatic inflammation (normal leukocyte counts) and negative urine cultures are classified as having prostatodynia. Despite their symptoms, these patients most likely do not have prostatic infection and should not be given antimicrobial agents.

REFERENCES

BAILEY RR: Single-dose therapy for uncomplicated urinary tract infections. NZ Med J 98:327, 1985

JOHNSON JR, STAMM WE: Diagnosis and treatment of acute urinary tract infections. Infect Dis Clin North Am 1:773, 1987

KOMAROFF AL: Acute dysuria in women. N Engl J Med 310:368, 1984

———: Urinalysis and urine culture in women with dysuria. Ann Intern Med 104:212, 1986

KRIEGER JN: Complications and treatment of urinary tract infections during pregnancy. Urol Clin North Am 13:685, 1986

KUNIN CM: Use of antimicrobial agents in treating urinary tract infection. Adv Nephrol 14:39, 1985

———: *Detection, Prevention and Management of Urinary Tract Infections*, 4th ed. Philadelphia, Lea & Febiger, 1987

LIPSKY BA: Urinary tract infections in men. Ann Intern Med 110:138, 1989

MEARES EM JR: Acute and chronic prostatitis: Diagnosis and treatment. Infect Dis Clin North Am 1:855, 1987

PEZZLO M: Detection of urinary tract infections by rapid methods. Clin Microbiol Rev 1:268, 1988

RONALD AR: Current concepts in the management of urinary tract infections in adults. Med Clin North Am 68:335, 1984

STAMM WE et al: Causes of the acute urethral syndrome in women. N Engl J Med 303:409, 1980

——— et al: Diagnosis of coliform infection in acutely dysuric women. N Engl J Med 307:463, 1982

——— et al: Urinary tract infections: From pathogenesis to treatment. J Infect Dis 159:400, 1989

SVANBORG-EDEN C et al: Host-parasite relationship in urinary tract infection. J Infect Dis 157:421, 1988

WARREN JW: Catheter-associated urinary tract infections. Infect Dis Clin North Am 1:823, 1987

96 INFECTIOUS ARTHRITIS

DANIEL ROTROSEN

NONGONOCOCCAL SEPTIC ARTHRITIS Acute bacterial arthritis is a common medical problem affecting individuals of all ages. Prompt recognition and treatment are important to avoid permanent articular disability.

Etiology, pathogenesis, and predisposing factors Approximately 75 percent of nongonococcal pyoarthroses are due to gram-positive cocci, particularly *Staphylococcus aureus*. Pneumococci and group A beta-hemolytic and viridans streptococci collectively account for less than half of these. Among immunocompromised individuals, group G streptococci are an infrequent cause of septic arthritis, and group B streptococci are an important cause of arthritis in neonates. *Staphylococcus epidermidis* is the leading cause of prosthetic joint infection.

Gram-negative bacilli account for approximately 20 percent of cases, typically in patients with obvious risk factors for gram-negative bacteremia. *Pseudomonas aeruginosa* is an important cause of septic arthritis in intravenous drug addicts and neonates. *Haemophilus influenzae* type B is a prominent cause of pyoarthrosis among children under age 5.

Septic arthritis usually results from direct hematogenous seeding of the synovium. Conditions which predispose to septic arthritis include infancy, immunosuppressive therapy, alcoholism, drug abuse, some chronic systemic illnesses, hemoglobinopathies, complement and immunoglobulin deficiencies, phagocytic cell dysfunction, chronic arthritis, and previous joint damage. Infection may occur as a complication of arthroscopy, intraarticular glucocorticoid injection, or prosthetic joint surgery. A history of minor joint trauma is a common but often overlooked feature in patients with suppurative arthritis. An extraarticular focus of infection (e.g., cutaneous abscesses) can be identified in about 25 percent of patients and can be useful in both establishing a cause and choosing antibiotics before joint fluid culture results are available.

The synovium is well vascularized and lacks a limiting basement membrane, allowing relatively free access of bloodborne microorganisms to the joint space once extravasation has occurred. In experimentally induced arthritis, microorganisms are found scattered throughout the synovium 1 to 2 h after inoculation. Within 1 to 2 days vascular congestion, leukocyte infiltration, and hyperplasia of the synovial lining cells are prominent. The host response may be sufficient to eradicate infection in some cases, but early changes usually progress to purulent effusion accompanied by microabscess formation within the synovium and subchondral bone. Increased intraarticular pressure causes ischemia and impairs cartilage biomechanics and nutrition; chondrolytic enzymes released from neutrophils contribute to the destruction of articular cartilage, subchondral bone, and joint capsule. Irreversible changes may ensue as a consequence of synovial lining cell proliferation, mononuclear cell infiltration, and the appearance of granulation tissue; such changes may appear as early as 1 week after infection begins.

Clinical and experimental observations suggest that host immune mechanisms play a critical role in the development and maintenance of synovial inflammation. Sterile bacterial products, including endotoxins, exotoxins, and cell wall peptidoglycan induce acute and chronic arthritis in laboratory animals. Deposition of immune complexes in synovium and periarticular tissues may be followed by a sterile synovitis during the convalescent phase of certain bacterial and viral infections. Individuals who develop postinfectious arthritis or Reiter's syndrome following *Shigella, Salmonella, Yersinia,* and *Campylobacter* infection of the gastrointestinal tract are more likely than matched controls to have the specific histocompatibility antigen HLA-B27.

Manifestations Nongonococcal septic arthritis presents as a monarticular synovitis with a predilection for large weight-bearing joints. The knee is the most frequently involved joint in children and adults, followed by the hip. The ankle, wrist, elbow, shoulder, sternoclavicular, and sacroiliac joints are involved less often. The interphalangeal joints are rarely affected in bacterial arthritis, except in patients with gonococccal synovitis or mycobacterial infection. Gram-positive coccal arthritis usually presents as an acute illness with severe constitutional symptoms accompanied by swelling, pain, warmth, and restricted motion of the involved joint. In septic arthritis of the hip, effusion may not be readily appreciated, and pain may be minimal or referred to the groin, buttock, lateral thigh, or anterior knee. Patients with suppurative arthritis usually seek medical attention within 3 to 4 days of the onset of symptoms. Signs of inflammation may be masked in patients taking glucocorticoids or other immunosuppressive medications and in those with chronic debilitating illnesses. Individuals with coexistent rheumatoid or gouty arthritis often attribute their symptoms to a flare-up of the underlying disease and consequently delay medical evaluation. In this setting a high degree of suspicion is warranted, and studies to exclude infection are important when articular symptoms fail to respond to anti-inflammatory agents.

If medical attention is sought early in the illness, a source of bacteremia is usually identified, and the responsible pathogen can be isolated from the blood in about 50 percent of cases. In contrast, gram-negative bacillary arthritis follows a more indolent course with moderate constitutional symptoms and less prominent articular complaints. These differences contribute to the more prolonged time to diagnosis in gram-negative bacillary arthritis (typically 3 weeks from the onset of symptoms) and to the high incidence of coexistent osteomyelitis at the time of diagnosis. Rarely, *S. aureus* may have a less acute presentation when it causes arthritis (see Chap. 100).

Prosthetic joint infection is associated with mild symptoms and an indolent course resulting in a mean diagnostic delay of 2 to 8 months. *S. epidermidis* and *S. aureus* account for most of these infections, but multiple organisms, gram-negative bacilli, and anaerobes are not uncommon. Infection occurs in 1 to 4 percent of prostheses followed for 10 years and is more frequent after revision of a previous total joint replacement. It invariably is accompanied by osteomyelitis at the site of implantation. Eradication of the infection usually requires removal of the prosthesis.

Certain pathogens are likely to cause infection at unusual sites. Spinal arthritis is most often associated with osteomyelitis of adjacent vertebral bodies. It is usually due to *S. aureus,* but *Brucella, Salmonella,* and *Mycobacterium tuberculosis* also preferentially involve the spine. Among intravenous drug addicts, *P. aeruginosa* infection can occur in the sternoclavicular and sacroiliac joints.

Laboratory findings and diagnosis Analysis of synovial fluid is essential in the evaluation of suspected bacterial arthritis. Fluid sufficient for complete analysis can usually be obtained by percutaneous arthrocentesis. Care should be taken not to contaminate the joint space by inserting the needle through an area of overlying cellulitis or through an infected bursa. Fluoroscopic guidance may facilitate aspiration of the hip, shoulder, spinal, or sacroiliac joints. When joints are difficult to aspirate, arthrotomy may be required to obtain fluid or synovial tissue. Synovial fluid in septic arthritis is usually turbid or grossly purulent. The synovial fluid leukocyte count is greater than 100,000 per microliter (range $<$ 10,000 to $>$ 300,000 per microliter, usually $>$ 90 percent polymorphonuclear neutrophils) in one-third to one-half of patients. In patients with unexpectedly low leukocyte counts on initial evaluation, repeat joint aspiration 12 to 24 h later almost always demonstrates leukocytosis. The synovial fluid leukocyte count and differential are of limited diagnostic utility due to considerable overlap with values in other acute inflammatory arthritides. However, serial counts are important in monitoring response to therapy.

Gram's stain of synovial fluid is important in establishing an etiologic diagnosis of septic arthritis. Stains are positive in 75 to 95 percent of gram-positive coccal and in approximately 50 percent of gram-negative bacillary infections. Regardless of the results of Gram's stain, synovial fluid should be cultured aerobically and anaerobically to identify the specific pathogen and provide data on antimicrobial sensitivity. Joint fluid cultures are positive in most patients with nongonococcal bacterial arthritis. If the patient has taken oral antibiotics prior to arthrocentesis, the microbiology laboratory should be notified, because growth of the organism may be delayed and cultures may require special handling. Blood cultures should be obtained, and a diligent search should be made for occult sources of bacteremia. Bacterial antigen detection by counterimmunoelectrophoresis has been advocated as a rapid diagnostic test for certain etiologic agents (e.g., *Streptococcus pneumoniae* and *H. influenzae*), but is not widely used.

In septic arthritis the synovial fluid glucose level may be low and lactate elevated, compared to the corresponding levels in serum, but neither test is sufficiently sensitive or specific to be of general diagnostic utility. Elevated synovial fluid protein and poor mucin clot are diagnostically nonspecific.

Unless arthritis arises by extension of adjacent osteomyelitis, distention of the joint capsule and periarticular soft tissue swelling are the only radiographic findings expected on initial evaluation. Nonetheless, early films are useful to establish a baseline for subsequent evaluation. Destructive changes are rarely noted radiologically before the second to third week of untreated infection. At that time, periosteal elevation, juxtaarticular osteoporosis, bony erosions on the articular surface, and joint space narrowing due to cartilage destruction may be apparent. In prosthetic joint infection radiographic evidences of implant loosening and ostemyelitis are usually seen.

In the setting of staphylococcal or gram-negative bacillary arthritis, computed tomography (CT) or magnetic resonance imaging (MRI) of involved joints is helpful, particularly when the sternoclavicular joint or the hip is involved. These joints are poorly visualized by conventional techniques, and CT or MRI may reveal extensive bony involvement and parasynovial abscesses when conventional x-ray films are negative. Such findings have important implications for surgical intervention and for the duration of antimicrobial therapy.

Radioisotope scans lack diagnostic specificity and may be positive in noninfectious inflammatory joint disease. However, scans are useful to identify inapparent foci of osteomyelitis and to bolster suspicions of low-grade infection in the hip, shoulder, spine, and sacroiliac joints.

Other conditions to be considered in the differential diagnosis of oligoarticular arthritis include septic bursitis (usually olecranon or prepatellar), juvenile rheumatoid arthritis, psoriatic arthritis, acute rheumatic fever, Reiter's syndrome, sarcoid arthropathy, trauma, villonodular synovitis, aseptic necrosis, and intermittent hydroarthrosis. Infection that can present as oligoarticular arthritis include Lyme disease and infections caused by mycobacteria and fungi.

Management and outcome Optimal management of suppurative arthritis includes parenteral antimicrobial therapy, joint drainage, and articular rest. Most antibiotics achieve therapeutic levels in the infected joint following parenteral administration. There is accordingly no rationale for intraarticular administration of antibiotics, and in fact, direct injection of certain antibiotics can induce chemical synovitis. The initial choice of antibiotics should be guided by Gram's stain of synovial fluid and revised as dictated by culture results. Antibiotic regimens for specific organisms are provided in the chapters dealing with these organisms and in Chap. 85, which details the properties of each antibiotic. When no organisms are seen on Gram's stain, the antimicrobial regimen should be tailored to cover the likely pathogens based on the patient's age and the clinical setting. Infants under 1 month of age should be treated with a semisynthetic penicillin and an aminoglycoside to provide coverage against *S. aureus*, gram-negative bacilli, and group B streptococci. In children under 5 years of age therapy should be targeted against *S. aureus* and ampicillin-resistant *H. influenza*. Children over 5 years and adults should receive a semisynthetic penicillin and an aminoglycoside until culture results are available. Vancomycin is the drug of choice in patients with serious penicillin allergy and may be required in prosthetic joint infection due to methicillin-resistant *S. epidermidis*. The results of single-drug therapy of gram-negative bacillary arthritis have been disappointing, despite in vitro sensitivity to the agents used. Because of the high rates of failure and relapse in this setting combination chemotherapy is generally advised. After an initial clinical response (and if in vitro sensitivities permit) substitution of a newer β-lactam or quinolone antibiotic may be advisable to avoid the toxicities of prolonged aminoglycoside therapy.

Most cases of streptococcal arthritis are cured by a 10- to 14-day course of antibiotics, whereas staphylococcal and gram-negative bacillary infections require longer treatment, usually 3 to 6 weeks, particularly with complicating osteomyelitis. Drainage of purulent joint fluid is essential to relieve pain, diminish the risk of loculation and pressure necrosis, and remove chondrolytic products that promote destructive changes within the joint. As with other closed space infections, drainage of acidic, purulent fluid improves the bactericidal activity of neutrophils, cell-wall-active antibiotics, and aminoglycosides. Percutaneous needle aspiration and joint irrigation can be performed daily or twice daily for the first 5 to 7 days of therapy. The development of loculations, continued culture positivity, or persistence of a purulent effusion beyond that time are indications that arthroscopy or open drainage may be required. When the hip joint is involved, surgical intervention is usually warranted from the outset, especially in children, due to the technical difficulty of repeated percutaneous aspiration and the risk of vascular compromise from elevated intracapsular pressure. Early exploratory arthrotomy and open drainage have been beneficial in septic arthritis of the shoulder and sternoclavicular joints. Persistently positive cultures despite adequate drainage are an indication for reculture of the fluid to exclude emergence of antibiotic-resistant strains.

During the acute phase the joint should be immobilized in a position that minimizes capsular tension, usually midway between full extension and flexion. Passive range-of-motion exercises should be started as the synovitis improves, but weight bearing should be avoided until pain and signs of inflammation are gone.

Most cases of streptococcal arthritis resolve without sequelae, whereas in staphylococcal and gram-negative bacillary arthritis the response is generally less salutary. In this setting healing may be delayed by a sterile, postinfectious synovitis. Despite microbiologic cure such patients may be left with limitation of motion and persistence of pain. Other major determinants of a poor outcome are failure to recognize and treat the infection within 7 days of onset and involvement of the hip joint. In children with hip or ankle arthritis impaired ambulation and shortening of the extremity are not uncommon.

GONOCCOCAL ARTHRITIS (See Chap. 110) Gonoccocal infection is the leading cause of bacterial arthritis in young adults and the most common form of infectious arthritis seen at urban medical centers. It may be a complication of sexual abuse in young children. In disseminated gonococcal infection an early arthritis-dermatitis syndrome is typically followed by a joint-localization stage. The early phase is characterized by constitutional symptoms, migratory tenosynovitis and arthralgias, vesiculopustular skin lesions, and minimal joint effusion. The knee, shoulder, wrist, and interphalangeal joints of the hands are commonly involved. Cultures of blood and skin lesions may be positive at this stage of the illness, whereas culture and Gram's stain of synovial fluid are usually negative. A presumptive diagnosis can be made if the gonococcus is isolated from a silent primary focus (e.g., urogenital tract, pharynx, or rectum). Without treatment, constitutional symptoms and dermatitis usually abate, but joint involvement progresses to a purulent mon- or pauciarticular arthritis. Synovial fluid cultures may be positive at this stage whereas blood cultures are almost always negative. In 30 to 40 percent of patients a biphasic pattern of illness is not observed, and some patients present with a monarticular purulent arthritis and few systemic manifestations. Terminal complement component deficiencies, menstruation, and pregnancy predispose to gonococcal dissemination.

The differential diagnosis of disseminated gonoccocal infection includes acute rheumatic fever, Reiter's syndrome, chronic meningococcemia, and *Streptobacillus moniliformis* infection. In Reiter's syndrome constitutional toxicity is usually less pronounced, there is often a history of symptomatic urethritis and conjunctivitis, and distinct, but subtle mucocutaneous lesions are usually present. Sacroiliitis and Achilles tendonitis are more common in Reiter's syndrome, but involvement of the upper extremity, especially the wrist, is unusual. A clinical response to antibiotics (in gonoccocal disease) or to salicylates (in rheumatic fever) may help to differentiate among these syndromes.

In the United States most gonococcal isolates causing disseminated infection are penicillin-sensitive, enabling treatment with oral antibiotics on an outpatient basis. Hospitalization and administration of parenteral antibiotics are warranted for unreliable patients and for those with purulent monarticular arthritis or uncertain diagnoses. In documented penicillin resistance ceftriaxone or spectinomycin is effective. Penicillin-resistant species are more common in the Philippines, southeast Asia, and Africa (see Chap. 110).

CHRONIC MONARTICULAR ARTHRITIS Certain mycobacteria and fungi cause chronic oligoarticular arthritis that is clinically and histologically distinct from other forms of septic arthritis.

Tuberculous arthritis (See Chap. 125) *Mycobacterium tuberculosis* causes a slowly progressive arthritis that is monarticular in up to 90 percent of cases. With the decline in primary tuberculosis in developed countries, spinal arthritis is rare, and involvement of the knee, hip, wrist, ankle, or small joints of the hand is more common. These sites become infected by reactivation of long-dormant lymphohematogenous foci. Rupture of such a focus (often in the epiphyseal region of long bones) into the joint space causes effusion and a progressive granulomatous reaction of synovial membranes, articular cartilage, and tendons. Localized pain may precede other signs of inflammation or x-ray changes by weeks or even months. The insidious nature of the infection usually delays diagnosis by weeks or months (the average time elapsed was 19 weeks from onset in one series). The granulomatous process eventually imparts a boggy, doughy feeling to the joint and periarticular structures. Cold abscesses and draining sinuses may develop. Constitutional symptoms are not prominent, and active pulmonary tuberculosis is unusual. Most patients are tuberculin-positive. Radiographs initially show subchondral osteoporosis and periarticular bone destruction with overlying periosteal thickening. Eventually, destructive changes are noted within the joint. The synovial fluid leukocyte count ranges from about 1000 to >100,000 per microliter (average about 15,000 per microliter) with a preponderance of polymorphonuclear neutrophils when counts are high, but frankly purulent fluid is uncommon. Acid-fast bacilli are not often seen on smears of synovial fluid (approximately 20 percent yield), but cultures of synovial fluid or tissue are positive in 80 to 90 percent of cases. Demonstration of characteristic granulomatous changes with or without caseation on synovial biopsy is sufficient evidence to initiate antituberculous therapy while awaiting culture and sensitivity results. Infection due to atypical mycobacteria (e.g., *M. kansasii, M. marinum, M. avium-intracellulare*) may produce a chronic granulomatous arthritis with similar clinical and histopathologic features. The correct diagnosis and choice of an appropriate antimicrobial regimen depend on isolation of the organism from synovial fluid or tissues. For treatment of tuberculosis and nontuberculous mycobacterial infection see Chaps. 125 and 127. In spinal tuberculosis surgery is usually reserved for drainage of abscesses or stabilization of the spine and is rarely required for treatment of other joints. Arthritis due to *Brucella* sp., *Nocardia asteroides,* and fungi may resemble mycobacterial infection.

Fungal arthritis Any of the invasive mycoses may infect bone and articular structures (see Chap. 151). With the exception of acute arthritis due to *Candida* sp. or blastomycosis, the fungal arthritides tend to be slowly progressive and may elude accurate diagnosis for months or years. All show a predilection for involvement of large weight-bearing joints, especially the knee. While common in blastomycotic arthritis, a history of serious underlying illness in other fungal arthritides is often absent, and joint infection usually occurs without obvious evidence of extraarticular dissemination.

In acute pulmonary *coccidioidomycosis,* benign, self-limited, sterile synovitis occurs as a component of the acute hypersensitivity syndrome known as "desert fever." Persistent coccidioidal synovitis may arise via direct hematogenous seeding of the synovium or via extension from an adjacent osteomyelitic focus. In the former case the disease tends to follow an indolent course with recurrent effusion, maintenance of joint space integrity, no evidence of osteomyelitis, and only late progression to a destructive villonodular arthritis with pannus formation. With extension from an adjacent bony focus effusion is less prominent, and destructive changes tend to occur earlier. Diagnosis depends on culture and histology of synovial tissue; joint fluid cultures are positive in <5 percent of cases.

Sporotrichotic arthritis usually occurs in the complete absence of the more familiar lymphocutaneous syndrome. There is a predilection for involvement of the small joints of the hand and wrist in addition to the knee. Articular disability is uncommon until late in the disease. The etiologic agent, *Sporothrix schenckii* is easily cultured from synovial fluid. As opposed to cutaneous sporotrichosis, articular disease is relatively refractory to iodide therapy, and response to amphotericin B may be slow.

Isolated articular involvement is unusual in *blastomycosis,* and patients usually present with a rapidly progressive "pulmonary-cutaneous-arthritic" syndrome. Involvement of multiple joints is the rule. In contrast to other granulomatous arthritides, joint fluid is frankly purulent in articular blastomycosis, and the organism is easily visualized on wet-mount microscopy of synovial aspirates.

Candida arthritis usually follows direct hematogenous seeding of synovium in patients with risk factors for disseminated candidiasis. The acute articular infection may spread to involved adjacent bone.

In *histoplasmosis* a migratory polyarthritis accompanied by erythema nodosum may be analogous to the acute hypersensitivity syndrome of coccidioidomycosis; osseous and articular involvement is exceedingly rare.

In *cryptococcosis* bone involvement is common with dissemination, but synovitis is unusual.

Successful management of fungal arthritis usually requires prolonged administration of amphotericin B; surgical debridement is helpful in cases with extensive pannus formation.

VIRAL ARTHRITIS Self-limited polyarthritis is a common manifestation of rubella, type B hepatitis, and arboviral diseases not found in the western hemisphere (chikungunya and o'nyong-nyong in Africa and Ross River arthritis in Australia). Synovitis is less common in mumps, varicella, adenovirus, and parvovirus infection. Destructive joint changes are uncommon in viral arthritis even with recurrent disease.

Arthritis occurs in natural *rubella* infection and following immunization with live, attenuated rubella virus. Approximately 15 percent of postpubertal women develop frank arthritis in the course of natural rubella infection. Large and small joints may be involved; the small joints of the hand and wrist are most severely affected. Occasional involvement of the distal interphalangeal joints helps to differentiate this syndrome from the onset of rheumatoid arthritis. The onset of arthritis in rubella usually occurs at the same time or within a few days of the rash and within 2 to 10 weeks after immunization. Rubella arthritis usually abates spontaneously within 1 to 2 weeks; recalcitrant cases respond to salicylates. Joint symptoms may recur for a year or more in natural rubella, but rarely after rubella immunization.

The synovitis that accompanies *type B hepatitis* resembles serum sickness with abrupt onset of fever and articular symptoms. Symmetric polyarthritis of the small joints of the hand may be associated with rheumatoid arthritis-like morning stiffness. The knee, shoulder, ankle, elbow, and wrist are also involved, but the joints of the feet are typically spared. Synovitis is usually accompanied by an urticarial rash, but the rash may be erythematous, maculopapular, or petechial. The possibility of hepatitis-associated arthritis is rarely entertained at the onset of the illness because synovitis usually occurs in the anicteric/prodromal phase. Over a third of patients never become jaundiced, but liver function tests invariably show evidence of hepatitis. In overt hepatitis the arthritis usually resolves. Immune complexes containing hepatitis B antigens are present in serum and synovium during the prodromal stage of hepatitis, lending support to the concept that this form of synovitis is immunologically mediated.

In contrast to rubella, the arthritis of *mumps* has a predilection for men. It generally follows complete subsidence of parotitis, may be accompanied by high fever, and is resistant to salicylates. In children and adults, *coxsackie* and *adenoviral* infection have been associated with recurrent fever, polyarthritis, and polyserositis resembling Still's variety of juvenile rheumatoid arthritis. *Parvoviruses* can also cause a self-limited acute polyarthritis, predominately in women.

SPIROCHETAL ARTHRITIS Articular disease occurs in congenital, secondary, and tertiary *syphilis* (see Chap. 128). Congenital syphilis is associated with metaphyseal osteochondritis of the long bones that abates spontaneously after 6 months of age and ongoing periostitis that continues after that age. At puberty, a typically painless bilateral synovitis of the knees and elbows (Clutton's joints) may develop. Synovial fluid shows a lymphocytic pleocytosis. Arthralgias, arthritis, and tenosynovitis may accompany the classic signs of secondary syphilis. Gummatous synovitis of the large joints occurs in tertiary syphilis. Neurogenic joint degeneration (Charcot's joint) occurs in neurosyphilis. Articular manifestations may also occur in the nonvenereal treponematoses.

Lyme disease (see also Chap. 132) is a multisystem disorder caused by a spirochete, *Borrelia burgdorferi,* that is transmitted by the bite of *Ixodes dammini* or related ticks. The hallmark of the disease is a characteristic rash, erythema chronicum migrans, during the early phase of infection. Weeks to months later, neurologic and cardiac abnormalities occur, accompanied by polyarthralgias and tenosynovitis. Joint manifestations may evolve to frank arthritis, particularly of the large joints, and recur for years. Prompt oral therapy with penicillin or tetracycline eradicates the rash, and generally prevents late manifestations. Diagnosis is usually made by serologic studies. Less than 5 percent of patients are seronegative but develop late manifestations, possibly related to a spirochetal "persister" state induced by early oral antibiotic therapy. Established late manifestations are cured by parenteral penicillin or ceftriaxone; response to therapy may take several months, and repeated treatment may be necessary.

REFERENCES

Bayer AS, Guze LB: Fungal arthritis. II. Coccidioidal synovitis: Clinical, diagnostic, therapeutic, and prognostic considerations. Semin Arthritis Rheum 8:200, 1979

Goldenberg DL, Reed JI: Bacterial arthritis. N Engl J Med 312:764, 1985

Steigbigel NH: Diagnosis and management of septic arthritis, in *Current Clinical Topics in Infectious Diseases*, JS Remington, MN Swartz (eds). New York, McGraw-Hill, 1983, vol 4, pp 1–29

97 OSTEOMYELITIS

JON T. MADER

DEFINITION Osteomyelitis refers to an infection of the bone, generally of the cortical and/or medullary portions. While many types of microorganisms may cause osteomyelitis, it is usually bacterial in origin.

PATHOGENESIS Long bone infections are either hematogenous or secondary to a contiguous focus of infection. Contiguous focus osteomyelitis can be subdivided into bone infections occurring in (1) patients who have relatively normal vascularity and in (2) patients with generalized vascular insufficiency. Both hematogenous and contiguous focus osteomyelitis may be acute or chronic processes.

Hematogenous osteomyelitis occurs mainly in infants and children. The metaphyses of the long bones (tibia, femur) are the most frequently involved. The terminal vessels of the growth plates form large sinusoids that are easy targets for infection. Initially, the acute infection is usually focal, resulting in a breakdown of leukocytes, increased bone pressure, decreased pH, and decreased oxygen tension. The cumulative effects of these physiologic factors compromise the medullary circulation and predispose to extension of the infection. Eventually, the infection may extend laterally through the Haversian and Volkmann canal systems, perforate the bony cortex, and lift the periosteum from the surface of the bone. When this occurs, both periosteal and endosteal circulation are lost and large segments of dead cortical and cancellous bone result. A single pathogen is almost always recovered from the bone in hematogenous osteomyelitis, with *Staphylococcus aureus* being the most commonly isolated organism.

Hematogenous osteomyelitis also occurs in adults. Typically, the long bone infection begins in the diaphysis and spreads to involve the entire medullary canal. Adult hematogenous osteomyelitis most commonly occurs in the vertebrae. The infection is usually monomicrobic with *S. aureus* and aerobic gram-negative rods having the highest incidence. There is often a history of urinary tract infection or intravenous drug abuse. The lumbar vertebral bodies are most often involved, followed in frequency by the thoracic and cervical vertebrae. Spread of the infection to adjacent vertebral bodies may occur rapidly via the rich venous networks in the spine.

When bacteria are introduced into bone by direct trauma or by extension of adjacent soft tissue infections, contiguous focus osteomyelitis results. Open fractures, joint infections, and chronic soft tissue infections are common causes. Osteomyelitis can also occur from contamination at surgery. Most infections of hardware and joint prostheses arise in this way. Unlike hematogenous osteomyelitis, multiple bacterial organisms are usually isolated from the infected bone. The bacteriology is diverse, but *S. aureus* and *S. epidermidis* are the most commonly isolated pathogens. In addition, aerobic gram-negative bacilli and anaerobic organisms are frequently isolated.

The small bones of the feet are common sites of contiguous focus osteomyelitis in patients with generalized vascular disease. Inadequate tissue perfusion predisposes these patients to infection by blunting the local inflammatory response. The infection commonly develops following minor trauma, infected nail beds, cellulitis, or trophic skin ulceration. Multiple aerobic and anaerobic bacteria are usually isolated from the infected bone.

PATHOLOGY Osteomyelitis may be acute or chronic. The acute disease is characteristically suppurative and is accompanied by edema, vascular congestion, and small vessel thrombosis. The vascular supply to the bone is compromised as the infection extends into the surrounding soft tissue. Large areas of dead bone (sequestra) may be formed when both the medullary and periosteal blood supplies are compromised. Despite an intense host response and/or antibiotic therapy, viable colonies of bacteria may be harbored within the necrotic and ischemic tissues. Once the antibiotics are discontinued or the host response declines, the organisms may again proliferate, which leads to a recurrence of the infection. The hallmarks of chronic osteomyelitis are a nidus of infected dead bone or scar tissue, an ischemic soft tissue envelope, and a refractory clinical course.

MANIFESTATIONS Some patients (particularly children) with hematogenous osteomyelitis present with abrupt fever, irritability, lethargy, and local signs of inflammation 3 weeks or less in duration. However, 50 percent of patients present with vague complaints including pain in the involved limb of 1 to 3 months' duration and minimal, if any, temperature elevation. The clinical signs of soft tissue extension often dominate the presenting findings and may lead to inappropriate diagnostic and therapeutic measures unless the clinical suspicion of osteomyelitis is considered.

The patient with hematogenous vertebral osteomyelitis presents with vague symptoms and signs: dull, constant back pain, spasms of the paravertebral muscles, point tenderness over the involved vertebral body, and low-grade or absent fever.

The clinical features of contiguous focus osteomyelitis include local pain, draining sinuses, tenderness, and erythema over the involved bone. The patient is often afebrile. In patients with vascular disease the clinical features are more subtle and are usually associated with foot ulcers.

Infection of a joint prosthesis may become evident shortly after surgery, especially if the infecting organism is virulent. Erythema and drainage at the operative site are common. More frequently, the onset is delayed, with persistent pain and loosening of the prosthesis developing 3 to 12 months after surgery. Local signs of infection are typically absent. Differentiating infections from noninfectious mechanical loosening of the prosthesis can be very difficult and can be substantiated only by the isolation of a pathogen by arthrocentesis or surgical culture.

DIAGNOSIS Bacterial osteomyelitis is confirmed by the identification of causative bacteria from bone or blood. However, chronic osteomyelitis is rarely accompanied by a bacteremia except in response to an acute extension of the infection into the soft tissues. Since sinus tract cultures are not reliable in identifying which organisms(s) will be isolated from the infected bone, antibiotic treatment of osteomyelitis should be based only on deep bone biopsy cultures.

Radiographic changes in acute hematogenous osteomyelitis are often nebulous. Initial radiographic changes include soft tissue swelling, periosteal thickening and/or elevation, and focal osteopenia. These subtle observations may be overlooked and occur at least 2 weeks following onset of the infection. Diagnostic lytic changes are more protracted and often accompany an indolent infection of several months' duration. In contiguous focus and chronic osteomyelitis the radiographic changes are even more vague, are often found in association with other nonspecific radiographic findings, and require a careful clinical correlation to achieve diagnostic significance.

An earlier diagnosis of osteomyelitis may be achieved with radionuclide imaging, such as technetium-99m diphosphonate, gallium-67 citrate, or indium-111 chloride scans. Although these studies may be definitive as early as 48 h after onset of infection, they may also be negative due to decreased blood flow. Positive scans may be difficult to interpret and require clinical correlation.

Computed tomography and magnetic resonance imaging (MRI) can be more useful than conventional radiographic approaches to define the extent of bone damage due to osteomyelitis. MRI is particularly helpful in defining abscesses and spinal cord impingement in vertebral osteomyelitis.

TREATMENT **Acute hematogenous osteomyelitis** In children, acute hematogenous osteomyelitis is primarily a medical disease which can be treated nonsurgically. In adults, debridement surgery is often required. Identification of the causative pathogen is essential. The infection will usually respond to specific antimicrobial therapy. Mismanagement with inappropriate antibiotic(s) or dosages results in disease extension, sequestra formation, and the development of a refractory infection. Surgical intervention is indicated in those patients in whom the infection has not responded to specific antimicrobial therapy within 48 h, or in those with evidence of a soft tissue abscess or a confirmed or suspected joint infection. The initial approach is to obtain appropriate culture material. A bone biopsy is essential unless blood cultures are positive and are accompanied by radiographic or bone scan findings consistent with osteomyelitis. Following cultures, a parenteral antimicrobial regimen is chosen which covers the clinically suspected pathogens. Gram's stains can direct the choice of initial antibiotic until culture results are known. In the event of a negative Gram's stain, initial treatment usually includes an antistaphylococcal penicillin or a cephalosporin with good antistaphylococcal activity (e.g., cefazolin). Once the organism is isolated, the antibacterial activity of different antibiotic classes can be determined by appropriate sensitivity methods (see Chap. 85). Appropriate parenteral antimicrobial therapy should be administered for 4 to 6 weeks dated from the initiation of therapy or following the last major debridement surgery. Occasionally oral antibiotic therapy can be utilized for treatment of childhood osteomyelitis. However, 2 weeks of parenteral antibiotic therapy are recommended prior to changing to an oral agent.

Osteomyelitis secondary to contiguous focus infection, chronic osteomyelitis Common denominators of these types of osteomyelitis are infected necrotic bone and poorly perfused soft tissue enveloping the bone. Adequate drainage, thorough debridement, obliteration of dead space, wound coverage with viable soft tissue, and specific antimicrobial coverage are essential to successful therapy. Following diagnostic evaluation, a bone biopsy should be performed to obtain aerobic and anaerobic cultures. However, if immediate debridement surgery is required, antibiotics that cover clinically suspected pathogens are mandated until the bacteriologic tissue data are reported. These antibiotics may be modified, if necessary, after results of the debridement cultures and sensitivities are known.

Surgical exposure should be direct and designed to avoid unnecessary devitalization of bone and soft tissue. The cortical and cancellous bone remaining in the wound after debridement surgery must bleed uniformly to ensure antibiotic perfusion and avoid continued sequestration. Repeat debridements may be necessary.

Appropriate management of the dead space created by debridement surgery is mandatory to arrest the disease and maintain the integrity of the skeletal part involved. The goal of dead space management is to replace dead bone and scar with durable vascularized tissue. Complete wound closure should be attained whenever possible. Local tissue flaps, free tissue flaps, vascularized bone grafts, bone transfers, and antibiotic beads may be used to fill dead space. Cancellous bone grafts may be placed beneath local or transferred tissues when structural augmentation is necessary. Careful preoperative planning is crucial to making efficient use of the patient's limited cancellous bone reserves. Finally, if motion is present, stability of the skeletal unit must be achieved. This is usually managed with external fixators (Hoffmann, Orthofix), which allow soft tissue access, or fixators (Ilizarov) that allow segmental resection and bone transfer.

Since the soft tissue envelope enclosing the debrided bone requires 3 to 4 weeks to become revascularized after debridement surgery, antibiotics are used to treat live infected bone and to safeguard soft tissue and bone undergoing revascularization. Parenteral antimicrobial therapy is administered for 4 to 6 weeks after the last major debridement surgery. However, the duration of antibiotic administration for osteomyelitis remains controversial. Long-term intravenous access catheters make outpatient intravenous treatment possible and decrease hospitalization time. Oral therapy with the quinolone class of antibiotics is currently being evaluated in adult patients.

If bony stability is present, treatment of osteomyelitis associated with hardware requires removal, thorough debridement, and antimicrobial therapy. If bony stability is not present, rigid bony stability must be established. Debridement of infected material plus antimicrobial agents are essential to permit union to occur. Once stability is reestablished, the hardware can be removed, the bone debrided, and another course of antimicrobials begun. Osteomyelitis associated with a joint prosthesis generally requires removal of the appliance, thorough debridement, and appropriate antimicrobial therapy.

Osteomyelitis secondary to contiguous focus infection with vascular disease Osteomyelitis associated with vascular insufficiency is difficult to treat because of the reduced ability of the host to participate in the eradication of the infection. Most of these infections occur in the feet of diabetic individuals. They are insidious and are often beyond simple salvage by the time the patient seeks medical therapy. Polymicrobial infection is common, and the presence of a foul odor or gas in the surrounding soft tissues is indicative of anaerobic bacteria (see Chap. 108).

Assessment of the vascular status of the tissue at the infection site is essential. Several methods may be used to determine perfusion adequacy. Doppler flow, thermograms, arteriograms, and pulse pressures (ischemic index) have been used. Cutaneous oxygen tensions plus pulse pressures are most commonly employed. Cutaneous oxygen tensions are obtained by a modified Clark electrode applied to the skin surface. Cutaneous oxygen tension values provide rough guidelines for determining the location of adequate tissue perfusion. The values are also helpful in assessing whether local debridement surgery can be performed and in selecting surgical margins where wound healing can be expected to occur in cases requiring amputations. Hyperbaric oxygen therapy may facilitate healing in areas having marginally satisfactory tensions.

Suppressive antibiotic therapy, local debridement surgery, or ablative surgery may be indicated in selected patients. Management decisions must consider tissue oxygen perfusion at the infection site, extent of the osteomyelitis, and patient preference. If definitive surgical intervention would result in unacceptable patient morbidity or disability, long suppressive therapy may be preferable. This is also an option when the patient refuses local debridement or ablative surgery. Despite suppressive antibiotic therapy, most patients will eventually require ablative surgery. For localized osteomyelitis with good perfusion, debridement surgery and a 4-week course of antibiotics may be sufficient. Extensive osteomyelitis with poor tissue oxygen perfusion usually requires ablative surgery with the amputation level being dictated by the vascular status of the tissues proximal to the site of infection.

REFERENCES

CALHOUN JH et al: Treatment of diabetic foot infections: Wagner classification, therapy, and outcome. Foot Ankle J, 9:101, 1988

CIERNY G, MADER JT: Adult chronic osteomyelitis. Orthop 7:1557, 1984

MACKOWIAK PA et al: Diagnostic value of sinus tract cultures in chronic osteomyelitis. JAMA 239:2772, 1978

RUTTLE PE et al: Chronic osteomyelitis treated with a muscle flap. Orthop Clin North Am 15:451, 1984

SAPICO FL, MONTGOMERIE JZ: Pyogenic vertebral osteomyelitis: Report of nine cases and review of the literature. Rev Infect Dis 1:754, 1979

WALDVOGEL FA et al: Osteomyelitis: A review of clinical features, therapeutic considerations, and unusual aspects. N Engl J Med 282:198, 260, 316, 1970

98 INFECTIONS CAUSED BY ANIMAL BITES AND SCRATCHES

ROB ROY MACGREGOR

Millions of humans suffer scratches and bites from domestic and wild animals every year. Fortunately, few result in significant infections. Rabies, the most severe complication, is discussed elsewhere (see Chap. 147). This section will review three syndromes: animal bite–related infections in general, rat-bite fever, and cat-scratch disease.

ANIMAL BITE INFECTIONS

DEFINITION These infections result from the inoculation of an animal's oral flora into tissue traumatized by a bite.

EPIDEMIOLOGY AND ETIOLOGY The more than 100 million dogs and cats in the United States inflict between 1 and 2 million bites each year. Over 1 percent of all pediatric emergency room visits are for treatment of animal bites and their complications, and approximately 10,000 require hospitalization. Dogs account for 75 to 90 percent of reported bites, cats account for 8 to 15 percent, and the remainder are due to rodents, monkeys, and other animals.

Most animal bites are by pets known to their victims. Children and young adults are affected most commonly. In children 60 to 80 percent of reported bites are to the head and neck; in adults 75 percent are on the extremities. Infection rates are highest in bites to the hand; rates also vary by animal (5 to 15 percent for dog bites and 40 to 60 percent for cat bites). The difference is thought to result from the character of the bites: dog bites tend to cause laceration and tissue crush injury and as such are likely to receive careful debridement and cleansing; cat bites may appear more trivial initially, and cat tooth punctures are more difficult to clean. Rat and monkey bites appear to cause a low frequency of infection when given proper wound care. The most common organisms causing infection are *Pasteurella multocida, Staphylococcus aureus,* streptococcal species, and obligate anaerobes, all normal mouth flora in cats and dogs. In addition, a slow-growing gram-negative bacillus designated DF-2 (dysgonic fermenter type 2, CDC classification) can cause life-threatening septicemia following dog bites and licks.

P. multocida is a small, nonsporulating, nonmotile gram-negative coccobacillus found in 25 to 50 percent of dog bites and in up to 80 percent of cat-bite infections. The organism produces small, gray, nonhemolytic colonies on blood agar and will not grow on MacConkey's agar. It ferments most sugars with the exception of lactose and is urease- and catalase-positive. It can be serotyped on the basis of capsular and somatic antigens. It can be cultured as a single pathogen from rapidly progressing cellulitis that develops within 12 to 24 h after a cat or dog bite (see below).

DF-2 is a gram-negative rod that grows slowly (4 to 10 days) in most blood culture systems and on chocolate agar or heart infusion agar supplemented with 5% rabbit blood in an increased CO_2 environment. On the latter medium organisms are 1 to 4 μm long and can be curved or filamentous in morphology. Owing to the difficulty in culturing, the 10 percent frequency of isolation from the canine oral cavity is probably an underestimate, as is the number of reported human infections. It has been recognized almost exclusively as a cause of septicemia and meningitis occurring usually 4 to 8 days after patients have sustained dog or cat bites and scratches. In the normal host it appears to be of low virulence, because 90 percent of reported cases are in patients at increased risk secondary to splenectomy, alcoholic liver disease, chronic lung disease, or other conditions known to compromise host resistance.

Other organisms have occasionally been identified as the cause of infection following animal bites and scratches: *Herpesvirus simile* (B-virus) is inoculated by the bite of clinically healthy monkeys and causes an acute, usually lethal encephalomyelitis. Two animal pox viruses are pathogenic in human beings: *bovine papular stomatitis virus,* which produces stomatitis and skin lesions in young cattle and causes small painless papules or verrucous nodules in humans, and *Orf virus,* which causes watery, papillomatous lesions on the mucous membranes of goats and sheep and a papulovesicular lesion, which occasionally may become generalized or progress to a hyperplastic nodular mass, at sites of inoculation in humans. *Lymphocytic choriomeningitis* can be contracted from handling mice and hamsters (see Chap. 149). *Brucella* (see Chap. 119) can be inoculated by handling infected animal tissue, and *tularemia* (see Chap. 120) has occurred following bites and scratches from infected animals. *Leptospirosis* (see Chap. 130) may occur after bites of dogs, mice, and rats (even though organisms normally are not found in saliva). *Erysipeloid,* or "fish-handler's disease," is an acute cellulitis resulting from inoculation of *Erysipelothrix rhusiopathiae* through skin scratches while dressing fish; occasionally it can progress to septicemia and endocarditis (see Chap. 103).

CLINICAL MANIFESTATIONS Patients sustaining animal bites generally present at two distinct times after injury; clinical and management concerns are different at each. One group comes for care within several hours of the bite, before infection has had time to develop; management issues involve hemostasis, cleansing, repair, and prophylaxis (see below). Other patients seek medical aid 8 h to a week or more following injury and present with obvious evidence of infection. In most cases signs and symptoms of infection (swelling, pain, dysfunction) are restricted to the injured part. Fever and leukocytosis are seen in only a third of patients. Blood cultures are usually sterile. Infections caused by *P. multocida,* either alone or in concert with other mouth flora, can produce rapid onset of swelling, pain, and loss of function, often with attendant lymphangitis. Particularly in the hand, infection can spread quickly along tendon sheaths and fascial planes, leading to tissue destruction and long-term disability. Tenosynovitis, septic arthritis, and osteomyelitis are associated complications. In patients with chronic liver disease, *P. multocida* can also cause bacteremia and spontaneous bacterial peritonitis following animal bites and scratches. The striking exception to the pattern of localized bite-induced cellulitis is the systemic presentation of DF-2 infections, in which high fever, prostration, shock, purpura, and meningitis can rapidly lead to death from disseminated intravascular coagulation and bacteremia, often with little or no evidence of local wound infection.

DIAGNOSIS AND TREATMENT In most cases, the diagnosis of wound infection is obvious, although the small puncture wounds inflicted by cats may be masked by marked cellulitis and tenosynovitis. Specific microbiologic diagnosis requires culturing pus and tissue from debridement. In contrast, DF-2 infections often occur sufficiently long after animal exposure to obscure the association. Therefore, DF-2 bacteremia should be considered in any patient presenting with fulminant bacteremic shock and disseminated intravascular coagulation who has a history of splenectomy, liver disease, chronic lung disease, or immunosuppression. Often, the organism can be seen on Gram stain of buffy coat smears but takes 4 to 10 days to grow in blood cultures.

Treatment of bites and scratches depends upon the time elapsed since the bite: the fresh wound (with no signs of infection) requires careful and copious saline irrigation (puncture wounds should be entered with a 20-gauge needle) followed by exploration, debridement of devitalized tissue, and removal of foreign material. Some authorities recommend against suturing bite wounds, because of the risk of infection. However, many surgeons prefer primary closure of wounds of the face, neck, and hands because of their potential for disfiguring, and the risk of infection is small if suturing is performed in association with careful wound cleansing and prophylactic antibiotic administration. Internal fixation of fractures is contraindicated, and lacerations of tendons and nerves are usually repaired in a second procedure. Tetanus prophylaxis should be given if immunization has lapsed or if immune status is unknown. If the patient is seen later, when infection is present or suspected, incision and drainage are necessary, with exploration of tendon sheaths and other locations of possible deeper loculated infection (see Chap. 91). These wounds are usually not closed until several days later. Elevation of the extremity will reduce swelling and promote healing.

Antibiotics must often be chosen on the basis of presumptive evidence: procaine penicillin G, 600,000 units intramuscularly every 12 h, or penicillin V, 500 mg orally every 6 h, is recommended initial treatment for *P. multocida,* streptococci, and most anaerobic mouth organisms. If the Gram stain suggests presence of staphylococci, a penicillinase-resistant penicillin should be added; however, because many *P. multocida* are resistant to penicillinase-resistant penicillins, they should not be used as monotherapy. Alternatively, the fixed combination of amoxicillin plus clavulinic acid, which has a spectrum of activity that includes all organisms commonly encountered in bite wounds, has been used successfully as a single agent. Cefoxitin may be used when empiric intravenous therapy is required. The recommended treatment in penicillin-allergic patients is a tetracycline, although these drugs should not be used in pregnant women or in children with developing teeth; in such patients erythromycin (even though up to 50 percent of *P. multocida* are not susceptible) and cotrimoxazole appear to be effective alternatives. The required duration of therapy is not established, and recommendations vary from 1 to 4 weeks. In vitro testing shows DF-2 to be susceptible to penicillins, cephalosporins, tetracyclines, erythromycin, and clindamycin and to be resistant to aminoglycosides. Intravenously administered penicillin G, in doses up to 20 million units daily, is recommended for suspected and proven septicemia with this organism.

PREVENTION No studies of the efficacy of prophylactic antibiotics have been decisive, owing to the small number of infections encountered. Nonetheless, because of the potential severe consequences, most authorities recommend treatment of all but trivial lacerations and abrasions of the hands and face with a penicillinase-resistant penicillin (with or without addition of penicillin itself), ampicillin-clavulinic acid, or tetracycline for several days.

RAT-BITE FEVER

DEFINITION Rat-bite fever (RBF) is a syndrome characterized by relapsing fever, rash, and arthralgias occurring days to weeks after a rat bite.

ETIOLOGY AND EPIDEMIOLOGY The syndrome has two causes: *Streptobacillus moniliformis* and *Spirillum minus;* the former is a pleomorphic gram-negative bacillus that grows slowly in liquid medium, causing typical "puffball" colonies over 2 to 7 days. Growth on trypticase soy agar requires enrichment with 20% serum and incubation in 8% CO_2. Its pleomorphic morphology is best demonstrated by Giemsa stain and includes short rods, filaments, coccobacillary chains, and yeast-like swellings, which give it its name. In anaerobic cultures, it can be mistaken for bacteroides or fusospirochetal species. *Spirillum minus* is a short, thick, and tightly coiled gram-negative spiral organism with polar flagella that create rapid, darting motility under dark-field examination. It has not been grown in culture and is best isolated by intraperitoneal inoculation of infected tissues and blood into mice or guinea pigs. Both organisms are normal flora in wild and laboratory rats; infections have been reported following contact with rodents, pigs, squirrels, cats, and dogs and as a result of ingestion of contaminated milk. Infection is an occupational hazard to laboratory workers. Risk of infection from an individual bite appears to be low: in one series of 50 consecutive rat bites treated with local cleansing alone, only 1 became infected, and none developed RBF. The true incidence of the disease is unknown, but it appears to be uncommon in the United States, where *Streptobacillus moniliformis* is the more common documented cause (which may simply indicate the relative ease of finding the two organisms in tissue and blood). In Japan, where RBF is known as *sodoku, Spirillum minus* is more common.

CLINICAL MANIFESTATIONS With both organisms the infection begins with a rat bite, usually to the face or upper extremity. In the streptobacillary form, the wound heals uneventfully, usually without regional adenopathy, but is followed 2 to 10 days later by the abrupt onset of rigors, high fever, headache, myalgias, and prostration. Several days later patients develop a morbilliform or petechial rash, either on the extremities (including palms and soles) or generalized. At the same time, over two-thirds of patients experience severe arthralgias or frank arthritis, usually affecting large joints, which can be either monarticular or migratory and polyarthralgic. Untreated, the acute symptoms remit after several days and can be followed by an irregular pattern of relapsing fevers and other constitutional symptoms lasting for weeks to months. Complications include septic arthritis, endocarditis, pericarditis, pneumonia, and metastatic abscess. In spirillary RBF, the incubation period is longer, usually between 7 and 21 days. The healed bite wound often suppurates at the time of generalized symptoms and is associated with lymphangitis and regional adenopathy. The rash consists of large, reddish-brown macules, and arthritis is uncommon. Untreated, a relapsing fever course ensues similar to that in the streptobacillary form. A mortality of 10 percent has been reported, usually from endocarditis, but prognosis in antibiotic-treated patients is excellent. When the streptobacillary form occurs in the absence of documented animal exposure or in epidemic form, it has been called Haverhill fever or *erythema arthriticum epidermicum,* named for an epidemic in 1926 caused by ingestion of unpasteurized, contaminated milk.

DIAGNOSIS Symptoms of acute fever and prostration several days to weeks after a rat bite should cause consideration of RBF. If the incubation period is less than a week and if the syndrome includes prominent joint manifestations, the streptobacillary form is likely; a longer incubation period, particularly if associated with suppuration at the healed bite site, lymphangitis, and adenopathy, favors the spirillary form. *Streptobacillus moniliformis* can be grown from joint fluid, blood, and other body fluids when cultured in serum-enriched broth. Blood culture medium should be inoculated with twice the normal volume of patient's blood (for serum enrichment), and the commonly used anticoagulant sodium polyanethol sulfonate (SPS; Liquoid) should be omitted, as it is inhibitory to the organism. Gram stain of joint effusions may show pleomorphic gram-negative rods. Isolation of *Spirillum minus* requires intraperitoneal inoculation of blood or other infected material into mice or guinea pigs followed by dark-field examination of the animal's blood and peritoneal fluid 1 to 3 weeks later; occasionally, the organisms can be observed in direct dark-field examination of material from the patient's bite site, regional node, or blood. In both forms the white blood count may be normal or elevated, and a biologic false-positive test for syphilis occurs in up to 25 percent of streptobacillary cases and in more than 50 percent of spirillary cases. Differential diagnosis of a syndrome of fever, rash, and arthritis can be broad, especially when the history of rat bite is not elicited, as in Haverhill fever. Infectious causes include Rocky Mountain spotted fever (especially when the rash is limited to the extremities), viral exanthems, Lyme disease, gonococcal arthritis, and secondary syphilis; immune disorders include rheumatoid arthritis, systemic lupus erythematosus, and drug reactions.

TREATMENT Both organisms are susceptible to penicillin, and a dose of 600,000 units of procaine penicillin given every 12 h for 7 to 10 days should be curative. When endocarditis is present, most experts advise a dose of 15 to 20 million units per day for 4 weeks. When penicillin cannot be used, tetracycline and streptomycin are effective alternatives. Although the risk of infection from an individual rat bite appears to be low, prophylactic administration of oral penicillin V for 1 to 2 days may abort incipient infection.

CAT-SCRATCH DISEASE

DEFINITION Cat-scratch disease (CSD) is an indolent, self-limited disease characterized by a local infection at the site of the scratch followed by regional adenopathy and variable systemic symptoms lasting for weeks to months. The pathogen is a gram-negative cell-wall-defective rod, strongly associated with cats.

ETIOLOGY Over the years a number of agents were proposed as causing CSD, including viruses, chlamydiae, mycobacteria, and other bacteria. Since 1983 attention has focused on a small, pleomorphic, gram-negative bacillus that has been seen in lymph nodes, skin, and conjunctivae of patients with CSD. Margileth and colleagues have summarized the evidence supporting the etiologic role of this organism: (1) The organism has been grown on biphasic brain-heart infusion media from lymph nodes taken from 10 of 19 patients with clinical CSD and not from patients with other diseases. (2) Organisms of similar appearance have been demonstrated by Warthin-Starry stain in nodes and skin lesions from infected patients. (3) Patients have a rise in the antibody titers to the organism. (4) Antibody raised against the organism in a rabbit reacted with CSD bacilli in human tissue sections. (5) The organism causes dermal lesions in armadillos similar to those of early CSD. Several immunologically distinct subtypes may exist. In culture, the organism is thin (0.2 to 0.5 μm in diameter), short (0.2 to 2.5 μm long), and slightly curved with bulbous ends, connected in aggregates by delicate filaments. Transmission electron micrography shows that organisms in culture and tissue sections lack portions of their cell walls, which may contribute to the difficulty in culturing them. Nonetheless, the failure to grow or stain the organism in a higher percentage of patients warrants caution as to whether it is the true pathogen of CSD.

EPIDEMIOLOGY CSD is primarily a disease of childhood, the majority of cases occurring in children under age 10 and more than 90 percent of cases under age 18. The range is worldwide; all races are affected; a late summer-autumn seasonality is discernible in temperate climates. Ninty percent or more of patients report contact with a cat, although anecdotal cases suggest transmission through other mammals or by puncture wounds from inanimate objects. Cats that transmit the infection are not ill, and the duration of infectiousness is unknown. This stems partially from the fact that the disease is not very communicable: less than 5 percent of affected families have more than one case.

Subclinical disease may be common; reaction to the CSD skin test is around 20 percent in cat owners versus 1.5 percent in people who have minimal contact with cats.

PATHOLOGY The microscopic appearance of infected lymph nodes shows characteristic suppurative granulomatous inflammation but is nonspecific; other diseases causing similar pathologic appearance include lymphogranuloma venereum, tularemia, brucellosis, sarcoid, mycobacterial infection, and even some lymphomas. The characteristic delicate pleomorphic organisms can be demonstrated by Warthin-Starry silver stain in the majority of infected lymph nodes.

DIAGNOSIS The diagnosis is suggested when, with or without systemic symptoms, tender regional adenopathy and a lesion compatible with an inoculation site develop within several weeks after exposure to a cat, particularly in children. The diagnosis is confirmed when criteria in Table 98-1 are met. The CSD skin test, although unstandardized and not available commercially, is reliable, with false-positive and false-negative rates in the 5 percent range. Antigen is prepared by diluting pus aspirated from a suppurative CSD node, heating it to 60°C for 8 h, and testing for sterility and viral antigens such as hepatitis B and human immunodeficiency virus. Failure to develop at least 5 mm of induration 48 to 72 h after intracutaneous inoculation of 0.1 mL of this material on two occasions at least 4 weeks apart makes the diagnosis very unlikely. Despite the crude nature of the test material, no serious side effects have been described.

TABLE 98-1 Criteria for the diagnosis of cat-scratch disease

Diagnosis confirmed if three of the first four or one of the first four plus number five are present:

1 History of cat contact and presence of a scratch or primary dermal or eye lesion
2 Positive cat-scratch disease skin test
3 Negative studies for other causes of lymphadenopathy
4 Characteristic histopathology of a biopsied lymph node
5 Presence of typical silver-staining bacteria in histopathologic sections of lymph nodes or primary skin or eye lesions

SOURCE: BL Hainer, Cat-scratch disease, J Fam Pract 25:497, 1987.

It appears that the responsible organism has been identified, and it is likely that specific CSD antigen will provide for standardized skin testing and measurement of antibody response, thereby simplifying diagnosis. Diagnostic biopsy of involved lymph nodes or skin lesions should be restricted to the occasional case with atypical aspects such as protracted symptoms or lack of exposure to cats. Silver stain techniques should demonstrate the organism. The differential diagnosis includes infectious causes of localized adenopathy such as infectious mononucleosis, mycobacterial infection, streptococcal and staphylococcal infection, syphilis, tularemia, toxoplasmosis, sporotrichosis, and other fungi and noninfectious disorders such as lymphoma, sarcoid, congenital cysts, and Kawasaki disease.

TREATMENT Antibiotic therapy has not been studied systematically, but anecdotal evidence suggests that it has not been effective. However, the presumed causative bacillus appears to be susceptible to cefoxitin, cefotaxime, and aminoglycoside antibiotics in vitro, agents largely untried to date in CSD. Because of the benign and self-limited nature of the disease, treatment is largely supportive. Limitation of activity should be dictated by the level of constitutional symptoms, and sequential monitoring will help determine when needle aspiration of suppurative lymph nodes is warranted. A second aspiration is necessary in about half of cases. Incision and drainage or excisional biopsy of affected nodes is not recommended routinely. Isolation of affected patients is not appropriate because person-to-person spread has not been shown.

REFERENCES

CARITHERS HA: Cat-scratch disease; an overview based on a study of 1,200 patients. Am J Dis Child 139:1124, 1985

ELLIOT DL et al: Pet-associated illness. N Engl J Med 313:985, 1985

ENGLISH CK et al: Cat-scratch disease. Isolation and culture of the bacterial agent. Am J Dis Child 139:1124, 1985

FEDER HM et al: Review of 59 patients hospitalized with animal bites. Pediatr Infect Dis 6:24, 1987

HICKLIN H et al: Dysgonic fermenter 2 septicemia. Rev Infect Dis 9:884, 1987

HOLROYD KJ et al: *Streptobacillus moniliformis* polyarthritis mimicking rheumatoid arthritis: An urban case of rat bite fever. Am J Med 85:711, 1988

KOEHLER JE et al: Cutaneous vascular lesions and disseminated cat-scratch disease in patients with the acquired immunodeficiency syndrome and AIDS-related complex. Ann Intern Med 109:449, 1988

MARGILETH AM et al: Systemic cat scratch disease: Report of 23 patients with prolonged or recurrent severe bacterial infection. J Infect Dis 155:390, 1987

MCDONOUGH JJ et al: Management of animal and human bites and resulting human infections, in *Current Clinical Topics in Infectious Diseases*, JS Remington, MN Swartz (eds). New York, McGraw-Hill, 1987, vol 8, pp 11–36

SHANSON DC et al: *Streptobacillus moniliformis* isolated from blood in four cases of Haverhill fever. Lancet 2:92, 1983

section 4 Diseases caused by gram-positive organisms

99 PNEUMOCOCCAL INFECTIONS

ROBERT AUSTRIAN

ETIOLOGY The pneumococcus *(Streptococcus pneumoniae)* is a gram-positive encapsulated coccus that usually grows in pairs or short chains. In the diplococcal form, the adjacent margins are rounded and the opposite ends slightly pointed, giving the organisms a lancet shape. In stained preparations of exudate, gram-negative forms are sometimes present. Pneumococcal colonies are surrounded by greenish discoloration on or in blood agar and are confused at times with other alpha-hemolytic streptococci to which they are closely related. Their isolation from respiratory secretions may be facilitated by inclusion of 5 μg gentamicin per milliliter in the medium. Pneumococci can be distinguished by their bile solubility and mouse virulence or by serologic typing. Another method with approximately 90 percent specificity, utilizing inhibition of pneumococci by Optochin-impregnated paper disks, is less cumbersome.

The capsular substances are complex polysaccharides and are the basis for dividing pneumococci into serotypes. Organisms exposed to type-specific antiserum show a positive capsular precipitin reaction, the Neufeld quellung reaction; by this means, 84 serotypes have been identified. All are pathogenic for human beings, but types or groups 1, 3, 4, 7, 8, 9, and 12 are encountered most frequently in clinical practice. Types or groups 6, 14, 19, and 23 often cause pneumonia and otitis media in children but are less common in adults.

Specific typing of pneumococci remains of great clinical importance if pneumococcus is to be identified with regularity, and recognition of pneumococcus has decreased significantly since the abandonment of capsular typing by most clinical laboratories. The detection of pneumococcal capsular polysaccharides in sputum and in other body fluids by immunologic methods such as counter-immunoelectrophoresis (CIE) or latex agglutination provides an alternative to bacteriologic techniques for the presumptive diagnosis of pneumococcal infection. Because of cross reactions between the polysaccharides of pneumococci and of other bacterial species, immunologic diagnosis is less specific than bacteriologic diagnosis.

PATHOGENESIS The mechanism by which pneumococci damage the mammalian host is obscure, and no toxin elaborated by the organism has been shown to play a major pathogenic role in pneumococcal infection, although components of the cell wall may cause inflammation. The capsular polysaccharides, though nontoxic, are known to be necessary factors in virulence and to offer some protection of the organism from phagocytosis.

Although "pneumococcal pharyngitis" is a doubtful clinical entity, invasion of nasopharyngeal tissue may occur in the infant and occasionally in the nonimmune adult and be followed by spread to the circulation via the cervical lymphatics. At times, secondary infection of serous cavities in the absence of demonstrable focal infection of the upper or lower respiratory tract may occur. The organisms multiply readily in vivo and may produce acute inflammation of the lungs, serous cavities, and endocardium.

The normal human respiratory tract is provided with a variety of mechanisms which guard the lungs from infection. The lower respiratory tract is protected by the glottis and larynx, and material passing these barriers stimulates the expulsive cough reflex. Removal of small particles impinging on the walls of the trachea and bronchi is facilitated by their mucociliary lining (see Chap. 207); and growth of bacteria reaching normal alveoli is inhibited by their relative dryness and by the phagocytic activity of alveolar macrophages. Any anatomic or physiologic derangement of these coordinated defenses tends to augment the susceptibility of the lungs to infection. Anesthesia, alcoholic intoxication, convulsions, and disturbed innervation of the larynx depress the cough reflex and may permit aspiration of infected material. Alterations in the tracheobronchial tree leading to anatomic changes in the epithelial lining or to localized obstruction increase the vulnerability of the lungs to infection. Pulmonary edema, local or generalized, resulting from viral infection, inhalation of irritant gases, cardiac failure, or contusion of the chest wall, provides a fluid menstruum in the alveoli for the growth of bacteria and their spread to adjacent areas of the lung. Viral infection of the respiratory epithelium with concomitant disruption of its component cells interferes significantly with the clearance of bacteria from the lungs, an observation in accord with the high incidence of pneumococcal pneumonia during epidemics of viral influenza and its frequent clinical association with sporadic viral respiratory infections.

Pneumonia usually begins in the right lower, right middle, or left lower lobe, those areas to which gravity is most likely to carry upper respiratory secretions aspirated during sleep. Bronchial embolization with infected mucinous secretions during the course of an upper respiratory infection appears to be the initiating factor in many cases of pneumococcal pneumonia. Protected initially from phagocytosis by mucinous material, the bacteria multiply and, in infected alveoli, evoke the outpouring of proteinaceous fluid which serves both as a nutrient and as a vehicle for spread to adjacent alveoli. Soon thereafter, polymorphonuclear leukocytes migrate from the pulmonary capillaries to phagocytize a part of the pneumococcal population before the appearance of detectable antibody. Delay in the polymorphonuclear leukocytic response occurs during alcoholic intoxication and certain forms of anesthesia, permitting spread of infection. Glucocorticoids may also interfere with leukocyte migration. Later, as the pneumonic lesion evolves, macrophages appear in the exudate and remove the debris of fibrin and cells. It is probable that antibody to the capsular polysaccharide of the invading pneumococcus makes its appearance locally in the lung before being detectable in the circulation. Such antibody increases the efficiency of phagocytosis approximately twofold and causes agglutination of the organisms and their adherence to alveolar walls, thereby slowing their dissemination in the lung. The outcome of infection depends, therefore, on the rate at which bacteria can multiply in the edema fluid and spread, and on the host's ability to immobilize and destroy them by phagocytosis. Individuals with hypogammaglobulinemia and patients with multiple myeloma (see Chap. 265) incapable of producing anticapsular antibody are prone to recurrent attacks of pneumococcal pneumonia. Repeated infection with the same pneumococcal type should always prompt a search for dysgammaglobulinemia.

Failure of local defense mechanisms in the lung results in lymphatic spread of pneumococci to the hilar lymph nodes. In the sinusoids of these organs, a sequence of events not unlike that in the lung ensues. If infection is not checked in this secondary line of defense, organisms find their way into the thoracic duct and then into the circulation. Although transient bacteremia may occur at the onset of many cases of pneumococcal pneumonia, it is detectable in only 20 to 30 percent of cases. Bacteremia, which reflects the body's inability to localize the pulmonary infection, is a poor prognostic sign and carries with it the danger of metastatic infection. The mortality of treated or untreated bacteremic pneumococcal pneumonia is four times that resulting from comparably managed nonbacteremic infections. Metastatic infection secondary to bacteremia may occur in the meninges, joints, or peritoneum or on the endocardium. Direct spread from the infected lung may give rise to empyema or to pericarditis.

Natural recovery from pneumococcal infection coincides usually, but not invariably, with the appearance of detectable type-specific antibody in the circulation and is often accompanied by a dramatic and abrupt fall in temperature, the so-called crisis. Antibody aids recovery by increasing the efficiency of phagocytosis and by limiting dissemination of the organisms. Bacteriostatic drugs, such as sulfonamides, facilitate control of the infection by limiting the size of the pneumococcal population, but the host's defense mechanisms are still required for the elimination of the bacteria. Bactericidal agents, such as penicillin, cause the death of pneumococci in the lung and are effective when some of the host's defense mechanisms are compromised. With the arrest of infection, the alveolar exudate undergoes liquefaction, the inflammatory debris is removed by expectoration and via the lymphatic channels, and the lung is restored to its normal state. Necrosis of pulmonary tissue as a result of pneumococcal infection is distinctly uncommon. Primary pneumococcal lung abscess is a rare clinical entity, although the diagnosis is mistakenly made at times when pneumococcal infection complicates lung abscess of other origins.

In addition to causing pneumonia and its metastatic sequelae, pneumococcus can extend from the nasopharynx to its adjacent structures, giving rise to otitis media, mastoiditis, paranasal sinusitis, or conjunctivitis. Soft tissue abscesses are rare but may occur.

PNEUMOCOCCAL PNEUMONIA

Pneumococcal pneumonia is a disease of considerable uniformity, in contrast to other infections such as typhoid fever and tuberculosis. The diseases produced by different pneumococcal serotypes show little variation in severity or in clinical manifestations. The prognosis in type 3 pneumococcal pneumonia is usually regarded as poor, probably because type 3 infections occur frequently in the aged and in patients with other debilitating diseases, such as diabetes and congestive heart failure. The usual lesion in adults is segmental or lobar in distribution, but in children and the aged, bronchopneumonia, characterized by patchy involvement, is frequent.

MANIFESTATIONS Pneumonia is often preceded for a few days by coryza or some other form of common respiratory disease. The onset is frequently so abrupt that the patient can state the exact hour that illness began. There is a sudden *shaking chill* in more than 80 percent of the cases and a rapid rise in temperature, with corresponding tachycardia and an increase in respiratory rate (tachypnea). Most patients with pneumococcal pneumonia have a single rigor unless antipyretic drugs are administered, and repeated chills should suggest another etiologic agent.

About 75 percent of patients develop severe *pleuritic pain* and *cough,* productive of pinkish or "rusty" mucoid sputum within a few hours. The chest pain is agonizing, and respirations become rapid, shallow, and grunting as the patient tries to splint the affected side. Many patients are mildly cyanotic as a result of hypoxia caused by $\dot{V}/\dot{Q}$ (ventilation-perfusion ratio) abnormality or shunt, which accompanies altered respiration, and show dilatation of the alae nasi when first seen. Patients appear acutely ill; but nausea, headache, and malaise are not prominent, and most individuals are alert. Pleuritic pain and dyspnea are the dominant complaints.

In the untreated disease, there are sustained fever of 39.2 to 40.5°C (103 to 105°F), continued pleuritic pain, cough, and expectoration; and *abdominal distention* is frequent. *Herpes labialis* is a common complication. After 7 to 10 days, there are diaphoresis, abrupt defervescence, and dramatic improvement in well-being, the "crisis."

In cases which terminate fatally, there is usually extensive pulmonary involvement, and dyspnea, cyanosis, and tachycardia are prominent. Circulatory collapse or a picture resembling adult respiratory distress syndrome has been observed. Death in a few patients is associated with empyema or some other suppurative complication such as meningitis or endocarditis.

Physical examination reveals restricted motion of the affected hemithorax. Tactile fremitus may be decreased during the initial day of illness but is usually increased when consolidation is fully established. Deviation of the trachea away from the affected lung suggests pleural effusion or empyema. The percussion note is dull, and if the lesion is in an upper lobe, impaired motion of the diaphragm can be detected on the affected side. Very early in the course of infection, breath sounds are diminished, but as the lesion evolves, they become tubular or bronchial in quality, and bronchophony and whispered pectoriloquy can be elicited. These findings are accompanied by fine crepitant rales.

EFFECT OF SPECIFIC CHEMOTHERAPY Pneumococcal pneumonia usually improves promptly when an appropriate antimicrobial drug is given. Within 12 to 36 h after initiation of treatment with penicillin, temperature, pulse, and respiration begin to fall and may reach normal values, pleuritic pain subsides, and the spread of the inflammatory process is halted. The temperature of approximately half the patients, however, requires 4 days or longer to become normal, and failure of the patient's temperature to reach normal in 24 to 48 h should not prompt a change in antibacterial therapy in the absence of other indications.

COMPLICATIONS The typical course of pneumococcal pneumonia can be modified by the development of one or more local or distant complications:

In the lung ATELECTASIS Atelectasis of all or part of a lobe may occur during the active stage of pneumonia or after treatment has been instituted. The patient may complain of sudden recurrence of pleuritic pain and show rapid respirations. Small areas of atelectasis are often detected by x-ray in the absence of symptoms. These areas usually clear with coughing and deep breathing, but bronchoscopic aspiration is occasionally necessary. If atelectasis is allowed to persist, the affected area becomes fibrotic and functionless.

DELAYED RESOLUTION Return of physical findings in the lung to normal after pneumococcal pneumonia is usually complete within 2 to 4 weeks. X-ray evidence of residual pulmonary consolidation, however, may persist as long as 8 weeks, and other radiologic manifestations of the infection (volume loss, stranding, and pleural disease) may persist for up to 18 weeks. The process of resolution may require a longer time in those over 50 years of age and in those with chronic obstructive airway disease or alcoholism.

ABSCESS Lung abscess is a rare sequel to pneumococcal infection, although pneumococcal pneumonia is a not uncommon complication of lung abscess of other origins. It is manifested by continued fever and profuse expectoration of purulent sputum. X-ray shows one or more cavities. This complication is exceedingly rare in patients who receive penicillin therapy and is most likely to follow infection with pneumococcus type 3.

In adjacent structures PLEURAL EFFUSION Pleural effusion detectable in lateral decubitus x-rays of the chest occurs in approximately half of patients with pneumococcal pneumonia and is associated with delay in the initiation of therapy and with bacteremia. Usually the effusion is sterile and is absorbed spontaneously within a week or two. At times, however, the effusion is large and requires aspiration or drainage.

EMPYEMA Before the introduction of effective chemotherapy, empyema occurred in 5 to 8 percent of patients with pneumococcal pneumonia; it is now observed in less than 1 percent of treated cases. It is manifested by persistent fever or pleuritic pain, together with signs of pleural effusion. In the early stages, the gross appearance of infected fluid may not differ from that of a sterile pleural effusion; later, there is a profuse outpouring of polymorphonuclear leukocytes and fibrin, resulting in an exudate of thick greenish pus containing large clots of fibrin. The quantity of exudate may become large enough to displace mediastinal structures. In neglected cases, this process leads to extensive pleural scarring, with limitation of thoracic movement. Rupture and drainage through the chest wall *(empyema necessitatis)* occur, but are rare. Metastatic *brain abscess* is an occasional complication of chronic empyema.

PERICARDITIS A particularly serious complication is spread of infection to the pericardial sac. This lesion is characterized by pain in the precordial region, a friction rub synchronous with the heartbeat, and distention of cervical veins, although one or all of these findings may be absent. The possibility of coexisting purulent pericarditis should be considered whenever a very ill patient with pneumonia develops empyema.

Metastatic infections *Arthritis* occurs more often in children than in adults. The affected joint is swollen, red, and painful, with a purulent effusion. It usually subsides promptly with systemic administration of penicillin, although aspiration and intraarticular injection of penicillin may be necessary in adults.

Acute bacterial endocarditis and *meningitis*, complications of pneumococcal pneumonia, are discussed subsequently.

Paralytic ileus Gaseous abdominal distention is commonly present and in severely ill patients may assume such serious proportions that the term *paralytic ileus* is justified. This complication further impairs respiratory movement by elevation of the diaphragm and constitutes a difficult problem in management. A rarer and more serious gastrointestinal complication is acute gastric dilatation.

Impaired liver function Alterations in hepatic function are common during the course of pneumococcal pneumonia, and mild jaundice is not at all rare. The pathogenesis of the jaundice is not entirely clear, although in some patients it appears to be related to glucose-6-phosphate dehydrogenase deficiency.

LABORATORY FINDINGS *Sputum* should be obtained in the physician's presence before the administration of antimicrobial drugs to ensure its quality. Although resort to transtracheal aspiration or lung puncture may be necessary on occasion to establish the cause of pneumonia, routine use of these invasive techniques is not recommended because of their attendant, albeit infrequent, complications. When stained by Gram's method, the sputum shows polymorphonuclear leukocytes and variable numbers of gram-positive cocci, singly and in pairs. These can be typed directly by the Neufeld quellung technique, and this procedure should be used to facilitate diagnosis whenever possible. The *blood culture* is positive for pneumococci during the first days of untreated illness in 20 to 30 percent of cases. The white blood cell count usually shows a polymorphonuclear *leukocytosis* ranging from 12×10^9/L to 25×10^9/L (12,000 to 25,000 cells per microliter). A normal white count or leukopenia is sometimes observed in patients with overwhelming infection and bacteremia. Occasionally, pneumococci may be seen directly in granulocytes of patients with bacteremia by examining the buffy coat after staining with Wright's stain. These patients often have asplenia. *X-ray of the chest* usually reveals a homogenous density in the affected area of the lung. In well-established cases, the density may occupy one or more entire lobes. Atypical patterns of consolidation may be seen in patients with underlying chronic pulmonary disease.

EXTRAPULMONARY PNEUMOCOCCAL INFECTION

PNEUMOCOCCAL MENINGITIS The pneumococcus is second only to the meningococcus as a cause of purulent meningitis in adults; in children, meningitis caused by *Haemophilus influenzae* is also more frequent than pneumococcal infection.

Pneumococcal meningitis can develop as a "primary" disease without preceding signs of infection elsewhere; as a complication of pneumococcal pneumonia; by extension from otitis, mastoiditis, or sinusitis; or following a skull fracture which creates an opening between the subarachnoid space and the nasal cavity or paranasal sinuses. Patients with pneumococcal endocarditis frequently develop meningeal infection. Patients with multiple myeloma and with sickle cell disease seem to be prone to pneumococcal infection of the meninges, just as they are to pneumonia.

The *manifestations* are of those of any acute pyogenic meningitis (see Chap. 354) and include chills, fever, headache, nuchal rigidity, Kernig's and Brudzinski's signs, delirium, and cranial nerve palsies. Evidence of otitis, sinusitis, or pneumonia should be carefully sought by physical and roentgenographic examination in all patients.

The *spinal fluid* is under increased pressure, appears cloudy, often with a greenish tint, and shows a high protein and low glucose content. Stained smears usually reveal gram-positive diplococci and polymorphonuclear leukocytes; in some patients, the number of cells in the spinal fluid is surprisingly small, and much of the cloudiness is produced by the bacterial content. The diagnosis can be established rapidly by identification of pneumococci in the spinal fluid by Gram's stain. Immunologic tests (CIE or latex agglutination) are positive in approximately 80 percent of culture-positive cases and may provide a presumptive bacterial cause of infection in some patients from whose spinal fluid no organism is recovered.

With appropriate chemotherapy, recovery can be expected in 70 percent of cases; the prognosis is better in children than in infants or in adults. Relapse may occur but is unusual if adequate treatment is carried out. Subarachnoid block, the result of accumulation of large amounts of thick exudate in the meningeal space and at the base of the brain, is an infrequent complication.

PNEUMOCOCCAL ENDOCARDITIS Endocarditis is a rare complication of pneumonia or meningitis. The clinical picture is that of acute bacterial endocarditis (see Chap. 90), with remittent fever, splenomegaly, and metastatic infection of the lungs, meninges, joints, eye, and other tissues. Petechiae are uncommon. The infection can attack normal valves and is particularly likely to occur on the aortic valve. The valvular infection is destructive, and loud murmurs and heart failure develop rapidly. Rupture or perforation of cusps or even rupture of the aorta may occur. The blood culture is consistently positive for the pneumococcus in the absence of treatment with antimicrobial drugs; yet at the same time antibodies to the infecting organism may be demonstrable in the blood, a combination of findings seldom observed except in endocarditis or brucellosis. Although the infection is relatively easy to cure with penicillin, damage to valve leaflets, especially to the cusps of the aortic valve, may be followed by rapidly progressive heart failure. Surgical repair or replacement of damaged valvular structures should be carried out early, before heart failure becomes intractable.

PNEUMOCOCCAL PERITONITIS Pneumococcal peritonitis is a rare disease and is probably the sequel to transient pneumococcal bacteremia, although, because of its somewhat greater frequency in young girls, it has been hypothesized that the organism may gain entry to the peritoneum via the vagina and fallopian tubes. Peritonitis was formerly a common complication of the nephrotic syndrome, particularly in children, but it occurs now with a frequency of less than 2 percent. In adults, the disease is seen in association with cirrhosis or with carcinoma of the liver. The diagnosis is made by examination of the ascitic fluid; blood cultures are often positive, and a polymorphonuclear leukocytosis is the rule.

TREATMENT

SPECIFIC ANTIMICROBIAL THERAPY Although resistance of pneumococci to antimicrobial drugs has not been regarded as a significant problem in the past, a small but increasing number of strains have been found to be resistant to one or all of the following agents: penicillins, cephalosporins, tetracyclines, chloramphenicol, erythromycin, clindamycin, co-trimoxazole, and aminoglycosides.

For this reason sensitivity of the infecting organism to the drug(s) to be used should be determined, particularly in treating extrapulmonary infection. In the absence of resistance or of hypersensitivity to it, penicillin G (benzylpenicillin) is the drug of choice for all manifestations of pneumococcal infection. Strains of pneumococcus manifesting increased resistance to penicillin have been recovered infrequently from humans; and although the level of such resistance does not often preclude treatment with this antibiotic, awareness of the phenomenon is necessary. A dose of 600,000 units daily provides a good margin of safety in treating adults with bacteremic or nonbacteremic infection in the absence of an extrapulmonary focus, but the occurrence of pneumococci showing increased resistance to penicillin makes the initiation of therapy with larger amounts desirable. Treatment may be started with doses of 600,000 units of aqueous crystalline penicillin G or procaine penicillin administered at 12-h intervals to be continued until the patient has been afebrile for 48 to 72 h. Pneumococcal pneumonia can be treated with an oral penicillin, preferably one resistant to gastric acid (see Chap. 85), in dosage equivalent to 2.4 to 4.8 million units of penicillin G. *Peritonitis* caused by sensitive strains responds usually within 36 to 48 h to 2 to 4 million units of penicillin daily.

Pneumococcal meningitis in adults should be treated with 18 to 24 million units of penicillin G daily intravenously. Larger amounts should not be used, to avoid neurotoxicity from excessive dosage. Intrathecal administration of penicillin is unnecessary, and supplementation of penicillin with broad-spectrum bacteriostatic drugs such as tetracyclines may exert a deleterious effect. All pneumococcal isolates from cerebrospinal fluid should be tested promptly for their sensitivity to antibacterial drugs. Vancomycin is the drug of choice for treatment of meningitis caused by pneumococci resistant to multiple antimicrobial agents.

Moderate doses of penicillin G are used to treat pneumococcal endocarditis—8 to 12 million units daily by intravenous infusion. Rapidly developing heart failure as a result of valvular injury and a tendency to form myocardial abscess, however, often lead to a fatal outcome despite the use of antibiotics. Prompt surgical repair or replacement of damaged heart valves should be considered when cardiac failure develops.

Cephalosporins in parenteral doses of 1 to 2 g daily are effective in pneumococcal pneumonia but must be administered with caution to those hypersensitive to penicillin. Many members of this class of β-lactam drugs cannot be used to treat meningitis because of their poor ability to penetrate the blood–cerebrospinal fluid barrier. Several of the newer cephalosporins, including cefotaxime and ceftriaxone, show promise of efficacy in treating pneumococcal meningitis although experience with each is limited. The tetracyclines in doses of 1 to 2 g daily, erythromycin in doses of 1.6 g daily, or clindamycin in doses of 1.2 g daily are effective treatment for pneumococcal pneumonia if it is caused by a sensitive strain, but they are recommended only for patients who have had untoward reactions to penicillins or cephalosporins. Despite its efficacy, chloramphenicol should not be used to treat pneumococcal infections other than meningitis in patients hypersensitive to penicillin who are infected with a drug-sensitive strain. For patients with illness caused by multiply drug-resistant pneumococci, vancomycin in doses of 2 g daily is the drug of choice. Sulfonamides have little place in the present-day treatment of pneumococcal pneumonia and are useless in endocarditis and meningitis. Aminoglycosides, such as gentamicin, tobramycin, and amikacin, should not be employed to treat pneumococcal infection.

Pneumococcal arthritis responds to systemic penicillin, but aspiration and intraarticular instillation of the drug may be necessary.

Empyema should be detected and treated as early as possible. When an effusion is found, fluid should be removed and examined for bacteria, leukocytes, glucose concentration, and pH. The presence of bacteria, pus, a pH below 7.0, and/or a pleural fluid glucose below 2.2 mmol/L (40 mg/dL) are indications for institution of closed-chest tube drainage. Failure to cure empyema early may be followed by pleural fibrosis and may necessitate subsequent surgical decortication of the lung to restore pulmonary function.

OTHER MEASURES Oxygen administered through a face mask should be used to treat significant cyanosis, cardiac failure, and delirium. In the presence of adult respiratory distress syndrome, positive end-expiratory pressure may be indicated. Codeine, 32 to 64 mg every 4 h, will usually control pleuritic pain. When pain is severe, it may require intercostal nerve block with 1 to 2% procaine for relief.

PROGNOSIS AND PREVENTION

Although the mortality from pneumococcal pneumonia has diminished significantly since the advent of antimicrobial drugs, available evidence indicates that the incidence of the disease has changed little, if at all. The fatality rate in patients over the age of 12 years with bacteremic pneumococcal pneumonia treated with an antibiotic is 18 percent, and in patients over the age of 50 and in those with underlying systemic illness, it is significantly higher.

Signs of poor prognosis in pneumonia include leukopenia, bacteremia, multilobar involvement, any extrapulmonary focus of pneumococcal infection, presence of preexisting systemic disease, circulatory collapse, and occurrence of the infection in the first year of life or after the age of 55. Infection with pneumococcus type 3 has a higher mortality rate than that caused by other pneumococcal types. Death is most likely to occur in individuals sustaining irreversible physiologic damage early in the course which is unaltered by antimicrobial therapy. Until the nature of the injury produced by pneumococcus is understood and ways are devised to repair it, vaccination will remain the principal means of protecting those at high risk of a fatal outcome.

A 23-valent vaccine containing the capsular polysaccharides of pneumococcal types 1, 2, 3, 4, 5, 6B, 7F, 8, 9N, 9V, 10A, 11A, 12F, 14, 15B, 17F, 18C, 19F, 19A, 20, 22F, 23F, and 33F, which include the serotypes or groups responsible for 90 percent of bacteremic infections in the United States, is recommended for prevention of pneumococcal infection caused by these serotypes in individuals at high risk of a fatal outcome. Those at higher-than-average risk are individuals over the age of 55 and patients with a variety of chronic systemic illnesses including heart disease, chronic bronchopulmonary disease, hepatic disease, renal insufficiency, diabetes, and a variety of malignancies. Persons of all ages with sickle cell disease have an increased risk of developing pneumococcal infection, and the vaccine is recommended for those with this disorder over the age of 2 years. Since anatomic or functional asplenia is associated with fulminant overwhelming pneumococcal septicemia with disseminated intravascular coagulation, giving rise to a clinical picture resembling that of the Waterhouse-Friderichsen syndrome, such individuals should also be immunized. However, the vaccine does not contain the antigens of all pneumococcal types, and infection caused by nonincluded types may occur occasionally in immunized subjects. Reactions to the vaccine are usually absent or mild, although in the occasional individual they may resemble those following immunization with typhoid vaccine: local pain, erythema, and elevation of temperature. Because of the persistence of pneumococcal antibodies after a single injection of vaccine, reimmunization is not necessary. The aggregate efficacy of the vaccine in preventing bacteremic infection is 65 to 70 percent in immunocompetent adults. It may afford little, if any, protection, however, to those with agamma- or dysgammaglobulinemia or to patients who have been subjected recently to intensive antitumor chemotherapy and radiation. In children, immunologic responsiveness to different capsular antigens develops at different times prior to puberty as a result of maturational characteristics of the human immune system and, in infancy, may be manifested only by antibodies of the IgM class. Currently, vaccines of capsular polysaccharide conjugated to proteins such as diphtheria toxoid, which are antigenic in infancy, are under development for pediatric populations. If circumstances dictate, pneumococcal vaccine may be administered concomitantly with influenza viral vaccine, provided each vaccine is injected from a separate syringe at a separate site.

REFERENCES

Applebaum PC: World-wide development of antibiotic resistance in pneumococci. Eur J Clin Microbiol 6:367, 1987

Austrian R: *Life with the Pneumococcus*. Philadelphia, University of Pennsylvania Press, 1985

———: Untreated pneumococcal bacteraemia of cryptic origin in the human adult with spontaneous recovery. S Afr Med J 70(Suppl):46, 1986

Bolan N et al: Pneumococcal vaccine efficacy in selected populations in the United States. Ann Intern Med 104:1, 1986

Fruchtman SM et al: Adult respiratory distress syndrome as a cause of death in pneumococcal pneumonia. Chest 83:598, 1983

Heffron R: *Pneumonia with Special Reference to Pneumococcus Lobar Pneumonia*. Cambridge, Harvard, 1979

Kaplan SL: Antigen detection in cerebrospinal fluid—pros and cons. Am J Med 75:109, 1983

Klugman KP, Koornhof HJ: Drug resistance patterns and serogroups or serotypes of pneumococcal isolates from cerebrospinal fluid or blood, 1979–1986. J Inf Dis 158:956, 1988

Paton JC et al: Antibody response to pneumococcal vaccine in children aged 5 to 15 years. Am J Dis Child 140:135, 1986

Research Committee, British Thoracic Society: Community-acquired pneumonia in adults in British hospitals in 1982–83: A study of aetiology, mortality, prognostic factors and outcome. Quart J Med 62:195, 1987

Shapiro ED, Clemens JD: A controlled evaluation of pneumococcal vaccine for patients at high risk of serious pneumococcal infections. Ann Intern Med 101:325, 1984

Stephen JJ et al: The radiographic resolution of *Streptococcus pneumoniae* pneumonia. N Engl J Med 293:798, 1975

Tuomanen E et al: Induction of pulmonary inflammation by components of the pneumococcal cell surface. Am Rev Resp Dis 135:869, 1987

Viladrich PF et al: Characteristics and antibiotic therapy of adult meningitis due to penicillin-resistant pneumococci. Am J Med 84:839, 1988

100 STAPHYLOCOCCAL INFECTIONS

RICHARD M. LOCKSLEY

The staphylococci, of which *Staphylococcus aureus* is the most important human pathogen, are hardy, gram-positive bacteria that colonize the skin of most human beings. If the skin or mucous membranes are disrupted by surgery or trauma, staphylococci may gain access to and proliferate in the underlying tissues, giving rise to a typically localized, superficial abscess. Although these cutaneous infections are most commonly harmless and self-limited, the multiplying organisms may invade the lymphatics and the blood, leading to the potentially serious complications of staphylococcal bacteremia. These complications include septic shock, which may be indistinguishable from that caused by gram-negative bacteria, and serious metastatic infections, including endocarditis (see Chap. 90), arthritis (see Chap. 96), osteomyelitis (see Chap. 97), pneumonia (see Chap. 207), and abscesses (see Chap. 91) in virtually any organ. Certain strains of *S. aureus* produce toxins that cause skin rashes or that mediate multisystem dysfunction, as in toxic shock syndrome. Coagulase-negative staphylococci, particularly *S. epidermidis*, are important nosocomial pathogens, with a particular predilection for infecting vascular catheters and prosthetic devices. *S. saprophyticus* is a common cause of urinary tract infection.

ETIOLOGY AND MICROBIOLOGY Staphylococci are gram-positive, nonmotile, aerobic or facultatively anaerobic, catalase-positive cocci within the family Micrococcaceae. The name derives from the typical clustering of organisms (the Greek *staphyle*, "bunch of grapes") observed microscopically in stained specimens taken from colonies grown on solid media. Pathogenic staphylococci are distinguished from nonpathogenic micrococci by the ability of staphylococci to ferment glucose anaerobically and by their sensitivity to lysostaphin endopeptidase. *S. aureus*, the most important human pathogen in the genus, is named for the golden color of colonies grown aerobically on solid media. All staphylococcal strains producing coagulase are designated *S. aureus*. In contrast to coagulase-negative staphylococci, *S. aureus* ferments mannitol, produces DNase, and displays greater susceptibility to lysostaphin. *S. aureus* strains are generally hemolytic when cultured on blood agar and exhibit greater expression of biochemical activity (production of coagulase, toxins, hemolysis) than coagulase-negative staphylococci.

There are 21 recognized species of coagulase-negative staphylococci. Twelve are part of the normal human flora, of which *S. epidermidis* and *S. saprophyticus* are the most important clinically.

Differentiation among strains of *S. aureus* or *S. epidermidis* has been used to identify a common source during epidemics or intrahospital outbreaks of staphylococcal disease. Strains may be distinguished by antimicrobial susceptibility profiles, patterns of lysis by staphylococcal bacteriophages (phage typing), and biochemical testing (biotyping) and molecular analysis of plasmids or of plasmid or chromosomal DNA. Of these three tests, antibiotic susceptibility testing has the least, and molecular analysis the most, discriminatory ability.

EPIDEMIOLOGY The coagulase-negative staphylococci are part of the normal flora of the skin, mucous membranes, and lower bowel; *S. epidermidis* is the commonest species isolated. *S. aureus* transiently colonizes the anterior nares in 70 to 90 percent of persons and may be recovered for relatively prolonged periods of time in 20 to 30 percent of them. Nasal carriage is often accompanied by secondary colonization of the skin. Independent colonization of the perineal area occurs in 5 to 20 percent of persons, and vaginal carriage has been demonstrated in 10 percent of menstruating females. Higher carriage rates of *S. aureus* have been documented in hospital employees (including physicians and nurses), hospitalized patients, persons with atopic dermatitis, and patients whose care requires frequent puncture of the skin, e.g., with insulin-dependent diabetes, dialysis-dependent renal failure, or frequent desensitization injections for allergies. Drug abusers who use needles also have enhanced *S. aureus* carriage rates. Presumably, disturbances in the local cutaneous barrier allow *S. aureus* to establish and maintain colonization successfully.

S. saprophyticus demonstrates enhanced adherence to urothelial cells compared to *S. epidermidis*. Approximately 5 percent of healthy males and females have low colony counts of *S. saprophyticus* in the urethral or periurethral areas (see Chap. 95).

Although staphylococci can survive in the environment for prolonged periods of time and airborne spread of organisms can be demonstrated, person-to-person transfer via contaminated hands is the most important mechanism for transmission of these organisms. Hospitalized patients with active staphylococcal infection or those who become heavily colonized, particularly at cutaneous sites (surgical wounds, burns, decubitus ulcers), constitute the greatest reservoir for nosocomially acquired infection. Such patients shed an enormous number of organisms, and the hands of hospital personnel caring for these patients are readily colonized. Failure to use aseptic technique and neglect of hand washing allows transmission of the organisms to the skin of other patients. Strains of both *S. aureus* and *S. epidermidis* may become endemic in areas of the hospital housing patients with large integumental defects, particularly when widespread antimicrobial use favors the acquisition of multiply resistant strains (burn units, intensive care units, bone marrow transplant units). Less frequently, otherwise healthy hospital employees who are nasal carriers have been implicated in nosocomial outbreaks. Upon careful examination, most of these carriers will have active dermatologic infections during the time that effective transmission of staphylococci is documented.

If infections arising from the urinary tract are excluded, *S. aureus* and *S. epidermidis* together have become the most common cause of nosocomial infection in United States hospitals. They are the most frequently isolated pathogens in both primary and secondary bacteremias and in cutaneous and surgical wound infections.

PATHOGENESIS Infection by staphylococci usually results from a combination of bacterial virulence factors and diminution in host defense. Important microbial factors include the ability of the staphylococcus to survive under harsh conditions, its cell wall constituents, the production of enzymes and toxins that promote tissue invasion, its capacity to persist intracellularly in certain phagocytes, and its potential to acquire resistance to antimicrobials. Important host factors include an intact mucocutaneous barrier, an adequate number of functional neutrophils, and removal of foreign bodies or devitalized tissues.

Microbial factors Cell wall components of *S. aureus* include a large peptidoglycan complex that confers rigidity on the organism and enables it to survive under unfavorable osmotic conditions, a unique teichoic acid linked to peptidoglycan, and protein A, found both attached to peptidoglycan over the outermost parts of the cell and released in soluble form. Both peptidoglycan and teichoic acid are capable of activating the complement cascade via the alternative pathway. Although important for opsonization of organisms for ingestion by phagocytes, complement activation may also play a role in the pathogenesis of shock and disseminated intravascular coagulation. Protein A binds in the Fc portion of certain classes of IgG as well as to the Fc receptor on phagocytes and may serve as a blocking factor preventing neutrophil ingestion of the organism. Specific receptors for laminin, the major glycoprotein of the vascular basement membrane, may mediate the widespread metastatic potential of *S. aureus*. Activation of tissue factor (procoagulant activity) occurs when endothelial cells and monocytes are incubated with *S. aureus*. Some strains of *S. aureus* may be coated by an antiphagocytic capsule that requires specific antibodies for ingestion. The cell wall of certain strains of *S. epidermidis* is also capable of activating complement; shock and disseminated intravascular coagulation during infections by these organisms have been described, although less frequently than with *S. aureus*. The capacity of *S. epidermidis* to adhere to intravascular cannulas and prosthetic devices may explain the propensity of these organisms to cause foreign body infections. These organisms bind fibronectin and other matrix proteins that coat catheters and secrete an exopolysaccharide slime that forms a protective biofilm over the colonizing organisms.

Certain enzymes produced by *S. aureus* may play a role in virulence. Catalase degrades hydrogen peroxide and may protect the organism during phagocytosis when it must withstand the phagocyte's respiratory burst. Coagulase is present in both soluble and cell-bound forms, and causes plasma to clot by formation of thrombinlike material. The high correlation between coagulase production and virulence suggests that this substance is important in the pathogenesis of staphylococcal infections, but its precise role as a determinant of pathogenicity has not been determined. Many strains also produce hyaluronidase, an enzyme that degrades hyaluronic acid in the connective tissue matrix and that may promote spreading of infection. A trypsinlike protease from some strains enhances influenza virus infection by proteolytic cleavage of the viral precursor hemagglutinin into its active fragments, and may contribute to the morbidity of such coinfections. *S. saprophyticus* produces urease, an enzyme capable of breaking down urea to ammonium, alkalinizing the urine and favoring the formation of struvite stones.

S. aureus may produce numerous extracellular toxins. The expression of multiple toxins, as in gram-negative bacilli, is coordinately regulated by an accessory gene regulator protein, presumably in response to physicochemical environmental stimuli. Toxins may be encoded by chromosomal or plasmid DNA. Four different red cell hemolysins—designated alpha, beta, gamma, and delta toxins—have been identified. Alpha toxin is also dermonecrotic when injected subcutaneously into animals. Delta toxin inhibits water absorption by elevating cyclic AMP in guinea pig ileum and may play a role in the acute watery diarrhea seen in some cases of staphylococcal infection. Leukocidin lyses granulocyte and macrophage membranes by producing membrane pores permeable to cations.

While the role of the above factors in virulence is incompletely understood, the exfoliatin toxins A and B, the staphylococcal enterotoxins, and the toxic shock syndrome toxin—TSST-1—have been implicated in disease. The exfoliatin toxins mediate the dermatologic manifestations of the staphylococcal scalded skin syndrome. The chromosomally mediated toxins cause intraepidermal cleavage of the skin at the stratum granulosum, leading to bullae formation and denudation. Antibodies to the toxins are protective in both humans and animals. Five serologically distinct enterotoxins (A through E) have been implicated in food poisoning due to *S. aureus*. The toxins enhance intestinal peristalsis and seem to induce vomiting by a direct effect on the central nervous system. Enterotoxins B and C may also mediate toxic shock syndrome (TSS), although this is more frequently due to TSST-1. TSST-1 is produced by over 90 percent of *S. aureus* recovered from women with menstrual TSS and over 60 percent of nonmenstrual cases. Most TSST-1 negative strains produce enterotoxin B and, rarely, enterotoxin C. TSST-1 is a 22-kDa protein that causes hypotension, conjunctival and cutaneous hyperemia, and fever when injected into rabbits; death may result from multisystem failure and mimics human TSS. TSST-1 is a potent stimulus for cytokine release by mononuclear cells: tumor necrosis factor (TNF) and interleukin 1 (IL-1) are released by monocytes, and lymphotoxin, IL-2, colony-stimulating factors, and interferon-γ are released by lymphocytes. Host cytokines presumably mediate most of the symptoms of TSS (see Chaps. 20 and 89). The *tst* gene encoding TSST-1 is present in 5 to 25 percent of clinical isolates of *S. aureus* as part of a large, mobile transposon-like element. Similar elements encode the enterotoxin B and C genes. Like TSST-1, enterotoxins B and C cause a TSS-like syndrome in animals, are pyrogenic, and are potent inducers of cytokine production by human T cells and macrophages.

Antimicrobial resistance by staphylococci favors their persistence in the hospital environment. Over 90 percent of both hospital and community strains of *S. aureus* causing infection are resistant to penicillin. Resistance is due to the production of β-lactamases, usually by plasmids. A subgroup of *S. aureus* hyperproduce β-lactamase in vitro and show borderline susceptibility to oxacillin that disappears when clavulanic acid (β-lactamase inhibitor) is added. Infections due to these organisms with "acquired resistance to oxacillin" can be treated safely with penicillinase-resistant β-lactam antimicrobial agents. The true penicillinase-resistant *S. aureus*, called methicillin-resistant *S. aureus* (MRSA), are resistant to all the β-lactam antimicrobics, as well as to the cephalosporins, despite the fact that standard disk susceptibility testing may indicate sensitivity to cephalosporin drugs. Resistance of MRSA is chromosomally mediated and involves production of an altered penicillin-binding protein (PBP 2a or PBP 2′) with a low binding affinity for β-lactams. Not uncommonly, MRSA has acquired R plasmids mediating some combination of resistance to erythromycin, tetracycline, chloramphenicol, clindamycin, and aminoglycosides. MRSA has become increasingly common worldwide, particularly in tertiary care referral hospitals. In the United States, approximately 5 percent of hospital isolates of *S. aureus* are MRSA; one-third of hospitals surveyed have experienced bacteremias due to MRSA. The isolation of these organisms has remained relatively constant since 1980. Outbreaks continue to occur periodically in the form of intrahospital epidemics. The community carriage rate of MRSA is low, although selected patient populations, like parenteral drug abusers, may have MRSA at the time of admission to the hospital. These isolates remain susceptible to vancomycin.

Tolerance of staphylococci to β-lactams is an in vitro phenomenon characterized by resistance to the lethal action of normally cidal antimicrobials. It is characterized by a marked discrepancy between the minimal inhibitory and the minimal bactericidal concentrations of the drug. The mechanism may relate to a defect in the normal activation of autolytic enzymes of the bacteria by cell wall-active antimicrobials. Demonstration of the trait is influenced markedly by physicochemical conditions. Although tolerance has been reported to influence the outcome of severe staphylococcal infection adversely, it has been difficult to incriminate tolerance to β-lactams as a significant cause of antibiotic failure. This may reflect the in vitro observation that continued treatment with β-lactams will kill tolerant *S. aureus,* although killing proceeds more slowly.

Most instances of *S. epidermidis* infection are nosocomially acquired and typically express greater variability and degrees of antimicrobial resistance than those of *S. aureus.* Virtually all isolates contain R plasmids that produce β-lactamase and are resistant to penicillin. Approximately one-third are resistant to aminoglycosides and two-thirds are resistant to tetracycline, erythromycin, clindamycin, and chloramphenicol. Hospital isolates of *S. epidermidis* containing multiple antimicrobial-resistant plasmids can serve as important reservoirs for the acquisition of resistance by *S. aureus* and *Enterococcus* species.

Methicillin resistance is common among *S. epidermidis* strains; over 80 percent of isolates from cases with prosthetic valve endocarditis in one study were methicillin-resistant. Conditions of temperature, pH, osmolality, and the presence of chelating agents and heavy metals all may influence the demonstration of resistance. Methicillin-resistant isolates may appear susceptible by routine susceptibility testing. The most reliable identification of these organisms is by their growth from a large inoculum (10^7 cells) spread on agar containing 6 μg/mL oxacillin. Cross-resistance to the other β-lactam antimicrobials and to the cephalosporins is always present, although as with MRSA, these bacteria may appear susceptible to cephalosporins using conventional disk testing. As with *S. aureus, S. epidermidis* strains remain susceptible to vancomycin, although resistance has occurred in strains of *S. haemolyticus.* Although the quinolone antibiotics are active against methicillin-resistant staphylococci, resistance has occurred when these drugs are used alone.

HOST FACTORS The importance of host factors in resisting staphylococcal infections is demonstrated by the observation that enormous numbers of bacteria are required to establish experimental infections in humans and animals. Areas where skin or mucosal continuity is broken provide portals of entry for staphylococci. More than 50 percent of serious staphylococcal infections of deep tissues arise from cutaneous foci; a smaller number originate from the respiratory, gastrointestinal, or less frequently, the genitourinary tract. Direct inoculation of organisms into the blood is an important route of infection in hospitalized patients with intravenous catheters and in drug abusers.

Staphylococci often invade the integument via plugged hair follicles and sebaceous glands, or areas involved by burns, wounds, abrasions, insect bites, or dermatitis. Colonization and invasion of the lungs may occur when the normal mucociliary clearance mechanisms are either bypassed, as occurs with endotracheal intubation, or depressed, as occurs following viral infections of the lung (influenza) or in patients with cystic fibrosis. Mucosal damage to the gastrointestinal tract following cytotoxic chemotherapy or radiotherapy predisposes to invasion from that site.

Once the integument has been breached, local bacterial multiplication is accompanied by inflammation and tissue necrosis at the site of infection. Neutrophils rapidly enter the area and ingest large numbers of staphylococci. Thrombosis of surrounding capillaries occurs; fibrin is deposited about the periphery; later, fibroblasts create a relatively avascular wall about the area. The fully developed staphylococcal abscess consists of a central core of dead and dying leukocytes and bacteria which gradually liquefies to form characteristic thick, creamy pus, surrounded by a fibroblastic wall. When host mechanisms fail to contain the cutaneous or submucosal infection, staphylococci may enter the lymphatics and the bloodstream. Common sites of metastatic seeding include the diaphyseal ends of long bones in children, and the lungs, kidneys, cardiac valves, myocardium, liver, spleen, and brain.

Polymorphonuclear leukocytes appear to be the major protective mechanism against staphylococcal disease. Persons with neutropenia or inherited or acquired defects of neutrophil chemotaxis, ingestion, or killing are particularly susceptible to staphylococcal infections. A low number of staphylococci are capable of surviving within phagocytes, which may account for the relatively slow response of staphylococcal infections to antimicrobials and the potential for relapse.

Although infections may occur in all age groups, serious staphylococcal infections most commonly afflict the young and old—particularly those with underlying debilitating disease. Primary staphylococcal pneumonia is common in infants but rare in adults. Acute staphylococcal osteomyelitis is almost exclusively a disease of children. Superficial staphylococcal pyoderma is more frequent in infants, whereas actual abscess formation occurs more often in adults. While these examples suggest some role for immunity in resistance against staphylococci, there has been no satisfactory demonstration that human staphylococcal disease is followed by effective immunity or that infection can be modified significantly by vaccination. Virtually 100 percent of adults possess antistaphylococcal antibodies in their serum. Except for the efficacy of neutralizing antibodies to toxins in staphylococcal toxin–mediated diseases, the role of humoral immunity in modifying or protecting against staphylococcal infection is unclear.

The presence of a foreign body such as a suture or a prosthetic device markedly decreases the inoculum of staphylococci required to produce experimental infection. Once established, such infections are very difficult to cure without removal of the foreign body. Strains of *S. epidermidis* are capable of adhering firmly to and invading plastic catheters and of secreting a protective glycocalyx covering the adherent colonies. Neutrophil function is also altered in the presence of a foreign body; phagocytosis and killing of *S. aureus* are diminished.

DIAGNOSIS The diagnosis of all staphylococcal infections is made by Gram's stain and culture of purulent material, either aspirated pus or involved tissue, or by culture of normally sterile body fluids. Typical clustering of organisms may not be seen in clinical specimens; individual cocci and even short chains of three or four organisms may be present. Bacteria in the static phase or within leukocytes may appear gram-negative. Abundant neutrophils, many containing intracellular organisms, are usually present, except in severely neutropenic patients.

SPECIFIC DISEASES **Superficial infections** Infection of hair follicles manifested as a collection of minute erythematous papules without involvement of the surrounding skin or deeper tissues is termed *folliculitis.* A more extensive and invasive follicular or sebaceous gland infection with some involvement of subcutaneous tissues is termed a *furuncle,* or *boil.* Itching and mild pain are followed by progressive local swelling and erythema, and the overlying skin becomes exquisitely painful on pressure or motion. Relief of pain occurs promptly after spontaneous or surgical drainage.

Furuncles occur most commonly in areas subjected to maceration or friction, poor personal hygiene, or involved by acne or dermatitis. The face, neck, axillae, buttocks, and thighs are common sites. Staphylococcal infection may involve the apocrine sweat glands in the axilla or groin (hidradenitis suppurativa). These infections may be deep-seated, slow to localize and drain, and are prone to recurrence and scarring.

Staphylococcal infections within the thick, fibrous, inelastic skin of the back of the neck and upper part of the back lead to formation of a *carbuncle.* The relative thickness and impermeability of the overlying skin lead to lateral extension and loculation, and a large, indurated, painful lesion with multiple ineffective drainage sites results. Carbuncles produce fever, leukocytosis, extreme pain, and prostration. Bacteremia is common.

Staphylococci frequently colonize impetiginous lesions, but most impetigo is due to group A streptococci. However, staphylococcal impetigo does occur, and while it cannot be clearly differentiated on the basis of its clinical features from streptococcal impetigo, it tends to produce multiple superficial, localized lesions at different stages of development, has a grayish rather than golden-yellow crust, and less often produces high fever.

Treatment of most superficial infections does not require the use of antibiotics. Local moist heat, attention to personal hygiene, and washing with germicidal soaps that leave an inhibitory residue on the skin (hexachlorophene, chlorhexidine, triclosan) are usually sufficient.

For more severe or recurrent disease, oral antibiotic therapy with dicloxacillin or cloxacillin (2 g/d in four divided doses) for 7 to 10 days may be effective. Incision and drainage should be utilized selectively. Disease presenting with prominent constitutional symptoms or facial or periorbital infection should be treated with intravenous doses of appropriate antimicrobials as outlined in the section on bacteremic disease.

Toxin-mediated staphylococcal diseases STAPHYLOCOCCAL SCALDED SKIN SYNDROME (SSSS) SSSS is a generalized exfoliative dermatitis complicating infection by toxin (exfoliatin)-producing strains of *S. aureus*. The disease typically occurs in newborns (Ritter's disease) and in children under the age of 5; it is rare in adults. Strains of *S. aureus* causing SSSS in the United States are frequently phage group II. The disease begins with a localized cutaneous infection often accompanied by a nonspecific viral-like prodrome. Fever and leukocytosis are mild. A scarlatiniform rash begins in the perioral area, becomes generalized over the trunk and extremities, and finally desquamates. The disease may consist of rash alone (staphylococcal scarlet fever), or large, flaccid bullae develop that may be localized (more common in adults) or generalized. The bullae burst, resulting in red, denuded skin resembling a burn. Friction applied to healthy areas of skin causes the epidermis to wrinkle and separate (Nikolsky's sign). *S. aureus* can usually be recovered from the skin and nasopharynx. Most adults with SSSS are immunosuppressed or have renal insufficiency. Blood cultures are frequently positive, and mortality is significant. Therapy includes antistaphylococcal antibiotics and local skin care. Recovery usually occurs in infants and children.

In adults, SSSS has been grouped with other severe scalding syndromes such as toxic epidermal necrolysis (Lyell's disease). Drug reactions are the most frequent cause of toxic epidermal necrolysis in adults, and the syndrome may be differentiated from SSSS by skin biopsy. Cleavage of the skin in drug-induced toxic epidermal necrolysis occurs at the basal cell layer resulting in full-thickness denudation, with a greater potential for superinfection and significant fluid and electrolyte loss. In SSSS, cleavage occurs within the epidermis. Kawasaki's disease and toxic shock syndrome should also be considered in the differential diagnosis of SSSS.

TOXIC SHOCK SYNDROME Toxic shock syndrome (TSS) was described in 1978 as a multisystem disease presenting with high fever, a "sunburn" rash that subsequently desquamated, and hypotension in children who had group I *S. aureus* isolated from mucosal or sequestered sites. In 1980 TSS became epidemic among young, primarily white, women, with onset during menstruation. A strong correlation was found between TSS and recovery of *S. aureus* from vaginal or cervical cultures of affected patients. The occurrence of a rash, the infrequency of bacteremia, and the association with *S. aureus* suggested a toxin-associated illness. Subsequently a marker toxin, TSST-1, that mediates most cases of this syndrome was identified. Staphylococcal enterotoxins B or C may also mediate TSS. The pathogenesis involves establishment of a toxin-producing strain in a nonimmune individual under conditions favoring toxin formation; i.e., an aerobic, nutrient environment favoring late-log to stationary phase growth of the organism. The attack rate of TSS among the 10 percent of persons lacking sufficient levels of antitoxin antibodies approaches 25 percent when infected with toxin-positive strains.

Epidemiologically, TSS was associated with the introduction of certain brands of hyperabsorbent tampons. Their prolonged intravaginal use enhances the aerobic surface area in the vagina favoring the growth of intravaginal *S. aureus* and TSST-1 production. Public education and removal of hyperabsorbent tampons from the market have resulted in a marked decrease in the number of reported cases of TSS. Although the majority of cases continue to occur among menstruating females, nonmenstrual TSS now accounts for up to 45 percent of TSS cases in the United States.

The diagnosis of TSS is based on clinical criteria that include high fever, a diffuse rash that desquamates on the palms and soles over the subsequent 1 to 2 weeks, hypotension that may be orthostatic, plus evidence of involvement in three or more organ systems. These commonly include gastrointestinal dysfunction (vomiting or diarrhea), renal or hepatic insufficiency, mucous membrane hyperemia, thrombocytopenia, myalgias with elevated creatine phosphokinase (CK) levels, and disorientation with a normal cerebrospinal fluid examination. Milder forms of the syndrome have been reported.

The onset is acute and typically occurs around the start of menses in a young woman using tampons or barrier contraception methods. The vaginal mucosa is hyperemic, and *S. aureus* can be cultured from the vaginal discharge. Blood cultures are usually negative. Clinical findings are the same in nonmenstrual-associated TSS. Cutaneous infections, postpartum vaginal and cesarean section wound infections, focal tissue infections (abscesses, empyema, osteomyelitis), postinfluenza pneumonia, and rarely primary staphylococcal bacteremia have been associated with TSS. Signs of infection may be minimal among patients with postoperative wound infections where the onset typically occurs on the second day after surgery. Nosocomial transmission has been described. The mortality rate of TSS is 3 percent and is most often due to refractory hypotension and the development of the adult respiratory distress syndrome (ARDS) with or without disseminated intravascular coagulation.

Treatment is directed at correcting shock and treating renal failure, pulmonary insufficiency, and disseminated intravascular coagulation when present. Antistaphylococcal antibiotics should be administered parenterally. Focal collections of *S. aureus* must be drained. Because neutralizing antibodies are widespread, the use of intravenous pooled gamma globulin is being investigated. Up to 30 percent of menstruating women with TSS may have recurrences with subsequent menses, although these are generally milder. The use of antistaphylococcal antibiotics to treat TSS and discontinuation of tampon use significantly decrease the likelihood of recurrences.

The differential diagnosis of TSS includes Rocky Mountain spotted fever, meningococcemia, streptococcal scarlet fever, toxic epidermal necrolysis, and Kawasaki's syndrome. A similar syndrome has been described following group A streptococcal infection.

Staphylococcal food poisoning See Chap. 92.

Invasive staphylococcal infections BACTEREMIA AND ENDOCARDITIS Bacteremia due to *S. aureus* may arise from any local infection, either at extravascular (cutaneous infections, burns, cellulitis, osteomyelitis, arthritis) or intravascular foci (intravenous catheters, dialysis access sites, intravenous drug abuse). Up to one-third of patients do not have an identifiable focus.

Rarely, patients with bacteremia die within 12 to 24 h with high fever, tachycardia, cyanosis, and vascular collapse. Disseminated intravascular coagulation may produce a disease mimicking meningococcemia. Commonly, the disease progresses more slowly, with hectic fever and metastatic abscess formation in the bones, kidneys, lungs, myocardium, spleen, brain, or other tissues.

A major complication of *S. aureus* bacteremia is endocarditis (see Chap. 90). *S. aureus* is the second most common cause of endocarditis and the commonest cause among drug addicts. Among nonaddicts, normal valves are involved in 30 to 60 percent of cases, and older, frequently hospitalized, patients with underlying medical disease are most often infected. The mitral, aortic, or both valves may be involved. The disease typically pursues an acute course with high fever, progressive anemia, and frequent embolic and extracardiac septic complications. Progressive valvular insufficiency leads to significant murmurs in 90 percent of patients. Valve ring and myocardial abscesses are common. The mortality rate is 20 to 30 percent. Infection of the aortic valve, the development of uncontrolled congestive heart failure, or evidence of central nervous system involvement are poor prognostic signs; these patients frequently require surgical intervention.

Among addicts, *S. aureus* frequently involves the tricuspid valve. Evidence for septic pulmonary emboli (chest pain, hemoptysis, nodular infiltrates) is common. Audible murmurs and peripheral stigmata of endocarditis are less common than in nonaddicts. Myalgias and back pain may be the major presenting symptoms and obfuscate the diagnosis. The mortality rate is 2 to 10 percent.

Differentiation of bacteremia from endocarditis may be difficult. Patients with normal heart valves with an identifiable, easily managed or removable primary focus of infection, who receive and respond promptly to appropriate antibiotic therapy, and who do not develop evidence of metastatic complications during the subsequent 2 weeks on therapy usually can be treated for bacteremia alone. Patients with underlying valvular disorders, with murmurs of valvular regurgitation, with community-acquired disease and no obvious focus, with infection secondary to drug abuse, with evidence for embolic events, or with echocardiographic evidence for vegetations should be treated for endocarditis. The presence of antibodies to the teichoic acid cell-wall component of *S. aureus* after 2 weeks of illness does not distinguish reliably between endocarditis or bacteremia with metastatic foci and uncomplicated bacteremia.

Three carefully collected blood cultures are adequate for the diagnosis in most instances; usually all are positive for *S. aureus*. More cultures may be required if the patient has previously received antibiotics. Purulent skin lesions and urine should also be cultured before instituting antibiotic therapy. The urine may be positive in up to a third of cases of staphylococcal bacteremia (with colony counts typically lower than 10^5 per milliliter); staphylococcal bacteriuria in this setting does not indicate metastatic renal infection.

Intravenous therapy should be initiated with a penicillinase-resistant agent. Nafcillin (1.5 g every 4 h) and oxacillin (2.0 g every 4 h) are preferred to methicillin because of the high incidence of interstitial nephritis with methicillin. Gentamicin (1 mg/kg every 8 h, adjusted for renal function) is frequently added for the first 48 to 72 h because of evidence for synergy with β-lactam antimicrobials against *S. aureus* and the tendency for patients treated with both drugs to defervesce more rapidly and to achieve earlier sterilization of the bloodstream. Rare isolates that do not produce β-lactamase should be treated with intravenous penicillin G (4×10^6 units every 4 h). First-generation cephalosporins (cephalothin, cefazolin) have also been used successfully in infections with both penicillinase-positive and -negative strains of *S. aureus*. Patients with serious penicillin allergy or with infections due to methicillin-resistant *S. aureus* should be treated with vancomycin 30 mg/kg per day in two or three divided doses, adjusted for renal function.

Cases of uncomplicated *S. aureus* bacteremia can be treated for 2 weeks. These patients should be followed carefully; relapses should be treated as endocarditis. Uncomplicated right-sided endocarditis in drug addicts has been successfully treated with 2 weeks of intravenous nafcillin plus tobramycin or gentamicin. All other cases of endocarditis should receive 4 to 6 weeks of parenteral antimicrobials. Prosthetic valve endocarditis should be treated with an appropriate penicillin or vancomycin, plus gentamicin, with or without rifampin, for 6 weeks. Most cases will require surgery as well.

The response to antimicrobials in staphylococcal endocarditis may be slow. The fever may not disappear until the second week of therapy. Persistent fever or signs of sepsis should prompt a search for metastatic abscesses that require drainage.

S. epidermidis is the most common isolate in primary nosocomial bacteremias and the most frequent organism infecting intravenous access devices. It has been recognized as a major cause of bacteremia among neutropenic cancer patients, arising either from long-term, indwelling central catheters or from the gastrointestinal tract. Continued fever, progressive sepsis, multiple pulmonary abscesses, and death may result if this complication is left untreated.

Although an uncommon cause of native valve endocarditis, *S. epidermidis* is the commonest cause of prosthetic valve endocarditis (40 percent of cases). Most cases are due to inoculation of organisms at the time of surgery but may not become clinically apparent until 1 year later. Infections frequently involve the valve ring and require surgical intervention. Over 50 percent of patients die.

Because coagulase-negative staphylococci are frequent blood culture contaminants, distinguishing infection from contamination can be difficult. Positive blood cultures demand careful inspection of catheter sites and repeat blood cultures, even in the absence of symptoms, in patients with indwelling catheters, or with prosthetic heart valves or vascular grafts. Speciation of multiple isolates may be useful if isolates can be demonstrated to be the same; plasmid analysis may be required. Catheters should be removed and cultured, although antibiotic therapy alone has been successful for treatment of bacteremic catheter-related infections.

Hospital-acquired *S. epidermidis* infections are usually multiply antibiotic resistant. Methicillin resistance is heterotypic and difficult to exclude. For these reasons, all serious *S. epidermidis* infections should be treated with vancomycin in doses used for *S. aureus*. Prosthetic valve endocarditis should be treated for 6 weeks with vancomycin plus gentamicin, with or without rifampin. Monitoring of renal function and ototoxicity is required.

OSTEOMYELITIS *S. aureus* is responsible for the majority of cases of acute osteomyelitis (see Chap. 97). This infection occurs most commonly in children under the age of 12, but adults are also susceptible to acute osteomyelitis, especially of the spine. Approximately 50 percent of patients give a history of a furuncle or superficial staphylococcal infection preceding osteomyelitis. In children, the frequent localization in the diaphyseal end of the long bones is thought to be due to the endarterial circulation of the diaphysis. Many patients give a history of preceding trauma to the involved area. Clavicular osteomyelitis has complicated septic thrombosis of a catheterized subclavian vein.

Once established, infection spreads through the newly formed juxtaepiphyseal bone to the periosteum or along the marrow cavity. If the infection reaches the subperiosteal space, the periosteum is lifted, a subperiosteal abscess forms, and rupture with infection of the subcutaneous tissues may occur. Rarely, the joint capsule is penetrated, producing pyogenic arthritis. There is death of bone, producing a sequestrum, followed by new bone formation, the involucrum. Occasionally indolent staphylococcal infections of bone may persist for years within dense granulation tissue about a central necrotic cavity, a so-called Brodie's abscess.

Osteomyelitis in children may present as an acute process beginning abruptly with chills, high fever, nausea, vomiting, and progressive pain at the site of bony involvement. Muscle spasm about the affected bone is a common early sign, and the child may refuse to move the affected limb. Leukocytosis is common. Blood cultures are positive for *S. aureus* in 50 to 60 percent of cases early in disease. The tissues overlying the involved bone become edematous and warm, and the skin becomes erythematous. Anemia develops during the course of untreated disease.

Staphylococcal vertebral osteomyelitis in the adult differs considerably from acute osteomyelitis in the child. The onset is less abrupt, and there is a greater tendency for bony fusion with obliteration of the disk space. The lumbar spine is most frequently affected.

Osteomyelitis should be suspected in any child with fever, limb pain, and leukocytosis. Similarly, back or neck pain in an adult, when accompanied by fever, should raise the possibility of vertebral osteomyelitis. A history of a preceding cutaneous infection, local tenderness over the bone, and culture of *S. aureus* from the blood are confirmatory. Roentgenograms are usually normal during the first week, but radionuclide scans may be abnormal. Bony rarefaction, local periosteal elevation, and new bone formation can frequently be seen during the second week. Needle aspiration or bone biopsy should be performed if necessary to obtain a specific etiologic diagnosis prior to institution of chemotherapy. In chronic osteomyelitis, sinus tracts are often present, but cultures of the sinus tracts are not reliable in the diagnosis.

Therapy should be initiated parenterally using a penicillinase-resistant semisynthetic penicillin as outlined for bacteremia and endocarditis and continued for 4 to 6 weeks. Cephalosporins and clindamycin have also been used. Uncomplicated osteomyelitis in children has been managed with 2 weeks of intravenous therapy followed by 2 to 4 weeks of oral therapy. Vancomycin can be used in penicillin-allergic patients and in infections due to methicillin-resistant organisms. Surgery may be required to remove devitalized bone and to drain soft tissue and periosteal abscesses. Neurologic findings due to epidural abscess and cord compression complicating vertebral osteomyelitis demand early surgical intervention. Aggressive treatment of acute osteomyelitis has decreased the incidence of chronic osteomyelitis, with its penchant for recurrent flare-ups and sinus formation. The cure rate for acute staphylococcal osteomyelitis is approximately 90 percent, and death is rare.

PNEUMONIA (See Chap. 207) *S. aureus* causes approximately 1 percent of community-acquired bacterial pneumonias. This disease occurs sporadically except during influenza outbreaks, when staphylococcal pneumonia is relatively more common, although still less frequent than pneumococcal pneumonia.

Primary staphylococcal pneumonia in infants and children frequently presents with high fever and cough. Multiple thin-walled abscesses, or pneumatoceles, are present on the chest roentgenogram. Empyema formation is common. Cough may be nonproductive, and blood cultures are usually negative, frequently necessitating empiric antistaphylococcal therapy. In older children and healthy adults staphylococcal pneumonia is generally preceded by an influenza-like respiratory infection (influenza, measles, or other viruses). Onset of staphylococcal involvement is abrupt, with chills, high fever, progressive dyspnea, cyanosis, cough, and pleural pain. The sputum may be bloody or frankly purulent.

Staphylococci frequently colonize the bronchiectatic airways in children with cystic fibrosis and may cause recurrent episodes of bronchopneumonia. Nosocomial staphylococcal pneumonia typically occurs in intubated patients in intensive care units and in debilitated patients who are prone to aspiration. Residents of nursing homes may have an increased incidence of staphylococcal pneumonia. Infections distal to an obstructing bronchogenic carcinoma may also be caused by *S. aureus*. These infections can begin insidiously, with increasing fever, tachycardia, and tachypnea the only indications of infection. The disease may also be less abrupt when pulmonary involvement occurs during the course of staphylococcal bacteremia, as in patients with right-sided endocarditis or septic thrombophlebitis. Cavitation and pleural effusions are common, but empyema is unusual.

The course of staphylococcal pneumonia may be stormy despite adequate antimicrobial therapy. Gradual defervescence starting 48 to 72 h after the initiation of therapy is typical.

Staphylococcal pneumonia must be differentiated from other pneumonias. The preceding influenza-like illness, rapid onset of pleural pain, cyanosis, and prostration out of proportion to physical findings should suggest primary staphylococcal pneumonia. Sputum Gram's stain showing masses of neutrophils and gram-positive intraleukocytic cocci provides supportive evidence. Leukocytosis is generally present. Blood cultures are positive in 20 to 30 percent of cases. When pneumonia develops suddenly or insidiously in debilitated hospital patients, staphylococci should be considered.

Parenteral therapy should be initiated with antistaphylococcal antimicrobials as outlined for serious bacteremia and endocarditis. Two weeks of intravenous therapy is usually adequate if complications do not develop. Empyema usually necessitates chest tube drainage and may be complicated by the formation of loculations or bronchopleural fistulas. Ultrasound or computed tomography scan may be required to identify loculated collections of pus for drainage.

URINARY TRACT INFECTION *S. saprophyticus* is, after *Escherichia coli*, the most common cause of primary, nonobstructive urinary tract infection in sexually active young women (see Chap. 95). It is responsible for 10 to 20 percent of infections in healthy outpatients. Symptoms of urgency, frequency, and burning are indistinguishable from urinary infections due to other agents. Fever is absent or low-grade. Although lower tract infection is most common, pyelonephritis has been reported.

The diagnosis is established by examination of the urinary sediment, which characteristically reveals pyuria, microscopic hematuria, and cocci in clumps. The organism may be identified by its resistance to novobiocin and nalidixic acid. *S. saprophyticus* grows readily on blood agar, but less well on MacConkey agar and may be missed by currently available rapid diagnostic methods that depend on nitrate reduction or glucose utilization. The criterion for greater than 10^5 bacteria per milliliter developed for gram-negative urinary tract infection is unreliable.

The organism is susceptible to most antimicrobials used for urinary tract infection, including ampicillin, trimethoprim, sulfonamides, and nitrofurantoin. Relapses after appropriate therapy should raise the consideration of infected renal calculi, which may be formed because of the organism's capacity to produce urease.

Isolation of *S. aureus* from a well-collected urine specimen should prompt consideration of staphylococcal bacteremia, which may have been complicated by renal, perinephric, or prostatic abscesses.

Other infections Infection of the vascular-access site with *S. aureus* is a major cause of morbidity and death among patients on hemodialysis. Chronic nasal carriage is the source of most infections. The use of 5-day courses of oral rifampin and topical bacitracin every 3 months significantly decreases the incidence of infection, and should be considered in hemodialysis centers where such infections are endemic. *S. epidermidis* and *S. aureus* rank first and second among pathogens infecting prosthetic devices and intravascular grafts. *S. epidermidis* infections tend to be more insidious and frequently pursue a prolonged course with high morbidity due in part to the temptation to regard positive cultures as contaminants. Subtle clinical findings are common—prosthetic hip infections may present with pain and loosening of the prosthesis, and cerebrospinal fluid shunt infections may present as hypocomplementemic glomerulonephritis due to circulating immune complexes. *S. epidermidis* is a common cause of endophthalmitis complicating ocular surgery. *S. aureus* is a frequent cause of mastitis among nursing mothers.

CONTROL OF HOSPITAL OUTBREAKS (See Chap. 85) Hospital outbreaks of staphylococcal disease may develop rapidly in burn units, intensive care units, or neonatal care units—areas housing debilitated patients under continuous antibiotic pressure. The index case is frequently a patient recently discharged or transferred from another hospital where the organism is endemic. The implicated strains of *S. aureus* are frequently methicillin-resistant (MRSA).

Control demands the rapid identification of the patient reservoir in the affected care units by cultures of wounds, nares, and perineum; urine cultures should be obtained from patients with indwelling urinary catheters. Isolation of culture-positive patients together with reinforcement of the need for proper aseptic technique and hand washing by hospital personnel decreases transmission. Housekeeping antisepsis using phenolic cleaning agents should be carried out in the rooms of colonized patients. Early discharge of colonized patients should be encouraged. Charts should be labeled and the patient returned to strict isolation upon readmission to the hospital until shown to be culture-negative.

Although nasal carriers among hospital personnel may transmit the organism, efficient dissemination is by cutaneous diseases (eczema, atopic dermatitis) that have become colonized with *S. aureus*. Such personnel should be removed from clinical duties until they become culture-negative either spontaneously or following therapy.

Decolonization of the skin and nares in patients and personnel has been accomplished by whole-body washing with antiseptic soaps that leave an inhibitory residue on the skin—hexachlorophene, chlorhexidine, or triclosan. Topical antibiotics are ineffective. Oral antibiotics may be required to abolish the carrier state. Rifampin (600 mg every day for 5 days) has been used successfully alone or, depending on the sensitivity of the staphylococcal isolate, combined with trimethoprim-sulfamethoxazole, doxycycline, or dicloxacillin to prevent the emergence of rifampin resistance.

REFERENCES

ARBUTHNOT J et al (eds): International Symposium on Toxic Shock Syndrome. Rev Infect Disease 11 (Suppl 1):S1, 1989

Brumfitt W, Hamilton-Miller J: Methicillin-resistant *Staphylococcus aureus*. N Engl J Med 320:1188, 1989

Chambers HF et al: Right-sided *Staphylococcus aureus* endocarditis in intravenous drug abusers: Two-week combination therapy. Ann Intern Med 109:619, 1988

Martin MA et al: Coagulase-negative staphylococcal bacteremia. Mortality and hospital stay. Ann Intern Med 110:9, 1989

Pfaller MA, Herwaldt LA: Laboratory, clinical and epidemiological aspects of coagulase-negative staphylococci. Clin Microbiol Rev 1:281, 1988

Todd JK: Staphylococcal toxin syndromes. Annu Rev Med 36:337, 1986

Yu VL et al: *Staphylococcus aureus* nasal carriage and infection in patients on hemodialysis. Efficacy of antibiotic prophylaxis. N Engl J Med 315:91, 1986

101 STREPTOCOCCAL INFECTIONS

ALAN BISNO

Streptococci are among the commonest bacterial pathogens of humans. They are responsible for a diverse spectrum of diseases including pharyngitis and tonsillitis, scarlet fever, erysipelas, impetigo, lymphangitis, and perinatal infections of mother and child. Certain representatives of this genus are prominent causes of endocarditis and urinary tract infections. In addition to their role in causing acute pyogenic infections, strains of *Streptococcus pyogenes* are capable of giving rise to the delayed nonsuppurative sequels of acute rheumatic fever and acute glomerulonephritis.

ETIOLOGY AND CLASSIFICATION Streptococci are spherical or ovoid bacterial cells which grow in pairs or chains of varying lengths. Most are facultative anaerobes. The organisms are gram-positive, usually nonmotile, non-spore-forming, and catalase-negative. No single system of classification suffices to differentiate this heterogeneous group of organisms. Instead, classification depends upon a combination of features, including patterns of hemolysis observed on blood agar plates, antigenic composition, growth characteristics, biochemical reactions, and genetic studies.

When cultivated on sheep blood agar plates, colonies of streptococci may exhibit complete (beta), partial (alpha), or no (gamma) hemolysis. The term *hemolytic streptococci* is currently applied to beta-hemolytic strains. Colonies of such strains are surrounded by clear colorless zones within which the red cells have been completely lysed. This pattern of hemolysis is characteristic of *S. pyogenes* and many other streptococci pathogenic for humans. Alpha-hemolytic colonies are surrounded by a zone of greenish discoloration, whence the often-used designation ''viridans streptococci.'' Strains of *S. pneumoniae* are alpha hemolytic, as are many other streptococci which normally inhabit the upper respiratory and gastrointestinal tracts.

Although classification of streptococci on the basis of hemolytic reactions is quite useful in certain clinical situations, more precise identification of streptococci is accomplished by differentiation into serogroups, as originally described by Lancefield, on the basis of antigenic differences in cell wall carbohydrates or teichoic acids. The majority of beta-hemolytic streptococci isolated from human infections belong to groups A to D and G. Certain alpha-hemolytic and nonhemolytic strains also contain group-specific antigens. The most important of these are the group D streptococci, including the so-called enterococci, among which many strains fail to show beta hemolysis.

Species designation is based upon growth characteristics under varying conditions of temperature, pH, and media composition. Some species do not possess group antigens, and a number of serogroups do not encompass any of the recognized species.

Anaerobic streptococci include members of the family Peptococceae, genus *Peptostreptococcus;* four species are recognized. Hemolytic reactions of these organisms are variable, and no satisfactory method of classifying them has been devised.

GROUP A STREPTOCOCCAL INFECTIONS

Streptococci of Lancefield's group A (*S. pyogenes*) are uniquely important because of the frequency with which they cause human infections and their role as precursors of rheumatic fever and glomerulonephritis.

ETIOLOGY The *group-specific carbohydrate* of group A streptococci is a polymer of rhamnose and *N*-acetylglucosamine. There are approximately 80 recognized and provisional group A serotypes. The typing system is based upon antigenic differences in a cell wall constituent known as *M protein,* which is the principal virulence factor of group A organisms. Strains rich in M protein are highly resistant to phagocytosis by polymorphonuclear leukocytes in vitro and are capable of initiating disease in humans and experimental animals. Strains lacking M protein are avirulent. The antiphagocytic effect of M protein is due, at least in part, to its ability to prevent opsonization of the organism by the complement system. This effect is enhanced by the ability of M protein to precipitate fibrinogen directly onto the bacterial surface. Acquired human immunity to streptococcal infection is based upon development of opsonic antibodies directed against the antiphagocytic moiety of M protein. Immunity is type-specific and lasts for many years, perhaps indefinitely. M proteins of certain types share antigenic determinants with certain constituents of the human heart, including sarcolemmal membrane and cardiac myosin.

T protein serves as the basis of a subsidiary typing system which has been useful in classifying strains not typable by the M system; unlike M protein, the T antigen plays no role in virulence. *Lipoteichoic acid,* a substance which has a marked affinity for biological membranes, has been found to play a crucial role in colonization by binding group A streptococci to fibronectin sites on the surface of human epithelial cells. The streptococcal *cell membrane* contains a number of antigenic structures, certain of which have been reported to share determinants with constituents of human heart and with basement membrane of the renal glomerulus. During the early logarithmic phase of replication, streptococci are enveloped in a *hyaluronic acid capsule* which serves to retard phagocytosis and, therefore, represents an accessory virulence factor. Highly encapsulated group A streptococcal strains produce mucoid colonies on sheep blood agar plates. Such strains have been observed in association with epidemics of acute rheumatic fever.

As streptococci grow in vitro or in vivo, they elaborate a number of extracellular products. Streptococcal pyrogenic exotoxins (erythrogenic toxins) which are induced by lysogeny with temperate bacteriophages are responsible for the rash of scarlet fever. There are three serologically distinct toxins, the effects of which may be neutralized by antibody. Two distinct hemolysins are elaborated. *Streptolysin O* is reversibly inhibited by oxygen (hence exerting its effect primarily on subsurface colonies) and irreversibly inhibited by cholesterol. It is produced by almost all group A strains as well as by many group C and G organisms. In clinical practice, titration of antistreptolysin O (ASO) antibodies in human serums is the most widely used serologic procedure to detect group A streptococcal infection. Streptolysin S differs from streptolysin O in being oxygen-stable and nonantigenic, but both hemolysins possess the capacity to damage membranes of polymorphonuclear leukocytes, platelets, and subcellular organelles. A number of other extracellular products exert effects which might serve to facilitate the organisms' survival in vivo by liquefying pus (streptokinase and deoxyribonucleases A to D) or by allowing spread through tissue planes (hyaluronidase and proteinase). Their role in streptococcal virulence remains unproved.

The two most frequent types of group A streptococcal infection are pharyngitis and pyoderma. They differ markedly in their epidemiologic, clinical, and bacteriologic characteristics.

STREPTOCOCCAL PHARYNGITIS Epidemiology The incidence of this ubiquitous infection is highest in children aged 5 to 15 years; males and females are affected equally. The great majority of such infections are due to group A streptococci, but strains of other serogroups, particularly group C or G, are involved occasionally. The organism is ordinarily transmitted directly from person to person, most likely by droplet spread, and crowding markedly facilitates interpersonal transmission. This may account for the increased incidence of streptococcal pharyngitis in northern latitudes during the colder months of the year, as well as for the explosive outbreaks which occur in military recruit camps and other crowded institutional settings. Common-source epidemics of streptococcal sore throat with high attack rates occasionally occur following contamination of a food item with beta-hemolytic streptococci.

Patients with acute streptococcal pharyngitis harbor large numbers of organisms in the anterior nares and throat. If antibiotics are not administered, the organisms may persist in the upper respiratory tract for weeks to months after symptoms have subsided. However, as the length of the carrier state increases, the organisms decrease in number, disappear from the anterior nasal secretions, and lose detectable M protein. Therefore, convalescent carriers are less likely than acutely ill patients to transmit group A streptococci to exposed individuals. Group A pharyngeal carriage rates vary with geographic location, season of the year, and age group. Among school-age children, rates of 15 to 20 percent have been reported; the carriage rate among adults is considerably lower.

Symptoms The usual incubation period of streptococcal pharyngitis is between 2 and 4 days. The classic syndrome, in older children and adults, is ushered in by the rather abrupt onset of sore throat, particularly by pain on swallowing. Associated symptoms include headache, malaise, feverishness, and anorexia. Chilliness is a frequent symptom, but true rigors are rare. Nausea, vomiting, and abdominal pain are common in children.

Physical signs The patient appears moderately ill with tachycardia and fever which frequently exceeds 38.3°C (101°F). There is diffuse erythema, edema, and lymphoid hyperplasia of the posterior pharynx. The uvula is edematous. The tonsils, if present, are enlarged, reddened, and covered by a punctate or coalescent exudate which may be yellow, gray, or white. Discrete areas of pinhead-size exudate may be present on the hypertrophied lymphoid follicles of the posterior pharynx. On the soft palate, small, red, raised follicular lesions with yellowish centers (''doughnut lesions'') are occasionally seen. The anterior cervical lymph nodes at the angles of the jaw are enlarged and tender. Cough and hoarseness, if present, are mild and, in the absence of the signs and symptoms indicated above, do not suggest the diagnosis of streptococcal pharyngitis. Laryngeal involvement with hoarseness or loss of voice is not a feature.

The full-blown clinical syndrome of acute exudative tonsillopharyngitis is seen frequently during explosive epidemics of streptococcal disease, particularly those occurring in institutional settings. In endemically occurring infections among civilians, however, the illness is frequently much milder and only about half the children with sore throats and positive cultures for group A streptococci will have tonsillar exudate, and a third or less may have fever greater than 38.3°C (101°F) or marked leukocytosis. Patients who have undergone tonsillectomy tend to experience a milder clinical syndrome. In infants, streptococcal upper respiratory infections tend to be less sharply localized to the lymphoid tissue of the faucial and posterior pharyngeal areas. Infections at this age are characterized by rhinorrhea with excoriation of the nares, low-grade fever, anorexia, and a protracted clinical course. Exudative pharyngitis in children under 3 is rarely streptococcal in etiology.

Course The course of streptococcal pharyngitis is usually brief and self-limited. Fever abates within a week, usually within 3 to 5 days. Constitutional symptoms and sore throat disappear with defervescence or shortly thereafter. Several weeks may be required, however, for the tonsils and lymph nodes to return to normal size.

SCARLET FEVER When streptococcal pharyngitis is due to a lysogenic strain producing pyrogenic (erythrogenic) toxin, and when the host does not possess neutralizing antibody to the toxin, scarlet fever may ensue. A preexisting state of hypersensitivity to streptococcal products may predispose to the development of scarlet fever.

The rash usually appears within 2 days after onset of sore throat, involves first the neck, upper chest, and back, then spreads over the remainder of the trunk and the extremities, and spares the palms and soles. The rash may be difficult to appreciate in black patients. It consists of a diffuse erythema, which blanches on pressure, with numerous 1- to 2-mm punctate elevations that impart a ''sandpaper'' texture to the skin. Discrete lesions are absent from the face, but there is a generalized facial flush which contrasts with the prominent circumoral pallor. The rash is more intense along skin folds, such as those of the antecubital fossae and axillary folds, and in these locations often produces linear striations of confluent petechiae known as *Pastia's lines,* which are due to increased capillary fragility.

The exanthem of scarlet fever is accompanied by an enanthem, consisting of punctate erythema and petechiae on the soft palate. Early in the disease, the tongue is covered with a white coat through which hypertrophied papillae protrude as islands of red (white strawberry tongue). By the fourth or fifth day the coating is gone and the entire tongue appears beefy red (red strawberry or raspberry tongue). In rare cases, scarlet fever may be complicated by jaundice, hydrops of the gallbladder, pleural effusion, and arthralgia.

The rash usually lasts 4 to 5 days and is followed by extensive desquamation which begins as early as a few days or as late as 3 to 4 weeks after onset of the disease and is often a striking feature of the convalescent phase of scarlet fever.

Although scarlet fever usually follows upper respiratory infection due to group A streptococci, rarely pyrogenic toxins are produced by streptococci of other groups and by certain strains of staphylococci. Moreover, scarlet fever may follow streptococcal impetigo or secondary streptococcal infection of superficial wounds or surgical incisions. The disease must be differentiated from various of the childhood exanthems (e.g., rubeola, rubella, exanthem subitum), toxic shock syndrome, Kawasaki disease, infectious mononucleosis (when the latter is associated with rash), miliaria, and drug eruptions. Management consists of adequate treatment of the infection.

Streptococcal pyrogenic exotoxin A has been reported to have an amino acid homology of nearly 50 percent with staphylococcal enterotoxin B, a putative mediator of non-menstrual toxic shock syndrome. This fact may explain the existence of a toxic shock–like syndrome due to *S. pyogenes*. The cases have occurred in adults, in several instances with a localized cellulitis or soft tissue infection. Clinical manifestations include diffuse erythroderma, hypotension, and dysfunction of multiple organs.

Complications Streptococcal pharyngitis may give rise to suppurative complications, among which acute otitis media and acute sinusitis are the most frequent. Suppurative cervical lymphadenitis, peritonsillar cellulitis, peritonsillar abscess, or retropharyngeal abscess may also occur. The abscesses themselves, however, usually contain a variety of oropharyngeal flora, including anaerobic bacteria, with or without group A streptococci. Certain other complications, common in the past, are almost never seen in the antibiotic era: (1) extension up the cribriform plate of the ethmoid or via the mastoid, giving rise to meningitis, brain abscess, or thrombosis of cerebral venous sinuses; and (2) bacteremia with metastatic foci of infection such as suppurative arthritis, endocarditis, osteomyelitis, or liver abscess. Streptococcal pharyngitis is associated with two delayed nonsuppurative sequels: acute rheumatic fever (ARF) and acute glomerulonephritis (AGN). These are discussed in Chaps. 187 and 227, respectively.

Diagnosis Sore throat due to group A streptococci must be differentiated from that caused by a number of other agents. *Diphtheria* is rare in immunized populations. It is characterized by the presence of an extensive diphtheritic membrane, and in severe cases by respiratory embarrassment due to laryngeal involvement, as well as by myocarditis and cranial nerve palsies. Cultures on Loeffler's medium will be positive for *Corynebacterium diphtheriae*. *C. hemolyticum* may cause exudative pharyngitis and a scarlatiniform rash which is clinically indistinguishable from that due to *S. pyogenes*. Most such infections occur in teenagers and young adults. The organism is difficult to recognize on sheep blood agar plates.

Gonococcal tonsillopharyngitis is suggested by a history of homosexuality or fellatio and confirmed by appropriate cultures. *Yersinia enterocolitica* is a rare but life-threatening cause of pharyngitis in adults. Some, but not all, patients have associated gastrointestinal symptoms. *Vincent's angina* (*fusobacterial membranous tonsillitis*) is characterized by sore throat and tonsillopharyngeal exudate. Unlike streptococcal sore throat, however, there is an insidious onset without constitutional symptoms, pharyngeal ulcerations are frequent, and the disease is usually unilateral.

The major differential diagnostic confusion is with viral upper respiratory infections, which occur more frequently than streptococcal infections. In many cases, the viral etiology may be suspected because of the more prominent catarrhal, "common cold–like" symptoms. *Adenoviruses* may cause an exudative pharyngitis which is indistinguishable clinically from that due to group A streptococci. *Infectious mononucleosis* also produces severe exudative pharyngitis with fever and at times is accompanied by a rash which may be confused with scarlet fever. The generalized lymphadenopathy, splenomegaly, prolonged fever, and presence of abnormal lymphocytes and heterophile antibodies in the peripheral blood serve to differentiate this entity. Pharyngitis due to group A coxsackieviruses (*herpangina*) or to primary infection with *herpes simplex* is characterized by formation of vesicles, which rupture and leave shallow ulcers. *Influenza* virus infections frequently occur in epidemics; they are accompanied by severe myalgias, bronchitis is a frequent clinical feature, and all age groups are affected. *Mycoplasma pneumoniae* infections may cause pharyngitis that at times may be exudative. Bullous myringitis, if present, should suggest this diagnosis.

Although use of algorithms incorporating combinations of epidemiologic data, symptoms, and signs may enhance diagnostic accuracy, in many instances it is impossible to differentiate streptococcal from nonstreptococcal sore throat on clinical grounds alone. For this reason, precise diagnosis requires identification of the infecting organism in the pharynx. This is achieved most reliably by a throat culture. In obtaining the culture, it is important to rub the swab over both tonsils or tonsillar fossae, the oropharynx, and the nasopharynx posterior to the uvula. The swab should be inoculated onto a sheep blood agar plate to allow evaluation of patterns of hemolysis after overnight incubation. If beta-hemolytic streptococci are isolated, they may be identified presumptively as group A if growth is inhibited around a low-potency (0.04-unit) bacitracin disk. Definitive identification may be accomplished by fluorescent antibody, agglutination, or precipitin techniques. A number of the positive cultures obtained, particularly those with relatively few organisms on the culture plate, will emanate from streptococcal carriers rather than cases of acute infection. It is not possible to differentiate cases from carriers on the basis of culture results, but culture does serve to exclude from antimicrobial therapy the bulk of patients with sore throat (approximately 70 percent) who have negative cultures for beta-hemolytic streptococci. A number of commercial kits are available which allow detection of group A antigen directly from throat swabs by immunologic means. These kits provide results within an hour or less. The direct antigen tests are highly specific, and the physician may proceed confidently on the basis of a positive result. Although the immunologic tests are in general quite sensitive, they fail to identify reliably patients with weakly positive cultures. It is likely, however, that many such patients are asymptomatic carriers. Nevertheless, it is advisable to confirm negative direct antigen tests with throat cultures. This is especially important in epidemiologic settings in which there is an appreciable risk of acute rheumatic fever.

In selecting patients for throat culture or antigen testing, it should be borne in mind that group A streptococcal pharyngitis and acute rheumatic fever are extremely rare in children under 3 in the United States. Likewise, first attacks of rheumatic fever are rare in older adults. Routine use of streptococcal diagnostic procedures is less cost-effective in these groups.

Assays of serum antibodies to streptococcal extracellular products (e.g., ASO, anti-DNase B) provide confirmatory evidence of recent streptococcal infection in patients suspected of having ARF or AGN, but such tests are of no value in the diagnosis of acute infection.

Treatment Therapy of streptococcal pharyngitis is directed primarily toward prevention of ARF and of suppurative sequelae. It is unclear whether treatment of the antecedent streptococcal infection will prevent development of AGN. Prevention of ARF correlates with eradication of the infecting organism from the pharynx, which requires prolonged antibiotic treatment. Penicillin is the drug of choice. It is inexpensive and nontoxic, and all group A streptococci have remained exquisitely sensitive to it. A single intramuscular injection of benzathine penicillin G, 600,000 units for children weighing 27 kg (60 lb) or less and 1.2 million units for all others, ensures a prolonged penicillinemia and is a highly effective form of therapy. Many physicians now elect oral therapy for compliant patients. This is an attractive alternative because the risk of severe allergic reactions is presumed to be less with oral than with intramuscular penicillin. A full 10 days of therapy is required, however, but is often difficult to achieve, because patients are usually asymptomatic well before the 10 days have elapsed. If oral therapy is utilized, penicillin V, 250 mg, three times daily, is the treatment of choice.

Penicillin-allergic individuals may be treated with oral erythromycin estolate, 20 to 40 mg per kilogram of body weight per day, or erythromycin ethyl succinate, 40 mg/kg per day, which should be administered in two to four equally divided portions. The total dose should not exceed 1 g/d. Treatment should be continued for 7 to 10 days.

Nearly all group A streptococci in the United States have remained susceptible to erythromycin, but extensive resistance has been reported in Japan. On the other hand, tetracycline-resistant strains are encountered with some frequency in the United States, and this drug should not be used. Sulfonamides are ineffective in eradication of established streptococcal infection, although they are useful prophylactically in preventing new pharyngeal acquisitions of group A streptococci and in preventing recurrences of ARF (see Chap. 187).

A variable percentage of patients, ranging from 5 to 30 percent, continue to harbor group A streptococci in the pharynx following a course of antimicrobial therapy. This may be due to noncompliance, reinfection, or true treatment failure. Because patients in this category are frequently streptococcal carriers rather than acutely infected individuals, and because the risk of rheumatic fever remains low in most U.S. populations, routine follow-up cultures are not currently recommended in asymptomatic individuals. Exceptions should be made, however, if there is a history of ARF in the family or in family contacts, and in those areas of the United States wherein marked increases in rheumatic fever incidence have recently been reported.

Appropriate antibiotic therapy is effective in preventing ARF, even when initiated as long as 9 days after the onset of acute pharyngitis. Therefore, in the patient seen early in the course of illness, the delay in initiating therapy occasioned by processing a throat culture is not ordinarily a matter of concern. Although treatment also speeds resolution of fever, sore throat, and systemic symptoms associated with streptococcal pharyngitis, the effect of antibiotics is in most cases not dramatic. Indeed, given the self-limited course of the illness, it is difficult to demonstrate clinical improvement in antibiotic-treated vs. placebo-treated patients if therapy is initiated more than 24 h after onset of symptoms. Unless patients have high fever, severe systemic toxicity, or evidence of suppurative complications, initiation of antimicrobial therapy can await the results of throat culture.

In patients judged to be more severely ill, therapy may be initiated at the time of the initial visit after a throat culture has been obtained. If oral antibiotic therapy is elected, the throat culture serves as a guide to the necessity of completing a full 10-day course or, alternatively, of recalling the patient for definitive therapy with an injection of benzathine penicillin G. If signs or symptoms are present, a positive direct antigen test warrants therapy at the time of initial evaluation.

Patients with more severe suppurative complications, such as mastoiditis or ethmoiditis, require larger doses of penicillin than those used for treatment of uncomplicated sore throat. When streptococcal upper respiratory infection is complicated by the development of abscesses associated with suppurative cervical adenitis or in the peritonsillar or retropharyngeal soft tissues, incision and drainage are usually required.

The role of tonsillectomy, if any, in the management of patients with frequent recurrences of acute pharyngitis or in the prevention of ARF remains undefined. Clinical episodes of pharyngitis occur less frequently and tend to be milder following tonsillectomy, but this may make detection and appropriate treatment of immunologically significant streptococcal infections more difficult.

Family contacts of patients with streptococcal sore throat frequently develop symptomatic infections or become asymptomatic pharyngeal carriers. Symptomatic secondary cases in families should be treated appropriately. Asymptomatic family contacts should be cultured in high-risk circumstances. These include the presence of a rheumatic subject in the family or of known cases of ARF occurring in the general area. In situations where the risk is lower, cultures of asymptomatic family contacts need not be performed routinely.

STREPTOCOCCAL SKIN INFECTIONS Erysipelas Also known as Saint Anthony's fire, erysipelas is an acute infection of the skin, with marked involvement of cutaneous lymphatic vessels. It is caused by group A streptococci, and, rarely, other streptococci and *Staphylococcus aureus*. The disease most frequently affects infants, young children, and elderly individuals. The commonest site of involvement is the face, where cutaneous infection originates from an upper respiratory source, presumably by way of small or inapparent breaks in the skin. Erysipelas may also result from streptococcal infection of wounds, surgical incisions, or even areas of dermatophytosis, in which case any portion of the body may be involved.

The onset is usually abrupt; initial symptoms include malaise, chilliness, feverishness, headache, and vomiting. The skin lesion may begin with itching and mild discomfort at the site of infection and is followed shortly thereafter by a small area of erythema which enlarges during the ensuing hours. The lesion spreads rapidly, reaching its maximum extent in 3 to 6 days. It is warm, pink to deep red, and has an advancing elevated margin which protrudes irregularly into the surrounding areas of normal skin. Vesicles and bullae may appear; these rupture leaving crusts on the surface. While the advancing margin remains inflamed, central clearing may be evident with a return of the skin to normal appearance or with residual pigmentation. The eruption may be less well demarcated in areas where the skin is loose, but edema and erythema are constant features. Facial erysipelas commonly involves the bridge of the nose and one or more cheeks in a "butterfly" distribution.

The disease process may be accompanied by high fever and bacteremia. Recovery is usually apparent by the end of a week, but this varies with the severity of the infection. The substantial mortality attending bacteremic cases of erysipelas in the preantibiotic era has been markedly reduced by penicillin. Fatalities still occur among children within the first few months of life and in elderly, debilitated, immunosuppressed individuals. The disease tends to recur, especially in areas of chronic lymphatic obstruction. The diagnosis of erysipelas is primarily clinical. Group A streptococci may at times be isolated from the respiratory tract, the bloodstream, or the lesion itself.

Pyoderma This term is used collectively to denote localized purulent streptococcal skin infections. Some pyoderma lesions represent obvious secondary infections of wounds or burns. For the most part, however, the term is used synonymously with streptococcal impetigo or impetigo contagiosa and refers to discrete purulent lesions which appear to be primary infections of the skin. Streptococcal impetigo differs from streptococcal pharyngitis in a number of particulars (Table 101-1). Epidemiologically, impetigo is more prevalent among underprivileged children residing in warm, humid climates such as the southeastern United States or the tropics. However, the disease may also occur during the summer in northern settings, such as the American Indian reservations of Minnesota. The peak incidence is in young children (2 to 6 years), and there is no definite sex or racial predisposition.

TABLE 101-1 Comparative features of pharyngitis and pyoderma due to group A streptococci

	Pharyngitis	Pyoderma
Predominant geographic distribution	Ubiquitous	Subtropic-tropic
Season (temperate zone)	Winter-spring	Summer-fall
Peak age group	5–15 years	2–5 years
Mode of spread	Direct contact (droplet)	Unknown (?insects)
Clinical illness	Acute	Indolent
Streptococcal types	Generally lower-numbered M types	Generally higher-numbered M types
ASO responses	Good	Weak
Type-specific antibody responses	Generally good	Variable, often poor
Nonsuppurative sequelae	Acute rheumatic fever, acute glomerulonephritis	Acute glomerulonephritis

SOURCE: Modified from Wannamaker LW, N Engl J Med 282:23, 1970

The mode of spread of streptococcal pyoderma is unknown, but personal contact and insect vectors such as *Hippelates* flies are probably both important. "Skin strains" of group A streptococci (i.e., strains of M and T types usually associated with pyoderma) are capable of contaminating unbroken skin, from where they may be inoculated intradermally by local scratches, abrasions, or insect bites. Nasal and pharyngeal carriage of skin strains is frequent in children with impetigo, but such carriage does not ordinarily occur until after establishment of cutaneous carriage or overt infection.

The pattern of immunologic responses to streptococcal impetigo differs from that associated with upper respiratory infection. In particular, the ASO response to impetigo is weak, perhaps because streptolysin O is inactivated by lipids present in the skin. However, antibody responses to anti-DNase B and anti-hyaluronidase, as well as to the Streptozyme slide hemagglutination reagent, are brisk. Type-specific anti-M responses are variable, depending in part upon the antigenicity of the infecting strain, but in general such responses are weaker than in pharyngeal infections. The role of type-specific antibodies in protection against reinfection in pyoderma has not been adequately studied.

Streptococcal impetigo occurs on exposed areas of the body, most frequently on the lower extremities. The lesions remain well-localized but are frequently multiple. They begin as papules but rapidly evolve into vesicles surrounded by an area of erythema. The vesicular lesions are rarely recognized clinically; they give rise to pustules which gradually enlarge, then break down over 4 to 6 days to form characteristic thick crusts. The lesions heal slowly, leaving depigmented areas. A deeply ulcerated form of impetigo is known as *ecthyma*. Although regional lymphadenitis often occurs, systemic symptoms are not ordinarily present.

In addition to the indolent, impetiginous skin infections of young children, a more severe and extensive form of pyoderma has been observed in combat troops serving in hot, wet environments such as the jungles of southeast Asia. In their most common form, they consist of multiple ecthymatous ulcers located on the ankle or dorsum of the foot. The ulcers are usually circular, punched-out lesions 0.5 to 3.0 cm in diameter, have borders, and are surrounded by a zone of erythema. They are filled with purulent material and covered with grayish-yellow adherent crusts. Secondary cellulitis or lymphadenitis may be present.

The diagnosis of streptococcal pyoderma is made by culture. Adequate cultures require removal of the surface crusts in order to obtain specimens from the base of the lesions. Although both *S. pyogenes* and *Staphylococcus aureus* may be isolated from the lesions, the former is the major pathogen. Morphologically characteristic lesions respond well to penicillin, even when penicillinase-resistant staphylococci are recovered. These lesions contrast with bullous impetigo, which is ordinarily due to *S. aureus* and not to streptococci. Antibiotic regimens are the same as those for pharyngitis, and benzathine penicillin G, oral penicillin V, or oral erythromycin all result in cure rates in excess of 95 percent. Topical antiseptics and antibiotics are of limited value. Prevention of pyoderma depends primarily upon adherence to good personal hygiene, with special attention to frequent scrubbing with soap and water.

Streptococcal pyoderma does not give rise to ARF. This observation remains unexplained, but may indicate a requirement for infection at the pharyngeal site, with its rich endowment of lymphoid tissue, in order to initiate the immunologic events leading to ARF. On the other hand, studies of populations in which ARF and AGN occur simultaneously indicate that the streptococcal strains responsible for each sequelum are distinct and suggest that "pyoderma strains" of group A streptococci may be nonrheumatogenic. When pyoderma is due to a nephritogenic strain of group A streptococcus, AGN may ensue. Indeed, pyoderma is by far the commonest antecedent of poststreptococcal glomerulonephritis in subtropical and tropical regions of the world. Strains of a number of M types (49, 55, 57, and others) have been associated with both sporadic cases and large epidemics of pyoderma-associated nephritis in diverse geographic areas. There are no conclusive data to indicate that treatment of an individual case of pyoderma will prevent the subsequent occurrence of AGN in that patient. Such treatment is important, however, in eradicating nephritogenic streptococci from the environment in epidemiologic settings in which these strains are prevalent.

Cellulitis Streptococcal cellulitis may occur in areas of tissue damage due to trauma, operative wounds, or stasis ulceration. Although such infections are frequently due to group A organisms, beta-hemolytic streptococci of groups G, B, or C may be responsible. Cellulitis is an acute inflammation of the skin and subcutaneous tissues marked by pain, tenderness, erythema, fever, and often regional lymphadenopathy. In contrast to erysipelas, the margins of the lesions are neither elevated nor sharply demarcated from the surrounding uninvolved tissue. Rarely such lesions may progress to frank gangrene. Certain patients who have undergone saphenous venectomy for coronary bypass surgery experience recurrent bouts of acute streptococcal cellulitis for months or years after surgery. The cellulitis always involves the saphenous donor extremity. Frequently the patients suffer from tinea pedis, and eradication of the superficial fungal infection, which may serve as a nidus for streptococcal colonization, may result in abolition of the recurrent attacks.

Cellulitis of the perianal area may be manifested by painful defecation or by pruritus; asymptomatic anal colonization has been the source of several outbreaks of hospital-acquired streptococcal infection. Vaginal colonization by group A streptococci has a number of features in common with perianal involvement. In both instances there is a close epidemiologic association with streptococcal upper respiratory infection. Anal and vaginal streptococcal infection may be either symptomatic or asymptomatic. Outbreaks of nosocomial streptococcal infection have been attributed to asymptomatic vaginal carriers.

LYMPHANGITIS, BACTEREMIA, AND PUERPERAL SEPSIS Local trauma, whether or not complicated by frank cellulitis, may give rise to *acute lymphangitis*. This entity is characterized by the appearance of red linear streaks extending from the portal of entry to the draining regional lymph nodes, which are enlarged and tender. Systemic symptoms, including chills, fever, malaise, and headache, are prominent, and the process may be accompanied by demonstrable bacteremia.

Streptococcal bacteremia, from whatever cause, may give rise to metastatic foci of infection, such as suppurative arthritis, osteomyelitis, peritonitis, endocarditis, meningitis, or visceral abscesses. Streptococcal bacteremia may complicate parenteral drug abuse; such infections are often associated with local abscesses at the injection site and/or infective endocarditis (see Chap. 90). The clinical course of streptococcal bacteremia may be fulminant and lead rapidly to prostration, shock, purpura fulminans, disseminated intravascular coagulation, and death.

Puerperal sepsis follows abortion or childbirth when streptococci invade the endometrium and surrounding structures and then the lymphatics and bloodstream. The process may be further complicated by pelvic cellulitis, septic pelvic thrombophlebitis, peritonitis, or pelvic abscess. The causative organism may be transmitted to the pregnant woman directly by medical personnel or attendants. Group B streptococci have supplanted other organisms as the most frequent cause of perinatal streptococcal infections of mother and child (see below). Anaerobic streptococci, along with other anaerobic organisms, have also been implicated (see Chap. 108).

PNEUMONIA AND EMPYEMA Pneumonia due to group A streptococci is uncommon and usually occurs following influenza, measles, pertussis, or varicella. The illness occurs in epidemic form in military recruit camps and is characterized by abrupt onset of fever, chills, myalgia, dyspnea, cough, pleuritic chest pain, and hemoptysis. Patients are severely ill and often cyanotic. Pathologically and radiologically, this is usually a bronchopneumonia, and lobar consolidation is uncommon. A characteristic feature of streptococcal pneumonia is the early and rapid accumulation of copious amounts of thin, serosanguinous empyema fluid. Bacteremia occurs in 10 to 15 percent of cases. Extension of the pneumonic process to the pericardium may give rise to a purulent pericarditis. Other potential complications include mediastinitis, pneumothorax, and bronchiectasis. Therapy consists of at least 4 to 6 million units of parenteral penicillin daily in the form of aqueous procaine penicillin G, given every 6 to 12 h intramuscularly, or intravenous aqueous crystalline penicillin G, and adequate drainage of empyema fluid, which usually requires insertion of a chest tube.

MYOSITIS, GANGRENE, AND SEPTIC BURSITIS Myositis due to group A streptococci is a rare disorder characterized by severe pain and marked signs of local inflammation in the infected area. The patients are usually bacteremic, and the clinical course is frequently rapid and fulminant. The mortality rate is extremely high. Aggressive surgical debridement and penicillin therapy are required. *Hemolytic streptococcal gangrene* may occur after trauma or surgery or without an obvious portal of entry. It is characterized by necrosis of subcutaneous and dermal tissues which spreads along fascial planes. This entity is a form of necrotizing fasciitis, and a similar clinical picture can result from infection due to a variety of anaerobic and facultatively aerobic bacteria, often in combination. *Septic bursitis* of the olecranon bursa, although usually caused by *Staphylococcus aureus*, may also be due to *S. pyogenes*.

GROUP B STREPTOCOCCAL INFECTIONS

Streptococci belonging to serogroup B have been of interest to veterinarians because of their association with bovine mastitis, an association which led to their species designation as *S. agalactiae*. The organisms are usually, but not uniformly, beta-hemolytic and are resistant to bacitracin. In addition to the presence of group B carbohydrate in their cell walls, *S. agalactiae* may be identified by biochemical means, including production of hippuricase and so-called CAMP factor and failure to hydrolyze bile esculin agar. Group B streptococci may be subdivided into serotypes by means of surface polysaccharides and protein antigens. The capsular antigens are virulence factors and immunity to them is type-specific.

Human strains of group B streptococci, which appear to be biologically distinct from bovine strains, frequently colonize the female genital tract as well as the throat and rectum. Asymptomatic vaginal carriage rates in postpubertal women generally have ranged between 6 and 25 percent, depending on the bacteriologic methods employed and on the socioeconomic status and geographic residence of the women sampled. The majority of serious group B infections occur as perinatal events. Maternal infections include chorioamnionitis, septic abortion, and puerperal sepsis. *Streptococcus agalactiae* now ranks with *Escherichia coli* as one of the two most frequent causes of neonatal sepsis and meningitis. Neonatal disease takes one of two forms. Early-onset disease, occurring within the first 10 days of life, is usually due to organisms acquired from the maternal genital tract. It involves primarily the lungs, probably as a result of aspiration of infected amniotic fluid, but the organism can be cultured from the blood, nasopharynx, skin, and myocardium. Early-onset group B streptococcal infection occurs in approximately two of every thousand live births (the incidence is higher following prolonged or complicated delivery) and is attended by a high mortality rate. Late-onset disease occurs in infants over 10 days old, may be due to nosocomial transmission of group B streptococci, is manifested primarily by meningitis and bacteremia, and has a lower mortality rate than early-onset disease. Although the serotypes involved in early-onset illness are variable, type III organisms predominate as the cause of late-onset meningeal infection. Transplacentally acquired antibodies to type III organisms may protect against late-onset disease: they are present in serums of most women delivering healthy babies but are usually lacking in serums of mothers whose offspring develop late-onset meningitis due to type III group B streptococci.

Group B streptococci also cause adult infections not associated with the puerperium. These are often opportunistic and involve debilitated patients with diabetes mellitus, malignancy, or other severe illnessses. Adult infections due to group B organisms include urinary tract infections, suppurative soft tissue infections, bacteremia, endocarditis, pyogenic arthritis, pneumonia, empyema, meningitis, and peritonitis. Although recovered from a small proportion of throat cultures, group B streptococci are rarely the cause of clinically significant pharyngitis. All strains are susceptible to penicillin, which is the drug of choice, although group B organisms have higher minimal inhibitory concentrations for penicillin than do group A strains. Life-threatening group B infections in neonates are often treated initially with aminoglycosides in addition to high doses of penicillin because this combination is synergistic in vitro and avoids the occasional occurrence of penicillin tolerance in group B strains. Most strains are sensitive to erythromycin, but tetracyclines should not be used without prior susceptibility testing because resistance to them is common.

OTHER STREPTOCOCCAL INFECTIONS

Although streptococci of groups C and G are human commensals, both are capable of causing pharyngitis, and epidemics of upper respiratory disease due to these organisms have been reported, particularly following ingestion of contaminated foods. Strains of both serogroups produce streptolysin O, and pharyngeal infections with groups C and G elicit rises in ASO titer. Streptococci of groups C and G are highly susceptible to penicillin.

There have been several outbreaks of human disease due to group C in which the vehicle was unpasteurized or inadequately pasteurized milk or cheese. Clinical manifestations have included pharyngitis, cervical adenitis, and disseminated deep tissue infections. In two outbreaks, cases of poststreptococcal glomerulonephritis ensued.

Group G streptococcal bacteremia often arises from cutaneous foci such as localized cellulitis or decubitus ulcers, and chronic lymphatic obstruction and venous insufficiency are important predisposing factors. The patients involved frequently have underlying conditions such as malignancy, alcoholism, or parenteral drug abuse. Bacteremia may lead to severe, life-threatening complications such as endocarditis, meningitis, or septic arthritis.

Lancefield's group D include both enterococcal and nonenterococcal species. The former have recently been recognized as a distinct genus, of which the major human pathogens are *Enterococcus faecalis* and *E. faecium*. Enterococci are frequent causes of urinary tract infection in patients with structural abnormalities of the urinary tract and are responsible for 10 percent or more of cases of bacterial endocarditis. They are isolated from infected decubitus ulcers and intraabdominal abscesses, usually in combination with other bacteria. These microorganisms are ordinarily alpha-hemolytic or nonhemolytic but may be beta-hemolytic. The treatment of severe enterococcal infections, particularly bacterial endocarditis, is complicated; the organisms are resistant to many antibiotics and are relatively resistant to the penicillins. In the therapy of enterococcal endocarditis, a combination of intravenous penicillin G or ampicillin in high doses plus an aminoglycoside should be used, because this combination exerts a synergistic effect in the killing of enterococci (see Chap. 90). Formerly, streptomycin was the aminoglycoside of choice, but high-level resistance (>2000 μg/mL) to streptomycin and kanamycin has been found in a significant number of enterococcal isolates and synergy is not observed in the presence of such high-level resistance. Gentamicin is the drug of choice along with penicillin or ampicillin in treatment of serious enterococcal infections due to organisms which are highly resistant to streptomycin. The combination of penicillin and tobramycin is not lethal in vitro for strains of *E. faecium*.

Fortunately, gentamicin remains an effective synergistic agent for treatment of most deep tissue enterococcal infections encountered in the United States. In treatment of individual cases, however, it is advisable to rule out the presence of high-level gentamicin resistance by in vitro testing. Treatment of life-threatening enterococcal infections in patients who cannot tolerate penicillin is difficult. The cephalosporins and clindamycin are of no value, but vancomycin, in combination with gentamicin, is likely to be effective. Strains of *E. faecalis* that produce beta lactamase have been described but are rare.

Nonenterococcal group D streptococci, of which *S. bovis* is the major pathogen, remain extremely sensitive to penicillin and are amenable to therapy with this agent alone. Bacteremia or endocarditis due to *S. bovis* has been associated with carcinoma of the colon. Enterococci can be differentiated from nonenterococcal group D streptococci by their ability to grow in 6.5% NaCl and by a positive PYR (pyroglutamyl aminopeptidase) test.

Streptococci of most groups have been isolated at least occasionally from infected heart valves, soft tissues, or visceral abscesses. Such infections may occur as "opportunists" following surgical manipulation or in patients with malignant disease. Group F streptococci occasionally are associated with abscess formation and bacteremia, and a number of instances of meningitis and bacteremia in humans due to streptococci of serogroup R, a group of organisms well-known as pathogens of swine, have been reported. In nearly all human cases there had been a history of contact with pigs.

Viridans streptococci are normal inhabitants of the oropharynx and gastrointestinal tract. They remain the most frequent causative agents of subacute bacterial endocarditis occurring on native heart valves (see Chap. 90). The taxonomy of these organisms is confused, but one classification scheme recognizes five species (in addition to *S. pneumoniae*): *salivarius, mitior, milleri, sanguis,* and *mutans*. Although viridans streptococci are not usually highly invasive, *S. milleri* is capable of causing serious pyogenic infections such as liver and brain abscesses, peritonitis, and empyema. Endocarditis due to *S. milleri* is more likely to be complicated by abscess formation in peripheral tissues than are similar infections due to other species of viridans streptococci. All the viridans species, including *S. milleri,* are susceptible to penicillin. Modest increases in the minimal inhibitory concentrations of oral streptococci to penicillin occur following prolonged oral or high-dose intravenous therapy.

Anaerobic streptococci (see Chap. 108) abound in the mouth, intestinal tract, and vagina. They may be found, often in combination with other anaerobic and aerobic microorganisms, in abscess cavities throughout the body. In the head and neck, anaerobic streptococci occur in infected paranasal sinuses, brain abscesses, dental abscesses, infections of the retropharyngeal or lateral pharyngeal spaces, and as Ludwig's angina. In the chest, these organisms occur in lung abscesses and empyema fluids. Abscesses of the liver and other intraabdominal viscera, as well as perirectal abscesses and pelvic abscesses in women, may be due in part to peptostreptococci. These organisms may also thrive in dead or devitalized muscle, skin, or subcutaneous tissue. *Anaerobic streptococcal myositis* is characterized by marked edema, crepitant myositis, pain, and the presence of chains of gram-positive cocci in a seropurulent exudate. *Progressive synergistic gangrene* usually develops about a surgical incision and consists of an ulcerated lesion surrounded by gangrenous skin. The infection is associated particularly with the use of through-and-through sutures after abdominal surgery and is thought most often to be due to the synergistic action of *Staph. aureus* and microaerophilic streptococci. *Chronic burrowing ulcer* is a deep soft tissue infection, caused by microaerophilic streptococci, which erodes through subcutaneous tissue to emerge as an ulcer at a distant site. Management of infections due to anaerobic and microaerophilic streptococci consists of drainage of abscesses, debridement of devitalized tissues, and high-dose intravenous penicillin therapy.

REFERENCES

Adams EM et al: Streptococcal myositis. Arch Intern Med 145:1020, 1985

American Heart Association, Committee on Rheumatic Fever Endocarditis and Kawasaki Disease: Prevention of rheumatic fever. Circulation 70:1082, 1988

Auckenthaler R et al: Group G streptococcal bacteremia: Clinical study and review of the literaure. Rev Infect Dis 5:196, 1983

Baddour LM, Bisno AL: Recurrent cellulitis after coronary bypass surgery: Association with superficial fungal infection in saphenous venectomy limbs. JAMA 251:1049, 1984

Barg NL et al: Group A streptococcal bacteremia in intravenous drug abusers. Am J Med 78:569, 1985

Brennan RO, Durack DT: The viridans streptococci in perspective, in *Current Clinical Topics in Infectious Diseases,* JS Remington, MN Swartz (eds). New York, McGraw-Hill, 1984

Cone LA et al: Clinical and bacteriologic observations of a toxic-shock like syndrome due to *Streptococcus pyogenes*. New Engl J Med 317:146, 1987

Edwards MS, Baker CJ: *Streptococcus agalactiae* (group B streptococci), in *Principles and Practice of Infectious Diseases,* 2d ed, GL Mandell et al (eds). New York, Wiley, 1985, p 1155

Hoffman S, Moellering RC Jr: The enterococcus: "Putting the bug in our ears." Ann Intern Med 106:757, 1987

Kellogg JA, Manzella JP: Detection of group A streptococci in the laboratory or physician's office. JAMA 255:2638, 1986

Miller RA et al: *Corynebacterium hemolyticum* as a cause of pharyngitis and scarlatiniform rash in young adults. Ann Intern Med 105:867, 1986

Stevens DL et al: Severe group A streptococcal infections associated with a toxic shock-like syndrome and scarlet fever toxin A. N Engl J Med 321:1, 1989

Stollerman GH: *Rheumatic Fever and Streptococcal Infection.* New York, Grune & Stratton, 1975

102 DIPHTHERIA

RANDALL K. HOLMES[1]

DEFINITION Diphtheria is a localized infection of mucous membranes or skin caused by *Corynebacterium diphtheriae*. A characteristic pseudomembrane may be present at the site of infection. Some strains of *C. diphtheriae* produce diphtheria toxin, a protein that can cause myocarditis, polyneuritis, and other systemic toxic effects. Respiratory diphtheria is usually caused by toxinogenic (tox^+) *C. diphtheriae,* but cutaneous diphtheria is frequently caused by nontoxinogenic (tox^-) strains.

ETIOLOGY *C. diphtheriae* is an aerobic, nonmotile, nonsporulating, irregularly staining, gram-positive rod. The bacteria are 2 to 6 μm long, 0.5 to 1 μm wide, club-shaped, and often arranged in clusters (Chinese letters) or parallel arrays (palisades). *C. diphtheriae* forms gray to black colonies on selective media containing potassium tellurite. Three biotypes, designated gravis, mitis, and intermedius, are distinguished on the basis of colonial morphology, hemolytic activity, sugar fermentation reactions, and other biochemical tests. Some strains of *C. diphtheriae* produce diphtheria toxin. Both tox^+ and tox^- strains cause infections, and tox^+ strains of all three biotypes can cause severe disease. Individual strains of *C. diphtheriae* within a biotype can be identified by phage typing, analyzing bacterial polypeptides or bacterial DNA restriction patterns, or performing hybridization tests with specific DNA probes.

The gene for diphtheria toxin is present in specific corynephages. Nontoxinogenic *C. diphtheriae* acquire the ability to produce diphtheria toxin by infection with tox^+ phages, a process termed *phage conversion*. Growth of *C. diphtheriae* under low-iron conditions, which mimic the environment of host tissues, induces diphtheria toxin synthesis.

IMMUNOLOGY Treatment of diphtheria toxin with formaldehyde converts it to a nontoxic product called diphtheria toxoid. Immunization with toxoid elicits antibodies (antitoxin) that neutralize the toxin and prevent respiratory diphtheria. Antitoxin does not prevent colonization by *C. diphtheriae* or eradicate the carrier state. If most individuals in a population have antitoxic immunity, the carrier rate for tox^+ strains of *C. diphtheriae* usually decreases to a low level. Thus, herd immunity reduces the risk that nonimmune individuals in the population will be exposed to tox^+ *C. diphtheriae*. Nonimmune individuals may contract diphtheria if they travel to regions where the disease is prevalent or if tox^+ strains of *C. diphtheriae* are introduced into their community.

No specific amount of antitoxin provides absolute protection against diphtheria. Both the attack rate and the mortality rate for diphtheria are much lower in individuals with >0.01 units of antitoxin per milliliter, so that level is often used for epidemiologic studies as an index of immunity. Antitoxic immunity can also be determined by the Schick test, in which standardized doses of diphtheria toxin and toxoid are injected intracutaneously at separate sites on the volar surface of the forearm. A tender, swollen, erythematous lesion reaching maximal intensity at 4 to 5 days at the site of the toxin injection only (a positive reaction) is a direct toxic effect of diphtheria toxin; the individual is not immune. No lesion at either site (a negative reaction) indicates that the toxin was neutralized by circulating antitoxin; the individual has antitoxic immunity. Tuberculin-like reactions at both sites that reach a maximum at 2 to 3 days and then fade (a pseudoreaction) indicates delayed hypersensitivity to toxin/toxoid in an individual with antitoxin. Delayed hypersensitivity reactions at both sites combined with a subsequent positive reaction at the site of toxin administration only (a combined reaction) indicates delayed hypersensitivity in an individual without a protective level of antitoxin.

EPIDEMIOLOGY Humans are the reservoir for *C. diphtheriae*. Transmission occurs primarily by close contact of diphtheria patients or carriers with susceptible individuals, but the risk of transmission from patients appears to be substantially greater than from asymptomatic carriers. Transmission involving fomites and indirect routes is less common, although *C. diphtheriae* can survive for weeks to months in the environment. The incubation period for respiratory diphtheria is typically 2 to 5 days and, rarely, up to 8 days. Cutaneous diphtheria is usually a secondary infection, and the signs of infection develop an average of 7 days (range 1 to >21 days) after the appearance of primary skin lesions.

In unimmunized populations in temperate climates diphtheria primarily involves the respiratory tract, occurs year round with peak incidence in the colder months, and is usually caused by tox^+ *C. diphtheriae*. Most infants are immune because of transplacental transfer of maternal IgG antitoxin, but they become susceptible by 6 to 12 months of age. Diphtheria is primarily a disease of children that affects up to 10 percent of individuals and sometimes occurs in devastating epidemics. Approximately 75 percent of individuals become immune by age 10 from clinical or subclinical

[1]The opinions expressed herein are those of the author and do not necessarily represent the views of the Department of Defense or the Uniformed Services University of the Health Sciences.

infection with *C. diphtheriae*. Mortality rates of 30 to 40 percent are common in untreated disease and sometimes exceed 50 percent in epidemics.

Treatment with antitoxin can reduce the case mortality rate to 5 to 10 percent.

In the United States routine immunization with toxoid introduced in the 1920s has resulted in a progressive decrease in disease and shift of cases to older age groups. More than 206,000 cases of diphtheria occurred in 1921; only 22 cases were reported from 1980 to 1987. Forty-eight percent of cases in 1971 to 1981 were in persons over 15 years of age. Despite high rates of immunization in children by school entry (96 percent) 25 to 50 percent of older adults are susceptible to diphtheria. In the United States large local outbreaks of diphtheria occurred in San Antonio, Texas (1969 to 1970, 201 cases) and Seattle, Washington (1972 to 1982, 1100 cases). Alcoholism, low socioeconomic status, crowded living conditions, and Native American ethnic background were significant risk factors in these and other recent diphtheria outbreaks.

In the tropics cutaneous diphtheria is more common than respiratory diphtheria, occurs throughout the year, and often occurs as a secondary infection complicating other dermatoses. Isolates of *C. diphtheriae* from skin lesions are more often tox^- than tox^+. A study in Rangoon, Burma, demonstrated *C. diphtheriae* (18.5 percent tox^+ strains) in more than 60 percent of bacterially infected skin lesions in patients under 12 years of age. Eighty percent of isolates were from impetiginous scabies, with most other isolates from impetiginous eczema or impetigo. Cutaneous diphtheria has also been increasingly recognized in temperate climates during the past two decades and accounted for 86 percent of the 1100 cases in Seattle.

Molecular epidemiologic studies demonstrated that the Seattle epidemic actually consisted of three discrete but overlapping outbreaks involving intermedius, gravis, and mitis strains. The intermedius and gravis strains were shown to be distinct clones of *C. diphtheriae* with loss of toxigenicity occuring in the gravis clone late in the epidemic (1978–1982). The mitis strains isolated throughout the epidemic were predominantly tox^- and represented multiple clones. A recent outbreak in Sweden (1984–1986) with high mortality (>20 percent) was found to be caused by a single tox^+ mitis strain that differed from *C. diphtheriae* strains isolated concurrently from carriers. These observations suggest that traits other than toxigenicity can contribute to virulence of *C. diphtheriae*. Evidence for initiation of an epidemic by phage conversion of tox^- to tox^+ strains in vivo in one individual with subsequent dissemination to other susceptible subjects was found in an outbreak in England.

PATHOLOGY AND PATHOGENESIS *C. diphtheriae* infects mucous membranes, most commonly in the respiratory tract, and also invades open skin lesions from insect bites or trauma. In infections caused by tox^+ *C. diphtheriae,* initial edema and hyperemia are often followed by epithelial necrosis and acute inflammation. Coagulation of the dense fibrinopurulent exudate produces a pseudomembrane, and the inflammatory reaction accompanied by vascular congestion extends into the underlying tissues, accompanied by vascular congestion. The pseudomembrane contains large numbers of *C. diphtheriae,* but the bacterium is rarely isolated from the blood or internal organs.

Diphtheria toxin acts both locally and systemically. Very small amounts cause dermonecrosis, as in the Schick test, and toxin presumably contributes to pseudomembrane formation. The lethal dose of diphtheria toxin for nonimmune humans and highly susceptible animals is about 0.1 μg/kg body weight. Absorbed toxin can cause myocarditis, neuritis, and focal necrosis in other organs including the kidneys, liver, and adrenal glands. Early changes in diphtheritic myocarditis include cloudy swelling of muscle fibers and interstitial edema. These are followed in succeeding weeks by hyaline and granular degeneration of muscle fibers, sometimes with fatty degeneration of the myocardium, progressing to myolysis and, finally, replacement of lost muscle by fibrosis. Thus, diphtheria can cause permanent cardiac damage. In diphtheritic polyneuritis pathologic changes include patchy breakdown of myelin sheaths in peripheral and autonomic nerves, but recovery of nerve damage is the rule if the patient survives.

Diphtheria toxin is produced by *C. diphtheriae* as an extracellular polypeptide. It is cleaved by proteases to form nicked toxin, consisting of fragments A and B which remain linked by a disulfide bond. Fragment B binds to specific receptors on plasma membranes of cells from humans or susceptible animals, and the bound toxin is internalized by receptor-mediated endocytosis. Fragment A is translocated across the endosomal membrane and released into the cytoplasm where it catalyzes the transfer of the adenosine diphosphate ribose moiety from nicotinamide adenine dinucleotide (NAD) to a modified histidine residue (diphthamide) on elongation factor 2 (EF-2), thereby inactivating EF-2 and inhibiting protein synthesis. One molecule of fragment A in the cytoplasm can kill a cell. Other metabolic alterations in intoxicated cells are secondary to inhibition of protein synthesis. In the intoxicated heart, depletion of carnitine occurs and may contribute to the pathogenesis of diphtheritic myocarditis. Diphtheria toxin and exotoxin A of *Pseudomonas aeruginosa* have the same enzymatic activity and their catalytic domains have homologous amino acid sequences. Nevertheless, their biologic effects differ because they bind to different cell surface receptors and exhibit different cellular tropisms.

CLINICAL MANIFESTATIONS Patients with *C. diphtheriae* in the respiratory tract are classified as diphtheria cases if they have symptoms consistent with local infection and as diphtheria carriers if they are asymptomatic. Signs and symptoms vary depending on the site and severity of the local infection, patient's age, preexisting nasopharyngeal disease, and concomitant systemic disease. Onset is often gradual, but most patients seek medical care within a few days of becoming ill. Sore throat is the most common symptom, but children are less likely than adults to complain of sore throat and more likely to have nausea and vomiting. Fever of 37.8 to 38.9°C (100 to 102°F) and dysphagia occur in about half the patients, but cough, hoarseness, chills, and rhinorrhea are less common. Systemic manifestations are primarily due to toxic effects of diphtheria toxin. Patients without toxicity feel well except for discomfort associated with the local infection, whereas severely toxic patients may have listlessness, pallor, and tachycardia that can progress rapidly to vascular collapse.

Primary infection in the respiratory tract is most often tonsillopharyngeal (one-half to two-thirds of cases), followed in decreasing order of frequency by laryngeal, nasal, and tracheobronchial infection. Multiple sites are frequently involved, and secondary spread of pharyngeal infection upward to the nasal mucosa or downward to the larynx and tracheobronchial tree is much more common than primary infection at those sites. Systemic toxicity is usually less severe in nasal diphtheria than in tonsillopharyngeal diphtheria and most severe when extensive pseudomembrane extends from the tonsils and pharynx into contiguous regions. A small percentage of patients present with malignant or "bull-neck" diphtheria with abrupt onset, extensive pseudomembrane formation, foul breath, massive swelling of the tonsils and uvula, thick speech, cervical lymphadenopathy, striking edematous swelling of the submandibular region and anterior neck, and severe toxicity.

In tonsillopharyngeal diphtheria, only erythema may be noted initially, but isolated spots of grey or white exudate are common. These often extend and coalesce within a day to form a confluent, sharply demarcated pseudomembrane which becomes progressively thicker, more tightly adherent to the underlying tissue, and darker gray in color. Unlike the exudate in streptococcal pharyngitis, the diphtheritic pseudomembrane often extends beyond the margin of the tonsils onto the tonsillar pillars, palate, or uvula. Dislodging the membrane is likely to cause bleeding. Estimates of the proportion of patients with pharyngeal diphtheria who develop typical pseudomembranes vary widely, from as few as one-third to almost all. The higher estimates may be biased by failure to consider and confirm the diagnosis of diphtheria in patients who do not develop pseudomembranes. Patients with nasal diphtheria often present with serosanguinous nasal discharge, which may be unilateral or bilateral and cause irritation of the nares or lip. Laryngeal diphtheria often presents with hoarseness and cough. Demonstration of laryngeal pseudomembrane by laryngoscopy is helpful for distinguishing diphtheria from other infectious forms of laryngitis. Primary or secondary diphtheritic infection occasionally involves other mucous membranes, including conjunctiva, genitourinary tract, and gastrointestinal tract.

Cutaneous diphtheria usually presents as an infection by *C. diphtheriae* of preexisting dermatoses involving, in decreasing order of frequency, the lower extremities, upper extremities, head, or trunk. The clinical features are similar to other secondary cutaneous bacterial infections. In the tropics cutaneous diphtheria occasionally presents with morphologically distinct "punched-out" ulcers that are covered by necrotic slough or membrane and have well demarcated edges.

COMPLICATIONS Obstruction of the respiratory tract, presenting as tachypnea, dyspnea, stridor, cyanosis, and use of accessory muscles of respiration, can be caused by extensive pseudomembrane formation and swelling during the first few days of the disease or by sloughed pseudomembrane that becomes lodged in the airway at a later stage in the disease. The risk of respiratory obstruction is greater when infection involves the larynx or tracheobronchial tree and is higher in children because of the small size of the airways.

Myocarditis and polyneuritis are the most prominent toxic manifestations of diphtheria. Their risk is proportional to the severity of local disease, and both can occur in individual patients. Myocarditis may present during the acute phase of illness, develop as the local disease is improving, or begin insidiously after several weeks. One-half to two-thirds of patients with typical diphtheria have subtle evidence of cardiac dysfunction, including electrocardiographic abnormalities, but clinically apparent myocarditis develops in 10 to 25 percent of patients and is usually more severe when the onset is early. Electrocardiographic abnormalities include ST-T wave changes, varying degrees of heart block, and arrhythymias, including atrial fibrillation, ventricular premature beats, ventricular tachycardia, or ventricular fibrillation. Clinical signs include diminished heart sounds, gallop rhythm, systolic murmurs, and, less commonly, acute or insidiously progressive congestive heart failure. Serum aspartate aminotransferase levels reflect the intensity of myocardial damage and can be used to monitor its course.

Polyneuritis is uncommon in mild diphtheria but occurs in approximately 10 percent of cases of average severity and in up to 75 percent of severe cases. Bulbar dysfunction typically develops during the first 2 weeks. Palatal and pharyngeal paralysis usually develop first. Swallowing is difficult; the voice is nasal; and ingested fluids may be regurgitated through the nose. With unilateral pharyngeal infection, ipsilateral palatal paralysis is more common than contralateral or bilateral paralysis. Additional bulbar signs may develop over several weeks, with oculomotor and ciliary paralysis occurring more often than facial or laryngeal paralysis. Peripheral polyneuritis typically begins from 1 to 3 months after the onset of diphtheria with proximal weakness of the extremities that spreads distally. Severity varies from mild weakness of the pelvic muscles with unsteady gait to total paralysis including failure of respiration. Paresthesias may occur, most often in a "glove-and-stocking" distribution. Polyneuritis usually resolves completely, with the time needed for improvement approximately equal to that taken for development of symptoms. Severe muscular weakness may develop 1 to 2 weeks before maximal abnormalities in peripheral nerve conduction velocity can be demonstrated, resulting in a striking dissociation between clinical and electrophysiologic findings. Cerebrospinal fluid most often shows moderately increased albumin, occasionally with pleocytosis, but the abnormalities in CSF do not determine the prognosis.

Pneumonia occurs in more than half of fatal cases of diphtheria. Less common complications include renal failure, encephalitis, cerebral infarction, pulmonary embolism, and bacteremia or endocarditis due to invasive infection by *C. diphtheriae*. Serum sickness may result from antitoxin therapy.

COURSE AND PROGNOSIS Most cases of diphtheria occur in nonimmunized patients. The attack rate, severity of disease, and risk of complications are much lower when diphtheria occurs in immunized patients. The pseudomembrane may continue to increase in size during the first day after administration of antitoxin. During the next several days to a week it becomes softer, less adherent, and nonconfluent and it eventually disappears as the normal mucosa is regenerated. In the preantibiotic era, *C. diphtheriae* persisted in the throat for about 2 weeks in half of patients and for 1 month or more in about one-fifth. Mortality increases with increasing severity of local disease, extent of pseudomembrane formation, and delay between onset of local disease and administration of antitoxin. Mortality is highest during the first week of illness; in patients with "bull-neck" diphtheria; in patients with myocarditis who develop ventricular tachycardia, atrial fibrillation, or complete heart block; in patients with laryngeal or tracheobronchial involvement; in infants and those over 60 years of age; and in alcoholics. In cutaneous diphtheria both the mortality rate and the risk of developing myocarditis or peripheral neuropathy are significantly lower than in respiratory diphtheria.

DIAGNOSIS A characteristic pseudomembrane on the mucosa of the oropharynx, palate, nasopharynx, nose, or larynx suggests diphtheria, but pseudomembrane is not uniformly present. Diphtheritic pseudomembrane must be distinguished from other pharyngeal exudates, including those of group A beta-hemolytic streptococcal infections, infectious mononucleosis, viral pharyngitides, fusospirochetal infection, and candidiasis. Diphtheria should be considered in patients with sore throat, cervical adenopathy or swelling, and low-grade fever, especially when accompanied by systemic toxicity, hoarseness, stridor, palatal paralysis, or serosanguinous nasal discharge, with or without demonstrable pseudomembrane. Treatment with diphtheria antitoxin should be initiated as soon as the clinical diagnosis of diphtheria is made. Definitive diagnosis of diphtheria depends on isolation of *C. diphtheriae* from local lesions. The laboratory should be notified that diphtheria is suspected to ensure use of media appropriate for isolation of *C. diphtheriae,* such as Tinsdale's tellurite agar or Loeffler's coagulated serum medium. Rapid presumptive diagnosis of *C. diphtheriae* can sometimes be made by methylene blue or fluorescent antibody staining of bacteria from direct swabs, or preferably after several hours of selective cultivation, but confirmation of biochemical reactions to differentiate *C. diphtheriae* from corynebacteria of the normal flora (diphtheroids) requires days. Toxigenicity tests should be performed on all isolates of *C. diphtheriae*. Group A beta-hemolytic streptococci and *Staphylococcus aureus* are also isolated frequently from patients with diphtheria.

Cutaneous diphtheria may present with a characteristic "punched-out" ulcer with a membrane, but it is more often indistinguishable from other inflammatory dermatoses. Diagnosis depends on a high degree of suspicion and on the use of laboratory media appropriate for isolation of *C. diphtheriae* from culture of specimens from cutaneous lesions. Throat cultures for *C. diphtheriae* should be obtained from all patients with cutaneous diphtheria.

TREATMENT The decision to treat with diphtheria antitoxin is based on the clinical diagnosis of diphtheria, without definitive laboratory confirmation, since each day of delay is associated with increased mortality. Because diphtheria antitoxin is produced in horses, it is necessary to obtain a history of possible allergy to horse serum and to perform a conjunctival or intracutaneous test with diluted antitoxin for immediate hypersensitivity. Epinephrine must be available to treat any severe allergic reactions immediately. Patients with immediate hypersensitivity should be desensitized before a full therapeutic dose of antitoxin is given. The dose of diphtheria antitoxin currently recommended by the Committee on Infectious Diseases of the American Academy of Pediatrics is based on the site of the primary infection and the duration and severity of disease: 20,000 to 40,000 units for disease involving the pharynx or larynx and of ≤ 48 h duration; 40,000 to 60,000 units for nasopharyngeal infections; and

80,000 to 100,000 units if the disease is extensive, has been present for 3 or more days, or is accompanied by brawny anterior cervical edema. Antitoxin is administered intravenously by infusion in saline over 60 min to neutralize unbound toxin rapidly. The approximately 10 percent risk of developing serum sickness is acceptable because of the established therapeutic value of antitoxin in decreasing mortality from respiratory diphtheria. During the early phase of the Seattle epidemic, all patients with cutaneous diphtheria were treated with 20,000 units of antitoxin. Later, when most isolates were known to be tox$^-$, antitoxin was withheld initially and administered only to patients from whom tox$^+$ strains of *C. diphtheriae* were isolated. The potential systemic complications from cutaneous diphtheria must be weighed against the potential adverse effects from antitoxin treatment, and authorities are not unanimous in recommending antitoxin therapy for cutaneous diphtheria.

Antibiotics have little demonstrated effect on healing of the local infection in diphtheria patients treated with antitoxin. The primary goal of antibiotic therapy for patients or carriers is, therefore, to eradicate *C. diphtheriae* and prevent its transmission from the patient to susceptible contacts. Commonly recommended regimens for treatment of adults with respiratory diphtheria are erythromycin (500 mg four times daily, parenterally or orally) or intramuscular procaine penicillin G (600,000 units at 12-h intervals) for 14 days. Patients with cutaneous diphtheria and carriers can be treated orally with erythromycin (500 mg four times daily) or rifampin (600 mg once daily) for 7 days. If compliance is in question, a single dose of benzathine penicillin G (1.2 to 2.4 million units intramuscularly) can be substituted. Eradication of *C. diphtheriae* should be documented by negative cultures taken at least 24 h after completion of antibiotic therapy on two or three successive days, and some authorities also recommend a repeat throat culture 2 weeks later. The small percentage of patients who continue to be infected with *C. diphtheriae* after treatment should receive an additional 10-day course of oral erythromycin or rifampin. Plasmid-mediated resistance to erythromycin of the MLS type in *C. diphtheriae* emerged temporarily during the Seattle epidemic but declined dramatically in prevalence after routine use of erythromycin was discontinued.

Patients with respiratory diphtheria or cutaneous diphtheria caused by tox$^+$ *C. diphtheriae* or strains of unknown toxinogenicity should be hospitalized, kept initially at bed rest, handled with respiratory and contact isolation procedures appropriate for the site of infection, and given supportive care as needed. Respiratory and cardiac function must be monitored closely. Early intubation or tracheostomy is recommended when the larynx is involved or signs of impending airway obstruction are present. Mechanical removal of a tracheobronchial membrane can sometimes be accomplished via the endotracheal tube or tracheostomy. Primary or secondary pneumonia should be diagnosed and treated promptly. Sedative or hypnotic drugs that may mask respiratory symptoms are contraindicated. Close electrocardiographic monitoring, treatment of arrhythmias, and electrical pacing for heart block are essential. Congestive heart failure should be treated as described in Chap. 182. Glucocorticoids do not reduce the risk of diphtheritic myocarditis or polyneuritis. Oral Therapy with DL-carnitine (100 mg/kg per day given in twice-daily doses for four days) may have a beneficial effect in diphtheritic myocarditis, but such therapy should be considered experimental until additional data are available. Ulcerative or ecthymatous cutaneous lesions should be treated with Burow solution to wet compresses after debridement of necrotic areas, and treatment for associated conditions such as pediculosis, scabies, or underlying dermatoses should be instituted.

PREVENTION Vaccines available in the United States for immunization against diphtheria include diphtheria and tetanus toxoids and pertussus vaccine adsorbed (DTP); diphtheria and tetanus toxoids adsorbed (DT) (for pediatric use); and tetanus and diphtheria toxoids adsorbed (Td) (for adult use). Each vaccine contains one dose in 0.5 mL and is administered intramuscularly. The adsorbent is alum, which functions as an adjuvant and enhances immunogenicity of the vaccines. Td contains less diphtheria toxoid than DPT or DT and causes fewer adverse reactions in adults.

Initial immunization against diphtheria requires completion of a primary series, and periodic booster doses throughout life are required to maintain immunity. The recommended primary series for immunization of children up to the seventh birthday is four doses of DTP: the first at 6 weeks to 2 months of age, two additional doses after successive intervals of 4 to 8 weeks, and a fourth dose at 6 to 12 months after the third. DT is substituted for DPT if pertussis vaccine is contraindicated. If primary immunization is delayed until after the seventh birthday, the primary series is three doses of Td: the second dose at 4 to 8 weeks after the first, and the third at 6 to 12 months after the second. If primary immunization is interrupted, the series should be completed, but there is no need to start a new series. Children who complete a primary series should receive one dose of DPT before entering kindergarten, unless the final dose of the primary series was given after the fourth birthday. Adults with an uncertain history of immunization should receive a primary series. Patients with diphtheria should be actively immunized after recovery. Booster doses of Td should be given at intervals of 10 years throughout life, preferably at the mid-decade ages of 15 years, 25 years, etc.

Close contacts of diphtheria patients should be cultured for *C. diphtheriae*, kept under surveillance for 1 week, and treated with appropriate antibiotics if cultures are positive. Previously immunized close contacts should receive an appropriate booster containing diphtheria toxoid if their last booster was given >5 years previously. If immunization status is uncertain, close contacts should receive an antibiotic regimen appropriate for carriers and primary immunization against diphtheria appropriate for their age.

REFERENCES

BJORKHOLM B et al: An outbreak of diphtheria among Swedish alcoholics. Infection 15:354, 1987

CENTERS FOR DISEASE CONTROL: Diphtheria, tetanus, and pertussis: Guidelines for vaccine prophylaxis and other preventive measures. Ann Intern Med 103:896, 1985

CHEN RT et al: Diphtheria in the United States, 1971–1981. Am J Public Health 75:1393, 1985

COYLE MB et al: The molecular epidemiology of three biotypes of *Corynebacterium diphtheriae* in the Seattle outbreak from 1972 1982. J Infect Dis 159:670, 1989

GORE I: Myocardial changes in fatal diphtheria. A summary of observations in 221 cases. Am J Med Sci 219:257, 1948

HARNISH JP et al: Diphtheria among alcoholic urban adults. A decade of experience in Seattle. Ann Intern Med 111:71, 1989

KJELDSEN K et al: Immunity against diphtheria and tetanus in the age group 30–70 years. Scand J Infect Dis 20:177, 1988

MACGREGOR RR: Other corynebacteria, in *Principles and Practice of Infectious Diseases*, G Mandell et al (eds), 3d ed. New York, Churchill Livingstone, 1990

MORTIMER EA JR: Diphtheria toxoid, in *Vaccines*, SA Plotkin, EA Mortimer, Jr (eds). Philadelphia, Saunders, 1988, p 31

OLSNES S et al: Diphtheria toxin entry: Protein translocation in the reverse direction. Trends Biochem Sci 13:348, 1988

RAMOS ACMF et al: The protective effect of carnitine in human diphtheric myocarditis. Pediatr Res 18:815, 1984

RAPPUOLI R et al: Molecular epidemiology of the 1984–1986 outbreak of diphtheria in Sweden. N Engl J Med 318:12, 1988

COMMITTEE ON INFECTIOUS DISEASES: Diphtheria, in *Report of the Committee on Infectious Diseases*, 21st ed. Elk Grove Village, IL. American Academy of Pediatrics, 1988, p 174

SINGH M et al: Diphtheria in Afganistan—a review of 155 cases. J Trop Med Hyg 88:373, 1985

WARD, WHJ: Diphtheria toxin: A novel cytocidal enzyme. Trends Biochem Sci 12:28, 1987

103 INFECTIONS CAUSED BY *LISTERIA MONOCYTOGENES* AND *ERYSIPELOTHRIX RHUSIOPATHIAE*

PAUL D. HOEPRICH

LISTERIA MONOCYTOGENES INFECTIONS

DEFINITION Listeriosis, a disease caused by *L. monocytogenes*, consists of many clinical syndromes. Perinatal infection, acquired either transplacentally or during parturition, is the most nearly unique form of listeriosis, while meningitis is the most frequent clinical manifestation.

ETIOLOGY *Listeria monocytogenes* are gram-positive, non-acid-fast, microaerophilic, motile bacilli that form smooth colonies but do not produce either capsules or spores. Several serotypes have been defined on the basis of O and H antigens. The epidemiologically essential aid of typing is available from the Centers for Disease Control. Of the 17 types, 1/2a, 1/2b, and 4b account for more than 70 percent of the cases worldwide. Weakly hemolytic gram-positive bacilli are presumed to be *L. monocytogenes* if they are motile (when grown at 20 to 25°C), reduce 2,3,5-triphenyltetrazolium chloride, hydrolyze esculin, and display characteristic animal pathogenicity: (1) The Anton test—3 to 5 days after inoculation into the conjunctival sac of a rabbit or a guinea pig, *L. monocytogenes* cause a keratoconjunctivitis; (2) general listeriosis (intravenous or intraperitoneal inoculation) typically provokes a monocytosis in rabbits, and focal hepatic necrosis in mice.

EPIDEMIOLOGY AND PATHOGENESIS Found on every continent save the Antarctic, *L. monocytogenes* are distinct from the nonhemolytic, nonpathogenic, bacilli (found mainly in soil, decaying matter, and feces) that are designated *L. innocua* or assigned to the new genus *Murraya*. *Listeria ivanovii* and *L. seeligeri* have rarely been associated with disease in humans, whereas *L. welshimeri* has not; all three are differentiable from *L. monocytogenes* by biochemical and augmentation hemolysis (CAMP) tests. Although typical *L. monocytogenes* have been isolated from silage, other vegetative sources, and 1 to 5 percent of specimens of human feces, listeriosis is uncommon and occurs sporadically with a frequency of 3.6 cases per million population per year in the United States. Listeriosis is more common in urban than rural dwellers, occurring most frequently in July and August (northern hemisphere). Ingestion of food or drink contaminated with *L. monocytogenes* is the usual mode of infection in adults, as exemplified by outbreaks associated with coleslaw, pasteurized milk, ice cream, and fresh Mexican-style cheese.

Infection by direct transfer of *L. monocytogenes* occurs in two circumstances: (1) as an occupational hazard in butchers, abattoir workers, and veterinarians; and (2) from the infected pregnant woman to her offspring either transplacentally or intrapartum. Transplacental perinatal infection results in disseminated fetal listeriosis. The fetus is usually stillborn or is prematurely ejected, virtually always with lethal listeriosis. Fetal listeriosis acquired during delivery is typically not clinically evident for 1 or 2 weeks post partum and usually presents as meningitis.

Listeriosis is preponderantly a disease of persons under 1 year and over 55 years of age. Persons in apparent good health may develop listeriosis. However, other diseases, particularly those with diminished cell-mediated immunity (listerias can survive intracellularly), facilitate the occurrence of listeriosis: for example, neoplasms (especially of the lymphoreticular system) and any conditions requiring treatment with pharmacologic doses of glucocorticoids, irradiation, or cytotoxic agents; alcoholism; cardiovascular disease; diabetes mellitus; and tuberculosis.

MANIFESTATIONS *Listeriosis of the newborn* ranges from meningitis that is clinically apparent within 1 month post partum to diffuse disseminated disease in aborted, premature, stillborn infants, and neonates, who die within minutes to days after birth. If clinical disease is delayed to 1 to 4 weeks post partum, it is generally localized to the central nervous system, as is the rule when children 1 month to 6 years of age are afflicted.

Infants born alive with listeriosis may or may not have fever; yet these babies are critically ill, with cardiorespiratory distress, vomiting, and diarrhea. Dark-red skin papules are frequent, particularly on the lower extremities. Hepatosplenomegaly may be present. This form of listeriosis is also known as septic or miliary granulomatosis. The findings at necropsy are characteristic and mimic those seen in listeriosis of rodents: widely disseminated abscesses varying in size from grossly visible to microscopic, involving, in order of decreasing frequency, liver, spleen, adrenal glands, lungs, pharynx, gastrointestinal tract, central nervous system, and skin. Typically, the lesions are abscesses, but classic granulomas may be seen, depending principally on the duration of infection before death. Microscopic examination of a Gram-stained smear of meconium from the normal newborn infant does not disclose bacteria; fetal listeriosis results in meconium laden with gram-positive bacilli. For this reason, examination of meconium by Gram's stain and by culture should be carried out whenever there is gross soiling of the amniotic liquid with meconium, prematurity, or unexplained fever in the mother before or at the onset of labor. This is particularly important because listeriosis in the pregnant woman may be asymptomatic or may cause a mild, nonspecific illness. A week to a month ante partum, there may have been malaise, a chill, diarrhea, pain in the back or flanks, and itching. Even when symptomatic, the disease is benign and self-limited in the mother; however, as symptoms subside, a decrease or cessation of fetal movement may be noted. Infection of the fetus may occur as early as the fifth month of gestation but occurs most often in the third trimester. Following delivery of infants with proved fetal listeriosis, cervical cultures are, or soon become, negative for *L. monocytogenes*; subsequent conception, gestation, and delivery are normal.

Meningitis accounts for about three-fourths of the cases verified by culture and is the predominant clinical form of listeriosis. Meningitis caused by *L. monocytogenes* cannot be distinguished on clinical grounds from meningitis caused by other bacteria.

Nonmeningeal listeriosis of the central nervous system is associated with fever, nausea and vomiting, headache, and listeremia; the cerebrospinal fluid is normal. Localizing neurologic signs may develop (especially if abscess forms), or the picture may be that of an encephalitis.

Typhoidal listeriosis, i.e., listeremia that has no identifiable source and is associated with high fever and severe prostrating illness, occurs most often in patients with cancers and immunosuppression. However, primary listeremia may also develop in patients with cirrhosis, alcoholism, pregnancy, and no discernible underlying disease.

Listerial endocarditis is generally a chronic process without singular manifestations. About half of the patients have no known predisposing cardiac disease.

Other rare forms of listeriosis include ocular infections, dermatitis, infections of serous cavities, and abscesses in various organs.

LABORATORY FINDINGS Although *L. monocytogenes* grow well on the usual culture media, etiologic diagnosis by isolation and identification may be hampered by failure of differentiation from *Corynebacterium* spp., *Erysipelothrix rhusiopathiae*, and *Streptococcus* spp. Recognition of listerial colonies in a mixed culture, as may result with vaginal or cervical specimens, is difficult and may be aided by using selective media and/or enrichment procedures.

Serodiagnosis by assay for agglutinins has not been useful because of the common finding of so-called natural antibodies. Such nonspecific reactions may reflect the known antigenic relationship between *Staphylococcus aureus* and several listerial serotypes, or contact with nonpathogenic *Listeria* spp. or *Murraya* spp. The humoral antibody response to listeriosis in humans is almost exclusively IgM throughout the disease, whereas staphylococci elicit IgG as well as IgM; i.e., treatment of sera with 2-mercaptoethanol may not eliminate nonspecific reactivity.

Monocytosis is not common in human listeriosis. Leukocytosis with neutrophilia, as in any acute bacterial infection, is seen in listerial meningitis, nonmeningeal infection of the central nervous system, primary listeremia, listerial endocarditis, and abscesses in hosts capable of mounting a granulocytic response. In most patients with listerial meningitis, the findings in the cerebrospinal fluid do not differ from those found in other bacterial meningitides; however, a relative increase in mononuclear cells may be seen in patients with underlying malignancies.

DIFFERENTIAL DIAGNOSIS Abortion, premature delivery, stillbirth, and neonatal death are more often due to causes other than listeriosis: Rh incompatibility, syphilis, or toxoplasmosis.

In patients with leptomeningitis, conjunctivitis, endocarditis, bacteremia, or polyserositis, reports of isolation of "diphtheroids" or "nonpathogens" must always be challenged. A statement that *L. monocytogenes* has been excluded is required.

TREATMENT *Listeria monocytogenes* are susceptible to several antimicrobials in vitro, including penicillin G, ampicillin, erythromycin, rifampin, streptomycin, gentamicin, tobramycin, amikacin, trimethoprim-sulfamethoxazole, and the tetracyclines. *Listeria* are resistant to all classes of cephalosporins. Tolerance, i.e., inhibition at low concentrations with much higher concentrations needed for killing, is characteristic with the penicillins, erythromycin, rifampin, trimethoprim-sulfamethoxazole, and streptomycin. Accordingly, combination therapy is necessary for maximally listericidal therapy, e.g., penicillin G [150 to 200 mg (240,000 to 320,000 units) per kilogram of body weight per day, intravenously, as six equal portions every 4 h] plus tobramycin (5 to 6 mg/kg per day, intravenously, as three equal portions every 8 h). Ampicillin and gentamicin (same dosages) may be substituted but offer no advantage. Such treatment is appropriate for listeriosis of the newborn (2 weeks), listeremia in pregnancy (2 weeks), primary listeremia (4 weeks), listerial endocarditis (4 to 6 weeks), and any form of listeriosis outside the central nervous system in immunosuppressed patients (4 to 6 weeks).

As gentamicin and tobramycin do not enter the central nervous system reliably, high-dosage therapy with penicillin G [200 to 300 mg (320,000 to 480,000 units) per kilogram of body weight per day, intravenously, as six equal portions every 4 h] is the primary treatment. Ampicillin may be substituted in the same dose, but the cephalosporins, including the newer derivatives, should not be used. Optimal treatment of patients who are allergic to the penicillins is uncertain; candidate antimicrobials include erythromycin (40 to 50 mg/kg per day, intravenously, as four equal portions every 6 h); doxycycline (3 mg/kg, intravenously as a loading dose, and 1.5 mg/kg per day, intravenously, as two equal portions every 12 h for maintenance); trimethoprim/sulfamethoxazole (15/75 mg/kg per day, intravenously, as 3 equal portions every 8 h). Treatment should be continued in full dosage by intravenous injection for 14 to 21 days after defervescence.

PROGNOSIS Prompt, vigorous antimicrobial treatment of the acute forms of listeriosis, excepting fetal listeriosis, is usually curative. On the basis of agglutinin titers, specific antibody disappears during the months following cure. However, reinfection has not been reported.

ERYSIPELOTHRIX RHUSIOPATHIAE INFECTIONS

DEFINITION Erysipeloid is the commonest and most nearly unique form of infection in humans caused by *Erysipelothrix rhusiopathiae*. Infective endocarditis and arthritis are rare forms of erysipelothricosis in humans.

ETIOLOGY As gram-positive, nonmotile, nonencapsulated, nonsporulating, microaerophilic bacilli, *E. rhusiopathiae* may be confused with nontoxinogenic *Corynebacterium* spp. and *Listeria monocytogenes*. However, *E. rhusiopathiae* is nonmotile and fails to grow on media selective for *Corynebacterium* spp. Also, unlike *L. monocytogenes, E. rhusiopathiae* only rarely causes conjunctivitis, following conjunctival inoculation, or monocytosis, after intravenous inoculation, in the rabbit. Because alpha hemolysis is commonly evident after 48 h of incubation of *E. rhusiopathiae,* confusion with streptococci may also occur. Isolates of *E. rhusiopathiae* appear to be serologically homogeneous. Although serodifferentiation from other gram-positive bacilli is possible, few laboratories are capable of definitive serodiagnosis.

EPIDEMIOLOGY AND PATHOGENESIS Primarily a saprobe, *E. rhusiopathiae* is worldwide in distribution. Humans are virtually always infected by traumatic dermal inoculation; erysipeloid is the usual result. The disease is almost wholly restricted to persons who in their occupations handle edible or nonedible dead animal products. If the bacilli are not successfully confined to the skin, bacteremia may result and may lead to infective endocarditis; in about two-thirds of the reported cases, there was no evidence of preexisting valvular heart disease and the aortic valve was involved in about 60 percent of the cases. Septic arthritis, usually in previously damaged joints, may also complicate bacteremia.

The seasonal incidence of erysipeloid parallels that of swine erysipelas, being highest in summer and early fall. Yet persons who tend pigs, even pigs ill with porcine erysipelas, do not commonly develop erysipeloid.

MANIFESTATIONS Erysipeloid begins 2 to 7 days after injury, often after the initial lesion has healed. An itching, burning, painful irritation may precede and always accompanies the appearance of the maculopapular, nonvesiculated, sharply defined, raised, purplish-red zone surrounding the site of entry. There is local swelling, and when, as is usual, a finger or the hand is involved, nearby joints may become stiff and painful. Centrifugal spread from the site of inoculation is apparent in a day or two. Movement is slow, 1 to 2 cm per 24 h maximally, and more rapid proximally than distally; involvement of the terminal phalanx of a finger is rare, while spread to other fingers and the hand distal to the wrist is common. With extension, the original center subsides without desquamation or suppuration. There are usually no systemic signs or symptoms; regional lymphangitis and lymphadenitis are rare. Untreated, the disease heals within 3 weeks in most patients, although relapse has been observed.

The manifestations of erysipelothrical endocarditis may be either acute or chronic, depending on the virulence of the infecting strain and on the state of resistance of the host. Usually, there are no classic erysipeloid skin lesions to suggest the disease at the time that endocarditis is clinically evident. However, a history of recent erysipeloid may be helpful.

Erysipelothrical arthritis is not clinically characteristic but usually can be related to erysipeloid or erysipelothrical bacteremia. Isolation of *E. rhusiopathiae* from synovial fluid has not been reported.

LABORATORY FINDINGS The usual culture media are adequate for the growth of *E. rhusiopathiae*. However, differentiation from diphtheroids, listerias, and streptococci depends primarily on the clinician's alerting the laboratory to the possibility of erysipelothricosis. In erysipeloid, *E. rhusiopathiae* are best recovered by incubating, in broth containing glucose, a full-thickness biopsy of skin removed from the advancing edge of a lesion. Culture of an aspirate obtained after injection of sterile, bacteriostat-free 0.9% NaCl solution into the periphery of a lesion is less likely to yield *E. rhusiopathiae*. With endocarditis and arthritis, the findings are in keeping with the respective clinical syndromes and are in no way characteristic for *E. rhusiopathiae,* whereas abrasion of a florid lesion with culture of the resultant exudate may be rewarding.

DIFFERENTIAL DIAGNOSIS The appearance and location of erysipeloid, its slow and limited spread, the lack of constitutional reaction, the history of occupation and injury, all serve to identify this disease. The afflicted skin in *erysipelas* is very erythematous, and the face and scalp are affected; there are regional lymphangitis and lymphadenitis, leukocytosis, fever, and malaise. Eczematous lesions may itch, but they display vesicles and little abnormal color. The various erythemas have a different location and do not usually itch or burn; they are more apt to be chronic and nonmigratory.

TREATMENT The penicillins, the cephalosporins, erythromycin, clindamycin, the tetracyclines, and chloramphenicol inhibit *E. rhusiopathiae* in vitro at concentrations practical in therapy. Penicillin G is the agent of choice. Erysipeloid is adequately treated by injection of 1.2 million units of benzathine penicillin G. Erythromycin (15 mg/kg per day in four equal portions taken orally for 5 to 7 days) is an alternative. Cure of erysipelothrical endocarditis has been effected by the daily injection of 2 to 20 million units of penicillin per day or cefazolin (65 to 75 mg/kg per day, intravenously, as four equal portions every 6 h) for 4 to 6 weeks; the dose can be monitored by determination of the bactericidal activity of serum from the patient against the infecting strain. Intractable cardiac failure may oblige surgical excision of an infected valve and insertion of a prosthesis. Erysipelothrical arthritis usually responds to repeated needle aspiration drainage plus penicillin or cefazolin in the dosage given for endocarditis. Antimicrobial therapy should be continued for at least one week after the effusion clears.

PROGNOSIS Penicillin therapy is highly effective in curing erysipelothrical infections. As with infective endocarditis from any cause, the prognosis is primarily a function of the severity of the valvular damage. Despite appropriate antimicrobial therapy, the mortality remains 30 to 40 percent; earlier diagnosis, and, perhaps, earlier resort to surgical excision and replacement of infected valves, may improve the outcome.

REFERENCES

CHERUBIN CE et al: Listeria and gram-negative bacillary meningitis in New York City, 1972–1979. Am J Med 71:199, 1981

CIESIELSKI CA et al: Listeriosis in the United States: 1980–1982. Arch Intern Med 148:1416, 1988

FLEMING DW et al: Pasteurized milk as a vehicle of infection in an outbreak of listeriosis. N Engl J Med 312:404, 1985

GORBY GL et al: *Erysipelothrix rhusiopathiae* endocarditis: Microbiologic, epidemiologic, and clinical features of an occupational disease. Rev Infect Dis 10:317, 1988

HOEPRICH PD: Listeriosis, in *Infectious Diseases*, 4th ed, PD Hoeprich (ed). Philadelphia, Lippincott-Harper, 1989, chap 56

———: Erysipeloid, in *Infectious Diseases*, 4th ed, PD Hoeprich (ed). Philadelphia, Lippincott-Harper, 1989, chap 112

LINNAN MD et al: Epidemic listeriosis associated with Mexican-style cheese. N Engl J Med 319:823, 1988

NELSON E. Five hundred cases of erysipeloid. Rocky Mount Med J 52:40, 1955

ROCOURT J, GRIMONT PAD: *Listeria welshimeri* sp. nov. and *Listeria seeligeri* sp. nov. Int J Syst Bacteriol 33:866, 1983

SCHLECH WF III et al: Epidemic listeriosis—evidence for transmission by food. N Engl J Med 308:203, 1983

SEELIGER HPR: *Listeriosis*. Basel, Karger, 1961

104 ANTHRAX

RANDALL K. HOLMES

DEFINITION Anthrax is an acute bacterial infection caused by *Bacillus anthracis* that occurs most frequently in herbivorous animals. Humans become infected when spores of *B. anthracis* are introduced into the body by contact with infected animals or contaminated animal products, insect bites, inhalation, or ingestion. In humans the most common form is cutaneous anthrax, characterized by development of a localized skin lesion with a central eschar surrounded by marked nonpitting edema. Inhalation anthrax (woolsorter's disease) typically produces hemorrhagic mediastinitis, rapidly progressive systemic infection, and a very high mortality rate. Gastrointestinal anthrax is rare and has a high mortality rate.

ETIOLOGY *B. anthracis* is a large (1 to 1.5 μm by 4 to 10 μm), nonmotile, encapsulated, chain-forming, aerobic gram-positive rod that forms centrally located, oval spores. Oxygen is required for sporulation but not for germination of spores, and sporulation does not occur in living animals. The individual bacteria in the chains are rectangular, giving them a boxcar-shaped appearance. On blood agar virulent *B. anthracis* usually forms nonhemolytic or weakly hemolytic, gray-white, rough colonies with irregular, comma-shaped projections, said to resemble a Medusa's head; but if the medium contains bicarbonate and incubation is carried out in the presence of excess CO_2 the colonies are smooth and mucoid. Virulent strains of *B. anthracis* are pathogenic for animals, including mice and guinea pigs. Known virulence factors include three proteins collectively called *anthrax toxin* (see below) and an antiphagocytic capsular polypeptide, composed of D-glutamic acid residues linked by peptide bonds involving the gamma carboxyl group. The genes that determine production of anthrax toxin and of capsular polypeptide are present on separate plasmids of *B. anthracis*. Determination of susceptibility to bacillus phage gamma and demonstration of species specific antigens by direct fluorescent antibody tests or by hemagglutination tests are helpful in laboratory identification of *B. anthracis*. Spores of *B. anthracis* can survive for years in dry earth but are destroyed by boiling for about 10 min, by treatment with oxidizing agents such as potassium permanganate or hydrogen peroxide, or by dilute formaldehyde. Most strains of *B. anthracis* are susceptible to penicillin.

EPIDEMIOLOGY The distribution of anthrax is worldwide. All animals are susceptible to varying degrees, but the disease is most prevalent among domestic herbivores, including cattle, sheep, horses, and goats, and wild herbivores.

Grazing animals become infected when they are foraging for food in areas contaminated with spores of *B. anthracis* under appropriate climatic conditions. Anthrax in herbivores tends to be severe, with high mortality. Terminally ill animals have overwhelming bacteremic infections and often bleed from the nose, mouth, and bowel, thereby contaminating soil or watering places with vegetative *B. anthracis* that can subsequently sporulate and persist in the environment. The carcasses of infected animals provide additional potential foci of contamination. Whether or not *B. anthracis* multiplies to any significant extent in the soil is controversial, and environmental factors which affect the probability that animals grazing in infected areas will become infected are not fully defined. Epidemics among animals may spread from an initial focus to contiguous geographic areas, consistent with the movement of infected animals. Biting flies have also been implicated as vectors for the spread of anthrax, and vultures that feed on infected carcasses are believed to be involved in the occasional spread of anthrax from an infected area to noncontiguous areas, probably by contaminating surface water pools.

The natural resistance of humans to anthrax is greater than that of herbivorous animals. It is difficult to determine the annual worldwide incidence of human anthrax because many cases do not receive medical attention and are not reported; estimates of 20,000 to 100,000 cases per year have been made. Human cases are classified as agricultural or industrial based on the epidemiologic setting in which they occur. Agricultural cases result most often from contact with animals that have anthrax (skinning, butchering, dissecting, etc.), from bites of contaminated or infected flies, and rarely from consumption of contaminated meat. Industrial cases are associated with exposure to contaminated hides, goat hair, wool, or bones that are used for commercial purposes. Anthrax in animals has been a longstanding problem in Iran, Turkey, Pakistan, and Sudan, and probability is high that animal products, especially goat hair, originating from these areas will be contaminated with anthrax spores.

Only four cases of anthrax occurred in the United States from 1984 through 1988, and gastrointestinal anthrax has never been documented in the United States. Large epidemics of anthrax occurred in Sverdlovsk in the Soviet Union in April, 1979, and in Zimbabwe between 1978 and the early 1980s. The outbreak in Zimbabwe involved more than 9700 cases of agricultural anthrax in 1979 and 1980. The massive outbreak in Zimbabwe occurred during wartime and was associated with disruption of the veterinary and medical infrastructure and cessation of anthrax vaccination programs (see below).

PATHOGENESIS *B. anthracis* is an extracellular pathogen that can evade phagocytosis, invade the bloodstream, multiply rapidly to a high population density in vivo, and kill rapidly. Capsular polypeptide and anthrax toxin are recognized as virulence factors of *B. anthracis*.

Anthrax toxin was discovered by demonstrating that transfer of sterile blood from guinea pigs dying of anthrax to uninfected guinea pigs kills the recipient animals and that death is prevented by specific immune serum.

Anthrax toxin consists of three separate soluble proteins called protective antigen (PA), edema factor (EF), and lethal factor (LF). Antibodies against PA protect experimental animals and man against anthrax. PA is the major component of the vaccine against anthrax used for humans in the United States. Loss of the plasmid that encodes anthrax toxin is the probable basis for attenuation of the strain of *B. anthracis* developed by Pasteur for his original experiments on immunization of animals against anthrax. Capsular polypeptide of *B. anthracis* is antiphagocytic. Loss of ability to produce capsule is the primary basis for attenuation of the live spore vaccine (Sterne strain) used for animals in the United States. These nonencapsulated strains produce anthrax toxin and elicit antitoxic antibodies but are less invasive than wild-type strains.

PA, EF, and LF have been purified and characterized and their structural genes cloned and sequenced. PA binds to receptors on the plasma membrane of target cells and is then cleaved by trypsin or a protease with similar specificity to produce two fragments. The smaller fragment is released, but the larger fragment remains on the cell surface and displays a binding site for EF or LF. The large fragment of PA on the cell surface serves, therefore, as a specific receptor for EF or LF; and it mediates entry of EF or LF into target cells by receptor-mediated endocytosis. EF is a calmodulin-dependent adenylate cyclase. The enzymatic activity of EF is only expressed within target cells, which provide the required calmodulin activator as well as the ATP substrate that is converted into cyclic AMP. The actions of cyclic AMP in the intoxicated cells are presumed to be responsible for the biological effects of EF, which include formation of the edema characteristic of anthrax lesions as well as inhibition of phagocytosis by polymorphonuclear leukocytes. PA-mediated entry of LF into susceptible target cells leads to cell death, but the mechanism of action of LF has not yet been determined.

Cutaneous anthrax is initiated by introducing spores of *B. anthracis* into the skin through cuts or abrasions or by biting flies. The spores germinate within hours, and the vegetative cells begin to multiply and produce the components of anthrax toxin. Histologically the lesion in cutaneous anthrax is characterized by necrosis, vascular congestion, hemorrhage, and gelatinous edema. The number of leukocytes is disproportionately small in comparison with the amount of tissue damage. The clinical description of this lesion as a ''malignant pustule'' is not in concordance with the pathologic findings.

In inhalation anthrax *B. anthracis* spores in airborne particles of less that 5 μm diameter are deposited directly into the alveoli or alveolar ducts. The spores are phagocytized by alveolar macrophages and some are carried to and germinate in mediastinal nodes. Hemorrhagic necrosis of the nodes, associated with hemorrhagic mediastinitis and development of overwhelming *B. anthracis* bacteremia, may develop rapidly. Secondary pneumonia sometimes occurs.

Gastrointestinal anthrax usually results from ingestion of inadequately cooked meat from animals with anthrax. Primary infection can be initiated in the intestine by germination of spores that survive passage through the stomach, but an oropharyngeal form of the disease has also been described. Lesions in the throat or intestine are usually accompanied by hemorrhagic lymphadenitis.

B. anthracis bacteremia can develop in any form of anthrax and occurs in almost all fatal cases. Autopsies reveal large numbers of bacteria in blood vessels, lymph nodes, and many organs.

CLINICAL MANIFESTATIONS Approximately 95 percent of human cases are cutaneous anthrax, and about 5 percent are inhalation anthrax. Gastrointestinal anthrax occurs rarely. Anthrax meningitis occurs in a small percentage of all cases but is a frequent complication of overwhelming *B. anthracis* bacteremia.

Cutaneous anthrax The cutaneous lesion in anthrax is most often found on exposed areas of skin. In Zimbabwe, lesions in children under 5 years old were significantly more likely to be on the head, neck, or face and less likely to be on the upper limbs than in adults. This correlated with the fact that children had less contact with carcasses of infected animals and were more likely to acquire infection by fly bites.

Within days after inoculation of *B. anthracis* spores into skin, a small, red macule appears. During the next week the lesion typically progresses through papular and vesicular or pustular stages, leading to formation of an ulcer with a blackened, necrotic eschar surrounded by a highly characteristic, expanding zone of brawny edema. The early lesion may be pruritic, and the fully developed lesion is painless. Small satellite vesicles may surround the original lesion, and painful nonspecific regional lymphadenitis is common. Most patients are afebrile, with mild or no constitutional symptoms, but in severe cases edema may be extensive and associated with septic shock. Spontaneous healing occurs in 80 to 90 percent of untreated cases, but edema may persist for weeks. In the 10 to 20 percent of untreated patients who develop progressive infection, bacteremia develops and is often associated with high fever and a rapidly fatal outcome. The differential diagnosis includes staphylococcal skin infections, tularemia, plague, and orf. Cutaneous anthrax should be considered in all patients who have painless ulcers associated with vesicles and edema as well as contact with animal products or animals.

Inhalation anthrax The presenting symptoms of inhalation anthrax (woolsorter's disease) are often similar to those of severe viral respiratory diseases, making early diagnosis difficult. After 1 to 3 days an acute phase supervenes, with increasing fever, dyspnea, stridor, hypoxia, and hypotension usually leading to death within 24 h. Occasionally patients present with the fulminant disease. A characteristic x-ray finding associated with the hemorrhagic mediastinitis is symmetrical mediastinal widening.

Gastrointestinal anthrax Symptoms of gastrointestinal anthrax are variable and include fever, nausea and vomiting, abdominal pain, bloody diarrhea, and sometimes rapidly developing ascites. Diarrhea is occasionally massive, causing hemoconcentration and severe contraction of intravascular volume. The major features of oropharyngeal anthrax are fever, sore throat, dysphagia, painful regional lymphadenopathy, and toxemia; respiratory distress may be present. The primary lesion is most often on the tonsils and features necrosis, hemorrhage and exudate formation.

LABORATORY DIAGNOSIS *B. anthracis* is present in large numbers in cutaneous lesions of anthrax and can be demonstrated by Gram's stain, direct fluorescent antibody staining, or culture unless the patient has been treated with antibiotics. A small proportion of patients with anthrax have bacteremia, but the disease may progress to a fatal outcome before cultures become positive. Patients with anthrax meningitis have bloody spinal fluid containing a large number of *B. anthracis* demonstrable by staining or culture. Virulence of suspected isolates of *B. anthracis* can be demonstrated by inoculating guinea pigs; death occurs within 24 h with positive cultures from heart blood. Patients with mild disease usually have normal leukocyte counts, but patients with disseminated disease typically have polymorphonuclear leukocytosis. Tests for antibody to *B. anthracis* are useful in confirming the diagnosis of anthrax.

TREATMENT Viable *B. anthracis* disappears from the lesions of cutaneous anthrax within 5 h in patients treated with parenteral penicillin G. Recommended therapy for adults is 2 million units of penicillin G at intervals of 6 h until edema subsides, followed by oral penicillin to complete a 7- to 10-d course of treatment. For penicillin-sensitive adults erythromycin or tetracycline (500 mg every 6 h) can be substituted. Chloramphenicol has also been used successfully. Antibiotics decrease local edema and systemic toxicity in patients with cutaneous anthrax but do not prevent eschar formation. Cutaneous lesions should be cleaned and covered, and used dressings should be decontaminated. For inhalation anthrax high-dose penicillin therapy (2 million units at 2-hourly intervals) is recommended, and a similar regimen is recommended for gastrointestinal anthrax or anthrax meningitis. A rational case can be made for passive immunization with anthrax antitoxin in addition to antibiotic therapy in severely ill patients with anthrax, but appropriate antitoxin is not commercially available.

PREVENTION Inhalation anthrax was virtually eliminated in England before 1940 by developing methods to decontaminate wool and goat hair and by improving working conditions for handlers of animal products. Nonliving vaccines consisting of alum precipitated or aluminum hydroxide adsorbed extracellular components of unencapsulated *B. anthracis* are available in the UK and USA for use in humans who are at risk for exposure to anthrax. The major active component of these vaccines is PA. Molecular engineering was recently used to produce a mutant form of PA that lacks the trypsin-sensitive sequence and cannot interact with EF or LF to mediate toxicity. The mutant PA is being tested as a potential new vaccine against anthrax. Immunization of domestic herbivores with spores of nonencapsulated strains of *B. anthracis* has a major role in decreasing the prevalence of anthrax in livestock both in developed and in developing countries. Living attenuated spore vaccines are not used for humans in the United States but are used both for humans and animals in the Soviet Union. Carcasses of animals that succumb to anthrax should be buried intact or cremated. Necropsies or butchering of infected animals should be avoided because sporulation of *B. anthracis* occurs only in the presence of oxygen.

PROGNOSIS The mortality rate is 10 to 20 percent for untreated cutaneous anthrax and is very low with appropriate antibiotic therapy. In contrast, the mortality rate of inhalation anthrax approaches 100 percent, and therapy is usually unsuccessful. The mortality rate in treated gastrointestinal anthrax is approximately 50 percent. Anthrax meningitis is usually fatal.

The opinions expressed herein are those of the author and do not necessarily represent the views of the Department of Defense or the Uniformed Services University of the Health Sciences.

REFERENCES

BRACHMAN PS: Inhalation anthrax. Ann NY Acad Sci 353:83, 1980

BRAGG TS, ROBERTSON UL: Nucleotide sequence and analysis of the lethal factor gene (lef) from *Bacillus anthracis*. Gene 81:45, 1989

DAVIES JCA: A major epidemic of anthrax in Zimbabwe, Part II. Distribution of cutaneous lesions. Central African J Med 28:291, 1982

———: A major epidemic of anthrax in Zimbabwe. The experience of the Beatrice Road Infectious Diseases Hospital, Harare. Central African J Med 31:176, 1985

DOGANAY M et al: Primary throat anthrax. A report of six cases. Scand J Infect Dis 18:415, 1983

———: A case of cutaneous anthrax with toxemic shock. Brit J Dermatol 117:659, 1987

GORDON VH et al: Adenylate cyclase toxins from *Bacillus anthracis* and *Bordetella pertussis*. Different processes for interaction with and entry into target cells. J Biol Chem 264:14792, 1989

HAMBELTON P et al: Anthrax: The disease in relation to vaccines. Vaccine 2:125, 1984

KNUDSON GB: Treatment of anthrax in man: History and current concepts. Military Medicine 151:71, 1986

LAFORCE FM: *Bacillus anthracis* (anthrax), in *Principles and Practice of Infectious Diseases*, 3d ed, GL Mandell et al (eds). New York, Churchill Livingstone, 1990, p 1593

MARSHALL L: Sverdlovsk: Anthrax capital? Science 240:383, 1988

O'BRIEN J et al: Effects of anthrax toxin components on human neutrophils. Infect Immun 45:306, 1986

SINGH Y et al: A deleted variant of *Bacillus anthracis* protective antigen is non-toxic and blocks anthrax toxin action in vivo. J Biol Chem 264:19103, 1989

105 TETANUS

ELIAS ABRUTYN

DEFINITION Tetanus is a neurologic disorder, characterized by increased muscle tone and spasms, that is caused by tetanospasmin, a powerful protein toxin elaborated by *Clostridium tetani*. Tetanus occurs in several clinical forms including generalized, neonatal, and localized disease.

MICROBIOLOGY The organism is an anaerobic, motile gram-positive rod that forms an oval, colorless, terminal spore creating a shape that resembles a tennis racket or drumstick. It is found worldwide in soil, in the inanimate environment, in animal feces, and occasionally in human feces. Spores may survive for years in some environments and are resistant to various disinfectants and boiling for 20 min. Vegetative cells, however, are easily inactivated and are susceptible to several antibiotics (penicillin, erythromycin, and others).

Tetanospasmin is formed in vegetative cells under plasmid control. It is a single polypeptide chain. With autolysis, the single-chain toxin is released and cleaved to form a heterodimer consisting of a heavy chain (93,000 mol wt) and a light chain (52,000 mol wt) joined by a disulfide bond. The amino acid structures of the two most powerful toxins known, botulinum and tetanus toxin, are partially homologous.

EPIDEMIOLOGY Tetanus occurs sporadically and almost always affects nonimmunized or partially immunized persons, or fully immunized individuals who fail to maintain adequate immunity with booster doses of vaccine. Although entirely preventable by immunization, worldwide the burden of disease is large. The disease is common where soil is cultivated, in rural areas, in warm climates, during summer months, and in males. In countries without a major immunization program, neonatal tetanus and tetanus in the young predominate; worldwide an estimated 800,000 neonates die each year. In the United States and other nations with successful immunization programs, neonatal tetanus rarely occurs and the disease affects other age groups and those in groups inadequately reached by immunization such as nonwhites. The elderly, in particular, are prominently involved. Under 100 cases have been reported to the Centers for Disease Control annually: 95 percent of cases occurred in persons over 20 years of age and 71 percent in individuals over 50.

In the United States, most tetanus occurs after an acute injury, such as a puncture wound or laceration, and is often acquired at home, either indoors or outdoors, frequently in a garden. The injury may be major, but often is trivial so medical attention is not sought. The disease may complicate chronic conditions such as skin ulcers, abscesses, and gangrene. Tetanus is also associated with burns, frostbite, ear infection, surgery, abortion, childbirth, and drug abuse, notably skin "popping." In some patients no portal of entry can be identified.

PATHOGENESIS Contamination of wounds with spores is probably frequent. Germination and toxin production, however, only occur in wounds with low oxidation-reduction potential such as those containing devitalized tissue, foreign bodies, or active infection. *Clostridium tetani* does not itself evoke inflammation.

Toxin released in the wound binds to peripheral motor neuron terminals, enters the axon, and is transported to the nerve cell body in the central nervous system by retrograde intraneuronal transport. It then crosses the synapse to enter the inhibitory interneurons where it acts to block neurotransmitter release, resulting in heightened motor activity. By a similar process the toxin causes increased sympathetic activity. Animal studies suggest that the toxin is disseminated via the bloodstream to other peripheral neurons; toxin in the blood does not cross the blood-brain barrier.

CLINICAL MANIFESTATIONS Generalized tetanus, the most common form, is characterized by increased muscle tone and generalized spasms. The median onset after injury is 7 days; 10 percent of cases occur within 3 days and 10 percent after 14 days.

Typically, the patient first notices increased tone in the masseter muscles (trismus or lockjaw). Dysphagia or stiffness or pain in the neck, shoulder, and back muscles may also be present. Soon other muscles are involved, producing a rigid abdomen and stiff proximal limb muscles; the hands and feet are relatively spared. Sustained contraction of the facial muscles produces a grimace or sneer (risus sardonicus), and contraction of the back muscles an arched back (opisthotonos). Some patients develop paroxysmal, violent, painful, generalized muscle spasms that may cause cyanosis and threaten ventilation. They occur repetitively and may be spontaneous or provoked by even the slightest stimulation. A constant threat during generalized spasms is reduced ventilation or apnea or laryngospasm. The severity of illness may be mild (muscle rigidity and few or no spasms), moderate (trismus, dysphagia, rigidity, and spasms), or severe (frequent explosive paroxysms). The patient may be febrile, although many have no fever; mentation is unimpaired. Deep tendon reflexes may be increased. Dysphagia or ileus may preclude oral feeding.

Sympathetic overactivity commonly complicates severe cases and is characterized by labile or sustained hypertension, tachycardia, hyperpyrexia, profuse sweating, arrhythmias, and increased plasma and urinary catecholamine levels. Late cardiovascular complications include hypotension and bradycardia which are easily reversed by physical stimulation such as suctioning. Hypotension, tachycardia, and hyperpyrexia are ominous signs.

Complications include pneumonia, fractures, muscle rupture, asphyxia, and unexplained cardiac arrest.

Neonatal tetanus usually occurs as generalized tetanus and usually is fatal. It develops in children born to inadequately immunized mothers, frequently after unsterile treatment of the umbilical cord or its stump. The onset generally occurs during the first 2 weeks of life. Poor feeding, rigidity, and spasms occur.

Local tetanus is an uncommon form in which manifestations are restricted to muscles near the wound; however, it may evolve to the generalized illness. The prognosis is excellent.

Cephalic tetanus, a rare form of local tetanus, follows head injury or ear infection. Trismus and dysfunction of one or more cranial nerves, often the seventh nerve, are found. The incubation period is a few days and the mortality is high.

DIAGNOSIS The diagnosis of tetanus is made entirely on the basis of clinical findings. Wound cultures should be done. However, *C. tetani* can be isolated from wounds of patients without tetanus, and frequently the organism cannot be recovered from the wounds of those with tetanus. The leukocyte count may be elevated. The cerebrospinal fluid examination is normal. Electromyograms may show continuous discharge of motor units and shortening or absence of the silent interval normally seen after an action potential. Nonspecific changes may be seen on the electrocardiogram. Muscle enzyme levels may be raised.

The differential diagnosis includes local conditions also producing trismus such as alveolar abscess, strychnine poisoning, dystonic drug reactions (such as phenothiazines and metoclopramide), and hypocalcemic tetany. Other conditions possibly confused with tetanus include meningitis/encephalitis, rabies, and an acute intraabdominal process (because of the rigid abdomen). The marked increased tone in central muscles (face, neck, chest, back, and abdomen) with superimposed generalized spasms and relative sparing of the hands and feet strongly suggest tetanus.

TREATMENT General measures The goals of therapy are to eliminate the source of toxin, neutralize unbound toxin, prevent muscle spasms, and provide support, especially respiratory support, until recovery. Patients should be admitted to a quiet room in an intensive care unit where observation and cardiopulmonary monitoring can be maintained continuously, but stimulation can be minimized. Protection of the airway is vital. Wounds should be explored, carefully cleansed, and thoroughly debrided.

Antibiotic therapy Although it is of questionable benefit, parenteral penicillin (10 to 12 million units daily for 10 days) is administered to eradicate vegetative cells, the source of the toxin. Clindamycin (150 to 300 mg every 6 h) or erythromycin (500 mg every 6 h) may be given as substitutes to patients with penicillin allergy. Specific therapy should be given for active infection caused by other organisms.

Antitoxin Given to neutralize circulating toxin and unbound toxin in the wound, antitoxin effectively lowers mortality; toxin already bound to neural tissue is unaffected. Tetanus immune globulin (human) (TIG) is the preparation of choice and should be given promptly. The dose is 3000 to 6000 units intramuscularly, usually in divided doses, because the volume is large. It may be best to administer antitoxin before manipulating the wound and perhaps to inject a dose proximal to the wound; the value of infiltrating the wound is unclear. Additional doses are unnecessary because the half-life of the antitoxin is long. Antibody does not penetrate the blood-brain barrier. Intrathecal administration has been attempted, but should be considered experimental. Equine tetanus antitoxin (TAT) is also available. It is cheaper, but the half-life is shorter and hypersensitivity and serum sickness are common; doses up to 100,000 units are given, part intramuscularly and part intravenously, but 10,000 units may suffice.

Control of muscle spasms Many agents, alone and in combination, have been used to treat the muscle spasms, which are painful and can threaten ventilation by causing laryngospasm or sustained contraction of ventilatory muscles. Ideal therapy would abolish spasmodic activity without causing oversedation and hypoventilation. Diazepam, a muscle relaxant that enhances presynaptic inhibition, is in wide use. The dose is titrated to as much as 120 mg/d or higher. Barbiturates and chlorpromazine are also used. Neuromuscular blockage (using pancuronium bromide or an equivalent agent) together with mechanical ventilation are highly effective for severe spasms, spasms that reduce ventilation, spasms unresponsive to medication, or hypoventilation from oversedation. Dantrolene and baclofen are being investigated as treatment to shorten the period of therapeutic paralysis.

Respiratory care Intubation or tracheostomy, with or without mechanical ventilation, may be required to avert aspiration in patients with trismus, disordered swallowing, dysphagia, or laryngospasm. The need should be anticipated, and the procedure performed electively and early.

Sympathetic overactivity The optimal therapy for sympathetic overactivity has not been defined. Beta blockers with alpha-blocking activity are used, although there are a few reports of associated profound hypotension and death. A simple alternative is morphine. Parenteral magnesium sulfate and epidural anesthesia have been used also. The relative efficacy of these four therapeutic modalities is unclear.

Vaccine Active immunization should be initiated because immunity is not induced by the small amount of toxin that produces disease.

ADDITIONAL MEASURES These include hydration to control insensible and other fluid losses which may be high, increased nutritional requirements which can be met by enteral or parenteral means, physiotherapy to prevent contractures, and heparin to prevent pulmonary emboli. Bowel, bladder, and renal function must be monitored. Gastrointestinal bleeding and decubitus ulcers must be prevented and intercurrent infection treated.

PREVENTION Active immunization All partially immunized and unimmunized adults should receive vaccine as should those recovering from tetanus. The primary series for adults consists of three doses: the first and second doses are given 4 to 8 weeks apart, and the third dose is given 6 to 12 months after the second. A booster dose is required every 10 years, and may be given at mid-decade ages, 35, 45, and so on. Combined tetanus and diphtheria toxoid adsorbed (for adult use) (Td) rather than single-antigen tetanus toxoid is preferred for persons over 7 years of age.

Wound management Proper wound management requires consideration of the need for (1) passive immunization with TIG and (2) active immunization with vaccine, preferably Td in those over age

7. For clean, minor wounds, Td is administered to persons who have (1) unknown tetanus immunization histories, (2) received less than three doses of adsorbed tetanus toxoid, (3) received three or more doses of adsorbed vaccine, but more than 10 years have elapsed since the last dose, and (4) received three doses of *fluid* (nonadsorbed) vaccine. The recommendations for contaminated or severe wounds are identical, except that vaccine should be given to those who received three or more doses of adsorbed tetanus toxoid, if more than 5 years have elapsed since the last dose. TIG is not recommended for clean, minor wounds, but is given for all other wounds if the vaccination history indicates unknown or partial immunization. The dose of TIG for passive immunization of wounds of average severity is 250 units intramuscularly, which produces a protective antibody level (0.01 antitoxin unit per ml) in the serum for at least 4 to 6 weeks; the dose of equine antitoxin is 3000 to 6000 units. Vaccine and tetanus antitoxin should be administered at separate sites in separate syringes.

Neonatal tetanus Preventive efforts include vaccine, even during pregnancy, and measures to increase the number of in-hospital births and training for nonmedical birth attendants.

PROGNOSIS The application of methods to support respiration has markedly improved the prognosis in tetanus; mortality rates as low as 10 percent have been reported from units accustomed to handling such cases. In the United States, the overall mortality for the years 1985 to 1986 was 31 percent; it was 42 percent in those over 50 years of age, but only 5 percent for those under 50 (no neonatal disease); untreated neonatal disease, however, also has a poor prognosis. The outcome is poor in those with a short incubation period, a short interval from the onset of symptoms to admission, or a short period from onset of symptoms to the first spasm (period of onset).

The course of tetanus extends over 4 to 6 weeks, and patients may require ventilatory support for 3 weeks during this period. Increased tone and minor spasms can last for months, but recovery is usually complete.

REFERENCES

BLECK TP: Pharmacology of tetanus. Clin Neuropharmacol 9:103, 1986

HINMAN AR et al: Neonatal tetanus: Potential for elimination in the world. Pediatr Infect Dis 6:813, 1987

MULLER H et al: Intrathecal baclofen in tetanus. Ann NY Acad Sci 531:167, 1988

ROCKE DA et al: Morphine in tetanus—The management of sympathetic nervous system overactivity. S Afr Med J 70:66, 1986

TRUJILLO MH et al: Impact of intensive care management on the prognosis of tetanus: Analysis of 641 cases. Chest 92:63, 1987

VIEIRA BI: Cephalic tetanus in an immunized patient: Clinical and electromyographic findings. Med J Austral 145:156, 1986

WESLEY AG, PATHER M: Tetanus in children: An 11-year review. Ann Trop Pediatr 7:32, 1987

106 BOTULISM

ELIAS ABRUTYN

DEFINITION Botulism is a paralytic disease that begins with cranial nerve involvement and progresses caudally to involve the extremities. It is caused by potent protein neurotoxins elaborated by *Clostridium botulinum.* The Centers for Disease Control (CDC) currently classifies cases as: (1) *food-borne botulism,* from ingestion of preformed toxin in food contaminated with *C. botulinum;* (2) *infant botulism,* from ingestion of spores and production of toxin in the intestine of infants; (3) *wound botulism,* from toxin produced in wounds contaminated with the organism; and (4) *indeterminate,* for patients over 1 year old with no recognized source for disease.

ETIOLOGY *C. botulinum,* a heterogeneous group of anaerobic gram-positive organisms that form subterminal spores, is found in soil and marine environments throughout the world and elaborates the most potent bacterial toxin known. Types A through G have been distinguished by the antigenic specificities of their toxins. Types with proteolytic activity can digest food and produce a spoiled appearance; nonproteolytic types leave the appearance of food unchanged.

Eight distinct toxin types (A, B, C_1, C_2, D, E, F, and G) have been described. All are neurotoxins, except for C_2, which is a cytotoxin of unknown significance. Toxicity is due to inhibition of acetylcholine release from cholinergic terminals at the motor end plate. The toxin resists degradation by acid and proteolytic enzymes but is inactivated by heat at 100°C for 10 min, as during routine home cooking. Spores, in contrast, are highly heat resistant, requiring exposure to 120°C for inactivation, as in steam sterilizers or pressure cookers.

Toxin types A, B, E, and rarely F cause human disease; type G has been associated with sudden death in a few patients in Switzerland; and types C and D cause animal disease.

EPIDEMIOLOGY Human botulism occurs worldwide. In the United States, the geographic distribution of cases by toxin type parallels the distribution of organism types found in the environment. Type A predominates west of the Rocky Mountains; type B is generally distributed, but is more common in the east; and type E is found in the Pacific northwest, Alaska, and the Great Lakes area. In the United States food-borne botulism has been associated primarily with home canned food, particularly vegetables, fruit, and condiments, and less commonly, with meat and fish. Type E outbreaks are frequently associated with fish products. Commercial products occasionally cause outbreaks, but some of these have resulted from improper handling after purchase. Outbreaks in restaurants, schools, and private homes have been traced to uncommon sources (commercial pot pies, beef stew, turkey loaf, sauteed onions, baked potatoes, and chopped garlic in oil). Food-borne botulism can occur when (1) a food to be preserved is contaminated with spores; (2) preservation does not inactivate the spores but kills other putrefactive bacteria that might inhibit growth of *C. botulinum* and also provides anaerobic conditions at a pH and temperature that allow germination and toxin production; and when (3) food is not heated before eating to a temperature that destroys toxin.

CLINICAL MANIFESTATIONS **Food-borne botulism** Following ingestion of food containing toxin, illness varies from a mild one for which no medical advice is sought to very severe disease which may result in death in 24 h. The incubation period is usually 18 to 36 h but depending upon toxin dose ranges from a few hours to several days. A symmetric descending paralysis is characteristic and can lead to respiratory failure and death. Cranial nerve involvement which almost always marks the onset of symptoms usually produces diplopia, dysarthria, and/or dysphagia; weakness progresses, often rapidly, from the head to involve the neck, arms, thorax, and legs. Nausea, vomiting, and abdominal pain may occur before or after onset of paralysis. Dizziness, blurred vision, dry mouth, and very dry, occasionally sore throat are common. Occasionally the weakness is asymmetric. Patients are generally alert and oriented, but may be drowsy, agitated, and anxious. Typically, fever is absent. Ptosis is frequent; the pupillary reflexes may be depressed, and fixed or dilated pupils are seen in half the patients. The gag reflex may be suppressed, and deep tendon reflexes may be normal or decreased. Paralytic ileus, severe constipation, and urinary retention are common.

Wound botulism When wounds are contaminated with *C. botulinum* spores, the spores may germinate to vegetative organisms that produce toxin. This rare condition resembles food-borne illness except that the incubation period is longer, averaging about 10 days, and gastrointestinal symptoms are absent. Wound botulism has been noted after traumatic wounds contaminated with soil, in chronic drug abusers, and after cesarean delivery. The illness has occurred even when antibiotics were given to prevent wound infection. When present, fever is probably from concurrent infection with other bacteria. The wound may appear benign.

Infant botulism In infant botulism, the most common form of disease, toxin is produced in and absorbed from the intestine following germination of ingested spores. The severity ranges from mild illness with failure to thrive to fulminant, severe paralysis with respiratory failure and may be one cause of sudden infant death. Ingestion of contaminated honey has been defined as one source of spores, leading to the recommendation that honey not be fed to children less than 12 months of age. Most cases cannot be attributed to a particular food source, and the mechanism of intestinal colonization with *C. botulinum* is undefined. It is not clear why disease develops in some infants and not others and why it is so age-dependent, with over 90 percent of cases occurring in infants under 6 months of age.

DIAGNOSIS Botulism must be considered in afebrile, mentally intact patients who have a symmetric descending paralysis without sensory findings. Conditions often confused with botulism include myasthenia gravis, which may be excluded by electromyography and appropriate antibody studies, and the Guillain-Barré syndrome, which is characterized by ascending paralysis, sensory abnormalities, and elevation in cerebrospinal fluid protein. The Miller-Fisher variant of Guillain-Barré—a descending paralysis—can be difficult to differentiate. Other conditions that may mimic botulism include poliomyelitis, tick paralysis, acute abdomen, pharyngitis, cerebrovascular accidents, and intoxications from drugs, mushrooms, or medications with anticholinesterase activities.

The demonstration of toxin in serum by bioassay in mice is definitive, but the test may be negative, particularly in wound and infant botulism. It is only performed by specific laboratories which can be identified by contacting regional public health authorities. The demonstration of toxin or the organism in vomitus, gastric fluid, or stool is strongly suggestive, because intestinal carriage is rare. Isolation of the organism from food without toxin is insufficient for diagnosis. Wound cultures showing the organism are suggestive. The edrophonium chloride (Tensilon) test for myasthenia gravis may be falsely positive in botulism but is usually less dramatic. Nerve conduction velocity is normal, but on electromyography, action potentials are decreased with a supramaximal stimulus and facilitation is found after repetitive stimulation at high frequency. The white blood cell count and sedimentation rate are normal.

TREATMENT Patients should be hospitalized and monitored closely both clinically and by spirometry, pulse oximetry, and measurement of arterial blood gases for incipient respiratory failure. Intubation and mechanical ventilation should be strongly considered when the vital capacity is less than 30 percent of predicted, especially when paralysis is progressing rapidly and hypoxemia with absolute or relative hypercarbia is present (see Chap. 219).

In food-borne illness trivalent (types A, B, and E) equine antitoxin should be administered as soon as possible after obtaining specimens for laboratory analysis. Laboratory confirmation, which may take days, is unnecessary before initiating treatment. After testing for hypersensitivity to horse serum, two vials are given, either both intravenously or one intravenously and one intramuscularly; the dose may be repeated in 2 to 4 h. Anaphylaxis and serum sickness are risks inherent in using the equine product, and in allergic patients desensitization may be necessary. If there is no ileus, cathartics and enemas may be given to purge the gut of toxin; emetics or gastric lavage are used also if the time since ingestion is brief, e.g., only a few hours. Antibiotics to eliminate an intestinal source for possible continued toxin production and guanidine hydrochloride to reverse paralysis are of unproven value. In the United States antitoxin and help in clinical management and laboratory confirmation are available at *any* time by calling the state health department or the Centers for Disease Control.

Treatment of infant botulism requires supportive care; neither antitoxin nor antibiotics have been shown to be beneficial. In wound botulism antitoxin is administered. The wound should be thoroughly explored and debrided and an antibiotic such as penicillin given to eradicate *C. botulinum* from the wound, although the benefit of this therapy is unproven; results of wound cultures should guide the use of other antibiotics.

PROGNOSIS Type A disease is generally more severe than type B, and mortality is higher above age 60. With improved respiratory and intensive care, the case-fatality rate in food-borne illness has fallen to about 7.5 percent and is low in infant botulism as well. Artificial respiratory support may be required for months in severe cases. Some patients experience residual weakness and autonomic dysfunction for as long as a year after disease onset.

REFERENCES

MacDonald K et al: The changing epidemiology of adult botulism in the United States. Am J Epidemol 124:794, 1986

McCroskey LM, Hatheway CL: Laboratory findings in four cases of adult botulism suggest colonization of the intestinal tract. J Clin Microbiol 26:1052, 1988

Mills DC, Arnon SS: The large intestine as the site of *Clostridium botulinum* colonization in human infant botulism. J Infect Dis 156:997, 1987

Smith LDS, Sugiyama H: *Botulism: The Organism, Its Toxins, the Disease*, 2d ed. Springfield, Charles C Thomas, 1988

Spika JS et al.: Risk factors for infant botulism in the United States. Am J Dis Child 143:828, 1989

St. Louis ME et al: Botulism from chopped garlic: Delayed recognition of a major outbreak. Ann Intern Med 108:363, 1988

Wainwright RB et al: Food-borne botulism in Alaska, 1947–1985: Epidemiology and clinical findings. J Infect Dis 157:1158, 1988

Wilcox P et al: Long-term follow-up of symptoms, pulmonary function, respiratory strength, and exercise performance after botulism. Am Rev Resp Dis 139:157, 1989

107 GAS GANGRENE AND OTHER CLOSTRIDIAL INFECTIONS

DENNIS L. KASPER

DEFINITION Bacteria of the genus *Clostridium* are gram-positive, spore-forming, obligate anaerobes that are ubiquitous in nature. There are over 60 recognized species of clostridia, many of which generally are considered saprophytic. Some of these species are pathogenic for humans and animals, particularly under conditions of lowered oxidation-reduction potential. Infections associated with these organisms range from localized wound contamination to overwhelming systemic disease. The four major disease categories for which clostridia are responsible include intestinal disorders, deep tissue suppurative infections, skin and soft tissue infections, and bacteremias (see Table 107-1). Toxins play a major role in some of these syndromes.

ETIOLOGY In humans, clostridia normally reside in the gastrointestinal tract and in the female genital tract, although they

TABLE 107-1 Classification of diseases caused by other clostridia

I Intestinal syndromes
- *A* Food poisoning
- *B* Enteritis necroticans
- *C* Antibiotic-associated colitis

II Suppurative deep tissue infections
- *A* Mixed bacterial infections
- *B* Only microorganism isolated

III Skin and soft tissue infections
- *A* Simple contamination
- *B* Local infection without systemic signs
- *C* Spreading cellulitis and fasciitis
- *D* Myonecrosis

IV Bacteremia
- *A* Transient bacteremia
- *B* Sepsis

occasionally can be isolated from the skin or the mouth. As with other pathogenic anaerobic bacteria, clostridia are quite aerotolerant. Of the known species of the genus *Clostridium,* at least 30 have been isolated from human infections. Clostridia characteristically produce abundant gas in artificial media and form subterminal endospores. *C. perfringens,* one of the most important of the species, is encapsulated, nonmotile, and rarely sporulates in artificial media; the spores usually can be destroyed by boiling. *C. tetani* and *C. botulinum* are discussed in Chaps. 105 and 106, respectively.

Clostridia are present in the normal colonic flora in concentrations of 10^9 to 10^{10} per gram. Of the 30 or more species that normally colonize humans, *C. ramosum* is the most common, followed by *C. perfringens*. These organisms are universally present in soil in concentrations of up to 10^4 per gram. Although clostridia morphologically are typical gram-positive organisms, many species appear to be gram-negative in clinical material or in stationary phase cultures. Therefore, Gram stains of cultures or clinical material should be interpreted with great care.

C. perfringens is the most common of the clostridial species isolated from tissue infections and bacteremias, followed in frequency by *C. novyi* and *C. septicum*. In the category of enteric infections, *C. difficile* is an important cause of antibiotic-associated colitis, and *C. perfringens* is associated with food poisoning and enteritis necroticans.

PATHOGENESIS Severe infections due to clostridial species are relatively uncommon despite the fact that clostridia can be cultured from most severe, traumatic wounds. Essential to the development of severe disease appears to be the presence of tissue necrosis and a low oxidation-reduction potential. *C. perfringens* requires about 14 amino acids and 6 or 7 additional growth factors for optimum growth. These nutrients are not found in appreciable concentrations in normal body fluids but are present in necrotic tissue. When *C. perfringens* grows in necrotic tissue, a zone of tissue damage due to the toxins elaborated by the organism allows for progressive growth. In contrast, when only a few bacteria leak into the bloodstream from a small defect in the intestinal wall, the organisms do not have the opportunity to multiply rapidly because blood as medium for growth is relatively deficient in certain amino acids and growth factors. Therefore, in a patient without tissue necrosis, bacteremia is usually benign.

C. perfringens possesses 17 possible virulence factors, including 12 active tissue toxins and enterotoxins. *C. perfringens* has been divided into five types (A through E) on the basis of four major toxins: alpha, beta, epsilon, and iota. The alpha toxin is a phospholipase C (lecithinase) that splits lecithin into phosphorylcholine and diglyceride. This alpha toxin has been associated with gas gangrene and is known to be hemolytic, destroy platelets and polymorphonuclear leukocytes, and cause widespread capillary damage. When injected intravenously, it causes massive intravascular hemolysis and damages liver mitochondria. Alpha toxin may be important in the initiation of muscle infections that may progress to gas gangrene. Experimentally, the higher the concentration of alpha toxin present in the culture fluid, the smaller the infecting dose of *C. perfringens* required to produce infection. The protective effect of antiserum is directly proportional to its content of alpha antitoxin. Beta, epsilon, and iota toxins are also known to increase capillary permeability.

C. difficile produces a cytotoxin and an enterotoxin. Toxigenic strains are more resistant to phagocytosis than nontoxigenic strains. The cytotoxin is potent in tissue culture assays and is a relatively sensitive and specific marker for *C. difficile*–induced enteric disease. The enterotoxin, designated toxin A, appears to be substantially more potent in biologic assays using animal models. Therefore, this toxin may play an important role in the expression of clinical disease. Toxin A binds to a carbohydrate receptor (Galα1–3Galβ1–4GlcNAc) on brush border membranes. Most cases of antibiotic-associated colitis are caused by antibiotic-mediated suppression of the endogenous flora and overgrowth of *C. difficile*. The bowel flora may also produce β-lactamases which destroy some antibiotics, like ampicillin, and allow the overgrowth of *C. difficile*.

CLINICAL MANIFESTATIONS Intestinal disorders FOOD POISONING *C. perfringens* is the second or third most common cause of food poisoning in the United States (see Chap. 92). Outbreaks generally have resulted from problems in the cooling and storage of foods cooked in bulk. The food sources primarily involved are meat, meat products, and poultry. Generally, the implicated meats have been cooked, allowed to cool, and then recooked the following day, often in a stew or hash. Strains of *C. perfringens* that contaminate meat manage to survive initial cooking. During reheating, the organisms sporulate and germinate. The disease is associated with an attack rate often as high as 70 percent. Symptoms of food poisoning from type A strains develop 8 to 24 h after ingestion of foods heavily contaminated with the organism. The primary symptoms include epigastric pain, nausea, and watery diarrhea lasting 12 to 24 h. Fever and vomiting are uncommon. Symptoms usually last less than 24 h. Diarrhea appears to be caused by a heat-labile protein enterotoxin. The enterotoxin inhibits glucose transport, damages the intestinal epithelium, and causes protein loss into the intestinal lumen.

ENTERITIS NECROTICANS Enteritis necroticans (*pigbel*), caused by type C strains of *C. perfringens,* has been the cause of necrotizing enteritis and death, occurring after a feast, in children and adults in New Guinea. A similar disease, *darmbrand,* was epidemic in Germany after World War II and was also reported from an evacuation site on the Thai-Kampuchean border. Clinical features include acute abdominal pain, bloody diarrhea, vomiting, shock, and peritonitis; death occurs in 40 percent of patients. Pathologically, there is an acute ulcerative process of the bowel restricted to the small intestine. The mucosa is lifted off the submucosa, forming large denuded areas. Pseudomembranes composed of sloughed epithelium are common, and gas may dissect into the submucosa. The source of the organisms may be the patient's own intestinal flora, because cultures of ingested pig have failed to yield the organism. Antitoxin against the beta toxin of *C. perfringens* has been of considerable benefit in changing the course of established disease and in a large-scale trial, children immunized with *C. perfringens* beta toxoid were protected.

ANTIBIOTIC-ASSOCIATED COLITIS Strains of *C. difficile* that produce toxins detectable in the stool have been identified as the major cause of colitis in patients with antibiotic-associated diarrhea. In order to diagnose this type of colitis, there should be no other identifiable cause of diarrhea and the onset of symptoms must occur either during antimicrobial administration or within 4 weeks after the implicated agent has been discontinued. The drugs implicated most commonly in *C. difficile* enterocolitis are clindamycin, ampicillin, and the cephalosporins. With the possible exceptions of vancomycin and parenterally administered aminoglycosides, nearly all antibiotics have been associated with this syndrome. Antibiotic-associated diarrhea is associated with up to 6 percent of clindamycin usage, and with 5 to 9 percent of ampicillin usage.

Antimicrobial-associated diarrhea can be divided into four anatomic categories: (1) normal colonic mucosa, (2) mild erythema with some edema, (3) granular, friable, or hemorrhagic mucosa, and (4) pseudomembrane formation. Most commonly, patients with antibiotic-associated diarrhea have a normal, minimally erythematous colonic mucosa with some edema. Occasionally colitis is more severe and is characterized by granular, friable, or hemorrhagic mucosa. Stool examination in these patients may reveal large numbers of red blood cells and some leukocytes. Biopsy shows subepithelial edema with round cell infiltration of the lamina propria and focal extravasation of erythrocytes. *C. difficile* toxin has been found in 15 to 46 percent of stools from patients in these first three categories, suggesting that other factors exist in the pathogenesis of antibiotic-associated diarrhea. The most characteristic form of antibiotic-associated colitis caused by *C. difficile* is pseudomembranous colitis (PMC). More than 95 percent of patients with documented PMC have positive stool toxin assays. Close inspection of pseudomembranes reveals exudative punctate raised plaques with skip areas or edematous hyperemic mucosa. These plaques can enlarge and coalesce over large segments of intestine in the later stages of disease. The clinical spectrum of antibiotic-associated PMC is diverse. Diarrhea is the common feature and is usually watery, voluminous, and without gross blood or mucus. Most patients have abdominal cramps and tenderness, fever, and leukocytosis. However, the symptoms may vary considerably. At one end of the spectrum are patients with annoying diarrhea but no systemic signs or symptoms, while at the other end there is severe systemic toxicity, fever to 40 or 40.6°C (104 or 105°F), and peripheral white blood cell counts of up to 50,000 per microliter. Fecal examination frequently reveals leukocytes. Without specific therapy, the course is highly variable. Some patients have prompt resolution of symptoms with discontinuation of the drug, while others have protracted diarrhea with large stool volumes for up to 8 weeks, with resultant hypoalbuminemia and electrolyte imbalance. Severely ill patients with toxic megacolon and colonic perforation have been reported. In those who are severely ill, mortality rates may be as high as 30 percent, while most patients with minimal symptoms have resolution of disease with discontinuation of antibiotics alone. In the majority of patients, symptoms begin 4 to 10 days after antibiotic therapy is initiated. However, about 25 percent of patients do not have symptoms until the implicated antimicrobial has been discontinued, in some cases as long as 4 weeks afterward. A few cases have been reported within hours after initiation of antibiotic therapy.

Diagnostic evaluation of patients with PMC should include examination of the stool for the presence of *C. difficile* cytotoxin. Although several assays are available, the tissue culture assay is the most practical and sensitive. The assay is performed by incubating stool filtrates with tissue culture cells and monitoring for a cytopathic effect which can be neutralized by antitoxin to either *C. sordellii* (which is cross-reactive with *C. difficile*, but does not cause PMC) or *C. difficile*. Endoscopy, although useful in establishing the presence of PMC, does not establish the etiology and should be reserved for more serious disease manifestations to exclude alternative diagnoses. Isolation of *C. difficile* from stool cultures is difficult, and *C. difficile* may be present as part of the "normal" flora in asymptomatic patients, particularly infants.

Suppurative deep tissue infection Clostridia are recovered frequently from various suppurative conditions in conjunction with other anaerobic and aerobic bacteria, but can also be the only organisms isolated. These conditions exist with severe local inflammation, but usually without systemic signs induced by clostridial toxins. These infections include intraabdominal sepsis, empyema, pelvic abscess, subcutaneous abscess, frostbite with gas gangrene, infected stumps in amputees, brain abscess, prostatic abscess, perianal abscess, conjunctivitis, infection of a renal cell carcinoma, and infected aortic grafts.

Clostridia are isolated in approximately two-thirds of patients with intraabdominal infections resulting from intestinal perforation. *C. ramosum, C. perfringens,* and *C. bifermentans* are the most commonly isolated species. The clinical presentation does not differ from that of other patients with similar infections in which clostridia are not cultured and there is no adverse effect on outcome (see Chap. 108).

An association has been made between malignancy and the isolation of *C. septicum* in the absence of grossly contaminated deep traumatic wounds. A major site for these malignancies is the gastrointestinal tract, particularly the colon. An association with leukemia or with other solid tumors also has been noted. Some of these patients present with *C. septicum* bacteremia and have a fulminant clinical course (discussed below). Others develop localized suppurative infection in the abdomen or the abdominal wall, without bacteremia. Presumably this infection arises from a silent perforation that leads to intraabdominal abscess formation.

Clostridia have been isolated from suppurative infections of the female genital tract, particularly tuboovarian and pelvic abscess. The major species involved has been *C. perfringens*. Most of these are mild suppurative infections without evidence of uterine gangrene. Isolation of *C. perfringens* has been reported in as many as 20 percent of diseased gallbladders at surgery. One clinical syndrome, emphysematous cholecystitis, is caused by clostridial species at least 50 percent of the time. In this syndrome there is gas formation in the biliary radicles and the wall of the gallbladder. It is seen most often in diabetic patients. Although the mortality rate in this entity is higher than in more common forms of cholecystitis, there is no evidence of myonecrosis.

Clostridia are among the many organisms found in empyema fluid or isolated by transtracheal aspiration from patients with lung abscesses. There is no clinical clue to the presence of clostridia (as opposed to other organisms) in these infections. *C. perfringens* has been reported as a cause of empyema arising from aspiration pneumonia, pulmonary emboli, and infarction. However, the majority of cases of clostridial empyema are secondary to trauma.

Skin and soft tissue infections Various categories of traumatic wound infections due to clostridia have been described: simple contamination, anaerobic cellulitis, fasciitis with or without systemic manifestations, and anaerobic myonecrosis.

SIMPLE CONTAMINATION Clostridia are cultured most often from wounds in the absence of clinical signs of sepsis. As many as 30 percent of battle wounds can be contaminated by clostridia without signs of suppuration, and 16 percent of penetrating abdominal wounds yield clostridia on culture despite treatment with cephalothin and kanamycin. In cases of trauma, clostridia are isolated with equal frequency from suppurative and well-healing wounds. Based on these findings, the diagnosis of clostridial infection should be clinical rather than bacteriologic.

LOCALIZED INFECTION OF THE SKIN AND SOFT TISSUE WITHOUT SYSTEMIC SIGNS This condition was originally referred to as anaerobic cellulitis. It is a localized infection involving the skin and soft tissue due to clostridia in pure or mixed culture. There are no systemic signs of toxicity, although the infection may invade locally, producing necrosis. These infections tend to be relatively indolent, spreading slowly to contiguous areas. Localized infections tend to be relatively free of pain and edema. Perhaps because of the lack of edema, gas that is limited to the wound and the immediately surrounding tissue may be more evident than in gas gangrene. In these localized infections gas is never found intramuscularly. Cellulitis, perirectal abscesses, and diabetic foot ulcers are typical infections from which clostridial species can be isolated. If inadequately treated, these localized infections advance by extension through subcutaneous tissue and fascial planes into muscle and may produce severe systemic disease with signs of toxemia.

A localized form of suppurative myositis has been described in heroin addicts. These patients develop local pain and tenderness in discrete areas (particularly the thigh and forearm) with the subsequent appearance of fluctuance and crepitance that require surgical drainage. The unusual aspect of these infections is that they remain localized without systemic signs of toxicity. Moreover these local areas are not necessarily sites of trauma or heroin injection. Pathologically there are subcutaneous abscesses, purulent myositis, and fasciitis, from which clostridia are recovered in pure culture; on occasion mixed infections involving aerobes and anaerobes are found.

SPREADING CELLULITIS AND FASCIITIS WITH SYSTEMIC TOXICITY This is diffuse spreading cellulitis and fasciitis, but myonecrosis is absent, and only mild inflammation is seen in muscle. These patients present with the abrupt onset of a syndrome which progresses rapidly through the fascial planes within hours. When suppuration and gas in soft tissues as well as overwhelming toxemia are present, the infection is rapidly fatal. On physical examination there is subcutaneous crepitance, but little localized pain. Surgery is of no proven value because there are no discretely involved tissues amenable to resection, as may be the case in myonecrosis. However, incision of the affected area should be performed, because in rapidly advancing fasciitis, it is still the cornerstone of therapy. The initial local lesion may be quite innocuous and arises from an area involved by tumor or other infection and not from injury. The systemic toxic effects include hemolysis and injury of capillary membranes. Usually, this infection is uniformly fatal within 48 h, despite intensive therapy involving antitoxin and exchange transfusion. This syndrome is seen most commonly in patients with carcinoma, especially of the sigmoid or the cecum. Presumably, the tumor invades the fascia, and tumoral contents leak into the abdominal wall. These patients present with extreme toxicity and occasionally with total-body crepitance. The syndrome differs from necrotizing fasciitis caused by other organisms in three respects: (1) rapid mortality, (2) rapid tissue invasion, and (3) the systemic effects of the toxin typified by massive hemolysis.

CLOSTRIDIAL MYONECROSIS (GAS GANGRENE) Clostridial myonecrosis occurs when bacteria invade healthy muscle from adjacent traumatized muscle or soft tissue. The infection originates in a wound contaminated with clostridia. Despite the fact that more than 30 percent of deep wounds are infected with clostridia, the incidence of clostridial myonecrosis is quite low. These infections occur in military or civilian settings. An essential factor in the genesis of gas gangrene appears to be trauma, particularly involving deep lacerated muscle wounds. The entity of clostridial myonecrosis is relatively uncommon after simple, through-and-through bullet wounds without shattering of bone, and relatively common following shrapnel fragmentation wounds, particularly when deep muscle is involved. In civilian cases, gas gangrene can occur after trauma, surgery, or intramuscular injection. The trauma need not be severe; however, the wound must be deep, necrotic, and without communication to the surface.

The incubation period of gas gangrene is usually short: almost always less than 3 days, and frequently less than 24 h. Eighty percent of cases are caused by *C. perfringens,* while *C. novyi, C. septicum,* and *C. histolyticum* cause most of the other cases. Typically, gas gangrene begins with the sudden appearance of pain in the region of the wound, which helps to differentiate it from spreading cellulitis. Once established, the pain steadily increases in severity, but remains localized to the infected area and only spreads if the infection spreads. Soon after pain develops, local swelling and edema, accompanied by a thin, often hemorrhagic exudate, appear. These patients frequently develop marked tachycardia, but elevation in temperature may be only minimal. Gas usually is not obvious at this early stage and may be completely absent. Frothiness of the wound exudate may be noted. The skin is tense, white, often marbled with blue, and cooler than normal. The symptoms progress rapidly; swelling, edema, and toxemia increase and a profuse serous discharge, which may have a peculiar sweetish smell, appears. Gram stain of the wound exudate shows many gram-positive rods with relatively few inflammatory cells.

At surgery, the muscle is characteristically pale, edematous, and does not contract when probed with the scalpel. The muscle appears beefy red and nonviable and can progress to become black, friable, and gangrenous. It is important to establish a diagnosis early, preferably by frozen section biopsy of muscle.

Despite hypotension, renal failure, and often body crepitance, patients with myonecrosis often have a heightened awareness of their surroundings until just before death, when they lapse into toxic delirium and coma. In untreated cases, as the local wounds progress, the skin becomes bronzed; bullae appear, become filled with dark red fluid, and are accompanied by dark patches of cutaneous gangrene. Gas appears in later phases but may not be as obvious as in anaerobic cellulitis. Jaundice is rarely seen in wound gas gangrene (in contrast to uterine infections) and when it does appear, is almost invariably associated with hemoglobinuria, hemoglobinemia, and septicemia. There have been reports of cases of clostridial myonecrosis without a history of trauma. These patients have bullous lesions and crepitance of the skin; they present with a rapidly worsening course which includes myonecrosis, especially of the extremities.

Bacteremia and clostridial septicemia The relatively common entity of transient bacteremia due to clostridia can arise in any hospitalized patient but is most common with a predisposing focus in the gastrointestinal tract, biliary tract, or uterus. Fever frequently resolves within 24 to 48 h without therapy. Despite the finding of clostridial bacteremia following septic abortions and the frequent isolation of clostridia from the lochia, most of these patients do not have evidence of septicemia. In one series of 60 patients with clostridial bacteremia, half of the cases could be associated with an infected site, while the other half had a totally unrelated illness, such as tuberculous pneumonia, meningitis, or benign gastroenteritis. Frequently, by the time the blood culture reports return, the patients are completely well and sometimes have been discharged. Therefore, when a blood culture report is positive for clostridia, the patient must be assessed clinically rather than simply treated for the positive blood culture.

Clostridial septicemia is an uncommon but almost invariably fatal illness occurring after clostridial infection primarily of the uterus, colon, or biliary tract. This entity must be differentiated from transient clostridial bacteremia, which is much more common than septicemia. *C. perfringens* causes the majority of septicemic infections, as well as the majority of cases of transient bacteremia. *C. septicum, C. sordellii,* and *C. novyi* account for most of the remainder of cases. Clostridia account for 1 to 2.5 percent of all positive blood cultures in major hospital centers.

The majority of cases of clostridial septicemia originate from the female genital tract following septic abortion. Introduction of a foreign body is a common antecedent event. In the uterus there may be residual necrotic fetal and placental tissues and traumatized endometrium that allow the growth of clostridia. Only a small fraction of cases of septic abortion (1 percent) are followed by serious septicemic illness.

In these patients, sepsis, fever, and chills begin from 1 to 3 days after the attempted abortion. The initial signs are malaise, headache, severe myalgias, abdominal pain, nausea, vomiting, and occasionally diarrhea. Frequently a bloody or brown vaginal discharge is noted. Patients may rapidly develop oliguria, hypotension, jaundice, and hemoglobinuria. The hemolysis, which is secondary to *C. perfringens* alpha toxin, causes a characteristic bronzing of the skin. As in myonecrosis, the mental status of severely ill patients is characterized by increased alertness and apprehension. Local examination of the pelvis reveals foul cervical discharge, occasionally with gas. Frequently laceration marks around the cervix or perforation of the cervical segment are evident. If the infection involves the myometrium or has spread to the adnexa, extreme tenderness, guarding, and an adnexal mass may be found.

Laboratory studies in septicemic patients reveal an elevated white count and may show pink, hemoglobin-tinged plasma. Anemia is proportional to the degree of hemolysis, and the hematocrit may be extremely low. Platelets may be reduced, and there is often evidence of disseminated intravascular coagulation. Oliguria or anuria, increasingly refractory hypotension, and hemorrhage and bruising may develop.

Clostridia may enter the bloodstream from the gastrointestinal or biliary tract. This occurrence is associated with ulcerative lesions or obstruction of the small or large intestine, necrotic or infiltrating malignancy, bowel surgery, or various abdominal catastrophes. The patient may present with an acute febrile illness with chills and fever, but no other signs of localized infection. Intravascular hemolysis occurs in as many as half the cases. Biliary or gastrointestinal symptoms, if present, may be the only clue to the etiology. Positive blood cultures provide the definitive clue for the diagnosis.

Patients with malignant disease also can develop rapidly fatal clostridial sepsis, particularly from a gastrointestinal focus. The most common species in this setting is *C. septicum.* Characteristic signs and symptoms include fever, tachycardia, hypotension, abdominal pain or tenderness, nausea, vomiting, and, preterminally, coma. The tachycardia may be out of proportion to the fever. Only about 20 to 30 percent of patients develop hemolysis. A striking feature of this syndrome is the rapidity of death, which frequently occurs in less than 12 h.

DIAGNOSIS The diagnosis of clostridial disease must be based primarily on clinical findings. Because of the presence of clostridia in many wounds, their mere isolation from any site, including the blood, does not necessarily indicate severe disease. Smears of wound exudates, uterine scrapings, or cervical discharge may show abundant large gram-positive rods as well as other organisms. Cultures should be placed in selective media and incubated anaerobically for identification of clostridia.

The urine of patients with severe clostridial sepsis may contain protein and casts, and some patients may develop severe uremia. Profound alterations of circulating erythrocytes are seen in severely toxemic patients. Patients have a hemolytic anemia, which develops extremely rapidly, along with hemoglobinemia, hemoglobinuria, and elevated levels of serum bilirubin. Spherocytosis, increased osmotic and mechanical red blood cell fragility, erythrophagocytosis, and methemoglobinemia have been described. Disseminated intravascular coagulation may be seen in patients with severe infection. In patients with severe septicemia, a Wright or Gram stain smear of peripheral blood or buffy coat may demonstrate clostridia.

X-ray examination sometimes provides an important clue to the diagnosis by revealing gas in muscles, subcutaneous tissue, or the uterus. However, the finding of gas is not pathognomonic for clostridial infection. Other bacteria, particularly anaerobes, mixed with aerobic organisms may produce gas.

The diagnosis of clostridial myonecrosis can be established by frozen section biopsy of muscle. The diagnosis of *C. difficile*–associated colitis is made by the identification of *C. difficile* toxin in stool.

TREATMENT The treatment of choice for clostridial infection is penicillin G, 20,000,000 units a day in adults. In cases of penicillin sensitivity or allergy, other antibiotics should be considered, but all should be tested for in vitro efficacy because of the occasional isolation of resistant strains. Chloramphenicol, 4 g/d, usually is an effective alternative. Clostridia are frequently, but not universally, susceptible in vitro to cefoxitin, carbenicillin, clindamycin, metronidazole, doxycycline, minocycline, tetracycline, third-generation cephalosporins, and vancomycin. For severe clostridial infections, sensitivity testing should be done before using an antimicrobial with unpredictable susceptibility. Simple contamination of a wound with clostridia should not be treated with antibiotics. Localized skin and soft tissue infection can be managed by debridement rather than with systemic antibiotics. Drugs are required when the process extends into adjacent tissue, or when fever and systemic signs of sepsis are present.

Suppurative infections should be treated with antibiotics. Frequently, broad-spectrum antibiotics must be used because of mixed flora in these infections. Aminoglycosides can be used for the aerobic gram-negative bacteria in mixed infections.

The use of a polyvalent gas gangrene antitoxin is still recommended by some authorities. At present the antitoxin is not produced in the United States, and most centers have discontinued its use in management of patients with suspected gas gangrene or clostridial postabortion sepsis because of questionable efficacy and the substantial risk of hypersentitivity to horse serum.

The use of hyperbaric oxygen in the treatment of gas gangrene is also controversial. Studies in humans are not well designed to answer questions on efficacy, but several knowledgeable authors believe that hyperbaric oxygen therapy has contributed to dramatic clinical improvement. It may, however, be associated with untoward effects due to oxygen toxicity and high atmospheric pressure. Some centers without hyperbaric chambers have reported acceptable mortality rates, indicating that expert surgical and medical management and control of complications are probably the most important factors in treating gas gangrene.

Treatment of *C. difficile* enterocolitis The treatment of *C. difficile*–associated colitis requires discontinuation of the offending antimicrobial agent. In some patients symptoms will resolve over a period of 2 weeks. However, specific therapy has been beneficial. The most widely used agent in the treatment of antibiotic-associated diarrhea ascribed to *C. difficile* is oral vancomycin. Most strains of *C. difficile* are susceptible to achievable concentrations of oral vancomycin. This antibiotic is poorly absorbed after oral administration and high levels appear in the stool. Dosing should begin with 125 mg orally four times a day for 7 to 10 days, but the dose may be increased to 500 mg orally four times a day. Oral metronidazole at a dose of 500 mg three times a day for 7 to 10 days is also effective. However, a few cases of *C. difficile* colitis have developed after oral metronidazole therapy for other infections. Because response to the two treatment regimens is comparable and metronidazole is less costly, it is reasonable to initiate treatment with metronidazole. If diarrhea persists, then therapy should be changed to oral vancomycin. Therapy with oral cholestyramine was initially reported to provide dramatic improvement in patients with pseudomembranous colitis (PMC). Subsequent studies have shown that cholestyramine, as well as other anionic resins, bind the cytotoxin produced by *C. difficile*. However, comparative trials in animals have shown that cholestyramine is distinctly inferior to oral vancomycin. Combination therapy with oral vancomycin and cholestyramine in refractory cases has been successful. Toxin production in PMC persists in 5 to 10 percent of treated patients. Relapses are reported in up to 20 percent of patients, but patients usually respond to a second course of oral vancomycin.

REFERENCES

BARTLETT JG et al: Antibiotic-associated pseudomembranous colitis due to toxin-producing clostridia. N Engl J Med 298:531, 1978

———, TAYLOR NS: Antibiotic-associated colitis, in *Medical Microbiology*, CSF Easman, J Jeljaszewicz (eds). London, Academic, 1982, pp 1–48

BORNSTEIN DL: Clostridial myonecrosis, in *Medical Microbiology and Infectious Diseases*, A Braude (ed). Philadelphia, Saunders, 1981, chap 239

DAILEY DC et al: Factors influencing the phagocytosis of *Clostridium difficile* by human polymorphonuclear leukocytes. Infect Immun 55:1541, 1987

FINEGOLD SM: *Anaerobic Bacteria in Human Disease*. New York, Academic, 1977

———: Anaerobic infections and *Clostridium difficile* colitis emerging during antibacterial therapy. Scand J Infect Dis (Suppl)49:160, 1986

GORBACH SL: Other *Clostridium* species (including gas gangrene), in *Principles and Practice of Infectious Diseases*, GL Mandell et al (eds). New York, Wiley, 1985

———, THADEPALLI H: Isolation of *Clostridium* in human infections: Evaluation of 114 cases. J Infect Dis 131:S81, 1975

JENDRZEJEWSKI JW et al: Nontraumatic clostridial myonecrosis. Am J Med 65:542, 1978

JOHNSON S et al: Enteritis necroticans among Khmer children at an evacuation site in Thailand. Lancet 2:496, 1987

KORANSKY JR et al: *Clostridium septicum* bacteremia. Am J Med 66:63, 1979

KRIVAN HC et al: Cell surface binding site for *Clostridium difficile* enterotoxin: Evidence for a glycoconjugate containing the sequence Gal alpha 1–3 Gal beta 1–4 Glc NAc. Infect Immun 53:573, 1986

PRITCHARD JA, WHALLEY PJ: Abortion complicated by *Clostridium perfringens* infection. Am J Gynecol 111:484, 1971

SMITH LDS: Virulence factors of *Clostridium perfringens*. Rev Infect Dis 1:254, 1979

TEASLEY DG et al: Prospective randomized trial of metronidazole versus vancomycin for *Clostridium difficile*–associated diarrhea and colitis. Lancet 2:1043, 1983

108 INFECTIONS DUE TO MIXED ANAEROBIC ORGANISMS

DENNIS L. KASPER

DEFINITIONS Anaerobic bacteria are organisms that require reduced oxygen tension for growth, failing to grow on the surface of solid media in 10% CO_2 in air. Microaerophilic bacteria can grow in 10% CO_2 in air or under anaerobic or aerobic conditions. Facultative bacteria can grow in the presence or absence of air. This chapter addresses infections caused by nonsporulating anaerobic bacteria. In general, anaerobes associated with human infections are relatively aerotolerant. They can survive for as long as 72 h in the presence of oxygen, although generally they will not multiply in this environment. Less pathogenic anaerobic bacteria, which are also part of the normal flora, die after brief contact with oxygen, even in low concentrations.

The nonsporulating anaerobic bacteria exist as normal flora on the mucosal surfaces of humans and animals. The major reservoirs of these bacteria are the mouth, gastrointestinal tract, skin, and the female genital tract. Of the oral flora, anaerobes are the predominant commensal organisms, ranging in concentrations from 10^9 per milliliter in saliva to 10^{12} in gingival scrapings. In the oral cavity the relative concentration of anaerobic to aerobic bacteria ranges from 1:1 on the surface of the tooth to 100 to 1000:1 in the gingival crevice. Anaerobic bacteria are not found in appreciable numbers in the normal intestine until the distal ileum. In the colon, the proportion of anaerobes increases significantly, as does the overall bacterial count. For example, in the colon there are 10^{11} to 10^{12} organisms per gram of stool, with a ratio of anaerobes to aerobes of approximately 1000:1. In the female genital tract there are approximately 10^9 organisms per milliliter of secretions, with a ratio of anaerobes to aerobes of approximately 10:1. Hundreds of species of anaerobic bacteria have been identified as part of the normal flora of humans. Identification of as many as 500 different anaerobic species in fecal specimens reflects the diversity of the anaerobic flora. Despite the complex array of bacteria which exist in the normal flora, relatively few species are isolated commonly from human infection.

Anaerobic infections occur when the harmonious relationship between the host and bacteria is disrupted. Any site in the body is susceptible to infection with these indigenous organisms when the mucosal barriers or skin are compromised by surgery, trauma, tumor, or ischemia or necrosis, which reduce local tissue redox potentials. Because the sites that are colonized by anaerobic bacteria contain many species of bacteria, disruption of anatomic barriers allows penetration of many organisms, resulting in mixed infections involving multiple species of anaerobes combined with facultative or microaerophilic organisms. Such mixed infections are seen in the head and neck (chronic sinusitis, chronic otitis media, Ludwig's angina, and periodontal abscesses). Brain abscesses and subdural empyema are the most frequent anaerobic infections of the central nervous system. Anaerobes are responsible for pleuropulmonary diseases such as aspiration pneumonia, necrotizing pneumonia, lung abscesses, or empyema. Anaerobes play an important role in various intraabdominal infections such as peritonitis and intraabdominal and liver abscesses. They are isolated frequently in female genital tract infections such as salpingitis, pelvic peritonitis, tuboovarian abscess, vulvovaginal abscesses, septic abortions, and endometritis. Anaerobic bacteria also are frequently found in infections of the skin, soft tissue, bones, and in bacteremia.

ETIOLOGY The major anaerobic gram-positive cocci producing disease are *Peptostreptococcus* species. The major species involved in infections are *P. magnus, P. asaccharolyticus, P. anaerobius,* and *P. prevotii.* Clostridia are gram-positive rods which are isolated from wounds, abscesses, abdominal infections, and bacteremias; they are discussed in Chap. 107. The principal anaerobic gram-negative bacilli are the *Bacteroides* family, which includes the *Bacteroides fragilis* group, fusobacteria, and the pigmented *Bacteroides*. The *B. fragilis* group contains the anaerobic pathogens most frequently isolated from clinical infections. Members of this group are part of the normal bowel flora. Several distinct species comprise the group, including *B. fragilis, B. thetaiotaomicron, B. distasonis, B. vulgatis,* and *B. ovatis*. Of this group *B. fragilis* is the most important clinical isolate. However, in the normal fecal flora, the frequency with which *B. fragilis* is isolated is low compared to other *Bacteroides* species. A second major group of *Bacteroides* are part of the indigenous oral flora. These are primarily pigment-producing bacteria which were previously classified under the species *B. melaninogenicus*. The terminology of this group has changed so that several distinct species are recognized, including *B. gingivalis, B. asaccharolyticus,* as well as *B. melaninogenicus*. In female genital tract infections, *B. bivius* and *B. disiens* are the most frequent isolates, although *B. fragilis* is common. Fusobacteria are also isolated from clinical infections, including necrotizing pneumonia and abscesses.

Infections due to anaerobic bacteria most frequently are mixed infections with more than one organism. They may be due to one or several anaerobic species, or a combination of anaerobic organisms and aerobic bacteria acting synergistically.

APPROACH TO THE PATIENT WITH ANAEROBIC BACTERIAL INFECTIONS There are several features to remember when approaching the patient with presumptive infection due to anaerobic bacteria. (1) Most of these organisms are harmless commensals, and very few cause disease. (2) In order for these organisms to cause infection, they must spread beyond the normal mucosal barriers. (3) Conditions favoring the propagation of these bacteria, particularly a lowered oxidation-reduction potential, are necessary. These include sites of trauma, tissue destruction, compromised vascular supply, or complication of preexisting infection that produces necrosis. (4) There is a complex array of infecting flora. For example, as many as 12 different types of organisms can be isolated from a suppurative site. (5) Anaerobic organisms tend to be found in abscess cavities or in necrotic tissue. The detection of an abscess in a patient which fails to yield organisms on routine culture is the clue that the abscess is likely to contain anaerobic bacteria. However, often smears of this "sterile pus" are teeming with bacteria on Gram stain. The malodorous nature of the pus should suggest anaerobe infections. Although some facultative organisms, such as *Staphylococcus aureus,* also are capable of causing abscesses, abscesses in organs or within deeper body tissues should call to mind anaerobic infection. (6) Treatment need not be directed at all of the organisms in the infectious site. However, some species in particular require specific therapy. The best example of this principle is the need to treat the *B. fragilis* group. Many of these synergistic infections can be cured with antibiotics directed at some, but not all, of the organisms. Antibiotic therapy, combined with drainage, disrupts the interdependent relationship among the bacteria and species which are resistant to the antibiotic do not survive without the co-infective organisms. (7) Manifestations of disseminated intravascular coagulation are unusual in patients with anaerobic infection.

EPIDEMIOLOGY Difficulties in obtaining appropriate cultures, contamination of cultures by aerobic bacteria or normal flora, and the lack of readily available reliable culture techniques have made accurate incidence or prevalence data on anaerobic infections unavailable. However, these infections are encountered frequently in hospitals with active surgical, trauma, and obstetric and gynecologic services. In some centers anaerobic bacteria, particularly *B. fragilis,* account for approximately 8 to 10 percent of positive blood cultures.

PATHOGENESIS Anaerobic bacterial infections usually occur when an anatomic barrier becomes disrupted and the local flora enter a site which was previously sterile. The bacteria which are isolated from infected sites have survived changes in Eh and exposure to host defenses. Because of the specific growth requirements of anaerobic organisms and their presence as commensals on mucosal surfaces, conditions must arise which allow these organisms to penetrate mucosal barriers and enter tissue with a lowered oxidation-reduction potential. Therefore, tissue ischemia, trauma, surgery, perforated viscus, shock, or aspiration provide environments conducive to the proliferation of anaerobes. Highly fastidious anaerobes lack the enzyme superoxide dismutase (SOD) that in other organisms reduces toxic superoxide radicals, thereby lessening the potentially lethal effects of superoxide. A general correlation exists between the intracellular concentration of SOD and the oxygen tolerance of anaerobic bacteria; organisms that contain SOD have a selective advantage after exposure to aerobic environments. For example, in the case of a perforated viscus, hundreds of species of anaerobic bacteria are spilled into the peritoneal cavity, but many of these organisms are unable to survive because the highly vascularized tissue provides an adequate oxygen supply. The entry of oxygen into the environment results in selection of aerotolerant organisms.

The ability of an organism to adhere to host tissues is important to the establishment of infection. Some oral *Bacteroides* species adhere to crevicular epithelium in the oral cavity. *B. melaninogenicus* actually attach to other microorganisms. *B. gingivalis* is a common isolate in periodontal disease. These organisms have been shown to have fimbriae which facilitate attachment. Some unencapsulated

Bacteroides strains appear to be piliated which may account for their ability to adhere.

Anaerobic bacteria produce a number of exoenzymes which are capable of enhancing their virulence. These enzymes include a heparinase elaborated by *B. fragilis* which may contribute to intravascular clotting and lead to a requirement for increased doses of heparin in patients on heparin therapy. Collagenase, produced by *B. gingivalis,* may enhance tissue destruction. Both *B. fragilis* and *B. melaninogenicus* possess lipopolysaccharides (endotoxins) which lack the biologic potency characteristic of endotoxins associated with aerobic gram-negative bacteria. The biologic inactivity of the endotoxin may account for the rarity of disseminated intravascular coagulation and purpura in *Bacteroides* bacteremia compared to facultative and aerobic gram-negative rod bacteremia.

CLINICAL MANIFESTATIONS **Anaerobic infections of the mouth, head, and neck** Infections of the mouth can be divided into those infections that arise from the supragingival or subgingival dental plaque. Supragingival plaque formation begins with the adherence of gram-positive bacteria to the tooth surface. This form of plaque is influenced by salivary and dietary components, oral hygiene, and local host factors. Once established, the acquisition of pathogenic bacteria as well as an increase in the amount of plaque is responsible for the ultimate development of gingivitis. Early bacteriologic changes in the supragingival plaque initiate an inflammatory response in the gingiva, including edema, swelling, and increase in gingival fluid and are responsible for the development of caries and endodontic (pulp) infections. Also, these changes contribute to the subsequent pathogenic alteration in the subgingival plaque which arise from poor or inadequate oral hygiene. Subgingival plaque is associated with periodontal disease and disseminated infection arising from the oral cavity. Bacteria that colonize the subgingival area are primarily anaerobic. The black-pigmented gram-negative anaerobic bacilli belonging to the *Bacteroides* group, principally *B. gingivalis* and *B. melaninogenicus,* are the most important. Infections in this area are frequently mixed and involve both anaerobic and aerobic bacteria. After establishment of local infection either in root canals or in the periodontal area, infection may extend into the mandible, causing osteomyelitis; to the maxillary sinuses; or to local tissues in the submandibular or submental spaces, depending upon which teeth are involved. Periodontitis also may result in spreading infection that can involve adjacent bone or soft tissues. This form of infection may be due either to oral *Bacteroides* or to *Fusobacterium.*

GINGIVITIS Gingivitis may become a necrotizing infection (trench mouth, Vincent's stomatitis). The onset of disease is usually sudden and is associated with tender bleeding gums, foul breath, and a bad taste. The gingival mucosa, especially the papillae between the teeth, become ulcerated and may be covered by a gray exudate which is removable with gentle pressure. These patients may become systemically ill, developing fever, cervical lymphadenopathy, and leukocytosis. Occasionally, ulcerative gingivitis can spread to the buccal mucosa, the teeth, and the mandible or maxilla, resulting in widespread destruction of bone and soft tissue. This infection is termed *acute necrotizing ulcerative mucositis* (cancrum oris, noma). It destroys tissue rapidly, causing the teeth to fall out and large areas of bone, even the whole mandible, to be sloughed. A strong putrid odor frequently is present, although the lesions are not painful. The gangrenous lesions eventually heal, leaving large disfiguring defects. This infection is seen most commonly following a debilitating illness, or in severely malnourished children in underdeveloped areas. It has been known to complicate leukemia or to develop in individuals with a genetic deficiency of catalase.

ACUTE NECROTIZING INFECTIONS OF THE PHARYNX These usually occur in association with ulcerative gingivitis. There are an extremely sore throat, foul breath, and a bad taste in the mouth, accompanied by a sensation of choking and fever. Examination of the pharynx demonstrates that the tonsillar pillars are swollen, red, and ulcerated and covered with a grayish membrane that peels easily. Lymphadenopathy and leukocytosis are common. The disease may last for only a few days or may persist for weeks if not treated. Lesions begin unilaterally but may spread to the other side of the pharynx or the larynx. Aspiration of the infected material by the patient can result in lung abscesses. Soft tissue infection of the oral-facial area may or may not be odontogenic in origin. *Ludwig's angina,* a periodontal infection usually arising from the third molar, may produce submandibular cellulitis that results in marked local swelling of tissues with pain, trismus, and superior and posterior displacement of the tongue. Submandibular swelling of the neck develops, which can impair swallowing and cause respiratory obstruction. In some cases tracheotomy may be life-saving.

FASCIAL INFECTIONS These arise from the spread of organisms originating in the upper airways to potential spaces formed by the fascial planes of the head and neck. Although there are few well-documented reports on the microbiology of these syndromes, anaerobes from the oral flora have been implicated in many cases. *Staph. aureus* and *Streptococcus pyogenes* infections may arise from boils or impetigo, whereas anaerobes are associated with space infections arising from diseases of the mucous membranes, dental manipulations, or occurring spontaneously.

SINUSITIS AND OTITIS The role of anaerobic bacteria in acute sinusitis may be underestimated because of improper collection of specimens. In chronic sinusitis anaerobic bacteria were found in 52 percent of specimens collected during external frontoethmoidotomy or radical antrotomy. Anaerobic bacteria are much more easily implicated in chronic suppurative otitis media than in acute otitis media. Purulent exudate from chronically draining ears has been found to contain anaerobes, particularly *Bacteroides* species, in up to 50 percent of patients. In contrast to other infections of the head and neck, *B. fragilis* has been isolated from up to 28 percent of patients with chronic otitis media.

COMPLICATIONS OF ANAEROBIC HEAD AND NECK INFECTIONS Contiguous spread of these infections craniad may result in osteomyelitis of the skull or mandible, or in intracranial infections such as brain abscesses or subdural empyema. Caudad spread can produce mediastinitis or pleuropulmonary infections. Hematogenous complications also may result from anaerobic infections of the head and neck. Bacteremia, which can occasionally be polymicrobial, can lead to endocarditis or other distant infections. When infections spread to produce suppurative thrombophlebitis of the internal jugular vein, a destructive syndrome with prolonged fever, bacteremia, septic emboli to both the lung and brain, and multiple metastatic foci of suppurative infection may develop. This syndrome has been reported with septicemia from species of *Fusobacterium* following exudative pharyngitis but is uncommon in this era of antimicrobial agents.

Central nervous system infections Brain abscesses are frequently associated with anaerobic bacteria (see Chap. 354). If optimal bacteriologic techniques are employed, as many as 85 percent of brain abscesses yield anaerobic bacteria. The anaerobic bacteria found most often in these infections are anaerobic gram-positive cocci, followed in frequency by fusobacteria and *Bacteroides* species. Frequently, facultative or microaerophilic streptococci and coliforms are involved in brain abscesses as mixed infections.

Pleuropulmonary infections Anaerobic pleuropulmonary infections result from the aspiration of oropharyngeal contents, which is often associated with an altered state of consciousness or absent gag reflex. There are four clinical syndromes associated with anaerobic pleuropulmonary infection produced by aspiration: simple aspiration pneumonia, necrotizing pneumonia, lung abscess, and empyema.

ANAEROBIC ASPIRATION PNEUMONITIS Anaerobic aspiration pneumonitis must be distinguished from two other types of aspiration pneumonitis, neither of which is bacterial. One aspiration syndrome results from aspiration of solids, usually food. Obstruction of major airways with resulting atelectasis is typical. Moderate nonspecific inflammation occurs. Therapy consists of removal of the foreign body.

A second aspiration syndrome is more easily confused with bacterial aspiration. This is the so-called Mendelson's syndrome, resulting from regurgitation of stomach contents and aspiration of chemical material, usually gastric juices. Pulmonary inflammation including destruction of alveolar lining with transudation of fluid into the alveolar space occurs with remarkable rapidity. Typically this syndrome develops within hours, often following anesthesia when the gag reflex is depressed. The patient becomes tachypneic, hypoxic, and febrile. The leukocyte count may rise, and the chest x-ray may evolve suddenly from normal to a complete whiteout bilaterally within 8 to 24 h. Minimal sputum production occurs. The pulmonary signs and symptoms can resolve quickly with symptomatic therapy or result in respiratory failure with subsequent development of bacterial superinfection over a period of days. Antibiotic therapy is not indicated unless bacterial infection supervenes. The signs of bacterial infection include sputum, persistent fever, leukocytosis, and clinical evidence of sepsis.

In contrast to these syndromes, bacterial aspiration pneumonia develops more slowly. It is seen in patients who are hospitalized and have a depressed gag reflex, elderly patients, or those with transient impaired consciousness in the wake of seizures or alcoholic blackouts. Patients who enter the hospital with this syndrome typically have been ill for several days, generally complain of low-grade fever, malaise, and sputum production. Usually the history reveals a predisposition for aspiration, such as alcohol overdose or residence in a nursing home. Sputum characteristically is not malodorous unless the process has been present for at least a week. Mixed bacterial flora with many polymorphonuclear leukocytes are present on Gram stain; reliable cultures can be obtained only by avoiding contamination with normal oral flora, i.e., by transtracheal aspiration. Chest x-rays show consolidation in dependent pulmonary segments. These are the basilar segments of the lower lobes if the patient aspirated while upright or sitting, or in the posterior segment of the upper lobe, usually on the right side, or in the superior segment of the lower lobe if aspiration has occurred in the supine position. Organisms isolated reflect the pharyngeal flora; *B. melaninogenicus, Fusobacterium* species, and anaerobic cocci are the most frequent isolates. The patient who aspirates in a hospital setting also may have mixed infection involving enteric gram-negative rods.

NECROTIZING PNEUMONITIS This is a form of anaerobic pneumonitis characterized by numerous small abscesses which spread to involve several pulmonary segments. The process can be indolent or fulminating. This syndrome is less common than either aspiration pneumonia or lung abscess, and includes features of both types of infection.

ANAEROBIC LUNG ABSCESSES These result from subacute anaerobic pulmonary infection. The clinical syndrome typically involves a history of constitutional symptoms including malaise, weight loss, fever, chills, and foul-smelling sputum which may occur over a period of weeks (see Chap. 207). Patients who develop lung abscesses characteristically have dental infection and periodontitis, but there are reports of lung abscesses in patients who are edentulous. Abscess cavities may be single or multiple, and generally occur in dependent pulmonary segments. Anaerobic abscesses must be distinguished from tuberculosis, neoplasia, and other causes of lung abscess, despite the fact that the clinical syndrome is usually typical. Oral anaerobes predominate, although *B. fragilis* is isolated in up to 10 percent of cases. *Staph. aureus* may be found as well. While in vitro resistance by *B. fragilis* to penicillin is common, this antibiotic generally is successful in treatment when combined with vigorous pulmonary toilet. Bronchoscopy is indicated only to rule out the presence of airway obstruction but should be delayed until the antimicrobial has begun to affect the disease process so that it does not spread the infection. Bronchoscopy has no role in enhancing drainage. Surgery is almost never indicated because of the danger of spilling the abscess contents into the lungs.

Empyema Empyema is a manifestation of long-standing anaerobic pulmonary infection. The clinical presentation resembles other anaerobic pulmonary infections including the presence of foul-smelling sputum. Patients may complain of pleuritic chest pain and marked chest wall tenderness.

Empyema may be masked by overlying pneumonitis and should be considered especially in cases of persistent fever in a patient receiving antibiotic therapy. Diligent physical examination and the use of ultrasound to localize a loculated empyema are important diagnostic tools. The presence of a foul-smelling exudate obtained by thoracentesis is typical. Drainage is required. Defervescence, a return to a feeling of well-being, and resolution of the process may require several months.

Extension from a subdiaphragmatic infection also may result in an anaerobic empyema. Septic pulmonary emboli may originate from intraabdominal or female genital tract infections and can produce anaerobic pneumonia.

Intraabdominal infections Because anaerobic bacteria outnumber aerobic bacteria in normal bowel flora by 100 to 1000:1, it is not surprising that disruption of the bowel wall will result in peritonitis with a preponderance of anaerobic bacteria. Colonic perforation releases large numbers of these bacteria and therefore entails a high risk of intraabdominal sepsis. Following peritonitis, abscesses may develop in any part of the peritoneal cavity and retroperitoneal spaces. The peritoneum reacts with a marked inflammatory response and effectively walls off the infection in a very short time. If an intraperitoneal abscess is localized, typical signs and symptoms appear (see Chap. 91). For example, *subphrenic abscess* may cause an ipsilateral sympathetic pleural effusion, and the patient may have pleuritic-type pain and splinting of the hemidiaphragm on the affected side. Constitutional symptoms include fever, chills, and malaise. There may be a history of abdominal surgery, trauma, or other conditions that predispose to disruption of the bowel wall. In contrast, more subtle clinical signs must be sought when an intraabdominal abscess is not readily localized. Peritonitis and abscess formation are closely related processes. Often following surgery to repair a bowel perforation, a patient may be febrile without localizing abdominal signs or general clinical deterioration. Persistent leukocytosis may be related to the operative procedure and/or resolving peritonitis. Profuse, cloudy, or foul-smelling wound drainage suggests the possibility of purulent anaerobic infection. Gram stain revealing a mixed fecal flora is frequently helpful. *B. fragilis* is isolated from approximately 70 percent of surgical wounds after trauma involving perforation of the lower gut, and a similar percentage of isolates follows elective colonic surgery. Antibiotics effective against *B. fragilis,* as well as facultative bacteria, are important in therapy, although they are not a replacement for surgical or percutaneous drainage. Appendicitis with perforation and abscess formation is the most common intraabdominal anaerobic infection. Diverticulitis involves nonsporulating anaerobes and can result in perforation followed by generalized peritonitis, but generally results in small walled-off infections that do not require surgical drainage. Abdominal ultrasound, gallium- or indium-labeled neutrophil scans, computed tomography (CT) scans, or magnetic resonance imaging may be helpful in localizing intraabdominal abscesses. Surgical exploration, however, may be necessary to establish the site of such an infection.

Among visceral abdominal infections involving nonsporulating anaerobes, the most common is *liver abscess;* nonsporulating anaerobes are isolated from approximately 50 percent of liver abscesses. Liver abscess results from both bacteremic spread (sometimes following blunt trauma with localized infarction of hepatic tissue) and from contiguous infection, especially within the peritoneal cavity. Infection may spread from the biliary tract or from the portal venous system (suppurative pyelophlebitis) which results from direct extension of pelvic or intraabdominal sepsis. Symptoms and signs often suggest infection that can be readily localized, but nonspecific symptoms of fever, chills, weight loss, nausea, and vomiting are also seen. Only half the patients have hepatomegaly, right upper quadrant abdominal tenderness, and jaundice. The diagnosis can be confirmed by ultrasound, CT scan, or radioisotopic scanning. Occasionally more than one diagnostic procedure may have to be utilized. More than 90 percent of patients with liver abscesses have a leukocytosis and elevation of the serum alkaline phosphatase and aspartyl transaminase.

Fifty percent have associated anemia, hypoalbuminemia, and elevated serum bilirubin. A basilar pulmonary infiltrate, pleural effusion, or elevated hemidiaphragm can be seen on chest x-ray. One-third of these patients have bacteremia. Open surgical drainage is indicated when an abscess is associated with other lesions requiring surgical drainage. Otherwise, percutaneous drainage using ultrasonography or CT scan to guide the catheter may be combined with antimicrobial therapy. If a liver abscess arises from contiguous gallbladder infection, cholecystectomy is essential.

Pelvic infections The vagina of a healthy woman is one of the major reservoirs of anaerobic and aerobic bacteria. In the normal flora of the female genital tract, anaerobes outnumber aerobes by a ratio of approximately 10:1. These anaerobes include anaerobic gram-positive cocci and *Bacteroides* species. Serious infections of the upper female tract contain organisms found in the normal vaginal flora. Anaerobes are isolated from the majority of such patients. The major pathogens consist of *B. fragilis, B. bivius, B. disiens, B. melaninogenicus,* anaerobic cocci, and clostridial species. Anaerobes frequently are encountered in tuboovarian abscess, septic abortion, pelvic abscess, endometritis, and postoperative wound infection, particularly following hysterectomy. Although these infections are frequently mixed, involving both anaerobes and coliforms, pure anaerobic infections without coliform or other facultative bacterial species occur more often in pelvic infections than intraabdominal infections. These infections are characterized by drainage of foul-smelling pus or blood from the uterus, generalized uterine or local pelvic tenderness, and continued fever and chills. Suppurative thrombophlebitis of the pelvic veins may complicate the infections and lead to repeated episodes of septic pulmonary emboli.

Skin and soft tissue infections Injury to skin, bone, or soft tissue by trauma, ischemia, or surgery creates a suitable environment for anaerobic infections. These infections are most frequently found when the site is prone to contamination with feces or upper airway secretions. Examples include wounds associated with intestinal surgery, decubitus ulcers, or human bites. Anaerobic bacteria can be isolated in cases of crepitant cellulitis, synergistic cellulitis, or gangrene and necrotizing fasciitis. These organisms have been isolated from cutaneous abscesses, rectal abscesses, and axillary sweat gland infections (hydradenitis suppurativa). Anaerobes frequently have been cultured from foot ulcers in diabetic patients.

These types of soft tissue or skin infections are usually polymicrobial. A mean of 4.8 bacterial species can be isolated with a roughly 3:2 ratio of anaerobes to aerobes. The most frequently isolated organisms include *Bacteroides* species, anaerobic streptococci, enterococci, clostridial species, and *Proteus* species. The presence of anaerobes in these types of infections is associated with a higher frequency of fever, foul-smelling lesions, or a visible foot ulcer.

Anaerobic bacterial *synergistic gangrene* (Meleney's) is exquisitely painful, red, and swollen, followed by induration. Erythema surrounds a central zone of necrosis. A granulating ulcer which may heal forms at the original center as necrosis and erythema extend outward. Symptoms are limited to pain. Fever is not typical. These infections most usually involve a combination of anaerobic cocci and *Staph. aureus*. Treatment includes surgical removal of necrotic tissue and antimicrobial therapy.

NECROTIZING FASCIITIS This is a rapidly spreading destructive disease of the fascia, usually attributed to group A streptococci, but it can be caused by anaerobic bacteria including *Peptostreptococcus* and *Bacteroides* species. Similarly, myonecrosis can be associated with mixed anaerobic infection. Fournier's gangrene is an anaerobic cellulitis involving the scrotum, perineum, and anterior abdominal wall in which mixed anaerobic organisms spread along deep external fascial planes and cause extensive loss of skin.

Bone and joint infections Although *actinomycosis* (see Chap. 152) accounts on a worldwide basis for the majority of anaerobic infections in bone, other organisms, including anaerobic or microaerophilic cocci, *Bacteroides* species, *Fusobacterium,* and *Clostridium* species, can be found. These infections frequently arise in the setting of adjacent soft tissue infections. Hematogenous seeding of bone is uncommon. Oral *Bacteroides* are seen in infections involving the maxilla and mandible, whereas *Clostridium* species have been reported as anaerobic pathogens in cases of osteomyelitis of the long bones, following fracture or trauma. Fusobacteria have been isolated in pure culture from osteomyelitis adjacent to the perinasal sinuses. Anaerobic and microaerophilic cocci have been reported as significant pathogens in infections involving the skull or mastoid.

In cases of anaerobic septic arthritis, the most common isolates are *Fusobacterium* species. Most of these patients have uncontrolled peritonsillar infections progressing to septic cervical venous thrombophlebitis and resulting in hematogenous dissemination which shows a predilection for the joints. Following the introduction of antibiotics, the isolation of *Fusobacterium* species from joints has been less common. Unlike anaerobic osteomyelitis, most cases of pyoarthritis caused by anaerobes are not polymicrobial and may be acquired hematogenously. Anaerobes are important pathogens in infections involving prosthetic joints; in these infections the causative organisms are part of the normal skin flora, such as anaerobic gram-positive cocci and *P. acnes*.

In patients with osteomyelitis (see Chap. 97), the most reliable source of culture is a bone biopsy obtained free from normal uninfected skin and subcutaneous tissue. If mixed flora is isolated from a bone biopsy, all isolates should be treated. When an anaerobic isolate is recognized as a major or sole pathogen involving a joint, the treatment regimen should be similar to treatment of arthritis caused by aerobic bacteria. Therapy includes management of underlying disease states, appropriate antimicrobial therapy, temporary joint immobilization, percutaneous drainage of effusions, and usually removal of infected prostheses or internal fixation devices. Surgical drainage and debridement such as sequestrectomy are essential for removal of necrotic tissue that would sustain anaerobic infections.

Bacteremia Transient bacteremia is a well-known event that occurs in healthy people when the anatomic mucosal barriers are injured (e.g., toothbrushing). These bacteremic episodes, which are often due to anaerobes, have no pathologic consequences. However, anaerobic bacteria compose nearly 10 to 15 percent of bacterial blood isolates from clinically ill patients when proper culture techniques are used. *B. fragilis* is the single most frequent anaerobic isolate. The portal of entry can usually be deduced along with the likely underlying problem that led to seeding of the bloodstream, by identification of the organism and understanding its place of normal residence. For example, mixed anaerobic bacteremia including *B. fragilis* implies colonic pathology with mucosal disruption from neoplasia, diverticulitis, or some other inflammatory lesion. The initial manifestations are determined by the portal of entry and reflect the localized condition. However, when bloodstream invasion occurs, patients can become extremely ill with rigors and hectic fevers ranging up to 40.6°C (105°F). The clinical picture may be quite similar to that seen in sepsis with aerobic gram-negative bacilli. Although other complications of anaerobic bacteremia such as septic thrombophlebitis and septic shock have been reported, the incidence of these complications in association with anaerobic bacteremia is low. Anaerobic bacteremia is potentially fatal and requires rapid diagnosis and appropriate therapy.

ENDOCARDITIS (See Chap. 90) Endocarditis due to anaerobes is uncommon. However, anaerobic streptococci, which are often classified incorrectly, are responsible for this disease more frequently than is appreciated. Gram-negative anaerobes are unusual causes of endocarditis.

DIAGNOSIS Because of the time and difficulty involved in the isolation of anaerobic bacteria, diagnosis of these infections must frequently be made on presumptive evidence. Certain clinical settings such as avascular, necrotic tissues with lowered oxidation-reduction potential favor the diagnosis of an anaerobic infection. When infections occur in proximity to mucosal surfaces normally harboring anaerobic flora, such as the gastrointestinal tract, female genital tract, or oropharynx, anaerobes should be considered as potential etiologic agents. A foul odor often is present since anaerobes produce certain organic acids as they proliferate in necrotic tissue. Although the presence of these odors is nearly pathognomonic for anaerobic infection, the absence of odor does not exclude these organisms as potential etiologic agents. Because anaerobes often coexist with other bacteria to form a mixed or synergistic infection, Gram-stained exudate frequently reveals numerous pleomorphic cocci and bacilli suggestive of anaerobes. Sometimes these organisms will have morphologic characteristics associated with specific species.

The presence of gas in tissues is highly suggestive, but not diagnostic, of anaerobes. Culture reports from obviously infected sites which yield no growth or only streptococci or a single aerobic species such as *E. coli,* when a Gram stain reveals mixed flora, imply that the anaerobic microorganisms failed to grow because of inadequate transport and/or culture techniques. Failure of a patient to respond to antibiotics that are not active against anaerobes, for example, aminoglycosides, and, in some circumstances, penicillin, cephalosporins, or tetracyclines, suggests the possibility of anaerobic infection.

There are three critical steps to diagnose anaerobic infection: (1) proper specimen collection, (2) rapid transportation of these specimens to the microbiology laboratory, preferably in anaerobic transport media, and (3) proper handling of these specimens by the laboratory. Collection of specimens must be performed by meticulously sampling infected sites avoiding contamination with normal flora. When there is a likely contamination of a specimen with normal flora, the specimen is unacceptable for processing by the bacteriology laboratory. Examples of unacceptable specimens for anaerobic culture include: (1) sputum collected by expectoration, or nasal tracheal suction, (2) bronchoscopy specimens, (3) direct collections through the vaginal vault, (4) collections of urine by voided specimen, and (5) feces. Specimens which can be cultured for anaerobes include blood, pleural fluid, transtracheal aspirates, pus obtained by direct aspiration from an abscess cavity, fluid obtained by culdocentesis, suprapubic bladder aspirates, cerebrospinal fluid, and lung puncture specimens.

Because even brief exposure to oxygen may kill some anaerobic organisms and result in failure to isolate them in the laboratory, abscess cavities which are aspirated with a syringe should have the air expelled and the needle capped with a sterile rubber stopper. Proper precautions should be utilized when handling contaminated needles. Specimens can be injected into transport bottles containing a reduced medium or brought immediately in syringes to the laboratory for direct culture on anaerobic media. In general, swabs should not be used. If a swab must be used, it should be placed in a reduced semisolid carrying medium before transport to the laboratory. Delays in transportation may lead to failure to isolate anaerobes due to exposure to oxygen, or overgrowth of facultative organisms which may eliminate or obscure the anaerobes that are present. All clinical specimens from suspected anaerobic infections should be Gram-stained and examined for organisms with characteristic morphology. It is not unusual for organisms to be observed on Gram stain but not isolated in culture. If purulent materials are found to be sterile, or organisms are seen on Gram stain, but do not grow in the culture, suspicion should be raised that anaerobes are involved.

TREATMENT Successful therapy of anaerobic infections involves a combination of appropriate antibiotics, surgical resection, and drainage. Perforations must be closed promptly, devitalized tissues removed, closed spaces drained, tissue compartments decompressed, and adequate blood supply established. Drainage of abscess cavities should be carried out as soon as fluctuation or localization occurs. While surgery was formerly required to establish drainage, with the advent of CT scans and ultrasound, diagnostic radiologists now are able to perform percutaneous drainage of a number of abscess sites.

Patients with infections due to anaerobic bacteria require appropriate antibiotics. Most laboratories lack facilities to do antimicrobial susceptibility testing on anaerobic bacteria. In these instances presumptive therapy must be given and the patient's response followed closely. The selection of initial antibiotic therapy should be based on knowledge of the pathogens likely to be present in a specific clinical setting, in combination with the Gram-stain findings which should suggest the likelihood of certain species of organisms. Because many anaerobic infections tend to be mixed with coliforms and other facultative organisms, it is advisable, in general, to use drugs active against both aerobic and anaerobic components. If anaerobes are suspected, the choices of antibiotics can be made reliably since patterns of antimicrobial susceptibility are usually predictable (see Chap. 85 and Table 108-1).

TABLE 108-1 Antimicrobial therapy for anaerobic bacterial infection

	Bacteroides fragilis group or other penicillin-resistant anaerobes (usual source below diaphragm)	Other anaerobes in mixed infection (usual source above diaphragm)
Proven first-line therapy	Metronidazole* Clindamycin* Cefoxitin	Penicillin† Metronidazole‡ Clindamycin Cefoxitin
Alternatives	Chloramphenicol	Chloramphenicol
New drugs with good in vitro activity, but limited clinical experience	Imipenem Ampicillin-sulbactam Ticarcillin-clavulanic acid	Imipenem Ampicillin-sulbactam Ticarcillin-clavulanic acid

* Usually need to be given along with aerobic gram-negative bacterial coverage.
† The drug of choice for serious systemic clostridial infections
‡ Usually need to be given with aerobic gram-positive coverage in infections originating above diaphragm.

Organisms belonging to the *B. fragilis* group or the species *B. bivius* are resistant to penicillin. In general they do not play a significant role in infections originating above the diaphragm, such as head and neck infections, pleuropulmonary infections, and central nervous system infections. However, septic processes originating below the diaphragm, including in the pelvic and abdominal cavity, frequently contain these bacteria and specific microbial therapy directed at penicillin-resistant anaerobic organisms should be employed. Treatment of infections arising from sources above the diaphragm with penicillin is accepted. Depending on the site of infection and the severity, the dose of penicillin recommended is variable. For the treatment of lung abscesses a dose of 6 to 12 million units of penicillin G per day for at least 4 weeks is recommended. Infrequently, infections arising from oral organisms will fail to respond to penicillin. In such cases these patients should be treated with drugs such as metronidazole or clindamycin which are effective against penicillin-resistant anaerobes. Occasional resistance of oral *Bacteroides* such as *B. melaninogenicus* to penicillin may account for some of these treatment failures.

Infections arising from a colonic source are likely to contain *B. fragilis*. Many therapeutic failures have been noted in patients with documented *B. fragilis* infection who are treated with penicillin or first-generation cephalosporins. In intraabdominal sepsis the use of antibiotics effective against anaerobes has clearly reduced the incidence of postoperative infection and serious infectious complications. The number of antimicrobial agents effective against *B. fragilis* has expanded and there are currently several choices which are useful (Table 108-1). In general, greater than 80 percent cure rates can be achieved in patients with *B. fragilis* infection when treated with appropriate antimicrobial therapy and drainage.

Several classes of antibiotics are active in the treatment of *Bacteroides* infection: (1) metronidazole; (2) clindamycin; (3) cefoxitin and selected other cephalosporins; (4) chloramphenicol; (5) broader spectrum penicillins when used in combination with β-lactamase inhibitors, such as ticarcillin-clavulanic acid, or ampicillin-sulbactam; and (6) imipenem. Of the newer types of antibiotics, the quinolines are notable for absence of activity against *B. fragilis*. In vitro metronidazole and clindamycin are the most active against *B.*

fragilis group organisms of any current classes of antibiotics. Resistance rates are high to tetracycline, cefoperazone, and cefotaxime and these drugs should not be used. Resistance to cefoxitin varies from 8 to 30 percent. In contrast, clindamycin resistance is encountered in approximately 5 percent of anaerobic isolates, and metronidazole resistance is uncommon. Cefotetan may be potentially useful for treatment of *B. fragilis* infection but is less active against non-*fragilis Bacteroides* species. In general, *B. fragilis* species are more sensitive to the third generation cephalosporins than other organisms of the *B. fragilis* group. In some patients treated with cefoxitin alone, treatment failures occur because of emergence of facultative gram-negative bacilli resistant to cefoxitin.

Resistance of *B. fragilis* has rarely been reported with metronidazole. This well-tolerated drug achieves significant serum levels and also can be found in high levels within abscess cavities. It should be considered first-line therapy against *B. fragilis* infection. The two other widely used drugs, clindamycin and cefoxitin, also could be considered as first-line therapy because despite the reports of in vitro resistance of *B. fragilis* to these agents, there are only scattered case reports of clinical failure. If a patient fails to respond to one of these drugs, consideration should be given to alternative therapy and to determining the resistance patterns among *B. fragilis* group isolates. Although in vitro resistance to chloramphenicol has not been reported, this drug does not appear to be as effective as others. Among new drugs, ampicillin-sulbactam, ticarcillin-clavulanic acid, and imipenem hold great promise in the treatment of *B. fragilis* infection.

Specific regimens must be tailored to the initial infecting site in clinical situations. Intraabdominal sepsis should be treated with an aminoglycoside plus either metronidazole, 7.5 mg/kg every 8 h, or clindamycin, 600 mg intravenously every 8 h. This regimen is the "gold standard" because it treats both facultative aerobic and strictly anaerobic gram-negative bacilli which are responsible for morbidity and mortality. If gram-positive bacteria are suspected, an appropriate penicillin should be added. Chloramphenicol can be used successfully in patients with anaerobic central nervous system infections at a dose of 30 to 60 mg/kg per day depending on the severity of illness. However, penicillin G and metronidazole also cross the blood-brain barrier and are bactericidal for many anaerobic organisms (see Chap. 354).

Nearly all the drugs mentioned have toxic side effects. These are described in detail in Chap. 85.

Anaerobic infections that have failed to respond to treatment or that relapse should be reassessed. Consideration should be given to additional surgical drainage or debridement. Superinfections with resistant gram-negative facultative or aerobic bacteria should be ruled out. Drug resistance must also be entertained particularly if chloramphenicol was the antibiotic used; repeated cultures should then yield the pathogenic organism.

Other supportive measures in the management of anaerobic infections include: careful attention to fluid and electrolyte balance since extensive local edema formation may lead to hypoalbuminemia; hemodynamic support for septic shock; immobilization of infected extremities; maintenance of adequate nutrition during chronic infections by parenteral hyperalimentation; relief of pain and anticoagulation with heparin for thrombophlebitis. Hyperbaric oxygen therapy is of no proven value.

REFERENCES

Bartlett JG, Finegold SM: Anaerobic infections of the lung and pleural space. Am Rev Resp Dis 110:56, 1974

Bieluch VM et al: Clinical importance of cefoxitin-resistant *Bacteroides fragilis* isolates. Diagn Microbiol Infect Dis 2:119, 1987

Finegold SM: *Anaerobic Bacteria in Human Disease*. New York, Academic, 1977

Gibbs RS: Microbiology of the female genital tract. Am J Obstet Gynecol 156:491, 1987

Gorbach SC: Anaerobic bacteria, in *Principles and Practices of Infectious Diseases*, 3d ed, GL Mandell et al (eds). New York, Wiley, 1990

———, Bartlett JG: Anaerobic infections. N Engl J Med 290:1177, 1974

Harding GKM et al: Prospective randomized comparative study of clindamycin, chloramphenicol and ticarcillin, each in combination with gentamicin in therapy for intraabdominal and female tract sepsis. J Infect Dis 142:384, 1980

Kasper DL et al: Virulence factors of anaerobic bacteria. Rev Infect Dis 1:246, 1979

——— et al: Capsular polysaccharides and lipopolysaccharides from two strains of *Bacteroides fragilis*. Rev Infect Dis 6:525, 1984

Levin S, Goodman LJ: Selected overview of nongynecologic surgical intraabdominal infections. Prophylaxis and therapy. Am J Med 79(5B):146, 1985

Mathisen GE et al: Brain abscess and cerebritis. Rev Infect Dis 6:5101, 1984

Nakata MN, Lewis RP: Anaerobic bacteria in bone and joint infections. Rev Infect Dis 6:5165, 1984

Newman MG: Anaerobic oral and dental infections. Rev Infect Dis 6:5107, 1984

Onderdonk A et al: Use of a model of intraabdominal sepsis for studies of the pathogenicity of *Bacteroides fragilis*. Rev Infect Dis 6:5191, 1984

Sutter VL et al: *Wadsworth Anaerobic Bacteriology Manual*, 3d ed. St Louis, Mosby, 1980

Wexler HM, Finegold SM: In vitro activity of imipenem against anaerobic bacteria. Rev Infect Dis 7:S417, 1985

Zaleznik DF, Kasper DL: *Bacteroides* species, in *Principles and Practice of Infectious Diseases*, 3d ed, GL Mandell et al (eds). New York, Wiley, 1990

———: Role of bacterial virulence factors in pathogenesis of anaerobic infections, in *Anaerobic Infections in Humans*, S. Finegold (ed). Orlando, FL, Academic, 1989

section 5 Diseases caused by gram-negative organisms

109 MENINGOCOCCAL INFECTIONS

J. McLEOD GRIFFISS

DEFINITION *Neisseria meningitidis* is an ordinary commensal of the human oropharynx that can cause a variety of diseases, most notably bacteremia and meningitis. Its pathogenic potential can be expressed as epidemic disease or as sporadic endemic cases and focal outbreaks.

ETIOLOGY Meningococci are gram-negative single cocci or diplococci with flattened adjacent sides. They grow well on media containing blood or serum at temperatures between 35 and 37°C in a moist atmosphere reduced in oxygen and containing 5 to 10 percent CO_2. The organism is recovered readily when fresh specimens are inoculated on warm chocolate agar and incubated 18 to 24 h in a candle jar or other apparatus that provides a suitable environment.

Neisseria make cytochrome oxidase, which is responsible for the positive "oxidase" test; species usually are differentiated by their ability to use simple and compound sugars as sources of energy. Typically, meningococci use both glucose and maltose. Meningococci differ from other *Neisseria* in that they are surrounded by a polysaccharide "capsule."

Meningococci are divided into serologic groups on the basis of antigenic differences among their capsular polysaccharides. Groups A, B, C, W, and Y cause most serious disease; other groups frequently colonize the oropharynx but only very rarely disseminate. The serogroups are further divided into serotypes and subtypes based on independent antigenic differences among outer membrane protein and glycolipid constituents.

EPIDEMIOLOGY The natural habitat of meningococci is the human throat. Transmission from person to person is through inhalation of droplets of infected oropharyngeal secretions. Colonization only rarely proceeds to disease, because specific antibodies and complement lyse the organisms as they enter the bloodstream and thereby provide an effective barrier to dissemination. The incidence of disseminated infection varies cyclically, with peaks of increased frequency occurring every 10 to 15 years and lasting 4 to 6 years. Each cycle spreads slowly and is called a "hyperendemic wave" to distinguish it from the truly endemic disease that occurs between waves. Hyperendemic waves are often punctuated by focal outbreaks. Widespread epidemics have been absent from temperate areas of the world since the end of World War II; hyperendemic waves continue to occur; the last was in 1981. The between-waves endemic incidence in temperate climates is a fairly constant 1 reported case per 100,000 population per year. The prevalence of meningococcal infection is also subject to seasonal influences; the lowest attack rate occurs in midsummer and the highest in winter and early spring.

Epidemic disease receives the greatest public attention. An epidemic begins as a focal outbreak in a demographically discrete population in which a strain of a single serotype, the "epidemic strain," emerges from among the endemic strains. In less developed areas the outbreak quickly spreads, develops high attack rates, and involves large segments of the community. It remains either multicentric or evolves in the same pattern as a hyperendemic wave. Each focal outbreak in multicentric epidemics lasts 1 to 3 years, while the epidemic as a whole may last 5 or more years. In developed areas foci usually involve economically deprived segments of the population and do not spread or develop into generalized epidemics.

Group A strains caused most epidemics in the United States in the first half of this century; since World War II, group B and C meningococci have caused outbreaks in both military and civilian populations. Hyperendemic waves are caused by group B, C, or W organisms that share a limited set of serotypes. Group A strains do not share serotypes with other groups and do not cause hyperendemic waves. Group W strains have been associated with endemic and hyperendemic disease only. Group Y organisms only cause sporadic disease in older children and teenagers. Endemic disease predominantly is caused by group B organisms of diverse serotypes.

The attack rate of endemic meningococcal disease is highest for children between 6 and 36 months of age. The age distribution of epidemic cases is always shifted to proportionately older individuals, and those of any age may be involved. The attack rate in household contacts of sporadic cases is up to 1000 times the overall endemic rate and may be as much as 15,000 times that of the general population in epidemic periods.

Carriers Between epidemics, 2 to 30 percent of individuals, depending on age, carry meningococci in their throats. When sporadic disease occurs, the carrier rate in close contacts may rise to 40 percent, and in closed populations or during epidemics, it may approach 100 percent. Despite this high carrier rate, the prevalence of meningococcal disease cannot be attributed to the prevailing carrier rate, because only a small proportion of the meningococci carried on the throats of those who share a patient's environment are of the same clonotype as the patient's and are able to cause disease. Case-to-case transmission of infection is rare; carriers, not patients, are the foci from which disease is spread. Although some individuals harbor meningococci for years, oropharyngeal infection is usually transient, and in 75 percent of carriers the organism disappears within a few weeks to a few months.

Immunity The occurrence of clinical disease is most dependent on the immunologic status of the host. Natural immunity is usually type-specific and develops in most individuals within the first two decades of life. Natural immunization may result from pharyngeal colonization during the first few years of life by a closely related bacterium, *Neisseria lactamica. N. lactamica* strains are genetically diverse but many share important outer membrane protein and lipooligosaccharide antigens with virulent strains of *N. meningitidis.* They are not encapsulated and therefore do not survive in the bloodstream to cause disseminated disease. *N. lactamica* colonizes the throat earlier in life than does *N. meningitidis;* colonized infants develop bactericidal antibodies that initiate complement-mediated lysis of a broad range of potentially pathogenic meningococci.

Colonization with *N. meningitidis* gradually replaces that with *N. lactamica* as the child grows older, and lactamica carriage is only rarely encountered in teenagers, in whom meningococcal carrier rates of 15 to 25 percent are the rule, regardless of season. Meningococcal carriage induces antibodies to the infecting strain as well as to other strains, thereby reinforcing and broadening naturally acquired immunity. Many enteric bacteria make capsules that are chemically similar to those of meningococci. Asymptomatic colonization with them can induce group-specific antibody. Second episodes of meningococcal disease are encountered. Deficiency of one of the terminal complement components, C6, C7, C8, or C9, is a risk factor for repeated episodes of bacteremia with pathogenic *Neisseria* and should always be sought in patients with second episodes.

PATHOGENESIS Meningococcal infection begins in the oropharynx. In most instances, this infection is subclinical, but occasionally mild symptoms develop. Dissemination from the pharynx is via the bloodstream, and generally is followed by clinical manifestations. Purulent meningitis, the most common manifestation, may predominate, or it may be associated with signs and symptoms of meningococcemia. Rarely, extensive inflammation may cause an acute diffuse encephalitis.

There is a correlation between susceptibility to meningococcal disease and the absence of complement-mediated bactericidal activity in serum. The pathogenetic mechanisms that account for the different epidemiologic forms of meningococcal disease all interfere with the generation of bactericidal activity by the membrane attack complex of complement (C5–9) (see Chap. 13). Hypogammaglobulinemia, deficiencies of complement components, and interference by the organisms' capsular polysaccharides with the effective deposition of the attack complex into its outer membrane account for endemic disease. Primary isolated IgM deficiency is a rare cause of susceptibility that is easy to detect and therefore disproportionately reported. Deficiencies of complement components are seen more frequently in patients than in the general population. They may be either primary or secondary. Approximately 1 in 1000 people are deficient in one or another of the five terminal components. Disseminated meningococcal and gonococcal infections occur with increased frequency in these patients. Inheritance of properdin deficiency and ineffective alternative pathway complement activity is sex-linked. Males in these pedigrees are at extremely high risk of fulminant meningococcal disease. Several systemic diseases can result in secondary deficiencies of complement components, primarily the early components of the classical pathway, and sporadic meningococcal disease. People with functional asplenia are also at increased risk of sporadic meningococcal disease, although pneumococcal disease is a much more common complication.

The generation of hyperendemic waves remains incompletely understood. An "out-of-phase" response to fluctuations in antibody levels in the population is a possible mechanism. Focal outbreaks during hyperendemic waves can be correlated with the presence of elevated levels of circulating, strain-specific IgA which blocks initiation of complement-mediated lysis by IgM or IgG, but the precise contribution of IgA-mediated susceptibility to hyperendemic waves remains unclear. When a sufficiently large part of the population has developed blocking serum IgA, conditions are established for an epidemic to occur. The environmental events that cause IgA levels to be elevated within the epidemic focus are not known with certainty, but epidemic disease has been correlated with prevalent enteric colonization with cross-reacting organisms. The extent of induction of blocking IgA in the epidemic focus may explain the extent and intensity of the epidemic as well as the failure of focal outbreaks to develop into generalized ones. Asplenia and coincidental diseases that interfere with the normal hepatic clearance of IgA, such as alcoholism, biliary tract disease, hemoglobinopathies, and hemosiderosis, increase susceptibility within the epidemic focus.

The meningococcal outer membrane contains lipooligosaccharides that are chemically and biologically similar to the lipopolysaccharide endotoxins of enteric bacilli. They induce tumor necrosis factor (TNF) and interleukin 1 (IL-1), which may be responsible for the hypotension and vascular collapse observed in fulminant meningococcemia and for the purpura and visceral hemorrhages associated with meningococcal bacteremia (see Chap. 89). Thrombosis of dermal venules, adrenal sinusoids, and renal glomerular capillaries is most commonly seen in patients who die of fulminant meningococcemia. The ability to form pili and release endotoxin from the outer membrane have been correlated with "virulence" and a poor prognosis, respectively.

CLINICAL MANIFESTATIONS Of patients with meningococcal disease 90 to 95 percent have meningococcemia and/or meningitis.

Meningococcemia Thirty to fifty percent of patients who develop overt disease have meningococcemia without meningitis. The onset of clinical illness may be abrupt, but patients usually have nonspecific prodromal symptoms of cough, headache, and sore throat followed by the sudden development of spiking fever, chills, arthralgias, and myalgias. Patients usually appear acutely ill with an inordinate degree of prostration. In addition to high fever, tachycardia, and tachypnea, mild hypotension may be present. However, clinical shock does not occur unless fulminant meningococcemia supervenes. In the course of meningococcal bacteremia, about three-fourths of the patients develop a characteristic petechial rash. Lesions are frequently sparse, and the axillae, flanks, wrists, and ankles are most commonly involved. Often petechiae are located in the center of lighter-colored macules, and they may become nodular as the disease progresses. The diagnosis of meningococcemia occasionally can be established by demonstrating gram-negative diplococci in scrapings from these nodular lesions. In severe cases, purpuric spots or large ecchymoses develop, and a widespread petechial or purpuric eruption suggests fulminating disease. However, the absence of rash does not necessarily indicate that the illness will be mild. The levels of circulating endotoxin, or of the cytokines it induces, are sensitive markers for the development of fulminant disease and a poor prognosis.

Fulminant meningococcemia, or the Waterhouse-Friderichsen syndrome, is meningococcemia associated with vasomotor collapse and shock. It occurs in the 10 to 20 percent of patients in whom high levels of endotoxin circulate. The onset is abrupt, and profound prostration frequently occurs within a few hours. Petechiae and purpuric lesions enlarge rapidly, and hemorrhage into the skin may be extensive. Early in the preshock stage, there is generalized vasoconstriction; patients are alert and pale, with circumoral cyanosis and cold extremities. Upon entering the shock stage, however, the cardiac output decreases, and the blood pressure falls; mentation decreases and coma may develop. Despite appropriate therapy, 40 to 60 percent of patients die from cardiac and/or respiratory failure. Patients who recover may have extensive sloughing of skin lesions or loss of digits because of gangrene.

Occult meningococcemia is an uncommon form of meningococcal infection that affects children between the ages of 3 and 24 months. It is characterized by fever and bacteremia without an obvious source. Infection usually resolves without treatment but may lead to the development of meningitis or other metastatic infection.

Chronic meningococcemia is a very rare form of meningococcal infection that lasts for weeks or months and is characterized by fever, rash, and arthritis or arthralgia. Typically, the fever is intermittent, and during afebrile periods, which may last several days, patients appear remarkably well. The usual maculopapular or polymorphous rash waxes and wanes with the fever. Petechial and nodular lesions are occasionally seen. Joint involvement is present in two-thirds of the patients, and splenomegaly is detected in about 20 percent. If treatment is delayed, meningitis, carditis, or nephritis may occur.

Meningitis Meningitis is a common form of meningococcal disease that occurs primarily in children from 6 months to 10 years. Fever, vomiting, headache, and confusion or lethargy are the most common symptoms; in about one-fourth of the patients, symptoms begin abruptly and rapidly increase in severity. The more typical patient, however, has symptoms of an upper respiratory tract infection followed by an illness that progresses over several days. Twenty to forty percent of patients have meningitis without clinical evidence of meningococcemia, and the diagnosis depends upon bacteriologic examination of the cerebrospinal fluid. However, when meningitis occurs in association with a petechial or purpuric rash, a presumptive diagnosis of meningococcal disease is warranted because this pattern of illness is seen only rarely in other infections.

Rarer manifestations The meningococcus may cause purulent conjunctivitis or sinusitis. Primary pneumonia occurs rarely, but secondary pneumonia not infrequently follows viral respiratory infections, particularly influenza. Bacterial endocarditis, primary pericarditis, arthritis, and osteomyelitis have also been reported. Meningococci can also produce genital infections clinically indistinguishable from gonococcal disease, including urethritis and endometritis.

LABORATORY FINDINGS Aside from bacteriologic data, laboratory studies are of little value in establishing a specific diagnosis of meningococcal infection. Polymorphonuclear leukocyte counts usually are elevated but may be normal or low in meningococcemia; a left shift usually is present. Patients with hemorrhagic manifestations may have low platelet counts and decreased levels of circulating clotting factors as a result of disseminated intravascular coagulation (see Chap. 62). In meningitis, the cerebrospinal fluid (CSF) pressure is increased; the fluid usually contains from 10,000 to 40,000 polymorphonuclear leukocytes per microliter; the protein content is increased, and the concentration of glucose is low (see Chap. 354).

Meningococci usually can be recovered from cultures of blood or spinal fluid and, on occasion, of material aspirated from skin lesions or joints. In addition, gram-negative diplococci may be seen in stains of nodular petechiae or the buffy coat of blood from patients with meningococcemia. In meningococcal meningitis, a smear of the spinal fluid is diagnostic in about half the patients but often shows only a few intracellular bacteria, which are located with difficulty, particularly early in the course of the infection, when organisms may be present in the absence of CSF abnormalities. The infecting organisms shed their capsular polysaccharide, which usually can be detected in CSF, joint fluid, serum, or urine with use of highly specific antibodies in counterimmunoelectrophoresis (CIE) or latex agglutination (LA) assays. The sensitivity of these assays is dependent on the antibodies used and is least for group B; LA is somewhat more sensitive and easier to perform. In general, the immunoassays are more sensitive than culture alone and in combination with the Gram stain will provide a diagnosis in over 98 percent of cases. They are particularly helpful early in infection and when the patient has been treated with antibiotics, causing negative cultures.

COMPLICATIONS Herpes labialis occurs in 5 to 20 percent of patients with meningococcal disease. Other complications, which result from neurologic damage or secondary foci of infection, are uncommon following appropriate treatment and are often transient. Seizures or deafness occur in 10 to 20 percent of patients during the acute stages of meningitis, but postmeningitic epilepsy is rare, and the frequency of permanent nerve damage is probably less than 5 percent. A number of patients complain of recurrent headache, emotional lability, insomnia, backache, memory loss, and difficulty in concentrating for months after an episode of meningitis. These symptoms usually disappear a year or two after the infection.

Septic arthritis is a not uncommon complication of meningococcemia that may accompany meningitis or occur as the only metastatic manifestation. The joint fluid usually contains many granulocytes (see Chap. 96), but meningococci are recovered infrequently. It can be diagnosed by Gram stain, CIE, or LA, or by recovery of the organism on culture. It is treated in the same way as meningitis; recovery without sequelae is to be expected.

Immune-complex arthritis occurs in about 10 percent of patients during convalescence. As a rule, multiple joints are involved, primarily the larger ones. Inflammation appears between days 7 and 15 of treatment when newly produced antibodies form insoluble complexes with the infecting organism's capsular polysaccharide. No specific therapy is indicated; permanent joint changes are rare.

Other pyogenic complications have become extremely uncommon since antibiotics have been used routinely. Bacterial endocarditis is quite rare, but a high proportion of patients who die of meningococcal infection have myocarditis. A pericardial friction rub or electrocardiographic changes of pericarditis are seen in about 5 percent of patients; rarely, purulent pericarditis may develop.

DIAGNOSIS The diagnosis of meningococcal disease depends upon recovering *N. meningitidis* or detecting antigens in blood, spinal fluid, joint fluid, urine, or petechial scrapings from patients with a typical clinical picture. Capsular polysaccharides of serogroups A, B, C, Y, and W can be detected in fluids by LA or CIE. Recovery of meningococci from the pharynx does not establish the diagnosis of meningococcal disease; throat cultures are not indicated.

Few diseases need to be considered seriously in the differential diagnosis of meningococcal disease. If meningococcal meningitis is not accompanied by rash or other manifestations of bacteremia, it is indistinguishable from meningitis caused by other common pathogens (see Chap. 354). Occasionally, the common viral exanthems, mycoplasma infection, Rocky Mountain spotted fever (see Chap. 153), and vascular purpuras (see Chaps. 58 and 276) may be confused with meningococcemia.

TREATMENT In the absence of fulminant meningococcemia the treatment of meningococcal disease is not difficult, and the mortality rate should not exceed 5 percent. Therapy should be instituted as early as possible. Penicillin G is the drug of choice, and should be administered intravenously. The usual dosage for treatment of meningitis in adults with normal renal function is 12 to 24 million units per day (2 to 4 million units intravenously every 4 h), and in the pediatric age group, 300,000 to 400,000 units per kilogram per day, intravenously every 4 h in divided doses. When treatment is continued for a minimum of 7 days, or 4 to 5 days after the patient becomes afebrile, relapse is extremely rare. Chloramphenicol is just as effective as penicillin and may be the drug of choice in less-developed countries. It should be used when a patient is allergic to penicillin in a dosage of 50 mg/kg or, in adults, 2.0 to 4.0 g/d in divided doses every 4 h given intravenously until the patient is able to take oral medication. Some of the third-generation cephalosporins, such as cefotaxime, ceftriaxone, or cefuroxime (see Chaps. 85 and 354), are also effective and are often used to initiate therapy when the etiology of meningitis is uncertain. A significant proportion of meningococci are resistant to sulfonamides, so these should not be used routinely unless the infecting organism is shown to be susceptible. Sulfadiazine (2 to 3 g initially followed by 1 g 6-hourly thereafter given intravenously until the patient can take oral medication) or trimethoprim/sulfamethoxazole (160/800 mg intravenously every 6 h) is effective treatment for susceptible strains. The dosages must be reduced in renal failure and in children, depending on age (see Chap. 85).

Patients with meningococcal infections require supportive treatment as well as antimicrobial therapy. Maintenance of fluid and electrolyte balance and prevention of respiratory complications in comatose patients are of primary concern. When shock occurs, visceral perfusion must be improved. Vasoactive drugs should be employed according to the pathophysiologic derangement (see Chaps. 39 and 89). When disseminated intravascular coagulation is recognized, treatment with heparin, whole blood, or fibrinogen can be tried, but these are not certain to be effective.

PROGNOSIS Before the introduction of antibiotics, meningococcal meningitis and meningococcemia were almost invariably fatal. With prompt and appropriate chemotherapy, the mortality rate of meningitis without fulminant meningococcemia has dropped to less than 10 percent in the United States, and neurologic sequelae are rare. The mortality of fulminant infection remains high primarily because patients are often in irreversible shock when treatment is instituted. Most deaths occur within 24 to 48 h of admission, and the capacity of the meningococcus to kill a previously healthy individual within a few hours remains one of the most awesome characteristics of this disease.

PREVENTION The capsular polysaccharides from organisms of serogroups A, C, Y, and W induce group-specific bactericidal antibody responses after subcutaneous injection. A tetravalent vaccine containing these antigens is available for use to prevent or control outbreaks. Routine immunization of recruits has eliminated nearly all disease among military personnel, but in the United States immunization is recommended routinely only for travelers to areas where epidemic disease is occurring and for individuals with complement deficiencies or splenic dysfunction. An effective group B vaccine has not been developed. Chemoprophylaxis should be administered to intimate (usually household) contacts of sporadic cases. If the organism isolated from the patient is sensitive to sulfonamides, 2 days of prophylaxis with one of these drugs is recommended. When sensitivities are not known or the organism is resistant to sulfonamides, rifampin in a dosage of 600 mg every 12 h for 2 days for adults and 5 to 10 mg/kg every 12 h for children can be expected to eradicate the carrier state temporarily and minimize spread of meningococci. Vaccination is over 99 percent effective in preventing secondary cases (as compared with approximately 89 percent effectiveness for rifampin chemoprophylaxis), and vaccination of household or other intimate contacts should be encouraged.

REFERENCES

Brandtzaeg P et al: Plasma endotoxin as a predictor of multiple organ failure and death in systemic meningococcal disease. J Infect Dis 159:195, 1989

Counts GW et al: Group A meningococcal disease in the U.S. Pacific Northwest: Epidemiology, clinical features, and effect of a vaccination control program. Rev Infect Dis 6:640, 1984

Crowe BA et al: Clonal and variable properties of *Neisseria meningitidis* isolated from cases and carriers during and after an epidemic in The Gambia, West Africa. J Infect Dis 159:686, 1989

Densen P et al: Familial properdin deficiency and fatal meningococcemia: Correction of the bactericidal defect by vaccination. N Engl J Med 316:922, 1987

Ellison RT et al: Prevalence of congenital or acquired complement deficiency in patients with sporadic meningococcal disease. N Engl J Med 308:913, 1983

Griffiss J McL: Epidemic meningococcal disease: Synthesis of a hypothetical immunoepidemiologic model. Rev Infect Dis 4:159, 1982

Jarvis GA et al: Sialic acid of group B *Neisseria meningitidis* regulates alternative complement pathway activation. Infect Immun 55:174, 1987

Kim JJ et al: *Neisseria lactamica* and *Neisseria meningitidis* share lipooligosaccharide epitopes but lack common capsular and class 1, 2, and 3 protein epitopes. Infect Immun 57:602, 1989

Wolf RE, Birbara CA: Meningococcal infections at an army training center. Am J Med 44:243, 1968

110 GONOCOCCAL INFECTIONS

KING K. HOLMES / STEPHEN A. MORSE

DEFINITION Gonorrhea, an infection of columnar and transitional epithelium caused by *Neisseria gonorrhoeae,* is the most common reportable communicable disease in the United States. Anatomic sites which can be infected directly by the gonococcus include the urethra, rectum, conjunctivas, pharynx, and endocervix. Local complications include endometritis, salpingitis, peritonitis, and bartholinitis in the female, and periurethral abscess and epididymitis in the male. Systemic manifestations of gonococcemia include arthritis, dermatitis, endocarditis, and meningitis as well as myopericarditis and hepatitis.

ETIOLOGY *Neisseria gonorrhoeae* is a gram-negative coccus usually found in pairs with flattened adjacent sides. It forms oxidase-positive colonies and is differentiated from other *Neisseria* by its

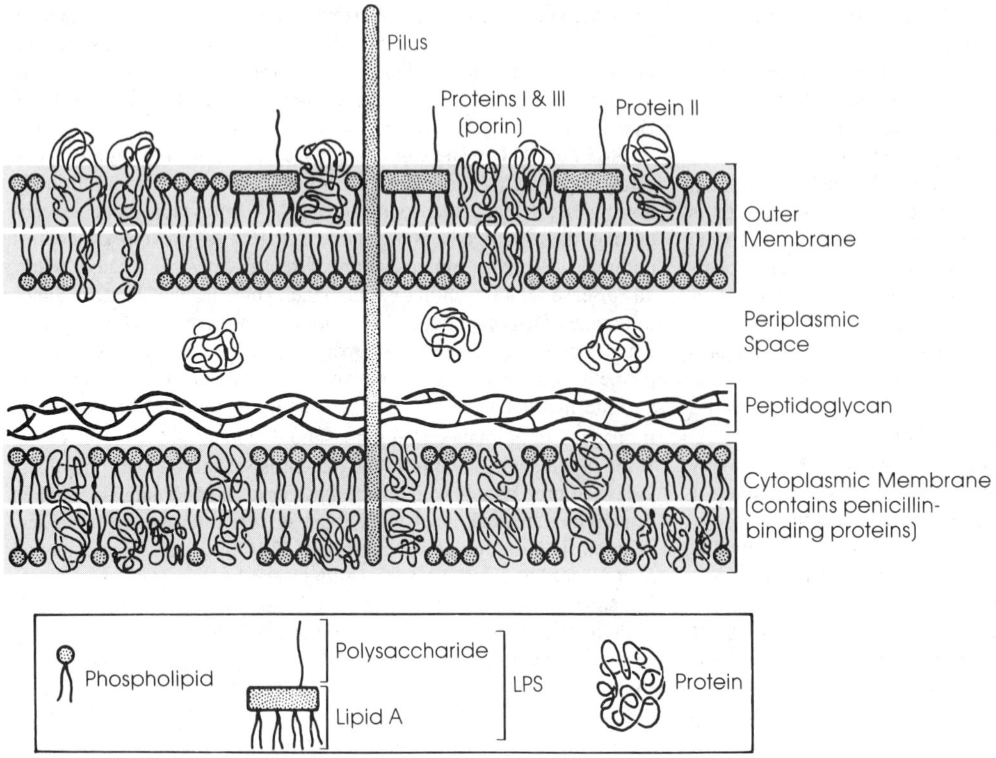

FIGURE 110-1 Diagram of the envelope of *N. gonorrhoeae*, showing structures thought to influence pathogenesis, antimicrobial susceptibility, and antigenicity.

ability to utilize glucose but not maltose, sucrose, or lactose, and by specific immunologic reactions.

Colonies examined within 20 h of inoculation from clinical specimens contain organisms covered by fimbriae (pili). As the colonies grow older, their appearance changes, reflecting the loss of pili. Piliated organisms cause infection and urethritis after inoculation into the urethras of male volunteers, whereas nonpiliated organisms do not. Pili mediate attachment to various epithelial cells and interfere with neutrophil phagocytosis. Each pilus is composed of repeating peptide subunits (pilin) which have a molecular weight of about 20,000. The pilin subunits consist of conserved and variable regions. Pili undergo both *antigenic* and *phase variation*. Chromosomal rearrangements, leading to expression of any one of a large number of incomplete (silent) pilin genes, lead to antigenic variation in pili (pil α, pil β, etc.). If the rearrangement involves a defective pilin gene, piliated gonococci (pil^+) produce nonpiliated variants (pil^-), a process known as *phase variation*. Antigenic variation of pilin may allow gonococci to adapt rapidly to attachment onto different types of epithelial surfaces and to evade the host's antibody response to pilin. Phase variation from pil^+ to pil^- may permit attachment and then persistence and spread.

The trilaminar outer membrane of the gonococcus contains several classes of proteins, including proteins I, II, and III, and lipopolysaccharide (Fig. 110-1). Like pili, protein II (now referred to as opacity-associated outer membrane proteins, or OPAs) also is thought to function as a ligand, mediating the attachment of gonococci to various types of human cells. As in the case with pili, individual strains of gonococci may or may not express OPAs. The serologic diversity of OPAs are relatively limited; up to seven or eight different OPAs may be expressed at different times by the same strain, and from zero to three may be expressed in the same gonococcal cell. The presence or absence of OPAs also influences colony opacity, and certain OPAs may be responsible for the clumping of gonococci that is so evident on Gram-stained smears of urethral exudate.

Opaque colonies contain organisms that express OPAs and predominate in isolates from the male urethra and in cervical isolates obtained from women in midcycle. Transparent colonies often lack OPAs and predominate in isolates from women during menses, and in isolates from blood, synovial fluid, or fallopian tubes.

Protein I (~32,000 mol wt) is quantitatively the major outer membrane protein. It appears to associate as a trimeric molecule, forming transmembrane channels (porins) that permit exchange of hydrophilic molecules through the outer membrane. Protein I also interacts with other outer membrane components, such as protein III and lipopolysaccharide (LPS), to form complex outer membrane structures. Protein molecules have been shown to move rapidly from gonococcal outer membranes to the more fluid cytoplasmic membrane of human cells. This process may initiate endocytosis of the gonococcus, the first step in gonococcal invasion of the epithelium.

The LPS of the gonococcus contains lipid A and an oligosaccharide. Gonococci have the ability to vary the composition of the oligosaccharide component of the LPS by a mechanism that is not well understood. One of the oligosaccharides is associated with serum resistance in *N. gonorrhoeae*. No capsular polysaccharide has been isolated, but high-molecular-weight surface polyphosphates have been demonstrated that may have functions similar to those of capsular polysaccharides in other organisms.

Gonococcal typing Gonococcal strains can be typed on the basis of nutritional requirements (auxotyping) or surface antigenic variation of protein I. Unlike pili and protein II, the protein I expressed by any single strain of gonococcus is antigenically stable, although there is considerable antigenic heterogeneity of protein I between strains. There are two structurally related forms of protein I, known as IA and IB, and individual strains contain either but not both. Protein IA and IB genes are alleles of the same gene. Monoclonal antibodies against different epitopes of protein IA and protein IB can be used to classify gonococci into a large number of serovariants, known as serovars IA1 to IA24, and IB1 to IB32.

EPIDEMIOLOGY The only natural hosts for *N. gonorrhoeae* are humans. In the United States the annual age-specific incidence rates tripled from 1963 to 1975, when over 1 million cases were reported and an equal number probably went unreported. During this period of epidemic gonorrhea, the incidence increased fastest in young white females. The incidence of gonorrhea has decreased from a peak of 473 cases per 100,000 in 1975 to about 300 per 100,000 in 1988.

Gonorrhea incidence and prevalence rates are known to be related to age, sex, sex preference, race, socioeconomic status, marital status, urban residence, and level of education—risk factors which influence sexual behavior, illness behavior, and accessibility of health care. Among sexually active individuals, the highest rates occur in teenagers, in nonwhites, in the poor and poorly educated, in large cities, and in unmarried persons—particularly those who live alone. Such individuals comprise a "core group" of "efficient transmitters" who play a disproportionate role in the spread of gonorrhea. Since 1985, the incidence of gonorrhea has continued to fall among white men and women, but has levelled off or increased among black men and women. There is some evidence that the spread of gonorrhea, like that of syphilis and chancroid, is associated with the crack cocaine epidemic and with exchange of sex by women for illegal drugs such as cocaine. The incidence of gonorrhea is highest in men, while the prevalence is highest in women. The prevalence rate is so high among women in the United States that routine endocervical cultures have been advocated for gonorrhea case detection in asymptomatic women age 30 or under who are considered to be at high risk because of sexual behavior or demographic factors cited above. However, greater reliance should be placed upon partner notification (contact tracing), which is far more efficient for control of gonorrhea, than upon routine endocervical culturing, which is expensive and does not focus on those most likely to transmit the infection. The single most important axiom about the epidemiology of this disease is that *gonorrhea is usually spread by carriers who have no symptoms or have ignored symptoms.* Symptomatic patients, male or female, have usually been recently infected by such carriers, who must in turn be traced and treated to prevent reinfection. *Men and women with symptomatic gonorrhea should always be interviewed to identify their recent sex contacts, who should be examined and treated if infected.* The growing association of gonorrhea, syphilis, and chancroid with the exchange of sex for drugs such as crack cocaine presents a new and unique challenge for sexually transmitted disease (STD) control and calls for intensified and innovative control efforts.

There are interesting regional differences in the antibiotic resistance of *N. gonorrhoeae*. In 1976, penicillinase-producing strains of *N. gonorrhoeae* (PPNG), completely resistant to penicillin and ampicillin, appeared almost simultaneously in two areas of the world: in England, where they had probably been imported from west Africa, and in the United States, where they had been imported from the Philippines. PPNG first became established and then spread in areas of the world where prostitution is exceptionally common and where access to subcurative antimicrobial therapy is unrestricted. PPNG now comprise 50 percent or more of all gonococci in many areas of Africa and Asia, and have by now become well established in many regions of the United States (e.g., Miami, New York, Los Angeles) and Europe. Plasmid-borne penicillin resistance results from the presence of a TEM-type β-lactamase gene on one of five small R factors which make up a very closely related family of plasmids. Plasmid-borne, tetracycline resistant *N. gonorrhoeae* (TRNG) is a highly resistant strain that results from the introduction of the streptococcal resistance determinant *tetM* into *N. gonorrhoeae,* where it resides on a plasmid derived in part from a conjugative plasmid. This new plasmid is self-transmissible and retains the capacity to mobilize some of the β-lactamase plasmids. TRNG are clinically resistant to tetracycline, minocycline, and doxycycline. Of equal importance has been the spread of gonococci with chromosomally mediated resistance to penicillin and tetracycline. These strains are referred to as chromosomally mediated resistant *Neisseria gonorrhoeae* (CMRNG). Auxotyping and monoclonal antibody serotyping have shown that in a midsized metropolitan city, as many as 60 to 100 different gonococcal strains are circulating, and new strains are being continuously introduced. Against this background, local outbreaks of PPNG, TRNG, or CMRNG belonging to a single auxotype-serovar class have been identified, and public health efforts have at times been successfully focused on the control of such strains.

IMMUNOLOGY AND PATHOGENESIS Epidemiologic data suggest that only about one-third of men become infected after a single exposure to gonorrhea, and under experimental conditions an inoculum of 10^3 organisms appears necessary to establish urethral infection in 50 percent of male volunteers. Factors that may confer resistance to infection are undefined. Components of the urethral or vaginal flora, such as *Candida albicans, Staphylococcus epidermidis,* and certain types of lactobacilli, can inhibit *N. gonorrhoeae* in vitro and may provide some natural resistance in vivo. Lactoferrin is present at mucosal surfaces, where it presumably competes with gonococci for iron, which is required for growth of the organism. However, when low environmental concentrations of iron are growth-limiting, gonococci produce iron repressible proteins, or FeRPs, that function in the removal of iron from lactoferrin or transferrin. Strains of gonococci requiring arginine, hypoxanthine, and uracil (AHU) for growth are generally unable to remove iron from lactoferrin, which could explain the tendency of such strains to cause asymptomatic mucosal infections. Gonococci infect mucus-secreting epithelial surfaces, and mucus could be a physical barrier or competitive inhibitor.

Attachment of gonococci to mucosal cells is mediated in part by pili and by protein II. Local antibody to pili or protein II can partially block attachment. Pili also impede phagocytosis of gonococci by neutrophils, and antibody to pili (as well as antibody to protein II) is opsonic. An enzyme produced by the pathogenic *Neisseria* IgA1 protease, which inactivates sIgA1, may interfere with IgA-mediated antiadherence activity, resulting in increased attachment.

Following attachment to columnar or transitional epithelium, gonococci penetrate through or between cells to reach the subepithelial connective tissue. Transfer of gonococcal protein I into the host cell may initiate endocytosis by the epithelial cell. Gonococcal LPS and peptidoglycan are toxic for fallopian tube organ cultures. Gonococci also produce several proteases, peptidases, phospholipases, and elastases which may play a role in pathogenesis. In subepithelial tissue, and in blood, gonococci presumably interact with serum antibody, including natural IgM antibody directed against LPS antigens, with generation of the chemotactic factor C5a and formation of the bactericidal C5b-C9 attack complex. Insertion of the attack complex into the outer membrane of serum-sensitive gonococci results in gonococcal cell lysis making antibody to LPS (like antibody to protein I) bactericidal. Although an attack complex is also formed when serum interacts with gonococci characterized by stable serum resistance, the insertion of the complex into the outer membrane of the organism has an abnormal configuration which does not result in rapid cell lysis. Furthermore, human serum also appears to contain non-complement-fixing IgG antibody directed against protein III which blocks the bactericidal action of IgM antibody for strains of gonococci with stable serum resistance.

Following phagocytosis by neutrophils, the susceptibility of gonococci to intracellular killing is controversial. During in vivo growth, gonococci apparently develop phenotypic serum resistance and resistance to neutrophil-mediated killing. The mechanisms responsible for these phenotypic changes are largely undefined but appear to involve the binding of host-derived CMP-*N*-acetyl neuraminic acid.

Spread of gonococci from the cervix to the endometrium and salpinges may be enhanced in women using an intrauterine device. Menstruation further increases the risk of intraluminal ascent from the cervix and also predisposes to gonococcal bacteremia.

CLINICAL MANIFESTATIONS The clinical spectrum of gonococcal infections depends upon the site of inoculation, the duration of infection, the virulence of the infecting strain, and the presence or absence of local or systemic spread of the organism. The influence of inoculum size, variations in host susceptibility, and of coinfection with *C. trachomatis* or other genital pathogens on clinical manifestations has not been well-defined.

Gonorrhea in the male The usual incubation period of gonococcal urethritis ("clap") in the male is 2 to 7 days following exposure, although longer intervals are not infrequent, and some men never develop symptoms. In one study, one auxotype with distinctive nutritional requirements was associated with 96 percent of asymptomatic infections and only 40 percent of symptomatic infections. Symptoms of urethritis include a purulent urethral discharge, usually associated with dysuria, frequent urination, and meatal erythema.

Although approximately 90 to 95 percent of men who acquire urethral gonococcal infection develop urethral discharge, most symptomatic men seek treatment and are removed from the infectious pool. The remaining men who never develop symptoms or who ignore their symptoms constitute about two-thirds of the infected men at any point in time, and they serve as the main source of spread of infection to women. Before antibiotic treatment became available, symptoms of urethritis persisted for an average of 8 weeks, and unilateral epididymitis occurred in 5 to 10 percent of untreated men. Epididymitis is now an uncommon complication (see below), and gonococcal prostatitis occurs rarely, if at all. Other local complications of gonococcal urethritis which are now unusual include inguinal lymphadenitis, edema of the penis due to dorsal lymphangitis or thrombophlebitis, submucous inflammatory "soft" infiltration of the urethral wall, periurethral abscess or fistula, unilateral inflammation or abscess of Cowper's gland (which lies between the thumb and forefinger when the forefinger is in the anal canal and the thumb is positioned anteriorly on the perineum), and, rarely, seminal vesiculitis.

In homosexual men, the frequency of gonococcal infection has fallen by 90 percent in many parts of the United States during the AIDS era of the 1980s. Gonococcal isolates from homosexual men tend to be more resistant to antimicrobials than are isolates from heterosexuals. This may be due to the fact that certain highly susceptible strains are rapidly killed by bile salts and fatty acids in feces and rarely occur in homosexual men, while gonococci possessing a gene for multidrug resistance (*mtr*) are resistant to bile salts and fatty acids and occur with increased frequency in homosexual men. Rectal infection may be asymptomatic from the outset or may produce anorectal pain, pruritus, tenesmus, and a bloody, mucopurulent rectal discharge. Proctoscopy and appropriate laboratory studies are essential to exclude several other conditions which cause similar symptoms (see Chap. 93). These symptoms may subside without treatment, leaving a chronic asymptomatic carrier state. Pharyngeal gonococcal infection occurs in approximately 20 percent of homosexual men or heterosexual women who engage in fellatio with men who have urethral infection, and in a smaller proportion of heterosexual men who engage in cunnilingus. Pharyngeal infection may produce exudative tonsillitis but frequently is asymptomatic; asymptomatic pharyngeal gonococcal infection usually clears spontaneously over several weeks, even without therapy.

Gonorrhea in the female Acute uncomplicated gonorrhea in the female often causes dysuria, frequent urination, increased vaginal discharge due to exudative endocervicitis, abnormal menstrual bleeding, and anorectal discomfort. While dysuria and frequency in young men arouse the suspicion of gonococcal urethritis, the same symptoms in a young woman are often automatically attributed to "cystitis." Actually, some of those without bacteriuria have gonococcal or chlamydial infection of the urethra. Young women with dysuria should have a thorough pelvic examination. Compression of the urethra through the anterior vaginal wall against the symphysis pubis may express urethral exudate which can be examined by Gram's stain and culture. Symptomatic young women with "sterile pyuria" (i.e., ≥ 10 neutrophils per $100\times$ microscopic field in the centrifuged sediment of clean-catch midstream urine; no uropathogens isolated from the urine) should be evaluated for gonococcal and chlamydial infection. Acute symptoms of gonococcal urethritis in the female may subside spontaneously or following subcurative therapy with sulfonamides or urinary antiseptics. The proportion of women with gonorrhea who never develop symptoms is undefined.

Asymptomatic gonococcal infection in the female involves the endocervix, urethra, anal canal, and pharynx, in decreasing order of frequency. Extension of infection from the endocervix to the fallopian tubes occurs in at least 15 percent of women with gonorrhea. This tends to occur soon after acquisition of infection or during menstruation and results in acute endometritis, with abnormal menstrual bleeding and midline low abdominal pain and tenderness, followed by *acute salpingitis,* the major complication of gonorrhea. Coexisting *C. trachomatis* infection may increase the rate of pelvic inflammatory disease (PID). Extension of infection to the pelvis may produce signs of pelvic peritonitis, accompanied by nausea and vomiting, and may lead to pelvic abscess. Early antibiotic treatment, before development of adnexal masses, restores normal tubal function and fertility in nearly all cases of gonococcal salpingitis. However, if prominent adnexal swelling has occurred before treatment is begun, bilateral tubal damage occurs in 15 to 25 percent.

Spread of gonococci or chlamydia into the upper abdomen may cause *perihepatitis* (Fitz-Hugh–Curtis syndrome) manifested by right upper quadrant or bilateral upper abdominal pain and tenderness, and occasionally by a hepatic friction rub.

Acute inflammation of Bartholin's gland is usually unilateral and frequently is due to gonococcal infection. The acutely infected duct is surrounded by a red halo and exudes pus at the posterior third of the labium majus. Occlusion of the duct results in formation of a Bartholin's abscess. Chronic Bartholin cysts are rarely caused by active gonococcal infection.

There is suggestive evidence that peripartum endocervical gonococcal infection is associated with premature rupture of membranes, preterm delivery, and postpartum endometritis.

Gonorrhea in children During childbirth, the gonococcus may infect the conjunctivas, pharynx, respiratory tract, or anal canal of the newborn. The risk of contamination increases with prolonged rupture of membranes. Prevention of gonococcal ophthalmia by prophylactic use of 1% silver nitrate eyedrops or ophthalmic preparations containing erythromycin or tetracycline is a cost-effective measure in most areas of the world, including the United States. Since neonates and young infants lack bactericidal IgM antibody against *N. gonorrhoeae,* they may be at increased risk for gonococcal bacteremia. During the first year of life, infection of the infant usually results from accidental contamination of the eye or vagina by an adult. Between 1 year of age and puberty, many cases of gonorrhea involve vulvovaginitis in females who have been molested, and medicolegal considerations necessitate a complete bacteriologic diagnosis and child welfare consultation. Auxotyping and serotyping of isolates from the sexual assault victim and accused assailant have been used as evidence in court.

Disseminated gonococcal infection The incidence of disseminated gonococcal infection (DGI) varies with time and place, in relation to the local incidence of infection with strains of gonococci that have a propensity to produce bacteremia. Approximately two-thirds of patients with DGI are women, and symptoms of bacteremia often begin during menses. The majority of men and women with gonococcemia do not have symptoms of urogenital, anorectal, or pharyngeal gonococcal infection.

Patients typically present either with symptoms and signs of gonococcemia, or with purulent arthritis affecting one or two joints. The onset of gonococcemia is characterized by fever, polyarthralgias, and papular, petechial, pustular, hemorrhagic, or necrotic skin lesions. Approximately 3 to 20 such lesions appear, usually on the distal extremities. Gonococci are demonstrable by immunofluorescent staining in about two-thirds of gonococcal skin lesions. The initial joint involvement is characteristically limited to tenosynovitis involving several joints asymmetrically. The wrists, fingers, knees, and ankles are most often involved. Circulating immune complexes have been demonstrated at this stage of infection in some studies. Serum complement levels are normal (except in those with complement deficiency), and the role of immune complexes, if any, is uncertain. Without treatment, the duration of gonococcemia is variable; the systemic manifestations of bacteremia may subside spontaneously within a week. Alternatively, septic arthritis ensues, often without prior symptoms of fever, polyarthralgias, or skin lesions. Pain and swelling then increase in one or, very occasionally, more joints, with accumulation of purulent synovial fluid, leading to progressive destruction of the joint if treatment is delayed.

IgM antibody to gonococcal lipopolysaccharide, present in normal human serum, is bactericidal for most strains of gonococci in the presence of complement. Gonococci isolated from patients with DGI have stable resistance to normal human serum. These strains usually contain outer membrane protein IA, and are highly susceptible to penicillin. They often require arginine, hypoxanthine, and uracil for growth, and belong to the AHU auxotype. Patients deficient in complement components C5, C6, C7, and C8 are uniquely susceptible to gonococcemia and meningococcemia because they cannot mount a serum bactericidal response to gonococci or meningococci. Strains isolated from these patients may not be resistant to normal human serum. However, gonococci isolated from DGI patients without complement deficiency are resistant to pooled normal human serum. Isolates from patients with tenosynovitis and skin lesions are even more serum-resistant than are isolates from patients with purulent arthritis, suggesting that the two different DGI syndromes may be determined by characteristics of the causative organism.

The probability of positive blood cultures decreases after 48 h of illness, and the probability of recovery of gonococci from synovial fluid increases with increasing duration of illness. Gonococci are infrequently recovered from early effusions containing less than 20,000 leukocytes per microliter, but are usually recovered from effusions containing more than 80,000 leukocytes per microliter. In the individual patient, gonococci are seldom recovered from blood and synovial fluid simultaneously.

Other common manifestations of disseminated gonococcal infection include mild myopericarditis and "toxic" hepatitis. Endocarditis and meningitis are infrequent but severe complications. Endocarditis is suggested by pathologic or changing heart murmurs, major embolic phenomena, severe myocarditis, deterioration of renal function, or an unusually large number of skin lesions.

DIFFERENTIAL DIAGNOSIS Gonococcal infection produces several common clinical syndromes which have multiple etiologies or which mimic other conditions. In particular, the epidemiology and clinical manifestations of *Chlamydia trachomatis* infections closely resemble those of gonococcal infections. The differential diagnosis of urethritis, epididymitis, and proctitis in men, vaginitis and cervicitis in women, and of acute arthritis in young adults is discussed in Chap. 93. The differential diagnosis of pelvic inflammatory disease is discussed in Chap. 94.

LABORATORY DIAGNOSIS A presumptive diagnosis of gonorrhea may be made if intracellular gram-negative diplococci are observed in leukocytes on Gram-stained smears of urethral or endocervical exudate. A diagnosis is equivocal if only extracellular or atypical gram-negative diplococci are seen, and is negative if no gram-negative diplococci are seen. When these criteria are employed by experienced microbiologists, the sensitivity and specificity of Gram's stain of the urethral exudate approach 100 percent. Presumptive diagnosis of gonorrhea cannot be made on the basis of gram-negative diplococci in pharyngeal smears because other *Neisseria* spp. are normal flora at this site. In areas where resistant gonococci are seen, culture should be performed to allow testing of isolates for antimicrobial resistance. The specificity of Gram's stain of purulent cervical exudate also is high, but the sensitivity is only about 50 percent. Selective media, i.e., Thayer-Martin (TM) medium, modified Thayer-Martin medium, and Martin-Lewis medium, which contain antibiotics to selectively inhibit most other organisms, are most useful for recovering the gonococcus from the urethra, endocervix, and pharynx. Rectal specimens are plated on modified Thayer-Martin medium or equivalent media containing trimethoprim lactate, which suppresses swarming organisms such as *Proteus* spp. The concentration of vancomycin in the selective medium should not exceed 3 μg/mL, and even this concentration may inhibit a small proportion of gonococci. After inoculation, the medium should be placed in a chamber with 70% humidity and an atmosphere containing 3 to 10% carbon dioxide to permit growth of the gonococcus. This can be accomplished in a candle jar, by generation of carbon dioxide chemically within packets that are sealed after inoculation, or within special CO_2 incubators. Inoculated media should be incubated at 35 to 37°C for 48 h, and putative gonococcal colonies should be confirmed by oxidase reaction, Gram's stain, sugar utilization tests, rapid enzyme tests, or agglutination reactions using antibodies that are specific for *N. gonorrhoeae*. The latter three tests are especially important for isolates from the pharynx and rectum and for cultures obtained from populations which have a low prevalence of gonorrhea, such as prenatal patients. DNA probes have been introduced for the confirmatory identification of *N. gonorrhoeae*. Limited comparisons indicate that they are at least equivalent in effectiveness to other confirmatory tests.

In men with incubating or chronic asymptomatic urethral infection without exudate, or as a test of cure following treatment, a very thin swab should be inserted 2 cm into the anterior urethra and used to inoculate TM or other selective medium. Cultures of the pharynx and rectum should be obtained from homosexual men with suspected gonorrhea.

The most efficient test for gonorrhea in women is the endocervical culture, which is positive on a single examination in approximately 80 to 90 percent of those with gonorrhea. This diagnostic yield can be increased by performing a second endocervical culture and by performing cultures of the rectum, urethra, and pharynx.

Standard blood culture broth medium (tryptic soy, Columbia, brain-heart infusion) should be used in culturing blood and is also recommended for culturing synovial fluid. The broth should be vented and incubated under increased CO_2 tension. Synovial fluid can also be plated onto chocolate agar rather than a selective medium because it is not likely to be contaminated with commensal bacteria. In pus from skin lesions, *N. gonorrhoeae* is demonstrable by immunofluorescent staining, but this test is seldom performed. Techniques designed to detect gonococcal infection by testing of a single serum for antibody to *N. gonorrhoeae* have been limited by inability to differentiate antibody due to past gonorrhea from antibody due to current infection, and by false-positive tests caused by cross-reactive antibody to *N. meningitidis*. For these reasons, serologic tests for gonorrhea have had a very low predictive value and are not used in clinical practice.

Another diagnostic approach is the detection of gonococcal antigen in urethral or cervical secretion by enzyme-linked immunosorbent assay (ELISA). In men with urethritis, the Gram stain is just as accurate, quicker, and cheaper. In women, such tests may be an acceptable alternative to culture for diagnosis of endocervical gonococcal infection in settings where culture is not feasible. However, the positive predictive value of antigen detection tests requires careful study, particularly in populations with a low prevalence of gonorrhea. The medical-legal and psychosocial implications of a false-positive diagnosis of gonorrhea can be troublesome.

TREATMENT Until 1989 the preferred drugs for gonococcal infection have been penicillin G, ampicillin or amoxicillin, tetracycline hydrochloride, and spectinomycin. Although long-acting forms of penicillin (such as benzathine penicillin G) are effective in syphilotherapy, they have *no place* in the treatment of gonorrhea. Penicillin V and the isoxazolyl penicillins are not recommended for the treatment of gonococcal infection. Similarly, first-generation cephalosporins are not used for gonorrhea. In 1989, the Centers for Disease Control published new guidelines for treatment of gonorrhea. These guidelines, which are presented in this chapter, are based upon several observations: the importance of single-dose efficacy; the increasing proportion of infections due to antibiotic-resistant strains of *N. gonorrhoeae*, including PPNG, TRNG, and strains with chromosomally mediated resistance to multiple antimicrobials; the high frequency of coexisting chlamydial infections in persons with gonorrhea; the absence of a cheap, rapid test for chlamydial infection; and the severity of complications of gonococcal and chlamydial infections. The guidelines do not represent a comprehensive list of all possible treatment regimens. As is shown in Table 110-1, a regimen combining a single intramuscular dose of ceftriaxone, together with a 7-day course of tetracycline or doxycycline, is recommended for uncomplicated urethral, endocervical, rectal, or pharyngeal gonococcal infections in heterosexual adults. This combination regimen can be expected to provide adequate therapy for gonorrhea at any site and

TABLE 110-1 Recommended treatment for gonococcal infection

Diagnosis	Treatment of choice
Uncomplicated urethral, endocervical, rectal, or pharyngeal infection	Ceftriaxone 250 mg single IM dose plus Doxycycline 100 mg PO twice daily for 7 days.
Treatment failure	True treatment failure with the above regimen has so far occurred rarely, if ever. Evaluate for reinfection, alternative diagnosis.
Alternative regimen	For patients unable to take ceftriaxone, use spectinomycin, 2-g single IM dose, plus doxycycline.
Gonorrhea in pregnancy	Ceftriaxone 250 mg single IM dose plus Erythromycin base 500 mg PO four times daily for 7 days. Equivalent dose of erythromycin stearate (500 mg) or ethylsuccinate (800 mg) can be used.
Disseminated gonococcal infection (DGI)	Hospitalization is recommended. Ceftriaxone 1 g IM or IV every 24 h or Ceftizoxime 1 g IV every 8 h or Cefotaxime 1 g IV every 8 h (see text for duration of inpatient and subsequent ambulatory therapy).
Gonococcal PID	Hospitalization is recommended. See Chap. 94 for recommended therapy.
Gonococcal epididymitis	See Chap. 93.
Pediatric gonococcal infections	
Infants	Ceftriaxone 25–50 mg/kg once daily or Cefotaxime 25 mg/kg twice daily. Usual duration of therapy is 7 days (longer for meningitis or endocarditis).
Children	Children who weigh 100 lb (45 kg) should receive adult doses; for those weighing less, see text.

will eliminate coexisting *C. trachomatis* infections. Tetracycline hydrochloride, 500 mg orally four times daily, can be substituted for doxycycline. Pregnant women and those unable to tolerate doxycycline or tetracycline can instead be given erythromycin base or stearate, 500 mg by mouth four times daily for 7 days, or erythromycin ethylsuccinate, 800 mg by mouth four times daily for 7 days, to accompany the ceftriaxone. All tetracyclines are ineffective as single-dose therapy for gonorrhea, and even a 7-day course of tetracycline has been ineffective in a growing proportion of patients, due to the spread of TRNG and the high proportion of strains with chromosomal resistance to tetracycline. Ceftriaxone can be prepared in 1% lidocaine as diluent (for intramuscular injection only) to reduce discomfort due to the injection. Other β-lactam antibiotics (cefotaxime, cefuroxime, ceftizoxime) and certain oxyquinolones (e.g., ciprofloxacin) are also very effective for resistant gonorrhea, but the long half-life of ceftriaxone, together with its in vitro activity, make it the optimal drug for single-dose therapy of gonorrhea. For patients who cannot take ceftriaxone, the preferred alternative is spectinomycin, 2 g intramuscularly as a single dose. Although spectinomycin resistance has emerged where that drug was used commonly for gonorrhea (e.g., in England and Korea), it has been rare in the United States. Other alternatives to ceftriaxone for uncomplicated urethral, endocervical, or rectal gonorrhea include ciprofloxacin, 500-mg single oral dose; cefuroxime axetil, 1-g single oral dose given simultaneously with probenecid, 1 g orally; cefotaxime, 1-g single intramuscular dose; or ceftizoxime, 500-mg single intramuscular dose.

All patients with gonorrhea should have a serologic test for syphilis at the time of diagnosis, and should be offered confidential testing for human immunodeficiency virus (HIV). Patients with incubating seronegative syphilis, without clinical signs of syphilis, are likely to be cured of syphilis by the recommended ceftriaxone-doxycycline regimen. However, patients with gonorrhea who also have syphilis or who are established contacts of someone with syphilis should be given additional treatment appropriate to the stage of syphilis (see Chap. 128).

Follow-up and treatment failure Treatment failure following combined ceftriaxone-doxycycline therapy is exceedingly rare; therefore, a follow-up culture is not essential. Patients should be advised to return for reexamination if any symptoms persist or recur after completion of treatment. Persistent or recurrent symptoms or signs after treatment for gonorrhea should be evaluated by culture for *N. gonorrhoeae* and a specific test for chlamydial infection. Any gonococcal isolate should be tested for antibiotic susceptibility. Additional treatment for gonorrhea should be with ceftriaxone, 250 mg intramuscularly, or with 2.0 g spectinomycin intramuscularly (except in areas where spectinomycin resistance is a problem). Recurrent gonococcal infections after treatment with the recommended schedule are almost certainly due to reinfection or indicate a need for improved sex partner referral and patient education.

Postgonococcal urethritis (PGU) usually becomes apparent about 2 to 3 weeks after treatment of gonorrhea with a penicillin or a cephalosporin. PGU often is caused by *C. trachomatis* which may have been acquired at the same time as gonorrhea but did not become clinically apparent until later because of the longer incubation period of chlamydial infection. When PGU occurs, it can be managed, like nongonococcal urethritis, with doxycycline, 100 mg orally twice daily, or tetracycline, 0.5 g four times a day, for at least 7 days. Similarly, mucopurulent cervicitis in women often persists or appears after treatment of gonorrhea with cephalosporin, penicillin, or spectinomycin, is often caused by *C. trachomatis,* and can be treated like PGU. Men and women exposed to gonorrhea should be examined, cultured, and treated with one of the recommended treatment schedules.

All pregnant women should be cultured for *N. gonorrhoeae* (and tested for *C. trachomatis* infection and syphilis) at the time of the first visit as an integral part of the prenatal care. A second culture late in the third trimester (as well as tests for chlamydial infection and syphilis) should be obtained from women at high risk of sexually transmitted disease.

The regimen of choice for gonorrhea in pregnancy is ceftriaxone, in a 250-mg single intramuscular dose, plus erythromycin for a possible coexisting chlamydial infection. Pregnant women allergic to β-lactams can be treated with a single dose of spectinomycin, 2.0 g intramuscularly, plus erythromycin. Doxycycline and tetracycline should not be used in pregnant women because of potential toxic effects for mother and fetus.

The management of pelvic inflammatory disease is discussed in Chap. 94.

Treatment of gonococcal arthritis can be accomplished satisfactorily with several regimens. Gonococci recovered from patients with gonococcal arthritis have been significantly less resistant to penicillin or tetracycline than isolates from patients with uncomplicated gonorrhea. However, several cases of DGI caused by PPNG have been reported. Because of the threat of endocarditis, meningitis, and joint sepsis, all patients with disseminated infection should be hospitalized and treated with ceftriaxone intravenously, 1 g once a day, or with the alternatives listed in Table 110-1. Reliable patients without endocarditis or meningitis can be discharged 24 to 48 h after symptoms resolve, to complete a total of 7 to 10 days' therapy with an oral regimen of cefuroxime axetil, 500 mg twice a day; amoxicillin, 500 mg, with clavulanic acid, 125 mg, three times a day; or (if not pregnant) ciprofloxacin, 500 mg twice a day. If the infecting gonococcus is shown to be penicillin-sensitive, treatment can be completed with oral amoxicillin, 500 mg three times a day, without clavulanic acid. Failure to improve with appropriate antimicrobial regimens as listed above strongly suggests a diagnosis other than disseminated gonococcal infection. Repeated joint aspiration or closed irrigation of the joint with sterile saline may be required to reduce inflammation in patients with high synovial fluid leukocyte counts. Open drainage is seldom, if ever, required for gonococcal arthritis, except in infants with hip infection. Temporary immobilization of the joint may reduce discomfort and may be useful during initial ambulation in patients with persistent effusions of the knee or ankle. Antibiotics should not be injected directly into the joint. Once the diagnosis of gonococcal arthritis is proven, then occasional patients may benefit from use of anti-inflammatory agents along with antimicrobial therapy. However, if the diagnosis is suspected, but not proven, then early use of anti-inflammatory drugs will prevent monitoring the response to antimicrobial therapy, which is usually rapid and often of diagnostic importance in gonococcal arthritis.

Meningitis and endocarditis caused by the gonococcus require high-dose intravenous therapy with an agent effective against the strain causing the disease: ceftriaxone, 1 g intravenously every 12 h, for 10 to 14 days for meningitis and for 1 month for endocarditis. Patients with gonococcal endocarditis or meningitis, and perhaps all patients with DGI, should be evaluated for complement deficiency.

Gonococcal conjunctivitis in the adult or in children over 20 kg should be managed as a medical emergency by irrigation of the conjunctiva with saline, together with ceftriaxone, 1 g in a single intramuscular dose. All patients must have careful ophthalmologic evaluation, including slit-lamp examination.

Pediatric gonococcal infection The infant born to a mother with gonorrhea is at high risk of infection and requires prophylactic treatment with a single injection of ceftriaxone, 50 mg/kg intravenously or intramuscularly, not to exceed 125 mg. Ceftriaxone should be given with caution to hyperbilirubinemic infants, especially premature babies. Topical prophylaxis for neonatal ophthalmia is not adequate treatment for infections at other sites. Infants with gonococcal infection at any site (e.g., eye) should be evaluated for DGI by examination and culture of blood and CSF. They should be treated for 7 days with ceftriaxone, 25 to 50 mg/kg in a single daily intravenous or intramuscular dose. Alternatively, cefotaxime can be used in a dose of 25 mg/kg twice daily intravenously. Limited data suggest that uncomplicated gonococcal ophthalmia in the infant can be cured with a single injection of ceftriaxone, 50 mg/kg, up to a dose of 125 mg. Irrigation of the eyes with saline or buffered ophthalmic solutions should be performed immediately and then repeated as often as necessary to eliminate discharge. Topical antibiotic preparations alone are not sufficient or required when appropriate systemic antibiotic therapy is given. Both of the parents of a newborn with gonococcal ophthalmia must be treated for gonorrhea. The parents and infant should also be tested for chlamydial infection.

Children who weigh 45 kg or more should be treated with adult regimens. Children who weigh less than 45 kg should be treated as follows: For uncomplicated vulvovaginitis, cervicitis, urethritis, proctitis, and pharyngitis, the recommended treatment is ceftriaxone, a 125-mg single intramuscular dose. The alternative regimen is spectinomycin, a 40 mg/kg single intramuscular dose. Children 8 years of age or older can also be given doxycycline, 100 mg twice a day for 7 days. Children with gonorrhea should be evaluated for coexisting syphilis and chlamydial infection.

Topical and/or systemic estrogen therapy is of no benefit in gonococcal vulvovaginitis. All children should have follow-up cultures, and the source of infection should be identified, examined, and treated. Child abuse should be carefully considered and evaluated. For treatment of complicated disease, the alternative regimens recommended for adults may be used in appropriate pediatric dosages.

Treatment of gonorrhea in developing countries The proportion of gonococcal infections caused by PPNG or CMRNG is highest in developing countries, which can least afford ceftriaxone, spectinomycin, or other new antimicrobials effective against these strains. Inexpensive alternatives to penicillin G and tetracycline, the traditional mainstays of gonorrhea therapy, have been disappointing. For example, a sulfonamide-trimethoprim combination which initially cured over 95 percent of cases of gonorrhea in African countries, fell to less than 75 percent efficacy within 2 years after it became a popular regimen in Kenya. One approach has been the use of 4.8 million units of procaine penicillin G intramuscularly plus 1.0 g probenecid orally (a standard regimen for non-PPNG infections) together with 125 mg of clavulanic acid (in the form of one capsule of amoxicillin-clavulanate) to inhibit gonococcal β-lactamase. This inexpensive regimen has been effective in small trials in Kenya, even against PPNG infections. Gentamicin, in a 280-mg single intramuscular dose, has also been used effectively in this setting. Newer cephalosporins in lower than recommended doses, to reduce cost, should be discouraged. There is a growing need for clinical trials with less expensive regimens, and for ongoing surveillance of in vitro sensitivity of *N. gonorrhoeae*.

PREVENTION AND CONTROL There is probably no more striking illustration than gonorrhea of the failure of a specific treatment alone to eradicate a communicable disease. Vaccination is not available. A field trial of a purified gonococcal pili vaccine in U.S. soldiers in Korea showed that the vaccine was not effective. Use of the condom can prevent transmission, and the extensive use of condoms for contraception may be responsible for the low rates of gonorrhea in some countries (e.g., Japan). Spermicidal preparations used with a diaphragm or impregnated with nonoxynol-9 cervical sponges probably offer some protection against gonorrhea and chlamydial infection. Prophylactic antibiotics (e.g., 200 mg minocycline or doxycycline taken soon after sexual exposure) reduce the risk of infection, but are not recommended for general use or for individuals with known exposure to gonorrhea, who should receive one of the regimens recommended for established gonorrhea.

To contain the increasing spread of antimicrobial-resistant gonococci, several measures are important: (1) routine use of diagnosis by cultures and testing of isolates for antimicrobial resistance or β-lactamase production; (2) routine use of ceftriaxone to prevent gonorrhea treatment failures; and (3) rapid identification and treatment of sexual partners of patients with gonorrhea, particularly partners of those with recurrent infection and those known to be infected with resistant gonococci.The most effective public health measure now available for control of gonorrhea is treatment of sexual partners of infected patients.

REFERENCES

Boslego JW et al: Effect of spectinomycin use on the prevalence of spectinomycin resistant and of penicillinase-producing *Neisseria gonorrhoeae*. N Engl J Med 317:272, 1987

Britigan BE, Sparling PF: Gonococcal infection: A model of molecular pathogenesis. N Engl J Med 312:1683, 1985

Centers for Disease Control: 1989 Sexually transmitted diseases treatment guidelines. Morb Mort Week Rep 38(Suppl 8):1, 1989

———: Policy guidelines for the detection, management, and control of antibiotic resistant strains of *Neisseria gonorrhoeae*. Morb Mort Week Rep 36(5S):1, 1987

Handsfield HH et al: Localized outbreak of penicillinase-producing *Neisseria gonorrhoeae:* Paradigm for introduction and spread of gonorrhea in a community. JAMA 261:2357, 1989

Hook EH III, Holmes KK: Gonococcal infections. Ann Intern Med 102:229, 1985

Knapp JS et al: Serologic classification of *Neisseria gonorrhoeae* using monoclonal antibodies directed against outer membrane protein I. J Infect Dis 150:44, 1985

Morse SA et al: High-level tetracycline resistance in *Neisseria gonorrhoeae* is result of acquisition of streptococcal *tetM* determinant. Antimicrob Agents Chemother 30:664, 1986

——— (eds): Perspectives on pathogenic *Neisseria* spp. Clin Microb Rev 2:1S, 1989

Plummer FA et al: Epidemiologic evidence for the development of serovar-specific immunity after gonococcal infection. J Clin Invest 83:1472, 1989

Rice PA et al: Immunoglobulin G antibodies directed against L protein III block killing of serum-resistant *Neisseria gonorrhoeae* by immune serum. J Exp Med 164:1735, 1986

Sparling PF: Biology of *Neisseria gonorrhoeae*, in *Sexually Transmitted Diseases*, 2d ed, KK Holmes et al (eds). New York, McGraw-Hill, 1990, pp 131–147

111 DISEASES CAUSED BY GRAM-NEGATIVE ENTERIC BACILLI

DENNIS R. SCHABERG / MARVIN TURCK

The Enterobacteriaceae are a group of gram-negative nonsporing rods which are aerobic but can grow under anaerobic conditions, and which are commonly found in the gastrointestinal tract. They are characterized biochemically by their ability to ferment glucose, their ability to reduce nitrates to nitrites, and the fact that they are oxidase-negative. The diverse genera in this family, including *Escherichia, Salmonella, Shigella, Klebsiella, Serratia, Enterobacter, Proteus, Morganella, Yersinia, Providencia,* and other less common genera, are differentiated by serologic tests and computerized analysis of biochemical reactions. It is important to make this differentiation, not only taxonomically but also because of epidemiologic and therapeutic implications.

Other gram-negative bacilli which are not members of the family Enterobacteriaceae may also be causes of infection. Important genera include *Pseudomonas, Acinetobacter,* and *Eikenella.*

ESCHERICHIA COLI INFECTIONS

ETIOLOGY *Escherichia coli* is a commensal in the gastrointestinal tract. It may spread from there to infect contiguous structures if normal anatomic barriers are interrupted, as occurs in appendiceal perforation. It is believed that the urinary tract is infected via urethral contamination, but direct hematogenous spread may also account for renal infection. Once infection has occurred in a primary focus, further spread to distant organs may occur via the bloodstream. A consequence of bacteremia that occurs potentially with all gram-negative bacilli is septic shock (Chap. 89). In more than 50 percent of *E. coli* infections, the urinary tract is the portal of entry; infections emanating from the hepatobiliary tree, peritoneal cavity, skin, and lung are also common. Some patients with *E. coli* bacteremia have no demonstrable portal of entry; they often are leukopenic. There may be other defects in host resistance, including diabetes mellitus, cirrhosis, and sickle cell anemia or recent administration of irradiation, cytotoxic drugs, glucocorticoids, or antibiotics. There is also epidemiologic evidence that *E. coli* and other Enterobacteriaceae tend to colonize the skin and mucous membranes of debilitated patients, possibly accounting for the increased frequency of these infections in patients with advanced illness.

EPIDEMIOLOGY Strains of *E. coli* are characterized by their somatic (O), flagellar (H), and capsular (K) antigens, and there are hundreds of different serologic varieties. Any of the strains is capable of causing disease. Clinical and epidemiologic studies have demonstrated that certain specific *E. coli* serotypes are more frequently incriminated in diarrheal disease of the infant and newborn as well as in outbreaks of enteric disease in adults. Strains incriminated in infantile diarrhea probably are disseminated within nurseries by symptomatic or asymptomatic infant carriers, mothers, and staff. Although fecal contamination is the usual mode of spread, airborne contamination and fomite spread may also occur.

Some epidemiologic studies have suggested that *E. coli* O4, O6, and O75 are responsible for most *E. coli* infections other than infantile diarrhea. It is unclear whether these strains actually are more virulent or merely are more prevalent than other somatic types.

Strains of *E. coli* with K1 antigen are recovered from an inordinate number of neonates with meningitis. These K antigens have been implicated in promoting adherence to host cells and in resisting phagocytosis.

MANIFESTATIONS **Urinary tract infections** *Escherichia coli* accounts for over 75 percent of urinary tract infections, including cystitis, pyelitis, pyelonephritis, and asymptomatic bacteriuria (Chap. 95). Strains cultured from patients with acute uncomplicated urinary tract infections are almost invariably *E. coli,* whereas other Enterobacteriaceae and strains of *Pseudomonas* become prevalent among patients with chronic infection.

Peritoneal and biliary infections *Escherichia coli* can usually be cultured from a perforated or inflamed appendix or from abscesses secondary to perforated diverticula, peptic ulcers, subphrenic or lesser sac abscesses, or mesenteric infarction. Often, other organisms, including anaerobic streptococci, clostridia, and *Bacteroides,* are found along with *E. coli.* Acute cholecystitis with gangrene and perforation is often associated with *E. coli* infection. An air-fluid level associated with stones or a circumferential layer of gas in the wall of the gallbladder may be detectable by x-ray and is characteristic of acute emphysematous cholecystitis. From the gallbladder, infection may ascend via the biliary tree to produce cholangitis and multiple liver abscesses. More rarely, *E. coli* infection in the peritoneal cavity may produce a septic thrombophlebitis of the portal vein (pylephlebitis), which in turn is followed by liver abscesses.

Bacteremia Invasion of the bloodstream is the most serious manifestation of *E. coli* infection; it is characterized usually by the sudden onset of fever and chills but sometimes only by mental confusion, dyspnea, or unexplained hypotension. It is most common in patients with urinary tract infection and biliary or intraperitoneal sepsis. In some patients no portal of entry is evident. Most cases occur in elderly males, presumably because of the high incidence of urethral instrumentation and catheterization in this group. Hyperventilation may be an early sign. Hypotension may be present from the onset but usually occurs within 12 to 16 h after bacteremia; if it is persistent, it is accompanied by oliguria and often by mental confusion, stupor, and coma, a syndrome known as *gram-negative* or *septic shock* (Chap. 89). Occasionally, *E. coli* bacteremia develops in patients with cirrhosis without an overt portal of entry. This has been attributed to portosystemic shunts both in and around the liver, impaired reticuloendothelial function, and diminution in humoral and cellular defense mechanisms. Persistence or reappearance of bacteremia with *E. coli* or other members of the Enterobacteriaceae on therapy, so-called breakthrough bacteremia, has a poor prognosis and suggests an intraabdominal focus for infection or undrained pus.

Other manifestations *Escherichia coli* may produce abscesses anywhere in the body. Subcutaneous infections are found at the site of insulin administration in diabetics, in ischemic extremities, and in surgical wounds. Perirectal phlegmons are not uncommon in patients with leukemia. Subcutaneous abscesses, especially among diabetics, are often characterized by formation of gas in tissue, which may be detected by crepitation or by x-ray and which must be differentiated from clostridial infection. This is most rapidly accomplished by Gram's stain. *Escherichia coli* may cause pneumonia de novo; also, *E. coli* are often cultured from sputum in pulmonary superinfections.

Neonatal infection Neonates, particularly premature infants, often develop *E. coli* bacteremia associated with meningitis and bloodborne pyelonephritis. Fecal soiling and absence of maternal gamma-globulin (IgM) antibody are two of the factors which render this group particularly susceptible to *E. coli* infections.

Gastroenteritis Some strains of *E. coli* can interact with intestinal mucosa by a variety of pathogenic mechanisms to produce gastroenteritis. Some strains are enterotoxigenic (ETEC) and can produce one of two toxins, one heat labile (LT) and similar to the toxin elaborated by *Vibrio cholerae* and the other heat stable (ST) (see also Chaps. 92 and 122). As a toxin-mediated process the diarrhea from ETEC generally is large in volume and watery. Other *E. coli* produce bloody diarrhea and are referred to as enterohemorrhagic (EHEC). These strains were first recognized in patrons of fast-food restaurants; *E. coli* O157:H7 was isolated from hamburger in one outbreak. These strains produce Shiga's toxin, also called verotoxin, because of the cytotoxicity it produces with vero cells in tissue culture. A third clinical picture that can be due to *E. coli* is a dysenteric type of stools with low volume but with abdominal cramps, blood, and mucus. These strains are enteroinvasive (EIEC) and carry a large plasmid also found in invasive *Shigella* strains. Finally, some patients, especially children under 2 years of age, develop gastroenteritis typified by nausea, vomiting, and watery diarrhea. Most outbreaks of this disease have occurred in nurseries and have been due to specific serotypes of enteropathogenic *E. coli* (EPEC). These strains appear to have special adherence for mucosal cells, a property that correlates with ability to cause diarrhea. The rapid dehydration, with its attendant high mortality, demands prompt recognition of this condition, isolation of the infants, and treatment of both patients and contacts.

LABORATORY FINDINGS There are no characteristic laboratory abnormalities. The white blood cell count is usually elevated, and there is a preponderance of granulocytes. At times, however, the white count is normal or low. When *E. coli* infection occurs in previously healthy individuals, anemia is absent, but more commonly there is anemia which is usually related to underlying disease. *Escherichia coli* grows readily in a variety of bacteriologic media and should be cultured from appropriate secretions and blood. In the presence of bacteremia there can be metabolic derangements, including azotemia, metabolic acidosis, hypokalemia, and hyperkalemia as well as a variety of coagulation defects.

DIAGNOSIS *E. coli* cannot be differentiated from most other gram-negative bacteria on Gram's stain, and culture followed by appropriate biochemical characterization is necessary to identify the organism precisely. Serologic typing of *E. coli* may be useful in individual patients with recurrent urinary tract infections in order to help differentiate between relapse and reinfection.

TREATMENT As with other infections, drainage of pus and removal of foreign bodies are essential. If *E. coli* is suspected as the etiologic agent in a particular infection, choice of an appropriate antimicrobial will depend upon the site and type of infection as well as upon its severity; outcome is often related to underlying disease. For example, in acute, uncomplicated urinary tract infection in females, the disease is frequently self-limited even without antimicrobial therapy, and there is no evidence that antibiotics are superior to sulfonamides. Conversely, sustained *E. coli* bacteremia is associated with a high incidence of shock, and the response and survival are highly dependent on the choice of the correct antimicrobial.

In most situations, antibiotics should be selected on the basis of in vitro susceptibility tests. Although no drug is uniformly active against all strains of *E. coli*, a number of agents are effective against the majority of clinical isolates. Resistance to ampicillin is close to 30 percent in most hospitals, and for severe infections, cephalosporins are recommended as the initial treatment. Third-generation cephalosporins have lower minimal inhibitory concentrations (MICs) for *E. coli*; this increased activity coupled with slightly enhanced CNS penetration make them useful for the therapy of meningitis due to *E. coli* (Chap. 354). Gentamicin and tobramycin have been employed effectively in the initial treatment of severe *E. coli* infections in doses of 5 mg/kg per day in divided doses every 8 h. Amikacin is very active against isolates which are resistant to the other aminoglycosides in doses of 15 mg/kg per day, divided to be administered every 8 to 12 h. Tetracyclines and chloramphenicol are still used in the treatment of *E. coli* infection, but better drugs are now available. Although combinations of antimicrobials have been recommended, there is little need to employ more than one agent in most situations. Nitrofurantoin (400 mg) and nalidixic acid (2 to 4 g) are reserved for treating patients with *E. coli* bacteriuria, and should not be employed when infection is suspected outside the urinary tract. Trimethoprim-sulfamethoxazole and the fluoroquinolones are also useful, especially in urinary tract infections (Chap. 85). Intravenous trimethoprim-sulfamethoxazole is effective for treating severe *E. coli* infections and can be substituted for aminoglycosides, cephalosporins, or ampicillin.

PREVENTION Isolation and antimicrobial therapy of infants and contacts are essential to abort epidemic infantile diarrhea. In adults, many *E. coli* infections are hospital-associated, and their incidence can be reduced by limiting use of indwelling urinary and intravenous catheters, by careful surgical aseptic technique, by appropriate isolation of infection-prone patients, and by judicious use of antibiotics, glucocorticoids, and cytotoxic agents.

KLEBSIELLA-ENTEROBACTER-SERRATIA INFECTIONS

ETIOLOGY Next to *E. coli*, strains of *Klebsiella, Enterobacter*, and *Serratia* are the most important enteric organisms infecting humans. These are also of the family Enterobacteriaceae. In many laboratories *Klebsiella* are more resistant to antibiotics than are *E. coli*, and their isolation from blood, purulent exudates, and urine is of more serious epidemiologic and prognostic significance. The Friedlander bacilli (*K. pneumoniae*) are encapsulated gram-negative bacilli found among the normal flora of the mouth and intestinal tracts. *Klebsiella* are closely related to the genera *Enterobacter* and *Serratia* and may be differentiated only by certain amino acid decarboxylase tests. In addition to differentiation by these biochemical tests, which identify the *Klebsiella, Enterobacter*, and *Serratia* groups, strains of *Klebsiella* usually are nonmotile and form large mucoid colonies on solid media, whereas the other species are typically motile. Strains of *Klebsiella* can be further distinguished on the basis of type-specific capsular antigens; more than 75 known capsular types have been identified. There is little evidence that certain types are more virulent than others, and the main role of capsular typing of *Klebsiella* is as an epidemiologic tool in nosocomial outbreaks of infection.

Klebsiella rhinoscleromatis is probably the causative agent of rhinoscleroma, and *K. ozenae* has been isolated occasionally from the noses of patients with ozena, a chronic severe rhinitis associated with turbinate atrophy and progressive anosmia. *Klebsiella oxytoca* is the new designation for indole-positive strains of *K. pneumoniae*.

PATHOGENESIS *Klebsiella, Enterobacter*, and *Serratia* are all capable of causing disease in diverse anatomic sites. However, results of clinical and epidemiologic studies suggest that differences in pathogenicity may exist among these genera and that precise taxonomic identification is of value. Although infections of the respiratory tract with *K. pneumoniae* have been emphasized most in the past, the urinary tract presently accounts for the majority of clinical isolates. In this site clinical manifestations and pathogenesis are similar to those of infections produced by *E. coli*, but *Klebsiella* is more frequently found in patients with complicated and obstructive urinary tract disease. Infections of the biliary tract, peritoneal cavity, middle ear, mastoids, paranasal sinuses, and meninges also are not uncommon. In these locations, *Klebsiella* is more frequent than either *Enterobacter* or *Serratia* and is more likely to produce an illness of greater severity. The apparent increased frequency of infection by *Serratia* represents an increase primarily due to nosocomial spread of this organism. *Enterobacter* species have been incriminated frequently in outbreaks of in-hospital bacteremia attributed to contaminated intravenous solutions.

MANIFESTATIONS Symptoms and signs of common infections caused by *Klebsiella*—namely, those involving the urinary tract, biliary tree, and peritoneal cavity—are indistinguishable from those caused by *E. coli*. These infections commonly occur in diabetics and in the form of superinfections in patients who have received antimicrobials to which these organisms are resistant. *Klebsiella* infection is also an important etiologic agent in septic shock. *Serratia* and *Enterobacter* are almost exclusively nosocomial pathogens. These organisms have been implicated as pathogens in a wide variety of infections, most frequently pneumonia, urinary tract infections, and bacteremia.

Pneumonia *Klebsiella* is well recognized as a pulmonary pathogen but probably accounts for less than 1 percent of all cases of community-acquired bacterial pneumonia. The disease is most common in men over 40 years of age and is most frequently found in alcoholics. Other factors associated with increased susceptibility include diabetes mellitus and chronic bronchopulmonary disease. Aspiration of oropharyngeal secretions containing *Klebsiella* organisms is the likely inciting factor among alcoholic patients. The clinical manifestations are indistinguishable from those of pneumococcal pneumonia (Chap. 99), with sudden onset of chills, fever, productive cough, and severe pleuritic chest pain. Patients are frequently delirious and prostrated, but this may also occur with pneumococcal infection. The pulmonary lesion is most frequent in the right upper lobe but often rapidly progresses and, if untreated, may spread from lobe to lobe. Cyanosis and dyspnea develop rapidly, and jaundice, vomiting, and diarrhea may be present. Physical findings consist primarily of consolidation, unless pleural effusion or necrotizing pneumonitis with rapid cavitation has intervened. The blood leukocyte count may be elevated but is often low, which probably is a reflection of severe infection in an alcoholic patient with poor bone marrow reserve and folate deficiency. Lung abscess and empyema are much more frequent than they are in pneumococcal pneumonia; they are related to the destructive capabilities of this organism. So-called characteristic radiographic features such as bulging fissures and loss of lung volume occur only occasionally; they also may be found in pneumococcal infection as well as in necrotizing pneumonia caused by other gram-negative species.

Klebsiella, Serratia, and *Enterobacter* are frequently seen in nosocomial pneumonia. Older patients become colonized with gram-negative bacilli in the oropharynx, and these organisms can then gain access to the respiratory tract and cause pneumonia or purulent bronchitis. Common-source outbreaks, with contamination of a variety of respiratory therapy devices, have been implicated in infections with these pathogens, especially *Serratia*. As a general rule, the most drug-resistant strains of *Serratia* are nonpigmented and account for the majority of nosocomial isolates. However, pigmented and multiply sensitive *Serratia* isolates are also seen in device-related infections. Rarely, infection with *Klebsiella* may progress, often in indolent fashion, to a chronic necrotizing pneumonitis resembling tuberculosis. The principal symptoms are productive cough, weakness, and anemia.

DIAGNOSIS Diagnosis of community-acquired pneumonia is established by an awareness of the clinical setting in which *Klebsiella* infections occur and by isolation of the organism. A presumptive diagnosis of *Klebsiella* pneumonia should be made on the basis of a Gram's stain of the sputum which shows a predominance of short, plump, gram-negative bacilli, frequently surrounded by a clear space because of the capsule. Often these gram-negative organisms occur together with gram-positive cocci, and because the gram-positives are easier to see, the gram-negative bacteria may be ignored and the diagnosis may be missed. This, in turn, may lead to potentially serious delays in instituting therapy. Additional proof of *Klebsiella* infection in the lung is the isolation of the organisms from blood and pleural exudate. In extrapulmonary infections, the organisms are readily seen in, or cultured from, pus or secretions of involved organs.

The diagnosis of nosocomial respiratory infection with these organisms may be more difficult, mainly because colonization has to be distinguished from infection. Careful evaluation of the clinical course is necessary in establishing a diagnosis. Transtracheal aspiration of sputum for culture and Gram's stain or bronchoscopy may be useful in difficult cases.

TREATMENT *Klebsiella, Enterobacter,* and *Serratia* have variable susceptibility to antimicrobial drugs, and cultures of these organisms need to be tested in vitro. Frequently, antimicrobial therapy needs to be begun before results of antibiotic susceptibility tests are available. In general, most strains of *Klebsiella* are susceptible to the aminoglycosides and the third-generation cephalosporins. *Klebsiella* isolates do not respond to most penicillin analogues, although many isolates are inhibited by ureidopenicillins, e.g., mezlocillin. *Serratia* isolates are frequently resistant to many antimicrobials, and resistance to gentamicin and tobramycin is being encountered with increasing frequency. Amikacin has been used effectively in these drug-resistant infections. The antimicrobial regimen of choice in the treatment of *Klebsiella, Enterobacter,* and *Serratia* infection will vary from one institution to another depending on the resistance patterns as well as upon the degree of clinical severity of infection. In severely ill patients, the combination of an aminoglycoside such as tobramycin or gentamicin (3 to 5 mg/kg per day) or amikacin (15 mg/kg per day) with cephalothin, cephapirin, or cefazolin (4 to 12 g/d) is usually preferred. Cefoxitin, third-generation cephalosporins, aztreonam, or imipenem-cilastatin also may be active against *Klebsiella, Enterobacter,* and *Serratia*. Occasionally, one or all of these compounds may be more active than the older cephalosporins, and in vitro susceptibility tests will be required to select the most appropriate agent. Trimethoprim-sulfamethoxazole is often an effective agent against *Klebsiella, Serratia,* and *Enterobacter* species resistant to other antimicrobials. Aztreonam can be used to treat these and other serious gram-negative infections in patients who have experienced IgE-based β-lactam hypersensitivity in the past (Chap. 85). Regardless of the antimicrobial regimen employed, treatment should be continued for a minimum of 10 to 14 days and prolonged if there is extensive cavitation. Pleural effusions must be drained; antibiotic therapy alone is not sufficient treatment for closed-space infections of the pleural cavity. At times, rib resection with open drainage may be necessary and should be considered if effusions recur.

PROGNOSIS Before the introduction of antimicrobials, the fatality rate from these infections varied from 50 to 80 percent, and death within 48 h was not infrequent. Even with antimicrobial treatment the course of these infections is quite variable and the prognosis must be guarded. For the most part, the prognosis reflects the age group involved and the frequent association of *Klebsiella* infections with alcoholism, malnutrition, and severe underlying disease.

PROTEUS, MORGANELLA, AND *PROVIDENCIA* INFECTIONS

ETIOLOGY The genus *Proteus* of the family Enterobacteriaceae consists of gram-negative bacilli which do not ferment lactose and are characterized by their active motility and spreading growth on solid media. Organisms once thought to be related and once classified as *Proteus* have been renamed based on detailed DNA studies. *Proteus morganii* has been reclassified as *Morganella morganii,* while some biogroups of *Proteus rettgeri* have been reclassified as *Providencia stuartii* and *Providencia rettgeri*. *Proteus mirabilis* and *Proteus vulgaris* retain their nomenclature; *Proteus mirabilis* causes 75 to 90 percent of human infections. It is distinguishable from the other organisms mentioned by its inability to form indole. All four split urea, with production of ammonia. Some strains of *Proteus vulgaris* share a common antigen with certain rickettsia, which accounts for the appearance of antibodies against *Proteus* organisms (Weil-Felix reaction) in typhus, scrub typhus, and Rocky Mountain spotted fever. The *Providencia* group of organisms resembles those of the genus *Proteus* closely except for some differences in biochemical tests.

EPIDEMIOLOGY AND PATHOGENESIS These organisms are normally found in soil, water, and sewage and are part of the normal fecal flora. Occasionally, they have been implicated as a cause of epidemic diarrhea in infants, but the evidence for this is inconclusive. They are frequently cultured from superficial wounds, draining ears, and sputum, particularly in patients who have received antibiotics; they replace the more susceptible flora eradicated by these drugs.

MANIFESTATIONS These organisms are rarely primary invaders but produce disease in locations previously infected by other pathogens. These locations include skin, ears and mastoid, sinuses, eyes, peritoneal cavity, bone, urinary tract, meninges, lung, and bloodstream.

Cutaneous infections These organisms can be isolated from surgical wounds, particularly after antimicrobial therapy, but they do not interfere with normal wound healing provided that the tissues are viable and foreign bodies are not present. Burns, varicose ulcers, and decubitus ulcers may become contaminated with these organisms, often in company with other gram-negative bacilli or staphylococci.

Infections of the ears and mastoid sinuses Otitis media and mastoiditis, especially with *Proteus mirabilis,* can result in extensive destruction of the middle ear and mastoid sinuses. Fetid otorrhea, cholesteatoma, and granulation tissue constitute a chronic focus of infection in the middle and inner ears and mastoid, and deafness ensues. Paralysis of the facial nerve is an occasional complication. The great danger of these infections lies in intracranial extension, leading to thrombosis of the lateral sinus, meningitis, brain abscess, and bacteremia.

Ocular infections These pathogens may cause corneal ulcers, usually following trauma to the eye, which occasionally terminate in panophthalmitis and destruction of the eyeball.

Peritonitis Because they are part of the normal intestinal flora, these organisms may be isolated from the peritoneal cavity following perforation of viscera or mesenteric infarction.

Urinary tract infections These organisms are a common cause of urinary tract infections, usually in patients with chronic bacteriuria, many of whom have had obstructive uropathy, a history of bladder instrumentation, and repeated courses of chemotherapy. They are often recovered from bacteriuric patients with renal or bladder calculi. This may be related to the urease activity which renders the urine alkaline and provides a fertile medium for formation of ammonium-magnesium-phosphate stones.

Bacteremia Bloodstream invasion is the most serious manifestation of infection with this organism. In 75 percent of cases, the urinary tract serves as the portal of entry; in the remainder, the biliary tree, gastrointestinal tract, ears and sinuses, and skin are the primary foci. Bacteremia is frequently preceded by cystoscopy, urethral catheterization, transurethral prostatic resection, or other operative procedures. Clinically, the signs, symptoms, and laboratory findings of sepsis—high fever, chills, shock, metastatic abscess, leukocytosis, and thrombocytopenia—are indistinguishable from those of bloodstream infections with *E. coli, Klebsiella,* or other gram-negative bacteria.

DIAGNOSIS The diagnosis of *Proteus, Morganella,* or *Providencia* infection depends on culture of the organism from blood, urine, or exudate and its identification by appropriate biochemical tests. It is especially important to separate *Proteus mirabilis,* the indole-negative species, from organisms that are indole-positive, because only *P. mirabilis* is susceptible to the action of penicillin and many other antibiotics. *Proteus* organisms are often present in mixed infections with other pathogens. Particular care should be exercised in the isolation of other organisms growing in the same medium with *Proteus mirabilis* or *Proteus vulgaris* lest they be masked by spreading growth. The spreading character of these bacteria also may make antibiotic sensitivity tests difficult to interpret.

TREATMENT Most strains of *Proteus mirabilis* are sensitive to penicillin in high concentration (10 units per milliliter or greater), ampicillin, carbenicillin, gentamicin, tobramycin, or amikacin, and the cephalosporin antibiotics. *Proteus mirabilis* bacteriuria can be readily eradicated with any of these drugs during treatment; ampicillin in dosage of 0.5 g every 4 to 6 h is highly effective. In severe infection, therapy should be parenteral: 6 to 12 g ampicillin or 20 million units of penicillin G plus tobramycin or gentamicin in divided doses of 5 mg/kg per day, if renal function is adequate. There is some evidence that an aminoglycoside is synergistic with ampicillin and penicillin G in *P. mirabilis* infections. In general, all strains of *P. mirabilis* are resistant to tetracycline. Most strains other than *P. mirabilis* are predictably sensitive only to aminoglycosides and the third-generation cephalosporins. Carbenicillin, ticarcillin, and the ureidopenicillins, imipenem-cilastatin, and aztreonam are effective against many isolates. Ideally, therapy should be based on in vitro susceptibility, or lacking this, an awareness of local resistance patterns. As with all other gram-negative infections, appropriate attention must be given to drainage of pus, maintenance of fluid and electrolyte status, and, if septic shock is present, treatment of circulatory collapse.

PSEUDOMONAS INFECTIONS

ETIOLOGY *Pseudomonas aeruginosa* is a motile gram-negative rod which generally is not encapsulated and forms no spores. It grows readily in all ordinary culture media, and on agar it forms irregular, soft, iridescent colonies which usually have a fluorescent yellow-green color because of diffusion into the medium of two pigments, pyocyanin and fluorescein. *Pseudomonas* produces acid but no gas in glucose, and it is proteolytic. It is oxidase-positive and produces ammonia from arginine. A number of different strains have been identified by immunofluorescent techniques or bacteriophage typing. There is no evidence that these strains vary in their virulence for humans. Other *Pseudomonas* species (*P. maltophilia, P. cepacia, P. fluorescens, P. testosteroni,* and *P. putida*) also may cause infection in human beings. For the most part, these organisms have been associated with common-source nosocomial outbreaks; in addition, they have been incriminated in bacteremia, endocarditis, and osteomyelitis in narcotic addicts.

EPIDEMIOLOGY *Pseudomonas* organisms are present on the skin of some normal persons, particularly in the axilla and anogenital regions. They are uncommon in the stools of adults not receiving antibiotics. In the majority of instances, *Pseudomonas* organisms are cultured as avirulent secondary contaminants in superficial wounds or from the sputum of patients treated with antibiotics. Ordinarily this is of little consequence because the organisms merely fill the bacteriologic vacuum left by the elimination of more sensitive bacteria. Occasionally, however, infections with *Pseudomonas* organisms occur in the ear, lung, skin, or urinary tract of patients, often after the primary pathogen has been eradicated by antibiotics. Serious infections are almost invariably associated with damage to local tissue or with diminished host resistance. Despite the many potential virulence factors shared by strains of *Pseudomonas,* the organism rarely causes disease in healthy persons. Patients compromised by cystic fibrosis and those with neutropenia appear at particular risk to severe infection with *P. aeruginosa.* Premature infants; children with congenital anomalies and patients with leukemia (who are usually receiving antibiotics, adrenal glucocorticoids or antineoplastic drugs); patients with burns; and geriatric patients with debilitating diseases are likely to develop *Pseudomonas* infections. Most often these infections occur in the hospital environment, and they generally are exogenous infections with the organism acquired from sources other than the patient's normal flora. In hospitals, the organisms have been cultured from a variety of sources that have in common an aqueous environment, including such items as sinks, antiseptic solutions, and aqueous medications. The organism is prevalent in urine receptacles and on catheters, and on the hands of hospital staff. In several outbreaks, *Pseudomonas* urinary tract infections appear to have been transmitted from patient to patient by human carriers. Similar epidemics have been reported in nurseries among premature infants, and cross-infection on burn wards is common. Although *P. aeruginosa* is found in the gastrointestinal tract of only approximately 5 percent of normal adults, carriage rates increase in hospitalized patients.

PATHOGENESIS The portal of entry of *Pseudomonas* organisms varies with the patient's age and underlying disease. In infancy and childhood, the skin, umbilical cord, and gastrointestinal tract predominate; in old age, the urinary tract is more often the primary focus. Often the infections remain localized to the skin or subcutaneous tissues. In burns, the region below the eschar may become massively infiltrated with bacteria and inflammatory cells and usually serves as the focus for bacteremia, the single most lethal complication. Hematogenous dissemination is characterized by hemorrhagic nodules in many areas, including the skin, heart, lungs, kidneys, and meninges. The histologic picture is one of necrosis and hemorrhage. Typically the walls of arterioles are heavily infiltrated with bacteria, and the vessels are partially or wholly thrombosed.

Most strains of *P. aeruginosa* produce a layer of slime which is rich in carbohydrate and shares heat-stable somatic antigenicity with the cell wall. Antibody against the specific serologic type of slime antigen affords protection to experimental challenge. Most isolates also produce a number of exotoxins. Exotoxin A, which shares many properties with diphtheria toxin, is the most potent toxin produced by *P. aeruginosa*. In life-threatening infection with *P. aeruginosa*, high antibody titers against exotoxin A correlate with increased survival.

MANIFESTATIONS *Pseudomonas* infections occur in many locations, including the skin, subcutaneous tissues, bone and joints, eyes, ears, mastoid and paranasal sinuses, meninges, and heart valves. Bacteremia without a detectable primary focus may also occur and should raise the question of contaminated intravenous medications, intravenous solutions, or antiseptics used for preparing an intravenous site, especially when *Pseudomonas* species other than *P. aeruginosa* are isolated.

Infections of the skin and subcutaneous tissues *Pseudomonas* organisms are frequently cultured from surgical wounds, varicose and decubitus ulcers, and burns, particularly following antibiotic therapy. Draining tuberculous or osteomyelitic sinuses may become secondarily infected. The mere presence of *Pseudomonas* in these sites is of little significance provided that bacterial multiplication deep in subcutaneous tissues does not occur and bacteremia does not ensue. Cutaneous infections usually heal after removal or slough of devitalized tissue. *Pseudomonas* organisms may be responsible for green nails in persons whose hands are excessively exposed to water, soap, and detergents, who have onychomycosis, or whose hands are subject to mechanical trauma. The organism can usually be cultured from the nail plate. It has been incriminated in whirlpool-associated dermatitis. The disease is benign and resolves spontaneously.

Osteomyelitis Osteomyelitis is unusual with *Pseudomonas* except as a complication of bacteremia, intravenous drug abuse, or puncture wounds. If a puncture wound, especially a nail puncture of the foot in a child, fails to respond to standard therapy within 3 to 4 days, complicating *Pseudomonas* osteomyelitis must be considered.

Infections of the ear, mastoid, and paranasal sinuses Otitis externa is the most common form of *Pseudomonas* infection which involves the ear. It is particularly troublesome in tropical climates and is characterized by chronic serosanguineous and purulent drainage from the external auditory canal. A rapidly progressive, severe infection due to *Pseudomonas* involving the ear, referred to as malignant otitis externa, can develop, especially in diabetics. In contrast to the usual otitis externa, this infection requires aggressive management including surgical debridement and parenteral antimicrobial therapy. Otitis media or mastoiditis usually occurs as a superinfection following eradication of gram-positive organisms by antimicrobial agents.

Infections of the eye Corneal ulceration is the most severe form of ocular *Pseudomonas* infection. It usually follows a traumatic abrasion and may terminate in panophthalmitis and destruction of the globe. Purulent conjunctivitis occurs as a manifestation of *Pseudomonas* infection in premature infants. Contamination of contact lenses or lens fluid may be an important means of infecting the eyes with *Pseudomonas*.

Urinary tract infections *Pseudomonas* organisms are common pathogens in the urinary tract and are usually found in patients with obstructive uropathy who have been subjected to repeated urethral manipulations or to urologic surgery. *Pseudomonas* bacteriuria is in no way unique and cannot be distinguished from infection with other organisms on clinical grounds.

Gastrointestinal tract *Pseudomonas* organisms have been implicated as a cause of epidemic diarrhea of infancy. In addition, a number of infants dying from neonatal sepsis have the classic necrotic, avascular ulcers of *Pseudomonas* bacteremia in the bowel at autopsy. A "typhoidal" form of *Pseudomonas* infection characterized by fever, myalgia, and diarrhea occurs predominantly in the tropics. This illness, also called 13-day fever or Shanghai fever, is self-limited, and the prognosis is good.

Respiratory tract Primary *Pseudomonas* pneumonia is infrequent, and culture of this organism from the sputum usually is indicative of aspiration of oropharyngeal contents with secondary infection following eradication of a more sensitive flora with antibiotics. The normal oropharyngeal flora of hospitalized patients is frequently replaced by gram-negative rods, including *Pseudomonas*, early in hospitalization. A variety of nosocomial events, most notably administration of sedative medications, endotracheal intubation, and intermittent positive pressure breathing treatments, can predispose to respiratory infection with *Pseudomonas*. Pulmonary infection is often associated with microabscesses. The organism is often isolated from the sputum of patients with bronchiectasis, chronic bronchitis, or cystic fibrosis who have lingering infections punctuated by multiple courses of chemotherapy, or from the stomata of tracheostomy sites. *Pseudomonas* bronchitis and bronchiolitis may be the terminal event in cystic fibrosis, and sputum isolates often have a characteristic mucoid colonial morphology when cultured on agar.

Meningitis Spontaneous *Pseudomonas* meningitis is unusual, but the bacilli may be introduced into the subarachnoid space by lumbar puncture, spinal anesthesia, intrathecal medication, or head trauma. Shunts performed for hydrocephalus may become contaminated with *Pseudomonas*, and revision or removal of the shunt offers the best hope of cure.

Bacteremia Bloodstream invasion tends to occur in debilitated patients, premature infants, children with congenital defects, patients with lymphomas, leukemias, or other malignant tumors, and elderly patients who have undergone surgery or instrumentation of the biliary or urinary tract. *Pseudomonas* bacteremia is an important cause of death in patients with severe burns. In adults, *Pseudomonas* bacteremia is indistinguishable from bloodstream infection with other bacterial species except for two findings: (1) ecthyma gangrenosum, the classic skin lesion, often located in the anogenital or axillary region as a round, indurated, purple-black area about 1 cm in diameter with an ulcerated center and a surrounding zone of erythema; and (2) rarely, the passage of green urine, presumably due to the hemoglobin pigment verdoglobin. Organisms usually can be cultured from cutaneous lesions and may provide an early clue to the diagnosis.

Bacterial endocarditis A number of cases of *Pseudomonas* subacute bacterial endocarditis have followed open-heart surgery. Usually the organisms become implanted on a silk suture or a synthetic patch employed for closure of septal defects. Reoperation with removal of the vegetation and foreign bodies offers the best hope of cure. *Pseudomonas* endocarditis has been found on normal heart valves in patients with burns and in drug addicts. Metastatic abscesses in bone, joint, brain, adrenal glands, and lungs are frequent consequences of *Pseudomonas* endocarditis (see Chap. 90).

TREATMENT Localized *Pseudomonas* infection can be treated by irrigation with 1% acetic acid or topical therapy with colistin or polymyxin B. Debridement and drainage of purulent material is essential when deeper tissues are involved. For deep-seated tissue infections and life-threatening infection, such as pneumonia or bacteremia, parenteral therapy must be employed. The aminoglycoside antibiotics tobramycin and gentamicin inhibit most strains of *Pseudomonas*. In patients with normal renal function, 5 mg/kg per day in divided doses will provide inhibitory levels. Amikacin is also active against *Pseudomonas* and is especially useful against strains which have developed enzyme-mediated drug resistance to tobramycin and gentamicin. It should be given in doses of 15 mg/kg per day in divided doses. Replacement of amikacin-sensitive by amikacin-resistant *Pseudomonas* has been reported in a few instances. Ticarcillin and mezlocillin are active against most strains of *Pseudomonas* in doses of 16 to 20 g/d. Piperacillin and azlocillin are active in vitro against some isolates not inhibited by ticarcillin. These isolates are usually nosocomial in origin. The combination of an aminoglycoside active against *Pseudomonas* plus an antipseudomonal penicillin is frequently employed to delay emergence of resistance during therapy and provides enhanced activity, especially in granulocytopenic patients with *Pseudomonas* infection. Ceftazidime plus an aminoglycoside makes for the most effective treatment for serious *Pseudomonas* infection. Asymptomatic bacteriuria, particularly when confined to the bladder, should be treated with the least toxic agent, which at times may be a sulfonamide or tetracycline. The fluoroquinolone antimicrobics such as norfloxacin or ciprofloxacin are very active against *P. aeruginosa* at urinary concentrations. Ciprofloxacin is also useful in prolonged oral treatment of osteomyelitis or pulmonary infections with *P. aeruginosa*. The antimicrobial susceptibility of *Pseudomonas,* except for *P. aeruginosa,* is variable, and some of these isolates may be resistant to aminoglycoside antibiotics. Some of the newer cephalosporins like cefoperazone and ceftazidime are also active in vitro against many isolates of *Pseudomonas*. Selective pressure of intense antimicrobial use in closed settings such as burn units or intensive care units has resulted sometimes in strains of *Pseudomonas* resistant to the usual β-lactams. Imipenem-cilastatin often remains active against such isolates, but should be combined with an effective aminoglycoside to avoid emergence of resistance.

PROPHYLAXIS *Pseudomonas* cross-infections in hospitals can be reduced by careful attention to aseptic techniques and good infection control practices (see Chap. 83). Systemic antibiotic prophylaxis aimed at preventing colonization and infection with *Pseudomonas* organisms has been notoriously unsuccessful and should be interdicted. A polyvalent vaccine for *Pseudomonas* has been developed, as well as hyperimmune gamma globulin. The latter is undergoing intensive evaluation in prophylaxis and therapy of serious *Pseudomonas* infections.

PROGNOSIS The mortality rate in *Pseudomonas* bacteremia is 75 percent and is highest in patients with shock or severe associated disease such as massive third-degree burns, leukemia, or prematurity. When bacteremia originates in the urinary tract and is not accompanied by shock, the prognosis is considerably better. Localized *Pseudomonas* infections do not present a threat to life unless hematogenous dissemination occurs.

ACINETOBACTER INFECTIONS

DEFINITION Organisms of the genus *Acinetobacter* are pleomorphic, gram-negative bacilli which are easily confused with members of the genus *Neisseria.* Severe infections with these organisms, including meningitis, bacterial endocarditis, pneumonia, and bacteremia, have been described with increasing frequency.

ETIOLOGY *Acinetobacter calcoaceticus* var. *lwoffi* was described by DeBord as *Mima polymorpha* in 1939. It is one of two well-characterized varieties of *Acinetobacter,* the other being *Acinetobacter calcoaceticus* var. *anitratus,* formerly called *Herellea vaginicola.* These organisms are pleomorphic, gram-negative, encapsulated, and nonmotile. They grow well on ordinary media, forming white, convex, smooth colonies. Diplococcal forms predominate in colonies grown on solid media; rods and filamentous forms are more common in liquid media. The species can be differentiated from the Enterobacteriaceae by their negative nitrate reaction and from members of the genus *Neisseria,* which they may resemble morphologically, by their simple growth requirements, their bacillary form in liquid media, and their usually negative oxidase reaction.

EPIDEMIOLOGY AND PATHOGENESIS *Acinetobacter* organisms are ubiquitous. Twenty-five percent of normal subjects are skin carriers of *Acinetobacter*. The striking association of *Acinetobacter* bacteremia with cutdowns or indwelling intravenous catheters favors the skin as a major portal of entry in human beings. *Acinetobacter* pneumonia, both as a primary infection and as a superinfection, also points to the respiratory tract as an important portal of entry. It appears that *Acinetobacter* organisms are normal human commensals of relatively low virulence which produce colonization much more frequently than infection. Infections seem to occur in patients subjected to the same epidemiologic pressures encountered with nosocomial, gram-negative bacilli; serious infections are produced under conditions of decreased host resistance, or in the presence of instrumentation, or with prior broad-spectrum antimicrobial therapy. An unexplained predominance of *Acinetobacter* pulmonary infections occurring in late summer has been noted. The role of these organisms as a cause of conjunctivitis, vaginitis, and urethritis requires further documentation.

MANIFESTATIONS Serious infections caused by *Acinetobacter* include (1) meningitis, (2) subacute and acute bacterial endocarditis, (3) pneumonia, (4) urinary tract infections, and (5) bacteremia. Usually, the signs and symptoms associated with infections in these sites are no different from those produced by other pathogens. Occasionally, *Acinetobacter* may be the cause of a fulminating bacteremia, with high fever, vascular collapse, petechiae, and ecchymoses, which is indistinguishable from fulminant meningococcemia. More often, however, bacteremia is associated with an overt portal of entry, such as infected cutdowns or indwelling intravenous catheters, surgical wounds, or burns; it may follow urethral or other surgical instrumentation. The clinical picture presented by these patients is dominated by endotoxemia, and the prognosis is poor.

DIAGNOSIS The diagnosis of *Acinetobacter* infection can be missed, either because the clinical bacteriology laboratory is unfamiliar with these organisms and reports them incorrectly or because they are considered contaminants. The confusion attending the taxonomic classification of these organisms has not simplified matters. For practical purposes, isolation of *Acinetobacter* from blood, spinal fluid, sputum, urine, or pus should be considered significant unless there is no evidence of infection on clinical grounds. Since *Acinetobacter* isolates are resistant to penicillin and members of the genus *Neisseria* are sensitive, differentiation of these organisms is of obvious importance.

TREATMENT Antibiotic sensitivities of *Acinetobacter* strains vary, but most strains are inhibited by gentamicin, tobramycin, amikacin, imipenem-cilastatin, the ureidopenicillins such as piperacillin, and aztreonam. Sensitivity to the tetracyclines is unpredictable, and most strains are resistant to penicillin, ampicillin, the cephalosporins, erythromycin, and chloramphenicol. For serious systemic infections, the appropriate antibiotic, generally an aminoglycoside, should be administered, and since these organisms may produce localized abscesses, surgical drainage may be necessary.

EIKENELLA INFECTIONS

ETIOLOGY *Eikenella corrodens* is a facultătively anaerobic or capnophilic gram-negative rod which is oxidase-positive. As colonies develop on blood agar, characteristic "pitting" or "corroding" of the agar is seen with many strains and generally requires 48 to 72 h of growth to develop.

EPIDEMIOLOGY *Eikenella corrodens* is an inhabitant of the mouth, upper respiratory tract, and gastrointestinal tract of mammals. Infections frequently involve bowel or oral contamination. A striking association between *Eikenella* infections and methylphenidate abuse has been noted, perhaps related to the low redox potential created by "skin popping" of this agent as well as a tendency for needles to become contaminated with oral secretions through needle licking.

MANIFESTATIONS The most common infection caused by *Eikenella* is that of skin or soft tissue. Endocarditis, pneumonia, osteomyelitis, and meningitis are reported but are rare. *Eikenella* infections frequently mimic infections caused by strict anaerobes such as *Bacteroides fragilis* or *Peptostreptococcus*. The infections are indolent and frequently mixed with aerobic gram-positive cocci, and drainage is often foul-smelling. Abscess formation is common.

TREATMENT *Eikenella corrodens* is susceptible to penicillin, ampicillin, carbenicillin, and tetracycline. Adequate drainage of purulent material is essential in the management of these infections. Ampicillin or penicillin coupled with surgical drainage generally provides a good response. Of note is the marked resistance of *Eikenella* to clindamycin, making the differentiation between *Eikenella* infections and those caused by mixed anaerobes even more important.

REFERENCES

Enterobacteriaceae: General

BOSCIA JA et al: Epidemiology of bacteriuria in an elderly ambulatory population. Am J Med 80:208, 1986
KARNAD A et al: Pneumonia caused by gram-negative bacilli. Am J Med 79:61, 1985
KREGER BE et al: Gram-negative bacteremia. Am J Med 68:332, 1980
MAKI DG: Nosocomial bacteremia: An epidemiologic overview. Am J Med 70:719, 1981
MOORE RD et al: Association of aminoglycoside plasma levels with therapeutic outcome in gram-negative pneumonia. Am J Med 77:657, 1984
TANCREDE CH, ANDREMONT AO: Bacterial translocation and gram-negative bacteremia in patients with hematological malignancies. J Infect Dis 152:99, 1985

Escherichia coli infections

GERACI JE et al: Endocarditis due to gram-negative bacteria. Mayo Clin Proc 57:145, 1982
LEVINE MM: *Escherichia coli* that cause diarrhea: Enterotoxigenic, enteropathogenic, enteroinvasive, enterohemorrhagic, and enteroadherent. J Infect Dis 155:377, 1987
OSTROFF SM et al: Infections with *Escherichia coli* 0157:H7 in Washington State. JAMA 262:355, 1989
RAHAL JJ, SIMBERKOFF MS: Host defense and antimicrobial therapy in adult gram-negative bacillary meningitis. Ann Intern Med 96:468, 1982

Klebsiella-Enterobacter-Serratia infections

COOPER R, MILLIS J: *Serratia* endocarditis. Arch Intern Med 140:199, 1980
MELTZ DJ, GRIECO MH: Characteristics of *Serratia marcescens* pneumonia. Arch Intern Med 132:359, 1973
RENNIE RP, DUNCAN IBR: Emergence of gentamicin-resistant *Klebsiella* in a general hospital. Antimicrob Agents Chemother 11:179, 1978

Proteus infections

BERGER SA: *Proteus* bacteremia in a general hospital. J Hosp Infect 6:293, 1985
IANNINI PB et al: Multidrug-resistant *P. rettgeri*. Ann Intern Med 55:161, 1976
SENIOR BW et al: The ureases of *Proteus* strains in relation to virulence for the urinary tract. J Med Microbiol 13:468, 1982

Pseudomonas infections

BAGEL J, GROSSMAN ME: Subcutaneous nodules in *Pseudomonas* sepsis. Am J Med 80:528, 1986
BODEY GP et al: Infections caused by *Pseudomonas aeruginosa*. Rev Infect Dis 5:279, 1983
GOULD IM, RISE R: *Pseudomonas aeruginosa:* Clinical manifestations and management. Lancet 2:1224, 1985
HILF M et al: Antibiotic Therapy for *Pseudomonas aeruginosa* bacteremia: Outcome correlations in a prospective study of 200 patients. Am J Med 87:540, 1989
MALONEY J et al: Analysis of amikacin-resistant *Pseudomonas aeruginosa* developing in patients receiving amikacin. Arch Intern Med 149:630, 1989
MORRISON AJ, WENZEL RP: Epidemiology of infection due to *Pseudomonas aeruginosa*. Rev Infect Dis 6(Suppl):S627, 1984
POLLACK M: The virulence of *Pseudomonas aeruginosa*. Rev Infect Dis 6(Suppl):S617, 1984

Acinetobacter infections

BERGOGNE-BEREZIN E et al: Epidemiology of nosocomial infections due to *Acinetobacter calcoaceticus*. J Hosp Infect 10:105, 1987
HARSTEIN AI et al: Multiple intensive care unit outbreak of *Acinetobacter calcoaceticus* subspecies *antitratus* respiratory infection and colonization associated with contaminated, reusable ventilator circuits and resuscitation bags. Am J Med 85:624, 1988

Eikenella infections

SURVANGOOL SL et al: Pathogenicity of *Eikenella corrodens* in humans. Arch Intern Med 143:2265, 1983

112 MELIOIDOSIS AND GLANDERS

JAY P. SANFORD

MELIOIDOSIS

DEFINITION Melioidosis is an infection of humans and animals with a protean clinical spectrum. Melioidosis, which means "a resemblance to distemper of asses," bears a striking resemblance to glanders both clinically and pathologically, but is epidemiologically dissimilar.

ETIOLOGY Melioidosis is caused by a gram-negative motile bacillus, *Pseudomonas pseudomallei,* which can be differentiated from *P. mallei* by bacteriologic and serologic means. *P. pseudomallei* (also known as Whitmore's bacillus) is a small, gram-negative, motile, aerobic bacillus. When it is stained with methylene blue, Wayson's, or Wright's stain, marked irregularities with a bipolar "safety pin" pattern are observed. It grows well on standard bacteriologic media, with a characteristic wrinkling of colony surfaces after 48 to 72 h of incubation. Two antigenic types have been distinguished, type I (Asian), found widely, including in Australia, and type II (Australian), found mainly in Australia. The two types are equally pathogenic.

EPIDEMIOLOGY The disease is endemic in southeast Asia where human and animal cases occur commonly. Disease in humans has been reported from adjacent areas including India, Borneo, the Philippines, Guam, Indonesia, Sri Lanka, New Guinea, and Australia (north Queensland, Northern Territory). Cases in humans or animals have been reported from Madagascar, Chad, Kenya, Central West Africa (Niger, Upper Volta), Iran, and Turkey. In 1976, *P. pseudomallei* was isolated from animals in the Paris zoo. Human melioidosis has been described only rarely in the western hemisphere (Panama, Ecuador, Mexico)—a neonatal case in Hawaii, a case in Georgia, and a possible case in Oklahoma. With these exceptions, confirmed melioidosis has occurred in United States or European residents only when they have traveled in endemic areas. As of January 1973, when all American forces had been withdrawn from Vietnam, there had been 343 cases with 36 deaths reported in United States Army personnel who were or had been in Vietnam.

Pseudomonas pseudomallei is a saprophyte which can be isolated from soil, ponds, rice paddies, and market produce in endemic areas. Its ubiquitous nature is illustrated by its isolation as a laboratory contaminant or following an intraarticular injection. *Pseudomonas pseudomallei* is capable of causing disease in epizootic form among sheep, goats, swine, and horses. Occasional isolates have also been reported from cows, rodents, dogs, cats, wallabies, and birds. Although animals are susceptible to the disease, they apparently do not represent a reservoir for human disease. Attempts to culture *P. pseudomallei* from the urine and feces of a large variety of healthy animals have been unsuccessful. Arthropod-borne infection does not occur naturally. Humans contract melioidosis by soil contamination of skin abrasions. Ingestion, nasal instillation, and inhalation are other probable methods of spread. In contrast to glanders, infections have been uncommon, but can occur, in laboratory workers. *P. pseudomallei* has been recovered from urine specimens of patients who had urethral catheters, while hospitalized in an endemic area. Person-to-person transmission of melioidosis is rare. Venereal transmission is extremely rare. Also, the development of melioidosis in a 2-day-old newborn in Hawaii and demonstration of a significant antibody titer in a nurse who had never been in an endemic area but who had worked on wards with melioidosis patients raises the question of spread from person-to-person within a hospital.

PATHOLOGY In acute infections, the majority of lesions occur in the lungs, with occasional abscesses in other organs. In subacute infections, lung abscesses tend to be more extensive, and lesions are found throughout the body, in the skin, subcutaneous tissue, meninges, brain, eye, heart, liver, kidney, spleen, bone, prostate, synovial membranes, and lymph nodes. The acute abscesses are characterized by an outer border of hemorrhage, a medial zone heavily infiltrated with polymorphonuclear leukocytes, and an inner core of necrotic debris containing large histiocytes with two or three nuclei that have been termed giant cells. A striking histologic feature has been the marked karyorrhexis. In chronic infections, the lesion consists of a central area of caseation necrosis, mononuclear and plasma cells, and granulation tissue. Calcification does not occur.

Melioidosis is associated with impaired cellular immunity; total lymphocyte counts are usually less than 1000 per microliter; the percentage of total T cells is less than 50 percent due to a decrease in T helper cells; and skin tests with dinitrochlorobenzene are negative.

The number of T suppressor cells is normal, as is the number of B cells.

CLINICAL MANIFESTATIONS The clinical manifestations of melioidosis are variable. The illness can present as an acute, subacute, or chronic process. The incubation period has not been defined; however, judging by the lapse of time between injury and the development of infection, it may be as short as 2 days. Following a laboratory accident, an incubation period of 3 days ensued. Clinically inapparent infections may remain latent for a number of years after an individual leaves an endemic area, with an interval of 26 years reported in one patient. Men are more often affected than women, a finding which is thought to represent occupational exposure. Melioidosis may be recognized as inapparent infection, asymptomatic pulmonary infiltration, acute localized suppurative infection, acute pulmonary infection, acute septicemic infection, or chronic suppurative infection.

Inapparent infection In Thailand, Vietnam, and Malaysia, 6 to 8 percent of healthy adult men have significant antibody titers against *P. pseudomallei,* with the prevalence reaching 20 percent in a group of Army recruits from the rice-growing states of western Malaysia. Only 1 percent of Thai women had positive reactions. None of the sera from a control group from the United States was positive. The prevalence of significant antibody titers has been reported as 2 percent for Europeans living in Vietnam and 1 to 9 percent in unselected patients in United States Army hospitals and in a group of normal uninjured soldiers who had served in Vietnam. Occasionally, asymptomatic infections have been discovered by routine chest x-ray. In a serologic survey of 275 Chinese patients in a Hong Kong tuberculosis sanatorium, 14 percent had hemagglutinin titers of ≧1:80.

Acute localized suppurative infection Infection by inoculation of a break in the skin usually results in a nodule with an area of acute lymphangitis and regional lymphadenitis. There are usually fever and generalized malaise. This form of infection may rapidly progress to the acute septicemic form.

Acute pulmonary infection The most common form of the disease has been pulmonary infection, which may represent a primary pneumonitis or hematogenous spread. The acute pulmonary infection can vary in severity from a mild bronchitis to overwhelming necrotizing pneumonia. The onset may be abrupt without prodromal symptoms or more gradual, with headache, anorexia, and generalized myalgia. Fever occurs in almost all patients, is often in excess of 38.9°C (102°F), and may be associated with rigors. Dull or pleuritic chest pain is common. Cough, with or without sputum, occurs. There may be mild pharyngitis. Tachypnea may be out of proportion to the fever and findings on physical or x-ray examination. Chest findings may be minimal but usually consist of rales in the area of pneumonitis. In the absence of dissemination, the spleen and liver are not palpable. Laboratory findings include total leukocyte counts ranging from normal to 20,000 cells per microliter. Mild normochromic, normocytic anemia may appear during the illness. The pneumonia usually involves the upper lobes with the radiographic appearance of consolidation. Thin-walled cavities, usually 2 to 7 cm in diameter, frequently occur. Without specific therapy, the temperature may become normal within a few days; however, the upper lobe cavitation persists, resulting in a radiographic appearance of tuberculosis. While uncommon, pleural effusions, a pleural mass, and bilateral hilar adenopathy have been reported. Progressive pulmonary spread or hematogenous dissemination with the development of septicemic manifestations may ensue.

Acute septicemic infection This is the form originally described primarily among narcotic addicts. Subsequent reports, however, have shown a predilection for debilitated patients with diabetes mellitus and alcoholism. The onset may be abrupt, with the dominant symptoms depending upon site of major involvement. In individuals with bacteremia complicating pneumonitis, symptoms may include disorientation, extreme dyspnea, severe headache, pharyngitis, watery diarrhea, and development of cutaneous pustular lesions on the head, trunk, or extremities. There is high fever, extreme tachypnea, a flushed skin, and cyanosis. Muscle tenderness may be striking. On examination of the chest, signs may be absent, or rales, rhonchi, and pleural rubs may be heard. The liver and spleen may be palpable. Signs of arthritis or meningitis may appear. Patients with the septicemic form usually have a rapidly progressive fatal course, which in many instances may be too fulminant to be altered by therapy. The leukocyte count may be normal or slightly increased. Chest radiographs most commonly show irregular nodular densities 4 to 10 mm in diameter disseminated throughout the lungs. These enlarge, coalesce, and often undergo cavitation as the disease progresses. Pleural effusion is rare. Other radiographic patterns include unilateral irregular mottled densities which become confluent.

Chronic suppurative infection Acute or chronic abscesses dominate the clinical picture. Individuals have been misdiagnosed as having tropical pyomyositis which is caused by staphylococci. Organs involved include skin, brain, lung, myocardium, liver, spleen, prostate, bones, joints, lymph nodes, and even the eye. These patients may be afebrile.

Recrudescent infection Activation of inapparent or quiescent infection may present as acute localized suppurative, acute pulmonary, acute septicemic, or chronic suppurative disease remote from the probable time of exposure (up to 26 years having been reported). Surgery, trauma, intercurrent illness such as severe influenza pneumonia, diabetic ketoacidosis, alcoholic debauches, or radiation therapy appeared to act as triggering events. Since *P. pseudomallei* is an intracellular parasite and is associated with suppression of T helper lymphocytes, it seems only a matter of time before melioidosis will be added to the list of infections which occur in individuals with HIV infections, especially in areas where *P. pseudomallei* is endemic.

DIAGNOSIS Melioidosis should be considered in the differential diagnosis of any febrile illness in an individual who has been in an endemic area, especially if the presenting features are those of fulminant respiratory failure, if multiple pustular or necrotic skin or subcutaneous lesions develop, or if there is a radiographic pattern of tuberculosis in a patient from whom tubercle bacilli cannot be isolated.

Microscopic examination of exudates shows poorly staining, small, gram-negative bacilli with characteristic staining irregularities and "safety pin" bipolar staining with methylene blue. *Pseudomonas pseudomallei* will grow on most laboratory media, including eosin methylene blue agar (EMB) or MacConkey's agar, in 24 to 48 h. The organisms can be differentiated from *P. mallei* and *P. aeruginosa* by standard bacteriologic procedures, although isolates may pose problems in identification with some commercial medium kits. The hemagglutination, direct agglutination test, and complement fixation test are aids in diagnosis if a fourfold or greater rise in titer is demonstrated in paired sera. Single low titers are difficult to interpret because of nonspecific responses. The complement fixation test is said to be specific with titers above 1:8 during the acute illness, but may cross-react with *P. mallei.* A negative complement fixation test does not exclude disease. The hemagglutination and agglutination tests show more cross reactions. Titers of 1:40 or more suggest infection. In one-third of patients, with both fulminating and subacute disease, the serology has been negative at the time the culture became positive.

TREATMENT Virtually all strains of *P. pseudomallei* produce β-lactamase. In the past, most isolates have been sensitive in vitro to the tetracyclines, chloramphenicol, novobiocin, kanamycin, amikacin, and trimethoprim-sulfamethoxazole. In vitro studies with newer antimicrobial agents have shown over 90 percent of strains susceptible to ceftazidime, cefotaxime, cefoperazone, piperacillin, imipenem, amoxicillin-clavulanate, ampicillin-sulbactam, ticarcillin-clavulanate, and coumermycin (coumamycin). The fluorinated 4-quinolones such as ciprofloxacin and the monobacteram aztreonam have poor activity against *P. pseudomallei.* In Thailand, multiple resistant strains (resistant to chloramphenicol, tetracycline, trimethoprim-sulfamethoxazole), presumably permeability mutants, have been isolated from patients on admission and have emerged during treatment. In patients with pneumonitis who are not severely ill, currently recommended therapy is trimethoprim-sulfamethoxazole (4 mg/kg trimethoprim, 20 mg/kg sulfamethoxazole) for 60 to 150 days. In patients who are allergic to sulfonamides or in areas of trimethoprim-sulfamethoxazole resistance, alternatives include ceftazidime, 3 g daily (50 mg/kg), or cefotaxime, 3 g daily (30 mg/kg). Following clinical response to a third-generation cephalosporin, completion of a course with amoxicillin-clavulanate, 500 mg orally every 8 h, appears rational based on in vitro data; however, clinical experience is lacking. If the patient is severely ill, two antimicrobials in combination should be given for 30 days followed by another 30 to 120 days of trimethoprim-sulfamethoxazole. Although experience with the third-generation antipseudomonal cephalosporins is limited, a combination of ceftazidime (100 mg/kg per day) and trimethoprim (20 mg/kg per day)-sulfamethoxazole (100 mg/kg per day) is appropriate unless resistance is demonstrated. Individuals with low-titer positive serologic tests but with no clinical evidence of infection do not require therapy. The mean interval for sputum cultures to become negative has been 6 weeks. If sputum cultures remain positive for 6 months, surgery with lobectomy should be considered. In patients with extrapulmonary suppurative lesions, therapy should be continued for 6 months to 1 year and the usual principles of surgical drainage should be followed. In desperately ill patients with severe pneumonitis or the septicemic form, multiple antibiotics should be administered by the parenteral route. Levamisole[1] (150 mg twice per week) has been used as an adjunct to antibiotic therapy in several patients with results that suggest it may be beneficial in the treatment of relapses.

PROGNOSIS Prior to antimicrobials, the mortality rate of apparent infection was 95 percent. With better diagnosis and more prolonged appropriate therapy, the mortality rate in all except the septicemic form is low. Even with vigorous appropriate antibiotics and supportive therapy, the mortality rate in patients with melioidosis septicemia is greater than 50 percent. Very few patients have had long-term follow-up, and the incidence of late relapses is approximately 20 percent.

PREVENTION There is no means of active immunization. In endemic areas, vigorous cleansing of abrasions and lacerations is recommended.

GLANDERS

DEFINITION Glanders is a serious infection of equine animals caused by *P. mallei,* which is transmitted occasionally to other domestic animals and to human beings.

ETIOLOGY *Pseudomonas mallei* is a small, slender, nonmotile, gram-negative bacillus. When it is stained with methylene blue, marked irregularities in staining are observed. Organisms grow on most common meat infusion media but require glycerol for optimum growth.

EPIDEMIOLOGY Glanders was at one time widespread throughout Europe, but owing to the introduction of control measures, its incidence has decreased steadily in most countries. The disease still occurs in Asia, Africa, and South America, but not in the United States and western Europe. Glanders has never been common in humans; the occasional infection, however, may be very serious. There have been no naturally acquired infections in the United States since 1938.

Glanders is primarily a disease of horses, mules, and donkeys, although goats, sheep, cats, and dogs sometimes naturally contract the disease. Pigs and cattle are resistant. In horses, the disease may be systemic, with prominent pulmonary involvement (*glanders*) or may be characterized by subcutaneous ulcerative lesions and lymphatic thickening with nodules (*farcy*). Inhalation, ingestion, and inoculation through breaks in the skin have been suggested as routes of infection in animals. In humans, the disease occurs primarily in individuals with close contact with horses, mules, or donkeys through inoculation of or a break in the skin or by exposing the nasal mucosa to contaminated discharges. A number of instances of airborne infection have been reported in laboratory workers.

[1] This drug has not been approved for this purpose by the Food and Drug Administration at the time of publication.

CLINICAL MANIFESTATIONS The manifestations, which frequently overlap, may be categorized as (1) acute localized suppurative infection, (2) acute pulmonary infection, (3) acute septicemic infection, and (4) chronic suppurative infection. Nearly 60 percent of patients have been between the ages of 20 and 40 years. The disease has been rare in women, probably because there is little opportunity for contact.

Infection acquired by inoculation through an abrasion in the skin usually results in a nodule with an area of acute lymphangitis. The incubation period is probably 1 to 5 days. In all types of acute glanders, there are usually fever, generalized malaise, and prostration.

Infection of the mucous membranes may result in a mucopurulent discharge involving the eye, nose, or lips followed by extensive ulcerating granulomatous lesions which may or may not be associated with systemic reactions. With systemic invasion, a generalized papular eruption which may become pustular is frequent. This septicemic form of disease is usually fatal in 7 to 10 days.

Infection by inhalation is followed by an incubation period of 10 to 14 days. The more common symptoms include fever, occasionally associated with rigors, generalized myalgia, fatigue, headache, and pleuritic chest pain. Other symptoms consist of photophobia, lacrimation, and diarrhea. Findings on physical examination are usually normal except for fever and occasional lymphadenopathy, especially in the cervical chain, and splenomegaly. Laboratory findings include mild leukocytosis with 60 to 80 percent neutrophilic leukocytes, but leukopenia with relative lymphocytosis has been recorded. In the acute pulmonary form, chest radiographs characteristically reveal circumscribed densities which suggest early lung abscesses. Other findings may include lobar or bronchopneumonia. In the chronic suppurative form of the disease, the most frequent finding consists of multiple subcutaneous and intramuscular abscesses which most often involve the arms or legs. Approximately one-half the patients will have associated fever, lymphadenopathy, and nasal discharge or ulceration. Visceral involvement including pulmonary or pleural, ocular, skeletal, hepatic, splenic, and meningeal or intracranial involvement occurs in some patients.

DIAGNOSIS Microscopic examination of exudates may reveal small gram-negative bacilli which stain irregularly with methylene blue; however, organisms generally are very scanty. *Pseudomonas mallei* and *P. pseudomallei* cannot be distinguished morphologically. Growth occurs on most meat infusion nutrient media. Blood cultures are usually negative except in the terminal stages of disease. Serologic tests show a rapidly rising agglutination titer, which reaches levels of 1:640 within 2 weeks. Serum from normal persons has been reported to show agglutination titers in dilutions up to 1:320. The complement fixation test is less sensitive but more specific and usually becomes positive during the third week; it is considered positive in dilutions of 1:20 or greater.

TREATMENT The limited number of recent infections in human beings has precluded evaluation of most of the antibiotic agents. Sulfadiazine has been found to be an effective agent in experimental animals and in humans. The dosage utilized has been approximately 100 mg/kg administered in divided doses. Treatment should be given for at least 30 days. Penicillin is ineffective. Tetracycline, chloramphenicol, the antipseudomonal aminoglycosides, carbenicillin, the third-generation antipseudomonal cephalosporins, and trimethoprim-sulfamethoxazole have not been evaluated. In the absence of clinical experience and pending in vitro susceptibility studies, it would seem most reasonable to utilize the regimens appropriate for patients with melioidosis. In the acute infections, appropriate supportive measures are essential, and in chronic suppurative infections, the usual principles of surgical drainage should be followed.

PROGNOSIS The prognosis depends upon the type of infection. The acute septicemic form has been uniformly fatal. The localized or chronic forms have a much better prognosis.

PREVENTION Next to acquisition from diseased horses, the commonest source of natural disease in human beings has been contact with human glanders. Isolation is indicated.

REFERENCES

Barnes PF et al: A case of melioidosis originating in North America. Am Rev Respir Dis 134:170, 1986

Chaowagul W et al: Melioidosis: A major cause of community-acquired septicemia in Northeastern Thailand. J Infect Dis 159:890, 1989

Dance DAB et al: Antibiotic resistance in *Pseudomonas pseudomallei*. Lancet 1:994, 1988

Dodin A, Galimand M: Whitmore's bacillus. Rec Med Vet 152:323, 1976

Everett ED, Nelson, R: Pulmonary melioidosis, observations in 39 cases. Am Rev Respir Dis 112:331, 1975

Gillespie SH et al: In vitro susceptibility of *Pseudomonas pseudomallei* to DNA gyrase inhibitors. J Antimicrob Chemother 20:612, 1987

Guard LR et al: Melioidosis in far north Queensland. Am J Trop Med Hyg 33:467, 1984

Jackson AE et al: Recrudescent melioidosis associated with diabetic ketoacidosis. Arch Intern Med 130:268, 1972

Lumbiganon P et al: Neonatal melioidosis report of 5 cases. Pediatr Infect Dis J 7:634, 1988

McCormick JB et al: Human-to-human transmission of *Pseudomonas pseudomallei*. Ann Intern Med 83:512, 1975

McEniry DW et al: Susceptibility of *Pseudomonas pseudomallei* to new beta-lactam and aminoglycoside antibiotics. J Antimicrob Chemother 21:171, 1988

Morrison RE et al: Melioidosis: A reminder. Am J Med 84:965, 1988

Schlech WF III et al: Laboratory-acquired infection with *Pseudomonas pseudomallei* (melioidosis). N Engl J Med 305:1133, 1981

So SY et al: Melioidosis: A serological survey in a tuberculosis sanatorium in Hong Kong. Trans Roy Soc Trop Med Hyg 81:1017, 1987

Tanphaichitra D, Srimuang S: Cellular immunity in tuberculosis, melioidosis, pasteurellosis, penicilliosis and role of levamisole and isoprinosine. Dev Biol Stand 57:117, 1984

Wanvarie S: Melioidosis: Certain interesting presentations and treatment. Trop Geo Med 36:165, 1984

Wall RA et al: A case of melioidosis in West Africa. J Infect Dis 152:424, 1985

Wilkinson L: Glanders: Medicine and veterinary medicine in common pursuit of a contagious disease. Med Hist 25:363, 1981

113 SALMONELLOSIS

GERALD T. KEUSCH

Organisms of the genus *Salmonella* are capable of causing a large variety of infections in humans, including typhoid (or enteric) fevers, focal systemic infections, septicemias, and gastroenteritis varying clinically from watery diarrhea to dysentery. Nontyphoidal salmonellosis usually refers to enteric disease caused by many members of the genus except *S. typhi*. Convalescent carriage of gastroenteritis strains is usually transient. A few subjects, generally young children under 5 years, may become long-term (longer than 1 year) asymptomatic carriers although they are not important in the spread of infection. Patients with *S. typhi* are more likely to become long-term carriers, for years or possibly for life, and they serve as reservoirs for the spread of infection.

ETIOLOGY The salmonellae are nonencapsulated gram-negative bacilli, almost always motile by means of peritrichous flagellae, expressing two or more forms of H antigens. They are generally lactose nonfermenters, and this property is used for initial selection in the clinical microbiology laboratory. The salmonellae ferment glucose, resulting in a typical acid butt and alkaline slant on triple sugar iron agar (TSI). They generally produce H_2S, which is detectable as a black reaction product and serves initially to distinguish isolates from *Shigella*, which also give an alkaline/acid TSI reaction. There are a very large number of *Salmonella* O and H antigens, allowing the separation of over 2200 different organisms on the basis of the patterns of the O and H antigens. As these isolates have often been named after the place they were first detected, *Salmonella* classification more closely resembles geography. On the basis of major somatic antigens, a limited number of serogroups have been defined, and most human pathogens are members of groups A to D.

More rational classification schemes have been introduced that divide the genus into three species. One scheme includes *S. cholerasuis*, the prototype species; *S. typhi*, the major cause of typhoid (enteric) fever; and *S. enteritidis*, a catchall designation for all of the remaining serotypes only some of which are pathogenic for humans. These serotypes do not have the taxonomic rank of species and should not be italicized, but for clinical and epidemiologic ease the convention is to use only the serotype name. Thus, *S. enteritidis* serotype typhimurium becomes *S. typhimurium*, and *S. enteritidis* serotype enteritidis becomes *S. enteritidis*.

Some salmonellae are highly host-adapted to humans (e.g., *S. typhi*, *S. paratyphi A*, and *S. paratyphi B*) while most animal-adapted species cause no human disease. Others infect both man and lower animals causing gastroenteritis or less commonly, localized or septicemic infections.

TYPHOID FEVER

Typhoid fever is a distinctive acute systemic febrile infection of the mononuclear phagocytes and deserves separate consideration. Since it may be caused by several *species* (*S. typhi*, *S. paratyphi A* and *paratyphi B*, and occasionally *S. typhimurium*), many clinicians prefer the term *enteric fever*. But because typhoid is fundamentally not an enteric disease, this term is also inappropriate. On balance, *typhoid fever* is still the best term, for it is understood by nearly all clinicians to describe a particular syndrome that is, in fact, due primarily to *S. typhi*.

EPIDEMIOLOGY Because the cause of clinical typhoid fever is almost always a human-adapted *Salmonella*, most cases can be traced to a human carrier. The proximate cause may be water (the most common route) or food contaminated by a human carrier. Chronic carriers are generally over 50 years old, are more commonly women, and often have gallstones. *S. typhi* reside in the bile, even within the interiors of stones, and intermittently reach the lumen of the bowel, when they are excreted in the stool, thereby contaminating water or food.

With improvements in environmental sanitation in the United States, the incidence of typhoid has gradually dropped. Compared with 1920 when almost 36,000 cases were detected, the annual number now is approximately 500. Over 80 percent of these are active typhoid cases, and the others are convalescent carriers. The median age of a case is around 24 years, while the median age of carriers is over 60 years. Data gathered by the Centers for Disease Control (CDC) show that the incidence in the United States dropped fivefold from 1955 to 1966, from 1 per 100,000 to 0.2 per 100,000 population, and has remained steady since then. At the same time, the proportion of infections acquired abroad has increased, from 33 percent in the 1960s to over 60 percent in the 1980s. Mexico is the leading source for Americans, accounting for 39 percent of cases from 1975 to 1984; almost 60 percent were acquired somewhere in the Americas. The next most common location (17 percent) is the Indian subcontinent. Students are most at risk. In England, the majority of cases are also acquired abroad, usually in India or Pakistan. Known hot-spots for typhoid include Alexandria, Egypt; Jakarta, Indonesia; and Santiago, Chile.

Typhoid contracted in the United States is primarily due to association with known or newly diagnosed carriers (30 percent) or from food-borne outbreaks (28 percent). The highest rates occur in states bordering Mexico. The groups most likely to be at risk are bacteriology laboratory workers, other medical personnel, and sewage workers, but they actually have relatively low rates and account for less than 5 percent of identified cases. However, the number of patients is clearly underestimated, and an unknown proportion of patients escape detection because appropriate cultures are not done or the patients have already taken antibiotics.

PATHOGENESIS Following ingestion of a suitable inoculum, *S. typhi* pass the gastric barrier to reach the small bowel. Experimental human infections with the Quailes strain have revealed that 10^3 organisms will not cause symptomatic disease but that 10^5 bacteria cause symptoms in 27 percent of volunteers. Higher doses result in more frequent illness, unless the organisms lack the ability to produce the Vi antigen. Animal studies suggest that *S. typhi* invade the host in the upper small bowel, resulting in a transient and asymptomatic bacteremia. The organisms are ingested by mononuclear phagocytes and must survive and multiply intracellularly to cause illness.

Persistent bacteremia initiates the clinical phase of infection. The ability of the inoculum to invade mononuclear cells and multiply intracellularly determines whether or not this secondary bacteremia occurs. The absence of bactericidal antibodies allows organisms to be phagocytized in a viable state. Intracellular survival is dependent upon microbial factors that promote resistance to killing and the state of specific T-lymphocyte–activated host cell–mediated immunity. Dose dependence of clinical disease appears to be governed by the balance between bacterial multiplication and acquired host extracellular and intracellular defenses. When the number of intracellular bacteria surpasses a critical threshold, secondary bacteremia occurs and results in the invasion of the gallbladder and Peyer's patches of the intestine. The sustained bacteremia is responsible for the persistent fever of clinical typhoid, while inflammatory responses to tissue invasion determine the pattern of clinical expression (cholecystitis, intestinal hemorrhage, or perforation). With invasion of the gallbladder and Peyer's patches, bacteria regain entry to the bowel lumen, and by the second week of clinical disease the prevalence of positive stool cultures increases. Seeding of the kidney leads to positive urine cultures but in a much lower percentage of patients. The lipopolysaccharide endotoxin of *S. typhi* may contribute to causing fever, leukopenia, and other systemic symptoms, but the occurrence of such symptoms in subjects made tolerant to endotoxin supports a role for other factors, such as cytokines released from infected mononuclear phagocytes, that can mediate inflammation (see Chap 20).

CLINICAL MANIFESTATIONS The incubation period is variable and depends on both the inoculum size and the state of host defenses. A range of 3 to 60 days has been reported. The disease usually presents with a steplike daily increase in temperature to 40 to 41°C, associated with headache, malaise, and chills. The hallmark of typhoid fever is prolonged, persistent fever (4 to 8 weeks in untreated patients). Mild and brief illness may occur, but in some patients acute, severe infection with disseminated intravascular coagulation and central nervous system involvement may result in death. In other patients, necrotizing cholecystitis or intestinal bleeding and perforation can occur in the third or fourth week of illness, when the patient is otherwise improving. In most, the onset of these complications is dramatic and clinically obvious. Intestinal perforation appears to be less common in children under 5 years of age.

Early intestinal manifestations include constipation, especially in adults, or mild diarrhea in children, associated with abdominal tenderness. Mild hepatosplenomegaly is detectable in the majority of patients. Bradycardia relative to the height of the fever may be a clinical clue to typhoid, but is present in a minority of patients. Epistaxis may occur in the early stages of illness. ''Rose spots,'' appearing as small, pale red, blanching, slightly raised macules, may be seen on the chest and abdomen during the first week. They can also evolve into nonblanching small hemorrhages that are difficult to see in dark skinned patients. While the major characteristics of untreated typhoid and persistent high fever, severe anorexia, weight loss, and changes in sensorium, a variety of other complications may be seen, including hepatitis, meningitis, nephritis, myocarditis, bronchitis, pneumonia, arthritis, osteomyelitis, parotitis and orchitis. The frequency of all of these complications, including hemorrhage and perforation, is reduced by prompt use of appropriate antibiotics.

Around 3 to 5 percent of patients become long-term asymptomatic carriers, some for life unless treated. Many carriers give no history of typhoid fever and probably had an undiagnosed mild infection.

LABORATORY FINDINGS In the early phases of typhoid fever the white blood cell count is usually in the range of 4000 to 5000 cells per microliter, and a left shift is present. This relative leukopenia in relation to the degree of fever may be a clue to the diagnosis. Rarely, severe leukopenia (<2000 cells per microliter) can occur. In the event of intestinal perforation or pyogenic complications, secondary leukocytosis develops. The anemia of blood loss may be superimposed on the anemia of chronic infection.

Definitive diagnosis depends on isolation of the organism or a serologic response. The recovery of organisms from blood is highest in the first week of illness, when it approaches 90 percent. Bacteremia is detectable in 50 percent in the third week and at a progressively lower frequency later on. Early in the illness culture of bone marrow aspirates will yield the organism in the majority of patients, even after brief prior antimicrobial treatment. Stool cultures are frequently negative in the first week but usually become positive in 75 percent of patients during the third week. By the eighth week, stools are positive in only 10 percent of patients, but in approximately 3 to 5 percent of patients will remain so for at least 1 year. The frequency of positive urine cultures parallels the yield from stools and may represent, in some patients, contamination with feces.

Serologic diagnosis is less reliable than culture. Most, but not all, patients will develop agglutinating antibodies to O, H, and Vi antigens (the Widal test). In the absence of recent immunization, a high titer of antibody to O antigen (>1:640) is useful but not specific. Other serogroup D salmonellae share the antigen used in the Widal test, as do some organisms in groups A and B. H antibodies may be found in even higher titer, but because of their broad cross reactivity are difficult to interpret. A fourfold rise in antibody in paired samples is a good criterion but is of little use in the acutely ill patients and may be blunted by early effective antimicrobial therapy. The earlier the baseline sample is obtained, the more likely a significant rise will be detected. Vi antibodies typically rise later, after three to four weeks of illness, and are of less use in the early diagnosis of infection.

DIFFERENTIAL DIAGNOSIS When all the classic clinical manifestations are present, including rose spots, prolonged fever, relative bradycardia, and leukopenia, the diagnosis of typhoid will be strongly suggested. However, most cases do not fit this ''typical'' profile. Differential diagnosis includes infections associated with prolonged fever such as the rickettsioses, brucellosis, tularemia, leptospirosis, miliary tuberculosis, viral hepatitis, infectious mononucleosis, cytomegalovirus infections, and malaria, as well as noninfectious causes such as lymphoma (see Chap. 20). In the United States, typhoid should be considered in any patient with prolonged, unexplained fever, especially after recent travel to places with endemic typhoid fever.

TREATMENT Since its introduction, chloramphenicol has been the antimicrobial gold standard for treatment. No drug has been better in promoting a favorable clinical response, and this usually becomes apparent within 24 to 48 h of the start of treatment in the appropriate dosages (3 to 4 g/d in adults or 50 mg/kg body weight per day in young children). The drug is given orally for 2 weeks, and the dose may be reduced to 2 g/d or 30 mg/kg per day when the patient becomes afebrile, which usually is not before day five of treatment. Other effective oral regimens include amoxicillin (4 to 6 g/d in four divided doses in adults or 100 mg/kg per day in children); trimethoprim-sulfamethoxazole (640 and 3200 mg, respectively, in two divided doses daily in adults or 185 mg/m^2 body surface area per day of the trimethoprim component for children); or in those over 17 years, a 4-fluoroquinolone such as ciprofloxacin or ofloxacin. Parenteral ampicillin (8 g/d in adults or 200 mg/kg per day in four divided doses in children) is also effective. Chloramphenicol or trimethoprim-sulfamethoxazole may be given intravenously if patients are unable to tolerate oral therapy. Initial studies with ceftriaxone (75 mg/kg per day) administered for 5 days indicate that it is effective treatment.

Chloramphenicol-resistant *S. typhi* first appeared in 1972 and were responsible for an epidemic in Mexico. Resistant strains are still encountered sporadically in Mexico, the Indian subcontinent, and in Southeast Asia and Indonesia. Resistance is plasmid-mediated and usually carries multiple common antibiotic resistances to sulfonamides, streptomycin, and tetracycline. Occasional isolates are doubly resistant to chloramphenicol and trimethoprim-sulfamethoxazole or ampicillin. The availability of 4-fluoroquinolones for adults simplifies the problem of treating nonresponders or those in whom single or double resistance to one of the more generally used antimicrobials is encountered.

Patients with severe typhoid who present with central nervous system manifestations and/or evidence of disseminated intravenous coagulation should be given intravenous glucocorticoids such as dexamethasone, 3 mg/kg as a loading dose over 30 min followed by 1 mg/kg every 6 h for 24 h, in addition to parenteral antimicrobials. Salicylates should be avoided to reduce the danger of intestinal hemorrhage. It is often recommended that the late complications of hemorrhage and perforations be managed conservatively with antibiotics and general support. This is largely because these occur most commonly in developing countries where patients frequently present late in the course of illness, are usually malnourished, and are poor surgical risks, and where there are limitations in surgical and postoperative care. Bowel perforations occurring in patients in countries with sophisticated medical facilities should be treated surgically as indicated by the clinical state and not by the microbiologic diagnosis. Selective angiography or radioisotopic scanning methods (see Chap. 46) to localize the bleeding site can facilitate operative repair. Small perforations may localize with supportive care and antibiotics alone. In developing countries, limited surgery to close the site of perforation, without bowel resection, may be the wisest choice.

The early use of effective antimicrobials is associated with a relatively high rate of relapse; relapse rates of 20 percent can be expected, compared with 5 to 10 percent in untreated patients. This is presumably because prompt therapy inhibits the development of an adequate immune response. Relapses are usually milder than the initial attack and will respond to the same antimicrobial used initially.

Successful treatment of chronic carriers can be difficult. Administration of 100 mg/kg per day of ampicillin or amoxicillin plus probenecid (30 mg/kg per day) or trimethoprim/sulfamethoxazole (160/800 mg) twice daily plus rifampin 600 mg once daily for at least 6 weeks is usually successful if there are no gallstones. Prolongation of antimicrobial therapy for 3 months can cure some carriers with gallstones; however, the most reliable treatment is cholecystectomy plus antimicrobials. Regimens using 4 weeks of treatment with the quinolones may be equally effective; however, experience with this approach is still limited.

PREVENTION AND CONTROL Worldwide experience has shown that improvement of environmental sanitation, including sewage disposal and water supplies, will sharply reduce the incidence of typhoid fever. Where this approach is not yet possible, and for travelers, immunization has been used. Killed, whole typhoid bacillus vaccine provides limited protection for several months, presumably by inducing bactericidal antibodies. The vaccine produces fever and pain and will induce O and H antibodies that give a positive Widal test and impeded diagnostic interpretation of serologic data.

Other vaccines have been used in an attempt to improve efficacy and reduce toxicity. A purified Vi vaccine given intramuscularly has been shown to provide equal efficacy to whole killed vaccines with minimal side effects. Studies are also proceeding with live oral vaccines. Two approaches have achieved some success, but not sufficient for routine use. These are a galactose epimerase mutant *S. typhi*, Ty 21a, and auxotrophic mutants selected for aromatic metabolites not available inside cells. Both vaccine prototypes invade mononuclear cells and stimulate immunity, but neither survive within cells and, therefore, are avirulent. Because of these properties, there are many attempts to use these strains as "piggyback" vectors to carry unrelated antigens for immunization purposes.

Typhoid is a reportable disease in the United States. Patients should be monitored for prolonged carriage and treated for this if necessary. Precautions in food handling by carriers and in disposal of their stools are obvious and important (see Chap. 83).

PROGNOSIS Appropriate therapy of typhoid fever, especially if patients present for medical care in the early stage of disease, is highly successful. The mortality rate should be under 1 percent and few complications should occur.

NONTYPHOIDAL SALMONELLOSIS

Infections caused by any *Salmonella* other than *S. typhi* are termed nontyphoidal salmonellosis. These infections can present as acute diarrhea, a septicemic syndrome, focal abscesses, meningitis, osteomyelitis, endocarditis, or mycotic aneurysm or can be asymptomatic.

EPIDEMIOLOGY The species *S. cholerasuis* and *S. enteritidis* include a diverse group of organisms with both host-adapted and nonhost-adapted serotypes. Two human-adapted serotypes, *S. paratyphi A* and *S. schottmuelleri* (more often called *S. paratyphi B*), have been discussed under typhoid fever. Of the more than 2200 known *S. enteritidis*, just ten account for 75 percent of all human disease isolates in the United States, and four serotypes (*S. typhimurium, enteritidis, heidelberg,* and *newport*) cause about two-thirds of all disease. *S. typhimurium* is the most frequent isolate, representing around 35 percent of all strains reported to the CDC. In past surveillance studies, periodic increases in recovery of certain serotypes have represented either introduction of a new transmission source or the occurrence of a large outbreak. For example, the number of *S. typhimurium* isolates increased from an average of 12,000 per year to over 28,000 in 1985 due to a massive outbreak related to consumption of contaminated milk in the Chicago area. A fivefold increase in *S. enteritidis* isolates between 1976 and 1986 was due to ingestion of contaminated grade A eggs primarily in the northeastern United States.

Careful analysis of surveillance data in the United States has shown that not only is the number of nontyphoidal *Salmonella* isolates increasing, but the incidence appears to be increasing as well, from 8 per 100,000 of the general population in 1965, to 12 per 100,000 in 1975, to around 18 per 100,000 by 1985. These data are biased in part by excess reporting of investigated outbreaks, and because infants, the elderly, and severely ill patients are the most likely to have cultures performed. While the incidence of disease in young children is five times higher than in older subjects, the rate is also somewhat higher in adults over 70 years. Between 1970 and 1986 the median age of infected individuals rose from 6 years to 20 years. The greatest increase has been in the 20- to 39-year-old population, suggesting that foods consumed by young adults are becoming important vehicles or that they are traveling more to endemic areas. A reasonable estimate of the total incidence of symptomatic *Salmonella* infection in the United States is 1 to 2 million cases per year. This degree of morbidity implies a significant economic impact in lost productivity and medical costs and, by extension, a serious and underestimated cause of mortality.

Because nontyphoidal *Salmonella* are so often nonhost-adapted, many kinds of domestic animals can harbor the organism and serve as the source for human infection. Conditions of raising, shipping, slaughtering, and marketing contribute to the spread of *Salmonella* in the food supply. Introduction of the organism into processed foods can result in widespread dissemination, and contamination of such common foods as eggs or milk leads to large-scale outbreaks. Dried or frozen foods preserve viable salmonellae. For these reasons, salmonellosis is more a disease of the industrialized world than of the developing world. Additional sources of human infection are animals sold as pets, including baby chicks or ducks and turtles, and medical products of animal origin, such as carmine dye (from insects); pancreatin; bile salts; or tissue extracts from thyroids, adrenals, stomachs, or rattlesnakes.

A potentially serious problem is the selection of antibiotic-resistant strains of salmonellae by unregulated drug use in animal husbandry. There are a number of instances where transmission to humans has occurred. Persistent and severe salmonellosis has also been recognized as a problem among patients with acquired immunodeficiency syndrome (AIDS) (see Chap. 264).

PATHOGENESIS As with *S. typhi*, the events following ingestion of the organism are determined by environmental factors (dose), microbial factors (serotype, invasion, and other virulence properties), and host factors (resistance). As few as 10^3 virulent organisms may cause disease, especially in patients with achlorhydria or having recent antimicrobial therapy. Systemic invasion is more likely in patients with "reticuloendothelial blockade" due to hemolysis (malaria, bartonellosis, leptospirosis, sickle cell anemia) or intracellular infections (histoplasmosis). The incidence of documented bacteremia varies from 5 to 45 percent, but is assumed to occur early in the course of many, and possibly all, *Salmonella* infections and is quickly cleared in most patients infected with *S. enteritidis* serotypes. Certain serotypes, such as *dublin, infantis, virchow, panama,* and *newport,* may be more invasive and more commonly isolated from blood. *S. typhimurium* is the most frequent blood isolate, but the rate of isolation is no more than the average for all nontyphoidal *Salmonella*. Systemic and focal tissue infections are secondary to bacteremia. *S. cholerasuis* is a highly invasive serotype that usually causes a septicemia syndrome and is most commonly isolated from blood but not from stool. Microbial factors, which determine the invasiveness of salmonellae, include motility and the presence of plasmid genes needed to establish progressive infection of mononuclear phagocytes. Such genes have been identified on a small common Eco R1 restriction fragment in plasmids of varying size in *S. dublin, S. enteritidis,* and *S. cholerasuis*.

The pathogenesis of *Salmonella* enteritis is not clear. Virulent strains appear to be invasive and able to induce inflammatory responses in the gut mucosa, but these properties are not sufficient to cause intestinal fluid secretion. This may depend on a heat-labile enterotoxin which is structurally, functionally, and immunologically related to the cholera and *E. coli* LT toxins. This toxin has now been cloned and expressed in *E. coli*. Heat-labile cytotoxins that act like Shiga toxins to inhibit intestinal protein synthesis may also be involved.

CLINICAL MANIFESTATIONS **Gastroenteritis** The incubation period of *Salmonella* gastroenteritis is generally short, 24 to 48 h. Sporadic illness is likely to go undiagnosed because cultures are not taken. Large outbreaks, often considered as "food poisoning" and characterized by self-limited fever and diarrhea, are more likely to be investigated and diagnosed. Diarrhea may be associated with nausea, vomiting, and abdominal cramps and occasionally becomes bloody or even dysenteric when the colon becomes involved. The stool contains many leukocytes when examined by direct microscopy, a clue to the invasive nature of the infection. The illness is generally mild and resolves without use of specific therapy, but may cause severe dehydration or disseminate and lead to death in debilitated elderly patients or neonates. Blood cultures often become positive as the patient is improving. Treatment may be discontinued after identification of the organism unless there is an underlying immunosuppressive disease (e.g., sickle cell disease, AIDS, malignancy such as a lymphoma or the patient is receiving glucocorticoid or immunosuppressive drug therapy). In these conditions treatment with an appropriate antibiotic should be administered for 7 to 10 days. Carriage in the stool of salmonellae that can cause gastroenteritis lasts several weeks after symptomatic disease and rarely exceeds 2 months.

Localized systemic infections Blood-borne salmonellae can invade any tissue or organ. The most common isolates are *S. typhimurium, S. enteritidis,* and *S. cholerasuis*. Localized infections usually follow intestinal infection, although there may be no prior diarrhea. Endocarditis is rare, but when it occurs there may be destructive cardiac lesions including valve perforations or ring or septal abscesses. Therapy requires both appropriate antimicrobials and surgery when necessary (see Chap. 90).

Arterial infection generally occurs in preexisting arteriosclerotic infrarenal aortic aneurysms, especially in men older than 50. *S. cholerasuis* accounts for about 20 percent of the isolates, in contrast to being found in <1 percent of patients with diarrhea due to salmonella infection, reflecting its capacity to cause systemic invasive disease. *S. typhimurium* accounts for ~25 percent of isolates in arterial infections, consistent with its high incidence in causing gastrointestinal salmonellosis (about 35 percent of all cases). In addition to treatment with antimicrobials, eradication usually requires prompt excision and drainage with bypass through uninvolved tissue. The disease should be suspected when elderly men develop prolonged fever following gastroenteritis, accompanied by back, abdomen, or chest pain; when bacteremia is present or recurrent after therapy for the initial illness; or when it occurs in patients with vertebral osteomyelitis or in those with prosthetic valves.

Cholecystitis, other *hepatobiliary infection*, or *splenic abscess* are the most common intraabdominal localized infections due to salmonellae. In addition to *S. typhimurium* and *S. enteritidis, S. typhi* is an important cause.

Urinary tract infections sometimes occur, especially in patients with urolithiasis, structural abnormalities, or immunosuppressive diseases or therapy. Salmonella urinary tract infection sometimes coexists with renal tuberculosis or *Schistosoma haematobium* infection.

Pneumonia or *empyema* caused by salmonella is rare and usually seen in patients with preexisting abnormalities of the lungs or pleura or with conditions that predispose to infection, including malignancy, diabetes, glucocorticoid use, sickle cell disease, or alcohol abuse.

Meningitis caused by salmonella is also rare and is most prevalent in young infants and children. Gram stains of cerebrospinal fluid are usually positive. Mortality rates of 40 to 60 percent are reported in children and adults, respectively. In survivors, residua include seizures, hydrocephalus, subdural empyemas, and permanent disabilities such as retardation, paresis, athetosis, or visual disturbances.

Septic arthritis due to salmonella is associated with positive joint-fluid cultures and should not be confused with reactive arthritis (a culture-negative inflammatory joint disease occurring after invasive diarrheas, especially in HLA-B27 or -B7 positive patients). Underlying conditions that are often present include glucocorticoid or immunosuppressive drug therapy, sickle cell disease, prosthetic joints, or aseptic necrosis. Drainage may be needed in addition to appropriate antibiotics.

Salmonella *osteomyelitis* is predictably associated with sickle cell disease, sickle-C disease, or sickle thalassemia. It generally affects long bones and occurs primarily in young patients; blood cultures are often positive (the most common isolate is *S. typhimurium*).

Bacteremia Sepsis, with prolonged fever and positive blood cultures but generally without prior diarrhea, occurs most commonly with *S. cholerasuis* infection. While this presentation is "typhoidal," typical manifestations of typhoid (rose spots, relative bradycardia, leukopenia) are absent, and the disease is more acute in onset and duration. *S. cholerasuis* sepsis is a severe disease, associated with high mortality.

Intermittent symptomatic *Salmonella* bacteremia is seen in patients with hepatosplenic or urinary schistosomiasis. Clinically severe *Salmonella* sepsis due to *S. typhimurium* also occurs in AIDS patients (see Chap. 264), is often recurrent, and may develop before the diagnosis of AIDS is made. The infection may be refractory to treatment or recurrent in spite of appropriate therapy. The incidence of salmonellosis in AIDS patients in the United States is now estimated to be between 46 and 384 per 100,000, which is 100 to 1000-fold greater than the incidence in the general population (0.3 per 100,000).

DIAGNOSIS Specific diagnosis depends on the isolation of the organisms from stool, blood, or tissue fluids. All clinical laboratories should be able to make the initial isolation and identify common serotypes. Uncommon serotypes usually must be sent to reference laboratories for identification.

TREATMENT Treatment for focal systemic infections requires selection of the most appropriate antibiotic and, at times, drainage or resection of infected tissue. Bactericidal antibiotics by the parenteral route are the usual choice and may include ampicillin in a dose of 6 to 12 g/d in adults or 100 mg/kg in young children in divided doses; chloramphenicol in a dose of 2 to 4 g/d in adults or 50 mg/kg in children in divided doses; or appropriate doses of third-generation cephalosporins such as ceftriaxone or cefotaxime when the organism is ampicillin-resistant (see Chap. 85). Because the experience with these latter drugs is not great, they cannot be recommended for routine use. The results with 4-fluoroquinolones suggest that these agents will become increasingly valuable because they are effective by the oral route.

The proper treatment of *Salmonella* gastroenteritis is not clear; antibiotics do not shorten illness but do increase the duration of convalescent carriage. For this reason it is generally recommended that no treatment other than supportive care and fluid replacement be administered. Early results suggest that 4-fluoroquinolones reduce the duration of illness and eradicate the organism from stool. However, until these drugs are shown to be safe this approach should not be routinely employed in children. When blood cultures are positive in the setting of otherwise uncomplicated gastroenteritis, prolonged treatment is usually reserved only for patients with underlying immunosuppressive disease. In an infant under 3 months of age with diarrhea, the stool should be cultured, a workup to localize the septic process initiated, and presumptive treatment begun with a third-generation cephalosporin until culture results are available. Fever is often absent in very young infants and is not a reliable indicator of systemic infection. Asymptomatic patients with salmonellae other than *S. typhi* in the stool should *not* receive antimicrobial treatment, since active disease may be produced and the carriage state prolonged.

PREVENTION AND CONTROL It is probably not possible to eradicate nontyphoidal salmonellosis since the organisms are so widespread in nature. Reduction in the use in animal feed of antimicrobials employed for human infection and improved animal rearing and marketing practices would be useful. Vigilance in food preparation and in quality testing of the known and commonly contaminated foods should help as well. It is recommended that eggs be fully cooked and not eaten raw or partially cooked. If universal body substance precautions are not routinely utilized, hospital staff caring for patients with salmonellosis should be placed on "enteric precautions," with gowning and gloving when handling stool and urine, and careful hand washing after patient contact (see Chap. 83).

During outbreaks, food handlers may be responsible for transmission. Much effort is given to the identification by stool culture of asymptomatic food handlers who are carriers during food-borne outbreaks, and they are usually kept from work until they become culture-negative. However, it is more important to determine what standards of practice are maintained to ensure proper environmental and personal hygiene of food handlers to prevent the problem from occurring. This is because carriage may be intermittant and is often not uniform within a single stool sample, and because any food contaminated with the organism would require improper handling to permit the growth of a sufficient inoculum to cause disease. Perhaps the only situation where it may be truly justifiable to restrict carriers from the workplace is in the course of a hospital outbreak or when there are workers who refuse to improve their personal hygiene.

The development of effective vaccines may be difficult because of the great number of serotypes involved in infection. Some progress has been made with galactose epimerase or aroA vaccine mutants of *S. typhimurium* for use in animals, and these may ultimately be tested in humans. Of all of the nontyphoidal salmonellae, it would be most useful to have vaccines for *S. cholerasuis* serotypes typhimurium and enteritidis.

REFERENCES

ACHARYA IL et al: Prevention of typhoid fever in Nepal with the Vi capsular polysaccharide vaccine of *Salmonella typhi*. N Engl J Med 317:1101, 1987

CHOPRA AK et al: Cloning and expression of the salmonella enterotoxin gene. J Bacteriol 169:5095, 1987

COHEN JI et al: Extra-intestinal manifestations of *Salmonella* infections. Medicine 66:349, 1987

FERRECCIO C et al: Efficacy of ciprofloxacin in the treatment of chronic typhoid carriers. J Infect Dis 157:1235, 1988

HARGRETT-BEAN NT et al: *Salmonella* isolates from humans in the United States, 1984–1986. Morbidity and Mortality Annual Surveillance Reports 37 No. SS-2:25, 1988

HOFFMAN SL et al: Reduction of mortality in chloramphenicol-treated severe typhoid fever by high-dose dexamethasone. N Engl J Med 310:82, 1984

RYAN CA et al: *Salmonella typhi* infections in the United States, 1975–1984: Increasing role of foreign travel. Rev Infect Dis 11:1, 1989

SPIKA JS et al: Chloramphenicol-resistant *Salmonella newport* traced through hamburger to dairy farms: A major persisting source of human salmonellosis in California. N Engl J Med 316:565, 1987

ST LOUIS ME et al: The emergence of grade-A eggs as a major source of *Salmonella enteriditis* infections: New implication for the control of salmonellosis. JAMA 259:2103, 1988

TOPLEY JM: Mild typhoid fever. Arch Dis Child 61:164, 1986

114 SHIGELLOSIS

GERALD T. KEUSCH

DEFINITION Shigellosis is an acute infectious inflammatory colitis due to one of the members of the genus *Shigella.* Although the disease is often referred to as "bacillary dysentery," many patients have only mild watery diarrhea and never develop dysenteric symptoms. The less severe illness predominates in industrialized countries such as the United States, whereas more severe, often fatal dysentery occurs in patients in developing countries.

ETIOLOGY The *Shigellae* are slender, gram-negative, nonmotile bacilli and are members of the family Enterobacteriaceae and tribe *Escherichae*. They are so closely related to *Escherichia coli* that the two genera cannot be distinguished by DNA hybridization methods. There are four *Shigella* species (*dysenteriae, flexneri, boydii* and *sonnei*) defined on the basis of surface somatic O antigens and carbohydrate fermentation patterns. Most are lactose-negative (*S. sonnei* are late lactose fermenters) and produce acid but not gas from glucose, resulting in a typical acid butt and alkaline slant in triple sugar iron agar (TSI), without H_2S production, in contrast to *Salmonella*. The genus is characterized by its ability to invade intestinal epithelial cells and to produce highly potent protein toxins that irreversibly inhibit eukaryotic cell protein synthesis by a specific enzymatic action.

EPIDEMIOLOGY It is estimated that at least 140 million cases and almost 600,000 deaths occur annually due to shigellosis in young children under the age of 5 years. The organism is found everywhere in the world, but is most common in developing countries where poor environmental sanitation and crowding facilitate transmission from person to person. The incidence in the United States is much lower, and less than 15,000 cases each year are reported to the Centers for Disease Control (CDC). This is no doubt a gross underestimate, as organisms from many patients are neither cultured nor identified. In industrialized countries and developing countries alike, most patients are young children. In the United States from 1974 to 1980, 93,516 cases were identified by means of a nationwide passive surveillance system. While the overall isolation rate was 4.7 per 100,000 population per year, among children aged 1 to 4 the rate was 22.3 per 100,000 children per year. In the United States, the disease is most common in the urban poor, in infants in day-care centers, and in retarded children institutionalized for custodial care. One high-risk group has also been identified: male homosexuals, who transmit infection by anal-oral sexual practices.

Since the description of the genus, major global shifts in prevalence of the four species have been noted. Until World War I, *S. dysenteriae* type 1 was the predominant isolate, frequently occurring in devastating epidemics with high mortality until it was replaced by *S. flexneri*. Since World War II, however, *S. flexneri* has been steadily replaced by *S. sonnei* in the industrialized countries. The reasons for these shifts are not clear. In Bangkok, Thailand, *S. sonnei* is now overtaking *S. flexneri,* whereas in the countryside *S. flexneri* strains still predominate. *S. boydii,* the fourth species, has remained largely confined to the Indian subcontinent and is uncommon elsewhere.

The genus is highly host-adapted and is a natural pathogen of only humans and a few subhuman primates. Transmission is fecal-oral from person to person and is generally via direct contact, although contaminated food, water, and fomites may serve as vectors. Direct contact is efficient and only a few hundred organisms suffice to transmit disease. For this reason, rapid spread can occur among confined populations kept in close contact, as, for example, in day-care centers, in institutions for the mentally retarded, on cruise ships, or among military personnel. Shigella is also one of several pathogens associated with "gay bowel syndrome." These cases are almost always due to *S. flexneri,* and homosexual young men may be a major reservoir for these organisms in the United States.

Shigellosis is associated with a high secondary household transmission rate. As many as 40 percent of children and 20 percent of adult household contacts of a case (generally a preschool child) will develop *Shigella* infection, which is usually symptomatic in children but asymptomatic in adults, who seem to have an acquired immunity. In contrast, epidemic disease affects all ages, with a clustering of severe and fatal cases in the very young and very old. Since 1969, epidemic *S. dysenteriae* type 1 has reappeared first in Latin America, then in the Indian subcontinent and elsewhere in Asia, and in central Africa. In each place, the disease has been accompanied by relatively high mortality rates until the cause was recognized and effective therapy initiated. Prolonged asymptomatic carriage is uncommon, and unless there is underlying malnutrition which is associated with prolonged fecal excretion, organisms are cleared in a few weeks.

PATHOGENESIS AND PATHOLOGY *Shigellae* are orally ingested and, though they are acid labile in the laboratory, they seem to have little difficulty in passing the gastric acid barrier. An essential step in pathogenesis is invasion of colonic epithelial cells and cell-to-cell spread of infection. Both invasion and cell-to-cell spread involve the initial attachment of the organism to colonic cells and then entry by an endocytic mechanism in which organisms are initially encased in and then escape from plasma-membrane enclosed vesicles. This not only provides the organism with a means to evade host defenses, but also allows effective local spread. Although invasion is initially innocuous, with subsequent intracellular multiplication, cell damage and death occur, resulting in characteristic mucosal ulcerations.

These virulence properties of the organism are determined by both chromosomal and plasmid genes. Studies with *Shigella–E. coli* hybrids, produced by introducing *E. coli* genes into *Shigella,* have demonstrated at least three chromosomal regions to be necessary—one bounded by the *xyl* and *rhl* loci, the *his* locus, and the *pur*E locus. The *xyl-rhl* region is known to code for aerobactin and iron-regulated outer membrane proteins (OMPs), while the *his* region controls specific side chains of lipopolysaccharide, which respectively may help the organism compete for iron with the host and protect it from host defenses. However, if these regions are transferred from *S. flexneri* to a recipient *E. coli* K12, the resulting recombinant hybrid is still avirulent until other genes present on the large 120- to 140-MDa plasmids in all virulent *Shigella* are transferred as well. These plasmids contain at least two loci within a 22-MDa region, the *ipa* (invasion plasmid antigen) region, which controls production of several OMPs, and the *inv* region, which is thought to control insertion of these OMPs into the outer membrane of the organism.

The large plasmids also carry other virulence-associated genes, such as *vir*F, which regulates surface charge (affecting forces of attraction between the gut cell and the bacterium), and *vir*G, which controls the production of a hemolysin that probably is involved in rapid escape of the organism from intracellular vesicles after invasion. Another gene, *ics,* codes for a 120-kDa OMP that polymerizes epithelial cell actin, allowing organisms to migrate along the actin network to the plasma membrane. From this location organisms can invade adjacent cells and spread locally. The multiple genes needed to induce the nonphagocytic colonic cell to mimic a phagocyte indicate the complexity of the process and the high degree of specialization of the organism.

A second property of apparent importance in virulence is the ability of *Shigellae* to produce protein toxins that cause cytotoxicity in susceptible cells. These toxins are composed of two distinct peptide subunits and seem to be related members of a family of Shiga toxins. The toxins have two highly conserved active regions. The first, located on the larger A subunit, is an *N*-glycosidase enzyme, which hydrolyzes adenine from specific sites of ribosomal RNA of the mammalian 60-S ribosomal subunit, resulting in the irreversible inhibition of protein synthesis. The second common region is a binding site on the B subunit that recognizes glycolipids terminating in a galactose $\alpha 1 \rightarrow 4$-galactose disaccharide. The glycolipid Gb3, containing a "gal-gal" trisaccharide, is a specific receptor present on toxin-sensitive rabbit intestinal epithelial cells. In this species, Gb3 is only expressed on villus cells, and toxin action is specific for these cells, sparing the crypts. It is assumed that Gb3 is the toxin receptor on human intestinal epithelial cells as well. Following binding to the rabbit intestinal cell surface, toxin is transported from the coated pits on the cell surface by receptor-mediated endocytosis. Inhibition of protein synthesis in villus cells leads to functional impairment in neutral sodium absorption, with no effect on crypt cell chloride secretion. Unopposed chloride secretion results in accumulation of electrolytes and water in the gut lumen. If the same process occurs in the human gut, the modest fluid loss of shigellosis can be accounted for. In contrast, the prodigious fluid losses due to cholera toxin are caused by the combined effects of inhibition of villus sodium absorption and increased crypt cell chloride secretion.

In shigellosis, the epithelial surface of the human colon shows extensive ulcerations, with an exudate consisting of desquamated colonic cells, polymorphonuclear leukocytes, and erythrocytes; the ulcerations may resemble a pseudomembrane in severely affected areas. Marked mucus depletion and increased mitotic activity is seen in the crypt regions, presumably as a response to the loss of surface colonic cells. The lamina propria is edematous and hemorrhagic and infiltrated with neutrophils and plasma cells. There is also swelling of capillary and venular endothelial cells, with margination of neutrophils. At the ultrastructural level, bacteria can be seen within vesicles as well as free in the cytoplasm.

Epidemiologic evidence indicates that immunity develops and is serotype specific. The nature of this immunity, however, is not known. Common surface OMPs involved in invasion are known to elicit serum antibodies; however, these are cross-reactive for many *Shigella* species and serotypes. The serotype-specific determinants are likely to be somatic antigens, and there is evidence of IgA-mediated mucosal anti-O antigen responses during convalescence from shigellosis. Cellular mechanisms have also been proposed that involve antibody-dependent cellular cytotoxicity responses by Fc receptor–positive lymphocytes and phagocytic cells.

CLINICAL MANIFESTATIONS The spectrum of clinical shigellosis was expressed in a study in which human volunteers ingested 10,000 *S. flexneri* type 2a. While approximately one-quarter of the volunteers never became ill, over the first 24 to 48 h approximately 25 percent of volunteers developed a transient fever, another 25 percent had fever and a self-limited watery diarrhea, and the remaining 25 percent had fever and watery diarrhea that progressed to bloody diarrhea and dysentery. In young children, in particular, the temperature can rapidly rise to 40 to 41°C, and sometimes result in typical febrile seizures. Dysentery is characterized by small-volume stools consisting of blood, mucus, and pus, abdominal cramps, and tenesmus, with 40 or more bowel movements each day. Painful straining often leads to rectal prolapse, especially in young children. The likelihood of severe dysentery is greatest in *S. dysenteriae* type 1 and *S. flexneri* infection and least likely in *S. sonnei*. With mild disease, patients generally recover without specific therapy in a few days to a week. Severe shigellosis can progress to toxic dilatation and colonic perforation, which may be fatal.

Endoscopy shows the mucosa to be hemorrhagic with mucous discharge and focal ulcerations, sometimes with overlying exudate. The majority of the lesions are in the distal colon and progressively diminish in the more proximal segments of large bowel. Mild dehydration is common in patients with watery diarrhea; severe dehydration is very rare. With extensive colonic involvement, protein-losing enteropathy occurs and can have very important adverse nutritional consequences for the already poorly nourished child.

A variety of *extraintestinal complications* of shigellosis have been described. The majority of these occur in patients in developing countries and are related to both the prevalence of *S. dysenteriae* type 1 and *S. flexneri* infection as well as the poor nutritional state of the patients. For example, bacteremia, thought to be relatively infrequent in the United States, occurs in up to 8 percent of patients hospitalized for shigellosis in Dacca, Bangladesh. The causative *Shigella* species is isolated in half the patients; other Enterobacteriaceae are found in the remainder. Bacteremia is associated with higher than usual mortality and is more common in infants under 1 year of age and in those with protein-energy malnutrition. Persistent and clinically severe *Shigella* bacteremia has been encountered in the United States in patients with the acquired immunodeficiency syndrome (AIDS) (see Chap. 264).

Hemolytic-uremic syndrome (HUS) may occur with *S. dysenteriae* type 1 infection. In the United States, the more likely cause of HUS is a hemorrhagic colitis–causing strain of *E. coli* producing high levels of Shiga-family toxins, such as *E. coli* 0157:H7. HUS usually develops toward the end of the first week of shigellosis, when the dysentery is already resolving. Oliguria and a marked drop in hematocrit (as much as a 10 percent decrease within 24 h) are the first signs and may progress to anuria and renal failure or severe anemia with congestive heart failure, respectively. With HUS, leukemoid reactions with leukocyte counts over 50,000 per microliter may occur; thrombocytopenia (30,000 to 100,000 platelets per microliter) is common. Profound hyponatremia and severe hypoglycemia may be present. Central nervous system abnormalities include encephalopathic symptoms, seizures, altered consciousness, and bizarre posturing.

Other less common extraintestinal manifestations include seizures in some patients and in others reactive arthritis, both usually due to infection with *S. flexneri* strains. In patients expressing histocompatibility antigen HLA-B270, the full triad of Reiter's syndrome sometimes develops (see Chap. 274). Pneumonia, meningitis, vaginitis in prepubertal girls, keratoconjunctivitis, and "rose spot" rashes are rare events.

DIAGNOSIS AND LABORATORY FINDINGS Shigellosis is the principal bacterial cause of dysentery and should be considered in every patient presenting with bloody diarrhea. However, in the United States, because *S. sonnei* is the most common species, most patients will present with fever and a nonbloody watery diarrhea, while many patients with bloody diarrhea will have enterohemorrhagic *E. coli* as the cause. The specific diagnosis is made by culturing *Shigella* from the stool; most laboratories do not process *E. coli* found in stool cultures. The yield of *Shigella* is increased by culturing organisms from only those patients with fecal leukocytes or bloody diarrhea. The organism is very labile and must be quickly transferred to plates or holding media (such as buffered glycerol saline) or it will not survive. Stool samples are preferable to swabs; when the latter are used, a rectal sample should be obtained. For culturing, more than one selective medium should be used, including MacConkey and one other, such as Hektoen Enteric, Tergitol-7-tetrazolium, xylose-lysine-deoxycholate, or SS agars.

Serology can be performed as antibodies to somatic antigens develop early in the acute phase of disease; however, serum tests are not generally available and are usually used only for epidemiologic studies.

The differential diagnosis includes other microbial causes of inflammatory colitis: enterohemorrhagic and enteroinvasive *E. coli, Campylobacter jejuni, Salmonella enteriditis* serotypes, *Yersinia enterocolitica, Clostridium difficile,* and the protozoan *Entamoeba histolytica*. Ulcerative colitis or Crohn's colitis are among the "noninfectious" causes (see Chap. 241). All except *E. histolytica* are associated with the presence of large numbers of fecal leukocytes. Amebiasis can be diagnosed by finding erythrophagocytic trophozoites in the stool (see Chap. 158).

Other laboratory studies usually disclose a moderate neutrophilic leukocytosis, anemia due to blood loss with hemorrhagic diarrhea, prerenal azotemia, and a hyperchloremic acidosis if watery diarrhea has been pronounced. Laboratory findings in shigellosis complicated by the HUS are discussed above.

TREATMENT The mild dehydration in shigellosis can usually be easily corrected. Depending upon the severity of illness and the patient's ability to tolerate oral fluids, replacement therapy can be administered intravenously or orally. The oral replacement therapy recommended is similar to that for cholera (see Chap. 122).

The role of antibiotic therapy is variable and dependent upon the organism and severity of disease. Since *S. sonnei* infection is usually self-limited, culture results generally do not become available until the patient is better and there is little clinical need for further therapy. The use of antibiotics in more severe cases with bloody diarrhea or dysentery will reduce the duration of illness and can shorten the duration of the carriage state. Resistance to sulfonamides, streptomycin, chloramphenicol, and tetracyclines is almost universal, and many *Shigella* are now also resistant to ampicillin and trimethoprim-sulfamethoxazole. Knowledge of the pattern of resistance in a given population, which can change with time, is useful. In the United States, either ampicillin, 50 to 100 mg/kg per day in children or 2 g/d in adults in divided doses, or trimethoprim/sulfamethoxazole, 8/40 mg/kg per day in children or 2 regular strength tablets twice a day in adults, given for 5 days is generally recommended. Amoxicillin should *not* be substituted for ampicillin since it is not effective treatment for shigellosis. In developing countries, where resistance to both of these drugs is commonplace, the drug of choice for the treatment of multiresistant *S. dysenteriae* type 1 infections has been nalidixic acid, 55 mg/kg per day for 5 days. The 4-fluoroquinolones (e.g., ciprofloxacin) are highly effective for all strains (see Chap. 85), but are currently too costly for the third world and in the United States are not yet approved for use in children under 17 because of the concern for cartilage toxicity. Alternative drugs shown to be effective include pivamdinocillin (not yet approved by the Food and Drug Administration in the United States) and cefoperazone. In small clinical trials, cephalexin has had no effect in limiting symptoms; single doses of ceftriaxone may be effective, but more information is needed. No antibiotic treatment is recommended for the convalescent carriage state since this is usually limited to only several weeks' duration. Patients with AIDS may develop chronic carriage of shigella and be subject to relapsing infection with bacteremia (see Chap. 264). This cycle may be interrupted by prolonged (several weeks) treatment with a quinolone.

The role of antimotility agents such as atropine sulfate and diphenoxulate (Lomotil) and loperamide (Imodium) remains unclear in the early phases of shigellosis. They have had a limited effect in relieving diarrhea; conversely, they have not provoked more severe disease through retention of organisms. There is no indication for their use in the dysenteric phase of disease, and they are not recommended.

Treatment of complications of shigellosis often differs in developed and developing countries. For example, antibiotic-unresponsive toxic megacolon, with or without perforation, is often managed by colectomy in the United States. Surgery is less often employed in developing countries because of lack of availability or difficulties in ileostomy management. Hemolytic-uremic syndrome often requires dialysis. In developing countries this is less commonly used because azotemia is slow to develop; also the risk of significant hyperkalemia is often diminished because of the preexisting deficiency in total body potassium with malnutrition and wasting of lean body mass. The management of hyponatremia is governed by its severity and the symptomatic state of the patient as outlined in Chap. 50. Infusion of glucose can reverse clinical manifestations due to hypoglycemia and responses can be monitored by finger-stick blood glucose tests if no biochemistry laboratory is available. Optimal nutritional management is needed to correct the deficiencies due to underlying malnutrition and the superimposed catabolic stress and protein-losing enteropathy of shigellosis. This should begin during the acute illness and may require months of nutritional support afterwards (see Chap. 75).

PREVENTION Direct contact transmission of shigellosis can be prevented by appropriate environmental and personal hygiene. Hand washing with soap and water, decontamination of water supplies, use of sanitary latrines or toilets, protection of food preparation and its storage can all reduce the primary and secondary transmission of *Shigella* infection. In the highly endemic developing countries, infants are protected during the period of exclusive breast feeding, and this should be encouraged. Any measures that also reduce the burden of malnutrition will have a favorable effect on the population as well. Hospitalized patients should be put on stool precautions to ensure safe disposal of infected excreta and linens, and hospital personnel must wash their hands and medical instruments such as stethoscopes after each contact with an infected patient. Children in day-care must be kept at home while clinically ill and ideally should have a negative stool culture before returning to the group. Food handlers who develop shigellosis should also be required to be culture-negative before being allowed to return to work. Antibiotic treatment is not indicated for the asymptomatic carriage state. No effective vaccine is available.

REFERENCES

Askenazi S et al: Convulsions in shigellosis: Evaluation of possible risk factors. Am J Dis Child 141:208, 1987

Baskin DH et al: Shigella bacteremia in patients with the acquired immune deficiency syndrome. Am J Gastroenterol 82:338, 1987

Bennish ML et al: Death in shigellosis. Incidence and risk factors in hospitalized patients. J Infect Dis 161:507, 1990

Clemens JD et al: Breast feeding as a determinant of severity in shigellosis. Am J Epidemiol 123:710, 1986

Clerc PL, Sansonetti PJ: Entry of *Shigella flexneri* into HeLa cells: Evidence of directed phagocytosis involving actin polymerization and myosin accumulation. Infect Immun 55:1681, 1987

Hale LH, Formal SB: Pathogenesis of Shigella infections. Pathol Immunopathol Res 6:117, 1987

Keusch GT, Bennish ML: Shigella, in *Enteric Infection: Mechanisms, Manifestations, and Management*. MJG Farthing, GT Keusch (eds). London, Chapman & Hall, 1988, pp 265–282

115 HAEMOPHILUS INFECTIONS

DAVID C. WAAGNER / GEORGE H. McCRACKEN, JR.

INTRODUCTION Bacteria of the genus *Haemophilus* were first observed by Robert Koch in conjunctival exudates. The genus name, *Haemophilus*, reflects the growth requirements of these organisms for accessory factors found in erythrocytes. Many *Haemophilus* species are part of the normal respiratory tract flora, while others are identified only in the presence of disease. Of the 16 species within the genus, *H. influenzae* is encountered most frequently as a human pathogen. *H. parainfluenzae, H. ducreyi, H. aegyptius, H. aphrophilus*, and *H. paraphrophilus* are also associated with disease in humans.

Members of the genus are small, nonmotile, non-spore-forming, gram-negative bacilli. *Haemophilus* species are aerobic or facultatively anaerobic, reduce nitrates, and produce variable carbohydrate fermentation. Marked pleomorphism is characteristic of all *Haemophilus* species and is most prominent in those requiring only the V factor for growth. In cultures of pathologic materials, the organisms are primarily coccobacillary. The pleomorphic appearance and inconsistent uptake of safranin dye may promote confusion with other pathogens, most notably pneumococci and meningococci. *Haemophilus* species require at least one or both of two preformed growth factors present in erythrocytes: a heat-stable X factor (protoporphyrin X) and/or a heat-labile V factor [nicotinamide adenine dinucleotide (NAD) or NAD phosphate].

HAEMOPHILUS INFLUENZAE

BACTERIOLOGY *H. influenzae* strains are subdivided into eight distinct biotypes on the basis of indole production and urease and ornithine decarboxylase activity. Biotype I is isolated most frequently from patients with meningitis. Healthy children can harbor simultaneously several biotypes of *H. influenzae*, while usually only one biotype is recovered from healthy adults. *H. influenzae* strains are further subdivided by the presence or absence of an antigenically distinct polysaccharide capsule, demonstrable by quellung reaction with specific antisera. Six distinct antigenic capsule serotypes, a to f, have been described. Encapsulated strains of serotype b frequently produce invasive disease. Type b strains are further subdivided by differences in outer membrane proteins (OMPs). Antibodies to designated OMPs P1, P2, and P6 are partially protective in animal models. Encapsulated serotypes other than type b and nonencapsulated strains are more commonly associated with colonization of mucosal surfaces and disease of contiguous sites such as the middle ear (otitis media) and sinuses.

The virulence of *H. influenzae* is enhanced by several features. The polyribose ribitol phosphate (PRP) capsule of type b strain is protective against phagocytosis and serum complement activity. Outer membrane vesicles composed of lipooligosaccharide (LOS) and other membrane constituents are present on the cell wall surface and are excreted in vitro as membrane blebs. Antibodies to *H. influenzae* type b PRP capsule cross-react with antigens of certain pneumococcal and enterobacterial capsular polysaccharides. Utilizing monoclonal antibodies directed against epitopes present in the oligosaccharide portion of *Haemophilus* endotoxin, four distinct antigenic groups have been identified among *H. influenzae* type b strains. These LOS epitopes appear to be highly conserved among different strains. *H. influenzae* LOS produces a paralytic effect on ciliary motility in respiratory epithelial cells and induces meningeal inflammation when inoculated intracisternally in rabbits. *H. influenzae* produce three distinct IgA proteases capable of disrupting peptide bonds within IgA molecules, thereby enhancing infection of mucosal surfaces.

Growth of *H. influenzae* in culture media requires the presence of both X and V factors under aerobic conditions. *H. influenzae* grows poorly on ordinary blood agar, which contains heat-labile V factor inhibitors. Peptic digestion of blood (Fildes medium) or mild heating (Levinthal's medium or chocolate agar) liberates sufficient quantities of both factors for growth. Growth is maximally enhanced at 37°C and, in some strains, by the addition of 10% CO_2. On Levinthal's medium, encapsulated strains demonstrate a characteristic iridescence with obliquely transmitted light. When cultured under anaerobic conditions, *H. influenzae* does not require X factor for growth.

EPIDEMIOLOGY *H. influenzae* is indigenous to humans, residing primarily in the upper respiratory tract. *H. influenzae* infections have a worldwide distribution and are considered endemic. Nonencapsulated strains of *H. influenzae* colonize the oropharynx shortly after birth. Up to 90 percent of preschool children are currently or have been colonized with nonencapsulated *H. influenzae;* colonization and frequency of disease decrease with age. In contrast, asymptomatic colonization with *H. influenzae* type b occurs in less than 5 percent of children and adults. Rates of carriage can be markedly higher in closed crowded communities, such as day care centers and in close contacts, such as family members of an infant with disease. Carriage of *H. influenzae* type b can persist for months, despite orally or parenterally administered antibiotics or the presence of circulating antibody. In approximately 80 percent of patients with systemic *H. influenzae* type b infections, the organism can be recovered from pharyngeal culture.

Invasive *H. influenzae* is primarily a disease of infants and young children. *H. influenzae* type b meningitis, the most common invasive form, has a peak incidence between 6 and 7 months of age. The Centers for Disease Control estimate that the attack rate for *H. influenzae* type b meningitis in the United States is 1.45 per 100,000 population. Approximately two-thirds of *H. influenzae* type b infections occur in children under 2 years of age: specifically 90 percent of cellulitis and septic arthritis cases, 80 percent of cases of meningitis, and 75 percent of pneumonias. The peak incidence for epiglottitis occurs between ages 2 to 4 years. This age-related epidemiologic pattern is different in other countries such as Finland. A seasonal incidence for *H. influenzae* infections with peaks in both fall and early spring has been documented. A fourfold increase in the reported incidence of *H. influenzae* type b infections has occurred in the past four decades; it is not clear whether this is due to better diagnostic methods or represents a true increase in disease rates.

Certain host factors contribute to an increased risk for invasive *H. influenzae* disease. These include low socioeconomic status, large family size, neutropenia, immunoglobulin deficiency, sickle cell anemia, asplenia, low birth weight, and CSF shunt placement. Transplant recipients and patients with malignancies undergoing immunosuppression have an increased susceptibility to *H. influenzae*. Patients undergoing therapy for Hodgkin's lymphoma are notably at risk and often fail to produce protective anti-PRP antibody titers following infection. Alcoholism in adults is associated with an increased risk of *H. influenzae* pneumonia. Native Americans have a higher incidence of *H. influenzae* infections with younger peak attack rates and higher rates of recurrence than do other populations in the United States. Household contacts under 4 years of age of patients with *H. influenzae* type b meningitis have an approximately 500-fold greater likelihood of developing *H. influenzae* disease than does the general population.

PATHOGENICITY *H. influenzae* is transmitted through contact or inhalation of infected respiratory secretions. After nasopharyngeal colonization, organisms may infect the entire respiratory tract, spread contiguously to adjacent structures, or invade the bloodstream and seed distant foci. At least 95 percent of systemic diseases caused by *H. influenzae* are caused by type b strains.

Organisms are thought to reach the intravascular space from the nasopharynx as a result of transport within phagocytes from the mucosa into lymphatic channels. In experimental models, antecedent viral infection potentiates nasopharyngeal colonization of *H. influenzae* type b and enhances adherence to tissue culture cells. Within the bloodstream, the PRP capsule of type b organisms resists phagocytosis and complement activity. During bacteremia organisms can spread to all serous structures, most notably the meninges, pleura, joint spaces, and pericardium. The site of entry into the CSF from bloodborne organisms is the highly vascularized choroid plexus. The occurrence of meningitis correlates directly with the duration and magnitude ($>10^3$ colony forming units) of the bacteremia.

IMMUNITY The increased susceptibility of infants and young children to *H. influenzae* infections has been directly attributed to lack of sufficient anti-PRP antibody. Serum anti-PRP titers in relation to age correlate directly with the age-dependent susceptibility to *H. influenzae*. Newborns transiently acquire anti-PRP IgG antibody transplacentally, which diminishes after the first months of life. Acquisition of natural immunity generally does not occur until 2 to 4 years of age, leaving children between the ages of 2 months to 2 years at greatest risk for invasive disease.

Acquisition of anti-PRP antibody does not solely result from colonization of *H. influenzae* on mucosal surfaces. Many children naturally develop anti-PRP antibodies despite a lack of exposure to type b strains. This can result from colonization with organisms containing cross-reacting capsular antigens such as intestinal infection with *Escherichia coli* K100 strains. Children under 2 years of age produce low or undetectable concentrations of anti-PRP antibodies in response to *H. influenzae* infection or to PRP capsular vaccine. Antisomatic antibodies to noncapsular protein antigens from exposure to nonencapsulated strains can be cross-reactive with encapsulated *H. influenzae* strains as well. Passive immunization with antibodies to epitopes on the oligosaccharide portion of *Haemophilus* LOS has conferred protection in experimental disease, but their presence in acute phase sera of some infants with *H. influenzae* infection suggests that they are not protective in the clinical setting.

CLINICAL ILLNESSES *H. influenzae* is the most common cause of bacteremic illness in the pediatric population. Meningitis accounts for greater than 50 percent of invasive *H. influenzae* diseases, followed by pneumonia (12 to 15 percent), epiglottitis (5 to 17 percent), cellulitis (6 to 15 percent), and isolated bacteremia (2 to 11 percent). Osteomyelitis, pyogenic arthritis, and pericarditis occur less commonly. Healthy adults seldom develop invasive *H. influenzae* illness, but nonencapsulated strains of *H. influenzae* appear to play an important role in exacerbations of chronic bronchitis.

Meningitis *H. influenzae* type b is the most common cause of bacterial meningitis in children between 3 months and 5 years of age and is associated with a case fatality rate of approximately 5 percent and a long-term morbidity rate of 15 to 30 percent. Meningitis can develop insidiously over several days, usually associated with an upper respiratory infection, or abruptly, progressing in a few hours. The signs and symptoms of *H. influenzae* meningitis are identical to those seen in bacterial meningitis caused by other pathogens. Nonspecific findings include fever, lethargy, irritability, anorexia, emesis, respiratory distress, and altered mental status. Older children and adults often have headache, stiff neck, and photophobia. The characteristic stiff neck with Kernig's and Brudzinski's signs are seen infrequently in children younger than 15 months of age. Focal neurologic findings can appear early, with up to one-third of patients having seizures before admission. Purpuric lesions identical to those seen in *Neisseria meningitidis* infection occur uncommonly and are usually associated with disseminated intravascular coagulation.

Epiglottitis Epiglottitis is characterized by the abrupt onset of epiglottic edema, which may progress rapidly to complete obstruction of the airway, representing a true medical emergency. *H. influenzae* type b is the principal cause of epiglottitis. The peak incidence occurs between 2 to 4 years of age. A genetic predisposition is suggested by a marked predominance in Caucasians, its unusual rarity in Native American and Eskimo populations, and the frequent association with certain HLA groups. *H. influenzae* bacteremia occurs in greater than 90 percent of patients with epiglottitis, yet extraepiglottic foci are uncommon.

Patients typically present with an abrupt onset of fever, sore throat, stridor, dyspnea, pooling of oral secretions, and drooling. They appear anxious, sitting in a prone position with their mouths open and their necks fully extended. Indirect visualization of the oropharynx with a tongue blade is contraindicated, as this maneuver can potentiate epiglottic edema resulting in acute respiratory obstruction. Adults can have a more insidious onset with sore throat and progressive dysphagia. Direct laryngoscopy should be performed in all patients only in a setting where immediate endotracheal intubation can be performed or an emergency tracheostomy placed if intubation is unsuccessful. The epiglottis is usually edematous with a cherry-red appearance, and the aryepiglottal folds and surrounding tissues are swollen and inflamed. Placement of an artificial airway (endotracheal tube or tracheostomy) is advocated because of the high mortality (up to 80 percent) when obstruction occurs. Radiographs of the lateral neck can demonstrate an enlarged epiglottis (the ''thumb'' sign).

Pneumonia Type b strains cause up to one-third of bacterial pneumonias in children between 4 months and 4 years of age. Many of the children with *H. influenzae* pneumonia have positive blood cultures, and almost half have evidence of additional foci of infection. *H. influenzae* pneumonia is clinically indistinguishable from *Streptococcus pneumoniae* infection. Radiographic appearance is more often segmented or lobar, although bronchopneumonia and interstitial patterns have been described. Pleural reaction with effusion or frank empyema is more common than with other pathogens. Pneumatocele formation occurs infrequently.

The exact incidence of pneumonia due to nonencapsulated strains of *H. influenzae* is unknown, as they are frequently found as part of the upper respiratory flora. Alcohol abuse significantly increases the risk of *H. influenzae* in adults. Some estimates place nonencapsulated *H. influenzae* strains as the second commonest cause of community acquired bacterial pneumonias in adults.

Cellulitis Cellulitis caused by *H. influenzae* primarily occurs in children under age 2 and predominantly in the buccal and periorbital areas. *H. influenzae* cellulitis has a rapid onset, develops within hours, and is associated with bacteremia in almost three-fourths of patients. Additional foci of infection are found in 10 percent of cases. The involved area often has a characteristic violaceous or reddish-blue appearance.

Septic arthritis *H. influenzae* type b strains are the most common cause of suppurative arthritis in young children. Cultures of joint fluid or blood will yield the pathogen in approximately 70 percent of cases. The presence of capsular antigen in joint fluid is usually diagnostic. Needle aspiration or open drainage of purulent material with antimicrobial therapy are the mainstays of management (see Chap. 96). Significant joint dysfunction has been described despite adequate antibiotic therapy.

Bacteremia without focal disease After *S. pneumoniae, H. influenzae* is the leading cause of bacteremia without localized disease in children less than 2 years of age. Older children and adults with asplenia, sickle cell disease, or immunodeficiency, or who are undergoing cancer chemotherapy are also at risk.

Pericarditis Purulent pericarditis caused by *H. influenzae* infrequently accompanies systemic *H. influenzae* disease. Pericarditis complicates *H. influenzae* pneumonia in approximately 5 percent of cases. Echocardiographic studies can identify the presence of excess fluid in the pericardial space which must be confirmed and managed by open drainage and antibiotic treatment (see Chap. 193).

Additional respiratory tract disease Nonencapsulated *H. influenzae* strains are a common cause of acute sinusitis and otitis media in all age groups and of chronic bronchial disease in adults. Greater than 90 percent of *H. influenzae* strains obtained from middle ear fluid in acute otitis media are nonencapsulated. Exacerbations of chronic bronchitis have been attributed to nonencapsulated *H. influenzae* strains, although their exact role is uncertain.

Other infections *H. influenzae* has been identified as a rare cause of osteomyelitis, endocarditis, endophthalmitis, pyelonephritis, mediastinitis, peritonitis, epididymitis, and tenosynovitis. Abscess formation is rare, but has been described in brain, lung, muscle, and peritonsillar tissue.

DIAGNOSIS A definitive diagnosis is made by recovery of *H. influenzae* from cultures of infected body tissues and fluids. Cultures of the nasopharynx are not useful. Examination and culture of the CSF must be considered in all infants and young children with evidence of systemic *H. influenzae* disease. Needle aspirations in areas of cellulitis should be performed at the site of maximal induration for highest yield.

Identification of organisms on Gram-stained smears of CSF correlates directly with bacterial density; 96 percent positive at a concentration $>10^5$ CFU/mL, 78 percent positive between 10^3 to 10^5 CFU/mL, and 0 at $\leq 10^3$ CFU/mL. The pleomorphic appearance of *H. influenzae* and its Gram stain variability can produce frequent misinterpretation, estimated at 15 percent in one series. Acridine orange stains can be useful in detecting intracellular bacteria and small numbers of organisms in body fluids. Approximately one-third of patients with bacterial meningitis receive antimicrobial therapy before hospital admission, substantially reducing the diagnostic reliability of the Gram-stained smear and the culture.

The detection of PRP antigen in body fluids can be used to diagnose *H. influenzae* infection before culture results are available, or when prior antibiotic therapy has sterilized cultures. The most frequently used techniques in order of decreasing sensitivity are latex particle agglutination (LPA), coagulation, and countercurrent immunoelectrophoresis. LPA is capable of detecting PRP antigen at bacterial concentrations of approximately 100 CFU/mL or greater. Despite the occurrence of cross-reacting antigens among other organisms, false-positive results are uncommon. Enzyme-linked immunosorbent assays for PRP have been developed but are more difficult and time-consuming, offering few benefits over LPA identification.

THERAPY Antibacterial agents that are bactericidal in vitro and achieve adequate bactericidal activity in body fluids should be used for systemic *H. influenzae* infections. Regional differences in antimicrobial susceptibilities must be considered in selecting appropriate therapy. The high prevalence of β-lactamase-producing strains of *H. influenzae* type b (15 to 50 percent in the United States) dictates that an assay for β-lactamase and disk susceptibilities be performed on all isolates. Organisms should also be tested for chloramphenicol resistance (prevalence <10 percent in United States) as a result of plasmid-mediated acetyltransferase.

Empiric therapy with ampicillin (200 to 300 mg/kg per day for children, 4 to 6 g/d for adults, intravenously in four or six divided doses), in combination with chloramphenicol (75 to 100 mg/kg per day for children, 4 g/d for adults, intravenously in four divided doses) until results of susceptibility studies are available, has been used effectively for more than a decade. Chloramphenicol is bactericidal against *Haemophilus* strains. The unpredictable metabolism of chloramphenicol in patients with hepatic dysfunction or hypotension, in young infants, and in those receiving anticonvulsant therapy requires monitoring of serum chloramphenicol concentrations to maintain safe and therapeutic levels.

The emergence of multiply resistant strains of *H. influenzae* has promoted the development of newer antimicrobials which provide alternatives to conventional therapy with ampicillin and chloramphenicol. Cefotaxime and ceftriaxone are β-lactamase-stable and achieve high bactericidal titers in all body fluids, including CSF, providing effective single-drug therapy for *H. influenzae* infections. Ceftriaxone has a long serum half-life (6 to 8 h), permitting the option of single daily doses (see Chap. 85). Other, newer cephalosporins shown to be effective in systemic *H. influenzae* disease include ceftazidime, cefuroxime, and ceftizoxime. In comparative trials cefotaxime or ceftriaxone are as effective as ampicillin and chloramphenicol for the therapy of meningitis and in many centers in the United States are used as primary treatment.

Outpatient therapy of less severe *H. influenzae* infections may be accomplished with a variety of oral antimicrobials. Amoxicillin is the therapy of choice for susceptible isolates. Alternative oral antibiotic selections for resistant organisms or in penicillin-sensitive patients include trimethoprim-sulfamethoxazole, erythromycin-sulfasoxazole, cefaclor, cefuroxime axetil, and chloramphenicol (for dosages see Chap. 85). The routine use of oral chloramphenicol is discouraged due to emergence of resistance and hematologic toxicity. Pharmacologic combinations of amoxicillin and ampicillin with β-lactamase inhibitors such as potassium clavulanate and sulbactam permit these agents to be used for therapy of β-lactamase-producing strains of *H. influenzae*. Although not approved yet for use in children, the oral quinolones, such as ciprofloxacin, have excellent activity against *H. influenzae*.

Duration of antimicrobial therapy is dependent on the disease process and the patient's response to treatment. Invasive *H. influenzae* disease requires intravenous antimicrobial therapy until all infectious foci are sterilized and the patient is afebrile and without clinical or laboratory evidence of infection. Patients with meningitis traditionally receive 10 to 14 days of therapy; however, recent studies indicate that uncomplicated *H. influenzae* meningitis can be treated for only 7 to 10 days.

In addition to antimicrobial therapy, supportive care of systemic *H. influenzae* infection is of critical importance. Immediate attention must be directed at airway maintenance, reduction of increased intracranial pressure and cerebral edema, and support of the respiratory and cardiovascular systems. Establishment of a secure airway is of the utmost urgency in epiglottitis. Dexamethasone given intravenously in a dose of 0.15 mg/kg every 6 h for the first 4 days of therapy significantly diminishes meningeal inflammation and the incidence of moderate or severe hearing loss of *H. influenzae* meningitis. Patients with systemic *H. influenzae* infection should be kept in respiratory isolation for 24 h following initiation of appropriate antibiotic therapy.

PREVENTION Large epidemiologic studies have demonstrated significantly increased attack rates in young household contacts of patients with systemic *H. influenzae* infection. Age-specific attack rates range from 6 percent in those under 1 year of age to 0.5 percent for those between ages 4 and 6. Only rifampin (rifampicin) has proved effective in eliminating nasopharyngeal carriage and in preventing secondary cases among household contacts.

Currently, the American Academy of Pediatrics recommends rifampin (20 mg/kg per day for children, 600 mg/d for adults, in a single daily dose for 4 days) be given to all household contacts (including adults and the index case) of an index case when at least one sibling is under 4 years of age. Rifampin prophylaxis of day care contacts is recommended only if two or more cases of invasive disease occur within a 60-day period.

The low immunogenicity of PRP in infants and young children has hampered development of an effective vaccine. Vaccines composed of purified *H. influenzae* PRP are immunogenic for older children and adults, but have little immunogenicity in those under 24 months of age. A more immunogenic vaccine composed of PRP covalently linked to diphtheria toxoid (PRP-D) was licensed for use in the United States in December 1987, based on evidence from Finland indicating protective efficacy in young infants and children. It is likely that other *Haemophilus* PRP conjugated vaccines will be approved for use. The American Academy of Pediatrics recommends immunization of all children at 18 months of age with one injection of the conjugate vaccine.

HAEMOPHILUS AEGYPTIUS

H. aegyptius, also known as the *Koch-Weeks* bacillus, closely resembles nonencapsulated *H. influenzae* and demonstrates a 78 percent DNA homology. *H. aegyptius* can be distinguished by hemagglutination activity, lack of indole production, and triacetyloleandomycin (troleandomycin) susceptibility.

This organism is associated with a purulent conjunctivitis of worldwide distribution. The conjunctivitis responds to local irrigation, and therapy with topical aminoglycoside, polymyxin, or sulfonamide ophthalmic preparations. *H. aegyptius* also has been identified as the etiologic agent of Brazilian purpuric fever (BPF). BPF is a fulminant disease of infants and children characterized by the acute onset of conjunctivitis, fever, emesis, and abdominal pain, with rapid progression to purpura, vascular collapse, peripheral necrosis, and death within 48 h of onset. First recognized in 1984, BPF is endemic in South America, and has a case fatality rate approaching 70 percent.

HAEMOPHILUS DUCREYI

H. ducreyi grows poorly on most media, requiring X but not V factor. Isolation of organisms from clinical specimens occurs in only 60 to 70 percent of cases, even with selective media. Gram-stained smears show gram-negative coccobacilli in chains or a ''school of fish'' pattern.

This organism causes chancroid, a sexually transmitted disease that occurs worldwide (see Chap. 93), most commonly in nonwhite uncircumcised men in poor socioeconomic conditions. Chancroid is manifested by painful, sharply demarcated ulcerations usually confined to the genitalia and perineal area. Suppurative inguinal lymphadenopathy develops in more than one-half of patients. Approximately 10 percent of patients with chancroid have concomitant primary syphilis. Clinical diagnosis can be confirmed by Gram stain and cultures of ulcers or lymph node aspirates. Most strains are resistant to ampicillin and many are resistant to sulfonamides and tetracycline. Erythromycin (2 g/d given orally in four divided doses) or trimethoprim/sulfamethoxasole (320 mg/1.6 g per day given orally in two divided doses) for a total of 10 days is the regimen of choice.

HAEMOPHILUS PARAINFLUENZAE

H. parainfluenzae is usually isolated as part of the microflora of the human nasopharynx and mouth. *H. parainfluenzae* requires V but not X factor, prompting confusion with *H. influenzae* when *H. influenzae* is incubated anaerobically as in stabbed cultures. A small percentage of isolates produce β-lactamase.

Infection with *H. parainfluenzae* may follow bloodstream invasion from dental manipulation. Risk factors include immune deficiency, alcoholism, and congenital or rheumatic valvular heart disease. Otitis media, pharyngitis, pneumonia, empyema, liver abscess, meningitis, endocarditis, and urinary tract infections have been described. Endocarditis is the most frequent manifestation of *H. parainfluenzae* infection, usually occurring in young or middle-aged adults with underlying valvular disease. Arterial embolization is more prominent than in endocarditis caused by other pathogens. Antimicrobial therapy consists of ampicillin or a third-generation cephalosporin often combined with an aminoglycoside.

HAEMOPHILUS APHROPHILUS

H. aphrophilus is part of normal human oral microflora. Optimal growth requirements include high CO_2 concentration and X factor (but not V factor)–enriched media. Most infections with *H. aphrophilus* follow oropharyngeal infection or trauma, resulting in bacteremia. *H. aphrophilus* causes endocarditis and brain abscess in patients with underlying heart disease. Sinusitis, pneumonia, emphysema, dental abscess, peritonitis, meningitis, osteomyelitis, and pyarthrosis caused by *H. aphrophilus* have been described. Most isolates are susceptible to ampicillin, third-generation cephalosporins, tetracycline, aminoglycosides, and chloramphenicol.

HAEMOPHILUS PARAPHROPHILUS

H. paraphrophilus is part of human oropharyngeal flora, requiring V factor (but not X) for growth. Reported disorders include endocarditis, osteomyelitis, and urinary tract infections.

REFERENCES

Haemophilus influenzae

AMERICAN ACADEMY OF PEDIATRICS COMMITTEE ON INFECTIOUS DISEASES: *Haemophilus influenzae* infections, in *1988 Red Book,* G Peter et al (eds). Elk Grove Village, IL, American Academic of Pediatrics, 1988, pp 204–210

BORENSTEIN DG, SIMON GL: *Haemophilus influenzae* septic arthritis in adults. A report of four cases and a review of the literature. Medicine 65:191, 1986

CROWE HM, LEVITZ RE: Invasive *Haemophilus influenzae* disease in adults. Arch Intern Med 147:241, 1987

GINSBURG CM ET AL: Report of 65 cases of *Haemophilus influenzae* type b pneumoniae. Pediatrics 64:283, 1979

KATZ SL, MORTIMER EA: Proceedings of a round table. *Haemophilus influenzae* type b: The disease and its prevention. Pediatr Infec Dis J 6:773, 1987

LEBEL MH et al: Dexamethasone therapy for bacterial meningitis: Results of two double-blind placebo controlled trials. N Engl J Med 319:964, 1988

MAYOSMITH MF et al: Acute epiglottitis in adults. An eight-year experience in the state of Rhode Island. N Engl J Med 314:1133, 1986

MURPHY TF, APICELLA MA: Nontypable *Haemophilus influenzae:* A review of clinical aspects, surface antigens, and the human immune response. Rev Infect Dis 9:1, 1987

MURPHY TO et al: Risk of subsequent disease among day care contacts of patients with systemic *Haemophilus influenzae* type b disease. N Engl J Med 316:1, 1987

WEINBERG GA, GRANOFF DA: Polysaccharide-protein conjugate vaccines for the prevention of *Haemophilus influenzae* type b disease. J Pediatr 113:621, 1988

Haemophilus aegyptius

BRAZILIAN PURPURIC FEVER STUDY GROUP: Brazilian purpuric fever; epidemic purpura fulminans associated with antecedent purulent conjunctivitis. Lancet 2:757, 1987

———: Biochemical, genetic, and epidemiologic characterization of *Haemophilus influenzae* biogroup aegyptius *(Haemophilus aegyptius)* strains associated with Brazilian purpuric fever. J Clin Microbiol 26:1524, 1988

Haemophilus ducreyi

FAST MV: Antimicrobial therapy of chancroid: An evaluation of five treatment regimens correlated with *in vitro* sensitivity. Sex Trans Dis 8:192, 1981

Haemophilus parainfluenzae

BLACK CT et al: *Haemophilus parainfluenzae: Haemophilus parainfluenzae* infections in children with report of a unique case. Rev Infect Dis 10:342, 1988

Haemophilus aphrophilus

BIEGER RC et al: *Haemophilus aphrophilus:* A microbiologic and clinical review of 42 cases. Medicine 57:345, 1978

Haemophilus paraphrophilus

KILIAN M, BIBERSTEIN EL: Genus II, *Haemophilus,* in *Bergey's Manual of Systemic Bacteriology,* NR Kreig, JG Holt (eds). Baltimore, Williams & Wilkins, 1984, vol 1, p 567

116 WHOOPING COUGH

BISHARA J. FREIJ / GEORGE H. McCRACKEN, JR.

DEFINITION Pertussis, or whooping cough, is an acute infection of the respiratory tract caused by *Bordetella pertussis.* This illness occurs worldwide and is most severe when it afflicts unimmunized infants. The term *pertussis* (meaning intensive cough) is generally preferred to whooping cough because many patients, especially infants, with this infection do not manifest the characteristic whoop. Despite the availability of protective vaccines, worldwide control of pertussis has yet to be achieved because of large populations of unimmunized infants and children in developing countries and, in industrialized countries, because of the intense controversy surrounding the use of pertussis vaccines as a result of their purported severe reactions.

MICROBIOLOGY Of the three *Bordetella* species known to infect humans, *B. pertussis* is by far the most common cause of whooping cough. *B. parapertussis, B. bronchiseptica,* and adenovirus types 1, 2, 3, 5, 12, and 19 are infrequent causes of the pertussis syndrome.

B. pertussis is a small, encapsulated, nonmotile, gram-negative coccobacillus. Special strains are required to demonstrate the capsule because capsular swelling in the presence of antiserum does not occur. When grown on Bordet-Gengou medium, *B. pertussis* colonies are smooth, convex, glistening, and translucent with a zone of surrounding hemolysis. *B. pertussis* can be distinguished from *B. parapertussis* and *B. bronchiseptica* by biochemical reactions such as nitrate reduction, citrate utilization, and urease production and by the presence of species-specific heat-labile capsular K antigens (K1 for *B. pertussis,* K12 for *B. bronchiseptica,* and K14 for *B. parapertussis*). *B. bronchiseptica* possesses lateral flagella and is the only motile *Bordetella* species. There is extensive DNA homology between the three *Bordetella* species, suggesting that they may represent different biotypes of the same organism.

B. pertussis produces many biologically active substances that may function as virulence factors, including lymphocytosis-promoting factor (LPF, also known as leukocytosis-promoting factor), histamine-sensitizing factor, islet-activating factor, pertussis toxin, and pertussigen. Other potential virulence factors include filamentous hemagglutinin (FHA), adenylate cyclase (AC), lipopolysaccharide (LPS), tracheal cytotoxin (TCT), hemolysin, heat-labile toxin, and agglutinogens.

PATHOGENESIS *B. pertussis* is typically transmitted to a new host by inhalation of airborne respiratory secretions from an infected individual. The organisms colonize the respiratory tract by adhering to ciliated epithelial cells. FHA, LPF, and agglutinogens appear to be important for the attachment process because specific antibodies against these factors protect experimental animals from respiratory infection by *B. pertussis.* Persistence of infection may be accomplished through impairment of host immune effector cell function by both AC (inhibition of phagocyte function) and LPF (altered lymphocyte production), as well as by disruption of normal clearance mechanisms by tracheal cytotoxin. Local respiratory tract tissue damage can be mediated by TCT, AC, hemolysin, and heat-labile toxin. The leukocytosis and lymphocytosis observed in this disease are systemic effects of LPF. The pathogenesis of pertussis encephalopathy is unclear. Other systemic manifestations may be due to pertussis LPS, but its role in pathogenicity is not well-defined.

EPIDEMIOLOGY It is difficult to estimate the true worldwide impact of pertussis because of problems in accurately diagnosing the illness and of underreporting of cases. Approximately 600,000 pertussis-related deaths are believed to occur each year; most of these involve unimmunized infants. The total number of reported pertussis cases in the United States has declined annually over the past 10 years from about 115,000 to 270,000 (with 5000 to 10,000 deaths) per year in the prevaccine era to about 1200 to 4200 (with 4 to 11 deaths per year). The number of reported cases per 100,000 population in the United States, however, has recently increased from a range of 0.54 to 0.95 during the years 1978 to 1982 to 0.96 to 1.74 for the years 1983 to 1987. Reported cases are thought to represent only 15 to 25 percent of actual cases.

Pertussis is a highly communicable infection. Secondary attack rates of 70 to 100 percent have been reported for susceptible household contacts and of 25 to 50 percent in schools. Humans are the only known natural host of *B. pertussis.* Although asymptomatic transient carriage of this organism has been noted in some household contacts of index patients, a chronic carrier state does not exist.

Pertussis is endemic in the United States. Localized geographic outbreaks of this disease continue to occur largely because of failure to immunize large numbers of susceptible individuals. Seasonal variations in the incidence of pertussis have been noted; autumn appears to be the season of lowest incidence.

The attack rates for females are greater than those for males, and these differences become more prominent with increasing age. No racial differences in attack rates have been noted. About half of all reported cases in the United States are in infants under 1 year of age; an estimated 15 percent are in individuals 15 years of age or older. Clinical disease in adolescents or adults may be atypical and is frequently misdiagnosed as bronchitis. Pertussis can occur in adults who received vaccine in infancy and childhood. Such individuals can potentially serve as important reservoirs for transmitting the infection to susceptible infants and children.

CLINICAL MANIFESTATIONS The incubation period for pertussis ranges from 5 to 21 days with a mean of 7 to 10 days. In infants and young children the disease can be divided into three symptomatic stages. The initial *catarrhal* stage is characterized by nonspecific upper respiratory symptoms such as sneezing, rhinorrhea, conjunctival injection, tearing, mild cough, and low-grade fever. This stage lasts 1 to 2 weeks and represents the most infectious period of this disease.

In the second or *paroxysmal* stage, there is progression to increasing bouts of severe coughing. Each paroxysm is characterized by 5 to 20 forceful coughs within a span of a few seconds. The characteristic whoop is produced when air is forcefully inhaled through a narrowed glottis. At the peak of disease activity, patients may experience 15 to more than 25 such paroxysms over a 24-h period, usually more often at night. The attacks may be prolonged to such an extent that patients become hypoxic. Ventilatory support is sometimes required, especially in young infants. Other physical findings during an attack may include cyanosis, neck vein congestion, bulging eyes, and protrusion of the tongue. The paroxysms may be provoked by yawning, sneezing, or eating. Vomiting frequently follows paroxysms. Fever is generally absent unless secondary suppurative complications develop. Patients usually appear normal between attacks. This stage lasts from 2 to 4 weeks or longer.

During the third or *convalescent* stage, the paroxysms become less frequent and less intense. This stage can last several months although a 3- to 4-week course is more usual. Patients are not usually infectious during this period despite continued coughing. After recovery, noxious stimuli or a viral respiratory infection can provoke recrudescence of the paroxysmal cough.

The disease in older children and adults is much milder and usually consists only of a prolonged bronchitis, which lasts several weeks or, rarely, months.

COMPLICATIONS Approximately 40 percent of infants and young children with pertussis require hospitalization; the frequency is highest for infants younger than 6 months of age (75 percent) and decreases with advancing age. The mortality rate is highest in infancy and an estimated 1.0 percent of all infants under 6 months die from complications of this disease.

Pneumonia is the most frequent complication of pertussis. It occurs in 12 percent of all young patients and in about 20 percent of those under 1 year of age. The pneumonia may be caused by *B. pertussis* itself but is more commonly caused by secondary bacterial pathogens such as *Haemophilus influenzae, Streptococcus pneumoniae, S. pyogenes,* or *Staphylococcus aureus.* The development of significant temperature elevation should prompt evaluation for superinfection by any of these bacteria. Other pulmonary complications of pertussis include interstitial or subcutaneous emphysema, pneumothorax, atelectasis, and bronchiectasis.

Central nervous system complications are serious but uncommon. They are most likely to occur during the paroxysmal stage, and infants appear to be the most susceptible. Seizures occur in about 1.7 percent of all reported pertussis cases, while encephalopathy is noted in approximately 0.5 percent. Seizures are usually generalized but focal convulsions can occur. Other acute neurologic abnormalities include hemiplegia, paraplegia, deafness, blindness, ataxia, and aphasia. The cerebrospinal fluid of these patients is typically normal, although a mild lymphocytic pleocytosis of 100 cells or less per microliter and/or a protein concentration of 1.0 g/L (100 mg/dL) can be found. The prognosis for patients with pertussis who develop neurologic complications is poor. Of those who develop pertussis encephalopathy, approximately a third die, a third survive with permanent sequelae, and a third survive with no apparent deficits. Long-term residua can include focal or generalized convulsions, focal paralysis, mental retardation, or behavioral abnormalities.

Otitis media is common. Hemorrhagic complications are rare and include epistaxis, petechiae, melena, subdural or epidural hematomas, subarachnoid or intraventricular bleeding, subconjunctival and scleral hemorrhages, as well as hemorrhagic bullous myringitis. Other infrequent complications include activation of latent tuberculosis, diaphragmatic rupture, umbilical hernia, rectal prolapse, ulceration of the frenulum of the tongue, and weight loss, with or without dehydration, from poor nutritional intake.

DIAGNOSIS A clinical diagnosis of pertussis in infants and young children is usually first suggested during the paroxysmal stage of the disease. The nonspecific respiratory signs and symptoms encountered during the catarrhal stage are not suggestive of pertussis unless a history of contact with a known case is elicited or they occur in the setting of an outbreak of this disease. Spasmodic cough is, however, not pathognomonic of pertussis and can be associated with other diseases such as bronchiolitis; chlamydial, viral, or mycoplasmal pneumonia; cystic fibrosis; tuberculosis; and such noninfectious entities as foreign bodies or extrinsic airway compression caused by lymphadenopathy or malignancies. These conditions can generally be differentiated from pertussis by clinical and laboratory findings, by the chest x-ray, and by the course of the disease. In older children and adults the disease may mimic prolonged bronchitis from other causes; however, it can be distinguished from chronic bronchitis (see Chap. 210) by its acute onset and self-limited course.

The white blood cell count can be helpful in establishing the diagnosis. Characteristically, marked elevations of the white blood cell count (20,000 to 50,000 or more cells per microliter) with a lymphocytosis of 60 percent or more are seen at the end of the catarrhal and during the paroxysmal stages of pertussis; the degree of the lymphocytosis may correlate with disease severity. Both T and B lymphocytes are increased in number. Lymphocytosis is seen in older children and adults with the disease and helps to differentiate pertussis from other cases of prolonged bronchitis.

The definitive diagnosis of pertussis is made by recovering *B. pertussis, B. parapertussis,* or *B. bronchiseptica* from nasopharyngeal swabs. Dacron or calcium alginate swabs are preferred to cotton swabs because the latter contain fatty acids that may inhibit the growth of *B. pertussis.* Specimens should be directly plated on selective media to maximize the chance of obtaining a positive culture. The best selective media for isolation of *B. pertussis* are Regan-Lowe, Bordet-Gengou, and modified Stainer-Scholte agar.

Bacterial isolation rates are highest when cultures are obtained within the first 3 to 4 weeks of the illness. Factors that contribute to low recovery rates of *B. pertussis* include a delay in specimen collection (e.g., only 15 to 20 percent of cases are culture-positive at 6 weeks), antimicrobial therapy (especially with erythromycin, tetracycline, or trimethoprim-sulfamethoxazole), previous pertussis immunization, incorrect collection procedures or delays in specimen transport, overgrowth of contaminating bacteria, and inexperienced laboratory personnel who may fail to recognize the organism in culture. *B. pertussis* can be isolated from as many as 80 to 90 percent of patients during the catarrhal stage and from 50 percent or less of those in the paroxysmal stage of the disease.

A direct fluorescent antibody (DFA) test utilizes a polyclonal fluorescein-labeled antibody against *B. pertussis* to stain and directly identify the organism in nasopharyngeal specimens; however, its sensitivity is variable, with both high rates of false-negative or false-positive results reported in different laboratories.

Enzyme-linked immunosorbent assay (ELISA), complement fixation, immunodiffusion, and other antibody assays are not helpful in the diagnosis of pertussis. The detection of antipertussis antibodies may indicate natural infection with this organism or prior immunization. The demonstration of fourfold or greater rises in IgG titers against *B. pertussis* antigens is infrequent even in culture-positive cases, because the acute phase serum is usually not obtained early enough in the disease. Serum IgA responses to pertussis are found only after natural infection; however, many infants with this disease fail to produce detectable pertussis-specific IgA antibodies. These antibodies may also persist in normal populations because of subclinical infection, making it difficult to differentiate a recent acute infection from past disease.

B. pertussis–specific secretory IgA antibodies can be detected by ELISA in nasopharyngeal secretions after natural infection with this organism, but not after immunization. These secretory IgA antibodies usually appear during the second or third week of the disease and can persist for 3 months or longer. This test may ultimately prove to be useful in the diagnosis of pertussis in culture-negative cases.

TREATMENT Supportive care is of paramount importance in the management of patients with pertussis. Those with potentially severe disease, especially infants under 6 months, should be hospitalized. Strict respiratory isolation for 5 days after initiation of appropriate antibiotics is recommended before patients can be considered noninfectious. Close nursing observation, gentle suctioning to remove respiratory secretions, avoidance of stimuli that can provoke paroxysms such as invasive procedures or tobacco smoke, provision of adequate nutritional intake, attention to fluid and electrolyte balance, oxygen administration to avoid hypoxia, and management of apnea episodes all contribute to a satisfactory outcome. Neither cough suppressants nor antihistamines are helpful in reducing the intensity or frequency of paroxysms. The use of glucocorticoids and $beta_2$-adrenergic agonists to reduce coughing paroxysms remains controversial.

Antimicrobial therapy provided in the incubation period or catarrhal stage may prevent or ameliorate the disease. Antibiotics are generally considered ineffective in modifying the clinical course of the disease once it reaches the paroxysmal stage, but are administered to these patients to reduce their infectivity and to prevent spread of the organisms. Erythromycin in a dosage of 40 to 50 mg/kg per day in four equally divided doses (maximum, 2 g/d) given orally is preferred for treatment and is continued for 14 days. Erythromycin will eliminate *B. pertussis* from the nasopharynx in 4 or fewer days. Bacteriologic relapse occurs, however, in 10 percent of patients treated for periods shorter than 2 weeks. Trimethoprim/sulfamethoxazole (8/40 mg/kg per day in two divided doses) can be used in patients who cannot tolerate erythromycin, but its efficacy has not been established.

PREVENTION **Management of contacts** Household and other close contacts, whether children or adults, should be prophylactically treated with erythromycin in a dosage of 40 to 50 mg/kg per day (maximum, 2 g/d) in four equally divided doses given orally for 14 days. Even fully immunized individuals should receive chemoprophylaxis. In addition, close contacts younger than 7 years of age who have received at least four doses of pertussis vaccine (usually in the form of the triple diphtheria-tetanus-pertussis, DTP, vaccine) should be given a booster dose of DTP unless one has been given within the preceding 3 years. Those under age 7 who have not yet been completely immunized should continue with the recommended vaccine schedule and receive erythromycin prophylaxis.

Day-care center attendees should be treated as close contacts and managed accordingly. Children with pertussis may be allowed to return to day care after 5 days of erythromycin therapy, assuming their general condition permits unrestricted activity. All close contacts should be observed for the development of respiratory symptoms for 14 days after exposure to the index case. Those developing symptoms should be evaluated by a physician and excluded from day care until the cause of their symptoms is identified and appropriately managed.

Vaccines Currently available pertussis vaccines are generally prepared from either whole-cell suspensions or partially purified cell products. Only the adsorbed whole-cell vaccines are used in the United States; by contrast, Japan uses only the acellular type of pertussis vaccines. The efficacy of whole-cell vaccines is believed to be 80 to 90 percent. The duration of protection is uncertain, but limited data suggest that the efficacy declines to 50 percent 4 to 7 years after the last dose and is almost absent after 12 years. The efficacy of the acellular vaccines also appears to be approximately 85 to 90 percent based on studies conducted in Japan principally in children 2 years of age and older. The duration of protection with the acellular product is unknown.

Completely immunized individuals can still develop pertussis, but disease is typically milder. Although improvements in housing as well as in the general health of the population have been suggested as the cause for the decline in incidence of pertussis, industrialized countries such as the United Kingdom, Japan, and Sweden experienced major pertussis epidemics shortly after routine pertussis immunization was stopped because of concerns regarding vaccine safety.

A number of adverse reactions have been associated with pertussis immunization. Transient local and systemic reactions are common and include redness (7 percent), swelling (9 percent), and pain (51 percent) at the injection site; fever to 38°C or greater (47 percent); and vomiting (6 percent). These reactions occur within a few hours of vaccination, are transient, and tend to increase in frequency with subsequent doses of vaccine. These reactions do not constitute a contraindication to future pertussis immunization. The administration of acetaminophen in a dose of 15 mg/kg at the time of vaccination and 4 and 8 h later will reduce the incidence of these reactions. Sterile abscesses at the site of injection are rare. Similar reactions have been reported for the acellular vaccines but they are usually less frequent and milder in nature.

A number of other uncommon but more severe adverse reactions have been associated with pertussis immunization. These include fever of 40.5°C or greater (0.3 percent), seizures (0.06 percent), persistent or unusual crying for 3 h or longer (1 percent), shock-like hyporesponsive state (0.06 percent), encephalopathy, and severe allergic reactions. Several other serious problems have been blamed on the pertussis vaccine, but careful evaluation indicates that they are merely temporal associations and do not represent a cause-and-effect relationship. Among these unsubstantiated events are infantile spasms and sudden infant death syndrome.

Absolute contraindications to further administration of pertussis vaccines include:

1 Encephalopathy within 7 days of vaccination
2 Seizures within 3 days
3 Persistent or unconsolable crying for 3 h or longer or a high-pitched cry that is unusual for that infant within 2 days
4 Collapse or a shock-like hyporesponsive episode within 48 h of vaccination
5 Fever of 40.5°C or greater within 48 h
6 An immediate severe allergic reaction or anaphylaxis

In addition to these contraindications, the pertussis vaccine may be omitted or delayed in patients with infantile spasms, uncontrolled epilepsy, or progressive encephalopathy of unknown etiology.

Routine pertussis vaccination is not recommended after the age of 7 because the risk of severe disease is extremely low and reactions to vaccination may be higher. Vaccine has been employed in adults during outbreaks within hospitals with a prominent incidence of local reactions (>50 percent) and rarely occurring skin rashes.

The pertussis vaccine is almost always given in conjunction with other immunizing agents such as diphtheria and tetanus toxoids. Five 0.5-mL intramuscular doses of DTP are recommended for primary immunization; the first is given at about 2 months of age, the second and third doses are given 2 and 4 months later. A fourth dose is given 6 to 12 months after the third dose, and a fifth booster dose is given at about 4 to 6 years of age at the time of school entry. In outbreaks, pertussis immunization can be started as early as 2 weeks of age and the 2 subsequent doses given 4 weeks apart. Children in whom the recommended schedule for pertussis immunization has been interrupted or deferred and who need to resume vaccination can receive the next dose on schedule, regardless of the interval from the previous dose. No modifications in the immunization schedule are needed for premature infants.

REFERENCES

Blennow M et al: Primary immunization of infants with an acellular pertussis vaccine in a double-blind randomized clinical trial. Pediatrics 82:293, 1988

Cherry JD et al: Report of the Task Force on Pertussis and Pertussis Immunization—1988. Pediatrics 81:939, 1988

Friedman RL: Pertussis: The disease and new diagnostic methods. Clin Microbiol Rev 1:365, 1988

Gillis J et al: Artificial ventilation in severe pertussis. Arch Dis Child 63:364, 1988

Hoffman HJ et al: Diphtheria-tetanus-pertussis immunization and sudden infant death: Results of the National Institute of Child Health and Human Development Cooperative Epidemiological Study of Sudden Infant Death Syndrome risk factors. Pediatrics 79:598, 1987

Linnemann CC Jr et al: Use of pertussis vaccine in an epidemic involving hospital staff. Lancet 2:540, 1975

Onorato IM, Wassilak SGF: Laboratory diagnosis of pertussis: The state of the art. Pediatr Infect Dis J 6:145, 1987

Robertson PW et al: *Bordetella pertussis* infection: A cause of persistent cough in adults. Med J Aust 146:522, 1987

Shields WD et al: Relationship of pertussis immunization to the onset of neurologic disorders: A retrospective epidemiologic study. J Pediatr 113:801, 1988

117 CHANCROID

ALLAN R. RONALD / FRANCIS A. PLUMMER

DEFINITION Chancroid, or soft chancre (ulcer molle), is an acute sexually transmitted infection characterized by painful genital ulcerations often associated with inflammatory inguinal adenopathy which may progress to suppuration. The diagnosis is established by isolation of *Haemophilus ducreyi* from the lesion or a suppurative node and by exclusion of syphilis, genital herpes, and other specific causes of genital ulceration.

ETIOLOGY The isolation of *H. ducreyi* from ulcers proves the microbial etiology of chancroid. Other organisms are often present, but there is no evidence that these are independent pathogens or require specific therapy. The clinical response to antimicrobial therapy parallels the susceptibility of *H. ducreyi*. In areas where chancroid is common, *H. ducreyi* can be isolated from up to 90 percent of ulcers that clinically appear to be chancroid. The organism is a gram-negative facultative aerobe which requires hemin (X factor) but not nicotinamide adenine dinucleotide (V factor) for growth. Although no unique biochemical or immunologic features are known, the colonial morphology of *H. ducreyi* is distinct in that the yellow-gray colonies can be moved intact across the agar surface. Some strains demonstrate a typical streptobacillary ''chaining'' appearance on Gram stain.

EPIDEMIOLOGY The incidence of chancroid is unknown, owing to inaccurate diagnosis and incomplete reporting. It is common in southeast Asia and Africa, and is more prevalent than syphilis in many countries. A resurgence of chancroid is occurring in many U.S. urban centers, and endemic foci have been identified in Florida, New York City, and Dallas. The annual incidence has increased sixfold during the past decade and is continuing to rise. Over 5000 cases were reported in 1987. Uncircumcised males are more susceptible to the disease. Prostitution plays a major role in transmission, and among merchant seamen and military troops whose sexual contacts are prostitutes, chancroid is more common than syphilis. The role of asymptomatic female carriers, without ulcers, in the transmission of *H. ducreyi* is uncertain. Over one-half of the secondary sex partners of men with chancroid develop clinical chancroid.

Studies from Africa provide substantial evidence that chancroid is a major cofactor that facilitates the heterosexual spread of human immunodeficiency virus (HIV-1). Prostitutes with chancroid are more susceptible to HIV-1 infection following heterosexual intercourse and they also transmit HIV-1 much more frequently to their clients in the presence of genital ulcers. Almost one-half of bidirectional heterosexual transmission of HIV-1 may be attributed to chancroid in some African communities. Control and eradication of chancroid is now recognized as an urgent priority to curtail heterosexual transmission of HIV-1.

CLINICAL MANIFESTATIONS After an incubation period of 3 to 10 days, a small tender papule appears which rapidly ulcerates. The classic chancroidal ulcer is superficial, ranging in diameter from a few millimeters to several centimeters. The edge is ragged and undermined. The ulcer base is covered by a necrotic exudate. The ulcers are often multiple and may merge to form giant or serpiginous ulcers. Occasionally, the lesions remain pustular and resemble folliculitis or pyogenic infection. In contrast to syphilis, the chancroidal ulcer in males is painful and not indurated. The most frequent areas of localization are the preputial orifice, the internal surface of the prepuce, and the frenulum in men, and the labia, fourchette, and perianal region in women. The lesions in females tend to be more superficial and less painful. Extragenital ulcers are rare.

Acute, painful, tender inflammatory inguinal adenopathy occurs in almost 50 percent of patients and is frequently unilateral. If the patient is untreated, the involved nodes become matted, forming a unilocular suppurative bubo. The overlying skin becomes erythematous and tense and finally ruptures, forming a deep single ulcer.

DIAGNOSIS The morphologic diagnosis of genital lesions is fraught with error, and many lesions diagnosed as chancroid are actually genital herpes or syphilis. In the United States, one study of 100 consecutive men with penile ulceration disclosed genital herpes in 22, syphilis in 17, and traumatic lesions in 8. Classic chancroidal ulcers were noted in 12, only 2 of whom had ulcers that yielded *H. ducreyi*. In Kenya, of 97 consecutive men with penile ulceration, 60 were infected with *H. ducreyi*, 11 had syphilis, and only 4 had genital herpes.

Primary genital infection with herpes simplex virus produces tender inguinal adenopathy, but can be distinguished by the history of onset with vesicular lesions or of recent exposure to herpes and the presence of systemic symptoms such as fever and myalgia. Chancroid rarely causes systemic symptoms.

The chancre of primary syphilis is indurated, and the associated adenopathy is bilateral, nontender, and nonsuppurative. To exclude syphilis, all patients with genital ulcers should have two dark-field examinations performed on separate days, together with monthly serologic tests for syphilis for 3 months.

Lymphogranuloma venereum (LGV) differs from chancroid in that the adenopathy develops after the ulcer is healed. It is indolent, often bilateral and nontender, and develops multilocular suppuration and fistulas.

The diagnosis of chancroid is confirmed by the isolation of *H. ducreyi* from an ulcer. Exudate should be directly plated onto chocolate agar enriched with 1% Isovitalex and 5% sheep serum, plus 3 mg/L of vancomycin. Colonies usually appear within 48 h of incubation in 5% CO_2 with 100% humidity but may require 4 to 5 days. No serologic tests are available for the diagnosis of chancroid.

TREATMENT Untreated chancroid can persist for months. Small lesions may heal within 2 to 4 weeks. Although sulfonamides and tetracyclines were effective treatment, the emergence of multiresistant strains ended their usefulness. Many isolates of *H. ducreyi* possess plasmids which mediate resistance to sulfonamides, tetracyclines, chloramphenicol, ampicillin, and kanamycin. Trimethoprim/sulfamethoxazole, 320/1600 mg daily, or erythromycin, 2 g daily, each for 1 week are the regimens recommended by the Centers for Disease Control. Trimethoprim/sulfamethoxazole will not interfere with the dark-field examination for *Treponema pallidum* or with the development of a positive serologic test for syphilis. Ciprofloxacin, 500 mg orally, twice daily for three days is also effective. The usual time to healing after onset of therapy is about 9 days. Several single-dose regimens including trimethoprim/sulfamethoxazole, 640/3200 mg, spectinomycin, 2 g intramuscularly, and ceftriaxone, 250 mg intramuscularly have proved effective for chancroid in Kenya. HIV-infected patients appear to respond less well to therapy; the efficacy of regimens for chancroid treatment in patients concomitantly infected with HIV requires further study. Fluctuant buboes should be aspirated to prevent rupture. Lymph node suppuration may progress despite otherwise effective therapy. Buboes larger than 5 cm in diameter almost always require aspiration.

Sexual contacts of patients with chancroid should be examined for ulcers, and treatment of contacts is recommended. Although the epidemiology of chancroid suggests that effective control measures, specifically designed for limited target populations such as prostitutes and known sexual contacts, could halt the spread of this disease, further prospective epidemiologic studies to demonstrate this are required.

REFERENCES

BOWMER MI et al: Single dose ceftriaxone for chancroid. Antimicrob Agents Chemother 31:67, 1988

GREENBLATT RM et al: Genital ulceration as a risk factor for human immunodeficiency virus infection. AIDS 2:47, 1988

McNicol PJ et al: The plasmids of *Haemophilus ducreyi*. Antimicrob Agents Chemother 14:561, 1984

Salzman RS et al: Chancroid ulcers that are not chancroid: Cause and epidemiology. Arch Dermatol 120:636, 1984

Schmid GP et al: Chancroid in the United States. Reestablishment of an old disease. JAMA 258:3265, 1987

Simonsen JN et al: Human immunodeficiency virus infection among men with sexually transmitted diseases: Experience from a centre in Africa. New Engl J Med 319:274, 1988

118 DONOVANOSIS (GRANULOMA INGUINALE)

KING K. HOLMES

DEFINITION Donovanosis (granuloma inguinale) is a mildly contagious, chronic, indolent, progressive, autoinoculable, ulcerative disease involving the skin and lymphatics of the genital or perianal areas. The disease may be sexually transmitted and is associated with the presence in affected tissues of an intracellular microorganism, identified morphologically as the Donovan body.

ETIOLOGY Donovanosis was described by McLeod in India in 1882, and in 1905 Donovan described the intracellular bodies which are thought to cause the disease. Encapsulated bacteria resembling Donovan bodies have been recovered from lesions and pseudobuboes of granuloma inguinale by inoculation of chick embryo yolk sacs or yolk-agar medium. These bacteria, which are known as *Calymmatobacterium granulomatis,* measure 1.5 by 0.7 μm. They are antigenically related to *Klebsiella* species but do not reproduce the disease when inoculated intradermally in humans. It is uncertain whether these isolates are responsible for the disease. Electron microscopic studies of Donovan bodies confirm their morphologic resemblance to gram-negative bacteria.

EPIDEMIOLOGY Donovanosis is endemic in the tropics, particularly in New Guinea and among Hindus in India, and in parts of central Australia, the Caribbean, and Africa. In the United States the disease is rare. Most cases occur in the southeastern states and involve homosexual men. In reported cases the sex ratio of males to females is nearly 10:1. The disease is uncommon in Caucasians. The reported frequency of donovanosis in conjugal partners of chronically infected patients ranges from 1 to 64 percent. Evidence for sexual transmission includes the age-specific incidence, which corresponds to that of other sexually transmitted diseases, the frequent concomitant presence of syphilis, and the predilection for genital involvement in heterosexuals and for anorectal infection in homosexually active men.

CLINICAL MANIFESTATIONS The incubation period ranges from 8 days to 12 weeks, but most lesions appear within 30 days after sexual exposure.

Donovanosis begins as a papule that ulcerates and develops into a painless elevated zone of clean, beefy-red, friable granulation tissue. The edges are irregular and spread by continuity or by autoinoculation of approximated skin surfaces. Secondary anaerobic infection may produce pain and a foul-smelling exudate. Less common complications of the disease include deep ulcerations, chronic cicatricial lesions, phimosis, lymphedema, and exuberant epithelial proliferation which grossly resembles carcinoma. In men, the lesions are usually located on the glans, prepuce, or shaft of the penis or the perianal area, while infection of the labia is most common in women. Lesions in women often arise at the fourchette and progress anteriorly in a V shape along the vulva. Extragenital lesions may occur, involving the face, neck, mouth, and other sites. The chronicity of the disease is of diagnostic importance, since several months often elapse before patients seek treatment. Extension to the inguinal region by autoinoculation, by continuity, or via the lymphatics results in diffuse intradermal and subcutaneous swelling or suppuration, known as "pseudobubo," because involvement of the underlying lymph nodes is minimal. Locally destructive lesions and secondary infection may produce severe morbidity or death. Fatal disseminated disease, involving the bones, joints, or liver, has been reported after several years of chronic local infection. The relationship of donovanosis to subsequent carcinoma of the genitalia is uncertain.

DIAGNOSIS Early donovanosis may be mistaken for the primary chancre or condyloma latum of syphilis. Epithelial proliferation resembling carcinoma in the genital or perianal region in a young individual should always raise the suspicion of donovanosis if unnecessary destructive surgery is to be avoided. Chronic ulcerative or cicatricial changes may resemble lymphogranuloma venereum.

Amebiasis can produce penile lesions resembling donovanosis. In the United States, *Haemophilus ducreyi* has frequently been isolated from lesions resembling donovanosis; this has been termed *pseudo-granuloma inguinale–chancroid.* Histologic studies in donovanosis reveal marked acanthosis and pseudoepitheliomatous hyperplasia. The dermis contains an inflammatory infiltrate consisting mainly of plasma cells and histiocytes. Because Donovan bodies are seldom detectable in sections stained with hematoxylin and eosin, these changes may lead to an erroneous diagnosis of carcinoma and to unnecessary destructive surgery. Although silver impregnation techniques are useful for demonstration of Donovan bodies in sections, the diagnosis is best made by examination of impression smears prepared from specimens obtained by punch biopsy of granulation tissue from the periphery of a lesion; the deep portion of the specimen is removed, crushed between two slides which are air-dried and fixed in methanol, and stained with Wright-Giemsa stain. With this method, Donovan bodies appear as very rounded coccobacilli, 1 by 2 μm in size, which lie within cystic spaces in the cytoplasm of large mononuclear cells. The capsule stains as a dense acidophilic zone surrounding the bacterium, which resembles a closed safety pin because of bipolar condensation of chromatin. The pathognomonic mononuclear cell is 25 to 90 μm in diameter and has many cystic areas containing Donovan bodies. Donovan bodies have also been identified in histiocytes in cervical Papanicolaou smears.

Perianal donovanosis may resemble condylomata lata of secondary syphilis. Other venereal diseases, particularly syphilis, very frequently coexist with donovanosis. Repeated dark-field examinations of lesions before treatment and a serologic test for syphilis should therefore be performed. In countries where donovanosis is endemic, the persistence of suspected condylomata lata after appropriate penicillin therapy for syphilis is highly suggestive of donovanosis. Other forms of genital ulcers (chancroid, syphilis, genital herpes) have been associated with increased risk of acquisition or transmission of human immunodeficiency virus. These diseases appear to be less responsive to therapy in HIV-seropositive individuals. Anecdotal cases of severe donovanosis associated with HIV infection have been reported, but the association has not been well studied.

TREATMENT The treatment of choice is tetracycline, 2 g daily, for at least 3 weeks, preferably continued until healing is complete. Healing is usually apparent within 3 weeks, as the lesions become pale and flatter and develop peripheral reepithelialization. Lack of objective clinical response within 7 days should lead to reassessment of the diagnosis and therapy. Donovan bodies disappear from lesions within a few days after onset of therapy. If tetracycline cannot be given, streptomycin may be used in a dose of 1 g intramuscularly every 12 h for 10 to 15 days. Chloramphenicol, 500 mg every 8 h orally, or gentamicin, 1 mg/kg twice daily, is used for cases which appear resistant to tetracycline. Co-trimoxazole (trimethoprim 160 mg, sulfamethoxazole 800 mg) twice daily for 10 days is also reported to be effective. In pregnant women, erythromycin, 500 mg every 6 h, may be effective.

REFERENCES

Hart G: Donovanosis, in *Sexually Transmitted Diseases*, 2d ed, KK Holmes et al (eds). New York, McGraw-Hill, 1990, chap 25, pp 273–277

KRAUS SJ et al: Pseudogranuloma inguinale caused by *Haemophilus ducreyi*. Arch Dermatol 118:494, 1982
KUBERSKI T: Granuloma inguinale (donovanosis). Sex Transm Dis 7:29, 1980
ROSEN T et al: Granuloma inguinale. J Am Acad Dermatol 11:433, 1984
SCHNEIDER J et al: Extragenital donovanosis: Three cases from Western Australia. Genitourinary Med 62:196, 1966

119 BRUCELLOSIS

DONALD KAYE

DEFINITION Brucellosis is an infection caused by bacteria of the genus *Brucella*. Human infection results from occupational contact with an infected animal or by ingestion of infected milk, milk products, or tissues. The symptoms of brucellosis are often nonspecific and include fever, malaise, and weight loss, often without physical findings.

ETIOLOGY There are four species of *Brucella* that cause infection in humans. The most pathogenic is *B. melitensis*, followed by *B. suis*, *B. abortus*, and *B. canis*. While each of these tends to produce infection in a specific animal host (*B. melitensis* in sheep and goats, *B. suis* in swine, *B. abortus* in cattle, and *B. canis* in dogs), cross-species infection occurs (e.g., *B. abortus* in sheep) and other animals may become infected.

Brucella are small, nonmotile, nonencapsulated, gram negative coccobacilli which do not form spores. *Brucella* grow best at 37°C under increased CO_2 tension and are separated from each other by biochemical and serologic techniques.

EPIDEMIOLOGY Animals acquire brucellosis either sexually or by ingesting contaminated milk or other animal products. Humans develop disease following ingestion of contaminated animal food products, by contact of *Brucella* with abraded skin, through the conjunctivae, or by inhalation. Person-to-person transmission rarely, if ever, occurs.

While there are 500,000 new cases of brucellosis reported annually worldwide, it has become a rare disease in the United States with fewer than 200 cases each year. However, it is estimated that only about 4 percent of cases are recognized and reported. *B. abortus* and *B. suis* cause most cases in the United States; *B. melitensis* and *B. canis* are rare. In the United States brucellosis is mainly an occupational disease with most cases occurring in working-age males who are abattoir workers, butchers, or farmers. Veterinarians may become infected by accidental inoculation of live attenuated *B. abortus* vaccine which causes mild disease. In most instances of brucellosis acquired in the United States from ingestion of contaminated milk products, the foods came from other parts of the world (Mexico, Mediterranean countries, the Far East, and South America).

Worldwide, *B. melitensis* is the most frequent cause of brucellosis. There are tremendous differences in the yearly incidence of human brucellosis in different countries, mainly depending on the extent of animal brucellosis. The areas with the highest prevalence are the Mediterranean countries, Asia, and Central and South America.

PATHOGENESIS AND PATHOLOGY After invading the body, *Brucella* are phagocytized by polymorphonuclear leukocytes and macrophages. Some *Brucella* are killed but others multiply within these cells and destroy them. Organisms spread via lymphatics to regional lymph nodes and, if not contained, to the bloodstream. Bacteremia may result in foci in cells of the reticuloendothelial system in the liver, spleen, and bone marrow and in other organs such as the kidneys. *Brucella* inside of phagocytic cells (as in the reticuloendothelial system and tissue macrophages) are protected against antibody and many antibiotics.

The reaction of tissues to *Brucella* is the formation of granulomas with epithelioid cells, giant cells, lymphocytes, and plasma cells. *B. abortus* usually causes mild disease with noncaseating granulomas in the liver and other reticuloendothelial organs. *B. suis* causes more severe disease with local suppurative complications and granulomas that may caseate. *B. melitensis* produces the most severe acute disease with symptoms that may be disabling. *B. canis* results in mild disease similar to that seen with *B. abortus*. Activated macrophages can kill *Brucella*, and this is the probable mechanism by which spontaneous cure and immunity occur. Granulomas in brucellosis eventually heal with fibrosis and often calcification.

Although brucellosis is a common cause of abortion in animals, there is no evidence that human abortions occur any more frequently with this disease than with other bacteremias.

MANIFESTATIONS Brucellosis may be asymptomatic with only serologic evidence of infection. Children are particularly prone to subclinical infection. The manifestations of symptomatic brucellosis may be divided into acute brucellosis, localized disease, and chronic brucellosis.

Acute brucellosis The incubation period of acute brucellosis usually varies between 7 and 21 days, but may be months. The onset is often insidious with a low-grade fever and no localizing complaints. Malaise, weakness, fatigue, headache, backache, myalgias, sweats, and chills are often prominent. Most patients are anorectic and lose weight. With *B. melitensis* infection the onset may be acute with high fever.

Typically, there are a multitude of complaints but a paucity of physical findings. When physical findings occur, the major manifestations are splenomegaly (which occurs in 10 to 20 percent of patients), lymphadenopathy (15 percent of patients), and hepatomegaly (less than 10 percent).

Localized brucellosis Localized disease may occur at almost any anatomic location, but osteomyelitis, splenic abscess, genitourinary tract infection, pulmonary disease, and endocarditis are among the more common. Osteomyelitis usually occurs in the vertebrae, with the lumbosacral area the most frequent site. There is a disc space infection with involvement of both adjacent vertebrae. Bone scans are positive early, followed by roentgenographic evidence of osteoporosis, anterior vertebral plate erosion, and formation of ''parrot-beaked'' osteophytes. Arthritis, which is much less common than osteomyelitis, most often involves the knee. Splenic abscesses may occur and result in areas of calcification. Epididymoorchitis and less often clinically apparent prostatic or renal infection may be observed. Neurologic complications are uncommon and include meningoencephalitis, myelitis, radiculitis, and peripheral neuropathy. Pleural effusion and pneumonia are occasional manifestations.

Endocarditis is the most common cause of mortality among patients with brucellosis. It has been reported predominantly in males, most often involves the aortic valve, has an indolent onset, results in bulky and ulcerative vegetations, is accompanied by a high rate of congestive heart failure and arterial embolization, and has usually required both valve replacement and antibiotic therapy to achieve cure.

Chronic brucellosis Chronic brucellosis is defined as ill health for more than 1 year following onset of brucellosis. It has mixed manifestations and includes patients with relapsing illness, with or without localized infection, as well as those who have no objective signs of infection (e.g., no fever) and no evidence of active brucellosis (by serology or culture). While the former clearly have brucellosis, it is doubtful that the latter have active brucellosis. Their complaints, fatigue and weakness, are more likely functional.

An unusual complication that occurs in veterinarians removing placentas from infected animals consists of an erythematous macular, papular, or postular rash on the hands and arms, which is presumed to be a hypersensitivity reaction to *Brucella* antigens.

DIAGNOSIS Brucellosis is a relatively rare disease, and there are many common illnesses that may mimic the most frequent presentation (i.e., fever without localizing symptoms or physical findings). Among them are infectious mononucleosis, toxoplasmosis, tuberculosis, hepatitis, systemic lupus erythematosus, typhoid fever, and many others. The clinical suspicion that the patient has brucellosis should be higher in farmers, abattoir workers, veterinarians, and others exposed to infected tissues or animal products. Most routine laboratory tests are not helpful. The white blood cell count is usually normal or low, and the erythrocyte sedimentation rate may be normal.

Cultures The definitive evidence of *Brucella* infection consists of isolating *Brucella* from the patient. However, culturing *Brucella* organisms may be dangerous to laboratory personnel. Therefore, specimens should be labelled as "suspected brucellosis" and should be processed only in laboratories that have Biosafety level 3 facilities. Up to half the untreated patients studied early in the course of infection will have *Brucella* in the blood when a culture is grown in trypticase soy broth for 1 to 3 weeks in the presence of 5 to 10% CO_2. Optimally, Casteñeda's medium (a biphasic trypticase soy broth and agar medium) should be used and incubated for 4 weeks. Bone marrow cultures are often positive in acute brucellosis when blood cultures are not. They are also more likely to remain positive later in the course of the disease and in spite of administration of antimicrobial agents. As the illness progresses, bacteremia is less frequent and organisms may then be isolated from infected lymph nodes or granulomas involving the spleen, liver, and bone. Altogether, only 15 to 20 percent of cases of brucellosis are confirmed by culture. In localized brucellosis, biopsy and isolation of *Brucella* may be necessary for diagnosis. In the majority of cases of brucellosis, the diagnosis is made serologically.

Serology The standard tube *Brucella* agglutination test (STA) has been used most in the diagnosis of brucellosis. It measures antibodies directed primarily at *Brucella* lipopolysaccharide antigens. A titer of ≥ 1:160 is considered positive and indicates past or present exposure to *Brucella* organisms or antigens that cross-react with *Brucella* species (*Brucella* skin tests, cholera vaccination, and infection with *Vibrio cholerae, Francisella tularensis,* or *Yersinia enterocolitica*). A fourfold or greater rise in titer of antibody in serum specimens drawn 1 to 4 weeks apart is indicative of recent exposure to *Brucella* or *Brucella*-like antigens. Paired specimens should be tested on the same day in the same laboratory. As measured by the STA, most patients develop a rise in titer within 1 to 2 weeks of illness, and by 3 weeks virtually all patients will show seroconversion. If there is strong clinical suspicion of brucellosis, dilutions as high as 1:1280 should be made, because false-negative tests due to blocking antibodies have been reported with blocking antibody titers as high as 1:640. True STA titers below 1:160 are strong evidence against active brucellosis.

The methods for serologic diagnosis of brucellosis use *B. abortus* antigens, because antibodies to *B. melitensis* and *B. suis* cross-react with *B. abortus*. However, antibodies to *B. canis* will not react with *B. abortus* antigen, and specialized serologic studies are necessary to detect these antibodies.

IgM antibody titers rise early in brucellosis (usually in the first week of infection), peak at about 3 months, and then fall gradually. However, high titers may persist for years. IgG antibodies appear 2 to 3 weeks after onset of illness, peak in about 8 weeks and persist as long as the infection is active. With cure, IgG antibody titers decrease rapidly and usually disappear within 1 year. The persistence of IgG antibody indicates continuing active infection. With relapse, both IgM and IgG titers increase. Use of 2-mercaptoethanol (2-ME) in the STA destroys the agglutinating activity of IgM antibodies and allows measurement of only the IgG-agglutinating antibody. In contrast to elevated IgM antibodies, a single titer of ≥ 1:160 in the 2-ME STA is good evidence of either current or very recent infection.

The *Brucella* skin test is only a measure of past infection. Because it may cause a rise in antibody titers, confusing the interpretation of the STA, it should not be performed.

TREATMENT The combination of tetracycline 30 mg/kg per day in four equally divided doses, orally, for 3 to 6 weeks plus streptomycin 15 mg/kg every 12 h intramuscularly for the first 2 weeks is considered the treatment of choice for brucellosis. The longer duration of tetracycline is recommended for patients with localized brucellosis. Patients who relapse are usually cured with retreatment. Tetracycline should not be used in pregnant women or children below the age of 8 because of the danger of staining developing teeth. Streptomycin may cause eighth-nerve toxicity, and the dose must be decreased in patients with renal insufficiency.

A variety of other regimens, including tetracycline plus gentamicin or rifampin in lieu of streptomycin, doxycycline instead of tetracycline, or trimethoprim-sulfamethoxazole alone, have been tried in an attempt to decrease relapses and toxicity but none have been superior to the tetracycline-streptomycin combination. When tetracycline plus streptomycin cannot be used, trimethoprim/sulfamethoxazole (480/2400 mg/d) for 4 weeks is a reasonable substitute, although relapses are common. Addition of rifampin (900 mg/d) to the basic tetracycline-streptomycin or trimethoprim-sulfamethoxazole regimen may improve results when response is poor or when meningitis or endocarditis is present. Successful therapy of endocarditis has usually required valve replacement in addition to one of the above antimicrobial regimens. Despite apparent in vitro activity against strains of *Brucella,* the role of the third-generation cephalosporins in brucellosis remains to be determined.

Abscesses should be drained when indicated. Splenectomy has been performed in some patients with splenomegaly and multiple relapses and has apparently been successful in preventing further relapses.

Prednisone in an oral dose of 60 mg/d tapered rapidly over a 5- to 7-day period may be helpful in patients with brucellosis characterized by severe debility, but is rarely necessary. Headache, backache, and generalized aches and pains should be treated with analgesics.

PROGNOSIS Even before the advent of antimicrobial treatment, the mortality rate of brucellosis was less than 5 percent and only 15 percent of patients had an illness exceeding 3 months in duration. With chemotherapy, the mortality rate is less than 2 percent and long illnesses and complications are rare. When the morbidity exceeds 1 to 2 months, other causes, previously unsuspected underlying disease, or a complication of brucellosis should be considered.

PREVENTION The key to elimination of brucellosis in humans is the eradication of animal brucellosis. This can be accomplished by immunization of animals with a live attenuated *Brucella* vaccine which produces immunity. No vaccine is available for human immunization in the United States. The risk of acquiring brucellosis can be decreased by use of pasteurized milk and pasteurized milk products, by guarding against exposure to tissue from infected animals, and by protecting potential portals of entry in high risk individuals (veterinarians, meat inspectors, slaughterhouse workers) with protective bandages over cuts and by the use of protective clothing, gloves, and goggles.

REFERENCES

ARIZA J et al: Comparative trial of rifampin-doxycycline versus tetracycline-streptomycin in the therapy of human brucellosis. Antimicrob Agents Chemother 28(4):548, 1985

——— :Comparative trial of co-trimoxazole versus tetracycline-streptomycin in treating human brucellosis. J Infect Dis 152(6):1358, 1985

FERNANDEZ-GUERRERO ML et al: Prosthetic valve endocarditis caused by *Brucella melitensis*. Arch Intern Med 147:1141, 1987

GOTUZZO E et al: An evaluation of diagnostic methods for brucellosis—the value of bone marrow culture. J Infect Dis 153(1):122, 1986

HEWITT WG, PAYNE D: Estimation of IgG and IgM *Brucella* antibodies in infected and non-infected persons by a radioimmune technique. J Clin Pathol 37:692, 1984

JEROUDI M et al: Brucella endocarditis. Br Heart J 58:279, 1987

POLT SS et al: Human brucellosis caused by *Brucella canis:* Clinical features and immune response. Ann Intern Med 97:717, 1982

SHARDA DC, LUBANI M: A study of brucellosis in childhood. Clin Pediatr 25(10):492, 1986

YOUNG EJ: Human brucellosis. Rev Infect Dis 5:821, 1983

——— et al: Phagocytosis and killing of *Brucella* by human polymorphonuclear neutrophils. J Infect Dis 151:682, 1985

120 TULAREMIA

DONALD KAYE

DEFINITION Tularemia (rabbit fever, deer fly fever) is an infection caused by *Francisella tularensis*. *F. tularensis* is found in many animals and is transmitted to human beings by direct contact or via an insect vector. The illness is characterized by an ulcerative lesion at the site of inoculation with regional lymphadenopathy, by pneumonia, or by fever without localizing findings.

ETIOLOGY *F. tularensis* is a small, nonmotile, pleomorphic, gram-negative aerobic coccobacillus. It grows poorly in many media but will grow well in glucose-cysteine blood agar, thioglycolate broth, and other media supplemented with cysteine. *F. tularensis* is found only in the northern hemisphere. There are two types of *F. tularensis*. Type A is distributed solely in North America, is virulent for humans and rabbits, produces citrulline ureidase, and ferments glycerol. Type B is found in North America, Europe, and Asia, causes no or mild disease in humans and rabbits, does not produce citrulline ureidase, and does not ferment glycerol. *F. tularensis* cross-reacts serologically with *Brucella* species and *Yersinia pestis*.

EPIDEMIOLOGY *F. tularensis* has been found in many mammals including rabbits, squirrels, muskrats, beavers, deer, cattle, and sheep, in birds, in amphibians, and in fish. Tularemia can result from skin contact with any of these species. Tularemia has also been caused by cat bite. Ticks and deer flies can transmit the bacterium. Ticks pass *F. tularensis* to their offspring via a transovarian route. The organism is found in tick feces but not in salivary glands. In the United States the disease can be carried by *Dermacentor andersoni* (Rocky Mountain wood tick), *Dermacentor variabilis* (American dog tick), *Dermacentor occidentalis* (Pacific Coast dog tick), and *Amblyomma americanum* (Lone Star tick). *F. tularensis* has also been recovered from streams.

In the United States most cases of tularemia result from skin contact with infected wild rabbits (especially cottontail rabbits) or tick feces. Infection occasionally results from ingestion or inhalation of infected material. Hunters and trappers are at greatest risk. Tularemia is most likely to occur in adult males, and person-to-person transmission rarely, if ever, occurs.

Tularemia has been reported from all parts of the United States, but mostly from Arkansas, Illinois, Missouri, Texas, Virginia, and Tennessee. Fewer than 200 cases are reported annually in the United States. Arthropod-borne disease occurs mainly in the spring and summer, and rabbit-produced infection mainly in the winter.

PATHOGENESIS AND PATHOLOGY In human infection, the most common portal of entry is through the skin or mucous membranes either directly through inapparent abrasions or via the bite of a tick or other arthropod. Inhalation or ingestion of *F. tularensis* can also result in infection. Fewer than 50 organisms will result in infection when injected into the skin or inhaled, whereas more than 10^8 are usually required to produce infection via the oral route.

Following inoculation into the skin, the bacteria multiply locally and after 2 to 5 days (occasionally 1 to 10 days) produce an erythematous, tender, or pruritic papule. The papule rapidly enlarges and forms an ulcer with a black base. The bacteria spread to regional lymph nodes producing lymphadenopathy, and further spread with bacteremia may occur. With bacteremia, organisms are cleared from the blood by phagocytic cells of the reticuloendothelial system (mainly in the liver and spleen) and may survive intracellularly for long periods of time.

Affected organs (liver, spleen, lymph nodes) demonstrate areas of focal necrosis initially surrounded mainly by polymorphonuclear leukocytes. Subsequently granulomas form with epithelioid cells and lymphocytes and sometimes multinucleated giant cells surrounding the areas of necrosis which may resemble caseation necrosis. Coalescence of granulomas can lead to formation of abscesses. Nodes may occasionally become fluctuant and even rupture. Healing occurs with fibrosis and calcification of the granulomas.

Contamination of the conjunctiva can result in infection of the eye with regional lymph node enlargement. Aerosolization and inhalation of *F. tularensis* can result in pneumonia. Pneumonia can also occur via the hematogenous route. There is an inflammatory reaction with foci of alveolar necrosis and initially polymorphonuclear leukocytic and later mononuclear cell infiltration with granuloma formation. Chest roentgenograms usually reveal bilateral patchy infiltrates rather than large areas of consolidation. Mediastinal or other regional lymphadenopathy may occur.

Pharyngitis with cervical lymphadenopathy or gastrointestinal tularemia with mesenteric lymphadenopathy may follow ingestion of large numbers of *F. tularensis*. Typhoidal tularemia, which is characterized by fever and no localizing signs, is uncommon; the portal of entry is unknown.

CLINICAL MANIFESTATIONS Tularemia usually has an incubation period of 2 to 5 days after which there is onset of one of a number of syndromes (listed below), all of which are usually associated with fever and chills and often with headache, myalgias, and malaise. Tender hepatosplenomegaly is common. About 20 percent of patients develop a generalized maculopapular rash which may occasionally become pustular, and some report erythema nodosum.

Ulceroglandular tularemia Most patients with tularemia (75 to 85 percent) develop infection secondary to inoculation of the skin. In cases related to rabbits the portal of entry is usually on the finger or hand. In tick-related cases, the site of inoculation is usually on the lower extremities, inguinal or axillary areas, scalp, abdomen, or chest.

At time of onset of illness the patient usually has an erythematous papule that may be tender or pruritic, or an ulcer is already present at the portal of entry of the organism. If there is a papule, it evolves over a period of several days to form a punched out ulcer with sharply dermarcated edges and a yellow exudate. The ulcer gradually develops a black base. The patient has very tender, large regional lymphadenopathy (usually axillary or epitrochlear with tularemia from rabbits, and inguinal or femoral lymphadenopathy with tick-borne disease). The nodes may become fluctuant and drain spontaneously. In 5 to 10 percent of patients, the skin lesion may be inapparent and the lymphadenopathy the only physical finding. This has been called "glandular tularemia."

Oculoglandular tularemia In about 1 percent of patients, the conjunctiva serves as the portal of entry for the organism. Purulent conjunctivitis with regional lymphadenopathy (preauricular, submandibular, or cervical) is present. Corneal perforation may occur.

Oropharyngeal and gastrointestinal tularemia Rarely tularemia occurs after ingestion of *F. tularensis* (usually in undercooked meat), resulting in acute exudative or membranous pharyngitis associated with cervical lymphadenopathy or ulcerative intestinal lesions with associated mesenteric lymphadenopathy, diarrhea, abdominal pain, nausea, vomiting, and gastrointestinal bleeding.

Pulmonary tularemia Involvement of the lung can result from inhalation of *F. tularensis* or as a part of the bacteremia caused by tularemia at another site. Inhalation pulmonary disease occurs most often in laboratory workers and is a serious infection with high mortality. Pulmonary involvement occurs in 10 to 15 percent of patients with ulceroglandular tularemia and in about half of the patients with typhoidal tularemia. The patient has cough, which is usually nonproductive, and may have dyspnea or pleuritic chest pain. Most often the physical examination is normal. Roentgenograms of the chest usually reveal bilateral patchy infiltrates which have been described as "ovoid densities." Lobar pneumonia may occur, and pleural effusion(s) with a polymorphonuclear leukocytic (rarely mononuclear) exudate may be present.

Typhoidal tularemia In about 10 percent of cases of tularemia fever develops without apparent skin lesion or lymphadenopathy. In the absence of a history of possible contact with a vector of the disease, diagnosis is extremely difficult.

Other manifestations Meningitis, pericarditis, peritonitis, endocarditis, and osteomyelitis have been reported. The meningitis causes a lymphocytic response in the spinal fluid.

DIAGNOSIS **Differential diagnosis** In patients with fever and large, tender lymphadenopathy the possibility of tularemia should be strongly considered, and an attempt should be made to determine if there was an appropriate animal or arthropod vector contact. The suspicion of tularemia should be especially high in hunters, trappers, game wardens, veterinarians, and laboratory workers. However, in up to 40 percent of patients with tularemia, no history of epidemiologic contact with an animal or arthropod vector can be elicited.

Ulceroglandular tularemia is often so characteristic that it does not present a problem in differential diagnosis, but on occasion it must be differentiated from other diseases. The skin lesion may resemble those seen in sporotrichosis, skin infection with coagulase-positive staphylococci or group A streptococci, syphilis, anthrax, rat bite fever (caused by *Spirillum minus*), rickettsial infections (such as scrub typhus), and *Mycobacterium marinum* infection. However, the regional lymphadenopathy in these diseases is usually not as impressive as in tularemia.

The lymphadenopathy of tularemia must be differentiated from that of plague (see Chap. 121), lymphogranuloma venereum (see Chap. 155), and cat-scratch fever (see Chap. 98). However, in these infections there is usually no local lesion resembling the ulcer of tularemia.

Typhoidal tularemia may resemble typhoid fever, other *Salmonella* bacteremias, rickettsial infections (such as Rocky Mountain spotted fever), brucellosis, infectious mononucleosis, toxoplasmosis, miliary tuberculosis, sarcoid, or hematologic malignancies. Tularemia pneumonia may resemble pneumonias caused by other bacteria as well as viral or *Mycoplasma* pneumonia.

Laboratory diagnosis Blood cultures are usually negative and the diagnosis is most frequently made serologically by agglutination methods. A significant rise in titer (i.e., fourfold or greater) in paired serum specimens over a 2- to 3-week period is diagnostic. Agglutinating antibody appears after 1 to 2 weeks of illness. Fifty percent of patients have antibody in the second week, and the rest develop antibody later in the course. Titers peak at 4 to 8 weeks and may remain elevated for years. A single agglutinating titer of $\geq$ 1:160 in a patient who has been ill for at least 2 weeks is highly suggestive of tularemia but may only indicate old infection. Antibodies to *F. tularensis* may cross-react with *Brucella,* but the titers to *Brucella* are usually much lower than the titers to *F. tularensis*. In the future enzyme-linked immunosorbent assay (ELISA) tests may offer an advantage because they tend to turn positive earlier than agglutinating antibody tests.

F. tularensis is rarely observed on Gram stains of skin lesions, sputum, or aspirates of nodes. However, the organisms can often be demonstrated by staining with a modified Dieterle stain or by fluorescent antibody staining techniques. Cultures of these materials or blood may be positive if processed on appropriate media, but there is a major risk of infection in laboratory personnel. Cultivation of *F. tularensis* should only be attempted in laboratories with adequate isolation techniques and experienced personnel.

Isolation of *F. tularensis* can be achieved by inoculation intraperitoneally into guinea pigs, which will die within 10 days, and by direct plating onto glucose-cysteine blood agar. Agents such as cycloheximide, polymyxin B, and penicillin are frequently added to media to suppress other organisms in specimens that may overgrow *F. tularensis*.

A delayed-type skin test (similar to the tuberculin test) with *F. tularensis* antigen or killed whole bacilli turns positive during the first week of illness, prior to the appearance of agglutinating antibody, and persists for years. However, the skin test antigen is not available commercially, and can boost titers of agglutinating antibodies.

The white blood cell count is usually normal, and the erythrocyte sedimentation rate may be normal as well. Pyuria is common.

TREATMENT Streptomycin, in a dose of 7.5 to 10 mg/kg every 12 h intramuscularly, is considered the drug of choice. In severe infections, 15 mg/kg every 12 h may be used for the first 48 to 72 h. Therapy is continued for 7 to 10 days. Gentamicin, in a dose of 1.7 mg/kg, intramuscularly or intravenously, every 8 h, is also effective. Virtually all strains are susceptible to streptomycin and gentamicin. Temperature response occurs within 2 days, but skin lesions and lymph nodes may take 1 to 2 weeks to heal. When therapy is not initiated until several weeks of illness have elapsed, the temperature response may be delayed. Relapses are very uncommon with streptomycin therapy.

Tetracycline or chloramphenicol, 30 mg/kg per day in four divided doses for 14 days, has also been used to treat tularemia. While response to these agents is good, the relapse rate is unacceptably high, occurring in up to 20 percent of patients.

If fluctuant nodes require aspiration or drainage, at least several days of antibiotic therapy should be given first to avoid exposure of medical personnel to aerosolization of infected material.

PREVENTION Prevention of tularemia is based on avoidance of exposure and vaccination of high-risk populations. Avoidance of skinning wild mammals, especially rabbits, and wearing gloves while handling rabbit carcasses will decrease the risk of transmission. Use of insect repellents and prompt removal of ticks will help prevent transmission by ticks in tick-infested areas.

A multiple-puncture intradermal vaccine (used in a fashion similar to vaccinia) made from live attenuated *F. tularensis* and available from the Centers for Disease Control, is effective in decreasing the frequency and severity of disease, but will not totally prevent tularemia. Protection is long-lasting. Veterinarians, hunters, trappers, game wardens, and others who are likely to come in contact with infected wild mammals are candidates for immunization. Laboratory workers who handle specimens containing *F. tularensis* should be immunized. Prophylactic treatment with streptomycin will prevent development of clinical disease in patients who are incubating *F. tularensis*.

PROGNOSIS If untreated, symptoms of tularemia usually last 1 to 4 weeks but may continue for months. The mortality of severe untreated infection (which includes all untreated tularemia pneumonia) can be as high as 30 percent. However, the overall mortality rate for untreated tularemia is less than 8 percent. Mortality is about 1 percent with appropriate therapy and is often associated with long delays in diagnosis and treatment. Following tularemia there is usually lifelong immunity.

REFERENCES

Evans ME et al: Tularemia: A 30-year experience with 88 cases. Medicine 64:251, 1985

Harper JL et al: Tularemic meningitis in a child with mononuclear pleocytosis. Pediatr Infect Dis 5:595, 1986

Kaiser AB et al: Tularemia and rhabdomyolysis. JAMA 253:241, 1985

Koskela P, Salminen A: Humoral immunity against *Francisella tularensis* after natural infection. J Clin Microbiol 22:973, 1985

Penn RL, Kinasewitz GT: Factors associated with a poor outcome in tularemia. Arch Intern Med 147:265, 1987

Sandstrom G et al: Antigen from *Francisella tularensis:* Nonidentity between determinants participating in cell-mediated and humoral reactions. Infect Immun 45:101, 1984

Sanford JP: Landmark perspective: Tularemia. JAMA 250:3225, 1983

121 PLAGUE AND OTHER *YERSINIA* INFECTIONS

DARWIN L. PALMER

PLAGUE

Plague is an acute infectious illness of humans, wild rodents, and their ectoparasites which is caused by the gram-negative bacillus *Yersinia pestis*. The disease persists because of its firm entrenchment in sylvatic rodent-flea ecosystems throughout the world. Wild rodent contact leads to sporadic human disease; the historically explosive urban epidemics resulted from transmission of disease into rats. Human bubonic plague follows bites by rodent fleas; after several days painful local adenopathy (the bubo) and sepsis spread to other organs, and death occurs. Primary plague pneumonia is transmitted between humans by cough-generated aerosols, has a fulminant course, and is almost universally fatal if untreated.

EPIDEMIOLOGY Sylvatic plague involves more than 200 species of wild rodents and is concentrated in the southwestern United States, the southern Soviet Union, India, Indochina, and South Africa. In the United States, ground squirrels, mice, voles, marmots, wood rats, prairie dogs, and chipmunks are potential carriers. Rodent disease is characterized by occurrence in the spring and summer, year-to-year variations in disease activity, chronicity in the populations involved, slow regional spread, and rare geographic regression. The disease dies off in some populations in cyclical fashion, leaving both resistant survivors and infected fleas seeking another host. Disease also persists in natural foci because of latent infection during animal hibernation, by prolonged viability of *Y. pestis* in soil of rodent burrows, by survival of infected fleas, and by persistent infection in relatively resistant rodents. Rodent predators may also spread plague; felines, such as domestic cats, generally die when infected with *Y. pestis*, while canines, such as foxes, coyotes, and dogs, often recover and may serve as serologic sentinels of wild rodent disease. Human disease can be readily acquired from domestic pets when the pets become infected or catch and return plague-infected rodents or their fleas to rural homes. Hares and rabbits are occasional nonrodent sources of the disease in humans, especially during the winter hunting season.

Rodent fleas are critical to the natural plague cycle and are implicated in about 85 percent of human cases. After infection, fleas develop obstruction of the foregut, causing regurgitation of plague bacilli during the next blood meal. The rat flea, *Xenopsylla cheopsis*, is an especially efficient plague vector both between rats and between rodents and humans. Transmission without fleas may occur by ingestion of infected carcasses by predators, possibly by contact with infected tissue through an open wound, or by inhalation of infected aerosols. Human body lice as well as ticks are also capable of inter-human or person-to-person transmission.

In the past three and one-half decades there has been a rising incidence of sporadic human plague originating in the western United States, with a death rate of 16 percent. This rate, double that seen in large outbreaks, reflects delay in the diagnosis or incorrect therapy due to travel during the incubation period out of plague endemic areas, or failure to elicit a history of animal exposure. Sporadic human plague occurs most frequently in the spring and summer, especially in males and children or youths under 20, reflecting their increased risk of wild rodent contact. While urban rat–related human outbreaks are now rare, they represent a continued threat; spread from sylvatic rodents into urban rats was documented as recently as 1983 in Los Angeles. Primary plague pneumonia arises as a secondary infection during bubonic/septicemic disease, with subsequent person-to-person spread via infectious aerosols. In closed quarters it is rapidly transmitted. A primary pneumonic plague outbreak in the United States last occurred in 1919, when 13 cases with 12 deaths (including two physicians and one nurse) developed before the disease was recognized and halted by case isolation. Cases of primary human pneumonic plague have also been acquired from domestic cats dying of plague pneumonia.

ETIOLOGY *Yersinia pestis* is a member of the family Enterobacteriaceae. It is a pleomorphic, gram-negative, nonmotile, aerobic bacillus which grows optimally at 28°C. The organism grows readily but slowly on routine media, and cultures should not be discarded before 72 h. Although weakly gram-negative, *Y. pestis* stains best with Giemsa's or Wayson's stain, with which it shows prominent bipolar "safety pin" microscopic morphology. The organism is a facultative intracellular parasite which maintains its virulence by the production of V and W antigens, enabling the organism to resist phagocytic intracellular killing, while production of capsular fraction 1 antigen partially protects the organism from phagocytosis by polymorphonuclear leukocytes. Other virulence factors include pesticin, fibrinolysin, coagulase, and a lipopolysaccharide endotoxin. The production of V and W antigens is plasmid-mediated, dependent on calcium, and may reflect the response of *Y. pestis* to its frequent intracellular location. No separate serotypes are recognized, but biotypes *antigua*, *orientalis*, and *mediaevalis* have geographic distributions which presumably mark previous epidemic spread. The organism is relatively resistant to drying and may maintain its viability in cool, moist conditions, such as the soil of an animal burrow, for many months. Antibiotic resistance can be developed in the laboratory, and both streptomycin- and tetracycline-resistant strains have been isolated from clinical specimens.

PATHOGENESIS After *Y. pestis* is inoculated into the skin by a flea bite, bacteria migrate to local lymph nodes, where they are taken up but not killed by mononuclear cells. Intracellular multiplication results in development of capsular envelopes containing fraction 1 protein; other toxins are elaborated. An acute inflammatory response is provoked in the lymph node in 2 to 6 days. At this stage the organisms are relatively resistant to phagocytosis by polymorphonuclear leukocytes because of the protection by capsules containing fraction 1 antigen and the lack of specific opsonic antibody. Characteristically, hemorrhagic necrosis of lymph nodes next occurs from which large numbers of bacteria gain access to the bloodstream and other organs. Extension along lymphatics involves both superficial nodes at the site of inoculation, the spleen, and nodes in the abdomen, mediastinum, or perihilar areas. The lung is secondarily infected in 10 to 20 percent, generally as a rapidly progressive, multilobar pneumonia, often with pleural exudate. The early acute inflammatory reaction is followed by lobar consolidation and hemorrhagic necrosis, and if death does not intervene, may progress to abscess formation. Fibrin thrombi may be extensive in the pulmonary vessels as well as in glomeruli and vessels of skin and other organs. Secondarily, the adult respiratory distress syndrome or a rise in pulmonary artery pressure may be seen. Pericarditis with a small amount of seropurulent exudate is frequent, and meningitis may occur late in untreated bacteremic plague. In 5 to 15 percent, the skin, predominantly of the extremities, is involved early on with petechiae and hemorrhages due to thrombocytopenia and vasculitis. Late in the disease, buboes may become fluctuant and occasionally may become superinfected with other bacteria. Endotoxemia may result in both endotoxin shock and disseminated intravascular coagulation.

MANIFESTATIONS Bubonic plague has an incubation period of 2 to 7 days from flea bite to onset of illness. Although many patients do not remember an insect contact, a small eschar may be found at the bite site. Patients present with a painful bubo and fever accompanied by headache, prostration, and abdominal distress. The bubo, a tender enlarged lymph node or nodes, ranges in size from 1 to 10 cm and is found in the groin in 70 percent; alternatively, buboes may develop in axillary or cervical nodes or in several lymphatic chains simultaneously. Buboes are extremely tender, not fixed to skin or underlying structures, and the overlying skin is often erythematous.

Fever and rigors are prominent and occasionally precede appearance of a bubo by 1 to 3 days. Gastrointestinal symptoms are present in more than half the patients, with abdominal pain often extending from the groin bubo and accompanied by anorexia, nausea, vomiting, and diarrhea, which may be bloody. Cutaneous petechiae and hemorrhages occur in 5 to 50 percent, and may be extensive late in the disease. Disseminated intravascular coagulation occurs in subclinical form in as many as 86 percent of patients, 5 to 10 percent of whom have clinical manifestations, including gangrene of the skin, fingers, toes, and penis. If untreated, bubonic disease may proceed without other organ system involvement to generalized sepsis, prostration, hypotension, and death within the next 2 to 10 days. Some patients have very prominent signs of sepsis with no demonstrable bubo. This represents a form of bubonic plague in which lymphatic involvement is limited to deep structures or where the buboes are so small as to be overlooked in the presence of overwhelming signs of infection. Septicemic disease may progress rapidly with chills, fever, rapid pulse, severe headache, nausea, vomiting, delirium, and death within 48 h. In such fulminant sepsis, bacteremia is so prominent that blood buffy coat may readily show *Y. pestis* on Gram stain.

Other than the lymphatics, the lung is the organ most commonly involved, with development of secondary pneumonia in 10 to 20 percent of all patients. Cough, fever, and tachypnea appear on days 2 to 3 of illness, accompanied by minimal pulmonary infiltrates. Later, or less commonly from the start, symptoms worsen rapidly with marked dyspnea, bloody sputum, and evidence of respiratory failure. There may be multilobar involvement, with variable degrees of consolidation, and the sputum may teem with *Y. pestis* and is highly contagious when disseminated by cough-generated aerosols. Primary plague pneumonia is a fulminant illness; time from the initial contact to death ranges from 2 to 6 days. The adult respiratory distress syndrome (ARDS), characterized by noncardiac pulmonary edema, anoxia, and respiratory failure, also occurs as a manifestation of plague sepsis and may be indistinguishable from plague pneumonia except for the absence of bacteria in respiratory secretions. Both *Y. pestis* pneumonia and the ARDS form of illness have a mortality in excess of 75 percent, despite appropriate antimicrobial and supportive therapy. Less commonly, marked perihilar adenopathy may present alone or accompany pneumonia.

Plague meningitis, as a late complication that occurs in 6 percent of untreated patients, is characterized by nuchal rigidity, headache, confusion, and coma, and is often preceded or accompanied by bacteremia. Most meningitis cases have been described in patients treated with antibiotics that do not readily cross the blood-brain barrier, such as tetracycline and streptomycin. Other contributory factors seem to be late or inadequate therapy. Meningitis due to plague is indistinguishable from that caused by other bacteria.

Rarely, patients with plague have a very mild illness manifested chiefly by low-grade fever and adenopathy. In this group are patients with tonsillar plague, who have positive throat cultures, serologic conversion, and minimal illness. Other less common late complications include persistent hectic fever despite appropriate therapy; fluctuance and spontaneous drainage from buboes; and pulmonary cavitation with abscess formation.

LABORATORY FINDINGS With the exception of definitive microbiologic studies, laboratory tests are of little diagnostic help. A polymorphonuclear leukocytosis of 15,000 to 20,000 cells per cubic millimeter is common, and the white cells may show toxic changes. Rarely, a marked leukemoid reaction with more than 100,000 white cells is seen. Modest elevations of serum glutamic oxaloacetic transaminase are common, but otherwise liver function studies are normal. Evidence of disseminated intravascular coagulation with low platelet counts, prolonged partial thromboplastin times, and positive fibrin degradation products is common. The electrocardiogram is usually normal but may show right axis deviation and peaked P waves indicative of acute cor pulmonale. The chest x-ray shows infiltrates, often with pleural effusion, in secondary or primary plague pneumonia or shows evidence of pulmonary edema in patients with ARDS. In meningitis, examination of cerebrospinal fluid demonstrates polymorphonuclear pleocytosis, low sugar, elevated protein, and gram-negative coccobacillary organisms, although culture may demonstrate *Y. pestis* more reliably.

Confirmation of the clinical suspicion of bubonic plague may be obtained by needle-aspiration of a bubo with direct staining of the aspirated material. With either Wayson's or Giemsa's stain, the characteristic bipolar-staining "safety pin" forms are seen. By fluorescent antibody staining, a presumptive diagnosis may be specifically confirmed in about 80 percent of cases. Cultures of aspirated material, as well as sputum, pleural fluid, and blood, will be positive in a high percentage of patients. Microscopic examination of buffy coat smear may show *Y. pestis* in septicemic cases. A serologic response with a fourfold or greater rise in titer is detected in the second week of illness by complement fixation, hemagglutination or indirect immunofluorescent antibody.

DIAGNOSIS Bubonic plague must be suspected in any febrile patient with painful adenopathy who has a history of wild animal exposure in a plague endemic area, but may be confused with other illnesses. Presentation with fever and a painful groin bubo can mimic granuloma venereum or syphilis or, when more severe, an acute abdominal crisis such as incarcerated inguinal hernia, appendicitis, or a ruptured viscus. Abdominal pain and bloody diarrhea can be mistaken for shigellosis or other acute diarrheal processes. With an axillary or cervical bubo, acute streptococcal or staphylococcal lymphadenitis, tularemia, cat-scratch fever, granuloma venereum, or syphilis need to be considered. Bubonic/septicemic disease with an absent or minimal bubo, suggests typhoid fever or bacteremia due to other causes. Primary or secondary pneumonic plague may mimic bacterial pneumonia from any cause.

When plague is suspected, diagnostic maneuvers must include aspiration of buboes with appropriate stains and cultures, as well as blood cultures and cultures from other sources. Cultures should not be discarded early because the organism grows slowly and may only appear in 48 to 72 h. A serologic rise by passive hemagglutination is evident by day 5 and peaks by day 14. Newer serologic methods such as enzyme-linked immunosorbent assay compare well in sensitivity to standard passive hemagglutination tests and are more rapid.

TREATMENT If plague is strongly suspected on clinical and/or epidemiologic grounds, therapy must be started immediately, prior to completion of diagnostic studies. Antibiotic and supportive treatment should reduce the 40 to 100 percent mortality of untreated bubonic or pneumonic plague to 5 to 10 percent. Effective antibiotics include streptomycin, tetracycline, and chloramphenicol. Streptomycin should be given initially in a dosage of 7.5 to 15 mg/kg every 12 h intramuscularly; tetracycline, intravenously in a dosage of 5 to 10 mg/kg every 6 h, may be started concurrently and streptomycin discontinued when the patient becomes afebrile. Larger doses, even in those with severe illness, offer no benefit. Tetracycline should be continued for a total of 3 to 4 days after the fever has disappeared. In less severely ill patients, tetracycline alone at 5 to 10 mg/kg every 6 h may be given either by mouth or intravenously. Chloramphenicol in a dose of 12.5 to 25 mg/kg given intravenously every 6 h should be substituted for tetracycline in patients with meningitis because of its better central nervous system penetration. While antibiotic-resistant organisms have appeared only rarely, gentamicin is as effective as streptomycin. Tetracycline or trimethoprim-sulfamethoxazole are effective for the prophylaxis of case contacts and should be given orally for 5 days. Local treatment of the bubo is not indicated unless fluctuance or spontaneous drainage occurs, when cultures should be obtained to detect staphylococci. Ventilatory support for patients with plague pneumonia or ARDS may be necessary and lifesaving.

PREVENTION AND CONTROL Individuals working in high-risk occupations in plague endemic areas or conducting laboratory work with *Y. pestis* should consider use of the formalin-killed whole-bacteria vaccine; however, the vaccine must be readministered every 6 months due to rapidly waning immunity. Alternatively, individuals briefly visiting a plague endemic area may take tetracycline or trimethoprim-sulfamethoxazole prophylaxis. Following the presumptive diagnosis of pneumonic plague, patients should be placed in respiratory isolation; simple hand-washing precautions suffice for bubonic cases. Contacts of a patient with plague pneumonia should be given oral tetracycline prophylaxis, 250 mg four times daily by mouth, and should be advised to seek medical attention if respiratory symptoms or fever develop. Possibly due to such precautions, transmission of primary plague pneumonia has not occurred in this country for many years.

The potential for spread of plague into urban rat populations from sylvatic rodent sources is an ever-present risk. Prevention depends on control of urban rat populations and their exclusion from dwellings as well as surveillance of sylvatic rodents and of their local predators. Picnickers, hikers, and others traveling into plague endemic regions during the spring-summer season should be warned that plague is a potential danger. They should avoid touching carcasses or sick rodents and should restrain and treat pets with flea-repellent powders. No practical measures exist for eliminating plague from wild rodent sources. Reducing rodent harborage around rural homes in endemic regions is important. Killing rodents around rural dwellings with rodenticides should be preceded by insect control to prevent displaced rodent fleas from seeking humans or domestic pets.

OTHER *YERSINIA* INFECTIONS (*Y. PSEUDOTUBERCULOSIS* AND *Y. ENTEROCOLITICA*)

ETIOLOGY *Y. enterocolitica* and *Y. pseudotuberculosis* are both non-lactose-fermenting, gram-negative, aerobic bacilli related to one another and to *Y. pestis* and are members of the Enterobacteriaceae. Both organisms grow slowly on media used for the detection of other enteric bacteria, and their detection can be enhanced by cold enrichment incubation at 20 to 25°C. Strains can be distinguished from one another and from *Y. pestis* on the basis of serologic and biochemical reactions as well as by antibiotic sensitivities. As in *Y. pestis,* both organisms elaborate W and V virulence factors and, with *Y. pseudotuberculosis,* virulence is also related to its ability to survive intracellularly. Both organisms produce an endotoxin and *Y. enterocolitica* elaborates a heat-stable enterotoxin which may be of significance in food-borne illness. A large number of serotypes of both organisms exist causing disease in many animal species, but most human infections are caused by a limited number of strains.

MANIFESTATIONS Although recognized most commonly in northern Europe and North America, *Y. enterocolitica* causes enteric infection worldwide and accounts for approximately 1 to 3 percent of all cases of acute bacterial enteritis. The origin of the disease is often unclear and outbreaks traced to both food and water have been reported; person-to-person as well as animal-to-person transmission is common. Manifestations of the disease vary with age. In infants and young children the predominant symptom is acute watery diarrhea lasting 3 to 14 days; 5 percent of children have blood in the stool. In older children and young adults, a syndrome of right lower quadrant pain accompanied by fever and moderate leukocytosis indistinguishable from acute appendicitis occurs. In adults, especially in women over age 40, erythema nodosum often follows enteritis by 1 to 2 weeks. Adults may develop a monarticular arthritis of the knee, foot, or hand with or without preceding enteritis. Rarely, a severe, disabling suppurative arthritis is seen. Among patients with arthritis, 65 percent have histocompatibility group HLA-B27. *Y. enterocolitica* also causes bacteremia, mostly in individuals with underlying illness such as diabetes mellitus, severe anemia, cirrhosis, or malignancy. Septicemic patients complain of headache, fever, and abdominal pain with or without diarrhea and frequently develop abscesses in multiple organs. Exudative pharyngitis with *Y. enterocolitica* was found in adult patients during the course of an outbreak of milk-borne yersiniosis.

Pseudotuberculosis is a rare illness acquired from humans or domestic and wild animals, presumably by fecal-oral contact. Most cases are sporadic and occur in the young, with males more commonly affected than females and with a peak in the winter months corresponding to the peak occurrence in animals. After ingestion, the organisms apparently penetrate the ileal mucosa, localize in the ileocecal lymph nodes, and produce an acute mesenteric adenitis, which is generally accompanied by vomiting, abdominal pain, and diarrhea. Fever is usually high and leukocytosis is common. At laparotomy the appendix appears normal, but enlarged mesenteric lymph nodes and inflammation of the terminal ileum may be seen. Complications appear in adults less commonly than with *Y. enterocolitica* but include arthritis, erythema nodosum, and septicemia.

DIAGNOSIS *Y. enterocolitica* and *Y. pseudotuberculosis* cause similar signs and symptoms but may have different reservoirs; the first is characterized primarily by diarrhea and the second by mesenteric adenitis. Therefore *Y. enterocolitica* causes disease similar to other bacterial diarrheas and must be distinguished from them by microbiologic means. Laboratory detection of the organism depends on special cultural techniques. The diagnosis is made best by isolation of the organism from stool in patients with enteritis, or atypical cases of appendicitis, erythema nodosum, or reactive arthritis. Cultures of the pharyngeal exudate, blood, peritoneal fluid, and other body fluids should be obtained where clinically indicated. Hemagglutination titers peak in 8 to 10 days and remain elevated for 18 months after infection. Cross-reactivity with some *Brucella, Salmonella,* and *Vibrio cholerae* antigens occurs. The diagnosis of *Y. pseudotuberculosis* is also made by culture of stool and mesenteric lymph nodes.

THERAPY AND PREVENTION *Y. enterocolitica* organisms are susceptible in vitro to aminoglycosides, chloramphenicol, tetracycline, trimethoprim-sulfamethoxazole, and the third-generation cephalosporins but are generally resistant to the penicillins and first-generation cephalosporins. However, the value of antimicrobial therapy is unclear, because most cases of enteritis are self-limited. Patients with very severe illness or septicemia should be treated, because treatment may shorten both the duration of disease and the shedding of organisms. *Y. pseudotuberculosis* is usually sensitive to ampicillin, tetracycline, choramphenicol, and cephalosporins. No controlled clinical trials demonstrate efficacy of treatment, although patients with septicemic disease should receive ampicillin or tetracycline, because severe infection has a high mortality. Prevention depends on hygienic measures such as careful food handling, availability of clean drinking water, and hand washing to prevent spread within families or other human contacts.

PASTEURELLA MULTOCIDA INFECTION (See Chap. 98)

REFERENCES

Plague

Barnes AM, Poland JD: Plague in the United States, 1983, Centers for Disease Control Surveillance Summaries, Publication 33 (no 1SS), 1984

Becker TB et al: Plague meningitis. A retrospective analysis of cases reported in the US, 1970–1979. West J Med 147(5):554, 1987

Butler T: A clinical study of bubonic plague: Observations on the 1970 Vietnam epidemic with emphasis on coagulation studies, skin histology, and electrocardiograms. Am J Med 53:268, 1972

Kaufman AF et al: Public health implications of plague in domestic cats. Am J Vet Assoc 179:875, 1981

Reed WP et al: Bubonic plague in the Southwestern United States—A review of recent experience. Medicine 49:465, 1970

Tomich PQ et al: Evidence for the extinction of plague in Hawaii. Am J Epidemiol 119: 261, 1984

Other *Yersinia* Infections

Boyce JM: *Yersinia* species, in *Principles and Practice of Infectious Diseases,* 2d ed, GL Mandell et al (eds). New York, Wiley, 1985, pp 1296–1301

Cover TL, Aber RC: *Yersinia enterocolitica.* N Engl J Med 321:16, 1989

Granfors K et al: Yersinia antigens in synovial-fluid cells from patients with reactive arthritis. N Engl J Med 320:216, 1989

Tacket CO et al: *Yersinia enterocolitica* pharyngitis. Ann Intern Med 99:40, 1983

Tertti R et al: An outbreak of *Yersinia pseudotuberculosis* infection. J Infect Dis 149:245, 1984

122 CHOLERA

GERALD T. KEUSCH

DEFINITION Cholera is an acute diarrheal disease due to a highly motile, curved gram-negative rod, *Vibrio cholerae,* and it can result in severe and rapidly progressive dehydration and death in a matter of hours unless quickly treated. As a result, ''cholera gravis'' is a much feared disease, especially when it occurs in epidemics or in worldwide pandemics associated with high mortality rates.

ETIOLOGY AND EPIDEMIOLOGY *V. cholerae* is a family of organisms, classified on the basis of their somatic O antigen. The major cause of clinical cholera belongs to O group 1 (O-1), which distinguishes it from the more than 70 other members of *V. cholerae* collectively known as non-O1 vibrios. While some of the latter cause diarrhea, only rarely is this cholera gravis. Eight other *Vibrio* species have been defined, of which *V. parahemolyticus, V. fluvialis, V. hollisae,* and *V. mimicus* also cause human diarrhea (see Chap. 92). *V. cholerae* exists in two biotypes, classical and El tor, that are distinguished on the basis of a number of diverse characteristics, such as phage susceptibility and hemolysin production. Both biotypes may be separated into serotypes known as Inaba and Ogawa, which are useful serologic markers for field epidemiologic studies.

Cholera is native to the Ganges delta in the Indian subcontinent, but since 1817, seven world pandemics have occurred. The last to reach the United States was in 1911, when the sixth pandemic made brief entry into New York and Massachusetts. In the past decade, sporadic endemic infection has been recognized along the Gulf coast of Louisiana and Texas, due to eating shellfish contaminated with free-living cholera vibrios. Small outbreaks on offshore oil rigs due to contaminated drinking water have occurred as well. In southern Asia, where the majority of cases in the world occur, fecal contamination of water from an infected human is the most common means of transmission, but contamination of food can contribute to intrafamilial spread. The infectious dose is relatively high, but is markedly reduced in hypocholorhydric subjects or when the gastric pH is buffered by a meal. In endemic areas, cholera is predominantly a pediatric disease, but it affects children and adults equally when the organism is newly introduced into a population. The seasonality of cholera in endemic areas is not fully explained, but may relate to environmental conditions that influence multiplication of vibrios and/or seasonal alterations in human behavior that affect their contact with water. Asymptomatic infections are frequent and are more common with El tor cholera. Young children under 2 years are less likely to develop severe cholera in endemic regions, which may be due in part to passive immunity from breast milk. For unexplained reasons, blood group status is significantly associated with cholera susceptibility; those with group O are at greater risk and those with group AB are at lesser risk.

PATHOGENESIS Once the organism is ingested and safely passes through the stomach, it colonizes the upper small bowel. There are a number of bacterial adhesins that may mediate this phenomenon. Once established, the organism produces the protein, cholera toxin (CT), the principal cause of the watery diarrhea of cholera. CT binds to glycolipid receptors on jejunal epithelial cells, specifically to G_{M1} ganglioside, by a sugar-specific recognition mechanism. CT is an enzyme that transfers ADP-ribose from nicotine adenine dinucleotide (NAD) to a target protein in the adenylate cyclase enzyme system of intestinal epithelial cells. This G protein, the GTP-binding regulatory component of adenylate cyclase, permanently upregulates the cyclase catalytic unit when ADP-ribosylated, resulting in production of high levels of cyclic AMP. In turn, this alters transport of Na and Cl in both the Na-absorbing villus cell and the Cl-secreting crypt cells, leading to accumulation of NaCl in the intestinal lumen. Because water will move passively to maintain osmolality, isotonic fluid accumulates in the lumen, and when the volume exceeds the capacity of the rest of the gut to reabsorb the fluid, watery diarrhea occurs. Dehydration, leading to shock, and loss of base, leading to acidosis, then develop unless these fluids and electrolytes are replaced adequately.

The nature of immunity to cholera is poorly understood but seems to be primarily antibacterial at the level of the mucosa itself and, to a lesser extent, related to antitoxin antibody of the secretory IgA class. Serum antibody is more a marker of prior exposure than an indication of protection.

CLINICAL MANIFESTATIONS After a 24 to 48 h incubation, the disease begins with the sudden onset of painless watery diarrhea that quickly becomes voluminous and is often quickly followed by vomiting. In severe cholera, adults can lose as much as 1 L/h and children 10 mL/kg per hour in the first 24 h. Without replacement, this fluid loss can cause lethal volume depletion. There is usually no fever, but muscle cramps may occur later due to potassium depletion. The stool has a characteristic appearance, a nonbilious, gray, slightly cloudy fluid with flecks of mucus and a somewhat sweet, inoffensive odor. Clinical symptoms parallel volume contraction, with thirst observed at 3 to 5 percent loss; postural hypotension, weakness, tachycardia, and decreased skin turgor at 5 to 8 percent; and oliguria, weak to absent pulses, sunken eyes and (in infants) sunken fontanelles, wrinkled (''washerwoman'') skin, and somnolence progressing to coma with fluid losses in excess of 10 percent of normal body weight. When clinical manifestations of volume depletion are treated with fluid and salt, the process is self-limited to a few days at most, and complications such as renal failure due to acute tubular necrosis can be averted.

Laboratory data usually reveal elevation of the hematocrit in nonanemic patients; mild neutrophilic leukocytosis; elevations of BUN and creatinine consistent with prerenal azotemia; normal sodium, potassium, and chloride; a markedly reduced bicarbonate (<15 mmol/L); and elevation of the anion gap due to coexistent increases in serum lactate, protein, and phosphates. When measured, arterial pH is usually low (about 7.2).

DIAGNOSIS Clinical suspicion of cholera can be proven by identification of the organism in stool. Dark-field microscopy by an experienced technician can directly detect the organism in a wet mount of fresh stool and even reveal serotype by immobilization with Inaba- or Ogawa-specific antisera. The best selective culture medium is thiosulfate–citrate–bile salt–sucrose (TCBS) agar, on which the organism grows as a flat yellow colony. In endemic areas there is little need for biochemical characterization, but this may be worthwhile where *V. cholerae* is an uncommon isolate. Standard biochemical testing for enterobacteriaceae will suffice. All vibrios are oxidase-positive, and *V. cholerae* can be distinguished from the otherwise similar *V. mimicus* by its ability to ferment sucrose. If a delay in processing samples is expected, it is recommended that Carey-Blair transport medium and/or alkaline-peptone water enrichment medium be inoculated as well.

TREATMENT Cholera is simple to treat, needing only the rapid and adequate replacement of fluids, electrolytes, and base. Mortality rates are usually less than 1 percent. It has been conclusively proven that fluid may be given by the oral route, using the glucose-Na cotransport mechanism to move Na across the gut mucosa together with an actively transported molecule such as glucose. Since Na losses in the stool are high, fluid containing 90 mmol/L Na has been recommended by the World Health Organization (WHO) (Table 122-1). This amount of Na is higher than is needed in other diarrheas, but the solution is safe if alternated with Na-free fluid such as breast milk or water. For the sake of simplicity, WHO advises use of this single solution instead of multiple different formulae tailored for different etiologies. Because severe acidosis is common in severely dehydrated patients (pH <7.2), 50% *N* saline with added bicarbonate (44 mmoL/L) is the preferred solution for intravenous administration. For severely dehydrated patients the total fluid deficit (usually

TABLE 122-1 Oral rehydration fluids recommended by the World Health Organization

	Concentration, mmol/L		
Component	Bicarbonate based	Citrate based	Super-ORS*
Sodium	90	90	90
Potassium	20	20	20
Chloride	80	80	80
Citrate	—	10	—
Bicarbonate	30	—	30
Glucose	111	111	111
Glycine	—	—	111†

* Super-ORS refers to the use of solutions containing two substrates that are actively cotransported across the intestinal mucosa together with sodium, such as glucose and glycine.

† In the developing world, 30–50 g of rice powder is being substituted for glucose, as it is an inexpensive source of small-chain oligosaccharides that provide substrate for facilitated cotransport with sodium but do not increase osmolarity. In addition, rice-based ORS seems to provide more nutritional benefits than standard ORS and may reduce the net fluid output of diarrheal stool, an effect not seen with ordinary ORS.

estimated as 10 percent of body weight) can be safely replaced intravenously within the first 4 h following admission. Half of this may be given within the first hour. After this, oral therapy can usually be initiated to maintain fluid balance and intake equal to output. However, patients with continued large volume diarrhea may require prolonged administration of intravenous fluids to maintain adequate volume status until the diarrhea stops. Severe hypokalemia may be present, but will respond to potassium given by either the intravenous or oral route. Without adequate staff to monitor patient progress, the oral route is safer and is physiologically regulated by thirst and urine output.

The use of antibiotics to which the organism is susceptible will diminish the duration and the amount of fluid loss and more rapidly clear the organism from the stool, but is not necessary to achieve complete cure. Tetracycline is efficacious, but is not recommended for children under 8 years of age because of side effects on bone and developing teeth. Other antibiotics, including chloramphenicol, trimethoprim-sulfamethoxazole, and ampicillin are also effective.

CONTROL In outbreaks, attention should first be given to identification of case contacts and treatment of incubating carriers. Next, epidemiologic study is needed to establish the modes of transmission to help define the best control strategy. At the same time establishment of rehydration centers is essential to reduce mortality. The role of killed whole cholera vaccine is less clear.

PREVENTION Provision of safe water, facilities for sanitary disposal of feces, improved nutrition, and attention to food preparation and storage in the household could significantly reduce the incidence of cholera. Much attention has been given to the development of a cholera vaccine in the past two decades, focusing particularly on use of a live oral vaccine strain. The traditional killed cholera vaccine, consisting of three injections of 5 billion dead *Vibrios,* provides little protection to nonimmune subjects while predictably causing side effects, including local pain, malaise, and fever. A new approach consisting of oral administration of killed whole bacterial cells together with the toxin B-subunit has provided promising results. In trials in Bangladesh, the combined vaccine conferred 85 percent protection, compared to 58 percent for killed whole cells vaccine, 4 months after administration. However, the benefit of adding the B-subunit toxin was no longer detectable by 8 months, and by the end of 1 year protection was equivalent for the two vaccines (around 60 percent). Increasing the number of killed bacteria given by mouth may also increase its protective efficacy. Until this or another vaccine is available, parenteral cholera vaccine is not recommended for Americans traveling in cholera-endemic areas unless required by the country to be visited. Careful hygiene and attention to eating and drinking habits to reduce the likelihood of encountering the organism are recommended.

REFERENCES

CLEMENS JD et al: Field trial of oral cholera vaccines in Bangladesh: Results of one year of follow-up. J Infect Dis 158:60, 1988

GLASS RI: Cholera and non-cholera vibrios, in *Enteric Infections: Mechanisms, Manifestations, Management,* MJG Farthing, GT Keusch (eds). London, Chapman & Hall, 1989, pp 317–325

LEVINE MM et al: Volunteer studies of deletion mutants of *Vibrio cholerae* O1 prepared by recombinant techniques. Infect Immun 56:262, 1988

MILLER CJ et al: Cholera epidemiology in developed and developing countries: New thoughts on transmission, seasonality, and control. Lancet 2:261, 1985

MORRIS JG JR, BLACK RE: Cholera and other vibrioses in the United States. N Engl J Med 312:343, 1985

WANG F et al: The acidosis of cholera. Contributions of hyperproteinemia, lactic acidemia and hyperphosphatemia to an increased serum anion gap. N Engl J Med 315:1591, 1986

WORLD HEALTH ORGANIZATION: *World Health Organization Guidelines for Cholera Control.* WHO/CDD/Ser/80.4 Revl, Geneva, 1986

123 BARTONELLOSIS

JAMES J. PLORDE

DEFINITION Bartonellosis (Carrión's disease) is an infection with *Bartonella bacilliformis.* Two well-defined clinical stages occur: an acute febrile anemia of rapid onset and high mortality, designated *Oroya fever,* and a benign eruptive form with chronic cutaneous lesions, called *verruga peruana.* Either of these types may be mild, and asymptomatic cases constitute the greatest epidemiologic hazard.

ETIOLOGY *Bartonella bacilliformis* is a small, motile, aerobic, pleomorphic, gram-negative coccobacillus which stains reddish violet with Giemsa's stain. It can be cultured on enriched media and does not produce a hemolysin. The organisms are sensitive to several antibiotics in vitro.

EPIDEMIOLOGY The disease is limited to certain valleys in the Andes Mountains comprising parts of Peru, Ecuador, and Colombia. It occurs in regions between the altitudes of 750 and 2500 m (2400 and 8000 ft) where the phlebotamine sandfly vector, *Lutzomyia,* propagates. Although *L. verrucarum* is the principal vector of the disease, other species are involved in Colombia as well. Asymptomatic cases and convalescent carriers are the only known reservoir of infection. A low-grade bacteremia may persist for years following resolution of symptoms, and *B. bacilliformis* can be recovered from the blood of 5 to 10 percent of the apparently normal population in an endemic area. Epidemics often coincide with immigration of workers from uninfected areas.

PATHOLOGY AND PATHOGENESIS The manifestations of the disease are thought to reflect the immune status of the host. In nonimmune individuals Oroya fever develops. Large numbers of the *Bartonella* bacteria enter the bloodstream, adhere to erythrocytes, and invade the endothelial cells of the capillaries and lymphatics where they multiply. Subsequent invasion and multiplication within erythrocytes result in their phagocytosis and destruction by the liver and spleen. The red blood cell life span is greatly shortened, and anemia develops. This is accentuated by a defective erythropoietic response early in the course of infection. The pathogenesis of the hemolytic anemia remains unknown. Agglutinins and hemolysins have not been found, and tests for mechanical fragility of red blood cells have given variable results. Invasion and swelling of capillary endothelial cells may lead to vascular occlusion and tissue infarcts. It is thought that an impairment of reticuloendothelial function secondary to massive phagocytosis of red blood cells and immune suppression are responsible for the frequency with which *Salmonella* and other coliform bacteremias, staphylococcal infections, tuberculosis, malaria, and amebiasis are seen in Oroya fever.

With developing immunity, the bacteria nearly disappear from the peripheral blood and capillary endothelium. After a latent period they reappear in the skin and subcutaneous tissue where they are apparently responsible for the development of the hemangioid lesions of verruga peruana. Second attacks of Carrión's disease are unusual. When they occur, they almost invariably present as verruga.

CLINICAL MANIFESTATIONS The incubation period is approximately 3 weeks but may be longer. The initial symptoms are fever and pains in the bones, joints, and muscles. At this point the disease often resembles influenza or malaria, but blood cultures are positive. After these prodromes, the patient usually develops one of the two classic forms of the infection.

Oroya fever This form is characterized by sudden onset of high fever, extreme pallor, weakness, and a precipitous drop in the number of red blood cells. The count may fall from normal to 1 million per microliter within 4 or 5 days. The anemia is characterized by normochromic macrocytes in the peripheral blood, striking polychromasia and polychromatophilia, nucleated red blood cells, Howell-Jolly bodies, Cabot rings, and basophilic stippling. There may also be a mild leukocytosis with a shift to the left. Organisms are numerous in the blood, and stained smears may show 90 percent of the erythrocytes heavily invaded. Salmonellosis, malaria, amebiasis, tuberculosis, and other intercurrent infections may occur and are an important factor in fatal cases.

Muscle and joint pain and headache are severe, and insomnia, delirium, and coma are the terminal manifestations. In untreated patients, the mortality rate may exceed 50 percent; death occurs within 10 days to 4 weeks. With treatment, or sometimes spontaneously, recovery results if the organisms decrease and fever abates. The red blood cell count stabilizes and approaches normal values in about 6 weeks, when convalescence begins.

Verruga peruana This form of the disease, characterized by a profuse skin eruption, may follow the anemic form or may occur in patients without previous symptoms. The verrugas vary in color from red to purple. They may be miliary, nodular, or eroding, and they range in size from 2 to 10 mm up to 3 or 4 cm in diameter. They may resemble the lesions of Kaposi's sarcoma. The three types of verruga may occur together; since eruption takes place in successive crops, verrugas of all types and in all stages of development may be found on the same patient. The chief sites involved are the limbs and face, and less frequently the genitalia, scalp, and mucosa of the mouth and pharynx. They may persist for 1 month to 2 years. The eruption is accompanied by pain, fever, and moderate anemia. Bartonellas may be demonstrated in the lesions and cultured from the blood.

DIAGNOSIS A clinical diagnosis of verruga peruana can be made with accuracy in endemic areas. It is confirmed by demonstrating the Giemsa-stained organism in biopsy specimens from representative lesions. During Oroya fever the organism is easily seen on peripheral blood smears. It may be recovered from blood cultures in all stages of the disease.

TREATMENT Oroya fever responds dramatically to a number of antibiotics including tetracycline and chloramphenicol. The latter in a dose of 2 g per day for 7 days is often preferred because of the frequency with which *Salmonella* infections complicate this disease. Fever disappears within 48 h, and the patient recovers rapidly. Transfusions may be required when the anemia is severe. Antibiotic therapy [rifampin (rifampicin) 600 mg/d for 6 days] of the verrugal stage may hasten the involution of these lesions. The use of DDT in both the interior and exterior of human dwellings is highly effective in controlling the night-biting sandflies. Insect repellents and bed netting afford personal protection.

REFERENCES

Arias-Stella J et al: Verruga peruana, mimicking malignant neoplasms. Am J Dermatopathol 9:279, 1987

Caudra MC: Salmonellosis complication in human bartonellosis. Tex Rep Biol Med 14:97, 1956

Dooley JR: Haemotropic bacteria in man. Lancet 2:1237, 1980

Garcia FU: Tissue reaction in Bartonellosis may suggest Kaposi's sarcoma. Arch Pathol Lab Med 109:703, 1985

Schultz MG: Daniel Carrión's experiment. N Engl J Med 278:1323, 1968

124 *LEGIONELLA* INFECTIONS

MICHAEL S. BERNSTEIN / RICHARD M. LOCKSLEY

DEFINITION The family Legionellaceae consists of over 25 species of fastidious gram-negative, aerobic bacilli. The organisms are ubiquitous in the environment and cause disease when a sufficient environmental inoculum is aerosolized and inhaled by a human host. The course of the subsequent disease is determined both by virulence factors of the bacterium and by the immune competence of the host. The organism in humans behaves as a facultative intracellular bacterium. Legionnaire's disease, a fulminant pneumonia caused by *Legionella pneumophila,* is the prototypic illness caused by these organisms. Pontiac fever is a self-limited, flulike syndrome that occurs in immunocompetent individuals. The spectrum of disease caused by these organisms is designated legionellosis.

HISTORY Legionnaire's disease refers to an epidemic of pneumonia that affected 221 people and caused 34 deaths during the American Legion Convention at the Bellevue-Stratford Hotel in Philadelphia during July and August 1976. Initially referred to as the Legionnaire's disease agent, the organism was shown to be a new species of bacterium and subsequently designated *L. pneumophila.* Serotyping revealed that this organism had been responsible for previous epidemics of pneumonia, including 20 cases of severe pneumonia among attendees at a convention in Philadelphia at the same hotel in 1974. Furthermore, in July 1968, 144 employees and visitors in a health department building in Pontiac, Michigan, developed a self-limited illness consisting of fever, myalgias, headache, and malaise, subsequently termed Pontiac fever. Exposure of guinea pigs to aerosols of water from the building's air conditioning system led to isolation of the organism, eventually identified as *L. pneumophila.*

The discovery of *L. pneumophila* led rapidly to the isolation of related organisms within the family Legionellaceae (Table 124-1). There are more than 34 species (29 named) and over 50 distinct serogroups (46 named). Many isolates cause pneumonia indistinguishable from that caused by the initial strain, designated *Legionella pneumophila* serotype 1. This isolate accounts for 50 percent of human infection, followed in frequency by serotype 6 (10 percent). *L. micdadei* (Pittsburgh pneumonia agent) accounts for 7 percent of cases. The serologically unrelated, unnamed legionellae are designated *Legionella*-like organisms (LLOs).

ETIOLOGY The legionellae are classified in a single genus, *Legionella,* within the family Legionellaceae. The legionellae are gram-negative, aerobic, nonencapsulated bacilli measuring 0.3 to 0.9 μm in width and 2 to 5 μm in length. They are non-spore-forming, and most are motile due to polar or subpolar flagellae. Electron microscopy reveals multiple fimbriae (pili) extending from the surface. Legionellae have complex growth requirements and do not grow on standard bacteriologic media. All species require supplementation of growth media with L-cysteine and ferric salts and grow best at pH 6.8 to 7.0. Legionellae display an unusual dependence on amino acids, as opposed to carbohydrates, for energy and carbon sources. The fatty acids of legionellae contain an unusually high proportion of branched-chain acids, permitting identification by gas-liquid chromatography.

In most clinical laboratories legionellae are recognized by their growth on selective media. Identification is confirmed by serologic reactivity with defined antisera. A commercially available slide

TABLE 124-1 Identified *Legionella*

Species (serogroups)	Pneumonia	Pontiac fever	DFA*
L. pneumophila (14)	X	1,6†	1–10
L. micdadei	X		X
L. bozemanii (2)	X		1
L. dumoffii	X	?	X
L. gormanii	X		X
L. longbeachae (2)	X		1,2
L. jordanis	X		X
L. oakridgensis	X		
L. wadsworthii	X		
L. feeleii (2)	X	X	
L. sainthelensi	X	?	
L. anisa	X	X	
L. maceachernii	X		
L. jamestownensis			
L. rubrilucens			
L. erythra			
L. hackeliae (2)	X		
L. spiritensis		?	
L. parisiensis			
L. cherrii	X		
L. steigerwaltii			
L. santicrucis			
L. israelensis			
L. cincinnatiensis	X		
L. quinlivanii			
L. birminghamensis	X		
L. moravica			
L. brunensis			
L. tucsonensis	X		

* Direct fluorescent antibody reagents available.
† Numbers refer to serogroups.

agglutination test identifies 22 *Legionella* species and 33 serogroups. Further identification of a *Legionella* isolate may require analysis in a reference laboratory. Biochemical analysis, autofluorescence, immunofluorescence staining, and gas-liquid chromatography are used to characterize different species and strains. Less widely available techniques include restriction endonuclease analysis, alloenzyme typing, and plasmid DNA profiling.

ECOLOGY AND TRANSMISSION Legionellae are ubiquitous in aquatic environments. Diverse natural *reservoirs* harbor these organisms, including mud, frozen streams, hot springs, and stagnant lakes. Certain algae provide all of the nutritional and growth requirements for *L. pneumophila*. Some amebas and ciliated protozoa ingest legionellae and support their intracellular multiplication, protecting the bacteria from disinfectants and other adverse conditions. Legionellaceae have no animal or human reservoir.

Amplifiers are man-made water supplies that favor the growth of legionellae. Growth is enhanced by elevated temperatures (36 to 70°C), a source of iron and simple nutrients, and low levels of other competing bacteria. Hot water systems and heat exchange units are frequently contaminated due to stagnation, infrequent decontamination, and the presence of sediment or decayed plumbing, all of which contribute to suboptimal levels of chlorine. Decomposing rubber gaskets and sealing washers are capable of supporting the growth of these organisms. Legionellae have been isolated from such diverse man-made aqueous environments as potable water, ice machines, hot tubs, and humidifiers.

Disseminators facilitate transmission to the human respiratory tract by generating infectious aerosols. Airborne transmission by environmentally generated aerosols was suggested by epidemiologic evidence and has been reproduced in experimental animals. Aerosolized *L. pneumophila* can survive for more than 2 h and have been isolated nearly 1 mile downwind of cooling towers. Infectious aerosol particles are less than 5 μm in diameter and can be inhaled directly into the alveoli. A variety of sources have been identified in outbreaks of Legionnaire's disease, including cooling towers, air conditioning systems, humidifiers, whirlpool baths, respiratory nebulizers, and showers. Aerosolized legionellae have been traced to contaminated soil disturbed by excavation and to industrial lubricants used to cool machinery.

Other routes of transmission may exist. Microaspiration of contaminated water has been suggested by epidemiologic studies. Wound infection by *L. pneumophila* has been reported from a contaminated whirlpool bath. There is no evidence of person-to-person transmission.

EPIDEMIOLOGY *Legionella* infections account for 1 to 3 percent of community-acquired pneumonias and, in some studies, up to one-fourth of "atypical" community-acquired pneumonias. *L. pneumophila* may be responsible for 10 percent of nosocomial pneumonias and as much as 30 percent during endemic hospital outbreaks. About half of adults show evidence of prior exposure to at least one *Legionella* species.

Legionella infections occur in epidemic outbreaks, sporadic cases, or highly endemic clusters related to sustained nosocomial outbreaks. Both pneumonic and nonpneumonic legionellosis exist in epidemic form but differ in their attack rates and incubation periods. *Legionella* pneumonia has an attack rate of 1 to 7 percent, whereas Pontiac fever affects 95 to 100 percent of those exposed. The incubation period for pneumonia is 2 to 12 days, while that for nonpneumonic outbreaks is 24 to 48 h. There is a higher incidence of legionellosis during summer, presumably due to warmer water temperatures and increased use of water cooling systems that transmit the organism.

Pneumonic legionellosis affects men three times as often as women and is uncommon in children. Other risk factors for pneumonic disease include cigarette smoking, heavy alcohol use, advanced age, chronic illness, and use of immunosuppressive medication. Renal transplant patients appear to be at particular risk. Nonpneumonic legionellosis has no demonstrable risk factors.

PATHOGENESIS AND PATHOLOGY Direct alveolar deposition of infectious aerosols containing legionellae is the predominant form of inoculation in *Legionella* infections. The short incubation period and the association with environmental aerosols are consistent with this mechanism. The inoculum of aerosolized bacteria and poorly defined variability in virulence among strains may be important in determining the outcome of infection. Common-source exposures can result in nonpneumonic illness or severe pneumonia in different individuals, depending on the extent of exposure to infectious aerosols.

Legionellae appear to be susceptible to clearance by the mucociliary apparatus. Asymptomatic colonization does not occur, and, during disease, pathologic findings are limited to the lower respiratory tract. Alveolar deposition via aerosol and factors, such as smoking, that impair mucociliary clearance permit the organism to establish infection within resident alveolar macrophages. In the human host, legionellae are facultative intracellular pathogens of monocytes and macrophages. The organisms activate complement by the classic pathway but are resistant to lysis. Mononuclear phagocytes ingest *L. pneumophila* by a mechanism termed *coiling phagocytosis* that is mediated by complement receptors CR1 and CR3. Ingested organisms inhibit fusion of the phagosome to primary and secondary lysosomes, blocking the transfer of microbicidal substances into the phagosome and interfering with acidification of the vacuole. The sequestered organisms divide by binary fission within unusual vacuoles studded by host ribosomes and surrounded by glycogen granules and mitochondria. Continued replication results in lysis of the mononuclear cell and spread to adjacent cells. Both neutrophils and monocytes are recruited to the developing inflammatory lesion but are unable to inhibit bacterial growth efficiently. Specific antibody is produced, but the organisms remain resistant to antibody-mediated complement lysis. Phagocytosis is enhanced by specific antibody, thus further targeting the bacteria to the intracellular environment.

From the initial site, infection spreads by endobronchial, hematogenous, or lymphatic routes or by contiguous invasion. Bacteremia occurs in as many as one-third of patients with legionellosis and is the most common source of extrapulmonary infection.

Infection is controlled coincident with the appearance of cell-mediated immunity, similar to that with other intracellular pathogens. Sensitized T lymphocytes secrete macrophage activating factors, primarily interferon-γ, that enable the cell to inhibit intracellular replication. Interleukin 2–activated natural killer cells are also capable of destroying *Legionella*-infected monocytes in vitro. Immunization using aerosolized avirulent *L. pneumophila* or subcutaneous injection of a secreted bacterial protein protects guinea pigs against otherwise lethal aerosol challenge. The importance of cell-mediated immunity is supported by the increased incidence and severity of legionellosis among immunosuppressed patients, including transplant recipients.

Macroscopically, bronchopneumonia ranges from a patchy lobular process to more extensive multilobar consolidation. Round, nodular lesions are sometimes present. Abscesses with central necrosis occur in 25 percent of fatal cases. Pleuritis and small serosanguinous pleural effusions are common, but empyema is rare. Microscopically, infection is characterized by intense alveolitis and bronchiolitis. Alveolar spaces are filled with polymorphonuclear leukocytes, macrophages, fibrin, and proteinaceous exudate. Many inflammatory cells have undergone leukocytoclasis leaving only nuclear debris and fibrin. Organisms can be visualized using the Gimenez stain, Dieterle silver impregnation stain, or direct fluorescent antibody and are predominantly located within phagocytes. Alveolar septae and interstitial spaces are thickened by edema and inflammatory cells. More severe disease occurs in immunocompromised patients, including diffuse alveolar damage with hyaline membrane formation. Pathologic changes do not extend proximal to terminal bronchioles, a finding consistent with inoculation by aerosol. Pathologic changes are usually limited to the lungs. Brain tissue is normal even in cases with neurologic abnormalities.

CLINICAL MANIFESTATIONS Legionnaire's disease and Pontiac fever are the two well-described syndromes. The complete spectrum of infection by Legionellaceae remains undefined, however, and probably includes asymptomatic seroconversion, mild self-resolving illness, and isolated extrapulmonary manifestations.

Pneumonic illness typically begins with an abrupt prodrome of malaise, headache, myalgia, and weakness. Fever and intermittent rigors appear 24 h later, with temperatures exceeding 40°C in more than half of patients. Nonproductive cough is common. About half of patients eventually produce thin or minimally purulent sputum, and one-third may have scant hemoptysis. Pleuritic chest pain and dyspnea can raise the suspicion of pulmonary embolism. Gastrointestinal symptoms include diarrhea, nausea, vomiting, and abdominal pain. Altered mental status suggesting toxic encephalopathy may include confusion, disorientation, lethargy, hallucinations, depression, delirium, obtundation, or coma. Seizures are rare, but cranial or peripheral neuropathy and cerebellar dysfunction are not uncommon. Physical examination usually shows a toxic appearance and high fever. Relative bradycardia is common. Lung examination reveals rales and consolidation, but the physical findings are mild when compared to radiographic findings. Complications and systemic manifestations include lung abscess, empyema, respiratory failure, hypotension, shock, rhabdomyolysis, disseminated intravascular coagulation (DIC), thrombotic thrombocytopenic purpura (TTP), and renal failure.

Pontiac fever is an acute, self-limited illness lasting 2 to 5 days. A prodrome of malaise, myalgia, and headache is followed rapidly by fever, chills, and, variably, cough, coryza, and sore throat. Diarrhea, nausea, and mild neurologic symptoms such as dizziness or photophobia may be present.

Legionellae may also cause extrapulmonary infections related to bacteremia at the time of pneumonia or local exposure to contaminated water. Pericarditis, myocarditis, pyelonephritis, pancreatitis, sinusitis, and hemodialysis fistula infections; abscesses in liver, skin, and the perirectal area; and postoperative wound infections have been reported. *L. pneumophila* and *L. dumoffii* can cause subacute and chronic prosthetic valve endocarditis with annular and myocardial abscesses. The organisms are nosocomially acquired during the perioperative period when the primary infection may cause a postpericardiotomy–like syndrome. Emboli are rare.

LABORATORY FINDINGS *Legionella* pneumonia is usually accompanied by leukocytosis with an increase in early granulocyte forms; the total leukocyte count exceeds 20,000 cells per microliter in 10 to 20 percent of cases. None of the laboratory abnormalities associated with pneumonic legionellosis is specific although hyponatremia occurs in 50 to 70 percent, more commonly than in other forms of pneumonia. Other laboratory findings may include hypophosphatemia, azotemia, microhematuria, proteinuria, and abnormal tests of liver function. Hematologic findings are typically normal unless the illness is complicated by DIC or TTP. Cerebrospinal fluid examination is usually normal although pleocytosis and elevated protein have been reported. Gram stain of the sputum may show inflammatory cells, but legionellae stain poorly or not at all in clinical specimens. *L. micdadei* is acid-fast by Kinyoun and modified Ziehl-Neelsen stains.

Early roentgenographic patterns include diffuse patchy infiltrates or ill-defined nodular densities. Pneumonia progresses to bilateral infiltrates in 50 percent of patients; a lobar-segmental pattern predominates. Small pleural effusions are present in 20 to 50 percent. Cavitation is uncommon but may occasionally be seen, particularly in immunosuppressed patients.

Leukocytosis is frequently the only laboratory abnormality in Pontiac fever.

DIAGNOSIS The diagnosis of *Legionella* infection may be made by culturing the organism, identifying its antigens or nucleic acids in tissue or secretions, or demonstrating a serologic response in the host (Table 124-2). A positive culture is diagnostic since no carrier state occurs. Cultures are performed on buffered charcoal yeast extract agar with α-ketoglutarate (BCYE-α agar), but 2 to 5 days may be required to identify the organism. BCYE-α agar is not selective, and supplementation with antibiotics or acidification is required for sputum samples to inhibit the growth of other bacteria. Typical results of the culture of clinical specimens are listed in Table 124-2. Blood cultures must be subcultured on BCYE-α agar after 24 h of aerobic incubation.

Legionellae may be visualized in clinical specimens by direct fluorescent antibody (DFA) staining. Clinical specimens are treated with fluorescein-conjugated rabbit antibody and examined by fluorescence microscopy. The test requires only 2 to 4 h. Commercially available DFA reagents detect over 90 percent of strains responsible for clinical disease (Table 124-1). However, the relatively low sensitivity (50 percent) and the need for an experienced technician are disadvantages. DFA may be less sensitive after a patient has received appropriate antibiotics.

Available tests for *Legionella* antigens in urine include an enzyme-linked immunosorbent assay, radioimmunoassay, and latex agglutination. The relative ease of specimen collection and assay performance may make this an attractive rapid test. However, antigenuria may persist for months, obscuring the distinction between acute and past infection. A radiolabeled nucleic acid hybridization kit is promising because it allows the detection of all *Legionella* species, although false-positive results have been reported. The radioactive isotope limits the shelf life of the assay.

Serum antibody is most commonly measured using the indirect fluorescent antibody (IFA) assay. Routinely available reagents detect antibody directed only against *L. pneumophila* serogroup 1, believed to account for half of human disease. A diagnosis of legionellosis is made by a fourfold rise in titer between acute and convalescent sera

TABLE 124-2 Laboratory tests in Legionnaire's disease

Test	Sensitivity, %	Specificity, %
Culture		
Sputum	60	100
Transtracheal	80	100
Lung biopsy	90	100
Blood	38	100
DFA	50	95
Urine antigen*	80	99
DNA probe	70	99
Serology (IFA)*	80	99

* *L. pneumophila* serogroup 1 only, indirect fluorescent antibody.

to at least 1:128, or a single titer of 1:256 or greater. Serum samples should be obtained acutely and after 3 weeks, although as many as one-fourth of patients may seroconvert within the first week of illness. Seroconversion develops in 80 percent of patients by 10 weeks.

While no clinical features of *Legionella* pneumonia are unique, the diagnosis should be suspected in a patient with severe pneumonia, high fever, nonproductive cough, hyponatremia, and altered mental status, particularly in the setting of immunosuppression. Each of the tests employed to diagnose legionellosis has its limitations. Combined approaches are recommended. No diagnostic test may be used to exclude the disease absolutely. Thus, clinical judgment must often prevail in decisions regarding therapy.

The diagnosis of Pontiac fever requires a compatible clinical illness, evidence of serologic conversion and, preferably, isolation of the organism from the environment. Viable legionnellae have never been isolated from a case of Pontiac fever, raising the possibility that the pathogenesis involves hypersensitivity to bacterial antigens rather than true infection.

TREATMENT Erythromycin is the antibiotic of choice for pneumonic legionellosis. For serious infection, patients should receive 4 g/d intravenously. Dosage reduction may be necessary in renal failure to avoid ototoxicity. Immunocompromised patients and those with severe disease should receive rifampin (rifampicin) concurrently in a dose of 600 mg/d. Immunosuppressive medications should be tapered when possible. Response to therapy occurs in 24 to 48 h, although fever may persist for up to a week. With improvement, erythromycin may be reduced to 2 g/d orally. Therapy should continue for 3 weeks; shorter courses have been associated with relapse. Doxycycline or trimethoprim-sulfamethoxazole are potential alternatives when erythromycin is not tolerated, or in the rare patients failing to respond to erythromycin. Ciprofloxacin and other quinolones appear to be effective, but clinical experience with these agents is small. Effective antibiotics are those that diffuse readily into phagocytic cells, suggesting that their role may be to arrest intracellular multiplication until the development of cellular immunity.

Legionella prosthetic valve endocarditis usually requires valve replacement and prolonged antibiotic therapy (3 to 12 months). Pontiac fever is a self-limited illness requiring no therapy.

PROGNOSIS AND IMMUNITY Overall case fatality rates for *Legionella* pneumonia are approximately 15 percent. Mortality is 80 percent among untreated immunosuppressed patients and is reduced to 25 percent with appropriate antibiotic treatment. Untreated immunocompetent hosts have a 25 percent mortality rate; with proper therapy only 7 percent succumb.

Patients who survive usually have no permanent sequelae. Full recovery of pulmonary function is usual, although pulmonary fibrosis with respiratory disability has been reported. Immunocompetent individuals who recover from infection are immune to reinfection with the same strain. Reinfection with an identical serotype has been reported in an immunocompromised patient.

PREVENTION AND CONTROL Understanding the chain of transmission of legionellae from natural reservoirs to man-made amplifiers and disseminators is important in devising control strategies. Surveillance efforts should concentrate on documenting human infection, rather than routinely screening the environment. During epidemic or endemic outbreaks, sentinel cases occur among immunosuppressed patients. Once detected, a careful search for the environmental source should be conducted. Multiple legionellae may be recovered from environmental cultures, many of which are not associated with human disease. Therefore, clinical isolates should be characterized so that control measures can focus on the source of pathogenic strains. Legionellosis is a reportable infection, and local health departments can provide assistance in the isolation and characterization of environmental strains.

Sources of environmental aerosols (disseminators), such as shower heads and air conditioning systems, must be identified so that transmission can be interrupted. Contaminated water systems (amplifiers) can be sterilized. Legionellae may be present in low titer in potable water systems, requiring culture of large volumes on selective media or following pretreatment with heat or acid to enhance recovery. Rusted plumbing and decayed rubber gaskets should be replaced. Sites of stagnation and sediment in water tanks may require elimination. Decontamination of potable water systems is accomplished by hyperchlorination (2 to 3 ppm) and/or intermittent heating to 60°C with flushing of distal outlets. During nosocomial outbreaks, prophylactic treatment of high-risk patients using oral erythromycin has been effective. Periodic monitoring of hospital water may be necessary to detect reemergence of the organism.

REFERENCES

CUNHA BA (ed): Legionnaire's disease. Semin Respir Infect 2:189, 1987

FANG GD et al: Disease due to the Legionellaceae (other than *Legionella pneumophila*). Historical, microbiological, clinical, and epidemiologic review. Medicine (Baltimore) 68:116, 1989

FRASER DW et al: Legionnaire's disease. Description of an epidemic of pneumonia. N Engl J Med 297:1189, 1977

MUDER RR et al: Mode of transmission of *Legionella pneumophila*. A critical review. Arch Intern Med 146:1607, 1986

TOMPKINS LS et al: Legionella prosthetic-valve endocarditis. N Engl J Med 318:530, 1988

WINN WC JR: Legionnaire's disease: Historical perspective. Clin Microbiol Rev 1:60, 1988

section 6 Mycobacterial diseases

125 TUBERCULOSIS

THOMAS M. DANIEL

DEFINITION Tuberculosis is a chronic bacterial infection caused by *Mycobacterium tuberculosis* that is characterized by the formation of granulomas in infected tissues and by cell-mediated hypersensitivity. The usual site of disease is the lungs, but other organs may be involved. In the absence of effective treatment for active disease, a chronic wasting course is usual and death ultimately supervenes. Most cases of tuberculous infection are asymptomatic.

ETIOLOGY *Mycobacterium tuberculosis,* the tubercle bacillus, is one of more than 30 well-characterized and many unclassified members of the genus *Mycobacterium.* Along with the closely related *M. bovis,* it causes tuberculosis. *M. leprae* is the etiologic agent of leprosy (see Chap. 126), and a number of other mycobacterial species produce less common human diseases (see Chap. 127). Most mycobacteria are not pathogenic for humans, and many are readily isolated from environmental sources.

Mycobacteria are distinguished by their surface lipids which render them acid-fast so that they cannot be decolorized with acid alcohol after staining. Because of this lipid, heat or detergents are usually necessary to accomplish primary staining.

Important to understanding the pathogenesis of tuberculosis is recognition that *M. tuberculosis* contains many immunoreactive substances. Surface lipids of mycobacteria and water-soluble components of cell wall peptidoglycan are important adjuvants that may exert their effects through their primary actions on host macrophages. *M. tuberculosis* survives the intracellular milieu of macrophages, and this intracellular persistence may be facilitated by cell wall lipids which inhibit phagosome-lysosome fusion. Mycobacteria contain an array of protein and polysaccharide antigens, some probably species-specific but others clearly sharing epitopes broadly throughout the genus. Cell-mediated hypersensitivity is characteristic of tuberculosis and is an important determinant of the disease's pathogenesis.

EPIDEMIOLOGY Tuberculosis has been disappearing rapidly from Europe and North America, but in the rest of the world it continues as an important cause of death. In 1986, a total of 22,768 cases of tuberculosis were reported in the United States, a case rate of 9.4 per 100,000 per year. The case rate had been falling at a rate of 5 to 6 percent per year, but since 1985 this trend has been interrupted by AIDS. It is estimated that 10,000,000 Americans have a positive tuberculin test but that fewer than 1 percent of American children are tuberculin reactors. Tuberculosis in North America tends to be a disease of the elderly, the urban poor, of minority groups, and of patients with AIDS. At all ages case rates among nonwhites tend to be twice those in whites. Hispanic, Haitian, and southeast Asian immigrants may have case rates as high as those of the countries from which they come, and in these individuals the frequency of disease among younger persons reflects its occurrence in those countries. Increasingly, tuberculosis in the United States is being seen in microepidemics, often centered in families.

Because in the United States tuberculosis has become a disease of the elderly, it is frequently seen in nursing homes. Although transmission of infection can occur at any age, most disease in older persons represents a legacy of previous times. The elderly of today were children when transmission of tubercle bacilli occurred much more frequently. Of those who were infected, many developed disease in young adulthood. Some, especially males, did not and are only now developing reactivation disease in their late years. However, an increasing portion of elderly persons has never been infected, and have acquired nosocomial new infections in nursing homes.

In much of the world transmission of tuberculous infection is declining, but in many impoverished nations this is not true. In some countries estimated new case rates are as high as 400 per 100,000 per year. As in North America and Europe, poverty and tuberculosis go hand in hand. In high-prevalence areas, tuberculosis is seen with equal prevalence in rural and urban settings, and afflicts chiefly young adults. In countries where human immunodeficiency virus (HIV) infection is endemic, tuberculosis is a frequent cause of morbidity in AIDS patients. A reasonable estimate of the magnitude of tuberculosis in the world is that half of the population of the world is infected with *M. tuberculosis,* that there are 30 million cases of active tuberculosis in the world, that 10 million new cases occur annually, and that 3 million die of tuberculosis each year. Tuberculosis probably causes 6 percent of all deaths worldwide.

TRANSMISSION *M. tuberculosis* is transmitted from person to person via the respiratory route. Although other routes of transmission are possible and have been documented on occasion, none is of major importance. Tubercle bacilli in respiratory secretions form nuclei for water droplets expelled during coughing, sneezing, and vocalizing. Small droplets evaporate within a short distance from the mouth, and thereafter desiccated bacilli remain airborne for long periods. Infection of a susceptible host occurs when a few of these bacilli are inhaled. The number of bacilli excreted by most infected persons is not large; typically, household contact of many months is required for transmission. However, laryngeal tuberculosis, endobronchial disease, recent transbronchial spread of tuberculosis, and extensive cavitary pulmonary disease are often highly contagious. Infectiousness correlates with the number of organisms in the expectorated sputum, extent of pulmonary disease, and frequency of cough. Mycobacteria are susceptible to ultraviolet irradiation, and outdoor transmission of infection rarely occurs in daylight. Adequate ventilation is the most important measure to reduce the infectiousness of the environment. Fomites are not important in the transmission of tuberculosis. Most patients become noninfectious within 2 weeks after the institution of appropriate chemotherapy because of a decrease in the number of organisms excreted and a decrease in cough.

Transmission of infection with *M. bovis* has long been associated with the consumption of contaminated cow's milk. This organism is no longer a major cause of human disease in most of the world.

PATHOGENESIS The initial entry of tubercle bacilli into the lungs or other site of a previously uninfected individual elicits a nonspecific acute inflammatory response which is rarely noted and is usually accompanied by few or no symptoms. Bacilli are then ingested by macrophages and transported to the regional lymph nodes. If spread of the organism is not contained at the level of regional lymph nodes, then tubercle bacilli reach the bloodstream and widespread dissemination ensues. Most lesions of disseminated tuberculosis heal, as do most primary pulmonary lesions, although they remain potential foci of later reactivation. Dissemination may result in miliary or meningeal tuberculosis—illnesses with potential for major morbidity and mortality, especially in infants and young children.

During the 2 to 8 weeks after primary infection, while bacilli continue to multiply in their intracellular environment, cell-mediated hypersensitivity develops in the infected host. Immunologically competent lymphocytes enter areas of infection, where they elaborate chemotactic factors, interleukins, and lymphokines. In response, monocytes enter the area and undergo transformation into macrophages and subsequently into specialized histiocytic cells which are organized into granulomas. Mycobacteria may persist within macrophages for many years despite increased lysozyme production within these cells, but their further multiplication and spread are usually confined. Healing then occurs, often with late calcification of the granulomas, sometimes leaving a residual lesion visible on chest radiograph. The combination of a calcified peripheral lung lesion and calcified hilar lymph node is known as a Ghon complex.

In the United States, 95 percent of individuals undergo complete healing of primary tuberculous lesions with no subsequent evidence of disease. In other populations, where infective inocula may be higher and where nutritional status and other host factors may be less propitious, failure of complete healing may occur in more than 5 percent of individuals. Famine and many intercurrent diseases adversely affect healing and threaten the stability of healed tuberculous lesions.

Tuberculosis—the clinical disease—develops in the minority who do not successfully contain their primary infections. In some individuals tuberculosis develops within weeks after primary infection; in most, organisms lie dormant for many years before entering a phase of exponential multiplication leading to disease. Among many, age can be identified as a significant factor determining the course of tuberculosis. In infants tuberculous infection frequently progresses rapidly to disease, and the risk of disseminated disease including meningitis and miliary tuberculosis is high. In children older than 1 or 2 years up to about the age of puberty, primary tuberculous lesions almost always heal; most of those destined to develop tuberculosis do so during adolescence or young adulthood. Individuals infected in adulthood are at greatest risk of developing tuberculosis within approximately 3 years following infection. Tuberculous disease is more common in young adult women, whereas it is more common in men later in life.

IMMUNOLOGY **Immunity** Humans display native immunity to tuberculosis, with substantial individual variation. Twin studies have demonstrated that tuberculosis is more likely to occur in both members of monozygotic sibships than in dizygotic sibships or other family relationships. Attempts to link susceptibility to tuberculosis to HLA phenotype have produced conflicting data. Although susceptibility to tuberculosis has been associated with race, the evidence is largely anecdotal and is not convincing. As noted, age is an important determinant of native immunity to tuberculosis. Although specific data on nutrition and tuberculosis immunity are lacking, the association of tuberculosis with famine is clear.

Acquired immunity follows primary tuberculous infection. Disease due to exogenous reinfection is probably rare in North America and Europe; it may be more frequent in populations of high prevalence where risk of repeated exposure is great. It is useful to recall that *immunity* in the classic use of the word refers to resistance to infection, whereas *hypersensitivity* describes a state of altered host reactivity. In this sense, immunity may also result from vaccination with bacillus Calmette-Guérin (BCG) or from infection with other species of mycobacteria.

Antigen-specific immunity is T-lymphocyte-dependent and can be transferred adoptively with lymphocytes. It closely parallels cutaneous-type delayed hypersensitivity in its development.

Tuberculin hypersensitivity Tuberculin hypersensitivity is antigen-specific in nature and follows primary infection. It is chiefly or perhaps entirely directed against protein antigens. It is mediated by T lymphocytes through secretion of lymphokines which act upon effector monocytes.

Mycobacterial antigens have been subjected to extensive immunochemical study. It is clear that there is no single dominant antigen, and that infected and artificially sensitized hosts develop hypersensitivity to an array of mycobacterial proteins. Tuberculin purified protein derivative (PPD), the antigen preparation most frequently employed clinically and epidemiologically to demonstrate tuberculin hypersensitivity, is a crude mixture of largely denatured antigens and is a poor representative of native antigens. Nevertheless, its use has yielded much information.

Antigen recognition by the sensitized host follows processing by macrophages and depends upon expression by the macrophage at its surface of antigen-specific epitopes in association with Ia antigen, a gene product of the major histocompatibility locus. This complex is recognized by specific T lymphocytes. Macrophage synthesis and secretion of interleukin 1 is also necessary for T-lymphocyte response to the presented antigen. Following antigen presentation, T-lymphocyte clonal expansion occurs. Specific subsets of T lymphocytes develop which have antigen-specific immunoregulatory functions and which modulate the immune response (see Chap. 13).

Immunoreactive lymphocytes secrete mediators, and in response macrophages become activated and serve as the principal effector cells of tuberculin hypersensitivity. Peripheral blood monocytes from tuberculous patients have been shown to have several features characteristic of activated macrophages, including increased hexose monophosphate shunt activity, augmented surface adhesiveness, expression of characteristic membrane structures, and increased bactericidal activity. Animal studies have demonstrated that these features are T-lymphocyte-dependent. Activated monocytes/macrophages are important immunoregulatory cells possessing suppressor functions.

In tuberculosis, aberrations of this carefully modulated state of hypersensitivity occur with some frequency and are recognizable in 15 percent of acutely ill patients. This has given rise to the suggestion that tuberculosis may present with an immunologic spectrum similar to that seen in leprosy but more subtly expressed. At one pole are patients with chronic cavitary disease, relatively chronic courses, and florid expression of tuberculin hypersensitivity. At the other pole are the less frequently seen patients with cutaneous anergy, a few of whom have absence of granuloma formation and all other manifestations of cellular hypersensitivity and have pancytopenia, widely disseminated disease, and a progressive downhill course. Although the delayed tuberculin skin reaction is the best known manifestation of tuberculin hypersensitivity (see below), granuloma formation is probably its central and most important expression because it is important in containing the spread of infection.

Production of antibodies to protein and polysaccharide antigens of mycobacteria is readily demonstrated in tuberculosis. There is no evidence that these antibodies play a role in immunity, hypersensitivity, or pathogenesis of tuberculosis.

CLINICAL MANIFESTATIONS **Primary tuberculosis** Primary tuberculous infection is usually asymptomatic. A nonspecific pneumonitis typically occurs in the lower or midlung zones. Hilar lymph node enlargement is usual and in children is sometimes sufficient to produce bronchial obstruction. In low-prevalence areas primary infection may not occur until adulthood. It may progress directly to clinical disease which has the pathologic features of reactivation disease. In these persons such perplexing presentations as subapical pneumonias are common.

Reactivation tuberculosis Reactivation tuberculosis is a chronic wasting disease, and in pulmonary tuberculosis constitutional manifestations are often more prominent than respiratory symptoms. Weight loss and low-grade fever are common. Many patients present with typical drenching night sweats over the upper half of the body several times a week.

Pulmonary tuberculosis Pulmonary tuberculosis has a predilection for the apical posterior segments of the upper lobes and the superior segments of the lower lobes of the lungs. The location has been attributed both to posture and to higher intraalveolar oxygen concentration in the uppermost portions of the lung. The extent of disease varies from minimal infiltrates that produce no clinical illness and that are barely discernible on chest radiographs to massive involvement with extensive cavitation and debilitating constitutional and respiratory symptoms. In the absence of effective therapy, pulmonary tuberculosis pursues a chronic and progressive course. There are often long periods of stability and relative well-being, but in most patients these give way to episodes of disease progression with involvement of increasing lung parenchyma.

The onset of pulmonary tuberculosis is usually insidious, and illness may not be noted by the patient for some time. However, it is incorrect to view this onset as one of slow progression. In fact, pulmonary tuberculosis usually reaches its full extent within a few weeks. About one-third of patients will live long lives with chronic illness interspersed with periods of relative well-being. However, the overall death rate of untreated pulmonary tuberculosis probably approaches 60 percent, and the median course to death is about 2½ years.

As pulmonary lesions progress, central necrosis occurs with development of caseation, so named because of the cheesy nature of necrotic material which only partly liquifies. Satellite lesions grow concomitantly. They can usually be recognized on chest x-ray films and are often helpful in distinguishing tuberculosis from pulmonary neoplasms. Necrotic material may empty into bronchi resulting in cavitation of the nodular disease. Other parts of the lung may be seeded transbronchially with the development of exudative lesions. In some patients tuberculous pneumonia develops in a lobar or segmental pulmonary distribution. Occasionally transbronchial spread following rupture of a tuberculous peribronchial lymph node into a bronchus leads to tuberculous pneumonia in the absence of other obvious disease. With the progression of pulmonary tuberculosis, the normal pulmonary architecture is lost. Fibrosis, volume loss, and upward contraction are typical. However, recently diseased areas may heal with relatively little destruction when effective chemotherapy is administered.

Pulmonary cavities may persist even though effective chemotherapy has resulted in apparent cure. In the absence of therapy, persistence of cavities is to be expected. Cavities may be a source of major hemoptysis, especially in the presence of continued active disease. Persistent terminal pulmonary arteries within cavities may be a source of profound bleeding (Rasmussen's aneurysm). Another cause of bleeding is an aspergilloma in a chronic tuberculous cavity, and bleeding in this instance may occur without persisting tuberculous disease. Rupture of a tuberculous cavity into the pleural space may lead to tuberculous empyema and bronchopleural fistula.

Chronic cough is the principal respiratory symptom. Sputum is usually scant and nonpurulent. Hemoptysis is frequent and is usually limited to blood streaking of the sputum. Massive, life-threatening hemoptysis is rare.

Findings on physical examination of the lung in patients with pulmonary tuberculosis are typically few and generally can be appreciated only in the presence of extensive disease. Rales which are accentuated or heard only posttussively are characteristic of apical disease. With extensive cavitation, amphoric breath sounds may be present. Dullness to percussion may sometimes be recognized in Krönig's isthmus and at the clavicles, reflecting extensive apical disease.

Extrapulmonary tuberculosis PLEURISY WITH EFFUSION Pleurisy with effusion results when the pleural space is seeded with *M. tuberculosis*. Following a peripheral primary infection, the pleural space may be contaminated by organisms that are transported lymphogenously to the pleura and hence across the surface of the lung to the hilum. Pleural effusion occurs, sometimes massively, usually with substantial pleuritic pain. The onset of symptoms is often abrupt. The effusion is most frequently, but not invariably, unilateral. Classically, tuberculous pleurisy with effusion occurs in younger individuals in the absence of pulmonary tuberculosis. However, in the United States this disease presents in many individuals past the age of 35 and simultaneous pulmonary tuberculosis is present in about one-third of patients. The effusion is exudative in nature, and a protein concentration greater than 3.0 g/dL is the most characteristic feature of the pleural fluid. Lymphocytes usually, but not invariably, predominate among the pleural fluid cells. Mesothelial cells are rare. Needle biopsy of the parietal pleura may reveal granulomas, confirming the diagnosis of tuberculous pleurisy. The tuberculin skin test is negative in one-third of patients, either because the disease presents early before tuberculin reactivity develops, or because this form of tuberculosis is particularly prone to aberrations of immunoregulation. Untreated, tuberculous pleurisy usually remits, but active pulmonary tuberculosis develops within 5 years in two-thirds of cases. Response to chemotherapy is good. Complete removal of pleural fluid is not necessary. There is rarely a need for surgical decortication.

Bronchopleural fistula and tuberculous empyema are catastrophic complications of untreated tuberculosis resulting from rupture of a pulmonary lesion into the pleural space. The diagnosis is usually not difficult, and acid-fast bacilli are usually readily demonstrated in the pleural exudate. Treatment consists of adequate surgical drainage and chemotherapy.

TUBERCULOUS PERICARDITIS AND PERITONITIS The pericardium and peritoneum may be the sites of tuberculosis. Pericarditis sometimes occurs in association with pleurisy and may represent an extension of that process. More commonly the pericardium is seeded by drainage from an infected lymph node. Exudative effusion occurs and patients present with fever and pericardial pain. A friction rub may be present. Cardiac tamponade occasionally occurs. Chronic constrictive pericarditis is a late sequel. The diagnosis of tuberculous pericarditis is often difficult and sometimes requires thoracotomy for pericardial biopsy.

Tuberculous peritonitis results from hematogenous seeding of the peritoneum or entry of bacilli from an abdominal lymphatic or genitourinary organ source. As with other serositis, an exudative effusion occurs. The onset is usually insidious, and the disease is often mistaken for hepatic cirrhosis in alcoholic patients. As with tuberculous pericarditis, the diagnosis is often difficult, and recovery of the organism from paracentesis fluid is possible only in a minority of cases. Surgical biopsy may be necessary for diagnosis.

LARYNGEAL AND ENDOBRONCHIAL TUBERCULOSIS Tuberculosis of the larynx is usually seen in association with far-advanced pulmonary disease. Occasionally it occurs with only minimal pulmonary involvement. It results from seeding of the mucosal surface during expectoration. The disease progresses from a superficial laryngitis to ulceration and granuloma formation. The epiglottis and hypopharynx are occasionally involved. Hoarseness is the principal symptom of tuberculous laryngitis. In a similar fashion the bronchial mucosa may be seeded, causing tuberculous bronchitis. Indeed, localized bronchitis in segmental bronchi leading to diseased portions of lung is common. Cough and minor hemoptysis are the chief clinical manifestations. Patients with tuberculous laryngitis and extensive bronchitis are usually highly infectious. These forms of disease respond rapidly to chemotherapy and have a favorable prognosis with treatment.

TUBERCULOUS ADENITIS Scrofula is chronic tuberculous lymphadenitis of the cervical lymph nodes. Any of the cervical nodes may be involved, but those high in the neck just below the mandible are the most frequent site of disease. Tuberculous nodes are usually rubbery and not tender. With progression, they become harder and matted. Chronic draining fistulas may develop, but these are rare, and the course of this form of tuberculosis is usually indolent. The diagnosis is commonly established by surgical biopsy. Lymph node biopsy specimens obtained for this purpose should always be submitted for culture as well as histologic examination, and chemotherapy should be instituted at or before the time of surgery to avoid postoperative fistulas in the surgical wound site. Lymph nodes other than those in the cervical regions are less commonly involved in tuberculosis and account for about 35 percent of tuberculous adenitis.

In children, *M. scrofulaceum* and *M. intracellulare* are frequently the cause of scrofula. The onset of this disease is usually before 5 years of age. As with tuberculosis, lymph nodes high in the neck are most frequently involved. A single enlarged node is commonly the presenting manifestation. Constitutional symptoms are absent, and the adenitis usually is not tender. Progression is common, with necrosis of the node and the development of fistulous sinus tracts. The organisms involved are usually not susceptible to drugs, and treatment, if necessary, is surgical excision. Spontaneous resolution is usual after puberty.

SKELETAL TUBERCULOSIS Bone and joint disease is a not infrequent manifestation of tuberculosis. Pott's disease, tuberculosis of the spine, usually involves the midthoracic spine. Tubercle bacilli reach the spine hematogenously or through lymphatic channels from the pleural space to paravertebral lymph nodes. Anterior erosion of vertebral bodies leads to collapse. The result is a sharply angulated kyphosis without scoliosis (gibbus deformity). Paraplegia may result. If there is no neurologic compromise, Pott's disease can be treated with chemotherapy. If the spine is unstable, surgical stabilization may be necessary. In the face of new paraparesis, immediate orthopedic consultation should be obtained. Paravertebral "cold abcesses" are a frequent concomitant of tuberculous spondylitis. They usually do not need to be drained, if adequate chemotherapy is given, unless they are very large. They may extend along fascial planes and point in the inguinal region or in other remote sites.

Tuberculosis of joints most frequently affects large weight-bearing joints such as the hips and knees. It responds well to immobilization and chemotherapy. Tuberculous synovitis may occur alone or in association with tuberculous arthritis.

GENITOURINARY TUBERCULOSIS Genitourinary tuberculosis may involve any part of either the male or female genitourinary system. Renal tuberculosis usually presents initially as microscopic pyuria and hematuria with a sterile urine culture. The diagnosis may be established by finding tubercle bacilli on culture of the urine. As the disease progresses, cavitation of the renal parenchyma occurs. In the past, nephrectomy was often performed for renal tuberculosis. However, with adequate chemotherapy surgical removal of a kidney is almost never necessary. The ureters and bladder may be infected by tubular spread of the organism, and ureteral stricture may result.

Tuberculous salpingitis often results in female sterility. Genital tuberculosis in the male most commonly involves the prostate, seminal vesicles, and epididymis. Prostatic and epididymal tuberculosis are characterized by nontender nodular induration detectable by physical examination. The presentation of genital tuberculosis in both males and females is insidious, with chronic or subacute symptoms. The diagnosis is usually made by culture of acid-fast bacilli.

MENINGEAL TUBERCULOSIS The leptomeninges are relatively frequently seeded by organisms which disseminate during primary infection. In young children, tuberculous meningitis may develop at this time. This chronic infection is manifested not only by meningeal signs but also frequently by cranial nerve signs, reflecting a tendency for basilar distribution of the infection. High protein content, low glucose, and lymphocytosis are characteristic of the cerebrospinal fluid. Prior to the advent of effective chemotherapy, this disease was almost always fatal. Chemotherapy with isoniazid, rifampin, and ethambutol is effective. Intrathecal drug administration is not necessary. Late reactivation of meningeal tuberculous foci may produce disease in adults who have no evidence of pulmonary tuberculosis. Tuberculomas of the meninges or brain may become evident in adult life many years after primary infection, and seizures are often their major clinical manifestation.

OCULAR TUBERCULOSIS Tuberculosis may involve almost any part of the eye. Chorioretinitis and uveitis are the most common manifestations. The diagnosis of tuberculosis of the eye is extremely difficult to establish, and most diagnoses are presumptive. The manifestations cannot be distinguished clinically from sarcoidosis or systemic mycoses, but phlyctenular keratitis strongly suggests tuberculosis. Phlyctenular lesions are thought to represent manifestations of tuberculin hypersensitivity rather than bacterial infection. Choroid tubercles are often present in patients with miliary tuberculosis, and their recognition may be helpful in the diagnosis of miliary tuberculosis. Ocular tuberculosis responds well to standard chemotherapeutic agents.

GASTROINTESTINAL TUBERCULOSIS The stomach is extremely resistant to tuberculous infection, and a large number of virulent tubercle bacilli can be swallowed without establishing an infection. Rarely, usually concomitantly with extensive cavitary pulmonary disease and severe debility, swallowed organisms reach the terminal ileum and cecum and tuberculous ileitis develops. Chronic diarrhea and fistula development are the principal manifestations, and the disease is difficult to distinguish from Crohn's disease. Tuberculosis of the liver can occur as an isolated event, but it is usually a manifestation of miliary tuberculosis.

ADRENAL TUBERCULOSIS Hematogenous seeding of the adrenal gland is probably fairly common, but disease due to this infection is rare and usually seen only in association with long-standing and extensive pulmonary tuberculosis. The cortex is most frequently involved and adrenal insufficiency may result. In contrast, carcinomatous involvement of the adrenal cortex, even though very extensive, rarely produces clinical adrenal insufficiency.

CUTANEOUS TUBERCULOSIS Tuberculous infection of the skin is rare in the absence of long-standing, untreated disease elsewhere. Lupus vulgaris is a granulomatous disease of the skin, and it responds well to treatment. Diagnosis is made by skin biopsy. Tuberculin hypersensitivity manifestations are common. Erythema nodosum may be present, although it much more commonly results from other granulomatous diseases including sarcoidosis and systemic mycoses. Tuberculids are poorly understood papular lesions of tuberculin hypersensitivity.

MILIARY TUBERCULOSIS Miliary tuberculosis results from widespread hematogenous dissemination. It often presents as a perplexing fever, sometimes with a double quotidian curve, often accompanied by anemia and splenomegaly. Miliary tuberculosis is apt to be more fulminating in children than in adults.

Classically, miliary tuberculosis develops following hematogenous dissemination at the time of primary infection, and patients present no antecedent history of tuberculosis. Lesions develop synchronously throughout the body. Patients become ill before radiographic changes, which take 4 to 6 weeks to become recognizable, appear. The typical radiologic findings are soft, uniformly distributed, fine nodules throughout both lung fields. They often can be recognized first on a lateral chest film or an underpenetrated anteroposterior radiograph. The diagnosis is difficult, and expectorated sputum rarely contains organisms. Transbronchial biopsy and liver biopsy are usually but not invariably positive. Bone marrow biopsy is positive in approximately two-thirds of patients.

When hematogenous dissemination occurs in a previously diseased individual, a much more fulminant course results. Prostration is common. Diffuse but ragged nodular infiltrates develop within a few weeks, and the sputum is often positive. The diagnosis is rarely difficult.

The subacute form and the rare chronic form of miliary tuberculosis often present major problems in diagnosis. This type of disease is usually attributed to repeated seeding of the blood stream from a tuberculous focus. A very rare form of disseminated tuberculosis occurs with widespread dissemination of disease, a massive number of bacteria in tissues, complete absence of granuloma formation, and pancytopenia. It is termed disseminated nonreactive tuberculosis and has a poor prognosis, even with chemotherapy.

Tuberculin anergy is common in miliary tuberculosis, and a negative skin test should not be a deterrent to considering this diagnosis. Anergy may or may not extend to other delayed hypersensitivity antigens. In vitro cultured leukocyte studies also demonstrate hyporesponsiveness, suggesting that this anergy is mediated by monocytes with suppressor function. With treatment and stabilization of patients with miliary tuberculosis, tuberculin hypersensitivity is restored.

Without treatment, the prognosis for miliary tuberculosis is grave. This disease responds well to chemotherapy, however, and can be treated with the same drug regimens employed for other forms of tuberculosis.

SILICOTUBERCULOSIS Tuberculosis occurs with increased frequency in patients with silicosis and possibly in patients with some other pneumoconioses. The diagnosis is often difficult because of confounding radiographic changes due to the underlying pneumoconiosis. Even with therapy, the prognosis is less favorable than in other patients. Patients with silicotuberculosis should be treated for longer than customary periods. Patients with silicosis who are tuberculin-positive should be considered for isoniazid prophylaxis even when they do not meet other criteria for this form of therapy. Isoniazid prophylaxis may be less effective in persons with silicosis.

TUBERCULOSIS IN AIDS Tuberculosis occurs in more than 50 percent of individuals previously infected with *M. tuberculosis* who subsequently become infected with HIV. It usually precedes the development of other opportunistic infections associated with AIDS by about 3 months. In central Africa and Haiti, 30 to 50 percent of tuberculosis patients are HIV seropositive; only about one-third of these patients have other opportunistic infections associated with AIDS. In the United States, tuberculosis is most frequently seen in AIDS patients who are intravenous drug users or who are immigrants from Haiti or central Africa. Nearly half of AIDS patients with tuberculosis have extrapulmonary forms of the disease, with tuberculous lymphadenitis predominating. Among AIDS patients with pulmonary tuberculosis, nearly half have atypical roentgenographic findings, with diffuse infiltration. Mycobacterial infections other than tuberculosis are frequently seen in patients with AIDS. In the United States approximately half of AIDS patients develop disseminated disease due to *M. avium-intracellulare*, usually late in the course of AIDS (see Chap. 127).

DIAGNOSIS Bacteriology The diagnosis of tuberculosis is established when tubercle bacilli are identified in the sputum, urine, body fluids, or tissues of the patient. For the majority of patients who have pulmonary tuberculosis, the diagnosis can be most readily established by sputum examination. The staining characteristics of *M. tuberculosis* allow its ready identification in clinical specimens, although it is usually present in small numbers so that prolonged study of stained slides is necessary. A slender (less than 0.5 μm diameter), curved, often polychromatically beaded rod, it frequently presents in clinical specimens as pairs or clumps of a few organisms lying side by side. When stained with fluorescent auramine-rhodamine, tubercle bacilli can be seen under usual high-dry (100×) magnification. A more definitive stain consists of carbol fuchsin; this stain requires meticulous scanning with oil immersion (1000×) microscopy. Sputum culture adds to the diagnostic yield and also permits the specific identification of acid-fast bacilli and the determination of drug susceptibility. Primary isolation from clinical specimens usually requires 4 to 8 weeks on classical media. Radiometric techniques using highly selective media allow cultivation in 1 or 2 weeks, but confirmation of the identity of an isolated organism may require additional time. Mycobacteria are aerobes. Modern culture techniques are excellent, and there is no longer reason to inoculate guinea pigs for primary isolation. Niacin production characterizes *M. tuberculosis* and helps to distinguish it from other species. Nucleic acid hybridization probes have been developed for the rapid identification of mycobacteria in cultures. Probes for direct use with clinical specimens are under investigation.

If expectorated sputum is not readily available for examination, expectoration may be induced or samples obtained by nasotracheal aspiration. Early morning gastric aspiration provides excellent material for culture and for smear examination. Although nonpathogenic mycobacteria are occasionally found in gastric aspirates, their number is so small as to preclude their appearance in smears of gastric aspirates. Bronchoscopy has a high yield in the diagnosis of tuberculosis, but in the absence of other considerations it should not be undertaken unless multiple attempts by simpler means have failed and the diagnosis remains obscure.

The diagnostic yield of sputum smear and culture is directly related to the extent of pulmonary disease. About one-third of patients in whom a positive sputum culture can be obtained will have acid-fast bacilli identified on an initial sputum smear. With repeated examinations on separate days, this figure rises to about two-thirds. There is rarely an indication for obtaining more than five sputum examinations. However, only about one-third of patients with minimal pulmonary tuberculosis will have a positive sputum smear, even after multiple examinations. If there is no lesion visible on the chest radiograph, then there is usually little reason to obtain sputum examinations for tubercle bacilli. Conversely, if a patient with extensive cavitary disease or an exudative pneumonic process has a negative sputum smear, diagnoses other than tuberculosis should be sought.

Serology Serologic tests for the diagnosis of tuberculosis remain experimental and are not routinely available. The most specific serologic tests have used highly purified antigens. Enzyme-linked immunosorbent assay (ELISA) techniques offer the potential for readily applied serologic tests for tuberculosis, and should have great value in the diagnosis of tuberculosis in children and in extrapulmonary disease where sputum is not available.

Radiology The chest x-ray is an important tool for both the diagnosis and evaluation of tuberculosis. Healed primary lesions may leave a small peripheral nodule which may calcify with the passing of years. The Ghon complex comprises a calcified peripheral nodule together with a calcified hilar lymph node. Similar lesions result from histoplasmosis, and it is not possible to distinguish between healed primary lesions of these two diseases radiologically. Calcification of right paratracheal lymph nodes is more commonly seen in histoplasmosis.

Multinodular infiltration in the apical posterior segments of the upper lobes and superior segments of the lower lobes is the most typical lesion of pulmonary tuberculosis. Cavitation is frequently present and is usually accompanied by substantial amounts of infiltration in the same pulmonary segments. Laminagrams are often helpful in recognizing satellite nodular lesions, which are characteristic of tuberculosis and not usually seen in carcinoma. Lordotic views may be of help in evaluating disease obscured by the intersection of the third or fourth posterior rib, second anterior rib, and clavicle. They are of little use in evaluating disease located elsewhere. As tuberculosis becomes inactive or heals, fibrotic scarring becomes apparent on the chest radiograph. There is frequently volume loss in the involved upper lobes, and upward and medial retraction of hilar markings is common. Fibrotic lesions may develop calcifications. The activity of tuberculosis may be judged from serial films. It is never wise to judge tuberculosis to be inactive on the basis of a single chest film.

Clinical pathology Other than bacteriologic examinations, clinical laboratory tests contribute relatively little to the diagnosis of tuberculosis. Peripheral blood monocytosis in the range of 8 to 12 percent is common. The erythrocyte sedimentation rate is usually elevated, and modest anemia may be present.

Tuberculin test The intracutaneous tuberculin skin test is a reliable means of recognizing prior mycobacterial infection. The preferred antigen is tuberculin purified protein derivative (PPD) and the intermediate-strength dose should be used. In North America this is 5 tuberculin units of material which is standardized by bioassay (bioequivalent) against reference antigen designated PPD-S. In other parts of the world, PPD lot RT-23, prepared in Denmark and widely distributed by the World Health Organization, is available. A gravimetric unit has been assigned to this material, and 2 units of this PPD are equivalent to 5 units of PPD-S. Diluents for PPD should contain polysorbate 80, which decreases loss of potency due to adsorption onto glass and plastic surfaces. Multiple puncture devices offer much convenience, but do so at the cost of decreased specificity. They can be recommended only as screening tests, and positive tests should be repeated using intracutaneous PPD.

The tuberculin test is usually applied on the forearm. Reactions should be read by measuring the transverse diameter of induration as detected by gentle palpation at 48 to 72 h. Patients with tuberculosis have normally distributed reaction sizes with the mean and mode at 17 mm. Infected but healthy, nondiseased individuals have similarly distributed reactions. Hence, a reaction to PPD is presumptive evidence of prior mycobacterial infection.

Tuberculin hypersensitivity may result from contact with nonpathogenic, environmental mycobacteria, and this nonspecific reactivity may confound the interpretation of tuberculin tests. Nonspecific tuberculin reactivity is rarely found in northern climates, and in such areas all reactivity to PPD can be considered to reflect infection with *M. tuberculosis*. In many warm and humid climatic zones, including all of the coastal areas of the southeastern United States, nonspecific tuberculin reactivity is common. In such regions it is customary to consider reactions smaller than 10 mm as not significant and attribute them to cross reactivity with environmental mycobacterial antigens. However, considering smaller reactions as not significant always incurs the risk of missing some reactions which bespeak infection with *M. tuberculosis*.

Repeated skin testing may boost reaction size, whether the primary reactivity was directed to *M. tuberculosis* or was nonspecific. Caution must be used in attributing a small increase in reactivity to new infection. It is well-established, however, that repeated skin testing with PPD does not lead to positive reactions in uninfected persons. Positive reactions do not occur as a result of allergy to components of the diluent. Tuberculin reactivity wanes with advancing age, and the booster phenomenon may be useful in this situation. For example, if an older person fails to react to initial testing, repeat testing with intermediate strength PPD may be done after 7 to 10 days. A reaction at this time should be accepted as significant.

PPD is also available in a second strength which contains 50 times the amount of PPD in intermediate-strength material. Except as a test for anergy, this product has little use. Because PPD at this strength so readily elicits nonspecific reactivity, a positive reaction to second-strength PPD is much more apt to give misinformation than to contribute to the correct diagnosis. A first-strength PPD is also available. It contains one-fifth the amount of PPD of intermediate PPD but is not useful clinically.

Anergy is the paradoxical absence of dermal tuberculin reactivity in infected persons. It occurs in association with a number of disease states and in immunosuppressed individuals. It also occurs in as many as 15 percent of tuberculous patients with newly active pulmonary disease. In these persons tuberculin reactivity reappears with stabilization of the disease process. One-half of patients with miliary tuberculosis and one-third of patients with newly diagnosed tuberculous pleurisy have negative tuberculin tests. It has become common practice in many medical centers to use a battery of delayed hypersensitivity antigens to serve as controls for tuberculin tests in demonstrating anergy. However, antigens standardized for this purpose are not available, and tuberculin anergy may be antigen-specific. False-negative tuberculin tests may result from technical errors including subcutaneous injection, use of outdated PPD, and permitting PPD to remain in syringes before use. Such errors should not be mistaken for anergy.

TREATMENT The modern treatment of tuberculosis is based on the administration of effective drugs. In the presence of adequate chemotherapy, hospitalization, rest, and improved diet do not contribute to achieving cures. In order to prevent the emergence of drug-resistant mutants which are present initially in very small numbers, two effective drugs are always required. Because of the slow generation time of mycobacteria and their long periods of metabolic inactivity, prolonged courses of drug therapy are always necessary. Treatment regimens do not differ for pulmonary and extrapulmonary tuberculosis.

Table 125-1 presents dosage and toxicity information on drugs currently in use for the treatment of tuberculosis. Table 125-2 describes several effective treatment regimens. Daily therapy with isoniazid and rifampin for 9 to 12 months represents the most effective regimen available and is capable of achieving a favorable outcome in 99 percent of patients. Many experts add ethambutol initially until the results of sensitivity tests become available. Daily therapy with isoniazid and ethambutol for 18 months is 90 to 95 percent effective, and is probably equal to isoniazid and rifampin in patients with minimal disease. In developing countries where drug costs are a limiting factor, the extremely low-cost combination of isoniazid and thioacetazone for 12 to 18 months provides a regimen which can achieve 80 to 90 percent cure rates.

An accepted hypothesis states that tubercle bacilli exist in tuberculous patients in three pools—a metabolically active extracellular pool and relatively metabolically inactive intracellular and necrotic caseum pools. Only rifampin is bactericidal for all of these pools, and it may not be necessary to continue rifampin-containing regimens for as long as other regimens which rely upon organisms entering the metabolically active pool to achieve sterilization. Isoniazid and streptomycin are both bactericidal against extracellular, metabolically active organisms. Against intracellular organisms, isoniazid and pyrazinamide are bactericidal and streptomycin is inactive. In clinical trials, pyrazinamide has been found to be particularly useful during the first 2 months of treatment. Ethambutol is only bacteriostatic.

TABLE 125-1 Drugs used in the treatment of tuberculosis

Drug	Usual daily adult dose	Major toxicity
Isoniazid	300 mg	Hepatitis, peripheral neuropathy, drug fever
Rifampin	600 mg	Hepatitis, influenza-like syndrome, thrombocytopenia (rare)
Streptomycin	0.75–1 g	Deafness, loss of vestibular function, loss of renal function
Pyrazinamide	1.5–2 g	Hepatitis, hyperuricemia
Ethambutol	15 mg/kg	Optic neuritis (extremely rare at this dose)
p-Aminosalicylic acid	12 g	Diarrhea, hepatitis, hypersensitivity reactions
Ethionamide	1 g	Hepatitis
Cycloserine	1 g	Depression, personality changes, psychosis, convulsions
Thioacetazone	150 mg	Exfoliative dermatitis, hepatitis
Kanamycin	1 g	Deafness, loss of renal function, loss of vestibular function (rare)
Capreomycin	1 g	Deafness, loss of vestibular function, loss of renal function
Viomycin	1 g	Deafness, loss of vestibular function, loss of renal function

TABLE 125-2 Effective drug regimens for the treatment of tuberculosis

Regimen (adult drug dose)	Comment
Isoniazid (300 mg) and rifampin (600 mg) daily for 9–12 months	The usual regimen for initial treatment of all patients unless drug resistance is suspected, in which case ethambutol 15 mg/kg should be added.
Isoniazid (300 mg) and ethambutol (15 mg/kg) daily for 12–18 months	The least toxic effective regimen. Suitable for patients with minimal disease. The regimen of choice in pregnant women.
Isoniazid (300 mg) and thioacetazone (150 mg) daily for 12–18 months	The least expensive effective regimen. Streptomycin (0.75–1 g) may be added daily for the first 8 weeks to increase effectiveness, but this doubles both cost and toxicity.
Isoniazid (300 mg), rifampin (600 mg), pyrazinamide (2 g), and streptomycin (1 g) or ethambutol (15 mg/kg) daily for 2 months followed by one of the following:	Initial intensive phase for short course regimens. Short course regimens have only been demonstrated to be effective under conditions of close patient supervision.
a Isoniazid (300 mg) and rifampin (600 gm) daily for 4 months	
b Isoniazid (300 mg) and thioacetazone (150 mg) daily for 6 months	Inexpensive.
c Isoniazid (300 mg), rifampin (600 mg), and streptomycin (1 g) twice weekly for 6 months	Suitable for fully supervised therapy.
Isoniazid (300 mg) and rifampin (600 mg) daily for 1 month followed by isoniazid (900 mg) and rifampin (600 mg) twice weekly for 8 months	Effectiveness demonstrated in ambulatory treatment programs in Arkansas. Has not been compared with other regimens in clinical trials.

The major problem in tuberculosis treatment programs is patient default. It is unusual for a tuberculosis clinic to achieve a default rate of less than 15 percent, and default rates of 40 to 60 percent are common. Unfortunately, these rates tend to be highest in those parts of the world where high tuberculosis prevalence is coupled with limited resources. Default not only leads to treatment failure but also to the emergence and transmission of drug-resistant organisms. Since most patient defaults occur within the first 6 months of the treatment program, short-course therapy has been employed to mitigate the consequences of default. This strategy will be successful only if the resources conserved by shortening treatment are used to maintain patient compliance. Completely supervised regimens are successful for noncompliant patients, but their widespread use is costly. Twice weekly drug administration is effective and facilitates patient supervision.

Short-course treatment programs are best considered as consisting of two phases. An initial 2-month intensive phase of daily therapy should include isoniazid, rifampin, pyrazinamide, and either streptomycin or ethambutol. A consolidation phase of daily therapy with isoniazid and one other drug should be given for at least 4 months, and preferably 6 months. In the United States, a regimen of isoniazid 300 mg and rifampin 600 mg daily for 1 month, followed by isoniazid 900 mg and rifampin 600 mg twice weekly for 8 months has been highly effective. Patients with AIDS should be treated in the same manner as immunocompetent individuals with tuberculosis. Response to therapy is favorable in these patients, although they have more frequent drug reactions, particularly skin rashes. The optimum duration of therapy for these patients is not known, although it is probably wise to avoid short-course regimens. AIDS patients should be followed for relapse after therapy for the rest of their lives.

Relapses after successful therapy should be less than 1 percent. Since these few relapses usually present with symptoms and are almost never found by routine x-rays, patients may be discharged from follow-up at the completion of therapy. Relapses are more frequent after short-course therapy, usually occurring within the first year, and follow-up for such patients for 1 or 2 years is justified.

Symptomatic improvement occurs within the first 2 to 3 weeks in most patients. Clearing of infiltrates on the chest radiograph may not occur within the first month but usually is readily recognized between the second and fourth months. Most patients reach a point of radiologic stability between 3 and 6 months. Therapy should be continued for 6 months after this point of stability is reached, even if this means prolonging the planned period of treatment. Sputum conversion occurs in most patients within the first 2 months. The fact that an individual patient responds more slowly than the norm should not necessarily be a cause for concern, provided the patient is taking effective drugs.

Since there are alternative effective drug regimens, toxicity becomes a factor in choice of therapy. Major individual drug toxicities are listed in Table 125-1; the toxicity of greatest concern is hepatitis. Toxicity sufficient to require change in regimen occurs in 3 to 5 percent of patients taking isoniazid and rifampin and in about 1.5 percent of patients taking isoniazid and ethambutol. The toxicity of isoniazid and thioacetazone appears to vary with the racial characteristics of the patient population. It reaches about 30 percent in oriental groups but is only 2 to 5 percent in other populations. Routine monitoring of serum enzymes or other blood tests reflecting liver disease is of little use and is not recommended. Normal values do not predict absence of toxicity, and serum enzymes in patients taking isoniazid may rise transiently to three times normal values without the subsequent development of hepatitis. A well-educated patient and an alert treatment supervisor are the principal safeguards against drug hepatitis. If medication is discontinued during the prodromal phase or promptly with the onset of jaundice, drug hepatitis can be expected to resolve without untoward incident. Isoniazid toxicity is probably due to toxic metabolites of acetyl isoniazid. Induction of cytochrome P_{450} enzymes by alcohol or long-acting barbiturates predisposes to isoniazid hepatitis. Isoniazid also causes a peripheral neuropathy which is preventable and reversible by the administration of pyridoxine. Patients with such predisposing factors as old age, diabetes, alcoholism, and malnutrition should be given pyridoxine concomitantly with isoniazid; the usual dose is 50 mg/d.

Isoniazid is safe in pregnant patients. Data are less complete for other drugs but suggest that ethambutol is the companion drug of choice. Rifampin should be used if the tuberculosis is disseminated or very extensive. Streptomycin should not be used in pregnancy because of the risk of fetal ototoxicity. Tuberculosis often pursues an unfavorable course during and just after pregnancy, and treatment of a pregnant woman should never be deferred. It is reasonable, however, to postpone isoniazid prophylaxis until just after delivery.

Patients with chronic renal failure also present special treatment problems, and these patients have tuberculosis case rates approximately 10 times those of the general population. Isoniazid is acetylated to an inactive form by the liver and then excreted by the kidney. Acetyl isoniazid is the precursor of hydrazines, which are probably hepatotoxic. Both isoniazid and acetyl isoniazid are not bound by plasma proteins and are dialyzable. In patients with renal failure isoniazid should be reduced to 5 mg/kg body weight (300 mg in adults) two or three times weekly. Patients on dialysis should receive the drug following each dialysis. Ethambutol behaves like isoniazid, except that it is excreted by the kidney as the active drug. As with isoniazid, the usual daily dose should be given at longer intervals, and administration should follow dialysis. Optic nerve toxicity of ethambutol appears to be related not to intermittent high drug levels but to sustained high drug levels. Patients with renal failure who are receiving ethambutol should have their color vision and visual acuity monitored regularly. Rifampin is protein-bound, nondialyzable, and excreted in the bile by the liver. No change in dose or interval is necessary in the presence of renal failure. Caution should be exercised in using rifampin in patients with hepatic failure.

Faced with relapse in a previously treated patient, a major concern should be the possibility of drug resistance, and resistance studies of the organism should be obtained in a competent reference laboratory. In one-third of patients who relapse after adequate regular drug therapy, the relapse is caused by drug-resistant organisms. If, however, the patient took the drug sporadically or the previous regimen was inadequate, then the likelihood of drug resistance is about two chances in three. Therapy for presumed drug-resistant tuberculosis should be instituted with two drugs which the patient has not taken previously, provided that one of these two new drugs is isoniazid or rifampin. Otherwise, four drugs should be used, including as many new drugs as possible. When resistance studies become available, the regimen should be modified appropriately. It is beneficial to continue isoniazid even when laboratory studies indicate drug resistance. In general, all re-treatment regimens should be closely supervised and directed by physicians with special experience with this problem.

Primary drug resistance should be suspected in patients who appear to have contracted their infection from patients with known drug resistance or with known noncompliance and in patients who come from areas where drug resistance is common. In the United States, this group includes immigrants from Haiti, southeast Asia, and many areas of Latin America. While laboratory resistance studies are pending, drug therapy should be dictated by the prior treatment of the suspected index case. In immigrant populations, most of the drug resistance of concern is to isoniazid. In this circumstance, therapy should be initiated with isoniazid, rifampin, and ethambutol. One of these drugs may be discontinued when resistance studies become available.

PREVENTION Chemoprophylaxis In one of the largest controlled clinical trials ever conducted, 1 year of isoniazid has been shown to be effective in reducing the incidence of tuberculosis in tuberculin-positive individuals presumed to have been infected with *M. tuberculosis*. The benefit of isoniazid prophylaxis has been demonstrated so clearly that the question of its use now hinges primarily on the risk of drug toxicity, chiefly hepatitis.

In administering isoniazid prophylaxis, highest priority should be assigned to treating household contacts of persons with active tuberculosis and to persons known to have become infected within the preceding year. The risks of developing tuberculosis in these two groups are, respectively, 0.5 percent per year and 3 percent during the first year. Particular attention should be given to treating children in these categories. Prophylaxis of childhood household contacts with isoniazid should be started immediately. After 3 months of therapy, the child should be skin-tested with intermediate-strength PPD. If the skin test is negative at that time, isoniazid may be discontinued. If it is positive, 12 months of prophylaxis should be completed.

Younger individuals benefit most from isoniazid prophylaxis because the drug is most effective when the infection is recent and because older individuals have often already outlived a substantial part of their risk. The risk of hepatitis rises with age, reaching approximately 2 percent by the seventh decade. Cost-benefit analyses with large data bases have shown that there is a 1:1 ratio of cases of tuberculosis prevented and hepatitis caused at age 45 when individuals without added risks are considered. Based on this calculation, there is a general consensus that all persons younger than age 35 with a positive tuberculin reaction should receive isoniazid 300 mg/d for 1 year.

It is also possible to develop criteria for the prophylactic use of isoniazid in older persons with remote tuberculosis, either known historically or evident radiographically, who have never received adequate chemotherapy. The annual risk of tuberculosis in such persons is at least 0.5 percent. Isoniazid 300 mg/d should be given for 1 year to all persons in this category who have a life expectancy greater than 10 years. In compliant adults with fibrotic residuals of untreated tuberculosis visible on roentgenograms, 1 year of isoniazid prophylaxis reduced disease during the subsequent 5 years by 93 percent, and 6 months of isoniazid reduced disease by 69 percent. Others at high risk for the development of tuberculosis include tuberculin-positive individuals with AIDS or Hodgkin's disease (both of which alter T-lymphocyte-mediated immunity), patients with silicosis (which affects macrophage function), and persons who are (1) receiving immunosuppressive agents or glucocorticoids chronically or (2) who suffer from renal failure. As with therapy for active tuberculosis, monitoring serum enzymes is not useful in patients receiving isoniazid prophylaxis.

BCG vaccination Bacillus Calmette-Guérin (BCG) is an attenuated strain of *M. bovis* which has been given to more than 2 billion persons as a vaccine against tuberculosis. It is clearly safe, but its efficacy is in some dispute. In some controlled studies it offered little or no protection. However, even then, the disseminated forms of tuberculosis which have such high mortalities among children were virtually eliminated. While final judgment on the efficacy of BCG must be reserved, its continued use in high-prevalence areas appears justified.

BCG vaccination induces tuberculin hypersensitivity. However, the dermal reaction to PPD is usually not as large as that which follows natural infection, usually does not persist as long, and varies from strain to strain of vaccine. Individuals with large PPD reactions persisting for many years after vaccination should be viewed as infected and considered for isoniazid prophylaxis.

CONTROL PROGRAMS In most low-prevalence areas, such as North America, resources are relatively abundant and disease occurrence is mostly sporadic. Increasingly, tuberculosis is being seen in microepidemics, often centered in family groups. Immigrant groups and residents and employees of nursing homes are at highest risk. Central to any program is an efficient case-reporting and registry system. Contact investigation must be carried out effectively and is especially important when index cases occur in children. The major modality for decreasing the spread of infection is chemotherapy for all infectious patients. Chemoprophylaxis is necessary for contacts.

At the other end of the spectrum are high-prevalence areas with few or no resources for tuberculosis control. The single, most effective measure in this setting is a network of ambulatory tuberculosis treatment centers that provide diagnosis by direct sputum smear and standardized drug therapy. Successful treatment must entail no cost to the patient. Tuberculosis diagnostic and treatment programs should be integrated into national health programs, under expert supervision. Treatment records should be maintained, but complex registries are of little value.

In high-prevalence areas, BCG vaccine should be offered to every individual under 15 or 20 without prior tuberculin testing. Older individuals can be assumed to have been infected already. Before a mass BCG campaign is initiated, planning should begin for continuing vaccination of newborns or young schoolchildren. Community-wide isoniazid prophylaxis programs have not been successful.

REFERENCES

AMERICAN THORACIC SOCIETY: Diagnostic standards and classification of tuberculosis and other mycobacterial diseases (14th ed). Am Rev Respir Dis 123:343, 1981

———: Treatment of tuberculosis and other mycobacterial diseases. Am Rev Respir Dis 128:336, 1983

CHAISSON RE et al: Tuberculosis in patients with the acquired immunodeficiency syndrome. Am Rev Respir Dis 136:570, 1987

COMSTOCK GW, EDWARDS PQ: The competing risks of tuberculosis and hepatitis for adult tuberculin reactors. Am Rev Respir Dis 111:573, 1975

——— et al: The tuberculin skin test. Am Rev Respir Dis 124:356, 1981

———: Epidemiology of tuberculosis. Am Rev Respir Dis 125(suppl):8, 1982

DUTT AK et al: Short-course chemotherapy for extrapulmonary tuberculosis. Ann Intern Med 104:7, 1986

EDWARDS LB et al: An atlas of sensitivity to tuberculin, PPD-B, and histoplasmin in the United States. Am Rev Respir Dis 99(suppl):1, 1969

FOX W: The chemotherapy of pulmonary tuberculosis: A review. Chest 76(suppl):785, 1979

GLASSROTH J et al: Tuberculosis in the 1980s. N Engl J Med 302:1441, 1980

GROSSET J: Bacteriologic basis of short-course chemotherapy for tuberculosis. Clin Chest Med 1:231, 1980

GRZYBOWSKI S, ENARSON DA: The fate of cases of pulmonary tuberculosis under various treatment programmes. Bull Int Union Tuberc 53:70, 1978

PITCHENIK AE et al: Human T-cell lymphotrophic virus-III (HTLV-III) seropositivity and related disease among 71 consecutive patients in whom tuberculosis was diagnosed. A prospective study. Am Rev Respir Dis 135:875, 1987

SELWYN PA et al: A prospective study of the risk of tuberculosis among intravenous users with human immunodeficiency virus infection. N Engl J Med 320:545, 1989

SNIDER DE, JR: The tuberculin skin test. Am Rev Respir Dis 125(suppl):108, 1982

STEAD WW et al: Tuberculosis as an endemic and nosocomial infection among the elderly in nursing homes. N Engl J Med 312:1483, 1985

TENDAM HG et al: Present knowledge of immunization against tuberculosis. Bull WHO 54:255, 1976

126 LEPROSY (HANSEN'S DISEASE)

RICHARD A. MILLER

DEFINITION Leprosy (Hansen's disease) is a chronic granulomatous infection of humans which attacks superficial tissues, especially the skin and peripheral nerves. The clinical and immunologic manifestations of disease form a continuum extending from polar *tuberculoid* leprosy to polar *lepromatous* leprosy. The borderline portion of the spectrum lies between these two extremes, and is usually subdivided into *borderline tuberculoid, borderline,* and *borderline lepromatous* classes. In addition, an early indeterminate form is seen, which may spontaneously remit or develop into overt leprosy.

ETIOLOGY *Mycobacterium leprae,* or Hansen's bacillus, is the causal agent of leprosy. It is an acid-fast rod assigned to the family Mycobacteriaceae on the basis of morphologic, biochemical, antigenic, and genetic similarities to other mycobacteria. Although it has not been cultivated in artificial media or tissue culture, it can be consistently propagated in the foot pads of mice. The bacillus multiplies exceedingly slowly, with an estimated optimal doubling time of 11 to 13 days during logarithmic growth in mouse foot pads. The mouse model has been used extensively for the study of antileprosy drugs, and the high bacterial yield from armadillos has been crucial for immunologic studies.

Lepromin is a suspension of killed *M. leprae* prepared from heavily infected human or armadillo tissue. Intradermal injection elicits, somewhat variably, a tuberculin-like reaction at 48 h (Fernandez's reaction) and more consistently, a papular reaction at 3 to 4 weeks (Mitsuda's reaction). The Mitsuda reaction is usually positive in tuberculoid patients and is always negative in lepromatous patients. However, because it is also positive in nearly all normal adults, even those residing in areas free of endemic leprosy, it has no diagnostic value. Lepromin is not commercially available.

EPIDEMIOLOGY There are probably 10 to 20 million persons affected with leprosy in the world. The disease is more common in tropical countries, in many of which the prevalence rate is 1 to 2 percent of the population. A warm environment is not critical for transmission, and leprosy also occurs in certain regions with cooler climates, such as Korea and central Mexico. Distribution of infected individuals within countries is very nonhomogeneous, and districts in which 20 percent of the population is affected can be found. The distribution of cases across the spectrum of leprosy also varies between countries, with lepromatous disease predominating in some countries, such as Mexico, and tuberculoid disease in others, such as India. Ninety percent of the cases diagnosed in the United States in the past two decades have occurred in immigrants from leprosy-endemic countries. Indigenous transmission occurs primarily in Hawaii, the Pacific Island territories, and sporadically along the Gulf coast. The incidence of leprosy in the United States has fallen from a peak of 360 cases in 1985.

Leprosy can present at any age, although cases in infants less than 1 year of age are extremely rare. The age-specific incidence peaks during childhood in most developing countries; up to 20 percent of cases occur in children under 10. Since leprosy is most prevalent in poorer socioeconomic groups, this may simply reflect the age distribution of the high-risk population. The sex ratio of leprosy presenting during childhood is 1:1, but males predominate by a 2:1 ratio in adults.

Direct human-to-human transmission is believed responsible for most cases of leprosy. Animal reservoirs exist among feral armadillos and possibly among nonhuman primates, but there is little evidence that they have an important role in the epidemiology of human disease. Familial spread is facilitated by the indolence of the clinical illness and the potential for transmission prior to the development of symptoms. Among close family contacts (spouse-spouse or spouse-child) of untreated lepromatous patients the risk of disease is increased approximately eightfold, and the attack rate can be as high as 10 percent. Development of clinical disease in contacts of tuberculoid patients is less common, although immunologic tests suggest that most of these contacts have been sensitized to *M. leprae*. The site of entry remains a matter of conjecture, but is probably either the skin or the mucosa of the upper respiratory tract. The chief portal of exit is thought to be the nasal mucosa of untreated lepromatous patients.

The incubation period is frequently 3 to 5 years, but has been reported to range from 6 months to several decades.

PATHOGENESIS The early events following the entry of *M. leprae* into the body have not been described in humans. The bacilli are surrounded by a dense, nearly inert lipid capsule, produce no exotoxins, and engender little inflammatory response. Immunologic and epidemiologic studies suggest that only a small fraction, possibly 10 to 20 percent, of those exposed to viable bacilli will develop signs of indeterminate leprosy and that only about 50 percent of those with indeterminate disease will progress to full-blown clinical leprosy.

The intensity of the specific cell-mediated immune response to *M. leprae* correlates with the clinical and histologic disease class. Individuals with polar tuberculoid disease have an intense cellular response to *M. leprae* and a low bacillary load, whereas patients with lepromatous leprosy have no detectable cellular immunity to the leprosy bacillus. There is evidence from family studies that specific HLA-associated genes may be linked to different classes of disease. HLA-DR2 is inherited preferentially by children with polar tuberculoid disease, whereas HLA-MT1 is associated with polar lepromatous disease. The effect of the HLA-associated genes is limited to influencing the type of leprosy, and there is no association between HLA haplotypes and overall susceptibility to leprosy.

The defect in cell-mediated immunity in lepromatous patients is extremely specific. They do not suffer increased morbidity following infection by pathogens such as viruses or parasites for which cellular immunity is important, and they do not have an increased risk of neoplasia. Tuberculin reactivity may be suppressed in untreated lepromatous disease, but usually returns with treatment, unlike the lepromin response, which remains negative. Patients with lepromatous leprosy have been shown to have an increased number of circulating $CD8^+$ (''suppressor'') lymphocytes which can be specifically activated by *M. leprae* antigens, and the lymphocytes present in their cutaneous granulomas are almost exclusively $CD8^+$. In contrast, $CD4^+4B4^+$ (''helper'') cells predominate among the T cells in the cutaneous lesions of tuberculoid patients. In lepromatous leprosy, cells of the monocyte-macrophage family become engorged with *M. leprae* and are unable to kill or digest the organisms. Intracellular accumulation of large amounts of the *M. leprae*–specific surface lipid, phenolic glycolipid I, may contribute to the macrophage dysfunction. However, when studied in vitro, monocytes from these patients respond normally to lymphokines and display normal phagocytic and microbicidal activity. These results suggest that an underlying defect in regulation of T-lymphocyte subpopulations is responsible for the immunologic tolerance characteristic of lepromatous leprosy.

Intense bacillemia is very common in lepromatous leprosy, and organisms can often be seen in stained smears of peripheral blood or buffy coats, but high fever and signs of systemic toxicity are absent. Even in the most advanced cases, destructive lesions are limited to the skin, peripheral nerves, anterior portions of the eyes, upper respiratory passages above the larynx, testes, and structures of the hands and feet. The trophism of *M. leprae* for these tissues may be due to the fact that they are all usually several degrees cooler than 37°C. Two sites of preferential involvement are the ulnar nerves near the elbow and the peroneal nerves where they pass around the head of the fibula; above and below these areas where these nerves take deeper courses, they are less severely involved. In patients with lepromatous leprosy, collections of bacilli are also found in the liver, spleen, and bone marrow. No visceral organ system dysfunction has been associated with the presence of these bacilli, and it is unclear whether they are capable of reproduction at core body temperatures.

CLINICOPATHOLOGIC CLASSIFICATION The manifestations of leprosy are many and variable. The classification in general use is based on clinical and histopathologic findings.

Lepromatous leprosy is one of the polar forms. The cutaneous involvement is extensive, diffuse, and bilaterally symmetric. Even apparently normal skin will usually contain bacilli demonstrable by staining. Peripheral nerves are heavily infected but often better preserved than in the tuberculoid form. Histologically, there is a diffuse granulomatous reaction with macrophages, large foam (Virchow's) cells, and many intracellular bacilli, frequently in spheroidal masses (globi). Epithelioid cells and giant cells are not found.

Tuberculoid leprosy is the other polar type. Skin lesions are single or few and are sharply demarcated. Neurologic involvement is relatively pronounced and may occur in the absence of cutaneous lesions (pure neural leprosy). The histologic picture consists of lymphocytes, epithelioid cells, and perhaps giant cells; bacilli are frequently absent or difficult to demonstrate.

Classification within the borderline region of the spectrum is less precise. Lesions tend to increase in number and heterogeneity, but decrease in individual size as the lepromatous pole is approached. The histopathology of the granulomas also changes from an epithelioid cell to a macrophage predominance. The presence and number of lymphocytes are variable and correlate poorly with the disease class. Bacilli are present in large numbers in the skin granulomas of borderline and borderline lepromatous patients. For this reason, these groups, together with polar lepromatous leprosy, are referred to as ''multibacillary leprosy.'' Borderline tuberculoid, polar tuberculoid, and indeterminate classes are grouped together as ''paucibacillary leprosy.'' The borderline disease states are unstable and may shift toward the lepromatous form in the untreated patient or toward the tuberculoid pole during treatment. Change of either polar type to the other is exceedingly rare. In all forms of leprosy peripheral nerve involvement is a constant feature. In any histologic section involvement of nerves will tend to be more severe than involvement of other tissues. Much of the neural destruction appears to result from the granulomatous reaction of the host, rather than from an innate neurotoxic property of the bacillus.

CLINICAL MANIFESTATIONS **Early leprosy** The first signs of leprosy are usually cutaneous. One or more hypopigmented or hyperpigmented macules or plaques may be seen. Often an anesthetic or paresthetic patch is the first symptom noted by the patient, but on careful examination skin involvement can also be found. When contacts are examined, a single skin lesion is often noted, especially in children; usually, this is a hypesthetic macule that may clear spontaneously in a year or two, but specific treatment is usually recommended. Sensation is often preserved in early lesions, particularly those on the face.

Tuberculoid leprosy Early tuberculoid leprosy is frequently manifested by a hypopigmented macule which is sharply demarcated and hypesthetic. Later the lesions are larger, and the margins are elevated and circinate or gyrate. There is peripheral spread and central healing. Fully developed lesions are densely anesthetic and have lost the normal skin organs (sweat glands and hair follicles). The lesions appear singly or are few in number and are not symmetric. Nerve involvement occurs early, and the superficial nerves leading from the lesions may be enlarged. The larger peripheral nerves (especially the ulnar, peroneal, and greater auricular nerves) may be palpably and visibly enlarged, particularly those closest to the skin lesion. There may be severe neuritic pain. Neural involvement leads to muscle atrophy, especially of the small muscles of the hand. Contractures of the hand and foot are frequent. Trauma, especially from burns and splinters and from excessive pressure, leads to secondary infection of the hands and to plantar ulcers. Later, resorption and loss of phalanges may supervene. When the facial nerves are involved, there may be lagophthalmos, exposure keratitis, and corneal ulceration leading to blindness.

Lepromatous leprosy The skin lesions are macules, nodules, plaques, or papules. The macules are often hypopigmented. The borders of the lesions are ill defined and the centers of raised lesions are indurated and convex (rather than concave as in tuberculoid disease). There is also diffuse infiltration between the lesions. The sites of predilection are the face (cheeks, nose, brows), ears, wrists, elbows, buttocks, and knees. Involvement with infiltration and little or no nodulation may progress so subtly that the disease goes unnoticed. Loss of the lateral portions of the eyebrows is common. Much later the skin of the face and forehead becomes thickened and corrugated (leonine facies), and the earlobes become pendulous.

Nasal "stuffiness," epistaxis, and obstructed breathing are common early symptoms. Complete nasal obstruction, laryngitis, and hoarseness are also frequent. Septal perforation and nasal collapse lead to saddlenose. Invasion of the anterior portion of the eye leads to keratitis and iridocyclitis. Painless inguinal and axillary lymphadenopathy occurs. In adult males infiltration and scarring of the testes lead to sterility. Gynecomastia is common.

Involvement of major nerve trunks is less prominent in the lepromatous form, but diffuse hypesthesia involving the peripheral portions of the extremities is common in advanced disease.

Borderline leprosy The skin lesions of borderline tuberculoid leprosy generally resemble those of tuberculoid disease, but are greater in number and have more poorly defined borders. Involvement of multiple peripheral nerve trunks is more common than in polar tuberculoid disease. Increasing variability in the appearance of the skin lesions is characteristic of borderline leprosy (sometimes referred to as "dimorphic" leprosy). Papules and plaques may coexist with macular lesions. Anesthesia is less prominent than in tuberculoid disease. The earlobes may be slightly thickened, but the eyebrows and nasal regions are spared.

REACTIONAL STATES The general course of leprosy is indolent, but it may be interrupted by two types of reaction. Both forms of reactions can occur in untreated patients, but more often emerge as complications of chemotherapy.

Erythema nodosum leprosum Erythema nodosum leprosum (ENL), or type 2 lepra reaction, occurs in lepromatous and borderline lepromatous patients, most frequently in the latter half of the initial year of treatment. Tender, inflamed subcutaneous nodules develop, usually in crops. Each nodule lasts a week or two, but new crops may appear. ENL may last only a week or two, or it may continue for long periods. Low-grade fever, lymphadenopathy, and arthralgias can accompany severe ENL. Histologically, ENL is characterized by polymorphonuclear infiltration and deposits of IgG and complement, resembling an Arthus reaction.

Reversal reaction Reversal reaction, or type 1 lepra reaction, can complicate all three borderline categories. Existing skin lesions develop erythema and swelling, and new lesions may appear. An early influx of lymphocytes into existing lesions is followed by edema and a shift toward tuberculoid histology. Cellular immunity increases. Reversal reactions can be differentiated from disease progression or relapse by mouse inoculations to test bacillary viability and by histologic studies. Downgrading reactions, which clinically mimic reversal reactions, are most common in untreated patients and in women during the third trimester of pregnancy. Skin biopsies reveal a shift toward lepromatous histology and reflect a decrease in cellular immunity.

COMPLICATIONS Leprosy is probably the most frequent cause of crippling of the hand in the world. Trauma and secondary chronic infections can lead to loss of digits or distal extremities. Blindness is also common.

The *Lucio phenomenon*, characterized by arteritis, is limited to patients with diffuse, infiltrative, nonnodular lepromatous disease. Severe cases clinically resemble other forms of necrotizing vasculitis and are associated with a high mortality rate.

Secondary amyloidosis is a complication of severe lepromatous disease, especially in chronic ENL.

DIAGNOSIS The demonstration of acid-fast bacilli in skin smears made by the scraped-incision method is strong evidence for leprosy, but in tuberculoid disease bacilli may not be demonstrable. Wherever possible, a skin biopsy specimen from the affected area should be sent to a pathologist knowledgeable in leprosy. The histologic involvement of peripheral nerves is pathognomonic, even in the absence of bacilli.

Hematologic and blood chemistry tests are of little help in establishing the diagnosis. Lepromatous patients frequently have mild anemia, elevated erythrocyte sedimentation rate, and hyperglobulinemia. Between 10 and 20 percent of lepromatous patients have low titer false-positive serologic tests for syphilis or autoantibodies directed against nuclear or cellular antigens.

A specific serodiagnostic test for leprosy has been developed. Based on the detection of antibody to the *M. leprae*–specific surface antigen, phenolic glycolipid I, this assay has a sensitivity of over 95 percent in polar lepromatous disease and about 30 percent in tuberculoid disease. The level of antibody appears to correlate with the bacillary load which explains both the high false-negative rate in polar tuberculoid disease and the persistence of seropositivity in lepromatous patients, in whom bacterial remnant forms can persist for many years. Despite these limitations, the near 100 percent specificity of this assay makes it potentially useful for confirming the diagnosis of leprosy and monitoring the response to therapy, and as an epidemiologic tool for studying disease incubation and transmission.

The differential diagnosis includes lupus erythematosus, lupus vulgaris, sarcoidosis, yaws, dermal leishmaniasis, and a host of banal skin diseases. The skin lesions of leprosy, especially of turberculoid disease, are characterized by hypesthesia, and peripheral nerve involvement can always be demonstrated. Peripheral neuropathy from other causes and syringomyelia may be confused with leprosy, although skin involvement is not a feature of other diseases causing peripheral neuropathy. The combination of a chronic skin disease and peripheral nerve involvement should always lead to the consideration of leprosy.

TREATMENT The management of leprosy involves a broad, multidisciplinary approach, including consultative services such as orthopedic surgery, ophthalmology, and physical therapy in addition to antimicrobial chemotherapy.

Specific chemotherapy *Dapsone* (4,4′-diaminodiphenylsulfone, DDS, diphenylsulfone), a folate antagonist, is the mainstay of therapy. The daily dosage is 50 to 100 mg in adults. Dapsone is very inexpensive, safe in pregnancy, and has a long serum half-life of about 24 h, allowing once daily administration. Major side effects are relatively uncommon, but include hemolysis, agranulocytosis, hepatitis, and potentially fatal exfoliative dermatitis. In lepromatous disease enough bacilli are killed during the first 10 to 12 weeks of dapsone monotherapy to render mouse foot pad inoculations negative. However, in this form of the disease nonviable bacilli disappear slowly and may be found in the tissues for 5 to 10 years. Moreover, a few viable bacilli (persisters) may survive in the tissues for many years and cause a relapse if treatment is discontinued.

Dapsone resistance is a problem of increasing concern. Secondary resistance is most common in lepromatous patients and presents as a clinical and bacteriologic relapse after several years of apparently successful, regular therapy. Sulfone resistance can be demonstrated by mouse foot pad inoculation. The frequency of this secondary resistance has been 2 to 30 percent in different countries, depending on the sulfone preparation used and the regularity of its administration. Primary dapsone resistance in as many as 30 percent of previously untreated patients has complicated empiric therapy in many parts of the world, but has remained uncommon in newly diagnosed patients in the United States. Because of the problems of dapsone-resistant bacilli and of persister bacilli, multiple drug therapy is now recommended for all multibacillary disease.

Rifampin is the most rapidly mycobactericidal drug known for *M. leprae*. The viability of skin bacilli falls to undetectable levels within 5 days following a single 1500-mg dose of oral rifampin. The usual dosage is 600 mg/d. The high cost of rifampin has limited its use in the developing world, and has led to regimens in which it is given at a dosage of 600 or 900 mg once per month. Until more clinical experience has been accumulated, however, many leprologists prefer to treat with daily or twice weekly rifampin. Rare cases of rifampin-resistant *M. leprae* have been reported. Rifampin has not been approved for the intermittent treatment of leprosy by the Food and Drug Administration.

Clofazimine is a compound derived from a phenazine dye. It is highly lipophilic and accumulates in the skin, the gastrointestinal tract, and in macrophages and monocytes. It is usually given in a dosage of 50 to 200 mg/d and has an apparent half-life of over 70 days. Major toxicity is restricted to the skin and the intestinal tract. The reddish skin pigmentation, often accompanied by ichthyosis, is unacceptable to many light-skinned patients and can lead to poor compliance. The intestinal toxicity is also dose-related and is reflected in diarrhea and cramping abdominal pain. Clofazimine is not safe for use during pregnancy.

Several other agents, including ethionamide, prothionamide, thiambutosine, and amithiozone, have limited activity against *M. leprae* and may be of value in multiple drug regimens. None of these drugs have been approved for this purpose by the Food and Drug Administration. Based on promising results in animal studies, clinical trials are underway with the quinolones, ofloxacin and pefloxacin, as well as with minocycline.

Therapy for multibacillary disease should consist of three drugs, usually dapsone, rifampin, and clofazimine. If the organism is known to be dapsone-sensitive, the combination of dapsone and rifampin may be adequate for borderline and borderline lepromatous cases, but the likelihood of secondary dapsone resistance makes the addition of a third drug advisable in lepromatous disease. Objective measures of response to therapy, including skin scrapings and biopsies, should be monitored and therapy continued at least until morphologically intact bacilli are consistently absent and the inflammatory cell infiltrate has resolved. The optimal duration of therapy is unknown, but a minimum of 2 years is recommended. Indefinite therapy may be required for lepromatous disease.

Therapeutic regimens containing two drugs, usually dapsone and rifampin, are adequate for paucibacillary leprosy. The World Health Organization recommends a 6-month course, which can be repeated if relapse occurs. Standard practice in the United States is to treat with dapsone and rifampin for the first 6 to 12 months (depending on the clinical response), followed by dapsone alone to complete a total of 24 months of therapy.

Evidence of clinical improvement should be visible by the second or third month of treatment. The clinical response to adequate therapy may be confused by intercurrent reactional states, but the disease stops progressing and the skin lesions gradually improve. Recovery from neurologic impairment is limited.

Treatment of reactional states Mild ENL is managed with antipyretics and analgesics. Severe cases can be rapidly controlled with high dosages of prednisone (60 to 120 mg/d). Antimicrobial therapy should be continued as glucocorticoid therapy promotes the viability of *M. leprae* in mice not given antileprosy drugs. Rifampin enhances the metabolism of glucocorticoids by the liver, necessitating administration of larger doses to achieve a given therapeutic effect. Thalidomide is the most effective drug for ENL. The usual initial dosage is 200 mg twice a day, which can be gradually tapered to a maintenance dosage of 50 to 100 mg/d for patients with chronic ENL. Thalidomide is absolutely contraindicated in women of child-bearing age because of its teratogenicity, but has proved relatively free of major side effects in other leprosy patients. This drug has not been approved by the Food and Drug Administration but is available through the Hansen's Disease Center, Carville, Louisiana, as an investigational agent. Clofazimine has anti-inflammatory properties as well as antimycobacterial activity and can be valuable in the treatment of chronic ENL, but requires at least 3 to 4 weeks to reach effective levels, making it of little use in acute attacks. Other classes of anti-inflammatory agents including antimalarials such as chloroquine and cytotoxic drugs have been used in difficult cases; in general these unusual situations should be managed in consultation with a leprosy specialist.

Reversal reactions are often acute and can lead to rapid and irreversible neurologic damage. Glucocorticoids are indicated for severe reversal reactions. Clofazimine is of some use in chronic situations, but it is generally necessary to continue glucocorticoids as well. Reversal reactions do not respond to thalidomide.

Other measures Many of the deformities and disabilities of leprosy are preventable. Plantar ulcers, which are very common, may be prevented by rigid-soled footwear or walking plaster casts, and contractures of the hand may be prevented by physical therapy and application of casts. Reconstructive surgery is sometimes helpful. Nerve and tendon transplants and release of contractures can give patients more functional ability. Vocational retraining is often necessary for those with permanent disability. Plastic repair of facial deformities assists acceptance of patients in society. The psychological trauma which resulted from prolonged segregation is now minimized by home therapy in virtually all cases.

Control Case finding and chemotherapy form the present basis of control. Infectiousness can be quickly suppressed with chemotherapy. Early detection of cases is especially important. In endemic countries this means establishing clinics or traveling teams. Family and other close contacts need regular examinations for leprosy. In the United States patients are eligible for treatment by the Public Health Service, and special clinics are located in several major cities, as well as an inpatient facility at the Hansen's Disease Center in Carville. Risk of transmission is very low, even in untreated patients, and no unusual infection control precautions are required when patients are hospitalized. Chemoprophylaxis with lowered doses of dapsone is effective, but contact screening by yearly physical examinations is preferred to empiric therapy in most situations. Vaccine trials with bacillus Calmette-Guérin in endemic areas continue despite conflicting results and modest efficacy. Two new experimental vaccines, one containing viable BCG and heat-killed *M. leprae*, and the second consisting of a cultivable mycobacterium (ICRC bacillus) are currently in field trials.

REFERENCES

Bloom BR, Godal T: Selective primary health care: Strategies for control of disease in the developing world. V. Leprosy. Rev Infect Dis 5:765, 1983

Bullock WE: Rifampin in the treatment of leprosy. Rev Infect Dis 5:S606, 1983

———: *Mycobacterium leprae* (leprosy), in *Principles and Practice of Infectious Diseases*, 2 ed, GL Mandell et al (eds). New York, Wiley, 1985, pp 1406–1413

Hastings RC (ed): *Leprosy*. New York, Churchill Livingstone, 1985

Modlin RL et al: Learning from lesions: Patterns of tissue inflammation in leprosy. Proc Natl Acad Sci USA 85:1213, 1988

Neill MA et al: Leprosy in the United States, 1971–1981. J Infect Dis 152:1064, 1985

Ridley DS, Joping WH: Classification of leprosy according to immunity: A five-group system. Int J Lepr 34:255, 1966

Serological tests for leprosy, editorial. Lancet 1:533, 1986

Shields ED et al: Genetic epidemiology of the susceptibility to leprosy. J Clin Invest 79:1139, 1987

Thomas DA et al: Armadillo exposure among Mexican-born patients with lepromatous leprosy. J Infect Dis 156:990, 1987

Vaccines against leprosy, editorial. Lancet 1:1183, 1987

127 OTHER MYCOBACTERIAL INFECTIONS

STANLEY D. FREEDMAN

INTRODUCTION Mycobacteria other than the tubercle bacilli were shown to be agents of human disease in the 1950s. A classification of these organisms based upon colonial morphology and growth characteristics was provided by Runyon. These bacteria are widely distributed in nature as saprophytes, primarily in soil and water. Animals can be infected and serve as reservoirs for infection of humans. Person-to-person transmission has not been documented. Epidemiologic studies using tuberculins from the various species demonstrated the extent of infection in the United States and other countries, as well as notable geographic differences. These organisms have been referred to as atypical mycobacteria or anonymous mycobacteria. Although the organisms are not always anonymous, the frequency with which they are found in the environment demands repeated isolation from a diseased area or isolation from blood or bone marrow before they can be accepted as the etiologic agent. With the steady improvement of laboratory techniques including radiometric cultures, species designations are now increasingly familiar and preferred in the study of these pathogens (Table 127-1). With increasing sophistication of medical practice and the emergence of newly recognized diseases, additional syndromes associated with different species have emerged and have assumed major importance.

MYCOBACTERIUM ULCERANS *M. ulcerans* is the etiologic agent of the Buruli or Bairnsdale ulcer. It grows only at 30 to 33°C. Colonies require 7 weeks to appear; isolation is enhanced by inoculation of mouse footpads. A disease of the tropics, it is concentrated in Australia and Africa. The first sign of infection with *M. ulcerans* is a small painless nodule developing into an extensive granulomatous ulceration usually affecting the extensor surfaces of the extremities. Characteristically, the ulcer is deep with a necrotic base and undermined edges. Tissue destruction may be due to a soluble bacterial toxin that may mute the host response. Wide surgical excision with skin grafting is curative; there are no clear data regarding chemotherapy.

MYCOBACTERIUM MARINUM This organism, previously called *M. balnei,* is a psychrophilic (30°C) photochromogen which inhabits fresh and salt water and causes disease in fish. Human infections are usually associated with some aquatic activity, like working in aquaria and swimming. The organism enters abraded skin and either forms a nodule, which can spread along lymphatics suggesting sporotrichosis, causes verrucous lesions, or, less commonly, ulcerates. The pathology consists of a granulomatous lesion usually without caseation—the so-called swimming pool or fishtank granuloma. Infection is frequently associated with a positive tuberculin test reflecting shared antigens with *M. tuberculosis.* Because the differential diagnosis includes sporotrichosis as well as other mycobacterial infections, appropriate cultures (30 to 32°C incubation) are critical. Infections of tendon sheaths and synovia have been described in association with penetrating injuries. Ulcerations similar to those caused by *M. ulcerans,* as well as disseminated skin lesions, have been reported in immunocompromised patients. Minor lesions can resolve spontaneously. The organism is often sensitive in vitro to rifampin and ethambutol, and these drugs have been curative. Tetracycline, especially minocycline, and trimethoprim-sulfamethoxazole have also been used with favorable results. Surgical debridement is sometimes required.

MYCOBACTERIUM KANSASII *M. kansasii* produces pigment upon exposure to light, grows at 37°C, and is a long, thick, acid-fast organism with prominent transverse banding. Infections are more common in the central United States, Texas, England, and Wales. The reasons for these geographic variations are unknown, but likely relate to subtle ecologic properties of these organisms. Person-to-person spread is not recognized. Reported cases reflect a preponderance of white adult men.

Pulmonary disease is the commonest expression of this organism, and the clinical picture closely resembles pulmonary tuberculosis although signs and symptoms are milder. Pneumoconiosis and chronic obstructive pulmonary disease (COPD) are considered predisposing conditions. Thin-walled cavities with minimal inflammatory reaction are characteristic. The usual situation, without treatment, is slow progression.

Disseminated disease is now recognized as an important manifestation of *M. kansasii* infections. Such hematogenous spread is associated with pancytopenia, hairy cell leukemia, malignancies, acquired immunodeficiency syndrome (AIDS), and bone marrow and renal transplantations. Fever, anemia, and signs and symptoms of multiple organ system involvement occur. The diagnosis is confirmed by appropriate cultures of involved tissues. Skin and soft tissue involvement is seen and may mimic *M. marinum* infections. Tenosynovitis, osteomyelitis, lymphadenitis, pericarditis, and genitourinary tract infections have been reported.

Diseases due to *M. kansasii* respond well to treatment. Rifampin appears to be the most effective drug and should be used in all initial regimens. Ethambutol and isoniazid are usually the other drugs administered. Over 95 percent of patients respond to this combined regimen. Retreatment programs should be guided by in vitro sensitivity testing, and rifampin used if the organism is sensitive.

MYCOBACTERIUM SCROFULACEUM This bacillus, which forms pigment even in the dark (scotochromogenic), is a major cause of lymphadenitis in children. Cervical nodes are usually involved, and associated systemic symptoms are rare. Definitive diagnosis requires culture, and definitive therapy requires total excision of the node and sinus tract, if present. There are a few reports of pulmonary disease and osseous and soft tissue infections; dissemination usually is associated with serious underlying conditions. Sensitivity patterns vary, and multiple-drug regimens have been used.

MYCOBACTERIUM SZULGAI At 37°C this organism is scotochromogenic and can be confused with more common tap water contam-

TABLE 127-1 Human mycobacterial pathogens other than *M. tuberculosis* and *M. leprae*

Mycobacterium	Pigmentation of culture*	Usual site of disease	Usual source of infection	Response to drugs
M. marinum	P	Skin	Swimming pools, aquaria, fish	Good
M. ulcerans	N	Skin	Tropical environment	Variable
M. avium-intracellulare	N	Lungs	Environment, animals?	Poor
M. kansasii	P	Lungs	Environment?	Good
M. xenopi	S	Lungs	Water, animals?	Variable
M. szulgai	S†	Lungs	?	Good
M. scrofulaceum	S	Lungs, lymph nodes	Water, soil	Poor
M. fortuitum	N	Skin (abscesses), lungs	Soil, dirt, water	Poor
M. chelonei	N	Skin (abscesses), lungs	Soil, dirt, water	Poor

* P = photochromogenic (develops yellow-orange pigment only when exposed to light); N = nonpigmented; S = scotochromogenic (develops yellow-orange pigment in the dark).
† Scotochromogenic at 37°C, photochromogenic at 25°C.

inants. It was initially recognized as an uncommon pulmonary pathogen producing disease similar to *M. tuberculosis*. Bursitis, lymphadenitis, tenosynovitis, and disseminated disease have also been reported. Most isolates are sensitive to rifampin and ethambutol.

MYCOBACTERIUM XENOPI *M. xenopi* is a slow-growing scotochromogen which infrequently causes tuberculosis-like pulmonary disease in humans usually with underlying diseases. Extrapulmonary disease is rare. However, reports of disseminated disease are becoming more common and include an association with AIDS (see below). Unlike a number of nontuberculous mycobacteria it is sensitive to most of the antituberculous drugs but combination therapy is required.

MYCOBACTERIUM AVIUM-INTRACELLULARE Although seroagglutination, thin-layer chromatography, and enzyme-linked immunosorbent assays can distinguish *M. avium* from *M. intracellulare*, distinction is difficult and they are considered as a complex (MAC). These ubiquitous organisms are particularly prevalent in the southeastern United States and, overall, are the most commonly isolated mycobacteria other than *M. tuberculosis*. Colonization and inapparent infection are common; knowledge of transmission is limited. The lungs are most commonly involved, and the clinical picture is similar to pulmonary tuberculosis. Underlying pulmonary disease, a possible genetic predilection, and age are risk factors. Solitary pulmonary nodules are not uncommon. It is important to be certain of the etiology and the pathogenic role of the organism isolated, because chemotherapy is often associated with morbidity.

Skin involvement and musculoskeletal infections including vertebral osteomyelitis resembling Pott's disease have been described. MAC is a major cause of lymphadenitis in children. Disseminated disease is also recognized in children, and in adults in association with severe underlying diseases. Fever, anemia, leukocytosis, hypergammaglobulinemia, and hepatosplenomegaly are prominent features.

There is a striking association between organisms of the *Mycobacterium avium* complex and AIDS (see Chap. 264). The manifestations are unique and reflect overwhelming infection in these patients with impaired immunity. There is mycobacteremia, and organisms abound in most organs and body secretions. There is a minimal cellular response, granulomatous or otherwise. Profound diarrhea with intestinal pathology that resembles Whipple's disease, due to macrophages packed with MAC, is present. In other organs these macrophages resemble lepra cells. Blood cultures using the lysis centrifugation system combined with the radiometric systems and using DNA probes for identification can quickly confirm the diagnosis in many patients. The organisms are readily seen and cultured from other involved sites using standard techniques.

Treatment is difficult and unsatisfactory. The organisms are usually resistant to most of the antimycobacterial agents. Yet multiple-drug therapy is recommended with some demonstrable benefit possibly reflecting synergy which is difficult to prove in vitro. Drugs chosen should include those antimicrobials to which the organism is sensitive. Three to six drugs are used concurrently, chosen from among isoniazid, ethambutol, rifampin, ethionamide, pyrazinamide, cycloserine, streptomycin, kanamycin, amikacin, and capreomycin. Of these, ethambutol, rifampin, ethionamide, cycloserine, and amikacin appear more effective. Clofazamine may be useful in immunocompetent patients. Surgical excision is the treatment of choice for lymphadenitis and is a reasonable alternative for a few other localized infections. Treatment of patients with AIDS is problematic and controversial; combinations including rifampin, ethambutol, clofazamine, amikacin, one of the quinolones, along with immunomodulators, may be beneficial for some patients.

MYCOBACTERIUM FORTUITUM* AND *CHELONEI The unique feature of these acid-fast bacteria is their rapid growth; initial growth may take 1 to 5 weeks, but subsequent subcultures grow within 5 days. Reflecting their meager nutritional requirements, they are readily cultured on most media. These two species account for virtually all the reported infections due to rapid growers. *M. fortuitum* is more frequently associated with posttraumatic and postsurgical skin and soft tissue infection. *M. chelonei* is a more common cause of pulmonary infections and disseminated disease. It has also been reported as a cause of chronic otitis media. Subspeciation is not necessary for clinical purposes. Widespread in nature and in hospital environments, and highly resistant to drugs, antiseptics, and disinfectants, rapid growers are important nosocomial pathogens.

Most human infections are associated with interruption of the integument and injury or alteration of the soft tissues. Inhalational pulmonary disease complicates underlying lung disease. Although a chronic granulomatous reaction with caseation may occur, the distinguishing feature is a suppurative process with microabscesses, and diphtheroid-like organisms on Gram stain. Infections have followed cardiothoracic surgery, augmentation mammoplasty, arthroplasty, injections, ocular surgery, and dialysis. Clinical manifestations include lymphadenitis, keratitis, osteomyelitis, meningitis, and endocarditis involving porcine, prosthetic, and natural valves. Hematogenous dissemination is uncommon, and affects primarily those with impaired host defenses.

Nodular erythematous skin lesions on the legs of renal transplant recipients are often due to *M. chelonei*.

Adequate debridement and drainage with removal of foreign bodies is indicated whenever possible. Many of these organisms are highly resistant to all antimicrobial agents. However, reflecting their growth characteristics, antimicrobial sensitivity testing is more reliable in determining appropriate chemotherapy than is the case with other atypical mycobacteria. Amikacin is most effective; other drugs reported to be of value include gentamicin, cefoxitin, doxycycline, minocycline, erythromycin, sulfonamides, rifampin, ethambutol, ciprofloxacin, imipenem, and clofazamine. Sulfonamides are more active against *M. fortuitum*, and erythromycin inhibits some *M. chelonei*. Because of the emergence of resistant organisms, two or three drugs may be preferable to one.

OTHER MYCOBACTERIA *M. haemophilum* is a skin pathogen. It is psychrophilic, but requires iron supplements for growth. Virtually all reported cases have occurred in immunosuppressed patients, including some with AIDS. *M. malmoense* causes chronic pulmonary disease usually in the setting of pneumoconiosis. With increasing laboratory and clinical sophistication, the list of diseases caused by nontuberculous mycobacteria continues to expand.

REFERENCES

Alberts WM, Chandler KW: Pulmonary disease caused by *Mycobacterium malmoense*. Am Rev Respir Dis 135:1375, 1987

Bennett C, Vardiman J: Disseminated atypical mycobacterial infection in patients with hairy cell leukemia. Am J Med 80:891, 1986

Chow SP, Ip FK: *Mycobacterium marinum* infection of the hand and wrist. Results of conservative treatment in twenty-four cases. J Bone Joint Surg [AM] 69:1161, 1987

Cooper JF et al: *Mycobacterium chelonei:* A cause of nodular skin lesions with a proclivity for renal transplant recipients. Am J Med 86:173, 1989

Hampson SJ, Portaels F: DNA probes demonstrate a single highly conserved strain of *Mycobacterium avium* infecting AIDS patients. Lancet 1:65, 1989

Maloney JM, Gregg CR: Infections caused by *Mycobacterium szulgai* in humans. Rev Infect Dis 9:1120, 1987

Parrot RG, Grosset JH: Post-surgical outcome of 57 patients with *Mycobacterium xenopi* pulmonary infection. Tubercle 69:47, 1988

Pimsler M, Sponsler TA: Immunosuppressive properties of the soluble toxin from *Mycobacterium ulcerans*. J Infect Dis 157:577, 1988

Roth RI, Owen RL: Intestinal infection with *Mycobacterium avium* in acquired immune deficiency syndrome (AIDS). Dig Dis Sci 30:497, 1985

Wallace RJ: Treatment of nonpulmonary infections due to *Mycobacterium fortuitum* and *Mycobacterium chelonei* on the basis of in vitro susceptibilities. J Infect Dis 152:500, 1985

———, Swenson JM: Spectrum of disease due to rapidly growing mycobacteria. Rev Infect Dis 5:657, 1983

Wong B, Edwards FF: Continuous high-grade *Mycobacterium avium-intracellulare* bacteremia in patients with the acquired immune deficiency syndrome. Am J Med 78:35, 1985

Woods GL, Washington JA: Mycobacteria other than *Mycobacterium tuberculosis:* Review of microbiologic and clinical aspects. Rev Infect Dis 9:275, 1987

section 7 Spirochetal diseases

128 SYPHILIS

SHEILA A. LUKEHART / KING K. HOLMES

DEFINITION Syphilis is a chronic systemic infection caused by *Treponema pallidum* subspecies *pallidum,* is usually sexually transmitted, and is characterized by episodes of active disease interrupted by periods of latency. Following an incubation period averaging 3 weeks, a primary lesion appears and is often associated with regional lymphadenopathy; a secondary bacteremic stage is associated with generalized mucocutaneous lesions and generalized lymphadenopathy, followed by a latent period of subclinical infection lasting many years. In about one-third of untreated cases, the tertiary stage is characterized by progressive destructive mucocutaneous musculoskeletal or parenchymal lesions, aortitis, or symptomatic central nervous system disease.

ETIOLOGY The discovery of *Treponema pallidum* in syphilitic material was made by Schaudinn and Hoffman in 1905. *Treponema pallidum* is one of the many spiral-shaped microorganisms which propel themselves by spinning around their longitudinal axis. The Spirochaetales include three genera which are pathogenic for humans and for a variety of other animals: the *Leptospira,* which cause human leptospirosis; the *Borrelia,* including *B. recurrentis* and *B. vincentii,* which cause relapsing fever and Vincent's angina, respectively, as well as *B. burgdorferi,* the causative agent of Lyme disease; and the *Treponema,* responsible for the diseases known as treponematoses. The *Treponema* include *T. pallidum* subspecies *pallidum* (hereafter called *T. pallidum*) which causes venereal syphilis, *T. pallidum* subspecies *pertenue* which causes yaws, *T. pallidum* subspecies *endemicum* which causes endemic syphilis or bejel, *T. carateum* which causes pinta (see Chap. 129), and *T. paraluiscuniculi,* the cause of rabbit syphilis. Other *Treponema* species are found in the human mouth, genital mucosa, and gastrointestinal tract but have no proven pathogenic role. These can be confused with *T. pallidum* on dark-field examination.

Treponema pallidum is a thin, delicate organism with 6 to 14 spirals and tapered ends, measuring 6 to 15 μm in total length and 0.2 μm in width. The cytoplasm is surrounded by a trilaminar cytoplasmic membrane, which in turn is surrounded by a delicate peptidoglycan layer providing some structural rigidity. The outer membrane is rich in lipid and contains relatively few integral membrane proteins. Six endoflagella wind around the cell body in a space between the inner cell wall and the outer membrane and may be the contractile elements responsible for motility. None of the four pathogenic treponemes has yet been cultured in vitro in quantity, and no convincing morphologic, serologic, or metabolic differences between them have been discerned. They are distinguished primarily according to the clinical syndrome they produce. The only known natural host for *T. pallidum* is the human. Many mammals can be infected with *T. pallidum,* but only humans, higher apes, and a few laboratory animals regularly develop syphilitic lesions. Virulent strains of *T. pallidum* are maintained in rabbits.

EPIDEMIOLOGY Nearly all cases of syphilis are acquired by sexual contact with infectious lesions (i.e., the chancre, mucous patch, skin rash, or condyloma latum). Less common modes of transmission include nonsexual personal contact and infection in utero or following blood transfusions.

The total reported number of cases of syphilis fell steadily from 575,593 in 1943 to a low of 64,621 in 1977, an 88 percent decrease, but has increased 60 percent in the past 11 years to 103,437 in 1988, with a 50 percent increase from 1986 through 1988. The number of new cases of infectious syphilis reached a peak in 1947, then fell to approximately 6000 in 1956; since then, there has been a rather steady increase in infectious syphilis punctuated by three periods of rapid growth: 10,000 more new cases by 1960 compared to 1956; 13,000 more new cases by 1982 compared to 1979; and from 1986 through 1988, an increase of 12,608 new infectious cases within only 2 years. In 1988, there were 40,117 reported cases of primary and secondary syphilis and 35,600 cases of early latent syphilis; the number of undiagnosed cases is estimated to be much greater.

The populations at highest risk for acquiring syphilis have changed. Between 1977 and 1982, approximately half of all patients with early syphilis in the United States were homosexual or bisexual men. Largely because of changing sexual practices in this population due to the AIDS epidemic, the proportion of early syphilis cases involving homosexual and bisexual men has decreased. The current epidemic of syphilis is occurring predominantly in black and Hispanic heterosexual men and women, largely in urban areas. In some cities, infectious syphilis is significantly correlated with exchange of sex for crack cocaine. The peak incidence of syphilis occurs in the age group 15 to 34. Although the reported incidence of syphilis is much higher in blacks and Hispanics than in whites and is higher in urban than in rural areas, these differences may reflect the fact that many members of urban minority groups are treated at public clinics, where case reporting is more complete. The case rates of early syphilis are highest in large urban population centers, including New York City, parts of Florida and Texas, Los Angeles, and the District of Columbia.

The incidence of congenital syphilis roughly parallels that of infectious syphilis in females. The number of reported cases of congenital syphilis in infants ≤1 year of age was lowest (107 cases) in 1978, when infectious syphilis was most prevalent in homosexual and bisexual men. The dramatic increase in primary and secondary syphilis in women from 1986 to 1988 has resulted in a proportional increase in the number of infants born with congenital syphilis, to 691 infants in 1988. Approximately one of two individuals named as contacts of infectious syphilis becomes infected. Many contacts will have already developed manifestations of syphilis when they are first seen, and about 30 percent of apparently uninfected contacts of infectious syphilis who are examined within 30 days of exposure will actually be in the incubation stage and will themselves develop infectious syphilis if not treated. Because of this, the identification and "epidemiologic" treatment of all recently exposed contacts has become an important aspect of syphilis control. Also important is the identification of syphilitics by serologic testing of pregnant women, hospital admissions, military inductees, and persons undergoing examination in physicians' offices. Of 45 million blood specimens examined during 1980 in the United States, 1.4 million tests were reactive, representing untreated syphilis, previously treated syphilis, or false-positive tests. Of all reported early syphilis cases of less than 1 year's duration in 1983, 47 percent were detected as a direct result of either contact tracing or serologic testing. More controversial are laws and regulations requiring routine premarital serologic testing for syphilis. Of 3.8 million premarital serologies performed in 1978, only 1 in 8461 was positive for infectious syphilis; the number positive for latent syphilis requiring treatment is probably larger, though national data are not available.

NATURAL COURSE AND PATHOGENESIS OF UNTREATED SYPHILIS *Treponema pallidum* rapidly penetrates intact mucous membranes or abraded skin and within a few hours enters the lymphatics and blood to produce systemic infection and metastatic foci long before the appearance of a primary lesion. Blood from a patient with incubating or early syphilis is infectious. The generation time of *T. pallidum* in vivo is estimated to be 30 to 33 h, and the incubation period of syphilis is inversely proportional to the number of organisms inoculated. The concentration of treponemes generally reaches at least 10^7 per gram of tissue before the appearance of a clinical lesion. In experimental infection in rabbits or humans, very low numbers of treponemes can initiate infection which leads to a discernible lesion only after several weeks, although histopathologic changes are evident earlier; intradermal injection of 10^6 organisms usually produces a lesion within 72 h. The number of organisms required for production of symptomatic infection in humans was determined by intradermal injection of three graded doses of *T. pallidum* simultaneously at separate inoculation sites into each of eight volunteers; based upon these results, the infectious dose 50 (ID_{50}) was calculated to be 57 organisms. The median incubation period in humans is about 21 days, suggesting an average inoculum of 500 to 1000 infectious organisms for naturally acquired disease. Experimental inoculations of humans and rabbits show that the period from inoculation until the primary lesion is discernible rarely exceeds 6 weeks. Subcurative therapy during the incubation period may delay the onset of the primary lesion, but it is not certain that this reduces the probability of ultimate development of symptomatic disease.

The primary lesion appears at the site of inoculation, usually persists for 2 to 6 weeks, and then heals spontaneously. Histopathology of primary lesions shows perivascular infiltration, chiefly by lymphocytes (including CD8+ and CD4+ cells), plasma cells, and histiocytes, with capillary endothelial proliferation, and subsequent obliteration of small blood vessels. At this time *T. pallidum* is demonstrable in the chancre in spaces between epithelial cells as well as within invaginations or phagosomes of epithelial cells, fibroblasts, plasma cells, and the endothelial cells of small capillaries, within lymphatic channels, and in the regional lymph nodes. Phagocytosis of organisms by macrophages ultimately causes their destruction.

The generalized parenchymal, constitutional, and mucocutaneous manifestations of secondary syphilis usually appear about 6 to 8 weeks after healing of the chancre, although 15 percent of patients with secondary syphilis have persisting or healing chancres. In other patients, secondary lesions may appear several months after the chancre has healed, and some patients may enter the latent stage without ever developing secondary lesions. Secondary maculopapular skin lesions show histopathologic features of hyperkeratosis of the epidermis, capillary proliferation with endothelial swelling in the superficial corium, and dermal papillae with transmigration of polymorphonuclear leukocytes, and in the deeper corium, perivascular infiltration by monocytes, plasma cells, and lymphocytes. Treponemes are found in many tissues including the aqueous humor of the eye and the cerebrospinal fluid. Cerebrospinal fluid abnormalities are detected in as many as 40 percent of patients during the secondary stage. Clinical hepatitis and immune complex–induced membranous glomerulonephritis are relatively rare but recognized manifestations of secondary syphilis; abnormal liver function tests may be demonstrated in up to 50 percent of patients with early syphilis. Generalized lymphadenopathy is present in 85 percent of patients with secondary syphilis and is characterized by marked follicular hyperplasia, with histiocytic infiltration and lymphocyte depletion of the paracortical areas, where treponema are present in greatest numbers. The reason for the paradoxical appearance of secondary manifestations in the face of high antibody titers (including immobilizing antibody) to *T. pallidum* is unknown. The secondary lesions subside within 2 to 6 weeks, and the patient enters the latent stage, which is detectable only by serologic testing. In the preantibiotic era, up to 25 percent of untreated patients experienced one or more subsequent generalized or localized mucocutaneous relapses at some time during the first 2 to 4 years after infection. Since 90 percent of such infectious relapses occur during the first year, identification and examination of sexual contacts are most important for patients with syphilis of less than 1 year's duration. Recurrent generalized rash is now rare.

In the preantibiotic era, about one-third of patients with untreated latent syphilis developed clinically apparent tertiary disease; today specific and coincidental therapy of early and latent syphilis have greatly reduced the incidence of apparent tertiary disease. In the past, the most common type of tertiary disease was the gumma, a usually benign granulomatous lesion. Today, gummas are very uncommon. The tertiary lesions are caused by obliterative small vessel endarteritis which usually involves the vasa vasorum of the ascending aorta and, less often, the central nervous system. Asymptomatic CNS involvement is demonstrable in up to 25 percent of patients with late latent syphilis. Factors which determine development and progression of tertiary disease are unknown.

The course of untreated syphilis has been studied retrospectively in a group of nearly 2000 patients with primary or secondary syphilis diagnosed clinically, before the dark-field and Wassermann tests came into use (the Oslo Study, 1891–1951); prospectively in 431 black men with seropositive latent syphilis of 3 or more years' duration (the Tuskegee Study, 1932–1972); and retrospectively in a review of 198 autopsies of patients with untreated syphilis (the Rosahn study).

In the Oslo Study, 24 percent of the patients developed relapsing secondary lesions within 4 years, and 28 percent eventually developed one or more manifestations of late syphilis. Cardiovascular syphilis, including aortitis, was detected in 10 percent, with no cases occurring in those infected before age 15; symptomatic neurosyphilis occurred in 7 percent, and 16 percent developed benign tertiary syphilis (gumma of the skin, mucous membranes, and skeleton). Syphilis was the primary cause of death in 15 percent of males and 8 percent of the females. Cardiovascular syphilis was found in 35 percent of men and 22 percent of women who eventually came to autopsy. In general, serious late complications were nearly twice as common in men as in women.

The Tuskegee Study showed that the death rate of untreated syphilitic black men, 25 to 50 years of age, was 17 percent greater than in nonsyphilitics, and 30 percent of all deaths were attributable to cardiovascular or central nervous system syphilis. The ethical issues raised by this study, begun in the preantibiotic era but continuing into the early 1970s, had a major influence on development of current guidelines for human medical experimentation. By far the most important factor in increased mortality was cardiovascular syphilis. Anatomic evidence of aortitis was found in 40 to 60 percent of autopsied syphilitics (versus 15 percent of controls), while CNS syphilis was found in only 4 percent. Hypertension was also increased in the syphilitics. These studies each show that about one-third of patients with untreated syphilis develop clinical or pathologic evidence of tertiary syphilis; about one-fourth die as a direct result of tertiary syphilis; and additional excess mortality not directly attributable to tertiary syphilis is also seen.

MANIFESTATIONS **Primary syphilis** The typical primary chancre usually begins as a single painless papule which rapidly becomes eroded and usually, but not always, is indurated, with a characteristic cartilagenous consistency on palpation of the edge and base of the ulcer (Fig. 128-1). Histologic examination of the ulcer shows lymphocytic and histiocytic infiltrates with obliterative endarteritis and periarteritis of small vessels. *Treponema pallidum* is seen by electron microscopy to lie in interstitial perivascular spaces and within invaginations or phagosomes of macrophages, neutrophils, endothelial cells, and plasma cells.

The chancre is usually located on the penis in heterosexual men while in homosexual men, it is often found in the anal canal or

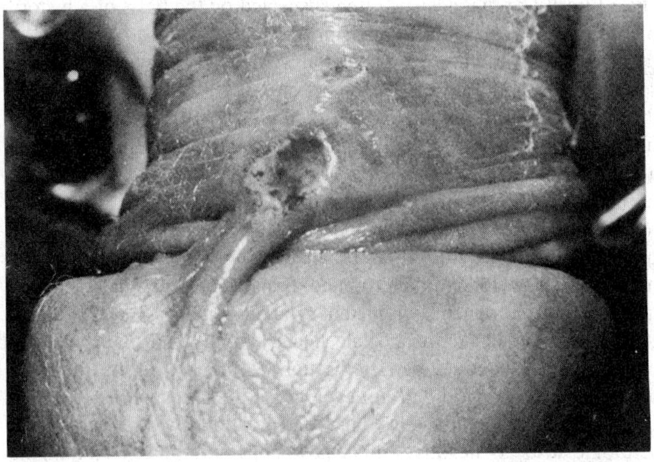

FIGURE 128-1 Primary chancre on the penis. *(Reprinted, with permission, from Sexually Transmitted Diseases, Prof. Dr. E. Stolz, Rotterdam, ©Boehringer Ingelheim International, 1977.)*

rectum, within the mouth, or on the external genitalia. In women, common primary sites are the cervix and labia. Consequently primary syphilis may go unrecognized in women or in homosexual men.

Atypical primary lesions are common. The clinical appearance depends upon the number of treponemes inoculated and upon the immunological status of the patient. A large inoculum produces a dark-field–positive ulcerative lesion in nonimmune human volunteers, but in individuals with a previous history of syphilis may produce either a small dark-field–negative papule, an asymptomatic but seropositive latent infection, or no response at all. A small inoculum usually produces only a papular lesion, even in nonimmune humans. Therefore, syphilis should be considered even in the evaluation of trivial or atypical, dark-field–negative, genital lesions. The most common genital lesions which must be differentiated from primary syphilis include traumatic superinfected lesions, genital herpes simplex virus infection (see Chap. 135), and chancroid (see Chap. 117). *Primary genital herpes* may produce inguinal adenopathy, but the nodes are tender and associated with multiple painful vesicles which later ulcerate, and which are often accompanied by systemic symptoms including fever; *recurrent genital herpes* typically begins with a cluster of painful vesicles, usually without associated adenopathy. *Chancroid* produces painful, superficial exudative, nonindurated, more often multiple ulcers; adenopathy is either unilateral or bilateral, is tender, and may suppurate.

Regional lymphadenopathy usually accompanies the primary syphilitic lesion, appearing within 1 week of the onset of the lesion. The nodes are firm, nonsuppurative, and painless. Inguinal lymphadenopathy is bilateral and may occur with anal as well as with external genital chancres, since lymphatic drainage of the anus involves inguinal nodes. Rectal chancres result in perirectal lymphadenopathy, while chancres of the cervix and vagina result in iliac or perirectal adenopathy. The chancre generally heals within 4 to 6 weeks (range 2 to 12 weeks), but the lymphadenopathy may persist for months.

Secondary syphilis The manifestations of the secondary stage are protean but usually include localized or diffuse symmetric mucocutaneous lesions and generalized nontender lymphadenopathy. The healing primary chancre is still present in 15 percent of cases. The skin rash consists of macular, papular, papulosquamous, and occasionally pustular syphilides, often with one or more forms present simultaneously. The eruption may be very subtle, and approximately 25 percent of patients with a discernible rash of secondary syphilis may be unaware that they have dermatologic manifestations. Initial lesions are bilaterally symmetric, pale red or pink, nonpruritic, discrete, round macules, 5 to 10 mm in diameter, distributed on the trunk and proximal extremities (Fig. 128-2). After several days or weeks red, papular lesions 3 to 10 mm in diameter also appear. These

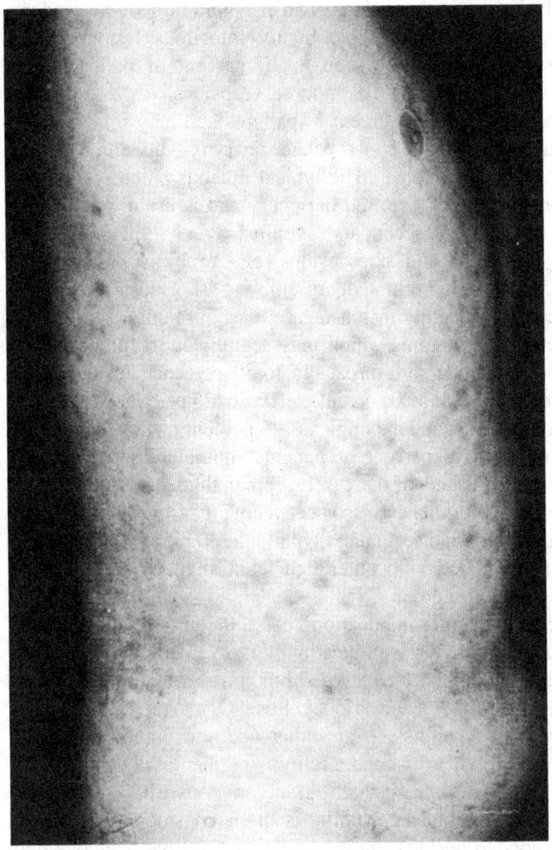

FIGURE 128-2 Maculopapular rash of secondary syphilis. *(Reprinted, with permission, from Sexually Transmitted Diseases, Prof. Dr. E. Stolz, Rotterdam, ©Boehringer Ingelheim International, 1977.)*

may progress to necrotic lesions (resembling pustules) in association with increasing endarteritis and perivascular mononuclear infiltration. These lesions are distributed widely, frequently involve the palms and soles (Fig 128-3), and may occur on the face and scalp. Tiny papular *follicular syphilides* involving hair follicles may result in patchy alopecia (alopecia areata) and loss of scalp hair, eyebrows, or beard in up to 5 percent of patients. Nonpatchy hair loss also occurs in secondary syphilis. Progressive endarteritis obliterans and ischemia result in superficial scaling of papules (*papulosquamous syphilides*) and eventually may lead to central necrosis (*pustular syphilides*). In warm, moist, intertriginous areas, including the perianal area, vulva, scrotum, and inner thighs, axillae, and the skin under

FIGURE 128-3 Secondary rash on palms and soles. [*From Ronald Roddy; reprinted, with permission, from Gynecology and Obstetrics, JW Sciarra (ed), New York, Harper & Row, 1985.*]

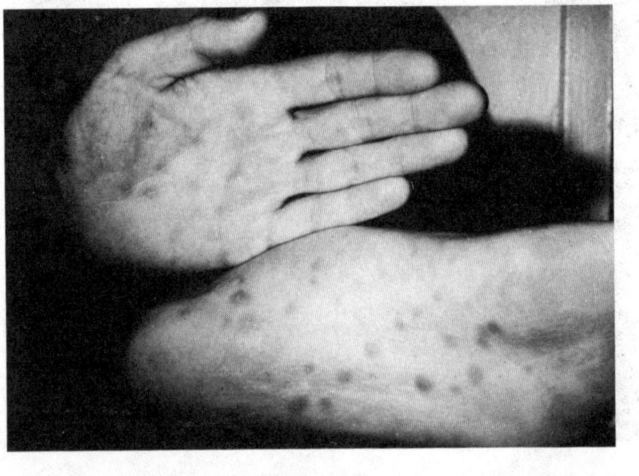

pendulous breasts, papules enlarge and become eroded, to produce broad, moist, pink or gray-white highly infectious lesions called *condylomata lata,* which are seen in 10 percent of patients with secondary syphilis. Superficial mucosal erosions, called *mucous patches,* occur in 10 to 15 percent of patients and may involve lips, oral mucosa, tongue (Fig. 128-4), palate, pharynx, vulva and vagina, glans penis, or inner prepuce. The typical mucous patch is a silver-gray erosion surrounded by a red periphery and is usually painless.

During relapses of secondary syphilis, condylomata lata are particularly common, and skin lesions tend to be asymmetrically distributed and more infiltrated, resembling skin lesions of late syphilis, perhaps reflecting increasing cellular immunity.

Constitutional symptoms which may accompany or precede secondary syphilis include sore throat (15 to 30 percent), fever (5 to 8 percent), weight loss (2 to 20 percent), malaise (25 percent), anorexia, headache (10 percent), and meningismus (5 percent). *Acute meningitis* occurs in only 1 to 2 percent of patients, but increased cells and protein have been found in the cerebrospinal fluid in 30 percent or more. *Treponema pallidum* has also been recovered from cerebrospinal fluid during primary and secondary syphilis in 30 percent of patients; this is often correlated with other CSF abnormalities, but may be seen in patients with normal CSF.

Other less common complications of secondary syphilis include hepatitis, nephropathy, gastrointestinal involvement (hypertrophic gastritis, patchy proctitis, ulcerative colitis, or a rectosigmoid mass), arthritis and periostitis, and iridocyclitis. Ocular findings which suggest secondary syphilis include otherwise unexplained pupillary abnormalities, optic neuritis, and a retinitis pigmentosa syndrome, as well as the classic iritis (especially granulomatous iritis) or uveitis. The diagnosis of secondary syphilis is often considered only after failure to respond to steroid therapy. Anterior uveitis has been reported in 5 to 10 percent of patients with secondary syphilis, and *T. pallidum* has been demonstrated in the aqueous humor from these cases. *Syphilitic hepatitis* is distinguished by an unusually high serum alkaline phosphatase and by a nonspecific histologic appearance which is unlike viral hepatitis and includes moderate inflammation with polymorphonuclear leukocytes and lymphocytes, some hepatocellular damage, and no cholestasis. The *renal involvement* is associated with proteinuria, an acute nephrotic syndrome, or rarely with hemorrhagic glomerulonephritis and is characterized by subepithelial electron-dense deposits and glomerular immune complexes, suggesting that this complication is a form of immune complex glomerulonephritis.

Latent syphilis A diagnosis of latent syphilis is established by the finding of a positive specific treponemal antibody test for syphilis, together with a normal cerebrospinal fluid examination and the absence of clinical manifestations of syphilis on physical examination and chest films. The diagnosis is often suspected on the basis of a history of primary or secondary lesions, history of exposure to syphilis, or delivery of an infant with congenital syphilis. A previous negative serologic test and a history of lesions or exposure may help establish the duration of latent infection. *Early latent* syphilis encompasses the first year after infection, while *late latent* syphilis, beginning 1 year after infection, in the untreated patient, is associated with relative immunity to infectious relapse and with increasing resistance to reinfection. *Treponema pallidum* may still intermittently seed the bloodstream during this stage; pregnant women with latent syphilis may infect the fetus in utero; and transfusion syphilis has been transmitted from patients with latent syphilis of many years' duration. It was thought that untreated late latent syphilis had three possible outcomes: (1) it could persist throughout the life of the infected individual; (2) it could end in development of late syphilis; or (3) it could end with spontaneous cure of infection, with reversion of serologic tests to negative. It is now apparent, however, that the more sensitive treponemal antibody tests rarely if ever become negative. About seventy percent of untreated patients with latent syphilis never develop clinically evident late syphilis, but the occurrence of spontaneous cure is in doubt.

FIGURE 128-4 Mucous patches on the tongue. [*From Ronald Roddy; reprinted, with permission, from Sexually Transmitted Diseases, 2d ed, KK Holmes et al (eds), New York, McGraw-Hill, 1990.*]

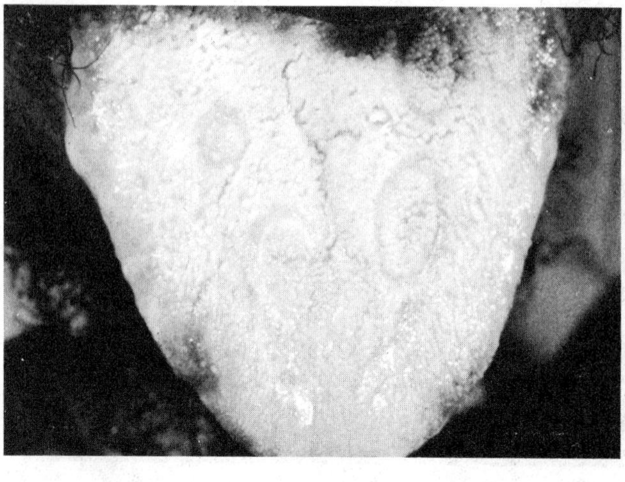

Late syphilis The onset of slowly progressive inflammatory disease leading to the tertiary stage begins early during the pathogenesis of syphilis, although it may not be clinically apparent for years. Evidence of early syphilitic aortitis is present soon after the secondary lesions subside, and it is patients who develop CSF abnormalities during the early stages of syphilis who appear to be at highest risk of late neurologic complications.

ASYMPTOMATIC NEUROSYPHILIS Central nervous system syphilis represents a continuum of early invasion, usually within the first weeks or months of infection, and asymptomatic involvement, which may or may not result in neurologic manifestations. Traditionally, the diagnosis of asymptomatic neurosyphilis has been made in patients who no longer have manifestations of primary or secondary syphilis, who lack neurologic symptoms and signs, and who have certain CSF abnormalities. Such abnormalities are found in up to one-quarter of patients with untreated late latent syphilis, and it is these patients who are known to be at risk for neurologic complications. However, evidence of CNS involvement can include isolation of *T. pallidum* from CSF even in the absence of other CSF abnormalities, and approximately 40 percent of patients with primary and secondary syphilis have had *T. pallidum* isolated from the CSF, abnormalities of the CSF consistent with asymptomatic neurosyphilis, or both. Although the therapeutic implications of these findings in early syphilis are uncertain, it seems appropriate to conclude that patients with early syphilis who have such findings do indeed have asymptomatic neurosyphilis. The risk of progression to symptomatic neurosyphilis is two or three times greater in whites than in blacks and is twice as common in men as in women. The risk of parenchymal neurosyphilis (tabes dorsalis or general paresis) is five times greater in men than in women. In patients with untreated asymptomatic neurosyphilis, the overall cumulative probability of progression to clinical neurosyphilis is about 20 percent in the first 10 years, but increases with passing time, and is highest in those who show the greatest degree of pleocytosis or protein elevation. Patients with untreated latent syphilis and normal CSF probably have no future risk of subsequently developing neurosyphilis.

SYMPTOMATIC NEUROSYPHILIS Although mixed features are common, the major clinical categories of symptomatic neurosyphilis include meningovascular and parenchymatous syphilis. The latter category includes general paresis and tabes dorsalis. The interval from infection to onset of symptoms is a few months to 12 years (average 7 years) for meningovascular syphilis, 20 years for general paresis, and 25 to 30 years for tabes dorsalis. However, many patients with symptomatic neurosyphilis, particularly in the antibiotic era, do not present a classic picture, but have mixed and subtle or incomplete syndromes. *Meningovascular syphilis* is associated with diffuse inflammation of the pia and arachnoid, together with evidence of focal or widespread arterial involvement of small, medium, or large vessels. The most common presentation is a stroke syndrome in a relatively young adult, involving the middle cerebral artery; however, unlike the usual thrombotic or embolic stroke syndrome of sudden onset, meningovascular syphilis often presents after a subacute encephalitic prodrome with headaches, vertigo, insomnia, and psychologic abnormalities followed by a gradually progressive vascular syndrome. The manifestations of *general paresis* reflect widespread parenchymal damage and include abnormalities corresponding to the mnemonic *paresis* [*p*ersonality, *a*ffect, *r*eflexes (hyperactive), *e*ye (e.g., Argyll Robertson pupils), *s*ensorium (illusions, delusions, hallucinations), *i*ntellect (decreased recent memory, orientation, calculations, judgment, insight), and *s*peech]. *Tabes dorsalis* presents symptoms and signs of demyelinization of the posterior columns, dorsal roots, and dorsal root ganglia. Symptoms include ataxic, wide-based gait and footslap, paresthesias, bladder disturbances, impotence, areflexia, and loss of position, deep pain, and temperature sensation. Trophic joint degeneration (Charcot's joints) and perforating ulceration of the feet can result from loss of pain sensation. The Argyll Robertson pupil, seen in both tabes dorsalis and paresis, is a small, irregular pupil which reacts to accommodation but not to light. *Optic atrophy* also occurs frequently in association with tabes.

CARDIOVASCULAR SYPHILIS Cardiovascular manifestations are limited to the large vessels in which the blood supply is provided by vasa vasorum. Endarteritis obliterans of the vasa vasorum produces medial necrosis with destruction of elastic tissue, particularly in the ascending and transverse segments of the aortic arch, resulting in uncomplicated aortitis, aortic regurgitation, saccular aneurysm, or coronary ostial stenosis. The onset of symptoms occurs from 10 to 40 years after infection. Cardiovascular complications are more common and occur at an earlier age in men than in women, and in blacks than in whites. The incidence of symptomatic cardiovascular complications in late untreated syphilis is approximately 10 percent, with aortic regurgitation being two to four times as common as aneurysm. However, syphilitic aortitis was demonstrated at autopsy in about one-half of black men with untreated syphilis.

Asymptomatic syphilitic aortitis may be suspected if linear calcification of the ascending aorta is demonstrated on chest x-ray films, since arteriosclerotic disease seldom produces this sign. Aortic dilatation and a tambour quality of the sound of aortic closure are unreliable signs of aortitis. Syphilitic aneurysms are usually saccular, occasionally fusiform, and do not lead to dissection. Approximately 1 in 10 aortic aneurysms of syphilitic origin may involve the abdominal aorta, but tend to occur above the renal arteries, whereas arteriosclerotic abdominal aneurysms usually are found below the renal arteries. With increasing age, the nervous system is also affected in up to 40 percent of patients with cardiovascular syphilis.

LATE LESIONS OF THE EYES Iritis associated with pain, photophobia, and dimness of vision or chorioretinitis occurs not only during secondary syphilis, but also as a relatively common manifestation of late syphilis. Adhesions of the iris to the anterior lens may produce a fixed pupil, not to be confused with Argyll Robertson pupil.

LATE BENIGN SYPHILIS (GUMMA) Gummas may be multiple or diffuse, but are usually solitary lesions which range from microscopic size to several centimeters in diameter, and histologically consist of granulomatous inflammation with central necrosis surrounded by mononuclear, epithelioid, and fibroblastic cells, occasional giant cells, and perivasculitis. Although *T. pallidum* is rarely demonstrated microscopically, it has reportedly been recovered from the lesions. The most commonly involved sites are the skin and skeletal systems, mouth and upper respiratory tract, larynx, liver, and stomach, although any organ may be involved. Gummas of skin produce painless nodular, papulosquamous, or ulcerative lesions, which are indurated, and form characteristic circles or arcs, with peripheral hyperpigmentation. The lesions are usually indolent, and may heal spontaneously with scarring, but may also be explosive in onset and are often destructive. These lesions may resemble many other chronic granulomatous conditions, including tuberculosis and sarcoidosis, leprosy, and deep fungal infections. Skeletal gummas involve long bones of the legs with greatest frequency, although any bone may be affected. Trauma may predispose to involvement of a specific site. Presenting symptoms usually include focal pain and tenderness. When sufficiently advanced to produce radiographic abnormalities, the findings may include periostitis or destructive or sclerosing osteitis. Gummas of the upper respiratory tract can lead to perforation of the nasal septum or palate. Gummatous hepatitis may produce epigastric pain and tenderness and low-grade fever, and may be associated with splenomegaly and anemia.

The histopathology and extensive tissue necrosis associated with gummas suggest that delayed hypersensitivity to *T. pallidum* produces these lesions. Certain individuals appear to develop an exaggerated delayed hypersensitivity response to *T. pallidum*, presumably mediated by sensitized T lymphocytes and macrophages. Since the histologic changes may be suggestive but are nonspecific, the diagnosis of late benign syphilis is confirmed by serologic testing and by therapeutic trial. Treatment with penicillin results in rapid healing of active gummatous lesions.

Congenital syphilis Transmission of *T. pallidum* from a syphilitic woman to her fetus across the placenta may occur at any stage of pregnancy, but the lesions of congenital syphilis develop generally after the fourth month of gestation, when immunologic competence begins to develop. This suggests that the pathogenesis of congenital syphilis may depend upon the immune response of the host rather than upon a direct toxic effect of *T. pallidum*. The risk of infection of the fetus during untreated early maternal syphilis is estimated to be 75 to 95 percent, decreasing to about 35 percent for maternal syphilis of longer than 2 years' duration, with the risk of fetal infection apparently continuing throughout late latent maternal syphilis. Adequate treatment of the mother before the sixteenth week of pregnancy should prevent fetal damage. Untreated maternal infection may result in up to 40 percent fetal loss (stillbirth is more common than abortion, because of the late onset of fetal pathology), prematurity, neonatal death, or nonfatal congenital syphilis. Of mothers with untreated syphilis of <2 years' duration, 21 percent aborted or had a stillbirth, 13 percent had infants who died within 2 months, 43 percent had infants with syphilis alive at 2 months, and 23 percent had nonsyphilitic infants. Only fulminant cases of congenital syphilis are clinically apparent in live infants at birth, and these babies have a very poor prognosis. The most common clinical problem is the healthy-appearing baby born to a mother who has a positive serologic test. Routine serologic testing in early pregnancy is considered cost effective in virtually all populations, even in areas of low prenatal prevalence of syphilis. In noncompliant individuals, rapid plasma reagin (RPR) screening should be performed when pregnancy is detected to ensure prompt treatment. Where the prevalence of syphilis is high, and in high-risk patients, syphilis serology should be repeated in the third trimester and at delivery.

The recent dramatic rise in incidence of primary and secondary syphilis in women in the United States, particularly in indigent urban black women, has been accompanied by more than a sixfold increase in congenital syphilis in infants ≤1 year of age from 107 cases in 1978 to 691 in 1988.

The manifestations of congenital syphilis can be divided into (1) early manifestations, which appear within the first 2 years of life, often between 2 and 10 weeks of age, are infectious, and resemble severe secondary syphilis in the adult; (2) late manifestations, which appear after 2 years and are noninfectious; and (3) the residual stigmata of congenital syphilis. During 1988, 92 percent of reported cases of congenital syphilis were diagnosed during the first year of life.

The earliest sign of congenital syphilis is usually rhinitis ("snuffles") soon followed by other mucocutaneous lesions. These may include bullae (syphilitic pemphigus), vesicles, superficial desquamation, petechiae, and later, papulosquamous lesions, mucous patches, and condylomata lata. The most common early manifestations are osteochondritis and osteitis, particularly involving the metaphyses of long bones, progressing in severity during the first 6 months of life, then spontaneously subsiding; and periostitis, which continues to progress after the first 6 months. Hepatosplenomegaly, lymphadenopathy, anemia, jaundice, thrombocytopenia, and leukocytosis are common. The anemia is usually hypoproliferative but may be hemolytic (paroxysmal cold hemoglobinuria due to Donath-Landsteiner antibody, an IgG antibody that binds to the P antigen of red cells at low temperatures). The nephrotic syndrome in early congenital syphilis, as in adult secondary syphilis, represents an immune complex–induced glomerulonephritis. A compilation of clinical presentations of congenital syphilis in 9 studies involving a total of 212 infants included abnormal bone x-rays (61 percent), hepatomegaly (51 percent), splenomegaly (49 percent), petechiae (41 percent), other skin rash (35 percent), anemia (34 percent), lymphadenopathy (32 percent), jaundice (30 percent), pseudoparalysis (28 percent), and snuffles (23 percent).

Neonatal congenital syphilis must be differentiated from other generalized congenital infections, including rubella, cytomegalovirus or herpes simplex virus infection, and toxoplasmosis, and also from erythroblastosis fetalis. Neonatal death is usually due to pulmonary hemorrhage, secondary bacterial infection, or severe hepatitis. Pathologic findings include interstitial and perivascular inflammation followed by variable fibroblastic proliferation, involving skin, bones, liver, kidneys, pancreas, spleen, lungs, and intestines, and by extramedullary hematopoiesis.

Late congenital syphilis is defined as congenital syphilis which remains untreated after 2 years of age. In perhaps 60 percent of cases, the infection remains subclinical, while the clinical spectrum in the remainder differs in certain respects from that of acquired late syphilis in the adult. For example, cardiovascular syphilis rarely develops in late congenital syphilis, whereas interstitial keratitis is much more common and occurs between ages 5 and 25. The onset is acute with photophobia, pain, and circumcorneal injection, followed by superficial and deep vascularization of the cornea, which progresses despite antibiotic therapy, and eventually becomes bilateral. The symptoms and signs may be suppressed with glucocorticoid therapy. Although treponemes have occasionally been demonstrated in aqueous humor in interstitial keratitis, the pathogenesis is obscure and is ascribed to "hypersensitivity." Other manifestations associated with interstitial keratitis are eighth-nerve deafness and recurrent arthropathy. Bilateral knee effusions are known as *Clutton's joints*. Examination of CSF discloses asymptomatic neurosyphilis in about one-third of untreated patients without other late clinical manifestations, and clinical neurosyphilis occurs in a quarter of untreated individuals with congenital syphilis over 6 years of age. The clinical manifestations of congenital neurosyphilis correspond to those seen in adult neurosyphilis. Gummatous periostitis occurs between ages 5 and 20 and, as in nonvenereal endemic childhood syphilis, tends to cause destructive lesions of the palate and nasal septum.

Characteristic stigmata include *Hutchinson's teeth*, the centrally notched, widely spaced, peg-shaped upper central incisors, and "mulberry" molars, sixth-year molars which have multiple, poorly developed cusps, numbering more than the usual four. The abnormal facies of congenital syphilis, which includes frontal bossing, saddlenose, and poorly developed maxilla, may also be seen in congenital ectodermal dysplasia. Saber shins, or anterior tibial bowing, are rare but were probably more common in the past when syphilitic periostitis of the anterior tibia was accompanied by vitamin D deficiency. *Rhagades* are linear scars at the angles of the mouth and nose caused by secondary bacterial infection of the early facial eruption. Other stigmata include unexplained nerve deafness, old chorioretinitis, optic atrophy, and corneal opacities due to past interstitial keratitis.

LABORATORY EXAMINATIONS **Dark-field examination technique** Dark-field examination is essential in evaluating cutaneous lesions, such as the chancre of primary syphilis, or condylomata lata of secondary syphilis. Although it is often difficult to demonstrate *T. pallidum* in dry maculopapular lesions in secondary syphilis by dark-field examination, the organism may be demonstrated by saline aspiration of lymph nodes during this stage. The surface of the suspected ulcerated lesion should be cleaned with saline and gauze, then gently abraded further with dry gauze, without production of bleeding. The lesion is then squeezed to express a serous transudate, and a drop of the transudate is picked up on the surface of a glass slide. A drop of saline (without bacteriostatic additives) may be mixed with the transudate if necessary, and this is then covered with a coverslip and examined immediately for *T. pallidum* with a dark-field or phase contrast microscope by an experienced individual. The identification of a single characteristic motile organism by a trained observer is sufficient for diagnosis. Examination of oral lesions by this method is not recommended, and it is also difficult to differentiate *T. pallidum* from other spirochetes that may be present in anal ulcers. A single negative examination does not exclude syphilis, since at least 10^4 treponemes per microliter of transudate must be present to be seen, and prior use of topical antiseptic or cleansing by the patient may obfuscate the results. Cleansing or use of topical medication should, therefore, be avoided, and ideally the dark-field examination should be repeated on three successive days before being considered negative.

Direct immunofluorescence Most syphilis is diagnosed in private physicians' offices where dark-field microscopy is not available; alternative methods for the identification of *T. pallidum* in exudate are needed. The direct fluorescent antibody *T. pallidum* (DFA-TP) test, available at central laboratories, uses fluorescein-conjugated polyclonal antitreponemal antibody for detection of *T. pallidum* in fixed smears prepared from suspect lesions. Because of cross-reactive antibodies which will also stain commensal nonpathogenic spirochetes, the antiserum is extensively absorbed with cultured treponemes in an effort to produce a specific reagent.

A refinement of this technique using a monoclonal antibody which is specific for only the pathogenic treponemes has been developed, but is not yet commercially available. It has been shown in clinical trials to be as sensitive and specific as dark-field microscopy for examination of suspicious lesions.

Demonstration of *T. pallidum* in tissue It is often necessary to demonstrate *T. pallidum* in tissue when clinical or histopathologic features suggest the diagnosis of syphilis. Although the organism can be found in tissue by appropriate silver stains, these should be interpreted with caution, because artifacts resembling *T. pallidum* are often seen. Treponemes can be demonstrated more reliably in tissue by immunofluorescence, using specific monoclonal or polyclonal antibodies against *T. pallidum*.

Serologic tests for syphilis The profusion of serologic tests for syphilis causes much unnecessary confusion. Syphilitic infection produces two types of antibodies, the nonspecific *reaginic* antibody and specific antitreponemal antibody, which are measured by the nontreponemal and treponemal tests, respectively (Table 128-1). The treponemal tests, as well as the nontreponemal tests, are reactive in persons with any treponemal infection, including yaws, pinta, and endemic syphilis.

The nontreponemal antibodies produced in syphilis contain both IgG and IgM immunoglobulins directed against a lipoidal antigen that results from the interaction of *T. pallidum* with host tissues, and possibly against a lipoidal antigen of *T. pallidum* itself. The term *reagin* is unfortunate, since the unrelated IgE antibody involved in

TABLE 128-1 Common serologic tests for syphilis

Nontreponemal (reagin) tests
- Microscopic flocculation: Venereal Disease Research Laboratory (VDRL)
- Macroscopic flocculation: rapid plasma reagin (RPR)

Treponemal tests
- Immunofluorescence: fluorescent treponemal antibody-absorption (FTA-ABS)
- Hemagglutination: *T. pallidum* hemagglutination assay (MHA-TP, HATTS, TPHA)
- Immobilization: *Treponema pallidum* immobilization (TPI)

certain allergic phenomena is also known as reagin. The most widely used nontreponemal or reagin antibody tests for syphilis are the RPR test, which can be automated (ART), and the Venereal Disease Research Laboratory (VDRL) slide test. Other less frequently used nontreponemal tests include the unheated serum reagin (USR) and the reagin screen test (RST). In these tests, antibody is detected by the microscopic (VDRL, USR) or macroscopic (RPR, RST) flocculation of the antigen suspension (Table 128-1).

The RPR is often more expensive than the VDRL test but is easier to perform and uses unheated serum; it is the test of choice for rapid serologic diagnosis in a clinic or office setting. The VDRL reagents are less expensive, but must be prepared fresh daily. Although the development of the simpler macroscopic tests has resulted in the replacement of the VDRL by the RPR for examination of serum in many laboratories, the VDRL test remains the standard test for use with cerebrospinal fluid.

RPR and VDRL tests are equally sensitive and may be used for initial screening or for quantitation of serum reagin antibody titer. The reagin titer reflects the activity of the disease: a fourfold or greater rise in titer may be seen during the evolution of primary syphilis; VDRL titers usually reach 1:32 or higher in secondary syphilis; a persistent fall in titer following treatment of early syphilis provides essential evidence of an adequate response to therapy. VDRL titers do not correspond directly to RPR titers, and sequential quantitative testing (as for response to therapy) must employ a single test.

There are three standard treponemal tests: the fluorescent treponemal antibody-absorption (FTA-ABS), the microhemagglutination assay for antibodies to *T. pallidum* (MHA-TP), and the hemagglutination treponemal test for syphilis (HATTS). A third hemagglutination test, the TPHA is not available in the United States.

For the FTA-ABS test, the patient's serum is first diluted with a substance containing nonpathogenic treponemal antigens (sorbent) to bind group-specific antibodies which may be produced against saprophytic oral and genital treponemes. The patient's absorbed serum is then placed on a slide which contains fixed *T. pallidum*. If specific antibody to *T. pallidum* is present in the patient's serum, it is bound to the dried treponemes and is then detected by the addition of fluorescein-labeled antihuman gamma globulin and subsequent examination of the slide by fluorescence microscopy. The *T. pallidum* hemagglutination tests (MHA-TP, HATTS, and TPHA) also use a sorbent-like diluent for binding treponemal group antibodies. *T. pallidum*–specific antibody is detected by agglutination of *T. pallidum*–coated sheep or turkey erythrocytes. These hemagglutination tests are more commonly used than the FTA-ABS test. The *T. pallidum* immobilization (TPI) test, in which immobilization of live *T. pallidum* is produced by immune serum plus complement, is the most specific treponemal test, but is more laborious, and in the United States is available only in research laboratories. Both the hemagglutination and FTA-ABS tests are very specific and, when used for confirmation of positive reaginic antibody tests, have a very high positive predictive value for the diagnosis of syphilis. However, even these tests give false-positive rates as high as 1 to 2 percent when used for screening normal populations.

The relative sensitivities of the VDRL, FTA-ABS, and MHA-TP tests in the various stages of syphilis are shown in Table 128-2. The nontreponemal tests are nonreactive in nearly one-third of patients with primary or late syphilis. In early primary syphilis, the detection of antibody can be maximized either by performing an FTA-ABS test or simply by repeating a VDRL test after 1 to 2 weeks if the initial VDRL was negative. However, obtaining a reagin antibody test alone is not sufficient in evaluating late symptomatic syphilis; the more sensitive FTA-ABS test should be obtained routinely in suspected late syphilis. The hemagglutination tests are even less sensitive than the reagin tests in primary syphilis, but are as sensitive as the FTA-ABS in other stages. All treponemal and nontreponemal tests are reactive during secondary syphilis, and a nonreactive result virtually excludes syphilis in a patient with otherwise compatible

TABLE 128-2 Reactivity of serodiagnostic tests in untreated syphilis

	Stage of disease, % positive*			
Test	Primary	Secondary	Latent	Tertiary
VDRL	59–87	100	73–91	37–94
FTA-ABS	86–100	99–100	96–99	96–100
MHA-TP	64–87	96–100	96–100	94–100

* Percentage figures provided should not be interpreted as absolute values because there are small numbers in certain categories and test results vary from study to study.

SOURCE: Modified (with permission) from H Jaffe, D Musher, Management of the reactive syphilis serology, in *Sexually Transmitted Diseases*, KK Holmes et al (eds) 2d ed. New York, McGraw-Hill, 1990, p 935.

mucocutaneous lesions. (Less than 1 percent of patients with secondary syphilis have a nonreactive or weakly reactive VDRL test with undiluted serum which becomes positive in higher dilutions—the *prozone* phenomenon.) While the nontreponemal tests will become negative or decline in titer following therapy for early syphilis, the treponemal tests will usually remain reactive after therapy and are not helpful in determining the infection status in persons with past syphilis.

The presence of specific IgM antibody has been proposed as a marker for active syphilis, with the claim that IgM disappears following adequate therapy. The rate at which IgM declines after therapy is quite variable from patient to patient, and the use of this criterion for cure is not universally accepted. No IgM test for syphilis has been approved for use by the Centers for Disease Control.

False-positive serologic tests for syphilis Because the antigen used in the nontreponemal tests is found in other tissues, the tests may be reactive in persons without treponemal infection, although rarely in titers exceeding 1:8. In a population which has been selected for screening because of clinical suspicion, history of exposure, or increased risk for sexually transmitted infections, the percentage of reactive tests which are falsely positive is less than 2 percent. False-positive reagin tests are classified as acute if they become negative within 6 months and may occur during a variety of acute infections, such as viral diseases, mycoplasma pneumonia, and malaria, and following certain immunizations. Chronic reactions, which persist 6 months or longer, occur in intravenous drug addiction, autoimmune diseases, and aging. False-positive reagin tests occur in 25 percent of narcotic addicts, and in 10 to 20 percent of patients with active systemic lupus erythematosus. The autoimmune nature of the false-positive reagin test is suggested by the occurrence of systemic lupus erythematosus or other connective tissue diseases in 15 to 45 percent of chronic false-positive reactors. Other antibodies which have been found with great frequency in sera from chronic false-positive reactors include antinuclear, antithyroid, and antimitochondrial antibodies, as well as rheumatoid factor and cryoglobulins. The Donath-Landsteiner antibody responsible for paroxysmal cold hemoglobinuria is an autoimmune hemolysin which appears in syphilis. The prevalence of false-positive reagin tests increases with advancing age, and 10 percent of people over 70 years of age have false-positive reactions. Other diseases associated with hyperglobulinemia, such as leprosy, may also produce chronic false-positive reactions.

In the patient with a false-positive reagin test, syphilis is excluded by obtaining a nonreactive treponemal test. A typical *reactive* FTA-ABS occurs infrequently in conditions other than syphilis. Although false-positive FTA-ABS tests have been reported in 15 percent of patients with active systemic lupus erythematosus, the fluorescent staining is often weak or has an atypical "beaded" appearance. For practical purposes, most clinicians need to be familiar with the three uses of serologic tests for syphilis: (1) for testing large numbers of sera for screening or diagnostic purposes (e.g., RPR or VDRL); (2) for quantitative measurement of reaginic antibody titer in order to assess the clinical activity of syphilis, or to follow the reagin titer in response to therapy (e.g., VDRL or RPR); and (3) for confirmation of the diagnosis of syphilis in a patient with a positive reagin antibody test or with a suspected clinical diagnosis of syphilis (e.g., FTA-ABS, MHA-TP, HATTS).

Evaluation for asymptomatic neurosyphilis Asymptomatic involvement of the central nervous system is detected by examination of cerebrospinal fluid. CSF abnormalities are very infrequent in the primary stage, but pleocytosis or elevated protein can be demonstrated in CSF from up to 40 percent of patients with secondary or latent syphilis. *T. pallidum* has been recovered by rabbit inoculation from up to 40 percent of those with secondary syphilis, but rarely from those with latent syphilis. The demonstration of *T. pallidum* in CSF is often associated with other CSF abnormalities; however, organisms can be recovered from patients without pleocytosis or elevated protein. In the prepenicillin era, the risk of developing clinical neurosyphilis was roughly proportional to the intensity of spinal fluid changes in early syphilis. CSF examination is essential in any seropositive patient with neurologic signs and symptoms and is recommended in all patients with untreated syphilis of unknown duration or of greater than 1 year's duration. The possibility that asymptomatic neurosyphilis is present in some patients with secondary and early latent disease is not addressed by these recommendations. Because standard penicillin G benzathine (benzathine benzylpenicillin) therapy for early syphilis fails to achieve treponemicidal levels in the CSF, some experts advise lumbar puncture in secondary and early latent syphilis, with follow-up examinations for patients with abnormalities.

CSF is examined for pleocytosis, increased protein concentration, and VDRL reactivity. The CSF-VDRL is very specific if the fluid is not contaminated with blood. The CSF-VDRL is relatively insensitive, however, and may be nonreactive even in progressive symptomatic neurosyphilis. Highest sensitivities are seen in meningovascular syphilis and paresis; lower sensitivities are seen in asymptomatic neurosyphilis and tabes dorsalis. The unabsorbed FTA test on cerebrospinal fluid is reactive far more often than the CSF-VDRL test in all stages of syphilis, but may reflect passive transfer of serum antibody into the CSF. Most specialists do not recommend performing an FTA test on spinal fluid. Similarly, the finding of a reactive CSF-FTA-ABS test without other cerebrospinal fluid abnormalities in a patient with nonspecific neurologic findings does not prove a diagnosis of neurosyphilis. Even in the absence of confirmatory CSF examination, a therapeutic trial of penicillin in doses adequate for neuro syphilis is warranted in any patient with a positive serum treponemal antibody test who also has neurologic findings consistent with neurosyphilis.

Attempts to identify a more sensitive and specific marker for neurosyphilis have included CSF oligoclonal banding and measurement of intrathecal production of antitreponemal IgM and IgG. CSF from 80 percent of patients with multiple sclerosis and approximately 40 percent of patients with other inflammatory CNS diseases (including neurosyphilis, bacterial meningitis, viral encephalitis, subacute sclerosing panencephalitis) have discrete oligoclonal immunoglobulin bands in the gamma globulin region following agarose gel electrophoresis of CSF. These antibodies are thought to be intrathecally produced and have specificity for the etiologic agent (e.g., *T. pallidum* in syphilis and measles virus in subacute sclerosing panencephalitis); however, an oligoclonal banding pattern per se is not specific for neurosyphilis in a seropositive patient.

Evaluation for syphilis in patients concurrently infected with human immunodeficiency virus (HIV) Because persons at highest risk for acquiring syphilis (inner city populations and homosexually active men) are also at high risk for acquisition of HIV, these infections are frequently found in the same patient. There is evidence that syphilis and other genital ulcer diseases may be important risk factors for acquisition and transmission of HIV infection. Several studies propose that the manifestations of syphilis may be altered in patients with concurrent HIV infection; and multiple cases of neurologic relapse following standard therapy have been reported in HIV-infected patients. *T. pallidum* has been isolated from the CSF of patients following therapy for early syphilis with penicillin G benzathine. One case of VDRL and FTA-ABS seronegative secondary syphilis has been reported in a patient with AIDS; this patient finally seroconverted prior to therapy after weeks of secondary manifestations. HIV-infected patients with unusually high VDRL or RPR titers have also been described. The implications of these studies are numerous and alarming, but the nature and extent of the interaction between HIV infection and syphilis has not been well defined. The frequency of unusual clinical and laboratory manifestations of syphilis in patients coinfected with HIV is unknown, and such changes may be dependent upon the stage of HIV infection and degree of immunosuppression.

The evaluation of all syphilis patients should include serologic testing for HIV, with the patient's consent. Conversely, persons with newly diagnosed HIV infection should be tested for syphilis. Examination of CSF for evidence of neurosyphilis is recommended by some authorities for all coinfected patients, regardless of the clinical stage of syphilis. If CSF abnormalities are found, or if CSF examination is not performed, therapy adequate for neurosyphilis should be administered regardless of the apparent stage of infection. Serologic testing following treatment is important for all patients with syphilis, and particularly for those also infected with HIV.

TREATMENT OF ACQUIRED SYPHILIS Penicillin G is the drug of choice for all stages of syphilis. *Treponema pallidum* is killed by very low concentrations of penicillin G, although a long period of exposure to penicillin is required for treatment because of the unusually slow rate of multiplication of the organism. The efficacy of penicillin for syphilis remains undiminished after nearly 50 years of use. Other antibiotics which are effective in syphilis include the tetracyclines, erythromycin, and the cephalosporins. Aminoglycosides and spectinomycin inhibit *T. pallidum* only in very large doses, and the sulfonamides and the quinolones are inactive. The optimal dose and duration of therapy have not been definitively established for any antimicrobial for any stage of syphilis.

It is necessary to achieve serum levels of penicillin G of 0.03 μg/mL or more for at least 7 days to cure early syphilis. Recurrence rates for a given regimen increase as infection progresses from incubating syphilis to seronegative primary to seropositive primary to secondary to late syphilis. Therefore it is probable, but unproved, that a longer duration of therapy is required to effect cure as the infection progresses. For these reasons some authorities use more prolonged penicillin therapy than that recommended by the U.S. Public Health Service when treating secondary, latent, or late syphilis.

The treatment regimens recommended for syphilis are summarized in Table 128-3 and described below.

Early syphilis Preventive (abortive, ''epidemiologic'') treatment is recommended for seronegative individuals without signs of syphilis who were exposed to infectious syphilis within the previous 6 weeks. Before treatment is given, every effort should be made to establish a diagnosis by examination and serologic testing. *The regimens recommended for preventive treatment are the same as those recommended for early syphilis.*

For patients without known exposure to syphilis but who are undergoing treatment for other STDs, most currently recommended STD regimens involving beta lactam or tetracycline antibiotics are probably also effective for very early incubating syphilis. It is likely that the regimen currently recommended for treating gonorrhea [ceftriaxone 250 mg intramuscularly followed by doxycycline or tetracycline orally for 1 week (see Chap. 110)] is effective against incubating syphilis.

Penicillin G benzathine is the most widely used form of treatment for early syphilis, including primary, secondary, and early latent syphilis, although it is more painful on injection than penicillin G procaine. A single dose of 2.4 million units cures over 95 percent of cases of primary syphilis. Because efficacy for secondary syphilis may be slightly lower, some physicians administer a second dose of 2.4 million units 1 week after the initial dose for secondary syphilis. There are reports of treatment failure following penicillin G benzathine in patients coinfected with HIV and early syphilis. Therapeutic recommendations should be guided by knowledge of CSF abnormal-

TABLE 128-3 Recommendations for therapy of syphilis*

Stage of syphilis	Patients without penicillin allergy	Patients with confirmed penicillin allergy
Primary, secondary, or early latent	Benzathine penicillin G, 2.4 million units single dose IM (1.2 million units in each buttock).	Tetracycline hydrochloride, 500 mg PO 4 times daily; or doxycycline, 100 mg PO twice daily, for two weeks.
Late latent (or latent of uncertain duration), cardiovascular, or benign tertiary	Lumbar puncture CSF normal: Benzathine penicillin G, 2.4 million units IM weekly for 3 weeks. CSF abnormal: Treat as neurosyphilis.	Lumbar puncture CSF normal: Tetracycline hydrochloride, 500 mg PO 4 times daily, or doxycycline, 100 mg PO twice daily, for 4 weeks. CSF abnormal: Treat as neurosyphilis.
Neurosyphilis† (asymptomatic or symptomatic)	Aqueous penicillin G, 12–24 million units per day IV for 10–14 days. *Or* Aqueous procaine penicillin G, 2.4 million units IM daily plus oral probenecid 500 mg 4 times each day, both for 10–14 days.	Confirm penicillin allergy by skin-testing. If confirmed, desensitize and treat with penicillin.
Syphilis in pregnancy	According to stage.	Confirm penicillin allergy by skin-testing. If confirmed, desensitize and treat with penicillin.

* See test for discussion of syphilis therapy in HIV-infected individuals.
† Some authorities recommend following these regimens with three doses of 2.4 million units of benazathine penicillin G, given IM one week apart. Benzathine penicillin G alone has given inferior results for treatment of neurosyphilis. Drugs other than penicillin are not recommended. Many patients who give a history of penicillin allergy prove negative when skin-tested for immediate hypersensitivity to penicillin and could be given aqueous crystalline penicillin G for CNS syphilis under close supervision in the hospital. Certain third generation cephalosporins (e.g., ceftriaxone, cefotaxime) have some promise for certain penicillin-allergic patients with CNS syphilis but require further evaluation.
SOURCE: These recommendations are modified from Centers for Disease Control, 1989.

ities in such patients. CSF examination in HIV-seropositive individuals with syphilis of any stage is recommended. Patients without HIV infection may also benefit from CSF examination. Some experts recommend treatment with regimens effective against neurosyphilis for all HIV-seropositive individuals with syphilis of any stage.

Late latent and late syphilis Recommended treatment for late latent syphilis with normal CSF, for cardiovascular syphilis, and for late benign syphilis (gumma) is penicillin G benzathine, 2.4 million units intramuscularly once a week for 3 successive weeks (7.2 million units total). Lumbar puncture should be performed in the evaluation of latent syphilis of more than 1 year's duration, in suspected neurosyphilis, and also in late complications other than symptomatic neurosyphilis, since asymptomatic neurosyphilis may coexist with other late complications. Abnormal cerebrospinal fluid findings can then be followed serially as a guide to therapy.

In older asymptomatic individuals, the yield of lumbar puncture is relatively low. CSF examination is most clearly indicated in the following situations: neurologic signs or symptoms; treatment failure; serum reagin titer ≥ 1:32; HIV antibody–positive; other evidence of active syphilis (e.g., aortitis, gumma, visual or hearing changes); or nonpenicillin therapy planned.

No studies of penicillin G benzathine for cardiovascular syphilis have been reported, and the efficacy of penicillin therapy in any form for cardiovascular syphilis has not been proved. The response of cardiovascular syphilis to penicillin is seldom dramatic because aortic aneurysm and aortic regurgitation cannot be reversed by antibiotic treatment, although further progression of these lesions may be arrested. In contrast, the response of benign tertiary syphilis and of meningovascular syphilis to penicillin G is usually impressive. The response of parenchymal neurosyphilis has been variable. In a cooperative study of the treatment of 1086 general paretics with penicillin, the frequency of clinical improvement or termination of progression ranged from 38 percent of those with severe involvement to 81 percent of those with mild involvement. Tabes dorsalis or optic atrophy responds less often. In general, treatment of inactive neurosyphilis in which neurologic damage has already occurred may not produce any clinical change, and retreatment of such cases is not warranted. However, persistence of cerebrospinal fluid pleocytosis, or recurrence of pleocytosis following initial response to treatment, indicates continuing active infection, which should respond to additional treatment. The 1989 Centers for Disease Control treatment guidelines for neurosyphilis are presented in Table 128-3. Because penicillin G benzathine given in doses of up to 7.2 million units to adults or 50,000 units per kilogram to infants does not produce detectable concentrations of penicillin G in cerebrospinal fluid, this form of penicillin is unreliable for the treatment of neurosyphilis in the adult or infant, and asymptomatic neurosyphilis has been found to relapse in up to one-quarter of patients treated with 2.4 million units of penicillin G benzathine. Therefore use of penicillin G benzathine alone for treatment of neurosyphilis is not recommended. On the other hand, administration of intravenous penicillin G in doses of 12 million units or more per day for 10 days or longer ensures treponemicidal concentrations of penicillin G in cerebrospinal fluid, and occasionally cures patients who failed to respond to conventional therapy. There are no data to support the use of antibiotics other than penicillin G for the treatment of neurosyphilis; however, some of the third-generation cephalosporins (e.g., ceftriaxone, cefotaxime) may deserve further evaluation. In patients with penicillin allergy documented by skin testing, desensitization may be the best course (see Chap. 90).

Management of syphilis in pregnancy Every pregnant woman should be tested with a nontreponemal test at her first prenatal visit, and women who are at high risk for acquiring sexually transmitted diseases should have a repeat test in the third trimester and at delivery. In the pregnant patient with presumed syphilis, evidenced by a reactive serology, with or without clinical manifestations, and with no history of treatment for syphilis, expeditious evaluation and initiation of treatment is essential. Therapy should be administered according to stage of the disease, as for nonpregnant patients. Patients should be warned of the risk of a Jarisch-Herxheimer reaction, which is often associated with mild premature contractions but rarely results in premature delivery.

Penicillin is the only recommended therapy for syphilis in pregnancy. If the patient has well-documented penicillin allergy, and this is confirmed by demonstration of an immediate wheal-and-flare response to skin testing with penicilloyl polylysine or penicillin G minor determinant mixture, desensitization should be carried out in a hospital using the 1989 STD guidelines issued by the Centers for Disease Control. After treatment, a quantitative reagin test should be repeated monthly throughout pregnancy, and if a fourfold rise in titer occurs, treatment should be repeated. Treated women who do not show a fourfold decrease in titer in a 3-month period should also be retreated.

Evaluation and management of congenital syphilis Newborn infants of mothers with reactive VDRL or FTA-ABS tests may themselves have reactive tests, whether or not they have become infected, because of transplacental transfer of maternal IgG antibody. Rising or persistent titers indicate infection, and the infant should be treated. If the seropositive mother received inadequate penicillin treatment or treatment other than penicillin, or her treatment status is unknown, or if the infant may be difficult to follow, the infant should be treated at birth. It is unwise to require proof of diagnosis before treatment in such cases. The CSF should be examined as a baseline before treatment of such infants. Penicillin is the only recommended drug for syphilis in infants. The calculation of penicillin dosage for treatment of late congenital syphilis is the same as that used in the infant, until dosage based upon weight reaches that used for adult neurosyphilis. Specific recommendations for treatment of infants can be found in the 1989 Centers for Disease Control treatment guidelines. Neonatal IgM antibody can be detected in cord or neonatal serums in a modified FTA-ABS test, employing fluorescein-labeled antihuman IgM to detect antitreponemal IgM antibody. However, the specificity of this test is questionable because of evidence that infants with a variety of congenital infections may produce IgM antibody to maternal allotypes of IgG (rheumatoid factor). IgM antibody detected in the IgM-FTA-ABS test may then be directed against maternal IgG antibody bound specifically to *T. pallidum,* rather than against *T. pallidum* itself. Because of the questionable sensitivity and specificity of this test, the IgM-FTA-ABS is not currently recommended. Instead, monthly quantitative reagin tests are performed on asymptomatic infants born to women who were treated adequately with penicillin during pregnancy.

Jarisch-Herxheimer reaction A dramatic reaction consisting of fever (average temperature elevation, 1.5°C), chills, myalgias, headache, tachycardia, increased respiratory rate, increased circulating neutrophil count (average total white blood cell count, 12,500 per microliter), and vasodilatation with mild hypotension, may occur following initiation of treatment for syphilis. This reaction occurs in approximately 50 percent of patients with primary syphilis, 90 percent with secondary, and 25 percent with early latent syphilis. The onset occurs within 2 h of treatment, the peak temperature occurs at about 7 h, and defervescence takes place within 12 to 24 h. The reaction is more delayed in neurosyphilis, with peak fever occurring after 12 to 14 h. In patients with secondary syphilis, an increase in erythema and edema of the mucocutaneous lesions occurs; occasionally subclinical or early mucocutaneous lesions may first become apparent during the reaction. The pathogenesis of this reaction is controversial. Patients should be warned to expect such symptoms, which can be managed by bed rest and aspirin. The Jarisch-Herxheimer reaction in neurosyphilis or cardiovascular syphilis has, on very rare occasions, been associated with acute progression of irreversible organ damage.

Follow-up evaluation of responses to therapy for all stages of syphilis The response of early syphilis to treatment should be determined by following the quantitative VDRL titer 1, 3, 6, and 12 months after treatment. More frequent serologic examination (1, 2, 3, 6, 9, and 12 months) is recommended for patients concurrently infected with HIV. Because the FTA-ABS and hemagglutination tests remain positive in nearly all patients treated for seropositive early syphilis, these tests are not useful in following the response to therapy. After successful treatment of seropositive primary or secondary syphilis, the VDRL titer progressively declines, becoming negative within 3 to 12 months in about 75 percent of seropositive primary cases and 40 percent of secondary cases. Two years after treatment for primary syphilis, nearly all patients have a negative VDRL, although 25 percent of secondary cases and a higher proportion of those treated for early latent syphilis maintain low reagin titers. If the VDRL becomes negative or reaches a fixed low titer within 1 or 2 years, performing a lumbar puncture is unnecessary at that time, since the spinal fluid examination is almost invariably normal and there is little risk of subsequent neurosyphilis. However, if a VDRL titer of 1:8 or more fails to fall at least fourfold within 12 months, if the VDRL titer rises fourfold, or if clinical symptoms persist or recur, retreatment is indicated. Every effort should be made to differentiate treatment failure from reinfection, and the CSF should be examined. Suspected treatment failures, especially those with abnormal CSF, should be treated as described for neurosyphilis. If the patient remains seropositive but asymptomatic after such retreatment, no further therapy is necessary. Patients treated for late latent syphilis frequently have a low-titered VDRL prior to therapy and may not demonstrate a fourfold drop following therapy with penicillin; about half of these patients remain seropositive in low titer for years following therapy. Retreatment is not warranted unless the titer rises or signs and symptoms of syphilis recur.

The activity of neurosyphilis correlates best with the degree of cerebrospinal fluid pleocytosis. Changes in the cerebrospinal fluid cell count, and to a lesser extent, in cerebrospinal fluid protein concentration, provide the most sensitive index of response to treatment. Spinal fluid examination should be performed every 3 to 6 months for 3 years after treatment of asymptomatic or symptomatic neurosyphilis. An elevated cerebrospinal fluid cell count falls to 10 or less per microliter within 3 to 12 months in 95 percent of adequately treated cases, and becomes normal in all cases within 2 to 4 years. Elevated levels of cerebrospinal fluid protein fall more slowly, and the CSF reagin titer declines slowly over a period of several years.

Persistence of treponemal forms The persistence of *T. pallidum* in the aqueous humor, CSF, lymph nodes, brain, inflamed temporal arteries, and other tissues following "adequate" penicillin treatment of latent or late syphilis has been suggested by dark-field microscopy, immunofluorescent antibody and silver staining techniques, and rabbit inoculation. Because the data on persisting treponemes are scanty, no modification of the treatment recommendations for latent or late syphilis seems warranted. Adherence to recommendations regarding CSF examination prior to selection of therapy should minimize the possibility of *T. pallidum* persistence.

IMMUNITY AND PREVENTION OF SYPHILIS Only about 50 percent of the named contacts of primary and secondary syphilis become infected, but the actual risk of infection from a single exposure is probably much lower. The rate of development of acquired resistance to *T. pallidum* following natural or experimental infection is quantitatively related to the amount of the antigenic stimulus, which depends upon both the size of the infecting inoculum and the duration of infection prior to treatment. The role of serum antibody in conferring immunity to syphilis remains controversial. Reagin antibody is not protective. Passively administered antibody from rabbits recovering from experimental syphilis prevents or delays appearance of clinical manifestations of syphilis; it does not prevent infection. Cellular immunity is considered to be of major importance in the healing of early lesions and control of syphilis infection. The cellular infiltration of early lesions is predominantly composed of T lymphocytes and macrophages, and specifically sensitized T lymphocytes develop early in the course of infection in humans and experimentally infected rabbits.

Inability to cultivate pathogenic treponemes in vitro has hindered analysis, purification, and concentration of treponemal antigens. Attempts to induce immunity to syphilis by vaccination have shown limited promise, although several specific antigens have been identified and characterized. The outer membrane of *T. pallidum* contains few integral membrane proteins, although many of the major antigens appear to be proteolipins, which may be associated via their lipid tail with the outer membrane. Repeated injection of rabbits with gamma-irradiated motile strains has conferred immunity to a rechallenge. The prevention of syphilis depends upon use of condoms, antiseptic prophylactic agents, and detection and treatment of infectious cases.

REFERENCES

Berry CD et al: Neurologic relapse after benzathine penicillin therapy for secondary syphilis in a patient with HIV infection. N Engl J Med 316:1587, 1987

Bryceson ADM: Clinical pathology of the Jarisch-Herxheimer reaction. J Infect Dis 133:696, 1976

Centers for Disease Control: Guidelines for the prevention and control of congenital syphilis. Morb Mort Week Rep (Suppl) 37(S-1):1, 1988

———: Recommendations for diagnosing and treating syphilis in HIV-infected individuals. Morb Mort Week Rep 37:600, 1988

———: 1989 Sexually transmitted diseases treatment guidelines. Morb Mort Week Rep 38(Suppl 8):1, 1989
Chapel T: The signs and symptoms of secondary syphilis. Sex Trans Dis 7:161, 1980
Fiumara NJ: Treatment of primary and secondary syphilis: Serologic response. JAMA 243:2500, 1980
Greene BM et al: Failure of penicillin G benzathine in the treatment of neurosyphilis. Arch Intern Med 140:1117, 1980
Hook EW III et al: Detection of *Treponema pallidum* in lesion exudate with a pathogen-specific monoclonal antibody. J Clin Microbiol 22:241, 1985
Hotson JR: Modern neurosyphilis: A partially treated chronic meningitis. West J Med 135:191, 1981
Luger A et al: Diagnosis of neurosyphilis by examination of the cerebrospinal fluid. Br J Vener Dis 57:232, 1981
Lukehart SA et al: Characterization of lymphocyte responsiveness in early experimental syphilis: II. Nature of cellular infiltration and *Treponema pallidum* distribution in testicular infection. J Immunol 124:461, 1980
——— et al: Invasion of the central nervous system by *Treponema pallidum*: Implications for diagnosis and treatment. Ann Intern Med 109:855, 1988
Mascola L et al: Congenital syphilis. Why is it still occurring? JAMA 252:17, 1984
Mohr JA et al: Neurosyphilis and penicillin in cerebrospinal fluid. JAMA 236:2208, 1976
Muller F, Moskophidis M: Estimation of the local production of antibodies to *Treponema pallidum* in the central nervous system of patients with neurosyphilis. Br J Vener Dis 59:80, 1983
Radolf JD et al: Outer membrane ultrastructure explains the limited antigenicity of virulent *Treponema pallidum*. Proc Natl Acad Sci 86:2051, 1989
Reimer CB et al: The specificity of fetal IgM: Antibody or anti-antibody? NY Acad Sci 254:77, 1975
Ross WH, Sutton HFS: Acquired syphilitic uveitis. Arch Ophthalmol 98:496, 1980
Simon RP: Neurosyphilis. Arch Neurol 42:606, 1985
Wendel GD et al: Penicillin allergy and desensitization in serious infections during pregnancy. N Engl J Med 312:1229, 1985

129 NONVENEREAL TREPONEMATOSES: YAWS, PINTA, AND ENDEMIC SYPHILIS

PETER L. PERINE

GENERAL CONSIDERATIONS Nonvenereal treponematoses occur in remote, impoverished areas of the world. Yaws, pinta, and endemic syphilis are distinguished from venereal syphilis solely by clinical and epidemiologic features. Yaws and pinta are caused by treponemes which are conventionally designated as unique species (*Treponema pertenue* causes yaws, and *T. carateum* pinta), but no significant morphologic or genetic differences have been demonstrated among *T. pertenue, T. carateum,* and *T. pallidum*. The etiologic agents of endemic syphilis and yaws are generally held to be identical with *T. pallidum* and have been designated as *T. pallidum* ssp. *endemicum* and ssp. *pertenue*, respectively. Pinta involves the skin alone; yaws affects skin and bones; and endemic syphilis involves the skin, bone, and mucous membranes. Each disease tends to progress by stages, but these are neither as distinct nor as predictable as in syphilis. Congenital infections and cardiovascular and central nervous system involvement occur rarely, if ever, in the nonvenereal treponematoses but are common in syphilis. It is unclear whether the clinical and epidemiologic differences among yaws, pinta, endemic syphilis, and venereal syphilis are solely determined by environmental and host factors or are attributable to undefined biologic differences among the causal treponemes. The relationship of the treponematoses is summarized in Table 129-1.

EPIDEMIOLOGY Treponemal antibodies are demonstrable in some proportion of nonhuman primates in regions of Africa where human yaws and endemic syphilis are common, and pathogenic treponemes have been found in skin lesions and lymph nodes of seropositive animals. These treponemes have produced yaws-like lesions in susceptible monkeys and hamsters.

Yaws and endemic syphilis are diseases of young children. Yaws occurs throughout the world between the tropics of Cancer and Capricorn, in humid, warm environments. Transmission of yaws among children is favored by scanty clothing, poor hygiene, and frequent skin trauma. Spread occurs by direct contact with infected lesions and perhaps by passive transfer of treponemes by insects. Endemic syphilis occurs in arid subtropical or temperate climates in Africa, the eastern Mediterranean, the Arabian peninsula, and central Asia. It is not observed in the western hemisphere. Skin-to-skin transmission is less important than in yaws; instead, infection of mucous membranes results from direct mouth-to-mouth contact or from contaminated fomites, such as shared drinking or eating utensils. Venereal syphilis can spread by nonvenereal contact among children and cause household outbreaks in modern cities when crowding and poverty favor transmission of *T. pallidum*.

Although cutaneous pigmentary changes resembling late stages of pinta occur in yaws or endemic syphilis, pinta is a separate, more benign disease which occurs only in the western hemisphere. The onset is typically later than in yaws or endemic syphilis, usually when the person is between 10 and 20 years of age. Pinta is not very contagious, and its mode of transmission is not well defined.

The WHO/UNICEF-assisted mass campaign for eradication of endemic nonvenereal treponematosis from 1948 to 1969 was an unusually successful public health campaign. Over 160 million people were examined in 46 countries, and approximately 50 million cases, contacts, and latent infections were treated. The impact of this program was remarkable. The prevalence of active yaws lesions was reduced from over 20 percent to less than 1 percent in many rural areas. In Bosnia, Yugoslavia, endemic syphilis was eradicated—the only example of eradication of an endemic treponematosis.

Relaxation of active surveillance activities after the mass campaigns has led to a resurgence of yaws, particularly in Africa. Yaws has not been eradicated in any large area. The Ivory Coast, Ghana, Togo,

TABLE 129-1 Etiology, epidemiology, and clinical manifestations of the treponematoses

	Venereal syphilis	Endemic syphilis	Yaws	Pinta
Organism	*T. pallidum* ssp. *pallidum*	*T. pallidum* ssp. *endemicum*	*T. pallidum* ssp. *pertenue*	*T. carateum*
Transmission	Sexual, transplacental*	Household contacts: mouth-to-mouth or via drinking, eating utensils	Skin-to-skin ? Insect vector	Skin-to-skin ? Insect vector
Usual age	Adult	Early childhood	Early childhood	Adolescent
Primary lesion	Cutaneous ulcer (chancre)	Rarely seen	Framboise (raspberry), or "mother yaw"	Nonulcerating papule with satellites
Secondary lesion	Mucocutaneous; occasional periostitis	Florid mucocutaneous lesions (mucous patch, split papule, condyloma latum); osteoperiostitis	Cutaneous papulosquamous lesions; osteoperiostitis	Pintides
Tertiary	Gumma, cardiovascular, and CNS lues	Destructive cutaneous osteoarticular gummas	Destructive cutaneous osteoarticular gummas	Dyschromic, achromic macules

* Since the nonvenereal treponematoses are usually acquired in childhood and treponemal bacteremia ceases with time, only in adult-onset venereal syphilis is there any likelihood of a mother giving birth to an infected child.

and Benin have large reservoirs of yaws and account for over 90 percent of cases reported to WHO since 1982. North of these countries, the Sahelian nations of Mali, Niger, Burkina Faso, and Senegal have prevalence rates in some areas of 10 to 15 percent for endemic syphilis. These rates exceed those reported before the mass treatment campaigns. Seroactivity and late manifestations of endemic syphilis continue to occur among nomads in Saudi Arabia. The resurgence of yaws and endemic syphilis led to a new yaws campaign in Ghana in 1980, and other national campaigns are planned to control resurgent yaws and endemic syphilis in Africa.

Antitreponemal and reaginic seroreactivity has been detected in a small percentage of children without clinical disease born after the mass campaigns in some areas (e.g., Nigeria, New Guinea, and Bosnia). This may represent attenuated or asymptomatic infection, or may simply reflect the decreased predictive value of serologic tests (probability that disease is present if the test is positive) when the prevalence of disease is sharply reduced.

In the Americas, foci of yaws persist in Haiti; Dominica, St. Lucia, and St. Vincent; Peru, Colombia, and Ecuador; a few areas of Brazil; and Guyana and Surinam. Pinta is confined to Central America and northern South America, where it appears to have regressed to remote Indian villages. Its prevalence today is probably less than 1 percent of that found 20 years ago.

BIOLOGIC RELATIONSHIPS Specific humoral antibodies to *T. pallidum* are produced in individuals with yaws, pinta, or endemic syphilis, but the time of appearance of antibodies after onset of infections is variable. The fluorescent treponemal antibody absorption (FTA-ABS) test, the *T. pallidum* hemagglutination test (TPHA), and the *T. pallidum* immobilization (TPI) test cannot differentiate among the treponematoses.

In addition to the clinical and epidemiologic differences among the treponematoses in humans, the range of susceptible animal hosts and some manifestations of experimental infection are also different. In particular, *T. carateum* has produced an infection in chimpanzees which resembles pinta, but attempts to infect other experimental animals have been unsuccessful. Individuals who have had yaws or pinta are considered relatively immune to syphilis, and persons with active pinta or syphilis cannot be superinfected with *T. pallidum* ssp. *pertenue* by experimental inoculation.

CLINICAL MANIFESTATIONS Yaws Also known as pian, framboesia, or bubas, yaws is a chronic infectious disease of childhood caused by *T. pallidum* ssp. *pertenue*. The disease is characterized by an initial skin lesion(s) followed by relapsing, nondestructive, secondary lesions of skin and bone. In the late stages, destructive lesions of skin, bone, and joints occur.

The incubation period following experimental inoculation of susceptible human beings is 3 to 4 weeks. Disruption of the skin by insect bites, abrasions, or injuries promotes acquisition of natural infection from infected contacts, most likely by fingers contaminated directly or indirectly with material from early yaws lesions. The initial early lesion is a single papule which is usually located on a leg. The lesion enlarges and becomes papillomatous (Fig. 129-1). This lesion also is known as a framboesioma (raspberry) or "mother yaw." It becomes superficially eroded and covered by a thin yellow crust of serous exudate containing *T. pertenue*. Erythema and induration do not occur. The lesion is mildly pruritic, and regional lymphadenopathy occurs. The initial lesion usually heals in 6 months. As a result of treponemal bacteremia and autoinoculation, a generalized secondary eruption of similar lesions appears either before or after the initial lesion has healed and is most extensive on the exposed surfaces of the body. These early cutaneous lesions of yaws have a variety of forms, including desquamative macular and papular as well as papillomatous types. Painful papillomata on the soles of the feet result in a crablike gait referred to as "crab yaws." Early lesions are infectious and heal slowly; they may result in scarring, hyperpigmentation, or depigmentation, resembling the pigmentary changes seen in pinta. Histologic findings are mononuclear-cell infiltration, acanthosis, hyperkeratosis, and the presence of many treponemes.

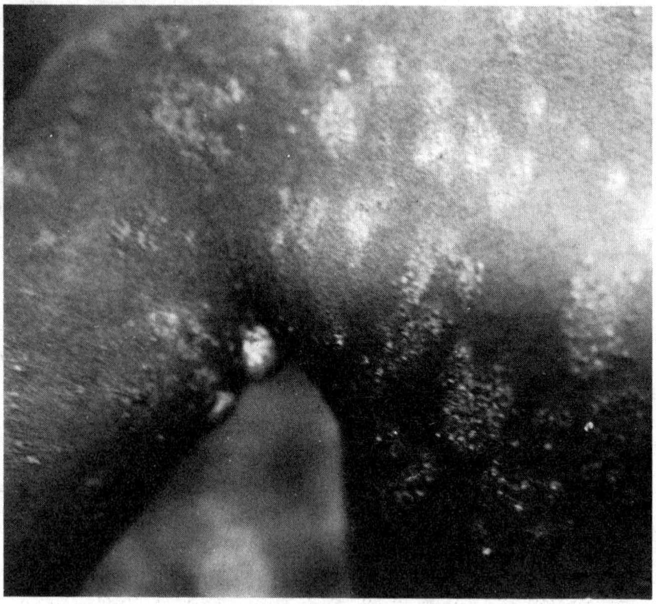

FIGURE 129-1 Young man with squamous micropapules of early yaws with papillomas in the left axilla and scapular area.

Other manifestations of early yaws include lymphadenopathy and nocturnal bone pain and polydactylitis due to periostitis. Fever and other constitutional symptoms are rare, however, unless lesions become secondarily infected. Infectious cutaneous relapses are characteristic during the first 5 years after infection. Late yaws lesions occur in about 10 percent of cases, starting 5 years or more after infection, and differ histologically from early lesions in showing endarteritis. Late lesions include gummas of the skin and long bones, particularly of the legs, hyperkeratoses of the soles and palms, osteitis, periostitis, juxtaarticular fibromatous nodes, and hydrarthrosis.

Late lesions of yaws are characteristically extensive and usually destructive. Destruction of the nose, maxilla, palate, and pharynx, termed *gangosa*, or *rhinopharyngitis mutilans*, occurs in late yaws, as well as in leprosy and leishmaniasis. Hypertrophic paranasal maxillary osteitis produces distinctive facies known as *goundou*.

The clinical features of yaws have become less reliable for diagnosis as the prevalence of yaws has decreased, necessitating the use of easily performed serologic tests, such as the rapid plasma reagin (RPR) card test. *T. pertenue* can be demonstrated by dark-field examination in early cutaneous lesions but should not be confused with other spirochetes found in tropical ulcers. The serum reagin antibody tests become positive after 1 month, and the FTA-ABS test is also positive.

Endemic syphilis Synonyms for endemic syphilis are Bejel, Siti, Dichuchwa, Njovera, and Skerljevo. It is a chronic nonvenereal, treponemal infection of childhood, characterized by early mucous membrane or mucocutaneous lesions, a latent period of indeterminate duration, and late complications including gummas of bone and skin. The causative organism is indistinguishable from *T. pallidum*. Endemic syphilis differs from congenital syphilis in that dental changes, interstitial keratitis, and neurosyphilis rarely, if ever, occur. Cardiovascular complications are considered rare in both endemic and congenital syphilis.

Primary cutaneous lesions are infrequent and when present are extragenital. The earliest manifestation of endemic syphilis is usually an intraoral mucous patch or mucocutaneous lesion resembling the split papules or condylomata of secondary syphilis. Periostitis is common. Regional lymphadenopathy occurs, but generalized lymphadenopathy is unusual. Treponemes are abundant in the moist early lesions and in aspirates from regional lymph nodes. After a variable latent period, late lesions may develop and are the most frequent clinical manifestations. These resemble the lesions of late benign syphilis and include osseous or cutaneous gummas. Destructive gummas, osteitis, and gangosa are more common than in late yaws. Gummas occur on the nipples of mothers who have themselves previously had endemic syphilis and who breastfeed infants with oral lesions. Both early and late forms of endemic syphilis thus may coexist in the same family. The tertiary lesions of endemic syphilis sometimes may be a consequence of repeated exposure of a previously sensitized host to reinfection.

Pinta Also known as mal del pinto, carate, azul, or purupuru, pinta is an infectious disease of the skin caused by *T. carateum*. This disease has three cutaneous stages characterized by marked changes in the skin color, does not involve osseous tissue or viscera, and causes no disability other than that associated with cosmetic disfigurement.

The initial lesion is a small papule which appears 7 to 30 days after exposure and is located most often on the extremities, face, neck, or buttocks. It increases in size slowly by peripheral extension and by coalescing with smaller satellite papules. Regional lymphadenopathy occurs. A secondary eruption not associated with generalized lymphadenopathy appears 1 month to 1 year after the appearance of the initial lesion. The secondary lesions are termed *pintides*, may be numerous, and evolve into a psoriatic or circinate configuration. Pintides are initially red but become deeply pigmented, reaching a slate-blue color after a period of time which is related to exposure to sun. Pigmentation occurs most rapidly on the exposed parts of the body. These pigmented lesions are known as dyschromic macules and contain treponemes which are located principally in the epidermis in older lesions. Histologically there is deposition of pigment in the dermis with decreased melanin pigment in the basal cell layer. Within 3 months to a year, most of the pintides show varying degrees of depigmentation, becoming brown and finally white and giving the skin a mottled appearance. The porcelain-white achromic lesions represent the "late" stage of the disease in which the epidermis is atrophic, and melanocytes and melanin are absent. *T. carateum* can be demonstrated in transudates from initial, early secondary, or dyschromic lesions. Reaginic and antitreponemal antibody tests are positive, but may take four times longer to become positive in pinta than in venereal syphilis.

TREATMENT Treatment is similar for all the endemic treponematoses. Intramuscular injection of 2.4 million units of benzathine penicillin G in adults and half this dose in children results in rapid resolution of lesions and prevents recurrence. Procaine penicillin G in oil and 2% aluminum monostearate (PAM) has been used extensively. In persons who are allergic to penicillin, tetracycline hydrochloride in a dose similar to that used for infectious syphilis (see Chap. 128) is effective. In areas where less than 5 percent of the population has active disease, cases are managed on an individual basis, and all contacts of infected persons are treated with antibiotics.

PREVENTION Although the nonvenereal treponematoses are less amenable to eradication than smallpox, the resurgence of yaws has led some authorities to suggest that the application of *selective epidemiologic control* as used in smallpox eradication be applied to yaws control. This strategy would emphasize ongoing active surveillance, investigation of outbreaks, and treatment of active cases and their contacts rather than mass treatment.

REFERENCES

BURKE JP et al (eds): International symposium on yaws and other endemic treponematoses. Rev Infect Dis 7:S217, 1985

FOHN MJ et al: Specificity of antibodies from patients with pinta for antigens of *T. pallidum* ssp. *pallidum*. J Infect Dis 157:32, 1988.

GUTHE T: Clinical, serological and epidemiological features of framboesia tropica (yaws) and its control in rural communities. Acta Derm Venereol 49:343, 1969

HOPKINS DR: Yaws in the Americas, 1950–1975. J Infect Dis 136:548, 1977

PERINE PL et al: *Handbook of Endemic Treponematoses*. WHO, Geneva, 1984

Treponematoses Research: Report of a WHO Scientific Group, WHO Technical Report Series 674, 1982

WORLD HEALTH ORGANIZATION: Endemic treponematoses. Week Epidem Rec 61:198, 1986

130 LEPTOSPIROSIS

JAY P. SANFORD

DEFINITION *Leptospirosis* is a term applied to disease caused by all leptospiras regardless of specific serotype. Correlation of clinical syndromes with infection by differing serotypes leads to the conclusion that a single serotype of *Leptospira* may be responsible for a variety of clinical features; conversely, a single syndrome, e.g., aseptic meningitis, may be caused by multiple serotypes. Hence there is a preference for the general term leptospirosis rather than the synonyms such as Weil's disease and canicola fever.

ETIOLOGY The genus *Leptospira* contains only one species, *L. interrogans*, which may be subdivided into two complexes, interrogans and biflexa. The interrogans complex includes the pathogenic strains, while the biflexa complex includes saprophytic strains. Within each complex the organisms show antigenic variations that are stable and allow them to be classed as serotypes (serovars). Serotypes with common antigens are arranged in serogroups (varieties). Despite contrary common usage, an example of the correct designation of *Leptospira* is as follows: Pomona serogroup of *L. interrogans* or *L. interrogans* var. pomona, not *L. pomona*. The interrogans complex now contains about 170 serotypes arranged in 18 serogroups (the number in parentheses refers to number of serotypes within the serogroup): Icterohemorrhagiae (18), Hebdomadis (30), Autumnalis (17), Canicola (12), Australis (12), Tarassovi (17), Pyrogenes (12), Bataviae (10), Javanica (8), Pomona (8), Ballum (3), Cynopteri (3), Celledoni (3), Grippotyphosa (5), Panama (2), Shermani (1), Ranarum (2), and Bufonis (1). At least 27 serotypes of *Leptospira* occur naturally in the United States.

EPIDEMIOLOGY Leptospirosis is thought to be the most widespread zoonosis in the world. Cases are regularly reported from all continents except Antarctica and are especially prevalent in the tropics. Although leptospirosis is not a common disease, it has been reported from all regions of the United States including arid areas such as Arizona. Between 1985 and 1988, 41 to 57 cases were reported annually. Infection in humans is an incidental occurrence and is not essential to the maintenance of leptospirosis. The disease occurs in a wide range of domestic and wild animal hosts, including poikilothermic vertebrates. In many species, such as opossums, skunks, raccoons, and foxes, infectivity ratios in the range of 10 to 50 percent are not unusual. Interspecies spread of specific serotypes of leptospiras between animal hosts is frequent, e.g., Pomona, a serotype principally associated with livestock, has been demonstrated in dogs. Infection in animals may vary from inapparent illness to severe fatal disease. Even asymptomatic animals may carry high numbers ($>10^{10}$ organisms per gram) in their kidneys. The carrier state, in which the host may shed leptospiras in its urine for months to years, may develop in many animals. Immunization of dogs may not prevent the carrier, or shedder, state.

Survival of pathogenic leptospiras in nature is governed by factors including pH of the urine of the host, pH of soil or water into which they are shed, and ambient temperature. Leptospiras in most "urine spots" in soil retain infectivity for 6 to 48 h. Acid urine permits only limited survival; however, if the urine is neutral or alkaline and is shed into a similar moist environment which has low salinity, is not badly polluted with microorganisms or detergents, and has a temperature above 22°C, leptospiras may survive for several weeks. Human infections can occur either by direct contact with urine or tissue of an infected animal or indirectly through contaminated water, soil, or vegetation. The usual portals of entry in humans are abraded skin, particularly about the feet, and exposed conjunctival, nasal, and oral mucous membranes. The previously held concept that organisms could penetrate intact skin has been questioned. While leptospiras have been isolated from ticks, these arthropods appear to be unimportant in transmission.

With the ubiquitous infection of animals, leptospirosis in human beings can occur in all age groups, at all seasons, and in both sexes. However, it is primarily a disease of teenage children and young adults (about one-half of patients are between the ages of 10 and 39), occurs predominantly in males (80 percent), and develops most frequently in hot weather (in the United States one-half of infections occur from July to October). The wide spectrum of animal hosts results in both urban and rural human disease. Leptospirosis has been considered an occupational disease; however, improved methods of rat control and better standards of hygiene have reduced the incidence among occupational groups such as coal miners and people who work in sewers. The epidemiologic pattern has changed; in the United States and the United Kingdom, water-associated and cattle-associated leptospirosis is most common. Less than 20 percent of patients have had direct contact with animals; they are mostly farmers, trappers, or abattoir workers. In the majority of patients exposure is incidental; two-thirds of cases occur in children, students, or housewives. Swimming or partial immersion in contaminated water, e.g., riding motorcycles through contaminated pools of water, has been implicated in one-fifth of patients and has accounted for most of the recognized common-source outbreaks. In Hawaii, one-fourth of cases have been associated with aquaculture industries, while in Italy leptospirosis remains common in the rice-growing areas of the Po River Valley.

PATHOLOGY In patients who have died with hepatorenal involvement (Weil's syndrome), the significant gross changes include hemorrhages and bile staining of tissues. The hemorrhages, which vary from petechial to ecchymotic, are widespread and are most prominent in skeletal muscle, kidneys, adrenals, liver, stomach, spleen, and lungs.

In skeletal muscle, focal, necrotic, and necrobiotic changes typical of leptospirosis occur. Biopsies early in the illness demonstrate swelling and vacuolation. Leptospiral antigen has been demonstrated in these lesions by the fluorescent antibody technique. Healing ensues by the formation of new myofibrils with minimal fibrosis. The renal lesions in the acute phase involve predominantly the tubules and vary from simple dilatation of distal convoluted tubules to degeneration, necrosis, and basement membrane rupture. Interstitial edema and cellular infiltrates consisting of lymphocytes, neutrophilic leukocytes, histiocytes, and plasma cells are uniformly present. Glomerular lesions either are absent or consist of mesangial hyperplasia and focal foot process fusion which are interpreted as representing nonspecific changes associated with acute inflammation and protein filtration. Microscopic alterations in the liver are not diagnostic and correlate poorly with the degree of functional impairment. The changes include cloudy swelling of parenchymal cells, disruption of liver cords, enlargement of Kupffer cells, and bile stasis in biliary canaliculi. The changes in the brain and meninges are also minimal and are not diagnostic. Microscopic evidence of myocarditis has been recorded. Pulmonary findings consist of a patchy, localized hemorrhagic pneumonitis. Special staining techniques utilizing silver impregnation methods have demonstrated organisms in the lumina of renal tubules but rarely in other organs.

CLINICAL MANIFESTATIONS General features The incubation period following immersion or accidental laboratory exposure has shown extremes of 2 to 26 days, the usual range being 7 to 13 days and the average 10 days.

Leptospirosis is a typically biphasic illness. *During the leptospiremic* or *first phase,* leptospiras are present in the blood and cerebrospinal fluid. The onset is typically abrupt, and initial symptoms include headache, which is usually frontal, less often retroorbital, but occasionally may be bitemporal or occipital. Severe muscle aching occurs in most patients, the muscles of the thighs and lumbar areas being most prominently involved, and often is accompanied by severe pain on palpation. The myalgia may be accompanied by extreme cutaneous hyperesthesia (causalgia). Chills followed by a rapidly rising temperature are prominent. Following the abrupt onset, the leptospiremic phase typically lasts 4 to 9 days. Features during this interval include recurrent chills, high spiking temperatures [usually 38.9°C (102°F) or greater], headache, and continued severe myalgia. Involvement of one organ system may predominate, often leading to initial misdiagnosis. Such symptom complexes most commonly include hepatitis, nephritis, atypical pneumonia, influenza, or "viral" gastroenteritis. Anorexia, nausea, and vomiting are encountered in one-half or more of the patients. Occasional patients have diarrhea. Pulmonary manifestations, usually either cough or chest pain, have varied in frequency of occurrence from less than 25 percent to 86 percent. Hemoptysis occurs but is rare. Examination during this phase reveals an acutely ill, febrile patient, with a relative bradycardia and normal blood pressure. Disturbances in sensorium may be encountered in up to 25 percent of patients. Transient cerebral ischemic attacks in children associated with leptospiral arteritis have been reported from China.

The most characteristic physical sign is conjunctival suffusion, which usually first appears on the third or fourth day. It may be lacking in some patients but more often is overlooked. It may be associated with photophobia, but serous or purulent secretion is unusual. Less common findings may include pharyngeal injection, cutaneous hemorrhages, and skin rashes that are usually macular, maculopapular, or urticarial and usually occur on the trunk. Uncommon findings are splenomegaly, hepatomegaly, lymphadenopathy, or jaundice. The first phase terminates after 4 to 9 days, usually with defervescence and improvement in symptoms. This coincides with the disappearance of leptospiras from the blood and cerebrospinal fluid.

The second phase has been characterized as the "immune" phase and correlates with the appearance of circulating IgM antibodies; the concentration of C3 in serum remains normal. The clinical manifestations of this phase show greater variability than those during the first phase. After a relatively asymptomatic period of 1 to 3 days, the fever and earlier symptoms recur and meningismus may develop. The fever rarely exceeds 38.9°C (102°F) and is usually of 1 to 3 days' duration. It is not uncommon for fever to be absent or quite transient. Even when symptoms or signs of meningeal irritation are absent, routine examination of cerebrospinal fluid after the seventh day has revealed pleocytosis in 50 to 90 percent of patients. Less common features include iridocyclitis, optic neuritis, and other nervous system manifestations, including encephalitis, myelitis, and peripheral neuropathy. Leptospirosis during pregnancy may be associated with an increased risk of fetal loss.

Specific features WEIL'S SYNDROME Weil's syndrome, which may be due to serotypes other than Icterohemorrhagiae, is defined as severe leptospirosis with jaundice, usually accompanied by azotemia, hemorrhages, anemia, disturbances in consciousness, and continued fever. There is uncertainty as to the pathogenesis of the syndrome, i.e., whether it represents direct toxic damage due to leptospiras or whether it is the consequence of immune response to leptospiral antigens. The consensus favors toxic damage.

The onset and first stage are identical with the less severe forms of leptospirosis. The distinctive features of Weil's syndrome appear from the third to the sixth days but do not reach their peak until well into the second stage. As in milder forms of leptospirosis, there is a tendency for defervescence about the seventh day; however, with recurrence, fever is marked and may persist for several weeks. Either renal or hepatic manifestations may predominate. Hepatic disturbances include tenderness in the right upper quadrant and hepatic enlargement, both of which are common when jaundice is present. Serum glutamic oxaloacetic transaminase (SGOT) values are rarely increased more than fivefold regardless of the degree of hyperbilirubinemia, which is predominantly conjugated. The predominant mechanism appears to be an intracellular block to bilirubin excretion.

HEMORRHAGIC FEVER WITH RENAL SYNDROME Studies on the epidemiology of Hantavirus (Chap. 148) have shown that for the initial 24 to 72 h there is significant overlap in the clinical features of leptospirosis, hemorrhagic fever with renal syndrome (HFRS), and scrub typhus (H.W. Lee, personal communication). In Korea, where all three diseases are prevalent, of the blood samples submitted for

Hantavirus serology 21 percent had antibody to *Leptospira* antigens and 6 percent to *Rickettsia tsutsugamushi*. Conversely, among 261 patients in Singapore clinically suspected of having leptospirosis, 3 percent had serologic evidence of Hantavirus infection. Hantavirus disease, which varies from mild (nephropathica epidemica) to severe (Balkan nephropathy), is common in Europe and Scandinavia. Because of the similarity in epidemiology and clinical presentation and the potential for dual infections, it has been recommended that blood be submitted for Hantavirus serology in all cases of suspected leptospirosis. Clinically the term *lepthangamushi syndrome* has been used to describe this overlap syndrome.

Renal manifestations of Weil's syndrome consist primarily of proteinuria, pyuria, hematuria, and azotemia. Dysuria is rare. Serious renal damage usually occurs in the form of acute tubular necrosis associated with oliguria. The peak elevation of blood urea nitrogen usually is seen on the fifth to seventh day. Hemorrhagic manifestations are most prevalent in this group of patients and include epistaxis, hemoptysis, gastrointestinal bleeding, hemorrhage into the adrenal glands, hemorrhagic pneumonitis, and subarachnoid hemorrhage. These have been explained on the basis of diffuse vasculitis with capillary injury. In addition, in some patients hypoprothrombinemia and thrombocytopenia have been observed.

ATYPICAL PNEUMONIA SYNDROME Pulmonary symptoms and signs are common in patients with leptospirosis; even the adult respiratory distress syndrome (ARDS) has been reported. While not fully appreciated in the United States, in other parts of the world leptospirosis is recognized as an important differential diagnostic consideration in the patient with fever, chills, headache, severe myalgia, and bilateral bronchopneumonia, with or without an associated "active" urine sediment. In Italy, respiratory or influenza-like symptoms were the only clinical signs of illness in 21 percent of over 300 patients with confirmed leptospirosis. Of 15 patients with leptospirosis reported from the Republic of Korea, 5 presented with bilateral pulmonary infiltrates. Given appropriate epidemiologic circumstances, leptospirosis should be added to the differential diagnosis of "atypical" pneumonia.

ASEPTIC MENINGITIS A leptospiral etiology has been incriminated in 5 to 13 percent of sporadic cases of aseptic meningitis. Pleocytosis is not present before the immune phase, but then develops rapidly. There are usually tens to hundreds of leukocytes, occasionally 1000, per microliter, among which neutrophils or mononuclear cells may predominate. CSF glucose concentration is almost always normal, but occasional instances of lowered glucose levels have been recorded. CSF protein may exceed 1 g/L (100 mg/dL) early in the course. Xanthochromic cerebrospinal fluid has been observed in the presence of jaundice. Each of the serotypes of leptospiras that are pathogenic for humans is probably capable of causing aseptic meningitis. The most prevalent serotypes have been Canicola, Icterohemorrhagiae, and Pomona.

MYOCARDITIS Cardiac arrhythmias including paroxysmal atrial fibrillation, atrial flutter, ventricular tachycardia, and premature ventricular contractions have been described but are usually of little clinical significance. However, on rare occasions definite cardiac dilatation with acute left ventricular failure has been observed. Associated manifestations have included jaundice, pulmonary infiltrates, arthritis, and skin rashes. The serotypes thus far incriminated have included Icterohemorrhagiae, Pomona, and Grippotyphosa.

CHILDREN Several clinical features which are not seen or are very rare in adults occur in children: hypertension, acalculous cholecystitis (five of nine children in one series), pancreatitis, abdominal causalgia, and peripheral desquamation of a rash that may be associated with gangrene and cardiopulmonary arrest. The features of desquamation, myocardial involvement, and hydrops of the gallbladder suggest Kawasaki syndrome [mucocutaneous lymph node syndrome (see Chap. 63)].

LABORATORY FEATURES Leukocyte counts vary from leukopenic levels to mild elevations in the anicteric patients. In patients with jaundice, leukocytosis as high as 70,000 cells per microliter may be present. However, regardless of the total leukocyte count, neutrophilia of greater than 70 percent is very frequently encountered during the first stage.

Hemolytic substances have been demonstrated in cultures of pathogenic leptospiras. In contrast to many hemolysins of bacterial origin which are not hemolytic in vivo, the leptospiral hemolysins appear to be active in vivo. In patients with jaundice, anemia may be severe and is most characteristically due to intravascular hemolysis. Other mechanisms of anemia include azotemia and blood loss secondary to hemorrhage. Anemia due to leptospirosis is unusual in anicteric patients.

Thrombocytopenia sufficient to be associated with bleeding (less than 30,000 platelets per microliter) may be encountered. Additional hematologic abnormalities include elevation of the erythrocyte sedimentation rate in over one-half of patients (usually less than 50 mm/h).

Urinalysis during the leptospiremic phase reveals mild proteinuria, casts, and an increase in cellular elements. In anicteric infections, these abnormalities rapidly disappear after the first week. Proteinuria and abnormalities in the urine sediment usually are not associated with elevations in blood urea nitrogen. Since the anicteric form of the disease often has gone undiagnosed, estimates of the frequency of azotemia and jaundice are probably high. Azotemia has been reported in approximately one-fourth of patients. In three-fourths of these patients, the blood urea nitrogen is less than 36 mmol/L (100 mg/dL). Azotemia is usually associated with jaundice. The serum bilirubin levels may reach 1110 μmol/L (65 mg/dL); however, in two-thirds of patients the levels are less than 340 μmol/L (20 mg/dL). During the first phase, one-half of the patients have increased serum creatine phosphokinase (CK) levels, with mean values of five times normal. Such increases are not seen in viral hepatitis, and a slight increase in transaminase with a definite increase in CK suggests leptospirosis rather than viral hepatitis.

DIAGNOSIS Diagnosis is based upon culture of the organism or serologic proof of its existence. The most common initial diagnostic impressions in patients with leptospirosis are meningitis, hepatitis, nephritis, fever of undetermined origin (FUO), influenza, Kawasaki syndrome, toxic shock syndrome, and Legionnaires' disease. Leptospiras may be isolated quite readily during the first phase from blood and cerebrospinal fluid or during the second phase from the urine. Leptospiras may be excreted in the urine for up to 11 months after the onset of illness and may persist despite antimicrobial therapy. Whole blood should be inoculated immediately into tubes containing semisolid medium, such as Fletcher's or EMJH medium. If culture medium is not available, leptospiras reportedly will remain viable up to 11 days in blood to which anticoagulants, preferably sodium oxalate, have been added. Animal inoculation (preferably either suckling hamsters or guinea pigs) may be used and is of particular value if specimens are contaminated. Direct examination of blood or urine by dark-field methods has been employed; *however, this method so frequently results in failure or misdiagnosis that it should not be employed.* Serologic methods are applicable during the second phase; antibodies appear from the sixth to the twelfth days of illness. Two serologic methods are commonly used: a macroscopic or slide agglutination test which is easy to perform but lacks specificity and sensitivity, and hence is suitable for screening only, and the microscopic agglutination test, which is more complicated but also more specific. An IgM-specific dot-ELISA (enzyme-linked immunosorbent assay) has been effective in diagnosing leptospirosis in an endemic area. Serologic criteria for diagnosis include a fourfold or greater rise in titer during the course of illness. Cross-agglutination reactions between various serotypes commonly occur so that the infection serotype often cannot be determined with certainty without isolation of leptospiras.

PROGNOSIS The prognosis is dependent upon both the virulence of the organism and the general condition of the patient. The mortality rate in reported cases in the United States has varied annually between 2.5 and 16.4 percent, averaging 7.1 percent. Age is the most significant host factor related to increased mortality. In a representative series, the mortality rate rose from 10 percent in men less than 50 years of age to 56 percent in those over 51 years of age. The virulence of the infecting leptospiras correlates best with the development of jaundice. In anicteric patients, mortality is extremely rare, but with the development of jaundice, the mortality rate in various series has ranged from 15 to 48 percent. The long-term prognosis following the acute renal lesion of leptospirosis is good. Glomerular filtration rates have returned to normal, usually within 2 months; however, a few patients show residual tubular dysfunction such as a defect in concentrating capacity.

TREATMENT A variety of antimicrobial drugs, including penicillin, streptomycin, the tetracycline congeners, chloramphenicol, and erythromycin, have been effective in vitro and in experimental leptospiral infections. Data concerning the efficacy of antibiotics in human beings have been conflicting. Within 4 to 6 h after initiation of penicillin G therapy, a Jarisch-Herxheimer type of reaction, which suggests antileptospiral activity, may occur. A controlled trial of intravenous penicillin (1.5 million units every 6 h for 7 days) clearly demonstrated shortening of duration of fever and creatinine elevation, shortening of hospitalization, and prevention of leptospiruria, even when treatment was started after the fifth day of illness. Doxycycline (100 mg orally taken twice daily for 7 days), when started within 4 days of onset of symptoms, significantly shortened the duration of fever and most other symptoms and decreased the frequency of leptospiruria in patients with mild illness. Doxycycline (200 mg orally taken once per week) is also highly effective in preventing disease in an area of high prevalence. Azotemia and jaundice require meticulous attention to fluid and electrolyte therapy. Since the renal damage is reversible, patients with azotemia should be considered for peritoneal hemodialysis. Exchange transfusion may be beneficial in the management of patients with extreme hyperbilirubinemia.

REFERENCES

CHUN SH et al: 15 cases of leptospirosis in the northern part of Kyoung Ki Do. Korean J Intern Med 32:76, 1987

CICERONI L et al: Recent trends in human leptospirosis in Italy. Eur J Epidemiol 4:49, 1988

FEIGIN RD, ANDERSON DC: Human leptospirosis. CRC Crit Rev Clin Lab Sci 5:413, 1975

GILKS CF et al: Failure of penicillin prophylaxis in laboratory acquired leptospirosis. Postgrad Med J 64:236, 1988

JOHNSON RC: *The Biology of Parasitic Spirochetes.* New York, Academic, 1976

JOHNSON WD JR et al: Serum creatine phosphokinase in leptospirosis. JAMA 233:981, 1975

KUDESIA G et al: Dual infection with *Leptospira* and Hantavirus. Lancet 1:1397, 1988

MCCLAIN JB et al: Doxycycline therapy for leptospirosis. Ann Intern Med 100:696, 1984

TAKAFUJI ET et al: An efficacy trial of doxycycline chemoprophylaxis against leptospirosis. N Engl J Med 310:497, 1984

WATT G et al: Placebo-controlled trial of intravenous penicillin for severe and late leptospirosis. Lancet 1:433, 1988

——— et al: Rapid diagnosis of leptospirosis: Prospective comparison of dot-ELISA and genus specific microscopic agglutination test at different stages of illness. J Infect Dis 157:840, 1988

WINEARLS CG et al: Acute renal failure due to leptospirosis: Clinical features and outcome in six cases. Q J Med 53:487, 1984

WONG ML et al: Leptospirosis: A childhood disease. J Pediatr 90:532, 1977

WORLD HEALTH ORGANIZATION: Tick-borne encephalitis and hemorrhagic fever with renal syndrome in Europe. EURO Reports and Studies No 104, Copenhagen 1986

131 RELAPSING FEVER

PETER L. PERINE

DEFINITION Relapsing fevers are a group of acute infections characterized by recurrent cycles of pyrexia which are separated by asymptomatic intervals of apparent recovery. They are caused by spirochetes of the genus *Borrelia* and occur in two epidemiologic varieties—louse-borne and tick-borne.

ETIOLOGY Borreliae are slender, helical-shaped, motile organisms measuring 7 to 20 μm long and 0.7 μm in diameter. Unlike other spirochetes, they are readily stained by aniline dyes. They are microaerophilic, and tick-borne strains grow well in Kelly's medium. Tick-borne *Borrelia* strains are named after their tick vectors, which in the United States include *B. hermsi, B. parkeri,* and *B. turicate.*

EPIDEMIOLOGY Louse-borne relapsing fever is transmitted from person to person solely by human body lice, which ingest blood infected with *B. recurrentis.* The spirochetes penetrate the wall of the intestine of the louse and multiply in its body cavity. Infection occurs when the louse is crushed against the bite site or an abrasion is caused by scratching. There is no known animal reservoir. The disease is endemic in remote areas of central and east Africa, the Peruvian Andes, and China, where poverty and crowding promote louse infestation. Like typhus, it is now present among the famine refugees in Ethiopia and Sudan. An occasional case of louse-borne relapsing fever has been imported into Europe and North America.

The tick vectors of relapsing fever belong to several species of the genus *Ornithodorus.* These long-lived, soft-shelled (argasid) ticks are reclusive, nocturnal biters which usually feed on ground squirrels and other small rodents. Their bite is painless and lasts for less than an hour. A small pruritic eschar may appear for a few days at the bite site. Ticks of both sexes are potentially infectious, and the spirochetes are transmitted by the female to her progeny. A rodent-tick reservoir of relapsing fever can persist near human dwellings or habitats for decades. Transmission to human beings occurs if the infected tick's saliva or coxial fluid contaminates its feeding site. Most cases in the United States occur during the spring and summer when ticks and rodents are active, particularly in western mountain states, from Texas to Colorado, Washington, Montana, and Idaho. Clusters of cases have often been linked to a tick-infested dwelling visited by travelers from different parts of the country.

PATHOGENESIS AND PATHOLOGY Once inoculated into a human, the borreliae reach the bloodstream, producing spirochetemia. Although most organs and tissues are invaded, the organisms remain and multiply primarily in the vascular system. Fever, the first manifestation of the disease, appears 3 to 12 days after infection. The severity of the fever and tissue injury is roughly correlated with the number of circulating spirochetes. Endothelial injury by borreliae is widespread, and subacute disseminated intravascular coagulation with thrombocytopenia and extravasation of blood into serosal membranes and skin is common. Immobilizing (opsonizing) antibodies appear after 3 to 5 days, and the organisms are rapidly cleared from the bloodstream by leukocyte phagocytosis, inducing a febrile crisis of short duration. Fever resolves, but a small number of a new antigenic variant of the spirochete survive in the blood or are sequestered in tissues. A new variant occurs spontaneously by genetic mutation with a frequency of once every 10^3 to 10^4 spirochetes and possesses surface proteins that are different from the infecting or preceding serotypes. They multiply and are detectable in the peripheral blood after a latent period of approximately 1 week, causing a second paroxysm of fever. The number of relapses is fewer in louse-borne than in tick-borne infections and is probably limited by the production of host antibodies directed against common, integral proteins possessed by each new variant.

MANIFESTATIONS Symptoms and signs are usually of greater severity in louse-borne relapsing fever and may vary in tick-borne infections depending on the particular species. After an incubation period of 3 to 18 days, the disease begins abruptly with the onset of high fever (39 to 40°C) which remains until the time of crisis. Patients appear acutely distressed, with some alteration in mental status. They complain of headache, muscle and joint pains, weakness, and anorexia. Nausea, vomiting, upper abdominal pain, and nonproductive cough are common. The pulse is increased in proportion to fever. Meningismus occurs in about 40 percent of patients. The liver and spleen are tender and enlarged in the majority of patients, especially in those with louse-borne disease. Jaundice, secondary to hepatocellular injury, occurs in between 10 and 80 percent of cases, appears late in the course of infection, and is more common in louse-borne disease.

Bleeding is common in both types of relapsing fever. In 10 to 60 percent of cases, a petechial or ecchymotic rash is present. Later, with the development of hepatitis, severe and prolonged epistaxis occurs in 25 percent of patients with louse-borne disease. Less common are hemoptysis, hematuria, and subconjunctival and retinal hemorrhages. Cerebral and gastrointestinal hemorrhage may occur as terminal events in fatal cases. Transient focal neurologic signs may be present without intracranial bleeding. Photophobia is common, and iritis or iridocyclitis leading to permanent visual impairment may develop in patients with tick-borne disease after several relapses.

Three to six days after the onset of symptoms, the attack resolves by crisis. It begins with a brief period of shaking chills which is followed by a transient but pronounced rise in temperature, heart rate, respiratory rate, and systolic blood pressure. This, in turn, is followed by reductions in temperature and peripheral vascular resistance, producing a hypotensive episode of several hours' duration. Most patients recover with return of vital signs to normal within 24 h, leaving the patient weak but comfortable. An identical crisis—the Jarisch-Herxheimer-like reaction—is precipitated by antibiotic therapy. The mediators of the crisis have not been identified, but phagocytosis of opsonized or antibiotically damaged spirochetes is the initiating event. An afebrile period of apparent recovery lasting 5 to 7 days ensues before the patient relapses with fever. In relapse, the symptoms are milder, shorter, and the crisis less severe than in the first attack. While only one or two relapses occur in louse-borne disease, multiple relapses over a period of several weeks are characteristic of tick-borne disease.

LABORATORY FINDINGS A moderate anemia is common. The leukocyte count is usually normal except for leukopenia at the peak of the crisis. The erythrocyte sedimentation rate is elevated. Thrombocytopenia with platelet counts below 150,000 per microliter and a prolonged bleeding time are seen regularly. Elevated serum aminotransferases, bilirubin, and prolonged prothrombin and partial thromboplastin times are common. Azotemia unrelated to extracellular fluid volume occurs in most patients with louse-borne disease. Electrocardiogram abnormalities include a prolonged QTc interval. The majority of patients with louse-borne and about 30 percent of those with tick-borne relapsing fever develop agglutinins to *Proteus* OXK antigens.

The definitive diagnosis is made by demonstrating borreliae in peripheral blood during a febrile episode by examining blood films stained with Giemsa's or Wright's stains. Repeated examinations may be required. Motile spirochetes can be visualized in wet mounts of freshly drawn blood by dark-field or phase-contrast microscopy. If direct methods are negative and tick-borne disease is suspected, blood may be injected into mice or rats and their blood examined frequently for the presence of spirochetes.

DIFFERENTIAL DIAGNOSIS Many acute febrile illnesses, including Lyme disease, rat-bite fever, salmonellosis, typhus, and Weil's disease, must be considered. Practically, there is seldom confusion if the travel history of the patient is considered and if blood films are examined carefully.

TREATMENT The peripheral blood is quickly cleared of spirochetes by treatment with penicillin, tetracyclines, erythromycin, or chloramphenicol. The first dose of any of these antimicrobial drugs usually provokes a Jarisch-Herxheimer-like reaction beginning 1 to 2 h after treatment is initiated. The severity of the reaction is greater and more predictable in louse-borne than in tick-borne relapsing fever, where it is potentially fatal. Treatment should be given in a hospital where supportive care can be given and vital signs can be monitored carefully. The hyperpyrexia can be treated with acetaminophen and tepid sponging. Most patients are hypovolemic and require 4 or more liters of isotonic saline during the first 24 h. Those with bleeding and jaundice should be given vitamin K; heparin is not effective in controlling the coagulopathy and should not be given.

The treatment of choice in louse-borne relapsing fever is tetracycline, chloramphenicol, or erythromycin stearate, 500 mg in a single oral or intravenous dose.

Tetracycline hydrochloride, 500 mg orally every 6 h for 10 days, is the recommended treatment for tick-borne relapsing fever. Doxycycline, 100 mg twice daily, is also effective. The dosage is halved for children under 12 years of age. Erythromycin stearate or chloramphenicol, 500 mg orally every 6 h for 10 days, can be given to patients who are allergic to tetracycline.

PROGNOSIS The untreated mortality rate in epidemics of louse-borne disease is between 30 to 70 percent. Appropriate treatment lowers mortality to less than 1 percent. Adverse signs are deep jaundice, delirium or coma, uncontrolled bleeding, and a marked prolongation of the QTc interval. Typhus, malaria, and enteric fever may occur simultaneously with louse-borne relapsing fever, and they probably contribute to the mortality rate, particularly during epidemics.

REFERENCES

Burgdorfer W: The enlarging spectrum of tick-borne spirotrichosis, RR Parker Memorial Address. Rev Infect Dis 8:932, 1986

Horton JM, Blaser MJ: The spectrum of relapsing fever in the Rocky Mountains. Arch Intern Med 145:871, 1985

Judge DM et al: Louse-borne relapsing fever in man. Arch Pathol 97:136, 1974

Perine PL, Teklu B: Antibiotic treatment of relapsing fever in Ethiopia: A report of 377 cases. Am J Trop Med Hyg 32:1096, 1983

Teklu B et al: Meptazinol diminishes the Jarisch-Herxheimer reaction of relapsing fever. Lancet 1:835, 1983

Warrell DM et al: Pathophysiology and immunology of the Jarisch-Herxheimer-like reaction in louse-borne relapsing fever: Comparison of tetracycline and slow release penicillin. J Infect Dis 147:898, 1983

132 LYME BORRELIOSIS

ALLEN C. STEERE

DEFINITION Lyme borreliosis, a tick-transmitted spirochetal illness, usually begins with a characteristic expanding skin lesion, erythema migrans (EM), accompanied by "flulike" or "meningitis-like" symptoms (stage 1). This phase of the disorder may be followed by frank meningitis, cranial or peripheral neuritis, carditis, or migratory musculoskeletal pain (stage 2), or by intermittent or chronic arthritis or chronic neurologic or skin abnormalities (stage 3).
3).

ETIOLOGY *Borrelia burgdorferi*, the causative agent of the disease, is 11 to 39 μm long. Organisms have 7 to 11 flagella, and their cytosine/guanine ratio is 27.3 to 30.5 percent. Like other *Borrelia*, they grow in Barbour, Stoenner, Kelly (BSK) medium. Isolates of *B. burgdorferi* have four to seven plasmids, one of which encodes for the organism's two major outer membrane proteins, the 31-kDa OspA protein and the 34-kDa OspB protein. These proteins appear to undergo antigenic variation during the course of the disease.

EPIDEMIOLOGY Lyme disease has worldwide distribution that correlates primarily with the geographic ranges of certain ixodid ticks—*Ixodes dammini, I. pacificus, I. ricinus,* and *I. persulcatus*. *I. dammini* is the principal vector in the northeastern United States from Massachusetts to Maryland and in the midwest in Wisconsin and Minnesota. In surveys of *I. dammini* in these states, 20 percent or more of the ticks have been infected with *B. burgdorferi*, and most of the cases of Lyme disease in the United States have occurred in these areas. *I. pacificus* is the vector in the western United States. The disease may be acquired throughout Europe—from Great Britain to Scandinavia to Russia—where *I. ricinus* is the vector; in Asia, where *I. persulcatus* is the vector; and in Australia. The ticks have different reservoirs; for *I. dammini*, the white-footed mouse is the preferred reservoir of the immature tick and the white-tailed deer of the mature tick.

Most new cases have onsets during the summer months. Cases have occurred in association with hiking, camping, or hunting trips or among people living in wooded or rural areas. Patients of any age and both sexes are affected. Cases have been reported in 33 states, and more than 1000 people now acquire the infection in the United States each summer.

PATHOGENESIS After injection into the skin, *B. burgdorferi* may migrate outward in the skin, producing EM, and may spread hematogenously to other organs. The spirochete has been cultured from blood, skin (EM), cerebrospinal fluid, and joint fluid and has been seen in most affected tissues. These findings and the response of all stages of the disease to antibiotic therapy suggest that the organism invades and persists in affected tissues throughout the illness.

Initially, the immune response seems to be suppressed. The mononuclear cells of patients respond minimally to *B. burgdorferi* antigens and less than normally to mitogens. Suppressor cell activity is greater than normal. After the first several weeks of infection, mononuclear cells generally have heightened responsiveness to *B. burgdorferi* antigens and to mitogens, less suppressor cell activity than normal, and evidence of B-cell hyperactivity—elevated total serum IgM levels, cryoprecipitates, and circulating immune complexes. The specific antibody response to the spirochete develops gradually over months to years and to an increasing array of spirochetal polypeptides. Specific IgM antibody titers to *B. burgdorferi* peak between the third and sixth week after disease onset; specific IgG antibody titers rise slowly and are generally highest months or years after when arthritis is present. By that time, antigen-reactive mononuclear cells and immune complexes are found in the fluid. Patients with chronic arthritis have an increased frequency of the B-cell alloantigens DR3 and DR4.

CLINICAL MANIFESTATIONS As with other spirochetal illnesses, Lyme disease occurs in stages, with remissions and exacerbations and different clinical manifestations at each stage. Stage 1 generally lasts for several weeks, stage 2 occurs during the following several months, and stage 3 occurs months to years after the onset of infection. Marked variation is possible in the clinical expression of the disease. Some patients without EM have the nonspecific symptoms associated with stage 1. In other patients, neurologic, cardiac, or joint involvement is the presenting sign of the illness. Antibiotic treatment at any point may modify or completely suppress the development and evolution of the characteristic stages.

Stage 1 After an incubation period of 3 to 32 days, EM, which occurs at the site of the tick bite, usually begins as a red macule or papule that expands to form a large annular lesion, usually with a bright red outer border and partial central clearing. Because of the small size of ixodid ticks, most patients do not remember the preceding tick bite. The center of the lesion sometimes becomes intensely erythematous and indurated, vesicular, or necrotic. In other instances, the expanding lesion remains an even, intense red; several red rings are found within the outside one; or the central area turns blue before it clears. Although the lesion can be located anywhere, the thigh, groin, and axilla are particularly common sites. The lesion is warm, but not often painful. Skin biopsies show perivascular infiltrates or lymphocytes and histiocytes. In some patients, the Lyme spirochete remains localized to this skin lesion and to regional lymph nodes and is sometimes accompanied by minor constitutional symptoms. In others, the organism spreads hematogenously to many different sites. Within days after the onset of EM, such patients often develop secondary annular skin lesions, which are similar in appearance to the initial lesion. Additional dermatologic manifestations include malar rash, diffuse erythema, urticaria, or evanescent lesions. Skin involvement is frequently accompanied by severe headache, mild neck stiffness, fever, chills, migratory musculoskeletal pain, arthralgias, and profound malaise and fatigue. Less common manifestations include generalized lymphadenopathy or splenomegaly, hepatitis, sore throat, nonproductive cough, conjunctivitis, iritis, or testicular swelling.

Except for fatigue and lethargy, which are often constant, the early signs and symptoms of Lyme disease are typically intermittent and changing. Even in untreated patients, the early symptoms usually improve or disappear within several weeks. However, fatigue and lethargy and sometimes vague musculoskeletal pain may last for months after the skin lesions have disappeared.

Stage 2 Symptoms suggestive of meningeal irritation may occur early in Lyme disease when EM is present but are usually not associated with a spinal fluid pleocytosis or objective neurologic deficit. After several weeks to months, about 15 percent of patients develop frank neurologic abnormalities, including meningitis, subtle encephalitic signs, cranial neuritis (including bilateral facial palsy), motor or sensory radiculoneuropathy, mononeuritis multiplex, chorea, or myelitis, alone or in various combinations. The usual pattern consists of fluctuating symptoms of meningitis accompanied by facial palsy and peripheral radiculoneuropathy. Cerebrospinal fluid shows a lymphocytic pleocytosis (about 100 cells per microliter), often with elevated protein, and normal or slightly low glucose. Neurologic abnormalities usually resolve completely within months, but chronic neurologic disease may occur later.

Within several weeks after the onset of illness, about 8 percent of patients develop cardiac involvement. The most common abnormality is fluctuating degrees of atrioventricular block (first-degree, Wenckebach, or complete heart block). Some patients have more diffuse cardiac involvement, including electrocardiographic changes of acute myopericarditis, left ventricular dysfunction on radionuclide scans, or, rarely, cardiomegaly or pancarditis. Cardiac involvement usually lasts only a few weeks but may recur.

During this stage, musculoskeletal pain is common. The typical pattern is migratory pain in joints, tendons, bursae, muscle, or bone, usually without joint swelling.

Stage 3 Within weeks to 2 years after the onset of infection, about 80 percent of patients in the United States who have received no antibiotic treatment develop joint symptoms ranging from subjective joint pain, to intermittent attacks of arthritis, to chronic erosive synovitis. Marked joint swelling does not usually begin until months after the onset of the illness. The typical pattern is intermittent attacks of oligoarticular arthritis in large joints, especially knees, lasting weeks to months in a given joint. Small joints and periarticular sites may also be affected. The total number of patients who continue to have recurrent attacks decreases by about 10 to 20 percent each year, but patients have been known to have recurrence for as long as 8 years. In a small percentage of patients, involvement in large joints becomes chronic, with erosion of cartilage and bone.

Joint fluid white cell counts range from 500 to 110,000 cells per microliter (average, 25,000 cells per microliter), mostly polymorphonuclear leukocytes. Tests for rheumatoid factor or antinuclear antibodies are usually negative. Synovial biopsies show fibrin deposits, villous hypertrophy, vascular proliferation, microangiopathic lesions, and a heavy infiltration of lymphocytes and plasma cells.

Although less common, chronic neurologic or skin involvement (acrodermatitis chronica atrophicans) may also occur months to years after the onset of infection. Some patients may have intermittent tingling paresthesias of their extremities for years. In severe cases, *B. burgdorferi* may cause slowly progressive encephalomyelitis, organic brain syndromes, spastic parapareses, transverse myelitis, or dementia. Acrodermatitis begins with red-violaceous lesions that become sclerotic or atrophic over a period of years.

TREATMENT For early Lyme disease, tetracycline, 250 mg four times a day, is effective therapy in adults. In vitro, *B. burgdorferi* is as sensitive to doxycycline and amoxicillin as to tetracycline. Phenoxymethylpenicillin, 500 mg four times a day, or erythromycin, 250 mg four times a day, are second- and third-choice alternatives. Therapy should be given for at least 10 days, and for up to 30 days, if symptoms persist or recur. In children, amoxicillin or phenoxymethylpenicillin are effective (50 mg/kg per day, but not more than

2g/d) in divided doses for the same duration, or, in cases of penicillin allergy, erythromycin, 30 mg/kg per day, in divided doses for 15 to 20 days, should be used. Approximately 15 percent of patients experience a Jarisch-Herxheimer-like reaction during the first 24 h of therapy.

Later in the illness, parenteral antibiotic therapy may be necessary. In patients with frank meningitis and cranial or peripheral neuropathies, intravenous penicillin G, 20 million units per day in divided doses for 14 days or intravenous ceftriaxone, 2 g/d, are usually effective. In patients with high-degree atrioventricular block or a PR interval of greater than 0.3 s, intravenous penicillin, 10 to 20 million units per day, or intravenous ceftriaxone, 2 g/d, for at least 10 days, and cardiac monitoring are recommended. In patients with complete heart block or congestive heart failure, glucocorticoids may be of benefit if the patient does not improve on antimicrobial therapy alone within 24 h. For established arthritis, doxycycline, 100 mg twice a day, or amoxicillin and probenecid, each 500 mg four times a day, given for 30 days, are effective in about 70 percent of patients. However, the response to therapy is frequently slow, and a repeat course of oral therapy or of intravenous penicillin or ceftriaxone may need to be given. A small percentage of patients with arthritis, particularly those with DR3 and DR4 HLA antigen, do not respond to antimicrobial therapy. Synovectomy may be successful in such patients.

PROGNOSIS The response to treatment is best early in the illness. When treated later, convalescence often requires months. Nearly half the patients with Lyme disease irrespective of the antibiotic given have minor recurrences of headaches, musculoskeletal pain, or lethargy. The recrudescences correlate significantly with the severity of the initial illness. Eventually, complete recovery ensues in the majority of patients.

REFERENCES

BARBOUR AG, HAYES SF: Biology of *Borrelia* species. Microbiol Rev 50:381, 1986

HALPERIN JJ et al: Lyme disease: Cause of treatable peripheral neuropathy. Neurology 37:1700, 1987

PACHNER AR, STEERE AC: The triad of neurologic manifestations of Lyme disease: Meningitis, cranial neuritis, and radiculoneuritis. Neurology 35:47, 1985

STEERE AC: Lyme borreliosis, in *Principles and Practice of Infectious Diseases*, 3d ed, GL Mandell et al (eds). New York, Churchill-Livingstone, 1990

———: Lyme disease. N Engl J Med 321:586, 1989

——— et al: Lyme carditis: Cardiac abnormalities of Lyme disease. Ann Intern Med 93:8, 1980

——— et al: The spirochetal etiology of Lyme disease. N Engl J Med 308:733, 1983

——— et al: The early clinical manifestations of Lyme disease. Ann Intern Med 99:76, 1983

——— et al: Treatment of the early manifestations of Lyme disease. Ann Intern Med 99:22, 1983

——— et al: The clinical evolution of Lyme arthritis. Ann Intern Med 107:725, 1987

section 8 Viral diseases

133 THE BIOLOGY OF VIRUSES

BERNARD N. FIELDS

STRUCTURE AND CLASSIFICATION OF VIRUSES A typical virus particle (*virion*) contains a core of nucleic acid of either DNA or RNA. There is considerable variability in the structure and size of viral nucleic acids (Table 133-1). The smallest molecular weight genomes, such as those of the parvoviridae, encode three or four proteins, whereas the larger genomes, such as those of the poxviridae, encode more than 50 structural proteins and enzymes. The number of proteins encoded by a viral genome may be greater than predicted from the genome's molecular weight because of the presence of multiple open reading frames and/or the presence of overlapping regions of nucleic acid that can be transcribed into several distinct mRNAs. Extensive nucleotide sequence data are available for part or all of the genomes of many viruses.

The viral nucleic acid is surrounded by either a single or double protein shell (*capsid*). The viral nucleic acid plus the capsid are referred to as the *nucleocapsid*. The viral capsids are composed of smaller repetitive subunits (*capsomers*) arranged in symmetric constructions. The repeating subunits facilitate assembly of viral proteins into mature virions and reduce the amount of genomic information required to encode structural proteins. Capsids are formed by self-assembly of their structural subunits.

The two fundamental patterns of capsid structural symmetry are icosahedral and helical. Some of the largest viruses, such as the poxviruses, have more complex structural patterns. The retroviruses appear to have icosahedral capsid symmetry and helical core symmetry. Viruses with icosahedral capsid symmetry generally follow principles of physical organization that specify the total allowable number of structural subunits. The nucleic acid in icosahedral viruses is usually in a condensed form and is geometrically independent of the surrounding capsid structure.

Animal viruses with helical symmetry have RNA genomes. A general feature of animal viruses is the binding of protein subunits of the capsid in a regular, periodic fashion along the viral RNA. This close interaction between the capsid proteins and nucleic acid is in sharp contrast to the loose interactions in viruses with icosahedral symmetry and imposes different constraints for viral assembly.

Many viruses have an envelope surrounding the nucleocapsid. The viral envelope is composed of viral-specific proteins and of lipids and carbohydrates derived from host cell membranes. The host cell components are added as the virus buds through the host cell nuclear membrane, endoplasmic reticulum, Golgi apparatus, or cytoplasmic membrane. Different viruses utilize distinctive types of host cell membranes for budding. The factors that determine this specificity are incompletely understood. In some cases viral-specific envelope proteins may include a matrix protein (*M protein*) which lines the inner side of the envelope and is in contact with the nucleocapsid. Viral-specific glycoproteins protrude from the outer surface of the envelope (e.g., as "spikes") and may in some cases contain hydrophobic domains, which span the lipid bilayer of the envelope, as well as internal domains which may contact the M proteins.

Viral proteins, referred to as *structural* or *virion proteins*, can form the viral capsid, can be a major component of viral envelopes, or can be associated with the viral nucleic acid (*core proteins*). A number of viruses contain surface glycoproteins that agglutinate red blood cells (*hemagglutinins*) by binding to receptors on the red cell surface. Many viruses contain proteins with enzymatic activity. In many cases these enzymes are required for the synthesis of messenger

TABLE 133-1 Structure of viral nucleic acid

Family	Example	Type of nucleic acid	Genome size, kilobases or kilobase pairs	Envelope	Capsid symmetry
Picornaviridae	Poliovirus	ss(+)RNA	7.2–8.4	No	I
Caliciviridae	Norwalk virus	ss(+)RNA	8	No	I
Togaviridae	Rubella virus	ss(+)RNA	12	Yes	I
Flaviviridae	Yellow fever virus	ss(+)RNA	10	Yes	UNK
Coronaviridae	Coronaviruses	ss(+)RNA	16–21	Yes	H
Rhabdoviridae	Rabies virus	ss(−)RNA	13–16	Yes	H
Filoviridae	Marburg virus	ss(−)RNA	13	Yes	H
Paramyxoviridae	Measles virus	ss(−)RNA	16–20	Yes	H
Orthomyxoviridae	Influenza viruses	8 ss(−)RNA segments*	14	Yes	H
Bunyaviridae	California encephalitis virus	3 circular ss(−)RNA segments	13–21	Yes	H
Arenaviridae	Lymphocytic choriomeningitis virus	2 circular ss(−)RNA segments	10–14	Yes	H
Reoviridae	Rotaviruses	10–12 dsRNA† segments	16–27	No	I
Retroviridae	HIV-1	2 identical ss(+)RNA segments	3–9	Yes	I-capsid H-nucleocapsid (probable)
Hepadnaviridae	Hepatitis B	dsDNA with ss portions	3	Yes	UNK
Parvoviridae	Human parvovirus B-19	ss(+) or (−) DNA	5	No	I
Papovaviridae	JC virus	Circular dsDNA	8	No	I
Adenoviridae	Human adenoviruses	dsDNA	36–38	No	I
Herpesviridae	Herpes simplex virus	dsDNA	120–220	Yes	I
Poxviridae	Vaccinia	dsDNA with covalently closed ends	130–280	Yes	Complex

* Influenza C = 7 segments.
† Reovirus, orbivirus = 10 segments; rotavirus = 11 segments; Colorado tick fever = 12 segments.
NOTE: ds = double-stranded; ss = single-stranded; (+) message sense; (−) anti-message sense; I = icosahedral; H = helical; UNK = unknown.
SOURCES: FA Murphy, in *Fundamental Virology*, BN Fields, DM Knipe (eds), New York, Raven, 1986, and KL Tyler, BN Fields, in *Laboratory Diagnosis of Infectious Diseases*, vol 2, EH Lennette et al (eds), New York, Springer-Verlag, 1988.

RNA (mRNA) of the appropriate (+) polarity for translation into protein or for replication of the viral genome. An RNA-dependent RNA polymerase activity is found in all (−) polarity RNA viruses. Poxviruses contain a DNA-dependent RNA polymerase. Retroviruses contain an RNA-dependent DNA polymerase commonly referred to as *reverse transcriptase*. Some viruses, including the poxviruses, reoviruses, paramyxoviruses, and rhabdoviruses, have RNA "capping enzymes" which modify viral mRNAs at their 5′ end by adding a 7-methylguanosine cap in 5′-5′-triphosphate linkage. Enzymes which polyadenylate the 3′ end of viral mRNAs may also be virally encoded. Additional virally encoded enzymes include protein kinases, nucleoside triphosphate phosphohydrolases, endonucleases, and RNAses.

The earliest classifications of viruses were based solely on their ability to pass through filters with small pore sizes. Subsequent classifications stressed pathogenic properties, specific organ tropisms (e.g., enteroviruses), or epidemiologic characteristics (e.g., arboviruses). Current classifications of viruses are based on a combination of genetic, physicochemical, and biologic factors. These include the type and structure of the viral nucleic acid, the nature of virion ultrastructure including size, type of capsid symmetry, capsid composition, and the presence or absence of an envelope, as well as the strategy used by the virus for genome replication. The reliance on morphologic criteria often means that electron-micrographic studies provide sufficient information to identify both the family and the genus to which a virus belongs. Subdivisions within major viral taxonomic groups may be based on immunologic, cytopathologic, pathogenetic, or epidemiologic features. The application of recombinant DNA techniques will require revision of these classifications based on degrees of genetic relatedness.

REPLICATION Replication refers to the process by which viruses infect susceptible cells, reproduce their genomic material and proteins, and assemble and release infectious progeny. The diversity among viruses in terms of structure and type of genomic material is reflected by the large number of replicative strategies.

The first stage of viral infection of target cells begins with adsorption of the virus particles and ends with the onset of formation of infectious progeny virus. This stage is often referred to as the *eclipse period* and varies from 1 to 5 h (e.g., picornaviruses, togaviruses, rhabdoviruses, orthomyxoviruses, herpesviruses) to 8 to 14 h (adenoviruses, papovaviruses). During this period there is a dramatic drop in the amount of infectious virus that can be recovered from disrupted cells.

Adsorption appears to be a process that is initially reversible, resulting from random collisions between viruses and target cells. It has been estimated that only one in 10^3 to 10^4 such collisions leads to tighter binding (*attachment*). Attachment is facilitated by the appropriate ionic and pH conditions but is largely temperature-independent and does not require energy. Adsorption of virus to a target cell may involve specific binding of viral proteins to receptors on the cell surface (also called attachment). The virion structure mediating cell attachment has been identified for a number of viruses. For enveloped viruses the viral attachment protein is typically one of the "spikes" inserted on the outer surface of the viral envelope such as the hemagglutinin (HA) of influenza viruses. Some enveloped viruses, such as the herpesviruses and vaccinia, may have more than one type of cell attachment protein. In nonenveloped viruses, surface polypeptides, such as the fiber protein of adenovirus and the hemagglutinin ($\sigma 1$) protein of reovirus, often function as the viral attachment proteins.

The exact nature of the cellular receptors for animal viruses is known in only a few specific cases. Even when the specific receptor is still unknown, it has been possible to identify "families" or classes of viral receptors using competition binding studies. Viruses of the same species, but different serotypes, may compete for the same receptor class (e.g., poliovirus serotypes 1, 2, 3) or for different receptor classes (e.g., human rhinovirus 2 and 14). Viruses from different families (e.g., coxsackievirus B3 and adenovirus 2) may also compete for the same class of receptor. These types of binding studies suggest that there are generally 10^4 to 10^6 viral binding sites (receptors) per cell.

Once attachment has occurred, the entire virion or a substructure containing the viral genome and any virion polymerases required for its initial transcription must be translocated across the plasma membrane of the cell. The rate of penetration varies depending on the nature of the virus, the type of cells being infected, and environmental factors such as temperature. Some nonenveloped viruses such as poliovirus and reovirus undergo a process of receptor-mediated endocytosis (*viropexis*) and appear in the cytoplasm inside endocytic vesicles. Other nonenveloped viruses may be able to cross the plasma membrane directly and appear free in the cytoplasm without entering endocytic vesicles.

Enveloped viruses also utilize at least two strategies for penetration. The first is exemplified by Semliki Forest virus (SFV). SFV, a togavirus, binds to specific cell surface receptors, which then aggregate at distinct sites on the plasma membrane (*coated pits*) and are internalized by receptor-mediated endocytosis. They subsequently appear inside clathrin-coated vesicles within the cell cytoplasm. Fusion between the viral envelope and the endosomal membrane causes release of the viral nucleocapsid into the cytoplasm. A second mechanism for penetration of enveloped viruses occurs with paramyxoviruses (e.g., Sendai). The viral envelope fuses directly with the cell plasma membrane, and the viral nucleocapsid is discharged free into the cytoplasm.

Uncoating is the process of removing or disaggregating part or all of the viral protein capsid in preparation for transcription and translation of the viral genome. In many cases penetration and uncoating are part of a single process. Some picornaviruses, for example, seem to undergo an alteration in capsid structure and integrity and loss of an internal protein as they are translocated across the plasma membrane. The structural alterations associated with loss of the protein may facilitate entry of the viral RNA into the cytoplasm.

Nonenveloped viruses which enter endosomes, such as adenovirus, may induce fusion of lysosomes with the endosome and have their capsid removed by lysosomal enzymes. In the case of reoviruses, intraendosomal proteases sequentially remove the three outer capsid proteins to produce a "subviral particle," a process which leads to activation of the viral transcriptase. Uncoating of poxviruses, such as vaccinia, first involves degradation of the outer protein coat by intraendosomal enzymes and then of the remaining "core," liberating the viral DNA. This step appears to require the synthesis of a virus-specified "uncoating protein."

A number of strategies have evolved for *transcription* of viral genomes into mRNA and *translation* of mRNA into protein. One approach is for viruses to contain mRNA that is translated into a large precursor polyprotein, which is then cleaved to produce the various virion proteins. This approach is exemplified by viruses such as the picornaviruses and togaviruses in which the nucleic acid is in the form of (+) polarity, single-stranded RNA (ssRNA) and serves as mRNA. It binds to large polyribosomes and is fully translated ($5' \rightarrow 3'$) to produce a single large polyprotein, which is then cleaved in a series of steps to produce the nonstructural, core, and capsid proteins. In the case of both the picornaviruses and the togaviruses a virally encoded RNA polymerase synthesizes a complementary RNA using the genomic RNA as template. In turn, the newly synthesized RNA serves as template for the synthesis of more genomic RNA. The new genomic RNAs may serve as mRNAs or as precursor RNA for progeny virions.

Viruses which contain linear or segmented RNA produce unique mRNAs for each viral protein rather than a single large mRNA molecule. A transcriptase enzyme contained in the virion (the virion polymerase) is required to produce mRNAs from the genomic RNA. The presence of multiple mRNAs allows regulation of the amount of each protein synthesized. A single region of genomic RNA may have multiple reading frames, each of which is transcribed into unique mRNAs, which are in turn translated into distinct proteins. Genomic (−)ssRNA is replicated via a (+)ssRNA intermediate, which then serves as a template to synthesize more (−)ss genomic RNA.

Reoviruses contain a RNA-dependent RNA polymerase that transcribes (+)ssRNAs from the (−) strand of each double-stranded (ds) RNA segment. These (+)ssRNAs are extruded from the viral core through channels in the core spike, and serve as mRNAs for translation into viral proteins. The viral RNA polymerase also synthesizes (+)ssRNAs, which in turn serve as templates for the complementary (−) strand during replication of the viral genome.

The retroviruses utilize a unique replicative strategy. Viral (+)ssRNA serves as a template for the virion RNA-dependent DNA polymerase (reverse transcriptase) and primer transfer RNAs (tRNAs). A ssDNA copy is produced which is initially hydrogen bonded to its complementary (+)ssRNA. A virally encoded ribonuclease digests the ssRNA, and a complementary DNA strand is synthesized. Then dsDNA is integrated into chromosomal DNA in the host cell nucleus. Transcription of this integrated viral DNA is under the control of the host cell transcriptases.

DNA-containing viruses are capable of using strategies similar to those in eukaryotic cells for replication during lytic infection. Papovaviruses, adenoviruses, and herpesviruses use replicative strategies in which transcription of viral DNA into mRNA occurs in the nucleus of the host cell and depends on host cell enzymes. In the case of papovaviruses (e.g., SV40), the initial proteins produced after infection are the *T antigens* (tumor antigens or *early proteins*). Some of the T-antigen proteins appear to interact with the viral genomic dsDNA by binding near the site of initiation of DNA replication. This binding facilitates DNA replication. Subsequently, mRNAs encoding the capsid polypeptides are transcribed (*late proteins*). The early mRNAs are all derived from only one of the two viral DNA strands (referred to as the E or *E*arly strand), and the late mRNAs from the other (the L or *L*ate strand). Adenoviruses also have early and late genes, but they are intermixed along both strands of the viral DNA rather than on separate strands.

In the replication of both papovaviruses and adenoviruses, early proteins appear to be primarily regulatory in nature and often pleiotropic in function. Late proteins include structural proteins. The individual mRNAs for both early and late proteins are often complementary to dispersed segments of the viral DNA, indicating that extensive splicing, with removal of intervening regions, has occurred. In many cases mRNAs are synthesized from overlapping regions of the viral DNA. This type of redundancy reduces the amount of viral DNA needed to encode viral proteins.

Poxviruses are the most complicated of the known animal viruses, and their replicative cycle is correspondingly complex. All the initial steps of transcription and translation appear to occur in the host cell cytoplasm, which requires that the virus contain its own DNA-dependent RNA polymerase to initiate transcription. One of the virus-encoded early proteins is responsible for the second stage of uncoating which makes the viral DNA fully accessible for transcription and replication. Replication, transcription, and later viral assembly all occur in virus-initiated "factories" within the host cell cytoplasm. Sequential groups of virus-specified proteins can be detected in infected cells. Early proteins include a number of enzymes (e.g., a DNA polymerase and a thymidine kinase), as well as some structural proteins. As infection proceeds, DNA replication begins, the synthesis of the early nonstructural proteins ceases, and the synthesis of late proteins begins. Many of the late proteins are structural proteins; other late proteins include enzymes and proteins that may play a role in viral assembly.

Once replication of the viral genome and synthesis of the viral proteins have been completed, intact virions must then be assembled and released from the host cells. Assembly of the nonenveloped viruses and the nucleocapsid of enveloped viruses often appears to proceed in a crystallization-like fashion which depends on the self-assembly of viral capsomers.

In most cases nonenveloped virions accumulate within the infected cell and are released together when the cell lyses. The events leading to cell disruption include inhibition of the synthesis of host cell protein, lipid, and nucleic acids, disorganization of the host cell cytoskeleton, and alteration of host cell membrane structure. Membrane disruption may result in increased cell permeability and in the release of proteolytic enzymes from lysosomes. The failure to replenish energy-rich substrate molecules inhibits the function of ion transport pumps and disturbs transport of essential nutrients and cellular waste products.

Enveloped viruses are typically released from infected cells by budding. This process may be lethal to the cell. In all cases virus-specified proteins are inserted into host cell membranes in a fashion that restructures the membrane by displacing some of its normal protein components. Viral capsids may then bind to virus-specified matrix proteins which line the cytoplasmic side of these altered patches of membrane. In the case of the smallest enveloped viruses, the togaviruses, the capsids bind to the intracytoplasmic domains of viral proteins inserted in the host cell membrane rather than to matrix proteins.

PATHOGENESIS The signs and symptoms of disease are the result of the culmination of a series of interactions between the virus and the host. A virus must first be able to enter the host, then undergo a period of primary replication, followed by spread to its final target tissue. Once a virus reaches its target organs, it must then infect and successfully replicate in a susceptible population of host cells. The outcome of this last step may be a productive infection with or without cell injury, latent infection, or persistent infection. To transmit infectious virus to the next host the virus must successfully avoid or overcome the host immune response and a wide variety of other host defense mechanisms. A great deal of viral replication can occur before any signs or symptoms of clinical illness are detectable. This "incubation period" can vary from a few days (e.g., influenza), to weeks (e.g., measles, varicella), to months (rabies, hepatitis), to years (slow viruses).

Most viral diseases result from exposure to exogenous virus. However, in some cases disease results from the reactivation of endogenous virus, which has been latent within specific host cells. Examples of infections caused by reactivated endogenous viruses include shingles (herpes zoster), progressive multifocal leukoencephalopathy (JC or BK papovaviruses), recurrent labial and genital herpes (herpes simplex), and some types of cytomegalovirus (CMV) infections.

In the majority of cases, transmission of viral illnesses occurs between members of a susceptible host population (*horizontal spread*). *Vertical spread* of infection occurs when the fetus becomes infected in utero through virus carried in the germ cell line, virus infecting the placenta, or virus in the maternal birth canal. Rubella virus, CMV, herpes simplex virus, varicella-zoster virus, and hepatitis B virus can all produce vertically transmitted congenital infections.

The age and genetic background of the host can have important implications for the outcome of viral infections. Newborns, for example, are particularly susceptible to severe, disseminated herpes simplex virus infections. In contrast, many of the exanthematous illnesses, poliovirus infection, and Epstein-Barr virus (EBV) infection are typically more severe in older individuals than in children. In mice, specific genes help determine susceptibility to certain viral infections. These genes may act through effects on the immune system, interferon production, or viral receptors. Inadequate host nutritional status may increase susceptibility to infections such as measles, perhaps by depressing cell-mediated immunity. The host can also influence viral infections in ways that are still poorly understood. Stress may trigger recurrent herpes labialis. Strenuous exercise may have an adverse effect on the course of polio.

Viral infection begins with *entry* into the host, which may occur via a number of routes. The stratum corneum of the skin provides both a physical barrier and a biologic barrier against the entry of viruses. Some viruses overcome the skin barrier by being directly inoculated via insect or animal bites or mechanical devices such as needles. The arthropod-borne viruses are directly inoculated into the bloodstream when an infected tick or mosquito takes a blood meal. Rabies virus and herpesvirus simiae (monkey B virus) enter tissues after an animal bite. Iatrogenic inoculation allows entry of a large number of viruses. Hepatitis B virus, CMV, and human immunodeficiency virus (HIV-1) may all be present in contaminated blood products used for transfusion. Infected corneal transplants, infected instruments used in neurosurgical procedures, and infected pituitary tissues used to prepare growth hormone have been implicated as causes of Creutzfeldt-Jakob disease. Parenteral vaccination using live attenuated virus represents another category of iatrogenic inoculation.

A large number of viruses enter the host by crossing mucosal barriers in the respiratory and gastrointestinal tracts. Respiratory infection can be either by means of aerosol droplets, nasal secretions, or saliva. Entry via either the respiratory or enteric routes requires that the virus overcome a formidable series of host defenses. In the lung, immunologic defenses include secretory IgA, natural killer (NK) cells, and macrophages. Nonspecific glycoprotein viral inhibitors are present in tracheobronchial mucus. Ciliated respiratory epithelial cells continually move mucus away from the lower respiratory tract. The harsh acidic environment of the stomach inactivates acid-labile viruses such as rhinoviruses. Bile salts, present in the lumen of the small intestine, can destroy the lipid envelope of many viruses and may account for the fact that entry via the gastrointestinal route is limited largely to nonenveloped viruses. Proteolytic enzymes and secretory IgA contribute to host antiviral defenses in the gastrointestinal tract. Specific viral capsid proteins may allow some viruses to withstand proteolytic digestion in the gut.

For some enteric viruses, passage across the mucosal barrier of the gut is mediated by a specific population of cells overlying Peyer's patches known as microfold (M) cells. These cells, and perhaps their analogues in bronchial lymphoid tissue, seem to facilitate transport of some viruses, including reoviruses and possibly enteroviruses, to the abluminal surface of the small intestine.

Venereal transmission with entry across the genitourinary or rectal mucosa appears to be important for herpes simplex virus type 2, CMV, hepatitis B virus, and HIV-1.

For some viruses, the processes of entry, primary replication, and tissue tropism all occur at the same anatomic site. Examples of this type of viral illness include the upper and lower respiratory infections caused by the rhinoviruses, ortho- and paramyxoviruses; the enteritis caused by rotaviruses; and the dermatologic lesions induced by human papillomavirus (warts) and paravaccinia virus (milker's nodules). In other cases a virus enters at one site and must subsequently spread to a distant area, such as the central nervous system, to produce disease. Enteroviruses enter via the gastrointestinal tract but must spread to the CNS to produce meningitis, encephalitis, and poliomyelitis. Measles virus and varicella virus enter the body through the respiratory tract but then spread to produce skin disease (exanthem) and often generalized organ involvement.

Neural, hematogenous, and lymphatic pathways are all utilized by viruses to spread to target tissues. Rabies virus, herpes simplex virus, herpesvirus simiae (monkey B), varicella-zoster virus, and the scrapie agent spread via nerves. Herpes simplex virus appears to enter nerves via receptors located primarily near synaptic endings rather than on the nerve cell body. Rabies virus accumulates at the motor end plate of the neuromuscular junction (NMJ) and may utilize the acetylcholine receptor (AChR) or a closely related structure to enter the distal axons of motor neurons. Other viruses including La Crosse bunyavirus and the togavirus Sindbis also accumulate at the NMJ, although their receptor molecules have not been identified. Rabies virus also infects muscle and spreads via motor and sensory nerves to the spinal cord. The kinetics of neural spread for rabies, herpes simplex, and polio strongly suggest that these agents utilize intraneuronal mechanisms involved with fast axonal transport. The scrapie agent, which appears to spread slowly along neural pathways, may be an example of movement via slow axonal transport. Infection of Schwann cells may provide another "neural" pathway to the CNS. Neural spread may be important not only as a pathway to the CNS but also for spread within the CNS and from the CNS to the periphery.

The olfactory pathway represents a special category of neural spread. The rod processes of olfactory receptor cells lie exposed in the olfactory mucosa. These cells synapse directly with the mitral cells in the olfactory bulb within the CNS. Under experimental conditions, intranasal or aerosol inoculations of rabies virus, herpes simplex virus, poliovirus, and some togaviruses can lead to CNS infection via the olfactory route. This route may provide a pathway to the CNS in humans for rabies, and possibly other viruses, in circumstances, such as in caves occupied by large numbers of rabid bats or in accidental laboratory-acquired infections, where high-titer aerosols are present. An olfactory route of spread might be one explanation for the localization of herpes simplex virus to the orbitofrontal and medial temporal cortex in cases of herpes simplex encephalitis.

Hematogenous spread is important for many viruses. A period of primary replication usually precedes the initial viremia and can be asymptomatic or result in prodromal symptoms. For enteric viruses, primary replication occurs in Peyer's patches and peritonsillar lymphatic tissue. Primary replication of respiratory viruses occurs in epithelial or alveolar cells and for many enteroviruses and togaviruses in skeletal muscle. In some cases virus travels from the site of initial multiplication via lymphatics to regional lymph nodes before entering the bloodstream. The initial (*primary*) viremia often disseminates virus to tissues such as the spleen and liver where continued multiplication in parenchymal cells leads to an amplified secondary viremia. Growth in endothelial cells may help sustain the viremic phase in some togavirus infections. Sustained secondary amplification of the viremia is required if a virus is to overcome clearance by reticuloendothelial cells.

Blood-borne virus can travel free or in association with cellular elements. Hepatitis B virus, picornaviruses, and togaviruses all travel free within plasma; Colorado tick fever virus and Rift valley fever virus are associated with red blood cells; EBV, CMV, rubella, and HIV are lymphocyte- or monocyte-associated.

In some cases viruses use different pathways of spread at different stages in the infectious cycle. Varicella-zoster virus disseminates to the skin by the hematogenous route to produce "chickenpox." The virus then spreads centripetally along nerves from the skin to neurons in the dorsal root ganglion where it remains latent. Reactivation results in centrifugal spread of virus down sensory nerves to their skin dermatome and the production of "shingles" (zoster). Neural spread of virus presumably accounts for recurrent episodes of oral and genital infection caused by herpes simplex virus. Poliovirus represents an example of a virus capable of spreading by both hematogenous and neural routes. The hematogenous route is generally accepted as the primary pathway to the CNS, although the virus may spread to the CNS via autonomic nerves in the gut. Axonal transport may play a role in the spread of poliovirus within the CNS.

Once a virus has spread from its site of primary replication to a target organ, it must infect a population of susceptible cells. This requires the interaction between specific viral structures (*viral attachment proteins*) and viral receptors on cells. Virus-encoded tissue-specific enhancers may in part mediate viral injury to specific cell populations. Lytic infection also requires that all of the subsequent steps in the viral replicative cycle be successfully completed.

HOST FACTORS **The antibody response** Most viruses make good antigens for stimulating the immune response because they contain a large number of foreign proteins, each of which may contain multiple antigenic sites. In addition, although the amount of viral antigenic material may initially be quite small, there is amplification in its quantity due to viral replication. Few of the antibodies play a significant role in protecting the host against infection, and in some cases they may themselves be implicated in disease pathogenesis.

The immunogenicity of viruses depends on the nature of the virus itself and on a variety of host factors. The slow virus agents responsible for kuru and Creutzfeldt-Jakob disease do not appear to provoke any detectable immune response in the host. The route of viral infection may also play a role in immunity. In experimental influenza infections, intravenous inoculation is more immunogenic than intraperitoneal inoculation, which in turn exceeds the subcutaneous route.

Antibodies which protect the host by destroying the infectivity of virus are referred to as neutralizing antibodies (Nab). Nabs usually are directed against epitopes present on viral proteins located on the surface of the virus particle. The binding of Nab to virus is generally a reversible reaction. Viral infectivity may be reduced because Nab inhibits attachment, penetration, or uncoating of virus; produces aggregation of virions; accelerates viral degradation in vesicles, or enhances viral opsonization and subsequent phagocytosis. In the case of poliovirus, Nab binding appears to induce a conformational rearrangement of the viral outer capsid which blocks viral uncoating but not attachment.

Complement Viruses can trigger activation of both the alternate and classic pathways of complement activation in the absence of an antibody response. Activated complement components (e.g., C3b) may act as opsonins that enhance phagocytosis of viruses. Activation of the alternate complement pathway, in combination with antibody, may produce lysis of enveloped viruses or virus-infected cells. Although the complement system plays a role in the protection against viral infection in animals, human complement deficiency states are not typically associated with an increase in the frequency or severity of viral illnesses.

Cell-mediated immunity Virus-infected cells can be lysed by lymphocytes and other cells through both antibody-dependent and antibody-independent pathways. NK cells are large granular lymphocytes that bind to infected target cells and then secrete cytotoxic molecules contained in azurophilic granular vesicles. NK activity is increased by interferons and possibly by some viral glycoproteins, and does not require antibody. NK cytotoxicity provides one of the earliest host defenses against viral infection (peak activity at 2 to 3 days) and precedes the appearance of antibody (7 days), cytotoxic T lymphocytes (CTL), and delayed type hypersensitivity (DTH). Activated NK cells have been identified in human viral infections caused by CMV, EBV, measles, and mumps virus.

Antibody-dependent lysis of infected cells can occur via antibody-dependent cell-mediated cytotoxicity (ADCC) or via antibody-independent CTLs. In ADCC reactions, virus-specific antibody bound to antigens on an infected cell interacts with Fc receptors for IgG on the surface of specialized lymphocytoid cells ["killer" (K) cells]. The binding of IgG to the Fc receptor activates the K cell and results in target cell killing. Macrophages, lymphocytes, and PMNs also have Fc receptors and may also participate in ADCC.

Lysis of infected cells mediated by CTLs is typically class I histocompatibility antigen restricted, although examples of class II restricted CTLs have been described. CTLs must be activated by antigen presented by macrophages or other antigen-presenting cells (APCs). The nature of the specific epitopes expressed on the surface of infected cells that CTLs recognize has been defined for some viruses, such as influenza. In contrast to the specificity of neutralizing antibodies, which typically recognize epitopes on intact viral surface proteins, CTLs recognize protein fragments derived from both viral surface and internal proteins. The pathways by which these peptides are processed, appear on the surface of infected cells, and interact with MHC antigens are subjects of active investigation.

Interferons Leukocytes produce more than a dozen alpha ("leukocyte") interferons that share about 70 percent amino acid sequence homology. Beta ("fibroblast") interferon is produced by fibroblasts and epithelial cells and has 30 percent homology to α-interferons. Both α- and β-interferons are acid-stable (pH = 2) and relatively heat resistant. "Immune" (γ-) interferon is produced by both sensitized and unsensitized T lymphocytes, has different physicochemical properties and different inducers, and uses a different cellular receptor from α- and β-interferons. Genes encoding interferons are located on human chromosomes 9(α and β), 2(β), 5(β), and 12(γ).

Interferons can be induced by both active and inactivated viruses, by double-stranded RNA, and by a number of other compounds. The amount of interferon produced may vary with different viruses. All the interferons have extremely high specific activity and are generally most active in cells of the species in which they are induced ("species-specific"), presumably because of variation in the nature of the interferon receptor. Interferon production appears to involve a derepression of cellular genes induced by the presence of viral nucleic acid in the host cell cytoplasm. This results in the rapid production of mRNAs for interferon and subsequent interferon synthesis.

Newly produced interferon is released into extracellular fluid and then binds to a specific receptor on adjacent cells. The gene encoding the glycoprotein receptor for α- and β-interferon appears to be on human chromosome 21. Binding of interferon to this receptor results in a complex variety of subsequent events. A protein kinase is synthesized which phosphorylates a protein synthesis initiation factor, resulting in inhibition of initiation complex formation and hence of viral protein synthesis. An induced 2,5-oligoisoadenylate synthetase produces 2,5-oligoadenylates, which in turn activate a cellular endonuclease (RNase L) which degrades viral mRNA. Methyltransferase reactions are inhibited, which decreases methylation of mRNAs and thereby interferes with viral protein synthesis. In addition to these actions there are changes in target cell surface antigens, resulting in enhanced expression of both class I and class II histocompatability antigens. Interferons also increase the activity of NK cells, CTLs, and cells involved in ADCC reactions. The relative importance of each of these activities in creating the interferon-induced antiviral state is not established.

Virus-induced immunopathology Viruses can combine with virus-specific antibodies to produce circulating immune complexes which may be involved in immunopathogenesis. Virus stimulation of B lymphocytes may result in the production of polyclonal antibodies to antigens unrelated to the inciting virus. Viruses can also induce cross-reacting antibodies to normal host structures which contain antigenic regions similar to those of the virus (*molecular mimicry*). These types of autoantibodies may also lead to immune-complex formation. Immune complexes can become trapped in basement membranes at a variety of sites including the skin, the kidney, the choroid plexus, and the walls of blood vessels. These immune complexes result in tissue injury by attracting and activating a variety of inflammatory mediators.

Autoantibodies produced by virus infection may also result in direct tissue injury. Autoantibodies to lymphocytes, platelets, smooth muscle, intermediate filaments, immunoglobulins and myelin basic protein are usually transient and of low titer. These autoantibodies could result from a variety of mechanisms including (1) incorporation of host antigens into viral structures or virus-induced alteration of host antigens, (2) virus-induced alterations in immunoregulatory systems, (3) cross-reactivity between virus antigens and normal host cell structures (molecular mimicry), and (4) eliciting anti-idiotypic antibodies which stimulate host cell receptors.

EPIDEMIOLOGY Viral epidemiology includes the study of the causes, distribution, frequency, modes of transmission, and spread of viral diseases. Accurate enumeration of the incidence and prevalence of viral diseases is an important aspect of epidemiology. Incidence can be defined as the number of *new* cases of a particular disease that appear during a defined period of time, and prevalence as the *total* number of cases. It is often useful to refer to incidence and prevalence *rates*, which are obtained by dividing incidence or prevalence numbers by the size of the total population at risk. Terms such as "epidemic" and "outbreak" are arbitrary and simply indicate that a greater than expected number of cases of a particular disease has occurred in a specific population, geographic location, or time period.

The appearance of an acute viral disease indicates that an infected host has come into contact with a susceptible individual under conditions that permit the transmission of a particular viral agent. The time interval between exposure to a virus and the development of signs and symptoms of disease is referred to as the "incubation period" and can vary from a few days (e.g., influenza) to years (slow virus diseases). Viral infection does not always lead to overt clinical disease. The percentage of those infected who develop overt disease ranges from 100 percent (e.g., rabies, measles) to 0 percent (BK, JC papovaviruses). In most cases symptomatic disease is less common in children than in adults (e.g., EBV mononucleosis, paralytic poliomyelitis, hepatitis A virus).

Transmission of a virus from an infected host to a susceptible individual can take a variety of forms. Human-to-human transmission can occur from an acutely ill individual, from a chronic carrier, or from mother to fetus. The method of spread can involve respiratory aerosols, fecal-oral contamination, sexual contact, or direct inoculation via infected needles or blood products.

Respiratory aerosolization usually occurs via coughing or sneezing. A sneeze may generate up to 2 million aerosol particles and a cough up to 90,000. The fate of these particles depends both on ambient environmental conditions (e.g., humidity, wind currents) and particle size. Small particles remain airborne longer and can escape the filtering action of the nose, which traps particles larger than 6 μm in diameter. The number of viral particles aerosolized may vary for different strains of the same virus.

For most viruses it is unclear how many viral particles are required to initiate a respiratory infection. For influenza A, adenovirus, or coxsackie A21, as few as 10 particles may be sufficient. Aerosolization is not the only possible route of respiratory transmission. EBV is typically spread by saliva during kissing. A critical pathway of spread for rhinoviruses, which cause the common cold, is from hands to eyes, nose, or mouth—a cycle which can be interrupted by hand washing.

Gastrointestinal transmission occurs when virus shed in feces contaminates food or water and is then ingested by a susceptible individual ("fecal-oral spread"). Stool-tainted hands, resulting from poor personal hygiene, provide another vehicle of spread for enteric viruses. The high incidence of enteric virus infections in infant day-care centers and institutions for the mentally retarded reflect the difficulty of maintaining hygiene in these settings.

In many types of viral disease the vector is an insect or infected animal. In dengue fever there is a continuing cycle between humans and infected mosquitoes. Dengue virus multiplies in the gut of the *Aedes aegypti* mosquito, spreads to its salivary glands, and is injected into a human during the mosquito's blood meal. The infected person develops a high-titer viremia which is sufficient to transmit virus to an uninfected mosquito during biting. In other arbovirus infections the human being is a "dead-end host" because the degree of viremia in infected individuals is insufficient to transmit infection to a new group of insect vectors. Examples of this type of cycle are provided by togaviruses, such as eastern, western, and St. Louis encephalitis viruses. The normal animal reservoirs for arboviruses include small birds and mammals. The horse, like humans, is usually a dead-end host, although in Venezuelan equine encephalitis, horses may be a reservoir of virus.

Some arthropod-borne infections do not require a viremic vertebrate intermediate host. Virus can be passed in transovarian fashion to the progeny of an infected tick or mosquito or by venereal transmission between male and female mosquitoes. Transovarian transmission may allow survival of arthropod viruses through the winter months.

Zoonotic infections illustrate another mechanism of disease transmission. In the case of rabies, transmission results from the bite of an infected animal. Many human infections occur when humans are exposed to the excreta (feces, urine, saliva) of infected rodents.

Examples include arenavirus infections and the hemorrhagic fevers with renal disease caused by the bunyaviruses.

Defective agents, such as the adeno-associated human parvoviruses (AAHP) and the delta hepatitis virus (hepatitis D), require coinfection with a "helper" virus. Infection with the delta virus is dependent on coincident infection with hepatitis B virus (HBV) and does not occur in its absence. Many details of the epidemiology of these viruses remain to be established. The defective adeno-associated human parvoviruses do not appear to alter significantly the disease produced by the helper adenovirus alone. Conversely, coinfection with HBV and the delta antigen frequently results in fulminant hepatitis.

DIAGNOSIS OF VIRAL DISEASES A reasonably accurate diagnosis of some viral illnesses, such as measles, can be made on clinical grounds alone. In other cases the best that can be done clinically is to identify a group of viruses that are likely pathogens for specific categories of illness. More definitive diagnosis is often necessary because of availability of antiviral agents with activity limited only to certain types of viruses. Definitive diagnosis requires isolation of the virus in animals or in tissue culture, identification of the virus or detection of virus-specified antigens or viral nucleic acids in tissues or body fluids, or documentation of specific serologic responses. The physician must ensure that the appropriate specimens are obtained for diagnostic studies during a suitable phase of the illness, that they are rapidly transported, and that adequate clinical information is provided to the diagnostic laboratories.

In the case of diarrheal or gastrointestinal illness where a viral etiology is suspected, a fresh stool sample is the specimen of choice for virus isolation. In diseases of the respiratory system, including pharyngitis, croup, bronchiolitis, and pneumonia, nasopharyngeal or tracheal *aspirates* provide the best specimens. Nasopharyngeal and throat *swabs* are less satisfactory. When a vesicular rash is present, a needle aspirate of vesicular fluid provides the optimum specimen. When the rash is petechial or maculopapular, both nasopharyngeal aspirates and a stool sample should be obtained. In patients with CNS diseases of suspected viral etiology, including meningitis, encephalitis, myelitis, and Guillain-Barré syndrome, a nasopharyngeal aspirate and stool and cerebrospinal fluid specimens should be obtained. A urine sample may be helpful when infection due to CMV, measles, mumps, or papovaviruses is suspected. Blood specimens may be useful for the detection of some arboviruses, herpesviruses, and LCM. Saliva has been used for the detection of rabies and mumps viruses. A brain biopsy specimen is often required for the definitive diagnosis of herpes simplex encephalitis, progressive multifocal leukoencephalopathy, subacute sclerosing panencephalitis (SSPE), progressive rubella panencephalitis, and slow virus diseases such as Creutzfeldt-Jakob disease.

Nasopharyngeal or rectal swab specimens should be placed in an appropriate transport medium. In general this consists of a few milliliters of a neutral isotonic salt solution to which a small amount of protein or animal serum has been added. Antibiotics should be added to inhibit bacterial contaminants. Specimens can be placed in a thermos flask filled with crushed ice if any delay in transport is anticipated. Ideally, specimens should be inoculated into the appropriate culture systems on arrival in the virology laboratory. Storage up to 48 h can often be safely done at refrigerator temperature (4°C), and longer storage should be at −70°C. Many viruses quickly lose infectivity if repeatedly frozen and thawed.

Isolation of virus from clinical specimens is done in cell cultures, embryonated eggs, and animals such as suckling mice. Cell culture techniques involve the use of primary cultures of cells prepared from organs of freshly killed animals (e.g., monkey kidney cells); human diploid cell lines such as WI-38 embryo fibroblasts; and continuous (heterodiploid) cell lines such as HeLa, HEp-2, BHK-21, and vero. Some viruses grow better on certain cell lines than others. Inoculation into the amniotic cavity or the allantoic cavity of embryonated chicken eggs is useful in the isolation of influenza virus. Intraperitoneal and intracerebral inoculation into neonatal mice may be necessary for isolation of coxsackie A viruses and may help in the isolation of many arboviruses, rabies virus, arenaviruses, and orbiviruses. Adult mice or guinea pigs can be used to isolate LCM virus. Identification of the agent responsible for slow virus diseases such as kuru and Creutzfeldt-Jakob disease may require intracerebral inoculation of higher primates such as chimpanzees. Special isolation techniques using brain tissue explants are required to identify measles virus in cases of SSPE, or rubella virus in patients with progressive rubella panencephalitis.

Once cell culture inoculation has been performed, the specimens are examined for distinctive patterns of cytopathic effect (CPE). Viruses such as HSV and many enteroviruses produce early CPE, whereas cultures may need to be followed for weeks and even subcultured to detect CPE due to CMV, rubella, and some adenoviruses. Cultured cells are examined for cell lysis and vacuolization. The presence of syncytia suggests HSV, RSV, measles, or mumps virus. Cytomegaly is seen with HSV, varicella-zoster virus (VZV), and CMV. Detection of inclusion bodies is aided by the use of Giemsa or other stains. Immunocytochemical staining of cell cultures to detect viral antigens using fluorescein or enzyme-conjugated specific antiviral antibodies can aid in the detection and identification of many viruses. Some viruses produce minimal or no detectable CPE. Ortho- and paramyxoviruses (influenza, parainfluenza, measles, mumps) can be detected by the ability of infected cultures to adsorb certain red blood cells (*hemadsorption*). Infection with rubella can be detected by the ability of infected cultures to block the CPE produced by infection with a second challenge virus (*interference*).

Identification of virus particles or antigens in tissue specimens provides another important method of viral diagnosis. Skin scrapings from the base of vesicles can be stained with Wright or Giemsa stain according to the Tzanck method to help identify HSV or VZV. Similar techniques may help identify CMV-infected cells in urine sediment or measles-infected cells in scrapings from Koplik spots. In some cases, examination of appropriately prepared specimens by electron microscopy (EM) is of diagnostic value; high concentrations of virus must be present. A special technique which concentrates virus in specimens by adsorbing excess fluid and salts on an agarose surface may enable detection of as few as 10^4 particles per milliliter (pseudoreplica technique). EM easily distinguishes between vaccinia and varicella-zoster viruses in vesicular fluid negatively stained with phosphotungstic acid, and may be extremely useful in identifying skin viruses such as human papilloma virus, orf virus, and molluscum contagiosum. The use of specific antisera to aggregate virus in prepared stool specimens facilitates EM detection of rotaviruses, hepatitis A virus, and the Norwalk agent. EM examination of brain biopsy specimens may allow identification of herpes simplex encephalitis, PML, and SSPE.

Detection of virus-specific antigens is facilitated by immunofluorescence and immunocytochemical techniques. These procedures are particularly valuable in diagnosing rabies, herpes infection, PML, and SSPE in brain biopsy specimens; herpes keratitis from corneal scrapings; HSV, VZV, and vaccinia infections from vesicle scrapings; parainfluenza, influenza, and RSV infections from nasopharyngeal aspirates; hepatitis B infections in liver biopsy specimens; and Colorado tick fever virus infection from blood clots. Viral antigens can be detected in these tissue specimens using virus-specific antibodies directly or indirectly coupled with fluorescein isothiocyanate (FITC), or enzymes including horseradish peroxidase (HRP), alkaline phosphatase (AP), and glucose oxidase (GO). Enzyme-linked antibody techniques offer the advantage of increased sensitivity, preservability of stained specimens, and detectability with conventional light microscopy. Coupling a biotin-linked antibody with avidin-linked FITC or enzymes promises to improve immunocytochemical techniques. Radioimmunoassays and immunoassays, in which viral antibody coupled to a solid support (ELISA) is used to detect viral antigens, have proved useful in the diagnosis of hepatitis A and B virus, rotavirus, and adenovirus infections.

The detection of a fourfold or greater increase in antibody titer to a specific viral agent in a patient's acute and convalescent (3 to 4 weeks later) sera can usually be considered diagnostic of acute infection. A single serum specimen is only occasionally useful in viral diagnosis. A high antibody titer against a rare agent in a typical clinical setting or a distinct pattern of antibody titers to viral antigens of specific types may provide presumptive evidence of acute infection. Blood for serology should be collected in anticoagulant- and preservative-free glass tubes, and allowed to clot. Serum should be separated out and stored frozen. A number of different types of antibodies including neutralizing (N), complement-fixing (CF), and hemagglutination-inhibiting (HI) antibodies are routinely assayed. The time course of these antibody responses and their sensitivity and specificity differ greatly.

Restriction enzyme analysis of the genomes of DNA viruses (e.g., HSV, VZV, CMV) and oligonucleotide fingerprinting of ribonuclease T_1 cleaved genomes of RNA viruses (e.g., influenza, dengue enteroviruses) are valuable in epidemiologic studies and in establishing the origin of certain types of viral isolates. In situ hybridization and the polymerase chain reaction technique may enable the detection of even single copies of virus genomes in tissue samples or cells from body fluids.

PREVENTION OF VIRAL ILLNESS **Vaccines** Currently available vaccines utilize inactivated virus, attenuated virus, or virus subunits to induce active immunization. Formalin- or β-propiolactone–inactivated vaccines are available for rabies, influenza, and polio. Strains used in the inactivated influenza whole-virus vaccine are specified yearly by the FDA. The vaccine is composed of formalin-inactivated natural isolates of influenza virus and laboratory-designed reassortant strains containing the hemagglutinin and neuraminidase genes of the influenza viruses that are currently circulating. As many as 60 to 80 percent of those immunized show a reduction in the frequency or severity of influenzal illness. Guillain-Barré syndrome occurred in 1 in 100,000 individuals vaccinated with the swine influenza vaccine in 1976 to 1977 but has not been associated with subsequent influenza vaccine preparations. Killed polio vaccine is used in Sweden, Finland, and the Netherlands, and in combination with live vaccine in Denmark, but has been supplanted by the Sabin live oral vaccine in the United States, except for use in immunodeficient individuals.

Inactivated virus vaccines have advantages and disadvantages compared to live vaccines. The absence of live virus results in immunization without active infection. Since there is no live virus present, reversion to virulence does not occur, although improperly prepared vaccines can contain virulent virus or adventitious viral contaminants (e.g., SV40, avian leukosis virus). Effective local immunity does not develop, so vaccinated individuals may still transmit virus to the community. In rare cases (measles, RSV), inactivated vaccines have resulted in atypical immunologic responses which potentiated rather than prevented subsequent natural infections.

The attenuated virus vaccines in current use have been developed from either naturally occurring attenuated viruses (e.g., poliovirus type 2 strain 712) or from viruses after serial passage in tissue culture cells or embryonated eggs. These passage-selected viruses have mutations when compared to their wild type parents. For example, the vaccine strain of poliovirus type 1 differs in 21 amino acids from the original parent virus. On some vaccine viruses, the largest number of mutations are located in genes coding for viral surface proteins such as VP1 (polio) or V3 (yellow fever). However, in the case of the type 1 polio vaccine strain, mutations responsible for attenuation appear to be distributed throughout the viral genome. In other cases (e.g., mumps) a clear marker for the vaccine virus strain has not been identified.

Following immunization with the oral Sabin polio vaccine, the vaccinated person excretes virus which can infect other individuals in the community. In rare cases, the excreted virus appears to be more virulent than the vaccine strain, and may account for some of the rare cases of paralytic polio in close contacts of vaccinees. Reversion to virulence by the vaccine strain of virus may also cause paralytic polio in vaccinees. Approximately 1 in 10 million vaccinated individuals develops paralytic polio, and there are 3 cases of paralytic polio per 10 million household and community contacts of recent vaccinees. These risks are small and are probably overestimates which include coincidental as well as causal associations. In rare settings, where exposure to polio occurs at a very young age, a combined program using both inactivated (killed) and attenuated vaccines may be of benefit (see also Chap. 144).

Live attenuated measles, mumps, and rubella vaccines can be administered together (MMR) without any loss in immunizing capacity (>90 percent). Of individuals who receive the measles vaccine alone (Schwarz strain), 10 to 30 percent have mild clinical reactions, and there are rare cases of encephalitis. It is not clear that the very rare cases of encephalitis in recipients of measles vaccine are related to the vaccine virus. On the contrary, by preventing natural measles, measles vaccine has been associated with a dramatic reduction in the incidence of SSPE. The attenuated Jeryl Lynn B strain is used in the live mumps virus vaccine. Adverse effects are rare and include allergic reactions as well as CNS complications. The most commonly used rubella vaccine strain (RA 27/3) was attenuated by multiple passages through the WI-38 line of cultured human diploid fibroblasts. The most notable complications are transient arthralgia and rare cases of arthritis.

A live attenuated vaccine for yellow fever has been prepared using virus derived from passage through chicken embryos. Of those vaccinated intradermally, 95 percent develop an immune response. Serious adverse reactions occur in fewer than 1 in 1 million cases.

A novel approach to vaccination is illustrated by the adenovirus vaccine. In this case the live vaccine virus strains (4, 7) are not attenuated, but the route of administration (via oral ingestion of an enteric coated tablet) results in an asymptomatic infection with subsequent immunity. Ingested virus does not reach the respiratory tract, but produces an intestinal infection that stimulates an immune response against subsequent adenovirus-induced respiratory infections.

Two vaccines utilize virus subunits rather than whole virus to induce immunity. The influenza subunit vaccine is composed of purified envelope glycoproteins. It appears to be less toxic than live whole virus vaccine but also less antigenic. The hepatitis B vaccine uses a formalin-treated antigen as an immunogen. Purified proteins from cloned viral DNA are used in hepatitis B vaccine that may be useful in a herpes vaccine. Synthetic polypeptides analogous to major antigenic sites on viral structural proteins may be of value either as vaccines or as primers that induce a primary immune response that requires a subsequent boost.

ANTIVIRAL THERAPY **Immune globulins** The role in antiviral therapy of immunoglobulins extracted from pooled lots of adult plasma is limited. Antibody titers to specific viruses in different pooled lots of gamma globulin vary over a tenfold range. Intramuscular administration of immune globulin at the time of exposure to hepatitis A virus can prevent infection or decrease the severity of subsequent illness. A similar beneficial effect has been reported for measles infection and possibly for hepatitis B infection.

Specific immune globulins are made from plasma with high antibody titer against specific viruses. When given within 72 h of exposure to varicella-zoster virus, varicella-zoster immune globulin can prevent or modify subsequent infection. Such therapy is of value in exposed immunocompromised individuals, pregnant women, infants of mothers who develop chickenpox, and newborns of nonimmune mothers exposed to chickenpox. Hepatitis B immune globulin is useful in preventing infection of individuals exposed to HBsAg-positive material (e.g., a needle stick) or of infants exposed to hepatitis B–infected mothers. Rabies immune globulin is an integral part of postexposure prophylaxis of rabies. Other immune globulins are available but are not widely used.

Antiviral chemotherapy See Chap. 86.

REFERENCES

EVANS AS (ed): *Viral Infections of Humans: Epidemiology and Control*, 2d ed. New York, Plenum, 1984
FIELDS BN et al (eds): *Virology*. New York, Raven, 1985
GALASSO GJ et al (eds): *Antiviral Agents and Chemotherapy*, 2d ed. New York, Raven, 1984
JOHNSON RT: *Viral Infections of the Nervous System*. New York, Raven, 1982
LENNETTE EH, HALONEN P, MURPHY FA (eds): *Laboratory Diagnosis of Infectious Diseases, Principles and Practice*, vol 2, *Viral, Rickettsial, and Chlamydial Diseases*. New York, Springer-Verlag, 1988
MIMS CA, WHITE DO: *Viral Pathogenesis and Immunology*. Oxford, Blackwell, 1984
NOTKINS AL, OLDSTONE MBA (eds): *Concepts in Viral Pathogenesis*. New York, Springer-Verlag, 1984
———: *Concepts in Viral Pathogenesis II*. New York, Springer-Verlag, 1986

134 THE HUMAN RETROVIRUSES

ROBERT C. GALLO / ANTHONY S. FAUCI

Retroviruses were first described at the beginning of the century as filterable agents that caused transmissible tumors in chickens; the first recognized mammalian retroviruses were isolated from mice with leukemia in the 1950s. However despite extensive investigation the first human retrovirus, HTLV-I, was not isolated until 1978. This became possible only after the discovery of RNA-to-DNA transcription by viruses and through the use of reverse transcriptase (RT) as a sensitive "footprint" for these viruses. In addition the obligate requirement of a T-cell growth factor, interleukin 2 (IL-2) (see Chap. 13), for growth of T cells in culture helped make isolation possible. There are now four human retroviruses belonging to two distinct groups: the human T-cell leukemia retroviruses, HTLV-I and HTLV-II, and the human immunodeficiency viruses, HIV-1 and HIV-2.

Although retroviruses are sometimes categorized as oncogenic viruses, lentiviruses, and spumaviruses, they may also be grouped by the disease they cause, their electron-microscopic appearance, and their biologic effects. In contrast to the infectious retroviruses some, called endogenous retroviruses, are transmitted in the germ line. Although there is limited homology of the genomes of animal retroviruses to some sequences in the human genome, there are no known human endogenous viruses. The spumaviruses are known for their ability to produce a characteristic foamy cytopathic effect in tissue culture, but their existence and biologic role in human beings is uncertain. The lentiviruses, first recognized in ungulates, are so far associated only with nonmalignant disease, particularly neurologic disorders (visna), immune-complex disease (equine infectious anemia virus), and encephalitis and arthritis (caprine arthritis encephalitis virus). These viruses are "slow-acting" only by comparison with viruses that cause acute infections such as influenza virus but not by comparison with other retroviruses. Retroviruses associated with malignant disease include HTLV-I and HTLV-II, some of the closely related simian viruses (STLV-I), feline leukemia virus (FeLV), bovine leukemia virus (BLV), gibbon ape leukemia virus (GaLV), and many avian and murine viruses. These viruses may also induce nonmalignant disease. For example, FeLV, which can cause T-cell leukemia, more frequently causes immunodeficiency in cats, mimicking the acquired immune deficiency syndrome (AIDS) of human beings. It appears that a change in the envelope of the virus is correlated with a change in the kind of disease induced by the virus.

GENERAL BIOLOGY OF RETROVIRUSES Retroviruses are enveloped viruses, usually about 100 nm in diameter, that form by budding from cell membranes (Fig. 134-1). An electron-dense central core surrounds two identical copies of the single-stranded viral RNA genome, making retroviruses diploid, which is unusual among viruses (see Chap. 133). However, it is the DNA polymerase, known as reverse transcriptase, that is the distinguishing feature of a retrovirus. Complexed to an RNA in the viral core, this enzyme catalyzes the transcription of the RNA genome into a double-stranded DNA form that migrates from the cytoplasm to the nucleus and integrates into the host cell DNA. In this form, known as the provirus, the viral genes remain integrated for the lifetime of the cell. They are duplicated with the cell DNA during the S phase of the cell cycle. Therefore, once established, infection of an organism is generally lifelong. When the provirus is expressed, viral RNA and proteins are found in the cell cytoplasm and assembled at the cell membrane, where budding and release of infectious virions completes the replication cycle (Fig. 134-2).

The molecular mechanisms by which retroviruses alter the life cycle of infected cells are strikingly diverse and often depend on the organization of the viral genome. All retroviruses contain three essential genes for virus replication: *gag*, *pol*, and *env* (Fig. 134-3). *Gag* codes for a polyprotein precursor that is cleaved by a viral protease into three or four structural proteins; *pol* codes for RT and the viral protease and integrase; *env* codes for the transmembrane and outer glycoprotein of the virus. The properties of the envelope have a major influence on the kind of cell the virus can infect, and production of antibodies against the envelope is one of the essential features sought in a vaccine. At either end of the provirus the long terminal repeats (LTR) are covalently joined to the cellular DNA;

FIGURE 134-1 Electron micrographs of the characterized human retrovirus. The viruses are shown as they replicate by budding from a cell membrane (*upper panels*) and as the mature infectious extracellular virion (*lower panels*).

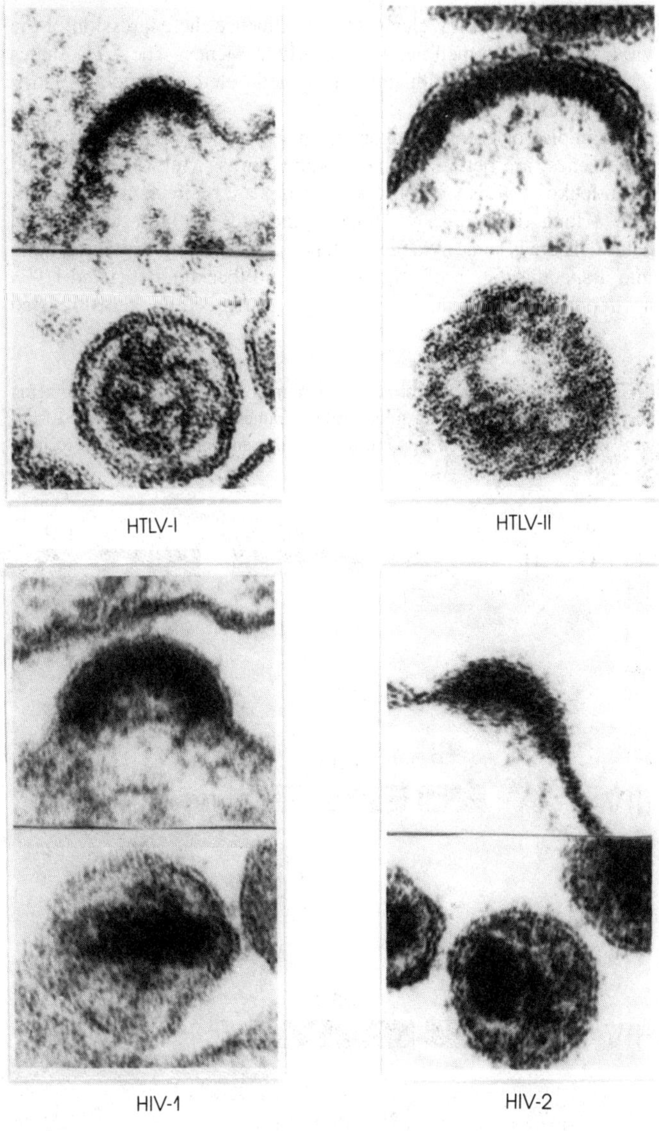

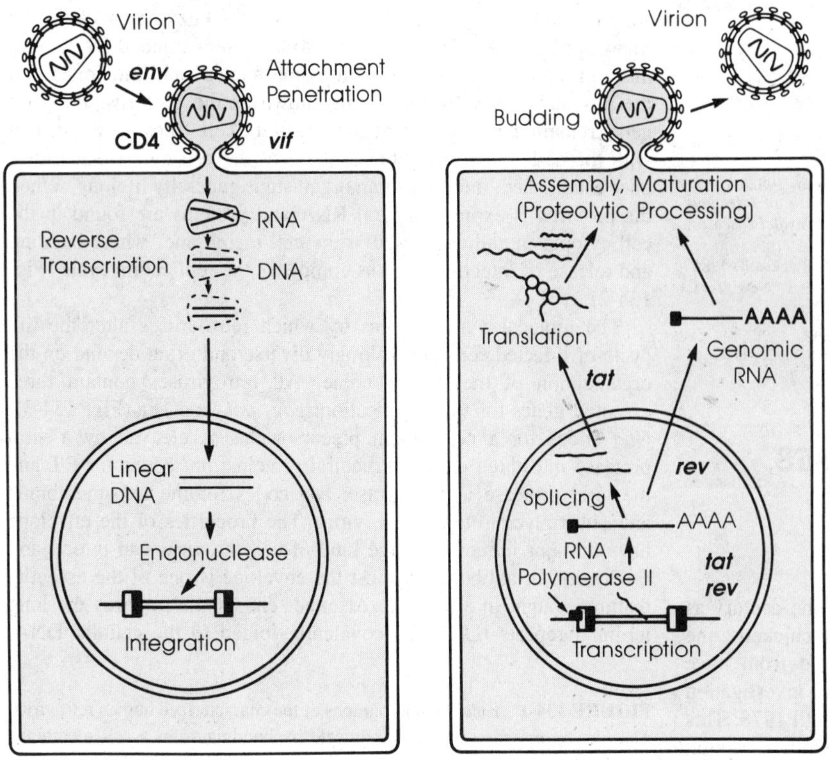

FIGURE 134-2 Life cycle of a retrovirus (as represented by HIV-1). Intact virions are endocytosed via a specific cellular receptor. The uncoated viral single-stranded RNA is then transcribed into double-stranded DNA, enters the cell nucleus, and integrates into the host genome. The DNA provirus in some conditions is unexpressed. In other cases it is transcribed, giving rise to viral RNA encoding viral proteins and genome-length viral RNA molecules which then reassemble with viral proteins to make complete virions. These progeny are released by budding from the cell membrane. All known infectious retroviruses follow these steps. The specific molecules described pertain only to HIV-1 (the CD4 receptor with *vif*, *tat*, and *rev* viral proteins).

they contain regulatory elements that influence the expression of the viral genes and sometimes nearby cellular genes. The LTR shares features in common with movable genetic elements such as retrotransposons.

Examples of chronic leukemia viruses, which contain only these three genes, are FeLV, murine leukemia virus (MuLV), GaLV, and avian leukosis virus (ALV). These viruses are replication competent, take a long time to cause disease, and are relatively common in nature. There is some evidence that they cause leukemia by integration into a specific region of a chromosome so that the associated LTRs act to promote continual expression of a nearby cellular gene involved in growth (a proto-oncogene) (see Chaps. 9 and 10). The best studied example of this *cis* mechanism is in chickens, where the LTR of avian leukosis virus promotes expression of the cellular proto-oncogene *myc,* believed to be the first step in the induction of B-cell leukemia by this virus. Since integration by retroviruses is random, a high rate of replication favors the chance of integration into regions sufficiently near the cellular oncogene as to effect its expression. There are no known human viruses of this type.

When a retrovirus acquires a host cell gene that rapidly transforms cells and induces acute malignancies, the virus is often called an *acute leukemia* or *sarcoma virus,* and the acquired gene (i.e., host

FIGURE 134-3 Genomic structure of human retroviruses. Viral proteins may be translated in each of three reading frames. RNA is transcribed from viral DNA and processed by viral and cellular enzymes giving rise to both genomic viral RNA and mRNA. Arrows indicate double spliced mRNA. LTR, long terminal repeat; *gag,* core proteins; *pol,* polymerase (RT); *env,* envelope. Viral genes shown in color code for regulatory proteins.

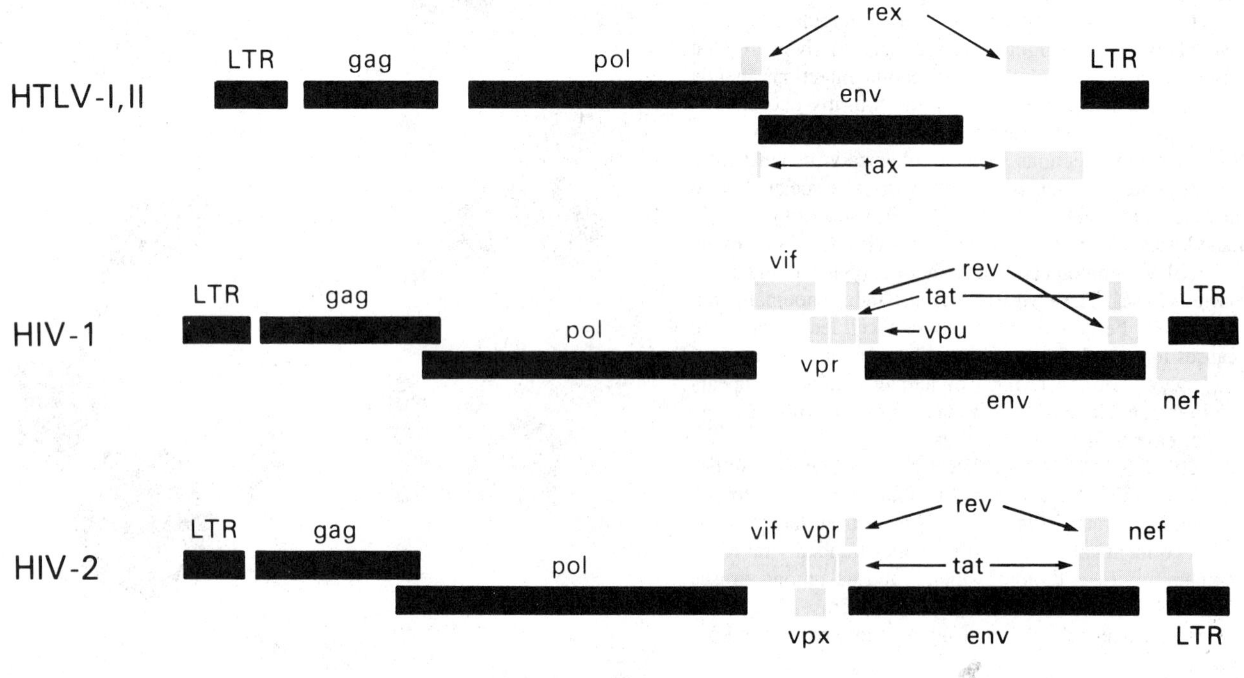

proto-oncogene) is called a *viral onc gene*. This type of change almost always leads to an incomplete viral genome which forms defective viral particles. The virus then needs the addition of a helper virus and in vitro manipulation for its propagation. Viruses with *onc* genes are thought to be rare in nature and are of interest in animals chiefly for investigating mechanisms of neoplastic transformation rather than as causes of naturally occurring cancer. An example of this appears with FeLV. In addition to the mechanism of specific integration near a proto-oncogene and subsequent activation of this gene, FeLV may cause malignancies by the relatively frequent acquisition of cell-derived oncogenes. Every cell infected by these viruses can be transformed (giving rise to polyclonal tumors) because the product of the viral *onc* gene directly transforms the cells. Therefore, a common site of integration or a second genetic event to trigger transformation is not needed. The development of the malignancy is usually rapid and sometimes occurs within months of infection. Human viruses of this type have never been found.

FEATURES OF HUMAN RETROVIRUSES The known human and some related animal retroviruses can be regarded as unique categories of retroviruses. Human T-lymphotropic (or leukemia) viruses (HTLV-I and HTLV-II) transform cells in culture, while human immunodeficiency viruses (HIV-1 and -2) are cytopathic in culture. While the two groups have little sequence homology, they have some striking similarities and differences.

In addition to the usual viral structural genes, all of the human retroviruses contain extra genes that provide regulatory signals essential to virus replication and to the biologic activities of the virus. Such genes were first found in HTLV-I and HTLV-II and more recently in HIV-2 and HIV-1, the well-known cause of AIDS.

One of these, called *tax*-1 in HTLV-I and *tat*-1 in HIV-1, codes for proteins that activate the expression of viral and some cellular genes. Another gene, *rex* in HTLV-I and *rev* in HIV-1, codes for proteins that favor the formation of unspliced or single-spliced viral mRNA; in their absence only small doubly spliced mRNAs are made. The *rev* protein is localized in the nucleus and appears to increase transport of the larger mRNA, which encodes for structural proteins, to the cytoplasm. Conversely, it diminishes the availability of the mRNA for *rev* itself and for the other regulatory proteins. For each virus these proteins are structurally distinct but have similar functions.

HIV-1 follows many of the same regulatory strategies as HTLV-I, but its genome is even more complex. By deletion analysis the function of several other genes has been evaluated. The *nef* gene product appears to be a negative regulator of viral production, while the *vif* gene affects the ability of virus particle(s) to infect target cells but does not affect viral replication. The *vpu* gene has been reported to enhance modestly the maturation and exit of virus from the cell in vitro, and the *vpr* gene has been reported to stimulate the promoter region of the virus. In reality, the functions of these genes are poorly understood and their in vivo relevance is unclear.

All of the four known human retroviruses preferentially infect the T4 lymphocyte, and the diseases they cause involve this cell, often resulting in profound biologic consequences. Ironically, the cellular receptor for HIV is the CD4 molecule itself (Fig. 134-2) (see Chap. 13 for discussion of the function of CD4.) The remarkably high affinity of gp120 envelope protein for this molecule probably determines the host range of the virus, the nature of cell target populations, the mode and ability of the virus to be efficiently transmitted, and contributes to the cytopathic effect both through the formation of syncytia and through effects upon virus production. A region of the transmembrane protein gp41 facilitates entry of the virus into the cell by helping to fuse the virus coat with the target cell membrane. The cellular receptor(s) for the HTLVs is not known, but its gene is on chromosome 17. HTLV-I can usually be transmitted only by cell-to-cell contact while the HIVs can be transmitted in this manner and as extracellular virus.

The monocyte-macrophage is also a major target for HIV-1. As for lymphocytes, entry requires attachment to CD4 molecules expressed on the cell surface and may be enhanced by Fc-receptor-mediated endocytosis. Infected monocytes are believed to play a major role in the disease by acting as reservoirs for the virus and as vehicles for its spread. Related cells are infected in the brain, lymph node, skin, lung, and gastrointestinal tract. Cytokine production by infected monocytes and T cells may play a direct role in the induction of malignancy, neurologic disease, and perhaps other clinical manifestations such as enteritis and lymphoid interstitial pneumonitis.

DISEASES ASSOCIATED WITH HTLV-I INFECTION HTLV-I rapidly induces transformation of human T cells in vitro; it has neither an *onc* gene nor a single integration site, yet results in monoclonal malignancies. The majority of HTLV-I–induced leukemias or lymphomas involve the T4+ cell. Infection of T4+ cells by HTLV-I or HTLV-II leads to the transformation of some of the infected cells, and the properties of such transformed cells are similar. The infected cells often exhibit extensive "cerebriform" lobulation of the nuclei and form giant multinucleated cells in culture. They constitutively express increased numbers of receptors for IL-2 (IL-2R) which can be found on circulating T4+ cells. This may be due to the *tax* gene product, which can up-regulate the receptor, transform T cells when transfected, and induce tumors in transgenic animals. The maintenance of malignancy is not believed to require additional viral gene products since the HTLV-I genes are usually not expressed in the leukemic cells in vivo by the time the leukemia is clinically evident. The reason that only some individuals develop malignancy is not known. Since cells other than T4 lymphocytes can be infected, the reason for the frequency of transformation of the T4+ cell is unclear. The relatively high incidence of adult T-cell leukemia/lymphoma (ATLL) (lifetime risk of 1 to 3 percent) independent of geographic location suggests that a specific environmental cofactor is not necessary to produce disease. In contrast, the development of lymphoma associated with EBV occurs at a much lower rate and only in certain areas such as the "Burkitt lymphoma belt" in Africa where specific environmental cofactors are present.

Leukemias/lymphomas caused by HTLV-I are characterized by an aggressive course, frequent hypercalcemia (associated with tumor necrosis factor β secretion), opportunistic infection and, in over one-half of the cases, leukemic skin infiltrates. HTLV-I may also be involved in T4 cell leukemias/lymphomas that exhibit a more chronic course (15 to 20 percent of cases) involving progression from polyclonal T-cell proliferation to an expansion of a particular clone to frank clinical malignancy. These malignancies may be indistinguishable pathologically or clinically from chronic T-cell lymphocytic leukemia (CLL), diffuse histiocytic lymphoma, large and mixed cell lymphomas, and mycosis fungoides or Sézary leukemias (see Chaps. 296 and 302). Typical ATL cases recognized worldwide are almost always HTLV-I-positive. In the United States only a small percentage of T-cell malignancies are HTLV-I-positive. In contrast, in endemic areas almost all T4 cell malignancies are virus-positive.

In areas of the world where HTLV-I is endemic, some B-cell lymphoid malignancies and certain other cancers are associated with HTLV-I infection more frequently than expected from the prevalence of the virus in the general population. In contrast to virus-positive T-cell leukemias, where the viral genes are integrated into the DNA of the leukemic cell, HTLV-I is not found in the DNA of these B-cell tumors. Instead, the virus is present in the normal T cells of these patients, and the role of the virus must be indirect. Several of these B-cell neoplasms have been shown to make specific antibody against HTLV-I, suggesting that years of stimulation of some B-cell populations by HTLV-I proteins may be involved in their malignant transformation.

The etiologic association of HTLV-I with ATL was firmly established by the epidemiology and serology in endemic areas and by the presence of proviral DNA integrated in a monoclonal manner in the tumor. This indicated that the first transformed cell contained the provirus rather than being infected later as an opportunistic infection. The ability of HTLV-I to immortalize target T cells in vitro is also consistent with its role in vivo as a transforming virus. Considerable data in animals show that exogenous type C retroviruses are usually leukemogenic. This finding predicted that HTLVs would also be leukemogenic in human beings.

A new aspect of HTLV-I has been revealed by the discovery of the association of this virus with a demyelinating disorder, tropical spastic paraparesis (TSP) (see Chap. 355). This syndrome has also been referred to as HTLV-I–associated myelopathy (HAM). It is a chronic progressive encephalomyelopathy with symmetric upper motor neuron disease, prominent lower extremity weakness, and hyperreflexia, with sphincter and sensory abnormalities that may resemble a spinal cord variant of multiple sclerosis. Central nervous system lesions are seen on MRI scans. The pathogenesis is not known, but high antibody responses to HTLV-I and improvement with glucocorticoids suggest an autoimmune disease mechanism. A few individuals have both ATL and neurologic disease. While the lifetime risk of developing ATL appears to be between 1 and 3 percent in HTLV-I–infected individuals, the attack rate of TSP in some areas such as Colombia may be higher. Several other neurologic diseases may be associated with HTLV-I infection in endemic areas including polymyositis, Bell's palsy, and Guillain-Barré syndrome.

Treatment There are two major considerations in the treatment of HTLV-I infection. First, the time from infection to disease may be 20 years or more. Second, when ATL develops, the virus is transcriptionally silent in the peripheral blood leukemic cells. Treatment for asymptomatic seropositive individuals at present is limited to periodic evaluation for neurologic and hematologic disease, screening family members at risk, and avoiding infection by breast feeding, sexual transmission, and transfusion donation. Thus far, no regimen of chemotherapy has been demonstrated to increase survival in ATL. Clinical trials with several experimental approaches are currently being evaluated including targeting of the IL-2 receptor on leukemic cells with toxin-coupled antibody. Since virus is not replicating, antiviral chemotherapy seems unlikely to be effective. Several reports have indicated that high-dose glucocorticoids benefit TSP patients, but well-controlled trials have not been done.

ORIGIN AND EPIDEMIOLOGY OF HTLV-I AND HTLV-II HTLV-I was originally discovered in two black patients with T-cell malignancies in the United States, and within 1 year it was associated with clusters of a newly described T-cell malignancy (ATL) in some southwestern islands of Japan and in Caribbean-born blacks. It may have been brought to both areas from Africa centuries ago by merchants and slave traders. HTLV-I occurs worldwide but tends to be highly geographically restricted or clustered. In endemic areas the fraction of infected individuals ranges from 5 to 25 percent. Transmission is by intimate contact, by blood or blood products, and by nursing mothers (and perhaps by infection of the developing fetus in utero). Because of increased travel, changes in sexual habits, intravenous drug abuse (blood-contaminated needles), and wide use of blood and blood products, the prevalence of HTLV in nonendemic areas may be increasing.

HTLV-II was originally isolated from a cell line derived from a patient with a T-cell variant of hairy cell leukemia and can be distinguished from HTLV-I by competition radioimmunoassay. The virus has subsequently been isolated from several patients with more chronic forms of T-cell malignancies. Overall it is about 55 percent identical at the nucleotide level to HTLV-I, and only a few biologic differences have been found between the two viruses.

Current routine serologic tests do not distinguish between antibodies to HTLV-I and HTLV-II. Seropositivity to HTLV-I has been found in surprisingly high frequency in drug addict populations also at risk for HIV infection. The risk of being HTLV-I–positive correlates with geographic location. In many areas of the country the dominant HTLV virus in the drug addict population is HTLV-II. At the present time, the role of HTLV-II in disease is unclear; there are suggestions that dual infection with HIV and one of the HTLVs may lead to accelerated emergence of AIDS.

DISEASES ASSOCIATED WITH HIV INFECTION (See also Chap. 264) The etiologic agent of AIDS is a retrovirus called HIV-1 (formerly HTLV-III/LAV). As the discovery of the tuberculosis bacillus or the spirochete of syphilis unified diverse disease manifestations, the spectrum of disease associated with AIDS has been interpreted in the context of the biology and epidemiology of HIV-1 infection. HIV-2, the most recently described human retrovirus, has about 40 percent genetic identity with HIV-1. It is even more closely related to some members of a group of viruses causing immune deficiency in simians [simian immune deficiency virus (SIV)]. It has been isolated from patients with immunodeficiency and has been detected serologically in western Africa in populations different from those with HIV-1 infection in whom AIDS is not endemic. It appears to be a relatively uncommon and inefficient cause of AIDS and is not spreading with the rapidity of HIV. Cofactors that increase virus replication or enhance T-cell killing are being investigated for their role in the progression of disease. Particular factors include viruses such as HTLV-I, human herpes virus (HHV-6), and cytomegalovirus (CMV) which can promote HIV expression and also directly infect T cells. HHV-6, a new herpes virus, can also kill T4 lymphocytes. However, only in the case of HTLV-I is more rapid progression to AIDS supported by epidemiologic data.

HIV-1–associated Kaposi's sarcoma (KS) HIV-1–infected patients have an increased incidence of certain B-cell lymphomas, Hodgkin's disease, certain carcinomas, and KS. The reason for the increase in these malignancies is not understood, but it is not necessarily associated with the degree of immune impairment. HIV-1 is not the direct cause of any of these tumors because viral sequences are not found in the DNA from the majority of tumor cells. For the B-cell lymphomas, the mechanism may be similar to the indirect role described above for HTLV-I. Direct culture of tissue from KS lesions suggests that the role of HIV in KS may be the induction of a growth factor produced by infected CD4+ cells. This factor activates vascular cells which release several cytokines; the continuous release of these cytokines may result in the mixed cell population of KS. Additional support for this model is the appearance of KS-like lesions in transgenic male mice expressing the *tat* protein.

MOLECULAR HETEROGENEITY OF HIV Analysis at the molecular level of various HIV isolates reveals variation of nucleotide sequences of certain parts of the genome, especially in the envelope gene. In different isolates the amino acid sequence of the envelope proteins ranges from very closely related (1 to 2 percent variation) to those that vary 25 to 30 percent. A single individual (and perhaps intimate contacts) is usually infected with a "swarm" of closely related viruses that may constitute a single "strain." Even a very small difference, called "microheterogeneity," may exert a profound influence on the biology of the virus. Variation probably develops with successive infections and does not occur during prolonged tissue culture of a single molecularly cloned virus, suggesting that these changes occur during transcription of the viral RNA genome to the DNA form and/or during the recombinational process when the DNA provirus integrates into the host cell DNA. RT tends to be error prone because, unlike cellular DNA polymerases, RT lacks a proofreading mechanism. The RT of HIV may be particularly error prone. Variation of other genes is generally far less than that of the envelope. It is possible that strain variation may account for a difference in the clinical course of an HIV infected person; experimental studies have revealed significant biologic variations among strains, including target cell tropism and response to neutralizing antibody. A variant that can avoid elimination by antibodies or cytotoxic T8+ cells could lead more easily to progressive disease. For example, selection pressure on cultured virus in the presence of human neutralizing antisera has resulted in a virus with one amino acid change that is no longer neutralized by the selecting sera.

PREVENTION AND TREATMENT OF RETROVIRUS INFECTION There are three major approaches to the control of human retroviral disease: vaccination; antiviral therapy; and education and public health measures (see Chap. 264). Vaccines have proved to be the least costly and most effective way of preventing infectious disease, especially those caused by viruses, but there are special problems with HIV: (1) Because of the integration of viral genes, a limited number of viral particles may be sufficient to establish infection, and therefore the demands on a vaccine may be very stringent. (2) T cells are the principal cells involved in protection against a virus, and these are the cells destroyed by the virus. (3) Envelope heterogeneity allows the escape from neutralizing antibodies; there are several conserved areas of the envelope gene which are being actively studied as subunit vaccines. (4) The nature of the protective immune response is not yet clear. Most infected individuals develop progressive disease despite the presence of neutralizing antibodies and cytotoxic T cells. The expectation is that immunization prior to infection may prevent disease. Some encouragement comes from the finding that for most infections of a single individual only one strain of the virus has been found. This suggests that an individual is infected only once despite repeated exposure. And (5) animal models for vaccine development against HIV are limited, but the development of animal systems with SIV, the related African green monkey virus that can produce AIDS in macaques, is likely to be very helpful.

Antiviral therapy is based on a detailed understanding of the viral replication cycle, and almost every definable step offers the possibility of interfering with replication of virus (see Chap. 264). Approaches are available beginning with HIV binding to the cell. Recombinant CD4 is being tested that acts as a "molecular decoy" for the virus by competing with cellular receptors for binding viral gp120 envelope proteins. Early studies in animals and humans have been encouraging with regard to toxicity, but no beneficial effects have as yet emerged. The most successful agents to date affect the next stage, formation of the DNA provirus, by inhibiting RT. These agents include AZT and other nucleoside analogues such as dideoxycytodine (ddC) and dideoxyinosine (ddI). The next targets are the synthesis, maturation, and transport from nucleus to cytoplasm of viral RNA from proviral DNA, for which inhibitors of *tat* and *rev* function are being studied. Viral mRNA must be translated, and on an experimental basis this step can be specifically inhibited with antisense DNA. Lastly, viral proteins must assemble to form new virus, and this depends on a specific viral protease. This protein has been crystallized, and inhibitors are under study.

Because infection with HIV probably always means integration of the viral genes into the DNA of the infected cells, it is likely that lifelong treatment will be required. To minimize toxicity and reduce the chance for viral resistance, it may be necessary to use a combination of compounds with different mechanisms of action. Another approach would be to kill infected cells; success would depend upon elimination of all infected cells. However, this may not be possible with human retroviruses because most infected cells do not express viral proteins and are therefore not distinguishable from uninfected cells. Moreover, infected macrophages appear to act as reservoirs for the virus and may release additional virions from intracellular vacuolar membranes when killed.

OTHER DISEASES ASSOCIATED WITH HUMAN RETROVIRAL INFECTION The possibility that several well-described human diseases are associated with retroviral infection should be carefully considered. While the promise of many candidate viruses has not been fulfilled, the number of retroviruses with diverse mechanisms of disease found in other species suggests a wide range of possibilities. A report of RT activity in non-A, non-B hepatitis has not been substantiated since a new flavivirus has been discovered as the probable cause. RT activity has been detected in patients with Kawasaki disease, but neither a virus nor viral sequences have been found and there has been no confirmation of the original reports. Mammary tumors in mice have been transmitted via breast milk infected with mammary tumor virus. Despite sporadic reports of electron-micrographic evidence of virus in human tumors, no human equivalent has been isolated and characterized. The presence of a retrovirus in some patients with mycosis fungoides that differs from HTLV-I–associated tumors has been reported as HTLV-V. Verification awaits further characterization of the candidate virus. Retroviruses are known to produce neurologic disease in some species (e.g., visna in sheep and MuLV in some mice); HIV-1 infects the central nervous system; and HTLV-I is associated with a demyelinating disease. A possible retroviral etiology of multiple sclerosis has been considered. Sequences related to HTLV-I have been reported in the peripheral blood of patients with multiple sclerosis by in situ hybridization or polymerase chain reaction. Differentiation of these sequences from those endogenous to cells and recovery of intact virus are needed to confirm the significance of these associations.

The discovery of the HTLV-I occurred at a time when many thought that there would be no human retroviruses. In the ensuing decade, four human retroviruses have been discovered and associated with several human diseases. These viruses have provided major insights into the pathogenesis of neoplastic, immunosuppressive, and neurologic disorders as well as some of the most difficult medical, social, and scientific challenges of the late twentieth century.

REFERENCES

BARRE-SINOUSSI F et al: Isolation of a T lymphotropic retrovirus from a patient at risk for acquired immune deficiency syndrome (AIDS). Science 220:868, 1983

BLATTNER W: Retroviruses, in *Viral Infections of Humans*, AS Evans (ed). New York, Plenum, 1989, pp 545–592

BRODER S, GALLO R: A pathogenic retrovirus (HTLV-III) linked to AIDS. N Engl J Med 311:1292, 1984

FAUCI AS: The human immunodeficiency virus: Infectivity and mechanisms of pathogenesis. Science 239:617, 1988

GALLO RC: The first human retrovirus. Sci Am 255:88, 1986

———, MONTAGNIER L: AIDS in 1988. Sci Am 259:41, 1988

——— et al: Frequent detection and isolation of cytopathic retroviruses (HTLV-III) from patients with AIDS and at risk for AIDS. Science 224:500, 1984

SALAHUDDIN SZ et al: Angiogenic properties of Kaposi's sarcoma-derived cells after long-term culture *in vitro*. Science 242:430, 1988

VARMUS H: Retroviruses. Science 240:1427, 1988

135 HERPES SIMPLEX VIRUSES

LAWRENCE COREY

DEFINITION Herpes simplex viruses (HSV-1, HSV-2) (*Herpesvirus hominis*) produce a variety of infections involving mucocutaneous surfaces, the central nervous system, and occasionally visceral organs. The advent of effective antiviral chemotherapy for HSV infections has made prompt recognition of these syndromes of clinical importance.

ETIOLOGY The genome of herpes simplex virus is a linear, double-stranded DNA molecule (about 100×10^6 in molecular weight) large enough to encode in excess of 60 gene products. The structure of the genome is unusual among DNA viruses because two unique nucleotide sequences are flanked by inverted repeated sequences. The two components can invert relative to each other, so that DNA isolated from the virus consists of four isomers differing in their orientation of the two components. The genomes of the HSV-1 and HSV-2 viruses are about 50 percent homologous. The homologous sequences are distributed over the entire genome map, and most (if not all) of the polypeptides specified by one viral type are antigenically related to polypeptides of the other viral type. Restriction endonuclease analysis of viral DNA can be utilized to distinguish between the two subtypes and among strains of the two subtypes. The variability of nucleotide sequences from clinical strains of HSV-1 and HSV-2 are such that HSV isolates obtained from two individuals can be differentiated by restriction enzyme patterns unless the isolates are from epidemiologically related sources such as sexual partners, mother-infant pairs, or common source outbreaks.

The viral genome is packaged within a regular icosahedral protein shell (capsid) composed of 162 capsomers. The outer covering of the virus is a lipid-containing membrane (envelope) derived from modified cell membrane, acquired as the DNA-containing capsid buds through the inner nuclear membrane of the host cell. Between the capsid and lipid bilayer of the envelope is the tegument, composed of a number of viral proteins whose properties and functions are largely unknown. Viral replication has both nuclear and cytoplasmic phases. The initial steps of replication include attachment, fusion between the viral envelope and a cell membrane to liberate the nucleocapsid into the cytoplasm of the cell, and disassembly of the nucleocapsid to release the viral DNA. Three classes of HSV genes have been defined. The genes designated α are expressed earliest in infection without any requirement for prior viral protein synthesis. Some of the α genes transcribe in latently infected cells. The HSV genes designated β require prior synthesis of an α protein but not viral DNA replication. The β proteins include regulatory proteins and enzymes required for DNA replication. Most current antiviral drugs interrupt β proteins such as the viral DNA polymerase enzyme. The third (γ) class of HSV genes require viral DNA replication for expression, and most of the structural proteins specified by the virus are γ proteins.

Following replication of the viral genome and synthesis of structural proteins, nucleocapsids are assembled in the nucleus of the cell. Envelopment occurs as the nucleocapsids bud through the inner nuclear membrane into the perinuclear space. In some cells, viral replication within the nucleus forms two types of inclusion bodies, type A basophilic Feulgen-positive bodies that contain viral DNA, and an eosinophilic inclusion body which is devoid of viral nucleic acid or protein, representing a "scar" of viral infection. Virions are then transported via the endoplasmic reticulum and the Golgi apparatus to the cell surface.

HSV infection of some neuronal cells does not result in cell death. Instead, viral genomes are maintained by the cell in a repressed state compatible with survival and normal activities of the cell, a process called *latency*. Subsequently, activation of the viral genome may occur resulting in viral replication and, in some cases, the redevelopment of herpetic lesions, a process termed *reactivation*. Whereas infectious virus rarely can be recovered from sensory or autonomic nervous system ganglia dissected from cadavers, maintenance and growth of the neural cells in tissue culture result in production of infectious virions, a process called *explantation*, and subsequent permissive infection of susceptible cells, a process called *cocultivation*. Virus replication was first detected in neurons during reactivation in vitro, suggesting that the neuron harbors the latent virus in vivo. Subsequently, viral DNA has been found in neural tissue at times when infectious virus cannot be isolated. HSV DNA extracted from latently infected neural tissue differs from HSV DNA in cells actively replicating virus. In latently infected cells only partial transcription of viral proteins occurs. Two RNA transcripts which overlap the immediate early (α) gene product, called ICP-o, are found in abundance in the nuclei of latently infected neurons. These RNA transcripts code in an "antisense" direction, suggesting that they may be a factor in inhibiting the subsequent transcription of β and γ proteins. Deletion mutants of this region have been made. While these viruses can become latent, the efficiency of their subsequent reactivation is reduced, suggesting that the "antisense" transcripts may play a role in maintaining rather than in establishing latency. Understanding molecular mechanisms of latency may lead to new therapies to prevent reactivation of HSV.

PATHOGENESIS Exposure to virus at mucosal surfaces or abraded skin permits entry of virus and initiation of replication in cells of the epidermis and dermis. Whether or not clinically apparent lesions develop, sufficient viral replication to permit infection of either sensory or autonomic nerve endings may occur. Whether latency always results from peripheral mucosal infection is unclear. Virus, or more likely, nucleocapsid, is then thought to be transported intraaxonally to the nerve cell bodies in ganglia. In humans, the time from inoculation of virus in peripheral tissue to spread to the ganglia is unknown. During the initial phase of infection, viral replication occurs in ganglia and contiguous neural tissue. Virus then spreads to other mucosal skin surfaces through centrifugal migration of infectious virions via peripheral sensory nerves. This spread of virus to the skin from peripheral sensory nerves helps explain the large surface area, the high frequency of new lesions distant from the initial crop of vesicles which are characteristic in patients with primary genital or oral-labial HSV, and the recovery of virus from neural tissue distant from neurons innervating the inoculation site. Contiguous spread of locally inoculated virus may also occur and allow further mucosal extension of disease.

Following resolution of primary disease, infectious virus can no longer be recovered in the ganglia, and the surface viral proteins are not expressed in detectable amounts. The mechanisms by which various stimuli cause reactivation of HSV infection are unknown. Ultraviolet light, immunosuppression, and trauma to the skin or ganglia are associated with reactivation.

Analysis of the HSV DNA from sequentially isolated strains of HSV or from multiple infected ganglia in any one individual has revealed identical restriction endonuclease patterns in most persons. Occasionally, and more frequently in immunocompromised persons, multiple strains of the same viral subtype can be detected in the same person, suggesting that exogenous infection with different strains of the same subtype is possible.

IMMUNITY Host responses to infection influence the acquisition of disease, severity of infection, resistance to development of latency, maintenance of latency, and frequency of HSV recurrences. Both antibody-mediated and cell-mediated reactions are clinically important. Immunocompromised patients with defects in cell-mediated immunity experience more severe and extensive HSV infections than those with deficits in humoral immunity such as agammaglobulinemia. Experimental ablation of lymphocytes indicates that T cells play a major role in preventing lethal disseminated disease, although antibodies help reduce virus titers in neural tissue. Some aspects of the pathogenesis of disease may also be related to the host immune response, e.g., stromal opacities associated with recurrent herpetic keratitis. The surface viral glycoproteins have been shown to be antigens recognized by antibodies mediating neutralization and immune-mediated cytolysis (antibody-dependent cell-mediated cytotoxicity, ADCC). Monoclonal antibodies specific for each of the known viral glycoproteins have, in experimental infections, conferred protection against subsequent neurologic disease or ganglionic latency. Multiple cell populations including natural killer (NK) cells, macrophages, a variety of T-lymphocyte populations, and lymphokines generated by these cells play a role in host defenses to HSV infections. In animals passive transfer of primed lymphocytes confers protection from subsequent challenge. Maximum protection usually requires the activation of multiple T-cell subpopulations including cytotoxic T cells and T cells responsible for delayed hypersensitivity. The latter cells may confer protection by the antigen-stimulated release of lymphokines (e.g., interferons) which may have a direct antiviral effect or activate other nonspecific effector cells. In humans the viral proteins to which the responses of cytotoxic T cells are directed are unknown.

EPIDEMIOLOGY Seroepidemiologic studies have shown that HSV infections are found worldwide. Much of the humoral immune response to HSV is to type-common antigenic determinants, making it difficult to detect HSV-2 antibodies in persons with prior HSV-1 infection and HSV-1 antibodies in those with prior HSV-2 infections. Serologic assays which utilize whole-virus antigen preparations such as complement fixation, neutralization, indirect immunofluorescent (IFA), passive hemagglutination (PHA), radioimmunoassay (RIA), and enzyme-linked immunosorbent assay (ELISA) do not reliably identify persons who are infected with both viral subtypes. Recently, serologic assays which identify antibodies to type-specific surface proteins of the two viruses have been developed. These assays can reliably distinguish the human antibody response between HSV-1 and HSV-2. These assays are based upon demonstrating antibodies to type-specific epitopes of the glycoprotein G of HSV-1 (gGl) and HSV-2 (gG2).

Infection with HSV-1 is acquired more frequently and earlier than infection with HSV-2. Over 90 percent of adults have antibodies to

HSV-1 by the fourth decade. In lower socioeconomic populations most persons will acquire HSV-1 infection before the third decade.

Antibodies to HSV-2 are not routinely detected until puberty, and antibody prevalence rates correlate with past sexual activity. Antibodies to HSV-2 are detected in 10 to 40 percent of the general U.S. population. In most routine obstetrical clinics 20 to 30 percent of pregnant women possess HSV-2 antibodies, although only 10 percent report a history of genital lesions. As many as 50 percent of heterosexual adults attending STD clinics possess HSV-2 antibodies. Antibody prevalence rates average about 5 percent higher in women than men.

HSV infections occur throughout the year. The incubation period ranges from 1 to 26 days (median 6 to 8 days). Contact with active ulcerative lesions or asymptomatically excreting patients can result in transmission. Asymptomatic salivary excretion of HSV-1 has been reported in 2 to 9 percent of adults and 5 to 8 percent of children. HSV-2 has been isolated from the genital tract of from 0.3 to 6 percent of males and 1.5 to 13 percent of females attending sexually transmitted disease clinics. The titer of HSV in cultures from lesions is 100 to 1000 times higher than from salivary or genital tract secretions in asymptomatically excreting persons. The efficiency of transmission is greater during symptomatic versus asymptomatic periods of viral excretion.

CLINICAL SPECTRUM HSV has been isolated from nearly all visceral or mucocutaneous sites. The clinical manifestations and course of HSV depend on the anatomic site of the infection, the age and immune status of the host, and the antigenic type of the virus. First episodes of HSV disease, especially primary infection (that is, first infections with either HSV-1 or HSV-2 in which the host lacks HSV antibodies in acute phase sera), are frequently accompanied by systemic signs and symptoms, involve both mucosal and extramucosal sites, have a longer duration of symptoms, a longer time from which virus is isolated from lesions, and a higher rate of complications than recurrent episodes of disease. Both viral subtypes can cause genital and oral-facial infections, and these infections are clinically indistinguishable. However, the frequency of future reactivations of infection is influenced by the anatomic site and virus type. Genital HSV-2 infection is twice as likely to reactivate and will recur 8 to 10 times more frequently than genital HSV-1 infection. Conversely, oral-labial HSV-1 infections will recur more frequently than oral-labial HSV-2 infections.

Oral-facial HSV infections Gingivostomatitis and pharyngitis are the most frequent clinical manifestations of first-episode HSV-1 infection, while recurrent herpes labialis is the most frequent clinical manifestation of reactivation HSV infection. HSV pharyngitis and gingivostomatitis usually result from primary infection and are most commonly seen in children and young adults. Clinical symptoms and signs include fever, malaise, myalgias, inability to eat, irritability, and cervical adenopathy, which may last from 3 to 14 days. Lesions may involve the hard and soft palate, gingiva, tongue, lip, and facial area. HSV-1 or HSV-2 infection of the pharynx usually results in exudative or ulcerative lesions of the posterior pharynx and/or tonsillar pillars. Concomitant lesions of the tongue, buccal mucosa, or gingiva may occur later in the course in one-third of cases. Fever lasting from 2 to 7 days and cervical adenopathy are common. The clinical differentiation of HSV pharyngitis from bacterial pharyngitis, *Mycoplasma pneumoniae* infections, and noninfectious causes of pharyngeal ulcerations such as Stevens-Johnson syndrome may be difficult. No substantial evidence suggests that reactivation oral-labial HSV infection is associated with symptomatic recurrent pharyngitis.

Reactivation of HSV from the trigeminal ganglia may be associated with asymptomatic excretion in the saliva, development of intraoral mucosal ulcerations, or herpetic ulcerations on the vermilion border of the lip or external facial skin. About 50 to 70 percent of seropositive patients undergoing trigeminal nerve root decompression and 10 to 15 percent of those undergoing dental extraction will develop oral-labial HSV infection a median of 3 days after these procedures.

In immunosuppressed patients infection may extend into mucosal and deep cutaneous layers. Friability, necrosis, bleeding, severe pain, and inability to eat or drink may result. HSV mucositis is clinically similar to mucosal lesions due to cytotoxic drug therapy, trauma, or fungal or bacterial infections. Persistent ulcerative HSV infections are one of the most common in patients with AIDS. Concomitant HSV and *Candida* infection also occur commonly. Systemic acyclovir therapy speeds the rate of healing and relieves the pain of mucosal HSV infections in immunosuppressed patients. Patients with atopic eczema may also develop severe oral-facial HSV infections (eczema herpeticum) which may rapidly involve extensive areas of skin and occasionally disseminate to visceral organs. Prompt resolution of extensive eczema herpeticum has been achieved with the administration of intravenous acyclovir. Erythema multiforme (EM) may also be associated with HSV infections, and some evidence suggests that it is the precipitating event in about 75 percent of cases of cutaneous EM. HSV antigen has been demonstrated in both circulatory immune complexes and in skin lesion biopsy of these patients. Patients with severe HSV-associated erythema multiforme may be candidates for chronic suppressive oral acyclovir therapy.

Genital HSV infections First-episode primary genital herpes is characterized by fever, headache, malaise, and myalgias. Pain, itching, dysuria, vaginal and urethral discharge, and tender inguinal lymph adenopathy are the predominant local symptoms. Characteristically widely spaced bilateral lesions of the external genitalia are seen. Lesions may be present in varying stages including vesicles, pustules, or painful erythematous ulcers. Involvement of the cervix and urethra are seen in over 80 percent of women with first-episode infections. First episodes of genital herpes in patients who have had prior HSV-1 infection are associated with less frequent systemic symptoms and faster healing than primary genital herpes. The clinical courses of acute first-episode genital herpes among patients with HSV-1 and HSV-2 infections are similar. However, the recurrence rates of genital disease differ. About 90 percent of patients with first-episode HSV-2 infection will have a recurrence within 12 months (median number of recurrences, four) compared to 55 percent of those with primary HSV-1 infections (median number of recurrences, less than one). Recurrence rates of genital HSV-2 infections vary greatly between individuals and over time within the same individual. HSV has been isolated from the urethra and urine of men and women without concomitant external genital lesions. A clear mucoid discharge and dysuria are characteristics of symptomatic HSV urethritis. HSV has been isolated from the urethra of 5 percent of women with the dysuria-frequency syndrome. Occasionally, genital tract disease manifested by HSV endometritis and salpingitis in women and HSV prostatitis in men may occur.

Rectal and perianal HSV infections due to HSV-1 and HSV-2 may be seen, especially among homosexual men and/or heterosexual women who engage in anorectal intercourse. Symptoms of HSV proctitis include anorectal pain, anorectal discharge, tenesmus, and constipation. Sigmoidoscopy reveals ulcerative lesions of the distal 10 cm of the rectal mucosa. Rectal biopsies show mucosal ulceration, necrosis, polymorphonuclear and lymphocytic infiltration of the lamina propria, and occasionally multinucleated intranuclear inclusion–bearing cells. Perianal herpetic lesions are also seen in immunosuppressed patients receiving cytotoxic therapy. HSV-1 strains, usually identical to those found in the oropharynx, are obtained from these lesions, suggesting the mode of spread is autoinoculation of the perianal area from HSV-infected saliva and/or finger lesions. Extensive perianal herpetic lesions and/or HSV proctitis may occur in patients with AIDS.

Herpetic whitlow Herpetic whitlow, HSV infection of the finger, may occur as a complication of primary oral or genital herpes by inoculation of virus via a break in the epidermal surface or by direct introduction of virus into the hand through occupational or other exposure. Clinical signs and symptoms include the abrupt onset of edema, erythema, and localized tenderness of the infected finger. Vesicular or pustular lesions of the fingertip indistinguishable from pyogenic bacterial infection are seen. Fever, lymphadenitis, and epitrochlear and axillary lymphadenopathy are common. Recurrences may occur. Prompt diagnosis to avoid unnecessary and potentially exacerbating surgical therapy and/or transmission is essential.

Herpetic eye infections HSV infection of the eye is the most frequent cause of corneal blindness in the United States. HSV keratitis presents with acute onset of pain, blurring of vision, chemosis, conjunctivitis, and characteristic dendritic lesions of the cornea. Use of topical corticosteroids may exacerbate symptoms and lead to involvement of deep structures of the eye. Debridement, topical antiviral, and/or interferon therapy hasten healing. However, recurrences are common and immunopathologic injury of the deeper structures of the eye may occur. Chorioretinitis, usually as a manifestation of disseminated HSV infection, may occur in neonates or those with AIDS. Acute necrotizing retinitis due to HSV is an uncommon but severe manifestation of HSV infection.

Central and peripheral nervous system infections with HSV-1 and HSV-2 HSV encephalitis is the most common identified cause of acute, sporadic viral encephalitis in the United States, comprising 10 to 20 percent of all cases. The estimated incidence is about 2.3 cases per million persons per year. Cases are distributed throughout the year, and the age distribution appears biphasic with peaks at between 5 and 30 and greater-than-50 years of age. HSV-1 accounts for more than 95 percent of cases. The pathogenesis of HSV encephalitis varies. In children and young adults primary HSV infection may result in encephalitis; presumably exogenously acquired virus enters the CNS by neurotropic spread from the periphery via the olfactory bulb. However, most adults with HSV encephalitis have clinical or serologic evidence of mucocutaneous HSV-1 infection prior to the onset of the CNS symptoms. In about 25 percent of the cases examined, the HSV-1 strains from the oropharynx and brain tissue of the same patient differ, suggesting that some cases may result from reinfection with another strain of HSV-1 that reached the CNS. Two theories have been proposed to explain the development of actively replicating HSV in localized areas of the CNS in persons from whom the ganglionic and CNS isolates are similar. Reactivation of latent trigeminal or autonomic nerve root HSV-1 infection may be associated with extension of virus into the CNS via nerves innervating the middle cranial fossa. HSV DNA has been demonstrated by DNA hybridization in human autopsy brain tissue. Reactivation of long standing latent CNS infection may be another potential mechanism for the development of HSV encephalitis.

The clinical hallmark of HSV encephalitis has been the acute onset of fever and focal neurologic, especially temporal lobe, symptoms. To date no reliable noninvasive radiologic or virologic technique has been developed to diagnose HSV encephalitis during its early clinical stages, and differentiation of HSV encephalitis from other viral encephalitides and other focal infections and noninfectious processes is difficult. An increase in CSF and serum antibodies to HSV does occur with most cases of HSV encephalitis. However, these antibody rises rarely are present prior to 10 days into the illness and, while useful retrospectively, are not helpful in establishing the clinical diagnosis early in the course of disease. Brain biopsy because of its high sensitivity, low complication rate, and ability to establish alternative potentially treatable diagnoses has been felt to be the most expeditious method to diagnose HSV encephalitis, but newly developed assays for HSV antigens or DNA in CSF may supplant it. Antiviral chemotherapy reduces the mortality of HSV encephalitis, and intravenous acyclovir is more effective than vidarabine. Even with therapy, however, neurologic sequelae are frequent.

HSV has been isolated from the cerebrospinal fluid of 0.5 to 3 percent of patients presenting to the hospital with aseptic meningitis. HSV meningitis is usually seen in association with primary genital HSV infection. HSV meningitis is an acute self-limited disease manifested by headache, fever, and mild photophobia, which lasts from 2 to 7 days. A lymphocytic pleocytosis in the CSF is characteristic. Neurologic sequelae are rare. Recurrent bouts of aseptic meningitis related to reactivation of HSV have been reported.

Autonomic nervous system dysfunction, especially of the sacral region, has been reported in association with both HSV and varicella-zoster infections. Numbness, tingling of the buttock or perineal areas, urinary retention, constipation, cerebrospinal fluid pleocytosis, and impotence in males may occur. Symptoms appear to resolve slowly over a period of days to weeks. Occasionally hypesthesia and/or weakness of the lower extremities may persist for many months. Rarely transverse myelitis manifested by a rapidly progressive symmetric paralysis of the lower extremities or a Guillain-Barré syndrome may occur after HSV infection. Similarly, peripheral nervous system involvement [idiopathic facial paralysis (Bell's palsy)] or cranial polyneuritis may also be related to reactivation of HSV-1 infection. Transitory hypesthesia of the area of skin innervated by the trigeminal nerve and vestibular system dysfunction as measured by electronystagmography are the predominant signs of disease. Studies to determine if antiviral chemotherapy may abort or alleviate the frequency and severity of these signs are unavailable.

Visceral infections HSV infection of visceral organs usually results from viremia, and multiple organ involvement is common. Occasionally, however, the clinical manifestations of HSV infections may involve only the esophagus, lung, or liver. HSV esophagitis may result from direct extension of oral-pharyngeal HSV infection into the esophagus or may occur de novo by reactivation of HSV and spread of virus to the esophageal mucosa via the vagus nerve. The predominant symptoms of HSV esophagitis are odynophagia, dysphagia, substernal pain, and weight loss. There are multiple oval ulcerations on an erythematous base with or without a patchy white pseudomembrane. The distal esophagus is most commonly involved. With extensive disease diffuse friability may spread to the entire esophagus. Neither endoscopic nor barium examination can differentiate HSV from *Candida* esophagitis, or from esophageal ulcerations due to thermal injury, radiation, and corrosives. Endoscopically obtained secretions for cytologic examination and culture provide the most accurate material for diagnosis. Anecdotal observations suggest resolution of the symptoms of HSV esophagitis with systemic antiviral chemotherapy.

HSV pneumonitis is uncommon except in severely immunosuppressed patients and may result from extension of herpetic tracheobronchitis into lung parenchyma. Focal necrotizing pneumonitis usually results. Hematogenous dissemination of virus from oral or genital mucocutaneous disease may also occur and produce a bilateral interstitial pneumonitis. Concomitant bacterial, fungal, and parasitic pathogens are common in HSV pneumonitis. As the mortality of HSV pneumonia in immunosuppressed patients is high (>80 percent), these patients should be candidates for antiviral chemotherapy. HSV has also been isolated from the lower respiratory tract of persons with acute respiratory distress syndrome (ARDS). However, the relationship between isolation of HSV and the pathogenesis of the respiratory distress syndrome is unclear.

HSV is an uncommon cause of hepatitis in immunocompetent patients. HSV infection of the liver is associated with fever, abrupt elevations of the bilirubin and serum transaminases, and leukopenia (white blood cells <4000 per microliter). Disseminated intravascular coagulation may also be present.

Other isolated but reported complications of HSV include monarticular arthritis, adrenal necrosis, idiopathic thrombocytopenia, and glomerulonephritis. Disseminated HSV infection in the immunocompetent patient is rare. In immunocompromised, burn, or malnourished patients, dissemination of HSV to other visceral organs such as adrenal glands, pancreas, small and large intestine, and bone marrow may occur occasionally. Rarely, primary HSV infection in pregnancy may disseminate and may be associated with mortality in both mother and fetus. This uncommon event is usually associated with acquisition of primary infection in the third trimester.

NEONATAL HSV INFECTION Neonates (<6 weeks of age) have the highest frequency of visceral and/or CNS infection of any HSV-infected patient population. Untreated, over 70 percent of neonatal herpes cases will disseminate or develop CNS infection. Without therapy, the overall mortality of neonatal herpes is 65 percent, and less than 10 percent of neonates with CNS infection experience normal development. While skin lesions are the most commonly recognized features of disease, many infants do not develop lesions until well into the course of disease. Seventy percent of neonatal HSV cases are caused by HSV-2 infection, almost all of which result from contact via infected genital secretions at the time of delivery. However, congenitally infected infants have been reported, usually from mothers who acquired primary HSV infection during pregnancy. Neonatal HSV-1 infections are usually acquired postnatally through contact with immediate family members with symptomatic or asymptomatic oral-labial HSV-1 infection or from nosocomial transmission within the hospital. Antiviral chemotherapy has reduced the mortality of neonatal herpes to 25 percent. However, the morbidity, especially in infants with HSV-2 CNS involvement, is still very high.

DIAGNOSIS Both clinical and laboratory criteria are useful for establishing the diagnosis of HSV infections. Clinical diagnosis can be made accurately where characteristic multiple vesicular lesions on an erythematous base are present. Scrapings of the base of the lesions and subsequent staining with Wright, Giemsa (Tzanck preparation), or Papanicolaou's stain will demonstrate characteristic giant cells or intranuclear inclusions of a herpesvirus infection. These cytologic techniques are often useful as a quick office procedure to confirm the diagnosis. Limitations of this method are that it does not differentiate between HSV and varicella-zoster infections and is only about 60 percent as sensitive as viral isolation. The laboratory confirmation of HSV infection is best performed by isolation of virus in tissue culture. HSV causes a discernible cytopathic effect in a variety of cell culture systems, and most specimens can be identified within 48 to 96 h after inoculation. Spin-amplified culture with subsequent staining for HSV antigen has shortened the time needed to identify HSV to less than 24 h. The sensitivity of viral isolation varies with the stage of lesions (higher in vesicular than in ulcerative lesions), whether the patient has a first or recurrent episode of the disease (higher in first episodes), and whether the sample is from an immunosuppressed or immunocompetent patient (more antigen in immunosuppressed). Immunofluorescent assays using monoclonal antibodies and some DNA hybridization procedures have approached the sensitivity of viral isolation for detecting HSV from genital or oral-labial lesions, but appear only about 50 percent as sensitive as viral isolation for the detection of asymptomatic HSV in cervical or salivary secretions. Laboratory confirmation allows for subtyping the virus, which may be useful epidemiologically as well as in helping to predict the frequency of reactivation after first-episode oral-labial or genital HSV infection. Restriction endonuclease analysis of viral DNA can also be used to differentiate between HSV-1 and HSV-2 as well as to differentiate between strains within the same subtypes, information which may be very useful in identifying common source outbreaks of HSV.

Acute and convalescent serum can be useful in documenting seroconversion during primary HSV-1 or HSV-2 infection. However, only 5 percent of patients with recurrent mucocutaneous HSV infections show a fourfold or greater rise in anti-HSV antibodies between acute and convalescent sera. Serologic assays have little utility in diagnosing acute mucocutaneous HSV infection and are best used to identify persons with past infection. Newly developed type-specific serologic assays can be utilized to identify asymptomatic carriers of HSV-1 or HSV-2 infection.

THERAPY Many aspects of mucocutaneous and visceral HSV infections are amenable to treatment with antiviral chemotherapy. For mucocutaneous infections acyclovir has been the mainstay of therapy. Several antivirals are available for topical use in HSV eye infections: idoxuridine, trifluorothymidine, and topical vidarabine. For HSV encephalitis, intravenous acyclovir is the treatment of choice. For neonatal HSV infections high-dose intravenous vidarabine and acyclovir are effective.

Acyclovir has been shown to be effective in shortening symptoms and the duration of lesions of mucocutaneous HSV infections in immunocompromised patients and first-episode genital herpes in immunocompetent patients (Table 135-1). Intravenous and oral acyclovir will also prevent reactivation of HSV in seropositive immunocompromised patients who are undergoing induction chemotherapy for acute leukemia or in the immediate posttransplant period.

Oral acyclovir has also been shown to speed the healing and resolution of symptoms in first and recurrent episodes of genital HSV-1 and HSV-2 infections. The benefit of treating acute episodes of recurrent genital disease with oral acyclovir is modest, and as such, routine use for recurrent episodes of disease, especially for mild episodes, is not recommended. Chronic daily suppressive therapy may be useful in reducing the frequency of reactivation disease among patients with very frequent genital herpes. Chronic suppressive oral acyclovir does not eliminate sacral ganglionic latency, and reactivation of genital herpes occurs after discontinuing therapy. Oral acyclovir is of benefit in primary gingivostomatitis but has limited benefit in the treatment of recurrent oral-labial lesions; lesions are not aborted and total healing time is not reduced. If started early, the duration of the ulcerative stage of the lip lesion may be reduced.

TABLE 135-1 Current antiviral chemotherapy of HSV infection

I Mucocutaneous HSV infections
- *A* Immunosuppressed patients
  - *1* Acute symptomatic first or recurrent episodes: IV acyclovir (5 mg/kg every 8 h) or oral acyclovir (400 mg PO 4 times per day for 7 to 10 days) relieves pain and speeds healing. With localized external lesions 5% topical acyclovir ointment applied 4 to 6 times daily may be beneficial.
  - *2* Suppression of reactivation disease: IV (5 mg/kg every 8 h) or oral acyclovir (400 mg PO 3 to 5 times per day) will when taken daily prevent recurrences during high-risk period, e.g., immediate post-transplantation period.
- *B* Immunocompetent patients
  - *1* Genital herpes
    - *a* First episodes: Oral acyclovir (200 mg PO 5 times per day for 10 to 14 days) is the treatment of choice. IV acyclovir (5 mg/kg every 8 h for 5 days) is given for severe disease or neurologic complications such as aseptic meningitis. Topical 5% ointment or cream applied 4 to 6 times daily for 7 to 10 days may be beneficial in patients without cervical, urethral, or pharyngeal involvement.
    - *b* Symptomatic recurrent genital herpes: Oral acyclovir (200 mg PO 5 times per day for 5 days) has modest benefit in shortening lesions and viral excretion time. Routine use for all episodes not recommended.
    - *c* Suppression of recurrent genital herpes: Daily oral acyclovir 200-mg capsules, 2 to 3 times daily or 400 mg PO 2 times per day will prevent reactivation of symptomatic recurrences; use at present limited to 6-month course in frequent recurrers.
  - *2* Oral-labial HSV
    - *a* First episode: Oral acyclovir 200 mg 4–5 times per day.
    - *b* Recurrent episodes: Topical acyclovir ointment is of no clinical benefit. Oral acyclovir has minimal benefit.
  - *3* Herpetic whitlow: Oral acyclovir 200 mg 5 times daily for 7–10 days.
  - *4* HSV proctitis: Oral acyclovir (400 mg PO 5 times per day) is useful in shortening course of infection. In immunosuppressed patients or in severe infection, IV acyclovir 5 mg/kg every 8 h may be useful.
- *C* Herpetic eye infections
  - *1* Acute keratitis: Topical trifluorothymidine, vidarabine, idoxuridine, acyclovir, and interferon are all beneficial. Debridement may be required; topical steroids may worsen disease.

II CNS HSV infection
- *A* HSV encephalitis: Intravenous acyclovir 10 mg/kg every 8 h (30 mg/kg per day) for 10 days or vidarabine (15 mg/kg per day) decrease mortality; acyclovir is the preferred agent.
- *B* HSV aseptic meningitis: No studies of systemic antiviral chemotherapy. If therapy is to be given IV, acyclovir at 15 to 30 mg/kg per day should be utilized.
- *C* Autonomic radiculopathy: No studies are available.

III Neonatal HSV infection: Intravenous vidarabine (30 mg/kg per day) or acyclovir (30 mg/kg per day). Neonates appear to tolerate this high dose of vidarabine.

IV Visceral HSV infections
- *A* HSV esophagitis: Systemic acyclovir (15 mg/kg per day) or vidarabine (15 mg/kg per day) should be considered.
- *B* HSV pneumonitis: No controlled studies: Systemic acyclovir (15 mg/kg per day) or vidarabine (15 mg/kg per day) should be considered.

V Disseminated HSV: No controlled studies, intravenous acyclovir or vidarabine should be attempted. No definite evidence that therapy will decrease mortality.

VI Erythema multiforme associated with HSV: Anecdotal observations suggest oral acyclovir capsules 2 to 3 times daily will suppress EM.

Both intravenous vidarabine 15 mg/kg per day over 12 h daily and intravenous acyclovir 30 mg/kg per day given as 10 mg/kg infusion over 1 h at 8-hourly intervals have been shown to be effective in reducing the mortality of HSV encephalitis. Primary determinants of outcome include young age and early therapy. Comparative trials of the two drugs for the treatment of HSV encephalitis have indicated a lower mortality rate and fewer neurologic sequelae with intravenous acyclovir. The major side effect associated with intravenous acyclovir is transient renal insufficiency usually due to crystallization of the compound in the renal parenchyma. This can be avoided if the medication is given slowly over 1 h and the patient is well-hydrated. Because CSF levels of acyclovir average only 30 to 50 percent of plasma levels, the dosage of acyclovir used for treatment of CNS infection (30 mg/kg per day) is double that used for treatment of mucocutaneous or visceral disease (15 mg/kg per day). Vidarabine at doses of 15 mg/kg per day tends to produce more hematopoietic and hepatic toxicity than acyclovir, but this is usually not a limiting problem in treating severe neonatal or CNS infections.

Acyclovir-resistant strains are being identified with increasing frequency. Almost all clinically significant acyclovir resistance has been seen in immunocompromised patients who have received multiple intermittent courses of therapy. Increasingly, patients with human immunodeficiency virus infection are noted to have persistent mucocutaneous HSV infection which is unresponsive to even very high dose acyclovir therapy. Most acyclovir-resistant strains of HSV have an altered substrate specificity for phosphorylating acyclovir. The frequent reactivation of virus and high virus titers in the lesions of immunocompromised patients in combination with the use of the medication selects out these resistant variants. In some patients, higher doses of acyclovir will be associated with clearing of lesions. In others, clinical disease will progress despite high-dose therapy. Therapy with an antiviral with another mechanism of action such as foscarnate or vidarabine may be useful (see Chap. 86).

PREVENTION The large reservoir of persons with asymptomatic HSV-1 and HSV-2 infections indicates that control of HSV disease through suppressive antiviral chemotherapy and/or educational programs will be limited. Control of HSV infection will require prevention of infection, a goal most likely achievable by vaccination. Effective HSV vaccines are not currently available. Heterologous vaccines such as smallpox, bacillus Calmette-Guérin, and influenza, which have been used as therapies for genital HSV infection, have been ineffective.

Barrier forms of contraception, especially condoms, may decrease transmission of disease especially during periods of asymptomatic viral excretion. Transmission of disease when lesions were present despite the use of a condom may still occur, and patients should be instructed to avoid sexual activity when genital lesions are present.

REFERENCES

COREY L: Genital herpes simplex virus infections: Clinical manifestations, course, and complications. Ann Intern Med 98:958, 1983

———, SPEAR P: Infections with herpes simplex viruses. N Engl J Med 314:686, 749, 1986

——— et al: Differences between herpes simplex virus type 1 and type 2 neonatal encephalitis in neurological outcome. Lancet 2:1, 1988

DORSKY DI, CRUMPACKER CS: Drugs five years later: Acyclovir. Ann Intern Med 107:859, 1987

DOUGLAS JM et al: A double-blind study of oral acyclovir for suppression of recurrences of genital herpes simplex virus infection. N Engl J Med 310:1551, 1984

ERLICH KS et al: Acyclovir-resistant herpes simplex virus infections in patients with the acquired immunodeficiency syndrome. N Engl J Med 320:293, 1989

SHEPP DH et al: Oral acyclovir therapy for mucocutaneous herpes simplex infections in immunocompromised marrow transplant recipients. Ann Intern Med 102:783, 1985

SPRUANCE SL et al: Early application of topical 15% idoxuridine in dimethyl sulfoxide shortens the course of herpes simplex labialis: A multicenter placebo-controlled trial. J Infect Dis 161:191, 1990

STRAUSS SE et al: Herpes simplex virus infection: Biology, treatment, and prevention. Ann Intern Med 103:404, 1985

136 VARICELLA-ZOSTER VIRUS INFECTIONS

RICHARD J. WHITLEY

DEFINITION Varicella-zoster virus (VZV) causes two distinct clinical entities: varicella, or chickenpox, and herpes zoster, or shingles. Chickenpox, a ubiquitous and extremely contagious infection, is usually a benign illness of childhood characterized by an exanthematous, vesicular rash. With reactivation of latent VZV, more common after the sixth decade of life, the disease presents as a dermatomal, vesicular rash which is usually associated with severe pain.

ETIOLOGY A clinical association between varicella and herpes zoster has been recognized for nearly 100 years. Early in the twentieth century, similarities in the histopathologic findings of skin lesions resulting from varicella and herpes zoster were demonstrated. Viral isolates from patients with chickenpox and herpes zoster demonstrated similar alterations in tissue culture, specifically the appearance of eosinophilic intranuclear inclusions and multinucleated giant cells, suggesting that the viruses were biologically similar. Restriction endonuclease analysis of viral DNA from a patient with chickenpox who subsequently developed herpes zoster verified the molecular identity of the two viruses responsible for these differing clinical presentations. Varicella-zoster virus is a member of the herpesvirus family, sharing such similar structural characteristics as a lipid envelope, surrounding a nucleocapsid with icosahedral symmetry, a total size of approximately 150 to 200 nm, and centrally located double-stranded DNA with a molecular weight of approximately 80 million. Only enveloped virions are infectious.

PATHOGENESIS AND PATHOLOGY **Primary infection** Transmission is likely by the respiratory route, followed by localized replication at an undefined site, and leading to seeding of the reticuloendothelial system with, ultimately, viremia. The occurrence of viremia in patients with chickenpox is supported by the diffuse and scattered nature of the skin lesions and can be verified in selected cases by the recovery of virus from the blood. Vesicles involve the corium and dermis with degenerative changes characterized by ballooning, multinucleated giant cells, and eosinophilic intranuclear inclusions. Infection may involve localized blood vessels of the skin, resulting in necrosis and epidermal hemorrhage. With disease evolution, vesicular fluid becomes cloudy with the recruitment of polymorphonuclear leukocytes, degenerated cells, and fibrin. Ultimately, the vesicles rupture and release their fluid contents, which include infectious virus, or are gradually reabsorbed.

Recurrent infection The mechanism of reactivation of VZV that results in herpes zoster is unknown. It is presumed that virus infects the dorsal root ganglia during chickenpox where it remains latent until reactivated. Histopathologic examination of the representative dorsal root ganglia during active herpes zoster demonstrates hemorrhage, edema, and lymphocytic infiltration.

Involvement with active VZV replication in other organs, such as the lung or brain, can occur during either chickenpox or herpes zoster but is uncommon in the immune-competent host. Lung involvement is characterized by interstitial pneumonitis, multinucleated giant cell formation, intranuclear inclusions, and pulmonary hemorrhage. Central nervous system (CNS) infection leads to histopathologic evidence of perivascular cuffing similar to that encountered with measles and other viral encephalitides. Focal hemorrhagic necrosis of the brain, characteristic of herpes simplex virus encephalitis, is uncommon with VZV infection.

EPIDEMIOLOGY AND CLINICAL PRESENTATION **Chickenpox** Humans are the only known reservoir for VZV. Chickenpox is highly contagious with an attack rate of at least 90 percent among susceptible or seronegative individuals. Both sexes and individuals of all races are infected equally. The virus is endemic in the population at large;

however, it becomes epidemic among susceptible individuals during seasonal periods, namely, late winter and early spring in the temperate zone. Children between the ages of 5 and 9 are most commonly affected and account for 50 percent of all cases. Most other cases occur between the ages of 1 to 4 and 10 to 14. Over the age of 15, approximately 10 percent of the population of the United States is susceptible to infection.

The incubation period of chickenpox ranges between 10 and 21 days but is usually between 14 and 17 days. Secondary attack rates in susceptible siblings within a household are between 70 and 90 percent. Patients are infectious approximately 48 h prior to the onset of the vesicular rash, during the period of vesicle formation, generally 4 to 5 days, and until all vesicles are crusted.

Clinically, chickenpox presents with a rash, low-grade fever, and malaise, although a few patients will develop a prodrome 1 to 2 days prior to the onset of the exanthem. In the immune-competent, this is usually a benign illness that is associated with lassitude and fever from 37.8 to 39.4°C (100 to 103°F) of 3 to 5 days' duration. The skin lesions, the hallmark of the infection, consist of maculopapules, vesicles, and scabs in varying stages of evolution. The evolution of lesions from maculopapules to vesicles occurs over a matter of hours to days. The lesions appear on the trunk and face and rapidly involve other areas of the body. Most are small and have an erythematous base with a diameter of 5 to 10 mm. Successive crops appear over a 2- to 4-day period. Lesions can also be found on the mucosa of the pharynx or the vagina. Their severity varies from individual to individual. Some individuals have very few lesions, while others can have as many as 2000. Younger children tend to have fewer vesicles compared to older individuals. Immunocompromised individuals, both children and adults, particularly those with leukemia, have more numerous lesions, often with a hemorrhagic base, and the lesions take longer to heal. These individuals also are at greater risk for visceral complications, which occur in 30 to 50 percent of cases and which are fatal in 15 percent.

The most common infectious complication of varicella is secondary bacterial superinfection of the skin, which is usually caused by *Streptococcus pyogenes* or *Staphylococcus aureus*. This may result from excoriation of skin lesions following scratching. Gram's stain of skin lesions should help clarify the etiology of unusually erythematous and pustulated lesions.

The most common extracutaneous site of involvement in children is the central nervous system and consists of acute cerebellar ataxia which generally appears approximately 21 days after the onset of the rash and rarely occurs in the preeruptive phase. The most prominent clinical finding is ataxia and meningeal irritation. The cerebrospinal fluid contains lymphocytes and elevated levels of protein. This is a benign complication of VZV infection in children and does not generally require hospitalization. Aseptic meningitis, encephalitis, transverse myelitis, and Reye's syndrome can also occur. Encephalitis is reported in 0.1 to 0.2 percent of children with chickenpox. No specific therapy is available for patients with central nervous system involvement caused by VZV.

Varicella pneumonia is the most serious complication following chickenpox, occurring more commonly in adults (up to 20 percent) than in children. It usually appears 3 to 5 days into the course of illness and is associated with tachypnea, cough, dyspnea, and fever. Cyanosis, pleuritic chest pain, and hemoptysis are frequent. Roentgenographic evidence of disease consists of nodular infiltrates and an interstitial pneumonitis. Resolution of pneumonitis parallels improvement of skin rash; however, patients may have persistent fever and compromised pulmonary function for weeks.

Other complications of chickenpox include myocarditis, corneal lesions, nephritis, arthritis, bleeding diatheses, acute glomerulonephritis, and hepatitis. Hepatic involvement, distinct from Reye's syndrome, is common in chickenpox and is usually characterized by an elevation of liver enzymes, particularly serum glutamic oxaloacetic transaminase (SGOT) and serum glutamic pyruvic transaminase (SGPT). Hepatic involvement is usually asymptomatic.

Perinatal varicella is associated with a high mortality rate when maternal disease develops within 5 days before delivery and 48 h post partum. Because the newborn does not receive protective transplacental antibodies and has an immature immune system, illness may be exaggerated. The mortality rate has been reported as high as 30 percent in this group. Congenital varicella with clinical manifestations at birth is extremely uncommon.

Herpes zoster Herpes zoster, a sporadic disease, is the consequence of reactivation of latent virus from the dorsal root ganglia. It occurs at all ages but mainly among the elderly. Most patients have no history of exposure to other individuals with VZV infection. The highest incidence is between 5 and 10 cases per 1000 persons for individuals in the sixth through the eighth decades of life. Approximately 2 percent of herpes zoster patients who do not receive immunosuppressive therapy will develop a second episode of infection. This figure is at least fivefold higher in immunocompromised individuals.

Herpes zoster, or "shingles," is characterized by a unilateral vesicular eruption within a dermatome, often associated with severe pain. The dermatomes from T3 to L3 are most frequently involved. If the ophthalmic branch of the trigeminal nerve is involved, zoster ophthalmicus results. The factors responsible for reactivation of virus are not known. In children, reactivation is usually benign, whereas in adults, acute neuritis and postherpetic neuralgia can be particularly debilitating. The onset of disease is heralded by pain within the dermatome that may precede lesions by 48 to 72 h, followed by an erythematous maculopapular rash which evolves rapidly to vesiculate. In the normal host, these lesions may remain few in number and continue to form only for a period of 3 to 5 days. The total duration of disease is generally between 7 and 10 days; however, it may take as long as 2 to 4 weeks before the skin returns to normal. In a few patients, characteristic localization of pain to a dermatome with serologic evidence of herpes zoster has been reported in the absence of skin lesions. When branches of the trigeminal nerve are involved, lesions may appear on the face, in the mouth, in the eye, or on the tongue. Lesions appear on the ear canal and tongue when the sensory branch of the facial nerve is involved (Ramsay Hunt syndrome).

The most debilitating complication of herpes zoster, both in the normal and in the immunocompromised host, is pain associated with acute neuritis and postherpetic neuralgia. Postherpetic neuralgia is uncommon in young individuals; however, at least 50 percent of patients over age 50 with zoster will report pain in the involved dermatome months after resolution of cutaneous disease. Changes in sensation within the dermatome, resulting in either hypo- or hyperesthesia, are common.

Central nervous system involvement following localized herpes zoster may occur. Many patients without signs of meningeal irritation will have cerebrospinal fluid pleocytosis and moderately elevated levels of CSF protein. Symptomatic meningoencephalitis is characterized by headache, fever, photophobia, meningitis, and vomiting. A rare manifestation of CNS involvement is granulomatous angiitis with contralateral hemiplegia, which can be diagnosed by cerebral arteriography. Other neurologic manifestations include transverse myelitis with or without motor paralysis.

As with chickenpox, herpes zoster in the immunocompromised host is more severe than in the normal individual. Lesion formation continues for over a week, and total scabbing does not develop in the majority of patients until 3 weeks into the course. Patients with Hodgkin's disease and non-Hodgkin's lymphoma are at greatest risk for progressive herpes zoster because cutaneous dissemination develops in about 40 percent of these patients. Among patients with cutaneous dissemination, there is a 5 to 10 percent increased risk of pneumonitis, meningoencephalitis, hepatitis, and other serious complications. However, even in immunocompromised patients disseminated zoster is rarely fatal.

Patients who have had a bone marrow transplant are at a particular risk of VZV infection. Thirty percent of cases of posttransplant VZV infection occur within 1 year (50 percent of these within 9 months), and 45 percent of such patients have cutaneous or visceral dissemination. The mortality rate is 10 percent, and postherpetic neuralgia, scarring, and bacterial superinfection are more frequent in VZV infections occurring within 9 months of a transplant. Among infected patients, concomitant graft-versus-host disease increases the chance for dissemination and/or a fatal outcome.

DIFFERENTIAL DIAGNOSIS The diagnosis of chickenpox is not difficult. The characteristic rash of chickenpox and the epidemiologic history of recent exposure should lead to prompt diagnosis. Other viral infections which can mimic chickenpox include disseminated herpes simplex virus infection in patients with atopic dermatitis, and the disseminated vesiculopapular lesions sometimes associated with coxsackievirus, echovirus, or atypical measles infections. These rashes are more commonly morbilliform with a hemorrhagic component rather than vesicular or vesiculopustular. Rickettsialpox can be confused with chickenpox; however, it can be easily distinguished by finding the "herald spot" at the site of the mite bite and a more pronounced headache. The serologic test is also useful in differentiating rickettsialpox from varicella.

Unilateral vesicular lesions in a dermatomal pattern should lead rapidly to the diagnosis of herpes zoster. Both herpes simplex virus infections and coxsackievirus infections can be a cause of dermatomal vesicular lesions. In such situations, a Tzanck smear with supportive diagnostic virology will be helpful in ensuring the proper diagnosis. In the prodromal stage of herpes zoster, the diagnosis can be exceedingly difficult and may only be achieved once lesions have appeared, or by retrospective serologic assessment.

LABORATORY FINDINGS Unequivocal confirmation of the diagnosis is possible only through the isolation of virus in susceptible tissue culture cell lines or by the demonstration of seroconversion or a fourfold or greater antibody rise when comparing acute and convalescent specimens. A rapid impression can be obtained by a Tzanck smear, performed by scraping the base of the lesions in an attempt to demonstrate multinucleated giant cells. Direct immunofluorescent staining of cells from the skin base or detection of viral antigens by other assays (immunoperoxidase) can also be utilized, although such tests are not commercially available. The most frequently employed serologic tools for assessing host response are immunofluorescent detection of antibodies to VZV membrane antigens, fluorescent antibody to membrane antigen (FAMA) test, immune adherence hemagglutination, or enzyme-linked immunosorbent assay (ELISA). The FAMA and ELISA tests appear to be the most sensitive.

PROPHYLAXIS In the normal host, prophylaxis and treatment of chickenpox are of little relevance since the disease is usually benign. However, because the immunocompromised individual is at significant risk for developing progressive varicella, modalities of prevention include passive immunization or experimental administration of a live attenuated vaccine. Immune prophylaxis can be accomplished by the administration of specific zoster immune globulin (ZIG), derived from patients with herpes zoster, varicella-zoster immune globulin (VZIG), or the intravenous formulation of zoster immune plasma (ZIP). Both ZIG and VZIG should be given within 96 h, but preferably within 72 h, of exposure in order to be effective. It is likely that ZIP can be given somewhat later. Indications for the administration of ZIG or VZIG are summarized in Table 136-1. VZIG should be administered to immunodeficient patients under 15 who have a negative or unknown history of chickenpox, who have not been vaccinated against VZV, and who have had a contact in a household, with a playmate for more than 1 h indoors, or in a shared hospital room. It should also be administered to the newborn whose mother had an onset of chickenpox within less than 5 days before delivery and 48 h post partum. The use of VZIG for susceptible individuals over 15 must be evaluated on an individual basis. There is no evidence that VZIG is useful for adults with chickenpox, including pregnant women.

Clinical trials in Japan and the United States have demonstrated the efficacy of live attenuated vaccine both in normal individuals and in immunocompromised hosts. A live attenuated VZV vaccine may be licensed in the United States in the future.

TABLE 136-1 Recommendations for VZIG utilization

I Exposure:
- *A* Both exposure to person with chickenpox or zoster as:
  - *1* Continuous household contact
  - *2* Playmate of >1-h duration indoors
  - *3* Hospital contact (same room or prolonged face-to-face)
  - *4* Newborn exposure whereby mother had onset of chickenpox <5 days before delivery to 48 h post partum
- *B* And time elapsed ≤96 h (preferably sooner)

II Candidates should:
- *A* Have significant exposure (see *I* above)
- *B* Be susceptible to VZV infection
- *C* Be <15 years of age (older immunocompromised patients require individual decision)
- *D* Have one of the following conditions:
  - *1* Leukemia or lymphoma
  - *2* Congenital or acquired immune deficiency
  - *3* Immunosuppressive treatment
  - *4* Newborn defined above (see *IA4*)

TREATMENT Medical management of chickenpox in the normal host is directed toward preventing avoidable complications. Obviously, good hygiene should include daily bathing and soaks. Secondary bacterial infection of the skin can be avoided by meticulous skin care, particularly with close cropping of fingernails. Pruritus can be decreased with topical dressings or the administration of antipruritic drugs. Tepid water baths and wet compresses are better than drying lotions for the relief of itching. Domeboro soaks for the management of herpes zoster can be both soothing and cleansing. Administration of aspirin should be avoided in children with chickenpox because of the recent association between aspirin derivatives and the development of Reye's syndrome.

Patients with varicella pneumonia may require removal of bronchial secretions and ventilatory support. Zoster ophthalmicus should be referred promptly and immediately to an ophthalmologist. Therapy consists of administration of analgesics for severe pain and the use of atropine. The role of parenteral administration of antivirals for the management of zoster ophthalmicus remains unclear, although both acyclovir and vidarabine have been utilized (see Chap. 86).

Both chickenpox and herpes zoster in the immunocompromised host can be treated successfully with intravenous vidarabine or acyclovir. When the former drug is administered to patients with either disease, healing of skin lesions is accelerated and visceral complications are likely to be decreased. For patients with herpes zoster, intravenous vidarabine therapy will also accelerate resolution of acute neuritis and decrease both the duration of postherpetic neuralgia and the frequency of cutaneous dissemination. The dose is 15 mg/kg per day once daily intravenously over 12 h at a concentration of 0.5 mg of standard intravenous fluids. While acyclovir is not yet approved for this indication by the Food and Drug Administration, it is used preferentially over vidarabine because of decreased toxicity, especially in immunocompromised patients. Intravenous acyclovir leads to the decreased occurrence of visceral complications but has no effect on healing of skin lesions or pain. The treatment of herpes zoster with oral acyclovir is experimental. Concomitant with the administration of intravenous acyclovir to the immunosuppressed host, it is desirable to attempt to wean patients from immunosuppressive treatment.

Management of acute neuritis and/or postherpetic neuralgia can be particularly difficult. In addition to the judicious use of analgesics, ranging from nonnarcotic to narcotic derivatives, drugs such as amitriptyline hydrochloride and fluphenazine hydrochloride have been reported to be beneficial for pain relief. Glucocorticoids have been reported in some studies to be useful when administered early in the course for prevention of postherpetic neuralgia. This approach remains controversial.

REFERENCES

BRUNELL PA et al: Prevention of varicella by zoster immune globulin. N Engl J Med 280:1191, 1969

ESSMAN V et al: Prednisone does not prevent postherpetic neuralgia. Lancet 2:126, 1987

GERSHON AA et al: Live attenuated varicella vaccine. JAMA 252:355, 1984

HOPE-SIMPSON RE: The nature of herpes zoster: A long-term study and a new hypothesis. Proc R Soc Med 58:9, 1965

LOCKSLEY RM et al: Infection with varicella-zoster virus after marrow transplantation. J Infect Dis 152:1172, 1985

PROBER CG et al: Acyclovir therapy of chickenpox in immunosuppressed children—a collaborative study. J Pediatr 101:622, 1982

SHEPP D et al: Treatment of varicella-zoster virus in severely immunocompromised patients: A randomized comparison of acyclovir and vidarabine. N Engl J Med 314:208, 1987

WEIBEL RE et al: Live attenuated varicella versus vaccine: Efficacy trial in healthy children. N Engl J Med 310:1409, 1984

WELLER TH: Varicella and herpes zoster: Changing concepts of the natural history, control, and importance of a not-so-benign virus. N Engl J Med 309:1362, 1434, 1983

WHITLEY RJ et al: Early vidarabine therapy to control the complications of herpes zoster in immunosuppressed patients. N Engl J Med 307:971, 1982

———: Vidarabine therapy of varicella in immunosuppressed patients. J Pediatr 1:125, 1982

———: Varicella-zoster virus infections, in *Antiviral Agents and Viral Diseases of Man 2*, GJ Galasso et al (eds). New York, Raven, 1984, pp 517–542

ZAIA JA et al: Evaluation of varicella-zoster immune globulin: Protection of immunosuppressed children after household exposure to varicella. J Infect Dis 147:737, 1983

137 EPSTEIN-BARR VIRUS INFECTIONS, INCLUDING INFECTIOUS MONONUCLEOSIS

ROBERT T. SCHOOLEY

DEFINITION Epstein-Barr virus (EBV) is a B lymphotropic human herpesvirus which is worldwide in distribution. Primary infection with EBV during childhood is usually subclinical. Between 25 and 70 percent of adolescents and adults who undergo a primary EBV infection develop the clinical syndrome of infectious mononucleosis. Infectious mononucleosis is defined by the clinical triad of fever, lymphadenopathy, and pharyngitis combined with the transient appearance of heterophil antibodies and an atypical lymphocytosis. EBV is also associated with nasopharyngeal carcinoma and certain B-cell lymphomas.

EPIDEMIOLOGY OF EBV INFECTIONS EBV is a ubiquitous agent that has been found in all population groups surveyed to date. The virus was initially described by Epstein, Achong, and Barr who noted, by electron microscopy, the presence of particles similar in morphology to herpes simplex virus in continuous cell lines which had arisen from tumor tissue obtained from patients with Burkitt's lymphoma. Following an observation by the Henles of antibodies to EBV in a patient with infectious mononucleosis, large-scale serologic surveys confirmed EBV as the etiologic agent for infectious mononucleosis.

EBV is transmitted primarily in saliva, or, less commonly, by blood transfusion. Primary infection tends to occur at an earlier age among lower socioeconomic groups and in developing countries. In industrialized countries approximately 50 percent of individuals have experienced a primary EBV infection by adolescence. These early infections are usually mild and nonspecific or clinically inapparent. A second wave of seroconversions to EBV occurs with the onset of the social activity associated with adolescence and young adulthood. Primary EBV infection among this age group accounts for most cases of infectious mononucleosis. The peak incidence of infectious mononucleosis occurs between 14 and 16 years of age for girls, and between 16 and 18 years of age for boys. By adulthood most individuals are EBV-seropositive.

EBV is shed from the oropharynx for up to 18 months following primary infection; thereafter it is shed intermittently by all EBV-seropositive individuals in the absence of a clinical illness. EBV can be isolated from the oropharyngeal washings of 15 to 25 percent of healthy EBV-seropositive individuals. Immunosuppressed individuals shed the virus more frequently. EBV can be isolated from 25 to 50 percent of the oropharyngeal washings obtained from renal allograft recipients and from virtually all patients with the acquired immunodeficiency syndrome (AIDS). Asymptomatic shedding of EBV by healthy individuals accounts for most of the spread to uninfected members of the population despite the fact that it is not highly contagious. Transmission is largely dependent on salivary contact (e.g., kissing). It is not likely to be transmitted by aerosol or fomites. Thus, isolation restrictions on patients with mononucleosis or individuals likely to be shedding EBV are not appropriate.

ETIOLOGY AND PATHOGENESIS OF INFECTIOUS MONONUCLEOSIS By electron microscopy the EB virus appears as an icosahedral nucleocapsid surrounded by a complex envelope and is indistinguishable from other members of the human herpesvirus group. The double-stranded EBV DNA has a molecular weight of approximately 101 × 10^6 and encodes for at least 30 polypeptides. There is no convincing evidence that there are strain differences among EBV isolates which account for the wide range of clinical conditions associated with EBV infection.

When EBV is transmitted by saliva, the initial site of replication is the oropharynx. EBV grows productively in B lymphocytes and oropharyngeal epithelial cells of patients with infectious mononucleosis; both cell types have specific surface receptors for EBV. During the acute phase of the illness, EBV antigens can be demonstrated within the nuclei of up to 20 percent of circulating B lymphocytes. After the infection subsides, the virus can be isolated from a small number of B lymphocytes of EBV-seropositive individuals and also resides within nasopharyngeal epithelial cells.

Virus-host interactions EBV infection has both direct and indirect effects on the cellular and humoral immune responses. Within 18 to 24 h after entry of EBV into B lymphocytes by means of the C3d receptor (also known as CD21), Epstein-Barr nuclear antigens (EBNA) are detectable within the nucleus of the infected cell. Expression of EBNA corresponds to the acquisition of the transformed or immortalized phenotype. EBV-infected B lymphocytes also express lymphocyte-determined membrane antigens (LYDMA) which serve as the putative target for the cellular immune response to virus-infected B lymphocytes. Immortalized B lymphocytes can be propagated continuously in vitro and are polyclonally stimulated by EBV to produce immunoglobulin. Antibodies reactive with sheep red blood cells (heterophil) and antibodies with several other specificities are manifestations of polyclonal immunoglobulin production and may mediate several of the complications of infectious mononucleosis. A minority of EBV-infected B lymphocytes enter the lytic cycle (production of mature progeny virus and death of the host cell) and produce EBV antigens that are detected during virus replication. These are divided into the early antigen complex (EA) and viral capsid antigens (VCA). The early antigen complex consists of two groups of antigens; (1) diffuse (EA-D), which are detectable in both the cytoplasm and the nucleus of cells in the lytic cycle, and (2) restricted (EA-R), which are demonstrable only in the cytoplasm. These antigens serve as markers of infection at the cellular level; the pattern of the antibody response to these antigens is useful diagnostically in the identification of EBV-associated disease states (Table 137-1). After the appearance of VCA the host cell dies and virions are released, which can infect and transform additional B lymphocytes.

An effective immune response to EBV involves humoral and cellular components. Neutralizing antibodies which inactivate cell-free virus and antibodies to VCA and EBNA appear during primary infection in all patients; antibodies to EA-D appear in most patients. The cellular immune response is largely responsible for controlling B-cell proliferation and polyclonal immunoglobulin production trig-

TABLE 137-1 EBV-specific antibodies

Antibody specificity	Time of appearance in IM	Persistence	Percent of IM patients with antibody	Comments
VCA:				
IgM	At clinical presentation	1–2 months	100	Best indicator of primary infection; not present with reactivation
IgG	At clinical presentation	Lifelong	100	Standard "EBV titer" reported by most commercial and state labs; major utility is as a marker for prior or current infection in epidemiologic studies
EA:				
EA-D	Peaks 3–4 weeks after onset	3–6 months	70	Presence correlates with more severe disease in patients with IM; present in nasopharyngeal carcinoma; IgA anti-EA-D antibodies useful for prediction of NPC in high-risk populations
EA-R	Several weeks after onset	Months to years		Present in high titer in African Burkitt's lymphoma; may be useful as an indicator of reactivation of EBV in immunosuppressed patients
EBNA	3–6 weeks after onset	Lifelong	100	Late appearance of anti-EBNA antibodies in IM makes seroconversion a useful marker for primary infection if IgM anti-VCA antibody studies are not available

NOTE: IM = infectious mononucleosis; VCA = viral capsid antigen; EA = early antigens; EA-D = diffuse early antigens; EA-R = restricted early antigens; EBNA = Epstein-Barr nuclear antigens; NPC = nasopharyngeal carcinoma.

gered by EBV and is composed primarily of T lymphocytes having functional and surface phenotypic characteristics of activated, suppressor-cytotoxic T lymphocytes (CD8+, Ia+). As the illness progresses, memory T lymphocytes capable of limiting proliferation of autologous EBV-infected B lymphocytes are demonstrable. These memory T lymphocytes persist for life. However, latent EBV remains in a small proportion of B lymphocytes and also in epithelial cells in the oropharynx.

During the primary immune response to EBV, global cellular immune hyporesponsiveness is readily demonstrable. This resolves after resolution of the illness, but reactivation of EBV is facilitated by conditions which interfere with the cellular immune response (immunosuppressive drugs, especially cyclosporin A, and disorders associated with cellular immunodeficiency, e.g., AIDS). EBV and cytomegalovirus (CMV) reactivation in immunosuppressed patients are frequently associated with a return of the immunoregulatory abnormalities characteristic of the primary immune response to these viruses. In the case of CMV, particularly, this hyporesponsiveness may contribute to many of the superinfections which frequently accompany CMV infections in immunocompromised hosts. The cellular hyporesponsiveness associated with EBV reactivation is generally less intense and less prolonged than that associated with CMV but may also contribute to morbidity in immunocompromised individuals.

CLINICAL MANIFESTATIONS **Symptoms and signs** After an incubation period of 4 to 8 weeks, prodromal symptoms of malaise, anorexia, and chills frequently precede the onset of pharyngitis, fever, and lymphadenopathy by several days. Severe pharyngitis is the symptom which most frequently prompts patients to seek medical attention. Occasionally patients will note only fever or lymphadenopathy or will present with one of the complications of infectious mononucleosis. Most patients also complain of headache and malaise. Abdominal pain is infrequent in the absence of splenic rupture.

Physical examination Fever is present in 90 percent of patients and may reach 39 to 40°C. Periorbital edema may be seen. The pharyngitis is usually diffuse; an exudate is observed in one-third of the cases. Palatal petechiae may also be observed. Posterior and/or anterior cervical adenopathy is noted in 90 percent of patients with infectious mononucleosis. Individual nodes are rarely painful but may be moderately tender to palpation. Hepatomegaly is infrequent, although mild hepatic tenderness is present in up to half the patients. Approximately half of all patients have splenomegaly, which is usually maximal in the second or third week of illness. In 5 percent of patients a macular, petechial, scarlatiniform, urticarial, or erythema multiforme-like rash may appear. Administration of ampicillin results in a pruritic, maculopapular eruption in 90 to 100 percent of patients.

Clinical course Infectious mononucleosis is a self-limited illness in the vast majority of cases. The pharyngitis is maximal for 5 to 7 days and then resolves over the subsequent 7 to 10 days. Fever usually persists for 7 to 14 days, but occasionally may continue somewhat longer. The course of the lymphadenopathy is variable, but rarely exceeds 3 weeks. The most persistent symptom is malaise. Most patients are well enough to return to work or school within 3 to 4 weeks, but occasional patients remain exhausted, have difficulty concentrating, and are unable to return to full activities for months. This subgroup is often found among those who present with a less acute onset without severe pharyngitis and high fever.

Occasional patients have been reported in which recurrent pharyngitis and fever is accompanied by persistent or resurgent heterophil antibodies. A group of patients has been described with nonspecific symptoms which may include malaise, fatigue, pharyngitis, fever, lymphadenopathy, and difficulty with higher cognitive function. These patients are usually heterophil-negative. The demonstration that some of these patients have anti-VCA and EA-R titers which are higher, and anti-EBNA titers which are lower, than median titers for the general population has led to the speculation that this symptom complex may be a manifestation of ongoing replication of EBV. However, healthy members of the general population not infrequently have antibodies to EA-R antigens, and one should be cautious about applying the diagnosis of chronic active EBV infection to patients with these nonspecific symptoms simply on the basis of the presence of anti-EA-R antibodies. Several studies have demonstrated the lack of utility of EBV-specific antibodies in the evaluation of most patients with chronic fatigue and malaise. A blinded placebo-controlled crossover study demonstrated no benefit from acyclovir therapy in this patient population. Occasional patients have been reported in whom mortality or severe morbidity (pneumonitis, fever, pancytopenia) is associated with evidence of ongoing EBV replication. Such patients are extremely rare, and specific antiviral therapy may be useful in their management.

Complications Complications of infectious mononucleosis occur infrequently but may be so dramatic as to be the predominant manifestation of the illness (Table 137-2). Hematologic complications include autoimmune hemolytic anemia, which may be mediated by

TABLE 137-2 Complications of infectious mononucleosis

Hematologic complications:
- Autoimmune hemolytic anemia
- Thrombocytopenia
- Granulocytopenia

Splenic rupture

Neurologic complications:
- Encephalitis
- Cranial nerve palsies, especially Bell's palsy
- Meningoencephalitis
- Guillain-Barré syndrome
- Seizures
- Mononeuritis multiplex
- Transverse myelitis
- Psychosis

Hepatic complications:
- Hepatitis

Cardiac complications:
- Pericarditis
- Myocarditis

Pulmonary complications:
- Airway obstruction
- Interstitial pneumonitis

IgM antibodies with anti-i specificity. Hemolytic anemia usually subsides over a 1- to 2-month period. Mild thrombocytopenia occurs in up to 50 percent of cases; profound thrombocytopenia is a rare, but well-recognized, complication and is frequently antibody-mediated. Mild granulocytopenia is frequently observed in uncomplicated infectious mononucleosis, and severe granulocytopenia associated with infection or death has been reported. Antibodies which react with granulocytes have been detected in up to 80 percent of patients and may contribute to the profound granulocytopenia which is occasionally observed. Both the thrombocytopenia and the granulocytopenia are usually self-limited and resolve over 3 to 6 weeks. Glucocorticoids have been advocated for treatment of both hemolytic anemia and thrombocytopenia associated with infectious mononucleosis, but efficacy has not been proved in controlled studies. Splenic rupture is an infrequent complication of infectious mononucleosis, often accompanied by the insidious or abrupt onset of abdominal pain, and is usually observed during the second or third week of illness. Surgery, usually splenectomy or splenorrhaphy, is the only effective management.

Neurologic complications of infectious mononucleosis may be the presenting or sole manifestation of the illness. Heterophil antibodies may be absent, and atypical lymphocytes may not be present at the onset of the neurologic event. The most frequent neurologic complications are cranial nerve palsies and encephalitis which may present initially with cerebellar findings. The onset of the encephalitis is usually abrupt. Cerebrospinal fluid findings are not diagnostic, and localization by noninvasive neurodiagnostic studies may suggest herpes simplex encephalitis. Eighty-five percent of patients with EBV-associated neurologic findings recover spontaneously.

Hepatitis is a common component of infectious mononucleosis. Almost 90 percent of patients have mild elevation of hepatic transaminases. Although more serious hepatic sequelae have been reported, severe or permanent hepatic dysfunction is exceedingly rare.

Cardiac abnormalities are uncommon but may include pericarditis, myocarditis, coronary artery spasm, or electrocardiographic abnormalities.

Airway obstruction from pharyngeal or paratracheal adenopathy can occur. This may require surgical intervention but is usually quite sensitive to glucocorticoid therapy. Pulmonary parenchymal abnormalities such as interstitial infiltrates are noted infrequently in adults but appear to be more common among children.

Infectious mononucleosis is rarely fatal. Neurologic complications, airway obstruction, and splenic rupture are the most frequent causes of death in previously healthy individuals with primary EBV infection. Sporadic or X-linked cases of overwhelming EBV infection accompanied by lymphoproliferation and hepatic dysfunction have been reported.

The X-linked condition, known as *X-linked lymphoproliferative (XLP) or Duncan's syndrome* (see Chap. 263), results in the death of 40 percent of affected males during primary EBV infection. In addition to overwhelming lymphoproliferation, XLP patients may manifest severe immunologic or hematologic sequelae such as agammaglobulinemia, aplastic anemia, or lymphocytic lymphoma. The pathophysiology of the XLP syndrome has not yet been completely elucidated, but an X-linked defect in the immune response to EBV may result in failure to control EBV replication or in disordered immunoregulation which leads to the other immunologic sequelae observed in this syndrome.

LABORATORY MANIFESTATIONS Heterophil antibodies Antibodies to sheep erythrocytes which can be removed by prior absorption with beef red blood cells, but not with guinea pig kidney, are termed heterophil antibodies. Heterophil antibodies are demonstrated in 50 percent of children and 90 to 95 percent of adolescents and adults with mononucleosis. Although the classic tube heterophil titer is still performed in many laboratories, the "monospot" test using a commerical kit is sensitive, specific, easily performed, and more routinely employed. The frequency of heterophil positivity associated with infectious mononucleosis depends upon the test used, the age of the patient population, and the time during the illness at which the test is performed. Monospot tests may be slightly more sensitive than heterophil titers. Ten to fifteen percent of patients with mononucleosis may be heterophil-negative if tested only during the first week of the illness. If the clinical suspicion of mononucleosis is high enough, retesting for heterophil antibodies during the second or third week of illness is warranted. Heterophil antibodies decline in titer after the acute illness has resolved but may be detectable for up to 9 months after the onset of the illness.

Atypical lymphocytosis A relative and absolute lymphocytosis is present in about 75 percent of cases of infectious mononucleosis. The lymphocytosis usually peaks in the second or third week of illness and is characterized by cells with atypical morphology. These atypical lymphocytes, which are primarily activated T lymphocytes, are larger than mature lymphocytes and often contain eccentrically placed lobulated nuclei with nucleoli, and vacuolated cytoplasm with rolled up edges. Mild neutropenia and thrombocytopenia are frequent. Other laboratory abnormalities include a mild polyclonal increase in immunoglobulins of the IgM, IgG, and IgA classes, and mild elevations of hepatocellular enzymes.

EBV-specific antibody response Antibodies to several EBV-specific antigens arise during primary EBV infection (Table 137-1). Proper utilization of EBV-specific antibody studies may facilitate the diagnosis of primary EBV infection in clinically atypical or heterophil-negative cases. IgM antibodies to the VCA are diagnostic of a primary EBV infection. IgG anti-VCA antibodies are present at clinical presentation in almost all patients and remain detectable for life. IgG anti-VCA antibodies are useful mainly as a test for susceptibility to EBV and are not useful for the diagnosis of primary infection. Approximately 70 percent of patients with infectious mononucleosis make antibodies to EA-D. Anti-EA-D antibodies usually peak 3 to 4 weeks after the onset of illness and usually disappear after recovery. Antibodies to EBNA appear 6 to 8 weeks into the illness and persist for life. The presence of IgM anti-VCA antibodies, and seroconversion to EBNA is diagnostic of a primary EBV infection. Patients with defects in cellular immunity may fail to make antibodies to EBNA.

DIAGNOSIS The diagnosis of infectious mononucleosis is not difficult in the vast majority of cases. The constellation of fever, pharyngitis, and lymphadenopathy coupled with an atypical lymphocytosis and heterophil antibodies is virtually always due to primary EBV infection and requires no further laboratory studies. Certain patients with EBV-induced mononucleosis, particularly preadolescents, or those with neurologic complications may be heterophil-negative or may lack an atypical lymphocytosis. Primary EBV infection can be diagnosed with certainty in these patients with the proper use of EBV-specific serologic studies (see above). Culturing EBV from oropharyngeal washings or peripheral blood mononuclear cells is laborious, and because of the ubiquity of the virus among EBV-seropositive individuals, it is not diagnostic of primary EBV infection.

Primary CMV infection is the illness most frequently confused with EBV-induced infectious mononucleosis. About two-thirds of adults with heterophil-negative mononucleosis have CMV-induced mononucleosis. Patients with CMV mononucleosis are, on the average, slightly older than those with EBV-induced infectious mononucleosis and usually have an illness characterized predominantly by fever and malaise. Pharyngitis and lymphadenopathy are less common than with infectious mononucleosis. CMV-induced mononucleosis is usually more insidious in onset and slower to resolve than EBV-induced mononucleosis. The diagnosis can be made by the isolation of CMV from the peripheral blood, and the demonstration of seroconversion or a fourfold or greater rise in antibody titer to CMV. Although CMV is also shed in saliva and urine by patients with CMV mononucleosis, demonstration of the agent in the blood is a more specific, but less sensitive, indicator of CMV-induced morbidity.

Severe pharyngitis may also be caused by another virus (e.g., herpes simplex) or by group A beta-hemolytic streptococci. Since group A beta-hemolytic streptococci can be isolated from the throat of up to 30 percent of patients with infectious mononucleosis, isolation of this organism does not rule out the diagnosis of infectious mononucleosis. Atypical lymphocytes may also be observed in a number of other conditions including rubella, hepatitis, toxoplasmosis, mumps, and drug reactions. These conditions rarely pose major differential diagnostic problems when careful attention is paid to the other clinical and laboratory features of these illnesses.

TREATMENT Infectious mononucleosis usually requires only supportive management. Patients should be advised to obtain adequate rest; there is no evidence that forced bed rest hastens recovery. Fever and pharyngitis are usually ameliorated by acetaminophen. Because of the infrequent complication of splenic rupture, patients should be advised to avoid contact sports for 6 to 8 weeks after the onset of illness. The timing of return to school or work is determined solely by symptoms. Patients with mild illness may not require any major changes in routine. Occasional patients with protracted illness may not return to a full school or work schedule for several months. Recovery from mononucleosis is often gradual and the malaise may wax and wane for some time.

Although glucocorticoids may hasten defervescence and the resolution of pharyngitis, they are indicated only for certain specific complications of mononucleosis; airway obstruction usually responds dramatically to parenteral glucocorticoids. Glucocorticoids may also hasten the recovery of patients with severe hemolytic anemia or thrombocytopenia. There is no evidence that glucocorticoids are beneficial for the neurologic complications of the illness. Occasional selected patients with protracted illness may benefit from a short course of prednisone, but glucocorticoids should be avoided in the majority of patients with infectious mononucleosis.

Acyclovir, interferon alpha, and 9-[2-hydroxy-1-(hydroxymethyl)ethoxy]methyl guanine (ganciclovir) are active inhibitors of EBV replication in vitro. Interferon alpha has antiviral activity and can decrease shedding of EBV by renal allograft recipients treated with antithymocyte globulin. Administration of intravenous or high-dose oral acyclovir halts oropharyngeal shedding of EBV in patients with acute infectious mononucleosis; however, clinical benefits are minimal or inapparent.

EBV-ASSOCIATED MALIGNANCY Since the initial description of EBV in patients with African Burkitt's lymphoma, the virus has been detected in association with several other malignancies. EBV DNA sequences have been detected in tumor tissue from more than 90 percent of patients with African Burkitt's lymphomas. American Burkitt's lymphoma, which often affects older children, and more often presents as an intraabdominal tumor, is EBV-associated in only 15 percent of cases. Anaplastic nasopharyngeal carcinoma, a common neoplasm in southeast China, is highly associated with EBV; virtually all adequately studied patients with this malignancy have evidence of EBV in tumor tissue.

There is increasing evidence that implicates EBV in the pathogenesis of certain cases of lymphocytic lymphoma in the immunoincompetent host (see Chap. 302). B-cell lymphoma is greatly overrepresented among malignancies developing in immunosuppressed individuals such as organ allograft recipients, patients with ataxia telangiectasia, and patients with AIDS. Immunologically privileged areas such as the central nervous system also appear to be particularly susceptible to B-cell lymphomas. Cardiac allograft recipients treated with cyclosporin A appear to be particularly susceptible to B-cell lymphoma. EBV sequences are detectable in up to half of the B-cell malignancies encountered in immunosuppressed individuals. Controversy exists as to whether the B-cell lymphoproliferation, which is initially polyclonal and may be driven by EBV reactivated in the setting of cellular immunodeficiency, is the first step in the development of these malignancies. The process, which is thought to be polyclonal initially, becomes oligoclonal or monoclonal with a second-step chromosomal translocation made more likely by the increased number of proliferating B lymphocytes. The biologic behavior of these tumors does not always correlate with clonality as defined by conventional techniques. Patients have been described who have succumbed to lymphoproliferative processes which appear to be polyclonal by surface immunoglobulin studies. More sensitive techniques of defining clonality, such as that utilizing immunoglobulin gene rearrangement, may reveal that a larger proportion of the polyclonal lymphomas are in fact oligo- or monoclonal. The response of these B-cell lymphomas to conventional chemotherapy is often disappointing. Some have advocated acyclovir therapy; others feel many of these lymphoproliferative syndromes are reversible if the immunosuppression is decreased. Studies of larger numbers of these patients for the presence of EBV sequences and for the progression from a polyclonal to an oligoclonal or monoclonal disorder will shed more light on the role of EBV in oncogenesis in both immunoincompetent and immunologically normal hosts.

REFERENCES

ANDIMAN W et al: Use of cloned probes to detect Epstein-Barr viral DNA in tissues of patients with neoplastic and lymphoproliferative diseases. J Infect Dis 148:967, 1983

GROSE C et al: Primary Epstein-Barr virus infections in acute neurologic diseases. N Engl J Med 292:392, 1975

HANTO DW et al: Epstein-Barr virus induced B-cell lymphoma after renal transplantation. Acyclovir therapy and transition from polyclonal to monoclonal B-cell proliferation. N Engl J Med 306:913, 1982

HENLE W et al: Epstein-Barr virus specific diagnostic tests in infectious mononucleosis. Hum Pathol 5:551, 1974

HOLMES GP et al: Chronic fatigue syndrome: A working case definition. Ann Intern Med 108:387, 1989

MILLER G et al: Selective lack of antibody to a component of EB nuclear antigen in patients with chronic active Epstein-Barr virus infection. J Infect Dis 156:26, 1987

SCHOOLEY RT et al: Chronic Epstein-Barr virus infection associated with fever and interstitial pneumonitis. Ann Intern Med 104:636, 1986

SIXBY JW et al: Epstein-Barr virus replication in oropharyngeal epithelial cells. N Engl J Med 310:1225, 1984

STRAUS SE et al: Treatment of the chronic fatigue syndrome with acyclovir: Lack of efficacy in a placebo-controlled trial. N Engl J Med 319:1692–1698, 1988

THORLEY-LAWSON, DA: Immunological responses to Epstein-Barr virus infection and the pathogenesis of EBV-induced diseases. Biochem Biophys Acta 948:263, 1988

138 CYTOMEGALOVIRUS INFECTION

MARTIN S. HIRSCH

DEFINITION Cytomegalovirus (CMV), which was initially isolated from patients with congenital cytomegalic inclusion disease, is now recognized as an important pathogen in all age groups. In addition to inducing severe birth defects, CMV causes a wide spectrum of disorders in older children and adults, ranging from an asymptomatic, subclinical infection to a mononucleosis syndrome in healthy individuals to disseminated disease in the immunocompromised. Human CMV is one of several related species-specific viruses that cause similar diseases in various animals. All are associated with the production of characteristic enlarged cells; hence the name cytomegalovirus.

ETIOLOGY CMV is a member of the herpesvirus group and contains double-stranded DNA, a protein capsid, and a lipoprotein envelope. Like other members of the herpesvirus group, CMV demonstrates icosahedral symmetry, replicates in the cell nucleus, and can cause either a lytic and productive or a latent infection. CMV can be distinguished from other herpesviruses by certain biologic properties such as host range and the type of cytopathology induced. Virus replication is associated with the production of large intranuclear inclusions and smaller cytoplasmic inclusions. The virus appears to replicate in a variety of cell types in vivo; in tissue culture it grows preferentially in fibroblasts. It is unclear whether CMV is oncogenic in vivo. However, the virus can rarely transform fibroblasts and genomic transforming fragments have been identified.

EPIDEMIOLOGY CMV has a worldwide distribution. Approximately 1 percent of newborns in the United States are infected with CMV, and the percentage is higher in many less-developed countries. Communal living and poor personal hygiene facilitate early spread. Perinatal and early childhood infections are common. Virus may be present in milk, saliva, feces, and urine. Transmission of CMV has been identified among young children in day-care centers and has been traced by restriction endonuclease techniques from infected toddler to pregnant mother to developing fetus.

The virus is not readily spread by casual contact but requires repeated or prolonged intimate exposure for transmission. In late adolescence and young adulthood, CMV is often transmitted sexually, and asymptomatic viral carriage in semen or cervical secretions is common. CMV antibody titers approach 100 percent in female prostitutes and in sexually active homosexual men. Sexually active adults may harbor several strains of CMV simultaneously. Transfusion of whole blood or certain blood products containing viable leukocytes may also transmit CMV with a frequency of 0.14 to 10 percent per unit transfused.

Once infected, an individual probably carries the virus for life. Most commonly these infections remain latent. However, with compromise of T-lymphocyte-mediated immunity, as occurs following organ transplantation or in association with lymphoid neoplasms and certain acquired immunodeficiencies in particular that caused by infection with the human immunodeficiency virus (HIV) (see Chap. 264), CMV reactivation syndromes develop frequently.

PATHOGENESIS Congenital CMV infection can follow either primary or reactivation infection of the mother. However, clinical disease in the fetus or newborn is almost exclusively limited to primary maternal infections. Factors determining the severity of congenital infection are unknown; a deficient capacity to produce precipitating antibodies and to mount T-cell responses to CMV are associated with more severe disease.

Primary infection in late childhood or adulthood is often associated with a vigorous T-lymphocyte response that may contribute to the development of a mononucleosis syndrome similar to that observed following Epstein-Barr virus infection (see Chap. 137). The hallmarks of such infections are the appearance of atypical lymphocytes in the peripheral blood; these cells are predominantly activated T lymphocytes of cytotoxic-suppressor phenotype. Polyclonal activation of B cells by the virus contributes to the development of rheumatoid factors and other autoantibodies during CMV mononucleosis.

Once acquired during symptomatic or asymptomatic primary infection, CMV persists indefinitely in tissues of the host. The sites of persistent or latent infection are unclear, but probably involve multiple cell types and various organs. Transmission following blood transfusion or organ transplantation is due to silent infections in these tissues. Autopsy studies suggest that lungs, salivary glands, and bowel may also be areas of latent infection.

If T-cell responses of the host become compromised by disease or by iatrogenic immunosuppression, latent virus can be reactivated to cause a variety of syndromes. Chronic antigenic stimulation, as occurs following tissue transplantation, in the presence of immunosuppression, appears to be an ideal setting for CMV activation and CMV-induced disease. Certain particularly potent suppressants of T-cell immunity, such as antithymocyte globulin, are associated with a high rate of clinical CMV syndromes, which may follow either primary or reactivation infection. CMV may itself contribute to further T-lymphocyte hyporesponsiveness, which often precedes superinfection with other opportunistic pathogens, such as *Pneumocystis carinii*. CMV and pneumocystis are frequently found together in immunosuppressed patients with severe interstitial pneumonia. CMV may function as a cofactor to activate latent HIV infection.

PATHOLOGY Cytomegalic cells in vivo are presumed to be infected epithelial cells. They are two to four times larger than surrounding cells and often contain an 8- to 10-μm intranuclear inclusion that is eccentrically placed and surrounded by a clear halo, resulting in an "owl's eye" appearance. Smaller granular cytoplasmic inclusions may also be demonstrated occasionally. Cytomegalic cells are found in a wide variety of organs including salivary glands, lung, liver, kidney, intestines, pancreas, adrenal glands, and the central nervous system.

The cellular inflammatory response to infection consists of plasma cells, lymphocytes, and monocyte-macrophages. Granulomatous reactions are occasionally observed, particularly in the liver. Immunopathologic reactions may contribute to CMV disease. Immune complexes have been described in infected infants, sometimes associated with CMV-related glomerulopathies. Immune-complex glomerulopathy has been observed in some CMV-infected patients following renal transplantation.

CLINICAL MANIFESTATIONS **Congenital CMV infection** Fetal infections range from inapparent to severe and disseminated. Cytomegalic inclusion disease develops in approximately 5 percent of infected fetuses and is seen almost exclusively in infants born to mothers who develop primary infections during pregnancy. Petechiae, hepatosplenomegaly, and jaundice are the most common presenting features (60 to 80 percent). Microcephaly with or without cerebral calcifications, intrauterine growth retardation, and prematurity are noted in 30 to 50 percent of patients. Inguinal hernias and chorioretinitis are observed less commonly. Laboratory abnormalities in decreasing order of frequency include increased serum IgM above 0.20 g/L (20 mg/dL), atypical lymphocytosis, elevated liver transaminases, thrombocytopenia, hyperbilirubinemia, and increased cerebrospinal fluid protein above 0.20 g/L (20 mg/dL). Prognosis among severely infected infants is poor, with mortality rates of 20 to 30 percent; few patients escape intellectual or hearing difficulties in later years. Differential diagnoses of cytomegalic inclusion disease in infants include syphilis, rubella, toxoplasmosis, herpes simplex or enterovirus infection, and bacterial sepsis.

Most congenital CMV infections are clinically inapparent at birth. Between 5 to 25 percent of asymptomatically infected infants develop significant psychomotor, hearing, ocular, or dental abnormalities over the next several years.

Perinatal CMV infection The newborn may acquire CMV at the time of delivery by passage through an infected birth canal or by postnatal contact with maternal milk or other secretions. Approximately 40 to 60 percent of infants who are breast-fed for over 1 month by seropositive mothers will become infected. Iatrogenic transmission can also result from neonatal blood transfusion. Screening of blood products prior to transfusion into low-birth-weight seronegative infants or seronegative pregnant women will decrease the risk of infection. The great majority of infants infected at or after delivery will remain asymptomatic. However, protracted interstitial pneumonitis has been associated with perinatally acquired CMV infection, particularly in premature infants, occasionally associated with *Chlamydia trachomatis*, *P. carinii*, or *Ureaplasma urealyticum* infections. Poor weight gain, adenopathy, rash, hepatitis, anemia, and atypical lymphocytosis may also be present, and CMV excretion often persists for months to years.

CMV mononucleosis The most common clinical manifestation of CMV infection in normal hosts beyond the neonatal period is a heterophil-antibody negative mononucleosis syndrome. This may occur spontaneously or following the transfusion of leukocyte-containing blood products. Although the syndrome occurs at all ages, sexually active young adults are most often involved. Incubation periods range from 20 to 60 days, and the illness generally lasts 2 to 6 weeks. Prolonged high fevers, sometimes accompanied by chills, profound fatigue, and malaise characterize this disorder. Myalgias, headache, and splenomegaly are frequent, but exudative pharyngitis and cervical lymphadenopathy are rare, in contrast to infectious mononucleosis caused by Epstein-Barr virus. Occasional patients will develop rubelliform rashes, often after exposure to ampicillin. Less commonly observed are interstitial or segmental pneumonia, myocarditis, pleuritis, arthritis, or encephalitis. Rarely, Guillain-Barré syndrome may complicate CMV mononucleosis. The characteristic laboratory abnormality is a peripheral blood relative lymphocytosis with greater than 10 percent atypical lymphocytes. Total leukocyte counts may be low, normal, or markedly elevated. Although significant jaundice is uncommon, moderately elevated serum transaminase and alkaline phosphatase levels are often present. Heterophil antibodies are absent; however, transient immunologic abnormalities are common. These may include the presence of cryoglobulins, rheumatoid factors, cold agglutinins, and antinuclear antibodies. Rarely, hemolytic anemia, thrombocytopenia, and granulocytopenia complicate recovery.

Most patients recover without sequelae, although postviral asthenia may persist for months. CMV excretion in urine, genital secretions, or saliva often continues for months to years. Rare patients have recurrent episodes of fever and malaise, sometimes associated with autonomic nervous system dysfunction, e.g., attacks of sweating or flushing.

CMV infection in the immunocompromised host CMV appears to be the most frequent and important viral pathogen complicating organ transplantation. In renal, cardiac, and liver transplant recipients, CMV induces a variety of syndromes including fever and leukopenia, hepatitis, pneumonitis, colitis, and retinitis. The maximal period of risk appears between 1 to 4 months after transplantation, although retinitis is often a later complication. The risk of disease appears greater following primary infection. In addition, restriction endonuclease studies indicate that seropositive transplant recipients are susceptible to reinfection with donor-derived CMV, often resulting in disease. Reactivation infection, although frequent, is less likely to be important clinically. Clinical disease is related to the degree of immunosuppression; patients receiving certain immunosuppressive agents, such as antithymocyte globulin, appear more likely to have severe infections than those receiving other agents, such as cyclosporine A.

CMV pneumonia occurs in nearly 15 to 20 percent of bone marrow transplant recipients, with a case fatality rate of 84 to 88 percent. The risk is greatest between 5 to 13 weeks after transplant, and several risk factors have been identified. These include type of immunosuppression, acute graft-versus-host disease, older age, viremia, seropositivity before transplantation, and granulocyte transfusions.

CMV has become recognized as an important pathogen in patients with the acquired immunodeficiency syndrome (AIDS) (see Chap. 264). CMV infection is nearly ubiquitous in this disorder and often causes retinitis or disseminated disease, contributing to death. CMV-induced immunosuppression probably also contributes to the T-lymphocyte deficiency initiated by the etiologic retrovirus.

CMV syndromes in the immunocompromised host often begin with prolonged fever, malaise, anorexia, fatigue, night sweats, and arthralgias or myalgias. Liver function abnormalities, leukopenia, thrombocytopenia, and atypical lymphocytosis may be observed during these episodes. The development of tachypnea, hypoxia, and unproductive cough signals respiratory involvement. Radiologic examination of the lung often demonstrates bilateral interstitial or reticulonodular infiltrates, beginning in the periphery of the lower lobes and spreading centrally and superiorly; localized segmental, nodular, or alveolar patterns are less commonly observed. Diagnosis requires lung biopsy, since neither peripheral virus excretion nor high antibody titers provides sufficient information to prove etiology. The differential diagnoses include *P. carinii,* other viral, bacterial, or fungal pathogens, pulmonary hemorrhage, and injury secondary to radiation or cytotoxic drugs.

Gastrointestinal CMV involvement may be localized or extensive and occurs almost exclusively in compromised hosts. Ulcers of the esophagus, stomach, small intestine, or colon may result in bleeding or perforation. CMV infection may lead to exacerbations of underlying ulcerative colitis. Hepatitis occurs frequently, and CMV-associated acalculous cholecystitis has been described.

CMV rarely causes meningoencephalitis in otherwise healthy individuals. Although CMV antigens and inclusions are observed occasionally in brains of patients dying from AIDS encephalopathy, the relative roles and interactions of CMV and HIV in this disorder are unclear.

CMV retinitis is an important cause of blindness in immunocompromised patients, including patients with AIDS and organ transplant recipients. Early lesions consist of small, opaque, white areas of granular retinal necrosis that spread in a centrifugal manner and are later accompanied by hemorrhages, vessel sheathing, and retinal edema (see Fig. A4-14). CMV must be distinguished from other causes of retinopathy including toxoplasmosis, candidiasis, and herpes simplex virus.

Fatal infections are often associated with persistent viremia and multiple organ system involvement. Progressive pulmonary infiltrates, pancytopenia, hyperamylasemia, and hypotension are characteristic, often with a terminal bacterial, fungal, or protozoan superinfection. Extensive adrenal necrosis with CMV inclusions is present at autopsy, as well as CMV involvement of many other organs.

In the renal transplant recipient, CMV also contributes to graft dysfunction by mechanisms other than direct viral cytopathic effects. An immune-complex glomerulopathy may accompany CMV infection and should be differentiated from true graft rejection, since the former does not respond well to increased immunosuppression. In addition, a protein encoded by the CMV genome contains sequence homology and immunologic cross-reactivity with a conserved domain of the HLA-DR antigen, suggesting an alternative mechanism for increased graft dysfunction associated with infection.

DIAGNOSIS The diagnosis of CMV infection cannot be made reliably on clinical grounds alone. Virus isolation from appropriate clinical specimens, together with demonstration of a fourfold or greater antibody rise or persistently elevated antibody titers, is the preferred diagnostic approach. Virus excretion or viremia is readily detected by culture of appropriate specimens on human fibroblast monolayers. If virus titers are high, as is frequently the case in congenital disseminated infection or in patients with AIDS, characteristic cytopathic effects may be detected within a few days. However, in some situations, e.g., CMV mononucleosis, virus titers are low and cytopathic effects may take several weeks to appear. Many laboratories expedite diagnosis by using an overnight tissue culture method (shell vial assay) with an immunofluorescence detection technique employing monoclonal antibodies to an immediate early CMV antigen. Virus isolation from urine or saliva by itself does not necessarily imply acute infection since excretion from these sites may continue for months to years following illness. Detection of CMV viremia is a better predictor of acute infection. Direct detection of CMV DNA or antigens in tissues or secretions does not yet appear of sufficient sensitivity or specificity to replace virus culture.

A variety of serologic assays (complement fixation, immunofluorescence, indirect hemagglutination, enzyme-linked immunosorbent assay) are available to detect antibody rises to CMV antigens. Antibody rises may not be detectable for up to 4 weeks after primary infection, and titers often remain high for years after infection. For this reason, single-sample antibody determinations are of no value in assessing the acuteness of infection. Detection of CMV-specific IgM is sometimes useful in the diagnosis of recent or active infection; circulating rheumatoid factors may result in occasional false-positive IgM tests.

PREVENTION AND TREATMENT Several prophylactic measures are useful to prevent CMV infection in patients at high risk. The use of blood from seronegative donors or blood that was frozen, thawed, and deglycerolized greatly decreases transfusion-associated transmission of CMV. Similarly, matching of kidney or bone marrow transplants by CMV serology, using only organs from seronegative donors for seronegative recipients, reduces primary infections following transplantation.

CMV immune globulin has been reported to reduce CMV-associated syndromes and fungal or parasitic superinfections in seronegative renal transplant recipients. Similar studies in bone marrow transplant recipients have been conducted; most, but not all, studies have shown benefit from prophylactic CMV immune globulin. Prophylactic acyclovir has been demonstrated to reduce CMV infection and disease in seronegative renal transplant recipients; acyclovir is not effective in treatment of active CMV disease, however.

Ganciclovir or DHPG (dihydroxypropoxymethylguanine) is a guanosine derivative with considerably more activity against CMV than its congener, acyclovir. Several trials in immunocompromised patients with life- or sight-threatening CMV infections suggested beneficial effects of intravenous ganciclovir, and it is now approved by the Federal Drug Administration in the United States for patients with CMV retinitis. Response rates of CMV retinitis or colitis range from 70 to 90 percent. CMV pneumonitis, particularly in bone marrow transplant recipients, responds less well, with improvement noted in ≤30 percent when ganciclovir is used alone; when ganciclovir is used in combination with CMV immune globulin, response rates of 50 to 70 percent have been noted. Peripheral blood neutropenia is the major toxic effect of ganciclovir and is sometimes dose-limiting. In many patients, particularly those with AIDS, clinical and virologic relapses of CMV infection occur once ganciclovir is discontinued. Therefore, prolonged maintenance regimens are recommended. Usual induction courses are 5 mg/kg twice daily for 14 days with maintenance regimens of 5 mg/kg for 5 to 7 days per week.

Phosphonoformate (foscarnet) also shows promise against CMV retinitis in patients with AIDS. Both foscarnet and ganciclovir are undergoing further evaluation in severe CMV infections.

REFERENCES

BALFOUR HH et al: A randomized, placebo-controlled trial of oral acyclovir for the prevention of cytomegalovirus disease in recipients of renal allografts. N Engl J Med 320:1381, 1989

BOWDEN RA et al: Cytomegalovirus immune globulin and seronegative blood products to prevent primary cytomegalovirus infection after marrow transplantation. N Engl J Med 314:1006, 1986

BUHLES WC et al: Ganciclovir treatment of life- or sight-threatening cytomegalovirus infection: Experience in 314 immunocompromised patients. Rev Infect Dis 10:S495, 1988

CHANDLER SH et al: Isolation of multiple strains of cytomegalovirus from women attending a clinic for sexually transmitted diseases. J Infect Dis 155:655, 1987

DREW WL: Diagnosis of cytomegalovirus infection. Rev Infect Dis 10:S468, 1988

DUMMER JS et al: Morbidity of cytomegalovirus infection in recipients of heart or heart-lung transplants who received cyclosporine. J Infect Dis 152:1182, 1985

EMMANUEL D et al: Cytomegalovirus pneumonia after bone marrow transplantation successfully treated with the combination of ganciclovir and high-dose intravenous immunoglobulin. Ann Intern Med 109:777, 1988

FELSENSTEIN D et al: Treatment of cytomegalovirus retinitis with 9-[2-hydroxy-1-(hydroxymethyl)ethoxymethyl] guanine (BWB759U). Ann Intern Med 103:377, 1985

GRUNDY JE et al: Symptomatic cytomegalovirus infection in seropositive kidney recipients: Reinfection with donor virus rather than reactivation of recipient virus. Lancet 2:132, 1988

HO M: *Cytomegalovirus: Biology and Infection.* New York, Plenum, 1982

HORWITZ CA et al: Clinical and laboratory evaluation of cytomegalovirus-induced mononucleosis in previously healthy patients. Medicine 65:124, 1986

JACOBSON MA, MILLS J: Serious cytomegalovirus disease in the acquired immunodeficiency syndrome (AIDS). Ann Intern Med 108:585, 1988

MEYERS JD et al: Risk factors for cytomegalovirus infection after human marrow transplantation. J Infect Dis 153:478, 1986

ONORATO IM et al: Epidemiology of cytomegaloviral infections: Recommendations for prevention and control. Rev Infect Dis 7:479, 1985

PASS RF et al: Young children as a probable source of maternal and congenital cytomegalovirus infection. N Engl J Med 316:1366, 1987

PREIKSAITIS JK et al: The risk of cytomegalovirus infection in seronegative transfusion recipients not receiving exogenous immunosuppression. J Infect Dis 157:523, 1988

REED EC et al: Treatment of cytomegalovirus pneumonia with ganciclovir and intravenous cytomegalovirus immunoglobulin in patients with bone marrow transplants. Ann Intern Med 109:783, 1988

SCHOOLEY RE et al: Association of herpesvirus infections with T-lymphocyte subset alterations, glomerulopathy, and opportunistic infections after renal transplantation. N Engl J Med 308:307, 1983

SKOLNIK PR, HIRSCH MS: Therapy and prevention of cytomegalovirus infections. In DeClerq E (ed): *Clinical Use of Antiviral Drugs.* Boston, Martinus Nijhoff 1988

SNYDERMAN DR et al: Use of cytomegalovirus immune globulin to prevent cytomegalovirus disease in renal transplant recipients. N Engl J Med 317:1049, 1987

139 INFLUENZA

RAPHAEL DOLIN

DEFINITION Influenza is an acute respiratory illness caused by infection with influenza viruses. The illness affects the upper and/or lower respiratory tracts, and is often accompanied by systemic signs and symptoms such as fever, headache, myalgia, and weakness. Outbreaks of illness of variable extent and severity occur nearly every winter. Such outbreaks result in significant morbidity in the general population and in increased mortality rates in certain "high-risk" patients, predominantly as a result of pulmonary complications.

ETIOLOGY Influenza viruses are members of the Orthomyxoviridae family. Influenza A and B viruses constitute one genus, and influenza C is the other genus. The designation of influenza viruses as types A, B, or C is based on antigenic characteristics of the nucleoprotein (NP) and matrix (M) protein antigens. Influenza A viruses are further subdivided (subtyped) on the basis of the surface hemagglutinin (H) and neuraminidase (N) antigens (see below). Individual strains are also designated according to the site of origin, isolate number, year of isolation, and subtype (e.g., influenza A/Victoria/3/79 H3N2). Influenza B and C viruses are similarly designated, but H and N antigens from these viruses do not receive subtype designations, since intratypic variations in H and N antigens of influenza B and C viruses are less extensive.

Most of the information regarding the molecular biology of influenza viruses has been generated from studies of influenza A viruses, and less is known about the replicative cycle of influenza B and C viruses. Morphologically, influenza viruses A, B, and C are similar. The virions are irregularly shaped spherical particles, 80 to 120 nm in diameter, and contain a lipid envelope from whose surface the hemagglutinin and neuraminidase glycoproteins project. The hemagglutinin serves as the site by which virus binds to cell receptors, while the neuraminidase degrades the receptor and probably plays a role in release of virus from infected cells after replication has taken place. Antibodies directed against the H antigen are the major determinants of immunity against influenza virus, while antineuraminidase antibodies limit viral spread and contribute to reduction of the infection. The inner surface of the lipid envelope contains the matrix proteins (M1 and M2), whose functions are incompletely understood but which may be involved in virus assembly and stabilization of the lipid envelope. The virion also contains the nucleoprotein (NP) with which the genome of the virus is associated, as well as three polymerase (P) proteins which are essential for transcription and synthesis of viral RNA. Three nonstructural (NS) proteins of unknown function are also present in infected cells.

The genome of influenza A virus consists of eight single-stranded segments of viral RNA, which code for the structural and nonstructural proteins. Because the genome is segmented, the opportunity for reassortment of genes during infection is high, and reassortment has been noted to occur frequently during infection of cells with more than one influenza A virus.

TABLE 139-1 Emergence of antigenic subtypes of influenza A associated with pandemic or epidemic disease

1889–90	H2N8*	Severe pandemic
1900–03	H3N8*	?Moderate epidemic
1918–19	H1N1† (formerly HswN1)	Severe pandemic
1933–35	H1N1† (formerly H0N1)	Mild epidemic
1946–47	H1N1	Mild epidemic
1957–58	H2N2	Severe pandemic
1968–69	H3N2	Moderate pandemic
1977–78‡	H1N1	Mild pandemic

* As determined by retrospective serologic survey of individuals alive during those years ("seroarcheology").
† Hemagglutinins formerly designated as Hsw and H0 are now classified as variants of H1.
‡ From this time until the present (1988–89), new antigenic subtypes of influenza A have not emerged. Rather, viruses of H1N1 or H3N2 subtypes have circulated either in alternating years or concurrently.

EPIDEMIOLOGY Influenza outbreaks occur virtually every year, although the extent and severity of such outbreaks vary widely. Localized outbreaks occur at variable intervals, usually every 1 to 3 years. Global epidemics or pandemics have occurred approximately every 10 to 15 years since the 1918–1919 pandemic (Table 139-1).

The most extensive and severe outbreaks are caused by influenza A viruses. In part, this is a result of the remarkable propensity of the hemagglutinin and neuraminidase antigens of influenza A virus to undergo periodic antigenic variation. Major antigenic variations are referred to as "antigenic shifts," which most likely occur from reassortment of genome segments between viral strains. Antigenic shifts may be associated with pandemics and are restricted to influenza A viruses. Minor variations are called "antigenic drifts" and likely arise from point mutations. These antigenic changes may involve the hemagglutinin alone, or both the hemagglutinin and the neuraminidase. In human infections, three major antigenic subtypes of hemagglutinins (H1, H2, and H3) and two neuraminidases (N1, N2) have been recognized. The hemagglutinins formerly designated as H0 and Hsw1 are now classified as variants of H1. An example of an antigenic shift which involved both the hemagglutinin and neuraminidase occurred in 1957, when the predominant influenza A virus subtype shifted from H1N1 to H2N2, and resulted in a severe pandemic, with an estimated 70,000 excess deaths in the United States alone. In 1968, an antigenic shift occurred which involved only the hemagglutinin (H2N2 to H3N2), and the subsequent pandemic was less severe than that seen in 1957. In 1977, an A/H1N1 virus emerged which caused a pandemic that primarily affected younger individuals, i.e., those born after 1957. As can be seen in Table 139-1, H1N1 viruses circulated from 1918 to 1956, so that individuals born prior to 1957 would be expected to possess some degree of immunity to H1N1 viruses. During most outbreaks of influenza A, a single subtype has circulated at a time. However, since 1977 both A/H1N1 and A/H3N2 viruses have circulated simultaneously resulting in outbreaks of varying severity. In some outbreaks influenza B viruses also circulated simultaneously with influenza A viruses.

The origin of pandemic strains is unknown. Because of the marked differences between the primary structures of the hemagglutinins of different subtypes of influenza A viruses (H1, H2, or H3), it is believed unlikely that antigenic shifts result from spontaneous mutations in the hemagglutinin gene. Because the segmented genome of influenza viruses may result in high rates of reassortment, it has been suggested that pandemic strains may emerge by reassortment of genes between human and animal influenza viruses. Influenza B viruses do not have an animal reservoir and do not undergo antigenic shifts, although antigenic drifting occurs.

Although pandemics provide the most dramatic evidence of the impact of influenza, illnesses that occur in between pandemics account for an even greater total in mortality and morbidity, albeit over a longer period of time. Since 1957, interpandemic illness has been associated with 10,000 or more "excess deaths" on 19 occasions in the United States, resulting in an accumulated mortality of more than 500,000 over that period of time. Influenza A viruses that circulate in between pandemics demonstrate antigenic drifts in the hemagglutinin antigen. These antigenic drifts apparently result from point mutations which involve the RNA segment which codes for the hemagglutinin. Amino acid analysis of "drifted" hemagglutinins indicates that changes in a single amino acid have little effect on the antigenic properties of the hemagglutinin. Epidemiologically significant strains, i.e., those which have potential for causing widespread outbreaks, have changes in amino acids in at least two of the four major antigenic sites in the HA molecule. Since two-point mutations are unlikely to occur simultaneously, it is believed that antigenic drifts result from point mutations which occur sequentially during the spread of virus from person to person. Antigenic drifts have occurred nearly annually since 1977 for A/H1N1 viruses, and since 1968 for A/H3N2 viruses.

Influenza A epidemics begin abruptly, reach a peak over a 2- to 3-week period, generally last for 2 to 3 months, and often subside almost as rapidly as they began. The first indication of influenza activity in a community is an increase in the number of children with febrile respiratory illnesses who present for medical attention. This is followed by increases in influenza-like illnesses among adults, and eventually by an increase in hospital admissions for patients with pneumonia, worsening of congestive heart failure, and exacerbations of chronic pulmonary disease. Rises in industrial and school absenteeism also occur at this time. An increase in the number of deaths caused by pneumonia and influenza ("excess mortality") is generally a late observation in an outbreak. Attack rates have been highly variable from outbreak to outbreak but most commonly are in the range of 10 to 20 percent of the general population. During the pandemic of 1957, it was estimated that the attack rate of clinical influenza exceeded 50 percent in urban populations, and that an additional 25 percent or more may have been subclinically infected with influenza A virus. Among institutionalized populations and in semiclosed settings where a large number of susceptible individuals are present, even higher attack rates have been reported.

Epidemics of influenza occur almost exclusively during the winter months in the northern and southern hemispheres. It is highly unusual to detect influenza A virus at times other than those in which an outbreak occurs, although rarely serologic rises have been noted at other times of the year. Where or how influenza A virus persists in between outbreaks is unknown. A possible explanation is that influenza A viruses are maintained in the human population on a worldwide basis by person-to-person transmission, and that large population clusters might be able to support a low level of interepidemic transmission. Alternatively, human strains may persist in animal reservoirs, but convincing evidence to support either explanation is not available. In the modern era, rapid modes of transportation may contribute to the transmission of viruses from widespread geographic locales.

The factors which result in the inception and termination of outbreaks of influenza are also incompletely understood. A major determinant of the extent and severity of an outbreak is the level of immunity present in the population at risk. When an antigenically novel influenza virus emerges to which little or no antibody is present in a community, extensive outbreaks may occur. When the absence of antibody is worldwide, epidemic disease may spread around the globe, resulting in a pandemic. Such pandemic waves can occur for several years, until immunity in the population reaches a high level. In the years following pandemic influenza, antigenic drifts among influenza viruses result in outbreaks of variable severity in populations that have high levels of immunity to the pandemic strain which circulated earlier. This situation persists until another antigenically novel pandemic strain emerges. On the other hand, outbreaks may also terminate despite the persistence of a large pool of susceptible individuals in the population. Occasionally, the emergence of a significantly different antigenic variant will result only in a localized outbreak. The "swine influenza outbreak" of 1976 in the United

States may be considered to be an example of this, although this outbreak may simply represent the introduction of a swine influenza virus into a crowded human population without spread beyond that setting. It has also been suggested that certain viruses, such as recently circulating A/H1N1 strains, may be intrinsically less virulent and cause less severe disease, even in immunologically virgin subjects, suggesting that other undefined factors besides the level of preexisting immunity play a role in the epidemiology of influenza.

Influenza B causes outbreaks which are generally less extensive and are associated with less severe disease than those caused by influenza A virus. The hemagglutinin and neuraminidase of influenza B virus undergo less frequent and less extensive variation than is seen in influenza A viruses, which may account, in part, for the observation of less extensive disease. Influenza B outbreaks are seen most frequently in schools and military camps, although occasional outbreaks in institutions in which elderly individuals reside have also been noted. The most serious complication of influenza B virus infection is Reye's syndrome (see below). Influenza C has been infrequently associated with human disease, although infection with influenza C virus is widespread.

The morbidity and mortality of influenza outbreaks continue to be substantial. Mortality occurs primarily in individuals with underlying diseases who have been characterized as being at "high risk" for complications of influenza. Excess hospitalizations for adults with "high risk" medical conditions have reached rates of 800 per 100,000 during recent outbreaks of influenza. These high-risk conditions are primarily chronic cardiac and pulmonary diseases, as well as increased age. Increased mortality rates have also been observed among individuals with chronic metabolic, renal, and certain immunosuppressive diseases, although to a lesser extent than among those with chronic cardiopulmonary diseases. In addition to the excess mortality, the morbidity of influenza in the general population is also extensive. For each of three outbreaks in the United States that were studied during the 1960s, it has been estimated that direct and indirect economic costs ranged from 1.5 to 3.5 billion dollars, and that today, such costs would be much greater.

PATHOGENESIS The initial event in influenza is infection of the respiratory epithelium with influenza virus, which is acquired from respiratory secretions of acutely infected individuals. In all likelihood, this occurs via aerosols generated by coughs and sneezes, although hand-to-hand, other personal contact, and even fomite transmission may occur. Experimental evidence suggests that infection by small-particle aerosol (less than 10-μm in diameter) is more efficient than that produced by larger droplets. Initially, viral infection involves the ciliated columnar epithelial cells, but it may also involve other respiratory tract cells, including alveolar cells, mucous gland cells, and macrophages. In infected cells, virus replication takes place within 4 to 6 h, after which infectious virus is released to infect adjacent or nearby cells. This results in spread of infection from a few foci to a large number of respiratory cells over several hours. In experimentally induced infection, the incubation period of illness has ranged from 18 to 72 h, depending on the size of the virus inoculum. Histopathologically, degenerative changes can be seen in infected ciliated cells, including granulation, vacuolization, swelling, and pyknotic nuclei. The cells eventually become necrotic and desquamate, and in some areas, previously columnar epithelium is replaced by flattened and metaplastic epithelial cells. The severity of illness is correlated with the quantity of virus shed in secretions, suggesting that the degree of viral replication itself may be an important mechanism in the pathogenesis of illness. Despite the frequent presence of systemic signs and symptoms such as fever, headache, and myalgias, influenza virus has only rarely been detected in extrapulmonary sites, including the bloodstream, and the pathogenesis of systemic symptoms in influenza remains unknown.

The host response to influenza infections involves a complex interplay of humoral antibody, local antibody, cell-mediated immune responses, interferon, and other host defenses. Serum antibody responses may be measured by a variety of techniques and can be detected by the second week after primary infection with influenza virus. Such antibodies may be measured by hemagglutination inhibition (HAI), complement fixation (CF), neutralization, enzyme-linked immunosorbent assays (ELISA), and antineuraminidase antibody assays. Antibodies directed against the hemagglutinin appear to be the most important mediators of immunity, and in several studies, HAI titers of 40 or greater have been associated with protection from infection. Secretory antibodies produced in the respiratory tract are predominantly of the IgA class, and also play a major role in protection against infection. Secretory antibody neutralization titers of 4 or higher have also been associated with protection. A variety of cell-mediated immune responses, both antigen-specific and nonantigen-specific, can be detected early after infection, depending upon prior immunity of the host. These responses include T-cell proliferative, T-cell cytotoxic, and natural killer cell activity. Interferons have been detected in respiratory secretions shortly after shedding of virus has begun, and rises in interferon titers coincide with decreases in virus shedding.

The host defense factors responsible for cessation of virus shedding and resolution of illness have not been defined specifically. Virus shedding generally stops within 2 to 5 days after symptoms first appear, at a time when serum and local antibody responses are often not detectable by conventional techniques, although antibody rises may be detected earlier by use of highly sensitive techniques, particularly in individuals with previous immunity to the virus. It has been suggested that interferon, cell-mediated immune responses, or nonspecific inflammatory responses may be important in the resolution of illness.

MANIFESTATIONS Influenza has been most frequently described as an illness characterized by the abrupt onset of systemic symptoms such as headache, feverishness, chilliness, myalgia, or malaise, accompanied by respiratory tract signs, particularly cough and sore throat. In many cases, the onset is so abrupt that patients can recall the precise time of the onset of illness. A typical case of naturally occurring influenza is depicted in Fig. 139-1. However, a wide spectrum of clinical presentations may occur. These can range from mild, afebrile respiratory illnesses similar to the common cold, with

FIGURE 139-1 Clinical characteristics of a naturally occurring case of influenza A in an otherwise healthy 28-year-old male. (*From R Dolin, Am Fam Phys 14:74, 1976.*)

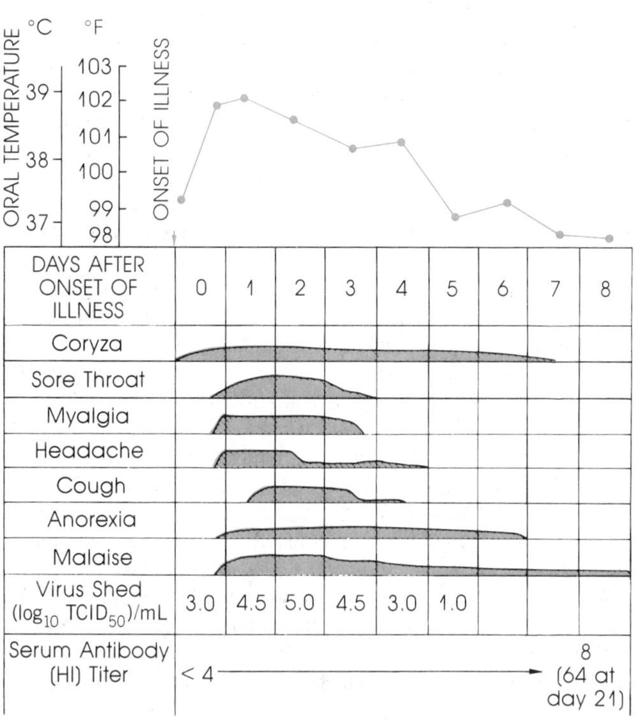

either gradual or abrupt onset, to illnesses in which severe prostration with relatively few respiratory signs and symptoms may be present. In the majority of cases which come to a physician's attention, fever is present and can range from 38°C to as high as 41°C. The temperature rises rapidly within the first 24 h of illness, and is generally followed by a gradual defervescence over a 2- to 3-day period, although, on occasion, fever may last for as long as a week. Patients complain of a feverish feeling and chilliness, but true rigors are rare. Headache, either generalized or frontal, is often a particularly troublesome complaint. Myalgias may involve any part of the body, but are most common in the legs and lumbosacral area. Arthralgias may also be present.

Respiratory complaints often become more prominent as systemic symptoms subside. Many patients complain of a sore throat or persistent cough which may last for a week or more, and which is often accompanied by substernal discomfort. Ocular signs and symptoms include pain on motion of the eyes, photophobia, and burning of the eyes.

Physical findings are usually minimal in cases of uncomplicated influenza. Early in the illness, the patient appears flushed and the skin is hot and dry, although diaphoresis and mottled extremities, particularly in older patients, may occur. Examination of the pharynx may be surprisingly unremarkable despite a severe sore throat, but injection of the mucous membranes and postnasal discharge can be present. Mild cervical lymphadenopathy may be noted, particularly in younger individuals. Chest examination is largely negative in uncomplicated influenza, although rhonchi, wheezes, and scattered rales have been reported with variable frequency in different outbreaks. Frank dyspnea, hyperpnea, cyanosis, diffuse rales, or signs of consolidation are evidence of pulmonary complications. Patients with apparently uncomplicated influenza have been reported to have a variety of mild ventilatory defects and increased alveolar-capillary diffusion gradients, indicating that subclinical pulmonary involvement may be more frequent than is appreciated.

In uncomplicated influenza, the acute illness generally resolves over a 2- to 5-day period, and most patients have largely recovered in 1 week. In a significant minority, however, symptoms of weakness or lassitude (''postinfluenzal asthenia'') may persist for several weeks, particularly in the elderly, and may prove troublesome for those who wish to return to full activity promptly. The pathogenetic basis for this ''asthenia'' is unknown, although pulmonary function abnormalities may persist for several weeks after uncomplicated influenza.

COMPLICATIONS OF INFLUENZA The most common complication of influenza is pneumonia, which may occur either as ''primary'' influenza viral pneumonia, secondary bacterial pneumonia, or mixed viral and bacterial pneumonia. Primary influenza viral pneumonia is the least common but most severe of the pneumonic complications. It presents as acute influenza which does not resolve, but instead relentlessly progresses with persistent fever, dyspnea, and eventual cyanosis. Sputum production is generally scanty but can contain blood, and few physical signs may be present early in the illness. In more advanced cases, diffuse rales may be noted, and chest x-ray findings consistent with diffuse interstitial infiltrates and/or acute respiratory distress syndrome may be present. In such cases arterial blood gases show marked hypoxia. Viral cultures, particularly if taken early in illness, show high titers of virus in respiratory secretions and in the lung parenchyma. Histopathology of fatal cases of primary viral pneumonia shows a marked inflammatory reaction in the alveolar septa, with edema and infiltration with lymphocytes, macrophages, occasional plasma cells, and variable numbers of neutrophils. Fibrin thrombi in alveolar capillaries, along with necrosis and hemorrhage, have also been noted. Eosinophilic hyaline membranes can also be found lining alveoli and alveolar ducts.

Primary influenza viral pneumonia has a predilection for individuals with cardiac disease, particularly those with mitral stenosis, but has also been reported in otherwise healthy young adults, as well as in older individuals with chronic pulmonary disorders. In some epidemics of influenza (notably 1918 and 1957), pregnancy increased the risk of the development of primary influenza pneumonia.

Secondary bacterial pneumonia is a complication in which bacterial infection develops following a case of acute influenza. With this illness, patients experience a period of improvement for 2 to 3 days after acute influenza, followed by a reappearance of fever, along with clinical signs and symptoms of bacterial pneumonia. These include cough, production of purulent sputum, and physical and x-ray signs of consolidation. The most common bacterial pathogens in this setting are *Streptococcus pneumoniae, Staphylococcus aureus,* or *Haemophilus influenzae,* organisms that can colonize the nasopharynx and that cause infection in the wake of changes in bronchopulmonary defenses. The etiology can often be determined by Gram stain and culture of an appropriately obtained sputum specimen. Secondary bacterial pneumonia occurs most frequently in high-risk individuals with chronic pulmonary and cardiac disease and in elderly individuals. Patients with secondary bacterial pneumonias will often respond to antibiotic therapy when it is instituted promptly.

Perhaps the most common of the pneumonic complications that occur during outbreaks of influenza are mixed viral and bacterial pneumonias. The clinical course of this complication contains features of both primary and secondary pneumonias. Patients may have a gradual progression of their acute illness, or may show a transient improvement followed by a clinical worsening, with eventual manifestion of the clinical features of a bacterial pneumonia. Sputum cultures may contain both influenza A virus and one of the bacterial pathogens described above. Patchy infiltrates or areas of consolidation may be noted by physical examination and chest x-ray. Patients with mixed viral and bacterial pneumonias generally have less widespread involvement of the lung than those with primary viral pneumonia, and their bacterial infections may respond to appropriate antibiotics. Mixed viral and bacterial pneumonias occur primarily in patients with chronic cardiovascular and pulmonary diseases.

In addition to the pulmonary complications of influenza, a number of extrapulmonary complications may occur. *Reye's syndrome* is a serious complication of influenza B, and to a lesser extent of influenza A virus infection, as well as of varicella-zoster virus infection. It occurs in children most commonly between the ages of 2 and 16, and follows several days after a generally unremarkable viral illness. Reye's syndrome is marked by the onset of nausea and vomiting for 1 to 2 days, after which central nervous system symptoms appear. These are most frequently changes in mental status, ranging from lethargy to coma, and can include delirium and seizures. Hepatomegaly is noted, along with a marked elevation of SGOT, SGPT, and LDH levels. Bilirubin values are only moderately elevated, so that the children are not jaundiced, but blood ammonia levels are elevated in virtually all patients. Hypoglycemia can occur, especially after varicella-zoster virus infection or after viral gastrointestinal illnesses. Children are usually afebrile, and while lumbar puncture generally shows an elevated pressure, the cerebrospinal fluid is quite unremarkable, indicating that an encephalopathy rather than a meningoencephalitis is present. The mortality of the syndrome is related to the state of consciousness on admission and has decreased from more than 40 percent, when the syndrome was originally described, to approximately 10 percent, reflecting earlier recognition and improved management of cerebral edema and hypoglycemia. Histopathology demonstrates little in the way of inflammatory changes in either the liver or the central nervous system. Liver biopsy shows diffuse fatty infiltration of hepatocytes, and swelling and pleomorphism in mitochondria. Cerebral edema and anoxic changes in neurons are the only pathologic changes detected in the central nervous system. The pathogenesis of Reye's syndrome is unknown, but the virus is almost never found in the affected liver and brain. An epidemiologic association with aspirin therapy for the antecedent viral infection has been noted, and the incidence of Reye's syndrome has decreased markedly with widespread warnings regarding the use of aspirin in children with acute viral respiratory infections.

Myositis, rhabdomyolysis, and myoglobinuria have also been reported as occasional complications of influenza infection. Although myalgias are exceedingly common in influenza, true myositis is rare. Patients with acute myositis have exquisite tenderness of the affected muscles, most commonly in the legs, and may not be able to tolerate even the slightest pressure, such as the touch of bed sheets. In the most severe cases, there is frank swelling and bogginess of muscles. Markedly elevated serum creatine phosphokinase and aldolase levels are present, and an occasional patient has developed renal failure from myoglobinuria. The pathogenesis of influenza-associated myositis is also unclear, although the presence of influenza virus in affected muscles has been reported.

Myocarditis and pericarditis in association with influenza virus infection was reported during the 1918–1919 pandemic, based largely on histopathologic findings, and has been infrequently documented since that time. ECG changes during acute influenza are commonly noted in patients who have cardiac disease but these have been most often ascribed to exacerbations of the underlying cardiac disease rather than to direct involvement of the myocardium with influenza virus.

Central nervous system disease has also been reported during influenza, including encephalitis, transverse myelitis, and Guillain-Barré syndrome. The etiologic relationship of influenza virus to such CNS illnesses remains unestablished.

In addition to complications involving the specific organ systems described above, every influenza outbreak includes a number of elderly and other high-risk individuals who develop influenza, and who subsequently experience a gradual deterioration of underlying cardiovascular, pulmonary, or renal function, occasionally leading to irreversible changes and death. These fatalities contribute to the overall toll of excess mortality associated with influenza A outbreaks.

LABORATORY FINDINGS Laboratory diagnosis is accomplished during the acute illness by isolation of virus from throat swabs, nasopharyngeal washes, or sputum. Virus is usually detected in tissue culture or less commonly in the amniotic cavity of chick embryos within 48 to 72 h after inoculation. Viral antigens may be detected somewhat earlier by use of immunodiagnostic techniques in tissue culture, or directly in exfoliated nasopharyngeal cells obtained by washings, although this technique is less sensitive than isolation of virus in tissue culture. The type of influenza virus (A or B) may be identified by either immunofluorescence or hemagglutination inhibition techniques, and the hemagglutinin subtype of influenza A virus (H1, H2, or H3) may be identified by hemagglutination inhibition using subtype-specific antisera. Serologic methods for diagnosis require comparison of antibody titers in sera obtained during the acute illness with those obtained 10 to 14 days after the onset of illness and are useful primarily in retrospect. Fourfold or greater rises as detected by hemagglutination inhibition, complement fixation, or significant rises by ELISA techniques are diagnostic of acute infection. Complement fixation tests are generally less sensitive than other serologic techniques, but since they detect type-specific antigens, they may be particularly useful when subtype-specific reagents are not available.

The remainder of other laboratory tests are generally not helpful in making a specific diagnosis of influenza virus infection. Leukocyte counts are variable, being frequently low early in illness, and normal or slightly elevated later. Severe leukopenia has been described in overwhelming viral or bacterial infection, while leukocytosis with counts of greater than 15,000 cells per microliter should raise the suspicion that secondary bacterial infection is present.

DIFFERENTIAL DIAGNOSIS On clinical grounds alone, an individual case of influenza may be difficult to differentiate from an acute respiratory illness caused by a variety of respiratory viruses or by *Mycoplasma pneumoniae*. Severe streptococcal pharyngitis or early bacterial pneumonia may mimic acute influenza, although bacterial pneumonias generally do not run a self-limited course. The presence of purulent sputum in which a bacterial pathogen can be detected by Gram stain is an important diagnostic feature in bacterial pneumonia. The fact that influenza occurs in characteristic outbreaks during the winter months may be helpful in making a clinical diagnosis. When local health authorities indicate that influenza activity is present in the community, the etiology of an acute febrile respiratory illness can be attributed to influenza with a high degree of certainty, particularly if the typical features of abrupt onset and systemic symptoms are present.

TREATMENT In uncomplicated cases of influenza, symptomatic therapy for headache, myalgia, and fever may be considered, employing either acetaminophen or salicylates, but salicylates should be avoided in children below 18 years of age because of the possible association of salicylates with Reye's syndrome. Since cough is ordinarily self-limited, treatment with cough suppressants generally is not indicated, although codeine-containing compounds may be employed if the cough is particularly troublesome. Patients should be advised to rest and maintain hydration during acute illness, and should return to full activity only gradually after the illness has resolved, particularly if illness has been severe.

The only specific antiviral therapy available for influenza is amantadine. Amantadine is active only against influenza A viruses and has been licensed for the prophylaxis and therapy of influenza A virus infections in the United States. If begun within 48 h of the onset of illness, amantadine reduces the duration of systemic and respiratory symptoms of influenza by approximately 50 percent, and in one study, was superior to aspirin. From 5 to 10 percent of individuals who receive amantadine will experience mild CNS side effects, primarily jitteriness, anxiety, insomnia, or difficulty in concentrating. These side effects disappear promptly upon cessation of the drug. The dose of amantadine for adults is 200 mg per day for 3 to 5 days or up to 48 h after illness has resolved. Because amantadine is excreted almost entirely by the kidneys, the dose should be reduced in individuals with renal insufficiency. Rimantadine, an experimental drug which is a closely related analogue of amantadine, appears to be equally efficacious and is associated with less frequent CNS side effects than is amantadine. Ribavirin, a nucleoside analogue with activity against a variety of viral agents, has been reported to be effective against both influenza A and B virus infections when administered as an aerosol, although it is relatively ineffective when administered orally.

Studies demonstrating the therapeutic efficacy of antiviral compounds in influenza have been carried out almost exclusively in uncomplicated disease in young adults, and it is not known whether such compounds are effective in the treatment of complications such as influenza pneumonia. Therapy for primary influenza pneumonia is directed at maintaining oxygenation and is most appropriately managed in an intensive care unit, with aggressive respiratory and hemodynamic support as needed. Bypass membrane oxygenators have been employed in this setting with variable results. When an acute respiratory distress syndrome develops, fluids must be administered cautiously, with close monitoring of blood gases and hemodynamic function.

Antibacterial drugs should be reserved for the therapy of bacterial complications of acute influenza such as secondary bacterial pneumonia. The choice of antibiotics should be guided by Gram stain and culture of appropriate specimens of respiratory secretions, such as sputum or transtracheal aspirates. If the etiology of a bacterial pneumonia is unclear from examination of respiratory secretions, empiric antibiotics should be selected which are effective against the most common bacterial pathogens in this setting, namely, *S. pneumoniae*, *S. aureus*, and *H. influenzae* (see Chaps. 99, 100, 115).

PROPHYLAXIS The major public health measure for prevention of influenza has been the use of inactivated influenza vaccines. These vaccines are derived from influenza A and B viruses which circulated during the previous influenza season. If the vaccine and currently circulating viruses are closely related, such vaccines would be expected to provide 50 to 80 percent protection against influenza. Currently available vaccines have been highly purified and are associated with few reactions. Up to 5 percent of individuals will experience low-grade fever and mild systemic symptoms 8 to 24 h after vaccination, and up to one-third may have mild redness or tenderness at the vaccination site. Since the vaccine is produced in eggs, individuals with true hypersensitivity to egg products should either be desensitized or should not receive vaccine. Although the 1976 swine influenza vaccine appears to have been associated with an increased frequency of Guillain-Barré syndrome, influenza vaccines administered since 1976 have not been associated with Guillain-Barré syndrome. Live attenuated (''cold-adapted'') influenza A vaccines have also been developed and appear to be promising in ongoing studies in adults and children. Such vaccines are administered intranasally and stimulate local antibody production more efficiently than conventional inactivated vaccines.

The U.S. Public Health Service recommends influenza vaccination for any individual older than 6 months who is at an increased risk for complications of influenza. These include individuals with chronic cardiovascular or pulmonary disorders (including asthma) and residents of nursing homes and other chronic care facilities. Other populations for whom the vaccine is recommended include otherwise healthy individuals over 65 years of age and individuals who have required regular medical attention for diabetes mellitus, renal disease, hemoglobinopathies, or immunosuppression. Individuals who provide care for high-risk patients or who come into frequent contact with such patients should also receive vaccine to reduce the likelihood of transmission of infection. Since commercially available vaccines are inactivated (''killed''), they may be administered safely to immunocompromised patients. Influenza vaccination is not associated with exacerbations of chronic nervous system diseases such as multiple sclerosis. Vaccination should be administered early in the autumn before influenza outbreaks occur, and should be administered on an annual basis to maintain immunity against the most current influenza virus strains.

Amantadine and rimantadine have also been demonstrated to be effective in the prophylaxis of influenza A. Studies have demonstrated 70 to 100 percent effectiveness of these drugs in preventing illness associated with influenza A virus infection. The major use for prophylaxis with amantadine or rimantadine is likely to be for high risk individuals who have not received influenza vaccine, or when the vaccines previously administered are relatively ineffective because of antigenic changes in the circulating virus. If vaccination is performed during an outbreak, amantadine can be administered simultaneously with inactivated vaccine, since it will not interfere with an immune response to the vaccine. There is also evidence that the protective effects of amantadine and vaccine may be additive. Amantadine has also been employed to control nosocomial outbreaks of influenza A. For prophylaxis, amantadine, or rimantadine should be instituted promptly when influenza A activity is detected and must be administered daily for the duration of the outbreak. The dosage most frequently employed has been 200 mg per day for adults, but the dose of amantadine should be reduced in patients with renal insufficiency and in the elderly.

REFERENCES

CENTERS FOR DISEASE CONTROL: Prevention and control of influenza. Morb Mort Week Rep 38:297, 1989

DOLIN R et al: A controlled trial of amantadine and rimantadine in the prophylaxis of influenza A infection. N Engl J Med 307:580, 1982

DOUGLAS RG JR (ed): Prevention, management, and control of influenza: A mandate for the 1980s. Am J Med 82 (suppl 6A), 1987

GLEZEN WP: Serious morbidity and mortality associated with influenza epidemics. Epidemiol Rev 4:25, 1982

LAMONTAGNE JR et al: Summary of clinical trials of inactivated influenza vaccines, 1978. Rev Infect Dis 5:723, 1983

MURPHY BR, WEBSTER RG: Orthomyxoviruses, in *Virology*, 2d ed, BN Fields (ed). New York, Raven, 1989, pp 1091-1152

140 COMMON VIRAL RESPIRATORY INFECTIONS

RAPHAEL DOLIN

GENERAL CONSIDERATIONS Acute viral respiratory illnesses are among the most common of human diseases, accounting for one-half or more of all acute illnesses. The incidence of acute respiratory disease in the United States is from 3 to 5.6 cases per person per year. The highest rates occur in children under 1 (6.1 to 8.3 cases per year) and the rates remain high until age 6, when a progressive decrease is noted. Adults have three to four illnesses per person per year. Morbidity from acute respiratory illnesses accounts for 30 to 50 percent of time lost from work by adults and from 60 to 80 percent of time lost from school by children.

It has been estimated that two-thirds to three-fourths of cases of acute respiratory illnesses are caused by viruses. More than 200 antigenically distinct viruses from 8 different genera have been reported to cause acute respiratory illness, and it is likely that additional agents will be described in the future. The vast majority of these viral infections involve the upper respiratory tract, but lower respiratory tract disease can also occur, particularly in younger age groups and in certain epidemiologic settings.

The illnesses caused by respiratory viruses traditionally have been divided into multiple distinct syndromes, such as the ''common cold,'' pharyngitis, croup (laryngotracheobronchitis), tracheitis, bronchiolitis, bronchitis, and pneumonia. These general categories of illnesses have a certain epidemiologic and clinical utility, e.g., croup occurs exclusively in very young children and has a characteristic clinical course. Some types of respiratory illnesses are more likely to be associated with certain viruses, e.g., the ''common cold'' with rhinoviruses, while others occupy characteristic epidemiologic niches, such as adenoviruses in military recruits. The syndromes most commonly associated with infection with the major respiratory virus groups are summarized in Table 140-1. Despite these associations, it is clear that most respiratory viruses have the potential to cause more than one type of respiratory illness, and frequently features of several types of illness may be present in the same patient. Moreover, the clinical illnesses induced by these viruses are rarely sufficiently distinctive to enable an etiologic diagnosis to be made on clinical grounds alone, although the epidemiologic setting increases the likelihood that one group of viruses rather than another may be involved. In general, laboratory methods must be relied upon to establish a specific viral diagnosis.

This chapter will review viral infections caused by five of the major groups of respiratory viruses: rhinoviruses, coronaviruses, respiratory syncytial viruses, parainfluenza viruses, and adenoviruses. Influenza viruses, which are a major cause of mortality as well as morbidity, are reviewed in Chap. 139. Herpesviruses, which occasionally cause pharyngitis and which also cause lower respiratory tract disease in immunosuppressed patients, are reviewed in Chap. 135. Enteroviruses, which account for occasional respiratory illnesses during the summer months, are reviewed in Chap. 144.

RHINOVIRUS INFECTIONS

ETIOLOGY Rhinoviruses are members of the Picornaviridae family, which are small (15 to 30 nm), nonenveloped viruses which contain a single-stranded RNA genome. In contrast to other members of the picornavirus family, such as enteroviruses, rhinoviruses are acid-labile and are almost completely inactivated at pH 3 or lower. Rhinoviruses grow preferentially at 33 to 34°C, which is the temperature of nasal passages in humans, rather than the higher temperature (37°C) of the lower respiratory tract. One hundred distinct serotypes of rhinoviruses are recognized.

TABLE 140-1 Illnesses associated with respiratory viruses

Frequency of respiratory syndromes associated with virus groups

Virus	Most frequent	Occasional	Infrequent
Rhinoviruses	Common cold	Exacerbation of chronic bronchitis and asthma	Pneumonia (children)
Coronaviruses	Common cold	Exacerbation of chronic bronchitis and asthma	Pneumonia and bronchiolitis
Respiratory syncytial virus	Pneumonia and bronchiolitis in young children	Common cold in adults	Pneumonia in elderly
Parainfluenza viruses	Croup and lower respiratory tract disease in young children	Pharyngitis and common cold	Tracheobronchitis in adults
Adenoviruses	Common cold and pharyngitis in children	Outbreaks of ARD in military recruits	Pneumonia in children and immunosuppressed patients
Influenza A viruses	"Influenza-like illness"†	Pneumonia and excess mortality in "high-risk" patients	Pneumonia in healthy individuals
Influenza B viruses	"Influenza-like illness"†	Rhinitis and pharyngitis alone	Pneumonia
Enteroviruses	Acute undifferentiated febrile illnesses‡	Rhinitis and pharyngitis	Pneumonia
Herpes simplex viruses	Gingivostomatitis‡ (children) Pharyngotonsillitis (adults)	Tracheitis and pneumonia in immunocompromised patients	Disseminated infection in immunocompromised patients

* Serotypes 4 and 7.
† Fever, cough, myalgia, malaise.
‡ May or may not have a respiratory component.

EPIDEMIOLOGY Rhinoviruses are a major cause of the common cold and have been isolated from 15 to 40 percent of adults with common cold–like illnesses. Infection rates are higher among infants and young children and decrease with increasing age. Rhinovirus infections occur throughout the year, but seasonal peaks occur in early fall and spring in temperate climates. Rhinovirus infections are most often introduced into families by preschool or grade school children below 6 years of age. Between 25 and 50 percent of initial illnesses in family settings are followed by secondary cases, with the highest attack rates occurring in the youngest siblings at home. Attack rates also increase with increasing size of families.

The spread of rhinoviruses appears to be by direct contact with infected secretions, usually respiratory droplets. In volunteer studies, transmission was most efficient by hand-to-hand contact, with subsequent self-inoculation of the conjunctival or nasal mucosa. Transmission appears to be much less efficient following exposure to large or small aerosolized particles. Virus can also be recovered from plastic surfaces inoculated 1 to 3 h previously, suggesting that environmental surfaces may also contribute to transmission. In studies conducted in married couples in which serum antibody was not present in either partner, transmission was associated with prolonged contact (122 h or more) during a 7-day period. Transmission was infrequent unless virus was recoverable from the donor's hands and nasal mucosa, at least 1000 $TCID_{50}$ of virus was present in nasal washes of the donor, and the donor was at least moderately symptomatic with the "cold." Despite anecdotal observations, exposure to cold temperatures, fatigue, or sleep deprivation has not been associated with increased rates of rhinovirus-induced illness in human volunteers.

Infection with rhinoviruses is worldwide in distribution, and by the time they reach adulthood, nearly all individuals have neutralizing antibodies to multiple serotypes, although the prevalence of antibody to any one serotype varies widely. Multiple serotypes circulate simultaneously, and generally no single serotype or group of serotypes has emerged as being more prevalent than others.

PATHOGENESIS Rhinoviruses infect cells via attachment to specific cellular receptors. Relatively limited information is available on the histopathology and pathogenesis of acute rhinovirus infections in humans. Biopsies performed in experimentally induced and in naturally occurring illness indicate that the nasal mucosa is edematous, often hyperemic, and during acute illness, is covered by a mucoid discharge. There is a mild infiltrate with inflammatory cells, including neutrophils, lymphocytes, plasma cells, and eosinophils. Mucus-secreting glands in the submucosa appear hyperactive; the nasal turbinates are engorged, which may lead to obstruction of nearby openings of sinus cavities.

The incubation period for rhinovirus illness is short, and generally ranges from 1 to 2 days. Virus shedding coincides with the onset of illness or may begin shortly before symptoms develop. The mechanisms of immunity to rhinovirus are not well worked out. In some studies, the presence of homotypic antibody significantly reduced the rates of subsequent infection and illness, but conflicting data exist as to the relative importance of serum and local antibody in protection from rhinovirus infection.

CLINICAL MANIFESTATIONS The most common clinical manifestations of rhinovirus infections are those of the common cold. Initially, illness begins with rhinorrhea and sneezing, accompanied by nasal congestion. Sore throat is frequently present and in some cases may be the initial complaint. Systemic signs and symptoms, such as malaise and headache, are mild or absent and fever is unusual. Illness generally lasts for 4 to 9 days, and resolves spontaneously without sequelae. In children, lower respiratory tract involvement may be seen, including bronchitis, bronchiolitis, and, on occasion, bronchopneumonia. Rhinoviruses may also cause exacerbations of asthma and chronic pulmonary disease in adults. The vast majority of rhinovirus infections resolve without sequelae, but complications related to obstruction of the eustachian tubes or sinus ostia, including otitis media or acute sinusitis, can occur.

DIAGNOSIS Although rhinoviruses are the most frequently recognized cause of the common cold, similar illnesses may be caused by a variety of other viruses, and the etiologic diagnosis cannot be made on clinical grounds alone. The diagnosis of rhinovirus infection is made by isolation of virus from nasal washes or nasal secretions in tissue culture. In practice, this procedure is rarely carried out because of the benign, self-limited nature of the illness. Because of the large number of serotypes of rhinovirus, diagnosis of rhinovirus infections by serum antibody tests is currently not practical. Common laboratory tests such as white cell count and sedimentation rate are not helpful in the diagnosis of rhinovirus infection.

TREATMENT AND PREVENTION Rhinovirus infections are generally mild and self-limited so that treatment is not necessary. Some patients may benefit from the use of analgesics and nasal decongestants, and reduction of activity is prudent if significant discomfort or fatigability is present. Specific antiviral therapy is not available. Application of interferon sprays intranasally has been effective in the prophylaxis of rhinovirus infections, but is also associated with local irritation of nasal mucosa. Prevention of rhinovirus infection by antibodies directed against rhinovirus receptors or by the use of the purified receptors themselves is under study. Experimental vaccines to certain rhinovirus serotypes have been prepared, but their utility is questionable because of the existence of the large number of serotypes and the uncertainty regarding the mechanisms of immunity. Thorough hand washing or barrier protection against autoinoculation may help to reduce transmission of infection.

CORONAVIRUS INFECTIONS

ETIOLOGY Coronaviruses are pleomorphic, single-stranded RNA viruses, 80 to 160 nm in diameter, with clublike projections emanating from the virus envelope, resulting in an appearance which resembles that of the solar "corona" from which their name is derived. Three distinct coronavirus serotypes, designated B814, 229E, and OC43, have been isolated from humans. Coronaviruses are fastidious and are difficult to culture in vitro. Some strains will grow only in human tracheal organ cultures rather than in tissue culture.

EPIDEMIOLOGY Only limited seroepidemiologic studies have been carried out in coronavirus infections. Seroprevalence studies of two of the serotypes, 229E and OC43, have yielded variable rates of serum antibodies, ranging from 12 to 80 percent in various populations. Overall, coronaviruses account for 10 to 20 percent of common colds. Coronavirus infections appear to be particularly prevalent in late fall, winter, and early spring, at a time when rhinovirus infections are less common. Depending on the serotype, a cyclical pattern for outbreaks of coronavirus infection has been suggested, which ranges from every 2 years for OC43, to every 2 to 4 years with 229E.

CLINICAL FEATURES The clinical features of illness caused by coronaviruses are similar to those caused by rhinoviruses. In volunteer studies, the mean incubation period of illness induced by coronaviruses (3 days) is somewhat longer than that caused by rhinoviruses, and the duration of illness is somewhat shorter, with a mean of 6 to 7 days. In some studies, the amount of nasal discharge was somewhat greater in colds induced by coronaviruses compared to those induced by rhinoviruses. Coronaviruses have also been recovered from infants with pneumonia and from military recruits with lower respiratory tract disease and have also been associated with worsening of chronic bronchitis. However, the overall significance of coronaviruses in lower respiratory tract disease in humans is unclear.

TREATMENT AND PREVENTION The approach to the treatment of common colds caused by coronaviruses is similar to that discussed above for rhinovirus-induced illnesses. Because of the uncertainty regarding the number and relative importance of coronavirus serotypes and the mechanisms of immunity, vaccines against coronaviruses have not been developed.

RESPIRATORY SYNCYTIAL VIRUS INFECTIONS

ETIOLOGY Respiratory syncytial virus (RSV) is a member of the Paramyxoviridae family and comprises the genus *Pneumovirus*. RSV is an enveloped virus approximately 150 to 300 nm in size, so named because virus replication leads to fusion of neighboring cells into large multinucleated syncytia. The single-stranded RNA genome codes for 10 virus-specific proteins. Viral RNA is contained in a helical nucleocapsid surrounded by a lipid envelope bearing two glycoproteins, one of which is the G protein by which the virus attaches to cells, and the other is the fusion protein which facilitates entry of virus into the cell by fusing host and viral membranes. Respiratory syncytial viruses have been considered to be of a single antigenic type, but it has been found that two distinct subtypes (A and B) exist. The epidemiologic and clinical significance of subtype differences are being investigated.

EPIDEMIOLOGY RSV is the major respiratory pathogen of young children and is the major cause of lower respiratory disease in infants. Infection with RSV is seen throughout the world, in annual epidemics which occur in either late fall, winter, or spring, and can last up to 5 months. The virus is rarely encountered during the summer. The highest rates of illness occur in infants between 1 and 6 months of age, with peak rates occurring between 2 and 3 months of age. The attack rates among susceptibles are extraordinarily high, approaching 100 percent in settings such as day-care centers where large numbers of susceptible infants are present. RSV accounts for 20 to 25 percent of hospital admissions for pneumonia of young infants and children, and up to 75 percent of cases of bronchiolitis in this age group. It has been estimated that more than half of infants who are at risk will become infected during an RSV epidemic.

In older children and adults, reinfection with RSV is frequent, but disease is milder than in infancy. A "common cold–like syndrome" is the illness most commonly associated with RSV infection in adults. Severe lower respiratory tract disease with pneumonitis can occur in elderly, often institutionalized, adults or those with immunocompromising disorders or treatment. RSV infection is more severe and prolonged in immunocompromised children. RSV is also an important nosocomial pathogen and can infect pediatric patients and up to 25 to 50 percent of the staff on pediatric wards during an RSV outbreak. The spread of virus among families is also efficient, and up to 40 percent of siblings may become infected when RSV is introduced into the family setting.

RSV is transmitted primarily by close contact with contaminated fingers or fomites, and by self-inoculation of the conjunctiva or anterior nares. Virus may also be spread by coarse aerosols produced by coughing or sneezing but is inefficiently spread by fine-particle aerosols. The incubation period of illness is approximately 4 to 6 days, and virus shedding may last for 2 weeks or longer in children and for shorter periods of time in adults.

PATHOGENESIS The characteristics of the immune response to RSV are not well elucidated. Because reinfection occurs frequently and is often associated with illness, the immunity that develops after single episodes of infection is not complete or long-lasting. However, the cumulative effect of multiple reinfections ameliorates subsequent disease and provides some temporary measure of protection against infection. Studies of experimentally induced disease in normal volunteers indicate that the presence of nasal IgA neutralizing antibody correlates more closely with protection than does the presence of serum antibody. Studies in infants, however, suggest that maternally acquired antibody provides some protection from lower respiratory tract disease, although severe illness may also occur in infants who have moderate levels of maternally derived serum antibody.

CLINICAL MANIFESTATIONS RSV infection leads to a wide spectrum of respiratory illnesses. In infants, 25 to 40 percent of infections result in lower respiratory tract involvement, including pneumonia, bronchiolitis, and tracheobronchitis. In infants, illness begins most frequently with rhinorrhea, low-grade fever, and mild systemic symptoms, often accompanied by cough and wheezing. Most patients gradually recover in 1 to 2 weeks. In more severe illness, tachypnea and dyspnea develop, and eventually frank hypoxia, cyanosis, and apnea can ensue. Physical examination may reveal diffuse wheezing, rhonchi, and rales. Chest x-ray shows hyperexpansion, peribronchial thickening, and variable infiltrates ranging from diffuse interstitial infiltrates to segmental or lobar consolidation. Illness may be particularly severe in children with congenital cardiac disease, bronchopulmonary dysplasia, or immunosuppression. One study documented a 37-percent mortality rate for infants with RSV pneumonia and congenital cardiac disease.

In adults, the most common symptoms of RSV infection are those of the common cold, with rhinorrhea, sore throat, and cough. Illness may occasionally be associated with moderate systemic symptoms such as malaise, headache, and fever. RSV has also been reported to cause febrile lower respiratory tract disease in adults, including severe pneumonia in the elderly.

LABORATORY FINDINGS AND DIAGNOSIS The diagnosis of RSV infection can be suspected on the basis of the epidemiologic setting, i.e., severe illness in infants during an outbreak of RSV in the community. Infections in older children and adults cannot be differentiated with certainty from those caused by other respiratory viruses. The specific diagnosis is established by isolation of RSV from respiratory secretions, including sputum, throat swabs, or nasopharyngeal washes. Virus is detected in tissue culture and identified specifically by immunologic reactions, employing immunofluorescence, enzyme-linked immunosorbent assay (ELISA), or other techniques. Immunofluorescence microscopy of nasal scrapings or washings provides a rapid diagnostic method that is in use in many diagnostic virology laboratories. Serologic tests which depend on fourfold or greater rises in complement fixing or neutralizing antibody titers are useful for diagnosis in older children and adults but are less sensitive in children under 4 months of age. Compared to complement fixation or neutralization tests, ELISA detects serum antibody with more sensitivity. As with other serologic tests, diagnosis requires comparison of acute and convalescent serum specimens and is therefore not useful during the acute illness.

TREATMENT AND PREVENTION Treatment of upper respiratory tract RSV infection consists primarily of symptomatic therapy similar to that for other upper respiratory tract viral infections. For lower respiratory tract infections, treatment consists of respiratory therapy, including hydration, suctioning of secretions, administration of humidified oxygen, and antibronchospastic agents as needed. If severe hypoxia is present, intubation and ventilatory assistance may be required. Studies of infants with RSV infection who were given aerosolized ribavirin, a nucleoside analogue which is active in vitro against RSV, have demonstrated a beneficial effect on the resolution of lower respiratory tract illness, including improvement of blood gases. Similar studies have not been performed in adults with RSV pneumonitis and its benefit in these patients is questionable.

Considerable interest exists in the development of an effective vaccine against RSV. Inactivated whole virus vaccines have been either ineffective or, in one study, potentiated the disease in infants. Other approaches to vaccine development include immunization with purified F and G surface glycoproteins of RSV, or generation of stable, live attenuated virus vaccines. In the settings where high rates of transmission occur, such as pediatric wards, barrier methods of protection of hands and conjunctiva may be useful in reducing the spread of virus.

PARAINFLUENZA VIRUS INFECTIONS

ETIOLOGY Parainfluenza viruses are members of the Paramyxoviridae family and comprise the genus *Paramyxovirus*. Parainfluenza viruses are 150 to 250 nm in diameter, enveloped, and contain a single-stranded RNA genome. The envelope is studded with two glycoproteins, one of which possesses both hemagglutinin and neuraminidase activity, while the other glycoprotein contains the fusion activity. The viral RNA genome is enclosed in a helical nucleocapsid and codes for seven virus-specific proteins. There are four distinct serotypes of parainfluenza viruses, all of which share certain common antigens with other members of the Paramyxoviridae family, including mumps and Newcastle disease virus.

EPIDEMIOLOGY Parainfluenza viruses are distributed throughout the world, although type 4 has been reported less widely, probably because it is more difficult to grow in tissue culture. Infection occurs in early childhood so that by 8 years of age, most children show antibodies to serotypes 1, 2, and 3. Parainfluenza types 1 and 2 cause epidemics during the fall, primarily in odd-numbered years. Type 3 infection has been detected during all seasons of the year, but epidemics of type 3 virus have occurred annually in the spring.

The contribution of parainfluenza infections to respiratory disease are variable according to both the location and year. In studies carried out in the United States, parainfluenza virus infections accounted for 4.3 to 22 percent of respiratory illnesses in children. In adults, parainfluenza infections are generally mild and account for less than 5 percent of respiratory illnesses. The major importance of parainfluenza viruses is as a cause of respiratory illness in young children, where they are second only to RSV as causes of lower respiratory tract illness. Like RSV, but unlike parainfluenza types 1 and 2, parainfluenza type 3 frequently causes illness during the first month of life, while passively acquired maternal antibody is still present. In contrast, parainfluenza type 1 is the most frequent cause of croup (laryngotracheobronchitis) in children, while serotype 2 causes similar, although generally less severe, disease. Parainfluenza type 3 is an important cause of bronchiolitis and pneumonia in infants, while illnesses associated with parainfluenza type 4 have been generally mild. Parainfluenza viruses are spread through infected respiratory secretions, primarily by person-to-person contact and/or by large droplets. In experimental studies, the incubation period has varied from 3 to 6 days but may be somewhat shorter in naturally occurring disease in children.

PATHOGENESIS Immunity to parainfluenza viruses is incompletely understood, but there is suggestive evidence that immunity to types 1 and 2 infections is mediated by local IgA antibodies in the respiratory tract. Passively acquired serum-neutralizing antibodies also confer some protection against infection with parainfluenza viruses types 1, 2, and, to a lesser degree, type 3.

CLINICAL MANIFESTATIONS Parainfluenza virus infections occur most frequently in children, in whom initial infection with serotypes 1, 2, and 3 is associated with an acute febrile illness in 50 to 80 percent of cases. Children may present with coryza, sore throat, hoarseness, and cough, which may or may not be croupy. In severe croup, fever persists, with worsening coryza and sore throat. A brassy or barking cough may be noted and may progress to frank stridor. In most children, recovery will occur over the next 1 to 2 days, although progressive airway obstruction and hypoxia may ensue occasionally. If bronchiolitis or pneumonia develops, progressive cough accompanied by wheezing, tachypnea, and intercostal retractions may be present. In this setting, a moderate increase in sputum production can be seen. Physical examination shows nasopharyngeal discharge and oropharyngeal injection, along with rhonchi, wheezes, or coarse breath sounds. Chest x-rays can show air trapping and, occasionally, interstitial infiltrates.

In older children and adults, parainfluenza infections tend to be milder, presenting most frequently as the common cold or hoarseness, with or without cough. Lower respiratory tract involvement in older children and adults is uncommon, but tracheobronchitis in adults has been reported. More severe and prolonged parainfluenza infection has been reported in children with severe immunosuppression.

LABORATORY FINDINGS AND DIAGNOSIS As with other respiratory viral diseases, the clinical syndromes caused by parainfluenza viruses are not sufficiently distinctive to permit a diagnosis to be made on clinical grounds alone, with the possible exception of croup in young children. A specific diagnosis is established by detection of virus in respiratory tract secretions, throat swabs, or nasopharyngeal washings. Virus is detected by growth in tissue culture, either by hemagglutination or by cytopathic effect, or by immunofluorescence of viral antigens in exfoliated cells from the respiratory tract. Serologic diagnosis can be made by fourfold or greater rises in acute and convalescent serum specimens as detected by hemagglutination inhibition, complement fixation, or neutralization tests. However, frequent heterotypic responses occur among the parainfluenza serotypes, so that identification of the serotype which causes the illness often cannot be made by serologic techniques alone.

Acute epiglottitis caused by *Haemophilus influenza*, type B (bacterial croup), must be differentiated from viral croup. Influenza A virus also is a common cause of croup during epidemic periods.

TREATMENT AND PREVENTION For upper respiratory tract illness, symptomatic therapy can be employed as discussed for other viral respiratory tract illnesses. If complications such as sinusitis, otitis, or superimposed bacterial bronchitis develop, appropriate antibiotics should be administered. Mild cases of croup should be treated with bed rest and moist air as generated by vaporizers. More severe cases require hospitalization and close observation for the development of respiratory distress. If acute respiratory distress develops, humidified oxygen and bronchodilators should be employed. There is no specific antiviral therapy available, although ribavirin has activity against parainfluenza viruses in vitro and is being evaluated clinically. Effective vaccines against parainfluenza viruses have not been developed.

ADENOVIRUS INFECTIONS

ETIOLOGY Adenoviruses are complex DNA viruses which are 70 to 80 nm in diameter. Human adenoviruses belong to the genus *Mastadenovirus,* of which 41 serotypes are recognized. Adenoviruses have a characteristic morphology consisting of an icosahedral shell composed of 20 equilateral triangular faces and 12 vertices. The protein coat ("capsid") consists of hexon subunits with group-specific and type-specific antigenic determinants, and penton subunits at each vertex primarily containing group-specific antigens. From each penton, a fiber with a knob at the end projects, which contains type-specific and some group-specific antigens. Adenoviruses have been divided into six or seven subgroups based on the homology of DNA genomes. The adenovirus genome is a linear double-stranded DNA which codes for structural and nonstructural polypeptides. The replicative cycle of adenovirus may result in either lytic infection of cells, or in the establishment of a latent infection (primarily involving lymphoid cells). Some adenovirus types can induce oncogenic transformation, and tumor formation has been observed in rodents, but despite intensive investigation, adenoviruses have not been associated with tumors in humans.

EPIDEMIOLOGY Adenovirus infections occur most frequently in infants and children. Infections occur throughout the year but are most commonly noted from fall to spring. Large-scale surveys have shown that adenoviruses account for 3 to 5 percent of acute respiratory infections in children. Infections are less frequent in adults and account for less than 2 percent of respiratory illness in civilians. Nearly 100 percent of adults have serum antibody against multiple serotypes, indicating that infection is common in childhood. Types 1, 2, 3, and 5 are the most frequent isolates obtained from children. Certain adenovirus serotypes, particularly 4 and 7, but also 3, 14, and 21, are associated with outbreaks of acute respiratory disease (ARD) in military recruits which occur in winter and spring. Transmission of adenovirus infection can occur by inhalation of aerosolized virus, by inoculation of virus in conjunctival sacs, and probably occurs by the fecal-oral route as well. Type-specific antibody generally develops after infection and is associated with protection against infection with the same serotype.

CLINICAL MANIFESTATIONS In children, adenoviruses cause a variety of clinical syndromes. The most common is an acute upper respiratory tract infection, with prominent rhinitis. On occasion, lower respiratory tract disease, including bronchiolitis and pneumonia, can also be seen. Adenoviruses, particularly types 3 and 7, cause pharyngoconjunctival fever, a characteristic acute febrile illness of children which occurs in outbreaks, most often in summer camps. The syndrome is marked by bilateral conjunctivitis in which the bulbar and palpebral conjunctiva have a granular appearance. Low-grade fever is frequently present, along with rhinitis, sore throat, and cervical adenopathy. The illness generally lasts for 1 to 2 weeks and resolves spontaneously. Febrile pharyngitis without conjunctivitis has also been associated with adenovirus infection. Adenoviruses have also been isolated from cases of whooping cough with or without *Bordetella pertussis;* the significance of adenovirus in that disease is unknown.

In adults, the most frequently reported illness has been ARD in military recruits caused by adenovirus types 4 and 7. This illness is marked by a prominent sore throat and the gradual onset of fever, often reaching 39°C on the second or third day of illness. Cough is almost always present, and coryza and regional lymphadenopathy are also frequently seen. Physical examination may show pharyngeal edema, injection, and tonsillar enlargement with little or no exudate. If pneumonia is present, auscultation of the chest and x-ray may indicate areas of patchy infiltration.

Adenoviruses have also been associated with a number of non-respiratory tract diseases, including acute diarrheal illness in young children caused by adenovirus types 40 and 41, and hemorrhagic cystitis caused by adenoviruses 11 and 21. Epidemic keratoconjunctivitis, caused most frequently by adenovirus types 8, 19, and 37, has been associated with contaminated common sources such as ophthalmic solutions and roller towels. Adenoviruses have also been associated with disseminated disease and pneumonia in immunosuppressed patients, including patients with acquired immunodeficiency syndrome (AIDS).

LABORATORY FINDINGS AND DIAGNOSIS Adenovirus infection should be suspected in the epidemiologic setting of ARD and in certain of the clinical syndromes such as pharyngoconjunctival fever or epidemic keratoconjunctivitis in which outbreaks of characteristic illnesses occur. In the majority of cases, however, illnesses caused by adenovirus infection cannot be differentiated from those caused by a number of other viral respiratory agents and *Mycoplasma pneumoniae*. A definitive diagnosis of adenovirus infection is established by culture or detection of virus from sites such as the conjunctiva and oropharynx or from sputum, urine, or stool. Virus may be detected in tissue culture by cytopathic changes, and specifically identified by immunofluorescence or other immunologic techniques. Adenovirus types 40 and 41, which have been associated with diarrheal disease in children, require special tissue culture cells for isolation, and these serotypes are most commonly detected by direct ELISA of stool. Serum antibody rises can be demonstrated by complement fixation, neutralization, ELISA, or radioimmunoassays. Hemagglutination inhibition tests may also be done for those adenoviruses which hemagglutinate red cells.

TREATMENT AND PREVENTION Only symptomatic and supportive therapy is available for adenovirus infections, and no clinically useful antiviral compounds have emerged. Live vaccines have been developed against adenovirus types 4 and 7 and are widely utilized to control this illness in military recruits. These vaccines consist of live, unattenuated virus which is administered in enteric coated capsules. Infection of the gastrointestinal tract with types 4 and 7 does not cause disease but stimulates local and systemic antibodies which protect against subsequent ARD with those serotypes. Vaccines prepared from purified subunits of adenovirus are currently under investigation.

REFERENCES

Rhinoviruses

D'Alessio DJ et al: Short-duration exposure and the transmission of rhinoviral colds. J Infect Dis 150:189, 1984

Gwaltney JM: Rhinoviruses, in *Viral Infections of Humans,* AS Evans (ed). New York, Plenum, 1982, pp 491–517

Rossman MG et al: Structure of a human common cold virus and functional relationships to other picornaviruses. Nature 317:145, 1985

Tyrrell DAJ: Common colds. Intervirology 25:177, 1986

Coronaviruses

Larson HE et al: Isolation of rhinoviruses and coronaviruses from 38 colds in adults. J Med Virol 5:221, 1980

McIntosh K: Coronaviruses, in *Virology,* 2d ed, BN Fields (ed). New York, Raven, 1989

Respiratory syncytial virus

Englund JA et al: Respiratory syncytial virus infection in immunocompromised adults. Ann Intern Med 109:203, 1988

Glezen WP et al: Risk of primary infection and reinfection with respiratory syncytial virus. Am J Dis Child 140:543, 1986

Hall CB et al: Aerosolized ribavirin treatment of infants with respiratory syncytial viral infection. A randomized double blind study. N Engl J Med 308:1443, 1983

Henderson FW et al: Respiratory syncytial virus infections, reinfections and immunity. N Engl J Med 300:530, 1979

Mufson MA et al: Respiratory syncytial virus epidemics: Variable dominance of subgroups A and B strains among children, 1981–1986. J Infect Dis 1:143, 1988

Parainfluenza viruses

Denny FW et al: Croup: An 11 year study in a pediatric practice. Pediatrics 71:871, 1983

Tyeryar FJ: Report of a workshop on respiratory syncytial virus and parainfluenza viruses. J Infect Dis 148:528, 1983

Wright PF: Parainfluenzaviruses, in *Textbook of Human Virology,* RB Belshe (ed). Littleton, MA, PSG Publishing, 1985, pp 1241–1255

Adenoviruses

BAUM SG: Adenoviruses, in *Principles and Practice of Infectious Diseases*, 3d ed, G Mandell et al (eds). New York, Wiley, 1990

FOX JP et al: The Seattle virus watch. VII. Observations of adenovirus infections. Am J Epidemiol 105:362, 1977

WIGAND R et al: Adenoviridiae: Second report. Intervirology 18:169, 1982

ZAHRADNIK JM et al: Adenovirus infection in the immunosuppressed patient. Am J Med 68:725, 1980

141 MEASLES (RUBEOLA)

C. GEORGE RAY

DEFINITION Measles, or rubeola, is an acute febrile eruption which has been one of the most common diseases of civilization. Despite the development of an effective vaccine it remains a worldwide health problem.

ETIOLOGY The measles virion is composed of a central core of ribonucleic acid with a helically arranged protein coat surrounded by a lipoprotein envelope with small, spikelike structures. The virion is 120 to 200 nm in diameter and is classified as a morbillivirus in the paramyxovirus family.

EPIDEMIOLOGY Measles occurs naturally only in human beings, although infection with the virus can be demonstrated in laboratory colonies of monkeys exposed to infected individuals. Before active immunization was available, epidemics of measles occurred in 2- to 3-year cycles, usually during the spring months, and about 95 percent of urban dwellers developed the disease before the age of 15. The virus is transmitted by transfer of nasopharyngeal secretions, either directly or in airborne droplets, to the respiratory mucous membranes or conjunctivae of susceptible individuals. Persons infected with the virus may transmit the disease during a period which extends from 5 days after exposure until 5 days after skin lesions have appeared. The virus is highly contagious, with secondary attack rates among susceptible household contacts usually exceeding 90 percent; asymptomatic primary infections are rare. Measles is typically a disease of childhood in populous areas, but may occur at any age in remote isolated communities if the disease is introduced. In the United States, there has been a distinct shift in age-specific attack rates, with outbreaks most usually occurring among teenagers and young adults. Infants are uncommonly affected under the age of 6 to 8 months, presumably because of the persistence of maternal antibody acquired by transplacental transmission. With increasingly effective attempts at control, the incidence of measles in the United States fell to the lowest level ever recorded in 1983. However, this trend was sharply reversed from 1984 to 1987, with increasing reports of outbreaks primarily among the 5- to 19-year age group. Transmission has occurred even though vaccination levels have exceeded 98 percent.

PATHOGENESIS AND PATHOLOGY It is probable that, after infection, measles virus multiplies in the epithelium of the respiratory tract and is disseminated by way of the blood to distant sites. For a few days before the rash appears, and for 1 or 2 days after, the virus can be isolated from blood or washed white blood cells, conjunctivae, lymphoid tissue, and respiratory mucous membranes and secretions. The virus can be obtained from urine for as long as 4 days after the onset of the eruptions. Virus replication in thymic Hassall's corpuscles, capillary endothelium, and hepatic duct epithelium also occurs.

The mucous membrane lesions (Koplik's spots) consist of vesicle formation and epithelial necrosis. Histology of the Koplik's spots reveals cytoplasmic and intranuclear inclusions, giant cells, and intercellular edema. Virion components can be detected in biopsy specimens of Koplik's spots and vascular endothelial cells in the areas of skin rash, suggesting that both the exanthem and enanthem are associated with local viral replication. Large multinucleated epithelial giant cells that show inclusion bodies within the nucleus and cytoplasm can be found during the prodrome and acute stages of illness in the buccal mucosa, pharynx, tracheobronchial mucosa, and occasionally in the urine. In addition, reticuloendothelial giant cells (Warthin-Finkeldey cells) are found in hyperplastic lymphoid tissues, including lymph nodes, tonsils, spleen, and thymus. During the viremic phase measles infects T and B lymphocytes, circulating monocyctes, and polymorphonuclear leukocytes without producing lytic changes. There are transient suppression of immunoglobulin synthesis, impaired natural killer cell activity, and diminished capability of polymorphonuclear leukocytes to generate oxygen radicals. The epithelium of the respiratory passages may become necrotic and slough off, leading to secondary bacterial infection; interstitial pneumonia with giant cell infiltration may be observed. Changes in the brain of patients with encephalitis resemble those seen in other postviral encephalitides and consist of focal hemorrhage, congestion, and perivenous demyelination. The pathogenesis is probably similar to experimental allergic encephalomyelitis.

MANIFESTATIONS The time from exposure to the development of the first symptoms of measles infection is usually 9 to 11 days, and from exposure to the appearance of rash about 2 weeks. The initial manifestations of the disease are malaise, irritability, fever as high as 40.6°C (105°F), conjunctivitis with excessive lacrimation, edema of the eyelids and photophobia, moderately severe hacking cough, and nasal discharge. The prodromal period usually lasts 3 to 4 days, with a range of 1 to 8 days before the onset of a rash. Koplik's spots—small, red, irregular lesions with blue-white centers—appear 1 or 2 days before the onset of the rash on the mucous membranes of the mouth and occasionally on the conjunctiva or intestinal mucosa. The findings of the prodromal illness subside or disappear within 1 or 2 days after the appearance of skin lesions, although the cough may persist throughout the course of the disease.

The red maculopapular rash of measles breaks out first on the forehead, spreads downward over the face, neck, and trunk, and appears on the feet on the third day. The density of lesions is greatest on the forehead, face, and shoulders, where coalescence of individual spots usually occurs. The lesions in each area persist for about 3 days and disappear in the same order in which they appeared, resulting in total duration of rash of about 6 days. As the maculopapules fade, a brown discoloration of the skin may be noticed, and finely granular desquamation may occur. In adults the duration of fever may be longer, the rash more prominent, and the incidence of complications higher.

The course of measles can be altered by the administration of gamma globulin soon after exposure. The incubation period may be prolonged for as long as 20 days. The prodromal period of the modified disease may be shorter; the fever, respiratory symptoms, and conjunctivitis milder; and the rash less marked; Koplik's spots may not be present. Rarely, an atypical, severe form of measles is seen in some persons who received inactivated measles vaccine several years before exposure. The prodromal period with prominent fever, headache, myalgias, and abdominal pain lasts for 1 or 2 days and is followed by an eruption which may be urticarial, maculopapular, hemorrhagic, and/or vesicular. In contrast to natural measles, the rash begins on the hands and feet and progresses toward the head. The rash is especially prominent on the legs and in the body creases. Peripheral edema and pneumonia have been prevalent in this form of atypical measles. The pneumonia is lobar or segmental; hilar lymphadenopathy and pleural effusion are frequent. Ill-defined nodular shadows may persist at the periphery of the lung for as long as 1 to 2 years.

COMPLICATIONS Measles, usually a benign self-limited disease, may be complicated by a number of illnesses. Viral involvement of the respiratory tract may lead to croup, bronchitis, bronchiolitis, or rarely to *interstitial giant cell pneumonia,* which is seen most often in children suffering from severe systemic disease such as leukemia, congenital or acquired immunodeficiency, or severe malnutrition, and which is characterized by severe respiratory symptoms, pulmonary infiltrations, and multinucleated giant cells in the pulmonary parenchyma. Pneumonitis may occur in the absence of the typical measles exanthem. *Conjunctivitis,* which is seen regularly in the course of uncomplicated measles, may occasionally progress to corneal ulceration, keratitis, and blindness. *Myocarditis,* characterized by transient changes in the electrocardiogram, occurs in about 20 percent of patients with measles, but clinical evidence of cardiac dysfunction is rare. Viral involvement of the mesenteric lymph nodes and appendix may result in abdominal pain and signs of peritoneal inflammation so severe that surgical exploration is considered. The situation is especially confusing if the evidence of appendiceal involvement becomes manifest during the preeruptive phase of the disease. *Hepatitis,* usually without clinical signs, also frequently occurs. It is usually detected by the presence of a transient elevation of SGOT or SGPT values during the acute phase of illness. *Acute glomerulonephritis* has also been transiently observed during the acute phase of illness. In adults, mild to moderate hypocalcemia and musculoskeletal symptoms with elevated CPK levels have each been reported to occur in one-third or more of cases. Measles infection of pregnant women results in death of the fetus in about 20 percent of the cases; however, a teratogenic effect such as that observed in rubella has not been demonstrated.

Superimposed bacterial pneumonia caused by streptococci, pneumococci, staphylococci, or *Haemophilus influenzae* is considerably more common than giant cell pneumonia and occasionally may progress to empyema or lung abscess. Bacterial otitis media is a frequent sequel of measles infection in children. In tropical areas, stomatitis, probably of bacterial origin, progressing to cancrum oris may be encountered during the course of the disease.

Clinically apparent *encephalomyelitis* occurs in 1 of 1000 patients with measles. It usually begins 4 to 7 days after the appearance of the eruption, but may precede the rash by 10 days or follow it by 24 days. It is characterized by high fever, headache, drowsiness, and coma, and in some patients by focal brain or spinal cord involvement. Death occurs in about 10 percent of affected individuals, and persistent signs of central nervous system damage, including mental changes, epilepsy, and paralysis, are encountered. Electroencephalographic abnormalities without other signs of central nervous system dysfunction may be demonstrated in 50 percent of patients with otherwise uncomplicated measles. A progressive, fatal encephalitis has been described in children with lymphatic malignancies treated with immunosuppressive drugs, with onset 1 to 6 months after an episode of measles. Other, more unusual neurologic complications include transverse myelitis and ascending myelitis. An extremely rare condition, *subacute sclerosing panencephalitis* (see Chap. 355), is probably a late complication of measles. *Thrombocytopenia* may occur 3 to 15 days after the onset of symptoms and results in purpura as well as bleeding from mouth, intestine, and genitourinary tract. Measles is also associated with transient suppression of delayed hypersensitivity to tuberculin, exacerbation of existing tuberculosis, and an increased incidence of new tuberculous infections.

LABORATORY FINDINGS Leukopenia is frequent in the prodromal phase of measles, and the appearance of leukocytosis suggests bacterial superinfection or another complication. Extreme lymphopenia (less than 2000 lymphocytes per microliter) is considered to be a poor prognostic sign. During the prodrome and in the early eruptive phase, multinucleated giant cells can be identified in stained preparations of sputum, nasal secretions, or urine, and the measles virus can be isolated by inoculation of the same materials onto appropriate cell cultures. Measles antigen can often be detected quickly by fluorescent antibody staining of infected respiratory or urinary epithelial cells. Complement fixation, enzyme immunoassay, immunofluorescent, and hemagglutination inhibition tests are available for serologic confirmation of measles. Spinal fluid protein of patients with encephalomyelitis ranges from 48 to 240 mg/dL, and lymphocyte counts are usually in a range of 5 to 99 per microliter, although counts as high as 1000 per microliter have been reported. Bacterial infection can be identified by appropriate cultures.

DIFFERENTIAL DIAGNOSIS With its prodrome, Koplik's spots, and characteristic rash, measles is infrequently confused with other diseases. Rubella is a milder disease of shorter duration with mild or no respiratory complaints. Infectious mononucleosis and toxoplasmosis can be identified by the presence of atypical lymphocytes and by serologic tests. Secondary syphilis may show skin lesions similar to the measles rash. Other infections which can sometimes mimic measles include those caused by adenoviruses, enteroviruses, *Mycoplasma pneumoniae, Staphylococcus aureus* (toxic shock syndrome), and *Streptococcus pyogenes* (scarlet fever). Drug reactions, particularly those associated with ampicillin and phenytoin, and Kawasaki syndrome can also produce a morbilliform rash. The atypical form of measles in patients previously immunized with inactivated vaccine may suggest Rocky Mountain spotted fever, varicella, scarlet fever, or meningococcemia.

PROPHYLAXIS Measles can be prevented by the administration of 0.25 mL/kg gamma globulin within 6 days of exposure. Passive immunization should be considered for any susceptible person exposed to the disease, but is especially important for children under 3 years of age, for pregnant women, for patients with tuberculosis, and for those patients in whom immune mechanisms are impaired. In this instance, a dose of 0.5 mL/kg gamma globulin (maximum of 15 mL) may be necessary. Prophylactic administration of antibiotics does not decrease the frequency or severity of bacterial superinfections.

Active immunity can be induced by the use of live, attenuated measles virus without spread to contacts of vaccinated individuals. Attenuated vaccine (Schwarz, Attenuvax) is associated with few local or systemic reactions. Vaccination induces antibody formation in more than 95 percent of susceptible individuals inoculated at age 15 months or older. The vaccine can induce protection if given before, or within 3 days after, exposure. Vaccination results in protection for at least 23 years, but the total duration of immunity is not known. Live measles vaccine should not be given to pregnant women, to patients with untreated tuberculosis, to patients with leukemia or lymphoma, or to those whose immune responsiveness is depressed. All children infected with human immunodeficiency virus should be immunized on schedule; the degree of protection is uncertain. Hypersensitivity reactions to the vaccine even among egg-sensitive individuals have been rare; however, the vaccine should not be given to persons known to be hypersensitive to vaccine components, such as trace amounts of antibiotics, and extreme caution should be observed in persons with a history of anaphylactic reactions following egg ingestion. Except in unusual circumstances, vaccination should not be given in the first 13 months of life. However, if epidemiologic circumstances suggest a risk to infants less than 15 months of age (where risk is defined as a county reporting more than 5 cases of measles among preschool-aged children each of the previous 5 years), the following is recommended: monovalent vaccine at 9 months of age or the first visit thereafter, followed by a dose of mumps-measles-rubella vaccine at 15 months of age. Measles vaccination has been very effective in decreasing the incidence of infection in the United States without producing serious side effects; however, there have been vaccine failures. These failures are related, in part, to early vaccination of infants who still have maternal neutralizing antibody, and perhaps to less-than-optimal vaccine storage and handling. There is evidence that vaccine manufactured before a new stabilizer was used in 1979 may have greater lability. It is therefore recommended that school-outbreak control measures include revaccination of all persons who received their most recent vaccination before 1980. If this is not practical, children vaccinated before 15 months of age should be revaccinated.

There is no indication for the use of *inactivated* vaccine because of severe atypical measles, which has been observed in persons immunized with it (see "Manifestations" above).

TREATMENT No therapy is indicated for uncomplicated measles. Gamma globulin, although effective in prophylaxis, is of no value once symptoms are evident. In countries where nutritional deficiencies are common, vitamin A supplementation on two successive days as soon as measles is diagnosed may reduce delayed mortality and blindness. Patients should be monitored for the development of bacterial superinfections, which require appropriate antibiotics on the basis of clinical and bacteriologic findings.

REFERENCES

Bloch AB et al: Measles outbreak in a pediatric practice: Airborne transmission in an office setting. Pediatrics 75:676, 1985

Centers for Disease Control: Measles prevention. Recommendation of the Immunization Practices Advisory Committee. Morb Mort Week Rep 36:409, 1987

———: Measles prevention: Supplementary statement. Morb Mort Week Rep 38:11, 1989

Fulginiti VA, Helfer RE: Atypical measles in adolescent siblings 16 years after killed measles virus vaccine. JAMA 244:804, 1980

Gavish D et al: Hepatitis and jaundice associated with measles in young adults. Arch Intern Med 143:674, 1983

Giladi M et al: Measles in adults: A prospective study of 291 consecutive cases. Brit Med J 295:1314, 1987

Gustafson TL et al: Measles outbreak in a fully immunized secondary-school population. N Engl J Med 317:771, 1987

Johnson RT et al: Measles encephalomyelitis—clinical and immunologic studies. N Engl J Med 310:137, 1984

Krause PH et al: Epidemic measles in young adults. Ann Intern Med 90:873, 1979

Lampe RM et al: Measles reimmunization in children immunized before 1 year of age. Am J Dis Child 139:33, 1985

Markowitz LE et al: Patterns of transmission in measles outbreaks in the United States, 1985–1986. N Engl J Med 320:75, 1989

Moench TR et al: Acute measles in patients with and without neurological involvement: Distribution of measles virus antigen and RNA. J Infect Dis 158:433, 1988

Mouallem M et al: Measles epidemic in young adults. Arch Intern Med 147:1111, 1987

Vitamin A for measles, editorial. Lancet 1:1067, 1987

142 RUBELLA ("GERMAN MEASLES") AND OTHER VIRAL EXANTHEMS

C. GEORGE RAY

RUBELLA

DEFINITION Rubella ("German measles," "3-day measles") is usually a benign febrile exanthem, but when it occurs in pregnant women it may lead to serious chronic fetal infection and malformations.

ETIOLOGY In the late 1930s and 1940s rubella was transmitted to humans and monkeys, and in 1962 a viral agent was recovered in cell cultures inoculated with nasopharyngeal secretions of infected persons. The rubella virion, 60 to 70 nm in diameter, is a somewhat spheroidal RNA virus which has been classified in the togavirus family.

PATHOGENESIS AND PATHOLOGY Rubella can be induced in susceptible persons by the instillation of virus into the nasopharynx, and natural infection is probably induced in the same way. Virus is present in blood, throat washings, and occasionally feces for several days before the exanthem becomes apparent. It can be detected in blood for 1 to 2 days, and in throat washings for as long as 7 days before appearance of rash, to 2 weeks after onset. Lymph nodes show edema and hyperplasia.

Congenital rubella results from transplacental transmission of virus to the fetus from an infected mother, and may be associated with growth retardation, infiltration of liver and spleen by hematopoietic tissue, interstitial pneumonia, a decreased number of megakaryocytes in the bone marrow, and various structural malformations of the cardiovascular and central nervous systems. The virus can persist in the fetus during intrauterine life and may be excreted for 6 to 31 months after birth.

EPIDEMIOLOGY Rubella is not as contagious as measles, and immunity to the disease is not so widespread. Estimates of susceptibility to rubella among unimmunized women of childbearing age range from 10 to 25 percent. Before the routine introduction of vaccine in 1969, epidemics occurred at 6- to 9-year intervals; however, this cyclical pattern is no longer seen. In 1964 more than 1.8 million cases of rubella were reported in the United States; in 1986, only 551 cases, an all-time low, were reported. Rubella was once most frequent among children 5 to 9 years of age, but with the advent of immunization programs often directed primarily at this age group as well as at preschoolers, a greater proportion of cases is now being reported among older schoolchildren (15 to 19 years) and young adults (20 to 24 years).

MANIFESTATIONS The time from exposure to the appearance of the rash of rubella is 14 to 21 days, usually about 18 days. In adults there may be a prodromal illness preceding the exanthem by 1 to 7 days. The prodrome consists of malaise, headache, fever, mild conjunctivitis, and lymphadenopathy. In children the rash may be the first manifestation of disease. It is apparent from serologic studies that 25 to 50 percent of infections are subclinical, or may result in only lymph node enlargement without skin lesions; however, rash without lymphadenopathy is uncommon. Respiratory symptoms are mild or absent. Small, red lesions (Forchheimer's spots) occasionally may be seen on the soft palate but are not pathognomonic of the disease.

The rash begins on the forehead and face and spreads downward to the trunk and extremities. The small maculopapular lesions, of lighter hue than those of measles, are usually discrete but may coalesce to form a diffuse erythema suggestive of scarlet fever. The rash may last from 1 to 5 days, but is most commonly present for 3 days. Enlarged, tender lymph nodes appear before the rash, are most impressive during the early eruptive phase, and may persist several days after the rash has disappeared. Splenomegaly or generalized lymphadenopathy may occur, but the postauricular and suboccipital nodes are most strikingly involved. Arthralgias and slight joint swellings may be a complication of rubella, especially in young women. The pain and swelling, involving wrists, fingers, and knees, are most marked during the period of rash and may persist for 1 to 14 days after other manifestations of rubella have disappeared. Recurring joint symptoms for a year or more have also been reported. Purpura with or without thrombocytopenia may occur and may be associated with hemorrhage. Encephalomyelitis following rubella resembles other postinfectious encephalitides and is much less common than encephalitis following measles. Testicular pain is also occasionally reported in young adults.

Congenital rubella The syndrome of congenital rubella has conventionally been thought to consist of heart malformations—patent ductus arteriosus, interventricular septal defect, or pulmonic stenosis; eye lesions—corneal clouding, cataracts, chorioretinitis, and microphthalmia; microcephaly; mental retardation; and deafness. In the American epidemic of 1964, thrombocytopenic purpura, hepatosplenomegaly, intrauterine growth retardation, interstitial pneumonia, myocarditis or myocardial necrosis, and metaphyseal bone lesions were encountered frequently in association with the previously recognized manifestations, leading to the term *expanded rubella syndrome*. Some infants have also been found to have significant humoral and/or cellular immunodeficiency, which generally resolves as chronic viral excretion diminishes and eventually ceases. Any combination of lesions may be seen in an individual infant, and the severity is highly variable.

Later complications include an apparent higher risk of subsequent development of diabetes mellitus. There are reports of patients with congenital rubella who develop a progressive, subacute panencephalitis, with onset in the second decade of life. It is characterized by intellectual deterioration, ataxia, seizures, and spasticity. T-cell abnormalities occur persisting into adulthood and are characterized by slightly decreased T4/T8 ratios and other minor subset defects.

Congenital rubella is usually the result of maternal infection during the first trimester of pregnancy, although well-documented cases have resulted from infection several days before conception; deafness may occur as a result of infection in the fourth month. The greatest risk to the fetus is when maternal infection develops 3 to 6 weeks after conception. Serologically identified, asymptomatic maternal rubella can also result in severe fetal disease. It is therefore desirable to ascertain the immune status of every woman, either before conception or as early in the pregnancy as possible, by history of previous immunization or by serologic testing. If rubella antibodies are present before or within 10 days after exposure, the patient is considered immune, and the risk of fetal damage is virtually nil. If antibodies are not detectable and exposure has occurred, acute and convalescent antibody titers should be determined simultaneously on serums obtained 2 to 4 weeks apart, depending upon the time after exposure when the acute sample was drawn.

DIAGNOSIS Rubella is frequently confused with other diseases associated with maculopapular exanthems, with infectious mononucleosis (see Chap. 137), as well as with drug eruptions and scarlet fever. *A certain diagnosis of rubella can be made only by virus isolation and identification, or by changes in antibody titers.* Rubella hemagglutination-inhibiting antibodies may be present by the second day of rash and increase in quantity over the next 10 to 21 days. Other serologic tests which are used for diagnosis or determination of immunity include complement fixation (CF), enzyme-linked immunosorbentassay (ELISA), fluorescence immunoassay (FIA), radioimmunoassay (RIA), and a variety of IgM-specific antibody tests. In addition, there are several inexpensive and rapid semiquantitative screening tests to determine immunity: latex agglutination, passive hemagglutination (PHA), and single radial hemolysis. Antibodies detected by ELISA, FIA, and RIA tend to parallel the hemagglutination-inhibiting antibodies, while the appearance of CF antibody lags behind the others by a period of 3 to 7 days and often does not disappear until 1 or 2 years after infection. The PHA antibody first appears even later (14 to 21 days after rash onset), but persists thereafter. The presence of IgM-specific antibodies suggests recent rubella infection (within 2 months); however, they have been known to persist as long as 1 year in some cases. There are no other laboratory findings helpful in the diagnosis of rubella, although lymphocytosis with atypical lymphocytes may occur.

Patients with the congenital rubella syndrome may lose antibodies at age 3 or 4 years. Therefore a negative serologic test in a child over 3 years does not exclude the possibility of congenital rubella. Congenital rubella should be differentiated by appropriate serologic tests from congenital syphilis (see Chap. 128), toxoplasmosis (see Chap. 162), and cytomegalic inclusion virus disease (see Chap. 138). IgM-specific antibodies are often found early in the first year of life in infants with congenital rubella, but virus isolation is the most reliable way to confirm the diagnosis.

PREVENTION In adults and children rubella is usually a mild disease with infrequent complications. However, the severity of congenital infection has prompted efforts to prevent the disease. Administration of gamma globulin to exposed persons can abort the clinical disease, but seroconversion and transmission of the disease from mother to fetus may occur despite the administration of large amounts of gamma globulin soon after exposure.

Active immunization with live attenuated rubella vaccines has been practiced in this country since 1969, especially among young children. The aim has been to decrease the frequency of the infection in the population and to decrease the chance that susceptible pregnant women will be exposed. Because of concern for a possibly enlarging pool of susceptible adolescents and adults, there has been increasing enthusiasm for serologic screening of pubertal females with no history of immunization, followed by selective immunization of those who are seronegative, with appropriate precautions, as noted below. Persons working in hospitals or clinics who might contract rubella from infected patients or who, if infected, might transmit the infection to pregnant patients should be required to have proof of immunity (either documented immunization or presence of serum antibody).

The attenuated virus can be detected in the respiratory secretions of vaccinees for as long as 4 weeks after immunization, but transmission to other susceptible individuals rarely, if ever, occurs, even in households where susceptible pregnant women are in contact with children who are being vaccinated. The vaccine induces detectable antibodies that persist for at least 16 years and probably longer, in about 95 percent of recipients. After heavy exposure in closed populations, vaccinated individuals sometimes develop subclinical infections (diagnosed by antibody rises and virus isolation). However, viremia has not been demonstrated in immunized persons, which suggests that previously vaccinated pregnant women will not infect their fetuses even if they acquire subclinical rubella.

Side effects of fever, rash, lymphadenopathy, polyneuropathy, or arthralgias occur very seldom in vaccinated children; joint pain and swelling or paresthesias are seen in less than 2 percent of women with vaccines prepared in human embryonic fibroblast cell cultures (RA 27/3 vaccine). The joint symptoms usually begin 1 to 3 weeks after vaccination, and may be confused with other forms of arthritis. *Rubella vaccine must never be given to pregnant women or to those who may become pregnant within 3 months of immunization.* Although no infant with the congenital rubella syndrome has been reported to have been born to a woman inadvertently vaccinated during pregnancy, the theoretical risk of vaccine virus–induced fetal damage remains. Vaccine is contraindicated in patients with immune-deficiency diseases other than children with HIV infection or who are taking immunosuppressive drugs.

OTHER VIRAL EXANTHEMS

In addition to the diseases such as measles, rubella, and chickenpox which historically have been associated with prominent skin lesions there are other virus infections in which skin manifestations may occur. Table 142-1 lists the most commonly recognized causes of maculopapular eruptions. Some of them, particularly the enteroviruses, can also occasionally cause papulovesicular or petechial rashes, others are capable of provoking erythema multiforme–like eruptions. One helpful aspect of the physical examination is the observation that viral-caused maculopapular (not vesicular) exanthems usually *relatively* spare the palms and soles. This is in contrast to eruptions associated with drug reactions, bacteria, *Mycoplasma,* and *Rickettsia,* in which a prominent palmar or plantar eruption is often noted.

EXANTHEM SUBITUM (ROSEOLA INFANTUM) Exanthem subitum is a benign disease of infants 6 months to 4 years of age that is characterized by a high fever and rash. The disease can be transmitted to humans and monkeys by the transfer of blood obtained from a patient during the first few days of illness. Several different agents, such as enteroviruses and adenoviruses, may produce a similar illness; however, human herpesvirus type 6 (HHV-6) has also been implicated as a major cause. The first manifestations of disease, after an estimated incubation period of 5 to 15 days, are the abrupt onset of irritability and fever, which last for 3 to 5 days; the temperature may be as high

TABLE 142-1 Causes of maculopapular eruptions

Viral	Other
Measles	*Mycoplasma pneumoniae*
Rubella	Syphilis
Exanthem subitum	Typhoid fever
Erythema infectiosum: human parvovirus B19	Bacterial toxins: streptococci and staphylococci
Enteroviruses: coxsackievirus, echovirus	Rat-bite fever
Infectious mononucleosis	*Rickettsia*
Adenoviruses	Live-virus vaccines
Reoviruses	Drug eruptions
Arboviruses	Mucocutaneous lymph node syndrome

as 40.6°C (105°F). There may be mild pharyngitis and slight lymph node enlargement; convulsions may occur during the height of the fever. On the fourth to fifth day of illness, there is a sudden drop in temperature to normal or below normal; several hours before or after defervescence the rash suddenly and surprisingly appears. It is characterized by faint 2- to 3-mm macules or maculopapules over the neck and trunk and may extend to the thighs and buttocks; it may last for only a few hours or may be present for a day or two. Leukopenia is frequently noted later in the febrile period. The disease is benign and not associated with complications, although rarely an infant may show sequelae as a result of febrile convulsions. In the early, preeruptive phase, the disease may be difficult to differentiate from an acute bacteremia, particularly from one associated with *Streptococcus pneumoniae*. Though a leukocytosis with an increase in band forms is often seen in bacteremias presenting in this fashion, blood cultures are necessary to make the diagnosis.

ERYTHEMA INFECTIOSUM (FIFTH DISEASE) Erythema infectiosum is a mild febrile exanthematous disease with little or no prodrome. The mean incubation period is estimated as approximately 4 to 12 days (median 7 days). The first manifestations are low-grade fever with varying degrees of conjunctivitis, upper respiratory complaints, cough, myalgia, itching, nausea, and diarrhea, followed in many cases by the appearance of indurated, confluent erythema over the cheeks, giving a "slapped face" appearance. A day or so later, a bilaterally symmetric eruption is seen on the arms, legs, and trunk, but rarely on the palms or soles. The lesions are maculopapular and tend to be confluent, forming slightly raised blotchy areas and reticular or lacy patterns. When it occurs, the rash usually lasts about a week, and during this time it may disappear, only to reappear in the same areas a few hours later. The waxing and waning eruption may occasionally persist for several weeks, and can be brought on by fever, heat, exercise, sunlight exposure, or emotional stress. Occasionally a hemorrhagic exanthem and enanthem with pustules and pseudopustules occur. Mild joint pain and swelling have been observed in a large proportion of adults with the disease, and some have had symptoms lasting from a few months to over 4 years. Some adults have had transient elevations in rheumatoid factor or ANA antibody tests. Erythema infectiosum affects all ages but is most common in children of school age and may occur in epidemic form. The etiologic agent has now been identified as a human parvovirus (B19) which also is considered to be the primary cause of aplastic crises in patients with chronic hemolytic anemias such as sickle cell disease and hereditary spherocytosis. This may be a result of the fact that the site of replication is the nucleus of an immature cell in the erythrocyte lineage, resulting in an impairment of normal erythrocyte development. Like rubella, active transplacental transmission of B19 virus can occur during primary infections, sometimes resulting in severe fetal anemia with hydrops fetalis. The frequency of this occurrence is as yet undetermined. The route of transmission of the natural disease is probably respiratory. Subclinical infection is common. Antibody to the virus has been demonstrated in 30 to 50 percent of healthy adults. Specific diagnosis is accomplished by detection of the virus particles in early acute-phase serum by electron microscopy, by demonstration of specific viral DNA in serum or pharyngeal secretions, or, more commonly, by detection of IgM-specific antibodies in sera collected in the acute or early convalescent phase of illness. A clinical diagnosis of this disease should be made with caution, since rubella and some enteroviruses have also been shown at times to cause a nearly identical syndrome.

ENTEROVIRAL EXANTHEMS Many individual enteroviruses have been associated with rash. Of these, polioviruses are rarely implicated. More commonly, echovirus serotypes 1 through 7, 9, 11, 12, 14, 16, 18, 19, 20, 25, and 30, coxsackievirus serotypes A4, A5, A6, A9, A10, A16, and B2, B3, and B5 have all been implicated. With the exception of hand-foot-and-mouth disease, usually associated with coxsackievirus A16 or enterovirus 71 infection (see Chap. 144), there is no set of clinical or epidemiologic features that aids in differentiating the specific enteroviral agent involved in a specific case. All are capable of producing maculopapular rashes which vary in intensity and duration, and can also occasionally produce petechial or papulovesicular exanthems and enanthems. In community and household outbreaks, younger children and infants are usually more likely to have exanthems, while other features of enteroviral infection, such as fever, myalgia, and aseptic meningitis, are more prominent among older children and young adults. Two enterovirus serotypes that have been particularly associated with outbreaks of febrile exanthems are echoviruses 9 and 16.

REFERENCES

Anderson MJ et al: Experimental parvoviral infection in humans. J Infect Dis 152:257, 1985

Asano Y et al: Viremia and neutralizing antibody response in infants with exanthem subitum. J Pediatr 114:535, 1989

Centers for Disease Control: Risks associated with human parvovirus B19 infection. Morb Mort Week Rep 38:81, 1989

Chu SY et al: Rubella antibody persistence after immunization. JAMA 259:3133, 1988

Clarke WL et al: Autoimmunity in congenital rubella syndrome. J Pediatr 104:370, 1984

Enders G et al: Outcome of confirmed periconceptional rubella. Lancet 1:1445, 1988

Herrmann KL: Available rubella serologic tests. Rev Infect Dis 7:S108, 1985

Hill HR, Ray CG: The differential diagnosis of viral exanthems and enanthems, in *Infections in Children*, RJ Wedgwood et al (eds). Philadelphia, Harper & Row, 1982, p 235

Konney JS et al: Risk of adverse outcomes of pregnancy after human parvovirus B19 infection. J Infect Dis 157:663, 1988

Kurtzman GJ et al: Chronic bone marrow failure due to persistent B19 parvovirus infection. N Engl J Med 317:287, 1987

Naides SJ et al: Human parvovirus B19–induced vesiculopustular skin eruption. Am J Med 84:968, 1988

Plummer FA et al: An erythema infectiosum-like illness caused by human parvovirus infection. N Engl J Med 313:74, 1985

Rabinowe SL et al: Congenital rubella. Monoclonal antibody–defined T cell abnormalities in young adults. Am J Med 81:779, 1986

Reid DM et al: Human parvovirus-associated arthritis: A clinical and laboratory description. Lancet 1:422, 1985

Semble EL et al: Human parvovirus arthropathy in two adults after contact with childhood erythema infectiosum. Am J Med 83:560, 1987

Thurn J: Human parvovirus B19: Historical and clinical review. Rev Infect Dis 10:1005, 1988

Tingle AJ et al: Failed rubella immunization in adults: Association with immunologic and virological abnormalities. J Infect Dis 151:330, 1985

Townsend JJ et al: Progressive rubella panencephalitis: Late onset after congenital rubella. N Engl J Med 292:990, 1975

143 SMALLPOX, VACCINIA, AND OTHER POXVIRUSES

HARVEY M. FRIEDMAN

INTRODUCTION Poxviruses that infect humans share the common feature of producing cutaneous vesicular eruptions. They are brick-shaped, double-stranded DNA viruses and are the largest of the animal viruses. Human pathogens include variola, vaccinia, monkeypox, cowpox, milker's node virus, and molluscum contagiosum. These viruses can be distinguished from one another by antigenic differences, clinical manifestations of infection, and pox morphology when inoculated onto chick embryo chorioallantoic membranes. Global eradication of smallpox and the concomitant reduction in smallpox vaccination programs have changed the epidemiology of variola and vaccinia and modified their importance in modern medicine.

SMALLPOX

DEFINITION Smallpox (variola major) is a highly contagious disease characterized by fever, a vesicular and pustular eruption, and a high mortality rate. A milder form (variola minor) may be caused by the same virus.

The global eradication of smallpox was officially announced in 1979, marking one of the greatest achievements of modern medicine. Over the past decade, smallpox has not reappeared. If this pattern persists, a disease that once accounted for 10 percent of all deaths will become an illness mainly of historical interest. Although smallpox may eventually disappear as a topic in future editions of textbooks of medicine, it seems prudent to continue to be prepared to recognize the disease and prevent its spread.

ETIOLOGY Variola virus, the causative agent of smallpox, is an orthopoxvirus within the Poxviridae family. Variola is a large (200 to 400 nm) DNA virus differing from other DNA viruses in that it lacks icosahedral symmetry. When viewed by electron microscopy it has a complex structure and appears brick-shaped. It has an outer membrane, two lateral bodies, and a dumbbell-shaped core that contains a single molecule of double-stranded DNA.

PATHOGENESIS AND PATHOLOGY The oropharynx of infected patients serves as the main source for virus spread. Contacts become infected by inhaling virus which enters the respiratory tract and multiplies locally, probably within macrophages. Virus is carried within macrophages into the circulation and to regional lymph nodes. Multiplication occurs within lymphoid organs and a secondary viremia develops. Virus localizes within small dermal blood vessels, leading to dilatation of capillaries, endothelial swelling, and mononuclear cell infiltration. Epidermal cells enlarge, and intraepidermal vesicles form in skin and mucous membranes. The vesicles rupture to form shallow ulcers, while the epidermal cells enlarge and extend into the corium. When stained with hematoxylin and eosin, the cytoplasm of infected cells contains faintly basophilic or acidophilic inclusions (Guarnieri bodies). Infiltration by granulocytes changes the vesicle into a pustule, which heals either by rupture or resorption. Extension of infection into the corium and sebaceous glands produces pockmarks, or scars, which, upon healing, are characteristic of smallpox infection. Focal infiltration of the liver, spleen, and lymph nodes with macrophages may occur.

Virus infection stimulates cytotoxic T-cell responses, neutralizing antibodies, and the production of interferons. These responses restrict viral replication and induce prolonged immunity if the patient recovers. The infection is likely to be most severe in impaired hosts, particularly those with T-cell deficits. Milder forms of the infection have been observed in immunized patients, although it remains unclear why variola minor may be produced by the same virus in the unimmunized.

EPIDEMIOLOGY Smallpox was described in Asia during the first century A.D. and in Europe and Africa around 700 A.D. Infection was carried to Central, South, and North America during the sixteenth and seventeenth centuries. Endemic variola major was eradicated from the United States in 1926, and variola minor during the 1940s. Eradication was slower in Asia, Africa, and parts of the Americas. The last naturally occurring smallpox infection occurred in Somalia, Africa, in October 1977. The last known case developed 1 year later in Birmingham, England, in September 1978 and was the result of a laboratory accident. Over the past decade smallpox has not reappeared. The ability to eradicate this disease by an effective worldwide vaccination program appears to be centrally related to the facts that man was the only known reservoir for the variola virus; that no asymptomatic carrier state existed, facilitating surveillance; and that early diagnosis and prevention of disease or modification of the course by rapid vaccination of contacts were possible.

In temperate climates, endemic smallpox occurred in winter and spring. It was mainly a disease of children and young adults. Spread in unvaccinated family contacts was approximately 58 percent compared with 4 percent in vaccinees. Patients were usually severely ill and confined to bed, which restricted transmission to immediate family contacts. Index cases rarely infected more than five patients, most commonly those sharing living quarters. Transmission intervals were 2 to 3 weeks apart, and new cases would appear in a community or region over many months.

CLINICAL FEATURES Smallpox was endemic in every country of the world and existed as two forms, variola major, which was a serious illness with a mortality rate of >20 percent in the unvaccinated, and variola minor, which was a milder infection with a mortality of <1 percent. Both were caused by the same virus. On an individual case basis, it may be difficult to distinguish variola minor from a mild case of variola major. The severity of an entire outbreak is generally required to differentiate the two. The evolution of rash in variola minor is more rapid, similar to accelerated smallpox.

Variola major has been classified into five clinical categories:

1 *Ordinary type:* This comprised >70 percent of cases. It is characterized by raised pustular skin lesions which can be divided into three categories: (a) *Confluent* rash present on face and forearms; (b) *semiconfluent* rash present on face with discrete rash elsewhere; (c) *discrete* rash on all involved areas with normal skin between pustules. In unvaccinated patients, mortality was 62 percent for confluent infection, 37 percent for semiconfluent, and 9 percent for discrete infection.
2 *Modified type:* This form of smallpox is similar to ordinary disease, except that the course is accelerated, and pustular lesions are smaller. Modified smallpox was common in vaccinated patients who developed lesions, in health care workers exposed by accidental inoculation, and in those intentionally infected by variolation, a procedure once widely used as a method of vaccination.
3 *Variola sine eruptione:* Patients have fever but no rash. This was seen in vaccinated patients or those previously infected. Laboratory testing is required for confirmation of the diagnosis.
4 *Flat type:* Pustules remain flat and are usually confluent or semiconfluent in distribution. This form of infection occurred mainly in children and was often fatal.
5 *Hemorrhagic type:* Skin lesions and mucous membranes become hemorrhagic. Pregnant women were predisposed to this form of smallpox, which was rare but severe. Profound prostration, heart failure, diffuse bleeding, and bone marrow suppression resulted, and most infections were fatal within 3 to 4 days, earning the name "sledgehammer smallpox."

In a typical case of ordinary type smallpox, the incubation period is 7 to 19 days, with a mean of 12. A preeruptive phase lasting 2 to 4 days is characterized by sudden onset of fever, severe headache, backache, and malaise. Vomiting occurs in 50 percent, and diarrhea in 10 percent of patients. The rash first appears as minute red spots on the tongue and palate and as small macules (herald spots) on the face. Spread is centrifugal, involving the face, proximal extremities, trunk, and then distal extremities. Intraoral rash evolves from papules to vesicles, which break down and release large amounts of virus. The enanthem is an important source of virus spread. On the skin, macules evolve to papules by day 2, vesicles by days 4 to 5, and pustules by day 7 of rash. Fever may recur during the pustular phase. Lesions, which range from few to thousands, have a shotty, hard feel to them. Crusts develop by day 14 and heal leaving depigmented areas.

LABORATORY FINDINGS **Virus isolation** Virus can be isolated from skin lesions (until scabs form), oropharynx, conjunctiva, and urine. Viremia precedes the rash and clears in most patients when the rash appears. Virus particles can be seen by negative-staining electron microscopy performed on fluid obtained from skin lesions. This form of diagnosis was used to identify cases during the intensified eradication programs carried out in the 1960s and 1970s.

Serology Antibodies appear by days 6 to 8 of infection. Antibody titer rises can be detected by testing paired serum samples drawn 2 to 3 weeks apart. Various methods have been used to measure antibodies, including hemagglutination inhibition, complement fixation, neutralization, and gel precipitation.

Hematology Granulocytopenia, thrombocytopenia, and lymphocytosis are common during the prodromal and early rash phase. Leukocytosis occurs with pustulation of the vesicles. A profile consistent with disseminated intravascular coagulation is seen in patients with hemorrhagic smallpox.

DIFFERENTIAL DIAGNOSIS Distinguishing varicella from smallpox was particularly difficult during epidemics of variola minor or when mild smallpox infection developed in vaccinated patients. Dense rash on the trunk and appearance of lesions in crops are features of varicella not seen in smallpox. Human monkeypox, seen in western and central Africa, is difficult to distinguish from smallpox. Monkeypox is associated with more lymphadenopathy than smallpox. In the past, virus isolation was required to differentiate the two. On occasion, virus isolation was also required to distinguish disseminated vaccinia infection from smallpox.

COMPLICATIONS AND SEQUELAE Complications include secondary bacterial infections of the skin, keratitis and corneal ulcerations, viral arthritis and osteomyelitis, bacterial pneumonia, orchitis, and encephalitis. Sequelae include blindness from corneal scarring, limb deformities, and pockmarks, which appear hypopigmented in dark-skinned individuals and hyperpigmented in light-skinned patients.

TREATMENT AND OUTCOME In the past, mortality was highest in infants and the elderly. Infection in pregnant women led to abortion rates of >60 percent. Vaccination during the first week of incubation modified the course of disease by protecting many and reducing the severity of infection in others. This constituted an important method for control of smallpox. Immunotherapy with vaccinia immune globulin given during the incubation period of infection modified disease; however, supplies were too limited for this form of therapy to be widely applicable. Several different thiosemicarbazones, a class of antiviral compounds, were tried for treatment, but no benefit was detected in controlled human trials. One thiosemicarbazone, metisazone, was found to be useful as preventive therapy following exposure. Vaccinia immune globulin was also effective in postexposure prophylaxis without the side effects of metisazone. The mainstay of treatment was good nursing care, which was often provided by family members at home or in hospitals.

CONTROL Attempts at control of smallpox began once it was noted that accidental exposure to smallpox by scratch on the skin resulted in less severe infection. This led to the practice of variolation, which began in China and India in the tenth century. Variolation involved intentional administration of pustular fluids or scabs to uninfected persons. In 1796, Edward Jenner showed that inoculation with cowpox virus protected against smallpox and carried less risk of illness than variolation. Subsequently, vaccination was modified to use of vaccinia virus for smallpox control. The origins of vaccinia virus are uncertain, but many strains existed which were apparently derived from either variola or cowpox virus. Successful vaccination provided high levels of protection for 5 years and some protection for 20 years. Periodic revaccination was necessary for optimal protection. Postexposure vaccination lowered the incidence and reduced the severity of infection when administered within 1 week after exposure.

In 1959, the World Health Assembly adopted a program aimed at global eradication of smallpox. The development of stable freeze-dried vaccine meant that vaccination programs could reach less developed tropical countries. Efforts were intensified by 1967 and were built on the principles of surveillance and containment involving case detection, quarantine of infected patients, and vaccination of contacts and others living in the immediate area. Surveillance and contact vaccination were extremely important for the eventual success of the program. This approach was successful because smallpox has a long incubation period that allows vaccination to modify the course of the illness. The lack of a reservoir for variola, other than humans, the ease of clinical diagnosis, and the fact that variola does not establish latent or persistent infection were important contributors to the success of the eradication program.

VACCINIA

DEFINITION AND ETIOLOGY Vaccinia is a localized skin infection caused by inoculation of vaccinia virus. In immunosuppressed patients it may occasionally disseminate and produce severe disease. Vaccinia virus is thought to be derived from either variola, cowpox, or perhaps a hydrid of the two. "Vaccination" with vaccinia induces immunity to variola and was the method used to control or prevent smallpox. Endemic smallpox was eradicated from the United States in 1949, which led to the eventual discontinuation of routine childhood immunization by 1972. Evidence of immunization against smallpox is no longer required for international travel. As a result, physicians today have little experience with vaccinia immunization or its complications.

COMPLICATIONS OF VACCINATION Vaccine is applied to the skin, which is punctured several times by a sterile needle to penetrate the epidermis. Primary vaccination results in formation of a papule in 4 to 5 days that becomes a vesicle 2 to 3 days later. Mild fever and localized lymphadenopathy are often present at this stage. Within 2 weeks a scab forms that leaves a scar when healing is complete. The response during revaccination is accelerated and generally is not associated with fever or lymphadenopathy.

Vaccinia virus never underwent controlled trials to establish safety and efficacy before licensing. Nevertheless, the vaccine was highly effective, despite considerable adverse effects. *Complications* included: (1) *Progressive vaccinia* (vaccinia gangrenosum) developed in patients who were agammaglobulinemic, T-cell deficient, or receiving immunosuppressive therapy. Destruction of local areas of skin, subcutaneous tissue, and other underlying structures occurred, with metastatic lesions appearing at other cutaneous sites and in viscera and bone. This complication developed in approximately 1 patient per million during primary or revaccination and was usually fatal over a period of several months. (2) *Eczema vaccinatum* involved wide cutaneous spread of vaccinia virus in vaccinees and their contacts who had eczema or other chronic skin diseases. It developed in 1 per 100,000 primary vaccinations or 1 per million revaccinations and was sometimes fatal; bacterial superinfection often complicated eczema vaccinatum. (3) *Generalized vaccinia,* characterized by satellite lesions around the inoculation site or more widely disseminated pox, occasionally occurred in immunocompetent individuals and developed in 3 per 100,000 primary vaccinations or 1 per million revaccinations. This complication had a good prognosis. (4) *Accidental inoculation,* especially of eyelids, perineum, and vulva, occurred in 3 per 100,000 to 1 million vaccinees. The consequences were generally not serious. (5) *Postvaccinial encephalitis* was a serious complication which occurred in 3 per 1 million patients after primary vaccination. It usually developed 6 to 15 days after vaccination and had a violent onset. Features included convulsions, hemiplegia, and aphasia. Spinal fluid analysis was normal except for increased pressure. Recovery was often incomplete, and neurologic sequelae ensued.

Contraindications to vaccination include B- or T-cell immune disorders, neoplasms of the reticuloendothelial system, concomitant use of immunosuppressive drugs, eczema, pregnancy, and disorders of the central nervous system. When complications developed due to uncontrolled or progressive vaccinia infection, some were treated effectively with vaccinia immune globulin. This treatment is not effective for postvaccinial encephalitis. A role for antivirals, such as thiosemicarbazones, has not been definitely established.

Interest has reemerged in vaccinia as a vehicle for vaccination. Genes from herpes simplex virus, hepatitis B virus, human immunodeficiency virus, and malaria have been introduced into the vaccinia genome. Proteins encoded by these genes are expressed in vitro during vaccinia infection, which indicates that this virus potentially could serve as a vector for multiple vaccines. Should this approach prove successful, then the same precautions should be followed as in vaccination to prevent smallpox.

OTHER POXVIRUSES

HUMAN MONKEYPOX The monkeypox virus is a member of the orthopox genus. Human monkeypox is a rare zoonosis that occurs in tropical rain forests of west and central Africa. This disease was first recognized in the 1960s during smallpox eradication efforts. Identification resulted from attempts to confirm suspected cases of smallpox by laboratory methods. Infection does not spread from person to person, which accounts for the low number of cases, less than 100, identified so far. The clinical features of infection are similar to smallpox, except that cervical and inguinal lymphadenopathy are more prominent in human monkeypox. The diagnosis can be established by the characteristic pox morphology when virus is inoculated onto chorioallantoic membrane cultures.

COWPOX Cowpox virus is another member of the genus *Orthopoxvirus*. Infection develops by hand contact with infected ulcers on the teats of cows. The virus is also found in wild rodents, which may serve as a reservoir for some human infections. After exposure, one or more skin lesions develop, most often on the hands. The evolution of a lesion is similar to that seen during primary smallpox vaccination: a vesicle progresses to a pustule that later scabs. The rash does not become generalized. It is often associated with lymphangitis and localized lymphadenopathy. The disease may be confused with milker's nodule (see below). Laboratory confirmation can be established by the characteristic pox that develop when virus is isolated on chorioallantoic membranes.

MILKER'S NODE VIRUS This infection is caused by a parapoxvirus and is sometimes referred to as pseudocowpox or paravaccinia. It is acquired by contact with infected cows. Lesions appear as red nodules that progress to firm purple papules. The lack of vesicles or pustules distinguish it from cowpox. Lesions are relatively painless and generally resolve in 4 to 6 weeks.

ORF This is a disease of sheep that is sometimes referred to as contagious pustular dermatitis. It is caused by a parapoxvirus. Human infection is acquired by contact with sheep infected around the mouth, nose, or eyes. Human infection usually occurs at abrasion sites on the hands. Single or multiple painful large vesicles develop and are often associated with lymphadenopathy. Resolution occurs within several weeks.

MOLLUSCUM CONTAGIOSUM This infection occurs only in humans and is caused by an unclassified poxvirus that cannot be cultured in vitro. Lesions occur anywhere on the body, except on the palms and soles, and appear as pearly, flesh-colored, raised, umbilicated nodules 2 to 5 mm in diameter. Lesions develop in crops, are painless, and resolve over a period of weeks to several years. Spread is probably by direct contact, which accounts for the commonly observed genital distribution of lesions in sexually active adults. An increased incidence of molluscum contagiosum is seen in patients infected with the human immunodeficiency virus. No specific therapy is available, although lesions can be removed by curettage.

REFERENCES

Baxby D: The origins of vaccinia virus. J Infect Dis 136:453, 1977

Breman JG, Arita I: The confirmation and maintenance of smallpox eradication. N Engl J Med 303:1263, 1980

Fenner F: Poxviruses, in *Virology*, 2d ed, BN Fields et al (eds). New York, Raven, 1990, pp 2113–2133

Fenner F et al: *Smallpox and Its Eradication*. World Health Organization, Geneva, 1988

Moss B: Poxviridae and their replication, in *Virology*, 2d ed, BN Fields et al (eds). New York, Raven, 1990, pp 2079–2111

144 ENTEROVIRUSES AND REOVIRUSES

C. GEORGE RAY

GENERAL CONSIDERATIONS

Enteroviruses consist of a major subgroup of picornaviruses that include the polioviruses, coxsackieviruses, echoviruses, and more recently discovered agents that are simply designated enteroviruses. The number of serotypes that infect humans is nearly 70, and more are likely to be found in the future. Their name is derived from their ability to infect intestinal tract epithelial and lymphoid tissues and to be shed into the feces.

Enteroviruses can cause paralytic disease, encephalitis and acute aseptic meningitis syndromes, pleurodynia, exanthems, pericarditis, myocarditis, nonspecific febrile illness, and occasional fulminant disease in the newborn. The spectrum of disease may be even broader. Some infections can lead to permanent damage, and others may trigger chronic, active disease processes.

Since these viruses have many features in common, they will first be considered as a group. Some of the special features of important serotypes will be discussed in detail later in this chapter.

CHARACTERISTICS OF ENTEROVIRUSES As a group, the picornaviruses are extremely small (22 to 30 nm in diameter), single-stranded RNA viruses with icosahedral symmetry. In contrast to the rhinoviruses, the enterovirus subgroup is resistant to ether, acid pH (3.0), and bile. Another feature is cationic stability; in the presence of magnesium chloride, the viruses become more resistant to thermal inactivation. They can survive for prolonged periods in sewage and even in chlorinated water if sufficient organic debris is present. Although some of the enterovirus serotypes share antigens, there are no significant serologic relationships between the major classes listed in Table 144-1; however, a single, highly conserved epitope may be shared by virtually all serotypes except enterovirus 72. Genetic variation within specific strains occurs, and mutants which exhibit antigenic drift and altered tropism for specific cell types have been recognized. Definitive identification of isolates usually requires neutralization tests.

Most of these agents can be isolated in primate (human or simian) cell cultures; however, some strains, such as several coxsackievirus group A serotypes, are grown with difficulty in cell cultures, and inoculation of newborn mice may be necessary for detection. Inoculation of newborn mice was one basis for the original classification of group A and B coxsackieviruses. After the mice have been inoculated, at 24 h of age or less, and observed for 2 to 12 days, group A viruses primarily have a widespread, inflammatory, necrotic effect on skeletal muscle, leading to flaccid paralysis and usually death; similar inoculation of group B viruses causes encephalitis, resulting in spasticity and occasionally convulsions. Other organs are variably affected, and histopathologic examination is sometimes helpful in distinguishing the two. Echoviruses and polioviruses rarely have an adverse effect on mice, unless special adaptation procedures are employed. The higher-numbered enteroviruses (types 68 to 72),

TABLE 144-1 Enteroviruses that infect humans

Class	Number of serotypes
Poliovirus	3
Coxsackievirus	
Group A	23*
Group B	6
Echovirus	31
Enterovirus	Types 68–72†

* Includes several subtypes; coxsackievirus A23 is the same as echovirus 9.
† The classification of the more recently described enteroviruses is based on overlapping biologic characteristics. These are identified numerically. Enterovirus 72 is hepatitis A virus.

which have overlapping growth and host characteristics, have been classified separately. Hepatitis A virus has been classified as enterovirus 72 and is discussed in Chap. 252.

Humans are the major natural host for the polioviruses, coxsackieviruses, and echoviruses. There are enteroviruses of other animals with a limited host range that does not appear to extend to humans. Conversely, viruses thought to be identical or related to human enteroviruses have been isolated from dogs and cats. Whether these agents cause disease in these animals is debatable, and there is no evidence of spread from animals to humans.

EPIDEMIOLOGY The enteroviruses have a worldwide distribution, and asymptomatic infection is common. The proportion of infected individuals who will develop illness varies from 2 to 100 percent, depending upon the serotype or strain involved, prior immune status, and the age of the patient. Secondary infections in households are common and range as high as 40 to 70 percent, depending upon factors such as family size, crowding, and sanitary conditions.

There is a seasonal predilection; epidemics are usually observed during the summer and fall. In subtropical and tropical climates, the duration of greatest transmission sometimes extends into the winter. In some years, certain serotypes emerge as dominant strains; they then may wane, only to reappear in epidemics years later. The emergence of dominant serotypes is unpredictable from year to year.

Direct or indirect fecal-oral transmission is considered the most common mode of spread. After infection, the virus persists in the oropharynx for 1 to 4 weeks, and it can be shed in the feces for 1 to 18 weeks. Sewage-contaminated water, contaminated foods, or insect vectors (flies, cockroaches) may occasionally be the source of infection. More commonly, however, spread is directly from person to person. Approximately two-thirds of all isolates are from children 9 years of age or younger.

Incubation periods vary, but relatively short intervals (2 to 10 days) are the rule. Illness is often seen concurrently in more than one family member, and the clinical features may vary within the household.

PATHOGENESIS AND PATHOLOGY After primary replication in the epithelial cells and lymphoid tissues in the upper respiratory and gastrointestinal tracts, viremic spread to other sites can occur. Potential target organs vary according to the virus strain and its tropism, but may include the central nervous system, heart, vascular endothelium, liver, pancreas, gonads, lungs, skeletal muscles, synovial tissues, skin, and mucous membranes. Histopathologic findings include cell necrosis and mononuclear cell inflammatory infiltrates; in the central nervous system, the inflammatory cells are localized most prominently in perivascular sites. The initial tissue damage is thought to result from the lytic cycle of virus replication. Viremia is usually undetectable by the time symptoms appear, and termination of virus replication commences with the appearance of circulating interferon, neutralizing antibody, and mononuclear cell infiltrations of infected tissue. The early antibody response is mainly immunoglobulin M–specific, and usually wanes 6 to 12 weeks after onset to be replaced by IgG-specific antibodies. The important role of antibodies in the termination of infection is supported by persistent enterovirus replication in patients with antibody-deficiency diseases.

Although initial acute tissue damage may be caused by the lytic effects of the virus on the cell, many of the secondary sequelae appear to be immunologically mediated. Enterovirus-caused poliomyelitis, disseminated disease of the newborn, aseptic meningitis, encephalitis, exanthems, and acute respiratory illnesses, thought to represent primary lytic infections, can usually be identified through routine methods of virus isolation and determination of specific antibody titer changes. On the other hand, syndromes such as myopericarditis, nephritis, and myositis have been associated with enteroviruses primarily by serologic evidence, and the use of cDNA probes to detect viral RNA in tissues. Viral isolation is the exception. The pathogenesis of these illnesses may be a cell-mediated immunologic response to tissue injury by the virus or to viral or virus-induced antigens that persist in the affected tissues.

Infection by a specific serotype in an immunologically normal host is followed by a humoral antibody response, which can often be detected by neutralization methods for many years thereafter. There is relative immunity to reinfection by the same serotype; however, reinfection has been reported, usually resulting in subclinical infection or mild illness. Although there is some antigenic sharing between serotypes in some of the enterovirus classes (for example, group B coxsackieviruses), there is no evidence of significant heterotypic immunity to infection by different serotypes.

LABORATORY DIAGNOSIS In acute enteroviral infections, the diagnosis is most readily established by virus isolation from throat swabs, stool or rectal swabs, body fluids, and occasionally tissues. Except in young infants, viremia is usually undetectable by the time symptoms appear. When there is central nervous system involvement, cerebrospinal fluid cultures taken during the acute phase of the disease may be positive in 10 to 85 percent of cases (except in poliovirus infections, in which virus recovery from this site is rare), depending upon the stage of illness and the serotype involved. Direct isolation of virus from affected tissues or body fluids in enclosed spaces (for example, pleural, pericardial, or cerebrospinal fluid) usually confirms the diagnosis. Isolation of an enterovirus from the throat is suggestive of an etiologic association because the virus is usually detectable at this site for only 2 days to 2 weeks after infection; isolation of virus from fecal specimens only must be interpreted more cautiously because asymptomatic shedding from the bowel may persist for as long as 4 months.

The diagnosis may be further supported by a fourfold or greater increase in neutralizing antibody titer in paired acute and convalescent serum samples. This method is expensive and cumbersome, requiring careful selection of serotypes for use as antigens. Serodiagnosis is generally reserved for critical situations in which the etiology is questionable, such as isolation of a virus only from a peripheral source such as the feces, or in illnesses such as myopericarditis, in which the yield on routine culture is low and the number of serotypes that might be expected to be involved is limited. Quantitative interpretations of antibody titers on single serum samples are rarely helpful because of the high prevalence and wide range of titers to different serotypes that can be found in healthy individuals. In acute poliovirus infections, complement-fixing antibody titer determinations on acute and convalescent sera can aid in diagnosis.

White blood cell counts and the erythrocyte sedimentation rates are usually only mildly elevated. If there is necrosis (e.g., liver, lung), a neutrophilic reaction may be noted. Hyperbilirubinemia and elevated transaminase and alkaline phosphatase levels may be seen in patients with hepatitis. Albuminuria often occurs transiently, but hematuria is rare.

PROPHYLAXIS AND TREATMENT Vaccines, which are available only for the prevention of poliovirus infections, will be discussed in detail below. Although proper disposal of feces and careful personal hygiene are recommended, the usual quarantine or isolation measures are relatively ineffective in controlling the spread of enteroviruses in the family or community.

None of the currently available antiviral agents or immune serum globulins has been effective in treatment or prophylaxis of enterovirus infections. The only exception may be the intravenous or intraventricular use of high-titered immunoglobulin in the treatment of chronic enteroviral encephalitis in antibody-deficient patients. Otherwise, treatment is entirely symptomatic and supportive. Glucocorticoids are contraindicated.

POLIOVIRUS INFECTIONS

The most important enteroviruses are the three poliovirus serotypes (types 1, 2, and 3). They first emerged as important causes of disease in developed temperate-zone countries during the latter part of the nineteenth century, and they continue to be a serious public health problem in developing countries.

The particular tropism of polioviruses for the central nervous system, which they usually reach by passage across the blood-CNS barrier, is perhaps favored by reflex dilatation of capillaries supplying the affected motor centers of the anterior horn of the brainstem or spinal cord. An alternate pathway may be via entry into motor neurons at peripheral neuromuscular junctions. Motor neurons are particularly vulnerable to infection and variable degrees of destruction. The histopathologic findings in the brainstem and spinal cord include necrosis of neuronal cells and perivascular "cuffing" by infiltration with mononuclear cells, primarily lymphocytes.

CLINICAL MANIFESTATIONS Most infections (perhaps 90 percent) are either subclinical or extremely mild. When disease does result, the incubation period can be from 4 to 35 days, but is usually between 7 and 14 days. The disease falls into three classes: The first, abortive poliomyelitis, is a nonspecific febrile illness of 2- to 3-day duration with no signs of CNS localization. A second group of patients will additionally develop aseptic meningitis. Recovery is rapid and complete, usually within a few days. The third class, paralytic poliomyelitis, is the major possible outcome of infection and is often preceded by a period of fever and "minor illness." Classically, after several days, symptoms disappear. In 5 to 10 days fever recurs, and signs of meningeal irritation and asymmetric flaccid paralysis ensue. Cramping muscle pain and spasm as well as coarse twitching in affected parts follows. The maximum extent of involvement is apparent within a few days after first paralysis. In children under 5 years, paralysis of one leg is most common. In patients 5 to 15 years of age, weakness of one arm or paraplegia is frequent, while in adults quadriplegia is more likely to occur. Urinary bladder and respiratory muscle dysfunction are also frequent in adults. Encephalitis is rare.

Tendon reflexes are diminished or absent. Sensation is intact, in contrast to the usually symmetric paralysis and mild sensory disturbance of the Guillain-Barré syndrome. Paralysis due to heavy metal poisoning may also be difficult to distinguish clinically from poliomyelitis.

Among paralytic cases, 6 to 25 percent may be bulbar. Myocarditis, hypertension, pulmonary edema, shock, nosocomial gram-negative or staphylococcal pneumonias, urinary tract infections, and emotional problems are among the complications of severe paralytic disease. Treatment is supportive. About 2 to 5 percent of children and 15 to 30 percent of adults with paralyzing infection die. As temporarily damaged neurons regain their function, recovery begins and may continue for as long as 6 months. Paralysis persisting beyond that time is permanent, and may be associated with complaints of severe pain in the affected areas which sometimes recur years after the illness.

Some patients develop progressive muscle weakness, usually beginning 20 to 30 years later. This is called post-poliomyelitis neuromuscular atrophy, or the "post-polio syndrome." Symptoms vary from mild to moderate deterioration of function, with fatigue, joint pain, and weakness that may stabilize or progress to muscle atrophy. It is not considered to be life-threatening. The pathogenesis appears to involve a dysfunction of surviving motor neurons with slow disintegration of axon terminals, leading to late denervation of muscle.

PREVENTION Two types of poliovirus vaccines are currently licensed in the United States: inactivated polio vaccine and live, oral, attenuated virus vaccine. Each contains the three serotypes of poliomyelitis virus.

Inactivated polio vaccine (IPV) remains the only vaccine used in some countries, notably Sweden, Finland, and the Netherlands, and its efficacy has been excellent. The current product is considered safe, with no significant deleterious side effects. In 1987, a more potent IPV, which is produced in human diploid cells, was licensed. This enhanced-potency IPV has been shown to produce 99 to 100 percent seropositivity for all three poliovirus types after two doses in infants. Primary vaccination with three subcutaneous doses (two doses 4 to 8 weeks apart, and the third 6 to 12 months later) is recommended for unimmunized children and adults. A booster dose at the time of school entry is recommended for children. The duration of protection is at least 5 years, and may be considerably longer.

Oral polio vaccine (OPV) is composed of live, attenuated viruses. The vaccine is given as a primary series of three doses (the first two doses usually 6 to 8 weeks apart, and the third 8 to 12 months later) and produces antibodies to all three serotypes in more than 95 percent of recipients. As with IPV, recall boosters are recommended to maintain adequate antibody levels. Like wild poliovirus, OPV viruses infect and replicate in the oropharynx and intestinal tract, and may be shed into the feces for 6 weeks or longer.

One disadvantage of OPV is the remote risk of vaccine-associated paralytic disease in some recipients, such as immunocompromised persons; susceptible adults are at a slightly higher risk than children. The incidence of vaccine-associated paralytic poliomyelitis is estimated at approximately 1 per 2.6 million doses distributed, and one per 520,000 after the first dose. Of the 138 cases of paralytic poliomyelitis reported in the United States from 1973 through 1984, 105 were vaccine-associated (35 in healthy recipients, 50 in close contacts, 14 with immune-deficiency conditions, and 6 with no history of vaccination or contact).

The major advantages of OPV include ease of administration and secondary immunization of nonimmune contacts through shedding of vaccine virus into the intestinal tract, resulting in more widespread immunity in the population. It is also theorized that during outbreaks, transient vaccine virus colonization results in the induction of mucosal immunity (primarily through secretory IgA), which may interfere with subsequent acquisition and spread of wild poliovirus.

The choice between IPV and OPV for routine primary immunization is widely debated; however, it is clear that both are highly effective vaccines, and that routine immunization with one or the other is important in the prevention of disease. Ideally, immunization should commence in infancy. A susceptible adult at risk of exposure to infection because of travel to an endemic area should receive complete immunization. Persons with immunodeficiency or altered immune status should not be exposed to OPV, either directly or by household contact, because of the increased risk of vaccine-associated paralysis.

Although there are no currently recognized areas of wild poliovirus prevalence in the United States, importation of these strains can readily occur from endemic areas in contiguous countries as well as from developing nations abroad. Once introduced into a community, the virus can spread rapidly among susceptible individuals. For this reason, continuing immunization programs are of utmost importance in preventing spread of this disease.

COXSACKIEVIRUSES AND ECHOVIRUSES

The coxsackieviruses and echoviruses are widespread throughout the world. The basic features of their epidemiology and pathogenesis appear to be the same as those of the polioviruses. Unlike polioviruses, they have a greater tendency to affect the meninges and occasionally the cerebrum, and only rarely do they affect anterior horn cells.

The consequences of infection with these agents are highly variable and related only in part to virus subgroup and serotype. Up to 60 percent of infections are subclinical. The main interest in these agents stems from their ability to cause more serious illness, which becomes most evident during epidemics.

Inapparent infection is common, but varies with the infecting strain and the host involved. The manifestations of illness range from mild to lethal and from acute to chronic. Table 144-2 lists the major syndromes and serotypes commonly associated with each. Considerable overlap occurs, however, and it is not surprising to find an enteroviral serotype associated with a specific syndrome which differs from that most often encountered. The group B coxsackieviruses generally have the greatest latitude with regard to tissue tropism.

ASEPTIC MENINGITIS (See Chap. 355) In terms of relative frequency, aseptic meningitis is the most important illness associated

TABLE 144-2 Clinical syndromes reported to be commonly associated with enterovirus serotypes

Syndrome	Coxsackievirus Group A	Coxsackievirus Group B	Echovirus and enterovirus (E)
Aseptic meningitis, encephalitis	2,4,7,9,10	1,2,3,4,5	4,6,9,11,16,30;E70,E71
Muscle weakness and paralysis (poliomyelitis-like disease)	7,9	2,3,4,5	2,4,6,9,11,30;E71
Cerebellar ataxia	2,4,9	3,4	4,6,9
Generalized disease (infants)	———	1,2,3,4,5	3,6,9,11,14,17,19
Exanthems and enanthems	4,5,6,9,10,16	2,3,4,5	2,4,5,6,9,11,16,18,25;E71
Pericarditis, myocarditis	4,16	2,3,4,5	1,6,8,9,19
Epidemic myalgia (pleurodynia), orchitis	9	1,2,3,4,5	1,6,9
Respiratory symptoms	9,16,21,24	1,3,4,5	4,9,11,20,25
Conjunctivitis	24	1,5	7;E70

with enterovirus infections. This syndrome can be mild and self-limiting; however, it is occasionally accompanied by encephalitis, which can lead to permanent sequelae, particularly in infants. Overall, enteroviruses cause the majority of all nonbacterial CNS infections now observed in the United States.

There may be a mild prodromal malaise, but major illness usually begins with fever, headache, and stiff neck. Kernig's and Brudzinski's signs may be present. Localizing sensory or motor deficits are unusual. Confusion and delirium are common. These acute findings may persist for 4 to 7 days. Cerebrospinal pleocytosis is usually less than 500 cells per microliter. Early, there may be as many as 90 percent polymorphonuclear leukocytes, but within 48 h the cellular response becomes completely mononuclear. Persistence of polymorphonuclear leukocytes in the cerebrospinal fluid suggests pyogenic meningitis or intracerebral, subdural, or epidural abscess. Gram's stain and appropriate spinal fluid cultures must be done to exclude bacterial meningitis, tuberculosis, or mycotic meningitis. Protein concentration in the cerebrospinal fluid is moderately elevated, but glucose is usually normal. Early in the illness enteroviruses may be isolated from spinal fluid, even in the absence of significant pleocytosis. It usually takes several weeks before the cerebrospinal fluid reverts to normal. An occasional patient may develop a transient syndrome of inappropriate secretion of antidiuretic hormone. In hypo- or agammaglobulinemic syndromes echoviruses have persisted in CSF for months to years, producing a progressive encephalitis or polymyositis.

For attempts at virus isolation, throat, stool, and cerebrospinal fluid specimens should be collected as early in the course as possible. Acute and convalescent sera can also be studied for rises in type-specific neutralizing antibodies in patients in whom viral isolation results are negative or equivocal.

It is not possible to distinguish clinically between aseptic meningitis due to various enteroviruses, arboviruses, Epstein-Barr virus, and mumps. Localizing findings, hemiplegia, oculogyric crises, coma, and bloody spinal fluid favor the diagnosis of type 1 herpes simplex virus encephalitis (see Chap. 135). Although enterovirus aseptic meningitis most often is self-limited and recovery in persons afflicted after the first year of life is usually complete, about 10 percent of patients have more serious involvement of the central nervous system. Minor muscle weakness with reflex changes may persist for weeks to months, but over 90 percent of patients recover completely within a year. Occasionally, choreiform movements, ataxia, nystagmus, transverse myelitis, Guillain-Barré syndrome, poliomyelitis-like symptoms, coma, bulbar involvement, and death occur.

OTHER ENTEROVIRAL ILLNESSES *Generalized disease of the newborn* is a highly lethal expression of enteroviral infection, in which the infant may be overwhelmed by simultaneous virus infection of the heart, liver, adrenals, brain, and other organs.

Acute myocarditis and/or pericarditis can be caused by a variety of viral agents; however, it is estimated that as many as 50 percent of cases are associated with infection by coxsackie B viruses. Such infections are usually self-limited, but can lead to a fatal outcome (arrhythmia or heart failure) or cause chronic heart disease (see Chaps. 192 and 193).

The exanthems may or may not be associated with CNS inflammation. The rashes usually resemble rubella, roseola infantum, or adenovirus macular or maculopapular exanthems, but may also appear as vesicular or hemangioma-like lesions. Hand-foot-and-mouth disease usually affects children and is characterized by a vesicular eruption over the extremities and the anterior oral cavity. Coxsackievirus A16 is the specific agent most frequently implicated, but others, such as enterovirus 71, can cause a similar illness.

Herpangina is an enanthematous (mucous membrane) disease characterized by the acute onset of fever and sore throat. Characteristic small vesicles or white papules (lymphonodules) surrounded by a red halo are seen over the posterior half of the palate, pharynx, and tonsillar areas. This mild, self-limiting (1 to 2 weeks) illness has usually been associated with infection by several different group A coxsackievirus serotypes.

Epidemic myalgia (pleurodynia, or Bornholm disease) is characterized by fever and sudden onset of intense upper abdominal or lower thoracic pain, often accompanied by a frontal headache. The pain may be aggravated by movement, such as breathing or coughing, and usually persists for 3 to 14 days. Coxsackie B viruses are most frequently implicated.

A variety of other illnesses may also result from infections by this subgroup. Epidemic acute hemorrhagic keratoconjunctivitis associated with enterovirus 70 has been reported in Asia and the United States, and disease resembling paralytic poliomyelitis caused by enterovirus 71 infection has occurred in Bulgaria, Australia, and the United States. There is some evidence that certain enteroviruses may participate in the pathogenesis of at least some cases of insulin-dependent diabetes mellitus, acute arthritis, polymyositis, hemolytic-uremic syndrome, and idiopathic acute nephritis.

REOVIRUS INFECTIONS

The reoviruses (respiratory enteric orphans) are naked virions that contain double-stranded RNA. They are extremely ubiquitous and have been found in humans, simians, cattle, rodents, and a variety of other hosts. Three serotypes are known to infect humans; however, their role and relative importance in causing disease remains uncertain. Sporadic cases of febrile upper respiratory infections, exanthems, pneumonia, hepatitis, encephalitis, and gastroenteritis have all been reported to be associated with these viruses. Reovirus type 3 has also been implicated as a possible cause of biliary atresia and neonatal hepatitis, but this relationship remains uncertain. Asymptomatic shedding of reoviruses also occurs, which makes it difficult to prove association with disease. Reoviruses can be isolated in cell cultures, particularly primary monkey kidney or human kidney monolayers.

REFERENCES

BOWLES NE et al: Detection of coxsackie-B-virus-specific RNA sequences in myocardial biopsy samples from patients with myocarditis and dilated cardiomyopathy. Lancet 1:1120, 1986

——— et al: Dermatomyositis, polymyositis, and coxsackie-B-virus infection. Lancet 1:1004, 1987

BROWN WR et al: Lack of correlation between infection with reovirus 3 and extrahepatic biliary atresia or neonatal hepatitis. J Pediatr 113:670, 1988

CASHMAN NR et al: Late denervation in patients with antecedent paralytic poliomyelitis. N Engl J Med 317:7, 1987

CHEMTOB S et al: Syndrome of inappropriate secretion of antidiuretic hormone in enteroviral meningitis. Am J Dis Child 139:292, 1985

CRENNAN JM et al: Echovirus polymyositis in patients with hypogammaglobulinemia. Failure of high-dose intravenous gamma-globulin therapy and review of the literature. Am J Med 81:35, 1986

DALAKIS MC et al: A long-term follow-up study of patients with post-poliomyelitis neuromuscular symptoms. N Engl J Med 314:959, 1986

JOSSELSON J et al: Acute rhabdomyolysis associated with an echovirus infection. Arch Intern Med 140:1671, 1980

KAPLAN MH et al: Group B coxsackievirus infections in infants younger than three months of age: A serious childhood illness. Rev Infect Dis 5:1019, 1983

MCBEAN AM et al: Serological response to oral polio vaccine and enhanced-potency inactivated polio vaccine. Am J Epidemiol 128:615, 1988

MCKINNEY RE JR et al: Chronic enteroviral meningoencephalitis in agammaglobulinemia patients. Rev Infect Dis 9:334, 1987

NKOWANE BM et al: Vaccine-associated paralytic poliomyelitis. JAMA 257:1335, 1987

SHARPE AH, FIELDS BN: Pathogenesis of viral infections: Basic concepts derived from the reovirus model. N Engl J Med 312:486, 1985

145 VIRAL GASTROENTERITIS

HARRY B. GREENBERG

INTRODUCTION In less developed countries, acute infectious diarrheal disease is a leading cause of morbidity in all age groups, and of mortality in infants and young children. In developed countries, acute diarrheal illness remains an important cause of morbidity among both children and adults. Two distinct groups of viruses—the rotaviruses and the Norwalk viruses—as well as a variety of bacterial pathogens (see Chap. 92) have emerged as important etiologic agents of gastroenteritis. The rotaviruses are primarily pathogens of young children. The Norwalk and related small round viruses affect predominantly older children and adults.

ROTAVIRUS Classification and characterization Rotaviruses are members of the Reoviridae family. The rotavirus virion consists of a 70-nm double-shelled icosahedral capsid which surrounds a genome composed of 11 segments of double-stranded RNA. The virus has two surface proteins which are both involved with viral neutralization. Because rotaviruses have a segmented genome, they are capable of undergoing gene reassortment at very high frequency. The role of gene reassortment in generating rotavirus antigenic diversity is not known. In humans, rotavirus infection is characterized by replication that is localized exclusively in the small intestinal epithelial cells.

Epidemiology Rotavirus infection occurs worldwide. By the age of 3, virtually every individual has been infected by rotaviruses at least once. In areas with a temperate climate, rotavirus infection is seasonal, occurring in the cooler winter months. In tropical areas rotavirus infection tends to occur throughout the year, with some increase in incidence during the cooler rainy season. Rotaviruses are the single most important cause of severe dehydrating diarrhea in infants and young children under 3 in both developed and less developed countries, and account for between 30 and 50 percent of all cases of diarrhea requiring hospitalization or intensive rehydration therapy. Although rotavirus infections are primarily confined to infants and small children, they are frequently associated with diarrhea in adults, particularly family members of affected infants, geriatric patients, and immunocompromised hosts. They account for up to 25 percent of traveler's diarrhea (see Chap. 92). Rotaviruses may also be responsible for some cases of acute and chronic diarrhea in patients with AIDS. Subclinical infections or mild gastrointestinal illnesses which do not require hospitalization account for the majority of rotavirus infections. Subclinical infections have also been documented in neonates; these infections were shown to protect against severe rotavirus gastroenteritis for up to 3 years. At least five distinct serotypes of human rotavirus have been described. The relationship of the frequency of infection with these serotypes to host immune status is unclear. A large variety of other mammals and avian species can be infected by rotavirus, but it does not appear that these animal rotavirus strains cause disease in humans under natural conditions. Rotaviruses are shed in very large numbers (up to 10^{10} particles per gram of feces) in the stool; it is presumed that transmission occurs via fecal-oral spread.

Pathophysiology Rotavirus infects and kills the mature villus tip cells of the small intestine. The mature epithelial cells are replaced by immature absorptive cells that cannot absorb carbohydrates or other nutrients efficiently. Rotavirus infection leads to an osmotic diarrhea due to nutrient malabsorption. Changes in intracellular cyclic adenosine monophosphate or guanosine monophosphate are not involved in the etiology of rotavirus diarrhea.

Manifestations These range from subclinical infections to mild diarrhea to severe, occasionally fatal, illness. Most information concerning the signs and symptoms of rotavirus infection has been derived from studies of hospitalized young children. The onset of illness is usually abrupt. Vomiting, followed by diarrhea, occurs in over 80 percent of affected children. About one-third of hospitalized children will have a temperature greater than 39°C (102.2°F). Gastrointestinal symptoms usually last between 2 and 6 days. Mucus is commonly found in the stool but white and red blood cells are present in less than 15 percent of cases. Rotavirus infection frequently occurs in conjunction with respiratory tract symptoms, but there is little evidence to indicate that rotavirus replicates in the respiratory tract. Rotavirus infection has been observed in association with a wide variety of other clinical syndromes, including sudden infant death syndrome, Reye's syndrome, encephalitis, aseptic meningitis, pneumonia, exanthem subitum, Kawasaki's syndrome, necrotizing enterocolitis, gastroenteritis (which may be accompanied by hemorrhage), intussusception, Henoch-Schönlein purpura, hemolytic uremic syndrome, disseminated intravascular coagulation, and Crohn's disease. The etiologic relationship between these clinical syndromes and rotavirus infection is probably coincidental rather than causal. Rotavirus infection may be especially severe, and even fatal, in immunocompromised children.

Clinical immunity Relative immunity to rotavirus illness is acquired following infection early in childhood. Immunity is not complete, and adults with low levels of antibody can be symptomatically infected. Local immunity appears to be the critical determinant in protection.

Diagnosis Because rotavirus is shed in large amounts in the stool, detection is relatively easy. A variety of specific commercial immunoassays are available to detect rotavirus antigen in fecal specimens. DNA probe diagnosis also appears to be sensitive and specific. There are no pathognomonic signs or symptoms of rotavirus infection, but rotavirus infection is more frequently associated with severe dehydration than other enteric bacterial or viral pathogens.

Treatment and prevention Despite the fact that rotavirus diarrhea is caused by intestinal epithelial cell lysis and death, it can be adequately treated by standard oral rehydration therapy. Only rarely is intravenous rehydration required. Since rotavirus infections have persisted in developed countries with advanced sanitation facilities and widely available clean water, it is unlikely that the viral infection will be preventable by hygienic measures alone. Progress with a number of candidate live attenuated vaccines suggests that prevention through vaccination may be feasible in the future.

NORWALK AND RELATED SMALL ROUND VIRUSES Classification and characterization A variety of round 27- to 32-nm particles, some with clearly defined ultrastructure, have been identified in the stools of individuals with acute nonbacterial gastroenteritis. These agents have not been definitely classified because they are shed in the stool in small amounts for only a few days, and they have not been adapted to cell culture or to animal models. The Norwalk virus represents the most extensively studied and best characterized member of this group of agents, which also includes such serologically distinct viruses as the Hawaii agent, the Snow Mountain agent, the W-Ditchling agent, and a number of agents described as either astrovirus-like or calicivirus-like. The Norwalk virus and the Snow Mountain virus appear to have a protein structure similar to typical caliciviruses, and it is likely that most of these 27-nm gastroenteritis agents will prove to be plus-stranded RNA viruses.

Epidemiology Norwalk infection occurs year-round and is common. From 58 to 70 percent of adults in both developed and less developed countries have antibodies to this virus. Antibody acquisition occurs at a considerably younger age in children in less developed countries than in those in developed areas, consistent with the presumption that Norwalk virus is spread by the fecal-oral route. In developed countries, the virus is responsible for approximately one-third of all epidemics of nonbacterial gastroenteritis. Norwalk virus has been incriminated in a variety of food-borne epidemics, and transmission vehicles have included oysters, green salad, and chocolate icing. The virus is a common cause of waterborne epidemics of gastroenteritis and has been shown to be the etiologic agent in nursing home, cruise ship, and institutional (summer camps and schools) outbreaks.

In less developed countries, the role of Norwalk virus infection in the etiology of diarrhea has not been thoroughly investigated. Preliminary studies indicate that Norwalk virus can cause mild diarrhea in young children, but it does not appear to cause severe illness in infants in either developed or less developed countries. The other serologically distinct small round gastroenteritis viruses must be studied in more detail before their epidemiology can be distinguished from Norwalk infection. It appears, however, that astroviruses and typical human caliciviruses are primarily pathogens of young children rather than adults.

Pathophysiology Following infection with Norwalk or Hawaii viruses, the proximal small intestinal architecture is altered with villus shortening, crypt hyperplasia, and lamina propria infiltration by polymorphonuclear and mononuclear cells. Changes are not observed in the stomach or colon. The cells in which viral replication occurs have not been identified. The histologic alterations are accompanied by mild steatorrhea, carbohydrate malabsorption, and decreased levels of some brush border enzymes. Changes in adenylate cyclase activity have not been observed.

Manifestations Norwalk illness has an incubation period of between 18 and 72 h. Disease is characterized by the abrupt onset of nausea and abdominal cramps followed by vomiting and/or diarrhea. Vomiting occurs more frequently in children than adults. Low-grade fever [above 37.5°C (99.5°F)] is seen in about half of affected individuals. Headache, myalgias, and abdominal pain are common. The white blood cell count is normal; rarely there is leukocytosis with a relative lymphopenia. Red and white cells are not found in the stool. The illness is usually mild and self-limited, lasting 24 to 48 h.

Clinical immunity For most people long-term (2 years or greater) resistance to Norwalk reinfection does not occur. In volunteers, there is a paradoxical relationship between the level of antibody to Norwalk virus and susceptibility to illness. Low levels of Norwalk antibody in the serum and intestine are associated with clinical resistance to illness. It appears, therefore, that immune mechanisms are not the primary determinants of protection from Norwalk virus.

Diagnosis, treatment, and prevention Radioimmunoassays and an enzyme-linked immunosorbentassay (ELISA) have been developed for Norwalk virus and several other 27- to 30-nm gastroenteritis agents. These tests are not yet available commercially. Norwalk illness is acute and self-limited; treatment is not usually required. In the rare case of severe vomiting or diarrhea, oral or intravenous rehydration is indicated. Because long-term immunity to Norwalk illness does not usually follow natural infection, it seems unlikely that a vaccine will be developed.

MISCELLANEOUS ENTERIC VIRAL PATHOGENS Enteric adenoviruses are a minor (~10 percent) cause of diarrheal illness in infants and children. These viruses differ from other adenovirus strains in a variety of ways including neutralization serotype, restriction endonuclease digestion pattern, and their ability to grow in tissue culture. The role of enteric adenovirus illness in adults or in less developed countries is not known.

Several strains of antigenically distinct rotaviruses, presently called "atypical rotaviruses" or group B and C rotaviruses, have been identified as the cause of occasional episodes of diarrhea in humans and animals.

Corona viruses are frequent causes of diarrheal disease in a variety of animals. Several investigators, using electron microscopy, have identified putative corona virus–like particles in the stools of patients with diarrhea. In most cases, however, these particles do not have the typical morphologic features of corona viruses and may represent bacterial breakdown products or cellular fragments.

REFERENCES

Black RE et al: A two-year study of bacterial, viral and parasitic agents associated with diarrhea in rural Bangladesh. J Infect Dis 142:660, 1980

Brandt CD et al: Pediatric viral gastroenteritis during eight years of study. J Clin Microbiol 18:71, 1983

Kapikian AZ et al: Rotaviruses, in *Virology*, B Fields (ed). New York, Raven Press, 1985, pp 863–906

——— et al: Norwalk group of viruses, in *Virology*, B Fields (ed). New York, Raven Press, 1985, pp 1495–1518

Kaplan JE et al: Epidemiology of Norwalk gastroenteritis and the role of Norwalk virus in outbreaks of acute non-bacterial gastroenteritis. Ann Intern Med 96:756, 1982

Morse DL et al: Widespread outbreaks of clam- and oyster-associated gastroenteritis. Role of Norwalk virus. N Engl J Med 314:678, 1986

Vesikari T et al: Protection of infants against rotavirus diarrhea by RIT 4237 attenuated bovine rotavirus strain vaccine. Lancet 1:977, 1984

146 MUMPS

C. GEORGE RAY

DEFINITION Mumps is an acute communicable disease of viral origin characterized by painful enlargement of the salivary glands and sometimes by involvement of the gonads, meninges, pancreas, and other organs.

ETIOLOGY The causative agent of mumps is a paramyxovirus of intermediate size (120 to 200 nm in diameter). It has a tight helical inner core (RNA) enclosed in an outer envelope of lipid and protein. The virus of mumps has two components capable of fixing complement. These are the soluble, or S, antigens derived from the nucleocapsid, and the V antigen derived from the surface hemagglutinin. The virus can be cultivated in chick embryos and in a variety of mammalian cell cultures.

EPIDEMIOLOGY Human beings are the only natural host for mumps. The disease is worldwide and is endemic in urban communities. Epidemics are relatively infrequent and are usually confined to closely associated groups who live in orphanages, army camps, or schools. The disease is most frequent in the spring, particularly during April and May. Although mumps is generally considered less "contagious" than measles and chickenpox, this difference may be more apparent than real because many mumps infections (at least 25 percent) tend to be inapparent clinically. In some surveys, 80 to 90 percent of an adult population had serologic evidence of previous infection with mumps. By 1985, the incidence of mumps in the United States had reached its lowest point since reporting began

(2982 cases). However, an alarming resurgence took place in the ensuing 2 years and almost 12,900 cases were reported in 1987.

Infections are rare before the age of 2 years and then increase in frequency, peaking at ages 10 to 19. Clinical mumps may be more common in males than in females. The virus is transmitted in infected salivary secretions, although its isolation from urine suggests that it may also spread via this route. Mumps virus is rarely isolated from stool. The saliva is infectious for approximately 6 days prior to the onset of parotitis, and virus has been recovered from this site for as long as 2 weeks after onset of parotid swelling. Viruria also persists for 2 to 3 weeks in some patients. Despite this prolonged secretion of virus, the peak of infectivity occurs a day or two before onset of parotitis and subsides rapidly after the appearance of glandular enlargement.

One attack of clinical or subclinical mumps confers lasting immunity, and second attacks are most unusual. Unilateral parotitis affords protection just as effectively as does bilateral disease.

PATHOGENESIS The virus enters via the respiratory route; during the incubation period of 12 to 25 days it presumably replicates in the upper respiratory tract and cervical lymph nodes, from which it is disseminated via the bloodstream to other organs, including the meninges, gonads, pancreas, breasts, thyroid, heart, liver, kidneys, and cranial nerves. The salivary adenitis is thought by many to be secondary to viremia, but primary spread from the respiratory tract has not been ruled out as an alternative mechanism.

MANIFESTATIONS **Salivary adenitis** The onset of parotitis is usually sudden, although it may be preceded by a prodromal period of malaise, anorexia, chilly sensations, feverishness, sore throat, and tenderness at the angle of the jaw. In many cases, however, parotid swelling is the first indication of illness. The glands enlarge progressively over a period of 1 to 3 days, and the swelling resolves within a week after maximal enlargement. The swollen gland extends from the ear to the lower portion of the mandibular ramus and to the inferior portion of the zygomatic arch, often displacing the ear upward and outward. The skin over the gland is usually not warm or erythematous, in contrast to bacterial parotitis. There may be reddening and pouting of the orifice of Stensen's duct. Usually, pain and tenderness are marked, although at times they are absent. The edema of mumps has been described as "gelatinous," and when the involved gland is tweaked, it rolls like jelly. Swelling may involve only the submaxillary and sublingual glands and may extend over the anterior part of the chest, producing *presternal edema*. Involvement of submaxillary glands alone can cause difficulty in distinguishing mumps from acute cervical adenitis. Swelling of the glottis occurs rarely but may require tracheostomy. Parotitis is bilateral in two-thirds of cases and remains confined to one side in the remainder. The second gland tends to swell as the first is subsiding, usually 4 to 5 days after onset. In general, parotitis is accompanied by a temperature of 37.8 to 39.4°C (100 to 103°F), malaise, headache, and anorexia, but systemic symptoms may be virtually absent, particularly in children. In most patients, the chief complaints refer to difficulty in eating, swallowing, and talking.

Epididymoorchitis Mumps is complicated by orchitis in 20 to 35 percent of postpubertal males. Testicular involvement usually appears 7 to 10 days after onset of parotitis, although it may precede it or appear simultaneously. Occasionally, orchitis occurs in the absence of parotitis. Gonadal involvement is bilateral in 3 to 17 percent of patients. Orchitis is heralded by recrudescence of malaise and appearance of chilly sensations, headache, nausea, and vomiting. Shaking chills and high fevers, with temperatures between 39.4 to 41.1°C (103 and 106°F), are frequent. The testicle becomes greatly swollen and acutely painful. The epididymis is often palpable as a swollen tender cord. Occasionally there may be epididymitis without orchitis. Swelling, pain, and tenderness persist for 3 to 7 days and gradually subside; lysis of fever usually parallels abatement of swelling. Occasionally, the temperature falls by crisis. Mumps orchitis is followed by progressive atrophy of the testicle in one-half the cases. Even after bilateral orchitis, sterility is unusual, provided no significant atrophy has taken place. However, if bilateral testicular atrophy occurs after mumps, sterility or subnormal sperm counts are quite common. Plasma testosterone levels are depressed during acute orchitis but return to normal with recovery. *Pulmonary infarction* has been noted to follow mumps orchitis. This may be the result of thrombosis of the veins in the prostatic and pelvic plexuses in association with the testicular inflammation. Priapism is a rare but painful complication of mumps orchitis.

Pancreatitis Pancreatic involvement is a potentially serious manifestation of mumps, which may rarely be complicated by shock or pseudocyst formation. It should be suspected in patients with abdominal pain and tenderness together with clinical or epidemiologic evidence of mumps. It is difficult to document, since hyperamylasemia, the hallmark of pancreatitis, is also often present in parotitis. Many times the symptoms resemble those of gastroenteritis. Although diabetes or pancreatic insufficiency rarely follows mumps pancreatitis, several children have developed "brittle" diabetes a few weeks after mumps.

Central nervous system involvement Approximately 60 percent of patients with clinical mumps have an increased number of cells, usually lymphocytes, in the cerebrospinal fluid (CSF), while 10 percent will have symptoms of meningitis: stiff neck, headache, and drowsiness. In typical cases, the onset of overt central nervous system signs and symptoms occurs 3 to 10 days after the onset of parotitis; however, CNS mumps may develop prior to the parotitis or 2 to 3 weeks later. In approximately 30 to 40 percent of laboratory-proven cases, there is *no* associated salivary gland involvement at any time in the course of illness. The CSF protein is moderately elevated, and CSF glucose tends to be normal, although in as many as 10 percent of patients low CSF glucose concentrations, in the range of 1.1 to 2.8 mmol/L (20 to 50 mg/dL), may be seen. True encephalitis is unusual, although it is responsible for most of the central nervous system sequelae, including behavioral disturbances, headaches, seizures, deafness (usually unilateral), and visual disturbances. Rarely, aqueductal stenosis and hydrocephalus have been reported as possible late sequelae to mumps encephalitis, but the association remains unproven. Mumps should also be recognized as capable of presenting a picture of mild paralytic poliomyelitis; definition of the cause depends on isolation of virus or serologic confirmation of mumps in the absence of changing antibody titers to poliomyelitis viruses. Rarely, mumps may produce a transverse myelitis, cerebellar ataxia, or the Guillain-Barré syndrome. Mumps meningitis, without clinical encephalitis, is generally thought to be benign.

Other manifestations Mumps virus tends to involve glandular tissues; inflammation of the lacrimal glands, thymus, thyroid, breasts, and ovaries occurs occasionally. *Oophoritis* may be recognized by persistence of pain in the lower part of the abdomen and fever. It does not result in sterility. Mumps virus has been implicated in the causation of subacute thyroiditis; the diagnosis can be made serologically, and occasionally the virus can be isolated from the thyroid gland. Myxedema following mumps thyroiditis has been reported. Ocular manifestations of mumps include dacryoadenitis, optic neuritis, keratitis, iritis, conjunctivitis, and episcleritis. Although these conditions may transiently interfere with vision, complete resolution is the rule. Mumps *myocarditis,* evidenced primarily by transient abnormalities in the electrocardiogram, is relatively common. On rare occasions it can be fatal but it does not usually produce symptomatic disease or impair cardiac function. Similarly, *hepatic* involvement may be manifested by mild abnormalities in liver function, but icterus and other clinical signs of hepatic damage are extremely rare. *Thrombocytopenic purpura* as a complication of mumps has been described, and an occasional patient has a leukemoid reaction involving predominantly lymphocytes. Tracheobronchitis and interstitial pneumonia have also been associated with mumps infection, particularly among young children.

A rare but interesting manifestation of mumps is *polyarthritis* which is often migratory. It is most common in males between the ages of 20 and 30. Joint symptoms begin 1 to 2 weeks after subsidence of parotitis; usually the large joints are involved. The illness lasts 1 to 6 weeks, and complete recovery is the rule. It is not clear whether arthritis is due to viremia or whether it is a "hypersensitivity reaction."

Acute hemorrhagic glomerulonephritis in the absence of streptococcosis has been reported after mumps. The relationship of these two diseases is not clear.

Late complications With the exception of the rare central nervous system complications and occasional patients who become sterile following bilateral testicular involvement, mumps leaves no sequelae. However, persistent mumps infection may be a cause of inclusion body myositis, a chronic inflammatory myopathy that occurs primarily in the sixth decade.There is no firm evidence that offspring with congenital defects are more common among mothers who have mumps during pregnancy. Likewise, the causal relationship between intrauterine mumps infection and endocardial fibroelastosis has not been clearly established. Mumps illness during the first trimester of pregnancy has been associated with an increased risk of spontaneous abortion.

LABORATORY FINDINGS In uncomplicated parotitis, the blood leukocyte count is normal, although there may be mild leukopenia with relative lymphocytosis. Patients with mumps orchitis, however, may have a marked leukocytosis with a shift to the left. In meningoencephalitis, the white blood cell count is usually within normal limits. The erythrocyte sedimentation rate is usually normal but may rise with testicular or pancreatic involvement. The serum amylase level is elevated both in pancreatitis and in salivary adenitis. It may also be elevated in some patients in whom the sole evidence of mumps is meningoencephalitis, and probably reflects subclinical involvement of the salivary glands. In contrast to the amylase, the serum lipase level is elevated only in pancreatitis, in which hyperglycemia and glucosuria also may occur. The cerebrospinal fluid contains 0 to 2000 cells per microliter, almost all mononuclear, although occasionally polymorphonuclear cells will predominate in the early stages. The pleocytosis in mumps meningitis tends to be greater than in aseptic meningitides caused by the polio-, coxsackie-, and echoviruses. There is no relationship between the cell count and the severity of central nervous system involvement. Transient hematuria and mild reversible abnormalities in renal function, including inability to concentrate the urine maximally and to clear creatinine, occur in association with the viruria of mumps.

DIAGNOSIS The definitive diagnosis of mumps depends on isolation of the virus from blood, throat swabs, secretions from Stensen's duct, cerebrospinal fluid, or urine. Immunofluorescence methods can detect positive cell cultures in 2 to 3 days rather than the 6 days required with standard methods. In addition, immunofluorescence can be utilized for rapid detection of the viral antigen directly in oropharyngeal cells. Serologic determination of acute infection or susceptibility can be done by a variety of methods. The best test is the enzyme-linked immunosorbent assay (ELISA). Immunofluorescent assays are also commonly available, and can be used for identification of IgM- and IgG-specific antibody responses. The complement fixation test can be employed to quantitate antibody responses to the S and V antigenic components for the diagnosis of acute or recent mumps infection. Antibodies to the S antigen develop rather rapidly, often reaching a peak within 1 week after the onset of symptoms, and usually disappear in 6 to 12 months. Complement-fixing antibodies to the V antigen reach a peak titer within 2 to 3 weeks after onset, remain elevated for at least 6 weeks, and then persist at lower levels for years afterward. Paired serums obtained 2 to 3 weeks apart are recommended. A fourfold increase in titer by any standard assay confirms recent infection. When an acute serum is not obtained until later in the course of illness, an elevation of antibodies to the S antigen which exceeds the V antibody titer or the presence of IgM-specific antibody suggests recent infection. The *skin test* consists of intradermal injection of killed mumps virus; previous exposure will result in a delayed reaction of the tuberculin type and an anamnestic antibody titer rise to mumps. The skin test is unreliable when used alone in determining the immune status of an individual, is useless in the diagnosis of acute mumps, and is no longer commercially available in the United States.

The diagnosis of mumps during an epidemic is usually obvious. Sporadic cases, however, must be distinguished from other causes of parotid enlargement. Parotitis may be caused by other viruses, notably parainfluenza, influenza, and coxsackieviruses. *Bacterial parotitis* usually occurs in debilitated patients with severe underlying diseases, such as uncontrolled diabetes mellitus, cerebrovascular accidents, or uremia. It may also follow surgical operations. The parotid glands are swollen, warm, and tender, and pus can be expressed from the orifices of Stensen's ducts. Marked polymorphonuclear leukocytosis is present. The disease is usually acquired in the hospital, and *Staphylococcus aureus* is the usual causative organism. Dehydration followed by inspissation of secretions in the salivary ducts is an important predisposing factor. *Calculus* in a salivary duct is usually detectable by palpation or by injection of radiopaque media into Stensen's duct. *Drug reactions* may produce tender swelling of the parotid and other salivary glands. "Iodine mumps" is the most common type; it may follow such procedures as intravenous urography. The antihypertensive agent guanethidine may also cause parotid enlargement and tenderness. A careful history usually serves to clarify the cause of these reactions. *Cervical adenitis* caused by streptococci, "bullneck" diphtheria, infectious mononucleosis, cat-scratch disease, sublingual cellulitis (Ludwig's angina), and cellulitis of the external auditory canal are usually easy to distinguish from mumps by careful examination. Parotid tumors and chronic infections such as actinomycosis tend to follow a more indolent course, with slowly progressive swelling. The common "mixed tumor" of the parotid is well-circumscribed, nontender, and very firm, almost cartilaginous on palpation. Parotid swelling and fever, often accompanied by lacrimal adenitis and uveitis (Mikulicz's syndrome), may occur in tuberculosis, leukemia, Hodgkin's disease, and lupus erythematosus. The onset may be sudden, but the process is usually painless and of long duration. "Uveoparotid fever" of similar type may be the first manifestation of sarcoidosis; in this disease parotid swelling is frequently accompanied by single or multiple palsies of cranial nerves, particularly the facial nerve, and is referred to as Heerfordt's syndrome. Presternal edema may also be a manifestation of malignant lymphoma involving retrosternal lymph nodes. Bilateral painless parotid swelling unassociated with fever is found in patients with Laennec's cirrhosis, chronic alcoholism, malnutrition, diabetes mellitus, pregnancy and lactation, and hypertriglyceridemia.

Sjögren's syndrome (see Chap. 273) is a chronic inflammation of the parotid and other salivary glands which is often associated with atrophy of the lacrimal glands and occurs most commonly in women past the menopause. With cessation of lacrimal and salivary function, there may be striking dryness of the conjunctiva and the cornea (keratoconjunctivitis sicca) and of the mouth (xerostomia). These patients may also have a variety of systemic manifestations, including rheumatoid arthritis, splenomegaly, leukopenia, and hemolytic anemia. The chronicity of the process and its occurrence in elderly women make confusion with mumps unlikely. Finally, benign hypertrophy of both masseter muscles, presumably due to habitual clenching and grinding of teeth, may be confused with painless parotid swelling.

The causes of aseptic meningitis are discussed in Chap. 355.

Orchitis occurring in the absence of parotitis is likely to remain undiagnosed. Serologic testing may later confirm the diagnosis of mumps. Orchitis may occur in association with acute bacterial prostatitis and seminal vesiculitis. It is a rare complication of gonorrhea. Occasionally testicular inflammation accompanies pleurodynia, leptospirosis, melioidosis, tuberculosis, relapsing fever, chickenpox, brucellosis, and lymphocytic choriomeningitis. *Chlamydia trachomatis* should also be considered in the differential diagnosis of epididymitis.

TREATMENT There is no specific treatment for infections with the mumps virus. Patients with parotitis should receive mouth care, analgesics, and a bland diet. Bed rest is advisable only as long as the patient is febrile; contrary to popular belief, physical activity has no influence on the development of orchitis or other complications. Patients with epididymoorchitis may be acutely ill and in great pain. Many forms of treatment, including surgical decompression of the testicle, infiltration of the spermatic cord with local anesthetics, estrogens, convalescent serum, and broad-spectrum antibiotics, have not been regularly effective. Despite failure to document their effectiveness in controlled studies, glucocorticoids have been of considerable benefit in diminishing fever and testicular pain and swelling, and in restoring the sense of well-being in a number of patients. It is important to give a large initial daily dose corresponding to 60 mg prednisone. Subsequently, administration of the hormone can be tapered over 7 to 10 days. Glucocorticoids have not exerted an adverse effect on concomitant pancreatitis or meningitis, although they have not benefited patients with meningeal involvement, and their withdrawal has usually been accompanied by a recrudescence of symptoms. They have not prevented the appearance of parotid involvement on the contralateral side. Mumps arthritis is usually mild and requires no treatment. Mumps thyroiditis may subside spontaneously, but excellent relief has been obtained with glucocorticoids.

PREVENTION A live attenuated mumps virus vaccine (Jeryl Lynn strain) has been highly effective in producing significant rises in mumps antibody in individuals who are seronegative prior to vaccination, and has afforded 75 to 95 percent protection to individuals subsequently exposed to mumps. The vaccine also has boosted antibody levels in vaccinated individuals who are seropositive. The vaccine produces an inapparent, noncommunicable infection. Parotitis after vaccination has been reported only rarely, and central nervous system dysfunction has not been proved to be a complication. It has conferred excellent protection for at least 17 years and has not interfered with vaccines against measles, rubella, and poliomyelitis or with smallpox vaccination given simultaneously. Protection has been demonstrated in both children and adults.

Live mumps vaccine can be administered at any time after 1 year of age, and should be considered particularly for children approaching puberty, adolescents, and adults born after 1956 who have not had clinical mumps or live mumps vaccine in the past. Individuals living in groups or in institutions should be vaccinated, particularly because it has been shown that physical isolation of mumps patients does not effectively prevent transmission of the infection.

Vaccination is contraindicated in babies under the age of 1 year because of the interfering effect of maternal antibody; in individuals with a history of hypersensitivity to vaccine components; in patients with febrile illnesses, leukemia, lymphoma, or generalized malignancies; in those receiving glucocorticoids, alkylating drugs, antimetabolites, or irradiation; and during pregnancy.

It is not known whether the vaccine will prevent infection when administered after exposure, but no contraindication to its use in this situation exists. Neither mumps immune globulin nor ordinary gamma globulin has been shown to be effective in postexposure prophylaxis, and neither is recommended.

REFERENCES

BEARD CM et al: The incidence and outcome of mumps orchitis in Rochester Minnesota 1935 to 1974. Mayo Clin Proc 52:3, 1977

CHOU SM: Inclusion body myositis: A chronic persistent mumps myositis? Hum Pathol 17:765, 1986

COCHI SL et al: Perspective on the relative resurgence of mumps in the United States. Am J Dis Child 142:499, 1988

GORDON SC, LAUTER CB: Mumps arthritis: Unusual presentation as adult Still's disease. Ann Intern Med 97:45, 1982

KAPLAN KM et al: Mumps in the workplace. JAMA 260:1434, 1988

LEVITT LP et al: Central nervous system mumps: A review of 64 cases. Neurology 20:829, 1970

SHEHAB ZM et al: Epidemiological standardization of a test for susceptibility to mumps. J Infect Dis 149:810, 1984

147 RABIES, RHABDOVIRUSES, AND MARBURG-LIKE AGENTS

LAWRENCE COREY

RABIES

DEFINITION Rabies is an acute viral disease of the central nervous system that affects all mammals and that is transmitted by infected secretions, usually saliva. Most exposures to rabies are through the bite of an infected animal, but on occasion a virus aerosol or the ingestion or transplantation of infected tissues may initiate the disease process.

ETIOLOGY The rabies virus is a bullet-shaped, enveloped, single-stranded ribonucleic acid virus of 75- to 80-nm diameter belonging to the rhabdovirus group. The envelope glycoproteins are arranged in knoblike structures, which cover the surface of the virion. The viral glycoproteins bind to acetylcholine receptors, contribute to the neurovirulence of rabies virus, elicit neutralizing and hemagglutination-inhibiting antibodies, and stimulate T-cell immunity. The nucleocapsid antigen induces a complement-fixing antibody. Neutralizing antibodies to the surface glycoproteins appear to be protective. Antirabies antibodies used in diagnostic immunofluorescent assays are generally directed against the nucleocapsid antigens. Isolates of rabies virus from different animal species and locales differ in their antigenic and biologic properties. These variations may account for differences in virulence between isolates. Interferon is induced by rabies virus, particularly in those tissues with high virus concentrations, and may play some role in retarding progressive infection.

EPIDEMIOLOGY Rabies exists in two epidemiologic forms: *urban,* propagated chiefly by unimmunized domestic dogs and/or cats, and *sylvatic,* propagated by skunks, foxes, raccoons, mongooses, wolves, and bats. Infection in domestic animals usually represents a "spillover" from sylvatic reservoirs of infection, and human beings can be infected by either. Hence, human infection tends to occur in locales where rabies is enzootic or epizootic, where there is a large population of unimmunized domestic animals, and where human contact with the outdoors is common. While only about 1000 rabies deaths are reported to the World Health Organization (WHO) each year, the worldwide incidence of rabies is approximated at over 30,000 cases per year. Southeast Asia, the Philippines, Africa, the Indian subcontinent, and tropical South America are areas where the disease is especially common. In some endemic areas 1 to 2 percent of autopsied patients show evidence of rabies. Increased spread of terrestrial rabies and increased travel to countries where urban rabies is present has made recognition of clinical rabies and its prevention of increasing importance. In the United States human rabies is exceedingly rare, and only 9 cases have been reported since 1980, 5 of which originated from exposures in countries where canine rabies was endemic.

In most areas of the world, the dog is the important vector of rabies virus for humans. However, the wolf (eastern Europe, arctic regions), the mongoose (South Africa, the Caribbean), the fox (western Europe), and the vampire bat (Latin America) may also be prominent vectors of the disease. Rodents and lagomorphs are rarely infected with rabies. In the United States, rabies in wildlife accounts for about 85 percent of the reported animal rabies, with dogs and cats comprising only about 2 and 3 percent, respectively. However, most cases of postexposure prophylaxis are associated with dog bites. Many human cases of rabies in U.S. citizens have resulted from domestic animal bites that occurred outside the country.

Several cases of human-to-human transmission of rabies through corneal transplantation have been documented.

PATHOGENESIS The first event is the introduction of live virus through the epidermis or onto a mucous membrane. Initial viral replication appears to occur within striated muscle cells at the site of inoculation. The peripheral nervous system is exposed at the neuromuscular and/or neurotendinal spindles. The virus then spreads centripetally up the nerve to the central nervous system, probably via peripheral nerve axoplasm. Experimentally, viremia has been shown to occur, but is not thought to play a role in naturally acquired disease. Once the virus reaches the central nervous system, it replicates almost exclusively within the gray matter and then passes centrifugally along autonomic nerves to reach other tissue—the salivary glands, adrenal medulla, kidney, lung, liver, skeletal muscle, skin, and heart. Passage into the salivary glands facilitates further transmission of the disease via infected saliva. The incubation period of rabies is exceedingly variable, ranging from 10 days to over 1 year (mean 1 to 2 months). The time period appears to depend upon the amount of virus introduced, the amount of tissue involved, host defense mechanisms, and the actual distance that the virus has to travel from the site of inoculation to the central nervous system. Host immune responses and viral strains may also influence disease expression. Cell-mediated immune responses were noted in patients with rabies encephalitis but were absent in patients with paralytic rabies.

The neuropathology of rabies resembles other viral diseases of the central nervous system: hyperemia, varying degrees of chromatolysis, nuclear pyknosis, and neuronophagia of the nerve cells; infiltration by lymphocytes and plasma cells of the Virchow-Robin space; microglial infiltration, and parenchymal areas of nerve cell destruction. The pathognomonic lesion of rabies is the Negri body. This eosinophilic mass, approximately 10 nm in size, is made up of a finely fibrillar matrix and rabies virus particles. Negri bodies are distributed throughout the brain, particularly in Ammon's horn, the cerebral cortex, the brainstem, the Purkinje cells of the cerebellum, and the dorsal spinal ganglia. Negri bodies are not demonstrated in at least 20 percent of rabies, and their absence in brain material does not rule out the diagnosis.

MANIFESTATIONS The clinical manifestations of rabies can be divided into four stages: (1) a nonspecific prodrome, (2) an acute encephalitis similar to other viral encephalitides, (3) a profound dysfunction of brainstem centers which produces the classic features of rabies encephalitis, and (4) rarely, recovery.

The prodromal period usually persists for 1 to 4 days and is marked by fever, headache, malaise, myalgias, increased fatigability, anorexia, nausea and vomiting, sore throat, and a nonproductive cough. The prodromal symptom suggestive of rabies is the complaint of paresthesias and/or fasciculations at or about the site of inoculation of virus and may be related to the multiplication of virus in the dorsal root ganglion of the sensory nerve supplying the area of the bite. This symptom is present in 50 to 80 percent of patients.

The encephalitic phase is usually ushered in by periods of excessive motor activity, excitation, and agitation. Quickly, confusion, hallucinations, combativeness, bizarre aberrations of thought, muscle spasms, meningismus, opisthotonic posturing, seizures, and focal paralysis appear. Characteristically, the periods of mental aberration are interspersed with completely lucid periods, but as the disease progresses, the lucid periods get shorter until the patient lapses into coma. Hyperesthesia, with excessive sensitivity to bright light, loud noise, touch, and even gentle breezes, is very common. On physical examination the temperature may be found to be as high as 40.6°C (105°F). Abnormalities of the autonomic nervous system include dilated, irregular pupils, increased lacrimation, salivation, perspiration, and postural hypotension. Evidence of upper motor neuron paralysis with weakness, increased deep tendon reflexes, and extensor plantar responses is the rule. Paralysis of the vocal cords is common.

The manifestations of brainstem dysfunction begin shortly after the onset of the encephalitic phase. Cranial nerve involvement causes diplopia, facial palsies, optic neuritis, and the characteristic difficulty with deglutition. The combination of excessive salivation and difficulty in swallowing produces the traditional picture of "foaming at the mouth." Hydrophobia, the painful, violent involuntary contraction of the diaphragm, accessory respiratory, pharyngeal, and laryngeal muscles initiated by swallowing liquids, is seen in about 50 percent of cases. Involvement of the amygdaloid nucleus may result in priapism and spontaneous ejaculation. The patient lapses into coma, and involvement of the respiratory center produces an apneic death. The prominence of early brainstem dysfunction distinguishes rabies from other viral encephalitides and accounts for the rapid downhill course. The median survival after the onset of symptoms is 4 days, with a maximum of 20, unless artificial supporting measures are instituted.

If intensive respiratory support is used, a number of late complications may appear and include inappropriate secretion of antidiuretic hormone, diabetes insipidus, cardiac arrythmias, vascular instability, adult respiratory distress syndrome, gastrointestinal bleeding, thrombocytopenia, and paralytic ileus. Recovery is very rare, and when it occurs, has been gradual.

Occasionally, rabies may present as an ascending paralysis resembling the Landry-Guillain-Barré syndrome (dumb rabies, *rage tranquille*). This clinical pattern occurs most frequently in those bitten by vampire bats or who have received postexposure rabies prophylaxis.

The difficulty of suspecting rabies when it is associated with ascending paralysis is illustrated by the documentation of person-to-person transmission of the virus by tissue transplantation. Corneal transplants from donors who died of presumed Landry-Guillain-Barré syndrome have produced clinical rabies and death in the recipient. Retrospective pathologic examinations of the brains of both patients demonstrated Negri bodies, and rabies virus was subsequently isolated from each donor's frozen eye.

LABORATORY FINDINGS Early in the disease the hemoglobin and routine blood chemistries are normal, but abnormalities occur as hypothalamic dysfunction, gastrointestinal bleeding, and other complications ensue. The peripheral white blood cell count is usually slightly elevated (12,000 to 17,000 per microliter) but may be normal or as high as 30,000 per microliter.

As in any viral infection, the specific diagnosis of rabies depends upon (1) the isolation of virus from infected secretions [saliva, rarely cerebrospinal fluid (CSF), or tissue (brain)], (2) the serologic demonstration of acute infection, or (3) the demonstration of viral antigen in infected tissue, e.g., corneal impression smears, skin biopsies, or brain. Samples of brain obtained either on postmortem examination or from brain biopsy should be subjected to (1) mouse inoculation studies for virus isolation, (2) fluorescent-antibody (FA) staining for viral antigen, and (3) histologic and/or electron-microscopic examination for Negri bodies. While the mouse inoculation studies for virus isolation and direct FA staining for viral antigen are quite reliable and sensitive, if the patient's life has been prolonged and high levels of neutralizing antibody are present in serum and CSF, "autosterilization" may occur, and these tests may be negative. The use of FA staining of skin biopsies, corneal impression smears, and saliva for evidence of rabies antigen has been helpful in diagnosing rabies during life. Confirmation of these findings either serologically or by demonstration of virus in brain should be sought.

If the patient has not received antirabies immunization, a fourfold rise in neutralizing antibody to rabies virus in serial serum samples is diagnostic. If the patient has received rabies vaccination, a clue to the diagnosis may be obtained from the absolute titers of serum-neutralizing antibody and the presence of neutralizing antibody to rabies in CSF. Postexposure rabies prophylaxis rarely produces CSF-neutralizing antibody to rabies. If present, it is usually in low titer, e.g., less than 1:64, whereas CSF titers in human rabies may vary from 1:200 to 1:160,000.

DIFFERENTIAL DIAGNOSIS There is little to distinguish rabies from other viral encephalitides, and the most helpful point in diagnosis is the history of exposure. Other problems to be considered include hysterical reactions to animal bites (pseudohydrophobia), Landry-Guillain-Barré syndrome, poliomyelitis, and allergic encephalomyelitis to rabies vaccine. The latter occurs most commonly after use of nerve tissue–derived vaccine and usually begins 1 to 4 weeks after vaccination.

PREVENTION AND TREATMENT Each year more than 1 million Americans are bitten by animals. In each instance, a decision must be made whether to initiate postexposure rabies prophylaxis. When deciding whether to institute rabies prophylaxis, the following considerations apply: (1) whether the individual came into physical contact with saliva or another substance likely to contain rabies virus; (2) whether rabies is known or suspected in the species and area associated with the exposure (e.g., all persons within the continental United States bitten by a bat that then escapes should receive postexposure prophylaxis); (3) the circumstances surrounding the exposure; and (4) the treatment alternative and complications. A guide for postexposure rabies prophylaxis is illustrated in Fig. 147-1.

If rabies is known to be present or suspected to be present in the animal species involved in a human exposure, the animal should be captured, if possible. Wild animals or any ill, unvaccinated, or stray domestic animal involved in a rabies exposure, particularly any animal involved in an unprovoked bite, exhibiting abnormal behavior, or suspected of being rabid, should be killed, and the head should be sent immediately to an appropriate laboratory for rabies FA examination. If examination of the brain by the FA technique is negative for rabies, it can be assumed that the saliva contains no virus, and the exposed person need not be treated. Persons exposed to escaped wild animals capable of carrying rabies (bats, skunks, coyotes, foxes, raccoons, etc.) in an area where rabies is known or suspected to be present should receive both passive and active immunization against rabies.

If a healthy dog or cat bites a person, the animal should be captured, confined, and observed for 10 days. If any illness or abnormal behavior develops in the animal during the observation period, it should be killed for FA examination.

Postexposure prophylaxis Once a decision regarding the necessity to initiate postexposure rabies prophylaxis has been made, the general principle of postexposure therapy is to minimize the amount of virus at the site of inoculation with local treatment of the wound and to establish an early and long-lasting neutralizing antibody titer to rabies virus. In most instances, this includes administration of globulin and vaccines. The following is a therapeutic regimen:

1 *Local wound therapy*. This is an important part of rabies prevention. The wound should be scrubbed with soap and then flushed with water. Both mechanical and chemical cleansing are important. Quaternary ammonium compounds such as 1 to 4% benzalkonium chloride or 1% cetrimonium bromide are useful because they inactivate the rabies virus. However, 0.1% benzalkonium solutions are less effective than 20% soap solutions. Usually tetanus toxoid and antibiotics should be administered.
2 *Passive immunization with antirabies antiserum* of either equine or human origin. Human rabies immune globulin (RIG) is preferred because equine antiserum may cause serum sickness. Fifty percent of the total dose of 20 units per kilogram for RIG and 40 units per kilogram for the equine antiserum is given by local infiltration of the wound, and the rest is administered intramuscularly into the gluteal region.
3 *Active immunization with antirabies vaccine*. Human diploid cell vaccine (HDCV) is the recommended rabies vaccine. HDCV is an inactivated whole-virus vaccine prepared from a laboratory strain of rabies virus grown in human diploid cell cultures. Severe reactions to HDCV are uncommon. Immediate hypersensitivity responses such as urticaria have been reported in approximately 1 in 650 recipients. Systemic reactions such as fever, headache, and nausea are generally mild and are reported in 1 to 4 percent of recipients. Local reactions such as swelling, erythema, and induration at the injection site occur in 15 to 20 percent of vaccinees.

Five 1-mL doses of HDCV are given intramuscularly as soon as possible after exposure. The first dose (day 0) should also be accompanied by antirabies serum (RIG) in the gluteal area. HDCV

FIGURE 147-1 Postexposure rabies prophylaxis algorithm.

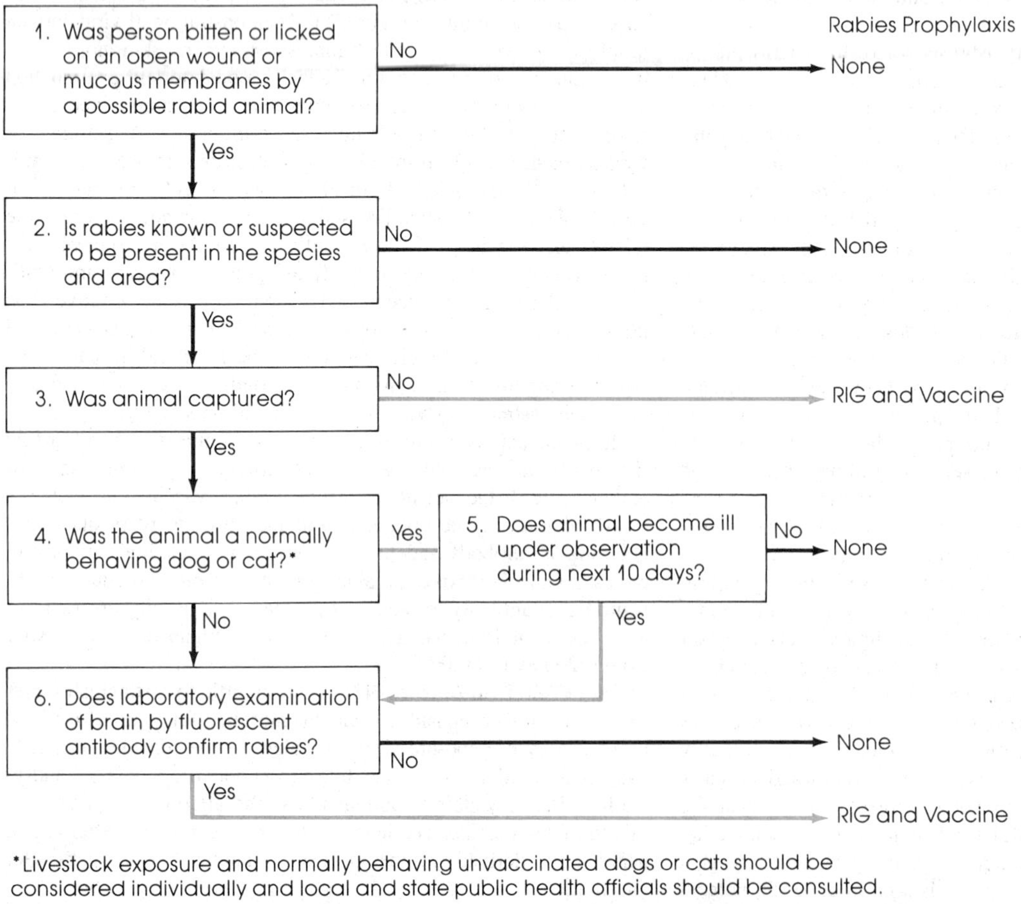

should be given intramuscularly in the deltoid area; five doses should be administered within 28 days on the following schedule: days 0, 3, 7, 14, and 28. The WHO also recommends a 21- and 90-day course.

The combination of RIG and HDCV produces high titers of neutralizing antibodies in almost all recipients. Only rarely has this regimen proved unsuccessful in preventing the subsequent development of rabies. The administration of vaccine alone appears to be associated with a higher failure rate than RIG and HDCV, especially in severe bite exposures. The combination of RIG plus 0.1-mL intradermal doses at eight sites on day 0, four sites on day 7, and one site on days 28 and 91 produces good antibody responses, although the clinical experience with this regimen is less than with intramuscular administration.

Preexposure prophylaxis Individuals with a high risk of contact with rabies virus—veterinarians, cave explorers, laboratory workers, and animal handlers—should have preexposure prophylaxis with rabies vaccine. HDCV is the preferred vaccine for preexposure prophylaxis; three IM or three 0.1-mL intradermal injections on days 0, 7, and 28 should be administered. A neutralizing antibody titer should be checked after vaccination. Concomitant chloroquine administration interferes with the antibody response to vaccine. Booster doses may be administered either as a single 1-mL intramuscular or 0.1-mL intradermal injection. Postexposure prophylaxis in individuals previously given preexposure therapy consists of HDCV vaccine alone (two IM doses of HDCV on days 0 and 3 are usually adequate).

Booster doses of HDCV are associated with fever, headache, muscle aches, and joint pains in about 20 percent of recipients. Up to 6 percent of persons receiving IM booster doses of HDCV have developed an immune-complex-like reaction characterized by urticaria, arthritis, nausea, vomiting, and, occasionally, angioedema. These reactions have been self-limited and appear to be less with infrequent administration of booster doses. Persons who work in high-risk areas should undergo periodic measurement of antibodies, and booster doses are recommended for those with low antibody titers. Those at very low risk may elect not to receive routine booster doses but only to receive active immunization with any substantive exposure.

MOKOLA VIRUS

Mokola virus was first isolated from wild shrews captured in Nigeria and subsequently was shown to be related morphologically and serologically to rabies. However, neither of the two reported cases of human disease (both children) demonstrated classic clinical features of rabies. One patient had a nonfatal illness characterized by fever, pharyngitis, and convulsions. Mokola virus was recovered from her cerebrospinal fluid. The second patient initially had fever, cough, and vomiting, followed in several days by drowsiness, confusion, and generalized flaccid weakness. Her cerebrospinal fluid was normal. She progressed to deep coma and died within 10 days of onset. Mokola virus was isolated from her brain, and histopathologic sections revealed finely granular cytoplasmic inclusions that were distinguishable from Negri bodies in many neurons.

VESICULAR STOMATITIS VIRUS

Vesicular stomatitis is a viral illness of animals which can occasionally infect humans. It presents as an acute self-limited influenza-like disease. The disease in animals is found in the United States and South America and affects chiefly domestic cattle, horses, swine, wild deer, raccoons, skunks, and bobcats.

In animals, vesicular stomatitis is characterized by the development of vesicles on the oral mucosa, particularly the tongue, udders, and heels. The mode of spread is probably by direct contact; however, epidemics tend to occur in warm weather, and the virus has been isolated from *Phlebotomus* sandflies in Panama and *Äedes* species in New Mexico, suggesting these as possible vectors. Two distinct serotypes, New Jersey and Indiana, have been recognized, and most of the outbreaks in North America have been attributed to the New Jersey strain. The disease is most common in laboratory workers, and in one report three-fourths of laboratory personnel handling experimentally infected animals or manipulating the virus developed neutralizing antibodies. The disease is transmissible, however, under natural conditions among workers having direct contact with infected animals, especially cattle. The incubation period ranges from 1 to 6 days. This is followed by the sudden onset of fever up to 40°C (104°F), chills, profuse sweating, myalgias, malaise, headache, and pain on ocular movement. One-third to one-half of patients have sore throat and cervical and/or submandibular adenopathy. Small raised vesicular lesions may appear on the buccal mucosa. Conjunctivitis and coryza are present in about 20 percent of cases. Occasionally, small subcorneal, intraepithelial vesicles may appear on the fingers, usually associated with direct inoculation of the virus. Symptoms generally last 3 to 4 days, but occasionally a diphasic course may occur. Inapparent infection is common, and among laboratory workers with serologic evidence of infection, only about one-half reported clinical symptoms. In some areas of Panama, 17 to 35 percent of the population have neutralizing antibodies against vesicular stomatitis virus.

The differential diagnosis includes hand-foot-and-mouth disease, herpangina, primary herpetic pharyngitis and other mucocutaneous syndromes, and influenza. Viral isolation from patients is not common; however, a rise in complement fixation and/or neutralizing antibodies to vesicular stomatitis virus between acute and convalescent serums will help to confirm the diagnosis. Treatment is nonspecific.

MARBURG VIRUS DISEASE

DEFINITION Marburg virus causes an acute systemic febrile illness characterized by the abrupt onset of headache, myalgias, pharyngitis, rash, and hemorrhagic manifestations. It was recognized first in 1967 when it caused simultaneous outbreaks in the Federal Republic of Germany and Yugoslavia among laboratory workers exposed to imported African green monkeys (*Cercopithecus aethiops*). Outbreaks have been reported from Kenya. The clinical manifestations are similar to other hemorrhagic fevers of the arenavirus class or flavivirus group (Argentina and Bolivian hemorrhagic fever, Chap. 149). The high case fatality rate and demonstrated ability for nosocomial spread has made recognition of this rare agent an important worldwide public health concern.

ETIOLOGY The Marburg virus has been isolated in guinea pig and various cell culture systems such as vervet monkey kidney. The virus particle contains lipid and RNA, and under the electron microscope the virus appears as an 80- to 100-nm elongated filamentous particle with occasional "blister-like excrescences." Marburg and Ebola viruses have been included in a new family of viruses called Filoviridae. These viruses are biosafety level 4 pathogens, and maximum biologic containment facilities are recommended.

EPIDEMIOLOGY The initial outbreak affected 31 patients in Marburg and Frankfurt, Germany, and Belgrade, Yugoslavia, and was epidemiologically linked to monkeys imported from the same source in Uganda. Virus was isolated from the blood and tissue of these monkeys. Of the 25 primary infections, there were seven deaths. Six secondary cases, involving two physicians, one nurse, a postmortem attendant, and the wife of a veterinarian, occurred. Person-to-person transmission was felt to take place via accidental needle sticks or abrasions, although respiratory and conjunctival infection could not be ruled out. The wife of one patient developed Marburg virus disease. Marburg virus was demonstrated in semen of the original patient, despite the presence of circulating antibody, and this secondary case is believed to have been acquired through sexual intercourse. The natural reservoir of Marburg virus is unknown.

Serologic survey for virus showed primates and guinea pigs to be susceptible to infection.

PATHOLOGY Marburg virus appears "pantropic" and produces lesions in almost all organs including lymphoid tissue, liver, spleen, pancreas, adrenals, thyroid, kidney, testes, skin, and brain. In lymphoid tissue focal necrosis with degeneration of lymphoid tissue is apparent. In the liver, eosinophilic cytoplasmic bodies resembling the Councilman bodies of yellow fever have been noted. The lungs may show interstitial pneumonitis, as well as vascular lesions in small arterioles indicative of endarteritis. Neuropathologic changes consist of multiple small hemorrhagic infarcts with glial proliferation.

CLINICAL MANIFESTATIONS After an incubation period of 3 to 9 days, patients develop the abrupt onset of frontal and temporal headache, malaise, myalgias, especially in the lumbar area, nausea, and vomiting. Fever of 39.4 to 40°C (103 to 104°F) is characteristic, and about half the patients have conjunctivitis. Between 1 and 3 days after onset, watery diarrhea, which is often severe, lethargy, and a change in mentation are noted. An enanthem of the palate and tonsils and cervical lymphadenopathy may also be noted during the first week of illness. The most reliable clinical feature is the appearance of nonpruritic maculopapular rash which begins on the fifth to seventh day on the face and neck and spreads centrifugally to involve the extremities. A fine desquamation of the affected skin, especially the palms and soles, appears 4 to 5 days later. Hemorrhagic manifestations, including gastrointestinal, renal, vaginal, and/or conjunctival hemorrhages, generally develop between days 5 and 7 of disease.

During the first week, the temperature continues in the vicinity of 40°C (104°F), falling by lysis during the second week, to increase again between the twelfth and fourteenth days. Other clinical signs apparent in the second week of disease include splenomegaly, hepatomegaly, facial edema, and scrotal or labial reddening. Complications include orchitis, which may lead to testicular atrophy, myocarditis with irregular pulse and electrocardiographic abnormalities, and pancreatitis. The overall case fatality rate has been about 25 percent, with death usually occurring during the eighth to sixteenth days of illness. Recovery is often protracted over a 3- to 4-week period, and during this period loss of hair, intermittent abdominal pain, poor appetite, and prolonged psychotic disturbances have been noted. Late sequelae including transverse myelitis and uveitis have been reported. Marburg virus has been isolated from the anterior eye chamber and semen nearly 3 months after onset of disease.

LABORATORY FINDINGS Abnormalities in granulocyte function are found, and leukopenia is detected as early as the first day, with leukocyte counts as low as 1000 per microliter and a neutrophilia by the fourth day. Subsequently, atypical lymphocytes, as well as neutrophils exhibiting the characteristic of the Pelger-Huet anomaly, may appear. Thrombocytopenia appears early and is most marked, often less than 10,000 cells per microliter, between the sixth and twelfth days. In fatal cases, evidence of disseminated intravascular coagulation can be demonstrated. Hypoproteinemia, proteinuria, and azotemia may occur. Elevations in serum glutamic oxaloacetic transaminase (SGOT) and alanine aminotransferase (SGPT) are usual. Lumbar puncture may be normal or reveal a minimal pleocytosis. The erythrocyte sedimentation rate is usually low.

DIAGNOSIS The characteristic clinical course and epidemiologic features are the basis of the diagnosis. Specific diagnosis requires isolation of the virus or serologic evidence of infection in paired serum samples. Viremia coincides with the febrile state of disease, and virus has been isolated from tissue as well as urine, semen, throat, and rectal swabs. Attempts to isolate virus must be carried out only in *specialized high-security laboratories*. All patients should be kept in strict isolation, and all specimens should be handled and shipped according to World Health Organization guidelines.

TREATMENT Patients have received a multiplicity of drugs without apparent influence on the course of the illness. Convalescent serum was administered to four patients, whose subsequent disease followed a mild course. However, similarly benign outcomes were observed in patients who did not receive serum.

EBOLA VIRUS

Between July and November 1976 simultaneous outbreaks of an acute febrile hemorrhagic disease occurred in southern Sudan and northern Zaire. "Secondary and tertiary" spread of infection, particularly among hospital staff, was noted. In the Sudan over 300 cases with 151 deaths and in Zaire 237 cases with 211 fatalities were reported. The virus isolated from these patients was morphologically similar to but antigenically distinct from the Marburg agent. The name Ebola virus, after the river in Zaire located near the epidemic, has been proposed. Biologic and antigenic differences between strains of Ebola viruses isolated in Zaire and Sudan may account for the differences in mortality between the two outbreaks. Sporadic cases of disease also appear to occur, and a serosurvey revealed a prevalence rate of 7 percent for antibodies to Ebola virus in endemic areas. As with other hemorrhagic fevers, neutrophil leukocytosis, hypofibrinoginemia, thrombocytopenia, and microangiopathic hemolytic anemia are features of the illness.

Ebola virus has been propagated in tissue culture (vero cells) and in suckling mice and guinea pigs. The source of the outbreak in both the Sudan and Zaire is unknown; however, as with other viral hemorrhagic fevers, peridomestic rodents are suspected as being a reservoir of the infection, and serologic evidence of Ebola virus infection was detected in a domestic guinea pig trapped in Zaire. Once established, nosocomial as well as community-acquired cases occur, especially among those with close and prolonged contact. Parenteral exposure to the virus through disinfected rather than sterilized needles may have played a role in transmission. Barrier nursing and strict isolation precautions using protective clothing appeared to decrease the number of nosocomial cases.

CLINICAL MANIFESTATIONS Clinically, the disease is similar to Marburg virus disease. The incubation period ranges from 4 to 6 days (mean is 7 days). Patients usually present on the fifth day of illness with a history of abrupt onset of headache, malaise, myalgias, high fever, diarrhea, abdominal pain, dehydration, and lethargy. Pleuritic chest pain, a dry hacking cough, and a pronounced pharyngitis were also noted. A maculopapular eruption develops between days 5 to 7 of illness. On black skins the rash is often faint and not recognized until desquamation occurs. Hematemesis, melena, and bleeding from the nose, gums, and vagina are common. Abortion and massive metrorrhagia was a frequent complication among pregnant women. Death usually occurs in the second week of illness and is preceded by severe blood loss and shock.

TREATMENT Patients should be isolated until virologic studies indicate they are free of virus, usually 21 days from onset of illness. Malaria parasites were frequently found in blood films of patients with Ebola virus infection in the Sudan indicating that the presence of parasitemia does not rule out concomitant viral illness. Treatment with plasma containing Ebola virus–specific antibodies has resulted in diminished levels of viremia; however, further tests are required to establish the effectiveness of this form of therapy. Requests for viral isolation as well as convalescent plasma should be addressed to WHO Regional Centers in Atlanta or Geneva.

REFERENCES

Rabies

BAER GM: Research towards rabies prevention: Overview. Rev Infect Dis 10 (Suppl 4):S576, 1988

———, Fishbein DB: Rabies post exposure prophylaxis. N Engl J Med 316:1270, 1987

BERNARD KW et al: Preexposure immunization with intradermal human diploid cell rabies vaccine. JAMA 257:1059, 1987

HOUFF SA et al: Human-to-human transmission of rabies virus by a corneal transplant. N Engl J Med 300:603, 1979

PAPPAIVANOU M et al: Antibody response to preexposure diploid-cell rabies vaccine given concurrently with chloroquine. N Engl J Med 314:280, 1986

Recommendations of the Public Health Service, Immunization Practices Advisory Committee (ACIP): Rabies prevention. United States. MMWR 38(13):205, 1989

SHILL M et al: Fatal rabies encephalitis despite appropriate post exposure prophylaxis. N Engl J Med 316:1257, 1987
WARRELL DA, WARRELL MJ: Human rabies and its prevention: An overview. Rev Infect Dis 10 (Suppl 4):S726, 1988

Mokola virus

FAMILUSI JB: Fatal human infection with Mokola virus. Am J Trop Med Hyg 21:959, 1972

Marburg virus

SIMPSON DH: Marburg and ebola virus infections: A guide for their diagnosis, management and control. Geneva, WHO Offset Publication 36, 1977
SMITH DH et al: Marburg-virus disease in Kenya. Lancet 1:816, 1982

Ebola virus

McCORMICK JB et al: Biologic differences between strains of Ebola virus from Zaire and Sudan. J Infect Dis 147:264, 1983
STANSFIELD SK: Antibody to Ebola virus in guinea pigs: Tandala, Zaire. J Infect Dis 146:483, 1982

148 ARBOVIRUS INFECTIONS

JAY P. SANFORD

Most viral infections in humans are either asymptomatic or present as undifferentiated illnesses characterized by fever, malaise, headache, and generalized myalgia. The similarities in clinical features between infections caused by viruses as dissimilar as the myxoviruses (e.g., influenza), the enteroviruses (e.g., poliovirus, coxsackievirus, echovirus), some of the herpesviruses (e.g., cytomegalovirus), and the arboviruses usually preclude an etiologic diagnosis based entirely on clinical manifestations without ancillary information regarding epidemiologic features and serologic findings. The purpose of this chapter is to define viral illness transmitted to humans by biting insects. Because the number of agents is large, mention will be made of those which have been best documented, have demonstrated unusual features, or seem to be of greatest potential public health importance.

DEFINITION AND CLASSIFICATION The definition of an arthropod-borne virus (arbovirus) was published in 1967 by the World Health Organization:

Arboviruses are viruses which are maintained in nature principally, or to an important extent, through biological transmission between susceptible vertebrate hosts by hematophagous arthropods; they multiply and produce viremia in the vertebrates, multiply in the tissues of arthropods, and are passed on to new vertebrates by the bites of arthropods after a period of extrinsic incubation.

From this definition it can be appreciated that the term *arbovirus* is used in the ecologic sense. Transmission by vectors is not correlated with virus architecture. Current approaches to taxonomy are based upon viral morphology, structure, and function. As a result, for taxonomic purposes, the term *arbovirus* has been eliminated.

The more than 250 antigenically distinct ''arboviruses'' are now grouped into six families (Table 148-1). The majority of agents contain single-stranded RNA, although some, such as the Reoviridae, contain double-stranded RNA.

''Arboviruses'' are of importance in both temperate and tropical zones. Representative viruses have been isolated in almost every geographic area outside the polar regions.

''Arbovirus'' infection of vertebrates is usually asymptomatic. The viremia stimulates an immune response which sharply limits the duration of the viremia. In ''arbovirus'' infections other than urban yellow fever, phlebotomus fever, chikungunya, o'nyong-nyong, mayaro, oropouche, dengue, and possibly Ross River virus, infection of humans represents an incidental occurrence which is tangential to the basic maintenance cycle of the virus. Hence, the isolation of

TABLE 148-1 Virus taxonomy and arboviruses-arenaviruses*

Family	Genus	Virus ''English vernacular name''†
Reoviridae	Orbivirus	Colorado tick fever‡ Orongo Kemerovo

Togaviridae	Alphavirus (group A)	Eastern equine encephalitis‡
		Venezuelan encephalitis‡
		Western equine encephalitis‡
		Sindbis
		Semliki Forest complex
		  Chikungunya‡
		  O'nyong-nyong
		  Ross River‡
		  Mayaro

	Flavivirus (group B)	*Associated with encephalitis*
		St. Louis encephalitis‡
		Japanese encephalitis‡
		Murray Valley encephalitis‡
		Tick-borne encephalitis complex‡
		  Russian spring-summer encephalitis
		  Central European encephalitis
		  Negishi
		  Powassan‡
		  Louping-ill
		Rocio

		Associated with fever-arthralgia-rash Dengue fever‡ West Nile fever‡ Nine other agents–not of major public health importance
		Associated with hemorrhagic fever Yellow fever‡ Dengue fever‡ Omsk hemorrhagic fever Kyasanur Forest disease
Rhabdoviridae	Vesiculovirus	Vesicular stomatitis Indiana‡ Vesicular stomatitis New Jersey‡ Cocal Chandipura Piry Isfahan
	Lyssavirus	Rabies‡ Mokola Duvenhage
Filoviridae		Marburg‡ Ebola‡

Bunyaviridae	Bunyavirus (16 serogroups)	Twenty-four agents may cause fever, fever-rash. None cause death. None in United States.
		California serogroup
		  LaCrosse‡
		  Snowshoe hare
		  Jamestown Canyon
		  California encephalitis
		  Tahyna
		  Inkoo

	Phlebovirus	Thirty-seven phleboviruses isolated from human beings; none cause death except Rift Valley fever virus. Sandfly fever–Naples‡ Sandfly fever–Sicilian‡ Rift Valley fever‡
	Nairovirus	Crimean-Congo hemorrhagic fever‡
	Not yet established	Hantaan‡ Puumala‡ Prospect Hill‡ Tchoupitoulas‡
Arenaviridae	Arenavirus	Lymphocytic choriomeningitis‡ Lassa‡ Machupo‡ Junin‡

* Only agents which have been shown to naturally infect humans are tabulated.
† Virus species have not yet been designated formally. The International Committee on Taxonomy of Viruses lists species under the term ''English vernacular name.''
‡ Viruses found in the United States and/or of major public health importance.

TABLE 148-2 Major clinical syndromes,* associated arboviruses-arenaviruses, and major geographic distribution

Virus	Geographic distribution
FEVER, ARTHRALGIA, RASH	
Chikungunya	Africa, southeast Asia
O'nyong-nyong	East Africa
Ross River	Australia, Fiji, Samoa, Cook Islands, New Guinea
Sindbis	Africa, U.S.S.R., Finland, Sweden
Mayaro	South and Central America
Dengue fever	Tropical Asia, Oceania, Africa, Australia, Americas
West Nile fever	Africa, Middle East, U.S.S.R., France, India, Indonesia
Lymphocytic choriomeningitis	United States, Germany, Hungary, Argentina
ENCEPHALITIS/ASEPTIC MENINGITIS	
Kemerovo	Central Europe
Eastern equine encephalitis	Atlantic, Gulf coasts, United States, upper New York, Caribbean, western Michigan
Venezuelan equine encephalitis	Northern South America, Central America, Mexico, Florida
Western equine encephalitis	United States, Canada, Central and South America
Semliki Forest	Africa
St. Louis encephalitis	United States, Caribbean
Japanese encephalitis	Japan, Korea, China, India, Philippines, southeast Asia, eastern U.S.S.R.
Murray Valley encephalitis	Australia
Rocio	Brazil
Omsk hemorrhagic fever	U.S.S.R.
Kyasanur Forest disease complex	India
Negishi	Japan
Powassan	New York, eastern Canada
Louping ill	United Kingdom, Ireland
Russian spring-summer encephalitis	U.S.S.R.
Central European encephalitis	Eastern Europe, Scandinavia, France, Switzerland
California group	North America
Tahyna	Europe
Inkoo	Europe
Phlebotomus fever	Mediterranean basin, Balkans, Near and Middle East, east Africa, central Asia, Pakistan, parts of India, southern China, Panama, Brazil
Rift Valley fever	South and east Africa
Lymphocytic choriomeningitis	United States, Germany, Hungary, Argentina
HEMORRHAGIC FEVER	
Yellow fever	South America, Africa
Dengue	Caribbean, southeast Asia
Chikungunya	Southeast Asia
Kyasanur Forest disease	India
Omsk hemorrhagic fever	U.S.S.R.
Crimean-Congo hemorrhagic fever	Africa, eastern Europe, Middle East, Asia
Hantaan	Korea, Japan, Scandinavia, U.S.S.R., central Europe
Marburg	Uganda, Kenya, Zimbabwe
Ebola	Zaire, Sudan
Lassa fever	West Africa
Machupo	Bolivia
Junin	Argentina

* Most agents are more often associated with undifferentiated febrile illness than with the specific syndromes. See text for exceptions.

virus from arthropod vectors or the detection of infection in the natural vertebrate host may provide a means for early detection and enable control of epizootic infection before significant spread to humans occurs.

Most human "arbovirus" infections are asymptomatic. When disease is produced, the spectrum of clinical illness is varied both in predominant features and in severity. Most commonly, disease is self-limited with symptoms of fever, headache, malaise, and myalgia. Associated lymphadenopathy may be a feature. "Arboviruses" which may cause three major clinical syndromes—arthralgia-arthritis, encephalitis–aseptic meningitis, or hemorrhagic disease—are tabulated in Table 148-2.

"ARBOVIRUS" INFECTIONS PRESENTING CHIEFLY WITH FEVER, MALAISE, HEADACHE, AND MYALGIA

PHLEBOTOMUS FEVER Phlebotomus (sandfly, pappataci, or 3-day) fever is an acute, relatively mild, self-limited infection caused by at least five immunologically distinct phleboviruses (Naples, Sicilian, Punta Toro, Chagres, and Candiru). Serologic evidence of human infection has been demonstrated for four additional agents (Bujaru, Cacao, Karimabad, and Salehabad). Humans, the only known host, probably serve as a dead-end host. Voles are suspected of being an endemic host in the Middle East.

Prevalence The disease occurs throughout the Mediterranean basin, the Balkans, the Near and Middle East, the eastern part of Africa, the Soviet republics of central Asia, Pakistan, parts of India, Panama, Brazil, and possibly certain parts of southern China. In the Middle East and central Asia native populations acquire the disease at an early age and develop and maintain high levels of immunity. Cases in Panama and Brazil are sporadic, occurring mainly in persons entering the forest. The apparent absence of phlebotomus fever in indigenous adult populations residing in areas where sandflies are abundant may present a deceptive picture of the actual risk to susceptible persons.

Epidemiology In the Middle East and central Asia, the disease occurs during the hot, dry season (summer or autumn months) and is transmitted to human beings by the bite of infected sandflies (*Phlebotomus papatasii*), which are small (2- to 3-mm) urban flies that can penetrate ordinary house screens. Only the female bites and usually does so during the night. In persons who are not sensitive, there is neither pain nor local irritation after the bite; hence only about 1 percent of patients will remember having been bitten. In contrast, most of the human-biting sandflies (*Lutzomyia* sp.) of tropical America are sylvan in their habits. Transovarial and transstadial transmission of the virus has been demonstrated and in view of the low-titered and transient viremia in humans suggests the phlebotomine fly is both vector and reservoir. In humans, the incubation period averages 3 to 5 days. Viremia is present for at least 24 h before the onset of fever, but is not detectable for more than 2 days after the onset of illness.

Clinical manifestations The onset of symptoms is abrupt in over 90 percent of patients, with the temperature rapidly rising to its highest point, which may vary from 37.8 to 40.1°C (100 to 105°F). Headache is nearly always present and often is accompanied by pain on moving the eyes and by retroorbital pain. Myalgia is common and may be localized to the chest, resembling pleurodynia, or to the abdomen. Other symptoms may include vomiting, photophobia, giddiness, neck stiffness, alteration or loss of taste, and arthralgia. Conjunctival injection is present in approximately one-third of patients. Small vesicles may be seen on the palate, and macular or urticarial rashes occur. The spleen is rarely palpable, and lymphadenopathy is absent. The pulse rate may be elevated in proportion to the temperature on the first day; thereafter bradycardia is often present. The fever persists 3 days in most patients, with gradual defervescence. Giddiness, weakness, and feelings of depression are frequently encountered during convalescence. Second attacks 2 to 12 weeks after the first occur in 15 percent of cases.

In common with other "arbovirus" infections, phlebotomus fever may be associated with *aseptic meningitis*. In one series, 12 percent of patients had symptoms and signs sufficient to warrant a lumbar puncture. Findings in these patients included pleocytosis, with an average cell count of 90 per microliter and a predominance of either polymorphonuclear or mononuclear leukocytes. Spinal fluid protein concentration ranged from 0.2 to 1.3 g/L (20 to 130 mg/dL). In another series mild papilledema was observed in a few patients with severe illness.

Laboratory findings The changes in leukocyte count constitute the only positive laboratory findings. Total leukocyte counts of less than 5000 per microliter are observed in 90 percent of patients if daily counts are done during the febrile period and convalescence. The leukopenia may not appear until the last day of fever or even after defervescence. The differential leukocyte count will reveal an absolute decrease in lymphocytes on the first day, accompanied by an increase in nonsegmented neutrophils. During the second or third day, the number of lymphocytes begins to return to normal and may constitute 40 to 65 percent of the total count. Concurrently, there is a reversal in proportion of segmented and band neutrophils. The differential count usually returns to normal within 5 to 8 days after defervescence. Erythrocyte values and urinalyses are usually normal.

Diagnosis In the absence of a specific serologic test, the diagnosis must be made on clinical and epidemiologic grounds.

Treatment The disease is self-limited, and no specific therapy is available. Symptomatic care, including bed rest, adequate fluid intake, and analgesia with aspirin, is recommended. Convalescence may require a week or longer.

Prognosis No fatalities have been recorded among tens of thousands of cases.

COLORADO TICK FEVER Colorado tick fever is one of the two tick-transmitted virus diseases of humans recognized in the United States and Canada, Powassan virus being the other. Though "mountain fever" had been described ever since the advent of immigrants to the Rocky Mountain region, it must be differentiated from mild Rocky Mountain spotted fever. Once the clinical picture of disease had been established, it was renamed Colorado tick fever. A second serotype of the Colorado tick fever serogroup (Eyach virus) was isolated from *Ixodes ricinus* ticks near the village of Eyach in West Germany.

Etiology Colorado tick fever virus is grouped as an "arbovirus" because it replicates in ticks. It is a double-stranded RNA virus belonging to the orbivirus genus of the Reoviridae family (see Table 148-1).

Prevalence The disease has been contracted in Colorado, Idaho, Nevada, Wyoming, Montana, Utah, eastern Oregon, Washington, California, northern Arizona and New Mexico, and Alberta and British Columbia. The possibility exists that Colorado tick fever may occur over a wider geographic area. Mild and clinically inapparent forms of the disease occur. Up to 15 percent of perennial campers have neutralizing antibodies. The number of cases of Colorado tick fever reported in Colorado is 20 times greater than that of Rocky Mountain spotted fever. In fact, almost one-half of the patients diagnosed as having Rocky Mountain spotted fever in Utah were subsequently shown to have Colorado tick fever.

Epidemiology Colorado tick fever is transmitted to humans by the adult hard-shelled wood tick, *Dermacentor andersoni*. The virus has been found in as many as 14 percent of this species of ticks collected in endemic areas. Transovarial transmission of the virus in the tick has been established. Illness occurs from late March through September, mostly in May and June. Virus can be recovered from blood for 2 weeks in most patients, for at least 1 month in nearly one-half, and from spinal fluid during the acute illness. The virus persists within erythrocytes of convalescent patients for as long as 120 days and can be readily isolated from washed erythrocytes 100 days following infection. Transfusion-associated Colorado tick fever has been reported.

Clinical manifestations The incubation period is usually 3 to 6 days, and in 90 percent a history of tick contact within 10 days of onset of illness can be obtained. Failure to obtain such a history militates against the diagnosis. Persons affected usually are those whose occupational or recreational activities bring them in contact with ticks. The disease may occur at any age, although 40 percent in one series were 20 to 29 years of age. The clinical picture is characterized by the sudden onset of severe aching of the muscles of the back and legs, chilliness without true rigors, a rapid increase in temperature, which usually reaches 38.9 to 40°C (102 to 104°F), headache with pain on ocular movement, retroorbital pain, and photophobia. Abdominal pain and vomiting occur in one-fourth of patients; diarrhea is rare. The physical findings are not specific. Tachycardia in proportion to the temperature, flushed facies, and variable conjunctival injection may be present. Occasionally the spleen is palpable. Rash occurs in only 5 percent of patients, but on occasion a petechial rash involving primarily the arms and legs or a maculopapular rash over the entire body may occur. Rarely, punched-out ulcers may form at the site of tick bite. The fever with the associated symptoms lasts about 2 days, then abruptly lyses to normal or subnormal, leaving the patient very weak. After an afebrile period of about 2 days, the fever recurs, may be higher than in the first phase, and may last as long as 3 days. One-half of patients show this saddleback pattern of temperature. Rarely there may be three febrile phases. Convalescence of more than 3 weeks is reported in 70 percent of patients over age 30, while symptoms last less than 1 week in 60 percent of patients under 20. Prolonged convalescence has no relationship to persistent viremia.

Evidence of central nervous system involvement has been recorded in a few patients. The findings are those of either an aseptic meningitis with stiffness of the neck or encephalitis with clouding of the sensorium, delirium, and coma. Rarer complications include epididymoorchitis and patchy pneumonitis.

Laboratory findings The most important laboratory feature is moderate to marked leukopenia, although in one-third of confirmed cases leukocyte counts remain about 4500 per microliter. On the first day of illness, the total leukocyte count may be at normal levels, but usually by the fifth or sixth day there has been a decrease to 2000 to 3000 per microliter. Characteristically there is a proportionate decrease in lymphocytes and granulocytes. Toxic changes in neutrophils are often conspicuous, and "virocyte" types of lymphocytes are frequently observed. Bone marrow examination reveals "maturation arrest" in the granulocytic series. Erythrocyte values remain normal. The blood picture returns to normal within a week after the fever subsides.

Diagnosis The diagnosis of Colorado tick fever is suspected on the basis of the epidemiologic history and clinical findings. Because of the infrequency of rash, patients who develop fever and rash after tick bites should be suspected of having Rocky Mountain spotted fever. The usual methods for confirming Colorado tick fever are mouse inoculation and fluorescent antibody (FA) staining of patients' erythrocytes; a combination of the two is best. Special handling of blood is not necessary for the FA test which remains positive for several weeks after clinical illness.

Treatment Treatment is entirely symptomatic.

Prognosis The prognosis is excellent.

Prevention Active immunity with an attenuated virus has been produced, but the immunization itself frequently produced mild disease. Colorado tick fever is best prevented by avoiding contact with the wood tick. Convalescent individuals should be excluded as blood donors for at least 6 months.

VENEZUELAN EQUINE ENCEPHALITIS Venezuelan equine encephalitis (VEE) was first noted in equines in Colombia in 1935.

Etiology Like other alphaviruses, the causative agent of VEE is a 40- to 45-nm, single-stranded RNA virus. Based on serologic tests and oligonucleotide fingerprints a complex of Venezuelan encephalitis viruses has been established: VE subtypes IA to IE, II (Everglades), III (Mucambo), and IV (Pixuna). IA was the original epidemic strain which occurred in Venezuela, and IB, which was recognized in Ecuador in 1963, spread through Central America into Mexico and was responsible for the epidemic in Mexico in 1971 which spread into southern Texas, with the occurrence of at least 76 laboratory-confirmed human cases. In early 1973, almost 4000 cases occurred in Peru.

Epidemiology VEE has been primarily a disease of equines and other mammals, although occasionally the agent has infected humans. Evidence of human infection (virus isolation or specific neutralizing antibodies) has been found in Colombia, Ecuador, Panama, Surinam, Guyana, French Guiana, Mexico, Brazil, Curaçao, Trinidad, Argentina, Peru, Florida, and Texas. Each subtype of VE virus is unique to its enzootic vector and does not replicate well in other vectors. Most common is an enzootic cycle between *Culex* mosquitoes and forest rodents. Enzootic VEE infects people who enter the rain forest or swamps, rubber tappers, forestry workers, and military personnel on jungle maneuvers. During an epizootic, many species of mosquitoes can transmit virus, especially *Aëdes, Mansonia,* and *Psorophora.* The virus has a wide host range in wild mammals, with at least 20 genera, including capuchin monkeys, rats, mice, opossum, jackrabbit, fox, and bats, being naturally infected. Domestic animals other than equines which have been shown to be infected include cattle and pigs in Mexico and goats and sheep in Venezuela. VEE appears to multiply well in mammals with high titers of virus in the blood; e.g., infected horses may have titers of up to $10^{7.5}$ mouse intraperitoneal lethal doses per milliliter of blood. Though 29 species of wild birds have been shown to be naturally infected with VEE (20 percent of which are colonial nestling herons and related species), whether the VEE-viremia levels in birds are high enough to infect vector mosquitoes is not known. During the initial 3 days of illness, viremia has been detected in approximately two-thirds of patients. The levels of viremia are sufficiently high that humans could serve as a reservoir. VEE virus also has been isolated by pharyngeal swab in a few patients, suggesting the potential for person-to-person transmission. The available observations make it reasonable to consider that the natural vector is a mosquito, with the primary reservoir being either wild or domestic terrestrial mammals. However, natural infection can probably take place without an arthropod vector. Laboratory infections have occurred and are probably due to inhalation of aerosols.

Clinical manifestations In humans, infection with VEE virus usually results in a mild acute febrile illness without neurologic complications. No age is spared, and there is no sex preponderance. The incubation period is 2 to 5 days, followed by the abrupt onset of headache, fever often associated with rigors, malaise, and myalgia. Other common symptoms may include nausea, vomiting, diarrhea, and sore throat. Uncommon features include photophobia, seizures, mental confusion, coma, tremors, and diplopia. Lymphadenopathy occurs in one-third of patients. On laboratory examination initial leukocyte counts are normal with 80 percent neutrophils. By the third day leukopenia occurs in two-thirds of patients. The cerebrospinal fluid may reveal pleocytosis with modest increases in protein and normal glucose concentration. Virus may be isolated both from blood and from cerebrospinal fluid. The symptoms usually last 3 to 5 days in mild cases and up to 8 days in more severe cases. A biphasic course of illness may be encountered, with recrudescence of symptoms on the sixth to the ninth day. In an epidemic in Venezuela in 1962, almost 16,000 cases of acute disease were evaluated; 38 percent were classified as encephalitis, but only 3 to 4 percent had severe neurologic abnormalities: convulsions, nystagmus, drowsiness, delirium, or meningitis. The mortality rate was estimated to be less than 0.5 percent, and nearly all deaths occurred in young children.

RIFT VALLEY FEVER Rift Valley fever is an acute disease principally of livestock, sheep, goats, cattle, and camels which is widespread throughout east and South Africa. It was first described in humans during an extensive epizootic of hepatitis in sheep in the Rift Valley in Kenya. During an epizootic in South Africa in 1950–1951, an estimated 20,000 humans became infected. Fatal human disease, four cases of hemorrhagic illness and hepatitis, was first reported during an epizootic in South Africa in 1975. In 1977 Rift Valley fever jumped the Sahara to Egypt with a major outbreak. Cases occurred in subsequent years until 1980; an estimated 200,000 cases with 598 reported deaths occurred in 1977.

Virus has been found in several species of mosquitoes: *Culex pipiens, Eretmapodites chrysogaster, Aëdes caballus, Aëdes circumluteolus,* and *Culex theileri. Culex pipiens* has been suggested as the vector in Egypt. While antibodies to Rift Valley fever have been found in wild field rats in Uganda, the reservoir is unknown. It has been suggested that the virus may be maintained by transovarial transmission in floodwater *Aëdes.* Although humans presumably can be infected by arthropods, many infections occur as a result of handling infected animal tissues. In addition, laboratory-acquired infections have been common, suggesting a respiratory route of transmission.

The incubation period is usually 3 to 6 days. The onset is abrupt, with malaise, chilly sensation or rigors, headache, retroorbital pain, and generalized aching and backache. The temperature rises rapidly to 38.3 to 40°C (101 to 104°F). Later complaints include anorexia, loss of taste, epigastric pain, and photophobia. Findings on examination are usually unremarkable except for flushing of the face and conjunctival injection. The temperature curve is often saddleback in type, with an initial elevation lasting 2 to 3 days, followed by a remission and second febrile period. Convalescence is typically rapid. Prior to the outbreak in Egypt, Rift Valley fever was a benign illness with almost no fatalities. In Egypt, approximately 1 percent of patients developed severe complications, such as encephalitis, retinopathy, or hemorrhagic manifestations. Encephalitis appeared as the acute infection waned and was severe with serious residua in some survivors. Generalized hemorrhages and icterus appeared as the disease evolved. Deaths from massive hepatic necrosis occurred 7 to 10 days after onset of illness. The fatality rate in severely ill patients may exceed 50 percent. Visual loss, including light perception, occurred 2 to 7 days after the onset of fever. Macular edema, hemorrhage, vasculitis, retinitis, and vascular occlusion were noted. One-half of patients had some permanent loss of visual acuity. A characteristic finding is an initial normal total leukocyte count followed by leukopenia with a decrease in neutrophils associated with an increase in band forms. The diagnosis is made by isolating the virus from the blood by inoculation of mice. Three-fourths of patients are viremic (up to 10^8 mouse intraperitoneal lethal doses per milliliter blood) when first seen. Neutralizing antibodies have been demonstrated as early as 4 days after onset. There is no specific treatment. A killed vaccine which had been stockpiled in the United States is being utilized.

ZIKA VIRUS Zika virus was first isolated from a captive rhesus monkey in Uganda and subsequently from wild mosquitoes. Serologic surveys reveal a prevalence of human infection up to 50 percent in central Africa and parts of Asia (Indonesia), but human disease is rarely reported. During investigation in eastern Nigeria of an outbreak of jaundice that was suspected of being yellow fever, Zika virus was isolated from one patient and two others had a rise in neutralizing antibodies. The symptoms in these patients included fever, arthralgia, and headache with retroorbital pain. Other findings were jaundice and albuminuria. The clinical syndrome appears to simulate mild yellow fever.

BUNYAVIRUSES The family Bunyaviridae consists almost entirely of viruses transmitted to vertebrate animals by arthropods. There are more than 200 viruses in the family, classified into five genera: Bunyavirus (formerly the Bunyamwera supergroup), Uukuvirus, Nairovirus, Phlebovirus, Hantavirus (Table 148-1). Most Bunyaviruses have not been associated with human infection or disease but 24 Bunyaviruses have been associated with febrile human disease which may or may not be associated with rashes. This includes the C group, Bunyamwera and Oropouche. The geographic distribution of C-group viruses includes Brazil, Trinidad, and Panama. Isolates have been obtained mostly from forest workers and laboratory technicians. Epidemics have not been recognized. The disease begins with headache, fever [with temperature up to 40.6°C (105°F)], and myalgia. Additional symptoms include malaise, photophobia, vertigo, and nausea. Illness is generally mild, lasting 2 to 4 days, and is occasionally followed by a relapse. No fatalities have been reported. Occasionally a prolonged period of convalescence ensues. Leukopenia, with total leukocyte counts as low as 2600 per microliter, is a common finding. Diagnosis has been established mainly by virus isolation.

Representative viruses of the Bunyamwera group are found in all inhabited continents except Australia. Only five viruses of the group—Bunyamwera itself, Germiston, Ilesha, Guaroa, and Wycomyia—have been associated with clinical disease. Serologic surveys give evidence of a high prevalence of inapparent infection in some areas. Clinical illness is characterized by low-grade fever, headache, and myalgia which last several days, and may be followed by weakness during convalescence. Infection due to Bunyamwera virus is associated often with arthralgia and sometimes with a rash. Since 1962 seven epidemics of Oropouche disease involving thousands of persons in Brazil, in the populated regions south of the Amazon River, have occurred during the rainy season. The epidemic vector is the midge of *Culicoides paraensis*. The incubation period is 4 to 8 days. Clinical features include abrupt onset of fever, usually to 39 to 40°C (102 to 104°F), with rigors. Symptoms, which include headache, photophobia, dizziness, myalgia, anorexia, nausea, and vomiting, last 2 to 5 days. Lymphadenopathy, splenomegaly, or rash have not been features. Laboratory findings include leukopenia with relative lymphocytosis. Urinalyses are normal. Mild elevations of transaminase may occur. Fatalities have not been reported.

"ARBOVIRUS" INFECTIONS PRESENTING CHIEFLY WITH FEVER, MALAISE, ARTHRALGIA, AND RASH

CHIKUNGUNYA In 1952 an epidemic of a disease occurred in Tanzania, which was given the name *chikungunya* ("that which bends up") because of the sudden onset of joint pains. An alphavirus of the Semliki Forest complex was isolated in 1956 both from serum of patients ill with the disease and from a pool of *A. aegypti* mosquitoes.

Chikungunya virus is responsible for a dengue-like illness in Africa, India, southeast Asia, New Guinea, and Guam, as well as for a rather mild form of hemorrhagic fever in Asian children. Outbreaks have been associated with high attack rates, with as many as 80 percent of inhabitants in some settlements becoming ill. In large epidemics, *Aëdes aegypti* is the vector. In Africa, virus is transmitted among monkeys and baboons by forest *Aëdes* mosquitoes, *A. africanus*. The cycle in southeast Asia has not been clearly defined, but humans may be the host.

After an incubation period of 3 to 12 days, the onset is typically abrupt, with a rapid rise in temperature to 38.9 to 40.6°C (102 to 105°F), often associated with a rigor and headache. Pain in large joints occurs early, incapacitating some individuals within a few minutes of onset. The arthralgia is often associated with objective arthritis. Sites of involvement include knees, ankles, shoulders, wrists, or proximal interphalangeal joints. Myalgia, especially backache, and malaise occur frequently. In 60 to 80 percent of patients a maculopapular eruption, which may appear at any time during the febrile course, is noted on the trunk or on the extensor surfaces of the extremities. Mild lymphadenopathy, predominantly in the axillary or inguinal areas, may be evident. Pharyngitis and conjunctival suffusion may be observed in a few patients. Fever continues for 1 to 10 days, and in some patients an afebrile interval of 1 to 3 days is followed by a second rise in temperature. The joint pains may continue after the temperature has returned to normal. In a few individuals joint pains have persisted for up to 4 months. Hematocrit values remain normal. Total leukocyte counts may be less than 5000 per microliter in some patients, while in others they remain normal. Urinalyses are normal. There is no specific antiviral treatment. Anti-inflammatory agents such as aspirin or indomethacin have been utilized. No second attacks have been recognized, and in the absence of the hemorrhagic fever syndrome, no deaths have been described.

MAYARO VIRUS DISEASE Outbreaks involving a number of persons have occurred in Brazil and Bolivia. Survey for antibodies in serums obtained from residents in Rio de Janeiro showed that almost one-third were positive. Mayaro virus has been isolated from a wild mosquito, *Mansonia venezuelansis*, and can be maintained serially in *A. aegypti* and *Anopheles quadrimaculatus*.

The incubation period has not been clearly defined but is about 1 week. Ages of patients have ranged from 2 to 62 years, with both sexes involved. Illness begins abruptly with fever, chills, severe frontal headache, myalgia, and dizziness. Temperatures usually exceed 40°C (104°F). Arthralgia occurs uniformly and is very prominent, occasionally incapacitating, and in some patients precedes the fever by a few hours. Involvement of the wrists, fingers, ankles, and toes predominates. Other initial symptoms (in less than one-third of patients) include nausea, vomiting, and diarrhea. Initial examination reveals inguinal lymphadenopathy (one-half of cases), swelling of affected joints (one-quarter of cases), and occasional conjunctival congestion. The initial clinical features last 3 to 5 days except the arthralgia, which may persist for 2 months. On about the fifth day a maculopapular rash develops over the chest, back, arms, and legs. Rash appeared in 90 percent of children and in one-half of adults and lasted about 3 days.

Laboratory findings include leukopenia with leukocyte counts as low as 2500 per microliter during the first week. Urinalysis revealed albuminuria (2+) in one-fourth of patients. Some patients showed slight elevations in serum glutamic oxaloacetic transaminase levels.

In Brazil, no relapses were observed and no deaths have been recognized. In Bolivia, more severe illness and several fatalities have been reported.

O'NYONG-NYONG FEVER O'nyong-nyong fever was first noted as an epidemic illness characterized by joint pains, rash, and lymphadenopathy in the northern province of Uganda in 1959. The agent is an alphavirus which shows close antigenic relationships with chikungunya viruses. The original outbreak was associated with an explosive epidemic which spread to Tanzania and other areas in east Africa. By 1961, 2 million cases were recorded. In some areas, 90 percent of the population had either clinical disease or inapparent infection. Local outbreaks extended over the entire year. All age groups were affected. The most likely vector is *Anopheles funestus*. The clinical features are similar to those of chikungunya virus infection. The disease disappeared in 1962. While the virus was isolated from *A. funestus* in Kenya in 1978, no further outbreaks have been recognized.

SINDBIS VIRUS Sindbis virus, once thought rarely to present as clinical disease, has been recognized in Africa (Uganda, Republic of South Africa), Australia, and Europe (U.S.S.R., Finland, and Sweden). In the U.S.S.R. it is known as Karelian fever, in Sweden as Okelbo disease, and in Finland as Pogosta disease. Clinically, fever is low-grade and accompanied by malaise, myalgia, and arthralgia involving joints and tendons. The most striking feature is a maculopapular rash appearing on the trunk and extremities but usually sparing the face. Unlike the rash of chikungunya or o'nyong-nyong, the rash often becomes vesicular, especially on the feet and hands.

ROSS RIVER VIRUS Epidemics of polyarthritis associated with rashes have been observed in Australia since 1928. Outbreaks occur almost entirely in the period December to June. Ross River virus infection was limited to Australia, New Guinea, and the Solomon Islands until 1979 when a major outbreak occurred in Fiji which spread to the Samoan, Cook, and some Melanesian Islands. In the Fiji outbreak in 1979, infection rates were equal at all ages and in both sexes, but clinical attack rates were 4 percent in patients under 20 years and 42 percent in adults, and the clinical attack rate of males to females was 1:1.7. The onset is characterized by headache, mild catarrh, and occasionally tenderness of the palms and soles. Initially fever may be absent or minimal [highest 38°C (100.4°F)]. In about one-half of patients, arthritis, involving mainly the small joints, wrists, and ankles and sometimes associated with swelling, and paresthesias precede a rash by 1 to 15 days. In the other half, the rash precedes the arthralgia. The rash, which lasts 2 to 10 days, is usually maculopapular, appears on the cheeks and forehead, occasionally spreads to the trunk, or may be restricted to the limbs.

The rash may be pruritic. Vesicles occur rarely. Tender lymphadenopathy occurs in one-fifth of the patients. Joint symptoms persist for 3 weeks to 3 months. The virus has been isolated from *Culex annulirostris* and *Aëdes vigilax*. Animals may serve as reservoir hosts in Australia. In the Pacific, person-mosquito-person transmission seems likely.

"ARBOVIRUS" INFECTIONS PRESENTING CHIEFLY WITH FEVER, MALAISE, LYMPHADENOPATHY, AND RASH

DENGUE FEVER Dengue is endemic over large areas of the tropics and subtropics, southeast Asia, the South Pacific, and Africa. Outbreaks of dengue have occurred in the Caribbean including Puerto Rico and the U.S. Virgin Islands since 1969. Approximately 3000 cases were reported in Mexico in 1979. Indigenous infection occurred in the United States for the first time in 35 years in 1980. Eleven cases have been recognized in residents of the Rio Grande valley of Texas. In the summer of 1981, 79,000 cases of dengue-like illness with 31 deaths were reported from Cuba. *Aëdes aegypti*, the vector, has reappeared along the U.S. Gulf Coast; hence, the threat of dengue along the Gulf Coast is real.

Etiology There are four distinct serogroups of dengue viruses, all of which are flaviviruses. In the Caribbean, type 1 was associated with the 1977–1978 outbreak, type 2 in 1968–1969, type 3 in 1963–1964, and type 4 was documented in the western hemisphere for the first time in 1981.

Epidemiology Dengue infections in nature involve primarily humans and *Aëdes* mosquitoes. Dengue transmission involving monkeys and forest *Aëdes* spp. has been documented in Malaysia and West Africa. *Aëdes aegypti* is the most important worldwide vector species. This species, as well as the less common vector species, is peridomestic, biting humans readily or even preferentially and breeding in small collections of water such as cisterns and backyard litter. Surveys in Texas have revealed containers with water in which *A. aegypti* were breeding in up to 25 percent of premises. They fly during the day. Humans appear to be uniformly susceptible, and susceptibility is not influenced by age, sex, or race. During outbreaks, attack rates may be very high; in Puerto Rico and the U.S. Virgin Islands, the overall rate of clinical illness was 20 percent, with infection rates as determined by serologic survey as high as 79 per 100.

Clinical manifestations Dengue viruses frequently produce inapparent infections in humans. When symptoms develop, three broad clinical patterns may be encountered: classic dengue, hemorrhagic fever (see below), and a mild atypical form. Classic dengue (breakbone fever) occurs primarily in nonimmune individuals, specifically nonindigenous adults and children. The usual incubation period is 5 to 8 days. Prodromal symptoms such as mild conjunctivitis or coryza may occur, followed in hours by the abrupt onset of a severe splitting headache, retroorbital pain, backache, especially in the lumbar area, and leg and joint pains. The headache is aggravated by movement. At least three-fourths of patients have ocular soreness, with pain on moving the eyes. A few have mild photophobia. Though true rigors are common during the course, they are usually not present at the onset. Additional symptoms include insomnia, anorexia with loss of taste or bitter taste, and weakness. Mild transient rhinopharyngitis occurs in as many as one-quarter of the individuals. Cough is almost never seen. Epistaxis has been observed. Examination reveals scleral injection (90 percent), tenderness upon pressure on the ocular globe, and nontender posterior cervical, epitrochlear, and inguinal lymphadenopathy. Over one-half of patients have an enanthem characterized initially by pinpoint-sized vesicles over the posterior half of the soft palate. The tongue is often coated. Skin rashes, varying from diffuse flushing to scarlatiniform and morbilliform, are frequently present over the thorax and inner aspects of the arms. These are transient and fade, only to be followed by a more definite maculopapular rash which appears on the trunk on the third to the fifth day and spreads peripherally. The rash may be pruritic and generally terminates with desquamation. Extreme bradycardia is not observed. Within 2 to 3 days after the onset, the temperature may decrease to nearly normal and other symptoms disappear. The remission typically lasts 2 days and is followed by return of fever and the other symptoms, although they are generally less severe than during the initial phase. This saddleback diphasic febrile course is considered characteristic, but often is not encountered. The febrile illness usually lasts 5 to 6 days and terminates abruptly. Complaints of fatigue for several weeks after infection are common.

In addition to this "classic" syndrome, an atypically mild illness may occur. Symptoms include fever, anorexia, headache, and myalgia. On examination, evanescent rashes may be seen, but lymphadenopathy is usually absent. The course is usually less than 72 h in duration.

At the onset both in classic and in mild dengue, the leukocyte counts may be low or normal; however, by the third to the fifth day, leukopenia, usually with counts of less than 5000 leukocytes per microliter, and neutropenia are the rule. Occasionally albuminuria of moderate degree occurs.

Diagnosis Inoculation of blood obtained within the first 3 to 5 days onto mosquito tissue cell cultures or inoculation into mosquitoes is used for primary viral isolation. Diagnosis can be made by serologic tests employing paired serums for hemagglutination inhibition tests and complement fixation tests. IgM antibodies are produced in primary dengue infections. Specific serologic diagnosis is complicated by cross-reactions with other flavivirus antibodies such as those following immunization with yellow fever vaccine.

Treatment Treatment is entirely symptomatic.

Prognosis In the absence of the dengue hemorrhagic fever or dengue shock syndrome, mortality is nil.

Prevention An attenuated vaccine for dengue type 2 is undergoing experimental evaluation. Control depends upon mosquito abatement.

WEST NILE FEVER West Nile virus is distributed throughout Africa, the Middle East, parts of Europe (Camargue, France), U.S.S.R., India, and Indonesia. It produces a clinical picture closely resembling dengue. Outbreaks of disease involving several hundred patients occurred in Israel in 1950 to 1952. In one outbreak, over 60 percent of the population developed overt disease.

Epidemiology The disease is highly endemic in Egypt but goes largely unrecognized. Presumably most of the adult population is immune, and the infection in childhood is an undifferentiated mild febrile illness, whereas in Israel it mainly affects adults. The infection occurs in the summer both in Israel and in Egypt. The transmission cycle in the Middle East is bird-mosquito-bird, with *Culex univittatus* and *Culex pipiens molestus* being the principal vectors. *Culex tritaeniorhynchus* is an important vector in Asia. Although humans and a variety of other vertebrates are infected by the virus, their involvement is tangential.

Clinical manifestations The incubation period is 1 to 6 days. Most of the patients in Israel have been young adults, with neither sex predominating. The onset is usually abrupt and without prodromal symptoms. The temperature quickly rises to 38.3 to 40°C (101 to 104°F), with chills occurring in one-third of patients. Symptoms include drowsiness, severe frontal headache, ocular pain, and pain in the abdomen and back. A small number of patients have anorexia, nausea, and dryness of the throat. Cough is uncommon. There are flushing of the face, conjunctival injection, and coating of the tongue. The prominent finding is general enlargement of lymph nodes, which are of moderate size but are not hard and are only slightly tender. Occipital, axillary, and inguinal nodes are usually involved. The spleen and liver are slightly enlarged in a small proportion of patients. In one-half of patients a rash may appear from the second to the fifth day of illness and may persist for several hours or until defervescence. The rash occurs predominantly over the trunk and consists of pale roseolar maculopapular lesions. The illness is self-limited and lasts 3 to 5 days in 80 percent of patients.

In a few patients, transitory meningeal involvement may be encountered. Spinal fluid examinations may reveal a pleocytosis and some increase in protein concentration.

Leukopenia occurs in the majority of patients, and total leukocyte counts are lower than 4000 per microliter in one-third. Differential counts vary from a moderate shift to the left to a slight lymphocytosis.

Convalescence is often prolonged, lasting 1 to 2 weeks, with prominent symptoms of fatigue. Enlargement of lymph nodes subsides over several months. Only rarely have complications, sequelae, or fatalities been seen in natural infections, although in one outbreak in a group of elderly patients a high proportion of patients developed meningoencephalitis, and four fatalities ensued.

Accurate diagnosis rests on virus isolation, which can be accomplished because viremia persists for as long as 6 days, or the demonstration of a rising specific antibody titer.

The treatment is symptomatic.

"ARBOVIRUS" INFECTIONS PRESENTING CHIEFLY WITH CENTRAL NERVOUS SYSTEM INVOLVEMENT

Four "arboviruses" are presently recognized as numerically important causes of central nervous system disease in the United States: St. Louis encephalitis virus (SLE), eastern equine encephalitis virus (EEE), western equine encephalitis virus (WEE), and the California serogroup (CE) viruses. The spectrum of infection caused by these agents includes inapparent infection, fever with headache, aseptic meningitis, and encephalitis. Some 1500 to 2000 cases of encephalitis are reported in the United States each year. In the absence of epidemics, 5 to 10 percent of these (75 to 200 cases) are confirmed as "arboviral" in etiology. In nonepidemic years, California serogroup viruses (predominantly LaCrosse virus) represent two-thirds to three-fourths of the cases. Because of epidemics of St. Louis and western equine encephalitis, which contribute a larger number of cases, the overall distribution in the 30 years between 1955 and 1984 has been: SLE 65 percent, CE 20 percent, WEE 13 percent, and EEE 2 percent.

Etiology Despite the diversity of specific viral etiologies (see Table 148-2), in individual patients the clinical manifestations of aseptic meningitis and encephalitis are very similar, and preclude an etiologic diagnosis without ancillary information regarding epidemiologic and serologic features (see Table 148-3). The clinical features of aseptic meningitis due to "arboviruses" are indistinguishable from those due to the more prevalent enteroviruses. Since transmission to humans in the United States and Canada involves arthropods, specifically mosquitoes, except for Powassan and Colorado tick fever, indigenously acquired disease occurs at times when mosquitoes are prevalent, such as late spring through early fall.

Clinical manifestations The clinical features of "arbovirus" encephalitis differ among age groups. In infants under 1 year of age, the only consistently noted symptoms are sudden onset of fever, which is often accompanied by convulsions. Convulsions may be either generalized or focal. Typically the fever ranges between 38.9 and 40°C (102 and 104°F). Other physical findings may include bulging of the fontanelle, rigidity of the extremities, and abnormalities in reflexes.

In children between 5 and 14 years of age, subjective symptoms are more easily elicited. Headache, fever, and drowsiness of 2 to 3 days' duration before medical attention is sought are common. The symptoms may then subside or become more intense and may be associated with nausea, vomiting, muscular pain, photophobia, and, less frequently, convulsions (less than 10 percent except in California encephalitis). The child is found to be acutely ill, febrile, and lethargic. Nuchal rigidity and intention tremors are often present, and on occasion muscular weakness can be demonstrated.

In adults, the initial symptoms commonly include the fairly abrupt onset of fever, nausea with vomiting, and severe headache. The headache is most often frontal but may be occipital or diffuse. Mental aberrations, represented by confusion and disorientation, usually appear within the subsequent 24 h. Other symptoms may include diffuse myalgia and photophobia. The abnormalities found on physical examination predominantly relate to the neurologic examination, although conjunctival suffusion is frequently seen and skin rashes may occur. Disturbances in mentation are among the most outstanding clinical features. These range from coma through severe disorientation to subtle abnormalities detected only by cerebral function tests such as the subtraction of serial 7s. A small proportion of patients show only lethargy, lying quietly, apparently asleep unless stimulated. Tremor is common and is observed more frequently in individuals over 40 years of age. The tremors vary in location and may be continuous or intention in type. Cranial nerve abnormalities resulting in oculomotor muscle paresis and nystagmus, facial weakness, and difficulty in deglutition may occur and are usually present within the initial several days. Objective sensory changes are unusual. Hemiparesis or monoparesis may occur. Reflex abnormalities are also common; these include exaggerated palmomental reflexes, and suck and snout reflexes. Superficial abdominal and cremasteric reflexes are usually absent. Changes in the tendon reflexes are variable and inconstant. The plantar response may be extensor and fluctuates almost hourly. Dysdiadochokinesia often exists.

The duration of the fever and neurologic symptoms and signs varies from several days to a month but usually ranges from 4 to 14 days. Clinical improvement generally follows the subsidence of the fever within several days unless irreversible anatomic changes have occurred.

Laboratory findings Erythrocytes are usually normal. Total leukocyte counts often reveal both a slight to moderate leukocytosis (occasionally greater than 20,000 leukocytes per microliter) and neutrophilia. Examination of the cerebrospinal fluid usually reveals several hundred cells per microliter, but on occasion cloudy cerebrospinal fluid with cells in excess of 1000 per microliter may be seen. Within the first several days of illness, polymorphonuclear neutrophils may predominate. The initial cerebrospinal fluid protein is usually

TABLE 148-3 Features of arboviral encephalitides common in the United States

Etiology	Geographic predominance in the United States	Urban/rural	Age, years	Sex	Unique clinical features	Mortality, %	Residua
California encephalitis	Midwest	Rural	5–10	M	Seizures	2	Seizures (one-fourth who had them in acute phase), behavioral problems (15%)
Eastern equine encephalitis	Eastern seaboard	Both	<5 >55	=	CSF may have >1000 WBC/μL	50	Children <10 years have emotional lability, retardation, convulsions
St. Louis encephalitis	Eastern and midwest	Both	>35	=	Dysuria	2–12	Ataxia, speech difficulties (5%)
Western equine encephalitis	Entire	Both	<1 >55	=	None	3	Children <3 months have behavioral problems, convulsions

only slightly elevated but on occasion may exceed 1.0 g/L (100 mg/dL). The level of spinal fluid sugar is normal; a significant decrease should raise serious consideration of an alternative diagnosis. As the illness progresses, mononuclear cells in the cerebrospinal fluid tend to increase so that they predominate and the protein concentration may increase. Other laboratory studies have been reported only sporadically, but abnormalities may include hyponatremia, often due to the inappropriate secretion of antidiuretic hormone, and elevations in serum creatine phosphokinase.

Diagnosis Specific diagnosis requires the isolation of the virus or detection of antibodies with a rising titer between the acute phase of disease and convalescence. Antibodies can be detected by hemagglutination inhibition, complement fixation, or virus neutralization techniques.

Treatment Treatment is entirely supportive and requires meticulous attention in the comatose patient.

LACROSSE ENCEPHALITIS A previously undescribed virus was isolated in 1943 from mosquitoes in Kern County, California. Since 1963, a large number of agents now designated as the California group of viruses have been isolated (Table 148-1). LaCrosse, snowshoe hare, Jamestown Canyon, and California encephalitis viruses cause human encephalitis in North America. Tahyna and Inkoo viruses are associated with febrile and, rarely, encephalitic disease in Europe. Since 1966 in the midwest United States, LaCrosse virus (California) encephalitis has been incriminated in 5 to 6 percent of cases of acute central nervous system disease, ranking above all agents except the enteroviruses.

Epidemiology LaCrosse virus infection occurs in the north central states, New York, in wooded areas of eastern Texas and Louisiana, and along the eastern seaboard. The virus is maintained by transovarial transmission in woodland mosquitoes, *Aëdes triseratus,* which breed in tree holes in hardwood forests and have adapted to discarded tires. The virus is present in seminal fluid of male mosquitoes and transmitted to the female. The virus overwinters in eggs of *A. triseratus.* Chipmunks and gray squirrels serve as amplifier hosts. LaCrosse virus (California) encephalitis occurs during the summer months (June to October), most often involving boys (60 percent) 5 to 10 years of age (60 percent) who live in rural areas.

Clinical manifestations Two clinical patterns of LaCrosse virus disease have been defined. One is a mild form with a 2- to 3-day prodrome of fever, headache, malaise, and gastrointestinal symptoms. About the third day the temperature increases to 40°C (104°F), and the patient becomes lethargic and develops meningeal signs. These findings abate gradually over a 7- to 8-day period without overt sequelae. The second pattern, a severe form which occurs in at least one-half of the patients, begins abruptly with fever, headache, and vomiting, followed shortly by lethargy and disorientation. During the first 2 to 4 days the course is rapidly progressive with the occurrence of seizures (50 to 60 percent), focal neurologic signs (20 percent), pathologic reflexes (10 percent), and coma (10 percent). Focal neurologic signs may include asymmetric flaccid paralysis. Uncommon findings have included arthralgia and rash. Clinical laboratory features include peripheral leukocyte counts ranging from 7000 to 30,000 per microliter (median 16,000 per microliter) with neutrophilia. Cerebrospinal fluid examination reveals 10 to 500 cells per microliter, usually with a predominance of mononuclear cells, protein concentrations of less than 1.0 g/L (100 mg/dL), and normal sugar concentrations. Electroencephalograms (EEGs) are abnormal in at least 80 percent of patients, revealing slow delta-wave activity. In one-half of the patients the abnormality is asymmetric, suggesting focal destructive lesions. Brain scans using [^{99}Tc]pertechnetate and computed tomography (CT) also may be abnormal, and temporal lobe localization has been observed. Beginning about the fourth day and proceeding over the next 3 to 7 days, there is progressive improvement, with almost all patients becoming afebrile, seizure-free, and ready for discharge from the hospital within 2 weeks after onset.

Diagnosis Serum and CSF should be tested for LaCrosse virus IgM antibodies. Serum capture IgM enzyme-linked immunosorbent assay (ELISA) tests detected 83 percent of cases on admission in LaCrosse encephalitis. Early specific diagnosis eliminates the need for brain biopsy to exclude herpes encephalitis which is suggested by the temporal lobe localization.

Treatment Initial seizure activity is frequently prolonged and difficult to control. The most effective anticonvulsant medication has been parenteral diazepam. Patients with the severe form of disease should be discharged on anticonvulsants such as phenobarbital for 6 to 12 months.

Prognosis The case fatality ratio is low (2 percent or less); however, one-third of patients may have abnormal neurologic findings at the time of discharge. During the early convalescent period, emotional lability and irritability are common. In one series, recurrent seizures occurred in one-quarter of the patients who had seizures during the acute phase. In this same series EEGs were abnormal in one-third of patients evaluated 1 to 8 years after their acute illness. In another series, 15 percent had sequelae, predominantly personality or behavioral problems.

OTHER CALIFORNIA GROUP ENCEPHALITIDES Jamestown Canyon encephalitis is uncommon, but in contrast to LaCrosse encephalitis usually occurs in adults. Snowshoe hare virus has been isolated from mosquitoes throughout Canada and from Alaska. Encephalitis has been reported from the eastern provinces. Clinical features of Tahyna virus disease, which has been seen in children in Europe, include fever, pharyngitis, pneumonitis, gastrointestinal symptoms, and aseptic meningitis. Neither mortality nor sequelae are reported.

EASTERN EQUINE ENCEPHALITIS Eastern equine encephalitis (EEE), an alphavirus, was first isolated in 1933 from the brain tissue of horses during an outbreak of equine illness in New Jersey. The first recognized human outbreak occurred in Massachusetts in 1938.

Epidemiology The virus is distributed along the eastern coast of the Americas from northeastern United States to Argentina. Foci have been found in the Syracuse region of New York, Ontario, Canada, western Michigan, and South Dakota. Viral isolations also have been reported in the Philippines, Thailand, Czechoslovakia, Poland, and the U.S.S.R., but the question of type specificity has not been resolved. In the northeastern United States, epidemics occur in the late summer and early fall. Epizootics in horses precede the occurrence of human cases by 1 to 2 weeks. The disease affects mainly infants, children, and adults over 55 years of age. There is no sex preponderance. Inapparent infection occurs in all age groups, suggesting that the decreased likelihood of developing overt infection in the 15- to 54-year age group is not the result of decreased exposure. The ratio of inapparent infection to overt encephalitis approximates 25:1.

The transmission of EEE involves *Culiseta melanura* mosquitoes and swamp-dwelling birds, e.g., red-winged blackbirds, sparrows, pheasants. Transmission by pecking has been shown in domestic pheasant flocks. *C. melanura* rarely feed on horses or humans, and other mosquitoes, especially *Aëdes sollicitans,* a salt-marsh mosquito which is an avid human feeder, have been postulated as the epidemic vector. The epidemiology of overwintering and maintenance between outbreaks remains unknown. Equine animals and human beings are "dead ends" in the transmission cycle, and infection in them is accidental.

Clinical manifestations Though human infections have been thought usually to result in serious, if not fatal, central nervous system involvement, the detection of inapparent infection as well as relatively mild disease establishes the occurrence of milder forms. In many patients, the cerebrospinal fluid is cloudy and contains in excess of 1000 cells per microliter.

Diagnosis ELISA tests for the detection of specific IgM antibodies in CSF or serum permit early diagnosis, although absence of IgM does not exclude infection. Confirmation can be obtained by a fourfold or more rise or fall in complement fixation (CF), hemagglutination inhibition, or virus neutralization tests.

Prognosis The mortality rate in clinical infection exceeds 50 percent. In the most severe cases, death occurs between the third and fifth days. Children under 10 years of age have a greater likelihood of surviving the acute illness, but they also have a greater likelihood of developing severe disabling residuals: mental retardation, convulsions, emotional lability, blindness, deafness, speech disorders, and hemiplegia.

ST. LOUIS ENCEPHALITIS St. Louis encephalitis (SLE) was first recognized as an entity during a major outbreak in St. Louis, Missouri, and the surrounding area in 1933. Subsequently, sporadic, unpredictable outbreaks have occurred in Houston (1964), Dallas (1966), Memphis (1974), northern Mississippi and Illinois (1975). The attack rate in Greenville, Mississippi, in 1975 was the highest which has been encountered, 10 per 10,000 population.

Epidemiology In the United States, epidemics of SLE fall into two epidemiologic patterns. One pattern is found in the west, where mixed outbreaks of western equine encephalitis and SLE have occurred primarily in irrigated rural areas. The vector has been *Culex tarsalis.* The second pattern occurred in the original St. Louis outbreak and the numerous subsequent epidemics in the midwest, Texas, New Jersey, and Florida. These outbreaks have been more urban in location and are characterized by occurrence of encephalitis in older persons. In such urban-suburban epidemics, the epidemic vectors have been mosquitoes of the *Culex pipiens-quinquefasciatus* complex with the exception of the Florida epidemic, in which *Culex nigripalpus* was incriminated. The presence of SLE virus outside the United States has been proved by isolations in Trinidad, Panama, Jamaica, Brazil, and Argentina. However, except for Jamaica, SLE has not been reported outside the United States. The basic transmission cycle is that of wild bird–mosquito–wild bird. The virus survives the winter in female mosquitoes which ingest a blood meal from a viremic bird before overwintering. The disease in humans usually appears in midsummer to early fall. In urban epidemics, there is no sex predominance while among sporadic cases in the west, men predominate 2:1 due to greater occupational exposure. The human represents an accidental host and plays no role in the basic transmission cycle. Serologic studies following most urban epidemics indicate that infection rates are similar in all age groups, and that the increasing age-specific attack rate for clinical encephalitis which is typical of urban St. Louis encephalitis is probably due to age differences in host susceptibility to overt disease rather than to a higher rate of infection.

Clinical manifestations Infection with SLE virus most commonly results in an inapparent infection. Of the patients with confirmed disease, approximately three-fourths have clinical encephalitis; the remainder present with aseptic meningitis, febrile headaches, or nonspecific illness. Virtually all patients over 40 years have encephalitic manifestations. Urinary frequency and dysuria have been symptoms in approximately 20 percent of patients despite sterile routine aerobic urine cultures. SLE virus antigen has been demonstrated in urine; this may account for the occurrence of urinary tract symptoms.

Diagnosis The occurrence of either encephalitis or aseptic meningitis as manifested by febrile illness with cerebrospinal fluid pleocytosis in the months of June through September in an adult, especially over 35 years of age, should raise the suspicion of St. Louis encephalitis. Because approximately 40 percent of patients with SLE have antibodies detectable by hemagglutination inhibition at the onset of illness, acute serum for serologic studies should be submitted promptly to a competent laboratory. ELISA tests for the detection of specific IgM antibodies in CSF or serum provide a means of early specific diagnosis.

Prognosis The case fatality ratio in the original St. Louis epidemic was 20 percent. In most subsequent outbreaks the mortality rate has varied from 2 to 12 percent. Subjective complaints, including nervousness, headaches, and easy fatigability and excitability, appear to be the most common residuals. Late organic defects such as speech defects, difficulty in walking, and disturbances in vision were demonstrated in approximately 5 percent of patients 3 years following infection.

WESTERN EQUINE ENCEPHALITIS Western equine encephalitis (WEE) virus is an alphavirus that was isolated in 1930 in California from horses with encephalitis. In 1938 it was recovered from a fatal human infection.

Epidemiology WEE virus has been isolated in the United States, Canada, Brazil, Guyana, and Argentina. Human disease has been diagnosed in the United States, Canada, and Brazil. In the United States, the virus is found in virtually all geographic areas. The central valley of California represents an important endemic area. The disease occurs mainly in early summer and midsummer. Wild birds, which develop viremia of sufficiently high titer to be able to infect mosquitoes that feed on them, are the basic reservoir. *Culex tarsalis* is the principal vector in the western United States. In areas east of the Appalachian Mountains, another vector may be operative. The virus has been repeatedly isolated from *Culiseta melanura;* however, the importance of this species has been questioned, since it is not primarily a human-biting mosquito. The overwintering mechanism is not known. The ratio of inapparent infection to disease, as evidenced by serologic survey studies, varies from 58:1 in children to 1150:1 in adults. Approximately one-fourth of patients are less than 1 year of age. The highest attack rates occur in persons 55 years or older.

Prognosis The fatality rate approximates 3 percent in laboratory-confirmed cases. The incidence and severity of sequelae are related to age. Sequelae among very young infants are frequent (appearing in 61 percent of a group of patients less than 3 months old) and severe; they consist of upper motor neuron impairment, involving the pyramidal tracts, extrapyramidal structures, and cerebellum, and result in behavioral problems and convulsions. Both the incidence and severity of sequelae diminish rapidly after 1 year of age. Adults may complain of nervousness, irritability, easy fatigability, and tremulousness for 6 months or longer after the acute illness. Probably not more than 5 percent of adults have sequelae which are sufficiently severe to be of practical significance. Postencephalitic seizures are rare.

JAPANESE ENCEPHALITIS The name Japanese B encephalitis was employed during an epidemic which occurred in 1924 to distinguish it from von Economo's disease, which was designated as type A encephalitis. The designation as Japanese B no longer seems useful, and the term Japanese encephalitis (JE) will be employed.

Epidemiology Japanese encephalitis virus infection is known to occur in eastern Siberia, China, Korea, Taiwan, Japan, Malaya, Vietnam, Thailand, Singapore, Guam, and India. Since the late 1960s JE has declined in Japan and China. JE remains a major problem in northern Thailand. In temperate climates, the disease shows a late-summer–early-fall seasonal incidence. In tropical climates there is no seasonal variation. The mosquito *Culex tritaeniorhynchus* is the major vector species. It is a rural mosquito which breeds in rice fields and preferentially bites large domestic animals, such as pigs, but also feeds on birds and humans. The human is an accidental host in the transmission cycle. In endemic areas, children ages 3 to 15 are primarily affected. Epidemics in nonendemic areas have affected all age groups, but young children and older adults predominate. The ratio of inapparent infection, as evidenced by a serologic survey study of Australian troops in Vietnam, was 210:1.

Clinical manifestations The incubation period is 5 to 15 days. As with SLE, illness may present as encephalitis, aseptic meningitis, or febrile headache. The occurrence of severe rigors at the onset has been noted in almost 90 percent of patients. On admission, most patients are alert, but deterioration of mental status occurs in about three-fourths of patients within 3 to 4 days. Localized paresis is found more often than with other "arboviral" encephalitides, e.g., in 31 percent of cases, with predominantly upper extremity involvement; however, it resolves rapidly with defervescence. Convulsions are frequent in children, but occur in less than 10 percent of adults. Severe hyperthermia may occur and require treatment. A peripheral leukocytosis with 50 to 90 percent neutrophils is common. Weight loss has been very striking. The failure of the temperature to lyse, appearance of diaphoresis, tachypnea, and the accumulation of bronchial secretions are grave prognostic signs.

Prognosis The immediate mortality rate has varied from 7 to 33 percent or higher. The occurrence of sequelae varies inversely with the fatality rate; in those series with high fatality rates (33 percent), sequelae occurred in 3 to 14 percent. In another series with a fatality rate of 7.4 percent, the rate of adverse sequelae was 32 percent. Individuals who had neurologic abnormalities during the acute phase but survived have no more than an 80 percent chance for complete recovery. Sequelae consist of seizures, persistent paralysis, ataxia, mental retardation, and behavioral disorders.

OTHER "ARBOVIRUSES" WITH CENTRAL NERVOUS SYSTEM INVOLVEMENT A large group of additional "arboviruses" have been associated with encephalitis or aseptic meningitis. Some of these agents are listed in Table 148-2. Though the epidemiologic picture of each of these agents is unique, the general features are sufficiently similar to require laboratory support for their differentiation.

"ARBOVIRUS" DISEASES PRESENTING CHIEFLY WITH HEMORRHAGIC MANIFESTATIONS

For 300 years, yellow fever was the only epidemic viral disease known to be accompanied by grave hemorrhagic manifestations. Since the 1930s diverse viral etiologies of the hemorrhagic fever syndrome have been recognized (Table 148-2). Additional agents include members of several families and genera: flavivirus, Filoviridae, phlebovirus, Nairovirus, Hantavirus, and arenavirus (see Chap. 149). Despite diverse etiologies, there are many similar clinical manifestations. The onset is usually sudden, with headache, backache, generalized myalgia, conjunctivitis, and prostration. From approximately the third day, the initial stage is followed by hypotension, and hemorrhagic manifestations may occur; these are characterized by bleeding gums, epistaxis, hemoptysis, hematemesis, melena, petechiae, ecchymoses, and hemorrhages into most visceral organs. Mild leukopenia develops early, but with the appearance of hemorrhagic manifestations, leukocytosis may occur. The pathophysiology of the cardinal signs is attributable to hematopoietic and capillary damage, with variable localization of lesions. On the basis of limited confirmatory observations, variable degrees of disseminated intravascular coagulation may be in part responsible for the pathophysiology of the hemorrhagic fever syndromes. Death usually occurs in the second week of disease, at which time a high titer of antibody has developed and the patient may have become afebrile. Death is usually associated with coma, which is due not to encephalitis but to an encephalopathy. The pathologic changes may be similar despite diverse viral etiologies, with midzonal hepatic necrosis and acidophilic cytoplasmic inclusions similar to the Councilman bodies of yellow fever.

YELLOW FEVER Yellow fever is an acute infectious disease of short duration and extremely variable severity; it is caused by a flavivirus and is followed by lifelong immunity. The classic triad of symptoms—jaundice, hemorrhages, and intense albuminuria—is present only in severe infections, which make up only a small proportion of the total.

Prevalence For more than 200 years, after the first identifiable outbreak occurred in Yucatan in 1648, yellow fever was one of the great plagues of the world. As late as 1905, New Orleans and other southern United States ports experienced at least 5000 cases and 1000 deaths. Because of the existence of the sylvatic form of the disease, protective measures must be maintained against human disease, as demonstrated by outbreaks in Central America from 1948 to 1957. In southern Ethiopia from 1962 to 1964 there were over 100,000 cases with some 30,000 deaths. From 1978 to 1980 there were outbreaks in Bolivia, Brazil, Colombia, Ecuador, Peru, and Venezuela. In 1979, yellow fever reappeared in Trinidad. During the same time period extensive epidemics were seen in Nigeria, Ghana, Senegal, and Gambia. In Gambia the attack rate was 2.6 to 4.4 percent with a case fatality rate of 19 percent. In 1983, epidemics occurred in Burkino Faso (formerly Upper Volta) and Ghana.

Epidemiology Human infection results from two basically different cycles of virus transmission, urban and sylvatic. The urban cycle is human-mosquito-human, i.e., *Aëdes aegypti*–transmitted yellow fever. After a 2-week extrinsic incubation period, mosquitoes can transmit infection. Sylvan yellow fever differs under various ecologic circumstances. In the rain forests of South and Central America, species of treetop *Haemagogus* or *Sabethes* mosquitoes maintain transmission in wild primates. Once infected, the mosquito vector remains infectious for life; hence it may serve as a reservoir as well as a vector. When humans come into proximity with the forest-canopy mosquitoes, sporadic cases or focal outbreaks may occur. With sylvan yellow fever, males predominate. Focal outbreaks may be quite extensive; in Brazil in 1973 at least 21,000 persons out of 1.5 million (1.4 percent) were infected. In east Africa, the mosquito-primate cycle is maintained by the forest-canopy mosquito, *A. africanus,* which seldom feeds on humans. The peridomestic mosquito *A. simpsoni* feeds upon primates entering the village gardens and can then in turn transmit the virus to humans. Once yellow fever is reintroduced into urban areas, the urban cycle can be reinitiated, with the potential for epidemic disease.

Clinical manifestations The incubation period is usually 3 to 6 days. In accidental laboratory- or hospital-acquired infections longer incubation periods (10 to 13 days) have been reported. In mild yellow fever the only symptoms may be the abrupt onset of fever and headache. Additional symptoms may include nausea, epistaxis, relative bradycardia known as Faget's sign [e.g., with a temperature of 38.9°C (102°F) the pulse may be only 48 to 52 beats per minute], and slight albuminuria. The mild illness lasts only 1 to 3 days and resembles influenza except that coryzal symptoms are lacking.

Moderately severe and malignant attacks of yellow fever are characterized by three distinct clinical periods: the period of infection, the period of remission, and the period of intoxication. Prodromal symptoms are usually absent. The onset is characteristically sudden, with headache, dizziness, and temperature elevations to 40°C (104°F) without a relative bradycardia. Young children may have febrile convulsions. The headache is followed quickly by pains in the neck, back, and legs. Often there is nausea with vomiting and retching. Examination reveals a flushed face and injection of the conjunctivae. The congestion of the eyes persists until the third day. The tongue characteristically shows bright-red margins and tip and a white furred center. Faget's sign appears by the second day. Epistaxis and gingival bleeding are common. On the third day of illness, the fever may fall by crisis and the patient enters remission, or, in the malignant form, copious hemorrhages, anuria, or delirium may occur. The stage of remission lasts from several hours to several days. In the third stage, the "classic" symptoms develop; the fever returns but the pulse remains slow. Jaundice becomes detectable about the third day; however, jaundice often is not prominent even in fatal illnesses. Increased epistaxis, melena, and uterine hemorrhages are common, but gross hematuria is rare. Of the classic signs, "black vomit" is more characteristic than is jaundice. Hematemesis usually does not occur before the fourth day and is often associated with a fatal outcome. Albuminuria, which rarely develops before the third day, occurs in 90 percent of patients and may be quite marked (3 to 20 g albumin per liter). In spite of this massive albuminuria, edema or ascites has not been reported. In malignant infections, coma frequently occurs 2 to 3 days before death. Shortly before death, which usually occurs between the fourth and the sixth days, the patient becomes delirious and wildly agitated. Though the duration of fever in the third stage is usually 5 to 7 days, the period of intoxication is the most variable of the stages and may last up to 2 weeks. Yellow fever is relatively free from complications, suppurative parotitis being the most striking of those which do occur. Clinical relapses are not characteristic of yellow fever.

Laboratory findings Early in the disease, progressive leukopenia may occur. By the fifth day, total leukocyte counts of 1500 to 2500 per microliter often are found, the decrease being due mostly to a decrease in neutrophils. Total leukocyte counts return to normal by the tenth day, and in fatal cases there may be a marked terminal leukocytosis. Hemoglobin values remain normal except terminally, when hemoconcentration or bleeding may occur. Platelet counts are normal or decreased. Prolongation of clotting, prothrombin, and partial thromboplastin times is marked in patients with jaundice. Increases in total and conjugated bilirubin occur. In icteric patients, marked elevations of serum glutamic oxaloacetic transaminase occur. Hypoglycemia has been seen in patients with severe hepatic damage. Electrocardiograms may show T-wave changes. The cerebrospinal fluid is normal.

Diagnosis Inoculation onto mosquito cell cultures or intrathoracically into mosquitoes are methods of choice for virus isolation from blood. Isolation is most likely from specimens obtained during the first 3 days of illness. Serologic methods include plaque reduction neutralization tests on paired sera and detection of yellow fever IgM antibodies and antigen usually by ELISA methods. The ELISA method enables confirmation in the field within 3 h.

Treatment The management has been symptomatic and supportive and should be based upon assessment and correction of the circulatory abnormalities. If evidence of disseminated intravascular coagulation is present, the administration of heparin should be considered. Close attention to fluids and electrolytes is essential. As with all of the hemorrhagic fevers, aspirin is contraindicated.

Prognosis The overall fatality rate in yellow fever is between 5 and 10 percent of clinical cases; it may be even less since many infections are mild or inapparent.

Prevention Effective control measures are available. Immunization has been effective in the prevention of outbreaks. With the occurrence of sylvatic outbreaks, work in the area of epizootic activity should be discontinued and intensive mosquito abatement measures should be instituted. These measures may provide the time necessary for a mass immunization program.

DENGUE HEMORRHAGIC FEVER All four dengue virus serotypes can cause dengue hemorrhagic fever (DHF) and dengue shock syndrome (DSS). Infection with dengue 1, 3, or 4 followed within a few years by dengue 2 may be especially important in the pathogenesis. There is consensus that DHF is an immunologically mediated disease. Enhanced growth of dengue 2 virus occurs in peripheral blood mononuclear phagocytes obtained from dengue immune donors or in cells from normal donors in the presence of subneutralizing concentrations of dengue or cross-reacting heterotypic flavivirus antibodies. Infectious virus-antibody complexes attach and enter mononuclear phagocytes by way of Fc receptors. Increased replication of virus in these cells may be followed by a secondary set of reactions: complement activation, mast cell degranulation, and activation of the kinin system.

Prevalence The reasons for the apparent sudden "appearance" of the syndrome in the past 30 years are completely obscure. However, during the 1922 epidemic of dengue fever in Louisiana, hemorrhagic manifestations, including epistaxis, bleeding gums, melena, menorrhagia, and even "black vomit," were observed. DHF is now a leading cause of morbidity and mortality in tropical Asia. Over 500,000 cases of DHF have been officially reported with major epidemics in the People's Republic of China, Vietnam, Indonesia, Thailand, and Cuba. In the Cuban outbreak in 1981, almost 350,000 persons developed dengue, approximately 10,000 had hemorrhagic manifestations, and 158 died (1.6 percent mortality). DHF in Asia is a disease of childhood with one peak observed in children under 1 year, and a second in children ages 3 to 5. The disease in infants is associated with primary infection in the presence of maternal antibody. Studies in Thailand have estimated the frequency of DSS as 11 cases per 1000 secondary dengue infections. DSS occurs more frequently in girls than boys. Dengue hemorrhagic fever occurs almost exclusively in indigenous populations; it has been observed only rarely in whites of European descent despite the frequent occurrence of classic dengue in this group.

Clinical manifestations Illness begins abruptly with a minor stage characterized by fever, cough, pharyngitis, headache, anorexia, nausea, vomiting, and abdominal pain which is often severe. This continues for 2 to 4 days. In contrast to classic dengue, myalgia, arthralgia, and bone pain are unusual. Physical signs include fever varying from 38.3 to 40.6°C (101 to 105°F), injection of the tonsils and pharynx, and palpable lymph nodes and liver. The initial state is followed by abrupt deterioration, with the rapid onset of lassitude and weakness (Table 148-4). On examination the child is found to be restless and to have cold clammy extremities with a warm trunk and a pallid face with circumoral cyanosis. Petechiae, most frequently located on the forehead and distal extremities, are seen in half the cases. Occasionally there may be a macular or maculopapular rash. The extremities are frequently cyanotic. Hypotension, with narrowing of the pulse pressure, and tachycardia occur. Pathologic reflexes may be present. Most fatalities occur in the fourth or fifth day of illness; melena, hematemesis, coma, or unresponsive shock are poor prognostic signs. Cyanosis, dyspnea, and convulsions are terminal manifestations. Following this critical period, survivors show steady and rapid improvement.

Laboratory findings In one study, hemoconcentration was found in one-fifth of the children. The majority had leukocyte counts between 5000 and 10,000 per microliter, with one-third showing a leukocytosis. Only 10 percent of children had a true leukopenia. The most characteristic findings were thrombocytopenia, rarely with blood platelets under 75,000 per microliter, positive tourniquet test, and prolonged bleeding time. Prothrombin time and partial thromboplastin times were usually near normal values. Depression of clotting factors V, VII, IX, and X may be present. Bone marrow examination may reveal maturation arrest of megakaryocytes. In Manila or Bangkok, hematuria has been infrequent even with other serious bleeding manifestations; however, in Tahiti, gross hematuria was common. Cerebrospinal fluid examinations are usually normal. Other abnormal laboratory findings may include hyponatremia, acidosis, elevated blood urea nitrogen levels, elevation in serum glutamic oxalacetic transaminase levels, mild hyperbilirubinemia, and hypoproteinemia. Electrocardiograms may reveal diffuse myocardial abnormalities. Two-thirds of patients have radiologic evidence of bronchopneumonia, with many showing pleural effusions.

Diagnosis The World Health Organization (WHO) has established criteria for the diagnosis of DHF: fever—acute onset, high, continuous, and lasting for 2 to 7 days; hemorrhagic manifestations including at least a positive tourniquet test and any of the following: petechiae, purpura, ecchymoses, epistaxis, bleeding gums, hematemesis, or melena; enlargement of the liver; thrombocytopenia, ≤100,000 per microliter; hemoconcentration, hematocrit increased by ≥20 percent. Criteria for DSS are a rapid, weak pulse with

TABLE 148-4 World Health Organization's clinical classification of dengue hemorrhagic fever

	Grade	Clinical features	Laboratory findings
DHF*	I	Fever, constitutional symptoms, positive tourniquet test	Hemoconcentration Thrombocytopenia
DHF*	II	Grade I plus spontaneous bleeding (e.g., skin, gums, gastrointestinal tract)	Hemoconcentration Thrombocytopenia
DHF*, DSS*	III	Grade II plus circulatory failure, agitation	Hemoconcentration Thrombocytopenia
DHF*, DSS*	IV	Grade II plus profound shock (blood pressure = 0)	Hemoconcentration Thrombocytopenia

* DHF, dengue hemorrhagic fever; DSS, dengue shock syndrome.

narrowing of the pulse pressure ($\leq$20 mmHg) or hypotension with cold, clammy skin and restlessness. The WHO classification includes a grading of severity (Table 148-4). Minor hemorrhagic manifestations may be seen during the course of classic dengue fever without meeting WHO criteria for DHF. These cases should be termed dengue fever with hemorrhage, not DHF.

Treatment The mainstay is correction of circulatory collapse while avoiding fluid overload. Administration of 5% glucose in 0.5 *N* saline at a rate of 40 mL/kg restored blood pressure within 1 to 2 h in one-half of patients. When stable, the rate of administration of intravenous fluids was slowed to 10 (mL/kg)/h. If improvement did not occur, plasma or a plasma expander (20 mL/kg) was administered. Transfusion of whole blood is not recommended. Oxygen should be administered. Glucocorticoids have been used, but doses of 25 mg/kg have not resulted in significant improvement. Since the evidence for severe disseminated intravascular coagulation is questionable, use of heparin is not clear-cut, although in a group of Filipino children with type 3 dengue virus, administration of heparin (1 mg sodium heparin per kilogram) was associated with a dramatic rise in number of platelets and level of plasma fibrinogen. Antibiotics are not indicated; sympathomimetic amines and salicylates are contraindicated. Recovery from vascular collapse usually occurs within 24 to 48 h, at which time diuretics and digitalis may be necessary. An uncontrolled trial of interferon was conducted during the 1981 epidemic in Cuba with some indication of efficacy.

Prognosis Mortality has varied from 1 to 23 percent. Deaths have been most common in infants under 1 year of age.

Prevention At present, vector control is the only method available to prevent hemorrhagic fever.

TICK-BORNE HEMORRHAGIC FEVERS Crimean-Congo hemorrhagic fever At the close of World War II, a new disease entity was recognized in the Crimea region of the U.S.S.R. Retrospective studies demonstrated that an almost identical syndrome had been recognized in the south central Asian republics of the U.S.S.R. for many years. Soviet workers repeatedly isolated virus strains during 1967 to 1969.

The virus of Crimean hemorrhagic fever (CHF) is antigenically identical with Congo virus, which was isolated from patients, cattle, and ticks in Kenya, Uganda, Zaire, and Nigeria. Crimean-Congo hemorrhagic fever (CCHF) virus is now known in South Africa, throughout most of subsaharan Africa, eastern Europe, the Middle East, and Asia as far as the Xinjiang province of China. CCHF occurs where *Hyalomma* ticks are found.

Approximately 30 cases of CCHF have been recorded annually in each of the known areas of occurrence in the U.S.S.R. The cases occur between April and September. The sex distribution of CCHF is equal, and 80 percent of the cases occur in the 20- to 60-year age group, with the majority occurring in dairy and agricultural workers. The major arthropod vectors for transmission to humans are ticks which belong to the genus *Hyalomma*. Cattle and wild hares appear to be important reservoirs, and rooks and other birds have been implicated. Once a case of human CCHF occurs, person-to-person transmission is possible. Nosocomial outbreaks have occurred in the U.S.S.R., Pakistan, India, and Iraq. Transmission is presumed to occur through direct contact with infected blood. There are no data to suggest airborne transmission.

After an incubation period of 3 to 6 days, the onset is abrupt, with temperatures to 40°C (104°F), dizziness, headache, and diffuse myalgia. The course of fever is occasionally biphasic, with an average duration of 8 days. Findings include flushing of the face, conjunctival injection, vomiting, and, on occasion, epigastric pain. Hepatomegaly occurs in half the patients. Splenomegaly has been reported in 2 to 25 percent of patients. Respiratory symptoms or signs are unusual. Hemorrhagic manifestations generally begin on the fourth day with petechiae on the oral mucosa and skin, epistaxis, gingival bleeding, hematemesis, and melena. Neurologic abnormalities, seen in 10 to 25 percent of patients, include nuchal rigidity, excitation, and coma. Laboratory findings show leukopenia, with the number of white blood cells falling as low as 1000 per microliter, and thrombocytopenia, which is often severe. Proteinuria and microscopic hematuria are common, but azotemia and oliguria are not. Convalescence may be prolonged. Death is usually attributed to shock or intercurrent infection. Sequelae include transient alopecia and mono- or polyneuritis.

The major approach to therapy has been supportive. Convalescent immune serum has shown promise if administered during the first 3 days of illness. Patients should be isolated with contact restricted to hospital staff and immediate family. Masks and gowns should be worn, and blood and body fluids handled as infectious. The reported mortality rate has varied between 9 and 50 percent.

Omsk hemorrhagic fever Omsk hemorrhagic fever (OHF) is an acute febrile disease which occurs in the Omsk and Novosibirsk oblasts in the U.S.S.R. and is caused by a flavivirus. The seasonal occurrence of OHF shows a biphasic pattern with peaks in May and August. The transmission cycle is uncertain. OHF is transmitted to humans either by the bite of infected ticks, *Ixodes apronophorus*, or by the handling of infected muskrats. The natural reservoir includes muskrats, other rodents, especially water voles, and ticks. Epidemics occurred from 1945 to 1948, but recently the disease has been less prevalent.

Following an incubation interval of 3 to 8 days, illness begins abruptly with fever, headache, and hemorrhagic manifestations, which include epistaxis and gastrointestinal and uterine bleeding. Rarely, neurologic abnormalities may occur. Laboratory features include leukopenia. In contrast to many of the other hemorrhagic fevers, OHF has a low case fatality rate (0.5 to 3.0 percent).

Kyasanur Forest disease Kyasanur Forest disease was first recognized in south India in 1957 as a discrete clinical entity shown to be due to a flavivirus. Kyasanur Forest disease occurs following occupational exposure to *Haemaphysalis spinigera* ticks in the tropical forests of western Mysore in southern India. The silent reservoir cycle which infects the primate- and bird-feeding *Haemaphysalis* ticks is now believed to be *Ixodes* ticks transmitted among small forest mammals, especially the shrew. Laboratory-associated infections have been common.

The major symptoms include abrupt onset of fever, headache, fatigue, myalgia (especially of the lumbar area and calf muscles), and retroorbital pain. Cough and abdominal pain occur in half the patients. Additional symptoms may include photophobia and polyarthralgia. Epistaxis and hematemesis are observed in some patients. On examination, findings include relative bradycardia, conjunctival injection, and generalized lymphadenopathy. Fine and coarse rales are frequently heard. Hepatosplenomegaly has been encountered occasionally. During the initial phase, generalized hyperesthesia of the skin occurs occasionally. The fever usually lasts from 6 to 11 days. After an afebrile period of 9 to 21 days, approximately half the patients may develop a second phase, which lasts from 2 to 12 days. This is manifested by recurrence of fever, severe headache, neck stiffness, mental disturbance, coarse tremors, giddiness, and abnormalities in reflexes, as well as by recurrence of many of the initial symptoms. No sequelae have been observed, but convalescence is often prolonged.

Only limited laboratory studies have been reported. During the initial phase, leukopenia is a constant feature, with a total leukocyte count of fewer than 3000 per microliter by the fourth to sixth day. The leukopenia is associated with neutropenia. During the second phase there is a mild leukocytosis. Lumbar puncture during the second phase has shown a pattern of aseptic meningitis. Diagnosis is based upon virus isolation from blood; this is readily accomplished, since viremia is prolonged. Serologic tests of paired serums also can be performed. The management is supportive. The mortality rate is approximately 5 percent.

HEMORRHAGIC FEVER WITH RENAL SYNDROME

Synonyms for this disease (HFRS) include Korean hemorrhagic fever, Far Eastern hemorrhagic fever, endemic or epidemic nephrosonephritis, Manchurian epidemic hemorrhagic fever, Songo fever, and Churilov's disease. A similar but milder disease in Scandinavia has been called nephropathia epidemica or epidemic nephritis (EN).

ETIOLOGY In 1976, the antigen of HFRS was reported in the lungs of the rodent *Apodemus agrarius coreae*. Diagnostic increases in immunofluorescent antibodies were demonstrated in 113 of 116 cases of severe HFRS. The agent designated Hantaan virus is a single-stranded RNA virus belonging to the family Bunyaviridae, genus Hantavirus (Table 148-1). The genus consists of at least four species: Hantaan virus (Korean hemorrhagic fever), Seoul virus, Puumala virus (nephropathia epidemica), and Prospect Hill virus (isolated from meadow voles in Maryland and associated with human diseases).

PREVALENCE In Korea between April 1951 and January 1953, 2070 cases of epidemic hemorrhagic fever were reported among United Nations personnel. The disease usually occurs as an isolated event; hence, overall attack rates have relatively less meaning. With this reservation, attack rates in two United States Army divisions stationed in Korea varied between 1.9 and 2.9 cases per 1000 persons per epidemic season. Approximately 800 cases per year have continued to occur; however, most cases are now seen in Korean civilians and military with less than 10 cases per year in U.S. military personnel. During the past 15 years, the disease has increased in prevalence in Korea, urban Japan, and in China. In the People's Republic of China over 100,000 cases of HFRS are reported annually; the incidence is increasing. Hundreds of cases of EN have occurred annually in Finland and other Scandinavian countries since the 1930s. In 1953 a severe form of HFRS was recognized in the Balkan countries, and in 1982 in Greece and France. Antibody studies indicate worldwide distribution. Antibodies in human sera have been found in Argentina, Brazil, Colombia, Europe, Canada, the United States, including Hawaii and Alaska, southeast Asia, Egypt, and central Africa.

EPIDEMIOLOGY The majority of cases occur in May to June and in October to November. These peaks coincide with rodent density population. Hantaan virus is present in rodent urine, feces, and saliva in high titer. Transmission from rodent to rodent is primarily respiratory, with transmission to people through inhalation of virus-containing dried excreta. There is no evidence for person-to-person transmission. The urban reservoir appears to be the house rat. Laboratory-acquired cases have occurred in the U.S.S.R., Korea, Japan, and Europe with rats implicated in Korea, Japan, and the U.K.

CLINICAL MANIFESTATIONS There are two forms of disease, a mild illness characteristically diagnosed in Scandinavia as epidemic nephritis (EN) and the more severe Far Eastern form, epidemic hemorrhagic fever.

EN is characterized by sudden onset of high fever, backache, headache, and abdominal pain. On the third or fourth day, hemorrhagic manifestations may occur and conjunctival hemorrhages, palatine petechiae, and a petechial rash appear on the trunk. About one patient in five is "toxic" and mentally obtunded. Oliguria and azotemia develop. Urinalysis reveals proteinuria, hematuria, and leukocyturia. After about 3 days the rash subsides, the patient develops polyuria, and recovers in several weeks.

Epidemic hemorrhagic fever The incubation period in epidemic hemorrhagic fever (EHF) is usually 10 to 25 days, with possible extremes of 7 and 36 days. Visitors who contract the disease in an endemic area may not develop illness until after their return home.

The clinical course of EHF may be divided into phases on the basis of the underlying physiologic aberrations: febrile, hypotensive, oliguric, diuretic, and convalescent. There is considerable variation among patients in the severity of the illness. In one study two-thirds of the 264 cases studied were classified as mild, while 14 percent were termed severe.

FEBRILE (INVASIVE) PHASE From 10 to 20 percent of patients describe vague prodromal symptoms resembling mild upper respiratory infections. The onset is then usually abrupt, often initiated by a chill and accompanied by fever, headache, backache, abdominal pain, and generalized myalgia. Anorexia and thirst are almost universal, while nausea and vomiting are common although not constant symptoms. The headache is most commonly frontal or retroorbital. Eye symptoms, especially mild photophobia and pain on movement of the eyes, are characteristic. Diarrhea is not a feature. Fever is present in almost all patients; the temperature ranges from 37.8 to 41.1°C (100 to 106°F), reaches a peak on the third or fourth day after onset, and falls by lysis on the fourth to seventh day. There is a relative bradycardia. Initially the blood pressure is normal. One of the most typical early findings is a diffuse reddening of the skin, most marked over the face and V area of the neck that may resemble a severe sunburn. The erythema blanches on pressure. Dermographism can be demonstrated in over 90 percent of patients at the same time as the flush. Slight edema of the upper eyelids causes a bleary-eyed appearance. Bulbar and palpebral conjunctivas show injection. Conjunctival petechiae may develop by the third or fifth day of illness. Subconjunctival hemorrhages may be striking. Intense pharyngeal reddening without significant sore throat is typical. The first location for petechiae is usually the palate, where they occur in half the patients. Within 12 to 24 h, petechiae appear at pressure areas such as the axillary folds, lateral chest wall, belt line, hips, and thighs. Retinal hemorrhages occur rarely. Cervical, axillary, and inguinal nodes are moderately enlarged but nontender. Abdominal and costovertebral tenderness is almost a constant finding. Splenomegaly is unusual and in Korea was generally attributable to malaria with which EHF coexisted in about 1 percent of patients. The degree of flush, fever, and conjunctival injection and the number of petechiae correlate quite well with the overall severity of illness.

Laboratory studies during this phase are often not striking. Initial hemoglobin and hematocrit values are usually normal. Prior to the fourth day, leukocyte counts range from 3600 to 6000 per microliter but are associated with neutrophilia. Early in the course urine specific gravity may be high. Albuminuria, which is an almost universal finding, appears, often abruptly, between the second and fifth days of illness. The urinary sediment reveals microscopic hematuria and hyaline, granular, red blood cell casts, and/or white blood cell casts. Erythrocyte sedimentation rates are normal during the first week. Capillary fragility tests are usually positive at the time of admission and become most abnormal by the ninth day. Electrocardiographic abnormalities may be seen in 15 to 30 percent of patients; these include sinus bradycardia and low or inverted T waves. Lumbar punctures may reveal gross blood in the spinal fluid.

HYPOTENSIVE PHASE On about the fifth day of illness, during the last 24 to 48 h of the febrile phase, hypotension or shock may occur. In mild cases, only a transient fall in blood pressure occurs; among moderately and severely ill patients shock may persist for 1 to 3 days. In 828 patients, 16.5 percent had clinical shock, and another 14 percent had hypotension without shock. Headache often diminishes, but thirst persists. In the beginning of the hypotensive phase, most patients have warm, dry skin and extremities. As the systolic blood pressure decreases and pulse pressure narrows, the skin becomes cool and moist. Tachycardia replaces the relative bradycardia.

At this stage, an increase in hematocrit with no change in total serum protein level is found. This is thought to reflect a loss of plasma through damaged capillaries. On about the fifth day, all patients develop marked proteinuria. The previously normal urine specific gravity begins to fall and in 2 to 3 days is usually around 1.010. Blood urea nitrogen concentrations begin to increase. Other laboratory findings include leukocytosis with white blood cell counts of 10,000 to 56,000 per microliter with neutrophilia and toxic granulation. The number of platelets often decreases to less than 70,000 per microliter.

OLIGURIC PHASE (HEMORRHAGIC OR TOXIC PHASE) About the eighth day of illness, blood pressure returns to the normal range and in some instances increases to hypertensive levels. While oliguria may have appeared during the shock phase, it now becomes a prominent feature. Oliguria develops even though hypotension was not recognized. Symptomatically patients continue to feel weak and thirsty and have more severe backache. Protracted vomiting and hiccups may ensue.

Blood urea nitrogen levels increase rapidly and are associated with hyperkalemia, hyperphosphatemia, and hypocalcemia. Metabolic acidosis is rarely severe. Although platelets begin to return to normal, hemorrhagic manifestations become more prominent and include petechiae, hematemesis (analogous to "black vomit" in yellow fever), melena, hemoptysis, gross hematuria, and hemorrhages into the central nervous system. The enlarged lymph nodes may now become tender.

With the onset of diuresis on about the seventh day in moderately ill patients and the ninth to eleventh day in severely ill patients, symptoms of fluid and electrolyte abnormalities and central nervous system or pulmonary complications may appear. Central nervous system symptoms include disorientation, extreme restlessness, lethargy, paranoid delusions, and hallucinations. Grand mal seizures, pulmonary edema, and pulmonary infection occur in some patients.

DIURETIC PHASE With the onset of diuresis, progressive improvement is the rule. Most patients begin to eat and regain their strength. In fatal cases the diuretic phase is associated with a daily urine output of less than 4 liters and often less than 2 liters, in contrast to larger volumes in surviving patients.

CONVALESCENT PHASE The convalescent phase lasts 3 to 6 weeks. Weight is regained slowly. Complaints include muscular weakness, intention tremor, and lack of stamina. Hyposthenuria and polyuria are present; however, within 2 months most patients are able to concentrate their urine to a specific gravity of 1.023 or greater after a 12-h period of water deprivation.

DIAGNOSIS Diagnosis is based on demonstration of specific IgM antibodies by ELISA or a fourfold change in immune adherence hemagglutination titers in paired sera. Studies on the epidemiology of Hantavirus have shown that during the initial 24 to 72 h (febrile phase) there is significant overlap in the clinical features of leptospirosis, HFRS, and scrub typhus. In Korea where all three diseases are prevalent, of blood samples submitted for Hantavirus serology, 21 percent had antibody to leptospira antigens and 6 percent to *Rickettsia tsutsugamushi*. Because of the similarity in epidemiology and clinical presentation and the potential for dual infections, it has been recommended that blood be submitted for Hantavirus serology in all cases of suspected leptospirosis (see Chap. 130).

TREATMENT Clinical management primarily revolves around meticulous supportive care. Trials with a variety of agents including antibiotics, glucocorticoids, antihistamines, convalescent serum, and alpha interferon were without significant beneficial effect during the Korean epidemics. In a controlled U.S./Chinese clinical trial in the People's Republic of China, ribavirin was shown to have efficacy.

PROGNOSIS The Soviet experience indicates a mortality rate of 3 to 32 percent; in China, the case fatality ratio was 7 to 15 percent. Between April 1951 and December 1976 the overall case fatality ratio in Korea was 6.6 percent.

Residua are uncommon. Of 783 surviving patients cared for at the Hemorrhagic Fever Center in Korea between April and December 1952, only 16 were unable to return to duty within a period of 4 months. Fifteen of these individuals still had hyposthenuria. Follow-up studies on former EHF patients 3 to 5 years later showed that they had many more subsequent hospital admissions for urologic problems than did a control group and that the relative frequency correlated with the severity of the acute episode of EHF.

REFERENCES

"Arboviruses": Definition and classification

FIELDS BN et al (eds): *Virology*. New York, Raven, 1985

"Arbovirus" infections characterized by fever, malaise, headaches, and myalgia

BOWEN GS et al: Clinical aspects of human Venezuelan equine encephalitis in Texas, 1971. Bull Pan Am Health Org 10:46, 1976

BRICENO ROSSIE AL: Rural epidemic encephalitis in Venezuela caused by a group A arbovirus (VEE). Prog Med Virol 9:176, 1967

CALISHER CH et al: Rio Grande—a new phlebotomus fever group virus from south Texas. Am J Trop Med Hyg 26:997, 1977

DIETZ WH JR et al: Ten clinical cases of human infection with Venezuelan equine encephalomyelitis virus, subtype I-D. Am J Trop Med Hyg 28:329, 1979

FLEMING J et al: Sandfly fever. Review of 664 cases. Lancet 1:443, 1947

GOODPASTURE HC et al: Colorado tick fever: Clinical, epidemiologic and laboratory aspects of 228 cases in Colorado in 1973–1974. Ann Intern Med 88:303, 1978

HUGHES LE et al: Persistence of Colorado tick fever virus in red blood cells. Am J Trop Med Hyg 23:530, 1974

LAUGHLIN LW et al: Epidemic Rift Valley fever in Egypt: Observations of the spectrum of human illness. Trans R Soc Trop Med Hyg 73:630, 1979

LENNETTE EH, KOPROWSKI H: Human infection with Venezuelan equine encephalomyelitis virus. JAMA 123:1088, 1943

SCHERER WF et al: Ecologic studies of Venezuelan encephalitis virus in Southeastern Mexico: VII. Infection of man. Am J Trop Med 21:79, 1972

SIAM AL et al: Rift Valley fever ocular manifestations: Observations during 1977 epidemic in Egypt. Br J Ophthalmol 64:366, 1980

VAN VELDEN et al: Rift Valley fever affecting humans in South Africa: A clinicopathologic study. S Afr Med J 29:867, 1977

"Arbovirus" infections presenting chiefly with fever, malaise, arthralgia, and rash

AASKOV JG et al: An epidemic of Ross River virus infection in Fiji, 1979. Am J Trop Med Hyg 30:1053, 1981

CLARK JA et al: Annually recurrent epidemic polyarthritis and Ross River virus activity in a coastal area of New South Wales. I. Occurrence of the disease. Am J Trop Med Hyg 22:543, 1973

DELLER JJ JR, RUSSELL PK: Chikungunya disease. Am J Trop Med 17:107, 1968

PINHEIRO FP et al: An outbreak of Mayaro virus disease in Belterra, Brazil: I. Clinical and virological findings. Am J Trop Med Hyg 30:674, 1981

ROBINSON MC: An epidemic of virus disease in Southern Province, Tanganyika territory in 1952–53: I. Clinical features. Trans R Soc Trop Med Hyg 49:28, 1955

SHORE H: O'nyong-nyong fever: An epidemic virus disease in East Africa: III. Some clinical and epidemiological observations in the Northern Province of Uganda. Trans R Soc Trop Med Hyg 55:361, 1961

"Arbovirus" infections presenting chiefly with fever, malaise, lymphadenopathy, and rash

ALVAREZ MD, RAMÍREZ-RONDA CH: Dengue and hepatic failure. Am J Med 79:670, 1985

CENTERS FOR DISEASE CONTROL: Dengue in the United States, 1983–1984. CDC Surveillance Summaries 34(255):555, 1985

MICKS DW, MOON WB: *Aëdes aegypti* in a Texas coastal county as an index of dengue fever receptivity and control. Am J Trop Med Hyg 29:1382, 1980

"Arbovirus" infections presenting chiefly with central nervous system involvement

BALFOUR HH JR et al: California arbovirus (LaCrosse) infections. Pediatrics 52:680, 1973

CENTERS FOR DISEASE CONTROL: Arboviral infections of the central nervous system—United States, 1987. Morb Mort Week Rep 37:506, 1988

DICKERSON RB et al: Diagnosis and immediate prognosis of Japanese B encephalitis. Observations based on more than 200 patients with detailed analysis of 65 serologically confirmed cases. Am J Med 12:277, 1952

EDELMAN R, PARYANONDA A: Human immunoglobulin M antibody in the serodiagnosis of Japanese encephalitis virus infections. Am J Epidemiol 98:29, 1973

FINLEY KH et al: Western equine and St. Louis encephalitis. Preliminary report of a clinical follow-up study in California. Neurology 5:223, 1955

GRABOW JD et al: The electroencephalogram and clinical sequelae of California arbovirus encephalitis. Neurology 19:394, 1969

HILTY MD et al: California encephalitis in children. Am J Dis Child 124:530, 1972

HOKE CH et al: Protection against Japanese encephalitis by inactivated vaccines. N Engl J Med 319:608, 1988

KETEL WB, OGNIBENE AJ: Japanese B encephalitis in Vietnam. Am J Med Sci 261:271, 1971

LUBY JP et al: The epidemiology of St. Louis encephalitis (SLE): A review. Ann Rev Med 20:329, 1969

———: Antigenemia in St. Louis encephalitis. Am J Trop Med Hyg 29:265, 1980

SCHNEIDER RJ et al: Clinical sequelae after Japanese encephalitis: One year follow-up study in Thailand. Southeast Asian J Trop Med Public Health 5:560, 1974

"Arbovirus" diseases presenting primarily with hemorrhagic manifestations

BURNEY MI et al: Nosocomial outbreak of viral hemorrhagic fever caused by Crimean hemorrhagic fever—Congo virus in Pakistan, January 1976. Am J Trop Med Hyg 29:941, 1980

CENTERS FOR DISEASE CONTROL: Viral hemorrhagic fever. Initial management of suspected and confirmed cases. Ann Intern Med 101:73, 1984

———: Korean hemorrhagic fever. JAMA 259:1622, 1988

DENNIS LH et al: The original hemorrhagic fever: Yellow fever. Blood 30:858, 1967

GARTNER L: Hantaan virus infection (Korean hemorrhagic fever) as a cause of acute renal failure. Dtsch Med Wochenschr 113:937, 1988

GUI XE et al: Hemorrhagic fever with renal syndrome: Treatment with recombinant alpha interferon. J Infect Dis 155:1047, 1987

HALSTEAD SB, O'ROURKE EF: Dengue viruses and mononuclear phagocytes: I. Infection enhancement by non-neutralizing antibody. J Exp Med 146:201, 1977
———: The pathogenesis of dengue: Molecular epidemiology in infectious disease. Am J Epidemiol 114:632, 1981
KLIKS SC et al: Antibody-dependant enhancement of dengue virus growth in human monocytes as a risk factor for dengue hemorrhagic fever. Am J Trop Med Hyg 40:444, 1989
KUDESIA G et al: Dual infection with leptospira and Hantavirus. Lancet 1:1397, 1988
LEE HW et al: Isolation of the etiologic agent of Korean hemorrhagic fever. J Infect Dis 137:298, 1978
MONATH TP et al: Yellow fever in the Gambia, 1978–1979: Epidemiologic aspects with observations on the occurrence of Orongo virus infections. Am J Trop Med Hyg 29:912, 1980
NELSON ER: Hemorrhagic fever in children in Thailand: Report of 69 cases. J Pediatr 56:101, 1960
PINHEIRO FP et al: An epidemic of yellow fever in Central Brazil 1972–1973: I. Epidemiological studies. Am J Trop Med Hyg 27:125, 1978
WORLD HEALTH ORGANIZATION: *Dengue hemorrhagic fever: Diagnosis, treatment and control.* Geneva, 1986
———: Hemorrhagic fever with renal syndrome: Memorandum from a WHO meeting. Bull WHO 61:269, 1983

149 ARENAVIRUS INFECTIONS

JAY P. SANFORD

DEFINITION AND CLASSIFICATION The term *arenavirus* is the proposed designation for a group of RNA viruses which have unique morphology. The virions are round, oval, or pleomorphic, with diameters between 60 and 350 nm, and contain an electron-dense membrane with projections and 2 to 10 inclusion-like dense particles (resembling ribosomes) that give the virion an appearance of having been sprinkled with sand (Latin *arenaceus,* "sandy"). Eleven distinct arenaviruses have been described (Table 149-1). All except Tacaribe are parasites of rodents, and most are unique to tropical America. A special property of arenaviruses that cause disease in humans, especially Machupo and lymphocytic choriomeningitis, is their capacity to induce persistent infection in their reservoir hosts with no ill effects and in the absence of an immune response.

LYMPHOCYTIC CHORIOMENINGITIS The first-recognized arenavirus was lymphocytic choriomeningitis (LCM) virus. It was recognized early that LCM was carried by apparently healthy laboratory mice. Clinically LCM has been considered primarily in the context of aseptic meningitis; however, it is associated with at least two clinical syndromes in humans: central nervous system and influenza-like illness which may be associated with rash, arthritis, or orchitis. LCM virus has provided a valuable model for the study of chronic, persistent, and generally symptomless viral infections in laboratory animals.

Prevalence In the United States human infection with LCM virus is rare; however, seroepidemiologic studies on specimens obtained in 1935 to 1940 from persons with no history of central nervous system disease from all parts of the United States revealed neutralizing antibodies in 10 to 28 percent. In recent years, the prevalence of infection seems to have decreased markedly.

Epidemiology The virus of LCM is worldwide in distribution. Foci of LCM virus have been defined in Germany, Hungary, and elsewhere in Europe. Scandinavia appears to be LCM virus–free as are most of the Americas except Argentina. Although infection can be induced in a variety of animals, mice are the major natural reservoir as well as the primary host in which latent, asymptomatic infection occurs. The latency of infection in the mouse depends upon immunologic tolerance. Animals infected in utero or shortly after birth excrete LCM virus for life without overt disease. Human infections are secondary to contact with an infected rodent. The mode of transmission is thought to be via airborne spread or contact with excrement from infected animals. In the past, most cases have arisen in persons living in rodent-infested houses, but lately outbreaks of LCM virus disease in humans have been reported from Germany and from the United States in which the source of infection was traced to laboratory animals and household pets, specifically hamsters which, like mice, can shed LCM virus in urine and stool. LCM occurs throughout the year but has been more frequent in the colder months. Person-to-person transmission has not been demonstrated.

Pathogenesis In natural infection, the portal of entry of the LCM virus is probably through the respiratory tract. Virus multiplication occurs initially in the respiratory epithelium, and an influenza-like illness develops. Dissemination of virus to extrapulmonary sites, presumably to reticuloendothelial cells with multiplication, and viremia occur. LCM virus crosses the blood-brain barrier. In mice, the resulting meningitis is attributed to a cell-mediated immune reaction. Support for this hypothesis derives from observations that disease but not infection can be prevented in experimental animals by neonatal thymectomy, irradiation, or immunodepressant drugs such as cyclophosphamide. Similar pathogenetic mechanisms may operate in humans, although isolation of LCM virus from the CSF of patients with aseptic meningitis is quite common.

Clinical manifestations The exact incubation period is not known. Following experimental inoculation of LCM virus into volunteers, fever occurred in 1½ to 3 days, while an influenza-like constellation of symptoms developed 5 to 10 days after exposure. An influenza-like illness is the commonest clinical pattern. In some patients the illness may be biphasic with subsequent aseptic meningitis or encephalomyelitis. Fever, usually from 38.3 to 40°C (101 to 104°F), associated with rigors, is uniformly noted. Other symptoms which are encountered in over one-half of patients include malaise, weakness, myalgia (especially lumbar aching), retroorbital headache, photophobia, anorexia, nausea, and light-headedness. Symptoms which occur in one-fourth to one-half of patients include sore throat, vomiting, and dysesthesias. Later, arthralgias, especially in the hands, occur. Less common complaints (up to one-quarter of patients) include aching pain in the chest, associated with pneumonitis; increased hair loss progressing to generalized alopecia, 2 or 3 weeks after the onset of illness; testicular pain or frank orchitis, usually unilateral, 1 to 3 weeks after onset; and parotid pain, which may lead to a misdiagnosis of mumps. Physical findings in the first week of illness are few. Patients often have a relative bradycardia. Pharyngeal injection without exudate is common (60 percent). Mild

TABLE 149-1 Classification of arenaviruses

Virus	Clinical disease	Reservoir	Known geographic range
Lymphocytic choriomeningitis	Aseptic meningitis, meningoencephalitis, influenzal syndrome, orchitis, arthritis	Mice, hamsters	Worldwide except Australia
Tacaribe		Bats	Trinidad
Junin	Argentinian hemorrhagic fever	*Calomys musculinus*	Argentina
Machupo	Bolivian hemorrhagic fever	*Calomys callosus*	Northeast Bolivia
Amapari			Brazil
Latino			Bolivia
Parana			Paraguay
Pichinde			Colombia
Tamiami			Florida
Lassa	Lassa fever	*Mastomys natalensis*	Nigeria, Liberia, Sierra Leone, Republic of Guinea, Central African Republic
Flexal		*Orzomys* sp.	Brazil

nontender cervical or axillary lymphadenopathy may occur. The initial phase lasts from 5 days to 3 weeks followed by improvement. After a remission of 1 to 2 days many patients relapse with recurrent fever and more prominent headache. Physical signs may include skin rashes, swelling of metacarpophalangeal and proximal interphalangeal joints, meningeal signs, orchitis, parotitis, and alopecia. Convalescence generally is of 1 to 4 weeks' duration, characterized by easy fatigability, an excessive need for sleep, dysesthesias, and occasional dizziness. Patients with aseptic meningitis almost always recover without sequelae. With encephalitis, 25 to 30 percent of patients have neurologic residua.

Laboratory findings Leukopenia and thrombocytopenia are almost uniform during the first week of illness. Although leukocyte counts usually vary between 2000 and 3000 per microliter, counts as low as 600 per microliter have been recorded. Differential counts generally show slight relative lymphocytosis. Platelet counts are usually between 50,000 and 100,000 per microliter. Anemia is not encountered. The erythrocyte sedimentation rate often is normal. Mild elevations of serum glutamic oxaloacetic transaminase (SGOT) and lactic dehydrogenase (LDH) may occur. Chest radiographs may suggest basilar pneumonias. In patients with meningeal signs, examination of the cerebrospinal fluid usually reveals several hundred cells per microliter, although cell counts in excess of 1000 per microliter are reported in half the patients in some series. Lymphocytes predominate (greater than 80 percent) even early. The initial cerebrospinal fluid protein is usually slightly elevated, but on occasion levels may exceed 1.5 g/L (150 mg/dL). Although a normal cerebrospinal fluid glucose level is considered the hallmark of viral meningitides, low CSF glucose has been observed in up to 27 percent of patients with LCM.

Diagnosis The diagnosis of LCM can be established with certainty by recovery of the virus from blood or spinal fluid. Complement-fixing antibodies are usually detectable 1 to 2 weeks after the onset of infection, peak at 5 to 8 weeks, and are gone by 6 months. Neutralizing antibodies appear after 6 to 8 weeks, increase in titer slowly, and remain high for years. Immunofluorescent studies have detected antibody to LCM virus earlier in the course of illness, and its appearance seems to parallel the development of the neurologic phase. The clinical manifestations of LCM cannot be differentiated from those produced by numerous other viruses.

Treatment There is no specific treatment.

ARGENTINIAN AND BOLIVIAN HEMORRHAGIC FEVERS The first cases of a new American hemorrhagic disease were seen near the Argentinian town of Junin near Buenos Aires in 1953. A virus was isolated from patients' blood and from local rodents and their mites. In 1959, cases of a disease thought to resemble severe epidemic typhus were noted among rural workers in northeastern Bolivia. The similarity between these syndromes was recognized. In 1963, the causal virus was isolated from patients and rodents and named the Machupo virus. Machupo virus is serologically related to but distinct from Junin virus.

Prevalence Junin virus infections have occurred in epidemic form since 1958 with between 100 and 3500 cases reported annually. The hemorrhagic disease in Bolivia has been particularly severe.

Epidemiology Argentinian hemorrhagic fever (AHF) occurs in sharply endemic seasonal form (February to August), mostly among male rural workers, especially those exposed to fields at the time of the maize harvest. Virus is transmitted in the urine of rodents with chronic infection and viruria. Humans acquire the virus through contact with items or foodstuffs which have been contaminated with infected rodent urine. The main reservoir is two species of cricetidae, *Calomys laucha* and *C. musculinus*.

Bolivian hemorrhagic fever (BHF) is similarly transmitted by the urine of *C. callosus* (a mouselike rodent) chronically infected with Machupo virus. Direct person-to-person transmission is possible and may have occurred in the outbreak in Cochabamba. Disease has not occurred in medical personnel attending infected patients.

Clinical features Argentinian hemorrhagic fever presents manifestations of renal, cardiovascular, and hematologic involvement. Inapparent infections are rare. The incubation period is estimated to be 7 to 16 days, followed by a gradual onset of chills, fever, headache, malaise, myalgia, anorexia, nausea, and vomiting. The temperature reaches 38.9 to 40°C (102 to 104°F), facial flushing may be prominent, and there is a painless enanthem of the pharynx. Lymphadenopathy and splenomegaly are not present. From 3 to 5 days after the onset, the signs and symptoms worsen, with the appearance of dehydration, hypotension to 50 to 100 mmHg, oliguria, and relative bradycardia. In the more severe cases, hemorrhagic manifestations, including bleeding from the gums, hematemesis, hematuria, and melena, occur. Progressive oliguria and tremor of the tongue and extremities may develop. Some patients develop psychic manifestations, with agitation, delirium, or stupor. Progressive shock, hypothermia, gallop rhythm, or gastrointestinal bleeding may occur from the seventh to tenth days. In fatal cases, pulmonary edema usually is the cause of death. During convalescence temporary alopecia has been noted. Erythrocyte counts are normal or elevated. The total leukocyte count drops to 1200 to 3400 blood cells per microliter. Thrombocytopenia may occur. Disseminated intravascular coagulation does not seem to be the mechanism responsible for the hemorrhagic manifestations. Complement components C2, C3, and C5 are decreased. The urine is dark with intense proteinuria. Blood urea nitrogen levels rise rapidly.

The clinical picture of Bolivian hemorrhagic fever is similar to Argentinian, although epistaxis and hematemesis at the onset is more common.

Diagnosis Antibody responses, including IgM antibodies, do not occur before 10 to 20 days.

Treatment Treatment consists of supportive measures, including peritoneal dialysis or hemodialysis-filtration to correct both the azotemia and the pulmonary edema. In AHF, a double-blind trial with immune plasma reduced mortality from 16 to 1 percent. However, fever and cerebellar signs occurred in patients treated with immune plasma. Preliminary studies suggest that ribavirin may be effective in experimental BHF in rhesus monkeys.

Prognosis The mortality rate among patients with Argentinian hemorrhagic fever is usually 3 to 15 percent, while that in Bolivian hemorrhagic fever is 5 to 30 percent.

Prevention In Bolivia, rodent control measures directed primarily against *C. callosus* populations in the houses has resulted in a prompt and dramatic cessation of human cases. In Argentina, the wide dispersal of infected hosts renders rodent control measures futile.

LASSA FEVER A virus disease which is both highly contagious and virulent occurred in a missionary nurse in Lassa, a town in northeast Nigeria, in 1969.

Epidemiology Since the initial outbreak at Lassa in 1969, during which one of the patients was transferred to New York City, there have been other outbreaks near Jos in northern Nigeria in 1970 (32 suspected cases with 10 deaths), in Zorzor, Liberia, in 1972 (11 cases with 4 deaths), and in the eastern province of Sierra Leone with 63 suspected cases admitted to two hospitals between 1970 and 1972. Lassa fever occurs as an endemic disease in eastern Sierra Leone. Population surveys showed more than one-half of older adults had antibodies. Other countries in west Africa having clinical or serologic evidence of Lassa fever include Senegal, Gambia, Guinea, Ghana, Burkina Faso (formerly Upper Volta), Mali, and Ivory Coast. Lassa-related viruses (Mopeia, Mobala) have been isolated from rodents in Mozambique, Zimbabwe, and the Central African Republic; however, they have not been associated with human illness. In Jos and Zorzor, outbreaks apparently resulted from person-to-person nosocomial spread from the index case to hospital workers or other patients. In Sierra Leone, the great majority of cases were acquired outside the hospital, although hospital workers were at risk. *Mastomys natalensis*, a multimammate rat widespread in Africa, is the animal reservoir, and primary human cases result from contamination of foodstuffs with rodent urine. Human-to-human transmission may occur through contact with urine, feces, vomitus, or saliva through droplets, and particularly through wounds contaminated with blood. Intrafamilial outbreaks have occurred around several cases. There are a number of cases which have been acquired through accidental autoinoculation with needles while starting intravenous fluids. At least one laboratory-acquired infection has occurred. In Sierra Leone 6 percent of the population surveyed had complement-fixing antibody against Lassa virus, while only 0.2 percent had recognized disease, suggesting mild disease or inapparent infection. In Liberia 10 percent of hospital personnel had antibodies.

Clinical features The incubation period is 1 to 24 days, and was 10 days following accidental inoculation. Patients have ranged from 5 months to 46 years of age; approximately two-thirds are women. Three of eight women in one series were 22 to 28 weeks pregnant during their illness. The apparent predilection for women may relate to exposure to contaminated food or work in hospitals rather than to differences in susceptibility. The onset of illness was described by most patients as insidious. The most frequent initial symptoms were fever (100 percent), chilliness and true rigors, headache (50 percent), malaise (100 percent), and myalgia (50 percent). Most patients did not seek medical attention for 4 to 9 days after onset. Symptoms of a systemic viral illness then developed with anorexia, nausea, vomiting, myalgia, and pain in the chest, epigastrium, and lumbar area. Headache was usually present. Early examination revealed fever and flushing of the face and V area of the neck. Pharyngitis developed early and became progressively more severe during the first week; examination in some cases revealed raised patches of whitish exudate occurring on the palatine arches, which occasionally coalesced into a pseudomembrane. Oral ulcerations have been noted in up to one-half of cases. Generalized nontender lymphadenopathy occurred in one-half of patients. During the second week severe lower abdominal pain and intractable vomiting were common, and facial and neck swelling with conjunctival edema and infection frequently developed. Occasionally patients had tinnitus, epistaxis, bleeding from the gums and venipuncture sites, maculopapular rashes, cough, and dizziness. During the acute stage, systolic blood pressures of less than 90 mmHg, with pulse pressures less than 20 mmHg, occurred in 60 to 80 percent of patients. Initially, relative bradycardia was common. During the second week, the patients who recovered defervesced while the patients who died often developed signs of shock, clouding of the sensorium, rales, signs of pleural effusion, agitation and, on occasion, grand mal seizures. The duration of illness in surviving patients ranged from 7 to 31 days (average 15 days), while that in fatal cases was 7 to 26 days (average 12 days). The mortality rates in Jos and Zorzor were 52 percent and 36 percent, respectively, while in Sierra Leone the rate was 8 percent. During convalescence occasional flurries of rapid involuntary eye movements (oculogyric crises) occurred. Late sequelae include deafness and alopecia.

Laboratory features The hematologic findings include relatively normal hematocrit values and early leukopenia (less than 4000 cells per microliter in 36 percent) with a relative neutrophilia and immature forms of leukocytes. In two cases in which it was recorded, the erythrocyte sedimentation rate was normal. Urinalyses revealed proteinuria, which was often massive. Chest radiographs may suggest basilar pneumonitis and pleural effusions. Electrocardiographic abnormalities compatible with diffuse myocardial disease have been encountered. Levels of serum enzymes, SGOT, creatinine phosphokinase (CPK), and LDH have been elevated. Lassa virus may be recovered from cerebrospinal fluid.

Diagnosis Diagnosis can be made by demonstrating a fourfold rise in antibody titer to Lassa virus between acute phase and convalescent phase serum specimens with the indirect fluorescent antibody technique or with Lassa IgM antibodies. The diagnosis is unlikely if IgM antibodies are absent by the fourteenth day of illness.

Treatment The management has been supportive. Infusion of immune plasma from convalescent patients resulted in a dramatic effect in three of four patients. Because of the self-limited nature of the disease, these results cannot be assessed easily. In a study of the antiviral agent ribavirin, 19 of 20 patients treated intravenously within 6 days of onset with a 2.0-g loading dose, followed by 1.0 g every 6 h for 4 days, then 0.5 g every 8 h for another 6 days, survived, whereas 11 of 18 who received no therapy, and 10 of 16 who received convalescent plasma died. In view of the hospital association and the presence of virus in pharyngeal secretions and urine, respiratory and enteric isolation and blood precautions are required. With reasonable isolation practices, nosocomial spread need not be as feared as previously.

OTHER HEMORRHAGIC FEVERS Ebola hemorrhagic fever and Marburg virus disease are caused by members of the family Filoviridae and are discussed in Chap. 147 and summarized in Table 148-1.

REFERENCES

Baum SG et al: Epidemic non-meningitic lymphocytic-choriomeningitis virus infection. N Engl J Med 274:934, 1966

Casals J: Arenaviruses. Yale J Biol Med 48:115, 1975

Centers for Disease Control: Viral hemorrhagic fever. Initial management of suspected and confirmed cases. Ann Intern Med 101:73, 1984

Fields BN et al (eds): *Virology*. New York, Raven, 1985

Frame JD et al: Lassa fever, a new virus disease of man from West Africa: I. Clinical description and pathological findings. Am J Trop Med Hyg 19:670, 1970

Johnson KM et al: Hemorrhagic fever of Southeast Asia and South America. A comparative approach. Prog Med Virol 9:105, 1967

McCormick JB et al: Lassa fever: Effective therapy with ribavirin. N Engl J Med 314:20, 1986

McKee KT Jr et al: Ribavirin prophylaxis and therapy for experimental Argentine hemorrhagic fever. Antimicrob Agents Chemother 32:1304, 1988

MacKenzie RB et al: Epidemic hemorrhagic fever in Bolivia: 1. A preliminary report of the epidemiologic and clinical findings in a new epidemic area in South America. Am J Trop Med Hyg 13:620, 1964

Mertens PE et al: Clinical presentation of Lassa fever cases during the hospital epidemic at Zorzor, Liberia, March–April 1972. Am J Trop Med Hyg 22:780, 1973

Monath TP et al: Lassa fever in the Eastern Province of Sierra Leone, 1970–1972: II. Clinical observations and virological studies on selected hospital cases. Am J Trop Med Hyg 23:1140, 1974

VanZee BE et al: Lymphocytic choriomeningitis in University hospital personnel. Clinical features. Am J Med 58:803, 1975

150 HUMAN PAPILLOMAVIRUS INFECTIONS

RICHARD C. REICHMAN

DEFINITION Human papillomaviruses (HPV) selectively infect the epithelium of skin or mucous membranes. These infections may be asymptomatic, produce warts, or be associated with a variety of both benign and malignant neoplasias.

ETIOLOGY HPV, members of the A genus of the family Papovaviridae, are nonenveloped viruses, 50 to 55 nm in diameter, with icosahedral capsids composed of 72 capsomeres. They contain a double-stranded, circular DNA genome of about 7900 base pairs. Papillomaviruses (PV) appear to be species specific, and HPV have not been propagated in tissue culture or in standard experimental animals. Significant quantities of virus are difficult to obtain, and HPV are incompletely characterized. Suitable HPV antigens have not been available, and work on the epidemiology, pathogenesis, immunology, and treatment of HPV-induced disease has been difficult to carry out. Structural viral proteins make up 88 percent of the mass of PV virions. A major capsid protein with a molecular weight of 56,000 and a minor capsid protein which migrates at 76,000 have been identified by sodium dodecyl sulfate polyacrylamide gel elec-

TABLE 150-1 Correlation of human papillomavirus (HPV) type with disease

Disease	Associated HPV types*
Deep plantar warts	1, 4
Common warts	1, 2, 4, 41
Common warts of meat handlers	7
Flat warts	3, 10, 27, 41
Intermediate warts	10, 26, 28
Epidermodysplasia verruciformis	5, 8, 9, 12, 14, 15, 17, 19–25, 36, 46, 47
Condylomata acuminata	6, 11, 40–45, 51
Intraepithelial neoplasias, unspecified	33, 35, 42–45, 51
Bowen's disease	16, 31
Bowenoid papulosis	16, 34, 39, 42
High-grade dysplasias	16, 18
Low-grade dysplasias	6, 11, 31, 45
Laryngeal papillomas	6, 11, 30
Focal epithelial hyperplasia of Heck	13, 32
Conjunctival papillomas	6, 11
Others	37, 38

*Types 29, 48–50, 52–60 have been identified but not published (data kindly supplied by Ethel-Michele de Villiers; HPV Reference Center, Heidelberg, FRG).

trophoresis. Four cellular histones are associated with the viral DNA. Type-specific antigenic determinants appear to be located on the virion surface and genus-specific determinants internally. Antisera produced by immunization of experimental animals with disrupted PV virions are broadly cross-reactive.

The genomic organization of all PV is similar. Types and subtypes are defined by degree of DNA hybridization under stringent conditions. DNA of a distinct PV type cross-hybridizes less than 50 percent with DNAs of other classified viruses. At least 60 types of HPV are recognized. Individual types are associated with specific kinds of warts (Table 150-1).

EPIDEMIOLOGY Seroepidemiologic studies of HPV infections have been hampered severely by lack of appropriate antigens, and there are few good studies of the incidence or prevalence of human warts in well-defined populations. Common warts are found in as many as 25 percent of some groups, and are most prevalent among young children. Plantar warts are also widely prevalent and occur most commonly among adolescents and young adults. The incidence of venereal warts (condylomata acuminata) has risen dramatically in the last 15 to 20 years, and condyloma acuminatum is one of the most common sexually transmitted diseases in the United States. HPV infection of the uterine cervix produces the most commonly detected squamous cell abnormalities on Papanicolaou smears.

CLINICAL MANIFESTATIONS Until the mid-1970s, it was generally believed that there was only one HPV and that clinical and pathologic differences among warts were a function of the nature of the squamous epithelium at the site of infection. With the discovery of multiple HPVs, it has become clear that the specific HPV is an important determinant of the nature of the lesion. Thus, clinical manifestations of HPV infection depend upon location of lesions and virus type. Common warts (verrucae vulgaris) usually occur on the hands, and are flesh-colored to brown, exophytic, hyperkeratotic papules. Plantar warts (verrucae plantaris) differ from most other warts by growing inward. They may be quite painful, and can be differentiated from callus by paring the surface to reveal thrombosed capillaries that bleed easily. Flat warts (verrucae plana) are most common among children and occur on the face, neck, chest, and flexor surfaces of forearms and legs.

Anogenital warts (condylomata acuminata, or venereal warts) occur on skin and mucosal surfaces of external genitalia and perianal areas. The differential diagnosis of anogenital warts includes condylomata lata of secondary syphilis, molluscum contagiosum, pearly penile papules, fibroepitheliomas, and a variety of benign and malignant mucocutaneous neoplasms. Anogenital warts are sexually transmitted, and have an incubation period of 1 to 6 months. In men, condylomata are found most frequently at the frenum or coronal sulcus, but they may affect any part of the penis. They occur commonly at the urethral meatus, and may extend proximally. Perianal warts are common among homosexual men, but appear in heterosexual men as well. In women, warts appear first at the posterior introitus and adjacent labia. They then spread to other parts of the vulva and commonly involve the perineum and anus. Condylomata frequently involve the vagina and cervix. These lesions may be present in the absence of external warts. Respiratory papillomatosis is uncommon, occurs predominantly in preschool children, and may result from acquisition of virus at the time of delivery through an infected birth canal. These lesions are typically multiple and may produce life-threatening airway obstruction. Disease in adults may be acquired by orogenital sexual contact.

Immunosuppressed patients, particularly those undergoing organ transplantation, often develop pityriasis versicolor–like lesions from which DNA of several HPV types has been extracted. Occasionally, such lesions appear to undergo malignant transformation.

Epidermodysplasia verruciformis is a rare, autosomal recessive disease characterized by the inability to terminate HPV infection and later development of cutaneous squamous cell malignancies. Lesions resemble flat warts or macules similar to those of pityriasis versicolor.

Complications of warts include itching and occasionally bleeding. Rarely, they may become secondarily infected with bacteria or fungi. Large masses of warts may produce mechanical problems such as obstruction of the birth canal. Epidemiologic, cytopathologic, virologic, and histologic data suggest an association of HPV infection with dysplasia and carcinoma of the uterine cervix. HPV nucleic acid sequences have been detected in cervical scrapings and biopsy specimens from most patients with these pathologic findings. Sequences homologous to certain HPV types have been found in 70 to 90 percent of specimens of cervical cancer tissue from patients in several geographic areas. Other genital tract malignancies have also been associated with these viruses.

PATHOGENESIS HPV infection is transmitted by close personal contact and is facilitated by minor trauma at the site of inoculation. It may result from direct contact with another individual, or, less commonly, by autoinoculation or via fomites. All types of squamous epithelium may be infected by HPV, and gross and histologic appearances of individual lesions vary with site of infection and virus type. Exophytic warts are characterized by papillomatosis, hyperkeratosis, and parakeratosis. Acanthosis, an increase in cellularity, occurs in the prickle cell layer in association with viral DNA synthesis. Late gene expression, manifested by appearance of structural proteins and assembled virions, is evident within nuclei of cells in the granular layer, where koilocytosis develops. Koilocytes are large round cells with pyknotic nuclei and large areas of perinuclear vacuolization surrounded by a ring of dense amphophilic cytoplasm. Histologically normal epithelium may contain HPV DNA. The presence of residual DNA after treatment often leads to recurrent disease.

Host defense responses to HPV infection are poorly understood. Most immunologic studies are difficult to interpret because crude and poorly characterized preparations have been employed as antigens. The potential importance of type-specific responses has not been adequately evaluated because appropriate antigenic materials are not widely available. Virus-specific IgM and IgG antibodies have been demonstrated in patients with and without clinical evidence of active infection. Cell-mediated immune responses to HPV antigens have also been measured, and patients with defects in cell-mediated immunity appear to be more susceptible than normals to HPV infections. Such patients occasionally develop extensive HPV disease.

DIAGNOSIS Most warts that are visible to the naked eye can be diagnosed correctly by history and physical examination alone. Colposcopy is invaluable in assessing vaginal and cervical lesions and is helpful in the diagnosis of oral and cutaneous HPV disease as well. Papanicolaou smears prepared from cervical scrapings often show cytologic evidence of HPV infection. Persistent or atypical lesions should be biopsied and examined by routine histologic methods. In addition, the genus-specific capsid antigen can be identified in tissue sections using immunologic techniques, and virus type can be determined by nucleic acid hybridization.

TREATMENT Therapy should be initiated with the knowledge that no treatment of proven safety and efficacy is currently available, and that many HPV lesions resolve spontaneously. Frequently used therapies include cryosurgery, application of caustic agents, electrodesiccation, surgical excision, and ablation with laser. Topical antimetabolites such as 5-fluorouracil have been used also. Failure as well as recurrence have been well-documented following all these methods of treatment. The high frequency of recurrence may be explained by the presence of HPV DNA in normal-appearing tissue adjacent to lesions, and in previously involved areas during periods of remission. For many years, topically applied podophyllum preparations have been used in treatment of condyloma acuminatum. However, use of these compounds is associated with resolution rates of less than 50 percent, and initial treatment of venereal warts with cryosurgery is preferable. Promising results have been observed in the treatment of respiratory papillomatosis and condyloma acuminatum with different interferon preparations.

At the present time, no effective methods of prevention are available for HPV infections other than avoiding contact with infectious lesions. Barrier methods of contraception may be helpful in preventing transmission of condyloma acuminatum and other HPV-associated diseases of the genital tract.

REFERENCES

HEALY G et al: Treatment of recurrent respiratory papillomatosis with human leukocyte interferon. N Engl J Med 319:401, 1988

HOWLEY PM: The role of papillomaviruses in human cancer, in *Important Advances in Oncology*, V de Vita, S Hellman, SA Rosenberg (eds). Philadelphia, Lippincott, 1987, pp 55–73

KOUTSY LA et al: Epidemiology of genital human papillomavirus infection. Epidemiologic Rev 10:122, 1988

MCCANCE DJ et al: Human papillomavirus type 16 alters human epithelial cell differentiation in vitro. Proc Natl Acad Sci USA 85:7169, 1988

REEVES WC et al: Human papillomavirus infection and cervical cancer in Latin America. N Engl J Med 320:1437, 1989

REICHMAN RC, BONNEZ W: Papillomaviruses, in *Principles and Practice of Infectious Diseases*, GL Mandell et al (eds) New York, Wiley 1990

——— et al: Treatment of condyloma acuminatum with three different interferons administered intralesionally. A double-blind, placebo-controlled trial. Ann Intern Med 108:675, 1988

SCHREIER AA et al: Prospects for human papillomavirus vaccines and immunotherapies. J Natl Cancer Inst 80:896, 1988

STEINBERG BM et al: Persistence and expression of human papillomavirus during interferon therapy. Arch Otolaryngol Head Neck Surg 114:27, 1988

STRIKE DG et al: Expression in *Escherichia coli* of seven DNA segments comprising the complete L1 and L2 open reading frames of human papillomavirus type 6b and localization of the "common antigen" region. J Gen Virol 70:543, 1989

ZUR HAUSEN H: Genital papillomavirus infections. Prog Med Virol 32:15, 1985

section 9 Infection caused by fungi and higher bacteria

151 FUNGAL INFECTIONS

JOHN E. BENNETT

INTRODUCTION Actinomycetes and fungi are considered together in this section, but this should not obscure profound differences between these two groups of organisms. The agents of actinomycosis, nocardiosis, and actinomycetoma are actinomycetes. These organisms are gram-positive higher bacteria that branch but have the diameter, antibiotic susceptibility, and ability to induce the neutrophilic inflammatory response of other bacteria. Actinomycetes resemble fungi in causing infections that may be extremely chronic and that are poorly transmissible from person to person. Few other similarities exist between fungi and actinomycetes. This introductory section will concern mycoses.

The diagnosis of a mycosis requires demonstration of the pathogenic fungus in appropriate patient specimens. Visualization of the fungus by smear or histology is a less precise and less sensitive diagnostic method than culture but is more rapid. Culture allows definitive identification of the pathogen and can detect a small number of organisms. False-positives occur with both methods. Artifacts may be mistaken for fungi in smears or histologic sections. *Candida albicans* can be isolated from the mouth, vagina, sputum, urine, or stool in the absence of candidiasis. *Aspergillus* and, occasionally, *Cryptococcus neoformans* appear in sputum of patients without a mycosis. Histology has the uniquely valuable potential of demonstrating the fungus within the area of inflammation. Only this method can show whether *Aspergillus* in the lung or paranasal sinus tissue exists as a pathogen or merely as a saprophyte growing in pooled secretions. Demonstration of fungi in tissue section usually requires special stains, such as methenamine silver.

Skin testing with fungal antigens has little diagnostic value in active infection. Serologic testing is very helpful in diagnosing coccidioidomycosis and cryptococcosis, as well as in following response to therapy of these mycoses. In histoplasmosis and paracoccidioidomycosis, serologic tests are useful in adding some support to the clinical diagnosis.

THE DEEP MYCOSES

CRYPTOCOCCOSIS Etiology Cryptococcosis is an infection caused by the yeastlike fungus *Cryptococcus neoformans*. *C. neoformans* reproduces by budding and forms round, yeastlike cells 4 to 6 μm in diameter. Within the host and on certain culture media, a large polysaccharide capsule surrounds each yeast cell. The fungus grows well as smooth, creamy white colonies on Sabouraud's or other simple media at 20 to 37°C. Certain culture media for ringworm contain cycloheximide, which inhibits *C. neoformans*. Identification is based on gross and microscopic appearance, biochemical tests, and growth at 37°C. The fungus has four capsular serotypes, designated A, B, C, and D.

Pathogenesis and pathology Infection is thought to be acquired by inhalation of fungus into the lungs. Pulmonary infection has a tendency toward spontaneous resolution and is frequently asymptomatic. Silent hematogenous spread to the brain leads to clusters of cryptococci in the perivascular areas of cortical gray matter, basal ganglia, and, to a lesser extent, other areas of the central nervous system. Inflammatory response around these foci is usually scant. In the more chronic cases, a dense basilar arachnoiditis occurs. Lung lesions show an intense granulomatous inflammation. Cryptococci are best seen in tissue by staining with methenamine silver or periodic acid Schiff. A strongly positive mucicarmine stain of the organism in tissue is diagnostic, but staining varies from intense to absent.

Cryptococcus neoformans has been isolated from several sites in nature, particularly weathered pigeon droppings. Patients are usually unaware of any unusual exposure to pigeon droppings. No significant case clustering, highly endemic areas, or racial or occupational predisposition is known. Infection before puberty is uncommon. The male/female ratio is about 2:1. Approximately three-fourths of the patients have a predisposing condition, such as lymphoma or sarcoidosis, or are receiving supraphysiologic doses of glucocorticoids. Approximately 7 percent of patients with the acquired immunodeficiency syndrome (AIDS) develop cryptococcosis. In these patients the mycosis disseminates and is difficult to cure. Neither neutropenia nor hypogammaglobulinemia seems to increase susceptibility to cryptococcosis. Transmission from animals to humans or from person to person has not been documented.

Clinical manifestations The majority of patients have *meningoencephalitis* at the time of diagnosis. This form of the infection is invariably fatal without appropriate therapy, and death occurs anywhere from 2 weeks to several years from onset of symptoms. Early manifestations include headache, nausea, staggering gait, dementia, irritability, confusion, and blurred vision. Both fever and nuchal rigidity are often mild or absent. Papilledema is present in one-third of the patients at the time of diagnosis. Cranial nerve palsies, typically asymmetric, occur in about one-fourth of the patients. Other lateralizing signs are rare. With progression of the infection, deepening coma and signs of brainstem compression appear. Autopsy often reveals cerebral edema in the more acute cases or hydrocephalus in more chronic cases.

Pulmonary cryptococcosis causes chest pain in about 40 percent of patients and cough in 20 percent. Chest x-ray shows one or more dense infiltrates, which are often well circumscribed. Cavitation, pleural effusions, or hilar adenopathy are infrequent. Calcification is not present, and fibrotic stranding is rarely noticeable.

Skin lesions are present in 10 percent of patients with cryptococcosis and the vast majority of patients with skin lesions have disseminated infection. One or a few asymptomatic tiny papular lesions appear, slowly enlarge, and tend to show central softening leading to ulceration. Osteolytic bone lesions occur in 4 percent of patients and usually present as a cold abscess. Rare manifestations of cryptococcosis include prostatitis, endophthalmitis, hepatitis, pericarditis, endocarditis, and renal abscess.

Diagnosis Cryptococcal meningoencephalitis must be distinguished from tuberculosis, neoplasm, coccidioidomycosis, histoplasmosis, candidiasis, viral meningitis, and sarcoidosis. Computed tomography (CT) scan or magnetic resonance imaging will occasionally show one or two focal areas of decreased density with contrast-enhancing margins. Lumbar puncture is the single most useful test. An india ink smear of centrifuged spinal fluid sediment reveals encapsulated yeast in one-half the cases, but artifacts resembling cryptococci may cause confusion. Cerebrospinal fluid glucose is reduced in half the cases, protein concentration is usually increased, and 20 to 600 leukocytes per microliter are typically present and consist predominantly of lymphocytes. Approximately 90 percent of patients with cryptococcal meningoencephalitis, including all those with a positive cerebrospinal fluid smear, will have capsular antigen detectable in cerebrospinal fluid or serum by latex agglutination. False-positive tests occur occasionally, making culture the definitive diagnostic test. *C. neoformans* is often present in urine from patients with meningoencephalitis. Fungemia occurs in 10 to 30 percent of patients, and is particularly common in AIDS patients.

Pulmonary cryptococcosis mimics malignancy by x-ray and symptoms. Sputum culture is positive in only 10 percent, and serum antigen tests are positive in only a third. Occasionally, *C. neoformans* appears in one or multiple sputum specimens as an endobronchial saprophyte. Biopsy is usually required for diagnosis of pulmonary cryptococcosis. Cutaneous cryptococcosis may be mistaken for a comedo, basal-cell carcinoma, or sarcoidosis. In AIDS patients, skin lesions may be numerous and mistaken for molluscum contagiosum. Biopsy reveals a myriad of cryptococci. Osseous cryptococcosis resembles tuberculosis.

Treatment Cryptococcal meningoencephalitis may be treated either with amphotericin B alone or in combination with flucytosine. Amphotericin B is given as 0.5 to 0.6 mg/kg per day when used alone or as 0.3 mg/kg per day in combination therapy. With either regimen, double-dose therapy on alternate days may be employed. Flucytosine is given initially as 37.5 mg/kg every 6 h to patients with normal renal function. Although nomograms are available for adjusting flucytosine dosage in the presence of reduced renal function, frequent measurement of serum levels and maintenance between 50 and 100 μg/mL offer the best chance of preventing toxicity. Even with this precaution, the problems of leukopenia, thrombocytopenia, diarrhea, and rash have been so common in AIDS patients that amphotericin B is usually given alone.

Duration of therapy is based upon the results of lumbar punctures. These are best done weekly until culture conversion is clearly documented. Six weeks of therapy may be adequate for patients with at least four weekly cultures of 2 to 4 mL CSF, whose india ink smear has become negative, and whose CSF glucose is normal. Approximately 50 to 70 percent of patients are cured. AIDS patients have proven so difficult to cure that most receive an intensive course of amphotericin B until CSF cultures are negative, and then require weekly intravenous injections of 1 mg/kg amphotericin B for the remainder of their lives. Average survival of AIDS patients after diagnosis of cryptococcosis has been about 8 months.

Hydrocephalus may be an early or late complication of cryptococcosis. Blindness, dementia, and personality change are other sequelae.

Patients with extraneural cryptococcosis most often require intravenous amphotericin B, with or without flucytosine. Observation or excision of lesions may suffice for some patients who are previously normal, who have a single focus in lung, skin, or bone, and who have no cryptococci in the cerebrospinal fluid, urine, or blood.

BLASTOMYCOSIS Etiology *Blastomyces dermatitidis* is a dimorphic fungus, growing at room temperature as a white or tan mold but growing within the host or at 37°C as budding, round yeastlike cells. The fungus is identified by its appearance, its dimorphism, and the appearance of small spores borne on hyphae of the mold form. When isolates of the two opposite mating types are grown closely together on specialized culture media, sporulating structures appear which characterize the perfect form, *Ajellomyces dermatitidis*.

Pathogenesis and pathology The infection is restricted by geography and age. Blastomycosis is uncommon in any locality, but the majority of cases occur in the southeast, central, and midatlantic areas of the United States, with occasional cases in other localities in the United States and Canada. Cases have also been encountered in Africa, Mexico, Central America, and, rarely, South America. Most patients are between 20 and 69 years old. The male/female ratio is about 10:1. There is no occupational predisposition.

Infection appears to be acquired by inhalation of the fungus from soil, decomposed vegetation, or rotting wood. Several case clusters have occurred during recreational activities in wooded areas along waterways. Infection is not transmissible from person to person. The initial pulmonary infection may heal spontaneously or become chronic. Spread to other portions of the lung, cavitation, or endobronchial lesions may appear in chronic cases. Whether or not the lung lesion resolves spontaneously, infection commonly spreads hematogenously to skin, subcutaneous tissue, bone, prostate, epididymis, or mucosa of the nose, mouth, or larynx. Less commonly, infection spreads to the brain, meninges, liver, lymph nodes, or spleen. Dissemination may not be evident for weeks or years after the appearance of the lung lesion. Progressive infection is only rarely attributable to an underlying disease or immunosuppressive treatment. The inflammatory response includes lymphocytes, giant cells, and neutrophils. Pseudoepitheliomatous hyperplasia may be striking and lead to a mistaken diagnosis of squamous cell carcinoma.

Clinical manifestations A small number of patients have an acute, self-limited pneumonia. Fever, productive cough, myalgia, and malaise usually have resolved within a month. Pulmonary infiltrates have cleared slowly as *B. dermatitidis* disappeared from the sputum.

The vast majority of patients with blastomycosis have an indolent onset and a chronically progressive course. Fever, cough, weight loss, lassitude, skin lesions, and chest ache are common symptoms. Skin lesions favor exposed areas and enlarge over many weeks from a pimple to a well-circumscribed, verrucous, crusted, or ulcerated lesion. Pain and regional lymphadenopathy are minimal. Large chronic lesions may show central healing with scarring and contracture. Mucous membrane lesions resemble squamous cell carcinoma. Chest x-ray is abnormal in two-thirds of cases, with one or more pneumonic or nodular infiltrates. Calcification, hilar adenopathy, and large pleural effusions are rare. Osteolytic lesions may occur in nearly any bone and present as cold abscess or a draining sinus. Extension to a contiguous joint may cause indolent swelling, pain, and restricted motion. Prostatic and epididymal lesions resemble tuberculosis clinically.

Diagnosis The diagnosis is made by demonstrating the fungus in culture of sputum, pus, or urine. In experienced hands, diagnosis by appearance of the organism in wet smear or histopathologic section is adequate. The fungus may be visible in a sputum cytology smear but is easily overlooked.

Treatment A few patients have been observed with transitory lung lesions, but no guidelines are known to distinguish these patients from those whose disease will progress locally or disseminate. Therefore, every patient should receive treatment. Intravenous amphotericin B is the drug of choice for patients with rapidly progressive infections, severe illness, or meningitis. Skin and noncavitary lung lesions should be treated for about 8 to 10 weeks. The recommended total dose for an adult is about 2.0 g. Cavitary lung disease or infection beyond the lung and skin should be treated for about 10 to 12 weeks with 2.5 g or more. Ketoconazole is an effective drug in patients with indolent nonmeningeal blastomycosis of mild to moderate severity and who take the drug reliably. The initial adult dose is 400 mg once daily, raised after a month to 600 or 800 mg daily if improvement is suboptimal. Therapy is continued for 6 to 12 months. The mortality rate in appropriately treated cases is 15 percent or less.

HISTOPLASMOSIS **Etiology** *Histoplasma capsulatum* is a dimorphic fungus that grows as a mold in nature or on Sabouraud's agar at room temperature. Hyphae bear both large and small spores, which are used for identification. *H. capsulatum* grows as a small budding yeast in host tissue and on enriched agar, such as blood cysteine glucose, at 37°C. Despite the name, the fungus is unencapsulated.

Pathogenesis and pathology Infection with *H. capsulatum* has been encountered in many areas of the world but is much more frequent in certain areas. Within the United States infection is most common in the southeastern, midatlantic, and central states. Endemic areas are probably determined by the availability of proper conditions in nature for growth of the fungus. *H. capsulatum* prefers moist surface soil, particularly when it is enriched by droppings of certain birds and bats. The fungus has not only been isolated repeatedly from such sites but many case clusters have occurred 5 to 18 days after groups were exposed to such dust, for example, by raking, cleaning dirt-floored chicken coops, bulldozing, or cave exploring. Judging by skin test reactivity in many endemic areas, 80 percent or more of residents over age 16 have been exposed.

Microconidia, or small spores, of *H. capsulatum* are small enough to reach the alveoli on inhalation and are transformed to budding forms. With time, an intense granulomatous reaction occurs. Caseation necrosis or calcification may mimic tuberculosis. The primary infection in children usually heals completely but may leave spotty calcification in the hilar nodes or lung. Transient dissemination may leave calcified granulomas in the spleen. In adults, a rounded mass of scar tissue, with or without central calcification, may remain in the lung. This has been called a *histoplasmoma*. Previous exposure is thought to confer some protection against reinfection, but infection in persons with prior positive skin tests clearly has occurred.

In a small proportion of patients, histoplasmosis becomes a progressive, potentially fatal infection. The disease occurs either as chronic fibrocavitary pneumonia or, less commonly, as disseminated infection. Patients with either form lack a history of acute primary pulmonary histoplasmosis. Chronic pulmonary infection favors otherwise healthy males over the age of 40. A history of cigarette use can be elicited from nearly all patients with chronic progressive pulmonary histoplasmosis. An acute, rapidly fatal course is most likely to be encountered in young children and immunosuppressed patients, including those with AIDS. A more chronic but equally lethal disseminated infection is more common in previously healthy adults.

Clinical manifestations The vast majority of infections are either asymptomatic or mild, and the diagnosis is elusive. Cough, fever, malaise, and chest x-ray findings of hilar adenopathy with or without one or more areas of pneumonitis occur. Erythema nodosum and erythema multiforme have been reported in a few outbreaks. Hilar adenopathy may cause temporary compression of the right middle lobe bronchus in children and young adults. Subacute pericarditis may occur, probably by extension from contiguous lymph nodes. Rarely, hilar nodes undergo a caseous, granulomatous reaction with perinodal fibrosis. Mediastinal structures become encased by progressive fibrosis, and, over many years, compression of the pulmonary veins, superior vena cava, pulmonary arteries, and esophagus may occur. Late in mediastinal disease only rare nonviable histoplasma can be found in caseous residua of lymph nodes.

Patients with *chronic pulmonary histoplasmosis* have a gradual onset over weeks or months of increasing productive cough, weight loss, and sometimes night sweats. Chest x-ray reveals uni- or bilateral fibronodular apical infiltrates. Approximately one-third of cases will stabilize or improve spontaneously early in the course. The remainder show insidious progression. Retraction and cavitation of the upper lobes occur with spread to the apex of the lower lobes and other areas of the lung. Emphysema and bullae formation further compromise pulmonary function. Death from cor pulmonale, bacterial pneumonia, or histoplasmosis occurs after months or years.

Acute disseminated histoplasmosis may be mistaken for miliary tuberculosis (see Chap. 125). Common findings include fever, emaciation, hepatosplenomegaly, lymphadenopathy, jaundice, anemia, leukopenia, and thrombocytopenia. All these features may occur in chronic dissemination as well, but the disease tends to be more localized. Indurated ulcers of the mouth, tongue, nose, or larynx occur in about a fourth of patients. Other focal findings include granulomatous hepatitis, Addison's disease, gastrointestinal ulceration, endocarditis, and chronic meningitis. Chest x-ray abnormalities occur in half the cases and show discrete nodules or a miliary pattern.

The presumed *ocular histoplasmosis* syndrome is a distinct clinical form of uveitis. Although a positive histoplasmin skin test is a requisite for diagnosis, none of these patients has had active histoplasmosis.

Diagnosis Histoplasmosis may be suspected by serologic tests and clinical manifestations, but definitive diagnosis requires demonstration of the organism by culture or histology. Serologic tests are performed on serum or CSF using either a culture filtrate called histoplasmin or whole yeast form cells. The results are interchangeable. Complement fixation is quantifiable and is the best test. An agar gel diffusion test with histoplasmin is useful but not quantifiable. An H band on agar gel testing is more diagnostic of active histoplasmosis than an M band. Frequent false-negatives and false-positives limit all current serologic tests. Serologic conversion is helpful but occurs rarely except in acute pulmonary histoplasmosis. High complement fixation titers, such as 1:32 or greater, are suggestive of the diagnosis, but no titer is diagnostic. Cross-reactions with serologic tests for blastomycosis are common. A 5-mm or more diameter area of induration 24 to 48 h after skin testing with histoplasmin has been very helpful in identifying prior exposure to *Histoplasma*, but false-negatives and false-positives are so frequent that skin testing has little value in the study of ill patients. Further, a positive skin test can cause seroconversion.

Culture of *H. capsulatum* from sputum is difficult but is the procedure of choice in chronic pulmonary histoplasmosis. Digestion by proteolytic enzymes and centrifugation of sputum are helpful. In disseminated histoplasmosis, cultures of bone marrow, blood, centrifuged urine sediment, and biopsy specimens are most often positive. Lysis centrifugation is the best method for blood culture. Histologic sections of bone marrow, liver, lymph node, lung, and mucosal lesions may yield the diagnosis.

Treatment Acute pulmonary histoplasmosis requires no therapy. Mediastinal fibrosis may benefit by surgery, but the ultimate prognosis is poor. All patients with disseminated or chronic fibronodular pulmonary histoplasmosis should receive chemotherapy. The indications for using ketoconazole, as well as the treatment regimen, are the same as those given in the section on "Blastomycosis." Amphotericin B is given as 0.4 to 0.5 mg/kg per day or double that on alternate days, and is continued for at least 10 weeks. AIDS patients with disseminated histoplasmosis respond poorly to ketoconazole and should be treated with amphotericin B. After an initial intensive course, these patients are often given weekly therapy with amphotericin B to prevent relapse. In chronic pulmonary histoplasmosis, chest x-ray abnormalities improve somewhat, but pulmonary function improves very little. Successful therapy prevents progression. Addisonian crisis is a preventable cause of death in disseminated histoplasmosis.

African histoplasmosis Patients have been encountered in Africa who seem to be infected with *H. capsulatum* except that the yeast form is larger. Clinical manifestations resemble blastomycosis more than histoplasmosis because skin and bone lesions are very common.

COCCIDIOIDOMYCOSIS Etiology *Coccidioides immitis* has two forms, growing as a white fluffy mold on most culture media but as a nonbudding spherical form, a spherule, in host tissue or under specialized conditions. Reproduction in the host tissue is by formation of small endospores within mature spherules. After rupture of the spherule, the released endospores enlarge, become spherules, and repeat the cycle. The fungus is identified by its appearance and by formation of thick-walled, barrel-shaped spores, called *arthrospores*, in the hyphae of the mold form.

Pathogenesis and pathology *C. immitis* is a soil saprophyte in certain arid regions of the United States, Mexico, Central America, and South America. Within the United States, most cases are acquired in California, Arizona, west Texas, and New Mexico. A few cases are acquired in bordering areas and by exposure to fomites from endemic areas, such as in cotton bales.

Infection in humans and animals results from inhalation of wind-borne arthrospores arising from soil sites. This primary pulmonary infection is symptomatic in only 40 percent of individuals, with symptoms ranging from a mild, influenza-like illness to severe pneumonia. Mild, self-limited infections may come to medical attention because of case clusters or hypersensitivity reactions: erythema nodosum, erythema multiforme, toxic erythema, arthralgia, arthritis, conjunctivitis, or episcleritis. Case clusters occur 10 to 14 days after a group of susceptible individuals is exposed to dust in an endemic area through such activities as unearthing Indian relics, rock hunting, military maneuvers, or construction. Wind storms can carry spores to adjacent nonendemic areas and cause case clusters. The usual course of primary pulmonary infection is complete healing, though an area of pneumonitis on x-ray may heal by forming a coinlike lesion, or coccidioidoma. Less commonly, a single thin-walled cavity remains as a chronic sequela in the area of consolidation. The consolidation may persist as a chronic pneumonia or progress to fibronodular, cavitary disease.

Pleural effusion may be the only manifestation of primary infection. Self-healing of this form is common.

An uncommon but dreaded complication of coccidioidomycosis is dissemination beyond the lung and hilar lymph nodes. Dissemination is more frequent in blacks, Filipinos, Native Americans, Mexican-Americans, and pregnant or immunosuppressed patients, including those with AIDS.

C. immitis incites a chronic granulomatous reaction in host tissue, often with caseation necrosis. Lung and hilar node lesions may show calcification. Both IgM and IgG antibodies against *C. immitis* are induced by infection but neither appears protective. The amount of specific IgG antibody is a rough measure of the antigenic mass, i.e., of the amount of infection, and a high titer is a poor prognostic sign. Appearance of delayed hypersensitivity to antigens of *C. immitis* is most common in those clinical forms of disease with a good prognosis, such as self-limited primary pulmonary disease. Negative skin tests to *Coccidioides* antigens occur in roughly half the patients with disseminated disease and portend a poor prognosis.

Clinical manifestations Symptomatic primary pulmonary infection is manifested by fever, cough, chest pain, malaise, and sometimes hypersensitivity reactions. Chest x-ray may show an infiltrate, hilar adenopathy, or pleural effusion. Peripheral blood may show a mild eosinophilia. Spontaneous improvement begins after several days to 2 weeks of illness and usually culminates in complete recovery.

The symptoms of a chronic thin-walled cavity include cough or hemoptysis in half the cases; the other patients are asymptomatic. Chronic progressive pulmonary coccidioidomycosis produces cough, sputum, variable degrees of fever, and weight loss. The first indications of dissemination usually appear during the primary infection. Reactivation with dissemination in later years occurs occasionally, especially if Hodgkin's disease, non-Hodgkin's lymphoma, renal transplantation, AIDS, or other immunosuppression has supervened. Dissemination should be suspected when fever, malaise, hilar or paratracheal lymphadenopathy, elevated sedimentation rate, and high complement fixation titers show abnormal persistence in patients with primary pulmonary coccidioidomycosis. With time, lesions appear in the bone, skin, subcutaneous tissue, meninges, joints, and other sites. Without therapy, dissemination may progress rapidly to death or wax and wane for years.

Diagnosis When coccidioidomycosis is suspected, sputum, urine, and pus should be examined for *C. immitis* by wet smear and culture. *The laboratory request should indicate clearly that coccidioidomycosis is suspected because the mold form must be handled with extreme care to prevent infection of laboratory personnel.* On biopsy, smaller spherules must be distinguished from nonbudding forms of *Blastomyces* and *Cryptococcus*, but appearance of the mature spherule is diagnostic.

Serologic tests are very helpful in coccidioidomycosis. Latex agglutination and agar gel diffusion tests are useful in screening sera for antibody to *Coccidioides*. The complement fixation test is used on cerebrospinal fluid and to confirm and quantitate serum antibody detected by screening tests. The number of cases with a positive complement fixation test will depend upon the severity of disease and upon the laboratory performing the test. Positive tests are least common in patients with solitary pulmonary cavities or primary pulmonary infection, while sera from patients with multiorgan disseminated disease are nearly all positive. Seroconversion is helpful in primary pulmonary coccidioidomycosis but may not occur for up to 8 weeks after onset. A positive complement fixation test in unconcentrated cerebrospinal fluid is diagnostic of meningitis. Rarely, a parameningeal focus will cause a positive CSF serology.

Conversion of the skin test from negative to positive ($\geq$5 mm induration at 24 or 48 h) with either coccidioidin or spherulin, the two commercially available antigens, may occur between the third and twenty-first days of symptoms in primary pulmonary coccidioidomycosis. Skin testing can also be helpful in epidemiologic studies, such as investigation of case clusters or definition of endemic areas.

The utility of skin testing as a diagnostic tool is limited by the presence of persistent positive tests resulting from remote exposures to *Coccidioides* and by the frequency of negative skin tests in many patients with either thin-walled cavities or disseminated coccidioidomycosis.

Treatment Primary pulmonary coccidioidomycosis usually resolves spontaneously. Some physicians give a few weeks of intravenous amphotericin B when patients show an unusually severe or protracted primary infection, hoping to abort disseminated or chronic pulmonary disease. There is no solid evidence to support this practice, but the stronger the suspicion of dissemination becomes in any given patient, the more logical this approach appears. Once evidence for dissemination becomes incontrovertible, amphotericin B may be palliative rather than curative. Incomplete recovery and relapse after apparent cure with amphotericin B have been distressingly common in both disseminated and chronic progressive pulmonary infection. The low toxicity and possibility of long-term oral therapy with ketoconazole have encouraged study of this drug in nonmeningeal coccidioidomycosis. Doses of 200 to 400 mg/d have resulted in improvement of some patients with skin, bone, and lung lesions. Patients failing to respond to this dose should have the dose escalated gradually in the 10 to 20 mg/kg per day range to assess clinical response and toxicity. Treatment is continued 12 months or more. A seriously ill or rapidly deteriorating patient should not be treated with ketoconazole. Such patients are given intravenous amphotericin B 0.5 to 0.7 mg/kg daily or 1.0 mg/kg on alternate days until infection appears relatively quiescent, often 10 or 12 weeks later. More prolonged courses may be changed to 1.0 mg/kg three times a week. Surgical debridement of bone lesions and drainage of abscesses contribute to cure. Resection of chronic progressive pulmonary lesions is a helpful adjunct to chemotherapy when infection is confined to the lung and to one lobe. A single thin-walled cavity tends to close spontaneously and ordinarily is not resected. Such a cavity responds poorly to chemotherapy. Coccidioidal meningitis is treated with long-term intrathecal amphotericin B. Hydrocephalus, a frequent complication, renders this therapy less effective. Fluconazole, an investigational agent, may be useful in such patients. The prognosis in all forms of chronic progressive coccidioidomycosis must be guarded.

THE OPPORTUNISTIC DEEP MYCOSES

CANDIDIASIS Etiology *Candida albicans* is the most common cause of candidiasis, but *C. tropicalis, C. parapsilosis, C. guilliermondii, C. krusei,* and a few other species can cause candidiasis and may even be fatal. *C. parapsilosis* is particularly notable for its ability to cause endocarditis. All *Candida* species pathogenic for humans are also encountered as commensals of humans, particularly in the mouth, stool, and vagina. These species grow rapidly at 25 to 37°C on simple media as oval budding cells. In specialized culture media, hyphae or elongated branching structures called *pseudohyphae* are formed. *C. albicans* can be identified presumptively by its ability to form germ tubes in serum or by the formation of thick-walled large spores, called *chlamydospores*. Final identification of all species requires biochemical tests.

Pathogenesis and pathology Either local or systemic factors may lead to tissue invasion by *Candida*. Chronic maceration predisposes to cutaneous candidiasis, as in diaper rash, intertrigo in obese patients, or paronychia in bartenders or cannery workers. Age is important because neonatal colonization often leads to oral candidiasis (thrush). Women in the third trimester of pregnancy are prone to vulvovaginal thrush. Patients with diabetes mellitus, AIDS, or hematologic malignancy, or who are receiving broad-spectrum antibiotics or high doses of adrenal corticosteroids, are especially susceptible to candidiasis. Breaks in the integrity of the skin or mucous membranes may provide access to deeper tissues. Examples include perforation of the gastrointestinal tract by trauma, surgery, and peptic ulceration; indwelling catheters for intravenous alimentation, peritoneal dialysis, and urinary tract drainage; severe burns; and intravenous drug abuse.

Candida grows within tissues in both yeast and pseudohyphal forms. Rarely, only one form is present. Visceral lesions are characterized by necrosis and a neutrophilic inflammatory response. Neutrophils kill *Candida* yeast cells and damage segments of pseudohyphae in vitro, and visceral candidiasis complicates neutropenia, chronic granulomatous disease, and myeloperoxidase deficiency, suggesting a major role for the neutrophil in host defense against this fungus. Visceral lesions show a preference for kidney, brain, spleen, heart, and liver.

Clinical manifestations *Oral thrush* presents as discrete and confluent adherent white plaques on the oral and pharyngeal mucosa, particularly in the mouth and tongue. These lesions are usually painless, but fissuring at the corners of the mouth can be painful. *Cutaneous candidiasis* presents as red, macerated intertriginous areas, paronychia, balanitis, or pruritus ani. Candidiasis of the perineal and scrotal skin may be accompanied by discrete pustular lesions on the inner aspects of the thighs. *Chronic mucocutaneous candidiasis* or *Candida granuloma* typically presents as circumscribed hyperkeratotic skin lesions, crumbling dystrophic nails, partial alopecia in areas of scalp lesions, and both oral and vaginal thrush. Systemic infection is very rare, but disfigurement of the face and hands can be severe. Other findings may include chronic epidermophytosis, dental dysplasia, and hypofunction of the parathyroid, adrenal, or thyroid glands. A variety of defects in T-cell function have been described in these patients. Vulvovaginal thrush causes pruritus, discharge, and sometimes pain on intercourse or urination. Speculum examination reveals an inflamed mucosa and a thin exudate, often with white curds.

From one to multiple small shallow ulcerations due to *Candida* may appear in the esophagus or gastrointestinal tract. Esophageal lesions favor the distal third and may cause dysphagia or substernal pain. Other such lesions tend to be asymptomatic but assume importance in the leukemic patient as a portal for disseminated candidiasis. Within the urinary tract, the most common lesions are either hematogenous renal abscesses, which can cause azotemia, or bladder thrush. Bladder invasion usually follows catheterization or instrumentation of a patient with diabetes mellitus or who is receiving broad-spectrum antibiotics. This lesion generally is asymptomatic and benign. Rarely, retrograde invasion of the renal pelvis leads to renal papillary necrosis.

Hematogenous dissemination of Candida presents with fever and toxicity but with few localizing findings. One or more retinal abscesses may appear and extend slowly into the vitreous humor. The patient may note orbital pain, blurred vision, scotoma, or opacities floating across the visual field. Pulmonary candidiasis is almost always hematogenous and is visible on chest x-ray only when the abscesses are numerous enough to cause a diffuse, vaguely nodular infiltrate. Candidiasis of the endocardium or around intracardiac prostheses resembles bacterial infection of these sites. Chronic *Candida* meningitis or arthritis may occur, from either disseminated disease or insertion of a prosthesis in the case of arthritis. Rare focal manifestations of disseminated disease include osteomyelitis, pustular skin lesions, myositis, and brain abscess.

Diagnosis Demonstration of pseudohyphae on wet smear with confirmation by culture is the procedure of choice for diagnosing superficial candidiasis. Scrapings for the smear may be obtained from skin, nails, and oral and vaginal mucosa. Culture alone is not diagnostic; however, recovery of *Candida* species from multiple superficial sites in immunosuppressed patients may portend visceral invasion.

Deeper lesions of *Candida* may be diagnosed by histologic section of biopsy specimens or by culture of cerebrospinal fluid, blood, joint fluid, or surgical specimens. Blood cultures in vented bottles or concentrated by lysis-centrifugation are very useful in *Candida* endocarditis and intravenous catheter-induced sepsis but are positive less often in other forms of disseminated disease. Serologic tests for antibody or antigen are not useful.

Treatment Cutaneous candidiasis of macerated areas responds to measures which reduce moisture and chafing plus a topically applied antifungal agent in a nonocclusive base. Nystatin, ciclopirox, and the imidazole creams such as clotrimazole and miconazole appear roughly equivalent. Nystatin and some imidazoles are available also for vaginal application. Oral candidiasis should be treated with clotrimazole troches or a nystatin suspension. Swallowing nystatin suspension, sucking on clotrimazole troches, or taking ketoconazole, 200 to 400 mg/d, may improve symptoms of esophageal candidiasis. When esophageal symptoms are pronounced, a 5- to 10-day course of intravenous amphotericin B, 0.3 mg/kg per day, may be beneficial. Bladder thrush responds to bladder irrigations with amphotericin B, 50 μg/mL for 5 days. In all forms of skin and mucosal candidiasis, relapse after successful treatment is common.

Intravenous amphotericin B is the drug of choice in disseminated candidiasis. The drug is usually given as 0.4 to 0.5 mg/kg every day or as a double dose on alternate days for several weeks. In patients with no contraindication to the use of flucytosine, administration of that drug in dosage of 100 to 150 mg/kg per day plus amphotericin B, 0.3 mg/kg per day, is an effective alternative. Ketoconazole in an adult dose of 200 mg daily is probably the drug of choice for chronic mucocutaneous candidiasis.

Candida isolated from a properly obtained blood culture should be considered significant; true false-positives are rare. Whether a patient with candidiasis should receive antifungal therapy will depend on the degree of illness and the likelihood of spontaneous recovery. For example, a febrile, severely immunosuppressed patient with one positive blood culture should receive prompt therapy because a rapidly fatal course is common. A nonimmunosuppressed patient acquiring candidiasis from an indwelling intravenous plastic catheter may recover spontaneously if the catheter is removed promptly. The species of *Candida* is irrelevant to this decision. Patients with candidiasis in whom antifungal therapy is withheld should be observed carefully for the development of endophthalmitis, endocarditis, arthritis, osteomyelitis, or other visceral lesions that require therapy.

ASPERGILLOSIS Etiology *Aspergillus fumigatus* is the most common pathogen, but *A. flavus, A. niger*, and several other species can cause disease. *Aspergillus* is a mold with septate hyphae about 2 to 4 μm in diameter. The fungus is identified by its gross and microscopic appearance in culture.

Pathogenesis and pathology All the common species of *Aspergillus* which cause disease in humans are ubiquitous in the environment, growing on dead leaves, stored grain, compost piles, hay, and other decaying vegetation. Inhalation of *Aspergillus* spores must be extremely common, but disease is rare. Invasion of lung tissue is almost entirely confined to immunosuppressed patients. Roughly 90 percent will have two of these three conditions: less than 500 granulocytes per microliter of peripheral blood, supraphysiologic doses of adrenal corticosteroids, and a history of cytotoxic drugs such as azathioprine. Infection in such patients is characterized by hyphal invasion of blood vessels, thrombosis, necrosis, and hemorrhagic infarction. Chronic granulomatous disease of childhood also predisposes to invasive pulmonary aspergillosis, but here the inflammatory response is granulomatous and blood vessel invasion is rare.

Massive inhalation of *Aspergillus* spores by normal persons can lead to an acute, diffuse, self-limited pneumonitis. Epithelioid granulomas with giant cells and central pyogenic areas containing hyphae are seen. Spontaneous recovery taking several weeks is the usual course.

Aspergillus can colonize the damaged bronchial tree, pulmonary cysts, or cavities of patients with underlying lung disease. Balls of hyphae within cysts or cavities may reach several centimeters in diameter and be visible on chest x-ray. Tissue invasion does not occur. The term *allergic bronchial aspergillosis* denotes the condition of patients with preexisting asthma who have eosinophilia, IgE antibody to *Aspergillus*, and fleeting pulmonary infiltrates from bronchial plugging (see Chap. 205).

Clinical manifestations *Endobronchial pulmonary aspergillosis* presents as chronic productive cough and often hemoptysis in a patient with prior chronic lung disease, such as tuberculosis, sarcoidosis, bronchiectasis, or histoplasmosis. *Aspergilloma* refers to a ball of hyphae within a lung cyst or cavity, usually in the upper lobe. *Aspergillus* may be spread from its endocavitary or endobronchial site to the pleura during the course of bacterial lung abscess or surgery.

Invasive aspergillosis in the immunosuppressed host presents as an acute pneumonia and has a tendency to cavitation. Infection progresses by hematogenous spread as well as extension to surrounding lung and other contiguous structures. Occasionally the portal of infection in the immunosuppressed host is the paranasal sinus, gastrointestinal tract, skin, or palate.

Aspergillus sinusitis in nonimmunosuppressed patients may take two forms. A ball of hyphae may form in a chronically obstructed paranasal sinus, without tissue invasion. Much less commonly, a chronic, fibrosing granulomatous inflammation with *Aspergillus* hyphae within tissue may begin in the sinus and spread slowly to the orbit and brain.

Growth of *Aspergillus* on cerumen and detritus within the external auditory canal is termed *otomycosis*. Trauma to the cornea may cause chronic *Aspergillus* keratitis. Endophthalmitis follows introduction of *Aspergillus* into the globe by trauma or surgery. *Aspergillus* may infect intracardiac or intravascular prostheses.

Diagnosis Repeated isolation of *Aspergillus* from sputum or demonstration of hyphae in sputum or bronchial brushing specimens suggests endobronchial colonization or infection. Even a single isolation of *Aspergillus* from the sputum of a neutropenic patient with pneumonia, particularly a child or nonsmoker, suggests the diagnosis of invasive aspergillosis. Fungus ball of the lung is usually detectable by chest x-ray. Antibody of the IgG class to *Aspergillus* antigens is demonstrable in the serum of many colonized patients and of virtually all patients with fungus ball.

Biopsy is usually required to diagnose invasive aspergillosis of the lung, paranasal sinus, or sites of dissemination. Blood cultures are rarely positive, even in patients with infected cardiac prosthetic valves. *Aspergillus* hyphae can be identified presumptively by histology, but culture is required for confirmation and determination of species.

Treatment Patients with severe hemoptysis due to fungus ball of the lung may benefit by lobectomy. Poor pulmonary function in residual lung and dense pleural adhesions around the lesion can complicate the resection. Systemic chemotherapy is of no value in endobronchial or endocavitary aspergillosis.

Intravenous amphotericin B has resulted in arrest or cure of invasive aspergillosis when immunosuppression is not severe. Combined flucytosine–amphotericin B may be useful in nonneutropenic patients with invasive aspergillosis.

MUCORMYCOSIS (ZYGOMYCOSIS, PHYCOMYCOSIS) Etiology Species of *Rhizopus, Rhizomucor*, and *Cunninghamella* are most common, but species of *Apophysomyces, Saksenaea, Mucor*, and *Absidia* occasionally cause mucormycosis. These molds have broad, rarely septate hyphae of uneven diameter, ranging from 6 to 50 μm. The fungus is inexplicably difficult to grow from infected tissue. When it occurs, growth is rapid and profuse on most media at room temperature. Identification is based upon gross and microscopic appearance of the mold.

Pathogenesis and pathology *Rhizopus* and *Rhizomucor* species are ubiquitous, appearing on decaying vegetation, dung, and foods of high sugar content. Infection is uncommon and is largely confined to patients with serious preexisting diseases. Mucormycosis originating in the paranasal sinuses and nose occurs predominantly in patients with poorly controlled diabetes mellitus. Patients with organ transplantation, hematologic malignancy, or who are receiving long-term deferoxamine therapy are predisposed to mucormycosis of either sinus or lung. Gastrointestinal mucormycosis occurs in a variety of conditions, including uremia, severe malnutrition, and diarrheal diseases. Infection is acquired from nature, with no person-to-person spread. In all forms of mucormycosis, vascular invasion by hyphae is prominent. Ischemic or hemorrhagic necrosis is the predominant histologic finding.

Clinical manifestations Mucormycosis originating in the nose and paranasal sinuses produces a characteristic clinical picture. Low-grade fever, dull sinus pain, and sometimes nasal congestion or a thin, bloody nasal discharge are followed in a few days by double vision, increasing fever, and obtundation. Examination reveals a unilateral generalized reduction of ocular motion, chemosis, and proptosis. The nasal turbinates on the involved side may be dusky red or necrotic. A sharply delineated area of necrosis, strictly respecting the midline, may appear in the hard palate. The skin of the cheek may become inflamed. Fungal invasion of the globe or ophthalmic artery leads to blindness. Opacification of one or more sinuses is found on CT scan or by NMR imaging. Carotid arteriogram may show invasion or obstruction of the carotid siphon. Coma is due to direct invasion of the frontal lobe. Early symptoms mimic bacterial sinusitis. Clouding of the sensorium may be attributed to diabetic acidosis. Cavernous sinus thrombosis may be considered when orbital invasion occurs. Without treatment, death may occur in a few days to a few weeks.

Pulmonary mucormycosis is a progressive severe pneumonia, accompanied by high fever and toxicity. The necrotic center of large infiltrates may cavitate. Hematogenous spread to other areas of the lung, as well as to brain and other organs, is common. Survival beyond 2 weeks is unusual. Gastrointestinal invasion presents as one or more ulcers which tend to perforate. Hematogenous dissemination can originate from the gastrointestinal tract, lung, or paranasal sinuses. Sometimes no portal of entry can be found.

Diagnosis Lesions of the lung and craniofacial structures are best diagnosed by biopsy and histologic section. Cultural confirmation should be attempted. Wet smear of crushed tissue can provide rapid diagnosis. Cultures of blood and cerebrospinal fluid are negative. Smear and culture of sputum may be positive during cavitation of a lung lesion.

Treatment Regulation of diabetes mellitus and decreasing the dose of immunosuppressive drugs aid in the treatment. Extensive debridement of craniofacial lesions appears to be very important. Orbital exenteration may be required. Intravenous amphotericin B is clearly of value in craniofacial mucormycosis and should be employed in the other forms of mucormycosis as well. Maximum tolerated doses are given until progression is halted. The drug is continued for a total of 10 to 12 weeks. Appropriate management results in cure of about half of the craniofacial infections. Survival of patients with pulmonary, gastrointestinal, or disseminated mucormycosis is rare.

SPOROTRICHOSIS Etiology *Sporothrix schenckii* lives as a saprophyte on plants in many areas of the world. In nature and on culture at room temperature the fungus grows as a mold, but within host tissue or at 37°C on enriched media it grows as a budding yeast. Identification is by appearance of the fungus in mold and yeast forms.

Pathogenesis and pathology Infection results when minor trauma inoculates the fungus into subcutaneous tissue. Nursery workers, florists, and gardeners acquire the illness from roses, sphagnum moss, and other plants. Infection may be limited to the site of inoculation (plaque sporotrichosis) or extend along proximal lymphatic channels (lymphangitic sporotrichosis). Spread beyond an extremity, the usual site of infection, is rare, and hematogenous dissemination from the skin remains unproven. The portal for osteoarticular, pulmonary, and other extracutaneous forms of sporotrichosis is unknown but is likely the lung.

Untreated sporotrichosis shows little evidence of self-healing and is capable of extreme chronicity. The inflammatory response contains both clusters of neutrophils and a marked granulomatous response with epithelioid cells and giant cells.

Clinical manifestations Lymphangitic sporotrichosis, by far the most common manifestation, forms a nearly painless red papule at the site of inoculation. Over the next several weeks, similar nodules form along proximal lymphatic channels. Nodules intermittently discharge small amounts of pus. Ulceration may occur. The proximal extension of these lesions, often with skip areas, is quite distinctive but may be mimicked by lesions of *Nocardia brasiliensis, Mycobacterium marinum,* or, on rare occasions, by *Leishmania brasiliensis* or *M. kansasii.*

Plaque sporotrichosis is a nontender red maculopapular granuloma confined to the site of inoculation. Osteoarticular sporotrichosis presents as mono- or polyarticular arthritis of indolent onset and progression over months or years, involving the elbows, knees, wrists, ankles, and, rarely, smaller joints of the extremities. Periarticular bone develops areas of demineralization on x-ray, and draining sinuses may appear over joints and bursae. Hematogenous spread to the skin may be observed during polyarticular disease, but none of the skin lesions shows lymphangitic spread. Immunosuppression predisposes to hematogenous spread. Pulmonary sporotrichosis usually presents as a single chronic cavitary upper-lobe lung lesion.

Diagnosis Culture of pus, joint fluid, sputum, or skin biopsy specimen is the preferred method of diagnosis. Appearance of *S. schenckii* in tissue is quite variable. In skin lesions, the organisms are hard to find.

Treatment Cutaneous sporotrichosis can be cured with oral administration of a saturated solution of potassium iodide, given in increasing divided daily doses up to 4.5 to 9 mL/d for adults, as tolerated. Gastrointestinal disturbance or acneiform rash over the cape area and face are common, but therapy should be continued for 1 month after resolution of all lesions. Patients with serious allergic reactions to iodides may respond to local heat, particularly when plaque sporotrichosis is the only form of disease. Itraconazole, an experimental drug, may be of value. Extracutaneous sporotrichosis rarely responds to iodides, but cures have been obtained in over half such patients with prolonged courses of intravenous amphotericin B.

RARER DEEP MYCOSES

PARACOCCIDIOIDOMYCOSIS Etiology Formerly called *South American blastomycosis,* this is the mycosis caused by *Paracoccidioides brasiliensis.* A dimorphic fungus, *P. brasiliensis* grows as a budding yeast but may be grown as either yeast or mold on a culture medium. Identification is by gross and microscopic appearance. A superficial resemblance to *Blastomyces dermatitidis* may cause misdiagnosis.

Pathogenesis and pathology Infection is thought to be acquired by inhalation of spores from environmental sources, but the reservoir in nature remains obscure. Pulmonary infection produces few symptoms initially. Hematogenous spread to the mucous membranes of the mouth and nose, the lymph nodes, and other sites brings the patient to medical attention. Fatal cases show spread to the adrenal, the gastrointestinal tract, and many other viscera.

Clinical manifestations Common symptoms include indurated ulcers of the mouth, oropharynx, larynx, and nose, enlarged and draining lymph nodes, lesions of the skin and genitalia, productive cough, weight loss, dyspnea, and sometimes fever. Acquisition of infection is restricted to South America, Central America, and Mexico, but the extreme indolence of this infection may lead to recognition many years after the patient has left the endemic area. Chest x-ray most often shows a bilateral patchy pneumonia.

Diagnosis Cultures of sputum, pus, and mucosal lesions are often diagnostic. The diagnosis can be made by smear or histologic section, though confirmation by culture is preferable. Serologic tests are useful in suggesting the diagnosis and monitoring therapy.

Treatment Milder cases may be cured by one year's treatment with oral ketoconazole, 200 to 400 mg daily. Itraconazole appears to give comparable results. More advanced cases are given intravenous amphotericin B, followed by ketoconazole.

PSEUDALLESCHERIASIS Etiology Also called *Petriellidium boydii, Pseudallescheria boydii* is a mold frequently found in soil. When the fungus is isolated in the imperfect state, it is called *Scedosporium apiospermum.*

Pathogenesis and pathology Wind-borne spores of *P. boydii,* arising in soil, are the presumed source of infection. The fungus grows as a mold within tissue, causing necrosis and abscess formation.

Clinical manifestations *P. boydii* resembles *Aspergillus* in its ability to colonize the endobronchial tree, to form fungus balls in the lung or paranasal sinuses, and to invade the cornea or globe following trauma or surgery and by its propensity to invade the immunosuppressed host. Hyphae of *P. boydii* in tissue may be difficult to distinguish from *Aspergillus*. Infection with *P. boydii* is much less common than with *Aspergillus. P. boydii* is the single most common cause in the United States of mycetoma. Intravascular hyphae, a hallmark of invasive aspergillosis, also can be found in pseudallescheriasis. Occasional normal patients have developed necrotizing pneumonia or abscesses in brain or other organs due to *P. boydii.*

Diagnosis Demonstration of hyphae in tissue and culture confirmation are required for diagnosis.

Treatment Intravenous miconazole or ketoconazole is recommended, but therapeutic response to all drugs has been poor.

TORULOPSOSIS Etiology *Torulopsis glabrata (Candida glabrata)* is a small yeast-like fungus, the same size as the yeast form of *Histoplasma capsulatum. T. glabrata* does not form hyphae or pseudohyphae. Identification is by biochemical tests.

Pathogenesis and pathology *T. glabrata* is a normal inhabitant of the human gastrointestinal tract and vagina. Within tissue, *T. glabrata* causes abscess formation with a neutrophilic inflammatory response. In immunosuppressed patients, a scanty or mononuclear inflammatory response may be seen.

Clinical manifestations Torulopsosis mimics many of the manifestations of candidiasis, but infection is less common and often less severe. Clinical entities include intravenous catheter–induced sepsis or endocarditis, gastrointestinal and disseminated infection in immunosuppressed patients, and retrograde infection of the urinary tract.

Diagnosis *Torulopsis* may be difficult to distinguish from yeast cells of *Candida* in histologic section. Culture is the most reliable diagnostic tool.

Treatment Therapeutic measures used in candidiasis appear appropriate for torulopsosis.

MYCETOMA Etiology *Actinomycetoma* refers to infection by actinomycetes of the genera *Nocardia, Streptomyces,* and *Actinomadura. Eumycetoma* is caused by true fungi of many different genera. The most common agent varies with the locality.

Pathogenesis and pathology The pathogens live in the soil and enter the skin through minor trauma. The most common site of infection is the foot. Infection runs a relentless course over many years, with destruction of contiguous bone and fascia. Grains are found in purulent foci, surrounded by fibrosis and a mononuclear cell inflammatory response.

Clinical manifestations *Mycetoma* is a chronic suppurative infection originating in subcutaneous tissue and characterized by the presence of grains, which are tightly clumped colonies of the causative agent. The infected site shows painless swelling, woody induration, and sinus tracts which discharge pus intermittently. Systemic symptoms and spread to distant sites in the body are not seen.

Diagnosis The clinical picture is characteristic, but confusion with chronic osteomyelitis or botryomycosis may occur. The diagnosis requires demonstration of grains in pus from the draining sinus or in biopsy sections. Many histologic sections may need to be examined to locate a grain.

Treatment Actinomycetoma may respond to prolonged combination chemotherapy, such as streptomycin and either dapsone or trimethoprim-sulfamethoxazole. Eumycetoma rarely has responded to chemotherapy. As a possible exception, some cases infected with *Madurella mycetomatis* have appeared to respond to ketoconazole.

CHROMOMYCOSIS This chronic subcutaneous mycosis is rarely seen in the United States but presents as a verrucoid, ulcerated, or crusted skin lesion. Disease originates when thorns or bits of vegetation introduce the fungus into the subcutaneous tissue. Infection spreads over ensuing months and years to contiguous tissue, causing very few symptoms. Appearance of the thick-walled dark-colored rounded forms ("copper pennies") in tissue is diagnostic. No satisfactory treatment is available.

DERMATOPHYTOSIS

Definition Dermatophytosis, also known as ringworm or tinea, is a chronic fungal infection of the skin, hair, or nails.

Etiology Species of *Trichophyton, Microsporum,* and *Epidermophyton* are called *dermatophytes*. They grow in and remain confined to the keratinous structures of the body. Other mycoses can show fungal invasion of keratinous structures, such as candidiasis, pityriasis versicolor, and tinea nigra, but are traditionally not termed *dermatophytoses*.

Pathology and pathogenesis Dermatophyte species are called anthropophilic, zoophilic, or geophilic, depending on whether their usual reservoir within nature appears to be humans, animals, or soil. Infectivity of all those sources is low, and group outbreaks are largely confined to an occasional case clustering of scalp infections in children. Acquisition of a dermatophytosis appears to be favored by minor trauma, maceration, and poor hygiene of the skin. Infection does not seem to confer solid immunity. Repeated infection with the same species is commonplace, particularly with anthropophilic species. Infrequency of scalp infection in adults has been attributed to local factors rather than immunity.

Invasion of the stratum corneum by dermatophytes may cause little inflammation, or, particularly with zoophilic fungi, inflammation can be intense. Shedding of the stratum corneum is increased by inflammation. To the extent that fungal growth cannot keep up with shedding, inflammation may help terminate infection. Conversely, infection is probably favored when shedding is reduced by glucocorticoids and cytotoxic drugs. Antifungal drugs interfere with the ability of fungal growth to keep up with shedding.

Clinical manifestations The disease varies with the site of infection and fungal species. Foot infection (athlete's foot, tinea pedis) may present as fissuring of the toe webs, scaling of the plantar surfaces, or vesicles around the toe webs and soles. Interdigital lesions may be pruritic or, when bacterial superinfection occurs, may be painful. Hand infection is less common but resembles foot infection. Scalp dermatophytosis (tinea capitis) is characterized by areas of alopecia and scaling. In so-called endothrix infection, the hair shaft breaks off at the skin surface, leaving the hairs visible as black dots in the scalp. With some forms of scalp infection an intense boggy suppuration occurs, called a *kerion*. Dermatophytosis of the glabrous skin (tinea corporis) presents as circumscribed lesions with a wide variety of appearances. Scales, vesicles, or pustules may appear. Inflammation may be minimal or intense. Central healing of less inflamed lesions may be seen. The serpiginous border of inflammation is the source of the name *ringworm*. Dermatophytosis of the bearded area (tinea barbae) appears as a pustular folliculitis. Onychomycosis (tinea unguium) presents as white discolored nails or thickened, chalky crumbling nails. Peeling and fissuring of the paronychia or keratotic debris under the nail edge may also be seen.

Diagnosis Discolored hairs, scales, and keratotic debris under infected nails should be collected for KOH smear and culture. In the scraping of skin lesions, a drop of water on the skin site may keep the removed scales from flying off and aid in their collection. Culture is important in distinguishing dermatophytes from *Candida* and fungal saprophytes growing in keratinaceous debris.

Treatment Mild or moderately severe lesions of the trunk, groin, and feet often respond to topical therapy with an imidazole or one of the other agents mentioned earlier in this chapter. Hyperkeratotic lesions of the palms and soles respond less well. Ringworm that is moderately severe or severe, that is unresponsive to topical therapy, or that involves the scalp, nails, or bearded area should be treated systemically. The drug of choice is griseofulvin. Either 500 mg of the microcrystalline form or 375 mg of the ultramicrocrystalline form is given once daily or divided into two doses, given with meals. Double this amount has been recommended for refractory infections. Treatment must be continued until all infected keratin is gone. Cutting of infected hair, epilating nails, and cleansing interdigital webs can expedite cure. Secondary bacterial infection of the foot may require soaks or antibacterial agents. Relapse of dermatophyte foot infections may be decreased by measures to keep the feet clean and dry. Griseofulvin-resistant cases may respond to oral ketoconazole, 200 to 400 mg daily.

REFERENCES

Therapy

Dameshmend TK, Warnock DW: Clinical pharmacokinetics of ketoconazole. Clin Pharmacokinetics 14:13, 1988

Heidemann HT et al: Amphotericin B nephrotoxicity in humans decreased by salt repletion. Am J Med 75:476, 1983

Kerridge D: Present status of antimycotics. Microbiol Sci 2:83, 1985

NIAID Mycoses Study Group: Treatment of blastomycosis and histoplasmosis with ketoconazole. Ann Intern Med 103:861, 1986

Saag MS, Dismukes WE: Azole antifungal agents: Emphasis on new triazoles. Antimicrob Agents Chemother 32:1, 1988

Cryptococcosis

Dismukes WE: Cryptococcal meningitis in patients with AIDS. J Infect Dis 157:624, 1988

——— et al: Treatment of cryptococcal meningitis with combination amphotericin B and flucytosine for four as compared with six weeks. N Engl J Med 317:334, 1987

Gal AA et al: The pathology of pulmonary cryptococcal infections in the acquired immunodeficiency syndrome. Arch Pathol Lab Med 110:502, 1986

Kovacs JA et al: Cryptococcosis in the acquired immunodeficiency syndrome. Ann Intern Med 103:533, 1985

Blastomycosis

Campbell GD, Chapman SW: Blastomycosis. Semin Respir Med 9:164, 1987

Klein BS et al: Two outbreaks of blastomycosis along rivers in Wisconsin: Isolation of *Blastomyces dermatitidis* from riverbank soil and evidence of its transmission along waterways. Am Rev Respir Dis 136:1333, 1987

Histoplasmosis

Goodwin RA et al: Histoplasmosis in normal hosts. Medicine 60:231, 1981

Johnson PC et al: Progressive disseminated histoplasmosis in patients with acquired immunodeficiency syndrome. Am J Med 85:152, 1988

Wheat LJ et al: Cavitary histoplasmosis occurring during two large urban outbreaks. Analysis of clinical, epidemiologic, roentgenographic, and laboratory features. Medicine 63:201, 1984

Coccidioidomycosis

Bouza E et al: Coccidioidal meningitis. An analysis of thirty-one cases and review of the literature. Medicine 60:139, 1980

Brenniman DA et al: Coccidioidomycosis in the acquired immunodeficiency syndrome. Ann Intern Med 106:372, 1987

Drutz DJ: Amphotericin B in the treatment of coccidioidomycosis. Drugs 26:337, 1983

Galgiani JN et al: Ketoconazole therapy of progressive coccidioidomycosis. Comparison of 400 and 800 mg doses and observations at higher doses. Am J Med 84:603, 1988

Candidiasis

Dupont B, Rouhet E: Cutaneous, ocular, and osteoarticular candidiasis in heroin addicts: New clinical and therapeutic aspects in 38 patients. J Infect Dis 152:577, 1985

Haron E et al: Hepatic candidiasis: An increasing problem in immunocompromised patients. Am J Med 83:17, 1987

Klein RS et al: Oral candidiasis in high-risk patients as the initial manifestation of the acquired immunodeficiency syndrome. N Engl J Med 311:354, 1984

Levine MS et al: *Candida* esophagitis; accuracy of radiographic diagnosis. Radiology 154:581, 1985

Odd FC: *Candida and Candidosis*. Baltimore, Saunders, 1988

Thaler M et al: Hepatic candidiasis in cancer patients: The evolving picture of the syndrome. Ann Intern Med 198:88, 1988

Aspergillosis

Gerson SL et al: Prolonged granulocytopenia: The major risk factor for invasive pulmonary aspergillosis in patients with acute leukemia. Ann Intern Med 100:345, 1984

Kuhlman JE et al: Invasive pulmonary aspergillosis in acute leukemia: Characteristic findings on CT, the CT halo sign, and the role of CT in early diagnosis. Radiology 157:611, 1985

Walsh TJ et al: *Candida* suppurative peripheral thrombophlebitis: Recognition, prevention, and management. Infect Control 7:16, 1986

Yu VL et al: Significance of isolation of *Aspergillus* from the respiratory tract in diagnosis of invasive pulmonary aspergillosis. Am J Med 81:249, 1986

Mucormycosis

Brennan RO et al: Cunninghamella: A newly recognized cause of rhinocerebral mucormycosis. Am J Clin Pathol 80:98, 1983

Lehrer RI et al: Mucormycosis. Ann Intern Med 93:93, 1980

Maniglia AL et al: Cephalic phycomycosis: A report of eight cases. Laryngoscope 92:755, 1982

Windus DW et al: Fetal *Rhizopus* infections in hemodialysis patients receiving deferoxamine. Ann Intern Med 107:678, 1987

Sporotrichosis

Bullpitt P, Weedon D: Sporotrichosis: A review of 39 cases. Pathology 10:249, 1978

England DM, Hochholzer L: Primary pulmonary sporotrichosis. Am J Surg Pathol 9:193, 1985

Friedman SJ, Doyle JA: Extracutaneous sporotrichosis. Int J Dermatol 22:171, 1983

Pluss JL, Opal SM: Pulmonary sporotrichosis: Review of treatment and outcome. Medicine 65:143, 1986

Urabe H, Honbo B: Sporotrichosis. Int J Dermatol 25:255, 1986

Paracoccidioidomycosis

Londero AT, Severo LC: The gamut of progressive pulmonary paracoccidioidomycosis. Mycopathologia 75:65, 1981

Restrepo A et al: Itraconazole in the treatment of parracoccidioidomycosis. A preliminary report. Rev Infect Dis 9(Suppl 1):51, 1987

Sugar AM et al: Paracoccidioidomycosis in the immunosuppressed host: Report of a case and review of the literature. Am Rev Respir Dis 129:340, 1984

Pseudallescheriasis

Alsip SG, Cobba CG: *Pseudallescheria boydii* infection of the central nervous system in a cardiac transplant recipient. South Med J 79:383, 1986

Galgiani JN et al: *Pseudallescheria boydii* infections treated with ketoconazole. Chest 86:219, 1984

Travis LB et al: Clinical significance of *Pseudallescheria boydii*: A review of 10 years' experience. Mayo Clin Proc 60:531, 1985

Yoo D et al: Brain abscesses due to *Pseudallescheria boydii* associated with primary nonHodgkin's lymphoma of the central nervous system: A case report and literature review. Rev Infect Dis 7:272, 1985

Torulopsosis

Kauffman CA, Tan JS: *Torulopsis glabrata* renal infection. Am J Med 57:217, 1974

Valdivieso M et al: Fungemia due to *Torulopsis glabrata* in the compromised host. Cancer 38:1750, 1976

Mycetoma

Gumaa SA et al: Mycetoma of the head and neck. Am J Trop Med Hyg 35:594, 1986

Tight RR, Bartlett MS: Actinomycetoma in the United States. Rev Infect Dis 3:1139, 1981

Chromomycosis

Londero AT, Ramos DC: Chromomycosis: A clinical and mycologic study of thirty-five cases observed in the hinterland of Rio Grande Do Sul, Brazil. Am J Trop Med Hyg 25:132, 1976

Dermatophytosis

Robertson MH et al: Ketoconazole in griseofulvin-resistant dermatophytosis. J Am Acad Dermatol 6:224, 1982

——— et al: Ketoconazole in griseofulvin-resistant dermatophytosis. J Am Acad Dermatol 6:224, 1982

Weismann K et al: White nails in AIDS/ARC due to *Trichophyton rubrum* infection. Clin Exp Dermatol 13:24, 1988

152 ACTINOMYCOSIS AND NOCARDIOSIS

JOHN E. BENNETT

ACTINOMYCOSIS

DEFINITION Actinomycosis is an indolent suppurative infection caused by certain anaerobic actinomycetes. The microorganisms grow within the tissue as grossly visible, tightly knit clusters, called *grains*.

ETIOLOGY *Actinomyces israelii* is the usual pathogen, with occasional cases due to other species of *Actinomyces* (*A. naeslundii, A. viscosus, A. odontolyticus, A. meyeri*) or *Arachnia propionica*. All can form branching gram-positive hyphae and are the same width as bacteria. Most species grow best in an atmosphere that is either anaerobic or contains 6 to 10% CO_2. Isolation of the causative agent is made difficult by the mixed flora usually present in actinomycotic abscesses.

PATHOLOGY AND PATHOGENESIS All agents of actinomycosis are commensals in the mouth and gastrointestinal tract of humans. The portal of entry appears to be either a break in the integrity of the mucosa or aspiration into the lung. Poor dental hygiene and dental abscess predispose to cervicofacial lesions. Within the gastrointestinal tract, the appendiceal area is the most common site. Infection presents as a chronic suppurative inflammation, usually in the cervicofacial, thoracic, or abdominal area. In histopathologic section, each grain is typically surrounded by polymorphonuclear neutrophils. The adjacent tissue shows subacute or chronic inflammation with extensive fibrosis and formation of sinus tracts. Giant cells are infrequent. Grains are a few millimeters in diameter. Several sections may have to be searched to find a grain. Grains may be observed grossly in pus or on bandages covering draining sinuses. These pale yellow, cheeselike particles can be crushed on a microscope slide and Gram-stained. Demonstration of gram-positive filaments in a smear of crushed grains or in histologic section helps distinguish actinomycosis from botryomycosis or eumycetoma.

Infection spreads by direct extension and hematogenously. Direct extension through the skin causes one or more chronic draining sinuses to appear in the abdomen, chest, or cervicofacial area. Hematogenous foci may appear in bone, brain, liver, or other organs.

CLINICAL MANIFESTATIONS *Cervicofacial actinomycosis* presents as a red or purplish, firmly indurated subcutaneous mass, typically in the submandibular area or in the anterior cervical triangle near the angle of the mandible. One or more draining sinuses may be present. Tenderness is slight or absent. Lethargy, weight loss, variable low-grade fever, anemia, and leukocytosis are infrequent in cervicofacial actinomycosis but common in *thoracic* and *abdominal actinomycosis*. Localizing findings in the latter forms include draining sinuses and, in thoracic actinomycosis, cough and purulent sputum. Pulmonic lesions may extend through the chest wall and present as an indolent subcutaneous abscess. Pain or a palpable mass may appear in abdominal actinomycosis. *Pelvic actinomycosis* may originate from either the female reproductive tract or the intestine, particularly the appendix. Women with an intrauterine device in place for more than 2 years appear to be at a slightly increased risk of pelvic actinomycosis. Tuboovarian abscess, ureteral obstruction, or, rarely, hepatic abscess have been reported. The indolent onset, variable low-grade fever, abdominal pain, and adnexal mass may lead to an erroneous diagnosis of pelvic inflammatory disease or tumor. In all forms of actinomycosis, disease typically has been present for weeks or months at time of diagnosis.

Chest x-ray may reveal an area of dense pneumonitis. Fibrosis, empyema, or cavitation may be seen. Periappendiceal abscess may appear as an extrinsic mass on barium enema or may be detected by ultrasonography or CT scan.

DIAGNOSIS Laboratory tests other than culture or histologic section are not helpful. Blood cultures are rarely positive. Isolation of *Actinomyces* or *Arachnia* species from the mouth, sputum, stool, or feculent draining sinuses is not diagnostic. Demonstration of a grain in pus or deep tissue is diagnostic if botryomycosis and mycetoma can be excluded. Nocardiosis can be distinguished by the absence of grains, identification of the organism in culture, and, usually, by the weak acid-fast staining of *Nocardia*.

TREATMENT Milder cases of actinomycosis, including most cervicofacial infections, respond well to penicillin V (2 to 4 g/d for adults) or one of the tetracyclines. Sulfonamides, metronidazole, oral cephalosporins, and oral antistaphylococcal penicillins are not recommended. More severe cases, including most thoracic and abdominal infections, should receive parenteral penicillin G for roughly 6 weeks (in adults 2 to 6 million units per day) followed by prolonged therapy with oral penicillin V or one of the tetracyclines. The likelihood of relapse is reduced if the total duration of therapy is 2 to 4 months in mild cases and up to 6 to 12 months in severe ones. Drug resistance has not been encountered in relapses. Curettage of bone lesions, surgical resection of necrotic tissue, and drainage of empyema, brain abscess, or other large collections of pus facilitate recovery but are usually not curative by themselves.

It is common in actinomycosis to isolate microbes other than actinomycetes from pus. In general, the antibiotic susceptibility of these secondary organisms does not have to be considered in the selection of therapeutic agents.

NOCARDIOSIS

DEFINITION Nocardiosis is an acute, subacute, or chronic infection, most often beginning in the lung.

ETIOLOGY *Nocardia asteroides, N. brasiliensis,* and *N. caviae* are the etiologic agents of two different diseases, nocardiosis and mycetoma. In the latter infection, the organism enters the skin by trauma, forms grains within tissue, and spreads slowly to contiguous tissue (see Chap. 151). While nocardiosis can result from local trauma, the organism usually enters via the lung, does not form grains, and is prone to hematogenous spread. Even though the etiologic agents of these diseases do overlap, *N. asteroides* causes most cases of nocardiosis and *N. brasiliensis* is the species usually isolated from mycetoma. *Nocardia otitidiscaviarum* is a rare cause of either disease. *Nocardia brasiliensis* and perhaps *N. asteroides* can also cause a lymphocutaneous disease closely resembling sporotrichosis; this infection differs from mycetoma by its lymphangitic spread and by the absence of grains.

Nocardia species are aerobic actinomycetes with branching hyphae the same width as bacteria. Hyphae are weakly gram-positive and weakly acid-fast. Growth appears in 2 to 5 days on blood agar, Sabouraud's agar, or other simple media. Incorporation of antibiotics into media to inhibit bacterial growth usually inhibits *Nocardia* as well. Colonies become rough and chalky with an orange or yellow hue. Identification of *Nocardia* species, including distinction between *Streptomyces, Actinomadura,* and *Nocardia,* is difficult and best assigned to a reference laboratory.

PATHOGENESIS AND PATHOLOGY *Nocardia* is a soil saprophyte widely distributed throughout the world. Infection is acquired from sites in nature, never from infected persons or animals. Males are infected two to three times more commonly than females. No age or exposure is known to predispose to nocardiosis. Many patients have serious preexisting conditions, such as adrenal corticosteroid therapy, cancer, pulmonary alveolar proteinosis, AIDS, or chronic granulomatous disease of childhood.

Lesions of nocardiosis show suppuration, necrosis, and abscess formation. Neutrophils are the predominant inflammatory cell. Branching hyphae are scattered throughout the lesion without formation of grains. Tissue Gram stain or overstained methenamine silver demonstrates the hyphae best. A modified Fite-Faraco stain of histologic sections can be used to demonstrate acid-fastness.

CLINICAL MANIFESTATIONS *Nocardia* pneumonia presents with fever and productive cough of several days' or up to several months' duration. The initial illness may resemble a bacterial pneumonia, but slow radiologic progression continues despite antibiotic therapy, often with cavitation of radiodense central areas. Hematogenous dissemination to brain and subcutaneous tissue is frequent. A pulmonary portal is usually but not always detectable clinically. Brain lesions are typically multiple abscesses. Purulent meningitis may result from rupture of an abscess into the ventricle. The subcutaneous lesion typically consists of one or a few indolent abscesses. Hematogenous dissemination to other organs occurs but is rarely detectable clinically.

DIAGNOSIS A progressive pneumonia with purulent sputum should suggest the diagnosis of nocardiosis, particularly if cavitation or spread to brain or subcutaneous tissue occurs. Sputum, pus, or bronchial lavage specimens should be examined by Gram stain and modified acid-fast stain. On Gram stain the hyphae are usually branching, beaded, and refractile. They are not strongly gram-positive but take the red counterstain even less well. Conventional acid-fast staining procedures such as Ziehl-Neelsen or a fluorochrome often do not stain *Nocardia*. Identification of branching, weakly acid-fast organisms in histologic section or smear of pus or sputum is sufficient to establish the diagnosis of nocardiosis. Cultural confirmation is highly desirable, but isolation of *Nocardia* from heavily contaminated specimens is difficult. Isolation of *Nocardia* from otherwise sterile pus is readily accomplished. *Nocardia* is rarely isolated from blood, but diphasic culture media or lysis centrifugation techniques facilitate isolation. When *Nocardia* is isolated from sputum, the diagnosis of nocardiosis should be suspected, but occasionally no disease can be detected.

TREATMENT Surgical drainage of empyema and abscesses in brain or subcutaneous tissue is helpful but not sufficient to achieve cure. Virtually all patients should receive prolonged chemotherapy. The treatment of choice is sulfisoxazole or trimethoprim-sulfamethoxazole. Sulfisoxazole therapy is begun orally or intravenously at 100 mg/kg per day in four divided doses. The dose is then adjusted downward to achieve a peak blood concentration of 10 to 15 mg/dL (100 to 150 μg/mL). Alternatively, trimethoprim-sulfamethoxazole can be given orally or intravenously as 50 mg/kg per day of the sulfamethoxazole component, divided into two doses per day. With either regimen, therapy is continued for 6 to 12 months, depending on the severity of the infection and the presence of immunosuppression. Addition of other antibiotics to sulfa drugs may be indicated in patients who show continued deterioration. Ampicillin 150 mg/kg per day, amikacin, imipenem, and minocycline have been used. In sulfa-allergic patients, minocycline has sometimes been successful in the absence of central nervous system involvement.

Survival has been reported in 92 percent of cases with isolated pulmonary nocardiosis compared to 52 percent in cases with brain abscess. Concomitant use of immunosuppressive therapy seems to impair the therapeutic response in nocardiosis.

REFERENCES

Actinomycosis

Bartels LJ, Vrabec DP: Cervicofacial actinomycosis—A variable disorder. Arch Otolaryngol 104:705, 1978

Benhof DF: Actinomycosis: Diagnostic and therapeutic considerations and a review of 32 cases. Laryngoscope 94:1198, 1984

Jackson AE et al: Ureteric obstruction secondary to pelvic actinomycosis. Br J Urol 62:85, 1988

Persson E: Genital actinomycosis and *Actinomyces israelii* in the female genital tract. Adv Contracept 3:115, 1987

Smego RA Jr: Actinomycosis of the central nervous system. Rev Infect Dis 9:855, 1987

Weese WC, Smith IM: A study of 57 cases of actinomycosis over a 36-year period. Arch Intern Med 135:1562, 1975

Nocardiosis

Adair JC et al: Nocardial cerebral abscess in the acquired immunodeficiency syndrome. Arch Neurol 44:548, 1987

Dewsnup DH, Wright CN: In vitro susceptibility of *Nocardia asteroides* to 25 antimicrobial agents. Antimicrob Agents Chemother 25:165, 1984

Gallis HA: The clinical spectrum of *Nocardia brasiliensis* infection in the United States. Rev Infect Dis 6:164, 1984

Gombert ME et al: Therapy of experimental cerebral nocardiosis with imipenem, amikacin, trimethoprim-sulfamethoxazole and minocycline. Antimicrob Agents Chemother 30:270, 1986

Petersen EA et al: Minocycline treatment of pulmonary nocardiosis. JAMA 250:930, 1983

Smego RA et al: Trimethoprim-sulfamethoxazole therapy for *Nocardia* infections. Arch Intern Med 143:711, 1983

section 10 Rickettsia, *Mycoplasma*, and *Chlamydia*

153 RICKETTSIAL DISEASES

THEODORE E. WOODWARD

INTRODUCTION The rickettsial diseases of humans consist of a variety of clinical entities caused by microorganisms of the family Rickettsiaceae. The rickettsias are obligate intracellular parasites about the size of bacteria and are usually seen microscopically as pleomorphic coccobacilli. Each of the rickettsias pathogenic for humans is capable of multiplying in one or more species of arthropod as well as in animals and humans. Indeed, the majority of the rickettsias are maintained in nature by a cycle which involves an insect vector and an animal reservoir, and infection of humans is unimportant in the cycle. Epidemic typhus presents a number of points of dissimilarity to most of the other rickettsioses. Until recently, the natural cycle of infection was thought to involve only humans and lice. The finding of a sylvatic reservoir in flying squirrels associated with a human illness which resembles classic typhus emphasizes that there are other mechanisms.

A compendium of information of the rickettsial diseases is given in Table 153-1.

Of all the afflictions of the human race the rickettsial diseases, particularly epidemic typhus, rank among the foremost as a cause of suffering and death. The record of deaths from epidemic typhus in this century in the Balkan countries and in Poland and Russia reached astounding figures. Typhus ravaged Russia and eastern Poland from 1915 to 1922, infecting 30 million inhabitants and causing an estimated 3 million deaths.

The past two decades have seen the development of excellent methods for the prevention and treatment of rickettsioses. In fact, these measures have been so successful that the rickettsioses have become of minor importance in the United States and in many other

TABLE 153-1 Rickettsial diseases

Disease: Type	Agent	Geographic distribution	Natural cycle: Arthropod	Natural cycle: Mammal	Principal means of transmission to humans	Serologic diagnosis: Weil-Felix reaction	Serologic diagnosis: CF, MA, and IFA reactions*
SPOTTED FEVER GROUP							
Rocky Mountain spotted fever	*R. rickettsii*	Western hemisphere	Ticks	Wild rodents, dogs	Tick bite	Positive OX-19 OX-2	Positive group- and type-specific
Boutonneuse fever	*R. conorii*	Africa, Europe, Middle East, India					
Queensland tick typhus	*R. australis*	Australia		Marsupials, wild rodents			
North Asian tick-borne rickettsiosis	*R. sibirica*	Siberia, Mongolia		Wild rodents			
Rickettsialpox	*R. akari*	United States, Russia, Africa(?)	Blood-sucking mite	House mouse, other rodents	Mite bite	Negative	
TYPHUS GROUP							
Endemic (murine)	*R. typhi*	Worldwide	Flea	Small rodents	Infected flea feces into broken skin	Positive OX-19	Positive group- and type-specific
Epidemic	*R. prowazekii*	Worldwide	Body louse	Humans Flying squirrels	Infected louse feces into broken skin	Positive OX-19	
	R. Canada	North America	Ticks			Positive OX-19	
Brill-Zinsser disease	*R. prowazekii*	Worldwide	Recurrence years after original attack of epidemic typhus			Usually negative	
Scrub	*R. tsutsugamushi*	Asia, Australia, Pacific islands	Trombiculid mites	Wild rodents	Mite bite	Positive OX-K	Positive in about 50% of patients
OTHER RICKETTSIAL DISEASES							
Q fever	*R. burnetii*	Worldwide	Ticks	Small mammals, cattle, sheep, goats	Inhalation of dried infected material	Negative	Positive
Trench fever	*R. quintana*†	Europe, Africa, North America	Body louse	Humans	Infected louse feces into broken skin	Negative	None available

* CF = complement fixation; MA = microscopic agglutination; IFA = immunofluorescent antibody.
† Some authorities no longer place the agent in the genus *Rickettsia* because it can be cultured on artificial media.

countries. Although conquered, these infections have not been eliminated, and they could again become rampant if the will to control them, the present high standards of sanitation, and the necessary industrial capacities for production of effective insecticides and therapeutic agents should be compromised.

PATHOGENESIS Rickettsial diseases develop after infection through the skin or the respiratory tract. Agents of the typhus and spotted fever group are introduced through the bite of the infected arthropod vector. Ticks and mites, which transmit the agents of spotted fever and scrub typhus, inoculate the rickettsias directly into the dermis during feeding. The louse and flea, which transmit epidemic and murine typhus, respectively, deposit infected feces on the skin; infection occurs when organisms are rubbed into the puncture wound made by the arthropod. The rickettsias of Q fever gain entry through the respiratory tract when infected dust is inhaled; the respiratory route is also occasionally implicated in epidemic typhus when infection results from inhalation of dried infected louse feces.

Although organisms probably multiply at the original site of entry in all instances, local lesions appear with regularity only in certain diseases, namely, the initial cutaneous lesions of scrub typhus, rickettsialpox, and boutonneuse fever, and the pneumonitis which develops in about half the persons with Q fever.

Volunteers infected with either scrub typhus or Q fever develop rickettsemia late in the incubation period, often some hours before the onset of fever. Similar events probably occur in all the rickettsial diseases; circulating rickettsias can be detected during the early febrile period in practically all patients. Little is known about the pathogenesis of infection during the midportion of the incubation period. However, it is reasonable to assume that during this time, in patients with typhus or spotted fever, a transient low-grade rickettsemia results from release of organisms multiplying at the initial site of infection and that this seeds infection in the endothelial cells of the vascular tree. Vascular lesions developing at such sites account for the pathologic changes, including the rash.

Rickettsias apparently invade and proliferate in the endothelial cells of small blood vessels. Endothelial cell destruction occurs from the proliferation of organisms and eventual disruption. Rickettsias may exert a cytotoxic effect on endothelial cells; in mice the rickettsial toxin causes remarkable increase in capillary permeability, independent of proliferation. The anatomic localization of multiple microscopic-sized lesions and the numerous foci of rickettsial vascular changes with rickettsias present coincide well with the organs examined microscopically such as the kidney, lung, heart, and liver. These findings confirm Wolbach's original conclusion that "the lesions of the blood vessel are due to the presence of the parasite." Absence of inflammatory cell reactions in fulminant Rocky Mountain spotted fever tends to exclude several host-mediated immunopathogenic mechanisms. The underlying cause of the toxic-febrile state which characterizes the rickettsial diseases remains unknown. Several rickettsial species contain type-specific toxins which are lethal for mice, and these may play a role in humans.

PATHOLOGIC PHYSIOLOGY Peripheral vascular collapse results in death in fulminating cases during the first week, with capillary dilatation and pooling of blood without increased capillary permeability or loss of fluid into extravascular spaces. Proliferative and thrombotic lesions develop in small vessels, resulting in necrosis and increased capillary permeability, with loss of water, electrolytes, proteins, and erythrocytes. This in turn results in a decrease in blood volume, together with an increase in the extravascular space and clinical edema. Edema, anoxia of the myocardium, and histologic evidence of myocarditis are disclosed by electrocardiographic abnormalities, including serious arrhythmias. Liver function is impaired. The azotemia which develops in seriously ill patients appears to be prerenal. Clinical manifestations resulting from the peripheral vascular collapse are oliguria and anuria, azotemia, anemia, hypoproteinemia, hyponatremia, edema, and coma. In spotted fever and typhus patients with hemorrhagic skin lesions, consumptive coagulopathy is present. All these alterations are absent or minimal in mild cases or in those who are given specific treatment early.

PATHOLOGY The basic changes in the spotted and typhus fever groups are vascular, with resultant widespread lesions in adjacent parenchymatous organs. They are most common in the skin, muscles, heart, lung, and brain. The most conspicuous and diverse are found in Rocky Mountain spotted fever, where swelling, proliferation, and degeneration of the endothelial cells occur, frequently with thrombus formation which partially or completely occludes the lumen. The muscle cells of the arterioles undergo swelling and fibrinoid changes. The adventitial tissues are infiltrated with mononuclear leukocytes, lymphocytes, and plasma cells. The vascular damage is scattered along arteries, veins, and capillaries, with normal architecture prevailing throughout most of the vascular bed. The changes in murine, epidemic, and scrub typhus fevers resemble those in Rocky Mountain spotted fever, but thrombosis is uncommon and involvement of the musculature is rare.

Interstitial myocarditis occurs in each of these diseases but is usually most extensive in Rocky Mountain spotted fever and in scrub typhus. In the brain glial nodules are found in all members of the group, but microinfarcts in the brain tissue or in the myocardium are most often observed in spotted fever.

Rickettsial pneumonitis occurs, at least to some extent, in many patients with spotted or typhus fever and is characteristic in patients with Q fever. The process is patchy and consists microscopically of areas of congestion and edema. Within the consolidated areas the alveoli are filled with compact fibrinocellular exudate containing lymphocytes, plasma cells, large mononuclear cells, and erythrocytes, but few, if any, polymorphonuclear leukocytes.

Rickettsias can occasionally be observed microscopically in sections of tissue. Failure to demonstrate them is of no diagnostic significance. They are readily identifiable by the immunofluorescent technique.

LABORATORY DIAGNOSIS Diagnostic procedures which depend on isolation of the etiologic agent from blood or other clinical material are expensive, time-consuming, and hazardous to laboratory personnel. Primary isolation of rickettsias by chick embryo inoculation or tissue culture usually fails because of the small number of organisms in the patient's blood. Rickettsias have been identified in stained cultured monocytes of infected monkeys and by direct or indirect immunofluorescence of infected animal tissues. Except in unusual circumstances, however, currently available serologic tests are adequate for laboratory confirmation of the clinical diagnosis in each of the rickettsial diseases. The demonstration of a rise in titer of specific antibody during convalescence is of prime importance in establishing laboratory confirmation. Table 153-2 summarizes the serologic results usually encountered in persons who have rickettsial diseases in the United States. The Weil-Felix test employing *Proteus* strains OX-19 and OX-2 gives positive results in patients with spotted fever and murine typhus and negative results in those with rickettsialpox and Q fever. It is useful as a screening procedure but cannot be relied upon to differentiate spotted fever from murine typhus. In patients with Brill-Zinsser disease the *Proteus* OX-19 reaction is usually negative or low in titer.

Serologic tests employing group-specific rickettsial antigens provide data which clearly differentiate the most common infections, i.e., epidemic typhus, murine typhus, Rocky Mountain spotted fever, and Q fever. Type-specific rickettsial antigens generally make it possible to distinguish rickettsialpox from spotted fever and Brill-Zinsser disease from murine typhus.

The type of immunoglobulin in acute (IgM) and late or recurrent (IgG) illness is helpful in identifying recrudescent typhus (Brill-Zinsser disease). In general, the Weil-Felix and complement fixation tests are useful for routine diagnosis; microscopic agglutination, immunofluorescent antibody, and hemagglutination reactions are valuable for specific identification.

Specific antibiotic therapy has little effect on the time of appearance of antibodies or on their ultimate titer, provided treatment is instituted some days after onset of the illness. However, if the illness is cut short by early and vigorous treatment, antibody production may be delayed for a week or so, and the maximum titers attained may be below those illustrated in Table 153-2. Under these circumstances a sample of blood taken 4 to 6 weeks after onset of illness should also be tested.

TABLE 153-2 Serologic diagnosis of rickettsial diseases in the United States

		Weil-Felix reaction				Complement fixation tests with type-specific antigen				
			Illustrative titer				Illustrative titer			
Group	Disease	Proteus	10th day	20th day	Cases with diagnostic titer	Rickettsial antigen	10th day	20th day	30th day	Cases with diagnostic titer
Spotted fever	Rocky Mountain spotted fever	OX-19 OX-2	40 20	320 160	Most	*R. rickettsii*	20	160	80	Most
	Rickettsialpox	OX-19 OX-2	0 0	0 0	None	*R. akari*	0	64	128	Most
Typhus	Murine typhus	OX-19 OX-2	160 10	640 40	Most	*R. typhi*	0	160	160	Most
	Epidemic typhus, squirrel related	OX-19 OX-2	160 10	640 40	Most	*R. prowazekii*	0	160	160	Most
	Brill-Zinsser disease	OX-19 OX-2	160 0	20 0	Infrequent	*R. prowazekii*	1280	640	320	Most
	Q fever	OX-19 OX-2	0 0	0 0	None	*R. burnetii*	10	80	160	Most

The immunofluorescent antibody test is very useful for detecting rickettsia in the tissues of patients with the typhus group of rickettsioses, the spotted fevers, and Q fever. Identifiable rickettsias have been visualized in skin lesions of patients with Rocky Mountain spotted fever as early as the fourth day of illness and as late as the tenth day. Rickettsias may be visualized in human tissues several days after administration of chloramphenicol or tetracycline. The technique also visualizes rickettsias in ticks and in animal tissues, including those fixed with paraffin.

Normochromic anemia occurs in patients severely ill with rickettsial diseases. The white blood cell count in Rocky Mountain spotted fever, rickettsialpox, murine and epidemic typhus, Brill-Zinsser disease, Q fever, and other rickettsial diseases is usually within the normal range; 6000 to 10,000 cells per microliter. Leukopenia is occasionally observed, and in the presence of complications, such as superimposed infections and extensive vascular lesions, moderate leukocytosis occurs. The differential blood cell count is usually normal. Thrombocytopenia occurs in severely ill spotted and scrub typhus fever patients with extensive vascular lesions; hypofibrinogenemia, prolonged prothrombin and partial thromboplastin times, and other clotting abnormalities occur.

TREATMENT Patients seriously ill with one of the diseases of the typhus–spotted fever group may show circulatory collapse, coma, oliguria and anuria, azotemia, anemia, hypoproteinemia, hypochloremia and hyponatremia, and edema. These alterations are often absent in the mildly ill, and in them management is much less complicated. The therapeutic principles necessary for treatment of all rickettsioses are (1) specific chemotherapy and (2) supportive care. Attention to both is mandatory for the seriously ill patient first recognized late in the disease. During the first week in the moderately ill patient, supportive therapy may need to be less energetic, because specific chemotherapy usually suffices. The early mild case may be successfully treated at home; more severely ill patients should receive hospital care.

Specific therapy Specific therapy is most effective when initiated during the early stages of disease coincident with the appearance of the rash. When therapy is delayed until the rash has become hemorrhagic and widespread, the response is less dramatic. The antibiotics of choice are chloramphenicol and the tetracyclines, which are effective because of their rickettsiostatic properties. They are not rickettsiocidal.

The following antibiotic regimen is considered optimal: for chloramphenicol, an initial dose of 50 mg per kilogram of body weight, and for tetracycline, 25 mg/kg. Subsequent daily doses are the same as the initial loading dose, with the requirement divided equally and given at 6- to 8-h intervals. Antibiotic treatment is continued until the patient has improved and has been afebrile approximately 24 h. In patients too ill to take oral medication, an intravenous preparation of one of the antimicrobials should be employed.

Adrenal cortical hormones may be needed for their antitoxemic effects in patients first observed late in the course of severe illness. Large doses for brief periods of about 3 days, in combination with specific antibiotics, are recommended in critically ill patients.

In uncomplicated cases of spotted fever, there is symptomatic improvement within 24 h and the temperature becomes normal in 60 to 72 h.

Supportive care Frequent turning of the patient relieves pressure from prominent bony parts and also militates against the development of aspiration pneumonia. Proper mouth care, with frequent swabbing of the oral cavity, may avert the development of parotitis and gingivitis. Sucking of the juice of a lemon or the oral use of glycerin or mineral oil is helpful. Usually food is well tolerated by patients with rickettsial disease, and the daily diet should provide 1 to 2 g protein per kilogram of normal body weight; the diet may need to be supplemented with oral or parenteral hyperalimentation (see Chap. 75).

When indicated, red cell transfusions given slowly are helpful. The support of the hypotensive patient with rickettsial disease is similar to other patients with shock (see Chap. 89). Dialysis is indicated when there is clear-cut evidence of acute renal failure.

ROCKY MOUNTAIN SPOTTED FEVER Definition Rocky Mountain spotted fever is an acute febrile illness caused by *Rickettsia rickettsii*. It is transmitted to humans by ticks. The disease is characterized by sudden onset with headache and chills and by fever which persists for 2 to 3 weeks. A characteristic exanthem appears on the extremities and trunk about the fourth day of illness. Delirium, shock, and renal failure occur in severely ill patients.

Etiology and epidemiology The causative microbe, *R. rickettsii*, is the prototype for the rickettsial group of agents. The minute organisms are purple when stained by Giemsa's method or red by Macchiavello's technique; most of them are gram-negative. These organisms often occur in pairs and possess a cell wall similar in structure and chemical composition to that of gram-negative bacteria; there are a cell membrane, cytoplasmic granules corresponding to ribosomes, and prokaryotic organization of nuclear material. The cell membrane is selectively permeable; the cell wall is the focus of important antigens and an endotoxin-like substance.

The rickettsias grow in the nucleus and the cytoplasm of infected cells of ticks, mammals, and embryonated eggs; the intranuclear situation of the organisms is shared by the other members of the spotted fever group, but not by rickettsias of the typhus group. *Rickettsia rickettsii* is readily distinguishable from the agents of the typhus fevers by cross-immunity tests in guinea pigs and by complement fixation tests employing antigens prepared from infected yolk sac tissues. The differentiation of *R. rickettsii* from closely related members of the spotted fever group frequently requires elaborate procedures. Strains of the agent of Rocky Mountain spotted fever vary considerably in their virulence for humans and animals.

The first reports of spotted fever in Idaho and Montana during the final decade of the last century led to the name Rocky Mountain spotted fever. However, the disease has been reported from all states (except Maine, Alaska, and Hawaii), as well as from Canada, Mexico, Colombia, and Brazil. Although related diseases are found on other continents, this particular infection is limited to the western hemisphere. In the years 1981, 1982, 1983, 1984, 1985, 1986, and 1987 there were 1176, 976, 1126, 848, 714, 760, and 604 cases reported. Why this decrease has occurred is not known. The mortality rate was about 20 percent in the days before specific therapy but has decreased to about 7 percent. More than half the cases occur in the south Atlantic and south central states, with the greatest number in North Carolina, Virginia, Georgia, Maryland, Tennessee, and Oklahoma.

An unusual outbreak of "urban" spotted fever occurred in New York City's Bronx borough during the summer of 1987. Eight percent of dog ticks were positive for *R. rickettsii*.

A number of species of ticks are found infected with *R. rickettsii* in nature, but only two are important in transmitting spotted fever to humans. These are *Dermacentor andersoni*, the wood tick, which is the principal vector in the west, and *D. variabilis*, the dog tick, which assumes this role in the east. *Amblyomma americanum*, the lone star tick, and *D. variabilis* are the common vectors in the west south central states. Infected female ticks transmit the agent transovarially to at least some of their offspring. Ticks which become infected, either through the egg or at one of the stages during their development cycle by feeding on an infected mammal, harbor the rickettsias throughout their lifetime, which may be several years, making the tick a reservoir as well as a vector. Small wild mammals are suspected of playing an important role in spreading the rickettsias in nature by infecting ticks which feed on them during rickettsemia.

Disease in humans is generally acquired from the bite of an infected tick. Transmission is unlikely unless the tick remains attached for a number of hours. Infection may also be acquired through abrasions in the skin which become contaminated with infected tick feces or tissue juices; hence, the hazard associated with crushing ticks between the fingers when removing them from persons or animals. The agent of Rocky Mountain spotted fever has been transmitted accidentally to humans by transfusion of blood taken from a donor just before onset of illness.

There are seasonal variations in the incidence of cases of spotted fever, as well as differences in age and sex distribution of cases. In each instance these differences are related to exposure to ticks. Most cases are seen during the period of maximal tick activity, i.e., April to September, and 60 percent of cases occur in individuals under 20 years of age. This age distribution is undoubtedly influenced by propinquity to the wood and dog ticks. The mortality rate increases with the age of the patient.

Rocky Mountain spotted fever has been acquired by laboratory workers via aerosol transmission, and special precautions are necessary when the agent is handled in the laboratory.

Clinical manifestations INCUBATION PERIOD AND PRODROMATA A history of tick bite is elicited in approximately 80 percent of patients. The incubation period varies between 3 and 12 days with a mean of 7 days. A short incubation period usually indicates a more serious infection.

ONSET In nonvaccinated persons, the onset is usually abrupt, with severe headache, a sudden shaking rigor, prostration, generalized myalgia, especially in the back and leg muscles, nausea with occasional vomiting, and fever which reaches 39.4 to 40°C (103 to 104°F) within the first 2 days. Pain in the abdominal muscles may be severe, and arthralgia is not uncommon. Deep muscle palpation often elicits tenderness. Occasionally the debut of illness in children and adults is mild, accompanied by lethargy, anorexia, headache, and low-grade fever. These symptoms are similar to those of many acute infectious diseases, making specific diagnosis difficult during the first few days.

PYREXIA Fever continues for approximately 15 to 20 days in untreated cases. The febrile course in children may be shorter. Hyperthermia of 40.5°C (105°F) or greater is of unfavorable prognostic significance, although fatalities may occur when the patient is hypothermic, with concurrent vasomotor collapse. Fever generally terminates by lysis over a period of several days, but rarely does so by crisis. Recurrent fever is uncommon except in the presence of secondary pyogenic complications.

The *headache* is generalized and excruciating, and frequently most intense over the frontal area. It persists throughout the first and second weeks of illness in untreated cases. Occasionally headache is mild. Malaise continues for the first week; irritability is notable, and the patient shuns distractions such as questioning and examination.

CUTANEOUS MANIFESTATIONS The rash which is present in practically all cases is the most characteristic and helpful diagnostic sign. It usually appears on the fourth febrile day; the range is 2 to 6 days. Faint-pink macules which fade on pressure have been noted on the first febrile day. The initial lesions are on the wrists, ankles, palms, soles, and forearms. The first lesions are macular, nonfixed, pink, irregularly defined, and measure 2 to 6 mm. A warm compress applied to the extremity accentuates the rash in the early stages. The exanthem is most prominent when the temperature is elevated. After 6 to 12 h, the rash extends centripetally to the axilla, buttocks, trunk, neck, and face. (This is in contrast to the eruption of typhus fever, which begins on the trunk and spreads centrifugally, rarely involving the face, palms, or soles.) The rash becomes maculopapular after 2 to 3 days (it may be felt by light palpation) and assumes a deeper red hue. By about the fourth day it is petechial and fails to fade on pressure. Not uncommonly, the hemorrhagic lesions coalesce to form large ecchymotic blemishes; these lesions tend to form over bony prominences and may ultimately slough to form indolent, slow-healing ulcers. Patients who have had the typical rash show brownish discolorations at the site for several weeks during convalescence. In milder cases, the rash does not become purpuric and may disappear within a few days. Antibiotic therapy may abort the early exanthem; the later fixed lesion fades less rapidly with specific therapy. Occasionally, a rash does not occur or is unnoticed, particularly in dark-skinned patients.

The application of tourniquets for several minutes, or the occasional taking of the blood pressure may provoke additional petechiae (Rumpel-Leede phenomenon), further evidence of capillary abnormalities.

CARDIOVASCULAR AND RESPIRATORY FEATURES During the early stages, the pulse is full and regular and is accelerated in proportion to the height of the temperature, and the blood pressure is well sustained. During the peak of illness in seriously ill patients, the pulse is rapid and feeble, and hypotension of 90 mmHg or less is common. If circulatory failure is sustained, the resultant hypoxia and shock lead to agitation and delirium and contribute to the formation of ecchymoses and gangrene of fingers, toes, genitalia, buttocks, earlobes, and nose. Cyanosis of the peripheral parts of the body is common. A reduction of the total blood volume is found occasionally. The ECG shows low voltage, minor ST-segment deflections, and, occasionally, delay in atrioventricular conduction. These changes are transient and nonspecific. Severely ill patients have a puffy appearance of the face, hands, ankles, feet, and lower parts of the sacrum. Occasionally a severe arrhythmia associated with myocarditis results in sudden death.

Respirations are either normal or slightly accelerated. Cough may be harassing and nonproductive, and localized pneumonitis may occur, but pulmonary consolidation is extremely rare. Pulmonary edema may develop after injudicious use of intravenous fluids.

HEPATIC AND RENAL MANIFESTATIONS In the majority of patients, there is little alteration in renal or hepatic function. The liver may be enlarged, but jaundice is unusual. Oliguria and anuria commonly occur in seriously ill patients. Azotemia is common; when marked, it is a very unfavorable sign. Abnormalities in liver function include hypoproteinemia, with reduction in the albumin fraction.

NEUROLOGIC MANIFESTATIONS The principal neurologic manifestations are headache, restlessness, and varying degrees of insomnia. Stiffness of the back is common. The cerebrospinal fluid is clear, with normal dynamics and normal chemical constituents. Occasionally, the CSF pressure is elevated; there may be a slight increase in mononuclear cells. Coma and muscular rigidity may occur. Athetoid movements, convulsive seizures, and hemiplegia are grave manifestations. Deafness during the active stages of the disease is not uncommon. As a rule, all neurologic signs abate without residua. Findings based upon follow-up examinations and electroencephalograms may be interpreted as indicative of minor residual brain damage for a year or more following recovery of some patients from Rocky Mountain spotted fever.

OTHER PHYSICAL MANIFESTATIONS Patients become dehydrated, with extreme dryness of lips, gums, tongue, and pharynx. The skin is hot and dry, the conjunctivas are frequently injected, and the eyes suffused. Photophobia is common in the early stages of illness. Petechial hemorrhages may be noted in the conjunctivas or in the retina. The spleen is enlarged in approximately one-half the cases and is firm and nontender. Usually there is abdominal distention and some degree of intestinal ileus. Occasionally the severity of abdominal discomfort may suggest the diagnosis of appendicitis or cholecystitis.

Course In patients with mild and moderately severe cases who are given no specific antibiotic therapy, the disease abates within 2 weeks, and convalescence is rapid. In fatal cases death usually occurs during the latter part of the second week as a result of toxemia, vasomotor collapse and shock, or renal failure. In a few patients, the course is fulminant with death occurring as early as the sixth day of illness.

In vaccinated individuals who contract the disease, the illness is mild, with a short febrile course and an atypical rash.

Prognosis If the serious manifestations of spotted fever are regarded as intrinsic parts of the disease, then complications are uncommon and consist mainly of secondary bacterial infections such as bronchopneumonia, otitis media, and parotitis. Thrombosis of major blood vessels may result in gangrene of a portion of an extremity. Hemiplegia and peripheral neuritis are rare sequelae.

The overall mortality rate for spotted fever was formerly about 20 percent. Death occurred in more than half of persons over 40 years of age, but the mortality rate was much lower in children and young adults. Since the introduction of the broad-spectrum antibiotics and the development of more precise knowledge regarding correction of the physiologic abnormalities which develop during the disease, fewer deaths occur. Some of the fatalities can be attributed to failure to consider spotted fever in the differential diagnosis and resultant delay in instituting appropriate treatment.

Differential diagnosis During the early stages of infection before the rash has appeared, differentiation from other acute infections is difficult. A history of tick bite while living or traveling in wooded or bushy sites known to be in a highly endemic area is helpful. The rash of meningococcemia (see Chap. 109) resembles Rocky Mountain spotted fever in certain aspects, because it is macular, maculopapular, or petechial in the chronic form, and petechial, confluent, or ecchymotic in the fulminant type. The meningococcal skin lesion is tender and develops with extreme rapidity in the fulminant form, whereas the rickettsial rash occurs on about the fourth day of disease and gradually becomes petechial. *Spotted fever is often confused with measles.* The exanthem of rubeola rapidly becomes confluent, while that of rubella *usually remains discrete.*

Murine typhus is a milder disease than Rocky Mountain spotted fever; the rash is less extensive, nonpurpuric, and nonconfluent, and renal and vascular complications are uncommon. Not infrequently differentiation of these two rickettsial infections must await the results of specific serologic tests. Epidemic typhus fever is capable of causing all the pronounced clinical, physiologic, and anatomic alterations seen in patients with Rocky Mountain spotted fever, i.e., hypotension, peripheral vascular collapse, cyanosis, skin necrosis and gangrene of digits, renal failure and azotemia, and neurologic manifestations. However, the rash of classic typhus is noted initially in the axillary folds of the trunk and later extends peripherally, rarely involving the palms, soles, or face. The serologic patterns in these two diseases are distinctive when specific rickettsial antigens are employed. Moreover, louse-borne typhus is now recognized in the United States as a flying squirrel–related illness which occurs sporadically and as Brill-Zinsser disease (recrudescent typhus fever). Rickettsialpox, although caused by a member of the spotted fever group, is usually readily differentiated from Rocky Mountain spotted fever by the initial lesion, the relative mildness of the illness, and the early vesiculation of the maculopapular rash. The Weil-Felix reaction is positive in Rocky Mountain spotted fever and in murine and epidemic typhus, but is negative in rickettsialpox. Agglutinins against *Proteus* OX-19 and OX-2 appear in the serum of patients with spotted fever, but only those against OX-19 are generally found in murine and epidemic typhus.

Complications *Pyogenic complications,* including otitis media and parotitis, are encountered in patients severely ill with Rocky Mountain spotted fever and other rickettsioses. These localized infections respond to therapy with appropriate antibiotics combined with surgical measures.

Pneumonitis may develop as a result of specific rickettsial action or as a bacterial superinfection. The sputum is scanty and should be examined to determine whether superimposed bacterial infection is present. Specific therapy is guided by the results of these laboratory studies. The pneumonitis generally responds to the antibiotic therapy the patient is receiving, but if staphylococcal pneumonia is suspected, a penicillinase-resistant penicillin or a cephalosporin should be added to the tetracycline or chloramphenicol.

Circulatory failure of peripheral or central origin is treated with careful administration of plasma expanders and fluids (see Chaps. 39 and 89). When the clinical signs reveal unmistakable evidence of cardiac failure, digitalis, diuretics, and other cardiac drugs should be employed as indicated (see Chap. 182).

Prevention Prevention is attained primarily by avoidance of tick-infested areas. When this is impractical, prophylactic measures include (1) spraying the ground with dieldrin or chlordane for area control of ticks (though there are environmental objections to the use of residual insecticides in area control of ticks, under special conditions such procedures may be warranted); (2) application of repellents such as diethyltoluamide or dimethylphthalate to clothing and exposed parts of the body, or in very heavily infested areas the wearing of clothing which interferes with the attachment of ticks, i.e., boots and a one-piece outer garment, preferably impregnated with repellent; and (3) daily inspection of the entire body, including the hairy parts, to detect and remove attached ticks. In removing attached ticks great care should be taken to avoid crushing the arthropod with resultant contamination of the bite wound. Gentle traction with tweezers applied close to the mouth parts may be necessary; the skin area should be disinfected with soap and water or other antiseptics. Similarly, precautions should be employed in removing engorged ticks from dogs and other animals, because infection through minor abrasions on the hands is possible. Improved vaccines containing inactivated *R. rickettsii* are under development and when available commercially should be used for those at great risk, namely, persons frequenting highly endemic areas and laboratory workers exposed to the agent. Because the broad-spectrum antibiotics are such excellent therapeutic agents in spotted fever, there has been less impetus for vaccination of persons who run only a minor risk of infection.

After a tick bite in a known endemic area, an exposed person should be observed for signs of fever, headache, prostration, and rash; therapy is very effective early in the infection.

MURINE (ENDEMIC) TYPHUS FEVER Definition Murine typhus fever is an acute febrile disease caused by *Rickettsia typhi (mooseri)* and transmitted to humans by fleas. The clinical illness is characterized by fever of 9 to 14 days, headache, a maculopapular rash appearing on the third to fifth day, and myalgia.

Etiology and epidemiology *R. typhi* resembles other rickettsias in morphologic properties, staining characteristics, and intracellular parasitism. Under the electron microscope *R. typhi* is seen to contain dense masses of nuclear material in a less dense homogeneous protoplasmic substance, the whole of which is surrounded by a limiting membrane. It differs from *R. rickettsii* in that it always multiplies within the cytoplasm of cells, in contrast to the intranuclear and cytoplasmic positions of spotted fever rickettsias.

Invasion of the body by *R. typhi* provokes specific and nonspecific immunologic responses. Utilizing highly purified antigens, specific antibodies may be demonstrated readily by complement fixation, microscopic agglutination, and immunofluorescent antibody reactions. The positive Weil-Felix reaction that occurs in this disease is nonspecific, because it is attributable to the presence of common carbohydrate antigens.

The common vector of *R. typhi* for rats and humans is the rat flea (*Xenopsylla cheopis*). In nature, the rat louse (*Polypax spinulosis*) may transmit the agent among rodents. Customarily, rat fleas become infected on ingestion of blood from diseased rats; the rickettsias multiply within the intestinal cells of the arthropod and are excreted in the feces. Infection in humans occurs after the flea bite and contamination of the broken skin by rickettsia-laden feces. Dried flea feces may also infect via the conjunctivas or the upper part of the respiratory tract.

Rats and mice are naturally infected with murine typhus, and although the rodent disease is nonfatal, viable rickettsias persist in the brain for variable periods.

Murine typhus is one of the most benign and widespread of the rickettsioses in the United States. Prevalent in the southeastern and Gulf Coast states, it has been identified in most of the other states and in harbor centers throughout the world wherever rats and fleas abound. In the early 1940s, 2000 to 5000 cases of murine typhus were reported annually. This contrasts to 67 and 69 cases reported in the United States in 1986 and 1987, respectively. This sharp reduction was achieved by control of rats and their fleas in known areas of high prevalence. In urban areas the disease is more prevalent during the summer and fall and occurs predominantly among persons working in proximity to granaries or food depots. There has been an extension to certain rural areas when changing agricultural practices have provided rats with ready access to adequate food supplies. Endemic typhus has been reported in laboratory workers. This emphasizes the importance of taking special precautions when working with rickettsial organisms in the laboratory.

Clinical manifestations INCUBATION PERIOD AND PRODROMATA The incubation period ranges from 8 to 16 days, with a mean of 10 days. Common prodromata are headache, backache, arthralgia, and chilly sensations. Nausea, malaise, and transient temperature rises may precede the true onset of disease.

ONSET AND GENERAL SYMPTOMS A frank shaking chill and repeated rigors are present at the onset, associated with a severe frontal headache and fever. This triad of headache, chill, and pyrexia is usually followed within a few hours by nausea and vomiting. Prostration, malaise, and weakness are sufficient to enforce cessation of activity in adults, in contrast to children, whose illness is less severe. Occasionally, mild symptoms make it difficult to define the actual onset.

PYREXIA The usual febrile course in murine typhus lasts for about 12 days in adults; the temperature ranges from 38.8 to 40°C (102 to 104°F) but may reach 40.5 to 41.1°C (105 to 106°F) in children. The temperature may reach high levels abruptly after onset or ascend in a stepwise manner during the first few days. With the appearance of the rash, fever is usually sustained, with partial daily remissions which occasionally reach normal levels in the morning. Defervescence is generally by lysis over several days but sometimes occurs by crisis. Transient mild fever of 37.7°C (100°F) is not uncommon during early convalescence. A few patients experience only low-grade fever throughout, but this does not necessarily connote a mild illness.

CUTANEOUS MANIFESTATIONS The early lesions, which are sparse and discrete, are hidden in the axillae and inner surface of the arm. Most patients then develop with surprising suddenness a generalized, dull-red macular rash of the upper part of the abdomen, shoulders, chest, arms, and thighs. The individual lesions are discrete and pea-sized, with an ill-defined border, and fade on pressure during the first 24 h. They later become maculopapular, in contrast to the exanthem of epidemic typhus, which is persistently macular. The distribution over the trunk with sparse involvement of the extremities, palms, soles, and face differs from the peripheral distribution and facial involvement of Rocky Mountain spotted fever. The murine rash generally appears initially on the fifth febrile day, but rarely it is seen concurrently with the onset of fever or develops as late as the seventh day.

Eighty percent of patients develop a rash which persists for 4 to 8 days and fades before defervescence. The cutaneous manifestations vary greatly in intensity and duration and may be fleeting. They are readily overlooked in dark-skinned patients, in whom they should be sought by light palpation and indirect lighting.

CARDIOVASCULAR AND RESPIRATORY FEATURES An irritating, nonproductive cough is frequent and is occasionally associated with moderate hemoptysis. Early in the second week, rales may be detected in the basilar lung areas. These changes are generally rickettsial rather than bacterial in origin and respond to the broad-spectrum antibiotics. Pulmonary congestion occurs in extremely ill and elderly patients.

Accelerated pulse and hypotension occur, although less frequently than in patients with epidemic typhus or Rocky Mountain spotted fever.

NEUROLOGIC MANIFESTATIONS Headache is the most common neurologic manifestation of murine typhus and may dominate the clinical picture. It is frontal and continues into the second week of illness. Stupor and prostration may occur in the second week, and in severe cases there may be delirium, extreme agitation, or coma. Coma in elderly patients after 2 weeks of illness presages death. Nuchal rigidity and general spasticity often suggest meningitis, although the spinal fluid is normal except for slight increases in pressure and the presence of lymphocytes (5 to 30 per microliter). Transient partial deafness occurs occasionally, but rarely is there localized neuritis or hemiplegia. Neurologic sequelae are unusual. Children experience minimal neurologic changes.

OTHER PHYSICAL MANIFESTATIONS During the first 2 days of illness the patient may be nauseated and vomit, but vomiting later in the illness should arouse suspicion of a complication. Abdominal pain is bothersome; when associated with diarrhea or ileus, it responds to intravenous alimentation. Hepatomegaly and jaundice are unusual. There is splenomegaly in approximately 25 percent of patients.

Photophobia, retroocular pain, and suffusion of the conjunctivas are common but are less severe than in the other typhus and spotted fevers.

Renal function is usually unaltered except in elderly patients with prolonged hypotension. Under these circumstances, azotemia may develop to the degree observed in epidemic typhus. In severe murine typhus, as in the epidemic typhus, hyponatremia and hypoalbuminemia are encountered.

Course After defervescence, murine typhus patients recover rapidly. Fatalities occur between the ninth and twelfth days in elderly or debilitated patients, usually as a result of circulatory and renal failure or intercurrent bacterial infection.

Prognosis The mortality rate in murine typhus was low even before the introduction of specific therapy (<1 percent).

Differential diagnosis Because murine typhus and Rocky Mountain spotted fever occur in many of the same states, the problem of differential diagnosis often arises. Flea-borne murine typhus, which is predominantly an urban disease, is more likely to occur in late summer and autumn. In contrast, spotted fever is a rural and suburban disease in which exposure to ticks is important. Most cases occur in the spring and summer.

Treatment and prevention Both chloramphenicol and the tetracycline antibiotics have controlled the disease (see above). Prevention of murine typhus in humans is attained by reducing the natural reservoir and vector by applying measures for eliminating rodents and employing appropriate insecticides in rat-infested areas to control fleas. Spraying of rat burrows with DDT effectively reduces the population of the vector.

EPIDEMIC (LOUSE-BORNE) TYPHUS FEVER **Definition** Classic epidemic typhus is a severe, febrile disease caused by *R. prowazekii* and transmitted to humans by the body louse. Intense headache, continuous pyrexia of about 2 weeks, a macular skin eruption appearing on about the fifth febrile day, malaise, and vascular and neurologic disturbances represent the principal clinical features. Confirmation of the diagnosis is made by demonstration of *Proteus* OX-19 agglutinins and of specific complement-fixing antibodies in convalescence. The broad-spectrum antibiotics are specific therapeutic agents.

Etiology and epidemiology The causative microbe, *R. prowazekii,* is closely related to *R. typhi,* which causes murine typhus; indeed, the two have a number of common antigens.

Human beings generally are infected when rickettsia-laden louse feces are rubbed into the broken skin; scratching the louse bite facilitates this process. *Pediculus humanus corporis,* which is peculiarly adapted to humans, is the only important vector of epidemic typhus. It dies of its infection and fails to transmit rickettsias to its offspring. *R. prowazekii* has been isolated from flying squirrels, and the organism probably infests their ectoparasites. Generally, however, the organism is maintained by a cycle involving human-louse-human. New epidemics apparently originate from patients with Brill-Zinsser disease (recurrent epidemic typhus). Flying squirrels can serve as a potential host to initiate an outbreak of epidemic typhus provided an avid human vector, such as the body louse, is prevalent. Pathogenic rickettsias reside for long periods in patients with epidemic typhus as well as Rocky Mountain spotted fever and scrub typhus. Lice readily become infected when fed on patients with recurrent typhus. Inhalation of dust containing dried louse feces may cause infection. An established nonhuman reservoir such as flying squirrels poses a serious threat.

If uncontrolled, epidemic typhus behaves as a cyclic disease in a susceptible population, extending over a 3-year period. During the first year there is a gradual seeding of cases throughout the group; during the second there is epidemic spread; and during the third the epidemic tapers off, because the majority of persons have become immune. Outbreaks of epidemic typhus last occurred in the United States in the nineteenth century, and its presence is now recognized in the form of Brill-Zinsser disease and flying squirrel–related typhus.

Clinical manifestations Epidemic typhus resembles murine typhus but is more severe. After an incubation period of about 7 days an abrupt onset of headache, chill, and rapidly mounting fever ushers in the illness. Headache, malaise, and prostration continue unabated until the rash appears on the fifth febrile day. It is initially macular in the axillary folds but ultimately invades the trunk and extremities as a pink, irregular macular lesion, which becomes fixed, petechial, and confluent in the later stages.

Neurologic features range from headache and general spasticity to extreme agitation, stupor, and coma. Circulatory disturbances consisting of tachycardia, hypotension, and cyanosis are more profound than those observed in murine typhus and are almost as severe as in Rocky Mountain spotted fever. Ultimately, in untreated cases, azotemia often reaches high levels as a result of vascular and renal failure, and death occurs late in the second week of illness. Thrombosis of major blood vessels and cutaneous gangrene develop in a manner similar to that seen in the virulent form of Rocky Mountain spotted fever.

The complications and sequelae of epidemic typhus are more severe than those in murine typhus, but not as severe as those in Rocky Mountain spotted fever. However, during certain outbreaks, epidemic typhus was fatal in 60 percent of those infected, and convalescence in survivors was prolonged. The use of chloramphenicol or tetracycline has almost eradicated mortality in this dread disease, provided therapy is instituted before irreversible organ system changes occur.

Differential diagnosis Differentiation of epidemic typhus from the various rickettsioses and other diseases with which it may be confused was described above. The disease is not known to occur in epidemic form in the absence of louse infestation in the general population. Under the conditions in which typhus epidemics are likely to occur, other diseases which may cause confusion include malaria, relapsing fever, pneumonia, and tuberculosis. Classic typhus contracted by a previously vaccinated person is usually mild and may be clinically indistinguishable from murine typhus except by serologic methods.

Treatment and prevention Both chloramphenicol and the tetracycline antibiotics have been found to be highly efficient therapeutic agents in epidemic typhus. Usually the patient becomes afebrile after 2 days of treatment. Under field conditions, 100 mg doxycycline in a single oral dose resulted in abatement of clinical manifestations and defervescence in epidemic typhus.

The most effective measures for controlling epidemic typhus are those which eliminate lice. DDT or lindane powder when dusted into clothing is suitable for this purpose. If resistant lice are found, malathion or carbaryl may prove effective.

A commercially available vaccine prepared from formalin-treated suspensions of infected yolk sac tissue is an effective immunizing agent.

BRILL-ZINSSER DISEASE (RECRUDESCENT TYPHUS) Brill-Zinsser disease is a recrudescent episode of epidemic typhus fever that occurs years after the initial attack. *R. prowazekii* have been isolated from lice fed on patients during the active stages of illness.

The clinical entity, not always mild, resembles epidemic typhus in the character of the rash, circulatory disturbances, and hepatic, renal, and nervous system changes. Recovery is the rule. The Weil-Felix reaction with the various *Proteus* antigens is usually negative, or positive in very low titer. The specific complement fixation, microscopic agglutination, and immunofluorescent antibody reactions are valuable in establishing the diagnosis. In Brill-Zinsser disease the specific complement-fixing antibodies appear as early as the fourth day after the onset of illness; antibodies are IgG, and the peak response is attained by the eighth to tenth days. Specific antibody titers in the primary attack of epidemic typhus begin later, about the eighth to twelfth day, with maximum titers on about the sixteenth day after onset. Treatment is the same as for other rickettsial infections.

SCRUB TYPHUS Definition Scrub typhus is limited to eastern and southeastern Asia, India, northern Australia, and the adjacent islands. It is caused by *R. tsutsugamushi* and is characterized by a primary lesion at the site of the bite of an infected mite, a fever of about 2 weeks' duration, a cutaneous rash which develops about the fifth day, and the appearance late in the second week of agglutinins against the OX-K strain of *Proteus* bacillus. The broad-spectrum antibiotics are specific therapeutic agents.

Etiology The agent of scrub typhus resembles other rickettsias in its physical properties but differs from them in antigenic structure, vector, and reservoir. The disease is transmitted by larvae of several species of mites, especially *Leptotrombidium* (*Trombicula*) *akamushi* and *L. deliense*. These tiny chiggers attach themselves to the skin and during the process of obtaining a meal of tissue juice may acquire infection from the host or transmit rickettsias to the vertebrate. The infection is maintained in nature by a cycle involving mites and small rodents and by transovarial transmission in mites; human infection represents an accident attributable to propinquity.

Clinical manifestations About 10 to 12 days after infection, illness begins abruptly with chilliness, severe headache, fever, conjunctival injection, and moderate generalized lymphadenopathy, which is most prominent in the nodes draining the area of the primary lesion. The initial lesion at the beginning of fever is evidenced by an erythematous indurated area 1 cm in diameter, surmounted by a multiloculated vesicle; within a few days the vesicle ulcerates and becomes covered with a black crust.

Fever increases progressively during the first week, generally reaching 40 to 40.5°C (104 to 105°F), but the pulse remains relatively slow, 70 to 100 beats per minute. The red macular rash, which begins on the trunk about the fifth day and spreads to the extremities, sometimes becomes maculopapular but usually fades in a few days. The course of the disease and the complications resemble those of endemic and epidemic typhus; however, interstitial myocarditis is more prominent than in the other typhus fevers.

Prognosis Before the introduction of chloramphenicol and tetracycline the mortality rate varied from 1 to 60 percent, depending on the geographic area and the virulence of the local strains of *R. tsutsugamushi,* and convalescence was prolonged. With modern therapeutic methods, deaths are rare and convalescence is short.

Differential diagnosis Scrub typhus must be differentiated from the other members of the typhus and the spotted fever group of diseases as well as from measles, typhoid fever, and the meningococcal infections. The geographic localization of scrub typhus, the primary lesion, and the occurrence of OX-K agglutinins are especially useful in establishing the diagnosis.

Treatment and prevention Chloramphenicol and the tetracycline antibiotics are extremely effective in scrub typhus. Scrub typhus is more amenable to drugs than are the other rickettsial infections, and patients with this disease regularly become afebrile and are decidedly improved within 24 to 36 h after beginning treatment, irrespective of the stage of disease. Antibiotic treatment may be discontinued after several afebrile days.

Relapse of clinical illness is unusual unless specific treatment is initiated early, such as before the fifth febrile day. Under these circumstances, recrudescence is obviated by giving the antibiotic for several days and resuming treatment about 5 days after cessation of the initial course of therapy.

Prevention of disease in the individual is accomplished by the application of miticidal chemicals (dibutyl phthalate, benzyl benzoate, diethyltoluamide, and others) to clothing and the skin. There is no satisfactory vaccine. Chemoprophylactic studies conducted in highly endemic infested areas of scrub typhus showed that single oral doses of chloramphenicol or tetracycline given every 5 days for a total of

35 days (seven doses with 5-day nontreatment intervals) prevent scrub typhus and result in active immunity. This procedure is recommended under special circumstances. A long-acting tetracycline (doxycycline) serves the same purpose.

TRENCH FEVER Trench fever is a rare febrile disease transmitted between humans by the body louse, *Pediculus humanus corporis*. It is characterized by a sudden onset with headache and severe pain in the muscles, bones, and joints. In most cases, the fever and other symptoms assume a relapsing character. Fatalities are rare. The disease is also known as shin bone fever, Volhynia fever, His-Werner disease, and quintan fever. Because of its rarity in the United States, textbooks of rickettsiology should be consulted for a detailed description.

RICKETTSIALPOX Definition Rickettsialpox is a mild, nonfatal, self-limited, febrile illness caused by *R. akari*, which is transmitted from mice to humans by mites. It is characterized by an initial skin lesion at the mite bite, a week's febrile course, and a papulovesicular rash.

Etiology and epidemiology Rickettsialpox was first recognized in New York City in 1946, and about 180 cases were reported annually for several years thereafter. It has been diagnosed in several other areas of the United States, and outbreaks have been reported in European Russia. The vector is a small, colorless mite, *Allodermanyssus sanguineus* (Hirst), which infests small mice and rodents. House mice serve as the reservoir of infection.

R. akari is morphologically and biologically similar to other rickettsias and is antigenically related to, but distinct from, *R. rickettsii*, the cause of Rocky Mountain spotted fever.

Clinical manifestations The initial skin lesion appears about 7 to 10 days after the mite bite as a firm red papule 1 to 1.5 cm in diameter. In a few days, the center vesiculates, and the papule is surrounded by an area of erythema. The regional lymph glands are moderately enlarged. The primary lesion, which is not painful, becomes covered with a black scab; it heals slowly, and a small scar is visible on separation of the crust.

The febrile phase begins 3 to 7 days after the initial lesion, and an exanthem may accompany the fever or begin several days later. The onset of fever is sudden, with chilly sensations or frank chills, headache, sweats, myalgia, anorexia, and photophobia. The pyrexia ranges from 39.4 to 40°C (103 to 104°F) and continues for about a week, occasionally with morning remissions.

The exanthem is maculopapular-vesicular, generalized in distribution, and may be abundant or scant. The lesions may involve the oral cavity but not the palms or soles. In a week, the vesicles dry and form scabs which eventually scale but leave no scar.

The constitutional symptoms are generally mild, and the course of illness is uncomplicated. No fatal cases have been reported.

The disease may be confused with chickenpox, which is different because it occurs usually in childhood and has no initial lesion and the papular cutaneous lesion is entirely transformed into a vesicle. Variola (smallpox) is accompanied by a more severe constitutional reaction, and the vesicles become pustules. The skin lesions of the other rickettsioses differ in their lack of vesiculation. The Weil-Felix reaction is usually negative in this rickettsial disease, but specific complement fixation, microscopic agglutination, and immunofluorescent antibody reactions are useful diagnostic aids even though there is considerable antigenic crossing with Rocky Mountain spotted fever.

Treatment and prevention Chloramphenicol and the tetracycline antibiotics are all effective for treating patients with rickettsialpox. The temperature reaches normal levels in about 2 days, and recovery is rapid.

Control measures should be directed toward elimination of house mice and the vector mites responsible for transmitting the disease.

OTHER TICK-BORNE RICKETTSIAL DISEASES Definition Boutonneuse fever, North Asian tick-borne rickettsiosis, and Queensland tick typhus, three diseases occurring in the eastern hemisphere, are caused by rickettsias closely related to one another and to the agent of Rocky Mountain spotted fever. Each is transmitted by the bite of an ixodid tick. These mild to moderately severe illnesses are characterized by an initial lesion (called *tache noire* in boutonneuse fever), a fever of several days to 2 weeks, and a generalized maculopapular erythematous rash which appears on about the fifth day and usually involves the palms and soles. Specific complement-fixing antibodies appear in the patients' sera during convalescence, but agglutinins to *Proteus* OX-19 (Weil-Felix reaction) are frequently found only in low titer.

Etiology and epidemiology The etiologic agents of these three diseases are all members of the spotted fever group of rickettsias. Together with *R. rickettsii* and *R. akari* they possess common group antigens which are readily demonstrated by agglutination, complement fixation, microscopic agglutination, and immunofluorescent antibody reactions.

Boutonneuse fever, which may be regarded as the prototype of the three, is caused by *R. conorii*. Modern serologic methods employing specific rickettsial antigens have shown this rickettsia to be the causative agent for a single widely disseminated disease known by various local names. Information on the distribution and etiology of the various tick-borne rickettsial diseases is contained in Table 153-1.

In general, the epidemiology of these tick-borne rickettsioses resembles that of spotted fever in the western hemisphere. Ixodid ticks and small wild animals maintain the rickettsias in nature; if humans intrude accidentally into the cycle, they become a dead end in the transmission chain. In certain areas, the cycle of boutonneuse fever involves domiciliary environments, with the brown dog tick, *Rhipicephalus sanguineus*, as the dominant vector.

Clinical manifestations These three tick-borne rickettsioses resemble one another closely. The clinical course is usually milder than that of spotted fever, with a shorter febrile period and fewer severe complications; fatalities are rare and generally limited to the aged and debilitated. The initial lesion, which is present in most cases at the onset of fever, heals slowly; the regional lymph nodes are enlarged. The rash usually remains papular and only in severe cases becomes hemorrhagic.

The clinical picture (including the primary lesion), the geographic location, and epidemiologic considerations are helpful in establishing the diagnosis. The typhus fevers, meningococcal infections, leptospirosis, and measles must be considered in the differential diagnosis; the Weil-Felix and complement fixation tests are of value here.

Treatment and prevention Chloramphenicol and the tetracyclines are effective therapeutic agents, patients generally become afebrile after 2 to 3 days of treatment, and recovery is rapid.

The major effective methods of control are concerned with avoidance of tick bites; these include application of repellents and prompt removal of attached ticks. Effective vaccines are not available commercially.

Q FEVER Definition Q fever is an acute infectious disease caused by *Coxiella burnetii* and characterized by a sudden onset of fever, malaise, headache, weakness, anorexia, and interstitial pneumonitis. Rickettsemia occurs during the febrile period, and specific complement-fixing antibodies are present during convalescence. In contrast to the other rickettsioses, the disease is not associated with a cutaneous exanthem or agglutinins for the *Proteus* bacteria (Weil-Felix reaction).

Etiology and epidemiology *C. burnetii* possesses the general properties of other rickettsias but is somewhat more resistant to inactivation in unfavorable environments and more pleomorphic than the others. Its infectivity after drying under natural conditions is of importance in the spread of infection to humans. *C. burnetii* has a wide host range in nature, but guinea pigs and embryonated eggs are the common laboratory hosts employed for its propagation.

C. burnetii undergoes antigenic phase variation similar to the rough-smooth dissociation of bacteria. Phase I organisms are found in nature; they possess a cell-wall-associated surface antigen that is probably related to virulence and is antiphagocytic. The phase II variant is a laboratory artifact that follows adaptation of phase I in chick embryos. Complement-fixing antibodies to phase I antigen reflect a recent acute infection; they appear in 7 to 10 days, peak at about 20 days, and slowly decline.

Human Q fever is contracted by inhalation of infected dusts, by handling infected materials, possibly by drinking milk contaminated with *C. burnetii,* and, in one instance, by blood transfusion. The disease in Australia is enzootic in animals, especially bandicoots, and is transmitted in nature by ticks. Rickettsia-laden tick feces may contaminate cattle hides, and inhalation of this material has caused infection in humans. In the United States, a number of species of ticks are naturally infected, among them *Dermacentor andersoni* and *Amblyomma americanum,* and in North Africa transovarial transmission of the agent in indigenous ticks has been demonstrated. Sheep, goats, and cows have been found to be naturally infected in North America and in Europe, and *C. burnetii* has been recovered from the milk of such animals. Milk, as well as infected excretions from livestock, probably accounts for certain outbreaks of human disease following inhalation by cows of infected dust from barns and pens. The airborne route of dried contaminated material is the most likely method of spread. A number of epidemics have occurred among laboratory workers engaged in studies on *C. burnetii.* The disease is not transmitted between humans.

Slaughterhouse workers are often exposed to infected aerosols; in 1985, five cases of hepatitis occurred at a meat packing plant that processed sheep in California. A serologic survey of approximately 100 employees, conducted to identify the extent of the outbreak, revealed a total of 31 persons with evidence of infection. The primary reservoirs of *C. burnetti* are cattle, sheep, goats, and ticks. Many wild and domestic animals are susceptible to infection. In Uruguay, there were 14 outbreaks of Q fever between 1975 and 1985, comprising 1358 clinically suspected cases, all of which occurred in workers at meat processing plants; 814 were serologically confirmed.

An ''urban'' outbreak of Q fever occurred in 12 poker players in Halifax, Nova Scotia. Presumably the disease was transmitted by a parturient cat.

Clinical manifestations After incubation of approximately 19 days (range 14 to 26 days), the disease begins with headache, chilly sensations, fever, malaise, myalgia, and anorexia. For several days, the temperature ranges from 38.3 to 40°C (101 to 104°F); the entire course rarely exceeds 2 weeks and usually ranges from 3 to 6 days. There may be wide fluctuations in the fever. Respiratory and gastrointestinal symptoms are not conspicuous in the early stages. Headache and fever predominate. A dry cough and chest pain occur after about 5 days, when rales are usually audible. Roentgenographic findings indistinguishable from those of primary atypical pneumonia are present usually by the third to fourth day of disease, first as patchy areas of consolidation involving a portion of one lobe, giving a homogeneous ground-glass appearance. Occasionally, a homogeneous localized infiltration may resemble a tumor mass. These manifestations persist beyond the febrile period and may appear in patients who are unaware of pulmonary involvement. Complications are rare, and coincident with defervescence the appetite begins to return. Convalescence progresses slowly for several weeks, during which time the principal disability is weakness. It is not uncommon for patients to lose 7 to 9 kg during the active stages of disease. The disease may be protracted in approximately 20 percent of cases, with fever persisting for longer than 4 weeks, particularly in elderly patients. Occasionally relapse occurs, especially in patients treated with antibiotics during the first several days of disease.

Hepatitis, with the development of clinically detectable icterus, occurs in approximately one-third of patients with the protracted form. This form of Q fever is characterized by fever, malaise, absence of headache or respiratory signs, and hepatomegaly with right upper quadrant pain. Liver biopsy specimens show diffuse granulomatous changes with multinucleated giant cells and scattered infiltrations of polymorphonuclear leukocytes, lymphocytes, and macrophages. *C. burnetii* may be demonstrated in such specimens with the fluorescent antibody technique. Q fever must be included in the differential diagnosis of patients with hepatitis and those with hepatic granulomas such as tuberculosis, sarcoidosis, histoplasmosis, brucellosis, tularemia, syphilis, and others.

Endocarditis with *C. burnetii* has been identified by smear and isolation of the rickettsia in vegetations on the heart valves obtained at operation or autopsy. The aortic valve is most commonly involved, often with large vegetations. It is important to suspect the possibility of Q fever in cases of apparent subacute bacterial endocarditis with persistently negative blood cultures. Operative intervention with replacement of damaged valves is usually necessary for recovery because the available antibiotics are not rickettsicidal. In some instances long-term antibiotic therapy has been successful.

A high complement-fixing antibody titer to phase I antigen is present in patients with endocarditis and granulomatous hepatitis.

Prognosis Few fatalities have been recorded and, except for the patient with protracted illness and hepatic involvement or endocarditis, the course of disease is generally uncomplicated and benign.

Treatment and control The tetracycline antibiotics and chloramphenicol are effective in the treatment of patients with Q fever. Most patients, when treated early in the course of disease, respond promptly and recover without relapses. The therapeutic procedures are comparable to those used in spotted fever.

Control of Q fever depends primarily on immunization of susceptible persons with specific vaccines. Vaccines made from phase I rickettsias are potent and afford considerable protection to slaughterhouse and dairy workers, herders, rendering-plant workers, woolsorters, tanners, laboratory workers, and others at risk. To avoid side reactions it is important that the vaccine be given only to persons who are skin test negative. Measures should be taken to avoid exposure to infected aerosols; milk from infected domestic livestock must be pasteurized or boiled.

REFERENCES

ANDREW R et al: Tick typhus in North Queensland. Med J Aust 2:253, 1946

BOZEMAN FM et al: Serologic evidence of *Rickettsia canada* infection in man. J Infect Dis 121:367, 1970

——— et al: Epidemic typhus rickettsiae isolated from flying squirrels. Nature 255:545, 1975

CENTERS FOR DISEASE CONTROL: Summary of notifiable diseases, United States, 1987. Morb Mort Week Rep 36:54, 1987

DERRICK EH: The epidemiology of Q fever: A review. Med J Aust 1:245, 1953

DESHAZO RD et al: Early diagnosis of Rocky Mountain spotted fever. Use of primary monocyte culture technique. JAMA 235:1353, 1976

FERGUSON IC et al: Clinical, virological and pathological findings in a fatal case of Q fever endocarditis. Br J Clin Pathol 15:235, 1962

GAMBRILL MR, WISSEMAN CL JR: Mechanisms of immunity in typhus infections. Infect Immun 8:519, 1973

HARRELL GT: Rickettsial involvement of the nervous system. Med Clin North Am 37:395, 1953

HATTWICK MAW et al: Rocky Mountain spotted fever: Epidemiology of an increasing problem. Ann Intern Med 84:732, 1976

KOSTER FT et al: Cellular immunity in Q fever: Specific lymphocyte unresponsiveness in Q fever endocarditis. J Infect Dis 152:1283, 1985

LANGLEY J et al: Poker player's pneumonia: An urban outbreak of Q fever following exposure to a parturient cat. N Engl J Med 319:354, 1988

MOULTON FR (ed): *The Rickettsial Diseases of Man.* Washington, DC, American Association for the Advancement of Science, 1948

MURRAY ES et al: Brill's disease: I. Clinical and laboratory diagnosis. JAMA 142:1059, 1950

———, SNYDER JC: Brill's disease: II. Etiology. Am J Hyg 53:22, 1951

ORMSBEE RA et al: The influence of phase on the protective potency of Q fever vaccine. J Immunol 92:404, 1964

——— et al: Serologic diagnosis of epidemic typhus fever. Am J Epidemiol 105:261, 1977

OSTER CN et al: Laboratory acquired Rocky Mountain spotted fever: The hazard of aerosol transmission. N Engl J Med 297:859, 1977

PEDERSEN CE et al: Demonstration of *Rickettsia rickettsii* in Rhesus monkeys by immune fluorescence microscopy. J Clin Microbiol 2:121, 1975

PHILIP RN et al: A comparison of serologic methods for diagnosis of Rocky Mountain spotted fever. Am J Epidemiol 105:56, 1977

ROSE HM: The clinical manifestations and laboratory diagnosis of rickettsialpox. Ann Intern Med 31:871, 1949

SALGO MP et al: A focus of Rocky Mountain Spotted Fever within New York City. N Engl J Med 318:345, 1988

SMADEL JE: Influence of antibiotics on immunologic responses in scrub typhus. Am J Med 17:246, 1954

——— (ed): *Symposium on Q Fever*, Medical Science Publication 6. Washington, DC, Walter Reed Army Institute of Research, 1959

SOMENSHINE DE et al: Epizootiology of epidemic typhus (*Rickettsia prowazekii*) in flying squirrels. Am J Trop Med Hyg 27:339, 1978

SOMMA-MOREIRA RE et al: Analysis of Q fever in Uruguay. Rev Infect Dis 9:386, 1987

VINSON JW: Etiology of trench fever in Mexico, in *Industry and Tropical Health*, vol V. Boston, Harvard School of Public Health, 1964, p 109

WALKER DH, CAIN BG: A method for specific diagnosis of Rocky Mountain spotted fever on fixed, paraffin-embedded tissue by immunofluorescence. J Infect Dis 137:206, 1978

———, BRADFORD WD: Rocky Mountain spotted fever in childhood, in *Perspectives in Pediatric Pathology*, vol 6, HS Rosenberg, J Bernstein (eds). New York, Masson Publishing, 1981, pp 35–61

WOODWARD TE: A historical account of the rickettsial diseases with a discussion of unsolved problems. J Infect Dis 127:583, 1973

———: Identification of *Rickettsia* in skin tissues. J Infect Dis 134:297, 1976

154 MYCOPLASMA INFECTIONS

WALLACE A. CLYDE, JR.

INTRODUCTION The mycoplasmas are a heterogeneous group of unusual bacteria belonging to microbial class Mollicutes (''soft skin''). They differ from classical bacteria by lacking rigid cell wall structures, being contained instead by trilaminar unit membranes. This property confers on mycoplasmas an inability to react with organic dyes, such as those in the Gram stain, and an absolute insensitivity to the penicillins, since there are no cell wall receptor sites for these antibiotics. The mycoplasma genome is roughly one-sixth the size of that in *Escherichia coli,* making them fastidious species requiring many precursor substances for growth in artificial media. With maximum dimensions of 0.15 to 0.5 μm, less than some of the larger viruses, mycoplasmas are the smallest organisms known that are capable of extracellular existence.

Mycoplasmas are ubiquitous in nature and cause a wide variety of diseases among animals, birds, plants, and insects. In humans the most important pathogen is *Mycoplasma pneumoniae,* a common cause of respiratory tract infections. *M. hominis* and *Ureaplasma urealyticum* also are implicated in disease involving mainly the genitourinary system. A newly described species having many pathogenic properties, *M. genitalium,* is of uncertain significance. In addition to these organisms there are eight other distinct species that are components of the normal microflora on the oropharyngeal and genital mucosal surfaces.

MYCOPLASMA PNEUMONIAE

DEFINITION *M. pneumoniae* produces an influenza-like respiratory illness of gradual onset with headache, malaise, fever, and cough. When pneumonia is present, physical findings may be minimal despite extensive changes seen in chest x-rays. Synonyms include Eaton agent pneumonia, cold hemagglutinin–positive pneumonia, atypical or primary atypical pneumonia, and ''walking'' pneumonia. Asymptomatic infections also occur, especially in young children and partially immune adults.

ETIOLOGY *M. pneumoniae* was discovered by Eaton in 1941 and related to the syndrome of atypical pneumonia. It is a minute, motile filament, measuring approximately 0.1 by 2 μm, that has one differentiated pole where a specialized adhesin (P1) mediates attachment to respiratory epithelial cells. Production of peroxide and an inhibitor of host cell catalase are thought to be major mediators of parasitized cell injury. The organism may be isolated from respiratory secretions using complex artificial media, requiring usually 1 to 3 weeks or more for growth and identification procedures. New rapid diagnostic techniques, based on antigen detection or nucleic acid probes used directly on specimens, appear promising.

EPIDEMIOLOGY Communicability of *M. pneumoniae* infections is thought to be via large droplets of respiratory secretions; close indoor contact such as in household, institutional, or dormitory settings facilitates spread. The incubation period has been estimated at 2 to 3 weeks. Disease occurs most commonly in elementary school children, adolescents, and young adults. Infections can be found during any season of the year, although epidemic disease tends to occur during the fall and early winter months in temperate countries. Many studies have shown a periodicity of 3 to 5 years in the occurrence of major outbreaks. In Seattle, Washington, it was found that the average incidence of disease across all years and age groups was 2/1000 population per year. This occurrence doubled during epidemic years and was higher in the age groups between 5 and 40 years. In adolescent patients, 15 to 20 percent of all pneumonias could be attributed to *M. pneumoniae.* The organism has been implicated in up to 50 percent of pneumonia episodes in college students and in 20 to 30 percent of cases occurring in military recruits.

CLINICAL MANIFESTATIONS The most common clinical syndrome associated with *M. pneumoniae* infections is that of an acute or subacute tracheobronchitis. Symptoms appearing over several days' time include headache, malaise, feverishness, scratchy sore throat, and dry cough. The cough may be paroxysmal, often disturbing sleep, and gradually becomes productive of mucoid or mucopurulent sputum. Physical findings may be minimal, other than temperature elevation rarely exceeding 38.9°C (102°F). If pneumonia is present, isolated crackles or areas of wheezing may be heard usually over one of the lower lobes. Areas of subsegmental atelectasis and small pleural effusions that rarely may be seen on chest x-rays are detectable by physical examination.

Most *M. pneumoniae* disease is mild and self-limited, running its course in 2 to 4 weeks without treatment. Appropriate antibiotics in controlled clinical trials have been shown to shorten significantly the duration of fever, days of hospitalization required, and x-ray manifestations. Rarely, severe, life-threatening, or fatal episodes can occur.

A wide variety of respiratory and nonrespiratory tract complications may be encountered. Otitis media may be seen in children, while sinusitis is commonly present in adults. Occasional patients develop the syndrome of bullous myringitis. Nondescript maculopapular skin rashes are frequent in children, and *M. pneumoniae* infections have been associated with erythema multiforme and the Stevens-Johnson syndrome. Central nervous system complications of meningoencephalitis, cerebellar ataxia, and various radiculopathies have been described. Other rare complications include monarticular arthritis, myocarditis, pericarditis, coagulopathies, hemolytic anemia, and noncardiogenic pulmonary edema.

ROENTGENOGRAPHIC FINDINGS X-ray manifestations of *M. pneumoniae* pneumonia are protean and nonspecific. The most frequent pattern is one of bronchial thickening with areas of interstitial infiltration and subsegmental atelectasis involving one of the lower lobes. Another common finding is the occurrence of ''platelike'' atelectasis, often seen to best advantage on lateral views. Other changes include areas of small nodular densities, which can be confused with tuberculosis, and hilar adenopathy suggesting a variety of other entities. Lobular or lobar consolidation and massive pleural effusions are uncommon.

LABORATORY FINDINGS Total blood leukocyte and differential cell counts are usually normal, but the erythrocyte sedimentation rate is often elevated and C-reactive proteins may be demonstrated. There are no characteristic findings in urinalysis, liver or renal function tests, serum electrolytes, or electrocardiograms, although abnormalities may be seen with some of the disease complications. Specific diagnostic tests include recovery of *M. pneumoniae* from respiratory secretions, or demonstration of fourfold titer changes between paired sera using a variety of methods of which the complement fixation technique is the most widely available. However, these test results are not available promptly enough to assist therapeutic decision making. New rapid diagnostic tests of two types have been marketed:

one depends upon detection of *M. pneumoniae* rRNA by a nucleic acid hybridization technique; a second detects a major protein present in the organisms. The usefulness of these rapid tests will be determined as greater clinical experience with them accrues. Another helpful test is cold hemagglutination serology, because of its rapidity and simplicity. These IgM class antibodies directed toward the I antigen of erythrocyte membranes develop during the first or second week of illness in up to 70 percent of patients with pneumonia, and may be present in high or rising titers when patients first present. Single titers of or above 64, or fourfold or greater titer changes in sera collected 5 or more days apart, are considered significant. "False"-positive cold hemagglutinin reactions may be seen in rubeola, infectious mononucleosis, adenovirus pneumonias, several tropical diseases, and, more rarely, in collagen vascular disease. As in some of these entities, polyclonal B-lymphocyte activation and T-cell suppression occurs during *M. pneumoniae* infections, which may explain the appearance of various host tissue autoantibodies and of transient anergy in some patients.

DIFFERENTIAL DIAGNOSIS Because of its common occurrence, *M. pneumoniae* should be considered in all cases of pneumonia. Generally patients with mycoplasma pneumonia have milder illnesses than those caused by classical bacteria, less dense pulmonary infiltrations on x-rays, and normal blood leukocyte values. Epidemiologic data are especially useful: age (5 to 40 years); season (fall months predominantly); year (3- to 5-year epidemic cycles); and contact history with other cases. Other infections requiring special consideration are influenza virus pneumonia or its secondary bacterial complications (during epidemic periods) (see Chap. 139), adenovirus pneumonias (see Chap. 140) (particularly in military recruits), and mild forms of community-acquired *Legionella pneumophilia* (see Chap. 124) pneumonia. A newly recognized agent, tentatively named *Chlamydia pneumoniae* (TWAR), may produce disease clinically indistinguishable from that due to *M. pneumoniae*.

TREATMENT Erythromycin and tetracycline derivatives are effective in reducing the morbidity of *M. pneumoniae* disease. For adults, erythromycin (0.5 g every 6 h orally), tetracycline (250 mg every 6 h orally), or doxycycline (100 mg once daily orally), in 10- to 14-day courses are usually prescribed. In severely ill patients intravenous erythromycin may be selected, but tetracycline is not recommended by this route. For children less than 8 to 10 years old erythromycin (30 to 50 mg/kg per day orally for 14 days) is the primary choice; tetracycline or doxycycline are alternatives for older patients. Relapses occasionally occur upon cessation of therapy but respond to retreatment. In cases where *Legionella* infection cannot be excluded, erythromycin should be chosen for therapy. If *Chlamydia pneumoniae* pneumonia is a consideration, the use of tetracycline or doxycycline is recommended.

OTHER MYCOPLASMAL INFECTIONS

A growing body of literature documents evidence of other human mycoplasma infections, including a variety of genitourinary syndromes in both sexes and in perinatal diseases. Mycoplasma infection should be considered in suppurative processes where classical bacterial cultures are negative; examples include urethritis, salpingitis, amnionitis, pyelonephritis, postpartum sepsis, and neonatal pneumonia or meningitis. Mycoplasmal abcesses or arthritis may occur in immunocompromised patients. Sexually transmitted diseases associated with mycoplasmas are considered in Chaps. 93 and 94.

In these infections the species most commonly encountered are *M. hominis* and *U. urealyticum*. Standard bacteriologic media may support growth of *M. hominis* as minute colonies, especially media for anaerobic bacteria that are incubated for several days. Selective media for *Ureaplasma* species are available that may permit their identification in 24 to 48 h. Cultural facilities for *Mycoplasma* species are available in some diagnostic microbiology laboratories, whereas serodiagnosis of infections other than those due to *M. pneumoniae* are not routine. Specimens may be transported on wet ice (within 24 h) or dry ice (greater than 24 h) to reference laboratories for assistance. For *M. hominis* infections, tetracycline or clindamycin are effective antibiotics; this species is insensitive to erythromycin. Erythromycin or tetracycline may be used for *Ureaplasma* infections. Resistance of both species to the recommended antibiotics occurs and is a problem requiring special laboratory guidance.

REFERENCES

Broughton RA: Infections due to *Mycoplasma pneumoniae* in childhood. Ped Infect Dis J 5:71, 1986

Cassell GH (ed): Ureaplasmas of humans: With emphasis upon maternal and neonatal infections. Ped Infect Dis J 5:S221, 1986

Clyde WA Jr: Mycoplasmal infections, in *Diagnostic Procedures for Bacterial Infections*, 7th ed, BB Wentworth (ed). Washington, DC, American Public Health Association, 1987, pp 391–405

Grayston JT et al: A new *Chlamydia psittaci* strain, TWAR, isolated in acute respiratory tract infections. N Engl J Med 315:161, 1986

Mårdh P-A et al (eds): International symposium on *Mycoplasma hominis*—a human pathogen. Sex Trans Dis 10(Suppl):225, 1983

McCracken GH Jr: Current status of antibiotic treatment for *Mycoplasma pneumoniae* disease. Ped Infect Dis J 5:167, 1986

Nagayama Y et al: Isolation of *Mycoplasma pneumoniae* from children with lower-respiratory-tract infections. J Infect Dis 157:911, 1988

155 CHLAMYDIAL INFECTIONS

WALTER E. STAMM / KING K. HOLMES

The genus *Chlamydia* contains three species, *C. psittaci, C. trachomatis,* and *C. pneumoniae* (formerly the TWAR agent). *C. psittaci* is widely distributed in nature, producing genital, conjunctival, intestinal, or respiratory infections in many mammalian and avian species. Genital infections with *C. psittaci* have been well characterized in several species and cause complications such as abortion and infertility. Although mammalian strains of *C. psittaci* are not known to infect humans, avian strains occasionally infect humans, causing pneumonia. *C. pneumoniae* is a fastidious chlamydial species that appears to be a frequent cause of upper respiratory tract infection and pneumonia, primarily in children and young adults. No animal reservoir has been identified for *C. pneumoniae*, and it appears to be a human pathogen spread by close personal contact.

C. trachomatis is exclusively a human pathogen and was recognized as the cause of trachoma in the 1940s. Since then, *C. trachomatis* has been recognized as a major sexually transmitted and perinatal infection.

Chlamydiae are obligate, intracellular parasites. They possess both DNA and RNA, have a cell wall and ribosomes similar to those of gram-negative bacteria, and are inhibited by antibiotics such as tetracycline. Chlamydiae are classified as bacteria belonging to their own order (Chlamydiales) and genus (*Chlamydia*).

A unique feature of all chlamydia is their complex reproductive cycle. Two forms of the microorganism—the extracellular elementary body and the intracellular reticulate body—participate in this cycle. The elementary body is adapted for extracellular survival and is the infective form transmitted from one person to another. Elementary bodies attach to susceptible target cells (usually columnar or transitional epithelial cells) via specific receptors and enter the cell within a phagosome. Within 8 h, the elementary bodies reorganize into reticulate bodies. These forms are adapted to intracellular survival and multiplication. They undergo binary fission, eventually producing numerous replicates contained within the membrane-bound "inclusion body" which occupies much of the infected host cell. Chlamydial inclusions resist lysosomal fusion until late in the developmental cycle. After 24 h, the reticulate bodies condense and form elementary bodies still contained within the inclusion. The inclusion then ruptures, releasing elementary bodies from the cell to initiate infection of adjacent cells.

C. psittaci, *C. pneumoniae*, and *C. trachomatis* share a genus-specific or group antigen. Antibody against this antigen is measured in the complement-fixation serologic test available in most state health departments. With a microimmunofluorescence test, *C. trachomatis* strains can be further characterized serologically on the basis of antibody produced against their major outer membrane protein. Using the serovar classification of Wang and Grayston, strains associated with trachoma have generally been those of the A, B, Ba, and C serovars, while serovars D through K have been largely associated with sexually transmitted and perinatally acquired infections. Serovars L_1, L_2, and L_3 produce lymphogranuloma venereum (LGV) and hemorrhagic proctocolitis. These LGV strains demonstrate unique biologic behavior in that they are more invasive than the other serovars, produce disease in lymphatic tissue, grow readily in cell culture systems and macrophages, and are fatal when inoculated intracerebrally in mice and monkeys. Non-LGV strains of *C. trachomatis* characteristically produce superficial infections involving the columnar epithelium of the eye, genitalia, and respiratory tract.

SEXUALLY TRANSMITTED AND PERINATAL *C. TRACHOMATIS* INFECTIONS

SPECTRUM OF *C. TRACHOMATIS* GENITAL INFECTIONS Genital infections caused by *C. trachomatis* are the most common sexually transmitted disease (STD) in the United States. An estimated 3 to 4 million cases occur each year. In adults the clinical spectrum of sexually transmitted *C. trachomatis* infections parallels the spectrum of gonococcal infections (Table 155-1). Chlamydial and gonococcal infections have been associated with urethritis in both sexes, with epididymitis, mucopurulent cervicitis, acute salpingitis, bartholinitis, proctitis, and the Fitz-Hugh–Curtis syndrome (perihepatitis), and both can be associated with systemic complications, particularly with arthritis. Simultaneous infection with *C. trachomatis* occurs in 30 to 50 percent of women with cervical gonococcal infection and in about 25 percent of heterosexual men with gonococcal urethritis.

EPIDEMIOLOGY Genital infections other than LGV are caused by *C. trachomatis* serovars D through K. The incidence of nongonococcal urethritis (NGU) increased dramatically during the 1960s and 1970s. During the 1980s, the incidence of NGU stabilized in the United States, even as the incidence of gonococcal urethritis fell, probably reflecting the relative lack of implementation of programs to control chlamydial infections.

TABLE 155-1 Clinical parallels between sexually transmitted infections due to *Neisseria gonorrhoeae* and *Chlamydia trachomatis*

	Resulting clinical syndrome	
Site of infection	*N. gonorrhoeae*	*C. trachomatis*
MEN		
Urethra	Urethritis	NGU, PGU
Epididymis	Epididymitis	Epididymitis
Rectum	Proctitis	Proctitis
Conjunctiva	Conjunctivitis	Conjunctivitis
Systemic	Disseminated gonococcal infection (DGI)	Reiter's syndrome
WOMEN		
Urethra	Acute urethral syndrome	Acute urethral syndrome
Bartholin's gland	Bartholinitis	Bartholinitis
Cervix	Cervicitis	Cervicitis
Endometrium	Endometritis	Endometritis
Fallopian tube	Salpingitis	Salpingitis
Conjunctiva	Conjunctivitis	Conjunctivitis
Liver capsule	Perihepatitis	Perihepatitis
Systemic	DGI	Reiter's syndrome

C. trachomatis has consistently been isolated from 30 to 50 percent of men with NGU. The peak age incidence of genital *C. trachomatis* infections is in the late teens and early twenties, resembling other sexually transmitted infections. The prevalence of chlamydial urethral infection in young men ranges from 3 to 5 percent of men seen in general medical settings, to over 10 percent of asymptomatic soldiers undergoing routine physical examination, to 15 to 20 percent of heterosexual men seen in STD clinics. Among homosexual men, urethral infection is less common than in heterosexual men, but rectal infections occur in homosexual men who practice receptive anorectal intercourse without condoms. The ratio of chlamydial to gonococcal urethritis is highest for heterosexual men and those with high socioeconomic status and lowest for homosexual men and indigent populations.

Cervical infection in women has ranged from approximately 5 percent of asymptomatic college students or prenatal patients in the United States, to over 10 percent of women seen in family planning clinics, to over 20 percent of women seen in STD clinics. In the United States, the prevalence of *C. trachomatis* in the cervix of pregnant women is 5 to 10 times higher than that of *Neisseria gonorrhoeae*. The prevalence of genital infection with either agent is highest in individuals who are single, nonwhite or Asian, and between ages 18 and 24. The proportion of infections that are asymptomatic appears to be higher for *C. trachomatis* than for *N. gonorrhoeae*, and symptomatic *C. trachomatis* infections are clinically less severe. It is suspected that mild or asymptomatic chlamydial infections of the fallopian tubes may nonetheless cause ongoing tubal damage and infertility. Furthermore, because the total number of *C. trachomatis* infections exceeds that of *N. gonorrhoeae* infections in industrialized countries, the total morbidity caused by *C. trachomatis* genital infections equals or exceeds that caused by *N. gonorrhoeae*. The prevalence of *C. trachomatis* is higher than that of *N. gonorrhoeae* in industrialized countries, in part because measures such as treatment of sex partners and routine cultures for case detection in asymptomatic individuals have been applied much more effectively for gonorrhea than for control of *C. trachomatis* infection.

CLINICAL MANIFESTATIONS Nongonococcal and postgonococcal urethritis Nongonococcal urethritis is a diagnosis of exclusion that is applied to men with symptoms and/or signs of urethritis who do not have gonorrhea. Postgonococcal urethritis (PGU) refers to nongonococcal urethritis which develops 2 to 3 weeks after treatment of gonococcal urethritis in men. *C. trachomatis* causes 30 to 50 percent of the cases of NGU and PGU in heterosexual men but is less commonly isolated from homosexual men with these syndromes. The cause of the remaining cases is uncertain, although considerable evidence suggests that *Ureaplasma urealyticum* causes some of these infections.

Nongonococcal urethritis is diagnosed by documentation of a leukocytic urethral exudate and by exclusion of gonorrhea by Gram's stain or culture. *C. trachomatis* urethritis is generally less severe than gonococcal urethritis, although in an individual patient these two forms of urethritis cannot be differentiated solely on clinical grounds. Symptoms include urethral discharge, dysuria (often whitish and mucoid rather than frankly purulent), and urethral itching. The examination may show meatal erythema and tenderness and a urethral exudate which is often demonstrable only by stripping the urethra. About one-third of male STD patients who have *C. trachomatis* urethral infection have no demonstrable signs or symptoms of urethritis. Asymptomatic chlamydial urethritis has been demonstrated in 5 to 10 percent of sexually active adolescent males screened in teen clinics. Such patients frequently have first-glass pyuria (15 leukocytes per 400 × microscopic field in the sediment of first-voided urine), a positive leukocyte esterase test, or an increased number of leukocytes on gram-stained smear prepared from a urogenital swab inserted 1 to 2 cm into the anterior urethra. The smear is first scanned at low power to identify areas of the slide containing the highest concentration of leukocytes. These areas are then examined under oil immersion (1000×). An average of four or more leukocytes in at least three of five 1000× (oil immersion) fields is indicative of urethritis and correlates with recovery of *C. trachomatis*. To differentiate between true urethritis and functional symptoms among symptomatic patients, or to make a presumptive diagnosis of *C. trachomatis* infection in asymptomatic men (e.g., male patients in STD clinics, sex partners of women with nongonococcal salpingitis or mucopurulent cervicitis, fathers of children with inclusion conjunctivitis), the examination of an endourethral specimen for increased leukocytes is useful if specific diagnostic tests for chlamydia are not available. Alternatively, noninvasive screening for urethritis can be accomplished by testing a first-void urine for pyuria either by microscopy or by the leukocyte esterase test.

Epididymitis *C. trachomatis* is the major cause of epididymitis in sexually active heterosexual men under 35 years of age who present with epididymitis. Coliform bacteria and *Pseudomonas aeruginosa* are the most common causes of epididymitis in men over 35. In homosexual men, sexually transmitted coliform infection acquired via rectal intercourse may cause epididymitis. Testicular torsion should be promptly excluded by radionuclide scan, Doppler flow study, or surgical exploration in a teenager or young adult who presents with acute unilateral testicular pain without urethritis. Testicular tumor or chronic infection (e.g., tuberculosis) should be excluded in the patient with unilateral intrascrotal pain and swelling who does not respond to appropriate antimicrobial therapy.

Reiter's syndrome *C. trachomatis* has been recovered from the urethra of up to 70 percent of men with untreated nondiarrheal Reiter's syndrome and associated urethritis. The syndrome consists of conjunctivitis, urethritis (or cervicitis in females), arthritis, and characteristic mucocutaneous lesions (see Chap. 274). In the absence of overt urethritis, it is important to exclude subclinical urethritis.

Proctitis *C. trachomatis* of either the genital immunotypes D through K or the LGV immunotype L_2 causes proctitis in homosexual men and heterosexual women who practice receptive anorectal intercourse. Either asymptomatic infection or mild proctitis not unlike gonococcal proctitis results from infection with immunotypes D through K. Clinically, these patients present with mild rectal pain, mucus discharge, tenesmus, and, occasionally, bleeding. Nearly all have neutrophils in their rectal Gram stain. Sigmoidoscopy in these non-LGV cases of chlamydial proctitis reveals mild, patchy mucosal friability and mucopurulent discharge, and the disease process is limited to the distal rectum. LGV strains produce a more severe ulcerative proctitis or proctocolitis which can be confused clinically with herpes simplex virus proctitis and which histologically resembles Crohn's disease in that giant-cell formation and granulomas can be seen (see Chap. 241).

Mucopurulent cervicitis *C. trachomatis* has been isolated from the cervix of 30 to 60 percent of women with gonorrhea or a history of contact with gonorrhea, from 30 to 70 percent of women whose male partners have nongonococcal urethritis, and from 10 to 20 percent of women attending STD clinics who do not have a history of contact with a partner with urethritis. Women who have cervical ectopy or who use oral contraceptives appear to have an increased prevalence of cervical infection with *C. trachomatis*.

Although some women with *C. trachomatis* infection of the cervix have no symptoms or signs, careful speculum examination shows that many have mucopurulent cervicitis. As discussed more fully in Chap. 94, mucopurulent cervicitis is associated with yellow mucopurulent discharge from the endocervical columnar epithelium, and with ≥30 neutrophils per 1000× microscopic field within strands of cervical mucus on a thinly smeared, Gram-stained preparation of endocervical exudate. Other characteristic findings include edema of the zone of cervical ectopy and a propensity of the mucosa to bleed on minor trauma as happens when specimens are collected with a swab. Pap smear shows increased neutrophils, as well as a characteristic pattern of mononuclear inflammatory cells, including plasma cells, transformed lymphocytes, and histiocytes. Cervical biopsy shows predominantly a mononuclear infiltrate of the subepithelial stroma, often with a follicular cervicitis.

Pelvic inflammatory disease (PID) *C. trachomatis* plays an important causative role in salpingitis. *C. trachomatis* infection has been demonstrated in laparoscopically verified salpingitis, recovered from the fallopian tubes in the absence of other pathogens, and serologic evidence of recent *C. trachomatis* infection has been found in women with PID. In the United States *C. trachomatis* has been identified in the fallopian tubes or endometrium in up to 50 percent of women with PID, and its role as an important etiologic agent in this syndrome is well accepted.

Pelvic inflammatory disease occurs via ascending intraluminal spread of *C. trachomatis* from the lower genital tract. Mucopurulent cervicitis is followed by endometritis, endosalpingitis, and finally pelvic peritonitis. Evidence of mucopurulent cervicitis is usually present in women with laparoscopically verified salpingitis. Similarly, endometritis, demonstrated by endometrial biopsy showing plasma cell infiltration of the endometrial epithelium, is present in most women with laparoscopically verified chlamydial (or gonococcal) salpingitis. Chlamydial endometritis also occurs in the absence of clinical evidence of salpingitis: approximately 40 to 50 percent of women with mucopurulent cervicitis have plasma cell endometritis. Histologic evidence of endometritis has been correlated with an "endometritis syndrome," consisting of vaginal bleeding, lower abdominal pain, and uterine tenderness in the absence of adnexal tenderness, and with peripheral blood leukocytosis. Since laparoscopy was not performed in these patients, it is not known what proportion of those with chlamydial endometritis without adnexal tenderness had salpingitis. However, chlamydial salpingitis apparently produces milder symptoms then does gonococcal salpingitis and is associated with less marked adnexal tenderness. The presence of mild adnexal or uterine tenderness in sexually active women with cervicitis should suggest PID.

Infertility associated with fallopian tube scarring has been strongly linked to antecedent *C. trachomatis* infection in serologic studies. Since many infertile women with tubal scarring and antichlamydial antibody in these studies had no history of prior PID, subclinical tubal infection may produce scarring. Ectopic pregnancy, which occurs in over 70,000 women in the United States annually, is also thought to be related to chlamydia-induced tubal scarring in many cases.

Perihepatitis, or the Fitz-Hugh–Curtis syndrome, was originally described as a complication of gonococcal PID. However, cultural and/or serologic evidence of *C. trachomatis* infection is found in three-quarters of women with this syndrome. *C. trachomatis* has also been cultured from exudate on the hepatic capsule in laparoscopically verified cases. This syndrome should be suspected whenever a young, sexually active woman presents with an illness resembling cholecystitis (fever and right upper quadrant pain of subacute or acute onset). Symptoms and signs of salpingitis may be minimal.

Urethral syndrome in women *C. trachomatis* has been found to be the most common pathogen isolated from college women with dysuria, frequency, and pyuria in the absence of uropathogens such as coliforms or *Staphylococcus saprophyticus* in *any* concentration in a clean-catch midstream urine specimen (see Chap. 95). *Chlamydia* can also be isolated from the urethra of women without symptoms of urethritis, and up to 25 percent of female STD clinic patients have had positive *C. trachomatis* cultures from the urethra only.

***C. trachomatis* infection in pregnancy** *C. trachomatis* in pregnancy has been associated in some studies (but not in others) with premature delivery and with postpartum endometritis. Whether these complications are in part attributable to *C. trachomatis* is not clear.

PERINATAL INFECTIONS: INCLUSION CONJUNCTIVITIS AND PNEUMONIA

EPIDEMIOLOGY Studies in the United States have demonstrated that 5 to 25 percent of pregnant women have *C. trachomatis* infections of the cervix. In these studies, approximately one-half to two-thirds of the children who were exposed during birth eventually showed laboratory evidence of *C. trachomatis* infection. Roughly half of the infants who developed laboratory evidence of infection (or 25 percent of the group exposed) developed clinical inclusion conjunctivitis. In addition to eye infection, *C. trachomatis* has been isolated frequently and persistently from the nasopharynx, the rectum, and the vagina, occasionally for periods exceeding 1 year in the absence of treatment. Pneumonia occurs in about 10 percent of children infected perinatally, and otitis media may in some cases result from perinatally acquired chlamydial infection.

INCLUSION CONJUNCTIVITIS OF THE NEWBORN (NEONATAL CHLAMYDIAL CONJUNCTIVITIS) In the newborn, chlamydial conjunctivitis generally has a longer incubation period than gonococcal conjunctivitis (usually 5 to 14 days vs. 1 to 3 days), but this is not reliable in the individual patient. The other common causes of conjunctivitis in newborns include *Staphylococcus aureus, Haemophilus influenzae, Streptococcus pneumoniae,* and herpes simplex virus. Neonatal chlamydial conjunctivitis has an acute onset and often produces a profuse mucopurulent discharge. However, it is impossible to differentiate chlamydial conjunctivitis from other forms of neonatal bacterial conjunctivitis clinically, and laboratory diagnosis is required. Inclusions within epithelial cells often can be demonstrated in Giemsa-stained conjunctival smears, but these smears are less sensitive than cultures or antigen detection tests. Similarly, Gram-stained smears may show gonococci, or occasional small gram-negative coccobacilli in *Haemophilus* conjunctivitis, but smears should be accompanied by cultures for these agents. Very rarely a trachoma-like eye disease occurs in children with chlamydial infection living in areas that do not have endemic trachoma. If neonatal chlamydial conjunctivitis is not treated appropriately with oral antimicrobials, it may be followed by chlamydial pneumonia.

INFANT PNEUMONIA *C. trachomatis* causes a distinctive pneumonia syndrome in infants. For details, standard textbooks of pediatrics should be consulted.

LYMPHOGRANULOMA VENEREUM

DEFINITION Lymphogranuloma venereum (LGV) is a sexually transmitted infection caused by *C. trachomatis* strains of the L_1, L_2, or L_3 serovars. Most cases are caused by L_2 infections. The acute disease in heterosexual men is characterized by a transient primary genital lesion followed by multilocular suppurative regional lymphadenopathy. Women, homosexual men, and, occasionally, heterosexual men may develop hemorrhagic proctitis with regional lymphadenitis. Acute LGV is almost always associated with systemic symptoms such as fever and leukocytosis and rarely with systemic complications such as meningoencephalitis. After a latent period of years, late complications include genital elephantiasis due to lymphatic involvement, strictures, and fistulas of the penis, urethra, and rectum.

EPIDEMIOLOGY LGV is usually sexually transmitted, but occasional transmission by nonsexual personal contact, fomites, or laboratory accidents has been documented. Laboratory work involving creation of aerosols of this organism (e.g., sonication, homogenization) must be conducted with appropriate biologic containment.

The peak incidence of LGV corresponds to the age of greatest sexual activity, the second and third decades of life. The worldwide incidence of LGV is falling, but the disease is still endemic and a major cause of morbidity in Asia, Africa, and South America. Only 303 cases were reported in the United States in 1987.

The frequency of infection following exposure is believed to be much less than that associated with gonorrhea and syphilis. Early manifestations are recognized far more often in men than in women, who usually present with late complications. In the United States, where the reported sex ratio is 3.4 males to 1 female, most cases have involved homosexually active men; travelers, seamen, and military personnel returning from abroad; and individuals of low socioeconomic status living in areas of low but continuing endemicity in the southeast. The main reservoir of infection is presumed to be asymptomatically infected individuals, although this has not been directly demonstrated.

CLINICAL MANIFESTATIONS In heterosexuals, a *primary genital lesion* occurs from 3 days to 3 weeks after exposure. It is a small, painless vesicle or nonindurated ulcer or papule located on the penis in men or on the labia, posterior vagina, or fourchette in women. The primary lesion is noticed by less than one-third of men with LGV and only rarely by women. It heals in a few days without scarring and even when noticed is usually not recognized as LGV except in retrospect. LGV strains of *C. trachomatis* have occasionally been recovered from genital ulcers, and also from the urethra of men and the endocervix of women who present with inguinal adenopathy, suggesting that these areas may be the primary site of infection in some cases.

In women and homosexual men, *primary anal or rectal infection* occurs following receptive anorectal intercourse. In women, rectal infection with LGV (or non-LGV) strains of *C. trachomatis* presumably can also arise either via contiguous spread of infected secretions along the perineum (as with rectal gonococcal infection in women) or perhaps by spread to the rectum via the pelvic lymphatics. From the site of the primary urethral, genital, anal, or rectal infection, the organism spreads via the regional lymphatics. Penile, vulvar, and anal infection can lead to inguinal and femoral lymphadenitis. Rectal infection produces hypogastric and deep iliac lymphadenitis. Upper vaginal or cervical infection results in enlargement of the obturator and iliac nodes. The most common presenting picture in heterosexual men is the *inguinal syndrome,* which is characterized by painful inguinal lymphadenopathy beginning 2 to 6 weeks after presumed exposure; rarely the onset occurs after a few months. The inguinal adenopathy is unilateral in two-thirds of cases, and palpable enlargement of the iliac and femoral nodes is often present on the same side as the enlarged inguinal nodes. The nodes are initially discrete, but progressive periadenitis results in a matted mass of nodes which become fluctuant and suppurative. The overlying skin becomes fixed, inflamed, and thinned and finally develops multiple draining fistulas. Extensive enlargement of chains of inguinal nodes above and below the inguinal ligament ("the sign of the groove") is common but is not specific, and is present in only a minority of cases. Histologically, infected nodes initially show characteristic small stellate abscesses surrounded by histiocytes. These abscesses coalesce to cause large, necrotic, suppurative foci. Spontaneous healing usually occurs after several months, leaving inguinal scars or granulomatous masses of varying size which persist for life. Massive pelvic lymphadenopathy in women or homosexual men may lead to exploratory laparotomy.

As cultures and serology for *C. trachomatis* are being used more often, increasing numbers of cases of LGV proctitis are being recognized in homosexual men. Such patients present with anorectal pain and mucopurulent, bloody rectal discharge. Although patients may complain of diarrhea, this usually represents frequent, painful, unsuccessful attempts at defecation (tenesmus). Sigmoidoscopy reveals ulcerative proctitis or proctocolitis, with purulent exudate and mucosal bleeding. Since the LGV agent is an obligate intracellular pathogen, the histopathologic findings in the rectal mucosa include granulomas with giant cells, along with crypt abscesses and extensive inflammation. These clinical, sigmoidoscopic, and histopathologic findings may closely resemble Crohn's disease of the rectum.

Constitutional symptoms are common during the stage of regional lymphadenopathy and, in the presence of proctitis, may include fever, chills, headache, meningismus, anorexia, myalgias, and arthralgias. These findings in the presence of lymphadenopathy are sometimes mistaken for malignant lymphoma. Other systemic complications are infrequent but include arthritis with sterile effusion, aseptic meningitis, meningoencephalitis, conjunctivitis, hepatitis, and erythema nodosum. Chlamydiae have been recovered from the cerebrospinal fluid, and in one case from the blood in a patient with severe constitutional symptoms, indicating the occurrence of disseminated infection. Laboratory infections due to suspected inhalation of aerosols have been associated with mediastinal lymphadenitis, pneumonitis, and pleural effusion.

Complications of untreated anorectal infection include perirectal abscess, fistula in ano, and rectovaginal, rectovesical, and ischiorectal fistulas. Secondary bacterial infection probably contributes to these complications. Rectal stricture is a late complication of anorectal infection and usually occurs 2 to 6 cm from the anal orifice, within reach on digital rectal examination. The stricture may extend proximally for several centimeters, leading to a mistaken clinical and radiographic diagnosis of carcinoma.

A small percentage of cases of LGV in men presents with chronic progressive infiltrative, ulcerative, or fistular lesions of the penis, urethra, or scrotum. Associated lymphatic obstruction may produce elephantiasis. Urethral stricture may occur and usually involves the posterior urethra, causing incontinence or difficulty with micturition.

APPROACH TO THE DIAGNOSIS AND TREATMENT OF *C. TRACHOMATIS* OCULOGENITAL INFECTIONS

Four types of laboratory procedures are available to confirm *C. trachomatis* infection. These are direct microscopic examination of tissue scrapings for typical intracytoplasmic inclusions, isolation of the organism, detection of chlamydial antigens by immunologic methods, and detection of antibody in the serum or in local secretions.

Except in conjunctivitis, direct microscopic examination of Giemsa-stained cell scrapings for typical inclusion has an unacceptably low sensitivity and false-positive interpretations by inexperienced observers are common.

Cell culture techniques have replaced the yolk sac of embryonated eggs for isolation of *C. trachomatis*. While LGV strains grow well in many cell lines, the other *C. trachomatis* strains are much more difficult to culture. Although culture remains the "gold standard" for diagnosis of chlamydial infection, it is expensive, technically demanding, and not widely available. Therefore, antigen detection methods have been developed that can be used instead of cultures. In the immunofluorescent slide test, potentially infected genital or ocular secretions are smeared on a slide, fixed, and stained with fluorescein-conjugated monoclonal antibody. When viewing the slide using a fluorescence microscope, the presence of fluorescing elementary bodies confirms the diagnosis. Compared with culture, this test is 85 to 90 percent sensitive and quite specific when used for confirmation of urethral, cervical, or ocular infection in high-risk patients with suspected *C. trachomatis* infection. The sensitivity of the test appears lower in low-risk populations. This plus the relatively labor-intensive nature of the test limit its value as a screening test. An enzyme-linked immunosorbent assay (ELISA) technique for chlamydial antigen detection has also been developed and provides another alternative to culture. Reported sensitivity and specificity of this test for genital infections has been 70 to 95 percent and 92 to 97 percent in high-risk populations. This test is well-suited to screening because large numbers of specimens can be easily processed.

Serologic tests have limited usefulness in the diagnosis of chlamydial oculogenital infections. The complement fixation (CF) test with the heat-stable genus-specific antigen has been used to diagnose LGV with some success, but it is insensitive in non-LGV *C. trachomatis* infections. The microimmunofluorescence (micro-IF) test with *C. trachomatis* antigens is more sensitive but is generally available only in research laboratories. The test measures antibodies by serovar specificity and by immunoglobulin class (IgM, IgG, IgA, secretory IgA) in both serum and local secretions. Serologic diagnosis using the micro-IF test may be useful in infant pneumonia (high-titer IgM antibody and/or fourfold titer rises can often be demonstrated), in women with chlamydial salpingitis (especially with Fitz-Hugh–Curtis syndrome), and in LGV.

Table 155-2 summarizes the diagnostic tests of choice for patients with suspected chlamydial infection. With few exceptions, the most suitable method for diagnosis is demonstration of the agent in tissue-cell culture or by antigen detection methods. Selection of the most appropriate of these tests depends upon local availability and expertise. Since *C. trachomatis* is an intracellular pathogen, adequate specimens for chlamydial culture must include epithelial cells. Cultures of pus result in fewer isolations of the organism. In urethritis, a thin-shafted urogenital swab should be inserted at least 2 cm into the urethra to obtain an appropriate specimen. When a cervical culture is taken, the external os should first be cleaned of debris and purulent material, and a plastic-shafted swab then inserted into the cervix, rotated slowly several times, and withdrawn. When conjunctival specimens are sought, the epithelium should be swabbed to remove cells, rather than simply purulent material. All specimens for chlamydial culture should be placed immediately into a transport medium and then either refrigerated if they will reach the laboratory within 12 to 18 h or frozen at $-70°C$ if longer storage is anticipated. A major advantage of antigen detection techniques is their less rigid transport requirements.

From a public health viewpoint, the most effective use of chlamydia diagnostic testing has not been established and will vary depending upon clinical population, local resources, and laboratory expertise. The Centers for Disease Control have recommended empiric treatment (without diagnostic testing if resources are not available for testing) of selected high-risk groups. These include men with NGU or sexually transmitted epididymitis; women with mucopurulent cervicitis (MPC) or PID; asymptomatic sex partners of patients with these syndromes; women and heterosexual men with gonorrhea (because of the high proportion of these patients who will also have *C. trachomatis* infection); and contacts of men or women with gonorrhea. Where funds for diagnostic testing are limited (e.g., in public clinics serving indigent patients), it has been rationalized that these groups will receive empiric therapy in any event, and hence diagnostic testing is not absolutely essential. However, it has several potential benefits in these patients, including confirmation of infection and support of the clinical diagnosis (especially in women with MPC and PID), enhancement of sex partner referral and compliance with drug therapy, determination of prognosis, and education of physicians (ability to correlate signs and symptoms with culture results). Where diagnostic testing must be rationed because of limited resources, highest priority should be given to screening asymptomatic high-risk women, especially those seen in high-risk settings (i.e., STD clinics, abortion clinics, family planning clinics), or individuals with a high-risk profile (young, multiple sex partners, lower socioeconomic status).

ANTIMICROBIAL SUSCEPTIBILITY In laboratory tests, death of inoculated mice and chick embryos, as well as growth in cell cultures, is prevented or inhibited by tetracyclines, erythromycin, rifampin (rifampicin), and certain of the fluoroquinolones; sulfonamides, clindamycin, and cycloserine are also active against *C. trachomatis*, but bacitracin and polymyxin B are less effective; penicillin and ampicillin suppress *Chlamydia* multiplication but do not eradicate the organism in vitro. The cephalosporins also appear relatively ineffective against *C. trachomatis*. Streptomycin, gentamicin, neomycin, kanamycin, vancomycin, ristocetin, spectinomycin, and nystatin are not effective at concentrations inhibitory for most bacteria and fungi. For treatment of human *C. trachomatis* infection, the tetracyclines, erythromycin, and sulfonamides are most useful.

TREATMENT In general, chlamydial infections cannot be eradicated by single-dose or short-term antimicrobial regimens. In most situations, at least 7 days and sometimes 2 to 3 weeks of antibiotic should be given. Failure after treatment of genital infections with a tetracycline usually indicates inadequate therapy, poor compliance, or reinfection. Tetracycline-resistant strains of *C. trachomatis* have not been described.

Therapy of *C. trachomatis* urethritis is more effective than therapy of other forms of NGU. *C. trachomatis* is eradicated from the urethra by treatment with tetracycline hydrochloride, 500 mg qid for 7 days, or doxycycline, 100 mg by mouth bid for 7 days. An effective alternative regimen is erythromycin, 500 mg qid for 7 days.

TABLE 155-2 Diagnostic tests in *C. trachomatis* infection

Infection	Suggestive signs/symptoms	Presumptive diagnosis*	Confirmatory test of choice
ADULT MALES			
Nongonococcal urethritis, postgonococcal urethritis	Discharge, dysuria	Gram stain with more than four neutrophils per oil immersion field, no gonococci	Urethral culture or antigen detection test for *C. trachomatis*
Epididymitis	Unilateral intrascrotal swelling, pain, tenderness; fever; nongonococcal urethritis	Gram stain with more than four neutrophils per oil immersion field, no gonococci	Urethral culture or antigen detection test for *C. trachomatis*
ADULT FEMALES			
Cervicitis	Mucopurulent cervical discharge, cervical edema, ectopy, bleeding	Cervical Gram stain with ≥30 neutrophils per oil immersion field in cervical mucus	Cervical culture or antigen detection test for *C. trachomatis*
Salpingitis	Evidence of pelvic inflammatory disease on examination	*C. trachomatis* should always be suspected in salpingitis	Cervical culture or antigen detection test for *C. trachomatis*
Urethritis	Dysuria and frequency without urgency or hematuria	Mucopurulent cervicitis, sterile pyuria, negative routine urine culture	Urethral and cervical cultures or antigen detection test for *C. trachomatis*
ADULTS OF EITHER SEX			
Proctitis	Rectal pain, discharge, tenesmus, blood; receptive anorectal intercourse	Negative gonococcal culture and Gram stain; ≥1 neutrophils in rectal Gram stain	Rectal culture or direct immunofluorescence test for *C. trachomatis*
Reiter's syndrome	Nongonococcal urethritis, arthritis, conjunctivitis, typical skin lesions	Gram stain with more than four neutrophils per oil immersion field, no gonococci	Urethral culture or antigen detection test for *C. trachomatis*
LGV	Regional adenopathy, primary lesion, proctitis, systemic symptoms	None	Isolation of LGV strain from node, rectum, occasionally from urethra or cervix; LGV CF-titer ≥1:64; micro-IF titer ≥1:512
NEONATES			
Conjunctivitis	Purulent conjunctival discharge 6 to 18 days postdelivery	Negative cultures and gram stains for gonococci, *Haemophilus* sp., pneumococci, staphylococci	Conjunctival culture or antigen detection test for *C. trachomatis;* Giemsa-stained scraping of conjunctival material can provide more rapid diagnosis but is less sensitive
Infant pneumonia	Afebrile, staccato cough, diffuse rales, bilateral hyperinflation, interstitial infiltrates	None	Chlamydial culture of sputum, pharynx, eye, rectum; micro-IF antibody to *C. trachomatis*—fourfold change in IgG or IgM antibody

* Although a presumptive diagnosis of chlamydial infection is often made in the syndromes listed when gonococci are not found, a positive test for *Neisseria gonorrhoeae* does not exclude *C. trachomatis,* which is very often also present in patients with gonorrhea.

Eradication of *C. trachomatis* from the cervix has been demonstrated with similar doses and durations of tetracycline, doxycycline, and erythromycin. Erythromycin base, 500 mg qid for 10 to 14 days, is the regimen of choice for pregnant women with *C. trachomatis* infection. Amoxicillin, 500 mg tid for 10 days, has also been used successfully in one study of pregnant women. Tetracycline hydrochloride, 500 mg qid for 14 days, produces clinical and microbiologic cure of epididymitis associated with *C. trachomatis* infection.

Treatment of sex partners Genital *C. trachomatis* infections have continued to increase in incidence, whereas gonococcal infections have steadily fallen in incidence over the same period. The increase in chlamydial infection probably is due to the inability to diagnose asymptomatic infection and also failure to diagnose and treat *C. trachomatis* infections in symptomatic patients or their sex partners. Cases of NGU, epididymitis, Reiter's syndrome, and mucopurulent endocervicitis are sometimes not treated with antimicrobials, and sex partners are treated even less often. *C. trachomatis* urethral or cervical infection has been well-documented in a high proportion of the sex partners of patients with NGU, epididymitis, Reiter's syndrome, salpingitis, or endocervicitis. This is analogous to the problem of asymptomatic gonococcal infection in sex partners of patients with gonorrhea. Confirmatory laboratory tests for *Chlamydia* should be obtained if possible, but antigen detection tests may be less sensitive in asymptomatic carriers. Even those without evidence of clinical disease who have been recently exposed to proven or possible chlamydial infection (for example, NGU) should be offered therapy.

In neonates with conjunctivitis or infants with pneumonia, erythromycin ethylsuccinate or estolate can be given orally in a dose of 50 mg/kg per day, preferably as 12.5 mg/kg qid, for 2 weeks. Careful attention must be given to compliance with therapy—a frequent problem. Relapses of eye infection are common following treatment with topical erythromycin or tetracycline ophthalmic ointment and may occur after oral erythromycin therapy also, so that follow-up cultures should be obtained after treatment. Both parents should be examined for *C. trachomatis* infection and, if diagnostic tests are not readily available, should be treated with a tetracycline.

TRACHOMA AND ADULT INCLUSION CONJUNCTIVITIS

DEFINITION Trachoma is a chronic conjunctivitis associated with infection by *C. trachomatis* serovars A, B, and C. It has produced an estimated 20 million cases of blindness throughout the world and remains an important preventable cause of blindness. Inclusion conjunctivitis is an acute ocular infection caused by sexually transmitted *C. trachomatis* strains (usually serovars D through K) in adults exposed to infected genital secretions and in their newborn offspring.

EPIDEMIOLOGY Epidemiologically, two types of eye disease are caused by *C. trachomatis*. In trachoma-endemic areas where the classic eye disease is seen, transmission is from eye to eye, via hands, towels, flies, and other fomites, and usually involves serovars A, B, or C. In nonendemic areas, organisms of serovars D through K can be transmitted from the genital tract to the eye, usually causing only the inclusion conjunctivitis syndrome with or without keratitis. Rarely the eye disease acquired in this way progresses with the development of pannus and scars similar to endemic trachoma. These cases may be referred to as paratrachoma to differentiate them epidemiologically from eye-to-eye transmitted endemic trachoma.

The worldwide incidence and severity of trachoma have decreased dramatically during the past 30 years in areas with improving hygienic and economic conditions. Endemic trachoma is still the major cause of preventable blindness in north Africa, sub-Saharan Africa, the Middle East, and parts of Asia. Transmission of the endemic disease occurs primarily through close personal contact, particularly among young children in rural communities. In endemic areas, trachoma is associated with repeated exposure and reinfection, but the infection can also be latent. In the United States a mild form of endemic trachoma still occurs in Mexican Americans as well as in immigrants from areas where trachoma is endemic. Acute relapse of old trachoma has been seen occasionally following treatment with cortisone eye ointment or in very old persons exposed in their youth.

CLINICAL MANIFESTATIONS Both endemic trachoma and adult inclusion conjunctivitis present initially as a conjunctivitis characterized by small lymphoid follicles in the conjunctiva. In regions with hyperendemic classic blinding trachoma, the disease usually starts insidiously before the age of 2 years. Reinfection is common and probably contributes to the pathogenesis of trachoma.

The cornea becomes involved with inflammatory leukocytic infiltration and superficial vascularization (pannus formation). As the inflammation continues, there is conjunctival scarring that eventually distorts the eyelids, causing them to turn inward so that the inturned lashes constantly abrade the eyeball (trichiasis and entropion); eventually the corneal epithelium is abraded and may then ulcerate with subsequent corneal scarring and blindness. Destruction of the conjunctival goblet cells, lacrimal ducts, and lacrimal gland may produce a "dry-eye" syndrome with resultant corneal opacity due to drying (xerosis) or secondary bacterial corneal ulcers.

Communities with blinding trachoma often experience seasonal epidemics of bacterial conjunctivitis with *Haemophilus influenzae* which contribute to the intensity of the inflammatory process. In such areas the active infectious process usually resolves spontaneously in affected persons between 10 and 15 years of age, but the conjunctival scars continue to shrink, producing trichiasis and entropion and subsequent corneal scarring in adults. In areas with milder and less prevalent disease the process may be much slower, with active disease continuing into adulthood; blindness is rare in these cases.

Eye infection with genital *C. trachomatis* strains, usually in sexually active young adults, presents with acute onset of unilateral follicular conjunctivitis and preauricular lymphadenopathy similar to acute adenovirus or herpesvirus conjunctivitis. If untreated, the disease may persist for 6 weeks to 2 years. It is frequently associated with corneal inflammation in the form of discrete opacities ("infiltrates"), punctate epithelial erosions, and minor degrees of superficial corneal vascularization. Very rarely conjunctival scarring and eyelid distortion occur, particularly in patients treated for many months with topical corticosteroids. Recurrent eye infections occur most often in patients whose sexual consorts are not treated with antimicrobials.

DIAGNOSIS The clinical diagnosis of classic trachoma can be made if two of the following signs are present:

1 Lymphoid follicles on the upper tarsal conjunctiva
2 Typical conjunctival scarring
3 Vascular pannus
4 Limbal follicles or their sequelae, Herbert's pits

The clinical diagnosis of endemic trachoma should be confirmed by laboratory tests in children with more marked degrees of inflammation. Intracytoplasmic chlamydial inclusions occur in 10 to 60 percent of Giemsa-stained conjunctival smears in such populations, but isolation in cell cultures is more sensitive. Follicular conjunctivitis in adult Europeans or Americans living in trachomatous regions is rarely trachoma.

Sporadic cases of adult inclusion conjunctivitis must be differentiated from adenovirus and herpes simplex virus keratoconjunctivitis during the first 15 days after onset, and later from other forms of chronic follicular conjunctivitis. Demonstration of chlamydial infection by Giemsa- or immunofluorescent-stained smears or by isolation in cell cultures constitutes definitive evidence of infection. Genital examination and tests for genital chlamydial infection are indicated. Serum antibody does not constitute evidence of chlamydial eye infection since many sexually active adults have serum antibody. A practical diagnostic procedure in cases with chronic follicular conjunctivitis is treatment for 6 days with an oral tetracycline or erythromycin; a marked symptomatic response within 3 to 4 days is highly suggestive of inclusion conjunctivitis, and treatment should be continued for at least 3 weeks.

DIFFERENTIAL DIAGNOSIS OF CONJUNCTIVITIS AND KERATOCONJUNCTIVITIS The eye and its adnexa may be infected during the course of many cutaneous and systemic viral diseases. Sometimes these ocular infections produce minor manifestations, such as the transient loss of accommodation in dengue and the milder forms of conjunctivitis in systemic adenovirus infections. Other virus infections, however, such as herpes simplex (see Chap. 135), herpes zoster (see Chap. 136), measles (see Chap. 141), and vaccinia (see Chap. 143), occasionally produce serious and permanent visual loss. In addition, congenital infections are an important cause of blindness, particularly rubella, which leads to cataracts and microphthalmus, cytomegalic inclusion disease with retinal involvement, and syphilis with interstitial keratitis. Among the viral infections limited to the outer eye and manifested as a follicular conjunctivitis are epidemic keratoconjunctivitis (EKC), herpes simplex keratoconjunctivitis, Newcastle disease virus (NDV) conjunctivitis, and acute hemorrhagic conjunctivitis.

TREATMENT Public health control programs for endemic trachoma have consisted of the mass application of tetracycline or erythromycin ointment to the eyes of all children in affected communities for 21 to 60 days or on an intermittent schedule. These programs also include surgical correction of inturned eyelids by a mobile surgical team that visits each locality. Oral erythromycin, but not oral tetracyclines, offers an alternative method of mass antibiotic treatment for trachoma of young children and pregnant women.

Adult inclusion conjunctivitis responds well to treatment with full doses of systemic tetracycline or erythromycin for 3 weeks. Treating all sexual consorts of the patient simultaneously is also necessary to prevent ocular reinfection and to avoid the genital diseases due to chlamydial infection. Topical antibiotic treatment is not required in patients treated with systemic antibiotics.

PREVENTION Efforts to develop a trachoma vaccine have not yet been successful. General hygienic measures associated with improved living standards are effective in the elimination of endemic trachoma. Adequate water supply for personal cleanliness may be a key factor. In some areas the reduction of flies in the household is important.

OTHER INFECTIONS CAUSED BY *C. TRACHOMATIS* IN ADULTS

C. trachomatis has been reported as an infrequent cause of subacute endocarditis, peritonitis, pleuritis, and possibly appendicitis, and may cause respiratory infections in older children and adults. Immunosuppressed patients with pneumonia have had, in some cases, either serologic or cultural evidence of *C. trachomatis* infection, but more data are necessary to define the role of *Chlamydia* in these patients.

PSITTACOSIS

DEFINITION Psittacosis is primarily an infectious disease of birds caused by *Chlamydia psittaci*. Transmission of infection from birds to humans results in a febrile illness characterized by pneumonitis and systemic manifestations. Inapparent infections or mild influenza-like illnesses may also occur. The term *ornithosis* is sometimes applied to infections contracted from birds other than parrots or parakeets, but *psittacosis* is the preferred generic term for all forms of the disease.

EPIDEMIOLOGY Almost any avian species can harbor *C. psittaci*. Psittacine birds (parrots, parakeets, budgerigars) are most commonly infected, but human cases have been traced to contact with pigeons, ducks, turkeys, chickens, and many other birds. Psittacosis may be considered an occupational disease of pet-shop owners, poultry workers, pigeon fanciers, taxidermists, veterinarians, and zoo attendants. Since 1973, there has been a steady increase in incidence, with cases occurring primarily among employees of poultry processing plants. It is suspected that many cases are undiagnosed and not reported. The disease appears to be more common in England, where budgerigars are popular household pets and where restrictions on the importation of these birds have been eased.

The agent is present in nasal secretions, excreta, tissues, and feathers of infected birds. Although the disease can be fatal, infected birds frequently show only minor evidence of illness, such as ruffled feathers, lethargy, and anorexia. Asymptomatic avian carriers are common, and complete recovery may be followed by continued shedding of the organism for many months.

Psittacosis is almost always transmitted to humans by the respiratory route. On rare occasions the disease may be acquired from the bite of a pet bird. Prolonged contact is not essential for transmission of the disease; a few minutes spent in an environment previously occupied by an infected bird has resulted in human infection. The severity of the disease in humans bears no apparent relationship to closeness or duration of contact, although sick birds are more likely to transmit infection than healthy ones. Transmission of a psittacosis-like agent between humans has occurred among hospital personnel, with severe and sometimes fatal infections. There is evidence that these "human" strains are more virulent than native avian organisms. There is no record of infection acquired by eating poultry products.

PATHOGENESIS The psittacosis agent gains entrance to the body through the upper part of the respiratory tract, spreads via the bloodstream, and eventually localizes in the pulmonary alveoli and in the reticuloendothelial cells of the spleen and liver. Invasion of the lung probably takes place by way of the bloodstream rather than by direct extension from the upper air passages. A lymphocytic inflammatory response occurs on both the interstitial and respiratory surfaces of the alveoli as well as in the perivascular spaces. The alveolar walls and interstitial tissues of the lung are thickened, edematous, necrotic, and occasionally hemorrhagic. Histologically, the affected areas show alveolar spaces filled with fluid, erythrocytes, and lymphocytes. The picture is not pathognomonic of psittacosis unless macrophages containing characteristic cytoplasmic inclusion bodies (LCL bodies) can be identified. The respiratory epithelium of the bronchi and bronchioles usually remains intact.

CLINICAL MANIFESTATIONS The clinical manifestations and course of psittacosis are extremely variable. After an incubation period of 7 to 14 days or longer, the disease may start abruptly with shaking chills and fever ranging as high as 40.5°C (105°F), but the onset is often gradual with increasing fever over a 3- to 4-day period. Headache is almost always a prominent symptom; it is usually diffuse and excruciating and often the patient's chief complaint.

Many patients present with a dry hacking cough which is usually nonproductive, but small amounts of mucoid or bloody sputum may be raised as the disease progresses. Cough may appear early in the course of the disease or as late as 5 days after the onset of fever. Chest pain, pleurisy with effusion, or a friction rub may all occur but are rare. Pericarditis and myocarditis have been reported. Most patients have a normal or slightly increased respiratory rate; marked dyspnea with cyanosis occurs only in severe psittacosis with extensive pulmonary involvement. In psittacosis, as in most nonbacterial pneumonias, the physical signs of pneumonitis tend to be less prominent than symptoms and x-ray findings would suggest. The initial examination may reveal fine, sibilant rales, or clinical evidence of pneumonia may be completely lacking. Rales usually become audible and more numerous as the illness progresses. Signs of frank pulmonary consolidation are usually absent. Symptoms of upper respiratory tract infection are not prominent, although mild sore throat, pharyngitis, and cervical adenopathy are often present; on occasion they may be the only manifestations of illness. Epistaxis is encountered early in the course of nearly one-fourth of the cases. Photophobia is also a common complaint.

There is commonly a complaint of generalized myalgia, and spasm and stiffness of the muscles of the back and neck may lead to an erroneous diagnosis of meningitis. Lethargy, mental depression, agitation, insomnia, and disorientation have been prominent features of the illness in some epidemics, but not in others; delirium and stupor occur near the end of the first week in severe cases. Occasional patients are comatose when first seen, and the diagnosis of psittacosis may be missed. Gastrointestinal complaints such as abdominal pain, nausea, vomiting, or diarrhea are present in some cases; constipation and abdominal distention sometimes occur as late complications. Icterus, the result of severe hepatic involvement, is a rare and ominous finding. A faint, macular rash (Horder's spots) simulating the rose spots of typhoid fever has been described.

Patients without cough or other clinical evidence of respiratory involvement present as fever of unknown origin (see Chap. 20). The pulse rate is slow in relation to the fever. When splenomegaly is present in a patient with acute pneumonitis, psittacosis should be considered; the reported incidence of splenomegaly ranges from 10 to 70 percent. Nontender hepatic enlargement also occurs, but jaundice is rare. Thrombophlebitis is not unusual during convalescence; indeed, pulmonary infarction is sometimes a late complication and may be fatal.

In untreated cases of psittacosis, sustained or mildly remittent fever persists for 10 days to 3 weeks, or occasionally as long as 3 months. Over this period, the respiratory manifestations gradually abate. Psittacosis contracted from parrots or parakeets is more likely to be a severe, prolonged illness than infections acquired from pigeons or barnyard fowl. Relapses occur but are rare. Occasional patients develop endocarditis, and *C. psittaci* infection should be considered in cases of culture-negative endocarditis. Secondary bacterial infections are uncommon. Immunity to reinfection is probably permanent.

LABORATORY FINDINGS The chest x-ray in psittacosis mimics that in a great variety of pulmonary diseases. The pneumonic lesions are usually patchy in appearance but can be hazy, diffuse, homogeneous, lobar, atelectatic, wedge-shaped, nodular, or miliary. The white blood cell count is normal or moderately decreased in the acute phase of the disease but may rise in convalescence. The erythrocyte sedimentation rate is frequently not elevated. Transient proteinuria is common. The cerebrospinal fluid sometimes contains a few mononuclear cells but is otherwise normal. Despite hepatomegaly, liver function tests are generally normal.

The diagnosis can be confirmed only by isolation of the causative microorganism or by serologic studies. The agent is present in the blood during the acute phase of the disease and in the bronchial secretions for weeks or sometimes years after infection, but it is difficult to isolate. Psittacosis is most readily diagnosed by the demonstration of a rising titer of complement-fixing antibody in serum. An acute and convalescent specimen should always be tested. *C. trachomatis*, *C. psittaci*, and *C. pneumoniae* share a common genus-specific "group" antigen, which is the basis of the complement fixation test and can lead to cross reactions in the micro-IF test as well. These three species have different protein antigens that are principal antigens in the micro-IF test. The prompt initiation of treatment with tetracycline has been shown to delay antibody rise in convalescence for several weeks or months. Interpretation of a single complement fixation test may be difficult because of the antigenic cross reaction between *C. psittaci*, *C. pneumoniae*, and *C. trachomatis*.

DIFFERENTIAL DIAGNOSIS A history of exposure to birds may be the only clinical basis for differentiating psittacosis from a great variety of infectious and noninfectious febrile disorders. A partial list of pulmonary diseases that may be confused with psittacosis includes *Mycoplasma* pneumonia, *C. pneumoniae* pneumonia, legionellosis (see Chap. 124), viral pneumonia, Q fever, coccidioidomycosis, tuberculosis, enteroviral infection, carcinoma of the lung with bronchial obstruction, and common bacterial pneumonias. In the early stages, before pneumonitis appears, psittacosis may be mistaken for influenza, typhoid fever, miliary tuberculosis, and infectious mononucleosis.

TREATMENT The tetracyclines are consistently effective in the treatment of psittacosis. Defervescence and alleviation of symptoms usually occur in 24 to 48 h after instituting therapy with 2 g daily in four divided doses. To avoid relapse, treatment should probably be continued for at least 7 days after defervescence. In severe cases, hospitalization and pulmonary intensive care may be indicated. Sulfonamides are not active against *C. psittaci*.

C. PNEUMONIAE INFECTIONS

A third and previously unrecognized chlamydial species, *C. pneumoniae,* has been described by Grayston and coworkers. *C. pneumoniae* shares genus-specific antigens with *C. trachomatis* and *C. psittaci* but is otherwise serologically distinct. *C. pneumoniae* can also be distinguished from the other two species on the basis of DNA hybridization and restriction endonuclease analyses. Although *C. pneumoniae* can be grown in a variety of cell cultures, it is considerably more difficult to culture than other chlamydiae, especially from clinical specimens. Fewer than 50 isolates have been obtained from patients worldwide.

Knowledge of the epidemiology of *C. pneumoniae* infections has been derived primarily from serologic studies. Infections begin to occur in late childhood and adolescence and continue to develop throughout adult life. Seroprevalence in many adult populations that have been tested throughout the world exceeds 40 percent and suggests that *C. pneumoniae* infections are ubiquitous. Secondary infections appear to occur in older adults. In Scandinavia, *C. pneumoniae* produces epidemics of pneumonia and respiratory illness followed by periods of infrequent infection. The incidence of infections that occur outside of epidemics remains poorly defined. Transmission is presumed to be from person to person.

The clinical spectrum of *C. pneumoniae* infection includes acute pharyngitis, sinusitis, bronchitis, and pneumonitis, primarily in young adults. The pneumonitis resembles *Mycoplasma pneumoniae* pneumonia because patients often have prominent antecedent upper respiratory tract symptoms, fever, nonproductive cough, mild to moderate degree of illness, absence of leukocytosis, minimal findings on chest auscultation, and small segmental infiltrates on chest x-ray. In elderly patients, pneumonia due to *C. pneumoniae* can be more severe and may necessitate hospitalization and respiratory support.

Diagnosis of *C. pneumoniae* is uncertain because cell culture techniques are probably too insensitive for routine clinical use and noncultural tests using antigen detection methods or DNA probes have not been developed. Acute and convalescent sera can be tested for chlamydial CF antibody to make a retrospective diagnosis. However, this test does not distinguish *C. pneumoniae* infection from infection due to *C. trachomatis* or *C. psittaci*. Although controlled treatment trials have not been conducted, *C. pneumoniae* is inhibited in vitro by erythromycin and tetracycline. Recommended therapy is 2 g/d of either agent for 10 to 14 days.

REFERENCES

ADGER H et al: Screening for *Chlamydia trachomatis* and *Neisseria gonorrhoeae* in adolescent males: Values of first catch urine examination. Lancet 2:944, 1984

ALEXANDER ER, HARRISON HR: Role of *Chlamydia trachomatis* in perinatal infection. Rev Infect Dis 5:713, 1983

BRUNHAM RC et al: Mucopurulent cervicitis—the ignored counterpart in women of urethritis in men. N Engl J Med 311:1, 1984

CENTERS FOR DISEASE CONTROL: *Chlamydia trachomatis* infections: Policy guidelines for prevention and control. Morb Mort Week Rep 34:535, 1985

COULTS II et al: Clinical and radiographic features of psittacosis infection. Thorax 40:530, 1985

GRAYSTON JT: *Chlamydia pneumoniae,* strain TWAR. Chest 95:664, 1989

——— et al: A new *Chlamydia psittaci* strain, TWAR, isolated in acute respiratory tract infections. N Engl J Med 315:161, 1986

HANDSFIELD HH et al: Criteria for selective screening for *Chlamydia trachomatis* infection in women attending family planning clinics. JAMA 255:1730, 1986

MÄRDH PA: Ascending chlamydial infection in the female tract, in *Chlamydial Infections,* D Oriel et al (eds). London, Cambridge University Press, 1986

MCCORMACK WM: Chlamydial infections in men, in *Chlamydial Infections*, D Oriel et al (eds). London, Cambridge University Press, 1986

SCHACHTER J et al: Experience with the routine use of erythromycin for chlamydial infections in pregnancy. N Engl J Med 314:276, 1986

STAMM WE: Diagnosis of *Chlamydia trachomatis* genitourinary infections. Ann Intern Med 108:710, 1988

——— et al: *Chlamydia trachomatis* urethral infections in men. Prevalence, risk factors, and clinical manifestations. Ann Intern Med 100:47, 1984

section 11 Protozoal and helminthic infections

156 THE IMMUNOLOGY OF PARASITES

JOHN R. DAVID

During the past decade interest in parasitic diseases of humans and in new approaches to their control has increased steadily. One reason for this is the enormous scope of the problem. Over a billion people in the world are affected by parasitic diseases. Although accurate statistics are difficult to obtain, it is estimated that over 200 million people have malaria, the most serious protozoan disease of humans, and that more than a million children die of malaria each year in Africa alone. Schistosomiasis, a disease caused by helminths that are transmitted by snails, affects 200 to 300 million persons. Filarial parasites affect an equal number of people, and one of these, *Onchocerca volvulus,* is the second major cause of blindness in the world. *Trypanosoma cruzi,* another protozoan, is the major cause of heart disease in South America, and hookworm infects over 800 million persons.

With the modernization of developing countries, many of these diseases are becoming more prevalent. For example, the pressure to provide energy for industrialization leads to building dams which have brought about profound changes in the local environment; the lake behind the Volta Dam has increased the coastline by 4000 miles, and the snails on its banks infected with schistosomes have increased the prevalence of schistosomiasis in people living on the lake's borders from a few percent to almost 100 percent. Improvement schemes for agriculture often involve extension of irrigation for the cultivation of rice. Some of these projects have been associated with increases in transmission of malaria by mosquitoes, which breed in the irrigation ditches. Another example of the unanticipated effects of progress can be seen in the Amazon basin, where the clearing of the forests in order to reclaim the land for industry and agriculture has greatly increased human contact with sandflies which live in these areas and transmit leishmaniasis.

Another reason for the increasing focus on these diseases by scientists and physicians is that the classic control measures are less than adequate. The most telling example of this is malaria. After World War II, there was great optimism that this disease could be eradicated by spraying homes with DDT and by treating the disease in humans with chloroquine. After an extensive eradication program was instituted in the early 1960s in Sri Lanka, only 18 cases of malaria were reported in that country. However, 5 years later there were over a half million cases. The failure of malaria eradication was due to at least three factors: (1) the surveillance stage of the eradication effort was not maintained; (2) mosquitoes became resistant to DDT; and (3) the parasite became resistant to chloroquine. Moreover, the cost of these control measures proved to be enormous.

The large number of people affected by parasitic diseases, the increasing environmental changes in the developing world, and the failure of classic control programs have stimulated the search for new approaches for the control of these disorders. One of these approaches is immunologic. Currently, immunologists are studying several aspects of parasites' interaction with the host. They are trying to delineate the mechanisms that parasites have evolved to evade the immune response of the host, to define which immune mechanisms they do not escape, and to learn which immune responses are the basis for the pathologic lesions. Immunology is also providing diagnostic tests and ultimately, it is hoped, will provide effective vaccines for some of these diseases. At present, there is not a single vaccine available to protect humans against parasites, despite the availability of several effective vaccines against animal parasitic diseases. For the purposes of this discussion, the most useful way to present the problems of vaccine development in these complex diseases is to give a relatively detailed description of what is being done in one disease, malaria, rather than a cursory summary of many.

MALARIA VACCINE Although investigators are trying to produce vaccines to many parasites, especially intensive work is under way on vaccines for *Plasmodium falciparum,* the most malignant malaria parasite. In order to understand the various approaches that are being pursued, it is necessary to review briefly the life cycle of the malaria parasite (see Chap. 159). When an infected mosquito bites a human, it injects the motile sporozoite, which is in its salivary gland. In less than half an hour, the sporozoite leaves the blood and invades the liver. It then goes through the exoerythrocytic cycle, undergoing asexual division by schizogony and producing many merozoites. These burst out of the liver cells into the blood and invade erythrocytes. Here, they differentiate into trophozoites, undergo division by schizogony, and burst, liberating more merozoites, which reinvade erythrocytes and continue the cycle. Some of the merozoites develop into the sexual stages, the gametocytes. When a mosquito bites an infected person, the gametocytes are taken up in the blood meal and rapidly come out of the erythrocytes. The male microgametes then fertilize the female macrogametes, forming the ookinete and then the oocyst. Further division within the oocyst leads to the infective stage, the sporozoite. Several of these stages can be targeted for immunologic attack by a vaccine.

Sporozoite vaccine Persons can become immune to *P. falciparum* via the sporozoite stage. This has been shown by allowing irradiated infected mosquitoes (containing irradiated sporozoites which cannot divide) to bite humans. Investigations have resulted in the characterization of a single sporozoite antigen. Monoclonal antibodies to this antigen can passively transfer resistance to malaria in rodents and monkeys. Using recombinant DNA technology, the gene coding for the protective sporozoite antigen of *P. falciparum* has been cloned. The protective epitope is made up of four amino acids repeated 23 times. Two trials of recombinant or synthetic sporozoite vaccines in humans had disappointing results; in general, the vaccines elicited poor antibody responses, and parasitemia was prevented in only a few individuals who had high titers of antibody. Studies suggest that the repeat portion of the circumsporozoite antigen may have limited immunogenicity; efforts are being made to improve immunogenicity by combining the repeat sequence with potent T-cell epitopes found elsewhere in the molecule. T-cell epitopes need to be used not only to enhance the antibody response but also because both γ-interferon, a T-cell lymphokine, and CD8 cytotoxic T cells play a protective role in the early stages of malaria in mice. Such epitopes should be on the natural molecule and not on an artificial carrier if the immunity from the vaccine is to be boosted in nature. The possibility of genetic restriction to these T-cell epitopes may complicate the development of an effective vaccine. Immunomodulators incorporated into the vaccine may be helpful in enhancing the immune response. The advantages of the sporozoite vaccine are that it may protect against different strains of *P. falciparum* and that it inhibits the early liver stages of the parasite. The disadvantage is that it may be an all-or-none phenomenon; if a few sporozoites evaded the immune response, the person might get malaria.

Blood-stage vaccine The host encounters merozoites for short periods as they leave one erythrocyte and invade another. Erythrocytes infected by parasites develop new antigens of parasite origin on their surfaces. Both merozoites and infected erythrocytes can be targets for a vaccine. Monoclonal antibodies to this stage in rodent malaria confer partial protection when transferred passively, and antigens isolated by means of these antibodies can induce protective immunity. There has been some success in protecting primates with blood-stage vaccines using recombinant or synthesized antigens combined with complete Freund's adjuvant. One study reported partial protection of humans using a combination of several synthetic peptides polymerized together. T cells have also been shown to play a role in immunity in mice during the blood stage.

Blood-stage vaccines have the advantage that they act against the parasite at the merozoite stage, which involves a longer interaction with the host than the sporozoite stage and also causes the symptoms and the pathology. Their disadvantages are that adjuvants are necessary in most cases, the vaccines may be strain-specific, and some of these antigens may exhibit variation.

Gamete vaccine If antibodies are raised against gametes in an animal, they will be taken up with the gametes when the mosquito bites and will then neutralize the gametes escaping from the erythrocytes in the mosquito. Several gamete antigens have been isolated, and some have been cloned. Monoclonal antibodies to these will prevent the fertilization of the gametes in the mosquito, thus blocking transmission. Studies suggest that natural antigamete antibodies to *P. vivax* may play a part in limiting the transmission of malaria. Because the antigamete vaccine would not protect the individual but might reduce transmission, it could be incorporated into a multivalent vaccine.

IMMUNE EVASION BY PARASITES Parasites have developed a variety of ingenious ways of evading the immune response of the host. Some of these are listed in Table 156-1. The most fascinating mechanism is that of antigenic variation by African trypanosomes, the flagellated protozoa transmitted by the tsetse fly that is the cause of sleeping sickness (see Chap. 161). The trypanosome has a thick surface coat, which is made up of many molecules of a single antigenic glycoprotein. When cloned organisms, all having the same surface antigen, are injected into certain animals, successive waves of parasitemia ensue similar to those seen when a human is bitten by an infected tsetse fly. The peak of each wave consists of organisms expressing a single variant surface glycoprotein antigen (VSG), and this VSG is different from VSGs expressed by organisms in previous peaks in the same animal. A cloned organism can produce over 100

TABLE 156-1 Some mechanisms of immune evasion

Parasite	Mechanism
Trypanosoma brucei	Antigenic variation
Toxoplasma	Lysosome-phagosome fusion prevented
Malaria, *Babesia*	Escape into host cells
Schistosomes	Host molecule acquisition
	Loss of surface antigens
	Intrinsic membrane changes
	Immune-complex blockade
Filaria, *Leishmania*	Specific T-cell suppression
Taenia, amebae	Inactivation of mediators of inflammation

different VSGs! Each peak of parasitemia induces soluble antibody directed at the major VSG. Presumably the antibody eliminates the organism with that specific VSG, but trypanosomes that can switch to another VSG escape. Analysis of the amino acid sequence of a number of VSGs indicates that they do not differ by only a few substitutions, which could be explained by point mutations; on the contrary, the amino acid sequence of each VSG is quite different.

Studies of the genes encoding the VSGs have shown that each VSG is encoded by a distinct gene. Every trypanosome, regardless of the VSG it is expressing, contains a copy of each VSG gene. Trypanosomes have several mechanisms for expressing a VSG. For example, the organism expressing a particular VSG gene may have an additional, duplicate copy of that gene; this is referred to as the *expression-linked copy*. Studies using restriction enzymes indicate that the expression-linked copy is moved to a new site in the trypanosome near the telomere that is gene-specific for expression. If each gene is visualized as a tape cassette in a library, to express the VSG the cassette is duplicated, the duplicate is removed from the library, inserted into a genetic tape deck, and expressed. Although recent studies have revealed alternatives to the formation of an expression-linked copy for VSG gene activation, the molecular mechanism of gene expression is still unclear.

It was thought initially that the driving force for antigenic variation was antibody to that antigen; however, it has been shown that antigenic variation can be triggered in the absence of antibody both in vitro and in vivo.

Some organisms have developed multiple ways of evading the immune response. Schistosomes, for instance, can lose surface antigens after they enter the host, can take up host antigens and masquerade as host tissue, can develop certain intrinsic membrane changes making them resistant to attack even when surface antigens are present, and can shed antigens which may block effector cells and antibodies. A number of parasites, *Toxoplasma* being one example, when engulfed by a macrophage, prevent the fusion of the phagosome with the lysosomes. Others, such as *Leishmania,* do not prevent fusion when engulfed but are resistant to toxic substances in the lysosomes of the macrophage. A lipophosphoglycan (LPG) molecule on the surface of *Leishmania* is thought to play a role in this immune evasion. Indeed, the length of the carbohydrate chains on the LPG molecule may determine whether the organism can resist lysis by the alternate complement pathway. Still other parasites, such as *Trypanosoma cruzi,* escape from the lysosomes into the cytoplasm.

A number of parasites such as filaria, *Leishmania,* and *Plasmodium* induce strong suppressor mechanisms, including T suppressor cells, which dampen or eliminate the host's effective immune response. Organisms evade lysis by the alternative complement pathway by a number of means, including the presentation of surface glycoproteins that bind the inactive fragment, iC3b, rather than the hemolytically active C3b. Some parasites can destroy mediators of inflammation involved in an effective immune response. For example, *Taenia* destroys complement components, and amebae produce factors that neutralize chemotaxins for macrophages. Other parasites such as *Ascaris* appear to have a surface coat that is antigenic and can induce an immune response but is, nevertheless, resistant to immune system attack.

Although some parasites can evade the immune response, they can induce an effective protective immune response to a subsequent infection by the same species. This is called *concomitant immunity* or *premunition*.

EFFECTOR MECHANISMS AGAINST PARASITES Mechanisms that may be effective against parasites include the following: antibodies, cells including cytotoxic T cells, T-cell–induced activated macrophages, natural killer cells, and a variety of cells that mediate antibody-dependent cell-mediated cytotoxicity. Amplifiers of the immune system such as lymphokines and complement are also involved.

Immunity against several parasites such as malaria, schistosomes, and *Trypanosoma cruzi* can be transferred by antibodies. Nevertheless, evidence obtained in a number of animal models suggests that cell-mediated immunity is also involved against these and other parasites, including the organisms causing malaria, leishmaniasis, toxoplasmosis, schistosomiasis, filariasis, and trichinosis. Studies in mice have shown that protective immunity to *Leishmania* is generally associated with the T-cell subset T_{H1}, which produces interleukin 2 (IL-2) and γ-interferon, whereas the T_{H2} subset, which produces IL-4 and IL-5, usually exacerbates the disease. It is less clear whether protective immunity develops against amebae, African trypanosomes, or hookworm. There appears to be no naturally acquired immunity to *Ascaris,* guinea worm, or pinworm.

Two immune mechanisms have been described which appear to be unique for helminths. These involve eosinophils in one case and IgE in the other.

EOSINOPHILS AND ANTIBODY-DEPENDENT CELL-MEDIATED CYTOTOXICITY (ADCC) It has been known for over 100 years that eosinophils are associated with helminth infections, but only in the past few years has it become known that these cells can function as killer cells. Specifically, highly purified preparations of eosinophils, when mixed with antibody-coated schistosomula of *Schistosoma mansoni* in vitro, killed the larvae. The antibody formed is of the IgG class, and the eosinophils attach to the Fc portion of the IgG by the cells' Fc receptor. Immune complexes or staphylococcal protein A, which can interfere with the binding of eosinophils to the Fc portion of the antibody, inhibit the reaction. Incubation at 37°C makes the interaction between eosinophils and antibody-coated schistosomula become irreversible. This is associated with degranulation and the release of major basic protein (MBP), the most abundant protein in the eosinophil granule, and eosinophil cationic protein (ECP) over the surface of the schistosomula. MBP and ECP, in turn, are toxic to the larvae. Eosinophils can also kill other helminths such as *Trichinella spiralis,* presumably by a similar mechanism.

Eosinophils from patients with eosinophilia exhibit an enhanced ability to kill antibody-coated schistosomula in vitro; they act as if they were activated. Moreover, a number of soluble substances such as granulocyte-monocyte colony stimulating factor (GM-CSF), tumor necrosis factor (TNF), and a monocyte-derived eosinophil cytotoxic enhancing factor (ECEF) can increase the eosinophil's capacity to kill in vitro. Eosinophils are activated in cancer patients treated with IL-2 and lymphokine-activated killer cells generated by IL-2. IL-5 stimulates eosinophilia. In mice, this lymphokine is produced by the T_{H2} subset of T cells. Mice given anti-IL-5 antibodies have very few eosinophils, providing a good model for studying the role of eosinophils in immunity.

ROLE FOR IgE The observation that IgE levels are elevated in some persons in the tropics, notably those infected with helminths, suggests that IgE may act to protect the host against parasites. The mediators released by triggered mast cells could affect the parasites directly, or, by increasing vascular permeability and releasing eosinophil chemotactic factors, they could lead to the accumulation of necessary antibodies (IgG) and cells to attack the parasite. IgE immune complexes can induce macrophage-mediated cytotoxicity to schistosomula. Rats made specifically IgE-deficient by the repeated injection of antiepsilon chain antibodies show markedly impaired resistance to *Trichinella* infection. IgE also plays an important role in pathology associated with parasites, such as in the tropical eosinophilia syndrome associated with filariasis; it mediates immediate hypersensitivity reactions triggered by parasites.

IMMUNOPATHOLOGY Immune mechanisms play a major role in the pathology induced by many parasites. Such mechanisms are the cause of the granulomatous reaction to eggs of *S. mansoni* which is the basis of the immunopathology of this disease; immune-complex renal disease in malaria and visceral leishmaniasis; heart disease due to *T. cruzi;* the obstructive and ocular disease in filariasis and onchocerciasis; the muscle pathology in trichinosis; the allergic reactions to ruptured hydatid cyst fluid; and the pulmonary complications to migrating nematode larvae. Just as suppressor mechanisms are involved in damping protective immunity, they are also involved in modulating the immunopathology. An example of this is the modulation of *S. mansoni* granulomas by T suppressor cells. Anti-idiotypic antibodies (see next section) can modify the host's response to the parasite. Some patients, including infants born to mothers with schistosomiasis, have anti-idiotypic T cells which react to antiegg antibodies. The precise role played by anti-idiotypic T cells and/or antigen transferred from mother to infant in the modulation of the child's immune response to the parasites needs further clarification.

MONOCLONAL AND ANTI-IDIOTYPIC ANTIBODIES Monoclonal antibodies to various stages of malaria parasites have been used to detect antigens that can induce protective immunity. In addition, passive protection has been demonstrated with monoclonal antibodies to the promastigote stage of *Leishmania mexicana* and to schistosomula of *S. mansoni.* Because of their specificity, monoclonal antibodies can also be used for diagnosis because they can be selected not to show the multiple cross-reactions with other parasites that are frequently found with sera from infected animals. For example, species-specific monoclonal antibodies have been developed which can distinguish between five different species of South American *Leishmania* without cross-reacting with *T. cruzi.* Antibodies in the serum of an infected patient will usually cross-react with all these parasites. Diagnostic tests using these antibodies have been developed.

An antibody to an antigen has a specific antigen unique to itself on the immunoglobulin. This antigen is called the *idiotype,* which is the unique amino acid sequence and configuration of the antigen-binding site of that antibody. For instance, it is possible to make an antibody to a particular monoclonal antibody; that antibody will then recognize the idiotype and is called an *anti-idiotypic antibody.* The monoclonal antibody will bind to the anti-idiotype or to the original antigen. If a monoclonal antibody to a parasite were used to induce an anti-idiotypic antibody, it should be possible to induce protective immunity with this anti-idiotype instead of using the antigen. This would have the advantage of bypassing the need to purify antigens and then to produce them in large quantities. This novel strategy for the production of a vaccine is under study. It has proved successful in producing immunity to schistosomiasis in rats.

The rapidly accelerating pace of discovery and definition of the regulatory systems of the immune response, together with the revolution in technology, may soon make it possible to induce stronger protective immunity artificially than that which is acquired naturally, and the prediction that vaccines can be produced against the diseases caused by a number of parasites is based on this assumption.

REFERENCES

DAVID JR: Host-parasite interface: Immune evasion, in *Tropical and Geographical Medicine,* 2d ed, KS Warren, AF Mahmoud (eds). New York, McGraw-Hill, 1990, p 117

DONELSON JE, TURNER MJ: How the trypanosome changes its coat. Sci Am 252(2):44, 1985

ENGLUND PT, SHER A (eds): *The Biology of Animal Parasitism.* New York, Plenum, 1986

HOMMELL M: Antigenic variation in malaria parasites. Immunol Today 6:28, 1985

MILLER LH et al: Research toward malaria vaccines. Science 234:1349, 1986

SILBERSTEIN DS, DAVID JR: The regulation of human eosinophil function by cytokines. Immunol Today 8:380, 1987

TRAGER W: *Living Together. The Biology of Animal Parasitism.* New York, Plenum, 1986

157 DIAGNOSIS OF PARASITIC INFECTIONS

JAMES J. PLORDE

SIGNIFICANCE OF PARASITIC INFECTIONS Parasitic diseases such as malaria, trypanosomiasis, leishmaniasis, schistosomiasis, and filariasis remain among the major causes of human sickness and death in the world. A number of technical, social, economic, and political phenomena have combined to produce a dramatic increase in the prevalence of some of these illnesses. This has been most devastating in the case of malaria. Growing resistance of the mosquito vector to insecticides, development of drug-resistant strains of *Plasmodium falciparum,* and cutbacks in many malaria control programs have led to a worldwide resurgence of this disease. At present, over 1 billion people reside in endemic areas; between 125 and 200 million of these are infected at any given time. In Africa, where the intensity of parasite transmission defies current control measures, malaria kills over 1 million children annually. The resurgence of malaria together with an increase in international travel has resulted in an upsurge in the number of infected patients who enter the United States. From 1969 to 1980 civilian malaria cases reported annually to the Centers for Disease Control have increased from 151 to 1864; in the seven subsequent years, the number has averaged 1000 cases annually. Over the same 18-year period, the number of infections involving U.S. citizens has climbed steadily from 90 to 421.

In Africa, from the Sahara in the north to the Kalahari Desert in the south, human strains of *Trypanosoma brucei* cause one of the most lethal of all human diseases, sleeping sickness. Animal strains of this species limit food supply in the same area through their impact on animal husbandry. In South America, a related organism, *T. cruzi,* infects several million people, leaving many with severe heart and gastrointestinal lesions (Chagas' disease).

Leishmaniasis is found in parts of Europe, Asia, Africa, and South and Central America where it may present as a chronic, highly lethal infection of the reticuloendothelial system (kala azar), a mutilating mucocutaneous infection (espundia), or a self limiting skin ulcer (oriental sore).

Schistosomiasis is the most serious of the helminthic infections, affecting an estimated 200 million individuals living between the tropics of Cancer and Capricorn. In many it produces bladder, intestinal, and/or liver disease which can eventually result in death. In many countries irrigation schemes have resulted in the dissemination of the disease to previously uninvolved areas, mitigating the economic gains of these projects. Although not transmitted in the continental United States, exogenously acquired schistosomiasis involves nearly a half million people now residing in this country.

Wuchereria bancrofti and *Brugia malayi,* two closely related filarial worms, obstruct lymphatic circulation and produce grotesque swellings of the legs, arms, and genitals in tropical populations. Onchocerciasis, another filarial infection, affects millions of people in Africa, leaving thousands blind.

Toxoplasmosis, pneumocystosis, giardiasis, cryptosporidiosis, and trichomoniasis are five cosmopolitan protozoan infections well known in the United States. The first infects perhaps one-third of the world's population. Although it is usually asymptomatic, congenital toxoplasmosis may result in abortion, stillbirth, prematurity, or severe neurologic defects. Even when there are no obvious signs at birth, chorioretinitis with visual impairment may occur years later. Mild or asymptomatic toxoplasma, pneumocystis, and cryptosporidia infections can result in fatal illness later in life during periods of immunosuppression.

In contrast, giardiasis and trichomoniasis seldom result in severe disability; nevertheless they cause morbidity in millions of otherwise healthy individuals. Both appear to be increasing in incidence, apparently the result of changing American lifestyles. Giardiasis is particularly frequent among day-care center attendees, hikers and campers in western states, and male homosexuals who practice anilingus, while the incidence of trichomoniasis is closely tied to the level of promiscuous heterosexual activity.

DIAGNOSIS Although some of the diseases mentioned above are uncommon in the United States, the continuous arrival of travelers and immigrants from endemic areas of the world makes it necessary to consider them in the differential diagnosis of many illnesses. Typically, neither the clinical manifestations nor the general laboratory findings observed in patients suffering from parasitic infections are sufficiently unique to raise this possibility in the mind of the clinician. Although eosinophilia has long been recognized as a clue to the presence of a hidden parasite, this phenomenon is characteristic only of helminthic infections. Even here its absence does not preclude this diagnosis. The eosinophilia reflects the terminal step in the host's immunologic response to worm antigens mounted during the stage of tissue migration and invasion. Once migration ceases and the worm matures to adulthood, eosinophilia may diminish or disappear.

PARASITE RECOVERY AND IDENTIFICATION Unless a careful travel, transfusion, and socioeconomic history is taken, the correct diagnosis may never be entertained. Once considered, however, the presence of a parasitic disease is easily confirmed. Most commonly, this is accomplished by the recovery and morphologic identification of the parasite in the stool, urine, sputum, blood, or tissues of the patient.

In intestinal infections, examination of a wet-mount and/or stained smear of the stool is usually adequate. Because many parasites are passed intermittently or in fluctuating numbers, the examination of a single stool specimen may detect only one-third to one-half of involved patients. The testing of three such specimens collected at intervals of 2 or 3 days will improve this yield substantially. Alternatively, a saline cathartic may be administered to evacuate the cecal area, where many protozoa are concentrated, and the entire purge examined. The stool must be free of interfering substances such as antidiarrheal or contrast agents, antacids, and antibiotics. If the appropriate specimens cannot be obtained prior to administration of such substances, testing should be performed 1 week or, in the case of antimicrobial agents, 3 weeks after their discontinuation. Occasionally, specimens other than stool must be examined. In small-bowel infections such as giardiasis and strongyloidiasis, the diagnosis, at times, can be established only by sampling the duodenal contents or by performing a jejunal biopsy. Similarly, eggs of *Enterobius* (pinworm) and *Taenia* (tapeworm) are frequently found on the perianal skin when absent from the feces. Recovery of large-bowel parasites such as *Entamoeba histolytica* and *Schistosoma mansoni* may require colonic intubation with aspiration or biopsy of suspect lesions. Whenever intestinal aspirates or soft to watery fecal specimens are collected, they should be immediately placed in a preservative such as polyvinyl alcohol (PVA) to prevent rapid disintegration of fragile protozoan trophozoites and allow the preparation of permanently stained smears. Protozoan cysts and helminthic ova found in formed stool will survive for 1 to 2 days at room temperature and indefinitely if placed in 5% formaldehyde.

Direct examination of the blood is useful for the detection of malaria parasites, leishmania, trypanosomes, and microfilaria. Preferably, fresh capillary blood should be used to prepare thin and thick blood smears and, when appropriate, wet mounts. Only specially prepared glass slides should be used, as traces of soda lime or potash on uncleaned slides may alter the pH of the stain, making recognition of parasites difficult. If an experienced technologist is not available to assist in the bedside preparation of smears, it is preferable to collect venous blood in an EDTA Vacutainer and send it to the laboratory. As in the case of intestinal parasites, organisms in the peripheral blood may fluctuate, requiring the collection of multiple specimens over a period of several days. Parasites dwelling within the tissues of the host are more difficult to identify. Some discharge their offspring into the sputum (lung flukes) where they can be found with appropriate concentration procedures. In others, larvae can be recovered with skin (*Onchocerca volvulus*) or muscle (*Trichinella spiralis*) biopsies.

Diagnostic procedures based on the recovery and morphologic identification of the parasite suffer from a number of limitations. The relative insensitivity of the techniques involved, the absence of diagnostic forms in excreta, blood, or tissue during the early stages of infection, and their irregular shedding thereafter often dictate the need for repetitive testing. In strongyloidiasis, for example, a dozen or more stool examinations may be required before rhabditiform larvae are eventually detected microscopically. Recovery of pathogens such as *Toxoplasma gondii* or *Taenia solium* from the central nervous system or other deep tissues may be difficult or even dangerous. The procedures themselves are labor intensive and require a level of technical expertise frequently unavailable to small clinical laboratories. Immunodiagnostic and nucleic acid hybridization techniques have begun to provide alternatives to these traditional methods.

Detection of circulating antibodies Although immunodiagnostic tests have long been available for a number of parasitic diseases, they have lacked the sensitivity and specificity of those developed for viral and bacterial agents. This has been particularly true for infections caused by helminths which are broadly cross-reactive with one another. Replacement of antigenically complex worm extracts and cryosections with highly purified stage- or fraction-specific antigens has improved the specificity of many of the tests for circulating antibodies. In malaria, as well as a few other diseases, synthesized, immunologically reactive peptides have been employed as test antigens. The use of such antigens in highly reactive test systems including enzyme-linked immunosorbent assays (ELISA), kinetic enzyme immunoassays (k-ELISA, FAST-ELISA), antibody capture ELISA, and immunoblot assays has provided a new generation of serologic tests with exquisite sensitivity and specificity. Currently, they are available through a limited number of reference laboratories. Table 157-1 lists the tests offered by the Centers for Disease Control (CDC). In Table 157-2, the diagnostic endpoint, sensitivity, and specificity of the most frequently requested CDC procedures are given.

Antigen detection Soluble antigens have been detected in the blood, body fluids, tissues, and excreta of a number of protozoan and helminthic diseases (Table 157-3). Early attempts at developing diagnostically useful antigen detection procedures focused on enteric protozoan infections, as microscopic examination of the stool for the causative agents is always tedious and frequently unsuccessful. Commercial immunofluorescent kits have been marketed for the detection of *Giardia* and *Crypotosporidium* in the stool and *Trichomonas vaginalis* in genitourinary secretions. Visually read enzyme immunoassays may soon be available for these and other enteric pathogens such as *Entamoeba histolytica*, circumventing the need for the highly trained technologists and expensive laboratory equipment that are required for immunofluorescent procedures. Although early studies indicate that the sensitivity and specificity of such tests is high, a number of technical problems remain to be addressed.

TABLE 157-1 Parasitic diseases for which serology is available

	Diagnostic usefulness	
Taxonomic group	High	Marginal
Protozoan	Amebiasis* Babesiosis* Chagas' disease* Leishmaniasis* Toxoplasmosis*	Malaria* Giardiasis Pneumocystosis
Helminthic	Cysticercosis* Echinococcosis* Paragonimiasis* Toxocariasis* Trichinosis*	Ascariasis Clonorchiasis Dracunculiasis Filariasis Schistosomiasis* Strongyloidiasis*

* Available at the Centers for Disease Control, Atlanta, Ga.

TABLE 157-2 Interpretation of tests frequently performed at the Centers for Disease Control

Disease	Test*	Diagnostic endpoint	Sensitivity†	Specificity†	Comments
Invasive amebiasis	IHA	≥1:256	70,[1] 95[2]	90[3]	*1* Intestinal infection. *2* Extraintestinal infection. *3* Titers may persist for years.
Cysticercosis	WBA[1]	+ or −	98[2]	100[2]	*1* 7 major bands. *2* Serum and CSF results identical.
Echinococcosis	IHA	≥1:256	60,[1] 88[2]	90–95[3,4]	*1* Lung or calcified cyst. *2* Liver or peritoneal. *3* Cross-reacts with cysticercosis. *4* Titer may persist for years.
	WBA[5]	+ or −	91[2]	100[6]	*5* 8-kDa antigen. *6* Cross-reacts with *E. multilocularis*.
Paragonimiasis	WBA[1]	+ or −	96	99	*1* 8-kDa protein, Chaffee antigen.
Schistosomiasis	FAST-ELISA[1]	≥10 U/μl	99,[2] 50[3]	99	*1* *S. mansoni* adult microsomal antigen. *2* *S. mansoni* infections. *3* *S. japonicum* infections.
	WBA[1]	+ or −	High	High	*1* Separate antigens for Sm, Sh, Sj.
Strongyloidiasis	ELISA	≥1:8	71[1]	80[2,3]	*1* *S. stercoralis* larval antigen. *2* No absolute reference standard *3* Cross-reacts with filariasis, ascariasis.
Toxocariasis					
Visceral	ELISA	≥1:32	78	92[1,2]	*1* Cross-reaction with ascariasis eliminated by preabsorption.
Ocular	ELISA	≥1:8	90	91[3]	*2* In children. *3* Patients with ocular disease.
Toxoplasmosis	IFA-IgG	≥1:16	High[1,2]	High[1,2]	*1* No absolute reference standard. *2* Antibodies may persist for years.
	Capture ELISA-IgM	≥1:4	High[1,3,4]	High[1,3]	*3* Antibodies may persist for months. *4* May be negative in immunocompromised patients.
Trichinosis	BFT	≥1:5	97[1]	90[2]	*1* Detected after third week of illness. *2* Titers may persist for years.

* IHA = Indirect hemagglutination; WBA = Western blot assay; ELISA = enzyme-linked immunosorbent assay; IFA = indirect fluorescent assay; BFT = bentonite flocculation.
† Superscript numbers refer to comments at right.
SOURCE: Division of Parasitic Diseases, CDC, 1989.

Rheumatoid factor and other copro-antibodies may produce false-positive results in some specimens. Antigens are rapidly destroyed by a variety of stool enzymes, restricting the use of these methods to fresh stool. Immunologic reagents may cross-react with one or more of the diverse complex of stool components. In solid-phase test systems, antibodies may desorb from plastic surfaces, affecting test sensitivity. There are a number of potential solutions to each of these problems, and it is expected that highly sensitive, specific, visually read immunoassays will be commercially available in the near future. A number of systems have been developed for the detection of malaria antigens in blood and *Toxoplasma gondii* antigens in tissue. Most of the malaria systems are less sensitive than the examination of a thick smear by a skilled technologist.

DNA probes Parasites, like other microorganisms, may be detected and identified in a clinical specimen by documenting the presence of genetic sequences unique to the parasite in question. The detection device is a DNA probe, a labeled nucleotide sequence complementary to a segment of parasitic genome unique to a particular strain, species, or genus. Addition of the probe to a positive specimen results in hybridization of the probe and parasite DNA with accompanying specimen labeling. The technology is highly specific, reproducible, inexpensive, and technically simple. Unlike immunodiagnostic tests, the effectiveness of DNA probes is not influenced by environmental or life-stage-dependent variations in antigenic expression. As the genome generally remains stable throughout the parasitic cycle, a single probe can often be used to identify any life stage of the pathogen.

TABLE 157-3 Diseases for which antigen detection procedures have been described

Protozoan diseases	Helminthic diseases
Amebiasis	Cysticercosis
Amebic meningoencephalitis	Echinococcosis
Chagas' disease	Lymphatic filariasis
Giardiasis	Onchocerciasis
Malaria	Schistosomiasis
Pneumocystosis	
Toxoplasmosis	
Trichomoniasis	

SOURCE: After Smith and Walls.

The effectiveness of DNA probes has been facilitated by the large number of short nucleotide sequences that are randomly repeated, often millions of times, throughout the parasitic genome. Those specific to the parasite sought can be cloned or synthesized. As probe sensitivity depends upon the copy number of the target sequences, highly repeated sequences are more likely to be detected in specimens containing small amounts of parasitic DNA. Methods of in vitro amplification of DNA sequences, as well as improvements in labeling techniques, will soon allow further increases in the sensitivity of individual probes.

DNA probes are available for the detection of *P. falciparum, Trypanosoma cruzi, T. brucei, Onchocerca* spp., and etiologic agents of lymphatic filariasis. Although used primarily by field epidemiologists for the detection of infected insect vectors, they are being increasingly applied to the detection of the parasites in vertebrate hosts. A diagnostic probe for *P. falciparum* has demonstrated a sensitivity that approaches that achieved by the traditional thick smear technique; filarial probes have been developed that can detect a single parasite in a DNA blot. The major limitations of DNA probes as diagnostic tools relate to technical aspects of the hybridization procedure itself, but these should be overcome in the near future.

REFERENCES

GAM AA et al: Comparative sensitivity and specificity of ELISA and IHA for serodiagnosis of strongyloidiasis with larval antigens. Am J Trop Med Hyg 37:157, 1987

HANCOCK K, TSANG VCW: Development and optimization of the FAST-ELISA for detecting antibodies to *Schistosoma mansoni*. J Immunol Methods 92:167, 1986

HERBRINK P et al: Interlaboratory evaluation of indirect enzyme-linked immunosorbent assay, antibody capture enzyme-linked immunosorbent assay, and immunoblotting for detection of immunoglobulin M antibodies to *Toxoplasma gondii*. J Clin Microbiol 25:100, 1987

MADDISON SE: Parasitic infections, in *Microbial Antigenodiagnosis*, Boca Raton, CRC Press, 2:110, 1987, vol 2

——— et al: A specific diagnostic antigen of *Echinococcus granulosus* with an apparent molecular weight of 8 kDa. Am J Trop Med Hyg 40:377, 1989

POST RJ, CRAMPTON JM: Probing the unknown. Parasitology Today 3:380, 1987

SLEMENDA SM et al: Diagnosis of paragonimiasis by immunoblot. Am J Trop Med Hyg 39:469, 1988

SMITH JW, WALLS KW: Rapid immunologic diagnosis of parasitic infections. Clin Microbiol Newsletter 10:89, 1988

TSANG VCW et al: An enzyme-linked immunoelectrotransfer blot assay and glycoprotein antigens for diagnosing human cysticercosis *(Taenia solium)*. J Infect Dis 159:50, 1989

158 AMEBIASIS

JAMES J. PLORDE

DEFINITION Amebiasis is an infection of the large intestine produced by *Entamoeba histolytica*. It is an asymptomatic carrier state in most individuals, but diseases ranging from chronic, mild diarrhea to fulminant dysentery may occur. Among extraintestinal complications, the most common is hepatic abscess, which may rupture into peritoneum, pleura, lung, or pericardium.

ETIOLOGY There are seven species of ameba that naturally parasitize the human mouth and intestine, but of these only *E. histolytica* causes disease. *Entamoeba coli* and *E. hartmanni* are the two species with which it is most likely to be confused in examination of stools.

E. histolytica exists in two forms: the motile trophozoite and the cyst. The trophozoite is the parasitic form and dwells in the lumen and/or wall of the colon, divides by binary fission, grows best under anaerobic conditions, and requires the presence of either bacteria or tissue substrates to satisfy its nutritional requirements. When diarrhea occurs, the trophozoites are passed unchanged in the liquid stool, where they can be distinguished by their size (10 to 20 μm in diameter), directional motility, sharply demarcated clear ectoplasm with slender finger-like pseudopodia, and finely granular endoplasm. In dysentery, the trophozoites are larger (up to 50 μm in diameter), and often contain ingested erythrocytes. In the absence of diarrhea, the trophozoites usually encyst before leaving the gut. The cysts have a chitinous wall which renders them highly resistant to environmental changes, chlorine concentrations found in water purification systems, and gastric acid. With rare exception they are responsible for transmission of disease. Young cysts have a single nucleus, a glycogen vacuole, and sausage-shaped collections of ribosomes known as chromatoid bodies. As the cyst matures, it absorbs its cytoplasmic inclusions and becomes quadrinucleate. The cysts of *E. histolytica* can be distinguished from those of *E. hartmanni* by their larger diameter (10 μm) and from those of *Entamoeba coli* by the presence of one to four nuclei with small centric karyosomes and fine peripheral chromatin and by their thick chromatoid bodies with round ends.

The electrophoretic mobility patterns of four enzymes found in trophozoites have been used to define 22 *E. histolytica* zymodemes. Amebas recovered from patients with invasive disease belong to just 9; all are characterized by the presence of advanced, paired hexokinase bands and/or a beta phosphoglucomutase without an accompanying alpha-phosphoglucomutase band. Although conversion between pathogenic and nonpathogenic zymodemes has been reported in cloned cultures, the zymodemes appear to be clinically stable markers of virulence.

Entamoeba histolytica can be cultivated in artificial media, a procedure that is essential for the determination of isoenzyme patterns and preparation of the purified antigens used in serologic testing. Its diagnostic value remains uncertain.

EPIDEMIOLOGY Although *E. histolytica* can sometimes infect animals, humans are the principal hosts and reservoir. Because trophozoites die rapidly after leaving the intestine, the asymptomatic cyst passer is the source of new infections; a chronic carrier may excrete several million organisms daily. The infective dose usually exceeds 10^3, but infection has followed the ingestion of a single cyst. These structures are transmitted by the fecal-oral route, usually through direct person-to-person contact. Poverty, ignorance, mental retardation, and other factors which impair personal hygiene facilitate the spread of the parasite. Oral-anal sexual contact produces high infection rates in male homosexuals. Food- and waterborne transmission occur in areas of the world with poor sanitation, including certain southern rural communities, Indian reservations, and migrant farm camps in the United States. Occasionally this results in common source outbreaks; these epidemics, however, are never as explosive as those produced by pathogenic intestinal bacteria. Symptomatic amebiasis is unusual below the age of 10 years in temperate climates, and both intestinal and hepatic lesions predominate in adult males to an extent that is not readily explainable on the basis of different rates of exposure to infection.

It has been estimated that 50 percent of inhabitants of some less well-developed nations, 10 percent of the world's population as a whole, and 1 percent of Americans are infected with *E. histolytica*. Invasive amebiasis, which produces an estimated 40 million disabling infections and 40,000 deaths annually, is concentrated in comparatively few parts of the world, most notably Mexico, western South America, south Asia, and west and southeastern Africa. This is presumably related to the concurrent presence in these geographic areas of virulent strains of *E. histolytica,* the hygienic and sanitary conditions necessary for their transmission, and, perhaps, malnutrition and immunodeficiency. Even in areas endemic for invasive disease, however, only 10 percent of infected patients harbor virulent zymodemes of *E. histolytica*. A minority of these experience clinical disease. In the United States the incidence of invasive amebiasis dropped sharply in the four decades preceding the 1970s. Between 1971 and 1974, an average of 3500 cases were reported annually to the Centers for Disease Control; since then the numbers have steadily increased. Isoenzyme studies of *E. histolytica* strains isolated from male homosexuals and inmates of mental hospitals in Great Britain indicate the overwhelming majority belong to nonpathogenic zymodemes, suggesting that virulent strains are now uncommon in developed countries. Although patients with dysentery and liver abscess can still be found in the impoverished segments of the American population, the bulk of the invasive disease diagnosed in the United States is now acquired outside the United States.

IMMUNITY Repeated intestinal infections are common. However, there are data suggesting the presence of protective immunity, particularly following invasive liver disease. There is no correlation between the presence of circulating antibodies and resistance to reinfection. It is likely that immunity is incomplete, develops only after recovery from invasive disease, and is cell-mediated.

PATHOGENESIS AND PATHOLOGY After ingestion, cysts undergo further nuclear division. In the small intestine, the cyst wall disintegrates, and trophozoites are released. The immature amebas are carried to the large intestine, where they live in the lumen of the gut feeding on bacteria and debris. Organisms belonging to nonpathogenic zymodemes are seldom responsible for sustained tissue invasion and destruction. In contrast, the almost universal presence of specific humoral antibodies in carriers of pathogenic zymodemes suggests that tissue invasion by these strains is the rule. Only in the minority, however, is this sufficiently extensive to produce symptoms. The factors modulating invasion are not completely understood, but the state of the host and the virulence of the infecting organism both play roles. High carbohydrate intake, corticosteroids, protein malnutrition, pregnancy, HIV infection, and other immunosuppressed states render the host more susceptible. High-molecular-weight glycoproteins present in colonic mucus bind avidly to an adhesion molecule on the surface of *E. histolytica* trophozoites, blocking their attachment to host cells. Changes in the composition or production of mucus may, therefore, alter the host's susceptibility to amebic invasion. Trophozoite virulence is enhanced by rapid animal passage; presumably, a similar phenomenon occurs in epidemiologic settings conducive to rapid spread of the protozoan from human to human. Direct association with certain strains of bacteria may also enhance the virulence of pathogenic strains, possibly by protecting the ameba from oxidant stress or through the exchange of genetic material.

The precise pathogenic mechanisms responsible for tissue invasion are not fully understood. The invasiveness of a strain correlates well with its phagocytic prowess, production of collagenase and an immunogenic cytotoxic protein, resistance to the host's inflammatory response, and, perhaps most importantly, its capacity to induce histolysis following direct cell-to-cell contact with host tissue. The latter phenomenon is initiated by a lectin-mediated adherence of the trophozoite to a target cell. Amebapore, a pore-forming protein, is released and polymerizes in the target cell membrane, forming large membrane holes. Cytolysis, which appears to require both intact microfilament function and amebic phospholipase A enzymes, rapidly follows. The lysis of neutrophils, which are attracted to, and killed by, *E. histolytica* trophozoites, may amplify tissue damage.

Amebic ulceration of the intestinal wall is characteristic. A small mucosal defect overlies a larger, burrowing area of necrosis in the submucosa and muscularis, producing a bottle-shaped lesion. There is little acute inflammatory response, and in contrast to the picture in bacillary dysentery, the mucosa between ulcers is normal. The sites of involvement in order of frequency are cecum and ascending colon, rectum, sigmoid, appendix, and terminal ileum. Involvement of the colonic musculature may lead to the formation of large masses of granulation tissue or *amebomas*. Amebas can enter the portal circulation and lodge in venules; liquefaction necrosis of liver tissue leads to the formation of an abscess cavity. Rarely, embolization results in lung, brain, or splenic abscess.

A soluble protein product of invasive strains of *E. histolytica* has been shown to induce HIV replication in infected lymphocytes. Conceivably, individuals infected with both pathogens might experience the accelerated development of AIDS (see Chap. 264).

CLINICAL MANIFESTATIONS **Asymptomatic cyst passer** In the majority of patients with this common form of amebiasis, *E. histolytica* probably lives as a commensal in the bowel lumen. Individuals infected in temperate climates are unlikely to harbor virulent strains. However, as invasion can occasionally occur, treatment of all cyst passers is warranted.

Symptomatic intestinal amebiasis In some patients there is intermittent diarrhea consisting of one to four foul-smelling loose or watery stools daily. The stools sometimes contain mucus and blood. Loose stools alternate with periods of relative normality and may persist for months or years. Flatulence and abnormal cramping are frequent. The only physical findings are occasional tender hepatomegaly and slight pain when the cecum and ascending colon are palpated. Sigmoidoscopy sometimes reveals typical ulcerations with areas of normal mucosa interspersed. The diagnosis depends upon finding the organism in the feces or in ulcers.

Fulminating attacks of amebic dysentery are less common. Waterborne outbreaks may occur, but fulminating dysentery is more likely to occur spontaneously in debilitated or immunocompromised individuals. Attacks may be precipitated by pregnancy or corticosteroids. The onset in half the cases is abrupt with high fever, between 40 and 40.6°C (104 and 105°F), severe abdominal cramps, and profuse, bloody diarrhea with tenesmus. There is diffuse abdominal tenderness, often so severe that peritonitis is suspected. Hepatomegaly is very frequent, and sigmoidoscopy almost always demonstrates extensive rectosigmoid ulceration. Trophozoites are numerous in stools and in material obtained directly from the ulcers.

In some cases there may be extensive destruction of the colonic mucosa and submucosa, massive hemorrhage or perforation of the bowel wall, with resultant peritonitis. Repeated severe attacks of intestinal amebiasis can lead to an ulcerative postdysenteric colitis. Penetration of trophozoites through the muscle wall of the bowel may result in the development of large masses of granulation tissue. When the entire circumference of the intestine is involved, there may then be partial obstruction, and a movable, tender, sausage-shaped mass is often palpable. This lesion, or ameboma, is most frequently seen in the cecum, where a palpable mass and radiologic demonstration of a ragged encroachment of the lumen may lead to a mistaken diagnosis of adenocarcinoma.

Hepatic amebiasis The term *amebic hepatitis* is used for a syndrome of tender hepatomegaly, right upper quadrant pain, fever, and leukocytosis in patients with amebic colitis. Hepatic biopsy reveals nonspecific periportal inflammation. The absence of ameba within the areas of inflammation, the rarity with which the syndrome is followed by an amebic liver abscess, and the resolution of the liver signs following treatment of the intestinal disease with luminal amebicides indicate that these manifestations are not secondary to spread of trophozoites from the intestine, but are rather a nonspecific accompaniment of amebic colitis.

Hepatic abscess may develop insidiously, with fever, sweats, weight loss, and no local signs other than painless or slightly tender hepatomegaly. In immunologically naive patients, there is more often an abrupt onset, with chills, fever to 40.6°C (105°F), nausea, vomiting, severe upper abdominal pain, and polymorphonuclear leukocytosis. Initially, cholecystitis, perforated ulcer, or acute pancreatitis may be suspected. Over 80 percent of patients with an insidious onset and half of those presenting with acute manifestations have a single abscess. Most commonly, this is localized in the posterior portion of the right lobe of the liver, because this lobe receives most of the blood draining the right colon through the "streaming" effect in portal vein flow. This location is responsible for several features that aid in diagnosis. *Point tenderness* in the posterolateral portion of a lower right intercostal space is frequent even in the absence of diffuse liver pain. Most abscesses enlarge upward, producing a bulge in the diaphragmatic dome, obliteration of the costophrenic gutter, small hydrothorax, basilar atelectasis, and pain referred to the right shoulder.

Liver function tests may be mildly to moderately disturbed and provide little diagnostic aid; the level of the serum glutamic oxaloacetic transaminase (SGOT), however, is of clinical value as it directly reflects the severity of disease. Jaundice is uncommon, and when present implies a grave prognosis. Radiologically, unruptured abscesses do not show a fluid level, and calcification of the liver parenchyma is very rare. Isotope liver scan utilizing two, or preferably three, projections is invaluable in confirming the presence and location of a liver abscess. It becomes positive within the first days of illness, often prior to other imaging techniques. Presumably these early changes reflect either a focal decrease in blood supply or injury to the Kupffer cells rather than liquefaction necrosis. Ultrasonic scanning and computed tomography, although becoming positive slightly later in the course of the disease, are ultimately as sensitive as isotopic scanning and provide confirmation of the cystic nature of the lesion. The defect seen on imaging commonly persists for several months after the complete recovery of the patient. Serologic tests are positive in over 90 percent of cases.

Needle puncture results in the withdrawal of "pus" which consists of liquefied, necrotic liver. Typically, it is thick and odorless, resembling "chocolate syrup" or "anchovy paste." It may, however, be thin in consistency and yellow or green in color. The pus contains no polymorphonuclear leukocytes (barring secondary bacterial infection) and, usually, no amebas. The parasites are localized in the cyst wall and may be demonstrated in the terminal portion of the aspirate or, at times, by a Vim-Silverman needle biopsy of the cyst wall following aspiration of the abscess.

Hepatic abscess complicates asymptomatic infection of the colon more often than symptomatic intestinal disease, another factor making recognition difficult. Trophozoites or cysts are demonstrable in the feces of only about one-third of patients with abscess, and fewer than one-half can recall significant diarrheal illness.

Pleuropulmonary amebiasis The right pleural cavity and lung are involved by direct extension from the liver in 10 to 20 percent of patients with liver abscess. Rarely, amebic lung abscess has resulted from embolization rather than direct extension. Manifestations are those of a consolidating pneumonia or lung abscess. If perforation into a bronchus occurs, patients expectorate large amounts of the typical exudate, some patients even commenting that the sputum "tastes like liver." Cough, pleural pain, fever, and leukocytosis are the rule, and secondary bacterial infection is frequent. Rupture into the free pleural space results in a massive pleural effusion; aspiration of "chocolate" fluid is diagnostic.

Other extraintestinal lesions Extension of an abscess from the left lobe of the liver to the pericardium is the most dangerous complication of hepatic abscess. It may be mistaken for tuberculous pericarditis or congestive cardiomyopathy. Less frequently, rapid cardiac tamponade occurs with ensuing dyspnea, shock, and death. *Peritonitis* is a result of perforation of colonic ulcer or rupture of liver abscess. Painful ulcers or condylomata of the genitalia, perianal skin, or abdominal wall (draining sinuses) are unusual complications which may be mistaken for syphilitic, tuberculous, or neoplastic lesions. They usually result from direct extension of intestinal disease; some are thought to result from sexual transmission. Metastatic brain abscess is rare, and an etiologic diagnosis is seldom made clinically. Splenic abscess has been reported but is very unusual.

DIFFERENTIAL DIAGNOSIS Intestinal amebiasis Patients with nondysenteric amebiasis are often misdiagnosed as having irritable bowel syndrome, diverticulitis, or regional enteritis. Ameboma may mimic colonic carcinoma or granulomatous disease, while the clinical spectrum of amebic dysentery overlaps those of shigellosis, salmonellosis, ulcerative colitis, and, in endemic areas, schistosomiasis. The invasive bacterial infections are usually more acute, severe, and self-limited than amebiasis. Stools from patients with shigellosis, salmonellosis, and ulcerative colitis contain large numbers of polymorphonuclear leukocytes, while those in amebic infection do not. Nevertheless, amebiasis may closely resemble any of the above diseases both clinically and radiologically and must be considered in the differential diagnosis of any chronic diarrhea or dysentery.

The identification of *E. histolytica* in the stool, however, does not eliminate other diagnostic possibilities. Amebic infection is often superimposed on or exacerbated by other colonic disease including schistosomiasis and cecal carcinoma. For this reason, patients with intestinal amebiasis and abdominal complaints still require stool culture, sigmoidoscopy, and a barium enema.

Hepatic abscess Once a filling defect has been demonstrated by isotope liver scanning, the differential diagnosis includes hepatic neoplasm, hydatid cyst, and pyogenic abscess. Neoplasms can usually be differentiated on the basis of their ultrasonic scanning characteristics, while the lack of constitutional manifestations and presence of an appropriate epidemiologic history is helpful in recognizing echinococcosis. The most difficult problem lies in the exclusion of a pyogenic abscess. An insidious onset in an adult male, a history of chronic diarrhea, significant pleuritic chest pain, and a single right lobe lesion favors the diagnosis of amebiasis. High fever, hyperbilirubinemia, multiple hepatic filling defects, and foul-smelling hepatic aspirate are more suggestive of pyogenic disease. Ultimately, the separation of the two diseases rests upon laboratory procedures.

LABORATORY DIAGNOSIS The diagnosis of intestinal amebiasis depends upon *identification of the organism in the stool or tissues*. Formed stools are microscopically examined initially in saline and iodine mounts for amebic cysts; concentration methods such as the formalin-ether technique increase the yield two- to threefold. Liquid or semiformed stools should be examined immediately in saline solution for the presence of motile hematophagous trophozoites. The addition of a supravital stain such as buffered methylene blue to the saline enhances nuclear detail and minimizes the possibility of confusing fecal leukocytes with amebic trophozoites. If there is any delay in examination of the stool, a portion of the specimen may be refrigerated for a few hours at 4°C, or placed in polyvinyl alcohol and 10% formalin. Definitive identification of *E. histolytica* requires the examination of permanently stained slides prepared from the material preserved with polyvinyl alcohol. An ocular micrometer is necessary to separate *E. hartmanni* from its larger relative. Four to six stool specimens may be required for diagnosis. If possible, the stool should be examined before the administration of antimicrobial, antidiarrheal, or antacid preparations because all these agents may interfere with the recovery of amebas. Likewise, enemas and radiographic procedures utilizing barium sulfate are best postponed until after a thorough search for *E. histolytica* has been made. A number of nonmicroscopic techniques have been developed for the rapid detection of *E. histolytica* in the stool. They include enzyme-linked immunosorbent and immunofluorescent assays for trophozoite and/or cyst antigens and DNA hybridization probes to tandemly repeated parasite nucleotide sequences. If commercially developed, they could provide a useful alternative to microscopic examination.

Sigmoidoscopy is of value in symptomatic cases. The mucosal lesions should be aspirated and the material examined for trophozoites as described above. Biopsy material obtained from such lesions and stained with periodic acid Schiff solution also will frequently reveal trophozoites.

The diagnosis of extraintestinal amebiasis is difficult. The parasite usually cannot be recovered from stool or tissue. Cultivation of amebas from feces or pus is possible but is not practical in most laboratories. *Serologic tests* employing purified antigens are positive in nearly all patients with proven amebic liver abscess and in a great majority of those with acute amebic dysentery. The persistence of significant antibody titers for months to years after complete cure makes serology, particularly in endemic areas, of more value in excluding the diagnosis than in confirming it. Of the available tests, the indirect hemagglutination and enzyme-linked immunosorbent assays appear to be the most sensitive; average time to positivity is 3 and 2 weeks, respectively. Indirect immunofluorescence, countercurrent electrophoresis, and agar gel diffusion are also highly reliable. A number of these testing procedures are now available as commercial kits, making serologic testing feasible for most laboratories.

TREATMENT Treatment should be aimed at relief of symptoms, replacement of fluid, electrolyte, and blood losses, and eradication of the organism. Amebas may be found in the lumen of the bowel, in the intestinal wall, or extraintestinally. Most amebicides are not effective at all sites or when used alone, and a combination of drugs is often necessary to achieve cure. The available drugs based on their site of action fall into two categories.

Luminal amebicides These oral agents act by direct contact with trophozoites dwelling in the bowel lumen but are ineffective against amebas in tissue. Of the large number of available drugs, diloxanide furoate is one of the most effective and well tolerated but is presently available in the United States only through the Centers for Disease Control. A response rate of 80 to 85 percent has been noted; flatulence appears to be the only major side effect.

Iodoquinol has been effective in 60 to 70 percent of cases. As with its analogue iodochlorhydroxyquin, myelooptic neuropathy has been reported after long-term use. However, no such case has been noted when the dosage was limited to that given in Table 158-1. The drug should not be used in patients with thyroid disease or preexisting optic neuropathy.

Tissue amebicides *Chloroquine phosphate* is a systemic amebicide which is useful in hepatic disease because of its high concentration in the liver. It has little activity elsewhere.

Emetine is an alkaloid derivative of ipecac. When given intramuscularly, it is highly effective in destroying trophozoites in tissue including those in the wall of the intestine. It is ineffective against luminal amebas. Emetine is relatively toxic and may produce vomiting, diarrhea, abdominal cramping, weakness, muscle pain, tachycardia, hypotension, precordial pain, and electrocardiographic abnormalities. The common ECG changes include T-wave inversion and prolongation

TABLE 158-1 Drug therapy of amebiasis

	Dosage
ASYMPTOMATIC INTESTINAL CARRIER	
Iodoquinol*	650 mg tid for 20 days
or diloxanide furoate†	500 mg tid for 10 days
MILD TO MODERATE INTESTINAL DISEASE	
Metronidazole	750 mg tid for 5–10 days
plus iodoquinol	As above
or diloxanide furoate	As above
or tetracycline	500 mg qid for 5 days
SEVERE INTESTINAL DISEASE	
Above regimen	
plus dehydroemetine†	1.0–1.5 mg/kg IM per day (maximum 90 mg/d) up to 5 d
or emetine	1 mg/kg IM per day (maximum 60 mg/d) for up to 5 days
EXTRAINTESTINAL DISEASE	
Metronidazole	As above
plus iodoquinol	
or chloroquine phosphate	1 g/d for 2 days, then 500 mg/d for 4 weeks
plus dehydroemetine†	As above for 10 days
or emetine	As above for 10 days

* Glenwood Laboratories, Inc, 83 North Summit St, Tenafly, NJ 07670.
† Investigational drug available through the Parasitic Drug Service, Centers for Disease Control, Atlanta, Ga, (404) 639-3670, nights and weekends 639-2888.

of the QTc interval. Rarely arrhythmias and prolongation of the QRS complex are seen. A synthetic derivative, dehydroemetine, is thought to be less toxic by virtue of its more rapid excretion and lower concentration in myocardial tissue. It is not free of toxicity, however, and patients treated with either drug should be at bed rest with ECG monitoring. Neither drug should be used in patients with renal, cardiac, or muscle disease, during pregnancy, or in children, unless other drugs fail.

Metronidazole is unique because it is effective against trophozoites at all sites, intestinally and extraintestinally. For intestinal amebiasis it is given in dosage of 750 mg three times daily for 5 to 10 days. Smaller doses are effective in hepatic amebiasis. Metronidazole has an Antabuse-like action, and alcohol should be avoided during its administration. The evidence that this drug is carcinogenic and possibly teratogenic in animals when given in large doses is disturbing but lacks confirmation in humans. Metronidazole should not be given in the first trimester of pregnancy.

Specific antiprotozoal therapy is outlined in Table 158-1.

In extraintestinal amebiasis including hepatic abscess, metronidazole is the drug of choice. In cases of relapse, impending rupture of an abscess, or in situations where the patient is unable to take oral medication, therapy with dehydroemetine or emetine should be instituted, and oral chloroquine added as soon as possible. Most authors prefer to add luminal amebicides to both the metronidazole and chloroquine-emetine programs. Treatment failures have been reported for both emetine-chloroquine and metronidazole. They appear to be unrelated to the organism's resistance.

There is debate over the value of routine aspiration of amebic liver abscesses. Certainly, if there is localized swelling over the liver, marked elevation of the diaphragm, severe localized liver tenderness, and failure to respond to systemic amebicides within 72 h, it should be done. Adequate drainage can usually be accomplished by needle alone, and surgical drainage is rarely necessary. The greatest hazard in needling an abscess is secondary bacterial infection.

PROGNOSIS Intestinal amebiasis usually responds readily and completely to appropriate drugs. Parasitologic relapses sometimes occur, and posttreatment stools should be checked monthly for 6 months. Repeated relapses, however, are usually a manifestation of reinfection, complicating illness, inadequate therapy, or incorrect diagnosis. The fatality rate is less than 5 percent.

Hepatic and pulmonary amebiasis are still accompanied by an appreciable mortality, but no reliable figures are available.

PREVENTION For the individual, avoidance of contaminated food and water, scalding of vegetables, and the use of iodine-releasing tablets in drinking water (chlorine, in the form of halazone, is ineffective) are important measures. Globaline tablets, containing tetraglycine hydroperiodide, are convenient and effective.

Improvements in general sanitation and the detection of cyst passers and their removal from food-handling duties are general measures in prophylaxis, but such segregation of carriers is rarely practiced. Community control of amebic disease by periodic mass treatment with metronidazole and diloxanide furoate has been successful in some areas. Personal chemoprophylaxis for travelers is not recommended.

PRIMARY AMEBIC MENINGOENCEPHALITIS AND KERATITIS

Primary amebic meningoencephalitis is caused by free-living amebas of the genus *Naegleria* or *Acanthamoeba*. The former most often affects children and young adults, appears to be acquired by swimming in fresh, warm water, and is almost invariably fatal. *Acanthamoeba* infections involve older immunocompromised individuals, and spontaneous recovery is sometimes seen.

Free-living amebas are ubiquitous in nature where they are commonly found in soil and water. Although generally considered harmless, some varieties are clearly pathogenic for the central nervous system of mammals. In those instances of human meningoencephalitis where the responsible organism has been isolated and cultured, it is usually an amoeboflagellate, *Naegleria fowleri*.

Over 140 *Naegleria* cases have been reported from different parts of the world. Serologic studies suggest that inapparent infections are much more common. Most of the 50 cases recognized in the United States have occurred in the southeastern states, particularly Florida, Georgia, and Virginia. Characteristically the patients have fallen ill during the summer months approximately 1 week after swimming in fresh or brackish water. The 16 Czechoslovakian cases followed swimming in an indoor pool with chlorinated water maintained at 24°C, and 6 cases have been acquired apparently after bathing in hot mineral water. In sub-Saharan Africa, cases appear to follow inhalation of airborne cysts during the dry, windy harmattan season. Histologic evidence suggests that the amebas reach the central nervous system directly via the nasal mucosa at the level of the cribriform plate. Clinically, the illness is rapid in onset, brief in duration, and inexorable in course. The initial symptom is a severe, persistent, frontal headache followed by nausea, vomiting, fever, and nuchal rigidity. Unusual tastes or smells may be noted. Later, drowsiness, confusion, convulsions, and coma appear. Focal neurologic findings may occur late in the course of the illness.

A more benign, chronic form of meningoencephalitis is produced by organisms of the genus *Acanthamoeba*. They appear to be disseminated to the brain and skin from the nasal sinuses or lungs. Clinical manifestations include cognitive abnormalities, focal neurologic findings, and coma. Patients with this clinical syndrome are frequently older, are immunocompromised, lack a history of freshwater swimming, and may recover spontaneously. Pathologically, the disease can be distinguished from *Naegleria* infections by the granulomatous nature of the inflammatory reaction and the presence of both trophozoites and cysts in the tissues. Unfortunately, the responsible organisms have seldom been recovered by culture and identified. It is possible that the free-living amebas of several species are involved. An increasing number of patients with *Acanthamoeba* keratitis have been reported. Infection usually follows eye trauma or prolonged use of soft contact lenses. The chronic progressive ulcerative disease can be distinguished from herpes simplex keratitis by a paracentral ring infiltrate, recurrent epithelial breakdown, severe pain, Progressive corneal damage usually results in blindness and/or corneal prolapse.

A careful examination of the cerebrospinal fluid is the single most helpful diagnostic procedure in patients with clinical evidence of meningitis. In *Naegleria* infections the fluid is usually bloody or sanguinopurulent and demonstrates an intense neutrophilic response. The protein is elevated and the glucose diminished. No organisms are demonstrated on Gram's stain or routine culture. Early examination of a wet preparation of unspun spinal fluid will usually reveal viable trophozoites. They are 10 to 20 μm in diameter, possess a granular cytoplasm, a distinct ectoplasm, and bulbous pseudopodia. If the specimen is allowed to cool, the trophozoites may become immobile and more difficult to recognize. The diagnosis is confirmed with direct fluorescent antibody (DFA) stains. Although the amebas may be easily grown on ordinary culture media which have been seeded with coliform bacteria, this is not helpful in clinical management, so rapidly progressive is the disease. In contrast, the spinal fluid in *Acanthamoeba* infections usually demonstrates a mononuclear response. Trophozoites have seldom been cultured or seen on wet mounts. A positive DFA stain has been seen in a few cases. Brain biopsy is diagnostic in approximately 75 percent of cases. *Acanthamoeba* keratitis is confirmed by demonstrating the typical double wrinkled wall cyst in corneal scrapings or biopsies. Culture, when available, is usually successful. Treatment with standard antiprotozoal agents seems completely ineffective. *Naegleria,* however, is highly sensitive to amphotericin B, miconazole, tetracycline, and rifampin. To date only four patients have survived a *Naegleria* infection. All were diagnosed early and treated, three with amphotericin B and the other with amphotericin B, miconazole, and rifampin. Intracisternal, as well as intravenous, administration of amphotericin is probably essential to rapidly obtain effective levels in the cerebrospinal fluid. The intraventricular dose is 0.5 to 1 mg for the first few days. The intravenous dose is similar to that for cryptococcal meningitis (see Chap. 87). *Acanthamoeba* are sensitive to sulfonamides, clotrimazole, 5-FC, and polymyxin B, in vitro but not clinically. Keratitis has responded to topical miconazole, propamidine isethionate (Brolene), and antibiotics followed by keratoplasty.

If the source of the infection can be determined, further *Naegleria* cases might be prevented by closing the area to bathing.

REFERENCES

Amebiasis

Adams EB, Macleod IN: Invasive amebiasis. Medicine 56:315, 1977

Denis M, Chadee K: Immunopathology of *Entamoeba histolytica* infections. Parasitology Today 4:247, 1988

Katzenstein D et al: New concepts of amebic liver abscess derived from hepatic imaging, serodiagnosis, and hepatic enzymes in 67 consecutive cases in San Diego. Medicine 61:237, 1982

Knobloch J, Mannweiler E: Development and persistence of antibodies to *Entamoeba histolytica* in patients with amebic liver abscess: Analysis of 216 cases. Am J Trop Med Hyg 32:727, 1983

Martinez-Palomo A: The pathogenesis of amoebiasis. Parasitology Today 3:111, 1987

Proctor EM et al: The electrophoretic isoenzyme patterns of strains of *Entamoeba histolytica* isolated in two major cities in Canada. Am J Trop Med Hyg 37:296, 1987

Ravdin JI: Pathogenesis of disease caused by *Entamoeba histolytica:* Studies of adherence, secreted toxins, and contact-dependent cytolysis. Rev Infect Dis 8:247, 1986

Salata RA, Ravdin JI: Review of the human immune mechanisms directed against *Entamoeba histolytica.* Rev Infect Dis 8:261, 1986

Thompson JE et al: Amebic liver abscess: A therapeutic approach. Rev Infect Dis 7:171, 1985

Walsh J: Problems in recognition and diagnosis of amebiasis: Estimation of the global magnitude of morbidity and mortality. Rev Infect Dis 8:228, 1986

Primary amebic meningoencephalitis

Auran JD et al: *Acanthamoeba* keratitis. A review of the literature. Cornea 6:2, 1987

Seidel JS et al: Successful treatment of primary amebic meningoencephalitis. N Engl J Med 306:346, 1982

Stehr-Green JK et al: *Acanthamoeba* keratitis in soft contact lens wearers. JAMA 258:57, 1987

Wiley CA et al: *Acanthamoeba* meningoencephalitis in a patient with AIDS. J Infect Dis 155:130, 1987

159 MALARIA

NICHOLAS J. WHITE / JAMES J. PLORDE

INTRODUCTION Malaria is a protozoan disease transmitted by the bite of *Anopheles* mosquitoes. It is the most important of the parasitic diseases of human beings, affecting approximately 200 million people and causing over 1 million deaths each year. Malaria has now been eradicated from North America, Europe, and Russia, but despite enormous control efforts, there has been a resurgence of the disease in many parts of the tropics. Added to this are the increasing problems of drug resistance. Malaria remains today, as it has for centuries, a major burden on tropical communities and a danger to travelers.

ETIOLOGY Four species of the genus *Plasmodium* infect humans (although occasional infections with primate malarias may occur). These are *P. vivax, P. ovale, P. malariae,* and *P. falciparum* (Table 159-1). Almost all deaths are caused by falciparum malaria. Human infection begins when a female anopheline mosquito inoculates plasmodial sporozoites from its salivary gland during a blood meal. These small motile forms are carried rapidly via the bloodstream to the liver where they target hepatic parenchymal cells, invade, and begin a period of asexual reproduction. By this process (known as intrahepatic or preerythrocytic schizogony), a single sporozoite eventually produces several thousand daughter merozoites. The swollen liver cell eventually bursts, discharging merozoites into the bloodstream, beginning the symptomatic blood stage of the infection. In *P. vivax* and *P. ovale* infections a proportion of the intrahepatic forms do not divide immediately, but remain dormant for months before reproduction begins. These sleeping forms, or hypnozoites, are the cause of the relapses that characterize infection with these two species.

After entry into the bloodstream merozoites rapidly invade erythrocytes. Attachment is mediated via a specific erythrocyte surface receptor. In *P. vivax* this is related to the Duffy blood group antigen Fy^a or Fy^b. Most west Africans, or people with origins in that region, carry the Duffy-negative FyFy phenotype and are therefore resistant to *P. vivax* malaria. The glycophorins, a family of membrane sialoglycoproteins, have been implicated as the red cell attachment sites for the merozoites of *P. falciparum.* During invasion the merozoite first orientates so that its apical end is apposed to the erythrocyte surface and then interiorizes itself so as to lie within an intraerythrocytic parasitophorous vacuole. During the early stage of development the small "ring forms" of the four parasite species appear similar under light microscopy. As the trophozoites enlarge, species-specific characteristics become evident, pigment becomes visible, and the parasite assumes an irregular or ameboid shape. By the end of the 48-h cycle (72 h for *P. malariae*) the parasite has grown to occupy most of the red cell. Multiple nuclear fission then takes place (schizogony), and the red cell ruptures to release from 6 to 24 daughter merozoites. Each of these is capable of invading a new red cell and repeating the cycle. After a series of such asexual cycles some of the parasites develop into morphologically distinct sexual forms (gametocytes) which are long-lived and relatively inert.

Following ingestion in the blood meal of a biting female anopheline mosquito, the male and female gametocytes fuse in the insect's midgut to form a zygote. This matures to form an ookinete, which penetrates and encysts in the mosquito gut wall. The resulting oocyst expands by asexual division until it bursts to liberate myriads of motile sporozoites, which then migrate to the salivary gland to await inoculation into another human at the next feeding.

The disease in human beings is caused by the direct effects of red cell invasion and destruction and the host reaction to this process.

EPIDEMIOLOGY Malaria occurs throughout most of the tropical regions of the world. *P. falciparum* predominates in Africa, New Guinea, and Haiti; *P. vivax* is more common in Central America and

TABLE 159-1 Human malaria parasites

	P. falciparum	*P. vivax*	*P. ovale*	*P. malariae*
Duration of intrahepatic phase (days)	$5\frac{1}{2}$	8	9	15
Number of merozoites released per infected hepatocyte	30,000	10,000	15,000	15,000
Duration of erythrocytic cycle (hours)	48	48	50	72
Red cell preference	Younger cells but can invade cells of all ages.	Reticulocytes	Reticulocytes	Older cells
Morphologic characteristics	Usually only ring forms. Parasitemia may exceed 2 percent with multiple infections of a single erythrocyte. Banana-shaped gametocytes.	Irregular-shaped large rings and trophozoites. Enlarged erythrocytes. Schüffner's dots.	Infected erythrocytes enlarged and oval. Schüffner's dots.	Band or rectangular forms of trophozoites common.
Pigment color	Black	Yellow-brown	Dark brown	Brown/black
Relapses	No	Yes	Yes	No

the Indian subcontinent. The prevalence of both species is approximately equal in South America, east Asia, and Oceania. *P. malariae* is found in most areas, but is much less common. *P. ovale* is relatively unusual outside Africa.

The epidemiology of malaria is complex and may vary considerably even within relatively small geographic areas. Endemicity is traditionally defined in terms of spleen rates in children (i.e., percentage of children with a palpable spleen) as hypoendemic < 10 percent, mesoendemic 11 to 50 percent, hyperendemic 51 to 75 percent, and holoendemic > 75 percent. In holo- and hyperendemic areas (Fig. 159-1) such as much of tropical Africa or coastal New Guinea, where there is intense *P. falciparum* transmission, people are infected repeatedly throughout their lives. There is considerable morbidity and mortality during childhood. Immunity is hard won, but by the time of adulthood malaria infections are largely asymptomatic. In areas where transmission is low, erratic, or focal, the chance of one infected person transmitting malaria to another is relatively small, full immunity is not acquired, and symptomatic disease may occur at all ages. This is termed ''unstable malaria'' in contrast to the ''stable'' malaria in holo- and hyperendemic areas. Even in areas with stable malaria, there is often seasonal variation coinciding with increased mosquito breeding during the rainy season. Malaria can behave like an epidemic disease in some areas, such as in north India and southeast Asia. This occurs when there are migrations (usually of refugees or workers) from a nonmalarious region to areas of high transmission. This usually produces considerable mortality at all ages.

The principal determinants of malaria epidemiology are the biting habits, longevity, and number (density) of the anopheline mosquito vectors. As a general approximation, malaria transmission is directly proportional to the density of the vector, the square of the number of human bites per day per mosquito, and the tenth power of the probability of the mosquito surviving for 1 day. Mosquito longevity

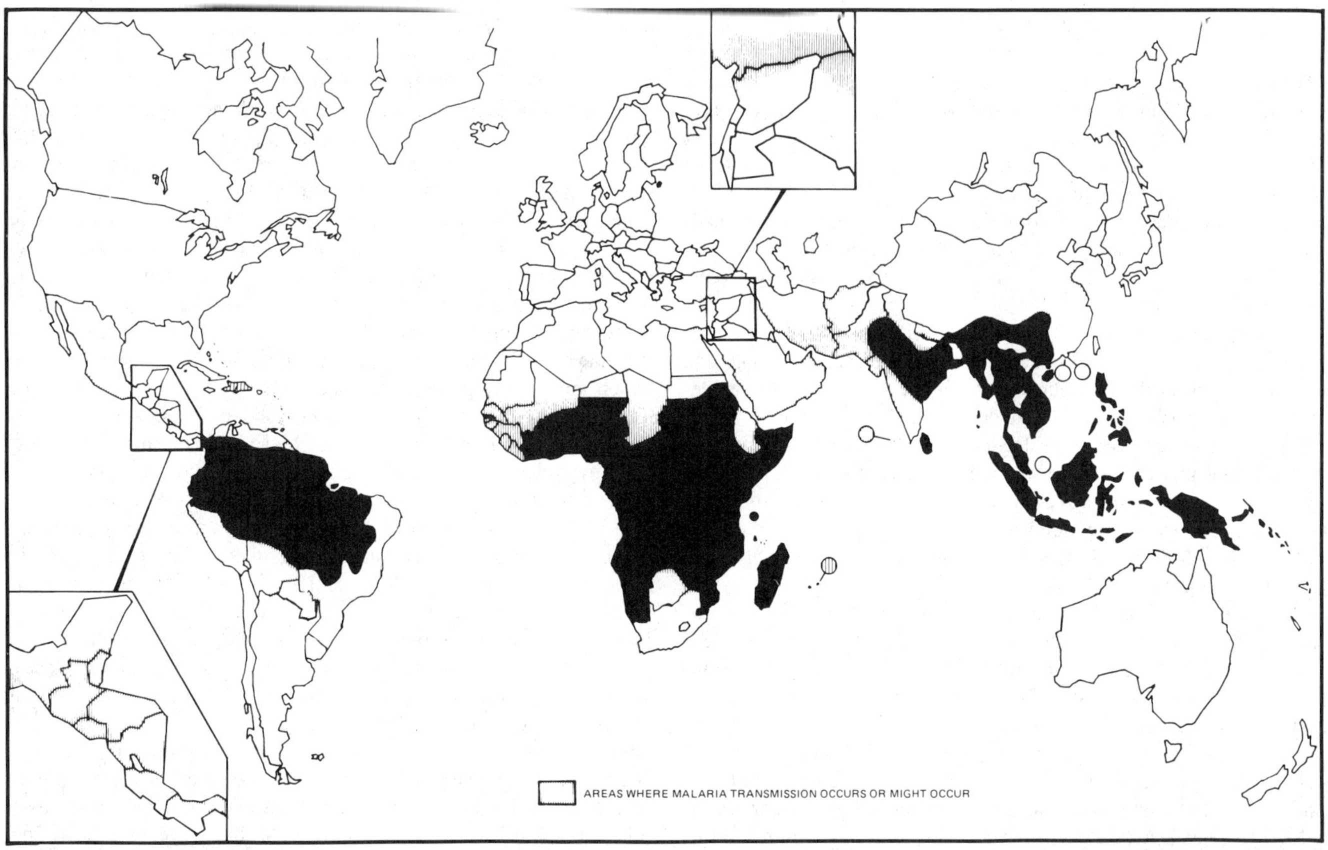

FIGURE 159-1 Distribution of chloroquine-resistant *Plasmodium falciparum,* 1988. Shaded area denotes regions where malaria occurs or might occur. *(Courtesy of Malaria Section, Centers for Disease Control.)*

is particularly important, because the extrinsic cycle from sporozoite ingestion to subsequent inoculation takes a minimum of 7 days (depending on ambient temperature) and in order to transmit malaria the mosquito must survive for longer than this. Therefore the most effective mosquito vectors are those (such as *A. gambiae* in west Africa) which are long-lived, occur in high densities, and bite humans frequently.

ERYTHROCYTE CHANGES After invasion, the growing parasite progressively consumes and degrades intracellular proteins, principally hemoglobin, and also alters the red-cell membrane by changing its transport properties, exposing cryptic surface antigens, and inserting new parasite-derived proteins. The red cell becomes more spherical and less deformable. In *P. falciparum* infections membrane protuberances appear on the erythrocyte surface in the second 24 h of the asexual cycle. These "knobs" overlie accretions of electron-dense, histidine-rich parasite proteins and extrude a high-molecular-weight, strain-specific, adhesive protein which mediates attachment to receptors on venular and capillary endothelium. These receptors are related to thrombospondin, its natural receptor, platelet glycoprotein 4, and other unidentified proteins. This process of "cytoadherence" is central to the pathogenesis of falciparum malaria. It results in sequestration of mature forms of the parasite in vital organs (particularly the brain and heart) where they interfere with microcirculatory flow and metabolism and continue development away from the principal host defense, i.e., by splenic processing and filtration. As a consequence, only the younger ring forms of the asexual parasites are seen in the peripheral blood in falciparum malaria, and the peripheral parasitemia is an underestimate of the true number of parasites within the body. In the other three "benign" malarias sequestration does not occur, and all stages of parasite development may be seen on peripheral blood smears. Whereas these species show a marked predilection for either old red cells or reticulocytes and parasitemias seldom exceed 2 percent, *P. falciparum* can invade erythrocytes of all ages, and very high parasitemias may occur.

HOST RESPONSE The initial response to infection in the non-immune subject is the activation of nonspecific host defense mechanisms. Splenic immunologic and filtrative clearance functions are augmented in malaria, and there is accelerated removal of both parasitized and uninfected erythrocytes. The parasitized cells escaping splenic removal are destroyed when the schizont ruptures. The material released induces activation of macrophages and release of mononuclear cell–derived cytokines (including tumor necrosis factor and interleukin 1) which cause fever and other pathologic effects. Temperatures of 40°C are schizonticidal, and this has the effect of synchronizing the parasite cycle and eventually producing the regular fever spikes and rigors that originally characterized the different malarias (quotidian, daily fever spike; tertian, every 2 days; quartan, every 3 days). These fever patterns are seldom seen in patients who receive effective antimalarial treatment.

The global distributions of sickle cell disease, thalassemia, and glucose-6-phosphate dehydrogenase deficiency closely resemble that of malaria before the introduction of control measures. This epidemiologic information strongly suggests that these genetic disorders affecting the red cell confer protection against death from falciparum malaria, and this has been confirmed in the case of HbA/S heterozygotes (sickle cell trait). The mechanism whereby these disorders protect against severe infection has not been clearly elucidated except in the case of Melanesian ovalocytosis, where the rigid erythrocytes resist merozoite invasion.

The specific immune response to malaria limits the rising parasitemia, and with exposure to sufficient strains, eventually confers protection from disease, but not from infection. Asymptomatic parasitemias are commonly found in adults living in holo- or hyperendemic areas. This state of premunition is specific for both the species and strain of infecting malaria parasite. Both humoral and cellular immunity are necessary, but the mechanisms are incompletely understood. Immune individuals have a polyclonal increase in serum IgM, IgG, and IgA (although much of this antibody is unrelated to protection). Antibodies against a variety of parasite stage–specific antigens (particularly those related to the red cell surface cytoadherence protein) presumably act in concert to limit in vivo parasite replication. Passively transferred IgG from immune adults has been shown to reduce parasitemia in children, and passive transfer of maternal antibody also presumably contributes to the relative protection from severe malaria in the first months of life. Several factors retard the development of cellular immunity. These include the absence of major histocompatibility antigens on the surface of infected red cells, which precludes direct T-cell recognition; malaria antigen–specific immune unresponsiveness; and the enormous strain diversity of malaria parasites and their ability to express variant antigens on the erythrocyte surface which change during the period of infection. Immunity against all strains is never achieved. Parasites may persist in the blood for months and, in the case of *P. malariae,* for many years if treatment is not given. The complexity of the immune response in malaria, the sophistication of the parasites' evasive mechanisms, and the lack of a good in vitro correlate with clinical immunity have all contributed to the slow progress toward an effective vaccine.

CLINICAL FEATURES The first symptoms of malaria are nonspecific; lack of well-being, headache, fatigue, and muscle aching followed by fever are all similar to those of a minor viral illness. In some patients headache, chest pain, abdominal pain, arthralgia, myalgia, or diarrhea may be prominent and suggest an alternative diagnosis. The classic malarial paroxysms in which fever spikes, chills, and rigors occur at regular intervals are rare. The fever is irregular at first and in nonimmune individuals or children often rises over 40°C accompanied by an appropriate tachycardia and, in some cases, delirium. Nausea, vomiting, and orthostatic hypotension are common. Although many clinical abnormalities have been described in acute malaria, most patients with uncomplicated infections have few abnormal findings other than mild anemia and, in some cases, a palpable spleen.

Severe falciparum malaria CEREBRAL MALARIA Coma is a characteristic and ominous feature of falciparum malaria and is associated with a mortality of 20 percent despite treatment. Lesser degrees of obtundation, delirium, or abnormal behavior should also be taken seriously. The onset may be gradual or sudden following a convulsion. Cerebral malaria is a diffuse symmetric encephalopathy. Focal neurologic signs are unusual. Although there may be some passive resistance to head flexion, signs of meningeal irritation are absent. The eyes may be divergent and a pout reflex is common, but other primitive reflexes are usually absent. The corneal reflexes are preserved except in deep coma. Muscle tone may be increased or decreased. The tendon reflexes are variable, and the plantars may be flexor or extensor. The abdominal and cremasteric reflexes are absent. Flexor or extensor posturing may occur. Approximately 15 percent of patients have retinal hemorrhages. Less than 5 percent have significant bleeding or other clinical evidence of disseminated intravascular coagulation. Anemia and jaundice are common. Convulsions, which are usually generalized, occur in 50 percent of adults and a higher proportion of children with cerebral malaria. Approximately 10 percent of children surviving cerebral malaria, particularly those with hypoglycemia, repeated seizures, and deep coma, will have some residual neurologic deficit following recovery of consciousness.

HYPOGLYCEMIA Hypoglycemia is an important and common complication of severe malaria and is associated with a poor prognosis. It is a particular problem in children and in pregnant women. Hypoglycemia results from failure of hepatic gluconeogenesis and increased consumption of glucose by both host and parasite. Plasma concentrations of the principal gluconeogenic substrates, lactate and alanine, are increased. To compound the situation, quinine, the drug of choice for severe chloroquine-resistant malaria, is a powerful stimulant to pancreatic insulin secretion. Hyperinsulinemic hypoglycemia is a particular problem in pregnant women receiving quinine treatment. In patients with severe disease the clinical diagnosis is difficult as the usual physical signs of hypoglycemia (sweating, gooseflesh, tachycardia) are absent and neurologic impairment cannot be distinguished from that caused by malaria.

LACTIC ACIDOSIS Lactic acidosis commonly coexists with hypoglycemia. Anaerobic glycolysis in tissues where sequestered parasitized erythrocytes interfere with microcirculatory flow, parasite lactate production, and a failure of hepatic lactate clearance combine to raise plasma lactate concentrations. The prognosis is poor. Hyperventilation is usually followed by circulatory failure refractory to volume expansion or inotropic drugs.

NONCARDIOGENIC PULMONARY EDEMA This may develop in adults with severe falciparum malaria even after several days' antimalarial therapy. The pathogenesis of this variant of the adult respiratory distress syndrome is unclear. The mortality is over 80 percent.

RENAL IMPAIRMENT This is common in adults with severe falciparum malaria but rare in children. It is a marker of severe disease and carries a high mortality. The pathogenesis of renal failure is unclear, but may be related to parasitized erythrocyte sequestration which interferes with renal microcirculatory flow and regional metabolism. Clinically and pathologically this syndrome behaves like acute tubular necrosis, and provided the acute phase of the disease can be overcome, renal function returns over a period of days or weeks (see Chap. 223).

HEMATOLOGIC ABNORMALITIES The pathophysiology of anemia in malaria is multifactorial. There are accelerated red cell destruction and removal by the spleen and bone marrow suppression with ineffective erythropoiesis. In severe malaria anemia develops rapidly, and transfusion is often required. Slight coagulation abnormalities are common in falciparum malaria, and mild thrombocytopenia is usual. In a small number of cases (less than 5 percent of patients with cerebral malaria) significant bleeding occurs with evidence of disseminated intravascular coagulation. Hematemesis, presumably from stress ulceration or acute gastric erosions, may also occur.

OTHER COMPLICATIONS Aspiration pneumonia following convulsions is an important cause of death in cerebral malaria. Malaria predisposes to bacterial superinfection. Catheter-induced urinary infections are common. Spontaneous gram-negative septicemia may occur in severe malaria, and *Salmonella* septicemias have been associated with *P. falciparum* infections in endemic areas.

Malaria in pregnancy Falciparum malaria is an important cause of fetal death. In hyper- and holoendemic areas malaria is associated with low birth weight, but in general the mothers remain asymptomatic despite intense parasitization of the placenta (due to sequestration of parasitized erythrocytes in the placental microcirculation).

In areas with unstable transmission, pregnant women are prone to severe infections, and are particularly vulnerable to develop high parasitemias with anemia, hypoglycemia, and acute pulmonary edema. Fetal distress, premature labor, and stillbirth commonly ensue, and congenital malaria can develop in the newborn.

Malaria in children Most of the estimated 1 million deaths from falciparum malaria each year occur in children. Convulsions, coma, hypoglycemia, metabolic acidosis, and severe anemia are relatively common in children with severe malaria, whereas acute renal failure and acute pulmonary edema are unusual. In general, children tolerate the antimalarial drugs well and respond rapidly to treatment.

Transfusion malaria Malaria can be transmitted by blood transfusion or needle sharing with infected intravenous drug addicts. *P. malariae* and *P. falciparum* have been the most common causes. The incubation period is often short because there is no preerythrocytic development. Clinical features and management are as in naturally acquired infections. Radical chemotherapy with primaquine in *P. vivax* and *P. ovale* infections is unnecessary.

CHRONIC COMPLICATIONS OF MALARIA Tropical splenomegaly (hyperreactive malarial splenomegaly) Chronic or repeated malaria infections produce hypergammaglobulinemia, a normochromic normocytic anemia, and, in certain situations, splenomegaly. Some residents of malaria-endemic areas exhibit an abnormal immunologic response to repeated infections which results in massive splenomegaly, hepatomegaly, marked elevations in serum IgM and malaria antibody, hepatic sinusoidal lymphocytosis, and, in Africa, peripheral (B-cell) lymphocytosis. On Flores Island, Indonesia, the condition is associated with the production of cytotoxic IgM antisuppressor lymphocyte (CD8+) antibodies. This leads to uninhibited B-cell production of IgM and the formation of cryoglobulins (IgM aggregates and immune complexes), which stimulates reticuloendothelial hyperplasia and clearance activity and eventually produces splenomegaly. Patients with hyperreactive malarial splenomegaly (HMS) present with an abdominal mass or complaints of a dragging sensation in the abdomen and occasional sharp abdominal pains suggesting perisplenitis. There is usually anemia and some degree of pancytopenia, but in most cases malaria parasites cannot be found in peripheral blood smears. There is increased vulnerability to respiratory and skin infections, and many patients die of overwhelming sepsis. HMS usually responds to effective antimalarial prophylaxis.

Quartan malaria nephropathy Chronic or repeated infections with *P. malariae* may cause soluble immune-complex injury to the renal glomeruli resulting in nephrotic syndrome. Other unidentified factors must be contributory, because only a very small proportion of infected patients develop renal disease. The histologic appearance is of a focal or segmental glomerulonephritis with splitting of the capillary basement membrane. Subendothelial dense deposits are seen on electron microscopy, and immunofluorescence reveals deposits of complement and immunoglobulins; in children *P. malariae* antigens can often be seen. Patients with a coarse granular pattern of basement membrane immunofluorescent deposits (predominantly IgG3) and selective proteinuria have a better prognosis than those with a fine granular, predominantly IgG2 pattern and nonselective proteinuria. Quartan nephropathy usually responds poorly to treatment with either antimalarials or glucocorticoids and cytotoxic drugs.

DIAGNOSIS The diagnosis of malaria rests on the demonstration of asexual forms of the parasite in peripheral blood smears stained with one of the Romanowsky stains (Wright's, Field's, Leishman's, or Giemsa at pH 7.2). Both thin and thick blood smears should be examined. The thin smear should be air-dried rapidly, fixed in anhydrous methanol, and stained, and the red cells in the tail of the film examined under oil immersion. The parasitemia is expressed as the number of parasitized erythrocytes in 1000 cells and then converted to the number per microliter. The relationship between parasitemia and prognosis is complex; in general, patients with parasitemias in excess of 10^5 per microliter are at an increased risk of a fatal outcome, but nonimmunes may die with much lower counts, and semi-immunes may tolerate parasitemias of three times this value with only minor symptoms.

The thick film should be of uneven thickness. The smear should be dried thoroughly and stained *without* fixing. As many layers of erythrocytes overlie each other and are then lysed during the staining procedure, the thick film has the advantage of concentrating the parasites, and therefore increasing the sensitivity of diagnosis. Both parasites and white cells are counted and the number of parasites per unit volume calculated from the total leukocyte count. A minimum of 200 white cells should be counted. Interpretation of thick films requires some experience because artifacts are common. Phagocytosed malaria pigment may be seen inside peripheral blood monocytes or polymorphonuclear leukocytes and may provide a clue to recent infection if malaria parasites are not seen. Occasionally parasites and pigment are evident in bone marrow aspirates or smears obtained from fluid expressed after intradermal puncture, but not on peripheral blood smears. Considerable advances have been made with DNA probes and flow cytometry in the diagnosis of malaria, and their sensitivity is approaching that of a trained microscopist.

Laboratory findings A normochromic normocytic anemia is usual. The leukocyte count is low to normal, although it may be raised in very severe infections. The erythrocyte sedimentation rate, plasma viscosity, and C-reactive protein levels are high. The platelet count is usually moderately reduced. In severe infections there may be prolongation of the prothrombin and partial thromboplastin times. Antithrombin III levels are reduced even in mild infection. In uncomplicated malaria, plasma concentration of electrolytes, blood urea nitrogen, and creatinine are usually normal. In severe malaria there may be a metabolic acidosis with low plasma concentrations of glucose, sodium, bicarbonate, calcium, magnesium, and albumin together with elevations in lactate, BUN, creatinine, muscle and liver enzymes, and conjugated and unconjugated bilirubin. Hypergammaglobulinemia is usual in immune and semi-immune subjects. Urinalysis is usually normal.

PREVENTION In most of the rural tropics, eradication of malaria is not feasible. Where possible, the disease is contained by judicious use of insecticides to kill the mosquito vector, and chemoprophylaxis in high-risk groups. All pregnant women at risk should receive prophylaxis, and prophylactic antimalarials should be given to children between the ages of 1 and 4 in areas where malaria causes high childhood mortality. Widespread use of bed nets, particularly if treated with permethrin (a residual pyrethroid), will considerably reduce the incidence of malaria. Despite massive investment toward development of a malaria vaccine, a safe, effective, and long-lasting vaccine is unlikely soon (see Chap. 156).

PERSONAL PROTECTION AGAINST MALARIA Simple measures to reduce the frequency of mosquito bites in malarious areas are very important. These include avoiding exposure at peak feeding times (usually dusk and dawn), and use of insect repellants, suitable clothing, and impregnated bed nets.

Chemoprophylaxis (Table 159-2) Few areas of therapeutics are as controversial as antimalarial drug prophylaxis. Recommendations for prophylaxis depend on a knowledge of local parasite drug sensitivity and the likelihood of acquiring malaria infection. Chemoprophylaxis is never entirely reliable, and malaria should always be considered in the differential diagnosis of fever in patients who have taken prophylactic antimalarial drugs. Chloroquine [5 mg base per kilogram per week (300 mg maximum) weekly] remains the drug of choice for the prevention of drug-sensitive *P. falciparum* and the other human malarias. It is generally well tolerated, although some patients are unable to take the drug because of dysphoria, headache, or, in dark-skinned patients, pruritus. It is considered relatively safe in pregnancy. With chronic administration a characteristic dose-related retinopathy develops; in adults cumulative doses over 100 g are associated with significant risk. Individuals receiving long-term chloroquine prophylaxis should therefore have regular ophthalmologic examinations. Idiosyncratic or allergic reactions are rare. Skeletal and cardiac myopathy may also occur but are more likely with the high doses used in the treatment of rheumatoid arthritis. Neuropsychiatric reactions and skin rashes are unusual. The related aminoquinoline amodiaquine has also been used, but is associated with a high risk of agranulocytosis and is not recommended. In the past the dihydrofolate reductase inhibitors pyrimethamine and proguanil (chloroguanide) have been used widely, but resistant strains of both *P. falciparum* and *P. vivax* have limited their use. Whereas the quinoline antimalarials such as chloroquine act on the erythrocyte stage of parasite development, the dihydrofolate reductase inhibitors also inhibit preerythrocytic growth (causal prophylactics) and development in the mosquito (sporontocidal activity). There has been a resurgence of interest in proguanil [1.5 to 3 mg/kg (200 mg maximum) daily] because it may retain efficacy against pyrimethamine-resistant strains of *P. falciparum,* and apart from rare cases of mouth ulceration, it is safe and well tolerated. Proguanil is considered the safest antimalarial prophylactic in pregnancy. The prophylactic use of the combination of pyrimethamine and sulfadoxine is not recommended because of an unacceptable incidence of severe toxicity, principally exfoliative dermatitis and other skin rashes, agranulocytosis, hepatitis, and pulmonary eosinophilia.

The combination of pyrimethamine with dapsone [0.2/1.5 mg/kg (25/200 mg maximum) weekly] is widely used in areas with chloroquine-resistant *P. falciparum* and is generally well tolerated, although there is increasing resistance and dapsone may cause methemoglobinemia, allergic reactions, and, with higher doses, a significant risk of agranulocytosis. In areas with multi-drug-resistant falciparum malaria there is no satisfactory, generally available prophylactic. Daily doxycycline (100 mg maximum) is effective and also has causal prophylactic activity. It is generally well tolerated but may cause *Monilia* infections, diarrhea, and photosensitivity and cannot be used in children or in pregnancy. Faced with the problems of variable drug resistance and the lack of safe and effective prophylactic antimalarials, the Centers for Disease Control have opted for pragmatism adopting a strategy of presumptive treatment for those at risk

TABLE 159-2 Prophylaxis and treatment of malaria

	Chloroquine-sensitive *P. falciparum, P. vivax, P. malariae,* and *P. ovale*	Chloroquine-resistant *P. falciparum*
Prophylaxis	Chloroquine 5 mg base/kg/wk (300 mg maximum) or proguanil 3 mg/kg/d (200 mg maximum).	No safe and reliable drug for all geographic areas. Strategies include combined chloroquine & proguanil or: 1. Chloroquine 10 mg base/kg/wk (600 mg maximum). 2. Doxycycline 1.5 mg/kg/d (100 mg maximum). 3. Presumptive treatment with either sulfadoxine-pyrimethamine or quinine.
	Mefloquine: See discussion on p. 788.	
Treatment of uncomplicated infections	Chloroquine 10 mg base/kg (600 mg maximum) stat followed by 5 mg/kg at 6 (600 mg maximum), 24, and 48 h (or 10 mg/kg daily for 3 days).	Quinine 10 mg salt/kg (650 mg maximum) q8h PO (5–7 days) together with tetracycline* 4 mg/kg (250 mg maximum) q6h (7 days), or in some areas pyrimethamine 1 mg/kg + sulfadoxine 20 mg/kg stat (75/1500 mg maximum).
Treatment of severe malaria†	Chloroquine 10 mg base/kg (600 mg maximum) infused IV at a constant rate over 8 h followed by 15 mg base/kg (900 mg maximum) infused over 24 h.	Quinine‡,§ 7 mg salt/kg (400 mg maximum) infused IV at a constant rate over 30 min, followed immediately by 10 mg salt/kg (600 mg maximum) over 4 h, and then, after an interval of 4 h, by infusions of 10 mg salt/kg (600 mg maximum) q8h for 7 days. (Infusion times 2–8 h.)
Hospital and nursing facilities		
Rural clinic without nursing facilities	Chloroquine 3.5 mg/kg base (200 mg maximum) q6h or 2.5 mg base q4h (150 mg maximum) by either SC or IM injection. Total dose 25 mg/kg (1500 mg maximum).	Quinine 20 mg salt/kg (1200 mg maximum) stat followed by 10 mg salt/kg q8h given by deep IM injection. The quinine concentration should be 60 mg salt/mL, and the first dose should be split into two, e.g., half the dose into each thigh.

* Tetracycline should not be given in pregnancy or to children under 8 years.
† Oral treatment should be substituted as soon as the patient recovers sufficiently to take fluids by mouth. Nasogastric administration of oral antimalarials should be attempted if patients are first seen in a situation where parenteral treatment is not possible pending transfer to hospital.
‡ Quinidine gluconate may be substituted if quinine is not available but electrocardiographic monitoring is advisable, and quinine should be substituted when possible. Loading dose 10 mg salt/kg infused over 1 h followed by continuous infusion given at rate of 0.02 mg/kg/min for 3 days.
§ A loading dose should not be given if quinine or quinidine has been given in the previous 24 h.

from multi-drug-resistant malaria. Adult travelers are advised to take three 25/500 mg tablets of sulfadoxine-pyrimethamine if they develop fever and have no recourse to medical facilities. Alternatives are weekly chloroquine and daily proguanil (Table 159-2), or weekly chloroquine and pyrimethamine-dapsone, with appropriate medical advice in case of fever.

Travelers should start taking antimalarial drugs at least 1 week before departure in order to detect untoward reactions and to provide therapeutic antimalarial blood concentrations when needed in the endemic area. Those persons starting chloroquine immediately before departure should take a loading dose [10 mg base per kilogram (600 mg maximum)]. Antimalarial prophylaxis should continue for 6 weeks after leaving an endemic area.

TREATMENT Patients in or from malarious areas who present with fever should have a blood smear to confirm the diagnosis and identify the species of infecting parasite. In endemic areas uncomplicated infections may be treated on an outpatient basis. Regimens for FDA-approved drugs are detailed in Table 159-2, and characteristics of various agents in Table 159-3. Three additional drugs yet to be approved for antimalarial use in the United States deserve mention; two are quinine analogues that can be substituted for that agent in some circumstances. The antiarrhythmic quinidine gluconate appears to be as rapidly schizonticidal as quinine and is more readily available. However, because it appears to be more cardiotoxic than quinine, its administration must be closely monitored if inadvertent arrhythmia and/or hypotension are to be avoided. Blood levels in excess of 6 μg/mL, QT interval greater than 0.6 s, or QRS widening beyond 25 percent of baseline are indications for slowing infusion rates. If arrhythmia or saline-unresponsive hypotension develop, the drug should be discontinued. Dosage is provided in Table 159-2. As the agent has not been approved for malaria, informed consent should be obtained prior to administration. Mefloquine, a newly developed oral 4-quinolinemethanol, also displays rapid schizonticidal activity against chloroquine-resistant strains of *P. falciparum.* Although effective as a prophylactic agent, there is concern that widespread use will accelerate the development of resistant strains and shorten its period of usefulness as a therapeutic agent in chloroquine-resistant falciparum infections. Its ease of administration and relative lack of toxicity has led to its replacement of quinine in some endemic areas. The third agent, halofantrine, is a well-tolerated, oral phenanthrenemethanol that is used in some parts of Africa. It is effective against both chloroquine-sensitive and chloroquine-resistant strains of falciparum malaria. Acetaminophen lowers fever and provides symptomatic relief and thereby reduces the propensity to vomit the oral antimalarial drugs. Pregnant women, young children, patients unable to tolerate oral therapy, and nonimmune subjects (e.g., travelers) with suspected malaria should be hospitalized.

If there is any doubt as to the identification of the malaria species, treatment for falciparum malaria should be given. If the smear is negative, this does not rule out malaria, and thick blood films should be checked 1 and 2 days later to exclude the diagnosis. Nonimmune subjects with malaria should have daily parasite counts performed until thick films are negative (parasite clearance). If the parasitemia does not fall below 25 percent of the admission value in 48 h, or has not cleared by 7 days, drug resistance should be suspected and treatment should be changed. If falciparum malaria has been contracted in an area of known drug sensitivity, chloroquine or sulfadoxine-pyrimethamine are preferable because they are better tolerated and simpler than quinine and tetracycline. If there is doubt about drug sensitivity, the latter combination should be prescribed.

Primaquine [0.2 mg base per kilogram (15 mg maximum)] should be given daily for 14 days in patients with *P. vivax* or *P. ovale*

TABLE 159-3 Antimalarial drugs

Drug	Pharmacokinetic properties	Antimalarial activity	Minor toxicity	Major toxicity
Quinine	Absorption: Oral: good Intramuscular: good Cl* $\downarrow$ and Vd† $\downarrow$ but plasma protein binding $\uparrow$ (90%) in malaria $t_{1/2}$: 16 h in malaria, 11 h in health	Rapid "schizonticide" Gametocytocidal against *P. vivax, P. ovale,* and *P. malaria*; no action on liver stages	Bitter-tasting Common: "cinchonism," tinnitus, high-tone hearing loss, nausea, vomiting, dysphoria, postural hypotension; prolongation of ECG QTc interval Rare: diarrhea, visual disturbance, rashes	Common: hypoglycemia Rare: hypotension, blindness, deafness, cardiac arrhythmias, thrombocytopenia, hemolysis, cholestatic hepatitis, neuromuscular paralysis
Chloroquine	Absorption: Oral: good Intramuscular: very rapid Subcutaneous: very rapid Complex pharmacokinetics Enormous Cl* and Vd† (unaffected by malaria) Distribution processes determine blood concentration profile in malaria $t_{1/2}$: 1–2 months	Rapid "schizonticide" Gametocytocidal against *P. vivax, P. ovale,* and *P. malaria*; no action on liver stages	Bitter-tasting Well-tolerated Common: nausea, dysphoria, pruritus in dark-skinned patients; postural hypotension Rare: accommodation difficulties, rash	Acute: hypotension shock (parenteral); cardiac arrhythmias; neuropsychiatric reactions Chronic: retinopathy (cumulative dose >100 g); skeletal and cardiac myopathy
Mefloquine:	See discussion on p. 788.			
Pyrimethamine	Absorption: Oral: good Intramuscular: insufficient data $t_{1/2}$: 4 days	Speed of action depends on stage of parasite development	Well-tolerated	Megaloblastic anemia Pancytopenia Pulmonary infiltration
Proguanil (chloroguanide)	Absorption: Oral: good Biotransformed to active metabolite cycloguanil $t_{1/2}$: 16 h	Causal prophylactic; not used for treatment	Well-tolerated Rare: mouth ulcers	Megaloblastic anemia in renal failure
Primaquine	Absorption: Oral: complete Active compound not known $t_{1/2}$: 7 h	Radical cure Eradicates exoerythrocytic forms of *P. vivax* and *P. ovale* Gametocytocidal against *P. falciparum*	Nausea, vomiting diarrhea, abdominal pain; hemolysis; methemoglobinemia	Massive hemolysis in subjects with severe G6PD deficiency

*Cl = systemic clearance.
†Vd = total apparent volume of distribution.

infections after laboratory tests for G6PD deficiency have proved negative. If the patient has one of the mild variants of G6PD deficiency, the primaquine can be given in a dose of 0.6 mg base per kilogram (45 mg maximum) once weekly for 6 weeks.

Severe falciparum malaria is a medical emergency requiring intensive nursing care and careful management. Patients should be weighed and, if comatose, nursed on their side and given a single parenteral dose of phenobarbital (3.5 to 5 mg/kg) to prevent convulsions. The immediate management is outlined in Table 159-4. Frequent evaluation is essential. Ancillary drugs such as high-dose glucocorticoids, mannitol, urea, heparin, and dextran are of no value. The choice of antimalarial drug depends on knowledge of the prevailing sensitivity of *P. falciparum* to antimalarials. If there is any doubt, quinine (or if not available, quinidine) should be given. Systemic clearance and apparent volume of distribution of these drugs are markedly reduced in severe malaria, and blood concentrations for a given dose are consequently higher. The optimum therapeutic range of quinine in severe malaria is not known with certainty, but plasma concentrations between 0.8 and 1.5 mg/dL are effective and do not cause serious toxicity. An initial loading dose is given to provide therapeutic concentrations as soon as possible but is not necessary if the patient has already started quinine treatment before admission to the hospital. If the patient remains seriously ill or in acute renal failure for 3 days, the maintenance doses should be reduced by one-third to one-half to prevent accumulation of quinine to toxic concentrations. The initial doses should never be reduced. If chloroquine is given, dose reduction is unnecessary even in the face of renal failure.

In unconscious patients the blood glucose should be measured every 6 h and blood glucose values below 2.2 mmol/L (40 mg/dL) treated with intravenous dextrose. Patients treated with intravenous quinine should receive a continuous infusion of dextrose. The parasite count and hematocrit should be measured every 12 h. Anemia develops rapidly; if the hematocrit falls below 20 percent, then whole blood (preferably fresh) or packed cells should be transfused slowly with careful attention to circulatory status and judicious use of small doses of a diuretic to prevent fluid overload. Renal function should be checked daily. Management of fluid balance is difficult in severe malaria because there is a thin dividing line between overhydration, leading to pulmonary edema, and underhydration, contributing to renal impairment. If necessary, pulmonary artery wedge pressure should be measured and maintained in the low-normal range. As soon as the patient can take fluids, oral antimalarials are substituted.

MEFLOQUINE Approved by the FDA in 1989 for prevention and treatment of *P. falciparum* and *P. vivax* malaria, the drug is active against all species including strains resistant to chloroquine and fansidar (some *P. falciparum* strains are resistant). Mefloquine HCl is well absorbed from the GI tract, metabolized in the liver, and excreted in the bile and feces. Doses of 500 to 1000 mg are effective, even against strains resistant to multiple drugs. Adverse effects are dose related and include vertigo, nausea, and lightheadedness. Confusion, convulsions, and psychosis have been reported. The drug may prolong cardiac conduction and is contraindicated in patients taking beta blockers and calcium channel blockers. It should not be used with quinine or quinidine nor by children or pregnant women. The dose for prophylaxis is one 250-mg tablet weekly for 4 weeks (beginning 1 week before travel), then one tablet every other week during a stay in a malarious area and for two doses afterward. For acute uncomplicated *P. falciparum* malaria treatment is a single oral dose of 1250 mg with 8 oz. of water.

COMPLICATIONS Acute renal failure If there is a rising blood urea nitrogen or creatinine level despite adequate rehydration, fluid administration should be restricted to keep pulmonary arterial wedge pressures from rising. The indications for dialysis are the same as those in other forms of hypercatabolic acute renal failure (see Chap. 223). Although peritoneal dialysis is adequate, secondary bacterial infections are common in the tropics, and hemodialysis is preferable. Some patients will pass small volumes of urine sufficient to allow control of fluid balance and may be managed conservatively if other indications for dialysis do not arise. Renal function usually improves in days, but may take weeks to recover fully.

Acute pulmonary edema Patients should be nursed at 45° and given oxygen and intravenous diuretics. Pulmonary artery wedge pressures may be normal, indicating increased pulmonary capillary permeability. Positive pressure ventilation should be instituted if these immediate measures fail (see Chap. 219).

Hypoglycemia An initial slow infusion of 50% dextrose (0.5 g dextrose per kilogram per hour) should be followed by an infusion of 10% dextrose (0.10 g dextrose per kilogram per hour). The blood glucose should be checked regularly thereafter, as recurrent hypoglycemia is common, particularly in patients receiving quinine or quinidine. In severely ill patients hypoglycemia commonly occurs together with a metabolic (lactic) acidosis, and may prove fatal.

Other complications Patients who develop spontaneous bleeding should be given fresh blood and intravenous vitamin K. Convulsions should be treated with intravenous (or rectal) diazepam. Aspiration pneumonia should be suspected in any unconscious patient with convulsions, particularly if there is persistent hyperventilation. Intravenous antimicrobials, pulmonary toilet, and oxygen should be administered. Hypoglycemia or gram-negative septicemia should be suspected in any patient who suddenly deteriorates for no immediately obvious reason while receiving antimalarial treatment.

TABLE 159-4 Immediate management of severe malaria

1. Weigh.
2. Check airway, nurse patient on side.
3. Make rapid clinical assessment.
4. Take venous blood for quantitative parasite count, hematocrit, blood glucose, blood urea nitrogen (or creatinine), blood culture, and blood group.
5. Take arterial blood for pH and gases if clinically indicated.
6. Start controlled-rate infusion of antimalarial.
7. Make brief clinical examination; assess state of hydration.
8. Check urine output and consider need for hemodynamic monitoring.
9. If core temperature exceeds 38.5°C, give rectal acetaminophen suppository and start tepid sponging and fanning.
10. If patient is comatose, perform diagnostic lumbar puncture and give single intravenous or intramuscular dose of phenobarbital (3.5 to 5 mg/kg).
11. Consider need for blood transfusion and treatment of complications such as hypoglycemia, bacterial superinfections, bleeding, etc.

REFERENCES

BRAY RS, GARNHAM PCC: Life cycle of primate malaria parasites. Br Med Bull 38:117, 1982

DAVID PH et al: Parasite sequestration in *Plasmodium falciparum* malaria: Spleen and antibody modulation of cytoadherence of infected erythrocytes. Proc Nat Acad Sci USA 80:5075, 1983

GALBRAITH RM et al: The human materno-fetal relationship in malaria. Trans R Soc Trop Med Hyg 74:52, 61, 1980

HOFFMAN SL et al: Reduction of suppressor T lymphocytes in the tropical splenomegaly syndrome. N Engl J Med 310:337, 1984

MOLINEAU XL, GRAMICCIA G: *The Garki Project. Research on the Epidemiology and Control of Malaria in the Sudan Savannah of West Africa*. Geneva, WHO, 1980

PASVOL G: Receptors on red cells for *Plasmodium falciparum* and their interaction with the merozoite. Philos Trans R Soc 307:189, 1984

PHILLIPS RE et al: Intravenous quinidine for the treatment of severe falciparum malaria. Clinical and pharmacokinetic studies. N Engl J Med 312:1273, 1985

SPITZ S: Pathology of acute falciparum malaria. Military Med 99:555, 1946

WARRELL DA et al: Dexamethasone proves deleterious in cerebral malaria. A double blind trial in 100 comatose patients. N Engl J Med 306:313, 1982

WHITE NJ: Drug treatment and prevention of malaria. Eur J Clin Pharmacol 34:1, 1988

——— et al: Severe hypoglycemia and hyperinsulinaemia in falciparum malaria. N Engl J Med 309:61, 1983

WORLD HEALTH ORGANIZATION, MALARIA ACTION PROGRAMME: Severe and complicated malaria. Trans R Soc Trop Med Hyg 80(Suppl):1,1986

160 LEISHMANIASIS

RICHARD M. LOCKSLEY

DEFINITION Leishmaniasis denotes disease caused by any of the number of species of protozoa in the genus *Leishmania*. There are four major clinical syndromes—visceral leishmaniasis (kala azar), cutaneous leishmaniasis of the old and new worlds, mucocutaneous leishmaniasis (espundia), and diffuse cutaneous leishmaniasis. Most commonly, these parasites are transmitted from animal reservoirs to human hosts by the bite of phlebotomine sandflies.

ETIOLOGY Different *Leishmania* species appear identical and are generally distinguished by clinical and geographic characteristics. Traditionally, speciation required determination of isoenzyme patterns, kinetoplast DNA buoyant densities, or specific phlebotomine vectors. Monoclonal antibodies, DNA hybridization, DNA restriction endonuclease fragment analysis, and chromosomal karyotyping using pulse-field electrophoresis are powerful new methods for distinguishing these parasites.

In the sandfly and in culture media, *Leishmania* exist as motile, spindle-shaped promastigotes (1.5 to 4 μm by 14 to 20 μm) with a single anterior flagellum. On inoculation into a mammalian host, the organisms enter mononuclear phagocytes, lose their flagella, and multiply as small (2 by 5 μm), oval, intracellular amastigotes (Leishman-Donovan bodies). In stained preparations a dark, slightly flattened nucleus and rod-shaped kinetoplast may be discerned.

EPIDEMIOLOGY Leishmaniasis is a zoonotic infection which involves the rodents, canines, and various forest mammals of every inhabited continent except Australia. The disease is spread when female sandflies of the genus *Phlebotomus* (old world) or *Lutzomyia* (new world) ingest amastigotes while taking a blood meal from an infected mammal. These transform into promastigotes within the insect's gut, migrate to the proboscis, and are deposited on the skin of the new host when the insect next engorges. Phlebotomines breed in warm, humid microclimates and are typically found in rodent burrows, termite hills, and rotting vegetation. Humans may acquire the disease when they encroach upon this sylvatic cycle. Establishment of infection in the domestic dog provides an important urban reservoir of leishmaniasis. Person-to-person transmission is infrequent except in the Indian form of kala azar. Rarely, transmission can occur by blood transfusion, contact inoculation, and coitus. It is estimated that worldwide over 12 million people are infected.

PATHOGENESIS Promastigotes are deposited on the skin into a small pool of blood drawn by the probing sandfly. Products from the fly salivary gland promote infectivity, in part via peptides that deactivate host macrophages. Complement is activated by the classical and/or alternative pathways, depending upon the species, and is deposited onto the major outer membrane molecules of the promastigote—a 63-kDa molecular weight glycoprotein (gp63) or lipophosphoglycan (LPG). LPG and gp63 either directly or through bound C3b or C3bi target the organisms to macrophages via the complement receptors CR3 and CR1. The promastigotes transform into amastigotes within phagolysosomes and replicate by binary fission. They eventually rupture the cell and invade adjacent macrophages.

The course of the subsequent disease is determined by the host's cellular immunity as well as the species of the parasite. In cutaneous leishmaniasis, there is a marked lymphocytic infiltration associated with a reduction in the number of parasites, the development of a delayed skin (leishmanin) reaction, and, frequently, spontaneous cure. In mucocutaneous disease, the complete or partial resolution of the primary lesion may be followed by metastatic mucocutaneous lesions at a later date. The destructiveness of the metastatic lesions is attributed to the development of hypersensitivity to parasite antigens. In diffuse cutaneous leishmaniasis there is no infiltration by lymphocytes or reduction in the number of parasites, the leishmanin reaction remains negative, and the skin lesions become chronic, progressive, and disseminated. The patients have a selective anergy to *Leishmania* antigens that is mediated at least in part by adherent suppressor cells. In visceral leishmaniasis the parasites spread to macrophages throughout the body, perhaps due to the greater resistance of *L. donovani* to the spontaneous cidal activity present in normal serum. Although antibodies are present, they are nonprotective. The ability of the organism to cause progressive disease may be related to the development in the host of suppressor T lymphocytes. Cure of leishmaniasis requires activation of infected macrophages by lymphokines released from sensitized T cells and confers immunity to the infecting strain.

DIAGNOSIS Diagnosis of leishmaniasis requires demonstrating the organism by smear or culture of aspirates or tissue. Although Novy-MacNeal-Nicolle (NNN) medium traditionally has been used to culture *Leishmania,* several commercially available liquid media offer improved storage capability and enhanced recovery of organisms. Cultures are maintained at 22 to 28°C for 21 days and examined microscopically for the presence of the motile promastigotes. Inoculation of hamsters with infected clinical material results in infections after a period of weeks.

Species-specific diagnosis of human cutaneous new world isolates has been achieved by hybridization of tissue touch blots with radiolabeled kinetoplast DNA probes, but the method is not readily available.

Antibodies are detectable in all forms of leishmaniasis. The direct agglutination test detects IgM antibody and is a sensitive indicator of acute disease. The test is group-specific, but the titer is generally greatest to the homologous strain. A positive test (> 1:32) varies from 97 percent in visceral leishmaniasis to 81 percent in new world cutaneous leishmaniasis. Direct agglutination antibodies decline and may disappear with cure. Complement fixation (positive > 1:8) and indirect immunofluorescence (positive > 1:16) titers[1] may persist for years after resolution of disease. Other serologic tests are less available.

VISCERAL LEISHMANIASIS (KALA AZAR) *Leishmania donovani* causes kala azar, a disease that may be endemic, epidemic, or sporadic. Although the characteristics of the disease are similar throughout the world, certain local peculiarities in its behavior justify the classification of visceral leishmaniasis into three main types. These differences are attributed principally to the length of time that the disease has been endemic in a population.

African kala azar is found in the eastern half of Africa from the Sahara in the north to the equator in the south. Sporadic cases have been reported from west Africa. It is a disease of older children and young adults (10 to 25 years); males are involved more commonly than females. It is endemic in dogs and several wild carnivores in many areas and is more resistant to therapy with antimony compounds than the forms of kala azar found in the rest of the world.

Mediterranean, or infantile, kala azar is seen primarily in the Mediterranean area, China, U.S.S.R., and Latin America. It is a disease of children under the age of 4, but adults, particularly travelers to endemic areas, are not spared. Dogs, jackals, and foxes serve as reservoirs. Rats have been identified as a potential reservoir in Italy. The strains responsible for the Eurasian and American disease are sometimes referred to as *L. infantum* and *L. chagasi,* respectively.

Indian kala azar has an age and sex distribution similar to African kala azar. Humans are the only known reservoir, and transmission is carried out by anthropophilic sandflies.

Manifestations The incubation period is generally about 3 months (3 weeks to 18 months). A primary cutaneous lesion (leishmanioma) is not uncommon in Africa. The onset of disease may be insidious or abrupt; the latter occurs more frequently in individuals from nonendemic areas. Failure to thrive is common among infected infants and children. Fever, typically nocturnal and occasionally double-quotidian, is almost universal and is accompanied by tachycardia without signs of toxemia. Diarrhea and cough are frequent. Nontender splenomegaly becomes dramatic by the third month. The liver enlarges

[1]Available from the Centers for Disease Control, Atlanta, Georgia.

less conspicuously. Cirrhosis and portal hypertension occur in about 10 percent of patients. Lymphadenopathy accompanies some cases of African kala azar. Asymptomatic and prolonged, subclinical forms of infection are common in endemic areas; malnutrition is a risk factor for the progression to full-blown disease. Fulminant kala azar has been described in patients with AIDS.

Pancytopenia is characteristic. Anemia is multifactorial: autoimmune hemolysis, splenomegaly, and gastrointestinal blood loss all contribute. The latter is exacerbated by thrombocytopenia. Agranulocytosis, cancrum oris, and superinfections complicate untreated cases. Extensive leishmanial infiltration of the gastrointestinal tract may lead to malabsorption. Hypoalbuminemia and polyclonal hypergammaglobulinemia (IgG and IgM) are constant features. Circulating immune complexes are frequently present. Immune-complex glomerulonephritis and interstitial nephritis have been described. Amyloidosis may occur in patients with chronic infections. Edema, cachexia, and hyperpigmentation (kala azar means "black fever") are late manifestations. Without treatment death occurs within 3 to 20 months in 90 to 95 percent of adults and 75 to 85 percent of children, usually from superinfections or gastrointestinal hemorrhage.

After successful treatment, 3 percent of African cases and up to 10 percent of Indian cases develop post–kala azar dermal leishmaniasis (PKDL), characterized by a spectrum of lesions ranging from depigmented macules to wartlike nodules over the face and extensor surfaces of the limbs. PKDL appears shortly after symptoms subside in African cases and typically disappears after several weeks. In the Indian disease, PKDL appears after a latent period of 1 to 2 years and may last for years, creating a persistent human reservoir.

Diagnosis Buffy coat preparations may demonstrate the parasite, particularly in Indian kala azar (90 percent). Bone marrow aspirate and biopsy are positive in over 85 percent of cases. In Kenya, splenic aspiration (95 percent) has proved quite safe and has been used serially to assess the response to therapy. In general, however, aspiration of the spleen or liver (75 percent) is not recommended because of the risk of hemorrhage. Aspirates or biopsy of enlarged lymph nodes will show parasites in 60 percent of cases. Suspicious skin lesions should be biopsied as well. The direct agglutination test is positive early in the disease. The leishmanin skin test becomes positive 6 to 8 weeks after recovery.[2] Other causes of fever in the tropics, including malaria, brucellosis, tuberculosis, typhoid, and hepatic abscess, can be distinguished by appropriate testing. PKDL must be differentiated from leprosy, syphilis, and yaws.

Treatment Transfusions and treatment of complicating superinfections must supplement specific therapy. Pentavalent antimonials are highly effective against *Leishmania* and are relatively nontoxic. Sodium antimony gluconate (Pentostam[1]; 100 mg Sb^{5+} per milliliter) is given intravenously or intramuscularly in a single daily dose of 10 mg/kg for adults and 20 mg/kg for patients under 18 years of age. Treatment should be given for at least 20 days in Indian kala azar and 30 days in other forms. Meglumine antimoniate (Glucantime; 85 mg Sb^{5+} per milliliter) can also be used. Therapy should be repeated using 20 mg/kg for 40 to 60 days in patients with relapses or incomplete responses. Periodic electrocardiographic monitoring is recommended during prolonged therapy. The addition of oral allopurinol (20 to 30 mg/kg per day in three divided doses) has been effective. Resistant cases must be treated with intravenous amphotericin B (0.5 to 1 mg/kg on alternate days) or pentamidine (3 to 4 mg/kg three times per week for 5 to 25 weeks, depending on the response). Adjunctive splenectomy has been successful in some cases of drug-resistant kala azar. Mortality remains 15 to 25 percent in advanced cases, although the cure rate is over 90 percent when therapy is given early. Follow-up at 3 and 12 months is recommended to detect relapses. PKDL should be treated in the same fashion as the initial illness. Recombinant human interferon-γ has shown promise as adjunctive therapy with pentavalent antimony in previous treatment failures or in seriously ill patients with kala azar.

[2]The leishmanin skin test (Montenegro test), performed by the intradermal injection of promastigote antigens, is nonstandardized and generally unavailable.

Prevention Preventive measures include early treatment of human cases, elimination of diseased dogs, and the use of DDT against sandflies. Application of insect repellents and the use of fine netting are important for travelers. There are no useful prophylactic agents.

CUTANEOUS AND MUCOCUTANEOUS LEISHMANIASIS This form of leishmaniasis is caused by a number of species in both the old world and the new world. Disease is characterized by the development of single or multiple localized lesions on exposed areas of skin that typically ulcerate. Although spontaneous healing is the rule for old world cutaneous leishmaniasis, this is less common in new world disease.

Old world cutaneous leishmaniasis *L. tropica* causes anthroponotic (urban, chronic, dry) cutaneous leishmaniasis, an endemic disease of children and young adults in areas bordering the Mediterranean, the Middle East, the southern U.S.S.R., and India. The principal reservoirs are humans, although domestic dogs are synanthropic hosts. The incubation period ranges from 2 to 24 months. Usually the lesion begins as a single, red pruritic papule on the face (oriental sore). The central area ulcerates and slowly enlarges centrifugally, reaching a size of approximately 2 cm. Lymphadenopathy is unusual. Healing occurs over 1 to 2 years and leaves a small depigmented scar. The disease can be complicated by the development of leishmaniasis recidiva, a condition marked by persistent facial lesions containing a scant number of parasites and by an exaggerated delayed hypersensitivity response to parasite antigens. Rarely, the organism may spread to the viscera.

L. major causes zoonotic (rural, acute, moist) cutaneous leishmaniasis, which is endemic to the desert areas of the Middle East, the southern U.S.S.R., and Africa. The reservoir is maintained in burrowing rodents. The incubation period ranges from 2 to 6 weeks. The initial lesions are often multiple and located on the lower extremities. Regional lymphadenopathy and satellite lesions are common. Healing with scarring occurs within 3 to 6 months. *L. major* has been implicated in cases of mucocutaneous leishmaniasis in Saudi Arabia. Although *L. major* confers immunity to *L. tropica*, the converse is not true.

L. aethiopica, maintained in rock hyraxes of the Ethiopian and Kenyan highlands, causes cutaneous leishmaniasis which may pursue a relatively prolonged course and can be complicated by the development of diffuse cutaneous leishmaniasis (see below).

DIAGNOSIS Lesions should first be cleansed with alcohol to reduce bacterial contamination, which hinders recovery of the organisms. Aspirates should be obtained from the outer edge of the ulcer. If the aspirated smears are negative, full-thickness skin biopsies from the ulcer margin should be taken for touch smears, histology, and culture. The direct agglutination test and the leishmanin skin test become positive within 4 to 6 weeks.

TREATMENT Specific therapy should be withheld in endemic areas until ulceration takes place, thereby conferring immunity. Exceptions include disfiguring or disabling lesions and lesions persisting for longer than 6 months. Treatment is with antimonials as described for kala azar, although shorter courses (10 days) are effective. Higher doses of antimony may be required for *L. aethiopica* infections (20 mg/kg twice a day for 30 days). Ulcers should be covered to prevent infection of vectors and other canine and human hosts.

New world cutaneous and mucocutaneous leishmaniasis Leishmania causing new world cutaneous disease is divided into subspecies within the *L. mexicana* and *L. braziliensis* groups. The natural reservoirs for these organisms include a wide variety of mammals inhabiting the forests of South and Central America. Organisms are transmitted to humans entering the jungle to gather chicle or to clear land. Disease is most prevalent in the Amazon basin but occurs in most countries of the area. *L. mexicana* species are endemic in south-central Texas.

L.m. mexicana causes chiclero's ulcer, or bay sore. Chicle gatherers who work in forests during the rainy season when sandflies are abundant develop isolated cutaneous lesions on the hand or head.

These show little tendency to ulcerate and generally heal spontaneously within 6 months. Ear lesions, however, persist for years and may cause extensive destruction of the pinna.

L.m. venezuelensis causes indolent nodular lesions, *L.m. garnhami* causes ulcerating lesions that usually heal spontaneously, and *L.m. amazonensis* causes persistent lesions that may be multiple and seldom heal spontaneously. *L.m. amazonensis* less frequently causes diffuse cutaneous leishmaniasis (see below) and, rarely, visceral leishmaniasis.

L.b. peruviana causes uta, a disease consisting of single or multiple ulcers typically on the face. Spontaneous healing within 3 months to a year is the rule. The reservoir is the domestic dog. The disease occurs on the western slopes of the Peruvian Andes at altitudes above 600 m (2000 ft). With widespread use of insecticides, the disease has become uncommon.

Mucocutaneous leishmaniasis, or espundia, is caused primarily by *L.b. braziliensis,* which typically produces one or several lesions on the lower extremities that undergo extensive ulceration; complete healing seldom occurs spontaneously. After months to years, metastatic lesions may appear in the nasopharynx in 2 to 5 percent of patients. Less frequently, lesions occur in the perineum. Multiple, large antecedent skin lesions and insufficient antimony therapy for the primary infection are risk factors. Nasal obstruction and epistaxis are frequent presenting symptoms. Extensive destruction of soft tissue structures ensues, with painful mutilating erosions (espundia). Fever, anemia, and weight loss are common. Death is caused by bacterial infection, inanition, aspiration, and respiratory obstruction.

L.b. panamensis causes nonhealing ulcerative lesions and *L.b. guyanensis* causes nodular lesions that persist and metastasize along lymphatics (pian bois). These strains may cause mucocutaneous leishmaniasis in Colombia.

DIAGNOSIS Speciation of the infecting organism should be attempted because of the marked differences in outcome. Skin biopsies are the preferred means of obtaining tissue for stains and culture. Parasites may be scant, particularly in mucocutaneous lesions. The direct agglutination test and the leishmanin skin test become positive within 4 to 6 weeks. Syphilis, yaws, blastomycosis, paracoccidioidomycosis, sporotrichosis, leprosy, and carcinoma must be considered in the differential diagnosis.

TREATMENT Inconspicuous lesions due to *L.b. peruviana* or *L. mexicana* subspecies other than *L.m. amazonensis* may heal spontaneously or be treated with intralesional injections of antimonials. Local heat (40 to 41°C) may accelerate healing. Disfiguring or disabling lesions, cartilaginous involvement or lymphatic spread, and lesions due to *L.m. amazonensis* or other *L. braziliensis* subspecies should be treated with systemic antimonials as described for kala azar.

Espundia should be treated with antimonials (20 mg/kg per day) for at least 30 days. Cases that fail to respond should be treated with amphotericin. Reconstructive facial prostheses should not be used until the disease has been in remission for at least 1 year without therapy. A rising antibody titer may predict relapse and indicate that further therapy is required.

Diffuse cutaneous leishmaniasis Diffuse cutaneous leishmaniasis is found in Venezuela, Brazil, and the Dominican Republic in the new world and in Ethiopia in the old world. Patients display a specific deficiency of cell-mediated immunity to leishmanial antigens. *L.m. pifanoi* (Venezuela), *L.m. amazonensis* (Brazil), members of the *L. mexicana* complex (Dominican Republic), and *L. aethiopica* (Africa) are responsible. Disease is characterized by massive dissemination of skin lesions without visceral involvement. The clinical picture often bears a striking resemblance to lepromatous leprosy. The diagnosis is not difficult, because the lesions contain large numbers of organisms. In contrast to all other types of cutaneous leishmaniasis, the leishmanin skin test remains negative. The disease is progressive and very refractory to treatment. High doses of antimony (20 mg/kg twice a day for 30 days) and multiple courses of amphotericin or pentamidine are often required to produce remission, but cures are rare.

REFERENCES

BADARO R et al: New perspectives on a subclinical form of visceral leishmaniasis. J Infect Dis 154:1003, 1986

——— et al: Treatment of visceral leishmaniasis with pentavalent antimony and interferon gamma. N Engl J Med 322:16, 1990

BALLOU WR et al: Safety and efficacy of high-dose sodium stibogluconate therapy of American cutaneous leishmaniasis. Lancet 2:13, 1987

BERENGUER J et al: Visceral leishmaniasis in patients infected with human immunodeficiency virus (HIV). Ann Intern Med 111:129, 1989

BERMAN JD: Chemotherapy for leishmaniasis: Biochemical mechanisms, clinical efficacy and future strategies. Rev Infect Dis 10:560, 1988

MARSDEN PD: Mucosal leishmaniasis ("espundia" Escomel, 1911). Trans R Soc Trop Med Hyg 80:859, 1986

PETERS W, KILLICK-KENDRICK R (eds): *The Leismaniases in Biology and Medicine.* London, Academic, 1987, vols I and II

WIRTH DF et al: Leishmaniasis and malaria: New tools for epidemiologic analysis. Science 234:975, 1986

161 TRYPANOSOMIASIS

LOUIS V. KIRCHHOFF

CHAGAS' DISEASE

DEFINITION Chagas' disease, or American trypanosomiasis, is a zoonosis caused by the protozoan parasite *Trypanosoma cruzi.* Acute Chagas' disease is generally a mild, febrile illness that results from initial infection with the organism. Following spontaneous resolution of the acute illness, most infected individuals remain for life in the indeterminate phase of chronic Chagas' disease, which is characterized by subpatent parasitemia, high levels of anti-*T. cruzi* antibodies, and an absence of symptoms. In a minority of chronically infected individuals, cardiac and gastrointestinal lesions result in serious morbidity and death.

LIFE CYCLE AND TRANSMISSION *Trypanosoma cruzi* is transmitted among its mammalian hosts by hematophagous triatomine insects, or reduviid bugs. The insects become infected by sucking blood from animals or humans who have circulating parasites. The ingested organisms multiply in the gut of the reduviids, and infective forms are discharged with the feces at the time of subsequent blood meals. Transmission to a second vertebrate host occurs when breaks in the skin, mucous membranes, or conjunctivae are contaminated with bug feces that contain infective parasites. *Trypanosoma cruzi* can also be transmitted by transfusion of blood donated by infected individuals, and congenital infection occurs as well.

PATHOLOGY An indurated inflammatory lesion, called a *chagoma,* often appears at the site of the parasite's entry. Local histologic changes include intracellular parasites in leukocytes and cells of subcutaneous tissues, interstitial edema, lymphocytic infiltration, and reactive hyperplasia of adjacent lymph nodes. After dissemination, muscles, including the myocardium, may be heavily parasitized. The characteristic pseudocysts seen in sections of infected tissues are intracellular aggregates of multiplying parasites.

The pathogenesis of chronic Chagas' disease is poorly understood. The heart is the organ most commonly affected, and changes include biventricular enlargement, thinning of the ventricular walls, apical aneurysms, and mural thrombi. Widespread lymphocytic infiltration, diffuse interstitial fibrosis, and atrophy of myocardial cells are often present, but parasites are rarely demonstrated in myocardial tissue. Conduction system involvement most frequently affects the right branch and the left anterior branch of the bundle of His. In chronic Chagas' disease of the gastrointestinal tract (megadisease), the esophagus and colon may be enormously dilated and hypertrophied. On microscopic examination focal inflammatory lesions with lymphocytic infiltration are seen, and the number of neurons in the myenteric plexus is reduced.

EPIDEMIOLOGY *Trypanosoma cruzi* is found only in the Americas. Wild and domestic mammals harboring *T. cruzi* and infected reduviids are found in spotty distributions from the southern United States to southern Argentina. Humans become involved in the cycle of transmission when infected vectors take up residence in the thatched roofs and walls of primitive wood and adobe houses common in much of Latin America. Thus, human. *T. cruzi* infection is primarily a health problem among the poor in rural areas of Central and South America. Most new *T. cruzi* infections in rural settings occur in children, but the incidence is unknown because most go undiagnosed. Thousands of individuals also become infected every year through blood transfusions in urban areas. It is estimated that 10 to 12 million people are chronically infected with *T. cruzi,* more than half of whom live in Brazil. Chronic Chagas' disease is a major cause of morbidity and mortality in many areas of Latin America, including Mexico, since many chronically infected individuals eventually develop symptomatic cardiac lesions or gastrointestinal disease.

Acute Chagas' disease is rare in the United States. Three cases of autochthonous transmission have been described, and two instances of transmission by blood transfusion have occurred. In addition, between 1971 and 1989, six laboratory-acquired infections and nine imported cases of acute Chagas' disease were reported to the Centers for Disease Control (CDC). In contrast, the prevalence of chronic *T. cruzi* infections in the United States has increased. Since the mid-1970s an enormous number of Central Americans have emigrated to the United States, and in one study in Washington, D.C., 5 percent of Salvadoran and Nicaraguan immigrants were found to have chronic *T. cruzi* infections. Conservative estimates place the total number of infected immigrants at more that 50,000. The presence of these carriers of *T. cruzi* poses a significant risk of transmission by blood transfusion, as evidenced by the occurrence of the two transfusion-associated cases.

CLINICAL COURSE The first signs of acute Chagas' disease occur at least 1 week after invasion by the parasites. When the organisms have entered through a break in the skin, an indurated area of erythema and swelling, a chagoma, accompanied by local lymphadenopathy may appear. Romaña's sign, the classic finding in acute Chagas' disease, consists of unilateral painless edema of the palpebrae and periocular tissues that can result when the conjunctiva is the portal of entry. These initial local signs are followed by malaise, fever, anorexia, and edema of the face and lower extremities. Generalized lymphadenopathy and mild hepatosplenomegaly may appear. Severe myocarditis develops rarely, and most deaths in acute Chagas' disease are due to heart failure. Neurologic signs are uncommon, but meningoencephalitis has been reported. The acute symptoms resolve spontaneously in virtually all patients, who then enter the asymptomatic or indeterminate phase of chronic *T. cruzi* infection.

Symptomatic chronic Chagas' disease becomes apparent years or decades after the initial infection. The heart is commonly involved, and symptoms are due to rhythm disturbances, cardiomyopathy, and thromboembolism. Right bundle branch block is the most common ECG abnormality, but other types of AV block, premature ventricular contractions, and tachy- and bradyarrhythmias are seen frequently. Cardiomyopathy often results in right-sided or biventricular heart failure, and embolization of mural thrombi to the brain or other areas may occur. Patients with megaesophagus suffer from dysphagia, odynophagia, chest pain, and regurgitation. Aspiration can occur, especially during sleep, and repeated episodes of aspiration pneumonitis are common. Weight loss, cachexia, and pulmonary infection can result in death. Patients with megacolon are plagued by abdominal pain and chronic constipation, and advanced megacolon can cause obstruction, perforation, septicemia, and death.

DIAGNOSIS The diagnosis of acute Chagas' disease is made by detecting parasites. Microscopic examination of fresh anticoagulated blood or of the buffy coat is the simplest way to see the motile organisms. Parasites can also be seen in Giemsa-stained thin and thick blood smears. When repeated attempts to visualize the organisms are unsuccessful, mouse inoculation and culture of blood on specialized media should be performed. As a last resort, xenodiagnosis should be attempted. In this technique, uninfected reduviid bugs are allowed to feed on the patient's blood. Approximately 30 days after the blood meal, the intestinal contents of the bugs are examined for parasites. When done properly, this method is positive in virtually all patients with acute Chagas' disease and in approximately half of those with chronic infections. Since early treatment of acute Chagas' disease is extremely important, however, the decision to initiate anti-*T. cruzi* therapy in a patient with negative wet preparations and smears must be made on clinical and epidemiologic grounds before the results of these indirect methods become available. Serologic testing is of limited usefulness in diagnosing acute Chagas' disease.

The diagnosis of chronic Chagas' disease is made by detecting serum antibodies that bind to *T. cruzi* antigens. Demonstration of the parasite is not of primary importance. A number of highly sensitive serologic tests for the detection of anti-*T. cruzi* antibodies are available, including complement fixation and immunofluorescence assays, and enzyme-linked immunosorbent assay (ELISA). However, a persistent problem with these conventional assays is the occurrence of false-positive reactions, typically with sera from patients with diseases such as leishmaniasis. For this reason, it is generally recommended that positivity in one assay be confirmed in two other tests, and that well-characterized positive and negative comparison sera be included in each run. A highly sensitive and specific method for detecting anti-*T. cruzi* antibodies that employs immunoprecipitation of radiolabeled *T. cruzi* antigens has been described. This assay effectively deals with the problem of false-positive reactions and is available as a confirmatory test in the author's laboratory, but it has not been adapted for mass screening.

TREATMENT Therapy for Chagas' disease is unsatisfactory. Nifurtimox is the only drug active against *T. cruzi* that is available in the United States. In acute Chagas' disease, nifurtimox markedly reduces the duration of symptoms and parasitemia and decreases mortality. Nevertheless, its ability to eradicate parasites is limited, since patients treated with nifurtimox during the acute phase may have positive xenodiagnoses after full courses of the drug. Nifurtimox treatment should be initiated as early as possible in the acute disease. Moreover, when laboratory accidents occur in which it appears likely that *T. cruzi* infection could become established, nifurtimox therapy should be initiated without waiting for clinical or parasitologic indications of infection.

The usefulness of nifurtimox in individuals with indeterminate phase or symptomatic chronic Chagas' disease has not been established. There is no evidence that patients in the indeterminate phase are less likely to develop symptomatic disease after treatment with nifurtimox, and likewise it has not been shown that it has any effect on symptomatic chronic disease. Moreover, posttreatment xenodiagnoses are also positive in many chronically infected patients given this drug. Hence, there is no indication for treating individuals with chronic *T. cruzi* infections with nifurtimox.

Common side effects of nifurtimox include abdominal pain, anorexia, nausea, vomiting, and weight loss. Neurologic symptoms may include restlessness, disorientation, insomnia, twitching, paresthesias, polyneuritis, and seizures. These symptoms usually disappear when the dosage is reduced or treatment is discontinued. The recommended dosage for adults is 8 to 10 mg/kg body weight per day. The dose for adolescents is 12.5 to 15 mg/kg body weight per day and for children 1 to 10 years of age is 15 to 20 mg/kg body weight per day. The drug should be given by mouth in four divided doses each day, and therapy should be continued for 90 to 120 days. In the United States, nifurtimox is available from the Drug Service of the CDC, Atlanta, Georgia [telephone no. 404-639-3670 (days), 404-639-2888 (nights)].

Benznidazole is a second agent used to treat Chagas' disease. Its efficacy is similar to that of nifurtimox, and side effects include peripheral neuropathy, rash, and granulocytopenia. The recommended oral dosage is 5 mg/kg body weight per day for 60 days. Benznidazole is used widely in Latin America, but it is not available in the United States.

PREVENTION Since drug therapy is unsatisfactory and vaccines are not available, the control of *T. cruzi* transmission in endemic countries must depend on reduction of domiciliary vector populations by spraying of insecticides and improvement in rural housing. Also, in endemic areas, expansion and improvement of programs for screening donated blood for the presence of *T. cruzi* are necessary to reduce transmission by transfusion. Tourists traveling in endemic areas should avoid sleeping in dilapidated houses or in dwellings with thatched roofs. Mosquito nets and insect repellent provide additional protection.

In the United States, blood donations should not be accepted from immigrants from regions in which Chagas' disease is endemic, unless serologic assays indicate that the donor is not infected with *T. cruzi*. Moreover, immigrants from endemic regions should be screened for serologic evidence of infection with the parasite. Identification of infected individuals in this group is important, not only to prevent transmission by blood transfusion, but also to enable physicians who care for these patients to undertake appropriate diagnostic monitoring and supportive therapy. Laboratory personnel should wear gloves and eye protection when working with *T. cruzi* and with infected vectors.

SLEEPING SICKNESS

DEFINITION Sleeping sickness, or African trypanosomiasis, is caused by flagellated protozoan parasites belonging to the *Trypanosoma brucei* complex and are transmitted to humans by tsetse flies. In untreated patients the trypanosomes first cause a febrile illness that is followed months or years later by progressive neurologic impairment and death.

THE PARASITES AND THEIR TRANSMISSION The east African (*rhodesiense*) and the west African (*gambiense*) forms of sleeping sickness are caused by two trypanosome subspecies, *T. brucei rhodesiense* and *T. brucei gambiense*. These subspecies are indistinguishable morphologically but cause illnesses that are epidemiologically and clinically distinct. The parasites are transmitted by bloodsucking tsetse flies of the genus *Glossina*. The insects acquire the infection when they ingest blood from infected mammalian hosts. After many cycles of multiplication in the midgut of the vector, the parasites migrate to the salivary glands, and transmission takes place when they are inoculated during a subsequent blood meal. The injected trypanosomes multiply in the blood and other extracellular spaces and evade immune destruction in mammalian hosts for long periods because they undergo antigenic variation, a process by which the antigenic structure of the surface coat of glycoproteins changes periodically.

PATHOGENESIS AND PATHOLOGY A self-limited inflammatory lesion (trypanosomal chancre) may appear a week or so after the bite of an infected tsetse fly. A systemic febrile illness then evolves as the parasites are disseminated through the lymphatics and bloodstream. Systemic African trypanosomiasis without central nervous system (CNS) involvement is generally referred to as stage I disease. In this stage, there is widespread lymphadenopathy and splenomegaly, reflecting marked lymphocytic and histiocytic proliferation and invasion of morular cells, which are plasmacytes that may be involved in the production of IgM. An endarteritis with perivascular infiltration of both parasites and lymphocytes may develop in lymph nodes and spleen. Myocarditis is common in stage I disease, especially with *T. b. rhodesiense* infection.

Hematologic manifestations in stage I trypanosomiasis include moderate leukocytosis, thrombocytopenia, and anemia. High levels of immunoglobulins, primarily polyclonal IgM, are a constant feature, and heterophile antibodies, anti-DNA antibodies, and rheumatoid factor are often detected. High levels of antigen-antibody complexes may play a role in the tissue damage and increased vascular permeability that facilitate dissemination of the parasites.

Stage II trypanosomiasis involves invasion of the CNS. The presence of trypanosomes in perivascular areas is accompanied by intense infiltration of mononuclear cells. Cerebrospinal fluid (CSF) abnormalities include increased pressure, elevated total protein concentration, and pleocytosis. Trypanosomes also are frequently present in the CSF.

EPIDEMIOLOGY The trypanosomes that cause sleeping sickness are found only in Africa. Approximately 50 million people are at risk for acquiring African trypanosomiasis, and about 20,000 new cases are reported each year. Humans are the major reservoir of *T. b. gambiense*, and infections occur in tropical rain forests of central and West africa. Gambiense trypanosomiasis is primarily a problem in rural populations, and tourists rarely become infected. Antelope species in savanna and woodland areas of central and east Africa are the principal reservoir of *T. b. rhodesiense*. Cattle also can become infected but generally succumb to the parasite. Humans acquire *T. b. rhodesiense* infection only incidentally, for the most part from contact with the tsetse flies that feed on wild animals. Thus, the disease is an occupational hazard for individuals who work in areas where infected game and vectors are present. In addition, occasional cases of *T. b. rhodesiense* infection occur among visitors to game parks in east Africa. During the past two decades 15 cases of imported African trypanosomiasis have been reported in the United States, most of which were caused by *T. b. rhodesiense*.

CLINICAL COURSE A painful trypanosomal chancre appears in some patients at the site where parasites were inoculated. Hematogenous and lymphatic dissemination (stage I disease) is marked by the onset of fever, and, typically, bouts of high temperatures lasting several days are separated by afebrile periods. Lymphadenopathy is prominent in gambiense trypanosomiasis. The nodes are discrete, movable, rubbery, and nontender. Cervical nodes are often visible, and enlargement of the nodes of the posterior cervical triangle, or Winterbottom's sign, is a classic finding in individuals infected with *T. b. gambiense*. Pruritus is frequent, and a circinate rash is often present. Inconstant findings include malaise, headache, arthralgias, weight loss, edema, hepatosplenomegaly, and tachycardia.

Central nervous system invasion (stage II disease) is characterized by the insidious development of protean neurologic manifestations, accompanied by progressive abnormalities in the CSF. A picture of progressive indifference and daytime somnolence (sleeping sickness) sometimes alternates with restlessness and insomnia at night. A listless gaze accompanies a loss of spontaneity, and speech may become halting and indistinct. Extrapyramidal signs may include choreiform movements, tremors, and fasciculations. Ataxia is frequent, and the patient may appear to have Parkinson's disease with a shuffling gait, hypertonia, and tremors. In the final phase, progressive neurologic impairment ends in coma and death.

The most striking difference between the west African and east African trypanosomiasis is that the latter illness tends to follow a more acute course. Typically in tourists, systemic signs of infection such as fever, malaise, and headache may appear before the end of the trip or shortly after return home. Persistent tachycardia unrelated to fever is common early in the course of rhodesiense trypanosomiasis, and death may result from arrhythmias and congestive heart failure before CNS disease develops. In general, untreated east African trypanosomiasis leads to death in a matter of weeks to months, often without a clear distinction between the lymphatic and CNS stages.

DIAGNOSIS A definitive diagnosis requires detection of the parasite. If a chancre is present, fluid should be expressed and examined directly under light microscopy for the highly motile trypanosomes. The fluid should also be fixed and stained with Giemsa. Material obtained by needle aspiration of lymph nodes early in the course of the illness should be examined similarly. Examination of wet preparations and of Giemsa-stained thin and thick films of serial samples of peripheral blood is also useful. If parasites are not found by these methods, the buffy coat from 10 to 15 mL of anticoagulated blood or the pellet obtained by centrifugation of the eluate from 25 to 50 mL of blood passed through a DEAE-cellulose column should be examined. Trypanosomes may also been seen in material aspirated from the bone marrow, and the aspirate can be inoculated into liquid culture medium, as can blood, lymph node aspirates, and CSF. Finally, *T. b. rhodesiense* infection can be detected by inoculation of these specimens into mice or rats, resulting in patent parasitemias in 1 to 2 weeks. This is a highly sensitive method for the detection of *T. b. rhodesiense*, but due to host specificity, *T. b. gambiense* cannot be detected by this technique.

Examination of the CSF is mandatory in all patients suspected of having African trypanosmiasis. An increase in the CSF cell count is the first abnormality to be detected, and increased opening pressure, total protein, and IgM levels develop later. Trypanosomes may be seen in the sediment of centrifuged CSF. Any CSF abnormality in an individual in whom trypanosomes have been found in specimens from other sites must be viewed as pathognomonic for CNS involvement, and specific treatment for CNS disease must be given.

A number of serologic assays are available to aid in the diagnosis of African trypanosomiasis, but their variable sensitivity and specificity mandates that treatment decisions be based on demonstration of the parasite. Such tests are of value for epidemiologic surveys.

TREATMENT The drugs traditionally used for treatment of African trypanosomiasis are suramin, pentamidine, and organic arsenicals. In addition, eflornithine has shown promise in the therapy of west African trypanosomiasis. Gambiense and rhodesiense trypanosomiases are treated similarly, and the type of therapy is determined by the presence or absence of CNS disease, side effects, and occasionally drug resistance. Suramin and pentamidine do not penetrate the CNS well, and the more toxic arsenicals must be used in patients with CNS involvement. Eflornithine penetrates the CNS well. In the United States, these drugs can be obtained from the CDC.

The drug of choice for treatment of patients with stage I African trypanosomiasis and normal CSF is suramin. A 100- to 200-mg test dose should be administered to detect hypersensitivity. The dosage for adults is 1 g intravenously on days 1, 3, 7, 14, and 21. The regimen for children is 20 mg/kg body weight intravenously on days 1, 3, 7, 14, and 21. The drug is given by slow intravenous infusion of a freshly prepared 10% aqueous solution. Suramin can cause serious side effects and must be administered under the close supervision of a physician. Approximately 1 patient in 20,000 has an immediate, severe, and potentially fatal reaction to the drug consisting of nausea, vomiting, shock, and seizures. Less severe reactions include fever, photophobia, pruritus, arthralgias, and skin eruptions. Renal damage is the most common, important side effect of suramin. Transient proteinuria often appears during treatment. Urinalysis should be done before each dose, and the drug should be discontinued if proteinuria increases or casts and red cells appear in the sediment. Suramin should not be used in patients with renal insufficiency.

Pentamidine isethionate is the alternative drug for patients with stage I trypanosomiasis. It is effective in the early stages of gambiense trypanosomiasis, but it has a lower cure rate than suramin. In addition, some *T. b. rhodesiense* infections are unresponsive to pentamidine. The dose for both adults and children is 4 mg/kg body weight per day intramuscularly or intravenously for 10 days. Frequent, immediate side effects include nausea, vomiting, tachycardia, and hypotension. These reactions are usually transient and do not warrant cessation of therapy. Other adverse reactions include nephrotoxicity, abnormal liver function tests, neutropenia, rashes, hypoglycemia, and sterile abscesses.

An arsenical, melarsoprol, is the drug of choice for African trypanosomiasis with CNS involvement. Melarsoprol will cure both stages of the disease, and thus it is also indicated for treatment of stage I patients in whom suramin and/or pentamidine have failed or are not tolerated. However, melarsoprol should never be the first choice for therapy of stage I disease, because of its relatively high toxicity. In adults the drug should be given in 3 courses of 3 days each. The dosage is 2 to 3.6 mg/kg body weight per day intravenously in 3 divided doses for 3 days, followed 1 week later by 3.6 mg/kg body weight per day, also in 3 divided doses for 3 days. The latter course is then repeated 10 to 21 days later. In debilitated patients, 2 to 4 days of suramin treatment is administered before starting melarsoprol, and an 18-mg initial dose of the latter drug, followed by progressive increases to the standard dose, has been recommended. For children, 18 to 25 mg/kg body weight total should be given over 1 month. A starting dose of 0.36 mg/kg body weight intravenously should be increased gradually to a maximum of 3.6 mg/kg at 1 to 5 day intervals for a total of 9 to 10 doses.

Melarsoprol is highly toxic and should be administered with great care. The incidence of reactive encephalopathy has been reported to be as high as 18 percent in some series. Clinical manifestations of reactive encephalopathy include high fever, headache, tremor, impaired speech, seizures, and even coma and death. Melarsoprol should be discontinued at the first sign of encephalopathy, but may be restarted cautiously with small doses a few days after the signs have resolved. Extravasation of the drug results in intense local reactions, and vomiting, abdominal pain, nephrotoxicity, and myocardial damage can occur.

The combination of the arsenical, tryparsamide, and suramin is the alternative treatment for patients with stage II disease who cannot tolerate melarsoprol. Tryparsamide is effective against *T. b. gambiense* but not *T. b. rhodesiense*. The dose of tryparsamide is one injection of 30 mg/kg body weight every 5 days for a total of 12 injections, and that for suramin is 10 mg/kg body weight intravenously every 5 days, also for a total of 12 injections. Tryparsamide can cause encephalopathy, fever, vomiting, abdominal pain, rash, tinnitus, and a variety of ocular symptoms.

Eflornithine is an experimental drug being used to treat gambiense trypanosomiasis. When given intravenously, it appears to be effective in both stages of the disease. The dosage is 20 to 30 g/d intravenously in 4 doses for 6 to 8 weeks. Eflornithine is also available as an oral preparation, but optimal dosage and duration of therapy have not been established. Side effects include diarrhea, anemia, thrombocytopenia, and seizures and hearing loss. The efficacy of eflornithine in *T. b. rhodesiense* has not been determined. The high dosage and long duration of therapy required are disadvantages that may make widespread use difficult.

PREVENTION The trypanosomiases constitute complex public health and epizootic problems in Africa. Considerable progress has been made in some areas through control programs that focus on eradication of vectors and drug treatment of infected humans, but there is no consensus on the best approach to solving the overall problem. Individuals can reduce the risk of acquiring trypanosomiasis by avoiding areas known to harbor infected insects, by wearing protective clothing, and by using insect repellent. Chemoprophylaxis is not recommended, and no vaccine is available to prevent transmission of the parasites.

REFERENCES

Chagas' disease

Brener Z: Biology of *Trypanosoma cruzi*. Ann Rev Microbiol 27:347, 1973

Goldsmith RS et al: Clinical and epidemiologic studies of Chagas' disease in rural communities in Oaxaca state, Mexico, and a seven-year follow up: I. Cerro de Air. Bull Pan Am Health Organ 19:120, 1985

Kirchhoff LV: Is *Trypanasoma cruzi* a new threat to our blood supply? Ann Intern Med 111:773, 1989

——— et al: American trypanosomiasis (Chagas' disease) in Central American immigrants. Am J Med 82:915, 1987

——— et al: Increased specificity of serodiagnosis of Chagas's disease by detection of antibody to the 72 and 90 kDa glycoproteins of *Trypanosoma cruzi*. J Infect Dis 155:561, 1987

Marr JJ, Docampo R: Chemotherapy for Chagas' disease: A perspective of current therapy and considerations for future research. Rev Infect Dis 8:884, 1986

Schiffler RJ et al: Indigenous Chagas' disease (American trypanosomiasis) in California. JAMA 251:2983, 1984

Schmunis GA: Chagas' disease and blood transfusion, in *Infection, Immunity and Blood Transfusion*, RY Dodd, LF Barker (eds). New York, Alan R. Liss, 1984, pp 127–145

Sleeping sickness

Donelson JE: Antigenic variation in African trypanosomes. Contrib Microbiol Immunol 8:138, 1987

JORDAN AM: *Trypanosomiasis Control and African Rural Development*. London, Longmans, 1986

POLTERA AA: Pathology of human African trypanosomiasis with reference to experimental African trypanosomiasis and infections of the central nervous system. Br Med Bull 41:169, 1985

SCHECHTER PJ et al: Therapeutic utility of selected enzyme-activated irreversible inhibitors, in *Enzymes as Targets for Drug Design*, MG Palfreyman et al (eds). San Diego, Academic Press, 1989, pp 201–210

VICKERMAN K: Development cycles and biology of pathogenic trypanosomes. Br Med Bull 41:105, 1985

162 TOXOPLASMOSIS

HENRY W. MURRAY

DEFINITION Toxoplasmosis is defined by the presence of clinical and/or pathologic evidence of *active* infection caused by the obligate intracellular protozoan *Toxoplasma gondii*. Using this definition, toxoplasmosis can and should be differentiated from the much more common asymptomatic infection typically associated with exposure to this pathogen.

THE ORGANISM AND ITS LIFE CYCLE *T. gondii* exists in three forms: trophozoite (tachyzoite), tissue cyst, and oocyst. The ingested cyst and oocyst contain thousands of trophozoites which are released in the gastrointestinal tract, initiate tissue infection, and are responsible for acute toxoplasmosis. Years later, trophozoites may be liberated in the tissues by cyst rupture leading to reactivated infection.

Trophozoites are oval or crescent-shaped and measure 3 by 7 μm. The trophozoite is an obligate intracellular form which requires a host cell for growth and, therefore, cannot survive or multiply extracellularly nor be maintained in culture medium alone. Trophozoites can invade and rapidly replicate within cytoplasmic vacuoles of any nucleated cell. After several rounds of intravacuolar division by endodyogeny, trophozoites rupture free from the host cell and proceed to infect adjacent cells. The proliferating trophozoites are responsible for and define acute infection. Intracellular replication and the parasitization of new cells do not slow until an effective immune response develops.

Cysts arise within host cells, range from 10 to 200 μm in diameter, and are filled with viable trophozoites. Cysts may form within as short a time as 1 week after infection; therefore, their initial development is probably not dependent on either the host's humoral or cellular immune response. In contrast, antigen-sensitized T cells appear critical for maintenance of the organism in the cyst form and for effective control over trophozoites potentially liberated in the tissues from periodic cyst breakdown. Cysts persist for life in the mammalian host and can be found in virtually any tissue, most commonly skeletal muscle, myocardium, and brain. Cysts are the pathologic hallmark of chronic (latent) infection and remain clinically silent in immunologically normal hosts. In contrast, cysts provide a ready endogenous source of trophozoites in patients who become immunosuppressed or T cell–deficient (AIDS), putting them at particular risk for developing reactivated infection (see Chap. 264). Trophozoites released from tissue cysts in immunologically intact individuals can create retinochoroiditis and rare cases of recurrent or persistent parasitemia.

Oocysts, 10 to 12 μm in diameter, are formed exclusively by a sexual cycle in the intestinal mucosal cells of cats which have ingested either cysts in poorly cooked meat or animal tissue or oocysts shed by other cats. Three to five days after such exposure, cats develop systemic infection and also begin to excrete up to millions of oocysts per day for as long as 3 weeks. After a cat has stopped shedding oocysts in its feces, the process seldom resumes. For oocysts to become infectious after excretion, they must first sporulate, a temperature-dependent process which requires several days at room temperature and fails to occur in the cold (4°C) or heat (37°C). Oocysts may persist in the environment in an infectious state for a year or more, however, if the conditions are favorable (e.g., in moist, warm soil).

EPIDEMIOLOGY Cats, small mammals, and birds serve as the likely natural reservoirs of *T. gondii,* but virtually any animal that has access to and ingests material contaminated by oocysts or cyst-containing tissue can become infected. Cysts can be found, for example, in 10 to 25 percent of lamb and 25 percent of pork prepared for human consumption and less often in beef. If meat is not properly heated during cooking to 60°C or frozen to below −20°C, cysts remain fully viable. The prevalence or frequency of *T. gondii* infection in humans varies considerably depending upon age and other factors including dietary habits, climate, and proximity to cats. In this country, positive serologic results increase with age at the rate of about 1 percent per year making 20 to 50 percent of adults seropositive depending upon the locale. In contrast, >90 percent of adults 30 to 40 years old may be seropositive to *T. gondii* in Central America, certain islands in the South Pacific, and France, where cats are plentiful or eating rare meat is customary. Outbreaks among families or closed groups may develop after a common source exposure, but human-to-human transmission does not occur.

TRANSMISSION There are three principal modes of transmission of *T. gondii*: ingestion of oocysts or cyst-containing material, transplacental spread, and inadvertent direct administration.

Ingestion of poorly cooked lamb, pork, or beef is the most likely mechanism of transmission in developed countries where cats are confined indoors and fed processed foods and where efforts are made to cover and refrigerate food. However, outdoor cats can ingest oocysts excreted by other cats or kill and eat infected small animals, acquire infection, and then shed oocysts in areas inside and outside the home that are accessible to both children and adults. Uncovered food may also become contaminated with oocysts transferred by insects such as flies or cockroaches.

Congenital toxoplasmosis in the fetus occurs if the mother acquires the infection during pregnancy. Maternal infection acquired during the 6 months prior to conception poses a possible but very low risk to the fetus; infection acquired more than 6 months before conception presents no risk. The likelihood that acute infection in a pregnant woman will be transmitted to the fetus increases with each trimester: 15 percent in the first, 30 percent in the second, and 60 percent in the third trimester. Congenital toxoplasmosis is most severe if acquired early on in the first trimester; most infants infected in the third trimester are asymptomatic at birth. Only 20 percent of pregnant women acutely infected with *T. gondii* show clinical signs of infection; most often the diagnosis is first suggested by the results of routine post-conception serologic testing which show high titers of specific antibody.

On rare occasions, *T. gondii* has also been transmitted by needle stick injury, laboratory or autopsy room accident, transplantation of infected organs (heart or kidney) into seronegative recipients, or by transfusion of whole blood, leukocytes, or platelets. Certain immunocompromised patients, such as those with chronic myelogenous leukemia, and, rarely, normal individuals may have recurrent asymptomatic parasitemia and transmit infection by donation of their blood products. In these patients, parasitemia may develop despite the presence of high titers of circulating specific antibody. *T. gondii* can survive for up to 50 days in refrigerated anticoagulated blood.

PATHOGENESIS AND PATHOLOGY Following ingestion of cysts or oocysts, trophozoites are released in the gastrointestinal tract and invade and multiply within mucosal cells. These cells are eventually disrupted by replicating organisms, the mucosal barrier is breached, and trophozoites disseminate lymphohematogenously to infect virtually any tissue or organ. Lymph nodes, skeletal muscle, myocardium, brain, the retina, and the placenta are particularly frequent and/or clinically important target organs. In infected tissues, trophozoites enter a variety of host cells (parenchymal, endothelial, epithelial, and macrophages), replicate in the cytoplasm, rupture the cell, and proceed to infect adjacent cells. In the immunologically intact individual, acute infection in all tissues is quite rapidly brought under control with the emergence of both humoral and cellular immune responses, trophozoites disappear, and the organisms encyst. However, in immunosuppressed or T cell–deficient patients (and, rarely, in otherwise healthy individuals), acute infection is not well controlled, and retinochoroiditis and potentially fatal encephalitis, pneumonitis, or myocarditis may develop.

Focal necrosis surrounded by an intense and largely mononuclear cell inflammatory response is seen in any tissue where constantly proliferating trophozoites have caused cell destruction. Larger and more destructive lesions are typically present in congenital infection, acute infection in immunodeficient patients, and in the unusual immunologically intact individual who develops progressive disseminated disease. In contrast to the histopathologic effects provoked by replicating trophozoites, the cyst form of *T. gondii* elicits no tissue inflammatory response.

In the immunocompetent individual, pathologic data concerning acute infection have been derived principally from lymph node examination since there is seldom an indication for biopsy or removal of other involved organs. Lymphadenitis resulting from *T. gondii* produces a characteristic and near-diagnostic histologic reaction consisting of exuberant follicular hyperplasia and irregular clusters of epithelioid histiocytes (macrophages) with eosinophilic cytoplasm which encroach upon the margins of germinal centers. Granulomas are typically not present. Trophozoites or cysts are seldom demonstrated in involved lymph nodes; however, mice inoculated with infected lymph node may subsequently yield the organism. Involvement of the eye produces single or multiple necrotic lesions in which both cysts and trophozoites are present along with inflammatory infiltrates made up of monocytes, lymphocytes, and plasma cells. Complications of the necrotizing retinitis occur largely in the posterior chamber, and include granulomatous choroiditis, iridocyclitis, cataracts, and glaucoma. Retinochoroiditis is probably initiated by trophozoites released from ruptured retinal cysts; a hypersensitivity reaction directed at retinal tissue has also been proposed.

Infection in immunocompromised patients, fetuses, and in infants with severe congenital disease has provided additional histopathologic data. Findings vary greatly from scattered cysts in virtually any organ to widespread areas of inflammation and necrosis with cysts and intra- and extracellular trophozoites often found at the periphery of destructive lesions. In disseminated disease associated with either primary or reactivated infection, the brain, heart, lungs, kidneys (glomerulonephritis), pancreas, spleen, and muscle may all be involved with single or multiple necrotic lesions approaching several centimeters in diameter. Central nervous system infection is accompanied by a mononuclear cell infiltrate and microglial nodule formation and can be associated with focal or diffuse necrotizing encephalitis, meningitis, or necrotic mass lesions (abscesses) with edema. Vasculitis and necrosis in periaqueductal and periventricular areas which may calcify are typical in congenital toxoplasmosis and may result in hydrocephalus.

HOST DEFENSE IMMUNOLOGIC RESPONSE In the healthy individual, *T. gondii* infection rapidly provokes both humoral and cellular immune responses which can be detected in the serum (specific IgM and IgG antibody) and in vitro by assays which measure T-cell responsiveness to *T. gondii* antigen. Both types of immune responses appear critical for the induction of initial control over the proliferating organism, and virtually all symptomatic patients with acute infection are seropositive when first seen. Activation of T cells also probably occurs soon after acute infection, but laboratory detection of specific reactivity to *T. gondii* antigen may require 6 to 8 weeks or longer. Specific IgG antibody lyses extracellular trophozoites in the presence of the alternative complement pathway, and opsonized organisms are susceptible to killing upon ingestion by mononuclear phagocytes. Experimental evidence also suggests that soluble products (lymphokines) secreted by antigen-sensitized CD4-positive helper T cells including interleukin 2 (IL-2) and interferon-gamma (IFN-γ) are crucial components of the successful response to *T. gondii* infection (see Chap. 13). IL-2 expands T-cell populations, activates T cells and natural killer cells, and stimulates the generation of IFN-γ. IFN-γ has pleiotropic and amplifying effects including the capacity to induce otherwise susceptible cells (e.g., the tissue macrophage and probably most parenchymal cells) to kill or inhibit the intracellular replication of *T. gondii* trophozoites. In vitro, peripheral blood T cells from healthy seropositive immune individuals readily proliferate and produce IL-2 and IFN-γ after stimulation with *T. gondii* antigen; cells from T cell–deficient seropositive AIDS patients with reactivated toxoplasmosis secrete neither lymphokine. In an animal model, treatment with either IL-2 or IFN-γ protects against acute toxoplasmosis, and conversely, administration of a neutralizing anti-IFN-γ monoclonal antibody converts an avirulent to a virulent infection. The critical role of such T-cell–dependent mechanisms has been clearly reemphasized by the reactivation of latent infection in iatrogenically immunosuppressed patients and in patients with AIDS despite the presence of circulating specific antibody. In otherwise healthy individuals, acute *T. gondii* infection may also induce substantial quantitative alterations in peripheral blood T-cell subsets, including depression of CD4-positive helper cells, increases in CD8-positive suppressor cells, and reduction in the CD4/CD8 cell ratio. Although such changes may be more pronounced in symptomatic patients and persist for 6 months or longer, their clinical significance is unclear since almost all healthy patients rapidly and spontaneously recover with no sequelae.

CLINICAL MANIFESTATIONS Data from serologic surveys indicate that acute, acquired toxoplasmosis probably goes unrecognized in 80 to 90 percent of healthy adults and children, and therefore is largely a self-limited, symptom-free infection. In immunologically intact individuals, the subsequent lifelong latent infection is of no consequence unless retinal cysts break down (retinochoroiditis) or protective T cell–dependent mechanisms become impaired permitting tissue infection to reactivate in any cyst-containing organ. Although fewer than 20 percent of pregnant women with acute toxoplasmosis are symptomatic or develop lymphadenopathy, transmission via placental infection to the fetus occurs relatively frequently (depending upon the trimester) and may produce congenital toxoplasmosis. The manifestations of the congenital disease are diverse and range from simply being seropositive at birth (but at risk for late neurologic sequelae or subsequent episodes of retinochoroiditis) to overt multiorgan dysfunction and congenital malformations, to prematurity and intrauterine death. The diagnosis and management of acute toxoplasmosis during pregnancy and the treatment of both symptomatic and asymptomatic congenital toxoplasmosis require special expertise.

Acute infection in the immunocompetent adult From 7 to 21 days after exposure, up to 20 percent of patients develop lymphadenopathy which may be asymptomatic or accompanied by a brief, systemic flulike illness. Cervical lymphadenopathy is the most common manifestation of *T. gondii* infection. Enlargement may involve one or several nodes, which are usually nontender. Anterior and posterior cervical and postauricular lymphadenopathy is most frequent, but any single node or node group may be enlarged including those in mediastinum and retroperitoneum. Generalized lymphadenopathy and splenomegaly occur in less than 30 percent of symptomatic patients. Although the majority of individuals with lymphadenopathy have no symptoms or other signs, between 20 and 40 percent have low-grade fever, headache, malaise, and fatigue. Fewer than 20 percent have arthralgias, myalgias, sore throat, abdominal pain, rash, or hepatomegaly. Unusual manifestations or complications in the normal host include high or prolonged fever and unilateral retinochoroiditis; transient pneumonitis and pleural effusion, hepatitis, pericarditis, myocarditis, Guillain-Barré syndrome, intracerebral mass lesions, and meningoencephalitis are all rare. Other than fatigue and minimal to moderate lymphadenopathy, both of which can persist or recur for months, the signs and symptoms of acute toxoplasmosis typically resolve within 1 to 3 weeks. A chronic syndrome of symptomatic lymphadenopathy occurs very infrequently.

Routine laboratory studies typically indicate a normal hemoglobin and white blood cell count, a modest lymphocytosis, <6 percent atypical lymphocytes, and either normal or only modest elevations in the sedimentation rate and hepatic transaminases. A Coombs-negative hemolytic anemia, striking atypical lymphocytosis (up to 40 to 50 percent), and electrocardiographic changes are seen only occasionally. The clinical manifestations of acute toxoplasmosis are not distinctive, and may be mimicked by a variety of disorders including lymphoma, mononucleosis due to Epstein-Barr virus or cytomegalovirus, tuberculosis, sarcoidosis, cat-scratch disease, AIDS, metastatic cancer, and virtually any disease associated with lymphadenopathy. Not infrequently, the diagnosis of toxoplasmosis is first made by lymph node biopsy in patients believed to have Hodgkin's disease.

Ocular infection Up to 35 percent of cases of chorioretinitis in all age groups is thought to be caused by *T. gondii* infection, and almost always but not exclusively reflects a late sequel of congenital infection. Ocular disease is characteristically associated with bilateral retinal lesions and usually occurs in individuals 10 to 30 years old; retinochoroiditis is unusual after the age of 40. The location and extent of retinal involvement determine both the degree of visual impairment (macular lesions) and symptoms which may include blurred vision, ocular pain, photophobia, scotoma, and epiphora. Funduscopic lesions are usually multiple, ill-defined yellow-white patches centrally located at the posterior pole. Separate lesions in clusters may be in various stages of development and simultaneously show yellow-white patches, pale atrophic gray plaques, or black pigmented scars. Panuveitis, papillitis, and optic atrophy may also be present. With treatment, inflammation subsides, but recovery of visual acuity may be incomplete, relapses are common up until the age of 40 years, and with relapses visual loss may be progressive. Other infections or inflammatory disorders which may cause somewhat similar types of ocular disease include cytomegalovirus, tuberculosis, syphilis, histoplasmosis, *Herpes simplex,* leprosy, and sarcoidosis.

Toxoplasmosis in the immunosuppressed and T cell–deficient patient Although acute *T. gondii* infection can occur in any immunocompromised patient who inadvertently ingests cysts or oocysts, reactivation of previously acquired (latent) infection is the pathogenetic mechanism usually encountered. Patients with Hodgkin's disease, any individual receiving corticosteroid or immunosuppressive agents (e.g., organ transplant recipients, those with hematologic malignancies), and patients with AIDS are at particular risk (see Chap. 264). In such settings, *acute* toxoplasmosis may be associated with a widely disseminated and rapidly fatal infection characterized by high fever, pneumonia, rash, hepatosplenomegaly, myocarditis, myositis, orchitis, and especially central nervous system involvement with intracerebral mass lesions or meningoencephalitis. Lymphadenopathy may not be present.

The signs and symptoms of *reactivated* toxoplasmosis in the immunodeficient patient depend upon the location(s) of cyst breakdown and the intensity of the resultant inflammatory response. Although liberated trophozoites may be found simultaneously in a variety of areas (e.g., lung, myocardium, muscle, testes, skin, ascitic fluid) and produce signs of organ dysfunction (pneumonitis, retinitis, orchitis), clinically apparent reactivated disease is largely limited to the central nervous system. This observation has been shown repeatedly by AIDS patients seropositive for *T. gondii* in whom intracerebral toxoplasmosis appears almost entirely due to reactivated infection and not infrequently is the first manifestation of AIDS. Up to 30 percent of patients infected with human immunodeficiency virus who have antibody to *T. gondii* have developed reactivated toxoplasmosis; conversely, between 25 and 80 percent of cases of encephalitis or brain abscess in AIDS patients are caused by *T. gondii*. Immunosuppressed non-AIDS patients may be more prone to develop reactivated infection outside the brain.

Intracerebral toxoplasmosis typically presents in a subacute fashion with headache, focal neurologic signs, seizures, or altered mental status which can progress to coma. Fever is not always present. In intracerebral toxoplasmosis associated with either acute or reactivated

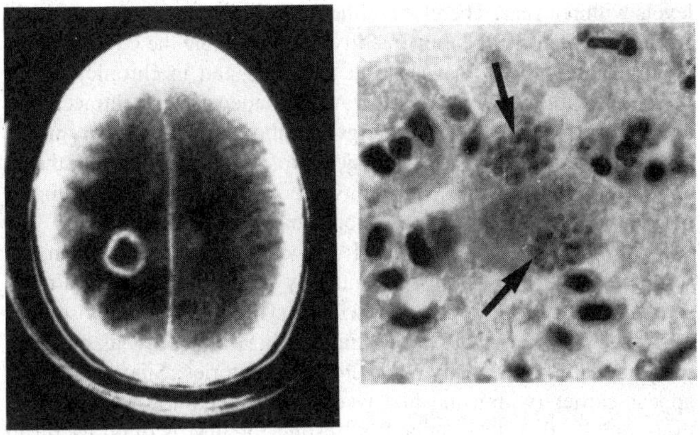

FIGURE 162-1 *Left:* Brain CT scan showing contrast-enhancing right cerebral lesion in a 35-year-old homosexual man. Biopsy demonstrated *T. gondii* cysts and free trophozoites on histologic examination. *Right:* Histologic appearance of replicating intracellular *T. gondii* trophozoites *(arrows)* in the brain biopsy of mass lesion in a patient with AIDS and neurologic signs (H & E, 600x).

infection, computed tomography (CT) of the brain may suggest encephalitis but more often shows single (Fig. 162-1) or numerous contrast-enhancing mass lesions of <2 cm in diameter with a predilection for the basal ganglia. Lesions can occur at any site in the brain, however, and may not show enhancement with contrast injection. Occasionally, the standard CT scan is normal early, in which case a follow-up scan, a double-dose-delay CT study, or magnetic resonance imaging (MRI) usually demonstrates the lesions. Cerebrospinal fluid changes include a modest mononuclear pleocytosis, moderately elevated protein, and only rarely a reduced glucose level. The diagnostic possibilities other than toxoplasmosis in an immunocompromised patient with intracerebral lesions are diverse: lymphoma, progressive multifocal leukoencephalopathy, histoplasmosis, mycobacterial infection, cryptococcosis, and encephalitis caused by cytomegalovirus and HIV. Therefore, brain biopsy (Fig. 162-1) should always be undertaken if clinically feasible. Stereotactic CT-guided needle biopsies provide a relatively safe approach with a high diagnostic yield, although excisional biopsies are usually more definitive. In AIDS patients a trial of anti-*Toxoplasma* treatment to assess response is appropriate before proceeding to brain biopsy.

DIAGNOSIS Infection with *T. gondii* is most frequently established by serologic testing for specific antibody; other methods include isolating the protozoan from clinical materials inoculated into tissue culture or mice, finding characteristic histopathologic changes (lymph node), and directly demonstrating trophozoites in either body fluids or cysts or in tissue sections. The presence of IgG antibody in the serum or cysts in the tissues may simply indicate prior infection and therefore does not imply any causal relationship to current signs or symptoms.

Serology Specific anti-*Toxoplasma* IgG antibody can be detected in the serum using the time-honored Sabin-Feldman dye test (SFDT), an indirect fluorescent antibody (IFA) test, or a complement fixation (CF) assay. Other techniques to measure IgG antibody are either not in general use or have not proved to be of particular value. In both the SFDT and IFA, positive titers (≥1:4) may be detected as early as 1 to 2 weeks after infection, are at or near their peak (≥1:1024, up to 1:64000 or greater) within 4 to 8 weeks, and begin to slowly decline after 6 to 12 months. IgG titers persist at low levels (1:16 to 1:256) for life. The rapid rise and peaking of SFDT and IFA titers accounts for the observation that 90 to 95 percent of symptomatic patients or those with lymphadenopathy have high titers (≥1:1024) when they first seek attention and also explains why diagnostic fourfold increases in SFDT or IFA titer can only be demonstrated in 20 percent of cases. Antibody detected by the CF test is generated less rapidly, appears in the serum 3 to 8 weeks after infection, rises over the next 2 to 8 months, and then declines to low or undetectable levels within a year. Therefore, although seroconversion or a fourfold increase in titer may be more readily detected using the CF test, titers may be absent both early in acute infection and in chronic (latent) infection. Up to 60 percent of AIDS patients with intracerebral toxoplasmosis have detectable IgG antibody to *T. gondii* in the cerebrospinal fluid, and in the majority of these patients, intrathecal antibody production can be demonstrated. This finding may support but does not prove that active toxoplasmosis is present.

Specific anti-*Toxoplasma* IgM antibody can be detected in the serum using an IgM fluorescent antibody (IgM-IFA) assay or a more sensitive and specific double-sandwich enzyme-linked immunosorbent technique (DS-IgM-ELISA). Testing for IgM antibody has not been well-standardized in many commercial laboratories. Since IgM titers appear earlier (within the first week after infection) and disappear more rapidly than IgG antibodies, testing for IgM is often useful in patients suspected of having acute infection. Within the first 6 months after the appearance of lymphadenopathy, sera from up to 80 percent of immunocompetent individuals show antibody in the IgM-IFA assay, and 90 percent are positive in the DS-IgM-ELISA. The absence of IgM antibody, however, does not exclude acute infection because 10 to 20 percent of patients with biopsy-proven acute-*Toxoplasma* lymphadenitis are seronegative for IgM. Between 4 and 6 months after infection, IgM-IFA titers decline to low or negative levels in 80 percent of cases. However, 50 percent of sera from acutely infected patients are still IgM antibody–positive 7 to 12 months later using the DS-IgM-ELISA, limiting the usefulness of an isolated positive titer in this test. Irrespective of the IgM or IgG test selected, acute and convalescent (4 weeks later) sera should always be obtained, frozen, and simultaneously assayed together for both IgM and IgG in the same laboratory. The presence of rheumatoid factor or antinuclear antibodies may cause false-positive reactions in both the IFA and the IgM-IFA tests.

In the immunologically intact individual, a serologic diagnosis of acute (recent) toxoplasmosis is suggested by a SFDT or IFA titer of ≥1:1024 and preferably confirmed by a fourfold rise in SFDT, IFA, or CF titer and a positive test for IgM antibody. In reactivated infection (retinochoroiditis in the normal host, intracerebral or disseminated disease in the immunosuppressed or HIV-infected patient), low serum titers (<1:1024) in the SFDT and IFA tests and absent CF and IgM titers are common. In these clinical settings, the role of serologic testing is primarily to document prior exposure to *T. gondii* by the presence of IgG antibodies. In a French study, however, sera from 20 percent of AIDS patients with *Toxoplasma* encephalitis contained IgM antibody, suggesting recent infection. These data directly contrast with the United States experience with AIDS patients (IgM antibody almost always absent) and presumably reflect the high prevalence of *T. gondii* infection (80 to 90 percent) in France. A negative (<1:4) SFDT or IFA test excludes *T. gondii* as the cause of ocular or intracerebral disease or other organ dysfunction. In congenital toxoplasmosis, maternal IgG antibody is readily passed to the fetus. However, stable or rising SFDT or IFA titers or a positive IgM test in an infant at risk or with consistent signs or symptoms strongly suggest congenital infection.

Isolation The isolation of *T. gondii* can be accomplished by injecting mice intraperitoneally with human material suspected of being infected—body fluids, buffy coat leukocytes, fetal blood clot, bone marrow, and homogenates of tissue including brain and placenta. The peritoneal fluid of inoculated mice is examined microscopically 1 to 2 weeks later for the presence of trophozoites; if none are found, mice are examined after 4 to 6 weeks for serum IgG antibody to *T. gondii* and brain cysts. In some laboratories, tissue cell cultures are also inoculated with clinical samples and examined for replicating trophozoites. Although asymptomatic parasitemia persisting for up to a year has been rarely reported, the isolation of *T. gondii* from blood or body fluids (cerebrospinal, amniotic, ascites) is considered diagnostic of acute toxoplasmosis. In contrast, the isolation of *T. gondii* from tissue homogenates does not necessarily confirm acute infection because such a result may simply reflect the presence of tissue cysts and latent infection.

Histologic diagnosis The finding of free or intracellular trophozoites (but not cysts) in tissue sections (Fig. 162-1), impression smears of tissue biopsies, or cytocentrifuge specimens of any fluid confirms the presence of acute infection. Cysts are also typically found in tissue sections, and if numerous, suggest but do not prove recent infection. Since trophozoites may be difficult to locate microscopically in conventionally stained sections, tissue likely to be infected should also be analyzed histocytochemically (immunoperoxidase assay) for the detection of trophozoites or cells bearing *T. gondii* antigen. In patients with lymphadenitis, the organism is seldom visualized; however, the histologic appearance of the lymph node tissue alone is sufficiently characteristic to permit an experienced pathologist to make the diagnosis. By itself, the inflammatory reaction in other tissues is not specific for *T. gondii* infection.

TREATMENT Pyrimethamine plus sulfadiazine The synergistic combination of pyrimethamine plus sulfadiazine, both of which inhibit folate synthesis, is active against trophozoites and is effective in treating patients with acute, reactivated, or congenital toxoplasmosis. The tissue cyst, however, is resistant to all currently available agents, and persists despite clinical responses to therapy. Once treatment is discontinued in the immunodeficient patient, relapse is common presumably because of continued breakdown of tissue cysts. In adults, oral pyrimethamine is initially administered as a 100 mg/d loading dose for 2 days and then continued at 25 mg/d given once daily thereafter. Because of its long half-life (4 to 5 days), pyrimethamine can be given every other day; however, in most immunodeficient patients, it is used daily and often increased to 50 to 75 mg/d for severe infections. Sulfadiazine is adminstered with an oral loading dose of 75 mg/kg (up to 4 g) given once followed by a total daily dose of 100 mg/kg (up to 8 g/d) administered orally in two or four divided doses. Trisulfapyrimidines in the same dosages can be substituted for sulfadiazine; other sulfonamides including sulfamethoxazole are less active. The most common adverse reaction to pyrimethamine is dose-related bone marrow suppression which may be exacerbated by sulfonamides but can be ameliorated by oral folinic acid (calcium leucovorin, 5 to 20 mg/d). Complete blood counts and platelet counts should be performed at least once or twice each week in all treated patients. Complications of sulfonamide therapy include hypersensitivity reactions (fever, rash, hepatitis) which are distressingly frequent in patients with AIDS, leukopenia, and crystalluria with potential urinary stone formation. An increased intake of fluids and high urine flow is important in sulfonamide-treated patients.

Other agents There are no uniformly accepted or clearly effective therapeutic alternatives to pyrimethamine plus sulfadiazine for the treatment of toxoplasmosis. Clindamycin, spiramycin, and trimethoprim-sulfamethoxazole each show either in vitro or in vivo anti-*Toxoplasma* effects, but are all less active and have not been systematically evaluated. However, accumulating clinical evidence suggests that clindamycin and spiramycin probably exert beneficial effects in reactivated and congenital toxoplasmosis, respectively (see below).

Indications for treatment Immunologically intact children or adults including those with lymphadenitis seldom require specific treatment for acute, acquired *T. gondii* infection. In the unusual, otherwise healthy individual with prolonged symptoms or signs suggesting vital organ involvement, 4 to 6 weeks of therapy is reasonable. Infections acquired by inadvertent direct inoculation (transfusion, laboratory accident) should also probably be similarly treated.

Retinochoroiditis Although ocular disease may remit spontaneously without specific therapy, 4 weeks of treatment with pyrimethamine and sulfadiazine results in demonstrable improvement in 70 percent of patients. Repeated courses of therapy may be required. Clindamycin, often recommended by ophthalmologists, is concentrated in the choroid and may also be effective. Control over retinal inflammation is critical in the presence of macular lesions, and systemic glucocorticoids are frequently used.

Acquired infection in pregnant women The incidence but not necessarily the severity of fetal infection can be reduced up to two- to threefold by treating pregnant women with acute toxoplasmosis. Although no one regimen has been proven to be superior, oral spiramycin (2 to 4 g/d), sulfadiazine alone, or alternating 3-week cycles of spiramycin and then sulfadiazine plus pyrimethamine (pyrimethamine is teratogenic and should only be used after the first trimester of pregnancy) all are probably effective in reducing transmission to and infection of the fetus. Some women opt for a therapeutic abortion. Irrespective of the presence of signs or symptoms of congenital toxoplasmosis, all infected infants should probably be treated to control active or subclinical infection and reduce the high likelihood of subsequent manifestations of symptomatic toxoplasmosis.

The immunodeficient patient Newly acquired or more likely reactivated toxoplasmosis always requires specific therapy in the immunosuppressed or T cell–deficient patient. For AIDS patients treated with pyrimethamine and sulfadiazine, between 60 and 80 percent show clear and rapid improvement and more than one-half of responding patients show complete resolution of clinical manifestations and brain CT scan abnormalities. In patients in whom immunosuppression can be relieved (e.g., discontinuing corticosteroid therapy), treatment is usually given for at least 4 weeks after all manifestations have resolved, which may take several months. Since the T cell–deficient state cannot be reversed in patients with AIDS, and at least 50 percent of these patients relapse once treatment is discontinued, anti-*Toxoplasma* therapy should be continued probably at full doses for life. The extraordinarily frequent drug toxicity observed in AIDS patients treated with pyrimethamine and sulfonamides often necessitates discontinuing the sulfonamide. In such cases, anecdotal information suggests that clindamycin (2.7 g/d intravenously, 1.2 to 1.8 g/d orally) can be given along with an increased dose of pyrimethamine (50 to 75 mg/d) to induce or maintain a clinical response. Relapses have occurred in patients treated with pyrimethamine or spiramycin alone, and there is insufficient experience to recommend clindamycin or trimethoprim-sulfamethoxazole alone. Addition of glucocorticoids is indicated only to reduce cerebral edema in patients with mass lesions; overall, their use has been neither beneficial nor apparently harmful. However, in patients with intracerebral disease thought but not proven to be caused by *T. gondii* (e.g., an AIDS patient seropositive to *T. gondii*, no brain biopsy), the clinical improvement induced by the use of glucocorticoids may obscure what is presumed to be a "diagnostic" response to anti-*Toxoplasma* therapy. Anti-seizure medications (e.g., phenytoin) are commonly added to treatment. Given the frequency with which toxoplasmosis develops in HIV-infected patients who have previously acquired (latent) *T. gondii* infection, it is essential to determine the efficacy of prophylactic agents (e.g., pyrimethamine-sulfadoxine) in preventing disease reactivation.

PREVENTION For seronegative pregnant women and immunodeficient patients, prevention of toxoplasmosis is important, and warnings to avoid eating undercooked meat and exposure to oocyst-containing materials are important. For seronegative immunodeficient patients as well as seronegative transplant recipients, it also seems reasonable to attempt to avoid direct inoculation by screening blood and organ donors for antibody to *T. gondii*. Although not universally accepted, recommendations for screening women two to three times during pregnancy if they are initially seronegative are also reasonable given the availability of therapy and consequences of untreated congenital infection.

REFERENCES

BROOKS RG et al: Role of serology in the diagnosis of toxoplasmic lymphadenopathy. Rev Infect Dis 9:1055, 1987

DAFFOS F et al: Prenatal management of 746 pregnancies at risk for congenital toxoplasmosis. N Engl J Med 318:271, 1988

DORFMAN RF, REMINGTON JS: Value of lymph node biopsy in the diagnosis of acute acquired toxoplasmosis. N Engl J Med 289:878, 1973

ISRAELSKI DM, REMINGTON JS: Toxoplasmic encephalitis in patients with AIDS. Infect Dis Clin North Am 2:429, 1988

LEPORT C et al: Treatment of central nervous system toxoplasmosis with pyrimethamine/sulfadiazine combination in 35 patients with the acquired immunodeficiency syndrome. Efficacy of long-term continuous therapy. Am J Med 84:94, 1988

LUFT BJ, REMINGTON JS: Toxoplasmic encephalitis. J Infect Dis 157:1, 1988

MASUR H et al: Outbreak of toxoplasmosis in a family and documentation of acquired retinochoroiditis. Am J Med 66:396, 1978

MCCABE RE et al: Clinical spectrum in 107 cases of toxoplasmic lymphadenopathy. Rev Infect Dis 9:754, 1987

———, REMINGTON JS: Toxoplasmosis: The time has come. N Engl J Med 318:313, 1988

MURRAY HW: Gamma interferon, the activated macrophage, and host defense against microbial challenge. Ann Intern Med 108:595, 1988

O'CONNOR GR: Manifestations and management of ocular toxoplasmosis. Bull NY Acad Med 50:192, 1974

RUSKIN J, REMINGTON JS: Toxoplasmosis in the compromised host. Ann Intern Med 84:193, 1976

163 PNEUMOCYSTIS CARINII PNEUMONIA

PETER D. WALZER

DEFINITION *Pneumocystis carinii* is an opportunistic pathogen whose natural habitat is the lung. The organism is an important cause of pneumonia in the compromised host.

ETIOLOGY The taxonomy of *P. carinii* is unsettled, but analysis of the organism's ribosomal RNA suggests that *P. carinii* is more closely related to fungi than to protozoa. Major developmental stages of the organism include the small (1- to 4-μm), pleomorphic trophozoite or trophic form; the 5- to 8-μm cyst, which has a thick cell wall and contains up to eight intracystic bodies; and the precyst, an intermediate stage. The life cycle of *P. carinii* probably involves asexual replication by the trophic form and sexual reproduction by the cyst which ends in release of the intracystic bodies; an intracellular stage has not been identified. Modest propagation of *P. carinii* of animal origin has been achieved in tissue culture. Ultrastructurally, *P. carinii* has a primitive organelle system, but little is known about its metabolism.

EPIDEMIOLOGY *P. carinii* has a worldwide distribution among humans and has been found in a variety of animals. Organisms for these hosts are morphologically identical, but species or strain differences exist. Data about environmental sources of *P. carinii* are lacking. Serologic surveys indicate that most normal children have been exposed to the organism by 3 to 4 years of age. Animal model experiments have demonstrated that *P. carinii* is transmitted by the airborne route. Human-to-human transmission has been suggested by the occurrence of outbreaks of pneumocystosis among institutionalized debilitated infants and in hospitals caring for immunosuppressed patients. Based on animal studies, the incubation period is thought to be 4 to 8 weeks.

PATHOGENESIS *P. carinii* pneumonia occurs in the following hosts: premature, malnourished infants; children with primary immunodeficiency diseases; patients receiving immunosuppressive therapy (particularly corticosteroids) for cancer, organ transplantation, and other disorders; and patients with the acquired immunodeficiency syndrome. AIDS is by far the most common underlying disease for *P. carinii;* conversely, *P. carinii* is the most common opportunistic infection in AIDS, occurring in at least 60 percent and perhaps up to 80 to 90 percent of patients during their lifetime (see Chap. 264).

Available data suggest that impaired cellular immunity is the major host predisposing factor in the development of pneumocystosis.

Antibodies are produced locally and systemically in response to exposure to *P. carinii*, but do not appear to have a protective role. *P. carinii* pneumonia which develops with the use of immunosuppressive drugs probably represents reactivation of latent infection. In some reports the incidence of the disease has been related to the intensity of the immunosuppression. *P. carinii* pneumonia which develops in patients with primary immunodeficiency diseases and AIDS either could arise from latent infection with the progressive breakdown of host defenses or could be acquired by contagion.

PATHOLOGY The histopathologic features of *P. carinii* pneumonia in humans and experimental animals are identical. Early in the infection the organisms line up along walls of alveoli in close apposition to the type I pneumocyte. The interaction of *P. carinii* with this alveolar cell plays a major role in the host-parasite relationship in the infection. The organisms propagate slowly and, as seen on methenamine silver–stained lung sections, gradually fill the alveolar spaces. With hematoxylin and eosin staining there is the typical foamy, vacuolated alveolar exudate which consists of organisms, host serum proteins, debris, and surfactant. On electron microscopy in the animal model there is a series of changes in alveolar microenvironment which culminate in damage to the type I cell.

The host inflammatory changes are mild and nonspecific, even with extensive infection. Hypertrophy of alveolar type II cells can frequently be found and has been interpreted as a reparative response. Alveolar macrophages are present but usually not prominent in phagocytosis of the organism. In most compromised hosts there is a mild mononuclear cell interstitial cell infiltrate; however, malnourished infants display an intense interstitial plasma cell infiltrate which was responsible for the disease's early name of "interstitial plasma cell pneumonia." Very rarely *P. carinii* can be found in tissue other than the lungs.

CLINICAL FEATURES Patients with *P. carinii* pneumonia complain of dyspnea, fever, and nonproductive cough. When corticosteroids have been administered, symptoms frequently begin after the dose has been tapered. The duration of illness until diagnosis is typically 1 to 2 weeks in non-AIDS patients, although considerable variation exists. Pneumocystosis in AIDS usually follows a more chronic and indolent course. Patients typically are ill for several weeks but sometimes may experience subtle respiratory symptoms for several months. As a consequence, *P. carinii* can be easily overlooked unless a careful history is taken. Physical findings include tachypnea, tachycardia, and cyanosis, but lung auscultation reveals few abnormalities. The white blood count is variable and usually governed by the patient's underlying disease. Arterial blood gases demonstrate hypoxemia, increased alveolar-arterial oxygen gradient ($P_{A_{O_2}} - P_{a_{O_2}}$), and respiratory alkalosis; changes in pulmonary function tests (e.g., vital capacity, diffusing capacity) are also present. These laboratory abnormalities are usually less severe in AIDS patients. The classic findings on chest radiograph consist of bilateral diffuse infiltrates beginning in the perihilar regions; with time, air bronchograms develop. Variants (e.g., nodular densities, unilateral infiltrates) to this picture have also been reported. Some patients may have a normal chest radiograph early in the course of the disease but demonstrate increased uptake on gallium scan.

DIAGNOSIS Since the clinical picture of *P. carinii* can be produced by many different infectious and noninfectious agents, diagnosis must be made by specific identification of the organism. Culture of human *P. carinii* is not yet feasible, and serology, whether based on antibody or antigen detection, is not reliable. Definitive diagnosis is made by histopathologic staining. Stains which selectively stain the cell wall of *P. carinii* cysts are the most popular. Methenamine silver is the prototype; but toluidine blue and cresyl echt violet are simpler, more rapid alternatives. Stains such as Giemsa's or Diff Quik stain both the trophozoite and cyst forms of *P. carinii;* these reagents also stain host tissues, and hence require a greater degree of experience for proper interpretation. *P. carinii* can also be stained by immunofluorescence and immunoperoxidase techniques.

Previously, *P. carinii* has been found infrequently in sputum; however, it has been shown that pneumocystosis can be diagnosed frequently in AIDS patients by examination of sputum induced by inhalation of a saline mist. This probably reflects the higher organism burden in AIDS patients as well as the improved proficiency of clinical laboratories. Fiberoptic bronchoscopy with bronchoalveolar lavage and/or transbronchial biopsy is the most commonly used procedure and has a high diagnostic yield in AIDS and non-AIDS patients. Open-lung biopsy, the most invasive technique, is usually performed when bronchoscopy is nondiagnostic or when infection with an additional organism is suspected.

COURSE AND PROGNOSIS Pneumocystosis is usually confined to the lungs, although cases of disseminated infection are receiving increasing attention. In the typical case of untreated *P. carinii* pneumonia, there is progressive respiratory embarrassment leading ultimately to death. Therapy is most effective when it is instituted early in the course of the disease before there is extensive alveolar damage. Prognosis is influenced by such factors as the patient's underlying disease and immune function, nutritional status, $P_{A_{O_2}} - P_{a_{O_2}}$, and concomitant infection with other opportunistic pathogens.

TREATMENT The two major drugs used in the treatment of *P. carinii* pneumonia have been trimethoprim-sulfamethoxazole (TMP-SMX) and pentamidine isethionate. These agents are equally effective, with an overall success rate of 70 to 80 percent. TMP-SMX acts by inhibiting folic acid synthesis, but the mode of action of pentamidine against *P. carinii* is unclear. TMP-SMX is administered orally or intravenously in a dose of 20 mg/kg per day TMP and 100 mg/kg per day SMX in four divided doses; this regimen should be modified to achieve optimum serum levels of 5 to 8 μg/mL TMP and 100 to 150 μg/mL SMX in adults. Pentamidine is given intramuscularly or by slow intravenous infusion in a dose of 4 mg/kg per day. Both drugs are administered for 14 days in non-AIDS patients and for 21 days in persons with AIDS.

TMP-SMX is well tolerated by non-AIDS patients, but over half of the AIDS patients experience serious adverse reactions including fever, rash, neutropenia, thrombocytopenia, and hepatitis. Pentamidine is a toxic drug for all recipients; major side effects include cardiovascular abnormalities, dysglycemias, azotemia, neutropenia, and sterile abscesses with intramuscular injection.

Clinical improvement usually begins after several days of therapy and is characterized by changes in fever, respiratory symptoms, and blood gases. Since persons with AIDS may respond even more slowly, it is prudent to wait at least 7 days in these patients before switching to another drug. The combination of TMP-SMX and pentamidine does not improve efficacy and may increase the risk of toxicity. Important general supportive measures include maintaining adequate oxygenation, nutrition, fluid and electrolyte balance, and tapering immunosuppressive drugs in non-AIDS patients to as low a dose as possible to control the underlying disease. The use of mechanical ventilation and other life support systems in persons with AIDS has provoked considerable debate and is best handled on an individualized basis. In cases of severe *P. carinii* pneumonia not responding to conventional therapy, glucocorticoids (e.g., methyl prednisolone) can be added with caution.

Alternative forms of therapy of pneumocystosis appear promising, but at the present time must be considered investigational. These include administration of pentamidine via aerosol, which results in high concentrations of the drug in the lungs with minimal systemic absorption; the use of trimetrexate, which is more active than TMP against *P. carinii* dihydrofolate reductase; dapsone, a sulfone which may be less toxic than SMX; α-difluoromethylornithine, which inhibits polyamine synthesis; and the combination of clindamycin and primaquine.

PREVENTION All patients who recover from pneumocystosis are at risk for recurrent episodes of the disease as long as the underlying immunosuppressive conditions persist. Persons with AIDS have the highest recurrence rate (about 50 percent at 1 year) despite the introduction of azidothymidine therapy; the mechanisms of these recurrences (i.e., relapse or reinfection) and their relationship to persisting organisms which are frequently present in follow-up bronchoscopy are unclear. TMP-SMX in the dose of 5 mg/kg per day TMP and 25 mg/kg per day SMX administered daily or three times a week has been highly effective in preventing *P. carinii* in non-AIDS patients; however, its use in AIDS patients has been limited by the high frequency of side effects. Aerosolized pentamidine is recommended as (secondary) prophylaxis for patients with previous bouts of *P. carinii* pneumonia as well as for patients with no history of pneumonia but with CD4+ T cells <200 per microliter. Other regimens including dapsone and pyramethamine-sulfadoxine are undergoing clinical evaluation and appear promising. Since none of these agents are lethal for *P. carinii,* they are only effective in chemoprophylaxis as long as they are being given. Specific environmental measures have not yet been developed, but it is prudent to separate patients with *P. carinii* infection from direct contact with other susceptible hosts.

REFERENCES

BRENNER M et al: Prognostic factors and life expectancy of patients with acquired immunodeficiency syndrome and *Pneumocystis carinii* pneumonia. Am Rev Respir Dis 136:1199, 1987

CARTER TR et al: *Pneumocystis carinii* infection of the small intestine in a patient with the acquired immunodeficiency syndrome. Am J Clin Pathol 89:679, 1988

CUSHION MT et al: Analysis of the developmental stages of *Pneumocystis carinii* in vitro. Lab Invest 58:324, 1988

EDMAN JC et al: Ribosomal RNA sequence shows *Pneumocystis carinii* to be a member of the fungi. Nature 334:519, 1988

FISCHL MA et al: Safety and efficacy of sulfamethoxazole and trimethoprim chemoprophylaxis for *Pneumocystis carinii* pneumonia in AIDS. JAMA 259:1185, 1988

HAGLER DN et al: Blastogenic responses to *Pneumocystis carinii* among patients with human immunodeficiency virus (HIV) infection. Clin Exp Immunol 74:7, 1988

KOVACS JA, MASUR H: *Pneumocystis carinii* pneumonia: Therapy and prophylaxis. J Infect Dis 158:254, 1988

MONTGOMERY AB et al: Aerosolized pentamidine as sole therapy for *Pneumocystis carinii* pneumonia in patients with acquired immunodeficiency syndrome. Lancet 2:480, 1987

MURRAY JF et al: Pulmonary complications of the acquired immunodeficiency syndrome: An update. Am Rev Respir Dis 135:504, 1987

SANKARY RM et al: Alveolar-capillary block in patients with AIDS and *Pneumocystis carinii* pneumonia. Am Rev Respir Dis 137:443, 1988

SATTLER FR et al: Trimethoprim-sulfamethoxazole compared with pentamidine for treatment of *Pneumocystis carinii* pneumonia in the acquired immunodeficiency syndrome. Ann Intern Med 109:280, 1988

STRINGER SL et al: *Pneumocystis carinii*: Sequence from ribosomal RNA implies a close relationship with fungi. Exp Parasitol 68:450, 1989

WALZER PD et al: *Pneumocystis carinii,* in *Parasitic Infections in the Compromised Host,* PD Walzer, RM Genta (eds). New York, Dekker, 1989, pp 83–178

164 BABESIOSIS

JAMES J. PLORDE

DEFINITION AND HISTORY Known since biblical times, this cosmopolitan infection of domestic and wild animals is caused by protozoa of the genus *Babesia.* These organisms are transmitted by ticks, multiply in red blood cells, and produce an acute febrile hemolytic anemia, the most prominent manifestation of which is hemoglobinuria.

EPIDEMIOLOGY AND CLINICAL MANIFESTATIONS The first human infection was described in Yugoslavia by Skrabalo in 1957. This and six other European cases were particularly severe with high fever, hemoglobinuria, jaundice, and renal failure. Both in their clinical presentation and in the presence of small intraerythrocytic parasites they closely resembled falciparum malaria with which they were originally confused. All seven occurred in splenectomized patients, and five ended fatally. The causative agents were bovine parasites (*B. bovis, B. divergens*). Some 120 cases have now been documented in the United States. Two California cases resembled the European infections and were thought to be caused by equine babesia. With the exception of single cases in Georgia and Wisconsin, all others have been acquired during the summer months on Cape Cod and the offshore islands lying between New York and Massachusetts, including Long Island, Fire Island, Shelter Island, Nantucket, and Martha's Vineyard. All of the New England and the single Wisconsin infection were caused by a rodent parasite, *B. microti,* and approximately 80 percent occurred in patients with intact spleens. The patients experienced an illness of several weeks characterized by the insidious onset of fever, chills, sweating, myalgia, and mild to moderate hemolytic anemia presumably caused by direct, parasite-induced damage to the erythrocytic membrane. The physical examination was usually negative except for occasional splenomegaly. In general, clinical manifestations have been more severe in asplenic subjects. Most patients were over 50 years of age, and all but two recovered. The carrier state persisted for weeks to months in some patients and in four resulted in subsequent transfusion-induced infections. Three of the four recipients were asplenic; the fourth was an elderly individual who represents the only fatality in the series. Serologic studies suggest that most patients infected with *B. microti* are asymptomatic; seroconversion rates of nearly 6 percent and point prevalence rates of 2 to 4.4 percent have been noted in endemic areas. All age groups seem equally susceptible. Like their symptomatic counterparts, patients with subclinical infections may remain parasitemic for several months.

B. microti has been found in field moles and deer mice in New York State, Wisconsin, Utah, and California. On the offshore islands of New England, however, the principal reservoir is the white-footed mouse. The northern deer tick, *Ixodes dammini,* which also serves as the vector in Lyme disease, is responsible for the transmission of *B. microti.* This hard-bodied tick takes a blood meal during each of its three developmental stages: larva, nymph, and adult. Rodents are the principal hosts of the first two stages while deer host the adult ticks. Only the nymphs, which feed from May through September, are capable of transmitting *B. microti* to humans. Since the engorged nymph measures 2 mm in diameter, infested patients may be oblivious to its presence. Transovarial transmission does not occur.

DIAGNOSIS The diagnosis depends on the demonstration of the intraerythrocytic parasite in Giemsa-stained peripheral blood smears. Like malaria parasites, these organisms measure 2 to 3 μm in diameter and demonstrate red-staining nuclear material with blue cytoplasm. In contrast to malaria parasites, however, neither gametocytes nor pigment are seen. As the parasites multiply by a nonsynchronous budding process, the organism displays marked pleomorphism; a single red cell may contain multiple parasites in different developmental stages. Unique basket shapes, tetrads, and trophozoites with multiple chromatin dots are helpful distinguishing features. In heavy infections, organisms can be seen outside red blood cells. Serologic diagnosis can be made with the indirect fluorescent antibody test or enzyme-linked immunosorbent assay. Because the disease is insidious in onset, most infected patients have titers ≥1024 at the time they present for medical care. There is no correlation between disease severity and the titer level; cross reactions with other *Babesia* species and malaria may be seen, but titers with homologous antigens are generally higher. Over 50 percent of patients with babesiosis have IgG- and IgM-specific antibodies to *Borrelia burgdorferi,* suggesting that simultaneous infections with these two organisms are more common than the limited number reported to date. Active infections have been demonstrated in smear-negative, serology-positive infections by inducing infection in experimental animals.

TREATMENT Mild disease should be managed symptomatically with antipyretics. If significant hemolysis ensues, transfusion may be warranted. In more severe infections specific therapy should be attempted. Although chloroquine provides symptomatic improvement, it appears to have little activity against this parasite. Oral quinine (650 mg tid for 7 days) plus clindamycin (600 mg tid for 7 days) has been successful in several patients. Antitrypanosomal agents also appear effective, and, in life-threatening infections, pentamidine should be considered. This agent appears to be effective in controlling the clinical manifestations of babesiosis and decreasing parasitemia; it may not eradicate the organism. Exchange transfusions are helpful in fulminant infections.

PREVENTION The prevention of *B. microti* infections in humans is difficult. Individuals summering on the offshore islands of New England should consider the use of insect repellents containing diethyltoluamide and examine themselves daily for the presence of the 2- to 3-mm nymphs. A pilot tick control program has been initiated on one of the islands. Asplenic patients should be advised to avoid endemic areas. To avoid transfusion-transmitted babesiosis, blood donors should be screened serologically for evidence of *B. microti* infection.

REFERENCES

BENECH JL et al: Serologic evidence for simultaneous transmission of Lyme disease and babesiosis. J Infect Dis 152:473, 1985

CHISHOLM ES et al: Indirect immunofluorescence test for human *Babesia microti* infection: Antigenic specificity. Am J Trop Med Hyg 35:921, 1986

JACOBY GA et al: Treatment of transfusion-transmitted babesiosis by exchange transfusion. N Engl J Med 303:1098, 1980

MARCUS LC et al: Fatal pancarditis in a patient with coexistent Lyme disease and babesiosis. Ann Intern Med 103:374, 1985

ROSNER F et al: Babesiosis in splenectomized adults: Review of 22 reported cases. Am J Med 76:696, 1984

RUEBUSH TK II et al: Development and persistence of antibody in persons with *Babesia microti*. Am J Trop Med Hyg 30:291, 1981

STEKETEE RW et al: Babesiosis in Wisconsin: A new focus of disease transmission. JAMA 253:2675, 1985

SUN T et al: Morphologic and clinical observations in human infection with *Babesia microti*. J Infect Dis 148:239, 1983

WITTER M et al: Successful chemotherapy of transfusion babesiosis. Ann Intern Med 96:601, 1982

165 GIARDIASIS

JAMES J. PLORDE

ETIOLOGY AND EPIDEMIOLOGY *Giardia lamblia* is a pear-shaped multiflagellar protozoan that parasitizes the human duodenum and the jejunum of humans and other animals, where it multiplies by longitudinal fission. Under a microscope, its pyriform shape, two nuclei, and central parabasal body give the organism the appearance of a face with two large eyes. It may actively browse the unstirred mucous layer at the bases of the microvilli or attach to the intestinal mucosa by means of a large ventral sucking disk. Unattached trophozoites may be carried in the fecal stream to the large bowel. If their passage through the gut is hurried, they will exit unchanged in the liquid stool and perish rapidly. With normal colonic transit times, however, the organisms retract their flagella, envelop themselves in a protective membrane, and undergo nuclear division. The resulting quadrinucleate cysts are infectious and may be transmitted to new hosts by a number of fecal-oral routes. Cysts deposited in cold water can survive for more than 2 months and have been shown to be resistant to chlorine concentrations (0.4 mg/L) routinely used in community purification systems. The ingestion of water contaminated with as few as 10 cysts is sufficient to establish human infection. Not surprisingly, waterborne outbreaks in humans have been documented repeatedly during the past two decades. In fact, *G. lamblia* is now the single most frequently defined cause of waterborne outbreaks of diarrhea in the United States. They have involved campers who have drunk from remote surface waters, skiers who have used well water, and ordinary citizens served by municipal systems with no or inadequate filtration equipment. Contamination of the water supply with raw sewage has been found in several outbreaks. In others, *G. lamblia*–infected beavers were located within the watershed, suggesting that these mammals may serve as alternate reservoirs. There have been two reports of *Giardia* transmission among swimming pool attendees. Waterborne cysts are also thought to be responsible for the high incidence of giardiasis in travelers returning from third-world countries. Food may also serve as a transmission vehicle in these areas as well.

Direct person-to-person spread occurs with some frequency. This is most dramatically evident among male homosexuals practicing anilingus, children attending day care centers, and the secondary cases seen in families of infected children. It may also explain apparent transmission from dogs to their masters.

Giardiasis is a cosmopolitan infection that is particularly common in areas with poor sanitation and among populations unable to maintain adequate levels of hygiene. The prevalence of giardiasis often exceeds 20 percent in developing countries. In the United States prevalence rates of 1 to 6 percent have been reported. Young children are three times more likely to be involved than adults, and among the institutionalized retarded, rates exceeding 50 percent have been reported. Giardiasis is also frequent in individuals with immunoglobulin deficiencies. It has been suggested that the parasite is able to persist in such patients because of a relative deficiency of secretory IgA. Similarly, the immune deficiencies accompanying protein-calorie malnutrition are thought to enhance the susceptibility of involved individuals to parasitization with *G. lamblia*.

Among adults, parasitism is common in parents of infected children, travelers to endemic areas, and campers who ingest untreated water, but the precise prevalence in these populations is unknown. Achlorhydric individuals may be more susceptible to infection. Several studies have emphasized the association between male homosexuality and intestinal parasitosis; infection rates for *G. lamblia* and/or *Entamoeba histolytica* have ranged from 11 to 40 percent.

PATHOLOGY AND PATHOGENESIS Clinical manifestations appear to be caused by an impairment of the absorptive capacity of the gut, particularly for fat and carbohydrates. The mechanism responsible for these changes is unknown. Mechanical blockage of the intestinal mucosa by large numbers of trophozoites, competition for essential nutrients, altered jejunal mobility with or without overgrowth of enteric bacteria or yeasts, pancreatic or biliary dysfunction, and organism-induced deconjugation of bile salts have been implicated. None, however, correlates well with disease severity, and eradication of associated microorganisms does not uniformly result in clinical improvement. Disaccharidase deficiency with lactose intolerance, altered levels of peptide hydrolyase and enteropeptidase, and decreased vitamin B_{12} absorption indicate that *G. lamblia* produces direct or indirect damage to the microvillar structure of the small bowel. Mechanical irritation of the fuzzy coat by the trophozoite's sucking disk might induce an accelerated turnover of the mucosal epithelium, resulting in functional immaturity of the transport systems. Excretion of a soluble toxin that interacts with the epithelial cell has been hypothesized, but never documented. Mucosal invasion may provoke a T cell–mediated insult to the jejunal mucosa. In experimentally infected nude mice immunologic reconstitution with lymphoid cells from previously infected animals results in marked mucosal changes including cellular infiltration and a decreased villus/crypt ratio. Similar pathologic findings have been reported in humans with giardial malabsorption. Both the structural changes and the malabsorption are reversible with specific therapy.

Although reinfection is common, the frequent occurrence of giardiasis in patients with immunologic defects, and the rarity with which it is seen in older adults, suggest that protective immunity, albeit incomplete, does develop with time. The diversity of surface antigens, secretory products, and DNA banding patterns in *Giardia* isolates could influence the effectiveness of the host immune response in preventing reinfection.

CLINICAL MANIFESTATIONS In endemic situations, over two-thirds of infected patients may be asymptomatic. This ratio is usually reversed in point-source outbreaks. From 1 to 3 weeks after exposure, the patient notes the explosive onset of watery diarrhea. The stool is foul smelling, greasy in appearance, and floats. There is neither blood nor mucus. Epigastric abdominal cramping is present. The formation of large quantities of intestinal gas produces distention, sulfuric eructation, and flatulence. Anorexia, nausea, vomiting, and low-grade fever may be present. Typically, acute symptoms continue for at least 5 to 7 days. In an occasional patient, they may persist for months, leading to significant malabsorption and weight loss. More commonly, the illness resolves spontaneously in 1 to 4 weeks or lapses into a chronic phase characterized by intermittent bouts of flatulence, epigastric pain, and the passage of mushy stools. It is not unusual for patients to present in this fashion without having experienced the more acute manifestations described above. Chronic giardiasis is associated with reduced growth in preschool children. Eventually, both parasites and symptoms disappear. Lactose intolerance, however, may persist, producing a clinical picture easily confused with the parasitologic disease and may result in unnecessary therapy.

DIAGNOSIS The diagnosis is made by identifying the cyst in formed feces or the trophozoite in diarrheal stools, duodenal secretions, or jejunal biopsies. In the majority of acute cases, the parasite can be demonstrated easily in a series of stool specimens collected and examined in the manner described for amebiasis (see Chap. 158). In acute illness, the onset of clinical manifestations may antedate the excretion of organisms by 5 to 7 days while in chronic infections the discharge of parasites is often scanty or intermittent, making laboratory confirmation more difficult. Many of these patients, however, can be diagnosed by examining specimens collected at weekly intervals for a period of 4 to 5 weeks. Alternatively, the duodenal contents can be sampled with a nylon string (Enterotest) or gastric tube and cultured by direct wet-mount preparation. Occasionally, jejunal biopsy is required to establish the diagnosis in patients with typical clinical manifestations. Immunodiagnostic methods for the rapid detection of *Giardia* antigen in feces appear both highly sensitive and specific, but are not commercially available. Enzyme-linked immunosorbent and indirect fluorescent serologic tests using axenically cultured *G. lamblia* have been developed. Their diagnostic usefulness remains to be established.

TREATMENT Treatment is usually carried out with quinacrine hydrochloride or metronidazole. Tinidazole, a more effective agent, is presently not available in the United States. Quinacrine, 0.1 g given three times daily for 5 days, eliminates the organisms in 70 to 95 percent of cases. Although the drug is usually well tolerated, it may produce gastrointestinal disturbances, exacerbate psoriasis, and, rarely, produce toxic psychosis. Metronidazole appears to be better tolerated and equally effective. A single oral dose of 2.0 g given on 3 consecutive days, 750 mg tid for 5 days, and 250 mg tid for 5 days give cure rates of 95, 95, and 70 percent, respectively. However, this drug is not currently licensed for giardiasis, and there is concern over its mutagenicity. Household contacts and sexual partners of infected patients should be examined; individuals harboring the parasite should be treated even if asymptomatic to prevent the spread to others. Pregnant women, however, should receive therapy only if severely symptomatic and never in the first trimester. Because parasitologic and clinical relapse can occur up to 7 weeks after the completion of therapy, long-term follow-up is essential.

PREVENTION Chemoprophylactic drugs are not effective in preventing the acquisition of giardiasis. Individuals visiting endemic areas should avoid the ingestion of potentially contaminated food and water. The latter may be made potable by boiling or by treating with a suitable halogen disinfectant. Most of the commercially available tablets appear effective when appropriate concentrations and contact times are utilized; they are temperature-dependent, and their dose should be increased when dealing with cold water. Custodial institutions for children should screen new admissions for the presence of *G. lamblia* and treat those found to be positive. Handwashing by children and staff must be emphasized. Community water purification systems should provide for adequate filtration as well as disinfection. Breast feeding appears to protect infants from giardiasis; this may be related to the known presence of antigiardial substances, including specific IgA antibodies, in breast milk.

REFERENCES

Black RE et al: Giardiasis in day-care centers—Evidence of person to person transmission. Pediatrics 60:486, 1977

Dykes AC et al: Municipal waterborne giardiasis: An epidemiologic investigation. Ann Intern Med 93:165, 1980

Gupta MC, Urrutia JJ: Effect of periodic antiascaris and antigiardia treatment on nutritional status of preschool children. Am J Clin Nutr 36:79, 1982

Jarroll EL Jr et al: *Giardia* cyst destruction: Effectiveness of six small-quantity water disinfection methods. Am J Trop Med Hyg 29:8, 1980

Nash TE et al: Experimental human infections with *Giardia lamblia*. J Infect Dis 156:974, 1987

Petersen LR et al: A food-borne outbreak of *Giardia lamblia*. J Infect Dis 157:846, 1988

Pickering LK, Engelkirk PG: *Giardia lamblia*. Ped Clin North Am 35:565, 1988

Stevens DP: Giardiasis: Host-pathogen biology. Rev Infect Dis 4:851, 1982

———: Selective primary health care: Strategies for control of disease in the developing world. XIX. Giardiasis. Rev Infect Dis 7:530, 1985

166 CRYPTOSPORIDIOSIS

JAMES J. PLORDE

DEFINITION Cryptosporidiosis is a diarrheal disease of vertebrates produced by protozoa of the genus *Cryptosporidium*. These parasites inhabit the microvillous border of the intestinal epithelium, where they produce clinical illness ranging from an acute, self-limited, watery diarrhea in normal individuals to chronic, severe, life-threatening gastroenteritis in the immunocompromised. Unknown as human pathogens prior to 1976, cryptosporidia now rank with *Salmonella, Shigella, Campylobacter,* enterotoxigenic *Escherichia coli,* rotavirus, and *Giardia lamblia* as major enteric pathogens of humans.

ETIOLOGY Regardless of animal host, most strains of this tiny parasite appear morphologically similar. Those capable of infecting humans and most domestic mammals have oocysts which measure 5 μm in diameter and are known as *C. parvum*. Cryptosporidia exhibit alternating cycles of sexual and asexual reproduction and are thereby classified as sporozoan protozoa. As is true for *Toxoplasma, Isospora,* and other members of the sporozoan subgroup known as Coccidia, both cycles are completed within the gastrointestinal tract of a single host. The infective forms or oocysts are shed into the intestinal lumen of the parasitized animal. These hardy structures are resistant to most disinfectants, chlorine concentrates generally present in municipal water supplies, and temperatures between −20°C and 60°C. In cool moist environments they may survive for months. Unlike those of *Toxoplasma* and *Isospora,* cryptosporidia oocysts are fully mature and immediately infective upon passage in the feces. Following ingestion by another animal, *sporozoites* are released from the oocyst, attach themselves to the epithelial surface, and begin a series of developmental changes. Although excluded from the cytoplasm of the epithelial cell, *trophozoites* and all subsequent developmental stages are surrounded by a double membrane of host origin and are, by definition, intracellular parasites. The trophozoites divide asexually by a process of multiple fission (*schizogony*) to form *meronts* containing eight daughter cells known as type I *merozoites*. Upon release from the meront, each merozoite attaches itself to another epithelial cell, where it repeats the schizogony cycle, producing another generation of type I merozoites. Eventually, meronts containing only four daughter cells are seen. Incapable of continued asexual reproduction, these type II merozoites are transformed into male (*microgamete*) and female (*macrogamete*) sexual forms. Following fertilization, the resulting *zygote* develops into an oocyst. The majority possess a thick, double-layered protective cell wall which ensures their intact passage in the feces and survival in the external environment. Approximately 20 percent of the oocysts, however, fail to develop such a wall. Their thin single cell membrane ruptures, releasing infective sporozoites directly into the intestinal lumen and initiating a new "autoinfective" cycle within the original host. In the normal host, the presence of innate or acquired immunity dampens both the cyclic production of type I merozoites and the formation of thin-walled oocysts, halting further parasite multiplication and terminating the acute infection. In the immunocompromised both presumably continue, explaining why such individuals develop severe, persistent infections in the absence of repeated reinfections.

EPIDEMIOLOGY Cryptosporidiosis appears to involve most vertebrate groups; the available prevalence studies demonstrate that although rare in adult animals, infection rates can be high in immature pets and farm stock. Experimental transmission of human *Cryptosporidium* strains to rodents, kittens, and puppies, and an outbreak of infection in human handlers of infected calves clearly suggest that domestic animals constitute an important reservoir of disease for humans. Disease outbreaks in day-care centers, hospitals, and urban family groups, however, indicate that most human infections result from person-to-person transmission rather than zoonotic spread. As in animals, human disease is more common in the young. In western countries, 0.6 to 4.3 percent of small children presenting to medical centers with gastroenteritis have been shown to harbor cryptosporidia oocysts; in third world countries the rates have varied from 3 to 30 percent. Up to 63 percent of children attending day-care centers during outbreaks of diarrhea have had oocysts detected in their stool. Infection rates in adults suffering from gastroenteritis are approximately one-third those reported for children and have been highest in family members of infected children, medical personnel caring for patients with cryptosporidiosis, AIDS patients, and travelers to foreign countries. Asymptomatic carriage is uncommon in the United States and Europe. However, in less well developed nations, oocysts have been found in up to 10 percent of diarrhea-free children, suggesting that early, repeated exposure may produce clinical immunity with persistent oocyst excretion. Other enteric pathogens, particularly *Giardia lamblia*, are recovered from a significant minority of infected patients. Since oocysts are found almost exclusively in stool, the principal transmission route is undoubtedly fecal-oral. In day-care centers and among male homosexual groups the spread is probably direct. The recovery of oocysts from both surface and drinking water and the documentation of at least two waterborne outbreaks makes it likely that indirect transmission via water, and possibly food and fomites, is not uncommon. The increase in infection rates seen during the summer months is compatible with this hypothesis. On rare occasions oocysts have been recovered from the pharynx or found in expectorated sputum, raising the possibility that cryptosporidiosis may be acquired through contact with the respiratory secretions of infected patients.

PATHOGENESIS AND PATHOLOGY Although the jejunum is most heavily involved, cryptosporidia have been found in the pharynx, bronchi, esophagus, stomach, duodenum, gallbladder, ileum, appendix, colon, and rectum of immunocompromised subjects. They appear as small, basophilic, spherical structures arranged in rows or clusters along the brush border of the epithelial cells. They color readily with Giemsa and hematoxylin-eosin, but not with acid-fast stains; they may be mistaken for epithelial blebs. Electron microscopy reveals the entire gamut of developmental forms including trophozoites, meronts, merozoites, and macrogametes. All are covered by a double membrane derived from the reflection, fusion, and attenuation of the microvilli over the parasite. By light microscopy, bowel changes appear minimal, consisting of mild-to-moderate villous atrophy, crypt enlargement, and a mononuclear infiltrate of the lamina propria.

The pathophysiology of the diarrhea that accompanies cryptosporidiosis is unknown, but malabsorption of fat and carbohydrate has been reported, particularly in AIDS patients, suggesting damage to the brush border. The profuse, watery diarrhea characteristic of the clinical disease raises the possibility of an enterotoxin, but none has been identified. The deep, intracellular location of some parasites may facilitate antigen processing with resultant immune-mediated damage. The vital role played by the host's immune status in the pathogenesis of the disease is further indicated by the enhanced susceptibility of the young to infection, the frequency with which clinical infection occurs during measles, and the prolonged, severe clinical disease seen in inmmunocompromised patients. Animal studies suggest that resistance to reinfection is mediated by T lymphocytes while the severity and duration of the primary infection are influenced by both cellular and humoral mechanisms.

CLINICAL MANIFESTATIONS **Immunocompetent hosts** Following an incubation period of 4 to 14 days, the patient notes the onset of an explosive, profuse, watery diarrhea accompanied by abdominal cramping. Typically, these manifestations persist for 5 to 11 days before rapidly abating; rarely, purging may continue for up to 4 weeks. When this happens, mild malabsorption with weight loss may be seen. Its shorter duration, more prominent abdominal pain and relative lack of flatulence help to distinguish cryptosporidiosis from the clinically similar *Giardia lamblia* infection. A small percentage of patients describe nausea, anorexia, low-grade fever, or vomiting. Routine laboratory work is unremarkable. Radiographic and endoscopic examinations of the gut either are normal or demonstrate mild, nonspecific abnormalities. Recovery is complete, and neither relapse nor reinfection has been reported.

Immunocompromised hosts Cryptosporidiosis has been described in patients with a broad range of immunodeficiencies. In third world countries, marasmus and other forms of childhood malnutrition have been most common. In the United States, AIDS, congenital hypogammaglobulinemia, measles, cancer chemotherapy, and immunosuppressive management of organ transplantation patients have been the abnormalities noted most frequently. In patients with these conditions, cryptosporidiosis is usually indolent in onset and prolonged in duration. The abdominal cramping and systemic manifestations are similar to those seen in normal hosts. The diarrhea, however, is characteristically more severe; fluid losses of up to 17 liters a day have been described. Unless the patient's immunologic defect is reversed, the disease usually continues in a persistent or remittent fashion for the duration of life. In two-thirds of patients, the diarrhea has lasted for more than 4 months; in a few it has persisted unabated for a number of years. Weight loss is often prominent. Patients occasionally experience cough and organisms have been identified on the bronchial epithelium of a few patients with progressive pneumonia. The prognosis depends upon the nature of the underlying immunologic abnormality; the 6-month survival rate in patients with AIDS is 50 percent. Although other intercurrent infections are usually the direct cause of death, malnutrition and complications of parenteral nutrition are often thought to play a contributory role.

DIAGNOSIS The diagnosis of cryptosporidiosis must be pursued in any immunocompromised patient who develops diarrhea. Before 1978, the diagnosis required small-bowel biopsy. The development of effective concentration and staining techniques, as well as the growing laboratory experience with this parasite, have made the recovery and identification of cryptosporidia oocysts from the stool the procedure of choice. Oocyst excretion is most intense during the first 4 or 5 days of illness, tapers during the second week, and generally stops within 1 or 2 weeks of the cessation of diarrhea; oocysts are rarely recovered from solid stool. Specimens should be examined immediately after passage or preserved in 2.5% potassium dichromate or 10% buffered formalin. Fresh and dichromate-preserved specimens are infectious and must be handled with care. The specimen may contain small amounts of mucus, but fecal erythrocytes or white cells are uncommon. Initially, an iodine wet mount can be made from the unconcentrated specimen and examined microscopically; the spherical 5-μm oocysts are differentiated from yeasts, which they resemble in size and morphology, by their failure to take up the iodine. As cryptosporidia oocysts are one of the few acid-fast particles found in feces, a presumptive identification can be made with any one of the many acid-fast staining procedures developed for mycobacteria. If the direct examinations are negative, the stool should be concentrated using either Sheather's sugar flotation or Ritchie's formalin-diethylacetate sedimentation procedure. The two are equally sensitive; use of both will improve yield in specimens with few oocysts. Supernatant from the former is examined by light or phase microscopy for the typical pink-tinged, refractile oocysts. Sediment from the formalin-diethylacetate procedure is acid-fast–stained before examination. Definitive identification of oocysts visualized by the methods described above can be afforded with commercially available, indirect immunofluorescent procedures utilizing crytosporidium-specific antibodies.

Highly sensitive and specific indirect immunofluorescent and enzyme-linked immunosorbent (ELISA) assays have been developed. IgG seroconversion occurs within 60 days of acute infection in both immunocompetent patients and those with AIDS; antibodies persist for at least 1 year. IgM antibodies rise and fall more quickly, but do not uniformly develop in patients with AIDS. Seroprevalence studies in developing nations have demonstrated that two-thirds of the population have detectable levels of specific IgG, indicating past infection. Positivity rates rose with advancing age, reaching a plateau in late childhood. The usefulness of such tests for the diagnosis of acute infection remains undetermined.

TREATMENT AND PREVENTION In the immunocompetent patient, the disease is self-limited, and attempts at specific antiparasitic therapy are not warranted. Oral, and occasionally parenteral, rehydration may be required in small children. In the immunocompromised host, the severity and chronicity of the diarrhea warrants therapeutic intervention. The only uniformly successful approach has been the reversal of underlying immunologic abnormalities. Withdrawal of cancer chemotherapy agents, discontinuation of immunosuppressive drugs, and successful bone marrow transplantation have all resulted in cure. Specific anticryptosporidial therapy has been attempted with a large number of drugs; most have been ineffective. Some patients have experienced an amelioration or complete resolution of symptoms following treatment with spiramycin, alpha-difluoromethylornithine (DFMO), oral bovine transfer factor, or trimetrexate, a folate antagonist; however, clinical failures have been common, and parasitologic cures have been reported in few. In patients who responded clinically but continued to excrete oocysts, relapses have followed discontinuation of the therapeutic agent. Because spontaneous remissions can occur, the value of these drugs in the treatment of cryptosporidiosis remains uncertain.

The stools of patients with cryptosporidiosis are infectious. Stool precautions should be instituted at the time the diagnosis is first suspected; for the immunosuppressed patient this should be whenever diarrhea, regardless of presumed etiology, is first noted. This is particularly important in cancer chemotherapy and transplantation units, where spread of the disease, directly or indirectly, from a symptomatic patient to other immunosuppressed patients can have life-threatening consequences.

REFERENCES

CURRENT WL: The biology of *cryptosporidium*. ASM News 54:605, 1988

D'ANTONIO RG et al: A waterborne outbreak of cryptosporidiosis in normal hosts. Ann Intern Med 103:886, 1985

HAYES EB et al: Large community outbreak of cryptosporidiosis due to contamination of a filtered public water supply. N Engl J Med 320:1372, 1989

JANOFF EN, RELLER LB: *Cryptosporidium* species, a protein parasite. J Clin Microbiol 25:967, 1987

KOCH KL et al: Cryptosporidiosis in hospital personnel. Evidence for person-to-person transmission. Ann Intern Med 102:593, 1985

ROBERTS WG et al: Prevalence of cryptosporidiosis in patients undergoing endoscopy: Evidence for an asymptomatic carrier state. Am J Med 87:537, 1989

SOAVE R: Cryptosporidiosis and isosporiasis in patients with AIDS. Infect Dis Clin North Am 2:485, 1988

TZIPORI S: Cryptosporidiosis in perspective. Adv Parasitol 27:63, 1988

UNGER BLP et al: Seroepidemiology of *cryptosporidium* infection in two Latin American populations. J Infect Dis 157:551, 1988

167 TRICHOMONIASIS AND OTHER PROTOZOAN INFECTIONS

JAMES J. PLORDE

TRICHOMONIASIS

Trichomoniasis is a venereal infection caused by the protozoan *Trichomonas vaginalis*. Of the many members of the genus *Trichomonas*, three are parasites of human beings: *T. hominis* in the intestine, *T. tenax* in the oral cavity, and *T. vaginalis*, the only established pathogen, in the vagina, urethra, and prostate. All three exist only in the trophozoite stage and resemble one another morphologically. *Trichomonas vaginalis* is the largest, however, and confusion in diagnosis is rare because of the anatomic specificity of their habits. Strains varying in size, growth rates, virulence, and antigenic characteristics have been described.

Trichomonas vaginalis is transmitted by sexual intercourse. Although the organism is viable for up to 24 h in urine, semen, and water and may survive on moist washcloths for a few hours, transmission by fomites is probably uncommon. Approximately 5 percent of children born to infected mothers acquire the infection. The parasite is cosmopolitan in its distribution. It is estimated that 3 million women in the United States and 180 million worldwide are infected annually; 30 to 70 percent of their male sexual partners are parasitized, at least transiently. Prevalence correlates directly with the number of sexual contacts. The incidence in adult virgins is zero; rates as high as 70 percent have been seen in prostitutes, individuals with other venereal disease, and sexual partners of infected patients. Women with trichomoniasis are, on the average, a decade older than those with gonorrhea. Although the peak incidence is between 16 and 35 years, there is a relatively high prevalence among the 30- to 40- and 40- to 50-year-old age groups.

In the female, trichomoniasis usually presents as a persistent vaginitis. It is estimated that half of women with *Trichomonas* are asymptomatic when first diagnosed. A third, however, go on to develop clinical manifestations within 6 months. In approximately two-thirds a discharge is present and is frequently accompanied by vulvar itching (50 percent), dyspareunia (50 percent), odor (10 percent), and dysuria. This acute stage may persist for a week or months, often fluctuating in intensity; it may worsen following menstruation. Eventually the discharge and other symptoms subside and may actually disappear completely, even though the patient still harbors trichomonads. Examination shows inflammation ranging from mild hyperemia of the vaginal vault and endocervix to extensive erosion, petechial hemorrhages, and perianal intertrigo. The finding of a granular, friable, reddened endocervix (strawberry cervix) is a highly characteristic, although uncommon, finding. A discharge, typically thin, gray to yellow, and frothy in nature, is found pooled in the posterior vaginal fornix.

The prostate and urethra are the usual sites of infection in the male. Most commonly the infection is completely asymptomatic, but may present as persistent or recurring nonspecific urethritis. Approximately 5 to 15 percent of all episodes of nongonococcal urethritis in males is caused by *T. vaginalis*. The prevalence is higher among those failing tetracycline therapy. Acute purulent urethritis occurs rarely.

The diagnosis is made by examining vaginal, prostatic, or urethral secretions for the presence of *Trichomonas*. The organism may also be found in the sedimented urine. A wet mount reveals squamous epithelial cells, polymorphonuclear nucleocytes, and *T. vaginalis* with its characteristic twitching motility; although highly specific when positive, it is often negative in asymptomatic women and in patients who have douched in the previous 24 h. Stained smears provide little additional help. Culture is more sensitive but is not generally available. Sensitive and specific latex agglutination, immunofluorescent, and enzyme immunoassays for *T. vaginalis* antigen that may prove useful in routine diagnostic laboratories have been developed.

Trichomonas is sometimes responsible for confusing changes in the cytologic pattern of exfoliated vaginal cells. Moreover, ordinary Papanicolaou preparations are not well suited to the diagnosis, and when trichomoniasis is suspected, fresh material should be looked at immediately.

Oral metronidazole (Flagyl), given either in dosage of 250 mg three times daily for 7 days or in a single 2-g dose, is an extremely effective therapeutic agent. Concurrent treatment of sexual partners is very important, particularly when single-dose therapy is given, if recurrent infection is to be avoided. A small number of *T. vaginalis* strains with high levels of resistance to metronidazole have been isolated from patients failing multiple courses of therapy.

The evidence that metronidazole is carcinogenic in rodents and mutagenic in bacteria mandates that the drug should not be used in the first trimester of pregnancy until further information on its teratogenicity is available. Because of the agent's antabuse-like action, alcohol consumption is contraindicated during therapy and for 24 h following its completion. Topical therapy with clotrimazole, an imidazole antifungal agent, can be employed in situations where systemic metronidazole therapy is contraindicated. The drug is applied intravaginally, in a dose of 100 mg daily for 6 days.

ISOSPORIASIS

This is an infrequently recognized disease characterized by fever, diarrhea, abdominal pain, and weight loss which results from ingestion of the oocysts of coccidia belonging to the genus *Isospora*. These sporozoan protozoa are widespread in the animal kingdom. *Isospora belli* and *Sacrocystis* (formerly *Isospora*) *hominis* have been shown to infect humans. Parasitization is much more common in children and is worldwide in distribution, particularly in tropical areas. In this country, a disproportionately large percentage of reported cases have occurred in patients with acquired immunodeficiency syndrome (AIDS).

Like the related plasmodia, there is both an asexual and sexual stage of multiplication in *I. belli* infections. However, both occur within a single host. Following the ingestion of an oocyst, *sporozoites* are released which invade the epithelial cells of the intestine to become trophozoites. These multiply asexually producing a large number of *merozoites,* which in turn invade other epithelial cells to continue the cycle. In some cells sexual gametocytes are produced. With the fertilization of the female gametocyte, an oocyst is formed which is then passed in the stool. Transmission is by the fecal-oral route. Volunteers develop symptoms about 1 week after the ingestion of viable oocysts. The illness usually has an acute onset with fever, headache, abdominal cramps, and diarrhea. Stools are often fatty and weight loss is common. Isosporiasis may be associated with a malabsorption syndrome and abnormalities of the mucosa in the small bowel. Symptoms, which presumably continue as long as the asexual cycle of multiplication continues, usually subside spontaneously within a few weeks. In the immunocompromised host, however, they are often severe, and may persist for months or even years, eventually resulting in death. Dissemination to the mesenteric and tracheobronchial lymph nodes with associated granulomatous inflammation has been reported in a patient with AIDS and cytomegalovirus enteritis.

A peripheral eosinophilia occurs in approximately half of the infected patients. The diagnosis can be made by examination of stool for oocysts. These are often scanty, and concentration techniques such as zinc sulfate flotation or the formol-ether method must usually be employed. Incubation of the stool for 2 days at room temperature improves the recovery rate. Duodenal aspiration and jejunal biopsy are less cumbersome and more reliable. The oocysts stain well with the acid-fast techniques described for the closely related *Cryptosporidium* species (see Chap. 166). *Isospora belli* infections have been successfully treated with combinations of pyrimethamine-sulfonamide and trimethoprim-sulfamethoxazole. The dose for the latter combination is 160/800 mg four times daily for 10 days, then three times daily for 3 weeks. In patients with AIDS or sulfonamide allergy, pyrimethamine alone, in the dose of 75 mg/d, can be used. Relapses in AIDS patients can be prevented by the daily administration of 25 mg.

Sarcocystis hominis oocysts are believed to be infectious only for pigs and cattle in which it produces tissue sarcocysts. Humans become infected by eating undercooked pork or beef containing the cysts. These liberate trophozoites which invade intestinal epithelial cells to undergo gametogony with the formation of new oocysts. The disease in humans is usually asymptomatic, but mild self-limited gastrointestinal manifestations have been described. Therapy is not required. The disease can be prevented by freezing raw beef and pork at −20°C (−4°F) for 24 h or cooking to an internal temperature of 65°C (150°F).

BALANTIDIASIS

Balantidium coli, the largest protozoan of human beings, inhabits the large intestine. In addition to producing an asymptomatic carrier state, it elicits disease ranging from mild recurrent diarrhea to fulminant ulceration with perforation and death. In many respects the disease is similar to amebiasis in its range of manifestations, exclusive of spread to the liver.

The illness has been reproduced by feeding the organism to volunteers. The diagnosis is made by finding the trophozoite or cyst in the stool, but repeated examinations may be required because shedding of *Balantidium* is intermittent. The disease is more likely to occur in tropical areas, particularly in Iran, New Guinea, and several Pacific islands. At least 60 cases have been reported in the United States. Swine and rats are frequent carriers of *B. coli* and may play an important role in the spread of the disease to humans. Outbreaks have been noted in mental institutions where coprophagy implicated direct person-to-person transmission.

The tetracyclines in ordinary doses are highly effective in treatment, as is iodoquinol (diiodohydroxyquinoline, INN) given in the dosage of 650 mg three times daily for 20 days. Metronidazole in the dosage used for amebiasis has also been effective (see Chap. 158).

DIENTAMEBIASIS

Dientamebiasis is an intestinal infection produced by a flagellated ameba, *Dientamoeba fragilis*. The genus and species names derive, respectively, from the binucleate nature of the trophozoite and the fragmented appearance of its nuclear chromatin. Like the related *Trichomonas* genus, the protozoan lacks a cyst stage. By virtue of its location in the large bowel, it has been thought to be spread from person to person by the fecal-oral route. However, the prevalence of the organism does not parallel that of other intestinal protozoa, its incidence in homosexual men does not correlate with the frequency of oral-anal sex, and the trophozoite is rapidly destroyed in both water and gastric juice. A mechanism of transmission compatible with these facts was suggested when *D. fragilis*–like structures were noted inside the eggs of pinworms. Several studies have demonstrated that coinfection with these two intestinal parasites is 9 to 20 times higher than that expected by random occurrence, reinforcing the possibility that the helminth eggs may serve as a vector for the protozoan trophozoite. *Dientamoeba fragilis* is a cosmopolitan parasite. Studies in this country report prevalence rates ranging from 1.4 to 18.6 percent. Rates are highest among children between 0 and 10 years of age, institutionalized individuals, communal groups, and missionaries serving in tropical areas. While *D. fragilis* was thought to be a harmless commensal of the colonic mucosal crypts, and probably is not capable of tissue invasion, it may act as a chronic irritant producing excess mucous secretion and hypermotility. Pathologic studies of surgically removed appendices shown to harbor *D. fragilis* demonstrated fibrosis that encroached upon the mucosal lymphoid tissue. Patients free of intestinal pathogens other than *D. fragilis* have reported a variety of clinical manifestations including diarrhea (58 percent) with blood or mucus (11 percent), abdominal pain (54 percent), and anal pruritus (11 percent).

The diagnosis is established by the identification of the parasite in stool. As the number of organisms varies greatly from day to day, at least three stool samples should be collected over a period of 3 to 6 days. Because the trophozoites are rapidly destroyed in the external environment, the stool should be examined immediately or preserved in polyvinyl alcohol. The use of permanent stains increases both the yield and identification accuracy of the examination. Tetracycline, iodoquinol, or metronidazole in the doses recommended for *Entamoeba histolytica* infections (see Chap. 158) have all been used. There are little data available on their relative efficacy.

BLASTOCYSTIS HOMINIS INFECTION

Previously considered a commensal yeast, it now appears that *Blastocystis hominis* is a protozoan that, at least on occasion, may act as an agent of human disease. Evidence of its protozoan nature includes the lack of a cell wall, the capacity for pseudopod formation and particulate matter ingestion, multiplication by binary fission or sporulation, and possession of a well-demarcated smooth and rough endoplasmic reticulum, membrane-bound central body, and protozoan-like mitochondria and Golgi apparatus. Physiologically the organism is a strict anaerobe that requires the presence of bacteria for growth; it grows best at a neutral pH and a temperature of 37°C (98.6°F). The organism is resistant to high concentrations of amphotericin B.

Surveys have generally found small numbers of this organism in 10 to 20 percent of human stools submitted for parasitologic studies; higher positivity rates and organism numbers have been reported in stools of AIDS patients and patients with other immunosuppressive diseases. Evidence of pathogenicity rests on the experimental induction of diarrhea in guinea pigs, its assocation with diarrhea in nonhuman primates, and a small number of reports describing human diarrheal disease, one fatal, for which no other cause could be established. Several studies attempting to evaluate the pathogenicity and clinical relevance of *B. hominis* have reported conflicting data on the rate of symptomatic enteritis in stool-positive patients, the frequency with which alternative explanations for diarrhea were available, the response of infected patients to therapy, and the correlation between resolution of symptoms and the disappearance of *B. hominis* from the stool. In the one study utilizing age- and sex-matched controls, the carriage of *B. hominis* was strongly associated with recent travel and the consumption of untreated water. Over 90 percent of patients without other enteric pathogens or apparent disease had gastrointestinal manifestations. Patients with high concentrations of *B. hominis* were significantly more likely to present with acute manifestations. Patients demonstrating a decrease in number, or a complete loss, of the parasite improved or became totally asymptomatic significantly more frequently than patients without a change in their parasite load. However, patients improved both parasitologically and clinically without therapy.

Routine stool examinations utilizing concentration and permanent staining procedures are adequate for the identification of *B. hominis*. Some authorities recommend treating symptomatic patients shown to have more than five organisms per oil immersion field if other causes of disease cannot be identified. Metronidazole and iodoquinol, used in the doses described for *E. histolytica* (see Chap. 158), appear to be suitable agents.

REFERENCES

Balantidiasis

GRAINGER CR: Endemic balantidiasis in the Seychelles. J R Soc Health 106:13, 1986
KNIGHT R: Giardiasis, isosporiasis and balantidiasis. Clin Gastroenterol 7:31, 1978
SCHMUTZHARD E, RAINER J: Acute balantidial dysentery associated with cholera: A case report. East Afr Med J 64:790, 1987

Blastocystis hominis infection

GARCIA LS et al: Clinical relevance of *Blastocystis hominis*. Lancet 1:1233, 1984
KAIN KC et al: Epidemiology and clinical features associated with *Blastocystis hominis* infection. Diagn Microbiol Infect Dis 8:235, 1987
MARKELL EK, UDKOW MP: *Blastocystis hominis:* Pathogen or fellow traveler. Am J Trop Med Hyg 35:1023, 1986
MILLER RA, MINSHEW BH: *Blastocystis hominis:* An organism in search of a disease. Rev Infect Dis 10:930, 1988

Dientamebiasis

SHEIN R, GELB A: Colitis due to *Dientamoeba fragilis*. Am J Gastroenterol 78:634, 1983
SPENCER MJ et al: *Dientamoeba fragilis*. Gastrointestinal protozoan infection in adults. Am J Gastroenterol 77:565, 1982
TURNER JA: Giardiasis and infections with *Dientamoeba fragilis*. Pediatr Clin North Am 32:865, 1985

Isosporiasis

COOK GC: Small-intestinal coccidiosis: An emergent clinical problem. J Infect Dis 16:213, 1988
DEHOVITZ JA et al: Clinical manifestations and therapy of *Isospora belli* infection in patients with the acquired immunodeficiency syndrome. N Engl J Med 315:87, 1986
RESTREPO C et al: Disseminated extraintestinal isosporiasis in a patient with acquired immune deficiency syndrome. Am J Pathol 87:536, 1987
WEISS LM et al: *Isospora belli* infection: Treatment with pyrimethamine. Ann Intern Med 109:474, 1988

Trichomoniasis

KRIEGER JN et al: Geographic variation among isolates of *Trichomonas vaginalis:* Demonstration of antigenic heterogeneity by using monoclonal antibodies and the indirect immunofluorescence technique. J Infect Dis 152:979, 1985
REIN MF, MÜLLER M: *Trichomonas vaginalis*, in *Sexually Transmitted Diseases*, 2d ed, KK Holmes et al (eds). New York, McGraw-Hill, 1990, pp 481–492
SEARS SD, O'HARE J: In vitro susceptibility of *Trichomonas vaginalis* to 50 antimicrobial agents. Antimicrob Agents Chemother 32:144, 1988
WLNER-HANSSEN P et al: Clinical manifestations of vaginal trichomoniasis. JAMA 261:571, 1989

168 TRICHINOSIS

JAMES J. PLORDE

DEFINITION Trichinosis is an intestinal and tissue infection of humans and other mammals caused by the nematode *Trichinella spiralis*. The disease is characterized by diarrhea during the development of the adults in the intestine and by myositis, fever, prostration, periorbital edema, eosinophilic leukocytosis, and, occasionally, evidence of myocarditis, pneumonitis, or encephalitis during the stage of larval migration in tissue.

ETIOLOGY Trichinosis in humans is contracted by ingestion of meat containing the encysted larvae of *T. spiralis*. The meat has almost always been domestic pork, but for the past several years about one-third of cases reported in this country have been attributed to feral meat, usually wild boar, bear, or walrus. This has been particularly frequent in the northern and western states. There are no intermediate hosts, and both the adult and larval stages develop in the same animal. Infection has been produced or observed in the bear, wild boar, wolf, coyote, fox, muskrat, horse, cow, dog, cat, rabbit, guinea pig, mouse, and marine mammals, in addition to the rat and the pig. Humans are particularly susceptible. Among pigs, infection is contracted following the feeding of uncooked scraps, less often by eating infected rats or the flesh of dead pigs. The incidence of infection in pigs has been reduced by laws requiring that garbage be cooked thoroughly before being fed. Rats also feed on uncooked pork scraps and, in addition, maintain a high incidence of infection by their cannibalism.

Soon after ingestion, the larvae are liberated from their cysts by gastric digestion and migrate into the intestinal mucosa, where maturation occurs. Following copulation the male dies, and within a week, the viviparous female is discharging larvae (100 by 6 μm), which enter the mucosal vascular channels and are distributed throughout the body. Larviposition continues for about 4 to 6 weeks, each female producing approximately 1500 offspring. The larvae enter skeletal muscle, coil, grow, and begin encysting within 3 weeks; calcification of cysts begins in 6 to 18 months. The life span of the encysted organism has been estimated at 5 to 10 years. The muscles of the diaphragm, tongue, and eye, and the deltoid, pectoral, gastrocnemius, and intercostal muscles are most often affected. Larvae carried to sites other than skeletal muscles do not encyst but disintegrate, often stimulating a granulomatous inflammatory reaction. The life cycle can be carried further only if a new host ingests the encysted larvae.

The description of a fatal case of trichinosis in an immunosuppressed patient emphasizes the importance of the immune response in limiting the intensity of infection. Apparently, it does so by acting directly on circulating larvae, inhibiting the reproduction of the female worms, and accelerating the expulsion of the adult parasites from the intestine. Eosinophils as well as B- and T-cell lymphocytes are involved in the response. The T cells appear to have a "helper" function in promoting the production of IgG and IgM antibodies which, in collaboration with eosinophils, induce fracture of the larval cuticle and disintegration of its internal structures. Once safely encysted in striated muscle, the larvae appear resistant to immunologic attack.

EPIDEMIOLOGY Trichinosis is particularly common in Europe and North America, but with the exception of Australia, India, and New Zealand, it is found worldwide. In the United States its prevalence as measured by finding cysts in human diaphragms at autopsy declined from 16.1 to 4.2 percent between 1930 and 1970. In the 1970 survey it was 1.8 percent in people under 45. The prevalence appears highest in the New England and mid-Atlantic states, Hawaii, and Alaska. It is estimated that 1.5 million Americans carry live trichinae in their musculature and that several thousand acquire new infections annually. The overwhelming majority of these infections are asymptomatic, and many of those that become clinically manifest are never correctly diagnosed. In 1986 only 51 cases were officially reported in the United States; over the last decade the case fatality rate has been 0.6 per 1000. Although pork products are not currently inspected for trichinosis, ready-to-eat products inspected by the U.S. Department of Agriculture are processed in a manner designed to destroy trichina larvae. Large outbreaks are usually caused by consumption of ready-to-eat pork sausage prepared in small commercial facilities or at home. The incidence appears highest among Americans of Italian, German, Polish, or Portuguese descent, presumably because of their inclination to make and eat pork sausage over the holiday season. Outbreaks have been reported among southeast Asian refugees living in the United States following the ingestion of undercooked pork obtained from private farms. Notable epidemics have also followed the ingestion of trichinae-infected wild pig in Hawaii and California and walrus in Alaska, the Canadian Arctic, and Greenland. Each year, a few cases are acquired from ground beef, attesting to the frequency with which this meat is adulterated with pork. Horsemeat has been implicated in several large outbreaks in France and Italy.

PATHOLOGY The adult female induces hyperemia, edema, and an eosinophilic inflammatory response in the submucosa of the small bowel. The most striking lesions are in the skeletal muscles, where there is a severe myositis with basophilic granular degeneration of the invaded muscle fiber. Adjacent fibers exhibit hyaline or hydropic degeneration, and the focus becomes infiltrated with neutrophilic and eosinophilic leukocytes, some lymphocytes, and mononuclear macrophages. Hyperemia, edema, and hemorrhages are constant features. Larvae do not encyst in cardiac muscle, but an intense myocarditis with eosinophilic infiltrates and focal necrosis has been observed in fatal cases. In cases of central nervous system involvement, there may be granulomatous nodules and vasculitis involving small arterioles and capillaries of the brain meninges, and eye. Although larvae may be present, encystment is unusual.

CLINICAL MANIFESTATIONS The severity of the clinical manifestations relates to the host's immune status, prior infection, and to the number of larvae disseminated to the tissues. Patients with severe disease usually harbor 50 to 100 larvae per gram of muscle, while those with 10 or less are often asymptomatic. The first symptoms usually appear within 1 to 2 days after ingestion of the uncooked or undercooked meat containing encysted larvae. At that time diarrhea, abdominal pain, nausea, and sometimes prostration and fever develop. Although generally brief, the intestinal phase appears to be common, severe, and prolonged in infections produced by arctic strains of trichina (*T. spiralis* var. *nativa*). The next stage, that of muscular invasion, is attenuated in *T. s. nativa* infections. Typically the muscular stage begins about the end of the first week and may last as long as 6 weeks. During this period, patients have fever, periorbital edema, conjunctivitis, muscle pain and tenderness, and often severe weakness. There may be a maculopapular rash which lasts for several days and subungual, subconjunctival, and retinal hemorrhages. More serious manifestations accompany lung, heart, or central nervous system invasion. Lung involvement is manifested by hemoptysis and consolidation on chest x-rays. Central nervous system involvement may be evident as polyneuritis, poliomyelitis, myasthenia, meningitis, encephalitis, focal or diffuse pareses, delirium, psychosis, and coma. Despite the severity of central nervous system involvement in some patients, the cerebrospinal fluid remains normal.

Myocarditis is characterized by persistent tachycardia or development of congestive heart failure. There are marked electrocardiographic alterations, including ST-T wave changes and conduction abnormalities in 20 percent of patients. High levels of circulating eosinophils may produce damage to the ventricular endothelium with superimposed thrombosis. A causal relationship between trichinosis and polyarteritis nodosa has been reported, presumably related to the presence of circulating immune complexes.

LABORATORY FINDINGS The most constant finding, and one of significance early in the course of the disease, is the eosinophilic leukocytosis (over 500 eosinophilic leukocytes per microliter) which generally appears before the end of the second week. In cases of moderate severity, the proportion of eosinophilic leukocytes peaks between 15 and 90 percent in the third or fourth week of illness. In severe cases, particularly terminally, the eosinophilic leukocytosis may disappear entirely. In severe trichinosis there may be marked hypoalbuminemia, probably because of protein leakage from damaged capillaries. During the fourth, fifth, and sixth weeks of the disease, concomitant with a rise in antibody, diffuse hypergammaglobulinemia occurs. Elevated levels of circulating IgE have been reported. There may be moderate rises in serum glutamic oxaloacetic transaminase, lactic dehydrogenase, aldolase, and creatine phosphokinase; electromyography may show evidence of altered motor function. Typically the sedimentation rate is slow.

The skin test to larval antigen becomes positive early in the third week of infection and may remain so for up to 20 years. The usual positive response is a wheal of 5 mm or more appearing within 30 min. The commercially available skin test preparations are not reliable and should not be used.

There are a variety of serologic tests for trichinosis, including the countercurrent electrophoresis test, the complement fixation test, the indirect hemagglutination test, the indirect fluorescent antibody test, and the bentonite flocculation test, which is probably the most widely used. A commercially available latex agglutination test is as sensitive but is less specific. These serologic tests all become positive during the third week of the disease and may remain positive for a few years. The highly sensitive enzyme-linked immunosorbent test is increasingly being used to detect specific antibody in the first week of infection. Since each may occasionally be falsely negative, two or more tests should be used; false negative results may be more common in *T. s. nativa* infections. The serologic tests are most valuable if they are negative initially and then turn positive or if there is a change in titer.

Muscle biopsy when carried out during the third week of infection remains the most useful test for demonstration of larvae or cysts. The deltoid or gastrocnemius muscles are the most useful sites for biopsy. A 1-g portion of the excised muscle should be compressed between glass slides and examined under a low-power microscope for the presence of larvae. Calcified cysts or larvae represent an old infection. The remainder of the biopsy should be submitted for routine processing because myositis is a significant finding even in the absence of larvae or cysts.

DIFFERENTIAL DIAGNOSIS Trichinosis must be differentiated from diseases that are characterized by eosinophilia (such as Hodgkin's disease, eosinophilic leukemia, and periarteritis nodosa) and from entities that are characterized by myopathy, such as dermatomyositis. When the central nervous system is involved, the diagnosis may be very difficult.

TREATMENT Thiabendazole (tiabendazole), in dosage of 25 mg/kg bid for 5 to 7 days (maximum 3 g/d), has resulted in apparent improvement in a number of patients, with relief of muscle pain and tenderness and with lysis of fever. The results have not been uniform and the drug may not be larvicidal. Moreover, the use of this drug in trichinosis has been associated with nausea, vomiting, abdominal discomfort, dermatitis, and drug fever. Mebendazole, given in the dosage of 400 mg tid for 2 weeks, appears to kill both adult worms and their larval offspring. Its side effects are minimal, but this drug should not be used in children or pregnant women.

Patients with "allergic" manifestations of trichinosis, including angioedema and urticaria as well as myocardial or central nervous system involvement, should be treated with prednisone in dosage of 20 to 60 mg per day. Response to steroids usually has been prompt, particularly in central nervous system trichinosis. Because steroids appear to prolong larval production, they should be given in conjunction with anthelmintics. Other measures should be directed at relief of pain and maintenance of adequate caloric and fluid intake.

PROGNOSIS The prognosis in trichinosis has improved markedly, and even when the central nervous system is involved, the mortality rate has fallen to under 10 percent. The overall mortality rate is now less than 1 percent.

PREVENTION The responsibility for control rests with the consumer. Adequate cooking of pork involves heating all portions of the meat to 77°C (170°F). Internal heating in microwave ovens is often uneven, allowing survival of larvae in apparently well-cooked meat. Meat demonstrating visibly pink juice has not been cooked adequately. Freezing procedures to kill porcine larvae require a temperature of −15°C for 20 days or −32°C for 24 h. Larvae isolated from arctic animals are more resistant to freezing. Proper smoking and pickling will also destroy the larvae. Important in control is the cooking of garbage fed to hogs. The enzyme-linked immunosorbent procedure described above is sufficiently sensitive, specific, and simple to be used for the routine inspection of pigs brought to slaughter. However, such screening tests have not been made mandatory.

REFERENCES

BAILY TM, SCHANTZ PM: Trichinosis surveillance, United States, 1986. MMWR CDC Surveill Summ 37:1, 1988

CAMPBELL WC (ed): *Trichinella and Trichinosis*. New York, Plenum, 1983

FOURESTIE V et al: Randomized trial of albendazole versus tiabendazole plus flubendazole during an outbreak of human trichinellosis. Parasitol Res 75:36, 1988

FRAYHA RA: Trichinosis-related polyarteritis nodosa. Am J Med 71:307, 1981

KAZURA JW, AIKAWA M: Host defense mechanisms against *Trichinella spiralis* infection in the mouse: Eosinophil mediated destruction of newborn larvae *in vitro*. J Immunol 124:355, 1980

KOLATA G: Testing for trichinosis: A new serological test should make it quick and easy to detect trichinosis in meat—a feat of no small economic importance. Science 227:621, 1985

MACLEAN JD et al: Trichinosis in the Canadian Arctic. Report of five outbreaks and a new clinical syndrome. J Infect Dis 160:513, 1989

METZLER MH et al: Second-degree atrioventricular block in acute trichinosis. Am J Dis Child 124:598, 1972

STEHR-GREEN JK, SHANTZ PM: Trichinosis in Southeast Asian refugees in the United States. Am J Pub Health 76:1238, 1986

169 FILARIASIS

BRUCE M. GREENE

Human filarial parasites infect an estimated 200 million persons and cause a range of disease manifestations that are relatively characteristic for individual parasite species. These include lymphadenitis, lymphangitis, elephantiasis, and other obstructive manifestations in the case of lymphatic filariasis, and blindness and dermatitis in the case of onchocerciasis. *Loa loa* causes transient subcutaneous swelling.

Although not associated with a high mortality rate, chronic filarial infection causes enormous suffering in a widely distributed population, and the socioeconomic impact due to long-term debility is extraordinarily great.

Adult filarial worms are threadlike, live in the subcutaneous tissues and lymphatics (or the peritoneum), and reproduce sexually to produce microfilariae, the first larval stage. Microfilariae are ingested by hematophagous arthropods, in which they develop into infective, or third-stage, larvae. Infective larvae molt in the vertebrate host and mature into male or female adult worms.

LYMPHATIC FILARIASIS

The three filarial parasites of humans that are associated with lymphatic filariasis are *Wuchereria bancrofti*, *Brugia malayi*, and *Brugia timori*, the latter being far less important than the other two. The threadlike adult parasites reside in the afferent lymphatic channels or lymph nodes, where they reproduce sexually to yield vast numbers of microfilariae, some of which circulate in the bloodstream. The adult females of *W. bancrofti* and *B. malayi* are approximately 4 to 10 cm in length. Bancrofti females are larger than the males; they measure about 4 and 1.5 cm, respectively. The adult parasites are quite thin, the females being approximately 250 to 150 μm in width. Adult parasites of *Brugia timori* are considerably smaller. Microfilariae are approximately 200 to 300 μm in length, and in all three species are sheathed. Infection is transmitted from person to person by mosquitoes, which ingest microfilariae while taking a blood meal. Microfilariae work their way through the wall of the proventriculus and midgut and penetrate into the thoracic muscles. They undergo two molts and over a period of approximately 2 weeks develop into infective larvae which then migrate to the tip of the labella, through which they escape at the time the blood meal is being taken. The infective larvae migrate into the tissues, and subsequently to the peripheral lymphatics, where they reside and develop into adult worms. Within the lymphatics, the male and female filariae mate, and microfilariae are discharged into the blood after 6 to 12 months. The adult parasites can live for decades in the human host.

EPIDEMIOLOGY *Wuchereria bancrofti* is the most widely distributed filarial parasite of humans, with distribution through equatorial Africa, the Indian subcontinent, southeast Asia, the western Pacific, the eastern Mediterranean region, and parts of South and Central America, as well as the Caribbean. The total number of persons infected with *W. bancrofti* is estimated to be 80 million. *B. malayi* has a much more restricted distribution, primarily involving southeast Asia and the western Pacific, with an additional focus in the southwestern coastal region of India. The total number of persons infected with the latter has been estimated at 9 million. *W. bancrofti* shows a markedly exaggerated concentration of microfilariae in the blood late at night (nocturnal periodicity) and is transmitted by *Culex* and, in urban areas, by *Anopheles* and *Aëdes* mosquitoes. There is also a subperiodic form (with less exaggerated fluctuations in microfilarial blood density) that occurs mainly in the eastern Pacific. *B. malayi* also demonstrates nocturnal periodicity and is transmitted primarily by *Anopheles* and *Mansonia* mosquitoes. A less common subperiodic form associated with an animal reservoir is transmitted by *Mansonia* and *Coquillettidia*. *B. timori* is nocturnally periodic and transmitted by *Anopheles* in Indonesia. Animal reservoirs are not thought to play a major role in epidemiology of lymphatic filariasis, although in Indonesia and Malaysia nonhuman primates may constitute an important reservoir of zoonotic filariasis that does play a part in human disease.

PATHOLOGY The principal pathologic changes in lymphatic filariasis result from chronic inflammatory damage to the lymphatics. Adult worms live in the afferent lymphatics or sinuses of the lymph nodes, and over a period of time, the lymphatics become thickened and tortuous and the lymph valves become damaged and incompetent. Histologically, there is infiltration with plasma cells, eosinophils, and macrophages in and around the affected vessels. There is endothelial and connective tissue proliferation, and eventually total lymphatic obstruction may occur. The overlying skin shows lymphedema, and chronic stasis changes with hard or brawny edema. Death of adult worms may hasten lymphatic obstruction.

PATHOGENESIS The presence of filarial parasites in the lymphatics elicits an inflammatory response. It is believed that most of the pathologic consequences of lymphatic filariasis relate to the immune response directed against the parasite, and the host immune response appears to be the major determinant of disease. In the lymphatics many highly immunogenic adult worm and microfilarial antigens are liberated; they are believed to cause the granulomatous and proliferative process that precedes obstruction. Whether microfilarial, adult worm, or infective larval antigens are of most importance in eliciting lymphatic inflammation is unknown. Superimposed bacterial infection may accelerate lymphatic blockage.

CLINICAL MANIFESTATIONS The major clinical presentation of lymphatic filariasis includes filarial fevers and lymphatic obstruction. In addition, asymptomatic individuals may be found to be microfilaremic. Tropical pulmonary eosinophilia is an uncommon presentation of infection by these parasites.

Filarial fevers are usually low-grade, but occasionally are severe and accompanied by chills. Other symptoms may include general malaise, headache, and vague pain. If the lymphangitis is superficial, pain along the lymphatics may be the predominant symptom. These episodes may occur several times a year, lasting up to a week at a time. Lymphadenitis often accompanies lymphangitis. On examination, the lymphatics are tender, thickened, firm, and red; the overlying skin is tender.

There are major differences in the clinical presentations most commonly seen in *W. bancrofti* versus *Brugia* infection. In bancroftian filariasis, the acute episodes most commonly affect the male genitalia leading to funiculitis, epididymitis, or orchitis. In contrast, lymphadenitis and lymphangitis of the extremities are more common in brugian than in bancroftian filariasis. This difference relates to the predilection that brugian filariasis has for involving the superficial inguinal nodes, typically one at a time, often with some concurrent lymphedema of the extremity. Occasional involvement of the upper extremities and, much less commonly, the breast and other areas is seen with both forms of lymphatic filariasis.

Chronic lymphatic obstruction leads to brawny edema, with thickening and hyperkeratosis of the skin. The skin becomes friable, easily abraded, and is subject to superinfection with bacteria and skin-dwelling fungi. Elephantiasis of the lower extremities in bancroftian filariasis typically involves the entire leg, while in brugian filariasis, the leg above the knee typically has a normal contour. Marked elephantiasis of the scrotum is a characteristic finding in bancroftian filariasis but tends not to occur in brugian filariasis.

Following the onset of patency, a number of individuals demonstrate asymptomatic microfilaremia. Such an individual may remain asymptomatic and spontaneously clear infection, or may develop the acute phase with recurrent lymphangitis and lymphadenitis described above.

Another category of illness associated with lymphatic filariasis is tropical eosinophilia, which is manifested primarily by respiratory symptoms including asthma, low-grade fever, and cough. This syndrome is found primarily in infected individuals from the Indian subcontinent. Marked eosinophilia, very high levels of serum IgE, and infiltrates on chest x-ray are characteristic. These individuals appear to be manifesting an abnormal immune response against the parasite, with trapping and destruction of microfilariae in the pulmonary capillaries. Pulmonary function testing demonstrates restrictive and sometimes obstructive defects.

DIAGNOSIS The diagnosis of lymphatic filariasis is made by finding microfilariae in the blood or, in the case of obstructive disease, by the clinical presentation. Usually microfilariae are not found in the latter setting. Other suggestive laboratory data include eosinophilia, particularly in association with acute symptoms and elevated titers of antifilarial antibodies. In addition to blood, microfilariae can occasionally be found in hydrocele fluid or urine. Chyluria is suggestive of bancroftian filariasis. The most efficient method for concentrating microfilariae in tissue fluids is by filtration through a 3- to 5-μm filter, through which blood cells pass freely but microfilariae are retained. Adult worms in the lymphatics are rarely found, except at autopsy.

In tropical eosinophilia, microfilariae are usually not found despite the presence of symptoms. High-titer antifilarial antibodies and the other clinical features mentioned above are usually present, and there is usually a response to diethylcarbamazine therapy (see below).

TREATMENT The treatment of choice for lymphatic filariasis is diethylcarbamazine citrate (DEC), 5 mg/kg daily in divided doses for 3 weeks. This treatment rapidly eliminates microfilariae from the blood and is partially effective against adult worms. However, side effects are quite common and may be severe. Systemic symptoms include malaise, myalgias, fever, chills, headache, dizziness, and arthralgias. Nausea and vomiting may occur. These side effects appear to be related to massive killing of microfilariae and are most prominent within the first 2 days following treatment. With heavy infection, a test dose of 25 to 50 mg DEC should be given. Because of the frequent adverse effects associated with DEC, other drugs are being actively investigated. Ivermectin, the drug of choice for onchocerciasis, also appears promising in treating lymphatic filariasis.

A course of treatment with DEC will eliminate microfilariae from the bloodstream, usually for several months. However, a single course of DEC usually does not eradicate adult worms, which may require long-term or repeated treatment. This may be indicated particularly in individuals who have left an endemic area and will not be subjected to continued reexposure.

Treatment of chronic lymphatic obstruction is difficult, but considerable improvement can be obtained in many individuals. Chronic therapy with 3 to 5 mg/kg per day of DEC is indicated to avoid further infection and to attempt to eradicate existing adult worms. In addition, surgical bypass shunts may be used to decompress the obstructed limb. Repeated bacterial infections should be avoided by meticulous skin care, and early treatment is essential. Surgical management of hydrocele frequently achieves marked success. The psychological trauma to the individual is frequently the overriding concern and should be dealt with positively.

Acutely inflamed lymph nodes may occasionally suppurate, but usually the ulceration heals spontaneously over approximately a week's time.

PREVENTION Avoidance of mosquito bites is usually not possible for residents of endemic areas, but visitors should make use of repellents and mosquito nets. Chronic administration of diethylcarbamazine has been effective in preventing disease.

ONCHOCERCIASIS

Onchocerciasis (river blindness) is caused by the filarial nematode *Onchocerca volvulus*. An estimated 20 million persons, located largely in equatorial Africa and Latin America, are infected by *O. volvulus*. Onchocerciasis is one of the four leading causes of blindness worldwide; in addition, it causes great suffering and disfiguration from dermatitis.

ETIOLOGY AND EPIDEMIOLOGY Infection in humans begins with inoculation of infective larvae into the skin by the bite of the female blackfly (*Simulium* species). Infective larvae develop into adult worms over a period estimated to be several months; the adult worms then coil up into roughly spherical bundles, typically containing two to three females and one to two males. After a prepatent period of from 7 to 34 months following introduction of infective larvae, the gravid female releases microfilariae, which then migrate out of the nodule and throughout the tissues of the host, concentrating in the dermis. Transmission of infection to other individuals is initiated by the bite of a female fly, which, along with a blood meal, ingests microfilariae from the host skin, some of which develop into infective larvae over a period of 6 to 8 days. Infective larvae are about 600 μm in length. Adult *O. volvulus* females are about 40 to 60 cm in length, and adult males 3 to 6 cm. *O. volvulus* microfilariae are unsheathed and measure 210 to 320 μm in length.

Simulium damnosum and its subspecies represent the predominant vector in most of the endemic areas of Africa and in south Arabia. In Central America, *S. ochraceum* is the principal vector.

Simuliids (blackflies) oviposit into free-flowing rivers and streams, particularly in rapids. The gravid female deposits eggs on sticks, rocks, and trailing vegetation or other superficial debris. Eggs hatch into larvae in 2 days; these migrate downstream and develop into pupae in 8 to 10 days. Pupae remain fixed to some stucture in the stream of water, and the adult fly emerges from the pupal shell in 2 days. Adult females are hematophagous, requiring a blood meal for initiation of a gonotrophic cycle. Female blackflies generally restrict their flight to within a few kilometers of larval and pupal habitats (commonly termed breeding sites) and bite most intensely in the immediate vicinity. However, blackflies can be carried long distances, perhaps hundreds of kilometers, in association with monsoon winds. There are an estimated 20 million persons worldwide infected with *O. volvulus*, the vast majority in equatorial Africa in a belt that extends for more than 6000 km from the far western Atlantic coast to the Red Sea. In Guatemala and Mexico there are about 70,000 infected persons, located at altitudes of 500 to 1500 m on the Pacific slope of the Sierra Madre; in Venezuela there are about 20,000 infected persons. Smaller foci have been found in Colombia, Brazil, Ecuador, Yemen, and Saudi Arabia. The occurrence of onchocerciasis is determined by the relation of the population to *Simulium* breeding sites. The level of endemicity depends upon distance from larval and pupal habitats, the hyperendemic zones lying within a few kilometers.

PATHOGENESIS The pathogenesis of the manifestations in onchocerciasis is largely unknown. The only exception is punctate keratitis, which on biopsy has been shown to represent an inflammatory focus surrounding dead or dying microfilariae. However, these lesions are transitory and resolve completely, and any direct relation of microfilariae to other tissue lesions remains speculative. Nevertheless, because of their vast number and wide distribution throughout the body, as well as the clinical correlation between microfilaria counts and complications, microfilariae are thought to cause, directly or indirectly, most of the disease manifestations. It is believed that the host immune response, including a contribution of immediate hypersensitivity (e.g., eosinophil degranulation), immune-complex deposition, products of activated lymphoid cells, and perhaps autoantibodies and cytotoxic T cells, is largely responsible for the disease.

CLINICAL MANIFESTATIONS The major disease manifestations are dermatitis, onchocercomata, lymphadenitis, and visual impairment or blindness. The frequency of these features varies according to duration and intensity of exposure and geographical location.

Skin The most frequent manifestation of onchocercal dermatitis is pruritus. The pruritus can be unrelenting and incapacitating, even though microfilariae in the skin may be sparse. In addition, transitory localized areas of edema and erythema may occur in any part of the body. Over a period of years, most persons with significant infections will develop premature and exaggerated wrinkling of the skin, which has been associated with accelerated loss of elastic fibers. Atrophy of the epidermis with loss of elastic fibers can lead to loose, redundant skin. Hypo- or hyperpigmentation may also occur.

A localized eczematoid dermatitis with hyperkeratosis, scaling, and pigmentary changes occurs with variable severity. Such lesions are commonly seen in the lower extremities but in some cases are quite extensive. They can become superinfected, particularly with repeated trauma or excoriation.

Onchocercomata These subcutaneous nodules, which may be visible or palpable, contain the adult worms. In Africa, they are found particularly over the coccyx and sacrum, the trochanter of the femur, and the lateral and anterior iliac crests. Other common locations include various bony prominences. In American onchocerciasis, nodules tend to be distributed preferentially about the head, neck, and shoulders. Nodules vary in size from barely palpable, measuring a few millimeters, to several centimeters in diameter. They are firm, nontender, and have variable mobility.

Lymph nodes In Africans, mild to moderate lymphadenopathy is frequent, particularly in the inguinal and femoral areas. Enlarged inguinal or femoral nodes and surrounding fluid may become dependent ("hanging groin") and may predispose to inguinal and femoral hernias.

Ocular tissues Visual impairment is the major complication of onchocerciasis and is usually seen only in persons with moderate or heavy levels of infection. Lesions occur in all parts of the eye. Conjunctivitis with photophobia is a common early finding, particularly in young persons. In the cornea, punctate keratitis occurs as an acute inflammatory infiltrate surrounding dying microfilariae, manifest as "snowflake" opacities. These lesions occur most frequently in younger age groups and resolve without apparent sequelae. Sclerosing keratitis occurs in approximately 5 percent of persons infected with savannah strains and 1 percent of those with the forest strain. Sclerosing keratitis is the leading cause of onchocercal blindness in the savannah areas of Africa. Sclerosing keratitis begins at the limbus and progresses inward, leading to irreversible visual impairment. Anterior uveitis and iridocyclitis occur in roughly 5 percent of all infected persons in Africa. In Central American onchocerciasis complications of anterior uveal tract involvement (e.g., pupillary deformity) are particularly prominent relative to other causes of visual impairment. Secondary glaucoma may occur. Characteristic chorioretinal lesions occur with atrophy of the retinal pigment epithelium and of the choriocapillaris and hyperpigmentation of the pigment epithelial layer. Chorioretinal lesions are more frequently a cause of blindness in the forest areas of Africa than is sclerosing keratitis. Constriction of the visual fields and frank optic atrophy may occur as part of the disease. Primary changes in the optic disk related to *O. volvulus* infection occur in about 2 percent of infected persons in Africa.

Systemic manifestations Some heavily infected individuals show wasting and generalized weakness, with loss of adipose tissue and muscle mass. In adults who become blind, there is a three- to fourfold increased mortality rate.

DIAGNOSIS Diagnosis of onchocerciasis is usually based on demonstration of microfilariae. A sclerocorneal punch is used to obtain an essentially blood-free skin biopsy which extends just below the epidermis to the tips of the dermal papillae. The biopsy tissue is weighed and incubated in tissue-culture medium or in saline in a flat-bottomed microtiter plate or on a glass slide. Emergent microfilariae are counted after 2 to 4 h or an overnight incubation. The skin-snip examination can provide both a definitive diagnosis and some quantification of the intensity of infection. One hundred or more microfilariae per milligram of skin indicates heavy infection and implies a significant risk of serious complications. Histopathologic examination of an excised nodule can yield the diagnosis, and a small percentage of individuals with negative skin biopsies will have palpable nodules which can be excised. Several serodiagnostic tests for onchocerciasis have been described, but their potential utility is unclear.

TREATMENT AND PREVENTION The major goals of therapy of infected individuals are to prevent irreversible ocular and skin lesions and to alleviate distressing symptoms, particularly pruritus.

Ivermectin, a semisynthetic macrocyclic lactone, has been extensively tested in human onchocerciasis over the past few years and is now considered the drug of choice. The advantages of this drug over DEC are: (1) it can be given in a single dose orally; (2) it causes little or no systemic and ocular reaction; and (3) it appears to suppress microfilariae in the skin and eye longer than does DEC, and therefore, can be given on a yearly basis.

Ivermectin (available from the Centers for Disease Control) is given orally on an empty stomach at least 2 h before the next meal in a single dose of 150 μg/kg. Following treatment, most persons have little or no reaction. Approximately 1 to 10 percent of persons will develop cutaneous edema and pruritus, with or without a maculopapular rash characteristic of the so-called Mazzotti reaction. Symptomatic hypotension develops in about one person in 10,000, and rarely may require intravenous fluids and additional supportive measures. Significant ocular reactions are rare.

Contraindications to ivermectin treatment include pregnancy; breast feeding within the first 3 months following delivery, central nervous system disorders including, in particular, meningitis or other illnesses that may increase penetration of ivermectin into the central nervous system; allergy to the drug; and age less than 5 years.

Diethylcarbamazine citrate (DEC) treatment results in rapid and massive killing of a majority of microfilariae over a period of a few days. In association with this microfilaricidal action, most individuals experience a number of adverse effects and, in some cases, serious complications. The early side effects (Mazzotti reaction) include pruritus, painful swelling of lymph nodes (particularly femoral, inguinal, and axillary nodes), fever, headache, rash, nausea and vomiting, and occasionally vertigo, arthralgias, and myalgias. Cardiovascular collapse has also been described. Frequent early ocular effects include conjunctivitis, punctate keratitis, limbitis, and anterior uveitis.

Because of the severity of the DEC reaction it is best to begin therapy with a test dose, e.g., 25 to 50 mg on the first day. If the test dose is tolerated, DEC is then continued for 2 weeks at 3 to 4 mg/kg per day in two daily doses. Moderate doses of corticosteroids, when started 24 to 48 h before therapy, significantly blunt the reaction. Because of the side effects and complications associated with DEC, it should be given only if ivermectin is contraindicated or unavailable and there is a clear need for treatment.

Suramin is a proven and potent macrofilaricidal agent, but it has major toxicity and must be given intravenously in repeated doses. Therefore, its use is restricted to the rare individual with moderate to heavy levels of infection who is leaving the endemic area and who cannot take repeated doses of ivermectin or DEC.

The potential of vector control as a means of containment of onchocerciasis is dependent on a number of local factors. These include the size, number, and accessibility of larval and pupal habitats; the proximity of other foci of onchocerciasis which may serve as a source of reinvading flies; the topography and vegetation; rainfall patterns; and the dynamics of transmission. Although vector control may be quite beneficial over a period of time in areas of high endemicity with breeding sites which are vulnerable to attack, a large proportion of endemic areas are not suited to this means of control based on current technology. It is possible to minimize *Simulium* bites by avoiding fly-infested areas in the morning and evening and by wearing protective garments. However, it is unlikely that such measures will achieve significant success for the indigenous populations in the near future.

There is no drug that has been shown to prevent infection with *O. volvulus.*

LOAISIS

Loa loa adult worms live in the subcutaneous tissues and evoke a characteristic edematous reaction. The adult females are approximately 4 to 7 cm in length and the males 3 cm. Microfilariae (sheathed) appear in the blood in maximal concentrations around midday. The infection is transmitted by biting *Chrysops* species. The disease is endemic across central Africa and is particularly prevalent in coastal west Africa around Nigeria and Cameroon.

The major disease manifestation in transient subcutaneous swelling (Calabar swelling), which characteristically affects the distal extremities or the soft tissues surrounding the eyes. This phenomenon is associated with migration of adult worms through the tissues. The swelling can be painful, but typically resolves in 1 to 2 days. A spectacular occurrence is the migration of an adult worm across the scleral or conjunctival tissues. In nonresidents of endemic areas, fever, urticaria, and marked eosinophilia occur, while residents tend to have less exaggerated reactions.

Treatment is surgical removal of migrating adult worms if accessible, or high doses of diethylcarbamazine citrate (400 to 600 mg/d for 3 weeks). Repeat dosing with diethylcarbamazine may be necessary. Because of occasional severe reactions to diethylcarbamazine, a test dose (e.g., 25 mg) is suggested. Once-weekly diethylcarbamazine (300 mg) has been demonstrated to prevent infection.

MANSONELLA INFECTIONS

MANSONELLA PERSTANS This parasite is widely distributed in tropical Africa and coastal South America, and is transmitted by *Culicoides* mosquitoes. The adult worms live in serosal cavities, primarily the peritoneal or, less commonly, the pleural cavity, and measure 4 to 8 cm in length. Microfilariae are unsheathed, with a predilection for nocturnal appearance in the blood (i.e., they are subperiodic). The infection may be associated with eosinophilia, but is not believed to cause definite symptomatology in many infected humans. However, particularly in visitors to endemic areas who become infected, edema, inflammation in serosal cavities, and fever may occur. Treatment with high-dose diethylcarbamazine as recommended for loaiasis may lead to cure. Mebendazole (100 mg bid for 30 days) has also been reported to be effective.

MANSONELLA STREPTOCERCA This filarial infection occurs in west Africa. The microfilariae may be found in the skin or blood and are 200 μm in length and unsheathed. The adult worms live in the dermis and measure approximately 3 cm. This infection may cause hypopigmented macules which resemble those of leprosy but are not anesthetic. Furthermore, pruritus due to *M. streptocerca* may suggest onchocerciasis, and the smaller microfilariae of *M. streptocerca* must be distinguished from *O. volvulus* on skin snips (see above). Treatment with diethylcarbamazine citrate (6 mg/kg for 10 days) is usually effective against microfilariae and adult worms.

MANSONELLA OZZARDI This parasite occurs in South and Central America and the Caribbean. Adult worms appear to live in the peritoneal cavity. Microfilariae are unsheathed and nonperiodic. There are few symptoms, although the occurrence of upper extremity and shoulder arthralgias has been reported in association with this infection. No drug has been proven effective.

DIROFILARIA IMMITIS Humans become infected with *D. immitis* (dog heartworm) as accidental hosts; the dog is the natural reservoir. Mosquitoes infected with *D. immitis* larvae are quite common in many urban areas throughout the United States, although the highest-intensity transmission occurs in the southeastern United States. This parasite is also found in Africa, Asia (including Japan), Australia, the Pacific Islands, and primarily southern Europe. The adult worms do not develop fully in humans, and circulating microfilariae are extremely rare. In humans, the infection may lead to cough, fever, and chest pain, signaling pulmonary infarction. A frequent radiographic finding is a solitary nodule resembling a neoplasm on chest x-ray. The diagnosis is usually made histopathologically after thoracotomy, when degenerating nematodes are found. No further treatment is necessary.

REFERENCES

ANDERSON J et al: Studies on onchocerciasis in the United Cameroon Republic: II. Comparison of onchocerciasis in rain-forest and sudan-savanna. Trans R Soc Trop Med Hyg 68:209, 1974

BAIRD JK et al: Adult *Mansonella perstans* in the abdominal cavity in nine Africans. Am J Trop Med Hyg 37:578, 1987

Ciba Foundation Symposium No. 127: *Filariasis*. Singapore, Wiley, 1987

CLARKE VDV et al: Filariasis: *Dipetalonema perstans* infections in Rhodesia. Cen African J Med 17:1, 1971

GREENE BM et al: Comparison of ivermectin and diethylcarbamizine in the treatment of onchocerciasis. N Engl J Med 313:133, 1985

KOCHAR AS et al: Human pulmonary dirofilariasis. Report of three cases and brief review of the literature. Am J Clin Pathol 84:19, 1985

MARINKELLE CH, GERMAN E et al: Mansonelliasis in the Comisaria del Vaupes of Columbia. Trop Geogr Med 22:101, 1970

MEYERS WM et al: Human streptocerciasis. Am J Trop Med Hyg 21:528, 1972

NUTMAN TB et al: Diethylcarbamazine prophylaxis for human loaisis. Results of a double-blind study. N Engl J Med 319:752, 1988

WHITE AT et al: Controlled trial and dose-finding study of ivermectin for treatment of onchocerciasis. J Infect Dis 156:463, 1987

WHO Expert Committee on Onchocerciasis: *Third Report*, Technical Report Series 752. Geneva, World Health Organization, 1987

YOGESHWAR D, NEAFIE RC et al: Human pulmonary dirofilariasis. A case report and review of the literature. Am Rev Respir Dis 112:437, 1975

170 SCHISTOSOMIASIS

THEODORE E. NASH

Three major schistosome species, *Schistosoma mansoni, Schistosoma haematobium,* and *Schistosoma japonicum,* and a number of less prevalent species of the genus *Schistosoma* infect humans. Both *S. mansoni* and *S. japonicum* adults reside in the venules of the intestine, and the major disease manifestations of these parasites are hepatic. *S. mansoni* is found in parts of South America (Brazil, Venezuela, and Surinam), some Caribbean islands, Africa, and the Middle East while infections with *S. japonicum* occur in the Far East, mostly in China and the Philippines. *S. haematobium* adults are found mostly in the venules of the urinary tract and cause lesions primarily of the ureters and bladder. Infections with this species occur in Africa and the Middle East. Of lesser importance are *S. mekongi,* a newly recognized parasite related to *S. japonicum* which is found along the Mekong River in Indochina, and *S. intercalatum,* found in certain areas of central West Africa. Worldwide, as many as 200 million persons may be infected, and infection of entire communities is common. However, most infected persons experience few, if any, signs and symptoms, and only a small minority develop significant disease.

LIFE CYCLE The schistosome species infecting humans all share the same basic life cycle but are unique in ways which account for some of the different clinical and pathologic findings. Important differences include the length of time before egg laying begins (prepatent period), location of the adult worms, number of eggs produced by each pair of worms, response by the host to the ova, and eventual fate of retained eggs. The morphology of the parasites and the types of intermediate host snail are also distinct. Humans become infected after contact with water containing the infective stage of the parasite, called a cercaria, which is a microscopic form of the schistosome possessing a forked tail used for swimming and a head which is the anlage of the worm. Cercariae penetrate the unbroken skin, with the help of secreted enzymes, and in the skin transform into schistosomules or developing schistosomes. After 2 to 3 days the schistosomules migrate to the lungs and then to the portal vein, probably by an intravascular route. In the portal vein the maturing male and female schistosomes pair and migrate to the venules of the mesentery, bladder, or ureters, depending on the species of schistosome, and begin to deposit eggs. The time spent in migration and maturation differs. *S. mansoni* and *S. japonicum* begin depositing eggs around 4 to 5 weeks after infection, while egg deposition begins after 2 to 3 months for *S. haematobium.* Adult worms are about 1 to 2 cm in length and migrate in the blood vessels without eliciting a local inflammatory reaction. Adult worms do not multiply in humans, and immunosuppressive therapy does not result in increased numbers of worms. Once released, eggs are either retained in the tissues at the site of deposition or swept back, mostly to the liver, by way of the venous portal system in the case of the intestinal schistosomes. Eggs are deposited mainly in the bladder and ureters by *S. haematobium.* A portion of the mature schistosome ova are extruded into the lumen of the intestines, bladder, or ureters and after contact with water, hatch, releasing a miracidium. This free-swimming ciliated stage seeks out the proper intermediate snail vector and burrows into the soft tissues of the snail. After 1 to 2 months, depending on the species, the miracidium develops into a primary and then secondary sporocyst which, after further development, begins releasing cercariae into the surrounding water. Thousands of cercariae can be released daily from each infected snail. Therefore one miracidium produces many cercariae, and this amplifies the number of infective parasites and the risk of infection. Cercariae are most infectious immediately after shedding and are not viable 48 h after release so storing water for 48 h before contact prevents exposure and infection. Unlike most other trematodes the sexes are separate in schistosomes, but this is only evident in the adult stage. Ova are laid only when males and females infect the same individual.

PATHOPHYSIOLOGY A number of factors govern the disease manifestations. These include the duration and intensity of infection, location of egg deposition, host genetics, concurrent infections, and other still undefined factors.

In individuals from endemic areas initial infection goes unnoticed. There are a number of possible reasons for this, including age of initial exposure, manner of exposure, and transfer of antigens, antibodies, and anti-idiotypes from the mother. In visitors to endemic areas initial infection with schistosomes commonly results in an acute febrile illness (Katayama fever or acute schistosomiasis) which is most likely a manifestation of the immune response to the developing schistosomes and eggs. There is a vigorous hypersensitivity response which becomes modulated. These individuals have elevated levels of eosinophils and immune complexes and react markedly to schistosome antigens as measured by lymphocyte blastogenesis. Despite ongoing infection, symptoms subside, as do blastogenic responses to schistosome antigens but not to unrelated antigens such as purified protein derivative of tuberculin (PPD). The exudative acute granulomatous response to schistosome eggs is also modulated.

A major factor in determining the development of disease in humans is the worm burden of the host, which determines the number of eggs produced. The inflammatory and fibrotic response to these eggs is responsible for most of the morbidity and mortality associated with schistosomiasis. Factors which limit parasite survival will limit the development of disease. In human schistosome infections it has not been clearly established that protective immunity develops, but immunity exists in experimental animals. In the first few days after infection the schistosomule is relatively susceptible to immune attack. A number of systems employing antibody and/or eosinophils, neutrophils, macrophages, and complement have been used to kill schistosomules in vitro. However, as the schistosomules mature, they become refractory to these immune responses. In addition, schistosomes coat their tegument with host proteins and evade recognition by the host. A number of antibodies which block effective killing may also result in enhanced parasite survival. Schistosomule and adult antigens have been defined with the hope of developing vaccines; the administration of murine monoclonal antibodies to some of these antigens has reduced worm burdens in challenge infections by about 50 percent, and immunization with one antigen has produced similar levels of protection. Successful vaccination with anti-idiotypes has also been reported.

All schistosome eggs elicit a granulomatous response which is best understood in *S. mansoni* infections. The host becomes sensitized to the egg proteins by a T-cell-mediated mechanism which induces a larger granuloma. However, with continued infection the granuloma decreases in size due to the recruitment of suppressor T cells, while antibody has no effect on granuloma size. The regulation of granulomas due to *S. japonicum* eggs differs from that of granulomas from *S. mansoni* eggs. Immune modulation is mediated by serum factors, including anti-idiotype networks, at least in the chronic stage of infection. Both eggs and granulomas release factors which induce fibroblast proliferation in vitro. The early cellular response induced by granulomas is followed by fibrosis in vivo; however, liver fibrosis in humans probably involves more than simple fusion of fibrotic granulomas. After years of continued infection, some heavily infected individuals develop end-stage fibrotic lesions, mainly portal fibrosis (Symmers' fibrosis), sometimes resulting in esophageal varices and splenomegaly in *S. mansoni, S. japonicum,* and *S. mekongi* infections, and fibrosis of the ureters and bladder in *S. haematobium* infections. After the development of portal fibrosis, eggs are shunted to the lungs via portal-systemic collateral veins resulting in cor pulmonale in about 15 percent of patients with Symmers' fibrosis. Immune complexes shunted to the systemic circulation cause glomerulonephritis.

Host genetic factors have been found to influence the development of Symmers' fibrosis although there is no general agreement as to which are important. Schistosomes even of the same species are also genetically diverse, as shown by endonuclease restriction analysis, but the effect of this on disease in humans is unknown.

CLINICAL SYNDROMES (See Table 170-1) **Acute schistosomiasis** Acute schistosomiasis, or Katayama fever, occurs following initial exposure and infection with *S. mansoni* and *S. japonicum.* It rarely follows infection with *S. haematobium.* Acute schistosomiasis is seldom recognized in endemic populations and therefore is noted primarily in visitors to endemic areas. Immediately following exposure, patients frequently complain of intense transient itching. From 2 to 6 weeks or longer after exposure the patient may complain of a variety of symptoms including fever, chills, headache, hives or angioedema, weakness, weight loss, nonproductive cough, abdominal pain, and diarrhea. Sometimes symptoms abate but return with increased intensity about the time egg laying commences. These symptoms gradually diminish but may last as long as 2 to 3 months. Other newly infected individuals may be asymptomatic or have only minimal symptoms. In these individuals the diagnosis is established only after further evaluation prompted by suggestive laboratory test results or exposure history. More severe symptoms occur with heavier infections, but light infections may cause severe illness. Central nervous system lesions may occur during acute schistosome infection. The diagnosis of acute schistosomiasis is suggested by the clinical findings and the presence of eosinophilia, which is sometimes greater than 50 percent. Leukocytosis, increased immune complexes, and elevated IgM, IgG, and IgE immunoglobulins are found commonly. Although immune complexes have been suggested to play a role in the pathophysiology of acute schistosomiasis, glomerulonephritis and vasculitis are not present. The specific diagnosis can be established, even before the shedding of ova, by the detection of antibodies to adult schistosome gut antigens, or after egg excretion (5 to 6 weeks following exposure), by appropriate serologic testing and the finding of eggs in the stool or rectal biopsy. Clinically, acute schistosomiasis is frequently misdiagnosed as typhoid fever but can be confused with any prolonged febrile illness. Although these patients seem to tolerate chemotherapy well, whether therapy shortens the course of disease or decreases symptoms is unclear. Glucocorticoids may be useful, but this has not been demonstrated in controlled studies.

TABLE 170-1 Clinical manifestations of schistosomiasis from various *Schistosoma* species*

Manifestation	*S. mansoni*	*S. japonicum*	*S. haematobium*
Acute toxemic schistosomiasis	+	+	+
Chronic asymptomatic schistosomiasis	+	+	+
Hepatosplenic schistosomiasis	+	+	0
Cor pulmonale	+	+	±
Glomerulonephritis (clinically significant)	+	+	0†
Colonic polyposis	+	+	±
Ectopic lesions			
Brain	±	+	±
Spinal cord	+	±	+
Skin	+	+	+
Chronic cystitis and ureteritis	0	0	+
Mass lesions, bladder and ureters	0	0	+
Bladder cancer	0	0	+
Association with salmonella	+	+	+
Prolonged fever	+	+	+
Urinary carrier stage	?	?	+
Swimmer's itch‡	+	+	+

* + = recognized complications of infections by this species; ± = findings much less prominent in individuals infected by this species; 0 = complications not present in infections by this species.
† Except with associated salmonella infections.
‡ Usually from schistosomes that do not infect humans.

Liver fibrosis The most important complication of intestinal schistosome infection is the development of periportal or Symmers' fibrosis and portal hypertension (hepatosplenic schistosomiasis). This pathognomonic finding occurs in *S. mansoni, S. japonicum,* and *S. mekongi* infections but has been best studied in *S. mansoni* infections, where it normally develops after 10 to 15 years of prolonged exposure and infection. The liver may be enlarged but in many cases is small, firm, and nodular, and the left lobe is characteristically prominent. Macroscopically, finger-sized bands of fibrosis ("pipe-stem" fibrosis) encompass the large portal tracts. The portal venous tracts are replaced with fibrous tissue sometimes leading to presinusoidal blockage, portal hypertension, splenomegaly, and esophageal and gastric varices. The intrahepatic pressure is normal. Hepatic function is generally well preserved, and patients commonly present with hematemesis and/or signs and symptoms of splenomegaly. Ascites, hepatic coma, edema, spider angiomas, gynecomastia, and other signs of liver failure occur less frequently than in alcoholic and postnecrotic cirrhosis. Despite repeated episodes of hematemesis, patients may do reasonably well.

In the past, the diagnosis of periportal fibrosis required a wedge biopsy of the liver; needle biopsy specimens are frequently inadequate. Ultrasonograms of the liver show characteristic findings. The fibrotic bands appear as dense echogenic areas surrounding the portal vein and its tributaries. Studies comparing wedge biopsies of the liver to ultrasonographic examination showed that the latter technique had a specificity and sensitivity of 100 percent. Ultrasonography should replace invasive biopsies as the method of choice to diagnose hepatic schistosomiasis.

Ultrasonographic evaluation of *S. mansoni*–infected populations in the Sudan revealed a much higher prevalence of periportal fibrosis than could be determined by physical examination. As many as half of the group studied lacked palpable splenomegaly, and a majority did not give a history of hematemesis.

Patients with periportal fibrosis may not have schistosome eggs in the feces because of previous treatment and/or attrition of adult worms without subsequent reinfection. Since schistosome infections are practically universal in many populations, the mere presence of schistosome eggs in the feces does not establish the diagnosis of schistosomal periportal fibrosis; other liver diseases may be present. It is not clear whether there is any benefit from shunting procedures or splenectomy although these procedures are used commonly. The mortality of patients with portal fibrosis has not been well studied, but in one group was 8.2 percent after 3.6 years.

Glomerulonephritis and pulmonary hypertension These two complications occur almost exclusively in patients with periportal fibrosis and portal hypertension. Pulmonary hypertension appears to be due to obliteration of pulmonary arterioles by granulomatous inflammation induced by shunted and embolized schistosome eggs. This is most frequently recognized with *S. mansoni* and *S. japonicum* infections but also occurs with *S. haematobium*. The association of glomerulonephritis and schistosomiasis has been noted in humans and in experimentally infected animals. This complication is manifested clinically as proteinuria and/or renal failure. Schistosome-specific antibodies and antigens have been detected in the glomeruli of infected patients.

Other complications Focal dense deposits of eggs of *S. mansoni* in the large intestine (and less commonly of *S. haematobium* and probably of *S. japonicum*) incite an exudative granulomatous response resulting in the formation of inflammatory polyps. Histologically, these consist of masses of eggs, inflammatory cells, and fibrosis. The major clinical presentation is bloody diarrhea, sometimes associated with protein-losing enteropathy and anemia. This type of involvement of the bowel is recognized primarily in Egypt and the Sudan. Gastrointestinal symptoms are not increased in most chronically infected patients compared to control populations, although blood in the stool is found more frequently in some studies. Granulomatous masses involving the bowel wall may mimic carcinoma of the bowel. Central nervous system (CNS) involvement with *S. mansoni* and *S. haematobium* has a predilection for the spinal cord, while the brain is involved more commonly in *S. japonicum* infections.

Patients infected with the three major species of schistosomes and subsequently infected with salmonella may develop a prolonged intermittent febrile illness. In *S. haematobium* infections prolonged excretion of salmonella in the urine is common. Many times treatment of the salmonella infection alone is not effective, and specific antischistosomal chemotherapy is also required. Salmonella may be protected from host immune responses by residing in schistosome gut or by adhering to the surface of the schistosome.

***SCHISTOSOMA MANSONI* Epidemiology and manifestations** *S. mansoni* is found in South America and certain islands of the Caribbean, Africa, and the Middle East. The prepatent period is about 4 to 5 weeks. The intermediate hosts are various species in the genus *Biomphalaria*.

Although infection is frequent and sometimes universal in endemic areas, the development of disease is relatively uncommon and depends on a number of factors which include the duration and intensity of infection. In endemic populations chronic infections are usual, many times lasting decades, and disease manifestations develop in a predictable manner. For the most part, the initial infection of persons living in endemic areas goes unnoticed. In endemic populations, throughout the first decade of life the intensity of infection as measured by the number of eggs excreted in the feces increases, and prevalence rates often approach 100 percent in highly endemic communities. Few if any symptoms are attributable to schistosomiasis during this time. The liver, particularly the left lobe, gradually enlarges and becomes firm. Between 10 and 15 years of age, some heavily infected persons develop splenomegaly which partly reflects the presence of portal fibrosis and portal hypertension. About the same time, the number of eggs in the feces decreases, and there is evidence to suggest that immune factors as well as decreased water contact are responsible for this. During the next three decades, persons with portal fibrosis and hypertension may experience repeated bouts of hematemesis secondary to esophageal varices or symptoms secondary to a massively enlarged spleen. Not infrequently, because of prior chemotherapy, decreased exposure, or increased host immunity, patients with end-stage portal fibrosis no longer excrete eggs. Adult schistosomes can survive 20 years or more in the human host but usually live 5 to 8 years. The prognosis and the potential for reversing complications of infection after appropriate chemotherapy depend on the stage of disease. Some regression of periportal fibrosis occurs after chemotherapy as judged by ultrasound examination, but in most individuals with periportal fibrosis and clinical manifestations, regression does not occur. Glomerulonephritis and cor pulmonale secondary to schistosomiasis occur exclusively in patients with portal fibrosis. Central nervous system involvement can occur at any stage of the infection and is not related to the intensity of infection.

Diagnosis The diagnosis of *S. mansoni* is established by identification of ova in the feces or tissues. The ova are 114 to 175 μm in length and 45 to 68 μm in width and have a prominent lateral spine. In light infections with less than 50 eggs per gram of feces, ova may not be detected in the stool without the use of techniques which sample large quantities of stool. Even in light infections, ova can usually be detected in rectal biopsies and are best identified by squashing a small amount of tissue between two glass slides and searching for ova microscopically.

Many serologic tests have been employed in the diagnosis of schistosomiasis. These tests are not standardized and differ in sensitivity and specificity. Most current tests have greater than 90 percent sensitivity, and a positive serology is indicative of a present or past infection. An immunofluorescent antibody test employing sections of adult schistosomes to determine the presence of antibodies to schistosome gut antigens has been extremely useful in identifying recently infected persons or those with acute schistosomiasis.

Treatment In the past, chemotherapy was offered only to more heavily infected individuals who were more likely to develop disease. Although the risks of continued infection have not been clearly defined, with the availability of easily administered and safe drugs, most infected persons are likely to benefit from treatment. Patients with active infections have live eggs, which can be identified microscopically by experienced parasitologists or by the presence of flame cells, or by their ability to hatch after contact with water. Although a number of drugs are available for the treatment of schistosomiasis mansoni, praziquantel and oxamniquine are the drugs of choice (Table 170-2). Both drugs are equally safe and effective in schistosomiasis mansoni found in the Caribbean and South America. Because some strains of *S. mansoni* in Africa are relatively resistant to oxamniquine, praziquantel is the better drug. Both drugs can be used in patients with portal fibrosis. The side effects of praziquantel and oxamniquine are frequent but transient and mild. For praziquantel they include abdominal pain, lethargy, diarrhea, and fever and for oxamniquine, dizziness, tiredness, nausea and vomiting, neuropsychiatric manifestations, and rarely convulsions.

***SCHISTOSOMA JAPONICUM* Epidemiology and clinical manifestations** *Schistosoma japonicum* is found in southeast Asia and is an important health concern in areas of China and the Philippines. The intermediate hosts are amphibious snails of the genus *Oncomelania*. Besides humans, numerous mammals such as cattle and water buffalo are naturally infected and serve as reservoirs of infection. The prepatent period is about 4 weeks.

The course of infection and clinical manifestations of *S. japonicum* are similar to those of *S. mansoni*, but the epidemiology and disease manifestations are less well studied. Experimental infections are more virulent, probably because each worm pair produces 10 times as many eggs as *S. mansoni*. The granulomas contain clusters of eggs and are larger and frequently show central necrosis. As in *S. mansoni* infections, periportal fibrosis is the major clinical manifestation. The other clinical syndromes described in *S. mansoni* also occur as

TABLE 170-2 Treatment of schistosomiasis

Species	Drug	Total dose* (mg per kilogram body weight)	Regimen
S. haematobium	Praziquantel	40	Single dose or two 20 mg/kg doses
	Metrifonate†	22.5–30	Single dose of 7.5 to 10 mg/kg body weight given every other week × 3
S. mansoni			
Americas and Caribbean	Oxamniquine	15	Single oral dose with food
	Praziquantel	40	Single or two 20 mg/kg doses 4 h apart with food
Africa and Middle East	Oxamniquine	60	15 mg/kg body weight twice a day for 2 days with food
	Praziquantel	40	Single dose or two 20 mg/kg doses 4 h apart with food
S. japonicum or *S. mekongi*	Praziquantel	60	20 mg/kg body weight every 4 h with food

* All recommended drugs are given orally.
† Available from the Parasitic Diseases Division, Centers for Infectious Diseases, Centers for Disease Control, Atlanta, GA 30333.

complications of this infection. However, there are some notable differences in disease manifestations, particularly CNS involvement. In acute schistosomiasis associated with *S. japonicum* infections, about 2 to 3 percent of patients experience CNS symptoms and signs that mimic acute encephalitis or a focal neurologic process. Computed tomography shows multiple enhancing lesions. In chronic infections, patients may present with focal lesions of the brain which mimic brain tumors. These lesions contain masses of eggs and granulomas. Uncontrolled studies suggest that treatment with antischistosomal drugs and glucocorticoids is effective.

Diagnosis The principles of diagnosis are similar to those of *S. mansoni* and require the demonstration of the typical ova in the tissues or feces of infected individuals. The eggs are oval in shape, 70 to 100 μm by 50 to 65 μm, and have a vestigial spine. Old, calcified, dead eggs are commonly retained in the tissues for long periods of time and do not indicate active infection.

Treatment Most infected persons should be treated. The only safe and effective therapy for *S. japonicum* infections is praziquantel (Table 170-2).

SCHISTOSOMA MEKONGI *Schistosoma mekongi* occurs in the Mekong River in Indochina (Laos, Cambodia, and Thailand). The intermediate host is an aquatic snail, *T. aperta*. The eggs are similar to *S. japonicum*'s but are slightly smaller and round, about 56 μm by 64 μm. Dogs and human beings are frequently naturally infected. The prepatent period is about 5 weeks. The disease manifestations appear to be similar to those of *S. japonicum* but are not fully documented. Praziquantel is effective therapy for this infection (Table 170-2).

SCHISTOSOMA HAEMATOBIUM **Epidemiology and clinical manifestations** *S. haematobium* infections occur in extensive areas of Africa and in the Middle East. The intermediate hosts are of the genus *Bulinus*. The prepatent period is 2 to 3 months. Natural infection is primarily limited to human beings.

As in *S. mansoni* infections, the prevalence and intensity of infection in endemic areas increases until 10 to 15 years of age. Thereafter, the intensity decreases markedly while the prevalence rate falls moderately. The signs and symptoms due to *S. haematobium*, owing to its predilection for the veins of the urinary tract, result from involvement of the ureters and bladder. In contrast to the asymptomatic period following initial infection with the intestinal schistosomes, dysuria and hematuria are frequently noted 2 to 3 months after infection. These findings may continue throughout the course of active infection. Initially, the eggs evoke an intense inflammatory and granulomatous response which may cause anatomic and/or functional obstruction, hydroureter and hydronephrosis, and masses in the bladder or ureters. Cystoscopic examination may reveal friable masses extending into the bladder, ulceration, petechiae, and granulomas. These early lesions are reversible after antischistosomal chemotherapy. Eggs shed into the urine are usually easily demonstrable. As the infection progresses, the inflammatory component lessens, possibly due to a modulating effect of the host's immune response, and fibrosis increases, most likely due to the accumulation of many old and some new lesions. Later most lesions consist of masses of dead and calcified eggs in fibrous tissue. When the concentration of calcified eggs in the tissues is large enough, radiographic opacification of the affected areas of the urinary tract becomes evident. Fibrotic lesions which cause hydroureter and hydronephrosis are not reversible by antischistosomal chemotherapy. Renal failure occurs in a surprisingly small proportion of infected individuals.

Portal fibrosis and clinically significant glomerulonephritis are not complications of this infection, but passage of eggs into the lungs may result in pulmonary hypertension. Prolonged excretion of salmonella in the urine and intermittent bacteremias are well documented. Urinary tract infections with other bacteria do not appear to be increased in frequency unless there is instrumentation of the urinary tract; however, they may be difficult to eradicate once established. Central nervous system infection most commonly involves the spinal cord, as in *S. mansoni* infections. Although eggs of *S. haematobium* are frequently detected in the feces in low numbers and are often found in rectal biopsies, intestinal polyposis is uncommon. In certain geographic areas squamous cell cancer of the bladder is felt to be associated with *S. haematobium* infection and is a significant cause of morbidity and mortality.

Diagnosis The diagnosis of *S. haematobium* is established by demonstrating the characteristic eggs in the tissues or urine. These are 112 to 170 μm by 40 to 70 μm, have a prominent terminal spine, and are easily seen in the urine. An increased number of eggs is excreted around midday, and microscopic examination of a centrifuged urine specimen collected at this time usually reveals ova. In light infections, examination of increased quantities of urine is sometimes required. Gross or microscopic hematuria is common in endemic populations, and its presence should always suggest the diagnosis in exposed individuals. Antibodies to *S. haematobium* can be detected using *S. mansoni* antigen preparations.

Treatment Infected persons should be treated. Dead and calcified eggs are common in tissue, are often seen in urine specimens, and should be differentiated from viable eggs. Although a number of drugs have been used to treat *S. haematobium*, praziquantel is the treatment of choice (Table 170-2). Metrifonate, a safe, orally administered agent, is also effective. Its major advantage is low cost, and the major disadvantage is that in order to cure infection it needs to be given in three doses 2 weeks apart.

SCHISTOSOMA INTERCALATUM *Schistosoma intercalatum* infection is limited to areas of West Africa. Eggs, 140 to 240 μm by 50 to 85 μm, are found in the stool and have a terminal spine. Few symptoms are attributable to this infection, and no cases of portal fibrosis have been reported. Praziquantel is effective treatment (Table 170-2).

SCHISTOSOME DERMATITIS (SWIMMER'S ITCH) When cercariae penetrate the skin, they may provoke a reaction known as schistosome dermatitis. Symptoms occur most commonly after penetration of nonhuman schistosomes of birds and mammals. In previously unexposed persons, the initial invasion causes transient itching and uncommonly urticaria followed by the development of macules within 24 h and papules after 24 h. Following repeated exposures, the signs and symptoms increase dramatically and occur earlier. Large pruritic, erythematous papules and, uncommonly, vesicles develop within 24 h. The lesions are most intense 2 to 3 days following exposure and subside after a few days. These lesions represent a delayed hypersensitivity reaction to the invading schistosome. Nonhuman schistosomes do not fully develop in humans, and the signs and symptoms are limited to the skin. A similar dermatitis also occurs after infection with human schistosomes.

Schistosome dermatitis occurs after exposure to fresh water in many areas of the world but is particularly common in the north central and western United States. A dermatitis following seawater exposure (clam digger's itch) has also been described.

Treatment is symptomatic. Since cercariae need some time to invade the skin (15 min or less), rapid removal of cercariae-containing droplets after water contact will decrease exposure. Limiting the numbers of the intermediate host snail in frequented areas can effectively control exposure.

CONTROL OF SCHISTOSOMIASIS Theoretically, schistosome infections can be controlled by a variety of methods, but their application has generally been only partially successful. Simple and effective health education measures such as the elimination of indiscriminate urination and defecation are difficult to implement in endemic areas. Elimination of the intermediate molluscan host can be accomplished with the use of molluscicides or by destroying the habitat of the snail. Both methods require dedication of resources and personnel often not readily available. Mass chemotherapy of populations has been tried, and repeated treatments will be needed depending on the degree of reinfection. Some advocate the treatment of those likely to develop serious disease (e.g., those heavily infected). The methods employed will depend on the nature of the endemic area and the resources available.

REFERENCES

CHEEVER AW, ANDRADE ZA: Pathological lesions associated with *Schistosoma mansoni* infection in man. Trans R Soc Trop Med Hyg 61:626, 1968

DAVIS A, WEGNER DHG: Multicenter trials of praziquantel in human schistosomiasis: Design and techniques. Bull WHO 57:767, 1979

FORSYTH DM: A longitudinal study of endemic urinary schistosomiasis in a small East African community. Bull WHO 40:771, 1969

HIAT RA et al: Factors in the pathogenesis of acute schistosomiasis mansoni. J Infect Dis 139:659, 1979

HOMEIDA M et al: Morbidity associated with *Schistosoma mansoni* infection as determined by ultrasound: A study in Gezira, Sudan. Am J Trop Med Hyg 39:196, 1988

———: Diagnosis of pathologically confirmed Symmers' periportal fibrosis by ultrasonography: A prospective blinded study. Am J Trop Med Hyg 39:86, 1988

JORDAN P, WEBBE G (eds): *Schistosomiasis, Epidemiology, Treatment and Control.* London, Heinemann Medical, 1982

LEHMAN JS et al: Urinary schistosomiasis in Egypt: Clinical, radiological, bacteriological, and parasitological correlations. Trans R Soc Trop Med Hyg 67:384, 1973

MCCUTCHAN TF et al: Differentiation of schistosome by species, strain, and sex by using cloned DNA markers. Proc Natl Acad Sci USA 81:889, 1984

NASH TE et al: Schistosome infections in humans: Perspective and recent findings. Ann Intern Med 97:740, 1982

——— et al: Treatment of *Schistosoma mekongi* with praziquantel: A double-blinded study. Am J Trop Med Hyg 3:977, 1982

ROLLINSON O, SIMPSON AJG (eds): *The Biology of Schistosomes. From Genes to Latrines.* New York, Academic, 1987

171 NEMATODES, CESTODES, AND HERMAPHRODITIC TREMATODES

JAMES J. PLORDE / PAUL G. RAMSEY

INTESTINAL NEMATODE INFECTIONS

ENTEROBIASIS Definition Enterobiasis (pinworm, seatworm, or threadworm infection, oxyuriasis) is an intestinal infection of humans caused by *Enterobius vermicularis* and characterized by perianal pruritus. It has been estimated that the worm infects 200 million people, 30 to 40 million of them in the United States and Canada.

Etiology The female averages 10 mm in length, the male 3 mm. They live with their heads attached to the mucosa of the cecum, appendix, and adjacent parts of the bowel. On average, an infected individual harbors 50 worms, but in areas of intense transmission thousands may be present. The gravid female migrates through the anal canal at night, deposits her 10,000 eggs on the perianal skin, and dies. In female patients the worm may enter the vagina and occasionally gain access to the peritoneal cavity through the fallopian tubes. Each egg contains an embryo which, within a few hours, develops into an infective larva. After the egg has been ingested, the larva is released in the small intestine and migrates down the bowel lumen to the cecum. In less than 1 month from the time of ingestion, newly developed gravid females are again discharging eggs. They are planoconvex and measure approximately 20 by 50 μm. The shell is clear and doubly contoured.

Epidemiology Humans are usually infected by the direct transfer of eggs from the anus to the mouth by way of contaminated fingers. Retroinfection, which is seen primarily in adults, may occasionally take place when eggs hatch in the perianal area and the larvae migrate back into the bowel to mature. The eggs, which are relatively resistant to desiccation, also contaminate nightclothes and bed linen, where they remain viable and infective for 2 to 3 weeks. Airborne transmission is possible, and spread within family and children's groups occurs readily. Prevalence rates in North America have been estimated at 30 percent, but may be higher in institutionalized individuals. The disease may be sexually transmitted among homosexuals. Enterobiasis is found in all climates.

Clinical manifestations Many infections are asymptomatic. The most common complaint is pruritus ani, which is most troublesome at night, being related to the migration of the gravid female worms. Irritability, insomnia, enuresis, and other minor complaints are probably secondary to the pruritus. Scratching may lead to perianal eczema or pyogenic infection. Vaginal discharge has been reported, and rarely a chronic granulomatous salpingitis or endometritis results from the presence of ectopic adults. An association between enterobiasis and cystitis in young females has been reported. This may result from the transport of enteric bacteria into the bladder by the migrating worm. Other rare ectopic locations include the lung, liver, and peritoneum. The worms can penetrate the bowel wall only if its continuity has been compromised by some other disease.

Laboratory findings Examination for ova of material obtained from the perianal skin by means of a cellophane tape swab is the preferable method for the detection of enterobiasis. The tape is folded sticky-side out over the end of a tongue blade, pressed firmly against the perianal area, and then spread on a glass slide and examined under the lower power of a microscope. The swab should be taken at home by the patient on three to five consecutive mornings prior to bathing and brought to the laboratory for examination. The diagnosis is sometimes made by finding adult worms in the perianal area or in the feces following a laxative or an enema. There is a strong association between infection with *Dientamoeba fragilis* and pinworm; discovery of this parasite in the stool should stimulate a search for pinworm.

Treatment All infected individuals in a family or communal group should be treated simultaneously. The frequently recommended sanitary measures aside from daily bathing and hand washing before meals and after stools are of dubious benefit. It is relatively easy to eradicate the worms, but reinfection is frequent. Retreatment does not appear necessary unless symptoms recur.

Two highly satisfactory drugs are available. Pyrantel pamoate given in a single oral dose of 11 mg/kg (maximum 1.0 g) is probably the drug of choice. Alternatively, a single 100-mg oral dose of mebendazole can be used. This drug is not recommended for infants or pregnant women. Pyrvinium pamoate is equally effective but less convenient. It is given orally as a single dose of 5 mg/kg in tablet or liquid form. This compound turns the stool red and may stain bedclothes or undergarments. In heavily contaminated environments, treatment with the above drugs may be repeated after an interval of 2 weeks to eliminate any new infections.

Prevention Methods of preventing autoinfection and dissemination within a group involving children are extremely difficult to enforce. Personal environmental hygiene should be stressed, and anthelmintic and symptomatic treatment of pruritus ani should be instituted. To control infection within a group, simultaneous treatment of all cases is mandatory.

TRICHURIASIS Definition Trichuriasis (whipworm infection, trichocephaliasis) is an intestinal infection of humans caused by *Trichuris trichiura* and is characterized by invasion of the colonic mucosa by the adult trichuris. Five to eight hundred million persons are thought to be infected with this parasite including 2.4 million in the United States. It may be the most commonly encountered helminthic infection in Americans returning from subtropical and tropical areas, where prevalence rates up to 80 percent have been reported.

Etiology The adult whipworms are found in the large intestine with their anterior ends deeply embedded in the mucosa. They are 30 to 50 mm in length and possess a threadlike anterior two-thirds with a stouter posterior third, giving them a whiplike structure. The female produces about 5000 eggs each day. They are characteristically football-shaped (20 to 50 μm), brown, thick-walled, with translucent knoblike ends. The eggs, like those of *Ascaris*, must incubate at least 3 weeks in soil before they become infective. After ingestion, the eggs hatch in the small intestine and the larvae become embedded in the intestinal villi. After several days they migrate to the large intestine where they mature in about 3 months. The adult worms may live for 4 to 8 years.

Epidemiology Whipworm is a cosmopolitan parasite but is most commonly found in the tropics, where the level of sanitation is low and environmental conditions necessary for the incubation of the eggs are optimal. In the United States, it is found throughout the rural areas of the southeast. Its distribution is similar to that of *Ascaris* and hookworm, but the eggs are less resistant to sunlight and drying than those of *Ascaris*. Because of their general lack of sanitary habits, children and the mentally retarded have the highest incidence of infection.

Pathogenesis and clinical manifestations Petechiae (subepithelial hemorrhages and superficial mucosal infiltration of eosinophilic lymphocytes) and plasma cells are seen at worm attachment sites in the gut. It has been estimated that infected patients lose 0.005 mL blood per worm per day. Symptomatic infection generally requires the presence of large numbers of adult whipworms and may be correlated in part with the degree of mucosal involvement. Typically, worm burdens sufficient to produce clinical disease are limited to 10 to 15 percent of infected individuals, primarily children 2 to 10 years of age. Burdens of 200 trichuris can produce growth retardation and three to four unformed stools daily, occasionally with mucus and blood. Infections with more than 800 worms often result in anemia, finger clubbing, abdominal pain, and dysentery. In heavier infections, the distribution of worms throughout the colon and rectum may result in rectal prolapse while straining at stool. Some investigators also feel that *Trichuris* infections predispose to amebic dysentery and bacterial gastroenteritis.

Laboratory findings In symptomatic infection, large numbers of eggs are present in the feces, and there may be eosinophilic leukocytosis and anemia. In light infections, concentration techniques may be necessary to recover the eggs. Quantitation of egg output is helpful since only counts above 3000 eggs per gram of feces are likely to be associated with symptoms. Stools should be cultured for bacterial pathogens and examined for the presence of *Entamoeba histolytica*.

Treatment Mebendazole in the oral dose of 100 mg twice daily for 3 days is the drug of choice. Its cure rate is 60 to 70 percent, and it achieves a 90 percent reduction in egg burden. The dose may have to be repeated in patients with heavy infections. It is not recommended for children under the age of 2 or pregnant women.

Prognosis Whipworm infection, unless characterized by severe diarrhea, blood loss, and systemic reaction, usually responds well to treatment. Posttreatment growth rates of children with heavy worm burden accelerate dramatically, even in the absence of nutritional supplements.

Prevention Measures recommended for ascariasis apply also to trichuriasis.

ASCARIASIS Definition Ascariasis is an infection of humans caused by *Ascaris lumbricoides* and characterized by an early pulmonary phase related to larval migration and a later, prolonged intestinal phase. It is estimated that 25 percent of the world's population, including 4 million Americans, are infected with this nematode.

Etiology The adult ascarids are large (15 to 40 cm in length), cylindric worms with blunt ends; they maintain themselves in the lumen of the jejunum by virtue of their muscular activity. Despite a life span of only 6 to 18 months, the female releases millions of eggs, both fertile and infertile, into the fecal stream; the daily output is estimated to be 200,000 per worm. Fertilized eggs are elliptic (30 to 40 μm by 50 to 60 μm) with an irregular, dense outer shell and a regular, translucent inner shell. They require a period of soil incubation before they become infective. Under optimum conditions of warmth and moisture this occurs in 2 to 3 weeks. The eggs may then remain viable for up to 6 years in temperate climates and may survive freezing. When an infective egg is ingested, the larva is liberated in the small intestine. It migrates through the wall and is carried by the bloodstream or lymphatics to the lung. After about 10 days in the pulmonary capillaries and alveoli, the larvae pass in turn up the bronchioles, bronchi, trachea, and epiglottis, are swallowed, and return to the jejunum. There they develop into mature adult worms within 2 to 3 months of ingestion. *Ascaris suum*, a roundworm of pigs, may occasionally complete a similar life cycle in humans.

Epidemiology Infection follows the ingestion of the embryonated eggs contained in contaminated food, or, more commonly, the introduction of the eggs into the mouth by the hands after contact with contaminated soil. Geophagia may produce massive infections. In endemic areas, the infection is maintained primarily by small children who defecate indiscriminately in the area of the home. In dry, windy climates, eggs may become airborne, get into the mouth, and be swallowed. Since the eggs are relatively resistant to desiccation and wide variations in temperature, the disease occurs worldwide. In the developing areas of the world where the lack of sanitary facilities exposes populations to the greatest risk, the prevalence of infection may be as high as 80 to 90 percent. Children are almost universally infected in these areas, with peak infection rates achieved by age 5. In temperate areas, the infection occurs in family clusters.

Pathogenesis and clinical manifestations Because of the extensive migration of which both the larvae and adults are capable, the manifestations may be diverse. Bronchopneumonia characterized by fever, cough, dyspnea, wheeze, eosinophilic leukocytosis, and migratory pulmonary infiltrates may occur during the passage of the larvae through the lung. This is most commonly seen in communities where *Ascaris* transmission is seasonal. The severity of symptoms is apparently related to both intensity of infection and the degree of sensitization resulting from previous exposures. Significant arterial oxygen desaturation and, rarely, death may occur. Adult worms may produce no symptoms if the infection is light and may be detected accidentally when the adult worm is vomited or passed in the stool. Heavier infections may cause abdominal pain and malabsorption of fat, protein, carbohydrate, and vitamins. In marginally nourished children this may produce growth retardation. Occasionally a bolus of worms may result in volvulus, intussusception, or intestinal obstruction in the ileocecal area. Children are most likely to have these complications because of their anatomically smaller intestine and larger worm loads. Up to 2000 worms have been found in children, although the usual load is less than 20. In the United States, where worm loads are usually modest, the incidence of obstruction is 2 per 1000 infected children per year. It often follows a febrile illness, spicy meal, anesthesia, or drug therapy which stimulates the worms to increase motility. Rarely, an adult worm will migrate into the appendix, bile ducts, or pancreatic ducts, causing obstruction and inflammation of these organs. Biliary tract obstruction may be associated with bacterial cholangitis and liver abscess. Worms may also penetrate the intestinal wall, particularly at a site of surgical anastomosis, and patients should be dewormed prior to elective surgery. Migration of the worms into the oral pharynx and mouth may lead to acute respiratory distress.

Laboratory findings The diagnosis is usually made by finding the ova in the feces. The fertilized eggs are usually numerous, characteristic, and not easily confused with those of other helminths. The occasional unisexual infection may pose diagnostic problems. The male produces no eggs, and the unfertilized ova produced by a single female may be atypical and difficult to recognize. Occasionally the worms may be seen after a barium meal, either as negative images or after ingesting barium themselves. In biliary ascariasis an intravenous cholangiogram will often demonstrate dilatation of the common duct and/or the negative image of the parasite. Ascaris pneumonia may be diagnosed by finding larvae and eosinophils in the sputum or gastric aspirate. Eggs will usually not be found until after the larvae have matured in the intestine. Eosinophilic leukocytosis is usually noted during larval migration, but diminishes and often disappears during the chronic intestinal phase of infection.

Treatment Only symptomatic treatment can be used during the period of pulmonary involvement by the migrating larvae. For removal of the adult worms from the intestines, either pyrantel pamoate or mebendazole should be used. Pyrantel is given as a single oral dose of 11 mg/kg (maximum 1.0 g). Mebendazole is given as described for trichuriasis and is the preferred agent if both *Ascaris* and *Trichuris* are present. An older agent, piperazine citrate, is highly effective, less expensive, but slightly more toxic than the above two agents. It is given in a single dose (75 mg/kg, maximum 3.5 g) after breakfast on two successive days. The drug must be administered with caution to patients with renal insufficiency and epilepsy, because impaired elimination may produce neurotoxic signs. In intestinal obstruction, nasogastric suction should be initiated. After vomiting is controlled, piperazine should be given through the nasogastric tube every 12 to 24 h in dosage of 65 mg/kg (maximum 1.0 g) for six doses. Usually surgery is not required.

Prognosis The prognosis in intestinal infection is generally good. When acute or chronic obstruction of ducts or hollow viscera has occurred, the immediate prognosis is determined by the promptness of diagnosis and treatment. The case fatality rate of intestinal obstruction in the United States is 3 percent. However, world-wide an estimated 20,000 people die of ascariasis annually.

Prevention Ascariasis is primarily a household infection of rural areas. All infections should be treated, personal hygiene stressed, and adequate toilet facilities provided. Mass therapy administered at 6-month intervals may be effective in controlling ascariasis in small communities.

TOXOCARIASIS (VISCERAL LARVA MIGRANS) Definition This is a human infection with the dog ascarid, *Toxocara canis. Bayliascaris procyonis,* an ascarid of raccoons, occasionally produces particularly severe human infection. These animal parasites are usually unable to complete their life cycle in humans, but may disseminate widely in the body, producing a variety of clinical manifestations, collectively referred to as *visceral larva migrans.*

Etiology and epidemiology The large adult toxocaral worms live in the intestine of dogs. Their eggs must be passed in the stool and incubate in soil for 2 to 3 weeks before they become infective. When ingested by a mammal, larvae are liberated in the intestine, penetrate the wall, and are carried in the blood to the liver, where most remain, and to the lung. If the host is a young puppy, the larvae burst into the alveoli and complete their life cycle in a manner analogous to *A. lumbricoides* in humans. In humans and fully grown dogs, *Toxocara* larvae, which are approximately one-half the size of those of *A. lumbricoides,* pass through the pulmonary capillaries to reach the systemic circulation. Larvae leave the circulatory system when their gradually increasing size approaches the diameter of the vessel through which they are traveling. They migrate extensively in the surrounding tissue; some may become dormant for years, only to resume migration at a later time. *Toxocara* infections of dogs are common and widespread. Transplacental and transmammary migration of larvae account for infection rates of 80 percent or more in young puppies; they can shed a large number of ova within 4 weeks of birth. Viable ova were found in 25 percent of soil samples taken from public parks in the United States and Great Britain. Although most of the 2000 documented human infections have occurred in the United States and Europe, cases have been reported from 48 countries around the world. Children from the age of 2 to 5 years, because of their sanitary habits, predilection to geophagia, and intimate association with domestic pets, are most frequently involved. The seroprevalence of childhood *Toxocara* infection in the United States varies from 3 to 25 percent; the rates are highest in the south and northeast.

Pathogenesis and clinical manifestations The larvae migrate freely in tissues, causing hemorrhage, necrosis, eosinophilic inflammatory reaction, and eventually granuloma formation. The most frequently involved organs are the liver, lungs, brain, eye, heart, and skeletal muscles. Symptoms and signs are related to the number and location of the granulomas as well as sensitization to the parasite antigen. Commonly, only asymptomatic eosinophilia marks the presence of infection. Symptomatic patients most frequently present with fever and tender hepatomegaly. Splenomegaly, skin rash, and recurrent pneumonitis with wheezing respirations may occur in more severe infections. Respiratory failure with death has been reported. Most fatalities, however, result from involvement of the myocardium or central nervous system; the latter may result in convulsions, behavior disorders, or focal neurological defects. There is often a history of dirt eating and contact with puppies. Leukocytosis with eosinophilia to high levels (over 60 percent) and hypergammaglobulinemia with raised levels of IgG, IgM, and IgE are common. These manifestations may persist for months or years. At surgery or autopsy the liver may be studded with small granulomas. An exudative or granulomatous endophthalmitis, which may be mistaken for retinoblastoma, is observed in older children and adults. Typically, this is unilateral and occurs in the absence of other clinical manifestations of visceral larva migrans. Decreased visual acuity, strabismus, or eye pain brings the patient to medical attention.

Diagnosis The diagnosis can usually be made on the basis of clinical findings. Infections with *A. lumbricoides,* hookworm, and *Strongyloides stercoralis,* as well as other nonhuman nematodes, may also on occasion present as visceral larva migrans, making the etiologic diagnosis difficult. Eosinophilic leukemia, trichinosis, trematode infections, and periarteritis nodosa must be ruled out. The adaptation of larval antigens to the enzyme-linked immunosorbent assay (ELISA) has provided a serologic test of diagnostic value. In one study, the sensitivity and specificity were 78 and 92 percent, respectively. A definitive diagnosis depends on the identification of the larvae in sputum or tissue granuloma. Biopsy of the liver with serial sections of the specimen may reveal eosinophilic granulomas or a *Toxocara* larva.

Treatment No uniformly effective therapy is available. Diethylcarbamazine as used in Bancroftian filariasis (see Chap. 169) is probably the drug of choice. Thiabendazole (tiabendazole) in dosage of 25 to 50 mg/kg for 7 to 10 days may be helpful. Glucocorticoids may be beneficial when respiratory difficulty is pronounced. Ocular larvae close to the macula may be destroyed with laser photocoagulation. Control measures are directed toward preventing ingestion of eggs. Removal and repeated worming of infected dogs must be considered. Animals less than 6 months of age should be wormed monthly; older ones every 2 or 3 months. Keeping raccoons as pets should be discouraged.

ANISAKIASIS Ascarids belonging to the family Anisakidae infect seals, dolphins, porpoises, whales, and other large sea mammals. Their larval stages are found in the flesh of squid and several marine fish including mackerel, herring, and salmon. The ascarids of the *Pseudoterranova* genus, however, are more commonly seen in bottom fish such as cod, halibut, and "Pacific red snapper." Humans are infected by eating raw, pickled, or slightly salted fish delicacies such as "green herring," sushi, sashimi, sunomono, ceviche, and gravlax, which contain the third-stage larvae. *Pseudoterranova* infections are usually confined to the stomach; they may be asymptomatic and noted only when the worm is coughed or vomited up. More characteristically, the larvae burrow into the mucosa of the stomach. Here they produce eosinophilic granulomatous tumors with edema, thickening, and induration which may be mistaken for gastric carcinoma or regional enteritis. The pathologic changes are thought to be the result of a hypersensitivity reaction. The patient develops recurrent waves of severe epigastric pain, nausea, and vomiting within a few hours of ingesting infected fish. Some patients note urticaria and tingling in the throat. Gastroscopically, 2- to 4-cm larvae can be seen penetrating the mucosa and can sometimes be removed. *Anisakis* larvae most frequently involve the intestine. Patients develop sudden abdominal pain 1 to 5 days after fish ingestion. The clinical picture may be severe enough to simulate an acute surgical abdomen. More commonly, colicky pain, diffuse abdominal tenderness, fever, and leukocytosis are seen. Occasionally, larvae may penetrate the intestinal wall to involve other abdominal organs. Perforations of the bowel with peritonitis have also been described. Peripheral eosinophilia is not always present, and a definitive diagnosis can be made only by the identification of larvae in tissue. Serologic tests are neither highly reliable nor generally available. The disease usually subsides spontaneously with conservative therapy. Occasionally, a chronic illness develops which requires surgical resection of the lesion.

Over 1000 cases have been recognized in the Netherlands and Japan; approximately 30 have been reported from North America, primarily following the ingestion of salmon or red snapper. The disease can be prevented by storing marine fish at $-20°C$ for a single day or by cooking it at normal cooking temperatures.

HOOKWORM DISEASE Definition Hookworm disease is a symptomatic infection caused by *Necator americanus, Ancylostoma duodenale,* or, less commonly, *A. ceylanicum*. Asymptomatic infection may be termed simply *hookworm infection,* and the individual with such infection is called a *carrier*.

Etiology *Ancylostoma duodenale,* also known as the "old world" hookworm, possesses four prominent hooklike teeth in its adult stage. The adults are about 1 cm long and inhabit the upper part of the human small intestine, where they attach to the mucosa by means of their mouth parts and suck blood. Each adult extracts approximately 0.20 mL blood daily. The adults migrate within the small intestine, and each site of attachment persists temporarily as a bleeding point. Following fertilization, the female liberates approximately 20,000 eggs per day. They measure about 40 by 60 μm and are usually in the two- to four-cell stage when discharged in the feces.

Necator americanus, the "new world" hookworm, has a buccal capsule containing dorsal and ventral plates rather than teeth. It is slightly smaller, deposits fewer eggs, and causes much less blood loss than *A. duodenale. Ancylostoma ceylanicum,* a hookworm of cats found in the Far East, may occasionally reach maturity in humans.

The life cycles of the hookworms are similar. Under appropriate conditions, the eggs hatch in 24 to 48 h, releasing free-living or rhabditiform larvae. Within a few days, these develop into infective or filariform larvae which may remain viable in the soil for several weeks. These, in turn, penetrate the skin to enter vessels which carry them to the lungs. The larvae leave the alveolar capillaries, enter the alveoli, ascend the respiratory tree, enter the pharynx, and are swallowed. They reach the intestine about 1 week after penetration of the skin and mature within 5 weeks. Larval development of *Ancylostoma* may be arrested or retarded in the human host. This may result in a prolonged latent period between the onset of infection and the appearance of gravid females in the intestine. Adults have been known to survive in the human intestine for as long as 14 years, but *A. duodenale* seldom persists beyond 6 to 8 years, and most *N. americanus* infections are eliminated within 2 to 4 years.

Epidemiology It has been estimated that hookworms infect 900 million people and cause the loss of 9 million liters of blood daily throughout the world from 45°N to 30°S latitude. *Necator americanus* is found predominantly in the tropical areas of Africa, Asia, and the Americas, while *A. duodenale* occurs in the Mediterranean Basin, the Middle East, northern India, China, and Japan. In many areas both species are found. In general, *Ancylostoma* presents a greater public health hazard than *N. americanus,* the species which is most prevalent in the southern United States, because it is more persistent in the environment, more harmful to the host, and less amenable to treatment. Conditions conducive to the development of the hookworm egg into infective filariform larvae are a mean temperature between 23 and 33°C, abundant rainfall, shade, and well-drained sandy soil. Hookworm infection occurs where there is opportunity for direct contact of the skin with soil contaminated by promiscuous defecation. *A. duodenale* disease may also be acquired by oral ingestion of infective larvae. Transmammary and transplacental transmission may also occur with this species; presumably this results from the activation of larvae whose development within the tissues of the host has been arrested or retarded. Because of greater exposure, males show a higher incidence of infection than females. Infections are particularly common in closed, heavily populated communities such as coffee or tea plantations.

Repeated infections of hookworm in dogs result in immunity and elimination of the parasite. It seems probable that a similar phenomenon occurs in human infections. When the possibility of reinfection is eliminated, the majority of worms is eliminated spontaneously within 1 or 2 years.

Pathogenesis and clinical manifestations During the invasion of the exposed skin by the larvae, there may be an erythematous maculopapular skin rash and edema with severe pruritus. These manifestations, which may persist for several days, are more marked in *N. americanus* infection. The lesions are most common about the feet, particularly between the toes, and have been termed "ground itch."

During migration through the lungs, cough, pneumonia, and, in severe infections, fever may occur. Usually, however, pulmonary involvement does not give rise to clinical symptoms.

Various gastrointestinal symptoms, ranging from vague epigastric distress and pica to typical ulcer pain, have been reported in association with hookworm infection. Roentgenographic studies may reveal nonspecific changes such as excessive peristalsis and "puddling," particularly in the proximal jejunum. However, gross and microscopic examination of the bowel itself reveals conspicuously little damage.

The major clinical manifestations of hookworm disease clearly are those of iron-deficiency anemia and hypoalbuminemia consequent to chronic intestinal blood loss. Whether anemia develops and how severe it becomes depends on the balance between iron lost in the gut and iron absorbed from the diet. The severity of the disease and the prognosis depend on the age of the patient, the magnitude of the worm burden, and the duration of the disease. Young children often have extreme anemia, with cardiac insufficiency and anasarca. These conditions may precipitate kwashiorkor. Those who survive to puberty show retarded physical, mental, and sexual development. Milder degrees of the disease, as seen in older children and adults, are characterized by lassitude, dyspnea, palpitation, tachycardia, constipation, and pallor of the skin and mucous membranes.

Asymptomatic infections outnumber symptomatic infections, considering all age groups, 20 to 40 times in endemic areas. The worm burden is small in asymptomatic infections, and the carrier state may be indicative of some degree of acquired host resistance.

Laboratory findings In symptomatic infection, hookworm eggs are usually numerous enough to be detected by microscopic examination of a direct or concentrated fecal smear. A quantitative egg count, using the cellophane thick smear (Kato) technique, allows an estimation of the intensity of infection. If a stool specimen is allowed to stand for several hours before examination, the eggs may hatch, releasing larvae which are easily confused with those of *Strongyloides*. The species of hookworm may be determined by the identification of the adult worm passed in the stool following treatment or by culturing the feces and identifying the third-stage larvae. This is seldom important in clinical practice. Abdominal and pulmonary symptoms appear before the eggs are discharged, although a presumptive diagnosis may be made on the basis of the clinical history and the eosinophilic leukocytosis.

Generally, the leukocyte count is normal. However, in some early cases, leukocytosis may be marked, with an eosinophilia as high as 70 or 80 percent. The anemia is characteristically hypochromic and microcytic.

Treatment In areas where reinfection is likely, administration of anthelmintics to patients with light infections (less than 2000 eggs per milliliter of feces) is probably not beneficial. A number of satisfactory anthelmintic agents are available, but two, pyrantel pamoate (see "Ascariasis" above) and mebendazole (see "Trichuriasis" above) are currently favored. Treatment can be repeated in a week if complete cure is desired and has not been accomplished. This is seldom necessary in endemic areas, where the aim of therapy is reduction of the worm load to an asymptomatic level.

The anemia requires iron replacement. When anemia is severe and there is malnutrition with anasarca, blood transfusions and a high-protein diet should be given before drug treatment is begun. Blood should be given in an amount sufficient to raise the hemoglobin level to 100 g/L (10 g/dL). In advanced cases it may be necessary to delay drug treatment for 2 to 3 weeks.

Prognosis The immediate prognosis is good. When opportunity for reinfection persists and nutrition cannot be maintained, a state of chronic debility develops. Maturation of children is impaired, and intercurrent disease is a serious problem in adults.

Prevention Many of the measures required are obvious but difficult to apply on a large scale. Even if facilities for proper disposal of feces are provided, it is no simple matter to sustain their use. Soil pollution must be eliminated. Avoidance of direct skin contact with the soil (by wearing shoes) is often not practical in endemic areas. Periodic mass treatment of the population has been used in some hookworm control programs. Dietary iron supplementation can prevent the development of anemia.

CUTANEOUS LARVA MIGRANS (CREEPING ERUPTION)

Definition Creeping eruption is an infection of human skin caused by the larvae of the dog and cat hookworm, *A. brasiliense*. The other dog hookworms, *A. caninum* and *Uncinaria stenocephala,* as well as the human parasites, *Strongyloides stercoralis* and *Necator americanus,* may also produce the disease. The larvae of *Gnathostoma spinigerum,* a nematode found in the Orient, and *Gasterophilus,* the horse botfly, may produce a similar cutaneous infection.

Etiology *Ancylostoma brasiliense* reaches adulthood regularly only in the dog and cat. The larvae emerging from eggs discharged in the feces develop to the filariform stage and then are capable of penetrating the skin. In humans, the larvae usually remain in the epidermis and migrate, producing an irregular erythematous tunnel visible on the skin surface.

Epidemiology and distribution Transmission to humans requires environmental temperature and humidity appropriate for development of the egg to the infective filariform larva stage. Beaches and other moist, sandy areas are hazardous, because animals choose such areas for defecation, and the *A. brasiliense* eggs develop well in such soil. In the United States infection is found in the southern Atlantic and Gulf states.

Pathogenesis and clinical manifestations The site of penetration of the skin by the larvae becomes apparent in a few hours. The migration of the larvae in the skin is accompanied by severe itching. Scratching may lead to bacterial infection. In the course of 1 week, the initial red papule develops into an irregular, erythematous, linear lesion which may attain a length of 15 to 20 cm. The larvae may persist for weeks to months without treatment.

Loeffler's syndrome has been observed in 26 of 52 cases of creeping eruption. Transient, migratory pulmonary infiltrations associated with an increased number of eosinophils in the blood and sputum were interpreted as an allergic reaction to the helminthic infection but may have reflected pulmonary migration of the larvae.

Laboratory findings Eosinophils occur in the lesion, but eosinophilic leukocytosis is slight, except when Loeffler's syndrome appears. The percentage of eosinophils in the blood may then rise to 50 percent and in the sputum to 90 percent. Only rarely are larvae found on skin biopsy.

Treatment Thiabendazole is the drug of choice; it should be given orally in the dosage suggested for strongyloidiasis (see below). It may be repeated if necessary. Alternatively, it may be applied topically as a 10% aqueous suspension. Topical administration avoids systemic toxicity. Superficial bacterial infections are improved by the application of wet dressings and elevation of the extremity. For intense itching, oral antihistaminics may be helpful.

Prognosis Untreated infections last several months. Treatment, which is usually sought because of severe pruritus, is usually successful.

Prevention Dogs and cats should be prevented from contaminating recreation areas and children's sandboxes.

TRICHOSTRONGYLIASIS Trichostrongyliasis is an intestinal infection of herbivorous animals, and incidentally humans, throughout the world. The disease is most common in Asia, the Middle East, and South America. In view of the high frequency of animal infections in the United States, the low incidence of human infections here is difficult to understand. The ova resemble those of the hookworm but are larger, have more pointed ends, and, when observed in a fresh fecal specimen, show a more advanced stage of segmentation (16- to 32-cell stage). Infection is acquired by ingestion of green leafy plants contaminated with third-stage larvae. On reaching the small intestine, they attach themselves to the mucosa and develop into adult worms within 4 weeks. The adult at that time sucks blood and maintains residence in the intestine for long periods. Most infections are asymptomatic, but massive infections may result in epigastric distress and anemia. The parasite owes its importance primarily to the resemblance of its ova to those of the hookworms. Moreover, because the trichostrongylidae do not respond to some of the anthelmintics effective in hookworm infection, it may be assumed incorrectly that refractory hookworm infection is present. The diagnosis depends on the finding of the ova in the feces. Since they are few, they are usually found only when a concentration method is used. In symptomatic infections, there may be leukocytosis with marked eosinophilia (80 percent). Thiabendazole 25 mg/kg twice daily for 2 or 3 days, or pyrantel pamoate as used in hookworm infections, is effective in symptomatic infections. Both are considered investigational drugs for this condition by the U.S. Food and Drug Administration.

STRONGYLOIDIASIS Definition Strongyloidiasis is an intestinal infection of humans caused by *Strongyloides stercoralis* or, on occasion, the primate species, *S. fuelleborni*. Extraintestinal involvement may occur in severe cases.

Etiology The tiny (2 mm in length) adult female resides and lays her eggs in the mucosa of the upper part of the jejunum. In heavy infections, the biliary and pancreatic ducts, the entire small bowel, and the colon may be parasitized. The eggs quickly hatch, releasing rhabditiform larvae which enter the lumen of the bowel and are passed in the feces. On reaching the soil, the larvae develop into the infective filariform stage. There, as in the case of the filariform larvae of hookworm, they penetrate the skin and small blood vessels of humans. They are then carried to the lungs where they leave the alveolar capillaries, ascend the respiratory tree, enter the pharynx, and are swallowed. On reaching the small intestine, they mature and burrow into the jejunal mucosa. Parasitic males have not been observed and it is likely that females reproduce parthenogenetically. Oviposition (up to 40 eggs per day) begins 17 to 28 days after the initial infection. In addition to the *direct* host-soil-host cycle, *Strongyloides* has two alternative cycles. In the first, or *indirect,* cycle, the rhabditiform larvae, after passing from the host, develop into free-living male and female adults which reside and reproduce in the soil, thus creating a reservoir of infection independent of the human host. Under certain environmental conditions, the free-living larvae are capable of transforming back into filariform larvae which initiate a new cycle in humans. In the second, or *autoinfection,* cycle, the rhabditiform larvae develop into filariform larvae before they are passed in the stool. They may then invade the intestinal mucosa or perianal skin of the same host without first going through a soil phase. This may explain the long persistence (20 to 30 years) of strongyloidiasis in patients who have left endemic areas and may also account for the extremely heavy worm loads in some individuals. Autoinfection appears to occur frequently in patients with achlorhydria, delayed intestinal transit time, and blind loops or diverticula. Contamination of the perianal area, clothing, or bedding with feces permits development of filariform larvae outside of the body and invasion of the perianal skin of the host or transmission to others by direct physical contact. The transformation of the filariform larvae outside the body is probably responsible for the frequency with which strongyloidiasis is seen in crowded, unsanitary institutions for the mentally retarded.

Epidemiology The usual mode of infection is the penetration of the skin by larvae. Some infections may result from ingestion of contaminated food and drink, and some are transmitted by contact. Transmission between sexual partners, however, appears to be uncommon. Transmammary passage in humans has been demonstrated for *S. fuelleborni.* The majority of the 80 million infected individuals reside in the tropics, where the warmth, moisture, and lack of sanitation favor its spread. Sporadic cases appear among Puerto Ricans and throughout the rural south of the continental United States. Homosexual men may be at increased risk. Chronic strongyloidiasis has been reported in Vietnam veterans.

Pathogenesis and clinical manifestations The initial cutaneous penetration of the filariform larvae usually produces no symptoms. However, *larva currens,* transitory skin eruptions characterized by blotchy erythema, serpiginous lesions, and urticaria, may be seen during episodes of autoinfection. These may recur at irregular intervals and are particularly common following recovery from an acute febrile illness. In these situations the lesions are generally found over the lower back and buttocks. Cough, dyspnea, gross hemoptysis, and bronchospasm may accompany migration through the lungs. Chest x-rays may show pulmonary infiltration at this time. The intestinal infestation is usually asymptomatic or productive only of vague abdominal complaints. In heavier infections, epigastric pain and tenderness, nausea, flatulence, vomiting, and diarrhea alternating with constipation may be observed. Peptic ulcer may be simulated, but food often aggravates the pain. The mucosal inflammation may be severe enough to produce subacute obstruction, segmental ileus, and impaired absorption. Chronic, relapsing intestinal and pulmonary manifestations have been noted in a few patients. A severe form of ulcerative colitis, accompanied by intestinal perforation and peritonitis, has also been encountered. In debilitated, immunodepressed, steroid-treated, alcoholic, and hemodialyzed patients, massive autoinfection with widespread dissemination of larvae to the extraintestinal organs including the central nervous system may occur. This hyperinfection is usually abrupt in onset with fever and severe abdominal pain; it is often associated with shock, pulmonary manifestations, severe enterocolitis, persistent gram-negative bacteremia, and occasionally gram-negative meningitis. Unrecognized, it usually leads to death. Disseminated strongyloidiasis should be considered in any compromised host with unexplained gram-negative bacteremia, abdominal complaints, and pulmonary infiltrates with or without eosinophilia.

Laboratory findings The definitive diagnosis can be made by identification of the larvae in the stool. Fresh fecal specimens should be examined to avoid confusion with hookworm infection; generally, fresh specimens contain *larvae* in strongyloidiasis infections, while in hookworm infection they contain *eggs.* Since the number of larvae in the stool is small and varies from day to day, several samples should be checked, using concentration and culture techniques. Microscopic examination of the duodenal aspirates and jejunal biopsies may also establish the diagnosis. Alternatively, a weighted string can be passed into the duodenum, allowed to remain for a short time, and then withdrawn. The bile-stained section of the string is stripped of fluid which is then examined for the presence of larvae. If pulmonary involvement is present, the sputum should be examined for larvae. An ELISA utilizing *S. stercoralis* larval antigens was shown to be positive in approximately 80 to 90 percent of patients and may have some diagnostic utility.

Eosinophilic leukocytosis is common, except in very severe cases. When eosinophilia occurs in association with peptic ulcer symptoms, strongyloidiasis should be suspected.

Treatment All infected patients should be treated to prevent the occurrence of severe invasive disease. The drug of choice is thiabendazole, which should be given orally in dosage of 25 mg/kg twice a day for 2 or 3 days. In disseminated strongyloidiasis, treatment should be continued for 7 days or more. Lightheadedness, nausea, and vomiting are common accompaniments of therapy with this agent. Delayed aminophylline excretion may result in toxicity. Hypersensitivity reactions may occur but usually respond to treatment with antihistamines. The stools should be rechecked at intervals of 3 months because the parasite is not easily eradicated and retreatment may be necessary.

Prognosis In the usual case, the prognosis is good. Since the occurrence of hyperinfection is unpredictable, every effort should be made to eradicate the infection in each case. In severe cases with hyperinfection, the prognosis is poor.

Prevention In general, the measures are those for the control of hookworm infection. In addition, it is well to remember that infection may be contracted by ingestion of contaminated food (especially uncooked vegetables) or of contaminated drinking water and by contact. Patients who have a history of residence in an endemic area or eosinophilia should be carefully checked for the presence of the parasite prior to the initiation of steroid or immunosuppressive therapy. Because the larvae may not appear in the stool for several weeks after the initiation of such therapy, repeated examinations of stool and upper intestinal aspirates are indicated. Since sputum, vomitus, stool, and body fluids of patients with disseminated disease may contain infective filariform larvae, gloves and gowns should be worn by hospital personnel caring for such patients.

INTESTINAL CAPILLARIASIS Definition Intestinal capillariasis is an infection of humans caused by the roundworm *Capillaria philippinensis* that is characterized by intractable diarrhea with a high mortality rate.

Etiology Adult *C. philippinensis* are small, measuring 2 to 4 mm in length. The peanut-shaped eggs have flattened bipolar plugs and an average size of 42 by 20 μm. The adults inhabit the mucosa of the small intestine, especially the jejunum. Adults, larval forms, and eggs are found in the stool.

Epidemiology The infection has been found almost exclusively in persons residing along the north and west coastal areas of Luzon, Philippines. Several cases from Thailand have also been reported. Since 1966 the disease has occurred in epidemic form, and more than 2000 cases and 100 deaths have been reported.

The mode of transmission and life cycle of the parasite are incompletely understood. The adult worm is thought to parasitize the gut of birds. Eggs passed in their excrement presumably embryonate in fresh water before being ingested by an intermediate fish or crustacean host. When humans ingest an infected intermediate host in the raw state, the first-stage larvae are released and develop to adulthood within their intestinal lumina. These rapidly produce new larvae which mature to a second generation of adults. Most of the females from this generation are oviparous, the resulting eggs passing in the stool. Some, however, remain larviparous, leading to another generation of intestinal adults.

Pathogenesis and manifestations Adult worms in large numbers invade the small-intestinal mucosa and cause a severe protein-losing enteropathy and malabsorption. Hypokalemia, hypocalcemia, and hypoproteinemia are the rule. Autopsy studies have failed to show extraintestinal spread of the parasite. Initial symptoms of intestinal "gurgling" (borborygmi) and recurrent vague abdominal pain are followed, usually within 2 to 3 weeks, by a voluminous watery diarrhea. Other findings, consistent with the basic pathophysiologic process, are anorexia, vomiting, weight loss, muscle wasting and weakness, hyporeflexia, and edema. Abdominal tenderness and distention may occur. The period between onset of symptoms and death is usually 2 to 3 months. Subclinical infection has not been noted.

Diagnosis The diagnosis is made by finding ova in the stool. The ova of *C. philippinensis* must be differentiated from those of *T. trichiura,* which are similar. Care must be taken that capillaria are not overlooked in patients with *Trichuris* infections because in the endemic area most patients with capillariasis have coexistent *Trichuris* infection.

Treatment Administration of mebendazole combined with fluid and electrolyte replacement leads to dramatic improvement; 400 mg per day in divided dosage should be given for 20 days to prevent relapse. Alternatively, thiabendazole, 25 mg/kg per day for 30 days, can be given.

TISSUE NEMATODE INFECTIONS

ANGIOSTRONGYLIASIS CANTONENSIS **Definition** *Angiostrongylus cantonensis,* the rat lungworm, is the etiologic agent of the common form of *eosinophilic meningitis* found in southeast Asia and the tropical areas of the Pacific.

Etiology The delicate filariform adults (20 mm in length) reside and lay their eggs in the pulmonary arterioles of rats and certain other rodents. After hatching, the larvae break into the alveoli, migrate up the respiratory tract, are swallowed, and pass in the feces. They develop into infective third-stage larvae within snails and slugs, their natural intermediate host. Viable third-stage organisms may also be found in land planarians, crabs, and freshwater prawns, which acquire the larvae by feeding on the tissues of infected mollusks. Humans, like rodents, become parasitized when they ingest raw intermediate or carrier hosts containing the infective stage. In rodents the larvae migrate to the brain where they grow into young adults. After a period of further maturation, the worms travel to the lungs and begin to deposit eggs. The nematode does not complete its life cycle in humans and dies after reaching the central nervous system.

Epidemiology The majority of human infections with *A. cantonensis* have been found in Thailand, Vietnam, Cambodia, Indonesia, the Philippines, Taiwan, Hawaii, and several smaller Pacific islands from Okinawa in the north to Tahiti in the south. Cases have been described in Puerto Rico, Cuba, Egypt, and the Ivory Coast.

Pathology and pathogenesis The nematode can produce extensive tissue damage by moving through the brain when alive and provokes a marked inflammatory reaction when dead. The pathologic lesions are characterized by (1) marked lymphocyte and eosinophilic infiltration of the meninges, (2) hemorrhagic worm tracts through the brainstem and spinal cord, (3) granuloma formation around dead parasites and necrotic debris which sheathes the worm, and (4) engorgement of almost all blood vessels, particularly the veins. Necrosis of vessel walls, aneurysmal dilatation of arteries, and perivascular hemorrhages have been noted. Living worms have been removed from the eyes of patients without central nervous system involvement.

Clinical manifestations The eosinophilic meningitis usually presents as severe headache of acute or insidious onset. Fever is usually mild or absent, and only 15 percent of patients show signs of meningeal irritation. Patients frequently complain of visual impairment and, in a majority of these, visual defects or blurring of the optic disk can be demonstrated. Paresthesias and exquisite pains of the trunk and lower extremities are a common complaint, and paralysis of the sixth and seventh nerves is seen in 3 to 7 percent of cases. Paralysis of the limbs, convulsions, and loss of consciousness are rare. Although some patients have experienced significant neurologic residua, the disease usually ends in complete spontaneous recovery. Death is rare. The cerebrospinal fluid contains several hundred cells per cubic millimeter and many eosinophils, and the protein is elevated. There may or may not be an eosinophilia in the peripheral blood.

Diagnosis The diagnosis is entertained on the basis of the clinical manifestations in an endemic area. Small areas of attenuation with surrounding hypodense collars may be seen on computed tomography (CT) scan of the brain. Rarely, the adult worm is found in the cerebrospinal fluid. Angiostrongyliasis must be differentiated from other ectopic worm infections of the central nervous system including strongyloidiasis, filariasis, paragonimiasis, hydatid disease, schistosomiasis japonicum, trichinosis, cysticercosis, toxocariasis, and gnathostomiasis. A case of visceral larva migrans with eosinophilic meningitis has been described, in which the raccoon ascarid, *Baylisascaris procyonis,* was implicated. The diagnosis can be confirmed with an ELISA for circulating antibodies.

Treatment and prevention Mebendazole, in the dose of 100 mg, is often administered twice daily for 5 days, but is of uncertain efficacy. Anthelmintic therapy has been thought by some authors to be dangerous since the simultaneous death of many worms might produce a severe inflammatory reaction. Steroids may be beneficial in severe cases. Prevention depends upon avoidance or proper cooking of such foods as snails, prawns, and crabs. Raw vegetables should be carefully inspected for the presence of planarians and mollusks before they are eaten. Freezing of crustaceans and mollusks at −15°C for 12 h will destroy infective larvae of *A. cantonensis.*

ANGIOSTRONGYLIASIS COSTARICENSIS *Angiostrongylus costaricensis* is a nematode that dwells in the mesenteric arteries of Central and South American rats. Larvae pass in the stool and develop in slugs, the intermediate hosts. Rats, and incidentally humans, are infected when they ingest slugs or vegetables contaminated with third-stage larvae deposited in the mucous trail of these mollusks. The larvae mature in the lymphatics and move to the mesenteric radicals of the cecum. Here they may cause arterial thrombosis, ischemic necrosis, ulceration, and eosinophilic granuloma formation. Infected patients present with fever, eosinophilic leukocytosis, abdominal pain, and a right lower quadrant mass. Occasionally, perforation of the bowel and generalized peritonitis occur. The fever may persist for up to 2 months. Children are more frequently involved than adults. Neither larvae nor eggs are seen in the stool of the human host. The diagnosis is usually established at the time of surgery. The value of specific anthelmintic therapy has not been established.

GNATHOSTOMIASIS **Definition** Gnathostomiasis is a tissue infection of humans caused by *Gnathostoma spinigerum.* Clinically it is manifest as cutaneous or visceral larva migrans, ocular infection, or a lethal eosinophilic meningitis.

Etiology and epidemiology The parasite, which is found throughout the Far East, lives encysted in the gastric mucosa of dogs, cats, and wild felines. The ova are passed to the external environment via the feces, hatch in water, and are ingested by *Cyclops,* the first intermediate hosts. These in turn are eaten by freshwater fish, frogs, snakes, and eels in whose flesh the infective third-stage larvae develop. Ducks and chickens fed on these second intermediate hosts may also come to harbor infective larvae. Human infections, which are most commonly seen in Thailand and Japan, occur when humans ingest infected uncooked fish (somfak, sashimi), duck, or chicken.

Pathogenesis and manifestations The parasite cannot complete its cycle in humans, and the immature worms migrate through the abdominal and thoracic organs producing localized areas of inflammation and hemorrhage. Clinically, this is manifest as fever, eosinophilic leukocytosis, urticaria, and pain. Typically, the systemic manifestations subside within a month as the worms make their way to the subcutaneous tissues. Here, their continued migration results in the production of transient serpiginous pruritic swellings, subcutaneous tunnels, and abscesses. If the worm invades the epidermis, the resulting lesions closely resemble those of cutanea larva migrans. Not uncommonly, the eye may be involved with orbital cellulitis, iritis, or uveitis. Migration into the central nervous system results in a lethal eosinophilic meningitis (see ''Angiostrongyliasis Cantonensis'' above). This presents as a radiculomyeloencephalitis with limb pain and paresis. The cerebrospinal fluid eosinophilic leukocytosis is present but less marked than in *Angiostrongylus* infections. The fluid is often xanthochromic. Death may occur from cerebral hemorrhage or destruction of vital centers.

Diagnosis and treatment Painless, recurrent migratory subcutaneous swellings and eosinophilic leukocytosis occurring in an endemic area make the diagnosis likely. It must be differentiated from cutanea larva migrans, however, and from angiostrongyliasis cantonensis when the central nervous system is involved. Areas of CNS hemorrhage appear as hyperdense areas on brain CT. Definitive diagnosis depends upon the removal and identification of the worm. The ELISA appears to be a useful diagnostic adjunct. Other than excision, there is no specific therapy of documented efficacy. However, mebendazole, 200 mg every 3 h for 6 days, is frequently administered with glucocorticoids in CNS disease. The disease can be prevented by the adequate cooking of fish, chicken, and duck in endemic areas.

DRACUNCULIASIS Definition Dracunculiasis is an infection of human connective and subcutaneous tissues by the guinea worm, *Dracunculus medinensis.*

Etiology and epidemiology Dracunculiasis affects about 10 million people in Africa, the Middle East, and the Indian subcontinent. Humans acquire the parasite when they ingest raw drinking water containing infected copepods (*Cyclops* spp.) which serve as the intermediate host. Shallow ponds, cisterns, and wells are the usual habitat of these crustaceans. In the stomach the copepod is digested and the larvae are released. The larva penetrates the intestinal wall and matures in the connective tissue of the retroperitoneal space. The adult male is small, seldom seen, and presumably dies after mating. In contrast, the female *Dracunculus* is one of the largest nematodes known—1 to 2 mm in diameter and 300 to 800 mm in length. The female reaches gravidity in approximately one year and then migrates to the subcutaneous tissue of the lower extremities. When the anterior end of the worm approaches the skin, a blister forms. This breaks down in a few days, forming a superficial ulcer. When the protruding portion of the worm comes in contact with water, the uterus prolapses through the body and discharges large numbers of motile rhabditiform larvae. Following ingestion by one of several species of *Cyclops,* the larvae undergo further development, becoming infective in 10 to 12 days. Mammals other than humans may be infected, but their importance as a disease reservoir is uncertain.

Pathogenesis and manifestations The infection is asymptomatic until the gravid female appears in the subcutaneous tissues, where it may, on occasion, be palpable. A few days before the formation of the blister, the patient frequently has fever, generalized urticaria, periorbital edema, and wheezing. Blister formation is accompanied by intense local pain and pruritus; like the systemic manifestations, this is thought to represent an allergic reaction to prematurely liberated larvae. The local lesion is usually found over the feet and ankles, making walking difficult, but may occur on the trunk or the upper extremities. Multiple infections are common. With the rupture of the blister and the release of embryos, the systemic manifestations abate, and the worm is slowly extruded over a period of 4 to 5 weeks. Secondary infection and cellulitis are common, particularly if the worm is ruptured during the process of extraction. In Nigeria, guinea worm ulcers are a common portal of entry for the spores of *Clostridium tetani.* The female worm often fails to reach the surface and discharge her larvae. In most of these cases, it dies without producing symptoms. The calcified appearance on roentgenograms is characteristic. Occasionally the worm may invade the deep tissues, causing serious symptoms, and sterile abscesses may follow the release of embryos. Invasion of joint spaces by the adult worm or larvae results in arthritis.

Diagnosis The clinical picture is characteristic. Placing a small amount of water on the worm results in discharge of larvae, which can then be examined microscopically.

Treatment and prevention If the outline of the worm can be clearly seen or palpated, it may sometimes be completely removed with a single incision. The gradual extraction of the worm can be accomplished by winding a few centimeters onto a stick each day. Thiabendazole in dosage of 25 mg/kg twice daily for 3 days or metronidazole 250 mg three times a day for 10 days is effective in the relief of symptoms, but there is serious question whether either agent hastens worm extrusion or death. Dracunculiasis can be prevented by the chemical treatment of drinking water or the provision of piped water.

CESTODE INFECTIONS

The tapeworms, or cestodes, are ribbon-shaped segmented hermaphroditic worms which inhabit the intestinal tract of many vertebrates. Unlike other helminths, they lack a digestive tract but absorb food through their entire surface. Tapeworms have a primitive nervous system, a muscular system, and excretory canals. Attachment to the host's intestinal mucosa is accomplished by sucking cups or grooves located on the head, or *scolex.* In some species, attachment is aided by hooklets located on the scolex. Behind the globular scolex lies a short, narrow neck from which segments or *proglottides* develop to form the chainlike *strobila* of the worm. The proglottides progressively mature as they are displaced further from the neck by new segments. As each section becomes gravid, eggs are released either through a uterine pore, by splitting open, or by disintegrating. Because the eggs of many tapeworms appear identical, species identification depends on the morphologic characteristics of the scolex or gravid proglottides.

Except for *Hymenolepis nana* the human tapeworms require one or more intermediate hosts for larval development. After ingestion by a susceptible intermediate host, eggs develop into larvae or *oncospheres* which are capable of penetrating the intestinal mucosa, migrating in tissues, and developing into encysted forms. A cyst with a single scolex is called a *cysticercus* or *cysticercoid* in the case of *H. nana.* A *coenurus* is a cyst which contains several scolices, and a *hydatid* is a structure with daughter cysts each containing several scolices. Ingestion of tissues containing cysts with viable scolices by a definitive host allows development of the larval stage into an adult tapeworm. Cestodes in the *Diphyllobothrium* genus have a more complex life cycle involving two intermediate hosts (see below).

Human tapeworm infections may be divided into two major clinical groups. In the first, humans act as the definitive host and harbor the adult tapeworm in their intestines. The important species in this group are *Taenia saginata, Diphyllobothrium* species, *Hymenolepis* species, and *Dipylidium caninum*. In the second group, humans are intermediate hosts and harbor the larval forms in their tissues. This is exemplified by echinococcosis, sparganosis, and coenurosis. *Taenia solium* is unique because humans may act as both the definitive and intermediate hosts.

TAENIASIS SAGINATA Epidemiology Intestinal infection in humans with *Taenia saginata* occurs in all countries where raw or undercooked beef is eaten. It is particularly prevalent in Ethiopia, Kenya, Yugoslavia, the Middle East, Mexico and parts of South America, and the U.S.S.R. Indigenously acquired infection is uncommon in the United States except in areas where cattle and humans are concentrated such as around feedlots in the southwest.

Etiology and pathogenesis Humans are the only definitive host for the adult stage of *T. saginata,* which inhabits the upper jejunum for as long as 25 years. The cestode is 3 to 10 m long and has a small, unarmed scolex with four prominent suckers and 1000 to 2000 proglottides. The gravid segments are longer than they are wide (5 by 20 mm) and have 15 to 30 lateral uterine branches (*T. solium* has 8 to 12). The eggs, which are indistinguishable from *T. solium* eggs, measure 30 by 40 μm, have a thick brown radially striated shell, and contain a fully developed embryo with three pairs of hooklets. After the egg-containing proglottides are deposited on soil or vegetation, they are ingested by cattle or other herbivores. The embryo is released in the intestine, invades the intestinal wall, and is carried by vascular channels to striated muscle in the hind limbs, diaphragm, and tongue, where it is transformed over a period of 3 to 4 months into an ovoid bladder worm, or cysticercus. This form, which may be viable for 1 to 3 years, measures about 5 by 10 mm and consists of one scolex suspended in a fluid-filled sac. After ingestion of the cyst in raw or undercooked beef by humans, an adult worm develops in the intestine in about 2 months.

Clinical manifestations Most patients have minimal or no symptoms. Mild epigastric discomfort, nausea, flatulence, or hunger sensations may occur. Weight loss, diarrhea, irritability, and an increase in appetite are more unusual. Movements of the worm are sometimes apparent, and occasionally proglottides may crawl through the anus, appearing in the bed linen or underclothing of the distraught host. Rarely, segments become impacted in the appendix or cystic or pancreatic duct, producing obstruction and inflammation of these organs.

Diagnosis After the adult tapeworm has been established for 2 to 3 months, several proglottides are shed daily in the stool. Eggs also may be found in the stool or on the perianal area if a proglottid ruptures during defecation. If proglottides or eggs are not found in the stool, the perianal region should be examined using a cellophane tape swab as for pinworm infection. Since egg morphology is not diagnostic, however, examination of mature proglottides or the scolex is still necessary to identify the tapeworm species correctly. Reliable serologic tests are not available.

Treatment Niclosamide (Yomesan) is a highly effective taenicide which kills the scolex and immature segments of the worm on contact. Four 0.5-g tablets are thoroughly chewed at one time and swallowed with a small amount of water. No preparation or purge is necessary, and few side effects have been reported. As the worm is digested before it is passed in the stool, no attempt should be made to recover the scolex. Stool should be examined at 3 and 6 months for test of cure. Alternatively, a single dose of praziquantel (10 mg/kg) is effective, but this agent has not been approved for treating taeniasis in the United States.

Prevention Thorough cooking of beef is the major means of preventing taeniasis saginata. Temperatures as low as 56°C for as little as 5 min will destroy cysticerci. Refrigeration and salting for prolonged periods or freezing at −10°C for 9 days also destroys the cysticercus. General preventive measures include adequate meat inspection and proper disposal of human feces.

TAENIASIS SOLIUM AND CYSTICERCOSIS *Taenia solium,* the pork tapeworm, inhabits the intestinal lumen of humans, its only definitive host. The hog is the usual intermediate host, although humans, dogs, cats, and sheep may harbor the larval form. When human tissue is invaded by the larval form, the condition is referred to as *cysticercosis.*

Epidemiology Taeniasis solium is worldwide but is most common in Mexico, Africa, southeast Asia, eastern Europe, and South America. *T. solium* has been found in swine in Colorado and New Mexico, and autochthonously acquired human disease has been recognized in the United States. Cysticercosis is more frequent in industrialized nations due to migration of infected persons from endemic areas.

Etiology and pathogenesis The adult worm is about 3 m in length, resides in the upper jejunum, and may live for decades. The globular scolex contains a rostellum with two rows of hooklets. There are usually fewer than 1000 proglottides. The gravid proglottid is about 6 by 12 mm and contains a uterus with 8 to 12 lateral branchings. The eggs are infective for both human and hog. Infection usually occurs by the fecal-oral route, but humans may be autoinfected when gravid segments are returned to the stomach by reverse peristalsis. In the intermediate host, the embryo is released from the egg, penetrates the intestinal wall, and is carried by vascular channels to all parts of the body. Localization with development over 60 to 90 days to the encysted larval stage (''bladder worm'') occurs primarily in striated muscle of the tongue, neck, and trunk. *Cysticerci cellulosae* are ovoid, gray-white opalescent structures about 1 cm in diameter, and *cysticerci racemosus* are irregular-shaped structures about 3 to 6 cm in diameter. Cysticerci can survive for 5 years. Humans become infected with the adult stage following ingestion of undercooked pork containing cysticerci.

Clinical manifestations Clinical manifestations of adult worm infestation resemble those with *T. saginata.* When humans serve as the intermediate host (cysticercosis), the clinical picture is entirely different. Cysticerci develop in the subcutaneous tissues, in muscles, in viscera, and, most importantly, in the eye and brain. Only a moderate tissue reaction occurs while the scolex is viable, but the dead larvae invoke a marked tissue response with muscular pains, weakness, fever, and eosinophilia. More inflammatory response is seen with racemose-type cysticerci than with cellulose-type. Symptoms in neurocysticercosis may be due to an acute encephalitic stage or due to brain cysts that are usually located in the cerebrum, ventricles, or subarachnoid space. The cerebral cysts are often less than 2 cm in diameter but may rarely be as large as 6 cm with the racemose type. Cerebral calcifications are seen in patients with dead parasites. Patients may have symptoms and signs of meningoencephalitis, including an eosinophilic cerebrospinal fluid pleocytosis, with the acute encephalitic stage or if cysticerci are widely distributed. Epilepsy, brain tumors, and other types of neurologic or psychiatric disorders may also be simulated. Clinical findings may change during the course of infection due to changes in the inflammatory response.

Diagnosis Infection with the adult worm can be detected by finding eggs in perianal scrapings or in the feces. To differentiate *T. solium* from *T. saginata,* proglottides or the scolex must be examined. Cysticercosis should be suspected in an individual who has lived in a hyperendemic area and who develops neurologic findings. Subcutaneous cysts may be found in approximately 50 percent of patients, and roentgenograms of soft tissue may show typical calcifications later in the course of cysticercosis. Contrast-enhanced CT scans and magnetic resonance imaging (MRI) are valuable for identifying brain lesions, which may appear as solid nodules or cystic or calcified lesions. In patients with the acute encephalitic stage, only hydrocephalus may be seen. Cerebrospinal fluid is often abnormal but not diagnostic. ELISA of serum and cerebrospinal fluid provides a sensitive serologic test for diagnosis of cysticercosis, but cross-reactive antibodies occur in some patients with other infections. Brain, subcutaneous nodule, or skin biopsy specimens permit a specific diagnosis.

Treatment The stage and location of the parasite determine the prognosis and treatment. For removal of the adult worm in the human intestine, niclosamide or praziquantel may be given as for *Taeniasis saginata*. However, because these drugs cause maceration of the proglottides with release of ova, cysticercosis could theoretically occur. To prevent this, some authorities recommend that a saline purge be administered 1 h after the medication.

Praziquantel has been used to treat neurocysticercosis associated with hydrocephalus with promising results, although the drug is not approved for this use in the United States. A dose of 50 mg of praziquantel per kilogram given daily in three divided doses for 15 days has been recommended. Treatment of neurocysticercosis with praziquantel may be associated with an exacerbation of symptoms in 90 percent of patients. Glucocorticoids have been used to ameliorate the exacerbations which presumably occur secondary to an inflammatory response to dying cysticerci. Other drugs including albendazole, flubendazole, and metrifonate may also be effective for neurocysticercosis. The optimal dose and duration of these agents, the long-term side effects, and the need for concomitant glucocorticoid treatment have not been studied adequately. There are two groups of patients with cysticercosis for whom praziquantel should not be considered. Treatment of ocular cysticercosis should be surgical. Patients with a seizure disorder, only calcifications on CT scan, and normal cerebrospinal fluid examination should be treated only with anticonvulsant medication.

HYMENOLEPIASIS NANA Epidemiology *Hymenolepis nana* (dwarf tapeworm) infection has been reported in temperate and tropical regions around the globe. It is the most common autochthonously acquired tapeworm in the United States, most of the infections occurring in the southern states. The infection is spread by the direct fecal-oral route and is particularly common in children and institutional populations.

Etiology and pathogenesis The life cycle is unique because both the larval and adult phases occur in the same host. The adult worm is small, about 2 cm, and lives for only a few weeks in the proximal ileum. Its proglottides are very small and are rarely seen in the stool. The gravid segments break apart in the fecal stream releasing spherical eggs. These measure 30 to 44 μm in diameter and have a double membrane enclosing the embryo which has six hooklets. The inner vitelline membrane has four to eight slender filaments arising from each pole. The eggs are immediately infective, and when ingested by a new host, the freed oncospheres penetrate the intestinal villi, becoming cysticercoids. Larvae migrate back into the intestinal lumen, attach to the mucosa, and mature into adult worms. The eggs may also hatch before passing in the stool, causing internal autoinfection with gradually increasing numbers of worms in the host.

Clinical manifestations Dwarf tapeworm infection may be asymptomatic even with many adult worms in the intestine. When infection is massive, abdominal cramps and diarrhea occur. Rarely, dizziness or seizures have been seen in children and have been attributed to a neurotoxic product of the worms.

Treatment Niclosamide, 2 g per day, must be given for 5 to 7 consecutive days. The dosage for children must be adjusted for body weight. The longer treatment course is necessary because niclosamide is not effective against the cysticercoid stage, and the encysted larvae continue to release organisms for 4 days. A repeat treatment course may be required in 2 weeks for patients with heavy infections. A single dose of praziquantel (25 mg/kg) may be more effective, but has not been licensed in the United States for this purpose.

Prevention With a single host involved and the eggs being immediately infective, eradication of the disease presents problems similar to those encountered with enterobiasis. Personal hygiene is imperative. In an institution, epidemics can be avoided by proper screening programs.

HYMENOLEPIASIS DIMINUTA *Hymenolepis diminuta* is a cestode of rats and mice that occasionally infects small children. Larval development occurs in a wide variety of insects including fleas and mealworms. Humans become infected with the adult worm when they ingest uncooked cereal foods contaminated by these insects. Infection is usually asymptomatic, and the diagnosis is made only when characteristic eggs are found in the stool. The eggs resemble those of *H. nana* but are longer and lack polar filaments. Niclosamide, as prescribed for *H. nana,* results in approximately a 90 percent cure rate.

DIPYLIDIASIS CANINUM *Dipylidium caninum* is the common tapeworm of cats and dogs. The orange-brown proglottid, which resembles a pumpkin seed, is often passed intact in the stool or migrates through the anal canal. This may cause animals harboring the parasite to drag their buttocks across the floor. The characteristic egg packets are then expelled by the proglottides and ingested by fleas to develop into infective larval forms. The definitive host becomes infected by swallowing involved fleas. Human infections occur primarily in small children who ingest fleas while playing with their pets. The diagnosis is made by recovering the characteristic proglottid or egg packet. Treatment is the same as for *T. saginata* described above. Periodic deworming of pets provides the best prevention.

DIPHYLLOBOTHRIASIS Epidemiology *Diphyllobothrium latum* and *Diphyllobothrium* species are common in the Baltic and Scandinavian countries, Japan, U.S.S.R., Switzerland, Italy, Chile, and central Africa. The infection occurs in the north central United States, Florida, and along the Pacific coast. Its prevalence is enhanced by the disposal of raw sewage into freshwater lakes. Anadromous Alaskan salmon have been implicated in an outbreak along the west coast. The popularity of raw fish dishes such as Japanese sushi and sashimi may lead to increased prevalence of the disease in the United States.

Etiology and pathogenesis The adult worm lies attached to the mucosa of the ileum and occasionally the jejunum by a pair of sucking grooves located on the scolex. It can live 20 years and achieve a length of more than 10 m. The 3000 to 4000 proglottides are wider than they are long. Unlike *Taenia,* the gravid segments are retained by the worm, and each day a million operculated ova are passed directly in the stool. On reaching water, the egg hatches, releasing a free-swimming embryo. This is eaten by small freshwater crustaceans belonging to the species *Cyclops* or *Diaptomus,* in which it develops into a *procercoid.* When the infected crustacean is swallowed by a fish, the larva migrates into the flesh and grows into a *plerocercoid,* or *sparganum,* larva. Humans acquire disease by ingesting raw infected fish. In 3 to 5 weeks the tapeworm matures in the intestine into an adult capable of discharging eggs. Several *Diphyllobothrium* species can infect humans, and *D. latum* cannot be distinguished from other species by its eggs or proglottides. Species determination requires examination of the scolex.

Clinical manifestations Most infections are asymptomatic or produce slight, transient abdominal discomfort. Rarely, there may be severe cramping abdominal pain, diarrhea or constipation, vomiting, weakness, and loss of weight. Intestinal obstruction has been reported in multiple infections. In 0.1 to 2 percent of infected patients, an anemia develops, and about 40 percent of fish tapeworm carriers will have low serum vitamin B_{12} levels. The anemia appears to result from the ability of the tapeworm to compete successfully with its host for vitamin B_{12} and resembles pernicious anemia including central nervous system involvement. A worm located high in the jejunum may take up 80 to 100 percent of labeled vitamin B_{12} ingested by a patient with anemia. These patients tend to be elderly, have diminished production of intrinsic factor, and have worms located in the proximal small bowel. Folate absorption may also be decreased and contribute to the anemia. Lysolecithin, a product of the tapeworm, may contribute to the severity of the disease. Neurologic manifestations are more common than in pernicious anemia and may occur in the absence of hematologic findings. Typically, they include paresthesias, impaired vibration sense, numbness, weakness, and, less commonly, central scotomas secondary to optic atrophy. These findings are reversible with proper treatment.

Diagnosis The characteristic eggs are present in the stool in large numbers, making the diagnosis easy. They measure 55 to 76 by 41 to 56 μm and possess a single shell with an operculum at one end and a knob on the other. Mild eosinophilia may be present.

Treatment Niclosamide or praziquantel as prescribed for taeniasis saginata will cure most infections. In the presence of macrocytic anemia, parenteral vitamin B_{12} should be given.

Prevention Fish tapeworm infection can be prevented by cooking to a temperature of at least 56°C for 5 min. Freezing at −10°C for 72 h or placing the fish in a brine solution with appropriate salt concentration and exposure time can also prevent disease. Commercially prepared lox is usually brined appropriately before smoking.

SPARGANOSIS The *sparganum,* or plerocercoid larva, of *Diphyllobothrium*-related tapeworms belonging to the genus *Spirometra* will develop in humans following ingestion (usually in drinking water) of a *Cyclops* bearing the procercoid larva. Sparganosis also follows ingestion of infected fish, snakes, or frogs or application of infected flesh as a poultice. The frog tissues contain the sparganum, which is capable of invading human tissues. The dog and cat are definitive hosts for *Spirometra.* The infection often presents as a painful subcutaneous swelling. Periorbital tissues may be involved with marked palpebral edema and destruction of the globe. A marked eosinophilia is usually present. The location of the larvae determines the prognosis of the infection in humans. Surgery and injection of ethyl alcohol with epinephrine-free procaine to kill worms is the preferred method of treatment.

COENUROSIS This is a rare infection of humans by the larval stage, or coenurus, of the dog tapeworm *Taenia multiceps.* As in cysticercosis, the subcutaneous tissue, eye, and central nervous system may be involved. In tropical areas the brain has often been invaded, and the cases have been fatal. The clinical presentation is that of a slowly growing space-occupying lesion. Diagnosis and treatment both rely on surgical excision of the lesion. Treatment with drugs including mebendazole has not been effective.

ECHINOCOCCIASIS Echinococciasis is a tissue infection of humans caused by the larval stage of *Echinococcus granulosus* or *E. multilocularis.* These species of echinococcus are distinct morphologically and biologically. In humans, *E. granulosus* produces cystic lesions primarily involving the liver and lungs, whereas *E. multilocularis* causes multilocular (alveolar) lesions that are locally invasive. A "sylvatic" form of *E. granulosus* differs in clinical findings from a "pastoral" form.

Epidemiology Canines are the definitive hosts for *E. granulosus.* Sheep, cattle, and, in the Middle East, camels are the common intermediates for the pastoral form. This form of the disease has its highest incidence in countries where sheep and cattle raising is carried out with the help of dogs, particularly in the Middle East, Australia, New Zealand, east and south Africa, South America, and central Europe. Approximately 200 cases per year of echinococciasis are diagnosed in the United States, but most are imported. Autochthonously acquired cases have been reported from a few well-defined populations, including Basque sheep farmers in California, southwestern Indians, and sheep raisers in Utah.

The sylvatic focus of *E. granulosus* exists primarily in Alaska and western Canada, where wolves act as the definitive host and caribou and moose as the intermediate. A second sylvatic cycle involving deer and coyotes has been reported from California. A domestic cycle can be established when humans kill the herbivores and feed their viscera to dogs.

In *E. multilocularis* infections, rodents such as deer mice are the natural intermediate hosts, while wolves, foxes, coyotes, and domestic dogs and cats may serve as definitive hosts. An urban cycle involving the cat and common house mouse has been described. Human infection in the United States is most common in Alaska but has also been described in Minnesota. Large series of patients with *E. multilocularis* have been reported from Siberia and Switzerland.

Etiology The adult *E. granulosus* is a small (5 mm) worm which resides in the jejunum of canines for 5 to 20 months. In addition to the scolex and neck, it has three proglottides, one immature, one mature, and one gravid. The gravid segment splits, either before or after passage in the stool, to release eggs which appear identical with those of *T. saginata.* When ingested by an appropriate intermediate host, the embryos escape from the eggs, penetrate the intestinal mucosa, and enter the portal circulation. Most are filtered out by the liver or lung, but some escape into the general circulation to involve brain, kidney, bones, and other tissues. The larvae that are not phagocytosed and destroyed develop into hydatid cysts which are unilocular and consist of an external laminated cuticula and an inner germinal layer. The laminated membrane in the sylvatic form may be semitranslucent in appearance and more fragile than in the pastoral type. Fluid fills and distends the cyst. Brood capsules and second- or third-generation daughter cysts develop from the germinal layer. "Hydatid sand" found in the cyst consists of scolices liberated from ruptured brood capsules. The cysts grow slowly over a period of years. In the pastoral type cysts often reach a diameter of over 10 cm, while cysts in the sylvatic form are usually only 3 to 5 cm. When the hydatid cyst is ingested by a canine, the cycle is complete.

The life cycle of *E. multilocularis* is similar except that small rodents serve as the natural intermediate host. However, the cyst is quite different. Humans do not provide optimal conditions for development of *E. multilocularis,* and the larval form remains in the proliferative phase. The hydatid cyst is always multilocular or alveolar in type. Its vesicles progressively invade the host tissue, usually the liver, by extension of processes from the germinal layer. In general, the growth pattern is like a neoplasm, and the lesions may metastasize when growth extends into blood vessels.

Clinical manifestations Echinococciasis is usually acquired in childhood, but a latent period of 5 to 20 years occurs before diagnosis. In one patient the latent period of a hepatic cyst was 75 years. Enlarging cysts usually produce tissue damage by mechanical means. The resulting symptoms depend upon the site, type, and rate of growth of the cystic lesions.

Patients with the sylvatic form of *E. granulosus* are usually asymptomatic at the time of diagnosis. Approximately 60 percent of the cysts are found in the lung and 40 percent in the liver. The cysts are diagnosed as an incidental finding on routine x-ray. Rarely, a patient may present with hemoptysis or a palpable mass in the liver. Morbidity and mortality are almost never seen.

With the pastoral type the ratio of pulmonary to liver cysts is reversed, and the hydatids may reach enormous size. In as many as 20 percent of patients, the pulmonary hydatid may rupture producing cough, chest pain, or hemoptysis. Hepatic lesions often present as abdominal pain or a palpable mass. Rupture through the diaphragm or into the peritoneal cavity can occur. Intrabiliary extrusion of calcified hepatic cysts has been reported in 5 to 15 percent of affected patients and mimics recurrent cholecystitis. Obstruction of the bile duct may result in jaundice. Rupture of a hydatid into the bile duct, peritoneal cavity, lung, pleura, or bronchus may produce fever, pruritus, urticarial rash, or an anaphylactoid reaction which may be fatal. Release of the numerous scolices leads to disseminated infection. Most patients initially have one or more hydatids in a single site, but in about 10 percent other tissues are involved. In bone, the cysts are semisolid, invade the medullary cavity, and slowly erode bone, producing pathologic fractures. Central nervous system involvement may produce epilepsy or blindness. Cardiac cysts can lead to conduction defects, pericarditis, and ventricular rupture. Hydatid antigen has been shown by fluorescent antibody in the glomerulus and has been related to membranous glomerulonephritis. Many other sites can be involved including spleen, ovary, prostate, and thyroid.

The alveolar cyst of *E. multilocularis* usually presents as a slowly growing hepatic tumor, with a minority of patients having metastatic disease to lung, brain, or other tissues. The natural course is one of malignant growth with massive destruction of the liver and extension into vital structures. If untreated, the disease is often fatal, but there is considerable individual variation in the course of the disease.

Diagnosis If a hydatid cyst ruptures or leaks fluid, an anaphylactoid reaction associated with eosinophilia and increased IgE levels may suggest the diagnosis. However, the clinical picture is usually not characteristic, and eosinophilia is seen in fewer than 25 percent of cases. Echinococciasis is most commonly discovered by routine x-ray. Pulmonary lesions usually are round, somewhat irregular masses of uniform density. They do not calcify. In contrast, hepatic cysts of *E. granulosus* show a smooth rim of calcification in about 50 percent of cases. Diffuse radiolucencies (2 to 4 mm) outlined by calcific densities may be seen in the liver with *E. multilocularis*. CT and ultrasound can be useful in demonstrating more details of the hydatid. In some cases of *E. granulosus*, simple, fluid-filled cysts indistinguishable from benign hepatic cysts are seen. In others, the findings of daughter cysts and hydatid sand strongly suggest echinococciasis. Thin eggshell calcification may indicate active disease. With alveolar hydatids, CT reveals indistinct solid masses, often with central necrosis, and plaque-like calcification. Angiography may be necessary prior to surgical therapy.

Specific diagnosis is best accomplished by histologic examination. In general, however, diagnostic aspiration should not be attempted because of potential anaphylactoid reactions to leakage of cyst fluid. Occasionally scolices may be found in sputum, stool, or urine and are shown by trichrome, Ziehl-Neelsen, and other stains. Serologic tests including indirect hemagglutination and latex agglutination are useful if positive, but many cyst carriers will not develop an immune response. Indirect hemagglutination should be positive in 90 percent of patients with hepatic cysts but in only 50 to 60 percent of those with pulmonary hydatids. ELISA provides the most sensitive and specific serologic diagnosis of hydatid disease. Following surgical removal of cysts, serologic tests may be helpful in screening for residual or recurrent disease.

Treatment Surgical treatment remains the standard therapy. Patients with small calcified hepatic cysts and pulmonary hydatids of the sylvatic type need to be operated on only if the cysts are symptomatic or enlarge dramatically over time. All others should have their cysts excised if possible, or sterilized and drained. With a large cyst, the contents should be sterilized with hypertonic saline before an attempt is made to open it. The entire endocyst should then be removed if possible, and all biliary or bronchial fistulas carefully closed. The residual space must be obliterated to prevent postoperative infection or prolonged drainage. Aspergillomas have been seen in residual cavities of pulmonary cysts.

Medical therapy with "high-dose" mebendazole (40 to 50 mg/kg per day in three divided doses) may be considered in patients with other medical problems that preclude surgery or in patients with extensive disease that makes surgical cure impossible. In selected patients, it may also be considered in conjunction with definitive surgery to reduce the risk of metastatic spread of viable organisms. In animal models, mebendazole is larvacidal for *E. granulosus* but not for *E. multilocularis*. In human trials, all forms of echinococciasis appear to respond to the agent, although the experience with *E. multilocularis* is limited. Significant side effects including neutropenia have been reported. The agent should be used only with the patient's informed consent. The absorption is erratic and drug levels should be followed. The drug is contraindicated in pregnancy. Other benzimidazoles such as flubendazole and albendazole also appear to be effective for echinococciasis.

Prevention The incidence of echinococciasis can be reduced by appropriate control measures as demonstrated in Iceland. Contact with infected dogs must be avoided, infected carcasses and offal should be burned or buried, and infected dogs should be treated with niclosamide or arecoline.

HERMAPHRODITIC TREMATODE INFECTIONS

The trematodes of humans are long-lived parasites that produce progressive damage to the tissues of their hosts. With the exception of schistosomes, they are similar in morphology and life cycle. The adult flukes are flat, leaflike hermaphrodites that vary in length from a few millimeters to several centimeters. Their digestive tract, unlike that of the nematodes, ends blindly. As their name indicates, they have two "holes" in the form of oral and ventral suckers which are used as organs of attachment and locomotion. The operculated eggs, which are passed in the feces or sputum, hatch in the water to produce a ciliated, free-swimming *miracidium*. The miracidium reaches and penetrates the tissue of an intermediate snail host to undergo a period of development, eventuating in the release of swarms of free-living *cercariae* from the snail. These thousands of tail-bearing larvae must, in turn, reach a second intermediate host, usually an aquatic animal or vegetation, where they encyst forming *metacercariae*. The definitive host is infected when he or she ingests the parasitized second intermediate host. The distribution of flukes is usually limited by the location of their molluscan intermediate host. With the exception of *Opisthorchis* and *Fasciola*, most hermaphroditic flukes are found only in tropical or subtropical areas.

PARAGONIMIASIS Definition Paragonimiasis (endemic hemoptysis) is a chronic infection of the lung caused by trematodes of the genus *Paragonimus*. Clinically, the disease is characterized by cough and hemoptysis. Ectopic worms may cause a variety of other manifestations.

Etiology and epidemiology Although *P. westermani*, which is widely distributed in the Far East, is the most common cause of human paragonimiasis, over 30 species, including *P. skrjabini*, *P. heterotremus* (China), *P. africanus* (central and west Africa), *P. mexicanus*, *P. ecuadoriensis*, and *P. caliensis* (Central and South America), may cause the disease. The short, plump adults (7 to 12 mm in length, 4 to 6 mm in width) have a life span of 4 to 5 years which they typically spend encysted, in pairs, within the lung parenchyma of the host. Their golden-brown operculated eggs (50 by 90 μm) reach the bronchioles from where they are coughed up and excreted in the sputum or swallowed and passed in the feces. They must embryonate several weeks in fresh water before hatching to release the miracidia.

The infection is acquired by ingestion of cysts in the second intermediate host, a freshwater shrimp, crab, or crayfish. The metacercariae excyst in the duodenum, burrow through the intestinal wall into the peritoneal cavity, and then usually migrate through the diaphragm and into the lung. The worms also may be found in the intestinal wall, liver, pancreas, kidney, epididymis, mesentery, skeletal muscle, subcutaneous tissues, and central nervous system, particularly the brain. The dog, cat, pig, rat, and wild carnivores are definitive hosts for the parasite in addition to humans. In some of these, very young adults can be found in their striated muscles. Human infection has been reported following the ingestion of this undercooked flesh.

It is estimated that there are over 3 million human infections, the vast majority in Asia, particularly China, Korea, Japan, Taiwan, the Philippines, and Southeast Asia. Approximately 1 percent of Indochinese immigrants to the United States harbor the trematode. Infections have also been reported from the Indian subcontinent, West Africa, Latin America, and the Pacific, including Samoa and the Solomon Islands. The incidence of paragonimiasis is often affected by food shortages or local customs. The metacercariae survive in vinegar, and lightly pickled or inadequately cooked food usually serves as the source of infection in the Far East. Children may acquire the disease in endemic areas while handling or eating raw crabs during play.

Pathogenesis and clinical manifestations During the migration of larvae, patients may experience fever, urticaria, abdominal pain, or diarrhea. An eosinophilic granuloma forms about the adult worm, eventually leading to the formation of a fibrous cyst. The pulmonary lesions which measure up to 1 cm in diameter frequently communicate with a bronchiole, resulting in secondary bacterial infection. Small, fibrous nodules representing reaction around deposited eggs also occur. Clinically the picture is one of chronic bronchitis and bronchiectasis with production of brownish sputum, hemoptysis, weight loss, nightsweats, low-grade fever, and occasionally finger clubbing. A poorly resolving pulmonary infiltrate, lung abscess, or pleural effusion may be present in heavy infections. Effusions are often large, may occur in the absence of parenchymal disease, and are typically exudative with eosinophils and cholesterol crystals. The roentgenographic findings vary with the stage of infection. Initially diffuse or segmental infiltrates, with or without pleural effusions, may be seen in lower or midlung fields. These are then gradually replaced by round 2- to 4-cm nodules which not infrequently cavitate. Eventually, cystic rings, fibrosis, and calcification occur, presenting a picture closely resembling tuberculosis, a disease which often coexists with paragonimiasis.

An abdominal mass, pain, and dysentery characterize intestinal or peritoneal infections. Ectopic worms in the liver or spleen may produce clinical manifestations of abscess formation. Involvement of the central nervous system usually presents acutely as a meningoencephalitis. Chronically, paralysis and epilepsy occur, usually the result of temporal or occipital lobe involvement. Homonymous hemianopsia, optic atrophy, and papilledema are common. The cerebrospinal fluid usually shows an eosinophilic leukocytosis and elevated protein. Cerebral calcifications are seen on x-ray in 50 percent of cases. *Paragonimus skrjabini* and, perhaps, *P. ecuadoriensis* infections are characterized by migratory subcutaneous nodules that contain adult flukes and that frequently ulcerate.

Laboratory findings Eosinophilia is a constant finding. CT scans of the head, chest, and abdomen provide the best demonstration of parasite cavities. Definitive diagnosis depends upon finding the characteristic operculated ova in the sputum, stool, pleural fluid, or tissue. Eggs may be rare or totally absent from the sputum during the first 3 months of infection but are eventually found in 75 to 85 percent of infected patients. Their presence correlates well with the roentgenographic appearance of cavities. Even later, however, repeated examinations using concentration techniques may be required for their recovery. Ziehl-Neelsen staining, often carried out for suspected tuberculosis, usually will not demonstrate the eggs. In fact, the sputum concentration techniques for tuberculosis may destroy the eggs that are present. Since many patients have concomitant tuberculosis, the diagnosis may be overlooked. Stool examination is frequently helpful in children. A number of serologic tests, including complement fixation, counterimmunoelectrophoresis, ELISA, and latex agglutination tests, are available; the results correlate well with active infection. They are particularly useful in extrapulmonary infections. The skin test does not distinguish present and past infections and is used primarily for epidemiologic purposes.

Treatment and prevention Praziquantel is the drug of choice. A total of 75 mg/kg is given in three divided doses for 1 or 2 days. Alternatively, bithionol may be administered. From 30 to 40 mg/kg in divided doses should be given every other day for a total of 10 to 15 treatment days. The symptoms disappear rapidly, and most infiltrates resolve within 3 months. Side effects are minor and consist of nausea, vomiting, and urticaria. Concomitant bacterial infection must be treated. Prevention of superinfection by the same parasite is important, because the disease is self-limiting.

The most practical control measure is the adequate cooking of all shellfish before they are eaten. Cooks should refrain from tasting shellfish during preparation and should wash their hands thoroughly thereafter.

CLONORCHIASIS Definition Clonorchiasis is an infection of the biliary passages caused by *Clonorchis sinensis*, the most important liver fluke of humans. Although the infection is usually asymptomatic, heavy worm loads may produce manifestations of biliary obstruction.

Etiology and epidemiology *Clonorchis sinensis* is a small fluke (5 by 15 mm) that lives as long as 50 years in the biliary tree of its host. Here the flukes feed on mucosal secretions and pass operculated eggs into the feces. On reaching fresh water, the eggs are ingested by the intermediate snail host. After multiplication and development within the snail, the cercariae are released and penetrate freshwater fish. Infections result from ingestion of the raw, dried, salted, or pickled flesh of freshwater fish containing encysted metacercariae. The larva is released in the duodenum. It enters the common bile duct and migrates to the second-order bile ducts, where it develops into the adult form in about 1 month. In addition to humans, dogs, cats, pigs, and rats serve as disease reservoirs. The main endemic areas are Korea, Japan, Taiwan, Hong Kong, southern China, and Vietnam where, in previous years, clonorchiasis was perpetuated by the practice of fertilizing fish ponds with manure and human feces. Improvements in the disposal of human feces have dramatically decreased transmission in most areas, but the infection rate has remained high due to the prolonged life span of the adult worm. Twenty-five percent of the population of Hong Kong and a small proportion of Chinese and southeast Asian immigrants to this country have been shown to be infected. The disease may also be acquired in the United States by the ingestion of infected, dried, frozen, or pickled fish imported from the Far East. Clinically apparent cases are restricted to the adult population in whom the accumulated worm load eventually produces pathologic effects.

Pathogenesis and clinical manifestations Light infections are usually asymptomatic, but worm loads of 500 to 1000 flukes often result in clinical manifestations. During the migration of the larvae, the patient may have fever, chills, tender hepatomegaly, mild jaundice, and eosinophilia. The mature worm causes proliferation of the biliary epithelium, increased mucin production, adenoma formation, chronic pericholangitis, and periductal fibrosis. Hepatic parenchymal damage and portal hypertension are not seen in uncomplicated infections. Recurrent attacks of suppurative cholangitis with or without intrahepatic choledocholithiasis may follow biliary obstruction with dead flukes. Hypoglycemic coma is a rare presenting manifestation. The occurrence of biliary stones in clonorchiasis is associated with an increased incidence of chronic *Salmonella typhi* carriage. Cholangiocarcinoma may occur in patients with severe, long standing infections. The adult worms may infest the pancreatic ducts, where they can cause squamous metaplasia, periductal fibrosis, and acute pancreatitis.

Laboratory diagnosis Clinical and epidemiologic findings often suggest the diagnosis. There may be elevation of the alkaline phosphatase, transaminase, and bilirubin levels during the acute phase of the disease, resulting in confusion with acute viral hepatitis. Eosinophilia is variable. Occasionally, a plain film of the abdomen will demonstrate intrahepatic calcification. Liver scan is usually negative in asymptomatic infections but may show multiple areas of diminished uptake in acute symptomatic disease. Percutaneous transhepatic cholangiography, sonography, and CT scans in these patients often reveal dilatation of the peripheral intrahepatic bile ducts and, on occasion, cholangiocarcinoma. The adult worms appear as round filling defects several millimeters in diameter. Definitive diagnosis depends on the demonstration of the eggs in the feces or the duodenal contents. They measure 29 by 16 μm, possess a conspicuous opercular rim as well as a posterior knob, and can be distinguished from the eggs of *Metagonimus, Heterophyes,* and *Opisthorchis* only with difficulty. An antigen extracted from adult worms can be used in a complement fixation or enzyme-linked immunosorbent test for the detection of the host's antibody response, but its diagnostic usefulness is questionable.

Treatment and prevention Praziquantel is an effective chemotherapeutic agent for clonorchiasis. It is administered in a dosage of 25 mg/kg tid for a single day. Acute cholangitis can usually be managed medically with antimicrobial agents. If obstruction persists, surgery with physical removal of worms and/or stones may be required. Thorough cooking of freshwater fish will prevent infection.

OPISTHORCHIASIS Opisthorchiasis is caused by *Opisthorchis felineus* or *O. viverrini* and is characterized by hepatic lesions produced by adult worms in the larger bile ducts. The life cycle resembles that of *C. sinensis*. The geographic distribution differs in that *O. felineus* is endemic in eastern and central Europe and in Siberia and occurs in some parts of Asia, while *O. viverrini* is found in Thailand and Laos. Cats and wild carnivores act as the principal reservoir hosts, and the infection is found most commonly along rivers and lakes which harbor an abundant fish life. Up to 90 percent of inhabitants of some villages in northeastern Thailand are purported to carry the parasite. The clinical picture is similar to that seen in clonorchiasis except that gallstones are rare. Cholangiocarcinoma occurs in approximately 50 percent of infected patients who come to autopsy. The diagnosis usually is based on the finding of the eggs in the feces or duodenal contents. Treatment as recommended for clonorchiasis may be used. Infection can be prevented by eating only well-cooked fish.

FASCIOLIASIS Fascioliasis is caused by *Fasciola hepatica*, which, like *Clonorchis*, inhabits the bile ducts of the definitive host. When fully matured, the adult measures about 3 by 1 cm and discharges large operculate eggs 140 by 70 μm which must embryonate in fresh water before hatching.

Fascioliasis produces so-called liver rot in sheep, the principal definitive host. The disease is most common in sheep- and cattle-raising countries but has been reported from many parts of the world. In North America it occurs in the southern and western United States, Central America, and in the Caribbean Islands, including Puerto Rico.

Infection is contracted by ingestion of the encysted forms of the fluke attached to edible aquatic plants such as watercress. The larvae excyst in the duodenum, migrate through the intestinal wall, pass into the peritoneal cavity, penetrate the liver capsule, and finally reach the bile ducts, where they mature. Occasionally larvae may migrate to and mature in ectopic locations including the pancreas, subcutaneous tissue, chest cavity, or brain.

Early clinical manifestations are related to the migration of the larval form to and within the liver. Epigastric pain, fever, diarrhea, jaundice, urticaria, pruritus, arthralgia, and eosinophilia may be observed during this stage. Fibrosis of the liver similar to that found in clonorchiasis appears only after prolonged residence of many adult worms in the bile ducts. Obstruction of the bile duct occurs frequently and may be the presenting manifestation of disease.

The diagnosis usually is based on the finding of the eggs in the feces or in the duodenal contents. It is difficult to distinguish the eggs from those of *Fasciolopsis buski*. Complement fixation, hemagglutination, and precipitin tests have been reported to be helpful. A skin test is also available.

Bithionol, as administered for paragonimiasis, appears to be superior to praziquantel for treatment.

To prevent infection, aquatic plants such as watercress should not be eaten, vegetables grown in fields irrigated with polluted water should be boiled, and safe drinking water should be provided.

FASCIOLOPSIASIS Fasciolopsiasis is caused by the large intestinal fluke *F. buski*, which inhabits the upper part of the intestine of its definitive host. The principal definitive host is the pig. China, Thailand, India, and other areas in the Far East are the major endemic loci. Infection of humans occurs following ingestion, or peeling with the teeth, of water chestnuts, water lotus, and other edible aquatic plants. The large adults attach themselves to the intestinal mucosa, and these sites may later ulcerate. The infection is usually asymptomatic. In heavy infections, diarrhea, abdominal pain, gastrointestinal hemorrhage, and intestinal obstruction may appear early. Later, asthenia with ascites and anasarca occurs. Diagnosis is based upon the history and the finding of eggs in the feces. The eggs resemble those of *Fasciola hepatica*. The prognosis in untreated heavy infections, especially in children, is poor. Praziquantel as given for clonorchiasis is the treatment of choice.

HETEROPHYIASIS AND METAGONIMIASIS *Heterophyes heterophyes* and *Metagonimus yakagawa* are small intestinal flukes of humans and other fish-eating mammals. They are found in the Far East and, in the case of *Heterophyes*, in the Philippines, India, Egypt, and Tunisia. Both are acquired by ingesting the raw or undercooked flesh of metacercarial-infected freshwater fish. The 2- to 3-mm adults attach themselves to the mucosa of the small intestine. If present in sufficient numbers, they may cause abdominal pain and/or diarrhea. Rarely the eggs have been found in sites such as the brain, spinal cord, or heart where they produce granulomatous lesions. Most commonly, they are passed in the stool where they very closely resemble those of *Clonorchis*. Both species can be treated with praziquantel as described for clonorchiasis. As the life span of these trematodes is limited to a year or less, treatment is not indicated unless the patient is symptomatic.

REFERENCES

Intestinal nematodes

Anisakiasis

KLIKS MM: Anisakiasis in the western United States: Four new case reports from California. Am J Trop Med Hyg 32:526, 1983

OSHIMA T: Anisakiasis—is the sushi bar guilty? Parasitology Today 3:44, 1987

Ascariasis

ARFAA F: Selective primary health care: Strategies for control of disease in the developing world. XII. Ascariasis and trichuriasis. Rev Infect Dis 6:364, 1984

PAWLOWSKI Z: Ascariasis: Host-parasite biology. Rev Infect Dis 4:806, 1982

Capillariasis

BASACA-SEVILLA V, CROSS JH: Attempts to modify treatment of intestinal capillariasis. Southeastern Asian J Trop Med Public Health 16:546, 1985

Enterobiasis

VERMUND SH, MACLEOD S: Is pinworm vanishing? Laboratory surveillance in a New York City medical center from 1971–1986. Am J Dis Child 142:566, 1988

WAGNER ED, EBY WC: Pinworm prevalence in California elementary school children, and diagnostic methods. Am J Trop Med Hyg 32:998, 1983

Hookworm

GILLIS HM: Selective primary health care: Strategies for control of disease in the developing world. XVII. Hookworm infection and anemia. Rev Infect Dis 7:111, 1985

LITTLE MD et al: *Ancylostoma* larva in a muscle fiber of man follow cutaneous larva migrans. Am J Trop Med Hyg 32:1285, 1983

Strongyloidiasis

IRGA-SIEGMAN Y et al: Syndrome of hyperinfection with *Strongyloides stercoralis*. Rev Infect Dis 3:397, 1981

NEVA FA et al: Biology and immunology of human strongyloidiasis. J Infect Dis 153:397, 1986

PELLETIER LL JR: Chronic strongyloidiasis in World War II Far East ex-prisoners of war. Am J Trop Med Hyg 33:55, 1984

Toxocariasis

GLICKMAN LT, SCHANTZ PM: Epidemiology and pathogenesis of zoonotic toxocariasis. Epidemiol Rev 3:230, 1981

TAYLOR MRH et al: The expanded spectrum of toxocaral disease. Lancet 1:692, 1988

WORLEY G et al: *Toxocara canis* infection: Clinical and epidemiological association with seropositivity in kindergarten children. J Infect Dis 149:591, 1984

Trichuriasis

COOPER ES, BUNDY DAP: *Trichuris* is not trivial. Parasitology today 4:301, 1988

FISHMAN JA, PERRONE TL: Colonic obstruction and perforation due to *Trichuris trichuria*. Am J Med 77:154, 1984

Miscellaneous tissue nematodes

Angiostrongyliasis

ANDERSON E et al: First report of *Angiostrongylus cantonensis* in Puerto Rico. Am J Trop Med Hyg 35:319, 1986

BIA F, BARRY M: Parasitic infections of the central nervous system. Neurologic Clinics 4:171, 1986

LORIA-CORTES R, LOBO-SANAHUJA JF: Clinical abdominal angiostrongylosis. A study of 116 children with intestinal eosinophilic granuloma caused by *Angiostrongylus costaricensis*. Am J Trop Med Hyg 29:538, 1980

WITTNER M et al: Eustrongylidiasis—a parasitic infection acquired by eating sushi. N Engl J Med 320:1124, 1989

Dracunculiasis

HOPKINS DR: Dracunculiasis eradication: A mid-decade status report. Am J Trop Med Hyg 37:115, 1987

Cestodes

Coenurosis

BENGER A et al: A human coenurus infection in Canada. Am J Trop Med Hyg 30:638, 1981

Cysticercosis

EARNEST MT et al: Neurocysticercosis in the United States: 35 cases and a review. Rev Infect Dis 9:961, 1987
NASCIMENTO E et al: Immunodiagnosis of human cysticercosis (*Taenia solium*) with antigens purified by monoclonal antibodies. J Clin Microbiol 25:1181, 1987
RAMOS DM et al: Diagnosis of neurocysticercosis by magnetic resonance imaging. Pediatr Infect Dis 5:470, 1986
RANGEL R et al: Cysticercotic encephalitis: A severe form in young females. Am J Trop Med Hyg 36:387, 1987

Echinococciasis

HIRA PR et al: Diagnosis of cystic hydatid disease: Role of aspiration cytology. Lancet 2:655, 1988
LANGER JL et al: Diagnosis and management of hydatid disease of the liver. A 15 year North American experience. Ann Surg 199:412, 1984
LANIER AP et al: Comparison of serologic tests for the diagnosis and follow-up of alveolar hydatid disease. Am J Trop Med Hyg 37:609, 1987
SCHANTZ PM: Effective medical treatment for hydatid disease? JAMA 253:2095, 1985
WILSON JF, RAUSCH RL: Alveolar hydatid disease. A review of clinical features of 33 indigenous cases of *E. multilocularis* infection in Alaskan Eskimos. Am J Trop Med Hyg 29:1340, 1980

Hermaphroditic trematodes

Clonorchiasis and Opisthorchiasis

FLAVELL DJ: Liver-fluke infection as an aetiologic factor in bile-duct carcinoma of man. Trans R Soc Trop Med Hyg 75:814, 1981
KOOMPIROCHANA C et al: Opisthorchiasis: A clinicopathologic study of 154 autopsy cases. Southeastern Asian J Trop Med 9:60, 1978
RIM H-J: The current pathobiology and chemotherapy of clonorchiasis. Korean J Parasitol 24 (suppl: Monograph Series 3):1, 1986
YANGCO BG et al: Clinical study evaluating efficacy of praziquantel in clonorchiasis. Antimicrob Agents Chemother 31:135, 1987

Fascioliasis and Fasciolopsiasis

FARID Z et al: Unsuccessful use of praziquantel to treat acute fascioliasis in children. J Infect Dis 154:920, 1986
JONES EA et al: Massive infection with *Fasciola hepatica* in man. Am J Med 63:842, 1977
PLANT AG et al: A clinical study of *Fasciolopsis buski* in Thailand. Trans R Soc Trop Med Hyg 63:470, 1969

Paragonimiasis

JOHNSON RJ et al: Paragonimiasis: Diagnosis and the use of praziquantel in treatment. Rev Infect Dis 7:200, 1985
YOKOGAWA M: *Paragonimus* and paragonimiasis, in *Advances in Parasitology*, B Dawes (ed). London, Academic, 1969, vol 7, p 375

172 SCABIES, CHIGGERS, AND OTHER ECTOPARASITES

JAMES J. PLORDE

SCABIES Scabies is a cosmopolitan skin infection commonly referred to as the "seven-year itch." It is caused by a burrowing mite, *Sarcoptes scabiei* var. *hominis,* and is transmitted from person to person by close bodily contact, particularly among family members and bed partners. The survival of mites for 2 or 3 days in bedding, clothing, and house dust makes it possible that fomite-spread disease occurs, at least occasionally. Although the disease is more common in the poor and unclean, sporadic cases involve individuals of all socioeconomic groups. Children under 15 years of age have the highest prevalence of scabies and are usually the first members of families to contract the disease. Those who spend nights with friends or exchange clothing with others are at increased risk. Institutional outbreaks in hospitals, nursing homes, mental institutions, and aboard naval vessels have been reported. There has been a worldwide resurgence of this infection over the past 20 years, and in the United States it currently involves 2 to 4 percent of patients seen by dermatologists.

The turtle-shaped female measures 0.4 mm in length and possesses four pairs of legs. With the help of the two anterior pairs and her mouth, she burrows into the superficial layer of the epidermis. Here she deposits two or three enormous eggs daily until she dies 30 to 60 days later. The newly hatched larvae mature to adulthood on the skin surface within 2 weeks to continue the cycle of infection. Although an involved person may harbor thousands or occasionally millions of adult mites, the average number of adult females per infection is 11.

Two-thirds of the burrows are found in the upper extremities, particularly on the interdigital spaces of the hands and the flexor surface of the wrists. In heavy infections, other sites are typically involved. These include the dorsal surfaces of the elbows, anterior axillary folds, female breasts, periumbilical area, penis, scrotum, and buttocks. In bedridden patients, lesions are often concentrated over pressure points. The face, head, palms, and soles are seldom involved in adults; in infants, any area of the skin can be involved. Characteristically, a burrow appears as a short dark wavy line which may end in a small vesicle, the site of the adult female.

Sensitization (type IV) to the mites and their products begins approximately 1 month after infection and results in a papular or eczematous reaction at the sites of involvement. Itching is often severe and tends to be more marked at night or after a hot bath. Scratching frequently leads to secondary infection with pustulation and lichenification. Acute glomerulonephritis has followed infection with nephritogenic strains of streptococci. Occasionally, reddish pruritic nodules are seen in the groin and axillary regions. Infected individuals with good personal hygiene usually have few lesions, and burrows may be difficult to identify. In mentally retarded, debilitated, or immunosuppressed patients, a particularly virulent infection known as *crusted (Norwegian) scabies* is sometimes seen. Millions of mites may be present, producing a highly infectious exfoliative dermatitis; crusted, psoriasiform plaques are common. Itching is often mild or absent. Scabies usually terminates spontaneously in a few months, but chronic cases occur.

The diagnosis should be considered in any patient presenting with a pruritic eruption, particularly if it involves several members of a living group. The occurrence of symmetric lesions at the sites of predilection should initiate a search for the characteristic burrows. These should be vigorously scraped with a sterile needle or scalpel blade, and the scrapings transferred to a drop of 10% potassium hydroxide on a glass slide. A coverslip is placed over the top, and the preparation examined for adults, larvae, and eggs. The diagnosis can also be made on histologic sections prepared from a punch biopsy. Considering the mode of disease transmission, adults shown to have scabies should also be checked for venereal disease.

All sexual contacts and household members should be treated simultaneously with the patient to prevent the occurrence of "ping-pong infections." The therapeutic agents are applied topically, covering the skin thinly but completely from the neck down. Although the patient is rendered noninfectious within 24 h, up to 2 months may be required for the clinical manifestations of the disease to disappear completely. Needless retreatment during this period can lead to contact dermatitis. Bed linen and clothes used by the patient the day prior to therapy should be washed in hot water.

A number of effective agents are available for use. Lindane

(gamma benzene hexachloride) is left on for 8 to 12 h and then thoroughly washed off. Care must be taken to keep it away from eyes and mucous membranes. It should not be used in infants or pregnant adults. Crotamiton (Eurax) is massaged into the skin, and a second dose applied 24 h later. Benzyl benzoate (25%) is administered in a similar fashion. Antihistamines or salicylates are helpful in counteracting pruritus. Topical steroids may potentiate the infection and should not be used. Antibiotics are required occasionally when there is a significant bacterial superinfection.

CHIGGER AND OTHER MITES The term *chigger* is used to refer to larvae of harvest mites belonging to the family Trombiculidae. The cosmopolitan adults feed on vegetable matter and deposit their eggs upon the ground. The tiny (0.4 mm) emergent larvae crawl along the ground and upward onto vegetation. Here, they await the passage of a vertebrate host, upon which they must feed before again dropping to the ground and molting. In humans, the chigger usually attaches about the ankles, but some advance along the skin until they are stopped by tight-fitting clothing. It then pierces the skin, releases a digestant to liquefy tissue cells, and feeds for 3 or 4 days. Within a few hours, the chigger's secretions have produced an intensely pruritic papule 0.5 to 2 cm in diameter. This usually vesiculates, resulting in a chickenpox-like lesion. Occasionally, subcutaneous bleeding results in a surrounding area of ecchymosis. The lesion and itching may persist for several weeks. In the United States, most clinical cases are seen during the summer months; in warm climates, the seasonal pattern is missing.

Grain mites as well as those of cats, dogs, fowl, and rodents may also feed on humans. Because these species are very small and the resulting skin lesions variable, diagnosis depends on the history of contact with the mite source. Treatment is directed at the relief of itching and the prevention of secondary infections. Insect repellents are highly effective prophylactic agents. Fumigation of mite sources may prevent recurrences.

FLEAS Fleas are small wingless laterally compressed ectoparasites of humans and other warm-blooded animals. They tend to be found on the hairy portions of the host where they feed and deposit their eggs. The active larvae, which hatch in 3 days, can be found on the host, in its nest, or in dust. They eventually pupate and may remain dormant for weeks or months before completing their development to adults. Medically, fleas serve as both vectors and agents of disease. Rodent fleas of the genus *Xenopsylla* are the most important. They are responsible for the transmission of both plague (*Yersinia pestis*) and murine typhus (*Rickettsia mooseri*) from animal reservoirs to humans. Humans may also acquire the rat tapeworm *Hymenolepis diminuta* by swallowing fleas containing the cysticeroid. The dog tapeworm *Dipylidium caninum* may be transmitted in a similar fashion. The bites of these and other species of fleas belonging to the family Pulicidae can induce an irritating dermatitis. In addition, the tungidae (*Tunga penetrans*) may burrow into the subcutaneous tissues, producing a painful and debilitating disease.

Flea dermatitis The fleas of humans (*Pulex irritans*), cats and dogs (*Cetenocephalides*), and rodents (*Xenopsylla*) may all induce dermatitis. In many individuals, the bites seem completely innocuous, but in sensitive persons, the saliva induces an erythematous raised pruritic papule. Repeated scratching may result in secondary infection with pustulation or ulceration. The intense pruritus, the ability of the flea to escape capture by virtue of its prodigious jumping ability, and the difficulty involved in crushing their hard chitinous bodies has led to many a frustrating nocturnal safari dedicated to the destruction of this unwanted bed partner. Control is effected by the use of frequent vacuuming to remove eggs, larvae, pupae, and adults from the environment. Insecticide sprays and dusting powders are also of help, but fleas have developed resistance to many of these. Dogs and cats should be washed, flea collars applied, and kennels dusted or sprayed with DDT or malathion. If rat runs can be located, they should also be dusted.

Tunga penetrans, sometimes referred to as a *jigger* or *chigoe flea*, is a burrowing flea found in the tropical areas of the Caribbean, South America, and Africa. These small (1 mm) free-living insects reside in sandy soil. The fertilized female burrows into the skin of the first warm-blooded animal encountered. In humans, they usually embed on the sole of the foot or under a toenail with only their anal pore exposed to the outside. Multiple infections are common. As the female becomes engorged with blood and eggs, a painful and pruritic pea-sized swelling is produced. Eventually, the overlying skin ulcerates, the flea dies, and the eggs are extruded. Secondary bacterial infections including tetanus and gas gangrene occur commonly. Autoamputation of the toes has been reported from Africa. The intact flea can usually be extracted by gently enlarging the entrance hole with a sterile needle and then applying pressure from the side. Alternatively, the lesion can be soaked in Lysol, the flea penetrated with a needle, and the lesion resoaked to kill the eggs and sterilize the wound. Antibiotics may be required to treat secondary bacterial infections.

PEDICULOSIS Lice are obligate human ectoparasites that complete their entire 30- to 40-day life cycle on the body of the host. *Pediculus humanus* var. *capitis* infests the head, *P. humanus* var. *corporis* the body and clothing, and *Phthirius pubis* (crab lice) the genital and occasionally other hairy areas of the body. All three are flattened dorsoventrally and measure 2 to 3 mm in length. The crab louse is broader and flatter than *Pediculus* and possesses powerful claws on its second and third legs, with which it clings to the pubic hair. The females lay five or six eggs daily, which they firmly attach to the hairs or, in the case of the body louse, the clothing of the host. These clearly visible tiny white nits hatch in 8 to 10 days. The resulting nymph matures to adulthood in an additional 2 weeks. Both the larvae and adults take two blood meals daily, leaving behind a small purpuric puncture site. With repeated exposure, the host develops an inflammatory hypersensitivity reaction manifested as a small red papule at each new feeding site. Pruritus results in scratching, a weeping dermatitis, and secondary infection. Chronic infections of the scalp may result in a fetid mass of matted hair and exudate. On the body and genital areas, the lesions may become lichenified and pigmented—so-called vagabond disease. Heavy infections with *P. pubis* may involve the eyebrows and eyelids leading to blepharitis.

Lice can be transferred from person to person by direct contact or via discarded clothing in which the body louse can survive for up to a week. Migration is stimulated by fever, making *P. humanus* var. *corporis* an efficient vector of relapsing fever (*Borrelia recurrentis*), typhus (*R. prowazekii*), and trench fever (*R. quintana*). *Phthirius pubis* is not known to be a vector of human disease.

Pediculosis corporis is typically seen in the poor and transient who are unable to maintain even minimal levels of personal hygiene. In contrast, head and pubic lice are found on patients of all socioeconomic classes and are currently enjoying a resurgence in the United States. *P. capitis* most frequently infests white schoolchildren; blacks are seldom involved. Pubic lice are more common among the sexually active; their presence should stimulate a search for venereal disease.

The diagnosis is suggested by the typical dermatitis and confirmed by finding the adults or nits on the hair or clothing of the patient. Treatment may be carried out with 1% pyrethrin (Nix—approved for head lice only), with piperonyl butoxide (RID), or lindane (1% gamma benzene hexachloride, Kwell). The latter agent may be absorbed through the skin, resulting in CNS toxicity if applied inappropriately. It should not be used in infants and pregnant women. In head infections, the hair should first be shampooed with ordinary soap. RID or Nix are then rubbed in for at least 10 min (Kwell shampoo, 4 min), the hair is rinsed, dried, and combed with a fine-tooth comb to remove the nits. If RID or Kwell have been used, the process should be repeated in 7 days. Combs and brushes should be heated in water to 65°C for 5 min or soaked in 2% Lysol. The clothing and bedding of the patient with body lice are heat-sterilized. The patient's body should be lathered for 10 min with RID or 4 min with Kwell and then rinsed thoroughly. The therapy may be repeated in 7 days. In crab louse infestations, RID or Kwell cream or lotion should be used on the involved areas and left for 24 h. In hirsute individuals, the treatment can be repeated in 1 week. If the eyelashes are involved, 0.25% physostigmine ophthalmic ointment is applied twice daily for 10 days. Lice and nits are carefully removed with a cotton-tipped applicator. Narrow-angle glaucoma should be ruled out before the physostigmine is used.

MYIASIS Infections with maggots or fly larvae are seen worldwide in a variety of animals. Human involvement occurs most frequently where people live in close contact with domestic animals. Many different species of flies are involved. In some, an animal host is required for larval development; in these, the larvae are capable of invading normal tissue or enter the body through the nose, mouth, or ears. Others are opportunists, depositing their eggs or larvae in the open wounds of debilitated patients. The clinical manifestations vary with the species of fly and site of involvement. Four of the more common clinical syndromes are described below.

Localized cutaneous myiasis In tropical America the lesions are produced by *Dermatobia hominis,* the human botfly. This remarkable forest-dwelling Diptera captures a mosquito or other blood-feeding insect on which to deposit its packet of eggs. When this unwilling vector then lands on a warm-blooded animal to feed, the eggs hatch and penetrate the feeding site. Within the skin of the host, the larva develops for 2 or 3 months. Finally, it emerges, drops to the ground, and pupates. The lesions are most frequently seen on unprotected areas of the body including the hands, feet, head, and neck. During the first week of infection, the pruritic lesion closely resembles a mosquito bite. As the larva grows and begins to move, it produces severe pain and itching. Tissue destruction and inflammation results in the development of a furuncle-like lesion. Generally, a central opening is present through which the posterior end of the larva protrudes. A dark serosanguinous discharge containing the feces of the insect may be noted.

In Africa, a similar lesion is produced by *Cordylobia anthropophaga* (tumbu fly). These flies deposit their eggs on sandy soil or laundry laid out to dry. The larvae hatch and invade the unbroken skin of humans or wild rodents, where they mature in 8 or 9 days. In either case, the larvae can be surgically extracted without difficulty. In tumbu fly infections, letting the larvae mature and drop off spontaneously may be appropriate. This process can occasionally be hastened by applying mineral oil to the central opening. This results in the suffocation of the larva and stimulates its early exodus.

Cutanea larva migrans This is usually caused by the large (1 to 2 cm) horse botflies belonging to the genus *Gasterophilus.* When the larvae hatch on the skin, they penetrate to the lower epidermis. Because they do not mature in humans, they may migrate in the skin for several months. Clinically, the infection presents as a pruritic serpiginous band of erythema closely resembling cutanea larva migrans produced by *Ancylostoma braziliense.* The diagnosis can be made by placing a small drop of mineral oil on the skin just in advance of the worm tract. This allows visualization of black backward-directed spines on its body segments. The parasite can be easily removed with a sharp needle. Occasionally, the larvae may penetrate the eye. A similar clinical picture is sometimes produced by the larvae of *Hypoderma* spp. (cattle botfly). These, however, often penetrate deeply into the subcutaneous tissue and produce more pain and less pruritus than *Gasterophilus* larvae.

Deep-tissue myiasis Screwflies of several genera can deposit large batches of eggs on unbroken skin or in wounds, ears, or the nose. After hatching, the larvae burrow into the tissues and develop for 2 or 3 weeks. The mature 1- to 2-cm larvae then drop to the ground and pupate. At times, they penetrate deep tissues, including the eye, nasal sinuses, and cranium, where they produce destructive foul-smelling lesions. Bacterial superinfection is common. In India and Africa, the flies are usually of genus *Chrysomyia.* In the western hemisphere, *Callitroga* spp. are involved. The occurrence of human cases in the United States often accompanies epizootics of screwworm activity. Flesh flies of the family Sarcophagidae have also been implicated in deep-tissue myiasis both in the United States and elsewhere. In all the above infections, the lesions should be surgically incised and debrided, the larvae removed, and secondary infections treated.

Intestinal myiasis When humans ingest food contaminated with the eggs or larvae of several genera of flies, some survive passage through the stomach and later mature in the intestine before they are extruded in the stool. In the United States, *Tubifera tenax* is the most frequently implicated species. Invasion of the intestinal mucosa may occur with *Sarcophaga* infections.

PENTASTOMIASIS Pentastomes, invertebrate endoparasites of reptiles, birds, and mammals, share a number of morphologic similarities with both the worms and arthropods. Although previously classified with each, they are now thought to constitute a phylum distinct from both, the Pentastomida. Adult worms resemble nematodes with an elongated, nonsegmented body varying in length from a few millimeters to several centimeters; separate sexes whose reproductive organs occupy the bulk of the body cavity; a straight, tubelike gut; and a chitinous cuticle. Their name (''five-mouthed'') resulted from the early misidentification of the four hooklets surrounding the mouth projection as additional mouths.

Adult worms are found in the respiratory tract of carnivores where they attach by their hooklets and feed on the host's epithelial cells, blood, and tissue fluid. Eggs released by the female are passed to the external environment in nasal discharge, saliva, or feces. Once ingested by herbivores, the eggs hatch in the gut of these intermediate hosts, releasing mitelike first-stage larvae; these penetrate the gut wall and encyst in a variety of tissues. After a series of molts, the third-stage larvae exit from the tissue cysts and return to the peritoneal cavity. When the definite host feeds on the tissues of the intermediate host, ingested third-stage larvae migrate to the respiratory tract where they mature to adulthood.

Most human infections are caused by one of two species, *Armillfer armillatus* and *Linguatula serrata.* The African python is the definite host of the first. Humans come in contact with the eggs while handling pythons or by ingesting contaminated drink or food. The larvae do not develop into adult worms in the human intermediate host and most infections remain asymptomatic. Occasionally, the enlargement of larval cysts, during the molting stage, produces mechanical pressure on vital organs, resulting in obstruction of bile ducts, gut, or bronchi. Migrating third-stage larvae may penetrate organs, inducing pneumonitis, pericarditis, meningitis, peritonitis, and prostatitis. The diagnosis is generally made at autopsy when the cysts are discovered in the liver, peritoneum, mesentery, or lung hilum. Dead, calcified larvae produce distinctive, 1-cm radiopaque lesions, shaped like cashew nuts, which may be apparent in abdominal or chest radiographs. Although serologic tests have been developed, their usefulness is uncertain. Treatment is indicated only when mechanical pressure on vital organs requires surgical removal of the larval cysts.

Human infection with *L. serrata* is found primarily in the Middle East, but isolated cases have been reported from Africa, Europe, and the Americas. The parasite is acquired when third-stage larvae are ingested in raw liver or lymph nodes of sheep or goats, generally at times of religious feasts. The larvae migrate to the nasopharynx where they produce pain and itching of the throat and ears, nasal discharge, lacrimation, hoarseness, dyspnea, dysphagia, cough, hemoptysis, and vomiting—a syndrome known as *halzoun* in the Middle East and *marrara* in the Sudan. Manifestations begin within minutes to hours of ingesting the infested tissues and usually persist for 7 to 10 days. Occasionally, respiratory obstruction requiring tracheostomy develops. Eustachian tube abscess, facial paralysis, and invasion of the ocular globe have also been reported. Rarely, the larvae mature to adulthood, producing nasal pressure, sneezing, and recurrent epistaxis. The diagnosis is established by demonstrating the 0.5- to 1.0-cm third-stage larvae in nasal discharge, sputum, or vomitus or, rarely, by the recovery of the adult worm following a violent attack of sneezing. Treatment is directed to the protection of the airway and antibiotic therapy of secondary bacterial infections.

A third species, *Reighardia sternae,* is thought to produce a cutanea larva migrans–like syndrome in Southeast Asians who ingest live lizards.

REFERENCES

CARSON DS et al: Pyrethrins combined with piperonyl butoxide (RID) vs 1% permethrin (NIX) in the treatment of head lice. Am J Dis Child 42:768, 1988

DRABICK JJ: Pentastomiasis. Rev Infect Dis 9:1087, 1987

HARWOOD RB, JAMES MT: Mylasis, in *Entomology in Human and Animal Health*. New York, Macmillan, 1979

KRINSKI WL: Dermatoses associated with the bites of mites and ticks (Arthropodia: Acari). Int J Dermatol 22:75, 1983

MAUNDER JW: Insecticides in pediculosis capitis. Arch Dis Child 64:69, 1989

REEVES JRT: Head lice and scabies in children. Pediatr Infect Dis J 6:598, 1987

SHELLEY WB et al: *Staphylococcus aureus* colonization of burrows in erythrodermic Norwegian scabies. A case study of iatrogenic contagion. J Am Acad Dermatol 19:673, 1988

VAN NESTE DJ: Human scabies in perspective. Int J Dermatol 27:10, 1988

PART SIX DISORDERS OF THE CARDIOVASCULAR SYSTEM

section 1 Disorders of the heart

173 CELLULAR AND MOLECULAR BIOLOGY OF CARDIOVASCULAR DISEASE

EUGENE BRAUNWALD

Because the principal function of the heart is to serve as a pump, clinical cardiology, since the era of William Harvey, has been deeply rooted in physiology and hemodynamics. The development of electrocardiography at the beginning of this century and the recognition of clinical disturbances of cardiac rhythm led to increasing interest in electrophysiology. Since both the mechanical and the electrical properties of the heart can be altered profoundly by drugs, pharmacology has also provided strong scientific underpinnings to clinical cardiology.

A fuller understanding of cardiac function and dysfunction will ulimately require studies at the cellular, molecular, and genetic levels. However, such investigations have been retarded by the absence of any cell line of adult, fully differentiated myocytes that can be readily grown in vitro, manipulated, and studied. Perhaps for this reason, cellular biology and molecular genetics have been slower to impact on cardiovascular disease than on some other branches of medicine, such as hematology, oncology, endocrinology, and infectious diseases. However, application of these techniques to cardiovascular science has now gained momentum, and these efforts are beginning to influence the care of patients with cardiovascular disease. Several examples of this influence are considered in this chapter and include advances in understanding myocardial cells, specifically the process of myocardial hypertrophy, the constituents of the bloodstream, such as apoproteins, and noncardiac cells, including vascular smooth-muscle cells, endothelial cells, and platelets. Discussed elsewhere (Chap. 289) are advances in thrombolytic therapy which have also resulted from studies at the cellular and molecular levels. The prominence of noncardiac cells in this discussion reflects the fact that the most prevalent forms of cardiovascular disease, hypertensive and ischemic heart disease, are diseases of the blood vessels, the myocardium itself being secondarily affected, as an "innocent bystander."

HYPERTROPHY

MYOCARDIAL HYPERTROPHY One of the most remarkable and important capacities of the heart is to adapt both acutely and chronically to changes in hemodynamic load. *Acute* adaptations are mediated by the two mechanisms discussed in Chap. 181: (1) an alteration in the number of cross-bridges that cycle between the actin and myosin myofilaments, depending on the length of the myocardial sarcomeres (this adaptation expresses, at the molecular level, Starling's law of the heart) and (2) changes in contractility mediated by the adrenergic neurotransmitter norepinephrine via beta-adrenergic receptors. The degree of activation of these receptors ultimately regulates the concentration of calcium ions around the contractile proteins and, thereby, myocardial contractility. In contrast, with *chronic* hemodynamic overload, as in hypertension, valvular heart disease, and many forms of congenital heart disease, *myocardial hypertrophy* is the major adaptive response. As the ventricle hypertrophies, new sarcomeres are added to each myocyte, protein synthesis is augmented, and sometimes protein degradation declines. The fraction of total cardiac protein composed of myofibrillar proteins increases in hypertrophy and subsequently declines as heart failure supervenes.

The mechanism responsible for the development of myocardial hypertrophy is the subject of intense investigation. The imposition of a pressure load on the ventricle is accompanied by an increase in the expression of messenger RNA (mRNA) that codes for various contractile proteins, and these increased levels of mRNA are responsible for the increase in myocardial protein synthesis. Proteins often occur in families of closely related isoforms, the expression of which is regulated in a tissue-specific and developmentally specific manner. In experimental animals the hypertrophic response involves the reappearance in the adult heart of contractile protein isoforms characteristic of the fetus such as the V_3 form of beta-myosin heavy chain ("slow myosin"), which has a low ATPase activity and promotes a slower, more sustained contraction requiring less energy than the V_1 form ("fast myosin"). The fetal isoforms of alpha-actin and tropomyosin and the mRNA of atrial natriuretic peptide (ANP, see later) are also reexpressed when left ventricular hypertrophy is induced. This reexpression of fetal protein genes appears to represent a general adaptive response.

In contrast to the cardiac hypertrophy resulting from hemodynamic overload, the hypertrophy of hyperthyroidism is *not* accompanied by the induction of fetal forms of contractile protein genes or of the ANP gene. Thyroid hormone acts directly via nuclear receptors to regulate myosin heavy chain gene expression at the transcriptional level, causing an accumulation of alpha-myosin heavy chain mRNA, and inhibits the expression of beta-myosin heavy chain mRNA, thereby increasing the level of myosin isoenzyme V_1 and bringing about a more rapid contraction. Hypothyroid hearts have higher levels of beta-myosin heavy chain mRNA and the V_3 myosin isoform, and lower levels of the mRNA encoding Ca^{2+} ATPase of sarcoplasmic reticulum.

Some of the changes in gene expression in ventricular hypertrophy involve proto-oncogenes, which are normal cellular homologues of transforming genes carried by oncogenic retroviruses (Chap. 10), and a gene that encodes one of the heat shock proteins (which appears to play a protective role during stress). Three major classes of proto-oncogenes are induced by pressure overload and are responsible for the acceleration of protein synthesis and of fetal isoforms: (1) one class encodes peptide growth factors, e.g., the c-*sis* proto-oncogene that encodes the beta chain of platelet-derived growth factor (PDGF, see later); (2) proto-oncogenes such as c-*myc* and c-*fos*, which code for nuclear proteins that regulate transcription of a variety of genes which influence the cell cycle; and (3) proto-oncogenes such as c-*ras*, which code for cytoplasmic proteins that bind to guanine nucleotides and regulate other intracellular signaling systems. The reinduction of genes normally expressed in fetal life, such as the fetal isoforms of myosin and ANP (in the ventricle), is a later event.

Stimuli that increase intracellular cyclic AMP and intracellular Ca^{2+} or alpha-adrenergic agonists that enhance the turnover of inositol phospholipids regulate the expression of the c-*fos* gene. The protein expressed by this gene may play a role in modulation of the response to neurotransmitters and drugs that affect the function of the heart acutely in the development of cardiac hypertrophy. Norepinephrine augments c-*myc* and c-*fos* mRNA expression, and stimulation of primary cultured neonatal cardiac myocytes by $alpha_1$-adrenergic agents causes their hypertrophy and induces the fetal isoforms of actin and myosin synthesis, possibly by increasing the expression of the c-*myc* and c-*fos* proto-oncogenes. This action of the alpha-adrenergic receptor on c-*myc* and c-*fos* may occur through an increase of phosphoinositide turnover and the activation of protein kinase C.

In addition to the growth of myocytes, the interstitium also participates in pressure overload hypertrophy, which is associated with hyperplasia of fibroblasts and the deposition of excess and altered types of extracellular collagen. The relief of hemodynamic overload, either surgical or pharmacologic, usually results in partial regression of myocyte hypertrophy, but not necessarily in regression of interstitial proliferation. Exactly how mechanical load is converted into growth, a process that might be termed *mechanogrowth coupling*, is poorly understood. When myocytes are stretched in vitro an increase in mRNA and protein synthesis takes place. Thus, myocytes appear to be able to *sense* external load and to undergo hypertrophy, perhaps triggered by the activation of *stretch-activated* channels through which an influx of cations occurs.

There are many potential applications to cardiology of the growing understanding of the mechanisms involved in myocyte hypertrophy. For example, the c-*myc* proto-oncogene is expressed in the heart of the Syrian hamster with hereditary idiopathic cardiomyopathy. Since this animal model resembles the human disorder, it will be of great interest to determine if the same might be true in the latter. Investigation of this phenomenon might also reveal the mechanism by which compensatory hypertrophy may lead to myocardial failure and could suggest measures to prevent this complication. Ultimately, this knowledge could also lead to the development of a method for stimulating myocardial hypertrophy or even myocyte hyperplasia after cell death has occurred consequent to myocardial infarction, viral myocarditis, and other conditions causing myocyte necrosis.

Efforts are also under way to identify genes causing hereditary forms of cardiomyopathy or cardiac hypertrophy using the technique of genetic linkage (or cosegregation) analysis (see Chap. 6). This technique allows identification of the genetic region responsible for a disease. It is used to map the loci of genes that are tightly linked to a specific phenotype by making use of restriction fragment length polymorphisms (RFLPs), which are due to DNA sequence differences between individuals. Such an approach has been used to localize the gene responsible for Duchenne's muscular dystrophy (Chap. 365) and for cystic fibrosis (Chap. 209), and the genes for these conditions, which often affect the heart directly or indirectly, have been cloned. A high-molecular-weight protein (dystrophin) is absent from the transverse tubules of skeletal muscle of patients with Duchenne's muscular dystrophy. Presumably its absence in the myocardium is responsible for the cardiomyopathy that frequently occurs in this condition. Similarly, a gene responsible for familial hypertrophic cardiomyopathy (Chap. 192) has been mapped to chromosome 14 using genetic linkage analyses. This should allow early (including prenatal) diagnosis.

VASCULAR WALL The renin-angiotensin system in the vascular wall may be involved in the development of hypertrophy of vascular smooth muscle. Angiotensinogen mRNA in blood vessel walls may be elevated in chronic hypertension. The addition of angiotensin II to cultures of vascular smooth-muscle cells causes the rapid activation of the c-*fos* proto-oncogene, which may mediate angiotensin II–induced hypertrophy in smooth-muscle cells in vivo. Indeed, angiotensin II induces hypertrophy of arterial smooth-muscle cells in vitro, in association with rapid induction in c-*fos*, c-*myc*, and c-*jun* mRNA levels followed by marked increases in the expression of the α chain of PDGF. This hypertrophy of vascular smooth muscle can be blocked by angiotensin-converting enzyme inhibitors. The gene for the PDGF receptor has been cloned; the PDGF receptor mediates the mitogenic effects of this substance on vascular smooth-muscle (and other) cells. The PDGF receptor has a structure similar to a family of growth factor receptors that have tyrosine kinase activity. The PDGF receptor interacts with the c-*ras* proto-oncogene product and activates phospholipase C.

Many growth factors in the cardiovascular system, such as angiotensin II, vasopressin, PDGF, and epidermal growth factor, are also vasoconstrictors. These considerations may be of significance in selecting or designing antihypertensive drugs. Indeed, angiotensin-converting enzyme inhibitors are more potent in causing regression of left ventricular hypertrophy than are direct-acting vasodilators such as hydralazine.

SPECIALIZED SARCOLEMMAL PROTEINS

ADRENERGIC AND MUSCARINIC RECEPTORS AND G PROTEINS (Fig. 173-1) Plasma membrane receptors mediate the interaction between ligands, including drugs, neurotransmitters, and cells, and basically constitute key transmembrane signalling systems (see Chaps. 11 and 68). There are important functional and topographic analogies and amino acid sequence homologues between the beta-adrenergic receptor, the muscarinic cholinergic receptor, and rhodopsin, the light receptor in the rods of the retina. These receptors are all glycoproteins with seven membrane-spanning domains (Fig. 173-2). A reduction in the density of $beta_1$-adrenergic receptors ("down regulation") occurs in chronic heart failure (Chap. 181) consequent to the heart's chronic exposure to the adrenergic agonist norepinephrine. Agonist-occupied receptors are preferentially phosphorylated, which leads to their dissociation from the sarcolemma and internalization in the myocyte.

After an agonist binds to a beta-adrenergic receptor, the receptor associates tightly with the G (guanine nucleotide regulatory) protein (Fig. 173-1), which in turn activates effectors such as adenylate cyclase or calcium channels (see also Chap. 68). Structure-function analyses of the beta-adrenergic receptor have defined the regions of the receptor involved in (1) binding ligands (drugs and neurotransmitters); (2) coupling to G proteins; and (3) desensitization. The ligand binding portion of the molecule lies in the transmembrane domains, and the third intracellular loop of the protein appears to be critical to the attachment of the receptor to the G protein. Beta-adrenergic and $alpha_1$-adrenergic receptors are coupled to different classes of G proteins. These proteins couple $alpha_1$ receptors to the activation of phospholipase C, which in turn breaks down a cell membrane phospholipid (PIP_2) into inositol trisphosphate (IP_3) and diacylglycerol; IP_3 liberates calcium from intracellular sites (see Chap. 11). G proteins may either augment or reduce the formation of the second messenger cyclic AMP. A stimulatory G protein (G_s) couples the beta-adrenergic receptor to adenylate cyclase, while an inhibitory G protein (G_i) causes inhibition of this enzyme (and therefore the formation of cyclic AMP) when muscarinic and adenosine receptors are stimulated. There is evidence that alterations in G proteins (reduced levels of G_s and increased levels of G_i) may play a role in the pathogenesis of heart failure; the mechanism responsible for these alterations remains to be elucidated.

Five muscarinic receptor cDNAs (complementary DNAs) have

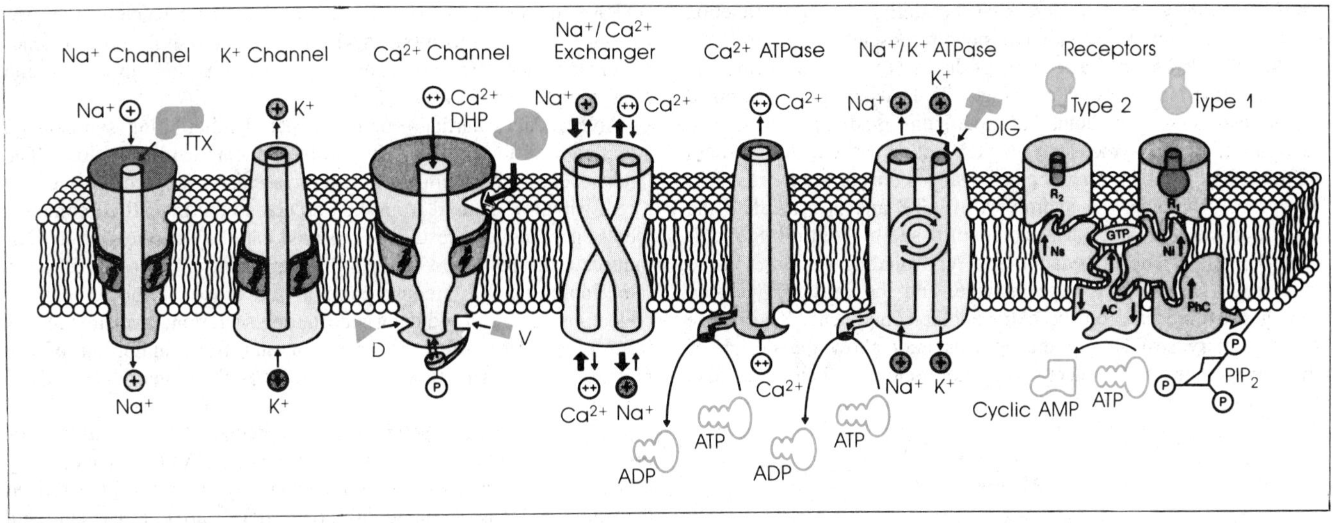

FIGURE 173-1 Ion transport through the sarcolemma of a myocyte. The Na^+ channel of the heart muscle cell opens briefly at the start of an action potential, permitting an influx of Na^+. The Na^+ channel can be blocked by tetrodotoxin (TTX) or by type I antiarrhythmic agents (see Chap. 185). Depolarization of the sarcolemma leads to Ca^{2+} influx through the Ca^{2+} channel, which is sensitive to the change in potential. The Ca^{2+} channel can be blocked by the calcium entry blockers. D, diltiazem; V, verapamil; DHP, dihydropyridines. Repolarization of the membrane results principally from the opening of K^+ channels and the efflux of K^+. Ca^{2+} is removed from the cell by the Na^+/Ca^{2+} exchanger and by a Ca^{2+}-ATPase (an energy-requiring process). The Na^+ pump (Na^+,K^+-ATPase) removes Na^+ which has flowed into the cell and returns K^+ to the cell by an energy-requiring process; it may be blocked by digitalis (DIG).

Two types of receptors modulate ionic pathways. Beta-adrenergic receptors (which are one kind of type 2 receptor) stimulate the production of the second messenger cyclic AMP which by causing phosphorylation (P) allows the Ca^{2+} channel to open. Muscarinic cholinergic receptors (one kind of type 1 receptor) inhibit cyclic AMP production and also activate phospholipase C, the enzyme producing the second messenger inositol trisphosphate (IP_3), which in smooth-muscle cells mobilizes intracellular calcium.

DIG, digitalis glycoside (Na^+,K^+-ATPase inhibitor); R_1 and R_2, binding proteins for the respective receptor types; AC, adenylate cyclase; Ni (AC-inhibiting) and Ns (AC-stimulating) nucleotide binding G proteins (G_i and G_s, respectively); PhC, phospholipase C; PIP_2, phosphotidylinositol diphosphate, a membrane phospholipid; P, phosphate. (*Reproduced with permission from U Ruegg, Sandorama, 2:5, 1987.*)

been cloned. These fall into two groups: the M_1 subtype predominates in the vasculature and neurons and the M_2 subtype, linked to adenylate cyclase, predominates in the heart.

The gene for the human beta$_2$-adrenergic receptor has been cloned; it is unusual in that it lacks introns within the coding region and in this respect it resembles the proto-oncogene c-*mas,* which also encodes the angiotensin II receptor. The large family of receptors that are coupled to G proteins probably arose from a common ancestral gene.

FIGURE 173-2 Structure of the human beta$_2$-adrenergic receptor as it may be organized within the membrane. Open circles represent amino acids that are identical to those of hamster beta$_2$-adrenergic receptor. (*Reproduced with permission from Dohlman et al, Biochemistry 26:2664, 1987.*)

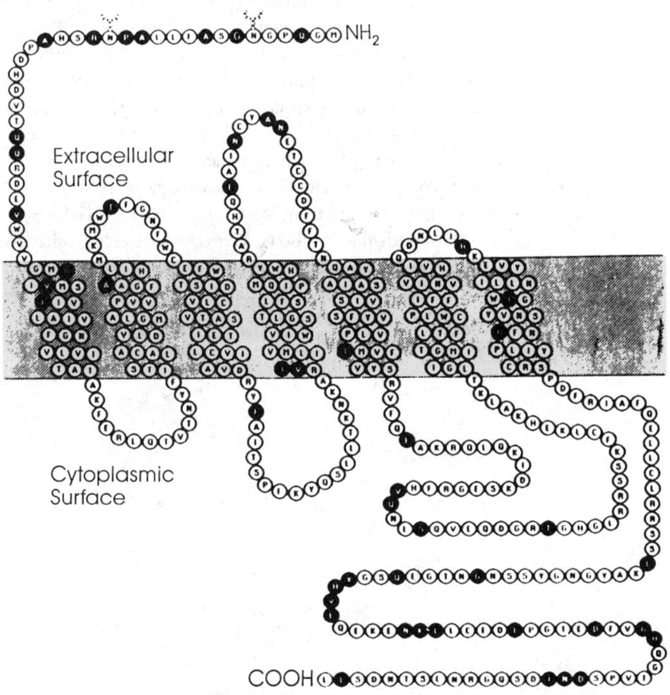

An understanding of the molecular structure of cardiac receptors and of the genes which encode them is likely to lead to more rational design of drugs that can modify cardiac function by acting on these receptors.

CALCIUM CHANNELS Calcium ions play a unique role in a variety of cellular functions, in particular, contraction of cardiac and vascular smooth muscle (Chap. 181). Calcium enters cardiac cells through voltage-sensitive calcium channels (Fig. 173-1) that are controlled by transmembrane electrical potentials and open during depolarization of the sarcolemma. The catalytic subunit of cyclic AMP–dependent protein kinase enhances the opening of calcium channels, thereby increasing influx of calcium into myocytes and enhancing the force of cardiac contraction. This explains, in part, the positive inotropic actions of the beta-adrenergic agonists and of the phosphodiesterase inhibitors, both of which enhance activity of cyclic AMP.

The (L-type) cardiac calcium channels appear to be large aqueous pores through which the calcium ions move, probably in single file. Their primary structure has been elucidated by cDNA cloning. These channels are quite selective for calcium ions under physiologic conditions and are composed of several subunits, the largest of which has a molecular weight of 243,000 Da and binds calcium channel antagonists. Prolongation of the action potential occurs often in hypertrophied myocytes and may be responsible for arrhythmias in patients with heart failure. This prolongation may be due to delays in the inactivation of the L-type calcium channels. Three physically associated, but distinct sites in the channels bind the three classes of calcium antagonists—nifedipine, verapamil, and diltiazem (Chap. 190). The cDNAs (DNAs complementary to their mRNA) encoding the calcium channels have been cloned, and their predicted sequences have been determined. This information should make possible the design of drugs to influence the function of these channels with greater specificity, thereby increasing the ability to control function of the myocardium and of vascular smooth muscle.

SARCOLEMMAL ATPase One of the most important membrane proteins is the Na^+,K^+-ATPase (Fig. 173-1) which plays a critical role in establishing sodium and potassium gradients across cell membranes. This enzyme catalyzes the reaction that extrudes sodium and transports potassium into the cell against concentration gradients. This process requires the hydrolysis of ATP and is critical to the function of cardiac (and other excitable) tissue by controlling membrane potentials. Phosphorylation and ATP binding sites are on the cytoplasmic component of the enzyme, and the cardiac glycoside binding site is located on the extracellular component. Knowledge of the primary structure of the enzyme may allow the design of inhibitors perhaps more potent and/or more selective than the cardiac glycosides.

ATRIAL NATRIURETIC PEPTIDE

In 1979 de Bold and his collaborators reported that extracts from atrial myocytes had potent vasodilatory and natriuretic properties. Subsequently it was shown that the active factor is a 28-amino-acid polypeptide named atrial natriuretic peptide (ANP). ANP is released from granules in atrial myocytes during atrial stretch and binds to receptors on the surfaces of cells in the kidney (renal vessels, glomeruli, and medulla), vascular bed, and adrenal gland. In the central nervous system, ANP acts in areas known to be involved in the control of vascular resistance and in the regulation of salt and water balance.

The interaction of ANP with its receptors activates plasma membrane–associated (particulate) guanylate cyclase leading to the accumulation of cyclic GMP, which in turn activates cyclic GMP–dependent protein kinases and thereby instigates the phosphorylation of a number of intracellular proteins. In vascular smooth muscle cyclic GMP causes relaxation by phosphorylating myosin light chains, while in renal tubular epithelial cells it inhibits the activity of sodium channels. In smooth-muscle cells, by stimulating cyclic GMP–dependent protein kinase, ANP enhances the activity of a Ca^{2+}-ATPase, thereby increasing the removal of ionic calcium and promoting vascular relaxation. ANP also inhibits basal and hormone-stimulated adenylate cyclase activity in vascular smooth-muscle and renal glomerular cells.

ANP reduces cardiac output, in part by inhibiting sympathetic stimulation of the heart and in part by reducing cardiac preload. The latter results from a reduction of intravascular volume consequent to a redistribution of fluid from the vascular to the interstitial compartments, perhaps as a result of increased capillary permeability. ANP induces natriuresis and diuresis by increasing glomerular filtration rate, inhibiting Na^+ reabsorption in the proximal tubule and the collecting duct, and reducing aldosterone secretion; the latter results from suppression of renin secretion and from inhibition of the biosynthesis and secretion of aldosterone by the glomerulosa cells of the adrenal cortex.

Collectively, these actions serve to reduce arterial and venous pressures and blood volume. As a consequence, ANP appears to play a role as a counterregulatory hormone in many disorders characterized by volume expansion, including congestive heart failure, acute and chronic renal failure, and nephrotic syndrome, hypertension, and hepatic disease.

The biosynthetic mechanisms for ANP have been defined (Fig. 173-3). The precursor of ANP in human atrial tissue is *preproANP*, a 151-amino-acid polypeptide encoded by a gene on the short arm of chromosome 1.

Factors that stimulate ANP secretion enhance the transcription of preproANP mRNA. Cleavage of the signal peptide from preproANP results in proANP, a 126-amino-acid peptide, which is the storage form of ANP and is converted to the active hormone at the time of its secretion from the atrial myocyte; the 28-amino-acid biologically active peptide is cleaved from the *C*-terminus of the storage form. ANP is synthesized in adult atrium, in normal fetal ventricle, and in adult ventricle which has been stimulated by glucocorticoids or stressed by left ventricular hypertrophy. As already described at the beginning of the chapter, such diseased ventricles have increased expression of ANP mRNA.

Additional stimuli affect the production and secretion of ANP. Glucocorticoids play a significant role in stimulating the secretion of

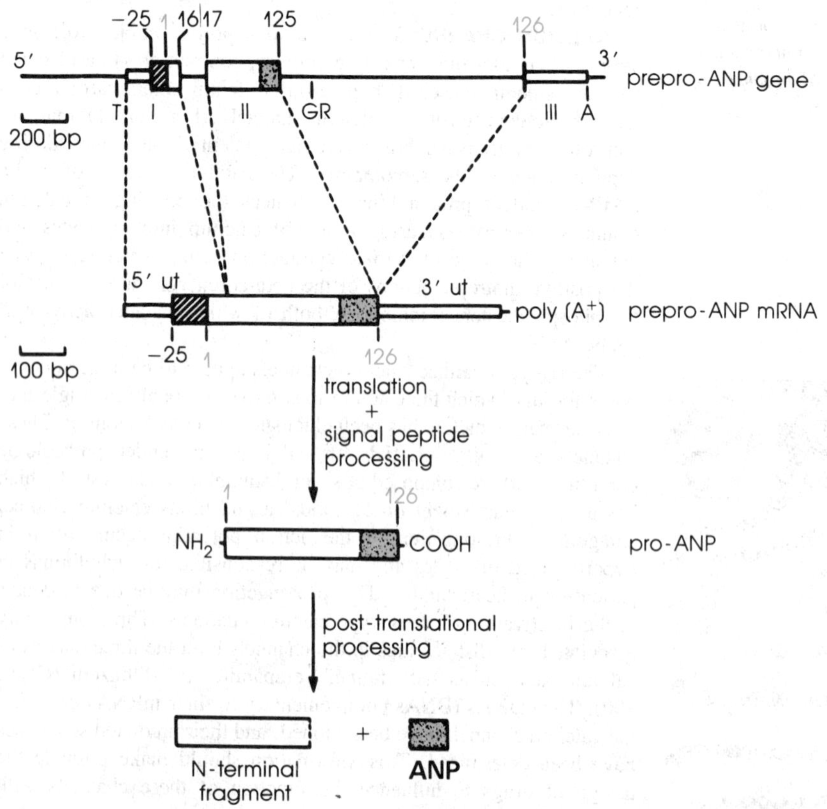

FIGURE 173-3 Schematic representation of the ANP gene, messenger RNA (mRNA), and precursor (pro-ANP). Arabic numberals indicate the positions of coding sequences to the respective amino acids in pro-ANP. The gene contains three coding regions or exons (I, II, III) and two intervening sequences (introns), as well as a typical iniation site (T) and poly-A tail (A). A putative glucocorticoid recognition site (GR) exists in the second intron. The mRNA contains untranslated regions (ut) at the 5′ and 3′ ends and also codes for a signal peptide (hatched region) which is typical for secreted proteins and is presumably cleaved cotranslationally. ANP (shaded region) is derived from the *C*-terminus (COOH) of pro-ANP, following hydrolytic cleavage between residue 98 and 99 in the heart but possibly at other points in extracardiac tissues. *(Reproduced with permission from SA Atlas, Recent Prog Horm Res 42:207–249, 1986.)*

ANP. There appears to be a glucocorticoid regulatory element near the ANP gene, and glucocorticoids increase its rate of transcription. Endothelin (see later), a potent vasoconstrictor released by endothelial cells, also increases the release of ANP from atrial myocytes; this may serve as a counterregulatory influence to the vasoconstrictor.

The elucidation of the structure of the ANP gene and the understanding of the mechanism by which ANP is synthesized, processed, and released represents a major advance in understanding the control of the circulation and regulation of blood volume. Analogues of ANP or substances that influence its synthesis and release or mimic its actions are being developed and should be useful in the treatment of a broad array of pathophysiologic states.

APOPROTEINS AND ATHEROGENESIS

Abnormalities in the number or function of the low-density lipoprotein (LDL) receptors are responsible for some forms of atherosclerosis (Chaps. 195 and 326). Abnormalities of the *apoproteins,* many of which are genetic, may play more frequent roles in atherogenesis. At least 10 apoproteins are embedded in the surface of the spherical lipoprotein particles that carry the lipids in the bloodstream and are encoded by genes localized to chromosomes 1, 2, 6, 11, and 19 (the LDL receptor gene is also on chromosome 19). Amino acid sequences suggest that several of these apoproteins are derived from a common ancestral gene. The major functions of apoproteins are to serve as (1) ligands that interact with cellular receptors for the lipoprotein particles, (2) cofactors of enzymes involved in lipid metabolism, and (3) structural components of the lipoproteins.

High-density lipoproteins (HDL) take up excess cholesterol from cells, and the concentration of circulating HDL is related inversely to the risk of the development of ischemic heart disease (Chaps. 195 and 326). Apoproteins AI, CIII, and AIV are three HDL apoproteins encoded by genes clustered on chromosome 11. Several disorders are associated with mutations of these apoproteins, leading to a defect in the synthesis or function of HDL and the development of premature atherosclerosis. For example, apo AI serves as a cofactor for the enzyme lecithin cholesterol acyl transferase (LCAT) which catalyzes the reaction that converts cholesterol taken up by the HDL particle into the form in which it is transported, i.e., cholesteryl ester. Some variants of apo AI are defective for this cofactor activity, thereby preventing the normal function of HDL and causing premature atherosclerosis.

Apo E is one of the principal constituents of very low density lipoproteins (VLDL) and of chylomicron remnants, the latter particles having great atherogenic activity. Three alleles of the apo E gene have been described. Subjects who are homozygous for the *e2* allele, which encodes apo E2, have decreased clearance of VLDL and chylomicron remnants from the circulation, presumably because apo E2 fails to bind normally to lipoprotein receptors. As a consequence, the *e2* allele plays a permissive role in the development of type III hyperlipoproteinemia, a condition associated with the development of xanthomas and premature atherosclerosis (Chap. 195). Patients who are homozygous for the *e4* allele, encoding for apo E4, have a reduced catabolism of LDL and premature atherosclerosis.

Elevation of the plasma concentration of Lp(a) (referred to as "lipoprotein little a") is another important risk factor for the development of premature atherosclerosis. Its protein components consist of apo B100 linked to apo(a). Six inherited apo(a) isoproteins and a series of alleles at a single gene locus control the apo(a) phenotypes and appear to determine the Lp(a) concentration. An interesting clue to the mechanism by which Lp(a) accelerates atherosclerosis has recently emerged. Through cDNA cloning and the deduced protein structure, it has been shown that apo(a) is a deformed relative of plasminogen, the precursor of the proteolytic enzyme plasmin, which dissolves fibrin clots (Chap. 288). Apo(a) contains 37 copies of kringle 4 (a portion of the plasminogen molecule in the shape of the Danish pastry known as *kringle*) followed by kringle 5 and the protease domain. This strong resemblance between a lipoprotein and plasminogen may provide a link between lipids, the clotting system, and atherogenesis. Microthrombi containing fibrin on the vessel wall become incorporated into atherosclerotic plaques. Kringle 4 of plasminogen normally binds to fibrin during fibrinolysis. Apo(a), with many copies of this kringle, could also bind to fibrin in microthrombi in the vessel wall. Following endothelial damage, Lp(a) may insinuate itself into the arterial wall, inhibiting the cleavage of fibrin in microthrombi by competing with plasminogen for access to fibrin.

Discussed above are three examples of how the genes encoding apolipoproteins can play a critical role in determining the risk for the development of atherosclerosis. It may prove to be cost-effective to attempt to identify genetic defects of apoproteins (as well as of the LDL receptor) in childhood and to use a preventive approach *selectively* on subjects identified by such genetic analyses, as opposed to the broad *shotgun* preventive approach that is currently in vogue and that is directed nonselectively at the entire population.

PLATELETS

Platelets (see Chap. 287) are intimately involved in three critical aspects of coronary artery disease: (1) they participate in the progression of the underlying atherogenic process; (2) they form the nidus of the coronary thrombus responsible for acute myocardial infarction; and (3) they may release vasoactive substances that can cause coronary vasoconstriction. Activated platelets secrete alpha granules that contain platelet factor 4, a procoagulant that neutralizes the action of heparin and several growth factors, including alpha and beta fibroblast growth factors and PDGF (see Chap. 9). The latter, a 30,000-Da protein, is also generated by macrophages and endothelial cells. PDGF acts on at least two specific membrane receptors which have been cloned. It is a powerful vasoconstrictor and a potent growth factor that stimulates DNA synthesis and proliferation of arterial smooth-muscle cells, an important step in atherogenesis.

PDGF may also be involved in malignant transformation. Its amino acid sequence is almost identical to that of a segment of transforming factor of the simian sarcoma virus (SSV), an acute transforming virus that induces the cells it invades to produce viral proteins, one of which, the v-*sis* gene product, causes monkey cells to undergo malignant transformation (Chap. 9).

Other substances released from aggregating platelets possess potent vasoactive properties; serotonin and thromboxane A_2 cause vasoconstriction, while ATP and ADP cause relaxation (through release of endothelium-derived relaxing factor, see below). The net effect of these influences depends on the presence of intact endothelium. In the normal endothelium the vasodilator influences dominate, while in the dysfunctional endothelium, as discussed below, the vasoconstrictor influences prevail.

ENDOTHELIUM

For many years the endothelium, the monolayer of cells in direct contact with blood, was considered to be a relatively inert, smooth boundary between the blood and the vascular wall (Fig. 173-4). In fact, endothelial cells are quite active metabolically and normally produce a number of substances that affect the vascular lumen as well as platelets.

The first and best known of the endothelial vasodilators is prostacyclin (PGI_2) (see Chap. 69), which also inhibits the adhesion and aggregation of platelets. The action of PGI_2 involves the activation of adenylate cyclase and formation of cyclic AMP. When stimulated by a large number of substances, including ATP and ADP, acetylcholine, thrombin, neurotransmitters, and serotonin, the normal endothelium also releases a labile, highly diffusible vasodilator, termed endothelium-derived relaxing factor (EDRF), which appears

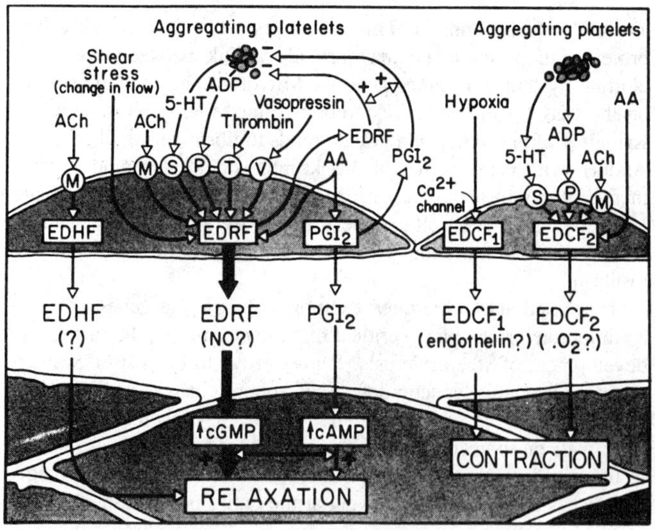

FIGURE 173-4 Current concepts of endothelium-derived factors and their modulation of vascular smooth-muscle contraction: Endothelium-derived relaxing factor (EDRF), a potent vasodilator of the underlying smooth muscle, increases cyclic GMP (cGMP) levels through activation of soluble guanylate cyclase. Prostacyclin (PGI_2) is another vasodilator released from the endothelium but whose effects depend on elevation of cyclic AMP (cAMP) through activation of adenylate cyclase. EDRF and PGI_2 may act synergistically in relaxing vascular smooth muscle and inhibiting platelet aggregation. The endothelial cells also secrete a hyperpolarizing factor (EDHF), the exact nature of which is unknown and which also has a vasodilator action. There are at least two endothelium-derived contracting factors; one is indomethacin-insensitive ($EDCF_1$) and may be endothelin, while the other is indomethacin-sensitive ($EDCF_2$) and may be superoxide anion. ACh, acetylcholine; 5-HT, 5-hydroxytryptamine (serotonin); ADP, adenosine diphosphate; AA, arachidonic acid; +, synergism or facilitation; −, inhibition; ?, exact nature unknown; M, muscarinic receptor; S, serotonergic receptor; P, purinergic receptor; T, thrombin receptor; V, vasopressinergic receptor. *(Reproduced with permission from P Vanhoutte and Shimokawa, Circulation 80:1, 1989.)*

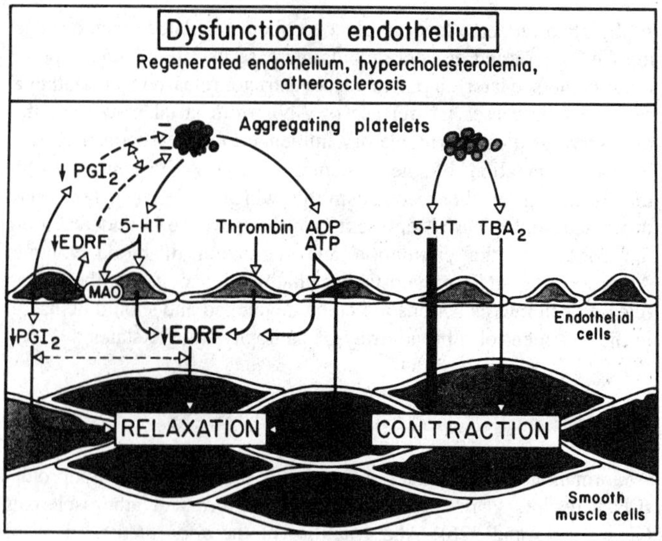

FIGURE 173-5 Responses of dysfunctional endothelium. The endothelium is dysfunctional when it is in a regenerated state, in the presence of hypercholesterolemia, hypertension, or atherosclerosis, releasing less endothelium-derived relaxing factor (EDRF), whereas the ability of the smooth muscle to contract is unaltered. As a result, in endothelial dysfunction smooth-muscle contraction predominates. In atherosclerosis, the production of both EDRF and prostacyclin (PGI_2) are reduced, and their synergistic actions against aggregating platelets may not occur, enhancing platelet aggregation. This may lead to thrombus formation, enhanced vascular contraction, and atherogenesis. 5-HT, 5-hydroxytryptamine (serotonin); ADP, adenosine diphosphate; ATP, adenosine triphosphate; TBA2, thromboxane A_2; MAO, monomine oxidase; ms, inhibition; +, synergism. *(Reproduced with permission from Vanhoutte and Shimokawa, Circulation 80:1, 1989.)*

to be nitric oxide (NO). Normal endothelium also releases EDRF when stimulated by the shear stress of flowing blood, thereby controlling the lumen of arteries and arterioles in relation to the blood flow through the vessel. EDRF stimulates soluble guanylate cyclase, which catalyzes the formation of cyclic GMP, which in turn relaxes vascular smooth muscle. EDRF also inhibits adhesion and aggregation of platelets, an action apparently also mediated by cyclic GMP. EDRF and prostacyclin interact synergistically to dilate blood vessels and inhibit platelet aggregation.

When the endothelium is destroyed or damaged (Fig. 173-5), as in atherosclerotic plaques, EDRF production may be impaired, thereby permitting coronary vasoconstriction in the vicinity of such plaques. Moreover, subtle damage to the endothelium, as in hypertension, some forms of hyperlipidemia, reperfusion after ischemia, and in regenerating endothelium after mechanical trauma, leads to defective release of EDRF. On the other hand, the eicosapentanoic acid in fish oils stimulates the production of EDRF, perhaps explaining the putative antiatherogenic properties of these substances.

Endothelium also synthesizes thrombomodulin, a glycoprotein with a molecular weight of 105,000 whose gene has been isolated. Thrombomodulin serves as an endothelial receptor for thrombin. When thrombin is bound to thrombomodulin, which is located on the luminal side of the vascular endothelium, it loses its procoagulant activity (conversion of fibrinogen to fibrin, stimulation of platelets), the rate at which it is inactivated by antithrombin III is accelerated, and its activation of protein C, an anticoagulant, is enhanced.

Endothelium also releases at least two vasoconstrictors, one a product of cyclooxygenase activity that appears to be responsible for hypoxia-induced vascular contraction. The other is a 21-amino-acid peptide called *endothelin,* an extremely potent vasoconstrictor. The expression of the gene for endothelin appears to be inhibited by the shear stress of flowing blood, a mechanism that appears to act in concert with the release of EDRF by the same stimulus to enhance vessel diameter as flow increases. In hypertension, EDRF release is impaired, whereas the release of endothelial-derived contracting factor(s) may be augmented, presumably aggravating this condition. Like PDGF, endothelin is both a vasoconstrictor and a smooth-muscle mitogen.

In early atherosclerosis, dysfunction of a G protein in endothelial cells may play a role in the failure of EDRF release. Endothelial injury or dysfunction also enhances platelet deposition on the arterial wall. If unopposed by EDRF and prostacyclin, serotonin and thromboxane A_2 released from the deposited platelets cause arterial constriction and spasm in the coronary arterial system. The adhesion and aggregation of platelets consequent to the defective production of EDRF enhances further the atherosclerotic process.

ANGIOGENESIS

Endothelial cells also secrete a group of growth factors that are mitogenic for endothelium and can induce formation of new blood vessels (angiogenesis). Angiogenic stimuli cause the elongation and proliferation of endothelial cells and the generation of new vessels. A group of angiogenic mitogens, which are heparin-binding peptides related to endothelial cell growth factors, have been identified. The amino acid sequences of several of these growth factors have been deduced by cloning and analysis of their genes.

Angiogenesis is of considerable pathogenetic significance. Folkman has postulated that the growth of tumors depends on an adequate blood supply, which in turn is dependent on the growth of new vessels into the tumors; the latter is stimulated by angiogenesis factors(s) secreted by the tumor. Inhibition of angiogenesis can cause tumor regression in animal models. Abnormal angiogenesis may be involved in diverse disease states, including diabetic retinopathy, neovascular glaucoma, rheumatoid arthritis, and psoriasis.

The development of new vessels in the heart, i.e., of the coronary collateral circulation, is of critical importance in protecting the myocardium from the consequences of coronary obstruction. The extent of the collateral circulation varies enormously among patients with similar degrees of coronary arterial narrowing, and this difference may be related in part to differences in the production of angiogenic factors. It has been speculated that the introduction of purified angiogenic factors directly into ischemic myocardium might enhance the development of collaterals, accelerate the healing of the necrotic tissue, and prevent infarct expansion and cardiac dilatation. Angiogenesis may also be deleterious. Coronary atheroma are highly vascularized by a fragile capillary network, and rupture of these newly formed capillaries when they are exposed to high intravascular pressures may lead to hemorrhage into atherosclerotic plaques and coronary occlusion.

CONCLUSIONS

The applications of cellular and molecular biology to studies of the myocardium, vascular wall, platelets, and lipoproteins have already increased greatly our understanding of the fundamental abnormalities in cardiovascular disease. In the future these approaches are likely to improve the diagnosis of patients with genetic disorders causing cardiac disease, help to identify individuals at risk of developing these disorders, thereby leading to the institution of preventive measures, and provide new agents for the treatment and prevention of cardiovascular diseases.

REFERENCES

Braunwald E: On future directions for cardiology: The Paul Dudley White lecture. Circulation 77:1:13, 1988

Brenner BM et al: The diverse biological actions of atrial natriuretic peptide. Physiol Rev (in press)

Catterall WA: Structure and function of voltage-sensitive ion channels. Science 242:50, 1988

Chien KR, Knowlton KU: Cardiovascular molecular biology. Circulation 80:2:219, 1989

Folkman J, Weisz PB: Control of angiogenesis, in *Biocatalysis and Biometrics*, JD Burrington, DS Clark (eds). Washington, DC, American Chemical Society, ACS Symposium Series 392, 1989, pp 19–32

Furchgott RF, Vanhoutte PM: Endothelium-derived relaxing and contracting factors. FASEB J 3:2007, 1989

Hathaway DR, March KL: Molecular biology: New avenues for the diagnosis and treatment of cardiovascular disease. J Am Coll Cardiol 13:265, 1989

Jarcho JA et al: Mapping a gene for familial hypertrophic cardiomyopathy to chromosome 14ql. N Engl J Med 321:1372, 1989

Katz AM: Molecular biology in cardiology, a paradigmatic shift. J Mol Cell Biol 20:355, 1988 (editorial)

Vanhoutte PM, Shimokawa H: Endothelium-derived relaxing factor and coronary vasospasm. Circulation 80:1, 1989

Venter JC, Triggle D (eds): *Structure and Physiology of the Slow Inward Calcium Channel*. New York, Alan R. Liss, 1987

174 APPROACH TO THE PATIENT WITH HEART DISEASE

EUGENE BRAUNWALD

The symptoms caused by heart disease result most commonly from myocardial ischemia, from disturbance of the contraction or relaxation of the myocardium, or from an abnormal cardiac rhythm or rate. Ischemia is manifest most frequently as chest discomfort, while reduction of the pumping ability of the heart commonly leads to weakness and fatigability or, when severe, produces cyanosis, hypotension, syncope, and elevated intravascular pressure behind a failing ventricle; the latter results in abnormal fluid accumulation, which in turn leads to dyspnea, orthopnea, and edema. Cardiac arrhythmias often develop suddenly, and the resulting signs and symptoms—palpitation, dyspnea, angina, hypotension, and syncope—generally occur abruptly and may disappear as rapidly as they develop.

A cardinal principle useful in the evaluation of the patient with suspected heart disease is that myocardial or coronary function which may be adequate at rest may be inadequate during exertion. Thus, a history of chest discomfort and/or dyspnea which appears only during activity is characteristic of heart disease, while the opposite pattern, i.e., the appearance of these symptoms at rest and their remission during exertion, is rarely observed in patients with organic heart disease.

Patients with cardiocirculatory disease may also be asymptomatic, both at rest and during exertion, but may present an abnormal physical finding, such as a heart murmur, elevated systemic arterial pressure, or an abnormality of the electrocardiogram or of the cardiac silhouette on the chest roentgenogram. Increasingly, patients are discovered to have asymptomatic ischemia on an exercise stress test or an ambulatory electrocardiogram.

Diseases of the heart and circulation are so common and the laity is so well acquainted with the major symptoms resulting from these disorders that patients, and occasionally physicians, erroneously attribute many noncardiac complaints to organic cardiovascular disease. Furthermore, the combination of the widespread fear of heart disease in the western world with the deep-seated emotional connotations concerning this organ's function results in the frequent development in persons with normal cardiovascular systems of symptoms which mimic those of organic disease. Sometimes it is difficult to interpret correctly the symptoms of patients with recognized organic cardiovascular disturbances. Such patients, in addition to having symptoms resulting from their disease, may also develop functional complaints referable to the cardiovascular system. The unraveling of symptoms and signs due to organic heart disease from those which are not directly related is an important and challenging task in these patients.

It must be recognized that dyspnea, one of the cardinal manifestations of diminished cardiac reserve, is not limited to disease of the heart, but is also characteristic of conditions as diverse as pulmonary disease, marked obesity, and anxiety (Chap. 36). Similarly, chest discomfort (Chap. 16) may result from a variety of causes other than myocardial ischemia. Whether heart disease is responsible for these symptoms can frequently be determined by carrying out a detailed clinical examination. Noninvasive testing using electrocardiography at rest and during exercise (Chap. 176), roentgenography, and echocardiography (Chap. 177) usually provide important additional information to permit the correct interpretation of symptoms; more specialized invasive examinations (catheterization and angiography) are occasionally necessary.

DIAGNOSIS In every branch of medicine the establishment of the prognosis and the development of a rational plan of management are based on a correct diagnostic appraisal. In patients with disorders of the cardiocirculatory system, particular care must be taken to establish not only a correct but also a *complete* diagnosis. As outlined by the New York Heart Association, the elements of a complete cardiac diagnosis include consideration of

1 *The underlying etiology*. Is the disease congenital, rheumatic, hypertensive, or ischemic in origin?
2 *The anatomic abnormalities*. Which chambers are enlarged? Which valves are affected? Is there pericardial involvement? Has there been a myocardial infarction?
3 *The physiologic disturbances*. Is an arrhythmia present? Is there evidence of congestive heart failure or of myocardial ischemia?
4 *The extent of functional disability*. How strenuous is the physical

activity required to elicit symptoms? The latter should be evaluated in the light of the intensity of therapy.

Two simple examples may serve to illustrate the importance of establishing a complete diagnosis: (1) The identification of myocardial ischemia as the cause of exertional chest discomfort is of great clinical importance. However, this diagnosis is insufficient to develop either a strategy of specific treatment or prognosis until the underlying disease process, e.g., coronary atherosclerosis or aortic stenosis, which is responsible for the myocardial ischemia, is identified and a judgment made as to whether severe anemia, thyrotoxicosis, or supraventricular tachycardia plays a contributory role. (2) Determining that heart disease is congenital provides an important starting point, but the decision about whether surgical treatment is advisable depends upon the specific anatomic defect present and often upon the nature of the physiologic disturbance and the functional impairment as well.

The establishment of a correct and complete cardiac diagnosis often requires the use of six different methods of examination: (1) history, (2) physical examination (Chap. 175), (3) electrocardiogram (Chap. 176), (4) chest roentgenogram (Chap. 177), (5) noninvasive graphic examinations (echocardiogram, radionuclide scanning techniques, and other newer "noninvasive" imaging techniques, Chaps. 177 and 178), and occasionally (6) specialized "invasive" examinations, such as cardiac catheterization, angiocardiography, and coronary arteriography (Chap. 179). In order to be most effective, the results obtained from each of these six modalities should be analyzed independently of one another as well as with the information derived from the other methods clearly in mind. Only in this way can one avoid overlooking a subtle, though extremely significant, finding. For example, an electrocardiogram should be obtained in every patient suspected of having heart disease. It may provide the critical clue in establishing the correct diagnosis, e.g., the finding of a moderate atrioventricular conduction disturbance in a patient with unexplained syncope, even when all other methods of examination reveal no abnormal findings. On the other hand, when combined intelligently with the results of other methods of examination, the electrocardiogram may provide essential confirmatory data. Thus, the knowledge that a patient has an apical diastolic rumbling murmur may direct particular attention to the P waves, and the recognition of left atrial enlargement electrocardiographically supports the suggestion that the murmur is caused by mitral stenosis. Under these circumstances the additional finding on the electrocardiogram of right ventricular hypertrophy suggests that pulmonary hypertension is present and that the mitral stenosis is severe.

Although the electrocardiogram is an invaluable aspect of every cardiovascular examination, with the exception of the identification of arrhythmias it rarely permits establishment of a specific diagnosis. In the absence of other abnormal findings, electrocardiographic changes must not be overinterpreted. The range of normal electrocardiographic findings is wide, and the tracing can be affected significantly by many noncardiac factors, such as age, body habitus, and serum electrolyte concentrations.

In obtaining the history of the patient with known or suspected cardiovascular disease, particular attention should be directed to the family history. Familial clustering is common in many forms of heart disease. Genetic transmission may occur, as in hypertrophic cardiomyopathy (Chap. 192) or Marfan's syndrome (Chap. 333). In patients with essential hypertension or coronary atherosclerosis the genetic component may be less obvious but is also of considerable importance. Familial clustering of cardiovascular diseases may occur not only on a genetic basis but may also be related to familial dietary or behavior patterns, such as excessive injection of salt or calories, or cigarette smoking.

When an attempt is made to ascertain the severity of functional impairment in a patient with heart disease, it is essential to determine the precise extent of activity and the rate at which it is performed before symptoms develop. Thus, breathlessness which occurs after running up two long flights of stairs denotes far less functional impairment than similar symptoms occurring after taking a few steps on the level. Also, the degree of customary physical activity at work and during recreation should be considered. The development of two-flight dyspnea in a marathon runner may be far more significant than the development of one-flight dyspnea in a previously sedentary person. Similarly, the history must include a detailed consideration of the patient's therapeutic regimen. For example, the persistence or development of edema, breathlessness, and other manifestations of heart failure in a patient whose diet is rigidly restricted in sodium content and who is receiving optimum doses of diuretics must be interpreted quite differently from the finding of edema in the absence of these measures. In an effort to ascertain the rate of progression of symptoms, and thereby of the severity of the underlying illness, it may be useful to ascertain what, if any, specific tasks the patient could carry out 1 year earlier which he or she cannot carry out now.

PITFALLS IN CARDIOVASCULAR MEDICINE Increasing subspecialization in internal medicine and the perfection of advanced diagnostic techniques in cardiology may sometimes be accompanied by several undesirable consequences, which can be summarized as follows:

1 Failure by the *noncardiologist* to recognize cardiac manifestations of systemic illnesses. The latter include but are not limited to (*a*) the Down syndrome (associated with endocardial cushion defect); (*b*) gonadal dysgenesis, i.e., Turner's syndrome (associated with a variety of congenital cardiovascular defects, particularly coarctation of the aorta); (*c*) bony abnormalities of the upper extremities (associated with atrial septal defect), the Holt-Oram syndrome; (*d*) muscular dystrophies (associated with cardiomyopathy); (*e*) hemochromatosis and glycogen storage disease (associated with myocardial infiltration); (*f*) congenital deafness (associated with prolonged QT interval and serious cardiac arrhythmias); (*g*) Raynaud's disease (associated with primary pulmonary hypertension and coronary vasospasm); (*h*) connective tissue disorders, i.e., Marfan's syndrome, Ehlers-Danlos syndrome, Hurler's syndrome, and related disorders of mucopolysaccharide metabolism (aortic dilatation, prolapsed mitral valve, a variety of arterial abnormalities); (*i*) chronic hemolytic anemia (cardiac dilatation); (*j*) Refsum's disease (myocardial failure and conduction defects); (*k*) acromegaly (accelerated coronary atherosclerosis, conduction defects, cardiomyopathy); (*l*) hyperthyroidism (heart failure, atrial fibrillation); (*m*) hypothyroidism (pericardial effusion, coronary artery disease); (*n*) rheumatoid arthritis (pericarditis, aortic valve disease); (*o*) Whipple's disease (pericarditis and endocarditis); (*p*) scleroderma (cor pulmonale, myocardial fibrosis, pericarditis); (*q*) systemic lupus erythematosus (valvulitis, myocarditis, pericarditis); (*r*) polymyositis (pericarditis, myocarditis); (*s*) sarcoidosis (arrhythmias, cardiomyopathy); (*t*) Fabry's disease (myocardial ischemia, heart failure); and (*u*) exfoliative dermatitis (high-output heart failure). In patients in whom these and other systemic disorders in which cardiovascular involvement may occur, a detailed cardiovascular examination should be carried out.

2 Failure by the cardiac specialist to recognize an underlying systemic illness, such as those listed above, among patients with a cardiac disorder. Patients known or suspected of having heart disease require a detailed general assessment and a search for the frequent noncardiac manifestations of systemic disorders with cardiovascular manifestations. Indeed, the cardiovascular abnormality may provide the clue critical to the recognition of these systemic disorders. Closely related is the failure to appreciate the profound effects of stress, such as that resulting from an intercurrent infection, from pregnancy, or from emotional disturbances, on cardiovascular performance and symptoms.

3 Overreliance on and overutilization of laboratory tests, particularly specialized invasive techniques for the examination of the cardiovascular system. Catheterization of the right and left sides of the heart, selective angiography, and coronary arteriography (Chap. 179) provide precise diagnostic information under many circumstances. For example, they aid in establishing a specific anatomic diagnosis and in determining the physiologic consequences of the abnormalities in patients with congenital heart disease and in patients with chest pain of uncertain etiology in whom coronary artery disease is suspected, and in determining the functional significance of valvular abnormalities in patients with rheumatic heart disease being considered for surgical treatment. Although a great deal of attention has been lavished on the newer specialized laboratory examinations, it should be recognized that they serve to *supplement,* not *supplant,* a careful examination carried out by clinical and noninvasive examination. There is an unfortunate tendency to carry out procedures such as coronary arteriography in patients with chest pain suspected of having coronary artery disease instead of taking a detailed and thoughtful history; although it may be established whether the coronary arteries are obstructed, the results often do not provide a definite answer to the question of whether a patient's complaint of chest pain is clearly attributable to coronary arteriosclerosis. Coronary arteriography is often carried out unnecessarily in patients with mild symptoms and signs of myocardial ischemia during exertion with normal left ventricular function who are not likely to be candidates for coronary bypass surgery. Similarly, catheterization of the left side of the heart is all too frequently employed to determine whether operative treatment of valvular disease is indicated, even before the patient has had a trial of medical therapy. Despite their enormous value, it must not be overlooked that these specialized examinations entail some small risk to the patient, involve discomfort and substantial cost, and place a strain on existing medical facilities. Therefore, *they should be carried out not as part of a "fishing expedition" or as evidence to the patient and the family that "everything is being done," but only if, after detailed clinical examination and assessment by noninvasive tests, the results of the invasive examination can be expected to modify or aid in the patient's management.*

TREATMENT After a complete diagnosis has been established, a number of therapeutic options are usually available. Several examples may be used to demonstrate some of the principles of modern cardiovascular therapeutics:

1 In the absence of evidence for the existence of heart disease a clear, definitive statement to that effect should be made and the patient should *not* be asked to return at intervals for repeated examinations. If there is no evidence for disease, such attention may lead to the patient developing an inappropriate and abnormal fixation on the heart.

2 If there is no evidence of cardiovascular disease but the patient has one or more risk factors for the development of ischemic heart disease (Chap. 195), a plan for their reduction should be developed and the patient should be retested at intervals to assess that he or she is complying and that these risk factors are in fact being reduced.

3 Asymptomatic or mildly symptomatic patients with established organic heart disease, e.g., valvular heart disease, should be evaluated periodically, e.g., every 6 to 12 months, by clinical and noninvasive examinations (Chap. 177). Early warning signs of deterioration of ventricular function can be detected in this manner and in appropriate patients may signify the need for cardiac catheterization and surgical treatment before the development of disabling symptoms, irreversible myocardial damage, and an excessive risk of surgical treatment (Chap. 188).

4 It is critical for the physician to establish clear criteria for deciding on the form of treatment (medical, angioplasty, or surgical revascularization) in patients with ischemic heart disease (Chap. 190). Surgical treatment represents a major therapeutic advance in the treatment of this most common form of heart disease, but operation has probably been employed too widely in the United States; the mere presence of angina pectoris and/or the demonstration of coronary arterial narrowing at angiography should not reflexly evoke a decision to treat the patient surgically. Instead, this form of treatment should be limited to those patients with ischemic heart disease in whom it has been demonstrated that surgical treatment is superior to medical treatment.

REFERENCES

BRAUNWALD E (ed): *Heart Disease,* 3d ed. Philadelphia, Saunders, 1988

FOWLER NO: *Cardiac Diagnosis and Treatment,* 3d ed. Hagerstown, Harper & Row, 1980

HORWITZ LD, GROVES BM (eds): *Signs and Symptoms in Cardiology.* Philadelphia, Lippincott, 1985

HURST JW et al (ed): *The Heart,* 7th ed. New York, McGraw-Hill, 1990

KANNEL WB: Contribution of the Framingham Study to preventive cardiology. *J Am Coll Cardiol* 15;1:206, 1990

NEW YORK HEART ASSOCIATION, INC, CRITERIA COMMITTEE: *Nomenclature and Criteria for Diagnosis of Diseases of the Heart and Great Vessels,* 8th ed. Boston, Little, Brown, 1981

PERLOFF JK (ed): *Physical Examination of the Heart and Circulation,* 2d ed. Philadelphia, Saunders, 1990

175 PHYSICAL EXAMINATION OF THE CARDIOVASCULAR SYSTEM

ROBERT A. O'ROURKE / EUGENE BRAUNWALD

An attentive physical examination remains a cost-effective method for assessing the status of the cardiovascular system and often provides important information relative to the appropriate selection of additional tests. The general physical appearance should first be assessed. The patient may appear tired because of a chronic low cardiac output; the respiratory rate may be rapid, indicating pulmonary venous congestion. Central cyanosis, often associated with clubbing of the fingers and toes, indicates right-to-left cardiac or extracardiac shunting or inadequate oxygenation of blood by the lungs. Cyanosis in the distal extremities, cool skin, and increased sweating result from vasoconstriction in patients with severe heart failure (Chap. 37). Noncardiovascular details can be equally important. For example, the diagnosis of infective endocarditis is highly likely in patients with petechiae, Osler's nodes, and Janeway lesions (Chap. 90).

The blood pressure should be taken in both arms and with the patient supine and upright; the heart rate should be timed for 1 min. Orthostatic hypotension and tachycardia may indicate a reduced blood volume, while resting tachycardia may be a clue to the presence of severe heart failure.

Careful examination of the optic fundi is essential (Chap. 196), and the retinal vessels may show evidence of systemic hypertension, arteriosclerosis, or embolism. The latter may result from atherosclerosis in larger arteries (e.g., carotid) or may represent a complication of valvular heart disease (e.g., endocarditis).

Palpation of the peripheral arterial pulses in the upper and lower extremities is necessary to define the adequacy of systemic blood flow and to detect the presence of occlusive arterial lesions. It is also important to examine both legs for evidence of edema, varicose veins, or thrombophlebitis (Chap. 198). The cardiovascular examination includes careful evaluation of both the carotid arterial and the jugular venous pulses, as well as deliberate precordial palpation and attentive cardiac auscultation. An understanding of the events of the cardiac cycle is vital to performing an accurate cardiovascular examination.

ARTERIAL PRESSURE PULSE The normal central aortic pulse wave is characterized by a fairly rapid rise to a somewhat rounded peak (Fig. 175-1). The anacrotic shoulder, present on the ascending limb, occurs at the time of peak rate of aortic flow just before maximum pressure is reached. The less steep descending limb is interrupted by a sharp downward deflection, synchronous with aortic valve closure, called the *incisura.* As the pulse wave is transmitted peripherally, the initial upstroke becomes steeper, the anacrotic

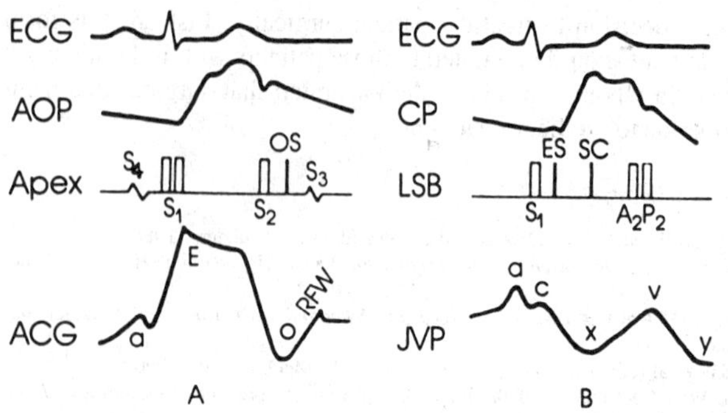

FIGURE 175-1 *A*. Schematic representation of electrocardiogram, aortic pressure pulse (AOP), phonocardiogram recorded at the apex, and apexcardiogram (ACG). On the phonocardiogram, S_1, S_2, S_3, and S_4 represent the first through fourth heart sounds; OS represents the opening snap of the mitral valve, which occurs coincident with the O point of the apexcardiogram. S_3 occurs coincident with the termination of the rapid-filling wave (RFW) of the ACG, while S_4 occurs coincident with the a wave of the ACG. *B*. Simultaneous recording of electrocardiogram, indirect carotid pulse (CP), phonocardiogram along the left sternal border (LSB), and indirect jugular venous pulse (JVP). ES, ejection sound; SC, systolic click.

shoulder becomes less apparent, and the incisura is replaced by the smoother dicrotic notch. Accordingly, palpation of a peripheral arterial pulse (e.g., radial) frequently gives less information than examination of a more central pulse (e.g., carotid) regarding alterations in left ventricular ejection or aortic valve function. However, certain findings such as the hyperkinetic pulse of aortic regurgitation or pulsus alternans are more readily evident in peripheral than in central arteries (Fig. 175-2). The carotid pulse usually is best examined with the sternocleidomastoid muscle relaxed and with the head rotated slightly toward the examiner. In examining the brachial arterial pulse, the examiner can support the subject's relaxed elbow with his or her right arm while compressing the brachial pulse with the thumb. The usual technique for palpating the pulse is to compress the artery with the thumb or forefinger until the maximum pulse is sensed. The examiner should apply varying degrees of pressure while concentrating on the separate phases of the pulse wave. This method, known as *trisection*, is useful for assessing the sharpness of the upstroke, systolic peak, and diastolic slope of the arterial pulse. In most normal persons a dicrotic wave is not palpable.

A small weak pulse, *pulsus parvus*, is frequently present in conditions with a diminished left ventricular stroke volume, a narrow pulse pressure, and increased peripheral vascular resistance (Fig. 175-2). A *hypokinetic* pulse may be due to hypovolemia, to left ventricular failure secondary to myocardial disease or myocardial infarction, to restrictive pericardial disease, or to mitral valve stenosis. In aortic valve stenosis the delayed systolic peak, *pulsus tardus*, is the result of mechanical obstruction to left ventricular ejection and is often accompanied by the transmission of a coarse systolic thrill. In contrast, a large bounding or *hyperkinetic* pulse is usually associated with an increased left ventricular stroke volume, a wide pulse pressure, and a decrease in peripheral vascular resistance. This occurs characteristically in patients with abnormally elevated stroke volumes as in complete heart block, hyperkinetic circulation due to anxiety, anemia, exercise, or fever, or in patients with an abnormally rapid runoff of blood from the arterial system (patent ductus arteriosus, peripheral arteriovenous fistula). Patients with mitral regurgitation or a ventricular septal defect may also have a bounding pulse, since vigorous left ventricular ejection produces a rapid upstroke in the arterial pulse even though the duration of systole and the forward stroke volume may be diminished. In aortic regurgitation the rapidly rising, bounding arterial pulse results from increased left ventricular stroke volume and the associated increased rate of ventricular ejection.

FIGURE 175-2 Schematic representation of arterial pulse waveforms that occur with alterations in cardiac hemodynamics which may result from normal physiologic responses or may be due to cardiac disease. S, systole; D, diastole. (*Modified from RA O'Rourke, in JW Hurst et al, eds. The Heart, 7th ed, New York, McGraw-Hill, 1990, with permission.*)

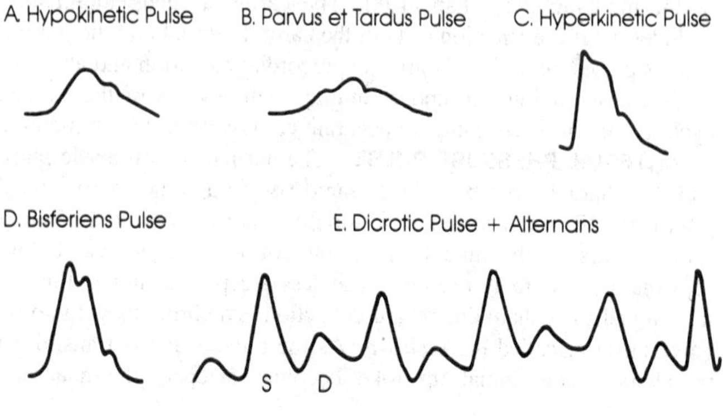

The *bisferiens pulse*, which consists of two systolic peaks, is characteristic of aortic regurgitation (with or without accompanying stenosis) and of hypertrophic cardiomyopathy (Chap. 192). In the latter the pulse wave upstroke rises rapidly and forcefully, producing the first systolic peak ("percussion wave"). A brief decline in pressure follows because of the sudden decrease in the rate of left ventricular ejection during midsystole, when severe obstruction often develops. This pressure trough is followed by a smaller and more slowly rising positive pulse wave ("tidal wave") produced by continued ventricular ejection and by reflected waves from the periphery. The *dicrotic pulse* has two palpable waves, one in systole and one in diastole. It occurs most frequently in patients with a very low stroke volume, particularly in those with dilated (congestive) cardiomyopathy.

Pulsus alternans refers to a pattern in which there is regular alteration of the pressure pulse amplitude, despite a regular rhythm (Fig. 175-2). It is due to alternating left ventricular contractile force, usually denotes severe left ventricular decompensation, and commonly occurs in patients who also have a loud third heart sound. Pulsus alternans may also occur during or following paroxysmal tachycardia or for several beats following a premature beat in patients without heart disease. In *pulsus bigeminus* there is also regular alteration of pressure pulse amplitude, but it is caused by a premature ventricular contraction that follows each regular beat. *Pulsus paradoxus* is an accentuation of the decrease in systolic arterial pressure accompanying the reduced amplitude of the arterial pulse which normally occurs during inspiration. In patients with pericardial tamponade (Chap. 193), airway obstruction, or superior vena cava obstruction, the decrease in systolic arterial pressure frequently exceeds the normal of 10 mmHg (1.33 kPa) and the peripheral pulse may disappear completely during inspiration.

Simultaneous palpation of the radial and femoral arterial pulses, which normally are virtually coincident, is important to rule out aortic coarctation, in which the latter is weaker and delayed (Chap. 186).

JUGULAR VENOUS PULSE (JVP) The two main objectives of the bedside examination of the neck veins are inspection of their waveform and estimation of the central venous pressure (CVP). In most patients, the right internal jugular vein is superior for both purposes, but occasionally examination of the other jugular vein or the venous pulsations in the supraclavicular fossae may yield more information. Usually, the maximum pulsation of the internal jugular vein is observed when the trunk is inclined by less than 30°. In patients with elevated venous pressure it may be necessary to elevate the trunk further, sometimes to as much as 90°. When the neck muscles are relaxed, shining a beam of light tangentially across the skin overlying the vein exposes the pulsations of the internal jugular vein. Simultaneous palpation of the left carotid artery aids the examiner in deciding which pulsations are venous and in relating the venous pulsations to their timing in the cardiac cycle.

The normal JVP reflects phasic pressure changes in the right

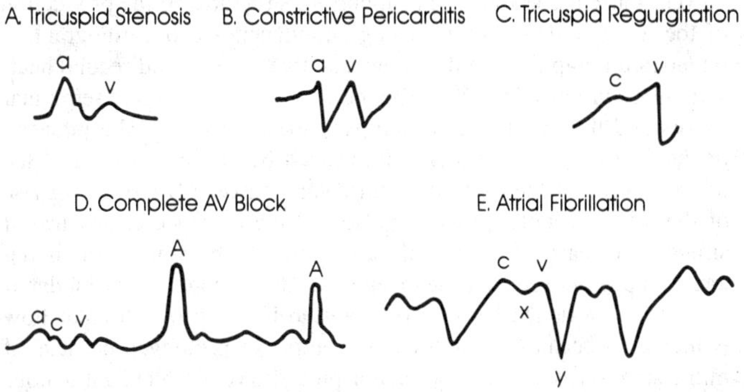

FIGURE 175-3 Abnormal jugular venous pulse waveforms commonly present in patients with cardiac disease and/or arrhythmias. See text. (*Modified from RA O'Rourke, in JW Hurst et al, eds. The Heart, 7th ed, New York, McGraw-Hill, 1990, with permission.*)

atrium and consists of two or sometimes three positive waves and two negative troughs (Fig. 175-1). The positive presystolic *a* wave is produced by venous distention due to right atrial contraction and is the dominant wave in the JVP, particularly during inspiration. Large *a* waves indicate that the right atrium is contracting against an increased resistance (Fig. 175-3), such as occurs with obstruction at the tricuspid valve (tricuspid stenosis) or more commonly with increased resistance to right ventricular filling (pulmonary hypertension or pulmonic stenosis). Large *a* waves also occur during arrhythmias whenever the right atrium contracts while the tricuspid valve is closed by right ventricular systole. Such "cannon" *a* waves may occur regularly (as during junctional rhythm) or irregularly (as in atrioventricular dissociation with ventricular tachycardia or complete heart block). The *a* wave is absent in patients with atrial fibrillation, and there is an increased temporal delay between the *a* wave and the carotid arterial pulse in patients with first-degree atrioventricular block.

The *c* wave, often but not invariably observed in the JVP, is a positive wave produced by the bulging of the tricuspid valve into the right atrium during right ventricular isovolumetric systole and by the impact of the carotid artery adjacent to the jugular vein. The *x* descent is due to a combination of atrial relaxation and the downward displacement of the tricuspid valve during ventricular systole. In patients with constrictive pericarditis (Fig. 175-3), there is often increased prominence of the *x* descent wave during systole, but this wave is reduced with right ventricular dilatation and often is reversed in tricuspid regurgitation. The positive, late systolic *v* wave results from the increasing volume of blood in the venae cavae and right atrium during ventricular systole when the tricuspid valve is closed. With mild tricuspid regurgitation the *v* wave becomes more prominent, and when tricuspid regurgitation becomes severe, the prominent *v* wave and the obliteration of the *x* descent result in a single large positive systolic wave ("ventricularization"). After the peak of the *v* wave is reached, the right atrial pressure diminishes because of the decreased bulging of the tricuspid valve into the right atrium as right ventricular pressure declines and the tricuspid valve opens (Fig. 175-3).

Following the summit of the *v* wave there is a negative descending limb, referred to as the *y* descent or "diastolic collapse," which is produced mainly by the tricuspid valve opening and the rapid inflow of blood into the right ventricle. A rapid, deep *y* descent in early diastole occurs with severe tricuspid regurgitation. A venous pulse characterized by a sharp *y* descent, a deep *y* trough, and a rapid ascent to the baseline is seen in patients with constrictive pericarditis or with severe failure of the right side of the heart and a high venous pressure. A slow *y* descent in the JVP suggests an obstruction to right ventricular filling, as occurs with tricuspid stenosis or right atrial myxoma.

For accurate estimation of the CVP, the right internal jugular vein is best utilized, with the sternal angle as the reference point, since in the average patient the center of the right atrium lies approximately 5 cm below the sternal angle, regardless of body position. The patient is examined at the optimum degree of trunk elevation for visualization of venous pulsations. The vertical distance between the top of the oscillating venous column and the level of the sternal angle is determined and generally found to be less than 3 cm (3 cm + 5 cm = 8 cm blood). The most common cause of an elevated venous pressure is an elevated right ventricular diastolic pressure. In patients suspected of having right ventricular failure who have a normal CVP at rest, the abdominojugular reflux test may be helpful. The palm of the hand is placed over the abdomen and firm pressure is applied for 10 s or more. Normally, the jugular venous pressure is not significantly altered, but with impaired function of the right side of the heart the upper level of venous pulsation usually increases. A positive abdominojugular test is best defined as an increase in JVP during 10 s of firm midabdominal compression followed by an abrupt drop in pressure of 4 cm blood upon release of the compression. The most common cause of a positive test is right heart failure secondary to elevated left heart filling pressures. Also, abdominal compression may elicit the typical JVP of tricuspid regurgitation when the resting pulse wave is normal. Kussmaul's sign, an increase rather than the normal decrease in the CVP during inspiration, is most commonly caused by severe right-sided heart failure; it is a frequent finding in patients with constrictive pericarditis or right ventricular infarction.

PRECORDIAL PALPATION The location, amplitude, duration, and direction of the cardiac impulse can usually be best appreciated by using the fingertips. The normal left ventricular apex impulse is located at or medial to the left midclavicular line in the fourth or fifth intercostal space and is a tapping, early systolic outward thrust localized to a point not more than 3 cm in diameter. It is due primarily to recoil of the heart as blood is ejected and should be evaluated with the patient supine and in the left lateral decubitus position. Left ventricular hypertrophy results in an exaggerated amplitude, duration, and often size of the normal left ventricular thrust. The impulse may be displaced laterally and downward into the sixth or seventh interspace, particularly in patients with a left ventricular volume load such as occurs in aortic regurgitation and in those with a dilated cardiomyopathy.

Additional abnormal features of the left ventricular apex include marked presystolic distention of the left ventricle, often accompanying a fourth heart sound in patients with an excessive left ventricular pressure load or myocardial ischemia/infarction, and a prominent early diastolic rapid-filling wave, often accompanying a third heart sound in patients with left ventricular failure or mitral valve regurgitation (Fig. 175-1). A double systolic impulse is frequently palpable in patients with hypertrophic cardiomyopathy.

Right ventricular hypertrophy results in a sustained systolic lift at the lower left parasternal area which starts in early systole and is synchronous with the left ventricular apical impulse. In patients with chronic obstructive pulmonary disease a right ventricular impulse may often be detected by sliding the fingers up under the rib cage just beneath the sternum. The enlarged right ventricle strikes the ends of the fingertips as an inferiorly directed movement.

Abnormal precordial pulsations occur during systole in patients with left ventricular dyssynergy due to ischemic heart disease or to diffuse myocardial disease from some other cause. These pulsations often occur in patients with a recent transmural myocardial infarction and may be present in some patients only during episodes of anginal pain. They are most commonly felt in the left midprecordium one or two interspaces above and/or 1 to 2 cm medial to the left ventricular apex. When a systolic bulge occurs in the region of the apex, it is difficult to distinguish it from the impulse of left ventricular hypertrophy.

A left parasternal lift is present frequently in patients with severe mitral regurgitation. This pulsation occurs distinctly later than the left ventricular apical impulse, is synchronous with the *v* wave in the left atrial pressure curve, and is due to anterior displacement of the right ventricle by an enlarged, expanding left atrium. A similar impulse occurs to the right of the sternum in some patients with severe tricuspid regurgitation and a giant right atrium. Pulsation of the right sternoclavicular joint may indicate a right-sided aortic arch or aneurysmal dilatation of the ascending aorta. Pulmonary artery pulsation is often visible and palpable in the second left intercostal space and may be normal in children or thin young adults. However, this pulsation usually denotes pulmonary hypertension, increased pulmonary blood flow, or poststenotic pulmonary artery dilatation.

Thrills are palpable, low-frequency vibrations associated with heart murmurs. The diastolic rumble of mitral stenosis and the systolic murmur of mitral regurgitation may be palpated at the cardiac apex. When the palm of the hand is placed over the precordium, the thrill of aortic stenosis crosses the palm of the hand toward the right side of the neck, while the thrill of pulmonic stenosis radiates more often to the left side of the neck. The thrill due to a ventricular septal defect is usually located in the third and fourth intercostal spaces near the left sternal border.

Percussion should be performed in each patient to identify normal or abnormal position of the heart, stomach, and liver. However, in patients with a normal cardiac situs, percussion adds little to careful inspection and palpation in the recognition of cardiac enlargement.

CARDIAC AUSCULTATION

To obtain maximal information from cardiac auscultation, the observer should keep in mind several principles: (1) It should be carried out in a quiet room to avoid the distractions caused by the noises of normal activity. (2) In order to hear a faint heart sound or murmur, attention must be focused on that phase of the cardiac cycle during which the auscultatory event may be expected to occur. (3) The accurate timing of a heart sound or murmur necessarily involves determining its relation to other observable events in the cardiac cycle—the carotid arterial pulse, the JVP, or the apical impulse. (4) To define the significance of a cardiac sound or murmur, it is often necessary to observe alterations in its timing or intensity during various physiologic and/or pharmacologic interventions (Table 175-1).

HEART SOUNDS The major components of heart sounds are vibrations associated with the abrupt acceleration or deceleration of blood within the cardiovascular system, but there is continuing controversy regarding the relative significance of the vibrations of valves, muscles, vessels, and supporting structures in the production of the heart sounds. Studies using simultaneous echocardiographic-phonocardiographic recordings indicate that the first and second heart sounds are produced primarily by the closure of the AV and semilunar valves and the events that accompany these closures. The intensity of the *first heart sound* (S_1) is influenced by (1) the position of the mitral leaflets at the onset of ventricular systole, (2) the rate of rise of the left ventricular pressure pulse, (3) the presence or absence of structural disease of the mitral valve, and (4) the amount of tissue, air, or fluid between the heart and the stethoscope. S_1 is louder if diastole is shortened because of tachycardia, if atrioventricular flow is increased because of high cardiac output or prolonged because of mitral stenosis, or if atrial contraction precedes ventricular contractions by a short PR interval. The loud S_1 in mitral stenosis usually signifies that the valve is pliable and that it remains open at the onset of isovolumetric contraction because of the elevated left atrial pressure. A reduction in the intensity of S_1 may be due to poor conduction of sound through the chest wall, a slow rise of the left ventricular pressure pulse, a long PR interval, or imperfect closure due to reduced valve substance, as in mitral regurgitation. S_1 is also soft when the anterior mitral leaflet is immobile because of rigidity and calcification even in the presence of predominant mitral stenosis.

Splitting of the two high-pitched components of S_1 by 10 to 30 ms is a normal phenomenon (Fig. 175-1). The first component of S_1 normally is attributed to mitral valve closure and the second to tricuspid valve closure. A widened split of S_1 is most often due to complete right bundle branch block and the resulting delay in onset of the right ventricular pressure pulse. Reversed splitting of the S_1 with the mitral component following the tricuspid component has occasionally been noted in complete left bundle branch block and frequently is present in patients with severe mitral stenosis or a left atrial myxoma.

Splitting of S_2 into audibly distinct aortic (A_2) and pulmonic (P_2) components occurs normally during inspiration when augmented inflow into the right ventricle increases its stroke volume and ejection period and delays closure of the pulmonic valve. P_2 is coincident with the incisura of the pulmonary artery pressure curve, which is separated from the right ventricular pressure tracing by an interval termed the "hangout time." The absolute value of this interval reflects the resistance to pulmonary blood flow and the impedance characteristics of the pulmonary vascular bed. This interval is prolonged, and physiologic splitting of S_2 is accentuated in conditions associated with right ventricular volume overload and a distensible

TABLE 175-1 Effects of physiologic and pharmacologic interventions on the intensity of heart murmurs and sounds*

Intervention	Changes in heart murmurs and sounds
Respiration	Systolic murmurs due to TR or pulmonic blood flow through a normal or stenotic valve and diastolic murmurs of TS or PR generally increase with inspiration as do right-sided S_3 and S_4. Left-sided murmurs and sounds usually are louder during expiration.
Valsalva maneuver	Most murmurs decrease in length and intensity. Two exceptions are the systolic murmur of HCM, which usually becomes much louder, and that of MVP, which becomes longer and often louder. Following release of the Valsalva, right-sided murmurs tend to return to control intensity earlier than left-sided murmurs.
Post VPB or AF	Murmurs originating at normal or stenotic semilunar valves increase in the cardiac cycle following a VPB or in the cycle after a long cycle length in AF. By contrast, systolic murmurs due to AV valve regurgitation do not change, diminish (papillary muscle dysfunction), or become shorter (MVP).
Positional changes	With *standing* most murmurs diminish, two exceptions being the murmur of HCM, which becomes louder, and that of MVP, which lengthens and often is intensified. With *squatting* most murmurs become louder but those of HCM and MVP usually soften and may disappear.
Exercise	Murmurs due to blood flow across normal or obstructed valves (e.g., PS, MS) become louder with both isotonic and submaximal isometric (handgrip) exercise. Murmurs of MR, VSD, and AR also increase with handgrip exercise. However, the murmur of HCM often decreases with near maximum handgrip exercise. Left-sided S_4 and S_3 are often accentuated by exercise, particularly when due to ischemic heart disease.
Pharmacologic interventions	During the initial relative hypotension following amyl nitrite inhalation, murmurs of MR, VSD, and AR decrease while murmurs of aortic stenosis or sclerosis increase. During the later tachycardia phase, murmurs of MS and right-sided lesions also increase. The response in MVP often is biphasic (softer then louder than control). The arterial constrictor phenylephrine tends to produce the opposite effects.
Transient arterial occlusion	Transient external compression of both arms by bilateral cuff inflation to 20 mmHg $>$ peak systolic pressure augments the murmurs of MR, VSD, and AR but not murmurs due to other causes.

* TR, tricuspid regurgitation; TS, tricuspid stenosis; PR, pulmonic regurgitation; HCM, hypertrophic cardiomyopathy; MVP, mitral valve prolapse; PS, pulmonic stenosis; MS, mitral stenosis; MR, mitral regurgitation; VSD, ventricular septal defect; AR, aortic regurgitation; VPB, ventricular premature beat; and AF, atrial fibrillation.

pulmonary vascular bed. However, in patients with an increase in pulmonary vascular resistance, the hangout time is markedly reduced and narrow splitting of S_2 is present. Splitting that persists with expiration, heard best at the pulmonic area or left sternal border, is usually abnormal when the patient is in the upright position. Such splitting may be due to delayed activation of the right ventricle (right bundle branch block), to prolongation of right ventricular contraction with an increased right ventricular pressure load (pulmonary embolism or pulmonic stenosis), or to delayed pulmonic valve closure because of right ventricular volume overload associated with diminished impedance of the pulmonary vascular bed and a prolonged hangout time (atrial septal defect). In pulmonary hypertension, P_2 is increased in intensity and splitting of the second heart sound may be diminished, normal, or accentuated, depending on the cause of the pulmonary hypertension, the pulmonary vascular resistance, and the presence or absence of right ventricular decompensation. Early aortic valve closure, occurring with mitral regurgitation or a ventricular septal defect, may also produce splitting that persists during expiration. It may also occur with constrictive pericarditis. In patients with large atrial septal defects the proportion of right atrial filling contributed by the left atrium and the venae cavae varies reciprocally during the respiratory cycle so that right atrial inflow remains relatively constant. Therefore, the volume and duration of right ventricular ejection are not significantly increased by inspiration, and there is little inspiratory exaggeration of the splitting of S_2. This phenomenon, termed "fixed splitting" of the second heart sound, is of considerable diagnostic value.

A delay in aortic valve closure causing P_2 to precede A_2 results in so-called reversed (paradoxic) splitting of S_2. Splitting is then maximal in expiration, and decreases during inspiration with the normal delay of pulmonic valve closure. The commonest causes of reversed splitting of S_2 are left bundle branch block and delayed excitation of the left ventricle from a right ventricular ectopic beat. Mechanical prolongation of left ventricular systole, resulting in reversed splitting of S_2, may be caused by severe aortic outflow obstruction, a large aorta-to-pulmonary artery shunt, systolic hypertension, and ischemic heart disease or cardiomyopathy with left ventricular failure. P_2 is normally softer than A_2 in the second left intercostal space; when P_2 is greater than A_2 in this area, it suggests pulmonary hypertension, except in patients with atrial septal defect.

The *third heart sound* is a low-pitched sound produced in the ventricle 0.14 to 0.16 s after A_2, at the termination of rapid filling. This sound is frequent in normal children and in patients with high cardiac output. However, in patients over 40 years of age, an S_3 usually indicates ventricular decompensation, AV valve regurgitation, or other conditions which increase the rate or volume of ventricular filling. The left-sided S_3 is best heard with the bell piece of the stethoscope at the left ventricular apex during expiration and with the patient in the left lateral position. The right-sided S_3 is best heard at the left sternal border or just beneath the xiphoid and is increased with inspiration. Often it is accompanied by the systolic murmur of functional tricuspid regurgitation. Third heart sounds often disappear with treatment of heart failure.

An earlier (0.10 to 0.12 s after A_2), higher-pitched third heart sound (pericardial knock) often occurs in patients with constrictive pericarditis; its presence is dependent upon the restrictive effect of the adherent pericardium, which halts diastolic filling abruptly.

The *opening snap* (OS) is a brief, high-pitched, early diastolic sound which is usually due to stenosis of an AV valve, more commonly the mitral valve. It is usually heard best at the lower left sternal border and radiates well to the base of the heart. The A_2-OS interval during exercise is inversely related to the height of the mean left atrial pressure, and ranges from 0.04 to 0.12 s. At the base an OS is often confused with P_2. However, careful auscultation at the upper left sternal border will reveal both components of the second heart sound, followed by the opening snap. The OS of tricuspid stenosis occurs later in diastole than the mitral OS. Since most patients with tricuspid stenosis also have severe mitral valve disease, the tricuspid OS is often overshadowed by the diastolic rumble and OS originating in the stenotic mitral valve. An OS also may occur when there is increased flow across an AV valve, such as exists with left-to-right intracardiac shunts and mitral or tricuspid regurgitation.

The *fourth heart sound* is a low-pitched, presystolic sound produced in the ventricle during the ventricular filling associated with an effective atrial contraction, and is heard best with the bell piece of the stethoscope. The sound is absent in patients with atrial fibrillation. The S_4 occurs when diminished ventricular compliance increases the resistance to ventricular filling, and it is present frequently in patients with systemic hypertension, aortic stenosis, hypertrophic cardiomyopathy, coronary artery disease, and acute mitral regurgitation. Most patients with an acute myocardial infarction and sinus rhythm have an audible S_4. The fourth heart sound is frequently accompanied by visible and palpable presystolic distention of the left ventricle. It is maximal in intensity at the left ventricular apex with the patient in the left lateral position, and is accentuated by mild isotonic or isometric exercise in the supine position. The right-sided S_4 is present in patients with right ventricular hypertrophy, secondary to either pulmonic stenosis or pulmonary hypertension, and frequently accompanies a prominent presystolic *a* wave in the JVP.

Audible fourth heart sounds also may be present during increased ventricular filling and normal ventricular compliance such as occurs in patients with severe anemia, thyrotoxicosis, or a peripheral arteriovenous fistula. An S_4 frequently accompanies delayed AV conduction even in the absence of clinically detectable heart disease. The incidence of an audible S_4 increases with increasing age. Whether an audible S_4 in adults without other evidence of cardiac disease is abnormal remains controversial.

The *ejection sound* is a sharp, high-pitched event occurring in early systole closely following the first heart sound. Ejection sounds occur in the presence of semilunar valve stenosis, i.e., opening snaps of the aortic or pulmonic valves, and in conditions associated with dilation of the aorta or pulmonary artery. The aortic ejection sound is usually heard best at the left ventricular apex and the second right interspace; the pulmonary ejection sound is of maximal intensity at the upper left sternal border. The latter, unlike most other right-sided acoustical events, is heard better during expiration.

Nonejection or midsystolic clicks, occurring with or without a late systolic murmur, often denote prolapse of one or both leaflets of the mitral valve. They may also be caused by tricuspid valve prolapse (Chap. 188). They probably result from functionally unequal length of the chordae tendineae of either or both AV valves and are heard best along the lower left sternal border and at the left ventricular apex. Systolic clicks may be single or multiple, and they may occur at any time in systole but usually later than the systolic ejection sound. Frequently the midsystolic click is misinterpreted as S_2, and the actual second heart sound is called an OS or S_3.

HEART MURMURS Cardiac murmurs result from vibrations set up in the bloodstream and the surrounding heart and great vessels as a result of turbulent blood flow, the formation of eddies, and cavitation (bubble formation as a result of sudden decrease in pressure).

The intensity or loudness of murmurs may be graded from I to VI. A grade I murmur is so faint that it can be heard only with special effort, and a grade VI murmur is audible with the stethoscope removed from contact with the chest. The configuration of a murmur may be crescendo, decrescendo, crescendo-decrescendo (diamond-shaped), or plateau. The precise time of onset and time of cessation of a murmur depend on the instant in the cardiac cycle at which an adequate pressure difference between two chambers appears and disappears (Fig. 175-4).

The location on the chest wall where the murmur is best heard and the areas to which it radiates can be helpful in identifying the cardiac structure from which the murmur originates. For example, the murmur of aortic valve stenosis is loudest usually in the second right intercostal space and radiates to the carotid arteries. By contrast, the murmur of mitral regurgitation is most often loudest at the cardiac apex and may radiate to the left sternal border and base of the heart

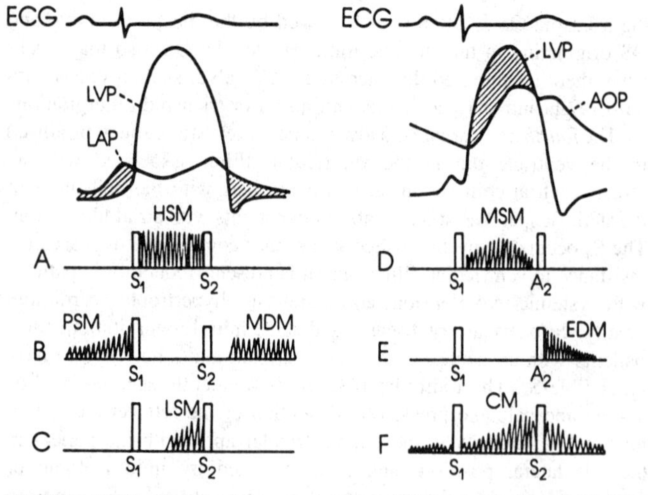

FIGURE 175-4 Schematic representation of ECG, aortic pressure (AOP), left ventricular pressure (LVP), and left atrial pressure (LAP). HSM is a holosystolic murmur; PSM, a presystolic murmur; MDM, a middiastolic murmur; MSM, a midsystolic murmur; EDM, an early diastolic murmur; LSM, a late systolic murmur; and CM, a continuous murmur.

when the posterior mitral leaflet is predominantly involved or to the axilla and back when the anterior leaflet is more severely affected. In the former case, the regurgitant blood is directed toward the posterior left atrial wall.

Often, it is difficult to classify with certainty a cardiac murmur based on its timing, configuration, location, radiation, pitch, or intensity. However, by noting changes in the characteristics of the murmur during maneuvers that alter cardiac hemodynamics, the auscultator often can identify its correct origin and significance (Table 175-1).

Accentuation of a murmur during inspiration which augments systemic venous return implies that it originates on the right side of the circulation; expiratory exaggeration has less significance. Prolonged expiratory pressure against a closed glottis, the Valsalva maneuver, reduces intensity of most murmurs by diminishing both right and left ventricular filling. The systolic murmur associated with *hypertrophic cardiomyopathy* and the late systolic murmur due to a *mitral valve prolapse* are exceptions and may be accentuated during the Valsalva maneuver. Murmurs due to flow across a normal or obstructed semilunar valve increase in intensity in the cycle following a premature ventricular beat or a long RR interval in atrial fibrillation. In contrast, murmurs due to AV valve regurgitation or a ventricular septal defect do not change appreciably during the beat following a prolonged diastole. Standing, which decreases heart size, accentuates the murmur of hypertrophic cardiomyopathy and occasionally the murmur due to mitral valve prolapse. Squatting, which increases both venous return and systemic arterial resistance, increases most murmurs, except those due to hypertrophic cardiomyopathy and mitral regurgitation due to a prolapsed mitral valve, which often decrease. Sustained handgrip exercise, which increases systemic arterial pressure and heart rate, often accentuates the murmurs of mitral regurgitation, aortic regurgitation, and mitral stenosis but usually diminishes those due to aortic stenosis or hypertrophic cardiomyopathy. Pharmacologic interventions include inhalation of amyl nitrite, which reduces systemic arterial pressure and increases blood flow, thereby increasing the intensity of murmurs due to valvular stenosis while diminishing those due to aortic or mitral regurgitation (Table 175-1). Transient external arterial occlusion by the inflation of bilateral arm cuffs to 20 mmHg (2.66 kPa) above systolic blood pressure for 5 s has been shown to intensify murmurs due to left-sided regurgitant lesions; this method is applicable to almost all patients and does not require administration of any drug.

Systolic murmurs *Holosystolic (pansystolic) murmurs* are generated when there is a flow between two chambers which have widely different pressures throughout systole, such as the left ventricle and either the left atrium or the right ventricle. The pressure gradient is established early in contraction and lasts until relaxation is almost complete. Therefore, holosystolic murmurs begin before aortic ejection, and at the area of maximal intensity they begin with S_1 and end after S_2. Holosystolic murmurs accompany mitral or tricuspid regurgitation, ventricular septal defect, and under certain circumstances, aortopulmonary shunts. Although the typical high-pitched murmur of mitral regurgitation usually continues throughout systole, the shape of the murmur may vary considerably. The holosystolic murmurs of mitral regurgitation and ventricular septal defect are augmented by transient exercise and are diminished by lowering the left ventricular systolic pressure by inhalation of amyl nitrite. The murmur of tricuspid regurgitation associated with pulmonary hypertension is holosystolic and frequently increases during inspiration, a feature of diagnostic importance. Not all patients with mitral or tricuspid regurgitation or ventricular septal defect have holosystolic murmurs (Chap. 188).

Midsystolic murmurs, often crescendo-decrescendo in shape, occur when blood is ejected across the aortic or pulmonic outflow tracts. The murmur starts shortly after S_1 when the ventricular pressure rises sufficiently to open the semilunar valve. Ejection then begins and with it the onset of the murmur; as ejection increases, the murmur is augmented, and as ejection declines, it diminishes. The murmur ends before the ventricular pressure falls enough to permit closure of the aortic or pulmonic leaflets. In the presence of normal semilunar valves an increased flow rate, as occurs in states of elevated cardiac output, ejection into a dilated vessel beyond the valve, or increased transmission of sound through a thin chest wall, may be responsible for the production of this murmur. Most benign, functional murmurs are midsystolic and originate from the pulmonary outflow tract. Valvular or subvalvular obstruction to either ventricle may also cause such a midsystolic murmur, the intensity being related to the flow.

The murmur of aortic stenosis is the prototype of the left-sided midsystolic murmur. The location and radiation of this murmur are influenced by the direction of the high-velocity jet within the aortic root. In *valvular aortic stenosis* the murmur is usually maximal in the second right intercostal space, with radiation into the neck. In *supravalvular aortic stenosis* the murmur is occasionally loudest even higher, with disproportionate radiation into the right carotid artery. In hypertrophic cardiomyopathy, the murmur originates within the left ventricular cavity, and is usually maximal at the lower left sternal edge and apex, with relatively little radiation to the carotids. When the aortic valve is immobile (calcified), the aortic closure sound (A_2) may be soft and inaudible so that the length and configuration of the murmur are difficult to determine. Midsystolic murmurs also occur in patients with mitral regurgitation or, less frequently, tricuspid regurgitation resulting from papillary muscle dysfunction. Murmurs due to mitral regurgitation are often confused with those originating in the aorta, particularly in elderly patients.

The patient's age and the area of maximal intensity aid in determining the significance of midsystolic murmurs. Thus, in a young adult with a thin chest and high velocity of blood flow, a faint or moderate midsystolic murmur heard only in the pulmonic area is usually without clinical significance, while a somewhat louder murmur in the aortic area may indicate congenital aortic stenosis. In elderly patients pulmonic flow murmurs are rare, while aortic systolic murmurs are frequent and may be due to aortic dilatation, to a significant degree of valvular aortic stenosis, or to nonstenotic deformity of the aortic valve. Midsystolic aortic and pulmonic murmurs are intensified by amyl nitrite inhalation and during the cardiac cycle following a premature ventricular beat, while those due to mitral regurgitation are unchanged or softer. Aortic systolic murmurs are diminished by interventions which increase aortic impedence, such as intravenous phenylephrine. Echocardiography or cardiac catheterization may be necessary to separate a prominent and exaggerated functional murmur from one due to congenital semilunar valve stenosis.

Early systolic murmurs begin with the first heart sound and end in midsystole. They may be due to a very small *ventricular septal defect, a large defect with pulmonary hypertension,* or *severe acute mitral* or *tricuspid regurgitation.* In large ventricular septal defects with pulmonary hypertension, the shunting at the end of systole may be small or absent, resulting in an early systolic murmur. A similar murmur may occur with very small muscular ventricular septal defects, the shunt being interrupted in late systole. An early systolic murmur is a feature of tricuspid regurgitation occurring in the absence of pulmonary hypertension. This lesion is common in drug addicts with infective endocarditis, in whom a tall regurgitant right atrial *v* wave reaches the level of the normal right ventricular pressure in late systole, confining the murmur to early systole. In patients with acute mitral regurgitation and a large *v* wave in a noncompliant left atrium, a loud early systolic murmur is frequently heard which diminishes as the pressure gradient between left ventricle and left atrium decreases in late systole (Chap. 188).

Late systolic murmurs are faint or moderately loud high-pitched apical murmurs, which start well after ejection and do not mask either heart sound. They are probably related to papillary muscle dysfunction caused by infarction or ischemia of these muscles or to their distortion by left ventricular dilatation. They may appear only during angina but are common in patients with myocardial infarction or diffuse myocardial disease. Late systolic murmurs following midsystolic clicks are associated with late systolic mitral regurgitation caused by prolapse of the mitral valve into the left atrium (Chap. 188).

Diastolic murmurs *Early diastolic murmurs* begin with or shortly after the second heart sound as soon as the corresponding ventricular pressure falls sufficiently below that in the aorta or pulmonary artery. The high-pitched murmurs of aortic regurgitation or pulmonic regurgitation due to pulmonary hypertension are generally decrescendo, since there is a progressive decline in the volume or rate of regurgitation during diastole. Faint, high-pitched murmurs of aortic regurgitation are difficult to hear unless they are specifically sought by applying firm pressure with the diaphragm over the left midsternal border while the patient sits, leans forward, and holds a breath in full expiration. The diastolic murmur of aortic regurgitation is enhanced by an acute elevation of the arterial pressure such as occurs with handgrip exercise; it diminishes with a decrease in arterial pressure as with amyl nitrite inhalation. The diastolic murmur of congenital pulmonic regurgitation without pulmonary hypertension is low- to medium-pitched. The onset of this murmur is delayed because at the onset of pulmonic valve closure the regurgitant flow is minimal, since the reverse pressure gradient responsible for the regurgitation is negligible at this time.

Middiastolic murmurs usually arise from the AV valves, occur during early ventricular filling, and are due to disproportion between valve orifice size and flow rate. Such murmurs may be loud despite only slight AV valve stenosis when there is normal or increased blood flow. Conversely, the murmur may be soft or even absent despite severe obstruction if the cardiac output is markedly reduced. When stenosis is marked, the diastolic murmur is prolonged and the duration of the murmur is more reliable than its intensity as an index of the severity of valve obstruction.

The low-pitched, middiastolic murmur of mitral stenosis characteristically follows the opening snap. It should be specifically sought by placing the bell of the stethoscope at the site of the left ventricular impulse, which is best localized with the patient on the left side. Frequently the murmur of mitral stenosis is present only at the left ventricular apex, and it may be increased in intensity by mild supine exercise or by inhalation of amyl nitrite. In tricuspid stenosis the middiastolic murmur is localized to a relatively limited area along the left sternal edge and may increase in intensity during inspiration.

Middiastolic murmurs may be generated across the mitral valve in ventricular septal defect, patent ductus arteriosus, or mitral regurgitation, and across the tricuspid valve in atrial septal defect or tricuspid regurgitation. These murmurs are related to the torrential flow across an AV valve, usually follow a third heart sound, and tend to occur with large left-to-right shunts or severe AV valve regurgitation. A soft middiastolic murmur may sometimes be heard in patients with acute rheumatic fever (Carey-Coombs murmur). It has been attributed to inflammation of the mitral valve cusps or excessive left atrial blood flow as a consequence of mitral regurgitation.

In acute aortic regurgitation, the left ventricular diastolic pressure may exceed the left atrial pressure, resulting in a middiastolic murmur due to "diastolic mitral regurgitation." In severe chronic aortic regurgitation a murmur is frequently present which may be either middiastolic or presystolic (Austin Flint murmur). This murmur appears to originate at the anterior mitral valve leaflet when blood simultaneously enters the left ventricle from both the aortic root and the left atrium.

Presystolic murmurs begin during the period of ventricular filling that follows atrial contraction and therefore occur in sinus rhythm. They are usually due to AV valve stenosis and have the same quality as the middiastolic filling rumble but are usually crescendo, reaching peak intensity at the time of a loud S_1. The presystolic murmur corresponds to the AV valve gradient, which may be minimal until the moment of right or left atrial contraction. It is the presystolic rather than the middiastolic murmur which is most characteristic of tricuspid stenosis and sinus rhythm. A right or left *atrial myxoma* may occasionally cause either middiastolic or presystolic murmurs that resemble the murmurs of mitral or tricuspid stenosis.

Continuous murmurs begin in systole, peak near S_2, and continue into all or part of diastole. These murmurs signify continuous flow due to communication between high- and low-pressure areas which persists through the end of systole and the beginning of diastole. A *patent ductus arteriosus* causes a continuous murmur as long as the pressure in the pulmonary artery is much below that in the aorta. The murmur is intensified by elevation of the systemic arterial pressure and is reduced by amyl nitrite inhalation. When pulmonary hypertension is present, the diastolic portion may disappear, leaving the murmur confined to systole. A continuous murmur is uncommon in aortopulmonary septal defects, since this malformation is generally associated with severe pulmonary hypertension. Surgically produced aortopulmonary connections and the subclavian–pulmonary artery anastomosis result in murmurs similar to that of a patent ductus.

Continuous murmurs may result from congenital or acquired *systemic arteriovenous fistula, coronary arteriovenous fistula,* anomalous origin of the left coronary artery from the pulmonary artery, and communications between the *sinus of Valsalva and the right side of the heart.* Continuous murmurs may also occur when high left atrial pressure results in continuous flow across a small defect in the atrial septum. Murmurs associated with *pulmonary arteriovenous fistulas* may be continuous but are usually only systolic. Continuous murmurs may also be due to disturbances of flow pattern in constricted systemic (e.g., renal) or pulmonary arteries when marked pressure differences between the two sides of the narrow segment persist; a continuous murmur in the back may be present in *coarctation of the aorta; pulmonary embolism* may cause continuous murmurs in partially occluded vessels.

In nonconstricted arteries continuous murmurs may be due to rapid flow through a tortuous bed. Such murmurs typically occur within the bronchial arterial collateral circulation in cyanotic patients with severe pulmonary outflow obstruction. The "mammary souffle," an innocent murmur heard during late pregnancy and early postpartum, may be systolic or continuous. The innocent cervical venous hum is a continuous murmur usually heard over the medial aspect of the right supraclavicular fossa with the patient upright. The hum is usually louder during diastole and can be instantaneously abolished by digital compression of the ipsilateral internal jugular vein. Transmission of a loud venous hum to the area below the clavicles may result in a mistaken diagnosis of patent ductus arteriosus.

The *pericardial friction rub,* which may have presystolic, systolic, and early diastolic scratchy components, may be confused with a murmur or extracardiac sound when heard only in systole. It is best appreciated with the patient upright and leaning forward and may be accentuated during inspiration.

REFERENCES

BARAGAN J et al (eds): *Dynamic Auscultation and Phonocardiography*. Maryland, Charles Press Publishers, 1979

BRAUNWALD E: Physical examination, in *Heart Disease*, 3d ed, E Braunwald (ed). Philadelphia, Saunders, 1988, p. 13.

CRAIGE E: Echophonocardiography and other noninvasive techniques to elucidate heart murmurs, in *Heart Disease*, 3d ed, E Braunwald (ed). Philadelphia, Saunders, 1988, p 65

———: Heart Sounds: Phonocardiography, carotid, apex and jugular venous pulse tracings; and systolic time intervals, in *Heart Disease*, 3d ed, E Braunwald (ed). Philadelphia, Saunders, 1988, p 41

DELL ITALIA LJ et al: Physical examination for exclusion of hemodynamically important right ventricular infarction. Ann Intern Med 99:608, 1983

EILEN SD, CRAWFORD MH, O'ROURKE RA: Accuracy of precordial palpation for detecting increased left ventricular volume. Ann Intern Med 99:628, 1983

EWY GA: The abdominojugular test: Technique and hemodynamic correlates. Ann Intern Med 109:456, 1988

FOWLER NO: Cardiac auscultation, in *Cardiac Diagnosis and Treatment*, 3d ed, NO Fowler (ed). Hagerstown, Harper & Row, 1980, p 62

LEMBO NJ et al: Bedside diagnosis of systolic murmurs. N Engl J Med 318:1572, 1988

PERLOFF JK (ed): *Physical Examination of the Heart and Circulation, 2d ed.* Philadelphia, Saunders, 1990

REDDY PS et al: Normal and abnormal heart sounds in cardiac diagnosis, Part II: Diastolic sounds. Curr Probl Cardiol 10(4):1, 1985

ROTHMAN A, GOLDBERGER AL: Aids to cardiac auscultation. Ann Intern Med 99:346, 1983

SHAVER JA et al: Normal and abnormal heart sounds in cardiac diagnosis, Part I: Systolic sounds. Curr Probl Cardiol 10(3):1, 1985

TAVEL ME: *Clinical Phonocardiography and External Pulse Recordings*, 4th ed. Chicago, Year Book, 1985

176 ELECTROCARDIOGRAPHY

ROBERT J. MYERBURG

INTRODUCTION The electrocardiogram (ECG) is a graphic description of the electrical activity of the heart, recorded from the body surface by electrodes positioned to reflect activity from a variety of spatial perspectives. The source of cardiac electrical activity resides within the working (contracting) myocardial cells, as well as within the specialized conducting tissue (SCT), as described in Chap. 184. However, only that activity generated by atrial and ventricular working muscle is recorded on the standard surface ECG. Electrical activity of the SCT can be deduced from features of the surface ECG, or recorded by signal averaging on the body surface or by intracardiac electrode catheters (see Chap. 185).

The magnitude and direction of the electrical activity recorded on the body surface are instantaneous averages of cumulative cell depolarizations or repolarizations occurring at a point in time. Although much of the electrical activity from individual cells is canceled out before reaching the body surface by opposing forces from other cells, the resultant recording is a reasonably reproducible and accurate approximation of net cardiac electrical activity. However, the signals recorded at the body surface do not identify specific sites of origin because a given vector at the body surface can be accounted for by innumerable combinations of cellular signals at their source in the heart.

Early in the development of the ECG, Einthoven popularized the concept that the human body represents a large volume conductor having the source of cardiac electrical activity at its center. While this theory is not strictly accurate, it provides the clinician with a practical point from which to work. As an extension of this concept, the *net* electrical activity at any instant in the cardiac cycle may be viewed as originating from a polarized point source at a theoretical "electrical center" of the heart. Since this "equivalent dipole" would have direction and magnitude, one might then extend the pattern into a sequence of instantaneous vectors recordable from the body surface. The application of this concept to ECG analysis is discussed below.

LEAD SYSTEMS The ECG lead system is composed of five electrodes, one on each of the four limbs and one placed at various sites on the precordium. Each lead is a continuous recording of the change in electrical potential during the cardiac cycle between two of the electrodes, or between one electrode and a combination of the others. The right-leg electrode is an inactive ground electrode in all leads.

The original lead system developed by Einthoven is based on assumptions of (1) the homogeneity of the body volume conductor, (2) the symmetry of the leads, and (3) a single equivalent dipole at the center of the volume conductor. The *standard limb leads* (I, II, and III) are composed of three bipolar permutations of the right arm (RA), left arm (LA), and left leg (LL) electrodes [Fig. 176-1*A* (1)]. Lead I records the potential difference between the LA and the RA,

FIGURE 176-1 Lead systems. *A*. Standard limb leads, showing (1) electrode positions, (2) the equilateral triangle of Einthoven, and (3) the conversion of the triangle to a triaxial reference system with positive (+) and negative (−) polarity. *B*. The unipolar chest leads, showing (1) the central terminal of Wilson (CTW) (or the indifferent electrode, i) and the chest electrode (C) (or the exploring electrode, E). The 5000 Ω between CTW and each limb electrode is not shown. The relationship between CTW and V_1 to V_6 in the horizontal plane is shown in part 2. *C*. The augmented unipolar limb leads, using the modified CTW. *D*. The hexaxial frontal plane reference system. Normal ranges are described in the text, and applications are derived in Figs. 176-5 and 176-6. RA, right arm; LA, left arm; LL, left leg; RL, right leg.

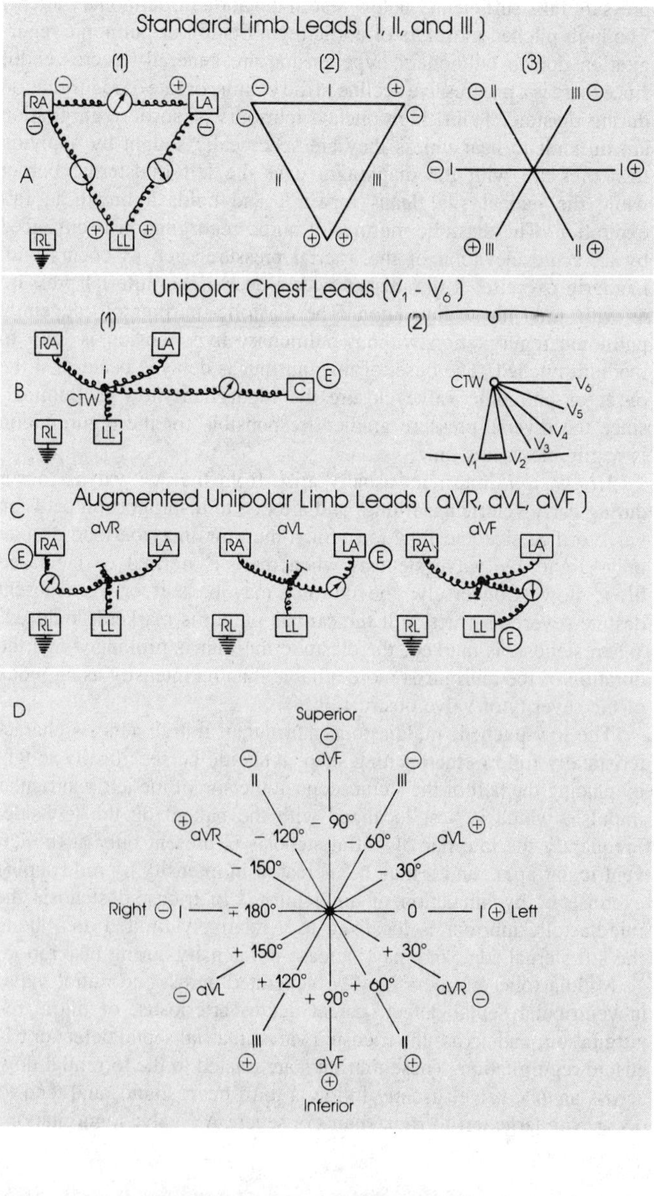

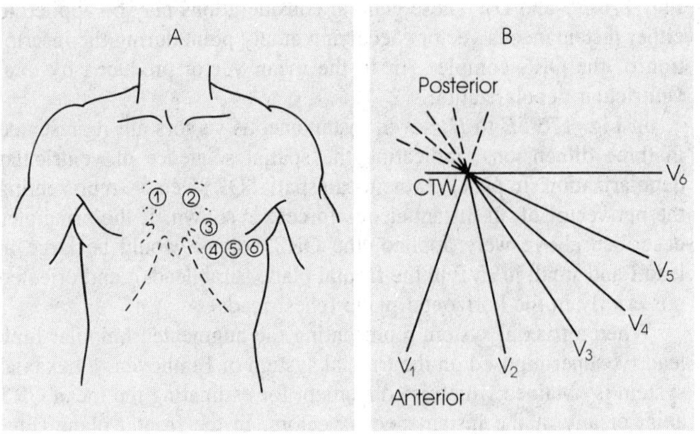

FIGURE 176-2 The unipolar chest leads. *A*. The position of the chest electrode for V_1 to V_6. *B*. The relationship between the CTW and the chest electrode (C) in the horizontal plane.

the positive electrode on the LA and the negative electrode on the RA [Fig. 176-1*A* (2)]. Lead II records the potential difference between the electrodes on the RA and the LL, the positive electrode on the LL. Lead III records the potential difference between the LA and the LL, with the positive electrode on the LL. It is likely that Einthoven arbitrarily selected the relationships between positive and negative electrodes in the three leads in order to have the major deflection of the QRS complex (see below) moving in an upward (positive) direction in most normal individuals.

The central terminal of Wilson (CTW) is constructed by connecting the RA, LA, and LL electrodes through 5000-Ω resistances, in order to cancel out the potentials from these three points. With the forces canceled out, the CTW theoretically remains inactive during the entire cardiac cycle, and an exploring electrode will function as a unipolar lead [Fig. 176-1*B* (1)]. The selection of the positions for the six *unipolar chest leads* [Figs. 176-1*B* (2) and 176-2] was based on the concept that the proximity of the heart to the anterior chest wall resulted in the unipolar chest leads functioning as "semidirect" leads, being influenced primarily by the tissue immediately beneath the electrode. While this concept does not have the quantitative significance originally desired, and the recordings do reflect the activity of the total heart, there is weighting of the voltages recorded by the tissue closest to the exploring electrode. The six standard chest leads (V_1 to V_6) are recorded by positioning the exploring chest electrode as follows: V_1 in the fourth intercostal space (4ICS) at the right sternal border; V_2 in the 4ICS at the left sternal border; V_4 in the 5ICS at the midclavicular line; V_3 midway between V_2 and V_4; V_5 at the left anterior axillary line at the level of V_4 horizontally; and V_6 at the left midaxillary line at the level of V_4 horizontally (Fig. 176-2). The exploring chest electrode is occasionally used in nonstandard positions for special purposes. V_4R, the equivalent position of V_4 on the *right* side of the chest, may be helpful in diagnosing right ventricular myocardial infarction (see below and Chap. 189) and right-sided leads (V_3R to V_6R) can be used to record ECGs in patients with dextrocardia (see Chap. 186). V_7 (left posterior axillary line) and V_8 to V_{10} (back) are used rarely to explore the left ventricle. The CTW is the indifferent electrode, and the exploring chest electrode is the active electrode for all chest leads.

Unipolar limb leads may be recorded by a system in which the CTW constitutes the indifferent electrode and the exploring electrode is one of the three active limb electrodes. These leads are referred to as VR, VL, and VF. By disconnecting the input to the CTW from the extremity being explored, the voltage of the unipolar limb leads is augmented by as much as 50 percent. This modification is universally used for clinical ECGs, and the leads are labeled aVR, aVL, and aVF (Fig. 176-1*C*).

In recent years, the clinical value of chest wall mapping has been studied by a number of investigators. Multiple electrodes (32 to 192)

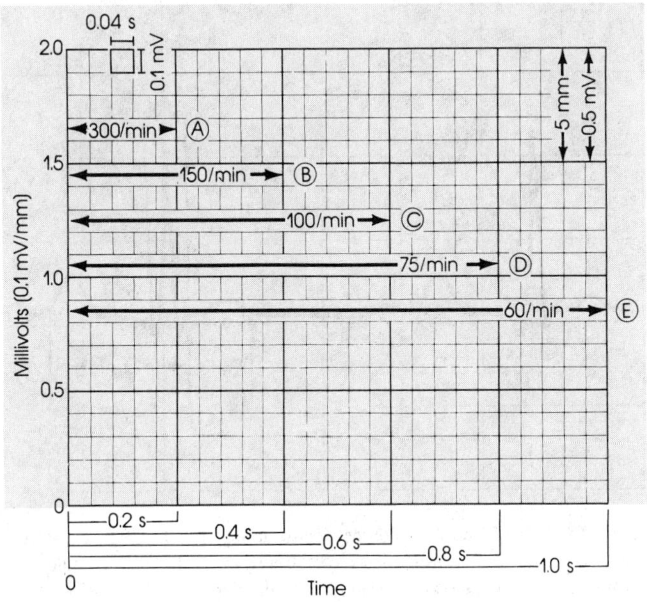

FIGURE 176-3 Standardization of the ECG. Standard time calibration is 1 mm = 0.04 s or 5 mm = 0.20 s. Standard voltage is 0.1 mV/mm. A repetitive event occurring every 5 mm (A) on time axis (0.20 s) is occurring at 300 per minute. A repetitive event occurring every 10 mm (B) (0.40 s) is occurring at 150 per minute. C, D, and E indicate that repetitive events at 0.60, 0.80, and 1.00 s are occurring at rates of 100, 75, and 60 per minute, respectively.

are used for simultaneous recording, and computer processing for data reduction and display. This procedure yields information not available from the standard 12-lead ECG. New insights into normal and abnormal depolarization and repolarization patterns are evolving, and the value of sequential changes in ST segments during acute myocardial infarction is being studied.

ELECTROCARDIOGRAPHIC WAVEFORMS, DURATIONS, AND INTERVALS Clinical ECGs are recorded on paper having a graphic background (Fig. 176-3) to permit rapid measurement of standardized time intervals and voltages. Time lines are 1 mm apart, with every fifth line intensified. Standard paper speed is 25 mm/s. Thus, 1 mm = 0.04 s (lighter lines), and 5 mm = 0.20 s (heavier lines). The horizontal lines, 1 mm apart, permit calibration of the voltage deflections of the ECG. Usual standardization is ↑ 10 mm = +1 mV (Fig. 176-3).

The P wave reflecting atrial depolarization is normally the initial wave of activity during the cardiac cycle (Fig. 176-4). Ventricular muscle depolarization is represented by the *QRS complex*. A Q wave is an initial negative wave; an R wave is an initial positive wave or a positive wave following a Q wave; and an S wave is a negative deflection following an R wave (Fig. 176-4). A QRS complex having a Q wave which returns to the baseline but does not produce a positive wave is labeled a QS complex, and the second R wave in a QRS complex having more than one R wave is labeled R′. The T wave represents ventricular muscle repolarization and is sometimes followed by a small wave, the U wave, the mechanism of which remains uncertain. Repolarization of atrial muscle is represented by the T_a (or T_p) wave, which occurs during the PR interval and QRS complex, and is usually difficult to identify. The interval between the end of the QRS complex and the onset of the T wave is the ST segment, representing the period of time between depolarization of the ventricles and the period of rapid repolarization of ventricular muscle.

The interval between the P wave and the QRS complex is the PR (or PQ) interval, measured from the *onset* of atrial depolarization (P) to the *onset* of ventricular depolarization (Q or R) (Fig. 176-4). The

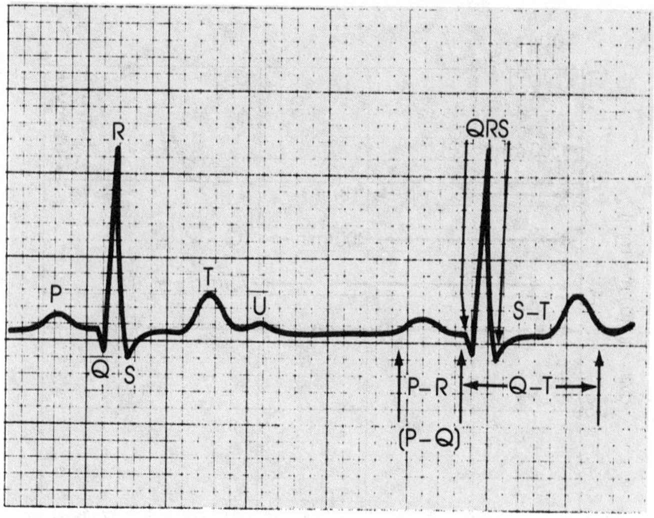

FIGURE 176-4 The waves of the electrocardiogram—P, QRS, T, and U—are indicated. The measurements of the PR interval, QRS complex, ST segment, and QT interval are identified on the right.

duration is 0.12 to 0.20 s in the adult. Since AV nodal activation begins before the end of depolarization of atrial muscle, the PR interval may be used as a rough approximation of AV conduction time.

The duration of the QRS complex (normal = 0.04 to 0.10 s) reflects the time required for depolarization of ventricular muscle. It may be slightly prolonged by regional block in a portion of the intraventricular SCT or by delayed conduction in a region of ventricular muscle. Block in a bundle branch prolongs the QRS to a greater extent. An approximation of the refractory period of the ventricles may be obtained by measuring the QT interval (from the onset of the QRS to the end of the T wave) (Fig. 176-4). The QT interval is rate-dependent, and may be altered by numerous pathophysiologic or pharmacologic influences. Bazett's formula may be used to calculate the QT interval corrected for heart rate (QT_c). The formula is:

$$QT_c = \frac{QT}{\sqrt{R\text{-}R}}$$

where R-R is the interval between two successive QRS complexes. QT_c is prolonged when it is ≥ 0.40 s in men and ≥ 0.45 s in women.

THE VECTOR CONCEPT AND ELECTRICAL AXIS The representation of a force by a graphic description of its direction and magnitude is referred to as a *vector*. In specific reference to cardiac electrical activity, a vector may be projected onto a two-dimensional plane as a scalar vector (Fig. 176-5*A* to *D*), or considered in three dimensions as a spatial vector (Fig. 176-5*E* to *H*). It may be used to represent instantaneous forces in the sequence of the cardiac electrical cycle (Fig. 176-5*A* and *E*), or it may represent either the mean or maximum axis during the cardiac cycle (Fig. 176-5*H*). Mean, maximum, and instantaneous vectors are most commonly applied to the analysis of the QRS complex, but the same principles may be applied to the P wave, ST segment, or T wave.

When an instantaneous electrical force recorded from the body surface is oriented in a direction perpendicular (or nearly so) to one of the leads (Fig. 176-5*C*, vector 6), the potential recorded by that lead at that instant will be minimum or isoelectric (Fig. 176-5*D*, point 6). Conversely, if the lead system is oriented parallel to the direction of an instantaneous electrical force (Fig. 176-5*C*, vector 4), the potential recorded by that lead will be maximum (Fig. 176-5*D*, point 4). An intermediate direction will record an intermediate voltage (for example, Fig. 176-5*C* and *D*, vector 2). If the instantaneous electrical force is oriented to the positive side of the lead, the deflection will be positive (4 in Fig. 176-5*C* and *D*); if the direction is oriented to the negative side, the deflection will be negative (1 in Fig. 176-5*C* and *D*). These general considerations may be applied to either instantaneous vectors occurring at any point during the inscription of the QRS complex, or to the mean vector produced by total ventricular depolarization.

In Fig. 176-5*E* to *H*, seven instantaneous vectors are represented in three dimensions, indicating the spatial sequence of ventricular depolarization. In panel *H*, the mean spatial QRS vector, representing the net vector of all instantaneous forces, is shown. If the principles described above were applied, the QRS voltage would be large in lead I and small in aVF in the frontal plane (limb leads), and oriented posteriorly in the horizontal plane (chest leads).

When a triaxial system representing the augmented unipolar limb leads is superimposed on the triaxial system of Einthoven, a hexaxial system is obtained which is convenient for estimating the mean QRS axis, or any of the instantaneous vectors, in the frontal plane (Fig. 176-1*D*). When the appropriate positive and negative voltage orientations are assigned to each of the leads, the hexaxial reference system becomes a simple means of scalar vector analysis, requiring a

FIGURE 176-5 *A*. Frontal plane scalar projection of six instantaneous QRS vectors. *B*. Vectors originating from a point source at the electrical center of the heart. *C*. Projection of the vectors on the lead I axis. *D*. Lead I QRS produced by the instantaneous vectors in panel *C* (see text). *E*. Spatial representation of ventricular depolarization. Seven instantaneous vectors in the sequence of depolarization indicated in spatial orientations. *F*. Spatial vectors originating from the electrical center of the heart. *G*. A line drawn through the terminations of the spatial vectors produces a spatial QRS loop (vector loop). *H*. The mean spatial QRS vector, average of all the instantaneous vectors—to the left, slightly inferiorly, and posteriorly. (See text.) *(From JW Hurst, RJ Myerburg, Introduction to Electrocardiography, 2d ed, New York, McGraw-Hill, 1973; modified and reproduced by permission of the publisher.)*

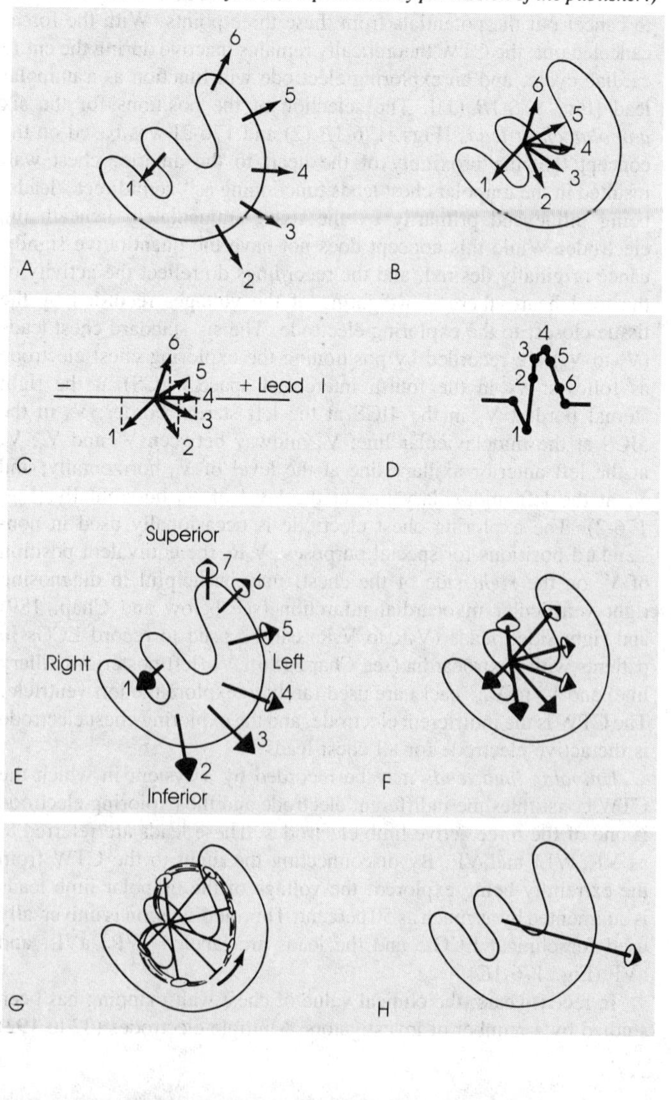

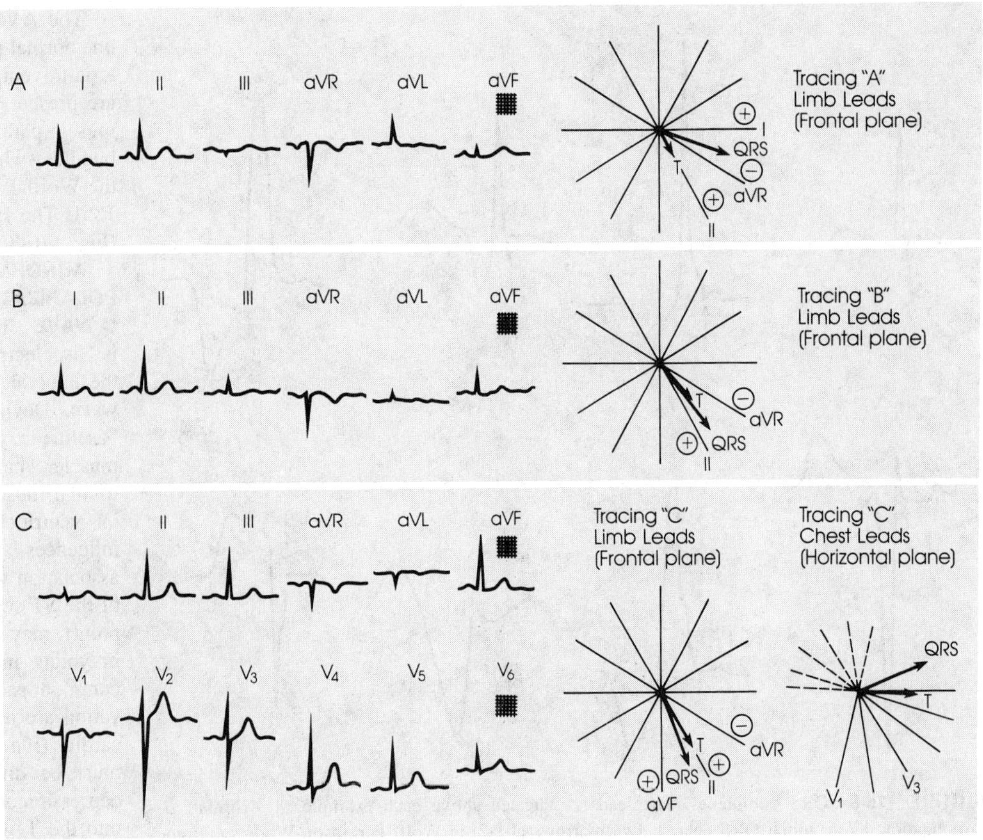

FIGURE 176-6 Three normal ECGs demonstrating: (*A*) horizontal, (*B*) intermediate, and (*C*) vertical mean frontal plane QRS axes constructed on the hexaxial system. In addition, the horizontal plane vector in *C* is constructed on an axial system and is posteriorly oriented. T-wave vectors are similarly constructed.

minimum of two leads for estimation of the mean axis. An ECG which reveals a maximum positive QRS deflection in lead I and an isoelectric deflection in aVF has a mean QRS vector oriented at 0°. Conversely, if the QRS voltage is positive and maximum in lead II and isoelectric in aVL, the mean vector is oriented at +60°. The mean QRS axis in the frontal plane in normal adults ranges from −30 to +110°. Overlap between normal and abnormal occurs in the range of +90 to +110°. Generally, an axis >+90° is referred to as *right axis deviation,* and more negative than −30° as *abnormal left axis deviation.* The determination of the mean QRS axis in the horizontal plane (Fig. 176-2*B*) is similarly derived, normal orientation being to the left and posteriorly.

Three normal ECGs are shown in Fig. 176-6. Analysis of the mean QRS axis in the *frontal plane* (I, II, III, aVR, aVL, aVF) reveals the axis of *A* to be oriented horizontally, of *C* to be oriented vertically, and of *B* to be oriented in an intermediate range. In *A* the net voltage of the QRS complex is largest in lead I, almost isoelectric in lead III, and low in aVF, placing the mean axis in a direction almost perpendicular to lead III. In *B*, the voltages in lead I and aVF are almost identical, and maximum in lead II and aVR. The mean QRS axis is between lead II (+) and aVR (−). In *C*, net voltage is largest in leads II and aVF and almost isoelectric in lead I, placing the mean QRS axis almost perpendicular to lead I. A similar approach is applied to QRS axis determination in the *horizontal plane.* In *C*, the lead in which the net forces are isoelectric is V_3. Therefore, as shown in the axial representation of the horizontal plane of tracing *C*, the QRS vector is oriented to the left and posteriorly. If this information is added to that obtained from the frontal plane axis, it is apparent that the mean QRS vector of electrocardiogram *C* is oriented inferiorly, to the left, and posteriorly. Similar principles may be applied to the analysis of the mean T-wave axis, which is normally oriented in the same general direction as the QRS axis. An angle between the QRS and T axes >45° in the frontal plane, or >60° in the horizontal plane, is abnormal.

ELECTRICAL ACTIVITY OF THE ATRIA The mean P-wave vector is normally directed to the left, inferiorly, and slightly anteriorly; the frontal plane P axis is usually oriented between +30 and +60°. Right atrial enlargement causes tall, peaked P waves (≥0.25 mV), most prominent in standard leads II and V_1 (Fig. 176-7). Left atrial enlargement causes broad, notched P waves in lead II, and inverted or biphasic P waves (with the inverted portion of the biphasic P wave broader and deeper than the upright portion) in lead V_1. The upper limit of normal for P-wave duration is 0.11 s, and the broad P wave of left atrial enlargement usually is ≥0.12 s. However, criteria for left atrial enlargement are nonspecific, similar changes occurring in intraatrial conduction disturbances (Fig. 176-7), and the two must be distinguished by techniques other than ECG.

ABNORMALITIES OF VENTRICULAR DEPOLARIZATION: QRS COMPLEX Since the QRS complex is the ECG representation of the sequence, time, and synchronization of total ventricular muscle depolarization, focal or diffuse abnormalities in ventricular muscle or in the SCT may cause changes in QRS form. Abnormalities may be confined to initial depolarization (Fig. 176-8*B*), terminal depolarization (Fig. 176-8*C*), or mid and late depolarization (Fig. 176-8*D*), or they may be diffuse (Fig. 176-8*E* to *G*).

The normal earliest site of activation is in the midportion of the left side of the interventricular septum, followed closely by a site on the lower portion of the right side of the interventricular septum and

FIGURE 176-7 P waves of right atrial enlargement (RAE) and left atrial enlargement (LAE).

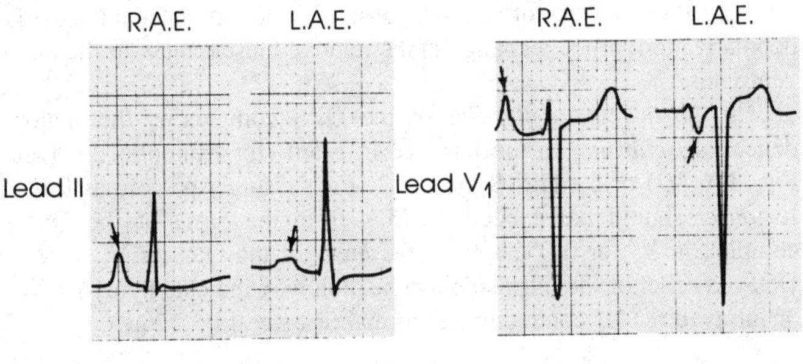

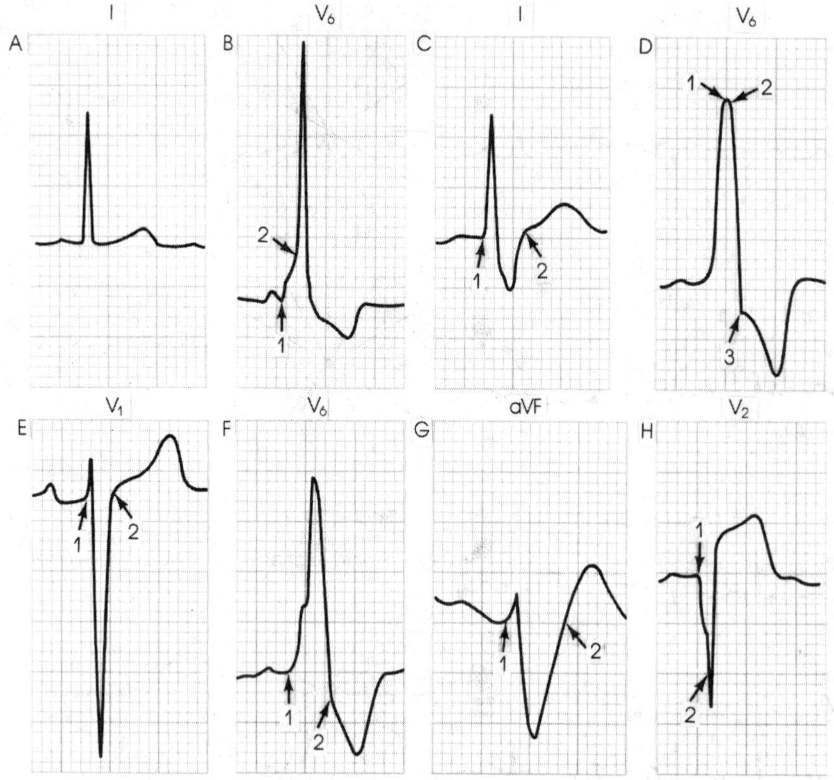

FIGURE 176-8 QRS complexes. The lead is indicated above each example. *A*. Normal. *B*. Prolongation due to initial QRS delay between arrows (1→2) in Wolff-Parkinson-White syndrome (see Chap. 184). *C*. Prolongation due to terminal delay (1→2) in right bundle branch block. *D*. Prolongation due to mid (1→2) and late (2→3) delay in left bundle branch block. *E*. Minor uniform prolongation (1→2) in left ventricular hypertrophy. *F*. Distortion of total QRS pattern (1→2) in a cardiomyopathy. *G*. Uniform prolongation (1→2) in an electrolyte abnormality. *H*. Pathologic Q wave (1→2) in myocardial infarction. Intrinsicoid deflection = 2→3 in *D* and S→2 in *E*.

the adjacent free wall endocardium. The dominant wavefront is that one arising on the left septum, which results in a small initial R wave in V_1 (anterior movement), and a small initial Q wave in I, aVL, and/or V_6 (rightward movement). Small initial Q waves in II, III, and aVF may be observed as an indication of a small superior movement of the initial wavefront. Normal septal Q waves are ≤0.02 s and of low amplitude. A normal R in V_1 is ≤0.4 mV.

After septal depolarization has been initiated, rapid endocardial propagation occurs through both ventricles. In the normal heart, the greater mass of the left ventricle predominates, and the magnitude and direction of the electrical vectors reflect this fact (Fig. 176-6). During normal depolarization, the sequence of instantaneous vectors rotates from rightward and anterior to leftward, posterior, and superior (Fig. 176-5*E* to *G*). Most individuals will have maximum QRS duration (i.e., the lead having the longest measurable QRS) of 0.05 to 0.08 s (normal range is 0.04 to 0.10 s). A QRS duration of 0.09 or 0.10 s may be a normal variant or may represent a conduction delay to limited regions of either ventricle (Fig. 176-8). QRS durations ≥0.12 s represent left or right bundle branch block or severe degrees of diffuse intraventricular conduction delay (Fig. 176-13).

Abnormal initial Q waves or an abnormal initial R in V_1 usually represents (1) a loss of muscle mass; (2) abnormal sequence of depolarization; or (3) a change in the relative muscle mass in the two ventricles.

The *intrinsicoid deflection* of the QRS complex is the major deflection *returning* to the baseline in a left (for example, 2→3 in Fig. 176-8*D*) or a right (S wave→2, Fig. 176-8*E*) precordial lead. Its *onset* should not exceed 0.035 s from the *onset* of the QRS complex in V_1, or 0.055 s from the *onset* of the QRS in V_5 or V_6. Delayed onset of the intrinsicoid deflection may indicate hypertrophy or intraventricular conduction abnormalities (see Fig. 176-8).

The AV node and His bundle constitute the one normal pathway for impulse conduction from atria to ventricles. However, *accessory pathways* are present in some hearts. These are bands of muscle parallel to the AV junction, named Kent bundles, which form the anatomic substrate for the Wolff-Parkinson-White syndrome (see Chap. 185). The ECG manifestation is the *delta wave* (Fig. 176-8*B*).

ABNORMALITIES OF VENTRICULAR REPOLARIZATION: ST SEGMENT, T WAVE, AND U WAVE In the normal ECG, the ST segment is "isoelectric," resting at the same potential as the interval between the T wave and the next P wave. Deviations of the ST segment from the baseline may occur as a result of injury to cardiac muscle, changes in the synchronization of ventricular muscle depolarization, overload or strain on ventricular muscle, or drug or electrolyte influences. Elevations of the ST segment, in association with an elevation of the takeoff point of the ST segment from the QRS complex (the J point), may occur as a normal variant, especially in young individuals (Fig. 176-9*A*). The most common pathologic causes of ST-segment elevation are acute myocardial infarction and pericarditis (Fig. 176-9*B* to *F*), and the normal variant must be differentiated from these. Horizontal depression or a downsloping ST segment merging into the T wave occurs as a result of ischemia, ventricular strain, changes in the pattern of ventricular depolarization, or drug effects (Fig. 176-9*H*, *I*, *M*, *N*, *Q*, and *R*).

Since the sequence of ventricular muscle *de*polarization is from endocardium to epicardium, and *re*polarization represents an electrical process opposite in direction to depolarization, the T wave would be in the opposite direction to the QRS complex if the sequence of repolarization were in the same direction as depolarization. However, T waves assume the same general direction as the major deflection of the QRS complex (see Fig. 176-6). It is assumed, therefore, that the direction of normal repolarization is opposite to the wave of depolarization—from epicardium to endocardium. T waves are considered abnormal when they are of low voltage, flat, or inverted in leads in which they are normally upright, or when they are abnormally tall and peaked. T-wave inversions are reflected vectorially by a widening of the angle between the QRS vector and the T vector (Fig. 176-6). Common causes of abnormalities of the T waves include ischemic heart disease, ventricular hypertrophy and strain, primary muscle disease, abnormal sequences of depolarization, electrolyte abnormalities, and drug influences (see Fig. 176-9*C*, *D*, *F*, *I*, *K*, *L*, and *N* to *R*), but the changes are often not specific.

The U wave is usually positive in leads in which the QRS complex is positive. The abnormal U wave is manifested as either an exaggeration of U-wave voltage, the appearance of a U wave in leads in which it is not normally seen, or inversion of a U wave. U-wave abnormalities occur in ischemic heart disease, left ventricular strain, and electrolyte disturbances. Unfortunately, the information they provide is usually nonspecific.

ECG MANIFESTATIONS OF VENTRICULAR HYPERTROPHY The normal dominance of the left ventricle on the features of the QRS complex is decreased or reversed in right ventricular hypertrophy (RVH) and exaggerated in left ventricular hypertrophy (LVH) (Fig. 176-10). RVH causes a shift of the net forces of depolarization from the left and posterior toward the right and anteriorly. On the ECG, this produces tall R waves in V_1 (≥0.5 mV), with an abnormal S wave in V_5 or V_6 (≥0.7 mV). In the frontal plane, the mean QRS axis shifts to the right of vertical (usually >110°). Less extreme

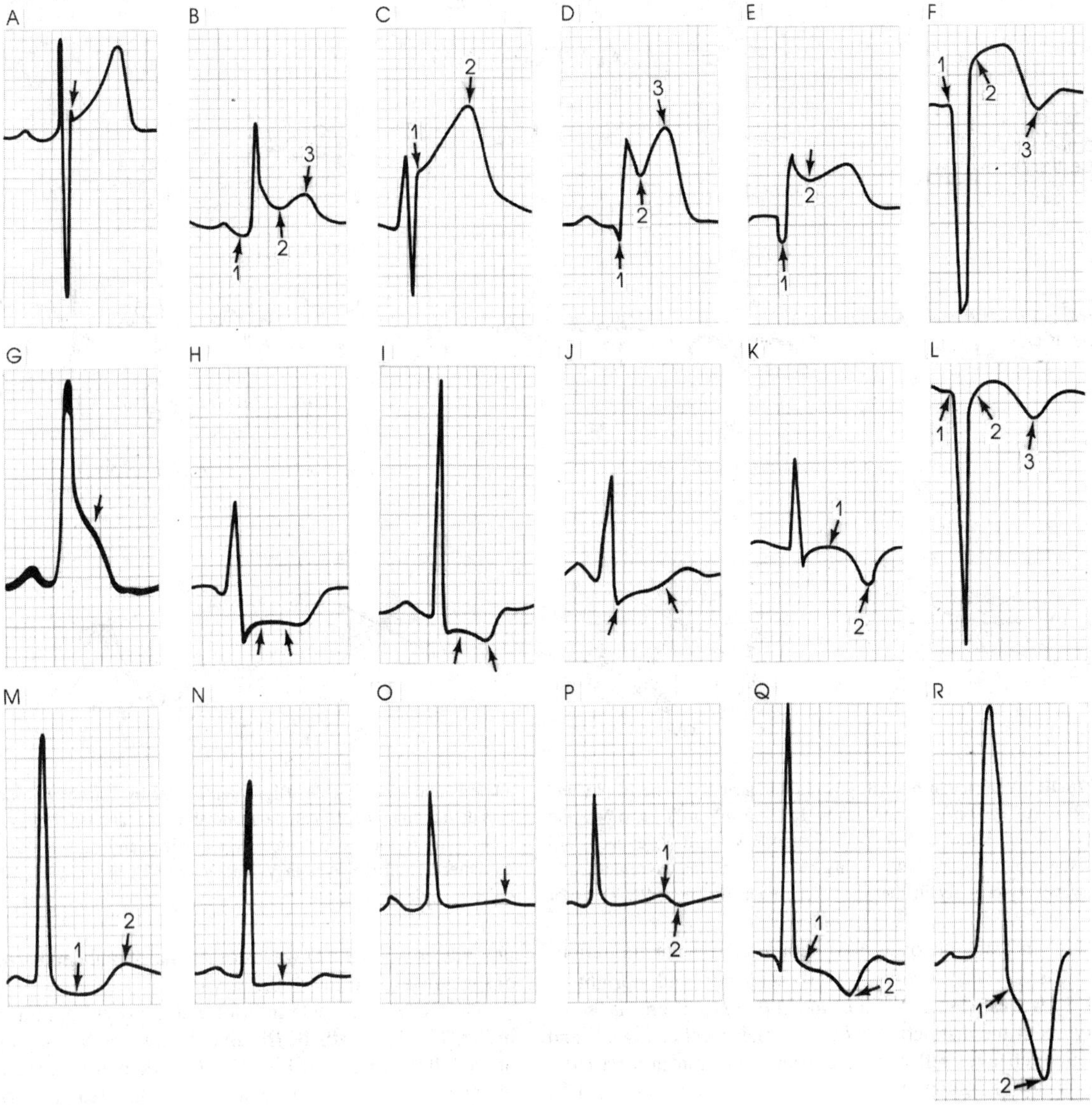

FIGURE 176-9 ST-segment and T-wave changes. Arrows in each panel indicate the major features of each complex. *A*. Early repolarization (J-point elevation), normal variant. *B*. Acute pericarditis: (1) depressed T_a; (2) elevated ST; (3) normal T. *C*. Early acute myocardial infarction (AMI): (1) elevated ST; (2) tall, peaked T wave; steep angle between 1 and 2. *D*. AMI: (1) small Q wave; (2) elevated ST segment; (3) tall, peaked T wave with steep 2→3 angle. *E*. AMI: (1) pathologic Q wave; (2) elevated ST segment. *F*. AMI: (1) Q wave; (2) elevated ST segment; (3) terminal T-wave inversion. *G*. Angina pectoris (Prinzmetal variant) with ST elevation during pain. *H* and *I*. Angina pectoris (usual form) with horizontal or downward sloping ST segment during pain or exercise. *J*. J-point depression with upsloping ST segment during exercise, normal response. *K*. Primary T-wave inversion (2) in ischemia or primary muscle disease. *L*. Myocardial infarction (healed): (1) pathologic Q; (2) ST returning to baseline; (3) symmetrically inverted T wave. *M*. Digitalis effect: (1) downward coving of ST segment, merging into (2) an upright T wave. *N* to *P*. Nonspecific ST-segment and T-wave changes often seen in chronic ischemic heart disease. *Q*. Left ventricular strain pattern with (1) downsloping ST segment and (2) asymmetrically inverted (secondary) T wave. *R*. Downsloping ST segment merging into a deeply inverted T wave in ventricular conduction abnormality.

degrees of RVH may result in preservation of a moderately deep S wave in V_1, with an R-wave voltage exceeding the S-wave voltage, or a normal R wave with a shallow S wave and prominent terminal S waves in V_5 and V_6. The primary QRS manifestation of LVH is an increase in voltage in those leads which reflect the electrical activity of the left ventricle. R waves in the standard limb leads may increase beyond the normal limit of 2.0 mV. Concomitantly, there is a tendency for a shift of the frontal plane QRS axis to the left. It is not likely that LVH alone will cause a shift in the QRS axis beyond −30°, but it commonly causes a shift in the range of 0 to −30° (Fig. 176-10). LVH causes a deep S wave in lead V_1 or V_2 (>2.5 mV) or an abnormal R wave in lead V_5 or V_6 (>2.5 mV). When T waves are normal, the presence of voltage criteria for LVH must be interpreted in terms of body habitus of an individual. Young, healthy, thin-chested individuals will frequently exceed the QRS voltage criteria for LVH in its absence. However, when the ST-segment and T-wave changes associated with "strain" are present (Figs. 176-9*Q* and 176-10), the diagnosis of LVH is clarified. Similarly, borderline voltage criteria are more specific for LVH when associated with the ST-segment and T-wave changes of left ventricular strain.

ACUTE MYOCARDIAL INFARCTION Three pathophysiologic events occur, either in sequence or simultaneously, in an acute myocardial infarction—ischemia, injury, and infarction. The ECG manifestations of these processes include changes in the T waves (ischemia), ST segments (injury), and QRS complexes (infarction). The earliest T-wave changes of acute myocardial ischemia are tall, peaked T waves ("hyperacute") (Fig. 176-9*C* and *D*), followed later by symmetrically inverted T waves (Fig. 176-9*F* and *K*). When the electrical integrity of the cell membranes is affected, currents of injury develop. The injury pattern on ECG during evolution of a transmural infarction is an elevation of the ST segments in the leads facing the infarcting area (Fig. 176-9*C* and *F*). The combination of ischemia and injury causes elevated ST segments, followed by either tall, peaked T waves (in the very early stages) or inverted T waves

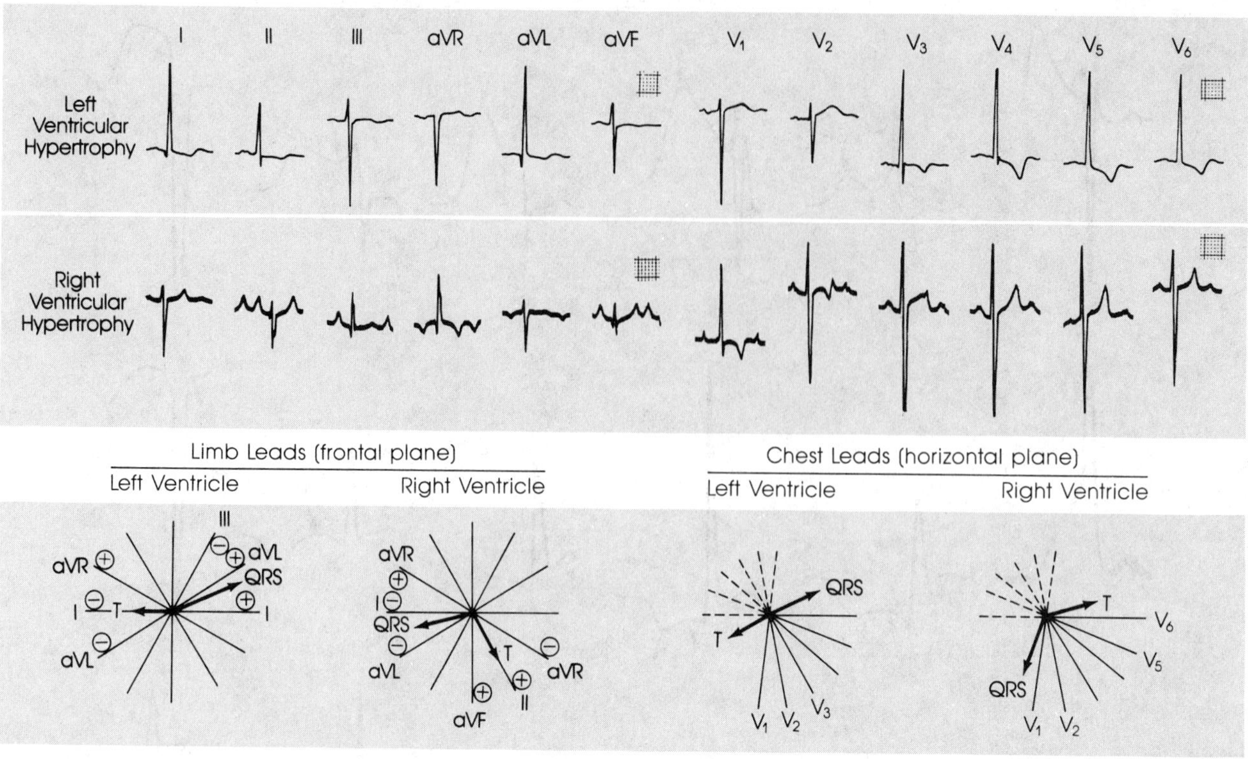

FIGURE 176-10 Ventricular hypertrophy. Left ventricular hypertrophy and strain with R wave >2.0 mV in limb leads; R >2.5 mV in V_5 and V_6, and S in V_1 >2.5 mV. The sum of S-V_1 or S-V_2 and R-V_5 or R-V_6 exceeds 3.5 mV. Strain is indicated by the downsloping ST segments and asymmetrically inverted T waves, especially in the lateral chest leads. The QRS-T vector angle is abnormally wide. Right ventricular hypertrophy is indicated by right axis deviation in the frontal plane and abnormal anterior forces in the horizontal plane. The former is indicated by a small R and deep S wave in lead I, and the latter by tall R waves in V_1 and V_2 with deep S waves in V_5 and V_6. The QRS-T angle is wide (strain).

(Fig. 176-11). In leads opposite the region of the acute infarction, reciprocal changes occur: depressed ST segments and upright or isoelectric T waves (Figs. 176-11 and 176-12). There is some controversy about the distinction between "reciprocal changes" and nearly identical changes reflecting coexistent ischemia in a vascular bed remote from the infarction, i.e., "ischemia at a distance." It is likely that remote ST depressions could be due to either. As the period of active injury resolves, the ST segments return to the baseline, but the inverted T waves may persist for days, months, or permanently (Fig. 176-9*L*). Pathologic Q waves are the QRS manifestation of a transmural myocardial infarction. Q waves are pathologic when they appear in a lead in which Q waves were previously not present, or when the Q waves of normal septal depolarization become exaggerated (>20 ms; >0.2 mV).

The ECG in an acute inferior wall myocardial infarction is shown in Fig. 176-11. Leads II, III, and aVF, which face the inferior surface of the left ventricle (see Fig. 176-1*D*), demonstrate the direct patterns of infarction (pathologic Q waves), injury (elevated ST segments), and ischemia (inversion of the T waves). Reciprocal changes (depressed ST, tall T) are demonstrated in aVL. The evolution of an acute anterior myocardial infarction is demonstrated in Fig. 176-12. The most obvious direct changes occur in aVL, V_2, and V_3, and reciprocal changes in II, III, and aVF. In the tracing of 4/11, ST elevations (most prominent in aVL, V_2, and V_3) are accompanied by "hyperacute" peaked T waves in V_2 and V_3. On 4/12, deeper Q waves are present in aVL and V_1 to V_3, and T waves have inverted in aVL and V_2 to V_5. ST elevations persist but less prominently. On 4/25, the pattern of a healing infarction—pathologic Q waves and

FIGURE 176-11 Acute inferior wall myocardial infarction. The ECG of 11/29 shows minor nonspecific ST-segment and T-wave changes. On 12/5 an acute myocardial infarction occurred. There are pathologic Q waves (1), ST-segment elevation (2), and terminal T-wave inversion (3) in leads II, III, and aVF indicating the location of the infarct on the inferior wall (see text). Reciprocal changes in aVL (small arrow). Increasing R-wave voltage with ST depression and increased voltage of the T wave in V_2 is characteristic of true posterior wall extension of the inferior infarction.

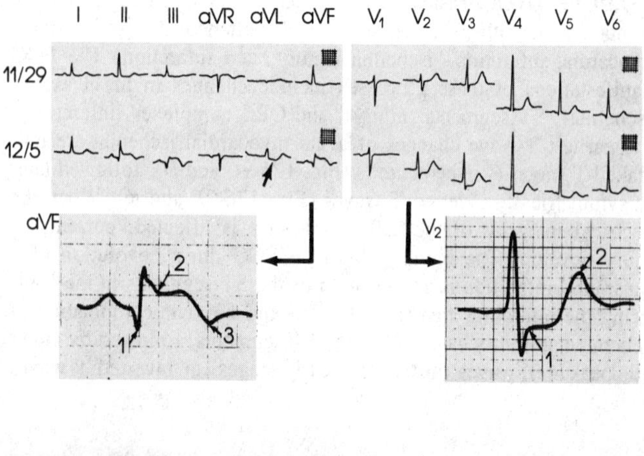

FIGURE 176-12 Acute anterior wall myocardial infarction. On 4/11, changes of a very early acute myocardial infarction in leads I, aVL, V_2, and V_3, with reciprocal changes in II, III, and aVF. On 4/12, ST segments remain elevated in the anterior leads, but T waves are inverted. On 4/25, a completed large anterior myocardial infarction is recorded—Q in I, aVL, V_1 to V_4.

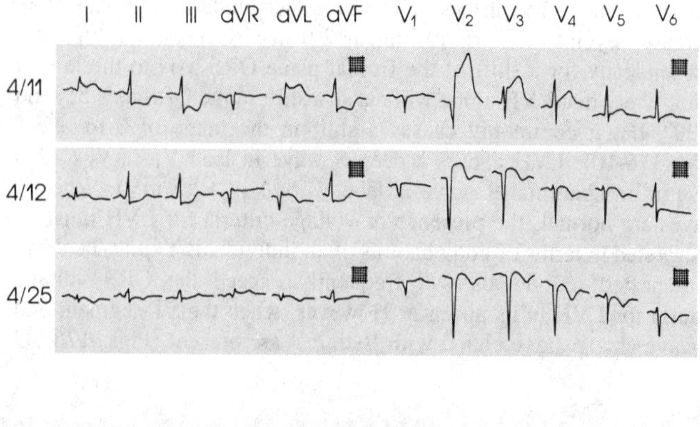

ischemic T waves—is present. Eventually, the T waves might become partially or completely normal, with persistence of the Q waves. An infarction of the true posterior wall of the left ventricle causes ECG changes opposite to those of an anterior infarction. Instead of Q waves, ST elevation, and T-wave inversion in the anterior precordial leads (V_1 and V_2), true posterior infarction is characterized by tall R waves, ST depression, and upright T waves in these leads. These infarctions usually occur in combination with inferior wall infarctions. Right ventricular myocardial infarction occurs infrequently and is almost always associated with inferior and/or posterior infarction of the left ventricle. Right ventricular infarction has no specific pattern on the standard 12-lead ECG; however, ST elevations on special right-sided precordial leads (V_4R to V_6R) may identify acute RV infarcts.

A nontransmural (subendocardial or subepicardial) myocardial infarction may cause persistent ST-segment and T-wave changes similar to those seen in transmural infarctions. However, abnormal Q waves do not appear in the QRS complex, although R-wave and/or S-wave voltages may change. The Q-wave criterion for distinguishing transmural and subendocardial infarctions is a useful ECG tool, but pathologic data have shown that exceptions do occur. It is clear that non-Q-wave patterns may reflect more than a subendocardial infarct. Large areas of intramural infarction, with only a shell of epicardium surviving, may not result in Q-wave formation. Thus, it is more accurate to distinguish between Q-wave and non-Q-wave infarctions, rather than transmural and subendocardial infarctions. The ST-segment and T-wave changes of non-Q-wave infarction are common in leads I, II, III, aVL, aVF, and/or V_4 to V_6. Similar, but transient, changes may occur during the pain of angina pectoris, in shock, after pulmonary embolism, and secondary to acute central nervous system lesions.

CHRONIC ISCHEMIC HEART DISEASE Other than Q waves of prior myocardial infarction, the ECG in chronic ischemic heart disease is often nonspecific. The patterns of chronic myocardial ischemia are intrinsically variable, and this fact is compounded by the problem of coexistent ECG changes related to pharmacologic interventions and/or LVH. Chronic ischemic heart disease causes a broad range of ST-segment and T-wave changes (Fig. 176-9*G* to *I*, *K*, *L*, and *N* to *P*). There may be moderate degrees of horizontal ST-segment depression or a downward sloping ST segment, flattening or inversion of T waves, and prominent U waves. It is difficult to define an abnormal ST-segment depression in precise quantitative terms. However, if the J point is more than 0.5 mm below the isoelectric line, the ST segment is horizontal or downsloping, and there is an associated T-wave abnormality, myocardial ischemia should be considered. The common clinical expression of chronic ischemic heart disease, angina pectoris, may be accompanied by a normal resting ECG or nonspecific ST-segment and T-wave changes. However, during spontaneous or exercise-induced pain, the ECG may demonstrate the horizontal or downward sloping ST-segment depressions shown in Fig. 176-9*H* and *I*, or rarely the variant pattern of spontaneous transient ST elevations (Prinzmetal variant) (Fig. 176-9*G*).

INTRAVENTRICULAR CONDUCTION DISTURBANCES The complex anatomy of the specialized conducting system of the ventricles, in conjunction with the focal nature of most cardiac diseases, is reflected in the multiplicity of ECG patterns which result from disorders of the sequence of activation of the ventricles. Disease of both the SCT and ventricular myocardium plays a role in the various patterns. The universal feature of ventricular conduction disturbances is a prolongation of the time required for depolarization of a portion of a ventricle, an entire ventricle, or both ventricles. Delayed or slow conduction may be diffuse or may be confined to a portion of the QRS complex (Fig. 176-8). Prolongation of the QRS may be modest, as in left ventricular hypertrophy, or extreme, as in cardiomyopathies or metabolic abnormalities (Fig. 176-8).

The classic bundle branch block patterns are associated with specific lesions in the left or right bundle branch in the majority of cases. Complete right bundle branch block (RBBB) (Fig. 176-13) is

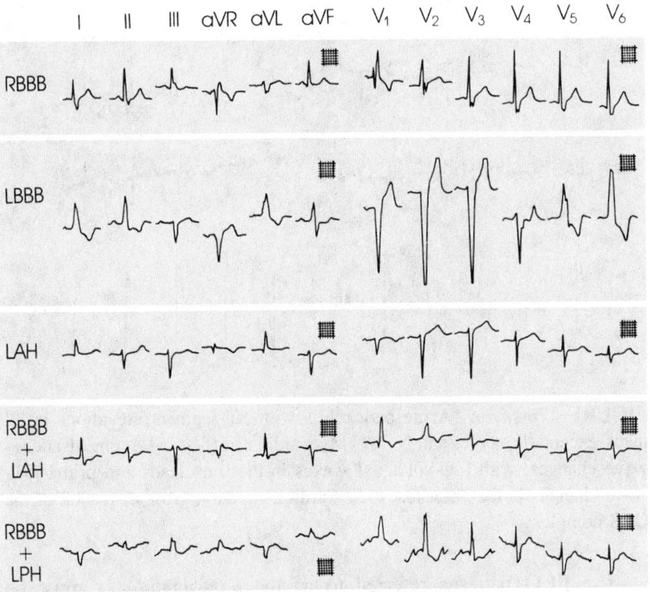

FIGURE 176-13 Intraventricular conduction abnormalities. Illustrated are right bundle branch block (RBBB); left bundle branch block (LBBB); left anterior hemiblock (LAH); right bundle branch block with left anterior hemiblock (RBBB + LAH); and right bundle branch block with left posterior hemiblock (RBBB + LPH) (see text).

characterized by prolongation of the QRS complex ($\geq$0.12 s) with the delayed activation of the right ventricle accounting for a terminal delay on the ECG. Since septal activation from the left bundle branch system normally precedes right ventricular activation, *the initial forces of ventricular depolarization are not disturbed in RBBB*, and the ability to identify coexistent pathologic Q waves is not hindered. The delayed activation of the right ventricle is reflected by the presence of terminal forces directed anteriorly and to the right. The rightward direction of the slow terminal forces is indicated by the broad terminal S wave in leads I, aVL, and V_6 (Fig. 176-13). The anterior orientation of these forces is indicated by a large terminal R wave (R′) in V_1. Since initial forces are not disturbed, the normal initial R wave in V_1 persists, followed by an S wave. Incomplete RBBB is present when the waveform criteria for RBBB (rSR′) are present, but the QRS duration is <0.12 s.

Left bundle branch block (LBBB) is also characterized by a QRS duration $\geq$0.12 s. However, since normal initial ventricular depolarization is dependent upon the LBB to deliver the impulses of initial depolarization to the left septum, the patterns produced by LBBB are more complex. Normal septal depolarization is disturbed, and delay of the normally dominant left ventricular forces produces a more generalized disturbance of QRS morphology. The septal Q wave in standard leads I, aVL, and V_6 is typically lost. In addition, the initial anterior force reflected by the small R wave in lead V_1 may be lost because of a less anterior orientation of the initial forces. The delay in left ventricular activation produces the greatest degree of slowing in the mid and late portion of the QRS complex. This often results in notching at the peak of the upstroke in leads I and V_6 (see Figs. 176-8*D* and 176-14), with a late intrinsicoid deflection (>0.055 s) in V_5 and V_6. Most cases of LBBB produce secondary T-wave abnormalities as demonstrated in Fig. 176-14. Because of the changes in the initial forces, and the secondary ST-segment and T-wave changes, it is usually difficult to evaluate the QRS-complex, ST-segment, and T-wave changes of coexistent ischemic heart disease. When the intrinsicoid deflection is delayed in leads V_5 or V_6, but the QRS duration is <0.12 s, incomplete LBBB may be present. LBBB may be associated with either a normal QRS axis (Fig. 176-13) or left axis deviation. Those with left axis deviation usually have more extensive conducting system disease and left ventricular dysfunction. As a group, they are older, have higher mortality rates, and more advanced structural disease.

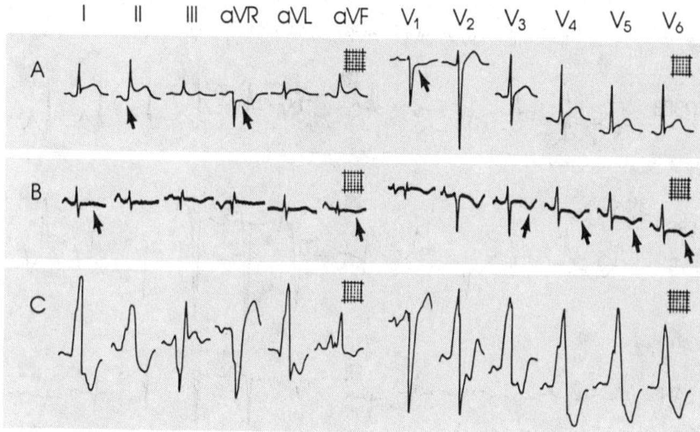

FIGURE 176-14 *A*. Acute pericarditis with ST-segment elevations in all leads except III, aVR, and V_1. *B*. Myocarditis: diffuse ST-segment and T-wave changes, with low-voltage T waves in the limb leads and primary T-wave changes in the chest leads. *C*. Cardiomyopathy: gross distortion of the QRS complex.

The ECG patterns referred to as the *left hemiblocks* must be distinguished from infarction or LVH patterns and from LBBB. *Left anterior hemiblock* (LAH) has been proposed to result from disease in the anterior radiation of fibers referred to as the anterior division of the LBB. *Left posterior hemiblock* (LPH) has been assumed to result from disease in the left posterior radiation. The complex nature of the LBB system has thus far defied a determination of whether focal proximal disease or diffuse distal disease in the distribution of these portions of the LBB is the mechanism responsible for the hemiblock patterns, although it is known that the pathologic process tends to be diffuse in those cases studied at autopsy.

LAH results in a moderate delay of activation of the superior portion of the left ventricular free wall, causing a modest prolongation of the QRS complex and shift of the front plane axis to the left. Initial septal depolarization is undisturbed (Fig. 176-13), and the QRS complex rarely exceeds 0.09 to 0.10 s. The differentiation between LAH and left ventricular hypertrophy (LVH) may occasionally be difficult. In general, LVH alone will not produce a left axis shift beyond $-30°$, and LAH will often produce left axis deviation $\geq -60°$. The key QRS features in left anterior hemiblock include small Q waves in leads I and aVL, with small initial R waves and deep S waves in leads II, III, and aVF.

LPH results in a moderate delay of activation of the posterior-inferior portion of the left ventricular free wall. Again, there is a modest prolongation of the QRS complex, but a shift of the frontal plane QRS axis to the *right*. Thus, the initial septal forces, though generally undisturbed, may be oriented more superiorly, producing small initial Q waves in leads II, III, and aVF. Since the specificity of the ECG manifestations of LPH is not very reliable, many clinicians will not make a diagnosis of isolated LPH without demonstrating a right axis shift on serial ECGs, plus definite exclusion of other causes of right axis shift. Of all the intraventricular conduction disturbances, isolated LPH is the most difficult to diagnose on ECG.

The hemiblocks frequently coexist with disease in the RBB system. The combination of RBBB, plus LAH or LPH, is referred to as *bifascicular block*—implying that two fascicles of the trifascicular model of the intraventricular SCT are diseased. This probably represents a pathophysiologic oversimplification, but it is useful for clinical purposes. Since RBBB alone does not produce abnormal left axis deviation, the coexistence of RBBB with abnormal left axis deviation (Fig. 176-13) is usually interpreted as LAH plus RBBB. Similarly, abnormal right axis deviation in association with RBBB is usually interpreted as the coexistence of LPH with RBBB, when the QRS criteria for LPH are met (Fig. 176-13). As is the case in isolated LPH, the diagnosis of LPH plus RBBB is difficult because a number of clinical settings may cause abnormal right axis deviation in conjunction with RBBB.

Trifascicular block describes abnormal conduction in all three divisions of the intraventricular SCT. The ECG diagnosis can be made only by inference when a patient has bifascicular block and a prolonged PR interval. Confirmation can be achieved only by intracardiac recordings (Chap. 184).

PERICARDITIS, MYOCARDITIS, AND THE CARDIOMYOPATHIES Acute pericarditis causes elevation of the ST segments in many leads without the reciprocal changes seen in acute myocardial infarction (Fig. 176-14*A*). ST-segment elevation may occur in all leads except aVR and rarely is present in V_1. After a period of days, the diffuse ST elevations return to the baseline, and T-wave inversions may occur. Coexistent ST elevations and T-wave inversions do not occur as often as they do in myocardial infarction (compare Figs. 176-11 and 176-14*A*). T-wave abnormalities may persist for weeks or months after the acute episode of pericarditis. If the pericarditis is accompanied by significant degrees of pericardial effusion, electrical alternans may occur. On alternate beats, ECG voltage shifts in magnitude. There also may be low voltage of the QRS complexes and T waves in all leads. Finally, the T_a waves may be transiently depressed because of atrial involvement by the inflammatory process [see Fig. 176-9*B* (1)].

The ECG changes of myocarditis (Chap. 192 and Fig. 176-14*B*) are often difficult to differentiate from the late phase of pericarditis, in which symmetric T-wave inversions are present. However, myocarditis may occur in many other settings, and an appreciation of the range of the ECG changes is important. Almost all systemic infections may produce minor myocardial involvement. Measles, mumps, influenza, hepatitis, infectious mononucleosis, and scarlet fever, just to name a few diseases, may be associated with ECG abnormalities and with histopathologic evidence of myocardial inflammation. When the myocardial involvement is subclinical, the ECG changes are usually subtle and nonspecific. There are minor T-wave changes, manifested as flattening or shallow inversion of the T waves in multiple leads (Fig. 176-9*O* and *P*). The conducting system may be involved, and prolongation of the PR interval may be noted. Resolution of these ECG changes over time is usual.

In clinically evident myocarditis, the ECG demonstrates symmetrically inverted T waves in most of the standard limb leads and in the lateral precordial leads (Fig. 176-14*B*). When the specialized conducting system is involved, bundle branch block or patterns of nonspecific intraventricular conduction defects may occur. Arrythmias are common. Resolution of ECG changes often lags behind clinical resolution of myocarditis.

The ECG may be helpful in distinguishing types of cardiomyopathies (Chap. 192). In the hypertrophic cardiomyopathies, the most common ECG pattern is LVH and strain (Fig. 176-10). When asymmetric septal hypertrophy is present, abnormal septal depolarization may be indicated by the presence of deep abnormal Q waves in leads I, aVL, V_5, and/or V_6, and a tall initial R wave may be present in V_1. In the congestive cardiomyopathies, nonspecific intraventricular conduction abnormalities, indicated by broad, notched QRS complexes without a specific bundle branch block pattern, are common (Fig. 176-14*C*). Nonspecific ST-segment and T-wave abnormalities are almost universal in congestive cardiomyopathies. In the restrictive cardiomyopathies, intraventricular conduction defects, low-voltage QRS complexes, or loss of R-wave progression across the precordium may occur.

ECG ABNORMALITIES IN METABOLIC AND ELECTROLYTE DISTURBANCES The electrically active tissues of the heart are particularly sensitive to changes in the extracellular concentration of K^+, and dramatic ECG changes may accompany abrupt changes in $[K^+]$. The initial effect of acute *hyper*kalemia is the appearance of tall, peaked T waves (Fig. 176-15). As the severity of hyperkalemia increases, the QRS complex widens and blends into the tall, peaked T waves, P-wave voltage decreases and may disappear entirely, and the PR interval is prolonged. As these changes evolve, there is marked prolongation of the QRS complex (Fig. 176-15) with the evolution of continuity between the S wave and T wave, ultimately producing a sine wave configuration. This pattern is a very late and

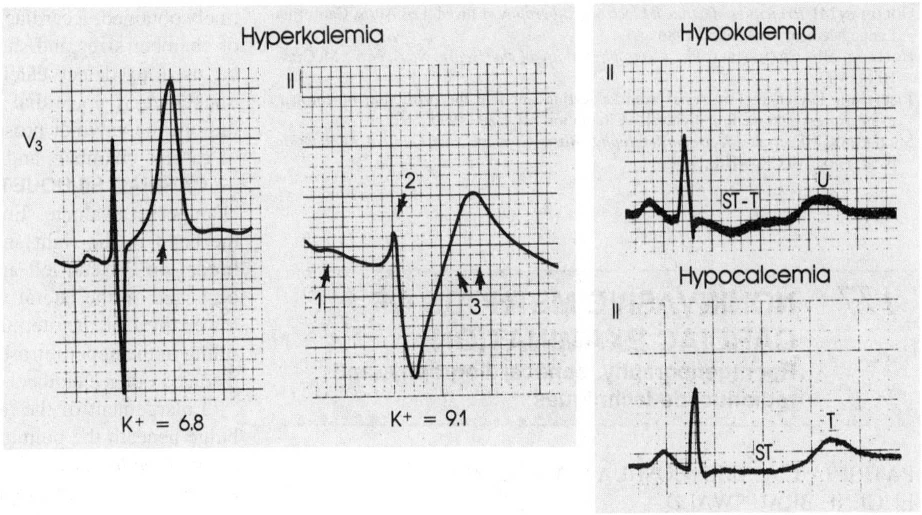

FIGURE 176-15 Electrolyte disturbances. *Hyperkalemia* ($K^+ = 6.8$) with tall, peaked T waves. Severe hyperkalemia ($K^+ = 9.1$) with (1) flattening of the P wave, and ↑ PR interval (1→2), (2) marked widening of the QRS complex (2→3), and (3) merging of the S wave into the T wave. *Hypokalemia* produces flat or inverted T waves with prominent U waves, causing prolonged "QU" interval, while hypocalcemia produces true prolongation of the ST segment with marked QT prolongation.

ominous manifestation of hyperkalemia. Equally dangerous is the occurrence of severe *hypo*kalemia, which also produces characteristic ECG changes. Instead of the tall, peaked T waves of hyperkalemia, hypokalemia produces a flattening or inversion of the T wave with concomitant prominence of the U wave. In its fully developed state, the ECG gives the appearance of a very long QT interval. Careful analysis reveals that the QT interval is not so prolonged, and the U wave has assumed the appearance of the T wave (Fig. 176-15). Thus, the major prolongation is a "QU" prolongation. This ECG manifestation of hypokalemia may forewarn of the occurrence of serious ventricular arrhythmias, especially in the presence of digitalis or class IA antiarrythmic drugs such as quinidine. One must be careful to differentiate the ECG effects of hypo*calcemia* from hypo*kalemia*. Whereas hypokalemia may produce the appearance of a long ST segment and late T wave because of flattening of the T wave and prominence of the U wave, hypocalcemia does, in fact, produce prolongation of the ST segment with a late T wave (Fig. 176-15). Hypocalcemia is not as immediately ominous as hypokalemia in regard to potentially serious ventricular arrhythmias. Most of the other electrolyte imbalances produce ECG changes too nonspecific to be clinically useful.

Abnormalities of metabolism, such as hyper- or hypothyroidism, Addison's disease, diabetic ketoacidosis, and infiltrative diseases, such as amyloidosis and hemochromatosis, all may produce ECG abnormalities which may be helpful in the recognition of the disease process but are often nonspecific.

Many drugs, especially the antiarrhythmics and psychotropics, can influence the ECG. The most common effects are on the AV junction (prolonged PR interval) and on repolarization (ST-T wave changes and prolonged QT intervals).

VECTORCARDIOGRAPHY

A vectorcardiogram (VCG) is a continuous loop representing the sequence of instantaneous electrical vectors in a two-dimensional plane (shown diagrammatically in Fig. 176-5*G*). This form of recording, requiring simultaneous voltage information from two leads, is achieved by recording one ECG lead on the vertical axis and replacing time by a second lead on the horizontal axis. The resulting loop is photographed on an oscilloscope screen. Most VCG systems today employ an XYZ lead system in which X is analogous to lead I (left-right), Y is analogous to lead aVF (superoinferior), and Z represents a lead in the anteroposterior orientation, most closely analogous to lead V_2. The XY plane records a vectorial loop in the frontal plane, projected on the hexaxial reference in Fig. 176-1*D*. The XZ plane records the horizontal loop in which the left-right orientation is plotted against the anteroposterior orientation on a reference system similar to that in Fig. 176-2*B*. In the YZ plane, the loop is in the sagittal orientation—the anteroposterior orientation (Z) plotted against the superoinferior orientation (Y). Recording in three planes provides information about spatial vectors, as in Fig. 176-5*F*. Loops consist of comma-shaped dots, the orientation of the comma indicating the direction of rotation, and the frequency of interruption providing a measurement of time. Closely grouped dots indicate a slow change in the magnitude and direction of the vector, while widely spread dots indicate rapid changes. Vectorial information of P waves, QRS complexes, ST segments, and T waves may be obtained.

The greatest value of the VCG today lies in the analysis of Q waves of uncertain significance and of certain intraventricular conduction abnormalities. When normal septal Q waves are absent in lead I or V_6, and no other evidence of septal infarction is present, the VCG may demonstrate either that the normal Q loop in the horizontal plane is absent, indicating a septal infarction or scarring, or conversely that the Q loop in the horizontal plane is morphologically normal but oriented directly anteriorly, accounting for the absence of the initial rightward forces. Similarly, the VCG can be helpful in assessing confusing initial forces or poor R-wave progression in the anterior precordial leads.

The VCG is particularly useful in identifying inferior wall myocardial infarctions. When the ECG is equivocal, the VCG may show the superior displacement of initial forces in the frontal plane and the clockwise rotation that is characteristic of inferior wall myocardial infarction. Furthermore, the difficulty in differentiating inferior wall infarctions from left anterior hemiblock on ECG, or recognizing their coexistence, may be aided by a VCG. In left anterior hemiblock, the initial forces are often normal, but there is superior displacement of the major portion of the frontal plane loop. However, the rotation is counterclockwise, in contrast to the clockwise rotation of inferior wall myocardial infarction. When the combination of inferior wall myocardial infarction and left anterior hemiblock is present, the infarction may be masked on the ECG; but the VCG may show the distinctly abnormal superiorly displaced initial forces of inferior wall myocardial infarction plus the counterclockwise rotation in the frontal plane characteristic of left anterior hemiblock.

REFERENCES

Castellanos A, Myerburg RJ: The resting electrocardiogram, in *The Heart*, 7th ed, JW Hurst et al (eds). New York, McGraw-Hill, 1990, p 265

Cooksey JD et al: *Clinical Vectorcardiography and Electrocardiography*, 2d ed. Chicago, Year Book, 1977

Fisch C (ed): *Cardiovascular Clinics*, vol 5, no 3: *Complex Electrocardiography I*. Philadelphia, Davis, 1973

———: Electrocardiography and vectorcardiography, in *Heart Disease*, 3d ed, E Braunwald (ed). Philadelphia, Saunders, 1988, p 180

GOLDMAN MJ: *Principles of Clinical Electrocardiography*, 12th ed. Los Altos, California, Lange Medical Publishers, 1986

HOFFMAN BF, CRANEFIELD PF: *Electrophysiology of the Heart*. New York, McGraw-Hill, 1960

JOSEPHSON RA et al: Can serial exercise testing improve the prediction of coronary events in asymptomatic individuals? Circulation 81; 1:20, 1990

SILVERMAN ME et al: *Electrocardiography: Basic Concepts and Clinical Application*. New York, McGraw-Hill, 1983

177 NONINVASIVE METHODS OF CARDIAC EXAMINATION
Roentgenography, echocardiography, and radionuclide techniques

PATRICIA C. COME / JOSHUA WYNNE / EUGENE BRAUNWALD

ROENTGENOGRAPHY

The chest roentgenogram provides pathoanatomic information about the size and configuration of the heart and great vessels and pathophysiologic information about pulmonary arterial and venous pressures and flow. Chamber dilatation usually produces changes in cardiac size and contour. Myocardial hypertrophy, in contrast, often results in wall thickening at the expense of cavity size, producing only a slight alteration of the cardiac silhouette. Although standard 6-ft posteroanterior (PA) and lateral chest roentgenograms are routinely obtained, a cardiac series (Fig. 177-1) permits better assessment of chamber sizes and shapes. Image-intensification fluoroscopy may be used to detect calcification, recognize pericardial effusion or thickening if epicardial fat can be identified, assess movement of radiopaque valvular prostheses, or define further the size and motion of cardiac chambers and great vessels.

CARDIAC SILHOUETTE The *right atrium* is the most difficult chamber to evaluate. Enlargement, however, may cause bulging of the heart to the right and an increased curvature of the right heart border on PA and left anterior oblique views. The *right ventricle* is best seen on the lateral view, where its anterior wall lies behind the lower third of the sternum. As it enlarges, it displaces lung tissue, filling in the upper retrosternal space. Further dilatation may passively displace other chambers, particularly the left ventricle.

Enlargement of the *left atrial appendage* may be suspected by a bulge beneath the pulmonary artery on the PA film. Dilatation of the body of the *left atrium* is best demonstrated by posterior displacement of the barium-filled esophagus in the lateral or right anterior oblique view. As the left atrium dilates further, its right border contacts right lung posteriorly, forming a second border or "double density" adjacent to the right atrial wall. The left bronchus may be displaced posteriorly and superiorly. The *left ventricle* enlarges inferiorly, posteriorly, and to the left, often increasing the cardiothoracic ratio (maximal cardiac diameter divided by maximal internal thoracic diameter, normally less than 0.50). The chest roentgenogram is a useful screening or initial test, but other imaging techniques, such as echocardiography, provide more definitive assessment of individual cardiac chambers.

PULMONARY VASCULATURE Since pulmonary vessel size is proportional to flow, vessels normally taper from central to peripheral

FIGURE 177-1 Posteroanterior (*A,B*), lateral (*C,D*), right anterior oblique (*E,F*), and left anterior oblique (*G,H*) views of the heart, demonstrating the positions of the cardiac chambers, valves, and interatrial and interventricular septa. AV = azygos vein; SVC = superior vena cava; RA = right atrium; IVC = inferior vena cava; TV = tricuspid valve; RV = right ventricle; MPA = main pulmonary artery; RPA = right pulmonary artery; LPA = left pulmonary artery; AO = aorta; LA = left atrium; LAA = left atrial appendage; LV = left ventricle; MV = mitral valve; IVS = interventricular septum; IAS = interatrial septum; RAA = right atrial appendage. [*From PC Come (ed), Diagnostic Cardiology. Reprinted with permission of Robert E. Dinsmore, M.D., and J.B. Lippincott Company.*]

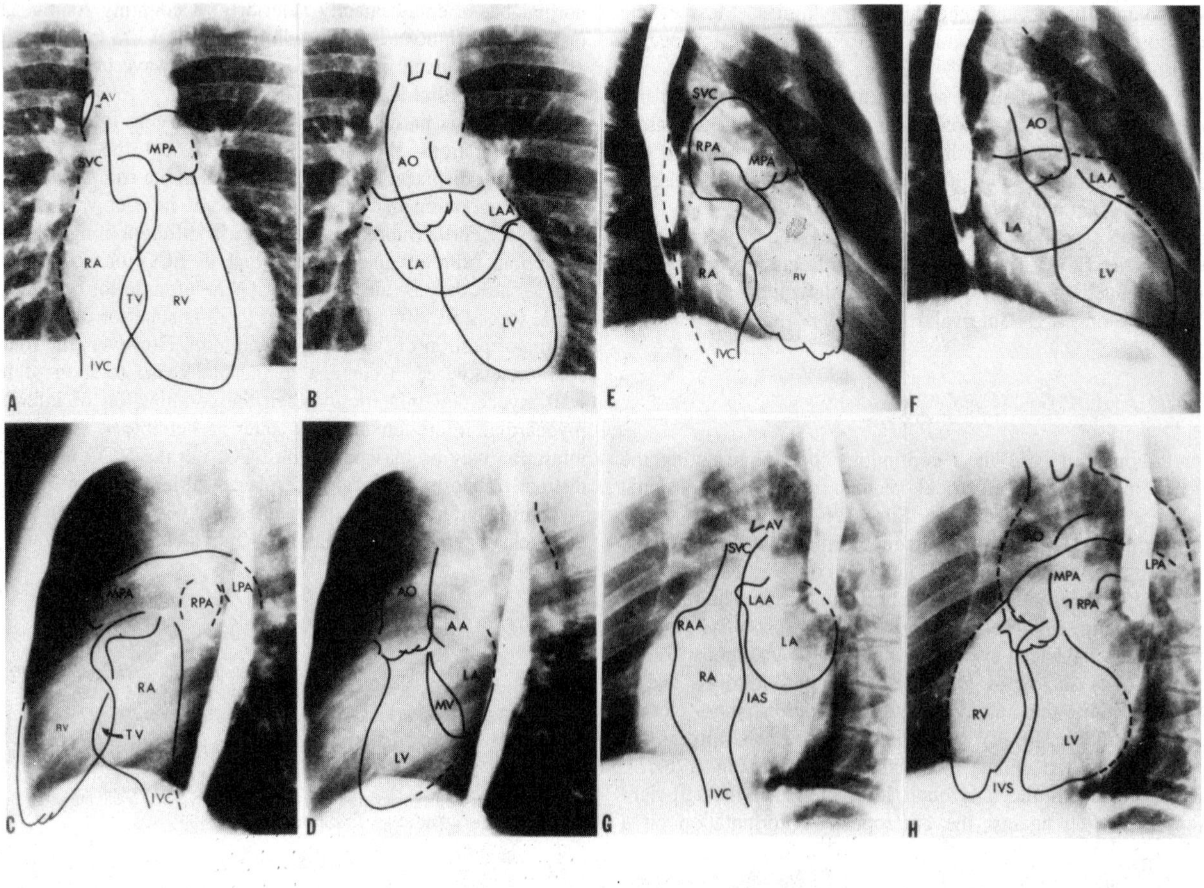

and from dependent to nondependent portions of the lungs. Increased flow, as with left-to-right shunts, results in enlargement and tortuosity of all vessels. Regional or global reduction of flow, due to pulmonary emboli, emphysematous blebs, or a right-to-left shunt, results in decreased vessel caliber.

Increases in pulmonary venous pressure produce perivascular edema in the dependent portions of the lungs, causing loss of vessel wall definition and redistribution of flow to nondependent areas. Further increases cause interstitial edema, with peribronchial cuffing, perihilar and peripheral lung haziness, and linear densities (Kerley B lines) perpendicular to the pleura. They represent fluid collection in the dependent interlobular septa. Alveolar pulmonary edema, with air bronchograms, may ultimately develop. There may be considerable temporal delay between hemodynamic changes and roentgenographic findings.

Pulmonary artery hypertension produces dilatation of the main pulmonary artery and its central branches. When associated with conditions increasing pulmonary arteriolar resistance, such as primary pulmonary hypertension, the distal pulmonary arteries often appear small ("pruned").

SPECIALIZED RADIOGRAPHIC METHODS *Digital subtraction angiography* (DSA) uses computer processing to digitize high-resolution fluoroscopic images. An image of the region of interest is subtracted from images obtained following intravenous, intracardiac, or intraarterial injection of contrast medium. Elimination of radiographic densities resulting from soft tissues and bone permits excellent definition of vascular structures using a concentration of contrast medium lower than that necessary for routine angiography. Vascular applications include recognition of vascular tumors, pulmonary emboli, and abnormalities of the aorta or of peripheral, cerebral, and renal arteries. Study of the heart permits assessment of ventricular function, intracardiac shunts, other congenital abnormalities, and bypass graft patency.

Computed tomography, *magnetic resonance imaging*, and *positron emission tomography* are also used to provide information about the heart and vessels. These techniques are discussed in Chap. 178.

ECHOCARDIOGRAPHY

Echocardiography uses ultrasound to image the heart and great vessels. A transducer containing a piezoelectric crystal, which interconverts electrical and mechanical (i.e., sound) energy, functions both as the transmitter of sound and as the receiver of reflected waves. Three types of studies are performed: M-mode, two-dimensional, and Doppler. In *M-mode echocardiography*, a single transducer, emitting 1000 to 2000 pulses per second along a single line, provides an "ice-pick" view of the heart, with excellent *temporal* resolution. When beam direction is changed, the heart can be scanned from the ventricles to the aorta and left atrium (Fig. 177-2). *Two-dimensional echocardiography* (Figs. 177-3 and 177-4) produces an image in two distance dimensions by steering the sound beam through an arc of up to 90° some 30 times per second. It provides excellent *spatial* resolution, permitting analysis of structural movement in real time from multiple transducer positions on the chest and upper abdomen. It is also possible to obtain imaging and Doppler echocardiographic studies via the esophagus, using a probe mounted at the tip of a flexible gastroscope. Transesophageal echocardiography appears most valuable in the assessment of prosthetic mitral valve function and in the detection of left atrial thrombus, aortic dissection, and complications of infective endocarditis.

Doppler echocardiography (Fig. 177-5) detects blood flow velocity and turbulence. When sound encounters moving red blood cells, the frequency of its reflected signal is altered. The magnitude of the change *(Doppler shift)* indicates the velocity V of blood flow with respect to the sound beam:

$$V = \frac{C \times (\text{Doppler shift})}{(2 \times \text{emitted frequency}) \cos \theta}$$

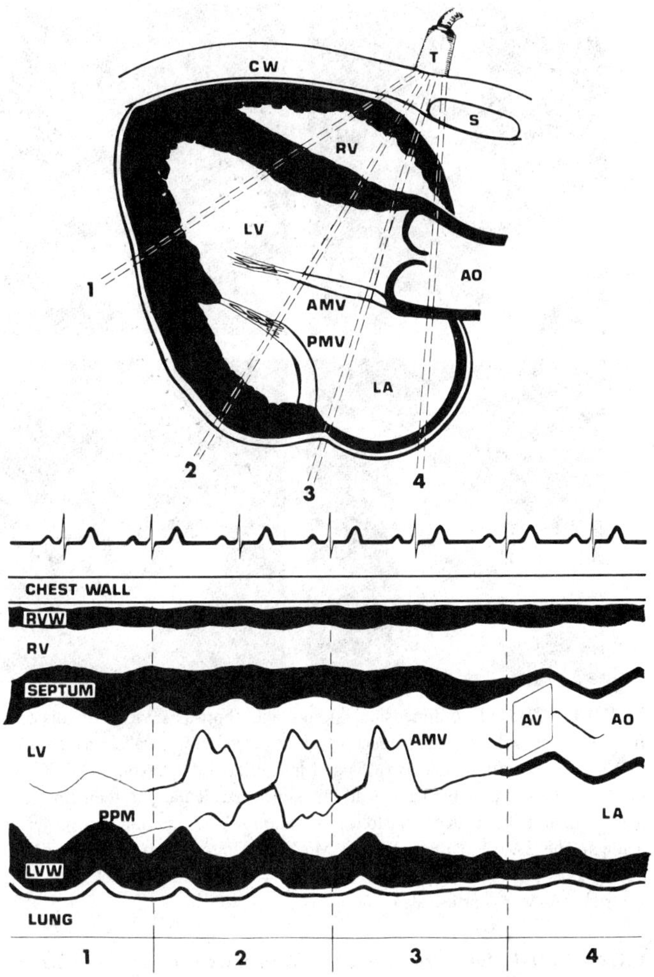

FIGURE 177-2 Schematic diagrams of an M-mode echocardiographic scan through a normal heart. A long-axis section of the heart is depicted in the upper diagram. The echocardiographic movement patterns that arise from the corresponding anatomic structures are illustrated in the bottom diagram. CW = chest wall; T = echocardiographic transducer, S = sternum; RV = right ventricle; LV = left ventricle; AO = aortic root; AMV = anterior mitral leaflet; PMV = posterior mitral leaflet; LA = left atrium; RVW = right ventricular wall; AV = aortic valve; PPM = posterior papillary muscle; LVW = left ventricular wall. [*From PC Come, Echocardiography in diagnosis and management of cardiovascular disease, Compr Ther 6(5):58, 1980. Courtesy of The Laux Company, Inc., Ayer, MA.*]

where C is the speed of sound in tissue, and θ is the angle between the Doppler beam and the mean axis of blood flow. An upward shift (increased frequency of the reflected sound) indicates blood motion toward the transducer and a downward shift, motion away. There are several types of Doppler studies, all of which can be performed using a single probe. Pulsed Doppler echocardiography, which uses a single crystal to assess flow velocity and turbulence within operator-selected areas of interest in the heart and great vessels, permits excellent spatial localization of flow disturbances resulting from valvular stenosis and regurgitation and from shunts. Quantitation of high-flow velocity requires a continuous wave transducer with two separate, adjacent crystals, one that continuously transmits sound and one that continuously receives reflected sound. Since continuous wave transducers cannot spatially localize flow disturbances, optimal assessment of flow within the heart and vessels generally requires both pulsed and continuous wave technology. Pressure gradients (P) across restrictive orifices such as cardiac valves can be calculated using the modified Bernoulli equation, $P = 4V^2$, where P is the pressure gradient in mmHg and V the velocity in m/s. Doppler color flow imaging is a complicated, combined imaging and Doppler technique in which blood flow direction, relative velocity, and turbulence are

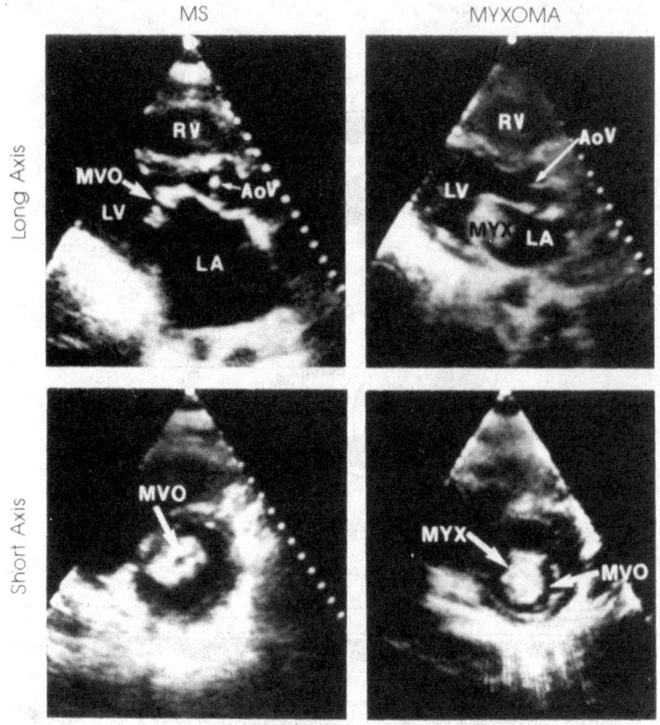

FIGURE 177-3 Two-dimensional long- and short-axis views in diastole from patients with marked reduction of effective mitral valve orifice area (MVO) due to mitral stenosis (MS) and left atrial (LA) myxoma (MYX). In the MS patient, the valve leaflets are thickened, particularly at their tips, and there is markedly reduced diastolic separation of the anterior and posterior leaflets. The LA is enlarged. The LA MYX is seen to prolapse into the MVO during diastole, causing obstruction. RV = right ventricle; LV = left ventricle; AoV = aortic valve.

depicted by various colors superimposed upon a two-dimensional image of the heart. The spatial information permits easier detection of shunts and of valvular regurgitation, especially of the periprosthetic type, and it may facilitate positioning of the sound beam for optimal pulsed and continuous wave Doppler interrogation of flow jets. Temporal resolution is limited by the low frame rate required for analysis. Combined Doppler and imaging techniques permit calculation of cardiac output. Unfortunately, not all patients can be successfully studied by echocardiography. Sound penetration may be suboptimal in many elderly, obese, and emphysematous patients.

VALVULAR HEART DISEASE Imaging echocardiography can detect abnormalities of valve thickness and movement responsible for stenosis and regurgitation. In addition, the heart's response to pressure or volume overload can be assessed in terms of chamber dilatation, hypertrophy, and wall movement. Doppler techniques permit evaluation of regurgitation and stenosis. (See also Chap. 188.)

Mitral stenosis The echocardiographic appearance of a restricted valve opening, due to leaflet thickening and commissural fusion, and of shortened, thickened chordae is virtually diagnostic of rheumatic deformity (Fig. 177-3, left). Planimetry of the mitral area in the diastolic short axis view and evaluation of the rate of falloff of the estimated transmitral diastolic pressure gradient by Doppler permit quite reliable estimation of valve area. Using the Doppler technique, mitral valve area (MVA) in square centimeters can be estimated with the equation, MVA = 220 divided by duration of time (in milliseconds) necessary for the peak diastolic pressure gradient to decrease by 50 percent. Other causes of inflow obstruction, such as atrial myxoma (Fig. 177-3, right) or thrombus, massive annular calcification, supravalvular ring, cor triatriatum, and parachute mitral valve may also be detected.

Mitral regurgitation Systolic mitral competence depends upon normal function of the mitral leaflets and their supporting structures, including the annulus, chordae tendineae, papillary muscles, and surrounding myocardium. Two-dimensional techniques are preferable

FIGURE 177-4 Long-axis parasternal views of the left ventricle in diastole and systole in a normal individual and in patients with dilated cardiomyopathy (CM) and hypertrophic cardiomyopathy (HCM). Normal diastolic wall thicknesses and normal systolic wall thickening and excursion are illustrated in the left panels. In the patient with dilated CM, left ventricular (LV) and left atrial (LA) diameters are increased, and there is markedly reduced systolic thickening and excursion of the septum (SEP) and posterior wall (PW). In the patient with HCM, the SEP is abnormally thick and highly echogenic. The LV cavity is small in diastole and almost disappears during systolic contraction. RV = right ventricle; MV = mitral valve; AoV = aortic valve.

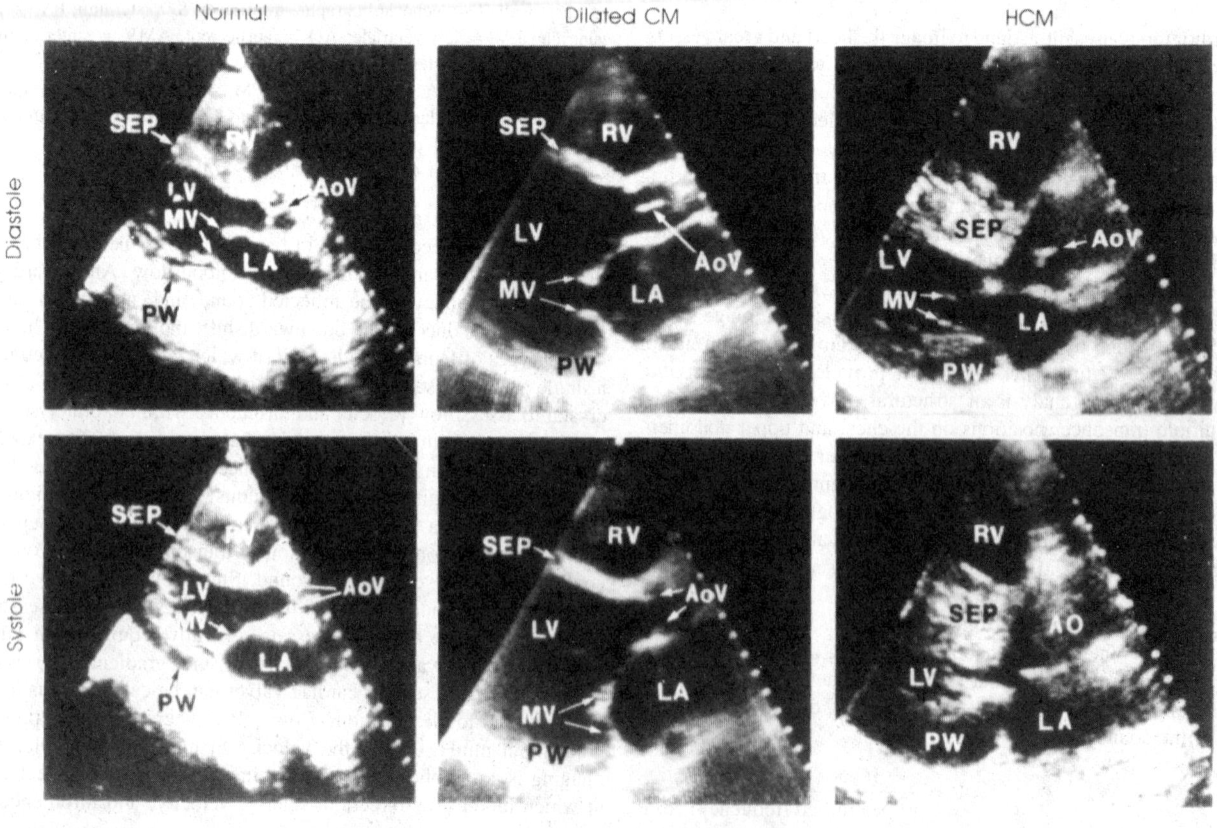

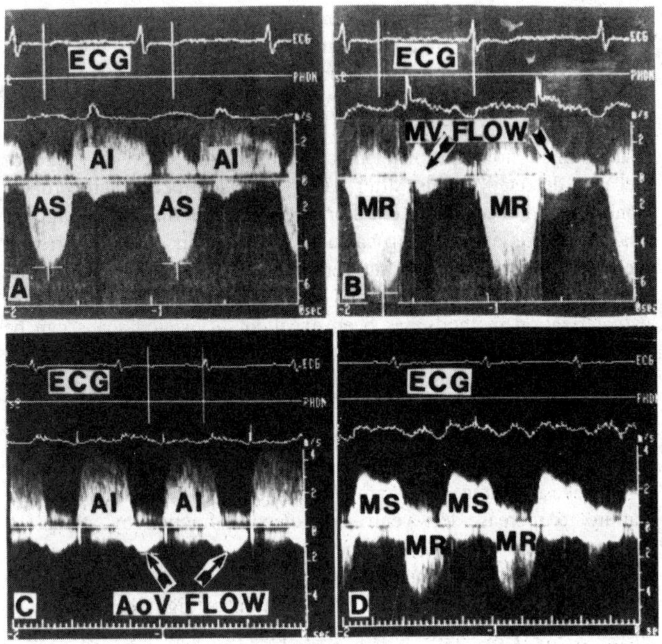

FIGURE 177-5 Continuous wave Doppler studies, performed with the probe positioned at the apex, from one patient (*A*, *B*) with aortic stenosis (AS), aortic insufficiency (AI), and mitral regurgitation (MR) and from another patient (*C*, *D*) with mital stenosis (MS), severe MR, and AI. Flow away from the transducer, in the AS and MR jets, is depicted below the center (zero flow) line, while flow toward the transducer, in the AI and MS jets, is depicted above the center line. Flow velocity (V) in meters per second is given on the right side of each panel. As expected from knowledge of points of crossover between aortic, left ventricular, and left atrial pressures, the AS signal is shorter in duration than the MR signal and has a lower velocity. The AI signal is of longer duration than the MS signal. Instantaneous pressure gradients (P) across the valves can be calculated using the equation, $P = 4V^2$. Peak V of 5.1 m/s in the AS jet indicates a peak left ventricular to aortic P of 104 mmHg, while the peak V of 6.8 m/s in the MR jet indicates a left ventricular to left atrial systolic P of 185 mmHg. Peak aortic to left ventricular diastolic P in the AI jet is 81 mmHg, and peak left atrial to left ventricular P in the MS jet is 40 mmHg. Mean gradient, calculated using an off-line computer system, in the MS jet was markedly elevated at 26 mmHg.

to M-mode in recognizing etiologies of mitral regurgitation, which include rheumatic disease, prolapse, flail leaflets resulting from chordal or papillary muscle rupture, annular calcification, atrioventricular canal defects, myxomas, endocarditis, hypertrophic cardiomyopathy, and ventricular dysfunction. Doppler mapping provides a gross estimate of the severity of regurgitation.

Aortic stenosis Subvalvular, valvular, and supravalvular obstruction can generally be detected by two-dimensional echocardiography. Systolic leaflet doming and an unusual number or size of cusps (two in a bicuspid valve) suggest congenital valve disease. Acquired fibrosis and calcification cause valve thickening. Normal leaflet separation excludes critical acquired aortic stenosis, but decreased separation is not specific for stenosis. Doppler detection of high-flow velocity across the valve, corresponding to a high transvalvular gradient, supports stenosis. Lesser flow velocities do not, however, exclude stenosis because both reduced stroke volume and inability to position the Doppler beam parallel to flow may appreciably decrease measured velocities. If velocity can be reliably measured, aortic valve area (AVA) can be quantitated using a continuity equation which assumes equal volume flow across the aortic valve and left ventricular (LV) outflow tract:

$$\text{AVA} = \frac{\text{(LV outflow tract area)(LV outflow tract velocity)}}{\text{velocity in aortic stenotic jet}}$$

Aortic regurgitation Aortic root dilatation and dissection can be distinguished from valve abnormalities causing regurgitation, including congenital disease, sclerosis, endocarditis, prolapse, and flail cusps. Two-dimensional techniques best define structural pathology, but M-mode techniques more readily detect both diastolic vibrations of the anterior mitral leaflet, a very sensitive sign of aortic regurgitation, and premature mitral closure, produced by the marked elevation of left ventricular diastolic pressure which may accompany severe, acute regurgitation. The presence and spatial extent of regurgitation is evaluated by Doppler study.

Tricuspid and pulmonary valve disease Two-dimensional scanning has improved visualization of right-sided valves. Changes in structure and movement may permit detection of rheumatic deformity, Ebstein's malformation, prolapse, flail cusps, endocarditis, congenital dysplasia, and thickening due to carcinoid, amyloid, Loeffler's endocarditis, or endocardial fibrosis. Systolic doming of the pulmonic valve is characteristic of pulmonic stenosis. Stenosis and regurgitation are assessed by Doppler techniques. The flow velocity in a tricuspid regurgitant jet can be used to estimate right ventricular and pulmonary arterial systolic pressures, permitting identification of pulmonary hypertension.

Prosthetic valves Mechanical prostheses are difficult to evaluate, because their intrinsically high echogenicity interferes with the recognition of vegetations and thrombi. Abnormal timing of valve opening and closure, best assessed using combined phonocardiography and M-mode techniques, and abnormalities on Doppler study may suggest dysfunction, but angiography and hemodynamic assessment are often necessary for full evaluation. Abnormalities of bioprostheses, including fibrosis, calcification, vegetations, and tears, are more easily recognized.

Endocarditis Valvular vegetations, characterized by masses of shaggy-appearing echoes, are evident in over half of patients with endocarditis. While their detection is associated with an increased risk of complications, many patients recover uneventfully with antibiotic therapy alone. (See also Chap. 90.)

Left ventricle M-mode echocardiography is widely used to measure left ventricular size, wall thickness, and function. The rate of wall thinning in diastole may permit assessment of diastolic function, and the percentage of shortening of the minor axis, normally greater than 28 percent, and the mean velocity of circumferential fiber shortening are useful measurements of systolic performance. These indexes of systolic performance are influenced, however, by preload and afterload as well as by myocardial contractility. Analyses of end-systolic pressure-dimension relations, which are independent of preload and incorporate afterload, provide better information regarding contractile function. Estimates of global ventricular performance, based on ice-pick M-mode views, are useful, however, only when ventricular shape is normal and systolic movement relatively symmetric in extent and timing. Two-dimensional echocardiography, which images the ventricle in a number of different planes, improves assessment of volumes and function, particularly in patients with asymmetric contraction resulting from ischemic heart disease. The left ventricular apex, the most common site of wall movement abnormalities and thrombi, can be adequately visualized only by two-dimensional techniques.

Echocardiography permits recognition of *cardiomyopathy* and classification into dilated, hypertrophic, and restrictive-obliterative types (Fig. 177-4). In dilated cardiomyopathy, both ventricles are generally enlarged and poorly contracting, and wall thicknesses are normal or only slightly increased. In contrast, appreciable ventricular hypertrophy, usually involving the septum asymmetrically, small ventricular size, enhanced systolic performance and impaired diastolic relaxation, characterize hypertrophic cardiomyopathy. Systolic anterior movement of the mitral valve to abut the septum and partial midsystolic closure of the aortic valve correlate with dynamic obstruction. Increased wall thickness also characterizes infiltrative disorders. In amyloidosis, the thick walls often appear "speckled" and there is diminished voltage on electrocardiogram (ECG).

Pericardial effusion Echocardiography can detect effusions as small as 15 to 20 mL, while certain findings, such as diastolic compression of the right atrium and ventricle, may suggest tamponade.

Cardiac masses Most masses involving the heart and pericardium are easily recognized. They include myxomas (Fig. 177-3), other primary and secondary tumors, and thrombi. The left atrium and its appendage are best studied by transesophageal echocardiography.

Congenital heart disease Since valvular abnormalities and relationships of atria, valves, ventricles, and great vessels can easily be recognized by two-dimensional echocardiography, this technique has revolutionized the diagnosis of congenital heart disease. Contrast and Doppler echocardiography, especially color flow mapping, facilitate detection of shunts and of valvular stenosis and regurgitation.

RADIONUCLIDE IMAGING OF THE HEART

There are four major clinical indications for radionuclide study of the heart: (1) assessment of systolic and diastolic ventricular function using radionuclide ventriculography; (2) identification and quantification of intracardiac shunts using radioangiocardiography; (3) assessment of myocardial perfusion using ionic tracers, principally thallium 201; and (4) detection of acute myocardial infarction with infarct-avid radionuclides.

VENTRICULAR PERFORMANCE Radionuclide ventriculography (RVG) uses a radioactive intravascular indicator to delineate heart chambers and great vessels (Fig. 177-6). The radionuclide, usually technetium 99m, is generally attached to red blood cells. RVGs may be performed using two different methods. In the *first-pass* technique, radiotracer is injected intravenously, and a scintillation camera tracks its transit through the right heart, lungs, and left heart. In the *equilibrium*, or *gated, method,* counts are recorded from several hundred cardiac cycles following uniform distribution of radiotracer throughout the blood pool. The scintigraphic information in each cycle is divided into multiple frames (often 30 or more), using the ECG as a timing reference. Counts from corresponding frames of each cycle are then summed by computer to provide images of the spatial distribution and density of counts over time. Images are generally obtained in at least two views [anterior and left anterior oblique (LAO)]. Gated scans are frequently obtained after first-pass scans, since no additional injection of radionuclide is required. Because detected counts, after background subtraction, are proportional to blood volume, equilibrium studies permit estimation of chamber volumes, enabling calculation of left and right ventricular ejection fractions, left-to-right ventricular stroke volume ratios, and rates of ventricular ejection and filling. Agreement with standard catheterization methods has been excellent. Repeated scans can be obtained up to 20 h after injection, permitting assessment of the effects of interventions, such as exercise and medications, on ventricular performance.

FIGURE 177-6 End-diastolic and end-systolic gated blood pool images from a normal individual (with estimated left and right ventricular ejection fractions of 69 and 45 percent, respectively) and from a patient with idiopathic dilated cardiomyopathy and marked, global reduction of left ventricular systolic function (left ventricular ejection fraction of 23 percent). In the patient with cardiomyopathy, there is very little change in left ventricular cavity size or count density from diastole to systole. The right ventricle, however, shows normal function, with an ejection fraction of 57 percent. RV = right ventricle; LV = left ventricle.

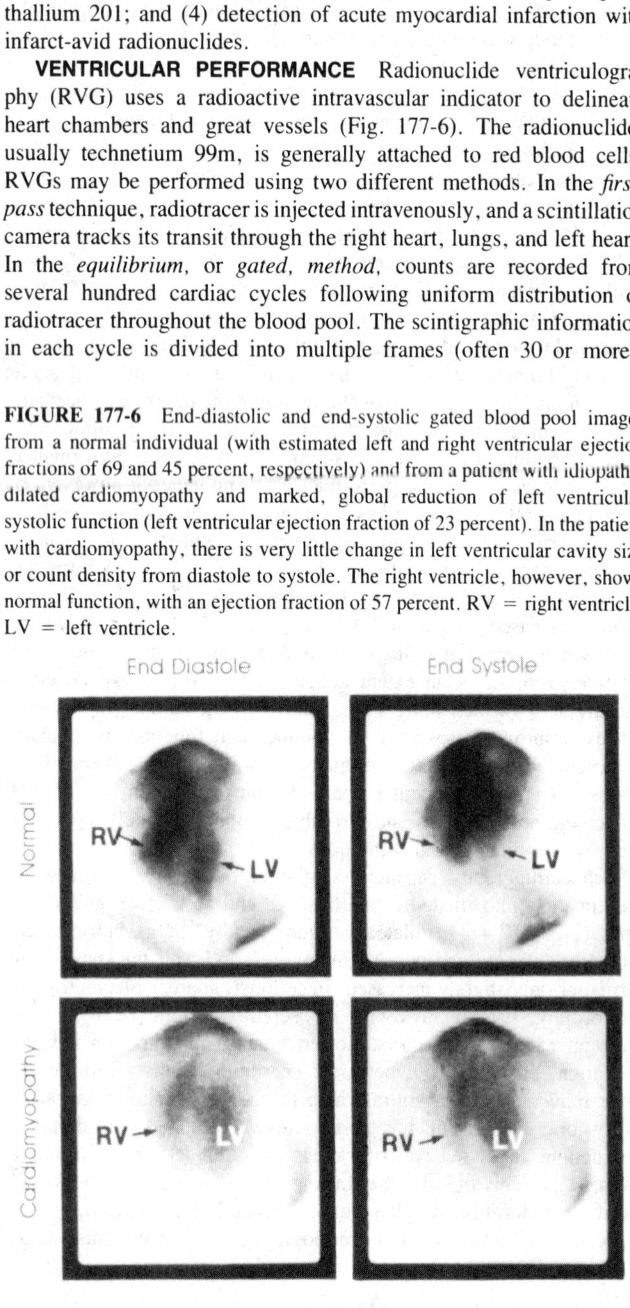

RVG may be used to detect patients with chronic ischemic heart disease. Since resting function may be normal, exercise is often used to provoke ischemia. Scans are obtained at rest and at peak exercise. Failure to increase left ventricular ejection fraction by at least 5 percent and development of one or more regional wall movement abnormalities have a sensitivity and specificity of approximately 90 and 60 percent, respectively, for detection of significant coronary disease. The test is most helpful in patients with an intermediate pretest probability of disease. Low resting ejection fractions after acute infarction have been correlated with increased short- and long-term morbidity and mortality. Mitral regurgitation, septal rupture, and aneurysms resulting from infarction may also be detected. RVG can assess systolic and diastolic function in patients with cardiomyopathy (Fig. 177-6) or volume overload. A reduced resting ejection fraction correlates with a poor prognosis in patients with mitral or aortic regurgitation, even after valve replacement. The added value of exercise RVG in detecting reduced myocardial reserve due to volume overload remains controversial. Thrombi and other tumors may be recognized, but RVG is less sensitive than echocardiography.

SHUNT SCINTIGRAPHY Assessment of left-to-right shunts utilizes a modification of the first-pass RVG in which the "region of interest" is focused over an area of lung. Following rapid injection of radiotracer into a large vein, usually the external jugular, the pulmonary time-activity curve is recorded by a gamma camera-computer system. Normally, counts increase sharply as the bolus reaches the lung underlying the detector. Following peak activity, there is a smooth descent and a later, smaller increase in counts representing normal recirculation of the radiotracer following systemic circulation. Left-to-right shunts cause premature interruption of the descent, due to early reappearance of radioactivity within the lung. Computer analysis of the areas under the curve permits reliable determination of the ratio of pulmonic-to-systemic blood flow. Right-to-left shunts may also be recognized and quantified.

MYOCARDIAL PERFUSION IMAGING Certain radiolabeled monovalent cations, especially the potassium analogue thallium 201 (half-life of 72 h), are widely used to assess myocardial perfusion since their active uptake by normal myocardial cells is proportional to regional blood flow. Areas of myocardial necrosis, fibrosis, and ischemia show reduced thallium accumulation ("cold spots") on images obtained soon after injection. Following its initial accumulation within cells, however, thallium 201 continues to exchange with the systemic pool. After several hours, all viable myocardial cells with intact membrane function will contain nearly equal concentrations.

Thallium 201 scintigraphy is most commonly used to detect exercise-induced ischemia (Fig. 177-7). Thallium is injected intravenously at peak exercise, and images are obtained in several projections 5 to 10 min later. Normal scans show relatively homogeneous distribution of activity, while those of patients with infarction or ischemia typically demonstrate one or more "cold spots." Due to continued exchange of thallium between viable cells and the systemic pool, however, initial defects due to ischemia "fill in" on repeat imaging several hours later. Areas of infarction demonstrate persistent reduction of uptake. Compared to routine exercise electrocardiogra-

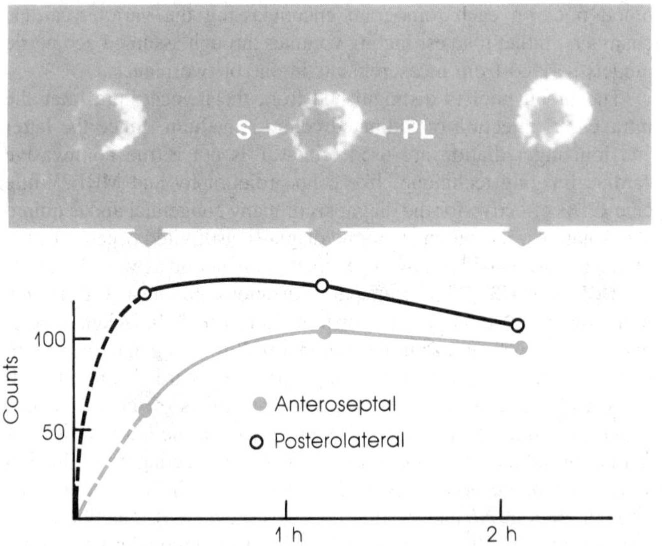

FIGURE 177-7 Serial thallium 201 scintigrams obtained in the 45° LAO projection in a patient undergoing exercise testing for evaluation of chest pain. The immediate postexercise image (*left*) demonstrates decreased perfusion of the septum. The 1- and 2-h delayed images (*middle and right*) demonstrate "filling in" of the defect, reflecting redistribution. The computer-derived time-activity curves (*bottom*) confirm the significant reduction in initial counts in the septum, relative to the posterolateral wall, and demonstrate near equalization of activity by 2 h. S = septum; PL = posterolateral wall. [*From PC Come (ed), Diagnostic Cardiology. Reprinted with permission of George A. Beller, M.D., and J.B. Lippincott Company.*]

phy, exercise thallium scintigraphy increases the sensitivity for detection of coronary disease from approximately 60 to 80 percent and increases specificity slightly from about 80 to 90 percent. It is most useful in patients with atypical chest pain in whom the exercise ECG is nondiagnostic or uninterpretable due to left bundle branch block, ventricular hypertrophy, or drug and electrolyte effects; in patients who fail to achieve 85 percent of predicted maximal heart rate; and in patients with a high likelihood of a false-positive exercise ECG study. Thallium scanning improves localization of ischemia and provides prognostic information, since the presence and number of redistributing defects correlate with the incidence of future cardiac events. Thallium scintigraphy has also been used to detect ischemia during pacing, dipyridamole-induced coronary vasodilatation, or spontaneous pain.

Thallium scanning does not distinguish new from old infarcts and is less accurate than serum enzyme analysis in detecting acute necrosis. It does, however, offer prognostic information. Patients with smaller defects have better survival rates. On submaximal exercise thallium tests following infarction, the presence of multiple or redistributing defects or increased lung uptake of thallium (probably representing transudation into the lung during periods of high pulmonary capillary pressure) identifies patients at higher risk for postinfarction morbidity and mortality.

Computed tomography using positron-emitting isotopes of potassium analogues permits quantitative assessment of radiotracer uptake. The short half-lives of such isotopes permit multiple studies over short periods of time, allowing assessment of changes in myocardial perfusion induced by therapeutic interventions.

POSITRON EMISSION TOMOGRAPHY See Chap. 178.

ACUTE INFARCT SCINTIGRAPHY Pyrophosphate appears to bind to calcium and organic macromolecules in irreversibly damaged myocardial cells. If coronary flow is sufficient for its delivery to necrotic myocardium (10 to 40 percent of normal flow is required), technetium 99m stannous pyrophosphate will bind there, producing an image with increased uptake ("hot spot"). Scans are most likely to be positive when injections are performed 48 to 72 h after suspected infarction, when the elevated creatine kinase activity has often returned to normal. The major clinical indication is the detection of acute infarction in those rare patients in whom traditional diagnostic methods cannot be interpreted or have provided equivocal results. Sensitivity and specificity for transmural infarcts are both about 90 percent. Uptake is often fainter and more poorly localized in subendocardial infarcts, and myocardial damage from causes other than coronary disease may result in a positive scan.

REFERENCES

Come PC (ed): *Diagnostic Cardiology: Noninvasive Imaging Techniques*. Philadelphia, Lippincott, 1985

Feigenbaum H: *Echocardiography*, 4th ed. Philadelphia, Lea & Febiger, 1986

Gerson MC (ed): *Cardiac Nuclear Medicine*. New York, McGraw-Hill, 1987

Hatle H, Angelsen B (eds): *Doppler Ultrasound in Cardiology: Physical Principles and Clinical Applications*, 2d ed. Philadelphia, Lea & Febiger, 1985

Holman BL: Nuclear cardiology, in *Heart Disease*, 3d ed, E Braunwald (ed). Philadelphia, Saunders, 1988, pp 83–139

Nanda NC (ed): *Doppler Echocardiography*. New York, Igaku-Shoin, 1985

Seward JB et al: Transesophageal echocardiography: Technique, anatomic correlations, implementation, and clinical applications. Mayo Clin Proc 63:649, 1988

178 NEW CARDIAC IMAGING TECHNIQUES

CHARLES B. HIGGINS

The strategy for applying cardiac imaging techniques for the diagnosis of cardiovascular disease is currently in transition. Echocardiography and cardiac scintigraphy (Chap. 177) have been used with increasing frequency during the past decade. Initially, these techniques were used for preliminary diagnosis but definitive therapy was generally based upon cardiac catheterization and angiography. Echocardiographic findings now have been accepted as sufficiently reliable and definitive for preoperative evaluation of some cardiac lesions. The emergence of the new noninvasive tomographic techniques, which include cine-computed tomography (cine-CT), magnetic resonance imaging (MRI), and positron emission tomography (PET), should encourage further the trend away from catheterization as a requisite for definitive therapy. The strength of cine-CT and MRI lies in their being comprehensive cardiac imaging techniques for evaluation of both cardiac anatomy and function. Because of the good contrast and spatial resolution and the capacity to image the entire heart in a tomographic fashion, quantitation of dimensions and function is achieved by cine-CT and MRI to a degree even exceeding that possible with cardiac angiography. Myocardial metabolism can now be assessed with positron emission tomography and magnetic resonance spectroscopy (MRS). Because these new techniques are still in the stage of development and evaluation, they are not available at many hospitals at the current time. The most readily available of the new techniques is MRI, but many of these instruments are still not fully adapted for cardiac diagnosis.

FAST COMPUTED TOMOGRAPHY (CINE-CT)

The unique design of the cine-CT scanner accomplishes the x-ray exposure for a complete tomogram in 50 ms. This short exposure time vitiates the degrading effects of cardiac motion. Moreover, tomograms at the same level can be obtained sequentially after a delay of only 8 ms and initiated by, as well as related precisely to, the time in the cardiac cycle. The multiple sequential images can all be obtained within a single cardiac cycle and thus provide a true real

TABLE 178-1 Principal indications for the new imaging modalities for cardiovascular diagnosis

Fast computed tomography
- *1* Thoracic aortic diseases
  - *a* Dissection
  - *b* Aneurysm
- *2* Pericardial disease
  - *a* Constrictive diseases
  - *b* Pericardial cysts, tumors
- *3* Paracardiac and intracardiac masses
  - *a* Primary tumors
  - *b* Secondary tumors
  - *c* Intracardiac thrombus
- *4* Coronary artery bypass graft patency
- *5* Complications of myocardial infarctions
  - *a* Left ventricular aneurysms
  - *b* Left ventricular thrombus
- *6* Analysis of ventricular function
  - *a* Global and regional left ventricular function (volume and wall thickness)
  - *b* Global right ventricular function (volume and wall thickness)
  - *c* Distribution of ventricular hypertrophy (assessment of hypertrophic cardiomyopathy)
  - *d* Ventricular function during interventions (exercise, drug interventions)
  - *e* Regional myocardial perfusion (under evaluation)

Magnetic resonance imaging
- *1* Thoracic aortic diseases
  - *a* Dissection
  - *b* Aneurysm
  - *c* Thrombus
  - *d* Aortitis
  - *e* Aortic hemorrhage
- *2* Pericardial diseases
  - *a* Constrictive disease
  - *b* Effusion, hemorrhagic vs. nonhemorrhagic
  - *c* Pericardial cyst, tumor
- *3* Paracardiac and intracardiac masses
  - *a* Primary tumors (myxoma, etc.)
  - *b* Secondary tumors (lung, mediastinal, metastatic)
  - *c* Intracardiac thrombus
- *4* Hypertrophic cardiomyopathy
  - *a* Variant forms (distribution of hypertrophy)
- *5* Complications of myocardial infarction
  - *a* Left ventricular aneurysm and pseudoaneurysm
  - *b* Left ventricular thrombus
- *6* Congenital heart disease
  - *a* Thoracic aortic anomalies
    - (*1*) Arch anomalies
    - (*2*) Coarctation
  - *b* Pulmonary arterial anomalies
    - (*1*) Pulmonary atresia (presence and size of central pulmonary arteries)
    - (*2*) Unilateral absence (atresia)
    - (*3*) Peripheral pulmonary stenoses
  - *c* Complex lesions
    - (*1*) Univentricular atrioventricular connections
    - (*2*) Volume of ventricles
    - (*3*) Presence and size of ventricular septum
    - (*4*) Status of extracardiac operative procedures; Fontan, Rastelli, Jatene, etc.
- *7* Analysis of ventricular function
  - *a* Ventricular volumes and mass
  - *b* Regional left ventricular function
  - *c* Detection and quantitation of valvular regurgitation

Positron emission tomography
- *1* Ischemic heart disease
  - *a* Recognition of viable myocardium
  - *b* Regional myocardial perfusion

time image; these images are laced together in a closed-loop cinematic format, termed a *cine-CT display*.

The tomograms are approximately 10 mm in thickness, so that 12 to 14 adjacent tomograms are required to encompass the average adult heart. Eight tomographic levels can be acquired during a single imaging sequence. The maximum number of images is 80 per sequence. When tomographic images encompassing the entire heart are required, cine-CT becomes a three-dimensional imaging technique. Consequently, highly accurate and reproducible measurements of ventricular volume are possible. Such precision is possible because chamber volumes can be measured directly by planimetry of the blood pool on each tomogram encompassing the various cardiac chambers, rather than estimating volumes through assumed geometric models derived from measurements in one or two planes.

The blood pool is distinguished from the myocardium after the intravenous injection of iodinated contrast medium. Since the latter and ionizing radiation are used, cine-CT is not a true noninvasive cardiac imaging technique, like echocardiography and MRI. While cine-CT is effective for the diagnosis of many congenital and acquired abnormalities, its role in anatomic diagnosis is limited because of the high diagnostic yield achieved by other totally noninvasive techniques.

INDICATIONS The principal indications for fast CT in the diagnosis of heart disease are given in Table 178-1. In ischemic heart disease, cine-CT demonstrates regional wall thinning and absence of systolic wall thickening at the site of prior myocardial infarction. It is most effective for demonstrating complications of infarction such as mural thrombi and true or false aneurysms of the left ventricle. A mural thrombus produces a filling defect projecting into the left ventricular blood pool; it is usually attached to the wall thinned by prior infarction. An aneurysm produces a regional evagination of the left ventricular wall in diastole and paradoxical motion during systole.

Cine-CT has a diagnostic accuracy of greater than 90 percent in the determination of patency of coronary arterial bypass grafts (Fig. 178-1). After intravenous injection of contrast medium, scans are exposed sequentially; the bypass grafts are opacified simultaneously with the ascending aorta. The technique is not usually capable of identifying stenosis of the graft or adequacy of blood flow through the graft, but there is hope that flow abnormalities might be detectable by analysis of contrast-dilution curves or contrast transit times in the grafts.

Cine-CT can be used in the evaluation of hypertrophic and congestive cardiomyopathies by quantitating ventricular volumes and myocardial mass. Because of the wide field of view and three-dimensional scope of this technique, it can depict the distribution of ventricular hypertrophy. This is particularly useful for definitive

FIGURE 178-1 Cine-CT images at the level of the proximal ascending aorta acquired on sequential heart beats during passage of contrast medium throughout the central cardiovascular structures. The bypass grafts to the right (arrow) and left anterior descending (arrow) coronary arteries opacify simultaneously with the ascending aorta (A). Images from upper left to lower right display sequential opacification from pulmonary artery to the aorta.

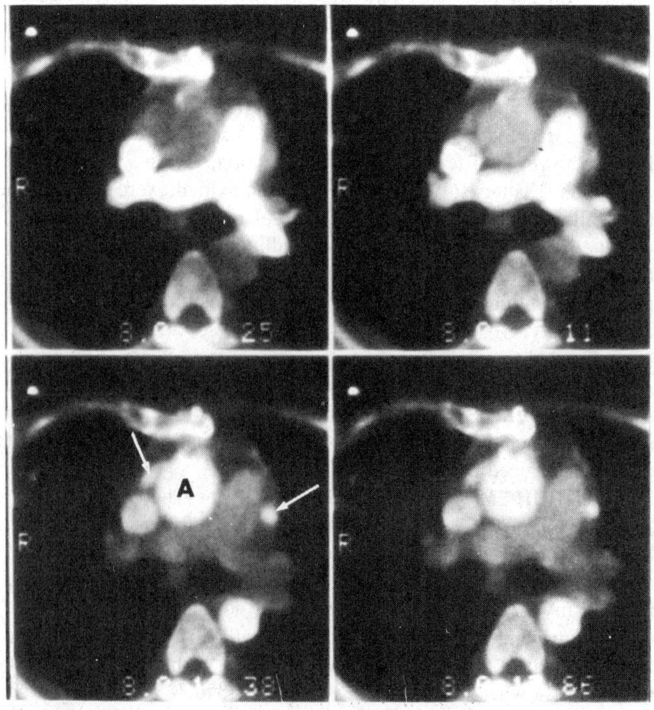

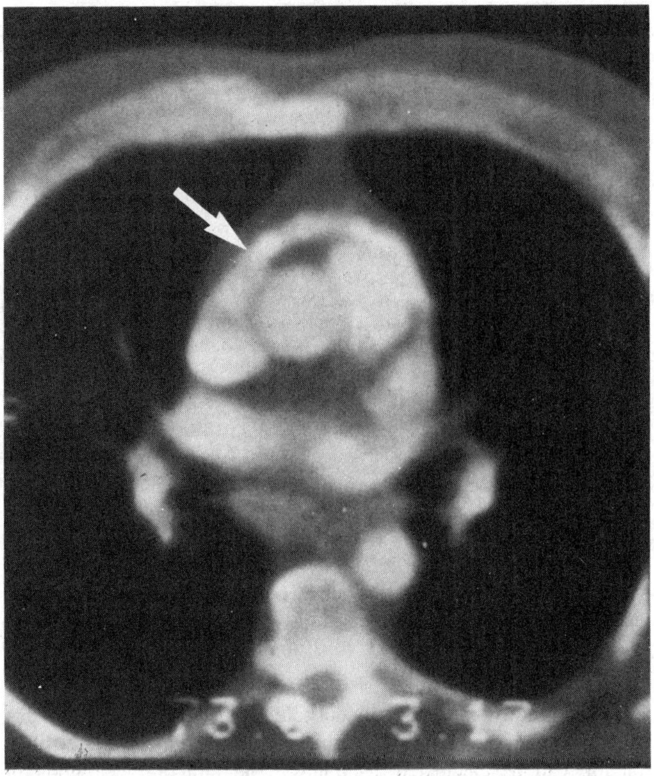

FIGURE 178-2 CT image shows calcification (arrow) and thickening of the pericardium in a patient with constrictive pericarditis.

assessment of the various forms of hypertrophic cardiomyopathy (Chap. 192).

The role of cine-CT in valvular heart disease is limited when compared to echo Doppler, with or without color flow mapping (Chap. 177) and cine-MRI. While both cine-MRI and echo Doppler can demonstrate the regurgitant flow and estimate its volume, cine-CT can evaluate only indirectly the severity of regurgitation (see below).

For the evaluation of pericardial disease, standard CT or cine-CT can be used to visualize and measure the thickness of the pericardium. The diagnosis of constrictive pericarditis is supported by demonstrating pericardial thickness exceeding 4 mm and, sometimes, calcification (Fig. 178-2). Other indirect signs of this disease shown by CT are: (1) dilated atria and inferior vena cava; (2) small ventricular chambers; and (3) a sigmoid-shaped ventricular septum. Pericardial thickening is also observed for a variable period of time after cardiac surgery and in patients experiencing the postpericardiotomy syndrome (Dressler's syndrome). CT can also be used to demonstrate pericardial effusions and pericardial masses. Standard CT has been used to evaluate intracardiac and paracardiac masses and to define possible cardiac involvement by mediastinal and lung tumors. The capability is considerably enhanced by cine-CT, although MRI seems to be superior to both standard and cine-CT for the evaluation of intra- and paracardiac masses.

The role of CT for the evaluation of congenital heart disease is very limited when considered in relation to the availability and success of echocardiography and MRI. While encouraging results have been shown for cine-CT, the results add little to echocardiography in the display of intracardiac anatomy and seem to be inferior to MRI for defining thoracic aortic and pulmonary arterial abnormalities.

Standard CT as well as cine-CT are effective for the diagnosis of diseases of the aorta (Chap. 197). The accuracy of CT for the diagnosis of aortic dissection exceeds 90 percent, and in some series it is nearly 100 percent. The definitive diagnosis of aortic dissection is based upon the demonstration of displacement of the inner portion of the aortic wall into the lumen (intimal flap) and/or differential enhancement of the true and false aortic channels.

EVALUATION OF CARDIAC FUNCTION WITH CINE-CT The fast CT scanners have the capability for the evaluation of cardiac function. The exposure time of 50 ms attained by cine-CT is adequate for quantitating many aspects of cardiac function. The three-dimensional nature of the technique permits precise measurement of chamber volume. Right and left ventricular volumes can be assessed with equal accuracy. A disparity in the stroke volumes of the two ventricles is caused by shunts and valvular regurgitation, which can be measured by cine-CT. Cine-CT can also be used for monitoring the effect of interventions on the right and left ventricles. Cine-CT performed at peak effort during supine bicycle exercise has been used to identify the *abnormal* response in patients with suspected coronary arterial stenoses. Most patients with severe lung disease and pulmonary arterial hypertension *also* display an abnormal response to exercise. Cine-CT has also been proposed as a method for measuring regional myocardial perfusion at rest and following interventions which increase myocardial blood flow, such as exercise and vasodilators. Perfusion is estimated by monitoring density values of the myocardium over time on CT scans exposed sequentially during peak opacification and wash-out of contrast medium from the myocardium.

MAGNETIC RESONANCE IMAGING (MRI)

This noninvasive technique uses no ionizing radiation or contrast medium for cardiovascular imaging. MR images are based upon the radiofrequency (RF) signal emitted by hydrogen nuclei of tissues after they have been perturbed by RF pulses in the presence of a strong magnetic field. The RF signal emitted has certain characteristics called *relaxation times:* T1 relaxation time (longitudinal magnetization) and T2 relaxation time (transverse magnetization). These properties are variable among tissues and are the predominant factors responsible for contrast among tissues. The signal intensity of one tissue compared to another (contrast) can be manipulated by varying the elapsed time between application of RF pulses (repetition time) and the time between an RF pulse and sampling the emitted signal (echo delay time).

The blood pool is generally a signal void, which provides high contrast between blood and the myocardial wall (Fig. 178-3). When the evaluation of cardiac structure is desired, the ECG gated spin-

FIGURE 178-3 ECG gated MR image acquired using the spin-echo technique in a short axis plane. There is increased thickness of the free wall of the right ventricle, indicating right ventricular hypertrophy. L = left ventricle; R = right ventricle. *(Reproduced with permission from CB Higgins, 1988.)*

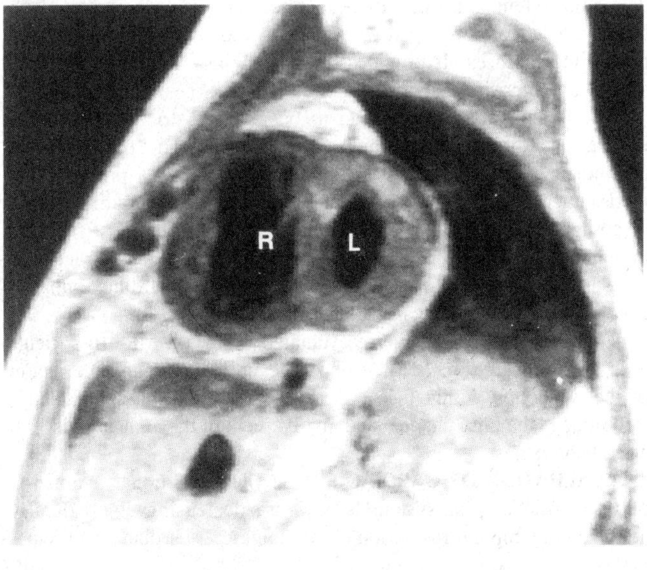

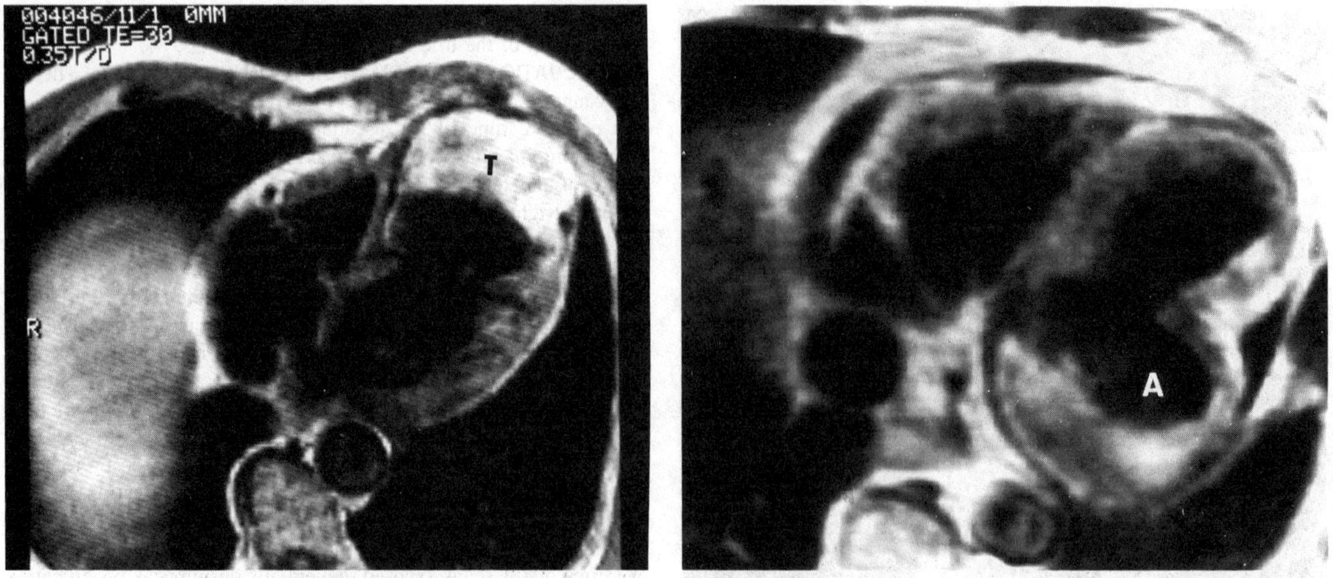

FIGURE 178-4 ECG gated spin-echo MR images acquired in transverse plane demonstrate complications of myocardial infarctions. True aneurysm and mural thrombus (T) (*left*). False aneurysm (A) (*right*). The ostium is nearly as wide as the fundus of the true aneurysm, while the ostium is smaller than the fundus for the false aneurysm.

echo technique, which provides static images with high signal-to-noise ratios, is used. When the primary goal is to assess cardiac contractile function, cine-MR imaging is used.

EVALUATION OF PATHOANATOMY MRI has been shown to be effective and useful in the diagnosis of a wide variety of cardiovascular abnormalities (Table 178-1). Patients with congenital heart disease are evaluated initially with the use of two-dimensional echocardiography, and in many congenital lesions MR is a secondary diagnostic technique in which the anatomy is displayed with the precision of angiography. In anomalies of the aortic arch and coarctation, MR can be considered the procedure of choice. MR imaging is also frequently the most useful study for the demonstration of pulmonary arterial abnormalities and for evaluating the status of the pulmonary arteries after systemic-pulmonary shunts have been surgically produced.

The major use of MRI in ischemic heart disease has been to demonstrate complications of acute myocardial infarction, such as true and false aneurysms of the left ventricle and intraventricular thrombi (Fig. 178-4). However, in the future, MR may assume a broader role in ischemic heart disease by demonstrating: (1) residual viable myocardium in a region involved by a previous infarct; (2) patency (or lack thereof) of coronary artery bypass grafts; and (3) regional perfusion using MR contrast media. MRI has been used to define the extent and distribution of abnormal muscle in patients with hypertrophic cardiomyopathy and for demonstrating a variety of pericardial diseases. It provides direct imaging of the pericardium, so that a diagnosis of abnormal pericardial thickness can be made.

MR imaging has been found to be effective for demonstrating intracardiac thrombi and tumors (Fig. 178-5). The utility of the technique has been shown in the demonstration of primary and metastatic cardiac tumors and tumors within the mediastinum invading or compressing central cardiovascular structures. The most frequent indication for the use of MR imaging in evaluating an intracardiac mass is when echocardiography raises a question regarding abnormal echogenicity within the cardiac chambers.

Thoracic aortic diseases are evaluated best with MR. In patients with aortic dissection, MRI displays the intimal flap and the extent of the dissection within the aorta (Fig. 178-6). It can also identify thrombus in the false channel and involvement of the arch and visceral arterial branches.

EVALUATION OF CARDIAC FUNCTION Functional evaluation of the cardiovascular system is now practical using cine-MR. By achieving a temporal resolution of 30 images per cardiac cycle, cine-MR successfully captures end diastole and end systole, such that end-diastolic and end-systolic volumes, stroke volume, and ejection fraction can be calculated accurately. The temporal resolution of cine-MRI does not capture a single cardiac cycle, but rather separates an ''average'' cycle, acquired over 256 cardiac cycles, into many component images. A good correlation has been found between left ventricular volumes calculated from cine-MRI and those measured by angiography. Measurement of left ventricular mass using MR imaging has shown a close correlation with postmortem measurements in animals and estimates from angiography in human beings. Accurate measurement of left ventricular mass is important, since changes in mass may be the most effective way to monitor the response to therapy in diseases causing left ventricular hypertrophy. Functional

FIGURE 178-5 ECG gated spin-echo MR image in transverse plane shows a mass (arrow) in the left atrium. (*Reproduced with permission from CB Higgins, 1988.*)

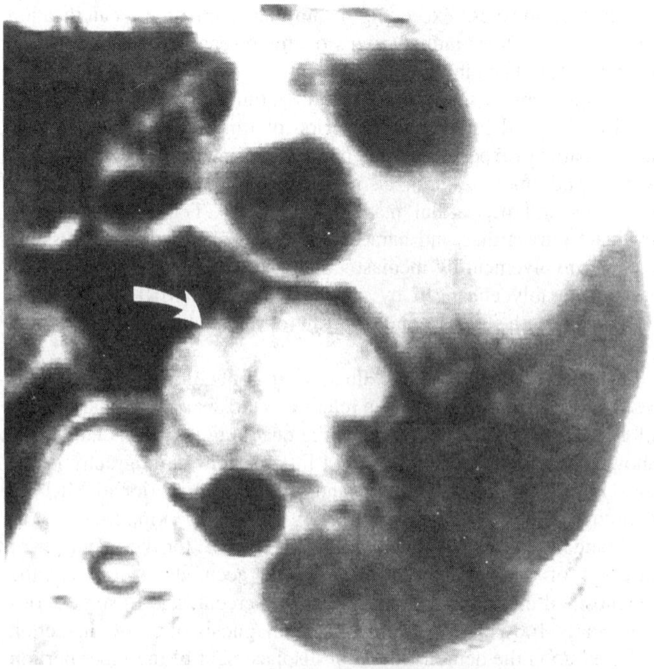

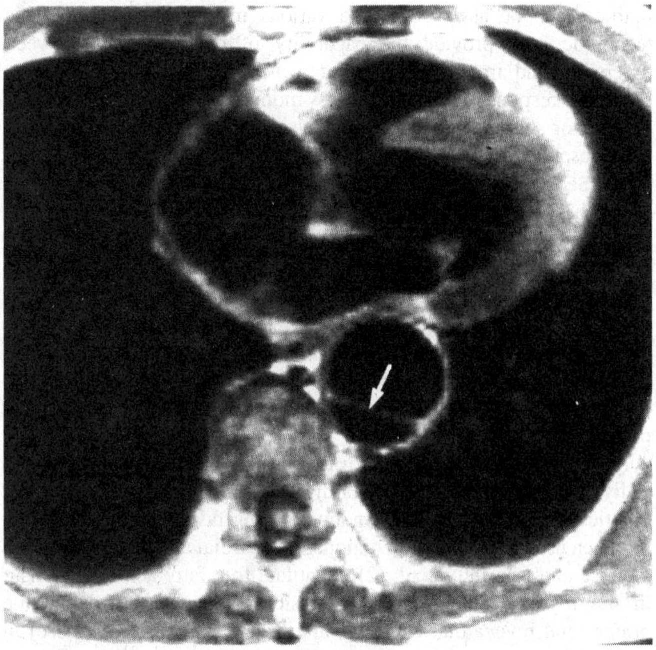

FIGURE 178-6 Aortic dissection. Transverse MR image shows intimal flap (arrow) separating true and false channels.

evaluation in ischemic heart disease by MR is achieved by monitoring wall thickening during the cardiac cycle. The site of previous myocardial infarction can be recognized by the absence or diminution of wall thickening during systole.

IDENTIFICATION AND QUANTITATION OF VALVULAR REGURGITATION The blood pool usually has a homogeneous high signal intensity throughout most of the cardiac cycle on cine-MR. Regurgitation through either the atrioventricular or semilunar valves is associated with a high-velocity jet which causes a signal void within the otherwise high-signal-intensity chamber (Fig. 178-7). This void

FIGURE 178-7 Cine-MRI (gradient refocused technique) in the coronal plane in aortic regurgitation. Images acquired in systole (*above*) and diastole (*below*). Note the signal void (arrow) emanating from the closed aortic valve. (*Reproduced from Sechtem et al, 1987.*)

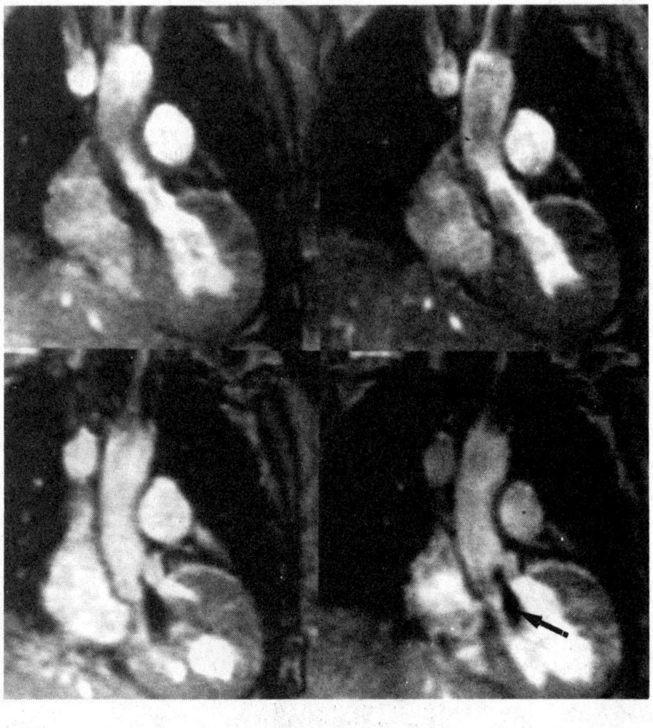

can be used to identify the presence of valvular regurgitation. In aortic regurgitation, the signal void is in continuity with the closed aortic valve, while in mitral regurgitation it is in continuity with the closed mitral valve. Quantitation of the severity of valvular regurgitation can be accomplished by measuring the right and left ventricular stroke volumes and using these measurements to calculate regurgitant fraction or regurgitant volume. The volume of the signal void caused by regurgitation can also be measured on the images and used to estimate the severity of regurgitation.

MR SPECTROSCOPY

MR spectroscopy is a new tool for the evaluation of myocardial metabolism which might eventually be used to assess the early response of the myocardium to various therapeutic and pharmacologic interventions, establish myocardial viability, assess beneficial or detrimental effects of reperfusion on the ischemically injured myocardium, and investigate the link between myocardial function and metabolism.

MR spectroscopy operates upon the same principle as MR imaging in that the nuclei of some atoms (those with an odd number of nuclear particles) resonate when radiofrequency energy is applied at a frequency specific for a particular atom. After this energy is applied, the nuclei resonate at a characteristic frequency so that the presence of a particular atom within a chemical compound or tissue can be identified by MR. In distinction to imaging, which is usually only sensitive to the presence of a certain atom within a compound, MR spectroscopy can provide a map of the various sites where an atom exists within a compound. MR spectroscopy depicts the very slight difference in resonant frequences of the same nuclei when it exists in different compounds. The slight variation in resonant frequencies of the same nuclei in various compounds is called *chemical shift*, and the graphic display of the various frequencies is the MR spectrum of the nuclei. An example of this is the MR spectrum of phosphorus 31 (^{31}P), where the multiple spectral peaks represent ^{31}P in the compounds inorganic phosphate, creatine phosphate, adenosine phosphate, etc. (Fig. 178-8). The MR spectra are displayed in a convention whereby the portion of the peak in the spectrum (horizontal axis) indicates the specific compounds, e.g., creatine phosphate, while the height of the peak (vertical axis) indicates the relative concentration of the compound.

FIGURE 178-8 Phosphorus 31 magnetic resonance spectrum from a normal subject. The important spectral peaks are inorganic phosphate, not seen; creatine phosphate (PCr); and the three for adenosine triphosphate (ATP). The 2,3-diphosphoglycerate (DPG) peak indicates that the signal is partially derived from intracavitary blood as well as from myocardium. PD = phosphodiester.

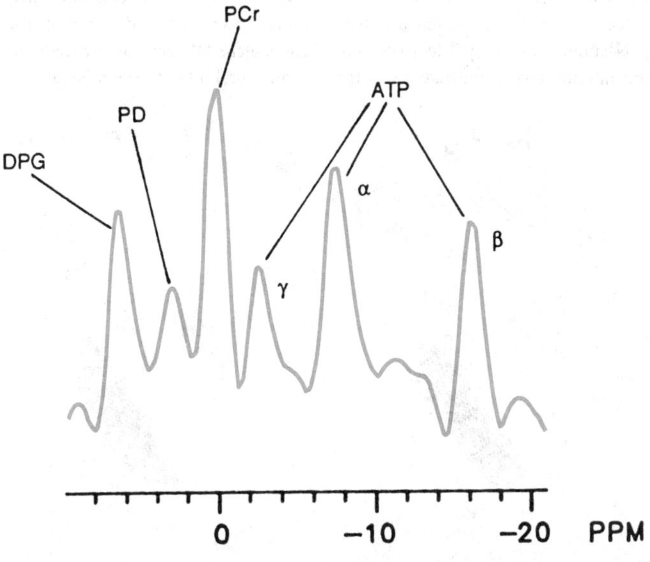

The nuclei for which MR spectroscopy seems to be the most useful for diagnostic purposes are hydrogen 1, carbon 13, and phosphorus 31. Hydrogen 1 (proton) spectroscopy has been used to detect lactate in ischemic tissue and lipid accumulation in ischemically injured tissue. Metabolism of energy substrates in the myocardium has been approached using carbon 13; the technique has the potential for monitoring the utilization of fat and glucose by the myocardium and the manner in which ischemia influences their utilization. At this time most attention has been devoted to phosphorus 31 MR spectroscopy as a method for studying high-energy phosphate stores in various myocardial disease states and alterations of high-energy phosphate stores in response to therapeutic interventions.

In experimental preparations, phosphorus 31 spectroscopy has been used to evaluate the influence of potentially toxic agents, such as adriamycin and ethanol, on the myocardium. Calcium channel antagonists have been found to enhance recovery of both function and high-energy phosphate stores of the ischemically injured myocardium. Phosphorus 31 MR spectroscopy may be used also in experimental preparations to determine whether ischemic myocardium which is reperfused is reversibly or irreversibly damaged. Abnormal ^{31}P spectra have been observed in patients with myocardial disease (Fig. 178-8). However, the sensitivity, specificity, and, indeed, the clinical utility of ^{31}P MR spectroscopy have yet to be established.

POSITRON EMISSION TOMOGRAPHY (PET)

PET is a technique in which tomographic images are produced in relation to the concentration and position of positron emitters within the heart or any other organ. The positron is a positively charged electron produced during positron decay of a nucleus. After the positron interacts with a neighboring electron, a pair of photons are emitted in opposite directions. Because the photons simultaneously travel at equal speeds along paths at 180° to one another, photon detectors arrayed in a circle around the body can compute the precise site of origin of the pair. A substantial number of positron emitters are available for evaluating blood flow and various aspects of metabolic activity of the myocardium. Blood flow can be measured with oxygen 15 (^{15}O)-, rubidium 82 (^{82}Rb)-, and nitrogen 13 (^{13}N)-labeled ammonia. Glucose utilization, fat utilization and metabolism, and myocardial oxygen consumption can be assessed by fluorine 18 (^{18}F)-labeled deoxyglucose, carbon 11 (^{11}C)-labeled palmitate, and ^{11}C-labeled acetate, respectively.

PET can evaluate regional myocardial blood flow and metabolism. The transverse tomograms provide distinct spatial separation between various regions of the left ventricle, so that the uptake of metabolic markers can be assigned to the various myocardial regions. This technique may provide the capability of distinguishing between reversibly and irreversibly injured ischemic myocardium and predicting its response to reperfusion. By monitoring changes in metabolic patterns or substrate uptake, it may also prove capable of monitoring early response to therapy.

ASSESSMENT OF REGIONAL MYOCARDIAL BLOOD FLOW Since the various regions of the left ventricle are separated from one another on the transverse tomographic images, PET scans using perfusion markers can be used to detect and localize coronary artery disease. Nitrogen 13 ammonia ($[^{13}N]H_3$) has been used to assess regional myocardial blood flow at rest and in a hyperemic state induced by the powerful vasodilator dipyridamole. This technique has shown regional reduction of the positron emitter in the presence of stenoses which reduce luminal diameter by more than 40 to 50 percent.

Myocardial metabolism An unique feature of PET is the capability to measure regional myocardial substrate uptake and metabolic kinetics in a noninvasive and nonperturbing fashion. Specifically, it has been used to (1) measure regional myocardial uptake of exogenous glucose and free fatty acid; (2) quantitate free fatty acid metabolism in the myocardium in various physiologic states; (3) define the preferential myocardial energy source (fatty acid versus glucose) in various physiologic states; and (4) evaluate myocardial chemical receptor sites.

PET employing $[^{13}N]H_3$ and $[^{18}F]DG$ (deoxyglucose) has been used to evaluate simultaneously regional myocardial perfusion and glucose uptake, respectively, in an effort to distinguish regions with a perfusion defect but containing viable myocardium from irreversibly infarcted myocardium. Using the combination of $[^{13}N]H_3$ (blood flow marker) and $[^{18}F]DG$ (glucose uptake), several patterns of segmental myocardial metabolic abnormalities have been described in patients with various forms of ischemic heart disease. One is a "blood flow–metabolism match," in which a defect in the regional myocardial distribution of both isotopes is present. This pattern is usually caused by myocardial scar or nonviable myocardium (Fig. 178-9*A*). A second pattern is a "blood flow–metabolism mismatch," in which there is a segmental defect in $[^{13}N]H_3$ without a deficit in $[^{18}F]DG$ (Fig. 178-9*B*). This indicates reduced perfusion to a myocardial region but continued uptake of glucose. Both patterns have been observed in patients with wall motion abnormalities in the left ventricular region displaying the perfusion defects. This mismatch pattern is considered to be associated with ischemic but viable myocardium since surgical revascularization of patients with this pattern causes improved wall motion in a majority of such segments. Moreover, a substantial percentage of patients showing the mismatch pattern after acute

FIGURE 178-9 Positron emission tomograms in two subjects: matched defects (*left*) and mismatched defects (*right*). Images show distribution for $[^{13}N]$ammonium and $[^{18}F]$deoxyglucose. The matched defects (arrowheads) in the anterior regions indicate a scar from a transmural infarct. The mismatched defects show reduced perfusion (arrow) but persistent glucose uptake (arrow) consistent with viable (salvageable) myocardium. (*Images provided courtesy of Heinrich Schelbert, MD.*)

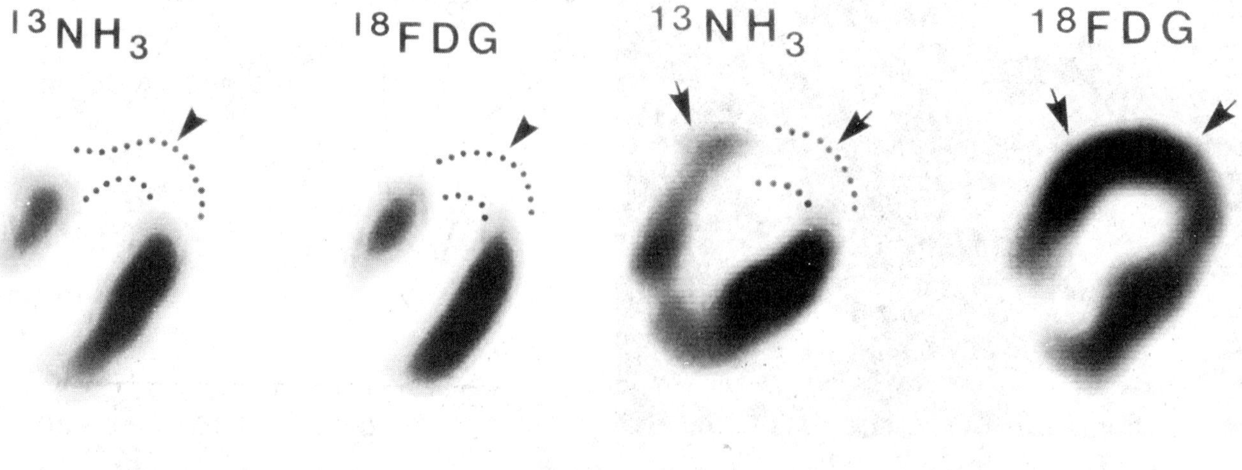

myocardial infarction have demonstrated some recovery of regional function. On the other hand, the match pattern has been associated with no recovery of function after revascularization of akinetic segments.

PET using the positron emitter [^{11}C]palmitic acid has identified the consequences of myocardial ischemia and infarction on myocardial free fatty acid metabolism. These studies revealed that exogenous ^{11}C-labeled palmitic acid can enter two metabolic pools within the myocardium: a rapidly metabolized pool in which the fatty acid is immediately oxidized to CO_2 or a storage pool of triglycerides. During myocardial ischemia, myocardial uptake of [^{11}C]palmitic acid and its distribution into the two pools are altered. The free fatty acid pathway most vulnerable to ischemia is β oxidation, and consequently the amount of [^{11}C]palmitic acid entering this pathway is decreased initially.

Prediction of successful salvage of myocardium after thrombolysis has been achieved by PET imaging of [^{11}C]palmitic acid uptake in the jeopardized myocardium. Successful thrombolysis is associated with resumption of uptake of [^{11}C]palmitic acid in the jeopardized region. The principal indications for PET at the current time are to detect ischemic myocardium and to demonstrate potentially salvageable (viable) myocardium in the presence of acute or chronic myocardial ischemia.

REFERENCES

Cine-CT

CAPUTO GR, LIPTON MJ: Evaluation of regional left ventricular function using cine CT, in *New Concepts in Cardiac Imaging*, GM Pohost et al (eds). Chicago, Yearbook Medical, 1988

STANFORD W et al: Sensitivity and specificity of assessing coronary bypass graft patency with ultrafast computed tomography. Results of a multicenter study. J Am Coll Cardiol 12:1, 1988

MR imaging

BARAKOS JA et al: Magnetic resonance imaging of cardiac and paracardiac masses. Pictoral essay. Am J Roentgenol 153:47, 1989

DIDIER D et al. Congenital heart disease: Gated MR imaging in 72 patients. Radiology 158:227, 1986

DOOMS GC, HIGGINS CB: MR imaging of cardiac thrombi. J Comput Assist Tomogr 10:415, 1986

HIGGINS CB: MR of the heart: Anatomy, physiology and metabolism. Am J Roentgenol 151:239, 1988

——— et al: Magnetic resonance imaging in hypertrophic cardiomyopathy. Am J Cardiol 55:1121, 1985

JOHNS JA et al: Quantitation of acute myocardial infarct size by nuclear magnetic resonance imaging. J Am Coll Cardiol 15:1, 1990

SECHTEM U et al: Cine MRI: Potential for the evaluation of cardiovascular function. Am J Roentgenol 148:239, 1987

——— et al: Mitral or aortic regurgitation: Quantification of regurgitant volumes in patients with cine MR imaging. Radiology 167:425, 1988

SOMMERHOFF BA et al: Aortic dissection: Sensitivity and specificity of MR imaging. Radiology 3:651, 1988

WHITE RD et al: Advances in imaging thoracic aortic disease. Invest Radiol 21:761, 1986

WINKLER M, HIGGINS CB: Suspected intracardiac masses: Evaluation with MR imaging. Radiology 165:117, 1987

MR spectroscopy

BUSER PT et al: Post ischemic recovery of mechanical performance and energy metabolism in the presence of left ventricular hypertrophy. A ^{31}P MRS study. Circ Res 1990

RICHARDS T et al: Proton NMR spectroscopy in canine myocardial infarction. Magn Reson Med 4:555, 1987

Positron emission tomography (PET)

SCHELBERT HR, BUXTON D: Insights into coronary artery disease gained from metabolic imaging. Circulation 78:496, 1988

TILLISCH J et al: Reversibility of wall motion abnormalities: Preoperative determination using positron tomography 18 fluorodeoxyglucose and $^{13}NH_3$. N Engl J Med 314:884, 1986

179 DIAGNOSTIC CARDIAC CATHETERIZATION AND ANGIOGRAPHY

WILLIAM GROSSMAN

Cardiac catheterization and angiography remain the gold standard for the assessment of both anatomy and physiology of the heart and vasculature. Initially developed in the animal laboratory, cardiac catheterization was first applied to humans in 1929 by Werner Forssmann, who at age 25 performed a right heart catheterization on himself. Forssmann's primary goal was to develop a therapeutic technique for the direct delivery of drugs into the heart. The potential of Forssmann's technique as a diagnostic tool was appreciated by others, especially André Cournand and Dickinson Richards in New York, who shared the Nobel prize with Forssmann in 1956 for the development of cardiac catheterization. Today, cardiac catheterization and angiography are performed as a combined procedure for diagnostic purposes, therapeutic intervention, or both. This chapter deals with cardiac catheterization as a diagnostic tool.

INDICATIONS FOR CARDIAC CATHETERIZATION Cardiac catheterization is recommended when there is a need to confirm the presence of a clinically suspected condition, define its anatomic and physiologic severity, and determine whether important associated conditions are present. This need most commonly arises when a patient is experiencing increased symptoms of cardiac dysfunction, or when objective measures suggest that rapid deterioration, myocardial infarction, or other adverse events are imminent.

There is debate as to whether cardiac catheterization is necessary in all patients being considered for cardiac surgery. Cardiac catheterization is the only technique currently capable of defining coronary anatomy with sufficient precision to provide the data base for decisions regarding coronary surgery or balloon angioplasty. In patients with other forms of heart disease (e.g., dilated cardiomyopathy, valvular heart disease), cardiac catheterization can provide hemodynamic characterization essential to the design of an appropriate medical regimen as well as assessment of prognosis. In some instances, decisions regarding cardiac surgery can be made without cardiac catheterization and angiography. Examples of such instances include children with simple congenital heart disease (e.g., patent ductus arteriosus, atrial septal defect), for whom a definitive noninvasive diagnosis is available.

Relative contraindications to cardiac catheterization are listed in Table 179-1.

A history of *allergic reaction* to radiographic contrast agents, which may range from urticaria to frank anaphylactic reaction, is an important relative contraindication to cardiac catheterization, which requires appropriate pretreatment. Generally, pretreatment with glucocorticoids (prednisone 20 to 40 mg every 6 h), conventional antihistamines (e.g., diphenhydramine 25 mg every 6 h), and H-2

TABLE 179-1 Relative contraindications to cardiac catheterization and angiography

1 Uncontrolled ventricular irritability: increased risk of ventricular tachycardia and fibrillation during catheterization if ventricular irritability is uncontrolled
2 Uncorrected hypokalemia or digitalis toxicity.
3 Uncorrected hypertension: predisposes to myocardial ischemia and/or heart failure during angiography
4 Intercurrent febrile illness
5 Decompensated heart failure: especially acute pulmonary edema, unless catheterization can be done with patient sitting up
6 Anticoagulated state: prothrombin time >18 s
7 Severe allergy to radiographic contrast agent
8 Severe renal insufficiency and/or anuria: unless dialysis is planned to remove fluid and radiographic contrast load

TABLE 179-2 Patient characteristics associated with increased mortality from cardiac catheterization

1 *Age:* Infants (<1 year old) and the elderly (>70 years old) are at increased risk of death during cardiac catheterization. Elderly women appear to be at higher risk than elderly men.
2 *Functional class:* Mortality in class IV patients is more than 10 times greater than in class I-II patients.
3 *Severity of coronary obstruction:* Mortality for patients with left main disease is more than 10 times greater than in patients with one- or two-vessel disease.
4 *Valvular heart disease:* Especially when severe and is combined with coronary disease is associated with a higher risk of death at cardiac catheterization than coronary artery disease alone.
5 *Left ventricular dysfunction:* Mortality in patients with left ventricular ejection <30 percent is more than 10 times greater than in patients with ejection fraction ≥50 percent.
6 *Severe noncardiac disease:* Patients with renal insufficiency, insulin-requiring diabetes, advanced cerebrovascular and/or peripheral vascular disease, and severe pulmonary insufficiency have an increased incidence of death and other major complications from cardiac catheterization.

antagonists (cimetidine 300 mg every 6 h), starting 18 to 24 h prior to the procedure, is adequate. Despite this pretreatment, occasional individuals will still develop anaphylactic reactions during radiographic contrast angiography, and intravenous epinephrine must be immediately available in such instances.

COMPLICATIONS OF CARDIAC CATHETERIZATION Since cardiac catheterization is an invasive technique, it should not be surprising that potential complications include death, myocardial infarction, stroke, perforation of the heart or great vessels, and local vascular problems. Table 179-2 lists those characteristics associated with increased risk of death from cardiac catheterization.

TECHNIQUES

Cardiac catheterization is performed with the patient in the fasting state and awake, although sedated. Typical sedatives include diazepam (Valium, 5 to 10 mg orally) and diphenhydramine (Benadryl, 25 to 50 mg orally). Prophylactic antibiotics are not necessary. If patients have been anticoagulated chronically with warfarin, this agent must be discontinued for at least 48 h prior to the procedure, and the prothrombin time must be less than 18 if the study is to be done safely. The technique of cardiac catheterization today involves either direct exposure of artery and vein (usually the brachial artery and vein in the antecubital fossa) or catheterization by percutaneous approach (usually involving the femoral vessels). Either technique can be used for right and/or left heart catheterization with coronary arteriography. The brachial approach has advantages in the patient with perpipheral vascular disease involving the abdominal aorta, iliac, or femoral arteries and suspected thrombosis of the femoral or iliac vein or inferior vena cava. Advantages of the percutaneous femoral approach are that arteriotomy and arterial repair are not required; the procedure can be performed repeatedly in the same patient at intervals; infection and thrombophlebitis at the catheterization site are quite rare, and no scar is left.

RIGHT HEART CATHETERIZATION This is most commonly performed under fluoroscopic guidance utilizing a balloon flotation catheter which is advanced from a suitable vein (brachial, femoral, subclavian, or internal jugular) into the superior vena cava, where blood is sampled for oximetry. The catheter is then advanced to the right atrium, where pressure is measured. The balloon is inflated with air or carbon dioxide and advanced to the right ventricle, pulmonary artery, and pulmonary artery wedge positions. Pressures are recorded in each position, and the balloon is then deflated so that pulmonary artery pressure is monitored and blood sampled from the catheter tip. With a thermistor-tipped balloon catheter, cardiac output can be measured utilizing cold saline injection and a small computer (thermodilution technique). Comparison of oxygen saturation in the vena cava, chambers of the right heart, and pulmonary artery blood permits assessment of the presence of a left-to-right shunt at the atrial, ventricular, or pulmonary artery level which will be manifested as an increase (''step-up'') in oxygen saturation of blood as it traverses these vessels and chambers.

The experienced operator will be alert for abnormalities in the course of the catheter during its passage through the right heart chambers, potentially providing information concerning the presence of congenital heart disease. For example, the catheter may pass directly from right to left atrium through an atrial septal defect, may enter an anomalous pulmonary vein draining into the right atrium, or may pass from the pulmonary artery directly into the aorta through a patent ductus arteriosus.

LEFT HEART CATHETERIZATION When left heart catheterization is done from the *brachial approach,* surgical cut-down is performed in the right (or left) antecubital fossa, with exposure of the brachial artery. An arteriotomy is made, and an appropriate catheter (e.g., Sones catheter) is advanced under fluoroscopic guidance to the central aorta, where pressure is measured and recorded. In many laboratories, peripheral arterial pressure is monitored by use of a radial artery line, and at this point in the procedure peripheral and central arterial pressures are compared. Next, the catheter is advanced in retrograde fashion across the aortic valve into the left ventricle where pressure is measured. If a right heart catheter is in place, this is an appropriate time for simultaneous measurement and recording of left heart, right heart, and peripheral arterial pressures together with determination of cardiac output by either thermodilution or Fick principle. These measures allow assessment of possible pressure gradients across the mitral and aortic valves, and catheter pullback on the right side permits assessment of possible gradients across pulmonic and tricuspid valves. Simultaneous measurement of pressures and cardiac output provides the data for calculation of systemic and pulmonary vascular resistances.

The *percutaneous femoral approach* to left heart catheterization involves puncture of the right (or left) femoral artery with a Seldinger needle, passage of a J-tipped guidewire retrograde to the abdominal aorta under fluoroscopic guidance, and placement of an intraarterial sheath with a side arm port for flushing. The side arm is attached to a pressure transducer and flush system, allowing continuous monitoring of peripheral arterial pressure. An appropriate catheter (e.g., pigtail catheter) is then advanced over a guidewire to the descending aorta, at which time the guidewire is removed and the catheter aspirated and flushed vigorously. Under pressure monitoring and fluoroscopic guidance, the catheter is advanced to the ascending aorta, where pressure is recorded simultaneously with peripheral arterial (sidearm) pressure. Subsequent steps in the procedure are identical to those listed for the brachial approach.

An additional method of left heart catheterization is the *transseptal approach.* This approach, which is not commonly employed today except for special diagnostic problems or for purposes of therapeutic intervention, involves a controlled puncture of the interatrial septum with a long stainless steel needle and advancement of a Teflon catheter over the needle into the left atrium. Rarely, direct catheterization of the left heart through the chest wall is necessary, by *left ventricular puncture* through a needle directed at the cardiac apex.

CARDIAC ANGIOGRAPHY

Cardiac angiography involves injection of radiopaque contrast agent into a specific cardiac chamber or vessel using either hand injection or power injection through an automated syringe. Contrast agents utilized today are broadly considered to be either nonionic or ionic; the newer, nonionic contrast agents have less myocardial depressant effect but are substantially more expensive than traditional ionic agents. Radiographic contrast injection is usually associated with vasodilatation and a sensation of marked warmth throughout the distribution of the injection.

CORONARY ANGIOGRAPHIC ANATOMY: REPRESENTATION IN STANDARD PRO

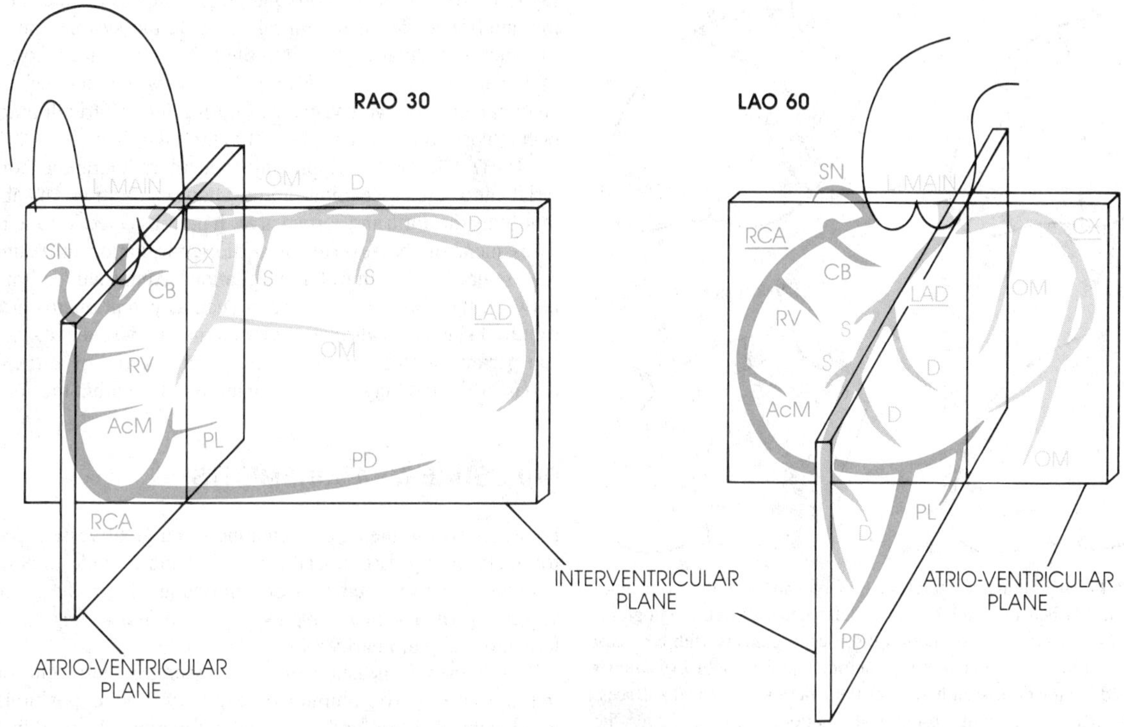

FIGURE 179-1 Representation of coronary anatomy relative to the interventricular and atrioventricular valve planes. Coronary branches are indicated as: L Main (left main), LAD (left anterior descending), D (diagonal), S (septal), CX (circumflex), OM (obtuse marginal), RCA (right coronary artery), CB (conus branch), SN (sinus node), AcM (acute marginal), PD (posterior descending, PL (posterolateral left ventricular). RAO, right anterior oblique, LAO, left anterior oblique. (*From DS Baim, W Grossman, in W Grossman, ed., 1986, with permission.*)

CORONARY ANGIOGRAPHY The commonest type of cardiac angiography currently performed involves selective injection of radiographic contrast agent into the coronary arteries. Placement of the catheter tips into the right and left coronary arteries is carried out under fluoroscopic guidance, and contrast agent is injected during recording of the radiographic image. Each coronary artery is usually viewed in several projections, to permit assessment of severity of stenosis and to minimize overlap of adjacent vessels. In addition to the detection of coronary artery stenoses, coronary angiography is useful for the detection of congenital abnormalities of the coronary circulation, coronary arteriovenous fistulas, and patency of coronary artery bypass grafts. Examples of normal and abnormal coronary anatomy are seen in Figs. 179-1 to 179-3.

LEFT VENTRICULOGRAPHY Injection of radiographic contrast directly into the left ventricular chamber is an important part of routine left heart catheterization, and yields important diagnostic information. Usually, a power injector is utilized to inject 30 to 45 mL of radiographic contrast into the left ventricular chamber at an injection rate appropriate for the particular catheter being used. Angiographic assessment of the left ventricular silhouette at end-

FIGURE 179-2 Coronary angiogram showing a right coronary artery (RCA) with a severe (95 percent) stenosis at its midpoint (*arrow*).

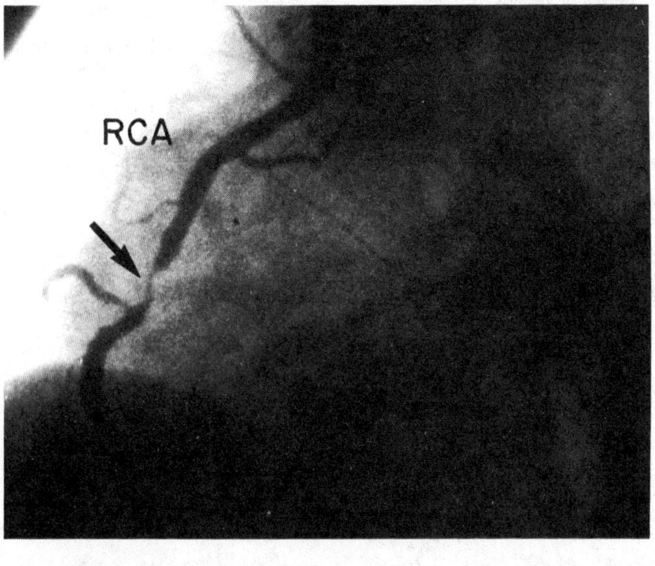

FIGURE 179-3 Coronary angiogram of a left coronary artery (LCA) with a tight stenosis in the proximal left anterior descending (LAD) artery (*black arrow*), immediately prior to the origin of a large septal branch. The circumflex artery (CX) has two moderately severe stenoses (*white arrows*).

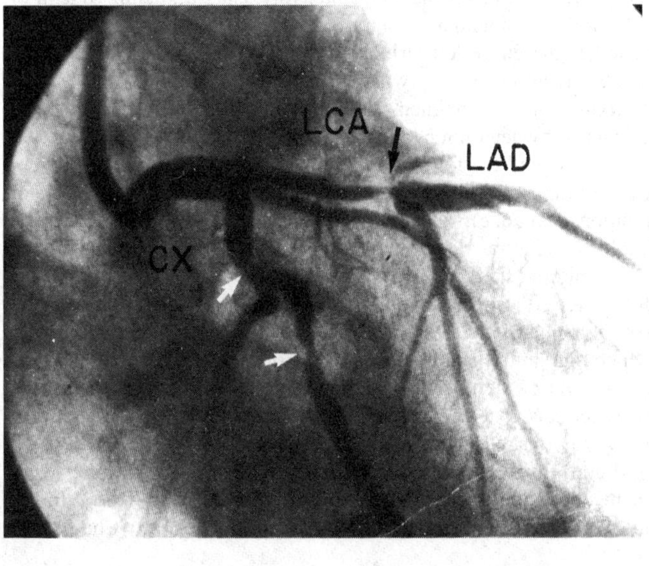

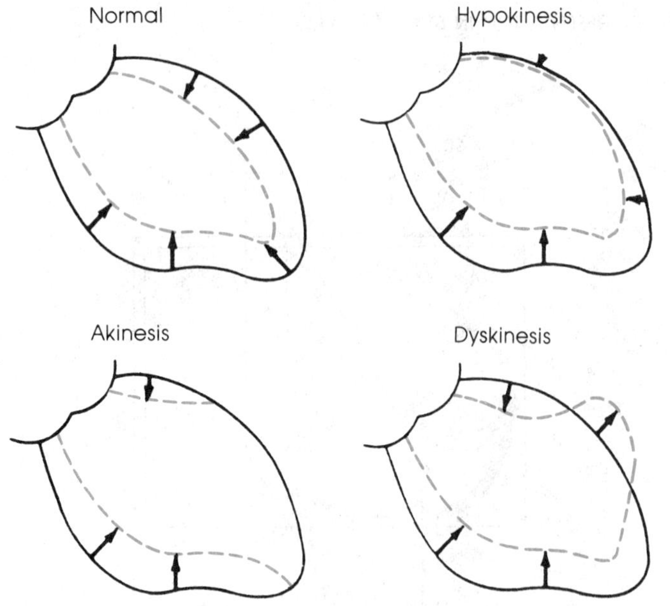

FIGURE 179-4 Diagrammatic representation of end-diastolic (solid line) and end-systolic (dashed line) silhouettes of left ventricular cineangiograms in various forms of localized wall motion disorder in patients with coronary heart disease. Normal wall motion is symmetric; a patient with *hypokinesis* exhibits reduced contraction, seen here over the anterior and apical surfaces; a patient with *akinesis* exhibits absent wall motion, seen here over the anteroapical surface; the patient with *dyskinesis* exhibits paradoxic bulging of a small portion of the anterior wall with systole.

diastole and end-systole permits calculation of left ventricular chamber volumes and ejection fraction, as well as assessment of regional wall motion abnormalities. The normal left ventricle ejects 50 to 80 percent of its end-diastolic volume with each beat; that is, its *ejection fraction* is 0.50 to 0.80. In adults, normal values for left ventricular volumes are: end-diastolic volume, 72 ± 15 mL/m^2 (mean ± standard deviation), and end-systolic volume, 20 ± 8 mL/m^2. Regional abnormalities of wall motion are illustrated in Fig. 179-4 and include diminished inward motion of a myocardial segment *(hypokinesis)*, no inward movement of a myocardial segment *(akinesis)*, and paradoxical systolic expansion of a regional myocardial segment *(dyskinesis)*.

Left ventriculography is usually performed in the right anterior oblique projection, which allows assessment of the mitral and aortic valves. Mitral regurgitation is easily visualized as the appearance of radiographic contrast in the left atrium during left ventricular systole. Its severity can be estimated qualitatively using a grading system of 1+ (mild, radiographic contrast clears with each beat and never opacifies the entire left atrium) to 4+ (severe, opacification of the entire left atrium occurs within one beat and contrast can be seen refluxing into the pulmonary veins). *Regurgitant fraction* can be calculated by determining the total left ventricular stroke volume (left ventricular end-diastolic volume minus end-systolic volume), subtracting the forward stroke volume (determined by Fick or indicator dilution technique), and dividing by the total stroke volume. The etiology of mitral regurgitation, such as myxomatous degeneration of the mitral leaflets and chordal rupture, may sometimes be identified from the left ventricular cineangiogram. Mitral and aortic stenosis can be *detected* by assessment of the speed and completeness with which the mitral and aortic leaflets open. Also important is an assessment of the thickness of the mitral and aortic leaflets, and the presence and extent of calcification. These findings, however, are usually not useful in estimating the *severity* of stenosis.

Left ventriculography also permits detection of abnormal communications such as ventricular septal defect (Chap. 186). In the most common form of hypertrophic cardiomyopathy (Chap. 192) (idiopathic hypertrophic subaortic stenosis, IHSS) left ventriculography in the left anterior oblique projection shows anterior motion of the anterior leaflet of the mitral valve during systole and bulging of the interventricular septum into the left ventricular cavity, especially in the subaortic region. Mural thrombi within the left ventricular chamber may be well visualized during left ventriculography. They occur most commonly in the left ventricular apex.

AORTOGRAPHY Rapid injection of radiographic contrast material into the ascending aorta allows detection of abnormality involving the aorta and aortic valve. It permits detection and qualitative assessment of the severity of aortic regurgitation utilizing a 1+ to 4+ scale, as for mitral regurgitation. Abnormal communications between the aorta and right heart such as patent ductus arteriosus or ruptured sinus of Valsalva aneurysm may be visualized. Aortography can permit identification of aortic aneurysm and of aortic dissection (Chap. 197) and may visualize an intimal flap within the aortic lumen.

PRESSURE MEASUREMENTS

Pressures within the cardiac chambers and great vessels are recorded routinely during cardiac catheterization and provide important information concerning function of ventricular myocardium and cardiac valves. Normal values for pressures measured during cardiac catheterization are summarized in Table 179-3.

Simultaneous measurement of pressures in left ventricle, aorta, and left atrium (or pulmonary capillary wedge position) permits assessment of mitral and aortic valve function. As seen in Fig. 179-5, left ventricular and aortic pressures are essentially equal during systole, while left atrial (pulmonary capillary wedge) and left ventricular pressures are equal during diastole in the normal heart. A pressure gradient between the left ventricle and aorta during systole may be due to obstruction at the level of the aortic valve (e.g., *calcific aortic stenosis*) or at the subaortic level (e.g., *hypertrophic obstructive cardiomyopathy*). A gradient between the left atrium (pulmonary capillary wedge) and left ventricle in diastole generally indicates *mitral stenosis*, although it may also be seen in rare conditions such as cor triatriatum and left atrial myxoma. An example of a large diastolic pressure gradient in a patient with mitral stenosis is seen in Fig. 179-6. As seen in Fig. 179-7, a prominent *v* wave in the pulmonary capillary wedge pressure will often increase substantially during modest exercise in a patient with significant mitral regurgitation. Severe *aortic regurgitation* produces a widening of the aortic pulse pressure, with equilibration of aortic and left ventricular

TABLE 179-3 Normal values for hemodynamic parameters

1 Pressures (mmHg)	
A Systemic arterial	
(*1*) Peak systolic/end-diastolic	100–140/60–90
(2) Mean	70–105
B Left ventricle	
(*1*) Peak systolic/end-diastolic	100–140/3–12
C Left atrium (or pulmonary capillary wedge)	
(*1*) Mean	2–10
(*2*) *a* wave	3–15
(*3*) *v* wave	3–15
D Pulmonary artery	
(*1*) Peak systolic/end-diastolic	15–30/4–12
(*2*) Mean	9–18
E Right ventricle	
(*1*) Peak systolic/end-diastolic	15–30/2–8
F Right atrium	
(*1*) Mean	2–8
(*2*) *a* wave	2–10
(*3*) *v* wave	2–10
2 Resistances [(dyn•s)/cm^5]	
(*1*) Systemic vascular resistance	700–1600
(*2*) Pulmonary vascular resistance	20–130
3 Cardiac output [(L/min)/m^2]	2.6–4.2
4 Oxygen consumption [(L/min)/m^2]	110–150
5 Arteriovenous oxygen difference (mL/L)	30–50

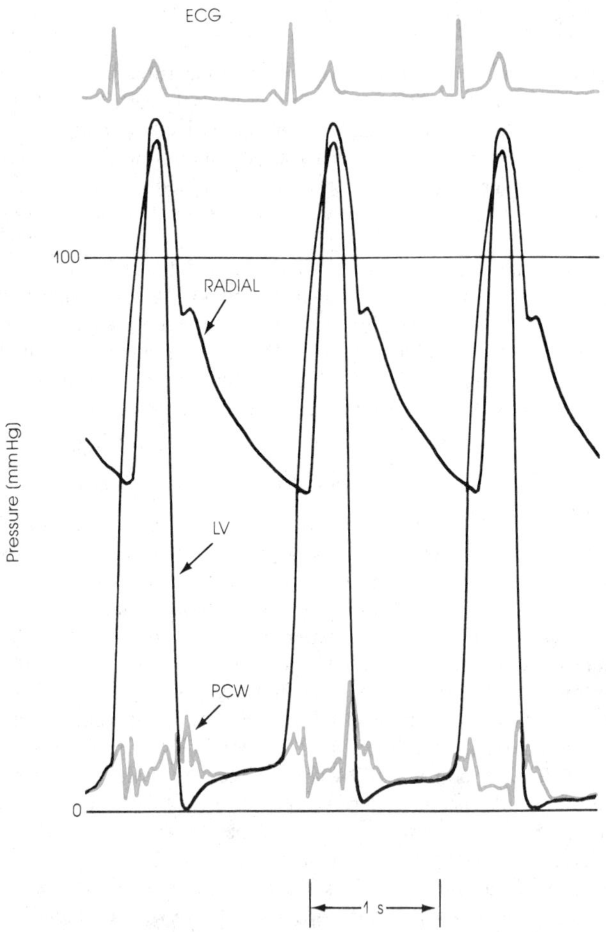

FIGURE 179-5 Left ventricular (LV), radial artery, and pulmonary capillary wedge (PCW) pressures in a patient with normal cardiovascular function. Note the absence of a pressure gradient between the LV and radial artery in systole and between the LV and PCW in diastole.

pressures in diastole (Fig. 179-8). Right-sided pressures exhibit characteristic deformity in the presence of valvular heart disease affecting the tricuspid or pulmonic valves. In patients with severe *tricuspid regurgitation,* right atrial pressure resembles closely in appearance the right ventricular pressure. Mean right atrial pressure

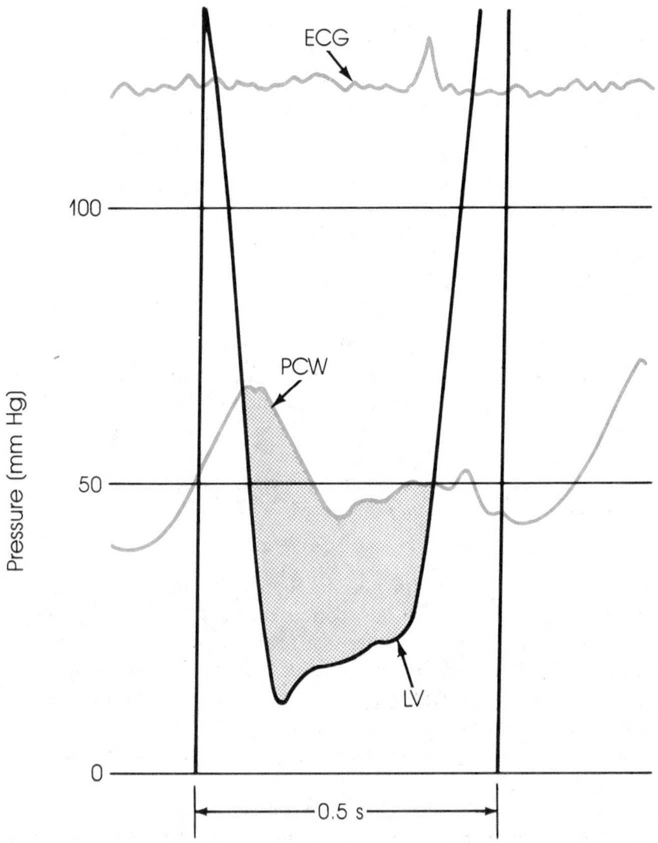

FIGURE 179-6 Pulmonary capillary wedge (PCW) and left ventricular (LV) pressure tracings in a 40-year-old woman with mitral stenosis. This patient also had systemic hypertension and significant elevation of her LV diastolic pressure. *(From BA Carabello, W Grossman, in W Grossman (ed), 1986, with permission.)*

and right ventricular end-diastolic pressure are both elevated in tricuspid regurgitation. In *tricuspid stenosis* there is a diastolic gradient between right atrium and ventricle.

Characteristic deformities of right and left ventricular diastolic pressures occur in patients with *cardiac tamponade* or *pericardial constriction.* In both conditions there is equalization of left and right ventricular diastolic pressures. However, in constrictive pericarditis,

FIGURE 179-7 Hemodynamic findings at rest and during exercise in a patient with mitral regurgitation. Left ventricular (LV), pulmonary capillary wedge (PCW), and radial artery pressure tracings are shown before (*left*) and during (*right*) the sixth minute of supine bicycle exercise. PCW mean pressure and *v* wave increase substantially with exercise. *(From BH Lorell, W Grossman, in W Grossman (ed), 1986, with permission.)*

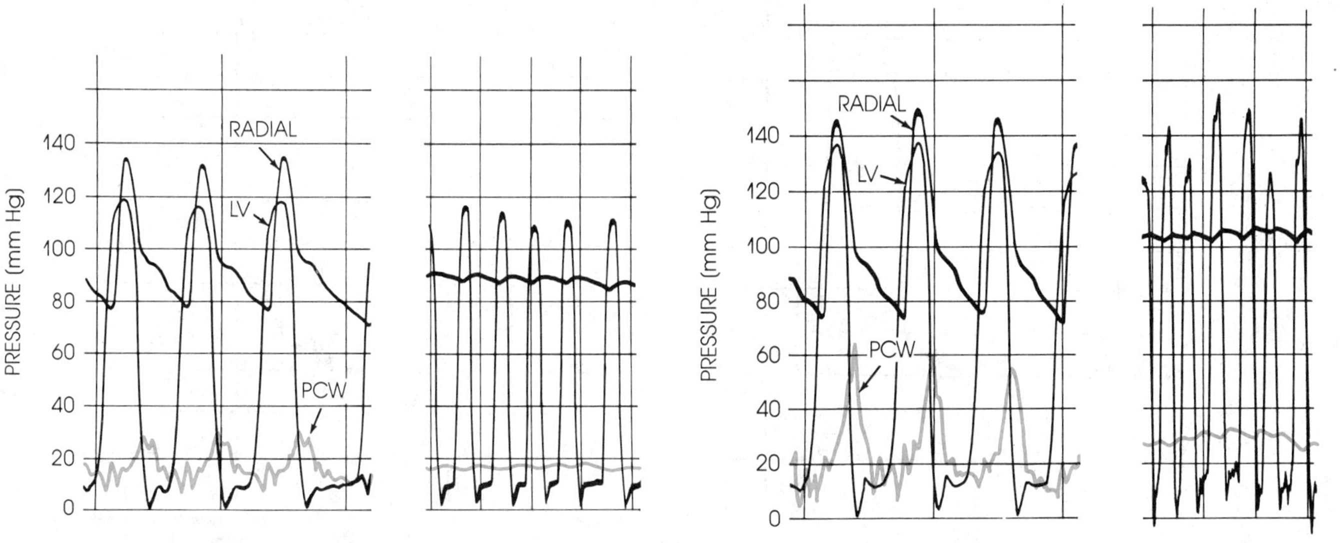

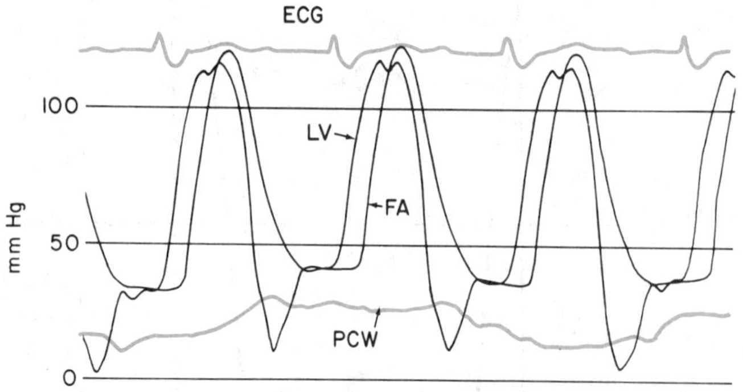

FIGURE 179-8 Severe aortic regurgitation. There is equilibration between the left ventricular (LV) and aortic or femoral artery (FA) pressures in diastole. Also, LV diastolic pressure exceeds pulmonary capillary wedge (PCW) pressure early in diastole, indicating premature closure of the mitral valve (a characteristic feature of severe aortic regurgitation). *(From W Grossman, in W Grossman (ed), 1986, with permission.)*

nearly all of ventricular filling occurs shortly after mitral and tricuspid valve opening; following this period of rapid filling, ventricular volumes cannot increase further due to the limit of the constricting pericardium. This abnormality produces an abrupt early ventricular diastolic pressure rise with a mid and late ventricular pressure plateau, giving the so-called square root sign (Fig. 179-9). In contrast, in tamponade there is equalization of diastolic pressures with a gradual increase throughout diastole.

Congestive heart failure due to myocardial contractile dysfunction is associated with characteristic alterations in the ventricular pressure waveforms seen at cardiac catheterization. Both isovolumic pressure rise and pressure decline are not nearly as steep as in the normal heart. The reduced slopes of pressure rise and decline are associated with an abbreviated ejection period, giving the left ventricular pressure tracing a triangular appearance (Fig. 179-10). Also, pressure decline does not continue to zero pressure, so that the minimal left ventricular diastolic pressure may be elevated. This hemodynamic finding correlates with an increased ventricular end-systolic volume, which is a sign of depressed contractile function of the left ventricular myocardium.

MEASUREMENT OF FLOW

Systemic and pulmonary blood flows may be measured by either the Fick or indicator-dilution methods. In the normal heart, these flows are equal and are termed *cardiac output*. Specialized techniques have made it possible to measure coronary artery blood flow (catheter-tip-mounted Doppler flowmeter), coronary sinus blood flow (thermodilution technique), and renal, cerebral, and femoral blood flows as well.

Cardiac output is most commonly measured today by the thermodilution technique, but the standard method, against which this technique and others are calibrated, remains the direct Fick oxygen method. In the direct Fick method, O_2 consumption is measured simultaneous with determination of arteriovenous oxygen difference across the lungs. Fick's principle states that

$$Q\,(\text{L/min}) = \frac{O_2\text{ consumption (mL/min)}}{\text{arteriovenous oxygen difference (mL/L)}}$$

In order to compare individuals of different body weights and sizes, O_2 consumption and cardiac output (Q) are commonly divided by body surface area. Normal values for O_2 consumption and cardiac output are given in Table 179-3. Cardiac output is calculated by dividing O_2 consumption by the arteriovenous O_2 difference across the lungs (estimated pulmonary venous–pulmonary arterial O_2 content); this actually measures *pulmonary blood flow* (Q_p). In patients with left-to-right shunts at the atrial, ventricular, or pulmonary artery levels, pulmonary blood flow exceeds systemic blood flow. In such cases, systemic blood flow (Q_s) is calculated by dividing O_2 consumption by the systemic arteriovenous O_2 difference. The latter is calculated as systemic arterial blood O_2 content minus mixed venous blood O_2 content, using blood from the chamber immediately proximal to the level of the shunt. The Fick method is most dependable when the cardiac output is low and the arteriovenous oxygen difference is large.

For indicator-dilution measurement of cardiac output using the thermodilution technique, a thermistor is mounted on the tip of a balloon-flotation catheter, and the catheter is advanced so that the balloon tip and thermistor are located in the pulmonary artery. Cold dextrose solution or saline is injected via a proximal port on the catheter into the vena cava or right atrium, and the change in

FIGURE 179-9 Left ventricular (LV), right ventricular (RV), and pulmonary capillary wedge (PCW) pressure tracings in a patient with severe constrictive pericarditis. Note the diastolic dip and plateau ("square root sign") pattern for left and right ventricular diastolic pressures left panel.

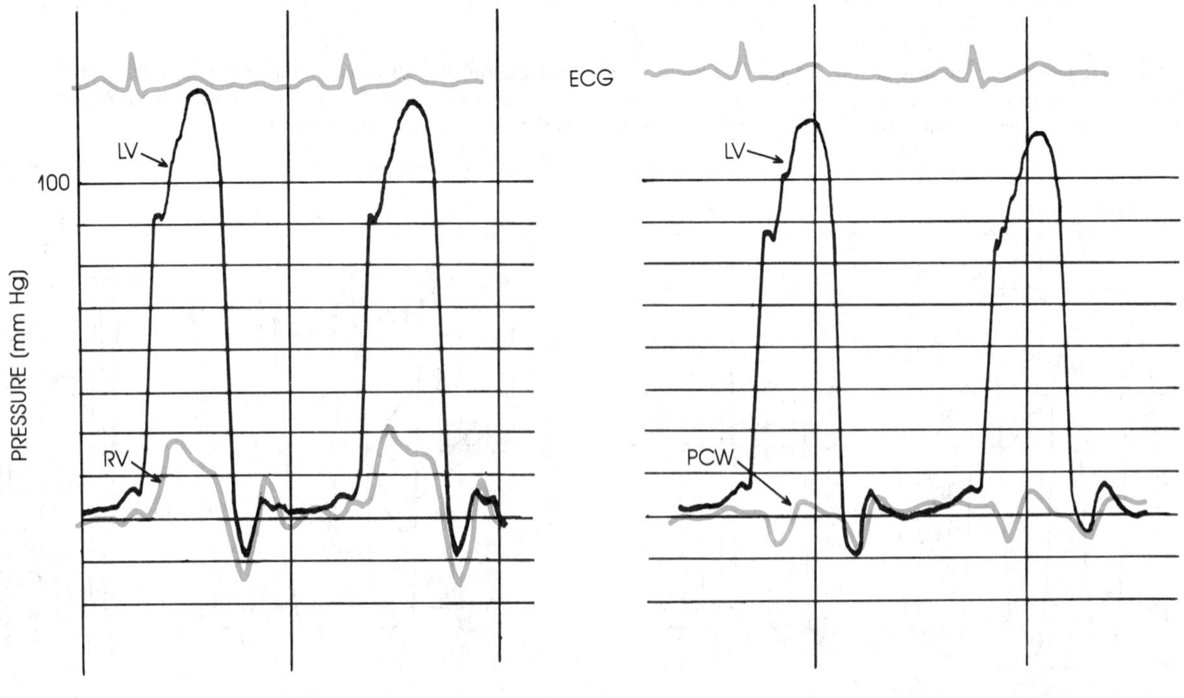

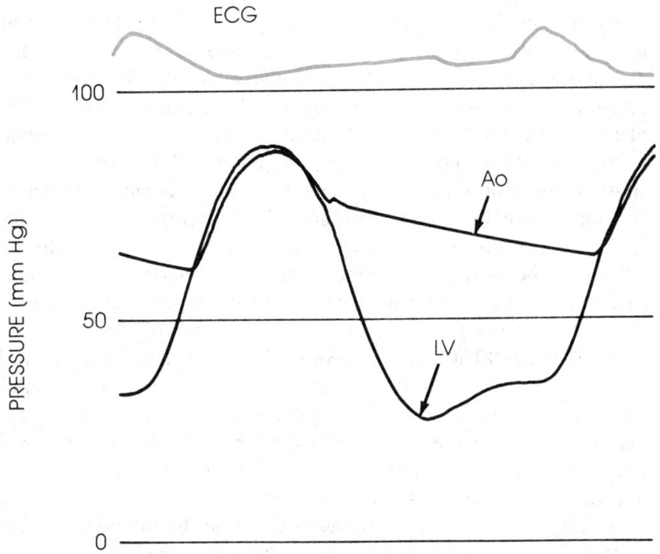

FIGURE 179-10 Left ventricular (LV) and aortic (Ao) pressures in a patient with advanced dilated cardiomyopathy. Marked slowing of the rates of left ventricular pressure rise and fall (impairment of contractility and relaxation) give the LV pressure pulse a triangular appearance. Also, the minimal value for left ventricular diastolic pressure is markedly elevated, suggesting an increased end-systolic volume and a reduced LV ejection fraction. *(From W Grossman, in W Grossman (ed), 1986, with permission.)*

temperature monitored at the thermistor is integrated mathematically. This integral is inversely proportional to the volume flow rate past the thermistor, and if the temperatures of the injectate and pulmonary artery blood are measured, cardiac output (actually pulmonary blood flow) can be calculated. In contrast to the Fick method, the indicator-dilution method is least reliable when the cardiac output is low.

Valve areas and resistances Using simultaneous measures of pressure and flow, the resistance to blood flow across cardiac valves as well as the pulmonary and systemic arteriolar beds may be estimated. Valve areas are calculated using the Gorlin formula:

$$A = \frac{\text{flow}}{K\sqrt{\Delta P}}$$

where A = valve orifice area (cm^2), *flow* is the blood flow (mL/s) across the stenotic valve, ΔP is the mean pressure gradient (mmHg) during the period of blood flow, and K is a constant (44.3 for the aortic valve and 37.7 for the mitral valve).

The resistance to blood flow through the systemic vascular bed is given as

$$\text{SVR} = 80(\text{MAP} - \text{RA})/\text{SBF}$$

where SVR is systemic vascular resistance (dyn·s/cm^5), MAP and RA are mean aortic and right atrial pressures (mmHg), 80 is a constant for converting to metric units, and SBF is systemic blood flow (L/min).

Resistance to blood flow through the pulmonary vascular bed is given as

$$\text{PVR} = 80(\text{PA} - \text{PCW or LA})/\text{PBF}$$

where PVR is pulmonary vascular resistance [(dyn·s)/cm^5], PA, PCW, and LA are pulmonary artery, pulmonary capillary wedge, and left atrial mean pressures (mmHg), and PBF is pulmonary blood flow (L/min). Normal values for pulmonary and systemic vascular resistances are given in Table 179-3.

REFERENCES

Grossman W, Barry WH: Cardiac catheterization, in *Heart Disease*, 3d ed, E Braunwald (ed). Philadelphia, Saunders, 1988, p 242

——— (ed): *Cardiac Catheterization and Angiography*, 3d ed. Philadelphia, Lea & Febiger, 1986

Kennedy JW et al: Complications associated with cardiac catheterization and angiography. Cathet Cardiovasc Diagn 8:5, 1982

Roberts WC: Reasons for cardiac catheterization before cardiac valve replacement. N Engl J Med 306:291, 1982

180 THERAPEUTIC APPLICATIONS OF CARDIAC CATHETERIZATION

WILLIAM GROSSMAN / DONALD S. BAIM

The development of catheter-based therapies for the treatment of cardiovascular disease has led to the creation of a new field: interventional cardiology. In current practice, interventional cardiology provides a safe and effective alternative to conventional surgery for many patients with coronary, valvular, and congenital heart disease (Table 180-1).

TREATMENT OF CORONARY STENOSES AND OCCLUSIONS WITH CORONARY ANGIOPLASTY

Percutaneous transluminal coronary angioplasty (PTCA) is an important form of therapy for coronary artery disease (see Chap. 189). More than 200,000 PTCA procedures were performed in the United States alone during 1988, nearly equal to the number of coronary bypass operations. Since PTCA is performed using local anesthesia, during a short (2- to 3-day) hospitalization, its use in suitable patients can greatly decrease expense and recovery time compared to coronary bypass surgery, although it carries a 0.4 to 1.0 percent procedure-related mortality, similar to that for elective coronary bypass surgery.

INDICATIONS The main indication for PTCA is the presence of one or more coronary stenoses that are felt to be responsible for a clinical syndrome warranting revascularization and that are approachable by balloon catheters (Fig. 180-1). Moreover, the risks and benefits for revascularization by PTCA should compare favorably to those of conventional surgery. Thus, significant left main stenosis or multivessel disease in which vessels supplying significant areas of viable myocardium are not approachable by PTCA (due to chronic total occlusion or other unfavorable anatomic features) constitute relative contraindications to PTCA if surgery is technically possible.

For most patients, the clinical syndrome being treated is moderately severe, chronic, stable angina that persists despite medical antianginal therapy. Approximately 15 to 20 percent of current PTCA patients, however, have only mild anginal symptoms despite suitable coronary anatomy and objective evidence of ischemia (i.e., an abnormal exercise test). At the other extreme, some patients have more pressing

TABLE 180-1 Therapeutic applications of cardiac catheterization

Techniques currently under clinical evaluation or in general use
Treatment of coronary stenoses and occlusions
Percutaneous transluminal coronary angioplasty (PTCA)
Laser techniques
Intravascular stent
Atherectomy
Treatment of valvular stenosis
Balloon valvuloplasty (aortic, mitral, pulmonic)
Treatment of congenital defects
Atrial septostomy
Umbrella closure of patent ductus arteriosus and defects in atrial or ventricular septum
Coil closure of undesired collateral vessels

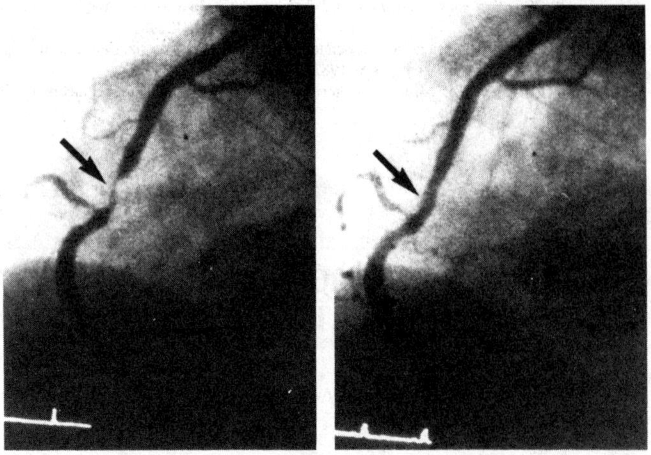

FIGURE 180-1 Right coronary angioplasty in a patient with unstable angina 6 weeks following successful dilatation. The lesion is shown before (*left panel*) and after (*right panel*) inflation of the PTCA balloon catheter.

indications for PTCA revascularization, including unstable angina or acute myocardial infarction (with or without prior thrombolytic therapy).

As the clinical indications for PTCA have broadened, so have its anatomic capabilities. Thus, PTCA is no longer restricted to proximal, discrete, subtotal, concentric, noncalcified lesions as was the case initially. Angioplasty catheters with smaller deflated profiles, controlled by highly steerable guidewires, are now available that can be advanced successfully across severe stenoses located virtually anywhere in the coronary tree. These balloon catheters tolerate inflation pressures up to 300 psi (20 atm), adequate to dilate even calcific lesions. Totally occluded coronary arteries (particularly those which have been occluded for less than 6 months) can be crossed and dilated effectively, although the success rate remains somewhat lower than for subtotal lesions (i.e., 60 percent versus 90 percent for subtotal stenotic lesions). In addition to lesions in the native coronary tree, lesions in saphenous vein or internal mammary artery bypass grafts can also be dilated successfully to treat postbypass angina. If multiple lesions are responsible for the clinical syndrome, most or all such lesions can generally be dilated during a single procedure.

RESULTS The current PTCA success rate (for reducing a target stenosis to <50 percent of its original diameter without producing an associated complication) exceeds 90 percent. About half of the failures result from inability to cross the target lesion with the guidewire or balloon catheter, particularly when that target lesion is a chronic total occlusion. The remaining failures are due to excessive local dissection (separation of coronary artery intima from media) resulting from attempted dilatation. While some local dissection is present in virtually all successful PTCA procedures, more extensive dissection (particularly in association with local thrombus formation or vasospasm) can lead to abrupt closure of the dilated segment soon after withdrawal of the balloon catheter. Routine use of vasodilators (nitrates and calcium channel antagonists), anticoagulation (heparin 10,000 to 15,000 units during the procedure), and antiplatelet therapy (aminosalicylic acid, 325 mg/d starting at least 24 h prior to PTCA and continued for 3 to 6 months after the procedure) helps to prevent abrupt closure due to spasm and/or thrombus formation. Closure due to dissection can frequently be reopened by repeat dilatation (Fig. 180-2), but if this is unsuccessful, emergency bypass surgery is required to restore blood flow and prevent myocardial infarction. Emergency bypass surgery is needed currently in only 2 percent of PTCA attempts, but this potential difficulty requires that angioplasty be performed only in hospitals where immediate cardiac surgery is available.

FOLLOW-UP After successful PTCA of all "culprit" lesions, marked improvement or complete resolution of the presenting ischemic syndrome should be evident. In approximately 20 to 30 percent of patients, however, evidence of ischemia returns within 6 months, due to so-called restenosis of the dilated segment. This appears to result from excessive local myointimal hyperplasia, triggered by platelet adhesion to the freshly dilated surface. To date, despite substantial effort, no mechanical or pharmacologic strategy has substantially reduced this restenosis rate. When recurrent ischemia develops more than 6 months after PTCA, this usually reflects progression of disease at another site, rather than restenosis. Repeat PTCA can be used to treat either restenosis or disease progression, so that only about 10 percent of PTCA patients require bypass surgery during the 5 years following a successful PTCA procedure.

NEWER NONBALLOON TECHNIQUES In an attempt to circumvent the existing limitations of balloon angioplasty, intensive evaluation of a variety of nonballoon techniques is currently under way. One or more of these newer techniques may aid in crossing total occlusions, dilating rigid or elastic lesions, stabilizing dissections, or reducing the incidence of restenosis.

Laser Laser energy (at wavelengths from the ultraviolet to the infrared) can be delivered to coronary lesions through optical fibers as small as 0.2 mm in diameter. Depending on the specific delivery parameters, this energy can produce direct ablation of an atherosclerotic plaque, associated with various degrees of local thermal injury. To date, however, no ablative laser technologies have proved adequate to distinguish plaque from normal vessel wall, leading to an unacceptable vessel perforation rate for safe application in the coronary arteries.

On the other hand, lasers can be used to deliver controlled thermal energy to the atherosclerotic plaque. Laser heating of a metal cap (the thermal probe) has been used successfully to cross occlusions in the peripheral circulation and is undergoing preliminary testing in the coronary arteries. Laser light can also be transmitted to the vessel wall from a diffusing fiber contained within a special balloon catheter (laser balloon angioplasty). This heats the vessel wall to 100°C, which appears to mold or weld the diseased wall into a desired configuration, so as to prevent or reverse abrupt closure. The smooth intimal surface which is left behind (and/or the thermal damage inflicted on the vascular smooth-muscle cells) has the potential to reduce restenosis, but this has yet to be demonstrated in clinical trials.

Intravascular stents Permanent metallic endoprostheses (stents) of several designs can be delivered into the peripheral and coronary circulation to aid in maintaining luminal patency. Over a period of weeks, these stents are covered by endothelial cells and incorporated into the vessel wall. Although stenting improves acute luminal

FIGURE 180-2 Abrupt closure of a mid-right coronary artery lesion following attempted dilatation in a patient with recurrent ischemia following rt-PA therapy for inferior wall infarction. The involved lesion is shown before dilatation (*left panel*), during abrupt closure immediately after initial dilatation (*center panel*, arrows indicate local dissection), and after stabilization by redilatation (*right panel*).

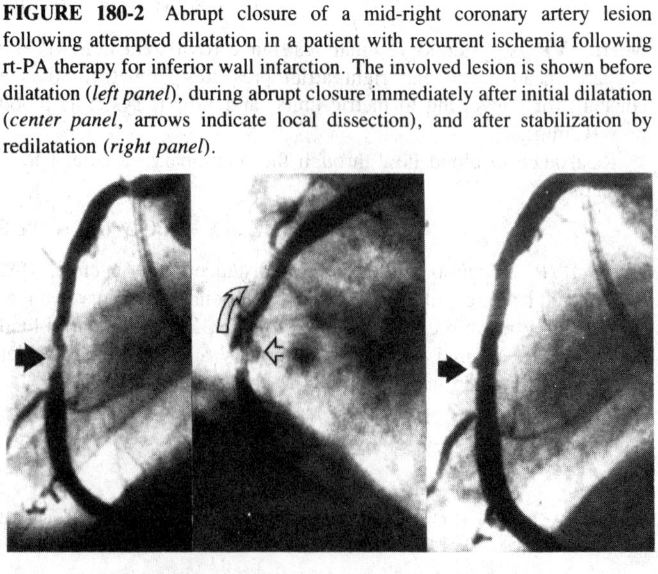

appearance and may be of value in managing elastic lesions or abrupt closure, reduction in restenosis has yet to be demonstrated. Moreover, stenting carries potential hazards, particularly local thrombosis and/or vasospasm.

Mechanical atherectomy catheters Unlike balloon angioplasty—which merely redistributes plaque to improve luminal caliber—atherectomy seeks to remove plaque material from the body. Several catheter designs have been developed, and preliminary testing in the peripheral and coronary circulations suggests that safe enlargement of lumen is possible with potentially less restenosis than is seen following balloon angioplasty.

TREATMENT OF VALVULAR STENOSIS: BALLOON VALVULOPLASTY

Following successful balloon dilatation of vascular stenoses, both pediatric and adult cardiologists applied balloon dilatation to the treatment of stenotic cardiac valves. While the initial use was in patients with congenital pulmonic and aortic stenosis, this technique has now been extended to patients with acquired rheumatic and calcific stenosis of the mitral and aortic valves.

PULMONIC VALVULOPLASTY Although congenital pulmonic stenosis is predominantly a pediatric disease, it is sometimes encountered in adult patients (see Chap. 186). Transvalvular gradients >50 mmHg may produce exertional symptoms or lead to progressive right ventricular hypertrophy or failure. Using a guidewire placed into the pulmonary artery from the femoral vein, one or more valvuloplasty balloons with a combined cross-sectional area as much as 20 percent larger than the pulmonic valve annulus are positioned within the stenotic valve and inflated with liquid contrast medium at pressures of 3 to 5 atm. This typically reduces the transvalvular gradient from 75 to 15 mmHg. More than 1000 procedures have been performed to date, and balloon pulmonary valvuloplasty now stands as the preferred therapy for this lesion.

MITRAL VALVULOPLASTY The predominant application of mitral valvuloplasty is in patients with rheumatic mitral stenosis, in whom stenosis results primarily from commissural fusion with associated leaflet thickening. Such patients previously would have undergone open or closed surgical commissurotomy, but are now treated almost exclusively by balloon valvuloplasty. Other patients (with left atrial thrombus, mitral regurgitation, subvalvular disease, or leaflet thickening or rigidity) have less satisfactory results with either surgical commissurotomy or balloon valvuloplasty and are better treated by surgical valve replacement.

The usual approach to mitral valvuloplasty is via transseptal puncture (right atrium to left atrium), followed by passage of a guidewire across the stenotic valve and into the left ventricle. One or more balloon catheters with a dilating area equivalent to a single 23- to 30-mm diameter balloon are advanced over this guidewire, and inflated within the stenotic valve. Successful dilatation separates fused commissures and enhances leaflet compliance, thus increasing the effective diastolic valve area from 0.9 to 2.0 cm^2 or more (Fig. 180-3). Although this is still restricted compared to the 3.5- to 5-cm^2 area of a normal mitral valve or the 4.5-cm^2 area of an inflated 25-mm balloon, this increase in valve area provides excellent symptomatic relief and is equivalent to the increase in orifice size resulting from surgical mitral commissurotomy or prosthetic mitral valve replacement.

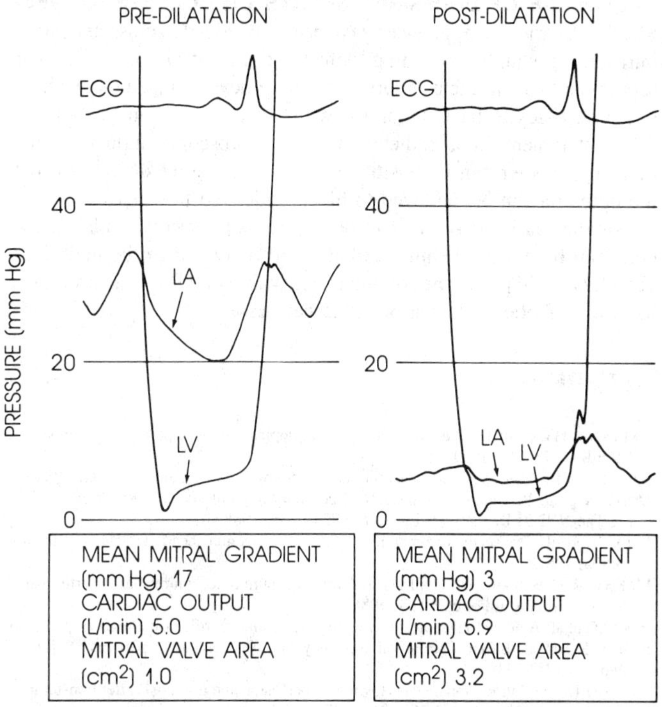

FIGURE 180-3 Hemodynamic results of mitral valvuloplasty in a 38-year-old woman with mitral stenosis. The transmitral [left atrium (LA)–to–left ventricle (LV)] gradient, cardiac output, and calculated mitral valve area are shown before (*left panel*) and after (*right panel*) balloon dilatation.

The main complications of mitral valvuloplasty relate to the potential for cardiac perforation during transseptal puncture (approximately 2 percent of patients) and the chance of systemic embolization (approximately 1 percent of patients) despite preprocedure echocardiographic exclusion of patients with left atrial thrombus.

AORTIC VALVULOPLASTY Balloon aortic valvuloplasty may be performed in children with congenital aortic stenosis and in adults with rheumatic or acquired calcific aortic stenosis. Some patients with rheumatic aortic stenosis have leaflet fusion, but the problem in acquired calcific aortic stenosis is rigidity of the valve leaflets themselves. In this latter group of patients, balloon valvuloplasty fractures leaflet calcium and provides new hinge points along which the valve leaflets can open.

The most prevalent approach to aortic valvuloplasty consists of femoral arterial puncture with retrograde passage of a guidewire and balloon (inflated diameter 18 to 23 mm) across the valve. Overdilatation of the valve annulus may cause leaflet avulsion and is generally avoided. Aortic valvuloplasty typically increases the effective systolic valve area from 0.6 to 1.0 cm^2. The resultant valve area is still small compared to the area of a normal aortic valve (3 to 4 cm^2) or to the effective area of an inflated 20-mm balloon (3.1 cm^2), but it does relieve symptoms at rest or during mild to moderate exertion in most patients with critical aortic stenosis. Unfortunately, the relatively small effective orifice achieved and the high incidence of valvular restenosis (up to 40 percent within 1 year after dilatation) make balloon aortic valvuloplasty most applicable to elderly patients who are poor risks for valve replacement, or as a "bridge" to valve replacement.

TREATMENT OF CONGENITAL MALFORMATIONS

Pediatric interventional cardiologists have developed a number of innovative techniques to correct or palliate congenital cardiac lesions. Some techniques are those described above—i.e., balloon dilatation of stenotic pulmonary arteries, surgical shunts, or balloon valvuloplasty—but others are unique to the pediatric population.

ATRIAL SEPTOSTOMY In some patients with cyanotic congenital heart disease, it is desirable to produce or enlarge an atrial septal defect in order to facilitate passage of oxygenated blood into the right heart. This can be achieved by passage of a balloon catheter from right to left atrium across a patent foramen ovale, followed by forceful withdrawal of the inflated balloon. Alternatively, a catheter with a concealed blade can be passed across the septum. The blade can then be deployed in the left atrium to incise the septum as the catheter is withdrawn. The resulting septal incision can be widened by conventional balloon septostomy.

CLOSURE OF UNDESIRED SHUNTS OR COLLATERAL VESSELS A variety of appliances have been developed to close undesired intracardiac shunts, including defects in the atrial or ventricular septum and patent ductus arteriosus. These devices resemble a single or double (back-to-back) umbrella, which can be folded into a cylinder for containment in a catheter. Under fluoroscopic guidance, the delivery catheter can be positioned across the target defect, so that the umbrella can be deployed to block undesired flow.

Smaller vascular shunts can be closed using special coils. These coils can be placed within a catheter and delivered to the undesired vessel. Once in place, the coil interferes with blood flow and promotes local thrombotic occlusion of the target vessel.

REFERENCES

ANDERSON HV et al: Usefulness of coronary angioplasty in asymptomatic patients. Am J Cardiol 65(1):35, 1990

BAIM DS (ed): A symposium: Interventional cardiology. Am J Cardiol 61:1G, 1988

DETRE K et al: Percutaneous transluminal coronary angioplasty in 1985–86 and 1977–81: The NHLBI Registry. N Engl J Med 318:265, 1988

LOCK JE et al: Transcatheter umbrella closure of congenital heart defects. Circulation 75:593, 1987

MCKAY RG: Balloon valvuloplasty for treating pulmonic, mitral, and aortic valve stenosis. Am J Cardiol 61:102G, 1988

PARK SC et al: A new atrial septostomy technique. Cathet Cardiovasc Diagn 1:195, 1975

SAFIAN RD et al: Balloon aortic valvuloplasty in 170 consecutive patients. N Engl J Med 319:125, 1988

SIGWART U et al: Intravascular stents to prevent occlusion and restenosis after transluminal angioplasty. N Engl J Med 316:701, 1987

SIMPSON JB et al: Transluminal atherectomy for occlusive peripheral vascular disease. Am J Cardiol 61:96G, 1988

WEINTRAUB WS et al: Changing use of coronary angioplasty and coronary bypass surgery in the treatment of chronic coronary artery disease. Am J Cardiol 65(3):183, 1990

181 NORMAL AND ABNORMAL MYOCARDIAL FUNCTION

EUGENE BRAUNWALD

CELLULAR BASIS OF CARDIAC CONTRACTION

The *myocardium* is composed of individual striated muscle cells (fibers), normally 10 to 15 μm in diameter and 30 to 60 μm in length (Fig. 181-1*A*). Each fiber contains multiple cross-banded strands (myofibrils), that run the length of the fiber and are, in turn, composed of serially repeating structures, the sarcomeres. The remainder of the cytoplasm, lying between the myofibrils, contains other cell constituents, such as the single centrally located nucleus, numerous mitochondria, and intracellular membrane system, the sarcoplasmic reticulum.

The *sarcomere*, the structural and functional unit of contraction, is delimited by two adjacent dark lines, the Z lines (Fig. 181-1). The distance between Z lines varies with the degree of contraction or stretch of the muscle and ranges between 1.6 and 2.2 μm. Within the confines of the sarcomere, alternating light and dark bands are seen, giving the myocardial fibers their striated appearance under the light microscope. At the center of the sarcomere is a dark band of constant width (1.5 μm), the A band, which is flanked by two lighter bands, the I bands, which are of variable width. The sarcomere of heart muscle, like that of skeletal muscle, is made up of two sets of myofilaments. Thicker filaments, composed principally of the protein myosin, traverse and are limited to the A band. They are about 10 nm (100 Å) in diameter, with tapered ends, and measure 1.5 to 1.6 μm in length. Thinner filaments, composed primarily of actin, course from the Z line through the I band into the A band. They are approximately 5 nm (50 Å) in diameter and 1.0 μm in length. Thus, there is overlapping of thick and thin filaments only within the A band, while the I band contains only thin filaments (Fig. 181-1). On electron-microscopic examination, bridges may be seen to extend between the thick and thin filaments within the A band.

THE CONTRACTILE PROCESS The "sliding" model for muscle rests on the fundamental observation that both the thick and thin filaments are constant in overall length, both at rest and during contraction. With activation of the sarcomere, repetitive interactions take place at the bridges between the actin and myosin filaments, and the actin filaments are propelled further into the A band. In the process, the A band remains constant in width, whereas the I band becomes more narrow and the Z lines move toward one another.

The myosin molecule is a complex, asymmetric fibrous protein with a molecular weight of about 500,000; it has a rod-like portion that is about 150 nm (1500 Å) in length with a globular portion at its end. This globular portion of the myosin contains adenosine triphosphatase (ATPase) activity and also forms the bridges between the myosin and actin. In forming the thick myofilament, the rod-like portions of the myosin molecules are laid down in an orderly, polarized manner, leaving the globular portions projecting outward so that they can interact with actin to generate force and shortening (Fig. 181-2*A*). Actin has a molecular weight of 47,000. The thin filament is composed of a double helix of two chains of actin molecules wound about each other, intimately associated with two regulatory proteins, tropomyosin and troponin (Fig. 181-2*B*); the latter can be separated into three components, troponins C, I, and T (Fig. 181-2*C*). In contrast to myosin, actin has no intrinsic enzymatic activity, but it has the ability to combine reversibly with myosin in the presence of ATP and Mg^{2+}, which activates the myosin ATPase. In relaxed muscle this interaction is inhibited by tropomyosin. During activation Ca^{2+} becomes attached to troponin C which results in a conformational change exposing the actin cross-bridge interaction sites. Physical changes in the cross-bridges result in sliding of the actin along the myosin filaments, ultimately causing muscle shortening and/or the development of tension. The splitting of ATP then dissociates the myosin cross-bridge from the actin. Linkages between actin and myosin filaments are made and broken cyclically as long as sufficient Ca^{2+} is present; these linkages are broken when Ca^{2+} concentration falls below a critical level, and the troponin-tropomysin complex once more prevents interactions between the myosin cross-bridges and the actin filaments. Ionic calcium is a principal mediator of the inotropic state of the heart; most positive inotropic drugs, including the digitalis glycosides and catecholamines, act by increasing the concentrations of Ca^{2+} in the vicinity of the myofilaments.

The *sarcoplasmic reticulum* (Fig. 181-1*B*), a complex network of anastomosing, membrane-lined intracellular channels, which invests the myofibrils and which is less profuse in cardiac than in skeletal muscle, consists of a series of interconnecting longitudinally disposed membrane tubules closely applied to the surfaces of the individual sarcomeres; it has no direct continuity with the outside of the cell. However, closely related to the sarcoplasmic reticulum, both structurally and functionally, are the transverse tubules or T system, formed by tubelike invaginations of the sarcolemma, which extend into the myocardial fiber, along the Z lines, i.e., the ends of the sarcomeres.

CARDIAC ACTIVATION At rest, the cardiac cell is polarized; i.e., the interior has a negative charge relative to the outside of the cell, with a transmembrane potential of −80 to −100 mV (Chap. 184). The sarcolemma, which in the resting state is largely impermeable to Na^+ and has a Na^+- and K^+-stimulated pump requiring adenosine triphosphate (ATP) that extrudes Na^+ from the cell, plays a critical role in establishing this resting potential. Thus, the inside of the cell has relatively high concentrations of K^+ with far lower concentrations of Na^+, while the extracellular milieu is high in $[Na^+]$ and low in $[K^+]$. At the same time, in the resting state, the extracellular $[Ca^{2+}]$ greatly exceeds the free intracellular $[Ca^{2+}]$.

During the plateau of the action potential (phase 2) there is a slow inward current which reflects primarily a movement of Ca^{2+} into the cell (Fig. 181-3), although the absolute quantity of Ca^{2+} that crosses

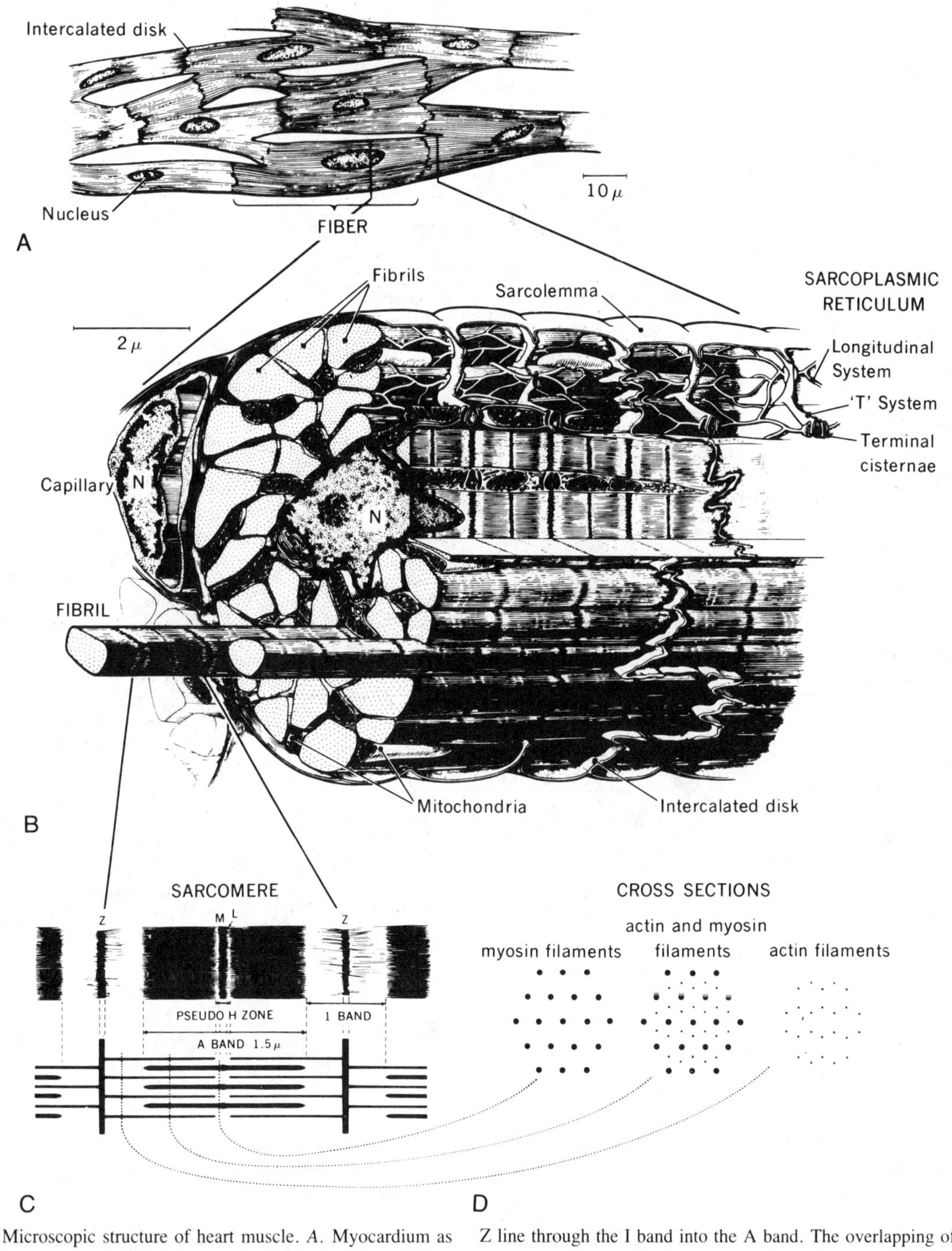

FIGURE 181-1 Microscopic structure of heart muscle. *A*. Myocardium as seen under the light microscope. Branching of fibers is evident. Each fiber, or cell, contains a centrally located nucleus. *B*. Myocardial cell, reconstructed from electron micrographs. Each cell is composed of multiple parallel fibrils. Each fibril is composed of serially connected sarcomeres (N, nucleus). *C*. Sarcomere from a myofibril, with diagrammatic representation of myofilaments. Thick filaments (1.5 μm long, composed of myosin) form the A band, and thin filaments (1 μm long, composed primarily of actin) extend from the Z line through the I band into the A band. The overlapping of thick and thin filaments is seen only in the A band. *D*. Cross sections of the sarcomere indicate the specific lattice arrangements of the myofilaments. In the center of the sarcomere only the thick, or myosin, filaments arranged in a hexagonal array are seen. In the distal portions of the A band, both thick and thin, or actin, filaments are found, with each thick filament surrounded by six thin filaments. In the I band only thin filaments are present. *(From Braunwald et al, 1976.)*

the surface membrane is relatively small and in and of itself appears to be incapable of bringing about full activation of the contractile apparatus. However, the depolarizing current not only extends across the surface of the cell but penetrates deeply into the cell by way of the ramifying T system. As a consequence of the transsarcolemmal movement of Ca^{2+}, much larger quantities of Ca^{2+} are released from the sarcoplasmic reticulum, a process termed "regenerative release" of Ca^{2+}.

The Ca^{2+} released from the sarcoplasmic reticulum then diffuses toward the sarcomere, and as already described, combines with troponin C, and, by repressing the inhibitor of contraction, activates the myofilaments to produce contraction. The sarcoplasmic reticulum then reaccumulates Ca^{2+}, an energy-requiring process, thereby lowering its concentration in the vicinity of the myofibrils to a level that inhibits the actin-myosin interaction which is responsible for contraction, and in this manner leads to relaxation. Thus, the cell membrane, transverse tubules, and sarcoplasmic reticulum, with their ability to transmit an action potential, to release and then reaccumulate Ca^{2+}, appear to play a fundamental role in the rhythmic contraction and relaxation of heart muscle.

The ATP formed from substrate oxidation is the principal source of energy for almost all of the mechanical work of contraction

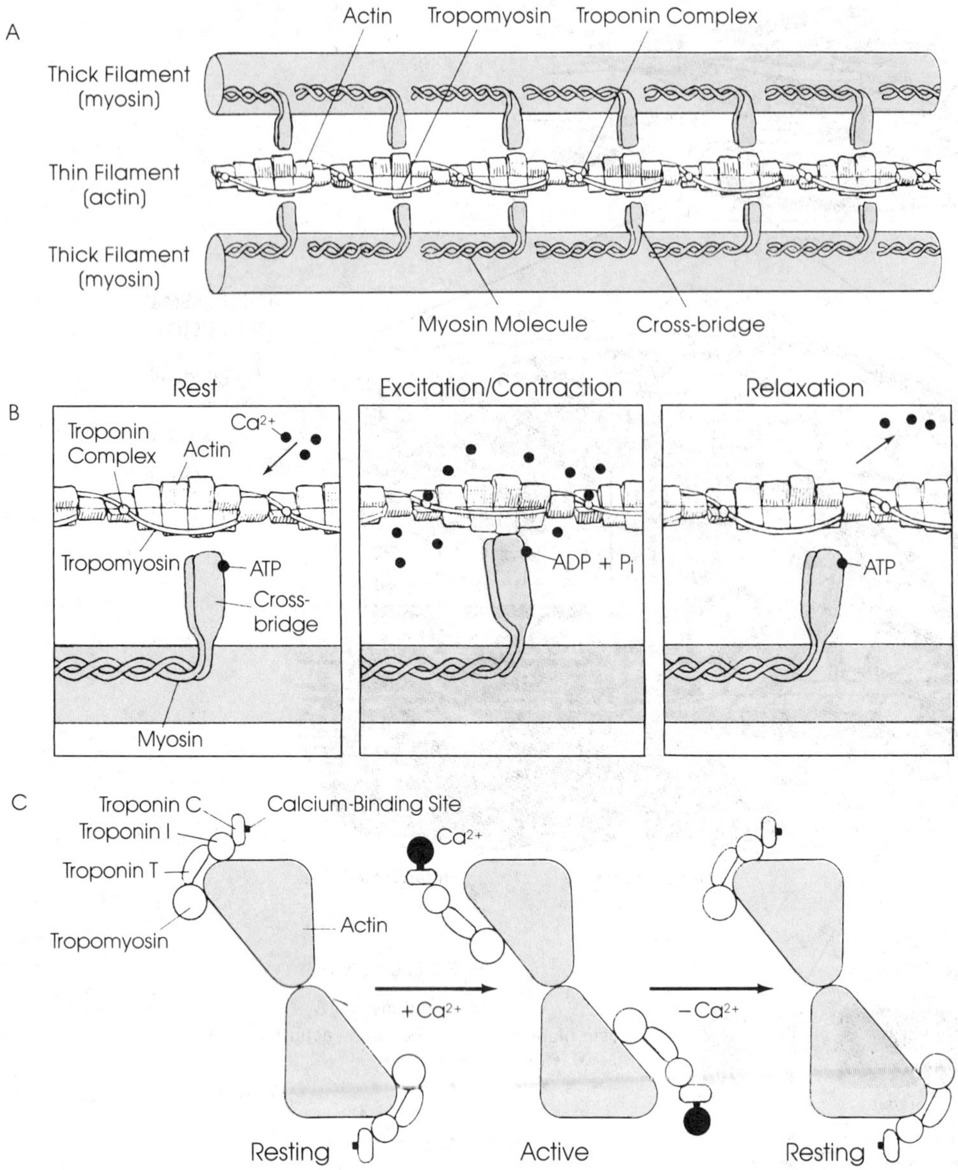

FIGURE 181-2 Contractile protein interactions and the role of calcium as activator messenger are shown schematically: *A*. Contractile proteins (myosin and actin) and regulatory proteins (troponin complex and tropomyosin) are shown in relative positions on myofilaments. *B*. Contraction takes place when the heads of myosin molecules, which form cross-bridges of thick filament, bind to actin, followed by shift in orientation of cross-bridge that pulls thin filament toward center of sarcomere. Activation requires calcium binding to troponin complex, reversing inhibition of interaction between myosin and actin. In the cycle of chemical reactions underlying contraction, hydrolysis of ATP produces the cross-bridge motion. Relaxation occurs when calcium becomes dissociated from troponin. *C*. Molecular rearrangements at the level of the thin filament involve regulatory proteins (tropomyosin and troponins C, I, T) in an allosteric effect. Calcium binding to troponin C loosens bond linking troponin I to actin; resulting dissociation of troponin T from actin backbone of thin filament displaces tropomyosin, exposing active sites for interaction with myosin. [*Reproduced by permission, from AM Katz, VE Smith, Hosp Prac, 19(1):69, 1984. Illustration by Bunji Tagawa.*]

performed by the myocardial cell. The high-energy phosphate stores in ATP are in equilibrium with those in the form of creatine phosphate. The activity of the myosin ATPase determines the rate of forming and breaking the actin-myosin cross-bridges and ultimately the velocity of muscle contraction.

THE ROLE OF MUSCLE LENGTH In all forms of striated muscle, including cardiac muscle, the force of contraction depends on initial muscle length. The sarcomere length associated with the most forceful contraction is approximately 2.2 μm. At this length the two sets of myofilaments of the sarcomere are most ideally situated to provide the greatest area for their interaction. In support of the sliding-filament hypothesis, force development diminishes in direct proportion to the decrease in the overlap between thick and thin filaments, and the resultant reduction in the number of reactive sites. The length of the sarcomere also appears to regulate the extent of activation of the contractile system, i.e., its sensitivity to Ca^{2+}, which is also greatest at approximately 2.2 μm. When sarcomere length is increased to 3.65 μm, the thin filaments are entirely withdrawn from the A band, and no tension can be developed. Similarly, when the sarcomeres are shorter than 2.0 μm, the thin filaments bypass one another, producing a double overlap of the thin filaments, a reduction of sensitivity of the contractile sites to Ca^{2+}, and the capacity for force development also declines.

The relation between the initial length of the muscle fibers and the developed force is of prime importance for the function of heart muscle. This forms the basis of the Frank-Starling relation (Starling's law of the heart), which states that, within limits, an augmentation of initial volume of the ventricle, which is a function of the initial length of the cardiac muscle, results in an increase in the force of ventricular contraction. It has been shown for heart muscle that along the ascending limb of the length–active tension curve sarcomere length is directly proportional to muscle length. As muscle length decreases to the point at which sarcomere length approaches 1.5 μm and at which developed tension approaches zero, the I bands at first narrow, then disappear while the A band remains constant in length. At this latter point, the Z lines abut the edges of the A bands. Thus, the sarcomere length–active tension curve forms the ultrastructural basis of Starling's law of the heart.

MYOCARDIAL MECHANICS

THE FORCE-VELOCITY CURVE The mechanical activity of all muscle may be expressed externally in two ways: shortening and the development of tension. Hill showed in skeletal muscle that the velocity of shortening is inversely related to the magnitude of tension development, an expression of the so-called force-velocity relation, now recognized to be a fundamental property of muscle. Expressed

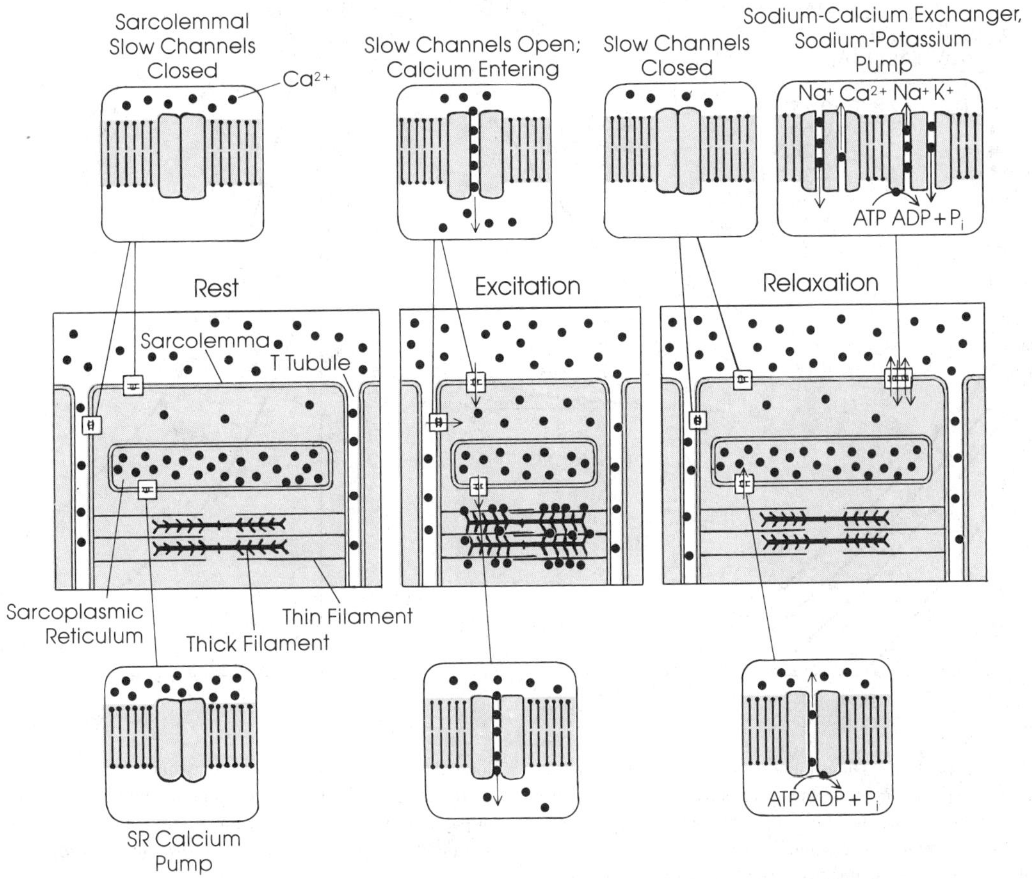

FIGURE 181-3 Calcium fluxes that activate contraction are downhill, and those that cause relaxation are uphill. As depicted in heart muscle at rest, calcium channels in the sarcolemmal membrane are closed, and intracellular calcium is stored in the sarcoplasmic reticulum. With excitation and membrane depolarization, voltage-sensitive sodium channels (not shown) and calcium channels in the sarcolemma open to allow rapid entry of extracellular sodium and calcium. Entry of calcium is now believed to cause release of calcium from the sarcoplasmic reticulum that initiates contraction. Reuptake of calcium by the sarcoplasmic reticulum by an ATP-dependent calcium pump is essential for the heart to relax. Importantly, contraction is activated mainly by passive calcium fluxes from the sarcoplasmic reticulum. By contrast, during diastole calcium must be pumped actively out of the cytosol to accomplish relaxation. Energy also must be expended during diastole to restore sodium and calcium gradients across the sarcolemma, which provide for the depolarizing ionic currents that generate the action potential. Sodium transport is accomplished by the sarcolemmal sodium pump (Na^+, K^+-ATPase), which utilizes ATP to pump sodium out of the cell in exchange for potassium. The resultant sodium gradient is largely responsible for active transport of calcium out of the cell during relaxation, via sodium-calcium exchange. [*Reproduced by permission from AM Katz, VE Smith, Hosp Prac, 19(1):69, 1984. Illustration by Bunji Tagawa.*]

simply, the greater the load the muscle is called upon to lift, the lower the velocity of shortening and vice versa. The force-velocity relation also applies to cardiac muscle. However, in this respect there is a basic difference between skeletal and cardiac muscle. Skeletal muscle has a single, essentially fixed, force-velocity curve; i.e., at any given muscle length, force and velocity are always related to each other in the same manner. The contractile activity of skeletal muscle is increased by the recruitment of additional muscle fibers, i.e., motor units, and by increasing the frequency of nerve impulses, while the contractile properties of each individual fiber remain constant. Although resting length also influences the characteristics of contraction, this variable remains essentially fixed in vivo because of the skeletal muscles' skeletal attachments. In contrast, the number of cardiac cells and within them the myofibrils and sarcomeres which become activated during each contraction is constant. However, the contractile activity of the myocardium may be readily altered under physiologic conditions by changes in resting fiber length and by changes in the inotropic state, i.e., the contractility, both of which shift the myocardial force-velocity curve.

Variations in myocardial contractile activity may be expressed as displacements of the force-velocity curve in two fundamental ways Figure 181-4*A* shows a family of force-velocity curves obtained from an isolated cardiac muscle; each curve was obtained at a different preload, i.e., with a different degree of stretch on the muscle. Note that changing the preload alters the intercept of the force-velocity curve on the horizontal axis; i.e., it increases the isometric force developed by the muscle. However, within limits, these alterations in preload do not appear to alter the velocity of shortening importantly, since all the curves extrapolate to the same intercept on the vertical axis. Thus, a change in initial length of heart muscle shifts the force-velocity curve primarily by altering the total force which can be developed by the muscle, as illustrated by the isometric length-tension curve, shown in the insert of Fig. 181-4*A*.

This type of shift in the force-velocity curve may be contrasted with that obtained when a positive inotropic agent, such as Ca^{2+}, digitalis, or norepinephrine (which act ultimately by increasing the concentration of Ca^{2+} in the vicinity of the myofilaments) is added to the muscle while the initial length is held constant (Fig. 181-4*B*). These agents not only increase the force which the muscle is capable of developing, i.e., the intercept of the force-velocity curve on the horizontal axis, therefore shifting the isometric length-tension curve upward, but they also increase the velocity of shortening of the unloaded muscle, i.e., the extrapolated intercept on the vertical axis.

It has been postulated that an increase in initial muscle length up to an optimal length brings about an increase in the number of effective force-generating sites as a consequence of a more advantageous overlap of interdigitating contractile filaments within the sarcomere as well as in the extent of activation of the contractile

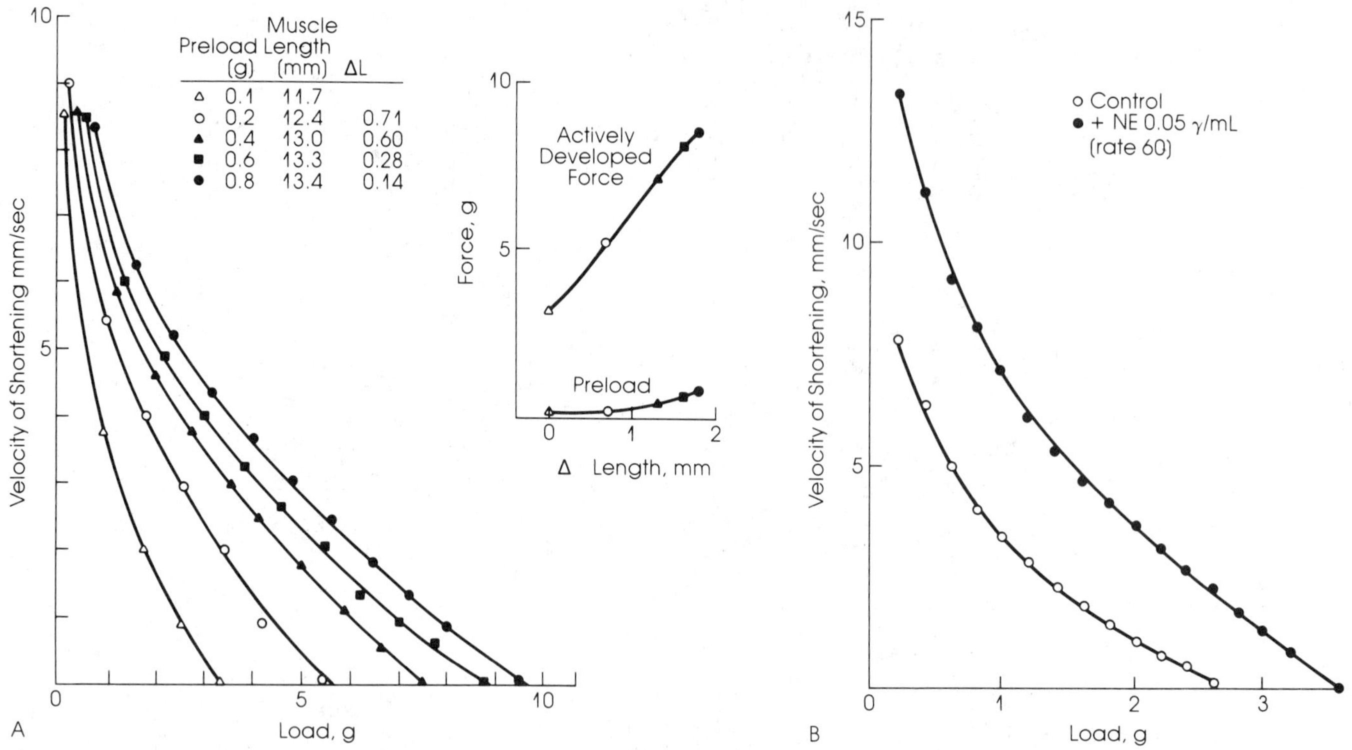

FIGURE 181-4 *A*. Effects of increasing initial muscle length on the force-velocity relation of cat papillary muscle. Initial velocity of shortening has been plotted as a function of load for five different muscle lengths. The maximum velocity of shortening is essentially unchanged, whereas the maximum force of contraction is augmented. The insert shows the places along the length-tension curves at which these force-velocity curves were determined. *B*. Effects of norepinephrine on the force-velocity relation of the cat papillary muscle. Both the maximum velocity of shortening and the force of contraction are increased. *(From Braunwald et al, 1976.)*

sites, i.e., their sensitivity to Ca^{2+}. A change in the inotropic state, characterized by an increase in the velocity of shortening of the unloaded muscle, can also result from an increase in the rate of cyclic force-generating processes at the contractile sites, without a change in the number of these sites, i.e., at a constant muscle length. Increased contractility appears to be related primarily to an increased availability of Ca^{2+} within the cell.

CONTRACTION OF THE INTACT VENTRICLE

Analysis of the heart as a pump has classically centered upon the relation between the filling pressure, or diastolic volume, of the ventricle (length of the muscle fibers) and its stroke volume (the Frank-Starling relation). In the heart-lung preparation the stroke volume is a function of diastolic fiber length at any given level of arterial resistance (afterload), and the failing heart delivers a smaller-than-normal stroke volume from a normal or elevated end-diastolic volume. The relation between the mean atrial or the ventricular end-diastolic pressure and the stroke work of the corresponding ventricle (the ventricular function curve) provides a useful definition of the level of the contractile, or inotropic, state of the ventricle. An increase in ventricular contractility is accompanied by a shift of the ventricular function curve upward and to the left, while depression of contractility is identified by downward and rightward displacement of this relation.

It has been observed that during the adrenergic stimulation of the myocardium accompanying a stress such as exercise, relatively little change in ventricular end-diastolic size occurs, while cardiac output, aortic flow velocity, stroke work, and the rate of ventricular pressure development are all augmented, sometimes greatly. Thus, neural and humorally mediated changes in myocardial contractility, heart rate, venous return, and peripheral vascular resistance may be of greater importance in circulatory adaptation than changes in ventricular end-diastolic volume and may mask the operation of the Frank-Starling mechanism.

The important influence of the adrenergic neurotransmitter substance norepinephrine (Chap. 67) on the mechanical properties of the myocardium has long been recognized. Direct stimulation of the cardiac adrenergic nerves augments ventricular function as a consequence of the release of norepinephrine from adrenergic nerve endings in the heart. These adrenergic effects are evidenced by tachycardia, a reduction in cardiac dimensions, increased velocity of ejection, and an enhanced rate of tension development.

CONTROL OF CARDIAC PERFORMANCE AND OUTPUT

The extent of shortening of mammalian heart muscle and, therefore, the stroke volume of the intact ventricle are, in the final analysis, determined by three influences: (1) the length of the muscle at the onset of contraction, i.e., the preload; (2) the inotropic state of the muscle, i.e., the position of its force-velocity-length relation; and (3) the tension which the muscle is called upon to develop during contraction, i.e., the afterload. Heart rate determines the cardiac output at any stroke volume as long as the other three influences are maintained.

VENTRICULAR END-DIASTOLIC VOLUME (PRELOAD) At any level of its inotropic state, the performance of the myocardium is influenced profoundly by ventricular end-diastolic fiber length and therefore by diastolic ventricular volume, i.e., by operation of the Frank-Starling mechanism. The following are the major determinants of ventricular preload in the intact organism:

Total blood volume When depleted, as in hemorrhage or prolonged vomiting, venous return to the heart declines (Chap. 39) and ventricular end-diastolic volume (preload) falls, as does ventricular performance, as reflected in ventricular work.

Distribution of blood volume At any given total blood volume, the ventricular end-diastolic volume is influenced by the distribution of blood between the intra- and extrathoracic compartments. This distribution in turn is influenced by the following:

1 *Body position.* Gravitational forces tend to pool blood in dependent portions. The upright posture augments extrathoracic at the expense of intrathoracic blood volume, and reduces ventricular work.
2 *Intrathoracic pressure.* Normally, mean intrathoracic pressure during the respiratory cycle is negative, a factor that acts to increase thoracic blood volume and ventricular end-diastolic volume and to enhance the return of blood to the heart, particularly during inspiration, when this pressure becomes more negative. Elevation of intrathoracic pressure, as occurs in a tension pneumothorax, during the Valsalva maneuver, in prolonged bouts of coughing, or with positive-pressure ventilation, tends to impede venous return to the heart and diminish intrathoracic blood volume and ultimately reduces stroke volume and ventricular work.
3 *Intrapericardial pressure.* When elevated, as in pericardial tamponade (Chap. 193), there is interference with cardiac filling, and the resultant reduction in ventricular diastolic volume lowers stroke volume and ventricular work.
4 *Venous tone.* The venous system is not a simple system of passive conduits between the systemic capillary bed and the right atrium. Instead, the smooth muscle in the walls of the venules and veins responds to a variety of neural and humoral stimuli. Venoconstriction occurs during muscular exercise, deep respiration, fright, or marked hypotension, tending to diminish extrathoracic and to augment intrathoracic and intraventricular blood volumes and ventricular performance.
5 *The pumping action of skeletal muscle.* During muscular exercise the contracting skeletal muscles squeeze blood out of the venous bed and, with the aid of the venous valves, displace it centrally, thereby increasing intrathoracic blood volume, ventricular end-diastolic volume, and ventricular work.

Atrial contraction Vigorous, appropriately timed atrial contraction augments ventricular filling and end-diastolic volume. The atrial contribution to ventricular filling is of particular importance in patients with ventricular hypertrophy, in whom the loss of atrial systole (as in atrial fibrillation) tends to reduce ventricular end-diastolic pressure and volume, ultimately lowering myocardial performance. The atrial contribution to ventricular filling may be reduced by atrioventricular dissociation, prolongation or abbreviation of the P-R interval, and depression of the inotropic state of the atrium.

INOTROPIC STATE (MYOCARDIAL CONTRACTILITY) A number of factors determine the level of ventricular performance at any given ventricular end-diastolic volume, i.e., the position of the ventricular function curve. These influences may be considered to operate by modifying myocardial force-velocity-length relations.

Adrenergic nerve activity (See also Chap. 67) The quantity of norepinephrine released by adrenergic nerve endings in the heart is, under ordinary circumstances, dependent on the adrenergic nerve impulse traffic, and alterations in the frequency of nerve impulses modify the quantity of norepinephrine released and acting upon the beta-adrenergic receptors in the myocardium. This mechanism is the most important one which acutely modifies the position of the force-velocity and ventricular function curves under physiologic conditions.

Circulating catecholamines (See also Chap. 67) The adrenal medulla and other sympathetic ganglia outside the heart, when stimulated by adrenergic nerve impulses, release catecholamines, which, when they reach the heart, augment the inotropic state and the frequency of contraction.

The force-frequency relation The position of the myocardial force-velocity curve is influenced also by the rate and rhythm of cardiac contraction; e.g., ventricular extrasystoles result in post-extrasystolic potentiation, presumably by increasing the Ca^{2+} which enters the cardiac cell.

Exogenously administered inotropic agents The cardiac glycosides, isoproterenol, dopamine, dobutamine, and other sympathomimetic agents, calcium, caffeine, theophylline, and their derivatives, all improve the myocardial force-velocity relation and therefore may be used therapeutically to augment ventricular performance at any given ventricular end-diastolic volume.

Physiologic depressants Included among these are severe myocardial hypoxia, hypercapnia, ischemia, and acidosis. Acting either singly or in combination, these influences exert a depressant effect on the myocardial force-velocity curve and lower the level of the left ventricular work at any given ventricular end-diastolic volume.

Pharmacologic depressants These include quinidine, procainamide, disopyramide, high doses of certain calcium antagonists, barbiturates, alcohol, and other local and general anesthetics, as well as many other drugs.

Loss of ventricular substance When a sufficiently large portion of ventricular myocardium becomes nonfunctional or necrotic, as occurs transiently during ischemia (Chap. 190) and permanently in myocardial infarction (Chap. 189), total ventricular performance at any given level of end-diastolic volume is depressed, even if the remaining myocardium functions normally or supranormally.

Intrinsic myocardial depression Although the fundamental mechanisms responsible for depression of myocardial contractility in chronic congestive heart failure still remain to be elucidated, it is now apparent that in this condition the inotropic state of each unit of myocardium is depressed and that the level of ventricular performance at any ventricular end-diastolic volume is thereby lowered.

VENTRICULAR AFTERLOAD The stroke volume is ultimately a function of the extent of ventricular fiber shortening. In the intact heart, as in isolated cardiac muscle, the velocity and extent of shortening of ventricular muscle fibers at any given level of diastolic fiber length and myocardial inotropic state are inversely related to the afterload imposed on the muscle. The afterload on the intact heart may be defined as the tension or stress developed in the wall of the ventricle during ejection. Therefore, the afterload on the ventricular muscle fibers also is dependent on the level of aortic pressure as well as on the volume and thickness of the ventricular cavity, since Laplace's law indicates that the tension of the myocardial fiber is a function of the product of the intracavitary ventricular pressure and ventricular radius divided by the wall thickness. Thus, at the same level of aortic pressure, the afterload faced by a dilated left ventricle is higher than that encountered by a ventricle of normal size. Furthermore, at any level of aortic pressure and left ventricular volume the afterload placed on any wall fiber varies inversely with wall thickness. The aortic pressure, in turn, is influenced largely by the peripheral vascular resistance, the physical characteristics of the arterial tree, and the volume of blood it contains at the onset of ejection. At any given ventricular end-diastolic volume and level of the inotropic state, the left ventricular stroke volume is related inversely to the afterload.

The critical role played by the ventricular afterload in cardiovascular regulation is summarized in Fig. 181-5. As already noted, increases in both preload and contractility increase myocardial fiber shortening, while increases in afterload reduce it. The extent of myocardial fiber shortening and left ventricular size are the determinants of stroke volume. Arterial pressure, in turn, is related to the product of cardiac output and systemic vascular resistance, while afterload is a function of left ventricular size and arterial pressure. An increase in arterial pressure induced by vasoconstriction, for example, augments afterload, which through a negative feedback depresses myocardial fiber shortening, stroke volume, and cardiac output; this in turn tends to restore arterial pressure to its previous level.

When left ventricular function becomes impaired and the chamber dilates, i.e., when there is no preload reserve, left ventricular afterload becomes increasingly important in determining cardiac performance. Increases in afterload may result from the influence on the arterial bed of neural, humoral, or structural changes which can occur in

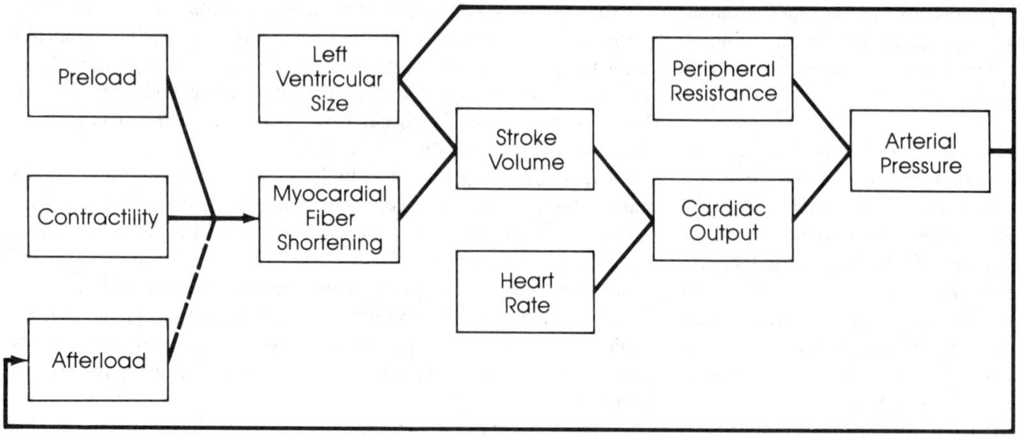

FIGURE 181-5 Scheme of interactions among various components that regulate cardiac activity. Solid lines indicate an augmenting effect; broken line represents an inhibiting effect. *(From Braunwald et al, 1976.)*

response to a fall in cardiac output. This increased afterload may reduce further cardiac output while myocardial oxygen requirements are increased. Treatment with vasodilators (Chap. 182) has the opposite effect. In this way, alterations in the peripheral vascular bed probably play an important role in the hemodynamic and metabolic events which usually are attributed to progressive impairment of the myocardium.

All of the influences acting on cardiac performance enumerated above interact in a complex fashion to maintain cardiac output at a level appropriate to the requirements of the metabolizing tissues, and in a normal person interference with one of these mechanisms may not influence the cardiac output. For example, a moderate reduction of blood volume *or* the loss of the atrial contribution to ventricular contraction can ordinarily be sustained without a reduction in the resting cardiac output. Presumably other factors, such as an increase in the frequency of adrenergic nerve impulses to the heart and an increase in heart rate, will, in a normal individual, augment contractility and sustain cardiac output. Mechanisms are also available that prevent elevation of the cardiac output when there is no physiologic demand for augmented flow. For example, augmentation of myocardial contractility by means of cardiac glycosides does not increase the cardiac output in normal humans. Thus, in analyzing the effect of an intervention on cardiac output, it is important to recognize that it is the preload, which in turn is related to the volume of blood available for filling the heart, rather than the inotropic state of the myocardium or the afterload which limits cardiac output in the normal individual and that an improvement of myocardial contractility by a drug such as digitalis or the reduction of afterload with nitroprusside would not be expected to elevate the output in a normal subject. On the other hand, in the presence of congestive heart failure, the cardiac output usually is limited by the depressed contractile state of the myocardium, and a positive inotropic drug and/or reduction of afterload would be expected to raise cardiac output, and, indeed, does so (Chap. 182).

EXERCISE The hemodynamic changes which normally occur during exercise in the upright position are complex (Fig. 181-6). The hyperventilation, the pumping action of the exercising muscles, and the venoconstriction which occur all tend to augment venous return and hence ventricular filling and preload. Simultaneously, the increase in the adrenergic nerve impulses to the myocardium, the increased concentration of circulating catecholamines, and the tachycardia which occur during exercise all combine to augment the contractile state of the myocardium (Fig. 181-6, curves 1 and 2) and lead to an elevation of stroke volume, with no change or even a decrease of end-diastolic

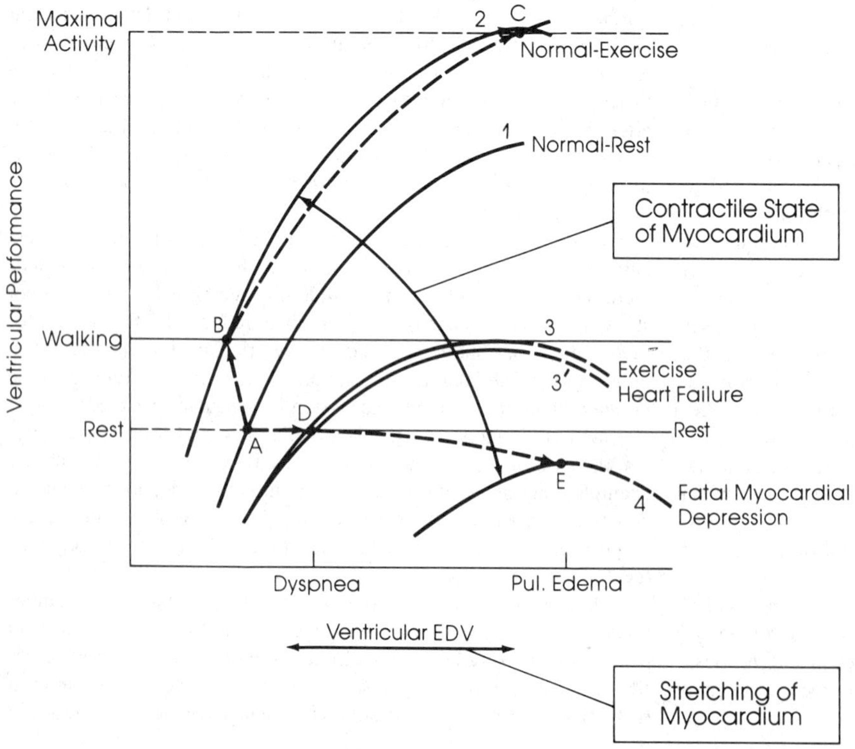

FIGURE 181-6 Diagram showing the interrelations among influences on ventricular end-diastolic volume (EDV) through stretching of the myocardium and the contractile state of the myocardium. Levels of ventricular EDV associated with filling pressures that result in dyspnea and pulmonary edema are shown on the abscissa. Levels of ventricular performance required when the subject is at rest, while walking, and during maximal activity are designated on the ordinate. The dotted lines are the descending limbs of the ventricular-performance curves, which are rarely seen during life but which show the level of ventricular performance if end-diastolic volume could be elevated to very high levels. For further explanation see text. *(From Braunwald et al, 1976.)*

pressure and volume (Fig. 181-6, points A and B). Vasodilatation occurs in the exercising muscles, thus tending to counteract the marked increase in arterial pressure which would otherwise occur as cardiac output rises. This ultimately allows the achievement of a greatly elevated cardiac output during exercise, at an arterial pressure only moderately higher than in the resting state.

THE FAILING HEART

Though heart failure may be readily described as a clinical syndrome, characterized by well-known symptoms and physical signs, a precise physiologic or biochemical definition is far more difficult. However, from the clinical point of view, heart failure may be considered to be the condition in which *an abnormality of cardiac function is responsible for the inability of the heart to pump blood at a rate commensurate with the requirements of the metabolizing tissues and/or can do so only from an abnormally elevated filling pressure.* Abnormalities during systole and/or diastole may be present in heart failure (Fig. 181-7). In so-called *systolic heart failure,* i.e., classic heart failure, an impaired inotropic state causes weakened systolic contraction, which leads, ultimately, to a reduction in stroke volume, inadequate ventricular emptying, cardiac dilatation, and often elevation of ventricular diastolic pressure. Idiopathic dilated cardiomyopathy (Chap. 192) is the prototype of systolic heart failure. In *diastolic heart failure* the principal abnormality involves impaired relaxation of the ventricle and leads to an elevation of ventricular diastolic pressure at a normal diastolic volume. Failure of relaxation can be functional, i.e., as during transient ischemia, or it can be caused by a stiffened, thickened ventricle. Typical conditions in which diastolic failure occurs are restrictive cardiomyopathy secondary to infiltrative conditions, such as amyloidosis or hemochromatosis, as well as hypertrophic cardiomyopathy (Chap. 192). In many patients with cardiac hypertrophy and dilatation, systolic and diastolic failure coexist; the ventricle both empties and fills abnormally. There may be cardiac dilatation, but the ventricle's pressure-volume relation is shifted, raising the ventricular diastolic pressure at any given volume.

Though a defect in myocardial contraction is characteristic of systolic heart failure, this defect may result from a primary abnormality in the heart muscle, as in cardiomyopathy, or it may be secondary to a chronic excessive work load as in hypertension and valvular heart disease, as well as in many forms of congenital heart disease. In ischemic heart disease systolic heart failure results from a loss in the quantity of normally contracting cells. It is important to distinguish heart failure from (1) states of circulatory insufficiency in which myocardial function is not primarily impaired, such as cardiac tamponade or hemorrhagic shock, (2) conditions in which there is circulatory congestion because of abnormal salt and water retention but in which there is no serious disturbance of the heart's function, and (3) conditions in which a normally contracting myocardium is suddenly presented with a load which exceeds its capacity, e.g., accelerated hypertension or rupture of a valve cusp secondary to infective endocarditis.

The intrinsic contractile state of myocardium removed from normal, hypertrophied, and failing animal hearts has been evaluated, and both ventricular hypertrophy and heart failure were shown to reduce the maximum isometric tension and velocity of shortening to subnormal levels; the changes are more marked in the myocardium of animals in which heart failure had been present than in those with hypertrophy alone. Papillary muscles removed from the left ventricles of patients with heart failure have also shown a depression of the maximum degree of active tension which they can develop. Electron-microscopic analysis of failing cat papillary muscles fixed at the apexes of the length–active tension curves revealed sarcomere lengths averaging 2.2 μm. Thus, the abnormalities of contractility do *not* appear to be produced by an alteration in the overlap of filaments within the sarcomere.

The failing ventricle may still eject a normal or nearly normal stroke volume despite considerable depression of function, when its end-diastolic volume increases, i.e., through the operation of the Frank-Starling mechanism. As outlined above, an increase in the initial volume of the ventricle is associated with stretching of the sarcomere, a process that augments the number of sites at which the actin and myosin filaments can interact and/or which increases their sensitivity to Ca^{2+}. Furthermore, the development of ventricular hypertrophy may be considered to provide additional contractile units, and thereby constitutes an important compensatory mechanism when the myocardium's intrinsic inotropic state is depressed.

ASSESSMENT OF CARDIAC PERFORMANCE Several techniques are available for defining impaired cardiac performance in intact humans. With the patient at rest, the cardiac output and stroke volume may be depressed, but not uncommonly these variables are within normal limits. A more sensitive index is the ejection fraction, i.e., the ratio of stroke volume to end-diastolic volume, which may be estimated by standard radiocontrast or radionuclide angiography (Chaps. 177 and 179), and which is frequently depressed in heart failure even when the stroke volume itself is normal. A limitation of the ejection fraction (and of cardiac output) in the assessment of

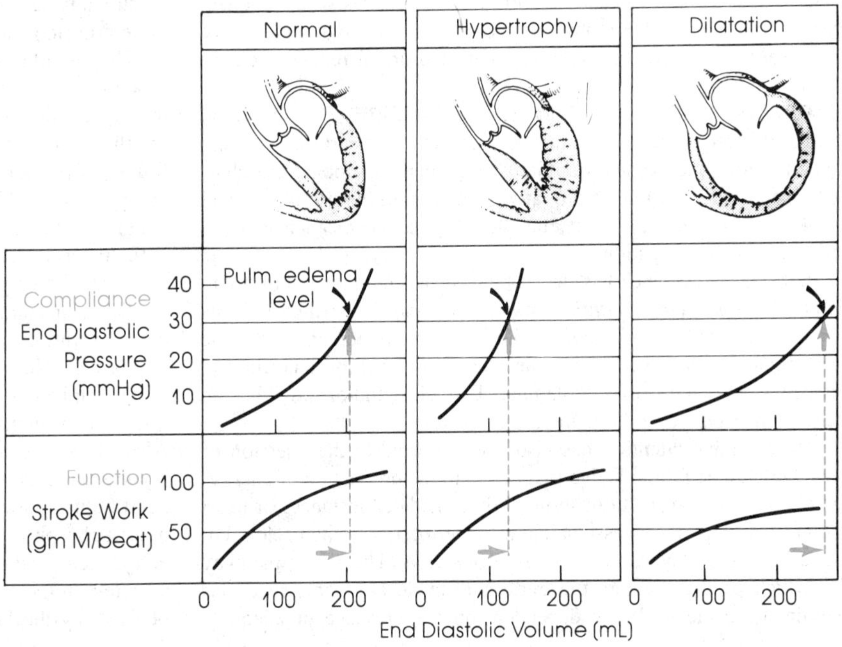

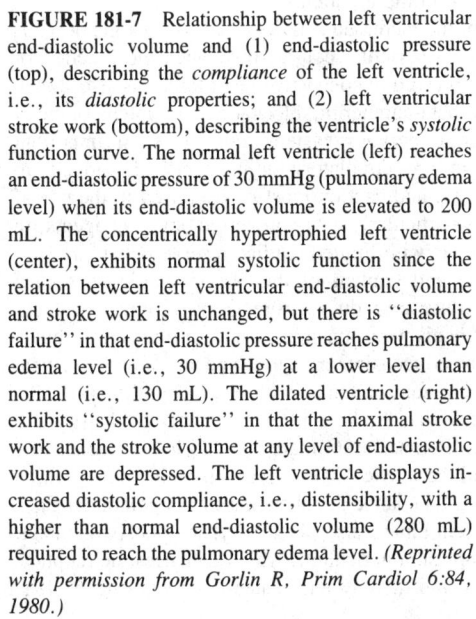

FIGURE 181-7 Relationship between left ventricular end-diastolic volume and (1) end-diastolic pressure (top), describing the *compliance* of the left ventricle, i.e., its *diastolic* properties; and (2) left ventricular stroke work (bottom), describing the ventricle's *systolic* function curve. The normal left ventricle (left) reaches an end-diastolic pressure of 30 mmHg (pulmonary edema level) when its end-diastolic volume is elevated to 200 mL. The concentrically hypertrophied left ventricle (center), exhibits normal systolic function since the relation between left ventricular end-diastolic volume and stroke work is unchanged, but there is "diastolic failure" in that end-diastolic pressure reaches pulmonary edema level (i.e., 30 mmHg) at a lower level than normal (i.e., 130 mL). The dilated ventricle (right) exhibits "systolic failure" in that the maximal stroke work and the stroke volume at any level of end-diastolic volume are depressed. The left ventricle displays increased diastolic compliance, i.e., distensibility, with a higher than normal end-diastolic volume (280 mL) required to reach the pulmonary edema level. *(Reprinted with permission from Gorlin R, Prim Cardiol 6:84, 1980.)*

cardiac function is that these variables are influenced by ventricular loading conditions. Thus, a depressed ejection fraction and lowered cardiac output may be observed in patients with normal ventricular function but reduced preload, as occurs in hypovolemia, or with acutely elevated arterial pressure. An even more sensitive method for detecting impaired ventricular performance is based on the measurement of the circulatory changes occurring during stresses such as exercise or increased afterload. Thus, left ventricular performance may be estimated accurately by measuring the left ventricular end-diastolic pressure, cardiac output, and total body O_2 consumption at rest and during exercise. In normal persons, the cardiac output rises by more than 500 mL/min for each 100-mL increase in minute O_2 consumption. The left ventricular end-diastolic pressure at rest is less than 12 mmHg and rises slightly, remains unchanged, or decreases slightly during exercise, while stroke volume usually rises, especially when exercise is carried out in the upright position. The failing left ventricle, on the other hand, is characterized by an elevation of end-diastolic pressure during exercise, which reaches a value exceeding 12 mmHg, accompanied by either no change or a fall in stroke volume and a subnormal increase in cardiac output related to the increase in minute O_2 consumption. Various degrees of impairment intermediate between the normal response and that of the failing left ventricle during the stress of exercise also have been described.

The potential value of stressing the left ventricle in assessing its performance is emphasized by the fact that the basal values for left ventricular end-diastolic pressure, cardiac index, and ventricular stroke work may be in the same range in patients with depressed ventricular function as in normal persons. The response to stress may prove useful not only in the detection of the impairment of myocardial function, but also in expressing the severity of this impairment quantitatively.

The performance of the left ventricle in humans may also be characterized by examining the instantaneous myocardial force-velocity relations and the extent of shortening during individual cardiac cycles. Angiocardiographic and echocardiographic studies (Chaps. 177 and 179) and analyses of the rate of change of intraventricular pressure (*dp/dt*) as a function of the simultaneously recorded pressure during isovolumetric contraction have shown that depressions in the velocity of myocardial fiber shortening and of tension development exist in patients with heart failure. In patients with ischemic heart disease these changes are often localized rather than diffuse. Thus, they are manifest by regional wall motion disorders, often in the face of normal global left ventricular function. The end-systolic left ventricular pressure-volume relationship is a particularly useful index of ventricular performance since it is independent of both preload and afterload. Noninvasive techniques, particularly echocardiography and radionuclide angiography, are of great value in the clinical assessment of myocardial function (Chap. 177).

CARDIAC METABOLISM IN HEART FAILURE The common forms of low-output heart failure, secondary to arteriosclerosis, hypertension, and certain valvular and congenital lesions, are characterized by an absolute or a relative reduction in the useful external work delivered by the heart, but the responsible mechanisms are under active investigation.

Substantial evidence has been obtained that in heart failure there is an *abnormality of excitation-contraction coupling*, which reduces the delivery of Ca^{2+} to the contractile sites, thereby impairing cardiac performance. However, the molecular basis of this abnormality, indeed its sites, i.e., the sarcolemma, T tubules, and/or sarcoplasmic reticulum, have yet to be defined.

Considerable attention has also been directed to the question of whether cardiac failure is due to a defect in the production of energy, its conservation, or its utilization. Only in isolated instances of heart failure, such as those associated with beriberi, are there clear-cut disturbances of myocardial *energy production*. The major pathway by which pyruvate enters the citric acid cycle and some reactions within the cycle itself are dependent on the presence of adequate concentrations of thiamine (Chap. 76). Thiamine deficiency results in diminished pyruvic acid utilization by heart slices, and in abnormally low pyruvate extraction coefficients in intact dogs and in humans.

In the second phase of cardiac metabolism, *energy conservation*, the energy of substrate oxidation is converted into the terminal-bond energy of creatine phosphate (CP) and of ATP, the immediate source of chemical energy utilized by heart muscle. This process, known as oxidative phosphorylation, occurs in the mitochondria. The effectiveness of the combined energy production-conservation mechanisms may be studied by measuring the stores of ATP and CP existing in the myocardium, while energy conservation may be evaluated by determining (1) the P/O ratio, i.e., the ratio of high-energy phosphate produced to oxygen consumed in the mitochondria, and (2) the degree of coupling between electron transport and the generation of high-energy phosphate compounds. Although controversy exists concerning the status of this phase of metabolism in heart failure, it now appears that severe impairment of myocardial performance may occur *without* disturbances of mitochondrial function or reduction of high-energy phosphate stores, although abnormalities in these processes have been shown to occur in some forms of experimental (and perhaps of clinical) heart failure.

In the absence of a definitive abnormality of energy liberation or conservation in the failing myocardium, attention has naturally been directed to the possibility that energy *utilization* is abnormal. An abnormality of energy liberation could certainly occur if the contractile proteins themselves were altered. A cardiac myosin isoenzyme characterized by immunologic and electrophoretic properties exhibiting a lower Ca^{2+}-dependent ATPase activity has been shown in some forms of experimentally produced heart failure, particularly those produced by mechanical overloading (Chap. 173). It is possible that this depression may be responsible for a defect in the breakdown of ATP, the process which leads to contraction.

THE ADRENERGIC NERVOUS SYSTEM IN HEART FAILURE In view of the importance of the adrenergic nervous system in stimulating the contractility of the normal myocardium, the activity of this system has also been studied intensively in patients with congestive heart failure. An index of the activity of this system, at rest and during exercise, is provided by measurements of the concentration of norepinephrine (NE) in arterial blood. Relatively small increases in the NE concentration occur during exercise in normal subjects. In patients with heart failure the levels of circulating NE may be markedly elevated at rest, indicating that the activity of the adrenergic nervous system is augmented at rest, and the prognosis varies inversely with the concentration. Also, much greater increments in circulating NE occur when patients with congestive heart failure exercise, again presumably because of an increased activity of the adrenergic nervous system during exercise in these patients.

The importance of the increased activity of the adrenergic nervous system in maintaining ventricular contractility when the function of the myocardium is depressed in congestive heart failure is also shown by the finding that beta-adrenergic blockade may intensify heart failure. The adrenergic nervous system thus plays an important compensatory role in the circulatory adjustments of patients to congestive heart failure, and caution must be exercised in the use of antiadrenergic drugs, particularly beta-adrenergic blocking agents, in the treatment of patients with limited cardiac reserve (Chap. 182).

The concentration and content of the NE in cardiac tissue of patients with heart failure are reduced, sometimes to only 10 percent of normal. The mechanism responsible is not entirely clear, but a prolonged increase in cardiac adrenergic tone appears to play a critical role and to interfere in some manner with the biosynthesis of NE. Also, there is evidence that the beta-adrenergic receptor density and myocardial cyclic AMP concentration are reduced in chronic, severe heart failure. Intracellular cyclic AMP activates protein kinase, which in turn phosphorylates Ca channels, enhancing transarcolemmal Ca^{2+} entry. Activated protein kinase also phosphorylates phospholamban, a protein in the sarcoplasmic reticulum, which enhances the reuptake of Ca^{2+} by the latter and thereby terminates contraction (Fig. 181-

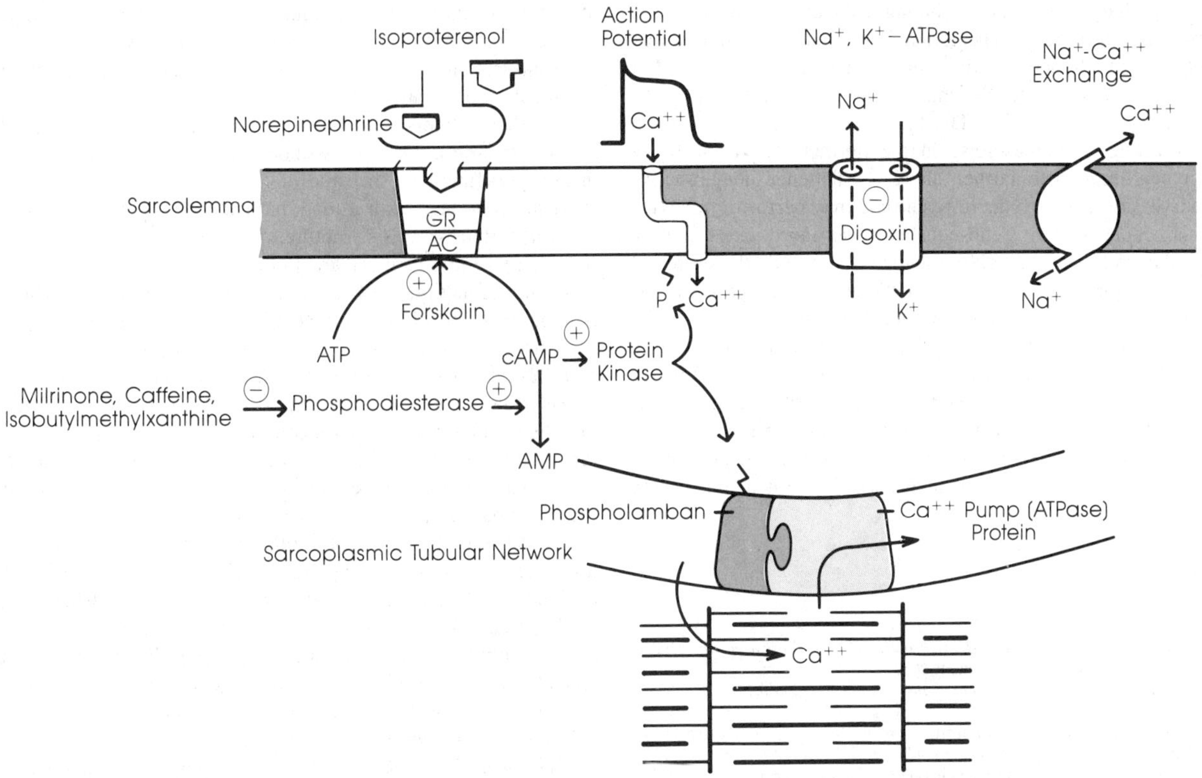

FIGURE 181-8 Schematic representation of influences on intramyocardial Ca^{2+} concentration and excitation-contraction coupling. The action potential is associated with intracellular entry of Na^+ and the extrusion of K^+ (not shown) and the entry of Ca^{2+} (shown). The Na^+-Ca^{2+} exchanger depends on concentration gradients and does not require ATP. Not shown is the energy-dependent sarcolemmal Ca^{2+} pump which extrudes Ca^{2+} from the cell. Isoproterenol and norepinephrine, the latter shown intraneuronally, stimulate the beta-adrenergic receptor in the outer sarcolemma. The beta receptor is coupled to G (guanine nucleotide–binding regulatory) proteins (GR), which in turn activate the catalytic adenylate cyclase (AC). The latter catalyzes the production of cyclic AMP from ATP. AC can be stimulated directly by the administration of *forskolin,* which bypasses both the beta receptor and the G proteins. Cyclic AMP activates protein kinase, which in turn enhances the phosphorylation of the Ca^{2+} channel, increasing transarcolemmal Ca^{2+} influx. Activated protein kinase also phosphorylates phospholamban, which in its phosphorylated form enhances the uptake of Ca^{2+} by the sarcoplasmic tubular network. Phosphodiesterase catalyzes the breakdown of cyclic AMP to AMP while milrinone, caffeine, and isobutylmethylxanthine inhibit phosphodiesterase, thereby augmenting cyclic AMP concentration. Digoxin inhibits the Na^+, K^+-ATPase in the sarcolemma, inhibiting Na^+ efflux from and K^+ influx into the cell. As a consequence the intracellular Na^+ concentration falls and Na^+-Ca^{2+} exchange is reduced, thereby raising intracellular Ca^{2+}. P represents phosphorylation. *(From Feldman MD et al, by permission of the American Heart Association, Inc.)*

8). A deficiency of intracellular cyclic AMP prolongs the action potential and the duration of contraction. The deficiency of intracellular cyclic AMP may be related in part to the "down-regulation" of myocardial $beta_1$ receptors which occurs in heart failure. Changes in the G (guanine regulatory) proteins, which couple the beta receptor to the catalytic adenylate cyclase (which is responsible for the production of cyclic AMP), may also play a role. There is some evidence that increased activity of an inhibitory subunit and reduced activity of the stimulatory subunit of the G proteins occur in heart failure.

In view of the strongly positive inotropic effect exerted by the NE released from these nerves, the adrenergic nervous system may be considered to provide an important potential source of support to the failing myocardium, as long as the number of myocardial beta adrenergic receptors and cyclic AMP concentrations are normal. However, the increments of heart rate and contractile force that occur in animals with experimental heart failure and cardiac NE depletion are abolished or markedly reduced with stimulation of the cardiac adrenergic nerves. Thus, it is likely that when congestive heart failure is accompanied by depletion of cardiac NE stores, the quantity of NE released by the adrenergic nerve endings in the heart is deficient relative to the impulse traffic along these nerves. Furthermore, whatever NE is released may not elicit a normal effect due to reduction of myocardial adrenergic receptor-effector mechanisms.

Cardiac stores of NE are not fundamentally necessary for maintaining the intrinsic contractile state of the myocardium. However, since the reduction of NE stores in heart failure is associated with a diminished release of neurotransmitter, this depletion of NE may be responsible for loss of the much-needed adrenergic support in the failing heart. In the later stages of heart failure, when the levels of circulating catecholamines are elevated and the cardiac NE stores depleted, the myocardium is largely dependent on a more generalized adrenergic stimulation derived from extracardiac sources, presumably the adrenal medulla; this would explain the deterioration of cardiac performance which may occur in patients with heart failure who are treated with beta-adrenergic blocking drugs. This generalized adrenergic stimulation resulting from circulating catecholamines may, however, also exert undesirable side effects, because it elevates vascular resistance and may present the heart with an afterload which is higher than optimal. It may also enhance the likelihood of ventricular arrhythmias. The survival of patients with congestive heart failure varies inversely with the concentration of circulating NE.

In the final analysis, in heart failure, the fundamental abnormality resides in depressions of the myocardial force-velocity relationship and of the length-active tension curve, reflecting reductions in the contractile state of the myocardium (Fig. 181-6, curves 1 to 3). In many instances, cardiac output and external ventricular performance at rest are within normal limits but are maintained at these levels only by an increased end-diastolic fiber length and an elevated ventricular end-diastolic volume, i.e., through the operation of the Frank-Starling mechanism (Fig. 181-6, points A to D). The elevation of left ventricular preload is associated with similar changes in the pulmonary capillary pressure, contributing to the dyspnea experienced by patients with heart failure. The normal improvement of contractility due to augmented adrenergic activity during exercise is attenuated or even prevented by NE depletion which occurs in severe heart failure (Fig. 181-6, curves 3 and 3′). The factors which tend to augment ventricular filling during exercise in the normal subject push the failing myocardium even farther along its flattened length-active tension curve, and although the left ventricle may perform somewhat better, this occurs only as a consequence of an inordinate elevation of ventricular end-diastolic volume and pressure and, therefore, of the pulmonary capillary pressure. The elevation of the latter intensifies dyspnea and therefore plays an important role in limiting the intensity of exercise which the patient can perform. Left ventricular failure becomes fatal when the myocardial length-active tension curve is depressed (Fig. 181-6, curve 4) to the point at which cardiac performance fails to satisfy the requirements of the peripheral tissues even at rest, and/or the left ventricular end-diastolic and pulmonary capillary pressures are elevated to levels which result in pulmonary edema (Fig. 181-6, point E).

REFERENCES

BRAUNWALD E et al (eds): *Congestive Heart Failure: Current Research and Clinical Applications*. New York, Grune & Stratton, 1982

——— et al: *Mechanisms of Contraction of the Normal and Failing Heart*, 2d ed. Boston, Little, Brown, 1976

——— et al: Contraction of the normal heart, in *Heart Disease*, 3d ed, E Braunwald (ed). Philadelphia, Saunders, 1988, pp. 383–425

BRISTOW MR et al: Myocardial α and β-adrenergic receptors in heart failure: Is cardiac-derived norepinephrine the regulatory signal? Eur Heart J 9(Suppl H):35, 1988

COHN JN et al: Plasma norepinephrine as a guide to prognosis in patients with chronic congestive heart failure. N Engl J Med 311:819, 1984

FELDMAN MD et al: Deficient production of cyclic AMP: Pharmacologic evidence of an important cause of contractile dysfunction in patients with end-stage heart failure. Circulation 75:331, 1987

FLEISCHER S, INNUI M: Regulation of muscle contraction and relaxation in heart. Prog Clin Biol Res 273:435, 1988

GROSSMAN W: Evaluation of systolic and diastolic function of the myocardium, in W Grossman (ed): *Cardiac Catheterization and Angiography*, 3d ed. Philadelphia, Lea & Febiger, 1986, p 301

KATZ AM: Cellular mechanisms in congestive heart failure. Am J Cardiol 62:3A, 1988

LOMPRE AM et al: Myosin isoenzyme redistribution in chronic heart overload. Nature 282:105, 1979

MORGAN JP, MORGAN KG: Intracellular calcium and cardiovascular function in heart failure: Effects of pharmacologic agents. Cardiovasc Drugs Ther 3(Suppl 3):959–970, 1989

——— et al: Abnormal intracellular calcium handling: A major cause of systolic and diastolic dysfunction in ventricular myocardium from patients with heart failure. Circulation 81(Suppl III):21–32, 1990

SPIRITO P et al: Noninvasive assessment of left ventricular diastolic function: Comparative analysis of Doppler echocardiographic and radionuclide angiographic techniques. J Am Col Cardiol 7:518, 1986

182 HEART FAILURE

EUGENE BRAUNWALD

Heart failure may be defined as the pathophysiologic state in which an abnormality of *cardiac* function is responsible for the failure of the heart to pump blood at a rate commensurate with the requirements of the metabolizing tissues *and/or* can do so only from an abnormally elevated filling pressure. Heart failure is frequently, but not always, caused by a defect in myocardial contraction, and then the term *myocardial failure* is appropriate. The latter may result from a primary abnormality in the heart muscle, as occurs in the cardiomyopathies (Chap. 192). Myocardial failure may also result from extramyocardial abnormalities, such as coronary atherosclerosis which leads to myocardial ischemia and infarction, as well as from abnormalities of the heart valves in which the heart muscle is damaged by the long-standing excessive hemodynamic burden imposed by the valvular abnormality, and/or by the rheumatic process (Chap. 187). In patients with chronic constrictive pericarditis, myocardial damage resulting from infiltration of the heart muscle by pericardial inflammation and calcification is common (Chap. 193).

In other patients with heart failure, however, a similar clinical syndrome is present, but without any detectable abnormality of *myocardial* function. In some of these patients the normal heart is suddenly presented with a load that exceeds its capacity, such as an acute hypertensive crisis, rupture of an aortic valve cusp, or massive pulmonary embolism. Heart failure, in the presence of normal myocardial function, also occurs in chronic conditions in which there is impairment of filling of the ventricles due to tricuspid and/or mitral stenosis, constrictive pericarditis without myocardial involvement, endocardial fibrosis, and ventricular hypertrophy.

Heart failure should be distinguished from (1) conditions in which there is circulatory congestion consequent to abnormal salt and water retention but in which there is no disturbance of cardiac function per se (the latter syndrome, termed the *congested state*, may result from the abnormal salt and water retention of renal failure, or from excess parenteral administration of fluids and electrolytes), and (2) from noncardiac causes of inadequate cardiac output, including shock due to hypovolemia and redistribution of blood volume (Chap. 39).

The ventricles respond to a chronically increased hemodynamic burden with the development of hypertrophy. With volume overload when the ventricle is called upon to deliver an elevated cardiac output, as in valvular regurgitation, it develops *eccentric* hypertrophy, i.e., cavity dilatation, with an increase in muscle mass so that the ratio between wall thickness and ventricular cavity size remains relatively constant. With pressure overload when the ventricle is called upon to develop increased pressure, as in valvular aortic stenosis, it develops *concentric* hypertrophy, in which the ratio between wall thickness and ventricular cavity size increases. In both conditions, a stable hyperfunctioning state may exist for many years but myocardial function may ultimately deteriorate, leading to heart failure.

CAUSES OF HEART FAILURE

In evaluating patients with heart failure, it is important to identify not only the *underlying cause* of the heart disease but the *precipitating cause* of heart failure as well. The cardiac abnormality produced by a congenital or acquired lesion such as valvular aortic stenosis may exist for many years and produce no clinical disability. Frequently, however, the manifestations of clinical heart failure appear for the first time in the course of some acute disturbance which places an additional load on a myocardium that chronically is excessively burdened and while compensated has no additional reserves, resulting in further deterioration of cardiac function. Identification of such precipitating causes is of critical importance because their prompt alleviation may be lifesaving. However, in the absence of underlying heart disease these acute disturbances do not usually, by themselves, lead to heart failure.

PRECIPITATING CAUSES

1 *Pulmonary embolism*. Patients with low cardiac output and physical inactivity are at increased risk of developing thrombi in the veins of the lower extremities or the pelvis. Pulmonary embolization may result in further elevation of pulmonary arterial pressure, which in turn may produce or intensify failure of the right ventricle. In the presence of pulmonary vascular congestion, such emboli may also cause infarction of the lung (Chap. 213).

2 *Infection*. Patients with pulmonary vascular congestion are also more susceptible to pulmonary infections, but any infection may precipitate heart failure. The resulting fever, tachycardia, hypoxemia, and the increased metabolic demands may place a further burden on the overloaded, but compensated, myocardium of a patient with chronic heart disease.

3 *Anemia*. In the presence of anemia the oxygen needs of the metabolizing tissues can be met only by an increase in the cardiac

output (Chap. 61); though such an increase in the cardiac output might be sustained by a normal heart, a diseased, overloaded, but otherwise compensated heart may be unable to augment sufficiently the volume of blood which it delivers to the periphery. In this manner the combination of anemia and previously compensated heart disease can lead to inadequate oxygen delivery and precipitate heart failure.

4 *Thyrotoxicosis and pregnancy.* As in anemia and fever, in thyrotoxicosis and pregnancy adequate tissue perfusion requires an increased cardiac output. The development or intensification of heart failure may actually be one of the first clinical manifestations of hyperthyroidism in a patient with underlying heart disease which was previously compensated (Chap. 316). Similarly, heart failure not infrequently occurs for the first time during pregnancy in women with rheumatic valvular disease in whom cardiac compensation may return following delivery.

5 *Arrhythmias.* In patients with underlying but compensated heart disease, arrhythmias are among the most frequent precipitating causes of heart failure. They exert a deleterious effect for a variety of reasons: (*a*) Tachyarrhythmias reduce the time period available for ventricular filling. In patients with coronary artery disease tachyarrhythmias may also cause ischemic myocardial dysfunction. (*b*) The dissociation between atrial and ventricular contractions characteristic of many arrhythmias results in the loss of the atrial booster pump mechanism, thereby tending to raise atrial pressures. (*c*) In any arrhythmia associated with abnormal intraventricular conduction, myocardial performance may become further impaired because of the loss of normal synchronicity of ventricular contraction. (*d*) The marked bradycardia associated with complete atrioventricular block requires a greatly elevated stroke volume if a marked reduction in cardiac output is to be prevented.

6 *Rheumatic and other forms of myocarditis.* Acute rheumatic fever and a variety of infectious or inflammatory processes affecting the myocardium may impair myocardial function in patients with or without preexisting heart disease (Chaps. 187 and 192).

7 *Infective endocarditis.* The additional valvular damage, anemia, fever, and myocarditis which often occur as a consequence of infective endocarditis may, singly or in concert, precipitate heart failure (Chap. 90).

8 *Physical, dietary, environmental, and emotional excesses.* The augmentation of sodium intake, the discontinuation of medications to treat heart failure, physical overexertion, excessive environmental heat or humidity, and emotional crises may all precipitate cardiac decompensation.

9 *Systemic hypertension.* Rapid elevation of arterial pressure, as may occur in some instances of hypertension of renal origin or upon discontinuation of antihypertensive medication, may result in cardiac decompensation (Chap. 196).

10 *Myocardial infarction.* In patients with chronic but compensated ischemic heart disease, a fresh infarct, sometimes otherwise silent clinically, may further impair ventricular function and precipitate heart failure (Chap. 189).

A systematic search for these precipitating causes should be made in every patient with the new development or recent intensification of heart failure, particularly if it is refractory to the usual methods of therapy. If properly recognized, the precipitating cause of heart failure can usually be treated more effectively than the underlying cause. Therefore, the prognosis in patients with heart failure in whom a precipitating cause can be identified, treated, and eliminated is more favorable than in patients in whom the underlying disease process has advanced to the point of producing heart failure.

FORMS OF HEART FAILURE

Heart failure may be described as *high-output* or *low-output, acute* or *chronic, right-sided* or *left-sided, forward* or *backward,* and *systolic* or *diastolic*. These descriptors are often useful in a clinical setting, particularly early in the patient's course, but late in the course the differences between some of these forms often become blurred.

HIGH-OUTPUT VERSUS LOW-OUTPUT HEART FAILURE It is useful to classify patients with heart failure into those with a low cardiac output, i.e., *low-output heart failure,* and those with an elevated cardiac output, i.e., *high-output heart failure*. The cardiac output is often depressed in patients with heart failure secondary to ischemic heart disease, hypertension, cardiomyopathy, valvular and pericardial disease, but tends to be elevated in patients with heart failure and hyperthyroidism, anemia, pregnancy, arteriovenous fistulas, beriberi, and Paget's disease. In clinical practice, however, low-output and high-output heart failure cannot always be readily distinguished. The normal range of cardiac output is wide [2.5 to 3.8 (liters/min)/m^2], and in many patients with so-called low-output heart failure the cardiac output may actually be just within the normal range at rest (although it is lower than it had been previously) and fails to rise normally during exertion. On the other hand, in patients with so-called high-output heart failure the output may not exceed the upper limits of normal (although it would have been found to be so had it been measured before heart failure supervened), but rather it may be close to the upper limit of normal. Regardless of the *absolute* level of the cardiac output, however, cardiac failure may be said to be present when the characteristic clinical manifestations described below are accompanied by a depression of the curve relating ventricular end-diastolic volume to cardiac performance (Fig. 181-6, p. 886).

An integral physiologic component of systolic heart failure (p. 892) is the finding that the heart does not deliver the quantity of oxygen required by the metabolizing tissues. In the absence of peripheral shunting of blood, such inadequate delivery of oxygen to the metabolizing tissues is reflected in an abnormal widening of the normal arterial–mixed venous oxygen difference [35 to 50 mL/L (3.5 to 5.0 mL/dL) in the basal state]. In mild cases, such an abnormality may not be present at rest but becomes evident only during exertion or other hypermetabolic states. In patients with the high-output cardiac states associated with arteriovenous fistula, beriberi, thyrotoxicosis, Paget's disease, etc., the arterial–mixed venous oxygen difference is normal or low. The mixed venous oxygen saturation is raised by the admixture of blood which has been diverted from the metabolizing tissues, and it may be presumed that even in these patients the delivery of oxygen to the latter is reduced despite the normal or even elevated mixed venous oxygen saturation. When heart failure occurs in such patients, the arterial–mixed venous oxygen difference, regardless of the absolute value, still exceeds the level which existed prior to the development of heart failure, and therefore the cardiac output, though normal or elevated, is lower than before heart failure supervened.

The mechanisms responsible for the development of heart failure in patients whose cardiac outputs are initially high are complex and depend on the underlying disease process. In most of these conditions the heart is called upon to pump abnormally large quantities of blood in order to deliver the normal quota of oxygen to the metabolizing tissues. The burden placed on the myocardium by the increased flow load resembles that produced by chronic regurgitant valvular lesions. In addition, thyrotoxicosis and beriberi may also impair myocardial metabolism directly, while severe anemia may interfere with myocardial function by producing myocardial anoxia.

ACUTE VERSUS CHRONIC HEART FAILURE The prototype of acute heart failure is the patient who suddenly develops a large myocardial infarction or rupture of a cardiac valve, while chronic heart failure is typically observed in patients with dilated cardiomyopathy or multivalvular heart disease which develops or progresses slowly. In acute failure, the sudden reduction in cardiac output often results in systemic hypotension without peripheral edema, while in chronic heart failure, arterial pressure tends to be well maintained, but there is accumulation of edema. Despite these differences in clinical presentation, there is no fundamental distinction between acute and chronic failure. For example, intensive efforts to prevent expansion of blood volume by means of dietary sodium restriction and the administration of diuretics will frequently delay the development of exertional dyspnea and edema in patients with chronic valvular heart disease, i.e., it will mask the clinical manifestations of chronic heart failure, until an acute episode, such as an arrhythmia or infection precipitates acute heart failure. Without intensive efforts to restrict blood volume the same patients would have been considered to have been suffering from chronic heart failure, even though their underlying myocardial disease was no further advanced.

RIGHT-SIDED VERSUS LEFT-SIDED HEART FAILURE Many of the clinical manifestations of heart failure result from the accumulation of excess fluid behind one or both ventricles (Chaps. 36 and 38). This fluid usually localizes upstream to (behind) the specific cardiac chamber which is initially affected. For example, patients in whom the left ventricle is mechanically overloaded (e.g., aortic stenosis) or weakened (e.g., postmyocardial infarction) develop dyspnea and orthopnea as a result of pulmonary congestion, a condition referred to as *left-sided heart failure*. In contrast, when the underlying abnormality affects the right ventricle primarily, e.g., valvular pulmonic stenosis or pulmonary hypertension secondary to pulmonary thromboembolism, symptoms resulting from pulmonary congestion such as orthopnea or paroxysmal nocturnal dyspnea are less common, and edema, congestive hepatomegaly, and systemic venous distention, i.e., clinical manifestations of *right-sided heart failure*, are more prominent. However, when heart failure has existed for months or years, such localization of excess fluid behind the failing ventricle may no longer exist. For example, patients with long-standing aortic valve disease or systemic hypertension may have ankle edema, congestive hepatomegaly, and systemic venous distention late in the course of their disease, even though the abnormal hemodynamic burden initially was placed on the left ventricle, in part because of the secondary pulmonary hypertension and resultant right-sided heart failure, but also because of the persistent retention of salt and water. It is also useful to recall that the muscle bundles composing both ventricles are continuous and both ventricles share a common wall, the interventricular septum. Also, biochemical changes which occur in heart failure and which may be involved in the impairment of myocardial function, such as norepinephrine depletion and alterations in the activity of myosin ATPase, occur in the myocardium of both ventricles, regardless of the specific chamber on which the abnormal hemodynamic burden is placed initially.

BACKWARD VERSUS FORWARD HEART FAILURE For many years a controversy has revolved around the question of the mechanism of the clinical manifestations resulting from heart failure. The concept of *backward heart failure*, propounded by James Hope in 1832, contends that when heart failure occurs, one or the other ventricle fails to discharge its contents normally, the end-diastolic volume of the ventricle rises, the pressures and volumes in the atrium and venous system behind the failing ventricle become elevated, and retention of sodium and water occurs as a consequence of the elevation of systemic venous and capillary pressures and the resultant transudation of fluid into the interstitial space (Chap. 38). In contrast, the proponents of the *forward heart failure* hypothesis, expounded by MacKenzie in 1913, maintain that the clinical manifestations of heart failure result directly from an inadequate discharge of blood into the arterial system. Salt and water retention, then, is a consequence of diminished renal perfusion and excessive proximal tubular sodium reabsorption and of excessive distal tubular reabsorption, through activation of the renin-angiotensin-aldosterone system.

A rigid distinction between *backward* and *forward heart failure* is artificial, since both mechanisms appear to operate to varying extents in most patients with heart failure. However, the rate of onset of heart failure often influences the clinical manifestations. For example, when a large portion of the left ventricle is suddenly destroyed, as in myocardial infarction, although stroke volume is reduced, the patient may die of either acute pulmonary edema, a manifestation of backward failure, or of failure of perfusion of the systemic tissues. Sometimes both mechanisms operate simultaneously. If the patient survives the acute insult, clinical manifestations resulting from a chronically depressed cardiac output, including the abnormal retention of fluid within the systemic vascular bed, might develop. Similarly, in the case of massive pulmonary embolism, the right ventricle may dilate and the systemic venous pressure may rise to high levels (backward failure), or the patient may develop shock secondary to low cardiac output (forward failure), but this low-output state may have to be maintained for some days before sodium and water retention sufficient to produce peripheral edema occurs.

SYSTOLIC VERSUS DIASTOLIC FAILURE The distinction between these two forms of heart failure, described on p. 887 and in Fig. 181–7, relates to whether the principal abnormality is the inability to expel sufficient blood (systolic failure) or to relax and fill normally (diastolic failure). The major clinical manifestations of systolic failure relate to an inadequate cardiac output with weakness, fatigue, and other symptoms of hypoperfusion, while in diastolic failure they relate principally to an elevation of filling pressures. In many patients, particularly those who have both ventricular hypertrophy *and* dilatation, abnormalities both of contraction and relaxation coexist.

REDISTRIBUTION OF CARDIAC OUTPUT The redistribution of cardiac output serves as an important compensatory mechanism when flow is reduced. This redistribution is most marked when a patient with heart failure exercises, but as heart failure advances, redistribution occurs even in the basal state. Blood flow is redistributed so that the delivery of oxygen to vital organs, such as the brain and myocardium, is maintained at normal or near-normal levels, while flow to less critical areas, such as the cutaneous and muscular beds and splanchnic viscera, is reduced. Vasoconstriction mediated by the sympathetic nervous system is largely responsible for this redistribution, which in turn may be responsible for many of the clinical manifestations of heart failure, such as fluid accumulation (reduction of renal flow), low-grade fever (reduction of cutaneous flow), and fatigue (reduction of muscle flow).

SALT AND WATER RETENTION (See also Chap. 38)

When the volume of blood pumped by the left ventricle into the systemic vascular bed is chronically reduced, and when one or both ventricles fail to expel the normal fraction of their end-diastolic volumes, a complex sequence of adjustments occurs which ultimately results in the abnormal accumulation of fluid. Though, on the one hand, many of the clinical manifestations of heart failure are secondary to this excessive retention of fluid, on the other, this abnormal fluid accumulation and the expansion of blood volume which accompanies it also constitute an important compensatory mechanism which tends to maintain cardiac output and therefore perfusion of the vital organs. Except in the terminal stages of heart failure, the ventricle operates on an ascending, albeit depressed and flattened, function curve (Fig. 181-6), and the augmented ventricular end-diastolic volume and pressure characteristic of heart failure must be regarded as helping to maintain the reduced cardiac output, despite causing pulmonary and/or systemic venous congestion.

In the presence of heart failure, effective filling of the systemic arterial bed is reduced, a condition which initiates the complex hemodynamic, renal, and hormonal adjustments that interact to promote reduced renal sodium and water excretion. Patients with severe heart failure may exhibit a reduced capacity to excrete a water load, which may result in dilutional hyponatremia. These abnormalities may be caused, in part, by excess antidiuretic hormone activity and/or factors that prevent sodium reabsorption in the distal tubule, such as avid proximal tubular reabsorption of sodium or the action of a diuretic acting on the distal tubule.

The importance of elevated systemic venous pressure and of the alterations of renal and adrenal function characteristic of heart failure vary in their relative importance in the production of edema in different patients with heart failure. The renin-angiotensin-aldosterone axis is activated most intensely by acute heart failure, and its activity tends to decline as heart failure becomes chronic. In patients with tricuspid valve disease or constrictive pericarditis the elevated venous pressure and the transudation of fluid from systemic capillaries appear to play the dominant role in edema formation. On the other hand, severe edema may be present in patients with ischemic or hypertensive heart disease, in whom systemic venous pressure is within normal limits or is only minimally elevated. In such patients, the retention of salt and water is probably due primarily to a redistribution of cardiac output and a concomitant reduction in renal perfusion, as well as activation of the renin-angiotensin-aldosterone axis. Regardless of the mechanisms involved in fluid retention, untreated patients with chronic congestive heart failure have elevations of total blood volume, interstitial fluid volume, and body sodium. These abnormalities diminish after clinical compensation has been achieved by treatment.

CLINICAL MANIFESTATIONS OF HEART FAILURE

Dyspnea Respiratory distress which occurs as the result of increased effort in breathing is the most common symptom of heart failure (Chap. 36). In early heart failure, dyspnea is observed only during activity, when it may simply represent an aggravation of the breathlessness which normally occurs under these circumstances. As heart failure advances, however, it appears with progressively less strenuous activity. Ultimately, breathlessness is present even when the patient is at rest. The principal difference between exertional dyspnea in normal persons and in cardiac patients is the degree of activity necessary to induce the symptom. Cardiac dyspnea is observed most frequently in patients with elevations of pulmonary venous and capillary pressures. Such patients usually have engorged pulmonary vessels and interstitial pulmonary edema, which reduces the compliance of the lungs and thereby increases the work of the respiratory muscles required to inflate the lungs. The activation of receptors in the lungs results in the rapid, shallow breathing of cardiac dyspnea. The oxygen cost of breathing is increased by the excessive work of the respiratory muscles. This is coupled with the diminished delivery of oxygen to these muscles, which occurs as a consequence of the reduced cardiac output, and which may contribute to fatigue of the respiratory muscles and the sensation of shortness of breath.

Orthopnea Dyspnea in the recumbent position is often a later manifestation of heart failure than exertional dyspnea. Orthopnea occurs in part because of the redistribution of fluid from the abdomen and lower extremities into the chest causing an increase in the pulmonary capillary hydrostatic pressure, as well as a result of elevation of the diaphragm. Patients with orthopnea generally report that they must elevate their heads on several pillows at night and frequently awaken short of breath or coughing (the so-called nocturnal cough) if their heads slip off the pillows. The sensation of breathlessness usually is relieved by sitting bolt upright, since this position reduces venous return and pulmonary capillary pressure, and many patients report that they find relief from sitting in front of an open window. As heart failure advances, orthopnea may become so severe that patients cannot lie down at all and must spend the entire night in a sitting position. On the other hand, in other patients with long-standing, severe left ventricular failure, symptoms of pulmonary congestion may actually diminish with time as the function of the right ventricle becomes impaired.

Paroxysmal (nocturnal) dyspnea This term refers to attacks of severe shortness of breath and coughing which generally occur at night, usually awaken the patient from sleep, and may be quite frightening. Though simple orthopnea may be relieved by sitting upright at the side of the bed with legs dependent, in the patient with paroxysmal nocturnal dyspnea coughing and wheezing often persist even in this position. The depression of the respiratory center during sleep may reduce ventilation sufficiently to lower arterial oxygen tension, particularly in patients with interstitial lung edema and reduced pulmonary compliance. Also, ventricular function may be further impaired at night because of reduced adrenergic stimulation of myocardial function. *Cardiac asthma* is closely related to paroxysmal nocturnal dyspnea and nocturnal cough and is characterized by wheezing secondary to bronchospasm—most prominent at night. *Acute pulmonary edema* (Chap. 36) is a severe form of cardiac asthma due to further elevation of pulmonary capillary pressure leading to alveolar edema, associated with extreme shortness of breath, rales over the lung fields, and the transudation and expectoration of blood-tinged fluid. If not treated promptly acute pulmonary edema may be fatal.

Cheyne-Stokes respiration Also known as *periodic* or *cyclic respiration*, Cheyne-Stokes respiration is characterized by diminished sensitivity of the respiratory center to arterial P_{CO_2}. There is an apneic phase, during which the arterial P_{O_2} falls and the arterial P_{CO_2} rises. These changes in the arterial blood stimulate the depressed respiratory center, resulting in hyperventilation and hypocapnia, followed in turn by apnea. Cheyne-Stokes respiration occurs most often in patients with cerebral atherosclerosis and other cerebral lesions, but the prolongation of the circulation time from the lung to the brain which occurs in heart failure, particularly in patients with hypertension and coronary artery disease and associated cerebral vascular disease, also appears to precipitate this form of breathing.

Fatigue and weakness These nonspecific but common symptoms of heart failure are related to the reduction of perfusion of skeletal muscle. Anorexia and nausea associated with abdominal pain and fullness are frequent complaints which may be related to the congested liver and portal venous system.

Cerebral symptoms In severe heart failure, particularly in elderly patients with accompanying cerebral arteriosclerosis, arterial hypoxemia, and reduced cerebral perfusion, there may be alterations in the mental state characterized by confusion, difficulty in concentration, impairment of memory, headache, insomnia, and anxiety. *Nocturia* is common in heart failure and may contribute to insomnia.

PHYSICAL FINDINGS In moderate heart failure the patient appears to be in no distress at rest except that he or she may be uncomfortable when lying flat for more than a few minutes. In more severe heart failure the pulse pressure may be diminished, reflecting a reduction in stroke volume, and occasionally the diastolic arterial pressure may be elevated as a consequence of generalized vasoconstriction. In acute heart failure hypotension may be prominent. There may be cyanosis of the lips and nail beds, sinus tachycardia, and the patient may insist on sitting upright. *Systemic venous pressure* is often abnormally elevated in heart failure and may be recognized by observing the extent of distention of the jugular veins. In the early stages of heart failure the venous pressure may be normal at rest but may become abnormally elevated during and immediately after exertion as well as with sustained pressure on the abdomen (positive abdominojugular reflux).

Third and fourth heart sounds (Chap. 175) are often audible but are not specific for heart failure, and *pulsus alternans*, i.e., a regular rhythm in which there is alternation of strong and weak cardiac contractions and therefore alternation in the strength of the peripheral pulses, may be present. Pulsus alternans may be detected by sphygmomanometry and in more severe instances by palpation; it frequently follows an extrasystole and is observed most commonly in patients with cardiomyopathy or with hypertensive or ischemic heart disease. It is caused by a reduction in the number of contractile units during weak contractions and/or by alternation in the ventricular end-diastolic volume.

Pulmonary rales Moist, inspiratory, crepitant rales and dullness to percussion over the lung bases are common in patients with heart failure and elevated pulmonary venous and capillary pressures. In patients with pulmonary edema, rales may be heard widely over both lung fields; they are frequently coarse and sibilant and may be accompanied by expiratory wheezing. Rales may, however, be caused by many conditions other than left ventricular failure. Patients with long-standing heart failure may have no rales because of increased lymphatic drainage of fluid.

Cardiac edema Cardiac edema is usually dependent, occurring in the legs symmetrically, particularly in the pretibial region and ankles in the evening in ambulatory patients, and in the sacral region of individuals at bed rest. Pitting edema of the arms and face occurs rarely and only late in the course of heart failure.

Hydrothorax and ascites Pleural effusion in congestive heart failure results from the elevation of pleural capillary pressure and transudation of fluid into the pleural cavities. Since the pleural veins drain into *both* the systemic and pulmonary veins, hydrothorax occurs most commonly with marked elevation of pressure in both venous systems, but may also be seen with marked elevation of pressure in either venous bed. It is more frequent in the right pleural cavity than the left. *Ascites* also occurs as a consequence of transudation and results from increased pressure in the hepatic veins and the veins draining the peritoneum (Chap. 48). Marked ascites occurs most frequently in patients with tricuspid valve disease and with constrictive pericarditis.

Congestive hepatomegaly An enlarged, tender, pulsating liver also accompanies systemic venous hypertension and is observed not only in the same conditions in which ascites occurs, but also in milder forms of heart failure from any cause. With prolonged, severe hepatomegaly, as in patients with tricuspid valve disease or chronic constrictive pericarditis, enlargement of the spleen may also occur.

Jaundice This is a late finding in congestive heart failure and is associated with elevations of both the direct- and indirect-reacting bilirubin; it results from impairment of hepatic function secondary to hepatic congestion and the hepatocellular hypoxia associated with central lobular atrophy. Serum transaminase concentrations are frequently elevated. If hepatic congestion occurs acutely, the jaundice may be severe and the enzymes strikingly raised.

Cardiac cachexia With severe chronic heart failure there may be serious weight loss and cachexia because of (1) elevation of the metabolic rate, which results in part from the extra work performed by the respiratory muscles, the increased oxygen needs of the hypertrophied heart, and the discomfort associated with severe heart failure; (2) anorexia, nausea, and vomiting due to central causes, to digitalis intoxication, or to congestive hepatomegaly and abdominal fullness; (3) some impairment of intestinal absorption due to congestion of the intestinal veins; and (4) rarely, in patients with particularly severe failure of the right side of the heart, a protein-losing enteropathy.

Other manifestations With reduction of blood flow the extremities may be cold, pale, and diaphoretic. Urine flow is depressed, and the urine contains protein and has a high specific gravity and a low concentration of sodium. In addition, prerenal azotemia may be present. In patients with long-standing severe heart failure impotence and depression are common.

ROENTGENOGRAPHIC FINDINGS In addition to the enlargement of the particular chambers characteristic of the lesion responsible for heart failure, distention of pulmonary veins is common in patients with heart failure and elevated pulmonary vascular pressures (Chap. 177). Also, pleural effusions may be present and associated with interlobar effusions.

DIFFERENTIAL DIAGNOSIS The diagnosis of congestive heart failure may be established by observing some combination of the clinical manifestations of heart failure, enumerated above, together with the findings characteristic of one of the etiologic forms of heart disease. Since chronic heart failure is often associated with cardiac enlargement, the diagnosis should be questioned, but is by no means excluded, when all chambers are normal in size. Two-dimensional echocardiography is particularly useful in assessing the dimensions of each cardiac chamber. Heart failure may be difficult to distinguish from pulmonary disease, and the differential diagnosis is discussed in Chap. 36. Pulmonary embolism also presents many of the manifestations of heart failure, but hemoptysis, pleuritic chest pain, a right ventricular lift, and the characteristic mismatch between ventilation and perfusion on lung scan should point to this diagnosis (Chap. 213).

Ankle edema may be due to varicose veins, cyclic edema, or gravitational effects (Chap. 38), but in these patients there is no jugular venous hypertension at rest or with pressure over the abdomen. Edema secondary to renal disease can usually be recognized by appropriate renal function tests and urinalysis and is rarely associated with elevation of the venous pressure. Enlargement of the liver and ascites occur in patients with hepatic cirrhosis, but may also be distinguished from heart failure by normal jugular venous pressure and absence of a positive abdominojugular reflux.

TREATMENT OF HEART FAILURE

The treatment of heart failure may be divided into three components: (1) removal of the precipitating cause, (2) correction of the underlying cause, and (3) control of the congestive heart failure state. The first two are discussed in subsequent chapters together with each specific disease entity or complication. An example is the treatment of pneumococcal pneumonia and acute heart failure followed by mitral valvotomy in a patient with mitral stenosis. In many instances surgical treatment will correct or at least improve the underlying cause. The third component of the treatment of heart failure may, in turn, also be divided into three categories: (1) reduction of cardiac work load, including both the preload and the afterload; (2) control of excessive salt and water retention; and (3) enhancement of myocardial contractility. The vigor with which each of these measures is pursued in any individual patient should depend upon the severity of the heart failure state. Following effective treatment, recurrence of the clinical manifestations of heart failure can often be prevented by continuing those measures that were originally effective. While a simple rule for the treatment of all patients with heart failure cannot be formulated because of the varied etiologies, hemodynamic features, and clinical manifestations of heart failure, insofar as the treatment of chronic congestive failure is concerned, simple measures such as moderate restriction of activity and sodium intake should be tried first. If these are insufficient, therapy with a combination of a diuretic, an angiotensin-converting enzyme inhibitor, and perhaps a digitalis glycoside is then begun. The next step is more rigorous restriction of salt intake and higher doses of loop diuretics sometimes accompanied by other diuretics. If heart failure persists, hospitalization with rigid salt restriction, bed rest, intravenous vasodilators, and positive inotropic agents comes next. In some patients the order in which these measures are applied may be altered.

REDUCTION OF CARDIAC WORK LOAD This consists of reducing physical activity, instituting emotional rest, and reducing afterload. Modest restriction of physical activity in mild cases and rest in bed or in a chair in severe failure remain cornerstones in the treatment of heart failure. Meals should be small in quantity, and every effort should be made to diminish the patient's anxiety. Physical and emotional rest tend to lower arterial pressure, and reduce the load on the myocardium by diminishing the requirements for cardiac output. These influences act in concert to diminish the need for redistribution of the cardiac output, and in many patients, particularly those with mild heart failure, simple bed rest and mild sedation often result in an effective diuresis.

Rest at home or in the hospital should be maintained for 1 to 2 weeks in patients with overt congestive failure and should be continued for several days after the patient's condition has stabilized. The hazards of phlebothrombosis and pulmonary embolism which occur with bed rest may be reduced with anticoagulants, leg exercises, and elastic stockings. In any event, *absolute* bed rest rarely is required, and the patient should be encouraged to sit in a chair and be given toilet privileges unless heart failure is extreme. Heavy sedation should be avoided, but small doses of tranquilizers may be helpful in calming the emotionally disturbed patient through the first few days of therapy and in permitting much-needed sleep. In patients with chronic, mild heart failure, bed rest on weekends will frequently allow continuation of gainful employment. Following recovery from heart failure, the patient's activities must be carefully assessed, and often his or her professional, family, and/or community responsibilities must be reduced. Intermittent rest during the day (e.g., a 1-h nap or enforced rest following lunch) and the avoidance of strenuous exertion are often helpful once compensation has been restored. Weight reduction by restriction of caloric intake in the obese patient with heart failure also diminishes cardiac work load and is an essential component of the therapeutic program.

CONTROL OF EXCESSIVE FLUID RETENTION Many of the clinical manifestations of heart failure result from hypervolemia and expansion of the interstitial fluid volume. By the time fluid retention due to heart failure first becomes clinically evident, most commonly as edema, considerable expansion of the extracellular space has already occurred, and heart failure usually is already advanced. Exertional dypsnea and orthopnea may be caused by displacement of fluid from the systemic to the pulmonary vascular bed. Treatment aimed at reducing extracellular fluid volume is dependent primarily on lowering total body sodium stores, while fluid restriction is of less importance. A negative sodium balance can be achieved by reducing the dietary intake and increasing the urinary excretion of this ion with the aid of diuretics. In severe heart failure mechanical removal of extracellular fluid by means of thoracentesis, paracentesis, and rarely hemodialysis or peritoneal dialysis may also be employed.

Diet In patients with mild heart failure, considerable improvement in symptoms may result from simply reducing the sodium intake, particularly if accompanied by periods of physical rest. In patients with more severe heart failure the sodium intake must be controlled more rigidly, and other measures, such as diuretics, vasodilators, and glycosides, are used. Even following recovery from a bout of heart failure, at least moderate sodium restriction should be maintained. The normal diet contains approximately 6 to 10 g sodium chloride; this intake can be reduced by half simply by excluding salt-rich foods and salt which is added at the table. Reduction of the ordinary dietary intake to approximately one-fourth of normal may be achieved if, in addition, all salt is omitted from cooking. In patients with severe heart failure, in whom the daily sodium chloride intake should be reduced to between 500 and 1000 mg, milk, cheese, bread, cereals, canned vegetables and soups, some salted cuts of meat, and some fresh vegetables, including spinach, celery, and beets, must be eliminated. A variety of fresh fruit, green vegetables, specially processed breads and milk, and salt substitutes are permissible, but it is difficult to keep such diets palatable. Water intake may be ad libitum in all but the most severe forms of congestive heart failure. Late in the course of heart failure, dilutional hyponatremia may develop in patients who are unable to excrete a water load, sometimes because of excessive secretion of antidiuretic hormone. In such cases water intake as well as sodium intake must be restricted.

Attention must also be directed to the caloric content of the diet. Substantial improvement can result from caloric restriction in obese patients with heart failure, in whom weight loss will reduce the load placed on the myocardium. On the other hand, in individuals with severe heart failure and cardiac cachexia, an attempt must be made to maintain nutritional intake and to avoid caloric and vitamin deficiencies.

Diuretics A variety of diuretic agents is available, and in patients with mild heart failure almost all are effective. However, in the more severe forms of heart failure, the selection of diuretics is more difficult, and any existing abnormalities in serum electrolytes must be taken into account. Overtreatment must be avoided, since the resultant hypovolemia may reduce cardiac output, interfere with renal function, and produce profound weakness and lethargy.

THIAZIDE DIURETICS These agents are widely used in clinical practice because of their effectiveness when administered orally. In patients with chronic heart failure of mild or moderate severity the continued administration of chlorothiazide or one of its many analogues abolishes or diminishes the need for rigid dietary sodium restriction, although salty foods and table salt should still be avoided. Thiazides are well absorbed following oral administration; chlorothiazide and hydrochlorothiazide reach their peak action in 4 h, and diuresis persists for approximately 12 h. Thiazide diuretics reduce the reabsorption of sodium and chloride in the first half of the distal convoluted tubule and a portion of the cortical ascending limb of the loop of Henle, and water follows the unreabsorbed salt. Thiazides fail to increase free water clearance, and in some instances reduce it, supporting the hypothesis that these drugs inhibit selective reabsorption of sodium chloride in the distal cortical diluting segment, at a site where the urine is normally diluted (Chap. 222). This may result in the excretion of a hypertonic urine and may contribute to dilutional hyponatremia. As a consequence of increased delivery of sodium to the distal nephron, sodium-potassium ion exchange is enhanced and kaliuresis results. In contrast to the loop diuretics which enhance calcium excretion, the thiazides have the opposite effect. These drugs are effective and useful in the treatment of heart failure as long as the glomerular filtration rate exceeds 50 percent of normal.

Chlorothiazide is administered in doses of up to 500 mg every 6 h. Many derivatives of this compound are available but differ principally in dosage and duration of action and therefore offer few, if any, significant advantages over the parent compound, except for chlorthalidone which may be administered once daily. Potassium depletion and metabolic alkalosis (the latter due to increased H^+ secretion as a substitute for the depleted intracellular stores of potassium and increased proximal tubular reabsorption of filtered HCO_3^- when there is relative depletion of the extracellular fluid volume) are the chief adverse metabolic effects following prolonged administration of the thiazides, of metolazone, and of the loop diuretics. Hypokalemia may seriously enhance the dangers of digitalis intoxication, induce fatigue and lethargy, and may be prevented by the oral supplementation of potassium chloride. However, the solution is not palatable and may be hazardous in patients with renal failure. Therefore, to prevent potassium depletion, in patients receiving thiazide diuretics, intermittent dosage schedules, e.g., omitting the diuretic every third day, and the addition of a potassium-retaining diuretic, such as a spironolactone or triamterene, may be preferable. Other side effects of thiazides include reduction of the excretion of uric acid, which may lead to hyperuricemia, and a hyperglycemic effect, which rarely may precipitate hyperosmolar coma in the poorly regulated diabetic. Skin rashes, thrombocytopenia, and granulocytopenia have also been reported.

METOLAZONE This quinethazone derivative has a site of action and potency similar to that of the thiazides, but has been reported to be effective in the presence of moderate renal failure. The usual dose is 5 to 10 mg/day.

FUROSEMIDE, BUMETANIDE, AND ETHACRYNIC ACID These "loop" diuretics are similar physiologically but differ chemically. These extremely powerful diuretics reversibly inhibit the reabsorption of sodium, potassium, and chloride in the thick ascending limb of Henle's loop, apparently by blocking a cotransport system in the luminal membrane. These agents may induce renal cortical vasodilatation and can produce rates of urine formation which may be as high as one-fourth of the glomerular filtration rate. While other diuretics lose their effectiveness as blood volume is restored to normal levels, the loop diuretics remain effective despite the elimination of excessive extracellular fluid volume. The major side effects of these agents are due to this marked diuretic potency, which on rare occasions may result in contraction of the plasma volume, circulatory collapse, reductions in the renal blood flow and glomerular filtration rate, and the development of prerenal azotemia. Metabolic alkalosis is produced by a large increase in the urinary excretion of chloride, hydrogen, and potassium ions. Hypokalemia (see discussion of thiazides, above) and hyponatremia may occur, and hyperuricemia and hyperglycemia are observed occasionally, as with thiazide diuretics. The reabsorption of free water is decreased.

All three drugs are readily absorbed orally and are excreted in the bile and urine. They are usually effective by mouth and intravenously. Weakness, nausea, and dizziness may complicate the administration of all three loop diuretics; ethacrynic acid has been associated with skin rash and granulocytopenia, as well as with transient or permanent deafness.

These extremely effective diuretics are useful in all forms of heart failure, particularly in otherwise refractory heart failure and pulmonary edema. They have been shown to be effective in patients with hypoalbuminemia, hyponatremia, hypochloremia, hypokalemia, and reductions in the glomerular filtration rate, and to produce a diuresis in patients in whom thiazide diuretics and aldosterone antagonists, alone and in combination, are ineffective.

In patients with refractory heart failure the action of furosemide, bumetanide, and ethacrynic acid may be potentiated by intravenous administration and the addition of thiazide diuretics, carbonic anhydrase inhibitors, osmotic diuretics, and the potassium-sparing diuretics—spironolactone, triamterene, and amiloride. These latter agents act on the cortical collecting ducts, are relatively weak, and therefore are rarely indicated as sole agents. However, their potassium-sparing properties make them particularly useful in conjunction with the more potent kaliuretic agents, the loop diuretics and thiazides. These agents fall into two classes, as noted below.

ALDOSTERONE ANTAGONISTS The 17-spironolactones resemble aldosterone structurally and act on the distal half of the convoluted tubule and the cortical portion of the collecting duct by competitive inhibition of aldosterone, thereby blocking the exchange between sodium and both potassium and hydrogen in the distal tubules and collecting ducts. These agents produce a sodium diuresis, and, in contrast to the thiazides, ethacrynic acid, and furosemide, they result in potassium retention. Although secondary hyperaldosteronism exists in some patients with congestive heart failure, the spironolactones are effective even in patients in whom the serum aldosterone concentration is within normal limits. Aldactone A may be administered in doses of 25 to 100 mg three to four times daily by mouth. The maximal effect of this regimen is not observed for approximately 4 days. Spironolactones are most effective when administered in combination with thiazide and loop diuretics. The opposing action of these drugs on urine and serum potassium makes possible a sodium diuresis without either hyper- or hypokalemia when spironolactone and one of these other agents are administered in combination. Also, since spironolactone, triamterene, and amiloride act on the distal tubule, they are particularly effective when used in combination with one of these other diuretics which acts more proximally.

Spironolactone, triamterene, and amiloride should not be administered alone to patients with hyperkalemia, renal failure, or hyponatremia. Reported complications include nausea, epigastric distress, mental confusion, drowsiness, gynecomastia, and erythematous eruptions.

TRIAMTERENE AND AMILORIDE These two drugs exert renal effects similar to those of the spironolactones; i.e., they block sodium reabsorption and secondarily inhibit potassium secretion in the distal tubules. However, their fundamental mechanism of action differs from those of the spironolactones, since they are active in adrenalectomized animals and their action does not depend on the presence of aldosterone. The effective dose of triamterene is 100 mg once or twice daily and that of amiloride is 5 mg daily. Side effects include nausea, vomiting, diarrhea, headache, granulocytopenia, eosinophilia, and skin rash. Both triamterene and the chemically unrelated diuretic amiloride resemble Aldactone A in that their diuretic potency is not great, but they are effective in preventing the hypokalemia characteristic of the administration of thiazides, furosemide, and ethacrynic acid. A number of diuretic preparations contain a combination of a thiazide and either triamterene or amiloride in a single capsule. They may be useful in patients who develop hypokalemia with a thiazide but should not be used in patients with impaired renal function and/or hyperkalemia.

CHOICE OF DIURETICS Orally administered thiazides or metolazone are the agents of choice in the treatment of chronic cardiac edema of mild to moderate degree in patients without hyperglycemia, hyperuricemia, or hypokalemia. Spironolactones, triamterene, and amiloride are not potent diuretics when used alone, but they potentiate other diuretics, particularly the thiazides and loop diuretics. However, in patients with heart failure and severe secondary hyperaldosteronism, spironolactone may be quite effective. Ethacrynic acid, bumetanide, or furosemide, given alone or with spironolactone or triamterene, are the agents of choice in patients with severe heart failure refractory to other diuretics. In very severe heart failure the combination of a thiazide, a loop diuretic, and a potassium-sparing diuretic (spironolactone, triamterene, or amiloride) is required.

VASODILATOR THERAPY In many patients with heart failure, left ventricular afterload is increased as a consequence of the several neural and humoral influences which act to constrict the peripheral vascular bed. These include increased activity of the adrenergic nervous system, elevation of circulating catecholamines, and activation of the renin-angiotensin system, and perhaps of increased circulating antidiuretic hormone as well. In addition to the vasoconstriction, the ventricular end-diastolic volume rises and as a consequence of the operation of Laplace's law, which relates myocardial wall tension to the product of intraventricular pressure and radius, the aortic impedance, i.e., the force which opposes left ventricular ejection, or the ventricular afterload, rises. The maintenance or even the elevation of arterial pressure is generally considered to be a useful compensatory mechanism that allows blood flow to vital organs to persist in the presence of hypovolemia and reduction of the total cardiac output. While this is the case in many forms of shock (Chap. 39), in the presence of severely impaired cardiac function, the increase in afterload may reduce cardiac output further.

As shown in Fig. 181-5, afterload is a major determinant of cardiac function. When cardiac function is normal, a moderate elevation in afterload does not alter stroke volume, because the resultant increase in left ventricular end-diastolic volume, i.e., preload, can be tolerated easily. However, when myocardial function is impaired, such an increase in preload evoked by an elevation of afterload may raise ventricular end-diastolic and pulmonary capillary pressures to levels that may produce severe pulmonary congestion or pulmonary edema. In many patients with heart failure, the ventricle is already operating at the peak, flat portion of its Frank-Starling curve (Fig. 181-6), and any additional increase in aortic impedance (afterload) will reduce stroke volume (p. 886). Conversely, a reduction of afterload will tend to restore hemodynamics to normal by elevating the stroke volume of the failing ventricle, and may reduce the elevated ventricular filling pressure.

The pharmacologic reduction of impedance to left ventricular ejection with vasodilator drugs represents an important adjunct in the management of heart failure. This approach may be particularly helpful but is by no means limited to patients with acute heart failure due to myocardial infarction (Chap. 189), valvular regurgitation, elevated systemic vascular resistance and/or arterial pressure, and marked cardiac dilatation. The reduction of afterload by means of a variety of vasodilators reduces left ventricular end-diastolic pressure, volume, and oxygen consumption, while raising stroke volume and cardiac output and causing only modest reduction in aortic pressure. Vasodilators should not be used in patients with hypotension.

In patients with both acute and chronic heart failure secondary to coronary artery disease, cardiomyopathy, or valvular regurgitation who are treated with vasodilators, cardiac output increases, the pulmonary wedge pressure falls, the signs and symptoms of heart failure are relieved, and a new steady state is achieved in which cardiac output is higher and afterload lower with no or only mild reduction of arterial pressure (Fig. 182-1). Furthermore, the reduction of elevated left end-diastolic pressure may improve subendocardial perfusion.

Vasodilator therapy is useful in the treatment of all forms of heart failure, ranging from the mild, chronic to the severe acute forms.

The several available vasodilators vary in their hemodynamic effects, locus and duration of action, and mode of administration.

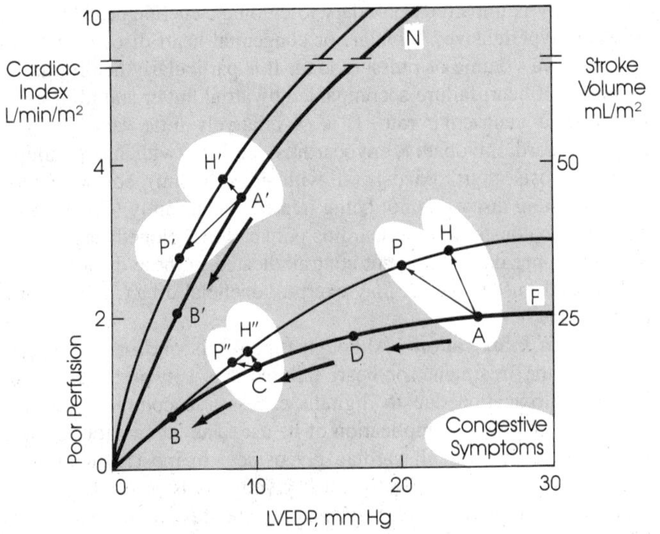

FIGURE 182-1 Effects of various vasodilators on the relationship between left ventricular end-diastolic pressure (LVEDP) and cardiac index or stroke volume in normal (N) and failing (F) hearts. H represents hydralazine or any other pure arterial dilator. It produces only a minimal increase in cardiac index in the normal subject (A′ → H′) or in the patient with heart failure with normal LVEDP (C → H″). In contrast, it elevates output in the patient with heart failure and elevated LVEDP (A → H). P represents a balanced vasodilator, such as sodium nitroprusside or prazosin. It reduces filling pressure in all patients, elevates cardiac output in patients with heart failure and elevated LVEDP (A → P), lowers cardiac output in normal subjects (A′ → P′), and has little effect on cardiac output in heart failure patients with normal filling pressures (C → P″). *(Reprinted with permission from TW Smith et al.)*

Some vasodilators, such as hydralazine, minoxidil, and the alpha-adrenergic blocking agents, act predominantly on the arterial bed and primarily increase stroke volume while others, such as nitroglycerin and isosorbide dinitrate, act almost entirely on the venous side of the circulation; the latter agents cause pooling of blood in the venous bed and act primarily to reduce ventricular filling pressures. Angiotensin-converting enzyme inhibitors, prazosin, and sodium nitroprusside are "balanced vasodilators" which act on both the arterial and venous beds. Some agents, such as sodium nitroprusside, must be administered by continuous intravenous infusion, nitroglycerin requires administration in ointment patch or intravenous forms when a prolonged effect is desired, while isosorbide dinitrate is most effective when it is administered by the sublingual route.

The ideal vasodilator for the treatment of *acute* heart failure should have a rapid onset and brief duration of action when administered by intravenous infusion; sodium nitroprusside qualifies as such a drug, but its use requires careful monitoring of the intraarterial pressure and electrocardiogram, and if possible of the pulmonary artery wedge pressure, in an intensive care unit. For the treatment of chronic congestive heart failure, the agent should be effective on oral administration, and its action should persist for at least 6 h. Angiotensin-converting enzyme inhibitors satisfy these requirements and have become the most useful and widely used vasodilators. It is advisable to commence therapy with very low doses, particularly in patients receiving diuretics, in order to avoid hypotension and gradually increase the dose.

Vasodilators are potent and effective in acutely improving the deranged hemodynamics of heart failure and there is evidence in favor of a beneficial chronic effect as well. Studies with angiotensin-converting enzyme inhibitors have demonstrated a favorable long-term reduction of symptoms and enhancement of exercise tolerance. Importantly, these drugs as well as the combination of hydralazine and isosorbide dinitrate prolong survival of patients with heart failure.

ENHANCEMENT OF MYOCARDIAL CONTRACTILITY—DIGITALIS The improvement of myocardial contractility by means of cardiac glycosides is an important component in the control of heart failure. The basic molecular structure of the digitalis glycosides is a steroid nucleus to which an unsaturated lactone ring is attached at C-17. These two elements together are called *aglycone* or *genin*, and it is this portion of the molecule which is responsible for the cardiotonic activity. The addition of sugar residues to this basic structure determines water solubility and pharmacokinetic properties for individual glycosides.

Pharmacokinetics In the absence of severe malabsorption, most digitalis glycosides are adequately absorbed from the intestinal tract even in the presence of vascular congestion secondary to heart failure. Oral absorption is close to complete within 2 h. The bioavailability (i.e., percent of intravenous dose) of orally administered glycoside varies. Considerable variability of bioavailability has been found in different commercial preparations of digoxin. The bioavailability of Lanoxin elixir is 70 to 85 percent, Lanoxin tablets 60 to 80 percent, and Lanoxicaps 90 to 100 percent. Digitoxin tablets have a bioavailability of virtually 100 percent. Cholesterol-lowering resins, antidiarrheal agents containing pectin and kaolin, nonabsorbable antacids, and neomycin can reduce the absorption of digoxin and digitoxin. Varying degrees of protein-binding of glycosides occur in the bloodstream (for example, 97 percent for digitoxin and 25 percent for digoxin), and though these differences may account in part for the varying durations of the effect of different glycosides, they are not related to the speed of action of these drugs. The plasma contains only approximately 1 percent of the body stores of digoxin; therefore, digoxin is not effectively removed from the body by dialysis, exchange transfusions, or during cardiopulmonary bypass, presumably because of tissue binding. The major fraction of the glycosides is directly bound by various tissues including the heart, in which the concentration is approximately 30 times that in the plasma for digoxin and 7 times for digitoxin; the latter is less polar and more lipid-soluble than digoxin.

Digoxin, which has a half-life of 1.6 days, is filtered in the glomeruli and secreted by the renal tubules; 85 percent is excreted in the urine, most in unchanged form; only 10 to 15 percent of digoxin is eliminated in the stool through biliary excretion in the presence of normal renal function. The ratio of digoxin clearance to endogenous creatinine clearance is 0.8, and the percentage of the body's total stores of digoxin lost per day can be calculated as (14 ± 0.2) × creatinine clearance in milliliters per minute. In patients with normal renal function a plateau concentration in the blood and tissue is reached after 5 days of daily maintenance treatment without a loading dose (Fig. 65-2). Therefore, significant reductions of the glomerular filtration rate reduce the elimination of digoxin (but not of digitoxin) and, therefore, may prolong digoxin's effect, allowing it to accumulate to toxic levels if it is administered in patients with impaired renal function. The administration of most diuretics does not alter the excretion of digoxin significantly, but spironolactone can inhibit tubular secretion of digoxin, resulting in significant accumulation of the drug. *Digitoxin,* with a half-life of approximately 5 days, is metabolized chiefly in the liver; only 15 percent is excreted in the urine unchanged and an equal fraction in the stool. Drugs such as phenobarbital and phenylbutazone that increase the activity of hepatic microsomal enzymes accelerate the metabolism of digitoxin. To reach a steady state, digitoxin requires maintenance doses for 3 to 4 weeks. *Ouabain* is very rapidly acting, exhibiting an onset of action in 5 to 10 min and a peak effect within 60 min following intravenous injection. It is poorly and irregularly absorbed from the gastrointestinal tract, is excreted by the kidneys, has a half-life of 21 h, and is useful in emergencies.

Mechanism of action The cardiac actions of all digitalis glycosides are alike. The clinical effects result from augmenting myocardial contractility and from prolonging the refractory period of the atrioventricular node, thereby slowing ventricular rate in patients with atrial fibrillation.

The most important effect of digitalis on cardiac muscle is to shift its force-velocity relation upward (Chap. 181). This positive inotropic effect is exhibited in normal, nonfailing hypertrophied as well as in failing hearts. In the absence of heart failure, however, when cardiac output is not limited by cardiac contractility, the drug does not elevate the output.

Excitation-contraction coupling is the membrane and intracellular process most likely involved in producing the positive inotropic effect of digitalis glycosides. These drugs inhibit transmembrane sodium and potassium movement by inhibition of the monovalent cation transport enzyme–coupled Na^+,K^+-ATPase. The latter, localized to the sarcolemma, appears to be the receptor for cardioactive glycosides whose action results in an increase in intracellular sodium content, and this in turn increases intracellular calcium concentration through a Na^+-Ca^{2+} exchange carrier mechanism (see Chap. 173). The increased myocardial uptake of calcium augments calcium released to the myofilaments during excitation (p. 881) and, therefore, invokes a positive inotropic response. There is a correlation between the degree of enzyme inhibition and the inotropic potency of the glycoside.

Cardiac glycosides also produce alterations in the electrical properties of both the contractile cells and the specialized automatic cells. While low concentrations of glycosides produce little effect on the action potential, high concentrations result in a reduction in the resting potential (phase 4, see Fig. 184-1) and an augmented rate of diastolic depolarization. The reduction in the resting potential brings the cell closer to the threshold for depolarization. These two effects lead to increased automaticity and ectopic impulse activity. With the lowering of the resting potential, the rate of rise of the action potential is reduced, resulting in a slowing of conduction velocity, which is conducive to the development of reentry. Thus, the known electrophysiologic effects of digitalis glycosides are capable of explaining the development of both reentry and ectopic foci and the resultant arrhythmias associated with digitalis intoxication.

The glycosides also prolong the effective *refractory period* of the atrioventricular node, largely as a result of an enhanced vagal effect. Digitalis also shortens the refractory period of the atrial and ventricular muscle. Small action potentials are propagated in a decremental fashion in the atrioventricular junction. Most do not reach the ventricles but leave some of the atrioventricular junctional cells in a refractory state. This helps to explain the slowing of ventricular rate produced by digitalis in supraventricular tachycardias. In atrial fibrillation, the slowing of ventricular rate is explained by prolongation of the effective refractory period of the atrioventricular node and increased concealed conduction. These actions reduce the frequency at which impulses penetrate the atrioventricular junction owing to both vagal and possibly direct effects of glycosides on junctional tissue.

Digitalis exerts a clinically significant negative chronotropic action, usually only in the setting of ventricular failure. In heart failure, slowing of the sinus rate following the administration of digitalis results also from withdrawal of sympathetic activity secondary to general improvement in circulatory status due to the positive inotropic effect of the glycoside. In the nonfailing heart the slowing effect is negligible, and digitalis should not be used for the treatment of sinus tachycardia unless heart failure is present. The apparent suppression of pacemaker activity which may take place following large doses of digitalis is probably due not to arrest of the pacemaker but rather to a sinoatrial block related to a depression of conduction of impulses out of the sinus node.

In addition, the digitalis glycosides also exert an action on the peripheral vasculature, causing venous and arterial constriction in normal individuals and reflex dilatation resulting from withdrawal of sympathetic constrictor activity in patients with congestive heart failure.

Use in heart failure By stimulating myocardial contractility, digitalis improves ventricular emptying; i.e., it increases cardiac output, augments the ejection fraction, promotes diuresis, and reduces the elevated diastolic pressure and volume and end-systolic volume of the failing ventricle with consequent reduction of symptoms resulting from pulmonary vascular congestion and elevated systemic venous pressure. It is most beneficial in patients in whom ventricular contractility is impaired secondary to chronic ischemic heart disease, or when hypertensive, valvular, or congenital heart disease imposes an excessive volume or pressure load. It is particularly helpful in the treatment of heart failure accompanied by atrial flutter and fibrillation and a rapid ventricular rate. It is of relatively little value in most forms of cardiomyopathy, myocarditis, beriberi with heart failure, mitral stenosis, thyrotoxicosis (all with sinus rhythm), cor pulmonale when the lung disease is not being treated concurrently (Chap. 191), and chronic constrictive pericarditis (Chap. 193). Nonetheless, when used in proper doses, it is not contraindicated in these disorders and is frequently used since it may exert a beneficial effect, albeit not a striking one.

Digitalis intoxication Although digitalis is one of the cornerstones of the treatment for heart failure, it is a two-edged sword, because intoxication due to digitalis excess is a common, serious, and potentially fatal complication of its use. The therapeutic-to-toxic ratios are similar for all cardiac glycosides. In most patients with heart failure the lethal dose of most glycosides is probably 5 to 10 times the minimal effective dose and only about twice the dose which leads to minor toxic manifestations. In addition, old age, acute myocardial infarction or ischemia, hypoxemia, magnesium depletion, renal insufficiency, hypercalcemia, electrical cardioversion, and hypothyroidism all may reduce the tolerance of the patient to the digitalis glycosides or provoke latent digitalis intoxication. The most common precipitating cause of digitalis intoxication, however, is depletion of potassium stores, which often occurs as a result of diuretic therapy and secondary hyperaldosteronism. Since it is not necessary for a patient to receive a maximally tolerated dose of digitalis to derive a beneficial effect, even small doses provide some therapeutic action; this point should be considered if these drugs are to be used in patients prone to toxicity.

Anorexia, nausea, and vomiting, which are among the earliest signs of digitalis intoxication, are caused by direct stimulation of centers in the medulla and are not of gastrointestinal origin. The most frequent disturbance of cardiac rhythm caused by digitalis is premature ventricular beats, which may take the form of bigeminy because of increased myocardial irritability or facilitation of reentry. Atrioventricular block of varying degrees of severity may occur. Nonparoxysmal atrial tachycardia with variable atrioventricular block is quite characteristic of digitalis intoxication. Sinus arrhythmia, sinoatrial block, sinus arrest, and atrioventricular junctional and multifocal ventricular tachycardia may also occur. These arrhythmias are due to action of the glycoside both on cardiac tissues and on the central nervous system. Chronic digitalis intoxication may be insidious in onset and characterized by exacerbations of heart failure, weight loss, cachexia, neuralgias, gynecomastia, yellow vision, and delirium. Digitalis-toxic cardiac arrhythmias precede extracardiac (gastrointestinal or central nervous system) toxicity in about one-half of cases.

Digitalis intoxication has been reported to occur in as many as 20 percent of hospitalized patients receiving a cardiac glycoside, which emphasizes the importance of recognizing this condition. The administration of quinidine to patients receiving digoxin raises the serum concentration of the latter by reducing both the renal and nonrenal elimination of digoxin and by reducing its volume of distribution and thereby increasing the propensity to digitalis intoxication. The calcium channel antagonist verapamil and the antiarrhythmic agent amiodarone also appear to raise serum digoxin levels. Therefore, serum digoxin concentrations and electrocardiograms should be followed carefully when these drugs are administered to digitalized patients. The radioimmunoassays for digoxin and digitoxin make possible the correlation of serum glycoside levels with the presence of toxicity. In patients receiving standard maintenance doses of digoxin and digitoxin and in whom no sign of intoxication is present, serum concentrations approximate 1 to 1.5 and 20 to 25 ng/mL, respectively. When signs of intoxication are present, serum levels of more than 2 and 30 ng/mL, respectively, of these glycosides are often found. Since many factors other than the serum concentration determine digitalis intoxication, and since there is considerable overlap in serum glycoside concentrations in patients with and without toxicity, these levels cannot be used as a sole guide to digitalis dosage. However, when taken together with findings on the clinical examination and electrocardiogram, they add useful information to the clinical evaluations of digitalis intoxication. In addition they will indicate whether a patient for whom the history of digitalis intake is in doubt has, in fact, been receiving the drug.

Treatment of digitalis intoxication When tachyarrhythmias result from digitalis intoxication, withdrawal of the drug and treatment with potassium, phenytoin, propranolol, or lidocaine are indicated. Potassium should be administered cautiously and by the oral route whenever possible if hypokalemia is present, but *small* doses may also be helpful when serum potassium levels are normal; *potassium must not be employed in the presence of atrioventricular block or hyperkalemia*. Propranolol should not be used to treat digitalis toxicity in the presence of severe heart failure or atrioventricular block but may be useful otherwise; lidocaine is effective in the treatment of digitalis-induced ventricular tachyarrhythmias in the absence of preceding atrioventricular block. A cardiac pacemaker may be required in digitalis-induced atrioventricular block. Electrical conversion may not only be ineffective in treating these arrhythmias but may induce more serious arrhythmias. However, it may be lifesaving in digitalis-induced ventricular fibrillation. Quinidine and procainamide are of limited value in the treatment of digitalis intoxication. Fab fragments of purified, intact digitalis antibodies represent a potentially lifesaving approach to the treatment of severe intoxication.

SYMPATHOMIMETIC AMINES (See also Chap. 67) Four sympathomimetic amines which act largely on beta-adrenergic receptors—epinephrine, isoproterenol (isoprenaline), dopamine, and dobutamine—improve myocardial contractility in various forms of heart failure. The latter two agents appear to be most effective; they must be administered by constant intravenous infusion and are useful in patients with intractable heart failure, particularly in those with a reversible component, such as exists in patients who have undergone cardiac surgery, and in some instances of myocardial infarction and shock or pulmonary edema. While they improve the hemodynamics in these conditions, it is not clear that they improve survival. Their administration must be accompanied by careful and continuous monitoring of the electrocardiogram, intraarterial pressure, and if possible pulmonary artery wedge pressure, in an intensive care unit.

Dopamine (p. 387), the naturally occurring immediate precursor of norepinephrine, has a combination of actions which make it particularly useful in the treatment of a variety of hypotensive states and congestive heart failure. At very low doses, that is, 1 to 2 (μg/kg)/min, it dilates renal and mesenteric blood vessels through stimulation of specific dopaminergic receptors, thereby augmenting renal and mesenteric blood flow and sodium excretion. In the range of 2 to 10 (μg/kg)/min, dopamine stimulates myocardial beta receptors but induces relatively little tachycardia, while at higher doses it also stimulates alpha-adrenergic receptors and elevates arterial pressure.

Dobutamine is a synthetic catecholamine which acts on $beta_1$, $beta_2$, and alpha receptors. It exerts a potent inotropic action, has only a modest cardioaccelerating effect, and lowers peripheral vascular resistance, but since it simultaneously raises cardiac output, it has little effect on systemic arterial pressure. Dobutamine, given in continuous infusions of 2.5 to 10 (μg/kg)/min, is useful in the treatment of acute heart failure without hypotension. Like the other sympathomimetic amines it may be particularly valuable in the management of patients requiring relatively short-term inotropic support—up to 1 week—in conditions which are reversible, such as the cardiac depression which sometimes follows open-heart surgery, or in patients with acute heart failure who are being prepared for operation. Adverse effects include sinus tachycardia, tachyarrhythmias, and hypertension.

A major problem with all sympathomimetics is the loss of responsiveness, apparently due to "downregulation" of adrenergic receptors, which becomes evident within 8 h of continuous administration.

Amrinone This bipyridine, a noncatecholamine, nonglycoside exerts both positive inotropic and vasodilator actions by inhibiting a specific phosphodiesterase. It is suitable for intravenous use only, and by simultaneously stimulating cardiac contractility and dilating the systemic vascular bed it reverses the major hemodynamic abnormalities associated with heart failure. Milrinone, a derivative of amrinone, and several other orally active phosphodiesterase inhibitors are under active investigation for chronic oral administration.

REFRACTORY HEART FAILURE When the response to ordinary treatment is inadequate, heart failure is considered to be refractory. Before assuming that this state simply reflects advanced, perhaps preterminal, myocardial depression, careful consideration must be given to several possibilities: (1) an underlying and overlooked cause of the heart disease that may be amenable to specific surgical or medical therapy, such as silent aortic or mitral stenosis, constrictive pericarditis, infective endocarditis, hypertension, or thyrotoxicosis; (2) one or a combination of the precipitating causes of heart failure, such as pulmonary or urinary tract infection, recurrent pulmonary emboli, arterial hypoxemia, anemia, or arrhythmia; and (3) complications of overly vigorous therapy, such as digitalis intoxication, hypovolemia, or electrolyte imbalance.

Recognition and proper treatment of the aforementioned complications are likely to make the patient responsive to therapy again. Perhaps the most common complication results from overzealous treatment with diuretics. When administered too rapidly, these drugs can produce sudden hypovolemia before edema fluid can be mobilized to replace the loss of blood volume, the result being a shocklike state with evidence of systemic hypoperfusion in the presence of edema. The chronically excessively diuresed patient may have exchanged the hazards of pulmonary edema and the inconvenience of systemic edema for a persistently depressed cardiac output with its associated weakness, lethargy, prerenal azotemia, and sometimes cardiac cachexia. Temporarily easing up on salt restriction and diuretic administration may overcome this difficulty, but as heart failure worsens, this course of action may lead to increased pulmonary congestion which is equally unacceptable.

Hyponatremia is a late manifestation of refractory heart failure. It, too, may be a complication of overaggressive diuresis leading to reduced glomerular filtration rate and decreased delivery of NaCl to the diluting sites in the distal tubule. Hyponatremia may also result from nonosmotic stimuli for the continued secretion of antidiuretic hormone. Therapy involves improvement of the cardiovascular status, if possible (sometimes requiring the administration of a sympathomimetic amine such as dopamine or dobutamine), as well as temporary cessation of diuretic therapy and restriction of oral water intake. Hypertonic saline is very rarely indicated because total body sodium is usually elevated, not depressed in heart failure.

The combination of an intravenously administered vasodilator, such as sodium nitroprusside, along with a potent sympathomimetic amine, such as dopamine or dobutamine, often results in an additive effect, raising cardiac output and lowering filling pressure. Intravenous amrinone, sometimes accompanied by the administration of a converting enzyme inhibitor, may also be useful in patients with refractory heart failure.

Cardiac transplantation When patients with heart failure become unresponsive to a combination of all of the aforementioned therapeutic measures, are in New York Heart Association class IV, and are deemed unlikely to survive 1 year, they should be considered for cardiac transplantation (see Chap. 183).

TREATMENT OF ACUTE PULMONARY EDEMA Pulmonary edema secondary to left ventricular failure or mitral stenosis is described in Chap. 36. It is life-threatening and must be considered a medical emergency. As is the case for the more chronic forms of heart failure, in the treatment of pulmonary edema, attention must be directed to identifying and removing any precipitating causes of decompensation, such as an arrhythmia or infection. However, because of the acute nature of the problem, a number of additional nonspecific measures are necessary. When possible, and if it does not delay treatment unduly, recording pulmonary vascular pressures through a Swan-Ganz catheter and intraarterial pressure directly is advisable. The first six measures listed below are ordinarily applied simultaneously or nearly so.

1 Morphine is administered intravenously repetitively, as needed, in doses from 2 to 5 mg. This drug reduces anxiety, reduces adrenergic vasoconstrictor stimuli to the arteriolar and venous beds, and thereby helps to break a vicious cycle. Naloxone should be available in case respiratory depression occurs.
2 Because the alveolar fluid interferes with oxygen diffusion, resulting in arterial hypoxemia, 100% oxygen should be administered, preferably under positive pressure. The latter increases intraalveolar pressure and therefore reduces transudation of fluid from the alveolar capillaries and impedes venous return to the thorax, reducing pulmonary capillary pressure.
3 The patient should be maintained in the sitting position, with the legs dangling along the side of the bed, if possible, which also tends to reduce venous return.
4 Intravenous loop diuretics, such as furosemide or ethacrynic acid (40 to 100 mg), or bumetanide (1 mg) will, by rapidly establishing a diuresis, reduce circulating blood volume and thereby hasten the relief of pulmonary edema. In addition when given intravenously, furosemide also exerts a venodilator action, reduces venous return, and reduces pulmonary edema even before the diuresis commences.
5 Afterload reduction is achieved with intravenous sodium nitroprusside at 20 to 30 μg/min in patients whose systolic arterial pressures exceed 100 mmHg.
6 If digitalis has not been administered previously, three-fourths of a full dose of a rapidly acting glycoside, such as ouabain, digoxin, or lanatoside C, should be administered intravenously.
7 Sometimes, aminophylline (theophylline ethylenediamine), 240 to 480 mg intravenously, is effective in diminishing bronchoconstriction, increasing renal blood flow and sodium excretion, and augmenting myocardial contractility.
8 If the above mentioned measures are not sufficient, rotating tourniquets should be applied to the extremities.

After these emergency therapeutic measures have been instituted, and the precipitating factors treated, the diagnosis of the underlying cardiac disorder responsible for the pulmonary edema must be established if it is not already known. After stabilization of the patient's condition a long-range strategy for prevention of future episodes of pulmonary edema must be established, and this may require surgical treatment.

PROGNOSIS

The prognosis in heart failure depends primarily on the nature of the underlying heart disease and on the presence or absence of a precipitating factor which can be treated. Also, the long-term prognosis for heart failure is most favorable when the underlying forms of heart disease can be treated. When one of the latter can be identified and removed, the outlook for immediate survival is far better than if heart failure occurs without any obvious precipitating cause. In the latter situation, survival usually ranges between 6 months and 5 years depending on the severity of the heart failure. The prognosis can also be estimated by observing the response to treatment. When clinical improvement occurs with only modest dietary sodium restriction and small doses of diuretics or digitalis, then the outlook is far better than if, in addition to these measures, intensive diuretic therapy and vasodilators are necessary. A large fraction of patients with congestive heart failure die suddenly, presumably of ventricular fibrillation. Unfortunately, there is no evidence that this complication can be prevented by the administration of antiarrhythmic agents.

REFERENCES

ARNOLD SB et al: Long-term digitalis therapy improves left ventricular function in heart failure. N Engl J Med 303:1443, 1980

BERGER BE, WARNOCK DG: Mechanisms of action and clinical use of diuretics, in *The Kidney*, 3d ed, BM Brenner, FC Rector (eds). Philadelphia, Saunders, 1986, p 433

BRAUNWALD E (ed): Newer positive inotropic agents. Circulation 73(Suppl III):1, 1986

——— et al (eds): *Congestive Heart Failure: Current Research and Clinical Applications.* New York, Grune & Stratton, 1982

BRISTOW MR: The adrenergic nervous system in heart failure. N Engl J Med 311:850, 1984

COHN JN (ed): *Drug Treatment of Heart Failure*, 2d ed. Secaucus, NJ, Advanced Therapeutics Communications International, 1988

——— et al (eds): Advances in congestive heart failure. Am J Cardiol (Suppl. A) 62:1, 1988

FIFER MA et al: Hemodynamic and renal effects of atrial natriuretic peptide in congestive heart failure. Am J Cardiol 65(3):211, 1990

FISCH C (guest ed): An account of the foxglove and some of its medical uses: 1785–1985. J Am Coll Cardiol 5 (Suppl A):1A, 1985

GOODMAN LS, GILMAN A (eds): Cardiovascular drugs, in *The Pharmacological Basis of Therapeutics*, 7th ed. New York, Macmillan, 1985, pp 716, 887

ISKANDRIAN AS et al: Predicting left ventricular function: Bedside examination. Prim Cardiol (Suppl) 10:3A, 1984

LEE WH, PACKER M: Prognostic importance of serum sodium concentration and its modification by converting-enzyme inhibition in patients with severe chronic heart failure. Circulation 73:257, 1986

MAKABALI C et al: Dobutamine and other sympathomimetic drugs for the treatment of low cardiac output failure. Semin Anesth 1:63, 1982

SIMON J et al: Pulmonary artery pressure changes during exercise and daily activities in chronic heart failure. J Am Coll Cardiol 15(1):52, 1990

SMITH TW (ed): *Digitalis Glycosides.* New York, Grune & Stratton, 1986

——— et al: Management of heart failure, in *Heart Disease*, 3d ed, E Braunwald (ed). Philadelphia, Saunders, 1988, p 485

SUKI WN et al: Physiology of diuretic action, in *The Kidney: Physiology and Pathophysiology*, 2d ed, DW Seldin, G Giebisch (eds). New York, Raven Press, 1985, p 2127

The Consensus Trial Study Group: Effects of enalapril on mortality in severe congestive heart failure: Results of the Cooperative North Scandinavian Enalapril Survival Study (Consensus). New Engl J Med 316:1429, 1987

183 CARDIAC TRANSPLANTATION

JOHN S. SCHROEDER

Orthotopic allograft cadaver cardiac transplantation as a treatment for end-stage cardiac disease achieved its twentieth anniversary on December 7, 1987. On that day in 1967 Dr. Christiaan Barnard accomplished the first successful cardiac transplant in man, quickly followed by Drs. Norman Shumway and Richard Lower at Stanford University. After an initial early wave of enthusiasm, the problems of immunosuppression slowed application of the procedure until the introduction of cyclosporine in 1980. A subsequent worldwide expansion of cardiac transplantation resulted in approximately 1500 cardiac transplants per year, with further increases limited only by the donor supply. Current 1- and 5-year survival rates of 60 and 70 percent indicate that cardiac transplant is the therapy of choice in patients with end-stage heart disease who are unlikely to survive the next 6 to 12 months. This chapter reviews the procedure, indications, short- and long-term immunosuppressive therapy, and complications.

Since the introduction of cyclosporine in 1980 and the development of "low-dose" triple immunosuppressive regimens using azathioprine and prednisone, 1-year survival is reported at 80 percent and 5-year survival at 60 to 70 percent. The longest survivor has now lived 19 years after transplantation and is functionally well. Therefore, these survival statistics must be compared to those for other medical or surgical therapies in considering alternative therapies for end-stage heart disease.

INDICATIONS AND SELECTION OF CANDIDATES The limited donor supply and relatively high cost of cardiac transplantation have restricted it to patients most likely to survive and resume a functional life after transplantation. It is estimated that only 2000 potential donors, for a pool of at least 20,000 candidates based on current guidelines, become available yearly in the United States. Attempts to increase donor awareness in both physicians and the public are being made. Optimal candidates for this procedure are those who would be expected to return to a functional life if their hearts were replaced. This requires a mentally vigorous, medically compliant person who has not suffered extensive other end-stage organ damage from cardiac failure or does not have other systemic disease such as severe diabetes mellitus and collagen vascular disease. Long-standing pulmonary hypertension or recurrent pulmonary emboli and infarction may result in irreversible pulmonary hypertension leading to intraoperative death. Several heart transplant centers have initiated cardiac transplantation for newborns with left ventricular hypoplasia, but long-term survival experience is still very limited.

Timing of the recommendation to undergo cardiac transplantation can be difficult and requires assessment of the patient's current disability, stability of course, and likelihood of surviving the next 6 to 12 months. Generally, left ventricular ejection fractions under 15 to 20 percent and presence of serious ventricular arrhythmias indicate a 1-year survival rate of 50 percent or less. Mechanical assistance devices, either a left ventricular assist or a totally implantable device, have been used to "bridge" the critically ill patient until a suitable donor can be found. This approach has been successful, but has been used relatively infrequently because of the potential for infection and the ethical problems of prioritizing distribution of available donor hearts. Tissue cross-matching between donor and recipient has generally not been done because of difficulty in obtaining good matches and lack of correlation between match and outcome. Size, ABO matching, negative lymphocyte cross-match, and avoidance of a transplantation from a cytomegalovirus (CMV)–positive donor to a CMV-negative recipient are more important.

OPERATIVE PROCEDURE The operative technique for orthotopic transplantation developed in animals in the early 1960s by Shumway and Lower remains little changed. In this technique, the surgeon removes the diseased heart but leaves the posterior wall of the right atrium in place and the superior and inferior venae cavae intact. The posterior wall of the left atrium is also left in situ with pulmonary veins intact. The donor heart is then removed in toto with the posterior wall of the right and left atria incised, which allows suturing of left atrial donor rim to recipient rim, and right atrial donor rim to recipient rim, with anastomosis of the aorta and pulmonary artery.

IMMUNOSUPPRESSION AND REJECTION Controlling rejection while avoiding the adverse side effects of immunosuppressive agents is pivotal to successful transplantation. Rejection is characterized by perivascular infiltration of killer T lymphocytes, which migrate into the myocardium and cause cellular necrosis if not checked. Since early rejection can be silent, it is important to detect it before necrosis occurs. Immunologic monitoring of activated T lymphocytes in peripheral blood offers clues to the timing of a rejection process but has not been sufficiently reliable to dictate antirejection therapy. Therefore, repeated percutaneous transvenous right ventricular endomyocardial biopsies via the right internal jugular vein are required for histologic determination of the state of immunosuppression and rejection.

Billingham et al. have graded the stages of rejection as: cannot rule out rejection, mild early rejection, moderate rejection, and severe rejection. Serial biopsies are taken every 1 to 2 weeks early after transplantation, with gradually widening intervals depending on the patient's course and rejection history. Prolongation of isovolumic relaxation time measured by echocardiography may also provide early clues to rejection.

Immunosuppressive therapy regimens vary but usually include triple therapy with cyclosporine, azathioprine, and prednisone. Prophylactic courses of OKT_3 or antithymocyte globulin may also be given early after transplantation. Careful monitoring of the adverse side effects of these agents is extremely important since they include nephrotoxicity, bone marrow suppression, and opportunistic infections.

EARLY COURSE AND COMPLICATIONS It is rare for a cardiac transplant patient to have a completely uncomplicated postoperative course. In the immediate postoperative period, right heart failure due to pulmonary vascular disease is most life-threatening. During the 2 to 3 weeks after transplantation the patient is hospitalized with meticulous monitoring for evidence of rejection and infections, repeated percutaneous transvenous endomyocardial biopsies, and adjustment of immunosuppressive drugs. During the ensuing 4 to 6 weeks, infectious complications, including bacterial, viral, and protozoan infections, are common. A successful transplant program requires a highly aggressive and sophisticated approach to diagnosis and therapy of infections in the immunocompromised host. Depending on the degree of cardiac cachexia preoperatively, the patient is usually functional at 1 week and discharged from the hospital at 2 to 3 weeks if no major complication occurs.

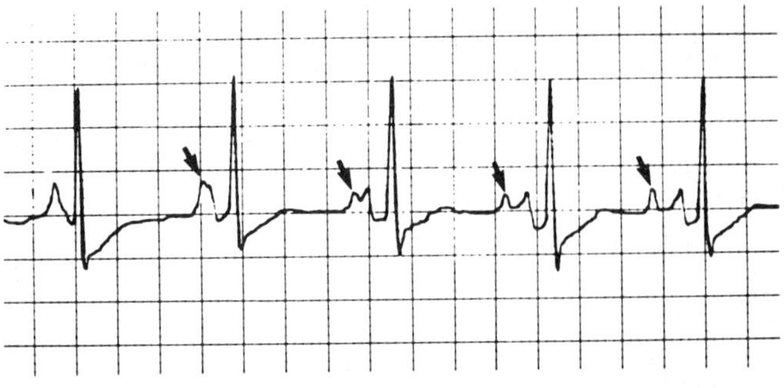

FIGURE 183-1 Electrocardiogram in a patient with a transplanted heart. The arrows denote the P wave generated by the recipient's atrium. The P wave just preceding the QRS complex is generated by the donor heart.

The average first-year cost ranges from $100,000 to $150,000, depending on the need for repeated hospitalization and cardiac biopsies, and is occasionally much higher. Yearly costs for immunosuppressive agents range from $5,000 to $10,000, in addition to the expense of medical surveillance for rejection or complications.

PHYSIOLOGY AND FUNCTION Since the allografted heart remains denervated, cardiac function differs from that of the innervated heart during both rest and exercise. The electrocardiogram in Fig. 183-1 shows two P waves. The P wave of the recipient's heart reflects the residual sinus node and posterior walls of the remaining native atria but is dissociated from the QRS, since the depolarization impulse does not cross the suture line. Although it does not control donor heart rate, the recipient's sinus node remains innervated and under the influence of the autonomic nervous system. The donor sinus node controls the rate of the transplanted heart. The donor heart's P wave has a regular PR interval, reflecting conduction to the ventricles. Since the controlling sinus node is denervated, it maintains a heart rate of 100 to 110 beats per minute, and rate increase depends on alterations in chronotropic agents perfusing the sinus node.

Ventricular function in response to isometric and isotonic exercise has been studied extensively. The early response to exercise is more dependent on the Frank-Starling mechanism and change in ventricular volume and filling pressure. As exercise proceeds and catecholamines are released with their positive inotropic effects, cardiac output begins to rise. The cardiac transplant recipient can achieve approximately 70 percent of the maximal cardiac output expected for his or her age, easily sufficient for the stresses of everyday life.

LATE COURSE AND COMPLICATIONS Although the rejection process partially subsides, lifelong administration of immunosuppressive drugs, albeit at lower doses, is still required and remains a hazard. Infectious complications and unsuspected rejection continue to occur, requiring ongoing surveillance and monitoring. Cardiac biopsies are performed at 3-month intervals to assess the response to rejection treatment. Table 183-1 shows the causes of death in patients surviving more than 1 year after transplantation in the Stanford program. In addition to the well-known hazards of long-term steroid usage, the immunosuppressed patient is at increased risk for neoplasia.

Accelerated coronary vascular disease appears to be one of the major factors limiting longer-term survival. The process is a fibrointimal hyperplasia which can go undetected by coronary arteriography

TABLE 183-1 Cause of death in patients surviving more than 1 year after cardiac transplantation in the Stanford Program

Cause of death	No. of patients
Graft atherosclerosis	14
Infection	16
Rejection	4
Lymphoproliferative disease	3
Nonlymphoid malignancy	5
Other	6
Cerebrovascular accident	1
Total deaths	49
Total at risk	228

at first and then cause diffuse atherosclerotic changes. Risk factors for its development include number of rejection episodes and elevated lipids, most likely reflecting rejection injury, as well as more commonly accepted causes of atherosclerosis. CMV infections have also been associated with higher frequency of this disease. Uncontrolled trials with anticoagulation, aspirin, and improved immunosuppression with cyclosporine have done little to lower this frequency; 40 to 50 percent of patients show arteriographic evidence of coronary vascular disease 5 years after transplantation. Retransplantation has been employed for some patients with severe graft atherosclerosis.

HEART-LUNG TRANSPLANTATION

Patients with congenital heart disease with Eisenmenger's complex (Chap. 186) or primary pulmonary hypertension (Chap. 212) are now considered for heart-lung transplantation. The surgical technique is similar to that for heart transplantation, except that the pulmonary venous attachments to the left atrium are left intact, and a tracheal anastomosis is required. The postoperative period is more complex, since the lungs may be rejected separately from the heart, requiring repeated endobronchoscopic biopsies when rejection is suspected. The immunosuppressive regimen is similar to that for heart transplants. Long-term survival has in the past been limited by obliterative bronchiolitis due to chronic unrecognized rejection; survival rates have been approximately 50 percent at 1 year and 30 percent at 2 years, but appear to be improving. More recently, heart-lung transplantation has been performed on patients with cystic fibrosis. Single-lung transplants are also potential options for these patients.

REFERENCES

COPELAND JG et al: Orthotopic total artificial heart bridge to transplantation: Preliminary results. J Heart Transplant 8:124, 1989

GAO SZ et al: Clinical and laboratory correlates of accelerated coronary artery disease in the cardiac transplant patient. Circulation 76(suppl V):56, 1987

GRATTAN MT et al: Cytomegalovirus infection is associated with cardiac allograft rejection and atherosclerosis. JAMA 261:3561, 1989

OAKS TE et al: Results of mechanical circulatory assistance before heart transplantation. J Heart Transplant 8:113, 1989

PICANO E et al: Electrocardiographic changes suggestive of myocardial ischemia elicited by dypyridamole infusion in acute rejection early after heart transplantation. Circulation 81(1):72, 1990

SAVIN WM et al: Response of cardiac transplant recipients to static and dynamic exercises. Heart Transplant 1:72, 1981

SCHROEDER JS, HUNT SA: Cardiac transplantation: Update 1987. JAMA 258:3142, 1987

STEVENSON LW et al: Poor survival of patients with idiopathic cardiomyopathy considered too well for transplantation. Am J Med 83:871, 1987

184 THE BRADYARRHYTHMIAS: DISORDERS OF SINUS NODE FUNCTION AND AV CONDUCTION DISTURBANCES

MARK E. JOSEPHSON / FRANCIS E. MARCHLINSKI / ALFRED E. BUXTON

ANATOMY OF THE CONDUCTING SYSTEM Under normal conditions the pacemaker function of the heart resides in the sinoatrial node, which lies at the junction of the right atrium and superior vena cava. The SA node is approximately $1\frac{1}{2}$ cm long and 2 to 3 mm wide and is supplied by the sinus node artery, which arises from either the right coronary artery (60 percent of cases) or the left circumflex coronary artery (40 percent). Once the impulse exits the sinus node and perinodal tissue, it traverses the atrium until it reaches the atrioventricular node. The blood supply of the AV node is derived from the posterior descending coronary artery (90 percent of cases), which lies at the base of the interatrial septum just above the tricuspid annulus and anterior to the coronary sinus. The electrophysiologic properties of the AV node result in slow conduction, which is responsible for the normal delay in AV conduction, i.e., the PR interval.

The bundle of His emerges from the AV node, enters the fibrous skeleton of the heart, and courses anteriorly across the membranous interventricular septum. It has a dual blood supply from the AV nodal artery and a branch of the anterior descending coronary artery. The branching (distal) portion of the bundle of His gives rise to a broad sheet of fibers that course over the left side of the interventricular septum to form the left bundle branch and a narrow cablelike structure on the right side that forms the right bundle branch. The arborization of both the right and left bundle branches gives rise to the distal His-Purkinje system, which ultimately extends throughout the endocardium of the right and left ventricles.

The sinus node, atrium, and AV node are significantly influenced by autonomic tone. Vagal influences depress automaticity of the sinus node, depress conduction, and prolong refractoriness in the tissue surrounding the sinus node, inhomogeneously decrease atrial refractoriness and slow atrial conduction, and prolong AV nodal conduction and refractoriness. Sympathetic influences exert the opposite effect.

ELECTROPHYSIOLOGIC PRINCIPLES

In the resting state, the interior of most cardiac cells, with the exception of the sinus and AV nodes, is approximately −80 to −90 mV, negative with respect to a reference extracellular electrode. The resting membrane potential is primarily determined by the concentration gradient of potassium across the cell membrane. Activation of cardiac cells results from movement of ions across the cell membrane, causing a transient depolarization known as the *action potential*. The ionic species responsible for the action potential varies among the cardiac tissues, and the configuration of the action potential is therefore unique to each tissue (Fig. 184-1).

The action potential of the His-Purkinje system and ventricular myocardium has five phases (Fig. 184-2). The rapid depolarizing current (phase 0) is mainly determined by an influx of sodium into myocardial cells followed by a secondary (slower) influx of calcium. The repolarization phases of the action potential (phases 1 to 3) are primarily related to outward flux of potassium. The resting membrane potential is phase 4.

The bradyarrhythmias result from abnormalities either of impulse formation, i.e., automaticity, or of conduction. *Automaticity,* which is normally observed in the sinus node, the specialized fibers of the His-Purkinje system, and some specialized atrial fibers, is the property

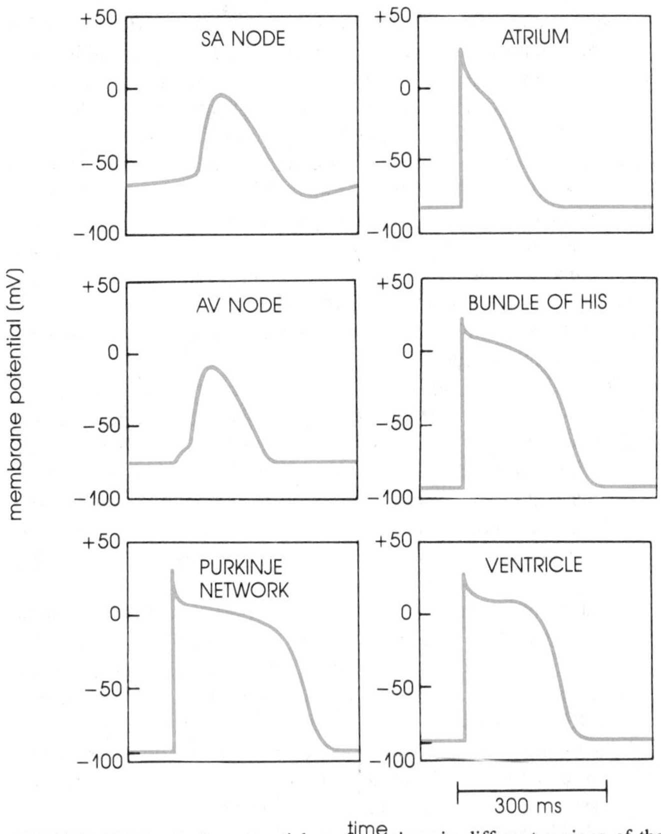

FIGURE 184-1 Action potential configurations in different regions of the mammalian heart. *(From AM Katz, Physiology of the Heart, New York, Raven, 1977.)*

of a cardiac cell to depolarize spontaneously during phase 4 of the action potential, leading to the generation of an impulse. To exhibit automaticity the resting membrane potential must decrease spontaneously until threshold potential is reached and an all-or-none regenerative response occurs. The ionic components producing spontaneous diastolic depolarization appear to involve the inward current of either sodium or calcium. The velocity of *conduction*, i.e., impulse propagation through cardiac tissues, depends on the magnitude of inward current, which is directly related to the rate of rise and amplitude of phase 0 of the action potential. The more positive the threshold potential and the slower the rate of depolarization toward threshold, the slower the rate of rise of phase 0 of the action potential and the slower the conduction velocity. Disease states or drugs may result in lower rates of rise of phase 0 at any given membrane potential.

Refractoriness is a property of cardiac cells which defines the period of recovery that cells require after being discharged before they can be reexcited by a stimulus. The *absolute refractory period* is defined by that portion of the action potential during which no stimulus, regardless of its strength, can evoke another response. The *effective refractory period* is that part of the action potential during which a stimulus can only evoke a local, nonpropagated response. The *relative refractory period* extends from the end of the effective refractory period to the time that the tissue is fully recovered. During this time a stimulus of greater than threshold strength is required to evoke a response which is propagated more slowly than normal. After completion of the action potential, excitability is recovered, and evoked responses have characteristics similar to the spontaneous normal response.

INTRACARDIAC RECORDINGS OF THE SPECIALIZED CONDUCTING SYSTEM Electrode catheters allow the recording of activation of portions of the specialized conducting system including the bundle of His. To obtain a recording from the bundle of His the electrode catheter is positioned across the tricuspid valve (Fig. 184-3). The interval from local atrial depolarization in the His bundle recording to the onset of depolarization of the His bundle deflection is called the AH interval (normal = 60 to 125 ms) and represents an indirect method of assessing AV nodal conduction time. The interval from the beginning of the His bundle deflection to the earliest onset of ventricular activation, as measured from any of multiple-surface electrocardiogram (ECG) leads or the intracardiac ventricular electrogram, is called the HV interval (normal = 35 to 55 ms) and represents conduction time through the His-Purkinje system. Electrode catheters can be positioned in the area of the sinus node to record high right atrial activity. Left atrial activity may be recorded directly via a catheter placed across a patent foramen ovale, or indirectly using a catheter inserted into the coronary sinus. The atrial activation sequence may be "mapped," and sites of intra- and interatrial conduction abnormalities may be ascertained.

FIGURE 184-2 Schematic representation of the action potential in normal ventricle depicting the direction, strength, and period of flow of the ionic currents underlying the action potential. The arrow's direction and size indicate whether current is inward- or outward-directed and the approximate current strength of the ion identified at the arrow's base. The horizontal position of the arrow corresponds to the same moment in the time course of action potential (see text). The five phases of the action potential are indicated by the numerals placed along the waveform. *(From Ten Eick et al; Progress in Cardiovascular Diseases 24(2):157, 1981; used with permission.)*

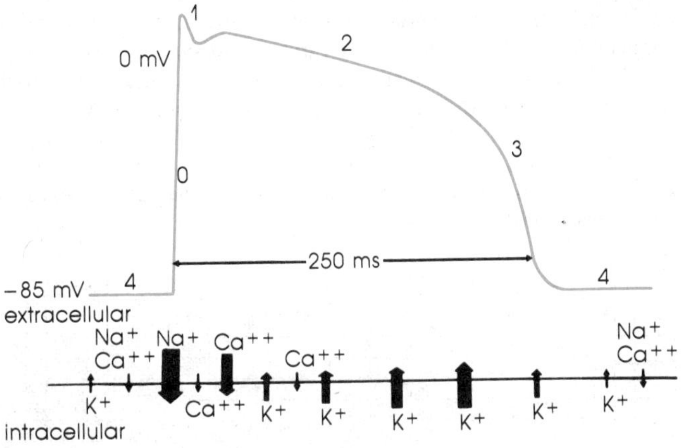

SINUS NODE DYSFUNCTION

The sinus node is normally the dominant cardiac pacemaker because its intrinsic discharge rate is the highest of all potential cardiac pacemakers. Its responsiveness to alterations in autonomic nervous system tone is responsible for the normal acceleration of heart rate during exercise and the slowing that occurs during rest and sleep. Increases in sinus rate normally result from an increase in sympathetic tone acting via beta-adrenergic receptors and/or decrease in parasympathetic tone acting via muscarinic receptors. Slowing of the heart rate is normally due to opposite alterations. In adults, the normal sinus rate under basal conditions is 60 to 100 beats per minute. Sinus bradycardia is said to exist when the sinus rate is less than 60 beats per minute, and sinus tachycardia when it exceeds 100 per minute. However, there is wide variation among individuals, and rates less than 60 per minute do not necessarily indicate pathologic states. For example, trained athletes often exhibit resting rates under 50 beats per minute due to increases in vagal tone. Normal elderly individuals may also show marked sinus bradycardia at rest.

ETIOLOGY Sinus node dysfunction most often is found in the elderly as an isolated phenomenon. Although interruption of the blood supply to the sinus node may produce dysfunction, the correlation between obstruction of the sinus node artery and clinical evidence of sinus node dysfunction is poor. Specific disease states associated with sinus node dysfunction include senile amyloidosis and other

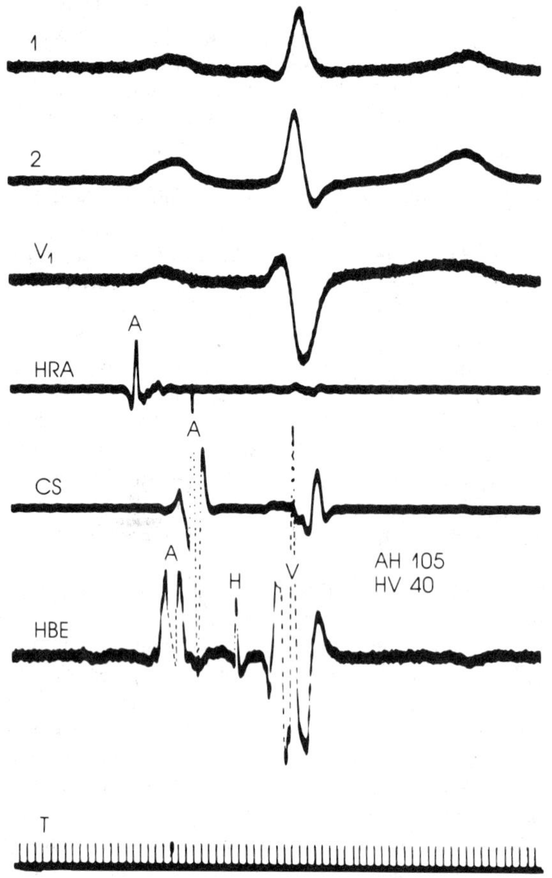

FIGURE 184-3 Normal intracardiac recording. Surface ECG leads I, II, and V_1 are displayed with intracardiac ECGs from the high right atrium (HRA), left atrium from the coronary sinus (CS), and AV junction to obtain a His bundle electrogram (HBE). T = time lines. Atrial activation begins in the high right atrium and spreads inferiorly to the low atrial septum, as recorded in the HBE, and the left atrium, as recorded in the CS. The AH and HV intervals represent AV nodal and His-Purkinje conduction times, respectively. Vertical lines = 0.10 s. (*From ME Josephson, SF Seides: Clinical Cardiac Electrophysiology: Techniques and Interpretations. Philadelphia, Lea & Febiger, 1979.*)

conditions associated with infiltration of the atrial myocardium. Sinus bradycardia is associated with hypothyroidism, advanced liver disease, hypothermia, typhoid fever, and brucellosis; it occurs during episodes of hypervagotonia (vasovagal syncope), severe hypoxia, hypercapnia, acidemia, and acute hypertension. However, in most cases of sinus node dysfunction a specific cause cannot be identified.

MANIFESTATIONS Although marked (≤50 beats per minute) sinus bradycardia may cause fatigue and other symptoms due to inadequate cardiac output, more commonly sinus node dysfunction is manifest as paroxysmal dizziness, presyncope, or syncope. These symptoms usually result from abrupt, prolonged sinus pauses caused by failure of sinus impulse formation (sinus arrest) or block of conduction of sinus impulses to the surrounding atrial tissue (sinus exit block). In either case, the ECG manifestation is a prolonged period (>3 s) of atrial asystole. In some patients sinus node dysfunction is accompanied by abnormalities in AV conduction. In addition to the absence of atrial activity, lower pacemakers fail to emerge during the sinus pauses, resulting in periods of ventricular asystole and syncope. Occasionally, sinus node dysfunction is manifested initially by the failure of the sinus rate to accelerate in response to conditions such as exercise or fever that normally cause increases in the sinus rate. In some patients sinus node dysfunction may become manifest only in the presence of certain cardioactive drugs: cardiac glycosides, beta-adrenergic blocking drugs, verapamil, quinidine, and other antiarrhythmic agents. These agents, which do not cause sinus node dysfunction in normal people, may unmask evidence of sinus node dysfunction in susceptible individuals.

The *sick sinus syndrome* refers to a combination of symptoms (dizziness, confusion, fatigue, syncope, and congestive heart failure) caused by sinus node dysfunction and manifested by marked sinus bradycardia, sinoatrial block, or sinus arrest. Because these symptoms are nonspecific and because ECG manifestations of sinus node dysfunction are not infrequently intermittent, it may be difficult to prove that such symptoms are actually caused by sinus node dysfunction.

Atrial tachyarrhythmias such as atrial fibrillation, flutter, or atrial tachycardia may be accompanied by sinus node dyfunction. The *bradycardia-tachycardia syndrome* refers to paroxysmal atrial arrhythmia which upon termination is followed by prolonged sinus pauses (Fig. 184-4) or in which there are alternating periods of tachyarrhythmia and bradyarrhythmia. Syncope or presyncope may result from failure of the sinus node to recover function following suppression of automaticity by atrial tachyarrhythmia.

DIAGNOSIS *First-degree sinoatrial exit block* denotes a prolonged conduction time from the sinus node to the surrounding atrial tissue. It cannot be recognized on a standard (surface) ECG but requires invasive intracardiac recordings (see below). *Second-degree sinoatrial exit block* denotes the intermittent failure of conduction of sinus impulses to the surrounding atrial tissue; it is manifested as the intermittent absence of P waves (Fig. 184-5). *Third-degree, or complete, sinoatrial block* is characterized by a lack of atrial activity or by the presence of an ectopic subsidiary atrial pacemaker. On the standard ECG, it cannot be distinguished from sinus arrest, but direct intracardiac recordings of sinus node activity permit this distinction. The *bradycardia-tachycardia syndrome* is manifested on the standard ECG as tachyarrhythmias (Fig. 184-4). Most often these are atrial flutter or fibrillation, although any tachycardia with retrograde conduction to the atria may cause overdrive suppression of the sinus node resulting in clinical appearance of this syndrome.

The most important step in the diagnosis is to correlate symptoms with ECG evidence of sinus node dysfunction. While ambulatory ECG (Holter) monitoring remains a mainstay in evaluating sinus node function, most episodes of syncope are paroxysmal and unpredictable. Single and even multiple 24-h Holter monitor recordings may fail to include a symptomatic episode. Therefore, noting the response to carotid sinus pressure and pharmacologic autonomic "denervation" of the heart is frequently helpful. Carotid sinus pressure is particularly useful in patients in whom paroxysmal dizziness or syncope is compatible with the hypersensitive carotid sinus syndrome (see Chap. 21). In such patients, the response can be dramatic, and sinus pauses in excess of 5 s may occur. Normally a sinus pause of ≤3 s results

FIGURE 184-4 Tachycardia-bradycardia syndrome. Rhythm strip of ECG lead II showing spontaneous cessation of supraventricular tachycardia followed by a 5.6-s pause prior to resumption of sinus activity. The patient was asymptomatic during supraventricular tachycardia, but the sinus pause caused severe light-headedness.

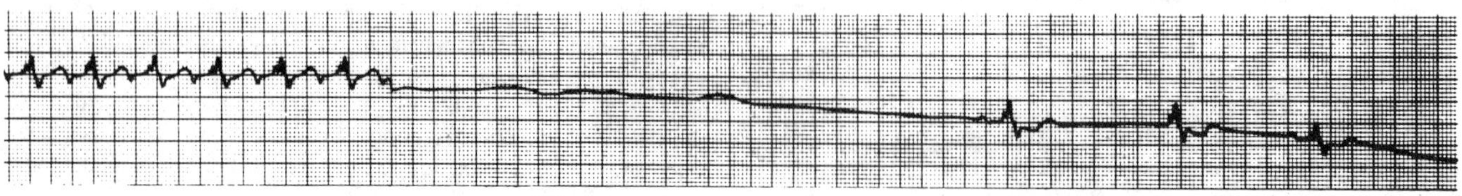

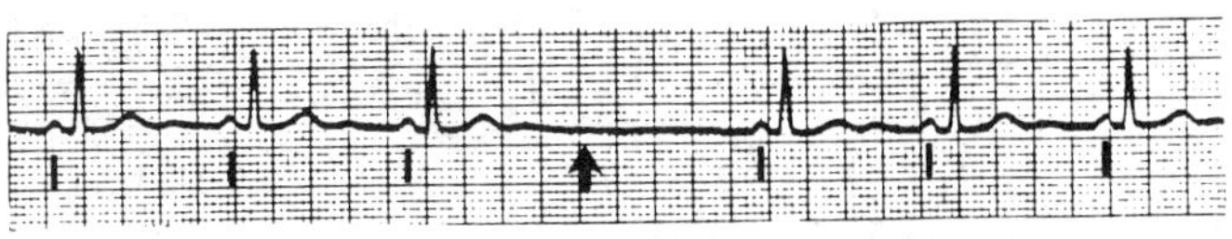

FIGURE 184-5 Second-degree sinoatrial exit block. Surface ECG denoting abrupt absence of P wave during sinus rhythm. Prior to the pause the sinus rate is regular. The interval of the pause is exactly twice the basal sinus cycle length. The arrow marks the appropriate location for the absent P wave.

from 5 s of unilateral carotid sinus massage. If atropine can prevent the effects of carotid sinus pressure, autonomic dysfunction, not primary (intrinsic) sinus node dysfunction, is responsible. The other noninvasive test of sinus node function involves the use of pharmacologic agents to manipulate the autonomic nervous system and assess the balance of parasympathetic and sympathetic activity on the sinus node. Physiologic or pharmacologic maneuvers which are vagomimetic (Valsalva maneuver or phenylephrine-induced hypertension), vagolytic (atropine), sympathomimetic (isoproterenol or hypotension by nitroprusside), or sympatholytic (beta-adrenergic blocking agents) can be utilized, singly and in combination. These studies are designed to test the response of the sinus node to autonomic stimulation and inhibition and thereby characterize the status of autonomic regulation of the sinus node. Abnormalities of the autonomic control of sinus function are particularly common in patients in whom the only presenting arrhythmia is sinus bradycardia.

Intrinsic heart rate This is a manifestation of the primary activity of the sinus node, and its determination requires chemical autonomic blockade of the heart. Complete autonomic blockade is achieved with 0.2 mg/kg propranolol intravenously, followed after 10 min by 0.04 mg/kg of atropine sulfate intravenously. Normal values of intrinsic heart rate (in beats per minute) are calculated by the formula $118.1 - (0.57 \times \text{age})$. The use of autonomic blockade can separate patients with asymptomatic sinus bradycardia into a group with primary sinus node dysfunction (slow intrinsic heart rate) and a group with autonomic imbalance (normal intrinsic heart rate). Autonomic blockade is particularly useful when combined with invasive assessment of sinus node function (see below). Autonomic blockade may depress conduction in patients with intrinsic disease of the conduction system and should be carried out only in a setting where arrhythmias can be monitored and rapidly treated.

Sinus node recovery time Sinus node recovery time is evaluated by assessing the response of the sinus node to rapid atrial pacing (Fig. 184-6). When atrial pacing is discontinued, a pause, the *sinus node recovery time,* occurs prior to resumption of spontaneous sinus rhythm. When the sinus recovery time is prolonged, the results of this test mimic the prolonged sinus pauses seen following termination of atrial tachyarrhythmias in the bradycardia-tachycardia syndrome (see Fig. 184-4). The corrected sinus node recovery time (sinus recovery time − sinus cycle length) normally is less than 550 ms and the uncorrected sinus node recovery time less than 150 percent of the spontaneous cycle length. In patients with symptomatic sinus node dysfunction, prolongation of the sinus node recovery time is often observed. Patients with abnormally slow intrinsic heart rates usually have abnormal sinus node recovery times, while those with normal intrinsic heart rates have normal recovery times.

FIGURE 184-6 Example of sinus node recovery time in a patient with symptomatic sinus node dysfunction. Cessation of atrial pacing at 150 beats per minute (cycle length 400 ms) results in a prolonged sinus pause (2.8 s). Surface ECG leads V_1 and V_6 are shown in addition to intracardiac recordings at the high right atrium (A), which demonstrates atrial pacing rate.

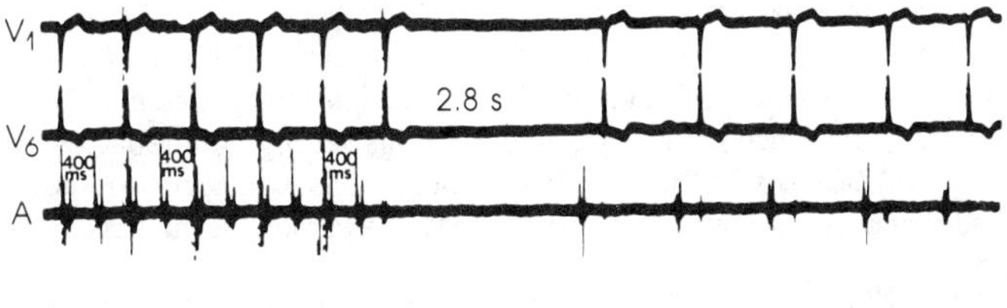

Sinoatrial conduction time Determination of the conduction time from the sinus node to the atrium allows for the differentiation of abnormalities of sinoatrial conduction from abnormalities of sinus impulse formation. The conduction time equals one-half of the difference between the pause following termination of brief periods of pacing and the sinus cycle length. Alternatively, the sinus node electrogram can be recorded directly by a catheter electrode placed near the sinoatrial node.

EVALUATION The electrophysiologic investigation of sinus node dysfunction should be undertaken in patients who have had symptoms compatible with sinus node dysfunction and in whom no documentation of the arrhythmia responsible for these symptoms has been obtained by prolonged Holter monitoring. Asymptomatic patients with sinus bradycardia need *not* be tested since no therapy is indicated. Similarly, symptomatic patients with ECG documentation of asystole, sinoatrial block or arrest, or the bradycardia-tachycardia syndrome do not require electrophysiologic tests for diagnosis. However, in symptomatic patients without documentation of an arrhythmia, electrophysiologic assessment of sinus node function can yield information that may be used to guide appropriate therapy. If a pacemaker is indicated, the side of pacemaker implantation for maximum hemodynamic effects can be guided by the results of electrophysiologic investigation. However, the results of tests of sinus node function must be interpreted with caution. Sinus node dysfunction coexists frequently with other disorders such as AV conduction disturbances which may cause symptoms such as syncope. Electrophysiologic evaluation of patients with symptoms such as undiagnosed syncope must not stop with the demonstration of abnormalities of sinus node dysfunction or carotid sinus hypersensitivity. Instead, complete evaluation, including His bundle recordings and programmed atrial and ventricular stimulation (see Chap. 185), is necessary to search for additional electrophysiologic abnormalities which could be responsible for symptoms.

TREATMENT Permanent pacemakers (page 907) are the mainstay of therapy for patients with symptomatic sinus node dysfunction. Patients with intermittent paroxysms of bradycardia or sinus arrest and with the cardioinhibitory form of the hypersensitive carotid sinus syndrome are usually adequately treated by demand ventricular pacemakers. These devices are reliable, relatively inexpensive, and suffice to prevent episodic symptoms due to abrupt bradycardia. Patients with symptomatic chronic sinus bradycardia or frequent prolonged episodes of sinus node dysfunction may do better with dual-chamber pacemakers that preserve the normal AV activation sequence. Although theoretically an atrial demand pacemaker should be adequate for patients with sinus node dysfunction, the frequent accompaniment of dysfunction in other portions of the cardiac conduction system usually mandates placement of a pacemaker capable of ventricular pacing.

AV CONDUCTION DISTURBANCES

The specialized cardiac conducting system normally ensures synchronous conduction of each sinus impulse from the atria to the ventricles. Abnormalities of conduction of the sinus impulse to the ventricles may portend the development of heart block, which can ultimately lead to syncope or cardiac arrest. In order to evaluate the clinical significance of conduction abnormalities the physician must assess (1) the site of conduction disturbance, (2) the risk of progression to complete block, and (3) the probability that a subsidiary escape rhythm arising distal to the site of block will be electrophysiologically and hemodynamically stable. This latter point is perhaps the most important since the rate and stability of the escape pacemaker determine what symptoms result from heart block. The escape pacemaker following AV nodal block is usually in the His bundle, which generally has a stable rate of 40 to 60 beats per minute and is associated with a QRS complex of normal duration (in the absence of a preexisting intraventricular conduction defect). This contrasts with escape rhythms arising in the distal His-Purkinje system, which have lower intrinsic rates (25 to 45 beats per minute), manifest wide QRS complexes with prolonged duration, and are unstable. Although prolonged QRS complexes are invariable when the distal His-Purkinje pacemakers form the escape mechanism, wide QRS complexes can also coexist with AV nodal block and a His bundle rhythm. Therefore, QRS morphology alone may not be adequate to identify the site of block.

ETIOLOGY The AV node is supplied by the parasympathetic and sympathetic nervous systems and is sensitive to variations in autonomic tone. Chronic slowing of AV nodal conduction may be seen in highly trained athletes who have hypervagotonia at rest. A variety of diseases can also influence AV nodal conduction. These include acute processes such as myocardial infarction (particularly inferior); coronary spasm (usually of the right coronary artery); digitalis intoxication; excesses of beta and/or calcium blockers; acute infections such as viral myocarditis; acute rheumatic fever; infectious mononucleosis; and miscellaneous disorders such as Lyme disease, sarcoidosis, amyloidosis, and neoplasms, particularly cardiac mesotheliomas. AV nodal block may also be congenital.

Two degenerative diseases are commonly responsible for damage to the specialized conducting system and produce AV block usually associated with bundle branch block (see Chap. 176). In *Lev's disease,* there is calcification and sclerosis of the fibrous cardiac skeleton, which frequently involves the aortic and mitral valves, the central fibrous body, and the summit of the ventricular septum. *Lenegre's disease* appears to be a primary sclerodegenerative disease within the conducting system itself with no involvement of the myocardium or the fibrous skeleton of the heart. These two diseases are probably the most common causes of isolated chronic heart block in adults. Hypertension and aortic and/or mitral stenosis are specific disorders that either accelerate the degeneration of the conducting system or have a direct effect by calcification and fibrosis involving the conducting system.

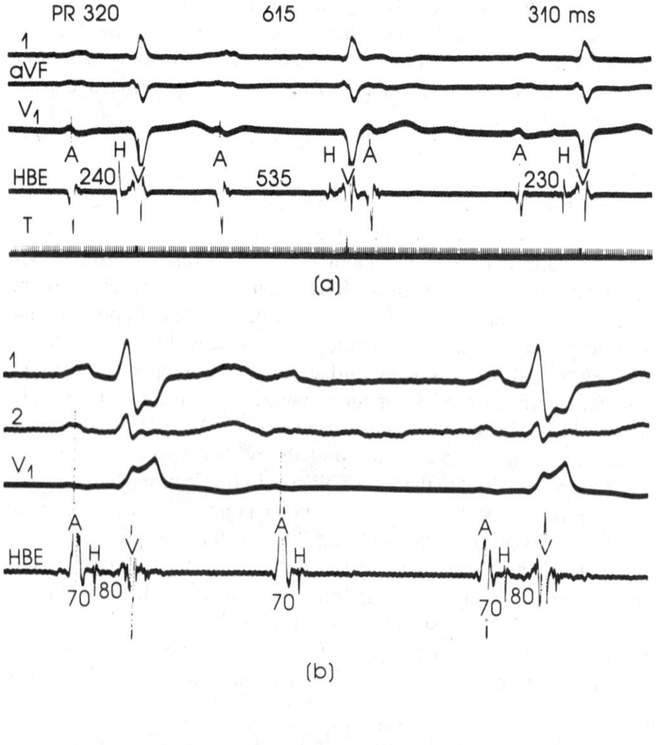

FIGURE 184-7 *A.* Mobitz type I second-degree AV block. Intracardiac recordings demonstrate that the PR prolongation (320, 615 ms) is localized to the AV node (AH 240, 535 ms, respectively). HBE = His bundle electrogram; A = atrium; H = His; V = ventricle. (*From ME Josephson, SF Seides: Clinical Cardiac Electrophysiology: Techniques and Interpretations. Philadelphia, Lea & Febiger, 1979.*) *B.* Mobitz type II second-degree AV block. Intracardiac recordings document block below the His bundle.

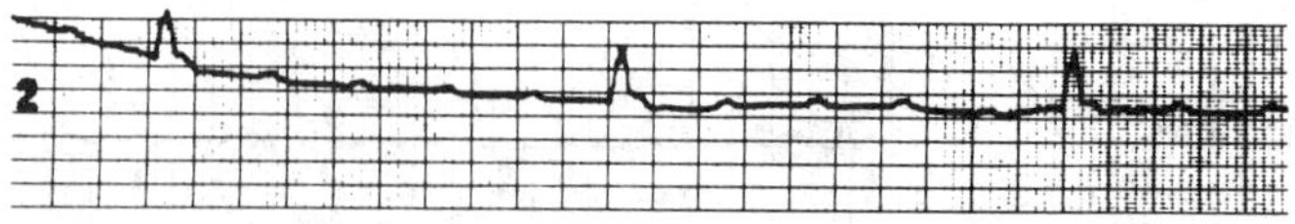

FIGURE 184-8 Third-degree AV block. Complete heart block with a slow, wide complex escape rhythm is present. Block in this instance is usually intra-His.

First-degree AV block, more properly termed *prolonged AV conduction,* is characterized by a PR interval >0.20 s. Since the PR interval is determined by atrial, AV nodal, and His-Purkinje activation, delay in any one or more of these structures can contribute to a prolonged PR interval. In the presence of a QRS complex of normal duration, a PR interval >0.24 s almost invariably is due to a delay within the AV node. If the QRS is prolonged, delays may be present at any of the levels mentioned above. Delay within the His-Purkinje system is always accompanied by a prolonged QRS duration in addition to a prolonged PR interval. However, as indicated below, it is only with intracardiac recordings that the exact site of delay can be determined.

Second-degree heart block (intermittent AV block) is present when some atrial impulses fail to conduct to the ventricles. Mobitz type I second-degree AV block (AV Wenckebach block) is characterized by progressive PR interval prolongation prior to block of an atrial impulse (Fig. 184-7*A*). The pause that follows is less than fully compensatory (i.e., is less than two normal sinus intervals), and the PR of the first conducted impulse is shorter than the last conducted atrial impulse prior to the blocked P wave. This type of block is almost always localized to the AV node and associated with a normal QRS duration. It is most often seen as a transient abnormality with inferior wall infarction or with drug intoxication, particularly digitalis, beta blockers, and occasionally calcium channel antagonists. This type of block can also be observed in normal individuals with heightened vagal tone. Although Mobitz type I block can progress to complete heart block, this is uncommon. Even when it does, however, the heart block is usually well tolerated because the escape pacemaker usually arises in the proximal His bundle and provides a stable rhythm. As a result, the presence of Mobitz type I second-degree AV block usually does not mandate aggressive therapy. Therapeutic decisions depend upon the ventricular response and the symptoms of the patient. If the ventricular rate is adequate and the patient is asymptomatic, observation is sufficient.

In Mobitz type II second-degree AV block, conduction fails suddenly and unexpectedly without a preceding change in PR intervals (Fig. 184-7*B*). It is usually due to disease of the His-Purkinje system and is most often associated with a prolonged QRS duration. It is important to recognize this type of block since it has a high incidence of progression to complete heart block with an unstable, slow, lower escape pacemaker. Therefore, pacemaker implantation is necessary in this condition. Mobitz type II block may occur in the setting of anteroseptal infarction or in the primary or secondary sclerodegenerative or calcific disorders of the fibrous skeleton of the heart. In so-called high-degree AV block there are periods of two or more consecutively blocked P waves. Regardless of the site of origin of the escape rhythm, if it is slow and the patient is symptomatic, a cardiac pacemaker is mandatory.

Third-degree AV block is present when no atrial impulse propagates to the ventricles. If the QRS complex of the escape rhythm is of normal duration, occurs at a rate of 40 to 55 beats per minute, and increases with atropine or exercise, AV nodal block is probable. Congenital complete AV block is usually localized to the AV node (Fig. 184-8). If the block is within the His bundle, the escape pacemaker usually is less responsive to these perturbations. If the escape rhythm of the QRS is wide and associated with rates ≤40, block is usually localized in, or distal to, the His bundle and mandates a pacemaker since the escape rhythm in this setting is unreliable.

AV DISSOCIATION AV dissociation exists whenever the atria and ventricles are under the control of two separate pacemakers and, while present in complete AV block, can occur in the absence of a primary conduction disturbance. AV dissociation unrelated to heart block may occur under two circumstances: First, it may develop with an AV junctional rhythm in response to severe sinus bradycardia. When the sinus rate and the escape rate are similar and the P waves occur just before, in, or following the QRS, *isorhythmic AV dissociation* is said to be present. Treatment usually consists of removal of the offending cause of sinus bradycardia (i.e., discontinuation of digitalis, beta blockers, or calcium antagonists), accelerating the sinus node by vagolytic agents, or insertion of a pacemaker if the escape rhythm is slow and results in symptoms. Second, AV dissociation can be caused by an enhanced lower (junctional or ventricular) pacemaker which competes with normal sinus rhythm and frequently exceeds it. This has been called *interference AV dissociation* because the rapid lower pacemaker results in bombardment of the AV node in a retrograde fashion, rendering it refractory to the normal sinus impulses. Thus, failure of antegrade conduction is a physiologic response in this circumstance. Interference dissociation commonly occurs during ventricular tachycardia accelerated junctional or ventricular rhythms seen with digitalis intoxication, myocardial ischemia and/or infarction, or local irritation following cardiac surgery. The accelerated rhythm should be treated with either antiarrhythmic drugs (see Chap. 185), removal of an offending drug, or correction of the metabolic abnormality or ischemia.

INTRACARDIAC ELECTROCARDIOGRAPHIC RECORDINGS IN DIAGNOSIS AND MANAGEMENT The main therapeutic decision in patients with AV conduction disturbance is whether or not a permanent pacemaker is required, and a number of circumstances exist in which His bundle electrocardiography can provide a useful diagnostic tool upon which to base this decision. It is unquestionable that patients with *symptomatic* second- or third-degree AV block should be paced, and therefore these patients do not require electrophysiologic study. However, intracardiac ECG recordings can be useful in at least the following three groups of patients:

1 Patients with syncope and bundle branch or bifascicular block without documentation of AV block. In such patients the demonstration of marked infra-His conduction disturbances, i.e., a prolonged HV interval (>100 ms) may usually be taken as an indication of the need for the insertion of the permanent pacemaker. With intervals ranging from 60 to 100 ms, the indications for pacing are equivocal. Block below the His bundle developing during atrial pacing at rates of less than 150 beats per minute and the development of an infra-His block or HV prolongation >100 ms following 1 g procainamide intravenously also signify that the patient is at high risk for the development of subsequent AV block and that a pacemaker is indicated. Complete electrophysiologic evaluation, including atrial and ventricular programmed stimulation, is indicated to help identify other possible cardiac etiologies for the syncope. Since the incidence of significant advanced AV block is low in *asymptomatic* patients who have bifascicular block, electrophysiologic evaluation or permanent pacemakers are not cost-effective. In this group observation appears most reasonable.

2 Patients with 2:1 atrioventricular conduction. Intracardiac recordings are necessary in order to ascertain the site of the conduction disturbance because the typical ECG features of Mobitz type I or Mobitz type II block cannot be discerned during a 2:1 pattern of AV conduction on the surface ECG. Intracardiac recordings may demonstrate that AV nodal block, intra-His block, infra-His block, or combinations of block may be responsible. A surface electrocardiogram finding that suggests an infra-His lesion is the presence of alternating bundle branch block associated with changing PR intervals. Intracardiac recordings in such patients confirm that the block is almost always in the His-Purkinje system. The finding of infra-His block in patients with asymptomatic second-degree AV block mandates pacemaker therapy because of the high likelihood of their developing symptomatic high-grade AV block and syncope.

3 Asymptomatic patients with third-degree AV block. In such patients electrophysiologic studies may be useful in assessing the stability of the junctional pacemaker. Pacing is indicated when the His bundle escape pacemaker is shown to be unstable by an inadequate response to exercise, atropine, or isoproterenol or by a prolonged junctional recovery time following ventricular pacing.

MANAGEMENT OF BRADYARRHYTHMIAS

PHARMACOLOGIC THERAPY Pharmacologic therapy is usually reserved for acute situations. Atropine (0.05 to 2.0 mg intravenously) and isoproterenol (1 to 4 μg/min intravenously) are useful in increasing heart rate and decreasing symptoms in patients with sinus bradycardia or AV block localized to the AV node. They have an insignificant effect on lower pacemakers. Recently theophylline has been suggested in patients with vasovagal syncope. Long-term therapy of bradyarrhythmias is best accomplished by pacemakers.

PACEMAKERS External energy sources can be used to stimulate the heart when disorders in impulse formation and/or transmission lead to symptomatic bradyarrhythmias. Pacer stimuli can be applied to the atria and/or ventricles. Indications for pacemakers inserted are listed in Table 184-1.

Temporary pacing This is usually instituted to provide immediate stabilization prior to permanent pacemaker placement or to provide pacemaker support when a bradycardia is precipitated by what is presumed to be a transient event such as ischemia or drug toxicity. Temporary pacing is usually achieved by the transvenous insertion of an electrode catheter with the catheter positioned in the right ventricular apex and attached to an external generator. This procedure is associated with a small risk of cardiac perforation, infection at the insertion site, and thromboembolism; the risk of the latter two complications increases markedly if the pacing wire is left in place for more than 48 h. The development of an entirely external transthoracic cardiac pacing system may preclude the need for transvenous pacing in selected patients. However, occasional failure of ventricular capture and significant discomfort related to the large current required for effective transthoracic ventricular stimulation precludes the uniform use of this approach.

Permanent pacing This mode of pacing is instituted for persistent or intermittent symptomatic bradycardia not related to a self-limiting precipitating factor or for documented infranodal second- or third-degree AV block. Permanent pacing leads are usually inserted transvenously through the subclavian or cephalic vein with the leads positioned in the right atrial appendage for atrial pacing and the right ventricular apex for ventricular pacing. The leads are then attached to the pulse generator, which is inserted into a subcutaneous pocket below the clavicle. Epicardial lead placement is used when: (1) transvenous access cannot be obtained; (2) the chest is already open, i.e., in the course of a cardiac operation; and (3) if adequate endocardial lead placement cannot be achieved. Most pacemaker generators are powered by lithium batteries. The life expectancy of the generator is related to (1) current output required for capture; (2) requirement for

TABLE 184-1 Indications for pacing

I Symptomatic carotid sinus hypersensitivity
- *A* Sinus node dysfunction
  - *1* Symptomatic sinus bradycardia
  - *2* Sinus pauses > 3 s
- *B* AV nodal block
  - *1* Symptomatic second-degree AV block (Mobitz I)
  - *2* Symptomatic complete heart block
- *C* Infranodal block
  - *1* New bifascicular block associated with acute infarction (usually anteroseptal)
  - *2* Alternating bundle branch block with changing PR
  - *3* HV > 100 ms in a patient with bifascicular block
  - *4* Block below the bundle of His with atrial pacing at rates ≤ 150 beats per minute
  - *5* 2 second-degree AV block (Mobitz II)
  - *6* Complete heart block

incessant or intermittent pacing; and (3) number of cardiac chambers paced. Life expectancy of the simple ventricular demand pacemaker can exceed 10 years.

Pacing code A code consisting of three to five letters has been developed for describing pacemaker type and function. The first letter indicates the chamber(s) paced and is designated *V* for ventricular pacing, *A* for atrial pacing, or *D* for dual-chamber (both atrial and ventricular) pacing. The second letter indicates the chamber in which electrical activity is sensed and is also indicated by *A*, *V*, or *D*. An additional designation, *O*, has been used when pacemaker discharge is not dependent on a sensed electrical activity. The third letter refers to the response to a sensed electrical signal. The letter *O* represents no response to an underlying electrical signal, usually related to the absence of associated sensing function; *I* represents inhibition of pacing function; *T* represents triggering of pacing function; and *D* indicates a dual response, i.e., spontaneous atrial and ventricular activity inhibiting atrial and ventricular pacing and atrial activity triggering a ventricular response. Additional fourth and fifth letters of the pacing code have been recommended to indicate whether the pacemaker is programmable and whether special antitachycardia functions are available. It follows from the described code that the standard VVI (ventricular demand pacemaker) paces the ventricle, senses the ventricle, and is inhibited by sensed spontaneous ventricular activity, while the DDD pulse generator is capable of sensing and pacing both the atria and ventricles and has a dual response to the sensed atrial and ventricular activity as described above.

Selection of the appropriate pacemaker and pacing mode depends on the clinical condition and the type of bradyarrhythmia being treated. The two most common pacing mode selections are DDD and VVI. DDD, or so-called universal pacing, provides AV sequential pacing, which is ideally suited for the relatively young and active patient who has intact sinus node function or intermittent dysfunction and high-grade persistent or intermittent AV block. The DDD mode will allow for physiologic atrial sensed and ventricular paced rates and improve exercise tolerance. AV synchrony and dual-chamber pacing may also be desirable in patients with borderline hemodynamic reserve who are dependent on atrial contribution to cardiac output and in those patients who develop the pacemaker syndrome (see below) in response to ventricular demand pacing. The DDD pacing mode is contraindicated in chronic atrial fibrillation or flutter, in which case rapid and irregular ventricular pacing will occur to the upper rate limit. In some cases this will produce a more rapid ventricular rate than the patient's own rate in the absence of a pacemaker. Chronotropic insufficiency is another contraindication since the pacemaker will act only as a "fixed rate" pacemaker at the new rate cutoff. In these situations, ventricular demand (VVI) or a rate adaptive pacemaker (see below) is indicated. The DDD pacing mode may also be contraindicated in patients with intermittent or persistent ventriculoatrial (VA) conduction, who may develop pacemaker-mediated tachycardia (see below).

In patients with impaired sinus node function or chronic atrial fibrillation, a sensor-driven, rate-adaptive pacemaker may be implanted. These pacemakers automatically adjust ventricular pacing rates to a sensed indicator of exertion (e.g., body vibration or blood temperature). This positive chronotropic response increases cardiac output and improves exercise tolerance.

Programmability of pacemakers This allows for modification of pacing function after implantation and for adaptation to changes in clinical needs. Pacemaker programming is accomplished by activation of the programming head positioned over the implanted pulse generator after making the desired changes in programmable parameters (Table 184-2). A radiofrequency system is routinely used to communicate the program to the pacemaker.

Complications Adverse effects of permanent pacing are usually associated with failure or malfunction of the pacing system. These problems are usually secondary to over- or undersensing, output failure, and/or lead fracture or displacement. Two other problems may occur. The *pacemaker syndrome* consists of fatigue, dizziness, syncope, and distressing pulsations in the neck and chest and can be associated with adverse hemodynamic effects. The pathophysiologic contributors to the pacemaker syndrome include (1) loss of atrial contribution to ventricular systole; (2) vasodepressor reflex initiated by cannon *a* waves which are caused by atrial contractions against a closed tricuspid valve observed in the jugular venous pulse (Chap. 175); and (3) systemic and pulmonary venous regurgitation due to atrial contraction against a closed AV valve. The symptoms associated with the pacemaker syndrome can be prevented by maintaining AV synchrony by dual-chamber pacing or, in the case of a ventricular demand pacemaker, by programming a hysteresis escape rate 15 to 20 beats per minute below that of the paced rate. As a result of this programming, sinus activity and thus atrial contraction will be less likely to occur at the same time as ventricular pacing and ventricular contraction. The second major problem peculiar to dual-chamber pacemakers is the development of *pacemaker-mediated tachycardia,* which is caused by ventriculoatrial conduction. In this instance, retrograde depolarization of the atria, resulting from a premature ventricular depolarization or a paced ventricular complex, is sensed and leads to subsequent triggering of ventricular pacing. This, in turn, can result in repetition of the phenomenon of ventriculoatrial conduction with the development of an endless-loop, pacemaker-mediated tachycardia. It may be corrected by programming the atrial refractory period.

TABLE 184-2 Programmable pacemaker functions

Rate*	Hysteresis
Energy output	Refractory period
Sensitivity	Mode of function
Lead polarity	AV delay

* Lower and upper rate limits apply to dual-chamber pacing.

REFERENCES

AUSTIN JL et al: Analysis of pacemaker malfunction and complications of temporary pacing in the coronary care unit. Am J Cardiol 49:301, 1982

DULK KD et al: The activitrax rate responsive pacemaker system. Am J Cardiol 61:107, 1988

ELLENBOGEN KA et al: New insights into pacemaker syndrome gained from hemodynamic, humoral and vascular responses during ventriculo-atrial pacing. Am J Cardiol 65(1):53, 1990

HUANG SK et al: Carotid sinus hypersensitivity in patients with unexplained syncope: clinical, electrophysiologic and long-term follow-up observations. Am Heart J 116:989, 1988

LANGENFELD H et al: Course of symptoms and spontaneous ECG in pacemaker patients: a 5-year follow-up study. PACE 11:2198, 1988

LUDMER PL, GOLDSCHLAGER N: Cardiac pacing in the 1980's. N Engl J Med 311:1671, 1984

NICOD P et al: Long-term outcome in patients with inferior myocardial infarction and complete atrioventricular block. J Am Coll Cardiol 12:589, 1988

PARSONETT V et al: Indications for dual chamber pacing. PACE 7:318, 1984

WIRTZFELD A et al: Physiologic pacing: Present status and future develoopments. PACE 10:41, 1987

ZOLL PM et al: External noninvasive temporary cardiac pacing: Clinical trials. Circulation 71:937, 1985

185 THE TACHYARRHYTHMIAS

MARK E. JOSEPHSON / ALFRED E. BUXTON / FRANCIS E. MARCHLINSKI

MECHANISMS OF TACHYARRHYTHMIAS

Tachyarrhythmias may be divided into disorders of impulse propagation and disorders of impulse formation. Disorders of impulse propagation (reentry) are generally considered to be the most common mechanism of sustained paroxysmal tachyarrhythmia. The requirements for initiating reentry include: (1) electrophysiologic inhomogeneity (i.e., differences in conduction and/or refractoriness) in two or more regions of the heart connected with each other to form a potentially closed loop; (2) unidirectional block in one pathway; (3) slow conduction over an alternative pathway, allowing time for the initially blocked pathway to recover excitability; and (4) reexcitation of the initially blocked pathway to complete a loop of activation. Repetitive circulation of the impulse over this loop can produce a sustained tachyarrhythmia. While anatomic obstacles may underlie reentry and provide an inexcitable center around which the impulse can circulate, they are not essential. Reentrant arrhythmias can be reproducibly initiated and terminated by premature complexes and rapid stimulation. The response of these arrhythmias to stimulation can help distinguish them from arrhythmias caused by triggered activity.

Disorders of impulse formation can be subdivided into tachyarrhythmias caused by enhanced automaticity and those caused by triggered activity. In addition to the sinus node, automatic pacemaker activity can be observed in specialized atrial fibers, fibers of the atrioventricular (AV) junction, and Purkinje fibers (see Chap. 184). Myocardial cells do not normally possess pacemaker activity. Enhancement of normal automaticity in latent pacemaker fibers or the development of abnormal automaticity due to partial depolarization of the resting membrane occurs as a consequence of a variety of pathophysiologic states, which include (1) increased endogenous or exogenous catecholamines; (2) electrolyte disturbances (e.g., hyperkalemia); (3) hypoxia or ischemia; (4) mechanical effects (e.g., stretch); and (5) drugs (e.g., digitalis). Tachycardia caused by automaticity cannot be started or stopped by pacing.

Triggered activity has been observed in atrial, ventricular, and His-Purkinje tissue under conditions such as increased local catecholamine concentration, hyperkalemia, hypercalcemia, and digitalis intoxication. All of these conditions produce an accumulation of intracellular calcium which causes depolarizations following the action potential, termed *afterdepolarizations*. With increasing amplitude of the afterdepolarizations, threshold can be reached and repetitive activity produced. In contrast to automatic rhythms, triggered activity requires preceding activity for initiation and therefore can be initiated by pacing. In contrast to tachyarrhythmias caused by automaticity and reentry, the response of triggered activity to overdrive pacing is acceleration.

The use of electrophysiologic (EP) studies, i.e., intracardiac recordings and programmed stimulation, has greatly expanded our understanding of the mechanisms of tachyarrhythmias. In addition to helping in the diagnosis of arrhythmias, these techniques may be of value in determining the most appropriate types of therapy. EP studies of tachycardias require the positioning of multiple electrode catheters at critical areas within the heart. These electrodes must be capable of both stimulating and recording from multiple sites in the atria and/or ventricles.

PREMATURE COMPLEXES

ATRIAL PREMATURE COMPLEXES (APCs) APCs can be found on 24-h Holter monitoring in over 60 percent of normal adults. APCs are usually asymptomatic and benign, although at times they may be associated with palpitations. In susceptible patients, they can initiate paroxysmal supraventricular tachycardias. APCs may originate from any location in either atrium, and they are recognized on the ECG as early P waves with a morphology which differs from the sinus P wave (Fig. 185-1*A*). While APCs usually conduct to the ventricles when they occur late in the cardiac cycle, relatively early APCs may reach the AV conduction system while it is still in its relative refractory period, resulting in a conduction delay manifested by prolonged PR interval following the premature P wave (Fig. 185-1*A*). Very early APCs may even block in the AV node if this structure is encountered during its effective refractory period. APCs, whether conducted or not, are usually followed by a pause before a return to sinus activity. Most commonly, an APC enters and resets the sinus node, so that the sum of the pre- and postextrasystolic PP intervals is less than the sum of two sinus PP intervals (Fig. 185-1*A*). In this case the pause is said to be less than fully compensatory. The QRS

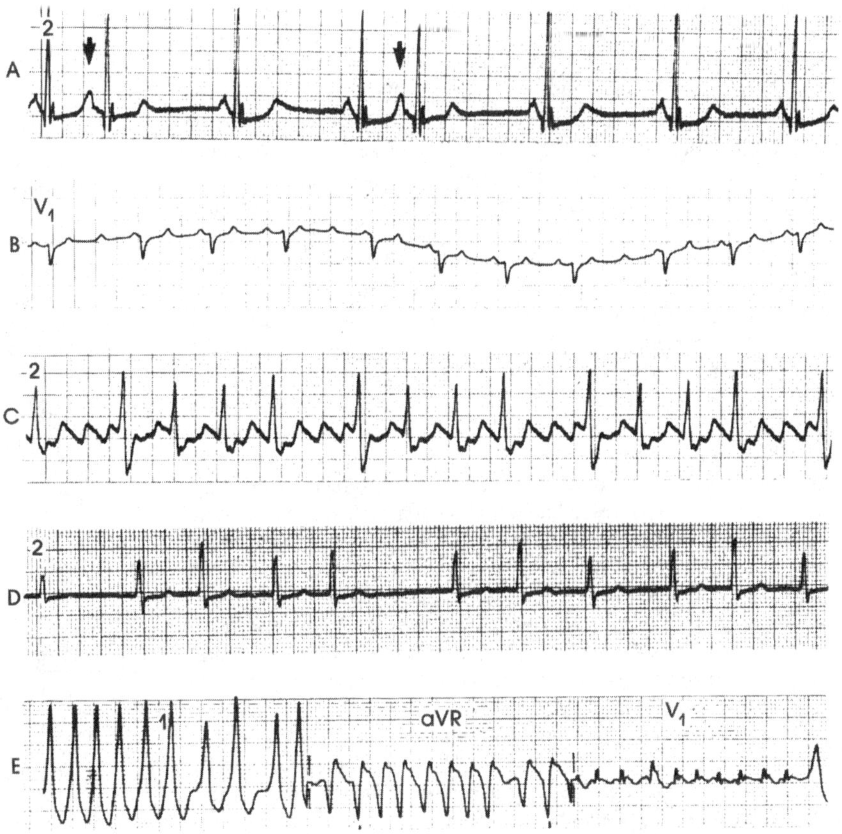

FIGURE 185-1 *A*. ECG lead II. Sinus rhythm with two atrial premature complexes (arrows). Note the difference in P-wave configuration between sinus and the premature atrial complexes. In addition, note that the PR interval of the premature complexes is prolonged, due to slowed conduction of the premature impulse through the AV conduction system. *B*. ECG lead V_1. Atrial tachycardia with varying degrees of AV block, typical of digitalis toxicity. *C*. ECG lead II. Atrial flutter. Note the characteristic sawtooth baseline seen in the inferior ECG leads during atrial flutter. Variable degrees of AV conduction block are present. *D*. ECG lead II. Atrial fibrillation. Note the irregular wavy baseline without discrete atrial activity. The ventricular response is irregularly irregular. *E*. ECG leads I, aVR, and V_1. Atrial fibrillation in a patient with Wolff-Parkinson-White syndrome. Note the extremely rapid, grossly irregular ventricular rate with wide, bizarre QRS complexes.

complex following most APCs is normal, although early APCs may be followed by aberrantly conducted QRS complexes.

Since most APCs are asymptomatic, treatment is not required. When they cause palpitations or trigger paroxysmal supraventricular tachycardias (see below), treatment may be useful. Factors that precipitate APCs such as alcohol, tobacco, or adrenergic stimulants should be identified and eliminated, and in their absence mild sedation or the use of a beta blocker may be tried. If this fails, quinidine, procainamide, or a similar agent may be used.

AV JUNCTIONAL COMPLEXES The site of origin of these complexes is thought to be in the bundle of His, since the AV node itself possesses no automaticity (page 906). AV junctional complexes are less common than either atrial or ventricular premature complexes and are more often associated with cardiac disease or digitalis intoxication. Junctional premature impulses can conduct both antegradely to the ventricles and retrogradely to the atrium and, on rare occasions, may fail to conduct in either direction. Premature AV junctional complexes can be recognized by normal-appearing QRS complexes that are not preceded by a P wave. Retrograde P waves (inverted in leads II, III, and aVF) may be observed after the QRS complex.

While often asymptomatic, junctional premature complexes may be associated with palpitations and cause cannon *a* waves which may result in distressing pulsations in the neck. When symptomatic, they should be treated like APCs.

VENTRICULAR PREMATURE COMPLEXES (VPCs) These are among the most common arrhythmias and occur in patients with and without heart disease. Of adult males $\geq$60 percent will exhibit VPCs during a 24-h Holter monitoring. In patients without heart disease, VPCs have not been shown to be associated with any increased incidence in mortality or morbidity. VPCs may occur in up to 80 percent of patients with previous myocardial infarction, and in this setting, if frequent ($>$10 per hour) and/or complex (occurring in couplets or triplets), they have been associated with increased mortality. However, cardiac mortality in such patients usually occurs in association with significantly impaired ventricular function. While frequent and complex ventricular ectopy is an independent risk factor, it is not as strong a risk factor as is impaired ventricular function. Moreover, even though ventricular tachycardia and/or fibrillation may be the basis for the sudden death in these patients, this does not a priori establish a cause-and-effect relation between spontaneous ectopy and life-threatening ventricular tachycardia or fibrillation. Very early cycle (R or T) VPCs have been stated by some to increase the risk of sudden death. Although this has been observed during acute ischemia and in the setting of QT prolongation, frequently ventricular tachycardia or fibrillation is precipitated by VPCs which occur after the T wave of the prior beat.

VPCs are recognized by wide (usually $>$0.14 s), bizarre QRS complexes that are not preceded by P waves (Fig. 185-2*A*). Often they bear a relatively fixed relationship to the preceding sinus complex and are thus considered fixed coupled VPCs. When fixed coupling is not present and the interval between VPCs has a common denominator, *ventricular parasystole* is said to be present (Fig. 185-3). Under these circumstances the VPCs are a manifestation of abnormal automaticity of a protected ventricular focus; because it is not penetrated by sinus impulses, it is not reset by them and the interectopic intervals remain relatively fixed ($\leq$120 ms variation of mean RR cycle length).

VPCs may occur singly; in patterns of bigeminy, in which every sinus beat is followed by a VPC; in trigeminy, in which two sinus beats are followed by a VPC; in quadrigeminy, etc. Two successive VPCs are termed *pairs* or *couplets*, while three or more consecutive VPCs are termed *ventricular tachycardia*. VPCs may have similar morphologies (monomorphic) or different morphologies (multiformed or polymorphic) (Fig. 185-2*C*).

Most commonly, VPCs are not conducted retrogradely to the atrium to reset the sinoatrial node. Thus, they produce a fully compensatory pause; i.e., the interval between conducted beats which bracket the VPC equals two basic RR intervals. Ventricular impulses

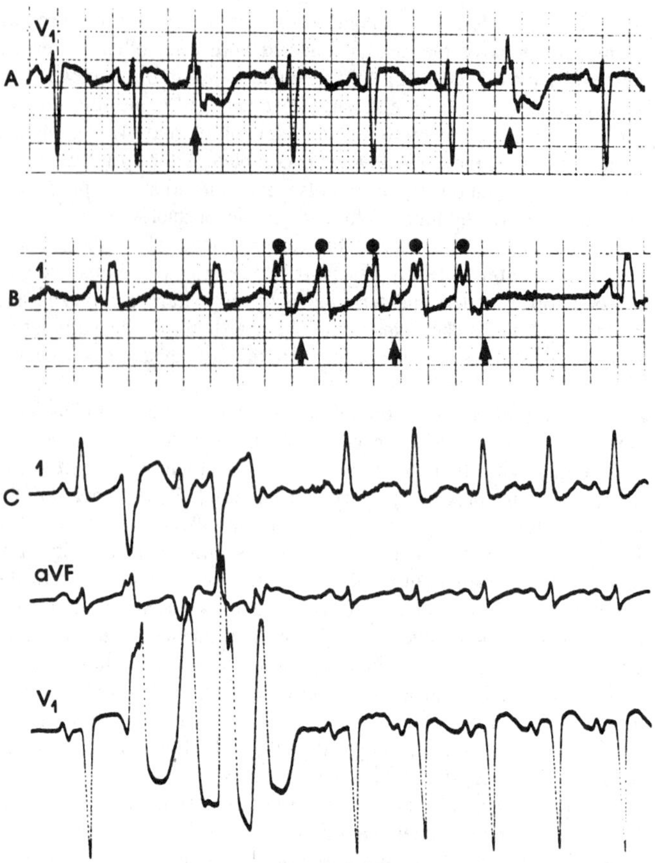

FIGURE 185-2 *A*. Single ventricular ectopy. During sinus rhythm two premature ventricular complexes (arrows) occur. Note that the QRS configuration is bizarre, different from that during sinus rhythm. The premature ventricular complexes are not preceded by P waves. The QRS width of the premature complexes is approximately 160 ms. The pause surrounding the premature complexes is fully compensatory, the sinus beat after the premature complex occurring on time. *B*. A 5-beat run of nonsustained ventricular tachycardia having a uniform morphology (dots). Although intraventricular conduction during sinus rhythm is slightly prolonged, during the run of ventricular tachycardia the QRS duration is further prolonged. Note that 2:1 VA conduction is present during ventricular tachycardia. Retrograde P waves are denoted by the arrows. *C*. Simultaneous recordings of ECG leads I, aVF, and V_1. A 4-beat run of polymorphic nonsustained ventricular tachycardia is demonstrated. No two consecutive QRS complexes are the same. Polymorphic VT is not associated with a prolonged QT interval in this case.

FIGURE 185-3 Ventricular parasystole. At varying sinus cycle lengths during exercise, interectopic intervals remain constant at 1620–1640 ms. However, the coupling intervals between sinus and ectopic complexes vary between 510 and 310 ms.

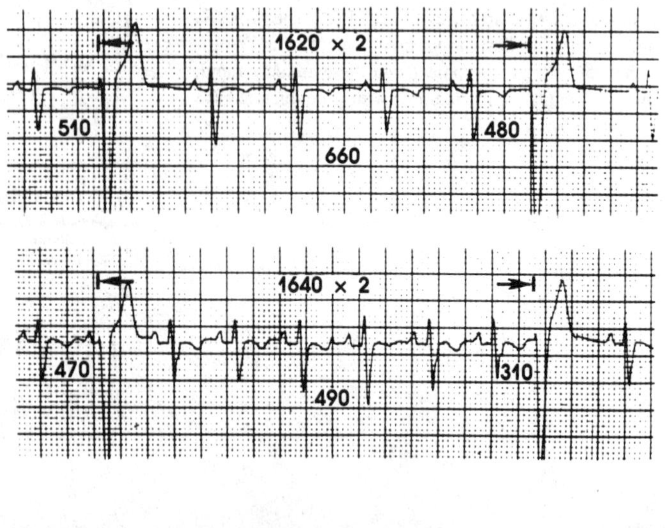

may also manifest retrograde conduction to the atrium and cause inverted P waves in leads II, III, and aVF. The pause that results may therefore be less than compensatory. In many instances, the QRS complex will not be associated with retrograde ventriculoatrial (VA) conduction but may block in the AV node. This renders the AV node refractory to the subsequent sinus beat and causes slowed conduction (i.e., prolonged PR interval) or block of the next sinus P wave. This prolonged PR interval is said to be a manifestation of concealed retrograde conduction of the ventricular impulse into the AV node. A VPC that does not produce any manifestation of retrograde concealed conduction and fails to influence the oncoming sinus impulse is termed an *interpolated VPC*.

VPCs can cause palpitations or neck pulsations secondary to either the occurrence of cannon *a* waves or the increased force of contraction due to postextrasystolic potentiation of ventricular contractility. Patients with frequent VPCs or bigeminy may develop syncope because the VPCs do not result in an adequate stroke volume and the cardiac output is reduced due to effective ''halving'' of the heart rate seen in patients with abnormal ventricular function.

Management In the absence of cardiac disease, isolated asymptomatic VPCs, regardless of configuration and frequency, need no treatment. When arrhythmias are symptomatic, the symptoms should first be addressed by either allaying the patient's anxiety, or if this is not successful, reducing the frequency of the VPCs with antiarrhythmic agents. Beta-adrenergic blockers may be successful in managing VPCs that occur primarily in the daytime or under stressful situations and in specific settings such as mitral valve prolapse and thyrotoxicosis. Quinidine or quinidine-like agents may be tried should this be unsuccessful. In patients with cardiac disease, frequent VPCs are often associated with an increased risk of sudden and nonsudden cardiac death, and many physicians attempt to eliminate or reduce the frequency of these VPCs in an attempt to reduce this risk. However, the cause-and-effect relationship of the VPCs to fatal events has not been established, and it has not been shown definitively that the suppression of VPCs with antiarrhythmic drugs prevents sudden death. In addition, it is important to recognize that the antiarrhythmic agents can also produce the lethal arrhythmias which they are given to prevent. Thus, therapy directed toward VPCs in the setting of chronic cardiac disease may result in an inappropriate and costly use of agents without proven efficacy and with potential side effects in many patients. The high incidence of side effects and the frequent exacerbation of arrhythmias caused by all antiarrhythmic drugs make it mandatory to monitor patients being treated with such agents.

In acute myocardial infarction the greatest incidence of primary ventricular fibrillation occurs within the first 24 h. Temporary prophylactic antiarrhythmic therapy has therefore been recommended for all patients with acute infarction, regardless of the presence or the degree of spontaneous ectopy.

TACHYCARDIAS

Tachycardias refer to arrhythmias with three or more complexes at rates exceeding 100 beats per minute; they occur more often in structurally diseased than in normal hearts. Those paroxysmal tachycardias that are initiated by APCs or VPCs are considered to be due to reentry except some of the digitalis-induced tachyarrhythmias, which are probably due to triggered activity (see below).

If the patient is hemodynamically stable, an attempt should be made to determine the mechanism and origin of the tachycardia since this will usually lead to an appropriate therapeutic decision. Information to be obtained from the ECG includes (1) the presence, frequency, morphology, and regularity of P waves and QRS complexes; (2) the relationship between atrial and ventricular activity; (3) a comparison of the QRS morphology during sinus rhythm and during the tachycardia; and (4) the response to carotid sinus massage or other vagal maneuvers. It is useful first to compare the ECG during the tachycardia with one recorded during sinus rhythm, and it is often desirable to record long rhythm strips using surface leads with the largest P waves, usually leads II or V_1. One can also utilize the electrodes situated at the end of a flexible pacing catheter inserted into the esophagus behind the left atrium to record atrial activity.

Carotid sinus pressure should only be applied while the patient is electrocardiographically monitored with resuscitative equipment available to manage the rare episode of asystole and/or ventricular fibrillation associated with this procedure. Carotid sinus massage should not be performed in patients with carotid arterial bruits. The patient should be positioned flat with the neck extended. Massage of one carotid bulb at a time should be performed by applying firm pressure just underneath the angle of the jaw for up to 5 s. Alternative vagomimetic maneuvers include the Valsalva maneuver, immersion of the face in cold water, and the administration of 5 to 10 mg edrophonium.

Observation of the jugular venous pulse can provide clues to the presence of atrial activity and its relationship to ventricular ectopy. Intermittent cannon *a* waves suggest AV dissociation, while persistent cannon *a* waves suggest 1:1 VA conduction. Flutter waves may be seen or no atrial activity may be apparent, as in the presence of atrial flutter and fibrillation, respectively. The arterial pulse may also manifest AV dissociation or atrial fibrillation by demonstrating variations in amplitude. A first heart sound of variable intensity during a regular rhythm also suggests AV dissociation or atrial fibrillation.

SINUS TACHYCARDIA In the adult, sinus tachycardia is said to be present when the heart rate exceeds 100 beats per minute; sinus tachycardia rarely exceeds 200 beats per minute and is not a primary arrhythmia; instead, it represents a physiologic response to a variety of stresses, such as fever, volume depletion, anxiety, exercise, thyrotoxicosis, hypoxemia, hypotension, or congestive heart failure. Sinus tachycardia has a gradual onset and offset. The ECG demonstrates P waves with sinus contour preceding each QRS complex. Carotid sinus pressure usually produces modest slowing with a gradual return to the previous rate upon cessation. This contrasts with the response of paroxysmal supraventricular tachycardias, which may slow slightly and terminate abruptly.

Sinus tachycardia should not be treated as a primary arrhythmia, since it is always a physiologic response to a demand placed on the heart. As such, the therapy should be directed to the primary disorder. This may involve institution of digitalis and/or diuretics for heart failure and oxygen for hypoxemia, treatment of thyrotoxicosis, volume repletion, aspirin for fever, or tranquilizers for emotional upset.

ATRIAL FIBRILLATION (AF) This common arrhythmia may occur in paroxysmal and persistent forms. It may be seen in normal subjects, particularly during emotional stress or following surgery, exercise, or acute alcoholic intoxication. It may also occur in patients with heart or lung disease who develop acute hypoxia, hypercapnia, or metabolic or hemodynamic derangements. Persistent AF usually occurs in patients with cardiovascular disease, most commonly rheumatic heart disease, nonrheumatic mitral valve disease, hypertensive cardiovascular disease, chronic lung disease, atrial septal defect, and a variety of miscellaneous cardiac abnormalities. AF may be the presenting finding in thyrotoxicosis. So-called lone AF, which occurs in patients without underlying heart disease, is considered to represent the tachycardia phase of the tachycardia-bradycardia syndrome (p. 904).

The morbidity associated with AF is related to (1) excessive rate of the ventricular response, which in turn may lead to hypotension or angina pectoris in susceptible individuals; (2) the pause following cessation of AF, which can cause syncope; (3) systemic embolization, which occurs most commonly in patients with rheumatic heart disease; (4) loss of the contribution of atrial contraction to cardiac output, which may cause fatigue; and (5) anxiety secondary to palpitations. In patients with severe cardiac dysfunction, particularly those with hypertrophied, noncompliant ventricles, the combination of the loss of the atrial contribution to ventricular filling and the abbreviated filling period due to the rapid ventricular rate in AF can produce marked hemodynamic embarrassment, resulting in hypotension, syncope, or heart failure. In patients with mitral stenosis in whom filling time is critical, development of AF with a rapid ventricular rate may precipitate pulmonary edema (see Chap. 188).

AF is characterized by disorganized atrial activity without discrete P waves on the surface ECG (Fig. 185-1*D*). Atrial activation is manifested by an undulating baseline or by more sharply inscribed atrial deflections of varying amplitude and frequency ranging from 350 to 600 per minute. The ventricular response is irregularly irregular. This results from the large number of atrial impulses which penetrate the AV node, making it partially refractory to subsequent impulses. This effect of nonconducted atrial impulses to influence the response to subsequent atrial impulses is termed *concealed conduction*. As a result, the ventricular response is relatively slow, considering the actual atrial rate. If AF converts to atrial flutter, which has a slower atrial rate, the effect of concealed conduction may be diminished and a paradoxic increase in the ventricular response may occur. The main factor determining the rate of the ventricular response is the functional refractory period of the AV node or the most rapid paced rate at which 1:1 conduction through the AV node can be observed.

If, in the presence of AF, the ventricular rhythm becomes regular and slow (e.g., 30 to 60 beats per minute), complete heart block is suggested, and if the ventricular rhythm is regular and rapid ($\geq$100 beats per minute), a tachycardia arising in the AV junction or ventricle should be suspected. Digitalis intoxication is a common cause of both of these phenomena.

Patients with AF exhibit a loss of *a* waves in the jugular venous pulse and variable pulse pressures in the carotid arterial pulse. The first heart sound usually varies in intensity. On echocardiography the left atrium is frequently enlarged, and in patients in whom the left atrial diameter exceeds 4.5 cm, it may not be possible to convert AF to sinus rhythm or to maintain the latter despite therapy.

Management In acute AF, a precipitating factor such as fever, pneumonia, alcoholic intoxication, thyrotoxicosis, pulmonary emboli, or pericarditis should be sought. When such a factor is present, therapy should be directed toward the primary abnormality. If the patient's clinical status is severely compromised, electrical cardioversion is the treatment of choice. In the absence of severe cardiovascular compromise, slowing of ventricular rate becomes the initial therapeutic goal. This may be accomplished with digitalis, calcium channel antagonists, or beta-adrenergic blockers, all of which prolong the refractory period of the AV node and slow conduction within it. Intravenous verapamil usually gives the most rapid response. However, in cases where catecholamine levels are likely to be elevated, beta blockers may be favored. Conversion to sinus rhythm may then be attempted, using quinidine or quinidine-like (type IA) agents (Table 185-1). It is important to slow AV node conduction prior to administering such drugs because their vagolytic effect and ability to convert AF to atrial flutter may reduce the concealed conduction and lead to an excessively rapid ventricular response. Beta-adrenergic blockers are especially useful in this regard. If medical therapy fails to convert AF, electrical cardioversion is useful; it generally requires 100 to 200 W·s of energy. Anticoagulation should be started at least 2 weeks prior to and continued for 2 weeks following any attempt at cardioversion, either pharmacologic or electrical, in patients with long-standing AF. Anticoagulation appears to decrease the incidence of systemic embolization associated with cardioversion. It is less likely for chronic AF to convert to or remain in sinus rhythm in the presence of long-standing rheumatic heart disease and/or when the atria are markedly enlarged. It is also unlikely for patients with lone AF to be converted to and maintained in sinus rhythm.

TABLE 185-1 Classification of antiarrhythmic drugs

Type I	Drugs that reduce maximal velocity of phase 0 depolarization ($\dot{V}_{max}$) due to block of inward Na^+ current in tissue with fast response action potentials
	A ↓ $\dot{V}_{max}$ at all heart rates and ↑ action potential duration, e.g., quinidine, procainamide, disopyramide
	B Little effect at slow rates on $\dot{V}_{max}$ in normal tissue, $\dot{V}_{max}$ in partially depolarized cells with fast response action potentials Effects increased at faster rates No change or ↓ in action potential duration, e.g., lidocaine, phenytoin, tocainide, mexiletine
	C ↓ $\dot{V}_{max}$ at normal rates in normal tissue Minimal effect on action potential duration, e.g., encainide, lorcainide, flecainide
Type II	Antisympathetic agents, e.g., propranolol and other beta-adrenergic blockers: ↓ SA nodal automaticity, ↑ AV nodal refractoriness, and ↓ AV nodal conduction velocity
Type III	Agents that prolong action potential duration in tissue with fast response action potentials, e.g., bretylium, amiodarone
Type IV	Calcium (slow) channel blocking agents: decrease conduction velocity and increase refractoriness in tissue with slow response action potentials, e.g., verapamil, diltiazem

If sinus rhythm is restored electrically or pharmacologically, quinidine or related agents may be used to prevent recurrence. In patients in whom cardioversion is unsuccessful or in whom AF is likely to recur, it is probably wisest to allow the patient to remain in AF and to control the ventricular response with calcium antagonists, beta-adrenergic blockers, or digitalis. Since they are always at risk of systemic embolization, chronic anticoagulation must be considered for such patients.

ATRIAL FLUTTER This arrhythmia occurs most often in patients with organic heart disease. Flutter may be paroxysmal, in which case there is usually a precipitating factor, such as pericarditis or acute respiratory failure, or it may be persistent. Atrial flutter (as well as AF) is very common during the first week following open heart surgery. Atrial flutter is usually less long-lived than is AF, although on occasion it may persist for months to years. Most commonly, if it lasts for more than a week, atrial flutter will convert to AF. Systemic embolization is less common in atrial flutter than AF.

Atrial flutter is characterized by an atrial rate between 250 and 350 beats per minute. Typically, the ventricular rate is half the atrial rate, i.e., approximately 150 beats per minute. If the atrial rate is slowed to <220 per minute by antiarrhythmic agents such as quinidine, which also possess vagolytic properties, the ventricular rate may rise suddenly because of the development of 1:1 AV conduction. Classically, flutter waves are seen as regular sawtooth-like atrial activity, most prominent in the inferior leads (Fig. 185-1*C*). When the ventricular response is regular and not a simple fraction of the atrial rate, complete AV block is present, which may be a manifestation of digitalis toxicity. Activation mapping suggests that atrial flutter is a form of atrial reentry localized to the low right atrium.

Management The most effective treatment of atrial flutter is direct current cardioversion, which can be accomplished at low energy (10 to 50 W·s) under mild sedation. In patients who develop atrial flutter following open-heart surgery or recurrent flutter in the setting of acute myocardial infarction, particularly when they are being treated with digitalis, atrial pacing (using temporary pacing wires implanted at the time of operation or a pacing lead inserted into the atrium pervenously) at rates of 115 to 130 percent of the atrial flutter rate can usually convert the atrial flutter to sinus rhythm. Atrial pacing may also result in the conversion of atrial flutter to AF, which allows for easier control of the ventricular response. If immediate conversion of atrial flutter is not mandated by the patient's clinical status, the ventricular response should first be slowed by blocking the AV node with a beta blocker, calcium antagonist, or digitalis; the latter drug occasionally converts atrial flutter into AF. Once AV nodal conduction is slowed with any of these drugs, an attempt to convert flutter to sinus rhythm using quinidine or quinidine-like agents should be made. Increasing doses of the drug selected are administered until the rhythm converts or side effects occur.

Quinidine, quinidine-like drugs, flecainide, and amiodarone (Table 185-2) may be useful in preventing recurrences of both atrial flutter and atrial fibrillation.

PAROXYSMAL SUPRAVENTRICULAR TACHYCARDIAS (PSVT) In most cases functional differences in conduction and refractoriness in the AV node or the presence of an AV bypass tract provide the substrate for the development of PSVT (previously termed *paroxysmal atrial tachycardia*). Electrophysiologic studies have demonstrated that reentry is the mechanism responsible for the vast majority of cases of PSVT (Fig. 185-4). Reentry has been localized to the sinus node, atrium, AV node, or to a macroreentrant circuit involving conduction in the antegrade direction through the AV node and retrograde through an AV bypass tract. Such a bypass tract may also conduct antegradely, in which case the Wolff-Parkinson-White (WPW) syndrome is said to be present. More frequently, however, the bypass tract manifests only retrograde conduction, and therefore it is termed a *concealed bypass tract* (Fig. 185-4*B*). In the absence of the WPW syndrome, reentry through the AV node or through a concealed bypass tract makes up more than 90 percent of all PSVTs.

AV NODAL REENTRANT TACHYCARDIA There is no age, sex, or disease predisposition for the development of AV nodal reentrant tachycardia, the most common cause of supraventricular tachycardia. It usually presents as a narrow QRS complex with regular rates ranging from 120 to 250 beats per minute. APCs that initiate the arrhythmia are almost always associated with a prolonged PR interval. Retrograde P waves may be absent, buried in the QRS complex, or appear as distortions at the terminal parts of the QRS complex (Fig. 185-4*A*).

AV nodal reentrant PSVT (Fig. 185-5) can be reproducibly initiated and terminated by appropriately timed atrial premature extrastimuli. The onset of the tachycardia is almost always associated with prolongation of the PR interval due to marked AV nodal conduction delay (prolonged AH interval) following the APC that is critical for the genesis of the arrhythmia. The sudden prolongation of the AH interval is consistent with the concept of dual AV nodal pathways: (1) A beta (fast) pathway, which exhibits rapid conduction and a long refractory period, and (2) an alpha (slow) pathway, which has a short refractory period but conducts slowly. During sinus rhythm only conduction over the fast pathway is manifest, resulting in a normal PR interval. The impulse which simultaneously conducts down the slow pathway reaches the His bundle after it has been depolarized and is therefore refractory. Atrial extrastimuli at a critical coupling interval are blocked in the beta pathway because of its longer refractory period and are conducted slowly through the alpha pathway. If conduction down the alpha pathway is slow enough to allow the previously refractory beta pathway time to recover excitability, a single atrial echo or sustained tachycardia ensues. A critical balance between conduction velocity and refractoriness within the node is required to sustain AV nodal reentry. Atrial and ventricular activation occur simultaneously, explaining why P waves may not be apparent on the surface ECG.

Clinical features AV nodal reentry may produce palpitations, syncope, and heart failure, depending on the rate and duration of the arrhythmia and the presence and severity of any underlying heart disease. Hypotension and syncope may occur because of the sudden loss of the atrial contribution to ventricular filling; this can also lead to a marked increase in atrial pressure, acute pulmonary edema, and a reduction in ventricular filling. Simultaneous atrial and ventricular contraction produces cannon *a* waves with each heartbeat.

Treatment In patients without hypotension, vagal maneuvers, particularly carotid sinus massage, can terminate the arrhythmia in 80 percent of cases. If hypotension is present, raising the blood pressure by the cautious use of intravenous phenylephrine may terminate the arrhythmia alone or in combination with carotid sinus pressure. If these maneuvers are unsuccessful, verapamil (2.5 to 10 mg intravenously) is the agent of choice. Propranolol (0.05 to 0.2 mg/kg, intravenously) or other beta blockers may be used to slow or terminate the tachycardia. Digitalis glycosides have a slower onset of action. When these drugs fail to terminate the tachycardia or when the tachycardia is recurrent, atrial or ventricular pacing via a temporary pacemaker inserted pervenously may be used to terminate the arrhythmia. However, if severe ischemia and/or hypotension is caused by the tachycardia, dc cardioversion should be considered.

AV nodal reentry can usually be prevented by the use of drugs that act primarily on the antegrade slow pathway (such as digitalis, beta blockers, or calcium antagonists) or on the fast pathway (such as quinidine-like agents and newer drugs such as encainide, flecainide, and amiodarone). Drugs most likely to avert recurrences prevent induction of the arrhythmias by programmed stimulation. This technique utilizes temporary pacemaker catheters connected to a physiologic stimulator capable of variable rate pacing and stimulation with one or more precisely timed premature impulses. If episodes of PSVT are frequent and produce disabling symptoms, therapy based on electrophysiologic studies is preferable to empiric drug trials. In symptomatic patients who require therapy, antitachycardia pacemakers may be preferable to the daily administration of antiarrhythmic drugs, particularly if there are long tachycardia-free intervals. Ablation of the AV junction (p. 923) has been developed as a method of controlling AV nodal reentry, but this approach should only be considered as a last resort, since it usually mandates insertion of a permanent ventricular pacemaker.

AV REENTRANT TACHYCARDIA PSVT due to AV reentry incorporates an AV bypass tract that conducts only retrogradely as part of the tachycardia circuit. Thus, the impulse passes antegradely from the atria through the AV node and His-Purkinje system to the ventricles, then retrogradely through the (concealed) bypass tract back to the atrium. Patients with this disorder manifest the same type of PSVT as do patients with the WPW syndrome (see below), but the bypass tract cannot conduct in an antegrade direction during sinus rhythm or other atrial tachyarrhythmias.

AV reentrant tachycardia can be initiated and terminated by either APCs or VPCs. Alternation of the QRS complexes and/or T wave occurs in approximately one-third of such tachycardias. Since atrial activation must follow ventricular activation during AV reentry, the P wave usually occurs after the QRS complex (Fig. 185-4*B*).

Atrial activation mapping is of major value in evaluating the origin of these tachycardias. Most concealed bypass tracts are left-sided. Thus, during supraventricular tachycardia or during ventricular pacing, the earliest activation sequence is recorded in the left atrium, usually via a catheter in the coronary sinus (Fig. 185-6). This eccentric atrial activation is quite distinct from the normal retrograde activation sequence in which the earliest activation of the atria is in the area of the AV junction. The ability of a ventricular stimulus to conduct to the atrium at a time when the bundle of His is refractory and the termination of the tachycardia by a ventricular stimulus that does not reach the atrium are diagnostic of retrograde conduction over a concealed bypass tract.

Treatment is similar to that for AV nodal reentry tachycardia. However, in addition to pharmacologic therapy, patients with reentrant tachycardias involving concealed bypass tracts may be candidates for surgical ablation (p. 923).

SINUS NODE REENTRY AND OTHER ATRIAL TACHYCARDIAS Reentry in the region of the sinus node or within the atria is invariably initiated by APCs. These arrhythmias are less common than AV nodal or AV reentry and are more often associated with underlying cardiac disease. During sinus node reentry the P-wave morphology is identical to that occurring in sinus rhythm, but the PR interval is prolonged. This is in contrast to sinus tachycardia, in which the PR interval tends to shorten. With intraatrial reentry the P-wave configuration differs from that during sinus rhythm, and the PR interval is prolonged (Fig. 185-4*C*).

Treatment Sinus node and atrial reentrant arrhythmias are managed like other reentrant PSVTs.

NONREENTRANT ATRIAL TACHYCARDIAS These may be a manifestation of digitalis intoxication or may be associated with severe pulmonary or cardiac disease, with hypokalemia, or with the administration of theophylline or adrenergic drugs. The latter frequently present as multifocal atrial tachycardias (MAT). By definition, MAT requires ≥ 3 consecutive P waves of different morphologies at rates greater than 100 bpm. MAT usually has an irregular ventricular rate because of varying A-V conduction. Treatment should be directed at the underlying disorder. The digitalis-induced arrhythmias may be

TABLE 185-2 Drugs used to treat cardiac tachyarrhythmias

Drug	Sinus node	Atrium and ventricle	AV node	His-Purkinje system	Atrioventricular bypass tracts
ELECTROPHYSIOLOGIC EFFECTS					
Digoxin and other cardiac glycosides (also see p. 897)	No change; patients with sinus node disease may develop sinus exit block or arrest	Controversial	Increase in ERP; decreased conduction velocity	No change	No change or decrease in ERP
Propranolol and other beta-adrenoreceptor blockers (also see p. 968)	Decreased sinus rate; increased sinus node recovery time	No change	Increase in ERP; decreased conduction velocity	No change	No change
Verapamil	Decreased sinus rate; sinus exit block in patients with sinus node disease	No change	Increase in ERP; decreased conduction velocity	No change	Indirect effects may decrease ERP when given IV
Quinidine	No change; may suppress sinus node in patients with underlying sinus node disease	Increased ERP; decreased conduction velocity	Decrease or no change in ERP, no change in conduction velocity	Decreased automaticity; decreased conduction velocity; increased ERP	Increased ERP may abolish all conduction
Procainamide	No change	Increased ERP; decreased conduction velocity	Decrease or no change in ERP; decrease or no change in conduction velocity	Decreased automaticity; decreased conduction velocity; increased ERP	Increased ERP may abolish all conduction
Disopyramide	No change	Increased ERP; decreased conduction velocity	Decrease or no change in ERP; no change in conduction velocity	Decreased automaticity; increased ERP; decrease conduction velocity	Increased ERP may abolish all conduction
Lidocaine	No change	No change in ERP	No change or decrease in ERP	No change or decrease in ERP	No change, decrease, or increase in ERP
Phenytoin	No change	No change in ERP	No change or decrease in ERP No change or increased conduction velocity	Decrease in ERP; decreased automaticity	
Tocainide	No change	No change	No change	No change; decreased automaticity	Increase in ERP
Bretylium	Initial increase in sinus rate followed by decrease	Increase in ERP	No change	No change	
Amiodarone	Decreased sinus rate	Increased ERP	Increased ERP; decreased conduction velocity	Increased ERP; decreased conduction velocity	Increased ERP
Mexiletine	No change; patients with sinus node disease may develop sinus arrest	No change	Variable and inconsistent effects on conduction and refractoriness	Increased ERP; no change or decreased conduction velocity	
Encainide	No change	Decreased conduction velocity; increase in ERP (oral therapy only)	Decreased conduction velocity; increase in ERP	Decreased conduction velocity	Decreased conduction velocity; increase in ERP; may abolish all conduction
Flecainide	No change; patients with sinus node disease may develop exit block or arrest	Decreased conduction velocity; increase in ERP	Decreased conduction velocity; increase in ERP	Decreased conduction velocity	Decreased conduction velocity; increase in ERP; may abolish all conduction

NOTE: AV = atrioventricular, ERP = effective refractory period, IV = intravenous, SVT = supraventricular tachycardia, VT = ventricular tachycardia, AF = atrial fibrillation, VF = ventricular fibrillation.

TABLE 185-2 Drugs used to treat cardiac tachyarrhythmias *(continued)*

Indications	Side effects and toxicity
CLINICAL EFFECTS	
Slowing of ventricular rate during AF, flutter, and other atrial tachycardias in the absence of preexcitation; SVT due to AV nodal reentry and AV reentry utilizing bypass tracts	Atrial tachycardia, VT, AV nodal block, accelerated junctional rhythms, atrial and ventricular premature depolarizations, VT, VF, anorexia, nausea, vomiting; acceleration of ventricular rate during AF/flutter in the presence of preexcitation causing VF
Slowing of ventricular rate during AF, atrial flutter, and other atrial tachycardias in the absence of preexcitation; SVT due to AV nodal reentry, rentry utilizing bypass tracts; arrhythmias induced by exercise; arrhythmias occurring in the presence of hyperthyroidism; polymorphic VT associated with congenital long QT syndrome	Sinus bradycardia, AV nodal block, congestive heart failure, bronchospasm, masking symptoms of hypoglycemia
Same as digoxin	Sinus arrest in patients with sinus node dysfunction; AV nodal block in patients with AV nodal dysfunction; exacerbation of congestive heart failure (may be potentiated in presence of beta-adrenergic blocking agents); elevation of digoxin levels; hypotension following IV administration; IV administration during AF/flutter in the presence of preexcitation may cause acceleration of ventricular response rate and VF or hemodynamic collapse; IV administration to patients with VT may cause hemodynamic collapse
Atrial and ventricular extrasystoles; atrial and ventricular tachyarrhythmias; all types of SVT; control of ventricular rate in patients with preexcitation and AF and flutter	Anorexia, nausea, vomiting, diarrhea; cinchonism: tinnitus, confusion, hearing and visual changes; thrombocytopenia, hemolytic anemia, rash; drug interactions: elevation of digoxin levels; phenytoin and phenobarbital will decrease quinidine levels; QT prolongation associated with polymorphic VT (torsade de pointes); conversion of nonsustained to sustained VT; acceleration of ventricular response to atrial flutter and fibrillation
Same as quinidine	Anorexia, nausea, confusion, hallucinations; agranulocytosis; lupus erythematosus-like syndrome; QT prolongation associated with polymorphic VT (torsade de pointes); marked elevations in the primary metabolite (NAPA) may be more likely to cause polymorphic VT; conversion of nonsustained into sustained VT; acceleration of ventricular response to atrial flutter and fibrillation
Same as quinidine	Anticholinergic actions including dry mouth, blurred vision, urinary retention or hesitancy, constipation, narrow angle glaucoma; congestive heart failure, especially in patients with abnormal ventricular function; QT prolongation associated with polymorphic VT (torsade de pointes)
VT and VF especially during acute ischemia and myocardial infarction	Dizziness, paresthesias, confusion, delirium, seizures, coma; may depress sinus node in patients with underlying sinus node disease; may suppress escape foci in patients with complete heart block; congestive heart failure or liver disease increase risk of side effects
Tachyarrhythmias induced by digitalis; occasionally effective for ventricular tachyarrhythmias not induced by digitalis alone or in combination with other antiarrhythmic agents; polymorphic VT associated with increased QT	Gingival hypertrophy, rash, blood dyscrasias, nystagmus, ataxia, stupor, coma, lupus erythematosus syndrome, lymph node hyperplasia, peripheral neuropathy, hypocalcemia, hyperglycemia, phlebitis and hypotension during IV administration
VT, VF, frequent VPCs	Ataxia, tremor, paresthesias, light-headedness, nausea, rash, lupus erythematosus syndrome, pulmonary fibrosis, bone marrow suppression; may exacerbate heart failure in patients with ventricular dysfunction
Refractory ventricular VT and VF, especially due to acute ischemia	Initially, transient hypertension; subsequently, hypotension increased in the upright position; the hypotensive effect can be prevented by tricyclic drugs; nausea, vomiting
Refractory atrial and ventricular tachyarrhythmias; refractory SVT due to AV nodal reentry and AV reentry utilizing bypass tracts; not approved by FDA for atrial arrhythmias	Marked sinus bradycardia, complete heart block; IV administration may cause hypotension; increased QT associated with polymorphic VT; increased T_4, hypo- and hyperthyroidism; peripheral neuropathy; proximal myopathy; pulmonary fibrosis; increased liver enzymes, hepatitis; photodermatitis, blue-gray skin discoloration; corneal microdeposits; elevation of digoxin levels; potentiation of oral anticoagulants
Ventricular tachyarrhythmias	Nausea, vomiting, ataxia, tremor, gait disturbances, rash
Refractory atrial and ventricular tachyarrhythmias; SVT due to AV node reentry and AV bypass tracts; not approved by FDA for supraventricular arrhythmias	Refractory polymorphic VT without increased QT if dose is increased too rapidly or in patients with abnormal left ventricular function; AV block in patients with abnormal conduction system; sinus arrest in patients with abnormal sinus node function; nausea, dizziness, blurred vision. May precipitate heart failure in patients with ventricular dysfunction
Same as encainide; not approved by FDA for supraventricular arrhythmias	Same as encainide

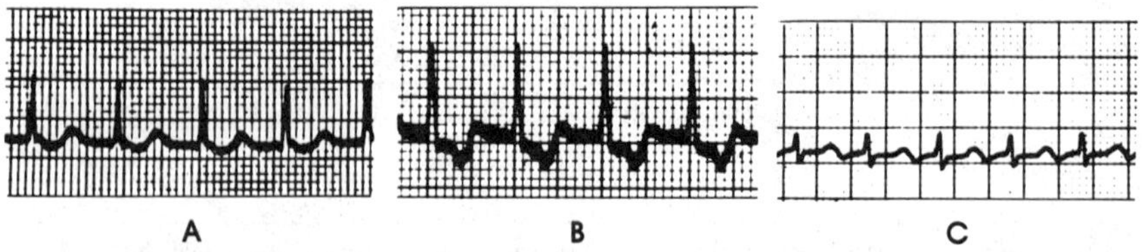

FIGURE 185-4 Examples of reentrant PSVT. *A*. AV nodal reentry. No P waves are visible. *B*. AV reentry using a concealed bypass tract. Inverted retrograde P waves are superimposed on the T wave. *C*. Intraatrial reentry. P waves precede the QRS complex.

caused by triggered activity and/or enhanced automaticity. In such atrial tachycardias with AV block secondary to digitalis intoxication (Fig. 185-1B), the atrial rate rarely exceeds 180 per minute, and typically 2:1 block is present. Atrial arrhythmias precipitated by digitalis can usually be treated by withdrawal of the drug.

Automatic atrial tachycardias not caused by digitalis are difficult to terminate, and in such cases the main goal of therapy should be to control the ventricular response, either by drugs which affect the AV node, such as digitalis, beta blockers, or calcium channel antagonists, or by ablation techniques. Surgery has been employed in resistant cases.

PREEXCITATION (WPW) SYNDROME The most frequently encountered type of ventricular preexcitation is that associated with AV bypass tracts. These connections are composed of strands of atrial-like muscle which may occur almost anywhere around the AV rings. The term *Wolff-Parkinson-White (WPW) syndrome* is applied to patients with both preexcitation on the ECG and paroxysmal tachycardias. AV bypass tracts can be associated with certain congenital abnormalities, the most important of which is Ebstein's anomaly.

AV bypass tracts that conduct in an antegrade direction produce a typical ECG pattern of a short PR interval (<0.12 s), a slurred upstroke of the QRS complex (delta wave), and a wide QRS complex. This pattern results from a fusion of activation of the ventricles over both the bypass tract and the AV nodal His-Purkinje system (Fig. 185-7). The relative contribution of activation over each system determines the amount of preexcitation.

During PSVT in WPW the impulse is usually conducted antegradely over the normal AV system and retrogradely through the bypass tract. The characteristics are identical to those described on p. 913. Rarely (approximately 5 percent), tachycardias occurring in patients with WPW will exhibit a reverse pattern with antegrade conduction through the bypass tract and retrograde conduction through the normal AV system. This produces a tachycardia with a wide QRS complex in which the ventricles are totally activated by the bypass tract. Atrial flutter and AF also occur commonly in patients with WPW syndrome. Since the bypass tract does not have the same decremental conducting properties as the AV node, the ventricular responses during atrial flutter or fibrillation may be unusually rapid (Fig. 185-1*E*) and may cause ventricular fibrillation.

The goals of electrophysiologic evaluation in patients suspected of having the WPW syndrome are (1) to confirm the diagnosis; (2) to localize the bypass tract and determine how many bypass tracts are present; (3) to demonstrate the role of the bypass tract in the genesis of the arrhythmias; (4) to determine the potential for the development of possibly life-threatening rates during atrial flutter or fibrillation; and (5) to evaluate therapeutic options, such as specific pharmacologic agents, pacing therapy, and surgery.

Management This should be aimed at (1) decreasing the occurrence of the APCs and VPCs responsible for the initiation of the

FIGURE 185-5 Mechanism of AV nodal reentry: The atrium, AV node (AVN), and His bundle are shown schematically. The AV node is longitudinally dissociated into two pathways, with different functional properties. The alpha pathway conducts relatively slowly while the beta pathway conducts rapidly (see text). In each panel of this diagram, heavy lines denote excitation in the AV node which is manifest on the surface electrocardiogram, while light lines denote conduction which is concealed and not apparent on the surface electrocardiogram. *A*. During sinus rhythm (NSR) the impulse from the atrium conducts down both pathways. However, only conduction over the fast (beta) pathway is manifest on the surface ECG, producing a normal PR interval of 0.16 s. *B*. An atrial premature depolarization (APD) blocks in the beta pathway. The impulse conducts over the alpha pathway to the His bundle and ventricles, producing a PR interval of 0.24 s. Because the impulse is premature, conduction over the alpha pathway occurs more slowly than it would during sinus rhythm. *C*. A more premature atrial impulse blocks in the beta pathway, conducting with increased delay in the alpha pathway, producing a PR interval of 0.28 s. The impulse conducts retrogradely up the beta pathway producing a single atrial echo. Sustained reentry is prevented by subsequent block in the alpha pathway. *D*. A still more premature atrial impulse blocks initially in the beta pathway, conducting over the alpha pathway with increasing delay producing a PR interval of 0.36 s. Retrograde conduction occurs over the beta pathway and reentry occurs, producing a sustained tachycardia (SVT).

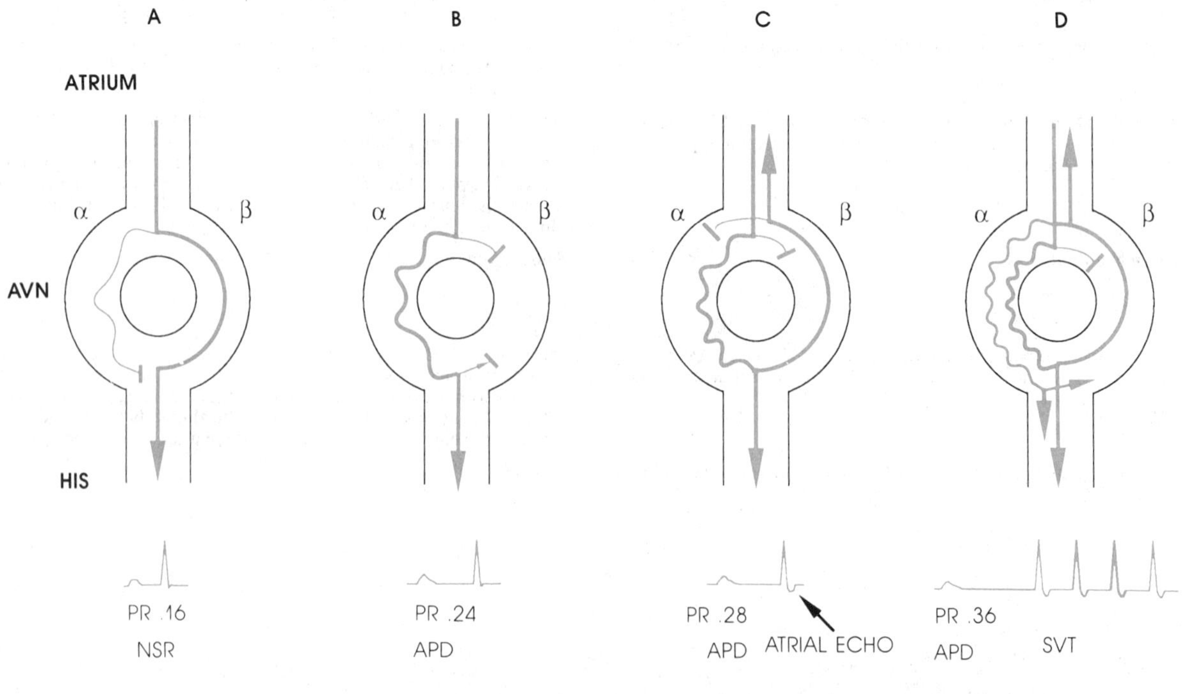

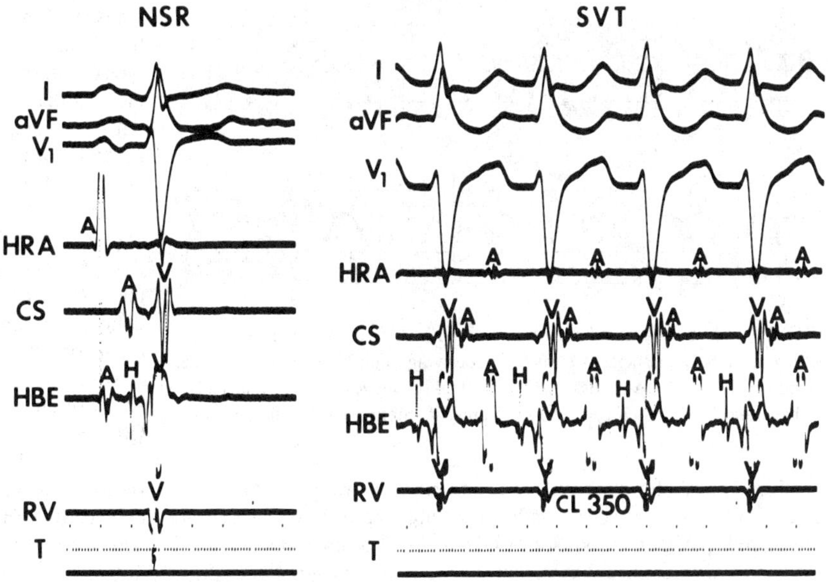

FIGURE 185-6 Intracardiac recordings during supraventricular tachycardia using a left-sided AV bypass tract. Intracardiac recordings during sinus rhythm (NSR) in supraventricular tachycardia (SVT) are shown. ECG leads I, aVF, and V_1 are displayed with electrograms from the high right atrium (HRA), coronary sinus (CS), His bundle (HBE), and right ventricle (RV). During NSR, the QRS complex and the AH and HV intervals are normal. During SVT the retrograde atrial activation sequence is abnormal. The earliest site of atrial activation is in the CS, which is followed by activation in the HBE and HRA. This activation sequence is diagnostic of a left-sided AV bypass tract conduction retrogradely from ventricle to atrium *[From ME Josephson, in Update IV, Harrison's Principles of Internal Medicine, KJ Isselbacher et al (eds), New York, McGraw-Hill, 1983; used with permission.]*

tachycardia; (2) increasing the refractory period of the bypass tract (refractory periods <250 ms are associated with rapid ventricular responses during AF); and (3) blocking conduction down the normal AV conduction system. Specific antiarrhythmic therapy can be assessed by electrophysiologic studies, as described on p. 921.

In patients with the WPW syndrome and AF, dc cardioversion should be carried out if there is a life-threatening, rapid ventricular response. Alternatively, lidocaine (3 to 5 mg/kg) or procainamide (15 mg/kg) administered intravenously over 15 to 20 min will usually slow the ventricular response. Caution should be employed when using digitalis or verapamil in patients with the WPW syndrome and AF, since these drugs can shorten the refractory period of the accessory pathway and can increase the ventricular rate, thereby placing the patient at increased risk for ventricular fibrillation. In addition to these drugs, beta blocking agents are of no utility in controlling the ventricular response during AF when conduction proceeds over the bypass tract. Although atrial or ventricular pacing can almost always terminate PSVT in patients with the WPW syndrome, they can induce AF. Successful surgical ablation of bypass tracts is possible in more than 90 percent of cases (p. 923) and offers a permanent cure of SVT and most AF associated with SVT.

Acute management of episodes of PSVT in patients with WPW syndrome is similar to that of PSVT in patients with concealed bypass tracts.

NONPAROXYSMAL JUNCTIONAL TACHYCARDIA This rhythm usually results from conditions that produce enhanced automaticity or triggered activity in the AV junction and is most commonly due to digitalis intoxication, inferior wall myocardial infarction, myocarditis, endogenous or exogenous catecholamine excess, acute rheumatic fever, or aftereffects of valve surgery.

The onset of nonparoxysmal junctional tachycardia is usually gradual with a ''warm-up'' period prior to stabilization of the rate, which can range from 70 to 150 per minute, with faster rates usually associated with digitalis intoxication. Nonparoxysmal junctional tachycardia is recognized by a QRS complex identical to that of sinus rhythm. The rate can be influenced by autonomic tone and can be increased by catecholamines, vagolytic agents, or exercise and slowed somewhat by carotid sinus pressure. When this rhythm is due to digitalis intoxication, it usually is associated with AV block and/or dissociation. Early after cardiac surgery, retrograde conduction is more likely to be present due to heightened sympathetic state.

Management This is directed toward elimination of the underlying etiologic factors. Since digitalis is the most common cause of this rhythm, discontinuation of this drug is indicated. If the rhythm is associated with other serious manifestations of digitalis intoxication, such as ventricular or atrial irritability, active intervention with lidocaine or a beta blocker may be useful, and in some instances use of digitalis antibodies (Fab fragments) should be considered. Cardioversion of this rhythm should not be attempted, particularly in the setting of digitalis intoxication. When AV conduction is intact, atrial pacing can capture and override the junctional focus and provide the AV synchrony necessary to maximize cardiac output. Nonparoxysmal junctional tachycardia usually is not a chronic, recurrent problem, and attention to the acute precipitating events can often resolve the tachycardia.

VENTRICULAR TACHYCARDIA (VT) *Sustained VT* is defined as *ventricular tachycardia* that persists for more than 30 s or requires termination because of hemodynamic collapse. VT generally accompanies some form of structural heart disease, most commonly chronic ischemic heart disease associated with a prior myocardial infarction. Sustained VT may also be associated with nonischemic cardiomy-

FIGURE 185-7 ECG in WPW syndrome. There is a short PR interval (0.11s), a wide QRS complex (0.12 s), and slurring on the upstroke of the QRS produced by early ventricular activation over the bypass tract (delta wave, d in lead I). The negative delta waves in V_1 are diagnostic of a right-sided bypass tract. Note the Q wave (negative delta wave) in lead III, mimicking myocardial infarction.

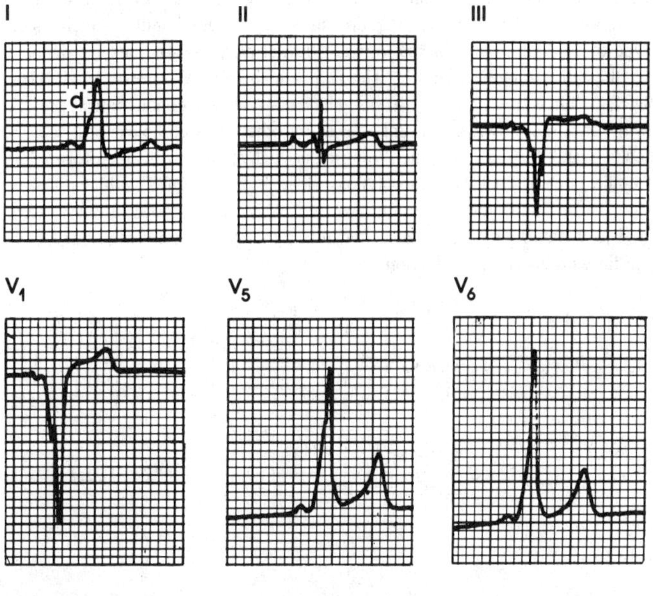

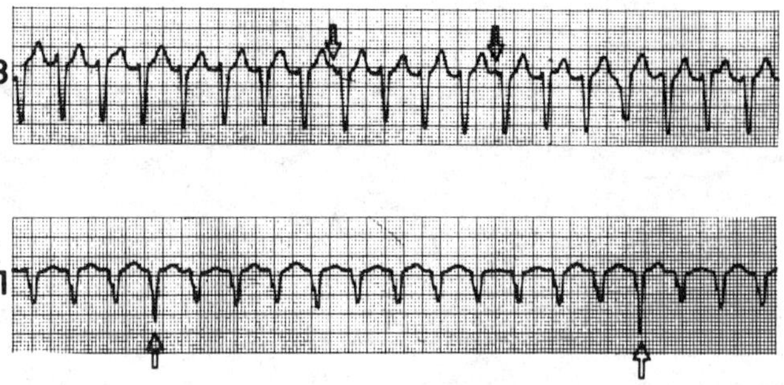

FIGURE 185-8 Ventricular tachycardia with AV dissociation. P waves which are totally dissociated from the underlying ventricular rhythm can be noted in lead III. AV dissociation is highly suggestive of ventricular tachycardia. In V_1 fusion complexes are present, confirming AV dissociation.

opathies, metabolic disorders, drug toxicity, or prolonged QT syndrome, and it occurs occasionally in the absence of heart disease or other predisposing factors. Nonsustained VT (3 beats to 30 s) is also associated with cardiac disease but occurs in its absence more often than the sustained arrhythmia. While nonsustained VT usually does not produce symptoms, sustained VT is almost always symptomatic and is often associated with marked hemodynamic embarrassment and/or the development of myocardial ischemia. A fixed anatomic substrate, not acute ischemia, is responsible for most recurrent episodes of sustained VT. Acute ischemia appears to have little role in the genesis of sustained uniform VT associated with chronic infarction but may play a role in the degeneration of stable VT into ventricular fibrillation (VF). Most episodes of VF begin with VT.

The ECG diagnosis of VT is suggested by a wide-complex tachycardia at a rate exceeding 100 per minute. While the rhythm is usually quite regular, slight irregularity may exist. Atrial activity may be dissociated from ventricular activity (Fig. 185-8), or the atria may be depolarized retrogradely. The onset of the tachycardia is generally abrupt, but in nonparoxysmal tachycardias it can be gradual. The QRS configuration during any episode of VT may be uniform (monomorphic) (Figs. 185-2*B* and 185-9), or it may vary from beat to beat (polymorphic) (Fig. 185-2*C*). *Bidirectional tachycardia* refers to VT that shows an alternation in QRS amplitude and direction. Paroxysmal VT is usually initiated by a VPC.

It is important to distinguish supraventricular tachycardia with aberration of intraventricular conduction from VT since the clinical implications and management of these two arrhythmias are totally different. It is always useful to have a 12-lead ECG recorded during sinus rhythm for comparison with that during the tachycardia. When the tracing obtained during sinus rhythm demonstrates a bundle branch block pattern with the same morphologic features as those during the tachycardia, the diagnosis of supraventricular tachycardia is favored. An infarction pattern on the sinus rhythm tracing suggests the potential presence of the anatomic substrate necessary for VT. Characteristics of the 12-lead ECG during the tachycardia that suggest a ventricular origin for the arrhythmia are (1) a QRS complex >0.14 s in the absence of antiarrhythmic therapy; (2) AV dissociation or variable retrograde conduction; (3) a superior QRS axis; (4) concordance of the QRS pattern in all precordial leads (i.e., all positive or all negative deflections); and (5) other QRS patterns with prolonged duration that are inconsistent with typical right or left bundle branch block patterns. A wide, complex, bizarre tachycardia that is very irregular suggests AF with conduction over an AV bypass tract (p. 916). Similarly, a QRS complex in excess of 0.20 s is uncommon during VT in the absence of drug therapy and is more common with preexcitation. Intravenous verapamil will stop most recalcitrant supraventricular tachycardias involving the AV junction, but it is rarely effective for ventricular tachycardia. Because of this property, verapamil has been utilized to attempt to differentiate supraventricular tachycardia with deviant conduction from ventricular tachycardia. However, this is extremely hazardous, since intravenous verapamil frequently precipitates cardiac arrest in patients with ventricular tachycardias.

The diagnosis of VT can be confirmed by analyzing the relationship between the electrogram recording from the His bundle and ventricular activity. In most cases of VT, the His deflection is not easily seen, but when visible, the interval from the His deflection to the onset of ventricular activation (HV interval) is less than that recorded during sinus rhythm, or negative due to retrograde activation over the His-Purkinje system, or it is dissociated from ventricular activation (Fig. 185-10). During SVT with aberrant conduction the HV interval is greater than or equal to that recorded during sinus rhythm. In patients with a wide QRS complex tachycardia, the diagnosis of VT is confirmed when atrial pacing at rates equal to or greater than that of the tachycardia produces normalization of the QRS complex with a normal HV interval. Regardless of QRS morphology [left or right bundle branch block patterns (Fig. 185-9)], VT due to ischemic heart disease arises from the *left* ventricle, in most instances near the subendocardium.

It has been possible to replicate sustained uniform VT in more than 95 percent of patients with this arrhythmia using programmed stimulation. In most patients the tachycardia is initiated with ventricular premature stimuli. A sustained monomorphic VT with a morphology identical to that of the spontaneous arrhythmia is the rule.

FIGURE 185-9 *A.* Sustained ventricular tachycardia having a uniform morphology. The QRS configuration in V_1 is a right bundle branch block type of configuration. Marked leftward frontal plane axis is present, denoted by the QS complex in lead II. The R/S ratio in lead V_6 is less than 1. The QRS width is greater than 140 ms. Note that 2:1 VA conduction is present with retrograde P waves present after every other QRS complex (best seen in leads I and V_1). *B.* Sustained ventricular tachycardia with a uniform, left bundle branch block type morphology (lead V_1). The QRS width is greater than 160 ms, and there are a Q wave in lead V_6 and a broad initial R wave in V_1, all favoring ventricular tachycardia rather than supraventricular tachycardia with aberrant conduction.

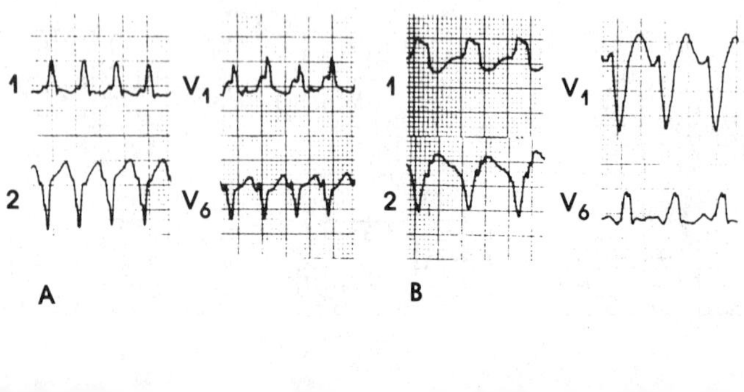

FIGURE 185-10 Intracardiac recordings distinguishing supraventricular tachycardia from ventricular tachycardia. ECG leads I, aVF, and V_1 are shown with a His bundle electrogram (HBE) and time line (TL). Wide QRS complex tachycardia with a right bundle branch block morphology are shown on the left and right panels. On the left, supraventricular tachycardia is diagnosed by the presence of His deflection (H) preceding each QRS complex, with normal HV interval. On the right, during ventricular tachycardia no His bundle deflections can be seen (arrow) and AV dissociation is observed (note single atrial deflection, A). *(From JA Kastor et al, N Engl J Med 304:1004, 1981; reprinted by permission.)*

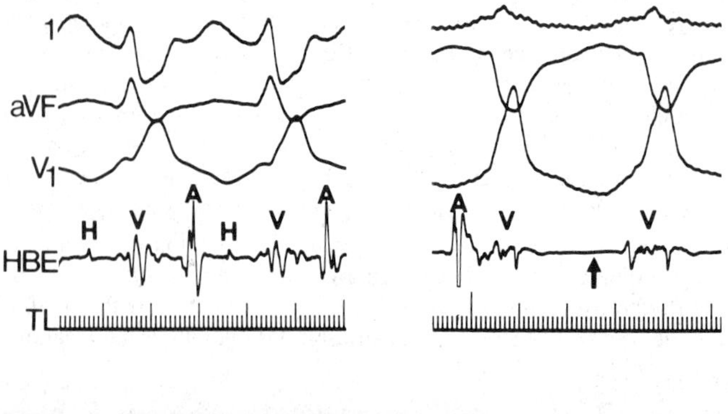

The clinical significance of polymorphic VT initiated by programmed stimulation is not clear. It has been shown that when more aggressive stimulation is performed (i.e., the use of three or four extrastimuli), polymorphic VT and even VF can be induced in some normal subjects and in patients who have never had a clinical arrhythmia.

Sustained uniform VT can be terminated by programmed stimulation or rapid pacing in at least 75 percent of patients; the remainder require cardioversion. The ability to initiate and terminate a sustained, uniform VT reproducibly permits assessment of pharmacologic and electrical therapy of these arrhythmias. Serial testing of antiarrhythmic agents over a period of several days can be accomplished and predicts the likelihood of success of the agents or devices tested (page 921).

The reproducible termination of VT by programmed stimulation permits evaluation of the effectiveness of antitachycardia pacemakers for long-term therapy of paroxysmal episodes of arrhythmia. Unfortunately, rapid pacing, the most effective form of therapy, can accelerate the tachycardia and/or produce ventricular fibrillation.

Clinical features Symptoms resulting from VT depend on the ventricular rate, duration of the tachycardia, and presence and extent of underlying cardiac disease. When the tachycardia is rapid and associated with severe myocardial dysfunction and cerebrovascular disease, hypotension and syncope are common. However, the presence of hemodynamic stability does not preclude a diagnosis of VT. The loss of the atrial contribution to ventricular filling and an abnormal sequence of ventricular activation are important factors producing a decreased cardiac output during VT.

The *prognosis* of VT depends on the underlying disease state. If sustained VT develops within the first 6 weeks following acute myocardial infarction, the prognosis is poor, with an 85 percent mortality rate at 1 year. Patients with nonsustained VT following myocardial infarction have a threefold greater risk of death than a comparable group of patients without this arrhythmia. However, a cause-and-effect relationship between the nonsustained tachycardia and subsequent sudden death has not been established.

Management The risk-benefit ratio of treating each specific type of VT should be considered before beginning therapy. This is important because antiarrhythmic agents can produce or exacerbate the very arrhythmias which they are given to prevent. In general, patients with VT but without organic heart disease have a benign course; such patients with asymptomatic, nonsustained VT need not be treated since their prognosis will not be affected. Patients with sustained VT in the absence of heart disease usually require therapy because the arrhythmia causes symptoms. These tachycardias may respond to beta blockers, verapamil, or quinidine-like agents. In patients with VT and organic heart disease, if marked hemodynamic embarrassment is present or if there is evidence of ischemia, congestive heart failure, or central nervous system hypoperfusion, the rhythm should be promptly terminated by dc cardioversion (see below). If the patient with organic heart disease tolerates the VT well, pharmacologic therapy may be tried. Procainamide is probably the most effective agent for acute therapy. It may or may not terminate the tachycardia, but almost always slows the rate. In stable patients in whom these drugs do not terminate the arrhythmia, a pacing catheter can be inserted pervenously into the right ventricular apex, and the tachycardia can be terminated by overdrive pacing.

Use of programmed stimulation is probably the most efficacious way to select the appropriate antiarrhythmic agent to prevent recurrent, sustained VT. In a controlled situation, drugs can be serially studied, and the drug that prevents initiation of the tachycardia can be selected; long-term successful prevention of the arrhythmia can then be expected in 90 percent of patients (see p. 921).

Antitachycardia pacing has been used as a means to terminate drug-resistant tachycardia. This usually requires that the tachycardia be stable and slow and the patient be aware of it. No automatic antitachycardia device has been approved for therapy of VT at the time of this writing because pacing during VT may accelerate tachycardia, converting a stable arrhythmia into an unstable one, resulting in severe hemodynamic compromise. However, availability of a new device, the automatic implantable cardioverter defibrillator (AICD) (see below) affords a "backup" means of terminating unstable arrhythmias. Radiofrequency pacemakers, which are best activated by a physician, have been used in occasional patients.

The advent of endocardial catheter and intraoperative mapping has led to the development of new surgical techniques for the management of VT. Activation mapping permits localization of the site of origin of the arrhythmia. In centers in which expertise in mapping is available, operation has been successfully employed to cure tachycardias in the majority of patients in whom it has been undertaken. Even though most patients with VT and ischemic heart disease have markedly impaired left ventricular function and multivessel coronary artery disease, the operative mortality rate has ranged between 8 and 15 percent. Following operation, 85 to 90 percent of survivors are controlled either off (two-thirds of patients) or on (one-third) antiarrhythmic agents that were previously ineffective in controlling these rhythms.

Specific types of VT TORSADE DE POINTES Torsade de pointes ("twisting of the points") (Fig. 185-11) refers to VT characterized by polymorphic QRS complexes that change in amplitude and cycle length, giving the appearance of oscillations around the baseline. This rhythm is by definition associated with QT prolongation. The latter may result from electrolyte disturbances (particularly hypokalemia and hypomagnesemia), use of a variety of antiarrhythmic drugs (especially quinidine), phenothiazines and tricyclic antidepressants, liquid protein diets, intracranial events, and bradyarrhythmias, particularly third-degree AV block. It may also occur as an isolated idiopathic congenital or acquired anomaly.

The electrocardiographic hallmark is polymorphic VT preceded by marked QR prolongation, often in excess of 0.60 s. These patients often have multiple episodes of nonsustained polymorphic VT associated with recurrent syncope, but they may also develop VF and sudden cardiac death.

Therapy should be directed at removing the precipitating factors, i.e., correcting metabolic abnormalities and removing drugs which have induced the prolonged QT interval. In the setting of drug-induced torsade de pointes, atrial or ventricular overdrive pacing and the administration of magnesium have also been useful in terminating and preventing the arrhythmia. For patients with the congenital prolonged QT interval syndrome, beta-adrenergic blocking agents have been the mainstay of therapy; agents which shorten the QT interval may also be useful (e.g., phenytoin). Cervicothoracic sympathectomy has been proposed as a form of therapy for congenital prolonged QT syndrome, but it is not often effective as the sole therapy.

Polymorphic tachycardias associated with normal QT intervals in patients with ischemic heart disease that are initiated by "R-on-T" VPCs are probably caused by reentry, and their treatment is totally different. This is not true "torsade de pointes." In such cases, quinidine-like agents may be the most effective form of therapy and should be administered in full antiarrhythmic doses. However, these arrhythmias may also result from acute, severe ischemia and will only respond to abolition of the ischemia, usually by revascularization.

FIGURE 185-11 Torsade de pointes. During sinus rhythm (lead II) a markedly prolonged QT interval was present. Lead V_1 shows polymorphic VT.

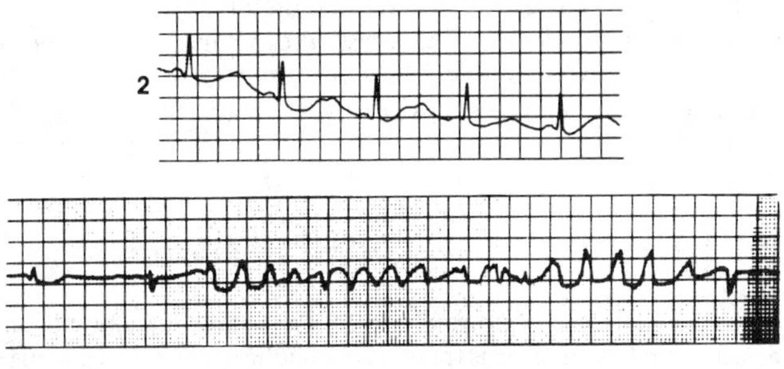

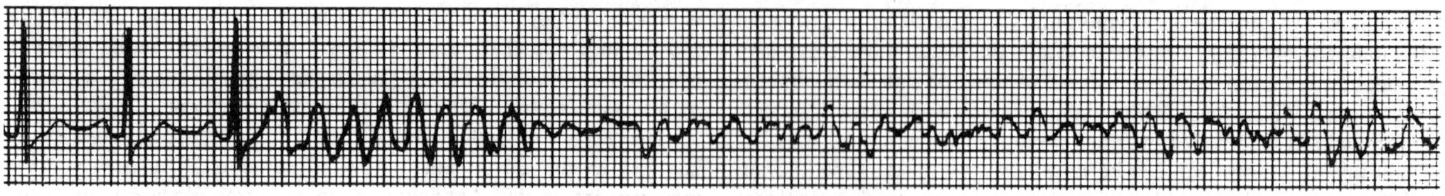

FIGURE 185-12 Ventricular fibrillation. In a patient with coronary disease ventricular fibrillation is initiated by a VPC that produces a rapid polymorphic ventricular tachycardia which rapidly degenerates to ventricular fibrillation (note the undulating baseline with indistinguishable systole and diastole).

ACCELERATED IDIOVENTRICULAR RHYTHM This arrhythmia, also termed slow VT, with a rate which ranges from 60 to 120 per minute, usually occurs in acute myocardial infarction, often during reperfusion. It may also be seen following cardiac operations, in patients with cardiomyopathy, rheumatic fever, or digitalis intoxication, as well as in patients with no evidence of heart disease. The rhythm is usually transient and rarely causes significant hemodynamic compromise or symptoms.

Treatment is rarely necessary and should usually be considered only if symptoms arise due to impaired hemodynamics, most commonly due to AV dissociation. In most cases, atropine can accelerate the sinus rate to overdrive the ventricular rhythm.

VENTRICULAR FLUTTER AND VENTRICULAR FIBRILLATION (VF) (Fig. 185-12; see also Chap. 40), Ventricular flutter and VF occur most often in patients with ischemic heart disease. They also occur following administration of antiarrhythmic drugs, particularly those which induce prolonged QT intervals and torsade de pointes (see above), with severe hypoxia or ischemia, and in patients with WPW who develop AF with an extremely rapid ventricular response (page 916). Electrical accidents frequently cause cardiac arrest due to the development of VF. The onset of these arrhythmias is rapidly followed by loss of consciousness and, if untreated, death. Episodes of cardiac arrest recorded during Holter monitoring reveal that approximately three-fourths of the sudden deaths are due to VT or VF.

In patients with VF, the onset almost always begins with a short run of rapid VT, which is initiated by a relatively late coupled VPC. In patients with acute myocardial infarction or ischemia, however, VF is usually precipitated by a single early ventricular complex beat falling on the T wave (the vulnerable period), which produces a rapid VT which degenerates into VF (Fig. 185-9).

The clinical setting in which VF occurs is important, since most patients who have primary VT within the first 48 h of the onset of acute infarction have a good prognosis, with a very low rate of recurrence or sudden cardiac death. In contrast, most patients who experience VF unassociated with the development of acute myocardial infarction have a recurrence rate of 20 to 30 percent in the year following the event (see Chap 40).

Ventricular flutter usually appears as a sine wave with a rate between 150 and 300 beats per minute. These oscillations make it impossible to assign a specific morphology to the arrhythmia and in some cases to distinguish it from rapid VT. VF is recognized by grossly irregular undulations of varying amplitudes, contours, and rates (Fig. 185-12). Electrophysiologic studies have demonstrated that regardless of the apparent gross irregularity on the surface ECG, VF usually starts out with the rapid repetitive sequence of VT which ultimately breaks down into multiple wavelets of reentry.

Electrophysiologic studies have been useful in patients who have been resuscitated from cardiac arrest. Programmed stimulation has demonstrated that in approximately 70 percent of such patients one can reproducibly initiate a sustained VT. Treatment is discussed in Chap. 40.

PHARMACOLOGIC ANTIARRHYTHMIC THERAPY

Prior to initiation of pharmacologic antiarrhythmic therapy, potential aggravating factors such as transient metabolic abnormalities, congestive heart failure, or acute ischemia must be corrected and in some cases may suffice to control arrhythmias. In addition, the potential role of drugs as a cause of exacerbating factor in the development of the arrhythmia must be considered.

Antiarrhythmic drugs are used in three principal situations: (1) to terminate an acute arrhythmia, (2) to prevent recurrence of an arrhythmia, and (3) to prevent a life-threatening arrhythmia for which the patient is perceived to be at risk, but which has never occurred.

Most currently available antiarrhythmic agents have a relatively low toxic/therapeutic ratio; all can exert proarrhythmic effects, and therefore they may exacerbate underlying arrhythmias. Serum levels can be determined for most currently available antiarrhythmic agents. Standards for therapeutic and toxic levels can serve only as a rough guide for selecting the appropriate dose in any individual patient. In the final analysis, the therapeutic level in a given patient is that concentration which achieves the desired antiarrhythmic effect, and the toxic level for each patient is that concentration at which undesirable side effects occur. Since many adverse effects are directly related to drug concentrations, the minimal serum level which achieves an effective antiarrhythmic response should be chosen.

In order to determine the therapeutic level for a patient, one must have a standard to judge drug efficacy. For a patient with an incessant arrhythmia, antiarrhythmic drugs may be administered empirically until the arrhythmia is suppressed. If a reproducible precipitating factor such as exercise can be identified, serial drug testing during such a provocative maneuver may be performed. Unfortunately, most arrhythmias are sporadic and occur unpredictably without identifiable precipitating factors. In these cases, if one waits to observe spontaneous recurrences on each antiarrhythmic drug, assessment of drug efficacy may require months. This type of assessment of efficacy may be adequate for arrhythmias which are not life-threatening. However, this mode of assessment is inadequate for arrhythmias that compromise hemodynamic stability, result in syncope, or cause cardiac arrest. In such cases two methods for determination of arrhythmic drug efficacy have been utilized. The first, which consists of continuous ECG monitoring in the control state and then in the presence of antiarrhythmic drugs, has been used in order to determine the effect that each drug has on spontaneous atrial or ventricular ectopy. This method presupposes that the mechanism responsible for sustained arrhythmias is the same as that causing isolated premature depolarizations (which may or may not be true) and that therefore eradication of isolated ectopy will correlate with prevention of sustained arrhythmias. This method has a number of limitations. First, patients frequently show marked degrees of spontaneous variation in frequency of ectopy, which may mimic antiarrhythmic drug effects. Second, 25 to 30 percent of patients with sustained ventricular arrhythmias such as VT or VF demonstrate only rare spontaneous ectopy. Finally, many patients demonstrate a dissociation between the effects of antiarrhythmic agents on spontaneous ectopy and the effects of the same agent on sustained arrhythmias.

An alternative method to assess drug efficacy is programmed stimulation. Numerous studies have demonstrated that most clinically occurring supraventricular and ventricular tachyarrhythmias may be reproducibly initiated and terminated safely using this technique. Studies are performed initially in a baseline state in the absence of antiarrhythmic drugs (Fig. 185-13). If the patient's clinical arrhythmia can be reproducibly initiated, then the ability of individual antiarrhythmic drugs to prevent reinduction of the arrhythmia can be

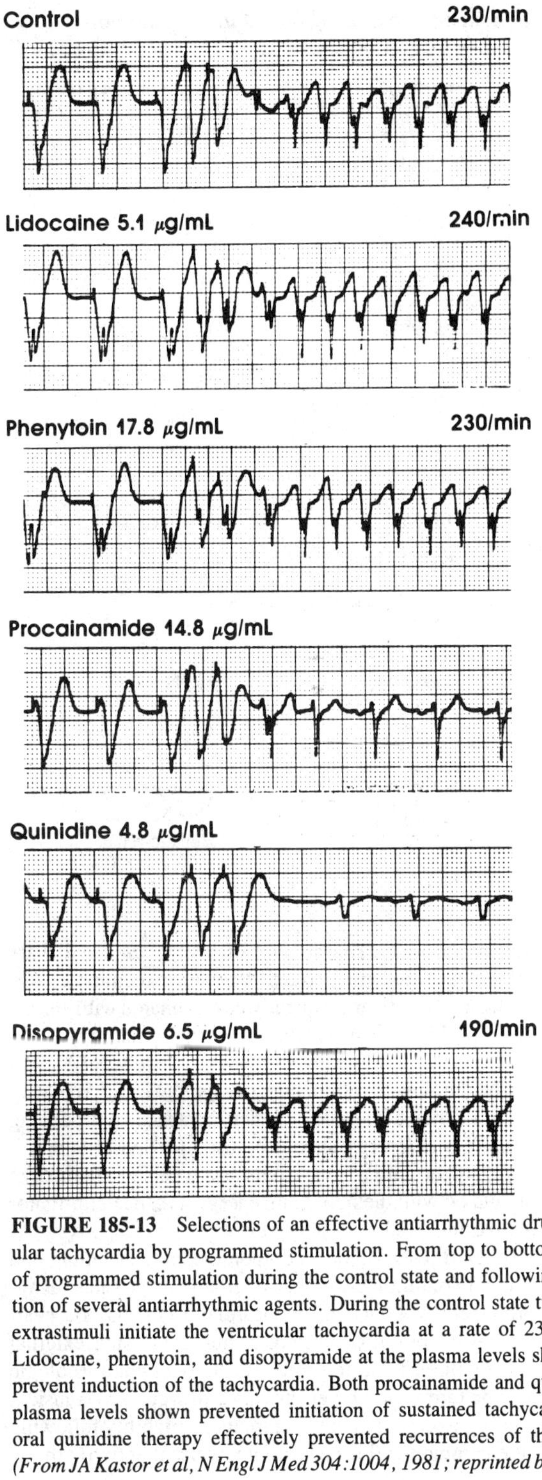

FIGURE 185-13 Selections of an effective antiarrhythmic drug for ventricular tachycardia by programmed stimulation. From top to bottom, the effects of programmed stimulation during the control state and following administration of several antiarrhythmic agents. During the control state two ventricular extrastimuli initiate the ventricular tachycardia at a rate of 230 per minute. Lidocaine, phenytoin, and disopyramide at the plasma levels shown failed to prevent induction of the tachycardia. Both procainamide and quinidine at the plasma levels shown prevented initiation of sustained tachycardia. Chronic oral quinidine therapy effectively prevented recurrences of the arrhythmia. *(From JA Kastor et al, N Engl J Med 304:1004, 1981; reprinted by permission.)*

assessed either after the drug is administered intravenously or after several days of oral loading in order to achieve a steady state serum concentration. Use of this method assumes that (1) the induced and spontaneous arrhythmias are identical, and (2) prevention of induction of arrhythmias will correlate with prevention or recurrent spontaneous tachycardias on the same drug regimen. This technique has been validated in patients with a variety of reentrant PSVTs, VT, and VF. The technique is safe when carefully performed, the potential complications being those of any intravascular catheterization. Appropriate interpretation of the results of programmed stimulation is critically dependent on correlating the patient's spontaneous arrhythmias with those induced in the laboratory, with regard to rate and morphology.

A number of classifications of antiarrhythmic drugs have been proposed, the most frequently used of which is a modification of that proposed by Vaughn-Williams (Table 185-1). This classification is based in part on the ability of antiarrhythmic drugs to modify the cardiac cellular (1) excitatory currents (Na^+ or Ca^{2+}), (2) action potential duration, and (3) automaticity (phase 4 depolarization). These effects of the drugs on isolated cardiac cells are thought to account for some of the antiarrhythmic properties of the drugs. Thus, depression of excitatory currents by type I and type IV antiarrhythmics results in slowing of conduction velocity and may interrupt arrhythmias by blocking conduction in areas of marginal excitability, where conduction velocity is already slow. Type III antiarrhythmics allegedly exert their action by increasing refractoriness through prolongation of the action potential duration. However, such classifications are limited in that the electrophysiologic effects of these drugs in vivo may differ from their effects on isolated cells. Also the effects of heart rate and fiber geometry are not considered. The uses and actions of currently available antiarrhythmic drugs are summarized in Tables 185-2 and 185-3.

ELECTRICAL THERAPY OF TACHYARRHYTHMIAS

PACEMAKERS Cardiac pacing can be used to terminate and in selected cases prevent recurrent supraventricular and ventricular arrhythmias. Because many tachyarrhythmias appear to be due to a reentrant mechanism with the impulse traveling in a circuit, a properly timed paced impulse can penetrate and prematurely depolarize part of the circuit, rendering it refractory to the next circulating wavefront, thereby interrupting the circus movement. Pacing therapy for arrhythmias is generally reserved for patients whose arrhythmias are refractory to the next circulating wavefront, thereby interrupting the circus movement. Pacing therapy for arrhythmias is generally reserved for patients whose arrhythmias are refractory to drug therapy and who remain hemodynamically stable during the tachycardia. All forms of pacing therapy require repeated demonstration of their effectiveness and reliability in terminating the arrhythmias during electrophysiologic testing prior to implantation of the pacing device.

The type of pacing device and modality selected for arrhythmia termination depend on (1) the rate of the tachycardia (rates >160 per minute are rarely terminated by a single premature stimulus); (2) the type of the arrhythmia (atrial flutter and VT are rarely terminated by single extrastimuli); and (3) concomitant drug therapy. Underdrive pacing, i.e., pacing at a rate slower than the tachycardia, can be used when a single premature stimulus has been demonstrated to reproducibly terminate a tachycardia. It is rarely used today since pacemakers are available which can deliver timed stimuli or an increasing number of stimuli.

Because many tachycardias cannot be terminated by single premature stimuli, pacemakers have been developed which allow for multiple extrastimuli (burst pacing) to be introduced. In reentrant tachycardias involving an accessory AV connection, sequential, near simultaneous activation of the heart from both the atria and the ventricle using a dual-chamber pacemaker will increase the likelihood of bidirectional block and termination of the tachycardia.

Cardiac pacing has also been used to prevent ventricular tachyarrhythmias. Polymorphic VT associated with a long QT interval and bradycardia (torsade de pointes, p. 919) is most likely to respond. Pacing the atrium and/or ventricle at rates between 90 and 120 per minute appears to increase the homogeneity of electrical recovery and markedly reduces the propensity for a recurrence of arrhythmias. Regardless of the arrhythmia being treated and the pacing mode selected, the potential for alterations in pacing requirements for termination of tachycardia and therefore programmability of pacing modes (e.g., underdrive, dual-demand, dual-chamber, burst), as well as rate and coupling interval of introduced extrastimuli, are probably essential features for pacemakers used to terminate tachycardias.

Pacemakers may be self-contained or energized by an external radiofrequency source. The self-contained pacemaker may function

TABLE 185-3 Dose, serum half-life ($t_{½}$) following oral administration, and route of metabolism of drugs used in treatment of arrhythmias

Drug	Mode of administration	$t_{½}$ (oral), h	Route of metabolism
Digoxin	IV, 0.75–1.5 mg Oral, 0.75–1.5 mg loading dose over 12–24 h Maintenance, 0.25–0.50 mg/d	36	Renal
Propranolol	IV, 0.5–1 mg/min to total dose of 0.15–0.2 mg/kg Oral, 10–200 mg q 6 h	3–6	Hepatic
Verapamil	IV, 2.5–10 mg over 1–2 min to total 0.15 mg/kg Oral, 80–120 mg q 6–8 h	3–8	Hepatic
Quinidine	IV, 20 mg/min to total 10–15 mg/kg Oral, 200–400 mg q 6 h	5–9	Hepatic
Procainamide	IV, 40–50 mg/min to total 10–20 mg/kg Oral, 500–1000 mg q 4 h	3–5	Hepatic-renal
Disopyramide	Oral, 100–300 mg q 6–8 h	8–9	Renal
Lidocaine	IV, 20–50 mg/min to total dose of 5 mg/kg loading followed by 1–4 mg/min	1–2	Hepatic
Phenytoin	IV, 20 mg/min total dose to 1000 mg Oral, 1000 mg loading over 24 h Maintenance, 100–400 mg/d	18–36	Hepatic
Tocainide	Oral, 400 to 600 mg q 8–12 h	10–17	Hepatic-renal
Bretylium	IV, 1–2 (mg/kg)/min to total load 5–10 mg/kg Maintenance, 0.5–2 mg/min	8–14	Renal
Amiodarone	IV, 5–10 mg/kg Oral, load 800–1400 mg/d for 1–2 weeks Maintenance, 100–600 mg/d	Unknown	Hepatic
Mexiletine	Oral, 100–300 mg q 6–8 h	9–12	Hepatic
Encainide	Oral, begin at 25 mg tid; at 3 to 5-day intervals may increase to 35 mg tid and then 50 mg tid	1–2 active metabolites: 3–4 and 6–12	Hepatic—active metabolite excreted by kidneys
Flecainide	Oral, begin at 50–100 mg bid; increase by no more than 50 mg not more often than every 4 days to a maximum of 400 mg daily	7–23	Hepatic-renal

automatically [i.e., it incorporates an arrhythmia recognition program (circuit)], or it may be activated by an external magnet. The major advantage of a fully automatic system is that there is no need for the patient to recognize the arrhythmia in order for termination to occur. The advantages of the externally activated system include (1) the decreased risk of unnecessary treatment because of faulty sensing; and (2) the opportunity to initiate monitoring at the time of attempted termination of arrhythmia. This type of monitoring is frequently helpful if pacing techniques are employed to terminate VT, given the risk of acceleration of the arrhythmia by pacing.

The limitations of pacing therapy are primarily related to (1) the changes in the characteristics of the arrhythmia over time such that programmed pacing parameters no longer terminate the tachycardia; and (2) the risk of acceleration of the tachycardia with the development of AF when stimulating the atrium and the development of rapid VT and VF when stimulating the ventricles. Future pacing generators which can also deliver a larger amount of energy and perform cardioversion and defibrillation of accelerated arrhythmias are likely to increase the applicability of pacing therapy for the treatment of arrhythmias.

CARDIOVERSION AND DEFIBRILLATION Electrical cardioversion and defibrillation remain the most reliable methods for terminating arrhythmias. By depolarizing all or at least a large portion of excitable myocardium in a near homogeneous fashion, the electrical shock can interrupt reentrant arrhythmias. External cardioversion is routinely performed by placing two paddles 12 cm in diameter in firm contact with the chest wall, with one paddle usually located to the right of the sternum at the level of the second rib and the other in the left midclavicular line in the fifth intercostal space. If the patient is conscious, a short-acting barbiturate to act as an anesthetic or an amnesic drug such as diazepam should be administered to prevent patient discomfort. A person skilled in maintaining an airway should be present. Energy is delivered synchronously with the QRS complex for all arrhythmias except ventricular flutter and VF, since asynchronous shocks can produce VF. The amount of energy used will vary with the type of tachycardia being treated. With the exception of AF, supraventricular tachycardias can frequently be terminated with energy levels in the range of 25 to 50 W·s, while AF usually requires ≥100 W·s for termination. For terminating VT, energy levels ≥100 W·s should probably be employed. While energies as low as 25 W·s may be successfully used, they also have a higher incidence of producing VF. At least 200 W·s of energy should be used for initial attempts at terminating VF. If the initial shock fails, all repeated attempts at defibrillation should be with the maximum energy that the defibrillator is capable of delivering (320 to 400 W·s).

Indications for cardioversion depend upon the clinical setting and the patient's general condition. Any tachycardia (except sinus tachycardia) that produces hypotension, myocardial ischemia, or heart failure warrants consideration of prompt termination using external cardioversion. Arrhythmias that fail to terminate with pharmacologic therapy may also be terminated by electrical cardioversion. Transient bradycardias and supraventricular and ventricular irritability following cardioversion are common and usually do not warrant antiarrhythmic intervention.

AUTOMATIC INTERNAL DEFIBRILLATION An automatic implanted cardioverter-defibrillator device has been developed to allow for prompt recognition and termination of life-threatening ventricular arrhythmias. The device delivers 25 to 33 W·s of energy. Clinical trials testing the function of the device in patients with drug-refractory ventricular arrhythmias have demonstrated survival from sudden death at 1 year ranging between 92 and 100 percent. Based on the results of the initial trials, it appears that an automatic sensing, implanted cardioverter-defibrillator will play an important role in management of life-threatening arrhythmias. At the time of this writing, use of this device should be reserved for patients with VT which is not hemodynamically tolerated or for patients with VF whose arrhythmias are refractory to drug therapy and who are not candidates for surgical intervention (see below). The most frequent problem with the device has been its inappropriate discharge in the absence of sustained ventricular arrhythmias. Additional potential problems include an increase in defibrillation threshold and decrease in tachycardia rates below the rate cut-off of the device in response to many antiarrhythmic drugs. Permanently implanted ventricular pacemakers may interfere with the device's ability to sense VF.

CATHETER ABLATION FOR ARRHYTHMIAS Catheter ablation of tachyarrhythmias, a technique that involves the delivery of large amounts of energy (25 to 400 W·s) through a catheter to effect closed-chest electroablation of the bundle of His, has been primarily used to interrupt AV conduction and prevent a rapid ventricular response to supraventricular arrhythmias. Although not yet approved by the Food and Drug Administration, catheter ablation of the AV junction has become the procedure of choice for creating AV block to control refractory supraventricular arrhythmias. However, the possible introduction of complete heart block necessitating a pacemaker and the small risk of sudden death associated with the procedure make catheter ablation a procedure of "last resort" at this time. This procedure is also under investigation for ablation of ventricular tachycardia and AV bypass tract tachycardia.

SURGICAL TREATMENT OF ARRHYTHMIAS

Programmed stimulation and endocardial activation mapping have provided a better understanding of the mechanisms and sites of origin of many supraventricular and ventricular tachyarrhythmias, so that in selected patients surgical treatment may be considered.

WOLFF-PARKINSON-WHITE SYNDROME Surgery may be preferable to other forms of therapy in some patients, particularly those with recurrent arrhythmias. Advances made in the localization and surgical ablation of bypass tracts now allow for an extremely high success rate with minimal morbidity. As a result, surgery can now be considered not only in patients with drug-refractory arrhythmias but also as a reasonable alternative in (1) patients with symptomatic arrhythmias who require long-term drug therapy; (2) patients with AF and a life-threatening rapid ventricular response; and (3) patients undergoing cardiac surgery for other reasons in whom a bypass tract is present.

SUPRAVENTRICULAR TACHYCARDIA AND OTHER ATRIAL ARRHYTHMIAS Although atrial flutter, AF, and PSVT are usually not life-threatening, they may be refractory to pharmacologic or pacing interventions. In such cases surgery may be considered as a method of removing the abnormal focus, interrupting the reentry circuits, and curing the tachycardia or controlling the ventricular response by creating AV block. In atrial flutter and AF the pathophysiologic substrate cannot be identified; thus, the only surgical option is to destroy the AV node–His bundle region by cryosurgery or transvenous catheter electroablation. Surgery, cryoablation, or electrode catheter ablation requires concomitant implantation of a permanent pacemaker. Focal atrial tachycardias have been treated surgically by discrete resection or ablation by cryothermal injury. Mapping the tachycardia is mandatory if a primary direct approach on the arrhythmia is to be performed. Surgery is for patients with arrhythmias refractory to other treatments and only when the tachycardia has been localized.

VENTRICULAR TACHYCARDIA The demonstration that VT due to ischemic heart disease can often be reliably induced by programmed stimulation and that the arrhythmia is localized to a small region of endocardium in the area of prior infarction has permitted the development of specific surgical techniques for the cure of the arrhythmia.

Preoperatively all morphologically distinct tachycardias that occur spontaneously are induced by programmed stimulation, and their respective sites of origin are determined by catheter activation mapping. Catheter mapping may be supplemented by intraoperative mapping, involving similar techniques. These studies have shown that tachycardias arise in the scar tissue near the endocardium.

Subendocardial resection and endocardial encircling ventriculotomy or cryoablation, the surgical techniques that have been applied to the management of ventricular tachycardia, are aimed at removing or isolating the pathophysiologic substrate of the arrhythmia, as identified by mapping. The major criterion for surgical success is the ability to localize the site from which the arrhythmias arise.

REFERENCES

ANDERSON JL: Effectiveness of sotalol for therapy of complex ventricular arrhythmias and comparisons with placebo and Class I antiarrhythmic drugs. Am J Cardiol 65(2):37, 1990

BAR FW et al: Differential diagnosis of tachycardia with narrow QRS complex (shorter than 0.12 seconds). Am J Cardiol 54:555, 1984

BHANDARI AK, SCHEINMAN M: The long QT syndrome. Mod Concepts Cardiovasc Dis 54:45, 1985

BOINEAU JP: Atrial flutter: A synthesis of concepts. Circulation 72:249, 1985

———, COX JL: Rationale for a direct surgical approach to control ventricular arrhythmias. Relation of specific intraoperative techniques for mechanism and location of arrhythmia circuit. Am J Cardiol 49:381, 1982

BREITHARDT G et al: *Nonpharmacological Therapy of Tachyarrhythmias*. Mt Kisco, NY, Futura, 1987

BRUGADA P, WELLENS HJJ (eds): *Cardiac Arrhythmias: Where To Go from Here?* Mt Kisco, NY, Futura, 1987

BURDITT DG, BENSON DW: *Cardiac Preexcitation Syndromes*. Boston, Martinus Nijhoff, 1986

FRAME LN, HOFFMAN BF: Mechanisms of tachycardia, in *Tachycardias*, B Surawicz (ed). Boston, Martinus Nijhoff, 1984

——— et al. Atrial reentry around an anatomic barrier with a partially refractory excitatory gap. Circ Res 58:495, 1986

JOSEPHSON ME: Paroxysmal supraventricular tachycardia: An electrophysiologic approach. Am J Cardiol 41:1123, 1978

———, SEIDES SF: *Clinical Cardiac Electrophysiology: Techniques and Interpretations*. Philadelphia, Lea & Febiger, 1979

———, WELLENS HJJ (eds): *Tachycardias: Mechanisms, Diagnosis, Treatment*. Philadelphia, Lea & Febiger, 1984

KUPPERMANN M, et al: An analysis of the cost effectiveness of the implantable defibrillator. Circulation 81(1):91, 1990

MANOLIS AS, ESTES, NAM III: Value of programmed ventricular stimulation in the evaluation and management of patients with nonsustained ventricular tachycardia associated with coronary artery disease. Am J Cardiol 65(3):201, 1990

WARD DE, CAMM AJ: *Clinical Electrophysiology of the Heart*. Baltimore, Edward Arnold, 1987

WINKLE RA, THOMAS A: The automatic implantable cardioverter defibrillator: The U.S. Experience, in *Cardiac Arrhythmias: Where to Go from Here?* Brugada P, Wellens HJJ (eds). Mt Kisco, NY, Futura, 1987

186 CONGENITAL HEART DISEASE

WILLIAM F. FRIEDMAN / JOHN S. CHILD

Congenital heart disease complicates approximately 1 percent of all live births. Substantial numbers of affected infants reach adulthood because of successful medical and/or surgical management, or because the alteration in cardiovascular physiology caused by the defect is well tolerated.

GENERAL CONSIDERATIONS

ETIOLOGY AND PREVENTION Congenital cardiovascular malformations are generally the result of aberrant embryonic development of a normal structure, or failure of such a structure to progress beyond an early stage of embryonic or fetal development. Malformations are due to complex multifactorial genetic and environmental causes. Recognized chromosomal aberrations and mutations of single genes account for less than 10 percent of all cardiac malformations (Table 186-1).

The presence of a cardiac malformation as one component of the multiple system involvement in Down's, Turner's, and the trisomy 13-15(D_1) and 17-18 (E) syndromes may be anticipated in occasional pregnancies by detection of abnormal chromosomes in fetal cells obtained from amniotic fluid or chorionic villus biopsy. Identification in such cells of the enzyme disorders characteristic of Hurler's

TABLE 186-1 Syndromes with associated cardiovascular involvement

Syndrome	Major cardiovascular manifestations	Major noncardiac abnormalities
HERITABLE AND POSSIBLY HERITABLE		
Ellis–van Creveld	Single atrium or atrial septal defect	Chondrodystrophic dwarfism, nail dysplasia, polydactyly
TAR (thrombocytopenia-absent radius)	Atrial septal defect, tetralogy of Fallot	Radial aplasia or hypoplasia, thrombocytopenia
Holt-Oram	Atrial septal defect (other defects common)	Skeletal upper limb defect, hypoplasia of clavicles
Kartagener	Dextrocardia	Situs inversus, sinusitis, bronchiectasis
Laurence-Moon-Biedl	Variable defects	Retinal pigmentation, obesity, polydactyly
Noonan	Pulmonary valve dysplasia, cardiomyopathy (usually hypertrophic)	Webbed neck, pectus excavatum, cryptorchidism
Tuberous sclerosis	Rhabdomyoma, cardiomyopathy	Phakomatosis, bone lesions, hamartomatous skin lesions
Multiple lentigines (leopard) syndrome	Pulmonic stenosis	Basal cell nevi, broad facies, rib anomalies
Rubenstein-Taybi	Patent ductus arteriosus (others)	Broad thumbs and toes, hypoplastic maxilla, slanted palpebral fissures
Familial deafness	Arrhythmias, sudden death	Sensorineural deafness
Osler-Rendu-Weber	Arteriovenous fistulas (lung, liver, mucous membranes)	Multiple telangiectasia
Apert	Ventricular septal defect	Craniosynostosis, midfacial hypoplasia, syndactyly
Incontinentia pigmenti	Patent ductus arteriosus	Irregular pigmented skin lesions, patchy alopecia, hypodontia
Alagille (arteriohepatic dysplasia)	Peripheral pulmonic stenosis, pulmonic stenosis	Biliary hypoplasia, vertebral anomalies, prominent forehead, deep-set eyes
DiGeorge	Interrupted aortic arch, tetralogy of Fallot, truncus arteriosus	Thymic hypoplasia or aplasia, parathyroid aplasia or hypoplasia, ear anomalies
Friedreich's ataxia	Cardiomyopathy and conduction defects	Ataxia, speech defect, degeneration of spinal cord dorsal columns
Muscular dystrophy	Cardiomyopathy	Pseudohypertrophy of calf muscles, weakness of trunk and proximal limb muscles
Cystic fibrosis	Cor pulmonale	Pancreatic insufficiency, malabsorption, chronic lung disease
Sickle cell anemia	Cardiomyopathy, mitral regurgitation	Hemoglobin SS
Conradi-Hünermann	Ventricular septal defect, patent ductus arteriosus	Asymmetric limb shortness, early punctate mineralization, large skin pores
Cockayne	Accelerated atherosclerosis	Cachectic dwarfism, retinal pigment abnormalities, photosensitivity dermatitis
Progeria	Accelerated atherosclerosis	Premature aging, alopecia, atrophy of subcutaneous fat, skeletal hypoplasia
CONNECTIVE TISSUE DISORDERS		
Cutis laxa	Peripheral pulmonic stenosis	Generalized disruption of elastic fibers, diminished skin resilience, hernias
Ehlers-Danlos	Arterial dilatation and rupture, mitral regurgitation	Hyperextensible joints, hyperelastic and friable skin
Marfan	Aortic dilatation, aortic and mitral incompetence	Gracile habitus, arachnodactyly with hyperextensibility, lens subluxation
Osteogenesis imperfecta	Aortic incompetence	Fragile bones, blue sclera
Pseudoxanthoma elasticum	Peripheral and coronary arterial disease	Degeneration of elastic fibers in skin, retinal angioid streaks
INBORN ERRORS OF METABOLISM		
Pompe's disease	Glycogen storage disease of heart	Acid maltase deficiency, muscular weakness
Homocystinuria	Aortic and pulmonary arterial dilatation, intravascular thrombosis	Cystathionine synthetase deficiency, lens subluxation, osteoporosis
Mucopolysaccharidosis:		
Hurler, Hunter	Multivalvular and coronary and great artery disease, cardiomyopathy	Hurler: Deficiency of α-L-iduronidase, corneal clouding, coarse features, growth and mental retardation Hunter: Deficiency of L-iduranosulfate sulfatase, coarse facies, clear cornea, growth and mental retardation
Morquio, Scheie, Maroteaux-Lamy	Aortic incompetence	Morquio: Deficiency of *N*-acetylhexosamine sulfate sulfatase, cloudy cornea, normal intelligence, severe bony changes involving vertebrae and epiphyses Scheie: Deficiency of α-L-iduronidase, cloudy cornea, normal intelligence, peculiar facies Maroteaux-Lamy: Deficiency of arylsulfatase B, cloudy cornea, osseous changes, normal intelligence

TABLE 186-1 Syndromes with associated cardiovascular involvement *(continued)*

Syndrome	Major cardiovascular manifestations	Major noncardiac abnormalities
CHROMOSOMAL ABNORMALITIES		
Trisomy 21 (Down's syndrome)	Endocardial cushion defect, atrial or ventricular septal defect, tetralogy of Fallot	Hypotonia, hyperextensible joints, mongoloid facies, mental retardation
Trisomy 13 (D)	Ventricular septal defect, patent ductus arteriosus, double-outlet right ventricle	Single midline intracerebral ventricle with midfacial defects, polydactyly, nail changes, mental retardation
Trisomy 18 (E)	Congenital polyvalvular dysplasia, ventricular septal defect, patent ductus arteriosus	Clenched hand, short sternum, low-arch dermal-ridge pattern on fingertips, mental retardation
Cri-du-chat (short-arm deletion-5)	Ventricular septal defect	Cat cry, microcephaly, antimongoloid slant of palpebral fissures, mental retardation
XO (Turner)	Coarctation of aorta, bicuspid aortic valve	Short female, broad chest, lymphedema, webbed neck
XXXY and XXXXX	Patent ductus arteriosus	XXXY: hypogenitalism, mental retardation, radial-ulnar synostosis XXXXX: small hands, incurving of fifth fingers, mental retardation
SPORADIC DISORDERS		
VATER association	Ventricular septal defect	Vertebral anomalies, anal atresia, tracheo-esophageal fistula, radial and renal anomalies
CHARGE association	Tetralogy of Fallot (other defects common)	Colobomas, choanal atresia, mental and growth deficiency, genital and ear anomalies
Williams	Supravalvular aortic stenosis, peripheral pulmonic stenosis	Mental deficiency, "elfin" facies, loquacious personality, hoarse voice
Cornelia de Lange	Ventricular septal defect	Micromelia, synophrys, mental and growth deficiency
Shprintzen (velocardiofacial)	Ventricular septal defect, tetralogy of Fallot, right aortic arch	Cleft palate, prominent nose, slender hands, learning disability
TERATOGENIC DISORDERS		
Rubella	Patent ductus arteriosus, pulmonic valvular and/or arterial stenosis, atrial septal defect	Cataracts, deafness, microcephaly
Alcohol-induced	Ventricular septal defect (other defects)	Microcephaly, growth and mental deficiency, short palpebral fissures, smooth philtrum, thin upper lip
Phenytoin-induced	Pulmonic stenosis, aortic stenosis, coarctation, patent ductus arteriosus	Hypertelorism, growth and mental deficiency, short phalanges, bowed upper lip
Thalidomide-induced	Variable	Phocomelia
Lithium-induced	Ebstein's anomaly, tricuspid atresia	None

syndrome, homocystinuria, or type II glycogen storage disease may also allow one to predict cardiac disease.

The feasibility of preventive programs will depend upon what is learned in the future about the cause of the majority of cardiovascular anomalies for which no cause is known. An effective rubella vaccine is available, and immunization of children with this vaccine may lessen maternal rubella and its cardiac consequences. Strict testing in animals of new drugs that can be teratogenic when taken early in pregnancy may reduce the chances of another thalidomide tragedy. In this regard, no medications should be taken during pregnancy without prior consultation with a physician. Physicians should be aware of known teratogens, as well as of drugs for which inadequate information exists as to teratogenic potential. Appropriate use of radiologic equipment and techniques for reducing gonadal and fetal radiation exposure should always be employed to reduce the hazards of birth defects.

PATHOPHYSIOLOGY The anatomic and physiologic changes in the heart and circulation due to any specific congenital cardiocirculatory lesion are not static, but rather progress from prenatal life to adulthood. Thus, malformations which are benign, or escape detection in childhood, may become clinically significant in the adult. For example, the functionally normal, congenitally bicuspid aortic valve may thicken and calcify with time, resulting in significant aortic stenosis; or the well-tolerated left-to-right shunt of an atrial septal defect may not result in cardiac decompensation, with or without pulmonary hypertension, until the fourth or fifth decade.

There are issues of particular concern to the *adult* with congenital heart disease that we will discuss separately in this chapter, including pulmonary hypertension and Eisenmenger syndrome of pulmonary vascular obstruction, the hematologic consequences of cyanotic heart disease, the special considerations of pregnancy in the woman with congenital heart disease, and problems involving employability and insurability.

Pulmonary hypertension This is a common accompaniment of many congenital cardiac lesions, and the status of the pulmonary vascular bed is often the principal determinant of the clinical manifestations, the course, and the feasibility of surgical repair. Increases in pulmonary arterial pressure result from elevation of pulmonary blood flow and/or resistance, the latter due sometimes to an increase in vascular tone but usually the result of obstructive, obliterative structural changes within the pulmonary vascular bed. Because pulmonary vascular obstructive disease can be the factor limiting a decision concerning the advisability of operation, it is important to quantify and compare pulmonary to systemic flows and resistances in patients with severe pulmonary hypertension. The causes of pulmonary vascular obstructive disease are unknow although increased pulmonary blood flow, increased pulmonary arterial blood pressure, elevated pulmonary venous pressure, polycythemia, systemic hypoxemia, acidosis, and the bronchial circulation have been implicated. The designation *Eisenmenger syndrome* is applied to patients with a large communication between the two circulations at the aortopulmonary, ventricular, or atrial levels and bidirectional or predominantly right-to-left shunts because of high-resistance and obstructive pulmonary hypertension. No specific treatment has proved beneficial for obstructive pulmonary vascular disease.

Erythrocytosis This is a physiologic response to chronic hypoxemia. The extremely high hematocrits observed in patients with marked arterial oxygen unsaturation cause a progressive increase in blood viscosity, especially beyond packed red blood cell volumes of 60 percent. Both the hematocrit and the circulating whole blood volume are increased in the polycythemia accompanying cyanotic congenital heart disease; the hypervolemia is the result of an increase in red cell volume. The latter provides an increased oxygen-carrying capacity and enhanced oxygen supply to the tissues. The compensatory polycythemia is often of such severity that it becomes a liability and produces adverse physiologic effects, such as thrombotic lesion in diverse organs and a hemorrhagic diathesis. In this regard, oral steroid contraceptives are contraindicated in the cyanotic female because of the enhanced risk of vascular thrombosis. Red cell volume reduction and replacement with plasma or albumin (erythropheresis) lowers blood viscosity and increases systemic blood flow and oxygen transport and so may be helpful in the management of patients with severe hypoxic polycythemia. Acute phlebotomy without fluid replacement is contraindicated. Repeated phlebotomy may cause depletion of iron stores and excessive production of microcytic erythrocytes that are less deformable, thereby raising blood viscosity and adversely influencing blood flow in the microcirculation, respectively.

PREGNANCY The presence of congenital heart disease or its consequences may pose special problems for the pregnant woman. Thus, pregnant women with pulmonary vascular obstruction, whether pre- or postoperative, are at risk of dying during delivery or in the immediate postpartum period. The cause of the increased mortality rate is poorly understood. A particularly high mortality rate has been reported for those undergoing a cesarean section, although such surgery should cause less cardiovascular stress than that of labor and vaginal delivery. Irrespective of approach to delivery, some simple guidelines include both continuous administration of oxygen and avoidance of inhalant anesthetic agents. Arterial blood gases and, if possible, pulmonary arterial and systemic blood pressure should be monitored serially throughout delivery and the early postpartum period. Some physicians advise early abortion in women with marked pulmonary vascular obstruction because of the risks of pregnancy, and all such women should receive counseling on birth control. Intrauterine devices should be avoided because of the risks of bleeding and infection; oral contraceptive agents are contraindicated because they are associated with a tendency to develop pulmonary vascular or cerebrovascular thrombosis. Use of a barrier method of birth control is preferable. Prevention of pregnancy is safer than any form of management during pregnancy, labor, delivery, and the postpartum period.

In women with regurgitant or obstructive left-side valvular lesions the increased volume and/or pressure load on the left atrium or left ventricle imposed by the augmentation in blood volume during pregnancy may result in pulmonary edema, requiring vigorous cardiac decongestive measures (Chap. 36). With medical control of the pulmonary edema, a normal vaginal delivery with careful local and ...idural anesthesia is preferable to nonvaginal delivery.

... problem exists in women whose congenital heart disease ...rrected with the use of a prosthetic cardiac valve and/or ...uch women are at risk for thromboembolism and/or ... of their conduits or valves, and are thus, usually, on anticoagulants. Early in pregnancy coumarin derivatives cause an increase in abortion and stillbirth and in craniofacial, neurologic, and other birth defects. Moreover, the transplacental passage of oral anticoagulants places the fetus at risk of intracranial hemorrhage during delivery. Accordingly, coumarin derivatives should be avoided early (before 10 weeks) and late (after 32 weeks) in pregnancy, and subcutaneous or intravenous heparin should be substituted, although heparin, to a lesser degree, also has been associated with adverse fetal outcome.

INFECTIVE ENDOCARDITIS (See also Chap. 90) Postsurgical patients with prosthetic heterograft or homograft valves or conduits are at particular risk of infective endocarditis. Although routine antimicrobial prophylaxis is recommended for all patients with congenital heart disease and for the majority of patients after operative repair of the lesion, it should be recognized that antibiotic prophylaxis is not uniformly effective. Nonetheless, it is recommended for all dental procedures, gastrointestinal and genitourinary surgery, and diagnostic procedures such as proctosigmoidoscopy and cystoscopy. The risk of endocarditis is undoubtedly related both to the magnitude of bacteremia and to the type of underlying heart disease. Since infection on a prosthetic heart valve or conduit may be devastating, combinations of antibiotics given prophylactically by parenteral route are advisable in these patients.

INSURABILITY Most patients with congenital heart disease must pay significantly more than standard life insurance rates, assuming their anomaly places them in a category that companies have determined is eligible for insurance. There is a paucity of actuarial survival data beyond adolescence for most cardiac lesions that have undergone operative repair. Accordingly, it is often difficult to convince insurance companies to offer insurance at reasonable cost to individual patients whose long term prognosis is quite good.

SPECIFIC CARDIAC DEFECTS

Various classifications of congenital cardiovascular lesions have been proposed, depending on hemodynamic, anatomic, and radiographic factors. Table 186-2 provides a classification of cardiac anomalies that recognizes the general categories of clinical presentation, functional consequences, and site of origin of congenital defects. The text of this section focuses selectively on the more common or important congenital cardiac malformations in adults, whereas Table 186-2 presents a comprehensive list of lesions. Cardiac lesions are organized into those which do or do not result in cyanosis. The acyanotic group is subdivided into malformations with and without a left-to-right shunt. The shunt lesions are segregated by the principal site of communication between the systemic and pulmonary circulations. The acyanotic lesions without a shunt are distinguished by the location of the lesion in the left or right heart and by inflow versus outflow regions on either side of the circulation. Cyanotic lesions are classified with respect to pulmonary blood flow, since the radiographic determination of the magnitude of the latter provides an insight into whether the cyanosis is the result of an obligatory admixture of systemic and pulmonary venous return (increased pulmonary blood flow) or of reduced pulmonary blood flow.

Categorizing the defect(s) in an individual patient requires an answer to a number of basic questions. Is the patient acyanotic or cyanotic? Is pulmonary arterial blood flow increased or not? Does the malformation originate in the left or right side of the heart? Which is the dominant ventricle? Is pulmonary hypertension present or not? With the above information as a foundation, using more refined diagnostic techniques such as echocardiography and Doppler imaging, magnetic resonance imaging, and/or hemodynamic study and angiocardiography leads to a precise anatomic and functional assessment.

TABLE 186-2 Classification of congenital heart disease

GENERAL

Congenitally corrected transposition of the great arteries
The cardiac malpositions
Congenital complete heart block

ACYANOTIC WITH LEFT-TO-RIGHT SHUNT

Atrial level shunt:
1 Atrial septal defect
a Ostium primum
b Ostium secundum
c Sinus venosus
2 Atrial septal defect with mitral stenosis (Lutembacher's syndrome)
3 Partial anomalous pulmonary venous connection

Ventricular level shunt:
1 Ventricular septal defect
a Inlet septum
b Muscular septum
c Perimembranous septum
d Infundibular septum
2 Ventricular septal defect with aortic regurgitation
3 Ventricular septal defect with left ventricular to right atrial shunt

Aortic root to right heart shunt:
1 Ruptured sinus of Valsalva aneurysm
2 Coronary arteriovenous fistula
3 Anomalous origin of the left coronary artery from the pulmonary trunk

Aortopulmonary level shunt:
1 Aortopulmonary window
2 Patent ductus arteriosus

Multiple level shunts:
1 Complete common atrioventricular canal
2 Ventricular septal defect with atrial septal defect
3 Ventricular septal defect with patent ductus arteriosus

ACYANOTIC WITHOUT A SHUNT

Left heart malformations:
1 Congenital obstruction to left atrial inflow
a Pulmonary vein stenosis
b Mitral stenosis
c Cor triatriatum
2 Mitral regurgitation
a Atrioventricular septal (Endocardial cushion)
b Congenitally corrected transposition of the great arteries
c Anomalous origin of the left coronary artery from the pulmonary trunk
d Miscellaneous (double-orifice mitral valve, congenital perforations, accessory commissures with anomalous chordal insertion, congenitally short or absent chordae, cleft posterior leaflet, parachute mitral valve, etc.)
3 Primary dilated endocardial fibroelastosis
4 Aortic stenosis
a Discrete subvalvular
b Valvular
c Supravalvular
5 Aortic valve regurgitation
6 Coarctation of the aorta

Right heart malformations:
1 Acyanotic Ebstein's anomaly of the tricuspid valve
2 Pulmonic stenosis
a Subinfundibular
b Infundibular
c Valvular
d Supravalvular (stenosis of pulmonary artery and its branches)
3 Congenital pulmonary valve regurgitation
4 Idiopathic dilatation of the pulmonary trunk

CYANOTIC

Increased pulmonary blood flow:
1 Complete transposition of the great arteries
2 Double-outlet right ventricle of the Taussig-Bing type
3 Truncus arteriosus
4 Total anomalous pulmonary venous connection
5 Single ventricle without pulmonic stenosis
6 Common atrium
7 Tetralogy of Fallot with pulmonary atresia and increased collateral arterial flow
8 Tricuspid atresia with large ventricular septal defect and no pulmonic stenosis
9 Hypoplastic left heart (aortic atresia, mitral atresia)

TABLE 186-2 Classification of congenital heart disease *(continued)*

CYANOTIC *(continued)*

Normal or decreased pulmonary blood flow:
1 Tricuspid atresia
2 Ebstein's anomaly with right-to-left atrial shunt
3 Pulmonary atresia with intact ventricular septum
4 Pulmonic stenosis or atresia with ventricular septal defect (tetralogy of Fallot)
5 Pulmonic stenosis with right-to-left atrial shunt
6 Complete transposition of the great arteries with pulmonic stenosis
7 Double-outlet right ventricle with pulmonic stenosis
8 Single ventricle with pulmonic stenosis
9 Pulmonary arteriovenous fistula
10 Vena caval to left atrial communication

SOURCE: Modified from JK Perloff, in *The Clinical Recognition of Congenital Heart Disease*, 3d ed. Philadelphia, Saunders, 1987.

ACYANOTIC CONGENITAL HEART DISEASE WITH A LEFT-TO-RIGHT SHUNT

ATRIAL SEPTAL DEFECT This is a commonly recognized cardiac anomaly in adults, and occurs more frequently in females than in males. Defects of the *sinus venosus* type occur high in the atrial septum near the entry of the superior vena cava, and are associated frequently with anomalous connection of pulmonary veins from the right lung to the junction of the superior vena cava and right atrium. Sinus venosus defects may also occur low in the atrial septum near the inferior vena cava orifice, associated with anomalous connection of the right inferior pulmonary vein to the right atrium. *Ostium primum* anomalies are a form of atrioventricular septal defect that lie immediately adjacent to the atrioventricular valves, either of which may be deformed and incompetent. Ostium primum defects occur commonly in patients with Down's syndrome, although the more complex atrioventricular septal defects with a common atrioventricular valve and a posterior defect of the basal portion of the interventricular septum are more characteristic of this chromosomal defect. Most often an atrial defect involves the fossa ovalis, is midseptal in location, and is of the *ostium secundum* type. This type of defect should not be confused with a *patent foramen ovale*. Anatomic obliteration of the foramen ovale ordinarily follows its functional closure soon after birth, but residual "probe patency" is a normal variant; atrial septal defect denotes a true deficiency of the atrial septum, and implies functional and anatomic patency. *Lutembacher's syndrome* is the term applied to the rare combination of atrial septal defect and mitral stenosis; this component of the malformation is usually the result of acquired rheumatic valvulitis.

The magnitude of the left-to-right shunt through an atrial septal defect depends on the size of the defect, the diastolic properties of both ventricles, and the relative impedance in the pulmonary and systemic circulations. The left-to-right shunt causes diastolic overloading of the right ventricle, and increased pulmonary blood flow.

Patients with atrial septal defect are usually asymptomatic in early life, although there may be some physical underdevelopment and an increased tendency for respiratory infections; cardiorespiratory symptoms occur in many older patients. Beyond the fourth decade, a significant number of patients develop atrial arrhythmias, pulmonary arterial hypertension, bidirectional and then right-to-left shunting of blood, and cardiac failure. Patients exposed to the chronic environmental hypoxia of high altitude tend to develop pulmonary hypertension at younger ages. In some older patients, left-to-right shunting across the defect increases as progressive systemic hypertension and/or coronary artery disease result in reduced compliance of the left ventricle.

Physical examination Examination usually reveals a prominent right ventricular cardiac impulse and palpable pulmonary artery pulsation. The first heart sound is normal or split, with accentuation of the tricuspid valve closure sound. Increased flow across the pulmonic valve is responsible for a midsystolic pulmonary ejection murmur. The second heart sound is widely split and is relatively fixed in relation to respiration. A middiastolic rumbling murmur, loudest at the fourth intercostal space and along the left sternal border, reflects increased flow across the tricuspid valve. In patients with ostium primum defects, an apical thrill and holosystolic murmur indicate associated mitral or tricuspid incompetence or a ventricular septal defect.

The physical findings are altered when an increase in the pulmonary vascular resistance results in diminution of the left-to-right shunt. Both the pulmonary and tricuspid murmurs decrease in intensity, the pulmonic component of the second heart sound and a systolic ejection sound are accentuated, the two components of the second heart sound may fuse, and a diastolic murmur of pulmonic incompetence appears. Cyanosis and clubbing accompany the development of a right-to-left shunt.

In adults with atrial fibrillation and an atrial septal defect, the physical findings may be confused with the findings of mitral stenosis with pulmonary hypertension, since the tricuspid flow murmur and widely split second heart sound may be mistakenly thought to represent the diastolic murmur of mitral stenosis and the mitral "opening snap," respectively.

Electrocardiogram In patients with an ostium secundum defect the ECG usually shows right axis deviation and an rSr′ pattern in the right precordial leads, representing delayed posterobasal activation of the ventricular septum. Right ventricular hypertrophy is common in children but not adults. An ectopic atrial pacemaker or first-degree heart block occurs occasionally in patients with defects of the sinus venosus type. In patients with an ostium primum defect, the right ventricular conduction defect is characteristically accompanied by left axis deviation and by superior orientation and counterclockwise rotation of the QRS loop in the frontal plane. Varying degrees of right ventricular and right atrial hypertrophy may occur with each type of defect, depending on the height of the pulmonary artery pressure; prolongation of the PR interval is most common with ostium primum defects. *Chest roentgenograms* reveal enlargement of the right atrium and ventricle, dilatation of the pulmonary artery and its branches, and increased pulmonary vascular marking. Left atrial enlargement is uncommon in the absence of atrial fibrillation.

Echocardiogram This shows pulmonary arterial and right ventricular dilatation, and anterior systolic (paradoxical) or flat interventricular septal motion if a significant right ventricular volume overload is present. The defect may be visualized directly from subcostal, right parasternal, or apical echocardiographic windows. In most institutions, two-dimensional echocardiography, supplemented by conventional or color Doppler flow examination, has supplanted cardiac catheterization as the confirmatory test for atrial septal defect. Cardiac catheterization is then employed if inconsistencies exist in the clinical data, if significant pulmonary hypertension or associated malformations are suspected, or if coronary artery disease is a possibility.

Management Operative repair, ideally in children between 3 and 6 years of age, should be advised for all patients with uncomplicated atrial septal defects in whom there is significant left-to-right shunting, i.e., with pulmonary-to-systemic flow ratios exceeding approximately 2.0:1.0. Excellent results may be anticipated, at low risk, even in patients beyond 40 years of age in the absence of pulmonary hypertension. The defect is closed, usually with a patch of prosthetic material with the patient on cardiopulmonary bypass. In patients with ...m defects cleft, deformed, and incompetent valves often ...r. Operation should not be carried out in patients with ...s and trivial left-to-right shunts, or in those with severe ...vascular disease without a significant left-to-right shunt.

Atrioventricular septal defects more complex than the ostium primum defect are associated with failure to thrive, heart failure, and pulmonary hypertension early in life, and require operative correction in infancy. Patients with atrial septal defect of the sinus venosus or ostium secundum types rarely die before the fifth decade. During the fifth and sixth decades the incidence of progressive symptoms, often leading to severe disability, increases substantially. Medical management should include prompt treatment of respiratory tract infections, antiarrhythmic medications for atrial fibrillation or supraventricular tachycardia, and the usual measures for hypertension, coronary disease, or heart failure (see Chap. 182), if these complications occur. Although the risk of infective endocarditis is quite low, antibiotics should be administered prophylactically prior to dental and other indicated diagnostic or surgical procedures (see Chap. 90).

VENTRICULAR SEPTAL DEFECT Defects of the ventricular septum are common as isolated defects and as one component of a combination of anomalies. The opening is usually single and situated in the membranous portion of the septum. The functional disturbance is dependent primarily on its size and on the status of the pulmonary vascular bed, rather than on the location of the defect. Only small or moderate-size defects are usually seen initially in adulthood since the vast majority of patients with isolated large defects come to medical and, often, surgical attention very early in life.

A wide spectrum exists in the natural history of ventricular septal defect, ranging from spontaneous closure to congestive cardiac failure and death in early infancy. Within this spectrum is the possible development of pulmonary vascular obstruction, right ventricular outflow tract obstruction, aortic regurgitation, and infective endocarditis. Spontaneous closure is more common in patients born with a small ventricular septal defect, and occurs in early childhood in most patients.

Patients with large ventricular septal defects and pulmonary hypertension are those at greatest risk for developing pulmonary vascular obstruction. Thus, large defects should be corrected surgically very early in life when pulmonary vascular disease is still reversible or not yet developed. In patients with severe pulmonary vascular obstruction (Eisenmenger syndrome), symptoms in adult life consist of exertional dyspnea, chest pain, syncope, and hemoptysis. The right-to-left shunt leads to cyanosis, clubbing, and erythrocytosis. In all patients, the degree to which pulmonary vascular resistance is elevated before operation is a critical factor determining prognosis. If the pulmonary vascular resistance is one-third or less of the systemic value, progression of pulmonary vascular disease after operation is unusual. However, if a moderate to severe increase in pulmonary vascular resistance exists preoperatively, either no change or a progression of pulmonary vascular disease is common postoperatively.

Right ventricular outflow tract obstruction develops in approximately 5 to 10 percent of patients who present in infancy with a moderate to large left-to-right shunt. With time, as subvalvular right ventricular outflow tract obstruction progresses, the findings in these patients begin to resemble more closely those of the cyanotic tetralogy of Fallot malformation.

In approximately 5 percent of patients, incompetence of the aortic valve results from insufficient cusp tissue or prolapse of the cusp through the interventricular defect; the aortic regurgitation then complicates and usually dominates the clinical course.

Two-dimensional *echocardiography* with conventional or color Doppler examination can usually define the number and location of defects in the ventricular septum, and detect associated anomalies. Hemodynamic and angiographic study may be employed to assess the status of the pulmonary vascular bed and clarify details of the altered anatomy.

Management Surgical treatment is not recommended for patients who have normal pulmonary arterial pressures with small shunts (pulmonary-to-systemic flow ratios of less than 1.5 to 2.0:1.0). Operative correction is indicated when there is a moderate to large left-to-right shunt with a pulmonary-to-systemic flow ratio that exceeds

1.5:1.0 or 2.0:1.0, in the absence of prohibitively high levels of pulmonary vascular resistance.

AORTIC ROOT TO RIGHT HEART SHUNTS Three malformations, congenital aneurysm of an aortic sinus of Valsalva with fistula, coronary arteriovenous fistula, and anomalous origin of the left coronary artery from the pulmonary trunk, are the most common causes of aortic root to right heart shunts. *Aneurysm of an aortic sinus of Valsalva,* particularly the right coronary sinus, consist of a separation or lack of fusion between the media of the aorta and the annulus fibrosis of the aortic valve. Rupture usually occurs in the third or fourth decade of life; the receiving chamber of the aortico-cardiac fistula is most often the right ventricle, but occasionally, when the noncoronary cusp is involved, the fistula drains into the right atrium. Abrupt rupture causes chest pain and creates bounding pulses, a continuous murmur accentuated in diastole, and volume overload of the heart. Diagnosis is confirmed by two-dimensional and Doppler echocardiographic studies; cardiac catheterization quantifies the left-to-right shunt, and thoracic aortography visualizes the fistula. Medical management is directed at cardiac failure, arrhythmias, or endocarditis. At operation, the aneurysm is closed and amputated and the aortic wall is reunited with the heart, either by direct suture or with a prosthesis.

Coronary arteriovenous fistula, an unusual anomaly, consists of a communication between a coronary artery and another cardiac chamber, usually the coronary sinus or right atrium or ventricle. The shunt is usually of small magnitude, and myocardial blood flow is not usually compromised. Potential complications include infective endocarditis, thrombus formation with occlusion or distal embolization, rupture of an aneurysmal fistula, and rarely, pulmonary hypertension and congestive failure. The finding of a loud, superficial, continuous murmur at the lower or midsternal border usually prompts a further evaluation of asymptomatic patients. Doppler echocardiography demonstrates the site of drainage; if the site of origin is proximal it may be detectable by two-dimensional echocardiography. Retrograde thoracic aortography or coronary arteriography permits identification of the size and anatomic features of the fistulous tract, which may be closed by suture obliteration.

The third anomaly causing a shunt from the aortic root to the right heart is *anomalous origin of the left coronary artery from the pulmonary artery*. As the elevated pulmonary vascular resistance declines immediately after birth, perfusion of the left coronary artery from the pulmonary artery ceases and the direction of flow in the anomalous vessel reverses. Total myocardial perfusion must pass through the right coronary artery and may be sufficient if adequate collateral channels develop between the two coronary circulations. Myocardial infarction and fibrosis commonly lead to death within the first year, though up to 20 percent of patients survive to adolescence and beyond without surgical correction. In older children or adults mitral regurgitation may result from dysfunction of ischemic or infarcted papillary muscles. The diagnosis of anomalous origin of the coronary artery is supported by the electrocardiographic findings of an anterolateral myocardial infarction. Aortic root or coronary angiography demonstrates the retrograde drainage of the coronary vessel into the pulmonary artery and the presence of a single right coronary artery arising from the aorta. Operative management of adults consists of coronary artery bypass with an internal mammary artery graft or saphenous vein–coronary artery graft. The outcome and prognosis are determined largely by the degree of preoperative myocardial damage.

PATENT DUCTUS ARTERIOSUS The ductus arteriosus is a vessel leading from the bifurcation of the pulmonary artery to the aorta just distal to the left subclavian artery. The vascular channel is open normally in the fetus, but closes immediately after birth. The flow across the ductus is determined by the pressure and resistance relationships between the systemic and pulmonary circulations, and by the cross-sectional area and length of the ductus. In most adults with this anomaly pulmonary pressures are normal and a gradient and shunt from aorta to pulmonary artery persist throughout the cardiac cycle, resulting in a characteristic thrill and a continuous "machinery" murmur with a late systolic accentuation at the upper left sternal edge. In adults who were born with a large left-to-right shunt through the ductus arteriosus, pulmonary vascular obstruction (Eisenmenger syndrome) with pulmonary hypertension, right-to-left shunting, and cyanosis have usually developed. Severe pulmonary vascular disease results in reversal of flow through the ductus, unoxygenated blood is shunted to the descending aorta, and the toes, but not the fingers become cyanotic and clubbed, a finding termed *differential cyanosis*. The leading causes of death in adults with patent ductus are cardiac failure and infective endocarditis; occasionally severe pulmonary vascular obstruction may cause aneurysmal dilatation, calcification, and rupture of the ductus. In the absence of severe pulmonary vascular disease and predominant left-to-right shunting of blood, the patent ductus should be surgically ligated or divided. Operation should be deferred for several months in patients treated successfully for infective endocarditis, because the ductus may remain somewhat edematous and friable.

ACYANOTIC CONGENITAL HEART DISEASE WITHOUT A SHUNT

CONGENITAL AORTIC STENOSIS Malformations that cause obstruction to left ventricular outflow include congenital valvular aortic stenosis, discrete subaortic stenosis, supervalvular aortic stenosis, and hypertrophic obstructive cardiomyopathy (Chap. 192).

Valvular aortic stenosis Valvular aortic stenosis occurs three to four times more often in males than in females. The congenital bicuspid aortic valve, which is not necessarily stenotic, is one of the most common congenital malformations of the heart, although it may go undetected in early life. Because bicuspid valves may become stenotic with time or be the site of infective endocarditis, the lesion may be difficult to distinguish in adults from acquired rheumatic or degenerative calcific aortic stenosis.

The dynamics of blood flow associated with a congenitally deformed, rigid aortic valve commonly lead to thickening of the cusps and, in later life, to calcification. Hemodynamically significant obstruction causes concentric hypertrophy of the left ventricular wall and dilatation of the ascending aorta.

The hemodynamic abnormalities are discussed in Chap. 188. A peak systolic pressure gradient exceeding 70 mmHg, in association with abnormal cardiac output, or an effective aortic orifice less than 0.6 cm^2 per square meter of body surface, is considered to represent critical obstruction to left ventricular outflow. In adults, the resting cardiac output is generally normal but often fails to rise normally during muscular exercise.

Many patients with congenital aortic stenosis are asymptomatic. Usually, a murmur is detected on a routine examination. Moderately severe obstruction should be suspected if there is a history of fatigability and exertional dyspnea. With severe obstruction, the inability of the left ventricle to increase its output and maintain cerebral flow during exercise may result in exertional syncope, and the disparity between the oxygen supply and myocardial oxygen requirements may cause angina. The symptomatic patient with valvular aortic stenosis generally has critical stenosis, although a lack of symptoms does not preclude the presence of moderately severe obstruction. Sudden death occurs in patients with critical stenosis, and ventricular arrhythmias, perhaps initiated by acute myocardial ischemia, may be responsible.

Hemodynamically significant obstruction is associated with a left ventricular lift and a precordial systolic thrill over the base of the heart, with transmission to the jugular notch and along the carotid arteries. Presystolic expansion is often palpable. A systolic aortic ejection sound, signifying opening of the aortic valve, is typically heard best at the cardiac apex when the valve is mobile, particularly with mild to moderate stenosis. A fourth heart sound is generally associated with severe obstruction. The systolic murmur starts after the completion of left ventricular isometric contraction, is rhomboid-shaped, loud, harsh, and best heard at the base of the heart. The murmur, like the thrill, radiates to the jugular notch and carotid vessels and to the apex. An early diastolic blowing murmur of aortic regurgitation may be present, but unless the valve has been eroded by infective endocarditis the regurgitation is usually not hemodynamically significant; rarely, in patients with a congenital bicuspid valve, severe aortic regurgitation may be the dominant hemodynamic lesion.

Electrocardiographic evidence of left ventricular hypertrophy tends to reflect the severity of obstruction, although a normal or near-normal electrocardiogram does not exclude severe aortic stenosis. The left ventricular "strain pattern" generally indicates that severe aortic stenosis is present. Two-dimensional echocardiography demonstrates the aortic valve morphology; Doppler echocardiography is the most accurate means of noninvasively estimating the magnitude of obstruction and valvular regurgitation if present. Cardiac catheterization and coronary angiography are indicated particularly if coronary artery disease is suspected.

The medical management of congenital valvular aortic stenosis includes prophylaxis against infective endocarditis and, in patients with diminished cardiac reserve, the administration of digitalis and diuretics and sodium restriction while awaiting operation. If severe aortic stenosis is present, strenuous physical activity should be avoided even when the patient is asymptomatic, and participation in competitive sports should probably be restricted in patients with milder degrees of obstruction. Aortic valve replacement is indicated in asymptomatic adults with severe obstruction, or in patients who are symptomatic with an aortic valve area less than 1.0 cm^2. If surgery is contraindicated because of a complicating medical problem such as malignancy, or renal or hepatic failure, balloon valvuloplasty may provide short term improvement.

Subaortic stenosis The most common form of subaortic stenosis is the *idiopathic hypertrophic* variety, also termed *hypertrophic cardiomyopathy,* which is present at birth in about one-third of the patients and is discussed in Chap. 192. Both clinically and physiologically, the *discrete* form of subaortic stenosis resembles valvular aortic stenosis. The lesion usually consists of a membranous diaphragm or fibrous ring encircling the left ventricular outflow tract just beneath the base of the aortic valve. Echocardiography demonstrates the subaortic obstruction; Doppler studies show turbulence proximal to the aortic valve and also detect and quantify aortic regurgitation. Treatment consists of excision of the membrane or fibrous ridge.

Supravalvular aortic stenosis This anomaly consists of a localized or diffuse narrowing of the ascending aorta originating just above the level of the coronary arteries at the superior margin of the sinuses of Valsalva. In contrast to other forms of aortic stenosis, the coronary arteries are subjected to the elevated pressures that exist within the left ventricle and are often dilated and tortuous.

COARCTATION OF THE AORTA Narrowing or constriction of the lumen of the aorta may occur anywhere along its length but is most common distal to the origin of the left subclavian artery near the insertion of the ligamentum arteriosum. Coarctation occurs in about 7 percent of patients with congenital heart disease and is twice as common in males as in females, although the lesion occurs frequently in patients with gonadal dysgenesis. Clinical manifestations depend on the site and extent of obstruction and the presence of associated cardiac anomalies, the most common of which is the bicuspid aortic valve. Aneurysmal dilatation within the arterial supply of the circle of Willis produces a high risk of sudden rupture and death.

[illegible]rity of children and young adults with isolated, discrete [illegible]re asymptomatic. Headache, epistaxis, cold extremities, [illegible]ation with exercise may occur, and attention is usually [illegible] the cardiovascular system when a heart murmur or hypertension in the upper extremities and absence, marked diminution, or delayed pulsations in the femoral arteries are detected on physical examination. Enlarged and pulsatile collateral vessels may be palpated in the intercostal spaces anteriorly, in the axillae, or posteriorly in the interscapular area. The upper extremities and thorax may be more developed than the lower extremities. A midsystolic murmur over the anterior part of the chest, back, and spinous processes may become continuous if the lumen is narrowed sufficiently to result in a high-velocity jet across the lesion throughout the cardiac cycle. Additional systolic and continuous murmurs over the lateral thoracic wall may reflect increased flow through dilated and tortuous collateral vessels. The electrocardiogram reveals left ventricular hypertrophy of varying degree. Roentgenograms may show a dilated left subclavian artery high on the left mediastinal border and a dilated ascending aorta. Indentation of the aorta at the site of coarctation and pre- and poststenotic dilatation (the "3" sign) along the left paramediastinal shadow are almost pathognomonic. Notching of the ribs, an important radiographic sign, is due to erosion by dilated collateral vessels. Two-dimensional echocardiography from para- or suprasternal windows identifies the site and length of coarctation, while Doppler studies record and quantify the pressure gradient. Magnetic resonance imaging or digital angiography allow visualization of the length and severity of the obstruction and the associated collateral arteries. In adults, cardiac catheterization is indicated primarily to evaluate the status of the coronary arteries.

The chief hazards result from severe hypertension and include the development of cerebral aneurysms and hemorrhage, rupture of the aorta, left ventricular failure, and infective endocarditis. Treatment is surgical; resection and end-to-end anastomosis or subclavian flap angioplasty are employed commonly, although it may be necessary to use a tubular graft, patch, or bypass conduit if the narrowed segment is long. Systemic hypertension postoperatively, in the absence of residual coarctation, appears to be related to the duration of preoperative hypertension.

PULMONARY STENOSIS WITH INTACT VENTRICULAR SEPTUM Obstruction to right ventricular outflow may be localized to the supravalvular, valvular, or subvalvular levels or occur at a combination of these sites. Multiple sites of narrowing of the peripheral pulmonary arteries are a feature of *rubella embryopathy* and may occur with both the familial and sporadic forms of supravalvular aortic stenosis. Valvular pulmonic stenosis is the most common form of isolated right ventricular obstruction.

The severity of the obstructing lesion, rather than the site of narrowing, is the most important determinant of the clinical course. In the presence of a normal cardiac output, a peak systolic transvalvular pressure gradient between 50 and 80 mmHg is considered to be moderate stenosis; levels below and above that range are classified as mild and severe, respectively. Patients with mild pulmonic stenosis are generally asymptomatic and demonstrate little or no progression in the severity of obstruction with age. In patients with more significant stenosis, the severity may increase with time. Symptoms vary with the degree of obstruction. Fatigue, dyspnea, right ventricular failure, and syncope may limit the activity of older patients, in whom moderate or severe obstruction may prevent an augmentation of cardiac output with exercise. In patients with severe obstruction, the systolic pressure in the right ventricle may exceed that in the left ventricle, since the ventricular septum is intact. Right ventricular ejection is prolonged with moderate or severe stenosis, and the sound of pulmonary valve closure is delayed and soft. Right ventricular hypertrophy reduces the compliance of that chamber, and a forceful right atrial contraction is necessary to augment right ventricular filling. A fourth heart sound, prominent *a* waves in the jugular venous pulse, and occasionally, presystolic pulsations of the liver reflect vigorous atrial contraction. The clinical diagnosis is supported by a right parasternal lift and harsh systolic ejection murmur and thrill at the upper left sternal border, typically preceded by a systolic ejection sound, if the obstruction is valvular. The holosystolic decrescendo murmur of tricuspid regurgitation may accompany severe pulmonic stenosis, especially in the presence of congestive heart failure. Cyanosis usually reflects venoarterial shunting through a patent foramen ovale or atrial septal defect. In patients with supravalvular or peripheral pulmonary arterial stenosis, the murmur is systolic or continuous and is best heard over the area of narrowing, with radiation to the peripheral lung fields.

The *electrocardiogram* may be helpful in assessing the degree of obstruction to right ventricular output. In mild cases, the electrocardiogram is often normal, whereas moderate and severe stenoses are associated with right axis deviation and right ventricular hypertrophy. A ventricular strain pattern, as well as high-amplitude P waves in leads II and V_1, indicating right atrial enlargement, is associated with severe stenosis. The chest roentgenogram with mild or moderate pulmonic stenosis often shows a heart of normal size and normal vascularity of the lungs. In the presence of valvular stenosis, poststenotic dilatation of the main and left pulmonary arteries may be evident. With severe obstruction and resultant right ventricular failure, right atrial and ventricular enlargement are generally evident. The pulmonary vascularity may be reduced with severe stenosis, right ventricular failure, and/or a venoarterial shunt at the atrial level.

Two dimensional *echocardiography* visualizes pulmonary valve morphology; the outflow tract pressure gradient can be estimated by Doppler ultrasonography. The cardiac catheter technique of balloon valvuloplasty (Chap. 179) is often effective. Direct surgical relief of moderate and severe obstruction may be accomplished at a low risk. Multiple stenosis of the peripheral pulmonary arteries are usually inoperable, but narrowing of a single branch or at the bifurcation of the main pulmonary trunk may be corrected.

CYANOTIC CONGENITAL HEART DISEASE WITH INCREASED PULMONARY BLOOD FLOW

COMPLETE TRANSPOSITION OF THE GREAT ARTERIES In this condition the aorta arises from the right ventricle to the right of and anterior to the pulmonary artery, which emerges from the left ventricle. This results in two separate and parallel circulations, and some communication between the two circulations must exist after birth to sustain life. Most patients have an interatrial communication, two-thirds have a patent ductus arteriosus, and about one-third have an associated ventricular septal defect. Transposition is more common in males and accounts for approximately 10 percent of cyanotic heart disease.

The course is determined by the degree of tissue hypoxia, the ability of each ventricle to sustain an increased work load in the presence of reduced coronary arterial oxygenation, the nature of the associated cardiovascular anomalies, and the status of the pulmonary vascular bed. Severe morphologic alterations develop in the pulmonary vascular bed by 1 to 2 years of age in most patients who also have an associated large ventricular septal defect or large patent ductus arteriosus in the absence of obstruction to left ventricular outflow.

Surgical treatment The creation or enlargement of an interatrial communication is the simplest procedure for providing increased intracardiac mixing of systemic and pulmonary venous blood; it may be achieved surgically or, preferably, by rupturing the valve of the foramen ovale with a balloon catheter during cardiac catheterization (Rashkind's procedure). Systemic-pulmonary artery anastomosis may be indicated in the patient with severe obstruction to left ventricular outflow and diminished pulmonary blood flow. Intracardiac repair may be accomplished by rearranging the venous returns so that the systemic venous blood is directed to the mitral valve and thence to the left ventricle and pulmonary artery, while the pulmonary venous blood is diverted through the tricuspid valve and right ventricle to the aorta (Mustard or Senning operation). Many surgeons now prefer to correct this malformation in infancy by transposing both coronary arteries to the posterior artery and transecting, contraposing, and anastomosing the aorta and pulmonary arteries (Jatene or arterial switch operation). For those patients with a ventricular septal defect in whom it is necessary to bypass a severely obstructed left ventricular outflow tract, corrective operation employs an intracardiac ventricular baffle and extracardia prosthetic conduit to replace the pulmonary artery (Rastelli's procedure). Patients with a large ventricular septal defect require closure of the ventricular septal defect and the atrial switch operation early in infancy. There are now many adults who underwent venous switch repair early in life who are experiencing the long-term complications of that operation, including arrhythmias, baffle leaks, or obstruction and reduced performance of the systemic right ventricle.

TOTAL ANOMALOUS PULMONARY VENOUS CONNECTION In this malformation all the pulmonary veins connect either to the right atrium directly or to the systemic veins or their tributaries. Because all venous blood returns to the right atrium, an interatrial communication is an integral part of this malformation. Most unoperated patients surviving to adult life have pulmonary vascular obstructive disease, a reduction in pulmonary blood flow, and cyanosis.

SINGLE VENTRICLE This designation applies to a family of complex lesions with both atrioventricular valves or a common atrioventricular valve opening to a single ventricular chamber. In most patients, the single ventricle morphologically resembles a left ventricular chamber that is separated from an infundibular outlet chamber by a bulboventricular septum; in these cases the anomaly is often referred to as double-inlet left ventricle. Associated anomalies are common and include abnormal great artery positional relationships, pulmonic valvular or subvalvular stenosis, and subaortic stenosis.

Depending upon the associated anomalies, the clinical presentation of single ventricle mimics other conditions in which cyanosis and decreased (or increased) pulmonary blood flow coexist, e.g., tetralogy of Fallot in the former instance and complete transposition of the great arteries in the latter. Survival to adolescence and adulthood depends upon a relatively normal pulmonary blood flow and good ventricular function. Correction of the defect usually consists of creation of a right atrial–pulmonary conduit (the Fontan procedure); some patients are candidates for a septation operation, in which the single ventricle is partitioned with a prosthetic patch.

CYANOTIC CONGENITAL HEART DISEASE WITH DECREASED PULMONARY BLOOD FLOW

TRICUSPID ATRESIA Atresia of the tricuspid valve, an interatrial communication, and, frequently, hypoplasia of the right ventricle and pulmonary artery exist in this malformation. Because of the small or nearly absent right ventricle, this anomaly is basically a "univentricular" heart with a single inlet (mitral) to the left ventricle. The clinical picture is usually dominated by severe cyanosis as a result of obligatory admixture of systemic and pulmonary venous blood in the left ventricle. The electrocardiogram characteristically shows right atrial enlargement, left axis deviation, and left ventricular hypertrophy.

Atrial septostomy and palliative operations to increase pulmonary blood flow, often by systemic arterial or venous–pulmonary artery anastomosis may allow survival to the second or third decade. A Fontan atriopulmonary connection may then allow functional correction in those patients with normal or low pulmonary arterial resistance pressure and good left ventricular function.

EBSTEIN'S ANOMALY This malformation is characterized by a downward displacement of the tricuspid valve into the right ventricle, due to anomalous attachment of the tricuspid leaflets. Tricuspid valve tissue is dysplastic; a variable portion of the septal and inferior cusps adhere to the right ventricular wall some distance away from the atrioventricular junction. The abnormally situated tricuspid orifice produces a portion of the right ventricle lying between the atriover tricular ring and the origin of the valve, which is continuous with the right atrial chamber. This proximal segment is "atrialized," and the distal ventricular chamber is small. The degree of impairment of right ventricular function depends primarily on the extent to which the right ventricular inflow portion is atrialized, and on the magnitude of tricuspid valve regurgitation. Most patients survive at least to the third decade. Although the clinical manifestations are variable, some patients come to initial attention because of progressive cyanosis from right-to-left atrial shunting, or symptoms due to tricuspid regurgitation and right ventricular dysfunction, or paroxysmal atrial tachyarrhythmias with or without bypass tracts (type B Wolff-Parkinson-White syndrome is common). Diagnostic findings by two-dimensional echocardiography include the abnormal positional relation between the tricuspid and mitral valves with apical displacement of the septal tricuspid leaflet. Tricuspid regurgitation is detected and quantified by Doppler examination. Surgical approaches have included prosthetic replacement of the tricuspid valve when the leaflets are tethered, or, in patients within elongated mobil anterior leaflet, creation of a competent, unicuspid valve by insertion of the elongated anterior leaflet into the original tricuspid annulus and plication of the atrialized right ventricle. Transection of bypass tracts may be necessary to abolish atrial tachyarrhythmias.

TETRALOGY OF FALLOT This malformation is responsible for about 10 percent of all forms of congenital heart disease and is the most common cause of cyanotic forms. The four components of the tetralogy of Fallot are ventricular septal defect, obstruction to right ventricular outflow, aortic override (straddle) of the ventricular septal defect, and right ventricular hypertrophy. The basic anomaly results from an anterior and superior deviation of the infundibular ventricular septum away from its usual location in the heart between the limbs of the trabecular septum. This displacement causes subpulmonary obstruction, aortic "override," and a large, nonrestrictive, malalignment-type ventricular septal defect.

The severity of obstruction to right ventricular outflow determines the clinical presentation. The severity of hypoplasia of the outflow tract of the right ventricle varies from mild to complete (pulmonary atresia). Pulmonary valve stenosis and supravalvular and peripheral pulmonary arterial obstruction may coexist; rarely there is unilateral absence of a pulmonary artery (usually the left). A right-sided aortic arch and descending aorta occur in about 25 percent of patients with tetralogy. The coronary arteries may have variations that are surgically important. The anterior descending artery sometimes originates from the right coronary artery, which may also give rise to a left branch coursing anterior to the infundibulum; a single left coronary artery may give rise to a branch that crosses the outflow tract of the right ventricle. Associated noncardiac anomalies are present in 20 to 30 percent of patients.

The relationship between the resistance to blood flow from the ventricles into the aorta and into the pulmonary vessels plays a major role in determining the hemodynamic and clinical picture. Thus, the severity of obstruction to right ventricular outflow is of fundamental significance. In many infants and children the obstruction is mild but progressive. When the obstruction is severe, the pulmonary blood flow is reduced markedly, and large volume of desaturated systemic venous blood is shunted from right to left across the ventricular septal defect. Severe cyanosis and polycythemia occur, and symptoms and sequelae of systemic hypoxemia are prominent.

The *electrocardiogram* ordinarily shows right ventricular and, less often, right atrial hypertrophy. Radiologic examination characteristically reveals a normal-sized, boot-shaped heart (*coeur en sabot*) with prominence of the right ventricle and a concavity in the region of the pulmonary conus. The pulmonary vascular markings are typically diminished, and the aortic arch and knob may be on the [illegible] Two-dimensional echocardiography from the parasternal [illegible]indows demonstrates the malalignment of the ventricular [illegible] and the subpulmonary stenosis. The presence or absence [illegible]t the origins of the main branch pulmonary arteries can also be assessed. Selective angiocardiography with right ventricular injection provides architectural details of the right ventricular outflow tract, pulmonary valve and annulus, and caliber of the main branches of the pulmonary artery; coronary arteriography identifies the anatomy and course of the coronary arteries.

Factors that may complicate the management of patients with tetralogy of Fallot include infective endocarditis, paradoxic embolism, polycythemia, coagulation defects, and cerebral infarction or abscess. Corrective operation is advisable at some point for almost all patients with this anomaly. Successful correction avoids progressive infundibular obstruction, delayed growth, and complications due to hypoxemia and polycythemia. The size of the pulmonary arteries rather than the age or size of the infant or child is the most important determinant in establishing candidacy for primary repair. Pronounced hypoplasia of the pulmonary arteries is a relative contraindication for an early corrective surgical procedure. When this problem is present, a palliative operation, such as creation of a systemic arterial–pulmonary arterial shunt, is carried out and is usually followed by complete correction, which can be carried out at a lower risk later in childhood.

OTHER FORMS OF CONGENITAL HEART DISEASE

CONGENITALLY CORRECTED TRANSPOSITION The two fundamental anatomic abnormalities in this malformation are transposition of the ascending aorta and pulmonary trunk and inversion of the ventricles. This arrangement results in desaturated systemic venous blood passing from the right atrium through the mitral valve to the left ventricle and into the pulmonary trunk; whereas arterialized pulmonary venous blood flows from the left atrium through the tricuspid valve to the right ventricle and into the aorta. Thus, the circulation is corrected functionally. The clinical presentation, course, and prognosis of patients with congenitally corrected transposition vary depending on the nature and severity of any complicating intracardiac anomalies. Ebstein-type anomalies of the left-side tricuspid atrioventricular valve, ventricular septal defect, obstruction to outflow from the venous ventricle, and congenital heart block are often associated with corrected transposition. The diagnosis of the malformation and associated lesions can often be established by two-dimensional echocardiography and Doppler examination.

MALPOSITIONS OF THE HEART Positional anomalies refer to conditions in which the cardiac apex is in the right side of the chest (dextrocardia), or at the midline (mesocardia), or in which there is a normal location of the heart in the left side of the chest but abnormal position of the viscera (isolated levocardia). Knowledge of the position of the abdominal organs and of the branching pattern of the main stem bronchi is important in categorizing these malpositions. When dextrocardia occurs *without* situs inversus, when the *visceral situs is indeterminate*, or if *isolated levocardia* is present, associated, often complex, multiple cardiac anomalies are usually present. In contrast, mirror-image dextrocardia is usually observed in a patient with complete situs inversus, a condition which occurs most frequently in individuals whose hearts are otherwise normal.

SURGICALLY MODIFIED CONGENITAL HEART DISEASE

Because of the enormous strides in cardiovascular surgical techniques that have occurred in the past 15 years, a large number of long-term survivors of corrective operations in infancy and childhood have reached adulthood. These patients are often challenging because of the diversity of anatomic, hemodynamic, and electrophysiologic residua and sequelae of cardiac operations.

TABLE 186-3 Potential late postoperative problems

Residual shunts
Residual ventricular outflow obstruction
Residual valvular anomalies
Systemic arterial hypertension
Pulmonary vascular obstruction
Arrhythmias and conduction defects
Myocardial dysfunction
Prosthetic valve malfunction
Prosthetic conduit obstruction
Infective endocarditis

The proper care of the survivor of operation for congenital heart disease requires that the clinician understand the details of the malformation prior to operation, pay meticulous attention to the details of the operative procedure, and recognize the postoperative residua (conditions left totally or partially uncorrected), sequelae (conditions caused by surgery), and the complications that may have resulted from the operation. With the exception of ligation and division of an uncomplicated patent ductus arteriosus, almost every other surgical repair of an anomaly leaves behind, or causes, some abnormality of the heart and circulation which may range from trivial to serious. Thus, even with results that are considered clinically to be good to excellent, continued long-term postoperative follow-up is advisable.

Table 186-3 lists the categories of common, late postoperative problems. Several of these residua, sequelae, and complications deserve special mention. Thus, cardiac operations importantly involving the atria, such as closure of atrial septal defect, or repair of total or partial anomalous pulmonary venous return, or venous switch corrections of complete transposition of the great arteries (the Mustard or Senning operations), may be followed years later by sinus node or atrioventricular node dysfunction or by atrial arrhythmias. Intraventricular surgery may also result in electrophysiologic consequences, including complete heart block necessitation pacemaker insertion to avoid sudden death. In addition, valvular problems may arise late after initial cardiac operation. An example is the progressive stenosis of an initially nonobstructive bicuspid aortic valve in the patient who underwent aortic coarctation repair. Such aortic valves may also be the site of infective endocarditis. After repair of the ostium primum atrial septal defect, the cleft mitral valve may become progressively incompetent. Low-pressure pulmonary regurgitation is common and well tolerated in most patients with repaired tetralogy of Fallot. However, in such patients with significant residual peripheral pulmonary arterial stenoses, severe pulmonary valvular regurgitation may result in right ventricular failure and tricuspid regurgitation. Tricuspid regurgitation may also be progressive in the post-operative patient with tetralogy of Fallot if right ventricular outflow tract obstruction was not relieved adequately at initial surgery. In many patients, inadequate relief of an obstructive lesion, or a residual regurgitant lesion, or a residual shunt will cause or hasten the onset of clinical signs and symptoms of myocardial dysfunction. In many patients, particularly those who were cyanotic for many years before operation, a preexisting compromise in ventricular performance is due to the original underlying malformation. A final category of postoperative problems involves the use of prosthetic valves, patches, or conduits in the operative repair. The special risks in such patients include infective endocarditis, thrombus formation, and premature degeneration and calcification of the prosthetic materials. There are many patients in whom extracardiac conduits are required to correct the circulation functionally, and often to carry blood to the lungs from the right atrium or right ventricle. These conduits may develop intraluminal obstruction and, if they incorporate a prosthetic valve, the latter may show progressive calcification and thickening.

REFERENCES

Borow KM, Braunwald E: Congenital heart disease in the adult, in *Heart Disease*, 3d ed, E Braunwald (ed). Philadelphia, Saunders, 1988, p 976

Engle MA, Perloff JK (eds): *Congenital Heart Disease After Surgery*, New York, Yorke, 1983

Fixler DE et al: Trends in congenital heart disease in Dallas County births 1971–1984. Circulation 81(1):37, 1990

Friedman WF: Congenital heart disease in infancy and childhood, in *Heart Disease*, 3d ed, E Braunwald (ed). Philadelphia, Saunders, 1988, p 896

Kirklin JW, Barratt-Boyes BG: *Cardiac Surgery*, New York, Wiley, 1986

Lock JE et al: The use of catheter intervention procedures for congenital heart disease. J Am Coll Cardiol 7:1420, 1986

Mitchell JH et al: 16th Bethesda Conference: Cardiovascular abnormalities in the athlete; Recommendations regarding eligibility for competition. J Am Coll Cardiol 6:1200, 1985

Perloff JK et al: From cyanotic infant to acyanotic adult—The odyssey of blue babies. West J Med 139:673, 1983

———: The UCLA Adult Congenital Heart Disease Program. Am J Cardiol 57:1190, 1986

———: *The Clinical Recognition of Congenital Heart Disease*, 3d ed. Philadelphia, Saunders, 1987

——— et al: Adults with cyanotic congenital heart disease: Hematologic management. Ann Intern Med 109:406, 1988

Roberts WC (ed): *Adult Congenital Heart Disease*. Philadelphia, Davis, 1987

Truesdell SC et al: Life insurance in children with cardiovascular disease. Pediatrics 77:687, 1986

187 RHEUMATIC FEVER

GENE H. STOLLERMAN

DEFINITION Rheumatic fever is an inflammatory disease which occurs as a delayed sequel to pharyngeal infection with group A streptococci. It involves principally the heart, joints, central nervous system, skin, and subcutaneous tissues. The usual manifestations in the acute form are migratory polyarthritis, fever, and carditis. Sydenham's chorea, subcutaneous nodules, and erythema marginatum may occur as other typical manifestations. No single symptom, sign, or laboratory test is pathognomonic of rheumatic fever, although several combinations of them are diagnostic. Although the name *acute rheumatic fever* emphasizes involvement of the joints, rheumatic fever owes its importance to the involvement of the heart, which can be fatal during the acute stage or lead to rheumatic heart disease, a chronic condition due to scarring and deformity of the heart valves.

ETIOLOGY AND PATHOGENESIS The etiologic relationship of group A streptococci to rheumatic fever can be summarized briefly, as follows. (1) Numerous clinical and epidemiologic studies have shown a close association of group A streptococcal infections and rheumatic fever. (2) Antecedent streptococcal infection can almost always be demonstrated immunologically in the acute stage of rheumatic fever by increased titers of antibodies to streptococcal antigens. Moreover, in long-term prospective follow-up studies, rheumatic fever recurs only as a result of intercurrent streptococcal infections. (3) Both primary and secondary attacks of the disease can be prevented by prompt treatment or prevention of streptococcal infections with antimicrobial therapy. The pharyngeal route of infection is necessary to initiate the rheumatic process. Streptococcal skin infections do not do so. Furthermore, strains of group A streptococci that have been clearly associated with outbreaks of rheumatic fever have high virulence properties, such as rich content of the type-specific surface M protein and large hyaluronate capsules (responsible for forming "mucoid" colonies). Such properties make them highly resistant to phagocytosis and cause vigorous immune responses. Such rheumatogenic strains have been associated most frequently with certain M-serotypes, such as types 3, 5, 18, 19, and 24.

The mechanism by which the group A streptococcus initiates the disease process remains unknown. A relatively small percentage of persons who suffer from streptococcal sore throats subsequently develop rheumatic fever. The organism is not demonstrable in the lesions when rheumatic fever appears several days or weeks after the acute streptococcal infection. No one product of the streptococcus has been incriminated as a cause of the lesions, either as a direct tissue toxin or as an antigen inducing hypersensitivity. Several streptococcal antigens have demonstrated cross-reactivity with cardiac and other tissues. Their direct relationship to pathogenesis is, however, unproven, and streptococcus-induced autoimmunity as a mechanism to explain the rheumatic process remains a popular but unestablished pathogenetic concept.

INCIDENCE AND EPIDEMIOLOGY Although rheumatic fever may occur at any age, it is extremely rare in infancy; it appears most commonly between the ages of 5 and 15 years, when streptococcal infection is most frequent and intense. Similarly, the geographic distribution, incidence, and severity of rheumatic fever are, in general, a reflection of the frequency and severity of streptococcal pharyngitis. The attack rate of rheumatic fever following exudative streptococcal pharyngitis in epidemics averages approximately 3 percent. When streptococcal pharyngitis is sporadic and mild or due to strains of lesser rheumatic potential, the attack rate of rheumatic fever may be very much lower. Strains of group A streptococci that cause epidemics of streptococcal pharyngitis are most likely to be rheumatogenic. Following such infections, the attack rate of rheumatic fever is directly correlated with the magnitude of the streptococcal immune response. Analysis of reported epidemics of acute rheumatic fever caused by a variety of serotypes shows some, such as type 5, to be overrepresented, and others to be conspicuously absent. In some populations, such as in Trinidad, strains responsible for rheumatic fever and acute glomerulonephritis are serotypically distinct.

Environmental, bacterial, and host factors which appear to play a role in the development of rheumatic fever are important primarily as they are related to the incidence and severity of preceding streptococcal infection. Such factors as latitude, altitude, dampness, economic factors, and age all affect the incidence of rheumatic fever because they are related to the incidence of streptococcal infection in general. Crowding is, however, the major environmental factor relating to the occurrence of this disease because, regardless of other variables, it promotes interpersonal spread of the most virulent group A streptococcal strains. Such crowding as occurs in military barracks, closed institutions, large families in small quarters, and those massed in the densely populated core of major urban centers is most likely to be associated with an increase in incidence of rheumatic fever.

The attack rate of rheumatic fever following streptococcal infections in patients who have had previous attacks of rheumatic fever is increased to as high as 5 to 50 percent and is also related to the virulence of the reactivating infection. Furthermore, the frequency of rheumatic recurrences following streptococcal infection is consistently greater in those with rheumatic heart disease than in those who escaped cardiac injury during prior attacks. The tendency to suffer recurrences of rheumatic fever following streptococcal infections declines with the passage of years since the preceding attack. It appears, therefore, that certain host variables, as well as probable qualitative and quantitative differences in the nature of the antecedent streptococcal infection, also influence the development of rheumatic fever. To what extent such variables are genetic or acquired has not been settled. It is common to obtain a family history of rheumatic fever as well as to encounter multiple cases among siblings of a single family. However, the concordance of rheumatic fever in identical twins is approximately 20 percent, suggesting only a limited penetrance of genetic predisposition to rheumatic fever. Although investigations of the distribution of haplotypes in rheumatic hosts have been limited in scope and number, there has been so far no consistent association of rheumatic fever, or any of its major manifestations, with any predominant histocompatibility locus antigens. Recently a B-lymphocyte allotypic antigen has been found to be strikingly overrepresented in patients with rheumatic heart disease. Its nature and relation to pathogenesis, however, is not yet known.

The mortality of acute rheumatic fever has been declining steadily for the past 30 years. It is still, however, a major cause of death and disability in children and adolescents in socioeconomically depressed areas of the world. The incidence of rheumatic fever has been decreasing dramatically in countries where housing and economic conditions have been improving steadily. The rate of decrease may have been accelerated by the wide use of antimicrobial therapy. The decrease also may be due to a change in the prevalence of rheumatogenic streptococcal strains. In the past few years, however, local outbreaks of rheumatic fever have occurred in the United States in two military populations, one at the San Diego Naval Base, California, and the other at Fort Leonard Wood, Missouri. Outbreaks have occurred also among schoolchildren in Utah, Ohio, and Pennsylvania. Middle class communities with relatively high standards of living and medical care have been affected. Further investigations of the streptococcal strains causing pharyngitis in these communities have resulted in the recovery of "mucoid" strains of group A streptococci belonging to M-types 3 and 18. These strains were once prevalent in well-studied epidemics of rheumatic fever in the 1940s and 1950s, particularly in military populations. They have rarely been seen since then. The explanation for the reappearance of these strains in middle class communities and in widely separated military bases is unclear and has caused a resurgence of interest in proper diagnosis and treatment of streptococcal sore throat. Rheumatic fever remains, however, a worldwide disease having its greatest incidence wherever poor economic conditions, overcrowding, and substandard housing are most common, and where such conditions promote the transmission of rheumatogenic streptococci.

PATHOLOGY The lesions of rheumatic fever are disseminated widely throughout the body, with special predilection for connective tissues. Focal inflammatory lesions occur particularly around small blood vessels.

Cardiovascular lesions The heart is the site of the most characteristic and consequential involvement, and all its layers—endocardium, myocardium, and pericardium—may be involved. This generalized involvement gives rise to the term *rheumatic pancarditis*. The most characteristic and specific pattern of rheumatic inflammation is found in the *myocardial Aschoff body*, a submiliary granuloma. This lesion, when present in its classic form, is generally considered to be pathognomonic of rheumatic fever. In many areas the inflammatory lesion is accompanied by swelling and fragmentation of the collagen fibers and alteration in the staining properties of the ground substances of the connective tissues. This change is described as *fibrinoid degeneration of collagen*, but its chemical basis has not been established. Aschoff bodies with less exudative and more productive changes may persist for many years as the lingering traces of chronic rheumatic inflammation in patients with rheumatic heart disease, long after rheumatic fever has become clinically quiescent. The persistence of such lesions is most common in patients who develop severe mitral stenosis. Eventually the Aschoff body is converted into a spindle-shaped or triangular scar lying between the muscle bundles and surrounding blood vessels.

Rheumatic endocarditis produces the verrucous valvulitis of acute rheumatic fever which leads to the most serious permanent cardiac damage. It may heal with fibrous thickening and adhesion of the valve commissures and chordae tendineae, leading to variable degrees of valvular regurgitation and stenosis. Deformity resulting in functional impairment of the heart occurs most commonly in the mitral and aortic valves, less frequently in the tricuspid, and almost never in the pulmonic valves. *Rheumatic pericarditis* (Chap. 193) produces a serofibrinous effusion, with the deposit of shaggy elements of fibrin on the surface of the heart. The pericardium may become calcified, but pericardial constriction does not occur.

Extracardiac lesions Involvement of the *joints* is characterized by exudative rather than proliferative changes, and healing of these structures occurs without significant scarring or deformity. *Subcutaneous nodules,* seen during the acute phase of the disease, are composed of granulomas with localized areas of "fibrinoid" swelling of subcutaneous collagen bundles, and perivascular collections of large cells with pale nuclei and prominent nucleoli. Synovitis is usually mild and nonspecific. *Pulmonary* and *pleural* lesions are less definite and less characteristic. Fibrinous pleurisy and rheumatic pneumonitis may occur with exudative and proliferative lesions but without definite Aschoff bodies. Patients with active *chorea* rarely die. The pathologic findings which have been reported in the central nervous system are not consistent, and no characteristic lesion has been reported to explain this clinical manifestation. During active chorea the spinal fluid remains normal, being free of cells, with no increase in total protein and no change in the relative concentration of various proteins.

CLINICAL FEATURES The major clinical manifestations by which rheumatic fever can be recognized are polyarthritis, carditis, chorea, erythema marginatum, and subcutaneous nodules.

Arthritis The classic attack of rheumatic fever appears as an acute migratory polyarthritis accompanied by signs and symptoms of an acute febrile illness. The large joints of the extremities are most frequently affected, but no joint is impervious to the inflammatory process; one may find arthritis of the hands and feet but only rarely of the spine or of the sternoclavicular or temporomandibular joints. Joint effusions occur but are not persistent. As pain and swelling subside in one joint, others tend to become involved. Although such "migratory" involvement is characteristic, it is not invariable, and several large joints may be inflamed at one time. To be acceptable as a criterion for the diagnosis of rheumatic fever, the polyarthritis should involve two or more joints, should be associated with at least two minor manifestations such as fever and elevation of sedimentation rate, and should be associated with high titer of antistreptolysin O or some other streptococcal antibody (Table 187-1). There is nothing distinctive about the arthritis of rheumatic fever, and other causes of migratory polyarthritis that may be associated only fortuitously with high streptococcal antibody levels must, of course, be excluded.

Acute rheumatic carditis Acute rheumatic carditis first manifests itself by the appearance of the heart murmurs of either mitral or aortic regurgitation, the former most frequently. Signs and symptoms of pericarditis and of congestive heart failure may supervene in more severe cases. Death may result from heart failure during the acute stage of the disease, or permanent valvular damage may be sustained which results ultimately in serious disability. Carditis may vary from a fulminating, fatal course to a low-grade, inapparent inflammation. *It is well to bear in mind that the vast majority of patients with carditis do not have symptoms referable to the heart.* The latter occur only in more severe cases when heart failure or pericardial effusions produce characteristic symptoms. For this reason, unless extracardiac manifestations, such as polyarthritis and chorea, are present, patients whose rheumatic fever is manifested only by carditis are frequently not diagnosed and in later life may be discovered to have rheumatic heart disease without a definite history of rheumatic fever.

When carditis is manifest, there is usually tachycardia disproportionate to the degree of fever, gallop rhythms are often heard, and the heart sounds may become fetal or "tic-tac" in quality. Occasionally, arrhythmias and/or a pericardial friction rub may be present.

TABLE 187-1 Jones criteria (revised)

Major manifestations	Minor manifestations
Carditis	Fever
Polyarthritis	Arthralgia
Chorea	Previous rheumatic fever or rheumatic heart disease
Erythema marginatum	Elevated ESR or positive CRP
Subcutaneous nodules	Prolonged PR interval

Two major criteria or one major and two minor criteria indicate a high probability of the presence of rheumatic fever with supporting evidence of preceding streptococcal infection: history of recent scarlet fever; positive throat culture for group A streptococcus; increased ASO titer or other streptococcal antibodies.

SOURCE: American Heart Association, 1965.

Prolongation of the conduction time may lead to dropped beats with varying degrees of heart block. Prolongation of the PR interval and other changes in the electrocardiogram are very common, but these findings, in the absence of clinical manifestations of carditis, have a benign prognosis. Therefore, changes in the electrocardiogram alone, unassociated with significant murmurs or cardiac enlargement, do not by themselves constitute an acceptable criterion for the diagnosis of rheumatic carditis. Pericarditis may cause precordial pain, and a friction rub may be audible.

A definite clinical diagnosis of carditis can be made if one or more of the following can be demonstrated: (1) the appearance of, or change in the character of, organic heart murmurs; (2) definite increase in heart size demonstrated by radiogram or fluoroscopy; (3) pericardial friction rub or effusion best demonstrated by echocardiography; or (4) signs of congestive heart failure. Rheumatic carditis is almost always associated with a significant murmur.

Subcutaneous nodules These are usually small, pea-sized, painless swellings over bony prominences and therefore frequently go unnoticed by the patient. The skin moves freely over them. Characteristic locations are the extensor tendons of the hands and feet, the elbows, margins of the patellae, the scalp, over the scapulae, and over the spinous processes of the vertebrae.

Chorea (Sydenham's chorea, chorea minor, Saint Vitus' dance) This is a disorder of the central nervous system characterized by sudden, aimless, irregular movements, often accompanied by muscle weakness and emotional instability. Chorea is a delayed manifestation of rheumatic fever, and other manifestations may or may not still be present at the time it appears. Polyarthritis, when part of the same attack, always subsides before chorea appears. Carditis is often discovered for the first time when the presenting feature of rheumatic fever is chorea. Chorea usually appears after a long latent period (up to several months) from the antecedent streptococcal infection and at a time when all other manifestations of rheumatic fever have abated. When no previous rheumatic manifestations are noted, such cases are called *pure chorea.*

The clinical onset of chorea is often gradual. Patients may be unusually nervous and fidgety and may have difficulty in writing, drawing, and handiwork. They may stumble or fall, drop things, and grimace. As symptoms become more severe, spasmodic movements extend to all parts of the body, and muscular weakness may become so marked that patients cannot walk, talk, or sit up. Often the weakness is severe enough to simulate paralysis. The irregular, jerky, spasmodic movements may become so violent that cribs and beds must be padded to prevent injury. Symptoms are exaggerated by excitement, effort, or fatigue but subside during sleep. Emotional instability is almost invariable in patients with chorea. All degrees of speech disturbance are seen. Central nervous system stimulants exacerbate and sedatives suppress choreiform activity.

Erythema marginatum This evanescent pink rash is characteristic of rheumatic fever. The erythematous areas often have clear centers and round or serpiginous margins. They vary greatly in size and occur mainly on the trunk and proximal part of the extremities, never on the face. The erythema is transient, migratory, and may be brought out by the application of heat; it is nonpruritic, not indurated, and blanches on pressure.

Minor clinical criteria These are clinical features which occur frequently in rheumatic fever but are also common to many other diseases and are therefore of minor diagnostic value. They include fever, arthralgia, abdominal pain, tachycardia, and epistaxis.

LABORATORY FINDINGS There is no specific laboratory test to indicate the presence of rheumatic fever. The appraisal of rheumatic activity by laboratory findings is, however, of value, since various tests may indicate *continued* rheumatic inflammation when clinical features are not apparent.

Streptococcal antibody tests to disclose preceding streptococcal infection Streptococcal antibody titers differentiate preceding streptococcal from other acute respiratory infections and are increased following asymptomatic as well as symptomatic streptococcal infections. These antibody levels are increased in the early stages of acute rheumatic fever. They may be declining, or low, if the interval between the acute streptococcal infection and the detection of rheumatic fever has been longer than 2 months, a situation which occurs most often in patients whose presenting rheumatic manifestation is chorea. However, patients whose only major manifestation is rheumatic carditis also may have low antibody titers when first seen. Their rheumatic attack may have been in progress several months before becoming symptomatic and recognized. Except in these two instances, *one should be reluctant to make the diagnosis of acute rheumatic fever in the absence of serologic evidence of a recent streptococcal infection.* The antistreptolysin O test (ASO) is the most widely used and best-standardized streptococcal antibody test. In general, single titers of at least 250 Todd units in adults and at least 333 units in children over 5 years of age are considered to be increased. Depending on the general prevalence of streptococcal infections, a varying percentage of the normal population may show titers of this magnitude.

About 20 percent of patients in the early stages of acute rheumatic fever, and most patients who present with chorea, have a low or borderline ASO titer. In these instances, it is advisable to obtain a different streptococcal antibody test such as anti-DNase B, or antihyaluronidase (AH). The antistreptozyme test (ASTZ) is a hemagglutination reaction to a concentrate of extracellular streptococcal antigens absorbed to red blood cells. It is a very sensitive indicator of recent streptococcal infection; virtually all patients with acute rheumatic fever have titers greater than 200 units per milliliter. The real value of the ASTZ test is in *ruling out* rheumatic fever when the titer is low in patients with isolated polyarthritis. To date, the specific antigens involved in the ASTZ test remain unidentified and therefore the test has not yet been adequately standardized. A rise in titer of two dilution tubes or more can be demonstrated for at least one of the specific streptococcal antibodies in almost all recurrent as well as primary attacks of rheumatic fever. Increased streptococcal antibodies, however, do not reflect rheumatic activity per se, and their rate of decline is independent of the course of the rheumatic attack.

Isolation of group A streptococci Some patients continue to harbor group A streptococci at the onset of acute rheumatic fever, but these organisms are usually present in small numbers and may be difficult to isolate by a single throat culture. The administration of penicillin or other antibiotics may also result in failure to isolate the infecting organism. In addition, a significant number of *normal* individuals, particularly children, may harbor group A streptococci in the upper respiratory tract. For these reasons, throat cultures are less satisfactory than antibody tests as supporting evidence of recent streptococcal infection.

Acute phase reactants These tests offer objective but nonspecific confirmation of the presence of an inflammatory process. *The erythrocyte sedimentation rate* (ESR) and the test for *C-reactive protein* (CRP) in serum are used most commonly. Unless the patient has received glucocorticoids or salicylates, these reactions are almost always abnormal in patients presenting with polyarthritis or acute carditis, whereas they are often normal in patients with chorea. Other laboratory findings which reflect inflammation include reactions such as leukocytosis, and increases in serum complement, mucoproteins, and $alpha_2$ and gamma globulins. Prolongation of the PR interval of the electrocardiogram, although neither specific for rheumatic fever nor diagnostic of serious cardiac involvement, is frequent in acute rheumatic fever (about 25 percent of all cases), and other nonspecific electrocardiographic changes are also common. Anemia, due to the suppression of erythropoiesis characteristic of chronic inflammatory diseases, is another feature of rheumatic activity.

COURSE AND PROGNOSIS The course of rheumatic fever varies greatly and is impossible to predict at the onset of the disease. In general, however, approximately 75 percent of acute rheumatic attacks subside within 6 weeks, 90 percent within 12 weeks, and less than 5 percent persist more than 6 months. These last usually consist of severe, intractable forms of rheumatic carditis or stubborn, prolonged attacks of Sydenham's chorea, both of which may persist for as long as several years. Once acute rheumatic fever has subsided and more than 2 months has elapsed after withdrawal of treatment with salicylates or glucocorticoids, rheumatic fever does not recur in the absence of new streptococcal infections. Recurrences are most common within the first 5 years of the initial attack and tend to decline with increasing duration of freedom from rheumatic activity. The frequency of recurrences is dependent upon the frequency and severity of streptococcal infection, the presence or absence of rheumatic heart disease following an attack, and the duration of freedom from the last attack.

Approximately 70 percent of patients who develop carditis do so within the first week of the disease, 85 percent within the first 12 weeks of the disease, and almost all within 6 months from the onset of the acute attack. Thereafter, if significant murmurs have not appeared, the prognosis for a patient in whom recurrences are prevented is excellent.

Chronic rheumatic carditis and the course of rheumatic heart disease The remarkable variability in the course of rheumatic carditis and rheumatic valvular disease stems from several factors: (1) the variability in the duration and severity of the rheumatic inflammation; (2) the amount of scarring of the valves and myocardium following the abatement of the acute inflammation; (3) the location and severity of the hemodynamic lesion due to valvular insufficiency or stenosis; (4) the frequency of recurrent bouts of carditis; and (5) the progression of valvular calcification and sclerosis, which occurs as a secondary phenomenon in a deformed or injured valve without recurrent or persistent rheumatic inflammation (as seen in congenital valvular disease or following healed acute bacterial endocarditis). These factors, and possibly others not yet appreciated, produce striking variations in the clinical syndromes of rheumatic heart disease.

Chronic rheumatic myocarditis In this syndrome, the presenting picture is one of chronic heart failure in a patient with a markedly dilated heart and with physical, roentgenographic, and electrocardiographic findings of mitral and/or aortic and sometimes tricuspid regurgitation. The differentiation of this syndrome from other forms of chronic myocarditis may be very difficult, if not impossible, when the associated extracardiac features of rheumatic fever (chorea, polyarthritis, and so forth) are not present (Chap. 192). Although rheumatic fever does not produce *isolated* myocarditis, and is almost invariably a pancarditis, the pericardial inflammation may not be clearly evident, and the mitral valvulitis may not be distinguishable from mitral regurgitation due to dilation of the mitral ring. In such cases one must search diligently for an evanescent friction rub, evidence of pericardial effusion, appearance of a soft aortic regurgitation murmur, and extracardiac clues such as fever responding promptly to salicylates, arthralgias, transient subcutaneous nodules, evanescent erythema marginatum, and subtle signs of chorea.

The course of chronic rheumatic carditis may be intractable and end fatally after months or even several years. Often, however, the patient improves rather suddenly and even recovers cardiac reserve dramatically in association with the disappearance of systemic manifestations of the inflammatory process. The heart may remain large, may decrease somewhat in size, or in occasional instances may return to normal size with varying degrees of residual valvular deformity. Such a course signals the termination of the "toxic" phase of the rheumatic process, and thereafter the course of rheumatic heart disease depends on the variables in healing cited above.

DIFFERENTIAL DIAGNOSIS Early cases of rheumatic fever may be confused with other diseases which begin with acute polyarthritis. It is wise to exclude *bacteremia* by blood cultures, particularly because such infections may be masked by penicillin given for presumed acute rheumatic fever. Polyarthritis due to *infective endocarditis* in a patient with preexisting rheumatic heart disease may be mistaken for a recurrence of acute rheumatic fever. If streptococcal antibodies are not increased, polyarthritis should be attributed to some cause other than rheumatic fever. Gonococcal polyarthritis may be distinguished from rheumatic fever by the dramatic response of the former to a therapeutic trial of penicillin. In rheumatoid arthritis, joint involvement will persist and characteristic joint deformities may appear. The latter are not seen in rheumatic fever. The rheumatoid factor so characteristic of rheumatoid arthritis is not present in rheumatic fever. Antibodies against nuclear components and other autoantibodies are absent in rheumatic fever. Rheumatic pericarditis and myocarditis, associated with cardiac enlargement and heart failure, are both almost invariably associated with valvular lesions which produce significant murmurs.

Overdiagnosis of rheumatic fever is a danger. Unless ill-defined febrile syndromes are clearly associated with a major manifestation of rheumatic fever, the diagnosis of rheumatic fever should not be made. A common error is the premature, vigorous administration of glucocorticoids or salicylates before the signs and symptoms of rheumatic fever are unmistakable. In the absence of a curative agent, one should not suppress the signs and symptoms of rheumatic fever until they are clearly expressed.

Particularly confusing in the differential diagnosis of rheumatic fever is the drug sensitivity with fever and polyarthritis which may occur after administration of penicillin for a previous pharyngitis. Urticaria or angioedema, if present, helps identify penicillin sensitivity in such cases. The abdominal pain of rheumatic fever may be mistaken for appendicitis, and the crisis of sickle cell anemia may also be associated with joint pain, enlargement of the heart, and cardiac murmurs. The rapidity with which the arthritis symptoms of rheumatic fever are controlled with salicylates is characteristic of this disease. Dramatic response to salicylates does not in itself, however, establish a diagnosis of rheumatic fever.

In order to help clarify the diagnosis of rheumatic fever, the American Heart Association has accepted and modified criteria usually referred to as the *Jones criteria* (Table 187-1). They are not to be used as a substitute for good medical judgment but are recommended as a guide for careful study of questionable cases. The finding of two major criteria, or of one major and two minor criteria, indicates a high probability of the presence of rheumatic fever if supported by evidence of a preceding streptococcal infection. The absence of the latter should always make the diagnosis questionable, except in the situation in which rheumatic fever is first discovered after a long latent period from the antecedent infection (Sydenham's chorea or low-grade carditis). Because the prognosis may differ according to the major manifestations, for recording purposes the diagnosis of rheumatic fever should be followed by a list of the major manifestations present, e.g., rheumatic fever manifested by polyarthritis and carditis (Table 187-2). An indication of the severity of carditis in terms of presence or absence of congestive heart failure and cardiomegaly is also advisable.

TREATMENT There is no specific cure for rheumatic fever, and no known measures change the course of the attack. Good supportive therapy, however, can reduce the mortality and morbidity of the disease.

Chemotherapy After rheumatic fever is first diagnosed, a course of penicillin should be given to eliminate group A streptococci. This course is advisable even if bacteriologic examination yields throat cultures negative for streptococci, since the organisms may be present in areas inaccessible to swabs. It is preferable to administer penicillin parenterally. An effective course is a single injection of 1.2 million units of benzathine penicillin intramuscularly or 600,000 units of procaine penicillin intramuscularly daily for 10 days. Attempts to reduce ultimate heart damage by administering penicillin early in the acute rheumatic attack in larger doses have not been successful. After completion of the therapeutic course of penicillin, continuous protection from reinfection with streptococci should be provided by instituting one of the prophylactic regimens described below.

Suppressive therapy For patients without carditis, treatment with glucocorticoids is unnecessary. Acute arthritis can be relieved with codeine or with salicylate, the latter being preferable to reduce fever and joint inflammation. When salicylate is used in the therapy of rheumatic fever, the dosage should be increased until the drug produces either a clinical effect or systemic toxicity characterized by tinnitus, headache, or hyperpnea. A starting dose of 100 to 125 mg/kg per day in children and 6 to 8 g in adults given in four or five divided doses is recommended. Of the various salicylate preparations ordinary aspirin is cheapest and most effective.

Many physicians prefer glucocorticoids to salicylates for the treatment of carditis, despite the lack of a demonstrated advantage of these adrenal hormones in controlled clinical trials. Glucocorticoids are more potent anti-inflammatory agents but are more likely to be followed by posttherapeutic "rebounds," and they have the additional disadvantage of more frequent side effects, particularly acne, hirsutism, and cushingoid changes in facies and habitus. For this reason it is preferable to begin treatment of patients who have carditis with salicylates; if these drugs fail to reduce fever and to ameliorate heart failure, therapy with glucocorticoids may be initiated promptly. Prednisone is administered in doses of 60 to 120 mg or higher when necessary in four divided doses daily. After the inflammation has been brought under control by either salicylates or glucocorticoids, treatment should be continued until the sedimentation rate approaches near-normal values and should be maintained for several weeks thereafter. To prevent poststeroid rebounds, an "overlap" course of salicylate therapy may be added when steroids are tapered off over a 2-week period. A useful method for tapering steroids is outlined in Chap. 317. Salicylates may then be continued for an additional 2 to 3 weeks. Rebounds of rheumatic activity are usually of short duration and, when mild, are best managed without resuming anti-inflammatory treatment, because a second or even a third rebound may occur when suppressive therapy is discontinued. About 5 percent of rheumatic attacks persist for 6 months or longer, either in the form of spontaneous acute recrudescences or as posttherapeutic rebounds. These "chronic" attacks are most likely to occur in patients with cardiac damage and with previous rheumatic episodes. Weekly tests for C-reactive protein in blood and for erythrocyte sedimentation rate are useful in following the healing process, particularly while treatment with glucocorticoids or salicylates is gradually withdrawn.

Treatment of chorea The signs and symptoms of chorea usually do not respond well to treatment with antirheumatic agents. Because the patient with chorea is frequently emotionally unstable and because the manifestations of chorea may be exaggerated by emotional trauma, complete mental and physical rest is essential. Patients with chorea should be kept in a quiet room and cared for by sympathetic attendants. Glucocorticoids or salicylates have little or no effect on chorea. Sedatives and tranquilizers, particularly diazepam and chlorpromazine, are useful. Chorea, no matter how severe, disappears during sleep, which should therefore be ensured by adequate sedation. Padded sideboards for the bed may be necessary to avoid injury to the patient. In the absence of other evidence of acute rheumatic disease, it is advisable to allow gradual resumption of physical activity when improvement is apparent rather than waiting for all choreiform movements to disappear, which may require many months.

Because of the great variability in the course of chorea, evaluating the effectiveness of various therapeutic measures is difficult. It is well to remember that chorea is a self-limited disease which is usually

TABLE 187-2 Ninety-nine cases of acute rheumatic fever indicated by three major manifestations of Jones Criteria

Major manifestations*	Percent
Carditis	14
Polyarthritis	14
Chorea	4
Carditis and polyarthritis	44
Carditis and chorea	14
Carditis, chorea, and polyarthritis	6
Polyarthritis and chorea	4
Total	**100**

*Categories are mutually exclusive.
SOURCE: Acute rheumatic fever—Utah. Morb Mort Week Rep 36:109, 1988

not followed by significant neurologic sequelae and that good results are almost invariably obtained by patient, attentive nursing care and by conservative medical management.

PREVENTION OF RECURRENCE The resurgence of localized outbreaks of rheumatic fever in the United States in recent years has been blamed, in part, upon less than faithful adherence to conventional recommendations for rigorous penicillin regimens known to be highly effective in the prevention of both primary and secondary rheumatic attacks. It is recommended, therefore, that these regimens continue to be employed. The most efficient regimen for continuous prophylaxis against group A streptococci is a monthly intramuscular injection of 1.2 million units of benzathine penicillin G. The disadvantages and discomfort of this regimen have to be weighed against the individual patient's susceptibility to recurrences. Those with rheumatic heart disease, recent rheumatic fever, and exposure to an environment in which the incidence of streptococcal infection is frequent deserve the most effective protection. As a second choice, prophylaxis may be administered orally with either 1 g sulfadiazine daily in a single dose or 200,000 units of penicillin given twice daily on an empty stomach. The duration of continuous prophylaxis cannot be fixed arbitrarily. Certainly, those under the age of 18 years should receive a continuous prophylactic regimen. A minimum period of 5 years is recommended for patients who develop rheumatic fever without carditis over the age of 18 years. The decision to continue prophylaxis beyond this period should take into account a number of variables. Patients with rheumatic heart disease are more susceptible to reactivation of rheumatic fever if they contract a streptococcal infection. Moreover, patients who have had carditis in a previous attack are much more likely to suffer carditis again in a subsequent attack. Climate, age, occupation, household situation, cardiac status, and length of time since the previous attack are all significant variables which influence the risk of recurrence. The decline in recurrence rates with increasing age is due to (1) decreased rate of streptococcal infection and (2) decrease in the rate of rheumatic reactivation following streptococcal infection in older rheumatic subjects. Despite this decreased rate, however, the risk of rheumatic recurrence in adults remains relatively high when the streptococcal disease encountered is severe or epidemic and particularly when rheumatic fever is known to be extant in the population to which a rheumatic subject is exposed.

PREVENTION OF INITIAL RHEUMATIC ATTACKS Early and adequate treatment of pharyngeal infection due to group A streptococci will prevent initial attacks of rheumatic fever. If clinical streptococcal disease were properly detected by throat cultures and adequately treated, the spread of infection in a given population would be prevented, the epidemiology of streptococcal disease would be modified markedly, and the incidence of rheumatic fever in the community would be diminished. In communities where group A streptococcal disease has been diagnosed early and treated well and where socioeconomic standards are high, the group A organisms cultured frequently from schoolchildren's throats may be of relatively low virulence and may cause rheumatic fever less frequently than do more virulent strains prevalent in many epidemics. The appearance of rheumatic fever in a community, however, signals the presence of rheumatogenic streptococci whose spread must be interrupted by use of effective penicillin regimens. In a closed population, such as a military base or an institution, an outbreak of rheumatic fever is best treated by mass penicillin prophylaxis, that is, treatment of all exposed individuals, whether or not symptomatic.

Streptococcal pharyngitis is adequately treated by a single intramuscular injection of 600,000 units of benzathine penicillin in children less than 10 years of age or 1.2 million units in older children and adults. Any alternate plan of parenteral therapy or combined parenteral and oral therapy should provide for treatment over a period of 10 days. If oral penicillin is employed, at least 800,000 units per day in four divided doses must be given for no less than 10 days to achieve results comparable with a single injection of benzathine penicillin. Erythromycin in daily doses of 1 g for 10 days may be substituted in penicillin-sensitive individuals. Tetracycline is not recommended because some strains of group A streptococci have acquired resistance to it. All group A streptococci have so far remained extremely sensitive to penicillin. When erythromycin has been used extensively in place of penicillin, as in Japan, erythromycin-resistant group A streptococci have emerged with high frequency. Penicillin therefore remains the treatment of choice for streptococcal sore throat.

REFERENCES

CENTERS FOR DISEASE CONTROL: Acute rheumatic fever—Utah. Morb Mort Week Rep 36:108, 1987

———: Acute rheumatic fever at a navy training center—San Diego, CA. Morb Mort Week Rep 37:101, 1988

———: Acute rheumatic fever among army trainees—Fort Leonard Wood, MO 1987–1988. Morb Mort Week Rep 37:519, 1988

AHA COMMITTEE ON RHEUMATIC FEVER AND BACTERIAL ENDOCARDITIS: Prevention of rheumatic fever. Circulation 70:1118A, 1984

AMERICAN HEART ASSOCIATION: Jones criteria (revised) for guidance in the diagnosis of rheumatic fever. Circulation 69:204A, 1984

BISNO AL et al: Contrasting epidemiology of acute rheumatic fever and acute glomerulonephritis. Nature of the Antecedent streptococcal infection. N Engl J Med 283:561, 1970

HOSIER DM et al: Resurgence of acute rheumatic fever. Am J Dis Child 141:730, 1987

JOINT REPORT OF UK-US COOPERATIVE STUDY: The natural history of rheumatic fever and rheumatic heart disease. 10 year report of a cooperative clinical trial of ACTH, cortisone and aspirin. Circulation 32:457, 1965

KAPLAN EL et al: Group A streptococci serotypes isolated from patients and sibling contacts during the resurgence of rheumatic fever in the United States in the mid-1980s. J Infect Dis 159:101, 1989

KHANNA AK et al: Presence of a non-HLA-B cell antigen in rheumatic fever patients and their families as defined by a monoclonal antibody. J Clin Invest 83:1710, 1989

LAND MA, BISNO AL: Acute rheumatic fever: A vanishing disease in suburbia. JAMA 249:895, 1983

MASSELL BF et al: Penicillin and the marked decrease in morbidity and mortality from rheumatic fever in the United States. N Eng J Med 318:280, 1988

READ S, ZABRISKIE JB (eds): *Streptococcal Diseases and the Immune Response*. New York, Academic, 1980

STOLLERMAN GH: The relative rheumatogenicity of strains of group A streptococci. Modern Concept Cardio Dis 44:35, 1975

———: Rheumatogenic group A streptococci and the return of rheumatic fever, in *Advances in Internal Medicine*, Vol. 35, Chicago, Year Book Medical Publishers, 1990

188 VALVULAR HEART DISEASE

EUGENE BRAUNWALD

The role of physical examination in the evaluation of patients with valvular disease is also considered in Chap. 175; of roentgenography, echocardiography, and other noninvasive techniques in Chap. 177; of electrocardiography in Chap. 176; of cardiac catheterization and angiography in Chap. 179; and of balloon valvuloplasty in Chap. 180.

MITRAL STENOSIS

ETIOLOGY AND PATHOLOGY Two-thirds of all patients with mitral stenosis (MS) are females. MS is generally rheumatic in origin. Pure or predominant MS occurs in approximately 40 percent of all patients with rheumatic heart disease. The valve leaflets are diffusely thickened by fibrous tissue and/or calcific deposits. The mitral commissures fuse, the chordae tendineae fuse and shorten, the valvular cusps become rigid, and these changes in turn lead to narrowing at the apex of the funnel-shaped valve. While the initial insult to the mitral valve is rheumatic, the later changes may be a nonspecific process resulting from trauma to the valve caused by altered flow patterns due to the initial deformity. Calcification of the stenotic mitral valve immobilizes the leaflets and narrows the orifice. Thrombus formation and arterial embolization may arise from the calcific valve itself. Rarely, MS is congenital in origin.

PATHOPHYSIOLOGY In normal adults the mitral valve orifice is 4 to 6 cm^2. In the presence of significant obstruction, i.e., when the orifice is less than one-half of normal, blood can flow from the left atrium to the left ventricle only if propelled by an abnormally elevated left atrioventricular pressure gradient (Fig. 196-6), the hemodynamic hallmark of MS. When the mitral valve opening is reduced to 1 cm^2, a left atrial pressure of approximately 25 mmHg is required to maintain a normal cardiac output. The elevated left atrial pressure in turn raises pulmonary venous and capillary pressures, reducing pulmonary compliance and causing exertional dyspnea. The first bouts of dyspnea are usually precipitated by clinical events which increase the rate of blood flow across the mitral orifice, which results in further elevation of the left atrial pressure (see below). In order to assess the severity of obstruction, it is essential to measure both the transvalvular pressure gradient and the flow rate (Chap. 179). The latter is dependent not only on the cardiac output but on the heart rate as well. An increase in heart rate shortens diastole proportionately more than systole, and diminishes the time available for flow across the mitral valve. Therefore, at any given level of cardiac output tachycardia augments the transvalvular gradient and elevates further the left atrial pressure.

The left ventricular diastolic pressure is normal in isolated MS; coexisting mitral regurgitation, aortic valve disease, the residua of damage produced by rheumatic myocarditis, systemic hypertension, or ischemic heart disease are sometimes responsible for elevations which reflect impaired left ventricular function and/or reduced left ventricular compliance. Left ventricular dysfunction, as reflected in reduced ejection fraction and circumferential fiber shortening rate, occurs in about one-fourth of patients with MS. This is a consequence of chronic reduction of preload and extension of the scarring from the valve into the adjacent myocardium. In pure MS and sinus rhythm, the mean left atrial and pulmonary artery wedge pressures are usually elevated and the pressure pulse shows a prominent atrial contraction (*a* wave) and a gradual pressure decline after mitral valve opening (*y* descent). In patients with mild to moderate MS without elevation of the pulmonary vascular resistance, the pulmonary arterial pressure may be near the upper limits of normal at rest and may rise with exercise. In severe MS and whenever the pulmonary vascular resistance is significantly increased, the pulmonary arterial pressure is elevated even when the patient is at rest, and in extreme cases it may exceed the systemic arterial pressure. Further elevations of left atrial, pulmonary capillary, and pulmonary arterial pressures occur during exercise. When the pulmonary arterial systolic pressure exceeds approximately 50 mmHg in patients with MS, or for that matter with any valvular lesion, the increased right ventricular afterload impedes the emptying of this chamber, and right ventricular end-diastolic pressure and volume usually rise as a compensatory mechanism.

Cardiac output This varies considerably. Thus, the hemodynamic response to a given degree of mitral obstruction may be characterized by a normal cardiac output at rest and a high left atrioventricular pressure gradient or, at the opposite end of the hemodynamic spectrum, by a reduced cardiac output and low transvalvular pressure gradient. In a small fraction of patients with moderately severe MS, the cardiac output is normal at rest and rises normally during exertion; under these circumstances, the high atrioventricular pressure gradient elevates the left atrial and pulmonary capillary pressures markedly, and this elevation is responsible for symptoms of relatively severe pulmonary congestion. In the majority of patients with moderate MS, however, the cardiac output is normal at rest but rises subnormally during exertion. In patients with severe MS, particularly those in whom the pulmonary vascular resistance is strikingly elevated, the cardiac output is subnormal at rest and may fail to rise or may even decline during activity. The depressed cardiac output in patients with MS is related primarily to the obstruction of the mitral orifice but may also be due to the impairment of the function of either ventricle.

Pulmonary hypertension The clinical and hemodynamic features of MS are influenced importantly by the level of the pulmonary artery pressure. Pulmonary hypertension results from (1) the passive backward transmission of the elevated left atrial pressure, (2) pulmonary arteriolar constriction, which presumably is triggered by left atrial and pulmonary venous hypertension (reactive pulmonary hypertension), and (3) organic obliterative changes in the pulmonary vascular bed. The elevation of pulmonary vascular resistance may be considered to be a complication of long-standing and severe MS; in time, the resultant severe pulmonary hypertension results in tricuspid and pulmonary incompetence as well as right-sided heart failure. However, the changes in the pulmonary vascular bed may also be considered to exert a protective effect; the elevated precapillary resistance reduces the likelihood of symptoms of pulmonary congestion by reducing the surge of blood into the pulmonary capillary bed which then dams up behind the stenotic mitral valve during activity. However, this protection occurs at the expense of a decreased cardiac output.

SYMPTOMS AND COMPLICATIONS In temperate climates the latent period between the initial attack of rheumatic carditis (in the increasingly rare circumstances in which a history of one can be elicited) and the development of symptoms due to MS is generally on the order of two decades; most patients begin to experience disability in the fourth decade. Once a patient with MS becomes seriously symptomatic, continuous progression of the disease to death usually occurs in 2 to 5 years unless the stenosis is relieved. In economically deprived areas, particularly on the Indian subcontinent, in Central America, and the Middle East, MS tends to progress more rapidly and frequently causes serious symptoms before the age of 20 years. On the other hand, slowly progressive MS in the elderly is being recognized with increasing frequency in the United States and western Europe.

When valvular obstruction is mild, many of the physical signs of MS may be present in the absence of any symptoms. However, even in those patients whose mitral orifices are large enough to accommodate a normal blood flow with only mild elevations of left atrial pressure, extreme exertion, excitement, fever, severe anemia, paroxysmal tachycardia, sexual intercourse, pregnancy, and thyrotoxicosis all may precipitate elevations of pulmonary capillary pressure and lead to dyspnea and cough. As stenosis progresses, the stresses that precipitate dyspnea become less severe, and the patient becomes limited in his or her daily activities. Redistribution of blood from the dependent portions of the body to the lungs, which occurs when the recumbent position is assumed, leads to orthopnea and paroxysmal nocturnal dyspnea. *Pulmonary edema* develops when there is a sudden surge in flow across a markedly narrowed mitral orifice (Chap. 36). When moderately severe MS has existed for several years, *atrial arrhythmias*—premature contractions, paroxysmal tachycardia, flutter, and fibrillation—occur with increasing frequency. The rapid ventricular rate associated with untreated or inadequately treated atrial fibrillation is frequently responsible for acute exacerbations of dyspnea. The development of permanent atrial fibrillation often marks a turning point in the patient's course and is generally associated with acceleration of the rate at which symptoms progress.

Hemoptysis (Chap. 35) results from rupture of pulmonary-bronchial venous connections secondary to pulmonary venous hypertension. It occurs most frequently in patients who have elevated left atrial pressures *without* markedly elevated pulmonary vascular resistances and is almost never fatal. True hemoptysis must be distinguished from the bloody sputum that occurs with pulmonary edema, pulmonary infarction, and bronchitis, three conditions that occur with increased frequency in the presence of MS.

As the condition progresses and the pulmonary vascular resistance rises or when tricuspid stenosis or regurgitation develops, symptoms secondary to pulmonary congestion may diminish, and the episodes of acute pulmonary edema and hemoptysis become reduced in frequency and severity. Elevation of pulmonary vascular resistance further increases right ventricular systolic pressure, leading to right ventricular failure, fatigue, abdominal discomfort due to hepatic congestion, and edema.

Recurrent pulmonary emboli, sometimes with infarction (Chap. 213), are an important cause of morbidity and mortality late in the course of MS, occurring most frequently in patients with right ventricular failure. *Pulmonary infections,* i.e., bronchitis, bronchopneumonia, and lobar pneumonia, commonly complicate untreated MS. *Infective endocarditis* (Chap. 90) is rare in *pure* MS but is not uncommon in patients with combined stenosis and regurgitation. *Chest pain* occurs in about 10 percent of patients with severe MS; it may be due to pulmonary hypertension or myocardial ischemia secondary to coronary atherosclerosis; often the cause cannot be discovered.

Pulmonary and pulmonary vascular changes In addition to the aforementioned changes in the pulmonary vascular bed, fibrous thickening of the walls of the alveoli and pulmonary capillaries occurs commonly in MS. The vital capacity, total lung capacity, maximal breathing capacity, and oxygen uptake per unit of ventilation are reduced (Chap. 201), and in patients with severe MS the latter fails to rise normally during exertion. The reduction of pulmonary compliance that occurs generally correlates directly with the severity of the dyspnea and with the heightened pulmonary capillary pressure, and these changes are intensified during exercise. In some patients airway resistance is abnormally increased. These alterations in pulmonary mechanics contribute to an increase in the work of breathing and play an important role in the genesis of dyspnea. The changes in the lungs are due, in part, to increased transudation of fluid from the pulmonary capillaries into the interstitial and alveolar spaces as a consequence of the elevated pulmonary capillary pressure. The distribution of blood flow and ventilation may be uneven; as in other conditions in which left atrial pressure is elevated, pulmonary blood flow in the erect position is displaced from the basal to the superior segments of the lung (Chap. 201). The diffusing capacity may be reduced, particularly during exertion, as a result of structural changes in the diffusing surface and reduction of the pulmonary capillary blood volume. The thickening of the alveolar and capillary walls impedes the transudation of fluid into the alveoli and the development of pulmonary edema at times when the pulmonary capillary pressure exceeds the plasma oncotic pressure. The increased capacity of the pulmonary lymphatic system to drain excess fluid also retards the development of pulmonary edema.

Thrombi and emboli *Thrombi* may form in the left atria, particularly in the enlarged atrial appendages of patients with MS. If they embolize, they do so most commonly to the brain, kidneys, spleen, and extremities. *Embolization* occurs much more frequently in patients with atrial fibrillation or unstable rhythms, in older patients, and in those with a reduced cardiac output, and it is seen in patients with relatively mild, as well as in those with severe, obstruction. Thus, systemic embolization may be the presenting complaint in otherwise asymptomatic patients with mild MS. At operation, thrombi are *not* found more frequently in the left atria of patients with a past history of embolization than in those without this complication, indicating that it is usually the freshly formed clots that dislodge. Patients who have had one or more systemic emboli have an increased predilection for further embolic episodes compared with patients with stenosis of comparable severity without previous embolization. Rarely, a large pedunculated thrombus or a free-floating clot may suddenly obstruct the stenotic mitral orifice. Such "ball valve" thrombi produce syncope, angina, and changing auscultatory signs with alterations in position, findings that resemble those produced by a left atrial myxoma (Chap. 194).

PHYSICAL FINDINGS (See also Chap. 175) **Inspection** Peripheral and facial *cyanosis* may occur in patients with extremely severe MS. In advanced cases there is a malar flush and the facies appear pinched and blue. The jugular venous pulse reveals prominent *a* waves due to vigorous right atrial systole in patients with sinus rhythm who have severe pulmonary hypertension or associated tricuspid stenosis. When atrial fibrillation is present, the jugular pulse reveals only a single expansion during systole (*c-v* wave). The systemic arterial pressure is usually normal or slightly low.

Palpation A right ventricular tap is present along the left sternal border, signifying an enlarged right ventricle. The first heart sound may be palpable in patients with pliable valve leaflets. In patients with pulmonary hypertension, the impact of pulmonary valve closure can usually be felt in the second and third left intercostal spaces just left of the sternum; the left ventricle is not palpable in severe, pure MS. A diastolic thrill is frequently present at the cardiac apex, particularly if the patient is turned into the left lateral recumbent position.

Auscultation The first heart sound (S_1) is generally accentuated and snapping, and since the mitral valve does not close until the left ventricular pressure reaches the level of the elevated left atrial pressure, this sound is often slightly delayed on phonocardiography, particularly in patients with severe stenosis. In patients with pulmonary hypertension, the pulmonary component of the second heart sound (P_2) is often accentuated, and the two components of the second heart sound are closely split. A pulmonary systolic ejection click may be heard in patients with severe pulmonary hypertension and marked dilatation of the pulmonary artery. The opening snap (OS) of the mitral valve is most readily audible in expiration at, or just medial to, the cardiac apex but may also be easily heard along the left sternal edge or at the base of the heart. This sound generally follows the sound of aortic valve closure (A_2) by 0.06 to 0.12 s, that is, it follows P_2. Since the OS occurs when the left ventricular pressure falls below the left atrial pressure, the time interval between A_2 closure and OS varies inversely with the severity of the MS. It tends to be short, that is, 0.06 to 0.07 s, in patients with severe obstruction and long, that is, 0.10 to 0.12 s, in patients with mild MS. The intensities of the OS and S_1 correlate with the mobility of the anterior mitral leaflet.

The OS usually ushers in a low-pitched, rumbling, diastolic murmur, heard best at the apex with the patient in the left lateral recumbent position and often accentuated by exercise carried out just before auscultation. In general, the duration of this murmur correlates with the severity of the stenosis. In patients with sinus rhythm the murmur often reappears or becomes reaccentuated during atrial systole, as atrial contraction reelevates the rate of blood flow across the narrowed orifice. Soft (grade I or II/VI) systolic murmurs are commonly heard at the apex or along the left sternal border in patients with pure MS and do not necessarily signify the presence of mitral regurgitation. Hepatomegaly, ankle edema, ascites, and pleural effusion, particularly in the right pleural cavity, may occur in patients with MS and right ventricular failure.

Associated lesions With severe pulmonary hypertension a loud pansystolic murmur produced by functional tricuspid regurgitation may be audible along the left sternal border. This murmur may be accentuated by inspiration, diminishes during forced expiration or during performance of the Valsalva maneuver, diminishes or disappears as compensation is restored, and must not be confused with the apical pansystolic murmur of mitral regurgitation, since management is quite different if mitral regurgitation is present.

The recognition of associated mitral regurgitation is of considerable clinical importance in patients with MS. A presystolic murmur and an accentuated first heart sound speak against the presence of serious associated mitral regurgitation, but when the first heart sound and/or the opening snap are soft or absent in a patient with mitral valve disease who also has an apical systolic murmur, it is likely that significant mitral regurgitation and/or serious calcification of the deformed mitral valve leaflets are present. A third heart sound at the apex often signifies that the mitral regurgitation is serious; this sound is generally duller and lower pitched and follows the opening snap. Occasionally, in patients with pure MS, physical signs may falsely suggest mitral regurgitation. Thus, in the presence of severe pulmonary hypertension and right ventricular failure, a third heart sound may originate from the right ventricle. The enlarged right ventricle may rotate the heart in a clockwise direction and form the cardiac apex, giving the examiner the erroneous impression of left ventricular enlargement. Under these circumstances the rumbling diastolic murmur and the other auscultatory features of MS become less prominent or may even disappear and be replaced by the systolic murmur of functional tricuspid regurgitation which is mistaken for mitral regurgitation. When cardiac output is markedly reduced in a patient with MS the typical auscultatory findings, including the diastolic rumbling murmur (silent MS), may not be detectable, but they may reappear as compensation is restored. Associated tricuspid stenosis also tends to obscure many of the physical signs of MS.

The Graham Steell murmur of pulmonary regurgitation, a high-pitched, diastolic, decrescendo blowing murmur along the left sternal border, results from dilatation of the pulmonary valve ring and occurs in patients with mitral valve disease and severe pulmonary hypertension. This murmur may be indistinguishable from the more common murmur produced by mild aortic regurgitation except that it is rarely audible at the second right intercostal space, and may disappear following successful surgical treatment of the MS.

Electrocardiogram In MS and sinus rhythm the P wave usually suggests left atrial enlargement (Chap. 176). It may become tall and peaked in lead II and upright in lead V_1 when severe pulmonary hypertension or tricuspid stenosis complicates MS and right atrial enlargement occurs. The QRS complex may be normal, even in patients with critical MS. However, with severe pulmonary hypertension, right axis deviation and right ventricular hypertrophy are usually found. When left ventricular hypertrophy is present in patients with MS, it generally indicates that an additional lesion which places a significant burden on the left ventricle, such as mitral regurgitation, aortic valve disease, or hypertension, is present.

Echocardiogram (See also Chap. 177) The echocardiogram is the most sensitive and specific noninvasive method for diagnosing MS. The M-mode tracing reveals that the anterior and posterior mitral leaflets do not separate widely in early diastole (i.e., less than 15 mm) and they maintain a fixed relation to each other throughout diastole. However, two-dimensional, color Doppler flow echocardiographic imaging and Doppler echocardiography provide critical information (see Figs. 177-3 and 177-5), including an estimate of the transvalvular gradient and of mitral orifice size, the presence and severity of accompanying mitral regurgitation, the extent of restriction of valve leaflets, their thickness, and the degree of distortion of the subvalvular apparatus. In addition, echocardiography provides an assessment of the size of the cardiac chambers, an estimation of the pulmonary artery pressure, and an indication of the presence and severity of associated tricuspid and pulmonic regurgitation.

Roentgenogram (Chap. 177) The earliest changes are straightening of the left border of the cardiac silhouette, prominence of the main pulmonary arteries, dilatation of the upper lobe pulmonary veins, and backward displacement of the esophagus by an enlarged left atrium. In patients with mild or moderate MS, the heart is not grossly enlarged. In severe MS, however, all chambers and vessels upstream to the narrowed valve are prominent, including the two atria, the pulmonary arteries and veins, right ventricle, and superior vena cava. Kerley B lines are fine, dense, opaque, horizontal lines which are most prominent in the lower and midlung fields and which result from distention of interlobular septa and lymphatics with edema when the resting mean left atrial pressure exceeds approximately 20 mmHg. As the pulmonary arterial pressure rises, the smaller pulmonary arteries become attenuated, at first in the lower, then in the mid-, and finally in the upper lung fields. Deposits of hemosiderin occur in the lungs of patients who have had multiple hemoptyses; the hemosiderin-containing macrophages fill the air spaces, and if they become confluent, result in a fine, diffuse nodulation most prominent in the lower lung fields.

DIFFERENTIAL DIAGNOSIS Significant mitral regurgitation may be associated with a prominent diastolic murmur at the apex, but this murmur commences slightly later than in patients with MS, and there is often clear-cut evidence of left ventricular enlargement on physical examination, roentgenography, and electrocardiography. In addition, an apical pansystolic murmur of at least grade III/VI intensity as well as a third heart sound should arouse the suspicion of significant associated regurgitation. Similarly, the apical middiastolic murmur associated with aortic regurgitation (Austin Flint murmur) may be mistaken for MS. However, in a patient with aortic regurgitation the absence of an opening snap or of presystolic accentuation if sinus rhythm is present points to the *absence* of MS. Tricuspid stenosis, a valvular lesion that occurs very rarely in the absence of MS, may mask many of the clinical features of MS. Echocardiography is particularly useful in detecting MS in patients who have or are suspected of having other valve lesions and in defining the severity of the various lesions.

Exertional dyspnea and recurrent pulmonary infections may be falsely ascribed to pulmonary emphysema in patients with both *chronic lung disease* and MS. Careful auscultation, however, will generally reveal the characteristic opening snap and rumbling diastolic murmur. Similarly, the hemoptysis that occurs in many otherwise asymptomatic patients with MS may be improperly attributed to bronchiectasis or tuberculosis. Actually, the latter condition is uncommon in patients with significant mitral obstruction.

Primary pulmonary hypertension (Chap. 212) results in a number of the clinical and laboratory features observed in MS. It occurs most frequently in young women; however, the OS and diastolic rumbling murmur are absent, there is no left atrial enlargement, and the pulmonary artery wedge and left atrial pressures are *normal*, as is the size of the left atrium on echocardiography. *Atrial septal defect* (Chap. 186) may also be mistaken for MS; in both conditions there is often clinical, electrocardiographic, and roentgenographic evidence of right ventricular enlargement and accentuation of the pulmonary vascularity. The widely split S_2 of atrial septal defect may be confused with the mitral OS, and the diastolic flow murmur across the tricuspid valve mistaken for the mitral diastolic murmur. However, the absence of left atrial enlargement and of Kerley B lines and the demonstration of fixed splitting of S_2 favor atrial septal defect over MS. *Cor triatriatum* is an unusual congenital malformation that consists of a fibrous ring within the left atrium. It results in elevation of the pulmonary venous, capillary, and arterial pressures. This lesion can be recognized most readily by means of left atrial angiography.

Left atrial myxoma (Chap. 194) may obstruct left atrial emptying, resulting in dyspnea, a diastolic murmur, and hemodynamic changes resembling those of MS. However, patients with left atrial myxoma often demonstrate findings suggestive of a systemic disease, with weight loss, fever, anemia, systemic emboli, and elevated erythrocyte sedimentation rate and serum IgG concentration. Usually an OS is not audible, there is no clinical evidence of associated aortic valve disease, and the auscultatory findings frequently change with body position. The diagnosis can be established by demonstrating a characteristic echo-producing mass in the left atrium by two-dimensional echocardiography and a lobulated filling defect by angiocardiography.

CARDIAC CATHETERIZATION AND ANGIOCARDIOGRAPHY Catheterization of the left side of the heart (Chap. 179) is extremely helpful in deciding whether valvulotomy is necessary in patients in whom it is difficult to estimate the severity of obstruction by clinical means and noninvasive tests. When combined with aortography and left ventricular angiocardiography, this procedure serves as the ultimate method for detecting and estimating associated mitral regurgitation and coexisting lesions such as aortic stenosis and regurgitation as well as left ventricular dysfunction. Left atrial thrombi and tumors may be detected or excluded by angiocardiography, particularly when the contrast medium is injected directly into the left atrium. These "invasive" methods are also helpful in the detection of accompanying conditions, such as coronary artery disease, that impair left ventricular function and would thereby contraindicate or reduce the effectiveness of mitral valvulotomy. Catheterization is not usually necessary to aid in the decision regarding surgery in young (<45 years for males; <50 for females) patients with typical findings of severe obstruction on clinical examination and echocardiography. In older patients coronary angiography is usually advisable preoperatively, in order to detect patients with critical coronary obstructions which should be bypassed at the time of operation. Catheterization and left ventricular angiography are also indicated in most patients who have undergone previous mitral valve operations and who have redeveloped serious symptoms; in such patients clinical assessment may be particularly difficult, and the hemodynamic studies allow determination of the severity of the lesion, intelligent planning of the operative procedure when it is indicated, and a more accurate estimate of the risk.

MANAGEMENT In the asymptomatic adolescent with mitral valve disease, penicillin prophylaxis of beta-hemolytic streptococcal infections (Chap. 187), prophylaxis for infective endocarditis (Chap. 90), and vocational counseling are important; physically strenuous occupations should be avoided so that premature retirement will not be necessary should symptoms develop later. In symptomatic patients some improvement usually occurs with restriction of sodium intake and maintenance doses of oral diuretics. Digitalis glycosides do not alter the hemodynamics and usually do not benefit patients with pure stenosis and sinus rhythm, but they are necessary for slowing the ventricular rate of patients with atrial fibrillation and for reducing the manifestations of right-sided heart failure in the advanced stages of the disease. Small doses of beta blockers (e.g., atenolol 25 to 50 mg qd) may be added when cardiac glycosides fail to control ventricular rate in patients with atrial fibrillation or flutter. Particular attention should be directed to detecting and treating any accompanying anemia and infections. Hemoptysis is treated by measures designed to diminish pulmonary venous pressure, including bed rest, the sitting position, salt restriction, and diuresis. Anticoagulants should be administered for at least 1 year in patients with MS who have suffered systemic and/or pulmonary embolization and those with atrial fibrillation.

If atrial fibrillation is of relatively recent origin in a patient whose MS is not severe enough to warrant surgical treatment, reversion to sinus rhythm pharmacologically or by means of electrical countershock is indicated. Usually this should be undertaken following 4 weeks of anticoagulant treatment. Conversion to sinus rhythm is rarely helpful in patients with severe MS, particularly those in whom the left atrium is especially enlarged or in whom atrial fibrillation has been present for more than 1 year, since reversion to atrial fibrillation is common.

Mitral valvulotomy Unless there is a specific contraindication, mitral valvulotomy is indicated in the symptomatic patient with pure MS whose effective orifice is less than approximately 1.2 cm^2. Operation not only usually results in striking symptomatic and hemodynamic improvement but also prolongs survival. In uncomplicated cases, the surgical mortality rate should be 0 to 2 percent. However, there is no evidence that surgical treatment improves the prognosis of patients with slight or no functional impairment. Therefore, unless recurrent systemic embolization has occurred, valvulotomy is *not* recommended for patients who are entirely asymptomatic, regardless of hemodynamic findings. When there is little symptomatic improvement following valvulotomy, it is likely that the procedure was ineffective, that it induced mitral regurgitation, or that associated valvular or myocardial disease was present. The recurrence of symptoms several years after what appeared to be a satisfactory initial result is usually due to an inadequate valvulotomy, but progression of other valvular lesions, the development of myocardial disease, restenosis of the mitral valve, or some combination of these conditions may also be responsible. In the *pregnant patient* with MS operative treatment should be carried out if pulmonary congestion occurs despite intensive medical treatment.

Percutaneous balloon valvuloplasty, described on p. 879, is an alternative to surgical mitral valvuloplasty in patients with pure or predominant rheumatic mitral stenosis. Young patients without extensive valvular calcification or subvalvular deformity are the optimal candidates for this procedure; in them the results approach those of closed surgical commissurotomy. It is particularly useful in pregnant women but may also be used in older patients with severe valvular deformity with serious extracardiac disease who are poor operative candidates.

An "open" operation using cardiopulmonary bypass is usually preferable to closed commissurotomy for patients with pure MS who have not been operated upon previously. In addition to opening the valve commissures, it is important to loosen any subvalvular fusion of papillary muscles and chordae tendineae and to remove large deposits of calcium, thereby improving valvular function, and to remove atrial thrombi. In patients with significant associated mitral regurgitation, those in whom the valve has been severely distorted by previous operative manipulation, or those in whom the surgeon does not find it possible to improve valve function significantly, the valve may have to be replaced with a prosthesis or a heterograft. Since the operative mortality of replacement of the mitral valve is still approximately 5 to 8 percent and since there are long-term complications of valve replacement, patients in whom preoperative evaluation suggests the possibility that replacement may be required should be operated on only if they have *critical* mitral stenosis, i.e., an orifice <1.0 cm^2, and are in the New York Heart Association class III, i.e., symptomatic with ordinary activity, despite optimal medical therapy.

VALVE REPLACEMENT The results of replacement of any valve are dependent primarily on (1) the patient's myocardial function at the time of operation, (2) the technical abilities of the operative team and the quality of the postoperative care, and (3) the durability, hemodynamic characteristics, and thrombogenicity of the prosthesis. Increased operative mortality is associated with the degree of preoperative functional disability and pulmonary hypertension. Late complications of replacement of any valve, which fortunately are declining in incidence, include paravalvular leakage, thromboemboli, bleeding due to anticoagulants, mechanical dysfunction of the prosthesis, and infective endocarditis.

The considerations regarding the choice between a bioprosthetic and artificial mechanical valve are similar in the mitral and aortic positions and in the treatment of stenotic, regurgitant, or mixed lesions. All patients who have undergone replacement of any valve with a mechanical prosthesis must be maintained permanently on anticoagulants. The primary advantage of bioprostheses (tissue valves) over mechanical prostheses is the reduction of thromboembolic complications and, except for patients with chronic atrial fibrillation, few such instances have been associated with their use. Bioprosthetic valves are *contraindicated* in younger patients (<35 years) because of accelerated deterioration and are particularly useful in the elderly (>65 years), in whom there is more concern about chronic anticoagulation than about long-term (>15 years) valve durability. These valves are also indicated in women who expect to become pregnant as well as others in whom anticoagulation may be contraindicated. In patients without such contraindications, particularly those under 60 years, a mechanical prosthesis may be preferable. Many surgeons now select the St. Jude prosthesis, a double-disk tilting prosthesis, for replacement of both aortic and mitral valves because of somewhat more favorable hemodynamic characteristics and a suggestion of lower thrombogenicity.

The overall 10-year survival of operative survivors following mitral valve replacement is approximately 60 percent. Long-term prognosis is worse in subgroups of older patients and those with marked disability and striking depression of the cardiac index preoperatively.

MITRAL REGURGITATION

ETIOLOGY Chronic rheumatic heart disease is the cause of severe mitral regurgitation (MR) in about one-third of cases. In contrast to MS, pure or predominantly rheumatic MR occurs more frequently in males. The rheumatic process produces rigidity, deformity, and retraction of the valve cusps and commissural fusion, as well as shortening, contraction, and fusion of the chordae tendineae.

MR may also occur as a congenital anomaly (Chap. 186), most commonly as (1) a defect of the endocardial cushions or in association with (2) corrected transposition, (3) endocardial fibroelastosis, and (4) the "parachute" mitral valve deformity. MR may occur with fibrosis of a papillary muscle in patients with healed myocardial infarction as well as in patients with a ventricular aneurysm involving the base of a papillary muscle. Transient regurgitation may also occur during periods of ischemia involving a papillary muscle or the adjacent myocardium and may accompany bouts of angina pectoris. MR may occur with marked left ventricular enlargement of any cause in which dilatation of the mitral annulus and lateral displacement of the papillary muscles interfere with coaptation of the valve leaflets. In hypertrophic cardiomyopathy the anterior leaflet of the mitral valve is displaced anteriorly during systole, leading to regurgitation (Chap. 192). Massive calcification of the mitral annulus of unknown cause, presumably degenerative, which occurs most commonly in elderly women, can also be responsible for significant MR. Systemic lupus erythematosus, rheumatoid arthritis, and ankylosing spondylitis are less common causes. *Acute* MR may occur secondary to infective endocarditis involving the valve or chordae tendineae, in acute myocardial infarction with rupture of a papillary muscle or one of its heads, as a consequence of trauma, or as a complication of cardiac surgery.

Abnormal elongation of chordae tendineae and/or redundant posterior cusps of the mitral valve with prolapse of the cusps into the left atrium, the so-called floppy valve, leading to the syndrome of midsystolic click and midsystolic murmur, also referred to as the *prolapsing mitral valve leaflet syndrome* (see below), is another important cause of MR.

Regardless of etiology, serious MR tends to be progressive, since enlargement of the left atrium places tension on the posterior mitral leaflet, pulling it away from the mitral orifice, thereby aggravating the valvular dysfunction. Similarly, the dilatation of the left ventricle increases the regurgitation, which in turn enlarges further the left atrium and ventricle, resulting in a vicious cycle; hence the aphorism, "mitral regurgitation begets mitral regurgitation."

PATHOPHYSIOLOGY The regurgitant mitral orifice may be considered to be in parallel with the aortic orifice, and therefore the resistance to left ventricular emptying is reduced in patients with MR. As a consequence, the left ventricle is decompressed into the left atrium during ejection, and with the reduction in left ventricular size there is a rapid decline in left ventricular tension i.e., a progressive reduction in left ventricular afterload, allowing a greater proportion of the contractile activity of the left ventricle to be expended in shortening. The initial compensation to MR consists of more complete systolic emptying of the left ventricle. However, a progressive increase in left ventricular end-diastolic volume occurs as the severity of the regurgitation increases and the function of the left ventricle deteriorates. The atrial contraction wave in the left atrial pressure pulse (a wave) is usually not as prominent as it is in MS, but the v wave is often much taller, since it is inscribed during ventricular systole, when the left atrium fills from the pulmonary veins as well as from the left ventricle. During early diastole, as the distended left atrium suddenly empties, there is a particularly rapid y descent as long as there is no associated MS (Fig. 179-7, p. 875). Left ventricular end-diastolic pressure may be slightly elevated. However, in chronic MR, there is often an increase in left ventricular compliance, so that ventricular volume may be increased with little elevation in end-diastolic pressure. The effective cardiac output usually declines in seriously symptomatic patients. Although a left atrioventricular pressure gradient persisting throughout diastole signifies the presence of significant associated MS, a brief, early diastolic gradient may occur in patients with pure regurgitation as a result of the torrential flow of blood across a normal-sized mitral orifice.

The prompt appearance of contrast material in the left atrium following its injection into the left ventricle signifies the presence and can be useful in the diagnosis of MR. The regurgitant volume can be measured by determining the difference between the total left ventricular stroke volume estimated angiocardiographically and the effective forward stroke volume determined by the Fick method (Chap. 179). The results of such studies suggest that the regurgitant volume may be of the same magnitude as the effective forward stroke volume or may even exceed it in patients with severe regurgitation. Qualitative, but clinically useful, estimates of the severity of regurgitation may be made by Doppler echocardiography, color Doppler flow echocardiographic imaging, and by observation on cineangiograms of the degree of left atrial opacification following the injection of contrast material into the left ventricle.

Patients with *severe* MR may be divided into three subgroups, depending on the compliance, i.e., the pressure-volume relationship, of the left atrium and pulmonary venous bed.

Group 1 *Normal or reduced compliance*. These patients usually have *acute* MR. There is little enlargement of the left atrium, but marked elevation of the left atrial pressure, particularly of the v wave. In these patients MR has usually developed suddenly, as when it follows rupture of chordae tendineae, infarction of one of the heads of a papillary muscle, or tear of a mitral leaflet. Pulmonary edema is common. After several months the pulmonary vascular resistance may become markedly elevated, presumably as a consequence of the left atrial hypertension, and right-sided heart failure may also occur; sinus rhythm is usually present.

Group 2 *Marked increase in compliance*. At the opposite end of the spectrum from group 1 are those patients with severe long-standing severe MR, massive enlargement of the left atrium, and normal or only slightly elevated left atrial pressure, pulmonary artery pressure, and pulmonary vascular resistance. These patients usually complain of severe fatigue and exhaustion secondary to a low cardiac output, while symptoms resulting from pulmonary congestion are less prominent; atrial fibrillation is almost invariably present. The association of a near-normal left atrial pressure with a markedly enlarged, thin-walled left atrium indicates that this chamber is far more compliant than normal. Thus, long-standing MR may, in some instances, alter the physical properties of the left atrial wall and thereby displace the atrial pressure-volume curve, allowing a greatly enlarged left atrium to have a normal atrial pressure.

Group 3 *Moderate increase in compliance*. By far the most common group are patients whose clinical and hemodynamic features are between those in the other two groups with variable degrees of enlargement of the left atrium and with significant elevation of the left atrial pressure. Symptoms are secondary to both reduced cardiac output and pulmonary congestion.

SYMPTOMS Only a fraction of patients with chronic MR ever experience any reduction of cardiac reserve, but in those who do become symptomatic, fatigue, exertional dyspnea, and orthopnea may be prominent complaints. Symptoms resulting from pulmonary congestion tend to be less episodic in nature in patients with chronic severe MR than MS, since fluctuations of the mean pulmonary capillary pressure are less marked. Indeed, acute paroxysmal pulmonary edema is quite rare in patients with chronic MR. Hemoptysis and systemic embolism also occur far less frequently in MR than in MS. On the other hand, fatigability, weakness, exhaustion, weight loss, and even cachexia are more prominent and occur most frequently in patients with MR and marked reduction of cardiac output. Right-sided heart failure, with painful hepatic congestion, ankle edema, distended neck veins, ascites, and tricuspid regurgitation, may be observed in patients with MR who have associated pulmonary vascular disease and marked pulmonary hypertension. In patients with *acute* severe MR, left ventricular failure with acute pulmonary edema and/or cardiovascular collapse is common.

PHYSICAL FINDINGS The arterial pressure is usually normal, and in severe MR the arterial pulse is often characterized by a sharp upstroke. The jugular venous pulse shows abnormally prominent a

waves in patients with sinus rhythm and marked pulmonary hypertension and prominent *v* waves in those with severe accompanying tricuspid regurgitation.

Palpation A systolic thrill is often palpable at the cardiac apex, the left ventricle is hyperdynamic with a brisk systolic impulse and a palpable rapid-filling wave, and the apex beat is often displaced laterally. When the left atrium is markedly enlarged, it may extend anteriorly, and its expansion may be palpable along the sternal border late during ventricular systole, resembling a right ventricular lift. The combination of the retraction of the left ventricle and expansion of the left atrium during systole may produce a characteristic rocking motion of the chest with each cardiac cycle. A right ventricular tap and the shock of pulmonary valve closure may be palpable in patients with marked pulmonary hypertension.

Auscultation The first heart sound is generally absent, soft, or buried in the systolic murmur, and an accentuated mitral closure sound is useful in excluding severe regurgitation. A pulmonary ejection sound is often audible in patients with associated pulmonary hypertension. Splitting of the second heart sound is usually normal, but in patients with severe MR, the aortic valve may close prematurely, resulting in wide splitting of the second heart sound. An OS indicates associated MS but does not exclude predominant regurgitation. A low-pitched third heart sound (S_3) occurring 0.12 to 0.17 s after the aortic valve closure sound, at the completion of the rapid-filling phase of the left ventricle, is believed to be caused by the sudden tensing of the papillary muscles, chordae tendineae, and valve leaflets and is an important auscultatory feature of severe MR. The absence of an S_3 indicates that if MR exists, it may not be severe. The S_3 may be followed, often after a brief interval, by a short, rumbling, diastolic murmur, even in the absence of MS. A fourth heart sound is often audible in patients with acute severe MR of recent onset who are in sinus rhythm. A presystolic murmur is not ordinarily heard in patients with pure MR and sinus rhythm but is present when there is significant associated MS.

A systolic murmur, grade III/VI in intensity or louder, is the most characteristic auscultatory finding in severe MR. It is usually holosystolic (Chap. 175), but it may be decrescendo when the tall *v* wave in the left atrial pressure pulse results in a reduced late systolic left ventricular–atrial pressure gradient in patients with acute severe MR. (The murmur commences in early to midsystole in mitral valve prolapse, see below.) Although the systolic murmur usually radiates into the axilla, in a minority of patients, particularly those with ruptured chordae tendineae or primary involvement of the posterior mitral leaflet, the regurgitant jet strikes the left atrial wall adjacent to the aortic root, and the systolic murmur is referred to the base of the heart and therefore may be confused with the murmur of aortic stenosis. In patients with ruptured chordae tendineae the systolic murmur may have a cooing or "sea gull" quality; in patients with a flail leaflet the murmur may have a musical quality.

Electrocardiogram In patients with sinus rhythm there is evidence of left atrial enlargement, but right atrial enlargement may also be present when pulmonary hypertension is extreme. Chronic, severe MR with left atrial enlargement is generally associated with atrial fibrillation. In many patients there is no clear-cut electrocardiographic evidence of enlargement of either ventricle. In others the signs of left ventricular hypertrophy are often present, although in patients with pulmonary hypertension combined ventricular hypertrophy or rarely pure right ventricular hypertrophy may be noted.

Echocardiogram The left atrium is usually enlarged and/or exhibits increased pulsations; the left ventricle may be hyperdynamic. With ruptured chordae tendineae or a flail leaflet coarse, erratic motion of the involved leaflets may be noted. Vegetations associated with infective endocarditis may be recognized. Incomplete coaptation of the anterior and posterior mitral leaflets, annular calcification, left ventricular dilatation, aneurysm, or dyskinesis, all of which may be of etiologic importance, can often be identified. Doppler echocardiography and color Doppler flow echocardiography imaging are the most accurate noninvasive techniques for the detection and estimation of MR (Fig. 177-5). The echocardiogram in patients with mitral valve prolapse is described below.

Roentgenogram The left atrium and left ventricle are the dominant chambers; in chronic cases the latter may be enlarged to aneurysmal proportions and forms the right border of the cardiac silhouette. Marked calcification of the mitral leaflets occurs commonly in patients with long-standing combined MR and MS but is uncommon in patients with pure MR. Contrast left ventriculography is useful in the quantification of MR.

TREATMENT Medical The nonsurgical management of MR is directed toward restricting those physical activities that regularly produce extreme fatigue and dyspnea, reducing sodium intake, and enhancing sodium excretion with the appropriate use of diuretics (Chap. 182). Vasodilators and digitalis glycosides increase the forward output of the failing left ventricle. Intravenous nitroprusside (p. 896) or nitroglycerin to reduce afterload and thereby the volume of regurgitant flow are useful in stabilizing patients with acute and/or severe MR. The same considerations as in patients with MS apply to the reversion of atrial fibrillation to sinus rhythm. In the late stages of heart failure anticoagulants and leg binders are used to diminish the likelihood of venous thrombi and pulmonary emboli.

Surgical In the selection of patients for surgical treatment, the chronic, often slowly progressive nature of the disease must be balanced against the immediate risks and long-term uncertainties attendant upon valve reconstruction or replacement. Patients with MR who are asymptomatic or who are limited only during strenuous exertion are not considered to be candidates for surgical treatment, since they may live for many years with little deterioration. On the other hand, unless there are contraindications, surgical treatment should be offered to patients with severe MR whose limitations do not allow them to work full time or to perform normal household activities despite optimal medical management. The risks of surgery rise sharply, the recovery of impaired left ventricular function is incomplete, and the long-term survival is reduced in patients with congestive heart failure. However, conservative management has little to offer these patients, so that operative treatment may be indicated even at these advanced stages of the disease, and occasionally the clinical and hemodynamic improvement following surgical treatment is dramatic. It is likely that the results of surgical treatment will continue to improve and will lead to recommendations of operative treatment for selected patients with MR before they become severely disabled. Though most patients who survive operation appear to be greatly improved, some degree of myocardial dysfunction may persist.

When surgical treatment is contemplated, right- and left-sided heart catheterization and selected left ventricular angiocardiography are generally indicated. These studies are helpful in confirming the presence of severe regurgitation and aid in the identification of patients with primary myocardial disease and relatively mild, functional MR, who usually do not benefit from operation. Hemodynamic studies are also helpful in detecting and assessing the severity of any associated valve lesions, which may have to be dealt with at the time of operation or which might limit the patient's ultimate improvement if they are left untreated. Coronary angiography identifies patients who require concomitant coronary revascularization.

Surgical treatment of MR, especially that caused by valves that are markedly deformed, with shrunken, calcified leaflets secondary to rheumatic fever, requires replacement of the valve with a prosthesis, although in an increasing fraction of patients, particularly those with severe annular dilatation, flail leaflets, mitral valve prolapse, ruptured chordae, or infective endocarditis, reconstruction of the mitral valve apparatus (mitral valvuloplasty) and/or mitral annuloplasty may be successful. Valve reconstruction should be carried out whenever feasible since it spares the patient the long-term adverse consequences of valve replacement (i.e., thromboembolic and hemorrhagic complications in the case of mechanical prostheses and late valve failure necessitating repeat valve replacement in the case of bioprostheses). Also, by preserving the integrity of the papillary muscles and subvalvular apparatus, mitral valvuloplasty maintains left ventricular function.

MITRAL VALVE PROLAPSE

Mitral valve prolapse (MVP) is also variously termed the *systolic click-murmur syndrome, Barlow's syndrome, floppy-valve syndrome,* and *billowing mitral leaflet syndrome,* a common, but highly variable, clinical syndrome resulting from diverse pathogenic mechanisms of the mitral valve apparatus. Among these are excessive or redundant mitral leaflet tissue, which is commonly involved with myxomatous degeneration and greatly increased concentration of acid mucopolysaccharide. It is a frequent finding in patients who have the typical features of Marfan's syndrome or cystic medial necrosis (Chap. 197), although in most patients myxomatous degeneration is confined to the mitral valve leaflets without other clinical or pathologic manifestations of disease; the posterior leaflet is usually more affected than the anterior, and the mitral valve annulus is often greatly enlarged. In many patients, elongated redundant chordae tendineae cause or contribute to the regurgitation. There are probably several subsets of these patients, who differ in regard to the etiology and hemodynamic and clinical sequelae of abnormal mitral valve function. In the majority of patients, the etiology is unknown, but MVP may be a genetically determined collagen tissue disorder. Fragmentation of collagen has been noted and an abnormality in the production of type III collagen has been incriminated in the etiology of the syndrome. MVP may be associated with thoracic skeletal deformities similar to but not as severe as those in Marfan's syndrome, including a high arched palate and alterations of the chest and thoracic spine. MVP may also occur as a sequel of acute rheumatic fever, in chronic rheumatic heart disease and following mitral valvulotomy, in ischemic heart disease, and cardiomyopathies, as well as in 20 percent of patients with ostium secundum atrial septal defect.

MVP is usually a benign abnormality that may progress to a stage involving significant regurgitation and ventricular dilatation in some individuals. In these, prolapse of the valve leads to excessive stress on the papillary muscles, which in turn leads to dysfunction and ischemia of the papillary muscles and subjacent ventricular myocardium; rupture of chordae tendineae and progressive annular dilatation also contribute to valvular regurgitation which then places more stress on the diseased mitral valve apparatus, thereby creating a vicious cycle. The electrocardiographic changes (see below) and ventricular arrhythmias appear to result from regional ventricular dysfunction related to increased stress placed on the papillary muscles.

MVP is more common in females and has been noted in a wide age range but most commonly between the ages of 14 and 30. Echocardiographic surveys have suggested that it may occur in as many as 7 percent of this group. There is an increased familial incidence suggesting an autosomal dominant form of inheritance. In many patients the echocardiographic abnormality is not accompanied by any other clinical manifestation of cardiac disease, and the significance of this finding is uncertain.

MVP encompasses a broad spectrum of severities, ranging from patients with only a systolic click and murmur and mild prolapse of the posterior leaflet of the mitral valve to those with severe MR due to chordal rupture and massive prolapse of both leaflets. In many patients, this condition progresses over years or decades.

Most of the patients are asymptomatic and remain so for their entire lives. Although severe MR is a relatively uncommon complication of MVP, the latter has become the most common cause of isolated *severe* MR. Arrythmias, most commonly ventricular premature contractions and paroxysmal supraventricular and ventricular tachycardia, have been reported and may cause palpitations, lightheadedness, and syncope. Sudden death is a very rare complication. Many patients have chest pain which is difficult to evaluate. It is often substernal, prolonged, poorly related to exertion, and rarely resembles typical angina pectoris. Transient cerebral ischemic attacks secondary to emboli from the roughened surface of the valve have been reported. Infective endocarditis may occur in patients with MR associated with MVP.

PHYSICAL EXAMINATION Auscultation The most common finding is the mid- or late (nonejection) systolic click, which occurs 0.14 s or more after the first heart sound and is thought to be generated by the sudden tensing of slack, elongated chordae tendineae or by the prolapsing mitral leaflet when it reaches its maximum excursion; systolic clicks may be multiple and are often followed by a high-pitched late systolic crescendo-decrescendo murmur, occasionally "whooping" or "honking," which is heard best at the apex. The click and murmur occur earlier with standing, the Valsalva maneuver, or inhalation of amyl nitrate, interventions which decrease left ventricular volume, exaggerating the propensity of mitral leaflet prolapse. Conversely, squatting and isometric exercise, which increase left ventricular end-diastolic volume, diminish the propensity for the mitral valve leaflets to prolapse, and the click-murmur complex is delayed and may even disappear. Some patients have a midsystolic click without the murmur; others have the murmur without a click.

LABORATORY EXAMINATION The *electrocardiogram* most commonly shows biphasic or inverted T waves in leads II, III, and aVF. The M-mode *echocardiogram* characteristically shows an abrupt posterior displacement of the posterior or sometimes of both mitral valve leaflets in mid- to late systole, immediately after the click, and during the systolic murmur. Two-dimensional echocardiography is particularly useful in identifying the abnormal position and prolapse of the mitral valve leaflets; a useful echocardiographic definition of MVP is systolic displacement of one or both mitral valve leaflets into the left atrium beyond the plane of the mitral annulus and imaged in the parasternal view. Thickening of the mitral valve leaflets identifies a subgroup of patients at higher risk of infective endocarditis and the development of severe MR. Doppler studies are helpful in revealing and evaluating accompanying MR. *Angiocardiography* generally shows prolapse of the posterior and sometimes of both mitral valve leaflets and, rarely, severe MR. Many patients have bulging of the posteroinferior wall of the left ventricle into the left ventricular cavity during systole and/or hypokinesis of the anterolateral left ventricular wall. Others display prolapse of other valves, particularly the tricuspid, in addition to the mitral.

TREATMENT The management of patients with MVP consists of reassurance of the asymptomatic patient, the prevention of infective endocarditis with antibiotic prophylaxis in patients with asystolic murmur and/or the typical echocardiographic features, and the relief of the atypical chest pain; beta blockers have been found to be helpful in this regard, although their use is empiric. Antiarrhythmic agents may be administered if frequent ventricular premature contractions or tachyarrhythmias have caused symptoms. If the patient is symptomatic secondary to severe MR, mitral valve repair or replacement is usually indicated. Antiplatelet aggregation agents (aspirin and dipyridamole) should be given to patients with transient ischemic attacks, and if these are not effective, anticoagulants should be employed.

AORTIC STENOSIS

Aortic stenosis (AS) occurs in about one-fourth of all patients with chronic valvular heart disease; approximately 80 percent of adult patients with symptomatic valvular AS are male.

ETIOLOGY AS may be congenital in origin, it may be secondary to rheumatic inflammation of the aortic valve, or it may be due to degenerative calcification of the aortic cusps of unknown cause. The *congenitally affected valve* may already be stenotic at birth (Chap. 186) and may gradually become more fibrotic and calcified during the first three decades of life, becoming progressively more stenotic. In others, the valve may also be congenitally bicuspid without serious narrowing of the aortic orifice during childhood; its abnormal architecture makes its leaflets susceptible to otherwise ordinary hemodynamic stresses, which ultimately lead to valvular thickening, calcification, increased rigidity, and narrowing of the aortic orifice.

Rheumatic endocarditis of the aortic leaflets produces commissural fusion, resulting sometimes in a bicuspid valve. This, in turn, also makes the leaflets more susceptible to trauma, and ultimately leads to calcification and further narrowing. By the time the obstruction to left ventricular outflow causes serious clinical disability, the valve is usually a rigid calcified mass, and careful examination may make it difficult or even impossible to determine whether the underlying process was rheumatic or congenital. Rheumatic AS is almost always associated with rheumatic involvement of the mitral valve. A rheumatic etiology is also favored by a history of active rheumatic fever and by associated severe aortic regurgitation.

Idiopathic calcific AS occurs most often in the elderly and is occasionally associated with fibrosis and fusion of the valve cusps; the pathologic process is considered to be a degenerative one—a "wear-and-tear" phenomenon. It may produce many of the characteristic physical signs of AS. However, the valvular obstruction is usually relatively mild and of little if any hemodynamic significance; it may, however, on occasion, produce critical obstruction.

OTHER FORMS OF OBSTRUCTION TO LEFT VENTRICULAR OUTFLOW Besides valvular AS, three other lesions may be responsible for obstruction to left ventricular outflow.

1 *Hypertrophic cardiomyopathy*. This is the most common of these conditions. It is characterized by marked hypertrophy of the left ventricle, involving in particular the interventricular septum of the left ventricular outflow tract, and may cause subaortic obstruction, as described in Chap. 192.
2 *Discrete congenital subvalvular AS*. This condition is produced by either a membranous diaphragm or a fibrous ridge just below the aortic valve (Chap. 186).
3 *Supravalvular AS*. This uncommon congenital anomaly is produced by narrowing of the ascending aorta or by a fibrous diaphragm with a small opening just above the aortic valve (Chap. 186).

PATHOPHYSIOLOGY The primary hemodynamic abnormality is obstruction to left ventricular outflow which leads to a systolic pressure gradient between the left ventricle and aorta. When severe obstruction is suddenly produced experimentally, the left ventricle responds by dilatation and reduction of stroke volume. However, in patients the obstruction may be present at birth and/or increase gradually over the course of many years, and left ventricular output is maintained by the presence of left ventricular hypertrophy. This serves as a useful compensatory mechanism since it reduces toward normal the systolic stress developed by each segment of myocardium. A large transaortic valvular pressure gradient may exist for many years without a reduction of cardiac output, left ventricular dilatation, or the development of any symptoms. As AS progresses in severity, the left ventricular systolic pressure continues to rise, but rarely exceeds 300 mmHg.

A peak systolic pressure gradient exceeding 50 mmHg in the face of a normal cardiac output or an effective aortic orifice less than 0.5 cm^2 per square meter of body surface area, i.e., less than approximately one-third of the normal orifice, is generally considered to represent critical obstruction to left ventricular outflow. The left ventricular pressure pulse exhibits a rounded summit as the contraction of this chamber becomes progressively more isometric. The elevated left ventricular end-diastolic pressure observed in many patients with severe AS does not necessarily signify the presence of left ventricular dilatation or failure, but may reflect diminished compliance of the hypertrophied left ventricular wall.

A large *a* wave in the left atrial pressure pulse is usually present with severe AS. Loss of an appropriately timed, vigorous atrial contraction, as occurs in atrial fibrillation or atrioventricular dissociation, may result in a rapid aggravation of symptoms.

Although the cardiac output at rest is within normal limits in the majority of patients with severe AS, it may fail to rise normally during exercise. Late in the course the cardiac output and left ventricular–aortic pressure gradient decline, and the mean left atrial, pulmonary artery wedge, pulmonary arterial, and right ventricular pressures become elevated.

The hypertrophied left ventricular muscle mass elevates myocardial oxygen requirements. In addition, even in the absence of obstructive coronary artery disease, there may be interference with coronary blood flow, because the pressure compressing the coronary arteries exceeds the coronary perfusion pressure. Metabolic evidence of myocardial ischemia, i.e., lactate production, can be demonstrated in patients with AS both in the presence and in the absence of coronary arterial narrowing, when myocardial oxygen needs are stimulated by isoproterenol.

A significant fraction of patients with rheumatic AS has associated mitral valve disease. AS intensifies the severity of mitral regurgitation by increasing the pressure driving blood from the left ventricle to the left atrium.

SYMPTOMS AS is rarely of hemodynamic or clinical importance until the valve orifice has narrowed to approximately one-third of normal. Severe AS may exist for many years without producing any symptoms because of the ability of the hypertrophied left ventricle to generate the elevated intraventricular pressures and the presence of a competent mitral valve behind the left ventricle.

Most patients with pure or predominant AS have gradually increasing obstruction for years but do not become symptomatic until the fifth to seventh decades. Exertional dyspnea, angina pectoris, and syncope are the three cardinal symptoms. Often there is a history of insidious progression of fatigue and dyspnea associated with gradual curtailment of activities. *Dyspnea* results primarily from elevation of the pulmonary capillary pressures, which in turn is caused by elevations of left atrial and left ventricular end-diastolic pressures, which are due in turn to left ventricular dilatation and/or reduced compliance. *Angina pectoris* usually develops somewhat later and reflects an imbalance between the augmented myocardial oxygen requirements and reduced oxygen availability; the former results from the increased myocardial mass and intraventricular pressure, while the latter may result from accompanying coronary artery disease which is not uncommon in patients with AS, as well as from compression of the coronary vessels by the hypertrophied myocardium. Therefore, angina may occur in severe AS without organic coronary obstruction; the *absence* of angina in such patients usually signifies that severe coronary obstructive disease is unlikely. *Exertional syncope* may result from a decline in arterial pressure caused by vasodilatation in the exercising muscles and inadequate vasoconstriction in nonexercising muscles in the face of a fixed cardiac output, or from a sudden fall in cardiac output produced by an arrhythmia.

Since the cardiac output at rest is usually well maintained until late in the course, marked fatigability, weakness, peripheral cyanosis, and other clinical manifestations of a low cardiac output are usually not prominent until this stage is reached. Orthopnea, paroxysmal nocturnal dyspnea, and pulmonary edema, i.e., symptoms of left ventricular failure, also occur only in the advanced stages of the disease. Severe pulmonary hypertension leading to right ventricular failure and systemic venous hypertension, hepatomegaly, atrial fibrillation, and tricuspid regurgitation are usually preterminal findings.

When AS and MS coexist, the latter lesion masks many of the clinical findings of the former. The reduction of cardiac output induced by MS lowers the pressure gradient across the aortic valve, diminishes the frequency of anginal episodes, and retards the development of severe left ventricular hypertrophy. On the other hand, symptoms considered more characteristic of MS, such as pulmonary congestion and hemoptysis, may be present. Physical, electrocardiographic, radiologic, and echocardiographic examinations in patients with combined AS and MS generally reveal more evidence of left ventricular enlargement than in patients with pure MS, and left heart catheterization is helpful in defining the relative importance of each valvular abnormality.

PHYSICAL FINDINGS AND GRAPHIC TRACINGS The systemic arterial pressure is usually within normal limits. In the late stages, however, when stroke volume declines, the systolic pressure may fall and the pulse pressure narrow. Systemic hypertension is unusual in patients with marked AS, and a basal systolic arterial pressure exceeding 200 mmHg practically excludes severe narrowing of this valve. The peripheral arterial pulse, as palpated in the carotid or brachial arteries, rises slowly to a delayed sustained peak. Indirect recordings of the carotid pulse exhibit a gradually ascending limb, often with a prominent anacrotic notch or shoulder on the upstroke, as well as a delayed peak, with coarse systolic vibrations. The left ventricular ejection period is prolonged, the preejection period is abbreviated, and the ratio of these two, i.e., the preejection period/systolic ejection period, is characteristically reduced. Late in the course of the disease, in the presence of heart failure, the ratio may be normal. A palpable double systolic arterial pulse, the so-called bisferiens pulse, excludes pure or predominant AS and signifies dominant or pure aortic regurgitation or obstructive hypertrophic cardiomyopathy (Chap. 192). In the late stages of valvular AS, when the pulse pressure is reduced, the pulse amplitude may be so small that the anacrotic nature of the pulse and the delay in its upstroke may become more difficult to appreciate. The jugular venous pulse may be normal, although in many patients the *a* wave is accentuated. This results from the diminished distensibility of the right ventricular cavity caused by the bulging, hypertrophied interventricular septum and/or the presence of pulmonary hypertension.

Palpation The apex beat is usually active and displaced inferiorly and laterally, reflecting the presence of left ventricular hypertrophy. A double apical impulse may be appreciated, particularly with the patient in the left lateral recumbent position; the first outward expansion occurs during atrial systole and reflects the important contribution made by atrial contraction to ventricular filling, while the second occurs during ventricular systole and usually is forceful and sustained during ejection. The right ventricle is usually palpable only when pulmonary hypertension develops in the late stages of the disease. A systolic thrill is generally present at the base of the heart, in the jugular notch, and along the carotid arteries, but occasionally it is palpable only during expiration and with the patient leaning forward. In patients who do not have marked pulmonary emphysema, a thick chest wall, thoracic deformity, or heart failure, the absence of a systolic thrill suggests that the aortic stenosis is relatively mild.

Auscultation The rhythm is generally regular until very late in the course; at other times, atrial fibrillation should suggest the possibility of associated mitral valve disease. An early systolic ejection sound, actually the OS of the aortic valve, is frequently audible in children and adolescents with congenital noncalcific valvular AS. This sound usually disappears when the valve becomes calcified and rigid. The sound of aortic valve closure can also be identified most frequently in patients with AS who have pliable valves, and calcification diminishes the intensity of this sound as well. As AS increases in severity, left ventricular systole may become prolonged so that the aortic valve closure sound no longer precedes the pulmonic valve closure sound, and the two components may become synchronous, or aortic valve closure may even follow pulmonic valve closure, causing paradoxic splitting of the second heart sound (Chap. 175). In patients with AS without a left intraventricular conduction defect, this finding usually signifies severe obstruction to left ventricular outflow. A fourth heart sound is audible at the apex in many patients with severe AS, and reflects the presence of left ventricular hypertrophy and an elevated left ventricular end-diastolic pressure; a third heart sound generally occurs when the left ventricle dilates and fails.

The murmur of AS is characteristically an ejection systolic murmur which commences shortly after the first heart sound, increases in intensity to reach a peak toward the middle of the ejection period, and diminishes progressively thereafter to end just before aortic valve closure (Chap. 175). The murmur is usually low-pitched, rough, and rasping in character and is loudest at the base of the heart, most commonly in the second right intercostal space. It is transmitted to the jugular notch and upward along the carotid arteries. In patients with mild degrees of obstruction or in those with severe stenosis with heart failure in whom the stroke volume and therefore the transvalvular flow rate is reduced, the murmur may be relatively soft and brief. However, in almost all patients with severe obstruction, the murmur is at least grade III/VI. Occasionally, the murmur is transmitted downward and to the apex and may be confused with the systolic murmur of MR; however, the latter is usually holosystolic.

Electrocardiogram This reveals left ventricular hypertrophy in the majority of patients with severe AS (Chap. 176). In advanced cases, ST-segment depression and T-wave inversion (left ventricular "strain") in standard leads I and aVL and in the left precordial leads are evident. However, there is no close correlation between the electrocardiogram and the hemodynamic severity of obstruction, and the absence of electrocardiographic signs of left ventricular hypertrophy does not exclude severe obstruction. Atrioventricular and intraventricular conduction defects, usually caused by infiltration with calcium and/or diffuse fibrotic involvement of the myocardium, are observed in 5 to 10 percent of patients. The presence of left atrial enlargement should suggest the possibility of associated mitral valve disease.

Echocardiogram This reveals left ventricular hypertrophy and in patients with valvular calcification, multiple, bright, thick, echoes from within the aortic root. While cusp calcification does not necessarily indicate significant valve stenosis, its absence can usually be used to *exclude* such a diagnosis after the age of 25. Eccentricity of the aortic valve cusps is characteristic of congenitally bicuspid valves. Left ventricular dilatation and reduced systolic shortening reflecting impairment of left ventricular function can be recognized. The transaortic valvular gradient can be estimated by Doppler echocardiography. Echocardiography is particularly useful for identifying valvular abnormalities such as MS and aortic regurgitation which sometimes accompany AS (Fig. 177-5), and for differentiating valvular from obstructive hypertrophic cardiomyopathy.

Roentgenogram The chest roentgenogram may show no or little overall cardiac enlargement for many years, since the development of concentric left ventricular hypertrophy is the initial response to obstruction to left ventricular outflow. Hypertrophy without dilatation may produce some rounding of the cardiac apex in the frontal projection and slight backward displacement in the lateral view; critical AS is often associated with poststenotic dilatation of the ascending aorta. Aortic calcification is usually readily apparent on fluoroscopic examination with an image intensifier or by echocardiography; *the absence of valvular calcification in an adult suggests that severe valvular AS is not present.* In later stages of the disease as the left ventricle dilates, there is increasing evidence of left ventricular enlargement, and there may also be roentgenographic signs of pulmonary congestion, as well as enlargement of the left atrium, pulmonary artery, right ventricle, and right atrium.

Catheterization and angiocardiography Catheterization of the left side of the heart and coronary arteriography should generally be carried out in patients suspected of having severe AS, particularly before a final decision concerning operative treatment is made. The goals are to (1) determine the severity of the aortic obstruction, often previously estimated by Doppler echocardiography, (2) assess the status of left ventricular function, and (3) determine the location of the left ventricular outflow obstruction. These investigations are especially indicated in the following:

1 Young, asymptomatic patients with noncalcific congenital AS (Chap. 186), in order to define the severity of obstruction to left ventricular outflow, since operation may be indicated in them even in the absence of symptoms if severe AS is present.
2 Patients in whom it is suspected that the obstruction to left ventricular outflow may not be at the aortic valve, but rather in the sub- or supravalvular regions.
3 Patients with clinical signs of AS and symptoms of myocardial ischemia, in whom associated coronary artery disease is suspected.

An effort should be made to determine whether aortic stenosis or coronary atherosclerosis is primarily responsible for the symptoms, and coronary arteriography should be carried out in addition to catheterization of the left side of the heart.

4 Patients with multivalvular disease, in whom the role played by each valvular deformity must be defined before operative treatment is planned.

Angiographic studies are helpful in defining the size of the left ventricular cavity, the thickness of the wall, the site of obstruction, the degree of deformity and mobility of the aortic valve cusps, the diameter of the ascending aorta, and the presence and degree of accompanying mitral and aortic regurgitation and of obstructive coronary disease. In patients with severe narrowing, a jet of contrast substance passing through the aortic orifice is readily visualized.

NATURAL HISTORY Death in patients with severe AS occurs most commonly in the seventh decade. Based on data obtained at postmortem examination, the average duration of various symptoms in patients *not treated surgically* was as follows: angina pectoris, 3 years; syncope, 3 years; dyspnea, 2 years; and congestive heart failure, 1.5 to 2 years. Moreover, in more than 80 percent of patients who died with AS, symptoms had existed for less than 4 years. Congestive heart failure was considered to be the cause of death in one-half to two-thirds of patients. Among adults dying with valvular AS, sudden death, which presumably results from an arrhythmia, occurred in 10 to 20 percent, and at an average age of 60 years.

TREATMENT Strenuous physical activity should be avoided even in the asymptomatic stage in patients with *severe* AS. Digitalis glycosides, sodium restriction, and the cautious administration of diuretics are indicated in the treatment of congestive heart failure, but care must be taken to avoid volume depletion. While nitroglycerin is helpful in relieving angina pectoris, vasodilator therapy for heart failure is usually of little value. The most critical decision in the management of AS, indeed of any valvular lesion, concerns the advisability of surgical treatment. The indications and results of operation, as well as the techniques, differ considerably, depending on the patient's age and the nature of the valvular deformity.

In children and adolescents with noncalcific congenital AS, considerable hemodynamic improvement can be anticipated from simple commissural incision under direct vision. This operation is recommended not only for symptomatic patients but also for asymptomatic children and adolescents with hemodynamic evidence of severe obstruction to left ventricular outflow, with a peak systolic pressure gradient exceeding 50 mmHg when the cardiac output is normal, or a calculated effective orifice less than 0.6 cm^2 per square meter of body surface area.

In the majority of adults with calcific AS, replacement of the valve is necessary. In most instances, it is prudent to postpone operation in patients with severe calcific AS who are asymptomatic, since their future course is difficult to predict and they may continue to do well for many years. However, they should be followed carefully by clinical examination for the development of symptoms and by the various noninvasive tests, such as echocardiograms and/or radionuclide angiograms (Chap. 177), for evidence of deteriorating left ventricular function; operation is generally indicated in patients with severe AS and left ventricular dysfunction, even if they are only mildly symptomatic. It is likely that as the results of surgical replacement of the aortic valve continue to improve, many asymptomatic patients with severe AS will become candidates for operation before their left ventricular function deteriorates. At the present, replacement of the aortic valve should be undertaken in patients with symptoms, even when relatively mild, that are believed to result primarily from AS and who have hemodynamic evidence of severe obstruction. In such patients the operative risk is relatively low (<5 percent) in centers with experience.

When angina pectoris, syncope, or left ventricular decompensation develops in adults with severe valvular AS, the outlook, despite medical treatment, is very poor and can be improved significantly by replacement of the aortic valve with a mechanical or bioprosthetic valve. Therefore, the risk entailed by operation in this group of patients although relatively high is still considerably lower than the risk involved by nonoperative treatment; moreover, the symptomatic improvement in many survivors of operation has been remarkable.

Operation should, if possible, be carried out before frank left ventricular failure supervenes; at this late stage, the operative risk is high (approximately 15 percent) and evidence of myocardial disease may persist even when the operation is technically successful. Furthermore, long-term postoperative survival also correlates inversely with preoperative functional disability. Nonetheless, in view of the very poor prognosis of such patients when they are treated medically, there is usually little choice but to advise immediate surgical treatment. In patients in whom severe AS and coronary artery disease coexist, relief of the AS and revascularization of the myocardium by means of aortocoronary bypass grafting may result in striking clinical and hemodynamic improvement. Since many patients with calcific AS are elderly, particular attention must be directed to the adequacy of hepatic, renal, and pulmonary function before valve replacement is recommended. The mortality rate depends to a substantial extent on the patient's preoperative clinical and hemodynamic state. The 10-year survival rate of operative survivors following aortic valve replacement is approximately 67 percent. Approximately 15 percent of bioprosthetic valves evidence primary valve failure in 10 years, requiring re-replacement, and an approximately equal percentage of patients with mechanical prostheses develop significant hemorrhagic complications as a consequence of treatment with anticoagulants. Fortunately, there is evidence that regression of left ventricular hypertrophy may occur following relief of obstruction.

Percutaneous balloon aortic valvuloplasty, described in Chap. 180, is an alternative to surgery in children and young adults with congenital aortic stenosis and in elderly patients with severe calcific aortic stenosis. Although the restenosis rate is high in the latter, the procedure may be useful in patients who are too ill or frail to undergo surgery, in patients with severe aortic stenosis and advanced extracardiac disease, as well as a "bridge to surgery" in patients with severe left ventricular dysfunction. The improvement in their left ventricular function following balloon valvuloplasty may make them suitable candidates for definitive operation, i.e. valve replacement.

AORTIC REGURGITATION

ETIOLOGY Approximately three-fourths of all patients with pure or predominant aortic regurgitation (AR) are males; however, females predominate among patients with AR who have associated mitral valve disease. In approximately two-thirds of patients with AR the disease is rheumatic in origin, resulting in a chronic form of the disorder with thickening, deformation, and shortening of the individual aortic valve cusps, changes which prevent their proper closure during diastole. A rheumatic etiology is less common in patients with isolated AR. Acute AR may also result from infective endocarditis, which may attack a valve previously affected by rheumatic disease, a congenitally deformed valve, or rarely a normal aortic valve, and may result in the perforation or erosion of one or more of the leaflets. Patients with discrete membranous subaortic stenosis often develop thickening of the aortic valve leaflets, which in turn leads to mild or moderate degrees of AR and makes these valves particularly susceptible to endocarditis. Aortic regurgitation may also occur in patients with congenital bicuspid aortic valves. Prolapse of an aortic cusp, resulting in progressive chronic AR, occurs in approximately 15 percent of patients with ventricular septal defect (Chap. 186). Congenital fenestrations of the aortic valve occasionally produce mild AR. Although traumatic rupture of the aortic valve is an uncommon cause of acute AR, it does represent the most frequent serious lesion observed in patients surviving nonpenetrating cardiac injuries. In patients with AR due to primary valvular disease, dilatation of the aortic annulus may occur secondarily and intensify the regurgitation.

AR, both acute and chronic, may also be due entirely to marked aortic dilatation, without primary involvement of the valve leaflets; widening of the aortic annulus and separation of the aortic leaflets are responsible for the aortic regurgitation. Syphilis and ankylosing rheumatoid spondylitis may be associated with cellular infiltration and scarring of the media of the thoracic aorta, leading to aortic dilatation, aneurysm formation, and severe regurgitation. In syphilis of the aorta (Chap. 197), the involvement of the intima may narrow the coronary ostia, which in turn may be responsible for myocardial ischemia. Cystic medial necrosis of the ascending aorta, which may or may not be associated with other manifestations of the Marfan syndrome, idiopathic dilatation of the aorta, and severe hypertension all may also widen the aortic annulus and lead to progressive AR. Occasionally, retrograde dissection of the aorta involving the aortic annulus produces aortic regurgitation.

The coexistence of hemodynamically significant AS with AR usually excludes all of the rarer forms of AR because it occurs almost exclusively in patients whose aortic regurgitation is on a rheumatic or congenital basis.

PATHOPHYSIOLOGY The total stroke volume expelled by the left ventricle (i.e., the sum of the effective forward stroke volume and the volume of blood which regurgitates back into the left ventricle) is increased in AR. In patients with wide-open (*free*) AR the volume of regurgitant flow may equal the effective forward stroke volume. In contrast to MR, in which a fraction of the left ventricular stroke volume is delivered into the low-pressure left atrium, in AR the entire left ventricular stroke volume must be ejected into a high-pressure zone, the aorta. The low aortic diastolic pressure (low afterload) facilitates ventricular emptying. However, an increase of the left ventricular end-diastolic volume (increased preload) constitutes the major hemodynamic compensation to aortic regurgitation. The dilatation of the left ventricle allows this chamber to expel a larger stroke volume without requiring any increase in the relative shortening of each myofibril. Therefore, severe AR may occur with a normal effective forward stroke volume and a normal ejection fraction [total (forward plus regurgitant) stroke volume/end-diastolic volume], together with an elevated left ventricular end-diastolic pressure and volume. However, through the operation of Laplace's law (which indicates that myocardial wall tension is the product of intracavitary pressure and left ventricular radius), left ventricular dilatation increases the left ventricular systolic tension required to develop any given level of systolic pressure. As left ventricular function deteriorates, the end-diastolic volume and the ejection fraction and forward stroke volume decline. Deterioration of left ventricular function often precedes the development of symptoms. Considerable thickening of the left ventricular wall also occurs with chronic AR, and at autopsy the hearts of these patients may be among the largest encountered, occasionally exceeding 1000 g in weight.

The reverse pressure gradient from aorta to left ventricle, which is responsible for the aortic regurgitant flow, falls progressively during diastole, accounting for the decrescendo nature of the diastolic murmur. Equilibration between aortic and left ventricular pressures may occur toward the end of diastole in patients with severe AR, particularly when the heart rate is slow, and the left ventricular end-diastolic pressure may be elevated, occasionally to extremely high levels (>40 mmHg). Rarely, the left ventricular pressure exceeds the left atrial pressure toward the end of diastole, and this reversed pressure gradient closes the mitral valve prematurely, or may cause diastolic mitral regurgitation.

In patients with free AR the effective forward cardiac output usually is normal or only slightly reduced at rest, but often it fails to rise normally during exertion. Early signs of left ventricular dysfunction include reductions of the fraction of systolic shortening and of the ejection fraction determined by echocardiography or radionuclide or contrast angiography. In advanced stages there may be considerable elevation of the left atrial, pulmonary artery wedge, pulmonary arterial, and right ventricular pressures, and lowering of the forward cardiac output at rest.

Myocardial ischemia may occur in patients with AR because both left ventricular dilatation and the elevated left ventricular systolic tension tend to augment myocardial oxygen requirements. However, the major portion of coronary blood flow occurs during diastole, when arterial pressure is subnormal, thereby reducing coronary perfusion pressure. The combination of increased oxygen demand and reduced supply may cause myocardial ischemia.

HISTORY A family history may frequently be elicited from patients with AR associated with the Marfan syndrome, and a history of a heart murmur heard early in life may be obtained from patients with congenital AR with or without a ventricular septal defect. Patients with AR of obscure cause should also be questioned about a positive serologic test for syphilis, and about prior chest trauma; a history compatible with infective endocarditis may sometimes be elicited from patients with rheumatic or congenital involvement of the aortic valve, and the infection often precipitates or seriously aggravates preexisting symptoms. Ankylosing spondylitis is usually self-evident.

The interval between the first episode of acute rheumatic fever and the development of hemodynamically significant AR averages approximately 7 years, and this period is followed by an asymptomatic interval of approximately 10 to 20 years, during which the severity of the AR usually increases. Thus, patients with severe AR may remain asymptomatic for many years.

In chronic severe AR, uncomfortable awareness of the heartbeat, especially on lying down, may be an early complaint. Sinus tachycardia during exertion or with emotion, or premature ventricular contractions, may produce particularly uncomfortable palpitations, as well as head pounding. These complaints may persist for many years before the development of exertional dyspnea, usually the first symptom of diminished cardiac reserve. This is followed by orthopnea, paroxysmal nocturnal dyspnea, and excessive diaphoresis. Chest pain occurs frequently, even in younger patients, and it is not necessary to invoke the presence of coronary artery disease to explain this symptom in patients with AR. It may be due to myocardial ischemia, or it may originate from excessive cardiac pounding on the chest wall. Anginal pain may develop at rest as well as during exertion. Nocturnal angina may be a particularly troublesome symptom, and it may be accompanied by marked diaphoresis. The anginal episodes may be prolonged and often do not respond satisfactorily to sublingual nitroglycerin. Late in the course of the disease, evidence of systemic fluid accumulation, including congestive hepatomegaly, ankle edema, and ascites, may develop. Patients with severe AR tolerate high fevers, infections, or cardiac arrhythmias poorly, and may die in pulmonary edema as a result of one of these complications.

In patients with acute severe AR, as may occur in trauma or infective endocarditis, the left ventricle rapidly exhausts its ability to dilate, and left ventricular diastolic pressure rises rapidly with associated elevations of left atrial and pulmonary capillary pressures.

PHYSICAL FINDINGS Even prior to the examination of the heart of the patient with free AR, the jarring of the entire body and the bobbing motion of the head with each systole can be appreciated, and the abrupt distention and collapse of the larger arteries are easily visible. The examination should be directed toward the detection of conditions predisposing to AR, such as the Marfan syndrome, rheumatoid spondylitis, syphilis, essential hypertension, and ventricular septal defect.

Arterial pulse A rapidly rising "water-hammer" pulse, which collapses suddenly as arterial pressure falls rapidly during late systole and diastole (Corrigan's pulse), and capillary pulsations (Quincke's pulse), an alternate flushing and paling of the skin at the root of the nail while pressure is applied to the tip of the nail, are characteristic of free AR. A booming, "pistol-shot" sound can be heard over the femoral arteries, and a to-and-fro murmur (Duroziez's sign) is audible if the femoral artery is lightly compressed with a stethoscope.

The arterial pulse pressure is widened, with an elevation of the systolic pressure, sometimes to as high as 300 mmHg, and a depression of the diastolic arterial pressure. The measurement of arterial diastolic pressure with a sphygmomanometer may be complicated by the fact that systolic sounds are frequently heard with the cuff completely deflated. However, the level of cuff pressure at the time of muffling of the Korotkoff sounds generally corresponds fairly closely to the true intraarterial diastolic pressure. The severity of AR does not always correlate directly with the arterial pulse pressure, and severe regurgitation may exist in patients with arterial pressures in the range of 140/60. As the disease progresses, and the left ventricular end-diastolic pressure rises markedly, the arterial diastolic pressure may actually rise also, since the aortic diastolic pressure cannot fall below the left ventricular end-diastolic pressure.

Palpation The apex beat is displaced laterally and inferiorly. The left ventricle is hyperdynamic in patients with free AR, and the systolic expansion and subsequent retraction of the apex are prominent and contrast sharply with the sustained systolic thrust characteristic of severe AS. A diastolic thrill is often palpable along the left sternal border, and a prominent systolic thrill may be palpable in the jugular notch and transmitted upward along the carotid arteries. This thrill and the accompanying systolic murmur are due to the markedly increased blood flow across the aortic orifice, and do not necessarily signify the coexistence of AS. In many patients with pure AR, or with combined AS and AR, palpation, or indirect recording of the carotid arterial pulse, reveals it to be bisferiens, i.e., with two systolic waves separated by a trough.

Auscultation In patients with severe regurgitation the aortic valve closure sound is usually diminished or absent. A third heart sound is common, and occasionally a fourth heart sound may also be heard. A loud systolic ejection sound is frequently audible; presumably it results from the sudden dilatation of the aorta by a greatly increased stroke volume. The murmur of AR is typically a high-pitched, blowing, decrescendo diastolic murmur which is usually heard best in the third left intercostal space. In patients with mild regurgitation this murmur is brief, but as the severity increases, the murmur generally becomes louder and longer, and in patients with free AR it is usually holodiastolic. When the murmur is soft, it can be heard best with the diaphragm of the stethoscope and with the patient sitting up, leaning forward, and with the breath held in forced expiration. As it increases in intensity it tends to radiate widely, particularly down the lower sternal edge. In patients in whom the regurgitation is caused by primary valvular disease, the diastolic murmur is usually louder along the left than the right sternal border. However, when the decrescendo diastolic murmur is heard best along the right sternal border, it suggests that the aortic regurgitation is caused by dilatation or an aneurysm of the aortic root. "Cooing" or musical diastolic murmurs suggest eversion of an aortic cusp vibrating in the regurgitant stream. A diastolic blowing murmur along the left sternal border is much more commonly caused by aortic than by pulmonic regurgitation. Unless it is trivial in magnitude, the AR is usually accompanied by peripheral signs such as a widened pulse pressure or a collapsing pulse. On the other hand, with the Graham Steell murmur of pulmonary regurgitation there usually is clinical evidence of severe pulmonary hypertension, including a loud and palpable pulmonary component of the second heart sound. In addition, the phonocardiogram reveals that the murmur of AR begins with the aortic second sound and therefore commences somewhat before the murmur of pulmonary regurgitation.

A midsystolic ejection murmur is frequently audible in AR. It is generally heard best at the base of the heart and is transmitted to the jugular notch and along the carotid vessels. This murmur may be as loud as grade V/VI without indicating the presence of organic obstruction; it is often higher pitched, shorter, and less rasping in quality than the ejection systolic murmur heard in patients with predominant AS. A third murmur which is frequently heard in patients with AR is the Austin Flint murmur, a soft, low-pitched, rumbling middiastolic or presystolic bruit. It is probably produced by the displacement of the anterior leaflet of the mitral valve by the aortic regurgitant stream but does not appear to be associated with hemodynamically significant obstruction to left ventricular filling; earlier onset of and longer Austin Flint murmurs correlate with more severe AR. Both the Austin Flint murmur and the rumbling diastolic murmur of MS are loudest at the apex, but the murmur of MS is usually accompanied by a loud first heart sound and immediately follows the opening snap of the mitral valve, while the Austin Flint murmur is often shorter in duration than the murmur of MS, and in patients with sinus rhythm the latter more frequently is characterized by presystolic accentuation. The auscultatory features of AR are intensified by isometric exercise such as strenuous handgrip, which augments systemic resistance, and reduced by inhalation of amyl nitrite, which evokes the opposite effect. A blowing holosystolic murmur at the apex, which is transmitted to the axilla, may also be heard in patients with aortic regurgitation who have marked left ventricular dilatation and functional mitral regurgitation.

In *acute* severe AR, the elevation of left ventricular end-diastolic pressure may lead to early closure of the mitral valve, an associated middiastolic sound, a soft or absent S_1, a pulse pressure that is not particularly wide, and a soft, short diastolic murmur.

Electrocardiogram In patients with mild AR there may be no electrocardiographic abnormalities, but with severe chronic AR the electrocardiographic signs of left ventricular hypertrophy become manifest (Chap. 176). In addition to the abnormally tall R waves over the left precordium and deep S waves over the right precordium, patients with severe aortic regurgitation frequently exhibit ST-segment depressions and T-wave inversions in leads I, aVL, V_5, and V_6 ("left ventricular strain"). Left axis deviation and/or QRS prolongation denote diffuse myocardial disease, generally associated with patchy fibrosis, and usually denote a poor prognosis.

Echocardiogram This reveals increased systolic excursion of the posterior left ventricular wall; the extent and velocity of wall motion are normal or even supernormal, until myocardial contractility declines. A rapid, high-frequency fluttering of the anterior mitral leaflet produced by the impact of the aortic regurgitant jet is a characteristic finding. The echocardiogram is also useful in detecting dilatation of the aortic annulus, and of the left atrium. Thickening of the aortic valve and failure of coaptation of the leaflets may also be noted. Color Doppler flow echocardiographic imaging is very sensitive in the detection of AR, and Doppler echocardiography is helpful in assessing its severity (Fig. 177-5).

Roentgenogram Moderate or severe degrees of chronic AR are associated with varying degrees of left ventricular enlargement. The apex is displaced downward and to the left in the frontal projection, and frequently the cardiac shadow extends below the left diaphragm. Left ventricular enlargement may also be apparent in the left anterior oblique and lateral projections, in which the left ventricle is displaced posteriorly and encroaches on the spine. In patients in whom primary valvular disease is responsible for the AR, the ascending aorta and aortic knob may be moderately dilated. When AR is caused by primary disease of the aortic wall, aneurysmal dilatation of the aorta may be noted roentgenographically, and the aorta may fill the retrosternal space in the lateral view.

Cardiac catheterization and angiography These tests should be carried out to aid in the decision regarding surgical treatment. In addition to providing an accurate measurement of the magnitude of regurgitation and the status of left ventricular function, the condition of the coronary arterial bed may be evaluated.

TREATMENT In deciding upon the advisability and proper timing of surgical treatment, two points should be kept in mind: (1) patients with chronic AR usually do not become symptomatic until *after* the development of myocardial dysfunction; and (2) surgical treatment often does not restore normal left ventricular function. Therefore, careful clinical follow-up and noninvasive testing, with echocardiography or radionuclide angiography, at approximately 6-month intervals, are necessary if operation is to be undertaken at the optimal time, i.e., with the onset of left ventricular dysfunction but prior to the development of severe symptoms. Operation can be deferred as long as the patient remains asymptomatic *and* retains normal left ventricular function.

Replacement of the aortic valve with a suitable mechanical or tissue prosthesis is generally necessary in patients with rheumatic AR and in many patients with other forms of regurgitation. Rarely, when a leaflet has been perforated during an episode of infective endocarditis, or torn from its attachments to the aortic annulus, surgical repair may be possible. When AR is due to aneurysmal dilatation of the annulus and ascending aorta, rather than to primary valvular involvement, it may be possible to reduce the regurgitation by narrowing the annulus or by excising a portion of the aortic root without replacing the valve. More frequently, however, regurgitation can be eliminated only by replacing the aortic valve, excising the aneurysm responsible for the regurgitation, and replacing the latter with a graft. This formidable procedure entails a higher risk than aortic valve replacement alone.

As in patients with other valvular abnormalities, both the operative risk of aortic valve replacement and late mortality are largely dependent on the stage of the disease and on myocardial function at the time of operation; patients with marked cardiac enlargement and prolonged left ventricular dysfunction have a late mortality of approximately 5 percent per year despite a technically satisfactory operation.

Although operation constitutes the principal treatment of aortic regurgitation, and should be carried out before the development of heart failure, the latter usually does respond initially to treatment with digitalis glycosides, salt restriction, diuretics, and vasodilators, especially angiotensin-converting enzyme inhibitors. Digitalis may also be indicated in patients with severe regurgitation and dilated left ventricles without symptoms of frank left ventricular failure. Cardiac arrhythmias and infections are poorly tolerated in patients with free AR, and must be treated promptly and vigorously. Although nitroglycerin and long-acting nitrates are not as helpful in relieving anginal pain as in patients with coronary artery disease or aortic stenosis, they are worth a trial. Patients with syphilitic aortitis should receive a full course of penicillin therapy (Chap. 128).

ACUTE AORTIC REGURGITATION Infective endocarditis, aortic dissection, and trauma are the most common causes of severe, acute AR. Since the left ventricle has not had time to dilate, stroke volume declines and ventricular diastolic pressure rises markedly; the arterial pulse pressure is often not markedly widened and the physical signs characteristic of severe chronic AR may be absent. Premature closure of the mitral valve is common and can be recognized by echocardiography. The first heart sound is soft or absent; the aortic diastolic murmur is characteristically brief. Patients present with pulmonary congestion and edema, and hypotension secondary to a low cardiac output. Acute, severe regurgitation requires prompt surgical treatment, which may be lifesaving.

TRICUSPID STENOSIS

Tricuspid stenosis (TS), a relatively uncommon valvular lesion, is generally rheumatic in origin and is much more common in women than in men. It does not usually occur as an isolated lesion or in patients with pure MR, but most commonly is observed in association with MS, and sometimes with combined MS and AS. Hemodynamically significant TS occurs in 5 to 10 percent of patients with severe MS; rheumatic TS is commonly associated with some degree of regurgitation.

PATHOPHYSIOLOGY A diastolic pressure gradient between the right atrium and ventricle is present. This gradient can be recorded most accurately and conveniently with a double-lumen cardiac catheter. It is augmented when the transvalvular blood flow increases during inspiration, and reduced during expiration. A *mean* diastolic pressure gradient exceeding 4 mmHg is usually sufficient to elevate the mean right atrial pressure to levels which result in systemic venous congestion and, unless sodium intake has been restricted or diuretics have been given, is associated with ascites and edema. In patients with sinus rhythm, the right atrial *a* wave may be extremely tall and may even approach the level of the right ventricular systolic pressure. The resting cardiac output is usually quite low and fails to rise during exercise. The low cardiac output is responsible for the normal or only slightly elevated left atrial, pulmonary arterial, and right ventricular systolic pressures despite the presence of even moderately severe MS.

SYMPTOMS Since MS generally precedes the development of TS, many patients initially have symptoms of pulmonary congestion. Amelioration of the latter should raise the possibility that TS may be developing. Characteristically, patients complain of relatively little dyspnea for the degree of hepatomegaly, ascites, and edema which they present. Weakness secondary to a low cardiac output and discomfort due to refractory edema, ascites, and marked hepatomegaly are common in patients with TS and/or regurgitation. In some patients TS may be suspected for the first time when symptoms of right ventricular failure persist after an adequate mitral valvulotomy.

PHYSICAL FINDINGS Since TS usually occurs in the presence of other obvious valvular disease, the diagnosis is often missed unless it is specifically considered and searched for. Severe TS is associated with marked hepatic congestion, often resulting in cirrhosis, jaundice, serious malnutrition, severe edema, and ascites. Congestive hepatomegaly and, in cases of severe tricuspid valve disease, splenomegaly are present. The jugular veins are distended, and in patients with sinus rhythm there may be giant *a* waves. The *v* waves are less conspicuous, and since tricuspid obstruction impedes right atrial emptying during diastole, there is a slow *y* descent. In patients with sinus rhythm there may be prominent presystolic pulsations of the enlarged liver as well.

The right ventricle and the shock of pulmonic valve closure are usually not easily palpable. Indeed, a giant *a* wave in the jugular venous pulse without palpatory evidence of pulmonary hypertension or right ventricular enlargement should immediately suggest the possibility of TS. On auscultation, the pulmonic closure sound is not accentuated, and occasionally an OS of the tricuspid valve may be heard or recorded phonocardiographically approximately 0.06 s after pulmonic valve closure. The diastolic murmur of TS has many of the qualities of the diastolic murmur of MS, and since TS almost always occurs in the presence of MS, the less-common valvular lesion may be missed. However, the tricuspid murmur is generally heard best along the left lower sternal margin and over the xiphoid process and is most prominent during presystole in sinus rhythm. In patients with sinus rhythm the presystolic component is often loudest. The murmur is augmented during inspiration, and it is reduced during expiration and particularly during the Valsalva maneuver, when tricuspid blood flow is reduced. This finding (Carvallo's sign) is often most easily elicited when the patient is in the erect position. The diastolic murmur is reduced in amplitude as the stethoscope is inched laterally, only to intensify or reappear as the mitral murmur at the apex.

Noninvasive examinations The features of right atrial enlargement (Chap. 176) include tall, peaked P waves in lead II, as well as prominent, upright P waves in lead V_1. The *absence* of electrocardiographic evidence of right ventricular hypertrophy in a patient with right-sided heart failure who is believed to have MS should suggest associated tricuspid valve disease. The chest roentgenograms in patients with combined TS and MS show particular prominence of the right atrium and superior vena cava without much enlargement of the pulmonary artery and with less evidence of pulmonary vascular congestion than occurs in patients with pure mitral valve disease. On echocardiographic examination the tricuspid valve is usually thickened; the transvalvular gradient can be estimated by Doppler echocardiography.

TREATMENT Patients with TS generally exhibit marked systemic venous congestion; intensive salt restriction and diuretic therapy are required during the preoperative period. Such a preparatory period may diminish hepatic congestion and thereby improve hepatic function sufficiently so that the risks of operation are diminished. Surgical treatment of the tricuspid valve is not ordinarily indicated at the time of mitral valve surgery in patients with *mild* TS. On the other hand, definitive surgical relief of the TS should be carried out, preferably at the time of mitral valvulotomy, in patients with moderate or severe TS who have mean diastolic pressure gradients exceeding 4 to 5 mmHg and tricuspid orifices less than 1.5 to 2.0 cm^2. TS is almost always accompanied by significant tricuspid regurgitation. Open-heart operations utilizing cardiopulmonary bypass may permit substantial improvement of tricuspid valve function. If this cannot be accomplished, the tricuspid valve may have to be replaced with a prosthesis, preferably a tissue valve.

TRICUSPID REGURGITATION

Most commonly, tricuspid regurgitation (TR) is functional and secondary to marked dilatation of the right ventricle and the tricuspid valve ring. Functional TR may complicate right ventricular enlargement of any cause, including inferior wall infarcts that involve the right ventricle, and it is commonly seen in the late stages of heart failure due to rheumatic or congenital heart disease with severe pulmonary hypertension, as well as in ischemic heart disease, cardiomyopathy, and cor pulmonale. It is in part reversible if pulmonary hypertension is relieved. Rheumatic fever may produce organic TR, often associated with TS. Less commonly, regurgitation results from congenitally deformed tricuspid valves, and it occurs with defects of the atrioventricular canal, as well as with Ebstein's malformation of the tricuspid valve (Chap. 186). Infarction of right ventricular papillary muscles, tricuspid valve prolapse, carcinoid heart disease, endomyocardial fibrosis, infective endocarditis, and trauma may also produce TR.

As is the case for TS, the clinical features of TR result primarily from systemic venous congestion and reduction of cardiac output. With the onset of TR in patients with pulmonary hypertension, as cardiac output declines, symptoms of pulmonary congestion diminish, but the clinical manifestations of right-sided heart failure become intensified. The neck veins are distended, with prominent *v* waves and marked hepatomegaly, ascites, pleural effusions, edema, systolic pulsations of the liver, and positive hepatojugular reflux are common. A prominent right ventricular pulsation along the left parasternal region and a blowing holosystolic murmur along the lower left sternal margin which is generally intensified during inspiration and reduced during expiration or the Valsalva maneuver are characteristic findings; atrial fibrillation is usually present.

The electrocardiogram usually shows changes characteristic of the lesion responsible for the enlargement of the right ventricle which leads to this form of valvular dysfunction. In the rare instances of isolated TR the electrocardiogram often shows incomplete right bundle branch block. Roentgenographic examination usually reveals enlargement of both the right atrium and ventricle. Echocardiography may be helpful by demonstrating right ventricular dilatation and prolapsing or flail tricuspid leaflets; the diagnosis of tricuspid regurgitation can be made by color flow echocardiography and the severity estimated by Doppler examination. The latter is also useful in estimating pulmonary artery pressure.

The cardiac output is usually markedly reduced, and the right atrial pressure pulse may exhibit no *x* descent during early systole, but a prominent *c-v* wave, with a rapid *y* descent. The mean right atrial and the right ventricular end-diastolic pressures are often elevated.

Isolated TR, without pulmonary hypertension, such as that occurring as a consequence of infective endocarditis or trauma, is usually well tolerated and does not require operation. Indeed, even total excision of an infected tricuspid valve is often well tolerated if the pulmonary artery pressure is normal. Treatment of the underlying cause of heart failure usually reduces the severity of functional TR. In patients with mitral valve disease and TR due to pulmonary hypertension and massive right ventricular enlargement, effective surgical correction of the mitral valvular abnormality results in lowering of the pulmonary vascular pressures and gradual reduction or disappearance of the TR without direct treatment of the tricuspid valve. However, recovery may be much more rapid in patients with severe secondary TR if, at the time of mitral valve replacement, tricuspid annuloplasty or, if necessary, tricuspid valve replacement is performed. Surgical treatment of the TR, consisting of either valve replacement or narrowing of the annulus, should be carried out in patients with severe regurgitation secondary to deformity of the tricuspid valve due to rheumatic fever, particularly those *without* severe pulmonary hypertension.

PULMONIC VALVE DISEASE

The pulmonic valve is affected by rheumatic fever far less frequently than the other valves and is uncommonly the seat of infective endocarditis. The most common acquired abnormality affecting the pulmonic valve is regurgitation secondary to dilatation of the pulmonic valve ring as a consequence of severe pulmonary hypertension of any cause. This produces the Graham Steell murmur, a high-pitched, decrescendo, diastolic blowing murmur along the left sternal border, which is difficult to differentiate from the far more common murmur produced by aortic regurgitation. It is of little hemodynamic significance; indeed surgical removal or destruction of the pulmonic valve by infective endocarditis does not produce heart failure unless serious pulmonary hypertension is also present.

Congenital pulmonic stenosis is discussed in Chap. 186.

REFERENCES

BOUDOULAS H, WOOLEY CF (eds): *The Mitral Valve Prolapse Syndrome*. Futura, Mount Kisco, NY 1988

BRAUNWALD E: Valvular heart disease, in *Heart Disease*, 3d ed, E Braunwald (ed). Philadelphia, Saunders, 1988, p 1023

COHEN SR et al: Tricuspid regurgitation in patients with acquired, chronic, pure mitral regurgitation: 1. Prevalence, diagnosis and comparison of preoperative clinical and hemodynamic features in patients with and without tricuspid regurgitation. J Thorac Cardiovasc Surg 94:481, 1987

CRAWFORD MH, KOUCHOUKOS NT (eds): Valvular heart disease. Current Opinion in Cardiology 4:189, 1989

FRANKL WS, BREST AN (eds):*Valvular Heart Disease: Comprehensive Evaluation and Management*. Philadelphia, FA Davis, 1986

FUSTER V et al: Prevention of thromboembolism induced by prosthetic heart valves. Semin Thromb Hemost 14:50, 1988

GALLOWAY AC et al: Current concepts of mitral valve reconstruction for mitral insufficiency. Circulation 78:1087, 1988

GREENBERG BH et al: Arterial dilators in mitral regurgitation: Effects on rest and exercise, hemodynamics and long-term clinical follow-up. Circulation 65:181, 1982

IONESCU MI, COHN LH (eds): *Mitral Valve Disease: Diagnosis and Treatment*. London, Butterworths, 1985

KIRKLIN JW, BARRATT-BOYES BG: Part III. Acquired valvular heart disease, in *Cardiac Surgery*, JW Kirklin, BG Barratt-Boyes (eds). New York, Wiley, 1986, p 323

LINGAMENI R et al: Tricuspid regurgitation: Clinical and angiographic assessment. Cath Cardiovasc Diag 5:7, 1979

MAHAPATRA RK et al: Rheumatic tricuspid stenosis. Indian Heart J 30:1381, 1978

MARKS AR et al: Identification of high-risk and low-risk subgroups of patients with mitral valve prolapse. N Engl J Med 320:1031, 1989

MASUYAMA T et al: Noninvasive evaluation of aortic regurgitation by continuous-wave Doppler echocardiography. Circulation 73:460, 1986

NAIR CK et al: Ten-year results with the St. Jude Medical Prosthesis. Am J Cardiol 65(3):217, 1990

OH JK et al: Prediction of the severity of aortic stenosis by Doppler aortic valve area determination: Prospective Doppler-catheterization correlation in 100 patients. J Am Coll Cardiol 11:1227, 1988

SAFIAN RD et al: Percutaneous aortic valvuloplasty in 170 connective patients. N Engl J Med 319:125, 1988

VAHANIAN A et al: Results of percutaneous mitral commissurotomy in 200 patients. Am J Cardiol 63:847, 1989

189 ACUTE MYOCARDIAL INFARCTION

RICHARD C. PASTERNAK / EUGENE BRAUNWALD

Myocardial infarction is one of the commonest diagnoses occurring in hospitalized patients in western countries. In the United States, approximately 1.5 million myocardial infarctions occur each year. Mortality with acute infarction is approximately 25 percent, with slightly more than half of the deaths occurring before the stricken individual reaches the hospital. Although survival following hospitalization has improved over the last decade and a half, an additional 5 to 10 percent of survivors die in the first year following myocardial infarction. Risk of excess mortality and recurrent nonfatal myocardial infarction persists in patients who recover.

CLINICAL PRESENTATION

Pain is the most common presenting complaint in patients with myocardial infarction. In some instances, the discomfort may be severe enough to be described as the worst pain the patient has ever experienced (Chap. 16). The pain of myocardial infarction is deep and visceral; adjectives commonly used to describe it are *heavy, squeezing,* and *crushing*. It is similar in character to the discomfort of angina pectoris but is usually more severe and lasts much longer. Typically the pain involves the central portion of the chest and/or epigastrium, and in about 30 percent of cases it radiates to the arms. Less common sites of radiation include the abdomen, back, lower jaw, and neck. The location of the pain beneath the xiphoid and patients' denial that they may be suffering a heart attack are chiefly responsible for the mistaken diagnosis of indigestion. The pain of myocardial infarction may radiate as high as the occipital area but not below the umbilicus. The pain is often accompanied by weakness, sweating, nausea, vomiting, giddiness, and anxiety. The discomfort usually commences with the patient at rest and exhibits circadian periodicity, occurring more commonly in the morning than at any other time of the day. Less than one-third of the time does the pain begin during a period of exertion; when it does, in contrast to angina pectoris, it does not usually subside with cessation of activity. Approximately one-half of patients with myocardial infarction exhibit the prodrome of unstable angina (Chap. 190).

Although pain is the most common presenting complaint, it is by no means always present; a minimum of 15 to 20 percent of myocardial infarcts are *painless*. The incidence of painless infarcts is greater in patients with diabetes mellitus, and it increases with age. In the elderly, myocardial infarction may present as sudden-onset breathlessness, which may progress to pulmonary edema. Other less common presentations, with or without pain, include sudden loss of consciousness, a confusional state, a sensation of profound weakness, the appearance of an arrhythmia, evidence of peripheral embolism, or merely an unexplained drop in arterial pressure. The pain of myocardial infarction can be similar to pain from acute pericarditis (Chap. 193), pulmonary embolism (Chap. 213), acute aortic dissection (Chap. 197), or costochondritis. These conditions should be considered in the differential diagnosis.

Patients at increased risk of developing acute myocardial infarction include those with unstable angina, multiple coronary risk factors (p. 239), and coronary artery spasm. Less common etiologic factors include hypercoagulability, coronary emboli, collagen vascular disease, coronary artery anomalies, and cocaine abuse.

PHYSICAL FINDINGS Most patients are anxious and restless, attempting to relieve the pain by moving about in bed, squirming, stretching, belching, or even inducing vomiting. Pallor is common and is often associated with perspiration and coolness of the extremities. The combination of substernal chest pain persistent for more than 30 min and diaphoresis strongly suggests acute myocardial infarction. Although many patients have a normal pulse rate and blood pressure, within the first hour of infarction about one-fourth of patients with anterior infarction have manifestations of sympathetic nervous system hyperactivity (tachycardia and/or hypertension), and up to one-half with inferior infarction show evidence of parasympathetic hyperactivity (bradycardia and/or hypotension).

The precordium is usually quiet, and the apical impulse may be difficult to palpate. In about one-fourth of patients with anterior wall infarction, an abnormal systolic pulsation develops in the periapical area within the first days of the illness and then may resolve. Other physical signs of ventricular dysfunction that may be present include, in decreasing incidence, fourth (S_4) and third (S_3) heart sounds, decreased intensity of heart sounds, and, rarely, paradoxical splitting of the second sound (Chap. 175). A transient apical systolic murmur, presumably due to mitral regurgitation secondary to papillary muscle dysfunction during acute infarction, may be midsystolic or late systolic in timing. A pericardial friction rub is heard in many patients with transmural myocardial infarction at some time in their course if they are examined frequently. Jugular venous distention occurs commonly in patients with right ventricular infarction. The carotid pulse is often slightly decreased in volume despite a normal upstroke. Temperature elevations in the range of 37 to 38°C may be observed during the first week following acute myocardial infarction; however, a temperature exceeding 38°C should prompt a search for other causes. The arterial pressure is variable; in most patients with transmural infarction systolic pressure declines approximately 10 to 15 mmHg from the preinfarction state.

LABORATORY FINDINGS

The laboratory tests of value in confirming the diagnosis of myocardial infarction may be divided into three groups: (1) nonspecific indexes of tissue necrosis and inflammation, (2) the electrocardiogram, and (3) serum enzyme changes.

The *nonspecific reaction* to myocardial injury is associated with polymorphonuclear leukocytosis, which appears within a few hours after the onset of pain, persists for 3 to 7 days, and often reaches levels of 12,000 to 15,000 leukocytes per microliter. The erythrocyte sedimentation rate rises more slowly than the white blood cell count, peaking during the first week, and sometimes remaining elevated for 1 or 2 weeks.

The *electrocardiographic manifestations* of acute myocardial infarction are described in Chap. 176. Although electrocardiographic/pathologic correlations are not excellent, transmural infarction is often diagnosed if the electrocardiogram demonstrates Q waves or loss of R waves; nontransmural infarction is considered to be present if the electrocardiogram shows only transient ST-segment and sustained T-wave changes. However, the latter changes are variable and nonspecific and should not form the sole basis for the diagnosis of infarction. Therefore, a more rational nomenclature for designating electrocardiographic infarction is now commonly in use, with the terms *Q-wave* or *non-Q-wave infarction* in place of the terms *transmural* or *nontransmural infarction,* respectively.

SERUM ENZYMES Enzymes are released in large quantities into the blood from necrotic heart muscle following myocardial infarction. The rate of liberation of specific enzymes differs following infarction, and the temporal pattern of enzyme release is of diagnostic importance. Creatine phosphokinase (CK) rises within 8 to 24 h, and generally returns to normal by 48 to 72 h, except in the case of large infarctions, when CK clearance is delayed. Lactic dehydrogenase (LDH) rises later (24 to 48 h) and remains elevated for as long as 7 to 14 days. The serum aminotransferase enzymes, AST and ALT (previously designated SGOT and SGPT), were utilized in the diagnosis of myocardial infarction for many years, but have fallen out of favor because it has been recognized that their time course of elevation is intermediate between CK and LDH, thus offering little advantage, and because of lack of tissue specificity. The MB isoenzyme of CK has the advantage over CK and LDH in that it is not present in significant concentrations in extracardiac tissue, and therefore it is more specific. CK-MB isoenzymes are particularly useful when skeletal muscle and/or brain damage are suspected since both of these tissues contain large quantities of the enzyme but none of the MB isoenzyme. The myocardial specificity of the MB isoenzyme determination depends on the technique used for measurement. Radioimmunoassay techniques are most specific, but the more commonly employed gel electrophoresis technique is significantly less specific and therefore prone to more frequent false positives. Five common LDH isoenzymes may be separated by starch-gel electrophoresis. Tissues differ with respect to the specific isoenzyme patterns; the rapidly migrating isoenzyme which predominates in the heart is referred to as LDH_1, while the slowly migrating components predominate in liver and skeletal muscle. LDH_1 rises before total LDH in patients with myocardial infarction and may rise when there is no change in total LDH. Therefore, increased LDH_1 is a more sensitive indicator of myocardial infarction than total LDH; sensitivity exceeds 95 percent. However, measurements of the LDH isoenzymes should be obtained only when the initial CK or CK-MB elevation might have been missed (after 48 h), for they are not more sensitive than CK-MB and therefore only increase cost without increasing diagnostic accuracy.

A two- to threefold elevation of total CK (not CK-MB) may follow an intramuscular injection. This may lead to the erroneous diagnosis of myocardial infarction in a patient who has been given an intramuscular injection of a narcotic for chest pain of noncardiac origin. Other potential sources of total CK elevation worthy of note are (1) muscular diseases including muscular dystrophy, myopathies, and polymyositis, (2) electrical cardioversion, (3) cardiac catheterization, (4) hypothyroidism, (5) stroke, (6) surgery, and (7) skeletal muscle damage secondary to trauma, convulsions, and prolonged immobilization. Cardiac surgery, myocarditis, and electrical cardioversion often result in elevation of serum levels of MB isoenzyme.

While it has long been recognized that the *total* quantity of enzyme released correlates with the size of the infarct, the *peak* enzyme concentration is only weakly correlated with infarct size. It has been demonstrated that the mass of heart muscle infarcted can be estimated from analysis of the concentration-time curve of the enzyme only if the kinetics of the release, degradation, disposal, etc., of the enzyme are known. Thus, while the *area* under the CK-MB time curve is related to infarct size, the *absolute* value of the peak CK-MB and its time to peak are related to the kinetics of CK-MB washout from myocardium. The opening of a coronary artery occlusion (either spontaneously, or by mechanical or pharmacologic means) in the early hours of myocardial infarction will cause early and higher peaking (at about 8 h following reperfusion) of the CK-MB time curve.

Characteristic rises occur in serum enzyme concentration in more than 95 percent of patients with clinically proven myocardial infarction. CK and LDH levels generally do not rise in unstable angina. Many patients with suspected infarction have baseline enzyme levels that are normal and increase threefold in a pattern consistent with infarction, although the absolute level of enzyme in the blood never exceeds the upper limits of normal. These have been termed "microinfarctions," and such patients have a prognosis intermediate between that of unstable angina and that of proven myocardial infarction. Isoenzyme studies are particularly helpful in this situation.

Several radionuclide imaging techniques are of value in the diagnosis or assessment of the patient with acute myocardial infarction (Chap. 178). Acute infarct scintigraphy ("hot-spot" imaging) is carried out with an infarct-avid imaging agent such as [^{99m}Tc] stannous pyrophosphate. Scans are usually positive 2 to 5 days after infarction, particularly in patients with transmural infarcts; although they aid in *localizing* infarcts and provide a measure of infarct size (chap. 177); these scans are less sensitive than CK determination for making the *diagnosis* of myocardial infarction. Myocardial perfusion imaging with thallium 201, which is taken up and concentrated by viable myocardium, reveals a defect ("cold spot") in most patients during the first few hours after development of a transmural infarct (p. 864). However, since it is not possible to distinguish acute infarcts from chronic scars, thallium scanning, although extremely *sensitive*, is not *specific* for *acute* myocardial infarction. Radionuclide ventriculography, carried out with ^{99m}Tc-labeled red blood cells (p. 864), frequently demonstrates wall motion disorders and reduction in ventricular ejection fraction in patients with acute myocardial infarction. While of value in assessing the hemodynamic consequences of infarction, and in aiding in the diagnosis of right ventricular infarction when the right ventricular ejection fraction is depressed, this technique is also quite nonspecific, since many cardiac abnormalities other than myocardial infarction alter the radionuclide ventriculogram. Two-dimensional echocardiography (Chap. 178) can also be of value in patients with acute myocardial infarction. Abnormalities of wall motion, particularly of the septal and inferior-posterior walls, are readily detectable. Although acute infarction cannot be distinguished from old myocardial scar or from acute severe ischemia, the ease and safety of the procedure make its use appealing as a screening tool. Echocardiography may be particularly useful in the diagnosis of right ventricular infarction, ventricular aneurysm, and left ventricular thrombus. Additionally, Doppler echocardiography is useful in the detection of a ventricular septal defect and mitral regurgitation, complications of acute myocardial infarction.

MANAGEMENT

Two general classes of complications have been defined: (1) electrical (arrhythmias) and (2) mechanical ("pump failure"). Ventricular fibrillation is the most common form of arrhythmic death in acute myocardial infarction. The vast majority of deaths due to ventricular fibrillation occur within the first 24 h of the onset of symptoms, and of these deaths, over half occur in the first hour. Although ventricular premature beats or ventricular tachycardia may precede an episode of ventricular fibrillation, the latter may occur without warning arrhythmias. Over the last 25 years, with careful monitoring and prompt attention to arrhythmias, the in-hospital mortality for acute myocardial infarction has been reduced from about 30 to less than 15 percent.

With the incidence of sudden in-hospital arrhythmic deaths markedly reduced, attention has turned to other major complications of acute myocardial infarction, i.e., pump failure and its prevention by attempts to limit infarct size. Nevertheless, pump failure remains the primary cause of in-hospital death from acute myocardial infarction. The extent of ischemic necrosis correlates well with the degree of pump failure and with mortality, both early, i.e., within 10 days of infarction, and later as well. A clinical classification dependent on the status of cardiac pump function originally proposed by Killip divides patients into four groups as follows: class I, no signs of pulmonary or venous congestion; class II, moderate heart failure as evidenced by rales at the lung bases, S_3 gallop, tachypnea, or signs of failure of the right side of the heart including venous and hepatic congestion; class III, severe heart failure, pulmonary edema; class IV, shock with systolic pressure less than 90 mmHg and evidence of peripheral constriction, diaphoresis, peripheral cyanosis, mental confusion, and oliguria. The expected hospital mortality rate of patients in these clinical classes when this classification was established was as follows: class I, 0 to 5 percent; class II, 10 to 20 percent; class III, 35 to 45 percent; and class IV, 85 to 95 percent. With recent advances in management, mortality has fallen, perhaps by as much as one-third, in each class.

GENERAL CONSIDERATIONS Given the information summarized above, the principal objectives of management of the patient with myocardial infarction are to prevent death from arrhythmia and to minimize the mass of infarcted tissue.

Arrhythmias can usually be managed successfully if trained personnel and appropriate equipment are available when this complication develops. Since mortality from arrhythmia is greatest during the first few hours after infarction, it is obvious that the effectiveness of treatment relates directly to the speed with which patients come under medical observation. The biggest delay usually is not in transportation to the hospital but rather between the onset of pain and the patient's decision to call for help. This delay can best be reduced by education of the public concerning the significance of chest pain and the importance of seeking early medical attention. Increasingly, monitoring and treatment are carried out by trained personnel in the ambulance, shortening even further the time between the onset of the infarction and appropriate care.

A number of "common sense" rules in the management of acute myocardial infarction deserve particular emphasis. It is essential to maintain an optimal balance between myocardial oxygen supply and demand in order to salvage as much of the jeopardized myocardium as possible. Therapeutic strategies that help to attain this goal include rest, analgesia, mild sedation, and a quiet atmosphere in order to reduce anxiety and thereby lower heart rate, a major determinant of myocardial oxygen consumption.

Marked sinus bradycardia (heart rate less than approximately 45 beats per minute) should be treated by leg elevation and atropine or by electrical pacing, particularly if the bradycardia is associated with a fall in blood pressure or with worsening ventricular arrhythmias. However, routine administration of atropine, with resultant increase in heart rate, to patients without serious bradycardia is not recommended. Patients with acute myocardial infarction who have a hyperdynamic state, i.e., tachycardia and elevation of arterial pressure, should be treated with a beta-adrenergic blocking agent. Initially, 0.1 mg/kg propranolol or 15 mg metoprolol given intravenously in three divided doses is safe, if there are no contraindications, such as heart failure, AV block, or history of asthma. All forms of tachyarrhythmias require prompt and direct treatment. Drugs that exert a positive inotropic effect, such as digitalis glycosides and cardioactive sympathomimetics, should be administered only if there is evidence of pronounced heart failure with a low cardiac output due to systolic dysfunction; they should not be given prophylactically. Of the various sympathomimetic amines available, isoproterenol with its chronotropic and vasodilator effects is the least desirable. Dobutamine (p. 899) and amrinone, which have less effect on heart rate and systemic vascular resistance, are more desirable when it is necessary to augment cardiac contractility. However, these drugs have vasodilating potential and may not be tolerated in patients with borderline or frank hypotension. Dopamine (p. 899) is useful in patients with left ventricular failure and systemic hypotension (systolic pressure <90 mmHg. Diuretics are indicated in the presence of pulmonary congestion and should, in fact, be used prior to cardiac stimulants unless the patient is hypovolemic or hypotensive.

All patients should inhale oxygen-enriched air (see below). Particular attention must be paid to preserving arterial oxygenation in patients with hypoxemia, as occurs in patients with chronic pulmonary disease, pneumonia, or left ventricular failure. *Severe* anemia, which can also extend the area of ischemic injury, should be corrected by cautious administration of packed red blood cells, sometimes accompanied by a diuretic. Associated conditions, particularly infections with accompanying tachycardia and elevated myocardial oxygen demand, require immediate attention. Systolic arterial pressure should not be allowed to deviate by more than 25 to 30 mmHg from the patient's usual level, unless untreated hypertension has been present, in which case a greater fall in arterial pressure is desirable.

CORONARY CARE UNITS These have resulted in improved care of patients with myocardial infarction, reduction in mortality rates, and major increases in knowledge about myocardial infarction. The unit should be equipped with a system which permits continuous monitoring of the cardiac rhythm of *each* patient and hemodynamic monitoring in *selected* patients. Defibrillators, respirators, and facilities for introducing pacing catheters and flow-directed balloon-tipped catheters should be available. Equally important is the organization of a highly trained team of nurses who can recognize arrhythmias, adjust the dosage of antiarrhythmic drugs, and perform cardiac resuscitation, including electroshock, when necessary.

The policies and procedures for admission to a coronary care unit should ensure that patients are admitted early in their illness when they may expect to derive maximum benefit from the care provided. In the past, all patients with suspected myocardial infarction were admitted to the coronary care unit. Currently, however, several factors have led to a change in this rule. The availability of electrocardiographic monitoring and trained personnel in "intermediate care units" has allowed admission of lower-risk patients (e.g., those not hemodynamically compromised or without active arrhythmias) to such units. For economic reasons, and to utilize limited facilities optimally, many institutions have developed guidelines to aid in triaging patients with suspected myocardial infarction. While most such patients in the United States are admitted to the hospital, in other countries, such as the United Kingdom, the patients at lowest risk may be cared for at home. Once admitted to the hospital the fraction of patients actually admitted to the coronary care unit may depend on a balance between the clinical status of the patient and bed availability. In some units beds are utilized primarily for patients with a complicated course, particularly those who require hemodynamic monitoring. Mortality rates for myocardial infarction treated in coronary care units vary from 5 to 20 percent, according to variations in admission policies, type of population served, nature of the hospital (tertiary care center versus community hospital), and other as yet unidentified factors.

REPERFUSION One of the most important developments in the care of patients with acute myocardial infarction derives from the recognition that early reperfusion of ischemic myocardium can potentially salvage tissue before it becomes irreversibly injured. Since most infarctions are caused by a relatively sudden thrombotic occlusion adjacent to an atherosclerotic plaque in a major epicardial coronary vessel, recent attention has been appropriately directed at techniques to pharmacologically or mechanically recanalize the "culprit" vessel. The thrombolytic agents, streptokinase, and tissue plasminogen activator (tPA) produced by recombinant DNA technology (Chap. 6), have been approved by the Federal Drug Administration for intravenous use in the setting of acute myocardial infarction. These agents, as well as other investigational ones, have been extensively studied in many clinical trials from which emerge important conclusions about the management of patients with acute myocardial infarction. Thrombolytic therapy can reduce in-hospital mortality for myocardial infarction by up to 50 percent when administered within the first hour of the onset of symptoms, with much of this benefit maintained for one or more years. Appropriately employed thrombolytic therapy appears to reduce infarct size and limit left ventricular dysfunction as well. Since salvage of myocardium can only occur before the myocardium is irreversibly injured, timing of thrombolytic therapy is of extreme importance in achieving maximum benefit. While an upper time limit has not been established, it is clear that "every minute counts" and that patients treated within 1 to 3 h of the onset of symptoms stand to benefit most. Although the reduction of mortality is more modest, institution of therapy remains of benefit in many patients seen 3 to 6 h after the onset of infarction, and some benefit appears possible up to 12 h (and perhaps even to 24 h) after, especially if chest discomfort is ongoing and ST segments remain elevated in electrocardiographic leads that do not yet demonstrate new Q waves. In addition to the possibility of early treatment, clinical factors that favor proceeding with thrombolytic therapy include: anterior wall injury, hemodynamically complicated infarction, widespread ECG evidence of myocardial jeopardy, and younger patient.

When compared directly, tPA is more effective than streptokinase at restoring coronary artery flow, but a difference in mortality has not been demonstrated. The current recommended total dose of tPA is 100 mg given as 60 mg intravenously over the first hour, beginning with a 5- to 10-mg bolus, followed by 20 mg each in the second and third hours. Streptokinase is administered as 1.5 million units intravenously over 1 h. Although the optimum adjunctive anticoagulant and antiplatelet regimen has not yet been firmly established, recent studies suggest that 80 to 325 mg of aspirin and 5000 units of heparin should be given with the institution of thrombolytic therapy. This should be followed by 325 mg of aspirin daily and a continuous infusion of heparin for 2 to 5 days.

Clear contraindications to the use of thrombolytic agents include a history of cerebrovascular accident, a recent (within 2 weeks) invasive or surgical procedure (or prolonged cardiopulmonary resuscitation), marked hypertension (systolic arterial pressure greater than 180 mmHg and/or diastolic pressure greater than 100 mmHg) at any time during the acute presentation, and active peptic ulcer disease. Other clinical reasons for an increased risk of bleeding (such as advanced age) should be sought for and the potential benefit of such therapy weighed against expected risk before the decision to administer a thrombolytic agent is made. Following thrombolytic therapy cardiac catheterization and coronary angiography should be carried out if there is evidence of coronary artery reocclusion (reelevation of ST segments, and/or recurrent chest pain) or if recurrent ischemia develops (such as recurrent angina in the early hospital course or a positive exercise stress test prior to discharge). Under these circumstances, and if the coronary anatomy is suitable, coronary angioplasty should be performed. Coronary artery bypass surgery should be reserved for a small minority of patients whose coronary anatomy is unsuitable for angioplasty but in whom revascularization appears to be advisable because of extensive jeopardized myocardium or recurrent ischemia.

Repeat administration of a thrombolytic agent is an alternative to early mechanical revascularization. Although there is little to suggest how this might be best undertaken, one reasonable strategy is to give a half dose of tPA (50 mg over 4 h) if reocclusion occurs 12 to 24 h after the agent is initially given and a repeat full dose (100 mg over 3 h) if such an event occurs more than 24 h later.

Acute primary percutaneous transluminal coronary angioplasty (PTCA), i.e., without preceding thrombolysis, has also been reported to be effective in restoring effective reperfusion in acute myocardial infarction, but this technique is very expensive in terms of personnel and facilities and probably should be limited to inpatients whose coronary anatomy is already known, e.g., in the setting of a post-cardiac catheterization coronary occlusion, and to patients in cardiogenic shock who can be brought to the catheterization laboratory within 3 h of the onset of symptoms.

The amount of myocardial tissue which becomes necrotic secondary to a coronary artery occlusion is determined by factors other than just the site of occlusion. One such important factor is the status of collateral blood supply to ischemic tissue. Myocardium well supplied by collaterals clearly has the capacity to survive hours longer than poorly collateralized areas. Infarct size is now known to vary with time and be affected by a number of therapeutic agents currently in use. The balance between myocardial oxygen supply and demand in areas rendered ischemic determines the ultimate fate of these areas of jeopardized myocardium. While no routine therapeutic approach to reduce infarct size in all patients is currently recommended, the realization that infarct size may be increased by interventions which adversely alter the supply-demand balance has prompted the reevaluation of previously accepted therapeutic maneuvers in the management of patients with acute infarction. Cardioactive sympathomimetic amines are used sparingly and only for clear-cut indications. The early administration of beta blockers, with or without thrombolytic therapy, appears to be of benefit.

TREATMENT OF THE PATIENT WITH AN UNCOMPLICATED INFARCTION

ANALGESIA Since myocardial infarction usually presents with severe pain, one of the important initial therapeutic objectives is the relief of pain. Morphine is an extremely effective analgesic for the pain associated with myocardial infarction. However, it may reduce sympathetically mediated arteriolar and venous constriction. The resultant venous pooling may produce a reduction in cardiac output and arterial pressure. This must be recognized but does not necessarily contraindicate its use. Hypotension associated with venous pooling usually responds promptly to elevation of the legs, but in some patients volume expansion with intravenous saline is required. The patient may experience diaphoresis and nausea, but these events usually pass and are replaced by a feeling of well-being associated with the relief of pain. Morphine also has a vagotonic effect and may cause bradycardia or advanced degrees of heart block, particularly in patients with posteroinferior infarction. These side effects of morphine usually respond to atropine (0.4 mg intravenously). Morphine is routinely administered by repetitive (every 5 min) intravenous injection of small doses of drug (2 to 4 mg) rather than by administration of a larger quantity by the subcutaneous route, by which absorption may be unpredictable. Meperidine hydrochloride or hydromorphone hydrochloride may be effectively employed in place of morphine.

Prior to administering morphine, sublingual nitroglycerin can be given safely to most patients with myocardial infarction. As long as hypotension does not occur, up to three 0.3-mg doses should be administered at about 5-min intervals. In addition to diminishing or abolishing chest discomfort, this form of therapy, once considered contraindicated in the setting of acute myocardial infarction, may be capable of both decreasing myocardial oxygen demand (by lowering preload) and increasing myocardial oxygen supply (by dilating infarct-related coronary vessels or collateral vessels). However, therapy with nitrates should be avoided in patients who present with a low systolic arterial pressure (<100 mmHg). The potential for an idiosyncratic reaction to nitrates, consisting of sudden marked hypotension and bradycardia, should be recognized. This problem, occurring more frequently in patients with inferior wall infarction, can usually be promptly reversed by the rapid administration of intravenous atropine. In patients whose initially favorable response to sublingual nitroglycerin is followed by the return of chest pain, particularly if accompanied by other evidence of ongoing ischemia such as further ST-segment or T-wave shifts, the use of intravenous nitroglycerin should be considered.

Intravenous beta blockers are also useful in the control of the pain of acute myocardial infarction. These drugs have been shown to control pain effectively in some patients, presumably by diminishing ischemia consequent to lowering myocardial oxygen demand. More importantly, there is some evidence that intravenous beta blockers reduce in-hospital mortality, particularly in high-risk patients. Dosing similar to that used to treat the hyperdynamic state (see above) may be utilized.

Glucocorticoids and nonsteroidal anti-inflammatory agents, with the exception of aspirin, should generally be avoided in the setting of acute myocardial infarction. They can impair infarct healing and increase the risk of myocardial rupture, and may produce a larger infarct scar. Additionally, they can increase coronary vascular resistance, thereby potentially reducing flow to ischemic myocardium.

OXYGEN The routine use of oxygen is supported by the observation that the arterial P_{O_2} is reduced in many patients with myocardial infarction and that oxygen inhalation reduces the area of ischemic injury in experimental animals. Although oxygen therapy has been associated with theoretically deleterious effects such as elevation of systemic vascular resistance and slight reduction of cardiac output, the weight of evidence favors its administration. It should be administered by face mask or nasal prongs for the first day or two after infarction.

ACTIVITY Factors which increase the work of the heart may increase the size of the infarct. Circumstances in which heart size, cardiac output, or myocardial contractility are increased should be avoided. It has been demonstrated that 6 to 8 weeks are required for complete healing, i.e., replacement of the infarcted myocardium by scar tissue. The purpose of reduced physical activity is to provide the most favorable possible circumstances for this healing.

Most patients with myocardial infarction should be admitted to a coronary care unit or suitable monitoring facility and remain there for 2 days under constant observation by trained personnel utilizing continuous electrocardiographic monitoring. A catheter should be introduced into a peripheral vein, firmly fixed so that it is not easily dislodged, and be kept open either by the slow infusion of isotonic glucose solution or by a closed heparin lock. In the absence of heart failure or other complications during the first 2 to 3 days, the patient should be in bed most of the day, with one or two periods of 15 to 30 min in a bedside chair. The patient may use a bedside commode and should be bathed but may eat unassisted. Bedside commode privileges are given to all hemodynamically stable patients with a stable rhythm from the first day. The bed should be equipped with a footboard, against which the patient should push both feet regularly to prevent venous stasis and thromboembolism and to maintain muscle tone in the legs.

By the third or fourth day the patient with an uncomplicated course should be spending at least 30 to 60 min in a chair twice a day. At this time the patient's blood pressure should be measured when standing in order to be aware of postural hypotension, which may be a problem when ambulation is begun. Standing and gradual ambulation are usually begun between the third and fifth days post infarction in patients with uncomplicated myocardial infarction. Ambulation is progressively increased, eventually including walks about the hospital floor. In many hospitals a cardiac rehabilitation program with progressive exercise is initiated in the hospital and continued after discharge. The total duration of hospitalization in uncomplicated cases is usually 6 to 11 days, but some physicians still hospitalize patients with Q-wave infarction for 2 weeks. Patients in clinical class II or higher may require 2 or more weeks of hospitalization, depending upon the rapidity with which heart failure resolves and the home situation to which the patient is returning. Many physicians perform a heart rate–limited exercise tolerance test just prior to discharge in selected patients with myocardial infarction. Such testing identifies high-risk patients as those who develop angina, ST-segment change, hypotension, or serious ventricular ectopic activity during or immediately following exercise. These patients require special attention, including measures such as antiarrhythmic drugs for ectopic activity, and beta-adrenergic blockers, long-acting nitrates, and/or calcium channel blocking agents for evidence of ischemia. If ischemia occurs at rest, or if during limited exercise ischemia and/or hypotension occur, coronary arteriography should be carried out. If a large quantity of viable myocardium, perfused by critically narrowed vessel(s), is found at angiography, then revascularization (either by angioplasty or by operation) may be required. Exercise tests also aid in formulating an individualized exercise prescription, which can be much more vigorous in patients who tolerate exercise without any of the above-mentioned adverse signs. Additionally, predischarge stress testing may provide an important psychological benefit related to building the patient's confidence through the demonstration of reasonable exercise tolerance. Furthermore, particularly when no arrhythmias or signs of ischemia are identified, the patient benefits by the physician's reassurance that objective evidence suggests no immediate jeopardy.

The remainder of the convalescent phase of myocardial infarction may be accomplished at home. From 2 to 6 weeks, the patient should be encouraged to increase activity by walking about the house and outdoors in good weather. Patients should still spend 8 to 10 h in bed each night. Additional rest periods in the morning and afternoon may be advisable for selected patients. Normal sexual activity may be resumed during this period.

From 6 to 8 weeks onward, the physician must regulate the patient's activity on the basis of his or her exercise tolerance. It is during this period of increasing activity that the patient may become aware of profound fatigue. Postural hypotension may still be a problem. Most patients will be able to return to work after 12 weeks, and many patients much earlier. A maximal exercise test is frequently performed after 6 to 8 weeks or prior to returning to work. A trend toward earlier ambulation, hospital discharge, and resumption of full activity for patients recuperating from acute myocardial infarction has developed in recent years.

DIET During the first 4 or 5 days, a low-calorie diet divided into multiple small feedings is preferred. Cardiac output increases following ingestion of food, and therefore the quantity of individual feedings should be kept low. If heart failure is present, sodium intake should be restricted. Since constipation is common, it is reasonable to give average or even increased amounts of bulk in the diet. In addition, the ingestion of potassium-rich foods should be encouraged in patients receiving diuretics. During the second week, increasing amounts of food may be introduced into the diet. At this time, the importance of restriction of calories, cholesterol, and saturated fat may be explained to the patient, and he or she can be started on an appropriate diet. Willingness to accept dietary restriction and to discontinue cigarette smoking is usually never greater than it is during this early period of convalescence.

BOWELS Bed rest of 3 to 5 days and the effect of the narcotics utilized for the relief of pain often lead to constipation. A bedside commode, rather than a bed pan, a diet rich in bulk, and the routine use of a stool softener such as dioctyl sodium sulfosuccinate, 200 mg daily, are recommended. If the patient remains constipated despite these measures, a laxative can be safely used. It is safe to perform a gentle rectal examination on patients with acute myocardial infarction.

SEDATION Most patients require sedation during hospitalization in order to withstand the period of enforced inactivity with tranquility. Diazepam 5 mg, oxazepam 15 to 30 mg, or lorazepam 0.5 to 2 mg, given three or four times daily, is usually effective. An additional dose of any of the above medications may be given at night to ensure adequate sleep. Temazepam 15 to 30 mg can also be used to induce sleep. Attention to this problem is especially important during the first few days in the coronary care unit, where the atmosphere of 24-h vigilance may interfere with the patient's sleep. However, sedation is no substitute for reassuring, quiet surroundings.

ANTICOAGULANTS AND ANTIPLATELET AGENTS Few topics have been more controversial than the use of anticoagulants in the routine treatment of acute myocardial infarction. The use of anticoagulant therapy to retard the process of coronary occlusion during the initial phases of the illness has undergone renewed interest as a result of the recognition that thrombosis plays an important role in the pathogenesis of acute myocardial infarction. Recent data from trials employing aspirin and/or thrombolytic agents have led to increased consensus about the appropriate treatment regimens. At the time of thrombolytic therapy, unless contraindications exist, most patients with possible or probable myocardial infarction should be started on aspirin, 160 or 325 mg daily. In the patient who is to receive a thrombolytic agent, a 5000-unit bolus of intravenous heparin should be administered, followed by a constant intravenous infusion beginning at 1000 units per hour adjusted to keep the partial thromboplastin time (PTT) at 1.5 to 2 times normal. Patients with acute myocardial infarction not undergoing thrombolytic therapy should also generally receive aspirin. This strategy has been shown to prevent some patients who present with unstable angina from progressing to myocardial infarction, and data suggest that in-hospital mortality is lowered even among patients who do develop myocardial infarction if they are given aspirin early in their course. Additionally, in order to prevent venous thrombosis, in patients *not* treated with thrombolytic therapy, small subcutaneous doses of heparin (5000 units every 8 to 12 h) should be employed as well. Once the patient is out of the intensive care area, oral anticoagulants should be reserved for patients with congestive heart failure which persists for more than 3 to 4 days or for those with large anterior infarctions in whom the risk of developing a left ventricular thrombus is greater.

The incidence of arterial embolism from a clot originating in the ventricle at the site of an infarction is small but definite. Two-dimensional echocardiography allows for the early detection of left ventricular thrombi in about one-third of patients with anterior wall infarction but rarely in patients with inferior or posterior infarction.

Arterial embolism often presents as a major complication, such as hemiparesis when the cerebral circulation is involved, or hypertension if the renal circulation is compromised. The low incidence of these complications, contrasted with their severity, renders it impractical to establish firm guidelines for the use of anticoagulant drugs as prophylaxis against arterial embolism in acute myocardial infarction. The likelihood of arterial embolism appears to increase with the extent of infarction and the resultant inflammation and endocardial stasis due to akinesis. Therefore the indication for anticoagulation as prophylaxis against arterial embolism increases with the extent of infarction. When a thrombus has been clearly demonstrated by echocardiographic or other techniques, systemic anticoagulation should be undertaken (in the absence of contraindications), for the incidence of embolic complications appears to be markedly lowered by such therapy. The appropriate duration of therapy is unknown, but probably should be carried out for 3 to 6 months.

BETA-ADRENERGIC BLOCKERS The chronic routine use of oral beta-adrenergic blockers for at least 2 years following acute myocardial infarction is supported by several well-conducted placebo-controlled trials which have demonstrated reductions in total mortality, sudden death, and in some instances, the reinfarction rate. While beta blockers are of benefit, even when started as late as 28 days following the acute event, additional benefit probably accrues to those patients who are started earlier, including patients receiving thrombolytic therapy. For patients presenting with the clear picture of a hyperdynamic state, in the absence of contraindications such as congestive heart failure, hypotension, bradycardia, atrioventricular block, or a history of asthma (p. 968), an intravenous dose of a beta blocker such as metoprolol may be given (5 mg every 5 to 10 min three times for a total dose of 15 mg, stopping between doses if any complications arise). This is usually followed by an oral dose regimen of metoprolol (50 to 100 mg bid). Later in the hospital course, a more slowly acting beta blocker, such as atenolol (50 to 100 mg qid) can be prescribed. Beta blocker therapy is probably indicated for most patients after myocardial infarction, except those for whom its use is specifically contraindicated (patients with heart failure, heart block, orthostatic hypotension, or severely compromised left ventricular function, but without symptoms of heart failure) and perhaps those whose excellent long-term prognosis (defined as mortality less than 1 percent per year) markedly diminishes any potential benefit (patients with normal ventricular function, no complex ventricular ectopy, no angina, and a negative maximal exercise stress test).

TREATMENT

ARRHYTHMIAS (See also Chaps. 184 and 185) The improved management of arrhythmias constitutes a most significant advance in the treatment of myocardial infarction.

Ventricular premature systoles Infrequent, sporadic ventricular premature depolarizations occur in almost all patients with infarction and do not require therapy. Suggested indications for suppression of ventricular ectopic beats are generally considered to be the following: (1) the presence of more than five isolated ectopic beats per minute, (2) the occurrence of consecutive or multifocal ventricular extrasystoles, and (3) the occurrence of ectopic ventricular beats early in diastole and hence superimposed on the T wave of the preceding beat (the so-called R-on-T phenomenon). Intravenous lidocaine has become the treatment of choice for such ventricular premature beats and other ventricular tachyarrhythmias because it acts rapidly and side effects disappear soon (15 to 20 min) after its administration is discontinued. Lidocaine is given as an intravenous bolus of 1 mg/kg to establish adequate blood levels quickly. This initial dose usually eliminates the ectopic activity, if present, and is followed by an infusion of 2 to 4 mg/min. An additional bolus of 0.5 mg/kg is given 10 min after the initial bolus if ectopy is still present. The dose should be reduced by half in patients with congestive heart failure, shock, or hepatic disease. Usually, ventricular premature beats spontaneously disappear after 72 to 96 h. If significant ventricular ectopic activity persists past this time, chronic antiarrhythmic therapy is often initiated although such therapy has not yet been demonstrated to improve survival. Prophylactic antiarrhythmic therapy, in the absence of clinically important ventricular ectopy, is contraindicated as such therapy may actually increase late mortality.

Procainamide, mexiletine, and quinidine are commonly used for the treatment of persistent ventricular ectopic activity. Several other agents are also available for suppression of ventricular ectopy; the choice must be based upon a physician's familiarity with the particular drug and upon patient tolerance. Beta-adrenergic blocking agents are also effective in abolishing ventricular ectopic activity in infarction patients. The latter agents should be used with great care in patients with left ventricular failure since they have a significant negative inotropic action. If the usual doses of these drugs (Chap. 185), singly or in combination, are not effective, blood levels should be measured to ensure that adequate blood concentrations are being obtained. Frequent clinical and electrocardiographic assessment of the patient for signs of drug toxicity is mandatory when higher doses of these agents are employed.

Ventricular tachycardia and ventricular fibrillation Within the first 24 h of myocardial infarction, ventricular tachycardia and fibrillation can occur without prior warning arrhythmias. The occurrence of such primary arrhythmias can be reduced by prophylactic administration of intravenous lidocaine. However, use in this manner has never been shown to reduce overall mortality with acute myocardial infarction. With earlier treatment of active ischemia, more frequent use of beta blocking agents, and the nearly universal success of electrical cardioversion or defibrillation, prophylactic antiarrhythmic drug therapy can no longer be routinely recommended. It should be reserved for patients who cannot reach a hospital or those treated in hospitals that lack the constant presence in the coronary care unit of a physician or nurse trained in the recognition and treatment of ventricular fibrillation. Sustained ventricular tachycardia is treated first with lidocaine, and if it cannot be terminated by one or two 50- to 100-mg doses, electroconversion should be employed (Chap. 185). Electroshock is used immediately in patients with ventricular fibrillation, or when ventricular tachycardia causes hemodynamic deterioration. If fibrillation has persisted for more than a few seconds, the first shock may be unsuccessful, and in this situation it is advisable to administer closed-chest massage and mouth-to-mouth respiration before attempting electroconversion again. Improvement of oxygenation and perfusion increase the likelihood of successful defibrillation. Bretylium is useful in the treatment of both refractory ventricular fibrillation and ventricular tachycardia. For ventricular fibrillation, bretylium is given as a 5-mg/kg bolus and defibrillation is again attempted. If the latter fails, a second bolus of 10 mg/kg is given to facilitate electroconversion of ventricular fibrillation. Ventricular tachycardia can be treated with bretylium 5 to 10 mg/kg injected slowly over 10 min. In either situation, the initial dose of bretylium may be followed by a continuous infusion of 2 mg/min if the arrhythmia is recurrent. Severe postural hypotension occurs after intravenous bretylium administration; therefore, patients should always be supine when and immediately after the drug is given, and intravenous fluids should be available for rapid administration if needed. Ventricular arrhythmias, including the unusual form of ventricular tachycardia known as *torsade de pointes* (Chap. 185), may occur in infarct patients as a consequence of other concurrent problems (such as hypoxia or hypokalemia) or due to the toxic effects of agents already being administered to the patient (such as digoxin or quinidine). A search for such secondary causes should always be undertaken.

Long-term survival is good in patients with *primary* ventricular fibrillation, i.e., ventricular fibrillation resulting as a primary response to acute ischemia and not associated with predisposing factors such as congestive heart failure, shock, bundle branch block, or ventricular aneurysm. In one series, 87 percent of patients with primary ventricular fibrillation left the hospital alive. This prognosis is in sharp contrast to that for patients who develop ventricular fibrillation *secondary* to severe pump failure. Only 29 percent of patients in this group survived.

In patients who develop ventricular tachycardia late in their hospital course, the mortality in 1 year may be as high as 85 percent. Such patients may warrant electrophysiologic study (Chap. 185).

Accelerated idioventricular rhythm Accelerated idioventricular rhythm (AIVR, ''slow ventricular tachycardia''), a ventricular rhythm with a rate of 60 to 100 beats per minute, occurs in 25 percent of patients with myocardial infarction. It is especially frequent in inferoposterior infarction, where it is usually associated with sinus bradycardia. It often occurs transiently during thrombolytic therapy at the time of reperfusion. The rate of AIVR is usually similar to that of the sinus rhythm which precedes and follows it, and this similarity of rate and the relatively minor hemodynamic effects make this rhythm difficult to detect other than by electrocardiographic monitoring. For the most part, this rhythm is benign and does not presage the development of classic ventricular tachycardia. Most AIVR does not require treatment if the patient is monitored carefully since degeneration into a more serious arrhythmia is rare, and if it occurs, the AIVR can generally be readily treated with a drug which decreases the ventricular escape rate, such as mexiletine, and/or one that increases the sinus rate (atropine).

Supraventricular arrhythmias Sinus tachycardia is the most common arrhythmia of this type. If it occurs secondary to other causes (such as anemia, fever, heart failure, or a metabolic derangement), the primary problem should be treated first. However, if sinus tachycardia appears to be due to sympathetic overstimulation, such as is seen as part of a hyperdynamic state, then treatment with a relatively short acting beta blocker, such as propranolol, should be considered. Other common arrhythmias in this group are junctional rhythm and tachycardia, atrial tachycardia, atrial flutter, and atrial fibrillation. These rhythm disturbances are often secondary to left ventricular failure. The administration of digoxin is usually the treatment of choice for supraventricular arrhythmias if heart failure is present. If heart failure is absent, verapamil (p. 968) is an ideal alternative, as this agent may also help control ischemia. If the abnormal rhythm persists for more than 2 h with a ventricular rate in excess of 120 beats per minute, or at any time when tachycardia induces heart failure, shock, or ischemia (as manifested by recurrent pain or ECG changes), electroshock should be utilized.

Junctional arrhythmias are of diverse etiology, are not indicative of any specific abnormality, and from a therapeutic viewpoint must be considered on an individual basis. Digitalis excess must be ruled out as a cause of junctional tachycardia. In some patients with severely compromised left ventricular function, the loss of appropriately timed atrial systole results in a marked decrease in cardiac output. Right atrial or coronary sinus pacing is indicated in such instances.

Sinus bradycardia The significance of bradycardia as a factor predisposing to ventricular fibrillation in acute myocardial infarction is controversial. While the incidence of ventricular tachycardia in patients with sustained bradycardia is twice that observed in patients with normal heart rates, sinus bradycardia has also been identified in hospitalized patients as an index of a favorable prognosis. Treatment of sinus bradycardia is indicated if significant ventricular ectopic activity is present or if hemodynamic compromise results from the slow heart rate. Elevation of the legs and/or the foot of the bed is frequently helpful in the treatment of sinus bradycardia. Atropine is the most useful drug for increasing heart rate and should be given intravenously in doses of 0.4 to 0.6 mg. If the rate remains below 60 beats per minute, additional doses of 0.2 mg, up to a total of 2.0 mg, may be given in divided doses. Persistent bradycardia (< 40 beats per minute) despite atropine may be treated with electrical pacing. Isoproterenol should be avoided.

Conduction disturbances Failure of conduction may develop at three different levels in the conduction system: the atrioventricular (AV) node, the bundle of His, or the more peripheral portions of the conduction system (Chap. 184). If the block occurs in the AV node, the escape rhythm usually originates in the AV junction and the QRS complexes are usually of normal duration; but when the block occurs distal to the AV node, the escape site is ventricular and the QRS configuration is abnormal and its duration is prolonged. Disturbances of conduction may occur in any one or two of the three peripheral branches (fascicles) of the conduction system (p. 858), and their recognition is of value in identifying patients at risk of developing complete heart block. When block occurs in any two of the three fascicles, bifascicular block is said to exist; complete AV block often develops in such patients. Thus, patients who develop the combination of right bundle branch block and either left anterior or left posterior hemiblock or patients with new left bundle branch block have a particularly high risk of progression to complete heart block.

The mortality rate of patients with complete AV block in association with anterior infarction (75 percent) is almost three times that of patients who develop AV block with inferior infarction (25 percent), and the risk of subsequent death in those who survive to leave the hospital is also increased in the former group. This difference is related to the fact that heart block in inferior infarction is usually caused by AV nodal ischemia. The AV node is a small discrete structure, and thus a small amount of ischemia or necrosis can result in AV nodal dysfunction. In anterior wall infarction, heart block is usually related to ischemic malfunction of all three fascicles of the conduction system and thus commonly results only from extensive myocardial necrosis.

Electrical pacing provides an effective means of increasing the heart rate of patients with bradycardia due to AV block, but it is not possible to be sure that such acceleration is always beneficial. For example, in patients with anterior wall infarction and complete heart block, the large size of the infarct is the major factor determining the outcome, and correction of the conduction deficit may not improve the poor prognosis in this group. Pacing does appear to be beneficial, however, in patients with inferoposterior infarction who have complete heart block associated with heart failure, hypotension, marked bradycardia, or significant ventricular ectopic activity. A subgroup of these patients, those with right ventricular infarction, often respond poorly to ventricular pacing because of the loss of the atrial ''kick.'' In such patients, dual chamber, atrioventricular sequential pacing may be required.

In the past, prophylactic placement of a pacing catheter has been advocated for patients with conduction disturbances known to be precursors of complete heart block. However, the recent availability of reliable noninvasive (external) temporary pacing devices makes it possible to pace conscious patients without insertion of a transvenous pacemaker lead. Therefore, routine use of prophylactic pacing is no longer necessary in most situations. Permanent pacing has been advocated for patients who develop the combination of persistent bifascicular and transient third-degree heart block during the acute phase of myocardial infarction. Retrospective studies in such patients suggest that the incidence of sudden death is decreased in those whom permanent pacing was instituted.

HEART FAILURE Some degree of transient impairment of left ventricular function occurs in over half of patients with myocardial infarction. The most common clinical signs are pulmonary rales and S_3 and S_4 gallop rhythms. Pulmonary congestion is also frequently seen on the chest roentgenogram. Elevation of left ventricular filling pressure and pulmonary artery pressure are the characteristic hemodynamic findings, but it should be appreciated that these findings may result from a reduction of diastolic ventricular compliance (diastolic failure) and/or a reduction of stroke volume with secondary cardiac dilatation (systolic failure) (Chap. 181). The therapy of heart failure in association with myocardial infarction is similar to that of heart failure secondary to other forms of heart disease, with a few exceptions (Chap. 182). The major difference concerns the use of cardiac glycosides. The benefit following the administration of digitalis in acute myocardial infarction is unimpressive. This is not surprising since the function of the noninfarcted tissue may be normal and digitalis would not be expected to improve the systolic or diastolic dysfunction of infarcted or ischemic tissue. On the other hand, diuretic agents are extremely effective in the treatment of heart failure following myocardial infarction, since they diminish pulmonary congestion in the presence of systolic and/or diastolic heart failure. A fall in left ventricular filling pressure and an improvement in orthopnea and dyspnea follow the intravenous administration of furosemide. This drug should be used with caution, however, as it can result in a massive diuresis with associated decrease in plasma volume, cardiac output, systemic blood pressure, and hence coronary perfusion. Nitrates in various forms may be used to decrease preload and congestive symptoms. Oral isosorbide dinitrate, topical nitroglycerin ointment, or, in patients with severe pulmonary congestion or pulmonary edema, intravenous nitroglycerin, all have the advantage over a diuretic of lowering preload through venodilatation without decreasing the total plasma volume. Additionally, nitrates may improve ventricular compliance if concurrent ischemia is present, since ischemia causes an elevation of left ventricular filling pressure. The patient with pulmonary edema is treated in the manner described in Chap. 182. Studies with vasodilators to reduce cardiac afterload indicate that the reduction in cardiac work, which results from the lowered afterload, may significantly improve left ventricular performance with a reduction of ventricular filling pressure and pulmonary congestion concomitant with an elevation of cardiac output.

Ventricular remodeling Soon after myocardial infarction, the left ventricle begins to dilate. Acutely, this occurs as the result of expansion of the infarct. Later, lengthening of the noninfarcted segments occurs as well. Overall chamber enlargement is related to the size of the infarction, with greater degrees of dilatation causing more marked hemodynamic impairment, more frequent heart failure, and a poorer prognosis as well. Recent data suggest that progressive dilatation, and its clinical consequences, may be attenuated by afterload-reducing therapy such as vasodilatation induced by the angiotensin converting enzyme inhibitor captopril. Thus, in patients with a depressed ejection fraction (less than 45%), particularly if signs of heart failure are present, consideration should be given to the institution of captopril therapy (beginning with 6.25 mg tid and advancing to 25 to 50 mg tid as tolerated).

Hemodynamic monitoring Hemodynamic evidence of abnormal left ventricular function becomes apparent when contraction is seriously impaired in 20 to 25 percent of the left ventricle. Infarction of 40 percent or more of the left ventricle usually results in the syndrome of cardiogenic shock (see below). Pulmonary capillary wedge pressure and pulmonary artery diastolic pressure correlate well with left ventricular diastolic pressure and are therefore often referred to as left ventricular filling pressures. Positioning of a balloon flotation catheter in the pulmonary artery enables the physician to monitor left ventricular filling pressure constantly, a technique which is useful in patients who exhibit clinical evidence of hemodynamic abnormalities or instability. However, in view of the complications that can occur, insertion of a pulmonary artery catheter should be limited to those patients with hemodynamic instability. Cardiac output can also be determined with a pulmonary artery catheter. With the addition of intraarterial pressure monitoring, systemic vascular resistance can be calculated as a guide to adjusting vasopressor and vasodilator therapy. Some patients with acute myocardial infarction have markedly elevated left ventricular filling pressures (>22 mmHg) and normal cardiac indexes [>2.6 and <3.6 (L/min)/m^2], while others have relatively low filling pressures (<15 mmHg) and reduced cardiac indexes. The former usually benefit from diuresis, while the latter respond to volume expansion by means of intravenous administration of colloid-containing solutions.

Cardiogenic shock—power failure In recent years efforts to reduce infarct size and prompt treatment of ongoing ischemia and other complications of myocardial infarction have reduced the incidence of cardiogenic shock.

It is useful to consider cardiogenic shock as a form of severe left ventricular failure. This syndrome is characterized by marked hypotension with systolic arterial pressure <80 mmHg and a marked reduction of cardiac index [<1.8 (L/min)/m^2] in the face of elevated left ventricular filling (pulmonary capillary wedge) pressure >18 mmHg. Hypotension alone is not a basis for the diagnosis of cardiogenic shock, because many patients who make an uneventful recovery will have serious hypotension (systolic pressure <80 mmHg) for several hours. Such patients often have low left ventricular filling pressures, and their hypotension usually resolves with the administration of intravenous fluids. The following *clinical* criteria for cardiogenic shock define a population of patients with a mortality rate of >70 percent: (1) systolic arterial blood pressure <90 mmHg which has declined by at least 30 mmHg below the previous level; (2) clinical signs of peripheral circulatory insufficiency, e.g., cold, moist skin and cyanosis; (3) dulled sensorium; (4) oliguria with urine flow of less than 20 mL/h; and (5) failure of improvement following relief of pain and administration of oxygen. Specifically *excluded* are patients with hypotension secondary to vasovagal reaction, hypovolemia, arrhythmia, drug reaction, or sepsis.

Cardiogenic shock may develop during the first hours of the infarct and be present at the time of initial hospitalization. Alternatively, it may appear after hospitalization—most commonly during the first day but sometimes as late as the sixth day. Risk factors for the in-hospital development of shock include advanced age, depressed left ventricular ejection fraction on admission, large infarct, history of diabetes mellitus, and previous myocardial infarction. Patients with several of these risk factors may be considered for cardiac catheterization and mechanical reperfusion (angioplasty or surgery) *before* the development of shock.

Pathophysiology of pump failure Marked reduction in the quantity of contracting myocardium is the cause of cardiogenic shock in myocardial infarction, although all organ systems are ultimately involved. The function of the heart is impaired by the initial insult; this results in a decrease in arterial pressure and hence in coronary blood flow because of its dependence on aortic perfusion pressure (Fig. 189-1). The reduction in coronary perfusion pressure and myocardial blood flow further impairs myocardial function and may increase the size of the myocardial infarction. Arrhythmias and metabolic acidosis also contribute to this deterioration because they

FIGURE 189-1 The sequence of events in the vicious cycle in which coronary artery obstruction leads to cardiogenic shock and progressive circulatory deterioration.

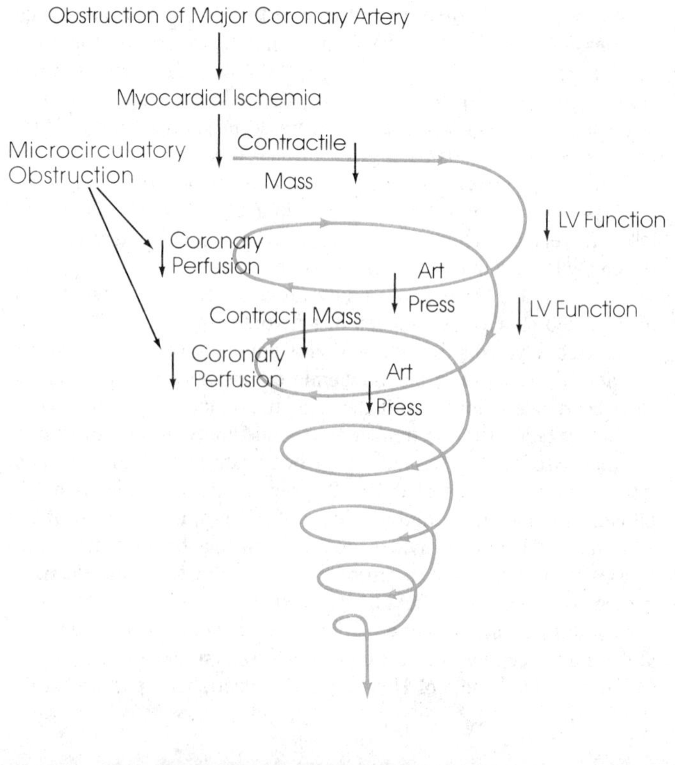

are the result of inadequate perfusion. It is this positive feedback loop which accounts for the high mortality rate associated with the shock syndrome.

Arterial blood pressure is a function of two factors—cardiac output and systemic vascular resistance—and a decrease in either without a compensatory rise in the other will result in a fall in arterial blood pressure. Cardiac output is lower in a population of patients with myocardial infarction and shock. However many patients with myocardial infarction without shock have cardiac outputs in the same range as those in patients with shock, and therefore it is not possible to characterize these patients on the basis of reductions of cardiac output alone. Systemic vascular resistance, the other factor important in determining blood pressure, may be either normal or increased in myocardial infarction. Normally, a fall in cardiac output is accompanied by a compensatory rise in systemic vascular resistance, but in patients with shock due to myocardial infarction, the appropriate elevation in resistance may fail to occur.

A simple schematic diagram depicting the relationship between left ventricular work and filling pressure is seen in Fig 189-2 The upper curve represents the familiar Frank-Starling relationship in the normal heart; the lower curve shows the relation which might be expected in the patient with shock secondary to myocardial infarction. It is obvious that, at all levels of end-diastolic pressure, the left ventricular work of the patient with myocardial infarction is depressed. At point C, the end-diastolic pressure is elevated, but at point B, it may be normal despite the fact that myocardial work is well below that expected of the normal heart at this diastolic pressure, as indicated by point A.

Treatment of pump failure The physiology and ominous prognosis associated with this condition dictate that all patients with shock should, if possible, have continuous monitoring of arterial pressure and of left ventricular filling pressure (as reflected in the pulmonary capillary wedge pressure measured with a pulmonary artery balloon catheter) as well as frequent determinations of cardiac output. All patients with the shock syndrome should receive oxygen continuously to help combat the hypoxemia which is universally present. When pulmonary edema coexists, endotracheal intubation may be necessary to ensure oxygenation. The relief of pain is important, as some vasodepressor reflex activity may be a response to severe pain. However, narcotics should be used cautiously in view of their propensity to lower arterial pressure.

The primary objective of treatment is to avoid the sequence depicted in Fig. 189-1, by attempting to maintain coronary perfusion by raising the arterial blood pressure with vasopressors (see below), intraaortic balloon counterpulsation, and manipulation of blood volume to a level that ensures an optimum left ventricular filling pressure (approximately 20 mmHg). The latter may require either infusion of crystalloid or diuresis.

FIGURE 189-2 Schematic representation of the Frank-Starling relationship as applied to patients with the shock syndrome in myocardial infarction.

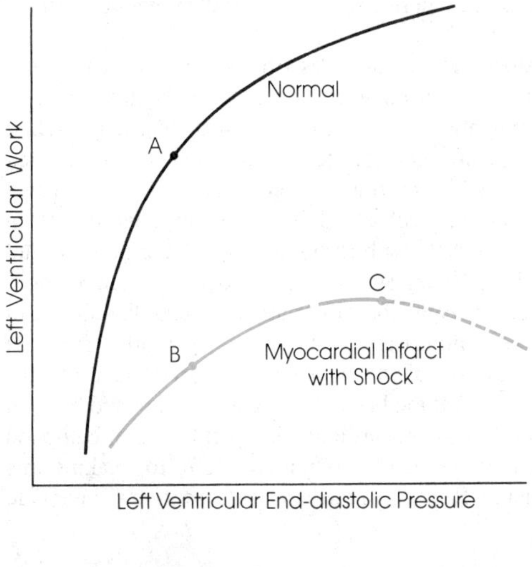

In patients seen within the first 4 h of the onset of infarction, reperfusion by thrombolytic therapy and/or PTCA (p. 877) may improve left ventricular function dramatically, thereby interrupting the cycle of hemodynamic deterioration.

Hypovolemia This is an easily corrected condition which may contribute to the hypotension and vascular collapse associated with myocardial infarction in some patients. Hypovolemia may be secondary to previous diuretic use, to reduced fluid intake during the early stages of the illness, and/or to vomiting associated with pain or medications. In addition, a state of *relative* hypovolemia may exist; i.e., with the acute reduction in contractile function and ventricular compliance resulting from infarction an increase in vascular volume is needed to maintain cardiac output. Owing to the acute nature of the process, there is insufficient time for compensatory fluid retention to accommodate this need, and relative hypovolemia in a normally hydrated patient results. Consequently, hypovolemia should be identified and corrected in patients with acute myocardial infarction and hypotension before embarking upon more vigorous forms of therapy. If left ventricular filling pressure is in the normal range, fluid should be administered until the cardiac output is maximized. This usually occurs at a left ventricular filling pressure of approximately 20 mmHg. However, the optimal left ventricular filling or pulmonary artery wedge pressure may vary considerably among different patients. Each patient's ideal level is reached by cautious fluid administration during careful monitoring of oxygenation and cardiac output. When the cardiac output plateaus (Fig. 189-2, point C), further increases in left ventricular filling pressure will only increase congestive symptoms and decrease systemic oxygenation. Central venous pressure measurements reflect right rather than left ventricular filling pressure and are inadequate in this situation, since left ventricular function is almost always affected much more adversely than is right ventricular function in acute myocardial infarction.

Vasopressors A variety of intravenous drugs may be used to augment arterial pressure and cardiac output in patients with cardiogenic shock. Unfortunately, all have important disadvantages or problems associated with their use, and none have been shown to change the outcome in patients with established shock. *Isoproterenol* is a synthetic sympathomimetic amine which is now rarely used in the treatment of shock due to myocardial infarction. Although this agent increases contractility, it also produces peripheral vasodilatation and increases heart rate. The resultant increase in myocardial oxygen consumption and reduction of coronary perfusion pressure may extend the area of ischemic injury. *Norepinephrine* is a potent alpha-adrenergic agent with powerful vasoconstrictive properties. It also possesses beta-adrenergic activity and therefore enhances contractility. Because the increase in afterload and contractility associated with its use causes a marked increase in myocardial oxygen consumption, it should be reserved for relatively desperate situations or for patients with cardiogenic shock and lowered systemic vascular resistance. It should be started at 2 to 4 μg/min. If pressure cannot be maintained with a dosage of 15 μg/min, it is unlikely that a further increase will be beneficial.

Dopamine (Chap. 67) is useful in many patients with power failure. At low doses [2 to 10 (μg/kg)/min] the drug has positive chronotropic and inotropic effects as a consequence of beta receptor stimulation. At higher doses, a vasoconstrictive effect results from alpha receptor stimulation. At lower doses dopamine [≤2 (μg/kg)/min] also has the unique effect of dilating the renal and splanchnic vascular beds and apparently has little effect on myocardial oxygen consumption. Intravenous dopamine is started at an infusion rate of 2 to 5 (μg/kg)/min with increments in dosage every 2 to 5 min up to a maximum of 20 to 50 (μg/kg)/min. Systolic arterial blood pressure should be maintained at approximately 90 mmHg. *Dobutamine* is a synthetic sympathomimetic amine with positive inotropic action and minimal positive chronotropic or peripheral vasoconstrictive activity in the usual dosage range [2.5 to 10 (μg/kg)/min]. It should not be employed when a vasoconstrictor effect is required. However, in patients with less profound degrees of hypotension, dobutamine may be an extremely useful agent, particularly if positive chronotropy is to be avoided.

Amrinone (see p. 899) is a positive inotropic agent without catecholamine structure or activity. It resembles dobutamine in its pharmacologic activity, although it has a potent vasodilating action. Initially a loading dose of 0.75 mg/kg is given over 2 to 3 min. If effective, this is followed by an infusion of 5 to 10 (μg/kg)/min, followed if necessary 30 min later by an additional bolus of 0.75 mg/kg. If necessary, the dose may then be increased up to 15 (μg/kg)/min for short periods.

Patients with global left ventricular ischemia as the cause of power failure and profound hypotension, such as those with critical left main coronary artery obstructive disease, may benefit from brief treatment with a pure vasoconstrictor in preference to a positive inotropic agent. In such cases coronary perfusion may be improved by the vasoconstrictor-induced increase in arterial pressure, whereas a positive inotropic agent may only increase ischemic injury in muscle that is incapable of performing more work. In this situation a pure vasoconstrictor such as *neosynephrine,* 10 to 100 μg/min, should be used, as briefly as possible, usually only as interim therapy while preparations are made for counterpulsation with an intraaortic balloon pump and/or emergency coronary artery surgery.

Cardiac glycosides (Chap. 182) Controlled studies have failed to demonstrate significant beneficial effects of cardiac glycoside therapy in the early phases (0 to 48 h) of acute myocardial infarction. Hemodynamic improvement has been documented at later times, but this effect, too, is marginal. Since cardiac glycosides cannot improve the function of necrotic myocardium and since pump failure is thought to be related to the total mass of infarcted tissue, digitalis therapy does not usually result in dramatic improvement in patients with acute myocardial infarction and sinus rhythm.

Aortic counterpulsation In cardiogenic shock mechanical assistance with an intraaortic balloon pumping system capable of augmenting both diastolic pressure and cardiac output can provide circulatory support. A sausage-shaped balloon at the end of a catheter is introduced percutaneously into the aorta via the femoral artery, and the balloon is inflated during early diastole, thereby enhancing both coronary blood flow and peripheral perfusion. The balloon collapses in early systole, thereby reducing the afterload against which left ventricular ejection takes place. Improvement in hemodynamic status has been observed with balloon pumping in a large number of patients, but long-term survival following this mode of therapy in patients with cardiogenic shock is still disappointing. The balloon counterpulsation system may best be reserved for patients whose condition merits mechanical (surgery or angioplasty) intervention (e.g., continuing ischemia, ventricular septal rupture, or mitral regurgitation) and in whom a successful result is likely to result in the reversal of cardiogenic shock. Intraaortic balloon pumping is contraindicated if aortic regurgitation is present or if aortic dissection is possible or suspected. The catheter introduced for balloon counterpulsation is large and frequently produces limb ischemia, particularly if peripheral vascular disease is present or if the catheter is inserted into a relatively small vessel (e.g., as would be present in an elderly female).

There is reason to believe that results of therapy of the shock syndrome secondary to myocardial infarction, while improving gradually as a result of meticulous attention to the details of therapy outlined above, will continue to be disappointing overall because a large fraction of patients with the syndrome have large areas of infarcted myocardium with severe, diffuse coronary atherosclerosis. Although occasional dramatic results have been reported with emergency revascularization surgery or coronary angioplasty, the overall results with these approaches, too, have been disappointing. It is hoped that the widespread and early application of thrombolytic therapy will reduce the amount of myocardium which becomes necrotic and thereby reduce the incidence of this syndrome. Also, revascularization in patients at high risk of developing shock in the hospital may have a similar effect.

Other complications MITRAL REGURGITATION Apical systolic murmurs of mitral regurgitation appear in more than one-fourth of patients during the first 5 days after the onset of a myocardial infarction, but mitral regurgitation is of hemodynamic importance in only a minority of these patients. In most patients the murmur is present during the acute phase of infarction, disappearing with recovery. The most common cause of mitral regurgitation following myocardial infarction is dysfunction of the papillary muscles of the left ventricle due to ischemia or infarction.

Mitral regurgitation may also be the result of alteration in the size or shape of the ventricle due to impaired contractility or to aneurysm formation. Either papillary muscle may rupture, the posterior one twice as frequently as the anterior. Left ventricular function may deteriorate dramatically with superimposition of mitral regurgitation. The differential diagnosis includes perforation of the ventricular septum (see below), and the differentiation from mitral regurgitation is conveniently made at the bedside by echocardiography and/or with a flow-directed balloon catheter. Large *v* waves may be recorded in the pulmonary capillary wedge position in patients with hemodynamically significant mitral regurgitation, and there is no oxygen "step up" as the catheter is advanced from the right atrium to the right ventricle. Surgical repair or replacement of the mitral valve may be followed by dramatic improvement in patients in whom acute heart failure results primarily from severe mitral regurgitation due to papillary muscle rupture or dysfunction and in whom myocardial function is relatively well preserved.

If aortic systolic pressure is lowered in patients with mitral regurgitation, a greater fraction of the left ventricular output will be ejected antegrade, thus lessening the regurgitant fraction. To this end, both intraaortic balloon counterpulsation, which lowers the aortic systolic pressure mechanically, and the infusion of sodium nitroprusside or nitroglycerin, which reduce systemic vascular resistance, have been used with success for the interim management of patients with severe mitral regurgitation in the setting of acute myocardial infarction. Ideally, definitive operative treatment should be postponed for 4 to 6 weeks after the infarct. However, if the patient's hemodynamic and/or clinical condition does not improve or stabilize, surgical treatment should be undertaken, even in the acute stage.

Cardiac rupture Myocardial rupture is a dramatic complication of myocardial infarction most likely to occur during the first week after the onset of symptoms; its frequency increases with the age of the patient. First infarction, no history of angina pectoris, and relatively large Q-wave infarcts are associated with a higher incidence of cardiac rupture. The clinical presentation may often be that of a sudden disappearance of the pulse, blood pressure, and consciousness while the electrocardiogram continues to show sinus rhythm (*apparent* electromechanical dissociation). The myocardium continues to contract, but forward flow is not maintained as blood escapes into the pericardium. Cardiac tamponade (Chap. 193) ensues, and closed-chest massage is ineffective. Although almost universally fatal, there have been instances in which cardiac rupture has been recognized and successfully treated by pericardiocentesis and emergency cardiac surgery.

Septal perforation The pathogenesis of perforation of the ventricular septum is similar to that of external rupture of the myocardium, but the therapeutic potential is greater. Patients with ventricular septal rupture present with severe heart failure in association with the sudden appearance of a pansystolic murmur, often accompanied by a parasternal thrill. It is often impossible to differentiate this condition from rupture of a papillary muscle with resultant mitral regurgitation, and a tall *v* wave in the pulmonary capillary wedge pressure in both conditions further complicates the differentiation. The diagnosis can be established by the demonstration of a left-to-right shunt (i.e., an oxygen step-up at the level of the right ventricle) by limited cardiac catheterization performed at the bedside using a flow-directed balloon catheter. Two-dimensional echocardiography, particularly if equipped with a Doppler flow probe, can be extremely useful for making this diagnosis at the bedside. Rupture of the ventricular septum is amenable to immediate surgical treatment, albeit at a significant risk, but this form of therapy is ordinarily indicated on an urgent basis in patients whose condition cannot be stabilized rapidly. A prolonged period of hemodynamic compromise may produce end-organ damage and other complications that can be avoided by early intervention including nitroprusside infusion and intraaortic balloon counterpulsation.

The physiology of acute mitral regurgitation and acute ventricular septal perforation are similar in that the level of aortic systolic pressure determines in part the regurgitant volume, the principal difference being the chamber into which the regurgitant fraction is ejected. In septal perforation, a fraction of left ventricular output is ejected into the right ventricle. In a manner analogous to mitral regurgitation, lowering of aortic systolic pressure by mechanical (intraaortic balloon counterpulsation) and/or pharmacologic (nitroglycerin or nitroprusside) means can decrease the hemodynamic compromise caused by perforation.

Ventricular aneurysm The term *ventricular aneurysm* is usually used to describe *dyskinesis* or local expansile paradoxical wall motion. Normally functioning myocardial fibers must shorten more if stroke volume and cardiac output are to be maintained in patients with ventricular aneurysm, and if they are unable to do so, overall ventricular function is impaired. Aneurysms are composed of scar tissue and neither predispose to nor are associated with cardiac rupture.

The complications of left ventricular aneurysm do not usually occur for weeks to months following myocardial infarction; they include congestive heart failure, arterial embolism, and ventricular arrhythmias. Apical aneurysms are the most common and the most easily detected by clinical examination. The physical finding of greatest value is a double, diffuse, or displaced apical impulse. The electrocardiographic finding of ST-segment elevation at rest is present in precordial leads in 25 percent of patients with either apical or anterior aneurysms. Ventricular aneurysms are readily detectable by two-dimensional echocardiography, which may also reveal a mural thrombus in aneurysms involving the anterior wall and/or apex. Rarely, myocardial rupture may be contained by a local area of pericardium, along with organizing thrombus and hematoma. Over time this *pseudoaneurysm* enlarges, maintaining communication with the left ventricular cavity via a narrow neck. Because spontaneous rupture of a pseudoaneurysm often occurs, if recognized, it should be surgically repaired.

Right ventricular infarction Approximately one-third of patients with inferoposterior infarction demonstrate at least a minor degree of right ventricular necrosis. An occasional patient with inferoposterior left ventricular infarction also has extensive right ventricular myocardial infarction. These patients often present with signs of severe right ventricular failure (jugular venous distention, Kussmaul's sign, hepatomegaly) with or without hypotension. ST-segment elevations of the right-sided precordial electrocardiographic leads, particularly lead V_4R, are present in the majority of patients with right ventricular infarction. Radionuclide ventriculography and two-dimensional echocardiography are also sensitive in the detection of right ventricular damage associated with acute myocardial infarction. Catheterization of the right side of the heart often reveals a distinctive hemodynamic pattern resembling cardiac tamponade or constrictive pericarditis (Chap. 193). Volume expansion is often successful in treating low cardiac output and hypotension associated with extensive right ventricular infarction.

Postinfarction ischemia and extension Recurrent angina develops in approximately 25 percent of patients hospitalized for acute myocardial infarction. This percentage is even higher in patients undergoing successful thrombolysis. Since recurrent or persistent ischemia often heralds extension of the original infarct and is associated with a doubling of risk following acute myocardial infarction, patients with these symptoms should be considered for prompt coronary arteriography and mechanical revascularization.

Infarct extension occurs in 5 to 10 percent of patients in the first 10 days following acute myocardial infarction, increasing to as many as 20 percent of patients following thrombolytic therapy. Hospital mortality is as much as four times greater in patients with infarct extension compared with those free of this complication. Careful monitoring for signs or symptoms of recurrent ischemia and early submaximal stress testing should be undertaken in order to identify patients at risk for extension [particularly those presenting with non-Q-wave infarction, with postinfarction angina, with a previous myocardial infarction, or with an early peaking CK-MB curve (less than 15 h)]. Early catheterization with coronary angiography should be considered for most patients with one or more risk factors for infarct extension. In such patients, revascularization (angioplasty or surgery) should be considered in order to prevent infarct extension.

Thromboembolism Clinically apparent thromboembolism complicates myocardial infarction in approximately 10 percent of cases, but embolic lesions are found in 45 percent of patients in necropsy series, suggesting that thromboembolism is often clinically silent. Thromboembolism is considered to be at least an important contributing cause of death in 25 percent of infarct patients who die following admission to the hospital. Arterial emboli originate from left ventricular mural thrombi, while most pulmonary emboli arise in the leg veins. Thromboembolism most commonly occurs in association with large infarcts in the presence of heart failure. Thromboembolism occurs extremely commonly in patients with echocardiographic evidence of a left ventricular thrombus, but only rarely if a thrombus is not present on the echocardiogram. Although well-controlled trials do not exist, the incidence of embolization appears to be decreased by anticoagulation.

Pericarditis (See also Chap. 193) Pericardial friction rubs and/or pericardial pain are frequently encountered in patients with acute transmural myocardial infarction. This complication can usually be managed with aspirin (650 mg qid). It is important to diagnose the chest pain of pericarditis accurately, since failure to appreciate it may lead to the erroneous diagnosis of recurrent ischemic pain and/or infarct extension with resultant inappropriate use of anticoagulants, nitrates, beta blockers, or coronary arteriography. No definite cause and effect relationship between administration of anticoagulants and pericarditis or tamponade has been proved. Nonetheless, the possibility that anticoagulants can cause tamponade in the presence of acute pericarditis is sufficiently high to contraindicate their use in patients with pericarditis, as manifested by either pain or persistent rub, unless there is a compelling indication.

Post-myocardial infarction syndrome—Dressler's syndrome (See also Chap. 193) This syndrome, characterized by fever and pleuropericardial chest pain, is thought to be due to an autoimmune pericarditis, pleuritis, and/or pneumonitis. It may begin from a few days to 6 weeks after myocardial infarction. The occurrence of Dressler's syndrome may be etiologically related to the early use of anticoagulants and appears to have decreased markedly in the last decade as long-term anticoagulants are used less frequently in acute myocardial infarction. The syndrome usually responds promptly to therapy with salicylates. On occasion, corticosteroids may be required to relieve discomfort of an unusual, refractory nature. Effusions associated with Dressler's syndrome may become hemorrhagic if anticoagulants are administered.

REFERENCES

Antman EM, Rutherford JD (eds): *Coronary Care Medicine: A Practical Approach*. Boston, Martinus Nijhoff, 1986

Coller BS: Platelets and thrombolytic therapy. *N Engl J Med* 322(1):33, 1990

Cunningham MJ, Pasternak RC: Acute myocardial infarction: In-hospital diagnostic decisions, in *Manual of Clinical Evaluation: Strategies for Cost-Effective Care*, MD Aronson, TL Delbanco (eds). Boston, Little, Brown, 1988

Davies MJ, Thomas AC: Plaque fissuring—The cause of acute myocardial infarction, sudden ischaemic death, and crescendo angina. Br Heart J 53:363, 1985

Goldman L et al: A computer protocol to predict myocardial infarction in emergency department patients with chest pain. N Engl J Med 318:797, 1988

Jain D et al: Clinical and prognostic significance of lung thallium uptake on rest imaging in acute myocardial infarction. Am J Cardiol 65(3):154, 1990

KRONE RJ et al and the MULTICENTER POSTINFARCTION RESEARCH GROUP: Low level exercise testing after myocardial infarction: Usefulness in enhancing clinical risk stratification. Circulation 71:80, 1985

LEE TH, GOLDMAN L: The coronary care unit turns 25: Historical trends and future directions. Ann Intern Med 108:887, 1988

———, ———: Serum enzyme assays in the diagnosis of acute myocardial infarction. Ann Intern Med 105:221, 1986

MULLER JE et al: Circadian variation in the frequency of onset of acute myocardial infarction. N Engl J Med 313:1315, 1985

——— et al and the MILIS STUDY GROUP: Myocardial infarct extension: Occurrence, outcome, and risk factors in the multicenter investigation of limitation of infarct size. Ann Intern Med 108:1, 1988

ONG L et al: Early prediction of mortality in patients with acute myocardial infarction: A prospective study of clinical and radionuclide risk factors. Am J Cardiol 57:33, 1986

PASTERNAK RC et al: Acute myocardial infarction, in *Heart Disease*, 3d ed, E Braunwald (ed). Philadelphia, Saunders, 1988, p 1222

PFEFFER MA et al: Effect of captopril on progressive ventricular dilatation after anterior myocardial infarction. N Engl J Med 310:80, 1988

ROIG E et al: In-hospital mortality rates from acute myocardial infarction by race in U.S. hospitals: Findings from the National Hospital Discharge Survey. Circulation 76:280, 1987

SIEGEL D et al: Risk factor modification after myocardial infarction. Ann Intern Med 109:213, 1988

SILVER MD, GOLDSCHLAGER N: Temporary transvenous cardiac pacing in the critical care setting. Chest 93:607, 1988

SCHULMAN SP et al: Prognostic cardiac catheterization variables in survivors of acute myocardial infarction: A five year prospective study. J Am Coll Cardiol 11:1164, 1988

STACK RS et al: Survival and cardiac event rates in the first year after emergency coronary angioplasty for acute myocardial infarction. J Am Coll Cardiol 11:1141, 1988

STONE PH et al and the MILIS STUDY GROUP: Prognostic significance of location and type of myocardial infarction: Independent adverse outcome associated with anterior location. J Am Coll Cardiol 11:453, 1988

THE STEERING COMMITTEE OF THE PHYSICIANS' HEALTH STUDY RESEARCH GROUP: Final report on the aspirin component of the ongoing Physicians' Health Study. N Engl J Med 19:129–35, 1989

TIMI STUDY GROUP: Comparison of invasive and conservative strategies after treatment with intravenous tissue plasminogen activator in acute myocardial infarction. Results of the Thombolysis in Myocardial Infarction (TIMI) Phase II Trial. N Engl J Med 320:618, 1989

———: Immediate versus delayed catheterization and angioplasty following thrombolytic therapy for acute myocardial infarction. TIMI IIA Results. JAMA 260:2849, 1988

TOPOL EJ et al and the THROMBOLYSIS AND ANGIOPLASTY in MYOCARDIAL INFARCTION STUDY GROUP: A randomized trial of immediate versus delayed elective angioplasty after intravenous tissue plasminogen activator in acute myocardial infarction. N Engl J Med 317:581, 1987

VOLPI A et al: In-hospital prognosis of patients with acute myocardial infarction complicated by primary ventricular fibrillation. N Engl J Med 317:257, 1987

WALL TC et al: Results of high dose intravenous urokinase for acute myocardial infarction. Am J Cardiol 65(3):124, 1990

190 ISCHEMIC HEART DISEASE

ANDREW P. SELWYN / EUGENE BRAUNWALD

Ischemia refers to a lack of oxygen due to inadequate perfusion. Ischemic heart disease is a condition of diverse etiologies, all having in common a disturbance of cardiac function due to an imbalance between oxygen supply and demand.

ETIOLOGY AND PATHOPHYSIOLOGY

The most common cause of ischemia is atherosclerotic disease of epicardial coronary arteries. By reducing the lumen of these vessels, atherosclerosis causes an absolute decrease in myocardial perfusion in the basal state or limits appropriate increases in perfusion when the demand for flow is augmented. Coronary blood flow can also be limited by arterial thrombi, spasm, and rarely coronary emboli as well as by ostial narrowing due to luetic aortitis. Congenital abnormalities, such as anomalous origin of the left anterior descending coronary artery from the pulmonary artery, may cause myocardial ischemia and infarction in infancy, but this cause is very rare in adults. Myocardial ischemia can also occur if myocardial oxygen demands are abnormally increased, as in severe ventricular hypertrophy due to hypertension or aortic stenosis. The latter can present with angina that is indistinguishable from that caused by coronary atherosclerosis. A reduction in the oxygen-carrying capacity of the blood, as in extremely severe anemia or in the presence of carboxyhemoglobin, is a rare cause of myocardial ischemia. Not infrequently, two or more causes of ischemia will coexist, such as an increase in oxygen demand due to left ventricular hypertrophy and a reduction in oxygen supply secondary to coronary atherosclerosis.

The normal coronary circulation is dominated and controlled by the myocardial requirements for oxygen. This need is met by the heart's ability to vary coronary vascular resistance (and therefore blood flow) considerably while the myocardium extracts a high and relatively fixed percentage of oxygen (Chap. 16). Normally, intramyocardial resistance arterioles demonstrate an immense capacity for dilation. With exercise and emotional stress, the changing oxygen needs affect coronary vascular resistance and in this manner regulate the supply of blood and oxygen (metabolic regulation). These same vessels adapt to physiologic alterations in blood pressure in order to maintain coronary blood flow at levels appropriate to myocardial needs (autoregulation). Although the large epicardial coronary arteries are capable of constriction and relaxation, in healthy persons they serve as conduits and are referred to as *conductance vessels,* while the intramyocardial arterioles normally exhibit striking changes in tone and are therefore referred to as *resistance vessels.*

CORONARY ATHEROSCLEROSIS (See also Chap. 195) Epicardial coronary arteries are a major site of atherosclerotic disease. Dysfunction of vascular endothelium and an abnormal interaction with blood monocytes and platelets lead to subintimal collections of abnormal fat, cells, and debris (i.e., atherosclerotic plaques), which develop at irregular rates in different segments of the epicardial coronary tree and lead eventually to segmental reductions in cross-sectional area. The relationship between pulsatile flow and luminal stenosis is complex, but experiments have shown that when a stenosis reduces the cross-sectional area by approximately 75 percent, a full range of increases in flow to meet increased myocardial demand is not possible. When the luminal area is reduced by more than approximately 80 percent, blood flow at rest may be reduced, and further minor decreases in the stenotic orifice can reduce coronary flow dramatically and cause myocardial ischemia.

Segmental atherosclerotic narrowing of epicardial coronary arteries is caused most commonly by the formation of a plaque, which is subject to fissuring, hemorrhage, and thrombosis. Any of these events can temporarily worsen the obstruction, reduce coronary blood flow, and cause clinical manifestations of myocardial ischemia, as described below. In addition, the location of the stenosis will influence the quantity of myocardium rendered ischemic and thus determine the severity of the clinical manifestations. Severe coronary narrowing and myocardial ischemia are frequently accompanied by the development of collateral vessels, especially when the narrowing develops gradually. When well developed, such vessels can provide sufficient blood flow to sustain the viability of the myocardium at rest but not during circumstances of increased demand.

Once severe stenosis of a proximal epicardial artery has reduced the cross-sectional area by more than approximately 70 percent, the distal resistance vessels will dilate to reduce vascular resistance and maintain coronary blood flow. A pressure gradient develops across the proximal stenosis, and poststenotic pressure falls. When the resistance vessels are maximally dilated, myocardial blood flow becomes dependent on the pressure in the coronary artery distal to the obstruction. In these circumstances alterations in myocardial oxygenation can be caused by changes in myocardial oxygen demand and changes in the caliber of the stenosed coronary artery due to physiologic vasomotion, pathologic spasm, or small platelet plugs. All these transient events can upset the critical balance between oxygen supply and demand and thus precipitate myocardial ischemia.

EFFECTS OF ISCHEMIA The inadequate oxygenation induced by coronary atherosclerosis may cause transient disturbances of the mechanical, biochemical, and electrical function of the myocardium. The abrupt development of ischemia usually affects a segment of left ventricular myocardium with almost instantaneous failure of normal muscle relaxation and contraction. The relatively poor perfusion of the subendocardium causes more intense ischemia of this portion of the wall. Ischemia of large segments of the ventricle will cause transient left ventricular failure, and if the papillary muscles are involved, mitral regurgitation can complicate this event. When ischemic events are transient, they may be associated with angina pectoris; if prolonged, they can lead to myocardial necrosis and scarring with or without the clinical picture of acute myocardial infarction (see Chap. 189). Coronary atherosclerosis is a focal process that causes nonuniform ischemia. As a result, focal disturbances of ventricular contractility cause segmental bulging or dyskinesia and can greatly reduce the efficiency of myocardial pump function.

Underlying these mechanical disturbances are a wide range of abnormalities in cell metabolism, function, and structure. When oxygenated, the normal myocardium metabolizes fatty acids and glucose to carbon dioxide and water. With severe oxygen deprivation, fatty acids cannot be oxidized, and glucose is broken down to lactate; intracellular pH is reduced as are the myocardial stores of high-energy phosphates, adenosine triphosphate (ATP), and creatine phosphate. Impaired cell membrane function leads to potassium leakage and the uptake of sodium by myocytes. The severity and duration of the imbalance between myocardial oxygen supply and demand will determine whether the damage is reversible or whether it is permanent, with subsequent myocardial necrosis.

Ischemia also causes characteristic electrocardiographic changes such as repolarization abnormalities, as evidenced by inversion of the T wave and later by displacement of the ST segment (Chap. 176). Transient ST-segment depression often reflects subendocardial ischemia, while transient ST-segment elevation is thought to be caused by more severe transmural ischemia. Another important consequence of myocardial ischemia is electrical instability, since this may lead to ventricular tachycardia or ventricular fibrillation (Chap. 185). Most patients who die suddenly from ischemic heart disease do so as a result of ischemia-induced malignant ventricular arrhythmias (Chap. 40).

CLINICAL MANIFESTATIONS

ASYMPTOMATIC VERSUS SYMPTOMATIC CORONARY ARTERY DISEASE Postmortem studies on accident victims and military casualties in western countries have shown that coronary atherosclerosis often begins to develop prior to age 20 and is widespread among adults who were asymptomatic during life. In addition, exercise stress tests in asymptomatic persons may show evidence of silent myocardial ischemia, i.e., exercise-induced electrocardiographic changes not accompanied by angina; coronary angiographic studies of such persons frequently reveal obstructive coronary artery disease. Postmortem examination of patients with obstructive coronary artery disease who had no history of any clinical manifestations of myocardial ischemia often shows macroscopic scars of myocardial infarction in regions supplied by diseased coronary arteries. According to population studies, approximately 25 percent of patients with acute myocardial infarction may not reach medical attention, and these patients carry the same adverse prognosis as those who present with the classic clinical syndrome (Chap. 189). Sudden death may be unheralded and is a common presenting manifestation of coronary disease (Chap. 40). Patients can also present with cardiomegaly and heart failure secondary to ischemic damage of the left ventricular myocardium that caused no symptoms prior to the development of heart failure; this condition is referred to as *ischemic cardiomyopathy*. In contrast to the asymptomatic phase of ischemic heart disease, the symptomatic phase is characterized by chest pain due to either angina pectoris or acute myocardial infarction (Chap. 189). Having entered the symptomatic phase, the patient may exhibit a stable or progressive course, revert to the asymptomatic stage, or suddenly die.

CHRONIC STABLE ANGINA PECTORIS This episodic clinical syndrome is due to transient myocardial ischemia. Various diseases that cause myocardial ischemia as well as the numerous pain syndromes with which it may be confused are discussed in Chap. 16. Males constitute approximately 80 percent of all patients with angina pectoris and an even greater fraction of those younger than 50 years of age. The typical patient with angina is a 50- to 60-year-old man who seeks medical help for troublesome or frightening chest discomfort, usually described as heaviness, pressure, squeezing, smothering, or choking and only rarely as frank pain. When the patient is asked to localize the sensation, he or she will typically press on the sternum, sometimes with a clenched fist, to indicate a squeezing, central, substernal discomfort. This symptom is usually crescendo-decrescendo in nature and lasts 1 to 5 min. Angina can radiate to the left shoulder and to both arms, and especially to the ulnar surfaces of the forearm and hand. It can also arise in or radiate to the back, neck, jaw, teeth, and epigastrium.

Although episodes of angina are typically caused by exertion (e.g., exercise, hurrying, or sexual activity) or emotion (e.g., stress, anger, fright, or frustration) and are relieved by rest, they may also occur at rest (see "Unstable Angina Pectoris," below) and at night while the patient is recumbent (angina decubitus). The patient may be awakened at night distressed by typical chest discomfort and dyspnea. The pathophysiology of nocturnal angina may be similar to that of paroxysmal nocturnal dyspnea (Chap. 182), i.e., the expansion of the intrathoracic blood volume that occurs with recumbency causes an increase in cardiac size and myocardial oxygen demand that lead to ischemia and transient left ventricular failure.

The threshold for the development of angina pectoris may vary by time of day and emotional state. A patient may report symptoms upon minor exertion in the morning (a short walk or shaving) yet by midday may be capable of much greater effort without symptoms. Angina may be precipitated by unfamiliar tasks, a heavy meal, or exposure to cold.

Sharp, fleeting chest pain or prolonged, dull aches localized to the left submammary area are rarely due to myocardial ischemia. However, angina pectoris may be atypical in location and may not be strictly related to provoking factors. In addition, this symptom may exacerbate and remit over days, weeks, or months, and its occurrence can be seasonal.

Systematic questioning of the patient with suspected ischemic heart disease is important to uncover a positive family history of ischemic heart disease, diabetes, hyperlipidemia, hypertension, cigarette smoking, and other risk factors for coronary atherosclerosis.

In *variant (Prinzmetal's) angina,* the chest discomfort characteristically occurs at rest or awakens the patient from sleep. It may be accompanied by palpitations or severe shortness of breath, explosive in onset, severe, and frightening. It may also be brought on by effort, although the workload at which it is precipitated usually varies considerably. Variant angina is caused by focal spasm of proximal epicardial coronary arteries; in approximately three-fourths of the patients atherosclerotic coronary artery obstruction is present, in which case the vasospasm occurs near the stenotic lesion.

Physical examination The physical examination is often normal. The patient's general appearance may reveal signs of risk factors associated with coronary atherosclerosis such as xanthelasma, xanthomas (Chap. 195), or diabetic skin lesions. There may also be signs of anemia, thyroid disease, and nicotine stains on the fingertips from cigarette smoking. Palpation can reveal thickened or absent peripheral arteries, signs of cardiac enlargement, and abnormal contraction of the cardiac impulse (left ventricular akinesia or dyskinesia). Examination of the fundi may reveal increased light reflexes and arteriovenous nicking as evidence of hypertension (an important risk factor for ischemic heart disease), while auscultation can uncover arterial bruits, a third and/or fourth heart sound, and, if acute ischemia or previous infarction has impaired papillary muscle function, a late apical systolic murmur due to mitral regurgitation. These auscultatory signs are best appreciated with the patient in the left decubitus position. Aortic stenosis, aortic regurgitation (Chap. 188), and hypertrophic cardiomyopathy (Chap. 192) must be excluded, since these disorders may cause angina even in the absence of coronary artery disease. Examination during an anginal attack is useful, since ischemia can cause transient left ventricular failure with the appearance of a third and/or fourth heart sound, a dyskinetic cardiac apex, mitral regurgitation, and even pulmonary edema.

Laboratory examination Although the diagnosis of ischemic heart disease can be made with confidence from a typical history, a number of simple laboratory tests can be most helpful. The urine should be examined for evidence of diabetes mellitus and renal disease, since both these conditions may accelerate atherosclerosis. Similarly, examination of the blood should include measurements of lipids (cholesterol—total, low density, and high density), glucose, creatinine, hematocrit, and, if indicated based on the physical examination, thyroid function. A chest x-ray is important, since it may show the consequences of ischemic heart disease, i.e., cardiac enlargement, ventricular aneurysm, or signs of heart failure. Calcification of the coronary arteries can sometimes be identified on chest fluoroscopy. These signs can support the diagnosis of coronary artery disease and are important in assessing the degree of cardiac damage and the effects of treatment for heart failure.

Electrocardiogram A normal ECG does not exclude the diagnosis of ischemic heart disease; however, certain characteristic abnormalities in tracings obtained at rest can confirm it. A 12-lead ECG recorded at rest is normal in about half the patients with typical angina pectoris, but there may be signs of an old myocardial infarction (Chap. 176). Serial tracings are particularly useful to look for past or evolving myocardial infarction. Although repolarization abnormalities, i.e., T-wave and ST-segment changes and intraventricular conduction disturbances at rest, are suggestive of ischemic heart disease, they are nonspecific, since they can also occur in pericardial, myocardial, and valvular heart disease or with anxiety, changes in posture, drugs, or esophageal disease. Typical ST-segment and T-wave changes that accompany episodes of angina pectoris and disappear thereafter are more specific. The most characteristic changes include displacement of the ST segment that is similar in every way to that induced during a stress test (see below). The ST segment is usually depressed during angina but may be elevated—sometimes strikingly so—as in the early stages of myocardial infarction and in Prinzmetal's angina.

Stress testing The most widely used test in the diagnosis of ischemic heart disease involves recording the 12-lead ECG before, during, and after exercise on a treadmill or using a bicycle ergometer. The test consists of a standardized incremental increase in external workload while the patient's ECG, symptoms, and arm blood pressure are continuously monitored. Performance is usually symptom-limited and the test is discontinued upon evidence of chest discomfort, severe shortness of breath, dizziness, fatigue, ST-segment depression of greater than 2 mm, a fall in systolic blood pressure exceeding 15 mmHg, or the development of ventricular tachyarrhythmias. This test seeks to establish the relationship between chest discomfort and the typical electrocardiographic signs of myocardial ischemia. The ischemic ST-segment response is generally defined as flat depression of the ST segment of more than 0.1 mV below the baseline (i.e., the PR segment) and lasting longer than 0.08 s. This type of depression is designated "square wave" or "plateau" and is flat or downsloping. Upsloping or junctional ST-segment changes are not considered characteristic of ischemia and do not constitute a positive test. Although T-wave abnormalities, conduction disturbances, and ventricular arrhythmias that develop during exercise should be noted, they are also not diagnostic. Negative exercise tests in which the target heart rate (85 percent of maximal heart rate for age and sex) is not achieved are considered to be nondiagnostic.

Based on the above criteria, the rate of false-positive diagnoses, using the coronary arteriogram as the gold standard, is approximately 15 percent, and a similar percentage of patients with severe, multivessel coronary artery disease will not have a positive test (false-negative). According to Bayes' theorem, the probability that ischemic heart disease exists in the patient or population under study (pretest probability) must be considered in light of the diagnostic features of the test in order to interpret a positive or negative test result (Fig. 2-3, p. 7). For example, a positive result on exercise indicates that the likelihood of coronary artery disease is 98 percent in patients with typical angina pectoris, 88 percent in those with atypical chest pain, 44 percent in those with nonanginal chest pain, and 33 percent in asymptomatic persons. The incidence of false-positive tests is increased in patients taking cardioactive drugs such as digitalis and quinidine, or in those with conduction disturbances, resting abnormalities of the ST segment and the T wave, myocardial hypertrophy, or abnormal serum potassium levels. It should be noted that the posterior surface of the heart is less accessible to the ECG and therefore more silent clinically.

The physician should be present throughout the exercise test, and it is important to measure total duration of exercise, the time to the onset of ischemic ST-segment change and chest discomfort, the external work performed, and the internal cardiac work performed; the last is represented by the heart rate–blood pressure product. The depth of the ST-segment depression and the time needed for recovery of these electrocardiographic changes are also important. Because the risks of exercise testing are small but real—estimated at one fatality and two nonfatal complications per 10,000 tests—equipment for resuscitation should be available. Modified (heart rate–limited rather than symptom-limited) exercise tests can be performed safely in patients as early as 10 days after myocardial infarction.

The normal response to exercise includes a progressive increase in heart rate and blood pressure. Failure of the blood pressure to increase or an actual decrease in blood pressure with signs of ischemia during the test is an important adverse prognostic sign, since it may reflect ischemia-induced global left ventricular dysfunction. The presence of pain or severe ST-segment depression at a low workload and ST-segment depression that persists for more than 5 min after the termination of exercise will increase the specificity of the test and indicate severe ischemic heart disease.

The exercise test can be enhanced by the intravenous administration of a radioisotope such as thallium 201 to assess regional myocardial perfusion by means of a gamma camera (p. 865). Images are recorded immediately after exercise (to identify acute ischemia) and 2 to 4 h later to discriminate between reversible ischemia and infarction (Fig. 177-7). Another radioisotope, most often technetium 99m, can be used to label the blood pool for gated radioisotope angiography. This technique (Fig. 177-6) can provide a measure of ventricular volume, ejection fraction, and regional ventricular wall motion at rest and during exercise, and can identify transient global and regional left ventricular dysfunction due to myocardial ischemia. A reduction in ejection fraction during exercise with the appearance of regional wall motion abnormalities is an important sign and suggests the presence of severe ischemia and/or multivessel coronary disease.

Although these tests were developed to detect myocardial ischemia and by inference coronary artery disease, the relationship between the presence and severity of these two conditions is complex. More recently, the severity of signs of ischemia in all the tests described above has been shown to correlate with risk for future adverse coronary events (myocardial infarction and death).

Two-dimensional echocardiography records cross-sectional images of the left ventricle and can identify regional wall motion abnormalities due to myocardial infarction (Chap. 177). In this way, this test can also be used as an aid in the diagnosis of ischemic heart disease.

Coronary arteriography (Chap. 179) This invasive diagnostic method outlines the coronary anatomy and can be used to detect important evidence of coronary atherosclerosis or to exclude this condition. By this means, one can assess the severity of obstructive lesions and both global and regional function of the left ventricle. Coronary arteriography is indicated in (1) patients with chronic stable or unstable angina pectoris who are refractory to medical therapy and who are being considered for revascularization, i.e., percutaneous transluminal coronary angioplasty or coronary artery bypass graft surgery; (2) patients with troublesome symptoms that present diagnostic difficulties in whom there is need to confirm or rule out the diagnosis of coronary artery disease; and (3) patients suspected of having left main stem or three-vessel coronary artery disease based on signs of severe ischemia on noninvasive testing, regardless of the presence or severity of symptoms.

Examples of other possible clinical situations include:

1 Patients with chest discomfort suggestive of angina pectoris but a negative exercise test who require a definitive diagnosis for guiding medical management, alleviating psychological stress, career or family planning, or insurance purposes.
2 Patients who have been admitted to the hospital several times for suspected acute myocardial infarction but in whom this diagnosis has not been established and in whom the presence or absence of coronary artery disease should be determined.
3 Patients with careers that involve the safety of others (e.g., airline pilots) who have questionable symptoms, suspicious or positive noninvasive tests, and in whom there are reasonable doubts about the state of the coronary arteries.
4 Patients with aortic stenosis or hypertrophic cardiomyopathy and angina in whom the pain could be due to coronary artery disease.
5 Male patients aged 45 and females aged 55 years of age or older who will undergo valve replacement and who may or may not have clinical evidence of myocardial ischemia.
6 Patients who are at high risk after myocardial infarction because of the recurrence of angina, heart failure, frequent ventricular premature contractions, or signs of ischemia in the stress test.
7 Patients with angina pectoris, regardless of severity, in whom noninvasive testing reveals signs of severe ischemia, i.e., early and/or marked (>2 mm) ST-segment depression, large or multiple perfusion defects and/or increased lung uptake on thallium-201 scintigrams following exercise, global left ventricular dysfunction precipitated by exercise, and/or exercise-induced hypotension.

PROGNOSIS

The principal prognostic indicators in patients with ischemic heart disease are the functional state of the left ventricle, the location and severity of coronary artery narrowing, and the severity or activity of myocardial ischemia. Angina pectoris of recent onset, unstable angina, angina unresponsive to medical therapy, or symptoms of congestive heart failure all indicate an increased risk for adverse coronary events. The same is true for physical signs of heart failure, episodes of pulmonary edema, or roentgenographic evidence of cardiac enlargement. An abnormal resting ECG or positive evidence of myocardial ischemia during a stress test also indicate increased risk. Most importantly, the following signs during noninvasive testing indicate a high risk for coronary events: a strongly positive exercise test showing onset of myocardial ischemia at low workloads, large or multiple perfusion defects or increased lung uptake during stress thallium scanning, a decrease in left ventricular ejection fraction during exercise on radionuclide ventriculography, hypotension with ischemia during stress testing, and episodes of asymptomatic ischemia recorded during continuous monitoring of the ECG in patients with unstable or stable angina pectoris and coronary artery disease.

On cardiac catheterization, elevations in left ventricular end-diastolic pressure and ventricular volume and a reduced ejection fraction are the most important signs of left ventricular dysfunction and are associated with a poor prognosis. Patients with chest discomfort but normal left ventricular function and normal coronary arteries have an excellent prognosis. In patients with normal left ventricular function and mild angina but with critical stenoses (≥70 percent luminal diameter) or one, two, or three epicardial coronary arteries, the 5-year mortality rates are approximately 2, 8, and 11 percent, respectively. Obstructive lesions of the proximal left anterior descending coronary artery are associated with a greater risk than are lesions of the right or left circumflex coronary artery, since the former vessel usually perfuses a greater quantity of myocardium. Critical stenosis of the left main coronary artery is associated with a mortality of about 15 percent per year.

With any degree of obstructive coronary artery disease, mortality is greatly increased when left ventricular function is impaired; conversely, at any level of left ventricular function, the prognosis is influenced importantly by the extent of myocardium perfused by the critically obstructed vessels. It is useful to consider that coronary atherosclerosis demonstrates its harmful potential by causing transient myocardial ischemia and characteristically destroys myocardium, thereby reducing cardiac reserve at an unpredictable rate. The larger the amount of myocardial necrosis, the less the heart is able to withstand additional damage and the poorer the prognosis. In this light, the various indices of ischemic damage, such as the ECG showing evidence of an old infarction and symptoms or signs of heart failure or cardiac enlargement, should be taken as indications of myocardial damage.

The segmental atherosclerotic plaques in epicardial arteries go through phases of cellular activity, degeneration, endothelial instability, abnormal vasomotion, platelet aggregation, and fissuring or hemorrhage. These factors can also temporarily worsen the stenosis and cause abnormal reactivity of the vessel wall thus exacerbating the manifestations of ischemia. The development of unstable angina and/or severe ischemia during stress testing reflects rapid progression.

MANAGEMENT

Each patient must be evaluated individually with respect to life patterns, risk factors, control of symptoms, and prevention of damage to left ventricular myocardium. The degree of the patient's disability and the specific physical and emotional stresses that precipitate pain must all be carefully recorded in order to set the proper goals for treatment. The management plan should consist of (1) explanation and reassurance, (2) reduction of risk factors in an attempt to slow the progression of coronary atherosclerosis, (3) treatment of coexisting conditions capable of aggravating angina, (4) sensible adaptations of activities to minimize anginal attacks, (5) a program of drug therapy, and (6) definition of end points that will indicate the need to consider mechanical revascularization.

EXPLANATION AND REASSURANCE Patients with ischemic heart disease need to understand their condition as best they can and to realize that a long and useful life is possible even though they suffer from angina pectoris or have experienced and recovered from an acute myocardial infarction. Offering case histories of persons in public life who have lived with coronary disease can be of great value when encouraging patients to resume or maintain activity and return to their occupation.

REDUCTION OF RISK FACTORS (SECONDARY PREVENTION) (See also Chap. 195) Clinical trials in selected patients seem to indicate that effective modification of risk factors (e.g., plasma lipid levels) can slow the growth of coronary atherosclerosis. Ideal weight should be attained and maintained, hypertension treated if present, and cigarette smoking forbidden. Diabetes mellitus and hyperlipidemia, when present, should be treated. Unless angina is provoked by strenuous activity, the patient should be encouraged to engage in steady, dynamic exercise such as walking; isometric exercise may be hazardous. By maintaining good physical condition, the patient will be able to perform physical work more efficiently and at a lower pulse rate, thus reducing the frequency of angina pectoris. Patients in good physical condition may also have a better chance of surviving a myocardial infarction.

ELIMINATION OF COEXISTING ILLNESS A number of illnesses that are not primarily cardiac in nature may either increase oxygen demand or decrease oxygen supply to the myocardium and may precipitate or exacerbate angina. In the former category, hypertension and hyperthyroidism may be treated successfully in order to reduce the frequency of anginal attacks. Decreased myocardial oxygen supply may be due to reduced oxygenation of the blood (e.g., in intrinsic pulmonary disease or, when carboxyhemoglobin is present, due to cigarette or cigar smoking) or decreased oxygen-carrying capacity (e.g., in anemia). Correction of these abnormalities, if present, may reduce or even eliminate anginal symptoms.

ADAPTATION OF ACTIVITIES Therapy of ischemic heart disease consists of eliminating the discrepancy between the demand of the heart muscle for oxygen and the ability of the coronary circulation to meet this demand. Most patients will understand this fundamental concept and utilize it in the rational programming of activity. Many tasks that ordinarily evoke angina may be accomplished without symptoms simply by reducing the speed at which they are performed. Patients must appreciate the diurnal variation in their tolerance of certain activities and should reduce their energy requirements in the morning and immediately after meals. Sometimes it is helpful to alter the eating pattern, taking small and more frequent meals.

It may be necessary to recommend a change in employment or residence to avoid physical stress; however, with the exception of manual laborers, most patients with ischemic heart disease can usually continue to function merely by allowing more time to complete each task. In some patients, anger and frustration may be the most important factors precipitating myocardial ischemia. If these cannot be avoided, training in stress management can be useful. A treadmill exercise test to determine the approximate heart rate at which ischemic electrocardiographic changes or symptoms develop may be helpful in the development of a specific exercise program. Ambulatory electrocardiography during daily activities may also be helpful in this regard.

DRUG THERAPY **Nitrates** This is the most valuable class of drugs in the management of angina pectoris. Nitrates act by causing systemic venodilation, thereby reducing myocardial wall tension and oxygen requirements, as well as by dilating the epicardial coronary vessels and increasing blood flow in collateral vessels. The activity of these agents depends on their absorption, which is most rapid and complete through the mucous membranes. For this reason, nitroglycerin is administered sublingually in tablets of 0.4 or 0.6 mg. Patients with angina should be instructed to take the medication both to relieve an attack and also in anticipation of stress that is likely to induce an attack. When the patient experiences discomfort on exertion, he or she should cease activity and place a tablet under the tongue. The discomfort generally disappears more rapidly with nitroglycerin than would be expected if the drug were not administered. Walking up a hill or flight of stairs or sexual intercourse may produce angina consistently, so that discomfort can often be prevented by the anticipatory use of nitroglycerin. The value of this prophylactic use of the drug cannot be overemphasized.

The dose of nitroglycerin should be sufficient to relieve discomfort but not so large as to produce hypotension, headache, or a feeling of pulsating fullness in the head. The last is the most common side effect of nitroglycerin and fortunately only rarely becomes disturbing at the doses usually required to relieve or prevent angina. Nitroglycerin deteriorates with exposure to air, moisture, and sunlight, so that if the drug neither relieves discomfort or headache nor produces a slight sensation of burning at the sublingual site of absorption, the preparation may be inactive and a fresh supply should be obtained. If relief is not achieved after the first dose of nitroglycerin, a second or third dose may be given, but the patient should be instructed not to continue to take the medication if the first few doses are ineffective. If discomfort continues for more than 7 to 10 min despite treatment, the patient should consult his or her physician or report promptly to a hospital emergency room for evaluation of possible unstable angina or acute myocardial infarction (Chap. 189).

Asking the patient with recently diagnosed angina pectoris to record the occurrence of pain relative to activity and other precipitating factors as well as nitroglycerin consumption is often helpful to the physician attempting to tailor a management program. Such a diary may also be valuable for detecting changes in the frequency or severity of discomfort that may signify the development of unstable angina pectoris and/or herald an impending myocardial infarction.

Unfortunately, none of the long-acting nitrates is as effective as sublingual nitroglycerin for the relief of angina. These preparations can be swallowed, chewed, or administered as a patch or paste by the transdermal route. They can provide effective plasma levels for up to 24 h, but the therapeutic response is highly variable, and tolerance often develops. Different preparations and/or administration during the daytime only should be tried in an attempt to relieve discomfort in the individual patient while avoiding side effects such as headache and dizziness. Individual dose titration is important in order to prevent side effects. Useful preparations include isosorbide dinitrate (5 to 20 mg sublingually every 3 h or 4 to 40 mg PO tid), nitroglycerin ointment (0.5 to 2.0 inches qid), or sustained-release transdermal patches (5 to 25 mg per day). Long-acting nitrates are relatively safe and can be used together with intermittent sublingual nitroglycerin to relieve discomfort and prevent attacks of angina.

Beta-adrenoceptor blockade (See also Chap. 67) Beta-adrenoceptor blockade represents an important component of the pharmacologic treatment of angina pectoris. These drugs reduce myocardial oxygen demand by inhibiting the increase in heart rate and myocardial contractility caused by adrenergic activity. Beta blockade reduces these variables most strikingly during exercise while causing only small reductions in heart rate, cardiac output, and arterial pressure at rest. Propranolol is usually administered in an initial dose of 20 to 40 mg four times a day and is increased as tolerated to 320 mg per day in divided doses; sometimes higher doses are required. Long-acting beta-blocking drugs (atenolol, 50 to 100 mg per day, and nadolol, 40 to 80 mg per day) offer the advantage of once-a-day dosage (see Table 67-1). The therapeutic aims include relief of angina and effective inhibition of exercise-induced increases in heart rate. These drugs can produce fatigue, impotence, cold extremities, intermittent claudication, and bradycardia and can worsen disturbed cardiac conduction, left ventricular failure, and bronchial asthma or intensify the hypoglycemia produced by oral hypoglycemic agents and insulin. Reducing the dose or even discontinuation of the drug may be necessary if these side effects develop and persist.

Calcium channel antagonists Nifedipine (10 to 40 mg qid), verapamil (80 to 120 mg tid), and diltiazem (30 to 90 mg qid) are all coronary vasodilators that produce variable and dose-dependent reductions in myocardial oxygen demand, contractility, and arterial pressure. These combined pharmacologic effects are of advantage and make these agents quite effective in the treatment of angina pectoris. Verapamil and diltiazem may produce symptomatic disturbances in cardiac conduction and bradyarrhythmias, exert negative inotropic actions, and are more likely to worsen left ventricular failure, particularly when used in combination with beta-adrenergic blockers in patients with underlying left ventricular dysfunction. Although useful effects are usually achieved when calcium channel antagonists are combined with beta-adrenoceptor blockers and nitrates, careful individual titration of dose is essential with these potent combinations. Variant (Prinzmetal's) angina responds particularly well to calcium channel antagonists, supplemented when necessary by nitrates. Population studies in asymptomatic adults have shown that aspirin (325 mg orally on alternate days) can decrease the incidence of myocardial infarction. Although this has not been established in all patients with known coronary disease, this prescription seems reasonable in the absence of side effects or contraindications.

Treatment of angina and heart failure Patients with angina pectoris and coronary artery disease may also have evidence of elevated ventricular diastolic pressures and volumes due to transient ischemia. This transient left ventricular failure with angina can be controlled by the judicious use of nitrates, calcium channel antagonists, and even beta blockers. For patients with established congestive heart failure the increased left ventricular wall tension raises myocardial oxygen demand. Treatment of congestive heart failure with digitalis and diuretics (Chap. 182) can help to decrease heart size, wall tension, and myocardial oxygen demands, which will help to control angina and ischemia. Nocturnal angina can often be relieved by these agents; however, there is no benefit—and possibly aggravation of angina—when these drugs are used in patients with a normal heart size and no evidence of heart failure. Nitrates are particularly useful and can improve the disturbed hemodynamics of congestive heart failure and relieve angina by preventing or reversing myocardial ischemia. The combination of congestive heart failure and angina in patients with coronary artery disease usually indicates a poor prognosis and warrants serious consideration of cardiac catheterization and mechanical revascularization, if possible.

Aspirin This should be given in a dose of 160 to 325 mg/d.

MECHANICAL REVASCULARIZATION

It is important to appreciate that the basic management of patients with a lifelong condition such as ischemic heart disease is medical. The years of medical management may be punctuated by mechanical revascularization procedures, as described below, but these interventions should not replace the continuing need to ease symptoms and modify risk factors.

PERCUTANEOUS TRANSLUMINAL CORONARY ANGIOPLASTY (PTCA) PTCA is a widely used method to achieve revascularization of the myocardium in patients with symptomatic ischemic heart disease and suitable proximal stenoses of epicardial coronary arteries. Whereas patients with stenosis of the left main coronary artery and those with distal three-vessel coronary artery disease who require revascularization are best treated with coronary artery bypass surgery, PTCA is widely employed in patients with symptoms due to proximal stenoses of one or two vessels, and even selected patients with three-vessel disease, and may offer many advantages over surgery.

The method is described in Chap. 179. After a flexible guidewire is advanced into a coronary artery and across the stenosis to be dilated, a miniature balloon catheter is advanced over the guidewire and into the stenosis followed by repeated inflations until the stenosis is decreased or relieved. The development of a range of steerable guidewires, low-profile balloon catheters, and the use of high inflation pressures have all helped to decrease complications, reach more distal lesions, and dilate more complex stenoses.

Indications and patient selection The most common clinical indication for PTCA is angina pectoris, stable or unstable, which should be accompanied by evidence of ischemia in an exercise test. This symptom should be sufficiently severe to warrant the consideration of bypass graft surgery. Some physicians will perform angioplasty on asymptomatic or mildly symptomatic patients with suitable stenosis of the left anterior descending coronary artery and severe ischemia on an exercise test, but the value of this procedure in improving outcome has not been established. PTCA can also be used to dilate stenoses in native coronary arteries and in bypass grafts in patients who have recurrent angina following coronary artery surgery. This is an important indication when considering the technical difficulties and the increased mortality that accompanies reoperation. Angioplasty has also been carried out in patients with recent total occlusion (within 3 months) of a coronary artery and severe angina; in this group the primary success rate is decreased to approximately 50 percent.

Risks Two and three vessels can be dilated in sequence with only a modest increase in risk. Female gender, left ventricular damage, stenosis of an artery perfusing a large segment of myocardium without collaterals, long eccentric or irregular stenoses, and calcified plaques all increase the likelihood of complications. The major complications are usually due to dissection or thrombosis with vessel occlusion, uncontrolled ischemia, and ventricular failure. In experienced hands, the overall mortality rate should be less than 1 percent, the need for emergency coronary surgery 3 to 5 percent, and myocardial infarction in approximately 3 percent of cases. Minor complications occur in 5 to 10 percent of patients and include occlusion of a branch of a coronary artery and complications of arterial catheterization.

Efficacy Primary success, i.e., adequate dilation with relief of angina, is achieved in 85 to 90 percent of cases. Recurrent stenosis of the dilated vessels occurs in 20 to 40 percent of cases within 6 months of the procedure, and angina will recur within 6 to 12 months in 25 percent of cases. This recurrence of symptoms and restenosis is more common in patients with unstable angina or with incomplete dilation of the stenosis. It is usual clinical practice to administer aspirin, and a calcium channel antagonist for months after the procedure. Although aspirin may help prevent acute coronary thrombosis during and immediately following PTCA, there are no controlled clinical trials that have demonstrated that these medications reduce the incidence of restenosis.

If patients do not develop restenosis or angina within the first year after angioplasty, the prognosis for maintaining improvement over the subsequent 4 years is excellent. If restenosis occurs, PTCA can be repeated with the same success and risks but the likelihood of restenosis increases with the third or more attempt.

Between 30 and 50 percent of patients with symptomatic coronary artery disease who require revascularization can be treated by PTCA and need not undergo coronary artery bypass grafting. Successful angioplasty is less invasive and expensive than coronary artery surgery, requires only 2 to 3 days in the hospital, and permits considerable savings in the cost of care. Successful PTCA also allows earlier return to work and the resumption of an active life.

CORONARY ARTERY BYPASS GRAFTING In this procedure, a section of a vein (usually the saphenous) is used to form a connection between the aorta and the coronary artery distal to the obstructive lesion. Alternatively, anastomosis of one or both of the internal mammary arteries to the coronary artery distal to the obstructive lesion may be employed.

Although some indications for coronary artery bypass surgery are controversial, certain areas of agreement exist:

1 The operation is relatively safe, with mortality rates less than 1 percent when the procedure is performed by an experienced surgical team in selected patients with normal left ventricular function.
2 Intraoperative and postoperative mortality increases with the degree of ventricular dysfunction and surgical inexperience. The effectiveness and risk of coronary artery bypass grafting vary widely depending on case selection and the skill and experience of the surgical team, so that the latter must be taken into account when a patient is being considered as a candidate for this procedure.
3 Occlusion is observed in 10 to 20 percent of *vein grafts* during the first year, the incidence is approximately 2 percent per year during 5- to 7-year follow-up and 5 percent per year thereafter. Long-term patency rates are considerably higher for internal mammary artery implantations; in patients with left anterior descending coronary artery obstruction, survival is better when coronary bypass involves the internal mammary artery rather than a saphenous vein.
4 Angina is abolished or unequivocally reduced in approximately 85 percent of patients following complete revascularization. Although this is usually associated with graft patency and restoration of blood flow, the pain may also have been alleviated as a result of infarction of the ischemic segment or a placebo effect.
5 Coronary artery bypass grafting does not appear to reduce the incidence of myocardial infarction in patients with chronic ischemic heart disease; perioperative myocardial infarction occurs in 5 to 10 percent of cases, but in most instances these infarcts are small.
6 Mortality is reduced by operation in patients with stenosis of the left main coronary artery. Some reduction in mortality is also achieved in patients with three-vessel coronary artery disease and impaired left ventricular function. However, there is no evidence that coronary artery surgery improves survival in patients with one- or two-vessel disease who have chronic stable angina and normal left ventricular function or in patients with one-vessel

disease and impaired left ventricular function. Evidence is conflicting concerning the effects of operation on survival in patients with impaired left ventricular function and obstructive disease of two coronary arteries, one of which is the proximal left anterior descending artery.

7 Other important considerations affecting outcome include the age and gender of the patient as well as accompanying medical problems such as diabetes mellitus, obesity, and renal disease.

Indications for coronary artery bypass grafting are usually based on the severity of symptoms, coronary anatomy, and ventricular function. The ideal candidate is male, less than 70 years of age, has no other complicating disease, has troublesome or disabling symptoms that are not adequately controlled by medical therapy, wishes to lead a more active life, and has severe stenoses of several epicardial coronary arteries with objective evidence of myocardial ischemia as a cause of the chest discomfort. Great symptomatic benefit can be anticipated in such patients. When the patient also has a disturbance of left ventricular function, coronary artery bypass grafting may, in addition, prolong life.

UNSTABLE ANGINA PECTORIS

The following three patient groups may be said to have unstable angina pectoris: (1) patients with new onset (<2 months) angina that is severe and/or frequent (≥3 episodes per day); (2) patients with accelerating angina, i.e., those with chronic stable angina who develop angina that is distinctly more frequent, severe, longer, or precipitated by less exertion than previously; (3) those with angina of any duration that occurs at rest. Unstable angina may be primary, i.e., occur in the absence of an extracardiac condition that has intensified myocardial ischemia, or it may be precipitated by a condition extrinsic to the coronary vascular bed that has intensified myocardial ischemia, such as anemia, fever, infection, tachyarrhythmias, emotional stress, or hypoxemia. Unstable angina may also develop shortly after myocardial infarction. Unstable angina, particularly when it is characterized by rest pain or occurs in the postinfarction state, carries an adverse prognosis, with significant risk of acute myocardial infarction or the development of intractable chronic stable angina.

When unstable angina is accompanied by objective electrocardiographic evidence of transient myocardial ischemia (ST-segment changes and/or T-wave inversions during episodes of chest pain), it is almost always associated with critical stenoses in one or more major epicardial coronary arteries. Less than 10 percent of patients with unstable angina have normal coronary arteries on arteriography. The atherosclerotic lesions may have a complicated morphology, with evidence of superimposed thrombosis in approximately 25 to 60 percent of cases. Segmental spasm in the vicinity of atherosclerotic plaques may also play a role in the development of unstable angina.

MANAGEMENT The patient should be admitted promptly to the hospital for observation, further diagnosis, and treatment. It is important to identify and treat concomitant conditions that can intensify ischemia, such as uncontrolled tachycardia, hypertension and diabetes mellitus, cardiomegaly, heart failure, arrhythmias, thyrotoxicosis, and any acute febrile illness. Acute myocardial infarction should be ruled out by means of serial ECGs and measurements of plasma cardiac enzyme activity.

Continuous electrocardiographic monitoring should be carried out and the patients should receive reassurance and sedation. Thrombus formation frequently complicates this condition. Therefore, intravenous heparin should be given for 3 to 5 days to maintain the partial thromboplastin time at 2 to 2.5 times control, followed by oral aspirin at a dose of 325 mg/d. Beta-adrenergic blocking drugs and calcium channel antagonists should be administered, but with caution and an awareness of all the possible side effects discussed above. Dosages must be titrated to avoid bradycardia, heart failure, and hypotension. Nitroglycerin should be given by the sublingual route. In addition, intravenous nitroglycerin is quite effective, although it requires continuous monitoring of intraarterial pressure. It is begun at a dosage of 5 μg/min and is raised in 5-μg/min increments to a level at which chest pain is abolished but systolic arterial pressure is maintained or reduced only slightly and other side effects are avoided.

The majority of patients improve with such treatment. However, the clinical outcome is highly variable. If angina and/or electrocardiographic evidence of ischemia do not diminish within 24 to 48 h of the comprehensive treatment described above in patients with no obvious contraindications for revascularization, then cardiac catheterization and coronary arteriography should be performed. If the anatomy is suitable, PTCA can be performed with surgical standby. If angioplasty cannot be done, coronary artery bypass grafting should be considered to relieve symptoms and myocardial ischemia and as a means of preventing myocardial damage. If the patient's symptoms and signs are controlled on medical therapy, a diagnostic exercise ECG should be obtained near the time of hospital discharge. If there is obvious evidence of myocardial ischemia, serious consideration should be given to catheterization and revascularization. It should be recognized that severe coronary artery disease is usually present in patients with unstable angina who respond to medical therapy, and although the unstable state may be controlled, it is often converted to severe chronic stable angina and ultimately requires mechanical revascularization.

ASYMPTOMATIC (SILENT) ISCHEMIA

Obstructive coronary artery disease, acute myocardial infarction, and transient myocardial ischemia are frequently asymptomatic. During continuous ambulatory electrocardiographic monitoring, the majority of ambulatory patients with typical chronic stable angina are found to have objective evidence of myocardial ischemia (ST-segment deviation) during episodes of chest discomfort while they are active outside the hospital, but many of these patients also appear to have more frequent episodes of asymptomatic ischemia. In addition, there is a large (but as yet unknown) number of totally asymptomatic people with severe coronary atherosclerosis who exhibit ST-segment changes during activity. Evidence of frequent episodes of ischemia (symptomatic and asymptomatic) during daily life appears to indicate an increased likelihood of adverse coronary events such as death and myocardial infarction. The widespread use of exercise electrocardiography during routine examinations has also defined some of these heretofore unrecognized patients with asymptomatic coronary artery disease. Longitudinal studies have demonstrated an increased incidence of coronary events (sudden death, myocardial infarction, and angina) in asymptomatic patients with positive exercise tests. In addition, patients who are asymptomatic after suffering a myocardial infarction are nonetheless at far greater risk for a second coronary event than is the general population. Patients who seek evaluation and who have asymptomatic ischemia should be subjected to a detailed noninvasive examination, utilizing stress electrocardiography and radionuclide scintigraphy.

MANAGEMENT The management of patients with asymptomatic ischemia must be individualized. Thus, the physician should consider the following: (1) the degree of positivity of the exercise test, particularly the stage of exercise at which electrocardiographic signs of ischemia appear, the magnitude and number of the perfusion defect(s) on thallium scintigraphy, and the change in left ventricular ejection fraction which occurs during ischemia and/or during exercise on radionuclide ventriculography; (2) the electrocardiographic leads showing a positive response, with changes in the anterior precordial leads indicating a less favorable prognosis than changes in the inferior leads; and (3) the patient's age, occupation, and general medical condition. Most would agree that an asymptomatic 45-year-old commercial airline pilot with 4-mm ST-segment depression in leads V_1 to V_4 during mild exercise should undergo coronary arteriography, whereas the asymptomatic, sedentary 75-year-old retiree with 1-mm ST-segment depression in leads II and III during maximal activity need not. However, there is no consensus about the appropriate procedure in the large majority of patients for whom the situation is less extreme. Patients with evidence of severe ischemia on noninvasive testing (as outlined earlier) should undergo coronary arteriography. Asymptomatic patients with three-vessel coronary disease and impaired left ventricular function may be considered appropriate candidates for coronary artery bypass surgery.

While the incidence of asymptomatic ischemia can be reduced by treatment with beta blockers, calcium channel antagonists, and long-acting nitrates it is not clear whether this is necessary or desirable in patients who have not suffered a myocardial infarction. However, there is evidence that beta-adrenoceptor blockade begun 7 to 35 days after acute myocardial infarction improves survival (Chap. 189). This therapy is recommended in asymptomatic patients as long as there are no contraindications such as heart failure, bradycardia, heart block, or asthma.

REFERENCES

ADAMS PC et al: Platelet/vessel wall interactions, rheologic factors and thrombogenic substrate in acute coronary syndromes: Preventive strategies. Am J Cardiol 60:9G, 1987

BELLER GA et al: Sensitivity, specificity and prognostic significance of noninvasive testing for occult or known coronary disease. Prog Cardiovasc Dis 24:241, 1987

BRAUNWALD E: Unstable angina—A classification. Circulation 80:410, 1989

BRAUNWALD E, SOBEL BE et al: Coronary blood flow and myocardial ischemia, in *Heart Disease*, 3d ed, E Braunwald (ed). Philadelphia, Saunders, 1988, p 1191

HEUSCH G: Alpha-adrenergic mechanisms in myocardial ischemia. Circulation 71(1):1, 1990

KING SB et al: Percutaneous transluminal angioplasty: The second decade. Am J Cardiol 62:2K, 1988

LADENHEIM ML et al: Incremental prognostic power of clinical history, exercise electrocardiography and coronary artery disease. Am J Cardiol 59:270, 1987

ROCCO MB et al: Prognostic importance of myocardial ischemia detected by ambulatory monitoring in patients with stable coronary artery disease. Circulation 78:877, 1988

RUTHERFORD JD et al: Chronic ischemic heart disease, in *Heart Disease*, 3d ed, E Braunwald (ed). Philadelphia, Saunders, 1988, p 1314

RYAN TJ et al: Guidelines for percutaneous transluminal coronary angioplasty. A report of the American College of Cardiology/American Heart Association Task Force on assessment of diagnostic and therapeutic cardiovascular procedures (Subcommittee on Percutaneous Transluminal Coronary Angioplasty). Circulation 78:486, 1988

SELWYN AP, GANZ P et al: Myocardial ischemia in coronary disease. N Engl J Med 318:1058, 1988

THEROUSE P et al: Aspirin, heparin or both to treat acute unstable angina. N Engl J Med 319:1105, 1988

VALLE GA: Silent ischemia: A clinical update. Chest 97(1):186, 1990

VARNAUSKAS E et al: Twelve-year follow-up of survival in the randomized European Coronary Surgery Study. N Engl J Med 319:332, 1988

191 COR PULMONALE

JOHN BUTLER

DEFINITIONS *Cor pulmonale* is the enlargement of the right ventricle due to the increase in its afterload that occurs in diseases of the thorax, lung, and pulmonary circulation; the presence of right ventricular failure is not necessary for cor pulmonale to be present. In this chapter, *right heart failure* is defined as a chronic increase in the end-diastolic transmural pressure of the right ventricle that is not expected from an increase in pulmonary blood flow. Since this definition specifies a sustained rise in transmural pressure, transient changes that normally occur with breathing and changes in posture are excluded. Right ventricular *preload* is defined as the end-diastolic transmural pressure of the ventricle; right ventricular *afterload* as the transmural pressure during systolic ejection.

NORMAL FUNCTION OF THE PULMONARY CIRCULATION

The pulmonary circulation is interposed between the right and the left ventricles for the purpose of gas exchange, the filtering out of particles, and the chemical "conditioning" of the blood (such as the conversion of angiotensin I to angiotensin II). It is an extraordinarily efficient, low-resistance system. Normally, flow through the pulmonary vascular bed depends not only on the right ventricle but also on respiratory movements and the contraction of the left ventricle. *Respiratory motion* facilitates pulmonary blood flow by aspirating blood into the thorax on inhalation; the blood is then propelled forward by the positive pressure of exhalation acting on a one way valved system. *Left ventricular systole* assists pulmonary blood flow because the left ventricular contraction augments ejection by tensing the right ventricular wall against the bulging ventricular septum; the driving pressure across the pulmonary circulation is increased because the left ventricular end-diastolic pressure and, therefore, the downstream pulmonary vascular pressure are reduced by an effective left ventricle; the systemic venous pressure, which causes venous return, is raised by the left ventricular output; and an efficient small left ventricle reduces the total volume of blood in the cardiac fossa and lowers the right atrial pressure to aid the returning systemic venous inflow.

The right ventricle ejects blood by a milking movement in contrast to the pumping action of the left ventricle. The stroke volume of the right ventricle, as of the left (Chap. 181), depends on its afterload, preload, rate, and myocardial contractility. The afterload due to the pulmonary artery pressure is low. It depends on alterations of pulmonary blood volume as much as on changes in pulmonary blood flow. The pulmonary artery pressure normally rises when blood is displaced into the chest at the start of exercise, on assuming recumbency, or with cold, anxiety, or pain. It is astonishing that a driving pressure of only about 0.5 kPa (5 cmH_2O) between the pulmonary artery [average 1.5 kPa (15 cmH_2O)] and the left atrium [average 1.0 kPa (10 cmH_2O)] drives the entire cardiac output of 6 L/min or more at rest, and up to 30 L/min during exercise, through a network of such minute capillary vessels in the pulmonary vasculature.

The vascular resistance R of the pulmonary circulation (p. 877) is calculated as the intravascular driving pressure [DP = pulmonary artery pressure minus downstream intravascular pressure] divided by flow rate $\dot{Q}$. The caliber of a distensible vessel depends on its transmural pressure. R increases when vessels collapse, narrow, or lengthen, or when the viscosity of the blood increases

$$R = \frac{Kl\mu}{r^4}$$

where K = constant
l = length
r = radius
μ = viscosity

A single value of R is obviously misleading because the relationship between driving pressure and flow is not linear through zero. There is an apparently decreasing "resistance" as flow increases because vessels are distended and recruited (Fig. 191-1).

The preload of the right ventricle is determined by the systemic venous return in relation to its contractility. Since the right ventricle constitutes a compliant reservoir for the heart, acute changes in venous return (e.g., its rise on inhalation and fall on exhalation) are accommodated with little change in pressure.

PATHOPHYSIOLOGY Sustained marked elevations in intrathoracic pressure, associated with mechanical ventilation and especially positive end-expiratory pressure (PEEP) cause intrathoracic vessels to narrow and can lead to such reductions in cardiac output as to endanger life.

Chronic dysfunction of the right ventricular myocardium is rarely a cause of right heart failure, since normally it is so thin-walled, and so much of its muscle function is provided by the left ventricle. It could be important when the muscle is hypertrophied in cor pulmonale because it can be affected by ischemic coronary artery disease. Acute right ventricular infarction, usually accompanying infarction of the inferior wall of the left ventricle (Chap. 189) but occasionally occurring

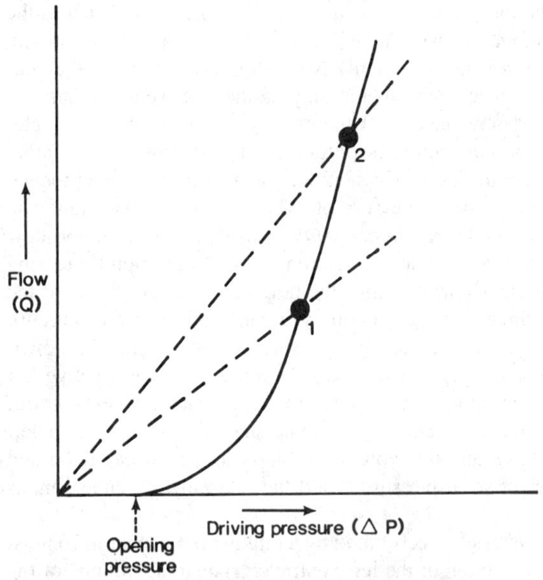

FIGURE 191-1 Relationship between flow and driving pressure (''vascular resistance'') in the pulmonary circulation. Note that it does not pass through zero at the origin since an opening pressure must be overcome before flow starts. Thus the calculated vascular resistance (reciprocal of relationship of flow to pressure, dashed lines) falls (1 → 2) as flow increases. *(Modified from Graham et al., 1983.)*

as an isolated event, is one of the causes of acute right ventricular failure.

The amount of right ventricular enlargement in cor pulmonale ranges from slight to severe depending on the increase of afterload and its duration. When there is pulmonary vascular or parenchymal lung disease and the resistance to pulmonary blood flow is increased, a periodic rise in cardiac output and afterload occurs with exercise which can elevate pulmonary artery pressure markedly. Afterload is chronically augmented when lung volume is enlarged, as in obstructive airflow disease, due to the lengthening of the pulmonary vessels and the flattening of the alveolar capillaries. Afterload can also increase when lung volume is reduced in restrictive lung diseases because pulmonary vessels are compressed and distorted. Right ventricular afterload rises with hypoxic vasoconstriction, an important cause of pulmonary hypertension. Hypoxic vasoconstriction in regions of the lung affected by disease is useful in distributing blood flow to normally ventilated regions. However, the elevation in pulmonary artery pressure becomes a significant stress when the lung disease is diffuse or when the entire lung becomes hypoxic due to hypoventilation. Hypoxic vasoconstriction results from alveolar, rather than intravascular hypoxia in the adult and is made worse by hypercarbia, probably because of the associated acidosis. When the hematocrit is markedly elevated, as in cyanotic congenital heart disease, an increase in blood viscosity can intensify the pulmonary hypertension.

CLINICAL SYNDROMES

The diseases causing cor pulmonale comprise those in which the pulmonary vasculature is primarily involved, and those in which the impediment to blood flow is secondary to diseases of the lung. The main syndromes and their physiologic responses are summarized in Table 191-1.

It has been estimated that about 50,000 people die each year from embolic pulmonary vascular disease in the United States (Chap. 213). Probably half die within the first hour from acute heart failure due to massive, or multiple, emboli. Chronic cor pulmonale due to recurrent emboli or to other vascular causes is rare. More than half of patients with severe obstructive lung diseases have cor pulmonale, so this may constitute 6 or 7 percent of all adult heart diseases in the United States. It constitutes a higher percentage of all forms of heart disease in countries such as the United Kingdom, where the incidence of obstructive lung disease is higher.

TABLE 191-1 Cor pulmonale

Mechanisms	Responses	Characteristics
PULMONARY VASCULAR DISEASES		
I Emboli, large or multiple	Fall in output due to acute obstruction	Acute cor pulmonale Right ventricular distention Shock
II Emboli, small; vasculitis; widespread lung damage (ARDS)	Pulmonary hypertension due to widespread hypoxia and microvascular obstruction High output	Subacute cor pulmonale Right ventricular distention Breathlessness and fever
III Emboli, medium and recurrent; primary pulmonary hypertension; diet or drug vasopathy	Pulmonary hypertension due to vascular obstruction Low or normal output	Chronic cor pulmonale Right heart hypertrophy Breathlessness
RESPIRATORY DISEASES		
I Obstructive		
A Chronic bronchitis and emphysema; chronic asthma	Pulmonary hypertension due to hypoxia, vascular stretching and loss Heart beat impeded externally by lung hyperinflation Normal or high output	Chronic cor pulmonale ''Blue bloater'' Underventilation
II Restrictive		
A Intrinsic: interstitial fibrosis, lung resection	Hypertension due to hypoxia, vascular distortion and loss Normal or low output	Chronic cor pulmonale Breathlessness Overventilation
B Extrinsic: obesity, myxedema, muscle weakness, kyphoscoliosis, upper airway obstruction, diminished respiratory drive, high altitude	Hypertension due to alveolar hypoxia Normal or high output	Chronic cor pulmonale Peripheral edema Underventilation

PULMONARY VASCULAR DISEASES In these conditions the right ventricular afterload is elevated as a consequence of the pulmonary vascular restriction to blood flow. The pulmonary hypertension may be severe, unlike the mild rise in pressure found in parenchymal pulmonary diseases. This form of chronic cor pulmonale usually results from repeated pulmonary emboli. Sometimes it is caused by pulmonary hypertension due to vasculitis, sometimes there is a chemically induced vasospasm, and sometimes it is due to unknown causes, when it is referred to as *primary pulmonary hypertension* (Chap. 212).

Thromboembolic pulmonary vascular hypertension is quite rare because of (1) the enormous capacity of the pulmonary vascular bed, so that when some vessels are obstructed, others are recruited; and (2) the normal rapid lysis of pulmonary emboli. The right ventricle begins to fail at systolic pressures exceeding approximately 40 to 45 mmHg. However, when emboli are recurrent, or when pulmonary vascular resistance rises gradually and right ventricular hypertrophy develops, higher pressures, sometimes above systemic arterial levels, may be generated.

Cor pulmonale due to pulmonary emboli This condition is associated with three distinct syndromes, depending on whether the emboli are very numerous and large, less numerous and medium-sized, or very small.

Acute cor pulmonale due to very numerous or large emboli causes a dramatic, low-output state, quite unlike chronic cor pulmonale. It can also occur with a moderate-sized embolism if the pulmonary circulation is critically compromised by previous pulmonary vascular disease. In acute cor pulmonale, there is frequently a marked fall in cardiac output since the right ventricle is unable to generate the pressure necessary to drive blood through the compromised pulmonary vascular bed. Acute cor pulmonale is suggested by the history of a sudden onset of severe dyspnea and collapse in a patient with, or predisposed to, venous thrombosis. The low cardiac output causes pallor, sweating, hypotension, and a rapid pulse of small amplitude. The neck veins are distended and often exhibit the prominent *v* waves of tricuspid regurgitation. The liver may also be pulsatile, distended, and tender. A systolic murmur of tricuspid regurgitation at the left sternal border may be accompanied by a presystolic (S_4) gallop rhythm. Blood gases frequently show hypoxemia due to ventilation/perfusion mismatching and a low Pa_{CO_2} due to hyperventilation. If sufficient blood flow is sustained over the critical first two or three hours, the natural thrombolytic response usually results in fragmentation of the clot to a sufficient extent that the patient can survive. Although it has been shown that treatment with thrombolytic agents lyses clots more rapidly than heparin (Chap. 213), this therapy is probably indicated only when blood flow is critically reduced and not improving.

Subacute cor pulmonale This condition is characterized by right ventricular distention and is associated with moderate pulmonary hypertension, most often due to multiple small emboli, pulmonary vascular obstruction caused by vasculitis, and/or hypoxia. Patients may present with malaise, dyspnea, and cyanosis. When septic microvascular embolization, or endotoxemia, occurs, an inflammatory edema develops, and hypoxic vasoconstriction is added to the embolic and thrombotic obstructions. In the adult respiratory distress syndrome (ARDS), the elevation in pulmonary artery pressure is usually not marked and cor pulmonale is not present. Because of the positive intrathoracic pressures of mechanical ventilation, the right ventricle is frequently small. However, sometimes the ventricle may be distended due to myocardial depression or because cardiac output is increased by hypoxia or the fever of sepsis.

Chronic cor pulmonale This condition can be caused by recurrent, medium-sized emboli that fail to lyse, particles from intravenous drug abuse, parasites, tumor tissue, or, rarely, pulmonary vascular compression caused by neoplastic diseases. *Primary pulmonary hypertension* (Chap. 212) causes chronic cor pulmonale, typically in young adult females. Chronic cor pulmonale can also be caused by any chronic widespread vasculitis such as occurs in association with the collagen vascular disorders, particularly the CREST syndrome (Chap. 271), or, occasionally, widespread radiation pneumonitis. Very rarely it is due to a vasoconstrictor arteriopathy associated with chemicals such as crotalaria, ingested as food, or drugs such as aminorex.

Symptoms and signs Breathlessness is a characteristic feature of pulmonary hypertension due to pulmonary vascular disease. In contrast to the orthopnea of left ventricular failure, it is particularly distressing during even mild exertion, and it is *not* relieved by sitting up. An unproductive cough is another frequent complaint. Occasionally there can be episodes with the production of pink, frothy sputum and radiologic changes suggestive of a patchy pulmonary edema. Anterior chest pain, due to acute dilation of the root of the pulmonary artery, can occur. The elevation in systemic venous pressure can cause hepatomegaly and ankle edema.

The patient has tachypnea that is evident on mild exertion and at rest; it may even persist during sleep. Occasionally there is cyanosis due to arterial hypoxemia and a low cardiac output. A right ventricular heave is felt in the epigastrium and a high-pitched pulmonary ejection click to the left of the upper sternum. There can be a soft midsystolic ejection murmur preceding a loud pulmonary second sound that is often palpable. The second (pulmonary) component of the second heart sound is intensified. Rarely, a diastolic murmur of pulmonary valve regurgitation is heard. There is a prominent *a* and a recognizable *v* wave in the jugular venous pulse and a systolic murmur of tricuspid regurgitation is common. The onset of right ventricular failure is reflected by an increase of venous pressure, the development of larger *v* waves associated with worse tricuspid regurgitation, a hepatojugular reflux, and a gallop rhythm with third and fourth heart sounds.

Special studies Noninvasive methods of cardiac diagnosis developed for the left heart are less useful when applied to the right side of the heart. The right ventricle is often hidden on the posteroanterior x-ray. Normally its cavity is so irregular that its volume cannot be quantitated angiographically or echocardiographically, and its muscle may be so thin that it has little influence on the ECG.

In pulmonary hypertension due to pulmonary vascular obstructions, *arterial blood gases* show hypoxia due to ventilation/perfusion mismatching and an increase in anatomic shunt. However, frequently the outstanding feature is the hypocarbia (due to the alveolar hyperventilation) that accompanies pulmonary artery hypertension. Usually there are no abnormalities on spirometry, but the ratio of dead space to tidal volume may be high, particularly when there are large vessel obstructions. The diffusing capacity of the lung is characteristically reduced when the vascular disease is severe enough to cause a capillary vasculitis and loss of capillary blood volume. Typically, exercise causes severe dyspnea with a marked fall in Pa_{O_2}. In practice, exercise testing may be a useful way to follow changes in the pulmonary hypertension of these patients because exercise ability is limited by cardiac output and the latter, in turn, by the severity of the pulmonary vascular obstruction.

The pulmonary trunk and hilar vessels are enlarged on *radiologic examination*. Widening of the hilum is judged from the ratio of the distance between the start of the first divisions of the right and left main pulmonary arteries divided by the transverse diameter of the thorax. A ratio >0.36 suggests pulmonary hypertension. Another indicator is simple widening of the descending right pulmonary artery shadow, usually under 16 mm, to over 20 mm. Ventilation and perfusion lung scans, and systemic venography showing deep vein thrombosis are helpful in confirming the diagnosis of embolic pulmonary vascular disease. The ECG is relatively insensitive, but is much more reliable in cor pulmonale due to pulmonary vascular diseases (in which the lung size and the position of the heart are normal) than in obstructive airflow disease. The usual findings are P pulmonale and right axis deviation.

Echocardiography allows the measurement of thickness of the right ventricular wall and, although volume changes cannot be measured, this technique can show enlargement of the right ventricular cavity in relation to that of the left ventricle. If the pulmonary valve can be imaged, its late opening, early closure, and tenseness during diastole may be used in estimating pulmonary artery pressure. Greater precision comes from the measurement of peak regurgitant tricuspid flow and pulmonic regurgitant flow with Doppler echocardiography, from which right ventricular systolic pressure can be calculated (Chap. 177).

Failure of the right ventricular ejection fraction (measured by radionuclide angiography) to increase normally on exercise appears to be a good indicator of pulmonary hypertension and/or intrinsic right ventricular dysfunction. Thallium 201 scintigraphy is also useful for diagnosing cor pulmonale, since the hypertrophied right ventricle is imaged (normally there is no visible right ventricular myocardium in relation to the marked uptake by the left ventricle).

Cardiac catheterization is necessary for the precise measurement of the pulmonary artery pressure, the calculation of pulmonary vascular resistance, and the response to oxygen and vasodilators. It is sometimes indicated to exclude congenital and left heart diseases and, in some instances, because angiography must be carried out to confirm the nature of the pulmonary vascular obstruction. Measurements of pressure and flow should be made during exercise to look for abnormal pressure increments or poor responses of cardiac output.

Lung biopsy can be useful in showing vasculitis in some types of specific pulmonary vascular disease such as the collagen vascular diseases, rheumatoid arthritis, and Wegener's granulomatosis.

RESPIRATORY DISEASES Cor pulmonale may be caused by both obstructive and restrictive lung diseases. In these syndromes the cor pulmonale is usually associated with only modest increments of pulmonary artery pressure. Cor pulmonale is much more commonly due to obstructive than to restrictive disease, partly because restrictive lung disorders have a much lower life expectancy once they reach the stage of cor pulmonale. Respiratory diseases are usually associated with local or generalized distortions of lung volume which affect the position and, perhaps, function of the heart, so that physical signs and special studies in this type of cor pulmonale tend to be blurred by noncardiac factors.

CHRONIC OBSTRUCTIVE LUNG DISEASE (COLD) (See Chap. 210) This is the most common cause of chronic cor pulmonale. The enlargement of the right ventricle is attributed to the mild-to-moderate pulmonary hypertension which is common in severe obstructive bronchitis and emphysema and rare (though not unknown) in asthma. Pulmonary artery systolic pressure is typically in the range of 30 to 50 mmHg, far below the systemic levels which appear to be tolerated in congenital heart disease and in normal people native to high altitudes.

The pulmonary hypertension is due to the generalized pulmonary vasoconstriction caused by the alveolar hypoxia and hypercarbia, the mechanical effects of the high lung volume on the pulmonary vessels, the loss of small vessels in the vascular bed in regions of emphysema, and the increased blood viscosity caused by the frequently associated polycythemia. Of these, the first is undoubtedly the most important. Pulmonary artery pressure rises further on exercise. The pulmonary artery pressure is decreased acutely by oxygen breathing, but not to normal, so chronic (home) oxygen therapy is often helpful. Cardiac output tends to be high in the absence of heart failure if hypoxia and hypercarbia are present. Because of the importance of hypoxic pulmonary vasoconstriction in causing pulmonary hypertension, the hypoventilating "blue bloater" patient with alveolar hypoxia and hypercarbia is characterized by cor pulmonale, while the emphysematous "pink puffer," without alveolar hypoxia, is less affected. Ischemic left heart disease is a frequent complication in these cigarette-smoking patients and there could be a rise in pulmonary artery pressure secondary, in part, to the increase in left atrial pressure resulting from left heart dysfunction. Almost half of all patients who die with cor pulmonale due to obstructive airflow disease also have left ventricular hypertrophy.

Right ventricular failure may be difficult to diagnose in obstructive lung disease. It appears to complicate cor pulmonale in the stage of ventilatory failure with hypoxia and hypercarbia. When there is a worsening of the airflow due to an increasing obstruction or asthmatic deterioration, the hypoxia and hypercarbia increase cardiac output by their direct vasodilator effects on systemic arterioles. Hypoxic pulmonary vasospasm is intensified, arrhythmias are common complications, and right heart failure ensues. The liver becomes palpable and tender because it is both swollen and displaced by the low diaphragm. A hepatojugular reflux is present. There is also a "square-wave" response to the Valsalva maneuver, a prolonged expiratory pressure against a closed glottis. This square wave response is a sustained rise in systemic blood pressure, with no bradycardia on releasing the positive pressure, rather than the normal rise and then fall in pressure with a characteristic bradycardia on release.

Any exacerbation of obstructive lung disease leads to a mechanical impediment to venous return which causes a difficult diagnostic problem in deciding whether or not right heart failure is present. The increase in obstruction to airflow is associated with prolonged exhalation, during which all of the intrathoracic pressures are more positive, and a high functional residual capacity that raises pressure around the heart relative to the normal subcostal pressures. The raised pressure around the heart impedes venous return and leads to a raised jugular venous pressure and peripheral edema. Yet this is not right ventricular failure since the transmural filling pressure and pulmonary blood flow response to a sustained stress are normal.

Pathology In obstructive airflow disease the right ventricular hypertrophy increases with time. The main pulmonary arteries are enlarged and the muscular pulmonary arteries show the development of prominent longitudinal muscle, together with prominent fibrosis and elastic changes, that continues into the arterioles, where the media also becomes muscularized. The small vessels and capillaries are distorted or disappear in regions of hyperinflation which sometimes greatly reduces the vascular bed.

Symptoms and signs The history of a productive cough and dyspnea, perhaps with wheezing, frequently reflects the severity of the addiction to cigarette smoking. Breathlessness limits the patient's ability in the minor stresses of daily living. Frequently there is a history of emergency hospital admissions because of respiratory infection, sometimes necessitating mechanical ventilation. There may have been increasing somnolence on breathing oxygen, or other symptoms of hypercarbia such as recurring headaches, confusion, and even vomiting which, combined with blurred optic discs (also due to cerebral vasodilation), constitutes the "pseudo tumor cerebri" syndrome. Hypoxia due to hypoventilation is usually worse at night, particularly when severe snoring leads to episodes of obstructive apnea (Chap. 217).

Physical findings These are of the obstructive airflow disease, together with a raised jugular venous pressure, a palpable liver, and ankle edema. Often there is nicotine staining of the fingers. The skin may be warm and the arterial pulse bounding in the high cardiac output state induced by hypoxia and hypercarbia. The chest distention due to the obstructive airflow and the rhonchi and wheezes due to the chronic bronchitis usually makes cardiac auscultation difficult. However, a protodiastolic (third) heart sound and a systolic murmur of tricuspid regurgitant may be audible. Signs of right heart failure are, as discussed above, difficult to separate from those due to severe airflow obstruction. However, a sudden worsening of peripheral edema and rise of systemic venous pressure when atrial fibrillation occurs or when pulmonary infection supervenes is usually considered as showing heart failure. This may be confirmed by the positive hepatojugular reflux and Valsalva responses described above. The distinction is important since patients can survive for years with the high systemic venous pressure and edema that are part of the airflow obstruction syndrome, yet usually have a poor prognosis after right heart failure develops.

Special studies *Pulmonary function studies* show marked airflow obstruction with severe hypoxemia and hypercarbia. Exercise is limited by ventilatory rather than cardiac dysfunction until right ventricular failure develops.

The *chest roentgenogram* reveals an increased total lung capacity (hyperinflation) which makes the degree of right heart enlargement difficult to assess. The central pulmonary arteries are large but the vessels are narrowed and disappear at the periphery, particularly in regions of the lungs which are markedly emphysematous. The ECG is relatively insensitive because the enlarged lungs characteristic of obstructive airflow disease are poor electrical conductors and the inspiratory position of the chest is associated with a vertical and leftwardly rotated position of the heart. If it does show right axis deviation, right ventricular hypertrophy, and right atrial enlargement as P pulmonale, with inferior shift of the P vector, there can be little doubt that cor pulmonale is present. Arrhythmias, particularly atrial fibrillation and multifocal atrial tachycardia, are common.

Echocardiographic imaging is often difficult because of the air in the distended lungs and the closeness of the densely reflective sternum, but may reveal an increased cross section of the right ventricular cavity and a greater thickness of the right ventricular wall. Myocardial scintigraphy shows an abnormally high ratio of right to left ventricular ^{201}Tl uptake; at present this is probably the most accurate noninvasive way of documenting an increased right ventricular muscle mass.

Right heart catheterization is usually unnecessary. It can be done at the bedside with a balloon-tipped, flow-directed, multichannel catheter fitted with thermocouples for measuring cardiac output by thermodilution (Chap. 179). The "balloon wedge" pressure measured through the catheter shows a normal left atrial pressure at rest in patients with uncomplicated cor pulmonale. However, cardiac catheterization is useful in assessing left ventricular function, the severity of the pulmonary hypertension and its response to oxygen breathing. An exercise study is helpful, particularly in excluding left heart dysfunction when a possible left heart abnormality has been found, for instance, by echocardiography.

Treatment This is aimed at correcting the alveolar hypoxia by judiciously increasing the inspired O_2 concentration (FI_{O_2}) (ventilation is, in part, driven by hypoxia in these patients) and by improving alveolar ventilation by relieving the airflow obstruction. When the lung disease improves and hypoxic vasospasm due to the alveolar hypoxia and hypercarbia are corrected, tachypnea, and thus overdistension due to gas trapping, lessens. The signs attributed to right heart failure are relieved. Bronchodilators and antibiotics lessen the airflow obstruction and diuretics relieve the edema.

In view of the possibility that part of the afterload of the ventricles is due to the external load from the necessary systolic distortion of the surrounding distended lungs, it is particularly interesting that recent studies have shown that the severity of the cor pulmonale in these patients is related more to the mechanical abnormalities of the lung function than the height of the pulmonary artery pressure.

RESTRICTIVE LUNG DISEASES Cor pulmonale in restrictive lung disease is associated with two different clinical syndromes: (1) hyperventilation in patients with "intrinsic" restrictive diseases or space-occupying intrathoracic lesions; and (2) hypoventilation in patients with "extrinsic" diseases, such as obesity, myxedema, or severe neuromuscular dysfunction. Pulmonary hypertension is due to the hypoxemia and to the increased pulmonary vascular resistance resulting from compression of the pulmonary circulation. Again, oxygen is the main treatment, but specific therapy may be available for some of the underlying lung diseases.

Combined obstructive airflow and restrictive lung disease has a particularly grim outlook. It frequently occurs in patients with a restrictive disease who smoke cigarettes.

PROGNOSIS Although prognosis in cor pulmonale is based on the degree of pulmonary hypertension, the presence of cor pulmonale is difficult to relate to the distress and morbidity of patients with obstructive airflow disease. However, it appears that death due to right ventricular failure per se is very rare compared with death due to the underlying pulmonary disease in these patients.

REFERENCES

GRAHAM R et al: Dopamine, Dobutamine and Phenotolamine effects on pulmonary vascular mechanics. J Appl Physiol 54:1277, 1983

MATHAY RA et al: Pulmonary artery hypertension in chronic obstructive pulmonary disease: Determination by chest radiography. Invest Radiol 16:95, 1981

MCDONALD IG, BUTLER J: Distribution of vascular resistance in the isolated, perfused dog lung. J Appl Physiol 23:463, 1967

MCFADDEN FR, BRAUNWALD E: Cor pulmonale and pulmonary thromboembolism, in *Heart Disease,* E Braunwald (ed). Philadelphia, Saunders, 1988, 3d ed, pp 1597–1616

PERMUTT S et al: Interaction between the circulatory and ventilatory pumps, in *Thorax, Part 3, vol 29: Lung Biology in Health and Disease,* C Roussos, PT Macklem (eds). New York, Marcel Dekker, 1985, pp 701–735

WIDIMSKY J: Non-invasive diagnosis of pulmonary hypertension in chronic lung diseases. Prog Resp Res 20:69, 1985

WILKINSON M et al: A pathophysiological study of 10 cases of hypoxic cor pulmonale. Q J Med, N.S. 66, 249:65, 1988

192 THE CARDIOMYOPATHIES AND MYOCARDITIDES

JOSHUA WYNNE / EUGENE BRAUNWALD

CARDIOMYOPATHY

The cardiomyopathies are diseases that involve the myocardium primarily and are not the result of hypertension or congenital, valvular, coronary, arterial, or pericardial abnormalities.[1] When the cardiomyopathies are classified on an etiologic basis, two fundamental forms are recognized: (1) a primary type, consisting of heart muscle disease of unknown cause; (2) a secondary type, consisting of myocardial disease of known cause, or associated with a disease involving other organ systems (Table 192-1). In many cases it is not possible to arrive at an etiologic diagnosis on clinical grounds, and thus it is often more desirable to classify the cardiomyopathies on the basis of differences in their pathophysiology and clinical presentation (Tables 192-2 and 192-3). The distinction between the functional categories is not absolute, however, and there is often some overlap.

DILATED (CONGESTIVE) CARDIOMYOPATHY Left and/or right ventricular systolic pump function is impaired, leading to cardiac enlargement and often producing symptoms of congestive heart failure. Mural thrombi are often present, particularly in the left ventricular apex. Histologic examination reveals extensive areas of interstitial and perivascular fibrosis, with minimal necrosis and cellular infiltration. Although no cause is apparent in many cases, dilated cardiomyopathy (formerly called congestive cardiomyopathy) is probably the end result of myocardial damage produced by a variety of toxic, metabolic, or infectious agents. There is increasing evidence to suggest that in at least some patients dilated cardiomyopathy may be the late sequel of acute viral myocarditis, possibly mediated through an immunologic mechanism. Although most commonly a disease of middle-aged men, it may occur in any patient population. A reversible form of dilated cardiomyopathy may be found with selenium deficiency, hypophosphatemia, hypocalcemia, and chronic uncontrolled tachycardia. A small number of patients have familial forms of the disease; in some, there is evidence of X-linked inheritance. *Right ventricular dysplasia* is a unique cardiomyopathy marked by progressive replacement of the right ventricular wall with adipose tissue. Often associated with ventricular arrhythmias, the clinical course is variable; sudden death is a constant threat.

Clinical manifestations Symptoms of left- and right-sided congestive failure, manifested by dyspnea on exertion, fatigue, orthopnea, paroxysmal nocturnal dyspnea, peripheral edema, and palpitations, develop gradually in most patients. Some patients have left ventricular dilatation for months or even years before becoming symptomatic. Although vague chest pain may be present, typical angina pectoris is unusual and suggests the presence of concomitant coronary artery disease.

Physical examination Variable degrees of cardiac enlargement and findings of congestive heart failure are noted. In patients with advanced disease, the pulse pressure is small, and the jugular venous pressure is elevated. Third and fourth heart sounds are common, and mitral or tricuspid regurgitation may occur. Diastolic murmurs, valvular calcification, hypertension, and changes of vascular disease in the optic fundi militate *against* the diagnosis of cardiomyopathy.

Laboratory examinations The chest roentgenogram demonstrates left ventricular enlargement, although generalized cardiomegaly is often seen, sometimes due to a concomitant pericardial effusion.

[1] Diffuse myocardial fibrosis secondary to multiple myocardial scars produced by extensive coronary arterial narrowing and occlusion can impair left ventricular function and is frequently referred to as ischemic cardiomyopathy. According to the definition given above, however, the term *cardiomyopathy* should be restricted to a condition *primarily* involving heart muscle. In ischemic "cardiomyopathy" the *primary* involvement is in the coronary vessels.

TABLE 192-1 Etiologic classification of cardiomyopathies

I Primary myocardial involvement
- *A* Idiopathic (D,R,H)
- *B* Familial (D,H)
- *C* Eosinophilic endomyocardial disease (R)
- *D* Endomyocardial fibrosis (R)

II Secondary myocardial involvement
- *A* Infective (D)
  - *1* Viral myocarditis
  - *2* Bacterial myocarditis
  - *3* Fungal myocarditis
  - *4* Protozoal myocarditis
  - *5* Metazoal myocarditis
- *B* Metabolic (D)
- *C* Familial storage disease (D,R)
  - *1* Glycogen storage disease
  - *2* Mucopolysaccharidoses
- *D* Deficiency (D)
  - *1* Electrolytes
  - *2* Nutritional
- *E* Connective tissue disorders (D)
  - *1* Systemic lupus erythematosus
  - *2* Polyarteritis nodosa
  - *3* Rheumatoid arthritis
  - *4* Progressive systemic sclerosis
  - *5* Dermatomyositis
- *F* Infiltrations and granulomas (R,D)
  - *1* Amyloidosis
  - *2* Sarcoidosis
  - *3* Malignancy
  - *4* Hemochromatosis
- *G* Neuromuscular (D)
  - *1* Muscular dystrophy
  - *2* Myotonic dystrophy
  - *3* Friedreich's ataxia (H,D)
  - *4* Refsum's disease
- *H* Sensitivity and toxic reactions (D)
  - *1* Alcohol
  - *2* Radiation
  - *3* Drugs
- *I* Peripartum heart disease (D)
- *J* Endocardial fibroelastosis (R)

NOTE: The principal clinical manifestation(s) of each etiologic grouping is denoted by D (dilated), R (restrictive), or H (hypertrophic) cardiomyopathy.
SOURCE: Adapted from the WHO/ISFC task force report on the definition and classification of cardiomyopathies, 1980.

TABLE 192-2 Clinical classification of cardiomyopathies

1 Dilated (congestive): Left and/or right ventricular enlargement, impaired systolic function, congestive heart failure, arrhythmias, emboli

2 Restrictive: Endomyocardial scarring or myocardial infiltration resulting in restriction to left and/or right ventricular filling

3 Hypertrophic: Disproportionate left ventricular hypertrophy, typically involving septum more than free wall, with or without an intraventricular systolic pressure gradient; usually of a nondilated left ventricular cavity

The lung fields may demonstrate evidence of pulmonary venous hypertension and interstitial or alveolar edema. The electrocardiogram often shows sinus tachycardia or atrial fibrillation, ventricular arrhythmias, left atrial enlargement, diffuse nonspecific ST-T-wave abnormalities, and sometimes intraventricular conduction defects. Echocardiography (Fig. 177-4) and radionuclide ventriculography (Fig. 177-6) show left ventricular enlargement, with normal or minimally thickened or thinned walls, and systolic dysfunction (reduced ejection fraction); a pericardial effusion is often noted. Radioisotopic imaging with gallium 67 may identify patients with dilated cardiomyopathy and myocarditis.

Hemodynamic studies reveal a cardiac output that may be normal, or moderately to severely reduced at rest; it does not increase normally with exercise. The left ventricular end-diastolic, left atrial, and pulmonary capillary wedge pressures usually are elevated; when failure of the right side of the heart supervenes, the right ventricular end-diastolic, right atrial, and central venous pressures are also elevated. Angiography reveals a dilated, diffusely hypokinetic left ventricle, often with some degree of mitral regurgitation; the coronary arteries are normal, thereby excluding so-called ischemic cardiomyopathy. Transvenous endomyocardial biopsy (Chap. 179) may be helpful in excluding certain conditions such as myocardial infiltration by amyloid; in some patients there is biopsy evidence of myocardial round cell inflammation, suggesting an inflammatory etiology and compatible with previous viral myocarditis.

Treatment Most patients pursue an inexorably downhill course, and the majority, particularly those over 55 years of age, die within 2 years of the onset of symptoms, but spontaneous improvement or stabilization occurs in a minority. Death is due to either congestive heart failure or ventricular arrhythmia; sudden death, presumably arrhythmic in etiology, is a constant threat. Systemic embolization is common, and all patients without contraindications should receive anticoagulants. Strenuous exertion should be interdicted. Treatment of heart failure in dilated cardiomyopathy primarily is directed toward improvement in symptoms; a modest improvement in longevity is achieved with specific vasodilator therapy (hydralazine-nitrate combination and enalapril). Standard therapy of heart failure with salt restriction, diuretics, digitalis, and vasodilators may produce symptomatic improvement, at least in the initial phases of the illness; however, these patients appear to be at increased risk of digitalis toxicity. Some patients with dilated cardiomyopathy who have evidence of myocardial inflammation have been treated with corticosteroids, often in association with azathioprine; others have been treated cautiously with gradually increasing doses of beta-adrenergic blockers. However, the indications and value of such experimental therapy remain controversial. Antiarrhythmic agents may be used to

TABLE 192-3 Laboratory evaluation of the cardiomyopathies

	Dilated (congestive)	Restrictive	Hypertrophic
Chest roentgenogram	Moderate to marked cardiac enlargement Pulmonary venous hypertension	Mild cardiac enlargement	Mild to moderate cardiac enlargement
Electrocardiogram	ST-segment and T-wave abnormalities	Low-voltage Conduction defects	ST-segment and T-wave abnormalities Left ventricular hypertrophy Abnormal Q waves
Echocardiogram	Left ventricular dilatation and dysfunction	Increased left ventricular wall thickness Normal systolic function	Asymmetric septal hypertrophy (ASH) Systolic anterior motion (SAM) of the mitral valve
Radionuclide studies	Left ventricular dilatation and dysfunction (RVG)	Normal systolic function (RVG)	Vigorous systolic function (RVG) Asymmetric septal hypertrophy (RVG or ^{201}Tl)
Cardiac catheterization	Left ventricular dilatation and dysfunction Elevated left- and often right-sided filling pressures Diminished cardiac output	Normal systolic function Elevated left- and right-sided filling pressures	Vigorous systolic function Dynamic left ventricular outflow obstruction Elevated left- and right-sided filling pressures

NOTE: RVG = radionuclide ventriculogram; ^{201}Tl = thallium 201.

treat symptomatic or serious arrhythmias, although they may be extremely resistant to the usual as well as investigational agents. Because of this, alternative experimental therapies, such as surgical interruption of the arrhythmic circuit or implantation of an automatic internal defibrillator, have gained favor. In patients with advanced disease who are refractory to medical therapy and who have no contraindications to the procedure, cardiac transplantation should be considered (Chap. 183).

Alcoholic cardiomyopathy Individuals who consume large quantities of alcohol over many years may develop a clinical picture identical to idiopathic dilated cardiomyopathy; indeed, alcoholic cardiomyopathy is the major form of secondary dilated cardiomyopathy in the western world. Ceasing alcohol consumption before severe heart failure has developed may halt the progression, or even reverse the course of this disease, unlike the idiopathic variety, which is marked by progressive deterioration. Alcoholics with advanced heart failure have a poor prognosis, particularly if they continue to drink; less than one-quarter survive 3 years. The key to the treatment of alcoholic cardiomyopathy is total and permanent abstinence. Although thiamine deficiency may be present in some of these patients, alcoholic cardiomyopathy is associated with a low cardiac output and systemic vasoconstriction. In contrast, beriberi heart disease (Chaps. 76 and 194) is characterized by elevated cardiac output and diminished peripheral vascular resistance, so that thiamine deficiency per se does not appear to cause alcoholic cardiomyopathy. A second presentation of alcoholic cardiotoxicity may be found in individuals without overt heart failure, and consists of recurrent supraventricular or ventricular tachyarrhythmias. Termed the "holiday heart syndrome," it typically appears after a drinking binge; atrial fibrillation is seen most frequently, followed by atrial flutter and ventricular premature depolarizations. Some patients develop left ventricular hypertrophy, perhaps related to concomitant systemic hypertension; they may present with symptoms of pulmonary congestion due to abnormal diastolic stiffness (diminished compliance) of the left ventricle.

Peripartum cardiomyopathy Cardiac dilatation and congestive heart failure of unexplained cause may develop during the last month of pregnancy or within the first few months after delivery. The etiology of this disorder is unknown but may relate to a preexisting cardiomyopathy that was not apparent prior to pregnancy. Necropsy shows cardiac enlargement, often with mural thrombi, along with histologic evidence of myocardial degeneration and fibrosis. The patient who develops peripartum cardiomyopathy is typically multiparous, black, and over the age of 30. While some patients are malnourished, there is no conclusive evidence that dietary deficiencies are etiologically involved. The symptoms, signs, and treatment are similar to those in patients with idiopathic dilated cardiomyopathy; pulmonary and systemic emboli are particularly common. The mortality rate may be as high as 25 to 50 percent. The prognosis in these patients appears to be closely related to whether the heart size returns to normal after the first episode of congestive heart failure. If it does, subsequent pregnancies may sometimes be well tolerated; if the heart remains enlarged, however, further pregnancies frequently produce increasing myocardial damage, ultimately leading to refractory congestive heart failure and death. Those who recover should be encouraged to avoid further pregnancies, particularly if cardiomegaly persists.

Neuromuscular disease (See also Chap. 365) Cardiac involvement is common in many of the muscular dystrophies. In *Duchenne's progressive muscular dystrophy,* myocardial involvement is most frequently indicated by a distinctive and unique electrocardiographic pattern consisting of tall R waves in right precordial leads with an R/S ratio greater than 1.0, often associated with deep Q waves in the limb and lateral precordial leads, and is not found in other forms of muscular dystrophy. These electrocardiographic abnormalities appear to result from selective transmural necrosis of the posterobasal left ventricle and associated papillary muscle. A variety of supraventricular and ventricular arrhythmias is frequently found. Rapidly progressive congestive heart failure may develop despite extended periods of apparent circulatory stability during which the only detectable abnormalities are in the electrocardiogram. *Myotonic dystrophy* is characterized by a variety of electrocardiographic abnormalities, especially disorders of impulse formation and particularly conduction, but other overt clinical evidence of heart disease is uncommon. Because of the abnormalities of impulse generation and conduction, syncope and sudden death are major hazards; in appropriate patients, insertion of a permanent pacemaker may be efficacious. In *limb-girdle* and *fascioscapulohumeral dystrophy,* cardiac involvement is uncommon and seldom severe. Involvement of the heart is very common in *Friedreich's ataxia* (manifested by abnormal electrocardiographic or echocardiographic findings), with as many as half of the patients developing cardiac symptoms. The electrocardiogram most commonly demonstrates ST-segment and T-wave abnormalities. The echocardiogram may demonstrate left ventricular hypertrophy, with either symmetric or asymmetric hypertrophy of the left ventricular septum compared with the free wall. Although morphologically similar to some cases of hypertrophic cardiomyopathy, cellular disarray is lacking.

Drugs A variety of pharmacologic agents may damage the myocardium acutely, producing a pattern of inflammation (myocarditis), or they may lead to chronic damage of the type seen with idiopathic dilated cardiomyopathy. Certain drugs produce only electrocardiographic abnormalities, while others may precipitate fulminant congestive heart failure and death. The anthracycline derivatives, particularly *doxorubicin* (Adriamycin), are powerful antineoplastic agents, which, when given in high doses (more than 550 mg/m^2 for doxorubicin), may produce fatal heart failure. The incidence of heart failure is related not only to the dose of the drug but to the presence or absence of several risk factors (cardiac irradiation, age greater than 70 years, underlying heart disease, hypertension, treatment with cyclophosphamide); at any dose patients with these risk factors have an eight- to tenfold greater frequency of developing heart failure than do patients lacking them. Radionuclide ventriculography (Chap. 177) may document preclinical deterioration of left ventricular function and allow appropriate dose adjustments; by so monitoring left ventricular function, it is often possible to continue doxorubicin even in patients at high risk for developing heart failure. Recent efforts to modify the dose schedule by giving the drug more slowly have further reduced the risk of cardiotoxicity. Some patients with congestive heart failure, even those with severe depression of left ventricular function, have demonstrated recovery of cardiac function with aggressive management with digitalis, diuretics, and vasodilators. High-dose *cyclophosphamide* may produce congestive heart failure acutely or within 2 weeks of administration; a characteristic histopathologic feature is myocardial edema and hemorrhagic necrosis. Rarely, patients treated with *5-fluorouracil* will develop chest pain and electrocardiographic changes of myocardial ischemia or infarction. Electrocardiographic changes and arrhythmias may result from treatment with tricyclic antidepressants, the phenothiazines, emetine, lithium, and various aerosol propellants. *Cocaine abuse* is associated with a variety of life-threatening cardiac complications, including sudden death, myocarditis, and acute myocardial infarction (resulting from coronary spasm and/or thrombosis with or without underlying coronary artery stenosis).

RESTRICTIVE CARDIOMYOPATHY The hallmark of the restrictive cardiomyopathies is abnormal diastolic function; the ventricular walls are excessively rigid and impede ventricular filling. Myocardial fibrosis, hypertrophy, or infiltration secondary to a variety of etiologies is usually responsible. The infiltrative diseases, which represent important etiologies for secondary restrictive cardiomyopathy, may also show some impairment of systolic function. Myocardial involvement with *amyloid* is a common cause of secondary restrictive cardiomyopathy, although restriction is also seen in hemochromatosis, glycogen deposition, endomyocardial fibrosis, fibroelastosis, the eosinophilias, neoplastic infiltration, and myocardial fibrosis of diverse causes. In many of these conditions, particularly those with substantial concomitant endocardial involvement, partial obliteration of the ventricular cavity by fibrous tissue and thrombus contributes to the abnormally increased resistance to ventricular filling. As a result of persistently elevated venous pressure these patients commonly have dependent edema, ascites, and an enlarged, tender liver. The jugular venous pressure is elevated and does not fall normally, or it may rise with inspiration (Kussmaul's sign). The heart sounds may be distant, and third and fourth heart sounds are common. In contrast to constrictive pericarditis, which these diseases resemble, the apex impulse is usually easily palpable. The electrocardiogram shows low-voltage, nonspecific ST-T-wave changes and various arrhythmias. Pericardial calcification on x-ray, which would suggest constrictive pericarditis, is absent. Echocardiography typically reveals symmetrically thickened left ventricular walls and normal or slightly reduced systolic function. Cardiac catheterization shows a decreased cardiac output, elevation of the right and left ventricular end-diastolic pressures, and a dip-and-plateau configuration of the diastolic portion of the ventricular pressure pulse resembling that seen in constrictive pericarditis.

Differentiation from constrictive pericarditis, at the bedside and even after cardiac catheterization, may be difficult or impossible (Chaps. 179 and 193). This distinction is of importance because the latter condition is potentially curable by operation. Helpful in the differentiation of these two diseases are right ventricular transvenous endomyocardial biopsy (by revealing interstitial infiltration or fibrosis in restrictive cardiomyopathy) and computed tomography or magnetic resonance imaging (by demonstrating a thickened pericardium in constrictive pericarditis).

Endomyocardial fibrosis This is a progressive disease of unknown etiology that occurs most commonly in children and young adults residing in tropical and subtropical Africa, particularly Uganda and Nigeria. The disease is characterized by fibrous endocardial lesions of the inflow portion of the right or left ventricle (or both) and often involves the atrioventricular valves, producing valvular regurgitation. The apex of the ventricles may be obliterated by a mass of thrombus and fibrous tissue. In many ways this disease resembles eosinophilic endomyocardial disease, although they occur in quite different geographic areas and age groups. Endomyocardial fibrosis is a frequent cause of heart failure in Africa, accounting for up to one-quarter of deaths due to heart disease.

The clinical picture depends upon which ventricle and atrioventricular valve show predominant involvement; left-sided involvement results in symptoms of pulmonary congestion, while predominant right-sided disease presents features of a restrictive cardiomyopathy. Medical treatment is often disappointing, and surgical excision of the fibrotic endocardium and replacement of the involved atrioventricular valve has led to substantial symptomatic improvement in a small number of patients.

Eosinophilic endomyocardial disease Also called *Loeffler's endocarditis* and *fibroplastic endocarditis*, this disease appears to be a subcategory of the hypereosinophilic syndrome in which the heart is predominantly involved. Typically, the endocardium of either or both ventricles thickens markedly, with involvement of the underlying myocardium. Large mural thrombi may develop in either ventricle, thereby compromising the size of the ventricular cavity and serving as a source of pulmonary and systemic emboli. Hepatosplenomegaly and localized eosinophilic infiltration of other organs are usually present. Routine management with digitalis, diuretics, afterload-reducing agents, and anticoagulation as indicated, in conjunction with glucocorticoids and cytotoxic drugs (hydroxyurea in particular), appears to have improved survival substantially.

Differential diagnosis Involvement of the heart is the most frequent cause of death in *primary amyloidosis* (Chap. 266), while clinically significant cardiac involvement is uncommon in the secondary form. Focal deposits of amyloid in elderly patients (*senile cardiac amyloidosis*) is common and usually clinically insignificant. In a minority of patients the clinical cardiac findings are identical to those of primary amyloidosis, the principal difference being the structural composition of the amyloid protein. Biopsy of the rectal mucosa, gingiva, liver, kidney, and myocardium permits the diagnosis to be made before death in over three-quarters of cases. The heart is firm, rubbery, and noncompliant, and four clinical presentations (alone or in combination) are seen: (1) diastolic dysfunction (restrictive cardiomyopathy); (2) systolic dysfunction; (3) arrhythmias; and (4) orthostatic hypotension. The two-dimensional echocardiogram may be helpful in making the diagnosis of amyloidosis and may show a thickened myocardial wall with a distinctive "speckled" appearance. *Hemochromatosis* (Chap. 327) should be suspected if cardiomyopathy occurs in the setting of diabetes mellitus, hepatic cirrhosis, and increased skin pigmentation. Phlebotomy may be of some benefit if employed early in the course of the disease. Continuous subcutaneous administration of deferoxamine may reduce body iron stores in advanced cases, but whether this produces clinical improvement is unclear. Myocardial *sarcoidosis* (Chap. 277) is generally associated with other manifestations of systemic disease and may have restrictive as well as congestive features, since cardiac infiltration by sarcoid granulomas results not only in increased stiffness of the myocardium but also in diminished systolic contractile function. A variety of arrhythmias, including atrioventricular block, have been noted. *Endocardial fibroelastosis* is a disease seen in infants, characterized by a thickened endocardium that shows proliferation of elastic tissue. It is most unusual in adult patients, although small patches of it may be found in patients with endomyocardial fibrosis.

HYPERTROPHIC CARDIOMYOPATHY This disease is characterized by left ventricular hypertrophy, typically of a nondilated chamber, without obvious antecedent cause. The hypertrophy is thus not secondary to a cardiovascular or systemic disease, such as hypertension or aortic stenosis, that places a hemodynamic burden on the left ventricle. Two commonly found features of the disease have attracted the greatest attention: (1) heterogeneous left ventricular (LV) hypertrophy, often with asymmetric septal hypertrophy (ASH), wherein the upper portion of the interventricular septum is preferentially hypertrophied compared to the posterobasal left ventricular free wall; and (2) a dynamic left ventricular outflow tract pressure gradient, related to narrowing of the subaortic area as a consequence of the midsystolic apposition of the anterior mitral valve leaflet against the hypertrophied septum, i.e., systolic anterior motion of the mitral valve (SAM). Initial studies of this disease emphasized the dynamic "obstructive" features, and it has been termed idiopathic hypertrophic subaortic stenosis (IHSS), hypertrophic obstructive cardiomyopathy (HOCM), and muscular subaortic stenosis. It has become clear, however, that only about one-quarter of patients with hypertrophic cardiomyopathy demonstrate an outflow tract gradient. The ubiquitous pathophysiologic abnormality is not systolic but rather *diastolic* dysfunction, characterized by increased stiffness of the hypertrophied muscle. This results in elevated diastolic filling pressures and is present despite a hyperdynamic left ventricle.

The pattern of hypertrophy is distinctive in hypertrophic cardiomyopathy and differs from that seen in secondary hypertrophy (as in hypertension). Most patients have striking regional variations in the extent of hypertrophy in different portions of the left ventricle, and the majority demonstrate a ventricular septum whose thickness is disproportionately increased when compared with the free wall. Other patients may demonstrate disproportionate involvement of the apex or left ventricular free wall; 10 percent or more of patients have concentric involvement of the ventricle. All, however, show a bizarre and disorganized arrangement of cardiac muscle cells in the septum, whether or not a gradient is present, along with a variable degree of myocardial fibrosis and abnormalities of the small intramural coronary arteries.

About half of all cases of hypertrophic cardiomyopathy appear to be transmitted as autosomal dominants with a variable degree of expression and penetrance; there is considerable variability in the extent of hypertrophy and symptoms even in close relatives. The remainder of cases appear to occur sporadically, but some may represent new mutations. Echocardiographic studies have confirmed that about one-third of the first-degree relatives (i.e., parents, siblings, and children) of patients with familial hypertrophic cardiomyopathy have evidence of the disease, although in many of these patients the extent of hypertrophy is mild, no outflow tract pressure gradient is present, and symptoms are not prominent. Since the hypertrophic characteristics may not be apparent in childhood and only first appear in adolescence, a single normal echocardiogram in a child does not entirely exclude the presence of the disease.

In contrast to the obstruction produced by a fixed narrowed orifice, such as valvular aortic stenosis, the pressure gradient in hypertrophic cardiomyopathy, when present, is dynamic and may change between examinations and even from beat to beat. Obstruction appears to result from further narrowing of an already small left ventricular outflow tract by systolic anterior motion of the mitral valve against the hypertrophied septum. While SAM may be found in a variety of other conditions besides hypertrophic cardiomyopathy, it is *always* found when obstruction is present in hypertrophic cardiomyopathy. Three basic mechanisms are involved in the production of the dynamic pressure gradient: (1) increased left ventricular contractility, which reduces ventricular systolic volume and increases the ejection velocity of the blood moving through the outflow tract, thus drawing the anterior mitral valve leaflet against the septum as a result of reduced distending pressure; (2) decreased ventricular volume (preload), which reduces further the size of the outflow tract; and (3) decreased aortic impedance and pressure (afterload), which increases the velocity of flow through the subaortic area and also reduces ventricular systolic volume. Interventions that increase myocardial contractility, such as exercise, isoproterenol, and digitalis glycosides, and those that reduce ventricular volume, such as the Valsalva maneuver, sudden standing, nitroglycerin, amyl nitrite, or tachycardia, all may cause an increase in the gradient and the murmur. Conversely, elevation of arterial pressure by phenylephrine, squatting, sustained handgrip, augmentation of venous return by passive leg raising, and expansion of the blood volume all increase ventricular volume and ameliorate the gradient and murmur. Sometimes the hypertrophied septum bulges into the outflow tract of the right ventricle, thereby impeding the ejection of blood from this chamber as well.

Clinical features Many patients with hypertrophic cardiomyopathy are asymptomatic and may be relatives of patients with known disease. Unfortunately, the first clinical manifestation of the disease may be sudden death, frequently occurring in children and young adults, often during or after physical exertion. In symptomatic patients the most common complaint is dyspnea, largely due to increased stiffness of the left ventricular walls, which impairs ventricular filling and leads to elevated left ventricular diastolic and left atrial pressures. Other symptoms include angina pectoris, fatigue, syncope, and near syncope (''graying-out spells''). Symptoms are not related to the presence or severity of an outflow gradient. Most patients with gradients demonstrate a double or triple apical impulse, a rapidly rising carotid arterial pulse, and a fourth heart sound. The hallmark of obstructive hypertrophic cardiomyopathy is a systolic murmur, which is typically harsh, diamond-shaped, and usually begins well after the first heart sound, since ejection is unimpeded early in systole. The murmur is best heard at the lower left sternal border as well as at the apex, where it is often more holosystolic and blowing in quality, no doubt due to the mitral regurgitation that usually accompanies obstructive hypertrophic cardiomyopathy.

Laboratory evaluation The *electrocardiogram* commonly shows left ventricular hypertrophy and widespread, deep, broad Q waves that suggest an old myocardial infarction but apparently result from the abnormal electrophysiologic properties of the hypertrophied septum. Many patients demonstrate arrhythmias, both atrial (supraventricular tachycardia or atrial fibrillation) as well as ventricular (ventricular tachycardia) during ambulatory (Holter) monitoring. *Chest roentgenography* may be normal, although a mild to moderate increase in the cardiac silhouette is common. The mainstay of the diagnosis of hypertrophic cardiomyopathy is the *echocardiogram*, which demonstrates left ventricular hypertrophy, often with the septum 1.3 or more times the thickness of the high posterior left ventricular free wall. The septum may demonstrate an unusual ground-glass appearance, probably related to its abnormal cellular architecture and myocardial fibrosis. Systolic anterior motion of the mitral valve is found in patients with pressure gradients. The left ventricular cavity is typically small in hypertrophic cardiomyopathy, with vigorous posterior wall motion, but reduced septal excursion. A rare form of hypertrophic cardiomyopathy, found principally in Japan, is characterized by massive apical hypertrophy, often associated with giant negative T waves on the electrocardiogram and a ''spade-shaped'' left ventricular cavity on angiography. The two-dimensional *echocardiogram* is particularly useful in identifying all of the characteristic changes, including the size and shape of the left ventricular cavity. The indirectly recorded *carotid arterial pulse* tracing rises unusually rapidly and often displays a ''spike-and-dome'' configuration when an outflow pressure gradient is present. *Radionuclide scintigraphy* with thallium 201 frequently reveals evidence of myocardial perfusion defects even in asymptomatic patients.

The two typical *hemodynamic* features are an elevated left ventricular diastolic pressure due to diminished left ventricular compliance and, when obstruction is present, a systolic pressure gradient between the body of the left ventricle and the subaortic region. When a gradient is not present, it often can be induced by provocative maneuvers such as infusion of isoproterenol, inhalation of amyl nitrite, or the Valsalva maneuver.

Treatment Beta-adrenergic blockers are often used and may ameliorate to some degree the symptoms of angina pectoris and syncope in one-third to one-half of patients. Resting intraventricular pressure gradients are usually unchanged, although these drugs may limit the increase in the gradient that occurs during exercise. It is not known whether beta-adrenergic blockers offer any protection against sudden death, which is presumably arrhythmic in origin. It is not established whether any antiarrhythmic agent is efficacious in this setting. However, the experimental agent amiodarone appears to be effective in reducing the frequency of supraventricular as well as life-threatening ventricular arrhythmias. The calcium channel antagonists are agents that may reduce the stiffness of the ventricle, reduce the elevated diastolic pressures, increase exercise tolerance, and, in some instances, reduce the severity of outflow tract gradients, although adverse side effects occur in about one-quarter of patients. Disopyramide has been used in some patients to reduce left ventricular contractility and the outflow gradient. Surgical myotomy/myectomy of the hypertrophied septum may result in lasting symptomatic improvement in about three-quarters of operated patients, but the mortality of approximately 5 percent limits the operation to severely symptomatic patients with large pressure gradients who are unresponsive to medical management. Digitalis, diuretics, nitrates, and beta-adrenergic agonists are best avoided if possible, particularly in patients with known left ventricular outflow tract pressure gradients.

Prognosis The natural history of hypertrophic cardiomyopathy is variable, although many patients demonstrate an improvement or stabilization of symptoms with time. Atrial fibrillation is common late in the course of the disease; its onset usually leads to a striking increase in symptoms, presumably due to loss of the atrial contribution to filling of the thickened ventricle. This rhythm, when sustained, is associated with a poor prognosis. Infective endocarditis occurs in less than 10 percent of patients, and endocarditis prophylaxis is indicated, particularly in patients with resting obstruction and mitral regurgitation. Progression of hypertrophic cardiomyopathy to left ventricular dilatation and dysfunction without an outflow gradient has been reported but is unusual; in about 5 to 10 percent of patients, however, some degree of left ventricular systolic impairment, wall thinning, and chamber enlargement occurs over time. The major cause of mortality in hypertrophic cardiomyopathy is sudden death, which may occur in asymptomatic patients or interrupt an otherwise stable course in symptomatic ones. Predictors of sudden death include: age less than 30 years, ventricular tachycardia on ambulatory monitoring, and a family history of sudden death. There is no correlation between the risk of sudden death and the severity of symptoms or the presence or severity of an outflow tract pressure gradient. Since sudden death often occurs during or just after physical exertion, strenuous exercise should be avoided in all patients, regardless of symptoms. Although hemodynamic factors may play a role, it is likely that most deaths, particularly those that are sudden, are due to ventricular arrhythmias.

MYOCARDITIS

Myocarditis is said to be present when the heart is involved in an inflammatory process. Most commonly the result of an infectious process, myocarditis may also be present in hypersensitivity states such as acute rheumatic fever (Chap. 187) or may be caused by radiation, chemicals, physical agents, and drugs. Myocarditis may be acute or chronic. In an unknown number of cases, acute myocarditis progresses to chronic dilated cardiomyopathy. While almost every infectious agent is capable of producing myocarditis, clinically significant acute myocarditis in the United States is caused most commonly by viruses. Coxsackievirus B is the most frequent cause of viral myocarditis, but coxsackievirus A, influenza, rubeola, rubella, polio-, adeno-, and echoviruses also cause the disease. In most cases, the presence of myocarditis is inferred only by the finding of transient electrocardiographic ST-T-wave abnormalities, but arrhythmias, heart failure, and death may occur in fulminant cases, particularly in infants and pregnant women. Myocarditis is frequently associated with acute pericarditis, particularly when it is caused by coxsackievirus B strains or echoviruses (Chap. 145).

Physical examination may be normal in patients who have only electrocardiographic abnormalities, although more severe cases may show a muffled first heart sound, along with a third heart sound and a murmur of mitral regurgitation. A pericardial friction rub may be audible in patients with associated pericarditis.

Experimental studies suggest that exercise may be deleterious in patients with myocarditis, and strenuous activity should be proscribed until the electrocardiogram has returned to normal. Prolonged bed rest has been advocated for more severe cases, although its efficacy remains to be established. Patients who develop congestive heart failure respond to the usual measures (digitalis, diuretics, salt restriction), but they appear to be unusually sensitive to digitalis. Arrhythmias are common and are occasionally difficult to manage. Deaths attributed to heart failure, tachyarrhythmias, and heart block have been reported, and it seems prudent to monitor the electrocardiogram of patients with arrhythmias, especially during the acute illness.

Though viral myocarditis is most often self-limited and without sequelae, active disease may recur, and it is likely that acute viral myocarditis occasionally progresses to a chronic form. Patients with viral myocarditis often give a history of a preceding upper respiratory febrile illness, and viral nasopharyngitis or tonsillitis may be evident clinically. The isolation of virus from the stool, pharyngeal washings, or other body fluids, and changes in specific antibody titers are helpful clinically. Some instances of apparent *idiopathic* dilated cardiomyopathy (page 975) appear to arise from mild or subclinical episodes of myocarditis. While corticosteroids may exacerbate heart damage in animals with acute viral myocarditis, a small number of humans with congestive heart failure and inflammatory myocarditis appear to respond to an experimental protocol utilizing immunosuppression with prednisone and azathioprine. Serial right ventricular endomyocardial biopsies have shown regression of inflammatory infiltrates in some patients so treated. However, the effects of this treatment program have not been rigorously compared to a comparable control group.

Bacterial myocarditis Bacterial involvement of the heart is uncommon, but when it does occur, it is usually as a complication of bacterial endocarditis (typically due to *Staphylococcus aureus* and enterococci). Myocardial abscess formation may involve the valve rings and interventricular septum. *Diphtheritic myocarditis* develops in over one-quarter of the patients with diphtheria, is one of the most serious complications, and is the most common cause of death due to diphtheria (Chap. 102). Cardiac damage is due to the liberation of a toxin that inhibits protein synthesis, and leads to a dilated, flabby, hypocontractile heart; the conducting system is frequently involved as well. Cardiomegaly and severe congestive heart failure typically appear after the first week of illness. ST-segment and T-wave abnormalities on the electrocardiogram are the rule, but atrial and ventricular arrhythmias, bundle branch block, and abnormalities of atrioventricular conduction are also common. Prompt therapy with antitoxin is crucial; antibiotic therapy is also indicated but is of less urgency.

Chagas' disease Chagas' disease, caused by the protozoan *Trypanosoma cruzi* and transmitted by an insect vector (Chap. 161), produces an extensive myocarditis that typically becomes evident years after the initial infection. It is one of the most common causes of heart disease encountered in Central and South America; in rural areas up to 20 percent of the population may be affected. Although only a minority of infected individuals have an acute illness, upwards of one-third develop chronic myocardial damage. Electrocardiographic evidence of cardiac involvement may appear in adolescence, although symptoms often do not appear until adulthood. The chronic form is characterized by dilatation of several cardiac chambers, fibrosis and thinning of the ventricular wall, aneurysm formation in the areas of thinning (especially at the apex), and mural thrombi. Chronic progressive heart failure, often predominantly right-sided, is the rule. The electrocardiogram typically shows right bundle branch block and left anterior hemiblock, which may progress to complete atrioventricular block. The echocardiogram may reveal a unique pattern of hypokinesis of the posterior left ventricular wall and relatively preserved septal motion. Ventricular arrhythmias are common and are seen particularly during and after exertion; oral amiodarone appears to be particularly effective in treating ventricular tachyarrhythmias. The cause of death is either intractable congestive heart failure or an arrhythmia. Therapy is directed toward amelioration of the congestive heart failure and arrhythmias; the latter may require implantation of a pacemaker. Medical therapy is often unsatisfactory or unavailable, however, and a more promising tactic has been the institution of public health measures, particularly the use of insecticides to eliminate the vector.

Toxoplasmic myocarditis (See also Chap. 162) This uncommon form of protozoal myocardial involvement occurs most frequently in immunosuppressed adults; congenital toxoplasmal infections are much more common, but myocarditis is not a prominent feature. Myocardial involvement may lead to cardiac dilatation, pericarditis, and pericardial effusion. Heart failure, arrhythmias, and conduction abnormalities may be seen. Because of the difficulty in diagnosing this condition, it may be a more common problem than is usually appreciated. Treatment is with pyrimethamine and sulfonamides, but the response to treatment is variable.

Giant cell myocarditis This rare myocarditis of unknown cause is characterized by the presence of multinucleated giant cells in the myocardium. It usually causes rapidly fatal congestive heart failure and arrhythmia in young to middle-aged adults. At necropsy, the distinctive features include cardiac enlargement, ventricular thrombi, grossly visible serpiginous areas of myocardial necrosis in both ventricles, and microscopic evidence of giant cells within an extensive inflammatory infiltrate. The cause of giant cell myocarditis remains obscure, although it occurs in association with thymoma, systemic lupus erythematosus, and thyrotoxicosis. No therapy has been shown to be efficacious.

Lyme carditis (See also Chap. 132) Lyme disease is caused by a tick-borne spirochete and is most common in the northeastern United States during the summer months. About 10 percent of patients develop symptomatic cardiac involvement, with conduction abnormalities the most common manifestations. Concomitant myopericarditis is not uncommon, and mild asymptomatic left ventricular dysfunction may occur. Penicillin is used to treat the accompanying skin rash, arthritis, and neurologic abnormalities. A temporary pacemaker may be needed for symptomatic heart block; the utility of glucocorticoids in reversing heart block is uncertain, but they are usually employed.

Human immunodeficiency virus myocarditis In addition to myocardial opportunistic infections by a wide variety of organisms and metastatic involvement by Kaposi's sarcoma, cardiac involvement in the acquired immunodeficiency syndrome (AIDS) (Chap. 264) often consists of a mild focal myocarditis. An occasional patient demonstrates advanced congestive heart failure with four-chamber cardiac enlargement. Therapy has been uniformly unsuccessful.

Radiation myocarditis A variety of acute and chronic cardiac complications may result from the use of ionizing radiation in the treatment of carcinoma of the lung or breast, lymphoma, or Hodgkin's disease. Only an occasional patient manifests acute cardiac abnormalities; typically such an abnormality consists of acute pericarditis. The most common presentation is that of chronic pericardial effusion or constriction occurring months or years after exposure (in rare cases up to 10 years) (Chap. 193). Myocardial fibrosis, resulting from damage to the microvasculature, often with formation of atherosclerotic plaques of the epicardial coronary arteries, is also common.

REFERENCES

BRAUNWALD E: Hypertrophic cardiomyopathy—continued progress. N Engl J Med 320:800, 1989

CHAUDARY S, JASKI BF: Fulminant mumps myocarditis. Ann Intern Med 110:569, 1989

COPLAN NL, BRUNO MS: Acquired immunodeficiency syndrome and heart disease: The present and the future. Am Heart J 117:1175, 1989

HEILBRUNN SM et al: Increased beta-receptor density and improved hemodynamic response to catecholamine stimulation during long-term metoprolol therapy in heart failure from dilated cardiomyopathy. Circulation 79:483, 1989

JARCHO JA et al: Mapping a gene for familial hypertrophic cardiomyopathy to chromosome 14ql. N Engl J Med 321:1372, 1990

KARAM R et al: Hypertensive hypertrophic cardiomyopathy or hypertrophic cardiomyopathy with hypertension? A study of 78 patients. J Am Coll Cardiol 13:580, 1989

KARCH SB, BILLINGHAM ME: The pathology and etiology of cocaine-induced heart disease. Arch Pathol Lab Med 112:225, 1988

KOUNIS NG et al: Hypersensitivity myocarditis. Ann Allergy 62:71, 1989

MCALISTER HF et al: Lyme carditis: An important cause of reversible heart block. Ann Intern Med 110:339, 1989

OLSHAUSEN KV et al: Long-term prognostic significance of ventricular arrhythmias in idiopathic dilated cardiomyopathy. Am J Cardiol 61:146, 1988

POPMA JJ et al: Diagnostic and prognostic utility of right-sided catheterization and endomyocardial biopsy in idiopathic dilated cardiomyopathy. Am J Cardiol 63:955, 1989

REZKALLA SH, KLONER RA: Management strategies in viral myocarditis. Am Heart J 117:706, 1989

ROMEO F et al: Predictors of sudden death in idiopathic dilated cardiomyopathy. Am J Cardiol 63:138, 1989

SPIRITO P et al: Clinical course and prognosis of hypertrophic cardiomyopathy in an outpatient population. N Engl J Med 320:749, 1989

STEWART JM et al: Symptomatic cardiac dysfunction in children with human immunodeficiency virus infection. Am Heart J 117:140, 1989

SUNNERHAGEN KS et al: Regional left ventricular wall motion abnormalities in dilated idiopathic cardiomyopathy. Am J Cardiol 65(1):364, 1990

Surgical treatment of hypertrophic obstructive cardiomyopathy. Lancet 1:358, 1989

THIENE G et al: Right ventricular cardiomyopathy and sudden death in young people. N Engl J Med 318:129, 1988

WEBB JG et al: Apical hypertrophic cardiomyopathy: Clinical follow-up and diagnostic correlates. J Am Coll Cardiol 15(1):83, 1990

WYNNE J, BRAUNWALD E: The cardiomyopathies and myocarditides, in *Heart Disease*, 3d ed, E Braunwald (ed). Philadelphia, Saunders, 1988, pp 1410–1469

193 PERICARDIAL DISEASE

EUGENE BRAUNWALD

NORMAL FUNCTIONS OF THE PERICARDIUM The visceral pericardium is a serous membrane, separated by a small amount of fluid, an ultrafiltrate of plasma, from a fibrous sac, the parietal pericardium. The pericardium prevents sudden dilatation of the cardiac chambers during exercise and hypervolemia, and as the result of the development of a negative intrapericardial pressure during ejection it facilitates atrial filling during ventricular systole. The pericardium also restricts the anatomic position of the heart, minimizes friction between the heart and surrounding structures, prevents displacement of the heart and kinking of the great vessels, and probably retards the spread of infections from the lungs and pleural cavities to the heart. Notwithstanding the foregoing, total absence of the pericardium does not produce obvious clinical disease. In partial left pericardial defects the main pulmonary artery and left atrium may bulge through the defect; rarely herniation and subsequent strangulation of the left atrium may cause sudden death.

ACUTE PERICARDITIS

It is useful to classify the types of pericarditis both clinically and etiologically (Table 193-1), as this disorder is by far the most common pathologic process involving the pericardium.

Pain, a pericardial friction rub, electrocardiographic changes, and pericardial effusion with cardiac tamponade and paradoxic pulse are cardinal manifestations of many forms of acute pericarditis and will be considered prior to a discussion of the most common forms of the disorder.

TABLE 193-1 Classification of pericarditis

I Clinical classification
- *A* Acute pericarditis (<6 weeks)
  - *1* Fibrinous
  - *2* Effusive (or bloody)
- *B* Subacute pericarditis (6 weeks to 6 months)
  - *1* Constrictive
  - *2* Effusive-constrictive
- *C* Chronic pericarditis (>6 months)
  - *1* Constrictive
  - *2* Effusive
  - *3* Adhesive (nonconstrictive)

II Etiologic classification
- *A* Infectious pericarditis
  - *1* Viral
  - *2* Pyogenic
  - *3* Tuberculous
  - *4* Mycotic
  - *5* Other infections (syphilitic, parasitic)
- *B* Noninfectious pericarditis
  - *1* Acute myocardial infarction
  - *2* Uremia
  - *3* Neoplasia
    - *a* Primary tumors (benign or malignant)
    - *b* Tumors metastatic to pericardium
  - *4* Myxedema
  - *5* Cholesterol
  - *6* Chylopericardium
  - *7* Trauma
    - *a* Penetrating chest wall
    - *b* Nonpenetrating
  - *8* Aortic aneurysm (with leakage into pericardial sac)
  - *9* Postirradiation
  - *10* Associated with atrial septal defect
  - *11* Associated with severe chronic anemia
  - *12* Infectious mononucleosis
  - *13* Familial Mediterranean fever
  - *14* Familial pericarditis
    - *a* Mulibrey nanism*
  - *15* Sarcoidosis
  - *16* Acute idiopathic
- *C* Pericarditis presumably related to hypersensitivity or autoimmunity
  - *1* Rheumatic fever
  - *2* Collagen vascular disease
    - *a* Systemic lupus erythematosus
    - *b* Rheumatoid arthritis
    - *c* Scleroderma
  - *3* Drug-induced
    - *a* Procainamide
    - *b* Hydralazine
    - *c* Other
  - *4* Postcardiac injury
    - *a* Postmyocardial infarction (Dressler's syndrome)
    - *b* Postpericardiotomy

* An autosomal recessive syndrome, characterized by growth failure, muscle hypotonia, hepatomegaly, ocular changes, enlarged cerebral ventricles, mental retardation, and chronic constrictive pericarditis.

Pain is an important but not invariable symptom in various forms of acute pericarditis; it is usually present in the acute infectious types and in many of the forms presumed to be related to hypersensitivity or autoimmunity. Pain is often absent in a slowly developing tuberculous, postirradiation, neoplastic or uremic pericarditis. The pain of pericarditis is often severe (Chap. 16). It is characteristically in the center of the chest, referred to the back and the trapezius ridge. Often the pain is pleuritic, i.e., sharp and aggravated by inspiration, coughing, and changes in body position, but sometimes it is a steady, constrictive pain, which radiates into either arm or both arms and resembles that of myocardial ischemia; confusion with myocardial infarction is common. Characteristically, however, the pericardial pain may be relieved by sitting up and leaning forward. The differentiation of acute myocardial infarction from acute pericarditis becomes even more perplexing when, with acute pericarditis, the serum transaminase and creatine kinase levels rise, presumably because of concomitant involvement of the epicardium. However, these enzyme elevations, if they occur, are quite modest, given the extensive electrocardiographic ST-segment elevation in pericarditis.

The *pericardial friction rub* is the most important physical sign; it may have up to three components per cardiac cycle, as described in Chap. 175, and can sometimes be elicited only when firm pressure with the diaphragm of the stethoscope is applied to the chest wall. It is heard most frequently during expiration with the patient in the sitting position, but an independent pleural friction rub may be audible during inspiration, with the patient leaning forward or in the left lateral decubitus position. The rub is often inconstant and transitory, and a loud to-and-fro leathery sound may disappear within a few hours, possibly to reappear the following day.

Moderate elevations of the MB fraction of creatine phosphokinase may occur and reflects accompanying myocarditis.

The *electrocardiogram* in acute pericarditis without massive effusion usually displays changes secondary to acute subepicardial inflammation (Fig. 176-14, p. 858). There is widespread elevation of the ST segments, involving two or three standard limb leads and V_2 to V_6, with reciprocal depressions only in aVR and sometimes V_1 and without significant changes in QRS complexes, except occasionally for some reduction in voltage. After several days, the ST segments return to normal and only then do the T waves become inverted. In contrast, in acute myocardial infarction, reciprocal depression of ST segments is usually more prominent; QRS changes occur, particularly the development of Q waves, and notching and loss of the amplitude of R waves; and T-wave inversions usually occur within hours *before* the ST segments have become isoelectric. Sequential electrocardiograms are useful in distinguishing acute pericarditis from acute myocardial infarction. Early repolarization is a normal variant and may also cause widespread ST-segment elevation, most prominent in left precordial leads. However, in this condition the T waves are usually tall and the ST/T ratio is under 0.25, but exceeds this number in acute pericarditis. Depression of the PQ segment (below the TP segment) also is common and reflects atrial involvement. With large pericardial effusions, the QRS voltage is reduced; atrial premature beats and atrial fibrillation are sometimes noted.

PERICARDIAL EFFUSION Usually associated with one or more of the above-mentioned manifestations of pericarditis and an enlargement of the cardiac silhouette, pericardial effusion is especially important clinically when it develops within a relatively short time, since it may lead to cardiac tamponade. Differentiation from cardiac enlargement may be difficult, but heart sounds tend to become faint; the friction rub may disappear or remain clearly audible, and the apex impulse may vanish, but sometimes it is palpable well medial to the left border of cardiac dullness. The chest roentgenogram may show a "water bottle" configuration of the cardiac silhouette, but it may also be normal or almost so. Lucent pericardial fat lines may be seen deep within the cardiopericardial silhouette. Fluoroscopic examination may show the ventricular pulsations to be diminished. When the effusion is large, an area of dullness and tubular breath sounds is often encountered at the angle of the left scapula, probably caused by compression of the lung (Ewart's sign).

Diagnosis of pericardial effusion Echocardiography (Chap. 177) is the most effective diagnostic laboratory technique available, since it is sensitive, specific, simple, innocuous, and noninvasive, and may be performed at the bedside. The presence of pericardial fluid is recorded as a relatively echo-free space between the posterior pericardium and left ventricular epicardium in patients with small effusions and such a space between the anterior right ventricle and the parietal pericardium just beneath the anterior chest wall with larger effusions (Fig. 193-1). In patients with large effusions the heart may swing freely within the pericardial sac; when severe, the extent of this motion alternates and may be associated with electrical alternans. Two-dimensional echocardiography allows localization and estimation of the quantity of pericardial fluid. In tamponade, during inspiration, right ventricular diameter increases while left ventricular diameter and mitral valve opening decrease. Often the right ventricular cavity is reduced and there is late diastolic inward motion (collapse) of the right ventricular free wall, and of the right atrium. The diagnosis

FIGURE 193-1 Two-dimensional (upper panel) and short-axis (lower panel) parasternal scans in systole in a patient with a large pericardial effusion surrounding the entire heart. Fluid is seen to extend behind the left atrium (white arrowhead) and anterior to the descending thoracic aorta (DA). AoV = aortic valve; LA = left atrium; LV = left ventricle; PE = pericardial effusion; RV = right ventricle. *(Modified from PC Come (ed), Diagnostic Cardiology: Noninvasive imaging techniques, Philadelphia, Lippincott, 1985.)*

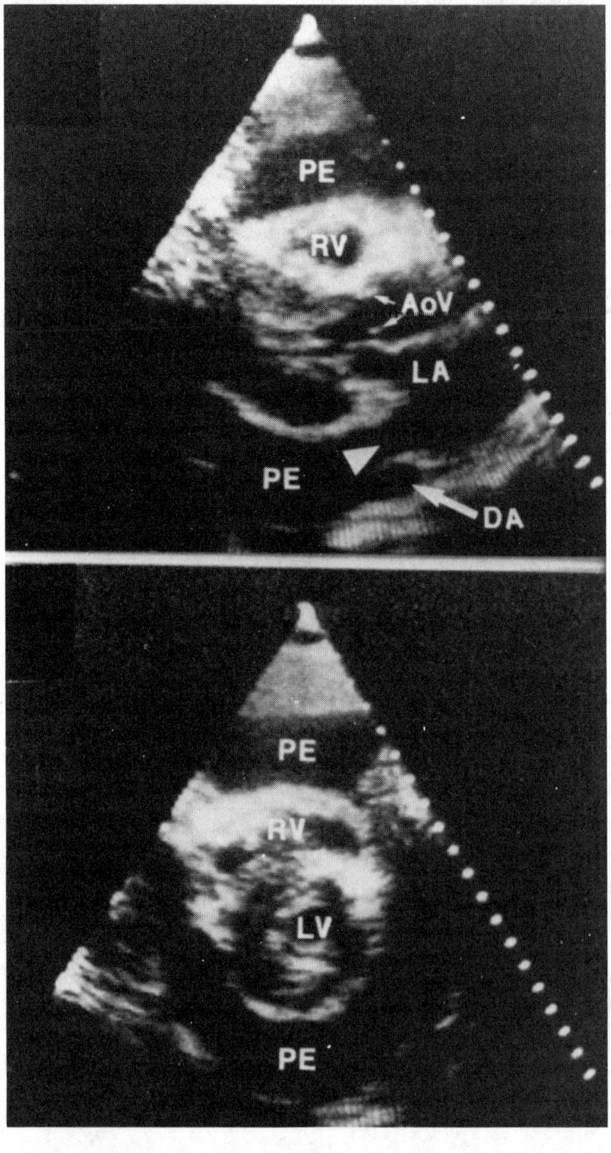

of pericardial fluid or thickening may be confirmed by one of the following:

1 *Cardiac catheterization*. A catheter is introduced into the right atrium and rotated so that its tip makes contact with the lateral right atrial wall. In the presence of an effusion, or pericardial thickening, the tip of the catheter is separated from the radiolucent lungs by an opaque band.
2 *Angiocardiography*. Contrast medium is injected rapidly into the right atrium; again the lateral wall is separated from the edge of the cardiac silhouette.

When it is deemed desirable to remove pericardial fluid for diagnostic and/or therapeutic purposes, a needle attached to a properly grounded electrocardiographic lead is inserted into the pericardial space, usually through a subxiphoid approach, and if possible using echocardiographic control. Intrapericardial pressure should be measured before fluid is withdrawn. Pericardial effusion nearly always has the physical characteristics of an exudate. Bloody fluid is commonly due to tuberculosis or tumor, but it may also be found in the effusion of rheumatic fever or in the post-cardiac injury syndrome (see below). Occasionally, bloody fluid may be found in the effusion of uremic pericarditis and in the hemopericardium following myocardial infarction, especially following the administration of anticoagulants.

CARDIAC TAMPONADE The accumulation of fluid in the pericardium in an amount sufficient to cause serious obstruction to the inflow of blood to the ventricles results in cardiac tamponade. The amount of fluid necessary to produce this critical state may be as small as 250 mL, when the fluid develops rapidly, or over 2000 mL in slowly developing effusions when the pericardium has had the opportunity to stretch and adapt to the increasing volume of fluid. The volume of fluid required to produce tamponade varies directly with the thickness of the ventricular myocardium and inversely with the thickness of the parietal pericardium. Tamponade results most often from bleeding into the pericardial space following cardiac operations, trauma (including cardiac perforation during diagnostic procedures), tuberculosis, tumor (most commonly carcinoma of the lung and breast and lymphoma), and aortic dissection, but it may occur in acute viral or idiopathic pericarditis, postirradiation pericarditis, renal failure during dialysis, and hemopericardium which may result when a patient with any form of acute pericarditis is treated with anticoagulants.

The clinical manifestations are due to the fall in cardiac output and to systemic venous congestion. However, the classic findings of falling arterial pressure, rising venous pressure, and a small quiet heart with faint heart sounds usually are seen only with severe tamponade usually occurring within minutes, as happens with cardiac trauma or rupture. More frequently, tamponade develops more slowly and the clinical manifestations, resembling those of heart failure, include dyspnea, orthopnea, hepatic engorgement, and jugular venous hypertension. A high index of suspicion is required, since, in many instances, no obvious cause for pericardial disease is apparent, and tamponade should be considered in any patient with hypotension and elevation of jugular venous pressure with a prominent x descent; often the y descent is diminutive or absent. A widening of the area of flatness to percussion across the anterior aspect of the chest wall, a paradoxical pulse (see below), relatively clear lung fields, diminished pulsations of the cardiac silhouette on fluoroscopy, enlargement of the cardiac silhouette in subacute or chronic tamponade, reduction in amplitude of the QRS complexes, and *electrical alternans* of the P, QRS, and T waves should raise the suspicion of cardiac tamponade.

A positive Kussmaul's sign (see below) is rare in cardiac tamponade, as is a pericardial knock. Their presence suggests that an organizing process and epicardial constriction are present in addition to effusion. Since immediate treatment of tamponade may be lifesaving, prompt measures to establish the diagnosis definitely, i.e., echocardiography followed by cardiac catheterization, should be undertaken. The latter reveals elevation of the right atrial pressure with prominence of the x but not of the y descent. When measured, the pericardial pressure is also elevated and equal to the right atrial pressure. There is ''equalization'' of pressures, i.e., the pulmonary artery wedge is equal, or close, to right atrial, right ventricular, and pulmonary artery diastolic pressures. The ''square root'' sign in the ventricular pressure pulses and the prominent y descent in atrial and jugular venous pressure are characteristic of constrictive pericarditis (see below) and are usually absent in tamponade. In an emergency, pericardiocentesis may be carried out without cardiac catheterization but preferably after confirmation of the clinical diagnosis by echocardiography.

Paradoxical pulse This important clue to the presence of cardiac tamponade consists of *a greater than normal (10 mmHg) inspiratory decrease in systolic arterial pressure*. When severe, it may be detected by palpating weakness or disappearance of the arterial pulse during inspiration, but usually sphygmomanometric measurement of systolic pressure during slow respiration is required (Fig. 193-2).

The mechanism of paradoxical pulse in cardiac tamponade is complex. Normally, the inspiratory decline in intrathoracic pressure enhances right ventricular filling by virtue of the increased pressure gradient between the extrathoracic veins and the chambers of the right side of the heart. As a consequence right ventricular diastolic volume and stroke output increase, and this increase is transmitted to the left side of the heart several cardiac cycles later, leading to an increase in systemic arterial pressure during the following expiration. Therefore, normally a small fall in left ventricular stroke volume and pressure occur during inspiration. Also, left ventricular afterload rises during inspiration as intrapericardial pressure falls, contributing to

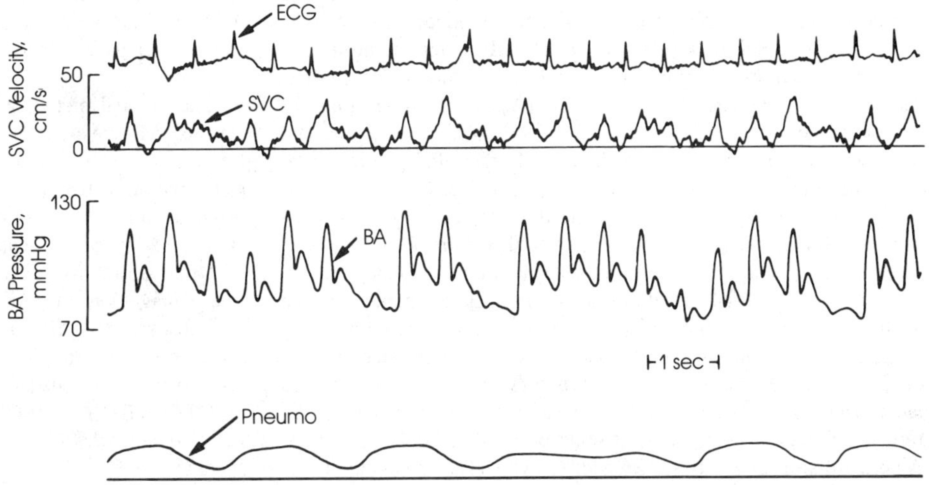

FIGURE 193-2 Simultaneous recording of electrocardiogram (ECG), blood flow velocity in the superior vena cava (SVC), brachial arterial pressure (BA), and the pneumogram (Pneumo) in a patient with cardiac compression and paradoxical pulse. A downward deflection of the pneumogram denotes inspiration, when SVC blood velocity rises and arterial pressure falls (paradoxical pulse). Arterial pressure is maintained during prolonged expiratory pause.

the small inspiratory decline in left ventricular stroke volume and arterial pressure. In cardiac tamponade, since both ventricles share a tight incompressible covering, i.e., the pericardial sac, the inspiratory increase in right ventricular volume compresses and reduces left ventricular volume substantially; leftward bulging of the interventricular septum further reduces the left ventricular cavity as the right ventricle enlarges during inspiration. Thus, in cardiac tamponade the inspiratory augmentation of right ventricular volume causes an exaggerated reciprocal reduction in left ventricular volume. Also, respiratory distress increases the fluctuations in intrathoracic pressure, which exaggerates the mechanism just described.

Low-pressure tamponade refers to mild tamponade in which the intrapericardial pressure is increased from its slightly subatmospheric levels to +5 to +10 mmHg; in some instances hypovolemia coexists. As a consequence the central venous pressure is normal or only slightly elevated while arterial pressure is unaffected. The patients are asymptomatic or complain of mild weakness and dyspnea. The diagnosis is aided by echocardiography, and both hemodynamic and clinical manifestations improve following mild pericardiocentesis.

Paradoxical pulse, a hallmark of cardiac tamponade, occurs in only approximately one-third of patients with *constrictive pericarditis*. It is important to bear in mind that paradoxical pulse is not pathognomonic of pericardial disease because it may be observed in various forms of restrictive cardiomyopathies (Chap. 192) and, in some cases of hypovolemic shock, chronic obstructive airways disease, and severe bronchial asthma.

TREATMENT All patients with acute pericarditis should be observed frequently and carefully for the possibility of a developing effusion or, if effusion is already present, for signs of tamponade. In the presence of an effusion, arterial and venous pressures and heart rate should be monitored continuously or followed carefully and serial echocardiograms obtained. When a diagnostic pericardiocentesis of a large effusion is carried out, an attempt should be made to remove as much fluid as possible. If manifestations of tamponade appear, pericardiocentesis must be carried out at once, since relief of the intrapericardial pressure may be lifesaving. A small catheter advanced over the needle inserted into the pericardial cavity may be left in place to allow draining of the pericardial space if fluid reaccumulates.

VIRAL OR IDIOPATHIC FORM OF ACUTE PERICARDITIS This disorder is an important clinical entity because of its frequency and because it may be confused with other more serious illnesses. In some cases an A or B coxsackievirus or the virus of influenza, echovirus type 8, mumps, herpes simplex, chickenpox, or adenovirus has been isolated from pericardial fluid and/or appropriate elevations in viral antibody titers have been noted; in other instances, acute pericarditis has occurred in association with illnesses of known viral origin and, presumably, was caused by the same agent. More commonly there is an antecedent infection of the respiratory tract, but in many patients such an association is not evident and viral isolation and serologic studies are negative. Most frequently, a viral causation cannot be established nor can it be excluded; the term *acute idiopathic pericarditis* is then appropriate. However, regardless of the specific causative factor, the clinical manifestations are similar. This form of acute pericarditis occurs at all ages but is more frequent in young adults; it is often associated with pleural effusions and pneumonitis. The appearance of fever and precordial pain at about the same time, often 10 to 12 days after a presumed viral illness, constitutes an important feature in the differentiation of acute pericarditis from myocardial infarction, in which pain precedes fever. The constitutional symptoms are usually mild to moderate, but occasionally the initial symptoms are stormy, the temperature rising to 40°C. The disease ordinarily runs its course in a few days to 2 weeks, but occasionally after the patient has apparently recovered he or she may have one or several recurrences, weeks or even months later. Tamponade is unusual and constrictive pericarditis develops rarely, although accumulation of some pericardial fluid is common. A pericardial friction rub is often audible. The ST segment alterations in the electrocardiogram are usually transitory, but the abnormal T waves may persist for several years or indefinitely and be a source of confusion in persons without a clear history of pericarditis. Pleuritis and pneumonitis frequently accompany pericarditis. The erythrocyte sedimentation rate is elevated. Granulocytosis followed by lymphocytosis is common.

There is no specific therapy, but anti-inflammatory treatment with aspirin, if necessary up to 900 mg qid, may be given. If this is ineffective, one of the nonsteroidal anti-inflammatory agents, such as indomethacin (25 to 75 mg qid) or a glucocorticoid (e.g., prednisone, 20 to 80 mg daily) effectively suppresses the clinical manifestations of the acute illness and may be useful in patients in whom the purulent and tuberculous forms of pericarditis have been excluded. After the patient has been asymptomatic and afebrile for about 1 week, the dose of the anti-inflammatory agent is gradually tapered. Occasionally progression to chronic constrictive pericarditis occurs. Recurrences occur in about one-fourth of patients, but the tendency to relapse decreases within 2 years after the initial episode. When recurrences continue beyond this period and are frequent, prolonged, and disabling, pericardiectomy may be effective in terminating the illness.

POST-CARDIAC INJURY SYNDROME An acute form of pericarditis may appear under a variety of circumstances which have one common feature: previous injury to the myocardium, with blood in the pericardial cavity. The syndrome has been observed when the injury has been induced in the course of a cardiac operation (postpericardiotomy syndrome). It may also follow myocardial infarction (Dressler's syndrome) (Chap. 189) or develop after trauma of the heart (Chap. 194), for example a stab wound, contusions after a nonpenetrating blow to the chest, or perforation of the heart with a pacemaker catheter.

The principal symptom is the pain of acute pericarditis, which usually develops 1 to 4 weeks following the cardiac injury but sometimes appears only after a lapse of months. Recurrences are common and may occur up to 2 years or more after the injury. Fever to 40°C, pericarditis, pleuritis, and pneumonitis are the outstanding features, the bout of illness usually subsiding in 1 or 2 weeks. The pericarditis, which appears to be the most constant lesion, may be of the fibrinous variety, or it may be a pericardial effusion, which is often serosanguineous and sometimes causes tamponade. Rarely, the pericarditis may be accompanied by arthralgias. Leukocytosis, an increased sedimentation rate, and electrocardiographic changes typical of acute pericarditis may also occur.

The mechanisms responsible for the clinical manifestations have not been identified, but there is a likelihood that they are the result of a hypersensitivity reaction in which the antigen originates from injured myocardial tissue and/or pericardium; the suggested designation of post-cardiac injury syndrome for this group of disorders implies that they may have a common pathogenetic mechanism. Circulating autoantibodies to myocardium occur frequently, but their precise role in this syndrome has not been defined. Viral infection may also play an etiologic role, since antiviral antibodies are often elevated in patients who develop this syndrome following cardiac surgery.

The clinical picture mimics acute viral or acute idiopathic pericarditis. Moreover, it is possible that the recurrences that occur so frequently in the latter condition are not always caused by an exacerbation of the original (presumably viral) infection, but that the original injury may have initiated the sequence of events that culminates in the post-cardiac injury syndrome.

Often no treatment is necessary aside from aspirin and analgesics. The management of pericardial effusion and tamponade has already been discussed. When the illness is followed by a series of disabling recurrences, therapy with a nonsteroidal anti-inflammatory agent or a glucocorticoid is usually effective.

DIFFERENTIAL DIAGNOSIS Differential diagnosis of *acute idiopathic pericarditis* is primarily one of exclusion, as there is no specific test for this disorder. Consequently all other disorders that may be associated with acute fibrinous pericarditis must be considered. When associated with *acute myocardial infarction,* acute fibrinous pericarditis may be confused with acute viral or idiopathic pericarditis; this complication of infarction, described on p. 963, is characterized by the occurrence of fever, pain, and a friction rub in the first 4 days following the development of the infarct (to be distinguished from the pericarditis in Dressler's syndrome, which occurs a week or two following myocardial infarction). Electrocardiographic abnormalities (such as the appearance of Q waves, brief ST-segment elevations with reciprocal changes, and earlier T-wave changes in myocardial infarction), the extent of the elevations of myocardial enzymes, and the total clinical picture are helpful in relating pericarditis to acute myocardial infarction. A common diagnostic error is assuming that acute viral or idiopathic pericarditis represents acute myocardial infarction and vice versa.

Acute pericarditis occurring as a component of the *post-cardiac injury* syndrome is most likely to be confused with acute idiopathic pericarditis. Pericarditis secondary to post-cardiac injury is differentiated from acute idiopathic pericarditis chiefly by timing. If it occurs within a few weeks of a myocardial infarction or a chest blow, it may be justified to conclude that the two are probably related. If the infarct has been silent or the chest blow forgotten, the relationship to the pericarditis may not be recognized.

It is important to distinguish *pericarditis due to collagen disease* from acute idiopathic pericarditis. Most important in the differential diagnosis is the pericarditis due to systemic lupus erythematosus (Chap. 269); often pain is present, sometimes the pericarditis appears as an asymptomatic effusion and rarely tamponade develops. Very rarely, when pericarditis occurs in the absence of other evidence of any underlying disorder, differentiation from acute viral and idiopathic pericarditis or tuberculous pericarditis may be made on discovery of lupus erythematosus (LE) cells, a rise in antinuclear antibodies, or by the specific methods for diagnosing tuberculosis (see below). Acute pericarditis is also an occasional complication of *rheumatoid arthritis, scleroderma,* and *polyarteritis nodosa,* but again, other evidence of these diseases is usually obvious. Asymptomatic pericardial effusion is also frequent in these disorders. It is important to question every patient with acute pericarditis about the ingestion of procainamide, hydralazine, isoniazid, cromolyn, and minoxidil, since these drugs can cause this syndrome.

The pericarditis of *acute rheumatic fever* is generally associated with evidence of severe pancarditis and with cardiac murmurs (Chap. 187). *Pyogenic (purulent) pericarditis* is usually secondary to cardiothoracic operations, immunosuppressive therapy, rupture of the esophagus into the pericardial sac, and rupture of a ring abscess in a patient with infective endocarditis and with septicemia complicating aseptic pericarditis. It is now uncommonly due to pneumococcal pneumonia and pleuritis, previously the most common cause. *Tuberculous pericarditis* (see Chap. 125) may present as an acute pericarditis, associated with fever, weight loss, and other clinical manifestations of active systemic tuberculosis; the diagnosis may be aided by a positive tuberculin test and evidence of pulmonary or mediastinal tuberculosis. Tubercle bacilli can be cultured from the pericardial space only infrequently, and a biopsy of the pericardium with bacteriologic and histologic examination may be required. Alternatively, tuberculous pericarditis may present as a chronic asymptomatic effusion, as subacute effusive-constrictive pericarditis, or frank chronic constrictive pericarditis (see below). *Uremic pericarditis* (Chap. 224) occurs in up to one-third of patients with chronic uremia, and is seen most frequently in patients undergoing chronic hemodialysis. It may be fibrinous or associated with a bloody effusion. A friction rub is common, but pain is usually absent. Treatment with an anti-inflammatory agent and intensification of hemodialysis are usually adequate therapy. Occasionally, tamponade occurs and pericardiocentesis is required. When uremic pericarditis is recurrent or persistent, pericardiectomy is necessary. Pericarditis due to *neoplastic diseases* results from irradiation or extension of primary or metastatic tumors (most commonly carcinoma of the lung and breast, malignant melanoma, and lymphoma) to the pericardium or from invasion by a lymphomatous or leukemic process; pain, atrial arrhythmias, and tamponade are complications which occur occasionally. *Mediastinal irradiation* for neoplasm may cause pericarditis after eradication of the tumor. Unusual causes of acute pericarditis include syphilis, fungus infection (histoplasmosis, blastomycosis, aspergillosis, and candidiasis), and parasitic infestation (amebiasis, toxoplasmosis, echinococcosis, trichinosis).

CHRONIC PERICARDIAL EFFUSIONS Chronic pericardial effusions are not infrequently encountered in patients without an antecedent history of acute pericarditis. They may cause few symptoms per se, and may be suspected by finding an enlarged cardiac silhouette on chest roentgenogram which may be obtained in the course of the workup of a patient with symptoms related to the underlying illness.

Tuberculosis This is a common cause of chronic pericardial effusion, although less so in the United States than in other parts of the world (Chap. 125). The symptoms are often those of a chronic, systemic illness in an individual with effusion. It is important to bear this condition in mind when a middle-aged or elderly person with fever has apparent enlargement of the cardiac silhouette of undetermined origin, with or without elevation of venous pressure. Weight loss, fever, and fatigability are sometimes observed. Inasmuch as effective specific methods of therapy have now reduced strikingly the mortality rate from the previous figures of about 70 percent, overlooking a tuberculous pericardial effusion is a serious error. Consequently, no method of examination should be omitted to establish this diagnosis. Included are chest roentgenograms for pulmonary tuberculosis and a search for tuberculosis in other organs; tuberculin skin tests, repeated after several weeks; cultures and smears of gastric washings and of pleural and pericardial fluid. Finally, if the diagnosis is still obscure, a pericardial biopsy, preferably by a limited thoracotomy, should be performed. If definitive evidence is then still lacking, but the specimen shows caseation necrosis, antituberculous chemotherapy for at least 24 months is justified (Chap. 125). Pericardiectomy should be carried out in order to prevent the development of constriction if the biopsy specimen shows a thickened pericardium.

Other causes of chronic pericardial effusion *Myxedema* may be responsible for a pericardial effusion that is sometimes massive but rarely, if ever, causes cardiac tamponade. The other manifestations of myxedema should clarify the diagnosis, but unfortunately, even when they are present, the diagnosis is frequently overlooked. It is important, therefore, to carry out appropriate tests for thyroid function (Chap. 316) in patients with an enlarged cardiac outline of undetermined origin. The cardiac silhouette is markedly enlarged and an echocardiogram is necessary to distinguish cardiomegaly from pericardial effusion. *Cholesterol pericardial disease* produces large pericardial effusions with a high cholesterol content, which may induce an inflammatory response and constrictive pericarditis.

Neoplasms, systemic lupus erythematosus, rheumatoid arthritis, mycotic infections, radiation therapy, pyogenic infections, severe chronic anemia, and chylopericardium may also cause chronic pericardial effusion and should be considered and specifically looked for in such patients.

Aspiration and analysis of the pericardial fluid are often helpful in diagnosis. In infections the organism can often be identified by smear or culture. Grossly sanguineous pericardial fluid results most commonly from a neoplasm, tuberculosis, uremia, or slow leakage from an aortic aneurysm.

CHRONIC CONSTRICTIVE PERICARDITIS

This disorder results when the healing of an acute fibrinous or serofibrinous pericarditis or a chronic pericardial effusion is followed by obliteration of the pericardial cavity with the formation of granulation tissue. This gradually contracts and forms a firm scar, encasing the heart and interfering with filling of the ventricles. In some reports, a high percentage of all cases has been of tuberculous origin. In other series, particularly those reported in the United States in the last two decades, tuberculosis has been an infrequent cause. The condition also may follow purulent infection, trauma, cardiac operation of any type, mediastinal irradiation, histoplasmosis, neoplastic disease, and acute viral or idiopathic pericarditis, rheumatoid arthritis, lupus erythematosus, and chronic renal failure with uremia treated by chronic dialysis. In many patients the cause of the pericardial disease is undetermined, and in them it is presumed that an asymptomatic or forgotten bout of viral pericarditis, acute or idiopathic, was the inciting event. Rarely, routine radiographic examination may reveal calcification of the pericardium in a person who is free of all symptoms referable to the heart. The heart may also be constricted and compressed by malignant tumors or organized blood clot in the pericardial cavity.

The basic physiologic abnormality in symptomatic patients with chronic constrictive pericarditis, as in those with cardiac tamponade, is the inability of the ventricles to fill adequately during diastole because of the limitations imposed by the rigid, thickened pericardium or the tense pericardial fluid. However, in constrictive pericarditis, ventricular filling is unimpeded during early diastole but is reduced abruptly when the elastic limit of the pericardium is reached; in cardiac tamponade, ventricular filling is impeded throughout diastole. Stroke volume is reduced, and the end-diastolic pressures in both ventricles, as well as the mean pressures in the atria, pulmonic veins, and systemic veins, are all elevated to about the same levels. Despite these hemodynamic changes myocardial function may be normal; instead, the ventricles may be considered to be underloaded. In constrictive pericarditis the central venous and right and left atrial pressure pulses display an M-shaped contour, with prominent x and y descents; the y descent is the most prominent deflection and is interrupted by a rapid rise in pressure during early diastole, when ventricular filling is impeded by the constricting pericardium. In cardiac tamponade the pressure contour differs in that the most prominent deflection is the x trough, while the y descent in the jugular venous pulse and the "square root" sign in the ventricular pressure pulse during diastole are usually absent. These characteristic changes are transmitted to the jugular veins, where they may be recognized by inspection or recorded. In constrictive pericarditis, both ventricular pressure pulses exhibit characteristic "square root" signs during diastole. These hemodynamic changes, although characteristic, are not pathognomonic of constrictive pericarditis but may also be observed in cardiomyopathies characterized by restriction of ventricular filling, as discussed in Chap. 192.

CLINICAL FINDINGS Weakness, fatigue, weight loss, and anorexia are common. The patients often appear to be chronically ill with decreased muscle mass and a protuberant abdomen; ankle edema may or may not be prominent. Contrary to a widely held impression, dyspnea, though absent or slight at rest, is often present on exertion, and orthopnea is common in chronic constrictive pericarditis, although it is not severe. Attacks of acute left ventricular failure (acute pulmonary edema) practically never occur. The cervical veins are distended and may remain so even after intensive diuretic treatment, and venous pressure may fail to decline during inspiration (Kussmaul's sign). In about one-third of the cases a paradoxical pulse may be observed. Congestive hepatomegaly is pronounced and may impair hepatic function; ascites is common and is usually more prominent than dependent edema. In about half of the patients, the heart is normal in size; if it is enlarged, the enlargement is rarely extreme. The apical pulse is reduced in intensity, retracts in systole, and moves outward in diastole. The heart sounds may be distant, an early third heart sound, i.e., a pericardial knock, occurring 0.06 to 0.12 s after aortic valve closure which coincides with a sudden deceleration in ventricular filling, is often conspicuous, and murmurs are usually absent. The apex beat is poorly defined, and cardiac pulsations under fluoroscopic examination are diminished. Because of the high sustained venous pressure, congestive splenomegaly may make the spleen palpable. In the absence of infective endocarditis or tricuspid valve disease, splenomegaly in a patient with congestive heart failure should arouse suspicion of constrictive pericarditis. Protein-losing gastroenteropathy due to impaired lymphatic drainage from the small intestine, and the nephrotic syndrome, or sometimes only marked proteinuria or hypoalbuminemia, may complicate chronic constrictive pericarditis. The electrocardiogram frequently displays low voltage of the QRS complex and diffuse flattening or inversion of the T waves. P mitrale may be present in patients with sinus rhythm; atrial fibrillation is present in about one-third of patients.

Systemic and/or pulmonary venous congestion is initially the result of impaired filling of the ventricles caused by the restrictive action of the inelastic pericardium. However, the fibrotic process may extend into the myocardium and cause myocardial scarring, and venous congestion may then be due to the combined effects of the myocardial and pericardial lesions. The interference with filling reduces the work of the heart and perhaps this leads to myocardial atrophy. The latter probably accounts for the delayed beneficial effects of operative treatment observed in some patients with advanced disease.

Inasmuch as the usual physical signs of cardiac disease (murmurs, cardiac enlargement) may be inconspicuous or absent in chronic constrictive pericarditis, hepatic enlargement and dysfunction associated with intractable ascites may lead to a mistaken diagnosis of cirrhosis of the liver. This error should be avoided if the neck veins are inspected carefully in all patients with ascites and hepatomegaly. *Given a clinical picture resembling that of cirrhosis, but with the added feature of distended neck veins, careful search for calcification of the pericardium by chest roentgenograms, fluoroscopy, and echocardiography should be carried out and may disclose a curable or remediable form of heart disease.* Calcification occurs in only about one-half of these patients and usually in those with long-standing pericardial constriction. Most patients with chronic constrictive pericarditis show pericardial thickening on echocardiographic examination. However, echocardiography cannot definitively exclude the diagnosis. Magnetic resonance imaging (MRI) is more precise in establishing or excluding the presence of a thickened pericardium (Chap. 178). Pericardial thickening and even pericardial calcification, however, are not synonymous with constrictive pericarditis since they may occur without seriously impairing ventricular filling. Very rarely, surgical exploration of the pericardium is necessary to establish the diagnosis.

DIFFERENTIAL DIAGNOSIS Like cor pulmonale (Chap. 191), chronic constrictive pericarditis may be associated with severe systemic venous hypertension but with little or no pulmonary congestion; the heart may not appear to be enlarged, and a striking inspiratory fall in arterial pressure may be present. However, in cor pulmonale advanced parenchymal pulmonary disease is usually evident and venous pressure *falls* during inspiration, i.e., Kusmaul's sign is negative. *Tricuspid stenosis* (p. 951) may also simulate the picture of chronic constrictive pericarditis; congestive hepatomegaly, splenomegaly, and ascites may be equally prominent, and the manifestations of left-sided heart failure may be inconspicuous. However, in tricuspid stenosis, the characteristic murmur, the almost universal coexistence of mitral stenosis, the absence of a paradoxic pulse, as well as the absence, in the jugular venous pulse, of the steep, deep y descent followed by a rapid ascent (manifested by the diastolic shock on palpation and its audible equivalent, the pericardial knock), facilitates the clinical differentiation.

It is of the greatest importance, though often difficult, to distinguish chronic constrictive pericarditis from various forms of heart disease which are characterized by a similar physiologic abnormality, i.e., restriction of ventricular filling, leading to a similar clinical picture. Described in Chap. 192, these include endomyocardial fibrosis; infiltrative cardiomyopathies such as amyloidosis, hemochromatosis, sarcoidosis, and scleroderma; and idiopathic myocardial hypertrophy. In the latter the marked thickening of the ventricular wall is responsible for the diminished compliance.

The features favoring the diagnosis of one of the above forms of cardiomyopathy are a well-defined apex beat, conspicuous enlargement of the heart, and pronounced orthopnea with attacks of acute left ventricular failure, left ventricular hypertrophy, gallop sounds (in place of a pericardial knock), bundle branch block, and in some cases significant Q waves in the electrocardiogram. The echocardiogram shows ventricular thickening, sometimes with a granular sparkling appearance. At catheterization, patients with chronic constrictive pericarditis usually have left atrial or pulmonary arterial wedge pressure equaling right atrial pressure, the latter often exceeding 15 mmHg despite intensive medical treatment for heart failure; the pulmonary artery systolic pressure is often less than 50 mmHg, and the right ventricular end-diastolic pressure often reaches one-third of the systolic pressure; the cardiac output is slightly depressed. In contrast, in patients with cardiomyopathy, the left atrial usually exceeds the right atrial pressure by more than 5 mmHg, the mean right atrial pressure often falls to below 15 mmHg following intensive treatment with diuretics, the pulmonary artery systolic pressure often exceeds 50 mmHg, and the right ventricular end-diastolic pressure is usually less than one-third of the systolic pressure, while the cardiac output is markedly depressed. The volumes of both ventricles, as determined by angiography or echocardiography, are characteristically reduced or normal in constrictive pericarditis, and the ejection fractions are normal or almost so; the left ventricular end-diastolic volume may also be normal in some cardiomyopathies but it is frequently elevated in others in which the ejection fraction is markedly reduced; the latter finding militates strongly against the diagnosis of constrictive pericarditis. The echocardiogram in chronic constrictive pericarditis characteristically shows pericardial thickening, i.e., a distinct echo posterior to the left ventricular wall, and paradoxical septal motion. The left ventricular wall moves sharply outward in early diastole and then remains flat. The definitive diagnosis of restrictive cardiomyopathy, when it is due to an infiltrative disease such as amyloidosis, can often be established by endomyocardial biopsy. MRI is very useful in distinguishing between restrictive cardiomyopathy and chronic constrictive pericarditis (p. 978).

It is important to emphasize that when a patient has progressive, disabling, and unresponsive congestive failure, and if he or she displays any of the phenomena of constrictive heart disease, the most careful and detailed clinical and laboratory studies must be carried out in order to detect or exclude constrictive pericarditis, which is potentially a curable condition. In some instances cardiac catheterization, selective angiocardiography, coronary arteriography, endomyocardial biopsy, and MRI may be required. However, in the rare instance when even these examinations do not yield a definitive diagnosis, surgical exploration of the pericardium is the only decisive method of determining whether constrictive pericarditis is responsible for the clinical manifestations of heart failure.

Occult constrictive disease Patients with this condition may have unexplained fatigue, dyspnea, and chest pain. No overt manifestations of pericardial disease are present, but following the rapid intravenous infusion of 1 liter of saline solution, the atrial and ventricular pressure pulses and diastolic equilibration of intracardiac pressures found in overt constrictive pericarditis occur. Although symptomatic improvement may follow pericardiectomy, this procedure should not be carried out in asymptomatic persons.

TREATMENT Pericardial resection is the only definitive treatment of constrictive pericarditis, but dietary sodium restriction and diuretics are useful during preoperative preparation. Digitalis may be beneficial in the prevention of heart failure when resection of the thickened pericardium permits an increased inflow into the ventricles and hence places an enhanced burden on an atrophic myocardium. The benefits derived from a complete cardiac decortication are often striking, and frequently the improvement, though slight at first, is progressive over a period of many months. The risk of this operation depends on the extent of penetration of the myocardium by the calcific process, by the severity of myocardial atrophy, and by the extent of secondary impairment of hepatic and/or renal function. Operative mortality is in the range of 7 to 10 percent. Therefore, surgical treatment should be carried out relatively early in the course.

Many instances of constrictive pericarditis are of tuberculous origin. Antituberculous therapy during the phase of effusion may prevent the development of constriction, and such therapy should be carried out before and after operation, if a tuberculous origin is suspected or cannot be excluded in a patient with chronic constrictive pericarditis (Chap. 125).

SUBACUTE EFFUSIVE-CONSTRICTIVE PERICARDITIS This form of pericardial disease is characterized by a combination of a tense effusion in the pericardial space, as well as constriction of the heart by thickened pericardium. It shares a number of features both with pericardial effusion producing cardiac compression and with pericardial constriction. It may be caused by tuberculosis, multiple attacks of acute idiopathic pericarditis, radiation, traumatic pericarditis, uremia, and scleroderma. The heart is generally enlarged, and there are a paradoxical pulse and a prominent *x* descent in the atrial pressure pulse. Following pericardiocentesis, the physiologic findings may change from those of cardiac tamponade to those of pericardial constriction, with a "square root" sign in the ventricular pressure pulse and a prominent *y* descent in the atrial and jugular venous pressure pulses. Furthermore, the intrapericardial pressure and the central venous pressure may decline, but not to normal. In many patients the condition progresses to the chronic constrictive form of the disease. Wide excision of both the visceral and parietal pericardium is usually effective.

OTHER DISORDERS OF THE PERICARDIUM

Pericardial cysts appear as rounded or lobulated deformities of the cardiac silhouette, most commonly at the right cardiophrenic angle. They do not cause symptoms, and their major clinical significance lies in the possibility of confusion with a tumor, ventricular aneurysm, or massive cardiomegaly. *Tumors* involving the pericardium are most commonly secondary to malignant neoplasms originating in or invading the mediastinum, including carcinoma of the bronchus and breast, lymphoma, and melanoma. The most common *primary* malignant tumor is the mesothelioma. The usual clinical picture of malignant pericardial tumor is an insidiously developing, often bloody, pericardial effusion. Surgical exploration is required to establish a definitive diagnosis and to carry out definitive or, more commonly, palliative treatment.

REFERENCES

Bush CA et al: Occult pericardial disease. Circulation 56:924, 1977

Fowler NO et al: Cardiac tamponade: A comparison of right versus left heart compression. J Am Coll Cardiol 12:187, 1988

Gold RG: Post-viral pericarditis. Eur Heart J 9:(G):175, 1988

Hancock EW: Subacute effusive-constrictive pericarditis. Circulation 43:183, 1971

Hatle LK et al: Differentiation of constrictive pericarditis and restrictive cardiomyopathy by Doppler echocardiography. Circulation 79:357, 1989

Lorell B, Braunwald E: Pericardial disease, in *Heart Disease,* 3d ed, E Braunwald (ed). Philadelphia, Saunders, 1988, pp 1484–1534

McCauhgan BC et al: Early and late results of pericardiectomy for constrictive pericarditis. J Thorac Cardiovasc Surg 89:340, 1985

Nishimura RA et al: Constrictive pericarditis: Assessment of current diagnostic procedures. Mayo Clin Proc 60:397, 1985

Ribeiro P et al: Constrictive pericarditis as a complication of coronary artery bypass surgery. Br Heart J 51:205, 1984

Sagrista-Sauleda J et al: Tuberculosis pericarditis: Ten year experience with a prospective protocol for diagnosis and treatment. J Am Coll Cardiol 11:724, 1988

Shabetai R: Pericardial and cardiac pressure. Circulation 77:1, 1988

194 CARDIAC TUMORS, CARDIAC MANIFESTATIONS OF SYSTEMIC DISEASES, AND TRAUMATIC CARDIAC INJURY

WILSON S. COLUCCI / EUGENE BRAUNWALD

TUMORS OF THE HEART

PRIMARY TUMORS Primary tumors of the heart are rare and are often classified as "benign" histologically (Table 194-1). However, since all cardiac tumors have the potential for causing life-threatening complications, and many are now curable by surgery, it is important that this diagnosis be made whenever possible. Approximately three-quarters are *histologically* benign, and the remainder are malignant, in almost all cases sarcomas.

Clinical presentation Cardiac tumors may present with a wide array of cardiac and noncardiac manifestations. There may be signs and symptoms of all the more common forms of heart disease, including chest pain, syncope, heart failure, murmurs, arrhythmias, conduction disturbances, and pericardial effusion or tamponade. The specific signs and symptoms produced are most closely related to the location of the tumor.

Myxoma Myxomas are the most common type of primary cardiac tumor, accounting for one-third to one-half of all cases. They occur at all ages and show no sex preference. Although the large majority of myxomas are sporadic, some are familial with autosomal dominant transmission or are part of a syndrome that involves a complex of abnormalities including lentigines or pigmented nevi, primary nodular adrenal cortical disease with or without Cushing's syndrome, myxomatous mammary fibroadenomas, testicular tumors, and/or pituitary adenomas with gigantism or acromegaly. Certain constellations of findings have been referred to as the *NAME syndrome* (nevi, atrial myxoma, myxoid neurofibroma, and ephelides) or the *LAMB syndrome* (lentigines, atrial myxoma, and blue nevi). Approximately 7 percent of cardiac myxomas are familial or part of the "complex myxoma" syndrome described above.

Most authorities consider the myxoma a true neoplasm, while others have suggested that it is formed by organization of an intracardiac thrombus attached to the endocardium. The large majority of sporadic myxomas are solitary and located in the atria, particularly the left, where they arise from the interatrial septum in the vicinity of the fossa ovalis. Sporadic myxomas may also occur in the ventricles or may be found in multiple locations. In contrast to sporadic myxomas, familial or "complex" myxomas tend to occur in younger individuals, are more often multiple in location, and are more likely to have postoperative recurrences, probably reflecting their multicentric nature (Table 194-2). Most are pedunculated on a fibrovascular stalk and average 4 to 8 cm in diameter. The most common clinical presentation resembles that of mitral valve disease, either stenosis as a result of tumor prolapse into the mitral orifice during diastole or regurgitation as a consequence of injury to the valve by tumor-induced trauma. Ventricular myxomas may cause outflow obstruction and may therefore mimic subaortic or subpulmonic stenosis. Characteristically, the symptoms and signs are highly dependent on position, intermittent, and sudden in onset as a result of changes in tumor position with gravity. On auscultation, a characteristic low-pitched sound, termed a "tumor plop," is audible during early or middiastole and is thought to result from the tumor abruptly stopping as it strikes the ventricular wall. Myxomas may also present with peripheral or pulmonary emboli, or any of several noncardiac signs and symptoms including fever, weight loss, cachexia, malaise, arthralgia, rash, clubbing, Raynaud's phenomenon, hypergammaglobulinemia, anemia, polycythemia, leukocytosis, elevated erythrocyte sedimentation rate, thrombocytopenia, or thrombocytosis. Not surprisingly, myxomas are frequently misdiagnosed as endocarditis, collagen vascular disease, or noncardiac tumor.

Both M-mode and two-dimensional echocardiography (Fig. 177-3, p. 862) are useful in the diagnosis of cardiac myxoma, the latter having the advantage of allowing determination of the site of tumor attachment and tumor size, important considerations in the planning of surgical excision. Computed tomography and magnetic resonance imaging may provide important information regarding the size, shape, and surface characteristics of the tumor. Because myxomas may be familial, echocardiographic screening of first-degree relatives is appropriate, particularly if the patient is young or has multiple tumors. While cardiac catheterization and angiography are often performed prior to surgery, catheterization of the chamber from which the tumor originates is attended by the risk of dislodgment of tumor emboli. In many centers catheterization is no longer considered mandatory when adequate noninvasive information is available.

Surgical excision utilizing cardiopulmonary bypass is indicated in all patients and is generally curative. Occasional reports of tumor recurrence are most likely due to inadequate excision of multiple tumor sites.

Other benign tumors Cardiac *lipomas,* although relatively common, are usually incidental findings at postmortem examination and seldom result in symptoms. However, they may grow as large as 15 cm and present with symptoms due to mechanical interference with cardiac function, arrhythmias, or conduction disturbances, or as an

TABLE 194-1 Relative incidence of primary tumors of the heart

Type	Percent
BENIGN	
Myxoma	30.5
Lipoma	10.5
Papillary fibroelastoma	9.9
Rhabdomyoma	8.5
Fibroma	4.0
Hemangioma	3.5
Teratoma	3.3
Mesothelioma of the AV node	2.8
Other benign tumors	2.1
Total	75.1
MALIGNANT	
Sarcomas	18.6
Lymphoma	1.6
Other malignant tumors	4.7
Total	24.9

SOURCE: Modified from HA McAllister, JJ Fenoglio, in *Atlas of Tumor Pathology*, Washington, Armed Forces Institute of Pathology, 1978, fasc 15, 2d series.

TABLE 194-2 Comparison of clinical features of sporadic myxoma and syndrome myxoma

Feature	Sporadic	Syndrome
Age (yr) (range)	56 (39–82)	25 (10–56)
Female/male ratio	2·7:1	1·8:1
Patients (no.)	70	44
Cardiac myxomas (no.)	72	103
Distributions of myxomas (%):		
Atrial/ventricular	100/0	87/13
Single/multiple	99/1	50/50
Biatrial	0	23
Recurrent	0	18
Familial	0	27
Freckling (%)	0	68
Noncardiac tumors (%)	0	57
Endocrine neoplasm (%)	0	30
Familial (%)	0	14

SOURCE: From HJ Vidaillet et al.

abnormality of the cardiac silhouette on chest x-ray. *Papillary fibroelastomas,* similarly, are relatively common findings on cardiac valves or the adjacent endothelium but seldom result in clinical symptoms. Occasionally, these growths may cause mechanical interference with valvular function. *Rhabdomyomas* and *fibromas,* the most frequent tumors in infants and children, most commonly occur in the ventricles, and therefore produce signs and symptoms by mechanical obstruction which may mimic valvular stenosis, congestive heart failure, restrictive or hypertrophic cardiomyopathy, and pericardial constriction. Rhabdomyomas are probably hamartomatous growths, are multiple in about 90 percent of cases, and may be associated with tuberous sclerosis, adenoma sebaceum, and benign kidney tumors. *Hemangiomas* and *mesotheliomas* are generally small tumors, most often intramyocardial in location, and may cause atrioventricular (AV) conduction disturbances and even sudden death as a result of their propensity for location in the region of the AV node.

Sarcomas Cardiac sarcomas may be of several histologic types, but in general are characterized by a rapidly downhill course leading to the patient's death in weeks to months from the time of presentation as a result of hemodynamic compromise, local invasion, or distant metastases. Sarcomas commonly involve the right side of the heart, and because of their rapid growth, invasion of the pericardial space and obstruction of the cardiac chambers or venae cavae are common. At the time of presentation these tumors have often spread too extensively for surgical excision. While there are scattered reports of palliation with surgery, radiotherapy, and/or chemotherapy, the overall experience with cardiac sarcomas is poor. The one exception to this appears to be cardiac lymphosarcomas, which may respond to a combination of chemo- and radiotherapy.

TUMORS METASTATIC TO THE HEART Tumors metastatic to the heart are several times more common than primary tumors, and as the life expectancy of patients with various forms of malignant neoplasms is extended by more effective therapy, it is likely that the frequency of cardiac metastases will also increase. Although cardiac metastases occur in 1 to 20 percent of all tumor types, the incidence is especially high in malignant melanoma, and to a somewhat lesser extent in leukemia and lymphoma. In absolute numbers, cardiac metastases are most common in carcinoma of the breast and lung, reflecting the high incidence of these cancers. Cardiac metastases almost always occur in the setting of widespread primary disease, and most often there is either primary or metastatic disease elsewhere in the thoracic cavity. Nevertheless, occasionally a cardiac metastasis may be the initial presentation of a tumor elsewhere in the body.

Cardiac metastases reach the heart via the bloodstream, lymphatics, or direct invasion and generally are small, firm nodules; although diffuse infiltrations may also occur, especially with sarcomas or hematologic neoplasms. The pericardium is most often involved, followed by myocardial involvement of any chamber, and, rarely, by involvement of the endocardium or cardiac valves.

Cardiac metastases result in clinical manifestations only about 10 percent of the time, and rarely are they the cause of death. In most patients they are *not* the cause of the presenting clinical features but occur in the setting of a previously recognized malignant neoplasm. While cardiac metastases may present a large number of nonspecific signs and symptoms, the most common are dyspnea, signs of acute pericarditis, cardiac tamponade, a rapid increase in the cardiac silhouette on chest x-ray, the new onset of an ectopic tachyarrhythmia, AV block, and congestive heart failure. As with primary cardiac tumors, the clinical presentation is more closely related to the location and size of the tumor than to its histologic type. Many of these signs and symptoms may also occur with myocarditis, pericarditis, or cardiomyopathy resulting from radiotherapy or chemotherapy.

The electrocardiographic findings are entirely nonspecific and may include ST-T-wave changes, decreased QRS voltage, arrhythmias, and conduction disturbances. On chest roentgenography the cardiac silhouette is most often normal but may reveal a pericardial effusion or bizarre contour. Echocardiography is useful for the diagnosis of pericardial effusion and the visualization of larger metastases. Computed tomography, magnetic resonance imaging, and radionuclide imaging with gallium or thallium may provide useful anatomic information. Angiography may delineate discrete lesions, and pericardiocentesis can allow a specific cytologic diagnosis. Since most patients with cardiac metastases have widespread disease, therapy generally consists of pericardiocentesis when there is hemodynamic compromise and treatment directed at the primary tumor. The removal of a malignant effusion by pericardiocentesis with or without concomitant instillation of a sclerosing agent (e.g., tetracycline) may palliate symptoms and delay or prevent reaccumulation of the effusion.

CARDIAC EFFECTS OF CANCER THERAPY See Chap. 192.

CARDIOVASCULAR MANIFESTATIONS OF SYSTEMIC DISEASES

DIABETES MELLITUS (See Chap. 319) In patients with insulin-dependent diabetes mellitus there is an increased incidence of large-vessel atherosclerosis and myocardial infarction, and diabetics are more likely to have an abnormal or absent pain response to myocardial ischemia, probably as a result of generalized autonomic nervous system dysfunction. Diabetic patients may also have myocardial dysfunction characteristic of a restrictive cardiomyopathy in the absence of large-vessel coronary artery disease, as evidenced by elevated left ventricular filling pressures. Histologically, these patients have increased amounts of collagen, glycoprotein, triglycerides, and cholesterol in the myocardial interstitium, and in some cases intimal thickening, hyaline deposition, and inflammatory changes have been observed in small intramural arteries. While these changes alone seldom result in clinical heart failure, it is likely that they contribute to the excessive cardiovascular morbidity and mortality of diabetics. There is some evidence that insulin therapy results in an amelioration of the myocardial dysfunction.

MALNUTRITION AND THIAMINE DEFICIENCY (BERIBERI) Malnutrition (See Chap. 71) In patients whose intake of protein, calories, or both is severely deficient, the heart may become thin, pale, and flabby with myofibrillar atrophy and interstitial edema. The systolic pressure and cardiac output are low and the pulse pressure narrow. Generalized edema is common and is due to a combination of factors, including reduced serum oncotic pressure and myocardial dysfunction. Such profound states of malnutrition, termed *marasmus* in the case of caloric deficiency or *kwashiorkor* in the case of relative protein deficiency, are most common in underdeveloped countries. However, significant nutritional heart disease may also occur in developed nations, particularly in patients with severe cardiac failure in whom gastrointestinal hypoperfusion and venous congestion may cause anorexia and malabsorption. Open-heart surgery poses an increased risk in such patients, who may benefit from preoperative intensive hyperalimentation. Deficient nutrients and minerals should be replaced gradually since rapid expansion of the intravascular space may stress the weakened heart and result in overt congestive heart failure.

Thiamine deficiency (See Chap. 76) In many cases, malnutrition is accompanied by thiamine deficiency, although this hypovitaminosis may also occur in the presence of an adequate protein and caloric intake, particularly in the Far East, where polished rice deficient in thiamine may be a major dietary component. The widespread use of thiamine-enriched flour in western nations confines this disease primarily to alcoholics and food faddists. Clinically, there is usually evidence of generalized malnutrition, peripheral neuropathy, glossitis, and anemia. The characteristic cardiovascular syndrome is that of high-output heart failure with tachycardia, increased cardiac output, and often elevated filling pressures in the left and right sides of the heart. It appears that the major cause of the high-output state is vasomotor depression, the precise mechanism of which is not understood, but which leads to a reduced systemic vascular resistance. The cardiac examination reveals a wide pulse pressure, tachycardia, a third heart sound, and, frequently, a systolic murmur at the apex. The electrocardiogram may show decreased voltage, a prolonged QT interval, and T-wave abnormalities; the chest x-ray generally shows a large heart with signs of congestive heart failure. The response to thiamine is often dramatic, with an increase in systemic vascular resistance, decrease in cardiac output, clearing of pulmonary congestion, and a reduction in heart size often occurring in 12 to 48 h. Although the response to digitalis and diuretics may be poor prior to thiamine therapy, these agents may be important *after* thiamine is given, since the left ventricle may not be capable of dealing with the increased workload presented by the return of vascular tone.

OBESITY (See Chap. 72) Although not defined as a disease per se, severe obesity is associated with an increase in cardiovascular morbidity and mortality, due in part to hypertension, glucose intolerance, and atherosclerotic coronary artery disease, all of which are more prevalent in obese patients. In addition, these patients have a distinct abnormality of the cardiovascular system characterized by increases in total and central blood volumes, cardiac output, and left ventricular filling pressure. It appears that cardiac output is elevated in order to help supply the metabolic needs of the excessive adipose tissue. Left ventricular filling pressure is often at the upper limits of normal and rises excessively with exercise. As a result of chronic volume and pressure overload, eccentric cardiac hypertrophy with cardiac dilation and abnormal ventricular function may develop. Pathologically, there is left and, in some cases, right ventricular hypertrophy and generalized cardiac enlargement, which is not due simply to fatty infiltration of the myocardium. Clinically, these patients may develop pulmonary congestion, peripheral edema, and exercise intolerance, findings which may be difficult to recognize in massively obese patients. Weight reduction is the most effective therapy and results in reduction in blood volume and in return of cardiac output toward normal. Digitalis, sodium restriction, and diuretics may also be useful. This form of heart disease should be distinguished from the Pickwickian syndrome (Chap. 217), which may share several of the cardiovascular features but, in addition, frequently has components of central apnea, hypoxemia, pulmonary hypertension, and cor pulmonale.

THYROID DISEASE (See Chap. 316) Thyroid hormone exerts a major influence on the cardiovascular system by a number of direct and indirect mechanisms, and not surprisingly, cardiovascular effects are prominent in both hypo- and hyperthyroidism. Thyroid hormone causes increases in total-body metabolism and oxygen consumption that indirectly place an increased workload on the heart. In addition, although the exact mechanism has not been defined, thyroid hormone exerts direct inotropic, chronotropic, and dromotropic effects that are similar to those seen with adrenergic stimulation (e.g., tachycardia, increased cardiac output). It has been shown that thyroid hormone increases the synthesis of myosin and of Na^+,K^+-ATPase, as well as the density of myocardial beta-adrenergic receptors.

Hyperthyroidism Excess thyroid hormone results in increases in heart rate, cardiac output, stroke volume, pulse pressure, and measures of left ventricular contractility. Patients may present with palpitations, systolic hypertension, fatigue, or, in patients with underlying heart disease, angina or heart failure. Sinus tachycardia is found in about 40 percent of patients, and atrial fibrillation in about 15 percent. Other findings include a hyperactive precordium, an increase in the intensity of the first heart sound and the pulmonic component of the second heart sound, and a third heart sound. An increased incidence of mitral valve prolapse has been associated with hyperthyroidism, and in some cases there may be a midsystolic murmur heard best at the left sternal border with or without a systolic ejection click. A systolic scratchy sound, the *Means-Lerman scratch*, may occasionally be heard at the left second intercostal space during expiration and is thought to result from the rubbing of the hyperdynamic pericardium against the pleura. Elderly patients with hyperthyroidism may present with only the cardiovascular manifestations of thyrotoxicosis, which may be resistant to therapy until the hyperthyroidism is controlled. Although there is some evidence that hyperthyroidism per se can result in myocardial dysfunction, angina pectoris and congestive heart failure are unusual, unless there is coexistent underlying heart disease, and in many cases will resolve with therapy of the hyperthyroidism.

Hypothyroidism There is a reduction in cardiac output, stroke volume, heart rate, blood pressure, and pulse pressure. In about one-third of patients there is a pericardial effusion which only rarely results in tamponade. Increased capillary permeability results in pleural and pericardial effusions, but only rarely results in tamponade. Other clinical signs include cardiomegaly, bradycardia, weak arterial pulses, and distant heart sounds. As a result of earlier detection and treatment of hypothyroidism, these overt signs are commonly absent, and the major findings may be exertional dyspnea and easy fatigability. Although the signs and symptoms of myxedema may suggest the diagnosis of congestive heart failure, in the absence of other cardiac disease, myocardial failure is uncommon. Biochemical abnormalities, including elevations of creatine kinase, serum glutamic oxaloacetic transaminase, and lactic dehydrogenase, may lead to a mistaken diagnosis of myocardial infarction. The electrocardiogram generally shows sinus bradycardia and low voltage and may show prolongation of the QT interval, decreased P-wave voltage, prolonged AV conduction time, intraventricular conduction disturbances, and nonspecific ST-T-wave abnormalities. Chest x-ray may show cardiomegaly, often with a ''water bottle'' configuration, pleural effusions, and, in some cases, evidence of congestive heart failure. Pathologically, the heart is pale, dilated, and flabby, often with myofibrillar swelling, loss of striations, and interstitial fibrosis.

Patients with hypothyroidism frequently have elevations of cholesterol and triglycerides and severe atherosclerotic coronary artery disease. Prior to treatment with thyroid hormone, patients with hypothyroidism frequently do not have angina pectoris, presumably because of the low metabolic demands made by their condition. However, such patients, especially when elderly, are prone to angina and myocardial infarction during replacement of thyroid hormone, and this should always be done with extreme care, starting with very low doses which are increased gradually.

MALIGNANT CARCINOID (See Chap. 262) These tumors elaborate a variety of vasoactive amines (e.g., serotonin), kinins, indoles, and other substances which are believed to be responsible for the diarrhea, flushing, and labile blood pressure seen in these patients. The cardiac lesions due to gastrointestinal carcinoids are almost exclusively in the right side of the heart and occur only when there are hepatic metastases, suggesting that the substance responsible for the cardiac lesions is inactivated by passage through the liver and lungs. Similar lesions occur in the left side of the heart when there is a right-to-left shunt or the tumor is located in the lungs. Fibrous plaques are found on the endothelium of the cardiac chambers, valves, and great vessels. These plaques, which result in distortion of the cardiac valves, consist of smooth muscle cells imbedded in a stroma of acid mucopolysaccharide and collagen, and presumably result from healing of endothelial injury. The clinical syndrome is most often that of tricuspid regurgitation, pulmonic stenosis, or both. In some cases a high-output state may occur, presumably as a result of a decrease in systemic vascular resistance due to a vasoactive substance released by the tumor. Progression of the cardiac lesions does not appear to be affected by treatment with serotonin antagonists, and in some severely symptomatic patients valve replacement is indicated. Coronary artery spasm, presumably due to a circulating vasoactive substance, may occur in patients with carcinoid syndrome.

PHEOCHROMOCYTOMA (See Chap. 318) In addition to causing hypertension, which may be labile or sustained, the high circulating levels of catecholamines may also cause direct myocardial injury. Focal myocardial necrosis and inflammatory cell infiltration are seen in about 50 percent of patients who die with pheochromocytoma and may contribute to clinically significant left ventricular failure and pulmonary edema. In addition, hypertension results in left ventricular hypertrophy.

RHEUMATOID ARTHRITIS AND THE COLLAGEN VASCULAR DISEASES **Rheumatoid arthritis** (See Chap. 270) There may be inflammation of any or all parts of the heart in patients with rheumatoid arthritis. *Pericarditis* is the most common cause of clinically apparent disease and may be found in 30 to 50 percent of all patients with rheumatoid arthritis, particularly those with subcutaneous nodules, if carefully searched for by echocardiography or at postmortem examination. However, only a small fraction of these patients will have clinical evidence of pericarditis, which usually follows a benign course, but occasionally may progress to cardiac tamponade or constrictive pericarditis. The pericardial fluid is generally an exudate, with decreased concentrations of complement and glucose and elevated cholesterol. Treatment is directed at the underlying rheumatoid arthritis and may include glucocorticoids. Pericardiectomy is usually required in cases of tamponade or persistent effusion. *Coronary arteritis* with intimal inflammation and edema is present in about 20 percent of cases but only rarely results in angina pectoris or myocardial infarction. The cardiac valves, most often the mitral and aortic, may be involved by inflammation and granuloma formation which in some cases may cause clinically significant regurgitation due to valve deformity. Myocarditis rarely results in cardiac dysfunction.

Seronegative arthropathies The seronegative arthropathies (Chaps. 274 and 283), ankylosing spondylitis, Reiter's syndrome, psoriatic arthritis, and the arthritides associated with ulcerative colitis and regional enteritis may be accompanied by a pancarditis and proximal aortitis; the latter may result in aortic regurgitation and may extend into the anterior mitral valve ring and/or AV node. Both aortic regurgitation and AV block are more common in patients with peripheral joint involvement and long-standing disease; and treatment with aortic valve replacement and permanent pacemaker placement may be required. Up to one-fifth of patients with peripheral joint involvement and disease for more than 30 years have significant aortic regurgitation. Occasionally, aortic regurgitation precedes the onset of arthritis, and, therefore, the diagnosis of a seronegative arthritis should be considered in young males with isolated aortic regurgitation.

Systemic lupus erythematosus (SLE) (See Chap. 269) Pericarditis is common, occurring in about two-thirds of patients, and generally pursues a benign course, although rarely tamponade or constriction may result. The characteristic *endocardial lesions* of SLE, described by Libman and Sacks, consist of wartlike lesions most often located at the angles of the AV valves or on the ventricular surface of the mitral valve. Hemodynamically important valvular regurgitation is rare. Myocarditis generally parallels the activity of the disease, and although common histologically, seldom results in clinical heart failure unless associated with hypertension. Although arteritis of large coronary arteries may rarely result in myocardial ischemia, there is also an increased frequency of coronary atherosclerosis which may be related to hypertension or glucocorticoid therapy.

TRAUMATIC HEART DISEASE

Cardiac damage may be due to both penetrating and nonpenetrating injuries. The most frequent cause of a *nonpenetrating injury* is impact of the chest against the steering wheel of an automobile. Serious injury of the heart may ensue even though no external sign of thoracic trauma is evident. Although the commonest injury is myocardial contusion, any structure of the heart may be affected by the trauma. If the valvular apparatus is ruptured, a loud heart murmur produced by valvular regurgitation may appear, followed by the development of rapidly progressive heart failure. The most serious consequence of nonpenetrating injury is rupture, either of the atria or of the ventricles, which is generally fatal. Hemopericardium may also follow tearing of a pericardial vessel or coronary artery.

Myocardial contusion may cause arrhythmias, bundle branch block, or electrocardiographic abnormalities resembling those of infarction, and so it is important to bear trauma in mind as a cause of otherwise unexplained electrocardiographic changes. Similarly, myocardial contusion may produce positive radionuclide scans and regional impairment of ventricular function, as occurs in myocardial infarction (Chap. 177). Pericardial effusion may occur weeks or even months after the accident. In these cases, the pericardial effusion is a manifestation of the postcardiac injury syndrome, which resembles the postpericardiotomy syndrome (Chap. 193).

Acute myocardial failure resulting from rupture of a valve usually requires operative correction. Myocardial infarction due to trauma is treated similarly to that due to ischemic heart disease (Chap. 189). Pericardial hemorrhage often leads to constriction which must be treated by decortication.

Penetrating injuries of the heart, produced by bullets or stab wounds, usually result in immediate or very rapid death because of hemopericardium or massive hemorrhage. However, sometimes the patient survives the acute incident and presents with a cardiac murmur and congestive heart failure. A left-to-right shunt due to traumatic ventricular septal defect, aortopulmonary artery fistula, or coronary arteriovenous fistula may be suspected and confirmed by cardiac catheterization and angiocardiography. Operation is indicated if hemodynamically significant abnormalities are present or if a foreign body, e.g., a bullet, is lodged in the heart. Immediate thoracotomy should be carried out if there is cardiac tamponade and/or shock, whether the trauma was penetrating or nonpenetrating. Pericardiocentesis may be helpful in patients with tamponade, but usually only as a holding maneuver. Patients who suffer penetrating injuries of the heart should be carefully examined several weeks after the event to rule out a ventricular septal defect or mitral regurgitation that may have gone undetected at the time of emergency surgery.

Rupture of the aorta is a common consequence of chest trauma. Indeed, rupture of the aorta at the isthmus or just above the aortic valve is the most common vascular deceleration injury. The clinical presentation is similar to that in aortic dissection (Chap. 197). The arterial pressure and pulse amplitude may be increased in the upper extremities and decreased in the lower extremities, and on chest roentgenogram there may be widening of the mediastinum. Occasionally, the rupture is limited by the aortic adventitia and results in a silent false aneurysm that may be discovered months or years after the injury. When great vessel rupture is due to a penetrating injury, there is usually a hemothorax and, less often, a hemopericardium. Hematoma formation may compress major vessels, and arteriovenous fistulae may be formed, sometimes resulting in high-output congestive heart failure.

REFERENCES

AYZENBERG O et al: Beriberi heart disease. S Afr Med J 68:263, 1985

COHN PF, BRAUNWALD E: Traumatic heart disease, in *Heart Disease*, 3d ed, E Braunwald (ed). Philadelphia, Saunders, 1988, p 1535

COLUCCI WS, BRAUNWALD E: Primary tumors of the heart, in *Heart Disease*, 3d ed, E Braunwald (ed). Philadelphia, Saunders, 1988, p 1470

DOHERTY NE, SIEGEL J: The cardiovascular manifestations of systemic lupus erythematosus. Am Heart J 110:1257, 1985

FEIN FS, SONNENBLICK EH: Diabetic cardiomyopathy. Progr Cardiovasc Dis 27:255, 1985

FYKE FE et al: Primary cardiac tumors: Experience with 30 consecutive patients since the introduction of two-dimensional echocardiography. J Am Coll Cardiol 5:1465, 1985

KLEIN I, LEVEY GS: New perspectives on thyroid hormone, catecholamines, and the heart. Am J Med 76:167, 1984

LOCKWOOD WB, BROGHAMER WL JR: The changing prevalence of secondary cardiac neoplasms as related to cancer therapy. Cancer 15:2659, 1980

MATTOX K et al: Cardiac evaluation following heart injury. J Trauma 25:758, 1985

ROSS EM, ROBERTS WC: The carcinoid syndrome: Comparison of 21 necropsy subjects with carcinoid heart disease to 15 necropsy subjects without carcinoid heart disease. Am J Med 79:339, 1985

VIDAILLET HJ et al: "Syndrome myxoma": A subset of patients with cardiac myxoma associated with pigmented skin lesions and peripheral and endocrine neoplasms. Br Heart J 57:247, 1987

STOLLERMAN E: Rheumatic fever, connective tissue disorders and heart disease, in *Heart Disease*, 2d ed, E Braunwald (ed). Philadelphia, Saunders, 1988, p 1641

section 2 Disorders of the vascular system

195 ATHEROSCLEROSIS AND OTHER FORMS OF ARTERIOSCLEROSIS

EDWIN L. BIERMAN

Arteriosclerosis, a generic term for thickening and hardening of the arterial wall, is responsible for the majority of deaths in the United States and most westernized societies. One type of arteriosclerosis is *atherosclerosis,* the disorder of the larger arteries that underlies most *coronary artery disease, aortic aneurysm,* and *arterial disease of the lower extremities* and also plays a major role in *cerebrovascular disease.* Atherosclerosis is by far the leading cause of death in the United States, both above and below age 65 (Table 195-1).

Other types of arteriosclerosis include focal calcific arteriosclerosis (*Mönckeberg's sclerosis*) and *arteriolosclerosis.* The major arterial diseases other than arteriosclerosis include *congenital structural defects, inflammatory* or granulomatous diseases (e.g., syphilitic aortitis), and disorders affecting mainly the smaller vessels, such as *hypersensitivity* or autoimmune diseases.

THE NORMAL ARTERY

STRUCTURE The normal artery wall consists of three reasonably well-defined layers: the intima, the media, and the adventitia.

Intima A single continuous layer of *endothelial cells* lines the lumen of all arteries. The intima is delimited on its outer aspect by a perforated tube of elastic tissue, the *internal elastic lamina.* This tube of elastic tissue is particularly prominent in the large elastic arteries and the medium-caliber muscular arteries, and it disappears in capillaries. The endothelial cells are attached to one another by a series of junctional complexes and are also attached, apparently somewhat tenuously, to an underlying meshwork of loose connective tissue, the *basal lamina.* These lining endothelial cells normally form a barrier that controls the entry of substances from the blood into the artery wall. Such substances usually enter the cells by specific transport systems. Normally, no other cell type is present in the intima of most arteries.

TABLE 195-1 Deaths by cause in the United States, 1986

	No. of deaths, thousands			
	Below age 65		Age 65 and above	
Causes of death	Male	Female	Male	Female
All causes	396	222	709	779
All cardiovascular diseases	119	54	357	438
Ischemic heart disease	71	25	203	222
Cerebrovascular disease	11	10	48	81
Hypertensive disease*	1	1	3	4
All infectious disease	5	3	1	2
All cancer	86	75	165	143
Accidents	52	17	13	12

* A substantial proportion of deaths of hypertensive persons occurs with ischemic heart disease or cerebrovascular disease; such deaths are classified in those categories.
SOURCE: National Center of Health Statistics, *Vital Statistics Report, Final Mortality Statistics, 1986.*

Media The media consists of only one cell type, the *smooth-muscle cell,* arranged in either a single layer (as in small muscular arteries) or multiple lamellae (as in elastic arteries). These cells are surrounded by small amounts of collagen and elastic fibers, which they elaborate, and usually take the pattern of diagonal concentric spirals through the vessel wall. They are closely apposed to one another and may be attached by junctional complexes. The smooth-muscle cell appears to be the major connective tissue–forming cell of the artery wall, producing collagen, elastic fibers, and proteoglycans. In that sense it is analogous to the fibroblast in skin, the osteoblast in bone, and the chondroblast in cartilage. The media is bounded on the luminal side by the *internal elastic lamina* and on the abluminal side by a less continuous sheet of elastic tissue, the *external elastic lamina.* In *elastic arteries,* like the aorta and the major pulmonary arteries, elastic lamellae are prominent. Such arteries expand and increase their elastic tension with the pulse of systole. In diastole, the elastic fibers recoil, helping to propel the blood distally and progressively damping the pulsatile character of flow toward more terminal vessels. In *muscular arteries,* in which smooth-muscle cells predominate, peripheral flow is regulated, particularly in arterioles, by contraction (vasoconstriction) and relaxation (vasodilatation). Located about midway through the media of most arteries is a ''nutritional watershed.'' The outer portion is nourished from the small blood vessels (vasa vasorum) in the adventitia; the inner layers receive their nutrients from the lumen.

Adventitia The outermost layer of the artery is the adventitia, which is delimited on the luminal aspect by the external elastic lamina. This external coat consists of a loose interwoven admixture of collagen bundles, elastic fibers, smooth-muscle cells, and fibroblasts. This layer also contains the vasa vasorum and nerves.

METABOLISM AND FUNCTION The artery wall is a metabolically active organ that must meet a steady demand for energy to maintain smooth-muscle tension and endothelial cell function and to repair and replenish tissue constituents. The mechanical forces on the arterial wall are complex, and considerable tensile stresses are imposed on it, mainly by hydraulic force. Shear or frictional stresses are especially prominent near the entrance regions of branches. The form and manner in which these forces are dissipated depend upon flow, the amount of elastic tension developed, and the tethering or external support provided by surrounding structures. Arteries are also permeable pipes, which constantly exchange fluid and solutes with the blood they carry.

Maintenance of the endothelial cell lining is critical. Endothelial cell turnover occurs at a slow rate but may be accelerated in focal areas by changing patterns of flow along the vessel wall. When intact, these cells selectively control the passage of circulating substances by active transport (endocytosis and exocytosis) through their cytoplasm, and they elaborate connective tissue components to form their own substratum. In addition, intact endothelial cells function to prevent clotting partly by elaboration of a particular prostaglandin (prostacyclin or PGI_2) that inhibits platelet function, thereby enhancing unimpeded flow of blood. When the lining is damaged, platelets adhere to it, in part as the result of production of a different class of prostaglandins, the thromboxanes, and form a clot; endothelial cells function in the clotting process by elaboration of key substances, including factor VIII.

The metabolism of arteries reflects the biochemistry of smooth-muscle cells. Arterial smooth-muscle cells form abundant collagen, elastic fibers, soluble and insoluble elastin, and glucosaminoglycans (mainly dermatan sulfate). Multiple anabolic and catabolic pathways are present. These cells metabolize glucose by both anaerobic and aerobic glycolysis. A variety of catabolic enzymes are present including fibrinolysins, mixed-function oxidases, and lysosomal hydrolases. Because of the prominence of lipids in atherosclerotic lesions, much attention has been directed to lipid metabolism in arteries. Arterial wall cells can synthesize fatty acids, cholesterol, phospholipids, and triglycerides from endogenous substrates to satisfy their structural needs (membrane replenishment), but smooth-muscle cells appear preferentially to utilize lipids from plasma lipoproteins transported into the wall. Circulating lipoproteins traverse endothelial cells in pinocytotic vesicles. Smooth-muscle cells possess specific high-affinity surface receptors for certain apoproteins on the surface of lipid-rich lipoproteins, thus facilitating the entry of lipoproteins into the cell by adsorptive endocytosis. As has been shown for cultured skin fibroblasts, in arterial smooth-muscle cells these vesicles fuse with lysosomes, resulting in catabolism of lipoprotein components (Chap. 326). Free cholesterol entering the cell in this manner inhibits endogenous cholesterol synthesis, facilitates its own esterification, and partially limits further entry of cholesterol by regulating the number of lipoprotein receptors. However, lipoprotein cholesterol can gain entry into arterial smooth muscle cells by receptor-independent pathways, potentially causing cholesterol ester accumulation.

Thus, many complex and interrelated metabolic processes are present in arterial wall cells. Although some of these may play a role in the production of arteriosclerosis, no one biochemical reaction can be singled out as culpable. Physiologic factors, such as transfer processes across the endothelial lining, the flux of oxygen and substrates from both the luminal and adventitial sides of the wall, and the reverse flow of catabolic products, need to be considered as well. The ability of the arterial wall to maintain the integrity of its endothelium, prevent platelet aggregation, prevent adherence of blood mononuclear cells, prevent cholesterol accumulation, and ensure the nutrition of its middle portion may be the critical determinants of the arteriosclerotic process.

CHANGES WITH AGING The major change that occurs with normal aging in the arterial wall in humans is a slow, apparently continuous, symmetric increase in the thickness of the intima. This intimal thickening results from a gradual accumulation of smooth-muscle cells (presumably resulting from migration of these cells from the media and their subsequent proliferation) surrounded by additional connective tissue. In the nondiseased artery wall, lipid content, mainly cholesterol ester and phospholipid (particularly sphingomyelin), also progressively increases with age. Phospholipid synthesis rises with aging (perhaps in response to the need for more membrane formation for plasma membranes, vesicles, lysosomes, and other intracellular organelles) followed by a compensatory increase in activity of all phospholipases except sphingomyelinase. While most of the phospholipid in the normal artery wall appears to be derived from in situ synthesis, the cholesterol ester that accumulates with aging appears to be derived from plasma, since it contains principally linoleic acid, the major plasma cholesterol ester fatty acid. Furthermore, low-density lipoproteins (LDL) are immunologically detectable in the intima of normal arteries in direct relation to their concentration in plasma. It has been estimated that between the second and sixth decade, the normal intima accumulates approximately 25 μmol (10 mg) cholesterol per gram of tissue. Thus, as the normal artery ages, smooth-muscle cells and connective tissue accumulate diffusely in the intima, leading to progressive thickening of this layer, coupled with progressive accumulation of sphingomyelin and cholesterol linoleate. This diffuse age-related intimal thickening is to be distinguished from focal discrete raised fibromuscular plaques, a characteristic feature of atherosclerosis.

Functionally, these changes with aging result in gradually increasing rigidity of vessels. The larger arteries may become dilated, elongated, and tortuous, and aneurysms may form in areas of an encroaching degenerating arteriosclerotic plaque. Such "wear-and-tear" changes are frequently proportional to the vessel diameter and correlated with branching, curvature, and anatomic points of attachment. The amount of external support also determines the ability of vessels, weakened by loss of elasticity, to withstand hydrostatic pressure. The unsupported cerebral arteries may be particularly vulnerable in this regard. Although senescence is accompanied by the intimal thickening that is a feature of localized atheromatosis, the changes of aging and arteriosclerosis appear to be separate and distinct processes.

NONATHEROMATOUS FORMS OF ARTERIOSCLEROSIS

Atherosclerosis involves primarily the intimal layer and occurs most commonly in the abdominal aorta and its large renal and lower extremity branches, the coronary arteries, and the cerebral vasculature. It may accompany or accelerate the other major forms of arteriosclerosis, *focal calcification* and *arteriolosclerosis* (Table 195-2).

FOCAL CALCIFICATION Not to be confused with atherosclerosis is focal calcification of the media, particularly in the medium-sized muscular arteries. This type of arteriosclerosis is called *Mönckeberg's sclerosis* and is common in the lower extremities, upper extremities, and the arterial supply of the genital tract in both sexes. This disorder is rare in individuals below age 50 and affects both sexes indiscriminately. The process involves degeneration of smooth-muscle cells, followed by calcium deposition. The vessels become hard and tortuous, so that palpable vessels such as the radial artery can be felt as rigid tubes. Its characteristic radiologic appearance consists of regular concentric calcifications in cross section and a railroad track in longitudinal section, commonly seen in vessels in the pelvis, legs, and feet. The medial changes alone do not narrow the lumen, have little effect on the circulation, and have relatively little clinical significance. However, in the lower extremities, medial arterial calcification is often associated with atherosclerosis, leading to arterial occlusion. These changes are common in the elderly and in patients on long-term corticosteroid therapy, but in individuals with diabetes mellitus, focal calcification may be accelerated and severe. It is much more common in diabetics with neuropathy, and sympathetic denervation of medial smooth muscle has been implicated in its etiology.

Focal calcification also can produce the arteriosclerotic aortic valve in the elderly. Progressive calcium deposition occurs on the aortic surface of normal trileaflet aortic valves with age, resulting in a spectrum of clinical findings ranging from an innocent systolic murmur to severe calcific aortic stenosis (Chap. 188).

ARTERIOLOSCLEROSIS This disorder involves hyaline and degenerative changes affecting both the intima and media of small

TABLE 195-2 Disorders associated with early arteriosclerosis

ATHEROSCLEROSIS
Diabetes mellitus
Hypertension
Familial hypercholesterolemia
Familial combined hyperlipidemia
Familial dysbetalipoproteinemia
Hypothyroidism
Werner's syndrome
Cholesterol ester storage disease
Systemic lupus erythematosus
NONATHEROMATOUS ARTERIOSCLEROSIS
Diabetes mellitus
Chronic renal insufficiency
Chronic vitamin D intoxication
Pseudoxanthoma elasticum
Idiopathic arterial calcification in infancy
Aortic valvular calcification in the elderly
Werner's syndrome
Homocystinuria

arteries and arterioles, particularly in the spleen, pancreas, adrenal, and kidney. In the kidney, but not necessarily elsewhere, arteriolosclerosis is almost invariably associated with hypertension. Lesser degrees of sustained hypertension characteristically cause *hyalinization* of renal arterioles; more severe or malignant hypertension produces a typical *fibrous and elastic hyperplasia*, and even necrosis, of the media and intima.

ATHEROSCLEROSIS

LESIONS Morbid anatomy Atherosclerosis is a patchy nodular type of arteriosclerosis. The lesions are commonly classified as *fatty streaks, fibrous plaques*, and *complicated lesions. Fatty streaks* may be the earliest lesions of atherosclerosis. They are characterized by an accumulation of lipid-filled smooth-muscle cells and macrophages (foam cells) and fibrous tissue in focal areas of the intima. They are stained distinctly by fat-soluble dyes but may be visible without staining as yellowish or whitish patches on the intimal surface. The lipid is mainly cholesterol oleate, partly derived from synthesis in situ. The fatty streak is usually sessile and causes little obstruction and no symptoms. The lesion is universal, appearing in various segments of the arterial tree at different ages beginning in the aorta in infancy. In all children, regardless of race, sex, or environment, fatty streaks are present in the aorta by age 10 and increase to occupy as much as 30 to 50 percent of the aortic surface by age 25, but they do not appear to extend further with aging. Despite a presumed relation between fatty streaks and fibrous atherosclerotic plaques, aortic fatty streaks are not correlated with the location and extent of fibrous lesions. In the coronary arteries, the extent of fatty streaks may be a better indicator of the development of clinically significant raised lesions later in life. They are usually observed by age 15 and continue to involve more surface area with increasing age. Fatty streaks in the cerebral arteries are also present in all populations, develop during the third and fourth decade, and are more extensive in those populations having a higher incidence of cerebrovascular disease. It is generally believed that fatty streaks may be reversible, but the evidence is inconclusive.

Fibrous plaques, also called raised lesions or pearly plaques, are palpably elevated areas of intimal thickening and represent the most characteristic lesion of advancing atherosclerosis. They do not share with fatty streaks the ubiquitous distribution among populations. These plaques first appear in the abdominal aorta, coronary arteries, and carotid arteries in the third decade and increase progressively with age. They appear in men before women, in the aorta before the coronary arteries, and much later in the vertebral and intracranial cerebral arteries. Reasons for the difference in susceptibility of various segments of the arterial tree and the nonuniform distribution of lesions are not known. Typically, the fibrous plaque is firm, elevated, and dome-shaped, with an opaque glistening surface that bulges into the lumen. It consists of a central core of extracellular lipid and necrotic cell debris ("gruel") covered by a fibromuscular layer or cap containing large numbers of smooth-muscle cells, macrophages, and collagen. Thus the plaque is much thicker than is normal intima. Although the lipid, like that of fatty streaks, is mainly cholesterol ester, the principal esterified fatty acid is linoleic rather than oleic. Thus plaque cholesterol ester composition differs from fatty streaks but resembles plasma lipoproteins.

The *complicated lesion* is a calcified fibrous plaque containing various degrees of necrosis, thrombosis, and ulceration. These are the lesions frequently associated with symptoms. With increasing necrosis and accumulation of gruel, the arterial wall progressively weakens, and rupture of the intima can occur, causing aneurysm and hemorrhage. Arterial emboli can form when fragments of plaque dislodge into the lumen. Stenosis and impaired organ function result from gradual occlusion as plaques thicken and thrombi form.

Localization Although the term *generalized atherosclerosis* is commonly used clinically, lesions are actually irregularly distributed; different vessels are involved at different ages and to varying degrees. The aorta, especially its abdominal portion, is involved earliest and most severely by atherosclerotic lesions, and it is the bellwether of lesions elsewhere. The *aorta* is usually most heavily involved in its abdominal portion, about the orifices of its branches (particularly at the level of the coronary and intercostal arteries), in the aortic arch, and frequently at its bifurcation into the iliac arteries. There is more atherosclerosis in the lower than in the upper limbs. In the legs, the incidence decreases peripherally, as the musculoelastic vessels give way to large muscular arteries and these become smaller vessels, such as the plantar or digital arteries. Plaques and thromboses are particularly common in the *femoral* artery, in Hunter's canal, and in the *popliteal* artery just above the knee joint. The *anterior* and *posterior tibial* arteries are often occluded together, but in different sites—the posterior where it rounds the internal malleolus and the anterior where it is superficial and becomes the dorsalis pedis artery. The peroneal artery, which is well embedded in muscle, often escapes when other major vessels are occluded, and it may be the main blood supply to the extremity (*peroneal leg*). Atherosclerosis in abdominal branches, except for the renal and mesenteric arteries, causes less difficulty than in coronary and cerebral vessels.

In the *coronary arteries*, raised lesions are most prominent in the main stems, the highest incidence being a short distance beyond the ostia. Atherosclerosis is nearly always found in the epicardial (extramural) portions of the vessels, while the intramural coronary arteries are spared. Coronary atherosclerosis is often diffuse. The degree to which the lumen is narrowed varies, but once the process is present, all the intima of the extramural portions of the vessel is usually involved. A single tiny plaque occluding an otherwise normal coronary artery is rare. Selective involvement of the coronary arteries may relate to the unique hemodynamic forces, unlike those of other major arteries, resulting from greater flow in diastole than systole. The implications of these flow patterns for atherogenesis are as yet unknown. Typical atheromatous fibrous plaques also develop in saphenous vein aortocoronary bypass grafts.

In the cervical and cerebral arteries the distribution of atherosclerosis is patchy, as it may be in other arteries. It first appears in the base of the brain in the carotid, basilar, and vertebral arteries. The proximal portion of the internal carotid artery in the neck is a site of special predilection. There is a concentration of lesions near bifurcations. Atherosclerosis in the *pulmonary artery* bears no relation to the severity of the disease in the aorta or other systemic arteries. There is some involvement in about half of adults over 50 years of age who have no reason to have pulmonary hypertension. Pulmonary hypertension per se, however, is associated with medial hypertrophy, intimal thickening, and great acceleration of atheroma formation.

THEORIES OF ATHEROGENESIS One generally accepted theory for the pathogenesis of atherosclerosis consistent with a variety of experimental evidence is the *reaction to injury* hypothesis. According to this idea the endothelial cells lining the intima are exposed to repeated or continuing insults to their integrity. The injury to the endothelium may be subtle or gross, resulting in a loss of the ability of the cells to function normally or to attach to one another and to the underlying connective tissue. In the extreme, the cells may desquamate. Examples of types of "injury" to the endothelium include chemical injury, as in chronic hypercholesterolemia or homocystinemia, mechanical stress associated with hypertension, and immunologic injury, as may be seen after cardiac or renal transplantation. Loss of functional endothelial cells at susceptible sites in the arterial tree would lead to exposure of the subendothelial tissue to increased concentrations of plasma constituents and a sequence of events including platelet adherence, platelet aggregation and formation of microthrombi, and release of platelet granular components, including a potent mitogenic factor. This platelet factor, in conjunction with other plasma constituents, including lipoproteins and hormones such as insulin, could stimulate both the migration of medial smooth-muscle cells into the intima and their proliferation at these sites of injury. These proliferating smooth-muscle cells would deposit a connective tissue matrix and accumulate lipid, a process that would be particularly enhanced with hyperlipidemia. Macrophages derived from circulating blood monocytes can also accumulate lipid.

Adherence of monocytes to altered endothelial cells and their migration into the arterial wall to become resident macrophages may be the earliest cellular abnormality in atherogenesis. Thus repeated or chronic injury could lead to a slowly progressing lesion involving a gradual increase in smooth-muscle cells, macrophages, connective tissue, and lipid. Areas where the shearing stress on endothelial cells is increased, such as branch points or bifurcation of vessels, would be at greater risk. As the lesions progress and the intima becomes thicker, blood flow over the sites will be altered and will potentially place the lining endothelial cells at even greater risk for further injury, leading to an inexorable cycle of events culminating in the complicated lesion. However, a single or a few injurious episodes may lead to a proliferative response that could regress, in contrast to continued or chronic injury. This hypothesis of reaction to injury thus is consistent with the known intimal thickening observed during normal aging, would explain how many of the etiologic factors implicated in atherogenesis might enhance lesion formation, might explain how inhibitors of platelet aggregation could interfere with lesion formation, and fosters some optimism regarding the possibility of interrupting progression or even producing regression of these lesions.

Other theories of atherogenesis are not mutually exclusive. The *monoclonal hypothesis* suggests, on the basis of single isoenzyme types found in lesions, that the intimal proliferative lesions result from the multiplication of single, individual smooth-muscle cells, as do benign tumors. In this manner, mitogenic, and possibly mutagenic, factors that might stimulate smooth-muscle cell proliferation would act on single cells. Focal *clonal senescence* may explain how intrinsic aging processes contribute to atherosclerosis. According to this theory, the intimal smooth-muscle cells that proliferate to form an atheroma are normally under feedback control by diffusible agents (mitosis inhibitors) formed by the smooth-muscle cells in the contiguous media, and this feedback control system tends to fail with age as these controlling cells die and are not adequately replaced. This is consistent with the recent observation that cultured human arterial smooth-muscle cells, like fibroblasts, show a decline in their ability to replicate as a function of donor age. If this loss of replicative potential applies to a controlling population of smooth-muscle cells, then cells that are usually suppressed would be able to proliferate.

The *lysosomal theory* suggests that altered lysosomal function might contribute to atherogenesis. Since lysosomal enzymes can accomplish the generalized degradation of cellular components required for continuing renewal, this system has been implicated in cellular aging and the accumulation of lipofuscin or "age pigment." It has been suggested that increased deposition of lipids in arterial smooth-muscle cells may be related in part to a relative deficiency in the activity of lysosomal cholesterol ester hydrolase. This would result in increased accumulation of cholesterol esters within the cells, perhaps accentuated by lipid overloading of lysosomes, eventually leading to cell death and extracellular lipid deposition. Consonant with this idea, patients with the rare cholesterol ester storage disease, caused by a defect in lysosomal cholesterol ester hydrolase, may have accelerated atherosclerosis. However, lipid droplets in foam cells are often cytoplasmic rather than lysosomal.

RECOGNITION OF ATHEROSCLEROSIS Angiographic visualization of deformity in the lumen of a vessel remains the best presumptive test of silent atherosclerosis. Coronary angiography now permits visualization and assessment of arteries as small as 0.5 mm in diameter. Several sophisticated noninvasive techniques have been developed for demonstrating its presence. Doppler probes for measuring velocity and amount of blood flow have been used noninvasively and adapted to determine vessel outlines. Ultrasonic techniques are not yet clinically useful for detection of plaques in the coronary arteries.

Functional tests based on pathophysiologic or metabolic effects of a narrowed arterial lumen often give indirect clues. Assessment of electrocardiographic changes induced after standardized exercise is a relatively simple noninvasive aid to the diagnosis of coronary atherosclerosis with significant narrowing. Similarly, myocardial perfusion defects demonstrable with imaging techniques using radionuclides are usually attributable to atherosclerosis (Chap. 178). Digital plethysmography with exercise often unmasks significant atherosclerotic involvement of lower extremity arteries.

Radiographic demonstration of calcification in the location of arteries does not always indicate the presence of atherosclerosis. Although calcified coronary vessels usually indicate atherosclerosis, complete luminal obstruction may occur in the absence of any calcification. Calcification or beading of peripheral arteries is not correlated directly with atherosclerosis, but more likely reflects medial sclerosis. Abnormalities in retinal arterioles evident upon funduscopic examination are not well correlated with atherosclerosis in arteries. Thus despite the availability of a variety of tests, detection of atherosclerosis usually awaits one of the clinical complications attending a critical decrease of blood flow in an involved vessel. As yet there is no blood test for atherosclerosis. Knowledge of the prevalence and incidence of arteriosclerosis and most of the inferences concerning its causes are derived from tabulations of the appearance of its complications.

Ischemic heart disease (IHD), synonymous with *coronary heart disease* or *arteriosclerotic heart disease* (Chap. 190), is the most reliable indicator of atherosclerosis available today. Practically all patients with myocardial infarction, as defined by electrocardiographic and enzyme changes, have coronary atherosclerosis. Rare exceptions are due to congenital anomalies of the coronary vessels, emboli, or ostial occlusion due to other types of cardiac or vascular disease. Nontraumatic *sudden death* (Chap. 40) makes up a sizable portion of all deaths eventually certified as due to IHD. At autopsy, evidence of fresh myocardial infarction or of *coronary thrombosis* is usually absent. While ventricular fibrillation may have been due to sudden closure of a partially compromised vessel by a small thrombus or embolus, or to *spasm,* none of these need have preceded a fatal arrhythmia. The majority of victims of sudden death have had a previous diagnosis of IHD; the number who had diabetes or hypertension is also significant. In epidemiologic studies of IHD, *angina pectoris* and electrocardiographic changes attributable to ischemia without infarction are considered "softer end points" and treated separately.

Cerebrovascular disease (stroke) is a less reliable criterion for the presence of atherosclerosis. It includes *cerebral hemorrhage* and *cerebral thrombosis* (Chap. 351). Cerebral thrombosis, including infarction or softening without evidence of embolus, is usually due to atherosclerosis. On the other hand, cerebral hemorrhage is most often the result of congenital aneurysms or of vascular defects peculiar to hypertension and diabetes. Dissections of the aorta (Chap. 197), *peripheral vascular disease* (Chap. 198), thrombosis of other major vessels, and ischemic renal disease (Chap. 230) likewise are not used to determine the prevalence of atherosclerosis in a population or as an index of atherosclerosis elsewhere. Therefore, from an epidemiologic standpoint, consideration of atherosclerosis focuses on IHD.

INCIDENCE AND PREVALENCE According to the National Health Examination Survey, about 5 million Americans have IHD. It is the leading cause of death in males after age 35 and in all persons after age 45. Premature deaths from IHD, arbitrarily defined as those appearing before age 65, occur preponderantly in men, and a third of all deaths from IHD in males occur before age 65. In fact nearly all the excess premature mortality in American males is due to IHD. Between the ages of 35 and 55 the death rate is five times higher in white men than in white women in the United States. The exceptions are women with hypertension, diabetes, hyperlipidemia, or premature (usually iatrogenic) menopause, who are at increased risk and often share the risk of the male. For both sexes, there is more than a fivefold increase in the average annual incidence of myocardial infarction between ages 40 and 60. A distressing higher mortality rate in younger nonwhite women is probably due mainly

TABLE 195-3 Age-adjusted death rates by cause in the United States, 1968 and 1986

Cause of death	Rate per 100,000 population 1968	1986	Percent change
All deaths	744	542	−27
All cardiovascular diseases	362	175	−52
Ischemic heart disease	242	119	−51
Cerebrovascular disease	71	31	−56
Rheumatic heart disease	7	2	−69
Cancer	129	133	+3

SOURCE: The National Center for Health Statistics, *Vital Statistics Report, Final Mortality Statistics, 1986.*

TABLE 195-4 Risk factors for atherosclerosis

Male sex
Family history of premature IHD (before age 55 in a parent or sibling)
Hyperlipidemia
Cigarette smoking (currently smoking more than 10 cigarettes per day)
Hypertension
Low HDL-cholesterol [below 0.9 mmol/L (35 mg/dL)]
Diabetes mellitus
Personal history of cerebrovascular disease or occlusive peripheral vascular disease
Severe obesity (>30% overweight)
High lipoprotein (a)

to a greater incidence of hypertension in blacks. There is less difference between men and women in the prevalence of angina pectoris than in that of myocardial infarction; after age 65 more women than men have angina without a history of infarction.

Changing death rates Death rates in the United States from IHD rose appreciably between 1940 and 1960. Mortality peaked in 1963 and started to decline, with the rate of decline accelerating in recent years for all ages, for both sexes, and for whites and nonwhites. This recent decline in mortality from coronary atherosclerosis (Table 195-3) is the first recorded in American history and is almost unique among industrialized countries. In other parts of the world, including the Soviet Union and many countries in Eastern Europe, IHD death rates are still climbing. By 1986 the reduction in IHD death rate averaged more than 30 percent. The trend cannot be attributed to a single cause, but there has been a concurrent change in living habits including reduced cigarette smoking among middle-aged men, decreased consumption of animal fats and cholesterol, better control of hypertension, and improved treatment of IHD.

International comparisons In most industrialized countries, IHD is the major single cause of premature cardiovascular deaths. There are, however, marked differences in premature death rates among them. The seven having the highest rates in men between 35 and 74 years of age are Finland, Scotland, Northern Ireland, Australia, New Zealand, England, and the United States. Much lower age-adjusted death rates from IHD are found in Latin America and Japan. The rates in Japan are about one-sixth of those in the United States. Subsamples obtained in many countries convey the strong impression that upper socioeconomic classes that have adopted the culture of western industrialized countries have far more IHD than do lower socioeconomic classes. Among the most obvious cultural differences between these groups are total calories, fat content of the diet, and amount of physical work. Extensive epidemiologic studies have not revealed the reasons for differences between cultures that are superficially similar. Migrants to the United States tend to have a higher risk of death from premature IHD than do age-matched relatives who remain at home. Although there are many instances in which different ethnic groups in the same locality have widely differing prevalences of IHD, the available data suggest that cultural factors are more important than genetic determination of IHD. Nevertheless, genetic heterogeneity undoubtedly underlies many of the striking differences in susceptibility seen among individuals sharing the same ethnic and cultural setting.

ETIOLOGIC FACTORS A number of conditions and habits present more frequently in individuals who develop atherosclerosis than in the general population; these factors have been termed *risk factors*. The majority of people below age 65 afflicted with atherosclerosis have one or more identifiable risk factors other than aging per se (Table 195-4). The risk factor concept implies that a person with at least one risk factor is more likely to develop a clinical atherosclerotic event and is likely to do so earlier than a person with no risk factors. The presence of multiple risk factors further accelerates atherosclerosis. They vary in terms of importance in the population of the United States. Hypercholesterolemia, hypertension, and cigarette smoking may be the most potent factors involved in causation of atherosclerosis. Risk factors also vary in terms of their potential reversibility with current techniques of preventive management.

Thus age, gender, and genetic factors are currently considered to be irreversible risk factors, whereas continually emerging evidence suggests that elimination of cigarette smoking and treatment of hypertension reverses the high risk for atherosclerosis attributable to those factors. A major multicenter trial has shown that reduction of hypercholesterolemia reduces the risk of IHD. Life insurance policyholder data suggest that reduction of marked obesity reduces total mortality, presumably by diminishing the sequelae of atherosclerosis. Other potentially reversible factors are currently under study.

These factors are not mutually exclusive since they clearly interact. For example, obesity, particularly of the abdominal type (assessed by the waist/hip circumference ratio), appears to be causally associated with hypertension, hyperglycemia, hypercholesterolemia, and hypertriglyceridemia. Genetic factors may play a role by exerting direct effects on arterial wall cell structure and metabolism, or they may act indirectly via such factors as hypertension, hyperlipidemia, diabetes, and obesity. Aging appears to be one of the more complex factors associated with the development of atherosclerosis, since many of the risk factors in themselves are related to aging, e.g., elevated blood pressure, hyperglycemia, and hyperlipidemia. Thus in addition to the possible involvement of intrinsic aging in atherogenesis (perhaps through effects on arterial wall metabolism), a variety of associated metabolic factors are also age-dependent.

Hyperlipidemia Both *hypercholesterolemia* and *hypertriglyceridemia* appear to be important risk factors for atherosclerosis. While there is no absolute quantitative definition of hyperlipidemia, statistical definitions, based on the upper 5 or 10 percent of the distribution of plasma lipid levels within a population, are often used. Such definitions are likely to detect affected individuals from families with one of the familial hyperlipidemias or having hyperlipidemia associated with other diseases or drugs; they also are useful for prediction of emergence of premature atherosclerosis and institution of preventive measures. However, these upper limits of "normality" are too high for defining those cholesterol and triglyceride levels that are correlated with increasing risk of IHD in whole populations. Thus, correlations between the cholesterol concentrations in young men in North America and the incidence of premature IHD indicate that an increasing risk can be detected when the cholesterol level is higher than 5.20 mmol/L (200 mg/dL), a value close to the median for men from 40 to 49 years of age in this population. Extrapolation of similar data from other populations suggests that a cholesterol level at birth averages 1.5 mmol/L (60 mg/dL). Within a month the average has risen to about 3 mmol/L (120 mg/dL) and by the first year to 4.5 mmol/L (175 mg/dL). A second rise begins in the third decade and continues to about age 50 in men and somewhat later in women.

A similar age-related increase in plasma triglyceride levels is also observed. The increases in cholesterol are associated mainly with a rise in *low-density lipoprotein* (LDL) concentrations, the increases in triglyceride with a rise in *very low density lipoproteins* (VLDL). Adiposity may play a key role in this age-associated rise in triglyceride and cholesterol levels since the increases in triglyceride, cholesterol, and body weight with age in whole populations occur concurrently. In primitive people who remain thin throughout adulthood, plasma lipids do not increase with age. Metabolic mechanisms have been postulated whereby abdominal obesity, which is associated with insulin resistance of peripheral tissues and compensatory hyperinsulinemia, promotes enhanced production of triglyceride- and cholesterol-rich lipoproteins by the liver. Current concepts of plasma lipoprotein transport suggest that accumulation of cholesterol in the circulation may in part be secondary to excessive production of triglyceride-rich lipoproteins.

Hypercholesterolemia is associated unequivocally with increased incidence of premature IHD; however, its importance varies in relation to age. In the Framingham Study, cholesterol levels in men below age 40 were closely related to the future development of IHD; this relation was much less pronounced in older individuals. In the Multiple Risk Factor Intervention Trial (MRFIT), men with cholesterol levels above about 6 mmol/L (240 mg/dL) had more than a threefold increase in risk of IHD death compared to men with cholesterol levels below about 5 mmol/L (200 mg/dL). There is a continuous gradient of risk as the cholesterol level ascends. These data are supported by comparisons of the prevalence of IHD and cholesterol (or LDL) in many other populations. The relationship of triglycerides and VLDL to IHD is confounded by a rise in cholesterol as VLDL increases. Nevertheless, in several, but not all, population studies, increased triglycerides (or VLDL) are independently correlated with premature IHD.

Hypertriglyceridemia may be associated with premature atherosclerosis in some specific disorders; this association may not be apparent in studies of whole populations. Patients with high VLDL who come from families with familial combined hyperlipidemia appear to be at the same increased risk as those affected members of these families with elevated LDL levels. In contrast, patients with comparably elevated VLDL levels who come from families with pure monogenic familial hypertriglyceridemia do not appear to have an increased risk. In addition, high VLDL may increase the risk for premature atherosclerosis when associated with other risk factors for coronary artery disease, such as in diabetics, and in patients on chronic hemodialysis who smoke and are hypertensive. Individuals in whom remnant lipoproteins accumulate, with resulting elevations in both cholesterol and triglycerides (Chap. 326), also seem to be at risk for early development of atherosclerosis.

Some of these relationships were clarified in a comprehensive study in Seattle of the role of the genetics of hyperlipidemia in clinical atherosclerosis in which 500 consecutive survivors of myocardial infarction were tested. Hyperlipidemia was present in about one-third of the group. Approximately one-half of the males and two-thirds of the females below age 50 had either hypertriglyceridemia, hypercholesterolemia, or both. On the other hand, in individuals over age 70 the prevalence of atherosclerotic coronary disease was very high, yet virtually no males (and only about one-fourth of the females) had hyperlipidemia. Thus, in both sexes there appeared to be a progressive decline with age in the association of hyperlipidemia with myocardial infarction. More than half of the hyperlipidemic atherosclerotic survivors appeared to have simple monogenic familial disorders inherited as an autosomal dominant trait (*familial combined hyperlipidemia, familial hypertriglyceridemia,* and *familial hypercholesterolemia,* in descending order of frequency, Table 195-5). These simply inherited hyperlipidemias (particularly hypercholesterolemia) were more frequent in myocardial infarction survivors below age 60 than in those who were older. In contrast, nonmonogenic forms of hyperlipidemia occurred with equal frequency above and below age 60. Thus it appears that genes associated with the simply inherited hyperlipidemias accelerate changes seen with age, leading to atherosclerosis at an earlier age than usual. All studies indicate that hyperlipidemia is a more meaningful risk factor below age 50 and that it operates independently of, and in addition to, hypertension, diabetes, obesity, and other factors. For men and women over age 65, there is no evidence of a correlation between hyperlipidemia and atherosclerosis or its complications.

TABLE 195-5 Frequency of hyperlipidemia in survivors of myocardial infarction

Disorder	% of total myocardial infarction survivors: Under age 60	Over age 60	Ratio
1 Monogenic hyperlipidemias	20.6	7.5	—
a Familial hypercholesterolemia	4.1	0.7	6:1
b Familial hypertriglyceridemia	5.2	2.7	2:1
c Familial combined hyperlipidemia	11.3	4.1	3:1
2 Polygenic hypercholesterolemia	5.5	5.5	1:1
3 Sporadic hypertriglyceridemia	5.8	6.9	1:1

SOURCE: Goldstein et al. 1973.

When the screening of individuals for hyperlipidemia occurs after a myocardial infarction, it is several decades too late, although interruption of further progression of atherosclerosis may be possible. Screening at birth or in childhood for genetic hyperlipidemia is not practical or useful except in the instance of familial hypercholesterolemia, which may affect about 1 in 1000 children. This is detectable by LDL elevations in cord blood when one already knows that a parent is affected. Other genetic or nongenetic primary hyperlipidemia is often not apparent until the third decade. *Today, screening measurement of blood cholesterol levels (nonfasting) is recommended for all adult patients. It is especially important in all young persons who have a family history of premature IHD.*

Hyperlipidemia is best confirmed by measurement of the concentration of total cholesterol and triglycerides and of high-density lipoprotein cholesterol in serum or plasma in a sample obtained after an overnight fast. The measurements should be made by a reliable laboratory that follows a program of standardization. Routine use of lipoprotein electrophoresis provides little additional information, is nonspecific, and is not recommended for screening or for management. In adults less than 65 years of age, a cholesterol concentration (C) greater than 6 mmol/L (240 mg/dL) or a triglyceride concentration (TG) greater than 2.8 mmol/L (250 mg/dL) clearly indicates hyperlipidemia sufficient to require some attention by the physician to the items listed in Table 195-6. Less severe degrees of hypercholesterolemia nevertheless can impart some degree of risk for IHD. The National Cholesterol Education Program has suggested that total cholesterol (C) > 6.2 mmol/L (240 mg/dL) is "high risk" and should prompt careful evaluation (Table 195-6), estimation of LDL cholesterol, and some approach to cholesterol lowering. Cholesterol between 5.2 and 6.1 mmol/dL (200 and 239 mg/dL) is borderline high. The presence of two or more risk factors (independent of C or TG levels) listed in Table 195-4, or preexisting IHD, puts these patients in the

TABLE 195-6 Factors to consider in patients with hyperlipidemia

1 Disorders to which hyperlipidemia is secondary
- *a* Uncontrolled diabetes mellitus (insulin deficiency)
- *b* Hypothyroidism
- *c* Uremia
- *d* Nephrotic syndrome (hypoproteinemia)
- *e* Obstructive liver disease
- *f* Dysproteinemia (multiple myeloma, lupus erythematosus)

2 Drugs producing or aggravating hyperlipidemia
- *a* Oral contraceptives
- *b* Estrogens
- *c* Glucocorticoids
- *d* Antihypertensives

3 Dietary factors
- *a* Caloric intake (recent weight gain)
- *b* Content of saturated fats and cholesterol
- *c* Alcohol intake

4 Genetic disorders (primary hyperlipidemias)
- *a* Family history of hyperlipidemia or xanthomas
- *b* History of pancreatitis or recurrent abdominal pain

TABLE 195-7 Guidelines for treatment of high blood cholesterol in adults

		Cholesterol, mmol/L (mg/dL)		
Decision	Basis	Desirable	Borderline-high	High
LDL estimation	Total C	<5.2 (200)	5.2–6.1 (200–239)*	>6.2 (240)
Treatment				
Diet	LDL-C	<3.4 (130)	3.4–4.1 (130–159)*	>4.2 (160)
Drug†	LDL-C			>5.1 (190) or >4.2 (160)*

* Becomes high-risk if definite IHD or >2 risk factors (see Table 195-4) are present.
† After a trial of diet alone.
SOURCE: National Cholesterol Education Program.

high-risk category. For treatment decisions, and when TG < 4.5 mmol/L (400 mg/dL), LDL cholesterol (LDL-C) levels can be estimated as total C − HDL-C − TG/5. Patients considered at high risk for IHD should be aggressively treated to lower blood cholesterol out of the high-risk range (Table 195-7). If C < 5 mmol/L (200 mg/dL), the tests need not be repeated for several years in an adult who maintains body weight and does not otherwise change in health or life-style. If causes of *secondary hyperlipidemia* or offending drugs are absent, attention to the origin of *primary hyperlipidemia* turns mainly to diet and genetic causes. Severe hyperlipidemia [C > 7.8 mmol/L (300 mg/dL) or TG > 5.6 mmol/L (500 mg/dL)] usually reflects a genetic disorder; when xanthomas are present, it practically always does. Diagnosis always includes examination of first-degree relatives and proceeds according to information contained in Chap. 326.

Reduction of hypercholesterolemia results in a decrease in progression of atherosclerosis in humans and other primates. Several controlled trials of different diets which have been accompanied by fall in mean cholesterol levels in small test populations have shown a favorable effect on incidence of the overall complications of IHD. The drug clofibrate given to a normal population reduced the incidence of nonfatal myocardial infarctions and was associated with a reduction of cholesterol levels; however, total mortality was not lowered. In the Lipid Research Clinics trial, the drug cholestyramine given to hypercholesterolemic asymptomatic men reduced morbidity and mortality from myocardial infarction in direct relation to the degree of cholesterol lowering; again, however, total mortality was not reduced. Lipid lowering by means of bile acid binding resins (with niacin and diet therapy) also decreases progression and even induces regression of coronary lesions as demonstrated by angiography in patients who have had coronary artery bypass graft surgery. Another fibric acid drug, gemfibrozil, has been shown to reduce mortality from IHD (but not total mortality) in association with lowered TG and C and raised HDL-C. Thus, the weight of evidence strongly favors conservative measures to reduce cholesterol levels in patients through middle age and aggressive measures in patients who are frankly hypercholesterolemic and are at high risk for progression of IHD.

The first step in treatment of primary hyperlipidemia is attention to diet. All patients with mild to moderate hyperlipidemia should first be brought to normal weight if they exceed it and then be maintained on a diet emphasizing decreases in intake of saturated fat and cholesterol. If hypertriglyceridemia is present, alcohol intake should be limited or eliminated. A single dietary approach to all forms of hyperlipidemia, including reduced intake of calories, cholesterol, and saturated fat, is appropriate for most patients. The degree of dietary restriction would be proportional to the degree and nature of the hyperlipidemia. The maximum effect of such a regimen will be observed within 3 months after body weight has stabilized. If at that time LDL-C is greater than 4.9 mmol/L (190 mg/dL), drugs such as a bile acid–binding resin (cholestyramine or colestipol) or nicotinic acid should be considered. If TG remains greater than 3.4 mmol/L (300 mg/dL), a fibric acid derivative (clofibrate or bezafibrate) may be tried. These two types of drugs may be used simultaneously if both C and TG are high. In patients with familial hypercholesterolemia (Chap. 326) combined therapy with a resin and nicotinic acid has achieved dramatic normalization of LDL cholesterol levels. New cholesterol synthesis inhibitors (e.g., lovastatin), which are more potent than resins, are currently being studied. However, further studies are needed to define the long-term efficiency of various hypolipidemic agents in the prevention of atherosclerosis and its sequelae in specific disorders. The long-term effects of these drugs used before puberty are unknown, and their use during pregnancy is not advocated. There is a paucity of data to justify their use in the elderly.

High-density lipoproteins (HDL) The level of HDL, a complex family of particles that carry about 20 percent of the total plasma cholesterol, is inversely associated with the development of premature atherosclerosis and therefore can be considered an "antirisk factor." HDL levels can be assessed simply by measurement of cholesterol in the supernatant fluid after the other lipoproteins in plasma have been precipitated. Thus individuals whose HDL cholesterol is elevated may be less likely to develop IHD; conversely, low HDL cholesterol is associated with increased risk of IHD. In the Framingham Study, low HDL cholesterol was a more potent lipid risk factor than was high cholesterol or LDL. At least five diverse population studies have confirmed a close correlation between IHD and low HDL, independent of other factors.

Consistent with differences in risk between the sexes, HDL cholesterol averages about 25 percent higher in women than in men. Estrogens tend to raise and androgens tend to lower HDL levels. In women, low HDL, particularly when associated with diabetes and obesity, markedly raises the risk of IHD. Octogenarians tend to have high HDL, which may be partly familial. Of interest for preventive measures, cigarette smoking decreases and regular strenuous exercise increases HDL cholesterol. Regular exercise increases HDL even in individuals after myocardial infarction. A small daily intake of alcohol has been associated with both reduced risk of IHD and high HDL levels. Mechanisms for these effects remain unknown.

The utility of HDL cholesterol measurements in individuals is limited since the analytical error in most laboratories exceeds the differences in HDL levels associated with risk. HDL measurements are most helpful for estimation of LDL cholesterol. Because of the close inverse relationship between plasma triglycerides (or VLDL) and HDL, HDL in most hypertriglyceridemic persons, with or without hypercholesterolemia, will be predictably low. Low HDL cholesterol is one of the factors that can place patients in a high-risk category for IHD (Table 195-7).

Hypertension (See Chap. 196) High blood pressure is an important risk factor for atherosclerosis, mainly IHD and cerebrovascular disease. The risk increases progressively with increasing blood pressure; in the Framingham Study, IHD incidence in middle-aged men with blood pressures exceeding 160/95 was more than five times that in normotensive men (blood pressure 140/90 or less). Hypertensive men and women are both affected, with the diastolic pressure perhaps being more important. In industrialized populations, blood pressure appears to increase inexorably with age; however, the nature of this age relation varies among populations, since there are remote primitive populations that age without any changes in blood pressure levels. The age-associated blood pressure increase might be related to physical activity or dietary factors, particularly sodium and total caloric content. In contrast to the other age-related risk factors, hypertension appears to increase atherosclerosis throughout the age span.

Conversely, the risk for atherosclerosis appears diminished by therapeutic reduction of blood pressure. Recent intervention studies have shown convincingly that reduction of diastolic levels that had been greater than 105 mmHg significantly reduces the incidence of strokes, IHD, and congestive heart failure in men. Even when patients with diastolic pressures between 90 and 105 mmHg are similarly maintained on adequate treatment, the incidence of some of these complications may be reduced. Special urgency for relief of hypertension obtains when hyperlipidemia, diabetes, or other risk factors are present.

Cigarette smoking Not only is cigarette smoking one of the more potent risk factors for atherosclerosis, it is also one of the factors that when reduced or eliminated clearly decreases the risk of developing atherosclerosis. Ample statistical evidence supports a mean increase of about 70 percent in the death rate, and a three- to fivefold increase in risk of IHD, in men who smoke one pack of cigarettes per day compared with nonsmokers. In general, the increase in death rate is proportional to the amount smoked and decreases with age. Excess morbidity from myocardial infarction is also present in women smokers, but the relationship is somewhat less firm than in men. However, there is an impressive accentuation of IHD mortality in women over age 35 taking oral contraceptives who in addition smoke cigarettes. In some atherosclerosis-prone populations, such as patients maintained on long-term hemodialysis, cigarette smoking interacts with other risk factors, resulting in a marked enhancement of atherosclerosis mortality. Such interaction is also likely for diabetic and hypertensive populations.

The association of smoking and increased IHD remains unexplained. Pipe and cigar smokers have a lesser increase in risk of IHD, presumably because less smoke is inhaled. Smokers dying of causes other than IHD have been found at autopsy to have more coronary atherosclerosis than nonsmokers. The major influence of smoking is upon the incidence of sudden death, however. Those who stop smoking show a prompt decline in risk and may reach the risk level of nonsmokers as early as after 1 year of abstention.

Hyperglycemia and diabetes mellitus (See Chap. 319) Studies in a variety of populations have shown an association of hyperglycemia with clinically evident atherosclerotic disease, suggesting a role of hyperglycemia in atherogenesis. In known diabetics, both insulin-dependent and non-insulin-dependent types, there is at least a twofold increase in incidence of myocardial infarction compared with nondiabetics. This risk is markedly increased in younger diabetics, and diabetic women are even more prone to IHD than are diabetic men. There is an increased tendency toward cerebral thrombosis and infarction but not toward cerebral hemorrhage in diabetes. Gangrene of the lower extremities has been variously estimated to be from 8 to 150 times as frequent in diabetics as in nondiabetics and is most often found in diabetics who smoke. Diabetes mellitus is associated with an increase in atherosclerosis observed at autopsy in a variety of populations worldwide, whether the prevalence of atherosclerosis in a particular population is high or low. The approximately twofold increase in the frequency of hypertension among diabetics, particularly adult females, may accentuate the risk. This relationship is presumably associated with abdominal obesity.

The risk for atherosclerotic disease, however, does not appear to be grossly related to the degree of hyperglycemia among diabetics. Results in the University Group Diabetes Program Study have suggested that reduction of blood glucose by insulin does not appear to influence mortality from established atherosclerosis during a 5-year period. Thus, hyperglycemia and atherosclerosis are associated, since there is an increased prevalence of large-vessel disease in known diabetics and, conversely, an increased prevalence of hyperglycemia in association with atherosclerotic disease. These associations remain unexplained and reversibility undocumented. Clinical and experimental studies also support a role for high circulating insulin levels in IHD. The capillary microangiopathy, pathognomonic of diabetes mellitus and causing important dysfunction of the kidneys and retina, has unknown clinical significance in relation to atherosclerotic disease in larger arteries.

Obesity In general, morbidity and mortality from IHD are higher in direct relation to the degree of overweight beyond about 30 percent. Furthermore, from data obtained in the Framingham Study, it appears that obesity may accelerate atherosclerosis since its effect is more apparent before age 50. Nevertheless, some of the major epidemiologic studies of coronary heart disease have not demonstrated an independent relationship between this condition and anything less than very severe obesity. Recent studies have shown a close relation between type of obesity (i.e., abdominal) and IHD. Furthermore, obesity is a disorder closely associated with four other potent risk factors, i.e., hypertriglyceridemia, hypercholesterolemia, hyperglycemia, and hypertension. The relationship between obesity and atherosclerosis is thus multifaceted; since in practice obesity does not occur "independently," it is of considerable importance as a risk factor.

Physical inactivity Study of the relationship of the prevalence of IHD to daily (occupational) physical activity is made difficult because so many variables are involved. Among prospective studies the Framingham data do indicate that the less sedentary an individual is, the less susceptible that individual is to sudden death. Physical work may be the major determinant of greatly differing incidences of IHD in southern black and white males in the United States and in populations that move from rural areas to urbanized environments. How physical activity may operate to decrease death from IHD, or possibly to decrease atherogenesis, is not known. Beyond the amelioration of hyperlipidemia by increasing caloric expenditure, no mechanism has been demonstrated. The meaning of the physical activity–induced increase in HDL, the antirisk factor for IHD, remains mysterious. Physical training has been shown to improve exercise performance in patients with IHD and angina pectoris. Regular physical activity is supported as a desirable element in a program of preventive health maintenance.

Stress and personality There is a valid clinical impression that psychic or emotional stress and anxiety are associated with precipitation of overt IHD and sudden death. Debate continues as to whether there may be distinct personality types prone to or relatively immune to premature IHD (the so-called personality types A and B) and whether the presumably more deleterious type is amenable to correction beyond elimination of cigarette smoking, adverse dietary patterns, and avoidance of stressful life situations. Many social and demographic analyses have so far failed to reach any agreement about the etiologic relationships of occupation and similar situational factors and the incidence of IHD.

Genetic factors Premature atherosclerosis often appears to be familial. In many instances this can be attributed to the inheritance of risk factors such as hypertension, diabetes mellitus, and hyperlipidemia. Occasionally, families with excessive premature vascular disease can be found in which none of the known risk factors appears to be operating. Genetic determinants of protective factors, such as HDL, and of nonlipid risk factors, such as apolipoprotein B, and lipoprotein (a), need to be understood; undoubtedly other important determinants remain to be discovered. Nevertheless, family history is one of the more important factors to be weighed in assessment of risk in helping the physician to avoid missing treatable risk factors and in institution of appropriate preventive measures.

ROLE OF DIET IN RISK FOR ATHEROSCLEROSIS The relationship of diet to IHD remains an area of intense interest and persistent controversy. In epidemiologic studies, no population habitually subsisting on a diet low in saturated fat and cholesterol has an appreciable amount of IHD. These populations also tend to have lower plasma lipid concentrations. There is a general upward shift of average cholesterol and triglyceride levels in highly developed countries, which is an effect of change in total culture and life-style as well as in diet. Dietary changes in migrant populations who move from more primitive to more industrialized societies commonly include increased intake of total calories, animal fats, cholesterol, and salt, leading to a diet-accentuated emergence of risk factors such as obesity, hyperlipidemia, diabetes, and hypertension. There is no question that the plasma cholesterol (and LDL) level is sensitive to the amount of saturated fat and cholesterol in the diet. The "average" adult male in the United States eats about 140 g fat per day and about 0.1 mmol (400 mg) cholesterol. The mixture of fats ingested usually contains about three times as much saturated fatty acids (mainly palmitic and stearic) as polyunsaturated fatty acids (mainly linoleic and linolenic). If a healthy young adult switches from this diet to one containing the same amount of total fat in which the ratio of polyunsaturates to saturates is closer to unity and the cholesterol content is less than 0.07 mmol (300 mg) per day, the cholesterol concentration will usually drop by 10 to 15 percent within 2 weeks and remain depressed on continuation of the diet.

The average cholesterol level in most populations is most closely related to the amount of animal fats (meat, eggs, and milk products, major sources of long-chain saturated fatty acids and cholesterol) in the diet. Increased animal fat consumption also tends to be correlated with a greater proportion of dietary fats being saturated and with lesser intake of complex carbohydrates and vegetable fibers; these are dietary changes that may lead to a rise in plasma cholesterol levels. The average triglyceride level is more sensitive to total caloric balance and to alcohol intake. It is important to note that physical activity, emotional stress, smoking, and intake of coffee or tea have only weak or indirect influences on total cholesterol and triglyceride concentrations.

In experimental animals added dietary cholesterol and fat are essential for the production of atherosclerosis. Typical American diets fed to nonhuman primates produce aortic and coronary atherosclerosis which is reversible when a cholesterol-free diet is fed. Controlled metabolic studies in humans show a direct relation between dietary and plasma cholesterol below intakes of about 0.15 mmol (600 mg) per day; no relation is observed at higher intakes when plasma cholesterol is already high. There appear to be marked genetic variations in the ability of dietary cholesterol to influence plasma cholesterol among individuals and among populations. The relation between dietary polyunsaturated/saturated fat ratio (P/S) and both cholesterol and triglyceride levels also has been amply established. The unique triglyceride-lowering effects of the particular long-chain polyunsaturated fatty acids in large ocean fish are currently under study.

A definitive prospective study of the effect of diet on IHD in the general population has never been undertaken. Nevertheless, preliminary reports of newer studies of alterations of diet in high-risk populations, coupled with published findings of studies in selected populations, provide strong evidence of a reversible relation among diet, plasma lipids, and IHD. On this basis, numerous authoritative nutrition councils have recommended prudent dietary modifications for the general population of western countries to be instituted early in life and to include a caloric intake adjusted to achieve and maintain ideal body weight, a reduction in total fat calories to 30 to 35 percent of total calories achieved by a substantial reduction in dietary saturated fat to less than 10 percent of total calories, and a reduction in cholesterol intake to less than 300 mg per day. Although a causal relationship in humans between sodium intake and hypertension has not been firmly established, avoidance of excessive dietary sodium also has been recommended.

RISK FACTORS AND MECHANISMS OF ATHEROGENESIS
Adiposity produces insulin resistance in peripheral tissues (mainly muscle and adipose), which leads to compensatory hyperinsulinemia. The liver is not resistant to some effects of insulin, and enhanced production of triglyceride-rich lipoproteins results, leading to elevated plasma triglyceride and cholesterol levels. Thus it has been demonstrated that body weight is related not only to triglyceride levels but also to cholesterol levels. Concomitantly, obesity is associated with increased total-body cholesterol synthesis. Obesity, particularly the abdominal type, produces higher circulating levels of insulin, both in the basal state and after stimulation with glucose or other secretagogues. Since obesity is related to atherosclerosis—both directly and via hypertension, hypertriglyceridemia, hypercholesterolemia, and hyperglycemia—it is not surprising that many studies show a relationship between serum insulin levels, particularly after oral glucose intake, and atherosclerotic disease of the coronary and peripheral arteries. A few studies, however, suggest that this association between insulin and atherosclerosis occurs independently of obesity. It has been postulated that insulin may directly affect arterial wall metabolism, leading to increased endogenous lipid synthesis and thus predisposing to atherosclerosis. Insulin has been shown to stimulate proliferation of arterial smooth-muscle cells, enhance binding of LDL and VLDL, and decrease binding of HDL to cells; it therefore may be one of the plasma factors involved in atheroma formation.

Hypertension may enhance atherogenesis by directly producing injury via mechanical stress on endothelial cells at specific high-pressure sites in the arterial tree. This would allow the sequence of events in the chronic injury hypothesis of atherogenesis to take place. In addition, hypertension might allow more lipoproteins to be transported through intact endothelial lining cells by altering permeability. Hypertension markedly increases lysosomal enzyme activity, presumably owing to stimulation of the cellular disposal system by the internalization of increased amounts of plasma substances. This might lead to increased cell degeneration and release of the highly destructive enzymes (within the lysosomes) into the arterial wall. Experimental hypertension also increases the thickness of the intimal smooth-muscle layer in the arterial wall and increases connective tissue elements. It is still not known if continued high pressure within the artery produces changes in the ability of smooth-muscle cells or stem cells to proliferate.

Diabetes could provide a unique contribution to atherogenesis. Although the fundamental genetic abnormality in human diabetes mellitus remains unknown, it has been suggested that genetic diabetes in humans represents a primary cellular abnormality intrinsic to all cells, resulting in a decreased life span of individual cells, which in turn results in increased cell turnover in tissues. If arterial endothelial and smooth-muscle cells are intrinsically defective in diabetes, accelerated atherogenesis can be readily postulated on the basis of any one of the current theories of pathogenesis. Platelet dysfunction in diabetes might also play a role.

The role of glucose in atheroma formation, if any, is poorly understood. Hyperglycemia is known to affect aortic wall metabolism. Sorbitol, a product of the insulin-independent aldose reductase pathway of glucose metabolism (the polyol pathway) accumulates in the arterial wall in the presence of high glucose concentrations, resulting in osmotic effects including increased cell water content and decreased oxygenation. Increased glucose also appears to stimulate proliferation of cultured arterial smooth-muscle cells. Glycosylation of apolipoproteins and other key proteins intrinsic to arterial wall cell function might also be involved.

The development of atherosclerosis accelerates in approximate quantitative relation to the degree of *hyperlipidemia*. A long-established theory suggests that the higher the circulating levels of lipoprotein, the more likely they are to gain entrance to the arterial wall. By an acceleration of the usual transendothelial transport, large concentrations of lipoproteins within the arterial wall could overwhelm the ability of smooth-muscle cells and monocyte-derived macrophages to metabolize them. Lipoproteins have been immunologically identified in atheroma, and in humans there is a close relationship between plasma cholesterol and arterial lipoprotein cholesterol concentration. Chemically modified or oxidized lipoproteins, possibly produced in hyperlipidemic disorders, could gain access to the scavenger arterial wall macrophages, leading to formation of foam cells as in xanthomas. It is possible that the lipid that accumulates in the arterial wall with increasing age results from infiltration of plasma lipoproteins. However, atheromatous lesions are associated with a more marked increase in arterial wall lipids, which may result in part from injury to the endothelium possibly produced by chronic hyperlipidemia, as demonstrated in cholesterol-fed monkeys. A further mechanism for accelerated atherogenesis in hyperlipidemia is related to the ability of LDL to stimulate proliferation of arterial smooth-muscle cells.

The effect of *chronic smoke inhalation* from cigarettes could result in repetitive injury to endothelial cells, thereby accelerating atherogenesis. Hypoxia stimulates proliferation of cultured human arterial smooth-muscle cells; thus, since cigarette smoking is associated with high levels of carboxyhemoglobin and low oxygen delivery to tissues, another mechanism for atherogenesis is suggested. Hypoxia could produce diminished lysosomal enzyme degradative ability, as evidenced by impaired degradation of LDL by smooth-muscle cells, causing LDL to accumulate in the cells. Consistent with this suggestion is the fact that aortic lesions that resemble atheroma have been produced in experimental animals by systemic hypoxia, and lipid accumulation in the arterial wall of cholesterol-fed rabbits and monkeys appears to be increased by hypoxia.

RISK FACTOR REVERSAL AND REGRESSION OF ATHEROSCLEROSIS Although the emergence of clinical consequences of atherosclerosis can be lessened, no convincing instance of regression or interruption of progression of atherosclerosis in asymptomatic individuals, determined by direct or indirect examination of lesions, by removal or reversal of any single risk factor or group of risk factors has yet been proved in humans. Nevertheless, feasibility of such demonstrations is now established, and the recent angiographic evidence in patients who have had coronary bypass surgery of interruption of lesion progression and even regression associated with lipid lowering is encouraging. Through mass-media educational efforts, whole communities can be influenced to reduce smoking, change diet, and lower blood pressure levels. Adult males in the United States have lowered cigarette consumption, although increases among teenage girls have kept total usage high. There has been a trend toward lower cholesterol and saturated fat consumption in the United States, coupled with increasing attention to reducing overweight and the use of exercise programs. Concomitantly, and perhaps causally, there has been the noted decline in IHD mortality. Treatment of hyperlipidemia in some instances has been shown to reduce atherosclerotic involvement of peripheral vessels by both invasive and noninvasive measurement. There is also some encouraging evidence in animals, most notably in primates, that relatively complicated plaques induced by hyperlipidemia will regress, and that further progression of atherosclerosis will cease when hyperlipidemia is removed. Therefore efforts to prevent atherogenesis, to interrupt progression, and perhaps to promote regression of existing lesions by risk factor reduction seem warranted.

PREVENTION Although premature IHD is overall the most costly and common of the untimely complications of atherosclerosis, preoccupation with IHD should not obscure the fact that angina pectoris and myocardial infarction are expressions of late-stage atherosclerotic lesions. Factors precipitating these clinical events may be independent of those leading to initiation of plaque formation or its progression to a complicated lesion. Steps taken to prevent recurrence of myocardial infarction or fatal arrhythmia, termed *secondary prevention,* will not necessarily be the same as those taken to delay or prevent formation of atherosclerosis (*primary prevention*). Since atherosclerotic plaques have been detected in the coronary arteries of American males as early as the second decade in autopsy studies of Korean and Vietnam war deaths, primary prevention of atherosclerosis must begin early in life, long before there is any suspicion of IHD.

Thus, *prevention of atherosclerosis, rather than treatment, is the goal.* Although an effective program has not been established with certainty, enough is known to act as a guide both in identification of those with a higher risk and in development of conservative measures that probably will reduce that risk. Thus prevention currently is equated with risk factor reduction.

The decline of American death rates from premature IHD today coincides with two trends in health practices. One is the increasing acceptance of the importance of detecting and attempting to correct some of the risk factors correlated with atherosclerosis. The other is a greater awareness of the dietary sources of cholesterol and saturated fats and a tendency of the public to restrict their intake somewhat. Whether these trends are causally related to the decline in death rate is not known. While a rigorous approach to changes in life-style for the general population may be debatable, it is desirable to continue finding and helping those most susceptible to early atherosclerosis. The physician's role in risk factor reduction involves treatment of hypertension and advice regarding diet, body weight, smoking, and exercise. Drug treatment of hyperlipidemia should be limited to those individuals at high risk who do not respond adequately to dietary management. Although preliminary trials are encouraging, the long-term value of antiplatelet drugs in reducing either the mortality rate or incidence of myocardial infarction in individuals with IHD remains unproved, and trials are continuing.

TREATMENT There is no agent proven to have any value in "treatment" of atherosclerosis unless it clearly reduces severe hyperlipidemia or obvious hypertension. In fact, there is no treatment of atherosclerosis, only of its complications. While end-stage treatment technology has reduced morbidity (Chap. 190), prevention remains the long-term goal of both research and medical practice.

REFERENCES

BIERMAN EL: Aging and atherosclerosis, in *Principles of Geriatric Medicine*, 2d ed, WR Hazzard et al (eds). New York, McGraw-Hill, 1990, Chap 45, pp 458–465

EVERHART JE et al: Medical arterial calcification and its association with mortality and complications of diabetes. Diabetologia 31:16, 1988

GORDON T et al: Diabetes, blood lipids, and the role of obesity in coronary heart disease risk for women. The Framingham Study. Ann Intern Med 87:393, 1977

KANNEL WB et al: Cholesterol in the prediction of atherosclerotic disease. New perspectives based on the Framingham Study. Ann Intern Med 90:85, 1979

LEAF A: Management of hypercholesterolemia: Are preventive interventions indicated? N Engl J Med 321(10):680, 1989

LEVY RI: Declining mortality in coronary heart disease. Arteriosclerosis 1:312, 1981

MARTIN MJ et al: Serum cholesterol, blood pressure, and mortality: Implications from a cohort of 361,662 men. Lancet 2:933, 1986

McGILL HC: Persistent problems in the pathogenesis of atherosclerosis. Arteriosclerosis 4:443, 1984

NATIONAL CHOLESTEROL EDUCATION PROGRAM: Report of the National Cholesterol Education Program Expert Panel on Detection, Evaluation and Treatment of High Blood Cholesterol in Adults. Arch Intern Med 148:36, 1988

PELL S, FAYERWEATHER WE: Trends in the incidence of myocardial infarction and in associated mortality and morbidity in a large employed population, 1957–1983. N Engl J Med 312:1005, 1985

ROSS R: The pathogenesis of atherosclerosis—an update. N Engl J Med 314:488, 1986

STEINBERG D: Lipoproteins and atherosclerosis: A look back and a look ahead. Arteriosclerosis 3:283, 1983

196 HYPERTENSIVE VASCULAR DISEASE

GORDON H. WILLIAMS

An elevated arterial pressure is probably the more important public health problem in developed countries—being common, asymptomatic, readily detectable, usually easily treatable, and often leading to lethal complications if left untreated. As a result of extensive educational programs in the late 1960s and 1970s by both private and governmental agencies, the number of undiagnosed and/or untreated patients has been significantly reduced to a level of less than 20 percent. This factor may be the most important one responsible for the decline in cardiovascular mortality which has taken place during the past 20 years (Chap. 195). Although our understanding of the pathophysiology of an elevated arterial pressure has increased, in 90 to 95 percent of cases the etiology (and thus potentially the prevention or cure) is still largely unknown. As a consequence, in most cases the hypertension is treated nonspecifically, resulting in a large number of minor side effects and a relatively high (~50 percent) noncompliance rate.

DEFINITION

Since there is no dividing line between normal and high blood pressure, arbitrary levels have been established to define those who have an increased risk of developing a morbid cardiovascular event and/or will clearly benefit from medical therapy. These definitions should consider not only the level of diastolic pressure but also systolic pressure, age, sex, and race. For example, patients with a diastolic pressure greater than 90 mmHg will have a significant reduction in morbidity and mortality with adequate therapy. These, then, are patients who have hypertension and who should be considered for treatment.

The level of *systolic* pressure is also important in assessing arterial pressure's influence on cardiovascular morbidity. Males with normal diastolic pressures (<82 mmHg) but elevated systolic pressures (>158 mmHg) have a $2\frac{1}{2}$-fold increase in their cardiovascular mortality rates when compared with individuals with similar diastolic pressures but whose systolic pressures are normal (<130 mmHg). However, reduction in mortality and morbidity with treatment has not been definitively documented in these patients. Other significant factors which modify blood pressure's influence on the frequency of morbid cardiovascular events are age, race, and sex with young black males being most adversely affected by hypertension.

When hypertension is suspected, blood pressure should be measured at least twice on two separate examinations. In adults, a *diastolic* pressure below 85 mmHg is considered to be normal; between 85 and 89 is high normal; 90 to 104 is mild hypertension; 105 to 114 moderate hypertension; 115 or greater is severe hypertension. When the diastolic pressure is below 90 mmHg, a *systolic* pressure below 140 mmHg indicates normal blood pressure; between 140 and 159 is borderline isolated systolic hypertension; 160 or higher is isolated systolic hypertension. Increasing use of 12- or 24-h blood pressure monitoring may provide additional useful information in patients who are difficult to classify. However, normal values for this procedure are not currently available.

Arterial pressure fluctuates in most persons, whether they are normotensive or hypertensive. Those who are classified as having *labile* hypertension are patients who sometimes, but not always, have arterial pressures within the hypertensive range. These patients are often considered to have borderline hypertension.

Sustained hypertension can become accelerated or enter a malignant phase. Though a patient with *malignant hypertension* often has a blood pressure above 200/140, it is papilledema, usually accompanied by retinal hemorrhages and exudates, and not the absolute pressure level, that defines this condition. *Accelerated hypertension* signifies a significant recent increase over previous hypertensive levels associated with evidence of vascular damage on funduscopic examination but without papilledema.

FREQUENCY The prevalence of hypertension depends on both the racial composition of the studied population and the criteria used to define the condition. In a white suburban population as used in the Framingham Study, nearly one-fifth have blood pressures greater than 160/95, while almost one-half have pressures greater than 140/90. An even higher prevalance has been documented in the nonwhite population.

ETIOLOGY

The cause of elevated arterial pressure is unknown in most cases. The prevalence of various forms of secondary hypertension depends on the nature of the population studied and how extensive the evaluation is. There are no available data to define the frequency of secondary hypertension in the general population, although in middle-aged males it has been reported to be 6 percent. On the other hand, in referral centers where patients undergo an extensive evaluation, it has been reported to be as high as 35 percent. The various forms of hypertension are outlined in Table 196-1, and their relative frequencies are given in Table 196-2.

ESSENTIAL HYPERTENSION Patients with arterial hypertension and no definable cause are said to have *primary, essential,* or *idiopathic hypertension*. Undoubtedly, the primary difficulty in uncovering the mechanism(s) responsible for the hypertension in these patients is attributable to the variety of systems that are involved in the regulation of arterial pressure—peripheral and/or central adrenergic, renal, hormonal, and vascular—and to the complexity of the relationships of these systems to one another. Several abnormalities have been described in patients with essential hypertension, often with a claim that one or more of these are primarily responsible for the hypertension. While it is still uncertain whether these individual abnormalities are primary or secondary, varying expressions of a single disease process or reflective of separate disease entities, the accumulating data increasingly support the latter hypothesis. Thus, just as pneumonia is caused by a variety of infectious agents, even though the clinical picture observed may be similar, so essential hypertension likely has a number of distinct causes. Therefore, the

TABLE 196-1 Classification of arterial hypertension

I Systolic hypertension with wide pulse pressure
- *A* Decreased compliance of aorta (arteriosclerosis)
- *B* Increased stroke volume
  - *1* Aortic regurgitation
  - *2* Thyrotoxicosis
  - *3* Hyperkinetic heart syndrome
  - *4* Fever
  - *5* Arteriovenous fistula
  - *6* Patent ductus arteriosus

II Systolic and diastolic hypertension (increased peripheral vascular resistance)
- *A* Renal
  - *1* Chronic pyelonephritis
  - *2* Acute and chronic glomerulonephritis
  - *3* Polycystic renal disease
  - *4* Renovascular stenosis or renal infarction
  - *5* Most other severe renal disease (arteriolar nephrosclerosis, diabetic nephropathy, etc.)
  - *6* Renin-producing tumors
- *B* Endocrine
  - *1* Oral contraceptives
  - *2* Adrenocortical hyperfunction
    - *a* Cushing's disease and syndrome
    - *b* Primary hyperaldosteronism
    - *c* Congenital or hereditary adrenogenital syndromes (17α-hydroxylase and 11β-hydroxylase defects)
  - *3* Pheochromocytoma
  - *4* Myxedema
  - *5* Acromegaly
- *C* Neurogenic
  - *1* Psychogenic
  - *2* "Diencephalic syndrome"
  - *3* Familial dysautonomia (Riley-Day)
  - *4* Polyneuritis (acute porphyria, lead poisoning)
  - *5* Increased intracranial pressure (acute)
  - *6* Spinal cord section (acute)
- *D* Miscellaneous
  - *1* Coarctation of aorta
  - *2* Increased intravascular volume (excessive transfusion, polycythemia vera)
  - *3* Polyarteritis nodosa
  - *4* Hypercalcemia
- *E* Unknown etiology
  - *1* Essential hypertension (>90% of all cases of hypertension)
  - *2* Toxemia of pregnancy
  - *3* Acute intermittent porphyria

TABLE 196-2 Prevalence of various forms of hypertension in the general population and in specialized referral clinics*

Diagnosis	General population, %	Specialty clinic, %
Essential hypertension	92–94	65–85
Renal hypertension:		
Parenchymal	2–3	4–5
Renovascular	1–2	4–16
Endocrine hypertension:		
Primary aldosteronism	0.3	0.5–12
Cushing's syndrome	<0.1	0.2
Pheochromocytoma	<0.1	0.2
Oral contraceptive–induced	2–4	1–2
Miscellaneous	0.2	1

* Estimates based on a number of reports in the literature.

distinction between primary and secondary hypertension has become blurred, and the approach to both the diagnosis and therapy of hypertensive patients has been modified. For example, as a group of patients with essential hypertension are separated into a distinct subset (e.g., low-renin essential hypertension), they have not been reclassified as a form of secondary hypertension but rather remain in the essential hypertensive group. In this chapter, we define those individuals with a specific organ defect responsible for hypertension as having a *secondary* form of hypertension. In contrast, individuals who may have generalized or functional abnormalities causing their hypertension are defined as having *essential* hypertension.

Heredity Genetic factors have long been assumed to be important in the genesis of hypertension. Data supporting this view can be found in animal studies as well as population studies in humans. One approach has been to assess the correlation of blood pressures within families (familial aggregation). From these studies the minimum size of the genetic factor can be expressed by a correlation coefficient of approximately 0.2. However, the variation in the size of the genetic factor in different studies reemphasizes the likely heterogeneous nature of the essential hypertensive population. Additionally, most studies support the concept that the inheritance is probably multifactorial or that a number of different genetic defects each have as one of their phenotypic expressions an elevated blood pressure.

Environment A number of environmental factors have been specifically implicated in the development of hypertension including salt intake, obesity, occupation, family size, and crowding. These factors have all been assumed to be important in the increase in blood pressure with age in more affluent societies, in contrast to the decline in blood pressure with age in more primitive cultures.

SALT-SENSITIVITY The environmental factor which has received the greatest attention is salt intake. Even this factor illustrates the heterogeneous nature of the essential hypertensive population in that the blood pressure in only approximately 60 percent of hypertensives is particularly responsive to the level of sodium intake. The etiologic basis for this special sensitivity to salt varies, with primary aldosteronism, bilateral renal artery stenosis, renal parenchymal disease, or low-renin essential hypertension accounting for about half of the patients. In the remainder, the pathophysiology is still uncertain, but recent postulated contributing factors include chloride, calcium, a generalized cellular membrane defect, and "nonmodulation" (see below).

Most studies assessing the role of salt in the hypertensive process have assumed that it is the sodium ion which is important. However, some investigators have suggested that the chloride ion may be equally important. This suggestion is based on the observation that feeding chloride-free sodium salts to salt-sensitive hypertensive animals fails to increase arterial pressure. Calcium has also been implicated in the pathogenesis of some forms of essential hypertension. A low calcium intake has been associated with an increase in blood pressure in epidemiologic studies; an increase in leukocyte cytosolic calcium levels has been reported in some hypertensives; and finally calcium entry blockers are effective antihypertensive agents. Several studies have reported a potential link between the salt-sensitive forms of hypertension and calcium. It has been postulated that with salt loading and a defect in the kidney's ability to excrete it, a secondary increase in circulating natriuretic factors may occur. One of these, the so-called digitalis-like natriuretic factor, inhibits ouabain-sensitive sodium-potassium ATPase and thereby leads to intracellular calcium accumulation and a hyperreactive vascular smooth muscle.

A third postulated explanation for salt-sensitive hypertension is a generalized membrane defect. This hypothesis derives most of its data from studies on circulating blood elements, particularly red blood cells, in which abnormalities in the transport of sodium across the cell membrane have been documented. Since both increases and decreases in the activity of different transport systems have been reported, it is likely that some abnormalities are primary and some secondary processes. It has been assumed that this abnormality reflects a defect in the cellular membrane and that this defect occurs in many, perhaps all cells of the body, particularly the vascular smooth muscle. Because of this defect, there is then an abnormal accumulation of calcium within vascular smooth muscle, resulting in a heightened vascular responsivity to vasoconstrictor agents. This defect has been proposed to be present in 35 to 50 percent of the essential hypertensive population based on studies using red cells. Other studies suggest that the abnormality in the red cell sodium transport is not a fixed abnormality but can be modified by environmental factors. Finally, the mechanisms underlying salt sensitivity in some patients may be a defect in the kidney's ability to excrete sodium appropriately, secondary to an abnormality in the control of the renal circulation and aldosterone secretion with changes in sodium intake. Sodium intake normally modulates adrenal and renal vascular responses to angiotensin II. With dietary sodium restriction, the adrenal response is enhanced and the renal vascular response reduced. Sodium loading has the opposite effect. In this subset of hypertensives this adjustment is absent, thus leading to the term "nonmodulators" to describe those patients in whom the excretion of a sodium load is impaired.

Each of these hypotheses has as a common final pathway an increase in cytosolic calcium resulting in increased vascular reactivity. However, as described above, several mechanisms might produce the increase in calcium accumulation.

Factors modifying the course of essential hypertension Age, race, sex, smoking, serum cholesterol, glucose intolerance, and weight may all alter the prognosis of this disease. The younger the patient when hypertension is first noted, the greater the reduction in life expectancy if left untreated. In the United States, urban blacks have about twice the prevalence rate for hypertension as whites and more than four times the hypertension-induced morbidity rate. At all ages and in both white and nonwhite populations, females with hypertension fare better than males. Yet, females with hypertension run the same relative risk of a morbid cardiovascular event compared with their normotensive counterparts as males do. Accelerated atherosclerosis is an invariable companion of hypertension. Thus, it is not surprising that independent risk factors associated with the development of atherosclerosis, e.g., an elevated serum cholesterol, glucose intolerance, and/or cigarette smoking, significantly enhance the effect of hypertension on mortality rates regardless of age, sex, or race (Chap. 195). There also is no question that there is a positive correlation between obesity and arterial pressure. A gain in weight is associated with an increased frequency of hypertension in subjects with normal pressures, and weight loss in obese subjects with hypertension lowers their arterial pressure and, if they are being treated, the intensity of therapy required to maintain them normotensive. However, there are no convincing data that obesity adversely affects the hypertension-associated mortality rate.

Natural history Because essential hypertension is a heterogeneous disorder, variables in addition to the level of arterial pressure modify its course. Thus, the probability of developing a morbid cardiovascular event with a given arterial pressure may vary by as much as twentyfold depending on whether associated risk factors are present (Table 196-3). Although exceptions have been reported, most untreated adults with hypertension will develop further increases in their arterial pressure with time. Furthermore, both from actuarial data and from experience in the era prior to effective therapy, it has been documented that untreated hypertension is associated with a shortening of life by 10 to 20 years, usually related to an acceleration of the atherosclerotic process, with the rate of acceleration in part related to the severity of the hypertension. Even individuals with relatively mild disease, i.e., without evidence of end organ damage, left untreated for 7 to 10 years have a high risk of developing significant complications. Nearly 30 percent will exhibit atherosclerotic complications, and more than 50 percent will have end organ damage related to the hypertension itself, e.g., cardiomegaly, congestive heart failure, retinopathy, a cerebrovascular accident, and/or renal insufficiency. Thus, even in its mild forms, hypertension is a progressively lethal disease, if left untreated.

TABLE 196-3 Factors indicating an adverse prognosis in hypertension

I Black race
II Youth
III Male
IV Persistent diastolic pressure >115 mmHg
V Smoking
VI Diabetes mellitus
VII Hypercholesterolemia
VIII Obesity
IX Evidence of end organ damage
  A Cardiac
    1 Cardiac enlargement
    2 ECG changes of ischemic or left ventricular strain
    3 Myocardial infarction
    4 Congestive heart failure
  B Eyes
    1 Retinal exudates and hemorrhages
    2 Papilledema
  C Renal: impaired renal function
  D Nervous system: cerebrovascular accident

SECONDARY HYPERTENSION

As noted earlier, in only a small minority of patients with an elevated arterial pressure can a specific cause be identified. Yet, they should not be ignored for at least two reasons: (1) with correction of the cause their hypertension may be cured, and (2) the secondary forms may provide insight into the etiology of essential hypertension. Nearly all the secondary forms are related to an alteration in hormone secretion and/or renal function and are discussed in detail in other chapters.

RENAL HYPERTENSION (See also Chap. 230) Hypertension produced by renal disease is the result of either (1) a derangement in the renal handling of sodium and fluids leading to volume expansion or (2) an alteration in renal secretion of vasoactive materials resulting in a systemic or local change in arteriolar tone. The main subdivisions of renal hypertension are renovascular hypertension, including preeclampsia and eclampsia, and renal parenchymal hypertension. A simple explanation for *renal vascular hypertension* is that decreased perfusion of renal tissue due to stenosis of a main or branch renal artery activates the renin-angiotensin system, described in Chap. 317. Circulating angiotensin II elevates arterial pressure by direct vasoconstriction, by stimulation of aldosterone secretion with resultant sodium retention, and/or by stimulating the adrenergic nervous system. In actual practice only about one-half of patients with renovascular hypertension have absolute elevations in renin activity in peripheral plasma, although when renin measurements are referenced against an index of sodium balance, a much higher fraction have inappropriately high values. The use of the competitive angiotensin antagonist, saralasin (1-sar, 8-ala, angiotensin II), has further clarified the role of angiotensin in the genesis of the hypertension in this disease. Nearly all patients with surgically correctable disease have exhibited a reduction of arterial pressure when given this agent in the sodium- or volume-depleted state.

Activation of the renin-angiotensin system also has been offered as an explanation for the hypertension in both acute and chronic *renal parenchymal disease*. In this formulation the only difference between renovascular and renal parenchymal hypertension is that the decreased perfusion of renal tissue in the latter case results from inflammatory and fibrotic changes involving multiple small intrarenal vessels. There are enough differences between the two conditions, however, to suggest that there are other mechanisms active in renal parenchymal disease: (1) peripheral plasma renin activity is elevated far less frequently in renal parenchymal than in renovascular hypertension; (2) cardiac output is said to be normal in the renal parenchymal type (unless uremia and anemia are present), but slightly elevated in renovascular hypertension; (3) circulatory responses to tilting and to the Valsalva maneuver are exaggerated in the latter condition; and (4) blood volume tends to be high in patients with severe renal parenchymal disease and low in patients with severe renovascular hypertension. Alternative explanations for the hypertension in renal parenchymal disease include the possibilities that the damaged kidneys (1) produce an unidentified vasopressor substance other than renin, (2) fail to produce a necessary humoral vasodilator substance (perhaps prostaglandin or bradykinin), (3) fail to inactivate circulating vasopressor substances, and/or (4) are ineffective in disposing of sodium, and the retained sodium is responsible for the hypertension as outlined earlier. Though all these explanations, including participation of the renin-angiotensin system, probably have some validity in individual patients, the hypothesis involving sodium retention is particularly attractive. It is supported by the observation that those patients with chronic pyelonephritis or polycystic renal disease who are salt wasters do not develop hypertension, and by the observation that removal of salt and water by dialysis or diuretics is effective in controlling arterial pressure in the majority of patients with renal parenchymal disease.

A rare form of renal hypertension results from the excess secretion of renin by juxtaglomerular cell tumors or nephroblastomas. The initial presentation is similar to that of hyperaldosteronism with hypertension, hypokalemia, and overproduction of aldosterone. However, in contrast to primary aldosteronism, peripheral renin activity is *elevated instead of subnormal*. This disease can be distinguished from other forms of secondary aldosteronism by the presence of normal renal function and with unilateral increases in renal vein renin concentration without a renal artery lesion.

ENDOCRINE HYPERTENSION **Adrenal hypertension** Hypertension is a feature of a variety of adrenal cortical abnormalities. In *primary aldosteronism* (Chap. 317) there is a clear relationship between the aldosterone-induced sodium retention and the hypertension. Normal individuals given aldosterone develop hypertension only if they also ingest sodium. Since aldosterone causes sodium retention by stimulating renal tubular exchange of sodium for potassium, hypokalemia is a prominent feature in most patients with primary aldosteronism, and therefore the measurement of serum potassium provides a simple screening test. The effect of sodium retention and volume expansion in chronically suppressing plasma renin activity is critically important for the definitive diagnosis. In most clinical situations plasma renin activity and plasma or urinary aldosterone levels parallel each other, but in patients with primary aldosteronism, aldosterone levels are high and relatively fixed because of autonomous aldosterone secretion, while plasma renin activity levels are suppressed and respond sluggishly to sodium depletion. Primary aldosteronism may be secondary either to a tumor or bilateral adrenal hyperplasia. It is important to distinguish between these two conditions preoperatively, as usually the hypertension in the latter is not modified by operation.

The sodium-retaining effect of large amounts of glucocorticoids also offers an explanation for the hypertension in severe cases of Cushing's syndrome (Chap. 317). Moreover, increased production of mineralocorticoids also has been documented in some patients with Cushing's syndrome. However, the hypertension in many cases of Cushing's syndrome does not seem volume-dependent, leading investigators to speculate that it may be secondary to glucocorticoid-induced production of renin substrate (angiotensin-mediated hypertension) or a steroid-induced change in vascular reactivity. In the forms of the adrenogenital syndrome due to C-11 or C-17 hydroxylase deficiency (Chap. 317) deoxycorticosterone accounts for the sodium retention and the resultant hypertension, which is accompanied by suppression of plasma renin activity.

In patients with pheochromocytoma (Chap. 318) increased secretion of epinephrine and norepinephrine by a tumor most often located in the adrenal medulla causes excessive stimulation of adrenergic receptors, which results in peripheral vasoconstriction and cardiac stimulation. This diagnosis is confirmed by demonstrating increased urinary excretion of epinephrine and norepinephrine or their metabolites.

Acromegaly (See also Chap. 313) Hypertension, coronary atherosclerosis, and cardiac hypertrophy are frequent complications of this condition.

Hypercalcemia (See also Chap. 339) The hypertension which occurs in up to one-third of patients with hyperparathyroidism ordinarily can be attributed to renal parenchymal damage due to nephrolithiasis and nephrocalcinosis. However, increased calcium levels can also have a direct vasoconstrictive effect. In some cases, the hypertension disappears when the hypercalcemia is corrected. Thus, paradoxically the increased serum calcium level in hyperparathyroidism raises blood pressure, while epidemiologic studies suggest that a high calcium intake lowers blood pressure. To further confuse the issue, calcium entry blocking agents are effective antihypertensive agents. Additional studies are needed to resolve these seemingly conflicting observations.

Oral contraceptives The most common cause of endocrine hypertension is that resulting from the use of estrogen-containing oral contraceptives. Indeed, this may be the most common form of secondary hypertension. The mechanism producing the hypertension is likely to be secondary to activation of the renin-angiotensin-aldosterone system. Thus, both volume (aldosterone) and vasoconstrictor (angiotensin II) factors are important. The estrogen component of oral contraceptive agents stimulates the hepatic synthesis of the renin substrate angiotensinogen, which in turn favors the increased production of angiotensin II and secondary aldosteronism. Women taking oral contraceptives have increased plasma concentrations of angiotensin II and aldosterone with some increase in arterial pressure. However, only about 5 percent actually have an increase in arterial pressure greater than 140/90, and in about half of these the hypertension will remit within 6 months of stopping the drug.

Why some women taking oral contraceptives develop hypertension and others do not is unclear but may be related to (1) increased vascular sensitivity to angiotensin II, (2) the presence of mild renal disease, (3) familial factors (over one-half have a positive family history for hypertension), (4) age (hypertension is significantly more prevalent in women over age 35), and/or (5) obesity. Indeed some investigators have suggested that the oral contraceptives are simply unmasking patients with essential hypertension.

COARCTATION OF THE AORTA (See also Chap. 186) The hypertension associated with coarctation may be caused by the constriction itself, or perhaps by the changes in the renal circulation which result in an unusual form of renal arterial hypertension. The diagnosis of coarctation is usually evident from physical examination and routine x-ray findings.

LOW-RENIN ESSENTIAL HYPERTENSION Approximately 20 percent of patients who by all other criteria have essential hypertension have suppressed plasma renin activity. This occurs more frequently in black than in white patients. Though these patients are not hypokalemic, they have been reported to have expanded extracellular fluid volumes, and it is tempting to implicate sodium retention and renin suppression due to excessive production of an unidentified mineralocorticoid. Involvement of the adrenal cortex is suggested by the observation that large doses of spironolactone, the mineralocorticoid antagonist, and the inhibition of steroidogenesis by aminoglutethimide can result in sodium loss and lowering of blood pressure in these patients. A search for other mineralocorticoids occasionally reveals increased secretion of 18-hydroxy-11-deoxycorticosterone, or 16-hydroxydehydroepiandrosterone, or 19-hydroxyandrostenedione in some patients. However, the frequency of these abnormalities is no greater than in patients with normal renin hypertension. Some studies have suggested that many of these patients have an increased sensitivity of their adrenal cortex to angiotensin II which may be the underlying mechanism. Since this altered sensitivity has been reported even in patients with normal renin hypertension, it is likely that patients with low-renin hypertension are not a distinct subset but rather form part of a continuum of patients with essential hypertension.

HIGH-RENIN ESSENTIAL HYPERTENSION Approximately 15 percent of patients with essential hypertension have plasma renin levels elevated above the normal range. It has been suggested that plasma renin plays an important role in the pathogenesis of the elevated blood pressure in these patients. However, most studies have documented that saralasin significantly reduces blood pressure in less than half of these patients. This has led some investigators to postulate that the elevated renin levels and blood pressure may both be secondary to an increased activity of the adrenergic system. It has been proposed that, in those patients with angiotensin-dependent high-renin hypertension whose arterial pressures are lowered by saralasin, the mechanism responsible for the increased renin and, therefore, the hypertension is a compensatory hyperreninemia secondary to a decreased adrenal responsiveness to angiotensin II. Additional studies have documented that patients with high-renin hypertension are the same as the nonmodulators described on p. 1003.

EFFECTS OF HYPERTENSION

Patients with hypertension die prematurely; the most common cause of death is heart disease, with stroke and renal failure also frequent, particularly in those with significant retinopathy.

EFFECTS ON HEART Cardiac compensation for the excessive work load imposed by increased systemic pressure is at first sustained by concentric left ventricular hypertrophy, characterized by an increase in wall thickness. Ultimately, the function of this chamber deteriorates, the cavity dilates, and the symptoms and signs of heart failure appear (Chap. 182). Angina pectoris may also occur because of the combination of accelerated coronary arterial disease and increased myocardial oxygen requirements as a consequence of the increased myocardial mass (Chap. 190). On physical examination the heart is enlarged and has a prominent left ventricular impulse. The sound of aortic closure is accentuated, and there may be a faint murmur of aortic regurgitation. Presystolic (atrial, fourth) heart sounds appear frequently in hypertensive heart disease, and a protodiastolic (ventricular, third heart) sound or summation gallop rhythm may be present. Electrocardiographic changes of left ventricular hypertrophy (Chap. 176) are common; evidence of ischemia or infarction may be observed late in the disease. The majority of deaths due to hypertension result from myocardial infarction or congestive heart failure.

NEUROLOGIC EFFECTS The neurologic effects of long-standing hypertension may be divided into retinal and central nervous system changes. Because the retina is the only tissue in which the arteries and arterioles can be examined directly, repeated ophthalmoscopic examination provides the opportunity to observe the progress of the vascular effects of hypertension (Table 196-4). The Keith-Wagener-Barker classification of the *retinal changes* in hypertension has provided a simple and excellent means for serial evaluation of hypertensive patients. Increasing severity of hypertension is associated with focal spasm and progressive general narrowing of the arterioles, as well as the appearance of hemorrhages, exudates, and papilledema. These retinal lesions often produce scotomata, blurred vision, and even blindness, especially in the presence of papilledema or hemorrhages of the macular area. Hypertensive lesions may develop acutely and, if therapy results in significant reduction of blood pressure, may show rapid resolution. Rarely, these lesions resolve without therapy. In contrast, retinal arteriolosclerosis results from endothelial and muscular proliferation, and it accurately reflects similar changes in other organs. Sclerotic changes do not develop as rapidly as hypertensive lesions, nor do they regress appreciably with therapy. As a consequence of increased wall thickness and rigidity, sclerotic arterioles distort and compress the veins as they cross within their common fibrous sheath, and the reflected light streak from the arterioles is changed by the increased opacity of the vessel wall.

Central nervous system dysfunction also occurs frequently in patients with hypertension. Occipital headaches, most often in the morning, are among the most prominent early symptoms of hypertension. Dizziness, lightheadedness, vertigo, tinnitus, and dimmed vision or syncope may also be observed, but the more serious manifestations are due to vascular occlusion, hemorrhage, or encephalopathy (Chap. 351). The pathogeneses of the former two disorders are quite different. *Cerebral infarction* is secondary to the

TABLE 196-4 Classification of hypertensive and arteriolosclerotic retinopathy

	Hypertension					Arteriolosclerosis	
	Arterioles						
Degree	General narrowing AV ratio*	Focal spasm†	Hemorrhages	Exudates	Papilledema	Arteriolar light reflex	AV crossing defects‡
Normal	3:4	1:1	0	0	0	Fine yellow line, red blood column	0
Grade I	1:2	1:1	0	0	0	Broadened yellow line, red blood column	Mild depression of vein
Grade II	1:3	2:3	0	0	0	Broad yellow line, "copper wire," blood column not visible	Depression or humping of vein
Grade III	1:4	1:3	+	+	0	Broad white line, "silver wire," blood column not visible	Right-angle deviation, tapering, and disappearance of vein under arteriole Distal dilatation of vein
Grade IV	Fine, fibrous cords	Obliteration of distal flow	+	+	+	Fibrous cords, blood column not visible	Same as grade III

* This is the ratio of arteriolar to venous diameters.
† This is the ratio of diameters of region of spasm to proximal arteriole.
‡ Arteriolar length and tortuosity increase with severity.

increased atherosclerosis observed in hypertensive patients, while *cerebral hemorrhage* is the result of both the elevated arterial pressure and the development of cerebral vascular microaneurysms (Charcot-Bouchard aneurysms). Only age and arterial pressure are known to influence the development of the microaneurysms. Thus, it is not surprising that the association of arterial pressure with cerebral hemorrhage is much better than with either cerebral or myocardial infarction.

Hypertensive encephalopathy consists of the following symptom complex: severe hypertension, disordered consciousness, increased intracranial pressure, retinopathy with papilledema, and seizures. The pathogenesis is uncertain but probably not related to arteriolar spasm or cerebral edema. Focal neurologic signs are infrequent, and if present, suggest that infarction, hemorrhage, or transient ischemic attacks are more likely diagnoses. Although some investigators have suggested that prompt lowering of arterial pressure in these patients may adversely affect cerebral blood flow, most studies indicate that this is not the case.

RENAL EFFECTS (See also Chap. 230) Arteriolosclerotic lesions of the afferent and efferent arterioles and the glomerular capillary tufts are the most common renal vascular lesions in hypertension and result in decreased glomerular filtration rate and tubular dysfunction. Proteinuria and microscopic hematuria occur because of glomerular lesions, and approximately 10 percent of the deaths secondary to hypertension result from renal failure. Blood loss in hypertension occurs not only from renal lesions; epistaxis, hemoptysis, and metrorrhagia also occur frequently in these patients.

APPROACH TO THE PATIENT WITH HYPERTENSION

In evaluating patients with hypertension, the initial history, physical examination, and laboratory tests should be directed at (1) uncovering correctable secondary forms of hypertension (Table 196-1), (2) establishing a pretreatment baseline, (3) assessing factors which may influence the type of therapy or which may be adversely modified by therapy, and (4) determining whether other risk factors for the development of arteriosclerotic cardiovascular disease are present (Chap. 195). Ideally, this evaluation would also determine the underlying mechanism(s) in essential hypertension, particularly if such information leads to a more specific therapeutic program. Unfortunately, at the present time this aspect of the evaluation is limited either by lack of knowledge of the underlying mechanisms, uncertainty as to the specificity of therapy for a distinct subset even if the underlying mechanisms are known, or the prohibitive expense in defining a subset of hypertensive patients even if specific therapy were available. However, with the accumulation of additional information a fifth component in the evaluation of patients with hypertension may become increasingly more important.

SYMPTOMS AND SIGNS The majority of patients with hypertension have no specific symptoms referable to their blood pressure elevation and will be identified only in the course of a physical examination. When symptoms do bring the patient to the physician, they fall into three categories. They are related to (1) the elevated pressure itself, (2) the hypertensive vascular disease, and (3) the underlying disease in the case of secondary hypertension. Though popularly considered a symptom of elevated arterial pressure, headache is characteristic only of severe hypertension; most commonly it is localized to the occipital region, is present when the patient awakens in the morning, and subsides spontaneously after several hours. Other possibly related complaints include dizziness, palpitations, easy fatigability, and impotency. Complaints referable to vascular disease include epistaxis, hematuria, blurring of vision owing to retinal changes, episodes of weakness or dizziness due to transient cerebral ischemia, angina pectoris, and dyspnea due to cardiac failure. Pain due to dissection of the aorta or to a leaking aneurysm is an occasional presenting symptom.

Examples of symptoms related to the underlying disease in secondary hypertension are polyuria, polydipsia, and muscle weakness secondary to hypokalemia in patients with primary aldosteronism, or weight gain and emotional lability in patients with Cushing's syndrome. The patient with a pheochromocytoma may present with episodic headaches, palpitations, diaphoresis, and postural dizziness.

CLINICAL EVALUATION History A strong family history of hypertension, along with the reported finding of intermittent pressure elevation in the past, favors the diagnosis of essential hypertension. Secondary hypertension often develops before the age of 35 or after the age of 55 years. The history of use of adrenal steroids or estrogens is of obvious significance. A history of repeated urinary tract infections suggests chronic pyelonephritis, although this condition may occur in the absence of symptoms; nocturia and polydipsia suggest renal or endocrine disease, while trauma to either flank or an episode of acute flank pain may be a clue to the presence of renal injury. A history of weight gain is compatible with Cushing's syndrome, and weight loss with pheochromocytoma. A number of aspects of the history aid in determining whether vascular disease has progressed to dangerous stages. These include angina pectoris and symptoms of cerebrovascular insufficiency, of congestive heart failure, and/or of peripheral vascular insufficiency. Other risk factors that should be elicited include cigarette smoking, diabetes mellitus, lipid disorders, and a family history of early deaths due to cardiovascular disease.

Physical examination The physical examination starts with the patient's general appearance. For instance, are the round face and trunkal obesity of Cushing's syndrome present? Is muscular development in the upper extremities out of proportion to that in the lower extremities, suggesting coarctation of the aorta? The next step is to compare the blood pressures and pulses in both upper extremities and in the supine and standing positions. A rise in diastolic pressure when the patient goes from the supine to the standing position is most compatible with essential hypertension; a fall, in the absence of antihypertensive medications, suggests secondary forms of hypertension. Detailed examination of the ocular fundi is mandatory, since funduscopic findings provide one of the best indications of the duration of hypertension and of prognosis. The Keith-Wagener-Barker classification of funduscopic changes (Table 196-4) is useful; the specific changes in each fundus should be recorded and a grade assigned. Palpation and auscultation of the carotid arteries for evidence of stenosis or occlusion are important; narrowing of a carotid artery may be a manifestation of hypertensive vascular disease, and it may also be a clue to the presence of a renal arterial lesion, since these two lesions may occur together. In examination of the heart and lungs, one should search for evidence of left ventricular hypertrophy and cardiac decompensation. Is there a left ventricular lift? Are third and fourth heart sounds present? Are there pulmonary rales? Chest examination also includes a search for extracardiac murmurs and palpable collateral vessels that may result from coarctation of the aorta.

The most important part of the abdominal examination is auscultation for bruits originating in stenotic renal arteries. Bruits due to renal arterial narrowing nearly always have a diastolic component or may be continuous and are best heard just to the right or left of the midline above the umbilicus, or in the flanks; they are present in many patients with renal artery stenosis due to fibrous dysplasia and in 40 to 50 percent of those with functionally significant stenosis due to arteriosclerosis. The abdomen also should be palpated for abdominal aneurysm and for the enlarged kidneys of polycystic renal disease. The femoral pulses must be carefully felt, and, if they are decreased and/or delayed in comparison to the radial pulse, the blood pressure in the lower extremities must be measured. Even if the femoral pulse is normal to palpation, arterial pressure in the lower extremities should be recorded at least once in patients in whom hypertension is discovered before the age of 30 years. Finally, examination of the extremities for edema and a search for evidence of a previous cerebrovascular accident and/or other intracranial pathology should be performed.

Laboratory investigation Controversy exists as to what laboratory studies should be performed in patients presenting with hypertension. In general, the disagreement resides in how extensively to evaluate the patient for secondary forms of hypertension or subsets of essential hypertension. In the following discussion laboratory studies are divided into those which should be performed in all patients with sustained hypertension (basic studies) and those which should be added if (1) from the initial evaluation a secondary form of hypertension is suggested and/or (2) arterial pressure is not controlled after initial therapy (secondary studies).

BASIC STUDIES Renal status is evaluated by assessing the presence of protein, blood, and glucose in the urine and measuring serum creatinine and/or blood urea nitrogen (BUN). Microscopic examination of the urine is also helpful. A serum potassium level is needed both as a screen for mineralocorticoid-induced hypertension and as a baseline prior to initiating diuretic therapy.

Other blood chemistries may also be useful, particularly since they can often be ordered as a battery of automated tests at minimal cost to the patient. For example, a blood glucose is helpful both because diabetes mellitus may be associated with accelerated arteriosclerosis, renal vascular disease, and diabetic nephropathy in patients with hypertension, and because primary aldosteronism, Cushing's syndrome, and pheochromocytoma all may be associated with hyperglycemia. Furthermore, since antihypertensive therapy with diuretics, for example, can raise the blood glucose level, it is important to establish a baseline. The possibility of hypercalcemia may also be investigated. Serum uric acid is useful because of the increased incidence of hyperuricemia in patients with renal and essential hypertension and because, as with blood glucose, the level subsequently may be raised by treatment with diuretics. Serum cholesterol and triglycerides may be measured to identify other factors which predispose to the development of arteriosclerosis. An electrocardiogram should be obtained in all cases as an assessment of cardiac status, particularly if left ventricular hypertrophy is present, and as a baseline. The chest roentgenogram may also be helpful by providing the opportunity to identify aortic dilatation or elongation and the rib notching that occurs in coarctation of the aorta.

SECONDARY STUDIES (Table 196-5) Certain clues from the history, physical examination, and basic laboratory studies may suggest an unusual cause for the hypertension and dictate the need for special studies. For example, the abrupt onset of severe hypertension and/or the onset of hypertension of any severity under the age of 25 or after the age of 50 years should lead to laboratory tests to exclude renovascular hypertension and pheochromocytoma. A history of headaches, palpitations, anxiety attacks, unusual sweating, hyperglycemia, and weight loss should also lead to tests to exclude pheochromocytoma. The presence of an abdominal bruit should lead to workup for renovascular hypertension, and the finding of bilateral upper abdominal masses on physical examination, consistent with polycystic renal disease, to the performance of an intravenous pyelogram. An elevated creatinine or blood urea nitrogen, associated with proteinuria and hematuria, should initiate a detailed workup for renal insufficiency (Chap. 222). Special studies for secondary hypertension are also indicated if there is therapeutic failure with the initial drug program. The specific diagnostic measures depend on the most likely causes of secondary hypertension.

Pheochromocytoma (See also Chap. 318) The easiest and best screening procedure for pheochromocytoma is the measurement of catecholamines or their metabolites in a 24-h urine collected during the time the patient is hypertensive. Measurement of plasma catecholamine levels may also be useful. These tests may be indicated even in patients who do not have episodic hypertension, since over half the patients with pheochromocytoma have fixed hypertension. Provocative tests are seldom if ever indicated, although occasionally a suppressive test may be useful.

Cushing's syndrome (See also Chap. 317) A 24-h urine test for cortisol or the administration of 1 mg dexamethasone at bedtime, followed by measurement of plasma cortisol at 7 to 10 A.M. is the best test for the presence of this condition. A urine cortisol less than 2750 nmol (100 μg) or suppression of the plasma cortisol level to below 140 nmol/L (5 μg/dL) effectively rules out Cushing's syndrome.

TABLE 196-5 Laboratory tests and special studies for evaluation of hypertension

I Basic studies
- *A* Always included
  - *1* Urine for protein, blood, and glucose
  - *2* Hematocrit
  - *3* Serum potassium
  - *4* Serum creatinine and/or blood urea nitrogen
  - *5* Electrocardiogram
- *B* Usually included, depending on cost and other factors
  - *1* Microscopic urinalysis
  - *2* White blood cell count
  - *3* Plasma/blood glucose, cholesterol, and triglycerides
  - *4* Serum calcium, phosphate, and uric acid
  - *5* Chest x-ray

II Special studies to screen for secondary hypertension
- *A* Renovascular: digital subtraction angiogram or rapid sequence IVP
- *B* Pheochromocytoma: 24-h urine for creatinine, metanephrines, and catecholamines or plasma catecholamines
- *C* Cushing's syndrome: overnight dexamethasone suppression test or 24-h urine cortisol

Renovascular hypertension (See also Chap. 230) The standard screening test for renal vascular hypertension has been the rapid-sequence intravenous pyelogram (IVP). Features suggestive of renal ischemia include (1) unilateral delayed appearance and excretion of contrast material, (2) a difference in kidney size greater than 1.5 cm, (3) irregular contour of the renal silhouette, suggesting partial infarction or atrophy, (4) indentations on the ureter or renal pelvis, possibly due to dilated ureteral arteries (collateral notching), and (5) hyperconcentration of contrast medium in the collecting system of the smaller kidney. When these criteria are used, the false-positive rate is 11 percent and the false-negative rate 12 percent. The digital subtraction angiogram has been received with considerable enthusiasm as a more precise screening test for renal vascular disease. Its ultimate place as a screening test is unclear, however, because of its relatively high cost and the need for an arterial rather than a venous injection. The isotope renogram and saralasin infusion test, both enthusiastically endorsed in the past as screening procedures, are now used infrequently either because of lower sensitivity and specificity or limited availability.

The definitive test of surgically correctable renal disease is the combination of a renal angiogram and renal vein renin determinations. The renal arteriogram both establishes the presence of a renal arterial lesion and aids in determining whether the lesion is due to atherosclerosis or to one of the fibrous or fibromuscular dysplasias. It does not, however, prove that the lesion is responsible for the hypertension, nor does it permit prediction of the chances of surgical cure; it must be noted that (1) renal artery stenosis is a frequent finding by angiography and at postmortem in normotensive individuals, and (2) essential hypertension is a common condition and may occur in combination with renal arterial stenosis which actually may not be responsible for the hypertension. Bilateral renal vein catheterization for measurement of plasma renin activity is, therefore, used to assess the functional significance of any lesion noted on arteriography. When one kidney is ischemic and the other is normal, all the renin released comes from the involved kidney. In the most straightforward situation, the ischemic kidney has a significantly higher venous plasma renin activity than the normal kidney by a factor of 1.5 or more. Moreover, the renal venous blood draining the uninvolved kidney exhibits levels similar to those in the inferior vena cava below the entrance of the renal veins. Significant benefit from operative correction may be anticipated in at least 80 percent of patients with the findings described above if care is taken to prepare the patient properly prior to renal vein blood sampling, i.e., discontinuing renin-suppressing drugs, such as beta blockers, for at least 10 days, placing the patient on a low sodium intake for 4 days, and/or giving a converting enzyme inhibitor for 24 h. When obstructing lesions in the *branches* of the renal arteries are demonstrated by arteriography, an attempt to obtain blood samples from the main *branches* of the renal vein should be made in an effort to identify a localized intrarenal arterial lesion responsible for the hypertension.

Primary aldosteronism (See also Chap. 317) These patients almost always exhibit hypokalemia. Diuretic therapy often complicates the picture when the hypokalemia is first observed and needs to be assessed. Given hypokalemia, the relation between plasma renin activity and the aldosterone level becomes the key to the diagnosis of primary aldosteronism. The aldosterone concentration or excretion is high and plasma renin activity is low in primary aldosteronism, and these levels are relatively unaffected by changes in sodium balance. A critical part of the evaluation after primary aldosteronism has been established is to determine whether unilateral or bilateral disease is present since surgical removal of the lesion usually reduces arterial pressure only in those with unilateral disease.

Plasma renin activity measurements Some studies have suggested that most hypertensive patients should have a plasma renin level measured and related to a 24-h urine sodium excretion rate to assess whether high, low, or normal levels are present. It has been proposed that this information may be important for both therapeutic and prognostic reasons. However, it is unclear, on the basis of presently available data and treatment programs, that these random measurements are really useful except in patients with findings suggestive of renal vascular disease or mineralocorticoid excess in whom lateralizing renal vein renin levels or suppressed peripheral renin levels may be of diagnostic and/or therapeutic significance.

TREATMENT

Virtually every patient with a diastolic arterial pressure which persistently exceeds 90 mmHg is a candidate for diagnostic studies and for subsequent treatment. Furthermore, at any given level of blood pressure elevation, the ultimate risk of developing hypertensive vascular complications is greater in men than in women, and in younger than in older persons. It may be argued, then, that it is hard to justify producing the uncomfortable side effects of therapy in, for example, an asymptomatic woman over 70 years of age with a diastolic pressure of 90 mmHg. On the other hand, it is easy to justify side effects in a man of 30 with a diastolic pressure exceeding 110 mmHg, because such a person may be expected to receive the greatest benefit from therapy. Fortunately, the choice of treatment is such that a satisfactory program to control arterial pressure with minimal side effects can be developed for most patients, particularly as more studies assessing the impact of specific therapeutic agents on the patient's quality of life are reported. A reasonable guideline would be that all patients with diastolic pressure repeatedly above 90 mmHg should be treated unless specific contraindications exist. There is controversy regarding the advisability of treating isolated *systolic* hypertension. Until the results of a well-controlled prospective study provide evidence to the contrary, treatment of isolated systolic hypertension may not be indicated. Patients with labile hypertension or isolated systolic hypertension who are not treated should have regular follow-up examinations at 6-month intervals, because of the frequent development of progressive and/or sustained hypertension.

The identification of an operable form of secondary hypertension does not automatically mean that surgical treatment is indicated. The decision depends upon the age and general health of the patient, the natural history of the lesion, and the response of the pressure to drug therapy. In patients with renovascular hypertension the feasibility of renal angioplasty, surgical repair versus nephrectomy, and the degree of overall renal function impairment must be considered. Age and general health are important in patients with renovascular hypertension due to arteriosclerosis, because there is no evidence that repair of the stenosis increases life expectancy in the elderly patient with other evidence of vascular disease. Knowledge of the natural history of the disease is especially important when approaching the decision in the young patient with renal-artery stenosis due to fibrous dysplasia. If the arteriographic appearance suggests that the stenosis is due to intimal or subadventitial fibroplasia, the lesion may be expected to progress and operation or angioplasty is required. Medial fibroplasia, on the other hand, often remains stable, and operation or angioplasty may not be necessary if pressure can be controlled by drug therapy. The decision regarding operation should also be considered carefully in patients with primary aldosteronism when bilateral adrenal venography does not demonstrate a tumor, because such patients may prove to have multinodular hyperplasia. This means that bilateral adrenalectomy would be required to eliminate the aldosterone excess, and, even then, hypertension usually persists. If hypokalemia can be controlled by spironolactone or other drug therapy, and arterial pressure lowered with antihypertensive agents, then it is reasonable to withhold operative treatment.

GENERAL MEASURES Nondrug therapeutic intervention is probably indicated in all patients with sustained hypertension and probably most with labile hypertension. The general measures employed include (1) relief of stress, (2) diet, (3) regular exercise, and (4) control of other risk factors contributing to the development of arteriosclerosis. Relief of emotional and environmental stress is one of the reasons for the improvement in hypertension that occurs when a patient is hospitalized. Though it is usually impossible to extricate the hypertensive patient from all internal and external stresses, he or she should be advised to avoid any unnecessary tensions. In rare instances, it may be appropriate to recommend a change of job or of life-style. Recently it has been suggested that relaxation techniques may also lower arterial pressure. However, it is uncertain that these techniques alone have much long-term effect.

Dietary management has three aspects:

1 Because of the documented efficacy of sodium restriction and volume contraction in lowering blood pressure, patients previously were instructed to curtail sodium intake drastically. Some investigators have suggested this is no longer necessary. They base their conclusion on two observations: (1) In many patients the blood pressure is not sensitive to the level of sodium intake, and (2) diuretics provide another method of decreasing body sodium stores in those individuals whose blood pressure may be sodium-sensitive. However, a number of reports have documented that while mild sodium restriction has little, if any, direct action on blood pressure, it significantly potentiates the efficacy of nearly all antihypertensive agents and thus, by allowing blood pressure control with lower doses of drugs, side effects are reduced. In addition, it is quite clear that in some hypertensive patients, as noted above, the level of sodium intake does influence the blood pressure. Thus, since there is no apparent risk to mild sodium restriction, the most practical approach now is to advise mild dietary sodium restriction (up to 5 g NaCl per day), which can be achieved by eliminating all additions of salt to food which is prepared normally. Some studies have also reported lowering of arterial pressure by *increasing* calcium intake. While the advisability of this form of dietary alteration is still controversial, since a moderately high calcium intake probably also reduces the extent of age-related osteoporosis, it is probably a useful adjunct.

2 Caloric restriction should be urged for the patient who is overweight. Some obese patients will show a significant reduction in pressure simply as a consequence of weight loss.

3 A restriction in intake of cholesterol and saturated fats is recommended since such a diet may diminish the incidence of arteriosclerotic complications. Regular exercise is indicated within the limits of the patient's cardiovascular status. Not only is exercise helpful in controlling weight, but in addition there is evidence that physical conditioning itself may lower arterial pressure. Isotonic exercises (jogging, swimming) are better than isometric exercises (weight lifting) since, if anything, the latter raises arterial pressure. The dietary management outlined above is aimed at the control of other risk factors. Probably the most significant additional step that could be taken in this area would be to convince the smoker to give up cigarettes.

DRUG THERAPY (Table 196-6) To make rational use of antihypertensive drugs, the sites and mechanisms of their action must be understood. In general, there are five classes of drugs: diuretics, antiadrenergic agents, vasodilators, calcium entry blockers, and angiotensin-converting enzyme (ACE) inhibitors.

Diuretics (See also Chap. 182) The thiazides are the most frequently used and most extensively investigated members of this group, and their early effect certainly is related to sodium diuresis and volume depletion. A reduction in peripheral vascular resistance also has been reported by some workers to be important in the long term. Traditionally, thiazide diuretics have formed the cornerstone of most therapeutic programs designed to lower arterial pressure and are usually effective within 3 to 4 days. However, in recent years increasing resistance to their routine use has occurred primarily because of their adverse metabolic effects, which include hypokalemia due to renal potassium loss, hyperuricemia due to uric acid retention, carbohydrate intolerance, and hyperlipidemia. The more potent loop-acting diuretics, furosemide and bumetanide, also have been shown to be antihypertensive but have been less extensively used for this purpose primarily because of their shorter duration of action. Spironolactone causes renal sodium loss by blocking the effect of endogenous mineralocorticoids, and therefore it may be more effective in patients whose mineralocorticoids are present in excess, e.g., primary or secondary aldosteronism. Although they do not compete directly with aldosterone, triamterene and amiloride act at the same site as spironolactone to impede sodium reabsorption and are effective in the same situations as spironolactone, except triamterene has little intrinsic antihypertensive effect. Their major disadvantage is that they can produce hyperkalemia, particularly in patients with impaired renal function. Any of these three potassium-sparing diuretics can also be given along with thiazide diuretics to minimize renal potassium loss.

Antiadrenergic agents (See also Chap. 67) These drugs act at one or more sites either centrally on the vasomotor center, in peripheral neurons modifying catecholamine release, or by blocking adrenergic receptor sites on target tissue. Drugs that appear to have predominant *central actions* are *clonidine, methyldopa, guanabenz,* and *guanfacine*. These drugs and their metabolites are predominantly alpha-receptor agonists. Stimulation of alpha$_2$ receptors in the vasomotor centers of the brain *reduces* sympathetic outflow, thereby reducing arterial pressure. Usually a fall in cardiac output and heart rate also occurs, more commonly with clonidine and guanabenz, but the baroreceptor reflex is intact. Thus, postural symptoms are absent. However, rebound hypertension may rarely occur when these drugs, particularly clonidine and guanabenz, are stopped. This is probably secondary to the increase in norepinephrine release which had been inhibited by these agents secondary to their agonist effect on presynaptic alpha receptors.

Another class of antiadrenergic agents is the *ganglionic blocking* drugs, which have little effect when the patient is supine but prevent reflex vasoconstriction in the upright position. Ganglionic blocking agents interfere with parasympathetic as well as sympathetic function, and this results in such side effects as impairment of visual accommodation, paralytic ileus, retention of urine, and failure of erection and ejaculation. Because of these problems, ganglionic blocking agents are now usually reserved for the rapid lowering of arterial pressure by parenteral administration of the short-acting agent *trimethaphan* in patients with severe hypertension.

Various drugs act at *postganglionic adrenergic nerve endings*. The *rauwolfia alkaloids* such as reserpine are the oldest members of the group; their long-term effect results from their ability to inhibit the storage of norepinephrine within the vesicles in adrenergic nerve endings, thus leading to depletion of catecholamine stores. The frequent side effects including depression, nasal congestion, diarrhea, impairment of sexual function, and increased gastric secretion have limited the use of these drugs. Reserpine is contraindicated in patients with current or past depression. *Guanethidine* and its shorter-acting analogue guanadrel block the release of norepinephrine from adrenergic nerve endings. They usually reduce cardiac output and lower systolic more than diastolic blood pressure. They also produce a greater postural effect than the other drugs that act at the nerve endings, and orthostatic hypotension is a frequent side effect particularly if other factors promoting vasodilation are present, e.g., heat, exercise, alcohol ingestion. However, centrally mediated side effects (sedation, depression) are infrequently observed since these drugs are poorly soluble in lipids and, therefore, do not readily enter the central nervous system.

The last group of drugs affecting the adrenergic system are those which block the *peripheral adrenergic receptors*, alpha, beta, or both (see also Chap. 67). *Phentolamine* and *phenoxybenzamine* block the action of norepinephrine at *alpha*-adrenergic receptor sites. While the above two compounds block both presynaptic (alpha$_2$) and postsynaptic (alpha$_1$) alpha receptors, the former action accounts for the tolerance which develops, while *prazosin* is more effective because it selectively blocks only *postsynaptic alpha* receptors, i.e., alpha$_1$ receptors. Thus, presynaptic alpha activity remains, suppressing norepinephrine release, and tolerance only infrequently occurs. Accordingly, prazosin produces less tachycardia but more postural

TABLE 196-6 Drugs used in treatment of hypertension—listed according to site of action

Site of action	Drug	Dosage	Indications	Contraindications	Frequent or peculiar side effects
DIURETICS					
Renal tubule	Thiazides: e.g., hydrochlorothiazide	Depends on specific drug Oral: 25 mg daily or twice daily	Mild hypertension, as adjunct in treatment of moderate to severe hypertension	Diabetes mellitus, hyperuricemia, primary aldosteronism	Potassium depletion, hyperglycemia, hyperuricemia, hypercholesterolemia, dermatitis, purpura, depression, hypercalcemia
	Loop acting: e.g., furosemide	Oral: 40–80 mg 2 or 3 times a day	Mild hypertension, as adjunct in severe or malignant hypertension particularly with renal failure	Hyperuricemia, primary aldosteronism	Potassium depletion, hyperuricemia, hyperglycemia, hypocalcemia, blood dyscrasias, rash, nausea, vomiting, diarrhea
	Potassium-sparing: Spironolactone	Oral: 25 mg 2 to 4 times daily	Hypertension due to hypermineralocorticoidism, adjunct to thiazide therapy	Renal failure	Hyperkalemia, diarrhea, gynecomastia, menstrual irregularities
	Triamterene	Oral: 50–100 mg 1 or 2 times daily	Hypertension due to hypermineralocorticoidism, adjunct to thiazide therapy	Renal failure	Hyperkalemia, nausea, vomiting, leg cramps, nephrolithiasis, GI disturbances
	Amiloride	Oral: 5–10 mg daily			
ANTIADRENERGIC AGENTS					
Central	Clonidine	Oral: 0.05–0.6 mg twice daily	Mild to moderate hypertension, renal disease with hypertension		Postural hypotension, drowsiness, dry mouth, rebound hypertension after abrupt withdrawal, insomnia
	Guanabenz	Oral: 4–16 mg twice daily			
	Guanfacine	Oral: 1–3 mg daily			
	Methyldopa (also acts by blocking sympathetic nerves)	Oral: 250–1000 mg twice daily IV: 250–1000 mg every 4–6 h (tolerance may develop)	Mild to moderate hypertension (oral), malignant hypertension (IV)	Pheochromocytoma, active hepatic disease (IV), during MAO inhibitor administration	Postural hypotension, sedation, fatigue, diarrhea, impaired ejaculation, fever, gynecomastia, lactation, positive Coombs tests (occasionally associated with hemolysis), chronic hepatitis, acute ulcerative colitis, lupuslike syndrome
Autonomic ganglia	Trimethaphan	IV: 1–6 mg/min	Severe or malignant hypertension	Severe coronary artery disease, cerebrovascular insufficiency, diabetes mellitus (on hypoglycemic therapy), glaucoma, prostatism	Postural hypotension, visual symptoms, dry mouth, constipation, urinary retention, impotence
Nerve endings	Rauwolfia alkaloids: Reserpine	Oral: 0.05–0.25 mg daily	Mild to moderate hypertension in young patient	Pheochromocytoma, peptic ulcer, depression, during MAO inhibitor administration	Depression, nightmares, nasal congestion, dyspepsia, diarrhea, impotence
	Guanethidine	Oral: 10–150 mg daily	Moderate to severe hypertension	Pheochromocytoma, severe coronary artery disease, cerebrovascular insufficiency, during MAO inhibitor administration	Postural hypotension, bradycardia, dry mouth, diarrhea, impaired ejaculation, fluid retention, asthma
	Guanadrel	Oral 5–75 mg twice daily			
Alpha receptors	Phentolamine	IV: 1–5 mg	Suspected or proved pheochromocytoma	Severe coronary artery disease	Tachycardia weakness, dizziness, flushing
	Phenoxybenzamine	Oral: 10–50 mg once or twice daily (tolerance may develop)	Proven pheochromocytoma		Postural hypotension, tachycardia, miosis, nasal congestion, dry mouth
	Prazosin	Oral: 1–10 mg twice daily	Mild to moderate hypertension	Use with caution in the elderly	Sudden syncope, headache, sedation dizziness, tachycardia anticholinergic effect, fluid retention
	Terazosin	Oral: 1–20 mg daily			

(continued)

hypotension than direct-acting vasodilators, e.g., hydralazine, and rarely can produce substantial hypotension following the first dose.

A variety of effective *beta-adrenergic receptor blocking agents* are available which block sympathetic effects on the heart and should be most effective in reducing cardiac output and in lowering arterial pressure when there is increased cardiac sympathetic nerve activity. In addition, they block the adrenergic nerve-mediated release of renin from the renal juxtaglomerular cells, and this action may be an important component of their blood pressure–lowering action. Beta-adrenergic blockers are particularly useful when employed in conjunction with vascular smooth-muscle relaxants, which tend to evoke a reflex increase in myocardial contractility, and with diuretics, the administration of which often results in an elevation of circulating renin activity. In practice, beta blockers appear to be effective even

TABLE 196-6 Drugs used in treatment of hypertension—listed according to site of action *(continued)*

Site of action	Drug	Dosage	Indications	Contraindications	Frequent or peculiar side effects
ANTIADRENERGIC AGENTS *(continued)*					
Beta receptors	Propranolol Metoprolol Nadolol Atenolol Timolol	Oral: 10–120 mg 2 to 4 times daily Oral: 25–150 mg twice daily Oral: 20–120 mg daily Oral 25–100 mg daily Oral: 5–15 mg twice daily	Mild to moderate hypertension (especially with evidence for hyperdynamic circulation), adjunct to hydralazine therapy	Congestive heart failure, asthma, diabetes mellitus (on hypoglycemic therapy), during MAO inhibitor administration, COPD, sick sinus syndrome, 2d or 3d degree heart block	Dizziness, depression, bronchospasm, nausea, vomiting, diarrhea, constipation, heart failure, fatigue, Raynaud's phenomenon, hallucinations, hypertriglyceridemia, hypercholesterolemia, psoriasis; sudden withdrawal may precipitate angina or myocardial injury in patients with heart disease
	Pindolol	Oral: 5–30 mg twice daily			Less resting bradycardia than other beta blockers
	Acebutolol	Oral: 200–600 mg twice daily			
	Labetalol	Oral: 100–600 mg twice daily IV: 2 mg/min			
VASODILATORS					
Vascular smooth muscle	Hydralazine	Oral: 10–75 mg 4 times daily IV or IM: 10–50 mg every 6 h (tolerance may develop)	As adjunct in treatment of moderate to severe hypertension (oral), malignant hypertension (IV or IM), renal disease with hypertension	Lupus erythematosus, severe coronary artery disease	Headache, tachycardia, angina pectoris, anorexia, nausea, vomiting, diarrhea, lupus-like syndrome, rash, fluid retention
	Minoxidil	Oral 2.5–40 mg twice daily	Severe hypertension	Severe coronary artery disease	Tachycardia, aggravates angina, marked fluid retention, hair growth on face and body, coarsening of facial features, possible pericardial effusions
	Diazoxide	IV: 1–3 mg/kg up to 150 mg rapidly	Severe or malignant hypertension	Diabetes mellitus, hyperuricemia, congestive heart failure	Hyperglycemia, hyperuricemia, sodium retention
	Nitroprusside	IV:0.5–8 (μg/kg)/min	Malignant hypertension		Apprehension, weakness, diaphoresis, nausea, vomiting, muscle twitching
ANGIOTENSIN-CONVERTING ENZYME INHIBITORS					
Converting enzyme	Captopril	Oral: 12.5–75 mg twice daily	Mild to severe hypertension, renal artery stenosis	Renal failure (reduction of dose), bilateral renal artery stenosis, pregnancy	Leukopenia, pancytopenia, hypotension, cough, angioedema, urticarial rash, fever, loss of taste, acute renal failure in bilateral renal artery stenosis
	Enalapril Enalaprilat Lysinopril	Oral: 2.5–40 mg daily IV: 0.625–1.25 mg over 5 minutes every 6–8 hrs Oral: 5–40 mg daily			Same as captopril, but little evidence for leukopenia, but increased frequency of cough and angioedema
CALCIUM CHANNEL ANTAGONISTS					
Vascular smooth muscle	Nifedipine	Oral: 10–30 mg 4 times daily	Mild to moderate hypertension	Heart failure, 2d or 3d degree heart block	Tachycardia, flushing, gastrointestinal disturbances, hyperkalemia, edema, headache
	Diltiazem Verapamil	Oral: 30–90 mg 4 times daily Oral: 30–120 mg 4 times daily or as SR form 120–480 mg daily			Same as nifidepine, except no tachycardia, but can cause heart block, constipation, and liver dysfunction

when there is no evidence of increased sympathetic tone with about one-half or more of all hypertensive patients showing a fall in pressure. However, these agents can precipitate congestive heart failure and asthma in susceptible individuals and must be used with caution in diabetics receiving hypoglycemic therapy because they inhibit the usual sympathetic responses to hypoglycemia. Cardioselective beta-blocking agents (so-called $beta_1$ blockers) have been developed (metoprolol, atenolol) which may be superior to nonselective beta blockers such as propranolol and timolol in patients with bronchospasm. Nadolol, a nonselective beta blocker, unlike other drugs of this class is excreted unchanged in the urine and has a half-life of 14 to 20 h. Therefore, only one dose a day is required. Atenolol also usually only needs to be given once a day. Pindolol and acebutolol are nonselective beta blockers with partial agonist activity and, therefore, produce less bradycardia. Labetalol exerts both alpha- and beta-adrenergic blocking actions. Thus, it lowers arterial pressure by the same complex actions as do beta blockers, but also directly by reducing systemic vascular resistance. Usually it has a more rapid onset of action but produces more postural symptoms and chronic sexual dysfunction than the other beta blockers.

Vasodilators *Hydralazine* is the most versatile of the drugs that cause direct relaxation of vascular smooth muscle; it is effective both orally and parenterally, acting mainly on arterial resistance, rather than on venous capacitance vessels, as evidenced by lack of postural changes. Unfortunately, the effect of hydralazine on peripheral resistance is partly negated by reflex increases in sympathetic discharge that raise heart rate and cardiac output. This limits the usefulness of hydralazine, especially in patients with severe coronary artery disease. However, the efficacy of hydralazine can be increased if it is given in conjunction with beta blockers or drugs such as methyldopa or clonidine, all of which block reflex sympathetic stimulation of the heart. A serious side effect of doses of hydralazine exceeding 300 mg per day has been the production of a lupus erythematosus-like syndrome.

Minoxidil is even more potent but unfortunately produces significant hirsutism and fluid retention and, therefore, is mainly limited to patients with severe hypertension and renal insufficiency.

Diazoxide, a thiazide derivative, is restricted in its application to acute situations. It is not a diuretic; in fact, it causes sodium retention. However, like other thiazides, it reduces carbohydrate tolerance. It must be given rapidly intravenously to guarantee effect. It begins to act immediately to lower blood pressure, and its effects may last for several hours. *Nitroprusside* given intravenously also acts as a direct vasodilator, with onset and offset of actions that are almost immediate. These latter two drugs are useful only for the treatment of hypertensive emergencies (Table 196-7).

Angiotensin-converting enzyme (ACE) inhibitors Drugs from several of the categories discussed above have been shown to possess an additional action resulting in inhibition of renin secretion. These include clonidine, reserpine, methyldopa, and beta blockers. A second group of drugs in this class are those which inhibit the enzyme converting angiotensin I into angiotensin II, e.g., captopril, enalapril, and lysinopril. These agents are useful because they not only inhibit the generation of a potent vasoconstrictor (angiotensin II) but also may retard the degradation of a potent vasodilator (bradykinin), alter prostaglandin production (most notably with captopril), and can modify the activity of the adrenergic nervous system. They are especially useful in renal or renovascular hypertension, as well as in accelerated and malignant hypertension. They are also as effective in mild, uncomplicated hypertension as beta blockers and thiazides—probably with fewer side effects, particularly those that adversely affect the patient's quality of life.

These drugs should be used with caution when the renin system is activated, e.g., with severe heart failure, prior diuretic therapy, or substantial salt restriction, in order to avoid profound hypotension. Usually diuretics are stopped 2 to 3 days before starting an ACE inhibitor and added back later if needed.

Calcium channel antagonists These drugs (diltiazem, nifedipine, and verapamil) modify the entry of calcium into cells by blocking the slow or voltage-dependent calcium channels, resulting in vasodilatation and in the case of nifedipine, usually reflex tachycardia. Diltiazem and verapamil both can slow atrioventricular conduction—a feature not observed with nifedipine. While calcium channel antagonists are also useful in angina pectoris (see Chap. 189), because of their negative inotropic actions they should be used with caution in hypertensive patients with heart failure.

APPROACH TO DRUG THERAPY (Fig. 196-1) The aim of drug therapy is to use the agents just described, alone or in combination, to return arterial pressure to normal levels with minimal side effects. Ideally, one would choose a therapeutic program which specifically corrects the underlying defect resulting in the elevated blood pressure, e.g., spironolactone for patients with primary aldosteronism. As our knowledge of the mechanisms underlying the hypertension in individual patients increases, more specific drug programs will become available. This presumably will result in normalization of blood pressure with fewer side effects. In the absence of that information an empiric approach is used, which takes into consideration efficacy, safety, impact on the quality of life, and ease of administration. When used in combination, drugs are chosen for their different sites of action. However, except for those patients with severe hypertension (average diastolic blood pressure greater than 130 mmHg) in whom intensive therapy with several agents simultaneously usually is required, most patients should *initially* be treated with a single agent. Since many effective antihypertensive agents are available, a number of useful therapeutic regimens have been developed, with the ideal program still unclear. Initial therapy with a diuretic or beta blocker has been the usual first approach. However, the Joint National Committee on Detection, Evaluation, and Treatment of Hypertension has recently added ACE inhibitors and calcium channel antagonists as first-line therapy, thus replacing the old stepped-care approach.

TABLE 196-7 Therapeutic agents used to treat malignant hypertension

Drug	Route	Time course of action: Onset	Peak	Duration	Oral preparation available
IMMEDIATE ONSET					
Diazoxide	IV bolus	1–3 min	2–4 min	4–12 h	No
Nitroprusside	Continuous IV	<1 min	1–2 min	2–5 min	No
Trimethaphan	Continuous IV	<1 min	1–2 min	2–5 min	No
DELAYED ONSET					
Enalaprilat	IV	10–15 min	3–4 h	6–24 h	Yes
Hydralazine	IV, IM	10–20 min	20–40 min	4–12 h	Yes
Labetalol	IV	5 min	20–30 min	3–6 h	Yes
Methyldopa	IV	1–3 h	3–5 h	2–12 h	Yes
Nifedipine	SL	5–15 min	30–60 min	3–6 h	Yes
Reserpine	IM	2–3 h	3–4 h	6–24 h	Yes

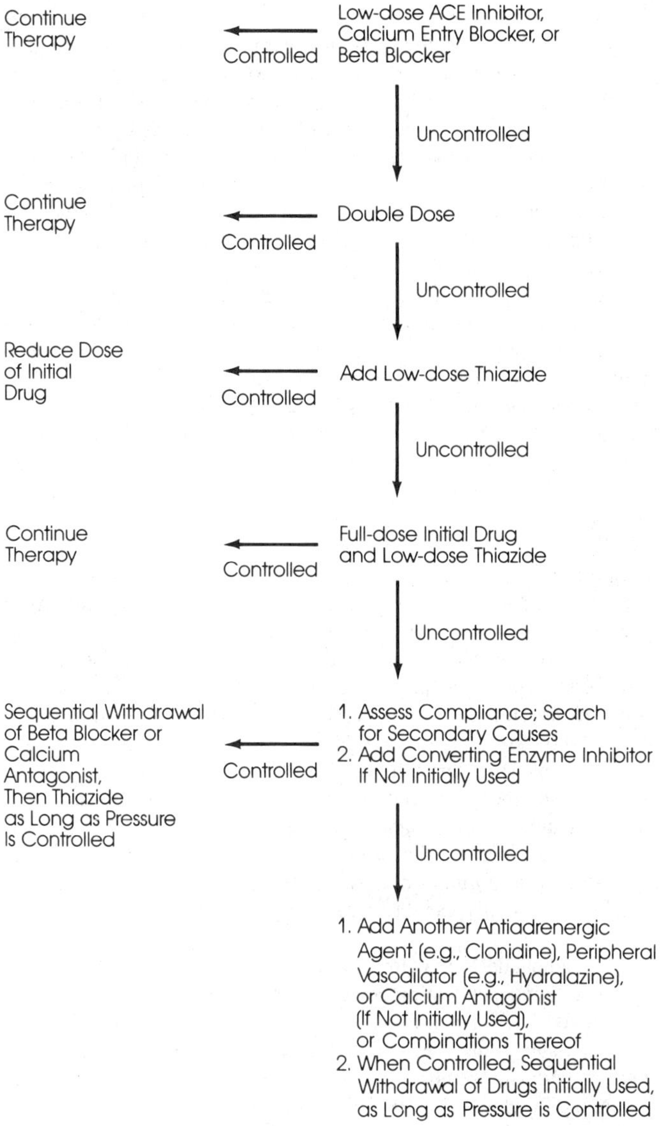

FIGURE 196-1 Schematic approach to the treatment of the patient with hypertension in whom a specific form of therapy is unavailable or unknown.

The physician is, therefore, required to choose from four classes of agents for initial therapy with little evidence that one is more effective than another. Because of their reduced side effects, some have suggested that an ACE inhibitor or calcium channel blocker be used first, with a slight preference for ACE inhibitors because of their longer duration of action and potentially less severe adverse effects. We agree with this suggestion. The reason for choosing one drug over the others is empiric although, in general, older individuals and blacks may be particularly responsive to diuretics while younger individuals and whites respond well to beta blockers, ACE inhibitors, and calcium channel antagonists.

The schema outlined in Fig. 196-1 takes into account the presently available data on effectiveness, adverse reactions, compliance, impact on quality of life, and economic impact (including cost, usage of health care resources, quality and quantity of work performance) in deciding when to use a given agent. This approach is applicable to all patients in whom an indication for a specific form of therapy is lacking. Because of its lower cost, low-dose thiazide therapy, e.g., 25 mg of hydrochlorothiazide (or its equivalent) daily, often has been the first choice. However, three major concerns with widespread thiazide usage have arisen: relatively poor compliance rates (approximately 80 percent) probably reflecting an adverse effect on the patient's quality of life; adverse metabolic effects (hypokalemia, hypomagnesemia, hyperglycemia, and possibly hypercholesterolemia); and potentially an increased frequency of cardiac arrhythmias including sudden death, probably secondary to the electrolyte disturbances. These concerns coupled with the eight- to tenfold increase in cost associated with the frequent need for potassium supplementation or a potassium-sparing diuretic have caused some to suggest that thiazides should play a more restricted role in initial antihypertensive therapy, limited to those individuals who are volume expanded. Thus, ACE inhibitors, beta blockers, and calcium channel antagonists are probably the preferred first line therapy for hypertension, with beta blockers being particularly useful in patients with a hyperactive hemodynamic state, e.g., hypertension with an elevated heart rate.

Under any circumstance, the agent should be started at a low dose, e.g., 25 mg of atenolol, 25 mg of captopril, 5 mg of enalapril, or 120 mg of diltiazem (or their equivalents) in divided doses as needed (Table 196-6). If arterial pressure is lowered to less than 140/90 with any of these agents, no further therapy is indicated (Fig. 196-1). If it is not, the next step is to double the dose of the primary agent. If still not controlled, then 25 mg of hydrochlorothiazide (or its equivalent) daily should be added. Thiazides potentiate the action of ACE inhibitors and probably of beta blockers and at least are additive to the antihypertensive effect of calcium channel antagonists. Combining diuretics with ACE inhibitors is particularly appealing since the adverse metabolic effects of the thiazide, in part, will be ameliorated by the ACE inhibitor. This is not true for beta blockers or calcium antagonists. Indeed, beta blockers and thiazides may actually potentiate each other's adverse effects insofar as electrolytes (hypokalemia) and metabolic actions (hypercholesterolemia) are concerned.

If therapy with two drugs does not achieve blood pressure control, the primary agent should be increased to full dose, e.g., 100 mg of captopril or atenolol, 20 mg of enalapril, or 360 mg of diltiazem. While larger doses than these can be used, it is probably advisable to switch to another medication rather than increase the dose further. Occasionally, increasing the thiazide to the equivalent of 50 mg of hydrochlorothiazide daily may bring about control of the hypertension; however, thiazide doses higher than this are seldom, if ever, warranted since they almost invariably produce significant side effects. If the blood pressure is still not controlled, then a detailed search for a secondary cause of hypertension as outlined above is indicated. If none is found, then a dietary assessment often will reveal a high sodium intake. With reduction in salt intake to 5 g per day or less, blood pressure often is controlled. If the blood pressure is still not controlled, then the primary agent should be switched, maintaining the thiazide. Caution should be used if an ACE inhibitor was not the original agent, since administration of such an agent to a patient who already is taking a diuretic may lead to profound hypotension. If none of the changes produce better control of arterial pressure, then the combination of a calcium channel antagonist and an ACE inhibitor or triple therapy usually with a diuretic, ACE inhibitor, and hydralazine may be effective.

If the blood pressure is controlled, then there should be stepwise reduction in the dose and/or withdrawal of some of the agents in order to determine the minimal therapeutic program that will maintain the blood pressure at 140/90 mmHg or less.

Fewer than 5 percent of patients will still be hypertensive at this point. In them, one first should consider the reasons for therapeutic failure as shown in Table 196-8. If none can be identified, then one of the other agents such as a vasodilator listed in Table 196-6 (e.g., hydralazine) or an antiadrenergic agent (e.g., prazosin or clonidine) should be added. If blood pressure is controlled, previous drugs are sequentially withdrawn in order to determine the minimal therapeutic program that maintains a normal blood pressure.

While the recommendations outlined above are satisfactory for a large majority of patients, it is important to use a flexible approach since individual patients may respond differently to individual drugs and drug combinations. For those patients requiring multiple drugs, once the appropriate combination has been found, the use of a single formulation with the appropriate combination of drugs may simplify

TABLE 196-8 Reasons for poor therapeutic response in patients with hypertension

1 Inadequate patient compliance
2 Volume expansion
  a Excessive sodium intake
  b Secondary to nondiuretic antihypertensive agent
3 Excessive weight gain
4 Inadequate doses
5 Drug antagonism
  a Cold remedies
  b Sympathomimetics
  c Oral contraceptives (estrogens)
  d Adrenal steroids
6 Secondary forms of hypertension

the regimen and thereby increase compliance. Every effort should be made to reduce the number of times each day the patients must interrupt his or her schedule for the medication. Pharmacologic treatment of essential hypertension is usually lifelong, and since most patients are asymptomatic, compliance with a complex regimen may be a serious problem, particularly if the therapeutic regimen has a negative impact on the quality of the patient's life.

Special considerations Four groups of patients with hypertension require special consideration because of associated conditions.

RENAL DISEASE Reduction of arterial pressure in hypertensive patients with impaired renal function is often accompanied initially by an increase in serum creatinine. This change does not represent further structural renal damage and should not deter continuation of therapy, since achievement of blood pressure control may eventually reduce the value toward normal. However, if serum creatinine increases in patients treated with a converting enzyme inhibitor, care needs to be exercised since these patients may have bilateral renal artery disease. Their renal function will continue to deteriorate as long as the converting enzyme inhibitor is given. Thus, converting enzyme inhibitors should be used cautiously in patients with impaired renal function and renal function should be assessed frequently (every 4 to 5 days) for the first 3 weeks. While converting enzyme inhibitors are contraindicated in patients with bilateral renal artery stenosis, these are the drugs of choice in patients with unilateral renal artery stenosis and a normally functioning contralateral kidney and perhaps in patients with chronic renal failure.

CORONARY ARTERY DISEASE In these patients who may also be taking cardiac glycosides, thiazides should be used judiciously and a reduction in serum potassium levels should be looked for and if found, should be corrected rapidly. Beta blockers should be withdrawn carefully, if at all, in these patients. Finally, calcium channel antagonists and converting enzyme inhibitors may be particularly useful in these patients since they minimize a number of potential adverse reactions accompanying other therapeutic agents, particularly nonspecific vasodilators.

DIABETES MELLITUS The diabetic patient with hypertension is particularly challenging since many of the agents used to lower blood pressure can affect glucose metabolism adversely. Converting enzyme inhibitors may be particularly useful in these individuals. They have no known adverse effects on glucose or lipid metabolism and may actually minimize the development of diabetic nephropathy by reducing renal vascular resistance and renal perfusion pressure—the primary factor underlying renal deterioration in these patients.

PREGNANCY The patient who is pregnant and hypertensive or who develops hypertension during pregnancy (pregnancy-induced hypertension, preeclampsia, eclampsia) is particularly difficult to treat. Because it is uncertain that autoregulation of uterine blood flow occurs, lowering blood pressure in the pregnant hypertensive may result in reduced placental and fetal perfusion. Thus, a conservative approach to lowering blood pressure is usually indicated. In the second and third trimesters, antihypertensives often are not indicated unless the diastolic pressure exceeds 95 mmHg. In general, severe salt restriction and/or diuretics are not given because of the associated increase in fetal wastage. Beta blockers need to be used cautiously for similar reasons. Methyldopa and hydralazine are the most frequent antihypertensives used since they have no known adverse effects on the fetus. Little is known about the safety of other antihypertensives in pregnancy except that nitroprusside and converting enzyme inhibitors may cause adverse effects on the fetus and should be avoided.

Probably fewer than one-third of hypertensive patients in the United States are being treated effectively. Only a small number of these failures is related to drug unresponsiveness. The majority is related to (1) failure to detect hypertension, (2) failure to institute effective treatment of the asymptomatic hypertensive subject, and (3) failure of the asymptomatic hypertensive subject to adhere to therapy. In order to improve this deficiency, patients must be educated to continue treatment once an effective regimen has been identified. Side effects and inconveniences of treatment must be minimized or counteracted in order to obtain the patient's continued cooperation.

MALIGNANT HYPERTENSION

In addition to marked blood pressure elevation in association with papilledema and retinal hemorrhages and exudates, the full-blown picture of malignant hypertension may include manifestations of hypertensive encephalopathy, such as severe headache, vomiting, visual disturbances (including transient blindness), transient paralyses, convulsions, stupor, and coma. These have been attributed to spasm of cerebral vessels and to cerebral edema. In some patients who have died, multiple small thrombi have been found in the cerebral vessels. Cardiac decompensation and rapidly declining renal function are other critical features of malignant hypertension. Oliguria may, in fact, be the presenting feature. The vascular lesion characteristic of malignant hypertension is fibrinoid necrosis of the walls of small arteries and arterioles, and this can be reversed by effective antihypertensive therapy.

The pathogenesis of malignant hypertension is unknown. However, at least two independent processes, dilatation of cerebral arteries and generalized arteriolar fibrinoid necrosis, contribute to the associated signs and symptoms. The cerebral arteries dilate because the normal autoregulation of cerebral blood flow decompensates secondary to the markedly elevated arterial pressure. As a result, cerebral blood flow is excessive, producing the encephalopathy associated with malignant hypertension. Many patients also show evidence of a microangiopathic hemolytic anemia; this secondary phenomenon could contribute to the deterioration of renal function. Most patients also have elevated levels of peripheral plasma renin activity and increased aldosterone production, and these may be involved in causing vascular damage.

About 1 percent of hypertensive patients develop the malignant phase, which occurs in the course of both essential and secondary hypertension. Rarely it is the first recognized manifestation of the blood pressure problem. The average age at diagnosis is 40, and men are more often affected than women. Prior to the availability of effective therapy, life expectancy after diagnosis of malignant hypertension was less than 2 years, with most deaths being due to renal failure, cerebral hemorrhage, or congestive heart failure. With the advent of effective antihypertensive therapy, at least half of the patients survive for more than 5 years.

Malignant hypertension is a medical emergency and requires immediate therapy. The initial aim of therapy should be to reduce diastolic pressure by one-third, but not below 95 mmHg. The drugs available for treatment of malignant hypertension can be divided into two groups on the basis of time of onset of action (Table 196-7). Those in the first group act within a few minutes but are not satisfactory for long-term management. If the patient is having convulsions, if arterial pressure must be reduced rapidly, then one from the immediate-acting group should be used. *Diazoxide* is the easiest to administer, for no individual titration of dosage is required. It primarily effects arteriolar and not venous tone. A dose of 300 mg is given rapidly intravenously, and the antihypertensive effect is noted in 1 to 3 min. The same dose can be repeated when the pressure begins to rise, usually after several hours. In an occasional patient, pressure may drop below normal levels after diazoxide administration. Because of this, some physicians use a modified program, giving 150 mg rather than 300 mg initially, followed by a second 150-mg dose in 5 min if the blood pressure response has been minimal. It should not be used in patients in whom aortic dissection or myocardial infarction is suspected. Because it can increase the force of myocardial contraction, often a beta blocker is given concomitantly. The other two agents in this group require continuous infusion and close monitoring. *Nitroprusside* is given by continuous intravenous infusion at a dose of 0.5 to 8.0 (μg/kg)/min. It is probably the agent of choice in this condition. It has the advantage over the ganglionic blockers of not being associated with the development of tachyphylaxis and can be utilized for days with few side effects. The dosage must be controlled with an infusion pump. *Trimethaphan,* a ganglionic blocker, is given at a rate of 1 to 15 mg/min. The patient should be in the sitting position, and the pressure should be monitored closely, preferably in an intensive care unit. Monitoring may be more complex than with nitroprusside, but trimethaphan may be better therapy in acute aortic dissection. An intravenous form of one ACE inhibitor, *enalaprilat,* has also proven effective in preliminary studies. Finally, intravenous *labetalol* may be particularly useful in patients with a myocardial infarct or angina since it prevents an increase in heart rate. However, it may be ineffective in patients previously treated with beta blockers and is contraindicated in patients with heart failure, asthma, bradycardia, or heart block.

Patients given any of these agents should also receive other medications effective for long-term control. Those in the second group in Table 196-7 require 30 min or more to obtain full effect but have the advantage of being satisfactory for subsequent oral administration and for long-term management of the patient's hypertension. If such a delay in attainment of full effect is acceptable, intravenous *methyldopa* is an effective drug with which to begin therapy if symptoms of encephalopathy are absent. A dose of 500 mg in 100 to 200 mL 5% dextrose in water is given intravenously over 30 min; if the effect is inadequate in 2 to 4 h, a second dose of 500 to 1000 mg is given. Additional intravenous doses may then be given every 6 h until the pressure is stabilized. Intravenous *hydralazine* is effective in many patients within 10 min; an effective protocol involves giving 10-mg doses intravenously every 10 to 15 min until the desired effect has been obtained or until a total of 50 mg has been administered. The total required for response may then be repeated intramuscularly or intravenously every 6 h. Hydralazine should be used with caution in patients with significant coronary artery disease and should be avoided in patients evidencing myocardial ischemia or aortic dissection. Sublingual *nifedipine* recently has been reported to be useful in some cases, although it may produce tachycardia and success has not been uniform.

Furosemide is an important adjunct to the therapy just discussed. Given either orally or intravenously, it serves to maintain sodium diuresis in the face of a falling arterial pressure and thus will speed recovery from encephalopathy and congestive heart failure as well as maintain sensitivity to the primary antihypertensive drug. Digitalis (Chap. 182) also is indicated if there is evidence of cardiac decompensation.

In patients with malignant hypertension in whom the existence of pheochromocytoma is suspected, urine should be collected for measurement of the products of catecholamine metabolism, and drugs which might release additional catecholamines, such as methyldopa, reserpine, and guanethidine, must be avoided. The parenteral drug of choice in these patients is phentolamine, administered with care to avoid a precipitous reduction in arterial pressure.

There is hope even for patients who fail to respond sufficiently to any of the forms of therapy and who show progressive deterioration in renal function. In some, a period of peritoneal dialysis or hemodialysis to deplete extracellular fluid has resulted in better blood pressure control and eventual improvement in renal function. In other patients with refractory hypertension and renal failure who do not respond to volume depletion or hypotensive therapy, including minoxidil, particularly those with marked elevation of plasma renin activity, bilateral nephrectomy has resulted in amelioration of hypertension; subsequently these patients have been maintained on chronic dialysis or have received renal homografts. However, bilateral nephrectomy should be avoided where possible since (1) the loss of renal erythropoietin will contribute to the associated anemia, (2) vitamin D metabolism may be adversely affected, and (3) all residual renal function will be lost.

REFERENCES

AMERY A et al: Mortality and morbidity results for the European working party on high blood pressure in the elderly trial. Lancet 1:1349, 1985

BERGLUND G et al: Prevalence of primary and secondary hypertension: Studies in a random population sample. Br Med J 2:554, 1976

BLAUSTEIN MP: Role of natriuretic factor in essential hypertension: An hypothesis. Ann Intern Med 98:785, 1983

BOUDOULAS H et al: Left ventricular mass and systolic performance in chronic systemic hypertension. Am J Cardiol 57:232, 1986

COOPE J, WARRENDER TS: Randomized trial of treatment of hypertension in elderly patients in primary care. Br Med J 293:1145, 1986

CURB JD et al: Antihypertensive drug side effects in the hypertension detection and follow-up program. Hypertension 11:51, 1988

DANNENBERG AL et al: Incidence of hypertension in the Framingham study. Am J Public Health 78:676, 1988

GOTTDIENER JS et al: Left ventricular hypertrophy in men with normal blood pressure: Relation to exaggerated blood pressure response to exercise. Ann Intern Med 112(3):161, 1990

HOLME I et al: Treatment of mild hypertension with diuretics. The importance of ECG abnormalities in the Oslo study and in MRFIT. JAMA 251:1298, 1984

JOINT NATIONAL COMMITTEE ON DETECTION, EVALUATION AND TREATMENT OF HIGH BLOOD PRESSURE: 1988 report. Arch Intern Med 148:1023, 1988

KAPLAN NM: Systemic hypertension: Therapy, in *Heart Disease,* 3d ed, E Braunwald (ed). Philadelphia, Saunders, 1988, p 862

KOTCHEN TA et al: Effect of chloride on renin and blood pressure responses to sodium chloride. Ann Intern Med 98:817, 1983

LITTENBERG B et al: Screening for hypertension. Ann Intern Med 112(3):192, 1990

MCCARRON DA: Calcium in the pathogenesis and therapy of human hypertension. Am J Med 78:27, 1985

OBERMAN A et al: Pharmacologic and nutritional treatment of mild hypertension: Changes in cardiovascular risk status. Ann Intern Med 112(2):89, 1990

SUBCOMMITTEE OF NON-PHARMACOLOGIC THERAPY OF THE JOINT NATIONAL COMMITTEE ON DETECTION, EVALUATION AND TREATMENT OF HIGH BLOOD PRESSURE: Nonpharmacological approaches to the control of high blood pressure: Final report. Hypertension 8:444, 1986

WEINBERGER MH et al: Definitions and characteristics of sodium sensitivity and blood pressure resistance. Hypertension 8:127, 1986

WILLIAMS GH: Quality of life and its impact on hypertensive patients. Am J Med 82:98–105, 1987

———: Converting enzyme inhibitors in the treatment of hypertension. New Engl J Med 319:1517–1525, 1989

———, HOLLENBERG NK: Pathophysiology of essential hypertension, in *Cardiology,* WW Parmley, J Chatterjee (eds). Philadelphia, Lippincott, 1987

WOODS JW: Oral contraceptives and hypertension. Hypertension 11:1, 1988

WORKING GROUP ON HYPERTENSION IN DIABETES: Statement on hypertension in diabetes mellitus: Final report. Arch Intern Med 147:830, 1987

WORKING GROUP ON HYPERTENSION IN THE ELDERLY, NATIONAL HIGH BLOOD PRESSURE EDUCATION PROGRAM: Statement on hypertension in the elderly. JAMA 256:70, 1986

197 DISEASES OF THE AORTA

VICTOR J. DZAU / MARK A. CREAGER

The aorta is the conduit through which the blood ejected from the left ventricle is delivered to the systemic arterial bed. In adults, its diameter is approximately 3 cm at the origin and 2.5 cm in the descending portion in the thorax. The aortic wall consists of a thin intima, a thick media, and an adventitia of smooth muscle cells, collagen, and elastic tissue. In addition to its conduit function, the viscoelastic and compliant properties of the aorta also subserve a

TABLE 197-1 Diseases of the aorta: classification and etiology

Aneurysm
  Atherosclerosis
  Cystic medial necrosis
  Syphilitic infection
  Mycotic infection
  Rheumatic aortitis
  Trauma
Aortic dissection
  Cystic medial necrosis
  Systemic hypertension
  Atherosclerosis
Aortic occlusion
  Atherosclerosis
  Thromboembolism
Aortitis
  Syphilitic aortitis
  Rheumatic aortitis
  Takayasu's arteritis and aortic arch syndromes
  Giant cell arteritis

buffering function. The aorta is distended during systole to enable a portion of the stroke volume to be stored and it recoils during diastole so that blood continues to flow to the periphery during diastole. Because of its continuous exposure to high pulsatile pressure and shear stress, the aorta is particularly prone to injury and disease resulting from mechanical trauma (Table 197-1).

ANEURYSMS

An aneurysm is defined as a pathologic dilatation of a segment of a blood vessel. A *true* aneurysm involves all three layers of the vessel wall and is distinguished from a *pseudoaneurysm* in which the intimal and medial layers are disrupted and the dilatation is lined by adventitia only and sometimes by perivascular clot. Aneurysms may also be classified according to their gross appearance. A *fusiform* aneurysm affects the entire circumference of a segment of the vessel resulting in a diffusely dilated lesion. In contrast, a *saccular* aneurysm involves only a portion of the circumference, resulting in an outpouching of the vessel wall.

The most common cause of aortic aneurysm is atherosclerosis. Other etiologies include cystic medial necrosis, syphilis or other bacterial infections, rheumatic aortitis, and trauma. Aortic aneurysms are also classified according to location, i.e., abdominal vs. thoracic. Those in the abdominal aorta are almost always due to atherosclerosis. Aneurysms of the ascending thoracic aorta may be caused by cystic medial necrosis, atherosclerosis, syphilis, bacterial infections, or rheumatoid arthritis. Aneurysms of the descending thoracic aorta are usually contiguous with infradiaphragmatic aneurysms and, as with the latter, are usually due to atherosclerosis.

Aortic aneurysms usually do not produce symptoms. However, as they expand they may become painful. Compression or erosion of adjacent tissue by aneurysms may also cause symptoms. The formation of mural thrombi within the aneurysm may predispose to peripheral embolization. Occasionally an aneurysm may leak, leading to extravasation of blood into the vessel wall and the periadventitial area and causing acute pain and local tenderness. This is usually a harbinger of rupture and represents a medical emergency. More often, acute rupture occurs without any prior warning and is always life-threatening.

ATHEROSCLEROTIC ANEURYSMS Seventy-five percent of atherosclerotic aneurysms are located in the distal abdominal aorta below the renal arteries. An abdominal aneurysm commonly produces no symptoms and is usually detected on routine examination as a palpable, pulsatile, and nontender mass or is an incidental finding on abdominal x-ray or ultrasound performed for other reasons. Some patients may complain of strong pulsations in the abdomen, others of low back pain. Rarely leakage of the aneurysm may result in severe pain and tenderness. Acute pain and hypotension occur with rupture of the aneurysm, requiring emergency operation.

Abdominal radiography may demonstrate the calcified outline of the aneurysm. The *diagnosis* is generally confirmed by ultrasound which can delineate the transverse and longitudinal dimensions of the aneurysm; mural thrombus may be detected. Ultrasound is useful for serial documentation of aneurysm size. Both computed tomography (CT) with contrast and magnetic resonance imaging (MRI) have been introduced for the detection and follow-up of aortic aneurysm. These relatively expensive techniques provide higher resolution than ultrasound and have replaced the latter in some centers. However, abdominal aortography remains the gold standard in evaluating patients with aneurysm for surgery. This technique is useful in documenting the extent of the aneurysm, especially its upper and lower limits, and the extent of associated atherosclerotic vascular disease. However, aortography may underestimate the diameter of an aneurysm since the presence of mural clots may reduce the luminal size.

The location and the severity of associated atherosclerotic vascular disease influence the overall prognosis. Frequently it is the severity of coronary artery and cerebral vascular diseases that determines the long-term prognosis in these patients. The most common cause of death of patients with aneurysms is rupture. The risk of rupture increases with the size of the aneurysm. The mortality of patients with abdominal aneurysms exceeding 6 cm in diameter is approximately 50 percent in 2 years, while in those with lesions between 4 and 6 cm, it is 25 percent.

Operative excision with replacement with a graft is indicated for patients with abdominal aneurysms greater than 6 cm in diameter, as well as in symptomatic patients and in those with rapidly expanding aneurysms irrespective of the absolute diameter. Except for patients with exceptionally high operative risk, operation is also usually recommended in patients with aneurysm diameter 5 to 6 cm. Serial noninvasive follow-up of smaller (<5 cm) aneurysms is an alternative to immediate surgery. In surgical candidates, a careful preoperative cardiac and general medical evaluation followed by appropriate therapy of complicating conditions are essential. With careful preoperative cardiac evaluation and postoperative care, which includes Swan-Ganz catheterization, operative mortality approximates 1 to 5 percent. Following acute rupture, the mortality of emergency operation is generally greater than 50 percent.

CYSTIC MEDIAL NECROSIS This is due to the degeneration of collagen and elastic fibers in the media of the aorta, which are replaced by multiple clefts of mucoid material. Cystic medial necrosis characteristically affects the proximal aorta, results in circumferential weakness and dilatation, and leads to the development of fusiform aneurysms involving the ascending aorta and the sinuses of Valsalva. This condition is particularly prevalent in patients with the Marfan syndrome (Chap. 333), but is also seen in pregnancy and hypertension and sometimes as an isolated condition in patients without any other condition. The clinical manifestations include expanding aneurysms, rupture, and aortic regurgitation. Operative repair is indicated to prevent rupture. Control of arterial pressure is an important part of the long-term management of this condition.

MYCOTIC ANEURYSM This rare condition develops as the result of staphylococcal, streptococcal, or salmonella infections of the aorta, usually at an atherosclerotic plaque. Blood cultures are usually positive and reveal the nature of the infecting agent. The aneurysms are usually saccular. Treatment requires parenteral antibiotics and surgical excision.

TRAUMA Aortic rupture may develop following penetrating injury or blunt trauma. Deceleration injury may tear the aortic isthmus at the site of insertion of the ligamentum arteriosum.

Other causes of aortic aneurysm, such as syphilitic infection and rheumatic vasculitis, are discussed later under aortitis.

AORTIC DISSECTION

Aortic dissection is caused by a circumferential or transverse tear of the intima, usually at the right lateral wall of the ascending aorta where the hydraulic shear is high. It has been speculated that the

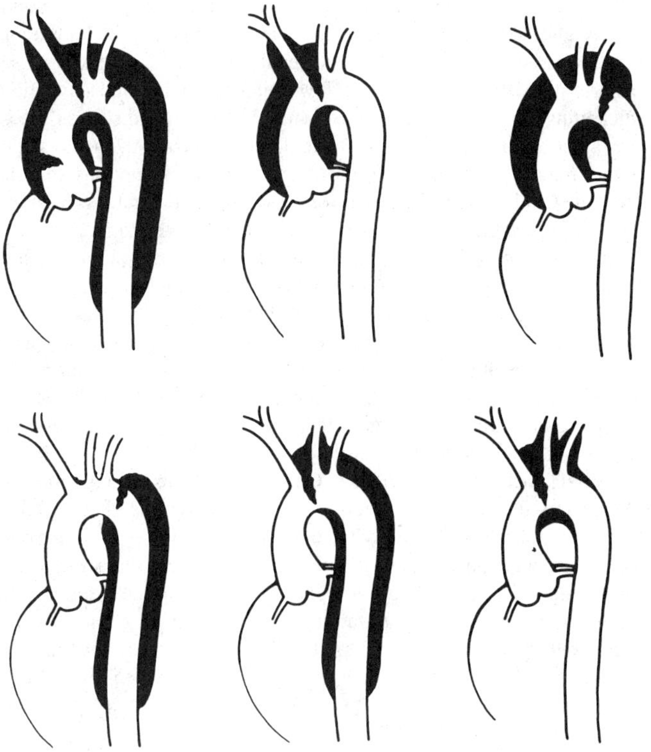

FIGURE 197-1 Classification of aortic dissections. Stanford classification: Top panels illustrate type A dissections that involve the ascending aorta independent of site of tear and distal extension; type B dissections (bottom panels) involve transverse and/or descending aorta without involvement of the ascending aorta. DeBakey classification: Type I dissection involves ascending to descending aorta (top left); type II dissection is limited to ascending or transverse aorta, without descending aorta (top center + top right); type III dissection involves descending aorta only (bottom left). *(From DC Miller, in RM Doroghazi, EE Slater (eds). Aortic Dissection. New York, McGraw-Hill, 1983, with permission.)*

initiating event is a medial hemorrhage that disrupts the intima. Another common site is the descending thoracic aorta just below the ligamentum arteriosum. The pulsatile aortic flow then dissects along the elastic lamellar plates of the aorta and creates a false lumen. The dissection usually propagates distally down the descending aorta and into its major branches, but it may also propagate proximally. In some cases a secondary distal intimal disruption occurs, resulting in the reentry of blood from the false to the true lumen.

DeBakey and coworkers classified aortic dissections as: type I, in which an intimal tear occurs in the ascending aorta and the dissection extends into the descending aorta; type II, in which the dissection is limited to the ascending aorta; and type III, in which the intimal tear is located in the descending area with distal propagation of the dissection (Figure 197-1). Another classification (Stanford) is that of type A, in which the dissection involves the ascending aorta, and type B, in which it is limited to the descending aorta.

The factors that predispose to aortic dissection include systemic hypertension, a coexisting condition in 70 percent of patients, and cystic medial necrosis. Aortic dissection is the major cause of morbidity and mortality in patients with the Marfan syndrome. The incidence is increased in patients with congenital aortic valve anomalies (e.g., bicuspid valve), coarctation of the aorta, and, in otherwise normal women, during the third trimester of pregnancy.

Clinical manifestations Acute aortic dissection presents with the sudden onset of pain (Chap. 16), which is often described as very severe and tearing, associated with diaphoresis. The pain may be localized to the front or back of the chest, often the interscapular region, and typically migrates with the propagation of the dissection. Other symptoms include syncope, dyspnea, and weakness. Physical findings may include hypertension or hypotension, loss of pulses, aortic regurgitation, pulmonary edema, and neurologic findings due to carotid artery obstruction (hemiplegia, hemianesthesia) or spinal cord ischemia (paraplegia). These clinical manifestations reflect complications resulting from the dissection occluding the major arteries. Bowel ischemia, hematuria, and myocardial ischemia have all been observed. Furthermore, clinical manifestations may result from the compression of adjacent structures (such as superior cervical ganglia, superior vena cava, bronchus, esophagus) by the expanding dissecting aneurysm and include Horner's syndrome, superior vena caval syndrome, hoarseness, dysphagia, and airway compromise. Hemopericardium and cardiac tamponade may complicate a type A lesion with retrograde dissection.

In dissections involving the ascending aorta, the chest x-ray often reveals a widened superior mediastinum. A pleural effusion (usually left-sided) may also be present. The electrocardiogram usually excludes acute myocardial ischemia unless a coronary artery is involved in the dissection. In dissections of the descending thoracic aorta, a widened mediastinum may also be observed on chest x-ray. In addition, the descending aorta may appear to be wider than the ascending portion. The diagnosis of aortic dissection is established by aortography which should be performed as soon as the diagnosis is seriously considered. It is important to identify the entry point, the intimal flap, and the false and true lumina and to establish the extent of dissection into the major arteries. Magnetic resonance imaging (Chap. 178) and CT with contrast have also been shown to be highly accurate in detecting aortic dissection. Two-dimensional echocardiography has also been helpful in some cases.

Treatment Medical therapy should be initiated as soon as the diagnosis is considered. The patient should be closely monitored. Unless hypotension is present, therapy should be aimed at reducing cardiac contractility and systemic arterial pressure, and thereby shear stress. Immediate parenteral administration of a beta-adrenergic blocker, unless contraindicated, should be accompanied by nitroprusside infusion. Recently, labetalol (p. 1011) has also been introduced as a parenteral agent in the acute therapy of dissection. If there is a contraindication to the use of beta blockers, parenteral reserpine may be substituted. Direct vasodilators, such as diazoxide and hydralazine, are contraindicated as these agents can increase hydraulic shear and may propagate dissection.

For ascending aortic dissection (type A), surgical correction, which includes reconstruction of the aortic wall, is the preferred treatment. Emergency operation carries a high operative mortality (up to 45 percent). Thus, if possible, stabilization of the patient's clinical status with semielective surgery 14 days or later is preferred. However, with continued pain and evidence of continuing dissection, despite medical therapy, emergency surgery is indicated. The major causes of perioperative mortality and morbidity include myocardial infarction, paraplegia, renal failure, tamponade, hemorrhage, and sepsis. In general, medical therapy is the preferred treatment for uncomplicated and stable distal dissection (type B) unless there is clinical evidence of propagation, compromise of major branches of the aorta, or continued pain.

Overall, the prognosis of aortic dissection is poor. Long-term therapy should include control of blood pressure and cardiac output with the use of beta-adrenergic blockers and other agents.

AORTIC OCCLUSION

CHRONIC ARTERIOSCLEROTIC OCCLUSIVE DISEASE

Chronic occlusive disease usually involves the distal abdominal aorta below the renal arteries. The disease extends frequently to the common iliac arteries but may spare the external iliac arteries. Because of the slowly progressive nature of the atherosclerotic process, the natural history of aortic occlusion is usually chronic and insidious. Claudication characteristically involves the lower back, buttocks, and thighs and may be associated with impotence in males (Leriche syndrome). The severity of the symptoms depends on the adequacy of collaterals.

With sufficient collateral blood flow a complete occlusion of the abdominal aorta may occur in some cases without the development of ischemic symptoms. The physical findings include absence of femoral and other distal pulses bilaterally and the detection of an audible bruit over the abdomen (usually at or below the umbilicus) and the common femoral arteries. Atrophic skin, loss of hair, and coolness of lower extremities are usually observed. In advanced ischemia, rubor on dependency and pallor on elevation can be seen.

The diagnosis is usually established by the physical examination and noninvasive testing, including leg pressure measurements, Doppler velocity analysis, and pulse volume recordings. The anatomy may be defined by abdominal aortography prior to revascularization. Operative treatment is indicated in patients with debilitating symptoms and/or with the development of leg ischemia.

ACUTE OCCLUSION The complication of acute occlusion occurring in the distal abdominal aorta represents a medical emergency as it threatens the viability of the lower extremities. It usually occurs as the result of an occlusive embolus that almost always originates from the heart. Rarely acute occlusion may occur as the result of in situ thrombosis in a preexisting severely narrowed segment of the aorta, or plaque rupture and hemorrhage into such an area.

The clinical picture is one of acute ischemia of the lower extremities. Severe rest pain, coolness, and pallor of the lower extremities and the absence of distal pulses bilaterally are the usual manifestations. Diagnosis should be established rapidly by aortography. Emergency thrombectomy or revascularization is indicated.

AORTITIS

Aortitis frequently affects the ascending aorta and may result in aneurysmal dilatation and aortic regurgitation; it occasionally obstructs branch vessels of the aorta.

SYPHILITIC AORTITIS This late manifestation of luetic infection (Chap. 128) usually affects the proximal ascending aorta, particularly the aortic root, resulting in aortic dilatation and aneurysm formation. Syphilitic aortitis may occasionally involve the aortic arch or the descending aorta. The aneurysms may be saccular or fusiform and are usually asymptomatic, but compression of and erosion into adjacent structures may result in symptoms; rupture may also occur.

The initial lesion is an obliterative endarteritis of the vasa vasorum, especially in the adventitia. This is an inflammatory response to the invasion of the adventitia by the spirochetes. Destruction of the aortic media occurs as the spirochetes spread into this layer, usually via the lymphatics of the vasa vasorum. Destruction of collagen and elastic tissues leads to dilatation of the aorta, scar formation, and calcification. These changes account for the characteristic radiographic appearance of a calcified ascending aortic aneurysm.

The disease typically presents as an incidental radiographic finding 15 to 30 years after initial infection. Symptoms may result from aortic regurgitation, from narrowing of coronary ostia due to syphilitic aortitis, from compression of adjacent structures (e.g., esophagus), or from rupture. Diagnosis is established by a positive serologic test, i.e., VDRL or fluorescent treponemal antibody (see Chap. 128). Treatment includes penicillin and surgical excision and repair.

RHEUMATIC AORTITIS Rheumatoid arthritis (Chap. 270), ankylosing spondylitis (Chap. 274), psoriatic arthritis (Chap. 283), Reiter's syndrome (Chap. 274), Behçet's syndrome (Chap. 275), relapsing polychondritis, and inflammatory bowel disorders may all be associated with aortitis involving the ascending aorta. The inflammatory lesions usually involve the ascending aorta, and may extend to the sinuses of Valsalva, the mitral valve leaflets, and adjacent myocardium. The clinical manifestations are aneurysm, aortic regurgitation, and involvement of the cardiac conduction system.

TAKAYASU'S ARTERITIS AND OTHER AORTIC ARCH SYNDROMES Inflammatory diseases of the aortic arch resulting in obstruction of the aorta and its major arteries characterize this major group of diseases. Takayasu's arteritis is also termed *pulseless disease* because of the frequent occlusion of the large arteries of the aorta. It may also involve the descending thoracic and abdominal aorta and occlude large branches such as the renal arteries. The pathology is a panarteritis with marked intimal hyperplasia, medial and adventitial thickening, and, in the chronic form, fibrosis. The disease is most prevalent in young females of Asian descent. During the acute stage, fever, malaise, weight loss, and other systemic symptoms may be evident. An elevation of the erythrocyte sedimentation rate is common. The chronic stages of the disease present with symptoms related to large artery occlusion, including upper extremity claudication, cerebral ischemia, syncope, etc. The chronic disease is intermittently active. Since the process is progressive and there is no definitive therapy, the prognosis is usually poor. Glucocorticoids and immunosuppressive agents have been reported to be effective in some patients during the acute phase. Occasionally anticoagulation prevents thrombosis and complete occlusion of a large artery. Surgical bypass of a critically stenotic artery may be necessary.

GIANT CELL ARTERITIS (See Chap. 276) This affects primarily large- and medium-sized arteries. The pathology is that of focal granulomatous lesions involving the entire arterial wall. It may be associated with polymyalgia rheumatica (Chap. 27). Obstruction of medium-sized arteries (e.g., temporal and ophthalmic arteries) and of major branches of the aorta and the development of aortitis and aortic regurgitation are some of the complications of the disease. High-dose corticosteroid therapy may be effective when given early.

REFERENCES

Bulkley BH, Roberts WC: Ankylosing spondylitis and aortic regurgitation. Circulation 48:1014, 1973

DeSanctis RW et al: Medical progress: Aortic dissection. N Engl J Med 317:1060, 1987

Estes JE Jr: Abdominal aortic aneurysm: A study of one hundred and two cases. Circulation 11:258, 1950

Larsen EW, Edwards WD: Risk factors for aortic dissection: A necropsy study of 161 cases. Am J Cardiol 53:849, 1984

Szilagyi DE et al: Contribution of abdominal aortic aneurysmectomy to prolongation of life. Ann Surg 164:678, 1966

Whittemore AD et al: Aortic aneurysm repair: Reduced operative mortality associated with maintenance of optimal cardiac performance. Ann Surg 192:414, 1980

198 VASCULAR DISEASES OF THE EXTREMITIES

MARK A. CREAGER / VICTOR J. DZAU

ARTERIAL DISORDERS

ATHEROSCLEROSIS OF THE EXTREMITIES Atherosclerosis (arteriosclerosis obliterans) is the leading cause of occlusive arterial disease of the extremities in patients over 40 years old; the highest incidence occurs in the sixth and seventh decades of life. As in patients with atherosclerosis of the coronary and cerebral vasculature, there is an increased prevalence of peripheral atherosclerotic occlusive disease in individuals with hypertension, hypercholesterolemia, diabetes mellitus, and in cigarette smokers. Atherosclerosis of the extremities is seen most frequently in elderly males.

Pathology (See Chap. 195) Segmental lesions causing stenosis or occlusion are usually localized in large- and medium-sized vessels. The pathology of the lesions includes atherosclerotic plaques with calcium deposition, thinning of the media, patchy destruction of muscle and elastic fibers, fragmentation of the internal elastic lamina, and thrombi comprised of platelets and fibrin. The primary sites of involvement are the abdominal aorta and iliac arteries in 30 percent of symptomatic patients, the femoral and popliteal arteries in 80 to 90 percent of patients, and the more distal vessels (including the tibial and peroneal arteries) in 40 to 50 percent of patients. Atherosclerotic lesions occur preferentially at arterial branch points, sites of increased turbulence, altered shear stress, and intimal injury. Involvement of the distal vasculature is most common in elderly individuals and patients with diabetes mellitus.

Clinical evaluation The most common symptom is intermittent claudication, which is defined as a pain, ache, cramp, numbness, or sense of fatigue in the muscles; it occurs during exercise but is relieved with rest. The site of claudication is distal to the location of the occlusive lesion. For example, buttock, hip, and thigh discomfort occur in patients with aortoiliac disease (Leriche syndrome), whereas calf claudication develops in patients with femoral-popliteal disease. Symptoms are far more common in the lower than in the upper extremities because of the higher incidence of obstructive lesions. In patients with severe arterial occlusive disease, rest pain may develop. Patients will complain of pain or a feeling of cold or numbness in the foot and toes. Frequently these symptoms occur at night when the legs are in a "neutral" position and improve when the legs are in a dependent position. With severe ischemia, rest pain may be persistent.

Important physical findings of chronic arterial insufficiency include decreased or absent pulses distal to the obstruction, the presence of bruits over the narrowed artery, and muscle atrophy. With more severe disease, hair loss, thickened nails, smooth and shiny skin, reduced skin temperature, and pallor or cyanosis are frequent physical signs. In addition, ulcers or gangrene may occur. Elevation of the legs and repeated flexing of the calf muscles produces pallor of the soles of the feet whereas rubor, secondary to reactive hyperemia, may develop when the legs are dependent. The duration of time for rubor to develop or for the veins in the foot to fill when the patient's legs are transferred from an elevated to a dependent position is related to the severity of the ischemia and the presence of collateral vessels. Patients with severe ischemia may develop peripheral edema, because frequently they keep their legs in a dependent position. Ischemic neuritis can result in numbness and hyporeflexia.

Noninvasive testing The history and physical examination are usually sufficient to establish the diagnosis of peripheral arterial occlusive disease. Objective assessment of the severity of disease is obtained by noninvasive techniques. These include digital pulse volume recordings, Doppler blood flow velocity, wave-form analysis, segmental pressure measurements, stress testing (usually using a treadmill), and tests of reactive hyperemia. In the presence of significant arterial occlusive disease, the volume displacement in the leg is decreased with each pulse and the Doppler velocity contour becomes progressively flatter.

Arterial pressure can be recorded noninvasively along the legs by serial placement of sphygmomanometric cuffs and use of a Doppler device to auscultate or record blood flow. Normally, blood pressures in the legs and arms are similar. Indeed, ankle pressures may be slightly higher than arm pressures due to pulse wave reflection. In the presence of hemodynamically significant stenoses the arterial pressure in the leg is decreased. Thus, if one were to obtain a ratio of the ankle and brachial artery pressures, it would be >1.0 in normal individuals and <1.0 in patients with arterial occlusive disease. A ratio of <0.5 is consistent with severe ischemia.

Treadmill testing allows the physician to assess functional limitations objectively. Decline of the ankle-brachial systolic pressure ratio immediately after exercise may provide further support for the diagnosis of arterial occlusive disease in patients with equivocal symptoms and findings on examination. Exercise testing also allows simultaneous evaluation for the presence of coronary artery disease.

Angiography should not be used for routine diagnostic testing, but is performed prior to potential revascularization. It is useful for defining the anatomy to assist operative planning and is also indicated if nonsurgical interventions are being considered, such as percutaneous transluminal angioplasty or thrombolysis.

Prognosis The natural history of patients with peripheral arterial occlusive disease is influenced primarily by the extent of coexistent coronary artery and cerebral vascular disease. Studies utilizing coronary angiography have estimated that approximately one-half of patients with symptomatic peripheral arterial occlusive disease also have significant coronary artery disease. Life table analysis has indicated that patients with claudication have a 72 percent 5-year and a 50 percent 10-year survival rate. The majority of deaths are either sudden or secondary to myocardial infarction. The likelihood of symptomatic progression of peripheral arterial occlusive disease appears less than the chance of succumbing to coronary artery disease. Approximately 70 percent of nondiabetic patients who present with mild to moderate claudication remain symptomatically stable. Improvement may occur in 10 to 15 percent of these patients; deterioration is likely to occur in the remainder with approximately 5 percent of the group ultimately undergoing amputation. Prognosis is worse in those patients who continue to smoke cigarettes or have diabetes mellitus.

Treatment Therapeutic options include supportive measures, pharmacologic treatment, nonoperative interventions, and surgery. Supportive measures include meticulous care of the feet. The feet should be kept clean and excessive drying should be prevented with the use of moisturizing creams. Well-fitting and protective shoes are advised to reduce trauma. Sandals and shoes made of synthetic materials that do not "breathe" should be avoided. Elastic support hose should be avoided since these reduce blood flow to the skin. In patients with ischemia at rest, shock blocks under the head of the bed together with a canopy over the feet may improve perfusion pressure and ameliorate some of the rest pain.

Treatment of associated factors that contribute to the development of atherosclerosis should be initiated. The importance of discontinuing cigarette smoking cannot be overemphasized. The physician must assume a major role in this lifestyle modification. It is important to control blood pressure in hypertensive patients but to avoid hypotensive levels. Treatment of hypercholesterolemia is advocated, although reduction in cholesterol levels has not been shown unequivocally to reverse peripheral atherosclerotic lesions. However, it has been shown to prevent or to slow progression of the disease. Patients with claudication should also be encouraged to exercise regularly and to progressively increasing levels. Daily walking to the onset of claudication may improve muscle efficiency and prolong walking distance. Patients should be advised not to walk "through their claudication," but to rest until the symptoms resolve before resuming ambulation. Other forms of exercise, such as bicycle riding and swimming, provide overall cardiovascular and psychologic benefit and often are tolerated better than walking.

PHARMACOLOGIC MANAGEMENT This form of treatment of patients with peripheral arterial occlusive disease has not been as successful as the medical treatment of coronary artery disease (Chap. 190). In particular, vasodilators, as a class, have not proven to be beneficial. During exercise, peripheral vasodilation occurs normally distal to sites of significant arterial stenoses. As a result, perfusion pressure falls, often to levels less than that generated in the interstitial tissue by the exercising muscle. Unless vasodilators are able to improve collateral blood flow, it is unlikely that they would improve perfusion pressure and thereby increase blood supply to the exercising muscle. Drugs such as alpha-adrenergic blocking agents, calcium channel antagonists, papaverine, and other vasodilators have not been shown to be effective in patients with occlusive arterial disease. Pentoxifylline, a substituted xanthine derivative, is reported to decrease blood viscosity and to increase red cell flexibility, thereby increasing blood flow to the microcirculation and enhancing tissue oxygenation. One placebo-controlled study demonstrated that pentoxifylline increased duration of exercise on the treadmill in patients with claudication. Additional studies are required to confirm this drug's efficacy in patients with peripheral arterial occlusive disease.

Platelet inhibitors, particularly aspirin, have been reported to decrease progression of atherosclerosis in patients with peripheral arterial occlusive disease. However, no study with aspirin has demonstrated any improvement in exercise capacity. The anticoagulants heparin and warfarin have not been shown to be effective in patients with *chronic* arterial occlusive disease but may be useful in *acute* arterial obstruction secondary to thrombosis or systemic embolism. Similarly, thrombolytic intervention using drugs such as streptokinase, urokinase, or recombinant tissue plasminogen activator may have a role in the treatment of acute arterial occlusion, but is not effective in patients with chronic arterial occlusion secondary to atherosclerosis.

REVASCULARIZATION Such procedures, including nonoperative as well as operative interventions, are usually reserved for patients with progressive, severe or disabling symptoms, ischemia at rest, and for those individuals who must be symptom-free because of their occupation. Angiography should be performed principally in those patients who are being considered for a revascularization procedure. Nonoperative interventions include percutaneous transluminal angioplasty (PTA) and the experimental procedures of laser angioplasty and atherectomy. PTA of the iliac artery is associated with a higher success rate than PTA of the femoral and popliteal arteries. Approximately 90 percent of iliac PTAs are initially successful and the 3-year patency rate is in excess of 70 percent. The initial success rate for femoral-popliteal PTA is approximately 80 percent with a 50 percent 3-year patency rate.

Several operative procedures are available for treating patients with aortoiliac and femoral-popliteal artery disease. The preferred operative procedure depends on the location and extent of the obstruction(s) and the general medical condition of the patient. Operative procedures for aortoiliac disease include aorto-bifemoral bypass, axillo-femoral bypass, femoral-femoral bypass, and aortoiliac endarterectomy. The most commonly utilized procedure is the aorto-bifemoral bypass, using knitted dacron grafts. Operative mortality ranges from 2 to 5 percent, mostly due to ischemic heart disease. Immediate graft patency approaches 99 percent and 5- and 10-year graft patency in survivors is in excess of 90 and 80 percent respectively. Operative complications include myocardial infarct and stroke, infection of the graft, peripheral embolization, and sexual dysfunction from interruption of autonomic nerves in the pelvis.

Operative therapy for femoral-popliteal artery disease includes in situ and reverse autogenous saphenous vein bypass grafts, polytetrafluoroethylene (PTFE) or other synthetic materials, and thromboendarterectomy. Operative mortality ranges from 1 to 3 percent. Long-term patency rate is dependent on the type of graft utilized, the location of the distal anastomosis, and the patency of run-off vessels beyond the anastomosis. Patency rates of femoral-popliteal saphenous vein bypass grafts at 1 year approach 90 percent and at 5 years 70 to 80 percent. In contrast, 5-year patency rates of infrapopliteal PTFE grafts are less than 30 percent. Lumbar sympathectomy alone or as an adjunct to aortofemoral reconstruction has fallen into disfavor. While this procedure may increase blood flow to the skin, it does not increase blood flow to muscle. There is no good clinical evidence that lumbar sympathectomy increases graft patency or improves limb survival.

THROMBOANGIITIS OBLITERANS Thromboangiitis obliterans (Buerger's disease) is an inflammatory occlusive vascular disorder involving small- and medium-sized arteries and veins in the distal upper and lower extremities. Cerebral, visceral, and coronary vessels may also be affected. This disorder develops most frequently in men under the age of 40. The prevalence is high in Asians and individuals whose lineage originates in eastern Europe. While the cause of thromboangiitis obliterans is not known, there is a definite relationship to cigarette smoking and an increased incidence of HLA-B5 and -A9 antigens in patients with this disorder.

In the initial stages of thromboangiitis obliterans, polymorphonuclear leukocytes infiltrate the wall of the small- and medium-sized arteries and veins. The internal elastic lamina is preserved and thrombus may develop in the vascular lumen. As the disease progresses, mononuclear cells, fibroblasts, and giant cells replace the neutrophils. Later stages are characterized by perivascular fibrosis and recanalization.

The clinical features of thromboangiitis obliterans often include a triad of claudication of the affected extremity, Raynaud's phenomenon (see below), and migratory superficial vein thrombophlebitis. Claudication is usually confined to the lower calves and feet or forearms and hands because this disorder primarily affects distal vessels. In the presence of severe digital ischemia, trophic nail changes, ulcerations and gangrene may develop at the tips of the fingers. The physical examination shows normal brachial and popliteal pulses, but reduced or absent radial, ulnar, and/or tibial pulses. Arteriography is helpful in making the diagnosis. Smooth tapering segmental lesions in the distal vessels are characteristic, as are collateral vessels at sites of vascular occlusion. Proximal atherosclerotic disease is usually absent. The diagnosis can be confirmed by excisional biopsy and pathologic examination of an involved vessel.

There is no specific treatment except abstention from tobacco. The prognosis is worse in individuals who continue to smoke but results are discouraging even in those who do stop smoking. Arterial bypass of the larger vessels may be used in selected instances, as well as local debridement, depending on symptoms and severity of ischemia. Antibiotics may be useful; anticoagulants and corticosteroids are not helpful. If these measures fail, amputation may be required.

ACUTE ARTERIAL OCCLUSION This results in the sudden cessation of blood flow to an extremity. The severity of ischemia and the viability of the extremity are dependent upon the location and extent of the occlusion and the presence and subsequent development of collateral blood vessels. There are two principal causes of acute arterial occlusion: embolism and thrombus in situ.

The most common sources of arterial emboli are the heart, aorta, and large arteries. Cardiac disorders that cause thromboembolism include atrial fibrillation, both chronic and paroxysmal, and acute myocardial infarction, ventricular aneurysm, cardiomyopathy, infectious and marantic endocarditis, prosthetic heart valves, and atrial myxoma. Emboli to the distal vessels may also originate from proximal sites of atherosclerosis and aneurysms of the aorta and large vessels. Less frequently, an arterial occlusion may result paradoxically from a venous thrombus that has entered the systemic circulation via a patent foramen ovale or other septal defect. Arterial emboli tend to lodge at the bifurcation of vessels because the caliber of the vessel decreases at these sites; in the lower extremities, emboli lodge most frequently in the femoral artery, followed by the iliac artery, aorta, and popliteal and tibioperoneal arteries.

Acute arterial thrombosis in situ occurs most frequently in atherosclerotic vessels at the site of a stenosis or aneurysm, and in arterial bypass grafts. Trauma to an artery may also result in the formation of an acute arterial thrombus. Arterial occlusion may complicate arterial punctures and placement of catheters. Less frequent causes include the thoracic outlet compression syndrome, causing subclavian artery occlusion, and entrapment of the popliteal artery by abnormal placement of the medial head of the gastrocnemius muscle. Polycythemia and hypercoagulable disorders (Chaps. 289 and 297) are also associated with acute arterial thrombosis.

Clinical features The symptoms of the acute arterial occlusion depend upon the location, duration, and severity of the obstruction. Often severe pain, paresthesias, numbness, and coldness develop in the involved extremity within 1 hour. Paralysis may occur with severe and persistent ischemia. Physical findings include loss of pulses distal to the occlusion; cyanosis or pallor; mottling; decrease in skin temperature; muscle stiffening; loss of sensation; weakness; and/or absent deep tendon reflexes. If acute arterial occlusion occurs in the presence of an adequate collateral circulation, as is often the case in acute graft occlusion, the symptoms and findings may be less impressive. In this situation, the patient complains about an abrupt decrease in the distance walked before claudication occurs, or of modest pain and paresthesias. Pallor and coolness are evident, but sensory and motor functions are generally preserved. The diagnosis of acute arterial occlusion is usually apparent from the clinical presentation. Arteriography is useful for confirming the diagnosis and demonstrating the location and extent of occlusion.

Treatment Once the diagnosis is made the patient should be anticoagulated with intravenous heparin to prevent propagation of the clot. In cases of severe ischemia of recent onset and particularly when limb viability is jeopardized, immediate intervention to ensure reperfusion is indicated. Surgical thromboembolectomy or arterial bypass procedures are used to restore blood flow to the ischemic extremity promptly, particularly when a large proximal vessel is occluded.

Intraarterial thrombolytic therapy is effective when acute arterial occlusion is caused by a thrombus in an atherosclerotic vessel or arterial bypass graft. Thrombolytic therapy also may be indicated when the patient's overall condition contraindicates surgical intervention or when smaller distal vessels are occluded, thus preventing surgical access. Intraarterial streptokinase is administered as a bolus injection of 25,000 to 250,000 IU followed by a continuous infusion of 5000 to 15,000 IU/h. One approach for administering intraarterial urokinase is to give a bolus of 60,000 to 120,000 IU followed by 240,000 IU/h for 2 h, 120,000 IU for 2 h, and then 60,000 IU/hour. Clinical trials are now in progress to assess the efficacy of intraarterial recombinant tissue plasminogen activator (rtPA). Meticulous observation for hemorrhagic complications is required during intraarterial thrombolytic therapy.

If the limb is not in jeopardy, a more conservative approach that includes observation and administration of anticoagulants may be taken. Anticoagulation prevents recurrent embolism and reduces the likelihood of thrombus propagation. It can be initiated with intravenous heparin and followed by oral warfarin. Recommended dosages are the same as those used in deep vein thrombosis (see p. 1024). Emboli resulting from infectious endocarditis, prosthetic heart valves, or atrial myxoma often require surgical intervention to remove the cause.

ATHEROEMBOLISM Atheroembolism constitutes a subset of acute arterial occlusion. In this condition, multiple small deposits of fibrin, platelet, and cholesterol debris embolize from proximal atherosclerotic lesions or aneurysmal sites. Atheroembolism may occur after intraarterial procedures. Since the emboli tend to lodge in the small vessels of the muscle and skin and may not occlude the large vessels, distal pulses usually remain palpable. Patients complain of acute pain and tenderness at the site of embolization. Digital vascular occlusion may result in ischemia and the "blue toe" syndrome; digital necrosis and gangrene may develop. Localized areas of tenderness, pallor, and livido reticularis (see later) occur at sites of emboli. Skin or muscle biopsy may demonstrate cholesterol crystals.

Ischemia resulting from atheroemboli is notoriously difficult to treat. Usually neither surgical revascularization procedures nor thrombolytic therapy are helpful because of the multiplicity, composition, and distal location of the emboli. Some evidence suggests that platelet inhibitors prevent atheroembolism. Surgical intervention to remove or bypass the atherosclerotic vessel or aneurysm that causes the recurrent atheroemboli may be necessary.

THORACIC OUTLET COMPRESSION SYNDROME This refers to a symptom complex resulting from compression of the neurovascular bundle at the thoracic outlet (artery, vein, or nerves) as it courses through the neck and shoulder. Cervical ribs, abnormalities of the scalenus anticus muscle, the proximity of the clavicle to the first rib, or abnormal insertion of the pectoralis minor muscle may compress the subclavian artery and brachial plexus as these structures pass from the thorax to the arm. Patients may develop shoulder and arm pain, weakness, paresthesias, claudication, Raynaud's phenomenon, and even ischemic tissue loss and gangrene. Examination is often normal unless provocative maneuvers are performed. Occasionally distal pulses are decreased or absent and digital cyanosis and ischemia may be evident. Tenderness may be present in the supraclavicular fossa. Several maneuvers are used to confirm the diagnosis of vascular compression and suggest the location of the abnormality. These include the scalene, costoclavicular, and hyperabduction maneuvers which may cause subclavian bruits and loss of pulses in the arm. A chest x-ray will indicate the presence of cervical ribs. The electromyogram will be abnormal if the brachial plexus is involved.

Most patients can be managed conservatively. They should be advised to avoid those positions that cause symptoms. Many patients benefit from shoulder girdle exercises. Surgical procedures such as removal of the first rib or resection of the scalenus anticus muscle are necessary occasionally for relief of symptoms or treatment of ischemia.

ARTERIOVENOUS FISTULA These abnormal communications between an artery and a vein, bypassing the capillary bed, may be congenital or acquired. Congenital arteriovenous fistulas are the result of persistent embryonic vessels that fail to differentiate into arteries and veins; these may be associated with birth marks, are located in almost every organ of the body, and frequently occur in the extremities. Acquired arteriovenous fistulas are either created to provide vascular access for hemodialysis or occur as a result of a penetrating injury such as a gunshot or knife wound or as a complication of arterial catheterization or surgical dissection. An infrequent cause of arteriovenous fistula is rupture of an arterial aneurysm into a vein.

The clinical features depend on the location and size of the fistula. Frequently a pulsatile mass is palpable, and a thrill and bruit lasting throughout systole and diastole are present over the fistula. With longstanding fistulas, clinical manifestations of chronic venous insufficiency, including peripheral edema, large tortuous varicose veins, and stasis pigmentation, become apparent because of the high venous pressure. Evidence of ischemia may occur in the distal portion of the extremity. Skin temperature is higher over the arteriovenous fistula. Large arteriovenous fistulas may result in an increased cardiac output with consequent cardiomegaly and high-output heart failure (Chap. 182).

Diagnosis is often evident from the physical examination. Compression of a large arteriovenous fistula may cause reflex slowing of the heart rate (Nicoladoni-Branham sign). Arteriography can confirm the diagnosis and is useful in demonstrating the site and size of the arteriovenous fistula. *Treatment* may involve surgery, radiotherapy, or embolization. Congenital arteriovenous fistulas are often difficult to treat because the communications may often be numerous and extensive and new ones frequently develop after ligation of the most obvious ones. Many of these lesions are best treated conservatively using elastic support hose to reduce the consequences of venous hypertension. Occasionally, embolization with autologous material, such as fat or muscle, or with hemostatic agents, such as gelatin sponges or silicon spheres, are used to obliterate the fistula. Acquired arteriovenous fistulas are usually amenable to surgical treatment that involves division or excision of the fistula. Occasionally this requires autogenous or synthetic grafting to reestablish continuity of the artery and vein.

RAYNAUD'S PHENOMENON Raynaud's phenomenon is characterized by episodic digital ischemia, manifested clinically by the sequential development of digital blanching, cyanosis, and rubor of the fingers or toes following cold exposure and subsequent rewarming. Emotional stress may also precipitate Raynaud's phenomenon. The color changes are usually well demarcated and are confined to the fingers or toes. Typically, one or more digits will appear white when the patient is exposed to a cold environment or touches a cold object. The blanching, or pallor, represents the ischemic phase of the phenomenon and is secondary to vasospasm of digital arteries. During the ischemic phase capillaries and venules dilate, and cyanosis results from the deoxygenated blood that is present in these vessels. Sensation of cold, numbness, or paresthesias of the digits often accompany the phases of pallor or cyanosis.

With rewarming, the digital vasospasm resolves, and blood flow into the dilated arterioles and capillaries increases dramatically. This "reactive hyperemia" imparts a bright red color to the digits. In addition to rubor and warmth, patients often experience a throbbing, painful sensation during the hyperemic phase. Although the triphasic color response is typical of Raynaud's phenomenon, some patients

TABLE 198-1 Classification of Raynaud's phenomena

Primary or idiopathic Raynaud's phenomenon: Raynaud's disease
Secondary Raynaud's phenomenon
- Collagen vascular diseases:
  - Scleroderma, systemic lupus erythematosus, rheumatoid arthritis, dermatomyositis, polymyositis
- Arterial occlusive diseases:
  - Atherosclerosis of the extremities, thromboangiitis obliterans, acute arterial occlusion, thoracic outlet syndrome
- Pulmonary hypertension
- Neurologic disorders
  - Invertebral disc disease, syringomyelia, spinal cord tumors, stroke, poliomyelitis, carpal tunnel syndrome
- Blood dyscrasias
  - Cold agglutinins, cryoglobulinemia, cryofibrinogenemia, myeloproliferative disorders, Waldenström's macroglobulinemia
- Trauma
  - Vibration injury, hammer hand syndrome, electric shock, cold injury, typing, piano playing
- Drugs
  - Ergot derivatives, methysergide, β-adrenergic receptor blockers, bleomycin, vinblastin, cisplatin

may develop only pallor and cyanosis; others may experience only cyanosis.

Pathophysiology Raynaud originally proposed that cold-induced, episodic digital ischemia was secondary to exaggerated reflex sympathetic vasoconstriction. This theory is supported by the fact that adrenergic-blocking drugs as well as sympathectomy decrease the frequency and severity of Raynaud's phenomenon in some patients. An alternative hypothesis is that there is enhanced digital vascular responsiveness to cold or to normal sympathetic stimuli. It is also possible that normal reflex sympathetic vasoconstriction is superimposed on local digital vascular disease, or that there is enhanced adrenergic neuroeffector activity.

Raynaud's phenomenon is broadly separated into two categories: the idiopathic variety termed *Raynaud's disease* and the secondary variety, which is associated with other disease states or known causes of vasospasm (Table 198-1).

Raynaud's disease This appellation is applied when the secondary causes of Raynaud's phenomenon have been excluded. Over 50 percent of patients with Raynaud's phenomenon have Raynaud's disease. Women are affected about five times more often than men and the age of presentation is usually between 20 and 40 years. The fingers are involved more frequently than the toes. Initial episodes may involve only one or two fingertips, but subsequent attacks may involve the entire finger and may include all of the fingers. The toes are affected in 40 percent of patients. Although vasospasm of the toes usually occurs in patients with symptoms in the fingers, it may happen alone. Rarely, the earlobes and the tip of the nose are involved. Raynaud's phenomenon occurs frequently in patients who also have migraine headaches or variant angina. These associations suggest that there may be a common predisposing cause for the vasospasm.

The physical examination is often entirely normal; the radial, ulnar, and pedal pulses are normal. The fingers and toes may be cool between attacks and may perspire excessively. Thickening and tightening of the digital subcutaneous tissue, i.e., *sclerodactyly*, develops in 10 percent of patients. Angiography of the digits for diagnostic purposes is not indicated.

Patients with Raynaud's disease, in general, appear to have the milder forms of Raynaud's phenomenon. Less than 1 percent of these patients lose a part of a digit. After the diagnosis is made the disease spontaneously improves in approximately 15 percent of patients and progresses in about 30 percent.

Secondary causes of Raynaud's phenomenon Raynaud's phenomenon occurs in 80 to 90 percent of patients with systemic sclerosis (scleroderma) and is the presenting symptom in 30 percent (Chap. 271). It may be the only symptom of scleroderma for many years. Abnormalities of the digital vessels may contribute to the development of Raynaud's phenomenon in this disorder. Ischemic fingertip ulcers may develop and progress to gangrene and autoamputation. About 20 percent of patients with systemic lupus erythematosus (SLE) have Raynaud's phenomenon (Chap. 269). Occasionally, persistent digital ischemia develops and may result in ulcers or gangrene. In most severe cases, the small vessels are occluded by a proliferative endarteritis. Raynaud's phenomenon occurs in about 30 percent of patients with dermatomyositis or polymyositis (Chap. 364). It frequently develops in patients with rheumatoid arthritis and may be related to the intimal proliferation that occurs in the digital arteries.

Atherosclerosis of the extremities is a frequent cause of Raynaud's phenomenon in men over 50 years of age. Thromboangiitis obliterans is an uncommon cause of Raynaud's phenomenon but should be considered in young men, particularly in those who are cigarette smokers. The development of cold-induced pallor in these disorders may be confined to one or two digits of the involved extremity. Occasionally, Raynaud's phenomenon may occur following acute occlusion of large- and medium-sized arteries by a thrombus or embolus. Embolization of atheroembolic debris may cause digital ischemia. The latter often involves one or two digits and should not be confused with Raynaud's phenomenon. In patients with the thoracic outlet syndrome, Raynaud's phenomenon may result from diminished intravascular pressure, stimulation of sympathetic fibers in the brachial plexus, or a combination of both. Raynaud's phenomenon occurs frequently in patients with primary pulmonary hypertension (Chap. 212); this is more than coincidental and may reflect a neurohumoral abnormality that affects both the pulmonary and digital circulations.

A variety of blood dyscrasias may be associated with Raynaud's phenomenon. Cold-induced precipitation of plasma proteins, hyperviscosity, and aggregation of red cells and platelets may occur in patients with cold agglutinins, cryoglobulinemia, or cryofibrinogenemia. Hyperviscosity syndromes that accompany myeloproliferative disorders and Waldenström's macroglobulinemia should also be considered in the initial evaluation of patients with Raynaud's phenomenon.

Raynaud's phenomenon occurs often in patients whose vocations require the use of vibrating hand tools such as chain saws or jackhammers. The frequency of Raynaud's phenomenon also seems to be increased in pianists and typists. Electric shock injury to the hands and frostbite may lead to the later development of Raynaud's phenomena.

Several drugs have been causally implicated in Raynaud's phenomenon. These include ergot preparations, methysergide, beta-adrenergic receptor antagonists, and the chemotherapeutic agents bleomycin, vinblastine, and cisplatin.

Treatment Most patients with Raynaud's phenomenon experience only mild and infrequent episodes. These patients need reassurance and should be instructed to dress warmly and avoid unnecessary cold exposure. In addition to gloves and mittens, patients should protect the trunk, head, and feet with warm clothing in order to prevent cold-induced reflex vasoconstriction. Tobacco use is contraindicated.

Drug treatment should be reserved for the severe cases. Adrenergic blocking agents have been the most frequently prescribed; reserpine, in doses of 0.25 to 0.5 mg orally once a day has been shown to increase nutritional blood flow to the fingers. A single infusion of intraarterial reserpine, 0.5 mg, into the brachial or radial artery has been reported to reduce pain and promote healing of ulcerations. Some but not all patients achieve satisfactory results with long-term reserpine therapy. Moreover, systemic use of the drug is limited by side effects of nasal stuffiness, lethargy, and depression. The post-synaptic $alpha_1$-adrenergic antagonist prazosin has been used with favorable responses. Other sympatholytic agents such as methyldopa, guanethidine, and phenoxybenzamine may be useful in some patients. The calcium channel antagonists, especially nifedipine (10 to 30 mg tid) and diltiazem (30 to 90 mg tid), have also been found to decrease the frequency and severity of Raynaud's phenomena. Occasionally surgical sympathectomy is helpful in patients who are unresponsive to medical therapy, but benefit is often transient.

ACROCYANOSIS In acrocyanosis there is arterial vasoconstriction and secondary dilatation of the capillaries and venules with resulting persistent cyanosis of the hands and, less frequently, the feet. Cyanosis may be intensified by exposure to a cold environment. Women are affected much more frequently than men and the age of onset is usually less than 30 years. Generally patients are asymptomatic but seek medical attention because of the discoloration. Examination reveals normal pulses, peripheral cyanosis, and moist palms. Trophic skin changes and ulcerations do *not* occur. The disorder can be distinguished from Raynaud's phenomenon because it is persistent and not episodic, the discoloration extends proximally from the digits, and blanching does not occur. Ischemia secondary to arterial occlusive disease can usually be excluded by the presence of normal pulses. Central cyanosis and decreased arterial oxygen saturation are not present. Patients should be reassured, and advised to dress warmly and avoid cold exposure. Pharmacologic intervention is not indicated.

LIVEDO RETICULARIS In this condition, localized areas of the extremities develop a mottled or net-like appearance of reddish to blue discoloration. The mottled appearance may be more prominent following cold exposure. The idiopathic form of this disorder occurs equally in men and women and the most common age of onset is in the third decade. Patients with the idiopathic form usually are asymptomatic and seek attention for cosmetic reasons. Livedo reticularis also occurs following atheroembolism (see above). Rarely, skin ulcerations develop. Patients should be reassured and advised to avoid cold environments. No drug treatment is indicated.

PERNIO (CHILBLAINS) Pernio is a vasculitic disorder that is associated with exposure to cold; acute forms have been described. Raised erythematous lesions develop on the lower part of the legs and feet in cold weather. These are associated with a pruritic and burning sensation and they may blister and ulcerate. Pathologic examination demonstrates angiitis characterized by intimal proliferation and perivascular infiltration of mononuclear and polymorphonuclear leukocytes. Giant cells may be present in the subcutaneous tissue. Patients should avoid exposure to cold, and ulcers should be kept clean and protected with sterile dressings. Sympatholytic drugs may be effective in some patients.

ERYTHROMELALGIA (ERYTHERMALGIA) This disorder is characterized by burning pain and erythema of the extremities. The feet are involved more frequently than the hands, and males are affected more frequently than females. Erythromelalgia may occur at any age but is most common in middle age. It may be primary or secondary to disorders such as polycythemia vera and hypertension. Patients complain of burning in the extremities, precipitated by exposure to a warm environment and aggravated by the dependent position. The symptoms are relieved by exposing the affected area to cool air or water or by elevation. Erythromelalgia can be distinguished from ischemia secondary to arterial occlusive disorders and peripheral neuropathy because the peripheral pulses are present and the neurologic examination is normal. There is no specific treatment; aspirin may produce relief. Treatment of associated disorders in secondary erythromelalgia may be helpful.

VENOUS DISORDERS

Veins in the extremities can be broadly classified as either superficial or deep. In the lower extremity, the superficial venous system includes the greater and lesser saphenous veins and their tributaries. The deep veins of the leg accompany the major arteries. Perforating veins connect the superficial and the deep systems at multiple locations. Bicuspid valves are present throughout the venous system to direct the flow of venous blood centrally.

VENOUS THROMBOSIS The presence of thrombus within a superficial or deep vein and the accompanying inflammatory response in the vessel wall is termed venous thrombosis or thrombophlebitis. Initially the thrombus is composed principally of platelets and fibrin. Red cells become interspersed with fibrin and the thrombus tends to propagate in the direction of blood flow. The inflammatory response in the vessel wall may be minimal or characterized by granulocyte infiltration, loss of endothelium, and edema.

The factors that predispose to venous thrombosis were initially described by Virchow in 1856 and include stasis, vascular damage, and hypercoagulability. Accordingly, a variety of clinical situations are associated with an increased risk of venous thrombosis (Table 198-2). Venous thrombosis may occur in more than 50 percent of patients having orthopedic surgical procedures, particularly those involving the hip or knee, and in 10 to 40 percent of patients who undergo abdominal or thoracic operations. The prevalence of venous thrombosis is particularly high in patients with cancer of the pancreas, lungs, genitourinary tract, stomach, and breast. Risk of thrombosis is increased following trauma, such as fractures of the spine, pelvis, femur, and tibia. Immobilization, regardless of the underlying disease, is a major predisposing cause of venous thrombosis. This may account for the relatively high incidence in patients with acute myocardial infarction or congestive heart failure. The incidence of venous thrombosis is increased during pregnancy and in individuals who use estrogens. A variety of clinical disorders that produce systemic hypercoagulability, including antithrombin III, protein C, and protein S deficiencies; systemic lupus erythematosus; myeloproliferative diseases; dysfibrinogenemia; and disseminated intravascular coagulation, may cause venous thrombosis. Venulitis occurring in thromboangiitis obliterans, Behçet's disease, and homocysteinuria also may cause venous thrombosis.

DEEP VENOUS THROMBOSIS The most important consequences of this disorder are pulmonary embolism (Chap. 213) and the syndrome of chronic venous insufficiency. Deep thrombosis of the iliac, femoral, or popliteal veins is suggested by unilateral leg swelling, warmth, and erythema. Tenderness may be present along the course of the involved veins, and a cord may be palpable. There may be increased tissue turgor, distention of superficial veins, and the appearance of prominent venous collaterals. In some patients, deoxygenated hemoglobin in stagnant veins imparts a cyanotic hue to the limb, a condition called *phlegmasia cerulea dolens*. In markedly edematous legs, the interstitial tissue pressure may exceed the capillary perfusion pressure, causing pallor, a condition designated *phlegmasia alba dolens*.

The diagnosis of deep venous thrombosis of the calf is often difficult to make at the bedside. This is because only one of the multiple veins may be involved, allowing adequate venous return through the remaining patent vessels. The most common complaint is calf pain. Examination may reveal posterior calf tenderness, warmth, increased tissue turgor or modest swelling, and rarely, a cord. Increased resistance or pain during dorsiflexion of the foot, *Homan's sign*, is an unreliable diagnostic sign.

Deep venous thrombosis occurs less frequently in the upper extremity than in the lower extremity, but the incidence is increasing

TABLE 198-2 Conditions associated with an increased risk for development of venous thrombosis

Surgery
  Orthopedic, thoracic, abdominal, and genitourinary procedures
Neoplasms
  Pancreas, lung, ovary, testes, urinary tract, breast, stomach
Trauma
  Fractures of spine, pelvis, femur, tibia
Immobilization
  Acute myocardial infarction, congestive heart failure, stroke, postoperative convalescence
Pregnancy
Estrogen use (for replacement or contraception)
Hypercoagulable states
  Deficiencies of antithrombin III, protein C, or protein S; circulating lupus anticoagulant; myeloproliferative diseases; dysfibrinogenemia; disseminated intravascular coagulation
Venulitis
  Thromboangiitis obliterans, Behçet's disease, homocysteinuria
Previous deep vein thrombosis

because of the greater utilization of subclavian vein catheters. The clinical features and complications are similar to those described for the leg.

Diagnosis Deep venous thrombosis can be diagnosed by venography. Contrast medium is injected into a superficial vein of the foot and directed to the deep system by the application of tourniquets. The presence of a filling defect or absence of filling of the deep veins is required to make the diagnosis.

A variety of noninvasive tests can also diagnose deep venous thrombosis at less discomfort and cost. Plethysmographic techniques used to measure changes in venous capacitance during physiologic maneuvers include impedance plethysmography (IPG) and phleborheography (PRG). The IPG uses skin electrodes and the PRG uses a series of air-filled cuffs to detect changes in leg volume. Venous obstruction blunts the normal changes in venous capacitance that occur during respiration or following inflation and deflation of a thigh cuff. The predictive value of these tests for detecting occlusive thrombi in proximal veins is approximately 90 percent. However, these tests are much less sensitive in the detection of deep venous thrombosis of the calves. A combination of ultrasonographic techniques, Doppler ultrasonography and B-mode (two-dimensional) imaging, termed duplex ultrasonography, is often useful. The Doppler ultrasound measures the velocity of blood flow in veins. This velocity is normally affected by respiration and by manual compression of the foot or calf. Flow abnormalities occur when deep venous obstruction is present. By imaging the deep veins using B-mode ultrasonography, the presence of thrombus can be detected by direct visualization or by inference when the vein does not collapse with compressive maneuvers. The positive predictive value of this diagnostic test approaches 95 percent for *proximal* deep vein thrombosis.

^{125}I-fibrinogen scanning is occasionally used for the diagnosis of deep venous thrombosis. Since this isotope is actively taken up by propagating venous thrombi, increases in radioactivity detected with a counter imply the presence of a thrombus. Fibrinogen scans detect more than 90 percent of calf vein thrombi but are less specific for proximal venous thrombi. A serious limitation of the technique is that it may take 48 to 72 h after administration of the isotope for a fibrinogen scan to become positive.

Deep vein thrombosis must be differentiated from a variety of disorders that cause unilateral leg pain or swelling, including muscle trauma or hemorrhage, ruptured popliteal cyst, and lymphedema. It may be difficult to distinguish swelling caused by the postphlebitic syndrome from that due to acute recurrent deep venous thrombosis. Leg pain may also result from nerve compression syndromes, arthritis, tendinitis, fractures, and arterial occlusive disorders. A careful history and physical examination can usually determine the cause of these symptoms.

Treatment Prevention of pulmonary embolism is the most important reason for treating patients with deep vein thrombosis, since in the early stages the thrombus may be loose and poorly adherent to the vessel wall. Patients should be placed in bed and the affected extremity should be elevated above the level of the heart until the edema and tenderness subside. Anticoagulants prevent thrombus propagation and allow the endogenous lytic system to operate. Heparin should be administered intravenously as an initial bolus of 5000 to 10,000 IU, followed by a continuous infusion of 1000 IU/h. The rate of the heparin infusion should be adjusted so that the activated partial thromboplastin time (APTT) is approximately twice the control value. Intermittent intravenous and subcutaneous injections of heparin have been used as alternative forms of therapy. In less than 5 percent of patients, heparin therapy may cause thrombocytopenia. Infrequently, these patients develop arterial thrombosis and ischemia. Heparin treatment should be maintained for at least 7 to 10 days. It is important to overlap heparin treatment with oral anticoagulant therapy for at least 4 to 5 days because the full anticoagulant effect of warfarin is delayed. The dose of warfarin should be adjusted to maintain the prothrombin time by 4 to 7 s beyond control values.

The use of anticoagulants for isolated deep vein thrombosis of the calf is controversial because the incidence of pulmonary embolism is very low. However, approximately 20 percent of calf thrombi propagate to the thigh, thereby increasing the risk of pulmonary embolism. Therefore, patients with calf vein thrombosis should either receive anticoagulants or be followed with serial noninvasive tests to determine whether proximal propagation has occurred.

Anticoagulant treatment should be continued for 3 to 12 months for patients with acute proximal deep vein thrombosis to decrease the chance of recurrence. The duration of anticoagulant treatment for patients with calf vein thrombosis should be at least 6 weeks. The duration of treatment is indefinite for patients with *recurrent* deep vein thrombosis and for those in whom associated causes, such as malignancy or hypercoagulability, have not been eliminated. If treatment with anticoagulants is contraindicated because of a bleeding diathesis or risk of hemorrhage, protection from pulmonary embolism can be achieved by mechanically interrupting the flow of blood through the inferior vena cava. Inferior vena cava plication generally has been replaced by percutaneous insertion of a filter.

Thrombolytic drugs such as streptokinase, urokinase, and tissue plasminogen activator also may be used, but there is no evidence that thrombolytic therapy is more effective than anticoagulants in preventing pulmonary embolism. However, early administration of thrombolytic drugs may preserve venous valves and decrease the potential for developing postphlebitic syndrome.

Prophylaxis should be considered in clinical situations where the risk of deep vein thrombosis is high. Low-dose heparin (5000 units 2 h prior to surgery and then 5000 units every 8 or 12 h postoperatively), often supplemented with dihydroergotamine (0.5 mg), warfarin, dextran, and external pneumatic compression are all useful. Low-dose heparin, however, does not reduce the risk of deep vein thrombosis following hip or knee surgery. Instead, warfarin, in doses that increase the prothrombin time to 1.5 to 2 times control values, is effective and can be started 48 to 72 h after surgery. External pneumatic compression devices applied to the legs are used to prevent deep vein thrombosis when even low doses of heparin may cause serious bleeding, such as during neurosurgery or transurethral resection of the prostate.

SUPERFICIAL VEIN THROMBOSIS Thrombosis of the greater or lesser saphenous veins or their tributaries, i.e., superficial vein thrombosis, does not result in pulmonary embolism or chronic venous insufficiency. It is associated with intravenous catheters and infusions, occurs in varicose veins, and may develop in association with deep vein thrombosis. Migrating superficial vein thrombosis is often a marker for a carcinoma and may also occur in patients with vasculitides, such as thromboangiitis obliterans. The clinical features of superficial vein thrombosis are easily distinguishable from those of deep vein thrombosis. Patients complain of pain localized to the site of the thrombus. Examination reveals a reddened, warm, and tender cord extending along a superficial vein. The surrounding area may be red and edematous.

Therapy is primarily supportive. Initially, patients can be placed at bed rest with leg elevation and application of warm compresses. Nonsteroidal anti-inflammatory drugs may provide analgesia, but also may obscure clinical evidence of thrombus propagation. If a thrombosis of the greater saphenous vein develops in the thigh and extends towards the saphenofemoral vein junction, it is reasonable to consider anticoagulant therapy to prevent extension of the thrombus into the deep system and a possible pulmonary embolism.

VARICOSE VEINS These are dilated tortuous superficial veins that result from defective structure and function of the valves of the saphenous veins, from intrinsic weakness of the vein wall, or rarely from arteriovenous fistulas. Varicose veins can be categorized as primary or secondary. Primary varicose veins originate in the superficial system and occur twice as frequently in women as men. Approximately half of patients have a family history of varicose veins. Secondary varicose veins result from deep venous insufficiency and incompetent perforating veins, or from deep venous occlusion causing enlargement of superficial veins that are serving as collaterals.

Patients with venous varicosities are often concerned about the cosmetic appearance of their legs. Symptoms consist of a dull ache or pressure sensation in the legs after prolonged standing; it is relieved with leg elevation. The legs feel heavy and occasionally mild ankle edema develops. Extensive venous varicosities may cause skin ulcerations near the ankle. Superficial venous thrombosis may be a recurring problem and rarely a varicosity ruptures and bleeds. Visual inspection of the legs in the dependent position usually confirms the presence of varicose veins.

Varicose veins can usually be treated with conservative measures. Symptoms often decrease when the legs are elevated periodically, when prolonged standing is avoided, and when elastic support hose are worn. External compression stockings provide a counterbalance to the hydrostatic pressure within the veins. Small symptomatic varicose veins may be treated with sclerotherapy in which a sclerosing solution is injected into the involved varicose vein and a compression bandage is applied. Surgical therapy usually involves extensive ligation and stripping of the greater and lesser saphenous veins and should be reserved for those patients who are very symptomatic, suffer recurrent superficial vein thrombosis, and/or develop skin ulceration. Surgical therapy may be indicated for cosmetic reasons.

CHRONIC VENOUS INSUFFICIENCY This may result from deep vein thrombosis and/or valvular incompetence. Following deep vein thrombosis, the delicate valve leaflets become thickened and contracted so that they are incapable of preventing retrograde flow of blood; the vein becomes rigid and thick-walled. Although most veins recanalize after an episode of thrombosis, the large proximal veins may remain occluded. Secondary incompetence develops in distal valves because high pressures distend the vein and separate the leaflets. Primary deep venous valvular dysfunction also may occur without previous thrombosis. Patients with venous insufficiency often complain of a dull ache in the leg that worsens with prolonged standing and resolves with leg elevation. Examination demonstrates increased leg circumference, edema, and superficial varicose veins. Erythema, dermatitis, and hyperpigmentation develop along the distal aspect of the leg, and skin ulceration may occur near the medial and lateral malleoli. Cellulitis may be a recurring problem.

Patients should be advised to avoid prolonged standing or sitting; frequent leg elevation is helpful. Graduated compression stockings should be worn during the day. These efforts should be intensified if skin ulcers develop. Ulcers should be treated with applications of wet to dry dressings and occasionally dilute topical antibiotic solutions. An Unna paste boot often is effective. Recurrent ulceration and severe edema may be treated by surgical interruption of incompetent communicating veins. Rarely surgical valvuloplasty and bypass of venous occlusions are employed.

LYMPHATIC DISORDERS

Lymphatic capillaries are blind-ended tubes formed by a single layer of endothelial cells. The absent or widely fenestrated basement membrane of lymphatic capillaries allows greater access to interstitial proteins and particles. Lymphatic capillaries merge to form larger vessels which contain smooth muscle and are capable of vasomotion. Small- and medium-sized lymphatic vessels empty into progressively larger channels which drain into the thoracic duct. The lymphatic circulation is involved in the absorption of interstitial fluid and in the response to infection.

LYMPHEDEMA Lymphedema may be categorized as primary or secondary (Table 198-3). The prevalence of primary lymphedema is approximately 1 per 10,000 individuals. Primary lymphedema may be secondary to agenesis, hypoplasia, or obstruction of the lymphatic vessels. It may be associated with Turner's syndrome, Noonan's syndrome, the yellow nail syndrome, the intestinal lymphangiectasia syndrome, and with lymphangiomyomatosis. Women are affected more frequently than are men. There are three clinical subtypes: *congenital lymphedema* which appears shortly after birth, *lymphedema praecox* which has its onset at the time of puberty, and *lymphedema tarda* which usually begins after the age of 35. Familial forms of congenital lymphedema (Milroy's disease) and lymphedema praecox (Meige's disease) may be inherited in an autosomal dominant manner with variable penetrance; autosomal or sex-linked recessive forms are less common.

TABLE 198-3 Classification of lymphedema

Primary
Congenital (includes Milroy's disease)
Lymphedema praecox (includes Meige's disease)
Lymphedema tarda
Secondary
Recurrent lymphangitis
Filariasis
Tuberculosis
Neoplasm
Surgery
Radiation therapy

Secondary lymphedema is an acquired condition resulting from damage to, or obstruction of, previously normal lymphatic channels (Table 198-3). Recurrent episodes of bacterial lymphangitis, usually caused by streptococci, are a very common cause of lymphedema. The most common cause of secondary lymphedema worldwide is filariasis (Chap. 169). Tumors, such as prostate cancer and lymphoma, also can obstruct lymphatic vessels. Both surgery and radiation therapy for breast carcinoma may cause lymphedema of the upper extremity. Less common causes include tuberculosis, contact dermatitis, lymphogranuloma venereum, rheumatoid arthritis, pregnancy, and self-induced or factitious lymphedema following application of tourniquets.

Lymphedema is generally a painless condition but patients may experience a chronic dull, heavy sensation in the leg and most often patients are concerned about the appearance of the leg. Lymphedema of the lower extremity, initially involving the foot, gradually progresses up the leg so that the entire limb becomes edematous. In the early stages of lymphedema, the edema is soft and pits easily with pressure. In the chronic stages of lymphedema, the limb has a woody texture and the tissues become indurated and fibrotic. At this stage, the edema may no longer be pitting. The limb loses its normal contour and the toes appear square. Lymphedema should be distinguished from other disorders that cause unilateral leg swelling, such as deep vein thrombosis and chronic venous insufficiency. In the latter, edema is softer and there is often evidence of a stasis dermatitis, hyperpigmentation, and superficial venous varicosities.

The evaluation of patients with lymphedema should include diagnostic studies to clarify the etiology. Abdominal and pelvic ultrasound and computed tomography can be used to detect obstructing lesions such as neoplasms. Lymphoscintigraphy and lymphangiography are rarely indicated but either can be used to confirm the diagnosis or differentiate primary from secondary lymphedema. Lymphoscintigraphy involves the injection of radioactively labeled technetium-containing colloid into the distal subcutaneous tissue of the affected extremity. Lymphangiography requires the isolation and cannulation of a distal lymphatic vessel and subsequent injection of contrast material. In primary lymphedema, lymphatic channels are absent, hypoplastic, or ectatic. In secondary lymphedema, lymphatic channels *usually* are dilated and the level of obstruction may be determined.

Treatment Patients with lymphedema of the lower extremities must be instructed to take meticulous care of their feet to prevent recurrent lymphangitis. Skin hygiene is important and emollients can be used to prevent drying. Prophylactic antibiotics are often helpful and fungal infection should be treated aggressively. Patients should be encouraged to participate in physical activity; frequent leg elevation can reduce the amount of edema. Patients can be fitted with graduated compression hose to reduce the amount of lymphedema that develops with upright posture. Occasionally, intermittent pneumatic compression devices can be applied at home to facilitate reduction of the edema. Diuretics are contraindicated and may cause depletion of intravascular volume and metabolic abnormalities. Recently, microsurgical lymphovenous anastomotic procedures have been performed to rechannel lymph flow from obstructed lymphatic vessels into the venous system.

REFERENCES

Bernstein EF: *Noninvasive Diagnostic Techniques in Vascular Disease,* 3d ed. St. Louis, Mosby, 1985

Browse NL: The diagnosis and management of primary lymphedema. J Vasc Surg 3:181, 1986

Coffman JD: Intermittent claudication and rest pain. Physiologic concepts and therapeutic approaches. Prog Cardiovasc Dis 22:59, 1979

———: *Raynaud's Phenomenon.* New York, Oxford, 1989

Doubilet P, Abrams HL: The cost of underutilization. Percutaneous transluminal angioplasty for peripheral vascular disease. N Engl J Med 310:95, 1984

Fairbairn JF II et al: *Peripheral Vascular Diseases,* 5th ed. Philadelphia, Saunders, 1980

Fogle MA et al: A comparison of in situ and reversed saphenous vein grafts for infrainguinal reconstruction. J Vasc Surg 5:46, 1987

Hirsh J et al: *Venous Thromboembolism.* New York, Grune & Stratton, 1981

Hull R et al: Adjusted subcutaneous heparin vs warfarin sodium in the long term treatment of venous thrombosis. N Engl J Med 306:189, 1982

Kakkar VV et al: Prevention of fatal postoperative pulmonary embolism by low doses of heparin. An international trial. Lancet 1:567, 1977

Loscalzo J et al: *The Textbook of Vascular Medicine and Biology.* Boston, Little, Brown, in press

Marder VJ, Sherry S: Thrombolytic therapy: Current status. N Engl J Med 318:1512, 1988

Moser KM, LeMoine JR: Is embolic risk conditioned by location of deep venous thrombosis. Ann Intern Med 94:439, 1981

Van Breda A et al: Urokinase vs. streptokinase in local thrombolysis. Radiology 165:109, 1987

PART SEVEN

DISORDERS OF THE RESPIRATORY SYSTEM

199 IMPACT OF CELL AND MOLECULAR BIOLOGY ON PULMONARY DISEASE

RONALD G. CRYSTAL

The major function of the lung is to exchange gases with the environment. As such, its essential role is mechanical—to bring the ambient air into close proximity to the output of the right heart, permitting efficient gas exchange at little energy cost. The traditional methods used to assess the lung in health and disease reflect this role, with chest x-rays used to evaluate lung anatomy and physiologic tests to assess lung function. These approaches define the type and extent of lung abnormalities associated with various categories of lung disease, but they give little insight into the underlying pathogenic processes.

These traditional methods have now been supplemented with the disciplines of cell and molecular biology. For this to become a reality, it was first necessary to have access to sufficient numbers of purified cellular and extracellular components of the lung so that they could be evaluated in vitro. Two developments made this possible: (1) techniques permitting the purification and in vitro culture of lung inflammatory and parenchymal cells; and (2) the use of the fiberoptic bronchoscope to sample the components of the epithelial surface of the lung by bronchoalveolar lavage.

The adaptation of tissue culture techniques to lung cells made it possible to study purified human lung alveolar macrophages and T lymphocytes, as well as lung parenchymal cells including bronchial and alveolar epithelial cells, endothelial cells, and mesenchymal cells.

Bronchoalveolar lavage (BAL) is a simple extension of fiberoptic bronchoscopy and typically yields 1 to 3 mL of epithelial lining fluid containing 10 to 30 $\times$ 10^6 inflammatory cells from normal individuals and up to 200 $\times$ 10^6 cells from subjects with chronic inflammatory diseases. Both the extracellular and cellular components can be assessed by the techniques of cellular and molecular biology.

Four disorders will be discussed to illustrate how these techniques have led to major advances in the understanding of human lung disease: idiopathic pulmonary fibrosis, chronic beryllium disease, $alpha_1$ antitrypsin deficiency, and cystic fibrosis.

IDIOPATHIC PULMONARY FIBROSIS (IPF) IPF is a chronic inflammatory fibrotic disorder localized to the lower respiratory tract and characterized by an alveolitis dominated by alveolar macrophages and neutrophils and, to a lesser extent, lymphocytes and eosinophils (see Chap. 211). The disease usually presents as dyspnea on exertion, the chest x-ray shows diffuse reticulonodular infiltrates, and analysis of lung function reveals restrictive abnormalities. Evaluation of the inflammatory cells recovered by BAL has lead to the concept that the cell responsible for directing the process of scar formation is the alveolar macrophage, a cell that normally defends the alveolar structures by phagocytosing infectious agents and particulates. In IPF, for reasons not completely understood but likely related to immune complexes formed in the local milieu, the alveolar macrophages express several genes that code for potent polypeptide mediators capable of recruiting fibroblasts and signaling them to proliferate. The consequence is that fibroblasts are abundant in the milieu of chronic damage. Since fibroblasts secrete a collagenous extracellular matrix, more collagen, i.e., a scar, forms.

Among the polypeptide mediators released by alveolar macrophages of IPF patients is fibronectin, a 220-kDa dimeric glycoprotein that interacts with the connective tissue matrix and with specific receptors on fibroblasts. Studies of fibronectin gene expression in alveolar macrophages demonstrate that fibronectin mRNA levels correlate with fibronectin release. Indeed, alveolar macrophages recovered from IPF patients contain more fibronectin mRNA than alveolar macrophages of normals (Fig. 199-1*A* and *B*).

Perhaps the most potent alveolar macrophage "growth factor" is platelet-derived growth factor (PDGF), a glycoprotein that in human alveolar macrophages is composed of dimers of A and B chains or homodimers of B chains. The genes for the A and B chains of PDGF are on different chromosomes and are modulated independently. Interestingly, the B chain is encoded by the *c-sis* gene, a cellular proto-oncogene on chromosome 22 with close homology to the *v-sis* gene, a transforming viral oncogene. Alveolar macrophages recovered from the lower respiratory tract of individuals with IPF express *c-sis* mRNA transcripts, and the PDGF protein product of the *c-sis* gene is released by these cells at a level fourfold greater than by normal macrophages (Fig. 199-1*C*). Thus, a gene homologous to a viral oncogene is expressed in an exaggerated fashion in one site and contributes to a localized proliferation of mesenchymal cells and eventual organ fibrosis. Furthermore, glucocorticoid therapy (the conventional treatment) does not affect PDGF release by the macrophages. Consequently, it is no surprise that most IPF patients continue to deteriorate even when treated in this fashion.

CHRONIC BERYLLIUM DISEASE Multiple exposures to airborne beryllium dusts, salts, or fumes can result, in susceptible individuals, in a chronic interstitial lung disorder characterized by the accumulation of lymphocytes and mononuclear phagocytes and the formation of noncaseating granulomas in the lower respiratory tract (see Chap. 206). The alveolitis is dominated by alveolar macrophages and T lymphocytes, in particular, activated CD4+ helper-inducer T cells, characteristic of the T cells in sites of chronic, delayed-type hypersensitivity reactions (Fig. 199-2*A*). Most noteworthy, the lung T cells proliferate in response to beryllium and do so to a greater extent than do blood T cells from the same individual, i.e., the antigen-specific T cells are compartmentalized to the site of the disease (Fig. 199-2*B*). Furthermore, the lung T cells proliferating in response to beryllium are confined to the helper-inducer subset. The proliferative response of these lung T cells is truly beryllium-specific in that the cells do not proliferate in response to other metal salts or to typical recall antigens such as tetanus toxoid or streptokinase.

Together, these observations define chronic beryllium disease as a chronic hypersensitivity disease in which beryllium-primed lung CD4+ T cells play a central role in its pathogenesis. Beryllium presumably acts as an antigen by combining (as a hapten) with one or more proteins. However, since chronic beryllium disease develops in only a small proportion of those exposed to the agent, individual susceptibility must play a major role in determining who is at risk. The proliferative response of lung T cells to beryllium provides a

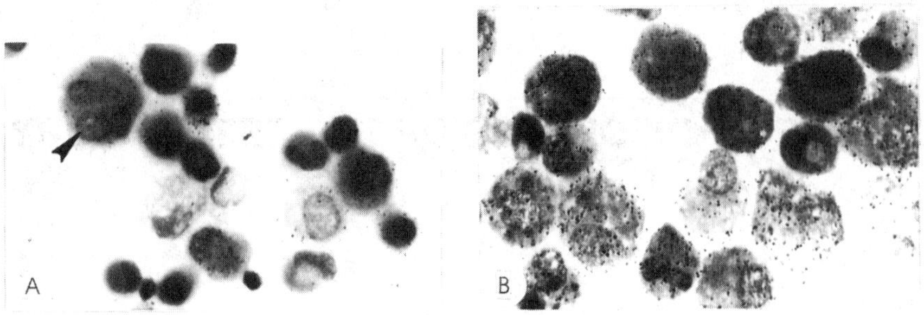

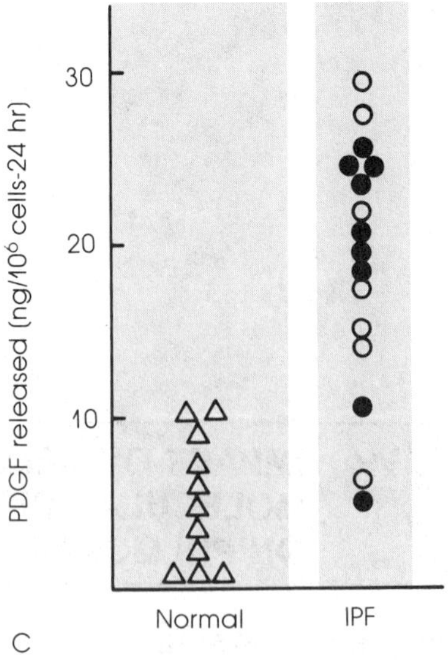

FIGURE 199-1 Exaggerated expression of alveolar macrophage genes coding for polypeptide mediators that modulate fibroblast accumulation in the alveolar walls of patients with idiopathic pulmonary fibrosis. *A*. Example of in situ hybridization analysis of fibronectin mRNA transcripts in alveolar macrophages of a normal individual. The mRNA transcripts in macrophages recovered by bronchoalveolar lavage were assessed with a ^{35}S-labeled fibronectin antisense cRNA probe and autoradiography. The grains above the macrophage (arrow) indicate fibronectin mRNA transcripts (×500). *B*. Similar to panel *A*, but with alveolar macrophages of a patient with IPF. On the average, there are twofold more fibronectin mRNA transcripts per macrophage than in normals (×500). *C*. Spontaneous exaggerated release of PDGF by alveolar macrophages recovered from the lower respiratory tract of individuals with IPF. Macrophages recovered by bronchoalveolar lavage were cultured for 24 h. Supernatants were evaluated for the presence of PDGF using a specific immunoassay. Each symbol represents one individual. For the IPF patients, closed circles represent untreated patients and open circles represent those receiving prednisone. Note that therapy has no effect on the release of this potent mediator.

diagnostic tool to identify individuals with this disorder, thus obviating the need for chemical analysis of the lung parenchyma.

ALPHA$_1$ ANTITRYPSIN DEFICIENCY Alpha$_1$ antitrypsin (α1AT) deficiency is a hereditary disorder characterized by reduced serum levels of α1AT, an antiprotease that provides the major defense for the lower respiratory tract against the ravages of neutrophil elastase, a powerful destructive protease. The loss of this protective screen of the fragile alveolar walls results in emphysema (Chap. 210).

The emphysema is the result of a variety of mutations in the α1AT gene on chromosome 14 (Fig. 199-3*A*). The two α1AT genes are codominantly expressed and together define the α1AT level in serum. The gene is pleomorphic with approximately 75 known alleles, of which at least 20 can cause a clinically relevant deficiency state. Most normal α1AT alleles are classified as M-type. Most α1AT is synthesized by liver hepatocytes; the enzyme is a typical secretory glycoprotein that is translated on the rough endoplasmic reticulum (RER), glycosylated in the cisternae of the RER, translocated to the Golgi, and then secreted (Fig. 199-3*B*). The two most common "deficiency" mutations are Z (exon V, Glu^{342} *G*AG → Lys *A*AG) and S (exon III, Glu^{264} G*A*A → Val G*T*A).

The Z mutation, carried by 1 in 50 Caucasians of European descent, causes hepatocytes of homozygotes to secrete only 10 to 15 percent of the normal amount of α1AT. Because the Glu^{342} → Lys substitution reverses the charge at this residue, the Z-type α1AT molecules aggregate in the RER, less α1AT is translocated to the Golgi, and hence α1AT deficiency results.

The S mutation, carried by up to 1 in 25 persons, causes a different derangement of α1AT processing. The hepatocytes degrade an

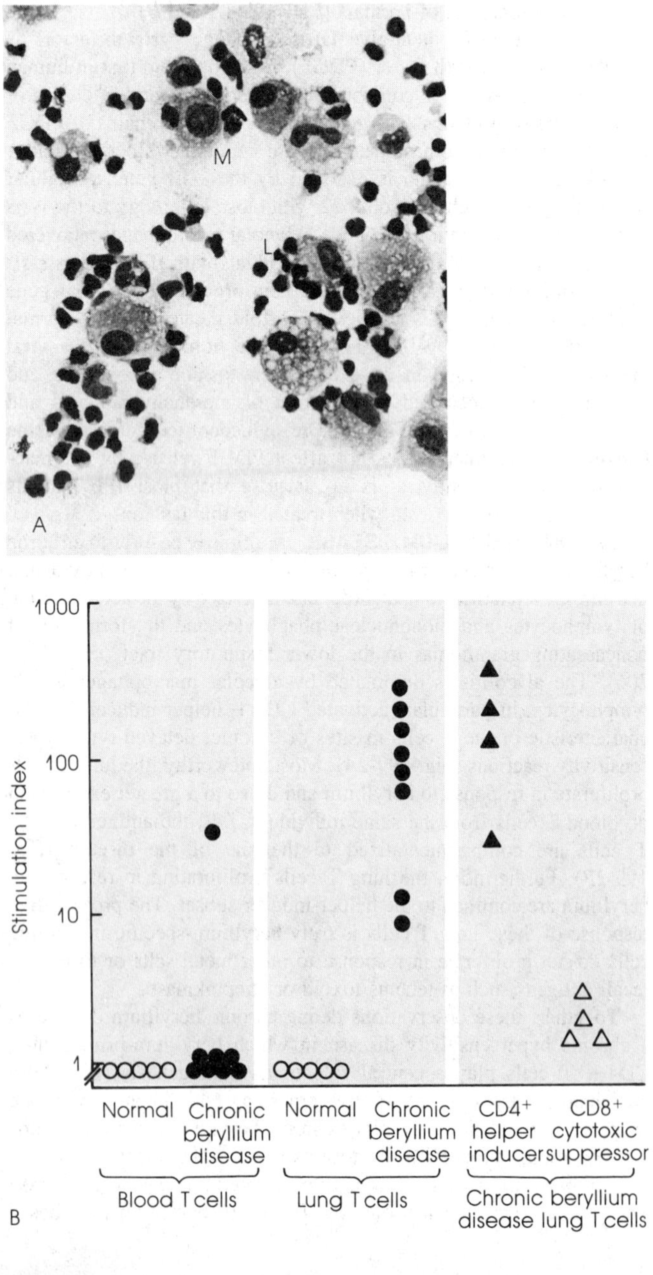

FIGURE 199-2 Beryllium-specific inflammatory processes in the lower respiratory tract of individuals with chronic beryllium disease. *A*. Inflammatory cells recovered by bronchoalveolar lavage of an individual with chronic beryllium disease. The alveolitis is dominated by lymphocytes (L) and alveolar macrophages (M) (×500). Flow cytometric analysis with appropriate monoclonal antibodies demonstrates that the lymphocytes are predominantly CD4$^+$ helper-inducer T lymphocytes. *B*. In vitro proliferation of blood and lung T lymphocytes of patients with chronic beryllium disease and normals in response to beryllium. The data are presented as a stimulation index (values >1 represent proliferation above control) and each symbol represents one individual. Normal blood and lung T cells rarely proliferate in response to beryllium. In contrast, lung, but not blood, T cells from individuals with chronic beryllium disease respond briskly to beryllium, with the CD4$^+$ helper-inducer T cells dominating the proliferative response.

increased proportion of the newly synthesized α1AT, resulting in less α1AT for secretion and hence the deficiency state. However, the relative "deficiency" associated with the S allele is less than that associated with Z. Consequently, S homozygotes are not at risk for emphysema, but SZ heterozygotes are at mild risk.

Z homozygotes have reduced α1AT in the lung and hence have a deficient screen against proteolytic attack by neutrophil elastase (Fig. 199-3*C*). While S homozygotes also have reduced α1AT levels, the amount is sufficient to afford protection, i.e., the "threshold" protective level is between that of S and Z homozygotes. Based on this concept, strategies to prevent the emphysema associated with α1AT deficiency have focused on augmenting the protective screen of the lower respiratory tract with α1AT. In this regard, intravenous administration of 60 mg/kg body weight of α1AT once a week results in α1AT serum levels sufficient to maintain lung levels above that necessary to provide sufficient antielastase protection to the alveoli, i.e., augmentation therapy reverses the biochemical abnormalities at the site of the target organ and thus is a rational approach to prevent the emphysema.

CYSTIC FIBROSIS (CF) CF is an autosomal recessive disorder of exocrine glands characterized in lung by accumulation of thick mucus, chronic bacterial infections, and chronic obstructive lung disease associated with severe bronchiectasis and parenchymal derangements (see Chap. 209). It is the most common lethal genetic disorder affecting Caucasian populations, with a heterozygote frequency of 1 in 20 to 25 individuals.

The technique of "chromosomal walking" was utilized to locate the cystic fibrosis gene to within approximately 300 kb in the q21-31 region of chromosome 7 (Fig. 199-4*A*). Family studies suggest that a single mutation of the CF gene is predominant. Even before the specific gene was identified, chromosomal markers were sufficiently close to permit accurate identification of CF homozygotes and of most heterozygotes and thus make possible genetic counseling.

Sequencing of the CF "gene" predicts that it codes for a protein of 168 kDa that spans the plasma membrane and contains a domain capable of binding adenosine triphosphate. Despite the fact that the function of the CF "protein" (called the *cystic fibrosis transmembrane conductance regulator*) is not known, it is possible to speculate about the pathogenesis of the disease (Fig. 199-4*B*). Measurement of potential differences across the tracheal epithelium of CF homozygotes has demonstrated a higher voltage than in normals, consistent with the known abnormality in electrolyte transport. In CF subjects who have received lung transplants the abnormal potential differences are no longer present. Cultured epithelial cells of CF patients exhibit abnormal potential differences similar to those observed in vivo. Importantly, the cultured epithelial cells are not capable of transporting Cl^- to the apical surfaces in a normal fashion. Together, these observations suggest that the abnormality of the CF gene is expressed in airway epithelial cells and implicate a dysfunction in the regulation of airway epithelial apical Cl^- channels as the fundamental abnormality. It is hypothesized that the defect in Cl^- channel function causes CF lung disease by modifying the quantity and composition of the airway epithelial fluid. Presumably, such changes alter the

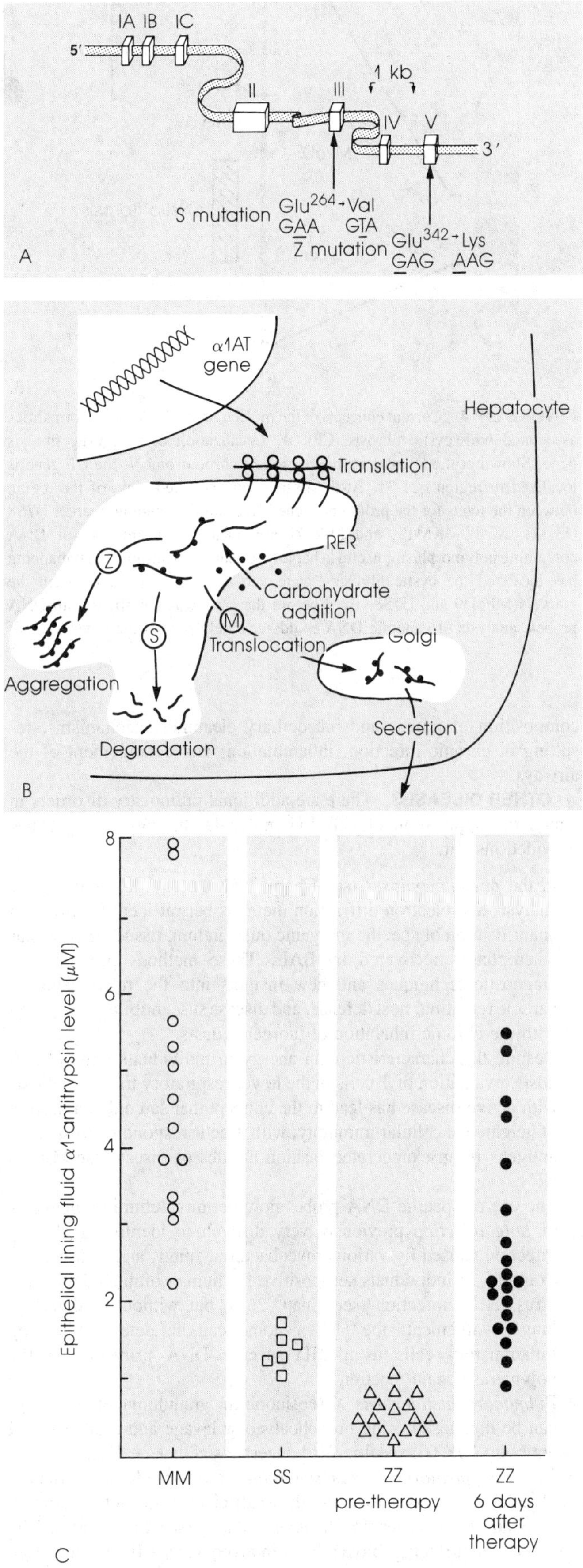

FIGURE 199-3 Pathogenesis and therapy of alpha$_1$ antitrypsin (α1AT) deficiency. *A.* Schematic of the 12.2-kb, 7-exon (I_A-I_C, II-V) α1AT gene. The two most common mutations of the normal M gene are S and Z. *B.* Synthesis and secretion of α1AT by hepatocytes. The normal M α1AT mRNA protein is translated on the rough endoplasmic reticulum (RER), carbohydrates are added, the molecule is translocated to the Golgi and secreted. The Z mutation results in aggregation of newly synthesized α1AT in the RER while the S mutation results in degradation. *C.* Consequences of mutations in the α1AT gene at the level of the alveoli. Shown are α1AT levels in alveolar epithelial lining fluid recovered by bronchoalveolar lavage. Each symbol represents a single individual. S and Z homozygotes have "deficient" amounts of α1AT in the lung, with the level for Z homozygotes below the threshold levels necessary to protect the lung. With once weekly intravenous augmentation therapy with purified human α1AT, the lung epithelial lining fluid α1AT level of Z homozygotes is restored above the protective threshold, thus protecting the lung from emphysema.

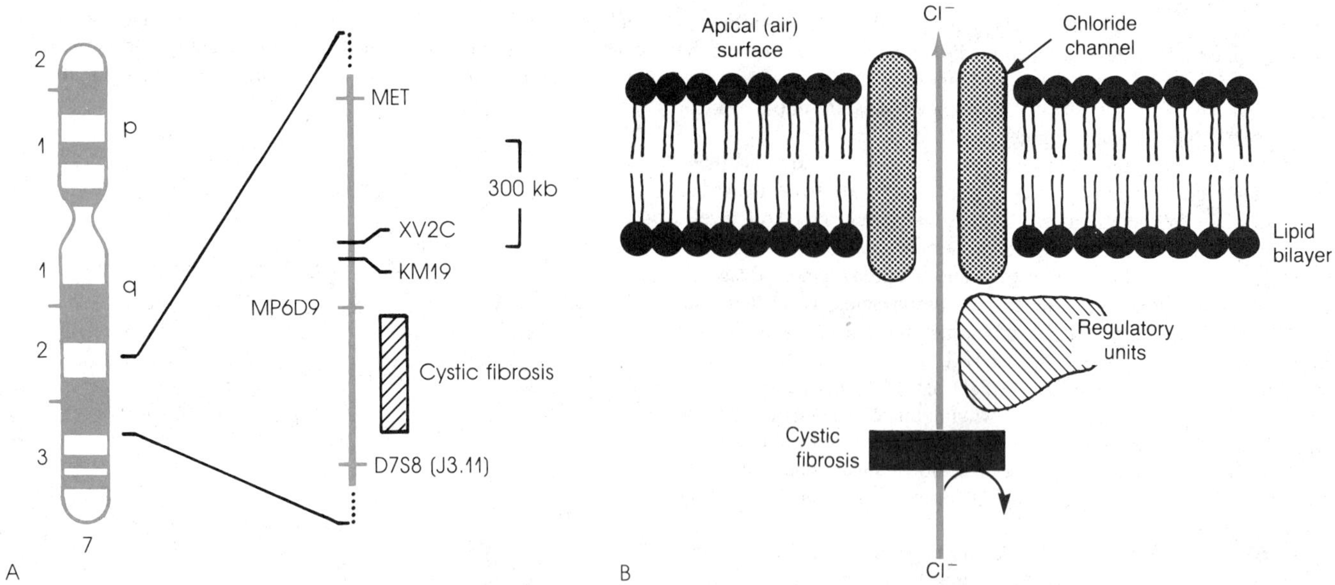

FIGURE 199-4 Current concepts of the molecular and biologic abnormalities associated with cystic fibrosis (CF). *A*. Localization of the cystic fibrosis gene. Shown at the left is a representation of chromosome 7; the CF gene is localized to region q21-31. At the right is an expanded view of the region between the locus for the proto-oncogene MET and the genomic marker D7S8 (J3.11); XV2C, KM19, and MP6D9 are other marker regions of DNA containing polymorphisms useful in haplotype analysis. Chromosomal mapping has localized the cystic fibrosis "gene" to a 250-kb region between the markers MP6D9 and D7S8. Even before the gene was identified with DNA probes, analysis of genomic DNA could accurately predict the inheritance of CF, permitting family planning. Now, specific probes have made accurate diagnosis rapid and simple. *B*. Schematic of the apical (air) membrane of an airway epithelial cell expressing the cystic fibrosis gene. In vivo measurements of electric potentials in the tracheal epithelium together with in vitro studies of cultured airway epithelial cells suggest the abnormality is related to the chloride channel on the apical surface of the epithelial cell, either directly involving a component of the channel or in regulatory units modulating its function. The control of Na^+, K^+, Cl^- through cotransporters and sodium-potassium pumps on the basolateral (serosal) surface of the epithelial cells appears normal, as does ion movement through tight junctions between cells.

composition of mucus and mucociliary clearance mechanisms, resulting in chronic infection, inflammation, and derangement of the airways.

OTHER DISEASES There are additional pulmonary disorders in which the application of cell and molecular biology methods has provided insight.

1 In the *pneumoconioses* (see Chap. 206), energy dispersive x-ray analysis and electron diffraction methods permit identification and quantification of specific inorganic dusts in lung tissue and alveolar macrophages recovered by BAL. These methods provide new diagnostic techniques and new insights into the relationship of particle retention, host defense, and disease susceptibility associated with the chronic inhalation of inorganic dusts.
2 Despite the characteristic skin anergy in individuals with *sarcoidosis,* evaluation of T cells in the lower respiratory tract of patients with active disease has lead to the concept that sarcoid is a disease of heightened cellular immunity, with T cells responding to specific antigens in an exaggerated fashion at sites of disease (see Chap. 277).
3 The use of specific DNA probes now permits definitive diagnosis of *lung infection* previously very difficult to identify, including infection caused by various mycobacteria, fungi, and viruses. For example, in individuals seropositive for human immunodeficiency virus (HIV) infection (see Chap. 264), but without evidence of lung involvement, the HIV genome can be detected in lung inflammatory cells using HIV-specific DNA primers and the polymerase chain reaction.
4 *Pulmonary histiocytosis X* (eosinophilic granuloma of the lung) can be diagnosed using bronchoalveolar lavage and a monoclonal antibody (OKT6) specific for Langerhans cells (see Chap. 211).
5 In the *respiratory distress syndrome of the newborn,* immature alveolar type II cells do not produce sufficient surfactant to maintain alveolar stability, leading to lung collapse (see Chap. 201). The control of surfactant biosynthesis in alveolar type II cells has been delineated using cell culture techniques, strategies have been developed to accelerate the expression of the surfactant system using pharmacologic agents, and the biochemical nature of surfactant has been fully defined. This definition has led to cloning of the apoproteins of surfactant, allowing in vitro reconstitution of an artificial surfactant for use in therapy.
6 In *asthma,* cell biology methodologies have led to the identification of a broad armamentarium of naturally occurring mediators that likely play a role in the pathogenesis of reversible airway disease, and several genes related to these mediators have been cloned and characterized (see Chap. 204).
7 Finally, capitalizing on the identification, cloning, and in vitro production of a variety of potent "inflammatory" polypeptides, much attention has been given to the concept that mediators such as tumor necrosis factor play a role in modulating the parenchymal dysfunction characteristic of the respiratory failure of *adult respiratory distress syndrome*.

CONCLUSIONS The application of modern cell and biology methods to investigate human disease depends on the capacity to obtain appropriate biologic materials relevant to the pathogenesis of the disease. For most diseases, the relevant biologic material must be obtained directly from the target organ, and this is a difficult task for internal organs. Utilizing cell culture techniques and the fiberoptic bronchoscope to gain access to the epithelial surface of the lung, many pulmonary disorders can now be investigated by the techniques of cell and molecular biology. As a consequence there has been a remarkable advance in the understanding of the pathogenesis of a variety of lung disorders and for several new insights into therapy.

REFERENCES

Adachi K et al: Evaluation of fibronectin gene expression by *in situ* hybridization: Differential expression of the fibronectin gene among populations of human alveolar macrophages. Am J Pathol 138:193, 1988

BRANTLY M et al: Molecular basis of α1-antitrypsin deficiency. Am J Med 84:13, 1988
CRYSTAL RG et al: Interstitial lung disease of unknown cause: Disorders characterized by chronic inflammation of the lower respiratory tract. N Engl J Med 310:154, 235, 1984
——— et al: The α1-antitrypsin gene and its mutations: Clinical consequences and strategies for therapy. Chest 95:196, 1989
MARTINET Y et al: Exaggerated spontaneous release of a platelet-derived growth factor by alveolar macrophages from patients with idiopathic pulmonary fibrosis. N Engl J Med 317(4):202, 1987
REYNOLDS HY: Bronchoalveolar lavage. Am Rev Respir Dis 135:250, 1987
RIORDAN JR et al: Identification of the cystic fibrosis gene: Cloning and characterization of complementary DNA. Science 245:1066, 1989
ROMMENS JM et al: Identification of the cystic fibrosis gene: Chromosome walking and jumping. Science 245:1059, 1989
SALTINI C et al: Chronic pulmonary berylliosis: Maintenance of the alveolitis by proliferation of beryllium-specific helper T-cells. N Engl J Med 230:1103, 1989
WELSH MJ, FICK RB: Cystic fibrosis. J Clin Invest 80:1523, 1987
WEWERS MD et al: Replacement therapy for alpha 1-antitrypsin deficiency associated with emphysema. N Engl J Med 316:1055, 1987
YAMAUCHI K et al: Modulation of fibronectin gene expression in human mononuclear phagocytes. J Clin Invest 80(6):1720, 1987

200 APPROACH TO THE PATIENT WITH DISEASE OF THE RESPIRATORY SYSTEM

EUGENE BRAUNWALD

As in other branches of medicine, a careful and detailed history and physical examination are the cornerstones for establishing an accurate diagnosis in patients with disorders of the respiratory system. In addition, the roentgenographic examination occupies a particularly important role in the evaluation of patients with lung disease. Since abnormalities of the respiratory system are frequently a manifestation of a systemic process, attention must be focused not only on the chest but also a comprehensive evaluation of the patient's entire health status is essential. For example, the presence of a pulmonary lesion on x-ray may be due to metastatic disease with the primary tumor elsewhere, and hemoptysis may be due to a disorder of hemostasis. Diffuse scleroderma may result in diffuse pulmonary infiltrative disease (Chap. 271), and multiple pulmonary cavities may be a manifestation of Wegener's granulomatosis (Chap. 276). All of the so-called collagen vascular diseases may have prominent pulmonary manifestations. Carcinoma of the lung (Chap. 215) may be accompanied by prominent extrathoracic manifestations, which may overshadow the pulmonary lesion. These include myopathy, peripheral neuropathy, hypertrophic pulmonary osteoarthropathy, and a variety of endocrine and metabolic manifestations, including Cushing's syndrome, the carcinoid syndrome, a hyperparathyroid-like picture, inappropriate secretion of antidiuretic hormone, gonadotropin (Chap. 309), and increased frequency of pulmonary infections.

HISTORY In eliciting the history of patients with pulmonary disease, it must be appreciated that an increasing fraction of the population is exposed to materials which are potentially toxic to the lung (Chap. 206). The history must therefore contain a detailed *occupational and personal history* with a description of exposure to hazards such as asbestos, coal, silica, beryllium, bagasse, iron oxide, tin oxide, cotton dust, titanium oxide, silver, nitrogen dioxide, animals, moldy hay, air conditioners, and furnace humidifiers. It is useful to construct a work history, which includes the patient's duties, duration of exposure, use of protective devices, and illness in fellow workers. The occupational history should include information on a job-by-job basis as well as the military service. Contact with both wild and domestic animals may result in pulmonary symptoms, such as bronchospasm in subjects allergic to pets, or, less commonly, acute pneumonitis in patients with psittacosis (Chap. 155), tularemia (Chap. 120), or Q fever. Because it is such an important risk factor for many forms of lung disease, history of tobacco consumption, especially cigarette smoking, must be sought and should be quantified, generally in "pack-years." It is important to record the residence and travel histories; histoplasmosis and coccidioidomyosis (Chap. 151) are indigenous to certain regions. The habits of the patient with pulmonary disease must be gone into. Aspiration pneumonia and pneumococcal and *Klebsiella* pneumonia are often seen in alcoholics; lung abscess occurs in intravenous drug abusers.

Pneumocystis carinii pneumonia and other lung infections are frequent complications of the acquired immunodeficiency syndrome (Chap. 264), and a history of intravenous drug abuse or of sexual relations with individuals at high risk for this condition should be obtained, especially in patients with a pulmonary infiltrate and fever. A record of the patient's *previous residence* is of considerable importance in the diagnosis of histoplasmosis (the south and midwestern United States), coccidioidomycosis (the southwestern United States), tropical eosinophilia, and South American blastomycosis. For example, pulmonary mass lesions in patients in the Mediterranean Basin may be due to hydatid cysts, hemoptysis in patients from central China may be caused by paragonimiasis (Chap. 171), and cor pulmonale in Egypt frequently results from schistosomiasis (Chap. 170).

It is vitally important to elicit a history of *drug exposure* since essentially every class of drugs can produce pulmonary toxicity (Chap. 205), and all parts of the respiratory apparatus can be affected, including the alveoli, tracheobronchial tree, mediastinum, pleural cavities, pulmonary vessels, respiratory muscles, and the medullary respiratory center. Examples include the interstitial infiltrative diseases caused by bleomycin, cyclophosphamide, methotrexate, and nitrofurantoin; noncardiogenic pulmonary edema caused by aspirin; bronchospasm caused by beta-adrenergic blockers and nonsteroidal anti-inflammatory drugs; pulmonary vasculitis from intravenous drug abuse; pulmonary thromboembolism in women receiving oral contraceptives; (drug-induced) systemic lupus erythematosus with pleural involvement caused by hydralazine and procainamide; and weakness of the respiratory muscles caused by the aminoglycoside antibiotics.

The *family history* should consider pulmonary diseases which may be genetic, such as cystic disease of the lung, pulmonary emphysema due to $alpha_1$ antitrypsin deficiency (Chap. 210), cystic fibrosis (Chap. 209), asthma (Chap. 204), hereditary telangiectasia, Kartagener's syndrome, and alveolar microlithiasis, as well as infections due to the tubercle bacilli, fungi, and schistosoma where exposure to involved family members is important.

Dyspnea is a cardinal manifestation of diseases involving the respiratory and cardiovascular systems (Chap. 36). A detailed physical examination of both organ systems is therefore mandatory in every patient with this symptom. Dyspnea secondary to cardiac disease is often recognized by the presence of other evidence of heart failure, such as cardiac enlargement, gallop rhythms, and cardiac murmurs. It may be difficult to differentiate paroxysmal nocturnal dyspnea due to pulmonary edema of cardiac origin from nocturnal attacks of bronchial asthma and from chronic pulmonary disease with pooling of the secretions in the recumbent position, but a detailed description of the circumstances in which this symptom occurs is most useful. Dyspnea also is a common functional complaint, and an important clue in the identification of this form is the observation that shortness of breath often occurs at rest and is relieved during exertion; the opposite is the case in patients in whom this symptom is secondary to disease of the lungs or heart. Equally important in the differential diagnosis is a careful elucidation of the relationship of dyspnea to other symptoms such as cough or angina pectoris.

Patients with diseases involving the respiratory system may also present with *chest pain* which is frequently caused by inflammation of the pleura, occurring in pneumonia, pulmonary thromboembolism, tuberculosis, and malignancy (Chap. 16). Pleuritic pain is usually localized to one side of the chest and is related to respiration and to movements of the thorax. Lesions confined to the pulmonary parenchyma do not produce pain, while diseases involving the organs in the mediastinum (Chap. 216) may cause local discomfort with radiation characteristic of the specific organ. Pain may also originate in or be referred to the chest wall; it may be due to intercostal neuritis, as in herpes zoster, or to compression of the intercostal nerves as they leave the spinal cord. Such pain is often superficial in character and may be related to coughing and straining. Thoracic pain may also be due to myositis, costochondral disturbances, myocardial ischemia, pericarditis, esophageal disease, and aortic dissection and aneurysm (Chap. 16). The most common causes of pain related to respiration are disorders of the chest wall, pleurisy, intercostal neuritis, and costochondral disease. The latter condition characteristically causes chest pain intensified by palpation. A major task is to distinguish chest pain due to abnormalities of the broncho-pulmonary system from that due to myocardial ischemia (see Chap. 16).

Cough and *expectoration* are also cardinal features of pulmonary disease (Chap. 35). Few patients can describe the severity of cough or quantity of expectoration reliably, and it is therefore desirable for the physician to inspect a 24-h collection of sputum. A cough productive of sputum is usually caused by an inflammatory process, while a nonproductive cough is caused by an irritative process. Cough is often precipitated by foreign materials irritating nerve endings in airways and is frequently caused by inflammation of the bronchi; the latter may be persistent (as in patients with a cigarette cough and chronic bronchitis) or acute (as in a variety of viral and bacterial infections). The time of occurrence of the cough and the character and quantity of expectorated material may point to the diagnosis. For example, bronchiectasis, lung abscess, and necrotizing pneumonia can produce purulent sputum which may have an offensive odor or be streaked with blood (Chaps. 207 and 208). In pulmonary edema, the sputum is pink, frothy, and watery (Chap. 36). Mucoid (translucent, viscid, shiny, white or gray) or mucopurulent (mucoid with flecks of yellow or green pus) sputum is characteristic of acute and chronic bronchitis. Sputum is bloody or rusty in pneumonia; it is thick, gelatinous, brick red, and laced with pus in *Klebsiella* pneumonia. Paroxysmal cough may also be the presenting feature in patients with bronchial asthma, in whom physical examination reveals wheezing respirations and squeaking musical sounds (Chap. 204), as well as in patients with left ventricular failure, in whom it generally occurs at night and in the recumbent position (Chap. 182). Pulmonary tuberculosis (Chap. 125), though less common than previously, remains a common cause of chronic cough, as does primary neoplasm of the lung (Chap. 215). A change in the character of a chronic cough, unaccompanied by an acute infection, should alert the physician to the need of carrying out a detailed examination.

Hemoptysis is often a frightening symptom (Chap. 35). Faint streaking of the sputum with blood may be observed in acute infections of the respiratory tract. However, many patients with bloody sputum have serious disease, such as pulmonary thromboembolism, tuberculosis, critical mitral stenosis, neoplasm of the lung, or bronchiectasis. In all instances it is necessary to exclude sources of blood in the nasopharynx and bleeding of gastric or esophageal origin. The character of the bloody expectorate should be defined, since it may be helpful in identifying the underlying disease process. Sputum which is frankly bloody without mucus or pus may be due to pulmonary thromboembolism (Chap. 213). When pus is present, pneumonia, bronchiectasis, or lung abscess should be considered. Dilute, pink, frothy sputum is observed in acute pulmonary edema (Chap. 36).

PHYSICAL EXAMINATION A careful examination of the thorax, including inspection, palpation, percussion, and auscultation, often provides the clue to the diagnosis of many common pulmonary disorders (Table 200-1). In addition, a meticulous *general physical examination* is mandatory in patients with disorders of the respiratory system. Enlarged lymph nodes in the cervical and supraclavicular regions should be sought. Disturbances of mentation or even coma occur in patients with acute carbon dioxide retention and hypoxemia. Telltale stains on the fingers point to heavy cigarette smoking; infected teeth and gums may occur in patients with aspiration pneumonitis and lung abscess; characteristic cutaneous lesions may point to sarcoidosis (Chap. 277), collagen vascular disease, Wegener's granulomatosis, and berylliosis, all of which may have prominent pulmonary manifestations. Clubbing of the fingers or, when advanced, osteoarthropathy (Chap. 284) may suggest carcinoma (Chap. 215) or suppurative disease (Chap. 207) of the lung; chronic hypoxemia, as occurs in patients with chronic bronchitis (Chap. 210); pulmonary arteriovenous fistula; or congenital heart disease with right-to-left shunt (Chap. 186). However, clubbing is also seen in some patients with biliary cirrhosis, regional enteritis, and ulcerative colitis. A careful search for infection in the teeth, gums, tonsils, or sinuses is recommended in patients suspected or known to have bronchiectasis or lung abscess. Neurologic findings including headache, drowsiness, papilledema, and other evidence of increased intracranial pressure may occur in patients with pulmonary disease who have hypoxemia and hypercapnia. Vascular collapse is a late complication of carbon dioxide intoxication and is characterized by hypotension, flushed skin, sweating, and tachycardia. A detailed examination of the cardiovascular system (Chap. 174) is mandatory in patients suspected of having respiratory disease and in patients with unexplained dyspnea, cough, or cyanosis because of the frequent difficulty of differentiating disorders of the respiratory and cardiovascular systems.

DIAGNOSTIC TESTS The *roentgenographic examination* of the chest represents the cornerstone of the diagnostic workup of the patient with suspected pulmonary disease, and it is the integration of the information obtained from the clinical examination and the roentgenogram which often provides the key to diagnosis. Every effort must be made to obtain past chest x-rays. Unfortunately, physical examination of the chest has been deemphasized, largely because of the recognition of the enormous value of radiographic

TABLE 200-1 Physical findings in some common pulmonary disorders

Disorder	Inspection	Palpation	Percussion	Auscultation
Bronchial asthma (acute attack)	Hyperinflation; use of accessory muscles	Impaired expansion; decreased fremitus	Hyperresonant; low diaphragm	Prolonged expiration; inspiratory and expiratory wheezes
Pneumothorax (complete)	Lag on affected side	Absent fremitus	Hyperresonant or tympanitic	Absent breath sounds
Pleural effusion (large)	Lag on affected side	Decreased fremitus; trachea and heart shifted away from affected side	Dullness or flatness	Absent breath sounds
Atelectasis (lobar obstruction)	Lag on affected side	Decreased fremitus; trachea and heart shifted toward affected side	Dullness or flatness	Absent breath sounds
Consolidation (pneumonia)	Possible lag or splinting on affected side	Increased fremitus	Dullness	Bronchial breath sounds; bronchophony; pectoriloquy; crackles

SOURCE: JF Murray, in *Textbook of Respiratory Medicine*, JF Murray, JA Nadel (eds), p 449.

techniques. However, abnormalities such as small or moderate amounts of fluid in the alveoli or in the mediastinum, bronchospasm, and pleural effusions can often be detected more accurately by physical examination than by chest roentgenography. Tracheal deviation can be readily recognized on physical examination and may be observed in obstruction of a major bronchus and in atelectasis.

Chest roentgenograms obtained in the lateral decubitus position frequently reveal small pleural effusions not evident in the upright posture. A number of other abnormalities may be associated with normal roentgenograms. These include solitary lesions less than 6 mm in diameter, acute pulmonary thromboembolism without infarction, early interstitial pneumonia, diffuse granulomatous disease such as miliary tuberculosis, interstitial disease such as scleroderma and systemic lupus erythematosus, bronchiectasis, acute chronic bronchitis, mild to moderate emphysema, endobronchial masses only partially obstructing the airways, and the majority of instances of hypoventilation due to disorders of the central nervous system or neuromuscular disease. On the other hand, gross abnormalities of thoracic structure; pulmonary, mediastinal, and pleural masses; parenchymal consolidation, cysts, cavities, and abnormalities of the pulmonary vascular bed are all detected more reliably by roentgenographic than by physical examination.

An abnormal chest roentgenogram may be the presenting feature in an asymptomatic patient. In such circumstances the physician must make every effort to obtain earlier films in order to determine whether the lesion is new or old. Laminography, computed tomography, magnetic resonance imaging (Chap. 202), angiocardiography, and pulmonary scintigraphy are additional procedures which may be helpful in establishing a diagnosis in a patient with an abnormality on the plain chest roentgenogram.

A variety of other diagnostic procedures are helpful in the workup of the patient with known or suspected pulmonary disease. These are discussed in Chap. 203 and include skin tests for tuberculosis; scratch or intradermal tests to detect atopic reactions; appropriate serum complement fixation tests; and examination and culture of the sputum, pleural fluid, and bronchial washings. Bronchoscopy, bronchial brushings, and bronchoscopic biopsy have been greatly facilitated by the development of the fiberoptic bronchoscope. Mediastinoscopy, scalene node and mediastinal node biopsy, and pleural and lung biopsy may also be instrumental in establishing a diagnosis in an otherwise asymptomatic patient. Particularly important points which must be investigated in the history of the asymptomatic patient with an abnormality discovered on a routine chest roentgenogram include exposure to individuals with tuberculosis; previous tuberculin and fungal skin tests; residence in or visits to areas where fungal disease is endemic; a history of smoking and of exposure to dusts; and symptoms of systemic disease such as fever, sweat, fatigue, and weight loss. Physiologic (lung function) studies (Chap. 201) are of limited value in establishing an etiologic diagnosis in the patient with pulmonary diseases. They are, however, very helpful in assessing the physiologic consequences of disorders of the respiratory system and chest wall, as well as in following the effects of their progression or remission. Simple functional tests, such as observing the patient climbing one or two flights of stairs, are often valuable in determining whether or not the patient is grossly disabled.

In the approach to a patient with pulmonary disease, consideration must be given to the observation that substantial changes in the relative incidence of disease affecting the respiratory system have taken place in the United States during the past three decades. The prevalence of chronic infectious disorders such as tuberculosis, lung abscess, and bronchiectasis have decreased. On the other hand, patients with chronic bronchitis and with emphysema now survive longer and form an increasing fraction of patients with chronic respiratory disease, as do patients with environmental lung disease and with drug-induced disease. Modern intercontinental travel has increased the appearance in the western world of parasitic infestations of the lung. Also, the reduction of immunologic competence which occurs in patients with the acquired immunodeficiency syndrome (Chap. 264) and in diabetics as well as in the treatment of patients with a variety of malignancies and those receiving immunosuppressive drugs has led to an increasing incidence of opportunistic infections of the lungs with a variety of microorganisms rarely pathogenic in the past.

REFERENCES

FISHMAN AP (ed): *Pulmonary Diseases and Disorders*, 2d ed. New York, McGraw-Hill, 1988

MURRAY JF: History and physical examination in *Textbook of Respiratory Medicine*, JF Murray, JA Nadel (eds). Philadelphia, WB Saunders, 1988, pp 431–451

BAUM GL, WOLINSKY E: *Textbook of Pulmonary Diseases*, 4th ed. Boston, Little, Brown, 1989

201 DISTURBANCES OF RESPIRATORY FUNCTION

STEVEN E. WEINBERGER / JEFFREY M. DRAZEN

The respiratory system includes the lungs, the central nervous system, the chest wall (with the diaphragm and intercostal muscles), and the pulmonary circulation. The CNS is the system controller, regulating the activity of the muscles of the chest wall, which serve as the respiratory system pump. As these components of the respiratory system act in concert to achieve gas exchange, malfunction of an individual component or alteration of the relationships among components can lead to disturbances in function. In this chapter, we consider three major aspects of disturbed respiratory function: (1) disturbances in ventilatory function, (2) disturbances in the pulmonary circulation, and (3) disturbances in gas exchange. Disorders relating to CNS control of ventilation are discussed in Chap. 217.

DISTURBANCES IN VENTILATORY FUNCTION

Ventilation is the process whereby the lungs provide fresh air to the alveoli. Measurements of ventilatory function in common diagnostic use consist of quantification of the air contained within the lungs under certain circumstances and the rate at which air can be expelled from the lungs. Two measurements of lung volume commonly used for respiratory diagnosis are total lung capacity (TLC) and residual volume (RV). The former is the volume of gas contained within the lungs after a maximal inspiration, while the latter is the volume of gas remaining within the lungs at the end of a maximal expiration. The volume of gas that is exhaled from the lungs in going from TLC to RV is called the vital capacity (VC) (Fig. 201-1).

Common clinical measurements of airflow are obtained from maneuvers in which the subject inspires to TLC and then forcibly exhales to RV. Three measurements are commonly made from a volume-time recording; i.e., a spirogram, obtained during such a forced expiratory maneuver: (1) the volume of gas exhaled during the first second of expiration (forced expiratory volume in 1 s or FEV_1); (2) the total volume exhaled (forced vital capacity of FVC); and (3) the average expiratory flow rate during the middle 50 percent of the vital capacity (maximal midexpiratory flow rate or MMFR; also called forced expiratory flow from 25 to 75 percent of the vital capacity, or $FEF_{25-75\%}$) (Fig. 201-2*A*).

PHYSIOLOGIC FEATURES The lungs are elastic structures, containing collagen and elastic fibers which resist expansion. In order for normal lungs to contain air, they must be distended by either a positive internal pressure, i.e., within the airways and alveolar spaces, or a negative external pressure, i.e., outside of the lung. The relationship between the volume of gas contained within the lungs

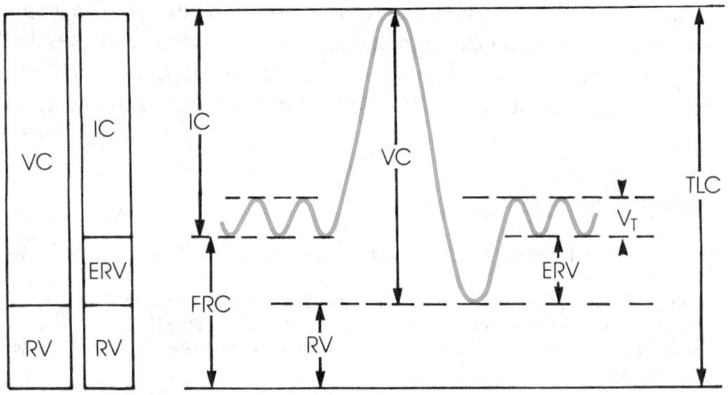

FIGURE 201-1 Lung volumes, shown by block diagrams (*left*) and by a spirographic tracing (*right*). TLC = total lung capacity; VC = vital capacity; RV = residual volume; IC = inspiratory capacity; ERV = expiratory reserve volume; FRC = functional residual capacity; V_T = tidal volume. (*From Weinberger*.)

and the distending pressure (transpulmonary pressure or P_{TP}, defined as internal pressure minus external pressure) is described by the pressure-volume curve of the lungs (Fig. 201-3*A*).

The chest wall is also an elastic structure, with properties similar to that of an expandable and compressible spring. The relationship between the volume enclosed by the chest wall and the distending pressure for the chest wall is described by the pressure-volume curve of the chest wall (Fig. 201-3*B*). For the chest wall to assume a volume different from its resting volume, the internal or external pressures acting on it must be altered. A positive distending pressure expands the chest wall, while a negative distending pressure compresses it.

Under normal circumstances, the lungs sit within the chest wall, so that the pressures and the forces acting on these structures are interrelated (Fig. 201-3*C*). At functional residual capacity (FRC), i.e., at the end of a normal exhalation, the lungs are partially inflated, so that their elastic recoil exerts a force tending to empty the lungs. At the same time, chest wall volume is such that its elastic recoil promotes outward expansion. Functional residual capacity occurs at the lung volume at which the tendency of the lungs to contract is opposed by the equal and opposite tendency of the chest wall to expand (Fig. 201-3*C*).

FIGURE 201-2 Spirographic tracings of forced expiration, comparing a normal tracing (*A*) and tracings in obstructive (*B*) and parenchymal restrictive (*C*) disease. Calculation of FVC, FEV_1, and MMFR is shown only for the normal tracing. Since there is no measure of absolute starting volume with spirometry, the curves are artificially positioned to show the relative starting lung volumes in the different conditions.

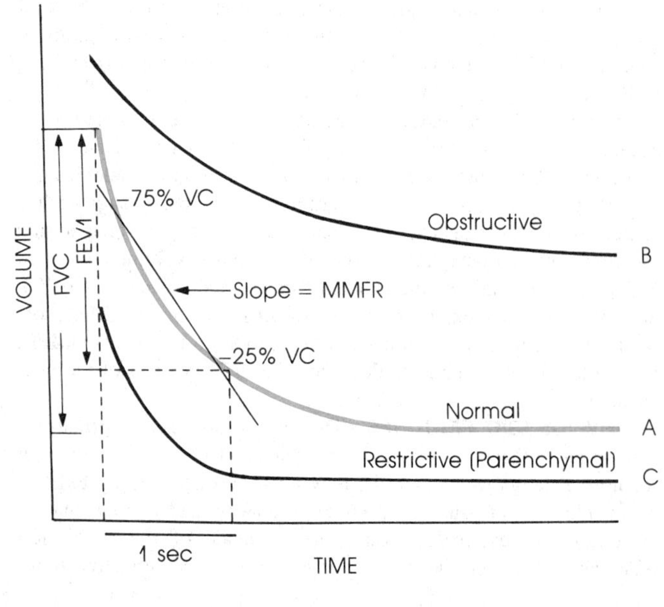

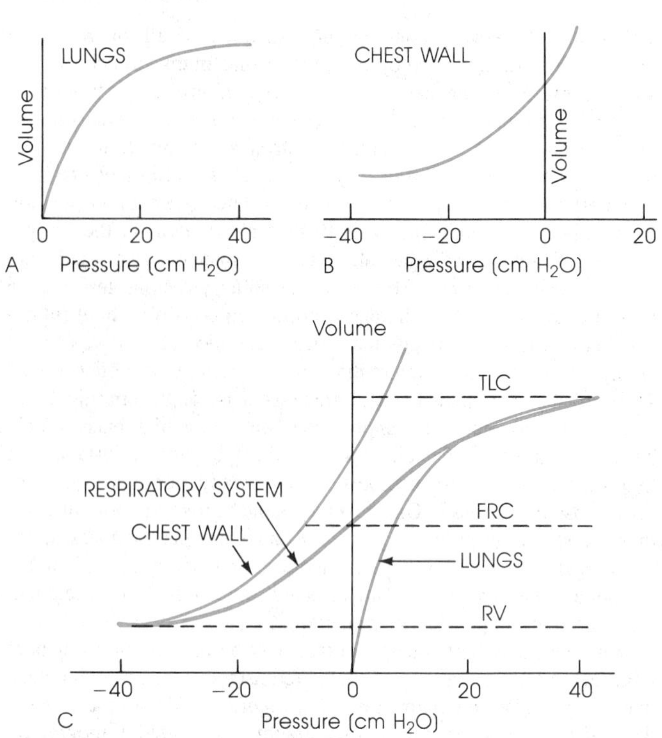

FIGURE 201-3 *A*. Pressure-volume curve of the lungs. *B*. Pressure-volume curve of the chest wall. *C*. Pressure-volume curve of the respiratory system, showing the superimposed component curves of the lungs and the chest wall. RV = residual volume; FRC = functional residual capacity; TLC = total lung capacity. (*From Weinberger*.)

In order for the lungs and the chest wall to achieve a volume other than the resting volume or FRC, either the pressures acting upon them can be changed passively, e.g., with a mechanical ventilator delivering positive pressure to the airways and alveoli, or the respiratory muscles can actively oppose the tendency of the lungs and the chest wall to return to FRC. During inhalation to volumes above FRC, the inspiratory muscles must actively overcome the tendency of the respiratory system to decrease volume back to FRC. During active exhalation below FRC, expiratory muscle activity must overcome the tendency of the respiratory system to increase volume back to FRC. At TLC, the force applied by the inspiratory muscles to expand the lungs is balanced by the inward recoil of the lungs. As a consequence, the major determinants of TLC are the stiffness of the lungs and inspiratory muscle strength. If the lungs become stiffer, i.e., less compliant, TLC is decreased. If the lungs become less stiff, i.e., more compliant, TLC is increased. If the inspiratory muscles are significantly weakened, they are less able to overcome the inward elastic recoil of the lungs, and TLC is lowered.

At RV, the force exerted by the expiratory muscles to decrease lung volume further is balanced by the outward recoil of the chest wall, which becomes extremely stiff at low lung volumes. Two factors influence the volume of gas contained within the lungs at RV. The first is the ability of the subject to exert a prolonged expiratory effort, which is related to muscle strength and to the ability to overcome sensory stimuli from the chest wall. The second is the ability of the lungs to empty to a small volume. In normal lungs, as P_{TP} is lowered, lung volume decreases. In lungs with diseased airways, as P_{TP} is lowered, flow-limitation or airway closure can limit the amount of gas that is expired. Consequently, both weak chest wall muscles or intrinsic airways disease can result in an elevation in measured RV.

Dynamic measurements of ventilatory function are made by having the subject inhale to TLC and then perform a forced expiratory maneuver. If a subject performs a series of such expiratory maneuvers using increasing muscular intensity, expiratory flow rates will increase until a certain level of effort is reached. Beyond this level, additional effort will not result in an increment in forced expiratory flow rates; this phenomenon is known as the *effort independence* of forced expiratory flow. The physiologic mechanisms determining the flow rates during this effort-independent phase of forced expiratory flow have been shown to be the elastic recoil of the lung, the airflow resistance of the airways between the alveolar zone and the physical site of flow limitation, and the airway wall compliance at the site of flow limitation. Physical processes which decrease elastic recoil, increase airflow resistance, or increase airway wall compliance will decrease the flow rate that can be achieved at any given lung volume. Conversely, processes that increase elastic recoil, decrease resistance, or stiffen airway walls increase the flow rate that can be achieved at any given lung volume.

MEASUREMENT OF VENTILATORY FUNCTION Ventilatory function is measured under static conditions for determination of lung volumes and under dynamic conditions for determination of forced expiratory flow rates. VC, expiratory reserve volume (ERV), and inspiratory capacity (IC) (Fig. 201-1) are measured by having the patient breathe into and out of a spirometer, a device capable of measuring expired or inspired gas volume while plotting volume as a function of time. Other volumes, specifically RV, FRC, and TLC, cannot be measured in this way because they include the volume of gas present within the lungs even after a maximal expiration. One of two techniques is commonly used to measure these volumes: helium dilution or body plethysmography. In the helium dilution method, the subject repeatedly breathes in and out from a reservoir of a known volume of gas containing a trace amount of helium. The helium is diluted by the gas previously present in the lungs and is not absorbed into the pulmonary circulation. From knowledge of reservoir volume and initial and final helium concentrations, the volume of gas present within the lungs can be calculated. With the helium dilution method, the volume of gas present within the lungs may be underestimated if there are slowly communicating airspaces, such as bullae. In this situation, lung volumes can be more accurately measured with a body plethysmograph, a sealed box in which the patient sits while panting against a closed mouthpiece. Because there is no airflow into or out of the plethysmograph, pressure changes within the thorax during panting cause compression and rarefaction of the gas within the lungs and simultaneous rarefaction and compression of gas within the plethysmograph. By measuring pressure changes in the plethysmograph and at the mouthpiece, the volume of gas present within the thorax can be calculated by using Boyle's law.

Lung volumes and measurements made during forced expiration are interpreted by comparing the values measured with the values expected based on the age, height, sex, and race of the patient. Regression curves have been constructed based on data obtained from large numbers of normal, nonsmoking individuals without any evidence of lung disease. Predicted values for a given patient can then be obtained by using the patient's age and height in the appropriate regression equation. As there is variability among normal individuals, values between 80 and 120 percent of predicted are generally considered to be normal. The normal ratio FEV_1/FVC is approximately 0.75 to 0.80, though this value does fall somewhat with advancing age. The MMFR is often a more sensitive measurement of early airflow obstruction, particularly in small airways. However, the MMFR must be interpreted cautiously in the patient with abnormally small lungs (low TLC and VC). In this setting, less volume is exhaled during forced expiration, and the MMFR may appear abnormal when compared with the predicted value for the patient's age, height, and sex, even though it is normal relative to the size of the patient's lungs.

It is also a common practice to plot expiratory flow rates against lung volume (rather than against time); the resulting *flow-volume curve* is useful in that flow rates are closely linked to lung volumes (Fig. 201-4). In addition, the spirometric values mentioned above can be calculated from the flow-volume curve. Commonly, flow rates during a maximal inspiratory effort performed as rapidly as possible are plotted as well, making the flow-volume curve into a *flow-volume loop*. At TLC, before expiratory flow starts, the flow rate is 0. During forced expiration, a high peak-flow rate is rapidly achieved. As expiration continues and lung volume approaches RV, the flow rate falls progressively, in a nearly linear fashion for a person with normal lung function. During maximal inspiration from RV to TLC, inspiratory flow is maximal at the midpoint of inspiration, so that the inspiratory portion of the loop is U-shaped or saddle-shaped. The flow rates achieved during maximal expiration can be analyzed quantitatively, by comparison of the flow rates at specified lung volumes with the predicted values, or qualitatively, by analysis of the shape of the descending limb of the expiratory curve.

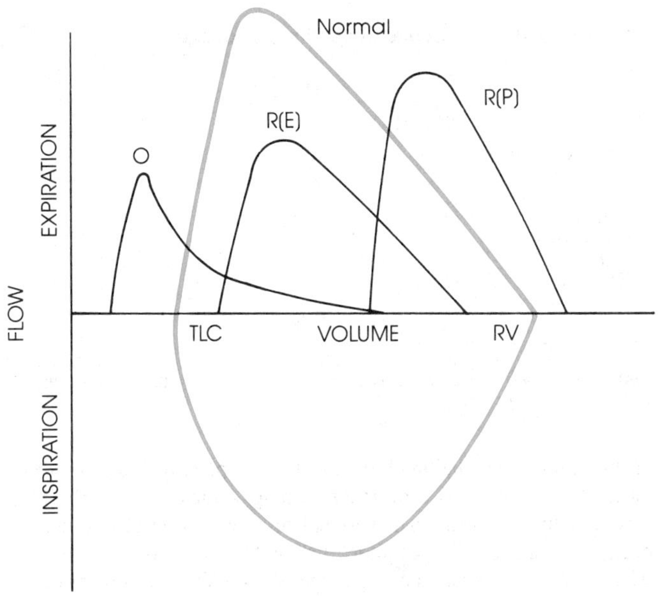

FIGURE 201-4 Flow-volume curves in different conditions: O = obstructive disease; R(P) = parenchymal restrictive disease; R(E) = extraparenchymal restrictive disease with limitation in inspiration and expiration. Forced expiration is plotted in all conditions; forced inspiration is shown only for the normal curve. TLC = total lung capacity; RV = residual volume.

PATTERNS OF ABNORMAL FUNCTION The two major patterns of abnormal ventilatory function, as measured by static lung volumes and spirometry, are restrictive and obstructive patterns. In the obstructive pattern, the hallmark is a decrease in expiratory flow rates. With fully established disease, the ratio FEV_1/FVC is decreased, as is the MMFR (Fig. 201-2, line *B*). The expiratory portion of the flow-volume loop demonstrates decreased flow rates for any given lung volume. Nonuniform emptying of airways is reflected by a coved (concave upward) configuration of the curve (Fig. 201-4). With early obstructive disease, which originates in the small airways, FEV_1/FVC may be normal; the only abnormalities noted on routine testing of pulmonary function may be a depression in MMFR and an abnormal configuration in the terminal portion of the forced expiratory flow-volume curve.

In *obstructive disease,* the TLC is normal or increased. When helium equilibration tests are used for measurement of lung volumes, the measured volume may be less than the actual volume, if helium was not well distributed to all airways and to all regions of the lung. Residual volume is elevated due to trapping of air during expiration, and the ratio RV/TLC is increased. Vital capacity is frequently decreased in obstructive disease, not because of low lung volumes, as is the case in restrictive disease, but because of the striking elevation in RV.

A *restrictive pattern* can be broadly subdivided into subgroups, depending on the location of the pathology—pulmonary parenchymal vs. extraparenchymal. For extraparenchymal disease, dysfunction can be predominantly in inspiration or in both inspiration plus expiration

TABLE 201-1 Alterations in ventilatory function

	TLC	RV	VC	FEV_1/FVC
Obstructive	N to ↑	↑	↓	↓ *
Restrictive				
Pulmonary parenchymal	↓	↓	↓	N to ↑
Extraparenchymal—inspiratory	↓	N to ↓	↓	N
Extraparenchymal—inspiratory + expiratory	↓	↑	↓	variable

* Mild obstructive (small airways) disease may have ↓ MMFR with normal FEV_1/FVC. For abbreviations see text.

(Table 201-1). The hallmark of a restrictive pattern, found in all of these subcategories, is a decrease in lung volumes, primarily TLC and VC. In pulmonary parenchymal disease, RV is also generally decreased, and forced expiratory flow rates are preserved. In fact, when FEV_1 is considered as a percent of the FVC, the flow rates are often supranormal, i.e., disproportionately high relative to the size of the lungs (Fig. 201-2, line *C*). The flow-volume curve may graphically demonstrate this disproportionate relationship between flow rates and lung volumes, since the expiratory portion of the curve appears relatively tall (preserved flow rates) but narrow (decreased lung volumes), as shown in Fig. 201-4.

In the extraparenchymal pattern characterized by *inspiratory dysfunction,* due to either inspiratory muscle weakness or a stiff chest wall, adequate distending forces are prevented from being exerted on an otherwise normal lung. As a result, achieved TLC values are less than predicted, RV is often not significantly affected, and expiratory flows are preserved. In the extraparenchymal pattern characterized by inspiratory and expiratory dysfunction, the ability to expire to a normal RV is also limited, either because of expiratory muscle weakness or a deformed chest wall that is abnormally rigid at volumes below FRC. Consequently, RV is often elevated, unlike the pattern observed in the other restrictive subcategories. The ratio FEV_1/FVC is variable and depends upon expiratory muscle strength. If expiratory muscle strength is significantly decreased, then the ability to expire rapidly is impaired, and FEV_1/FVC may be decreased even though there is no airflow obstruction. If expiratory muscle strength is normal but the chest wall is abnormally stiff below FRC, then FEV_1/FVC may be increased.

In Table 201-1, the expected alterations in ventilatory function as indicated by pulmonary function testing are summarized. One reason to establish a ventilatory diagnosis is to categorize the functional disorder. This in turn can provide diagnostic information as outlined in Table 201-2. Note that lung disease can be present without abnormal ventilatory function, but the presence of specific diagnostic findings is an aid in differential diagnosis.

TABLE 201-2 Common respiratory diseases by diagnostic categories

Obstructive
- Asthma
- Chronic obstructive lung disease (chronic bronchitis, emphysema)
- Bronchiectasis
- Cystic fibrosis
- Bronchiolitis

Restrictive—parenchymal
- Sarcoidosis
- Idiopathic pulmonary fibrosis
- Pneumoconiosis
- Drug- or radiation-induced interstitial lung disease

Restrictive—extraparenchymal
- Neuromuscular
  - Diaphragmatic weakness/paralysis
  - Myasthenia gravis*
  - Guillain-Barré syndrome*
  - Muscular dystrophies*
  - Cervical spine injury*
- Chest wall
  - Kyphoscoliosis
  - Obesity
  - Ankylosing spondylitis*

* Can have inspiratory and expiratory limitation (see text).

DISTURBANCES IN THE PULMONARY CIRCULATION

PHYSIOLOGIC FEATURES The pulmonary vasculature normally must handle the entire output of the right ventricle, approximately 5 L/min in a normal adult at rest. The comparatively thin-walled vessels of the pulmonary arterial system provide relatively little resistance to flow, and are capable of handling this large volume of blood at low perfusion pressures compared with those of the systemic circulation. The normal mean pulmonary artery pressure of 15 mmHg is much less than the normal mean aortic pressure of approximately 95 mmHg. Regional pulmonary blood flow within the lung is dependent upon hydrostatic forces. In the upright person, pulmonary arterial pressure is lowest at the apex of the lung and highest at the lung bases. As a result, in the upright position, perfusion is least at the apex and greatest at the lung bases. When cardiac output increases, as occurs during exercise, the pulmonary vasculature is capable of recruiting previously unperfused vessels and distending underperfused vessels. As a result, the pulmonary vascular system is capable of handling the increase in flow with a decrease in pulmonary vascular resistance, so that the increment in mean pulmonary arterial pressure is small.

METHODS OF MEASUREMENT Assessment of circulatory function within the pulmonary vasculature depends upon measuring pulmonary vascular pressures and cardiac output. Clinically, these measurements are commonly made in intensive care units capable of invasive monitoring and in cardiac catheterization laboratories. With a flow-directed pulmonary arterial (Swan-Ganz) catheter, pulmonary arterial and pulmonary capillary wedge pressures can be measured directly, and cardiac output can be obtained by the thermodilution method. Pulmonary vascular resistance can then be calculated according to the equation:

$$PVR = 80(PAP - PCW)/CO$$

where PVR = pulmonary vascular resistance
PAP = mean pulmonary arterial pressure (mmHg)
PCW = pulmonary capillary wedge pressure (mmHg)
CO = cardiac output (L/min)

The normal value for pulmonary vascular resistance is approximately 50 to 150 $(dyn \cdot s)/cm^5$.

MECHANISMS OF ABNORMAL FUNCTION (See Chap. 191) With disease, pulmonary vascular resistance may increase by a variety of mechanisms. Pulmonary arterial and arteriolar vasoconstriction is a prominent response to alveolar hypoxia. Pulmonary vascular resistance also increases if intraluminal thrombi or proliferation of smooth muscle within vessel walls diminishes the luminal cross-sectional area. If small pulmonary vessels are destroyed, either by scarring or by loss of alveolar walls, the total cross-sectional area of the pulmonary vascular bed diminishes, and pulmonary vascular resistance increases. When pulmonary vascular resistance is elevated, pulmonary arterial pressure rises to maintain normal cardiac output, or cardiac output falls if pulmonary arterial pressure does not increase.

CLINICAL CORRELATION Disturbances in function of the pulmonary vasculature as a result of primary cardiac disease, either congenital heart disease or conditions which elevate left atrial pressure such as mitral stenosis, are beyond the scope of this chapter and are discussed in Chaps. 186 and 188, respectively. Instead, the focus will be on the pulmonary vasculature as its function is affected by diseases primarily involving the respiratory system, including the pulmonary vessels themselves.

All diseases of the respiratory system causing hypoxemia are potentially capable of increasing pulmonary vascular resistance, since alveolar hypoxia is a very potent stimulus for pulmonary vasoconstriction. The more prolonged and intense the hypoxic stimulus, the more likely that a significant increase in pulmonary vascular resistance and pulmonary hypertension will result. In practice, patients with hypoxemia caused by chronic obstructive lung disease, interstitial lung disease, chest wall disease, and by the obesity hypoventilation–sleep apnea syndrome are particularly prone to developing pulmonary hypertension. If there are additional structural changes in the pulmonary vasculature secondary to the underlying process, these will increase the likelihood of developing pulmonary hypertension.

With diseases primarily affecting the pulmonary vessels, a decrease in the cross-sectional area of the pulmonary vascular bed is primarily responsible for increased pulmonary vascular resistance, while hypoxemia generally plays a lesser role. In the case of recurrent pulmonary emboli, parts of the pulmonary arterial system are occluded by intraluminal thrombi originating in the systemic venous system. With primary pulmonary hypertension (Chap. 212) or with pulmonary vascular disease secondary to scleroderma, the small pulmonary arteries and arterioles are affected by a generalized obliterative process that narrows and occludes these vessels. Pulmonary vascular resistance increases, and significant pulmonary hypertension often results.

DISTURBANCES IN GAS EXCHANGE

PHYSIOLOGIC FEATURES The primary functions of the respiratory system are to remove the appropriate amount of CO_2 from blood entering the pulmonary circulation and to provide adequate O_2 to blood leaving the pulmonary circulation. In order for these functions to be carried out properly, there must be adequate provision of fresh air to the alveoli for delivery of O_2 and removal of CO_2 (ventilation), adequate circulation of blood through the pulmonary vasculature (perfusion), adequate movement of gas between alveoli and pulmonary capillaries (diffusion), and appropriate contact between alveolar gas and pulmonary capillary blood (ventilation-perfusion matching).

A normal individual at rest inspires approximately 12 to 16 times per minute, each breath having a tidal volume of approximately 500 mL. A portion (approximately 30 percent) of each breath does not reach the alveoli, but remains in the conducting airways of the lung. This component of each breath, which is not generally available for gas exchange, is called the anatomic dead space component. The remaining 70 percent reaches and rapidly mixes with the gas resident in the alveolar zone and can participate in gas exchange. In this example, total ventilation each minute is approximately 7 L, composed of 2 L/min of dead space ventilation and 5 L/min of alveolar ventilation. In certain disease settings, some alveoli are ventilated but not perfused, so that additional ventilation is wasted beyond that portion related to the anatomic dead space. If total dead space ventilation is increased but total minute ventilation is unchanged, then alveolar ventilation must fall correspondingly.

GAS EXCHANGE This is dependent upon alveolar ventilation rather than total minute ventilation, as outlined below. The partial pressure of CO_2 in arterial blood (Pa_{CO_2}) is directly proportional to the amount of CO_2 produced per minute ($\dot{V}_{CO_2}$) and inversely proportional to alveolar ventilation ($\dot{V}_A$), according to the relationship:

$$Pa_{CO_2} = 0.863 \times \dot{V}_{CO_2}/\dot{V}_A$$

where $\dot{V}_{CO_2}$ is expressed in mL/min, $\dot{V}_A$ in L/min, and Pa_{CO_2} in mmHg. At fixed $\dot{V}_{CO_2}$, when alveolar ventilation increases, Pa_{CO_2} falls, and when alveolar ventilation decreases, Pa_{CO_2} rises. Maintaining a normal level of O_2 in the alveoli (and consequently in arterial blood) also depends upon provision of adequate alveolar ventilation to replenish alveolar O_2. This principle will become more apparent from the alveolar gas equation below.

Both O_2 and CO_2 diffuse readily down their respective concentration gradients through the alveolar wall and pulmonary capillary endothelium. Under normal circumstances this process is rapid, and equilibration of both gases is complete within one-third of the transit time of erythrocytes through the pulmonary capillary bed. Even in disease states where diffusion of gases is impaired, it is unlikely to be so severe that diffusion equilibration is not reached. Consequently, a diffusion abnormality rarely results in arterial hypoxemia at rest. If erythrocyte transit time in the pulmonary circulation is shortened, as occurs with exercise, and diffusion is impaired, then diffusion limitation may contribute to hypoxemia. Exercise testing can often demonstrate such physiologically significant abnormalities due to impaired diffusion. Even though diffusion limitation rarely makes a clinically significant contribution to resting hypoxemia, clinical measurements of what is known as *diffusing capacity* (see below) can be a useful measure of the integrity of the alveolar-capillary membrane.

Ventilation-perfusion matching In addition to the absolute level of ventilation and perfusion reaching the lung, gas exchange is critically dependent on the proper matching of ventilation and perfusion. The spectrum of possible ventilation-perfusion ($\dot{V}/\dot{Q}$) ratios within an alveolar-capillary unit ranges from zero, in which ventilation is totally absent and the unit behaves as a shunt, to infinity, in which perfusion is totally absent and the unit behaves as dead space. The P_{O_2} and P_{CO_2} of blood leaving each alveolar-capillary unit depend on the gas tension (blood and air) entering that unit and on the $\dot{V}/\dot{Q}$ ratio of that particular unit. At one extreme, when an alveolar-capillary unit has a $\dot{V}/\dot{Q}$ ratio $= 0$ and behaves as a shunt, blood leaving the unit has the composition of mixed venous blood entering the pulmonary capillaries. Under normal circumstances $P\bar{v}_{O_2} \sim 40$ mmHg and $P\bar{v}_{CO_2} \sim 46$ mmHg. At the other extreme, when an alveolar-capillary unit has a high $\dot{V}/\dot{Q}$ ratio and thus behaves almost like dead space, the small amount of blood leaving the unit has partial pressures of O_2 and CO_2 ($P_{O_2} \sim 150$ mmHg, $P_{CO_2} \sim 0$ mmHg while breathing room air) approaching the composition of inspired gas.

In the ideal situation, all alveolar-capillary units have equal matching of ventilation and perfusion, i.e., with a ratio of approximately 1 when each is expressed in L/min. But, even in the normal individual, some $\dot{V}/\dot{Q}$ mismatching is present, as there is normally a gradient of blood flow from the apices to the bases of the lungs. Moreover, there is a similar gradient of ventilation from the apices to the bases, but the gradient is less marked for ventilation than for perfusion. As a result, ventilation-perfusion ratios are higher at the lung apices than at the lung bases. Therefore, blood coming from the apices has a higher P_{O_2} and lower P_{CO_2} than blood coming from the bases. The net P_{O_2} and P_{CO_2} of the resulting mixture of blood coming from all areas of the lung is a weighted average of the individual components, which takes into account the relative amount of blood from each unit and the O_2 and CO_2 *content* of blood coming from each unit. Because of the sigmoid shape of the oxyhemoglobin dissociation curve, it is important to distinguish between the partial pressure and the content of O_2 in blood. Hemoglobin is almost fully saturated at a $P_{O_2} = 60$ mmHg, and little additional O_2 is carried by hemoglobin even with substantial elevations of P_{O_2} above 60 mmHg (see Fig. 290-4, p. 1517). On the other hand, significant O_2 desaturation of hemoglobin occurs once P_{O_2} falls below 60 mmHg onto the steep descending limb of the curve. As a result, blood coming from regions of the lung with a high $\dot{V}/\dot{Q}$ ratio, a high P_{O_2}, but only a small elevation in O_2 content, cannot compensate for blood coming from regions with a low $\dot{V}/\dot{Q}$ ratio, a low P_{O_2}, and a significant decrease in O_2 content. Although $\dot{V}/\dot{Q}$ mismatching can influence P_{CO_2}, this effect is less marked and often is overcome by an increase in overall minute ventilation.

MEASUREMENT OF GAS EXCHANGE **Arterial blood gases** The most commonly used measures of gas exchange are the partial pressures of O_2 and CO_2 in arterial blood, i.e., Pa_{O_2} and Pa_{CO_2}, respectively. These partial pressures do not measure directly the quantity of O_2 and CO_2 in blood, but rather the driving pressure for the gas to be carried in blood. The actual quantity or content of each of these gases in blood depends upon the solubility of the gas in plasma and the ability of any component of blood to react with or to bind the gas of interest. Since hemoglobin is capable of binding large amounts of O_2, oxygenated hemoglobin is the primary form in which O_2 is transported in blood. The actual content of O_2 in blood therefore depends both on the hemoglobin concentration and on the P_{O_2}. The P_{O_2} determines what percentage of hemoglobin is saturated with O_2, based upon the position on the oxyhemoglobin dissociation curve. Oxygen content in normal blood (at 37°C, pH 7.4) can be determined by adding the amount of O_2 dissolved in plasma to the amount bound to hemoglobin, according to the equation

$$O_2 \text{ content} = 1.34 \times (\text{hemoglobin}) \times \text{saturation} + 0.0031 \times P_{O_2}$$

since each gram of hemoglobin is capable of carrying 1.34 mL O_2 when fully saturated, and the amount of O_2 that can be dissolved in plasma is proportional to the P_{O_2}, with 0.0031 mL O_2 dissolved per deciliter of blood per mmHg P_{O_2}. In arterial blood, the amount of O_2 transported dissolved in plasma (approximately 0.3 mL O_2/dL blood) is trivial compared with the amount bound to hemoglobin (approximately 20 mL O_2/dL blood).

Most commonly, P_{O_2} is the measurement used to quantitate the adequacy of oxygenation of arterial blood. Arterial O_2 saturation can also be measured by oximetry and is particularly important in selected clinical conditions. For example, in patients with carbon monoxide exposure, carbon monoxide preferentially displaces O_2 from hemoglobin, essentially making a portion of hemoglobin unavailable for binding to O_2. In this circumstance, carbon monoxide saturation is high and O_2 saturation is low, even though the driving pressure for O_2 to bind to hemoglobin, reflected by P_{O_2}, is normal. Measurement of O_2 saturation, in order to determine O_2 content, is also important when mixed venous blood is sampled from a pulmonary arterial catheter to calculate cardiac output by the Fick technique. In mixed venous blood, the P_{O_2} is normally about 40 mmHg, but small changes in P_{O_2} may reflect relatively large changes in O_2 saturation.

A useful calculation in the assessment of oxygenation is the alveolar-arterial O_2 difference ($P_{A_{O_2}}$–Pa_{O_2}), commonly called the alveolar-arterial O_2 gradient (or A-a gradient). This calculation takes into account the fact that alveolar and, hence, arterial P_{O_2} can be expected to change depending on the level of alveolar ventilation, reflected by the arterial P_{CO_2}. When a patient hyperventilates and has a low P_{CO_2}, alveolar and arterial P_{O_2} will rise; conversely, hypoventilation and a high P_{CO_2} are accompanied by a decrease in alveolar and arterial P_{O_2}. These changes in arterial P_{O_2} are independent of abnormalities in O_2 transfer at the alveolar-capillary level, and reflect only the dependence of alveolar P_{O_2} on the level of alveolar ventilation.

In order to determine the alveolar-arterial O_2 difference, the alveolar P_{O_2} ($P_{A_{O_2}}$) must first be calculated. The equation most commonly used for this purpose, a simplified form of the alveolar gas equation, is

$$P_{A_{O_2}} = F_{I_{O_2}} \times (P_B - P_{H_2O}) - Pa_{CO_2}/R$$

where $F_{I_{O_2}}$ = fractional concentration of inspired O_2 (~0.21 when breathing room air)

P_B = barometric pressure (approximately 760 mmHg at sea level)

P_{H_2O} = water vapor pressure (47 mmHg when air is fully saturated at 37°C)

R = respiratory quotient (the ratio of CO_2 production to O_2 consumption, usually assumed to be 0.8)

If the above values are substituted into the equation for the patient breathing air at sea level, the equation becomes

$$P_{A_{O_2}} = 150 - 1.25 Pa_{CO_2}$$

The alveolar-arterial O_2 difference can then be calculated by subtracting measured Pa_{O_2} from calculated $P_{A_{O_2}}$. In a healthy young person breathing air, the $P_{A_{O_2}}$–Pa_{O_2} is normally less than 15 mmHg; this value increases with age and may be as high as 30 mmHg in elderly patients.

Adequacy of CO_2 elimination is measured by the partial pressure of CO_2 in arterial blood, i. e., Pa_{CO_2}. A more complete understanding of the mechanisms and chronicity of abnormal levels of P_{CO_2} also requires measurement of pH and/or bicarbonate (HCO_3^-), since P_{CO_2} and the patient's acid-base status are so closely intertwined (see Chap. 51).

Diffusing capacity The ability of gas to diffuse across the alveolar-capillary membrane is ordinarily assessed by the diffusing capacity of the lung for carbon monoxide (DL_{CO}). In this test, a small concentration of carbon monoxide is inhaled, usually in a single breath that is held for approximately 10 s. The carbon monoxide is diluted by the gas already present in the alveoli, and is also taken up by hemoglobin as the erythrocytes course through the pulmonary capillary system. The concentration of carbon monoxide in exhaled gas is measured, and DL_{CO} is calculated as the quantity of carbon monoxide absorbed per min per mmHg pressure gradient from the alveoli to the pulmonary capillaries. The value obtained for DL_{CO} depends upon the alveolar-capillary surface area available for gas exchange and upon the pulmonary capillary blood volume. In addition, the thickness of the alveolar-capillary membrane, the degree of $\dot{V}/\dot{Q}$ mismatching, and the patient's hemoglobin level will affect the measurement. The value for DL_{CO}, ideally corrected for hemoglobin, can then be compared with a predicted value, based either on age, height, and sex or on the lung volume at which the value was obtained. Because of the effect of hemoglobin levels on DL_{CO}, the measured DL_{CO} is frequently corrected to take the patient's hemoglobin level into account.

MECHANISMS OF ABNORMAL FUNCTION Arterial blood gases Hypoxemia is a common manifestation of a variety of diseases affecting the lungs or other parts of the respiratory system. The broad clinical problem of hypoxemia is often best characterized according to the underlying mechanism. The four basic mechanisms of hypoxemia are (1) decrease in inspired P_{O_2}, (2) hypoventilation, (3) shunt, and (4) $\dot{V}/\dot{Q}$ mismatching. Diffusion block contributes to hypoxemia only under selected clinical circumstances and is not usually included among the general categories of hypoxemia. Determining the underlying mechanism for hypoxemia depends upon measurement of the Pa_{CO_2}, calculation of the $P_{A_{O_2}}$–Pa_{O_2}, and knowledge of the response to supplemental O_2. A flow chart summarizing the approach to the hypoxemic patient is found in Fig. 201-5.

Decrease in the inspired P_{O_2} and hypoventilation both cause hypoxemia by lowering $P_{A_{O_2}}$ and therefore Pa_{O_2}. In each case, gas exchange at the alveolar-capillary level is occurring normally, and $P_{A_{O_2}}$–Pa_{O_2} is not elevated. Hypoxemia due to depression in inspired P_{O_2} can be diagnosed by knowledge of the clinical situation. Inspired P_{O_2} is lowered either because the patient is at a high altitude, where barometric pressure is low, or, much less commonly, because the patient is breathing a gas mixture containing less than 21 percent O_2. The hallmark of hypoventilation as a cause of hypoxemia is an elevation in Pa_{CO_2}. This is associated with an increase in $P_{A_{CO_2}}$ and a fall in $P_{A_{O_2}}$. When hypoxemia is due purely to a low inspired P_{O_2} or to alveolar hypoventilation, $P_{A_{O_2}}$–Pa_{O_2} is normal. If $P_{A_{O_2}}$–Pa_{O_2} and Pa_{CO_2} are both elevated, then an additional mechanism, such as $\dot{V}/\dot{Q}$ mismatching or shunt, is contributing to hypoxemia.

Shunting is a cause of hypoxemia when desaturated blood effectively bypasses oxygenation at the alveolar-capillary level. This occurs either because of a structural problem that allows desaturated blood to bypass the normal site of gas exchange, or because ventilation to perfused alveoli is absent. Shunting is associated with an elevation in the $P_{A_{O_2}}$–Pa_{O_2}. When shunting is an important contributing factor to hypoxemia, the lowered P_{O_2} is relatively refractory to improvement by supplemental O_2.

Finally, the largest clinical category of hypoxemia is $\dot{V}/\dot{Q}$ mismatching. With $\dot{V}/\dot{Q}$ mismatching, regions with low $\dot{V}/\dot{Q}$ ratios contribute blood with a low P_{O_2} and a low O_2 content. Corresponding regions with high $\dot{V}/\dot{Q}$ ratios contribute blood with a high P_{O_2}. However, because blood is already almost fully saturated with a normal P_{O_2}, elevation of the P_{O_2} to a high value does not significantly

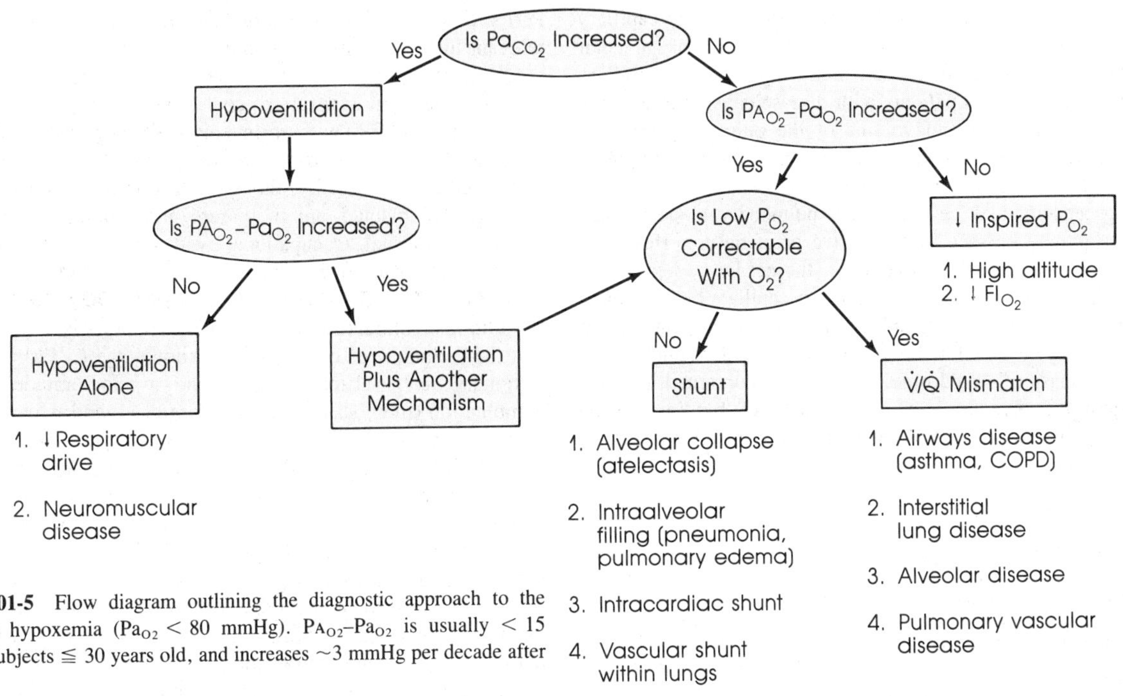

FIGURE 201-5 Flow diagram outlining the diagnostic approach to the patient with hypoxemia ($Pa_{O_2} < 80$ mmHg). PA_{O_2}–Pa_{O_2} is usually < 15 mmHg for subjects $\leqq 30$ years old, and increases ~3 mmHg per decade after age 30.

increase O_2 saturation or content, and therefore cannot compensate for the reduction of O_2 saturation and content in blood coming from regions with a low $\dot{V}/\dot{Q}$ ratio. When $\dot{V}/\dot{Q}$ mismatch is the primary cause of hypoxemia, PA_{O_2}–Pa_{O_2} is elevated, and P_{CO_2} is generally normal. Supplemental O_2 corrects the hypoxemia by raising the P_{O_2} in blood coming from regions with a low $\dot{V}/\dot{Q}$ ratio; this response distinguishes hypoxemia due to $\dot{V}/\dot{Q}$ mismatch from that due to true shunt.

The essential mechanism underlying all cases of hypercapnia is inadequate alveolar ventilation for the amount of CO_2 produced. It is conceptually useful to characterize CO_2 retention further, based on a more detailed examination of the potential contributing factors. These include: (1) increased CO_2 production; (2) decreased ventilatory drive ("won't breathe"); (3) malfunction of the respiratory pump or increased airways resistance, making it more difficult to sustain adequate ventilation ("can't breathe"); and (4) inefficiency of gas exchange (increased dead space or $\dot{V}/\dot{Q}$ mismatch) necessitating a compensatory increase in overall minute ventilation. In practice, more than one of these mechanisms is commonly responsible for hypercapnia, as increased minute ventilation is capable of compensating for increased CO_2 production and for inefficiencies of gas exchange.

Diffusing capacity Although the two main components affecting DL_{CO}, i.e., the membrane component and the pulmonary capillary blood volume, can be measured separately, this separation is made infrequently in clinical practice. Rather, the measurement is used in a more general way to assess the functional integrity of the alveolar-capillary membrane, which includes the pulmonary capillary bed. Diseases purely affecting the airways generally do not lower DL_{CO}, whereas diseases affecting alveolar walls or the pulmonary capillary bed will have an effect on DL_{CO}. Even though DL_{CO} is a useful marker to assess whether disease affecting the alveolar-capillary bed is present, an abnormal DL_{CO} does not necessarily imply that diffusion limitation is responsible for hypoxemia in a particular patient.

CLINICAL CORRELATIONS Arterial blood gases Useful clinical correlations can be made with the mechanisms underlying hypoxemia (Fig. 201-5). A lowered inspired P_{O_2} contributes to hypoxemia either at high altitude or if the concentration of inspired O_2 is less than 21 percent. The latter problem occurs if a patient receiving anesthesia or ventilatory support is inadvertently given a low-O_2 gas mixture to breathe, or if O_2 is consumed from ambient gas, as can occur during smoke inhalation from a fire. The primary feature of hypoventilation as a cause of hypoxemia is an elevation in Pa_{CO_2}. The clinical correlates with hypoventilation are discussed in Chap. 217.

Shunt as a cause of hypoxemia can reflect transfer of blood from the right to the left side of the heart without it ever entering the pulmonary circulation, as occurs with an intracardiac shunt. This problem occurs most commonly in the setting of cyanotic congenital heart disease, when an interatrial or interventricular septal defect is associated with pulmonary hypertension, so that shunting is in the right-to-left rather than left-to-right direction. Shunting of blood through the pulmonary parenchyma is most frequently due to disease causing absence of ventilation to perfused alveoli. This can occur if the alveoli are atelectatic or if they are filled with fluid, as in pulmonary edema (both cardiogenic and noncardiogenic) or with extensive intraalveolar exudation of fluid due to pneumonia. Less commonly, vascular anomalies with arteriovenous shunting in the lung can cause hypoxemia. These anomalies can be hereditary, as found with hereditary hemorrhagic telangiectasia (Osler-Rendu-Weber syndrome), or acquired, as in pulmonary vascular malformations secondary to hepatic cirrhosis, which are similar to the commonly recognized cutaneous vascular malformations ("spider hemangiomas").

Ventilation-perfusion mismatch is the most common cause of hypoxemia clinically. Most of the processes affecting either the airways or the pulmonary parenchyma are distributed unevenly throughout the lungs and do not necessarily affect ventilation and perfusion equally. Some areas of lung may have good perfusion and poor ventilation, whereas others have poor perfusion and relatively good ventilation. Important examples of airways diseases in which $\dot{V}/\dot{Q}$ mismatch causes hypoxemia are asthma and chronic obstructive lung disease. Parenchymal lung diseases causing $\dot{V}/\dot{Q}$ mismatch and hypoxemia include interstitial lung disease and pneumonia.

Clinically important alterations in CO_2 elimination range from excessive ventilation and hypocapnia to inadequate CO_2 elimination and hypercapnia. These clinical problems are discussed in Chap. 217.

Diffusing capacity Measurement of DL_{CO} may be useful for assessing disease affecting the alveolar-capillary bed or the pulmonary vasculature. In practice, three main categories of disease are associated with lowered DL_{CO}—interstitial lung disease, emphysema, and pulmonary vascular disease. With interstitial lung disease, scarring of alveolar-capillary units diminishes the area of the alveolar-capillary bed as well as pulmonary blood volume. With emphysema, alveolar walls are destroyed, so that the surface area of the alveolar-capillary bed is again diminished. In patients with disease causing a decrease in the cross-sectional area and volume of the pulmonary vascular bed, such as recurrent pulmonary emboli or primary pulmonary hypertension, DL_{CO} is commonly diminished.

Diffusing capacity may be elevated if pulmonary blood volume is increased, as may be seen in congestive heart failure. However, once interstitial and alveolar edema ensue, the net DL_{CO} depends on the opposing influences of increased pulmonary capillary blood volume elevating DL_{CO} and pulmonary edema decreasing it. Finding an elevated DL_{CO} may be useful in the diagnosis of alveolar hemorrhage, such as in Goodpasture's syndrome. Hemoglobin contained in erythrocytes within the alveolar lumen is capable of binding carbon monoxide, so that exhaled carbon monoxide concentration is diminished and the measured DL_{CO} is increased.

REFERENCES

GOLD WM, BOUSHEY HA: Pulmonary function testing, in *Textbook of Respiratory Medicine*, JF Murray, JA Nadel (eds). Philadelphia, Saunders, 1988, pp 611–682

WEINBERGER SE: *Principles of Pulmonary Medicine*. Philadelphia, Saunders, 1986

WEST JB: *Pulmonary Pathophysiology—The Essentials*, 3d ed. Baltimore, Williams & Wilkins, 1987

WEST JB: *Respiratory Physiology—The Essentials*, 3d ed. Baltimore, Williams & Wilkins, 1985

202 IMAGING IN PULMONARY DISEASE

PAUL J. FRIEDMAN

Radiologic examination of the lungs and pleura has grown beyond the capability—great as it is—of the plain chest film or radiograph and includes the imaging modalities of computed tomography, nuclear magnetic resonance, ultrasound, and nuclear medicine. This chapter will focus on their applications, best understood in relation to the traditional chest film.

THE BASIC PRINCIPLES OF CLINICAL IMAGING

Defining the problem The first step in the imaging examination is to define the problem clearly enough to indicate what new information needs to be provided by an imaging study.

Consultation The next step is to decide if a plain chest radiograph (CR) will suffice, whether special radiographic views are necessary, or if the problem demands more expensive and time-consuming techniques. In this era of growing specialization, rapidly changing technology, and cost consciousness, it is increasingly useful to get radiologic consultation for this step.

Getting the results The value of a radiographic report often depends on whether the radiologist was aware of the question being asked. It has been shown that radiologic interpretation is far more accurate when an appropriate history is provided. Even with a history the false-negative error rate (the "misses") is 30 to 40 percent on average, when measured in controlled situations. It is therefore important to (1) provide a history; (2) read the report carefully but skeptically; (3) look at the films yourself; and (4) review them with a radiologist.

Screening The routine posteroanterior (PA) and lateral CR are an exception to problem-based imaging, but admission films are needed only if there is suspicion of cardiac or pulmonary disease. Periodic health examinations do not require a CR unless there is a relevant history or physical finding.

OCCUPATIONAL HEALTH SCREENING Evaluating the extent of lung damage from exposure to coal or silica dust has been achieved by standardized CR, with an ingenious scoring system for pneumoconiosis. Health risks from exposure to asbestos dust are currently monitored by radiography, though with improved industrial hygiene the expected plaques are more rare and pulmonary fibrosis from asbestos is unusual. Occupational exposures to agents more likely to cause asthma than pneumoconiosis should not be monitored by CR.

APPLICATIONS OF IMAGING TECHNOLOGY, NEW AND OLD

Variations on chest radiography Chest radiologists uniformly agree that the technique of choice is high kilovoltage (>120 pkV), with a stationary scatter-absorbing grid, and a wide-latitude film-screen combination (more shades of gray, less black-and-white).

Portable films Though clearly necessary in many cases, the portable CR is deficient in detail resolution, latitude, penetration, and the normal gravitational gradient necessary for physiologic interpretation. It also has increased geometric distortion, more lung is obscured by heart or diaphragm, and it does not provide a lateral view. Lateral decubitus or prone positions may be useful in bedside radiography to show parts of the lung otherwise obscured by effusion; the lateral decubitus and other horizontal-beam films are good for demonstrating pneumothorax or fluid levels in the lung or pleural space. Portable radiographic examinations are also useful in assessing the positions of tubes and catheters commonly used in the intensive care unit.

Conventional tomography Essentially obsolete for most chest work, tomography is still used for studying the hilar regions, but far more information can be obtained about the hilar structures and the adjacent mediastinum from computed tomography (CT) or magnetic resonance (MR) imaging. Screening the lungs for metastases, formerly a major application of conventional tomography, is better done with CT. Conventional tomography should be used only in facilities where more advanced technology is not available.

COMPUTED TOMOGRAPHY

The x-ray absorption of each point (pixel) in a cross section of the body can be calculated by measuring the absorption of many fine x-ray beams at many angles within the plane of the cross section. The calculated numbers are displayed as radiographic densities with far more shades of gray than with CR (Fig. 202-1). In addition, CT eliminates the superimposition of structures that makes CR anatomy so difficult, and though the images are "noisy," there is less problem in detecting an abnormality because of obscuration by normal structures with CT than with CR. However, a set of images is needed to encompass the chest, since each represents only the information in a 1-cm thick transverse cross section. Each set of data is collected during suspended respiration, taking 1 to 4 s, and requires patient cooperation in taking and holding a comparable breath each time for good results.

MEDIASTINAL CT After less than a decade of use in the chest, CT is well established as the diagnostic procedure of choice for studying the mediastinum (Fig. 202-1*B*). The most common use is the assessment of lymph node size in the staging of lung cancer (Chap. 215). Detection of enlarged nodes may lead to biopsy, since enlargement of nodes by inflammation cannot be distinguished from that by tumor spread using only CT images. Most investigators find the false-negative error rate comparable to that of mediastinoscopy and somewhat better than cervical mediastinoscopy with left-sided lung cancers.

Lumps and bumps of the mediastinum, detected on CR, are readily analyzed using CT. Mediastinal cysts, tumors, fat, and calcification are readily distinguished because of the good density resolution. CT is also excellent for distinguishing vascular from nonvascular structures and for recognizing vascular anatomic variants or aneurysms.

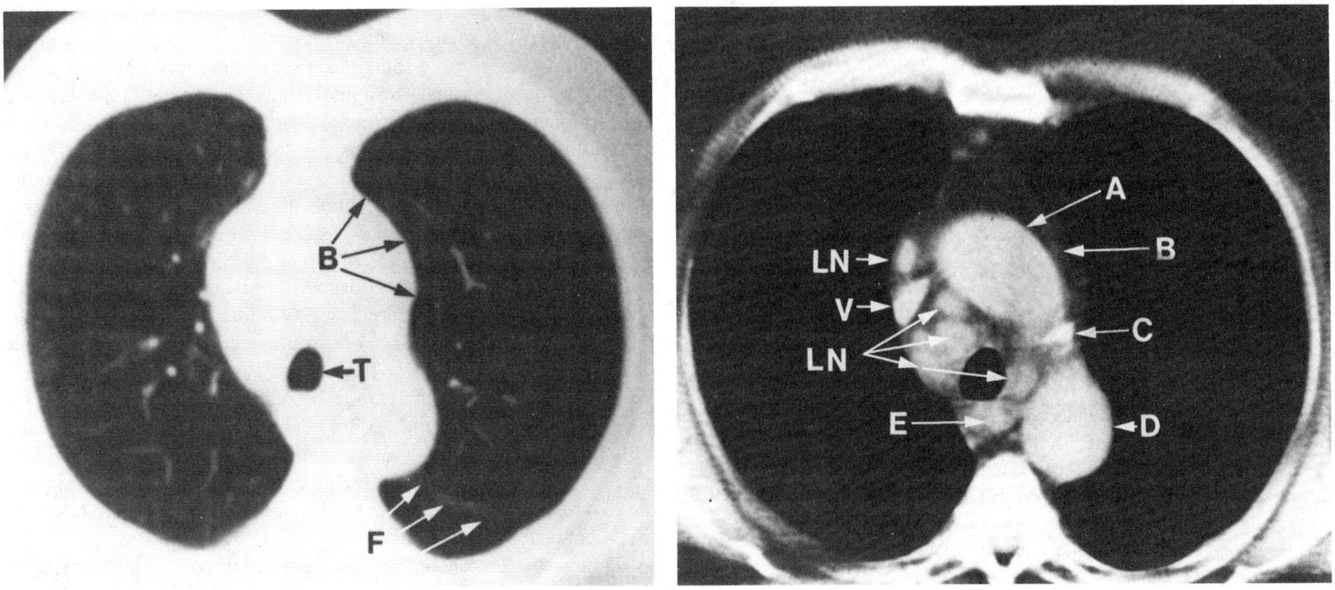

FIGURE 202-1 Normal CT of the chest, supine, standard 1 cm section, after intravenous contrast material. *A*. Typical "lung window" settings, with normal pulmonary vessels and the top of the oblique fissure (F) of the left lung visible. The dark circle within the mediastinum is the tracheal air column (T). Note bulge (B) along left mediastinum. *B*. Mediastinal settings show a clear delineation between the enlarged lymphomatous nodes (LN) and the surrounding fat. The soft tissue structure dorsal to the trachea is the esophagus (E). The major vessels visible are the superior vena cava (V) and ascending (A) and descending (D) aorta; small veins are also seen in the fat in front of the spine, behind the esophagus, and ventrally, behind the sternum, as well as in the generous layer of subcutaneous fat. The calcification (C) is a plaque in the aortic arch rather than a calcified lymph node. The mediastinal bulge (B) alongside the ascending aorta on the left is simply mediastinal fat, not an enlarged node.

CT is the best method for revealing fibrosing mediastinitis, since the important calcification is invisible with MR imaging.

CONTRAST MATERIAL There is no consensus about the indications for using intravenous contrast material in chest CT. Some institutions use contrast material universally and may even use the high dose–rapid infusion method known as *dynamic CT*. Others use contrast material regularly in studies of vessels or tumors but not for routine lung cancer staging. Injection of traditional hypertonic contrast media adds to the cost and risk of the study, since allergic and idiosyncratic reactions occur regularly. Serious reactions are uncommon, however, and death occurs no more than about once in every 40,000 intravenous injections. Newer agents are less toxic but are still several times as expensive.

CT OF THE PLEURA CT imaging resolves complex abnormalities which might involve the lung or pleura or both. For example, the diagnosis of bronchopleural fistula requires distinguishing pleural pockets from lung abscesses or cysts.

Tumors of the pleura are demonstrated in the transverse plane much more clearly than on CR, where they are hard to distinguish from inflammatory pleural thickening. The true extent of malignant mesothelioma or metastatic adenocarcinoma is therefore best shown on CT. The solid and fluid components of a pleural collection, which are the same density on CR, can be usefully distinguished on CT because of its greater density resolution (Fig. 202-2). Another asbestos-related application is the detection of pleural plaques and calcifications (Chap. 206). Though routine health screening of asbestos-exposed workers relies on the posteroanterior CR, sometimes it is necessary to use the much greater sensitivity of CT to detect pleural plaques or the characteristic small pleural calcifications.

CT OF THE LUNG AND AIRWAYS Since the CR has such excellent resolution and shows the air/tissue density differences so well, this application of CT has been the slowest to develop. The trachea and main bronchi are shown well in cross section (Fig. 202-2), and CT shows the mediastinal extent of endobronchial lesions, though longitudinal images of the trachea would be more useful clinically. Intrinsic tumors or deformity from other mediastinal primary or secondary neoplasms are demonstrable, but do not provide an indication for CT unless endoscopy is contraindicated. CT has much greater sensitivity for bronchial abnormality (thickening, dilatation, mucoid impaction) than CR. CT has practically replaced bronchography in screening for surgical bronchiectasis (Chap. 208), missing only minimal or localized cylindrical bronchiectasis.

Details of both alveolar and interstitial lung diseases can be

FIGURE 202-2 High-resolution CT, supine, 1.5 mm section, with edge-sharpening technique and standard "lung window." Patient with chronic thromboembolic pulmonary hypertension. Right pleural effusion (E). Airways are shown well, from the carina of the trachea (T) to segmental bronchi (arrowheads). Many visible peripheral pulmonary vessels are smaller than normal. Background vascularity is reduced in most regions, as contrasted to the subsegmental regions of more normal vascularity shown by the lighter density in the anterior segment of the right upper lobe (R) and, less clearly, in the axillary subsegment on the left (L). High-resolution CT can provide useful anatomic information about medium-sized vessels and bronchi. *(Courtesy of L. Olson.)*

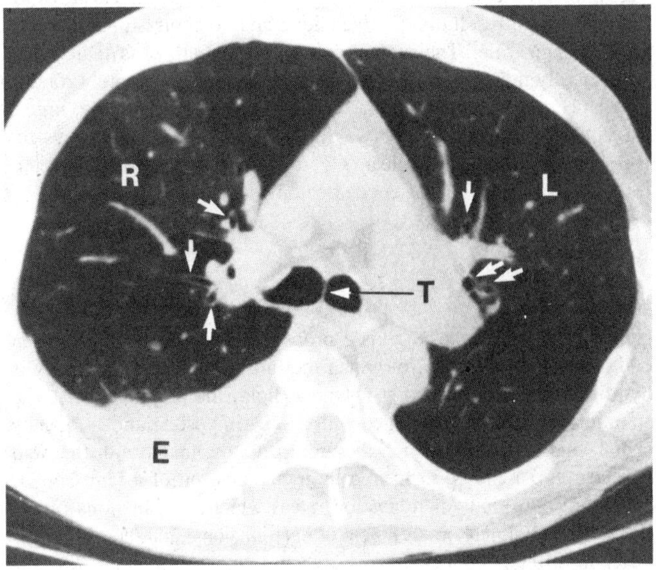

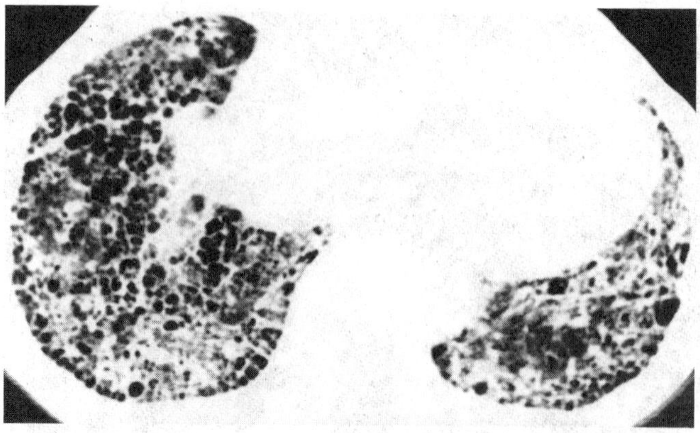

FIGURE 202-3 High-resolution CT, prone, 1.5 mm section, with edge-sharpening image processing, shown as a light "lung window." Chronic interstitial fibrosis with severe honeycombing: a graphic portrayal, comparable to looking directly at a lung specimen. High-resolution CT can show detailed gross pathologic findings in many lung diseases, with great sensitivity for alveolar filling, for interstitial alterations of various kinds, and for emphysema. *(Courtesy of I. Feuerstein.)*

demonstrated on CT. The utility of studying parenchymal abnormalities is still unclear, since characteristic changes have been described in only a few diseases such as carcinomatosis, interstitial fibrosis (Fig. 202-3), and emphysema.

HIGH-RESOLUTION CT The demonstration of parenchymal and bronchial abnormalities is enhanced by using high-resolution CT (Figs. 202-2 and 202-3). The geometric resolution of ordinary CT is nearly tenfold less than CR, but high-resolution brings it up to within a factor of two or three. The method uses a thin image plane, usually 1 to 2 mm instead of the conventional 10 mm, to reduce volume averaging of densities; often a smaller field of view to provide more pixels of computer resolution per unit area of lung; and a higher contrast or edge-enhancing image calculation. The result is comparable to a pathologist's naked-eye view of a slice of lung (Fig. 202-3). The trade-off is that the number of these thin slices that can be made is limited by radiation exposure, which precludes covering the entire lung; the method is used to sample the lung, like a noninvasive biopsy. Firm clinical indications have not developed yet, though this experimental technique should prove useful in the differential diagnosis of suspected interstitial lung diseases and is a preferred technique for excluding bronchiectasis.

LIMITED CT STUDIES CT scans of the chest initially were complete, top to bottom, without and with contrast injection. With more confidence in the anatomy as displayed on the scan and widened indications for using CT, studies of a limited part of the chest, using regular or high-resolution CT technique and no contrast, should play an increasing role. Their cost can be substantially less than a full scan, hardly more than adding a couple of oblique views to a routine CR. Uncertain CR findings can often be solved rapidly using limited CT studies, in preference to waiting a few costly hospital days for the diagnosis to become clear. CT densitometry is useful in determining the presence or absence of calcification in solitary pulmonary nodules.

MAGNETIC RESONANCE IMAGING

Nuclear magnetic resonance is a property of atomic nuclei with an odd number of nucleons, of which the most abundant in the body is hydrogen. While in a strong magnetic field, the alignment of these spinning nuclei can be changed with a superimposed radio-frequency signal, and the rate at which they return to alignment with the field ("relaxation") can be measured by their emission of a faint signal. There are two kinds of relaxation rates, which are functions of the atomic and chemical environment of each nucleus, and therefore they differ in different tissues.

By ingenious use of gradients, relaxation rates can be measured simultaneously at many points within a three-dimensional volume, which allows them to be shown as a set of gray scale images, either in the transverse, coronal, or sagittal plane. The timing of the imposed radio-frequency signal determines which of the relaxation rates predominates, and therefore the constructed images have different shades of gray for the same tissue, though the underlying anatomic structure is unchanged. At this time, there is only limited standardization of technique, especially since optimum differentiation of specific abnormalities requires different machine settings.

Transverse magnetic resonance (MR) images look much like CT images except for the different substitutions of light and dark for different tissues (Fig. 202-4). For example, fat is darker than water on CT, but is the brightest tissue on "T_1-weighted" MR images. Water (e.g., cerebrospinal fluid) becomes as bright as fat on T_2-weighted MR images (Fig. 202-4). The values, T_1 and T_2, are the half-times of the relaxation rates mentioned above, and are therefore a property of the tissue itself. The flexibility of eliciting and displaying the two relaxation rates provides MR images with even more effective tissue characterization contrast than CT.

Though the protons in blood have a strong MR signal because of the atomic environment of the iron and should therefore appear bright, flowing blood is seen as black, a signal void, on images. During the pause after the radio-frequency signal is triggered, while waiting to measure relaxation signals, the blood containing the altered protons has time to flow out of the plane of interest and is replaced by blood that is emitting no signal. Therefore, normal blood vessels as well as bronchi appear black on MR images (Fig. 202-4), but the distinction between nodes and vessels in the hilar regions is greatly facilitated compared to CT. There are artifactual signals from blood vessels, however, when blood flow is slow, notably on scans gated to diastole in the cardiac cycle (which are essential for studying the heart and hilar regions of the mediastinum) and on multisection simultaneous scans, when altered protons from one section will arrive at another level just in time for their signal to be detected. Finally, new methods of faster scanning result in images with flowing blood looking bright, as in an angiogram. The technology is evolving.

At present, MR scanning has important limitations compared with CT. A wide variety of artifacts complicate the interpretation of MR

FIGURE 202-4 Patient with ectopic ACTH syndrome caused by a bronchial carcinoid. Magnetic resonance image shows one bright region (high signal) in the posterior part of the left lower lobe (T). Normal pulmonary vessels are not visible because the MR signal of moving blood is emitted beyond the plane of the image. The carcinoid tumor was indistinguishable from vessels on the CT scan. This is a T_2-weighted image, as revealed by the bright appearance of the cerebrospinal fluid (C). The image is noisier than a CT image. The heart is blurred because of its motion (not a pulse-gated image), but the greater tissue resolution makes the tumor (T) visible compared to CT. There is absence of signal from the flowing blood in the descending aorta (d). *(Courtesy of I. Feuerstein and J. Doppman.)*

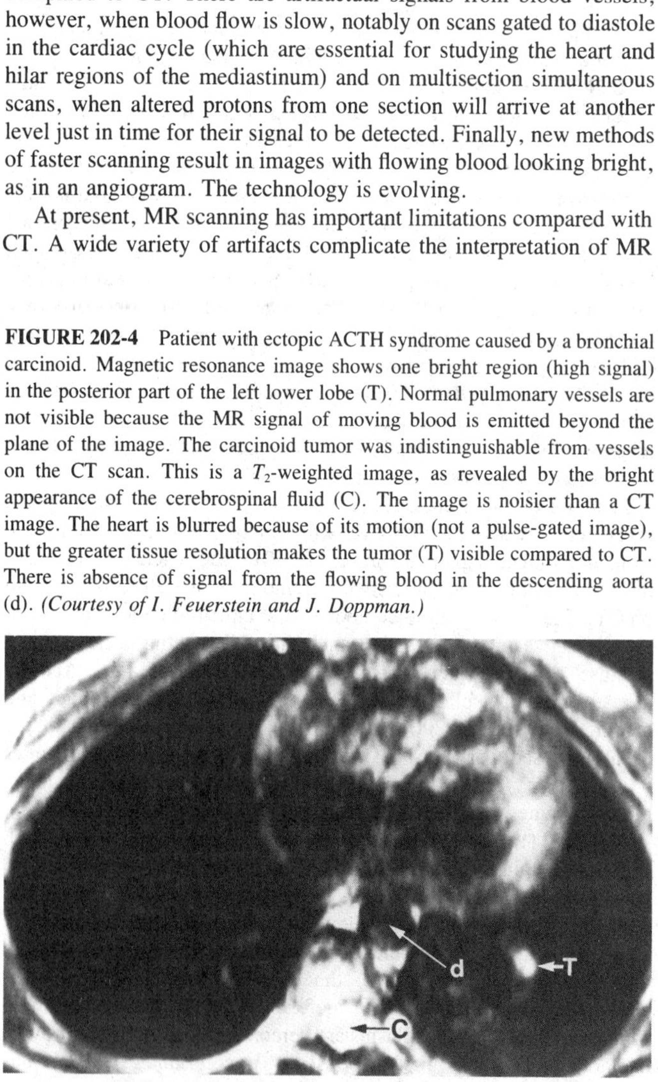

images and the images are also noisier and less uniform than those of CT. The geometric resolution of whole-body scans is inferior to CT, though superficial small regions can be shown with superb detail using special surface antennae to detect the faint relaxation signals. The advantage of being able to display data in any planar direction is weakened by the necessity (at present) of leaving a gap between the image slices. The collection of data (except with experimental fast-scan techniques) requires several minutes, which means that there are breathing artifacts in addition to those from cardiac motion. The narrow magnet tunnel into which the patient is inserted promotes claustrophobia, and the changes in the magnetic field cause a distressing noise. Ferromagnetic materials, including those in the patient, cannot be brought into the magnet room safely, for they will fly toward the center of the magnet. Other metal in the patient will merely ruin the image in its vicinity. Finally, the cost of MR scanning is substantial, approximately twice that of a contrast CT.

MR APPLICATIONS Gated cardiac studies are of great promise (Chap. 178), but are outside the scope of this discussion. The spine can be displayed with the perspective of an anatomic diagram, because of the availability of sagittal projections. This enables MR scanning to be particularly useful in questions of paraspinal, intraspinal, or intraosseous tumor. Tumors in the mediastinum can be analyzed by their T_1 and T_2 properties, but the hope for a way to distinguish inflammatory enlargement of nodes from that of tumor has not been realized yet. As noted, MR imaging is more sensitive than CT for distinguishing nonvascular tissue in the complex hilar regions and in the central portions of the lung (Fig. 202-4), but is probably less satisfactory in the mediastinum. Detection of intravascular pulmonary emboli or thrombi has been demonstrated experimentally, but clinical application is still remote.

Use of sagittal and coronal or oblique images in the mediastinum facilitates study of the arteries, so that MR scanning of the aorta is the preferred noninvasive way to detect aortic dissection or aneurysm (Chap. 197). These projections should be ideal for studying the trachea, but the trachea and bronchi are poorly displayed, with an artifactual narrowing of the lumen. The lungs and pleura do not usually benefit from MR study, in comparison with CT. The staging of lung cancer by mediastinal scanning has about the same effectiveness using MR as CT.

SPECTROSCOPY When chemists use MR to analyze mixtures and determine chemical structure, they study many nuclei in addition to hydrogen. Only hydrogen is sufficiently abundant in the body to provide enough signal to form images, but other substances can be quantitated in a volume that would be unsuitable for imaging. The most important is phosphorus, which has different resonant frequencies in its various molecular positions as part of ATP, AMP, creatine phosphate, inorganic phosphorus, etc. A limited number of relatively abundant cellular metabolites can also be measured by detecting protons with specific resonance values, if the very strong proton signal from water is suppressed. Metabolic processes can therefore be monitored by in vivo MR spectroscopy, a research technique of potential future clinical application.

NUCLEAR MEDICINE IMAGING

Injected or inhaled radioisotopes (radionuclides) incorporated into carefully chosen substances can provide anatomic, physiologic, and pathologic information from their distribution and disposition, as revealed on gamma camera images. Nuclear medicine remains the primary technique for the clinical problem of pulmonary thromboembolism (Chaps. 203 and 213) and the regional assessment of obstructive lung diseases.

ULTRASOUND IN THE CHEST

Imaging with ultrasound requires the computerized reconstruction of series of echoes of high-frequency sound emitted at various angles from a piezoelectric crystal transducer. The echoes arise as the radiating sound encounters surfaces of different acoustic impedance at right angles to its path. Ultrasound does not pass through air or bone, so the lungs themselves and the ribs are major limitations on its usefulness in the chest. A fluid collection such as a cyst or abscess will be echo-free, or *sonolucent,* unless it has debris in it, and will transmit sound and deeper echoes without attenuation. In solid tissues, the signal is attenuated as the sound is absorbed, so that the echoes become weaker as their depth in the tissue increases. Air-containing lung has no echo beyond the pleural interface at its surface, although consolidated lung may look like solid tissue.

APPLICATIONS The principal application of ultrasonography in the mediastinum is cardiac, discussed in detail in Chap. 177, including the detection of pericardial fluid and cysts. Bronchogenic cysts, in their most common subcarinal location, may also be confirmed to be fluid-containing by ultrasound. The most common pulmonary application is detection of fluid or pus in the pleural space. For diagnosis, ultrasound is convenient, since it can be performed with bedside apparatus, but it is not as accurate as CT (or MR) as it may confuse homogeneous pleural fibrosis or pulmonary consolidation with sonolucent pleural fluid. If the pleural fluid collection is loculated or small in amount, then localization by ultrasound enhances the safety and usefulness of thoracentesis.

INTERVENTIONAL RADIOLOGY

Advances in imaging with ultrasound and CT have brought with them a renaissance of percutaneous procedures for biopsy and drainage. Though fluoroscopically guided percutaneous needle biopsy of the lungs has been established for at least 20 years, CT has made it possible to pursue smaller targets and those close to vital structures. Under CT control, needle biopsy of enlarged nodes in the mediastinum can replace mediastinoscopic node biopsy, particularly when inoperability is being established by biopsy.

A more recent interventional innovation is drainage of pleural effusions, pneumothorax, and empyema in the thorax and abscesses in the abdomen by catheters inserted over guidewires that have been introduced through percutaneous needles, using techniques originally developed for angiography. The fluid or air pocket is localized and the needle position confirmed using ultrasound or CT, the specific technique depending on the ease with which the fluid can be delineated with ultrasound. Even lung abscesses can be drained percutaneously. Transcatheter embolization with particulate matter, coils, or detachable balloons has become widely used in the treatment of massive hemoptysis and arteriovenous malformations of the lung. Considerable savings are achieved in risk, pain, recovery time, and cost by avoiding major surgery with these methods.

REFERENCES

Carroll FE Jr: Lungs, in *Magnetic Resonance Imaging,* CL Partain et al (eds). Philadelphia, Saunders, 1988

Fraser RG et al: *Diagnosis of Diseases of the Chest,* 3d ed. Philadelphia, Saunders, 1988

Friedman PJ: Practical radiology of the hila and mediastinum. Postgrad Radiol 1:269, 1981

Haaga JR, Alfidi RJ (eds): *Computed Tomography of the Whole Body,* 2nd ed. St. Louis, Mosby, 1988

Higgins CB, Hricak H: *Magnetic Resonance Imaging of the Body.* New York, Raven, 1987

Proto AV: Mediastinal anatomy: Emphasis on conventional images with anatomic and computed tomographic correlations. J Thorac Imag 2:1, 1987

Sagel SS, Stanley RJ: *Computed Body Tomography with MRI correlation,* 2nd ed. New York, Raven, 1989

Van Sonnenberg E et al: CT- and ultrasound-guided catheter drainage of empyemas after chest-tube failure. Radiology 151:349, 1984.

Webb WR: Magnetic resonance imaging of the hila and mediastinum. Cardiovasc Intervent Radiol 8:306, 1986

———: *Mediastinum and hila,* in *Magnetic Resonance Imaging,* CL Partain et al (eds). Philadelphia, Saunders, 1988

203 DIAGNOSTIC PROCEDURES IN RESPIRATORY DISEASES

KENNETH M. MOSER

In seeking a definitive diagnosis in the patient with respiratory disease, a wide choice of diagnostic procedures is available. These procedures vary considerably, not only in diagnostic reliability and specificity, but also in terms of the discomfort and hazard to the patient. Hence, an orderly sequence of test selection is mandatory. This sequence should begin with procedures involving little risk and, only if necessary, move on to those which entail higher morbidity and potential mortality.

NONINVASIVE PROCEDURES

RADIOGRAPHIC PROCEDURES (See also Chap. 202) The *chest roentgenogram* serves two major roles in the search for a diagnosis in the patient with respiratory disease: *detector* and *guide*. Occasionally, in its role as a detector, the routine chest roentgenogram initiates the diagnostic search by disclosing an abnormality in an asymptomatic individual. However, routine chest roentgenography (e.g., as an element of all hospital admissions) is neither necessary nor cost-effective. Therefore, more commonly, it detects pulmonary involvement in someone already ill. Rarely, detection may coincide with diagnosis; e.g., in spontaneous pneumothorax or when a radiopaque foreign body has been aspirated.

Far more frequently, however, the roentgenogram, having detected potential disease, provides a guide to the selection of subsequent diagnostic procedures. Many radiographic findings are quite characteristic of certain diseases. A number of radiographic patterns are sufficiently repetitive to warrant descriptive names, such as bilateral hilar adenopathy, solitary pulmonary nodule, diffuse interstitial infiltrate, alveolar filling pattern, multinodular lesion, and honeycomb lung. Thus, a particular radiographic finding, combined with other pertinent data, often permits establishment of a reasonable list of possible diagnoses. For example, the roentgenographic detection of bilateral hilar adenopathy in an asymptomatic, 26-year-old black male immediately places sarcoidosis at the top of the list. A chest roentgenogram disclosing upper lobe cavities in a febrile male whose brother recently was admitted to a tuberculosis sanitarium would make tuberculosis the most likely entity. Or a "diffuse interstitial" infiltrate—for which more than 100 causes exist—may yield a prompt diagnosis of varicella pneumonia when combined with the classic skin lesions. Multinodular lesions, with some cavitating, in a patient with sinusitis and red cell casts on urinalysis makes Wegener's granulomatosis a primary diagnostic possibility. However, no roentgenographic pattern is sufficiently specific to *establish* a diagnosis. Lung cancer (primary and metastatic) can present many roentgenographic patterns, as can both infectious and noninfectious lung disorders. For example, cardiogenic pulmonary edema may present as a perihilar or diffuse alveolar filling pattern, as an interstitial process and, rarely, as a lobar infiltrate or interlobar collection of fluid ("pseudotumor")—all with or without a pleural effusion.

In some instances, special radiographic techniques may provide valuable diagnostic insights.

Fluoroscopy allows visualization of the thoracic contents in a dynamic rather than static manner and also permits a wide range of special views. It also indicates whether a lesion is pulsatile, what its precise location in the thorax is, whether the hemidiaphragms move normally, i.e., whether they are fixed or move paradoxically, and how various zones of the lung behave during inspiration and expiration. Thus, fluoroscopy can define whether a roentgenographic density is actually in a rib or in the pleura rather than in the parenchyma; and may distinguish between a unilateral hyperlucent lung due to emphysema (mediastinum shifts toward the normal lung on expiration) or to unilateral pulmonary arterial obstruction (no shift).

Thoracic *computed tomography* (*CT*) *scanning* has essentially replaced standard tomography (laminography, planigraphy). Both techniques provide a sequence of images, each representing a "slice of the lung" at a different depth. Ordinarily, "cuts" are made at 0.5- to 1.0-cm distances through the areas of interest. These procedures can identify a number of features which are not appreciated on the "routine" roentgenogram, including calcium in a solitary nodule (which if diffuse or in concentric rings signifies a benign etiology); a cavity within a mass lesion; and the presence of hilar, paratracheal, and subcarinal node enlargement. The CT scan is particularly useful in the definition of pleural disease (e.g., differentiating fluid from tumor; identifying calcium in asbestos-exposed individuals); with contrast injections, in differentiating tissue masses from vascular structures; and in identifying small parenchymal nodules. However, to some extent, the sensitivity of CT is a mixed blessing because it is still not known how many "normal" individuals have pleural or parenchymal abnormalities by CT and how these small, benign, hitherto undetected lesions can be distinguished from neoplastic lesions.

Magnetic resonance (MR) imaging remains, in terms of its value in pulmonary diseases, an investigational technique. It has potential value in achieving fine definition of mediastinal lesions and, perhaps, in defining embolic occlusion of major pulmonary arteries.

SKIN TESTS Having arrived at a tentative list of diagnostic possibilities based on the history, physical examination, and radiographic appearance, the physician should move to other procedures. One of the simplest and most commonly overlooked is the application of *skin tests* with specific antigens. Antigens are now available to assist in the diagnosis of tuberculosis, histoplasmosis, coccidioidomycosis, blastomycosis, trichinosis, toxoplasmosis, and aspergillosis. These tests vary with respect to sensitivity and cross-reactivity, and attention to scrupulous technique in performance and interpretation is vital. Also, some antigens (e.g., histoplasmosis) may confound serologic tests performed subsequently. A positive skin test indicates only that the antigen has been encountered previously by the host; it does not, regardless of reaction intensity, imply active disease. Furthermore, drugs or diseases which depress cell-mediated immunity (e.g., prednisone, cyclophosphamide, lymphomas, sarcoidosis, disseminated tuberculosis, or coccidioidomycosis) may cause skin anergy. Indeed, a negative battery of skin tests, if it incorporates antigens such as mumps, streptokinase-streptodornase, *Trichophyton,* and *Candida,* suggests that a cause of skin anergy should be sought.

SEROLOGIC TESTS These tests also may be useful in the diagnosis of histoplasmosis, blastomycosis, coccidioidomycosis, toxoplasmosis, *Mycoplasma* pneumonia, Legionnaires' disease, a variety of other infectious diseases involving the lungs, and certain immunologically mediated lung diseases (e.g., lupus erythematosus). Often, more extensive diagnostic procedures can be avoided if appropriate serologic tests are obtained. However, there is substantial interinstitutional variability with respect to the sensitivity, specificity, and types of serologic tests available. Therefore, their appropriate use requires close interaction with the responsible laboratory.

SPUTUM EXAMINATION Another rapid, innocuous diagnostic procedure is *sputum examination.* It is important that the specimen contain sputum, not saliva, the latter being identified by the presence of squamous (mouth) rather than epithelial (bronchial) cells. The gross nature of the sputum—color, odor, and the presence of blood—may provide valuable clues; e.g., foul sputum suggesting anaerobic pulmonary infection, and blood, in any amount, indicating an abnormality that mandates further investigation. Carefully stained smears of the sputum should be examined next, for these may disclose the causative organism in many bacterial pneumonias, tuberculosis, *Pneumocystis* pneumonia, and in some fungus infections. Sputum eosinophilia can suggest the presence of reversible airway disease responsive to glucocorticoids; hemosiderin-laden macrophages suggest the possibility of Goodpasture's syndrome. Often valuable time is lost because the sputum smear is not examined and results of culture are awaited instead. Sputum samples can be obtained from patients who are not coughing by having them inhale a heated mixture of a mildly irritative solution that induces cough. Such induced samples have been particularly useful in the diagnosis of *P. carinii* pneumonia and in obtaining cytologic specimens for the diagnosis of carcinoma of the lung (Chap. 215). Careful handling of such specimens and interpretive expertise heavily determine the diagnostic yield.

Culture of expectorated sputum (spontaneous or induced) has fallen into disrepute because of uncertain yield and, particularly, because of frequent and unavoidable contamination by the oropharyngeal bacterial flora. Although such cultures are invaluable for identification of organisms responsible for tuberculous and fungus infections, their utility in detection of other bacterial agents responsible for pulmonary infection is often uncertain and can be misleading, particularly in patients who are immunocompromised, intubated, or receiving antimicrobial therapy. Five procedures, described below, are now gaining wide acceptance because they limit oropharyngeal contamination and/or can be used to obtain representative samples of lung secretions from the area of lung involvement: (1) catheter-brush sampling, (2) bronchoalveolar lavage, (3) transtracheal aspiration, (4) transbronchial lung biopsy, and (5) percutaneous needle aspiration of the lung.

PULMONARY FUNCTION TESTS (See also Chap. 201) Certain "patterns" of derangement in spirometric tests, arterial blood gases, diffusing capacity, and other functional parameters are particularly suggestive of certain pulmonary diseases. For example, diffuse interstitial fibrotic diseases of the lungs (Chap. 211) produce a "restrictive" spirometric defect, reduced pulmonary compliance, a reduced diffusing capacity, and an alveolar-arterial oxygen tension difference which is widened at rest and widens further with exercise. Emphysema (Chap. 210) characteristically causes expiratory obstruction, lung hyperinflation, decreased static elastic recoil (increased compliance), and a reduced diffusing capacity.

PULMONARY SCINTIPHOTOGRAPHY Scintiphotographs ("scans") of intrathoracic structures are obtained by a variety of "scanning" devices which record the pattern of intrathoracic radioactivity after intravenous injection or inhalation of gamma-emitting radionuclides. Direct photographic or computer-derived images, or digital data, reflecting radionuclide distribution are used for diagnostic purposes. The most commonly used images are those which reflect the distribution of pulmonary blood flow (perfusion) and ventilation. Such scans have multiple diagnostic applications. For example, a normal perfusion scan excludes the diagnosis of acute pulmonary embolism (Chap. 213). When perfusion scans showing defects are combined with ventilation scans, ventilation-perfusion patterns are provided which assist in the diagnosis of parenchymal lung diseases and vascular occlusive disorders, including pulmonary embolism.

Another type of scan involves intravenous injection of radionuclides which have an affinity for intrathoracic inflammatory and neoplastic tissues. Gallium 67 is the most useful of such radionuclides now available. Concentration of such agents, defined by scanning, may permit detection of neoplastic or inflammatory disease in the lungs or mediastinal lymph nodes. Uptake by the lungs may, in some patients, reflect the intensity of inflammatory activity associated with diffuse interstitial pneumonitis, sarcoidosis, and granulomatous infections. Inapparent extrapulmonary foci of granulomatous or neoplastic diseases also may be detected by body scanning.

New radionuclides continue to emerge which, when complexed with such materials as platelets, white blood cells (e.g., indium 111), fibrinogen, and albumin, may allow imaging of intrathoracic vessels, thrombi, inflammation, and neoplasms. Tomographic and other image-processing methods are emerging which may further extend the value of these techniques.

All the above procedures involve minimal risks and discomfort to the patient. Where applicable, these approaches should be considered before the more invasive techniques discussed below are considered, unless the condition of the patient demands immediate diagnosis.

INVASIVE PROCEDURES

BRONCHOSCOPY The primary objectives of bronchoscopy include direct visualization of the tracheobronchial tree, including abnormalities such as tumors or granulomatous lesions; biopsy of suggestive or obvious endobronchial lesions; and lavage, brushing, or biopsy of lung regions for cultural and cytologic examinations. Both the *diagnostic reach of* and *accessibility to* bronchoscopy have been expanded by the flexible fiberoptic bronchoscope (FOB). This can be understood best by comparing the FOB with the "standard" rigid bronchoscope.

The rigid bronchoscope is a wide-bore metal tube which incorporates a lighted mirror-lens system. The FOB is composed of fiberoptic bundles which provide both illumination and visualization pathways. A small channel with a diameter of 1 to 3 mm traverses the FOB, through which instruments can be passed, fluids delivered, and suction applied. The rigid bronchoscope comes in various external diameters limited only by the feasibility of introducing the rigid device orally and through the larynx. Biopsy and other procedures are carried out through the rather capacious interior of the rigid tube. The FOB also is available in various external diameters, but all are substantially smaller than rigid bronchoscopes (since no "wall" exists in the FOB). The distal tip of the FOB can be *flexed* easily to 90° and usually to 130° or more from the vertical.

Thus, the rigid bronchoscope permits visualization only of lobar bronchi and the orifices of some segmental bronchi. The flexible, smaller FOB extends the range of *view* to all segmental and subsegmental bronchi and the range for *biopsy and sampling* to the pulmonary parenchyma itself. A biopsy forceps, catheter, or brush passed through the FOB can be directed well beyond the tip of the bronchoscope itself, permitting *transbronchial lung biopsy, brushings,* or *aspiration of secretions* for culture and cytologic examination from the most distal regions of the lung. Indeed, both forceps and brush can reach and perforate the pleura, leading to pneumothorax. Therefore, when the lesion being approached is distal, fluoroscopic guidance is essential. Not only does this permit placement of the FOB, forceps, catheter, or brush directly into the area of interest, but also it ensures that the pleura will not be inadvertently reached and punctured. The FOB also allows *regional* lung lavage to obtain materials for cytologic examination and culture. The use of specially designed catheters (see below) placed through the FOB is quite useful in obtaining representative, noncontaminated secretions for culture, thus avoiding the problems mentioned previously with expectorated sputum.

Thus, the FOB has sharply increased the limited diagnostic reach previously available with rigid bronchoscopy. Equally important, the FOB has made bronchoscopy more available to the physician and more acceptable to the patient. The performance of rigid bronchoscopy requires the supine position for peroral insertion of the device; can be performed safely by a relatively few trained physicians; and is often carried out under general anesthesia in an operating room. Therefore, it has been a procedure requiring significant preparation and hence delay. Fiberoptic bronchoscopy can be performed in the sitting or supine position, since the FOB is easily inserted transnasally; can be performed by a large number of trained pulmonary specialists as well as surgeons; usually requires only local anesthesia; and can be performed safely on the wards, in diagnostic rooms equipped with a "dentist-type" chair, and in intensive care units. The FOB can be used easily in intubated patients on ventilators with simple "side-arm" adapters attached to the endotracheal tube. Therefore, when bronchoscopy is indicated, it is not surprising that fiberoptic bronchoscopy is now commonly the first choice. The roomier rigid bronchoscope is now usually reserved for situations in which the small biopsy-suction channel in the FOB may be inadequate (e.g., for removal of large foreign bodies, for laser surgery). The FOB also has a widening range of therapeutic applications including aspiration or lavage of secretions in patients with airway obstruction or atelectasis due to retained secretions; obstruction of bleeding areas of the lung, with a wedged FOB itself or with a balloon catheter passed via the

FOB, in patients who are poor surgical risks; removal of small foreign bodies; and placement of radionuclides in tumors. Transtracheal needle aspiration of paratracheal and subcarinal nodes also can be performed via the FOB, a procedure which is particularly useful in the staging of carcinoma of the lung.

The hazards of bronchoscopy are modest but should be recognized. In addition to the risk of general anesthesia which rigid bronchoscopy usually requires, they can include hypoxemia, laryngospasm, bronchospasm, pneumothorax, and, of course, bleeding following biopsy. Proper management before, during, and after bronchoscopy should prevent most of these complications. There is no absolute contraindication to FOB. Even in the presence of massive hemoptysis, FOB with appropriate precautions can yield useful information. Patients with bronchospasm (or a history of bronchospasm) are at particular risk of acute enhancement of spasm and should be approached after good preparation and with resources for intubation-ventilation at hand. The primary contraindication to both rigid and fiberoptic bronchoscopy is the same: performance by inexperienced personnel. Lack of experience sharply reduces diagnostic and therapeutic yield while increasing risks.

BRONCHOGRAPHY In this method, radiopaque material is instilled into the tracheobronchial tree via a catheter or bronchoscope. Positioning of the patient and catheter permits the material to coat all portions of the tracheobronchial tree for a sufficient period so that their outline can be recorded on chest roentgenograms. Bronchography is indicated for the diagnosis of bronchiectasis, for the identification of obstruction in distal bronchi, and for the detection of other types of congenital and acquired forms of tracheobronchial distortion or malformation. Like FOB, bronchography may induce bronchospasm; also, the irritative effects of the contrast medium may persist for some days. In many situations in which bronchography was used in the past (e.g., for the diagnosis of bronchiectasis), it is being replaced by chest CT.

TRANSTRACHEAL, CATHETER-BRUSH, AND PERCUTANEOUS NEEDLE ASPIRATION OF THE LUNG All three of these procedures are used to obtain material for culture and microscopic examination. In the case of culture, all three techniques bypass the oropharyngeal flora, though transtracheal aspiration is the least certain in this regard.

Transtracheal aspiration involves needle puncture of the cricothyroid membrane, insertion of a plastic cannula, and instillation of a saline solution, followed by suctioning of a sample. The procedure cannot be performed in intubated patients; contamination rates are high in previously intubated patients or those who have aspirated oropharyngeal contents. Because the procedure entails risks, although these are minimized by meticulous technique and experience, clear indications for its use should exist. These include apparent pulmonary infections in patients who are unable to cough, in whom cough is nonproductive, or in whom there has been a lack of response to therapy based on smears or cultures from expectorated sputum.

In these same contexts, *catheter-brush devices* specially designed with a distal plug to avoid oropharyngeal contamination can be used. These are manipulated (through an FOB or without it) under fluoroscopic guidance into the involved lung area. The distal absorbable plug is then ejected and the inner brush or catheter advanced for sampling. Finally, an alternative procedure is direct percutaneous aspiration, which can be performed using a small (23- or 25-gauge), thin-walled, *noncutting* needle. The needle, connected to a syringe, is introduced percutaneously into the area of the lung of interest; 2 to 3 mL saline is injected and then aspirated into the syringe and the needle withdrawn. Both the catheter-brush and needle approaches are high-yield, low-contamination procedures. In experienced hands, the risks are low, consisting chiefly of pneumothorax and bleeding. Patients should be carefully monitored for both.

The presence of a hemorrhagic diathesis is a relative contraindication to all three of the above procedures.

BRONCHOALVEOLAR LAVAGE (BAL) This procedure is usually performed by lightly wedging a fiberoptic bronchoscope in distal airways, gently irrigating the air spaces beyond with saline, and analyzing the cells obtained. A "liquid biopsy" of the contents of the distal air spaces is obtained. The procedure has value in the diagnosis of *P. carinii* pneumonia and other infections, in alveolar proteinosis, and in some patients with interstitial pneumonitis of uncertain cause. Maximum diagnostic yield requires careful techniques and expert sample processing.

THORACENTESIS AND PLEURAL BIOPSY Thoracentesis should be performed to obtain pleural fluid in all pleural effusions of uncertain etiology and may be indicated for relief of symptoms in some patients with effusion of known cause. In effusions of uncertain cause, closed (needle) pleural biopsy should be performed as part of the same procedure.

When pleural fluid is small in amount or when its presence or location is uncertain from routine or lateral decubitus roentgenograms, performance of the thoracentesis and biopsy under fluoroscopic, ultrasound, or CT scan guidance enhances both yield and safety. Pleural fluid obtained should be examined for specific gravity, white blood cell count and differential, protein and glucose concentrations, lactic acid dehydrogenase (LDH), pH, P_{CO_2} (sample collected anaerobically), and amylase. Gram stain, cultures, and exfoliative cytologic specimens should be obtained; and in some instances, rheumatoid factor and complement levels are measured. The gross appearance of the fluid, the quantity obtained, and the precise location of the thoracentesis should be recorded. A combination of a pleural fluid LDH above 200 IU, a pleural fluid/serum protein ratio greater than 0.5, and a pleural fluid/serum LDH ratio greater than 0.6 all indicate that an "exudative" rather than "transudative" process is present. A low pH (<7.20) often indicates that an empyema, probably requiring tube drainage, is present (Chap. 216). Specific diagnostic findings in pleural fluid may include the opalescent, pearly fluid characteristic of chylothorax; positive smears or cultures for tuberculosis or other infections; a marked elevation of amylase indicative of effusion secondary to pancreatitis or a ruptured esophagus; and the very low glucose values often seen in effusions associated with rheumatoid arthritis.

As already noted, closed (needle) pleural biopsy should follow thoracentesis whenever the diagnosis is uncertain. It is important to leave some fluid in the pleural space as this makes biopsy easier and safer. Bleeding, pneumothorax, and bronchopleural fistula induced by cutting through the visceral pleura are all more likely in the absence of fluid, and a satisfactory biopsy specimen is less likely to be obtained. Several special needles are available for biopsy of the parietal pleura. All have a cutting edge and some device for retaining the biopsy. The needle is inserted into the pleural effusion, then withdrawn until it is seated on the parietal pleura, from which a biopsy is obtained with the cutting edge. Usually, three biopsies are taken from different sites at the same session. Care should be exercised to place the needle in a position least likely to impinge on the intercostal vessels. All fluid to be used for diagnosis should be removed before biopsy since postbiopsy bleeding may obscure the true character of the fluid.

Pleuroscopy, using a modified FOB inserted through an intercostal trocar, also can be used for both direct inspection and biopsy of the pleura. In the absence of a pleural effusion, two other options exist for obtaining tissue from pleural-based lesions: aspiration needle biopsy and open biopsy. The technique for aspiration biopsy is the same as that described above, although some physicians use "cutting" needles (see "Lung Biopsy" below). Open pleural biopsy involves a limited thoracotomy, requiring anesthesia. A small intercostal incision is made, and the parietal pleura is biopsied under direct visualization. The incision is then closed, often without an intercostal tube. Open biopsy has several advantages because a larger specimen is obtained and the pleura and underlying lung can be seen and palpated. When pleural involvement is "spotty," open biopsy increases the possibility of establishing a diagnosis.

PULMONARY AND BRONCHIAL ANGIOGRAPHY Visualization of the pulmonary arteries by *pulmonary angiography* is achieved by direct, rapid injection of radiopaque materials into the main pulmonary artery or its branches, preferably via cardiac catheterization. Nonionic radiopaque materials, while more expensive, reduce the frequency and severity of unwanted respiratory and hemodynamic responses (e.g., cough, elevation in pulmonary arterial pressure). Multiple, large films can be obtained by an automatic filmchanger; or motion picture or video film (cineangiography) can be used. If visualization of smaller pulmonary vessels is required, magnification techniques can be used. Digital subtraction pulmonary angiography, providing computer-derived images of digital data, may allow imaging of the larger pulmonary arteries with contrast injected more proximally (into superior or inferior vena cava or peripheral vein) or at lower concentrations; however, motion artifacts limit its sensitivity and specificity. Angiography is frequently used to detect pulmonary emboli and a variety of congenital and acquired lesions of the pulmonary vessels. The procedure carries some risk, particularly in patients with pulmonary hypertension, and clear indication for it must exist as well as personnel experienced in its performance and interpretation.

Angioscopy, an experimental technique for direct visualization of the right cardiac chambers and pulmonary arterial system, can be accomplished by insertion of a fiberoptic device via a peripheral vein. The diagnostic role of this procedure in embolic and other disorders remains to be defined.

Bronchial arteriography is of value to identify and control (embolotherapy) otherwise obscure bleeding sites in the lungs. Transarterial placement of a catheter into the orifices or parent vessels of bronchial arteries can be accomplished by experienced operators. Radiopaque material is then injected so that these arteries can be visualized. If a bleeding site is identified, emboli can be injected via the catheter as a means for halting hemoptysis.

MEDIASTINOSCOPY AND MEDIASTINOTOMY Another favored site for biopsy is the lymph nodes in the mediastinum. Because they receive lymphatic drainage from the lungs, these nodes often disclose intrathoracic diseases such as carcinoma, granulomatous infections, and sarcoidosis. As noted above, transtracheal needle aspiration of mediastinal nodes via the FOB is one approach to such nodes. Another is mediastinoscopy, which involves insertion of a lighted mirror-lens system, much like a bronchoscope, through an incision at the base of the neck anteriorly. The instrument is advanced under visual control into the mediastinum, where inspection and biopsy can be carried out. Because of its higher yield of diagnostic lymph nodes, mediastinoscopy has virtually replaced biopsy of the *scalene fat pad* for nodes of interest on the right side of the mediastinum. However, for anatomic reasons, mediastinoscopy on the left is less satisfactory and more hazardous. Nodes in this location are usually approached through a limited left anterior thoracotomy (mediastinotomy) or, occasionally, by scalene fat pad biopsy. Needle aspiration, mediastinoscopy, and mediastinotomy are low-risk, high-yield procedures. They are invaluable in the "staging" of patients with known or suspected pulmonary malignancy.

LUNG BIOPSY Finally, if the diagnosis still remains unclear, biopsy of the lung may be required. Again, "closed" and "open" approaches are available. Closed biopsies are of three types: transbronchial, aspiration, and "cutting needle." Transbronchial biopsy, carried out through the fiberoptic bronchoscope, is a highly useful procedure, particularly since larger forceps have been introduced and the taking of multiple biopsies during one procedure has become routine.

However, when lesions are small and/or anatomically located beyond the reach of the FOB, direct aspiration needle biopsy is often more rewarding. *Aspiration* biopsy, mentioned previously, provides cytologic material but does not actually obtain a specimen of lung whose architecture can be examined, a feature which may be necessary to establish a diagnosis. Various "cutting" needles are available which do provide a "core" of the involved lung. However, this approach has waned in popularity because of the high incidence of pneumothorax and bleeding, occasional deaths due to air embolism, and the small size of the biopsy specimen, which may limit diagnostic interpretation. Fluoroscopic guidance is essential in all these closed approaches, and they are contraindicated if pulmonary hypertension or a hemorrhagic diathesis is present.

Open-lung biopsy, requiring thoracotomy, is the final diagnostic resort. It is, however, a relatively safe procedure even in patients with respiratory failure, hemorrhagic diathesis, or pulmonary hypertension if meticulous surgical and anesthetic techniques are observed. Direct visualization allows selection of an optimum biopsy site, and of course, a specimen of adequate size is obtained. In selecting among these closed and open options, consideration of local expertise in their performance is a key factor.

All specimens obtained by biopsy should be both cultured and processed for pathologic examination.

REFERENCES

BORDELON JY JR et al: The telescoping plugged catheter in suspected anaerobic infections: A controlled series. Am Rev Respir Dis 128:465, 1983

BORDOW RA, MOSER KM: *Manual of Clinical Problems in Pulmonary Medicine*. Boston, Little, Brown, 1985

HASLAM PL: Bronchoalveolar lavage. Semin Respir Med 6:55, 1984

NAIDICH P et al (eds): *Computed Tomography of the Thorax*. New York, Raven Press, 1984

NICOD P et al: Pulmonary angiography in severe chronic pulmonary hypertension. Ann Intern Med 107:565, 1987

SHURE D (ed): *Diagnostic Technics: Clinics in Chest Medicine*. Philadelphia, Saunders, 1987

TURNER-WARWICK M, HASLAM PL: The value of serial bronchoalveolar lavage in assessing the clinical progress of patients with cryptogenic fibrosing alveolitis. Am Rev Respir Dis 135:26, 1987

WESSELIUS LJ et al: Computer-assisted versus usual lung gallium-67 index in normals and patients with interstitial lung disorders. Am Rev Respir Dis 128:1084, 1983

204 ASTHMA

E. R. McFADDEN, JR.

DEFINITION Asthma is a disease of airways that is characterized by increased responsiveness of the tracheobronchial tree to a multiplicity of stimuli. Asthma is manifested physiologically by a widespread narrowing of the air passages, which may be relieved spontaneously or as a result of therapy, and clinically by paroxysms of dyspnea, cough, and wheezing. It is an episodic disease, acute exacerbations being interspersed with symptom-free periods. Typically, most attacks are short-lived, lasting minutes to hours, and after them the patient seems to recover completely clinically. However, there can be a phase in which the patient experiences some degree of airway obstruction daily. This phase can be mild, with or without superimposed severe episodes, or much more serious, with severe obstruction persisting for days or weeks, a condition known as *status asthmaticus*.

PREVALENCE AND ETIOLOGY The prevalence and incidence of asthma is difficult to assess with certainty because of the lack of reliable population-based figures which have used uniform diagnostic criteria. However, it has been suggested that approximately 5 percent of adults and 7 to 10 percent of children in the United States and Australia have the disorder. Bronchial asthma occurs at all ages but predominantly in early life. About one-half of the cases develop before age 10 and another third occur before age 40. In childhood, there is a 2:1 male/female preponderance, which equalizes by age 30.

From an etiologic standpoint, asthma is a heterogeneous disease, and attempts to define it in etiologic or pathologic terms have proved difficult. It is useful for epidemiologic and clinical purposes to classify the forms of this disease by the principal stimuli that incite or are associated with acute episodes. However, it is important to emphasize that the distinction between various types of asthma may often be artificial, and the response of a given subclassification usually can be initiated by more than one type of stimulus. With this reservation in mind, one can describe two broad groups: allergic and idiosyncratic.

Allergic asthma is often associated with a personal and/or family history of allergic diseases such as rhinitis, urticaria, and eczema; positive wheal-and-flare skin reactions to intradermal injection of extracts of airborne antigens; increased levels of IgE in the serum; and/or positive response to provocation tests involving the inhalation of specific antigen.

A significant segment of the asthmatic population will present with negative family or personal histories of allergy, negative skin tests, and normal serum levels of IgE, and therefore cannot be classified on the basis of defined immunologic mechanisms. These we term *idiosyncratic*. Many of these will develop a typical symptom complex upon contracting an upper respiratory illness. The initial insult may be little more than a common cold, but after several days the patient begins to develop paroxysms of wheezing and dyspnea that can last for days to months. These individuals should not be confused with persons in whom the symptoms of bronchospasm are superimposed upon chronic bronchitis or bronchiectasis (see Chap. 210).

Unfortunately, many patients will not clearly fit into either of the above categories but will fall into a mixed group with features of each. In general, those patients whose onset of disease is in early life will tend to have a strong allergic component to their illness, while those who develop their asthma late tend to be nonallergic or to have mixed etiologies.

PATHOGENESIS OF ASTHMA The common denominator underlying the asthmatic diathesis is a nonspecific hyperirritability of the tracheobronchial tree. In asthmatics it correlates well with the clinical features of the illness. When airway reactivity is high, lung function becomes more unstable, symptoms are more severe and persistent, the acute response to bronchodilators is larger, and the amount of therapy required to control the patient's complaints increases. In addition, the magnitude of diurnal fluctuations in lung function becomes greater and the patient tends to awaken at night or in the early morning with breathlessness.

In both normal and asthmatic subjects, airway reactivity is known to rise following viral infections of the respiratory tract and exposure to oxidant air pollutants such as ozone and nitrogen dioxide. Viruses have more profound consequences, and following a seemingly trivial upper respiratory tract infection, airway responsivity may remain elevated for many weeks. In contrast, with exposure to ozone airway reactivity remains high for only a few days. Airway reactivity has also been shown to increase in normal individuals with the exogenous administration of platelet activating factor. Allergens can cause airway responsiveness to rise within minutes, and to remain elevated for weeks. If the dose of antigen is high enough, acute episodes of obstruction may occur daily for a prolonged period of time following a single exposure.

A number of causes have been postulated for the increased airway reactivity of asthma; however, the basic mechanism remains unknown. The most popular hypothesis at present is that of airway inflammation. Following exposure to an initiating stimulus, mast cells, basophils, and macrophages can be activated to release a variety of mediators which produce direct effects on airway smooth muscle and capillary permeability, thereby evoking an intense local reaction which can then be followed by a more chronic one. The latter may be brought about by the release of chemotactic factors which recruit cellular elements to the site of injury. In addition, it is thought that the acute and chronic effects of mediator release and cellular infiltration may result in epithelial damage with involvement of neural endings within the airways and the activation of an axon reflex. In this fashion, an essentially local phenomenon can be amplified to have widespread effects throughout the tracheobronchial tree.

The stimuli that increase airway responsiveness and incite acute episodes of asthma can be grouped into seven major categories: allergenic, pharmacologic, environmental, occupational, infectious, exercise-related, and emotional.

Allergens Allergic asthma is dependent upon an IgE response controlled by T and B lymphocytes and activated by the interaction of antigen with mast cell–bound IgE molecules. Most of the allergens that provoke asthma are airborne, and in order to induce a state of sensitivity, they must be reasonably abundant for considerable periods of time. Once sensitization has occurred, however, the patient can then exhibit exquisite responsivity, so that minute amounts of the offending agent can produce significant exacerbations of the disease. Immunologic mechanisms appear to be causally related to the development of asthma in 25 to 35 percent of all cases, and contributory in perhaps another third. Allergic asthma is frequently seasonal, and it is most often observed in children and young adults. A nonseasonal form may result from allergy to feathers, animal danders, molds, and other antigens present continuously in the environment. Exposure to antigen typically produces an immediate response in which airway obstruction develops in minutes and then resolves. In 30 to 50 percent of patients a second wave of bronchoconstriction, the so-called late reaction, develops 6 to 10 h later. In a minority only a late reaction occurs. In some individuals following a single exposure marked cyclic changes in airway lability may recur daily for a variable period.

The mechanism by which an inhaled antigen can provoke an acute episode of asthma is unknown but seems to depend, in part, upon antigen-antibody interactions on the surface of pulmonary mast cells with the subsequent generation and release of the mediators of immediate hypersensitivity. Current postulates hold that very small antigenic particles penetrate the lung's defenses and come in contact with mast cells that are interdigitating with the epithelium at the luminal surface of the central airways. The subsequent elaboration of mediators then produces the sequence outlined above. The mediators released—histamine; bradykinin; the leukotrienes C, D, and E; platelet activating factor; prostaglandins PGG_2, $PGF_{2\alpha}$, and PGD_2, and thromboxane A_2—produce an intense inflammatory reaction with bronchoconstriction, vascular congestion, and edema formation. In addition to their ability to produce prolonged contraction of airway smooth muscle and mucosal edema, the leukotrienes also produce some of the other pathophysiologic features of asthma such as increased mucus production and impaired mucociliary transport mechanisms. The chemotactic factors that are elaborated, such as eosinophil and neutrophil chemotactic factors of anaphylaxis and leukotriene B_4, bring eosinophils, platelets, and polymorphonuclear leukocytes to the site of the reaction. One of the most important of these may be the eosinophil; when activated, these cells can produce leukotriene C_4 and platelet activating factor and thereby contribute directly to airway narrowing and edema. They also can cause mast cells to release histamine and chemotactic factors which could set up a self-sustaining cycle in which additional secondary effector cells including more eosinophils are brought to the site of the reaction. Equally important, degranulation of eosinophils can release major basic protein and eosinophil cationic protein into the airways, thus causing cilia to stop beating and a disruption of mucosal integrity with exfoliation of cells into the bronchial lumen in the form of Creola bodies.

Pharmacologic stimuli The drugs most commonly associated with the induction of acute episodes of asthma are aspirin, coloring agents such as tartrazine, beta-adrenergic antagonists, and sulfiting agents. The typical aspirin-sensitive respiratory syndrome primarily affects adults, although the condition may be seen in childhood. This problem usually begins with perennial vasomotor rhinitis that is followed by a hyperplastic rhinosinusitis with nasal polyps. Progressive asthma then appears. On exposure to even very small quantities of aspirin, affected individuals typically develop ocular and nasal congestion and acute, often severe, episodes of airway obstruction. The prevalence of aspirin sensitivity in asthmatic subjects varies from study to study, but many authorities feel that 10 percent is a reasonable figure. There is a great deal of cross reactivity between aspirin and other nonsteroidal anti-inflammatory compounds. Indomethacin, fenoprofen, naproxen, zomepirac sodium, ibuprofen, mefenamic acid, and phenylbutazone are particularly important in this regard. On the other hand, acetaminophen, sodium salicylate, choline salicylate, salicylamide, and propoxyphene are well tolerated. The exact frequency of cross reactivity to tartrazine and other dyes in aspirin-sensitive asthmatic subjects is also controversial, and again 10 percent is the commonly accepted figure. This peculiar complication of aspirin-sensitive asthma is particularly insidious, however, in that tartrazine and other potentially troublesome dyes are widely present in the environment and may be unknowingly ingested by sensitive patients.

Patients with aspirin sensitivity can be desensitized by daily administration of the drug. Following this form of therapy cross tolerance also develops to other nonsteroidal anti-inflammatory agents. The mechanism by which aspirin and other such drugs produce bronchospasm is unknown; however, immediate hypersensitivity does not seem to be involved.

Beta-adrenergic antagonists regularly produce airway obstruction in asthmatics as well as in others with heightened airway reactivity and should be avoided in such individuals. Even the selective $beta_1$ agents have this propensity, particularly at higher doses. In fact, even the local use of $beta_1$ blockers in the eye for the treatment of glaucoma has been associated with worsening asthma.

Sulfiting agents, such as potassium metabisulfite, potassium and sodium bisulfite, sodium sulfite, and sulfur dioxide, which are widely used in the food and pharmaceutical industry as sanitizing and preservative agents, can also produce acute airway obstruction in sensitive individuals. Exposure usually follows ingestion of food or beverages containing these compounds, e.g., salads, fresh fruit, potatoes, shellfish, and wine. Exacerbation of asthma has been reported following the use of sulfite-containing topical ophthalmic solutions, intravenous glucocorticoids, and some inhalational bronchodilator solutions. The incidence and mechanism of action of this phenomenon are unknown. When suspected, the diagnosis can be confirmed by either oral or inhalational provocations.

Environment and air pollution (See Chap. 206) Environmental causes of asthma are usually related to climatic conditions that promote the concentration of atmospheric pollutants and antigens. These conditions tend to develop in heavy industrial or densely populated urban areas and are frequently associated with thermal inversions or other situations associated with stagnant air masses. In these circumstances, although the general population can develop respiratory symptoms, patients with asthma and other respiratory diseases tend to be more severely affected. The air pollutants known to have this effect are ozone, nitrogen dioxide, and sulfur dioxide. The last needs to be present in high concentrations and produces its greatest effects during periods of high ventilation.

Occupational factors (See Chap. 206) Occupational-related asthma is a significant health problem, and acute and chronic airway obstruction has been reported to follow exposure to a large number of compounds used in many types of industrial processes: bronchoconstriction can result from working with, or exposure to, *metal salts* (platinum, chrome, and nickel); *wood and vegetable dusts* (oak, western red cedar, grain, flour, castor bean, green coffee bean, mako, gum acacia, karay gum, and tragacanth); *pharmaceutical agents* (antibiotics, piperazine, and cimetidine); *industrial chemicals and plastics* (toluene diisocyanate, phthalic acid anhydride, trimellitic anhydride, persulfates, ethylenediamine, paraphenylenediamine, and various dyes); *biologic enzymes* (laundry detergents and pancreatic enzymes); and *animal and insect dusts, serums, and secretions*. It is important to recognize that exposure to sensitizing chemicals, particularly those used in paints, solvents, and plastics, can also occur during leisure or non-work-related activities.

The underlying mechanisms for this airway obstruction appear to be three in number: (1) in some cases the offending agent results in the formation of a specific IgE, and the cause seems immunologic (the immunologic reaction can be immediate, late, or dual); (2) materials being employed, in other cases, cause a direct liberation of bronchoconstrictor substances; and (3) work-related irritant substances, in still other cases, directly or reflexly stimulate the airways of either latent or frank asthmatics. With occupational exposures, other than those that give an immediate and dual immunologic reaction, the patients give a characteristic cyclic history. They are well when they arrive at work; symptoms develop toward the end of the shift, progress after leaving the work site, and then regress. Absence from work during weekends or vacation periods brings about a remission. Frequently, there are similar symptoms in fellow employees.

Infections Respiratory infections are the most common of the stimuli that evoke acute exacerbations of asthma. Well-controlled investigations have demonstrated that respiratory viruses and not bacteria or allergy are the major etiologic factors. In young children, the most important infectious agents are respiratory syncytial virus and parainfluenza virus. In older children and adults, rhinovirus and influenza virus predominate as pathogens. Simple colonization of the tracheobronchial tree is insufficient to evoke acute episodes of bronchospasm, and attacks of asthma occur only when symptoms of an ongoing respiratory tract infection are, or have been, present. The mechanism by which viruses induce asthma is unknown, but it is probable that the resulting inflammatory changes in the airway mucosa alter host defenses and make the tracheobronchial tree more susceptible to exogenous stimuli. Supporting evidence for this concept is derived from the fact that the airway responsiveness of even normal (nonasthmatic) subjects to nonspecific stimuli is transiently increased after a viral infection. Increased airway responsiveness can last from 2 to 8 weeks after the infection in both normals and asthmatics.

Exercise Asthma can also be induced or made worse by physical exertion. Provocation of bronchospasm by exercise is probably operative to some extent in every asthmatic patient, and in some it may be the only trigger mechanism that will produce symptoms. In the latter circumstance, when such patients are followed for sufficient periods of time, they often develop recurring episodes of airway obstruction independent of exercise: thus, the onset of this problem can frequently serve as the first manifestation of the full-blown asthmatic syndrome. The mechanism by which exercise produces acute exacerbations of asthma is related to the thermal changes that develop in the intrathoracic airways as heat and water are transferred from the mucosa to the inspired air to bring the latter to body conditions before it reaches the alveoli. The higher the ventilation and the colder, hence drier, the inspired air, the more the airway temperature falls, and so there is a significant interaction between the stress of the exercise task, the climatic environment in which it is performed, and the magnitude of the postexertional obstruction. Thus, for the same inspired air conditions, running will produce a more severe attack of asthma than will walking. Conversely, for a given task, the inhalation of cold air during its performance will markedly enhance the response, while warm, humid air will blunt or abolish it. Consequently, activities such as ice hockey, cross-country skiing, or ice skating are more provocative than is swimming in an indoor heated pool. The mechanism by which airway thermal changes evoke obstruction may be related to the hyperemia and engorgement of the microvasculature of the bronchial circulation brought about by rapid rewarming after the loss of heat described above.

Emotional stress Abundant objective data now exist which demonstrate that psychological factors can interact with the asthmatic diathesis to worsen or ameliorate the disease process. The pathways and nature of the interactions are complex but have been shown to be operational to some extent in almost half of the patients studied. Changes in airway caliber seem to be mediated through modification of vagal efferent activity. The most frequently studied variable has been that of suggestion, and the weight of current evidence is that it can be quite an important influence in selected asthmatics. When psychically responsive individuals are given the appropriate suggestion, they can actually decrease or increase the pharmacologic effects of adrenergic and cholinergic stimuli on their airways. The extent to which psychological factors participate in the induction and/or continuation of any given acute exacerbation is unknown but probably varies from patient to patient and in the same patient from episode to episode.

PATHOLOGY In a patient who has died of acute asthma, the most striking feature of the lungs at necropsy is their gross overdistention and failure to collapse when the pleural cavities are opened. When the lungs are cut, numerous gelatinous plugs of exudate are found in the majority of the bronchial branches down to the terminal bronchiole. Histologic examination shows hypertrophy of the bronchial smooth muscle, hyperplasia of mucosal and submucosal vessels, mucosal edema, denudation of the surface epithelium, pronounced thickening of the basement membrane, and eosinophilic infiltrates in the bronchial wall. In asthmatic patients who die from trauma and causes other than asthma itself, mucous casts, basement membrane thickening, and eosinophilic infiltrates are frequently observed. In both situations there is an absence of any of the well-recognized forms of destructive emphysema.

PATHOPHYSIOLOGY AND CLINICAL CORRELATES The pathophysiologic hallmark of asthma is a reduction in airway diameter brought about by contraction of smooth muscle, edema of the bronchial wall, and thick tenacious secretions. Although the relative contributions of each component to the patient's ventilatory impairment are unknown, the net result is an increase in airway resistance, decreased forced expiratory volumes and flow rates, hyperinflation of the lungs and thorax, increased work of breathing, alterations in respiratory muscle function, changes in elastic recoil, abnormal distribution of both ventilation and pulmonary blood flow, mismatched ratios, and altered arterial blood gases. Thus, although asthma is considered to be primarily a disease of airways, virtually all aspects of pulmonary function are compromised during an acute attack. In addition, in very symptomatic patients there frequently is electrocardiographic evidence of right ventricular hypertrophy, and pulmonary hypertension can be found. Quantification of the changes that develop during an acute episode of asthma demonstrate that when a patient presents for therapy, his or her forced vital capacity tends to be $\leq$50 percent of normal. The 1-s forced expiratory volume (FEV_1) averages 30 percent of predicted, while the maximum and minimum midexpiratory flow rates are reduced to 20 percent or less of expected. In keeping with the alterations in mechanics, the associated air-trapping is substantial. In acutely ill patients, residual volume (RV) frequently approaches 400 percent of normal, while functional residual capacity doubles. The patients tend to report that their attacks have ended clinically when their RV has fallen to 200 percent of its predicted value and when the FEV_1 rises to 50 percent.

Hypoxia is a universal finding during acute exacerbations, but frank ventilatory failure is relatively uncommon, being observed in 10 to 15 percent of patients presenting for therapy. Most asthmatics have hypocapnia and a respiratory alkalosis. Statistically, the finding of normal arterial carbon dioxide tension tends to be associated with quite severe levels of obstruction and consequently, when found in a symptomatic individual, should be viewed as impending respiratory failure and treated as such. Equally, the presence of metabolic acidosis in the setting of acute asthma heralds severe obstruction. Usually, there are no clinical counterparts to the derangements in blood gases. Cyanosis is a very late sign. Thus, a dangerous level of hypoxia can go undetected. Likewise the signs which are attributable to carbon dioxide retention such as sweating, tachycardia, and wide pulse pressure or to acidosis such as tachypnea do not tend to be of great value in predicting the presence of hypercapnia or hydrogen ion excess in individual patients, for they are too frequently seen in anxious patients with more moderate disease to be of much use. Consequently, trying to judge the state of an acutely ill patient's ventilatory status on clinical grounds alone can be extremely hazardous and should not be relied upon with any confidence. Arterial blood gas tensions, therefore, must be measured.

The symptoms of asthma consist of a triad of dyspnea, cough, and wheezing, the latter often being regarded as the *sine qua non*. In its most typical form asthma is an episodic disease, and all three symptoms coexist. Attacks often occur at night, for reasons which are not clear but may relate to fluctuations in airway receptor thresholds that may result from circadian variations in the circulating levels of endogenous catecholamines and histamine. Attacks may also abruptly follow exposure to a specific allergen, physical exertion, a viral respiratory infection, or emotional excitement. At the onset the patient experiences a sense of constriction in the chest, often with a nonproductive cough. Respiration becomes audibly harsh, and wheezing in both phases of respiration becomes prominent, expiration becomes prolonged, and patients frequently have tachypnea, tachycardia, and mild systolic hypertension. The lungs rapidly become overinflated, and the anterior-posterior diameter of the thorax increases. If the attack is severe or prolonged, the accessory muscles become visibly active and frequently a paradoxical pulse will develop. These two signs have been found to be extremely valuable in indicating the severity of the obstruction. In the presence of either, pulmonary function tends to be significantly more impaired than in its absence. It is important to note that the development of these signs depends upon the generation of large negative intrathoracic pressures. Thus, if the patient's breathing is shallow, these signs could be absent even though obstruction is quite severe. The other signs and symptoms of asthma imperfectly reflect the physiologic alterations that are present, so much so that if one relies upon the loss of subjective complaints, or even the sign of wheezing, as being the end point at which therapy for an acute attack should be terminated, an enormous reservoir of residual disease is missed.

Termination of the episode is frequently marked by a cough producing thick stringy mucus which often takes the form of casts of the distal airways (Curschmann's spirals), and when examined microscopically often shows eosinophils and Charcot-Leyden crystals. In extreme situations, wheezing may markedly lessen or even disappear completely, cough may become extremely ineffective, and the patient may begin a gasping type of respiratory pattern. These findings imply extensive mucous plugging and impending suffocation. Ventilatory assistance by mechanical means may be required. Atelectasis due to inspissated secretions may occasionally occur with asthmatic attacks. Other complications such as spontaneous pneumothorax and/or pneumomediastinum are rare.

Less typically, a patient with asthma may complain of intermittent episodes of nonproductive cough or dyspnea only on exertion. Unlike other asthmatics when examined during their symptomatic periods, these patients tend to have normal breath sounds but may wheeze after repeated forced exhalations and/or may show dynamic ventilatory impairments when tested in the laboratory. In the absence of both, a bronchoprovocation may be required to make the diagnosis.

The differentiation of asthma from other diseases associated with dyspnea and wheezing is usually not difficult, particularly if the patient is seen during an acute episode. The physical findings and symptoms listed above, and the history of periodic attacks, are quite characteristic. A personal or family history of allergic diseases such as eczema, rhinitis, or urticaria is valuable contributory evidence. *Upper airway obstruction by tumor* or *laryngeal edema* can occasionally be confused with asthma. Typically, such a patient will present with stridor, and the harsh respiratory sounds can be localized to the area of the trachea. Diffuse wheezing throughout both lung fields is usually absent. However, differentiation can sometimes be difficult, and indirect laryngoscopy or bronchoscopy may be required. Asthmalike symptoms in patients with glottic dysfunction have been described. These individuals close their glottis during inspiration and produce episodic attacks of severe airway obstruction, yet they do not respond to standard therapy. Frequently they produce enough obstruction to develop carbon dioxide retention. However, unlike asthma the arterial oxygen tension is well preserved, and the alveolar-arterial gradient for oxygen narrows during the episode and does not widen as is the case with lower airway obstruction. To establish the diagnosis of glottic dysfunction, the glottis should be examined when the patient is symptomatic. A normal examination at this time excludes the diagnosis; normal findings during asymptomatic periods do not.

Persistent wheezing localized to one area of the chest in association with paroxysms of cough indicates *endobronchial disease* such as foreign-body aspiration, neoplasms, or bronchial stenosis.

The signs and symptoms of *acute left ventricular failure* can occasionally mimic asthma, but the findings of moist basilar rales, gallop rhythms, blood-tinged sputum, and other signs of heart failure (Chap. 182) allow the appropriate diagnosis to be reached.

Recurrent episodes of bronchospasm can occur with *carcinoid tumors* (Chap. 262), *recurrent pulmonary emboli* (Chap. 213), and *chronic bronchitis* (Chap. 210). In the last there are no true symptom-free periods in that one can usually obtain a history of chronic cough and sputum production as a background upon which acute attacks of wheezing are superimposed. Recurrent emboli, particularly in young women on oral contraceptives, are occasionally very difficult to separate from asthma. Frequently, these patients will present with episodes of breathlessness, particularly on exertion, and they can sometimes wheeze. Pulmonary function studies may show evidence of peripheral airway obstruction (Chap. 201), and when these changes are present, lung scans may also be abnormal. The therapeutic response to bronchodilators, discontinuation of the contraceptives, and institution of anticoagulant therapy may be helpful, but pulmonary angiography may be necessary in order to establish the correct diagnosis.

Eosinophilic pneumonias (Chap. 205) are often associated with asthmatic symptoms as are various chemical pneumonias and exposures to insecticides and cholinergic drugs. Bronchospasm can occasionally be a manifestation of *systemic vasculitis* with pulmonary involvement.

LABORATORY FINDINGS It is difficult to establish the diagnosis of asthma in the laboratory, for no single test is conclusive. Positive wheal-and-flare reactions to skin tests can be demonstrated to various allergens, but that finding does not necessarily correlate with the intrapulmonary events. Sputum and blood eosinophilia and measurement of serum IgE levels are also helpful but are not specific for asthma. Chest roentgenograms showing hyperinflation are nondiagnostic, as are tests of pulmonary function. The latter, however, are quite useful in that one can measure the degree of obstruction present, document its reversible nature, and, when combined with provocational challenges, demonstrate the airway hyperirritability so characteristic of this disease. Furthermore, the performance of forced vital capacity maneuvers is very helpful in the evaluation of acute asthmatic attacks. A reduction in the FEV_1 to less than 25 percent of that predicted or to less than 0.75 liters with little or no response following the administration of a bronchodilator indicates that the patient should receive very careful surveillance in conjunction with intensive treatment.

THERAPY Elimination of the causative agent(s) from the environment of an allergic asthmatic is the most successful means available for treating this condition (for details on avoidance see Chap. 267). Desensitization or immunotherapy with extracts of the suspected allergens has enjoyed widespread favor, but controlled studies are limited and have not proved it to be highly effective.

Acute episodes of bronchial asthma represent one of the most common respiratory emergencies seen in the practice of medicine, and it is essential that the physician recognize which episodes of airway obstruction are life threatening and which patients demand what level of care. This can be readily accomplished by assessing selected clinical parameters in combination with measures of expiratory flow and gas exchange. The presence of a paradoxical pulse, use of accessory muscles, and marked hyperinflation of the thorax signify severe airway obstruction, and failure of these signs to remit within short order following aggressive therapy mandates objective monitoring of the patient using arterial blood gases and some index of pulmonary mechanics.

In general, there is a direct correlation between the severity of the obstruction with which the patient presents and the time that it takes to resolve it. Those individuals with the most impairment typically have multiple causes for their airway narrowing and require the most extensive therapy for resolution. In these circumstances, if the clinical signs of a paradoxical pulse and accessory muscle use are diminishing, and/or if peak expiratory flow rate is increasing, there is no need to change medications or doses. One need only to continue to follow the patient. If, however, peak flow is falling or if the magnitude of the pulsus paradoxicus is increasing, serial measures of arterial blood gases are required as well as a reconsideration of the therapeutic modalities being employed. If the patient has hypocarbia, one can afford to continue the current approaches a while longer. On the other hand, if the Pa_{CO_2} is within the normal range, or if it is elevated, the patient should be monitored in an intensive care setting and therapy should be intensified in order to reverse or arrest the patient's respiratory failure.

Drug treatment The drugs used in the treatment of asthma may be conveniently grouped into five major categories: beta-adrenergic agonists, methylxanthines, glucocorticoids, chromones, and anticholinergics. No one group is effective against all of the pathologic processes producing the disease, and since the degree of relief of airway obstruction is frequently incomplete with the use of a single agent, multiple drug regimens are commonplace.

ADRENERGIC STIMULANTS The drugs in this category consist of the catecholamines, resorcinols, and saligenins. These agents are analogues and produce airway dilatation through stimulation of beta receptors with the resultant formation of cyclic AMP. The catecholamines in widespread clinical use are epinephrine, isoproterenol, isoetharine, rimiterol, and hexoprenaline. The latter two are not available in the United States. As a group these compounds are short-acting and effective only by inhalational or parenteral routes. Epinephrine and isoproterenol are not $beta_2$-selective and have considerable chronotropic and inotropic cardiac effects. Epinephrine also has substantial alpha-stimulating effects. The usual dose is 0.3 to 0.5 mL of a 1:1000 solution administered subcutaneously. Isoproterenol is devoid of alpha activity and is the most potent agent of this group. It is usually administered in a 1:200 solution by inhalation. Controlled studies have shown that repetitive doses of epinephrine or isoproterenol are considerably more efficacious than the use of methylxanthines in the therapy of acute exacerbations of asthma. Isoetharine is the most $beta_2$-selective compound of this class, but is a relatively weak bronchodilator. It is employed as an aerosol and supplied as a 1% solution. The pharmacologies of hexoprenaline and rimiterol are similar to isoetharine.

The commonly used resorcinols are metaproterenol, terbutaline, and fenoterol, and the most widely known saligenin is albuterol, or salbutamol. With the exception of metaproterenol, these drugs are highly selective for the respiratory tract and virtually devoid of significant cardiac effects except in high doses. They are active by all routes of administration, and because their chemical structures allow them to bypass the metabolic processes used to degrade the catecholamines, their effects are long-lasting, exceeding 6 h in many studies.

Multiple studies now exist that demonstrate that the sympathomimetics are the drugs of choice in treating acute episodes of asthma. Based upon in vivo and in vitro data, there is little question that there is a range of potency among the currently available adrenergic agonists. However, the clinical importance of these observations is unclear, and in the main, differences in potency and duration between agents can be eliminated by adjusting doses and/or administration schedules. Non-$beta_2$ selective drugs tend to produce greater side effects such as tachycardia and nervousness, and most authorities recommend using long acting selective $beta_2$ agonists as initial therapy. The major side effect of the latter class is tremor.

The method by which beta agonists are administered is of great importance since it influences both the clinical response and the metabolic fate. Inhalation is the route of choice in that it increases the bronchial selectivity of these drugs and allows maximal bronchodilation to occur with fewer side effects than other routes of administration. This is true not just in maintenance therapy but also during the treatment of severe acute obstruction. In the past it was fashionable to treat episodes of severe asthma with intravenous sympathomimetics such as isoproterenol. This approach no longer appears justifiable. Isoproterenol infusions clearly can induce myocardial damage and even the $beta_2$ selective agents such as terbutaline and albuterol when given intravenously offer no advantages over the inhaled route.

METHYLXANTHINES Theophylline, and its various salts, are medium potency bronchodilators. Like the beta agonists, they improve the movement of airway mucus and may decrease the release of mediators. Although efficacious, the drugs in this class are not as potent as the sympathomimetics, and they have a narrower therapeutic-toxic window. The mechanism responsible for the bronchodilator effect of the methylxanthines is unknown. It was formerly thought that these drugs increased cyclic AMP by the inhibition of phosphodiesterase. However, the available evidence does not support this concept. The therapeutic plasma concentrations of theophylline lie between 10 and 20 μg/mL. But the dose required to achieve this level varies widely from patient to patient due to differences in the metabolism of the drug. Theophylline clearance, and thus dosage requirements, is decreased substantially in neonates and the elderly and those with acute and chronic hepatic dysfunction, cardiac decompensation, and cor pulmonale. Clearance is also decreased during febrile illnesses. Clearance is increased in children. In addition a number of important drug interactions can alter theophylline metabolism. Clearance falls with the concurrent use of erythromycin and troleandomycin, allopurinol, cimetidine, and propranolol. It rises with cigarettes, marijuana, phenobarbital, and phenytoin or any other drug that has the capability of inducing hepatic microsomal enzymes.

For maintenance therapy long-acting theophylline compounds are available and are usually given twice per day or once daily. The dose is adjusted on the basis of the clinical response with the aid of serum theophylline levels. There is some evidence that single dose administration in the evening may reduce nocturnal symptoms. In contrast to the large number of oral compounds, aminophylline is the only compound available for intravenous use. The recommendations for intravenous therapy in children aged 9 to 16 and young adult smokers not currently receiving theophylline products are as follows: a loading dose of 6 mg/kg is given followed by an infusion of 1.0 mg/kg per hour for the next 12 h and then 0.8 mg/kg per hour thereafter. In nonsmoking adults, older patients, and those with cor pulmonale, congestive heart failure, and liver disease, the loading dose remains the same but the maintenance dose is reduced to between 0.1 and 0.5 mg/kg per hour. In those patients already receiving theophylline, the loading dose is frequently withheld or in extreme situations given in a reduced amount at 0.5 mg/kg.

The most common side effects of theophylline are nervousness, nausea, vomiting, anorexia, and headache. At plasma levels greater than 30 μg/mL there is a risk of seizures and cardiac arrhythmias.

GLUCOCORTICOIDS Glucocorticoids have been used for many years in the treatment of asthma, but controversy still surrounds such basic issues as their specific indication and dose. Glucocorticoids are not bronchodilators, and their major use is in reducing airway inflammation. Although it is difficult to provide precise recommendations because objective data are lacking, there are several situations in the management of acute and chronic asthma in which all would agree that steroids should be employed. In acute illness, that is, when severe airway obstruction is not resolving, or is even worsening despite intense optimal bronchodilator therapy, and in chronic disease, steroids are most helpful when there has been failure of a previously optimal regimen with frequent recurrences of symptoms of progressive severity.

The dose that one should use is a matter of debate. Most would agree that sufficient quantities should be administered to achieve a plasma cortisol level of 100 μg/dL, but objective data supporting this figure do not yet exist. However, data are accumulating that indicate that very high doses do not offer advantage over more conventional amounts. For example, 6 mg/kg per day of hydrocortisone has been shown to produce the same effects as 80 mg/kg per day in status asthmaticus, and 15 to 20 mg of methylprednisolone every 6 h has the same consequences as doses eight to ten times greater. In most acute situations the intravenous administration of 4 mg/kg of hydrocortisone (or equivalent) as a loading dose, followed several hours later by an infusion regulated to deliver 3 mg/kg every 6 h will suffice. It should be emphasized that the effects of steroids in acute asthma are not immediate and may not be seen for 6 h or more after their initial administration. Consequently, it is mandatory to continue vigorous bronchodilator therapy during this interval. After 24 to 72 h, depending upon response, the patient can be switched to oral agents. A usual starting point is 40 to 60 mg prednisone as a single daily morning dose. The amount can then be reduced by half every third to fifth day. More rapid tapering frequently results in recurrent obstruction. In situations in which it appears that continued steroid therapy will be needed, an alternate-day schedule should be instituted to minimize side effects. This is particularly important in children, since continuous corticosteroid administration interrupts growth. Long-acting preparations such as dexamethasone should not be used in this approach for they defeat the purpose of alternate-day schedules by causing prolonged suppression of the pituitary-adrenal axis.

Several inhaled steroids of high topical potency are available and greatly facilitate the withdrawal of oral agents. They are also useful in reducing airway reactivity and as an alternative to oral glucocorticoids in situations where asthma symptoms are escalating. The former effect is quite important and data are accumulating that a reduction in airway reactivity can result in decreased morbidity. Hyperadrenal corticism and adrenal suppression are not major issues, and the most frequent side effect is symptomatic oropharyngeal candidiasis. This can be controlled by the use of a spacing device on the metered-dose inhaler.

CHROMONES Cromolyn sodium is not a bronchodilator. Its major therapeutic effect is the inhibition of degranulation of mast cells, thereby preventing the release of the chemical mediators of anaphylaxis. The drug does not inhibit the combination of antigen with antibody, nor does it affect the fixation of IgE to mast cells. Cromolyn has been shown to be of use in atopic and nonatopic asthmatics, and it blunts exercise-induced asthma in both children and adults. Numerous trials have shown that about 75 percent of patients derive worthwhile benefits from the drug in terms of reduction of medications and improvement in symptoms. Cromolyn, like inhaled steroids, can lower airway reactivity, and both drugs together may produce additive effects. Therapy with cromolyn is best initiated between attacks or in periods of relative remission. If no response is noted by 4 to 6 weeks, the drug can be discontinued. A newer agent, nedocromil, with a greater spectrum of activity, is available in Europe.

ANTICHOLINERGICS Anticholinergic drugs, such as atropine sulfate, are known to produce bronchodilatation in patients with asthma, but their use has been limited by systemic side effects. Nonabsorbable quaternary ammonium (atropine methylnitrate and ipratropium bromide) aerosol agents have undergone extensive trials and have been found to be both effective and remarkably free of untoward effects. They may be of particular benefit for patients with coexistent heart disease, in whom use of methylxanthines and beta stimulants may be dangerous. Furthermore, evidence is accumulating that addition of anticholinergics may enhance the bronchodilatation achieved by sympathomimetics. However, they are less potent and are slow to act (60 to 90 min may be required before peak bronchodilatation is achieved).

MISCELLANEOUS Opiates, sedatives, and tranquilizers should be absolutely avoided in the acutely ill asthmatic because the risk of depressing alveolar ventilation is great and respiratory arrest has been reported to occur shortly after their use. Admittedly most individuals are anxious and frightened, but experience has shown that they can be calmed equally well by the physician's presence and reassurances. Beta-adrenergic blockers and parasympathetic agonists should be avoided, or used with great caution, for they can cause marked deterioration in lung function.

Expectorants and mucolytic agents have enjoyed great vogue in the past, but they do not add significantly to the treatment of the acute or chronic phases of this disease. Mucolytic agents such as acetylcysteine may actually produce bronchospasm when administered to susceptible asthmatics. This can be overcome by aerosolizing them in solution with a beta-adrenergic agent. The use of intravenous fluids in the treatment of acute asthma has also been advocated. There is little evidence to indicate that this adjunct hastens recovery.

SPECIAL INSTRUCTIONS The treatment of patients with asthma who have coexisting conditions such as heart disease or pregnancy does not differ materially from that outlined above. Inhaled therapy with $beta_2$ selective agents is the mainstay, and the doses administered should be the lowest possible quantities required to produce the desired therapeutic effects. Such patients should routinely be given cromolyn and/or inhaled steroids to prevent acute episodes.

PROGNOSIS AND CLINICAL COURSE Death from asthma is uncommon. Statistics for the United States indicate a death rate of approximately 0.3 per 100,000 persons. In the last several years, there has been concern that asthma death rates are increasing. The data, however, are not sufficiently compelling to result in uniform acceptance.

Information on the clinical course of asthma suggests a good prognosis for 50 to 80 percent of all patients, particularly those whose disease is mild and develops in childhood. The number of children still having asthma 7 to 10 years after the initial diagnosis varies from 26 to 78 percent with an average of 46 percent; however, the percentage who continue to have severe disease is relatively low (6 to 19 percent). The natural course of asthma in adult life has been little investigated. Some studies suggest that spontaneous remissions occur in approximately 20 percent of those who develop the disease as adults and 40 percent or so can be expected to improve with less frequent and severe attacks as they grow older.

REFERENCES

BURROWS B: The natural history of asthma. J Allergy Clin Immunol 80:373, 1987

FANTA CH, MCFADDEN ER JR: Status Asthmaticus, in *Current Therapy in Internal Medicine*, TM Bayless et al (eds). Philadelphia, Decker, 1984, pp 6–10

KALINER MA, MCFADDEN ER JR: Bronchial asthma, in *Immunological Diseases*, M Samter et al (eds). Boston, Little Brown, 1988, pp 1067–1118

MCFADDEN ER JR: Asthma: Airway dynamics, cardiac function, and clinical correlates, in *Allergy: Principles and Practice*, E Middleton et al (eds). St Louis, CV Mosby, 1988, pp 1018–1036

SHELLER JR: Asthma: Emerging concepts and potential therapies. Am J Med Sci 293:298, 1987

205 HYPERSENSITIVITY PNEUMONITIS

GARY W. HUNNINGHAKE/HAL B. RICHERSON

DEFINITION Hypersensitivity pneumonitis (HP), or extrinsic allergic alveolitis, is an immunologically induced inflammation of the lung parenchyma, involving alveolar walls and terminal airways, secondary to repeated inhalation of a variety of organic dusts and other agents by a susceptible host. In contrast to many of the other interstitial lung diseases, the etiology of this interstitial and alveolar filling disease is known. Although a number of etiologic agents have been identified, most are rare, and a few well-documented syndromes are associated with the vast majority of cases. The diagnosis of HP requires a constellation of clinical, radiographic, physiologic, pathologic, and immunologic criteria, each of which by itself is rarely pathognomonic, and the preferred treatment is avoidance of the causative antigen.

ETIOLOGY Agents implicated as causes of HP include those listed in Table 205-1. Many cases of HP occurring in various occupations involve exposure to similar agents, particularly the thermophilic actinomycetes. Except for exotic occupational exposures, the usual sources of causative antigens are "moldy" hay, silage, or grain; pet birds; and heating, cooling, and humidification systems. Simple chemicals, such as isocyanates, may also cause hypersensitivity pneumonitis.

PATHOGENESIS The finding that precipitating antibodies against extracts of moldy hay were demonstrable in most patients with farmer's lung led to the early conclusion that HP was an immune-complex-mediated reaction. Subsequent investigations of HP in human beings and animal models provided evidence for the importance of cell-mediated hypersensitivity. The very early (acute) reaction is characterized by an increase in polymorphonuclear leukocytes in the alveoli and small airways. This early lesion is followed by an influx of mononuclear cells into the lung and the formation of granulomas. The latter lesion appears to be a classic delayed hypersensitivity reaction to repeated inhalation of antigen and adjuvant-active materials.

Bronchoalveolar lavage in patients with HP consistently demonstrates an increase in T lymphocytes in lavage fluid (a finding which is also observed in patients with other granulomatous lung disorders). Patients with recent or continual exposure to antigen may also have an increase in polymorphonuclear leukocytes in lavage fluid. Increased numbers of mast cells have also been reported. In most patients examined during recovery from acute disease, the T lymphocytes in lavage fluid are predominantly the suppressor-cytotoxic T-cell subset, which expresses surface antigens (CD8) detected by OKT8 or Leu 2a monoclonal antibodies. In patients with very recent exposure to antigen, however, the numbers of CD4-bearing helper T cells ($OKT4^+$ or Leu $3a^+$) may increase in lavage fluid. Similar findings may be present in similarly exposed, asymptomatic individuals. These observations suggest that there is an active modulation of granuloma formation in the lung by immunoregulatory T cells in this disorder.

CLINICAL PRESENTATION The *clinical picture* varies from patient to patient and is related to the frequency and intensity of exposure to the causative antigen and perhaps other host factors. The presentation can be *acute, subacute,* or *chronic*. In the *acute form*, symptoms such as cough, fever, chills, malaise, and dyspnea may occur 6 to 8 h after exposure to the antigen and usually clear within a few days if there is no further exposure to antigen. The *subacute form* often appears insidiously over a period of weeks marked by cough and dyspnea and may progress to cyanosis and severe dyspnea requiring hospitalization. In some patients, a subacute form of the disease may persist after an acute presentation of the disorder, especially if there is continued exposure to antigen. In most patients with the acute or subacute form of HP, the symptoms, signs, and other manifestations of HP disappear within days, weeks, or months if the causative agent is no longer inhaled. Transformation to a chronic form of the disease may occur in patients with continued antigen exposure, but the frequency of such progression is uncertain. The *chronic form* may also present as a gradually progressive interstitial disease associated with cough and exertional dyspnea without a prior history consistent with acute or subacute manifestations. Such a gradual onset frequently occurs with low-dose exposure to the antigen.

DIAGNOSIS Following acute exposure to antigen, neutrophilia and lymphopenia are frequently present. Eosinophilia is not a feature. All forms of the disease may be associated with elevations in erythrocyte sedimentation rate, C-reactive protein, rheumatoid factor, and serum immunoglobulins. Antinuclear antibodies are rarely present.

Examination for *serum precipitins* against suspected antigens, such as those listed in Table 205-1, is an important part of the diagnostic workup. If found, precipitins indicate sufficient exposure to the causative agent for generation of an immunologic response. The diagnosis of HP is not established solely by the presence of

TABLE 205-1 Selected examples of hypersensitivity pneumonitis (HP)

Disease	Antigen	Source of antigen
Bagassosis	Thermophilic actinomycetes	"Moldy" bagasse (sugar cane)
Bird fancier's, breeder's, or handler's lung	Parakeet, budgerigar, pigeon, chicken, turkey proteins	Avian droppings or feathers
Cephalosporium HP	Contaminated basement (sewage)	Cephalosporium
Cheese washer's lung	*Penicillium casei*	Moldy cheese
Chemical worker's lung	Isocyanates	Polyurethane foam, varnishes, lacquer, foundry casting
Coffee worker's lung	Coffee bean dust	Coffee beans
Compost lung	*Aspergillus*	Compost
Detergent worker's disease	*Bacillus subtilis* enzymes	Detergent
Familial HP	*Bacillus subtilis*	Contaminated wood dust in walls
Farmer's lung	Thermophilic actinomycetes*	"Moldy" hay, grain, silage
Fish meal worker's lung	Fish meal dust	Fish meal
Furrier's lung	Animal fur dust	Animal pelts
Hot tub lung	*Cladosporium* sp.	Mold on ceiling
Humidifier or air-conditioner lung (ventilation pneumonitis)	*Aureobasidium pullulans* or other microorganisms	Contaminated water in humidification and forced-air air-conditioning systems
Japanese summer house HP	*Trichosporon cutaneum*	House dust? Bird droppings
Laboratory worker's HP	Male rat urine	Laboratory rat
Lycoperdonosis	*Lycoperdon* puffballs	*Puffball* spores
Malt worker's lung	*Aspergillus fumigatus* or *A. clavatus*	Moldy barley
Maple bark disease	*Cryptostroma corticale*	Maple bark
Miller's lung	*Sitophilus granarius* (wheat weevil)	Infested wheat flour
Mushroom worker's lung	Thermophilic actinomycetes,* other	Mushroom compost
Paulis HP	Paulis reagent	Laboratory reagent
Pituitary snuff taker's lung	Animal proteins	Heterologous pituitary snuff
Potato riddler's lung	Thermophilic actinomycetes,* *Aspergillus*	"Moldy" hay around potatoes
Sauna taker's lung	*Auerobasidium* sp., other	Contaminated sauna water
Sequoiosis	*Aureobasidium, Graphium* sp.	Redwood sawdust
Streptomyces albus HP	*Streptomyces albus*	Contaminated fertilizer
Suberosis	Cork dust mold	Cork dust
Tap water lung	Unknown	Contaminated tap water
Thatched roof disease	*Sacchoromonospora viridis*	Dried grasses and leaves
Tobacco worker's disease	*Aspergillus* sp.	Mold on tobacco
Winegrower's lung	*Botrytis cinerea*	Mold on grapes
Wood trimmer's disease	*Rhizopus* sp., *Mucor* sp.	Contaminated wood trimmings
Woodman's disease	*Pencillium* sp.	Oak and maple trees
Woodworker's lung	Wood dust; *Alternaria*	Oak, cedar, and mahogany dusts; pine and spruce pulp

*Thermophilic actinomycetes species include *Micropolyspora faeni, Thermoactinomyces vulgaris, T. saccharrii, T. viridis,* and *T. candidus.*

precipitins, however, since precipitins merely indicate a significant exposure to an antigen source. Precipitins are found in sera of many individuals exposed to appropriate antigens who demonstrate no other evidence of HP. False-negative results may occur because of poor-quality antigens or an inappropriate choice of antigens. Extraction of antigens from the patient's environment may at times be helpful.

No specific or distinctive *chest roentgenogram* occurs in HP. It can be normal even in symptomatic patients. The acute or subacute phase may be associated with poorly defined, patchy, or diffuse infiltrates or with discrete, nodular infiltrates. In the chronic phase, the chest x-ray usually shows a diffuse reticulonodular infiltrate. Honeycombing may eventually develop as the condition progresses. Abnormalities rarely seen in hypersensitivity pneumonitis include pleural effusion or thickening, and hilar adenopathy.

Pulmonary function studies in all forms of HP may show a restrictive pattern with loss of lung volumes, impaired diffusion capacity, decreased compliance, and an exercise-induced hypoxemia. A resting hypoxemia may be found. Functional abnormalities may gradually increase in severity or may occur rapidly following acute or subacute exposure to antigen. As the chronic stage progresses, changes consistent with airway obstruction may also become increasingly prominent.

Bronchoalveolar lavage is used in some centers to aid in diagnostic evaluation, and the characteristic features of the lavage fluid are described above.

Lung biopsy may be indicated in patients without sufficient other criteria to make a definitive diagnosis. The initial biopsy procedure is usually a transbronchial biopsy. In some patients, an open-lung biopsy may be necessary, since this procedure will provide adequate material for pathologic studies whereas transbronchial biopsy may not. Although the histopathology is distinctive, it may not be pathognomonic of HP. When the biopsy is taken during the active phase of disease, typical findings include an interstitial alveolar infiltrate consisting of plasma cells, lymphocytes, and occasional eosinophils and neutrophils, usually with accompanying granulomas. Interstitial fibrosis may be present but most often is mild in earlier stages of the disease. Some degree of bronchiolitis is found in about half the cases, whereas vasculitis is not a feature of the disorder.

The lack of standardized, nonirritating antigens and of proven controlled protocols makes *skin testing* and *inhalational challenge* useful only for experimental purposes. Similarly, *in vitro tests of cell-mediated (delayed) hypersensitivity* have not been shown to consistently correlate with clinical HP and cannot be recommended in the routine diagnostic workup.

In summary, the diagnosis in most cases is established by (1) consistent history, physical findings, pulmonary function tests, and chest x-ray, (2) exposure to a recognized antigen, and (3) finding an antibody to that antigen. In a few circumstances, bronchoalveolar lavage and/or lung biopsy may be needed. Provocation tests are research procedures and are not indicated.

Chronic HP may often be difficult to distinguish from a number of other interstitial lung disorders such as idiopathic pulmonary fibrosis, interstitial lung disease associated with a collagen vascular disorder, and drug-induced lung diseases. A negative history for use of appropriate drugs and no evidence of a systemic disorder usually exclude the presence of drug-induced lung disease or a collagen vascular disorder. In some patients, a lung biopsy may be required to differentiate chronic HP from idiopathic pulmonary fibrosis.

The lung disease associated with acute or subacute HP may clinically resemble other disorders which present with systemic symptoms and recurrent pulmonary infiltrates. These disorders include the collagen vascular disorders, drug-induced lung disease, allergic bronchopulmonary aspergillosis, and other eosinophilic pneumonias. Eosinophilic pneumonia is often associated with asthma and is typified by peripheral eosinophilia; neither of these is a feature of HP. Allergic bronchopulmonary aspergillosis is sometimes confused with HP because of the presence of precipitating antibodies to *Aspergillus fumigatus*. It is an obstructive rather than a restrictive lung disease, however, that is associated with allergic (atopic) asthma.

TREATMENT Because effective treatment depends largely on avoiding the antigen, identification of the causative agent and its source is essential. This is usually possible if the physician takes a careful environmental and occupational history or, if necessary, visits the patient's environment.

The simplest way to avoid the incriminated agent is to remove the patient from the environment or the source of the agent from the patient's environment. This recommendation cannot be taken lightly when it completely changes the life-style or livelihood of the patient. In many cases, however, the source of exposure (birds, humidifiers) can easily be removed. If occupational exposure is involved, an initial attempt can be made at antigen avoidance maneuvers least disruptive to the patient's livelihood, which usually means avoiding areas associated with heavy exposure and wearing an appropriate mask. This will not suffice for small-molecular-weight agents such as isocyanates, which require elaborate filtration devices. Pollen masks, personal dust respirators, airstream helmets, and ventilated helmets with a supply of fresh air are increasingly efficient means of purifying inhaled air. If symptoms recur or physiologic abnormalities progress in spite of these measures, then more effective measures to avoid antigen exposure must be pursued.

Compromises with environmental control pertain only to the acute, recurrent, transient clinical form of HP and must be accompanied by careful follow-up. Subacute forms are ordinarily the result of a heavy, sustained exposure. The chronic form typically results from low-grade exposure over many months to years, and the lung disease may already be partially irreversible. These patients should be advised to avoid completely all possible contact with the offending agent.

Patients with the *acute*, recurrent form of HP usually recover without need for glucocorticoids. *Subacute* HP may be associated with severe symptoms and marked physiologic impairment, and may continue to progress for several days despite hospitalization. Urgent establishment of the diagnosis and prompt institution of glucocorticoid treatment are indicated in such patients. Such therapy may also hasten recovery in patients with lesser involvement. Prednisone at a dosage of 1 mg/kg per day or its equivalent is continued for 7 to 14 days, and then tapered over the ensuing 2 to 6 weeks at a rate which depends on the patient's clinical status.

Patients with *chronic* extrinsic allergic alveolitis may gradually recover without therapy following environmental control. In many patients, however, a trial of prednisone may be useful to obtain maximal reversibility of the lung disease. Following initial prednisone therapy (1 mg/kg per day for 2 to 4 weeks), the drug is tapered to the lowest dosage that will maintain the functional status of the patient. Many patients will not require or benefit from long-term therapy if there is no further exposure to antigen.

THE EOSINOPHILIC PNEUMONIAS

The eosinophilic pneumonias are composed of distinct individual syndromes characterized by eosinophilic pulmonary infiltrates and, commonly, peripheral blood eosinophilia. Since Loeffler's initial description of a transient, benign syndrome of migratory pulmonary infiltrates and peripheral blood eosinophilia of unknown cause, this group of disorders has been enlarged to include diseases of known and unknown etiology (Table 205-2). These diseases may be considered as examples of hypersensitivity lung disease but are not to be confused with hypersensitivity pneumonitis (extrinsic allergic alveolitis) in which eosinophilia is not a feature.

When an eosinophilic pneumonia is associated with bronchial asthma, it is important to determine if the patient has extrinsic (allergic, atopic) asthma and has wheal-and-flare skin reactivity to *Aspergillus* allergens. If so, other criteria should be sought for diagnosis of *allergic bronchopulmonary aspergillosis* (ABPA) (Table 205-3). *A. fumigatus* is the most common etiologic agent, although other *Aspergillus* species have also been implicated. The chest roentgenogram in ABPA may show transient, recurrent infiltrates or may suggest the presence of proximal bronchiectasis. The bronchial asthma of ABPA likely involves an IgE-mediated hypersensitivity whereas the bronchiectasis associated with this disorder is thought to result from a deposition of immune complexes in proximal airways. Adequate treatment usually requires the long-term use of systemic glucocorticoids.

TABLE 205-2 The eosinophilic pneumonias

1 Etiology known
- *a* Allergic bronchopulmonary aspergillosis
- *b* Parasitic infestations
- *c* Drug reactions

2 Idiopathic
- *a* Loeffler's syndrome
- *b* Chronic eosinophilic pneumonia
- *c* Allergic granulomatosis of Churg and Strauss
- *d* Hypereosinophilic syndrome

Tropical eosinophilia is usually caused by filarial infection; however, eosinophilic pneumonias also occur with other parasites such as *Ascaris, Ancyclostoma* species, *Toxocara* species, and *Strongyloides stercoralis*. Tropical eosinophilia due to *Wuchereria bancrofti* or *W. malayi* occurs most commonly in southern Asia, Africa, and South America, and is treated successfully with diethylcarbamazine.

Drug-induced eosinophilic pneumonias are typified by acute reactions to nitrofurantoin which may begin 2 h to 10 days after nitrofurantoin is started, with symptoms of dry cough, fever, chills, and dyspnea; an eosinophilic pleural effusion accompanying patchy or diffuse pulmonary infiltrates may also occur. Other drugs associated with eosinophilic pneumonias include sulfonamides, penicillin, chlorpropamide, thiazides, tricyclic antidepressants, hydralazine, mephenesin, mecamylamine, nickel carbonyl vapor, gold salts, isoniazid, para-aminosalicylic acid, and others. Treatment consists of withdrawal of the incriminated drugs and the use of glucocorticoids, if necessary.

The idiopathic eosinophilic pneumonias consist of a group of diseases of varying severity. *Loeffler's syndrome* is a benign, acute eosinophilic pneumonia characterized by migrating pulmonary infiltrates and minimal clinical manifestations. *Chronic eosinophilic pneumonia* presents with significant systemic symptoms including fever, chills, night sweats, cough, anorexia, and weight loss lasting several weeks to months. The chest x-ray frequently shows peripheral infiltrates which have been described as a photographic negative of pulmonary edema. Some patients also have bronchial asthma which

TABLE 205-3 Diagnostic features of allergic bronchopulmonary aspergillosis (ABPA)

MAIN DIAGNOSTIC CRITERIA

1 Bronchial asthma
2 Pulmonary infiltrates
3 Peripheral eosinophilia (> 1000 per cubic microliter)
4 Immediate wheal-and-flare response to *Aspergillus fumigatus*
5 Serum precipitins to *A. fumigatus*
6 Elevated serum IgE
7 Central bronchiectasis

OTHER DIAGNOSTIC FEATURES

1 History of brownish plugs in sputum
2 Culture of *A. fumigatus* from sputum
3 Elevated IgE (and IgG) class antibodies specific for *A. fumigatus*

is of the intrinsic or nonallergic type. Dramatic clearing of symptoms and chest x-rays is often noted within 48 h after initiation of glucocorticoid therapy.

Allergic angiitis and granulomatosis of Churg and Strauss is a multisystem vasculitic disorder that frequently involves the skin, kidney, and nervous system in addition to the lung (Chap. 276). The disorder may occur at any age and favors persons with a history of bronchial asthma. The asthma often is progressive until the onset of fever and exaggerated eosinophilia at which time the symptoms of asthma may ease. The illness may be fulminating and the prognosis grave unless treated aggressively with glucocorticoids and immunosuppressive therapy.

The hypereosinophilic syndrome is characterized by a peripheral blood eosinophilia over 1500 eosinophils per microliter for 6 months or longer; lack of evidence for parasitic, allergic, or other known causes of eosinophilia; and signs or symptoms of multisystem organ dysfunction. Consistent features are blood and bone marrow eosinophilia with tissue infiltration by relatively mature eosinophils. The organs affected typically include the heart, lungs, liver, spleen, skin, and nervous system. Therapy of the disorder consists of glucocorticoids and/or hydroxyurea plus therapy as needed for cardiac dysfunction, which is frequently responsible for much of the morbidity and mortality in this syndrome.

REFERENCES

Hypersensitivity pneumonitis

Haslam PL et al: Mast cells, atypical lymphocytes, and neutrophils in bronchoalveolar lavage in extrinsic allergic alveolitis: Comparison with other interstitial lung disease. Am Rev Respir Dis 135:35, 1987

Hunninghake GW, Bedell GN: Interstitial lung disease: Concepts of pathogenesis. Semin Respir Med 6:31, 1984

——— et al: Inflammatory and immune processes in the human lung in health and disease: Evaluation by bronchopulmonary lavage. Am J Pathol 97:149, 1979

Leatherman JW et al: Lung T cells in hypersensitivity pneumonitis. Ann Intern Med 100:390, 1984

Richerson HB: Hypersensitivity pneumonitis (extrinsic allergic alveolitis), in *Pulmonary Diseases and Disorders*, 2d ed, AP Fishman (ed). New York, McGraw-Hill, 1988, p 667

———: Hypersensitivity pneumonitis—pathology and pathogenesis. Clin Rev Allergy 1:469, 1983

Salvaggio JE: Hypersensitivity pneumonitis. J Allergy Clin Immunol 79:558, 1987

Semenzato G et al: Different types of cytotoxic lymphocytes recovered from the lungs of patients with hypersensitivity pneumonitis. Am Rev Respir Dis 137:70, 1988

The eosinophilic pneumonias

Greenberger PA, Patterson R: Allergic bronchopulmonary aspergillosis: A model of bronchopulmonary disease with defined serologic, radiologic, pathologic and clinical findings from asthma to fatal destructive lung disease. Chest 91:165S, 1987

Malo JL et al: Studies in chronic allergic bronchopulmonary aspergillosis. 1. Clinical and physiological findings. 2. Radiological findings. 3. Immunological findings. 4. Comparison with a group of asthmatics. Thorax 32:254, 262, 269, 275, 1977

Maycock RL, Saldana MJ: Eosinophilic pneumonia, in *Pulmonary Diseases and Disorders*, 2d ed, AP Fishman (ed). New York, McGraw-Hill, 1988, p 683

Schatz M et al: The eosinophil and the lung. Arch Intern Med 142:1515, 1982

Schoenberger CI, Crystal RG: Drug-induced lung disease, in *Update IV: Harrison's Principles of Internal Medicine*, KJ Isselbacher et al (eds). New York, McGraw-Hill, 1983, p 49

Slavin RG: Allergic bronchopulmonary aspergillosis. Clin Rev Allergy 3:167, 1985

206 ENVIRONMENTAL LUNG DISEASES

FRANK E. SPEIZER

This chapter is designed to provide perspectives on ways to assess pulmonary diseases for which environmental causes are suspected. This assessment is important because removal of the patient from a harmful environment is often the only intervention that might prevent further significant deterioration or lead to improvement in a patient's condition. Furthermore, the identification of an environmentally associated disease in a single patient may lead to primary preventive strategies in other similarly exposed people who have not yet developed disease. Unless the physician specifically considers environmental exposures, these diseases and their causes will go undetected.

The exact magnitude of the problem is unknown, but there is no question that large numbers of people are at risk of developing serious respiratory disease as a result of occupational or environmental exposures. For example, even if only 5 percent (a conservative estimate) of workers currently exposed to asbestos, cotton dust, or silica are to suffer from respiratory disease as a result of their exposure, this represents more than 100,000 individuals in the United States.

Although industries are required to spend substantial amounts of capital in efforts to protect their workers, occupationally related respiratory diseases continue to occur. These diseases are often attributed to exposures in the distant past at a time when we were not aware of or at least did not consider worker protection to the degree that we do today. We have, as a society, elected to pay compensation to affected individuals, and the physician is often called upon to judge not only the physical condition of such a patient but also the degree to which the illness can be related to, or aggravated by, a particular occupational exposure.

HISTORY AND PHYSICAL EXAMINATION The patient history is of paramount importance in assessing any potential occupational or environmental exposure. Often one is dealing with potential exposures in industries or environmental settings in which the physician has little personal experience. The physician must, therefore, ask the patient to describe a suspected environmental exposure in detail.

Inquiry into specific work practices should include questions about specific contaminants involved, the availability and use of personal respiratory protection devices, the size and ventilation of workspaces, the numbers of other workers potentially at risk of exposure, and whether other coworkers have similar complaints. In addition, the patient must be questioned about alternative sources for potentially toxic exposures, including hobbies or other environmental exposures at home. Short-term exposures to potential toxic agents in the distant past also must be considered. This information can be best elicited by a detailed occupational history which inquires about every job (beginning even with part-time jobs during schooling), about the nature of the work, the materials handled, and the duration and chronologic years of employment.

Many people are aware of the potential hazards in their workplaces, and recent legislation has made it a requirement in many states that employees be informed about potentially hazardous exposures. These requirements include the provision of specific educational materials (including Material Safety Data Sheets), personal protective equipment and instructions in their use, and information on environmental control procedures. Reminders posted in the workplace may warn workers about hazardous substances. Protective clothing, lockers, and shower facilities may be considered necessary parts of the job. However, even in these ideal settings, the introduction of new processes, particularly when related to the use of new chemical compounds, may change exposure significantly, and often only the employee on the production line is aware of the change. For the physician who regularly sees patients from a particular industry, a visit to the work site can be very instructive.

The physical examination of patients with environmentally related lung diseases may help to determine the nature and severity of the pulmonary condition. Unfortunately, the pulmonary response to most injurious agents is the development of a limited number of nonspecific physical signs. These findings do not point to the specific causative agent, and other types of information must be used to arrive at an etiologic diagnosis.

PULMONARY FUNCTION TESTS AND CHEST RADIOGRAPH The use of pulmonary function tests and radiographic examinations of the chest can provide insight into the nature of the exposures which have led to the current condition of the patient and the level of impairment. Many mineral dusts produce characteristic alterations in the mechanics of breathing and lung volumes which clearly indicate a restrictive pattern (Chaps. 201 and 211). Exposures to a number of organic dusts or chemical agents capable of producing occupational asthma result in pronounced obstructive patterns of pulmonary dysfunction that may be reversible (Chap. 204). Standardized approaches for measuring the mechanics of breathing and diffusion across the alveolar membrane (Chap. 201) have been proposed for screening large industrial groups. Measurement of change in forced expiratory volume (FEV_1) before and after a working shift can be used to detect an acute bronchoconstrictive response. An acute decrement of FEV_1 over the Monday work shift is a characteristic feature of cotton textile workers with byssinosis.

For many years the chest radiograph has been used to detect and monitor the pulmonary response to mineral dusts. To provide a standardized method of recording judgments about the kind and severity of radiographic abnormalities, the International Labour Organization (ILO) International Classification of Radiographs of Pneumoconioses was developed. The ILO scheme involves classifying chest roentgenograms according to the nature and size of opacities seen and the extent of involvement of the parenchyma. However, judgments based only on chest radiographs may over- or underestimate the functional impact of pneumoconiosis. With dusts causing rounded, regular opacities, such as in coal worker's pneumoconiosis, the degree of involvement on the chest radiograph may be extensive, while pulmonary function may be only minimally impaired. In contrast, in pneumoconiosis causing linear, irregular opacities, as seen in asbestosis, the radiograph may lead to underestimation of the severity of the impairment. It is possible to have a history of exposure, moderately reduced forced vital capacity (FVC), and a reduced diffusion in asbestosis with a relatively normal chest radiograph. The radiographic findings of irregular or linear opacities are simply more difficult to separate from normal markings until relatively late in the disease. When shadows become large (radiographic lesions greater than 1 cm in diameter), the condition is termed *complicated pneumoconiosis,* sometimes called *progressive massive fibrosis* (PMF). Chest CT scanning can sometimes contribute additional useful information. However, the additional cost and radiation involved militate against using this technique except in cases where clinical and radiographic data are in conflict.

Other diagnostic procedures of use in identifying environmentally induced lung disease include evaluating heavy metal exposures (arsenic, cadmium in battery plant workers); bacteriologic studies (tuberculosis in medical care personnel, anthrax in wool sorters); fungal studies (coccidioidomycosis in southwestern farm workers, histoplasmosis in poultry or pigeon handlers); or serologic studies (psittacosis in pet shop workers or owners of sick birds, Q fever in tanners or slaughterhouse workers). Ultimately, a lung biopsy may be required both to make a morphologic diagnosis of the underlying pulmonary disease and to attempt to identify the specific etiologic agent.

MEASUREMENT OF EXPOSURE If reliable environmental sampling data are available, these sources of information should be used in assessing a patient's exposure. Since many of the chronic diseases result from exposure over many years, current environmental measurements should be combined with work histories to arrive at estimates of past exposure. However, the dose of any environmental agent is a complex interaction of chemical reaction, both at the emission source and in the ambient atmosphere, and physiologic factors, including ventilation rate and depth, which may affect transport and deposition of aerosols and gases in the lung. Even in acute conditions, when monitoring of exposure may be possible, little may be known about the actual dose received by the lung. Most of the research on health effects of air pollutants (discussed later in this chapter) has relied upon fixed-station monitoring of outdoor air, often at locations somewhat distant from the residences of the people being studied. In addition, most people spend less than 20 percent of their time outdoors. Efforts to determine the penetration rate of outdoor contaminants into the indoors suggest that these penetration rates are highly pollutant specific. Therefore, outdoor measurements can be used only in a relative sense, and they cannot be relied upon to estimate actual dose.

In situations where individual exposure to specific agents has been determined, either in a work setting or for ambient air pollutants, transport of these agents through the airways may be an important factor affecting dose. The upper airways are remarkably effective filters of both particles and gases. For example, virtually 100 percent of sulfur dioxide, a highly soluble gas, is absorbed in the upper airways during quiet breathing, and even during exercise sulfur dioxide is unlikely to penetrate beyond the large bronchi. On the other hand, nitrogen dioxide, which is less soluble, may reach the bronchioles and alveoli in sufficient quantities to result in an acute life-threatening disease in farmers exposed even briefly to the gas evolved from moldy hay in silos (silo filler's disease).

Particle size and chemistry of air contaminants also must be considered. Particles above 10 to 15 μm, because of their settling velocities in air, do not penetrate beyond the upper airways. These larger particles are often referred to as "fugitive dusts" and include pollens, other windblown dusts, and dusts resulting from mechanical industrial processes. They have little or no role in chronic respiratory disease except as possibly related to cancer (see below).

Particles below 10 μm in size are created by the burning of fossil fuel or high-temperature industrial processes resulting in condensation products from gases, fumes, or vapors. These particles are divided into two size fractions on the basis of their chemical characteristics. Particles approximately 2.5 to 10 μm (coarse-mode fraction) contain crustal elements, such as silica, aluminum, and iron. These particles mostly deposit relatively high in the tracheobronchial tree. Particles less than approximately 2.5 μm (fine-mode fraction or accumulation mode) contain sulfates, nitrates, and organic compounds. The deposition of the fine-mode particles is more often in the terminal bronchioles and alveoli. The smallest particles, those less than 0.1 μm in size, remain in the airstream and deposit in the lung only on a random basis as they come into contact with the alveolar walls through thermal forces and/or Brownian movement.

Besides the size characteristics of particles and the solubility of gases, the actual chemical composition, mechanical properties, and immunogenicity or infectivity of inhaled material determine in large part the nature of the diseases found among exposed persons.

OCCUPATIONAL EXPOSURES AND PULMONARY DISEASE

INORGANIC DUSTS **Asbestos exposure** Except in localized regions with single industrial exposures, such as coal-mining or granite-quarrying regions, the most frequent inorganic dust–related chronic pulmonary diseases are associated with industries using *asbestiform fibers.* Asbestos is a generic term for several different mineral silicates, including chrysolite, amosite, anthophyllite, and crocidolite. Approximately 9.1 million workers in the United States who had exposure to the various forms of asbestos fibers were estimated to be alive in 1980 and therefore subsequently at risk of asbestos-related diseases. Besides mining, milling, and manufacturing of asbestos products, the exceptional thermal and electric insulation properties of asbestos led to its widespread use in construction, leading to exposure of pipe fitters, boiler makers, and other workers in the building trades. In addition, asbestos is used in the manufacture of fire-smothering blankets and safety garments, as filler for plastic materials, in cement and floor tiles, and in friction materials, such as brake and clutch linings.

Exposure to asbestos is not limited to persons who directly handle the material. Cases of asbestos-related diseases have been encountered in individuals with only moderate exposure, such as the painter or electrician who works alongside the insulation worker in a shipyard, or the housewife who does no more than shake out and wash her husband's work clothes. Community exposure has probably resulted from the use of asbestos-containing material sprayed on steel girders in many large buildings as a safety feature to prevent buckling in case of fire. Clusters of cases of mesothelioma have been noted in the neighborhood of an asbestos plant in London and in the communities near asbestos mines in South Africa.

Asbestos was first used extensively in the 1940s. Starting in 1975 it has been mostly replaced with man-made mineral fibers, such as fiberglass or slag wool. However, asbestos is still used in the manufacture of brake linings, and remains as pipe and boiler insulation in hundreds of thousands of workplaces and homes. Despite current regulations mandating adequate training for any worker potentially exposed to asbestos, exposure probably continues among inexperienced demolition workers. The major health effects from exposure to asbestos are pulmonary fibrosis (asbestosis) and cancers of the respiratory tract and pleura and, rarely, peritoneum.

Asbestosis is a diffuse interstitial fibrosing disease of the lung which is directly related to the intensity and duration of exposure. Except for a history of exposure to asbestos (generally in a work setting), asbestosis resembles the other forms of diffuse interstitial fibrosis (Chap. 211). Usually at least 10 years of moderate to severe exposure has occurred before the disease becomes manifest.

Physiologic studies reveal a restrictive pattern with a decrease in lung volumes. Flow rates are commonly reduced less than would be predicted on the basis of the volume reduction. An early sign of severe disease may be a reduction in diffusing capacity.

Pulmonary fibrosis may occur following sufficient exposure to any of the asbestiform fiber types. The fibrotic lesions do not appear to relate to either shape or chemical composition of any fiber type. Recent studies indicate that during phagocytosis of the asbestos fiber, the membrane of the macrophage is damaged, which results in the release of lysosomes containing enzymes which may act to damage the lung parenchyma. The clinical manifestations are typical of those physical findings in any patient with pulmonary fibrosis (Chap. 211).

The chest radiograph can be used to determine a number of manifestations of asbestos exposure, as well as to identify specific lesions. Past exposure is specifically indicated by pleural plaques, which are characterized by either thickening or calcification along the parietal pleura, particularly along the lower lung fields, the diaphragm, and the cardiac border. Without additional manifestations, pleural plaques imply only exposure, not pulmonary impairment. Benign pleural effusions may occur, particularly in patients with abestosis, but are not necessarily restricted to those with overt disease. The fluid is sterile, but may be a serous or blood-stained exudate and may occur bilaterally. The effusion may be slowly progressive or may resolve spontaneously.

The radiographic diagnosis of asbestosis depends upon the presence of irregular or linear opacities, usually first noted in the lower lung fields and spreading into the middle and upper lung fields as the disease progresses. An indistinct heart border or a "ground glass" appearance in the lung fields is seen in some cases. As the fibrotic changes in the parenchyma begin to coalesce, the patient develops obliteration of entire acinar units with eventual formation of the classical honeycombed lung, which appears on chest radiographs as coarse infiltrates with small (about 7- to 10-μm) air spaces. No specific therapy is available in the management of patients with asbestosis. The supportive care is that of any patient with diffuse interstitial fibrosis from any cause.

In general, newly diagnosed cases will have resulted from exposure levels that were present many years before and, in spite of the patients' having left the industry, are attributable to that former exposure. Since the patient may be eligible for compensation within a specific time frame after the diagnosis of an asbestos-related disease is made, the physician making the diagnosis should be certain to inform the patient promptly. On occasion, the physician may have reason to suspect ongoing exposure from a patient's current job description or actual monitoring data. In such cases, federal or state health authorities may need to be notified. Present-day occupational safety and health regulations, if followed properly, protect workers from exposure. Because the association of smoking and asbestosis increases the risk of developing lung cancer (see below), it is extremely important to advise such patients to stop smoking.

Lung cancer (Chap. 215), either squamous cell or adenocarcinoma, is the most frequent cancer associated with asbestos exposure. The excess frequency of lung cancer in asbestos workers is associated with a minimum lapse of 15 to 19 years between first exposure and development of the disease. Persons with more exposure are at greater risk of disease. In addition, there appears to be a significant multiplicative effect which leads to a far greater risk of lung cancer in persons who are cigarette smokers and have asbestos exposure than would be expected by taking the sum of both risks. Efforts to consider these high-risk individuals for special surveillance studies, including sputum cytologic examinations and repeated chest x-rays as frequently as every 4 to 6 months, suggest that cancers can be detected at an earlier stage and that the survival of these patients may be prolonged.

Mesotheliomas (Chap. 216), both pleural and peritoneal, are also associated with asbestos exposure. In contrast to lung cancer there does not appear to be any association with smoking. Relatively short-term exposures of 1 to 2 years or less occurring some 20 to 25 years in the past have been associated with the development of mesotheliomas (which stresses the point of obtaining a complete environmental exposure history). The risk for this type of tumor peaks 30 to 35 years after initial exposure. Although approximately 50 percent of mesotheliomas metastasize, the tumor generally is locally invasive, and death usually results from local extension. Most patients present with effusions that may obscure the underlying pleural tumor. In contrast to other causes of effusion, because of the restriction placed on the chest wall no shift of mediastinal structures toward the opposite chest will be seen. The major diagnostic problem is differentiation from peripherally spreading pulmonary adenocarcinoma or adenocarcinoma metastatic to pleura from an extrathoracic primary site. Although a needle biopsy may be diagnostic, an open biopsy is often necessary and even when performed may not provide a definitive diagnosis of the origin of the tumor.

One concern in making a definitive diagnosis of a mesothelioma relates to potential compensation to the survivors of a patient with this usually fatal disease. Since epidemiologic studies have shown that more than 80 percent of mesotheliomas may be associated with asbestos exposure, documented mesothelioma in a worker with occupational exposure to asbestos may be compensable in many parts of the United States.

Other naturally occurring asbestiform material (e.g., erionite, a fibrous zeolite) induces mesotheliomas in test animals and has been associated with an excess incidence of lung cancer and mesotheliomas in a population in central Turkey exposed to it in volcanic rock. Man-made mineral fibers (MMMF) have similar physiochemical properties to naturally occurring asbestiform fibers. However, recent studies of exposure suggest that if excess risks of lung cancer do occur, they are less than with naturally occurring fibers. To date no cases of mesotheliomas from MMMF without exposure to asbestos have been reported. Part of the difficulty in assessing the effects of MMMF is that they have been used for relatively shorter periods and generally at lower exposure levels than for asbestos. Fortunately, recent concern has led to better worker protection.

Silicosis In spite of the technical adequacy of existing protective equipment, *free silica* (SiO_2), or crystalline quartz, is still a major occupational hazard. In the United States estimates of potential numbers of exposed workers range between 1.2 to 3 million people. The major occupational exposures include mining, stone cutting, abrasive industries, foundry workers, packers of silica flour, and quarrying, particularly of granite. Most often the progressive pulmonary fibrosis (silicosis) occurs in a dose-response fashion after many years of exposure.

Workers exposed to sandblasting in confined spaces, tunneling through rock with high quartz content (15 to 25 percent), and engaged in the manufacture of abrasive soaps may develop acute silicosis with as little as 10 months' exposure. The disease may be rapidly fatal in less than 2 years in spite of the worker being removed from exposure. A radiographic picture of profuse miliary infiltration or consolidation is characteristic of acute silicosis.

In long-term, relatively less intense exposure, radiographic changes of rounded, small opacities in the upper lobes with retraction and hilar adenopathy classically appear after 15 to 20 years of exposure. Calcification of hilar nodes may occur in as many as 20 percent of cases and produces the characteristic "eggshell" pattern. These changes may be preceded by or be associated with a reticular pattern of irregular densities which are uniformly present throughout the upper lung zones.

The nodular fibrosis may be progressive in the absence of further exposure, with coalescence and formation of nonsegmental conglomerates of irregular masses in excess of 1 cm in diameter. These masses become quite large and are characteristic of progressive massive fibrosis (PMF). Significant functional impairment with both restrictive and obstructive components may be associated with this form of silicosis. In the late stages of the disease ventilatory failure may develop. Patients with silicosis are at greater risk of acquiring *Mycobacterium tuberculosis* infections (silicotuberculosis), although tuberculosis is not always involved in the progression of the disease to PMF. Because the frequency with which tuberculosis has been found at autopsy in patients with PMF exceeds considerably the frequency of premorbid diagnosis, treatment for tuberculosis is indicated in any patient with silicosis and a positive tuberculin test.

Other less hazardous silicates include fuller's earth, kaolin, mica, diatomaceous earths, silica gel, soapstone, carbonate dusts, and cement dusts. The production of fibrosis in workers exposed to these agents is believed to be related to either the free silica content of these dusts or, for substances which contain no free silica, to the potentially large dust loads to which these workers may be exposed.

Other silicates, including *talc dusts,* may be contaminated with asbestos and/or free silica. Accidental exposure to significant quantities of talc may result in an acute syndrome with cough, cyanosis, and labored breathing (acute talcosis). Severe progressive fibrosis with respiratory failure may ensue within a few years. Far more common is the fibrosis and/or pleural or lung cancer associated with chronic exposure in rubber workers who use commercial talc as a lubricant in tire molds. Pure talc does not produce fibrosis; thus, it is difficult to sort out whether the effects are due to the contamination of commercial talc by asbestos or by free silica.

Coal worker's pneumoconiosis (CWP) *Coal dust* is associated with CWP, which has enormous social, economic, and medical significance in every nation in which coal mining is an important industry. Simple radiographically identified CWP is seen in 12 percent of all miners and in as many as 50 percent of anthracite miners with more than 20 years' work on the coal face. The prevalence of disease is lower in workers in bituminous coal mines. Since much of the western United States coal is bituminous, CWP is less prevalent in that region.

Much of the symptomatology associated with simple CWP appears to be similar and additive to the effects of cigarette smoking on the development of chronic bronchitis and obstructive lung disease (Chap. 210). In the early stages of simple CWP, radiographic abnormalities consist of small, irregular opacities (reticular pattern). With prolonged exposure, one sees small, rounded, regular opacities, 1 to 5 mm in diameter (nodular pattern). Calcification is generally not seen, although approximately 10 percent of older anthracite miners have calcified nodules.

Complicated CWP is manifested by the appearance on the chest radiograph of nodules ranging from 1 cm in diameter to the size of an entire lobe, generally confined to the upper half of the lungs. This condition, considered a form of PMF, is accompanied by a significant reduction in diffusing capacity and with premature mortality. In contrast to patients with silicosis, only a relatively small percentage of underground miners with simple CWP (5 to 15 percent, depending on the type of coal) develop PMF.

The mechanism whereby PMF occurs in CWP is not fully understood. Several hypotheses have been proposed, including (1) sufficient free silica is present in the dust; (2) normal clearance mechanisms are unable to clear the excessive dust loads; (3) an interplay occurs between an intrinsic immunologic mechanism and the dust and/or damaged lung tissue; and (4) atypical reactions to *Mycobacterium tuberculosis* occur. As previously described, PMF in silicosis is associated with prolonged duration and high intensity of exposure to free silica. Heavy exposure to carbon particles free of silica occurs in carbon black, graphite, and charcoal workers. The prolonged exposure of these workers may result in sufficient accumulation of carbon in the lung to produce PMF. The mechanism appears to relate to a breakdown of the clearance capacity of the airways.

Caplan's syndrome, which includes seropositive rheumatoid arthritis with characteristic PMF, is consistent with an immunopathologic mechanism. The syndrome was first described in coal miners but subsequently has been found in a number of pneumoconioses. Similarly, the high prevalence of antinuclear antibodies in sandblasting workers with silicosis and the elevation of gamma globulin levels in silicotic individuals suggest an immunologic mechanism. Although mycobacterial infections are found more often in coal miners than PMF is found in silicotic patients, tuberculosis does not appear to be associated with most of the cases of PMF in coal miners.

Berylliosis Beryllium may produce an acute pneumonitis or, far more commonly, a chronic interstitial pneumonitis. Unless one inquires specifically about occupational exposures to beryllium in the manufacture of alloys, ceramics, high-technology electronics, and, before the 1950s, in the production of fluorescent lights, one may miss entirely the etiologic relationship to an occupational exposure. Nonspecific pulmonary function tests may be normal or may indicate evidence of restrictive disease. Between 2 and 15 years of exposure, depending on its intensity, is required for the disease to become manifest. On open lung biopsy granulomatous formation similar to that seen in sarcoidosis (Chap. 277) may make differentiation impossible unless tissue levels of beryllium are measured.

Rarely, other hard metals, including aluminum powders, chromium, cobalt, titanium dioxide, and tungsten, may produce an interstitial pneumonitis.

Other inorganic dusts Other dusts are considered *nuisance dusts* because their major impact seems to be reduction in visibility and irritation of eyes, ears, nasal passages, and other mucous membranes. If they penetrate to the lower airways, they do not affect the architecture of the terminal bronchioles or acinar spaces or destroy collagen. Generally, clinical effects are reversible. Pulmonary function tests are usually normal unless another disease process coexists. If radiodense, macular collections of these dusts may produce striking radiographic pictures which are so characteristic that patients with a history of significant exposure are easily diagnosed as having the condition which bears the name reflecting the nature of the dust. Examples are iron and iron oxides from welding or silver finishing (*siderosis*); tin oxide used in metallurgy, color stabilization, printing, and the manufacture of porcelain, glass, and fabric (*stannosis*); and barium sulfate used as a catalyst for organic reactions, drilling mud components, and electroplating (*baritosis*). Other metal dusts producing similar radiodense pictures include *cerium dioxide* and *antimony salts*.

Most of the inorganic dusts discussed thus far are associated with the production of either dust macules or interstitial fibrotic changes in the lung. Another set of dusts (see Table 206-1), along with some of the dusts previously discussed, is associated with chronic mucous hypersecretion (chronic bronchitis), with or without reduction of expiratory flow rates. These conditions may be caused by cigarette smoking, and any effort to attribute some component of the disease to occupational and environmental exposures must take cigarette smoking into account. Most studies suggest an additive effect of dust

TABLE 206-1 Selected occupational dusts believed to be associated with mucous hypersecretion and/or obstructive airway disease and other respiratory diseases*

Agent (Exposure)	Mucous hypersecretion	Obstruction	Other conditions†
INORGANIC DUST			
Antimony (Storage batteries, solder, ceramics, glass, plastics)	X		P
Arsenic (Manufacture of pesticides, pigments, glass, alloys)	X		C
Barium and compounds including BaO, $BaSO_4$, $BaCO_3$ (Catalyst, drilling mud, electroplating)	X		P
Cadmium dust (Electroplating, battery manufacture, welding, smelting, aluminum soldering)	X	X	P
Cement dust (Construction trades, manufacture of cement blocks)	X	X	
Chromium and CrO_3, CrF_2 (Corrosion inhibitor pigment, metallurgy, electroplating)	X		C
Coal dust (Mining)	X		P
Coke oven emissions (Retort house, coke ovens)	X	X	P, C
Graphite (Steelmaking, lubricants, pencils, paints, stove polish)	X	X	P
Iron dust (Steel and nonferrous foundry workers, welding)	X		P
Mica (Insulation, roofing shingles, oil refining, rubber manufacturing)	X		P
Phosphorus, elemental chlorides, sulfides (Manufacture of fireworks, agricultural chemicals, insecticides, pesticides)	X	X	
Rock dusts (Miners, tunnelers, quarry workers)	X		P
Vanadium pentoxide (Welding electrodes, additive to steel, byproduct in ash from oil burning)	X	X	
ORGANIC DUST (see Chap. 205)			
Cotton dust, flax, hemp (Manufacture of yarns for linen, rope, cotton; ginning, cottonseed crushing; waste fiber processing)	X	X	
Grain dusts (Farmers, workers in grain elevators, barge and grain ship crewmembers)	X	X	
Moldy hay (Farmers, other animal attendants)	X		HP

* The table excludes agents associated with asthma as the primary disease (see Chap. 204).
† Other conditions include hypersensitivity pneumonitis (HP), pneumoconiosis (P), and cancers (C).
NOTE: X indicates that mucous hypersecretion or obstruction are associated with exposure.

exposure and smoking. The pattern of the effect is similar to that of cigarette smoking, suggesting that small airways may be the initial site of pathologic response to those cases associated with the development of obstructive lung disease. Cigarette smoke is usually the more noxious agent, and dust effects may be discernible only in nonsmokers.

ORGANIC DUSTS Some of the specific diseases associated with organic dusts are discussed in detail in the chapters on asthma (Chap. 204) and on hypersensitivity pneumonitis (Chap. 205). Many of these diseases are named for the specific setting in which the disease is found, e.g., farmer's lung, malt worker's disease, or mushroom worker's disease. Occupational and other environmental exposures must be sought when these conditions are suspected. Often the temporal relation of symptoms to exposure furnishes the best evidence for the diagnosis. Three occupational groups are singled out for discussion because they represent the largest proportion of people affected by the diseases resulting from organic dusts.

Cotton dust (byssinosis) Estimates of the number of exposed persons in the United States vary, but probably over 800,000 are exposed occupationally to cotton, flax, or hemp in the production of yarns for cotton, linen, and rope making. Although this discussion focuses on cotton, the same syndrome to a somewhat lesser degree has been reported in exposure to flax, hemp, and jute.

Although cotton dust–related disease was first described in the seventeenth century, it is only in the last 40 years that the disease has been recognized as a worldwide problem in the textile industry. Exposure occurs throughout the manufacturing process but is most pronounced in those portions of the factory involved with the treatment of the cotton prior to spinning—i.e., blowing, mixing, and carding (straightening of fibers). Cases reported from spinning rooms are believed to be due to secondary contamination from carding rooms. Recent attempts to control dust levels by use of exhaust hoods, general increase in ventilation, and wetting procedures in some settings have been highly successful. However, respiratory protective equipment appears to be required during certain operations to prevent workers from being exposed to levels of dust that exceed the current United States cotton dust standard.

Byssinosis is characterized clinically as occasional (early stage) and then regular (late stage) chest tightness toward the end of the first day of the workweek (Monday chest tightness). In epidemiologic studies, up to 80 percent of carding room employees may show a significant drop in their FEV_1 over the course of a Monday shift, depending on the level of exposure in the carding room air.

Initially the symptoms do not recur on subsequent days of the week. However, in 10 to 25 percent of workers, the disease may be progressive with chest tightness recurring or persisting throughout the workweek. After more than 10 years of exposure, workers with recurrent symptoms are more likely to have an obstructive pattern on pulmonary function testing. These higher grades of impairment are seen in workers exposed both to high levels of dust and for greater durations. There is an additive effect of cotton dust exposure plus cigarette smoking. The highest grades of impairment are generally seen in smokers.

Treatment in the early stages of the disease is directed toward reversing the bronchospasm with bronchodilators; however, the chest tightness appears at least in part to relate to histamine release, and antihistamines have been shown to lessen anticipated fall in FEV_1 the first day of the week. Clearly, reduction of dust exposure is of primary importance. All workers with persistent symptoms or significantly reduced levels of pulmonary function should be moved to areas of lower risk of exposure. Regular surveillance of pulmonary function in the industry has made it easier to identify affected persons. Persons with reduced pulmonary function, a personal history of respiratory allergy, and positive history of continued cigarette smoking should be considered at increased risk of developing byssinosis in association with working in the cotton industry.

Grain dust Although the exact number of workers at risk in the United States is not known, at least 500,000 people work in grain elevators, and over 2 million farmers are potentially at risk. The presentation of disease in grain elevator employees or workers in flour or feed mills is virtually identical to the characteristic finding in cigarette smokers, i.e., persistent cough, mucus hypersecretion, wheeze and dyspnea on exertion, and reduced FEV_1 and FEV_1/FVC ratio (Chap. 201).

Dust concentrations in grain elevators vary greatly but appear to be in excess of 10,000 $\mu g/m^3$ with approximately one-third of the particles by weight being in the respirable range. The effect of grain dust exposure is additive to that of cigarette smoking with approximately 50 percent of workers who smoke having symptoms. Among nonsmoking grain elevator operators, approximately one-quarter have mucous hypersecretion, about five times the number that would be expected in unexposed nonsmokers. However, evidence of obstruction on pulmonary function studies is observed only in workers who smoke. It is not clear if this results from an enhancement of cigarette smoking effect in exposed workers or if smokers are more susceptible to the effects of grain dust.

Farmer's lung This condition results from exposure to moldy hay containing spores of thermophilic actinomycetes that produce a hypersensitivity pneumonitis (Chap. 205). There are few good population-based estimates of the frequency of occurrence of this condition in the United States. However, among farmers in Great Britain the rate of disease ranges from approximately 10 to 50 per 1000. The prevalence of disease varies in association with rainfall, which determines the amount of fungal growth, and with differences in agricultural practices related to turning and stacking hay.

The patient with acute farmer's lung presents 4 to 8 h after exposure with fever, chills, malaise, cough, and dyspnea without wheezing. The history of exposure is obviously essential to separate this disease from similar symptoms that might occur in influenza or pneumonia. In the chronic form of the disease, the history of repeated attacks after similar exposure is important to separate this syndrome from other causes of patchy fibrosis, e.g., sarcoidosis.

A wide variety of other organic dusts are associated with the occurrence of hypersensitivity pneumonitis (Chap. 205). For those patients who present with hypersensitivity pneumonitis, specific and careful inquiry about occupations, hobbies, or other home environmental exposures will, in most cases, reveal the source of the etiologic agent.

ASSESSMENT OF DISABILITY Significant reduction of dust levels in coal mines has resulted from federal legislation, enacted in the United States in 1969, which requires that respirable dust levels in underground mines be reduced to less than 2000 $\mu g/m^3$. This same legislation authorized payment to coal miners (or their survivors) totally disabled by CWP. The criteria for disability from CWP remain unclear and arbitrary. Much of the difficulty relates to the inability to determine in an individual with simple CWP what proportion of an observed respiratory impairment is related to coal dust and what proportion is due to cigarette smoking. The laws as currently interpreted suggest that to be eligible for payment of a claim, one need only show that an underlying condition (i.e., chronic bronchitis with obstruction, presumably due to cigarette smoking) is aggravated by CWP. Thus, it becomes critical that physicians involved in occupational lung disease claim cases be aware of detailed exposure histories of their patients, both in terms of occupational exposures and other environmental exposures (cigarette smoking). In addition, these physicians must understand that the extent to which the level of physiologic impairment incapacitates an individual may not be the sole criterion for determining disability. To assess disability properly may require input not only from physicians but also from experts in ergonomics and vocational rehabilitation, lawyers, and employer and employee representatives.

TOXIC CHEMICALS Exposure to toxic chemicals affecting the lung generally occurs in the form of gases and vapors. A common accident is one in which the victim is trapped in a confined space where the chemicals have accumulated to toxic levels. In addition to the specific toxic effects of the chemical, the victim will often sustain considerable anoxia, which can play a dominant role in determining whether the individual recovers.

Table 206-2 lists a variety of toxic agents which can produce acute and sometimes life-threatening reactions in the lung. All of these agents in sufficient concentrations have been demonstrated, at least in animal studies, to affect the lower airways and disrupt alveolar architecture, either acutely or as a result of chronic exposure. Some of these agents may be generated acutely in the environment. For example, when plastics burn, a number of compounds, including hydrogen cyanide and hydrochloric acid, may be formed and released. The effects and treatment of exposure to these toxic gases are discussed elsewhere (Chap. 374).

Fire fighters and fire victims are at risk of *smoke inhalation,* a numerically important cause of acute cardiorespiratory failure. Smoke inhalation kills more fire victims than does thermal injury. Carbon monoxide poisoning with resulting significant hypoxemia can be life-threatening (Chap. 374). Fire fighters may inappropriately use the ''blackness'' of the smoke to indicate the degree to which incomplete combustion and, thus, elevation of carbon monoxide levels are present. The increased use of synthetic materials (plastic, polyurethanes), which, when burned, may release a variety of other toxic agents, must be considered when evaluating smoke inhalation victims. Exposed victims may suffer some degree of lower respiratory tract inflammation, similar to that seen with exposure to other irritant gases, e.g., chlorine. Severe cases may develop pulmonary edema.

Fire fighters and victims also may be exposed to large quantities of particulate smoke. Significant long-term effects are not clearly associated with this particulate exposure except as related to the production of irritating effects on the upper airways. Studies attempting to demonstrate either an increased risk of cardiovascular events, presumably from recurrent exposure to carbon monoxide, or excess incidence of chronic respiratory disease from repeated smoke inhalation, are inconclusive, partly because of the difficulties in measuring exposure. Recent studies suggest increased airways responsiveness in firefighters with repeated episodes of smoke inhalation.

Some agents used in the manufacture of synthetic materials such as plastics, polyurethanes, and other polymers have resulted in some workers being sensitized to extremely low levels of *isocyanates, aromatic amines,* or *aldehydes.* Repeated exposure to these agents causes some workers to develop chronic cough and sputum production, asthma, or episodes of low-grade fever and malaise. Occasionally, as in byssinosis, these symptoms occur early in the workweek, but usually recur without workweek periodicity. In the case of exposure to diisocyanate in the production of polyurethane, chronic and persistent asthma in selected individuals appears to result from exposure to concentrations well below the recognized industrial standard. Methods to identify susceptible individuals are needed. At present, challenge testing is being used to determine if a given patient is sensitive. These challenges can be carried out in special environmental chambers where the physician can simulate the work exposure. Alternatively, nonspecific challenges with either pharmacologic agents, such as methacholine and histamine, or isocapneic cold air breathing are being used to identify patients with hyperreactive airways. The usefulness of this nonspecific approach as a method to screen potential sensitive workers has yet to be established.

An unusual route of exposure occurs in *polymer fume fever.* Polymers, notably fluorocarbons, which at normal temperatures produce no reaction, may be transmitted from a worker's hands to his or her cigarettes. Upon burning the cigarette, the polymer is volatilized, and the inhaled agent causes a characteristic syndrome of fever, chills, malaise, and occasionally mild wheezing. The same condition occurs in workers exposed to heated polymers without cigarette use. The syndrome is obviously controlled by proper attention to hygiene in the workplace. A similar self-limited, influenza-like syndrome—*metal fume fever*—results from acute exposure to fumes or smoke of zinc, copper, magnesium, and other volatilized metals. The syndrome may begin several hours after work and resolves within 24 h, only to return on repeated exposure. A proper occupational history should make the diagnosis evident.

ENVIRONMENTAL RESPIRATORY CARCINOGENS Historically, it has been the astute clinician who has recognized a higher incidence of malignant tumors associated with certain environmental exposures. When these observations are linked to an occupational setting, they must be pursued by epidemiologic studies of relatively large groups of both current and former workers. Often the concentration and/or exact nature of the substances contained in the putative exposures cannot be determined. Rarely, the possibility that a substance can play an etiologic role in cancer is supported by observing that a few cases of a very rare tumor in a particular group represent ''an epidemic.'' Examples of this are nasal sinus and lung

TABLE 206-2 Selected common toxic chemical agents

Agents	Selected exposures	Acute effects from high or accidental exposure	Chronic effects from relatively low exposure
Acid fumes; H_2SO_4, HNO_3	Manufacture of fertilizers, chlorinated organic compounds, dyes, explosives, rubber products, metal etching, plastics	Mucous membrane irritation, followed by chemical pneumonitis 2–3 days	No data
Ammonia	Refrigeration, petroleum refining, manufacture of fertilizers, explosives, plastics, and other chemicals	Same as for acid fumes	Chronic bronchitis
Cyanides	Electroplating, extraction of gold or silver, manufacture of mirrors, fumigants, photo supplies	Increase in respiratory rate followed by respiratory arrest, lactic acidosis, pulmonary edema, death	No data
Diazomethane	Methylating agent for acid compounds; laboratory workers	Violent coughing, dyspnea, wheezing, pulmonary edema	No data
Formaldehyde	Manufacture of resins, leathers, rubber, metals, & woods; laboratory workers, embalmers; emission from urethane foam insulation	Same as for acid fumes	Cancers in one species of animals; no data on humans
Halides (Cl, Br, F)	Bleaching in pulp, paper, textile industry; manufacture of chemical compounds; synthetic rubber, plastics, disinfectant, rocket fuel, gasoline	Mucous membrane irritation, pulmonary edema; possible reduced FVC 1–2 yrs after exposure	Dryness of mucous membrane, epistaxis, dental fluorosis, tracheobronchitis
Hydrogen sulfide	By-product of many industrial processes, oil, other petroleum processes and storage	Low exposure: conjunctival irritation; higher: respiratory paralysis similar to cyanides	Chronic bronchitis, recurrent pneumonitis
Isocyanates (TDI, HDI, MDI)	Production of polyurethane foams, plastics, adhesives, surface coatings	Mucous membrane irritation, dyspnea, cough, wheeze, pulmonary edema	Upper respiratory tract irritation, cough, asthma, allergic alveolitis
Nitrogen dioxide	Silage, metal etching, explosives, rocket fuels, welding, by-product of burning fossil fuels	Cough, dyspnea, pulmonary edema may be delayed 4–12 h; possible result from acute exposure: bronchiolitis obliterans in 2–6 wks	Emphysema in animals, ? chronic bronchitis
Ozone	Arc welding, flour bleaching, deodorizing, emissions from copying equipment, photochemical air pollutant	Mucous membrane irritant, pulmonary hemorrhage and edema, reduced pulmonary function transiently in children exposed to summer haze	Chronic eye irritation
Phosgene	Organic compound, metallurgy, volatization of chlorine-containing compounds	Delayed onset of bronchiolitis and pulmonary edema	Chronic bronchitis
Phthalic anhydride	Manufacture of resin esters, polyester resins, thermoactivated adhesives	Nasal irritation, cough	Asthma, chronic bronchitis
Sulfur dioxide	Manufacture of sulfuric acid, bleaches, coating of nonferrous metals, food processing, refrigerant, burning of fossil fuels, wood pulp industry	Mucous membrane irritant, epistaxis	? Chronic bronchitis

cancer in nickel workers, angiosarcomas in vinyl chloride workers, and adenocarcinomas of the nose in woodworkers.

Only in those few cases in which animal studies have been carried out can one confirm that a given suspected agent is really a carcinogen. For example, bis(chloromethyl) ether (BCME) has been shown to produce tumors in animals and oat cell cancer of the lung in humans. In this particular case, BCME, used as a chemical intermediary in the manufacture of a number of organic compounds, was known to produce tumors in animals almost before the substance was introduced into industry. (This case is one of the prime examples of why federal legislation was enacted in the United States in the 1970s to control the release of toxic substances, particularly new chemicals.)

In addition to the asbestos trades, other occupational exposures associated with either proven or suspected respiratory carcinogens include acrylonitrile, arsenic compounds, beryllium (animal studies only), BCME, chromium, coke ovens (exposure to polycyclic hydrocarbons), iron oxide, isopropyl oil (nasal sinuses), mustard gas, the various ores used to produce pure nickel, talc (possible asbestos contamination in both mining and milling), vinyl chloride, welding, wood used in woodworking (nasal cancer only), and uranium. The occurrence of excess cancers in uranium miners raises the possibility that there exists a large number of workers at risk by virtue of exposure to similar radiation hazards. This includes not only workers involved in processing uranium, up to and including its use in nuclear power plants and in military nuclear hardware, but also workers exposed in underground mining operations where radon daughters may be emitted from rock formations. In the latter case, the levels of exposure are generally considered to be relatively low; however, specific consideration must be given to the possibility of excess exposure for any hard rock miner.

GENERAL ENVIRONMENTAL EXPOSURES

AIR POLLUTION Dramatic and disastrous episodes of air pollution inversion have been documented in many industrialized centers in the world. Each of these episodes has been associated with excess acute mortality in the very old, the very young, and in those with chronic cardiopulmonary diseases. The most dramatic event was the London fog of 1952, in which approximately 4000 excess deaths occurred over a 2-week period following 5 days of severe cold and dense fog. Similar episodes in the United States, although less dramatic in terms of total deaths, occurred in Donora, Pennsylvania, in 1948, and in New York City in the 1960s. In these episodes, generally associated with cold temperature and air stagnation, patients with underlying cardiopulmonary disease were most severely affected.

In addition to significant excess mortality during these episodes, a large number of people required medical care for cardiorespiratory complaints. Subsequent follow-up studies failed to implicate these episodic disasters in the etiology of chronic respiratory disease in adults. On the other hand, many epidemiologic studies of both international and regional differences in the prevalences of chronic respiratory disease suggest that long-term exposures in polluted areas in the early to middle part of the twentieth century were associated with excess chronic respiratory disease.

In 1970, the U.S. federal government established air quality standards for several pollutants believed to be responsible for excess cardiorespiratory diseases. Primary standards regulated by the Environmental Protection Agency (EPA) designed to protect the public health with an adequate margin of safety exist for sulfur dioxide, total suspended particulates, nitrogen dioxide, ozone, lead, and carbon monoxide. These standards vary in their averaging times and levels, in part related to the differences in the known physiologic responses and epidemiologic evidence for each pollutant.

Pollutants are generated from both stationary sources (power plants and industrial complexes) and mobile sources (automobiles), and none of the pollutants occur in isolation. Thus, except for the change in carboxyhemoglobin from carbon monoxide exposure, it becomes extremely difficult to relate any specific health effect to any single pollutant. Furthermore, pollutants may be changed by chemical reactions after being emitted. For example, reducing agents, such as sulfur dioxide and particulate matter from a power plant stack, may react in air to produce acid sulfates and aerosols, the precursors of acid rain, which can be transported long distances in the atmosphere. Oxidizing substances, such as oxides of nitrogen and oxidants from automobile exhaust, may react with sunlight to produce ozone. Although originally a problem confined to the southwestern part of the United States, in recent years, at least during the summertime, elevated ozone and sulfate levels can occur throughout the United States. Both acute and chronic effects of these exposures are currently under investigation.

The symptoms and diseases associated with air pollution are the same as the nononcogenic conditions commonly associated with cigarette smoking. In addition, respiratory illness in early childhood has been associated with chronic exposure to only modestly elevated levels of SO_2 and total suspended particulates. It is not known whether persistent chronic exposure to a relatively constant level of pollutant(s) and recurrent short-term peak exposures which average to the same mean level have different effects. For a patient with significant cardiopulmonary impairment, one can only advise the individual to stay indoors during periods when pollution exceeds current standards.

INDOOR EXPOSURE Because of increased concern about energy costs, efforts to become energy efficient have led to reduced air exchange rates in indoor environments. The effects of these efforts have been to increase exposures to a variety of air contaminants heretofore not considered important. Two examples of potential health effects from exposure to indoor pollutants are discussed to indicate the magnitude of possible problems.

Until recently, little attention, beyond its nuisance effect, was given to the effects of *passive cigarette smoking*. The implication was that passive smoking exposures were too low to be of any consequence. Now studies have shown that the respirable particulate load in any household is directly proportional to the number of cigarette smokers living in the home. Increases in prevalence of respiratory illnesses and reduced levels of pulmonary function measured with simple spirometry have been found in children of smoking parents in a number of studies. The long-term consequences in terms of nononcogenic respiratory diseases are unknown. Two expert panels, however, have concluded that lung cancer risk is significantly higher in nonsmokers with long-standing residence in the households of smokers.

A novel source of indoor exposure to *formaldehyde* results from the curing process involved in the placement of urea-formaldehyde insulating foam or in several wood products used in modern furniture and the construction of mobile homes. Natural "degassing" of formaldehyde occurs during the first few months after the foam has been blown into the walls, with concentrations of formaldehyde as high as 5 ppm rapidly dropping off to less than 0.1 ppm. Chronic exposure to low levels of urea-formaldehyde (generally less than 1 ppm) may result if the foam is improperly installed. Patients apparently sensitive to concentrations of formaldehyde generally well below 1 ppm will complain of upper airway irritation with occasional epistaxis and sore throats. Lower respiratory complaints, such as chest pain and wheeze, however, are uncommon, and often the most disturbing complaints are mild memory and mood disorders. Formaldehyde is a proven animal carcinogen. Whether it causes cancer in humans is not established.

Radon gas is believed to be a risk factor for lung cancer. The main radon product (randon 222) is a gas that results from the decay series of uranium 238 with the immediate precursor being radium 226. The amount of radium in earth materials determines how much radon gas will be emitted. Outdoors the concentrations are trivial. Indoors levels are dependent on the ventilation rate and the size of space into which the gas is emitted. Levels associated with excess lung cancer risk may be present in as many as 10 percent of the houses in the United States. Where smoking exists in the household, the problem is potentially greater since the molecular size of radon particles readily attaches to smoke particles that are inhaled. Fortunately the technology is available for assessing and reducing the level of exposure.

PORTAL OF ENTRY The lung is a primary source of entry into the body for a number of toxic agents that affect other organ systems. For example, the lung is the route of entry for benzene (bone marrow), carbon disulfide (cardiovascular and nervous systems), cadmium (kidney), and mercury (kidney, central nervous system). Thus, in any disease state of obscure origin, it is important to consider possible inhaled environmental agents. Such consideration can sometimes furnish the clue needed to identify a specific external cause for a disorder that might otherwise be labeled "idiopathic."

REFERENCES

Becklake MR et al: The relationship between acute and chronic airway responses to occupational exposures. Curr Pulmonol 9:25, 1988

Cochrane AL, Moore FA: A 20-year follow-up of men aged 55–64 including coal miners and foundry workers in Stavley. Br J Ind Med 37:226, 1980

Craighead JE, Mossman BT: The pathogenesis of asbestos-associated diseases. N Engl J Med 306:1446, 1982

Guidelines for the Use of International Labour Office Classification of Radiographs of Pneumoconiosis. Occupational Safety and Health Sciences 22 (Revised 1980). Geneva, ILO, 1980

Koskinen H: Symptoms and clinical findings in patients with silicosis. Scan J Work Environ Health 11:101, 1985

Larunerys RR: Occupational toxicology, in *Casarett and Doull's Toxicology, The Basic Science of Poison*, 3d ed, CD Kloassen, MD Amden, J Doull (eds). New York, MacMillan, 1986, chap 29

National Research Council: *Asbestiform Fibers, Nonoccupational Health Risks*. National Academy Press, Washington DC, 1984, chaps 2, 5, 6

Parkes WR: *Occupational Lung Disorders*, 2d ed. London, Butterworth, 1982

Peto R, Schneiderman M (eds): *Quantification of Occupational Cancer*, Banbury Report, 9. Cold Spring Harbor, 1981

Rom WN (ed): *Environmental and Occupational Medicine*. Boston, Little, Brown, 1983, chaps 13, 20

Simonato L et al: The man-made mineral fiber European historical cohort study. Extension of the follow up. Scan J Work Environ Health 12:Suppl 1, 34, 1986

Weill J: Occupational pulmonary diseases and acute and accidental exposures to irritant gases, in *Pulmonary Diseases and Disorders*, 2d ed, A P Fishman (ed). New York, McGraw-Hill, 1987, chap. 54

207 PNEUMONIA AND LUNG ABSCESS

HERBERT Y. REYNOLDS

PNEUMONIA

DEFINITION Pneumonia is inflammation affecting the parenchyma of the lung—that portion distal to the conducting airways and involving the respiratory bronchioles and the alveolar units. Histologically, pneumonitis or an inflammatory reaction causes alveolitis and accumulation of an exudate and is most often due to infection. With spread to the interstitium around alveoli, consolidation and a degree of impaired gas exchange occur in the involved lung tissue. With successful inactivation of the infecting agent, resolution occurs and normal lung structure is usually restored. Exceptions to complete healing occur with certain necrotizing pneumonias, as caused by staphylococci or gram-negative bacteria, after which scars or fibrosis may develop in the lung. Bronchopneumonia denotes patchy and diffuse areas of involvement and often implies that a less severe form of disease exists because signs and radiographic evidence of consolidation are absent. Pneumonia is a commonly encountered disease and, in one form or another, continues to be a leading cause of death in the United States.

PATHOGENESIS **Microorganisms** These reach lung tissue in several ways: (1) by direct inhalation of infectious particles from ambient air, (2) by aspiration of secretions from the mouth and nasopharynx, (3) by deposition in lung vasculature following hematogenous spread from another site, and rarely, (4) by penetration of lung tissue or spread from a contiguous site. Aspiration of microbes colonizing the naso-oropharynx provides the most frequent entry to the lung. The normal microbial flora of the upper respiratory tract is a complex mixture of aerobic bacteria such as *Streptococcus* sp., *Streptococcus pneumoniae, Branhamella catarrhalis, Corynebacteria, Neisseria* sp. (including *N. meningitidis*), *Staphylococcus* sp., and *Haemophilus* sp. Aerobic gram-negative bacilli, such as *Pseudomonas aeruginosa, Klebsiella pneumoniae,* or *Escherichia coli,* are harbored there rarely in healthy people. Anaerobic bacteria, localized in crevices of the gums and teeth, are very numerous and can reach 10^8 organisms per milliliter of saliva (see Chap. 108). Viruses are not usual flora.

Pulmonary infection may follow acquisition of a virulent new strain in the nasooropharynx or an unusually large inoculum of microbes in the lung. The normally symbiotic relationship between colonizing bacteria on the nasooropharyngeal mucosa can be affected by a number of host conditions that promote selection of different pathogenic organisms. Cigarette smoking and chronic bronchitis favor colonization with *S. pneumoniae, H. influenzae,* and, perhaps, *Legionella pneumophila;* alcoholism, poorly controlled diabetes mellitus, uremia, prior use of antibiotics, poor nutrition, and many critical illnesses favor acquisition of aerobic gram-negative bacilli. The stress of hospitalization, confinement to a high-level-care nursing facility or intensive care unit, surgery, and treatment with antineoplastic chemotherapy or immunosuppressive drugs all promote rapid colonization with potentially pathogenic organisms. Nosocomial pneumonia can occur in a sizeable percentage of such patients (5 to 25 percent), and its morbidity and mortality are appreciable.

Host defense mechanisms Although a common disease, pneumonia is a relatively rare occurrence in normal people. This attests to the effectiveness of the respiratory host defense system—a complex mixture of anatomic barriers and cleansing mechanisms present in the nasopharynx and upper airways and local cellular and humoral factors in the terminal air-exchange units (alveoli). Normal lungs are generally kept sterile below the first major bronchial divisions.

In the upper respiratory tract and large airways, *mechanical mechanisms* exclude particulate material. These mechanisms include: (1) anatomic barriers, such as the epiglottis and tight apical cellular junctions between epithelial lining cells of the mucosa; (2) reflex closure of the glottis; (3) frequent branching of the pulmonary tree, which leads to aerodynamic filtering of inspired air; (4) mucociliary clearance of particulates that impact on the mucosa; and (5) the cough response. When infectious agents, bacteria in particular, elude these defenses and are deposited in the alveoli, another group of host factors takes over. The terminal units (alveolar ducts and alveoli) do not contain ciliated epithelium and mucus-secreting cells (goblet cells and mucous glands) and coughing does not effectively clear material from the alveoli. Clearance is dependent on phagocytic cells and humoral factors. These mechanisms are shown in Fig. 207-1.

OPSONINS When bacteria or particles reach the alveolar surface, most are rapidly ingested by phagocytes. Although alveolar macrophages avidly phagocytose some inert particles, they usually ingest viable bacteria more slowly. Coating or opsonizing the organisms will enhance phagocytosis approximately tenfold. Nonimmune opsonins are found in the film of fluid on the alveolar surface (lipoprotein surfactant from type II pneumocytes and large fragments of the glycoprotein, fibronectin, produced locally by alveolar macrophages or delivered from intravascular sources). Immune opsonins include IgG antibody and a complement factor, C3b, that augment attachment to specific plasma membrane receptors (see Chap. 13). These opsonins are produced locally or are delivered as part of systemic humoral immunity.

IgG and its subclasses are present in bronchoalveolar lavage (BAL) fluid from normal subjects in approximately the same proportions as found in serum (see Chap. 13). The IgG2 subclass contains antibodies made to capsular polysaccharides of respiratory pathogens such as *S. pneumoniae* and *H. influenzae,* to teichoic acid present in *Staphylococcus aureus,* and to gram-negative lipopolysaccharides. Cytophilic or adherent IgG on alveolar macrophage plasma membranes is of the IgG1 and IgG4 subclasses. Macrophage Fc gamma receptors are most numerous for IgG3 and to a lesser amount, IgG1. IgG2 and IgG4 receptors are masked or buried.

In the airways the complement system can be activated along the alternative pathway. This can lead to lysis of a susceptible organism or to generation of opsonic C3b. Once phagocytosis has occurred, intracellular killing proceeds, but often at a slower rate than that measured in polymorphonuclear leukocytes (PMNs) and by less well-

FIGURE 207-1 Alveolar host defense mechanisms (see text for details). Abbreviations: AM = alveolar macrophage; PMN = polymorphonuclear leukocytes; T-lym = T lymphocyte; INFγ = γ-interferon; MIF = migration inhibitory factor; TNF = tumor necrosis factor; IL-1 = interleukin 1.

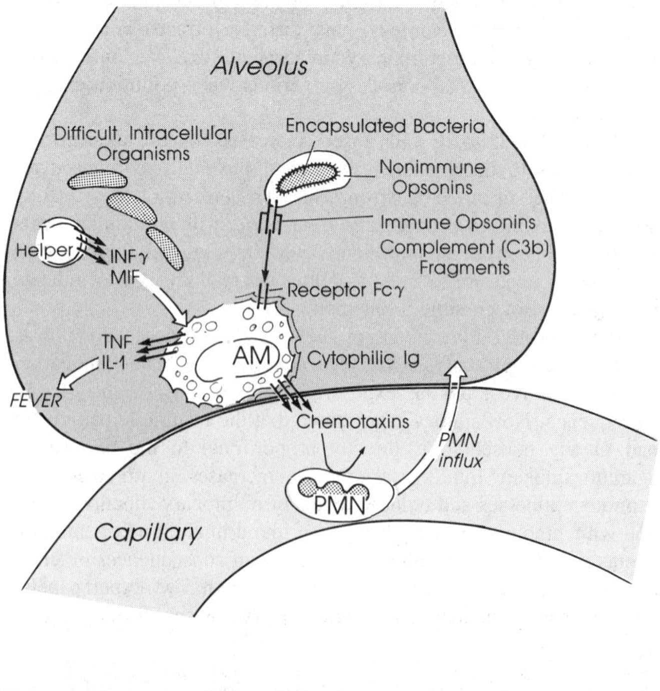

defined mechanisms involving both oxygen-dependent and -independent pathways. In contrast to PMNs, macrophages usually lack myeloperoxidase; production of superoxide and H_2O_2 are enhanced by macrophage "activation" (see Chaps. 13 and 81).

MACROPHAGE-LYMPHOCYTE INTERACTIONS In addition to phagocytosis, subsequent containment and destruction of microbes hinge on the effectiveness of the macrophages to kill the organisms and the development of an inflammatory reaction. Alveolar macrophages are long-lived tissue cells that can survive months to years and presumably are capable of handling repeated microbial challenges. Because they are motile cells, they can migrate quickly to other alveoli through the pores of Kohn or move to more proximal areas of the respiratory tract. Macrophages are instrumental in degrading antigenic material and presenting it to appropriate alveolar lymphocytes that, in turn, may initiate specific immune responses (see Chap. 13). In addition, macrophages gain entry into lung lymphatics in respiratory bronchioles and are transported to regional lymph nodes that are sites of humoral and cellular immune responses for the lung. The many secretory products of macrophages are essential participants in the immune effector system and can contribute to chronic inflammation and to fibrogenesis or granuloma formation (see Chap. 81). Lymphocytes are important in regulation of lung macrophage functions related to cellular activation and inflammation. They are also directly involved in the formation and regulation of antibody responses and activation of dormant cytotoxic lymphocytes (see Chap. 13).

Lymphocytes retrieved from normal alveoli account for about 10 percent of airway cells. Seventy percent of these are T lymphocytes and proportions of the major subpopulations are similar to those in peripheral blood. Among the helper T cells is a small percentage of HLA-DR–positive lymphocytes (7 percent) that secrete the major amount of interleukin 2. Killer T cells may be dormant but can be activated by γ-interferon. Several important cytokines produced by T lymphocytes activate alveolar macrophages (Fig. 207-1) and include γ-interferon and macrophage-inhibitory factor. Acquired cell-mediated immunity (CMI) is necessary if the macrophage population is to contain or kill certain intracellular microbes. Examples include: *Mycobacterium tuberculosis* and other species, *L. pneumophila, Pneumocystis carinii, Listeria monocytogenes,* and cytomegalovirus. Because of suppression of CMI pneumonias caused by *P. carinii,* various fungi, *M. tuberculosis,* and cytomegalovirus are common in patients receiving high doses of glucocorticoids or with the acquired immunodeficiency syndrome (AIDS) (see Chap. 264).

INFLAMMATORY MECHANISMS PMNs are usually separated from alveolar spaces by three planes: tissue-capillary endothelium, interstitial space, and alveolar epithelium. PMN movement by chemotaxis into the alveoli is an orderly reaction initiated from the alveolar side. Several pathways can be involved. Macrophages help promote the acute inflammatory response, including chemotaxis. Production of chemotactic factors, particularly leukotriene B4, from macrophages can attract PMNs from pulmonary capillaries and venules and alter pulmonary capillary permeability. Other chemotactic and capillary permeability–altering factors include C3a and C5a and components of the kinin systems (see Chap. 81). The combined action of these agents promotes the accumulation of PMNs, fluid, and other humoral substances in alveoli. With the appearance of an inflammatory response, clinical illness usually occurs and a chest roentgenogram reveals an infiltrate. Production of interleukin 1 (IL-1) and tumor necrosis factor by alveolar macrophages can contribute to many of the systemic effects of pneumonia—such as chills and fever, malaise, and myalgias (see Chap. 20).

Ultimately the lung tissues may become consolidated. Release of proteolytic enzymes (e.g., PMN-derived elastase) can contribute to lung injury. Their neutralization by several inhibitor proteins, $alpha_1$ antiprotease, and possibly $alpha_2$ macroglobulin can minimize destruction of lung tissue. Pending successful containment of the infection, resolution and healing eventually occur. Little is known about the processes that halt the acute inflammatory reaction in pneumonia and initiate recovery.

CLINICAL MANIFESTATIONS The major symptoms of pneumonia are usually cough, fever, production of sputum, chest pain, and dyspnea. Pneumonia can develop acutely in a previously healthy person, or can be discovered almost incidentally from a chest radiograph of a chronically ill patient without major symptoms, but with another underlying disease. Coryza or mild upper respiratory symptoms and malaise often precede the onset of pneumonia. Typically, a pyogenic bacterial pneumonia, as caused by *S. pneumoniae,* follows a viral upper respiratory tract infection and has an abrupt onset with chills, a sustained fever, cough which will become productive of mucopurulent sputum, and chest aching or pleuritic pain. In contrast, a viral or mycoplasmal pneumonia also may have a prodromal upper respiratory tract phase, but malaise, headache, and cough linger for days; coughing and fever gradually increase, but pleuritic chest pain and respiratory distress are not usual. The symptoms produced by these major etiologic forms of pneumonia may overlap so that a suspected diagnosis cannot be made with confidence from the patient's initial presentation. Furthermore, the patient's overall condition and ability to cooperate and communicate can affect how the illness may present to the physician.

Young adults often have the classic acute symptoms that readily point to the lower respiratory tract. Occasionally, a lower lobe infection can irritate the diaphragmatic surface so that upper abdominal pain, referred pain to the shoulder, or eructation and hiccups are part of the symptom complex and can divert attention away from the lung to another diagnosis. Elderly or severely ill patients may have little cough, scant sputum production, little evidence of respiratory symptoms, and a deceptive absence of fever. In a hospitalized or immunocompromised patient, the major initial manifestations may be limited to fever, tachypnea, agitation, or altered mentation because of changes in oxygenation. Pneumonia may be apparent only after systematically excluding infection in other organ systems.

Important historical information includes knowledge of hemoptysis, chills, pleuritic chest pain, or use of antibiotics; risk factors or prior or underlying illnesses that increase susceptibility to a specific microbial infection (see Chap. 82); special epidemiologic or travel considerations, i.e., contact with ill family members, pets or other animals; recurrences of pneumonia.

PHYSICAL FINDINGS The breathing pattern and the position assumed in bed can indicate the patient's discomfort, reveal tachypnea, and demonstrate splinting of the chest to minimize pleuritic pain.

Percussion and auscultation of the chest may reveal signs of lung consolidation (dullness, inspiratory crackles, or bronchial breath sounds). However, the lung examination may be normal, particularly with interstitial pneumonias, even though radiographic changes can be seen. Appearance of the skin and mucous membranes can help assess fluid status, indicate jaundice or cyanosis, or reveal needle tracks in users of illicit drugs. The presence of clubbing may indicate underlying lung disease. The condition of the teeth and gingiva and adequacy of the gag reflex may provide a clue to aspiration. The cardiac examination may reveal murmurs consistent with associated endocarditis or pleuropericardial rubs. Upper abdominal tenderness may reflect diaphragmatic irritation resulting from inflamed pleural surfaces, rather than an intraabdominal process. Abdominal distention due to paralytic illness is common in bacterial pneumonia, particularly if it involves the lower lobes. An altered mental status may be due to high fever, hypoxemia, or a complicating meningitis.

DIAGNOSTIC STUDIES The *chest radiograph* is essential to confirm the presence of pneumonitis and its location, but its appearance will not accurately predict the etiology. A well-penetrated frontal film that allows good visualization of the retrocardiac area on the left and a lateral view film are desirable. Certain radiographic appearances are more typical of some organisms than others. Pneumonias tend to conform to one of three pathologic and radiographic patterns (Fig. 207-2): (1) alveolar or air space pneumonia, (2) interstitial pneumonia, or (3) bronchopneumonia. In air space pneumonia the organism causes an inflammatory exudate that involves many contiguous alveoli. Segmental boundaries are not preserved, and the bronchi, relatively

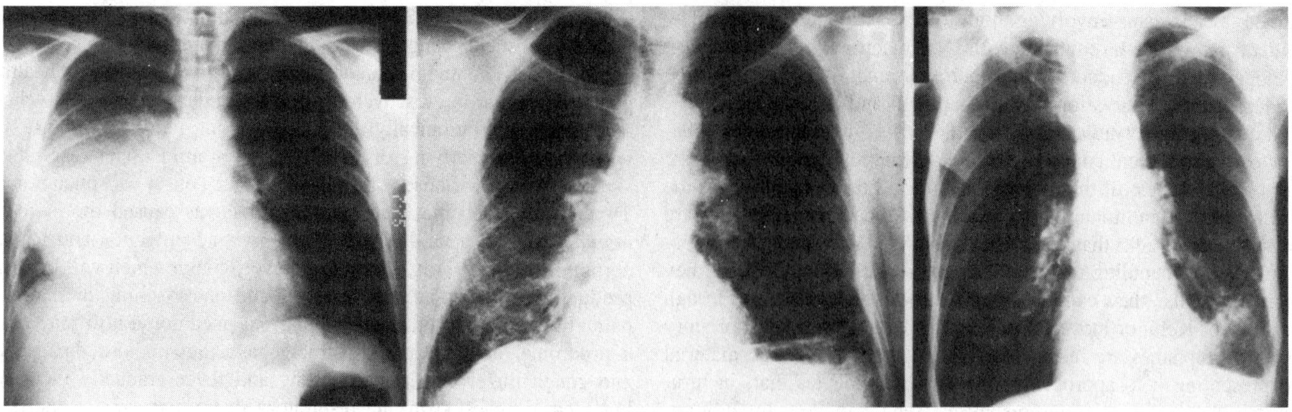

A B C

FIGURE 207-2 Roentgenographic appearances of pneumonia. *A*. Air space pneumonia. There is a dense, homogeneous, nonsegmental consolidation in the right lower lobe with a visible air bronchogram. *B*. Interstitial pneumonia. A linear or reticular pattern involves the lower lung fields bilaterally, more on the right. *C*. Bronchopneumonia. A segmental infiltrate without a visible air bronchogram appears in the left lower lung field.

uninvolved, remain patent. The radiologic result is nonsegmental consolidation with air bronchograms. A classic example is pneumococcal pneumonia. *Mycoplasma pneumoniae, P. carinii,* and viruses often cause an interstitial pneumonia, where inflammation is predominantly in the interalveolar septa, producing a reticular radiographic appearance. In bronchopneumonia, inflammation is restricted to the conducting airways, especially terminal and respiratory bronchioles, and the surrounding alveoli. Atelectasis may be present and air bronchograms are absent. *Staphylococcal pneumonia* is a typical example. The chest radiograph may also reveal diseases that can mimic pneumonia, such as pulmonary emboli with infarction (see Chap. 213), congestive heart failure (see Chap. 36), or neoplasms. Appropriate diagnostic studies should be carried out to exclude these possibilities, if indicated.

Bacterial pneumonias typically are associated with leukocytosis with a high percentage of PMNs and with a ''left shift'' (see Chap. 81), whereas changes in leukocyte counts may be minimal in viral and other pneumonias. The adequacy of the bone marrow reserves, use of glucocorticoid or cytotoxic therapy, and conditions such as alcoholism and renal or liver failure may have independent effects that make the white blood count a less predictable indicator of the nature of the inflammatory response. Arterial blood gases often reveal hypocarbia and respiratory alkalosis from hyperventilation and hypoxemia from perfusion of involved nonventilated alveoli. Respiratory and metabolic acidosis could be present from complicating severe bronchospasm, respiratory failure, or systemic sepsis.

Microscopic examination and *culture of respiratory secretions* are essential for the rational treatment of pneumonia; a vigorous attempt must be made to obtain adequate specimens. Several blood cultures should be obtained since they may reveal the etiologic agent and, if positive, can affect the prognosis and potential for metastatic infection.

A freshly obtained specimen of expectorated sputum should be prepared for a Gram's stain and culture (see Chap. 80). Examination of a wet-mounted specimen (purulent fleck of sputum emulsified with a few drops of saline on a microscopic slide, a coverslip placed over it, and viewed at 100×) can permit a decision about the adequacy of the sample from the cell types present. A sputum specimen representative of the lower respiratory tract will have PMNs and possibly alveolar macrophages visible and very few oral squamous epithelial cells (less than one or two per high-power field). Use of a mixture of anticapsular antibodies to cause capsular swelling or a quellung reaction for species of *S. pneumoniae* in a wet specimen can improve accuracy of sputum analysis.

If the patient is not producing sputum, an attempt to induce secretions by ultrasonic nebulization of water or saline particles is reasonable. Such particles (which may vary in size between 0.8 and 10 μm in diameter) serve as an irritant and stimulate most subjects to cough. As an example, *P. carinii* can be identified in the induced sputum of about 80 percent of patients with this pneumonia who have AIDS and in a smaller percentage of patients with non-HIV disease (see Chaps. 163 and 264). Attempts to obtain lung secretions by passing a small catheter through the nose or mouth rarely get beyond the vocal cords of an alert patient and may only obtain a sample of oropharyngeal fluids. This practice should be discouraged.

If it is impossible to induce an adequate respiratory sample, other, more invasive measures should be considered. The situation arises most often in the debilitated, chronically ill patient or the immunosuppressed host. Factors such as patient tolerance, hematologic parameters, probability of opportunistic infection, and expertise with a particular procedure all affect the choice of procedures; these might include transtracheal aspiration, fiberoptic bronchoscopy, percutaneous transthoracic needle aspiration, thoracentesis, or open-lung biopsy.

Percutaneous transtracheal aspiration is a direct approach that eliminates much of the contaminating oral microbial flora, but it carries a risk to the patient and is now rarely employed in most centers. A needle containing a polyethylene catheter is inserted through the cricothyroid membrane into the airway lumen, and material is aspirated after a small injection of saline solution which makes the patient cough. Although transtracheal specimens can become contaminated with mouth flora, both anaerobic and aerobic cultures should be done. Minor complications include air leak leading to subcutaneous or mediastinal emphysema, or blood-tinged sputum. Serious complications from subcutaneous emphysema and tracheal hemorrhage occur in less than 0.5 percent of procedures performed by experienced practitioners. This procedure should not be carried out by inexperienced operators or in uncooperative patients or those with thrombocytopenia or other coagulation disorders, since it may induce fatal hemorrhage or serious injury.

Fiberoptic bronchoscopy with BAL and a protected brush catheter provides another approach. The risk of bronchoscopy is small, even in patients with extensive pneumonia. Administration of supplemental oxygen during the procedure is necessary. Use of oximetry to monitor its effect is recommended. Platelet transfusions should be given to correct thrombocytopenia. A direct view of the affected lung anatomy, particularly if a loss of volume in the lung lobe accompanies the infection, may disclose an endobronchial obstruction. Removal of secretions or a mucus plug could make the procedure of therapeutic as well as diagnostic value. Usually, the lavage fluid or catheter brush culture will contain the offending pathogen; however, microbial cultures from the bronchoscopy specimens also contain contaminating flora from the nasopharynx, and interpretation can be confusing. Transbronchial biopsy can be added to the procedure to provide lung tissue for culture and histology. Multiple biopsies of pieces 2 to 3 mm in size are usually obtained from at least two segments of a lobe if a diffuse infiltrate is present.

Depending upon the pathogen, the combination of catheter brush and transbronchial biopsy cultures from immunocompromised hosts with lung infection will yield a specific etiologic diagnosis in 50 to 95 percent of cases.

Complications arising from bronchoscopy include hemorrhage and/or pneumothorax in about 5 percent of cases. Occasionally, a chest tube will be needed to treat the pneumothorax. About 25 percent of patients develop a postbronchoscopy fever about 4 to 8 h after the procedure. This usually lasts less than 24 h and is not a complicating pneumonia but a febrile reaction, due perhaps to cellular mediators produced in the lavaged lung segment (see Chap. 20). This episode can usually be managed with antipyretic therapy alone and without an additional antibiotic.

Percutaneous transthoracic needle aspiration is a diagnostic modality that is sometimes helpful in pneumonia, although needle aspiration guided by computed tomography (CT) is performed more frequently to diagnose discrete lung lesions. Spread of microorganisms along the needle track or soilage of pleural surfaces rarely occur, but pneumothorax is a complication.

With primary bacterial pneumonia a parapneumonic effusion may occur in 10 to 30 percent of cases; pleural effusions of small size can occur with *Mycoplasma* and *Legionella* infection as well, and pleural tuberculosis characteristically causes effusions (see Chap. 125). Decubitus chest radiographs or ultrasonography is used to confirm the presence of fluid in the pleural space. A diagnostic *thoracentesis* is indicated to determine whether the fluid contains organisms and/or has the characteristics of an empyema. Cellular analysis and certain chemical tests (pH, lactic dehydrogenase, glucose, and total protein) will identify pleural fluid to be a transudate or exudate (see Chap. 216). Empyema can develop with pneumonitis or lung abscess in adjacent lung tissue; the fluid is exudative and like pus. Microorganisms may be seen on stained smear and usually grow from cultures. If an empyema exists, repeated thoracentesis to drain the fluid or use of an indwelling chest tube to effect continuous drainage is usually necessary to hasten healing and to prevent or minimize future pleural adhesions.

If a parapneumonic effusion develops in the course of pneumonia, thoracentesis is indicated if: (1) fever has persisted for 72 h after beginning treatment with appropriate antibiotics; (2) a large effusion develops that is contributing to discomfort and impairing breathing or is increasing in size; and (3) there is evidence that once freely movable fluid has become loculated. In the absence of these findings, small effusions usually disappear, the patient continues to improve, and thoracentesis is usually not indicated.

Needle biopsy of the pleura should be included with a thoracentesis if malignancy or tuberculosis is suspected, or prior pleural fluid cellular analysis suggests an unsuspected primary pleural disease (see Chap. 216).

If bronchoscopy is unrevealing or contraindicated, diagnostic *open-lung biopsy* is often necessary in the immunocompromised patient with an advancing, pulmonary infiltrate (see Chap. 82). Problems with the procedure include delay until severe hypoxemia or other complications make the risk excessive; or handling of the tissue is poorly coordinated between the operator, the microbiologist, and the pathologist, and an optimal analysis is not performed. The radiologist or pathologist can often suggest the best area of lung to biopsy, and the microbiology laboratory can be prepared to ensure that the most appropriate cultures are processed quickly. A properly performed and handled open-lung biopsy will reveal a specific etiology for pulmonary infiltrates in over 90 percent of patients.

THERAPY The history, physical examination, chest radiograph, Gram stain of sputum, and other diagnostic measures will provide knowledge about predisposing factors of the illness, potential causes, and probable extent of pneumonia. These factors and the results of microbiologic studies will determine initial and subsequent therapy. The differential diagnosis will vary according to the status of certain host defenses and the epidemiologic setting. The more common microbiologically identifiable causes of a community-acquired pneumonia include *S. pneumoniae* (60 to 75 percent) (see Chap. 99), *Mycoplasma pneumoniae* (1 to 2 percent) (see Chap. 154), *Staph. aureus* (1 to 2 percent) (see Chap. 100), and *L. pneumophila* (2 to 15 percent) (see Chap. 124). No etiologic agent may be clearly defined in 20 to 40 percent of cases. *Haemophilus influenzae* (see Chap. 115) is an unusual cause of primary pneumonia and is more likely to be part of an infectious exacerbation of bronchitis in a person with chronic lung disease. With exposure to infected animals or birds rare causes of pneumonia, including *Coxiella burnetii* (Q fever) (see Chap. 153), *Chlamydia psittaci* (see Chap. 155), and *Francisella tularensis* (see Chap. 120), should be considered. Pneumonia can complicate a viral exanthem such as varicella (see Chap. 136) and, rarely, measles (see Chap. 141). Adenovirus (see Chap. 140) can be a cause of epidemic pneumonia in a young adult. In endemic areas, *Histoplasma capsulatum* and *Coccidioides immitis* (see Chap. 151) need to be considered as causes of acute illness. Respiratory infections, especially with *P. carinii,* are often the presentation of AIDS (see Chaps. 163 and 264).

A nosocomial pneumonia that develops during a patient's confinement to a specialized nursing home unit or hospital is likely to be caused by aerobic gram-negative enteric bacilli (see Chap. 111) or *Staph. aureus*. Similarly, hospitalized patients who have impaired host defenses or who are immunocompromised because of an underlying disease or therapy are at increased risk for pneumonias caused by organisms spread hematogenously from other body sites. Neutropenia and prolonged antibiotic use predispose to infection with fungi such as *Aspergillus fumigatus* (see Chap. 151).

Treatment entails appropriate support with fluids, antipyretic drugs, oxygen, airway suction or gravity (postural) drainage, and bronchodilator drugs if bronchospasm is present (see Chap. 204). Antibiotic therapy remains the cornerstone of medical management.

The initial antimicrobial therapy should be chosen on the basis of interpretation of clinical findings and in severely ill patients must be heavily weighed toward protecting the patient against the most dangerous of the conceivable infectious agents. Results of cultures and antibiotic susceptibilities for common bacterial pathogens take several days. Organisms that are not grown easily may require a diagnosis based on rising antibody titers in acute and convalescent serum (e.g., Q fever) or recognition by specific immunofluorescence (*Legionella* sp. in sputum). As a consequence, an element of uncertainty is often present, and initial antibiotic therapy is somewhat empiric. Three principles of antimicrobial therapy deserve emphasis: (1) all necessary specimens for appropriate bacteriologic cultures should be obtained before therapy is initiated so that there is a reasonable chance to recover the organism; (2) initial drug therapy should be as specific as the evidence pointing to the etiologic agent allows, yet sufficiently broad to cover the common microorganisms; and (3) a few days of broad-spectrum antimicrobial treatment usually will not cause superinfection or selection of drug-resistant bacteria; however, final antimicrobial treatment should be adjusted to use specific narrow-spectrum drugs, if possible, when the results of cultures and susceptibilities are available.

Certain categories of pneumonia suggest a choice of antibiotics for initial therapy. For a community-acquired pneumonia (CAP) in a previously healthy young or middle-aged adult, erythromycin (500 mg intravenously every 6 h) would be effective for most strains of *S. pneumoniae, L. pneumophila,* and *M. pneumoniae,* but not suitable for *Haemophilus* sp. and *Staph. aureus*. Cefotaxime (1 to 2 g intravenously every 8 h), or ceftizoxime (2 g intravenously every 12 h), or cefuroxime (750 mg intravenously every 8 h) would provide therapy for *S. pneumoniae, Haemophilus* sp., and *Staph. aureus,* but not for *Legionella*. In older adults with CAP, the probability increases that gram-negative bacteria are the cause, i.e., *K. pneumoniae, H. influenzae,* and *Enterobacter aerogenes,* favoring the use of the cephalosporins cited above. Reduced dosages will be required with renal failure (see Chap. 85).

Initial treatment for nosocomial pneumonia should consider aerobic gram-negative bacilli such as *K. pneumoniae, Pseudomonas aeru-*

ginosa, Serratia marcescens, or *Staph. aureus* as potential causes. In a nonimmunosuppressed adult with nosocomial pneumonia, initial therapy with a third-generation cephalosporin such as cefotaxime, ceftizoxime, ceftazidime (1 to 2 g intravenously every 8 to 12 h), or cefoperazone (1 to 2 g intravenously every 12 h) is acceptable. If the patient is neutropenic, it is preferable to use two antibiotics, an aminoglycoside such as gentamicin (1 to 1.5 mg/kg intravenously every 8 h), tobramycin (1 to 1.5 mg/kg intravenously every 8 h), or amikacin (5 mg/kg intravenously every 8 h) with ceftazidime or a semisynthetic broad-spectrum penicillin such as ticarcillin (40 mg/kg intravenously every 4 h) or piperacillin (40 mg/kg intravenously every 6 h); synergistic action will be provided against the most deadly bacterium in this patient setting, *Pseudomonas aeruginosa.* Reduced dosages are necessary in renal failure (see Chap. 85). If the neutropenic patient has already received extensive antimicrobial therapy, then infection with fungi is more likely and amphotericin B should be utilized (see Chaps. 82 and 151).

Aspiration pneumonia as part of a CAP is polymicrobial and will contain a variety of anaerobic flora such as *Bacteroides melaninogenicus, Fusobacterium nucleatum,* and anaerobic streptococci; several antibiotic regimens have been successfully employed (see Chap. 108). These include penicillin G, (1.0 million units intravenously every 4 to 6 h), or clindamycin (600 mg intravenously every 8 h). Amoxicillin or ampicillin (as 500 to 750 mg orally every 6 h) combined with metronidazole (as 500 mg orally every 6 h) is an effective oral regimen, especially if a lung abcess had developed that will require prolonged treatment. If aspiration occurs within the hospital, then treatment should be directed toward enteric gram-negative bacilli and *Staph. aureus* with a third-generation cephalosporin as outlined above.

Once the patient's therapy is underway, attention must be focused on possible complications. A resurgence of fever after an initial period of defervescence is a frequent clue to a complication. Poor coughing and an accumulation of secretions or a mucus plug can obstruct an airway, leading to partial collapse of a lobe or segment of lung. Chest percussion, gravity drainage, and/or endotracheal suction to remove secretions and help reexpand the atelectatic segment should be tried for 24 h before resorting to bronchoscopy. The development of loculated pleural fluid usually requires thoracentesis and possible chest tube drainage. Secondary bacterial infection following a viral pneumonia or superinfection occurring after broad-spectrum antimicrobial therapy may cause fever and worsening of the patient's condition; repeat culturing of the sputum and blood is necessary to confirm the diagnosis. Drug allergy may cause lingering fever, sometimes accompanied by mild eosinophilia and rash; improvement after discontinuation or substitution in the antibiotic regimen will aid in establishing this diagnosis. Finally, evidence of resolution of the pneumonic process must be observed radiographically. In uncomplicated cases repeat radiographs are indicated at 3 to 5 day intervals for the first week, with a follow-up chest x-ray 1 month after discharge or completion of treatment. In severely ill patients or those who do not respond promptly to treatment, radiography should be performed more frequently. Failure of the pneumonia to resolve may require sputum cytologies and bronchoscopy to rule out a partially obstructing airway lesion or an endobronchial tumor, or to establish more precisely the microbial etiology.

LUNG ABSCESS

DEFINITION AND PATHOGENESIS Lung abscesses form as a complication of a localized area of pneumonia or when a neoplasm becomes necrotic and contains purulent material that cannot drain easily from the area because of partial or complete bronchial obstruction. When the local pulmonary artery blood supply is occluded by emboli or by vasculitis (e.g., Wegener's granulomatosis) or is inadequate to support a rapidly growing neoplasm (primary bronchogenic carcinoma, usually squamous cell carcinoma), necrosis and cavity formation may occur. Existing bullae and cysts can become infected or develop secondary air-fluid levels when surrounding infection exists and resemble an abscess. When large areas of inflamed, fibrotic lung tissue coalesce, as found in advanced silicosis, vascular insufficiency may lead to cavity formation (see Table 207-1). Although the terms abscess and cavity tend to be used interchangeably, abscess is preferable because it implies the presence of necrosis, inflammation, or associated infection. A cavity is often a radiographic description that may be used to suggest a more static or quiescent process.

TABLE 207-1 Lung abscesses classified according to cause

I Necrotizing infections
- *A* Pyogenic bacteria (*Staphylococcus aureus, Klebsiella pneumoniae, Pseudomonas aeruginosa,* group A streptococcus, *Legionella* sp., *Bacteroides, Fusobacterium,* anaerobic and microaerophilic cocci and streptococci, other anaerobes including *Actinomyces* sp., *Nocardia* sp.)
- *B* Mycobacteria (*Mycobacterium tuberculosis, M. kansasii, M. avium-intracellulare*)
- *C* Fungi (*Histoplasma capsulatum, Coccidioides immitis, Aspergillus* sp.
- *D* Parasites (amebas, lung flukes)

II Cavitary infarction
- *A* Bland embolism
- *B* Septic embolism (*Staph. aureus,* various anaerobes, *Candida* sp.)
- *C* Vasculitis (Wegener's granulomatosis)

III Cavitary malignancy
- *A* Primary bronchogenic carcinoma
- *B* Metastatic malignancies (very uncommon)

IV Other
- *A* Infected cysts
- *B* Necrotic conglomerate lesions (silicosis, coal miner's pneumoconiosis)

In the context of pneumonia, tissue necrosis may be due to properties of the infecting organisms. Infection with *Staph. aureus,* especially when bacteremic with septic lung emboli, can produce multiple abscesses that may evolve into pneumatoceles (see Chap. 100). Gram-negative bacilli, such as *Pseudomonas aeruginosa,* secrete exotoxins that can create vasculitis in addition to pneumonitis (see Chap. 111). Cavitation may develop as a complication of *Legionella* pneumonia (Chap. 124). In contrast, pneumococci, *H. influenzae, M. pneumoniae,* and viral infections almost never cause abscess formation. An abscess resulting from aspiration of nasopharyngeal secretions or gastroesophageal reflux is polymicrobial, with a prevalence of aerobic and facultatively anaerobic organisms (see Chap. 108). These mixed infections can be fulminant or indolent; airway obstruction by particulate material may facilitate abscess formation.

CLINICAL PRESENTATION A pulmonary abscess may evolve as part of a severe and rapidly progressing pneumonia. Its appearance is recognized radiographically and is accompanied by delayed resolution or worsening of the patient's anticipated clinical course, with persisting fever, copious expectoration of sputum, possibly hemoptysis, pleurisy, and even a pneumothorax. Sometimes, with an established pneumonia, it can be difficult to distinguish between a parenchymal abscess and/or a contiguous pleural effusion and empyema. Septic pulmonary emboli can cause multiple areas of infiltration on the radiograph and appear as patches of bronchopneumonia; later cavitation may occur. Staphylococcal endocarditis of the tricuspid or pulmonary valves, which is most often a complication of the use of illicit intravenous drugs, is the usual cause. Fever, chest pain, and occasionally hemoptysis are prominent manifestations. A cavity within the pneumonic area may be more evident with CT views of the lung.

A chronic lung abscess is often less dramatic in presentation: Cough, productive of foul-smelling and -tasting sputum; dyspnea; intermittent fever; weight loss; anorexia; and chest pain are the predominant features. Aspiration of oral or gastric secretions is the usual cause. Poor dentition with periodontal disease and conditions that promote aspiration are the common predisposing factors. Typical locations in the lung for aspiration-caused abscesses are the posterior segment of the upper lobe and superior segment of the right lower lobe. Endobronchial obstruction from a tumor must be considered as well, particularly if the right middle lobe is involved. The characteristic presentations of pulmonary tuberculosis, or necrotizing pulmonary infection caused by fungi, nocardia, or actinomyces species are discussed in Chaps. 151 and 152, respectively.

Physical examination may vary to include signs of consolidation with bronchial breath sounds, rales, and dullness or cavernous or amphoric breath sounds. Clubbing can occur and may develop in a few weeks. The chest radiograph often reveals a radiolucency in an opaque area of consolidation. An air-fluid level establishes that partial airway patency exists. Because the differentiation between a parenchymal abscess, an empyema, a bronchopleural fistula creating an empyema, an infected cyst, or a fluid level in an emphysematous bulla can be difficult, special radiographic views or CT scanning may be needed for clarification. Further laboratory evaluation including sputum analysis, cultures, and blood tests is similar to that described for pneumonia. Sputum cytologies should be obtained. The role of bronchoscopy in the initial evaluation of an abscess is controversial. Cultures obtained by bronchoalveolar lavage and protected catheters have limitations, but it may be useful to view the endobronchial anatomy to rule out obstruction. Bronchoscopy in the presence of a large fluid-filled cavity must be done cautiously because a sudden discharge of fluid into the airways is a hazard. Bronchoscopy is also indicated in an abscess that does not close in 4 to 6 weeks following appropriate treatment.

TREATMENT Antibiotic choice is predicated on identification of the organisms or the most likely ones present. The antibiotic choices suggested for aspiration pneumonia are appropriate for aspiration-caused abscess and are discussed in detail in Chap. 108. Other measures are similar to those described for treatment of pneumonia, with the additional goals of promoting good drainage of secretions and providing adequate nutrition. Pleural space drainage may be required for loculated fluid and empyema if these complicate the lung abscess. Surgical resection is rarely needed for a persistent abscess cavity; however, massive hemoptysis, localized malignancy, and possibly bronchiectasis may require this approach.

REFERENCES

Pneumonia

MANGI RJ et al: Cefoperazone *versus* combination antibiotic therapy of nosocomial pneumonia. Am J Med 84:68, 1988

PENNINGTON JE (ed): Hospital-acquired pneumonias. Semin Resp Infect 2:1, 1987

REYNOLDS HY: Bacterial adherence to respiratory tract mucosa—a dynamic interaction leading to colonization. Semin Resp Med 2:8, 1987

———: Lung inflammation: Normal host defense or a complication of some diseases. Ann Rev Med 38:295, 1987

———: Immunoglobulin G and its function in the human respiratory tract. Mayo Clin Proc 63:161, 1988

———: Pulmonary host defense. Chest 95S:223, 1989

VERGHESE A, BERK SL: Bacterial pneumonia in the elderly. Medicine 62:271, 1983

Lung abscess

JOHANSON WG et al: Aspiration pneumonia, anaerobic infections, and lung abscess. Med Clin North Am 64:385, 1980

MAHLER DA, D'ESOPO ND: Peri-emphysematous lung infection. Clin Chest Med 2:51, 1981

SCHACTER EN: Suppurative lung disease: Old problems revisited. Clin Chest Med 2:41, 1981

208 BRONCHIECTASIS AND BRONCHOLITHIASIS

HERBERT Y. REYNOLDS / RICHARD K. ROOT

BRONCHIECTASIS

DEFINITION Bronchiectasis is the permanent abnormal dilatation of one or more bronchi. Ectasia, or expansion and dilatation, can develop in any segment of the cartilage-containing tracheobronchial conducting airways when persisting inflammation in the lumen and adjacent wall causes destruction of the ciliated epithelium and submucosa and degeneration of elastic and muscular tissue. The diagnosis of bronchiectasis is suspected in patients with chronic cough with excessive expectoration of phlegm or purulent mucus or in those who have diffuse or localized recurrent bronchopulmonary infections, especially if associated with recurrent sinusitis and otitis media. The clinical picture may be difficult to distinguish from chronic bronchitis, however, and the two conditions may coexist. The diagnosis of bronchiectasis can be confirmed by bronchography, but tracheobronchitis, pneumonia, or atelectasis can produce bronchographic findings consistent with bronchiectasis which, unlike the findings in bronchiectasis, reverse with successful treatment. Traditionally, bronchiectasis has been classified on the basis of structural abnormalities seen on bronchography and is divided into localized and diffuse forms.

ETIOLOGY AND PATHOGENESIS Inflammation usually initiates the destructive process that results in bronchiectasis. Such injury can be caused by a primary microbial infection or by localized obstruction from either an intrinsic lesion in an airway, bronchial stenosis, or external compression. Stagnation of secretions in the presence of obstruction leads to secondary infection with inflammation and accumulation of leukocytes. The cumulative effects of proteolytic enzymes (collagenase and elastase) and toxic oxygen radical species released by neutrophils (see Chap. 81), as well as other products of inflammation, contribute to tissue necrosis. The effects of increased pressure due to retained inspissated secretions in the lumen may contribute to mucosal injury. Pathology often reveals exudative debris in and occluding the dilated bronchi.

The general size or segmental level of bronchi involved has provided descriptive terms for the pathologic findings of bronchiectasis. *Saccular* or *cystic* bronchiectasis affects major or proximal bronchi that end in large sacs by the fourth generation of branching. *Cylindrical* or *fusiform* dilatation is found in the sixth to eighth generation, produces an uneven involvement, and is probably a less severe form of disease. Clinically, the cylindrical type is a "dry" bronchiectasis with a less productive cough and fewer secretions. Varicose bronchiectasis is intermediate between saccular and cylindrical in form. If fibrosis has developed in the peribronchial area or extensively in the parenchyma thereby forming cysts, a telescoping or wrinkling effect in the subtending bronchi and bronchioles can be produced that is described as *traction* bronchiectasis. It is more often found with end-stage fibrocystic interstitial fibrosis; infection and excessive formation of secretions are unusual. The anatomic lesions of bronchiectasis may be visualized with bronchography or inferred from the appearance of bronchial structure in the chest radiograph or ultrathin (0.5-cm) sections of computed tomographic (CT) scans. Overlapping of all lesions can be found in any patient; thus, the anatomic pattern is not useful for etiologic diagnosis or correlation with clinical severity and has little therapeutic or prognostic significance.

With well-developed bronchiectasis, the bronchial artery circulation becomes more pronounced; vessels may be hypertrophied and more vulnerable to rupture. Whether the lack of supporting tissue for the vessels or increased exposure to irritation and pressure changes induced by coughing makes hemoptysis more likely is uncertain; certainly this problem is important clinically.

Localized bronchiectasis This entity is caused by a variety of bronchopulmonary infections or by the obstruction of bronchi. Measles and whooping cough were important causes before the development of effective immunization; currently, infection with adenovirus or respiratory syncytial virus leads to bronchiectasis in a small percentage of children with these conditions. Pulmonary tuberculosis was once a frequent cause but is now rare in the United States. More effective treatment of severe, necrotizing bacterial pneumonias with antibiotics has helped to minimize residual airway injury, reducing the frequency of resultant bronchiectasis. Childhood respiratory infection as the inciting cause of bronchiectasis remains prominent in developing countries or among the disadvantaged in places where immunization and health care are scarce. Localized bronchiectasis may result from obstruction by aspirated foreign bodies; these can usually be retrieved promptly with fiberoptic bronchoscopy, and irreversible injury is less likely now than before the availability of this modality. Local endobronchial obstruction from a primary tumor or metastases or external bronchial compression from enlarged hilar lymph nodes remains an important cause of postobstructive pneumonitis and/or atelectasis that can lead to bronchiectasis. Recurrent aspiration of orogastric secretions can be an important cause of localized bronchiectasis in patients with neurologic impairment. Rarely, a congenital abnormality in bronchial formation can create a cul-de-sac or bronchial malacia, thus causing localized bronchiectasis.

Diffuse bronchiectasis Bronchiectasis involving multiple lobes is usually the consequence of inherited or acquired defects in the defense mechanisms which normally protect the airways from infection or inflammation (see Chap. 207). The acquired conditions may include those which lead to repeated aspiration of orogastric contents (altered states of consciousness, neuromuscular impairment of swallowing or cough, gastroesophageal sphincter incompetence, and nasogastric intubation) or which cause chronic bronchitis (see Chap. 210) or, rarely, asthma (Chap. 204). The congenital conditions may involve alterations in the function of the mucociliary blanket or other aspects of pulmonary host defense. The congenital disorders are often associated with repeated respiratory tract infections including sinusitis, otitis media, and pneumonias or, in the case of immunoglobulin deficiencies, with systemic bacterial infections (see Chap. 263). Specific congenital disorders causing diffuse bronchiectasis include cystic fibrosis, the dyskinetic ciliary syndromes, Young's syndrome (sinopulmonary infections and obstructive azospermia), the hypogammaglobulinemias, or deficiencies of specific IgG subclasses. Less likely causes are congenital forms of tracheobronchomegaly; a cartilage disorder which leads to short stature, thoracic deformities, and bronchomalacia (Williams-Campbell syndrome); and α_1-antitrypsin deficiency.

DISORDERS OF MUCOCILIARY FUNCTION Intrinsic defects in the ultrastructure of cilia throughout the body can impair ciliary motion in several organ systems, particularly ciliated epithelium in the nasal and conducting airways and in the fallopian tubes; sperm are also immotile. Three basic defects have been identified in the doublet tubular structure of cilia—absent inner or outer dynein arms (causing Kartagener's syndrome), absent radial spokes, and absence of the central doublet of the axoneme of the cilium. As ciliary function is not entirely absent but lacks coordination, these are now described as *dyskinetic* (rather than *immotile*) ciliary syndromes. These congenital illnesses feature recurrent sinopulmonary infections, dextrocardia or situs inversus (in about half the cases of Kartagener's syndrome), and infertility. Recurrent bronchitis and pneumonias leading to diffuse bronchiectasis are a consequence of impaired removal of airway secretions normally aspirated during sleep.

The pathogenesis of cystic fibrosis and the mechanisms by which bronchiectasis might occur as a complication are discussed in Chap. 209.

IMMUNODEFICIENCY DISORDERS An absence of immunoglobulins, systemically and in the airway secretions, predisposes to sinopulmonary infections that ultimately lead to bronchiectasis. The absence of IgA and/or IgG neutralizing antibodies against viruses in tracheobronchial secretions or IgG opsonizing antibodies against encapsulated bacteria creates the conditions for recurrent infections. Secretory IgA is the principal immunoglobulin present in upper airway secretions and in those from the trachea and major bronchi (see Chaps. 13 and 207). Isolated absence of IgA may not have any infectious consequences unless associated with deficiencies of IgG2 and IgG4 (see Chap. 263). Common variable hypogammaglobulinemia, which involves all immunoglobulin classes, can develop acutely at any age (see Chap. 263). Selective deficiencies of IgG2 and/or IgG4 occur also and are associated with recurrent sinopulmonary infections which may result in diffuse bronchiectasis. While pneumonias are common in neutropenic subjects and those with neutrophil dysfunction (see Chap. 81), bronchiectasis does not appear to be as frequent or prominent as in the immunoglobulin disorders.

CLINICAL MANIFESTATIONS A raspy, frequent cough that produces purulent sputum in amounts that can total several hundred milliliters daily is a cardinal manifestation of bronchiectasis. Chronic low-grade respiratory infection can be interspersed with bouts of more severe bronchitis and bronchopneumonia accompanied by fever and chest pain. The sputum may vary in daily volume, appearance, and thickness; in some patients these characteristics may not correlate well with exacerbations or resolution of acute infection. Flecks of blood may be periodically admixed with the sputum, and frank hemoptysis can occur. Although hemoptysis is worrisome, it usually subsides quickly, and it does not necessarily portend a major hemorrhage.

Constitutional or systemic symptoms and signs are variable and include intermittent fever, lassitude, fatigue, and poor appetite. These are more pronounced with acute exacerbations of pulmonary infection. Dyspnea is variable and depends upon the extent of lung involvement as well as the presence or absence of acute infection. Wheezing due to associated asthma or bronchospasm may be a feature. Colonization of the bronchiectatic airways with *Aspergillus* species or, rarely, other fungi can precipitate acute asthmatic episodes due to an allergic IgE-mediated mechanism (see Chap. 51). This is accompanied by coughing up of gelatinous, rubbery mucous plugs containing many eosinophils; fungal hyphae may be seen.

Bronchiectasis that is associated with conditions leading to recurrent sinusitis and otitis media may have prominent symptomatic involvement of these organs. Postnasal secretions are increased, throat clearing is common, tinnitus, diminished hearing, frontal headache, and maxillary and dental pain may occur. All patients with bronchiectasis are prone to exacerbations of acute bacterial pneumonia (see Chap. 207). In fact, if pneumonia occurs repeatedly in an isolated or dependent lung segment, bronchiectasis should be suspected.

Physical findings will vary depending upon whether an underlying systemic disease is present and upon the extent of the pulmonary involvement. Many patients with limited localized bronchiectasis appear healthy and have minimal or no physical abnormalities. With more extensive disease chest auscultation will reveal coarse crackles over the affected areas, and wheezing may be present. With complicating pneumonia or atelectasis, diminished breath sounds and dullness to percussion may be found. With advanced disease, clubbing of fingers and toes is common and nailbed cyanosis may be evident. With end-stage disease, signs of secondary pulmonary hypertension and cor pulmonale usually develop (see Chap. 191).

LABORATORY STUDIES AND DIAGNOSTIC EVALUATION Results of laboratory and chest imaging studies vary with the underlying systemic disease and type of bronchiectasis. The total white blood cell count may be mildly elevated with a neutrophilic leukocytosis; this will be more pronounced and a left shift of neutrophils may be present with complicating pneumonia or sepsis. The erythrocyte sedimentation rate is often elevated. Anemia is rare. Arterial blood gas values may show a respiratory alkalosis or hypoxemia; they may be altered further by complicating pneumonia or bronchospasm (see Chap. 207). Initially, with diffuse bronchiectasis, pulmonary function tests may show obstruction, but with advanced disease and after many infections, a restrictive pattern evolves. Sputum cultures often disclose only mixed oral flora, and the intermittent presence of pathogens such as *Haemophilus influenzae, Streptococcus pneumoniae, Staphylococcus aureus,* or gram-negative enteric bacilli. A foul odor to the sputum suggests a predominance of anaerobes. Mucoid strains of *Pseudomonas auruginosa* are commonly and persistently isolated in patients with the later stages of cystic fibrosis (CF) (see Chap. 209).

In advanced cases, conventional radiographs may reveal 1- to 2-cm cystic-appearing lesions with or without fluid levels consistent with saccular bronchiectasis. Often the chest film shows linear streaks (tram tracks), on-end thickened bronchi, or signet-ring deformity, and groups of small curvilinear shadows, called grape clusters; these findings can be subtle. Lung CT scanning using ultrathin sections is a sensitive way to detect bronchiectasis, especially the saccular form, and to define its distribution. Bronchography is now rarely needed to document bronchiectasis, and when used should not be performed until several months have elapsed after an acute pneumonia to avoid misdiagnosis of reversible bronchiectasis.

Fiberoptic bronchoscopy is usually required to evaluate recurrent, segmental disease and atelectasis or collapsed areas to eliminate endobronchial obstruction. It is not the recommended way, however, to visualize bronchiectatic areas, particularly if these are distal to the third or fourth generation of bronchi and out of reach.

With diffuse bronchiectasis attention should be paid to defining the associated disorders. Impaired swallowing, cough, or gastroesophageal reflux should be evident from the history and physical examination. A family history of affected siblings, infant deaths, kindred with similar symptoms, or problems with infertility can reveal mucociliary or immune-deficiency disorders. Preliminary screening tests should include: analysis of electrolytes contained in a sample of sweat (see Chap. 209); quantitative serum immunoglobulins, including subclasses of IgG, and assessment of sperm motility.

Patients with asthma and suspected allergic bronchopulmonary aspergillosis should have the sputum cultured for *Aspergillus,* measurements of serum IgE values (usually in excess of 2500 ng/mL), and serologic studies for *Aspergillus* precipitins (positive in >90 percent). In referral centers additional studies might include measurement of secretory IgA in parotid fluid or nasal washings, assessment of ciliary clearance with an aerosolized, isotopic tracer; and biopsy of nasal mucosal for electron-microscopic cross-sectional views of cilia to define ultrastructure.

TREATMENT Treatment is directed at controlling complicating infections and providing effective drainage of secretions.

With bacterial infection often responsible for initiating bronchiectasis as well as causing acute exacerbations with complicating pneumonitis, antibiotic treatment remains a mainstay in prevention and management. During exacerbations, microbial cultures will yield a mixture of bacteria, and it may be difficult to identify a discrete pathogen, with the exception of *P. aeruginosa* in patients with advanced CF. When no specific pathogen is identified and the patient is not so ill as to require hospitalization, use of an oral agent such as amoxicillin, ampicillin, tetracycline, trimethoprim-sulfamethoxazole, or the fixed combination of amoxicillin and clavulanic acid (Augmentin) are all reasonable initial choices (for dosages see Chap. 85). Parenteral antibiotics are usually reserved for more seriously ill patients with pneumonitis. Again the initial choice should be guided by results of Gram stain evaluation of the sputum and altered by culture results which reveal specific pathogens. When *S. aureus* is present or suspected, a penicillinase-resistant penicillin (nafcillin or oxacillin) or a cephalosporin (e.g., cefazolin) should be utilized. Infections with *P. aeruginosa,* as are common in patients with advanced CF, should be treated with a combination of an antipseudomonal penicillin or ceftazidime and an aminoglycoside such as tobramycin administered parenterally until a response occurs (see Chaps. 85 and 111). Favorable responses are usually defined by a decrease in and thinning of sputum and the resolution of systemic symptoms. These effects generally occur over 5 to 7 days. Clearing of radiologic evidence of pneumonitis may take weeks. In some patients treatment may need to be prolonged for several weeks. Since the sputum culture is not likely to be sterilized by treatment, repeat culturing is indicated only in the event of suspected superinfection with resistant organisms. Antibiotic treatment is usually reserved for acute exacerbations since prolonged and prophylactic use of antibiotics has not been shown to prevent exacerbations and may lead to the development of resistant organisms. Nebulized antibiotics have not been shown to be effective in treating acute exacerbations or as prophylaxis.

Respiratory therapy, in the form of chest percussion and gravity drainage, can promote removal of thick secretions. If bronchospasm is a complicating factor, therapy with inhaled bronchodilators is indicated (see Chaps. 204 and 210). Oral theophylline has been employed as an adjunct to enhance respiratory muscle performance and perhaps ciliary activity; however, its benefits in this regard are unproven. Expectorants and mucolytic agents are usually not helpful. Bronchoscopy may be required to remove inspissated secretions. If allergic bronchopulmonary aspergillosis is suspected, a trial of moderate doses of oral glucocorticoids (20 mg prednisone daily) may be employed to help reduce airway inflammation. Larger doses of oral or parenteral glucocorticoids may be required if asthma unresponsive to bronchodilators supervenes (Chap. 204). Immunoglobulin deficiency should be treated with human immune serum globulin (see Chap. 263).

Smoking of cigarettes should be interdicted. There should be yearly vaccination against influenza as well as vaccination against pneumococcal infection. Episodes of sinusitis should be promptly treated and may require joint management with an otolaryngologist for sinus drainage procedures and relief of nasal obstruction. Nasal oxygen may be required on a chronic basis to maintain adequate oxygenation. A program of graded exercise, routine deep breathing, and maintenance of good nutrition should be part of general management.

If a localized area of bronchiectasis is found to be the site of recurring infections, hemorrhage, or other symptoms, surgical removal of the segment or lobe or an approach to correct a partial obstruction may be indicated. CT scanning and perhaps bronchography should be performed to exclude a more generalized process. Pulmonary function studies should be performed before surgery to determine the capacity of the patient to tolerate lung resection and to estimate pulmonary reserve after operation. With aggressive deployment of antibiotics and other respiratory therapy procedures, resection surgery is rarely necessary. Severe bronchial hemorrhage may be controlled by bronchial artery embolization rather than surgery. Conversely with very extensive pulmonary involvement and lung destruction, transplantation surgery may offer the only hope for survival.

PREVENTION Prevention of bronchiectasis is promoted by prompt diagnosis and antimicrobial treatment of bronchopulmonary bacterial infections and by vaccination against measles and pertussis. Chronic bronchitis and asthma should be managed as outlined in Chaps. 204 and 210. Localized bronchiectasis due to obstruction can be prevented by prompt removal of foreign bodies, preferably by fiberoptic bronchoscopy; other causes of local obstruction should be surgically treated if feasible. For chronic aspiration of orogastric secretions, correction of the underlying cause should be carried out if possible. In some cases of swallowing disorders a feeding gastrostomy or even laryngeal closure with tracheostomy may be necessary. Immunoglobulin therapy should be administered to IgG-deficient patients as outlined in Chap. 263. Patients and their families with dyskinetic ciliary syndromes or CF should receive appropriate genetic counseling.

BRONCHOLITHIASIS

A broncholith represents a calcified fragment of tissue that is loose within the bronchial lumen. Broncholiths usually form from disorders that lead to calcification of pulmonary tissue or of lymph nodes which then impinge upon and erode into a bronchus. Most commonly, pulmonary calcification follows an infection that elicits a granulomatous response such as tuberculosis, histoplasmosis, or coccidioidomycosis. Tuberculosis is the leading cause of calcified pulmonary granulomas worldwide; however, in the United States histoplasmosis is probably more common. With bronchiectasis necrosis and calcification of bronchial cartilage may occur leading to fragmentation and the formation of broncholiths. Rarely, aspirated food or other tissues may be retained in the airway for a long time and become calcified.

Movements of the calcified particles into or within the airway cause the clinical manifestations of broncholithiasis: paroxysms of cough, symptomatic postobstructive bronchopulmonary infection, and episodic hemoptysis. The cough can be productive of a mixture of gritty, sandy particles or small stones admixed with purulent phlegm and blood.

Broncholithiasis should be considered in patients who have these symptoms, particularly if the chest x-ray discloses multiple calcifications in the lung and in hilar or mediastinal lymph nodes. Examination of the sputum may reveal calcified particles. CT scanning of the chest can be helpful in more precisely localizing areas of calcification. Some episodes of broncholithiasis are self-limited and require no further diagnostic evaluation or treatment. With persistence of symptoms, particularly if there is postobstructive infection, atelectasis, or significant hemoptysis, bronchoscopy is indicated to visualize the area of obstruction and, if possible, to extract the stone. Antibiotics as outlined for the treatment of bronchiectasis should be administered to treat associated infection. Rarely, thoracotomy and resection of involved pulmonary segments is required to manage persistent bronchial obstruction or massive hemoptysis.

REFERENCES

Bronchiectasis

Barker AF, Bardana EJ: Bronchiectasis: Update of an orphan disease. Am Rev Respir Dis 137:969, 1988

Reynolds HY: Host defense impairments that lead to respiratory infections. Clin Chest Med 8:339, 1987

Schuyler MR: Allergic bronchopulmonary aspergillosis. Clin Chest Med 4:15, 1983

Sturgess JM, Turner JAP: Recurrent illness due to immotile cilia syndrome. J Respir Dis 3.48 1982

Swartz MN: Bronchiectasis, in *Pulmonary Disease and Disorders*, 2d ed, AP Fishman (ed). New York McGraw-Hill, 1988, pp 1553–1581

Broncholithiasis

Cole FH et al: Management of broncholithiasis: Is thoracotomy necessary? Ann Thoracic Surg 42:255, 1986

Haines JD: Coughing up a stone. What to do about broncholithiasis. Postgrad Med 83:83, 1988

209 CYSTIC FIBROSIS

HARVEY R. COLTEN

Cystic fibrosis (CF) is an inherited multisystem disorder which is characterized by an abnormality in exocrine gland function. Nearly all patients develop chronic progressive disease of the respiratory system. Pulmonary disease is the most common cause of death and morbidity in patients with cystic fibrosis. Pancreatic dysfunction (exocrine or endocrine) occurs in 85 percent of patients; hepatobiliary and genitourinary disease are also frequent. Prior to the 1930s the syndrome was confused with several other disorders with signs and symptoms of intestinal malabsorption.

CF is common in populations of European origin. Estimates of the incidence of the disorder range from about 1/500 in Amish (Ohio) to 1/90,000 in Hawaiian Orientals. For the white American population the disease occurs in 1/1600 to 1/2000 live births. The disease is recognized less frequently in black Africans. From the autosomal recessive mode of inheritance the gene frequency in white Americans is estimated at 1/20. A series of DNA probes that detect sequences close to the "CF gene" on the long arm of chromosome 7 have been used to detect restriction fragment length polymorphisms and to isolate the "cystic fibrosis gene," permitting antenatal diagnosis and carrier detection. The use of these genetic data, coupled with cell physiologic studies indicating a defect in regulation of a chloride channel in epithelia facilitated a better understanding of the molecular pathophysiology of cystic fibrosis. Based on studies of several hundred families, it is clear that a three-base-pair deletion resulting in loss of a phenylalanine at position 508 accounts for 30 to 75 percent of CF cases in different populations. Other mutations within this gene are responsible for most, if not all, of the remaining CF cases.

Currently, the median survival for patients with CF is about 20 years, and many patients survive to the third and fourth decades. A few have survived to age 50 and beyond. Even though survival of CF patients has improved, the mutation is semilethal. More than 98 percent of males with CF are infertile (see below), and fertility is reduced in women with the disease. This, together with the high incidence of the disease, suggests a selective advantage for the individual heterozygous for the CF gene, but this remains speculative in the absence of precise information about the gene defect.

CLINICAL MANIFESTATIONS General The majority of CF patients are diagnosed in infancy or childhood, but some escape detection until adulthood. Table 209-1 summarizes the multiple

TABLE 209-1 Principal clinical manifestations of cystic fibrosis

I Respiratory/cardiovascular
- *A* Bronchitis, bronchopneumonia, bronchiectasis, lung abscesses, aspergillosis (allergic)
- *B* Atelectasis
- *C* Sinusitis, nasal polyposis
- *D* Pulmonary hypertension
- *E* Cor pulmonale and congestive heart failure
- *F* Hemoptysis
- *G* Pneumothorax
- *H* Respiratory failure

II Gastrointestinal
- *A* Intestinal
  - *1* Meconium ileus
  - *2* Volvulus
  - *3* Ileal atresia
  - *4* Rectal prolapse
  - *5* Intussusception
  - *6* Fecal impaction
  - *7* Pneumatosis intestinalis
- *B* Pancreatic
  - *1* Nutritional deficit and growth failure due to pancreatic insufficiency
  - *2* Steatorrhea
  - *3* Diabetes mellitus
  - *4* Recurrent pancreatitis
- *C* Hepatobiliary
  - *1* Atrophic gallbladder, cholelithiasis
  - *2* Loss of bile salts
  - *3* Focal biliary cirrhosis
  - *4* Portal hypertension
    - *a* Esophageal varices
    - *b* Hypersplenism
    - *c* Hemorrhoids

III Reproductive system
- *A* Males: sterility; absent or defective vas deferens, epididymis, and seminal vesicles in about 99 percent of males
- *B* Females: decreased fertility; increased viscosity of vaginal secretions

IV Skeletal
- *A* Retardation of bone age
- *B* Demineralization
- *C* Hypertrophic osteoarthropathy

V Other
- *A* Salt depletion
- *B* Heat stroke
- *C* Salivary gland hypertrophy
- *D* Retinal hemorrhage
- *E* Hypertrophy of apocrine glands

clinical features of this disease. Substantial pancreatic disease is more common in patients diagnosed early in life, because acute intestinal obstruction (meconium ileus at birth) or malnutrition and poor growth or development alerts the pediatrician and family. Patients with minimal or absent gastrointestinal complaints and atypical respiratory symptoms may be diagnosed for the first time when adult. The finding of microorganisms typically isolated from sputum of CF patients (a mucoid form of *Pseudomonas aeruginosa*) or male infertility in association with evidence of obstructive pulmonary disease suggests CF in a previously undiagnosed adult.

Respiratory All levels of the respiratory tract may be affected in CF. Nasal polyposis, sinusitis, and lower respiratory tract disease are common. Abnormalities in water and electrolyte transport across the respiratory epithelium are said to be uniquely abnormal in patients with CF. Primary qualitative or quantitative alterations in mucous secretion that are characteristic for CF have been suggested, but most if not all that have been experimentally determined appear similar to findings in patients with chronic bronchitis or bronchiectasis of diverse etiologies. Autopsy studies of infants dying of meconium ileus suggest that the lungs of newborns with CF are normal. The earliest pulmonary changes are hypertrophy of bronchial glands followed by mucous plugging and obstruction of small airways. Subsequent infection leads to a bronchiolitis, and centripetal progression of endobronchial disease results in chronic bronchitis, bronchiectasis, and peribronchial inflammation. The release of toxic oxygen species and proteolytic enzymes by bacterial and inflammatory cells probably contributes to the progression of airway disease. Specific and nonspecific systemic host defenses are normal or increased, though chronic inflammatory disease may lead to mechanical interference with local defense mechanisms.

Three major bacterial organisms chronically colonize or infect the airways of patients with CF. *Staphylococcus aureus* and *Haemophilus influenzae* are recovered from sputum in a minority, and *P. aeruginosa*, especially mucoid forms, are detected in more than 90 percent of CF patients. Once the *P. aeruginosa* is acquired, the organism is rarely if ever eliminated. Other bacteria (mucoid forms of *Escherichia coli*, *Legionella*, etc.) and other microorganisms, including viruses, mycoplasma, and fungi, may be present in the sputum of patients with CF. Colonization with *Pseudomonas cepacia* may herald a more unfavorable short-term prognosis. The mucoid *Pseudomonas* strains are detected almost exclusively in the CF population. Even family members of patients with CF are not colonized by this organism, so that recovery of a mucoid form of *P. aeruginosa* from patients with chronic pulmonary disease should prompt further diagnostic studies to rule out CF.

Acute and chronic pulmonary parenchymal involvement leads to loss of tissue, extensive fibrosis, and changes in lung and airway mechanics. The inflammatory and structural changes in airways and lung parenchyma lead to airway obstruction, hyperinflation, and ventilation-perfusion imbalance. The upper lobes are generally more involved than lower lobes. Pleural involvement is rare, and extrathoracic infection with respiratory pathogens is virtually absent. Secondary changes in pulmonary and bronchial vasculature in patients with advanced respiratory disease may lead to the substantial hemoptysis often observed in older patients. Pulmonary hypertension develops frequently in CF patients with severe airway obstruction and hypoxemia, resulting in progressive right ventricular failure (cor pulmonale). Clubbing is seen in nearly all patients.

TREATMENT Treatment of CF pulmonary disease is directed toward increasing mechanical drainage, as in patients with chronic bronchitis (Chap. 210), with the use of chest physiotherapy, exercise programs, etc. Control of bacterial infection or colonization is effected by antibiotic therapy specific for the common bacterial organisms isolated from CF sputum. Antibiotic-resistant strains of *P. aeruginosa* are frequently isolated from patients with advanced disease, but in general intravenously administered aminoglycosides in combination with modified penicillins or cephalosporins are employed for treatment of pulmonary exacerbations. Preliminary studies support the use of aerosolized antibiotics (generally aminoglycosides) in the management of chronic pulmonary infection with *Pseudomonas aeruginosa*, but the success of this approach is highly dependent on technical details of the delivery system. Management of the bronchospastic component of the disease involves the use of systemic and aerosolized bronchodilators. Occasionally surgery (e.g., lobectomy) is required when infection or tissue destruction is localized. Prompt attention to and specific therapy of complications of pulmonary disease have been important factors in the improved survival of patients with CF. Small pneumothoraxes can generally be managed expectantly, while many will respond to tube thoracostomy alone. However, the best evidence suggests that this approach is associated with high recurrence rates. Therefore most episodes are treated with pleural sclerosis (with agents such as tetracycline or quinacrine), open pleurectomy, or pleurodesis. Massive hemoptysis is treated most safely and effectively by bronchial artery embolization via a percutaneous catheter. Congestive heart failure is managed as described elsewhere (Chaps. 182 and 191). Finally, for patients with advanced pulmonary disease, lung or heart-lung transplantation has been employed on an experimental basis at a limited number of institutions.

Gastrointestinal Pancreatic insufficiency leading to fat and protein malabsorption is a feature in the majority of cases (Chap. 261). Deficiencies of fat-soluble vitamins, caloric deprivation, failure to grow and develop, and other manifestations such as rectal prolapse occur in patients with untreated pancreatic insufficiency. About 5 percent of patients with CF are born with meconium ileus, i.e., intestinal obstruction secondary to inspissated meconium in the terminal ileum. Occasionally perforation and meconium peritonitis can occur. Treatment of pancreatic insufficiency with oral pancreatic enzymes corrects most of the deficits. For instance, it decreases the number and bulk of stools; the amount of flatulence, abdominal pain, and distention; and it largely corrects the malabsorption and hence corrects the nutritional deficiencies.

In patients with intact or partial pancreatic exocrine function, recurrent acute pancreatitis may occur. A minority of patients (2 to 5 percent) develop overt diabetes mellitus requiring exogenous insulin, but subclinical abnormalities in glucose metabolism can be detected in a much larger group of CF patients. The longer survival of patients with CF may allow the development of typical diabetic complications such as retinal and glomerular lesions. These should prompt more aggressive efforts to maintain optimal diabetic control.

Hepatobiliary disease is common in older patients. There is chronic cholestasis, inflammation, fibrosis, and even cirrhosis. All of the features of portal hypertension have been recognized. Extrahepatic disease of the biliary system is common.

Genitourinary Abnormalities of the genitourinary tract are present in 98 percent of males. These are due to an interruption in wolffian duct structures (atresia of the vas deferens) which results in azoospermia and decreased ejaculate volume (Chap. 321). Sexual development and potency are unaffected by the genitourinary abnormalities. Women have abnormal cervical mucus. Sexual development, the menstrual cycle, and fertility in women are less affected by direct effects of the mutation than by the effects of poor nutrition and/or chronic pulmonary disease. Women with CF can conceive and deliver healthy infants, but the maternal and fetal risks are functions of the extent of pulmonary disease and its complications. Close monitoring and prompt therapy in centers expert in high-risk obstetrical management are indicated.

Sweat glands The abnormality in the eccrine sweat gland function provides the most reliable diagnostic test for CF at present. Sodium, potassium, and chloride are elevated in sweat of patients with CF. The chloride concentration exceeds 70 mmol per liter, and the sodium concentration is greater than 60 mmol per liter in sweat of nearly all patients, though some individuals with "borderline values" may have many other manifestations of the disease. The corresponding values for chloride and sodium in normals rarely exceed 50 and 40 mmol per liter, respectively. Sweat electrolytes are measured most reliably by the pilocarpine iontophoresis method.

Even when qualitative screening methods are used, the diagnosis cannot be made without a quantitative sweat electrolyte measurement. The increased electrolyte content results from a failure of reabsorption in the sweat duct. Electrolyte losses may lead to significant salt depletion, especially in young children.

CONCLUSION Increasing survival of patients with typical findings of CF as well as patients undiagnosed until adult life requires an increased awareness of this disorder among physicians. The relatively high prevalence of this disorder and the enormous resources required to treat patients with CF has stimulated research activity to define the basic genetic defect responsible for the protean clinical manifestations of CF.

REFERENCES

BOAT TF et al: Cystic fibrosis, in CR Scriver et al (eds): *The Metabolic Basis of Inherited Disease*, 6th ed. New York, McGraw-Hill, 1989, pp 2649–2680

DAVIS PB: Cystic fibrosis. Semin Resp Med 6:243, 1985

DI SANT'AGNESE PA, DAVIS PB: Cystic fibrosis in adults: 75 cases and a review of 232 cases in the literature. Am J Med 66:121, 1979

FELLOWS KE et al: Bronchial artery embolization in cystic fibrosis: Technique and long-term results. J Pediatr 95:959, 1979

KEREM B et al: Identification of the cystic fibrosis gene: Genetic analysis. Science 245:1073, 1989

KNOWLES M et al: Increased bioelectrical potential difference across respiratory epithelia in cystic fibrosis. N Engl J Med 305:1489, 1981

PARK RW, GRAND RJ: Gastrointestinal manifestations of cystic fibrosis: A review. Gastroenterol 81:1143, 1981

RIORDAN JR et al: Identification of the cystic fibrosis gene: Cloning and characterization of complementary DNA. Science 245:1066, 1989

ROMMENS JM et al: Identification of the cystic fibrosis gene: Chromosome walking and jumping. Science 245:1059, 1989

SCANLIN TF: Cystic fibrosis (including assessment of pulmonary performance), in *Pulmonary Diseases and Disorders*, 2d ed, AP Fishman (ed). New York, McGraw-Hill, 1987, chap 76

SHWACHMAN H et al: The sweat test: Sodium and chloride values. J Pediatr 98:576, 1981

210 CHRONIC BRONCHITIS, EMPHYSEMA, AND AIRWAYS OBSTRUCTION

ROLAND H. INGRAM, JR.

Chronic bronchitis and emphysema are two distinct processes, often present in combination in patients with chronic airways obstruction. The diagnosis of chronic bronchitis is made by history, chronic airways obstruction is assessed physiologically, and emphysema can be diagnosed with certainty only by histologic examination of sections of whole lung fixed at inflation. Although the relationships between clinical characteristics, physiologic derangements, and morphologic changes have been diligently studied for many years, reasonably certain and uniform clinical criteria are still not available. Definitions and classifications have evolved, but these are not universally accepted. Nonetheless, the following definitions along with brief qualifications and descriptions are currently used by most persons involved in the diagnosis, treatment, and epidemiology of the chronic obstructive airways syndromes.

DEFINITIONS *Chronic bronchitis* is a condition associated with excessive tracheobronchial mucus production sufficient to cause cough with expectoration for at least 3 months of the year for more than 2 consecutive years. Several subclassifications have been proposed. *Simple chronic bronchitis* describes a condition characterized by mucoid sputum production. *Chronic mucopurulent bronchitis* is characterized by persistent or recurrent purulence of sputum in the absence of localized suppurative diseases such as bronchiectasis. Since there may or may not be obstruction as assessed by the use of the forced expiratory vital capacity maneuver, *chronic bronchitis with obstruction* deserves a separate classification. There is a further subset of patients with chronic bronchitis and obstruction who experience severe dyspnea and wheezing in association with inhaled irritants or during acute respiratory infections. Such patients are said to have *chronic infective asthma* or *chronic asthmatic bronchitis*. Since there is considerable but not complete reversibility of airflow obstruction with bronchodilator treatment and abatement of inflammation and since hyperresponsiveness of airways to nonspecific stimuli is seen in this group of patients, confusion is possible between patients with this condition and those with asthma who may also have *chronic airways obstruction* (Chap. 204). The differentiation is based mainly upon the history of the clinical illness. The patient with chronic asthmatic bronchitis has a long history of cough and sputum production with a later onset of wheezing, whereas the asthmatic with chronic obstruction gives a long history of wheezing with later onset of chronic productive cough.

Emphysema is defined as distention of the air spaces distal to the terminal bronchiole with destruction of alveolar septa. *Chronic obstructive lung disease* is defined as a condition in which there is chronic obstruction to airflow due to chronic bronchitis and/or emphysema (see below). Although the degree of obstruction may be less when the patient is free from respiratory infection and may improve somewhat with bronchodilator drugs, significant obstruction is always present.

PREVALENCE Approximately 20 percent of adult males have chronic bronchitis, yet only a minority of these are clinically disabled. According to all surveys males are more often affected than females. With increased cigarette smoking in women, however, the prevalence of bronchitis in them is increasing. Although cigarette smoking is the single most important etiologic factor, occupational and environmental exposures are now receiving more attention, mainly as contributors to the effects of cigarette smoking (Chap. 206).

Since no criteria have been agreed upon for making the diagnosis of emphysema during life, the incidence data are derived solely from postmortem surveys. It is rare to find adult lungs completely free of emphysema. There is a distinct increase in the extent of emphysema in the fifth decade with further increases through the seventh decade and little increase after that. Approximately two-thirds of adult males and one-fourth of females (most without recognized dysfunction) will have well-defined emphysema, which is often limited in extent. Therefore, the majority of those with emphysema will not have had disability or even symptoms associated with it. The situation is analogous to atherosclerosis in that the morphologic changes are far more frequent than the clinical manifestations attributable to the changes.

PATHOLOGY *Chronic bronchitis* is associated with hyperplasia and hypertrophy of the mucus-producing glands found in the submucosa of large cartilaginous airways. Quantitation of this anatomic change, known as the *Reid index,* is based upon the ratio of the thickness of the submucosal glands to that of the bronchial wall. In persons without a history of chronic bronchitis the mean ratio is 0.44 with a standard deviation ± 0.09, whereas in those with such a history the mean ratio is 0.52 ± 0.08. Although a low index is *rarely* associated with symptoms and a high index is commonly associated with symptoms during life, there is a great deal of overlap. Therefore many persons will have morphologic changes in large airways without having had chronic bronchitis.

Perhaps more important than the abnormalities in large airways are the changes often found in the small noncartilaginous airways. Goblet-cell hyperplasia, mucosal and submucosal inflammatory cells, and edema, peribronchial fibrosis, intraluminal mucus plugs, and increased smooth muscle are characteristic findings in small airways. The frequency of these latter findings in relation to premortem clinical and functional status has not been determined. However, in lungs from patients with chronic obstructive lung disease which have been studied at postmortem, the major site of airflow obstruction has been shown to be in the small airways.

Emphysema is classified according to the pattern of involvement of the gas-exchanging units (acini) of the lung distal to the terminal bronchiole. Although several morphologic patterns have been described, the two most important in the context of this discussion are those involving the respiratory bronchioles and alveolar ducts in the center of the acinus (centriacinar emphysema) and those involving the entire acinus (panacinar emphysema). Quite often both morphologic patterns are present in a single lung of a patient dying from chronic obstructive lung disease, although one type may predominate over the other.

With centriacinar emphysema the distention and destruction are mainly limited to the respiratory bronchiole and alveolar ducts, with relatively less change peripherally in the acinus. Because of the large functional reserve in the lung, many units must be involved in order for overall dysfunction to be detectable. The centrally destroyed regions of the acinus have a high ventilation/perfusion ratio because the capillaries are missing yet ventilation continues. This results in increased wasted ventilation (*Vd/Vt*), while the peripheral portions of the acinus have crowded and small alveoli with intact, perfused capillaries giving a low ventilation/perfusion ratio. This results in wasted blood flow to give a high alveolar-arterial P_{O_2} difference ($PA_{O_2} - Pa_{O_2}$) (Chap. 201). Mild degrees of centriacinar emphysema, often limited to the lung apices, are extremely common in lungs from persons above age 50 and are practically considered a normal finding.

Panacinar emphysema involves both the central and peripheral portions of the acinus which results, if the process is extensive, in a reduction of the alveolar-capillary gas exchange surface and loss of elastic recoil properties. When emphysema is severe, it may be difficult to distinguish between the two types which most often coexist in the same lung.

CONTRIBUTORY FACTORS Smoking Cigarette smoking is the most commonly identified correlate with both chronic bronchitis during life and extent of emphysema at postmortem. Experimental studies have shown that prolonged cigarette smoking impairs ciliary movement, inhibits function of alveolar macrophages, and leads to hypertrophy and hyperplasia of mucus-secreting glands; massive exposure in dogs can produce emphysematous changes. In addition to these chronic effects, it is probable that smoke inhibits antiproteases and causes polymorphonuclear leukocytes to release proteolytic enzymes acutely. Inhaled cigarette smoke can produce an acute increase in airways resistance due to vagally mediated smooth-muscle constriction, presumably by way of stimulating submucosal irritant receptors. The relationship of such recurrent episodes of acute bronchial constriction to the development and progression of chronic airways obstruction is uncertain. Recent studies, however, indicate that increased airways responsiveness is associated with more rapid progression in those with chronic airways obstruction.

It is now well established that some young asymptomatic smokers have considerable obstruction in small airways without there being either an increase of airway resistance or a diminution in the forced expiratory volume in 1 s. Since small airways, because of their large total cross-sectional areas, contribute very little to overall airflow resistance, more sensitive tests must be used to detect mild degrees of small-airways obstruction. Some tests, such as a decrease in compliance and resistance at rapid breathing rates, are based upon nonuniform behavior of the lung which is apparent only at increased frequencies. Obstruction of small airways also results in airways closure at higher lung volumes than in persons of the same age with unobstructed airways (Chap. 201). The measurements of closing volume and frequency dependence of resistance and compliance require special equipment not often available to clinicians. However, the simple spirogram is useful since flow rates at or below the mid-vital capacity range are often diminished in persons with mild small-airways obstruction. It has been shown that obstruction of small airways is the earliest demonstrable mechanical defect in young cigarette smokers and that the obstruction may disappear after cessation of smoking. It is possible, but has not been established with certainty, that those with small-airways obstruction are at greater risk of developing disabling chronic airways obstruction at some future time.

Not only is cigarette smoking the most common single factor leading to chronic airways obstruction, it also interacts with virtually every other contributory factor to be discussed below.

Air pollution The incidence and mortality rates of both chronic bronchitis and emphysema may be higher in heavily industrialized urban areas. Exacerbations of bronchitis are clearly related to periods of heavy pollution with sulfur dioxide (SO_2) and particulate matter. While nitrogen dioxide (NO_2) can produce small-airways obstruction (bronchiolitis) in experimental animals exposed to high concentrations, there are no data convincingly implicating NO_2, at even the highest pollutant levels, in the pathogenesis or worsening of airways obstruction in humans (Chap. 206).

Occupation Chronic bronchitis is more prevalent in workers who engage in occupations exposing them to either inorganic or organic dusts or to noxious gases. Epidemiologic surveys have succeeded in demonstrating an accelerated decline in lung function in many such workers—e.g., workers in plastics plants exposed to toluene diisocyanate and carding room workers in cotton mills (Chap. 206)—suggesting that their occupational exposure contributes to their future disability.

Infection Morbidity, mortality, and frequency of acute respiratory illnesses are higher in patients with chronic bronchitis. Many attempts have been made to relate these illnesses to infection with viruses, mycoplasmas, and bacteria. However, only the rhinovirus is found more often during exacerbations; that is to say, pathogenic bacteria, mycoplasmas, and viruses other than rhinovirus are found just as often between as during exacerbations. It is intuitively appealing to assign some role to respiratory infections in the pathogenesis and progression of chronic obstructive lung disease, and although this question is under study, there has been no conclusion to date. Recent epidemiologic studies, however, implicate acute respiratory illness as one of the major factors associated with the etiology as well as the progression of chronic airways obstruction. It has been shown that cigarette smokers may either transitorily develop or worsen small-airways obstruction in association with even mild viral respiratory infections. There is also some evidence that severe viral pneumonia early in life may lead to chronic obstruction, predominantly in small airways.

Familial and genetic factors Familial aggregation of chronic bronchitis has been well demonstrated in the past. Recent surveys have shown that children of smoking parents may experience more frequent and severe respiratory illnesses and have a higher prevalence of chronic respiratory symptoms. In addition, nonsmokers who remain in the presence of cigarette smokers (passive smokers) have increased blood levels of carbon monoxide which indicate that they are significantly exposed to smoke. Another well-documented form of indoor air pollution relates to the use of natural gas for cooking. The role of such pollution, however, remains controversial. Thus a part of the familial aggregation may be related to home air pollution. However, some studies of monozygotic twins have suggested some genetic predisposition to the development of chronic bronchitis independent of personal or familial smoking habits and other indoor air pollution. The exact genetic mode of transmission, if it exists at all, is uncertain.

The protease inhibitor $alpha_1$ antitrypsin is an acute-phase reactant, and normally the serum levels rise in association with many inflammatory reactions and with estrogen administration. Either deficient or absent serum levels of $alpha_1$ antitrypsin are found in some patients with the early onset of emphysema. By use of the techniques of acid starch gel and immunoelectrophoresis, genetic typing of the protease inhibitor (Pi) types has been possible. Most of the normal population have two M genes, designated as Pi type MM, and have serum $alpha_1$-antitrypsin levels in excess of 2.5 g/L. Several genes are associated with alterations in levels of serum $alpha_1$ antitrypsin, but the commonest ones associated with emphysema are the Z and S genes. Individuals who are homozygous ZZ or SS have serum levels often near 0 but always less than 0.5 g/L and develop severe panacinar emphysema in the third and fourth decades of life. The panacinar process predominates at the lung bases. Progressive dyspnea with minimal cough characterizes the clinical presentation, although chronic bronchitis is prominent in smokers. Given that alpha$_1$-protease inhibitors can be chemically synthesized or biologically produced in significant quantities and can be shown with intravenous infusion to restore the protease-antiprotease balance in liquid lavaged from the lungs of ZZ patients, it has been suggested that replacement therapy should be of value in preventing the development of emphysema; limited clinical trials are underway. The MZ and MS heterozygotes have intermediate levels of serum alpha$_1$ antitrypsin (i.e., between 0.5 and 2.5 g/L); hence the genetic expression is that of an autosomal codominant allele. It is a matter of some controversy whether the heterozygous state is associated with lung function abnormalities. Published studies are in direct conflict on this point, and further data are needed to be certain. The matter is of some importance, since the heterozygous state is common, with incidence estimates varying between 5 and 14 percent of the general population.

The precise way in which antitrypsin deficiency produces emphysema is unclear. In addition to inhibition of trypsin, alpha$_1$ antitrypsin is an effective inhibitor of elastase and several other proteolytic enzymes. There is experimental evidence that the structural integrity of lung elastin depends upon this antienzyme, which protects the lung from proteases released from leukocytes. It is tempting to speculate that recurrent inflammatory reactions related to infection and pollutants play some role in pathogenesis by calling forth leukocytes whose released proteases are uninhibited and are free to cause the damage.

The role of proteolytic enzymes in the induction of emphysema is not restricted to patients with alpha$_1$-antitrypsin deficiency. Evidence is accumulating that proteolytic enzymes derived from neutrophilic leukocytes and alveolar macrophages can produce emphysema even in subjects with normal circulating levels of antiproteases. It is possible that local concentrations of proteolytic enzymes may exceed the inhibitory capacity of antiproteases, that some proteases present are not susceptible to the available antiproteases, or that some of the proteolytic enzymes may be physically inaccessible to the antiprotease activity. The ultimate clinical utility of exogenously produced protease inhibitors currently under development will undoubtedly depend upon which of the protease-antiprotease interactions predominates in the production of emphysema.

PATHOPHYSIOLOGY On the basis of the use of flow rates from forced expiratory vital capacity maneuvers and more sophisticated measures of airways resistance and elastic recoil properties of the lung, it has become clear that both chronic bronchitis and emphysema can exist without evidence of obstruction. However, by the time a patient begins to experience dyspnea as a result of these processes, obstruction is always demonstrable. Since chronic bronchitis and emphysema are usually combined, it might appear fruitless to determine the role of each in producing an individual patient's disability. However, one process may dominate over the other, and to the extent that inflammatory airways disease, secretions, and bronchospasm are present, there are therapeutic possibilities with some hope for improvement. Therefore it is of value to understand the mechanisms of airways obstruction in order to guide therapy and anticipate results.

Both chronic bronchitis and emphysema result in airways narrowing. In addition to the primary airways processes of chronic bronchitis, loss of elastic recoil of the lung in emphysema accounts for a decrease in airways caliber through loss of radial traction on airways. Narrowing of airways is often associated with both an increase in airways resistance and a diminution in maximal expiratory flow rates.

There are occasions in which a normal or only slightly elevated airways resistance is accompanied by low maximal expiratory flow rates. Under such circumstances an increase in the dynamic collapsibility of intrathoracic airways during forced exhalation is a possible explanation. Also in this context, the elastic recoil pressure of the lung must be considered in a slightly different way. In addition to providing radial support to airways during quiet breathing, the elastic recoil properties of the lung serve as a major determinant of maximal expiratory flow rates. The static recoil pressure of the lung is the difference between alveolar and intrapleural pressure. During forced exhalations, when alveolar and intrapleural pressures are high, there are points in the airway at which bronchial pressure equals pleural pressure. Flow does not increase with higher pleural pressure after these points become fixed so that the effective driving pressure between alveoli and such points is the elastic recoil pressure of the lung (Fig. 210-1). Hence maximal expiratory flow rates represent a complex and dynamic interplay between airways caliber, elastic recoil pressures, and collapsibility of airways. As a direct consequence of the altered pressure-airflow relationships, the work of breathing is increased in bronchitis and emphysema. Since flow-resistive work is flow rate–dependent, there is a disproportionate increase in the work of breathing with increased ventilation.

The designated subdivisions of the lung volume outlined in Chap. 201 are abnormal to varying degrees in both bronchitis and emphysema. The residual volume (RV) and functional residual capacity (FRC) are almost always higher than normal. Since the normal FRC is the volume at which the inward recoil of the lung is balanced by the outward recoil of the chest wall, loss of elastic recoil of the lung would clearly result in a higher static FRC. In addition, prolongation of expiration in association with obstruction would lead to a dynamic increase in FRC if inspiration is initiated before the respiratory system

FIGURE 210-1 *A.* A schematic diagram of the lung and intrathoracic airways with no airflow. The alveolar pressure (Palv) is greater than pleural pressure (Ppl) by an amount equal to the elastic recoil pressure of the lung (Pel)—i.e., Palv is the algebraic sum of Ppl + Pel. With no airflow Palv = P atmospheric, and for all of the intrathoracic airways, pressure outside is less than the pressure inside due to the Pel. *B.* The same schematic lung during forced exhalation when pleural pressure becomes quite positive. Palv is still greater than Ppl by an amount equal to Pel. However, there is a pressure drop along the airway associated with flow, and at some point Ppl equals local bronchial pressure (so-called equal pressure point, EPP). Mouthward from this point, Ppl exceeds local bronchial pressure and hence acts to compress the airways. *C.* Pressure within the airways from alveoli to the intrathoracic trachea is shown as a dashed line (---) and Ppl is shown as a constant (———). Therefore, the driving pressure from alveoli to EPP is equal to Pel, and a decrease in Pel (i.e., loss of elastic recoil) would mean a smaller driving pressure and smaller flow rates.

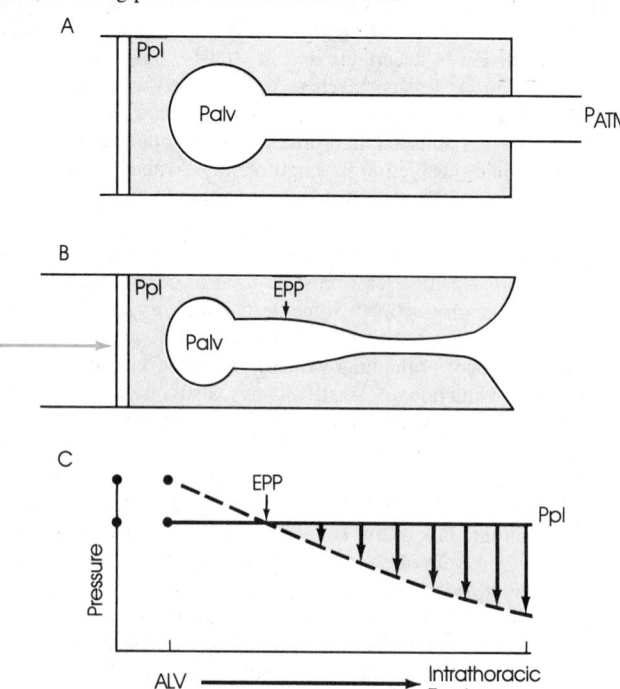

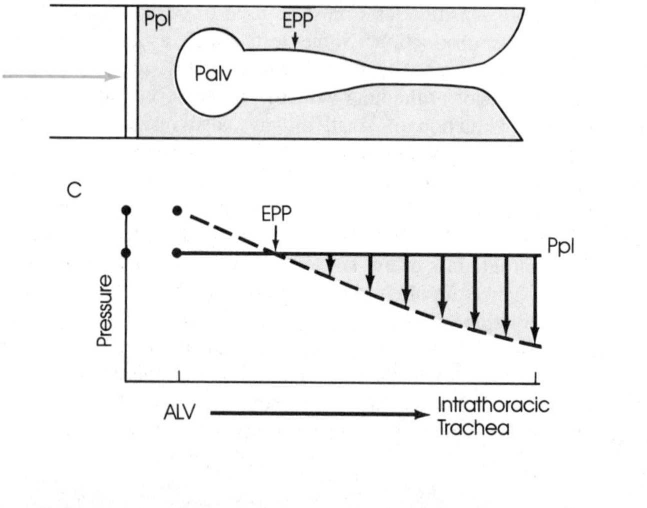

reaches its static balance point. Elevations of total lung capacity (TLC) are frequent. The exact cause is uncertain, but increases in TLC are often found in association with decreases in the elastic recoil of the lung. The vital capacity is frequently decreased, yet significant airways obstruction can be present with a normal to near-normal vital capacity.

The consequences of the airways and parenchymal processes are far more extensive than just the mechanical alterations discussed above. Maldistribution of inspired gas and blood flow is always present to some extent. When the mismatching is severe, impairment of gas exchange is reflected in abnormalities of arterial blood gases. There are regions of the lung with ventilation in excess of perfusion which increase the wasted ventilation ratio (that is, *Vd/Vt;* Chap. 201). At a normal resting CO_2 production, the net effective alveolar ventilation, as reflected by the arterial P_{CO_2}, may be excessive, normal, or insufficient depending upon the relationship of the overall minute volume to the wasted ventilation ratio. The net contribution of regions with perfusion in excess of ventilation can be assessed by either estimating or measuring the alveolar-arterial P_{O_2} difference (that is, $PA_{O_2} - Pa_{O_2}$; Chap. 201). Whatever the clinical syndrome associated with chronic bronchitis and emphysema, there are to some degree increases in both wasted ventilation and wasted blood flow.

The clinical manifestations depend, in large part, upon the ventilatory response to the disordered lung function. Some patients, at the cost of extremely high effort of breathing and chronic dyspnea, will maintain a strikingly increased minute volume, which results both in a normal to low arterial P_{CO_2}, despite the high *Vd/Vt,* and a relatively high arterial P_{O_2}, despite the high difference, $PA_{O_2} - Pa_{O_2}$. Other patients with only modest increases in effort of breathing and less dyspnea will maintain a normal to only moderately elevated minute volume at the cost of accepting a high arterial P_{CO_2} and a severely depressed arterial P_{O_2}.

Factors which account for clear differences in ventilatory responses between patients have been studied and debated for years. The bulk of available evidence suggests that those patients who maintain relatively normal or low arterial P_{CO_2} levels are those with an increased ventilatory drive relative to their blood gas values and those who chronically maintain high arterial P_{CO_2} and lower P_{O_2} levels have a diminished ventilatory drive in relation to their more severely deranged blood gas values. It is not at all certain whether individual differences are accounted for by variations in peripheral or central chemoreceptor sensitivity or through other afferent pathways. Perhaps of more immediate value is the fact that patients with predominant emphysema are either normally or excessively responsive both to hypercapnia and to exercise, whereas those with predominant bronchitis are less responsive to both, despite similar degrees of airways obstruction by spirometry.

The pulmonary circulation malfunctions not only in terms of regional distribution of blood flow but in terms of abnormal overall pressure-flow relationships. There is often mild to severe pulmonary hypertension at rest with further increases disproportionate to cardiac output elevations during exercise. A reduction in the total cross-sectional area of the pulmonary vascular bed can be attributed to anatomic changes and constriction of vascular smooth muscle in pulmonary arteries and arterioles as well as destruction of alveolar septa with loss of capillaries. Rarely does loss of capillaries alone lead to severe pulmonary hypertension with cor pulmonale, except as a near-terminal event. Of more importance is the constriction of pulmonary vessels in response to alveolar hypoxia. The constriction is reversible upon increase in alveolar P_{O_2} with therapy. There is a synergism between hypoxia and acidosis which assumes importance during episodes of acute or chronic respiratory insufficiency. Chronic hypoxia leads not only to pulmonary vascular constriction but also to secondary erythrocytosis. The latter, although not proved to be a significant contributor to pulmonary hypertension, could add an unfavorable rheologic load. As discussed in Chap. 191, the chronic afterload on the right ventricle leads to hypertrophy and, in association with disordered blood gases, ultimately to failure.

CLINICAL-FUNCTIONAL CORRELATIONS Dyspnea and impairment of physical work capacity are characteristic only of severe to moderately severe airways obstruction. There is considerable variation among patients, and those with predominant emphysema have greater dyspnea and restriction of physical activity with lesser degrees of obstruction than those in whom chronic bronchitis predominates. The majority of patients have functionally mixed disease, will usually experience exertional dyspnea when the forced expiratory volume in 1 s (FEV_1) falls below 50 percent of that predicted, and will have dyspnea at rest when the FEV_1 is less than 25 percent of that predicted. In addition to dyspnea at rest, carbon dioxide retention and cor pulmonale frequently occur when the FEV_1 falls to 25 percent of that predicted. However, those with predominant bronchitis often have carbon dioxide retention and cor pulmonale with FEV_1 values above 25 percent of normal, in contrast to patients with predominant emphysema whose FEV_1 usually falls well below that level before the onset of carbon dioxide retention and cor pulmonale. With a respiratory infection, small changes in the degree of obstruction can make a large difference in symptoms and gas exchange. Thus small therapeutic gains have rewarding results.

In general, the more severe the obstruction, the poorer the prognosis. Despite the general relationship, 20 to 30 percent of patients with severe obstruction and carbon dioxide retention will survive beyond 5 years.

CLINICAL SYNDROMES It is clear that the clinical presentation can vary in severity from simple chronic bronchitis without disability to the severely disabled state with chronic respiratory failure. From a practical standpoint, it is well to consider that any symptom or any measurable abnormality may foreshadow the development of severe disabling disease; hence cessation of smoking and avoidance of environmental irritants and toxins are to be advised. However, the advice to modify behavior and life patterns is rarely taken, and most physicians are called upon to categorize and treat patients with fully developed, chronic airways obstruction. Thus the approach taken here is to describe two polar opposite types of fully developed, chronic obstructive pulmonary disease with the realization that the majority of patients will have some features of both types. The salient features of each type are outlined in Table 210-1.

Predominant emphysema These patients often give a long history of exertional dyspnea with minimal cough which is productive of only small amounts of mucoid sputum. Mucopurulent exacerbations

TABLE 210-1 Chronic obstructive lung disease: Salient features of the two types

	Predominant emphysema	Predominant bronchitis
Age at time of diagnosis, y	60±	50±
Dyspnea	Severe	Mild
Cough	After dyspnea starts	Before dyspnea starts
Sputum	Scanty, mucoid	Copious, purulent
Bronchial infections	Less frequent	More frequent
Respiratory insufficiency episodes	Often terminal	Repeated
Chest film	"Hyperinflation" ± bullous changes, small heart	Increased bronchovascular markings at bases, large heart
Chronic Pa_{CO_2}, mmHg	35–40	50–60
Chronic Pa_{O_2}, mmHg	65–75	45–60
Hematocrit, %	35–45	50–55
Pulmonary hypertension:		
Rest	None to mild	Moderate to severe
Exercise	Moderate	Worsens
Cor pulmonale	Rare, except terminally	Common
Elastic recoil	Severely decreased	Normal
Resistance	Normal to slight increase	High
Diffusing capacity	Decreased	Normal to slight decrease

in association with infections are not frequent. The body build is asthenic with evidence of weight loss. The patient appears distressed with obvious use of accessory muscles of respiration which serve to lift the sternum in an anterosuperior direction with each inspiration. There is tachypnea with a relatively prolonged expiration through pursed lips, or expiration is begun with a grunting sound. While sitting, these patients often lean forward, extending the arms to brace themselves. The neck veins may be distended during expiration, yet they collapse briskly with inspiration. The lower intercostal spaces retract with each inspiration, and by palpation the lower lateral chest wall can be felt to move inward. The percussion note is hyperresonant, and by auscultation the breath sounds are diminished, with faint, high-pitched rhonchi heard toward the end of expiration. The cardiac impulse, if at all visible, is seen only in the xiphoid and subxiphoid regions, and cardiac dullness is either absent or severely reduced. By palpation there is frequently a sustained forward and downward right ventricular impulse in the subxiphoid region, and a presystolic gallop accentuated during inspiration is commonly heard.

The arterial P_{O_2} is often in the mid-70s (mmHg), and the P_{CO_2} is low to normal. Because of the maintained increase in minute volume and the maintenance of arterial P_{O_2} sufficient to nearly saturate hemoglobin, these patients have been referred to as "pink puffers." Their increased ventilatory drive probably accounts for their relatively preserved oxygenation and lack of hypercapnia; however, this increased drive with attendant increases in ventilation undoubtedly contributes to the severity of their dyspnea.

The TLC and RV are invariably increased, the vital capacity is low, and the maximal expiratory flow rates are diminished. The elastic recoil properties of the lung are severely impaired, and in direct proportion to this impairment, the capacity of the lung to transfer carbon monoxide is lowered.

On radiographic examination the diaphragms are low and flattened, the bronchovascular shadows do not extend to the periphery of the lung, and the cardiac silhouette is lengthened and narrowed. These findings in association with a large retrosternal translucency on lateral chest radiographs are interpreted as hyperinflation, which correlates well with increases in TLC and loss of elastic recoil. Peripheral attenuation of bronchovascular markings and increased retrosternal lucency correlate best with subsequent postmortem demonstration of extensive and severe emphysema which is predominantly of the panacinar type. Recently computed tomography (CT) has been shown to localize and quantitate emphysema. However, determining the localization of such regions most often is of little practical value and the overall quantitative assessments from elastic recoil properties and carbon monoxide transfer are just as good. Hence use of CT scans for this purpose is not ordinarily employed.

It is fortunate that the patient with predominant emphysema is less prone to mucopurulent relapses than is the patient with predominant bronchitis, since such relapses frequently lead to severe respiratory failure and death. That is to say, right-sided heart failure and hypercapnic respiratory failure are often terminal events in those patients with predominant emphysema. In the absence of such relapses, the clinical course is characterized by severe and progressive dyspnea for which little can be done. The physician's role is to seek out and treat any factor that is possibly reversible and strive to avoid pollutants and infections.

Predominant bronchitis The patient with predominant bronchitis usually has an impressive history of cough and sputum production for many years with an immodest history of cigarette smoking. Initially the cough is present only in the winter months, and the patient is apt to seek medical attention, if at all, only during the more severe of the frequent mucopurulent relapses. Over the years the cough progresses from hibernal to perennial, and mucopurulent relapses increase in frequency, duration, and severity. After beginning to experience exertional dyspnea, the patient often seeks medical help and will be found to have a severe degree of obstruction. Occasionally such a patient will seek out a physician only after the onset of peripheral edema secondary to overt right ventricular failure. More rarely the initial medical contact is made by family members who present the physician with a deeply cyanotic, edematous, and stuporous patient with acute respiratory insufficiency.

The patient with predominant bronchitis is often overweight and cyanotic. There is usually no apparent distress at rest, the respiratory rate is normal or only slightly increased, and there is no apparent usage of accessory muscles. The chest percussion note is normally resonant, and by auscultation, one can usually hear coarse rhonchi and wheezes which change in location and intensity after a deep and productive cough. There may be a sustained heave along the lower left sternal border which indicates right ventricular hypertrophy. In the presence of right ventricular failure there are often an early diastolic gallop and occasionally a holosystolic murmur, both of which are accentuated by inspiration. The latter finding is indicative of functional tricuspid regurgitation which is frequently accompanied by neck vein distention characterized by large *v* waves and brisk *y* descents. With right ventricular failure the cyanosis deepens and peripheral edema becomes prominent. Clubbing of the digits is unusual.

With or without right ventricular failure, the minute volume is only slightly increased due to an overall diminution in ventilatory drive which modulates the level of dyspnea. However, failure to increase minute volume greatly in the face of significant proportions of wasted ventilation and blood flow results in severely deranged arterial blood gases, with arterial P_{CO_2} values which are chronically increased to the range of the high 40s to low 50s (mmHg). The lowered P_{O_2} produces desaturation of hemoglobin, serves to stimulate erythropoiesis, and results in hypoxic pulmonary vasoconstriction. Desaturation and erythrocytosis combine to produce the cyanosis, and hypoxic pulmonary vasoconstriction accentuates the right-sided heart failure. Because of cyanosis and edema secondary to heart failure, such patients have been referred to as "blue bloaters." It has been proposed, with some supporting data, that one of the pathophysiologic events in the blue bloaters is the occurrence of repeated episodes of severe nocturnal oxygen desaturation in association with episodes of sleep apnea or periods of worsening hypoventilation. Such sleep-related ventilatory events worsen the degree of pulmonary hypertension and secondary erythrocytosis.

The TLC is often normal, and there is a moderate elevation of RV. The vital capacity is mildly diminished, and maximal expiratory flow rates are invariably low. The elastic recoil properties of the lung are normal or only slightly impaired, and the capacity of the lung to transfer carbon monoxide is either normal or minimally decreased.

On radiographic examination the diaphragms are well rounded, the bronchovascular markings are increased in the lower lung fields, and the cardiac silhouette is somewhat enlarged. In association with right ventricular failure the cardiac silhouette enlarges further, pulmonary arteries become more prominent, and an antigravity distribution of perfusion is apparent.

Despite well-planned management (see below) the patient with predominant bronchitis may experience many episodes of respiratory failure from which recovery is frequent with proper therapy (see p. 1080). The ability to recover from such repeated episodes in those patients is in striking contrast to the frequently fatal outcome of such events in those with predominant emphysema. Ultimately, the lungs at postmortem will be found to have severe bronchitic changes in both large and small airways and only moderate emphysema, predominantly of the centriacinar variety.

It should be reemphasized that the above syndromes are described as polar ends of a continuous spectrum of clinical features. Hence most patients will have some characteristics of each syndrome. The usefulness of recognizing and understanding the pathophysiologic bases for these lies in the planning of appropriate management strategies for each patient.

PRINCIPLES OF MANAGEMENT Intelligent management must be based upon as complete knowledge as possible of the degree of obstruction, the extent of disability, and the relative reversibility of the patient's illness. To the extent that obstructive processes in the airways are contributory, there is a chance for treatment to be effective. Since emphysema is an irreversible process, prevention of progression and avoidance of acute insults constitute the main approach. History, physical examination, and chest radiographs should be supplemented by tests of lung function performed during a symptomatically stable period. Ideally, complete spirometry, plethysmographic lung volumes, transfer of carbon monoxide, arterial blood gases, and lung elastic recoil properties should be measured. Spirometry and lung volumes should be remeasured after the administration of bronchodilators in order to assess the degree of acutely reversible airways obstruction. Failure to see an acute change with bronchodilator drugs does not rule out the possibility of improvement with more prolonged administration of these agents. In instances in which the degree of exertional dyspnea appears to be disproportionately greater than the degree of obstruction, measurements of blood gases, minute volume, CO_2 production, and O_2 consumption during exercise are indicated in order to determine whether impaired lung function is sufficient to account for the symptoms. After the initial assessment the physician has some idea of the relative emphasis to be placed upon patient education, rehabilitative and preventive measures, and direct therapeutic interventions in management of the patient and the illness.

Cessation of smoking is the only certain means of influencing the progression of the chronic obstructive airways syndromes, and although such behavior modification is most effective at early stages of the disease processes, it is effective in slowing the rate of decline in lung function, even when such function is severely compromised. In the instances in which occupational or environmental exposures are thought to play a significant role, change of occupation or relocation of dwelling is advisable. The validity of such advice should be carefully considered since the impact on both the patient and the family is likely to be great. A simpler environmental change is that of eliminating aerosol sprays such as deodorants, hair sprays, and insecticides from the household. Hair sprays have been shown to produce acute airways responses even in normal subjects. Other preventive measures include yearly vaccination against the common or expected influenza virus strains. The patient should be given pneumococcal polysaccharide vaccine only once. Recognition of severe Arthus-type immunologic reactions following repeat pneumococcal vaccination has led to this "once-in-a-lifetime" recommendation.

Infections cannot be totally avoided, and the patient should be made aware that increasing purulence, viscosity, or volume of secretions signals the onset of an infection which should be treated early. The commonest pathogenic bacteria found are *Haemophilus influenzae* and *Streptococcus pneumoniae*. As mentioned above, however, the role of such bacteria is in question since they are just as often isolated during periods of relative clinical quiescence. Nonetheless, tetracycline or ampicillin should be given for a 7- to 10-day course. It is practical to have the patient keep a 7- to 10-day supply of antibiotics at home and to begin treatment at the onset of symptoms. In Great Britain it is common practice to give continuous antibiotic therapy during winter months in order to prevent mucopurulent relapses. Although there is evidence that viruses are frequent causes of mucopurulent relapses, clinical studies have shown that the standard antibiotic regimens decrease the duration and severity of infective episodes unrelated to culturable bacterial pathogens. Microscopic examination and culture of sputum are indicated if there are chills, fever, or chest pain or if purulence fails to respond to usually administered antibiotics.

It has been shown repeatedly that exercise programs, although not accompanied by measurable improvement in lung function, result in increased exercise tolerance and an improved sense of well-being. The improvement is usually task-specific, so that most physicians advise walking in preference to the use of special apparatus, such as stationary bicycles or wall gyms.

If malnutrition as assessed by body weight less than 85 percent of ideal is present, oral dietary supplements can result in improved muscle strength, less fatigability, and lessening of breathlessness. A carefully taken dietary history and elimination of other serious causes for low body weight and weight loss should precede the start of any major nutritional supplement effort. As with exercise programs, there is not a direct and measurable effect on lung function from treating malnutrition; yet subjective relief and objective improvement in strength and exercise performance have been of great benefit in such patients.

Bronchodilator drugs are often quite helpful in alleviating symptoms, especially in those patients who respond to them acutely in the laboratory. These drugs form three categories: the methylxanthines, sympathomimetics with strong beta$_2$-adrenergic-stimulating properties, and anticholinergics. Theophylline, the most commonly used methylxanthine, can be given orally, rectally, or parenterally; in addition to bronchodilatation, it stimulates respiration and has cardiotonic and diuretic properties. Selective beta$_2$-stimulating drugs such as albuterol and metaproterenol can be given both orally and by aerosol with fewer cardiac side effects than are experienced with isoproterenol. Anticholinergic agents such as atropine have been avoided in the past because of their tendency to desiccate secretions; however, ipratropium bromide, an anticholinergic agent in metered dose inhaler form, is an extremely effective bronchodilator in chronic bronchitic patients. It is considered by many to be the bronchodilator of choice for these patients.

The use of systemic glucocorticoids is, at our present state of knowledge, based upon very little scientific data from properly controlled clinical trials. Since these agents have time- and dose-related side effects that vary from deleterious to catastrophic, the almost invariable subjective benefit must be supported by objective measurements. There is little room for doubt in the minds of physicians that some patients respond well, even dramatically, to these agents in both objective and subjective terms. The real problem is how to select those patients most likely to benefit. Eosinophilia in the sputum, rather than in the blood, appears in some instances to identify that subgroup in advance. However, the best guidelines are, first, to try these agents only after maximal bronchodilator and bronchopulmonary drainage measures have been tried without success; second, to begin prednisone 30 mg once per day; third, to confirm the objective change in terms of spirometry and gas exchange, stopping these agents if no objective benefit is seen; and fourth, to decrease to the smallest dose that will maintain the improved level of function. The role, if any, of inhaled glucocorticoid agents for these patients, in contrast to asthmatic patients, has not been established in the syndromes with chronic obstruction.

Bronchopulmonary drainage should be maintained in patients with hypersecretion. If the coughing mechanism is ineffective or if paroxysms of coughing are exhausting, postural drainage is often a useful adjunct. Although liquefaction of secretions by means of orally administered expectorants or aerosol delivery of mucolytic agents is an appealing idea, it has never been shown by properly designed trials to be more effective than simple maintenance of total-body hydration.

Intermittent positive pressure breathing (IPPB) devices were formerly advocated for home management. The various rationales included diminution in the work of breathing, promotion of bronchopulmonary drainage, and more efficient delivery of bronchodilator drugs. The first of the rationales has been shown to have no basis in fact, and the goals of the last two have been shown to be as well accomplished by postural drainage and use of less elaborate aerosol generators. Hence the use of IPPB for home management cannot be justified.

When arterial hypoxia is persistent and severe (Pa_{O_2} of 55 to 60 mmHg) in association with cor pulmonale (see Chap. 191) and signs of right heart failure, continuous oxygen therapy is indicated. If the Pa_{O_2} is persistently <55 mmHg, with or without cor pulmonale, continuous oxygen supplementation should also be prescribed. The available data indicate that supplemental oxygen improves both exercise tolerance and neuropsychological function and alleviates pulmonary hypertension and right heart failure. In patients with severe hypoxemia the need for hospitalization occurs less frequently and life span is lengthened by the use of supplemental oxygen. In view of the expense of such therapy and the dangers of uncontrolled oxygen delivery (see below), it should be given only when it can be carefully monitored and its beneficial effects objectively verified.

Since most patients with chronic airways obstruction, especially those with features of predominant bronchitis, can be shown to decrease their Pa_{O_2} values significantly during sleep, most prominently during the REM phase, nocturnal oxygen administration has been suggested. While the rationale is clear and the results quite good, a recent cooperative clinical trial that compared nocturnal with continuous O_2 supplementation in severely hypoxic patients found that continuous O_2 administration was associated with a significantly lower mortality rate. Patients in both treatment groups experienced neuropsychological and hemodynamic benefits. Thus, supplemental nocturnal oxygen is better than none, but continuous oxygen is better than nocturnal in such severely ill patients.

Secondary erythrocytosis with the hematocrit in excess of 0.50 is most easily viewed as a mechanism allowing greater oxygen delivery to compensate for the chronically lowered arterial Pa_{O_2}; hence improvement in oxygenation through improved lung function or by oxygen administration is the most physiologic means to reverse erythrocytosis. Since erythrocytosis results in elevation of blood viscosity at all shear rates, the proposal has been made that pulmonary vascular hypertension is aggravated by its presence. Although no study has demonstrated an objective improvement in hemodynamics, lung mechanics, or gas exchange at rest following phlebotomy, ventilatory and cardiovascular function during exercise improve. Some patients who complain of headaches and a sense of head fullness show a favorable subjective response to periodic phlebotomy when the hematocrit is in excess of 0.55 percent. In support of this subjective improvement is the demonstration that, following phlebotomy, cerebral blood flow, previously diminished, returns toward normal.

ACUTE RESPIRATORY FAILURE

DIAGNOSIS Although it may be strongly suspected on clinical grounds, the firm diagnosis of acute respiratory failure in chronic airways obstruction is based upon measurements of arterial blood gas (Pa_{O_2}, Pa_{CO_2}) and pH values that must be interpreted in relation to the patient's chronic status. Since many patients will have chronically lowered Pa_{O_2} levels and increased Pa_{CO_2} values, the diagnosis is based upon the degree of change from the usual state of the individual patient. With regard to oxygenation, an acute decrease in Pa_{O_2} from a usual mid-70 range to the low 60s (mmHg) is just as indicative of acute respiratory failure as is an acute drop from a chronic mid-50 range to the mid-40s (mmHg). Thus a drop in Pa_{O_2} equal to or greater than 10 to 15 mmHg indicates acute failure.

Since renal compensation for chronic hypercapnia results in adjustment of arterial pH to near-normal values, the acuteness of the increase in Pa_{CO_2} can often be judged by the pH, unless there is a concomitant metabolic acidemia. As a practical guide, any level of hypercapnia associated with an arterial pH value less than 7.30 should be considered as acute respiratory failure.

PRECIPITATING FACTORS Increases in volume, viscosity, and/or purulence of secretions, presumably due to infection of the tracheobronchial tree, are the most common antecedents of acute respiratory failure in chronic obstructive lung disease. Increasing airways obstruction with airways inflammation and secretion, especially in association with a relatively blunted ventilatory drive, leads to worsening hypoxia and increasing CO_2 retention. Agitation, insomnia, and increasing dyspnea with impending respiratory failure are occasionally treated, mistakenly, with either sedatives or narcotics, and these, too, may precipitate frank respiratory failure. In fact such depressant drugs which impair ventilatory drive should be avoided at all times in patients with severe chronic obstructive lung disease. Major episodes of air pollution can also lead to respiratory failure, and the physicians responsible for patients with severe bronchitis and emphysema should be alert to these environmental events.

Pneumonia, thromboembolism, left ventricular failure, and pneumothorax occasionally precipitate acute respiratory failure and are extremely difficult to detect unless considered and specifically sought. As a minimum, chest radiographs, electrocardiograms, and sputum examinations should be obtained in addition to arterial blood gas measurements in all patients with respiratory failure.

TREATMENT OF RESPIRATORY FAILURE The treatment of respiratory failure consists of two simultaneous processes: (1) maintaining acceptable levels of oxygenation and ventilation; and (2) treatment of infection, removal of secretions, and reversing any airway constriction present.

With regard to the first, these patients *need* oxygen when they are severely hypoxic, and while fears of respiratory depression due to the removal of the hypoxic respiratory stimulus are realistic, O_2 must be used, yet in the smallest concentration possible, to give a Pa_{O_2} in the mid-50-mmHg range while the patient's Pa_{CO_2}, pH, and clinical status are carefully monitored. It is best to begin with only modest increases in FI_{O_2} to approximately 0.24 (cf. air at 0.21), which can be accomplished using nasal prongs with O_2 flows at 1 to 2 liters per minute or, more precisely, with the use of a 0.24 Venturi mask. These latter masks, based upon Bernoulli's principle, deliver a fixed concentration of O_2 irrespective of the O_2 flow rate by entraining air in direct proportion to O_2 flow rate. They are high-flow masks (oxygen plus air entrained from the room), each designed for a specific FI_{O_2} (0.24, 0.28, 0.35, 0.40). Even small increases in Pa_{O_2} when starting from low levels result in significant increases in arterial oxygen content due to the shape of the oxygen-hemoglobin saturation curve over this range (Chap. 290). With improved oxygenation some patients will concomitantly increase their Pa_{CO_2} values. The standard explanation has been that this increase is due to the removal of the hypoxic drive to ventilation leading to further hypoventilation. While this is the most important mechanism, recent data indicate that worsening ventilation-perfusion relationships (Chap. 201) occur with O_2 treatment. This is attributed to reversal of hypoxic pulmonary arterial constriction in the more initially hypoxic, less well ventilated regions, which in turn leads to decreased perfusion of initially less hypoxic, better ventilated regions. The result is an increase in the wasted ventilation ratio (*Vd/Vt*, Chap. 201) leading to a smaller effective alveolar ventilation. In either case, the FI_{O_2} should be increased as little as possible to achieve a Pa_{O_2} in the mid-50-mmHg range. Some increase in Pa_{CO_2} can be expected and should not cause alarm if the patient is alert. The majority of patients can be managed in this conservative way with excellent results. However, occasionally large increases in Pa_{CO_2} occur and lead to stupor and coma. This can be explained by CO_2-induced cerebral vascular dilatation with increased intracranial pressure, including the development of papilledema, combined with the effect of hypercapnia and hypoxia on cerebral function. It must be emphasized that if stupor and coma supervene, stopping the administration of oxygen is the *worst possible* course of action. When CO_2 narcosis is present, respirations are sufficiently depressed from the CO_2 itself so that the patient will no longer respond to the rapidly worsening hypoxia, and fatal arrhythmias, generalized seizures, and death may ensue. The only alternative is to intubate the trachea and provide mechanical ventilatory support. Mechanical ventilators are described in Chap. 219.

Once mechanical ventilation has been instituted, the tidal volume and frequency should be set gradually to decrease the Pa_{CO_2} only down to the chronically elevated level rather than attempt to decrease it to or below a normal value. Since such patients have renal compensation for their chronic hypercapnia, Pa_{CO_2} values at or below the normal level result in significant alkalemia which in turn can lead to severe tachyarrhythmias and generalized seizures.

As mentioned above, maintaining oxygenation and ventilation serves to buy time while secretion removal, bronchial dilatation, and treatment of infection are instituted. Removal of secretions is accomplished by urging the patient to cough or by passing suction catheters into the trachea which, in addition to removing secretions that are present, stimulate cough that brings more secretions up to the region of the catheter tip. The advantage, if any, from the use of mucolytic agents in this process has yet to be demonstrated. However, $beta_2$-adrenergic bronchodilating agents have been shown to increase the rate of transport of particles by the mucociliary blanket, and, thus, in addition to bronchodilatation, such agents should improve the clearance of airway secretions. Postural drainage and chest percussion are other often-used adjuncts that have been shown, especially when secretions are voluminous, to improve tracheobronchial clearance, to increase sputum volume beyond that produced by cough, and to reduce airways obstruction.

Bronchodilatation with aminophylline given orally or by infusion and $beta_2$-adrenergic agonists by inhalation or subcutaneous injection has assumed a prominent role in treatment of acute respiratory failure in chronic airways obstruction. In addition to bronchodilatation these agents improve bronchopulmonary clearance and may help induce diuresis and hemodynamic improvement when there is cor pulmonale with failure (Chap. 191). Unless there is clearly an acute pneumonia, the use of antibiotics is more controversial in the setting of acute respiratory failure than in mucopurulent relapses without failure. Nonetheless, broad-spectrum antibiotics, if no single agent is suspected or isolated, or erythromycin, if legionellae or mycoplasmas are suspected, should be added to the regimen.

Complications arising in the course of treatment for acute respiratory failure are cardiac arrhythmias, most often multifocal supraventricular tachycardias, left ventricular failure, pulmonary emboli, and gastrointestinal hemorrhage from stress ulceration. Cardiac arrhythmias resulting from rapid decreases in oxygenation or increases in pH due to overventilation can be readily avoided. However, when giving multiple drugs having cardiotonic properties, the question always arises as to whether the arrhythmias are related to these. Keeping serum theophylline levels in the 10 to 20 mg per liter range and using relatively selective beta agonists, such as isoetharine by inhalation, can minimize these effects.

Left ventricular failure, usually attributable to coronary atherosclerosis with acute myocardial infarction, systemic hypertension, or aortic valvular disease, is difficult to detect in the presence of cor pulmonale. Fortunately, improving lung function and oxygenation most often reverse the pulmonary hypertension and right ventricular failure (Chap. 191) and induce a brisk diuresis. If signs of congestive failure persist or worsen after providing adequate oxygenation, consideration must be given to left ventricular failure; an assessment in such patients is best made through echocardiography or radioventriculography since the usual physical and radiographic findings are obscured in such patients. Only in the presence of adequate gas exchange and only with either the firm demonstration of, or strong clinical suspicion of, left ventricular failure should digitalis be used. Diuretic agents should also be reserved for left ventricular failure. They almost invariably produce hypokalemic, hypochloremic metabolic alkalemia that results in depression of ventilatory drive and interference with removal from mechanical ventilatory support.

Pulmonary emboli are suspected to be common in the setting of acute respiratory failure and are extremely difficult to detect since the lung scan is totally nonspecific and signs of cor pulmonale fluctuate in concert with the degree of lung dysfunction. Hence low-dose heparin prophylaxis should be used to prevent this complication. Gastrointestinal hemorrhage commonly complicates acute respiratory failure and is thought to be due to stress ulceration of the gastric mucosa. Awareness of this complication enhances the ability to detect it and act quickly. Antacids, coating agents such as sucralfate, nasogastric suction, and/or cimetidine have been used to diminish the frequency.

For those patients who have required mechanical ventilatory support, the process of removal from that support is largely empirical. In general, improving gas exchange and lung mechanics along with alertness and responsiveness of the patient signal that the support can be removed. Data such as maximal voluntary inspiratory mouth pressures greater than 20 cmH_2O, vital capacity greater than 10 mL per kilogram of body weight, and spontaneous tidal volume greater than 5 mL per kilogram of body weight are reassuring. However, many patients can be removed from such support with lesser values than these.

Failure to maintain gas exchange after removal of mechanical ventilatory support can usually be explained. *First* on the list is the continued administration or persistence of sedative and tranquilizing drugs that may have been prescribed earlier for agitation. These should be discontinued and time allowed for their metabolism. *Second* is the possibility that the endotracheal tube is of small bore and imposes a resistive load. If so, it should be replaced by a larger one. *Third* is worsening airways obstruction and accumulation of secretions; continued bronchial dilatation and airway suctioning avoid these. *Fourth* is a metabolic alkalemia, with or without diuretic therapy, that should be treated with potassium chloride. *Fifth* is having maintained a Pa_{O_2} and Pa_{CO_2} while being on mechanical ventilation that are too high and too low, respectively. This can be avoided by using an FI_{O_2} just sufficient to keep the Pa_{O_2} around 60 mmHg and using the assist mode with small enough tidal volumes to keep the Pa_{CO_2} at the expected chronic level (i.e., that associated with a normal or slightly low arterial pH) before discontinuing mechanical support. *Sixth* is poor nutrition, hypokalemia, or neuromuscular disease, making the patient too weak to maintain breathing or resulting in fatigue of the respiratory muscles. Nutrition, of course, is a longer range problem that should be anticipated, while hypokalemia is often handled along with the metabolic alkalemia. Muscle fatigue, especially diaphragmatic, has received a great deal of attention. From a practical standpoint, paradoxical (inward) movement of the upper abdomen with inspiration is the key clinical finding. Experimental evidence suggests that therapeutic levels of aminophylline or $beta_2$ agonists, such as fenoterol, reverse the manifestations of fatigue but the role of respiratory stimulants continues to be debated and the data to be inconclusive. In those patients with severely blunted ventilatory drive and improving lung function, stimulants may be tried cautiously. If there is severe metabolic alkalemia, acetazolamide can be tried as a stimulant while chloride replacement is being carried out. Medroxyprogesterone, a central stimulant, or almitrine, a peripheral chemoreceptor stimulant, appear to be safe and, in some instances, effective. Hypothyroidism is a metabolic condition with neuromuscular consequences and is difficult to detect in this clinical setting. Thus any prolonged and difficult weaning process should lead to the assessment of thyroid function.

PROGNOSIS On the average, data collected on large populations demonstrate a slow and relentless diminution in ventilatory function in patients with chronic airways obstruction. Although slow, the decrement in function with time far exceeds the rate of change seen with normal aging. In general, the likelihood of episodes of acute respiratory failure increases when the FEV_1 falls below 25 percent of predicted normal values. Although the in-hospital mortality rate averages 30 percent for a single episode and the 5-year survival rate after the initial episode of respiratory failure averages only 15 to 20 percent, the clinical syndrome is extremely important in determining both the short- and long-range prognosis. As noted above, those patients with predominant emphysema have a poorer prognosis after the onset of respiratory failure than do those with predominant bronchitis. In either case long-term oxygen treatment in those with severe hypoxemia results in prolongation of life and improvement in the quality of life.

BULLOUS EMPHYSEMA Confluent air spaces with diameters in excess of 1 cm are occasionally congenital but most often are found in association with generalized emphysema or progressive fibrotic processes. Gradual increases in size of such air spaces (or bullae) result from traction applied by regions with better elastic recoil properties, and such regions lose volume as the bullae become enlarged. If disability is severe, if the bulla is extremely large, and if either lobar gas sampling or ventilation and perfusion scans demonstrate that sufficient function remains in the nonbullous regions, surgical excision of the bulla may lead to functional improvement. Usually, however, improvement is relatively transitory because other emphysematous regions gradually enlarge into bullae after surgery.

VARIANTS OF EMPHYSEMA In addition to the centriacinar and panacinar forms of emphysema described above, other structural patterns have been described but are functionally less important. Often there is overdistention and alveolar septal destruction in lung regions surrounding scar tissue (paracicatricial or scar emphysema) or along the borders of the acinus (paraseptal emphysema). The latter form, when it occurs at the visceral pleural surface, may predispose to episodes of spontaneous pneumothorax (Chap. 216). Infants rarely develop a check valve mechanism in a lobar bronchus which leads to rapid and life-threatening overdistention (congenital lobar emphysema). Unilateral emphysema may be an incidental radiographic finding (Macleod's or Swyer-James's syndromes). Since, in this condition, the airways are normal in number and structure but the alveoli are reduced in number, this form of unilateral emphysema has been attributed to disease occurring before the age of 8 years when alveoli are normally increasing in number. Overdistention and alveolar septal destruction are not present, and so this condition does not fit the definition of true emphysema. Most often the pulmonary artery on the affected side is hypoplastic. Although usually an incidental finding, the affected lung may become repeatedly infected so that surgical excision may be indicated.

MISCELLANEOUS DIFFUSE OBSTRUCTIVE SYNDROMES *Bronchiolitis obliterans* is a term applied to widespread inflammatory and fibrotic obstruction of small airways. Initially this syndrome was thought to be restricted to those persons who had suffered severe viral infections in childhood, particularly those due to parainfluenza virus. However, recently this syndrome has also been described in adult patients with rheumatoid arthritis. The response to bronchodilator treatment is poor, as would be expected from the histopathologic findings, and fatal respiratory failure often ensues within 2 years. There have been reports suggesting a relationship between penicillamine therapy and the development of bronchiolitis obliterans in patients with rheumatoid arthritis; however, it is clear that this syndrome can develop in patients who have never received penicillamine.

A syndrome with similar histopathology has been described in recipients of autologous bone marrow transplants. Although most often interstitial pneumonitis and fibrosis are sequelae, it has been documented that some patients develop a bronchiolitis obliterans picture. It appears that the development of this process occurs most often in the setting of a chronic graft-versus-host syndrome; however, it is clear that diffuse airways obstruction has developed without evidence of this syndrome in bone marrow recipients.

Cystic fibrosis in the adult with chronic airways obstruction is discussed elsewhere (Chap. 209).

REFERENCES

ANTHONISEN NR: Home oxygen therapy, in *Update VI: Principles of Internal Medicine*, RG Petersdorf et al (eds). New York, McGraw-Hill, 1985, p 203

BLOCK ER: Oxygen therapy, in *Update: Pulmonary Diseases and Disorders*, AP Fishman (ed). New York, McGraw-Hill, 1982, p 349

CAMPBELL AH et al: Factors affecting the decline of ventilatory function in chronic bronchitis. Thorax 40:741, 1985

CATTERAL JR et al: Mechanism of transient nocturnal hypoxemia in hypoxic chronic bronchitis and emphysema. J Appl Physiol 59:1698, 1985

COHEN AB (ed): Proteases and antiproteases in the lung. Am Rev Resp Dis 127 (Suppl):S1, 1983

CHETTY KG et al: Improved exercise tolerance of the polycythemic lung patient following phlebotomy. Am J Med 74:415, 1983

EFTHIMOU J et al: The effect of supplementary oral nutrition in poorly nourished patients with chronic obstructive pulmonary disease. Am Rev Resp Dis 137:1075, 1988

FISHMAN AP: The spectrum of chronic obstructive disease of the airways, in *Pulmonary Diseases and Disorders*, 2d ed, AP Fishman (ed). New York, McGraw-Hill, 1987, Chap 68

LAROS CD et al: Bullectomy for giant bullae in emphysema. J Thorac Cardiovasc Surg 91:63, 1986

PUSA T, TCHERZEWSKI H: Analysis of proteolytic enzymes and their natural inhibitors in serum and bronchial lavage fluid in atopic bronchial asthma, chronic bronchitis and pneumonia. Allerg Immunol 31:169, 1985

THURLBECK WM: A pathologist's approach to clinical bronchitis and emphysema, in *Update: Pulmonary Diseases and Disorders*, AP Fishman (ed). New York, McGraw-Hill, 1982, p 137

211 INTERSTITIAL LUNG DISEASES

HERBERT Y. REYNOLDS

The interstitial lung diseases (ILDs) are a heterogeneous group of conditions that involve the alveolar walls and perialveolar tissue. The ILDs are nonmalignant and are not caused by any defined infectious agents. Although an acute phase of illness may occur, the onset is often insidious, and the disease is usually chronic in duration. The initial response of the host to the disease process is inflammation in the air spaces and alveolar walls, causing an acute phase of intraluminal and mural alveolitis. If the disease is chronic and smoldering, inflammation will spread to adjacent portions of the interstitium and vasculature and eventually produce interstitial fibrosis. The resultant scarring and distortion of lung tissue leads to significant derangement of gas exchange and ventilatory function. Inflammation can also involve the conducting airways, and bronchiolitis obliterans associated with an organizing pneumonia is probably part of the spectrum of an ILD.

This diverse group of diseases have many features in common, including similarity of symptoms, comparable appearance of chest radiographs, consistent alterations in pulmonary physiology, and typical histologic features. However, ILDs have been difficult to classify, because approximately 180 known individual diseases are characterized by interstitial lung involvement, either as primary disease or as a significant part of a multiorgan process, as occurs in the collagen vascular diseases. The chest radiograph is of limited aid in classification since it can have a similar appearance in many of the ILDs as well as in other unrelated lung diseases. One useful approach for classification is to separate ILDs into two groups, those with known causes and those with unknown causes; each of these groups can be divided into subgroups according to the presence or absence of histologic evidence of granulomas in interstitial or vascular areas (Table 211-1). For each ILD there may be an acute phase, and there is usually a chronic one as well.

Among the ILDs of known cause, the largest group comprises occupational and environmental inhalant exposures; these include diseases due to inhalation of inorganic dusts (Chap. 206), organic dusts, and various irritative or noxious gases (Chap. 205). The number of ILDs of unknown cause is also very large. The major ones within this category are idiopathic pulmonary fibrosis (IPF), sarcoidosis, and the ILD often associated with collagen vascular disorders. ILD secondary to inorganic dust exposure usually can be recognized if the occupational history is pursued. For the myriad (Table 211-1) of other diffuse ILDs, however, a precise diagnosis is obtained with difficulty, usually only after interpretation of an open-lung biopsy specimen; most of these diseases are relatively rare.

Although the initiating agent(s) or circumstances of the various ILDs may be diverse, and many are unknown, the immunopathogenic responses of lung tissue are limited, so that the initial mechanisms of injury, the development of alveolitis, and the attempts at repair sometimes leading to fibrosis will have common features. Idiopathic pulmonary fibrosis is discussed as the prototype ILD, as it is encountered relatively frequently and much of the recent research on mechanisms of lung fibrosis has focused on this disease.

TABLE 211-1 Major categories of alveolar and interstitial inflammatory lung diseases (ILDs)

Known cause	Unknown cause
LUNG RESPONSE: ALVEOLITIS, INTERSTITIAL INFLAMMATION, AND FIBROSIS	
Asbestos Fumes, gases Drugs (antibiotics) and chemotherapy drugs Radiation Aspiration pneumonia Residual of adult respiratory distress syndrome	Idiopathic pulmonary fibrosis Collagen vascular diseases Systemic lupus erythematosus, rheumatoid arthritis, ankylosing spondylitis, systemic sclerosis, Sjögren's syndrome, polymyositis-dermatomyositis Pulmonary hemorrhage syndromes Goodpasture's syndrome, idiopathic pulmonary hemosiderosis Pulmonary alveolar proteinosis Lymphocytic infiltrative disorders (lymphocytic interstitial pneumonitis) Eosinophilic pneumonias Lymphangioleiomyomatosis Amyloidosis Inherited diseases Tuberous sclerosis, neurofibromatosis, Niemann-Pick disease, Gaucher's disease, Hermansky-Pudlak syndrome Gastrointestinal or liver diseases (Crohn's disease, primary biliary cirrhosis, chronic active hepatitis, ulcerative colitis) Graft vs. host disease (bone marrow transplantation)
LUNG RESPONSE: AS ABOVE BUT WITH GRANULOMA	
Hypersensitivity pneumonitis (organic dusts) Inorganic dusts: beryllium silica	Sarcoidosis Langerhans cell granulomatosis (eosinophilic granuloma) Granulomatous vasculitides Wegener's granulomatosis, allergic granulomatosis of Churg-Strauss, lymphomatoid granulomatosis Bronchocentric granulomatosis

IDIOPATHIC PULMONARY FIBROSIS (IPF)

Many patients who present with nonproductive cough, progressive dyspnea, a chest radiograph showing lower lung zone reticular shadows, and pulmonary function tests showing a restrictive pattern (Chap. 201) will be said to have IPF after the diagnostic evaluation is completed. This condition is also known as *cryptogenic fibrosing alveolitis*. Although the terms *idiopathic* and *cryptogenic* mean that the etiologic agent is unknown, this is not a nebulous, wastebasket diagnosis or just a diagnosis of exclusion but rather a well-defined clinical entity.

IMMUNOPATHOGENESIS Several parts of the alveolar structure are affected in IPF, including the alveolar walls lined with type I and type II pneumocytes and the interstitial supporting structure composed of mesenchymal cells, especially fibroblasts and myofibroblasts, collagen, and various adhesive proteoglycans. The capillary endothelium may also be involved. The disease process does not affect the upper or conducting airways, but bronchiolitis of respiratory bronchioles may be present and alveolar units are always involved.

Normally, overlying or interspersed in the alveoli are a variety of immune cells including alveolar macrophages, dendritic macrophages, interstitial monocytes, lymphocytes, and inflammatory cells, such as polymorphonuclear leukocytes (PMNs) and eosinophils. The cellular content of normal bronchoalveolar lavage (BAL) fluid consists of approximately 80 percent alveolar macrophages, 10 percent lymphocytes (of which 70 percent are T lymphocytes), 1 to 5 percent B lymphocytes or plasma cells, 1 to 3 percent polymorphonuclear leukocytes, and 1 percent eosinophils.

In the earliest, reversible forms of alveolar injury, leakiness of the alveolar type I cells and the adjacent capillary endothelial cells occurs, causing alveolar and interstitial edema and the formation of intraalveolar hyaline membranes. With persistence of the disease, increased alveolar-capillary permeability and desquamation of intraalveolar cells (alveolitis), mural inflammation, and interstitial fibrosis are present on biopsy. This process is also reflected in the composition of cells and enzymes recovered in BAL fluid (Table 211-2) and in cellular components present in lung biopsy tissue. The presence and severity of the disease process are spotty in distribution; a continuum of inflammatory and fibrotic changes can be found throughout the affected lung.

Figure 211-1 depicts schematically immunopathogenic mechanisms that interconnect the intraalveolar (luminal) and alveolar mural tissue with the interstitial space and capillary vascular areas. The inciting agent or stimulus is often unknown but is likely an antigen that can initiate an immunoglobulin response. This is reflected by an increased ratio of IgG subclasses IgG1 and G3, an increased number of IgG-releasing cells, and perhaps the formation of immune complexes. IgG may function as an opsonin or as part of an immune complex that interacts with the surface of the alveolar macrophage.

An increased number of macrophages, which are activated phagocytes capable of producing many cytokines that affect other lung cells, are a hallmark of the alveolitis. These macrophage cytokines or mediators could operate in two directions. First, through the production of chemotaxins, which may include leukotriene LTB_4, inflammatory cells such as PMNs and eosinophils are attracted into the alveoli. An increased percentage of PMNs (20 percent or more) and eosinophils (1 to 4 percent) in the profile of BAL cells is usual in IPF. Lymphocytes are not usually increased, unless the IPF is part of a collagen vascular disease. Enzymes or oxidant radicals from inflammatory cells and histamine may cause local injury or alter the permeability of type I cells. Second, macrophages are also capable of secreting substances that stimulate mesenchymal cells. For fibroblasts to replicate in the interstitium and in the alveolar walls, they must first be attracted and adhere to a connective tissue matrix and then be primed to enter the G_1 phase of a growth cycle to proliferate.

Several products from alveolar macrophages can participate in these steps. Platelet-derived growth factor (PDGF) (see p. 60) is a

TABLE 211-2 Cellular and immunologic changes in various IPF specimens

BLOOD
IgG (IgG1,3) elevated immune complexes, cryoglobulins
Serologic titers (low)
T lymphocytes (sensitized to type I collagen)
BRONCHOALVEOLAR FLUID
Alveolitis characterized by increased percentage of PMNs (20%) and eosinophils (2–4%), but lymphocytes can be increased also (20%)
Alveolar macrophages: activated macrophages and their secretory components are numerous:
Chemotaxins to attract PMNs and muscle cells
Plasminogen activator
Macrophage-derived growth factor
Fibronectin
Platelet-derived growth factor (by c-*sis* oncogene)
Steroid receptors increased; mitotic index increased
Collagenase (PMN origin)
IgG increased (G3, G1 subclasses)
Immune complexes detectable
IgG-releasing cells present
Histamine elevated
LUNG TISSUE
Interstitial inflammation
Plasma cells, muscle cells, fibroblasts increased
Collagen synthesis increased
Fibrosis but no granuloma
Bronchiolitis obliterans can develop

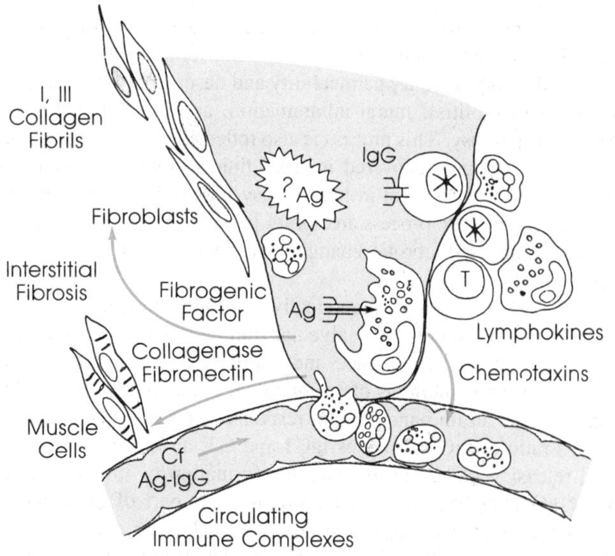

FIGURE 211-1 Immunologic mechanisms within the alveolar space, alveolar walls, and interstitium that can lead to inflammation and eventual fibrosis. The focus is on the alveolor macrophage, which is activated, possibly by an immune complex and an as yet unidentified antigen (Ag). Through mediators such as chemotaxins, the macrophage attracts PMNs and other cells from the circulation to the alveolar space, or it can initiate fibrogenesis with various mediators that can stimulate fibroblasts and muscle cells to proliferate. Interstitial fibrosis may result. *(From Reynolds, 1986.)*

chemoattractant for mesenchymal cells and a stimulus for fibroblasts to change from resting cells to cells entering G_1. Although PDGF is not produced by normal monocytes or macrophages, alveolar macrophages obtained from patients with IPF make it abundantly. This is correlated with c-*sis*, a proto-oncogene that codes for the beta chain of PDGF, which is increased in IPF-derived macrophages and which may drive the exaggerated release of PDGF. This mediator acts as a chemoattractant and a growth factor for fibroblasts. Later in the fibroblast replication cycle, alveolar macrophage-derived growth factor (AMDGF) can accelerate proliferation. Insulin and other cellular or metabolic substances are also needed in these growth-regulatory steps. Smooth-muscle cells can also proliferate. With continued activity of macrophages, fibrosis becomes more widespread and may involve the vasculature. Obliteration of functional alveolar structures occurs with scar tissue formation, and cystic areas develop from retraction of the terminal airways that once subtended the alveolar unit.

CLINICAL PRESENTATION History On the average, patients are 50 years old, although the range spans infancy to old age. Several family clusters have been reported, and it is possible that genetic factors may determine susceptibility to the disease. The first clinical manifestations of ILD are dyspnea, effort intolerance, and a dry cough without other obvious cause. A detailed work history is essential. For example, casual exposure to asbestos many years previously may provide a crucial clue to the etiology. Work-related compensation may influence complaints for some individuals.

Approximately one-third of patients can pinpoint their awareness of dyspnea to the aftermath of a viral respiratory illness. Usually months or years elapse between the onset of exertional dyspnea and its progression perhaps to the point of breathlessness at rest. Dyspnea and frequent coughing are often accompanied by other constitutional symptoms such as fatigue, anorexia, weight loss, and arthralgias.

Physical findings Initially, the physical examination may not be revealing and auscultation of the chest may be normal. As the disease advances, dry rales, or coarse crackles on inspiration, are usually heard at the lung bases. There may be tachypnea at rest, cyanosis, and clubbing of the fingers and toes, usually without hypertrophic osteoarthropathy. In later stages, cor pulmonale (Chap. 191) is evident, with findings of pulmonary hypertension, such as an accentuated pulmonic second sound or a right-sided lift, and eventually signs of right heart failure. The right ventricular ejection fraction determined by radionuclide ventriculography is often depressed in the face of normal left ventricular performance.

LABORATORY AND DIAGNOSTIC TESTS Imaging studies The chest radiograph usually reveals a pattern of diffuse reticular markings, prominent in the lower lung zones. Several radiographic patterns can be seen which correlate roughly with the duration of the disease. Early, a hazy ''ground glass'' appearance of the lower lung fields coincides with the stage of acute alveolitis. Later, curvilinear shadows predominate and may coalesce into nodular infiltrates. With end-stage disease, the linear opacities are seen in all lung fields, the lung fields appear contracted, and ring-shaped opacities resulting from cystic and bronchiectatic changes are obvious, creating the *honeycombed* or *swiss cheese* appearance of the lung. Biopsy-proven forms of diffuse IPF occasionally occur in patients with normal chest radiographs despite significant exercise intolerance, abnormal pulmonary function tests, including a reduced diffusing capacity, and dry rales.

Use of gallium 67 citrate scanning can be helpful in assessing inflammation of the lung parenchyma, as its uptake may correlate with the presence of PMNs in the airways and lung tissue. CT scanning, utilizing ultrathin cuts of 0.5 cm, is a sensitive means of documenting tissue infiltration and the presence of bronchiectasis or pleural changes.

Laboratory examination The erythrocyte sedimentation rate is usually elevated, circulating immune-complex titers and serum immunoglobulin levels may be increased, and cryoimmunoglobulins may be present. Serologic tests to screen for collagen vascular diseases are necessary to exclude these diagnoses. Although serum rheumatoid factor, antinuclear antibodies, depressed levels of complement, and other parameters of autoimmune diseases may be detected in approximately 10 percent of patients with IPF, the titers are generally quite low.

Lung function tests In patients with advanced disease, reductions in total lung capacity, vital capacity, and residual volume are found (Chap. 201). Usually evidence of airway obstruction is minimal and the FEV_1/FVC ratio is normal or increased. A restrictive respiratory functional pattern is usually present, reflecting the stiff, noncompliant lungs characteristic of IPF and its common aftermath, fibrosis. There is usually resting arterial hypoxemia, but the carbon dioxide tension is normal or decreased. Blood pH is normal. The alveolar-arterial oxygen gradient during exercise is elevated, and exercise tolerance is reduced. The carbon monoxide diffusing capacity is usually reduced by 30 to 50 percent. Changes in these variables are useful in monitoring the course of the illness and in assessing the effectiveness of treatment.

Bronchoscopy Direct investigation of the airways by fiberoptic bronchoscopy is part of the evaluation, and four to six transbronchial biopsies are taken to obtain lung tissue for diagnosis. These provide a sufficient quantity of tissue for a definitive pathologic diagnosis in approximately one-fourth of all cases of IPF. In some diffuse granulomatous interstitial diseases, such as sarcoidosis (Chap. 277), transbronchial biopsy will provide a tissue diagnosis in about 80 percent of cases. Bronchoscopy also permits bronchoalveolar lavage, which provides useful information about cells and proteins in the airways that generally correlates with histologic changes in the interstitial and alveolar tissues. An analysis of BAL fluid and cells can reveal a number of changes in IPF (Table 211-2).

Lung biopsy The importance of an adequate sample of lung tissue to permit a full histologic evaluation, good microbial cultures, immunofluorescence and electron-microscopic studies, and analysis of inorganic substances cannot be overemphasized. Therefore, if a transbronchial biopsy does not yield sufficient tissue for a confident diagnosis, open-lung biopsy should be considered. It is prudent to substantiate a tissue diagnosis before embarking on immunosuppressive therapy with its attendant complications.

DIAGNOSTIC APPROACH AND STAGING OF DISEASE ACTIVITY Following the clinical examination, chest radiograph, pulmonary function tests [lung volumes, FEV_1/FVC, and diffusing capacity (Chap. 201)], and arterial blood gas determination, the functional disability from the lung disease can be estimated. However, a histologic analysis of lung tissue should be made before the disease is diagnosed definitively. Fiberoptic bronchoscopy is usually the first invasive procedure and is important for ruling out infection, malignancy, and other specific diseases. Although transbronchial biopsy has a lower diagnostic yield in IPF than in sarcoidosis and other granulomatous diseases, it is nevertheless a useful, low-risk procedure with a 20 to 30 percent success rate for obtaining an adequate sample for a confident pathologic diagnosis. BAL for cellular and protein analysis may be useful in judging the nature of alveolar inflammation and immunologic activity (Table 211-2). However, the value of the periodic use of BAL analysis to monitor disease activity or its response to therapy has not been established. Use of gallium 67 lung scanning does not add diagnostic accuracy but may be an indication of general cellular activity in the lung.

If the diagnosis is still in doubt after the bronchoscopy and related procedures, an open-lung biopsy should be considered. The referring physician and the thoracic surgeon should cooperate in choosing the most representative area of the lung for biopsy, and the proper microbial cultures and immunologic studies can be obtained.

THERAPY Treatment is usually offered to patients with IPF, even to patients with advanced fibrotic disease. About 2 weeks after the open-lung biopsy, a trial of oral prednisone can be instituted in a dose of 1 mg/kg daily and continued for 8 to 12 weeks. If lung disease shows objective improvement, the dose is tapered to a maintenance level. Should the disease not respond or be progressive, the dosage of prednisone can be increased, but immunosuppression with cyclophosphamide should be considered. Cyclophosphamide is given at a dose of about 1.0 mg/kg daily (50 to 75 mg) with the patient continuing on a daily maintenance dose of oral prednisone (0.25 mg/kg). The dosages of cyclophosphamide may be increased as necessary by 50-mg increments at 7 to 10-day intervals. The objective is to reduce the white blood cell count to approximately half the normal baseline value, causing a distinct drop in the total blood lymphocyte count. However, a minimum count of 1000 polymorphonuclear leukocytes per microliter should be maintained.

Several other measures may help respiratory function. It is imperative that patients discontinue cigarette smoking. Since there is frequently a marked drop in Pa_{O_2} with exercise, supplemental oxygen therapy may be useful, sometimes using transtracheal catheter oxygen delivery. As the pulmonary vascular bed is destroyed by progressive fibrosis, pulmonary hypertension and cor pulmonale can develop; right-sided congestive heart failure can be difficult to control. Judicious use of diuretics is advised, and digitalis may be required, although adequate oxygenation is probably the best treatment for right heart failure (Chap. 191). Some patients may also develop obstruction to airflow and wheezing and coughing which may respond to bronchodilators. Infection may occur during immunosuppressive therapy and should be treated promptly and aggressively. Prophylactic use of pneumococcal and influenza vaccines is indicated. If refractory disease limited to the chest is present, the possibility of lung transplantation should be considered. Recent successes with single-lung transplantation for ILD make this therapy a reality for some patients.

INDIVIDUAL FORMS OF ILD

ILD ASSOCIATED WITH COLLAGEN VASCULAR DISORDERS

In these diseases, various pulmonary structures can be affected, especially the pleura, so that ILD is but one manifestation of intrathoracic involvement and often a minor part of the multiorgan process. Analysis of BAL fluid and cells from patients with ILD associated with rheumatoid arthritis and systemic sclerosis is similar to that found in IPF (Table 211-2) and suggests similar pathogenetic mechanisms for fibrosis. A lymphocytic alveolitis may accompany some cases of ILD in rheumatoid disease and is a harbinger of a better response to immunosuppressive therapy.

Systemic lupus erythematosus (SLE) (See Chap. 269) About half of patients with SLE ultimately develop overt lung disease. Pleuritis, pleural effusion(s), or acute pneumonitis are the most frequent forms of lung disease, while a chronic, progressive ILD is uncommon. Although pleuropulmonary involvement may not be evident clinically, pulmonary function testing, particularly the diffusing capacity for carbon monoxide, reveals abnormalities in many patients.

Rheumatoid arthritis (See Chap. 270) A variety of pulmonary manifestations can occur, including pleural disease (pleural effusion and subpleural nodules), parenchymal nodular infiltrates associated with pneumoconiosis in miners (Caplan's syndrome), and diffuse interstitial fibrosis. The ILD can develop before joint disease becomes evident, particularly in men, and is accompanied by high titers of rheumatoid factor. Rarely, upper airway obstruction can occur from arthritis of the cricoarytenoid joint. Patients with rheumatoid arthritis who are receiving treatment with methotrexate or gold may develop ILD that represents a drug hypersensitivity, which must be differentiated from a preexisting or developing ILD associated with the underlying disease. Penicillamine therapy in patients with rheumatoid arthritis has been implicated in causing bronchiolitis obliterans (p. 1082).

Ankylosing spondylitis (See Chap. 274) Bilateral upper lobe fibrosis, which can be complicated by fibrocavitary disease, may develop late in the course.

Systemic sclerosis (See Chap. 271) Radiographic evidence of lung involvement develops in a majority of patients, but its severity or progression is variable. Because distal esophageal motor dysfunction is present in many patients, reflux with regurgitation and chronic aspiration is common. In addition, cutaneous scleroderma can involve the anterior chest wall and abdomen, causing restrictive lung function.

Sjögren's syndrome (See Chap. 273) General dryness and lack of airways secretions cause the major problems of hoarseness, cough, and bronchitis. Presence of an ILD in these patients may signify a lymphocytic infiltrate in lung tissue which can behave as a low-grade lymphoma.

Polymyositis and dermatomyositis (See Chap. 364) Although ILD is reported to occur in only 5 to 10 percent of patients, its presence is more common in the subgroup of patients with an anti-Jo-1 antibody that is directed to tRNA synthetase. Weakness of respiratory muscles contributing to aspiration pneumonitis is a common occurrence.

SYNDROMES OF ILD WITH PULMONARY HEMORRHAGE

Recurrent hemoptysis, dyspnea, and hypoxemia in the presence of a chest radiographic pattern of diffuse alveolar opacities should raise the possibility of alveolar hemorrhage. An association between vasculitis involving the kidney (lung-renal syndromes) or other organ systems should be investigated. Alveolar hemorrhage occurs rarely in all collagen vascular disorders, but it is described most often with systemic lupus erythematosus. It can occur with systemic vasculitis and is described as an initial presentation of Wegener's granulomatosis; with Behçet's disease, in which aneurysm formation and rupture of small muscular arteries is a manifestation of necrotizing vasculitis; in allergic Churg-Strauss granulomatosis; in Henoch-Schönlein purpura syndrome; and in essential (mixed) cryoimmunoglobulinemia. Exposure to the toxic aerosol trimellitic anhydride may cause alveolar hemorrhage. Serologic tests for antinuclear antibody, anti-glomerular basement membrane antibody, and complement to document a vasculitis and immunologic disorder are the first steps, but renal biopsy and possibly lung biopsy may be required for a definitive diagnosis. Some specific syndromes in this category will be discussed next.

Goodpasture's syndrome (See Chap. 228) Pulmonary hemorrhage and glomerulonephritis are the features of this disease in which most patients have antibodies to renal glomerular and lung alveolar basement membranes.

Idiopathic pulmonary hemosiderosis Diffuse alveolar hemorrhage can occur in the absence of other organ involvement or an obvious immunologic cause and is therefore a diagnosis of exclusion after considering the many causes of alveolar bleeding associated with collagen vascular and vasculitic diseases. A lung biopsy is usually necessary to document the lack of inflammatory injury in the lung tissues and to exclude other diseases with confidence. The clinical course can be variable, ranging from a recurrent and fulminant one with development of progressive interstitial fibrosis to minimal disease that may remit without sequelae. Children and young adults are usually affected. Glucocorticoid treatment is useful for control of bleeding acutely but is not a predictable long-term remedy for keeping the disease suppressed and preventing recurrence.

PULMONARY ALVEOLAR PROTEINOSIS Similar clinical symptoms and the general appearance of the chest radiograph, showing diffuse alveolar consolidation and/or nodular shadows typically radiating from the hilar regions, place pulmonary alveolar proteinosis (PAP) in the ILD category. Histologically the alveoli are filled with granular material that stains with periodic acid Schiff reagent, but they exhibit no inflammation and have relatively normal septal structure. Strictly speaking, then, PAP is an intraalveolar process which resembles, but is not, an ILD. Because the proteinaceous response can be associated with inhaled dust exposure (silica and aluminum), malignancy, and chronic infection, termed *secondary PAP*, these disorders should be differentiated from primary PAP by lung biopsy. The intraalveolar material is a combination of surfactant phospholipid produced by type II pneumocytes and of other proteins and immunoglobulins found in alveolar lining fluid. The cytoplasm of alveolar macrophages appears engorged with inclusions. The "stuffed" macrophages with large phagolysosomes have diminished microbial killing capacity in vitro, but lung infections with unusual organisms are not frequent. Whole-lung lavage(s) will provide relief to many patients with dyspnea and progressive deterioration of arterial oxygenation and may also provide long-term benefit.

LYMPHOCYTIC INFILTRATIVE DISORDERS This is a group of disorders that feature lymphocyte and plasma cell infiltration of the lung parenchyma and either are benign or can behave as low-grade lymphomas. Within the spectrum of chronic interstitial pneumonias, referred to as IPFs, a subset has been described with lung histology that shows diffuse interstitial infiltration with lymphocytes and plasma cells. In some of these patients an autoimmune disease or dysproteinemia exists. However, lymphocytic interstitial pneumonia (LIP) is probably not a distinct entity, belongs within the IPF group, and can be associated with Sjögren's syndrome. LIP has been reported in patients, particularly children, with AIDS.

Included among these disorders is immunoblastic lymphadenopathy, also termed *angioimmunoblastic lymphadenopathy*, which usually is a fulminant lymphoma-like disease that may have an element of ILD in some cases. *Lymphomatoid granulomatosis* can be included, but its granulomatous response also places it with the granulomatous ILDs (Table 211-1).

EOSINOPHILIC PNEUMONIAS (See Chap. 205) These pneumonias encompass a spectrum of diseases in which lung hypersensitivity plays a role and in which a specific cause may or may not be identified. For example, with extrinsic asthma and exposure to fungal antigens, allergic bronchopulmonary mycosis can develop; filarial and other parasitic infections can cause tropical pulmonary eosinophilia; many common drugs can induce eosinophilic pneumonia. Chronic eosinophilic pneumonia has features that make it difficult to distinguish from IPF and other forms of progressive ILD. The disease, which more commonly affects older females, has several radiologic characteristics that are helpful in diagnosis: (1) a peripheral pattern of dense lung infiltrates that appear to cross anatomic lobar boundaries with sparing of the central lung regions; (2) regression but reappearance of infiltrates in the same lung locations; and (3) extreme sensitivity of the infiltrates (and disease symptoms) to modest doses of oral glucocorticoids. The diagnosis can be established by lung biopsy, which shows an eosinophilic inflammatory process.

LYMPHANGIOLEIOMYOMATOSIS Immature smooth-muscle cells can proliferate in lung tissue around and throughout bronchial, vascular, and lymphatic structures, causing local obstruction or creating constricting lesions that develop into cysts. Lymphatics and lymph nodes in other organs are also usually affected. Because this disorder occurs predominantly in females of reproductive age, an association between estrogens and the disease is probable. Pulmonary symptoms consist of dyspnea, cough, and hemoptysis; a more overt presentation occurs with spontaneous pneumothorax, which can be recurrent, or with chylous effusion. In addition, the chest radiograph shows reticulonodular shadows and small cyst-like areas or honeycombing throughout the lung fields. In contrast to most forms of ILD, lung volumes are normal or increased, as is also the case with Langerhans cell granulomatosis (see below). Therapy for progressive lung disease has not been particularly effective. Pneumothoraxes and effusions may require chemical or surgical pleurodesis. Treatment with progesterone combined with ovariectomy has been used. Lung transplantation may be considered for some patients.

AMYLOIDOSIS (See Chap. 266) Deposits of amyloid in the form of plaques or nodules can develop at all sites of the respiratory tract. Tracheal and endobronchial mucosal plaques or incidental parenchymal nodules can be difficult to diagnose clinically, but they usually coexist with extrapulmonary manifestations of primary or, less commonly, secondary amyloidosis. Lung biopsy is necessary for definitive diagnosis. As part of primary systemic amyloidosis or a plasma cell dyscrasia, an ILD may occur from amyloid deposits in alveolar septa and associated blood vessels, producing dyspnea, radiographic findings of diffuse reticulonodular shadows, and restrictive pulmonary function.

INHERITED DISORDERS ASSOCIATED WITH ILD Pulmonary infiltrates and respiratory symptoms typical of mild ILD can develop in related family members and in several inherited diseases. These include the phacomatoses (Chap. 358) tuberous sclerosis and neurofibromatosis and the lysosomal storage diseases (Chap. 331), such as Niemann-Pick disease and Gaucher's disease. The *Hermansky-Pudlak syndrome* is an autosomal recessive disorder, in which granulomatous colitis and ILD may occur. It is characterized by oculocutaneous albinism, bleeding diathesis from platelet dysfunction, and the accumulation of a chromolipid, lipofuscin material in cells of the reticuloendothelial system. The pulmonary fibrosis is similar to IPF, but the alveolar macrophages may contain cytoplasmic ceroid-like inclusions.

GASTROINTESTINAL AND LIVER DISEASE Rarely, inflammatory bowel disease and chronic hepatitis may be associated with a mild form of ILD. Crohn's disease, which has a number of similarities with sarcoidosis, may also be accompanied by asymptomatic lymphocytic alveolitis.

GRAFT VS. HOST DISEASE (GVHD) (See Chap. 299) Some degree of GVHD occurs in all patients receiving bone marrow transplantation. However, in about 10 percent a chronic phase may ensue with the onset of dry cough, mucositis, dyspnea, and airflow obstruction in the small airways, as demonstrated by pulmonary function testing. Chest radiographs reveal peribronchiolar infiltrates, and lung biopsy shows focal areas of interstitial infiltration with a mixture of lymphocytes and PMNs. The lesions are consistent with bronchiolitis; no vasculitis is present. Some recipients of heart-lung transplants also develop bronchiolitis. Bronchiolitis in chronic GVHD may stabilize and disappear or may be progressive and fatal. Treatment includes increasing the doses of the immunosuppressive drugs together with bronchodilators and antibiotics. Infection, especially with viral agents, is a common complication.

ILD WITH A GRANULOMATOUS RESPONSE IN LUNG TISSUE OR VASCULAR STRUCTURES Inhalation of organic dusts, which causes hypersensitivity pneumonitis, or of inorganic particles such as silica, which causes alveolitis and elicits a granulomatous inflammatory reaction leading to ILD, produces diseases of known etiology (Table 211-1) that are discussed in Chaps. 205 and 206. Sarcoidosis (Chap. 277) is prominent among granulomatous diseases of *unknown cause* in which ILD is an important feature.

Langerhans cell granulomatosis (eosinophilic granuloma or histiocytosis X) (See Chap. 63) This condition is being recognized with increasing frequency and may account for about 1 to 5 percent of ILD of unknown etiology. Previously, the proliferation of tissue macrophages (histiocytes) was thought to be characteristic of this disease that affects the lung, bones, and viscera. Now it is recognized that the precursor cell is the *dendritic cell,* which has potent stimulatory and accessory cell immune function, is normally found in the interstitium and alveolar septal areas, and is distinctly different from a tissue macrophage. The dendritic cell can evolve into the Langerhans cell, characterized by a specific CD1a surface antigen that reacts with a monoclonal antibody identified as T_6, and by intracytoplasmic organelles seen by electron microscopy that are called X bodies or Birbeck granules. Langerhans cells can be identified in skin and are present in bronchiolar epithelium of normal lung. Cigarette smoking or a similar irritant seems to be a stimulus for their proliferation. An increased number of these cells can be recovered in BAL from normal smokers, patients with bronchoalveolar carcinoma, and patients with IPF. However, in Langerhans cell granulomatosis of the lung, 3 percent or more of the BAL cells may be so identified, which greatly exceeds the percentage found in these other disorders. However, the Langerhans cells are not pathognomonic for this disease. The number of alveolar macrophages is also increased. Early in the disease a focus of Langerhans and surrounding inflammatory cells can be found adjacent to respiratory and terminal bronchioles, causing bronchiolitis. Later, alveolar structures are involved in progressive interstitial inflammation and fibrosis. In advanced disease, lung histology does *not* reveal the discrete typical granulomas that are found in sarcoidosis and hypersensitivity pneumonitis, nor are eosinophils greatly increased—two reasons that the prior appellation, "eosinophilic granuloma," was really a misnomer.

The pulmonary form of this disease occurs in young and middle-aged adults, usually males, and in those who use tobacco heavily; it may remain focal or involve one or several bony sites (long bones, spine, skull, or jaw). Occasionally, multifocal disease can affect the posterior pituitary gland, causing diabetes insipidus, a condition that is termed *Hand-Schüller-Christian disease*. In infants, *Letterer-Siwe disease* is a more fulminant visceral form of this disorder that mimics a malignant lymphoma. In adults, the presenting symptoms and signs do not distinguish this disease from other forms of ILD unless signs of a bone lesion exist. A spontaneous pneumothorax may herald the disease. Chest radiographs will show diffuse micronodular shadows and cystic spaces, sparing the costophrenic angles and preserving lung volume, as occurs in lymphangioleiomyomatosis. Pulmonary function tests may disclose a combination of obstructive and restrictive defects. As the disease progresses, greater airway obstruction may develop, and the chest radiograph can resemble that in advanced chronic obstructive lung disease. Treatment involves a mandatory cessation of tobacco use, which may cause the pulmonary disease to stabilize or regress. Glucocorticoids usually are not helpful. Penicillamine has been used in an attempt to prevent fibrosis with variable success. Local bone lesions may require radiation. For patients with increasing symptoms of airway obstruction, supportive therapy and bronchodilators may be tried, but their success has been modest.

Granulomatous vasculitis (See Chap. 276) Certain forms of vasculitis, accompanied by a granulomatous response, can involve the respiratory tract as part of a multiorgan process or can occasionally be localized to the respiratory tract, as occurs with a predominantly pulmonary form of Wegener's granulomatosis in which glomerulonephritis may not be prominent. It is very important to differentiate these conditions from lymphomatoid granulomatosis. Allergic angiitis and the granulomatosis of Churg and Strauss are forms of granulomatous vasculitis affecting many organs but especially the lungs; a history of asthma and the presence of eosinophilia are distinguishing features.

Lymphomatoid granulomatosis (See Chaps. 63 and 276) This involves primarily the lungs and less frequently the skin, central and peripheral nervous systems, and kidneys with an infiltration of lymphocytoid, plasmalike cells and macrophages creating a necrotic granulomatous inflammatory reaction, especially in or near blood vessels. The disease can progress as a lymphoproliferative disorder and evolve into malignant lymphoma in as many as 50 percent of patients. Treatment of lymphomatoid granulomatosis with glucocorticoids and cyclophosphamide may induce a remission, and if this occurs, subsequent relapse and development of lymphoma are not likely.

BRONCHOCENTRIC GRANULOMATOSIS In contrast to the necrotizing granulomatous reaction in lung vessels, i.e., angiocentric vasculitis, granulomatous destruction of bronchioles occurs in this condition. There is usually associated parenchymal inflammation causing ILD. Eosinophils can be present if asthma and hypersensitivity to fungal antigens within the bronchi have occurred. In other cases without these associated conditions, hypersensitivity to other microbial antigens is postulated. Bronchocentric granulomatosis must be differentiated from hypersensitivity pneumonitis caused by inhalation of organic dusts (see Chaps. 205 and 206).

REFERENCES

Idiopathic pulmonary fibrosis

Crystal RG et al: Interstitial lung diseases of unknown cause: Disorders characterized by chronic inflammation of the lower respiratory tract. N Engl J Med 310:154, 235, 1984

Epler GR et al: Bronchiolitis obliterans with organizing pneumonia. N Engl J Med 312:152, 1985

Reynolds HY: Idiopathic interstitial pulmonary fibrosis: Contribution of bronchoalveolar lavage analysis. Chest 89:139, 1986

———: Idiopathic pulmonary fibrosis, in *Current Therapy in Allergy, Immunology, and Rheumatology*, LM Lichtenstein, AS Fauci (eds). Toronto, Decker, 1988, vol 3, pp 214–220

Toronto Lung Transplant Group: Experience with single-lung transplantation for pulmonary fibrosis. JAMA 259:2258, 1988

Other interstitial lung diseases

Adamson D et al: Successful treatment of pulmonary lymphangiomyomatosis with oophorectomy and progesterone. Am Rev Respir Dis 132:916, 1985

Allen JN et al: Acute eosinophilic pneumonia as a reversible cause of noninfectious respiratory failure. N Engl J Med 321:569, 1989

Bitterman PB et al: Familial idiopathic pulmonary fibrosis. N Engl J Med 314:1343, 1986

Chan CK et al: Small-airways disease in recipients of allogenic bone marrow transplants. Medicine 66:327, 1987

Fauci AS et al: Lymphomatoid granulomatosis—prospective clinical and therapeutic experience over 10 years. N Engl J Med 306:68, 1982

Hance AJ et al: Pulmonary and extrapulmonary manifestations of Langerhans cell granulomatosis (histiocytosis X). Semin Respir Med 9:349, 1988

Kariman K et al: Pulmonary alveolar proteinosis: Prospective clinical experience in 23 patients for 15 years. Lung 162:223, 1984

Reynolds HY: Bronchoalveolar lavage. Am Rev Respir Dis 135:250, 1987

Rossi GA et al: Evidence for chronic inflammation as a component of interstitial lung disease associated with progressive systemic sclerosis. Am Rev Respir Dis 131:612, 1985

Seggen JS et al: Bronchiolitis obliterans. Chest 83:169, 1983

Strimlan CV et al: Lymphocytic interstitial pneumonitis. Ann Intern Med 88:616, 1978

212 PRIMARY PULMONARY HYPERTENSION

STUART RICH

Primary pulmonary hypertension is an uncommon disease characterized by increased pulmonary artery pressure and pulmonary vascular resistance without an obvious cause. The diagnosis can be made only after all etiologies for pulmonary hypertension have been excluded. There is a female-to-male preponderance (1.7:1), with patients most commonly presenting in the third and fourth decades, although the age range is from infancy to greater than 60 years. Because the predominant symptom of primary pulmonary hypertension is dyspnea, which can have an insidious onset in an otherwise healthy person, the disease is typically diagnosed late in its course. By that time the clinical and laboratory findings of severe pulmonary hypertension are usually present.

PATHOLOGY Three histologic patterns have been described in patients with primary pulmonary hypertension. *Plexogenic pulmonary arteriopathy* is the result of severe pulmonary hypertension from a variety of etiologies and is found in 30 to 60 percent of patients with primary pulmonary hypertension. It is more prevalent in younger women. The histology is characterized by changes in the pulmonary arteriolar bed including medial hypertrophy, concentric laminar intimal fibrosis, and plexiform lesions. Although the exact cause for the plexiform lesions remains unknown, they are only found when the pulmonary hypertension originates at the precapillary level. Plexogenic pulmonary arteriopathy also occurs in patients with pulmonary hypertension associated with congenital heart disease, with cirrhosis of the liver, and in pulmonary hypertension of collagen vascular disease. Some patients who present with primary pulmonary hypertension with high titers of antinuclear antibodies probably have a collagen vascular disease confined to the pulmonary vascular bed.

Thrombotic pulmonary arteriopathy accounts for approximately 40 to 50 percent of the cases of primary pulmonary hypertension and affects men and women equally. Histologically it is characterized by eccentric intimal fibrosis with medial hypertrophy, fibroelastic intimal pads in the arteries and arterioles, and scattered evidence of old recanalized thrombus appearing as fibrous webs. Although it has been proposed that recurrent microembolism is the cause for these lesions, no source for the emboli has been consistently found in these patients. Injury to the pulmonary vascular endothelium can create a procoagulant environment within the pulmonary arterial bed that might predispose to the development of thrombosis in situ, and abnormalities in fibrinolysis have recently been described in some patients. Whether the microthrombi represent a primary or secondary phenomenon is unknown, as microthrombi are also found in some patients with plexogenic pulmonary arteriopathy. Thrombotic pulmonary arteriopathy is also seen in patients with atrial septal defects and elevated pulmonary vascular resistance.

Pulmonary venoocclusive disease occurs in less than 10 percent of patients with primary pulmonary hypertension. Histologically it is manifest by widespread intimal proliferation and fibrosis of the intrapulmonary veins and venules, occasionally extending to the arteriolar bed. The pulmonary venous obstruction explains the increased pulmonary capillary wedge pressure observed in patients with advanced disease. These patients may develop orthopnea that can mimic left ventricular failure.

It is difficult to distinguish these three subsets of primary pulmonary hypertension on clinical grounds, as the symptoms are similar and the severity of the pulmonary hypertension is comparable in all three types. A chest radiograph and perfusion lung scan may be helpful, however. Patients with plexogenic pulmonary arteriopathy have normal perfusion lung scans, whereas those with thrombotic pulmonary arteriopathy and venoocclusive disease have an abnormal, patchy distribution of the radionuclide tracer. Patients with venoocclusive disease also have increased bronchovascular markings at the lung bases on chest radiograph.

ETIOLOGY The underlying cause for primary pulmonary hypertension is unknown. The high frequency of antinuclear antibodies suggests that some cases may be immunologically mediated, but specific etiologic agents for any of the three subtypes have not been identified. Insight into possible mechanisms was provided from the experience in Europe in the late 1960s in which the number of patients with unexplained pulmonary hypertension increased with the introduction of aminorex fumarate, an amphetamine-like drug used for appetite suppression. Use by susceptible individuals caused development of chronic pulmonary hypertension, the mechanism possibly pulmonary vasoconstriction from endothelial injury. Histologically, plexogenic pulmonary arteriopathy has been described in such cases. The median survival of patients with pulmonary hypertension from aminorex was almost three times longer than that of patients with primary pulmonary hypertension. While some patients improved when the aminorex was discontinued, others had a progressive downhill course, even though the causative agent had been withdrawn.

Pregnancy and oral contraceptives had been proposed as etiologic factors, but this has not been substantiated by other studies. Their frequent association is more likely related to the prevalence of primary pulmonary hypertension in young women.

PATHOPHYSIOLOGY The underlying hemodynamic derangement in primary pulmonary hypertension is an increased resistance to pulmonary blood flow. Early in the disease there is a marked elevation in pulmonary artery pressure with relatively normal cardiac function. Over time the cardiac output becomes progressively reduced rather than the pulmonary artery pressure becoming progressively increased. Initially the pulmonary arteries may respond to vasodilators, but as the disease progresses, the elevated pulmonary vascular resistance becomes fixed. The pulmonary capillary wedge pressure remains normal until the late stages when it tends to rise in response to impaired diastolic filling of the left ventricle due to the altered configuration of the intraventricular septum. Eventually, as the right ventricle fails, the right atrial and right ventricular end-diastolic pressures rise in an attempt to compensate for the myocardial depression that has developed in response to chronic severe right ventricular pressure overload.

Pulmonary function is usually normal in primary pulmonary hypertension, although a mild restrictive pattern (see Chap. 201) is sometimes seen. Hypoxemia is common and is believed to be due to mismatching between pulmonary ventilation and perfusion, magnified by a low cardiac output. Occasional patients develop a patent foramen ovale which can also contribute to systemic arterial desaturation.

DIAGNOSIS A thorough diagnostic evaluation to look for all potential etiologies should be undertaken (see Fig. 212-1 and Table

FIGURE 212-1 An algorithm for the workup of a patient with unexplained pulmonary hypertension. (*Adapted with permission from S Rich.*)

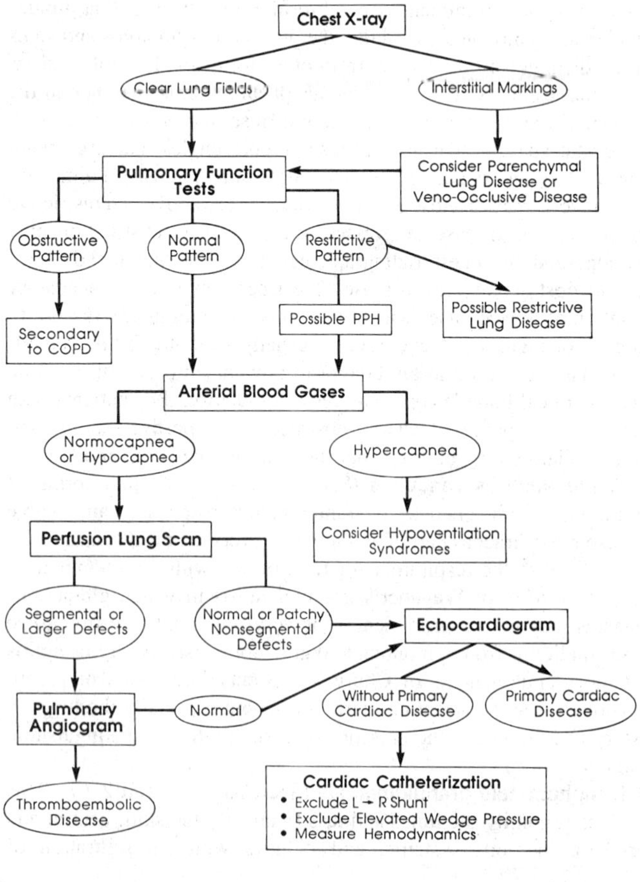

TABLE 212-1 Secondary causes of chronic pulmonary hypertension

Persistent fetal circulation
Congenital heart disease
Valvular heart disease
Primary myocardial disease
Pulmonary thromboembolic disease
Obstructive lung disease
Interstitial lung disease
Arterial hypoxemia with hypercapnea
Collagen vascular disease
Parasitic disease involving the lung
Sickle cell anemia
Intravenous drug abuse
Granulomatous lung disease
Chronic liver disease
Pulmonary artery stenosis
Pulmonary venous hypertension
Aminorex fumarate ingestion

SOURCE: From S Rich, Prog Cardiovasc Dis 31:205, 1988; used with permission.

212-1). The history usually reveals the gradual onset of shortness of breath with effort, progressing until the patient is dyspneic with minimal activity. The average duration from symptom onset until diagnosis is 2.5 years. Other common symptoms are fatigue, angina pectoris which likely represents right ventricular ischemia, syncope, near syncope, and peripheral edema. Approximately 7 percent of the cases are familial with the features of an autosomal dominant defect with variable expression.

The physical examination is characteristic. Increased jugular venous pressure, a reduced carotid pulse, and an easily palpable right ventricular lift are typical. Most patients have an increased pulmonic component of the second heart sound and right-sided third and fourth heart sounds. Tricuspid and pulmonic regurgitation and peripheral cyanosis and edema may be noted. Clubbing is not a feature.

The chest x-ray generally shows enlarged central pulmonary arteries and clear lung fields. The electrocardiogram usually reveals right axis deviation and right ventricular hypertrophy. The echocardiogram demonstrates right ventricular enlargement, a reduction in left ventricular cavity size, and abnormal septal configuration consistent with right ventricular pressure overload. Doppler studies have revealed a marked dependence upon atrial systole for ventricular filling. This would imply that atrial fibrillation could result in inadequate left ventricular filling and might be one cause for sudden death, as no patient with primary pulmonary hypertension and atrial fibrillation has been described. A mild restrictive pattern on pulmonary function tests is consistent with pulmonary hypertension and does not necessarily indicate restrictive lung disease. Hypoxemia, hypocapnia, and an abnormal diffusing capacity for carbon monoxide are almost invariable findings. Evidence of airways obstruction suggests a secondary etiology for the pulmonary hypertension. A perfusion lung scan may be normal or abnormal with multiple diffuse patchy filling defects of a nonsegmental nature and not suggestive of pulmonary thromboembolism. If the lung scan reveals perfusion defects of a segmental or subsegmental nature, a pulmonary angiogram must be done. Severe pulmonary hypertension in a patient with a high-probability lung scan should suggest a chronic process and not acute pulmonary embolism, as the nonconditioned right ventricle is unable to generate high systolic pressures acutely in the face of pulmonary thromboembolism. Chronic thromboembolic obstruction of the large pulmonary arteries can mimic primary pulmonary hypertension (see Chap. 213) but can be amenable to treatment with surgical thromboendarterectomy. Defining the precise location and extent of the clots is imperative for surgical removal.

There is risk in performing pulmonary angiography in patients with primary pulmonary hypertension, particularly in the presence of right ventricular failure with elevated right ventricular end-diastolic pressure. In these patients it is recommended that selective or subselective injections with smaller amounts of contrast be made to minimize the risks, and the use of low-osmolar, nonionic contrast may also diminish risk. One mechanism for cardiac arrest in this setting is hypotension and bradycardia that may be vagally mediated; the pretreatment of selected patients with 1 mg atropine is also advocated.

Cardiac catheterization is mandatory to characterize the disease and exclude an underlying cardiac shunt as the etiology. The use of balloon-flotation catheters, especially those with removable guidewires, can facilitate right heart catheterization, which can be technically difficult. A right-to-left shunt might be attributable to a patent foramen ovale, but any left-to-right shunting implies the presence of a congenital defect. Though it may be difficult to obtain an accurate pulmonary capillary wedge pressure tracing in some patients, the wedge pressure is not falsely elevated. If recordings suggest that the wedge pressure is increased, left heart catheterization should also be performed to exclude mitral stenosis or increased left ventricular end-diastolic pressures as the cause. Although the diagnostic evaluation of these patients can be hazardous, experience from a national multicenter study revealed no mortality or serious morbidity in more than 300 patients whose evaluation included pulmonary angiography and cardiac catheterization. It is not necessary to perform an open lung biopsy in these patients to make an accurate diagnosis. If the diagnostic evaluation is undertaken as outlined, a correct diagnosis will almost always be made.

On occasion a patient may have marked elevations in pulmonary artery pressure and a relatively mild disease that is known to cause pulmonary hypertension. It would be a mistake to characterize these patients as having primary pulmonary hypertension on the belief that the pulmonary hypertension is out of proportion to the underlying associated condition. Since the pulmonary vascular bed has variable vasoreactivity, these cases probably reflect an exaggerated pulmonary vasoconstrictive response to the associated condition. Thus, severe pulmonary hypertension can coexist with mild chronic obstructive pulmonary disease, small intracardiac shunts, mild mitral stenosis, and even ischemic heart disease. The distinction, however, is important since the treatment of pulmonary hypertension should always be focused toward the underlying etiology.

NATURAL HISTORY The natural history of primary pulmonary hypertension is unknown because the initial disease is largely asymptomatic. Several series have reported a mean survival of 2 to 3 years for patients from the time of diagnosis. Occasional patients survive more than 10 years. Functional class is a strong predictor of survival, as patients who are functional class II and III have a mean survival of 3.5 years compared to those who are functional class IV in whom the mean survival is 6 months. The cause of death is usually right ventricular failure or sudden death; sudden death appears to be a late feature of the disease. Increased right atrial pressure above 15 mmHg and reduced cardiac index below 2 $(L/min)/m^2$ are hemodynamic predictors of a poor prognosis.

MANAGEMENT The treatment of primary pulmonary hypertension is unsatisfactory. Because the pulmonary vascular resistance increases dramatically with exercise, patients should be cautioned against participating in activities that demand increased physical stress. The use of digoxin remains controversial, as no studies have documented a benefit or detriment. Diuretic therapy may relieve dyspnea and peripheral edema and may be useful in reducing right ventricular volume overload in the presence of tricuspid regurgitation.

The main focus of therapy is vasodilator drugs. Virtually every class of vasodilator drug has been investigated, including beta-adrenergic agonists, alpha-adrenergic blockers, smooth-muscle vasodilators, nitrates, angiotensin converting enzyme inhibitors, and calcium channel antagonists. Most studies reporting favorable acute effects document a reduction in the pulmonary vascular resistance that is manifest by an increase in cardiac output, without a reduction in the mean pulmonary artery pressure. Although patients may feel better initially from increased oxygen transport to the systemic tissues, this results in increased stroke work of the right ventricle, which can result in worsening of right ventricular function and precipitate right ventricular failure over time. For vasodilators to have sustained beneficial effects, they must lower the pulmonary artery pressure substantially while preserving cardiac output and systemic blood pressure. To date no study has documented that vasodilators prolong life. However, the calcium channel antagonists are effective over the short term in some patients. When given in high doses that are titrated to the hemodynamic response, dramatic reductions in pulmonary artery pressure and pulmonary vascular resistance may be associated with improvement in symptoms and regression of right ventricular hypertrophy. However, less than half of the patients with primary pulmonary hypertension respond to this regimen. It is not known whether the response depends upon the histologic subtype, but the therapy is more successful in patients who are diagnosed early and have less advanced disease.

The administration of vasodilators can have serious acute and chronic adverse effects. Maintenance of adequate systemic blood pressure is crucial since right ventricular coronary blood flow is already compromised due to the loss of the normal systolic gradient for myocardial perfusion between the aorta and right ventricle. Vasodilator drugs can provoke acute right ventricular ischemia, and deaths have been reported. For these reasons the pharmacologic evaluation of primary pulmonary hypertension should always be undertaken with direct monitoring of systemic and pulmonary arterial pressures and cardiac output. Infusions of the pulmonary and systemic vasodilator prostacyclin have been utilized to test pulmonary vasoreactivity of patients with primary pulmonary hypertension. Preliminary studies suggest that the response to prostacyclin may be predictive of the response to oral calcium blockers at higher doses.

Anticoagulant therapy has also been advocated based upon the evidence that thrombosis in situ is common. One retrospective study suggested that anticoagulants increase the survival of patients with primary pulmonary hypertension. Anticoagulants should not be expected to cause regression of the disease, however.

Patients who fail to respond to vasodilator drugs should be considered as possible candidates for heart-lung transplantation (see Chap. 183). The operation is best reserved for patients who are in the advanced stages of the disease in whom it may be predicted that survival is likely to be less than 1 year. A number of patients with primary pulmonary hypertension have undergone heart-lung transplantation, and to date recurrence of the disease has not been reported in a transplanted patient.

REFERENCES

Bjornsson J, Edwards WD: Primary pulmonary hypertension: A histopathologic study of 80 cases. Mayo Clin Proc 60:16, 1985

Fuster V et al: Primary pulmonary hypertension: Natural history and the importance of thrombosis. Circulation 70:580, 1984

Packer M: Vasodilator therapy for primary pulmonary hypertension. Ann Intern Med 103:258, 1985

Reitz BA: Heart-lung transplantation, in *Pulmonary Diseases and Disorders*, 2d ed, AP Fishman (ed). New York, McGraw-Hill, 1987, part 18

Rich S: Primary pulmonary hypertension. Prog Cardiovasc Dis 31:205, 1988

——— et al: High-dose calcium blocking therapy for primary pulmonary hypertension: Evidence for long-term reduction in pulmonary artery pressure and regression of right ventricular hypertrophy. Circulation 76:135, 1987

——— et al: Primary pulmonary hypertension: A national prospective study. Ann Intern Med 107:216, 1987

——— et al: Primary pulmonary hypertension: Radiographic and scintigraphic patterns of histologic subtypes. Ann Intern Med 105:499, 1986

——— et al: Pulmonary hypertension from chronic pulmonary thromboembolism. Ann Intern Med 108:425, 1988

Rubin LJ et al: Prostacyclin-induced pulmonary vasodilation in primary pulmonary hypertension. Circulation 66:334, 1982

213 PULMONARY THROMBOEMBOLISM

KENNETH M. MOSER

Pulmonary thromboembolism (PTE) is a leading cause of morbidity and mortality and can appear in many clinical contexts. Epidemiologic surveys indicate that PTE is responsible for more than 50,000 deaths in the United States annually. Many patients dying of PTE have serious underlying illnesses such as cancer and congestive heart failure. However, available data suggest that less than 10 percent of all pulmonary emboli result in death. Thus, the incidence of fatal plus nonfatal emboli probably exceeds 500,000 annually. This overall incidence seems verified by autopsy statistics. Evidence of recent or old embolism is detected in 25 to 30 percent of routine autopsies; with special techniques, this figure exceeds 60 percent. Even these data underestimate incidence, since many emboli resolve without trace and are not found at postmortem examination. The high incidence of PTE at autopsy contrasts sharply with the incidence of antemortem diagnosis. Available information suggests that an antemortem diagnosis has been made in only 10 to 30 percent of all cases in which old or recent embolism is demonstrated at autopsy.

VENOUS THROMBOSIS

PATHOGENESIS Available data indicate that more than 95 percent of pulmonary emboli arise from thrombi in the deep venous system of the lower extremities. Furthermore, it appears that the larger leg veins (popliteal vein and above) are by far the most common source of those pulmonary emboli which reach clinical attention. Thrombi occurring in the right cardiac chambers or in other veins account for the remainder. In situ pulmonary arterial thrombosis is rare. Thus, embolism should be viewed as a *complication* of deep venous thrombosis (DVT) in the lower extremity veins. Finally, some 90 percent of the deaths due to embolism occur within an hour or two—before a diagnostic-therapeutic plan can be implemented. These facts have several important implications with respect to PTE: (1) prevention of DVT is the most effective approach to prevention of, and death due to, embolism; (2) prompt treatment of DVT may limit the frequency of embolism; (3) techniques which identify the patient at high risk of DVT and allow prompt diagnosis are the key to reduction of embolic risk.

The three factors which promote DVT (and, therefore, embolic risk), as defined by Virchow in the nineteenth century, are stasis, abnormalities of the vessel wall, and alterations in the blood coagulation system. Coagulation alterations have been studied extensively, but as yet there is no reliable test for a state of "hypercoagulability," i.e., a test which will predict the risk of DVT. However, there is a growing list of conditions in which thrombotic risk is increased: deficiencies of antithrombin III, protein C, protein S, and components of the fibrinolytic system; presence of a lupus anticoagulant; and homocystinuria. But such discrete abnormalities are uncommon in the population that develops DVT and are usually discovered after the event. Therefore, the risk of DVT is best assessed by recognizing the presence of known "clinical" risk factors. Conditions associated with a high risk of venous thromboembolism include any surgical procedure requiring 30 min or more of general anesthesia, the postpartum period, left and right ventricular failure, fractures or other injuries of the lower extremities, chronic deep venous insufficiency of the legs, prolonged bed rest, carcinoma, obesity, and the use of estrogens.

NATURAL HISTORY In the contexts noted above, deep venous thrombi usually develop in the region of a venous valve. Platelets aggregate, forming a nidus (white thrombus), followed by development of a large fibrin (red) thrombus. The process is apparently a rapid one; large, extensive thrombi can develop within minutes. Growth occurs by continued fibrin and platelet accretion. Beyond formation, two processes may contribute to resolution: fibrinolysis and organization. Fibrinolysis may result in complete resolution within hours to several days. Any remaining thrombus undergoes organization, leaving behind a fibrotic zone that becomes reendothelialized. Valves are often rendered incompetent by this process, and modest or extensive luminal narrowing may occur. Once thrombus growth has halted, available data indicate that fibrinolysis/organization reaches a stable state in 7 to 10 days. It is during the first few days after formation, therefore, that embolic risk is highest.

DETECTION The clinical diagnosis of DVT is difficult. DVT is frequently present in the absence of clinical signs (e.g., pain, heat, swelling), and it is absent in 50 percent of patients in whom clinical signs or symptoms suggest its presence. Therefore a number of diagnostic tests have been developed. The gold standard is *ascending contrast venography;* but the application of this test is limited by technical and logistic considerations, and repetitive venography is impractical. Among available noninvasive techniques, two have been well-validated against venography: (1) impedance plethysmography (IPG), which detects venous outflow obstruction, is highly sensitive to acute above-knee thrombosis, but fails to detect many below-knee thrombi; and (2) the radiofibrinogen method, which is very sensitive to thrombus formation in calf veins and lower thigh veins, but not sensitive to thrombi which form in the upper thigh or above (also, 24 h is required for a definitive answer). The combination of IPG and radiofibrinogen leg scanning is equal in accuracy to contrast venography. Other available techniques await validation including Doppler ultrasound ("Duplex") studies, which are highly operator-dependent; radiovenography; and the use of other radiolabeled materials (^{111}In-platelets, antifibrin antibodies).

PROPHYLAXIS Application of these noninvasive approaches to the early diagnosis and follow-up of patients at high risk of DVT has led to significant changes in the approach to the prevention of DVT (and therefore of PTE). One validated prophylactic method is the use of small doses of subcutaneous heparin. Multiple studies, utilizing chiefly radiolabeled fibrinogen, have shown the high incidence of DVT in certain groups: patients over the age of 40 years with fractures of the pelvis and/or lower extremities; patients with myocardial infarction and/or severe congestive heart failure; patients undergoing major abdominal, thoracic, or gynecologic surgery. Furthermore, in the last group of patients, investigations have demonstrated a significant reduction in the incidence of DVT, PTE, and lethal PTE when heparin is given subcutaneously, in a dose of 5000 units every 12 h, beginning *before* operation (or on admission to the hospital) and continued until the patient is ambulatory. There is general agreement that this prophylactic approach, which has limited effect on coagulation tests and is associated with little risk of hemorrhage, should also be applied to *medical* patients at high risk of DVT and PTE. In the case of acute myocardial infarction, high risk would be imposed by the development of congestive failure, the presence of severe obesity, chronic venous insufficiency, or a prior history of DVT or PTE. Devices which compress the calf intermittently (usually once a minute) appear an effective alternative for prophylaxis in patients at risk of hemorrhage with low-dose heparin (neurosurgery, spinal cord trauma) or in whom low-dose heparin has proved ineffective (hip surgery, prostate surgery). Warfarin, started at the conclusion of lower extremity surgery, also is effective. Combinations (e.g., heparin plus venous compressive devices) are being explored in patients at particularly high risk. With these multiple options, some prophylaxis is available for almost every patient at risk of DVT.

NATURAL HISTORY OF PULMONARY EMBOLISM

THE ACUTE EVENTS The immediate result of thromboembolism is complete or partial obstruction of the pulmonary arterial blood flow to the distal lung. This obstruction leads to a series of pathophysiologic events which can be categorized as the "respiratory" and "hemodynamic" consequences of PTE.

Respiratory consequences Embolic obstruction produces a zone of the lung which is ventilated but not perfused—an intrapulmonary "dead space" (Chap. 201). Because it cannot participate in the process of gas exchange, ventilation of this nonperfused area is "wasted," in the functional sense. A potential consequence of embolic obstruction is constriction of the air spaces and airways in the affected lung zone. This pneumoconstriction, which might be viewed as a homeostatic mechanism to reduce wasted ventilation, appears to be due to the marked bronchoalveolar hypocapnia that results from cessation of pulmonary capillary blood flow, because it is abolished by inhalation of carbon dioxide–enriched air. While it occurs in animal experiments in which a double-lumen tube separates the ventilation from each lung, it probably occurs very rarely in patients who inhale dead space air (rich in carbon dioxide) into embolized lung zones.

Another disturbance caused by embolic obstruction—loss of alveolar surfactant—does not occur immediately. This surface-active lipoprotein is required to maintain alveolar stability. In its absence, alveolar collapse occurs. Cessation of pulmonary capillary blood flow leads to reduction in surfactant within 2 or 3 h, which becomes severe at 12 to 15 h. Frank atelectasis—the morphologic expression of alveolar instability—can be detected 24 to 48 h after interruption of blood flow.

Arterial hypoxemia is a common, though by no means universal, consequence of embolism. Several mechanisms can contribute to hypoxemia: ventilation-perfusion disturbances; cardiac failure with a lowered mixed venous P_{O_2} (widened arteriovenous difference); and obligatory perfusion through hypoventilated lung zones. Such obligatory perfusion develops because elevation of pulmonary arterial pressure due to embolic obstruction can overcome the vasoconstriction normally present in hypoventilated lung zones.

Hemodynamic consequences The primary hemodynamic consequence of thromboembolic obstruction is a reduction in the cross-sectional area of the pulmonary arterial bed. This loss of vascular capacity increases the resistance to pulmonary blood flow, which, if marked, leads to pulmonary hypertension and acute failure of the right ventricle. Tachycardia and often a decline in cardiac output also occur.

The factors that determine the severity of these hemodynamic changes have been the subject of continued debate. There is agreement that the *extent of embolic obstruction* is a key factor. However, the reserve capacity of the pulmonary arteriocapillary bed is so extensive that more than 50 percent of the vascular area must be obstructed before significant elevation in pulmonary arterial pressure results. Because pulmonary hypertension occurs in some patients with occlusion of lesser extent, investigators have searched for reflex or humoral vasoconstrictor mechanisms associated with embolism. Despite long and careful search for such mechanisms, their extent and frequency in human PTE remains unknown. Hence, some workers maintain that the degree of embolic obstruction itself is the only determinant of hemodynamic impairment. They suggest that instances of apparent disparity between the extent of embolism and clinical response reflect only clinical underestimation of the magnitude of the embolism. Other investigators, however, have presented compelling evidence to support the occurrence of pulmonary vasoconstriction with embolism. Some have demonstrated that constriction is associated with obstruction of the smaller, but not the larger, pulmonary arterial vessels. Another thesis holds that serotonin or thromboxane, known pulmonary vasoconstrictive-bronchoconstrictive substances, are released from platelets, which coat fresh emboli as they lodge in the pulmonary tree. This thesis introduces the attractive concept that an embolus might be regarded, in part, as a packet with pharmacologic, as well as obstructive, potential. A consensus view is that, while the extent of embolism is a key factor, humoral and/or reflex influences probably operate in certain patients and compromise the pulmonary circulation to a greater extent than might be expected on an anatomic basis alone.

The cardiopulmonary status of the patient prior to embolism is also critical in determining the clinical severity of embolism. A small embolus may have limited impact upon an otherwise healthy individual but may have serious consequences in someone with advanced cardiac or pulmonary disease.

Both experimental and clinical studies have established that infarction—death of lung tissue—rarely accompanies embolic occlusion. It is likely that less than 10 percent of emboli in humans lead to infarction. That infarction rarely follows embolism should occasion little surprise. The lung has three avenues for obtaining oxygen: the pulmonary arterial circulation, the bronchial arterial circulation, and the airways. Thus, infarction occurs infrequently, and its appearance usually is associated with compromise of bronchial arterial flow and/or airways to the involved area. Such compromise is promoted by the existence of other cardiac or pulmonary diseases, such as left ventricular failure, mitral stenosis, and chronic obstructive lung disease. Thus, infarction may occur in 30 percent or more of such patients, while it is quite rare in individuals who are free of cardiopulmonary disease.

BEYOND THE ACUTE STATE The vast majority of pulmonary emboli resolve, and resolve rather quickly. Resolution of fresh emboli begins within the first few days and is well advanced in 10 to 14 days. As in DVT, two mechanisms promote restoration of vascular patency: the fibrinolytic system and the process of organization. However, the fibrinolytic system appears capable of more rapid dissolution of emboli than of venous thrombi.

The availability of these two efficient mechanisms raises the question as to why not all emboli resolve. There may be some impairment of the intrinsic fibrinolytic system. The emboli may have been well organized prior to their lodgment in the lung so that they are subject to neither fibrinolytic attack nor further organization. Alternatively, some emboli may be recurrent, so that their failure to resolve is more apparent than real.

Another important element of the natural history of thromboembolism is the development of bronchial arterial collateral circulation. If pulmonary arterial obstruction persists, bronchial arterial flow increases substantially over a period of several weeks, restoring flow to the capillary bed. With the return of flow, surfactant production is restored, so that alveolar stability is regained and atelectasis resolves.

DIAGNOSTIC FEATURES

While sequential studies of patients with venous thrombosis have demonstrated that embolism, often of substantial magnitude, can occur without causing symptoms, *sudden onset of unexplained dyspnea* is the most common, and often the only symptom of pulmonary embolism. *Pleuritic chest pain and hemoptysis are present only when infarction has occurred* and, because bland embolism rarely leads to infarction, are usually absent. With extensive embolism, severe substernal oppressive discomfort may be present, probably due to right ventricular ischemia. Patients also may present with syncope, suggesting a neurologic disorder. Other "occult" presentations in which embolism should be considered include repetitive bouts of otherwise unexplained supraventricular tachyarrhythmias; sudden onset or worsening of congestive heart failure (Chap. 182); sudden deterioration in the patient with chronic obstructive lung disease; and as an alternative to the diagnosis of "psychic" (anxiety-associated) hyperventilation. The most reliable symptom, however, is breathlessness. Severe, persistent dyspnea is an ominous sign, for it usually indicates extensive embolic occlusion.

PHYSICAL EXAMINATION Findings on physical examination, like the history, may be deceptively normal. Examination of the lungs may disclose a few atelectatic rales; localized wheezes rarely are heard. A pleural friction rub or evidence of pleural effusion will not be present unless infarction has occurred.

On cardiac examination, the single consistent finding is tachycardia. Only in the rare cases of massive embolism will signs such as a right ventricular gallop, a palpable "lift" over the right ventricle (along the left sternal border), a loud pulmonary closure sound, or prominent *a* waves in the jugular venous pulse be found. A scratchy systolic ejection-type murmur may be heard in the pulmonic area. Also, a systolic or continuous murmur accentuated by inspiration may be audible over the lung fields. These murmurs appear to be generated by turbulence of flow in vessels partially obstructed by emboli since they disappear after resection or resolution of emboli. They should be carefully sought in any patient suspected of having PTE. Wide splitting of the second heart sound may be present. This indicates extensive embolic obstruction and implies both severe pulmonary hypertension and right ventricular failure. As embolic resolution occurs, this finding disappears. Absence of an accentuated pulmonic closure sound is not a reliable guide to the severity of PTE, since when embolism is sufficiently massive to reduce cardiac output, pulmonary arterial pressure falls, and the pulmonary closure sound may be normal or diminished.

The detection of *deep venous thrombosis* qualifies as an excellent clue to the diagnosis of embolism, but its absence does not exclude embolism, because the entire venous thrombus may embolize. Even when sought with diligence, *clinical* evidence of thrombophlebitis is found in less than half of patients with PTE. *Fever* in patients with pulmonary embolism is uncommon without complicating infection or infarction. With infarction, fever of 37.5 to 38.5°C (oral) is the rule; but temperature elevations to 39°C or above may occur, making the differentiation between pulmonary infarction and infection difficult.

On clinical grounds alone, then, a firm diagnosis of embolism cannot be made; the clinical *suspicion* of embolism requires confirmation by laboratory studies (Fig. 213-1).

LABORATORY STUDIES Routine laboratory studies contribute little toward the diagnosis. Leukocytosis and elevation of the sedimentation rate are rarely present in the absence of infarction. A variety of other blood tests, such as assay for specific fibrinopeptides, fibrin degradation products, or enzymes, have been proposed; none has been shown to be diagnostically sensitive or specific.

Aside from tachycardia, the *electrocardiogram* is normal in most patients. With extensive embolization, there may be evidence of acute pulmonary hypertension (rightward shift of the QRS axis, a tall, peaked P wave), and ST-T changes indicative of right ventricular strain (Chap. 176). These changes are often transient, lasting minutes to hours, but when persistent, suggest severe pulmonary vascular obstruction.

The *chest roentgenogram* may show a parenchymal infiltrate and evidence of a pleural effusion if *infarction* has occurred. Characteristically, the infiltrates caused by infarction abut against the pleura. However, their shape varies, and they do not usually appear until 12 to 36 h after the embolism has occurred. The effusion, which often precedes the infiltrate, is characteristically small. Thoracentesis usually, but by no means invariably, yields hemorrhagic fluid, with the characteristics of an exudate.

The radiographic findings with embolism alone are more subtle. Elevation of the hemidiaphragm may occur. *Differences in diameter between vessels that should be of equivalent size* should raise the suspicion of embolism. For example, embolic obstruction of the right main pulmonary artery can lead to dilation of the left main pulmonary artery because that vessel must accept the entire pulmonary flow. There may be *abrupt "cutoff"* of a vessel; i.e., as the vessel is traced distally, it suddenly disappears. Clot has the same radiodensity as blood, accounting for the proximal shadow; the absence of flow beyond the clot explains the sudden radiographic "disappearance" of the vessel.

Organization of a clot within a pulmonary artery may lead to retraction of the vessel's walls and a so-called rattail configuration, in which the vessel is relatively normal proximally and suddenly tapers to a sharp point. Finally, there may be *abnormal radiolucency* in some lung zones due to absent or decreased flow. Such abnormally

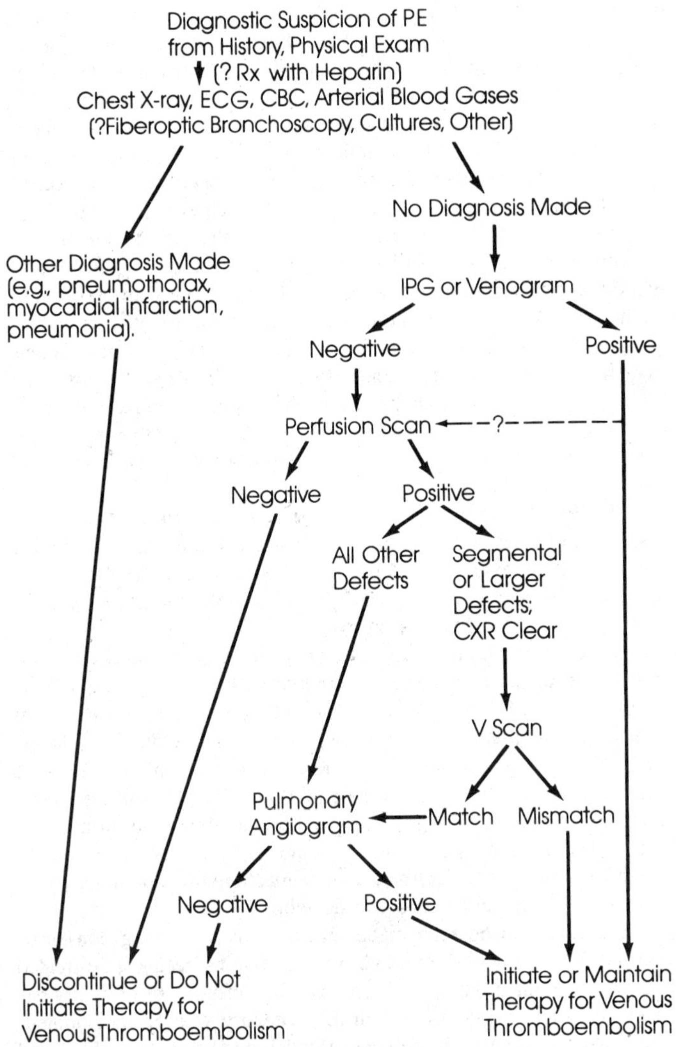

FIGURE 213-1 Flow chart used in diagnosis of pulmonary embolism (PE). IPG, impedance plethysmogram; V scan, ventilation scan.

lucent areas, indicative of proximal arterial obstruction, are best appreciated by examining comparable areas in the two lung fields.

Even in embolization without infarction, the roentgenogram may show small infiltrates, which appear in about 24 h and reflect atelectasis secondary to surfactant depletion. They are not associated with effusion, may fail to touch a pleural surface, and disappear without the linear scarring characteristic of infarction. It should be emphasized that a *normal chest roentgenogram does not exclude the diagnosis of PTE*. Indeed, a *normal* chest roentgenogram is the *most common* finding in embolic disease.

Analysis of arterial blood gases Massive embolism is commonly associated with arterial hypoxemia, hypocapnia, and respiratory alkalosis. In addition, the difference between alveolar P_{CO_2} and arterial P_{CO_2} ($PA_{CO_2} - Pa_{CO_2}$) may be widened owing to the increase in alveolar dead space (Chap. 201). However, a normal P_{O_2} does not exclude the diagnosis.

The laboratory tests discussed thus far are often negative in PTE and are relatively nonspecific. Therefore, it is usually necessary to proceed to two more definitive techniques: pulmonary perfusion and ventilation radiophotoscans and the pulmonary angiogram.

Pulmonary perfusion and ventilation scintiphotography Perfusion scintiphotographs (photoscans) are obtained by gamma camera imaging of the distribution of intravenously injected, gamma-emitting radionuclides. The most commonly used radionuclides are microspheres or macroaggregates of albumin (MAA), labeled with a gamma-emitting isotope such as technetium 99m. The radioactive particles, 50 to 100 μm in diameter, are trapped in the pulmonary capillary bed because the pulmonary capillaries approximate 10 μm in diameter. Alternatively, xenon 133 gas, dissolved in saline solution, may be used, but patients must hold their breath. The distribution of labeled particles entrapped in capillaries, or of xenon 133 evolved from them, accurately depicts the distribution of pulmonary blood flow.

The camera-generated perfusion image can be recorded on radiographic film, on special photographic film, on a television screen, or on videotape. Normal scans exhibit homogeneous distribution of radioactivity, smooth margins, and a configuration which corresponds to the normal anatomy of the lungs. Any deviation from these characteristics requires explanation because it represents an abnormality in blood flow distribution.

The perfusion lung photoscan is quite valuable in the diagnosis of embolism. A properly performed perfusion scan which is *normal* excludes the diagnosis of clinically significant pulmonary embolism, as indicated by reports of the excellent outcomes of persons suspected of embolism, who had normal scans and who were not treated. On the other hand, a scan demonstrating zones of absent or sharply decreased radioactivity in the patient whose other findings are compatible with PTE keeps the diagnosis of embolism among the possibilities. Scanning is simple, safe, and rapid. It can be repeated to define the resolution, or recurrence, of obstructive vascular phenomena. Like any laboratory test, however, the photoscan must be applied and interpreted with care. It is important, for example, to obtain multiple scan views because lesions not apparent in one view may be easily detected in others. Furthermore, the lung photoscan demonstrates only abnormalities of the *distribution of blood flow*. It does not provide anatomic information. Many disorders other than PTE are associated with abnormalities in the distribution of pulmonary blood flow. Any disease process, such as pneumonia, atelectasis, or pneumothorax, which reduces the ventilation of a lung zone will decrease its perfusion. Parenchymal diseases, such as emphysema, sarcoidosis, bronchogenic carcinoma, and tuberculosis, can all produce scan defects. Therefore a perfusion defect lacks specificity. One approach to enhancing specificity is the performance of a ventilation scan, best achieved by having patients breathe a radioactive gas such as xenon 127 or xenon 133. To assist in deciding whether a ventilation scan may be useful and when pulmonary angiography is required, two factors should be considered: the size of the perfusion defect(s) and the chest roentgenographic findings. If all defects are subsegmental in size *or* if all defects (of any size) are limited to areas of roentgenographic infiltration, ventilation scanning will not be useful, and pulmonary angiography is required, if a definitive diagnosis is necessary. If defect(s) are segmental or larger in size, and one or more are in areas clear by x-ray, a ventilation scan should be done. If the radioactive gas enters (''washes in'') and is cleared (''washes out'') from the area(s) of perfusion defect(s), this ''mismatch'' of ventilation and perfusion is characteristic of vascular obstruction (Fig. 213-2). Pulmonary vascular obstruction is present in 90 percent or

FIGURE 213-2 Perfusion scan (left), posterior view, shows multiple segmental and larger perfusion defects in right upper and lower lobes, left lower lobe, and lingula. Ventilation scan (right) is normal at equilibrium. Xenon 133 washed in and out normally. Multiple emboli were confirmed angiographically.

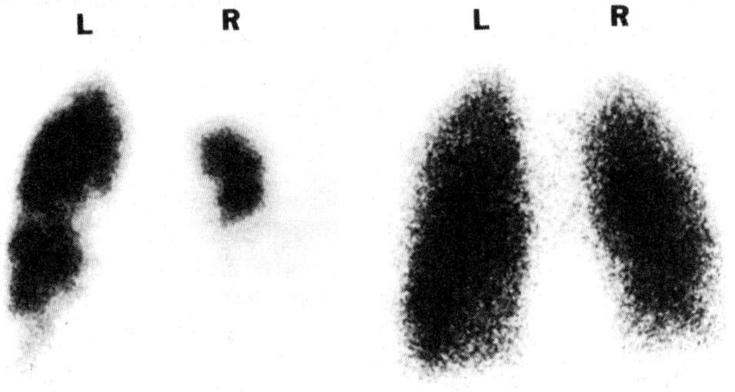

more of patients with this pattern. However, if ventilation is also abnormal (i.e., ventilation-perfusion "match" is present), no reliable diagnostic conclusion can be reached; pulmonary angiography is required. (It may not be required if DVT is present and already mandates therapy.) In some centers, ^{99m}Tc-DTPA particles are used for ventilation studies; this approach provides multiple views but does not allow "wash-out" evaluation.

Pulmonary angiography This is the only established means for providing anatomic information about the pulmonary vasculature. Radiopaque material is injected, preferably through a cardiac catheter advanced into the pulmonary artery. Cardiac catheterization and angiography require specialized personnel, and a reasonable period for preparation and performance, and they entail more risk than the procedures discussed above. However, angiography provides a visual image of the pulmonary vessels, and catheterization can provide potentially important hemodynamic data (pulmonary artery and wedge pressures, cardiac output). Interpretive limitations of angiography are of three types: (1) *Injection artifacts* may occur which suggest absence of flow to a vessel. Injection should be repeated whenever the question of such artifacts exists. (2) The inability to evaluate the patency of small vessels is another limitation. Emboli in vessels below the resolving capability of the method cannot be detected with certainty, although magnification techniques can extend resolving capability. (3) Interpretive errors may also be a consequence of *not looking for the proper type of defect*. There are only two findings diagnostic of acute embolism. One is the *abrupt "cutoff"* of a vessel at the point of embolic impaction. However, complete embolic obstruction is uncommon. Therefore, *filling defects* are the most frequent finding; i.e., the embolus creates a "negative" shadow as the radiopaque material flows around it. The major contraindication to angiography is the absence of personnel who are experienced in both performing the procedure and interpreting the results. Serious diagnostic errors are commonplace if optimal techniques are not used or the complexities of interpretation are not appreciated. However, the risks of angiography are low in experienced hands. Injection of large boluses of contrast medium into the main pulmonary artery should be avoided in favor of small injections into vessels supplying lung regions identified as abnormal on the perfusion scan.

How far one should proceed down the diagnostic pathway outlined above depends on many factors, the major ones being the presence or absence of documented venous thrombosis, the severity of the patient's symptoms, and the hazards of contemplated therapy. In each condition, there is a need for precise diagnosis. If IPG or venography already has documented deep venous thrombosis of the popliteal vein or above, one is committed to anticoagulant therapy; thus, proceeding beyond perfusion scanning is rarely necessary. This means that evaluation for venous thrombosis is an essential part of the evaluation of the embolic suspect. Unfortunately, the absence of venous thrombosis cannot be used to exclude the diagnosis of pulmonary embolism. More than 20 percent of patients with embolism have no evidence of venous thrombosis, apparently because the entire venous thrombus has embolized. Therefore, in such patients, if symptoms are severe and/or the hazards of therapy are substantial, diagnostic precision is mandatory, and there should be no hesitancy in proceeding to angiography. Substantial hazards of therapy which mandate angiography include a high risk of bleeding on, or absolute contraindication to, anticoagulant therapy and consideration of embolectomy, thrombolytic therapy, or vena caval interruption.

TREATMENT

Initial intravenous administration of heparin is the therapy of choice for PTE. With a strong *suspicion* of embolism based on clinical and routine laboratory tests, such therapy should be instituted immediately, without awaiting diagnostic confirmation, unless the initial dose of heparin places the patient at clear risk (i.e., in patients with recent or active bleeding or a known hemostatic defect). Except in such patients, heparin therapy should not await diagnostic confirmation; one can always stop therapy if such confirmation is not forthcoming.

There is consensus regarding the goals of therapy in both DVT and PTE: (1) immediate inhibition of the growth of thromboemboli, (2) promotion of thromboembolic resolution, and (3) prevention of recurrence. Heparin achieves the first goal; it encourages the second by allowing fibrinolytic dissolution to be achieved unopposed by thrombus growth; and it assists in, although it does not ensure, prevention of recurrence. In addition, heparin inhibits platelet aggregation (and therefore potential release of thromboxane and serotonin) at the embolic site, and its anticoagulant action is promptly reversible.

There is *not* consensus, however, regarding (1) heparin regimens which best combine safety and efficacy; (2) the need for, and type of, tests for monitoring coagulation behavior during heparin therapy; (3) how long, and with what agents, antithrombotic therapy should be maintained; or (4) in which patients thrombolytic therapy should antedate antithrombotic therapy.

REGIMENS In DVT, three methods of heparin administration have been advocated by various investigators: continuous intravenous, intermittent intravenous, intermittent subcutaneous. Continuous intravenous heparin is usually given in a dose of approximately 1000 units per hour. Intermittent intravenous heparin is commonly given in a dose of approximately 5000 units every 4 h or 7500 every 6 h. Subcutaneous heparin has been recommended at a dose of 5000 units every 4 h, 10,000 every 8 h, or 20,000 every 12 h. Studies exist which indicate that each of these regimens is more efficacious, safer, or both. Therefore, at this time, one can conclude only that *each* of these regimens (which approximate 30,000 units per 24 h) represents an acceptable treatment regimen. However, the continuous intravenous regimen, delivered by an infusion pump, is by far the most popular in the United States. *Intramuscular* injection of heparin is to be avoided because hematomas will develop.

It should also be recognized that there is a growing consensus that DVT that remains confined to the calf veins need *not* be treated with anticoagulant therapy. No increase in morbidity or mortality has been reported among patients in this category who are not treated. However, since 15 to 20 percent of calf-limited thrombi will extend to the popliteal veins and above during a 10- to 12-day period, such patients *must* be followed by serial IPG tests until this period has elapsed. If they cannot be followed in this manner, they should be treated.

In PTE, the same options for heparin therapy exist. The only additional question is whether an initial large intravenous bolus (10,000 to 20,000 units) should be given to inhibit the aggregation (and release reaction) of platelets adherent to the embolus. Most workers advocate such a dose, with one of the "standard" regimens being started 2 to 4 h later.

MONITORING The value of clotting times (CT), partial thromboplastin times (PTT), or other coagulation tests to monitor the safety and efficacy of heparin remains a complex issue. With regard to safety, the risk of hemorrhage (the principal complication of heparin therapy) is not clearly related to coagulation test alterations; rather, it appears related to factors such as the coexistence of other diseases associated with bleeding risk (gastric or duodenal ulcer, coagulopathies, uremia) and advanced age. Likewise, achievement of the desired effect of heparin (cessation of thrombus growth in vivo) has not been related consistently to coagulation tests. Therefore, it is questionable whether monitoring with such tests is superior to empiric use of one of the regimens described above. While animal investigations have disclosed that maintaining the PTT above 1.5 times control does prevent growth of venous thrombi, limited data are not available documenting this in human patients. If done improperly or poorly timed, the CT or PTT tests are worthless and may be misleading. Furthermore, even with continuous intravenous therapy, the CT and PTT may vary substantially during a 24-h period. Despite these vagaries, a majority of experts currently recommend attempting to keep the CT or PTT, measured *just prior to the next* intermittent dose, at or above 1.5 times the baseline CT or PTT and at 1.5 to 2.0 times control with continuous infusion.

DURATION OF THERAPY In DVT, full anticoagulant protection is usually maintained for 7 to 10 days, the rationale being that this is the period required for dissolution and/or organization of the thrombus. In PTE, for the same reasons, a similar duration of therapy is advised. Bed rest is indicated until cardiopulmonary or leg symptoms subside. Carefully applied elastic support hose should be used (to encourage venous flow) as soon as leg pain, if present, subsides and the patient is ambulated.

During and beyond the acute phase there are several options for achieving proper anticoagulant protection. In deciding among these options, it should be recognized that the major question being addressed is: Does the patient need continued protection against the risk of *recurrent* DVT (and, therefore, PTE)? If the risk factor(s) that precipitated the acute episode of DVT-PTE is no longer present, the patient is asymptomatic, and the IPG is normal, it is acceptable to reduce heparin to a lower dose starting on day 7, ambulate the patient, and, if no symptoms develop, discontinue heparin on day 9 or 10. If these criteria are not met, as is the case in most patients, prolonged prophylactic therapy is warranted. Two options exist for such prophylaxis. The most common one is to initiate a prothrombinopenic agent (e.g., warfarin) as soon as the decision for long-term protection is made. Often, this can be done on day 2 or 3 of heparin therapy. Prothrombinopenic drugs are not suitable for initial therapy in thromboembolism, as their onset of action is too slow. Their only role is in maintaining anticoagulant protection for prolonged periods. If they are initiated early in the acute treatment course, the patient must be "in range," as defined by a prothrombin time of 1.5 to 1.8 times the control time for 3 to 5 days *before heparin is discontinued.* A second option for long-term protection is the use of self-injected subcutaneous heparin. Current data suggest that a dose of 7500 to 10,000 units every 12 h is adequate, is well-tolerated, and need not be monitored with coagulation tests.

There is no consensus regarding the period for which anticoagulant protection should be maintained beyond hospital discharge because firm data on this point are lacking. If *reversible* risk factors are present (e.g., immobilization after a leg fracture), therapy should be continued until the risk factors present have resolved. If the risk factors present are nonreversible (e.g., severe left and/or right ventricular failure), if the IPG remains positive, or if major lung scan defects persist at discharge, empiric decisions are made. At a minimum, 3 months of therapy seems wise, because recurrence is relatively common during this period. Beyond 3 months, however, continuation depends upon the balance among specific risk factors exhibited by the patient, IPG results, lung scan results, and the risks of continued therapy. In some instances, this balance may warrant lifetime maintenance on anticoagulant drugs.

Thrombolytic therapy The place of *thrombolytic (fibrinolytic)* agents (Chap. 189) in the management of acute venous thromboembolism remains to be defined. There is no question that available agents (streptokinase, urokinase), as well as the second-generation (tissue plasminogen activator, tPA) and potential third-generation agents, can hasten the resolution of venous thrombi and pulmonary emboli. They do not replace antithrombotic therapy. When used, thrombolytic agents must be followed by a standard course of antithrombotic therapy. Despite extensive study, it has not been established that such agents alter short-term or long-term morbidity, mortality, or recurrence rates among patients with DVT or PTE. These drugs, despite high fibrin specificity in the case of tPA, are associated with hemorrhagic risk in patients who have had, or require, any invasive procedure (e.g., vein puncture, arterial puncture, angiography, Swan-Ganz catheterization); and in patients with localized vascular lesions due to recent operation, trauma, or concomitant disease (e.g., peptic ulcer, stroke). If thrombolytic agents prove to have a therapeutic advantage, it would appear to be (1) in patients with extensive, large-vein DVT (e.g., iliofemoral); and (2) in patients with massive embolism and persistent systemic hypotension in whom embolectomy would otherwise be contemplated.

Surgical therapy for DVT (thrombectomy) is now rarely considered because the results have not been encouraging. In PTE, surgical therapy should be reserved for those patients in whom heparin therapy is deemed inadequate or impractical. Anticoagulant therapy may be contraindicated by the presence of a bleeding diathesis, or the patient may be in such critical condition that it is felt unwise to await a response to medical therapy. In such instances *venous interruption* and *pulmonary embolectomy* must be considered.

The objective of venous interruption is to prevent immediate recurrence of embolism from lower extremity venous thrombi. While multiple ligation and clipping procedures have been used in the past, these have been largely supplanted by the use of filters placed in the inferior vena cava by a transvenous approach (jugular, femoral veins). Ligation of the inferior vena cava requires surgery, obstructs venous return acutely, and encourages collateral vein formation which bypasses the ligation. Clips require surgery for placement, may obstruct caval flow, and may thrombose. The filters, typified by the Greenfield filter, which has been the most widely used in recent years, are inserted transvenously, do not obstruct caval flow, protect against emboli greater than 2 mm in diameter, and are rarely subject to thrombosis.

There are two major indications for placement of a caval filter: (1) as a lifesaving procedure in patients with massive embolism who could not tolerate an embolic recurrence; and (2) to prevent embolism in patients with documented venous thrombosis in whom anticoagulant therapy is contraindicated.

There is one instance, however, in which prompt caval ligation is the therapy of choice: septic thrombophlebitis of pelvic origin with multiple septic pulmonary emboli. If these patients do not respond promptly to a heparin-antibiotic regimen, they may die unless caval (and left ovarian vein) ligation is carried out promptly.

Two criteria should be met before emergency pulmonary embolectomy is performed: (1) there must be evidence of severe hemodynamic compromise due to embolism, particularly sustained systemic hypotension, which is not responsive to supportive measures; and (2) the personnel and equipment required for embolectomy carried out with the aid of cardiopulmonary bypass must be available. Even with these criteria satisfied, it now appears likely that management of such patients by alternative approaches (placement of a caval filter plus heparin therapy; thrombolytic therapy) will be associated with lower mortality rates than is emergency embolectomy.

SPECIAL CONSIDERATIONS Total resolution of emboli does not always occur. Why some patients (perhaps 0.1 percent) fail to resolve their emboli is not yet known. However, if residual vascular obstruction is substantial, the patient may present, months or years after the actual embolic events, with dyspnea and pulmonary hypertension of uncertain cause, often with right ventricular failure. Such patients commonly are misdiagnosed, for months or years, as having "asthma," "chronic lung disease," "primary" pulmonary hypertension (Chap. 212), or cor pulmonale of unclear etiology (Chap. 191).

Such patients should be studied by appropriate techniques, since emboli in the main or lobar arteries can be surgically removed (thromboendarterectomy), allowing cure of this otherwise fatal form of pulmonary hypertensive disease. This entity, once an autopsy curiosity, is more common than previously appreciated: some 200 patients have been reported to have undergone thromboendarterectomy. Because surgical mortality is heavily conditioned by the severity of right ventricular dysfunction at the time of operation, early recognition is important.

PROGNOSIS IN PULMONARY EMBOLISM The prognosis of the patient with pulmonary embolism *in whom therapy is promptly instituted* is excellent. As stated at the outset of this chapter, less than 1 embolic event in 10 is lethal. The majority of these deaths occur suddenly and can be avoided only by prophylaxis (see above). The remainder appear to be due to embolic extension or recurrence, which therapy can moderate. Thus, for patients who survive long enough to reach medical attention and receive heparin, the outlook is quite good. Morbidity following embolism is uncommon since embolic resolution is the rule, and few patients develop the pulmonary hypertensive problem noted above.

Limited reliable data are available regarding recurrence rates in the months and years after a single embolic event (with or without prolonged postembolic anticoagulant therapy). In the absence of risk factors, or a positive IPG, recurrence appears to be uncommon, but more precise data are needed.

Whether the therapeutic approaches discussed here will be altered by new agents, such as low-molecular-weight heparin and newer thrombolytic agents, remains to be seen.

NONTHROMBOTIC EMBOLISM

Because the lung vasculature serves as a filter of the venous circulation, it is the recipient of diverse materials which can gain entry into venous blood, including bone marrow, foreign bodies, parasites, and tumor cells. The most frequently encountered form of nonthrombotic embolism is *fat embolism*. This dramatic and controversial entity follows the introduction of neutral fat into the venous circulation, most commonly after bone trauma or fracture (marrow fat), but occasionally after trauma to adipose tissue or liver infiltrated by fat. The clinical sequence is characteristic. After a latent period of 12 to 36 h or more, during which the patient is asymptomatic, sudden cardiopulmonary and neurologic deterioration appears. Mental aberrations, delirium, and coma develop. Dyspnea, tachypnea, and tachycardia occur, and the chest roentgenographic and physiologic components of the "adult respiratory distress syndrome" appear (see Chap. 218). Anemia and thrombocytopenia are common, as are petechiae on the upper thorax and arms. The pathogenesis of the syndrome is not clear, but it seems likely that two events occur: release of free fatty acids (by action of lipases on the neutral fat), which induces a toxic vasculitis, followed by platelet-fibrin thrombosis; and actual obstruction of small pulmonary arteries by macroaggregates of fat. Several forms of therapy have been proposed (corticosteroids, heparin, ethanol), but none has proved effective; treatment remains supportive and mortality rate high.

Another dramatic form of nonthrombotic embolism is *amniotic fluid embolism*. This occurs during both spontaneous delivery and cesarean section. Sudden and massive obstruction of the pulmonary microvasculature occurs, leading to shock and, often, death. With survival of the initial phase of the disease, the picture of disseminated intravascular coagulation appears. The syndrome is due to the entrance of a significant quantity of amniotic fluid into the venous circulation. This fluid is a potent thromboplastic agent which induces thrombosis in the pulmonary vasculature and elsewhere. The fluid also contains particulates which lodge in the lung. Treatment consists of supportive measures.

Nonembolic pulmonary arterial obstruction due to *vasculitis* has become a common problem among intravenous drug users. This vasculitis, caused by the drugs per se or materials (e.g., talc) mixed with the drugs, can induce thrombosis. This entity may be difficult to distinguish from PTE. Repetitive episodes may lead to irreversible and severe pulmonary hypertension.

REFERENCES

FEDULLO PF et al: ^{111}-Indium labelled platelets: Effect of heparin on uptake by venous thrombi and relationship to the activated partial thromboplastin time. Circulation 66:632, 1982

FISHMAN AP, KELLEY MA: Pulmonary thromboembolism (including prophylaxis, treatment, sickle cell disease and multiple pulmonary thrombi), in *Pulmonary Diseases and Disorders*, 2d ed, AP Fishman (ed). New York, McGraw-Hill, 1987, chap 66.

GOLDHABER SZ (ed): *Pulmonary Embolism and Deep Venous Thrombosis*. Philadelphia, Saunders, 1985

HUISMAN MV et al: Serial impedance plethysmography for suspected deep venous thrombosis in outpatients. N Engl J Med 314:823, 1986

HULL R et al: Pulmonary angiography, ventilation lung scanning and venography for clinically suspected pulmonary embolism in the abnormal perfusion scan. Ann Intern Med 98:891, 1983

——— et al: Adjusted subcutaneous heparin versus warfarin sodium in the long-term treatment of venous thrombosis. N Engl J Med 305:189, 1982

——— et al: Combined use of leg scanning and impedance plethysmography in suspected venous thrombosis. N Engl J Med 296:1497, 1977

KAKKAR VV et al: Prevention of post-operative embolism by low-dose heparin: An international multicenter trial. Lancet 2:45, 1975

KIPPER MS et al: Long-term follow-up of patients with suspected pulmonary embolism and a normal lung scan. Chest 82:411, 1982

MERCANDETTI A et al: Influence of perfusion and ventilation scans on therapeutic decision-making and outcome among embolic suspects. West J Med 142:208, 1985

MOSER KM et al: Thromboendarterectomy for chronic, major vessel thromboembolic pulmonary hypertension: Immediate and long-term results in 42 patients. Ann Intern Med 107:560, 1987

———, FEDULLO PF: Venous thromboembolism: Three simple decisions. Chest 83:117, 256, 1983

NIH Consensus Conference: Prevention of venous thrombosis and pulmonary embolism. JAMA 256:744, 1986

PHILBRICK JT, BECKER DM: Calf deep venous thrombosis: A wolf in sheep's clothing? Arch Intern Med 148:2131, 1988

SALZMAN EW et al: Intraoperative external pneumatic calf compression to afford long-term prophylaxis against deep vein thrombosis in urologic patients. Surgery 87:239, 1980

SASAHARA AA, DALEN JE: Controversy: Should fibrinolytic drugs be used to treat acute pulmonary embolism? J Cardiovasc Med 5:793, 1980

WESSLER S et al: *Dimensions of Warfarin Prophylaxis*. New York, Plenum, 1987

214 DISEASES OF THE UPPER RESPIRATORY TRACT

ROBERT LEBOVICS

The upper respiratory tract includes the nose and mouth, the paranasal sinuses, the ears and mastoids, the pharynx, and larynx. Its functions include the exchange and filtering of air, the intake of food and liquids and their separation from the air stream entering the tracheobronchial tree, the expression of speech, and the senses of taste, smell, and hearing. Respiratory ciliated epithelium lines those portions involved in air exchange and filtration; squamous cells line the oral cavity, tongue, and oropharynx. A complex neural network and collection of lymphoid tissues are involved in the operation of the senses and local immunity, respectively. This chapter will consider disorders involving specific regions of the upper respiratory tract. Disorders of taste, smell, and hearing and vestibular function are covered elsewhere (see Chaps. 24 and 26).

NOSE

EXTERNAL NASAL DISORDERS The nose is subject to the same skin diseases as those affecting the face. *Furunculosis* is common around the nasal vestibule in the region of the hair follicles. *Staphylococcus aureus* is the usual organism. Infection in that site can be dangerous because of the potential for spread to the cavernous sinus via draining veins. Treatment should be prompt and consists of local heat and antibiotics with antistaphylococcal activity (see Chap. 100). If there is marked local edema, fever, and signs of generalized sepsis, hospitalization and parenteral antibiotic therapy are necessary, with close evaluation for sinus or intracranial involvement. Incision and drainage of large lesions are usually required. Impetigo and erysipelas caused by group A *Streptococcus* can affect the outer nose; their recognition and management are discussed in Chap. 101.

Rhinophyma is a disease caused by chronic inflammation and hypertrophy of the skin, producing bulbous violaceous nasal tips, commonly in alcoholic men. Pathologically, sebaceous gland hypertrophy occurs with scarring and acanthosis. Treatment, when warranted, is surgical.

EPISTAXIS The nose receives major arterial vessels from both the internal and external carotid artery systems. Most nosebleeds come from Kiesselbach's plexus on the nasal septum. Disorders that produce a generalized bleeding diathesis such as the acute leukemias, thrombocytopenia, aplastic anemia or severe liver disease have general evidence of bruising, petechiae, or bleeding, but rarely can present as isolated epistaxis. Similarly, anticoagulant and antiplatelet drugs usually cause a more generalized bleeding diathesis, but epistaxis may be prominent. While hypertension does not cause epistaxis directly, it can perpetuate a nosebleed; prompt control of blood pressure is an essential part of treatment. A history of delayed nosebleeds after trauma often indicates bleeding from the anterior and posterior ethmoidal artery systems. Foreign body reactions, substance abuse (e.g., cocaine), and local infection may cause nosebleeds. Rare causes of repeated bouts of epistaxis include Osler-Weber-Rendu syndrome or von Willebrand's disease. A positive family history of epistaxis or gastrointestinal bleeding may suggest the diagnosis.

Treatment In many cases pressure or a small amount of packing will suffice to stop an anterior bleed. Additional medical management of acute but not life-threatening nosebleeds includes gentle suctioning of blood clots from the nose, locating the bleeding site, and electric or chemical cautery after anesthetizing the nose topically. Topical vasoconstrictors such as phenylephrine or oxymetazoline hydrochloride may facilitate control, as may local pressure. Underlying hematologic disorders should be identified and, if required, platelets and/or fresh frozen plasma should be administered (see Chap. 62). If these measures are not sufficient, firm petroleum-coated gauze packings need to be placed. Administration of an oral antibiotic such as trimethoprim-sulfamethoxazole or amoxicillin-clavulanic acid is usually recommended to prevent a secondary sinus infection, although efficacy has not been proven. In some cases of severe posterior bleeding, a "posterior pack" is required. This requires hospitalization and the administration of prophylactic intravenous antibiotics because of obstruction of the sinus ostia. Since the packing can cause hypoxemia secondary to a nasopulmonary reflex, careful monitoring of the arterial oxygen tension is necessary with pulse oximetry or arterial blood gas determination. Supplemental oxygen delivered by face mask may be required. Surgical management is reserved for patients who continue to bleed despite appropriate anterior and posterior packing, and patients who have severe recurrent bleeding after the removal of a posterior nasal pack.

NASAL DISCHARGE AND OBSTRUCTION **Rhinitis** Acute, self-limited nasal inflammation, or rhinitis, causing discharge and obstruction is usually due to acute viral upper respiratory tract infection. Chronic rhinitis may take several forms: *Vasomotor rhinitis* is characterized by an autonomic imbalance with increased parasympathetic tone involving the nasal mucosa. Usually there is no history of allergy and nasal smears may show nonspecific inflammatory cells; the etiology is unknown. Treatment includes decongestants and topical steroids and in severe cases may require surgical resection of the inferior turbinate or (rarely) interruption of the vidian nerve. *Allergic rhinitis* is often associated with a history of allergies. Nasal polyps may be present and in a small number of patients may be associated with hypersensitivity to aspirin. Medical treatment includes topical steroid sprays, oral decongestant and/or antihistaminic preparations, and desensitization to allergens (see Chap. 267). *Atrophic rhinitis* is characterized by foul odor and epistaxis with nasal obstruction. Examination reveals crusting, debris, and necrosis of the normal tissues and turbinates. Causes include excessive surgical resection of the turbinates, various types of infections, and granulomatous diseases such as Wegener's granulomatosis. Treatment requires management of the underlying disease, as well as nasal douches with saline. If the underlying cause is corrected, surgical reconstruction may be accomplished. *Rhinitis medicamentosa* refers to reactive swelling of the nasal turbinates, nasal obstruction, and increased watery secretions caused by the imprudent use of topical decongestants, specifically imidazoles and sympathomimetics. Treatment consists of termination of topical decongestants and administration of oral decongestants and topical steroids. A short course of systemic steroids may be helpful.

Cerebrospinal fluid rhinorrhea CSF rhinorrhea may follow trauma to the nose or mid-face, blunt cranial injury (e.g., basal skull fracture) causing cribriform plate fracture, or complicated nasal or transphenoidal surgery. It is characterized by a clear nasal discharge and may be complicated by acute or recurrent bacterial meningitis (see Chap. 354). The diagnosis is often confirmed by testing the fluid for glucose. The use of antibiotics to prevent infection is controversial since it is not clear that they are effective and they may change the nature of the infecting organism. Surgical treatment is necessary if spontaneous closure of the leak does not occur. Prior to definitive surgery, intravenous metrizamide coupled with computed tomographic (CT) study or fluorescein injections may demonstrate the site of the leak.

Miscellaneous disorders Less common infections and granulomatous, neoplastic, or vasculitic disorders may cause persistent discharge, obstruction, or necrotizing lesions. The infections include nasal diphtheria (Chap. 102), tuberculosis, leprosy, syphilis [with "congenital snuffles" (Chap. 128)]; glanders (Chap. 112); infection with *Klebsiella rhinoscleromatis;* histoplasmosis, cryptococcosis, and blastomycosis (Chap. 151); and mucocutaneous leishmaniasis (Chap. 160). Neoplasms include squamous cell carcinoma, malignant melanoma, lymphoma, and mycosis fungoides. Granulomatous necrotizing lesions with nasal septal destruction include Wegener's granulomatosis (Chap. 276), sarcoidosis (Chap. 277) and midline granuloma (Chap. 279). Diagnosis of these various disorders is established by culture, and histologic characteristics of biopsy materials. Treatment is outlined in the individual chapters on these diseases.

Nasal septal perforation A septal perforation is commonly the result of trauma, including nasal septal surgery and transphenoidal surgery of the pituitary gland. Perforation may be self-induced by nose picking and by substance abuse, specifically cocaine. Various granulomatous diseases, heavy metal poisoning, syphilis, leprosy, and foreign bodies are additional causes. The size of the perforation determines the clinical symptomatology such as respiratory whistling. Foreign bodies cause local inflammation, nasal obstruction, secondary infection of either the skin or paranasal sinuses, and local necrosis of the nasal tissue that can lead to septal perforation.

NASAL POLYPS AND PAPILLOMAS *Nasal polyps* are the most common mass lesion in the nose or paranasal sinuses and may be confused with neoplasms. Most patients will have associated allergic rhinitis; rarely nasal polyps occur after trauma or in cystic fibrosis. Samter's triad is rare and consists of asthma, nasal polyps, and acute hypersensitivity reactions to aspirin or nonsteroidal anti-inflammatory agents. Patients with polyps may have few symptoms or have rhinorrhea, obstruction, and anosmia. The polyps are usually seen on direct intranasal examination, and in contrast to normal nasal tissue there is no innervation so that polyps are painless on probing or manipulation. Treatment consists of surgical removal and therapy of the underlying allergic rhinitis, including glucocorticoid nasal sprays or low doses of oral glucocorticoids.

Squamous papillomas are relatively common tumors in the nose and are usually found anteriorly to overlie the alar mucosa or the nasal vestibule. These lesions can cause nasal obstruction and hemorrhage and may involve the paranasal sinuses. Thorough surgical removal is required, as these tumors frequently recur. A subtype known as the *inverting papilloma* is usually unilateral and affects men predominantly. The inverting papilloma is histologically benign but may be locally aggressive. Approximately 10 percent of inverting papillomas are associated with malignant transformation into squamous cell cancers. Such tumors occur in older individuals, but it is not clear if these malignancies represent actual malignant degeneration or only occur in conjunction with the inverting papilloma.

ANOSMIA See Chap. 24.

THE PARANASAL SINUSES

ANATOMY AND DEVELOPMENT The paranasal sinuses are cavities within the facial skeleton that are lined by ciliated respiratory epithelium and drain into the nose. The maxillary and ethmoid sinuses are present at birth; the ethmoid labyrinth grows and expands with age, so that the anterior ethmoid cells usually project above the orbital rim to develop into the frontal sinuses. Unilateral agenesis of one of the frontal sinuses is common; 4 percent of normal individuals will have bilateral agenesis. The sphenoid sinuses are the last to develop and often do not mature until patients reach their early twenties. The pituitary is located posteriorly and superiorly and may often bulge into the superior wall of the sphenoid sinus.

SINUSITIS **Acute sinusitis** Acute sinusitis frequently follows a viral infection of the upper respiratory tract. Rhinovirus, adenovirus, influenza, and parainfluenza virus may be recovered with bacteria in about one-fifth of cases. *Streptococcus pneumoniae* and *Haemophilus influenzae* (usually unencapsulated) account for approximately half of the bacteria isolated by direct sinus puncture and aspiration. Group A *Streptococcus, Staphylococcus aureus,* and *Branhamella catarrhalis* are found less frequently. Anaerobic mouth flora (see Chap. 108) are isolated in approximately 5 percent of cases and may be associated with dental disease. Sinusitis that develops in hospitalized patients, particularly following prolonged nasotracheal intubation, and sinusitis in patients on immunosuppressive or antimicrobial treatment has a higher frequency of gram-negative enteric bacteria.

Symptoms include fever, local pain, obstruction of the nasal cavity, secondary anosmia, and a purulent nasal discharge. Point-tenderness may be present over the affected sinus and transillumination of light may be diminished. In ethmoid sinusitis orbital cellulitis or blepharitis may herald intraorbital complications. The white blood cell count is elevated, with a left shift in the differential count. CT scan is most useful for confirming ethmoid or sphenoid infection and can define the extent of involvement of other sinuses.

Maxillary sinusitis can generally be treated on an outpatient basis. Therapy consists of systemic decongestants and oral antibiotics. Amoxicillin-clavulanic acid, trimethoprim-sulfamethoxazole, or cefaclor are all reasonable choices and are replacing ampicillin or amoxicillin because of the increasing frequency of β-lactamase-producing *H. influenzae* and *B. catarrhalis*. More acutely ill patients and those with complicating medical disorders such as diabetes mellitus or immunosuppressive therapy may require intravenous antibiotics. Needle aspiration of the maxillary sinus may be indicated to determine the precise microbial etiology of sinusitis in patients with a poor response to antimicrobials, persisting air-fluid levels, and facial pain.

Frontal sinusitis can present in a manner similar to maxillary sinusitis. However, because of the proximity of the frontal sinuses to the anterior cranial fossa the use of intravenous antibiotics is recommended. Additionally, serial neurologic evaluations may be required. If symptoms do not improve within 48 h after beginning therapy, surgical drainage of the affected sinus is recommended. Acute *sphenoid sinusitis* presents classically with retroorbital pain. Air-fluid levels on standard radiographs or CT scans should be diagnostic. Acute *ethmoid sinusitis* may be more difficult to diagnose clinically, although upper eyelid swelling should raise the index of suspicion.

In acute bacterial sinusitis, topical decongestant sprays (oxymetazoline, phenylephrine), used sparingly, and systemic decongestants are useful adjuncts to antimicrobials in treating the infection and restoring proper drainage. Suspected intracranial complications from acute sinusitis require immediate surgical drainage (see below).

Chronic sinusitis This common disorder has several etiologies. It can be allergic in nature or secondary to anatomic abnormalities, such as a deviated nasal septum. Symptoms of chronic sinusitis may be more vague and transient compared to the acute processes. However, a chronic purulent discharge associated with postnasal drainage, facial pain, and the sensation of pressure within the face or eye are common. Thickening of the sinus mucosa is usually present on x-rays; air-fluid levels are absent except in the case of exacerbations of acute sinusitis. Chronic sinusitis is associated more often with anaerobic organisms than are acute infections. If antibiotics, topical decongestants, and oral decongestants fail to improve the symptoms, sinus lavage may be indicated. Intranasal steroids are used in patients with known allergies and allergic rhinitis. Some patients with chronic or recurring sinusitis will have disorders of immunoglobulin production (Chap. 263), dyskinetic cilia (Chap. 208), or Wegener's granulomatosis (Chap. 276). If symptoms still persist, sinus surgery may be required to establish proper ventilation and drainage of the affected sinuses.

Complications of bacterial sinusitis EXTRACRANIAL COMPLICATIONS These most often involve the orbit. The medial border of the orbit is also the lateral border of the ethmoid labyrinth. Acute ethmoiditis can result in infection traversing the separating thin plate of bone to cause an *orbital cellulitis*. Infection in the other sinuses may also lead to orbital cellulitis. Orbital cellulitis may be either *preseptal* or *postseptal,* is accompanied by pain and lid edema, and may be a major threat to vision or a means of extension into the central nervous system. Preseptal orbital cellulitis requires prompt hospitalization and intravenous antibiotic therapy. Urgent ophthalmologic examination is necessary to assess visual acuity. Postseptal orbital cellulitis results from infection traversing the orbital septum; it requires emergency *surgical* treatment. Signs of postseptal infection include chemosis, conjunctival infection, and proptosis. Extraocular movements may become impaired, ultimately progressing to a frozen globe with the rapid development of blindness.

The *superior orbital fissure syndrome* is a complication of infection of the sphenoid sinus. Patients usually present with a palsied abducens nerve (VI) followed by lesions of cranial nerves III, IV, and V, orbital pain, exophthalmos, and ophthalmoplegia. Treatment involves documentation of sphenoid sinusitis and rapid surgical exploration.

Frontal sinus infection may extend into the anterior table of the frontal bone and cause osteomyelitis. The presentation includes fever, frontal headache, leukocytosis, and cool doughy, tender edema over the affected frontal sinus (''Pott's puffy tumor''). CT scanning is indicated to document the extent of the infection and in particular potential intracranial involvement (epidural, subdural, or frontal lobe brain abscess).

INTRACRANIAL COMPLICATIONS These include meningitis; epidural, subdural, or brain abscess; and cavernous sinus thrombosis. They are discussed in Chap. 354.

Fungal sinusitis This disorder is discussed in Chap. 151.

SINUS NEOPLASMS Neoplastic diseases of the paranasal sinuses are rare. Benign osteomas most commonly involve the frontal bone and may be a complication of chronic sinus disease. Malignancies include carcinoma of the maxillary sinus and sarcoma. Woodworkers, nickel workers, and patients with chronic sinusitis are at increased risk for developing carcinoma of the maxillary sinuses. Symptoms of neoplasms can include repeated acute sinusitis and/or recurrent epistaxis. Sinus films and/or CT scans are used to establish their existence. Biopsies are necessary for diagnosis.

EAR

OTITIS MEDIA **Acute otitis media** Viral upper respiratory tract infection is the most common predisposing factor to acute otitis media. The hallmark of middle ear infection is pain. A sense of fullness, purulent otorrhea, hearing loss, vertigo or tinnitus, fever, and leukocytosis may be present. Otoscopic examination will confirm the diagnosis of acute otitis media, by demonstrating a red, dull, and bulging or perforated tympanic membrane. *S. pneumoniae* (approximately 35 percent) and *H. influenzae* (approximately 20 percent) are the most frequent bacteria in middle ear effusions in acute otitis media. The majority of *H. influenzae* infections are due to the nontypeable strains. In children, infection by *H. influenzae* type b (about 10 percent of cases) can cause severe systemic toxicity and may be associated with meningitis (see Chaps. 115 and 354). Other common bacteria include *B. catarrhalis*, group A *Streptococcus*, and *Staph. aureus*. Mixed anaerobic bacteria can occasionally cause acute otitis media. Respiratory viruses are implicated in the pathogenesis but are rarely cultured. Respiratory syncytial and influenza viruses are among the more frequently incriminated agents.

Treatment of acute otitis media includes the use of antibiotics such as: amoxicillin-clavulanic acid, trimethoprim-sulfamethoxazole, or cefaclor. Antihistamines are not effective. Occasionally tympanocentesis is required for bacteriologic diagnosis in refractory cases. In persistent infection, a myringotomy with or without the insertion of a ventilating tube may be necessary. Severe pain, infection in immunologically compromised patients, or failure of antibiotic therapy are indications for surgical drainage of the middle ear space.

OTITIS MEDIA WITH CHRONIC EFFUSION Serous otitis media with chronic effusion is a leading cause of hearing loss in children and occasionally in adults. Otoscopic examination will show a retracted tympanic membrane associated with fluid in the middle ear cavity. Standard audiometry and tympanometry can reveal a conductive hearing loss and flat tympanogram consistent with restrictive disease in the middle ear space.

Therapy can be divided into conservative and surgical approaches. Decongestants and antihistamines have been advocated in the treatment of serous effusions, although their usefulness is unproven. Glucocorticoids and antibiotics have been used as well as mechanical insufflation via the eustachian tube (politerization). Control of predisposing factors is also indicated: i.e., the treatment of allergy, nasal infection, or chronic sinus infection. Occasionally the use of ventilating tubes is required for treatment of a chronic effusion in the middle ear with or without infection. This provides drainage for a potentially infected middle ear and will improve a conductive hearing loss caused by the accumulation of serous fluid in the middle ear.

Chronic otitis media The bacterial flora in chronic otitis media is variable. *Pseudomonas aeruginosa* and *Staph. aureus* are the most commonly isolated organisms, followed by *Escherichia coli* and *Proteus* species. Chronic foul-smelling otorrhea is associated with anaerobic infection. Chronic suppuration of the middle ear may be associated with perforation of the tympanic membrane and cholesteatoma (predominantly keratin debris) formation. Imaging with conventional x-rays or CT will show signs of mucosal thickening in the middle ear space as well as in the mastoid cavity. Cholesteatoma may penetrate into the temporal bone and, rarely, the cranial cavity. Treatment is directed at eradicating the infection with a combination of local care, antibacterial ear drops, and often systemic antibiotics. Surgical removal of a cholesteatoma is required.

MASTOIDITIS The mastoid air cells are in direct continuity with the middle ear space unless blocked by an intervening mass. Cholesteatoma, either acquired or congenital, may obstruct the natural drainage of the mastoid air cells. Because of the direct communication between the two cavities, every otitis media is in the truest sense a mastoiditis. The organisms causing mastoid infections are generally the ones that cause acute middle ear infections. Radiographs of the mastoid air cells frequently demonstrate fluid or mucosal thickening within the honeycomb labyrinth of the mastoid. This indicates chronic infection, and treatment is similar to that of acute otitis media.

Emergent simple mastoidectomy is indicated when there is high fever and leukocytosis with radiographic evidence of destruction of trabeculae and the honeycomb of the mastoid air cells. Signs of acute otitis media are usually also present. A subperiosteal abscess may be associated, in which case examination will reveal an ear that is displaced inferiorly and laterally with a red fluctuant mass behind the pinna. When suspected clinically, CT scanning will usually confirm the diagnosis.

COMPLICATIONS OF OTITIS MEDIA AND MASTOIDITIS Extracranial complications include conductive, mixed, and sensorineural hearing loss. Labyrinthitis manifested by vertigo as well as weakness or complete paralysis of the ipsilateral facial nerve may be direct complications of a middle ear infection. A syndrome consisting of otalgia, a draining middle ear, and paralysis of the ipsilateral sixth cranial nerve reflects infection of the petrous apex of the temporal bone (Gradenigo's syndrome). Therapy is medical, with surgical intervention reserved for refractory cases. Intracranial complications of otitis media include meningitis, brain abscess, epidural abscess, lateral sinus thrombophlebitis, and otitic hydrocephalus (see Chap. 364).

EXTERNAL OTITIS The external auditory canals are lined by skin and are subject to the same diseases of skin as the rest of the body. Psoriasis may be the cause of an external otitis. Glands within the external auditory canal secrete cerumen, which acidifies the external auditory canal and minimizes the overgrowth of bacteria. *Otitis externa* (swimmer's ear) is most common in the summer months and is thought to arise from a change in the milieu of the external auditory canal by increased alkalinization. This leads to the overgrowth of bacteria, most commonly *Staphylococcus*, *Streptococcus*, and *Pseudomonas* species. Treatment includes topical antibacterial ear drops, although occasionally systemic antibiotics are required. Mycotic infections that cause otitis externa refractory to antibacterial treatment are diagnosed by smears and culture and are treated with topical antifungal ear drops. *Herpes zoster* in the external auditory canal can cause an associated loss of the sensory and motor functions of the nerve VII (Ramsay-Hunt syndrome) (see Chaps. 136 and 360).

Necrotizing (malignant) otitis externa This progressive necrotizing infection results in osteomyelitis of the temporal bone and is almost always caused by *P. aeruginosa*. Occasionally the soft tissues and the cartilage of the pinna are also involved. The disorder occurs most commonly in patients with insulin dependent diabetes mellitus. The diagnosis should be suspected in patients with severe refractory otorrhea and disproportional pain. Physical examination will often reveal granulation tissue in the posterior ear canal wall that is eroding into the temporal bone. The auricle and surrounding scalp may be swollen, tender, and necrotic. CT, bone, and occasionally indium 111 leukocyte scans are useful for making the diagnosis. Treatment consists of local care including debridement and antibacterial ear drops combined with intravenous antibiotics directed against *P. aeruginosa* (Chap. 111). Good control of coexisting *diabetes mellitus* may hasten recovery (Chap. 319). Occasionally radical debridement of the temporal bone is required.

Perichondritis Perichondritis is an infection or inflammation of the cartilage of the pinna. The most common organism found in infectious perichondritis is *P. aeruginosa*. The lobule is spared infection because it contains no cartilage. *Relapsing polychondritis* is an inflammatory disease of the external ear that initially may mimic infection and needs to be distinguished from perichondritis (see Chap. 284).

THE PHARYNX

ACUTE PHARYNGITIS The cause of acute pharyngitis is almost always infection, although for pharyngeal inflammation and ulceration it may be agranulocytosis or injury by chemicals or radiation. The major symptom of acute pharyngitis regardless of etiology is sore throat, with or without attendant difficulty in swallowing. Examination will reveal erythema and congestion of the mucosa with hypertrophy of the lymphoid tissue including the tonsils. Exudate if present is suggestive of infection by group A *Streptococcus*. The differential diagnosis of acute exudative pharyngitis is discussed in detail in Chap. 101. Exudate may be seen with a variety of viral infections, in particular those caused by Epstein-Barr virus (Chap. 137), herpes simplex virus (Chap. 135), or adenovirus (Chap. 140). Other organisms that produce an exudate include the gonococcus (Chap. 110), *Corynebacterium diphtheriae* (Chap. 102), *Mycoplasma pneumoniae* (Chap. 154), and the TWAR strains of *Chlamydia* (Chap. 155). Infection with respiratory syncytial virus and parainfluenza and influenza viruses may also cause sore throat without exudate, whereas in rhinovirus infections (Chap. 140) a "scratchy" throat may be a prominent feature. The diagnosis and treatment of the specific causes are covered in the individual chapters.

COMPLICATIONS Chronic or acute infection of the naso- or oropharynx and its lymphoid tissue may lead to a variety of pyogenic complications that require emergent surgical drainage or removal. These include recurrent tonsillitis and peritonsillar and retropharyngeal abscesses and are discussed in Chaps. 91 and 101. Ludwig's angina, which is *not* a pharyngeal infection but rather a mixed bacterial infection of the sublingual or submandibular space, is discussed in Chaps. 91 and 108.

PHARYNGEAL TUMORS The nasopharynx can be the site of a variety of neoplasms. These include lymphomas, lymphoepitheliomas (Schmenke's tumor), squamous cell carcinoma, and anaplastic carcinoma. Less common tumors include amelanotic melanoma, rhabdomyosarcoma, and extramedullary plasmacytomas (often associated with multiple myeloma). Pharyngitis and lymphoid hypertrophy may cause obstruction, particularly in children. In adults, symptoms of obstruction, particularly when chronic, should raise concern about a possible neoplasm. Voice changes may be present with hyponasality. A conductive hearing loss may be due to blockage of the distal eustachian tube.

The most common neoplasm of the oropharynx is a squamous cell carcinoma. Clinical signs and symptoms include dysphagia, odynophagia, halitosis, weight loss, and in advanced cases, respiratory obstruction. Risk factors include excessive alcohol intake and cigarette smoking. Endoscopy and biopsy are required for diagnosis and staging. Therapy may include surgery, radiation, or combined modality treatments depending on the stage of the tumor and the status of the lymph nodes in the neck. Benign and malignant tumors of the minor salivary glands can present in the pharynx. Lymphomas, including Hodgkin's disease, may cause unilateral tonsillar swelling (see Chap. 302).

ORAL CAVITY DISORDERS

Disorders of the oral cavity are reviewed in Chap. 41.

THE LARYNX

SIGNS AND SYMPTOMS OF LARYNGEAL DISEASE Persistent unexplained change in the voice, i.e., hoarseness or weakness, is pathognomonic of laryngeal disorders. Other symptoms include cough that may be dry or associated with the production of clear, purulent, or blood-streaked sputum; pain that may refer to other branches of the vagus nerve, manifested by otalgia, and upper respiratory obstruction causing stridor. Dysphagia and odynophagia may be associated with neoplastic lesions of the larynx. Besides evaluation of the neck, oropharynx, and gag and swallowing reflexes, physical examination should include an indirect mirror examination and, if available, flexible fiberoptic endoscopy. Vocal cord dysfunction, mass lesions, mucosal ulceration, infection of the larynx, structural abnormalities, and occasionally subglottic lesions will be evident on these examinations. Definitive diagnosis requires biopsy usually under anesthesia.

DISORDERS OF VOCAL CORD FUNCTION (see Chap. 360) The vagus nerve can be damaged at the nuclear level in the brainstem; in the neck, where it loops around either the aorta on the left or the subclavian artery on the right; or in the tracheo-esophageal groove as it proceeds superiorly to innervate the intrinsic laryngeal musculature. The superior laryngeal nerve branches from the vagus nerve relatively high in the neck as part of the neurovascular pedicle that contains the superior thyroid artery. A lesion distal to this branching will result in isolated recurrent laryngeal nerve damage that causes paralysis of the posterior cricoarytenoid muscle and fixes the vocal cord on the affected side in a paramedian position. With combined dysfunction of both the recurrent and superior laryngeal nerves the vocal cord is paralyzed in an intermediate position, producing a faint, breathy voice, but a larger airway for the inspiration of air. With isolated superior laryngeal nerve dysfunction paralysis of the cricothyroid muscle occurs, the vocal cord on the affected side abducts, but the larynx is only slightly rotated and the vocal cord appears bowed.

Careful physical examination will help define the possible anatomic lesions causing either unilteral or bilateral vocal cord paralysis. Bilateral paramedian vocal cord paralysis is a surgical emergency. Although the voice may be preserved, stridor can be life-threatening. Emergency tracheotomy or endotracheal intubation is the usual treatment.

LARYNGEAL INFECTIONS Acute epiglottitis Rapidly progressive cellulitis of the epiglottis and surrounding tissues in the supraglottic airway can cause acute airway obstruction. In infants and children the causative agent is most commonly *H. influenzae* type b and bacteremia is frequent (see Chap. 115).

In adolescents and adults with acute bacterial epiglottitis, the clinical presentation may be less fulminant and other organisms have been implicated in some cases (e.g., *S. pneumoniae, Staph. aureus*). Frequently the patient complains of dysphagia, odynophagia, and fever that has progressed over one to two days. Depending on the degree of respiratory obstruction, stridor may or may not be present, but hoarseness and loss of voice power are almost universal findings. As in children, the adult with epiglottitis usually prefers to lean forward, drooling oral secretions. Because the caliber of the airway is larger in the adult, intubation or tracheotomy may not be necessary, but the possibility of complete airway obstruction dictates management. An edematous, cherry red epiglottis and surrounding pharyngeal mucosa are characteristic findings on fiberoptic examination, which in adults is the best way to confirm the diagnosis. In infants and children this approach is contraindicated because of the threat of acute airway obstruction (see Chap. 115). A lateral film of the neck may reveal an enlarged epiglottis—the so-called "thumb sign."

Until the possibility of airway obstruction has passed the adult patient is best managed by admission to an intensive care unit where adequate clinical monitoring is available. Fiberoptic examination in adults with a nasopharyngoscope should be performed only after preparations have been made to secure the airway by endotracheal intubation or, if necessary, tracheostomy. After blood and throat cultures are obtained, appropriate antibiotic treatment is initiated with either a combination of ampicillin and chloramphenicol, cefuroxime, or another third-generation cephalosporin, such as cefotaxime, administered intravenously (see Chaps. 85 and 115). Oxygen should be administered as dictated by O_2 saturations on pulse oximetry or arterial blood gas determination. Humidified air by face tent is advisable. If respiratory obstruction worsens, endotracheal intubation is required. Glucocorticoids have been administered as part of the treatment but with unproven benefit. Resolution of clinical manifestations usually occurs over 36 to 48 h. A child should not be extubated nor a patient removed from an intensive care setting unless the acute cellulitis has resolved, as confirmed by endoscopy.

Croup (laryngotracheobronchitis) Croup is a syndrome produced by acute infection of the lower air passages and is most commonly seen in children below age 3. The most common pathogen is the *Parainfluenza* virus (Chap. 140), but a variety of respiratory viruses and *Mycoplasma pneumoniae* can produce acute laryngotracheobronchitis and the croup syndrome. The pathophysiology is primarily one of circumferential mucosal inflammation in the subglottic larynx and trachea with variable involvement and spasm of the vocal cords; the epiglottis is not involved. The clinical hallmarks, namely, a barking or brassy cough with or without stridor and hoarseness, are discussed in Chap. 140. Croup can be distinguished readily from epiglottitis by lateral films of the neck which show no epiglottal edema, or by careful direct examination. Management of severe croup requires hospitalization, close observation, humidification, oxygenation as dictated by pulse oximetry, and rarely intubation. Glucocorticoid administration has been advocated by some, but the benefits are questionable.

Tuberculous laryngitis Tuberculous laryngitis is usually associated with active pulmonary tuberculosis. Characteristic manifestations include hoarseness, cough, and blood-tinged sputum; because of the large number of organisms in the sputum it is usually highly contagious. The most common site of disease in the larynx is in the interarytenoid fold (in the posterior portion of the larynx). Because granulomas tend to be subepithelial, *deep submucosal biopsies* may be essential for diagnosis. Treatment is the same as for pulmonary tuberculosis (Chap. 125), and symptomatic measures include voice rest and analgesics for pain. Occasionally tracheostomy is needed to protect the airway.

Fungal infections of the larynx The most commonly found mycotic infections of the larynx are histoplasmosis, candidiasis, and blastomycosis. Symptoms can include hoarseness, cough, dyspnea, dysphagia, and odynophagia. Examination may reveal oral and esophageal thrush with candidiasis or nodules on the vocal cords with or without ulceration (histoplasmosis or blastomycosis). With the latter, diagnosis is confirmed by biopsy showing microabscesses in an epithelium infiltrated with giant cells, mononuclear cells, and yeast (Chap. 151). Treatment with systemic antifungal agents is necessary. While not a fungus, actinomycosis may involve the pharynx and larynx from adjacent mandibular or tonsillar infection. The diagnosis and treatment are discussed in Chap. 152.

Other laryngeal infections Other infections which may involve the larynx include tertiary syphilis (Chap. 128), lepromatous leprosy (Chap. 126), diphtheria (Chap. 102), and glanders (Chap. 112). Biopsy is usually required for the diagnosis of syphilis and leprosy, both of which may produce infiltrating nodular lesions. Other diagnostic measures and treatment are discussed in the individual chapters on these agents.

PERICHONDRITIS *Perichondritis* in the larynx due to pyogenic bacterial infection or an inflammatory process may be difficult to distinguish from traumatic injury, certain neoplasms, or injury induced by radiation. The thyroid cartilage is the most common cartilage affected and an abscess may form beneath the mucoperichondrium. Symptoms and signs include pain, tenderness, and swelling that are usually slowly progressive but occasionally very acute. Hoarseness, airway compromise, dysphagia, and odynophagia require prompt radiographic evaluation to exclude the possibility of a foreign body. The airway should then be secured in the operating room. Treatment may require antibiotics or glucocorticoids and debridement of laryngeal granulations.

INFLAMMATORY DISORDERS OF THE LARYNX Ulcers and granulomas of the true vocal cords may result from a variety of types of abuse, including excessive use of the voice. Reflux esophagitis may cause contact ulcers of the vocal cords over the posterior larynx and the arytenoids. Persistent hoarseness is the most common manifestation. In reflux eosophagitis, both throat and gastric pain are common, and a history of gastric ulcer disease is common. On physical examination the classical lesion involves ulceration of the mucosa over the arytenoid cartilages. Treatment requires management of the underlying esophageal or gastric disease (Chaps. 237 and 238). Treatment of the larynx is symptomatic, with voice rest and speech therapy.

Vocal cord nodules Vocal abuse can cause vocal cord or "singer's" nodules. Sinusitis, upper respiratory tract infections, and allergy are known precipitating factors. Tobacco and alcohol may add to irritation. The diagnosis is made by direct or indirect (mirror) laryngoscopy. Treatment for children consists of voice therapy and parental counseling, and for adults voice rest and treatment of precipitating disorders. Occasionally operative removal of the nodules is required.

Sarcoid Sarcoidosis may rarely cause granulomatous disease of the epiglottis and surrounding structures of the vocal cords with sparing of the cords. Hoarseness and airway obstruction may be present (see Chap. 277).

Cricoarytenoid joint arthritis The cricoarytenoid joint is an articular joint which may be involved by systemic arthritis such as gout and rheumatoid arthritis. With rheumatoid arthritis of the cricoarytenoid joint, pain, aggravated by speech, or dysphagia associated with hoarseness are the most common symptoms. On physical examination a bright red swelling of the arytenoid is a common finding, and the vocal cords may be fixed. Evidence of systemic rheumatoid arthritis is usually present (see Chap. 270). Besides treatment for systemic rheumatoid disease, tracheostomy may be required if airway obstruction occurs.

LARYNGEAL STENOSIS Stenosis of the larynx is typically divided into supraglottic, glottic, and subglottic types. Many patients have stenosis at more than one level. Stenosis can be caused by ingestion of caustic materials, endotracheal intubation, irradiation, inflammatory or granulomatous disease, or infection. The etiology is usually apparent by history but with infiltrative processes may require biopsy for diagnosis. Most patients have some hoarseness, and, if the stenosis is severe, stridor and significant airway obstruction may be present. Symptomatic subglottic stenosis following endotracheal intubation is more common in children and may be progressive. Useful diagnostic studies include lateral neck x-rays with linear tomography to determine the site and extent of the stenosis, and confirmation by direct laryngoscopy. Flow-volume-loop studies will reveal upper airway obstruction (see Chap. 201). Management ranges from manual dilatation to surgical reconstruction, depending on the location and degree of the stenosis. With acute severe respiratory obstruction tracheostomy can be lifesaving and is generally preferred over intubation.

FOREIGN BODIES Choking on foods and other foreign bodies causes over 2000 deaths per year in the United States, and is the sixth most common cause of accidental death. Most foreign body aspiration occurs in children under four years of age. The aspiration in such cases is infrequently observed and may not be suspected initially. Peanuts seem to be the most common foreign body aspirated by children, followed by other food stuffs and metallic objects. Most of the foreign bodies lodge within the bronchial tree and about 5 percent get stuck in the larynx. In adults aspiration of poorly chewed food (the so-called "cafe coronary," often associated with inebriation, poor dentition, or swallowing disorders) is the most common cause of acute obstruction. Symptoms can include "sticking" pain localized to the larynx, laryngeal spasm, change in voice quality up to complete aphonia, stridor, and dyspnea, or complete lack of air movement despite attempted respiratory excursions. Perforation of the larynx by sharp objects may lead to infection. For acute obstruction with aphonia and no air movement forced pressure to the epigastrium—the *Heimlich maneuver*—is indicated to dislodge the material. Foreign bodies retained in the tracheobronchial tree require prompt endoscopic removal.

NEOPLASMS OF THE LARYNX Benign tumors The most common type of benign laryngeal tumor is the papilloma. Other tumors include hemangioma, angiofibroma, chemodectoma, neurofibroma, chondroma, and granular cell myoblastoma. As with many other laryngeal disorders, the presentation is with hoarseness. Dyspnea, dysphagia, and pain are late findings. Fiberoptic endoscopy can be done in an outpatient setting to evaluate hoarseness. If a laryngeal tumor is seen, formal endoscopic evaluation and biopsy are necessary. The histopathology is generally diagnostic and dictates subsequent treatment.

PAPILLOMA The papilloma is a benign tumor of the larynx that is caused by the human papilloma virus (Chap. 150) of which three predominant serotypes are involved in laryngeal disease. At present there is some debate as to whether there are two clinical forms: an adult form and a juvenile form. Generally, the adult form tends to be unifocal and easier to treat. Juvenile laryngeal papillomatosis is often multifocal and occurs in preschool children. Extensive laryngeal and tracheal involvement may cause stridor, and routine examination can be difficult. Endoscopic evaluation in the operating room with biopsy is needed for diagnosis.

The proper treatment of laryngeal papillomatosis is controversial, and recurrence is common. The mainstay of therapy is the carbon dioxide laser and several operative procedures may be required in order to extirpate the lesions. Papillomas can also be removed by mechanical debridement with a cupped forceps, cryotherapy, wide surgical excision (which is more commonly performed in the oropharynx and the oral cavity), and by argon laser treatment after photosensitization. Children with laryngotracheal papillomatosis may require long-term tracheostomies. Systemic α-interferon increases the rate of remission and decreases that of recurrence within the first 6 months of treatment, but long-term remission is rare with interferon alone. Because of the possibility of malignant degeneration, radiation should be avoided.

Laryngeal malignancies Squamous cell carcinoma, the most common neoplasm of the larynx, usually presents after the fifth decade of life and is associated with tobacco and alcohol use. Less common malignancies include neuroendocrine tumors, tumors of the minor salivary glands, and neoplasms of mesodermal origin. Hoarseness is the most prominent manifestation of cancers of the vocal cords; origin from other laryngeal locations may be asymptomatic until late in the course, when stridor and/or dyspnea develop. Pain can be scratchy, vague, and nonspecific or it may present as ipsilateral otalgia referred by the vagus nerve. Dysphagia may be produced by laryngeal tumors that have spread out of the larynx to invade either the base of the tongue or the walls of the adjacent hypopharynx. Odynophagia, chronic cough, and hemoptysis may also occur. Halitosis from tumor necrosis, metastatic cervical adenopathy, and weight loss are late features of this disease.

Laryngeal cancer is diagnosed by direct laryngoscopy, pharyngoscopy, and biopsy. The extent of spread beyond the site of origin can be assessed by physical examination and radiographic studies including CT and MRI. A staging system that categorizes the location, size, and extent of spread of malignancies has been utilized to develop appropriate therapeutic approaches and for prognostic purposes. Small stage 1 lesions are localized to the vocal cord and can be cured by radiation in over 90 percent of cases. Partial laryngectomy may be curative for more extensive localized disease, with radiation reserved for recurrences. Total laryngectomy is employed for advanced cancer and is combined with radical neck dissection if the tumor has spread to draining lymph nodes. Radiation can be employed either as adjunctive initial treatment or reserved for recurrences. Decisions as to which therapeutic approach to employ are usually best made by a multidisciplinary tumor board. As with other squamous cell cancers, metabolic complications such as hypercalcemia or hyponatremia may complicate advanced disease (see Chap. 309). Extensive surgery and external beam irradiation may lead to hypoparathyroidism and/or hypothyroidism.

REFERENCES

BALLENGER JJ: Acquired ultrastructural alterations of respiratory cilia and clinical disease: A review. Ann Otol Rhinol Laryngol 97:253, 1988

ENGLISH GM (ed): *Otolaryngology*, revised edition. New York, Harper & Row, 1989

FRICK WE, BUSSE WW: Respiratory infections: Their role in airway responsiveness and pathogenesis of asthma. Clin Chest Med 9:539, 1988

GWALTNEY JM: Sinusitis, in *Principles and Practice of Infectious Diseases*, 3d ed, GL Mandell et al (eds). New York, Churchill Livingstone, 1990, pp 510–514

HEALY G et al: Treatment of recurrent respiratory papillomatosis with human leukocyte interferon. N Engl J Med 319:401, 1988

HUOVINEN P et al: Pharyngitis in adults; the presence and coexistence of viruses and bacterial organisms. Ann Intern Med 110:612, 1989

LUCENT FE, HYAMS VJ: Inflammatory and neoplastic disorders of the nasal mucosa. Clin Dermatol 5:35, 1987

NACLERIO RM: The pathophysiology of allergic rhinitis: Impact of therapeutic intervention. J Allergy Clin Immunol 82:927, 1988

Nasal obstruction. Otolaryngol Clin North Am 22: 2, 1989

PARSONS JT et al: Hyperfractionation for head and neck cancer. Int J Radiat Oncol Biol Phys 14:649, 1988

TOGIAS A et al: Studies on allergic and nonallergic nasal inflammation. J Allergy Clin Immunol 81:782, 1988

WENIG BM et al: Moderately differentiated neuroendocrine carcinoma of the larynx: A clinicopathologic study of 57 cases. Cancer 62:2658, 1988

215 NEOPLASMS OF THE LUNG

JOHN D. MINNA

Each year, primary carcinoma of the lung affects more than 100,000 males and 50,000 females in the United States, most of whom die within 1 year of diagnosis, making it the leading cause of cancer death. The peak incidence of lung cancer occurs between ages 55 and 65 years. The overall incidence is increasing, causing the age-adjusted lung cancer death rate to double every 15 years. However, the effects of antismoking efforts started 10 to 20 years ago have finally started to be seen in a flattening of the incidence rate of lung cancer in white males while, unfortunately, the rate in females is still increasing. At the time of diagnosis, only 20 percent of all lung cancer patients will have local disease, while 25 percent will have disease spread to regional lymph nodes, and 55 percent will have distant metastatic cancer. Even in those patients with supposedly localized disease, overall 5-year survival is only 30 percent for males and 50 percent for females, and this survival rate has not changed significantly over the past 20 years. Thus, primary carcinoma of the lung is a major health problem with a generally grim prognosis. However, an orderly approach to diagnosis, staging, and treatment based on knowledge of the clinical behavior of lung cancer allows selection of the best therapy for either potential cure or optimal palliation of individual patients. This approach should be multidisciplinary, involving interaction of internists, chest physicians, medical, radiation, and surgical oncologists, pathologists, and supportive care personnel.

PATHOLOGY

The histologic classification of primary lung neoplasms recommended by the World Health Organization in 1977 should be used. Four major cell types make up 95 percent of all primary lung neoplasms. These are squamous or epidermoid carcinoma, small cell (also called "oat cell") carcinoma, adenocarcinoma (including bronchioloalveolar), and large cell (also called large cell anaplastic) carcinoma. The remainder include combined epidermoid and adenocarcinomas, carcinoids, bronchial gland tumors (including cylindromas and mucoepidermoid tumors), and mesotheliomas, as well as rarer tumor types. The various cell types have different natural histories and responses to therapy, and thus a correct histologic diagnosis by an experienced pathologist is the first step to correct treatment. In the past 10 years, for unknown reasons, the incidence of adenocarcinoma is rising while that of epidermoid cancer is falling.

Major treatment decisions are made on the basis of the crucial distinction between histologic classification of a tumor as a small cell carcinoma or one of the "non-small cell" varieties (which include epidermoid, adenocarcinoma, large cell carcinoma, bronchioloalveolar carcinoma, and mixed versions of these). Some of these distinctions are summarized in Tables 215-1 and 215-2. In general, small cell carcinoma has spread beyond the bounds of resectional surgery at the time of presentation and is primarily managed with chemotherapy with or without radiotherapy. In contrast, non-small cell cancers found to be localized at the time of presentation should be considered for a curative attempt with either surgery or radiotherapy. However, the response of non-small cell cancers to chemotherapy usually is not dramatic, making such therapy less important in metastatic disease than it is in nearly all small cell lung cancer patients.

Ninety percent of patients with lung cancer of all histologic types are cigarette smokers, while the rare nonsmoking patient who develops lung cancer usually has adenocarcinoma. However, in nonsmokers with adenocarcinoma involving the lung, the possibility of other primary sites, particularly breast cancer in women, should be considered. Epidermoid and small cell cancers usually present as central

TABLE 215-1 Incidence, frequency of metastases, and surgical resectability of the major lung cancer histologic types

Cell type	Incidence in autopsy series, %	Necropsy frequency of distant metastases when clinically localized, %*	Resectability rate (AJC study), %†	5-Year survival after curative resection, %
Non-small cell carcinoma:				
Epidermoid	33	17	60	37
Adenocarcinoma	25	40	38	27
Large cell carcinoma	16	14	38	27
Small cell carcinoma	25	63	11	<1

* Determined from autopsy studies of patients dying of causes other than cancer within 30 days following an apparent curative surgical resection.
† AJC = American Joint Committee Study for Cancer Staging and End Results Reporting, indicating percentage of cases thought to undergo a curative resection.
SOURCE: Adapted from JD Minna et al, 1989.

masses with endobronchial growth, while adenocarcinomas and large cell cancers tend to present as peripheral nodules or masses with pleural involvement. Epidermoid and large cell cancers cavitate in 20 to 30 percent of cases. Bronchioloalveolar carcinoma can present as a single mass, a diffuse, multinodular lesion, or as a fluffy infiltrate.

ETIOLOGY

The large majority of lung cancers are caused by carcinogens and tumor promoters ingested via cigarette smoking. There is a dose-response relationship between the lung cancer death rate and the total amount (often expressed in "cigarette pack-years") of cigarettes smoked, such that the risk is increased sixty- to seventyfold for the man smoking two packs a day for 20 years compared to the nonsmoker. Conversely, the chance of developing lung cancer decreases with cessation of smoking but may never return to the nonsmoker level. The increase in lung cancer in women is also associated with a rise in female cigarette smoking. As a preventive measure, efforts to get persons to stop smoking should continue. However, this is extremely difficult as the smoking habit represents a powerful addiction to nicotine. Therefore, it is equally important to prevent people from starting to smoke. Probably there is a cocarcinogenic effect of smoking and industrial or environmental pollutants such as radon gas from natural sources in the ground.

The current poor prognosis for most patients with lung cancer requires the continued performance of well-designed clinical trials to test new forms of therapy. These include further adjuvant and neoadjuvant trials combined with surgery and radiotherapy; prospective testing of tumor sensitivity in vitro to drugs, radiation therapy, and biologic response modifiers; tests of anti-growth factor therapy; and application of newer methods using monoclonal antibodies for early detection. The key intervention remains prevention, and broad antismoking efforts must continue. However, the detection of genetic lesions predisposing to malignancy would be a major step forward in focusing preventive efforts, early diagnosis, and eventually targeting therapy at the products that make lung cancer cells malignant.

While human lung cancer is not thought of as a genetic disease, a variety of molecular genetic studies have shown that lung cancer cells have acquired a number of genetic lesions including activation of dominant oncogenes and inactivation of the newly discovered tumor suppressor or recessive oncogenes (Chap. 300). In fact, it appears that to become clinically evident, lung cancer cells have to accumulate a large number (perhaps 10 or more) of such lesions. For the dominant oncogenes these include: point mutations in the coding regions of the *ras* family of oncogenes (particularly in the K-*ras* gene in adenocarcinoma of the lung); amplification, rearrangement, and/or loss of transcriptional control of *myc* family oncogenes (c-, N-,

TABLE 215-2 Comparison between small cell and non-small cell lung cancers

	Small cell	Non-small cell
Histology	Scant cytoplasm; small hyperchromatic nuclei with fine chromatin pattern; nucleoli indistinct; diffuse sheets of cells	Abundant cytoplasm; pleomorphic nuclei with coarse chromatin pattern; nucleoli often prominent; glands or squamous architecture
General neuroendocrine properties:		
Dense core granules	Present	Absent*
L-Dopa decarboxylase activity	High	Absent
Chromogranin	Present	Absent
Synaptophysin	Present	Absent
Neuron-specific enolase	High	Low
Creatine kinase BB isozyme	High	Low
Leu-7, HNK-1 antigens	Present	Absent
Peptide hormone production:		
Gastrin releasing peptide gene products	Present	Absent
Other neuropeptides	ACTH, AVP, calcitonin, ANF	PTH
Other markers:		
HLA, β_2-microglobulin	Absent/low	Present
Intermediate filament pattern	"SCLC"	"Non-SCLC"
Neurofilaments	Present	Absent
EGF receptors	Low or absent	Present
Mucin	Absent	Present in adenocarcinomas
Surfactant associate proteins	Absent	Often present
Carcinoembryonic antigen	Present	Present
Cytogenetics:		
3p(14–23) deletion	Present 100%	Present in 40–50%
rb gene abnormality	Present in majority	Present in minority
Other deletions (e.g., 17p)	Present	Present
Response to radiotherapy	Objective shrinkage in 80–90%; often complete response	Objective shrinkage in 30–50%; uncommonly complete
Response to combination chemotherapy:		
Overall regression rate	90%	30–40%
Complete regression rate	50%	5%
Overall 5-year survival rates	5%	8%

*Ten percent of non-small cell lung cancers have populations of cells expressing neuroendocrine markers, and these are best demonstrated by immunohistochemical stains.

and L-*myc*), with changes in c-*myc* found in non-small cell cancers while changes in all *myc* family members are found in small cell lung cancer; high-level, deregulated expression of the c-*raf* serine-threonine kinase activity; and high-level, deregulated expression of members of the *jun* family of oncogenes, which act as transcription factors and mediate cellular responses to tumor promoters. For the recessive oncogenes, cytogenetic and restriction fragment length polymorphism (RFLP) analysis has shown a prominent deletion involving chromosome region 3p(14–23) present in all small cell and 40 to 50 percent of non-small cell lung cancers; other deletions involving chromosome region 17p in small cell lung cancer; and most specifically, abnormalities of the *rb* gene (in chromosome region

13q14) in small cell lung cancer. In fact, the *rb* gene exhibits abnormalities in DNA, RNA, or protein in perhaps all small cell lung cancers and some non-small cell lung cancers.

The large number of genetic lesions could be acquired by several mechanisms. Cell biologic studies have shown that lung cancer cells produce a large number of peptide hormones which can act to stimulate their growth in an "autocrine" fashion. These include gastrin releasing peptide and transferrin in small cell lung cancer and insulin-like growth factors in all types of lung cancer. The production of these factors, and in addition, the high level of expression of *jun* family oncogenes, provides a setting for tumor promotion (outgrowth of cells with genetic lesions) in bronchial epithelium after genetic lesions have been initiated by carcinogens in cigarette smoke or the environment. Other possible sources for these genetic lesions include familial inheritance or lesions acquired during development. While lung cancer does not have a clear pattern of Mendelian inheritance, there are several indications of a potential for familial association. These include the inheritance of the high-debrisoquine metabolic phenotype; studies that show that first-degree relatives of lung cancer probands have a significant (two- to threefold) excess risk of lung cancer or other cancers, many of which are not smoking-related; and the strong risk of developing lung cancer that has been shown to be linked with development of chronic obstructive pulmonary disease.

CLINICAL MANIFESTATIONS AND MODE OF PRESENTATION

Lung cancer gives rise to signs and symptoms from local tumor growth, invasion or obstruction of adjacent structures, growth in regional nodes via lymphatic spread, growth in distant metastatic sites after hematogenous dissemination, or as a remote effect (paraneoplastic syndrome) usually resulting from peptide hormone secretion by the tumor. Appropriate identification of these signs and symptoms as tumor-related will guide further evaluation and therapy and be of prognostic importance.

If programs screening asymptomatic patients are excluded, 5 to 15 percent of patients are detected while asymptomatic, usually on a routine chest radiograph, while the vast majority of patients present with some sign or symptom. Signs and symptoms secondary to central or endobronchial growth of the primary tumor include cough, hemoptysis, wheeze and stridor, dyspnea, and pneumonitis (fever and productive cough) from obstruction. Signs and symptoms secondary to the peripheral growth of the primary tumor include pain from pleural or chest wall involvement, cough, dyspnea on a restrictive basis, and symptoms of lung abscess resulting from tumor cavitation. Signs and symptoms related to the regional spread of tumor in the thorax by contiguity or by metastasis to regional lymph nodes include tracheal obstruction, esophageal compression with dysphagia, recurrent laryngeal nerve paralysis with hoarseness, phrenic nerve paralysis with elevation of the hemidiaphragm and dyspnea, and sympathetic nerve invasion and paralysis with Horner's syndrome. *Pancoast's, or superior sulcus tumor, syndrome* results from local extension of a tumor (usually epidermoid) growing in the apex of the lung with involvement of the eighth cervical and first and second thoracic nerves, with shoulder pain which characteristically radiates in the ulnar distribution of the arm, often with radiologic destruction of the first and second ribs. Often Horner's syndrome and Pancoast's syndrome will coexist. Other problems of regional spread include *superior vena cava syndrome* from vascular obstruction; pericardial and cardiac extension with resultant tamponade, arrhythmia, or cardiac failure; lymphatic obstruction with resultant pleural effusion; and lymphangitic spread through the lungs with hypoxemia and dyspnea. In addition, bronchioloalveolar carcinoma can spread transbronchially, producing tumor growing along multiple alveolar surfaces with resultant impairment of oxygen transfer, respiratory insufficiency, dyspnea, hypoxemia, and production of large amounts of sputum.

Extrathoracic metastatic disease is found at autopsy in over 50 percent of patients with epidermoid carcinoma, 80 percent of patients with adeno- and large cell carcinoma, and over 95 percent of patients with small cell cancer. These autopsy studies have found lung cancer metastases in virtually every organ system. Thus, the majority of lung cancer patients eventually need therapy to palliate symptoms. Common clinical problems related to extrathoracic metastatic lung cancer include brain metastases with neurologic deficits; bone metastases with pain and pathologic fractures; bone marrow invasion with cytopenias or leukoerythroblastosis; liver metastases causing biochemical liver dysfunction, anorexia, biliary obstruction, and pain; lymph node metastases in the supraclavicular region and occasionally in the axilla and groin that can be painful and ulcerate; and spinal cord compression syndromes from epidural or bone metastases.

Paraneoplastic syndromes are common in lung cancer patients and may be the presenting finding or first sign of recurrence. In addition, paraneoplastic syndromes may mimic metastatic disease and, unless detected, lead to inappropriate palliative rather than curative treatment. Often the paraneoplastic syndrome may be relieved with successful treatment of the tumor, and tumor treatment is the basis for correcting such syndromes. In some cases the pathophysiology of the paraneoplastic syndrome is known, particularly when a hormone with biologic activity is secreted by a tumor (Chap. 309). However, in many cases the pathophysiology is unknown. *Systemic symptoms* of anorexia, cachexia, and weight loss (seen in 30 percent of patients), with fever, and suppressed immunity, are paraneoplastic syndromes of unknown etiology. *Endocrine syndromes* are seen in 12 percent of patients and have the best understood pathophysiology, including hypercalcemia and hypophosphatemia resulting from ectopic parathyroid hormone or PTH-related peptide production by epidermoid cancer; hyponatremia with the syndrome of inappropriate secretion of antidiuretic hormone or possibly atrial natriuretic factor by small cell cancer; and ectopic secretion of ACTH by small cell cancer, which usually results in additional electrolyte disturbances, especially hypokalemia, rather than the changes in body habitus seen in Cushing's syndrome from a pituitary adenoma.

Skeletal connective tissue syndromes include clubbing in 30 percent (usually non-small cell) and hypertrophic pulmonary osteoarthropathy in 1 to 10 percent (usually adenocarcinomas) with periostitis and clubbing giving pain, tenderness, and swelling over the affected bones, and a positive bone scan. *Neurologic-myopathic syndromes* are seen in only 1 percent of patients but are dramatic and include the myasthenic *Eaton-Lambert syndrome* with small cell cancer, while peripheral neuropathies, subacute cerebellar degeneration, cortical degeneration, and polymyositis are seen with all lung cancer types. *Coagulation and thrombotic and hematologic manifestations* occur in 1 to 8 percent of patients and include migratory venous thrombophlebitis (*Trousseau's syndrome*); nonbacterial thrombotic (marantic) endocarditis with arterial emboli; disseminated intravascular coagulation with hemorrhage; and anemia, granulocytosis, and leukoerythroblastosis. *Cutaneous manifestations* such as dermatomyositis and acanthosis nigricans are uncommon (1 percent or less) as are the *renal manifestations* of nephrotic syndrome or glomerulonephritis (1 percent or less).

DIAGNOSIS AND STAGING

EARLY DIAGNOSIS Screening persons at high risk (males over 45 years of age smoking 40 or more cigarettes per day) for lung cancer with sputum cytologies and chest radiographs every 4 months has shown a prevalence rate of lung cancer in asymptomatic patients of four to eight cases per 1000 persons. With follow-up screening, four new cases of lung cancer are found per 1000 persons followed per year. These lung cancers are detected 72 percent of the time by radiographs alone, 20 percent by cytology alone, while 6 percent are detected by both methods. In contrast to nonscreened patients, 90 percent of these screened patients who develop lung cancer are asymptomatic, 62 percent have resectable lung cancer, and 53 percent of all the new cases are postsurgical stage I (see below) with a 5-year survival probability of 45 percent. However, in a large, multi-institutional, prospective randomized trial there was no difference in the survival rate between the screened and the nonscreened group of smoking males ≥45 years old. This was because of the presence of metastases in the majority of patients even when tumors were detected at a very early stage.

ESTABLISHING A TISSUE DIAGNOSIS OF LUNG CANCER Once signs, symptoms, or screening studies suggest lung cancer, it is necessary to establish a tissue diagnosis of malignancy, determine the histologic cell type, and stage the patient for appropriate treatment. In the initial evaluation of each patient, tumor tissue should be obtained so that a histologic diagnosis of cancer and tumor cell type can be firmly made. Distinction of small cell from non-small cell lung cancer is crucial and is often difficult in cytology preparations. Therefore, cytologic diagnoses from washings or needle aspirates should be reserved for very high risk patients or patients relapsing with cancer after initial treatment. Tumor tissue can be obtained from a bronchial biopsy or transbronchial forceps biopsy at fiberoptic bronchoscopy; from node biopsy at mediastinoscopy; from the operative specimen at the time of definitive surgical resection; from percutaneous biopsy of an enlarged lymph node, soft tissue mass, lytic bone lesion, bone marrow, or pleural lesion; or from an adequate cell block from a malignant pleural effusion.

STAGING PATIENTS WITH LUNG CANCER Lung cancer staging consists of two parts: first, a determination of the location of tumor (anatomic staging) and second, an assessment of a patient's ability to withstand various antitumor treatments (physiologic staging). For example, in a patient with non-small cell lung cancer it is crucial to determine if the tumor can be resected by a standard surgical procedure such as a lobectomy or pneumonectomy (determination of "resectability") based on the anatomic stage of the tumor and whether the patient could tolerate such a surgical procedure (determination of "operability") based on the cardiopulmonary condition of the patient.

Non-small cell lung cancer The TNM international stage system (ISS) developed by the American Joint Committee (AJC) on End Results Reporting, and modified by an international commission, should be used in non-small cell lung cancer, particularly in preparing patients for curative attempts with surgery or radiotherapy (Table 215-3). The various T (tumor size), N (regional node involvement), and M (presence or absence of distant metastasis) factors are combined to form different stage groups and, in addition, there is a group covering occult carcinoma detected on screening cytology exam with no other evidence of tumor (Table 215-3).

Small cell lung cancer A simple two-stage system adapted from the Veterans Administration Lung Cancer Study Group is used. In this two-stage system, *limited stage disease* (about 30 percent of all small cell cancer patients) is defined as disease confined to one hemithorax and regional lymph nodes (including mediastinal, contralateral hilar, and usually ipsilateral supraclavicular nodes), while *extensive stage disease* (about 70 percent of all patients) is defined as disease beyond this. Employed in staging are clinical studies such as physical examination, x-rays, scans, and bone marrow examination. In part, the definition of *limited stage* relates to whether the known tumor can be encompassed within a tolerable radiation therapy port. Thus, contralateral supraclavicular nodes, recurrent laryngeal nerve involvement, and superior vena caval obstruction can all be limited stage disease. However, cardiac tamponade, malignant pleural effusion, and bilateral pulmonary parenchymal involvement are generally scored as extensive stage disease because of the size of the radiation therapy port required to cover all known disease.

GENERAL STAGING PROCEDURES (Table 215-4) All lung cancer patients should have a complete history and physical examination, with evaluation of all other medical problems and a determination of performance status and weight loss, both of which have

TABLE 215-3 TNM classification of lung cancer using the new International Staging System (ISS)

PRIMARY TUMOR (T)

T0	No evidence of a primary tumor.
TX	Occult cancer seen in bronchial washing cytologies but not seen on x-ray or fiberoptic bronchoscopy.
TIS	Carcinoma in situ.
T1	Tumor ≤3 cm in greatest dimension, surrounded by lung or visceral pleura, and without evidence of invasion proximal to a lobar bronchus at bronchoscopy. (Uncommon superficial tumors of any size with invasive components limited to the bronchial wall that extend proximal to the main bronchus are also classified as T1.)
T2	Tumor >3 cm in greatest dimension *or* a tumor of any size that either invades the visceral pleura or has associated atelectasis–obstructive pneumonitis extending to the hilar region. At bronchoscopy, the proximal extent of demonstrable tumor must be within a lobar bronchus or at least 2 cm distal to the carina. Any associated atelectasis or obstructive pneumonitis must involve less than an entire lung.
T3	A tumor of any size with direct extension into the chest wall (including superior sulcus tumors), diaphragm, mediastinal pleura, or pericardium without involving heart, great vessels, trachea, esophagus, or vertebral body *or* a tumor in the main bronchus within 2 cm of the carina without involving the carina.
T4	A tumor of any size with invasion of the mediastinum or involving heart, great vessels, trachea, esophagus, vertebral body, or carina *or* the presence of a malignant pleural effusion. (Pleural effusions that are not bloody and not exudative with several negative cytopathologic examinations are not scored as a malignant effusion for staging purposes.)

REGIONAL LYMPH NODES (N)

N0	No demonstrable metastasis to regional lymph nodes.
N1	Metastasis to lymph nodes in the peribronchial or ipsilateral hilar region, or both, including direct extension.
N2	Metastasis to ipsilateral mediastinal or subcarinal lymph nodes.
N3	Metastasis to contralateral mediastinal, contralateral hilar, ipsilateral or contralateral scalene, or supraclavicular lymph nodes.

DISTANT METASTASIS (M)

M0	No known distant metastasis.
M1	Distant metastasis present with site specified (e.g., brain).

STAGE GROUPING USING THE NEW ISS

Occult carcinoma	TX	N0	M0
Stage 0	TIS	Carcinoma in situ	
Stage I	T1	N0	M0
	T2	N0	M0
Stage II	T1	N1	M0
	T2	N1	M0
Stage IIIa	T3	N0	M0
	T3	N1	M0
	T1–3	N2	M0
Stage IIIb	Any T	N3	M0
	T4	Any N	M0
Stage IV	Any T	Any N	M1

SOURCE: Adapted from CF Mountain.

great prognostic value. An ear, nose, and throat examination is also necessary because of the frequent occurrence of second cancers in this area. While not done in every patient, fiberoptic bronchoscopy remains a cornerstone of lung cancer staging and follow-up, providing material for pathologic examination, and information on tumor size, location, degree of bronchial obstruction, and recurrence.

Chest roentgenograms are needed to evaluate tumor size and nodal involvement, and it is very useful to obtain old x-ray films for comparison. Chest computed tomography (CT) scans are now widely used in the staging and follow-up of lung cancer patients. CT scans are of use in non-small cell lung cancer in preoperative staging to detect mediastinal nodes and pleural extension, and in the planning of curative radiation therapy to allow design of fields to encompass all known tumor volume while avoiding as much normal tissue as possible. However, definitive characterization of mediastinal nodal

TABLE 215-4 Pretreatment staging procedures for lung cancer patients

ALL PATIENTS

Complete history & physical examination
Determination of performance status and weight loss
Ear, nose, and throat examination
Complete blood count with platelet determination
Serum electrolytes, glucose, calcium, phosphorus, renal and liver function tests
Electrocardiogram
Skin test for tuberculosis
Chest x-ray
Computed tomography scan of brain, chest, abdomen, and radionuclide scan of bone if any of the above studies suggest presence of tumor metastasis in these organs
X-rays of suspicious bony lesions detected by scan or symptom
Barium swallow radiographic examination if esophageal symptoms exist
Pulmonary function studies and arterial blood gas measurements if signs or symptoms of respiratory insufficiency are present
Biopsy of accessible lesions suspicious for cancer if a histologic diagnosis is not yet made or if treatment or staging decisions would be based on whether or not a lesion contained cancer

PATIENTS PRESENTING WITH NO OBVIOUS CONTRAINDICATION TO CURATIVE SURGERY OR RADIOTHERAPY

All above and:

Fiberoptic bronchoscopy with washings, brushings, and biopsy of suspicious areas
Pulmonary function tests and arterial blood gas measurements
Coagulation tests
Computed tomographic scans of brain, chest, and abdomen
If surgical resection is planned: surgical evaluation of the mediastinum at mediastinoscopy or at thoracotomy
If the patient is a poor surgical risk or a candidate for curative radiotherapy: Transthoracic fine-needle aspiration biopsy or transbronchial forceps biopsy of peripheral lesions if material from routine fiberoptic bronchoscopy is negative.

PATIENTS PRESENTING WITH DISEASE THAT IS NOT CURABLE BY EITHER SURGERY OR RADIOTHERAPY*

For non-small cell lung cancer or unknown, all under "All Patients" and:

Fiberoptic bronchoscopy if indicated by hemoptysis, obstruction, pneumonitis, or no histologic diagnosis of cancer
Biopsy of accessible lesions suspicious for tumor to obtain a histologic diagnosis or if therapy would be altered by finding of tumor
Transthoracic fine-needle aspiration biopsy or transbronchial forceps biopsy of peripheral lesions if fiberoptic bronchoscopy is negative and no other material exists for a histologic diagnosis
Diagnostic and therapeutic thoracentesis if a pleural effusion is present

For proven small cell lung cancer, all under "All Patients" and:

Fiberoptic bronchoscopy with washings and biopsy
Chest, abdomen, and brain CT scans useful but not mandatory
Bone marrow aspiration and biopsy

* Patients with non-small cell lung cancer and extrathoracic metastatic disease, malignant pleural effusion, or intrathoracic disease beyond the bounds of a tolerable radiotherapy port.

involvement should depend upon histologic proof when planning curative treatment. In small cell lung cancer, CT scans are used for chest radiation treatment planning and assessing the response to chemotherapy and radiation therapy. In following patients after surgery or radiotherapy, procedures which can make interpretation of conventional chest x-rays difficult, CT scans can provide good evidence of tumor recurrence.

If signs or symptoms suggest organ involvement by tumor, appropriate CT or radionuclide scans (e.g., brain, liver, or bone) are performed, as well as radiographs of any suspicious bony lesions. Routine scans are not obtained in the asymptomatic patient because of the high frequency of false-positive and false-negative studies. Any accessible lesions suspicious for cancer should be biopsied if a histologic diagnosis has not already been made, or if treatment decisions would be based on whether or not the lesion contained cancer.

In patients presenting with a mass lesion on chest x-ray and no obvious contraindications to a curative approach with surgery or radiotherapy after the initial evaluation, the mediastinum must be investigated. Approaches vary between different centers and include: (1) performing chest CT scan, and if this is positive, mediastinoscopy; (2) proceeding directly to mediastinoscopy (right-sided tumors) or lateral mediastinotomy (left-sided lesions) on all patients; (3) proceeding directly to thoracotomy with staging of the mediastinum at this time. In patients presenting with disease confined to the chest but not resectable, thus making them candidates for curative radiotherapy, other tests are only done as indicated to evaluate specific symptoms. In patients presenting with non-small cell cancer that is not curable by either surgery, radiotherapy, or their combination, all of the general procedures are done plus fiberoptic bronchoscopy as indicated to evaluate hemoptysis, obstruction, or pneumonitis; as well as diagnostic-therapeutic thoracentesis with cytologic examination if fluid is present.

STAGING OF SMALL CELL LUNG CANCER Pretreatment staging for patients with histologically documented small cell lung cancer includes the initial general lung cancer evaluation as well as fiberoptic bronchoscopy with washings and biopsies to determine the tumor extent before therapy; brain CT scan, since 10 percent of patients have metastases; bone marrow biopsy and aspiration, since 20 to 30 percent of patients have tumor in the bone marrow; and CT or radionuclide scans of liver and bone if symptoms or other findings are suggestive of disease involvement in these areas. Chest and abdominal CT scans are very useful but not mandatory to evaluate and follow tumor response to therapy. Percutaneous or peritoneoscopy-directed liver biopsy may be performed if other findings are suggestive but not diagnostic of the presence of tumor in the liver, and if tumor involvement here would alter the planned therapy.

If signs or symptoms of spinal cord compression or leptomeningitis develop at any time in lung cancer patients of any histologic type, a myelogram or magnetic resonance scan and examination of the cerebrospinal fluid cytology are performed to determine the need for local therapy to the site of compression (usually with radiotherapy) and for intrathecal chemotherapy (usually with methotrexate) if malignant cells are detected. In addition, a brain CT scan is performed to search for brain metastases that are often associated with spinal cord or leptomeningeal metastases.

DETERMINATION OF RESECTABILITY AND OPERABILITY In patients with non-small cell lung cancer, the following are major contraindications to curative attempts by surgery or radiotherapy alone using standard treatment methods: extrathoracic distant metastases; superior vena cava syndrome; vocal cord and, in most cases, phrenic nerve paralysis; malignant pleural effusion; cardiac tamponade; tumor within 2 cm of the carina (not curable by surgery but potentially curable by radiotherapy); metastasis to the contralateral lung; bilateral endobronchial tumor (potentially curable by radiotherapy); metastasis to the supraclavicular lymph nodes; lymph node metastasis in the contralateral mediastinum (potentially curable by radiotherapy); involvement of the main stem pulmonary artery; and a histologic diagnosis of small cell lung cancer.

PHYSIOLOGIC STAGING Patients with lung cancer often have cardiopulmonary and other problems related to chronic obstructive pulmonary disease as well as other medical problems. To improve their preoperative condition, correctable problems (e.g., anemia, electrolyte and fluid disorders, infections, and arrhythmias) should be addressed, smoking stopped, and appropriate chest therapy instituted. Since it is not always possible to predict whether a lobectomy or pneumonectomy will be required until the time of operation, a conservative approach is to restrict resectional surgery to patients who could potentially tolerate a pneumonectomy. In addition to nonambulatory performance status, a myocardial infarction within the past 3 months is a contraindication to thoracic surgery because 20 percent of patients will die of reinfarction alone, while an infarction in the past 6 months is a relative contraindication. Other major contraindications include: uncontrolled major arrhythmias; maximum breathing capacities of less than 40 percent predicted; an FEV_1 less than 1 L; CO_2 retention (which is more serious than hypoxemia); and severe pulmonary hypertension. Recommending surgery when the FEV_1 is 1.1 to 2.4 L requires careful judgment, while an FEV_1 over 2.5 L will usually permit a pneumonectomy. In patients with borderline pulmonary status or a question of pulmonary hypertension, split pulmonary function testing by ventilation-perfusion lung scans can define physiologic operability. The activity from quantitative scans is summed for each lung in the anterior and posterior view, and the ratio of the normal to total lung activity multiplied by the FEV_1. Pneumonectomy is physiologically tolerable if this predicted value is greater than 1 L.

TREATMENT

After a histologic diagnosis is obtained and appropriate anatomic and physiologic staging studies are completed, the overall treatment approach to patients with lung cancer may be formulated (Table 215-5).

NON-SMALL CELL LUNG CANCER: LOCALIZED DISEASE In patients with non-small cell lung cancer of stages I and II (Table 215-3) who can tolerate operation, the treatment of choice is pulmonary resection. In stage IIIa cases with favorable age, cardiopulmonary function, and anatomy, resection should also be considered. If a complete resection is possible, the 5-year survival rate for N1 disease is about 50 percent, while it is about 30 percent for N2 disease. However, only 20 percent of all patients who have N2 disease are technically resectable, and in most cases these resectable patients are only discovered to have N2 disease at thoracotomy. Patients with contralateral or bilateral positive mediastinal (N3) nodes, extracapsular nodal involvement, or fixed nodes are not currently considered resectable. New approaches to convert patients from unresectable to resectable status include: chest wall resections for direct extension of tumor; tracheal sleeve pneumonectomy; and sleeve lobectomy for lesions near the carina. Neoadjuvant (preoperative) chemotherapy, while experimental, gives tumor response rates of 50 to 60 percent and converts many responding patients to resectability.

The extent of resection is a matter of surgical judgment based on findings at exploration. In general, conservative resection that encompasses all known tumor gives survival equal to that obtained with more extensive procedures. Thus, lobectomy is preferred to pneumonectomy, while wedge resections and segmentectomies are reserved for patients with poor pulmonary reserve and small peripheral lesions. Approximately 43 percent of all lung cancer patients will undergo thoracotomy. Of these, 76 percent will have a definitive resection, 12 percent will only be explored for disease extent, and 12 percent will have a palliative procedure with known disease left behind. The fraction of long-term survivors following definitive surgical therapy is remarkably consistent throughout major centers performing lung cancer surgery in the United States. Approximately 30 percent of all patients resected for cure survive 5 years, and 15 percent survive 10 years. The 30-day hospital mortality following pulmonary resection at major centers is also very consistent, 3 percent for lobectomy and 6 percent for pneumonectomy. As a function of postsurgical treatment stage the 5-year survival data are (1) epidermoid: stage I, 54 percent, stage II, 35 percent, stage IIIa N0–N1, 19 percent, stage IIIa N2, 13 percent; (2) adenocarcinoma and large cell carcinoma: stage I, 51 percent, stage II, 18 percent, stage IIIa N0–N1, 10 percent, stage IIIa N2, 2 percent. Thus, the majority of patients who were initially thought to have a "curative" resection ultimately died of metastatic disease (usually within 2 years of surgery).

MANAGEMENT OF OCCULT AND STAGE 0 CARCINOMAS When sputum cytology screening indicates malignant cells but a normal chest radiograph is found (TX tumor stage), the lesion must be localized. Over 90 percent can be localized by meticulous examination of the bronchial tree with a fiberoptic bronchoscope under general anesthesia and collection of a series of differential brushings and biopsies. Often carcinoma in situ or multicentric lesions are found in these patients. Current recommendations are for the most conservative surgical resection, allowing removal of the cancer and conservation of lung parenchyma even if the bronchial margins are positive for carcinoma in situ. The 5-year overall survival for these occult cancers is approximately 60 percent. Close follow-up of these patients is indicated because of the high incidence of second primary lung cancers (approximately 5 percent per patient per year). A new approach to in situ or multicentric lesions uses systemically administered hematoporphyrin (which localizes to tumors and sensitizes them to light) followed by bronchoscopic phototherapy.

SOLITARY PULMONARY NODULE When a patient presents with an asymptomatic, solitary pulmonary nodule (defined as an x-ray density completely surrounded by normal aerated lung, with circumscribed margins, of any shape, usually 1 to 6 cm in greatest diameter), a decision to resect or follow the nodule must be made. Approximately 35 percent of all such lesions in adults will be malignant, the majority being primary lung cancer, while less than 1 percent are malignant in nonsmoking patients under 35 years of age. A complete history, including a smoking history, physical examination, routine laboratory tests, fiberoptic bronchoscopy, and old chest x-rays are obtained. If no diagnosis is immediately apparent, the following risk factors would all argue strongly in favor of proceeding with resection to establish a histologic diagnosis: history of cigarette smoking; age 35 years or older; a relatively large-sized lesion; lack of calcification; chest symptoms; associated atelectasis, pneumonitis, or adenopathy; and growth of the lesion compared to old x-rays. At present, only two radiographic criteria are strongly reliable for benignity of a solitary pulmonary nodule: lack of growth over a period greater than 2 years and certain characteristic patterns of calcification. Calcification alone does not exclude malignancy. However, a dense central nidus, multiple punctate foci, "bull's eye" (granuloma), and "popcorn ball" (hamartoma) calcifications are all highly suggestive of a benign lesion.

When old x-rays are not available and the characteristic calcification patterns are absent, the following approach is reasonable: nonsmoking patients under 35 years can be followed with serial chest x-rays every 3 months for 1 year and then yearly. If any significant growth is found, a histologic diagnosis is needed. For patients over 35 and all patients with a smoking history, a histologic diagnosis must be made.

TABLE 215-5 Summary of treatment approach to lung cancer patients

NON-SMALL CELL LUNG CANCER
Resectable (stages I, II, IIIa, and selected T3, N2 lesions)
Surgery
Radiotherapy for "nonoperable" patients
Postoperative radiotherapy for N2 disease
Nonresectable (N2 and M1)
Confined to chest: high-dose chest radiotherapy (RT) if possible
Extrathoracic: RT to symptomatic local sites; chemotherapy (CT) (for good-performance-status patients, with evaluable lesions)
SMALL CELL LUNG CANCER
Limited stage (good performance status)
Combination chemotherapy + chest RT
Extensive stage (good performance status)
Combination chemotherapy
Complete tumor responders (all stages)
Prophylactic cranial RT
Poor-performance-status patients (all stages)
Modified dose combination chemotherapy
Palliative RT
ALL PATIENTS
Radiotherapy for brain metastases, spinal cord compression, weight-bearing lytic bony lesions, symptomatic local lesions (nerve paralyses, obstructed airway, hemoptysis in non-small cell lung cancer and in small cell cancer not responding to chemotherapy)
Appropriate diagnosis and treatment of other medical problems and supportive care during chemotherapy
Encouragement to stop smoking

This can either occur at the time of nodule resection or, if the patient is a poor operative risk, via transthoracic fine-needle biopsy. Some institutions would use preoperative fine-needle aspiration on all such lesions; however, all positive lesions will have to proceed to resection, and negative cytologic findings will in most cases have to be confirmed by histology on a resected specimen. While much has been made of sparing patients an operation, the high probability of finding a malignancy (particularly in smokers over 35) and the excellent chance for surgical cure when the tumor is small, all suggest an aggressive approach to these lesions.

RADIOTHERAPY Those patients who are stage III, as well as those with stages I and II disease who refuse surgery or appear not to be candidates for pulmonary resection for medical reasons, should be considered for radiation therapy with curative intent. The decision to administer high-dose and potentially curative radiotherapy is based upon the extent of disease and the volume of the chest that requires irradiation. Patients with distant metastases, positive supraclavicular nodes, pleural effusion, or cardiac involvement are generally not considered for such curative radiation treatment. The median survival for unresectable patients with non-small cell lung cancer localized to the chest undergoing primary radiotherapy with curative intent is less than 1 year. However, 6 percent of these patients are alive at 5 years and cured when treated with radiotherapy alone. In addition to potential cure, radiotherapy, by controlling the primary tumor, may increase the quality and length of life of noncured patients. Treatment usually involves midplane doses of 55,000 to 60,000 mGy (5500 to 6000 rad), and the major concern is the amount of lung parenchyma and other organs in the thorax included within the treatment plan, including the spinal cord, heart, and esophagus. Patients with a major degree of underlying pulmonary disease may have to have the treatment plan compromised because of the deleterious effect of radiation on pulmonary function. Either split course or continuous fraction radiotherapy can be given with similar survival results. The development of radiation pneumonitis is proportional to the dose of radiation and volume of lung incorporated within the radiation field. The full clinical syndrome (dyspnea, fever, and radiographic infiltrate corresponding to the treatment port) occurs in 5 percent of cases. Acute radiation esophagitis occurs during treatment but usually is self-limited, while spinal cord injury should be avoided by careful treatment planning.

COMBINED MODALITY THERAPY Recent randomized trials have shown survival benefit for adjuvant chemotherapy given after surgical resection. However, this will have to be confirmed before adjuvant chemotherapy after surgery or radiotherapy is recommended for general use. Many centers give high-dose, postoperative radiation if postsurgical staging documents nodal disease. However, randomized trials of postoperative radiotherapy, while showing improved local tumor control, have not shown survival benefit.

Carcinomas of the superior pulmonary sulcus producing *Pancoast's syndrome* are often treated with combined radiotherapy and surgery. These patients should have the usual preoperative staging procedures, including mediastinoscopy as well as CT scans to determine tumor extent and neurologic examination with electromyography to document neurologic findings. Often a histologic diagnosis is not made, and with the constellation of tumor location and pain distribution the diagnostic accuracy for cancer is better than 90 percent. If mediastinoscopy is negative, two curative approaches may be used in treating a Pancoast's syndrome tumor. In the first, preoperative irradiation [30,000 mGy (3000 rad) in 10 treatments] is given to the area followed by an en bloc resection of the tumor and involved chest wall 3 to 6 weeks later. At 3 years, survival figures of 42 percent for epidermoid and 21 percent for adeno- and large cell carcinomas have been reported. The second approach involves radiotherapy alone in curative doses and standard fractionation with similar survival to combined modality therapy reported.

Data have now appeared suggesting a high frequency of brain metastases as isolated sites of relapse in patients with adenocarcinoma of the lung otherwise cured by surgery or radiotherapy. While there is no proven role for "prophylactic" cranial irradiation, it is not unreasonable to follow potentially cured, asymptomatic adenocarcinoma patients with frequent brain CT scans to detect such recurrence at the earliest possible time so that radiotherapy can be given.

DISSEMINATED NON-SMALL CELL LUNG CANCER The 70 percent of patients who have unresectable non-small cell cancer have a poor prognosis. For example, median survivals of 34, 25, 17, 8, and 4 weeks are seen for patients with performance status scores of 0 (asymptomatic), 1 (symptomatic, fully ambulatory), 2 (in bed <50 percent of the time), 3 (in bed >50 percent of the time), and 4 (bedridden), respectively. Standard medical management, the judicious use of pain medications, and the appropriate use of radiotherapy form the cornerstone of management. Patients whose primary tumors are causing symptoms such as bronchial obstruction with pneumonitis, hemoptysis, or upper airway or superior vena caval (SVC) obstruction should, in general, have radiotherapy to the primary tumor. The case for prophylactic treatment of the asymptomatic patient is to prevent major symptoms from occurring within the thorax. However, if the patient can be followed closely, deferring treatment until the development of symptoms is appropriate. Usually a course of 30,000 to 40,000 mGy (3000 to 4000 rad) over 2 to 4 weeks is given to the tumor. The frequencies of relief by radiation therapy of intrathoracic symptoms are hemoptysis, 84 percent; SVC syndrome, 80 percent; dyspnea, 60 percent; cough, 60 percent; atelectasis, 23 percent; and vocal cord paralysis, 6 percent. Other symptoms of metastatic disease treated with radiotherapy include cardiac tamponade (treated with pericardiocentesis and radiation therapy to the entire cardiac silhouette); painful bony metastases (with relief in 66 percent of cases); brain or spinal cord compression; and brachial plexus involvement. Usually, with brain and cord compression, dexamethasone (25 to 100 mg total per day in four divided doses) is also given and then rapidly tapered to the lowest dosage which relieves neurologic symptoms. In all cases, the key to effective palliation is to detect the complication and begin radiotherapy at the earliest possible time. Pleural effusions are common and are usually treated with thoracentesis as needed, but without radiotherapy. If they recur and are symptomatic, chest tube drainage with a sclerosing agent such as intrapleural tetracycline is used. The chest is first completely drained. Then 1000 mg of tetracycline is dissolved in 100 mL of normal saline, and 50 mL of 1% xylocaine added, and this is injected via the chest tube. The chest tube is clamped and the patient rotated onto different sides to distribute the sclerosing agent. Then 24 to 48 h later the chest tube is pulled when there is little drainage (usually less than 100 mL per 12 h). Symptomatic intrabronchial lesions that recur after surgery or radiotherapy, or the development of such lesions in patients with severely compromised pulmonary function, are difficult to treat with conventional therapy. However, neodymium-YAG (yttrium-aluminum-garnet) laser therapy administered via a flexible fiberoptic bronchoscope (usually under general anesthesia) can provide palliation to 80 to 90 percent of patients even when the tumor has relapsed after radiotherapy. In addition, patients can be retreated with YAG laser therapy.

The use of chemotherapy for non-small cell lung cancer requires careful judgment to balance potential benefits and toxicity. However, recent results suggest modest survival benefit from such combination chemotherapy. Approximately 30 to 40 percent of patients will have objective tumor response to combination chemotherapy. However, a complete clinical regression of tumor (a "complete response") occurs in less than 5 percent of cases. Those patients whose tumors respond to chemotherapy have significantly longer survivals (around 30 to 40 weeks median survival) compared to those patients who do not respond to therapy (10 to 20 weeks median). The problem is that the responding patients also have better prognostic features (such as good performance status), and it is difficult to separate the effect of these on survival from that of chemotherapy. However, in patients with good performance status, response to chemotherapy is also associated with prolonged survival, and in some cases, relief of symptoms. Nevertheless, such combination chemotherapy can have severe side effects including treatment-related mortality. Thus, in those patients with non-small cell lung cancer who desire chemotherapy, it is reasonable to give chemotherapy if the patient is fully ambulatory, has an evaluable tumor mass (to follow response to therapy), has not received prior chemotherapy, and is able to understand and accept the potential benefits and toxicities from such therapy. The chemotherapy should be delivered by an experienced physician or medical oncologist, who should use one of the published standard regimens, such as "CAP" [cyclophosphamide, doxorubicin (Adriamycin), cisplatin]; etoposide + cisplatin; or mitomycin C + vinblastine + cisplatin.

SMALL CELL LUNG CANCER Untreated patients with small cell lung cancer have median survivals of only 6 to 17 weeks, while patients treated with combination chemotherapy have median survivals of 40 to 70 weeks. Thus, the correct integration of chemotherapy with or without radiotherapy or surgery is the cornerstone of the treatment of small cell cancer. The goal of treatment is to obtain a complete clinical regression of tumor documented by repeating the initial positive staging procedures, particularly fiberoptic bronchoscopy with washings and biopsy. The initial response, determined 6 to 12 weeks after the start of therapy, predicts both median and long-term survival and potential cure. Patients obtaining a complete clinical regression of tumor survive longer than patients with only partial regression (tumor shrinkage of more than 50 percent of visible disease with no sign of tumor progression elsewhere), who in turn survive longer than patients with no response. In addition, all long-term (over 3 years) survivors come from the complete response group.

Following initial staging, patients are grouped into the limited or extensive disease stages and classified as being physiologically able or not able to tolerate combination chemotherapy or combined modality chemoradiotherapy. The overall mortality rate from initial combination chemotherapy even in these selected patients is about 5 percent at major centers. This figure is comparable to the operative mortality rate for pulmonary resection and indicates the need for physiologic staging of patients before chemotherapy. Such therapy should be reserved for ambulatory patients, with no prior chemotherapy or radiotherapy, no other major medical problems, and adequate heart, liver, renal, and bone marrow function. The arterial P_{O_2} on room air should be above 6.6 kPa (50 mmHg), and there should be no CO_2 retention. All patients with some or more of these limitations must have their initial chemoradio- or chemotherapy modified to prevent undue toxicity. In all patients the chemoradiotherapy must be coupled with supportive care for infectious, hemorrhagic, and other medical complications. This induction period is best supervised by a medical oncologist. Meticulous attention to the details of therapy and the day to day management of the patient through the initial 6 to 12 weeks of treatment is essential if therapy-related mortality is to be kept low.

Chemotherapy A variety of effective combination chemotherapy regimens have been reported for small cell lung cancer, including CAV (cyclophosphamide + doxorubicin + vincristine); CAVP-16 (cyclophosphamide + doxorubicin + VP-16); and VP-16 (etoposide) + cisplatin. At present there is no evidence that any one regimen is better than another if adequate drug dose and schedules are used. The initial combination chemotherapy often results in moderate to severe granulocytopenia (e.g., granulocyte counts less than 500 to 1500 per microliter) and thrombocytopenia (platelets less than 50,000 to 100,000 per microliter). Following the initial "induction" therapy, patients should be restaged to determine if they have entered a "complete clinical remission," indicated by complete disappearance of all clinically evident lesions and paraneoplastic syndromes, or a "partial remission"; or have "no response" or tumor progression (seen in 10 percent of patients or less). Following this, "maintenance" chemotherapy is given to responding patients for periods of 6 to 12 months in 3-, 4-, or 6-week cycles, depending on the chemotherapy regimen used. Appropriate drug dose modifications are made to keep the white blood count above 2000 per microliter and the platelet count above 50,000 per microliter. The patients are restaged between 6 and 12 months, depending on the individual regimens; if they are still in a complete remission, chemotherapy is stopped. The value of more prolonged chemotherapy is not documented. Patients with a partial tumor regression are generally kept on chemotherapy until the time of objective tumor progression and then switched to new chemotherapy (either with known activity or on an experimental protocol). Patients not responding or with objective tumor progression should be switched to new chemotherapy, preferably with a non-cross-resistant combination in an attempt to get an objective tumor response.

High-dose [40,000 mGy (4000 rad)] radiotherapy to the whole brain should be given to patients with documented brain metastases. Prophylactic cranial irradiation (PCI) may be given to patients with complete responses, as this will significantly decrease the development of brain metastases (occurring in 60 to 80 percent of patients living 2 or more years who do not receive such prophylactic radiotherapy), but such prophylactic therapy has not been shown to prolong survival. Because some studies indicate possible deficits in cognitive ability that could be related to PCI, long-term quality of life after PCI needs to be further studied. In the case of symptomatic progressive lesions in the chest or at other critical sites, if radiotherapy has not yet been given to these areas, it may be administered in full doses [e.g., 40,000 mGy (4000 rad) to the chest tumor mass].

There are definite toxicities of both an acute and chronic nature that should be expected with combined modality chemoradiotherapy, particularly if chemo- and radiotherapy are given concurrently. However, retrospective analysis of long-term survivors and analysis of local failures in the chest following chemotherapy alone suggest that chest radiotherapy is of benefit, and thus it is currently recommended for limited stage patients. Patients should be selected (limited stage disease with PS 0–1 and initial good pulmonary function) such that radiotherapy can be given in full doses, by conventional fractionation, and in a manner that will not sacrifice too much lung. The radiation oncologist must be prepared to deliver tailored radiotherapy with shaping of fields during treatment, much the same as is done for Hodgkin's disease. In extensive stage disease, the routine use of initial chest radiotherapy usually is not advocated. However, in favorable patients (e.g., those with PS 0–1, good pulmonary function, and only one site of extensive disease) radiotherapy can be considered. In all patients, if chemotherapy is inadequate to relieve local tumor symptoms, a course of radiotherapy can be added.

Several centers around the world have reported potential cure rates of 15 to 25 percent for limited stage disease and 1 to 5 percent for extensive stage disease. Overall, approximately 50 percent of patients with limited stage and 30 percent with extensive stage disease will enter a complete remission, and 90 to 95 percent of all patients will have some objective tumor shrinkage (complete or partial response). These responses increase the median survival from 2 to 4 months for untreated patients to 10 to 12 months for extensive stage and 14 to 18 months for limited stage patients. In addition, most patients have relief of their tumor-related symptoms and improvement of performance status. However, the maintenance of good performance status by the patient while receiving outpatient chemotherapy requires judgment and skill on the part of the medical oncologist delivering the chemotherapy so as to avoid undue therapeutic toxicity. New treatments such as new drug combinations, very intensive initial or "reinduction" therapy with autologous bone marrow infusion, as well as novel forms of combining chemo- and radiotherapy and surgery should all be reserved for approved clinical protocols.

While surgical resection is not routinely recommended for small cell lung cancer, occasional small cell cancer patients will either meet the usual AJC requirements for resectability (stage I or II with negative mediastinal nodes) or only have a histologic diagnosis made on review of the resected surgical specimen. Such patients have been reported to have high cure rates (above 25 percent) if adjuvant combination chemotherapy is used. Thus, such uncommon, resectable small cell lung cancer patients are candidates for combined modality surgery and chemotherapy.

BENIGN LUNG NEOPLASMS

The benign neoplasms of the lung, representing less than 5 percent of all primary tumors, include bronchial adenomas and hamartomas (90 percent of such lesions) and a group of very uncommon neoplasms (chondromas, fibromas, lipomas, hemangiomas, leiomyomas, teratomas, pseudolymphomas, and endometriosis). The diagnostic and primary treatment approach is basically the same for all of these neoplasms. They can present as central masses causing airway obstruction, cough, hemoptysis, and pneumonitis with or without x-ray findings but be accessible to fiberoptic bronchoscopy. Alternatively, they can present without symptoms as solitary pulmonary nodules and thus will be evaluated as part of a solitary pulmonary nodule workup. In all cases, the extent of surgery must be determined at operation, and a conservative procedure with appropriate reconstructions is usually performed.

BRONCHIAL ADENOMAS Bronchial adenomas (80 percent of which are central) are slowly growing intrabronchial lesions that represent 50 percent of all benign pulmonary neoplasms. Eighty to ninety percent are carcinoids, 10 to 15 percent are adenocystic tumors (or cylindromas), and 2 to 3 percent are mucoepidermoid tumors. Adenomas present in patients 15 to 60 years old (average age 45) as intrabronchial lesions and are often symptomatic for several years. Patients may have chronic cough, recurrent hemoptysis, or obstruction with atelectasis, lobar collapse, or pneumonitis and abscess formation. Bronchial carcinoids, which usually follow a benign course, and small cell lung cancers, which are highly malignant, are both derived from the same normal bronchial epithelial component, the Kulchitsky cell. This cell is part of the amine precursor uptake and decarboxylation (APUD) system. Carcinoids, like small cell lung cancers, may secrete other hormones such as ACTH or arginine vasopressin and thus cause paraneoplastic syndromes which resolve with resection. In addition, bronchial carcinoids when metastatic (usually to the liver) may produce the carcinoid syndrome, with cutaneous flush, bronchoconstriction, diarrhea, and cardiac valvular lesions (see Chap. 262), which small cell lung cancer does not. Occasionally pathologists may have difficulty in distinguishing carcinoids from small cell lung cancers. Carcinoid tumors appearing more aggressive histologically (referred to as "atypical carcinoids") metastasize in 70 percent of cases to regional nodes, liver, or bone, compared to only a 5 percent metastasis rate of carcinoids with typical histology.

Bronchial adenomas of all types, because of their endobronchial and often central location, are usually visible via fiberoptic bronchoscopy, and tissue for histologic diagnosis is obtained in this manner. Because they are hypervascular, they can bleed profusely after bronchoscopic biopsy, and this should be anticipated. Bronchial adenomas must be dealt with as potentially malignant and thus require removal not only for symptom relief but also because they can be locally invasive or recurrent, potentially can metastasize, or may produce paraneoplastic syndromes. Surgical excision is the primary treatment for all types of bronchial adenomas. The extent of surgery is determined at operation and should be as conservative as possible. Often bronchotomy with local excision, sleeve resection, segmental resection, or lobectomy is sufficient. Five-year survival rates following surgical resection are 95 percent, decreasing to 70 percent if regional nodes are involved. The treatment of metastatic pulmonary carcinoids is currently unclear because they can either be indolent, growing slowly over several years, or behave more like small cell lung carcinoma. Assessment of the tempo and the histology of the disease in the individual patient is necessary to determine if and when chemotherapy or radiotherapy is indicated.

HAMARTOMAS Pulmonary hamartomas have a peak incidence at age 60 and are more frequent in men than in women. Histologically, they contain normal pulmonary tissue components (smooth muscle and collagen) in a disorganized fashion. They are usually peripheral, clinically silent, and benign in their behavior. While it would be advantageous to avoid thoracotomy in these older patients, unless the radiographic findings are pathognomonic of hamartoma with "popcorn" calcification, the lesions will usually have to be resected for diagnosis, particularly if the patient is a smoker.

METASTATIC PULMONARY TUMORS

The lung is frequently the site of metastatic disease from primary cancers outside the lung. Usually such metastatic disease is considered incurable. However, two special situations may arise. First is the development of a solitary pulmonary shadow on chest x-ray in a patient known to have an extrathoracic neoplasm. This may represent a metastasis or a new primary lung cancer. Because the natural history of lung cancer is worse than for most other primary tumors, it is wise to approach the single pulmonary nodule in a patient with a known extrathoracic tumor as though the nodule were a primary lung cancer, particularly if the patient is over 35 years of age and a smoker. This means a vigorous evaluation looking for other sites of active cancer and, if none are found, surgical resection of the nodule. Second, multiple pulmonary nodules may be resected for cure as well. This is usually recommended if, after careful staging, (1) the patient can tolerate the contemplated pulmonary resection; (2) the primary tumor has been definitively and successfully treated; and (3) all known metastatic disease can be encompassed by the projected pulmonary resection. The key is selection and screening of patients to exclude patients with uncontrolled primary tumors and extrapulmonary metastases. Primary tumors whose pulmonary metastases have been successfully resected for cure include osteogenic and soft tissue sarcomas; colon, rectal, uterine, cervix, and corpus tumors; head and neck, breast, testis, and salivary gland cancer; melanoma; and bladder and kidney tumors. Five-year survival rates of 20 to 30 percent have been found in carefully selected patients, and the most dramatic results have been seen in osteogenic sarcomas, where resection of pulmonary metastases (sometimes requiring several thoracotomies) is becoming a standard curative treatment approach.

REFERENCES

BENOWITZ NL: Pharmacologic aspects of cigarette smoking and nicotine addiction. N Engl J Med 319:1318, 1988

BRUTINEL WM et al: A two-year experience with the neodymium-YAG laser in endobronchial obstruction. Chest 8:159, 1987

BUNN PA JR: Lung cancer. Semin Oncol 15(1):318, 1988

FINKELSTEIN DM et al: Long-term survivors in metastatic non-small cell lung cancer: An Eastern Cooperative Oncology Group Study. J Clin Oncol 4:702, 1986

FONTANA RS: Screening for lung cancer, recent experience in the United States. Cancer Treat Res 28:91, 1986

LUNG CANCER STUDY GROUP: Effects of postoperative mediastinal radiation on completely resected stage II and stage III epidermoid cancer of the lung. N Engl J Med 315:1377, 1986

MARTINI N et al: Comparative merits of conventional, computed tomographic, and magnetic resonance imaging in assessing mediastinal involvement in surgically confirmed lung carcinoma. J Thorac Cardiovasc Surg 90:639, 1985

MINNA JD et al: Lung cancer, in *The Principles and Practice of Oncology*, 3d ed, VT DeVita et al (eds). Philadelphia, Lippincott, 1989

——— et al: Genetic changes involved in the pathogenesis of human lung cancer including oncogene activation, chromosomal deletions, and autocrine growth factor production, in *Accomplishments in Cancer Research 1987*, JG Fortner, JE Rhoads (eds). General Motors Cancer Research Foundation, Philadelphia, Lippincott, 1988, p 155

MOUNTAIN CF: Prognostic implications of the International Staging System for Lung Cancer: A new international staging system for lung cancer. Chest 89:225s, 1986; Semin Oncol 15:236, 1988

RUCKDESCHEL JC et al: A randomized trial of the four most active regimens for metastatic non-small cell lung cancer. J Clin Oncol 4:14, 1986

SEIFTER EJ, IHDE DC: Therapy of small cell lung cancer: A perspective on two decades of clinical research. Semin Oncol 15:278, 1988

216 DISORDERS OF THE PLEURA, MEDIASTINUM, AND DIAPHRAGM

DAVID J. PIERSON

THE PLEURA

STRUCTURE AND FUNCTION The visceral and parietal pleurae consist of single layers of mesothelial cells, along with blood vessels, lymphatics, and connective tissue, that are separated by the pleural space. The latter is one of the body's "potential spaces," meaning that its volume is essentially zero unless some disease process causes fluid or solid tissue to accumulate there. Parietal pleura lines the chest cavity—chest wall, diaphragm, and mediastinum—and contains sensory fibers; visceral pleura covers the entire surface of both lungs and contains no pain fibers. Pleural fluid is elaborated from both the parietal and visceral pleural membranes, which in humans are both supplied by systemic vessels. Absorption is principally (approximately 90 percent) by lymphatics, which also absorb particles, large proteins, and cells. The remainder is absorbed by convection across the mesothelium into the lung or chest wall.

The pleural space is like an interstitial space, and excessive fluid can collect there (pleural effusion) according to the Frank-Starling relationship among hydrostatic pressure, osmotic pressure, and capillary permeability: excessive back-pressure from the visceral surface (e.g., congestive heart failure), a profound decrease in serum proteins (e.g., nephrotic syndrome), and pulmonary inflammation or lymphatic obstruction (e.g., pneumonia or infiltrating tumor) can all be associated with pleural effusion.

CLINICAL MANIFESTATIONS OF PLEURAL DISEASE *Pleuritic pain* is caused by irritation of sensory fibers in the parietal pleura and is typically produced or worsened by deep inhalation, cough, or other movement of the thorax. It is most often unilateral, sharp, and felt over the involved area, although it can be referred to the shoulder, neck, or abdomen. Pleuritic pain is often associated with splinting of the chest wall and with rapid, shallow breathing. Malignant tumors involving the parietal pleura typically cause steady, dull pain rather than the intermittent, lancinating pain of acute pleural inflammation. Pleural inflammation is often accompanied by a friction rub, a scratchy, rubbing sound heard on auscultation over the affected area during both inspiration and expiration. Friction rubs are often transitory and typically disappear as fluid accumulates in the pleural space.

Pleural effusion causes compression of adjacent lung tissue, producing dyspnea in proportion both to its size and to the functional status of the underlying lung. When an effusion is very large and symptoms are severe, removal of only 300 to 500 mL by thoracentesis may markedly decrease the patient's dyspnea. Physical signs of pleural effusion include diminished chest excursion over the effusion (when large), reduced tactile fremitus, dullness to percussion, diminished or absent breath sounds over the effusion, and bronchial breath sounds, sometimes with *E-to-A change,* from the lung just superior to the fluid level.

Symptoms of *pneumothorax* include pleuritic pain and dyspnea, although these vary considerably among individuals and some are virtually asymptomatic. Physical examination is less helpful than with pleural effusion, and the classic physical signs of pneumothorax (enlargement and diminished motion of the affected hemithorax, hyperresonance to percussion, and distant breath sounds) are often demonstrable only after the examiner has seen the patient's chest radiograph. The exception is tension pneumothorax, in which severe respiratory distress, hypotension, and tracheal deviation away from the affected side are often present.

Pleural tumors produce a dull pain, localized percussion dullness, and, when very large, the characteristic signs of pleural effusion.

DIAGNOSTIC TECHNIQUES Detection of pleural effusion on the chest radiograph depends upon the size of the effusion, the patient's position, and the technique and quality of the film. Effusions of 250 mL or more may go undetected on an upright film, and much larger volumes can be inapparent in a supine film. A film taken in the lateral decubitus position, with the affected side down, can detect a much smaller effusion (100 to 150 mL). Blunting of the costophrenic angle is the most common radiographic sign on an upright film; others are an increase in the distance between stomach bubble and lower left lung margin, a meniscus-like tracking of fluid up the lateral borders of the lungfields, and wider than normal interlobar fissures.

Pleural effusions may produce a restrictive defect on pulmonary function testing (reduced total lung capacity and vital capacity with normal ratio of forced expiratory volume in one second to forced vital capacity; Chap. 201), and its severity is related to the degree to which the underlying lung is compressed.

Thoracentesis (needle aspiration of pleural fluid) is the primary means of evaluating pleural fluid; as discussed below, its findings are used in determining the most likely diagnosis and to guide further investigation. It should be performed in all cases of undiagnosed pleural effusion, and whenever unusual or atypical features are present in effusion of "known" cause (e.g., fever or leukocytosis in congestive heart failure). In acute pneumonia, pleural effusion more than 1 cm in thickness on lateral decubitus radiograph should be tapped promptly, or, if small, followed using frequent repeat films with thoracentesis if an increase in size occurs.

Closed pleural biopsy, using any of several needles designed for this purpose, is unnecessary if the fluid is a transudate but indicated in any undiagnosed exudative effusion (see next section). Sufficient fluid should be present to separate the two pleural surfaces in order to reduce the likelihood of lung puncture. Ultrasound guidance can be helpful when the effusion is small or loculated. Several specimens should be taken, and a repeat procedure may be necessary to document diagnoses such as tuberculosis and certain malignancies. In cases in which an exudative pleural effusion remains undiagnosed despite needle pleural biopsy, pleuroscopy (thoracoscopy) under general anesthesia may be helpful. In experienced hands this procedure can frequently obviate thoracotomy.

PLEURAL EFFUSION Clinical evaluation of a patient with pleural effusion relies heavily upon examination of fluid obtained by thoracentesis. Effusions are most conveniently separated into transudates (ultrafiltrates of plasma resulting from increased hydrostatic pressure or profoundly decreased serum oncotic pressure) and exudates (protein-rich effusions resulting from increased capillary permeability), as characterized further in Table 216-1. An exudate is present whenever the total fluid/serum protein ratio exceeds 0.5 or the pleural fluid lactic dehydrogenase level exceeds 60 percent of the serum level.

TABLE 216-1 Evaluation of pleural fluid

	Transudate	Exudate
Typical appearance	Clear	Clear, cloudy, or bloody
Protein		
Absolute value	<3.0 g/dL	>3.0 g/dL*
Pleural fluid/serum ratio	<0.5	>0.5
Lactic dehydrogenase		
Absolute value	<200 IU/L	>200 IU/L
Pleural fluid/serum ratio	<0.6	>0.6
Glucose	>60 mg/dL (usually same as in blood)	Variable; often <60 mg/dL
Leukocytes	<1000/mL	>1000/mL
Polymorphonuclear	<50%	Usually >50% in acute inflammation
Erythrocytes	<5000/mL†	Variable
Pleural biopsy indicated?	No	Parapneumonic/other acute inflammation: no; chronic/subacute or undiagnosed effusion: yes

*Less in hypoproteinemic states.
†Assuming atraumatic tap.

Differential diagnosis Presence of a transudative pleural effusion generally denotes a systemic condition rather than pleural disease, whereas an exudate usually implies pathology involving the pleura itself. Aside from demonstration of organisms or malignant cells in the fluid, however, few findings are pathognomonic for specific diagnoses. Erythrocyte counts exceeding 100,000 per milliliter, when not associated with trauma, are most often seen in malignancy and pulmonary embolism. Pleural fluid eosinophilia (>10 percent of all cells) may be seen in resolving infection, hydropneumothorax, asbestos-related effusion, and other conditions. A low glucose concentration (<60 mg/dL) suggests empyema, malignancy, and tuberculosis, but this is variable; very low levels (<15 mg/dL) are characteristic of rheumatoid effusions.

Pleural fluid pH has enjoyed considerable popularity as a diagnostic aid. Its main use is in distinguishing complicated (e.g., infected) from benign parapneumonic effusions, and even here it has not proved as valuable as originally suggested. A value of <7.00 units in a patient with pneumonia indicates the presence of empyema, but nearly always when this occurs, the Gram stain is positive or the fluid is frankly purulent. Values of less than 7.20 units are often found in empyema, but do not always indicate the need for thoracostomy tube drainage. Pleural fluid pH is sufficiently variable and nonspecific in conditions other than pneumonia to be of dubious clinical value.

Table 216-2 lists the principal causes of pleural effusion, in roughly descending order of frequency, along with characteristics of the effusion in each. Congestive heart failure causes more effusions than any other condition, with parapneumonic effusion, malignancy-associated effusion, and effusion associated with pulmonary embolism next in frequency.

Pleural effusion in malignancy Most malignancy-associated pleural effusions occur in patients with lung cancer (35 percent of such effusions), breast cancer (25 percent), or lymphoma (10 percent). Pleural effusion in patients with malignancy is usually due to a local effect of the tumor, such as lymphatic obstruction or bronchial obstruction with pneumonia or atelectasis. However, it can also be a result of systemic effects of tumor elsewhere (e.g., pulmonary embolism secondary to hypercoagulability) or of therapy. The presence of malignant cells in the pleural effusion of a patient with lung cancer signifies inoperability, and tumor-related effusion in other malignancies generally implies a poor prognosis. Therapy depends upon the patient's symptoms. If the patient is asymptomatic, treatment may not be necessary. For mild symptoms thoracentesis may suffice. However, recurrent, symptomatic effusions usually require more definitive therapy. Chemical pleurodesis with tetracycline hydrochloride (20 mg/kg, instilled after chest tube drainage of the effusion, with clamping of the tube for 1 to 2 h) is the procedure of choice in most cases and is often successful. Thoracotomy with pleurectomy or pleural abrasion has a high success rate but is a major procedure with significant mortality. Systemic chemotherapy is generally ineffective, as is radiotherapy unless mediastinal lymph node enlargement is causing the effusion.

Chylothorax Pleural effusion due to leakage of chyle (thoracic duct lymph) into the pleural space is usually associated with lymphoma, lung cancer with mediastinal spread, or mediastinal fibrosis and may also be seen following trauma. The fluid is a milky-appearing exudate, usually with demonstrable fat globules on Sudan III staining and a total fat content of 1 to 4 g/dL. The cholesterol concentration is low. Therapy is usually unsuccessful in chylothorax associated with malignancy, although radiotherapy may be beneficial in some cases. Surgery becomes necessary in posttraumatic chylothorax if chyle drainage persists for more than 10 days.

Pseudochylothorax, a rare condition with similar gross appearance but high cholesterol content and demonstrable cholesterol crystals, is seen in long-standing benign effusions such as those due to tuberculosis or rheumatoid arthritis.

Hemothorax This is defined as a grossly bloody pleural effusion, with hematocrit at least 25 percent of that in the peripheral blood. Its usual cause is penetrating or nonpenetrating chest trauma, but it may also be iatrogenic (following central line placement, thoracentesis, or pleural biopsy, especially in patients with coagulopathy) or may occur in association with spontaneous pneumothorax. Therapy consists of thoracostomy tube drainage, both to remove the blood and to monitor the rate of bleeding; massive or persistent blood loss

TABLE 216-2 Characteristics of pleural effusion in different disorders*

Condition	Typical findings
Congestive heart failure	Transudate; protein may increase with diuresis or chronicity; right side more frequent but often bilateral; may localize in fissure (pseudotumor)
Pneumonia	Exudate; bacterial infections: in ⅓ of patients (more with pneumococcus and gram-negatives), cells mainly polymorphonuclears; viral infections: less common, usually small, cells mainly mononuclear; may be eosinophilic (>10%) in either; designated an empyema when organisms or gross purulence present
Malignancy	Exudate: lymphocytic, often hemorrhagic, with malignant cells in fluid or on pleural biopsy; often large and symptomatic; frequency: lung > breast > lymphoma > others
Pulmonary embolism	Exudate (75%) or transudate (25%); may be hemorrhagic; occurs in ⅓ to ½ of patients
Tuberculosis	Exudate: lymphocyte-predominant, high-protein; eosinophilia (>10%) rare; unilateral; small to moderate in majority; usually no associated parenchymal abnormality on chest radiograph; tubercle bacilli demonstrable in 10% on smear, 25% on culture, 50–75% on pleural biopsy; presentation either acute (<1 week, fever, chest pain) or subacute; can be asymptomatic
Cirrhosis	Transudate; usually right-sided; can be massive and symptomatic, even without marked ascites
Rheumatoid arthritis	Exudate; leukocyte count variable; glucose often very low (<15 mg/dL); LDH may be very high; may contain high cholesterol level and/or crystals; effusion occurs in 5% of patients, more commonly in men; may persist for months and require repeated drainage
Systemic lupus erythematosus	Exudate; leukocyte count variable; glucose near serum level; fluid complement levels (C3, C4 components) typically low; LE cells may be present; effusion occurs in ⅓ to ½ of patients; often bilateral, usually small and of short duration
Drug-induced effusion	Exudate; in drug-induced lupus, characteristics are similar to those in naturally occurring lupus; uncommon otherwise; often eosinophilic
Dressler's syndrome	Exudate; in setting of pleuropericarditis following myocardial infarction, trauma, or surgery involving pericardium
Benign asbestos-related effusion	Exudate: cells variable, often serosanguineous; may be eosinophilic (>10%); sometimes bilateral; can recur; usually small to moderate in size; asymptomatic in ⅔; related to amount of exposure; shorter lag time than with other asbestos-related conditions
Pancreatitis	Exudate with high amylase (of pancreatic origin); usually small-to-moderate size; typically left-sided but may be bilateral
Intraabdominal abscess	Exudate; leukocyte count (polymorphonuclears) often very high; glucose >60 mg/dL; sterile
Esophageal perforation	Rapidly increasing exudate, often with air-fluid level; epithelial cells, sometimes with food particles; high amylase (of salivary origin); may be on either side or bilateral; usually acute presentation with severe pain, toxicity, prostration

*In roughly descending order of frequency in clinical practice.

(e.g., >200 mL/h for >4 to 6 h) generally indicates the need for thoracotomy.

Empyema Pleural empyema (empyema thoracis) consists of a pleural fluid collection that is infected and/or frank pus. It is usually due to contiguous bacterial infection of the lung, but can also occur following external contamination (penetrating trauma, chest tube placement, or other surgical procedure) or esophageal perforation. Empyema can also develop as a complication of bacteremia from a distant source. Successful therapy requires prompt, complete drainage in addition to appropriate antibiotics administered systemically. Although needle aspiration may be attempted in early empyema if it is small and the fluid is thin, repeated aspiration and at least daily radiographic examinations will be required until it is certain that this has been successful. Chest tube drainage should be the initial therapy in most instances. Promptness is important, as loculation of the fluid sometimes develops within hours. If this happens, or if the patient does not defervesce within a few days, early limited thoracotomy, with resection of a small section of rib and establishment of assured drainage, is the therapy of choice. This approach appears to decrease morbidity and length of hospitalization as compared to "conservative" management with the ever-present hazard of fibrothorax despite the use of multiple chest tubes, instillation of fibrinolytic agents, and repeated drainage of loculations.

PNEUMOTHORAX Lung inflation is maintained so long as the pleural surfaces remain in complete contact. However, if air enters the pleural space from any source (pneumothorax), the lung will collapse in proportion to its natural elastic recoil (less than normal in emphysema, more in pulmonary fibrosis) and the quantity of air that accumulates. Tension pneumothorax occurs when pleural air collects under pressure, as when a flap of tissue permits air to enter the pleural space during deep breathing, coughing, or positive-pressure breathing but prevents it from leaving. Intrapleural pressures of more than 15 to 20 cmH_2O displace the mediastinum and compromise venous return to the heart, creating a true medical emergency.

Primary (simple) spontaneous pneumothorax This is a disorder most commonly affecting tall, slender men between 20 and 40 years of age and is believed to occur when subpleural blebs at the lung apices rupture directly into the pleural space. Although the pathophysiology is uncertain, the blebs may be a consequence of the increased traction placed on the uppermost parts of the lung during maximal inflation. From 30 to 50 percent of affected individuals experience a recurrence (75 percent ipsilateral, 25 percent contralateral), and after one recurrence subsequent episodes are much more likely. Chest pain and dyspnea are the usual symptoms, the former often beginning abruptly while the patient is at rest and tending to lessen as the pneumothorax increases in size. Severe, incapacitating symptoms are rare, as is tension pneumothorax.

Management is designed both to reexpand the affected lung and to decrease the likelihood of a recurrence on that side. Whether and how to drain the pleural air collection depends upon the size of the pneumothorax. Very small primary spontaneous pneumothoraces (< 10 to 15 percent of the diameter of the hemithorax on chest radiograph) may be observed without treatment so long as the patient's symptoms are mild and stable, although it may take a week or more for the air to be resorbed. The air is absorbed significantly faster if the patient breathes O_2-enriched gas. For larger air collections the choice is between simple aspiration and tube thoracostomy. Simple aspiration of a first primary pneumothorax, using a standard polyethylene intravenous catheter or commercial kit prepackaged with catheter and one-way flutter valve, is favored by many clinicians and permits the patient to return to normal activity sooner than formal chest tube drainage. When the pneumothorax is a recurrence or occupies >50 percent of the hemithorax, tube thoracostomy is the treatment of choice, with connection to a water seal once the air has been evacuated by suction. The tube should be left in place for 24 h after the lung has fully reexpanded without further air leak, clamped for another 24 h, and then removed if there is no radiographic evidence of recurrence. Although it is not indicated in a first episode, patients with recurrent primary spontaneous pneumothorax should probably be treated with intrapleural instillation of tetracycline hydrochloride or another sclerosing agent in an attempt to produce pleurodesis. Open thoracotomy should be considered if air leak persists after several days of tube drainage under suction, or if the condition recurs despite an attempt at chemical pleurodesis.

Secondary (complicated) spontaneous pneumothorax Unlike primary spontaneous pneumothorax, a generally benign condition which occurs in otherwise healthy young individuals, development of pneumothorax in a patient with underlying pulmonary disease is more serious and frequently life-threatening. Virtually all patients have dyspnea, most experience chest pain, and cyanosis and hypotension occur in perhaps 10 percent. Chronic obstructive pulmonary disease is the most common associated condition, although secondary pneumothorax is also a recognized feature of asthma, cystic fibrosis, idiopathic pulmonary fibrosis, tuberculosis, sarcoidosis, lung abscess, *Pneumocystis carinii* pneumonia, and several rarer pulmonary diseases. It is also common in the adult respiratory distress syndrome. In each instance the primary event is believed to be overdistention and rupture of an alveolus with dissection of air into the pleural space. The rupture may be directly across the visceral pleura, or air may dissect into an adjacent bronchovascular sheath, with subsequent centripetal air dissection to the root of the lung, and thence into the mediastinum and pleural space. This diagnosis should be considered whenever a patient with chronic lung disease develops sudden clinical deterioration. Tube thoracostomy should be performed promptly in all cases. Failure of complete lung reexpansion and persistent bronchopleural air leak (bronchopleural fistula) are more common than with primary spontaneous pneumothorax. Sclerosis of the pleural surfaces using tetracycline or another agent should probably be done after the first episode, because of the seriousness of the condition.

Traumatic pneumothorax This may follow either penetrating or nonpenetrating chest trauma. The air may reach the pleural space by alveolar overdistention and rupture, direct laceration of the lung by fractured rib or foreign object, or by entry of air directly through the chest wall. Treatment is by tube thoracostomy. If there is a large air leak and the lung fails to reexpand with suction, injury to the trachea or main bronchus should be suspected. Hydropneumothorax after closed-chest injury may be a sign of esophageal rupture, a diagnosis further suggested if the fluid contains high levels of amylase.

Iatrogenic pneumothorax Probably more common than all forms of spontaneous pneumothorax combined, this develops as a result of direct puncture or laceration of the visceral pleura (during attempts at central line placement, percutaneous lung aspiration, thoracentesis, or closed pleural biopsy), transbronchial lung disruption (bronchoscopic forceps biopsy or brushing), or direct alveolar overdistention (anesthesia, cardiopulmonary resuscitation, or mechanical ventilation). The diagnosis should be suspected in a patient who develops respiratory distress or hemodynamic deterioration following any of the above procedures. It is also commonly detected for the first time on a postprocedure or routine chest radiograph. Treatment differs from that for spontaneous pneumothorax in that prevention of recurrence is not a concern. Pneumothorax developing in a patient on mechanical ventilation should always be treated with chest tube drainage if the patient cannot be removed from the ventilator. Other patients may be observed without treatment if the pneumothorax is small and asymptomatic, or the air may be aspirated using a small catheter as described for primary spontaneous pneumothorax. Tube thoracostomy may be required if the latter is unsuccessful.

Catamenial pneumothorax is a rare condition in which spontaneous pneumothorax (usually right-sided) occurs in women over 25 to 30 years of age in association with menstruation. Whether it is the result of minute endometrial implants or of passage of air from the peritoneal cavity via a small diaphragmatic rent is controversial. The diagnosis should be considered if spontaneous pneumothorax develops within 48 h of the onset of a menstrual period. Ovulation-suppressing drugs are the preferred treatment, as the condition characteristically recurs and otherwise requires surgical exploration. Pleurodesis may be the treatment of choice, especially if the woman wants to conceive.

TUMORS OF THE PLEURA Most neoplastic disease involving the pleura is metastatic. Less common but increasing in incidence is *primary pleural mesothelioma,* a tumor that may also occur in the peritoneum. Both benign localized and diffuse malignant pleural mesotheliomas occur. The rare benign form may be asymptomatic, produce chest pain and cough, or be associated with a rheumatic-like syndrome. It remains localized, has a smooth, rounded radiographic appearance, and resembles a fibroma histologically. Surgical resection is curative. *Malignant mesothelioma* is a highly malignant neoplasm associated in the great majority of cases with prior asbestos exposure (Chap. 206). The latter may have been brief, and the usual lag time between exposure and clinical onset exceeds 25 years. Mesothelioma causes dull, persistent chest pain, dyspnea, and cough, and there is often a bloody pleural effusion. While malignant cells in fluid or pleural tissue can usually be demonstrated, the precise identification of the tumor as a mesothelioma is much more difficult. The diagnosis can be made on cytologic examination of pleural fluid in only about 10 percent of cases, and from closed pleural biopsy in 25 to 30 percent; even with thoracotomy the diagnosis cannot always be made with certainty prior to autopsy. Survival from the time of diagnosis averages less than 1 year, and no clearly effective therapy exists. Radiotherapy, local or systemic chemotherapy, radical pleuropneumonectomy, and various combinations of these have failed to show convincing benefit.

THE MEDIASTINUM

Most clinicians divide the mediastinum into anterior, middle, and posterior compartments as seen on the lateral chest radiograph (Fig. 216-1). The anterior compartment consists of everything lying superior to and forward of the heart shadow. Its normal contents include the thymus gland, substernal extensions of thyroid and parathyroid glands, the aortic arch and its main branches, the innominate veins, and lymphatics and lymph nodes in addition to loose areolar tissue. Posterior and inferior to the anterior compartment is the middle mediastinum, which contains the heart, pericardium, trachea and main bronchi, the pulmonary hila, the phrenic and vagus nerves, and lymph nodes. The posterior mediastinum occupies the space seen within the margins of the thoracic vertebrae on lateral projection; it normally contains the esophagus, descending aorta, azygos and hemiazygos veins, thoracic duct, vagus nerve, sympathetic chains, and lymph nodes. Assigning these structures to the three compartments is in agreement with embryonic development, and helps to understand how disease processes involving the mediastinum are manifested clinically.

FIGURE 216-1 Division of the mediastinum into anterior, middle, and posterior compartments, as visualized in the lateral projection. (*From Pierson.*)

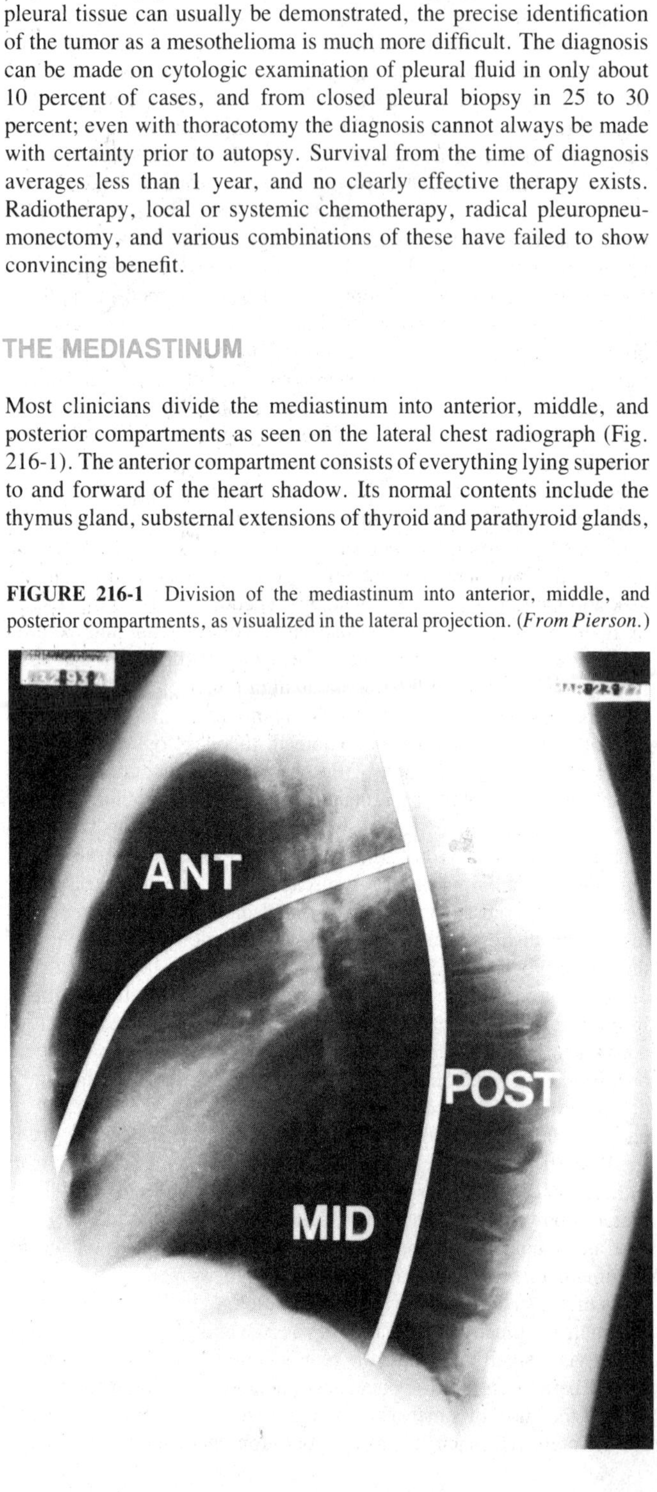

Methods of investigating the mediastinum include imaging by conventional radiography, computed tomography, magnetic resonance imaging, and radionuclide scanning. Techniques for obtaining mediastinal tissue, usually necessary for diagnosis of a mediastinal mass, include several procedures of varying invasiveness. Transbronchial needle aspiration of subcarinal or paratracheal lymph nodes via the fiberoptic bronchoscope may help to establish unresectability in patients with lung cancer. For many years the "gold standard" for mediastinal investigation has been suprasternal mediastinoscopy, which allows visualization and biopsy of lymph nodes and other masses in the superior portion of the anterior mediastinum. This procedure is complemented by anterior mediastinotomy, which permits access to structures in the subaortic fossa via an incision in the left second intercostal space. Although there are numerous possible complications, in experienced hands these procedures offer an alternative to formal surgical exploration with low morbidity and mortality.

MEDIASTINITIS Inflammation of the mediastinal structures is usually infectious in etiology and is best classified into "acute" and "chronic" categories.

Acute mediastinitis Once rare and invariably fatal, acute mediastinitis is more frequently encountered in the era of endoscopy and median sternotomy, and treatment is more often successful. There are several routes of infection. Perforation of the esophagus can occur, either "spontaneously" following forceful vomiting with a full stomach (*Boerhaave's syndrome*), as a result of penetrating trauma or instrumentation, or by an eroding carcinoma. The trachea can also be disrupted by any of the last three of these. Infection can also extend directly into the mediastinum from lung, pleura, and elsewhere both above and below the diaphragm. The onset of acute mediastinitis is typically sudden and dramatic, with chills, fever, apprehension, and prostration. Tachycardia, tachypnea, and systemic toxicity are prominent findings, and subcutaneous emphysema may be present. *Hamman's sign* (a crunching sound heard over the anterior chest in synchrony with cardiac systole) is characteristic but not invariably present. Radiographic hallmarks include mediastinal widening, air in the mediastinum and soft tissues, and pneumo- or hydropneumothorax. Therapy consists of prompt surgical drainage of both mediastinum and pleural cavities, along with appropriate antibiotics. Mortality may be as high as 75 percent when surgery is delayed, but can be reduced to 25 percent or less if drainage is achieved within 24 h of the precipitating event.

Mediastinitis following cardiac surgery has become an important entity during the last 20 years, occurring after 1 to 2 percent of procedures in several large series. It tends to be a less fulminating condition than acute mediastinitis in other settings. Most patients have drainage from the sternotomy incision and other localized signs of infection, and the diagnosis is generally made by reexploration of the wound. Treatment consists of surgical debridement and establishment of adequate drainage in addition to appropriate antibiotic therapy.

Chronic mediastinitis Granulomatous mediastinitis and mediastinal fibrosis represent the ends of a spectrum of chronic inflammation that causes varying degrees of host reaction and progresses in some cases to a largely acellular fibrosis. Granulomatous mediastinitis, most often due to histoplasmosis or tuberculosis, is usually asymptomatic and is detected as a mediastinal mass on chest radiograph. The end stage of mediastinal fibrosis can be caused not only by these infections but also by drugs (especially methysergide), so-called multisystem fibrosing disorder, silicosis, malignancy, syphilis, radiation, and other processes. Unlike the earlier form, this condition presents with symptoms, of which those of superior vena caval obstruction predominate. Compression of the esophagus, tracheobronchial tree, pulmonary vessels, and mediastinal nerves can also occur. Patients with chronic mediastinitis present with the superior vena caval syndrome (giddiness, headache, epistaxis, facial puffiness, cyanosis, and distended veins in face, neck, and arms), or with mediastinal widening detected on chest radiograph. Computed tomography reveals the extent of involvement but often cannot distinguish between benign and malignant processes, and in most cases flexible (fiberoptic) bronchoscopy, followed by surgical exploration, is required. No therapy is of definite help. Amphotericin and other specific therapies for presumed causes of chronic mediastinitis are generally ineffective, and the benefit of surgical "debulking" in areas of extensive fibrosis has not been shown.

PNEUMOMEDIASTINUM (MEDIASTINAL EMPHYSEMA) Air may appear within the tissue planes of the mediastinum spontaneously, in association with blunt or penetrating trauma, following instrumentation of the airways or esophagus, or because of disease above the thoracic outlet or below the diaphragm. Spontaneous pneumomediastinum occurs with sharply raised intrathoracic pressure, as in strenuous vomiting or coughing, or marked pressure swings from positive to negative, as in acute severe asthma. Alveolar overdistention and a pressure gradient from alveolus to bronchovascular sheath lead to dissection of air via the interstitium to the hila and mediastinum. From there, if it does not rupture into the pleural space and cause a pneumothorax, the air may spread into the subcutaneous tissue of the neck, chest, and elsewhere. Retrosternal pain and dyspnea are the usual symptoms, although there may be none, and physical examination may reveal Hamman's sign and subcutaneous emphysema. Chest radiographs in the posteroanterior and lateral positions confirm the diagnosis. Unlike spontaneous pneumothorax, spontaneous mediastinum does not recur and requires no treatment beyond reassurance and symptomatic relief of discomfort. Hemodynamic compromise and even cardiovascular collapse have been reported, but this is very rare. Fever and leukocytosis may occur, but do not require treatment if the patient otherwise feels well.

TUMORS AND CYSTS The most practical means of classifying mass lesions in the mediastinum is according to their location, as shown in Table 216-3. Overall, the most common etiologies for a mediastinal mass in an adult are neurogenic tumors, thymomas, and developmental cysts, which together account for approximately 60 percent of all cases. Lymphomas and germ cell tumors such as teratoma and seminoma account for another 25 percent, and the other 15 percent is made up of a large number of reported lesions.

TABLE 216-3 Tumors and cysts of the mediastinum

Masses occurring in the anterior mediastinum
Thymoma
Germ cell tumors: teratoma; seminoma; embryonal cell carcinoma; choriocarcinoma
Lymphoma
Mesenchymal tumors: lipoma; fibroma; others
Thyroid
Parathyroid
Masses occurring in the middle mediastinum
Lymph nodes: lymphoma; metastatic cancer; granulomatous disease
Developmental cysts: pericardial; bronchogenic; enteric
Vascular masses and enlargements
Diaphragmatic hernias
Masses occurring in the posterior mediastinum
Neurogenic tumors
Arising from peripheral nerves: neurofibroma; neurilemmoma; neurosarcoma
Arising from sympathetic ganglia: ganglioneuroma; ganglioneuroblastoma; neuroblastoma; sympathicoblastoma
Arising from paraganglionic tissue: pheochromocytoma; paraganglioma (chemodectoma)
Esophageal lesions: neoplasms; achalasia; hiatal hernia
Diaphragmatic hernias
Miscellaneous conditions: primary carcinoma or sarcoma; pancreatic pseudocyst; thoracic duct cyst; extramedullary hematopoiesis; meningocele

At least half of all mediastinal masses are asymptomatic, and of these some 90 percent prove to be benign. On the other hand, of masses that produce symptoms for which the patient consults a physician, at least half are malignant. Symptoms are usually those caused by invasion or compression of surrounding tissues or organs by the tumor. Such complaints frequently include cough, dyspnea, recurrent respiratory infections, dysphagia, and chest pain. Superior vena caval syndrome, hoarseness due to vocal cord paralysis, Horner's syndrome, phrenic nerve involvement, and spinal cord compression are other presentations. Unique to mediastinal tumors as a group is the frequency with which they are associated with systemic syndromes. These include myasthenia gravis (thymoma), pure red cell aplasia (thymoma), Cushing's syndrome (thymoma; carcinoid), gynecomastia (certain germ cell tumors), hypertension (pheochromocytoma, ganglioneuroma), and hypercalcemia (lymphoma, parathyroid adenoma), among others.

Aside from a very few circumstances, such as the demonstration of teeth in a teratoma or functioning thyroid tissue on radionuclide scan, none of the causes of a mediastinal mass is sufficiently specific in its features to permit a diagnosis to be made noninvasively. Thus, the main focus of diagnostic evaluation is an orderly preparation for obtaining a tissue diagnosis. Unless the diagnosis is discovered in the general evaluation of the patient, as in lymphoma or widespread carcinoma, tissue from the mass will have to be obtained. Needle aspiration or biopsy suffers from the limitations of sampling error in lesions that are frequently heterogeneous, and also from insufficient material for a definitive diagnosis in many cases. Because most lesions should be removed, even if benign, surgical exploration is considered by many to be the most expeditious approach.

THE DIAPHRAGM

A continuous sheet of muscle and tendon, normally broken only by openings for the principal structures passing from the thorax into the abdomen, the diaphragm is the main muscle of inspiration. The right and left halves are innervated separately, the motor supply exclusively via the phrenic nerves (C3 to C5), and the sensory input jointly from the phrenics and the lower intercostals. When the dome-shaped diaphragm contracts, it displaces the abdominal contents downward and the rib cage upward and outward, creating negative pressure in the chest and allowing air to flow passively into the lungs. The flattened diaphragm is characteristic of a hyperinflated condition; contraction of the diaphragm actually pulls the lower ribs inward. The principal disorders of the diaphragm are paralysis of one or both of its halves and hernias or eventrations producing localized bulges or masses.

DIAPHRAGMATIC PARALYSIS Unilateral diaphragmatic paralysis is caused by interruption of the phrenic nerve, occasionally by trauma but most commonly by invading tumor (chiefly bronchogenic carcinoma). Often it may prove to be idiopathic, despite extensive diagnostic evaluation. Unilateral diaphragmatic paralysis is usually asymptomatic, discovered on a routine film or during evaluation of lung cancer, although some patients complain of dyspnea. Pulmonary function is only mildly affected. The diagnosis is confirmed when an elevated hemidiaphragm is shown on fluoroscopy to move paradoxically (that is, upward) during the "sniff" maneuver. No treatment is known.

Although less common, bilateral diaphragmatic paralysis is a much more debilitating condition, and frequently leads to hypercapnic respiratory failure. It may occur because of cervical spinal cord trauma, cold cardioplegia during cardiac surgery, motor neuron disease, polyneuropathy, poliomyelitis, or mediastinal malignancy.

Most patients complain of severe dyspnea, worse when supine, and paradoxical (inward) motion of the abdomen is observed during inspiration when the patient is in the supine position. The vital capacity is severely reduced, more so in the supine position, but the "sniff test" under fluoroscopy may not reveal abnormal motion. Measurement of transdiaphragmatic pressure changes during inspiration, using esophageal and gastric balloons, can help to confirm the diagnosis. Assisted ventilation for all or part of each day is the treatment of choice; this may be accomplished without tracheostomy using a rocking bed, corset-type positive-pressure wrap, or negative-pressure ventilator. Electrophrenic respiration (diaphragm pacing), reported by a small number of investigators to be successful in long-term management, has proved to be ineffective, uncomfortable, or otherwise unsatisfactory for many patients.

DIAPHRAGMATIC HERNIAS AND EVENTRATIONS Herniation of the stomach or other viscera into the chest through the esophageal hiatus is by far the most common of the diaphragmatic hernias and eventrations (see Chap. 237). Hernias through the foramen of Bochdalek occur in the posterolateral chest, usually on the left, and are most often seen in infants. They may contain fat, the upper pole of the kidney, or occasionally the spleen. Anterior diaphragmatic hernias through the foramina of Morgagni occur most often in patients with increased intraabdominal pressure or marked obesity. Nearly always asymptomatic, they may contain omental fat, bowel, stomach, or even liver. Radiographically they appear as an anterior rounded density in the region of the right cardiophrenic angle. Diagnosis may be aided by radiographic contrast studies or by computed tomography. Although strangulation of the hernia's contents has been reported, both types of diaphragmatic hernia are nearly always asymptomatic and require no treatment. However, surgical exploration may become necessary to exclude other diagnoses. Eventration of the diaphragm is a localized elevation of a hemidiaphragm, evident on physical examination or chest radiograph, caused either by incomplete muscle development or localized atrophy. Most often seen in obese adults, it is typically asymptomatic.

REFERENCES

CELLI BR: Respiratory muscle function. Clin Chest Med 7:567, 1986

LIGHT RW: *Pleural Diseases*. Philadelphia, Lea & Febiger, 1983

———: Pneumothorax, in *Textbook of Respiratory Medicine*, JF Murray, JA Nadel (eds). Philadelphia, Saunders, 1988, pp 1745–1759

PIERSON DJ: Disorders of the mediastinum, in *Textbook of Respiratory Medicine*, JF Murray, JA Nadel (eds). Philadelphia, Saunders, 1988, pp 1781–1829

SAHN SA: Malignant pleural effusions, in *Pulmonary Diseases and Disorders*, 2d ed, AP Fishman (ed). New York, McGraw-Hill, 1988, pp 2159–2170

SARR MG et al: Mediastinal infection after cardiac surgery. Ann Thorac Surg 38:415, 1984

SILVERMAN NA, SABISTON DC: Mediastinal masses. Surg Clin North Am 60:757, 1980

TARVER RD et al: Imaging the diaphragm and its disorders. J Thorac Imag 4:1, 1989

WINTERBAUER RH: Nonneoplastic pleural effusions, in *Pulmonary Diseases and Disorders*, 2d ed, AP Fishman (ed). New York, McGraw-Hill, 1988, 2139–2157

217 DISORDERS OF VENTILATION

ELIOT A. PHILLIPSON

HYPOVENTILATION

DEFINITION AND ETIOLOGY Alveolar hypoventilation exists by definition when arterial P_{CO_2} (Pa_{CO_2}) increases above the normal range of 37 to 43 mmHg, but in clinically important hypoventilation syndromes Pa_{CO_2} is generally in the range of 50 to 80 mmHg. Hypoventilation disorders can be acute or chronic. The acute disorders, which represent life-threatening emergencies, are discussed in Chap. 218; this chapter deals with chronic hypoventilation syndromes.

TABLE 217-1 Chronic hypoventilation syndromes

Mechanism	Site of defect	Disorder
Impaired respiratory drive	Peripheral and central chemoreceptors	Carotid body dysfunction, trauma Prolonged hypoxia Metabolic alkalosis
	Brainstem respiratory neurons	Bulbar poliomyelitis, encephalitis Brainstem infarction, hemorrhage, trauma Brainstem demyelination, degeneration Chronic drug administration Primary alveolar hypoventilation syndrome
Defective respiratory neuromuscular system	Spinal cord and peripheral nerves	High cervical trauma Poliomyelitis Motor neuron disease Peripheral neuropathy
	Respiratory muscles	Myasthenia gravis Muscular dystrophy Chronic myopathy
Impaired ventilatory apparatus	Chest wall	Kyphoscoliosis Fibrothorax Thoracoplasty Ankylosing spondylitis Obesity-hypoventilation
	Airways and lungs	Laryngeal and tracheal stenosis Obstructive sleep apnea Cystic fibrosis Chronic obstructive pulmonary disease

SOURCE: Phillipson.

Chronic hypoventilation can result from numerous disease entities (Table 217-1), but in all cases the underlying mechanism involves a defect in either the metabolic respiratory control system, the respiratory neuromuscular system, or the ventilatory apparatus. Disorders associated with impaired respiratory drive, defects in the respiratory neuromuscular system, and upper airway obstruction produce an increase in Pa_{CO_2}, despite normal lungs, because of a reduction in overall minute volume of ventilation, and hence in alveolar ventilation. In contrast, disorders of the chest wall, lower airways, and lungs typically produce an increase in Pa_{CO_2}, often despite a normal or even increased minute volume of ventilation, because of severe ventilation-perfusion mismatching that results in net alveolar hypoventilation.

Several hypoventilation syndromes involve combined disturbances in two elements of the respiratory systems. For example, patients with chronic obstructive pulmonary disease may hypoventilate not simply because of impaired ventilatory mechanics but also because of a reduced central respiratory drive, which can be inherent or secondary to a coexisting metabolic alkalosis (related to diuretic and steroid therapy).

PHYSIOLOGICAL AND CLINICAL FEATURES Regardless of cause, the hallmark of all alveolar hypoventilation syndromes is an increase in alveolar P_{CO_2} (PA_{CO_2}) and therefore in Pa_{CO_2} (Fig. 217-1). The resulting respiratory acidosis eventually leads to a compensatory increase in plasma HCO_3^- concentration and a decrease in Cl^- concentration. The increase in PA_{CO_2} produces an obligatory decrease in PA_{O_2}, resulting in hypoxemia. If severe, the hypoxemia manifests clinically as cyanosis and can stimulate erythropoiesis and induce secondary polycythemia. The combination of chronic hypoxemia and hypercapnia may also induce pulmonary vasoconstriction, leading eventually to pulmonary hypertension, right ventricular hypertrophy, and congestive heart failure. The disturbances in arterial blood gases are typically magnified during sleep because of a further reduction in central respiratory drive. The resulting increased nocturnal hypercapnia may cause cerebral vasodilation leading to morning headache;

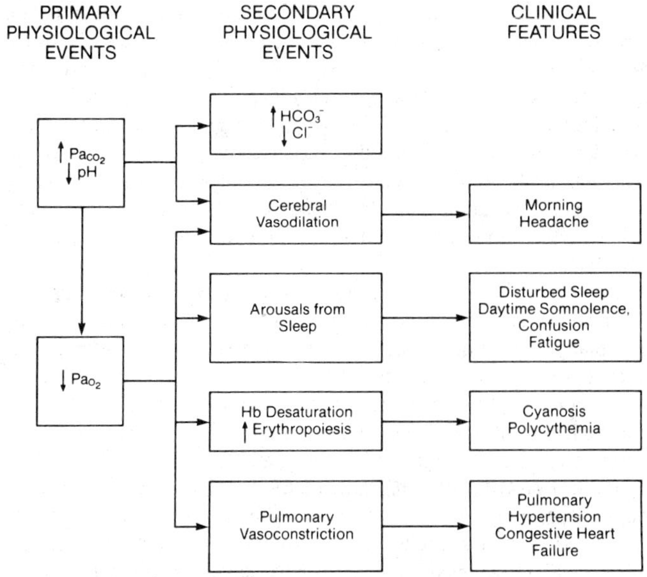

FIGURE 217-1 Physiologic and clinical features of alveolar hypoventilation. *(After EA Phillipson.)*

sleep quality may also be severely impaired, resulting in morning fatigue, daytime somnolence, mental confusion, and intellectual impairment. Other clinical features associated with hypoventilation syndromes are related to the specific underlying disease (Table 217-1).

DIAGNOSIS Investigation of the patient with chronic hypoventilation involves several laboratory tests that will usually localize the disorder to either the respiratory control system, the neuromuscular system, or the ventilatory apparatus (Fig. 217-2). Defects in the control system impair responses to chemical stimuli, including ventilatory, occlusion pressure, and diaphragmatic electromyographic (EMGdi) responses. During sleep, hypoventilation is usually more marked, and central apneas and hypopneas are common. However, because the behavioral respiratory control system (which is anatomically distinct from the metabolic control system), the neuromuscular system, and the ventilatory apparatus are intact, such patients can usually hyperventilate voluntarily, generate normal inspiratory and expiratory muscle pressures (PImax, PEmax, respectively) against an occluded airway, generate normal lung volumes and flow rates on routine spirometry, and have normal respiratory system resistance and compliance and a normal alveolar-arterial P_{O_2} [(A-a) P_{O_2}] difference. Patients with defects in the respiratory neuromuscular system also have impaired responses to chemical stimuli, but in addition are unable to hyperventilate voluntarily or to generate normal static respiratory muscle pressures, lung volumes, and flow rates. However, at least in the early stages of the disease the resistance and compliance of the respiratory system and the alveolar-arterial oxygen difference are normal.

In contrast to patients with disorders of the respiratory control or neuromuscular systems, patients with disorders of the chest wall, lungs, and airways typically demonstrate abnormalities of respiratory system resistance and compliance, and have a widened (A-a) P_{O_2}. Because of the impaired mechanics of breathing, routine spirometric tests are abnormal, as is the ventilatory response to chemical stimuli. However, because the neuromuscular system is intact, tests that are independent of resistance and compliance are usually normal, including tests of respiratory muscle strength and tests of respiratory control that do not involve airflow.

TREATMENT The management of chronic hypoventilation must be individualized to the patient's particular disorder, circumstances, and needs and should include measures directed to the underlying disease. Coexistent metabolic alkalosis should be corrected, including elevations of HCO_3^- that are inappropriately high for the degree of chronic hypercapnia. Administration of supplemental oxygen is effective in attenuating hypoxemia, polycythemia, and pulmonary hypertension, but can aggravate CO_2 retention and the associated

FIGURE 217-2 Pattern of laboratory test results in alveolar hypoventilation syndromes, based on the site of defect. Ventil = ventilation; P.1 = mouth pressure generated after 0.1 s of inspiration against an occluded airway; EMGdi = diaphragmatic EMG; PImax, PEmax = maximum inspiratory or expiratory pressure that can be generated against an occluded airway; (A-a) P_{O_2} = alveolar-arterial P_{O_2} difference; N = normal. Defects in the metabolic control system impair central respiratory drive in response to chemical stimuli (CO_2 or hypoxia); therefore responses of EMGdi, P.1, and minute volume of ventilation are reduced and hypoventilation during sleep is aggravated. In contrast, tests of voluntary respiratory control, muscle strength, lung mechanics, and gas exchange [(A-a) P_{O_2}] are normal. Defects in the respiratory neuromuscular system impair muscle strength; therefore all tests dependent on muscular activity (voluntary or in response to metabolic stimuli) are abnormal, but lung resistance, lung compliance, and gas exchange are normal. Defects in the ventilatory apparatus usually impair gas exchange. Because resistance and compliance are also impaired, all tests dependent on ventilation (whether voluntary or in response to chemical stimuli) are abnormal; in contrast, tests of muscle activity or strength that do not involve airflow (that is, P.1, EMGdi, PImax, PEmax) are normal. *(After EA Phillipson.)*

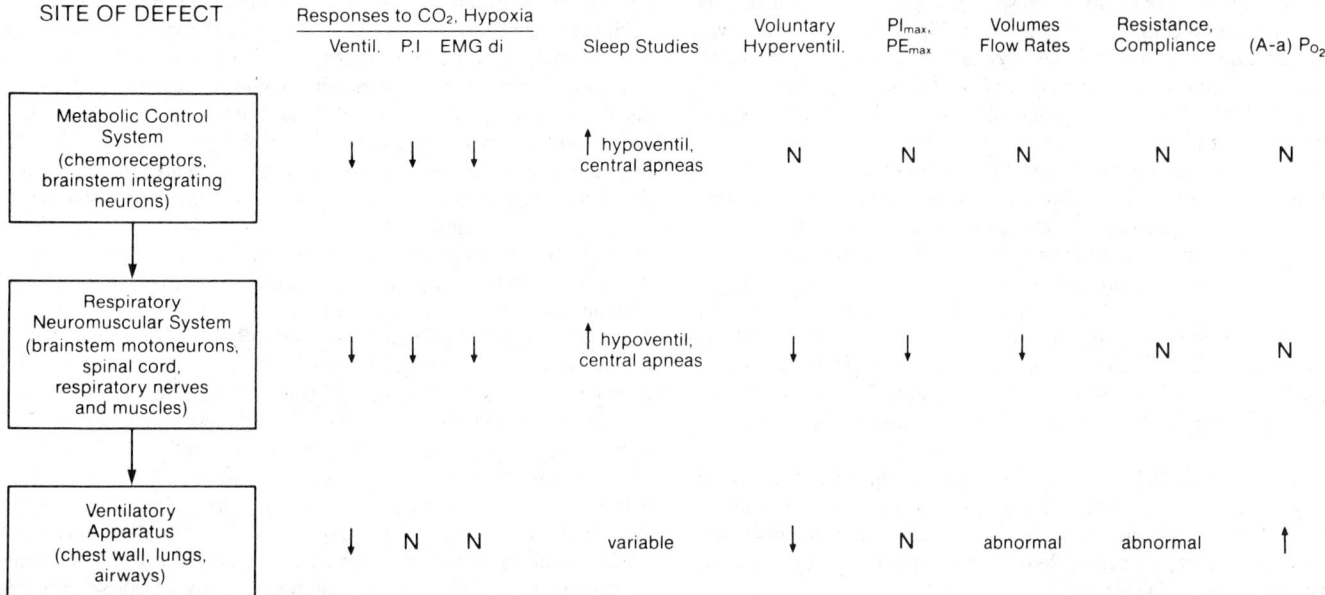

SITE OF DEFECT	Responses to CO_2, Hypoxia			Sleep Studies	Voluntary Hyperventil.	PI_{max}, PE_{max}	Volumes Flow Rates	Resistance, Compliance	(A-a) P_{O_2}
	Ventil.	P.I	EMG di						
Metabolic Control System (chemoreceptors, brainstem integrating neurons)	↓	↓	↓	↑ hypoventil, central apneas	N	N	N	N	N
↓									
Respiratory Neuromuscular System (brainstem motoneurons, spinal cord, respiratory nerves and muscles)	↓	↓	↓	↑ hypoventil, central apneas	↓	↓	↓	N	N
↓									
Ventilatory Apparatus (chest wall, lungs, airways)	↓	N	N	variable	↓	N	abnormal	abnormal	↑

neurologic symptoms. For this reason supplemental oxygen must be prescribed judiciously and the results monitored carefully. Pharmacologic agents that stimulate respiration (particularly progesterone) are of benefit in some patients, but generally results are disappointing.

Most patients with chronic hypoventilation related to impairment of respiratory drive or neuromuscular disease eventually require mechanical ventilatory assistance for effective management. When hypoventilation is severe, treatment may be required on a 24-h basis, but in many patients ventilatory assistance only during sleep produces dramatic clinical improvement and lowering of daytime Pa_{CO_2}. In patients with reduced respiratory drive but intact respiratory lower motor neurons, phrenic nerves, and respiratory muscles, diaphragmatic pacing through an implanted phrenic electrode can be very effective. However, for patients with defects in the respiratory nerves and muscles, electrophrenic pacing is contraindicated. Such patients can usually be managed effectively with either intermittent negative pressure ventilation in a cuirass, or intermittent positive pressure ventilation delivered through a tracheostomy or nosemask. For patients who require ventilatory assistance only during sleep, positive pressure ventilation through a nosemask is the preferred method because it obviates a tracheostomy and avoids the problem of upper airway occlusion that can arise in a negative pressure ventilator.

Hypoventilation related to restrictive disorders of the chest wall (Table 217-1) can also be managed effectively with nocturnal intermittent positive pressure ventilation through a nosemask or tracheostomy. Nocturnal ventilatory assistance has also been advocated for patients with hypercapnic chronic obstructive lung disease, as a means of alleviating possible chronic respiratory muscle fatigue, but the efficacy of such an approach has yet to be confirmed.

HYPOVENTILATION SYNDROMES

PRIMARY ALVEOLAR HYPOVENTILATION Primary alveolar hypoventilation (PAH) is a disorder of unknown cause, characterized by chronic hypercapnia and hypoxemia in the absence of identifiable neuromuscular disease or mechanical ventilatory impairment. The disorder is thought to arise from a defect in the metabolic respiratory control system, but few neuropathologic studies have been reported in such patients. Isolated PAH is relatively rare, and although it occurs in all age groups, the majority of reported cases have been in males aged 20 to 50 years. The disorder typically develops insidiously, and often first comes to attention when severe respiratory depression follows administration of standard doses of sedatives or anesthetics. As the degree of hypoventilation increases, patients typically develop lethargy, fatigue, daytime somnolence, disturbed sleep, and morning headaches; and eventually cyanosis, polycythemia, pulmonary hypertension, and congestive heart failure (Fig. 217-1). Despite severe arterial blood gas derangements, dyspnea is uncommon, presumably because of impaired chemoreception and ventilatory drive. If left untreated, PAH is usually progressive over a period of months to years and ultimately fatal.

The key diagnostic finding in PAH is a chronic respiratory acidosis in the absence of respiratory muscle weakness or impaired ventilatory mechanics (Fig. 217-2). Because patients can hyperventilate voluntarily and reduce Pa_{CO_2} to normal or even hypocapnic levels, hypercapnia may not be demonstrable in a single arterial blood sample, but the presence of an elevated plasma HCO_3^- should draw attention to the underlying chronic disturbance. Despite normal ventilatory mechanics and respiratory muscle strength, ventilatory responses to chemical stimuli are reduced or absent (Fig. 217-2), and breath-holding time may be markedly prolonged without any sensation of dyspnea.

Patients with PAH maintain rhythmic respiration when awake, although the level of ventilation is below normal. However, during sleep there is typically a further deterioration in ventilation with frequent episodes of central hypopnea or apnea, a disturbance that has been termed *Ondine's curse.*

PAH must be distinguished from other central hypoventilation syndromes that are secondary to underlying neurologic disease of the brainstem or chemoreceptors (Table 217-1). This distinction requires a careful neurologic investigation for evidence of brainstem or autonomic disturbances. Unrecognized respiratory neuromuscular disorders, particularly those that produce diaphragmatic weakness, are often misdiagnosed as PAH. However, such disorders can usually be suspected on clinical grounds (see below) and can be confirmed by the finding of reduced voluntary hyperventilation, as well as PImax and PEmax.

Some patients with PAH respond favorably to respiratory stimulant medications and to supplemental oxygen. However, the majority eventually require mechanical ventilatory assistance. Excellent long-term benefits have been reported with diaphragmatic pacing by electrophrenic stimulation and with negative or positive pressure mechanical ventilation. The administration of such treatment only during sleep is sufficient in most patients.

RESPIRATORY NEUROMUSCULAR DISORDERS Several primary disorders of the spinal cord, peripheral respiratory nerves, and respiratory muscles produce a chronic hypoventilation syndrome (Table 217-1). Hypoventilation usually develops gradually over a period of months to years, and often first comes to attention when a relatively trivial increase in mechanical ventilatory load (such as mild airways obstruction) produces severe respiratory failure. In some of the disorders (such as motor neuron disease, myasthenia gravis, and muscular dystrophy) involvement of the respiratory nerves or muscles is usually a later feature of a more widespread disease. In other disorders respiratory involvement can be an early or even isolated feature, and hence the underlying problem is often not suspected. Included in this category are the postpolio syndrome [a form of chronic respiratory insufficiency that develops 20 to 30 years following recovery from poliomyelitis (Chap. 355)], the myopathy associated with adult acid maltase deficiency, and idiopathic diaphragmatic paralysis.

Generally respiratory neuromuscular disorders do not result in chronic hypoventilation unless there is significant weakness of the diaphragm. Distinguishing features of bilateral disphragmatic weakness include orthopnea, paradoxical movement of the abdomen in the supine posture, and paradoxical diaphragmatic movement under fluoroscopy. However, the absence of these features does not exclude diaphragmatic weakness. Important laboratory features are a rapid deterioration of ventilation during a maximum voluntary ventilation maneuver and reduced PImax and PEmax (Fig. 217-2). More sophisticated investigations reveal reduced or absent transdiaphragmatic pressures, calculated from simultaneous measurement of esophageal and gastric pressures; reduced diaphragmatic EMG responses (recorded from an esophageal electrode) to transcutaneous phrenic nerve stimulation; and marked hypopnea and arterial oxygen desaturation during rapid eye movement (REM) sleep, when there is normally a physiologic inhibition of all nondiaphragmatic respiratory muscles and breathing becomes critically dependent on diaphragmatic activity.

The management of chronic alveolar hypoventilation due to respiratory neuromuscular disease involves treatment of the underlying disorder, where feasible, and mechanical ventilatory assistance, as described for the primary alveolar hypoventilation syndrome. However, electrophrenic diaphragmatic pacing is contraindicated in these disorders, except for high cervical spinal cord lesions in which the phrenic lower motor neurons and nerves are intact.

OBESITY-HYPOVENTILATION SYNDROME Massive obesity represents a mechanical load to the respiratory system because the added weight on the rib cage and abdomen serves to reduce the compliance of the chest wall. As a result the functional residual capacity (i.e., end-expiratory lung volume) is reduced, particularly in the recumbent posture. An important consequence of breathing at a low lung volume is that some airways, particularly those in the lung bases, may be closed throughout part or even all of each tidal breath, resulting in underventilation of the lung bases and widening of the (A-a) P_{O_2}. Nevertheless, in the majority of obese subjects

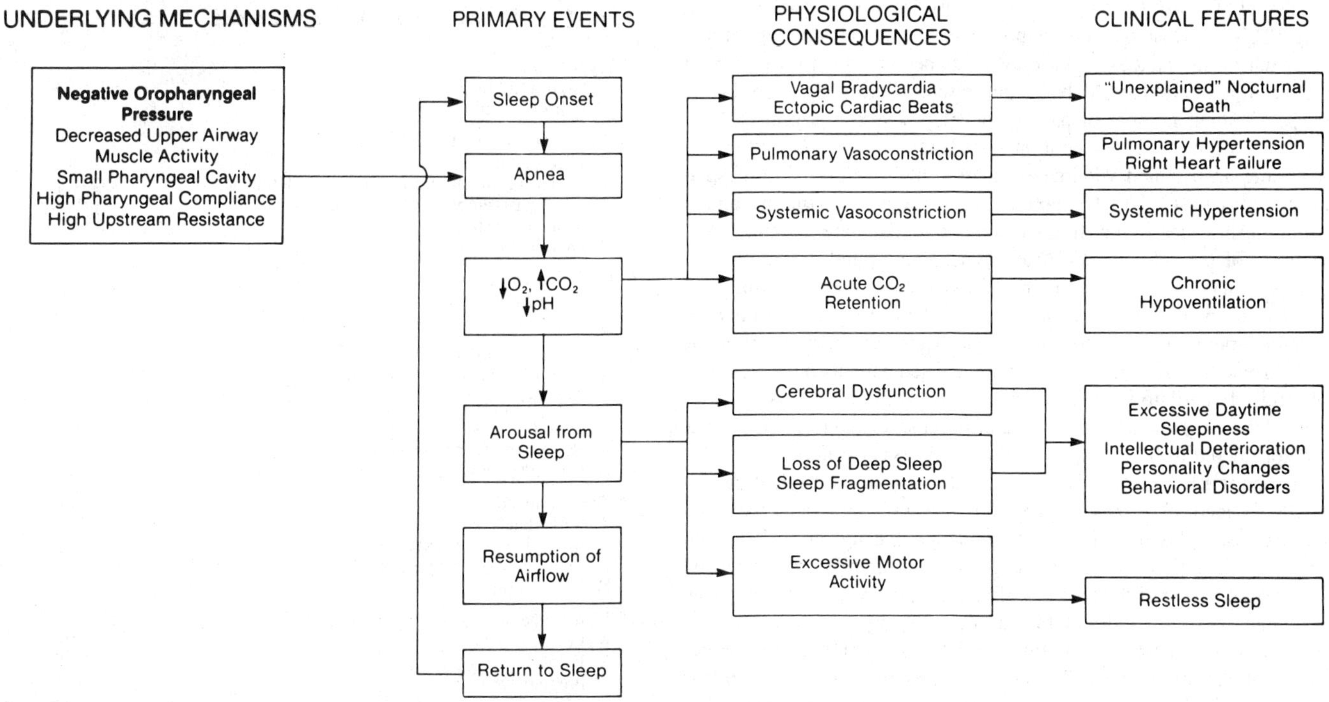

FIGURE 217-3 The primary sequence of events, underlying mechanisms, physiologic responses, and clinical features of obstructive sleep apnea. *(After EA Phillipson, Med North Am 23: 2314, 1982.)*

central respiratory drive is increased sufficiently to maintain a normal Pa_{CO_2}. However, a small proportion of obese subjects develop chronic hypercapnia, hypoxemia, and eventually polycythemia, pulmonary hypertension, and right heart failure. Those patients who also develop daytime somnolence have been designated as having the *Pickwickian syndrome* (see Chap. 34). In many such patients obstructive sleep apnea is a prominent feature, and even in those patients without sleep apnea, sleep-induced hypoventilation is an important element of the disorder and contributes to its progression. Most patients demonstrate a decrease in central respiratory drive which may be inherent or acquired, and many have mild to moderate degrees of airflow obstruction, usually related to smoking. Based on these considerations, several therapeutic measures can be of considerable benefit, including weight loss, cessation of smoking, elimination of obstructive sleep apnea, and enhancement of respiratory drive by medications such as progesterone.

SLEEP APNEA Sleep apnea is defined as an intermittent cessation of airflow at the nose and mouth during sleep. By convention apneas of at least 10 s duration have been considered important, but in most patients the apneas are 20 to 30 s in duration, and may be as long as 2 to 3 min. There is uncertainty as to the minimum number of apneas that should be considered clinically important, although by the time most patients come to attention they have at least 10 to 15 events per hour of sleep.

Sleep apneas have been classified into three types: central, obstructive, and mixed. In central sleep apnea (CSA) the neural drive to all the respiratory muscles is transiently abolished. In contrast, in obstructive sleep apnea (OSA) airflow ceases despite continuing respiratory drive because of occlusion of the oropharyngeal airway. Mixed apneas, which consist of a central apnea followed by an obstructive component, are a variant of OSA.

OBSTRUCTIVE SLEEP APNEA (OSA) Pathogenesis The definitive event in OSA is occlusion of the upper airway at the level of the oropharynx (Fig. 217-3). The resulting apnea leads to progressive asphyxia until there is a brief arousal from sleep, whereupon airway patency is restored and airflow resumes. The patient then returns to sleep and the sequence of events is repeated, often up to 400 to 500 times per night.

The immediate factor leading to collapse of the upper airway in OSA is the generation of a critical subatmospheric pressure during inspiration that exceeds the ability of the airway dilator and abductor muscles to maintain airway stability (Fig. 217-3). Sleep plays a permissive but crucial role by reducing the activity of the muscles of the upper airways. Alcohol is frequently an important cofactor because of its selective depressant influence on these muscles. In most patients the patency of the airway is also compromised structurally and therefore predisposed to occlusion. In a minority of patients the structural compromise is due to obvious anatomic disturbances, such as adenotonsillar hypertrophy, retrognathia, and macroglossia. However, in the majority of patients the structural defect is simply a subtle reduction in airway size that can often be appreciated clinically as ''pharyngeal crowding'' and that can usually be demonstrated by imaging or acoustic reflection techniques. Obesity frequently contributes to the reduction in size of the upper airways. More sophisticated studies also demonstrate a high airway compliance—i.e., the airway is ''floppy'' and therefore prone to collapse. In some patients a high upstream (i.e., nasal) resistance contributes to collapse of the upper airway by increasing the subatmospheric pressure generated in the pharynx during inspiration.

Pathophysiological and clinical features The narrowing of the upper airways during sleep, which predisposes to OSA, inevitably results in snoring. In most patients, snoring antedates the development of obstructive events by many years. However, the majority of snoring individuals do not have an OSA disorder; hence snoring alone does not warrant an investigation for OSA.

The recurrent episodes of nocturnal asphyxia and of arousal from sleep that characterize OSA lead to a series of secondary physiologic events, which in turn give rise to the clinical complications of the syndrome (Fig. 217-3). The most common manifestations are neuropsychiatric and behavioral disturbances that are thought to arise from the fragmentation of sleep and loss of slow-wave sleep induced by the recurrent arousal responses. The most pervasive manifestation is excessive daytime sleepiness. OSA is now recognized as a leading cause of daytime sleepiness and is being increasingly implicated as a risk factor for motor vehicle and industrial accidents. Other related symptoms include intellectual impairment, memory loss, personality disturbances, and impotence.

The other major manifestations are cardiorespiratory in nature and are thought to arise from the recurrent episodes of nocturnal asphyxia (Fig. 217-3). Most patients demonstrate a cyclical slowing of the heart during the apneas to 30 to 50 beats per minute, followed by a tachycardia of 90 to 120 beats per minute during the ventilatory phase. A small number of patients develop severe bradycardia with asystoles of 8 to 12 s duration, or dangerous tachyarrhythmias, including unsustained ventricular tachycardia. The presence of such arrhythmias has led to the notion that OSA may result in sudden death during sleep, but firm corroborative data are lacking. The majority of patients with OSA are hypertensive, and emerging data *suggest* that OSA contributes to the development of their hypertension. Finally, a small proportion of patients (10 to 15 percent) develop sustained pulmonary hypertension, right heart failure, polycythemia, and chronic hypercapnia and hypoxemia. Such patients have evidence of reduced ventilatory drive and many have diffuse airways obstruction. All such patients are obese and because of daytime sleepiness are considered to be examples of the Pickwickian syndrome.

Diagnosis Although OSA occurs at any age, the typical patient is a male aged 30 to 60 years who presents with a history of snoring and excessive daytime sleepiness, moderate obesity, and often mild to moderate hypertension. The diagnosis can often be confirmed by direct observation of the patient during sleep, or by the demonstration of cyclic arterial O_2 desaturation during sleep by ear oximetry, and of a cyclic brady/tachycardia by overnight Holter monitoring. However, the sensitivity of such simplified tests in diagnosing OSA is uncertain. Furthermore, while such tests can be helpful in diagnosing a sleep apnea disorder, they are not useful in identifying or excluding other possible causes of daytime sleepiness (narcolepsy, nocturnal myoclonus, nonrestorative sleep, phase-shifts syndromes). Therefore the definitive investigation for suspected OSA is polysomnography, a detailed overnight sleep study that includes recording of (1) electrographic variables that permit the identification of sleep and its various stages; (2) ventilatory variables that permit the identification of apneas and their classification as central or obstructive; (3) arterial O_2 saturation by ear oximetry; and (4) heart rate. The key diagnostic finding in OSA are episodes of airflow cessation at the nose and mouth despite evidence of continuing respiratory effort.

Treatment Several approaches to treatment of OSA have been advocated (Table 217-2). Patients with mild to moderate OSA can often be managed effectively by modest weight reduction if obese, avoidance of alcohol, improvement of nasal patency, and avoidance of sleeping in the supine posture. In some patients with more severe OSA, tricyclic medications, particularly protriptyline (20 to 30 mg at bedtime), have been beneficial in relieving daytime sleepiness and reducing the frequency of obstructive events. The role of nocturnal supplemental oxygen in managing OSA is uncertain. In some patients oxygen reduces the number of apneas, whereas in other patients it lengthens the duration of apneas. The most widely used treatments in severe OSA are uvulopalatopharyngoplasty and nasal continuous positive airway pressure (CPAP) during sleep. Uvulopalatopharyngoplasty is a surgical procedure designed to increase the pharyngeal lumen by resecting redundant soft tissue. When applied to unselected patients with OSA it produces long-term benefits in only about 50 percent of cases. More recent attempts to select patients based on the specific site of upper airway occlusion have yielded a higher success rate. Nasal CPAP, which prevents upper airway occlusion by splinting the pharyngeal airway with a positive pressure delivered through a nosemask, is currently the most successful approach to treatment, being well-tolerated and effective in over 80 percent of patients. For the few patients with severe OSA in whom all other treatment approaches fail, tracheostomy provides immediate relief.

TABLE 217-2 Management of obstructive sleep apnea (OSA)

Mechanism	Mild to moderate OSA	Severe OSA
↑ Upper airway muscle tone	Avoidance of alcohol, sedatives	Tricyclics
↑ Upper airway lumen size	Weight reduction Avoidance of supine posture	Uvulopalatopharyngoplasty
↓ Upper airway subatmospheric pressure	Improved nasal patency	Nasal continuous positive airway pressure
Bypass occlusion		Tracheostomy

SOURCE: Phillipson.

TABLE 217-3 Hyperventilation syndromes

I Hypoxemia
- *A* High altitude
- *B* Pulmonary disease

II Pulmonary disorders
- *A* Pneumonia
- *B* Interstitial pneumonitis, fibrosis, edema
- *C* Pulmonary emboli, vascular disease
- *D* Bronchial asthma
- *E* Pneumothorax

III Cardiovascular disorders
- *A* Congestive heart failure
- *B* Hypotension

IV Metabolic disorders
- *A* Acidosis (diabetic, renal, lactic)
- *B* Hepatic failure

V Neurologic disorders
- *A* Psychogenic or anxiety hyperventilation
- *B* Central nervous system infection, tumors

VI Drug-induced
- *A* Salicylates
- *B* Methylxanthine derivatives
- *C* Beta-adrenergic agonists
- *D* Progesterone

VII Miscellaneous
- *A* Fever, sepsis
- *B* Pain
- *C* Pregnancy

CENTRAL SLEEP APNEA (CSA) Pathogenesis The definitive event in CSA is transient abolition of central drive to the ventilatory muscles. The resulting apnea leads to a primary sequence of events similar to those of OSA (Fig. 217-3). Several underlying mechanisms can result in cessation of respiratory drive during sleep. First are defects in the metabolic respiratory control system and respiratory neuromuscular apparatus. Such defects usually produce a chronic alveolar hypoventilation syndrome (in addition to CSA) which becomes more severe during sleep when the stimulatory effect of wakefulness on breathing is abolished. In contrast are CSA disorders that arise from transient instabilities in an otherwise intact respiratory control system. Common to all these disorders in a P_{CO_2} level during sleep that falls transiently below the critical P_{CO_2} required for respiratory rhythm generation. The most frequent instability of this type occurs at sleep onset, because the P_{CO_2} level of wakefulness is often lower than that required for rhythm generation in sleep; hence an apnea develops at sleep onset until P_{CO_2} rises to the critical level. However, if the central nervous system state fluctuates at sleep onset between "asleep" and "awake," a pattern of periodic breathing develops as respiration follows the changes in state. During each cycle the waning phase of ventilation includes an hypopnea or outright central apnea (Cheyne-Stokes respiration). Hypoxia, whether due to high altitude or to underlying cardiorespiratory disease, enhances the tendency to periodic breathing and CSA, because of the associated hyperventilation that may drive P_{CO_2} levels during wakefulness well below the critical value required for respiratory rhythm generation during sleep. Hyperventilation due to CNS disease produces periodic breathing and CSA by a similar mechanism. Circulatory slowing secondary to cardiac failure may also induce ventilatory instability by prolonging the time lag between changes in blood gas values by ventilation and the detection of those changes by the peripheral and central chemoreceptors (Chap. 182). Consequently the ventilatory system overshoots the mark before reversing direction, resulting in periodic breathing that frequently includes central apneas.

Pathophysiological and clinical features Many healthy individuals demonstrate a small number of central apneas during sleep, particularly at sleep onset and in REM sleep. These apneas are not associated with any physiologic or clinical disturbances. In patients with clinically important CSA, the primary sequence of events that characterizes the disorder leads to prominent physiologic and clinical consequences (Fig. 217-3). In those patients whose CSA is a component of an alveolar hypoventilation syndrome, daytime hypercapnia and hypoxemia are usually evident, and the clinical picture is dominated by a history of recurrent respiratory failure, polycythemia, pulmonary hypertension, and right heart failure. Complaints of sleeping poorly, morning headache, and daytime fatigue and sleepiness are also prominent. In contrast, in patients whose CSA results from an instability in respiratory drive, the clinical picture is dominated by features related to sleep disturbance, including recurrent nocturnal awakenings, morning fatigue, and daytime sleepiness.

Diagnosis Initially, many patients with CSA are suspected clinically of having OSA because of a history of snoring, sleep disturbance, and daytime sleepiness. However, obesity and hypertension are less prominent in CSA than OSA. Definitive diagnosis of CSA requires a polysomnographic study, with the *key observation being recurrent apneas that are not accompanied by respiratory effort*. Measurements of transcutaneous P_{CO_2} are particularly useful in CSA. Those patients with a defect in respiratory control or neuromuscular function typically demonstrate an elevated P_{CO_2} that tends to increase progressively during the night, particularly during REM sleep. In contrast, patients with instabilities in the respiratory control system often demonstrate a mild degree of hypocapnia, which is an integral pathogenetic feature of their disorder (see above).

Treatment The management of patients whose CSA is a component of an alveolar hypoventilation syndrome is essentially the same as the management of the underlying hypoventilation disorder. Management of patients whose CSA arises from an instability of respiratory drive is more problematic. Patients with hypoxemia usually respond favorably to nocturnal supplemental oxygen. Others have responded to acidification with acetazolamide, and recent reports indicate a good response to nasal CPAP (as for OSA) in some patients. The precise mechanism by which CPAP abolishes central apneas is not clear.

HYPERVENTILATION AND ITS SYNDROMES

DEFINITION AND ETIOLOGY Alveolar hyperventilation exists when PA_{CO_2} decreases below the normal range of 37 to 43 mmHg. Hyperventilation is not synonymous with hyperpnea, which refers to an increased minute volume of ventilation without reference to PA_{CO_2}. Although hyperventilation is frequently associated with dyspnea, patients who are hyperventilating do not necessarily complain of shortness of breath; and conversely, patients with dyspnea need not be hyperventilating.

Numerous disease entities can be associated with alveolar hyperventilation (Table 217-3), but in all cases the underlying mechanism involves an increase in respiratory drive. Thus hypoxemia drives ventilation by stimulating the peripheral chemoreceptors, and several pulmonary disorders and congestive heart failure drive ventilation by stimulating afferent vagal receptors in the lungs and airways. Low cardiac output and hypotension stimulate the peripheral chemoreceptors and inhibit the baroreceptors, both of which increase ventilation. Metabolic acidosis, a potent respiratory stimulant, excites both the peripheral and central chemoreceptors and increases the sensitivity of the peripheral chemoreceptors to coexistent hypoxemia. Hepatic failure can also produce hyperventilation, presumably as a result of metabolic stimuli acting on the peripheral and central chemoreceptors.

Several neurologic disorders are thought to drive ventilation through the behavioral respiratory control system. Included in this category are psychogenic or anxiety hyperventilation and severe cerebrovascular insufficiency, which may interfere with the inhibitory influence normally exerted by cortical structures on the brainstem respiratory neurons. Rarely, disorders of the midbrain and hypothalamus induce hyperventilation, and it is conceivable that fever and sepsis also cause hyperventilation through effects on these structures. Several drugs cause hyperventilation by stimulating the central or peripheral chemoreceptors or by direct action on the brainstem respiratory neurons. Chronic hyperventilation is a normal feature of pregnancy and results from the effects of progesterone and other hormones acting on the respiratory neurons.

PHYSIOLOGICAL AND CLINICAL FEATURES Because hyperventilation is associated with increased respiratory drive, muscle effort, and minute volume of ventilation, the most frequent symptom associated with hyperventilation is dyspnea. However, there is considerable discrepancy between the degree of hyperventilation, as measured by PA_{CO_2}, and the degree of associated dyspnea. In patients whose hypocapnia is associated with alkalemia, neurologic symptoms may be present, including dizziness, visual impairment, syncope, and seizure activity (secondary to cerebral vasoconstriction); parasthesias, carpopedal spasm, and tetany (secondary to decreased free serum calcium); and muscle weakness (secondary to hypophosphatemia). Severe alkalemia can also induce cardiac arrhythmias and evidence of myocardial ischemia. Patients with a primary respiratory alkalosis are also prone to periodic breathing and central sleep apnea.

DIAGNOSIS In most patients with a hyperventilation syndrome, the cause is readily apparent on the basis of history, physical examination, and knowledge of coexisting medical disorders (Table 217-3). In patients in whom the cause is not clinically apparent, investigation begins with arterial blood gas analysis, which establishes the presence of alveolar hyperventilation (decreased PA_{CO_2}) and its severity. Equally important is the arterial pH, which generally allows the disorder to be classified as either a primary respiratory alkalosis (elevated pH) or a primary metabolic acidosis (decreased pH). Also of importance is the Pa_{O_2} and calculation of the (A-a) P_{O_2} since a widened alveolar-arterial oxygen difference suggests a pulmonary disorder as the underlying cause. The finding of a reduced plasma HCO_3^- establishes the chronic nature of the disorder and points towards an organic cause. Measurements of ventilation and arterial or transcutaneous P_{CO_2} during sleep are very useful in suspected psychogenic hyperventilation, since such patients do not maintain the hyperventilation during sleep.

The disorders that most frequently give rise to unexplained hyperventilation are pulmonary vascular disease (particularly chronic or recurrent thromboembolism) and psychogenic or anxiety hyperventilation. Hyperventilation due to pulmonary vascular disease is associated with exertional dyspnea, a widened (A-a) P_{O_2} and maintenance of hyperventilation during exercise. In contrast, patients with psychogenic hyperventilation typically complain of dyspnea at rest and not during mild exercise, and of the need to sigh frequently. They are also more apt to complain of dizziness, sweating, palpitations, and paresthesias. During mild to moderate exercise their hyperventilation tends to disappear and (A-a) P_{O_2} is normal, but heart rate and cardiac output may be increased relative to metabolic rate.

TREATMENT Alveolar hyperventilation is usually of relatively minor clinical consequence and therefore is generally managed by appropriate treatment of the underlying cause. In the few patients in whom alkalemia is thought to be inducing significant cerebral vasoconstriction, parasthesias, tetany, or cardiac disturbances, inhalation of a low concentration of CO_2 can be very beneficial. For patients with disabling psychogenic hyperventilation, careful explanation of the basis of their symptoms can be reassuring and is often sufficient. Others have benefited from beta-adrenergic antagonists or an exercise program. Specific treatment for anxiety may also be indicated.

REFERENCES

CHERNIACK NS, LONGOBARDO GS: Abnormalities in respiratory rhythm, in *Handbook of Physiology*, section 3: *The Respiratory System*, vol 2, *Control of Breathing*, NS Cherniack, JG Widdicombe (eds). Bethesda, MD, Am Physiol Soc, 1986, pp 729–749

PHILLIPSON EA: Hypoventilation syndromes, in *Textbook of Respiratory Medicine*, JF Murray, JA Nadel (eds). Philadelphia, Saunders, 1988, chap 84, pp. 1831–1840

———: Sleep disorders, in *Textbook of Respiratory Medicine*, JF Murray, JA Nadel (eds). Philadelphia, Saunders, 1988, chap 85, pp 1841–1860

———, BOWES G: Control of breathing during sleep, in *Handbook of Physiology*, section 3: *The Respiratory System*, vol 2, *Control of Breathing*, NS Cherniack, JG Widdicombe (eds). Bethesda, MD, Am Physiol Soc 1986, pp 649–689

PLUM F, LEIGH RJ: Abnormalities of central mechanisms, in *Regulation of Respiration, Part 2*, TF Hornbein (ed), *Lung Biology in Health and Disease*, vol 17. New York, Marcel Dekker, 1981, pp 989–1067

THAWLEY SE (ed): Sleep apnea disorders. Med Clin North Am 69(6), 1985

218 ADULT RESPIRATORY DISTRESS SYNDROME

ROLAND H. INGRAM, JR.

Adult respiratory distress syndrome (ARDS) is a descriptive term that has been applied to many acute, diffuse infiltrative lung lesions of diverse etiologies when they are accompanied by severe arterial hypoxemia. The term was chosen because of several clinical and pathologic similarities between such acute illnesses in adults and the neonatal respiratory distress syndrome. However, in the neonatal form, immaturity of alveolar surfactant production and a highly compliant chest wall are primarily involved in the pathophysiology, whereas in the adult, alveolar surfactant changes are secondary to the primary process, and the chest wall is not compliant. Despite the large number of causes (Table 218-1), the clinical characteristics, respiratory pathophysiologic derangement, and current techniques for management of these acute abnormalities are remarkably similar. It has been argued that the "lumping" of such processes of different etiologies obscures the unique features of each in terms of pathogenesis, prevention, and specificity of treatment. The conditions listed do not always lead to respiratory failure and specific treatment of the underlying processes will often be different. Therefore, the reader is urged to refer to the appropriate sections of this text for the special characteristics of each condition and to recognize that only the common features at the onset of respiratory failure will be covered in this chapter. Moreover, many of the listed conditions are often present in combination and may come into play at different times in the clinical course of the adult respiratory distress syndrome.

PATHOPHYSIOLOGY Regardless of the initiating process, ARDS is invariably associated with increased liquid in the lungs. It is a form of pulmonary edema, although distinct from cardiogenic pulmonary edema because pulmonary capillary pressure is not elevated (Chap. 36). Since hydrostatic pressures are not elevated, there is increased permeability of the alveolocapillary membranes that occurs via direct chemical injury in the case of inhaled toxic gases or aspirated acid or indirectly through activation and aggregation of formed elements of the blood within pulmonary capillaries in the case of septicemia and/or endotoxemia. Although platelet aggregation occurs, the major offenders appear to be monocytic phagocytes and polymorphonuclear leukocytes that adhere to endothelial surfaces and undergo a respiratory burst to inflict oxidant injury and release mediators of inflammation such as leukotrienes, thromboxanes, and prostaglandins. The monocytic phagocytes, mainly macrophages in the alveoli and those lining the vasculature, also release oxidants, mediators, and a series of degradative enzymes and peptides that directly damage endothelial and alveolar surfaces and cause polymorphonuclear leukocytes to release their lysosomal enzymes. Initially the injury to the alveolocapillary membrane results in leakage of liquid, macromolecules, and cellular components from the blood vessels into the interstitial space and, with increasing severity, into the alveoli. The increasing vascular permeability to proteins (decreased reflection coefficient σ, discussed in Chap. 36) leaves the hydrostatic gradient unopposed so that even mild elevations in capillary pressures greatly increase interstitial and alveolar edema. Alveolar collapse occurs secondary to the effect of the alveolar liquid, especially its fibrinogen, that interferes with normal surfactant activity and because of possible impairment of further surfactant production by injury to the granular pneumocytes. Though radiographically diffuse, the regional dysfunction is nonhomogeneous; it leads to severe ventilation-perfusion imbalance and the shunting of blood through regions in which alveoli are collapsed or filled with liquid. The lungs become less compliant—i.e., stiffen because of interstitial edema, alveolar collapse, and increase in surface forces. Because of the decreased compliance, large inspiratory pressures must be generated by the respiratory muscles so that the work of breathing is elevated. The large mechanical load may lead to fatigue of the muscles of breathing with resulting diminution in tidal volumes and worsening gas exchange. Both hypoxemia and the stimulation of receptors in the stiff lung parenchyma cause an increase in respiratory frequency, decrease in tidal volume, and deterioration in gas exchange.

PATHOLOGY In the absence of specific demonstrable pathogens, the pathology is remarkably similar among the various conditions leading to ARDS, since the lung has a limited number of ways in which it reacts to a large number of injuries. Grossly, the lungs are heavy, edematous, and nearly airless with regions of hemorrhage, atelectasis, and consolidation. By light microscopy there is edema and cellular infiltration of interalveolar septa and interstitial spaces surrounding airways and blood vessels, atelectasis and hyaline membranes in many regions, engorgement of vessels with red blood cells, and aggregates of platelets and polymorphonuclear leukocytes along with interstitial and alveolar hemorrhage. In addition to loss of alveolar type I pneumocytes, both hyperplasia and dysplasia of the granular (type II) pneumocytes are often present.

If the illness has been prolonged beyond 10 days, there is often a surprising amount of fibrosis in addition to the acute changes. In instances of recovery and subsequent death from another cause, significant interstitial fibrosis and emphysematous changes may be found in the lung. Many patients, however, will recover completely and have normal pulmonary function with no respiratory symptoms. Hence aggressive clinical management is both indicated and often rewarding.

CLINICAL CHARACTERISTICS At the time of initial injury and for several hours thereafter the patient may be free of respiratory symptoms or signs. The earliest sign often is an increase in respiratory frequency followed shortly by dyspnea. Arterial blood gas measurement in the earlier period will disclose a depressed P_{O_2} despite a decreased P_{CO_2} so that the alveolar-arterial difference for oxygen (Chap. 201) is increased. At this early stage, administration of oxygen results in a significant increase in the arterial P_{O_2}. The brisk rise in

TABLE 218-1 Conditions which may lead to the adult respiratory distress syndrome

1 Diffuse pulmonary infections (e.g., viral, bacterial, fungal, *Pneumocystis*)
2 Aspiration (e.g., gastric contents with Mendelson's syndrome, water with near drowning)
3 Inhalation of toxins and irritants (e.g., chlorine gas, NO_2, smoke, ozone, high concentrations of oxygen)
4 Narcotic overdose pulmonary edema (e.g., heroin, methadone, morphine, dextropropoxyphene)
5 Nonnarcotic drug effects (e.g., nitrofurantoin)
6 Immunologic response to host antigens (e.g., Goodpasture's syndrome, systemic lupus erythematosus)
7 Effects of nonthoracic trauma with hypotension
8 In association with systemic reactions to processes initiated outside the lung (e.g., gram-negative septicemia, hemorrhagic pancreatitis, amniotic fluid embolism, fat embolism)
9 Postcardiopulmonary bypass ("pump lung," "postperfusion lung")

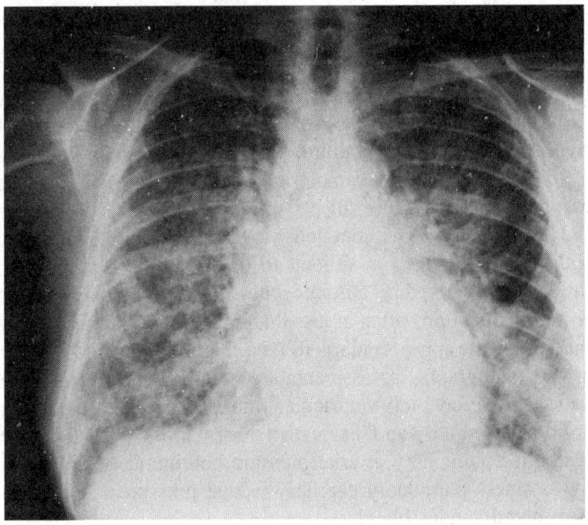

FIGURE 218-1 A standard posteroanterior chest radiograph from a patient with the adult respiratory distress syndrome secondary to a severe viral pneumonitis. Such a diffuse radiographic change is typical of all conditions listed in Table 218-1 when they are severe enough to cause acute hypoxemic respiratory failure. A similar radiographic picture is also seen in pulmonary edema due to left ventricular failure (Chap. 36). Often in such acutely ill patients, the radiograph must be taken with a portable unit and the film exposed from the anterior direction. Both the anteroposterior exposure and the failure to take a deep inspiration result in an apparent enlargement of the cardiac silhouette which further obscures the reliable detection of left ventricular failure.

P_{O_2} indicates that ventilation-perfusion mismatching and, possibly, diffusion impairment account for the widened alveolar-arterial P_{O_2} difference ($PA_{O_2} - Pa_{O_2}$) initially. Physical examination may be unremarkable, although a few fine inspiratory rales may be audible. Radiographically the lung fields may be clear or demonstrate only minimal and scattered interstitial infiltrates. With progression, the patient becomes cyanotic and increasingly dyspneic and tachypneic. Rales may become more prominent and easily heard throughout both lung fields along with regions of tubular breath sounds; the chest radiograph demonstrates diffuse, extensive bilateral interstitial and alveolar infiltrates (Fig. 218-1). At this point hypoxemia cannot be corrected simply by increasing the oxygen concentration of the inspired gas, and mechanical ventilatory support must be started. Right-to-left shunting of blood through collapsed or filled alveoli becomes the major mechanism for arterial hypoxemia at this more advanced stage. In contrast to ventilation-perfusion mismatching and diffusion impairment, with right-to-left shunts, $PA_{O_2} - Pa_{O_2}$ remains high with breathing of pure oxygen. Positive end-expiratory pressure (PEEP) serves to increase lung volume, which in turn opens collapsed alveoli and decreases shunting. With further progression, and if mechanical ventilator and PEEP therapy are delayed, the combination of increasing tachypnea and decreasing tidal volumes results in alveolar hypoventilation, a rising P_{CO_2}, and worsening hypoxemia; these represent an ominous constellation of findings.

MANAGEMENT OF HYPOXEMIC RESPIRATORY FAILURE The brief description given above contains the salient principles of management, integrated with the clinical events that lead to escalation of therapeutic interventions. Implicit in that description is that the simplest method and the lowest inspired fraction of oxygen (FI_{O_2}) should be used to give the desired result. The oxyhemoglobin dissociation curve gives some guide to the most desirable level of Pa_{O_2}. At a P_{O_2} of 60 mmHg hemoglobin is approximately 90 percent saturated. Therefore, a reasonable objective is to achieve that Pa_{O_2}, since higher levels add little to oxygenation and introduce the risk of oxygen toxicity to the lung. In contrast to respiratory failure complicating chronic airways obstruction (Chap. 210), depression of ventilation is not an important factor in hypoxemic respiratory failure.

There are multiple means for delivering O_2, in order of increasing effectiveness: soft nasal prongs, simple face masks, and face masks with inspiratory reservoir bags. The effective FI_{O_2} (that is actually entering the trachea) will be determined by the concentration of O_2 delivered from the tank or wall device, its flow rate, and the minute ventilation of the patient. In the hypoxemic form of respiratory failure, it is reasonable to start with moderate flow rates (5 to 10 liters per minute of 100% O_2) and monitor arterial blood gases, adjusting flow rates and O_2 concentrations depending upon results.

If adequate oxygenation cannot be maintained with these less invasive measures, endotracheal intubation should be done and mechanical ventilatory support should be instituted (see Chap. 219). The rationale behind mechanical ventilatory support in a patient who is hyperventilating is *not* to increase ventilation but to increase mean lung volume, thereby opening previously closed airways and improving oxygenation. This is accomplished by using large tidal volumes (approximately 10 to 15 mL per kilogram of lean body weight) at a slower breathing rate (12 to 15 breaths per minute) than the spontaneous one of the patient. Most often, at this juncture, the respiratory system is sufficiently stiff that high inflation pressures are required and a volume-cycled ventilator (in contrast to the pressure-cycled ones) is needed. If the patient makes expiratory efforts during the inflation cycle, peak inspiratory pressures will increase, possibly enough to activate the high-pressure pop-off valve, which results in delivery to the patient of a smaller tidal volume than selected. Under these circumstances during controlled ventilation, consideration is often given to sedation and/or neuromuscular paralysis. However, an alternative is to institute synchronized intermittent mandatory ventilation (SIMV). In the SIMV mode, the patient is allowed to breathe spontaneously with periodic delivery of mandatory breaths that are synchronized with spontaneous inspiratory efforts. If the spontaneous breathing rate is so rapid that expiratory efforts occur before the mandatory breath is fully delivered, sedation and/or paralysis should be used with controlled ventilation.

Should the Pa_{O_2} be greater than 60 mmHg, the next step is to lower the FI_{O_2}. If the FI_{O_2} can be lowered to 0.6 or less with a Pa_{O_2} equal to or greater than 60 mmHg the mechanical ventilation should proceed at that FI_{O_2} as long as necessary. There are two indications for the addition of PEEP, the rationale for which is to increase lung volume further, thereby opening previously closed alveoli. First, if the FI_{O_2} cannot be lowered to or below 0.6, then PEEP should be added to allow a decrease of the FI_{O_2} below the toxic range. Second, if the Pa_{O_2} cannot be increased to or above 60 mmHg with an FI_{O_2} of 1.0, PEEP should be added. The optimal magnitude of the PEEP is determined by the response of the Pa_{O_2} and the extent of the cardiovascular alterations resulting from the higher pressure. The major alteration is a decrease in cardiac output due to two mechanisms. First, increased intrapleural pressures serve to impede venous return directly, an effect which is, to a variable extent, offset by peripheral venoconstriction. Second, increases in lung volume may increase pulmonary vascular resistance, leading to increased pressure and dilatation of the right ventricle, which in turn displaces the interventricular septum toward the left. This displacement decreases left ventricular diastolic compliance; hence less filling leads to smaller stroke volumes. An additional mechanism for decreased diastolic filling of the ventricles is direct compression of the heart by the stiffened lung. The optimal levels of PEEP are those associated with the greatest delivery of O_2 to the body; the latter is the product of cardiac output and arterial oxygen content.

Patients who are critically ill may simultaneously develop both deterioration of arterial oxygenation, due to increased lung fluid and/or a fall in mixed venous oxygen levels, and precarious hemodynamics, due to the pressure effects of mechanical ventilation and/or cardiac dysfunction with either a contracted or an expanded intravascular volume. Ventilator adjustments (see Chap. 219) are not often helpful because higher inflation pressures reflect worsening lung function. In this situation of falling blood pressure, urinary output, and arterial oxygenation, the decision to expand intravascular volume by infusion or to decrease it by diuresis is difficult. Body weight change is rarely a reliable indicator of blood volume since there is often fluid retention from positive intrathoracic pressures produced by the ventilator (see Chap. 219) plus "third space" fluid sequestration, especially with sepsis. Nor is physical examination of much help since rales are usual in any case and portable anteroposterior chest radiographs do not allow accurate assessment of subtle changes in cardiac size. Therefore a flow-directed right heart balloon-tipped (Swan-Ganz) catheter is often used for monitoring pulmonary arterial and capillary wedge pressures and measuring changes in cardiac output by the thermodilution technique. Recognition of over-damping and accelerative artifacts in the pulmonary arterial pressure signal and learning the criteria for true wedging are essential if serious misinterpretations are to be avoided. Even with accurate pressure measurements, there is an additional precaution that must be taken with regard to interpretation of intrathoracic vascular pressures referenced to atmosphere when PEEP is being used. If pleural pressure is greater than atmospheric, as is most often the case with PEEP, the transmural (i.e., intravascular minus pleural) pressure will be overestimated and could lead to errors in both assessment and management. Since the lungs are stiff only a portion of the applied PEEP is transmitted to the pleural space. A reasonable estimate of the transmural pressure is gained by examining vascular pressures just before inflation and subtracting from these pressures an amount equal to one-half the value of PEEP. In view of the leaky alveolocapillary membrane it is best to keep the pulmonary capillary wedge pressure as low as is compatible with a reasonable cardiac output, arterial pressure, and urinary output. Inotropic and selective vasoactive agents (e.g., dopamine, p. 387) have been used with some success to achieve this, but require careful monitoring to assess effects and adjust doses.

Mixed venous blood P_{O_2} values have long been considered to indicate the adequacy of oxygen delivery relative to demand. A low value (e.g., <20 mmHg) surely indicates that there is tissue hypoxemia irrespective of measured cardiac output and Pa_{O_2}. However, a high value does not exclude serious tissue hypoxemia, especially in gram-negative septicemia, in which systemic low-resistance shunts can develop and leave several capillary beds underperfused.

Body position may also affect the degree of arterial oxygenation. Although patients with ARDS have diffuse lung disease, there may be some regional variation in the extent of disease such that one side is more severely involved than the other. In this instance the less involved lung should be the more dependent one when the patient is in a lateral position. Since the distribution of pulmonary blood flow is so heavily determined by gravity (Chap. 201), having the more involved lung, with its minimal ventilation, in the more dependent position results in a measurable increase in intrapulmonary shunting which may be manifested by a striking fall in Pa_{O_2}. The possible contribution of a positional effect on arterial oxygenation should always be considered before escalating therapeutic interventions.

Occasionally PEEP must be gradually increased to levels in excess of 20 cmH_2O in an attempt to maintain arterial oxygenation. At these high levels of PEEP there may be a paradoxic decrease in Pa_{O_2}. The explanation for this paradox is as follows: high levels of PEEP may not open some of the closed airways but will overdistend those alveolar units already open. Overdistention of units increases the vascular resistance in these regions and results in more blood perfusing regions with closed airways, thereby increasing the degree of shunt. The only alternative is to decrease PEEP to a level associated with the greatest delivery of oxygen to the body (product of cardiac output and arterial oxygen content).

In the situations where maximal PEEP with Fi_{O_2} of 1.0 does not supply sufficient oxygen, the possibility of utilizing extracorporeal membrane oxygenators (ECMO) has been both considered and tried. Despite the logical appeal of this form of supportive therapy, a randomized, large prospective study of ECMO therapy has demonstrated that, while it can support gas exchange, there is no effect on survival in acute hypoxemic respiratory failure.

COMPLICATIONS Increasing severity of the clinical illness and continued radiographic progressions in association with the primary process often obscure complications that arise during the course of acute hypoxemic respiratory failure. The development of *left ventricular failure* is a good example of a common, easily missed complication. This is because all patients are likely to have diffuse rales and rhonchi, even without left ventricular failure, and these sounds also serve to make it difficult to detect gallop rhythms. An additional difficulty is that portable chest films are taken in the anteroposterior direction, often at less than full lung inflation, so that the cardiac silhouette appears enlarged. As a consequence, the ordinary physical and radiographic assessments are not always reliable. With deterioration, therefore, left ventricular failure should be suspected; it is helpful to insert a Swan-Ganz catheter (see above) which can be used to monitor pulmonary arterial pressure continuously and intermittently to assess pulmonary capillary wedge pressure and oxygen content of mixed venous blood.

With a diffuse radiographic pattern, a secondary bacterial infection is easily overlooked; therefore, frequent sputum smears and cultures should be obtained, especially when there is fever. With many conditions—e.g., gram-negative septicemia, acute hemorrhagic pancreatitis, and "shock lung"—there may be associated *disseminated intravascular coagulation,* which leads to gastrointestinal and intrapulmonary hemorrhage (Chap. 289). Frequent monitoring of platelet count, fibrinogen level, and partial thromboplastin and prothrombin times is helpful in the early detection of this complication and in guiding treatment.

Bronchial obstruction by endotracheal or tracheostomy tubes is common. When these tubes are too long or poorly anchored, they may slide into one main bronchus, usually the right one because of its less angulated origin from the trachea. The tube then blocks ventilation of the other main bronchus, and atelectasis may ensue. This event usually causes abrupt deterioration in the patient with respiratory failure. It is detected readily by physical examination, which reveals the absence of breath sounds over the occluded lung. The tube should immediately be pulled back slowly if this complication is suspected. In the course of treating ARDS with mechanical ventilators and high inflation pressures, *pneumothorax* or *pneumomediastinum* may develop and may be impossible to detect except radiologically. Occasionally the presence of subcutaneous emphysema provides a clinical clue. Any deterioration should lead to consideration of this complication, repetition of the chest radiograph, and immediate institution treatment of pneumothorax, if present. If deterioration is sudden, *tension pneumothorax* should be suspected; if physical signs are present, a pleural catheter should be inserted immediately without radiographic confirmation. High oxygen concentrations (>0.60) for prolonged periods can produce both the lesions and the clinical picture of ARDS. Therefore, the *minimal* oxygen concentration associated with acceptable arterial oxygenation should always be used.

Discontinuation of mechanical ventilatory support The ability of the patient to maintain adequate gas exchange without the support of a mechanical ventilator is most often heralded by a decreasing Fi_{O_2} requirement, smaller inflation pressures for mandatory or assisted breathing, and a fall in spontaneous respiratory rate (see Chap. 219).

PROGNOSIS Given the diversity of the etiologies and the frequency of associated diseases, it is difficult, if not impossible, to give meaningful prognostic figures for ARDS. If all recently published series are taken together, the mortality rate is between 50 and 60 percent. This represents an improved survival rate over the nearly 100 percent mortality rate of a few years ago and is a result of the application of modern treatment techniques described above. If ARDS is due to drug overdose, the mortality rate is low; if associated with shock, the chances of a fatal outcome are much greater. It has become apparent that multiple organ system failure (e.g., renal, hepatic) supervenes when there is an extrapulmonic source of sepsis in need of surgical drainage and that almost all such patients die despite maximal support of the respiratory and cardiovascular systems. Other etiologies and associated diseases fall between these two extremes. The following factors appear to be associated with a poor outcome: an increase in $PA_{O_2} - Pa_{O_2}$, requiring increasing inspired O_2 concentrations and PEEP; decreasing compliance, requiring greater inflation pressures; either low or falling colloid osmotic pressures; and the onset of systemic arterial hypotension not responding to intravascular volume replacement.

In survivors with previously normal lung function, the long-term prognosis for recovery appears to be remarkably good. Lung volumes and arterial blood gases have been shown to return to normal levels within 4 to 6 months after respiratory failure. There are instances, however, when the fibrotic residua are sufficiently great that complete recovery is unlikely.

REFERENCES

COHEN AB et al: A peptide from alveolar macrophages that releases neutrophil enzymes into the lungs in patients with the adult respiratory distress syndrome. Am Rev Respir Dis 137:1151, 1988

GLAUSER FL et al: Worsening oxygenation in the mechanically ventilated patient. Am Rev Respir Dis 138:458, 1988

HOGG JC: Neutrophil kinetics and lung injury. Physiol Rev 67(4):1249, 1987

MATTHAY MA, CHATTERJEE K: Bedside catheterization of the pulmonary artery: Risks compared with benefits. Ann Intern Med 109:826, 1988

MATUSCHAK GM, RINALDO JE: Organ interactions in the adult respiratory distress syndrome during sepsis. Chest 94(2):400, 1988

PETTY TL: The use, abuse, and mystique of positive end-expiratory pressure. Am Rev Respir Dis 138:475, 1988

PINGLETON SK: Complications of acute respiratory failure. Am Rev Respir Dis 137:1463, 1988

RAFFIN TA: ARDS: Mechanisms and management. Hosp Pract 22(11):65, 1987

REYNOLDS HY: Lung inflammation: Normal host defense or a complication of some diseases? Annu Rev Med 38:295, 1987

219 MECHANICAL VENTILATORY SUPPORT

PAUL N. LANKEN

TYPES OF MECHANICAL VENTILATORY SUPPORT

All types of mechanical ventilatory support share a common life-sustaining therapeutic goal: to support respiratory gas exchange as safely and comfortably as possible in patients with respiratory failure, while the underlying condition responds to therapy or resolves spontaneously.

POSITIVE PRESSURE VENTILATORS Positive pressure ventilators are characterized by positive inspiratory airway pressures, i.e., greater than atmospheric, and, as a rule, all are used with cuffed tracheal tubes in order to prevent excessive leak of tidal volume around the tube during inflation. Currently, most adult patients are supported by *volume-cycled* mechanical ventilators in which inspiration ceases after a certain tidal volume has been delivered. As a rule, this method of ventilation reliably delivers preset tidal volumes despite severe and/or fluctuating derangements of respiratory mechanics. All volume-cycled ventilators also have inspiratory pressure alarms that function as "pop-off" valves if peak airway pressures exceed a certain value; this results in decreased tidal volumes delivered in an effort to diminish the risk of barotrauma (injury of the lung from high pressure). Much less commonly used in adults are *pressure-cycled* mechanical ventilators in which inspiration ceases once a preset inspiratory pressure is reached. The major limitation of this type of ventilator is its inability to deliver constant tidal volume when the patient's respiratory mechanics change as discussed below.

NEGATIVE PRESSURE VENTILATORS Negative pressure mechanical ventilators mimic spontaneous inspiration by applying subatmospheric pressure to expand the chest cavity and to make alveolar pressure negative. Examples include the venerable iron lung, or Drinker respirator, as well as more comfortable current versions (cuirass respirators) that enclose just the patient's trunk. Most operate as pressure-cycled ventilators with the same limitations as noted above; on the other hand, they can be used with uncuffed tracheal tubes or, in selected cases, with no tracheal tubes at all.

PHYSIOLOGIC PRINCIPLES OF MECHANICAL VENTILATION

STATIC PRESSURE-VOLUME RELATIONSHIPS In positive pressure ventilation, tidal volumes distend both the lungs and their enclosing structure—the chest bellows (chest wall and diaphragm). The relationship between tidal volumes and their distending pressures at end-inspiration defines the static compliance (Cst) of the respiratory system, i.e., the lungs and chest wall, where Cst equals the ratio of the change in volume to change in pressure (Fig. 219-1*A*). The normal range of Cst is 50 to 100 mL per cmH_2O.

DYNAMIC PRESSURE-VOLUME RELATIONSHIPS During a positive pressure inflation, the pressure at the proximal end of the tube, i.e., proximal airway pressure, exceeds alveolar pressure and provides the pressure gradient for airflow into the lungs. Note that the proximal airway pressure has two components: (1) alveolar pressure which is determined by the *static* pressure volume curve (Fig. 219-1*A*) for any degree of lung inflation, and (2) the pressure drop due to resistance by the airways to airflow. The proximal airway pressure during inflation is described by the dynamic pressure-volume curve of the respiratory system (Fig. 219-1*B*).

High peak proximal airway pressures can result from excessively high resistance to airflow, as occurs in severe asthma (Fig. 219-1*C*), or from abnormally low static compliance, as occurs in pulmonary edema (Fig. 219-1*D*). From Fig. 219-1 one can also see how the same peak pressure may deliver markedly different tidal volumes depending on the type and degree of alteration in lung mechanics; for this reason pressure-cycled ventilators are used infrequently in adult patients with respiratory failure.

INDICATIONS FOR MECHANICAL VENTILATION

Specific indications for mechanical ventilation vary according to the underlying mechanism causing the patient's respiratory failure. The latter can result from impairment of the respiratory system which has traditionally been divided into four functional components: (1) central neural drive; (2) the chest bellows, including peripheral nervous system and the respiratory muscles; (3) airways; and (4) alveoli.

CENTRAL NEURAL DRIVE Examples of patients with impaired central neural drive are those with self-administered narcotic or sedative drug overdoses, with excessive iatrogenic sedative therapy, and, rarely, those with strokes involving the brainstem. The trachea should be intubated to prevent aspiration if there is a diminished or lost gag reflex. A mechanical ventilator can then be used to monitor the respiratory rate and spontaneous tidal volumes as well as for therapy of subsequent hypoventilation.

CHEST BELLOWS (INCLUDES PERIPHERAL NERVOUS SYSTEM AND RESPIRATORY MUSCLES) Patients with respiratory failure due to disorders of chest bellows commonly include those with neuromuscular weakness, caused, for example, by myasthenia gravis (Chap. 366) or the Guillain-Barré syndrome (Chap. 363), as well as those with chest wall problems such as flail chest or severe kyphoscoliosis. As a general rule, when the vital capacity is less than 1 L, or 15 mL/kg body weight, elective intubation should be done and mechanical ventilation begun. Lower vital capacities (<10 mL/kg) and/or an arterial P_{CO_2} (Pa_{CO_2}) above 45 mmHg are indications for immediate intubation and mechanical ventilation.

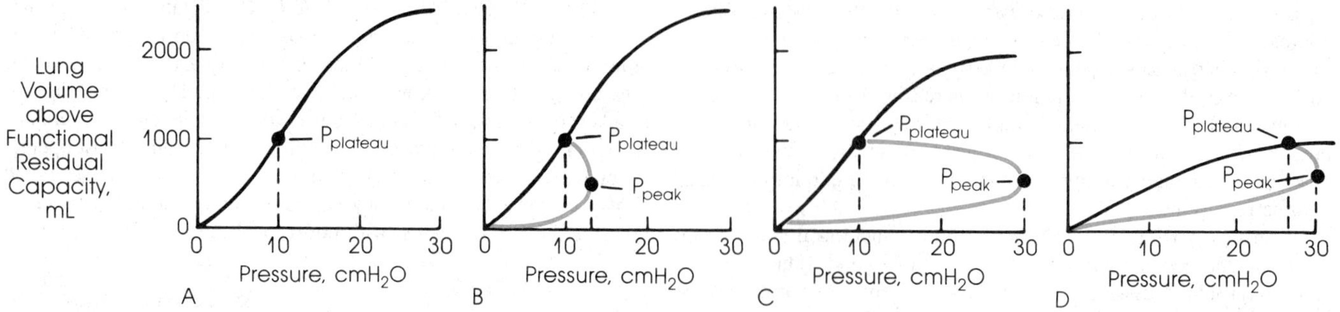

FIGURE 219-1 Schematic representations of pressure-volume curves of respiratory system (lungs and chest wall) during positive pressure mechanical ventilation. *A*. Static pressure-volume curve. $P_{plateau}$ is the alveolar pressure at end-inspiration after a 1000-mL tidal volume. It is measured by momentarily delaying the start of expiration after inflation by a tidal volume and allowing the gauge pressure to "plateau" at an end-inspiratory value. The slope of the curve from the origin to $P_{plateau}$ represents *static compliance*, which in this example is 100 mL per cmH_2O (Cst = change in volume ÷ change in pressure = 1000 mL ÷ 10 cmH_2O = 100 mL per cmH_2O). *B*. Dynamic pressure-volume curve added to the static pressure-volume curve. The peak proximal airway pressure (P_{peak}) is displayed during inspiration on the ventilator's pressure gauge. The pressure difference between the dynamic and static pressure-volume curves at the same lung volume represents the pressure drop due to resistance to airflow by the artificial and natural airways. P_{peak} is only 2 to 4 cmH_2O higher than $P_{plateau}$ in patients with normal airway resistance. *C*. Static and dynamic pressure-volume curves in a patient with severe asthma. Greatly increased P_{peak} is from airway obstruction. $P_{plateau}$ remains unchanged because static compliance is normal. *D*. Static and dynamic pressure-volume curves in a patient with pulmonary edema. Both P_{peak} and $P_{plateau}$ are increased because of decreased static compliance. In this disorder, because P_{peak} is only modestly elevated above $P_{plateau}$ (airway resistance being relatively normal), some clinicians have used P_{peak} instead of $P_{plateau}$ as the denominator in the ratio for respiratory system compliance. This latter ratio has been designated *dynamic compliance*. (*Adapted from Lanken.*)

AIRWAYS Indications for intubation and mechanical ventilation in patients with severe asthma (Chap. 204) depend on the level of Pa_{CO_2}: (1) Hypercapnia, i.e., $Pa_{CO_2} > 45$ mmHg, unresponsive to pharmacologic therapy almost always indicates the need for emergency intubation and mechanical ventilation; or (2) normocapnia, i.e., $Pa_{CO_2} = 40$ mmHg, may be associated with respiratory muscle fatigue or increasingly severe airways obstruction and is also an indication for intubation and mechanical ventilation. Since early in most asthmatic episodes the Pa_{CO_2} is low (30 to 33 mmHg) due to alveolar hyperventilation, a Pa_{CO_2} of 40 mmHg often represents a deteriorating clinical status with incipient respiratory failure. A normal Pa_{CO_2} in this situation has been termed *the cross-over point* to heighten clinicians' awareness of its ominous importance. In contrast, in patients with chronic obstructive pulmonary disease (COPD) (Chap. 210), initiation of mechanical ventilation should be for acute respiratory distress associated with a severe respiratory acidosis, e.g., arterial pH < 7.25, rather than for hypercapnia alone, since even quite high Pa_{CO_2} levels may be chronic and well tolerated.

ALVEOLI Examples of respiratory failure due to impairment of the alveolar component of the respiratory system include cardiogenic pulmonary edema, noncardiogenic pulmonary edema, also known as the adult respiratory distress syndrome (ARDS), extensive pneumonias, and diffuse alveolar hemorrhage syndromes. Diffuse alveolar flooding due to any cause results in an increased right-to-left shunt across the lungs, usually greater than 20 percent, and severe hypoxemic respiratory failure. Mechanical ventilation is urgently indicated in patients with these types of disorders if hypercapnia develops or if hypoxemia remains life-threatening, e.g., $Pa_{O_2} < 50$ mmHg, despite therapy with 100% oxygen delivered by a tight-fitting face mask. Positive end-expiratory pressure (PEEP) is often added to mechanical ventilation to decrease the right-to-left shunt and improve the hypoxemia. PEEP is also used in these patients to allow a reduction in fractional inspired oxygen FI_{O_2} in order to avoid oxygen toxicity. The rationale for the use of PEEP is to increase the end-expiratory lung volume, i.e., functional residual capacity, with attendant opening of previously collapsed and unventilated alveoli that were the cause of the high right-to-left shunt.

CARE OF PATIENTS RECEIVING MECHANICAL VENTILATION

GENERAL MEDICAL CARE Patients receiving mechanical ventilation to treat acute respiratory failure of any cause are usually clinically unstable and may be critically ill. In such patients, undetected disconnection from the ventilator may be lethal. Because of these considerations, acutely ill patients needing mechanical ventilation are admitted routinely to an intensive care unit (ICU) or other suitable special care unit that meets the needs of these patients in terms of availability of appropriate equipment and properly trained professional personnel.

Medical care of acutely ill ventilator-dependent patients is as challenging as it is comprehensive, requiring a broad knowledge of general internal medicine as well as of critical care medicine. The patients' medical care should be closely integrated with specialized care provided by others on the ICU health care team: the nursing staff, respiratory therapists, physical and occupational therapists, and others. Such collaborative ICU care represents an holistic approach to patient care including medical, emotional, and social aspects.

Three specific components of general ICU care should be given to all ventilator-dependent patients and deserve special mention: (1) systemic or local therapy to prevent stress erosions of the gastric mucosa; (2) appropriate nutrition based on assessments of nutritional status, resting energy expenditures, and anticipated duration of mechanical ventilation; and (3) careful monitoring of fluid balance and body weight since positive pressure ventilation predisposes to water and sodium retention. The mechanism of the latter observation relates to reduced cardiac output and possibly to decreased secretion of atrial natriuretic peptide (ANP).

PATIENT MONITORING DURING MECHANICAL VENTILATION All patients on mechanical ventilators should have continuous ECG monitoring as well as frequent measurements of vital signs, serum electrolytes, urine output, and fluid balance. The ICU team should also follow closely the patient's mental and neurologic status, respiratory secretions, and the integrity of the patient's skin and mucous membranes. Ventilator parameters and tracheal cuff pressures should also be monitored frequently. Determinations of arterial pH, P_{CO_2} and P_{O_2} should be made at appropriate intervals to assess alveolar ventilation and arterial oxygenation. Continuous pulse oximetry and end-tidal P_{CO_2} monitoring are often useful in selected patients during periods of respiratory instability or during weaning trials.

PATIENT CARE PROBLEMS ARISING FROM MECHANICAL VENTILATION **Artificial airways** In most patients mechanical ventilation is begun via naso- or endotracheal tubes; some of these patients go on to have tracheostomies—usually when the mechanical ventilatory support is anticipated to be of long duration. Tracheostomies are done after 2 or 3 weeks of mechanical ventilation not to decrease tracheal complications, since both classes of artificial airways have comparable complication rates, but rather to improve patient comfort and provide a more secure airway for patients needing chronic ventilator support. This support may be carried out at home or in a long-term care facility. Either type of tube should be used with the now-standard high-volume ''floppy'' cuff, which should be inflated to a sufficient pressure to allow just a slight (~50 mL) leak during inflation (minimal leak technique) or to occlude the trachea just enough to prevent any leak (minimal occlusion technique) in order to try to prevent severe tracheal wall damage at the cuff site.

Adverse hemodynamic consequences Positive pressure ventilation raises pleural pressure during inspiration which, in turn, decreases systemic venous blood return to the right atrium and, therefore, cardiac output. This effect may cause significant hypotension in the presence of blood volume depletion or in situations in which the mean alveolar pressure (and hence pleural pressure) is relatively high over the entire respiratory cycle. The latter occurs frequently during mechanical ventilation when there is: (1) a high inspiration-to-expiration (I:E) ratio, e.g., 1:1 or more; (2) addition of therapeutic positive end-expiratory pressure (PEEP) (Fig. 219-2); or (3) the presence of occult (non-therapeutic) positive end-expiratory pressure, also called auto-PEEP (Fig. 219-2). Occult PEEP occurs frequently in patients with severe airways obstruction and may cause profound hypotension that should be treated by intravascular volume expansion, increasing the time for expiration, and/or changing from assist mode to intermittent mandatory ventilation (IMV) mode.

FIGURE 219-2 Schematic representations of theoretical alveolar pressure wave forms and the ventilator's pressure gauge (right-hand side of figure) displaying proximal airway pressure (pressure in the ventilator's tubing near the proximal end of the tracheal tube) during mechanical ventilation, showing the effect of therapeutic positive end-expiratory pressure (PEEP) and occult PEEP (auto-PEEP). At the start of inspiration (insp) the negative deflections (small arrows) indicate the patient's spontaneous inspiratory effort which initiates the assisted breath. *A.* In the assist mode with no therapeutic PEEP added and in the absence of auto-PEEP; note that alveolar pressure falls rapidly to zero (large arrow) during passive expiration. At end-expiration, both the alveolar pressure and proximal airway pressure are zero. *B.* In the assist mode after the addition of 10 cmH_2O of PEEP; note that alveolar pressure again falls rapidly (large arrow) during passive expiration but to a new stable baseline of 10 cmH_2O. At end-expiration both the alveolar and proximal airway pressures are 10 cmH_2O. *C.* In the assist mode, a patient with severe airways obstruction has 10 cmH_2O of occult PEEP (auto-PEEP) due to a prolonged time for alveolar emptying. Note that the alveolar pressure never falls to a stable baseline (large arrow) during passive expiration before the next inspiration starts. At end-expiration, alveolar pressure is 10 cmH_2O but the proximal airway pressure gauge displays 0 cmH_2O, reflecting atmospheric pressure due to the circuit's open exhalation valve and not the alveolar pressure—hence the term occult PEEP. However, if the expiratory tubing is abruptly occluded at end-expiration, the gauge would rise from 0 cmH_2O to 10 cmH_2O, indicating the presence and magnitude of the auto-PEEP.

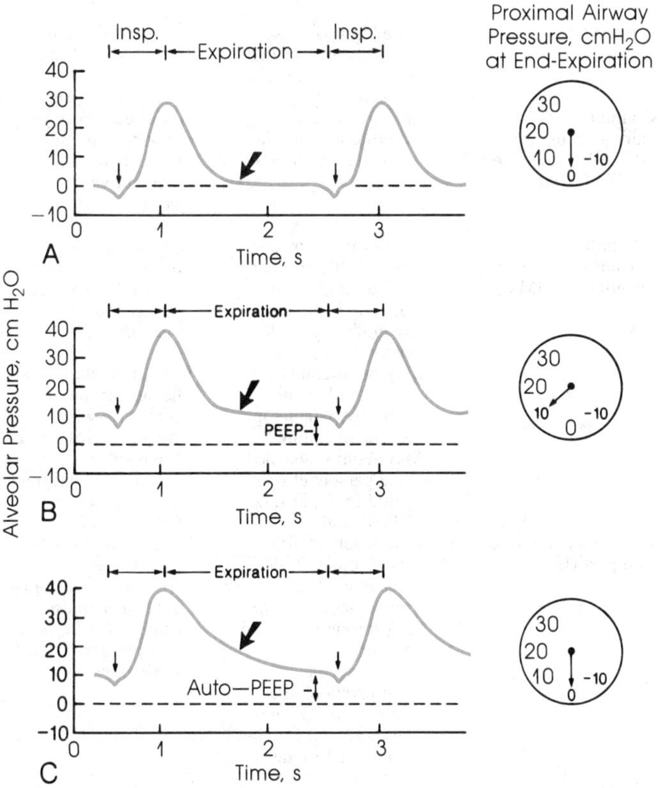

Barotrauma Injury to the lung by high distending pressures and volumes, i.e., barotrauma, not uncommonly occurs in ventilator-dependent patients, especially in those receiving high airway pressures. Barotrauma includes asymptomatic pneumothorax and tension pneumothorax with cardiovascular collapse, as well as the presence of air in the mediastinum (*pneumomediastinum*) or in the subcutaneous tissues in the neck or thorax (*subcutaneous emphysema*). Prevention of barotrauma is attempted by lowering peak airway pressures; this is achieved by decreasing tidal volume or inspiratory flow rates while maintaining alveolar ventilation. High peak airway pressures are often caused by poor synchrony between an anxious patient's spontaneous breathing efforts and the mechanical ventilator. This is treated as much as possible by reassurance and, if necessary, by sedation alone or sedation with pharmacologic paralysis.

The diagnosis of barotrauma can be elusive by clinical examination and, for this reason, daily chest radiographs of critically ill patients on mechanical ventilators are recommended. Therapy of severe barotrauma, e.g., tension pneumothorax, requires chest tube drainage and suction.

WEANING FROM MECHANICAL VENTILATORY SUPPORT

Success in weaning, the process of removing patients from mechanical ventilatory support, generally depends more on successful therapy or resolution of the precipitating cause of the respiratory failure than on the weaning technique utilized. For this reason, knowledge of the cause of the patient's respiratory failure, and whether the process has been reversed, is important in determining when to begin weaning. The weaning process should be done in steps as follows: (1) assessment prior to weaning; (2) trials of progressively less ventilator dependence, resulting in total ventilatory independence; and (3) removal of the tracheal tube, i.e., extubation.

ASSESSMENT PRIOR TO WEANING Preweaning physiologic assessment should address the basic question of whether the level of ventilation that patients can sustain (ventilatory supply) is equal to or greater than the ventilation that is needed to maintain their level of P_{CO_2} (ventilatory demand). Factors determining the balance between ventilatory supply and demand (Table 219-1) are reflected by a set of weaning parameters (Table 219-2) whose values have been found to be reasonably good predictors for success or failure in weaning. As a cautionary note, these weaning parameters should not be regarded as absolute criteria to predict weanability, but rather as one aspect of a preweaning assessment best understood in the context of the patient's overall clinical condition.

As noted above, the overall *clinical assessment* of the patient prior to weaning is equally as, if not more, important than the patient's weaning parameters. For example, it is imperative that the patient be relatively stable hemodynamically and not experiencing frequent life-threatening arrhythmias. In addition, the patient's neurologic status should be stable, with sufficient gag and cough reflexes to permit extubation. Other major organ system failure may preclude weaning through various mechanisms, e.g., metabolic acidosis in patients with renal failure, or a heightened drive to breathe in patients with hepatic failure.

TRIALS OF WEANING There are four commonly used weaning techniques: (1) ''T-piece'' trials; (2) the nearly equivalent ventilator

TABLE 219-1 Major factors determining the balance between ventilatory supply and demand

I Factors limiting ventilatory supply*
- *A* Respiratory muscle weakness (e.g., fatigue)
- *B* Unfavorable length-tension relationship (e.g., due to lung hyperinflation)
- *C* Airways obstruction (e.g., asthma)
- *D* Restricted lung volumes (e.g., pneumonia)

II Factors raising ventilatory demand†
- *A* High physiologic dead space-tidal volume ratio (V_D/V_T) (e.g., emphysema)
- *B* Elevated minute oxygen consumption and hence CO_2 production (e.g., sepsis)
- *C* Respiratory quotient (RQ) greater than 1.0 (e.g., excessive carbohydrate feeding)
- *D* Maintaining arterial P_{CO_2} below 36 mmHg (e.g., due to metabolic acidosis)

* The maximal sustainable ventilation (MSV) which is usually equal to ~½ maximal voluntary ventilation (MVV).
† The spontaneous minute ventilation ($\dot{V}_E$) needed to maintain a certain arterial P_{CO_2} set by the patient's central neuronal drive. If this $\dot{V}_E$ is greater than the patient's maximal sustainable ventilation, the patient will develop respiratory muscle fatigue at that $\dot{V}_E$.

TABLE 219-2 Various parameters useful for weaning from mechanical ventilators

Parameter	Value predicting failure	Value predicting success
I Respiratory muscle function		
A Maximal inspiratory pressure	< −20 mmHg	> −30 mmHg
II Ventilatory demand		
A Spontaneous respiratory rate	>35/min	<30/min
B Minute ventilation ($\dot{V}_E$)	>10 L/min	<10 L/min
C V_D/V_T*	≥0.6	<0.4
III Ventilatory ability		
A Vital capacity	<10 mL/kg	≥15 mL/kg
B Maximal voluntary ventilation	<2 × resting $\dot{V}_E$	≥2 × resting $\dot{V}_E$
IV Oxygenation		
A Intrapulmonary right-to-left shunt	>20%	<20%

* Physiologic dead space-tidal volume ratio.
SOURCE: Lanken.

mode of continuous positive airway pressure (CPAP) used without any PEEP, i.e., CPAP trials; (3) intermittent mandatory ventilation (Fig. 219-3); and (4) inspiratory pressure support ventilation (Fig. 219-3). Some major advantages and disadvantages of each of these four techniques are listed in Table 219-3. As a general rule, during any type of weaning trial the patients' clinical status needs to be assessed frequently; if patients become clinically unstable or acutely distressed, the trial should be stopped and the patients should be hand ventilated (''bagged'') or returned to the ventilator.

FIGURE 219-3 Schematic representation of proximal airway pressure wave forms during assisted ventilation and two modes of weaning. *A*. During mechanical ventilation in the assist mode, the patient ''triggers'' each breath by a short inspiratory effort (T) preceding the ventilator breath (Assist) at a rate of 15 per min. *B*. During synchronized intermittent mandatory ventilation (SIMV), the patient breathes spontaneously (Spont) at a rate of 20 per min, also from the ventilator's demand valve, and also receives unassisted ventilator-delivered tidal volumes (IMV) at a preset rate of approximately 7 per min. The SIMV breaths are synchronized to avoid ''stacking'' a ventilator breath on top of a spontaneous breath. *C*. During inspiratory pressure support ventilation, the patient breathes spontaneously at a rate of 20 per min from the ventilator's demand valve, as in the example of SIMV above, but the inspiratory effort is aided by the ventilator maintaining the proximal airway pressure relatively constant at 10 cmH_2O during the entire inspiration (IPS).

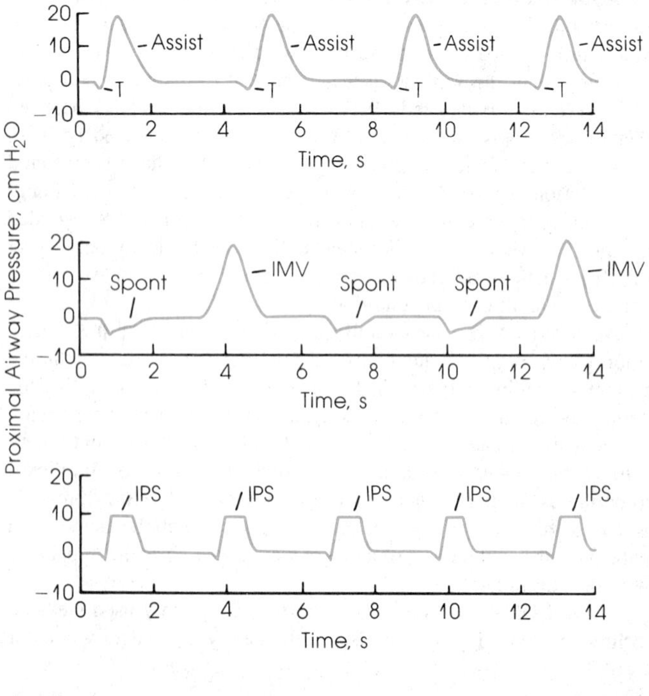

Preweaning patient education, encouragement, and similar measures to support the patient's psychological needs before and during weaning are important adjuncts to any weaning technique.

In a *T-piece trial*, the patient is disconnected from the mechanical ventilator and breathes spontaneously with the tracheal tube connected to a humidified gas source via a plastic connector called a T-piece. These periods of spontaneous breathing should be of a specific duration, and not to the point of fatigue; the periods are increased progressively depending on the patient's ventilatory capacity and endurance. Some newer ventilators have an additional mode that more closely resembles a T-piece trial by providing continuous gas flow through the inspiratory and expiratory circuits; patients inspire from this bias flow, rather than from a demand valve.

In a *CPAP trial* for weaning, commonly utilized without any

TABLE 219-3 Comparison of advantages and disadvantages of four commonly used weaning techniques

Technique	Major advantages	Major disadvantages
T-piece trial	No additional work of breathing needed to open ventilator's demand valve	No exhaled volume monitoring or other alarms No automatic sighs
Continuous positive airway pressure (CPAP) mode, i.e., a CPAP trial	Still connected to ventilator's circuits with full monitor's alarms	Additional work of breathing required to open ventilator's demand valve May lack sighs on some ventilators
Intermittent mandatory ventilation (IMV)	Allows for transition from 100% mechanical to 100% spontaneous ventilation as gradually as desired May be tolerated better hemodynamically by patients in left heart failure May require less bedside personnel compared to T-piece or CPAP trials	Additional work of breathing to open demand valve during spontaneous breaths Rate of weaning may be slower due to slow step-wise decreases in IMV rate May result in less bedside observations than T-piece or CPAP trials
Inspiratory pressure support (IPS)	Low levels of IPS (5–10 cmH_2O) decrease work of spontaneous breathing through artificial airway High levels of IPS (≥20 cmH_2O) may be more comfortable than assist mode	Tidal volumes with high levels of IPS will vary if respiratory mechanics change (analogous to a pressure-cycled ventilator)

additional PEEP, the patient remains connected to the ventilator, which provides the safety of the ventilator's alarm systems as well as psychological reassurance to the patient.

In weaning by use of *intermittent mandatory ventilation* (IMV), the ventilator's tidal volumes are delivered at progressively lower rates. IMV weaning may be a rapid or slow process. In a typical "slow" wean the starting rate is usually just less than the rate during the assist mode, and at the completion of the weaning period, which may be several days to weeks in duration, the finishing rates are $\frac{1}{2}$ to 1 per min (which probably function mostly as sighs). These "mandatory" ventilatory tidal volumes are synchronized so as not to be given simultaneously with the patient's own tidal volume. In an IMV wean, patients can breathe spontaneously at their own tidal volume and rate (Fig. 219-3) and thus can take over their own ventilation at rates as gradually as appropriate.

In *inspiratory pressure support* (IPS) weaning, the patient's spontaneous tidal volumes are augmented by application of a certain level of positive pressure during spontaneous inspirations. In this mode, the volume-cycled ventilator functions analogously to a pressure-cycled ventilator in the assist mode. High levels ($\geq$20 cmH_2O) of IPS in patients with unstable respiratory mechanics will result in variable tidal volumes because of the problems noted above with the use of pressure-cycled ventilators in this type of patient.

Extubation The final step in the weaning process is extubation of the tracheal tube from the patient. However, some patients may be totally weanable from the ventilator, i.e., they can breathe spontaneously, but cannot be extubated because of problems with upper airway obstruction or excessive airway secretions, or because of the need to protect the airway from massive aspiration in patients with poor or absent gag reflexes.

Following extubation, swallowing function may take from several hours to several days or longer to return to normal, and a slow, cautious approach to oral intake is advisable.

REFERENCES

BROCHARD L et al: Improved efficacy of spontaneous breathing with inspiratory pressure support. Am Rev Respir Dis 136:411, 1987

LANKEN PN: Mechanical ventilation, in *Pulmonary Diseases and Disorders*, 2d ed, AP Fishman (ed). New York, McGraw-Hill, 1988, chap. 155

LUCE JM et al: Intermittent mandatory ventilation. Chest 79:678, 1981

PEPE PE, MARINI JJ: Occult positive end-expiratory pressure in mechanically ventilated patients with airflow obstruction. Am Rev Respir Dis 126:166, 1982

PINGLETON SK: Complications of acute respiratory failure. Am Rev Respir Dis 137:1463, 1988

TOBIN MJ: Respiratory monitoring in the intensive care unit. Am Rev Respir Dis 138:1625, 1988

PART EIGHT DISORDERS OF THE KIDNEY AND URINARY TRACT

220 IMPACT OF MOLECULAR BIOLOGY ON NEPHROLOGY

SETH L. ALPER / HARVEY F. LODISH

Molecular biology has had two major impacts on nephrology: the cloning and sequencing of cDNAs and genes encoding proteins that play key roles in electrolyte homeostasis has provided new insight into renal function in health and disease, and the chromosomal mapping of mutations affecting the kidney has made possible new approaches to the prevention and treatment of hereditary diseases of the kidney. In addition, new animal models of kidney disease have been created with single genetic lesions. It is now clear that the techniques of modern biology will recast our understanding of renal development, renal injury, and the progression of chronic renal disease.

PROTEIN SEQUENCES FROM DNA CLONING A partial list of proteins of importance to renal function is given in Table 220-1. Some of the proteins comprise isoforms encoded by families of related genes, while others are products of alternative RNA transcripts from single genes. Sequence analysis of these isoforms has uncovered greater protein diversity than had been suspected by biochemical or physiologic analysis. Some of the isoforms are expressed in specific cell types, specific subcellular compartments, at specific times during development, or in response to hormonal or metabolic stimuli. Individual, engineered mutations in single domains of multidomain, multifunctional proteins have allowed structure-function relationships to be addressed at the single amino acid level even for proteins of low abundance.

MOLECULAR GENETICS OF KIDNEY DISEASE The number of genetic diseases of the kidney and of electrolyte metabolism for which the molecular basis has been elucidated is small: diabetes insipidus in the Brattleboro rat, the salt-wasting form of congenital adrenal hyperplasia secondary to steroid 21-hydroxylase deficiency, and hypocalcemic vitamin D–resistant rickets (Table 220-2).

The Brattleboro rat lacks circulating vasopressin and is therefore a useful model of central diabetes insipidus (see Chap. 315). This deficiency in the rat arises from the deletion of a single guanosine residue in the neurophysin coding region of the vasopressin-neurophysin-glycoprotein precursor gene. The single base deletion shifts the reading frame by which RNA is transcribed from the gene and creates a novel carboxy-terminal amino acid sequence without a stop codon. The result is normal baseline RNA transcription and splicing, deficient enhancement of mRNA level by dehydration, and impaired accumulation of the altered hormone precursor. The latter defect may be due to failure of the ribosome to release the mRNA in the absence of a stop codon or to instability of the altered protein translation product.

Adrenal steroid 21-hydroxylase deficiency results in decreased synthesis of mineralocorticoids and glucocorticoids, ACTH-mediated adrenal hyperplasia, and androgen excess (see Chaps. 317 and 324). The 21-hydroxylase is a cytochrome P_{450} enzyme, encoded by a gene on chromosome 6. One or more copies of a pseudogene are located near the coding gene. The pseudogene sequence differs from the functional gene in an 8-bp deletion in exon 3, a single base insertion in exon 7, a point mutation in exon 8, and four base changes in the putative promoter region. The pseudogene is not transcribed. The deficiency syndrome can arise from unequal gene crossover, from conversion of the functional gene to a pseudogene, or from single amino acid substitutions in the enzyme.

Hypocalcemic vitamin D–responsive rickets (see Chap. 340) is an autosomal recessive disorder characterized by target organ resistance to the action of 1,25-dihydroxy vitamin D and caused by altered function of the 1,25-dihydroxy vitamin D_3 receptor. In two affected families the receptors exhibited a unique single base change, resulting in an amino acid substitution in one of the DNA-binding zinc finger structures of the vitamin D receptor. In other instances the disorder

TABLE 220-1 Selected cDNA clones encoding proteins of importance to renal function

Transport proteins
Na^+-K^+ ATPases
Ca^{2+} ATPases
H^+-K^+ ATPase
H^+ ATPase 31-kDa subunit
Na^+-glucose symporter
Glucose carriers
Anion exchangers
Na^+/H^+ antiporter
K^+ channels
Putative urea carrier
Multiple drug carrier
Hormones and signal transducers
EGF, EGF receptor
PDGF receptor
Insulin receptor
TGF-β
IL-1 receptor
IL-2 receptors
Catecholamine and muscarinic receptors
1,25-$(OH)_2$ vitamin D receptor
Aldosterone and glucocorticoid receptors
Thyroxine and vitamin A receptors
ANF and ANF receptor
Vasopressin and oxytocin
Parathyroid hormone-like protein
Erythropoietin and erythropoietin receptor
Renin
Angiotensinogen and angiotensin receptor
Kallikrein
Protein kinases
G proteins
Phospholipases
Other proteins
Carbonic anhydrases
Angiotensin converting enzyme
Tamm-Horsfall protein
Fructose-1-P aldolase B
28-kd Ca^{2+} binding protein
Sm-D autoantigen
gp330 Heymann nephritis antigen
p30 nephritic antigen
Heparan sulfate proteoglycan core protein
Fibronectin and fibronectin receptor
Laminin and laminin receptor

SOURCE: After Alper and Lodish.

TABLE 220-2 Some inherited diseases of renal function or electrolyte metabolism that have been mapped to chromosomal loci

Disease	Affected gene product	Locus
Renal Cell Carcinoma		3p21→
von Hippel-Lindau syndrome		3p25
Congenital adrenal hyperplasia	Cytochrome P_{450} 21-OHase*	6p21.3
Cystic fibrosis	Cl^- channel or its regulator	7q22.3-q23.1
Isolated aldosterone deficiency	Corticosterone methyl oxidase II (cytochrome P_{450} II-OHase)?*	
Osteopetrosis–renal tubular acidosis–cerebral calcification syndrome	Carbonic anhydrase II†	8q22
Familial Mediterranean fever		9
Tuberous sclerosis		9q11-q22
Fructose intolerance	Fructose-1-phosphate aldolase B*	9q22
Nail-patella syndrome		9q34
Wilms' tumor		11p13
Vitamin D-Responsive rickets	$1,25(OH)_2$ vitamin D receptor	12
Hemodialysis-related amyloidosis		15q21-q22
Adult polycystic kidney disease		16p13.31-p13.12
Urolithiasis (2,8-dihydroxyadenine)	Adenosine phosphoribosyl-transferase	16q24
Diabetes insipidus		20
Hypophosphatemia		Xp22
Hypomagnesemia		Xp22
Fabry disease		Xq22
Alport's disease		Xq22-q25
Lowe oculocerebrorenal syndrome		Xq25
Lesch-Nyhan syndrome	Hypoxanthine-guanine phosphoribosyl-transferase*	Xq26-q27.2
Nephrogenic diabetes insipidus		Xq28
Proximal renal tubular acidosis		X
Orofaciodigital syndrome		X
Gout type II		X
Pseudohypoparathyroidism		X

Symbols: * molecular basis for mutations(s) described; † normal gene has been cloned but molecular basis for mutation(s) not yet described.

SOURCE: Compiled from: McKusick VA, *The Morbid Anatomy of the Human Genome*. Howard Hughes Medical Institute, 1988. (After Alper and Lodish.)

appears to be due to the presence of a premature termination codon that causes the formation of a short and nonfunctional receptor protein.

The autosomal recessive syndrome of osteopetrosis with mixed renal tubular acidosis and cerebral calcification (see Chap. 345) is tightly linked to a deficiency of carbonic anhydrase II (CAII). The disease and CAII both map to chromosome band 8q22, where the gene is also tightly linked to the genes for two other carbonic anhydrase enzymes. CAII is the only one of these carbonic anhydrases expressed in kidney and in brain. The mouse with CAII deficiency, created by ethylnitrosourea mutagenesis of whole animals and detected by isozyme screening, is runted and has alkaline urine but lacks osteopetrosis and cerebral calcification. The molecular defect in both human and murine deficiencies remains to be determined. Table 220-2 lists several additional diseases in which the altered or deficient protein is known but in which the molecular genetic defect associated with disease has not been reported. In addition, several diseases are listed for which only an approximate chromosomal location of the affected gene is available.

LINKAGE ANALYSIS AND ADULT POLYCYSTIC KIDNEY DISEASE It is possible in many instances to determine the chromosomal location of a disease locus and to clone the gene responsible in the absence of knowledge of the underlying biochemical defect that causes the disease (see Chap. 6). The numerous differences in DNA sequence among individuals (polymorphisms) are most easily detected when they alter the length of a DNA restriction fragment, resulting in a restriction fragment length polymorphism (RFLP) in the population. The combination of family linkage studies with molecular cloning of these DNA markers has led to the construction of genetic linkage maps with cloned polymorphic DNA markers arrayed at intervals along the lengths of each chromosome. With a collection of these RFLP markers and a large, multigenerational family affected with an autosomal dominant disease or multiple families in which one or more members is affected by an autosomal recessive mutation, the chromosomal locus of the disease gene can be determined by establishing genetic linkage with markers residing close to it. The first autosomal disease mapped by linkage to RFLP markers was Huntington's disease on chromosome 4. Using the same approach, Reeders et al localized to the short arm of chromosome 16 the genetic locus whose mutation causes autosomal dominant adult polycystic kidney disease (see Chap. 231). This locus is closely linked to the α-globin gene cluster. The inheritance of the α-globin locus can be followed by means of a RFLP that is so polymorphic that only 1 percent of people are homozygous at that locus. Detection of this RFLP allows the inheritance of each parentally contributed copy of chromosome 16 (carrying its α-globin allele) to be followed individually. Figure 220-1 shows that in one Dutch family, allele C of this polymorphic locus cosegregates with polycystic disease while the other alleles, D, G, J, and H, segregate independently, consistent with close linkage of the polymorphic locus to polycystic disease.

Adult polycystic disease (APKD) in Northern Europe may be caused by a single genetic locus since 28 families from England, Scotland, the Netherlands, and Finland all displayed close linkage of the disease to the α-globin cluster. However, two families of Italian origin with adult polycystic disease have demonstrated no linkage of the mutant gene to the α-globin cluster. Thus, mutations in at least two different genes are capable of causing APKD.

TRANSGENIC MICE AND ANIMAL MODELS OF KIDNEY DISEASE The development of the capacity to introduce foreign genes into the germ lines of mice has made it possible to construct animal models for several human diseases. A foreign gene can cause disease either by its own inappropriate expression or by disrupting an endogenous gene. Genes can be introduced into mice in several ways. Cloned DNA can be directly injected into a pronucleus of a fertilized mouse egg, or embryos at any of several developmental stages can

FIGURE 220-1 Autoradiograph of a Southern blot of restriction enzyme-digested genomic DNA from individuals of a single family cohort, displaying alleles C, D, G, J, and H of the polymorphic locus tightly linked to the α-globlin locus. Of these, only allele C cosegregates with polycystic disease (APKD). *(After ST Reeders et al.)*

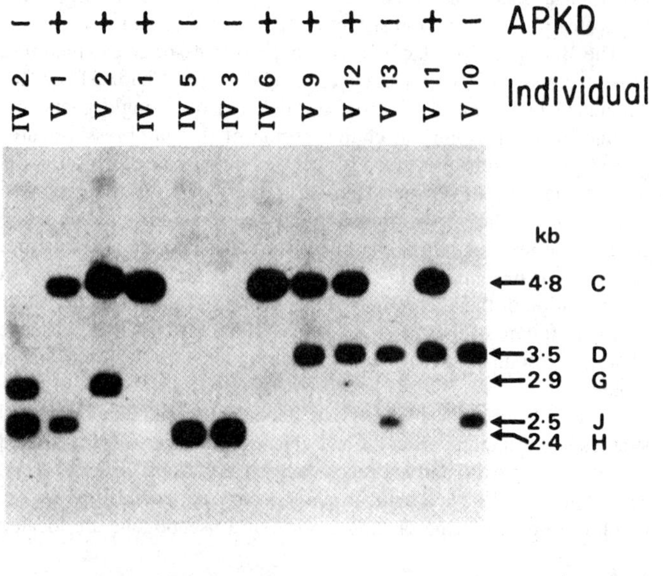

be infected by replication-deficient, integrating retroviruses. Alternatively, cultured embryonic stem cells can be injected into host blastocysts, where they colonize the embryo and contribute to the germ line of the resulting chimeric animals. The stem cells can be selected in cell culture for altered expression of the gene of interest before blastocyst injection.

Several lines of transgenic mice develop disorders of the kidney. Mice that carry the SV40 large T antigen (a viral oncogene) adjacent to SV40 viral enhancer sequences die from choroid plexus ependymoma at 5 months of age. The large T-antigen protein is expressed in the tumors and at lower level in kidney and thymus. Kidney tubules that express large T antigen develop epithelial cell proliferation with occasional cystic dilatation. Large T antigen was not clearly present in glomerular cells, but the mice developed progressive glomerular sclerosis with increasing proteinuria and nonspecific glomerular IgG deposits.

Ectopic expression of the Thy-1 surface protein member of the immunoglobulin superfamily in the kidneys of transgenic mice is also associated with glomerular disease. The function of the protein is unknown, but in some tissues it may play a role in cell-cell recognition or in proliferation. Though mouse kidney lacks Thy-1, it is present in human and rat kidney.

Mice that carry a chimeric Thy-1 gene whose 5′ flanking sequences and protein coding sequences are of murine origin and whose 3′ flanking sequence is of human origin expressed murine Thy-1 in glomerular podocytes. These mice develop severe proteinuria and segmental glomerulosclerosis with foot process swelling and vacuolation, mesangial and subendothelial deposits, occasional mesangial proliferation, and nonspecific deposits of IgG, IgM, and C3 in the mesangium. The onset of proteinuria coincided with an increase in Thy-1 mRNA expression in glomerular podocytes. These experiments suggest that a glomerular podocyte specific enhancer sequence in the 3′ flanking region of the human Thy-1 gene promotes expression of the Thy-1 gene in proximal tubule epithelium only when the sequence is removed from its normal context.

Retroviral infection of preimplantation embryos usually results in insertional inactivation of native genes for creation of mutant phenotypes. Once a phenotype of interest is found and a line of mice established, the inactivated gene can be cloned by screening a genomic library with a retroviral probe. One transgenic mouse line created in this way yielded homozygotes for the retroviral insertion, and these animals died at age 8 weeks with anemia, hypercholesterolemia, and proteinuric renal failure. At 5 to 6 weeks the mice developed a mesangioproliferative glomerulonephritis marked by mesangial thickening, fibrin deposition, and foot process fusion followed later by tubular dilatation, protein inspissation, and a monocytic interstitial infiltrate without evidence of vasculitis. The gene whose disruption leads to this pathology is under investigation.

UROLOGIC CANCER Molecular biology has increased the understanding of urologic cancers in three principal areas: pathogenesis, hypercalcemia of malignancy, and resistance to chemotherapy. Two varieties of oncogenes are associated with malignant transformation, "dominant" and "recessive" (see also Chap. 10). Dominant oncogenes encode growth-promoting proteins. A single functional copy of a dominant oncogene confers some aspects of the malignant phenotype. H-*ras*, the first dominant oncogene to be discovered, was identified in a cell line derived from a human urinary bladder carcinoma. Recessive oncogenes are postulated to be "antioncogenes" or negative regulators of cell growth. The best example of a recessive oncogene is the retinoblastoma (*Rb*) gene on chromosome 13. Loss of function of both normal *Rb* alleles contributes to the formation of retinoblastoma and in some cases osteosarcoma. In sporadic retinoblastoma, these loss-of-function events are both somatic mutations. In hereditary retinoblastoma the germ line already carries an inactivating mutation of *Rb* on one copy of chromosome 13. Retinal cells in which the second copy of the *Rb* gene is inactivated give rise to retinoblastomas.

Hereditary Wilms' tumor may arise by a similar mechanism involving a putative antioncogene locus on chromosome 11. Antioncogenes have been proposed to play similar roles in nonfamilial tumors of the urinary tract. For example, somatic deletions of portions of chromosome 11 occur in some cases of transitional cell carcinoma, and most renal cell carcinomas contain deletions of chromosome 3, often in the setting of unbalanced translocations of a variety of other chromosome fragments to the same region of chromosome 3. A search for the smallest chromosomal deletions associated with Wilms' tumor and with renal cell carcinoma may lead to the cloning of genes that share some of the growth-inhibitory or tumor-suppressor properties of the retinoblastoma gene.

Renal cell carcinoma is often associated with paraneoplastic syndromes (see Chap. 309). The humoral hypercalcemia of renal cell carcinoma is mediated by the secreted peptide products of the parathyroid hormone-like peptide gene, PTH-LP. PTH-LP acts by binding to PTH receptors and activating adenylate cyclase. The PTH-LP cDNA has been cloned from a renal cell carcinoma cell line, and an alternatively spliced PTH-LP cDNA encoding a different *C*-terminal amino acid sequence was cloned from a lung carcinoma cell line. The PTH-LP *N*-terminal 13 amino acids share 62 percent identity with PTH, but the proteins are different in sequence thereafter and in length.

Renal cell carcinoma is generally insensitive to chemotherapeutic drugs, possibly because the kidney is a site of high-level expression of the multiple drug resistance gene (*mdr*-1). The *mdr*-1 protein is a plasma membrane glycoprotein of the proximal tubule brush border and functions in tumor cells as an ATP-dependent, efflux pump for a variety of pharmacologic agents. Several related *mdr* genes, which undergo alternative splicing, spontaneous point mutations, and gene amplification, contribute to variable resistance in different tumors.

Drug resistance in renal cell carcinoma is associated with high levels of expression of *mdr*-1 mRNA. This drug resistance is reversed by high-dose verapamil and quinidine, agents that block *mdr*-1. Thus, newer antagonists of drug efflux may make it possible to treat renal cell carcinoma with drugs such as adriamycin and vinca alkaloids that are ordinarily ineffective when the *mdr*-1 protein is functional.

REFERENCES

ALPER SL, LODISH HF: Molecular biology of renal function, in *The Kidney*, 4th ed, BM Brenner, FC Rector, Jr (eds). Philadelphia, in press

FOJO AT et al: Intrinsic drug resistance in human kidney cancer is associated with expression of a human multidrug-resistance gene. J Clin Oncol 5:1922, 1987

JAENISCH R: Transgenic animals. Science 240:1468, 1988

KOVACS G et al: Consistent chromosome 3p deletion and loss of heterozygosity in renal cell carcinoma. Proc Natl Acad Sci USA 85:1571, 1988

MACKAY et al: Glomerulosclerosis and renal cysts in mice transgenic for the early region of SV40. Kidney Int 32:827, 1987

MALLOY PJ et al: Point mutations in the human vitamin D receptor gene associated with hypocalcemic rickets. Science 242:1702, 1988

MILLER WL: Gene conversions, deletions, and polymorphisms in congenital adrenal hyperplasia. Am J Hum Genet 42:4, 1988

REEDERS ST et al: A highly polymorphic DNA marker linked to adult polycystic kidney disease on chromosome 16. Nature 317:542, 1985

RICHTER D: Molecular events in expression of vasopressin and oxytocin and their cognate receptors. Am J Physiol 255:F207, 1988

SLY WS et al: Carbonic anhydrase II deficiency in 12 families with the autosomal recessive syndrome of osteopetrosis with renal tubular acidosis and cerebral calcification. N Engl J Med 313:139, 1985

221 APPROACH TO THE PATIENT WITH DISEASES OF THE KIDNEYS AND URINARY TRACT

FREDRIC L. COE / BARRY M. BRENNER

Diseases of the kidneys and urinary tract frequently give rise to consistent arrays or clusters of clinical signs, symptoms, and laboratory findings called *syndromes*. Syndromes are useful diagnostically because each has fewer causes than the individual clinical signs and symptoms it contains. For example, any injured capillary bed from glomerulus to the urethral meatus can cause hematuria, but only glomerular injury can also cause heavy albuminuria and erythrocyte casts (Chap. 49), and only a few of the diseases that injure the glomerular capillaries enough to cause hematuria and proteinuria also cause a rapid fall in glomerular filtration rate. Routine clinical evaluation is often sufficient to suggest that a particular syndrome may be present (Table 221-1), but additional laboratory measurements beyond the routine, as well as radiologic and/or urologic evaluation and sequential clinical observations, are usually required to establish the diagnosis. This chapter presents the general features of the syndromes and the clinical and laboratory data required for their recognition and outlines the diseases that cause them. Succeeding chapters in this section describe the diseases and their treatment in detail.

ACUTE (ARF) AND RAPIDLY PROGRESSIVE RENAL FAILURE (RPRF) Whether the glomerular filtration rate falls over a period of days (acute renal failure) or weeks (rapidly progressive renal failure) is a useful distinction, because the causes of these two syndromes are somewhat different (Tables 221-1 and 221-2). For example, acute tubular necrosis, from sepsis, nephrotoxic materials, shock, or other cause (see Chap. 223), presents itself as and is the usual cause of acute renal failure, whereas extracapillary proliferative (crescentic) glomerulonephritis, due to immunologic injury or to vasculitis, is an important cause of rapidly progressive, but not acute, renal failure (Chap. 227).

Proof for the existence of either syndrome requires serial determination of the glomerular filtration rate (GFR) or blood urea nitrogen or serum creatinine level. Anuria or oliguria (Chap. 49) strongly suggest acute renal failure, as life cannot be sustained for long with such inadequate renal function. Symptoms and signs of uremia of recent onset suggest rapidly progressive or acute renal failure, but could also result from chronic renal failure that has only recently become life-threatening. Although edema, hypertension, and abnormalities of electrolytes and the urine sediment (Table 221-1) are frequent in acute and rapidly progressive renal failure, they occur in other syndromes as well and are not specific.

The causes of these two important syndromes number about 36, but only 18 (indicated by T, Table 221-2) typically cause acute renal failure, and 8 cause rapidly progressive renal failure. Urinary obstruction, acute tubular necrosis, some forms of vasculitis, major renal vascular accidents, and endogenous and exogenous nephrotoxins are the usual causes of acute renal failure. Vasculitis and crescentic forms

TABLE 221-1 Initial clinical and laboratory data base for defining major syndromes in nephrology

Syndromes	Important clues to diagnosis	Findings which are common but not of diagnostic value	Location of discussion of diseases causing syndrome
Acute or rapidly progressive renal failure	Anuria Oliguria Documented recent decline in GFR	Hypertension, hematuria Proteinuria, pyuria Casts, edema	Chaps. 223, 227, 229, 230, 233
Acute nephritis	Hematuria, RBC casts Azotemia, oliguria Edema, hypertension	Proteinuria Pyuria Circulatory congestion	Chaps. 226 to 228
Chronic renal failure	Azotemia for > 3 months Prolonged symptoms or signs of uremia Symptoms or signs of renal osteodystrophy Kidneys reduced in size bilaterally Broad casts in urinary sediment	Hematuria, proteinuria Casts, oliguria Polyuria, nocturia Edema, hypertension Electrolyte disorders	Chaps. 222, 224
Nephrotic syndrome	Proteinuria > 3.5 g per 1.73 m^2 per 24 h Hypoalbuminemia Hyperlipidemia Lipiduria	Casts Edema	Chaps. 223, 228
Asymptomatic urinary abnormalities	Hematuria Proteinuria (below nephrotic range) Sterile pyuria, casts		Chap. 227
Urinary tract infection	Bacteriuria > 10^5 colonies per milliliter Other infectious agent documented in urine Pyuria, leukocyte casts Frequency, urgency Bladder tenderness, flank tenderness	Hematuria Mild azotemia Mild proteinuria Fever	Chap. 95
Renal tubule defects	Electrolyte disorders Polyuria, nocturia Symptoms or signs of renal osteodystrophy Large kidneys Renal transport defects	Hematuria "Tubular" proteinuria Enuresis	Chaps. 229, 231
Hypertension	Systolic/diastolic hypertension	Proteinuria Casts Azotemia	Chaps. 39, 196, 230
Nephrolithiasis	Previous history of stone passage or removal Previous history of stone seen by x-ray Renal colic	Hematuria Pyuria Frequency, urgency	Chap. 232
Urinary tract obstruction	Azotemia, oliguria, anuria Polyuria, nocturia, urinary retention Slowing of urinary stream Large prostate, large kidneys Flank tenderness, full bladder after voiding	Hematuria Pyuria Enuresis, dysuria	Chap. 233

TABLE 221-2 Syndromes produced by diseases of the kidneys and urinary tract

	Syndromes					
Diseases (Chap.)	ARF	RPRF	AN	CRF	NS	AUA
Bilateral arterial occlusion (230)	T					
Acute tubular necrosis (223)	T					
Bilateral acute renal vein thrombosis (230)	T					
Acute uric acid nephropathy (229)	T					
Hypovolemia (223)	T					
Cardiovascular collapse (223)	T					
Acute bilateral upper tract obstruction (233)	T					
Hypercalcemic nephropathy (229)	T			O		
Hemolytic uremic syndrome (230)	T	O	O			
Acute urinary retention (233)						
Malignant nephrosclerosis (230)	T	O				
Essential mixed cyroimmunoglobulinemia (228)	T	O	O	O	O	
Nephrotoxic drugs and chemicals (223, 229)	T			O		
Oxalate nephropathy (229)	T			O		
Cortical necrosis (223)	T			O		
Postpartum glomerulosclerosis (223)	T			O		
Hypersensitivity nephropathy (229)	T		O			P,H,L
Scleroderma (230)	T					P
Idiopathic rapidly progressive GN (227)	O	T	T		R	
Goodpasture's syndrome (227)	O	T	T	O		P,H
Non-Goodpasture's anti-GBM disease (227)	O	T	T	O		P,H
Acute bacterial endocarditis or visceral sepsis (227)		T	T	O	O	
Microscopic polyarteritis nodosa (228, 230)		T	T			
Wegener's granulomatosis (228, 230)		T	T			
Allergic granulomatosis (276)		T	T			
Acute radiation nephritis (229)		T	T			P
Poststreptococcal glomerulonephritis (227)		R	T	O	R	P,H
Nonstreptococcal postinfectious GN (227)		R	T	R	R	P,H
Macroscopic polyarteritis nodosa (276, 228, 230)				T		P,H
Diffuse proliferative lupus nephritis (228)	R	O	R	T	O	P,H,L
Chronic radiation nephritis (229)				T	O	
Balkan nephropathy (229)				T		P*,H
Analgesic nephropathy (229)				T		L,H
Heavy metals (lead, cadmium, mercury) (229)				T		P*
Cystinosis (229)				T		P*
Chronic obstructive uropathy (233)				T		H
Adult polycystic renal disease (231)				T		H,P
Medullary cystic renal disease (231)				T		
Gouty nephropathy (229)				T		
Minimal change disease (227)					T	
Idiopathic membranous nephropathy (227)				O	T	P,H
Membranoproliferative glomerulonephritis (227)		R	O	O	T	P,H
Renal amyloidosis (228)				O	T	P
Membranous lupus nephropathy (228)				O	T	P
Renal vein thrombosis (230)	O			O	T	
Rheumatoid arthritis (228)					T	
Congenital nephrotic syndrome (228)				O	T	
Dermatomyositis (227)					T	
Dermatitis herpetiformis (227)				O	T	P
Medullary sponge kidney (231)						T:H
Nephrolithiasis (226)						T:H
Neoplasms (234)						T:H
Arteriolar nephrosclerosis (230)				O		T:P
Waldenström's macroglobulinemia (228)	O					T:P
Multiple myeloma (228)	O	O		O	O	T:P
Reflux nephropathy (95, 230)				O	O	T:P
Diabetic nephropathy (228, 327)				O	O	T:P
Toxemia of pregnancy (230)						T:P
Orthostatic proteinuria (227)						T:P
Sarcoid nephropathy (228)						T:P
Hypokalemic nephropathy (229)						T:P
Berger's (IgA) nephropathy (227)	R	R	O	O	O	T:H,P
Henoch-Schönlein purpura (228)		O	O	R	O	T:H,P
Fabry's disease (228)				O		T:H,P
Alport's syndrome (228)				O		T:H,P
Sickle cell nephropathy (228)				O	R	T:H,P
Subacute bacterial endocarditis (90)						T:H,P
Minimal and mesangial lupus nephritis (228)						T:P,H
Mesangial proliferative GN (227)				R	O	T:P,H
Mixed connective tissue disease (228)					R	T:P,H
Chronic glomerulonephritis (224)				O		T:P,H
Nail patella syndrome (228)				R		T:P,H
Focal glomerulosclerosis (227)		R	O	O	O	T:P,H,L
Focal and segmental lupus nephritis (228)				O	O	T:P,H,L
Sjögren's syndrome (228)						T:L,P
Urinary and renal infection (95)						T:L,H

NOTE: T, typical presentation; O, occurs frequently, but not invariably; R, occurs rarely; P*, tubular proteinuria; P, proteinuria; H, hematuria; L, leukocyturia; ARF, acute renal failure; RPRF, rapidly progressive renal failure; AN, acute nephritis; CRF, chronic renal failure; NS, nephrotic syndrome; AUA, asymptomatic urinary abnormality.

of glomerulonephritis are the main causes of rapidly progressive renal failure. Hemolytic-uremic syndrome, malignant nephrosclerosis, and essential mixed cryoimmunoglobulinemia occasionally present as rapidly progressive renal failure. Idiopathic rapidly progressive glomerulonephritis—the prototype of a disease that produces rapidly progressive renal failure—sometimes causes acute renal failure. Chronic renal failure may occur in some patients with diseases that typically cause acute renal failure. Nevertheless, despite some variability of disease presentations, the finding of acute or rapidly progressive renal failure narrows the range of causes.

ACUTE NEPHRITIS (AN) A number of diseases involve the glomeruli and, to a generally lesser extent, the tubules in an acute but transient inflammatory process, manifested clinically by acute reduction in GFR, rapidly progressive renal failure, and salt and water retention. Expansion of the extracellular volume, if marked, causes hypertension, pulmonary vascular congestion, and facial and peripheral edema (Chap. 227). Since the causes of this syndrome all can damage the glomerular wall enough to permit red blood cells and plasma proteins to enter the urinary space and appear in the urine, gross or microscopic hematuria, red blood cell casts, and proteinuria are necessary for the diagnosis of acute nephritis, and their absence suggests other diagnostic possibilities. Acute nephritis itself is a transient inflammatory process, so its clinical and laboratory manifestations wax and wane over days to weeks. Many of the diseases that cause acute nephritis also cause acute or rapidly progressive renal failure (Table 221-2).

The fact that many diseases produce both acute nephritis and acute or rapidly progressive renal failure, some produce only acute nephritis, and some produce acute or chronic renal failure without acute nephritis is useful in diagnosis. Only two diseases, poststreptococcal glomerulonephritis and nonstreptococcal postinfectious glomerulonephritis, typically cause acute nephritis alone, and only three of the diseases that typically cause acute renal failure, idiopathic rapidly progressive glomerulonephritis, Goodpasture's syndrome, and non-Goodpasture's antiglomerular basement membrane (anti-GBM) disease, also cause acute nephritis (Table 221-2). On the other hand, most of the diseases that cause acute nephritis also cause rapidly progressive renal failure.

Acute glomerulonephritis following infection with group A streptococci is the prototype of a disease that causes acute nephritis alone (Chap. 227). Immune complexes deposit in the subepithelial region of the glomerular capillary wall, between the basement membrane and the visceral epithelial cells that separate the membrane from the urinary space, and provoke an intense but transient inflammatory process. GFR falls, but returns to normal within weeks to months in the vast majority of affected patients. Deposition of immune complexes is also believed to be the cause of acute nephritis following other bacterial and viral infections, and of lupus nephritis, membranoproliferative glomerulonephritis, Henoch-Schönlein purpura, and Berger's disease, i.e., IgA nephropathy. That the typical presentations of the last four diseases are chronic renal failure, nephrotic syndrome, and asymptomatic urinary abnormalities illustrates the weakness of relationships between pathogenesis and final clinical manifestations.

Renal biopsy is usually required for the evaluation of patients with acute nephritis, whether or not acute or rapidly progressive renal failure is also present. The usual histologic picture is proliferative glomerulonephritis, often with extracapillary crescent formation, but prognosis and treatment are influenced strongly by the precise histologic and ultrastructural pattern, as well as the types of immune complexes and immunoglobulins deposited in the renal tissues.

CHRONIC RENAL FAILURE (CRF) Chronic renal failure is a syndrome which results from progressive and irreversible destruction of nephrons, regardless of cause (Chap. 224). This syndrome may be considered to exist when GFR is found to be reduced and is known to have been reduced for at least 3 to 6 months (Table 221-1). Often a gradual decline in GFR can be documented over a period of years. Proof of chronicity is also provided by the demonstration of bilateral reduction of kidney size by abdominal scout film, ultrasonography, intravenous pyelography, or tomography. Other findings consistent with long-standing renal failure, such as renal osteodystrophy or signs and symptoms of uremia, also help to establish this syndrome. Several laboratory abnormalities are often regarded as reliable indicators of chronicity of renal disease, such as anemia, hyperphosphatemia, or hypocalcemia, but these are not specific and may be misleading (Chap. 222). In contrast, the finding of broad casts in the urinary sediment (Chap. 49) is specific for chronic renal failure, the wide diameters of these casts reflecting the compensatory dilatation and hypertrophy of surviving nephrons. Proteinuria is a frequent but nonspecific finding, as is hematuria. Chronic obstructive uropathy, polycystic and medullary cystic diseases, analgesic nephropathy, and the inactive end stage of any chronic tubulointerstitial nephropathy are excellent examples of conditions in which the urine often contains little or no protein, cells, or casts even though nephron destruction has progressed to the stage of chronic renal failure.

When ARF occurs and there is also clear evidence of CRF, the acute component must be evaluated as if CRF were not present, largely because the acute component is potentially reversible. In most instances, depletion of extracellular fluid volume accounts for the acute deterioration of renal function, but other factors such as urinary tract obstruction, drug-induced nephrotoxicity, or exacerbation of the underlying renal disease may also be responsible (Chap. 224).

NEPHROTIC SYNDROME (NS) This syndrome is generally held to be present when a patient excretes more than 3.5 g protein per 1.73 m^2 surface area per 24 h that consists mainly of albumin (massive proteinuria) and has reduced serum albumin concentration, edema, and hyperlipidemia (Table 221-1). Massive proteinuria alone has come to define the syndrome since this finding connotes serious renal disease whether or not the protein losses lead to hypoalbuminemia, lipid disturbances, or edema (Chap. 49). Provided the proteins appearing in the urine are not abnormal paraproteins readily excreted by the normal kidney (e.g., immunoglobulin light chains in multiple myeloma), massive proteinuria is invariably a sign of injury to the glomeruli.

Common causes of the nephrotic syndrome include minimal change disease, idiopathic membranous glomerulopathy, focal glomerulosclerosis, and diabetic glomerulosclerosis (Chaps. 227 and 228). Because these diseases typically cause less inflammation than those that cause acute nephritis, the urine contains fewer cellular elements, and acute changes in GFR and urine volume are uncommon. Hematuria may be a frequent manifestation of some forms of nephrotic syndrome, however, especially chronic membranoproliferative glomerulonephritis (Chap. 227). The presence of many cellular or granular casts should suggest lupus nephritis (Chap. 228) or one of the other causes of acute nephritis associated with massive proteinuria such as essential mixed cryoimmunoglobulinemia, acute bacterial endocarditis, visceral sepsis, and Henoch-Schönlein purpura (Table 221-2).

ASYMPTOMATIC URINARY ABNORMALITIES (AUA) As indicated in Table 221-2, mild degrees of microscopic hematuria, pyuria, casts, or less than 3.5 g protein per 1.73 m^2 surface area per 24 h may be present in the urine of a patient lacking concurrent evidence of other nephrologic syndromes. By exclusion, these patients are best considered to belong to the syndrome of asymptomatic urinary abnormalities. Isolated hematuria or proteinuria, or unexplained pyuria, are the most frequent abnormalities that occur in this syndrome.

Isolated hematuria, without proteinuria or casts, may be the sole clue to the presence of neoplasm, stone, or infection (e.g., tuberculosis) in any part of the urinary tract (Chaps. 49, 226, 232, and 234). Isolated hematuria may also arise from renal papillae in analgesic and sickle cell nephropathies (Chaps. 229 and 230). Persistent isolated hematuria often requires intravenous pyelography, cystoscopy, and, occasionally, renal arteriography to identify the source of bleeding. *Nephronal hematuria,* in which red blood cells or hemoglobin pigment is present in casts, indicates damage to the nephron (Chap. 49). It occurs without proteinuria, mainly in benign recurrent hematuria and Berger's disease (Chap. 227). *Nephronal hematuria and proteinuria* occur together in many specific renal diseases that may eventually lead to chronic renal failure (Chap. 224). In general, the combination of nephronal hematuria and proteinuria suggests a worse prognosis than either one alone.

Isolated proteinuria, without red blood cells or other formed elements in the urinary sediment, is characteristic of many renal diseases which manifest little or no inflammatory reaction within the glomeruli (e.g., diabetes mellitus, amyloidosis). Less than nephrotic-range proteinuria is common in mild forms of all the diseases that can cause overt nephrotic syndrome (Chaps. 227 and 228). "Tubular" proteinuria (Chap. 49) is the rule in cystinosis, in heavy metal intoxication from cadmium, lead, or mercury, and in the peculiar Balkan nephropathy localized to a small region along the Danube River (Chap. 229).

Pyuria (leukocyturia) may also be a sole urinary abnormality and frequently reflects infection or inflammation of the lower urinary tract rather than intrinsic parenchymal renal disease. Nevertheless, prominent pyuria can occur in any inflammatory disease of the kidneys, especially tubulointerstitial nephritis, lupus nephritis, pyelonephritis, and renal transplant rejection, but usually in association with mild proteinuria or hematuria. The finding of leukocyte casts (Chap. 49) establishes the kidney as the site of the inflammatory reaction.

Pyuria associated with urine that is sterile on routine bacteriologic culture presents a special problem. Certain causes of "sterile pyuria" that are clinically obvious include (1) recent bacterial urinary infection being treated with antibiotics, (2) glucocorticoid therapy, (3) acute febrile episodes, (4) cyclophosphamide administration, (5) pregnancy, (6) renal transplant rejection, (7) recent genitourinary trauma, and (8) prostatitis and cystourethritis. Leukocytes from vaginal secretions may contaminate the urine, so a midstream, clean-catch urine sample should be collected to substantiate a urinary origin. Pyuria associated with proteinuria, nephronal hematuria (Chap. 49), or casts probably signifies inflammatory disease of the renal glomeruli, tubules, interstitium, or microcirculation, and evaluation should focus not upon the pyuria but upon identifying the nature of the renal disease.

Persistent sterile pyuria that cannot be ascribed to any of the foregoing causes has a narrow differential diagnosis. Unusual infections, such as tuberculosis, fungi, atypical mycobacteria, *Haemophilus influenzae,* anaerobic bacteria, fastidious bacteria that grow only on enriched media, and L forms, all must be sought. Intravenous pyelography is needed to detect causes such as urinary tract calculi, papillary necrosis, and renal infiltration by lymphoma or myeloma cells. The latter is usually suspected because of other evidence of myeloma or lymphoma, for both rarely involve only the kidneys. If all tests are negative, cystoscopy may reveal cystitis or trigone inflammation.

URINARY TRACT INFECTION (UTI) This syndrome is defined by the demonstration in urine of pathogenic organisms, either bacteria, tubercle bacilli, or fungi (Chap. 95). When urine specimens are obtained for culture, the condition under which the urine is collected must minimize contamination from external genitourinary surfaces. Women should void into a wide-mouthed sterile container after preliminary cleansing of the vulva with a moist, sterile gauze pledget. In men, midstream collection is usually adequate. Bacterial colony counts of 10^5 organisms per milliliter or greater in urine generally indicate urinary tract colonization and infection. Levels above 10^2 colonies per milliliter are sufficient to indicate infection in symptomatic patients (Table 221-1) and in urine samples obtained by suprapubic aspiration or bladder catheter (Chap. 229). When the urinary tract is anatomically normal, *Escherichia coli* is the usual bacterial pathogen. After prolonged antibiotic treatment of persistent infections, particularly when urinary drainage is impaired or stones are present, *Klebsiella, Enterobacter,* and *Proteus* species predominate.

As discussed in Chap. 95, the presence of a positive urine culture need not imply that an organism is producing tissue inflammation or injury. In some patients, tissue effects may be trivial; in others, injury may be occurring even though symptoms or urinary abnormalities are not present at the time of evaluation. When bacteriuria is associated with tissue inflammation or injury, clinical manifestations usually depend upon the site(s) involved. Dysuria, frequency, urgency, and suprapubic tenderness are common symptoms of bladder and urethral inflammation (Chap. 49 and Table 221-1). Prostatitis also leads to frequency, dysuria, and urgency, and the prostate may be boggy and tender on rectal examination. Flank pain, chills, fever, nausea and vomiting, hypotension from sepsis, and leukocyte casts all suggest true renal parenchymal infection, i.e., pyelonephritis; their absence, however, does not exclude pyelonephritis.

RENAL TUBULE DEFECTS (RTD) This syndrome encompasses a large number of acquired and hereditary disorders, all of which tend to affect tubules more than glomeruli. Hereditary anatomic defects, including such entities as polycystic renal disease, medullary cystic disease, and medullary sponge kidney, are readily detected by intravenous pyelography, which is usually performed because of hematuria, bacteriuria, flank pain, or unexplained azotemia (Chap. 231).

Defects in tubule transport functions, on the other hand, tend not to be associated with prominent renal anatomic defects and arise either as inherited traits (Chap. 231) or during the course of acquired renal disease (Chap. 229). In general, these functional defects impair secretion and/or reabsorption of electrolytes and organic solutes, or limit urinary concentrating and diluting ability (Table 221-1). Typical manifestations of such functional disturbances include polyuria and nocturia (Chap. 49), metabolic acidosis (Chap. 51), and various disorders of fluid and electrolyte balance (Chap. 50). Such defects are defined by direct physiologic measurements; their elucidation requires a sound understanding of normal renal physiology.

HYPERTENSION (H) Hypertension is considered to exist when the average of a series of reliable blood pressure measurements exceeds 140 mmHg systolic or 90 mmHg diastolic (Table 221-1). The pathogenetic mechanisms, clinical and laboratory manifestations, and therapeutic approaches are discussed in detail elsewhere (Chaps. 39 and 196). In addition, a number of renal complications of hypertension are reviewed in Chap. 230, as is the entity of renal artery stenosis, an infrequent but potentially curable cause of hypertension.

NEPHROLITHIASIS (N) This syndrome is established with certainty when a stone is passed, visualized by x-ray, or removed at surgery or cystoscopy (Table 221-1 and Chap. 232). Less certain, but highly suggestive, evidence of nephrolithiasis exists in the patient with renal colic, painful hematuria, or unexplained pyuria, dysuria, and urinary frequency (Chap. 49). Colic varies in its symptomatology but usually begins suddenly in one flank, radiates downward toward the groin, and is excruciatingly painful.

Most renal stones are composed of calcium, uric acid, cystine, or struvite (magnesium ammonium phosphate). All are radiopaque except for those composed solely of uric acid and are, therefore, visible by routine abdominal radiography. Uric acid stones appear as radiolucent filling defects and can be mistaken for tumor or blood clot.

URINARY TRACT OBSTRUCTION (UTO) Documentation of the various structural or functional causes of urinary tract obstruction usually requires radiologic or surgical visualization. The manifestations of obstruction, which initiate the search for its causes, are numerous (Table 221-1) and are reviewed in Chap. 233. Anuria in an adult is almost always due to obstruction of bladder outflow. Less commonly, blockage of upper urinary drainage from both kidneys, or from a solitary functioning kidney, accounts for total or near-total cessation of urine flow. A large bladder after voiding is a sign of outflow obstruction, usually due to urethral stricture, tumor, stone, neurogenic causes, or prostatic hypertrophy. Nocturia, frequency and overflow incontinence, and slowing or hesitancy of micturition are also suggestive of outflow obstruction (Chap. 49). Upper tract obstruction often produces few clinical manifestations. When it is incomplete or unilateral, urine volume may be normal, or even elevated because of a loss of renal concentrating ability. Urinary stasis secondary to obstruction commonly predisposes to recurrent urinary tract infection, chronic obstruction to progressive loss of renal function (Table 221-2).

REFERENCES

BLACK DAK: Diagnosis and renal disease, in *Renal Disease*, 4th ed, DAK Black (ed). St. Louis, Blackwell, 1980

CAMERON JS: The natural history of glomerulonephritis, in *Renal Disease*, 4th ed, DAK Black (ed). St. Louis, Blackwell, 1980, p 329

COE FL, BUSHINSKY DA: Clinical and laboratory assessment of patients with renal and urinary tract disease, in *Clinical Nephrology*, BM Brenner, F Coe, and FC Rector Jr (eds). Philadelphia, Saunders, 1987, p 1

222 DISTURBANCES OF RENAL FUNCTION

BARRY M. BRENNER / THOMAS H. HOSTETTER / STEVEN C. HEBERT

Near constancy of the composition of the internal environment, including the volume, tonicity, and compartmental distribution of the body fluids, is a state essential to survival. With day-to-day variations in amount as well as composition of food and fluids, preservation of the internal environment requires the continuous excretion of these substances (and/or their by-products) in amounts that balance the quantities acquired by ingestion and metabolic transformation. Although losses from skin, lungs, and intestine normally contribute to this excretory capacity, by far the greatest responsibility for solute and water excretion is borne by the kidneys.

The kidneys operate primarily to maintain the composition and volume of the *extracellular* fluid compartment. The continuous exchange of water and solutes across all cell membranes, however, permits the kidneys to contribute indirectly to the regulation of the volume, composition, and tonicity of the *intracellular* fluids as well. To accomplish these tasks, the kidney has evolved physiologic mechanisms that enable the individual to excrete any excesses of water and nonmetabolized solute contained in the diet, as well as the nonvolatile end products of nitrogen metabolism, such as urea and creatinine. By contrast, when faced with deficits of water and/or any of the other major constituents of the body fluids, renal excretion of these substances can be curtailed, reducing the likelihood of severe volume or solute depletion. The purpose of this chapter is to review the major excretory functions of the normal kidney and to examine the way these functions are affected by disorders that impair the operations of this organ in humans.

MECHANISMS OF RENAL EXCRETORY FUNCTION WITH NORMAL AND REDUCED NEPHRON MASS

The volume of urine excreted per day (about 1.5 L, or roughly 1 mL/min) is the small residuum of two very large, and in many ways opposing, processes—namely, *ultrafiltration* of 180 L or more fluid per day (approximately 125 mL/min) across glomerular capillaries on the one hand and, on the other, *reclamation* (or *reabsorption*) of more than 99 percent of this ultrafiltrate by transport processes operating in the renal tubules. The remarkable feat of the initial step in this process in humans is underscored by the fact that, under resting conditions, about 20 percent of the cardiac output passes through the kidneys, which comprise less than 1 percent of body weight. Hence, per unit weight of tissue, the rate of blood flow to the kidneys is greater than that to other solid organs, including heart, brain, and liver.

GLOMERULAR ULTRAFILTRATION Urine formation begins with the elaboration of a protein-free ultrafiltrate of plasma across the walls of the glomerular capillaries. The rate of ultrafiltration (glomerular filtration rate, GFR) is determined by three factors: (1) the balance of pressures acting across the capillary wall (the glomerular capillary hydrostatic and Bowman's space oncotic pressures tend to favor filtration, while glomerular capillary oncotic and Bowman's space hydrostatic pressures tend to retard it), (2) the rate at which plasma flows through the glomeruli, and (3) the permeability and the total surface area of the filtering capillaries. A decrease in GFR can be expected when (1) glomerular hydrostatic pressure is reduced (as in hypotensive shock), (2) tubule (hence, Bowman's space) hydrostatic pressure is increased (ureteral or bladder neck obstruction), (3) plasma oncotic pressure rises to unusually high levels (hemoconcentration due to dehydration; multiple myeloma or other dysproteinemias), (4) renal (hence, glomerular) blood and plasma flow are decreased (circulatory collapse, profound heart failure), and (5) permeability and/or total filtering surface area is reduced (acute or chronic glomerulonephritis).

Despite the extraordinarily high rate of water movement across the glomerular capillary wall, all but the smallest of the circulating plasma proteins are normally excluded from passage through this barrier. Molecules the size of inulin (approximately 5200 mol wt) or smaller normally appear in glomerular urine in the same concentrations as in plasma water, whereas the transport of substances of increasingly greater size diminishes progressively, normally approaching very low values as the size of serum albumin is approached. The *glomerular capillary basement membrane* and the *slitlike diaphragms* that connect adjacent epithelial cell foot processes on the urinary aspect of the glomerular capillary wall (Fig. 49-1) serve as major barriers to protein filtration. In addition to these mechanical gates, *electrostatic factors* also serve to retard the filtration of plasma proteins, especially albumin. The albumin molecule behaves as a polyanion in physiologic solution, and is therefore retarded by the anionic glycoproteins in the various component layers of the glomerular wall. With disruption of these mechanical and electrostatic barriers, as seen in many forms of glomerular injury (see Chaps. 226 to 228), large quantities of plasma proteins gain access to the urine.

BIOLOGIC CONSEQUENCES OF SUSTAINED REDUCTIONS IN GFR Measurement of total GFR of both kidneys provides a sensitive and commonly employed index of overall renal excretory function. When renal excretory function is impaired, either acutely or chronically, one or more of the determinants of GFR in affected nephrons is altered unfavorably so that total GFR declines. The magnitude of the decline is determined by the sum of the impairments of function of individual glomeruli. Initially, the effect of such impairments in single-nephron GFR (SNGFR), no matter how small, is to reduce the total rate of excretion of water and those solutes normally contained in the glomerular ultrafiltrate. In the steady state, these reduced rates of filtration, when accompanied by comparably reduced rates of excretion, lead to *retention* and *accumulation* of the unexcreted substances in the body fluids. Further reduction in GFR augments the degree to which these substances are retained.

Figure 222-1 depicts the major patterns of response to these impairments in filtration. The degree of reduction in total GFR is plotted on the abscissa, expressed as a percentage of normal (100 percent). For the various solutes normally contained in glomerular filtrate, three general types of response are common, depicted by curves A, B, and C. Curve A describes the pattern seen with substances, such as creatinine and urea, which normally depend largely on glomerular filtration for their excretion into the urine; i.e., secretion fails to influence urinary excretion appreciably. Therefore, as GFR falls, plasma levels of creatinine, urea, and other substances normally excreted largely by filtration rise progressively, albeit in the nonlinear manner illustrated.

The clinical course of chronic renal failure (CRF) usually also conforms to the pattern described by curve A. Patients with CRF usually pass from a long asymptomatic period of "compensation" to a more accelerated and clinically symptomatic terminal phase. In other words, chronic forms of renal injury that lead to slow but inexorable destruction of nephron mass usually lead to progressive but modest elevations in creatinine and urea levels in plasma, but

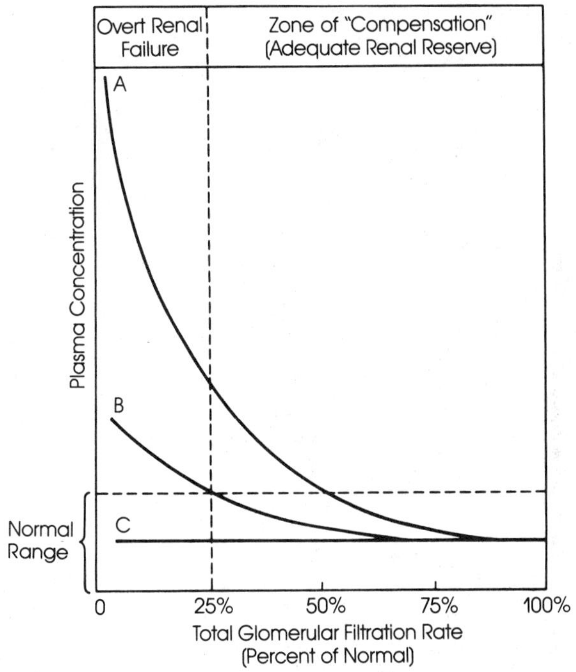

FIGURE 222-1 Representative patterns of adaptation for different types of solutes in body fluids in chronic renal failure. (*After NS Bricker et al, in Brenner and Rector, 3d ed.*)

not to levels beyond the range of normal, despite loss of as much as 50 percent of total GFR. With further loss of nephron mass, and further reduction in GFR, however (even though the rate of nephron destruction may not be accelerated), the limits of renal reserve are exceeded, and continued accumulation of curve A–type solutes leads to plasma concentrations clearly beyond the range of normal (Fig. 222-1). Because these retained solutes are believed to exert "toxic" effects on virtually all organ systems, manifestations of CRF now become overt. As a result, for patients with reduced renal mass, even small additional decrements in total GFR may spell the difference between "compensation" and overt uremia.

The accumulation of curve A–type solutes with progressive renal failure continues until external balance for these solutes is achieved, that is, until acquisition and/or production rates and excretion rates are exactly matched. In the case of creatinine, for example, assuming a constant rate of creatinine production, a 50 percent reduction in GFR results in an approximate doubling of the plasma creatinine concentration. The latter restores the filtered load of creatinine (that is, GFR × plasma creatinine concentration) to normal, and urinary excretion rate again becomes equivalent to the rate of creatinine production. Unfortunately, since no mechanism exists in human beings for augmenting creatinine excretion beyond this level, elimination of retained creatinine is not possible, and plasma concentration remains twice normal. With progressive reduction in GFR, plasma creatinine levels continue to rise, due both to the most recent loss of nephron excretory function and to the retention associated with earlier nephron destruction (Fig. 222-1). *In practice, so long as the net rates of acquisition and production* (i.e., *liver function and muscle mass*) *remain reasonably constant, the inverse relationship between plasma concentrations of solutes such as creatinine and urea and GFR is sufficiently reliable and predictable to allow plasma levels of the solutes to serve as useful clinical indexes of GFR.*

In contrast to solutes of the curve A type, plasma levels of substances such as phosphate, urate, and potassium (K^+) and hydrogen (H^+) ions usually fail to rise above the normal range until GFR falls to a small percentage of normal. With progressive renal failure this pattern of response, depicted by curve B in Fig. 222-1, reflects the participation of tubule transport mechanisms that contribute to the excretion of these substances. In other words, *as GFR declines, the tubules facilitate the excretion of progressively greater fractions of the filtered load of these solutes, either by enhancing their net secretion and/or by diminishing their net reabsorption.* Plasma levels of curve B–type solutes, therefore, rise much less than do those of curve A because, with progressive reduction in GFR, *excretion rate per nephron* and, therefore, *fractional excretion* both increase. Eventually, however, enhanced fractional excretion can no longer offset the reduction in the filtered load of these solutes caused by a markedly diminished GFR, and plasma levels rise above the normal range (Fig. 222-1). For urate, phosphate, and K^+, at least, increased fractional excretion usually serves to maintain normal plasma levels until GFR falls to less than one-fourth of normal.

Finally, for certain solutes, such as sodium chloride (NaCl), concentrations in plasma remain virtually constant, and at normal levels, throughout the entire course of CRF, despite continued ingestion of these substances in normal amounts. Such solutes conform to the pattern described by curve C in Fig. 222-1. The extent of compensation is nearly complete and represents a fundamental adaptation to renal injury. To illustrate the magnitude of the adaptation involved, it is useful to compare the excretion of Na^+ in an individual with normal renal excretory function (GFR of 125 mL/min) with that in an individual with advanced renal insufficiency (GFR of 2 mL/min). Both subjects are allowed to ingest a diet containing 7 g salt per day (120 mmol Na^+). With a normal serum Na^+ concentration of 140 mmol/L, external Na^+ balance is achieved in the normal individual by excreting approximately 0.5 percent of the filtered load of Na^+. By contrast, for external balance to be maintained in the patient with CRF, fractional excretion of Na^+ must rise to 30 percent. *In other words, external balance for Na^+ demands that the same quantity of Na^+ (120 mmol) be excreted into the urine each day in the subject with CRF as in the normal subject.* Given the drastic reduction in GFR faced by the patient with CRF, external balance can be achieved only by a progressive transformation of the Na^+ reabsorptive processes in surviving tubules, so that a progressively larger fraction of the filtered load of Na^+ escapes reabsorption and appears in final urine. In short, *the rate of excretion of Na^+ per surviving nephron increases in inverse proportion to the composite GFR of surviving nephrons.*

MECHANISMS OF TUBULE TRANSPORT WITH NORMAL AND REDUCED NEPHRON MASS Loss of renal function with nearly all forms of progressive renal disease is usually attended by a progressive distortion of renal morphology and architecture. Despite this structural disarray, glomerular and tubule functions often remain as closely integrated (i.e., *glomerulotubular balance*) in the diseased kidney as they do in the normal organ, at least until the final stages of CRF. A fundamental feature of this *intact nephron hypothesis* is that following loss of nephron mass, residual renal function derives primarily from the operation of surviving healthy nephrons, while the diseased nephrons are believed to cease functioning. Despite progressive nephron destruction, there is considerable evidence to suggest that many of the mechanisms that contribute to the maintenance of solute and water balance differ only quantitatively, and not qualitatively, from those believed to govern fluid and solute homeostasis under normal physiologic conditions. The most important of these are considered below.

Tubule transport of sodium chloride and water in health Most of the filtered water and Na^+ salts are reabsorbed by the tubules, leaving small and variable amounts, equivalent on a day-to-day basis to the quantities ingested, to reach the final urine. About two-thirds of the glomerular ultrafiltrate is reabsorbed in the *proximal tubule* with little change in the osmolality or Na^+ concentration of the unreabsorbed fraction (Fig. 222-2). In other words, fluid reabsorption in the proximal tubule is nearly *isosmotic* and is coupled to the active transport of Na^+. Since Cl^- and HCO_3^- are the primary anions in the extracellular fluid, most of the filtered Na^+ is reabsorbed with these anions. In the early convoluted portion of the proximal tubule, bicarbonate is the principal anion accompanying the reabsorption of sodium. This process occurs via a Na^+/H^+ exchange mechanism at

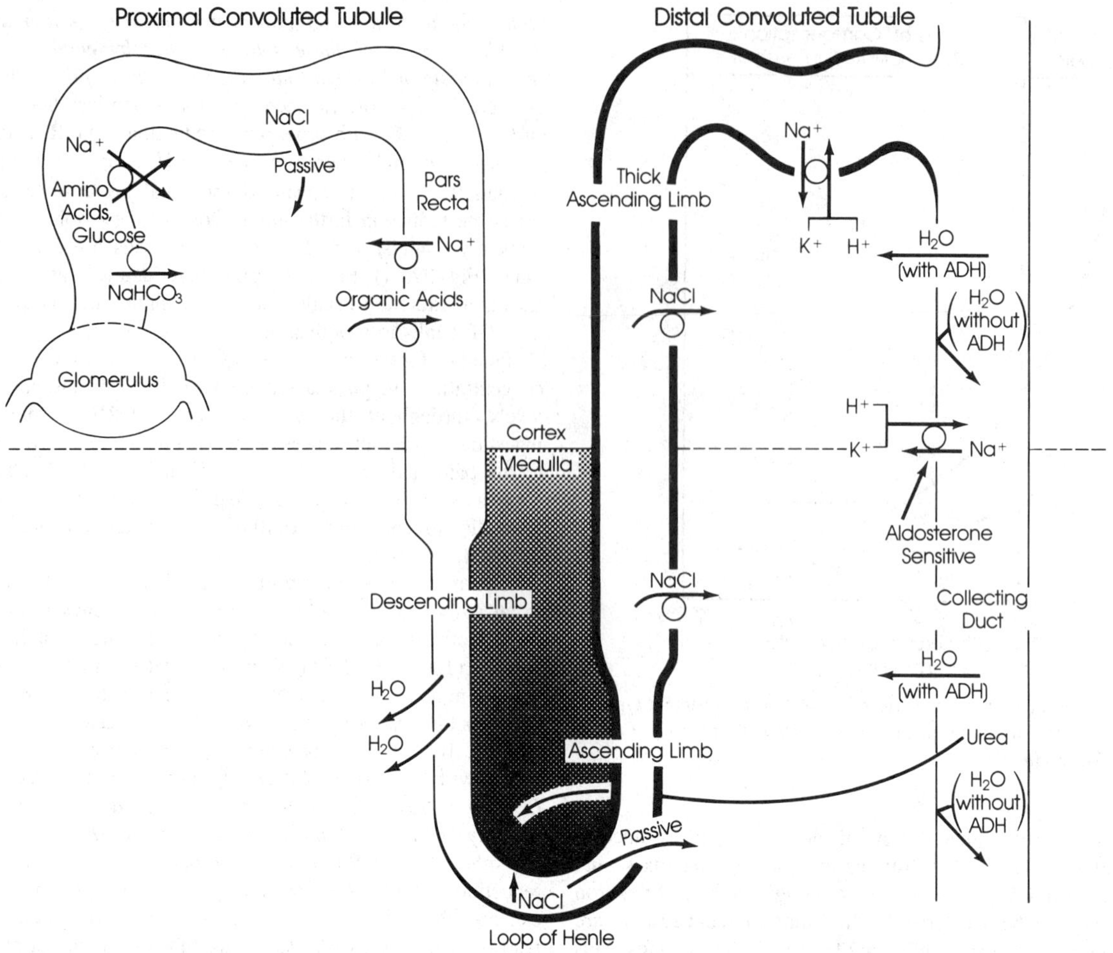

FIGURE 222-2 Transport functions of the various anatomic segments of the mammalian nephron. Fluid reabsorption across the proximal tubule is isosmotic and accounts for reabsorption of approximately two-thirds of the filtered Na^+ and H_2O. The major portions of the filtered HCO_3^-, amino acids, and glucose are reabsorbed in the early proximal convoluted tubule. Reabsorption of glucose and amino acids is coupled to Na^+ transport and thereby generates a negative potential difference within the tubule lumen. At the same time, HCO_3^- is reabsorbed by a nonelectrogenic mechanism, via H^+ secretion. The active transport of these solutes results in transepithelial concentration and effective osmotic pressure gradients promoting H_2O flow across the proximal tubule, into the peritubular capillaries. The rise in tubule fluid Cl^- concentration is a necessary reciprocal consequence of the decreased luminal HCO_3^- concentration. The resultant high concentration of Cl^- becomes an important force for the outward passive transport of Cl^- down its concentration gradient, resulting in a lumen-positive potential difference in the late proximal convoluted tubule. The pars recta of the proximal tubule is capable of active electrogenic transport of Na^+ independent of organic solute transport. Under normal conditions, approximately one-third of the glomerular filtrate enters the descending limb of Henle's loop. Because the thin descending limb is incapable of active outward NaCl transport and is characterized by low permeability to Na^+ but high H_2O permeability, H_2O is abstracted passively as the fluid approaches the bend of Henle's loop. Hypertonic fluid with a greater NaCl concentration but lower urea concentration than the surrounding medullary interstitium thus enters the thin ascending limb of Henle. This segment differs from the descending limb in that it is largely impermeable to H_2O and urea but highly permeable to NaCl. These characteristics allow for passive diffusion of NaCl out of the ascending limb. Active electrogenic NaCl transport across the water-impermeable thick ascending limb of Henle allows for separation of solute and water. In consequence tubule fluid becomes dilute, and the medullary interstitium hypertonic. Irrespective of the final osmolality of the urine, the fluid that enters the distal convoluted tubule is always hypoosmotic. This segment exhibits active Na^+ reabsorption. All but the terminal portion of the distal convoluted tubule is water impermeable, even in the presence of ADH. Aldosterone exerts its effect in this segment by enhancing Na^+ reabsorption, which is variably coupled to K^+ and H^+ secretion. The cortical and papillary portions of the collecting duct are sites where ADH exerts its principal effect. The permeability of these segments to H_2O in the absence of ADH is very low but can be greatly enhanced in the presence of ADH. These segments are also characterized by active Na^+ reabsorption, which appears to depend on the presence of mineralocorticoid. In the absence of ADH, the collecting tubule is water impermeable so that hypotonic tubule fluid courses through it. However, in the presence of ADH, water is avidly reabsorbed here, resulting in hypertonic final urine.

the luminal brush border and is dependent upon both cystolic and brush border carbonic anhydrase. Glucose, amino acids, and other organic solutes (e.g., lactate) are also extensively reabsorbed in the proximal convoluted tubule by a cotransport process that links the cellular entry of these organic substrates with Na^+. Three processes appear to operate in parallel to couple water (i.e., volume) absorption with solute absorption in the proximal tubule. First, given the remarkably high water permeability of this nephron segment, very small transepithelial osmolality differences, that is, *luminal hypotonicity* on the order of 2 to 3 mosmol, produced by solute absorption, could drive volume absorption. Second, due to the *preferential* absorption of HCO_3^- and organic solutes in the early portions of the proximal tubule, the concentrations of these substances decrease while that of Cl^- increases along the length of the proximal tubule. Volume absorption would occur if the rate of Na^+ and Cl^- diffusion down their respective electrochemical gradients were more rapid than the back diffusion of sodium bicarbonate into the lumen. Finally, an *effective osmotic gradient* would be established (despite equal macroscopic osmolalities of luminal and peritubular fluids) if the effective osmolality produced by Cl^- in the lumen were greater than that for bicarbonate in the peritubular fluid.

The rate of reabsorption of fluid from proximal convoluted tubules and peritubular interstitium is sensitive to the effects of *physical factors,* i.e., the hydrostatic and colloid osmotic (or oncotic) pressures acting across the walls of the peritubular capillaries. Because the plasma proteins in glomerular capillaries are concentrated by ultrafiltration, there is a marked rise in the oncotic pressure as plasma flows along the glomerular capillary network. This step-up in plasma oncotic pressure is transmitted largely unchanged to the peritubular capillaries, via the efferent arterioles. These resistance vessels cause a substantial drop in hydrostatic pressure, however, so that when the plasma reaches the peritubular capillaries, oncotic pressure greatly exceeds hydrostatic pressure. These *Starling forces* are therefore oriented in an *uptake mode,* in contrast to the *filtration mode* at the glomerulus, where hydrostatic pressure exceeds oncotic. The extent to which oncotic pressure exceeds hydrostatic pressure in the peritubular capillary network is thought to modulate the overall rate of reabsorption of fluid by the proximal tubules. Therefore, when peritubular oncotic pressure falls, or hydrostatic pressure rises, uptake of fluid by these capillaries is reduced. As a result, fluid is retained in the interstitial space, altering the hydrostatic pressure in the space, and ultimately retarding the egress of fluid from the lateral intercellular channels. Without an adequate route of drainage, fluid in the channels leaks back into the tubule lumen and diminishes *net fluid reabsorption* by this tubule segment. The opposite occurs in states in which peritubular oncotic pressure increases (increased filtration fraction) or hydrostatic pressure decreases (enhanced efferent arteriolar tone). Under these circumstances, peritubular capillary uptake of reabsorbate is augmented, leading ultimately to *enhanced net fluid reabsorption* by the proximal tubule.

In contrast to the proximal tubule, active outward transport of NaCl from tubule lumen to peritubular blood has not been established for the *thin limbs of Henle's loop.* However, passive outward salt transport does occur, as indicated in Fig. 222-2. In the next segment of the nephron, the *medullary thick ascending limb of Henle,* the concentration of NaCl is reduced below the level that prevails at the beginning of this segment. Here Cl^- absorption occurs by an active process involving a furosemide-sensitive $Na^+:K^+:2Cl^-$ cotransport mechanism in the luminal membrane, with one-half of Na^+ absorption proceeding passively, driven by the lumen-positive transepithelial voltage. Since the ascending limb of Henle is always impermeable to water, net NaCl reabsorption not only generates hypotonic tubule fluid, but also gives rise to the high NaCl concentration of the outer medullary interstitium (Fig. 222-2). In certain animals vasopressin (ADH) enhances NaCl absorption but not water permeability in the medullary portion of the thick ascending limb, but an effect of this hormone on this segment in human beings is uncertain.

The fluid leaving the thick ascending limb of Henle is normally low in NaCl concentration, a condition largely independent of the organism's diet or state of hydration. In the *distal convoluted tubule,* water reabsorption is variable, depending on the state of hydration or, more specifically, on the presence or absence of the ADH in plasma. In the absence of ADH, this and more distal nephron segments are impermeable to water, so that the hypotonic fluid entering this segment is excreted as *dilute urine.* Indeed, continued salt reabsorption along the distal convoluted tubule results in further dilution of the urine. In the presence of ADH, the permeability of the late portion of this segment to water increases, and as a result, the osmolality of the late distal tubule fluid rises to a value close to that of plasma. NaCl continues to be reabsorbed from the tubule lumen, against moderately steep chemical and electrical gradients. The reabsorptive process for NaCl at this site is enhanced by *aldosterone.*

The *cortical collecting tubule* possesses an extremely low permeability to water in the absence of ADH, whereas this permeability increases greatly in the presence of the hormone. The sensitivity of this segment to ADH appears to be more pronounced than that of the distal convoluted tubule. As with the distal convoluted tubule, the cortical collecting tubule is capable of further active reabsorption of NaCl.

The terminal segment of the distal nephron is the highly branched *papillary collecting duct.* Continued electrolyte transport in this segment results in the large ion concentration differences that normally exist between urine and plasma. As in the cortical collecting tubule, Na^+ transport appears to be active since reabsorption proceeds against sizable electrochemical gradients. The rate of Na^+ transport in this segment depends on the diet and on the load of Na^+ delivered from more proximal segments, and is affected by aldosterone. The permeability of this segment to water also increases markedly in the presence of ADH.

Effects of reduced nephron mass on sodium chloride transport in surviving nephrons With reductions in nephron mass the remaining healthy or less damaged nephrons may hypertrophy so that GFR is increased toward normal. For example, a patient who has a unilateral nephrectomy for renal cell carcinoma or for donation for transplantation loses one-half of the nephron mass, and GFR is reduced by 50 percent at the time of surgery. However, several months after the nephrectomy GFR may return to 80 percent of the preoperative value for two kidneys. This requires that the blood flow, GFR, and transport functions of individual remaining nephrons increase above normal values. This "compensatory hypertrophy" is evident by the large glomeruli and tubular structures observed on histologic sections of the kidney and by increases in many of the biochemical processes associated with tubule transport (e.g., Na^+, K^+-ATPase). Similar hypertrophic changes occur in nephrons from kidneys damaged by other processes (e.g., glomerulonephritis); however, as nephron damage progresses, the hypertrophy of single nephrons can no longer make up for the magnitude of nephron loss, and total GFR falls.

With progressive destruction of nephrons, *maintenance of external balance for NaCl requires that fractional salt excretion increase as GFR decreases.* Very likely several mechanisms contribute to this adaptive increase in fractional salt excretion. With losses of functioning nephron units, peritubular capillary hydrostatic and oncotic pressures are probably altered in directions that serve to suppress proximal tubule reabsorption of NaCl and water. For example, a rise in peritubular capillary hydrostatic pressure, which tends to inhibit net proximal fluid reabsorption, might be anticipated with arterial hypertension, a common feature of renal insufficiency. Similarly, peritubular oncotic pressure might be expected to decline with renal injury, owing both to reductions in filtration fraction and to hypoalbuminemia. While such alterations in peritubular factors clearly account for diminution in proximal fluid reabsorption in response to falling levels of GFR in animals, such alterations have not been established with certainty in humans. Aldosterone, normally an important determinant of Na^+ reabsorption in distal portions of the nephron, is probably not a major factor responsible for reducing fractional Na^+ reabsorption, since aldosterone levels in plasma are rarely reduced in CRF. Furthermore, external Na^+ balance is preserved in bilaterally adrenalectomized uremic dogs maintained on fixed doses of mineralocorticoid. Yet another factor contributing to the suppression of fractional NaCl reabsorption in CRF may relate to the retention of solutes as GFR declines. In addition to urea and creatinine, a host of *organic acids* (including *hippurates*) also accumulate. These substances are normally excreted by both filtration and tubule secretion; the latter process involves a carrier-mediated organic acid transport system in proximal tubule epithelia. When GFR is reduced and plasma levels of these organic acids increase, sufficient fluid may accompany the secretion of these organic anions into the proximal tubule lumen (by osmosis) to diminish net fluid reabsorption, and even favor net fluid secretion. Evidence in support of this mechanism derives from studies in which uremic sera were capable of inducing net fluid secretion in isolated proximal tubules of rabbits in vitro.

Several substances that regulate NaCl transport across the tubules may also participate in the enhanced fractional excretion of salt in renal insufficiency. Atrial natriuretic peptide is released from the cardiac atria in response to plasma volume expansion and atrial distention. This hormone effects a natriuresis by reducing net sodium reabsorption through its complementary actions on active collecting duct Na^+ transport and on physical factors within the adjacent vasa recta. Thus, atrial natriuretic peptide likely participates in the uremic adaptation to salt balance. In addition, prostaglandin E reduces NaCl reabsorption from the thick ascending limb. Since prostaglandin E production per nephron appears to rise in renal insufficiency, the local action of this prostaglandin may also contribute to natriuresis in the setting of reduced renal mass. Finally, other inhibitors of ion transport appear in uremic serum including an inhibitor(s) of the Na^+, K^+-ATPase. This factor(s) has not been fully characterized, and whether it represents an adaptation for maintenance of homeostasis or an unregulated accumulation of a toxin is also uncertain.

Serum and urine from patients and dogs with uremia contain factors capable of inhibiting NaCl transport across frog skin, toad bladder, and rat renal tubule. Accumulation of natriuretic factors in uremia may not be without cost; the "trade-off" for maintenance of external Na^+ balance is the possibility of abnormalities occurring in Na^+ transport across cell membranes, which often occurs in advanced renal insufficiency. This possibility is discussed in greater detail in Chap. 224.

The obligatorily high rate of solute excretion per surviving nephron (so-called osmotic diuresis due to urea and other retained solutes) may also contribute to enhancing fractional NaCl excretion, much as occurs in normal subjects following administration of nonreabsorbable solutes such as mannitol. Finally, certain forms of CRF tend to be associated with unusually pronounced salt losses in urine. These *salt-wasting nephropathies* include chronic pyelonephritis and other tubulointerstitial diseases (see Chap. 229) as well as polycystic and medullary cystic diseases. These disorders have in common greater destruction of medullary and interstitial than cortical and glomerular portions of the renal parenchyma. Preferential impairment of tubule reabsorptive function, rather than a primary reduction in GFR, may, therefore, underlie the salt-losing tendency in these disorders. A number of clinical derangements associated with the altered renal handling of NaCl in CRF (including hypo- and hypervolemia, hypertension, etc.) are considered in Chap. 224.

Effects of reduced nephron mass on water reabsorption in surviving nephrons As with NaCl, there is a progressive increase in the fractional excretion of water with advancing renal insufficiency, so that even the patient with a total GFR of 5 mL/min or less can usually maintain external water balance. The adaptations in the handling of water by the tubules of the diseased kidney are of importance in the pathogenesis of the urinary concentrating defect and, hence, of the polyuria and nocturia seen commonly in CRF (see Chap. 49). To appreciate the mechanisms involved, the responses of a normal and a uremic subject in maintaining external water balance need to be compared. Assuming that both subjects ingest the same diet and also the same amount of fluid, total solute and volume excretion in each subject should be identical as well. If the *obligatory solute load* to be excreted in each is assumed to be 600 mosmol per day, and urine osmolality is 300 mosmol/kg, a urine volume of 2 L/d will be required to excrete the total solute load in each subject. If GFR in normal and uremic subjects is 180 and 4 L/d, respectively, urinary volume excretion of 2 L/d represents excretion of slightly more than 1 percent of the filtered water in the normal individual, compared with a much larger value, 50 percent, in the uremic subject. Since the range of urine osmolalities that the diseased kidney can achieve (250 to 350 mosmol/kg) is much narrower than in the normal (40 to 1200 mosmol/kg), the individual with normal function is able to excrete the obligatory daily solute load of 600 mosmol in as little as 500 mL urine per day or as much as 15 L/d, compared with the much narrower range in the patient with renal insufficiency, from about 1.7 to 2.4 L/d.

In CRF, the limited ability to concentrate the urine usually correlates closely with other measures of impaired renal function. Isosthenuria is, therefore, a nearly universal finding when GFR falls below 25 mL/min. At this level of GFR and below, urine osmolality does not rise even with supraphysiologic parenteral doses of vasopressin, suggesting that the concentrating defect is related not only to loss of diseased nephrons but also to impaired concentrating ability in surviving nephrons. As has been discussed, with diminution in functioning nephron mass, there is a concurrent increase in fractional excretion of a number of solutes. As a consequence, solute diuresis per nephron obligates a nearly isosmotic amount of water and prevents the elaboration of either hypotonic or hypertonic urine. Disease-induced abnormalities of the architecture of the renal medulla (loops of Henle, vasa recta), aberrations in renal medullary blood flow, and defective transport of NaCl in the ascending limb of Henle undoubtedly also contribute to this defect in urine concentration. Finally, there is suggestive evidence that uremia per se may impair the responsiveness of terminal nephron segments to vasopressin.

Since patients with renal insufficiency are usually unable to excrete concentrated urine, they must have access to adequate amounts of water in order to ensure the excretion of total daily solute loads. For this reason, restriction of fluid intake may prove extremely hazardous in patients with CRF. Likewise, impairment of diluting capacity may prevent many patients from excreting large amounts of ingested fluids. The consequences of the abnormal water excretion patterns in CRF, including the tendencies to development of hypo- and hyper-natremia, are considered in Chaps. 50 and 224.

Tubule transport of phosphate with normal and reduced nephron mass Under normal physiologic conditions, about 80 to 90 percent of the filtered load of phosphate is reabsorbed, mainly in the proximal tubule. *Parathyroid hormone* (*PTH*), by augmenting phosphate excretion via inhibition of this proximal reabsorptive process (Chap. 339), plays a key role in phosphate homeostasis. In normal humans, when dietary phosphate intake increases, a *transient* rise in plasma phosphate concentration is usually observed. This results in a similarly transient reduction in the plasma ionized calcium concentration (due largely to calcium phosphate deposition in bone), which, in turn, stimulates PTH secretion. By enhancing fractional phosphate excretion, PTH restores external phosphate balance and normophosphatemia. This then enables plasma ionized calcium levels to return to normal, thereby removing the stimulus to PTH release, and restoring all elements of the phosphate control system to the original steady state.

With advancing renal disease, and constant dietary intake of phosphate, external phosphate balance is achieved by progressive reduction in fractional phosphate reabsorption. Enhanced PTH secretion is an important determinant of this phosphaturic response to reduced nephron mass. With each succeeding decrement in GFR, the total amount of phosphate filtered by surviving glomeruli is reduced, leading to transient retention of phosphate and, therefore, a rise (albeit small) in the phosphate concentration in extracellular fluid, including plasma. This rise in plasma phosphate concentration leads to a reciprocal small decline in plasma ionized calcium concentration and a corresponding increase in PTH secretion. Although the phosphaturic response of surviving tubules to this elevation in circulating PTH is thought to restore plasma phosphate and, therefore, calcium levels to normal (at least in the "compensated" stage of CRF described by the relatively flat portion of curve B in Fig. 222-1), the biologic cost of this return to normophosphatemia and normocalcemia is a *persistent elevation in the plasma PTH level.* With successive decrements in GFR, each stage in this overall process is repeated, but at an ever-increasing cost, namely, *progressive elevation in the circulating level of PTH*.

Alterations in vitamin D metabolism also contribute to the elevated PTH levels in renal failure. The kidneys are normally the major site of *metabolic conversion of vitamin D to its active metabolites.* As discussed in Chap. 339, precursors of the active form of vitamin D, synthesized in skin or acquired from foods, undergo initial hydroxylation in the liver to form 25-hydroxyvitamin D [25(OH)D]. The kidney is the site of a second important hydroxylation step, formation of 1,25-dihydroxyvitamin D [$1,25(OH)_2D$]. This activated form of vitamin D acts directly on the parathyroid gland to suppress PTH secretion as well as to enhance intestinal calcium and phosphate absorption and promote resorption of these ions from bone. In addition, 1,25(OH)$_2$D probably opposes the phosphaturic action of PTH at the level of the renal tubule by augmenting, rather than diminishing, phosphate reabsorption. With advancing renal disease, reduction in renal mass causes vitamin D hydroxylation to be impaired; phosphate retention also suppresses this important hydroxylation reaction. Not only are the circulating levels of 1,25(OH)$_2$D diminished in uremia, but the receptors that mediate its action within the parathyroid cells are diminished. These two effects disinhibit parathyroid hormone secretion and thereby increase circulating PTH levels. Reduction in circulating 1,25(OH)$_2$D levels, by suppressing calcium absorption from gut, contributes further to the development of the hypocalcemia and PTH excess of CRF, the consequences of which are considered in Chap. 224.

At least two additional processes are thought to contribute to elevated PTH levels in renal failure. One relates to the skeletal resistance to the calcemic effect of PTH seen in uremia. This resistance necessitates a greater than normal level of circulating PTH to effect an increment in serum calcium concentration. The other derives from the finding that reductions in renal mass impair the ability of the kidneys to degrade circulating PTH. The fact that phosphate conforms more to a curve B– than curve C–type solute in Fig. 222-1 indicates that these forms of adaptation are limited; ultimately phosphate retention occurs when GFR falls below about 25 mL/min.

Since PTH exerts major biologic effects on bone, as well as renal tubules, the external balance of phosphate in CRF is achieved at the expense of elevated PTH levels, which, in turn, account for many of the bone changes of renal osteodystrophy (i.e., *secondary hyperparathyroidism*, Fig. 224-1). In support of this ingenious *trade-off hypothesis*, studies in animals with CRF suggest that when dietary phosphate intake is reduced in proportion to the reduction in GFR, external balance of phosphate no longer requires augmentation of fractional phosphate excretion in surviving nephrons. Accordingly, circulating PTH levels no longer rise, and the typical bone changes of secondary hyperparathyroidism are diminished, if not prevented.

Hydrogen and bicarbonate transport with normal and reduced nephron mass As discussed in Chap. 51, the pH of extracellular fluid is normally maintained within a narrow range, 7.36 to 7.44, despite day-to-day variations in the quantity of acids entering the body fluids from dietary and metabolic sources (approximately 1 mmol H^+ per kilogram of body weight per day). These acids consume both intracellular and extracellular buffers, of which bicarbonate (HCO_3^-) is the most important in the intracellular compartment. Such buffering minimizes the changes in pH that would otherwise occur. The HCO_3^- buffer system would be of little long-term benefit were it not for homeostatic mechanisms, however, since with unrelenting acquisition of nonvolatile acids from dietary and metabolic sources, buffering capacity would ultimately be exhausted, eventually culminating in fatal acidosis. The kidneys normally function to prevent this possibility by *regenerating* HCO_3^- and, thereby, maintaining the concentration of HCO_3^- in the plasma. In addition to generating HCO_3^-, the kidneys also *reclaim* essentially all the HCO_3^- present in the glomerular ultrafiltrate. This reabsorptive process takes place largely in the proximal tubule and is virtually complete below a critical serum HCO_3^- concentration—the threshold concentration—which in humans is normally about 26 mmol/L, identical to the concentration of HCO_3^- in plasma. As a consequence, urinary wastage of HCO_3^- is prevented. Alternatively, when plasma HCO_3^- concentration rises above this threshold level, reabsorption of HCO_3^- becomes less complete, and the excess HCO_3^- escapes into the final urine, returning the plasma HCO_3^- concentration to the threshold level. Despite reabsorption of all the filtered HCO_3^-, metabolic acidosis would still ensue if HCO_3^- consumed in buffering nonvolatile strong acids were not constantly regenerated.

The *reabsorption* of filtered HCO_3^- in the proximal tubule occurs by the following mechanism. In proximal tubule cells, H^+, formed by the splitting of water into H^+ and OH^-, is secreted into the tubule lumen, very likely in exchange for Na^+. The OH^- ion, under the influence of *carbonic anhydrase*, combines with CO_2 to form HCO_3^-, which moves across the peritubular cell membrane via an electrogenic $Na(HCO_3)_2$ cotransporter to enter the extracellular HCO_3^- pool. The H^+ secreted into the tubule lumen combines with a filtered HCO_3^-, forming H_2CO_3. Dehydration of the latter in the proximal tubule lumen leads to the formation of CO_2 which also diffuses from lumen to peritubular blood. As a result, *a filtered HCO_3^- ion is reclaimed.* Secreted H^+ ions are also free to combine with non-HCO_3^- buffers (e.g., phosphate or ammonia) in the tubule fluid and are excreted in these forms in the final urine. HCO_3^-, the other original product of the breakdown of H_2CO_3, formed within the tubule cell, enters the peritubular blood, and *an HCO_3^- ion is regenerated.*

Hydrogen ions in the urine are bound primarily to filtered buffers (e.g., phosphate) in an amount (the so-called titratable acid) equivalent to the amount of alkali required to titrate the pH of the urine to the pH of blood. It is usually not possible, however, to excrete all the daily acid load as titratable acid alone. To serve as an additional buffer, the cells of the renal tubules generate ammonia (NH_3), largely from the hydrolysis of glutamine. NH_3 diffuses from these cells into the tubule lumen, where it combines with H^+ to form NH_4^+. As noted above, each mole of NH_4^+ excreted into the urine is associated with the regeneration of 1 mol of HCO_3^-. *Ammoniagenesis*, a process which occurs within proximal tubule cells, is responsive to the acid-base needs of the individual. When faced with an acute acid burden and an increased need for HCO_3^- regeneration, the rate of renal ammonia synthesis increases sharply.

The quantity of hydrogen ions excreted as titratable acid and NH_4^+ is equal to the quantity of HCO_3^- regenerated in tubule cells and added to the plasma. Under steady-state conditions, the quantity of net acid excreted into the urine (the sum of titratable acid and NH_4^+ minus HCO_3^-) must equal the quantity of acid gained by the extracellular fluid from all sources. Metabolic acidosis and alkalosis result when this delicate balance is perturbed, the former the result of *insufficient* net acid excretion, the latter due to *excessive* acid excretion.

Progressive loss of renal function usually causes little or no change in arterial pH, plasma bicarbonate concentration, or arterial carbon dioxide tension (P_{CO_2}) until GFR falls below 50 percent of normal. Thereafter, all three quantities tend to decline as *metabolic acidosis* ensues. In general, the metabolic acidosis of CRF is not due to overproduction of endogenous acids, but is largely a reflection of the reduction in renal mass, which limits the amount of NH_3 (and therefore HCO_3^-) that can be generated. Although surviving nephrons are probably capable of generating supernormal quantities of NH_3 *per nephron*, the diminished nephron population causes overall NH_3 production to be reduced to an extent inadequate to permit sufficient buffering of H^+ in urine. Though patients with CRF may acidify the urine normally (i.e., urine pH as low as 4.5), the defect in NH_3 production limits total daily acid excretion to 30 to 40 mmol, or one-half to two-thirds the quantity of nonvolatile acid formed in the same time period. Metabolic acidosis is the inevitable consequence of this positive balance for H^+, which in most patients with stable CRF is relatively mild and nonprogressive (arterial pH of approximately 7.33 to 7.37).

Given this substantial daily accumulation of H^+, and the typically stable and nonprogressive nature of the resulting acidosis, including the observed relative constancy of the plasma HCO_3^- concentration (albeit at reduced levels of 14 to 20 mmol/L), it follows that some large tissue source of buffering must account for the stability of the acidosis in CRF. Bone is the most likely candidate, particularly in view of its large reservoir of alkaline salts (calcium phosphate and calcium carbonate). Dissolution of this buffer source probably contributes to the osteodystrophy of CRF (see Fig. 224-1).

Although the acidosis of CRF is a consequence of the reduction in total renal mass and is therefore tubular in origin, it nevertheless depends to a large extent on the level of GFR. When GFR is reduced to only a moderate extent (i.e., to about 50 percent of normal), retention of anions, principally sulfates and phosphates, is not pronounced, so that as the plasma HCO_3^- level falls owing to tubule dysfunction, retention of Cl^- by the kidneys leads to the development of *hyperchloremic acidosis*. At this stage, therefore, *the anion gap is normal*. With further reduction in GFR and more pronounced azotemia, however, retention of phosphates, sulfates, and other *unmeasured* anions is the rule, and plasma Cl^- concentration falls to normal levels despite the reduction in plasma HCO_3^- concentration. *A moderate to large anion gap therefore develops.*

Tubule potassium transport with normal and reduced nephron mass As with H^+, the concentration of K^+ in extracellular fluid is normally maintained within a relatively narrow range, 4 to 5 mmol/L. Ninety-five percent or more of total-body K^+ is in the intracellular fluid compartment, where the intracellular concentration is approximately 160 mmol/L. Normal individuals maintain external K^+ balance by excreting into the urine an amount of K^+ per day equivalent to the amount ingested, minus the relatively small amounts lost in stool and sweat. K^+ is freely filtered at the glomerulus, although the amount excreted usually represents no more than about 20 percent of the quantity filtered. The great bulk of the filtered K^+ is *reabsorbed* in the early portions of the nephron, about two-thirds in the proximal tubule, and an additional 20 to 25 percent in the loop of Henle. A K^+ *secretory process* operates in the distal tubule and terminal nephron segments. This process is largely dependent on Na^+ reabsorption and the accompanying lumen-negative voltage creating an electrical gradient across the tubule wall, favoring K^+ secretion into the lumen of distal tubule and collecting duct.

The ability to maintain external K^+ balance and normal plasma K^+ concentration as well, until relatively late in the course of CRF, is a consequence primarily of a progressive increase in fractional excretion of K^+. Greatly enhanced rates of K^+ secretion in distal portions of surviving tubules appear to underlie this adaptation. The augmented secretion rate of aldosterone is believed to contribute to enhanced tubule secretion of K^+. In addition both the increased distal tubule flow rates in residual functioning nephrons due to the osmotic diuresis and the enhanced luminal electronegativity created by the increased concentration of highly impermeable anions such as phosphate and sulfate enhance K^+ excretion. Aldosterone also stimulates net entry of K^+ into the lumen of the colon, a mechanism known to be enhanced in CRF. More detailed discussions of the abnormalities in K^+ homeostasis in acute and chronic forms of renal failure are given in Chaps. 223 and 224.

REFERENCES

BALLERMANN BJ, BRENNER BM: Biologically active atrial peptides. J Clin Invest 76:2041, 1985

BRENNER BM, RECTOR FC JR (eds): *The Kidney*, 3d ed. Philadelphia, Saunders, 1986

BRICKER NS: On the pathogenesis of the uremic state: An exposition of the "trade-off" hypothesis. N Engl J Med 286:1093, 1972

FEINFELD DA, SHERWOOD LM: Parathyroid hormone and $1,25(OH)_2D_3$ in chronic renal failure. Kidney Int 33:1049, 1988

HAYSLETT JP: Functional adaptation to reduction in renal mass. Physiol Rev 59:137, 1979

HOSTETTER TH, BRENNER BM: Glomerular adaptations to renal injury, in *Contemporary Issues in Nephrology*, vol 8: *Chronic Renal Failure*. New York, Churchill Livingstone, 1981

KAJI D, KAHN T: Na^+-K^+ pump in chronic renal failure. Am J Physiol 252:F785, 1987

MAXWELL MH et al: *Clinical Disorders of Fluid and Electrolyte Metabolism*, 4th ed. New York, McGraw-Hill, 1987

ROSE BD: *Clinical Physiology of Acid-Base and Electrolyte Disorders*, 2d ed. New York, McGraw-Hill, 1984

WARNOCK DG: Uremic acidosis. Kidney Int 34:278, 1988

223 ACUTE RENAL FAILURE

ROBERT J. ANDERSON / ROBERT W. SCHRIER

Acute renal failure is defined as a rapid deterioration in renal function sufficient to result in accumulation of nitrogenous wastes in the body. Approximately 5 percent of all hospitalized patients develop acute renal failure. In some clinical settings such as intensive care units, acute renal failure occurs in up to 20 percent of patients. Development of acute renal failure increases the likelihood of a fatal outcome by eightfold in hospitalized patients, and mortality rates of oliguric and nonoliguric varieties of acute renal failure range from 20 to 90 percent. The high frequency and mortality demand a logical approach to early diagnosis and prompt therapy of acute renal failure.

PRESENTING MANIFESTATIONS Acute renal failure is usually recognized by finding a rising blood urea nitrogen and/or serum creatinine concentration during biochemical monitoring of the seriously ill patient. It is noteworthy that reductions in glomerular filtration rates of 20 to 40 percent occur before significant increases in serum creatinine concentrations can be detected. A falling urine output is also frequently associated with acute renal failure. However, many patients with acute renal failure are not oliguric, and the presence of urinary flow rates >20 to 30 mL/h does not exclude the presence of acute renal failure. Sometimes acute renal failure presents because of other clinical (e.g., abnormal mental status, gastrointestinal symptoms, fluid overload, pericarditis) or laboratory (e.g., anemia, hyperkalemia, metabolic acidosis, hypocalcemia, hyperphosphatemia, abnormal urinalysis) manifestations of loss of renal function.

DIFFERENTIAL DIAGNOSIS (See Table 223-1) Urine formation begins with glomerular ultrafiltration of blood delivered to the kidneys, proceeds through tubular processing of the ultrafiltrate by secretion and absorption, and ends by excretion of urine through the ureters, bladder, and urethra. It follows that acute renal failure can be due to decreased renal perfusion (prerenal azotomia), renal parenchymal disorders (renal azotemia), or obstruction to urine flow (postrenal azotemia).

Prerenal azotemia causes 40 to 80 percent of cases of acute renal failure. Prerenal azotemia, if appropriately treated, is readily reversible. Inadequately treated, prolonged renal hypoperfusion can lead to ischemic acute tubular necrosis with significant morbidity and mortality. A decrease in renal perfusion sufficient to lower glomerular capillary perfusion pressure usually occurs in the setting of either extracellular fluid volume loss (e.g., gastrointestinal hemorrhage, burns, diarrhea, diuretics) or sequestration (e.g., pancreatitis, peritonitis, muscle crush injury). Prerenal azotemia can also result from marked reduction in cardiac output (e.g., cardiogenic shock and severe congestive heart failure), peripheral vasodilation (e.g., sepsis), or profound renal vasoconstriction as occurs in severe liver disease (hepatorenal syndrome) and sepsis. A careful review of intake and output, serial weights, hemodynamic parameters, and clinical events is important for the recognition of prerenal azotemia. Physical examination including assessment of blood pressure and pulse rate, jugular venous pressure, cardiac function, skin turgor, and mucous membranes should be undertaken in all patients with acute renal failure.

Two types of commonly used pharmacologic agents can cause acute renal failure on a hemodynamic basis. Nonsteroidal anti-inflammatory agents decrease the synthesis of renal vasodilatory prostaglandins (e.g., prostacyclin, prostaglandin E_2). In settings of an increase in endogenous renal vasoconstrictors (e.g., circulating norepinephrine and angiotensin II) and increased renal adrenergic neural tone, a compensatory rise in renal vasodilatory prostaglandins occurs. Thus, in these settings, nonsteroidal anti-inflammatory agents can result in profound renal vasoconstriction and acute renal failure. Nonsteroidal anti-inflammatory agents should be used cautiously in any patient with diminished renal perfusion. Such states include

TABLE 223-1 Major causes of acute renal failure

Disorder	Example
PRERENAL FAILURE	
Hypovolemia	Skin, gastrointestinal, or renal volume loss; hemorrhage; sequestration of extracellular fluid (burns, pancreatitis, peritonitis)
Cardiovascular failure	Impaired cardiac output (infarction, tamponade); vascular pooling (anaphylaxis, sepsis, drugs)
POSTRENAL FAILURE	
Extrarenal obstruction	Urethral occlusion; bladder, pelvic, prostatic, or retroperitoneal neoplasms; prostatism; surgical accident; medications; calculi; pus; blood clots
Intrarenal obstruction	Crystals (uric acid, oxalic acid, sulfonamides, methotrexate)
Bladder rupture	Trauma
SPECIFIC RENAL DISEASES	
Vascular diseases	Vasculitis; malignant hypertension; thrombotic thrombocytopenic purpura; scleroderma; arterial and/or venous occlusion
Glomerulonephritis	Immune-complex disease; antiglomerular basement membrane disease
Interstitial nephritis	Drugs; hypercalcemia; infections, idiopathic
ACUTE TUBULAR NECROSIS	
Postischemic	All conditions listed above for prerenal failure
Pigment-induced	Hemolysis (transfusion reaction, malaria); rhabdomyolysis (trauma, muscle disease, coma, heat stroke, severe exercise, potassium or phosphate depletion)
Toxin-induced	Antibiotics; contrast material; anesthetic agents; heavy metals; organic solvents
Pregnancy-related	Septic abortion; uterine hemorrhage; eclampsia

volume depletion, shock, edematous disorders (such as cirrhosis of the liver, heart failure, and nephrotic syndrome), underlying renal insufficiency, and advanced age. Angiotensin-converting enzyme inhibitors can also decrease glomerular capillary perfusion pressure. With the agents, a decrease in systemic arterial, and thus renal perfusion, pressure combined with efferent glomerular arteriolar dilation can result in acute renal failure. These agents are particularly prone to induce acute renal failure in patients with bilateral renal artery stenosis, unilateral renal artery stenosis without a contralateral kidney, or other high-renin disorder states (e.g., volume depletion and edematous disorders).

Postrenal causes account for 10 percent or less of all cases of acute renal failure. Since obstruction to urine flow is usually amenable to treatment, it must be considered in every patient with deteriorating renal function. Bladder neck obstruction due to prostatic disease or denervation (e.g., neuropathy or anticholinergic medications) is a relatively common cause of postrenal azotemia and can be evaluated by suprapubic palpation and percussion for an enlarged bladder as well as by postvoid bladder catheterization to measure residual volume. Obstruction of the upper urinary tract is a less common cause of renal failure since it requires simultaneous obstruction of both ureters or unilateral ureteric obstruction with severe disease or absence of the contralateral kidney. Causes of bilateral urinary tract obstruction include retroperitoneal fibrosis and space-occupying processes such as tumor or abscess, surgical accident (e.g., ureteral ligation), or bilateral intraureteric occlusion (stones, papillary tissue, blood clots, or pus). A careful rectal and pelvic examination is essential in evaluation for postobstruction renal failure. A plain film of the abdomen may reveal retroperitoneal disease or radiopaque calculi (90 percent of kidney stones). If obstruction of the upper urinary tract cannot be excluded by ultrasound, infusion pyelography, or computed tomographic scanning, investigation of the patency of the ureter(s) by retrograde pyelography may be required. Obstruction to urine flow can also occur within the kidney. Such intrarenal obstruction is usually due to intratubular precipitation of poorly soluble material such as uric acid (tumor chemotherapy), oxalic acid (ethylene glycol overdose, methoxyflurane anesthesia, small-bowel bypass surgery), methotrexate (insoluble metabolites), acyclovir, sulfonamides (outdated, long-acting insoluble compounds), or, perhaps, myeloma proteins.

After pre- and postrenal forms of azotemia have been excluded, it is appropriate to focus on renal causes of azotemia. Disorders of the large renal arteries such as thrombosis, emboli, and dissection and disorders of the smaller renal arterial vessels including vasculitis, malignant hypertension, hemolytic-uremic syndrome, thrombotic thrombocytopenic purpura, disseminated intravascular coagulation, and scleroderma can all present as acute renal failure. These disorders usually have prominent extrarenal manifestations and a microangiopathic pattern of red blood cell destruction evident on peripheral blood smear examination. Acute glomerulonephritis (discussed in Chap. 227) is another occasional cause of acute renal failure, particularly in younger patients. Acute interstitial nephritis in the setting of drug hypersensitivity can cause acute renal failure, usually associated with unexplained fever, skin rash, arthralgias, and peripheral eosinophilia. Commonly used therapeutic agents that can induce acute renal failure due to acute interstititial nephritis include furosemide, penicillin, phenytoin, sulfonamides, rifampin, nonsteroidal anti-inflammatory drugs, trimethoprim, cimetidine, and captopril.

ACUTE TUBULAR NECROSIS After exclusion of renal vascular, glomerular, and interstitial causes of acute renal failure, there remains a large group of patients commonly referred to as having acute tubular necrosis. While overt tubular necrosis has not always been found on renal biopsy or autopsy of such patients, tubular dysfunction is a uniform hallmark of this form of acute renal failure.

Sixty percent of cases of acute tubular necrosis are related to surgery or trauma. Forty percent occur in a medical setting, and 1 to 2 percent are related to pregnancy. The most common cause is *renal ischemia*. Conditions associated with renal ischemia include severe hemorrhage, profound volume depletion, intraoperative hypotension, cardiogenic shock, sepsis, and operative procedures associated with interruption of renal circulation. The duration of the ischemia is important in the development of acute tubular necrosis. If ischemia is brief, then correction can restore renal function (i.e., prerenal azotemia). With longer duration of renal hypoperfusion, acute tubular necrosis may supervene.

Nephrotoxic agents can also cause acute tubular necrosis. In the past, heavy metals, organic solvents, and glycols were common factors. Although these toxins are now less frequent, their occasional occurrence illustrates the importance of seeking a history of occupational and environmental toxin exposure in each patient with acute renal failure. Aminoglycoside antibiotics and radiographic contrast agents are now the leading nephrotoxic causes of acute renal failure. Indeed, acute tubular necrosis occurs in 10 to 20 percent of patients receiving a course of an aminoglycoside. The renal failure associated with these drugs is enhanced by depletion of intravascular volume, advancing age, the presence of underlying renal disease, potassium depletion, and the concomitant use of other nephrotoxic agents or potent diuretics. Radiographic contrast agents have little nephrotoxicity in healthy individuals. However, in patients with underlying renal disease, particularly patients with diabetic nephropathy, contrast exposure is associated with a 10 to 40 percent frequency of acute tubular necrosis. Some anesthetic agents (methoxyflurane and enflurane) also may induce acute renal failure.

Release of large amounts of myoglobin into the circulation is another common cause of acute tubular necrosis. Rhabdomyolysis and myoglobinuria are often due to extensive trauma with crush injuries, but nontraumatic rhabdomyolysis can also be associated with increased muscle oxygen consumption (heat stroke, severe exercise, and seizures), decreased muscle energy production (hypokalemia, hypophosphatemia, and genetic enzymatic deficiencies), muscle ischemia (arterial insufficiency, drug overdosage with resultant coma and muscle compression, cocaine overdose), infections (influenza, Legionnaires' disease), and direct toxins (alcohol). Questioning of patients with acute renal failure for muscular symptoms as well as examination for tender, swollen muscles is therefore important, although many patients may have muscle necrosis without muscle symptoms. The exact mechanism whereby myoglobinuria results in acute renal failure is uncertain. Myoglobin is not directly nephrotoxic, but direct nephrotoxicity of other muscle breakdown products, as well as tubular obstruction due to myoglobin precipitation and cast formation, has been proposed as the mechanism of inquiry. Most patients with rhabdomyolysis-associated acute renal failure also have concomitant depletion of intravascular volume and renal hypoperfusion.

Intravascular hemolysis may also cause acute tubular necrosis. Although pure hemoglobin per se is not a potent nephrotoxin, toxic substances from red blood cell stroma and concomitant renal hypoperfusion may act synergistically to induce acute renal failure. Lastly, it is not always possible to establish a definite etiology for some cases of acute tubular necrosis. In many cases, multiple etiologies are likely, as in patients with shock who are volume-depleted, have received blood transfusions, are septic, and have received nephrotoxic antibiotics.

PATHOPHYSIOLOGY (Fig. 223-1) Current pathogenic theories of acute tubular necrosis suggest either a tubular or a vascular basis for renal failure. One tubular theory suggests that casts and cellular debris obstruct tubular lumina with resultant increases in intratubular pressure sufficient to decrease net filtration pressure. Alternatively, some investigators feel that "back-leak" of glomerular filtrate across damaged renal tubular epithelium is responsible for azotemia in acute tubular necrosis. Proponents of a vascular basis for acute tubular necrosis suggest that marked decreases in renal perfusion pressure, severe afferent arteriolar constriction, or efferent arteriolar dilatation reduce glomerular plasma flow and hydrostatic pressure sufficiently to diminish glomerular filtration. This vascular theory has led some proponents to suggest that *vasomotor nephropathy* might be the preferred term for such cases. Another theory of acute renal failure suggests that alterations in the permeability properties of the glomerular capillary wall are responsible for acute renal failure. Alternatively, some signal in the distal tubule at the macula densa may initiate a tubuloglomerular feedback mechanism leading to a fall in glomerular filtration pressure. On balance, it seems likely that both tubular and vascular events interact to cause acute renal failure. For example, ischemia may cause a lower glomerular capillary pressure, which then predisposes to slow tubular flow. Ischemic cellular necrosis with release of apical membrane into the tubular lumen may result in sludging debris and ultimately in secondary tubular obstruction. Additional studies are required to define the relative importance of such factors and to define mechanisms that are involved in the initiation (early) and maintenance (late) phases of acute renal failure.

FIGURE 223-1 Potential pathogenic schema in acute renal failure.

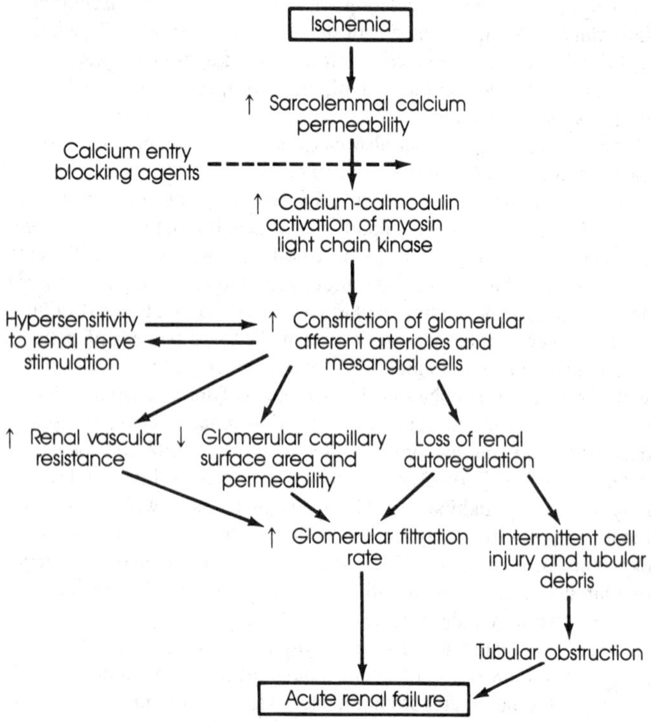

PATHOLOGY The histopathologic alterations in kidneys of patients with clinical features of acute tubular necrosis vary from no or minimal abnormalities on light microscopy to tubular necrosis with disrupted, necrotic, or regenerating tubular epithelium, intratubular casts, interstitial edema, and interstitial cellular infiltration. Tubular collapse and dilated tubules both may be present. Unless either disseminated intravascular coagulation or severe, prolonged ischemic lesions are present, intrarenal blood vessels and glomeruli are normal by light and electron microscopy. Microdissection studies demonstrate two general types of renal lesions. Direct nephrotoxic injury causes a uniform, diffuse necrosis of proximal tubular cells, especially of proximal convoluted and straight tubules. The tubular basement membrane is unaltered. In contrast, following renal ischemia, mild, patchy necrosis tends to be most marked in tubular segments at the corticomedullary junction. The juxtamedullary proximal straight tubule and medullary thick ascending limb of Henle appear particularly vulnerable. Disruption of tubular basement membrane is also observed. Despite these histologic differences, the clinical course of nephrotoxic and ischemic acute renal failure is similar. A lack of correlation between renal histopathologic changes and renal functional parameters is common. Renal biopsies performed after recovery from acute renal failure either demonstrate minor abnormalities or are normal.

DIAGNOSTIC APPROACH (See Table 223-1) The diagnosis of acute tubular necrosis is one of exclusion since prerenal (renal hypoperfusion), postrenal (obstruction of urine flow), and other intrarenal disorders (glomerulonephritis, renal interstitial and vascular diseases) may all lead to deteriorating renal function. In contrast to acute tubular necrosis, however, prerenal, postrenal, and other intrarenal vascular, glomerular, or interstitial disorders may be specifically treatable.

The initial presentation of the patient with end-stage chronic renal failure may be confused with acute renal failure when there is no information about renal function prior to presentation. Under these circumstances, the presence of uremic osteodystrophy, uremic neuropathy, bilateral small kidneys on abdominal films or ultrasound, and unexplained anemia suggests chronic renal failure. However, some end-stage renal diseases, such as amyloidosis, polycystic kidney disease, diabetic glomerulosclerosis, scleroderma, and rapidly progressive glomerulonephritis, may present with normal-sized or enlarged kidneys, making it necessary for continued observation and sometimes renal biopsy to distinguish between potentially reversible forms of acute renal failure and end-stage chronic renal failure.

The pattern of urine flow may provide a diagnostic clue as to the cause of declining renal function. Complete anuria (no urine by catheterization) is rare in acute tubular necrosis. Potential causes of total anuria include complete bilateral ureteric obstruction, diffuse cortical necrosis, rapidly progressive glomerulonephritis, and bilateral renal artery occlusion. Wide fluctuations in daily urine output suggest intermittent obstructive uropathy. Polyuria (>3 L per day) can be a hallmark of partial urinary tract obstruction and is secondary to the accompanying defect in renal concentrating ability. Although oliguria (<400 mL per day) has been considered to be a cardinal feature of

TABLE 223-2 Urine findings in prerenal azotemia and acute renal failure

Laboratory test	Prerenal azotemia	Acute renal failure
Urine osmolality (mosmol/kg)	>500	<400
Urine sodium (mmol/L)	<20	>40
Urine/plasma creatinine	>40	<20
Fractional excretion* of filtered sodium	<1	2
Urine sediment	Normal or occasional hyaline and granular casts	Brown granular casts, cellular debris

$$*\frac{\text{Urine Na/serum Na}}{\text{Urine creatinine/serum creatinine}} \times 100.$$

acute tubular necrosis, many patients have urine volumes of greater than 1 L per day. This situation is termed nonoliguric acute renal failure.

Examination of the urinary sediment is also of value in the differential diagnosis of acute impairment of renal function. Sediment containing few formed elements or only hyaline casts suggests prerenal azotemia or obstructive uropathy. With acute tubular necrosis, brownish pigmented cellular casts and renal tubular epithelial cells are present in over 75 percent of patients. Red blood cell casts suggest the presence of glomerular or vascular inflammatory diseases of the kidney and are rarely, if ever, present with acute tubular necrosis. The presence of large numbers of polymorphonuclear leukocytes, singly or in clumps, suggests acute diffuse interstitial nephritis or papillary necrosis. Eosinophilic casts on Hansel's stain of urine sediment support a diagnosis of acute hypersensitivity interstitial nephritis. The combination of brownish pigmented granular casts and positive occult blood tests on urine in the absence of hematuria indicates either hemoglobinuria or myoglobinuria. In acute renal failure, the finding in fresh, warm urine of large numbers of uric acid crystals may suggest a diagnosis of acute uric acid nephropathy, while large numbers of oxalic acid or hippuric acid crystals suggests ethylene glycol toxicity. The presence of large numbers of broad casts (greater than two to three white blood cells in diameter) suggests chronic renal disease.

Chemical analysis of urine composition is also helpful in differentiating acute tubular necrosis from prerenal azotemia in the oliguric patient (Table 223-2). Other disorders associated with abrupt deterioration in renal function and intact renal tubular integrity, such as glomerulonephritis, vasculitis, and early (few hours) obstructive uropathy, may cause urine chemical values similar to those encountered in prerenal azotemia. Prior administration of diuretic agents, osmotic diuresis due to mannitol, glycosuria, bicarbonaturia, and ketonuria may interfere with renal tubular reabsorption of sodium and water and thus alter urinary chemical indexes. A urinary uric acid/creatinine concentration ratio of greater than 1 is compatible with acute uric acid nephropathy as a cause of the acute renal failure.

The cause of declining renal function may not be readily apparent. In some cases, features considered atypical for acute tubular necrosis (gradual onset of renal failure; anuria in the absence of obstructive uropathy; the presence of marked hypertension, heavy proteinuria, significant hematuria, underlying systemic disease, and prolonged oliguria) will be present. Since such atypical features may indicate the presence of a potentially treatable form of renal parenchymal disease, e.g., Wegener's disease, systemic lupus erythematosus, Goodpasture's syndrome, or rapidly progressive glomerulonephritis, a diagnostic renal biopsy may be indicated when the cause of renal failure is not apparent or such atypical features are present.

CLINICAL COURSE The clinical course in acute tubular necrosis can be divided into an initiating phase, a maintenance phase, and a recovery phase. The initiating phase is the period of time between the precipitating event and the appearance of acute renal failure which is no longer reversible by alteration in extrarenal factors. Recognition of the initiating phase of acute renal failure is extremely important since early correction of the underlying cause of renal failure may theoretically prevent the development of the maintenance phase. However, the initiating phase of acute renal failure may be evident to the clinician only in retrospect because it lacks characteristic signs and symptoms.

Oliguria has been considered the cardinal feature of the initiating and maintenance phases of acute tubular necrosis. However, up to 40 to 50 percent of all patients with acute tubular necrosis are nonoliguric (urine volume >400 mL per day). Progressive acute renal failure without oliguria can result from any type of renal insult, including both ischemic and toxic insults, and this form of renal failure appears to be particularly frequent following nephrotoxic (e.g., aminoglycoside) drug injury. Progressive azotemia occurs in nonoliguric patients owing to the marked impairment in glomerular filtration rate and renal concentrating capacity. For example, maximal urine osmolality of the nonoliguric patient averages only 350 mosmol per kilogram of water. Therefore, with a urine output of 1000 mL per day, a maximum of 350 mosmol solute can be excreted daily. In acute renal failure, daily solute loads may be increased from normal values of 600 mosmol to values as high as 1000 mosmol. Thus, a positive solute (predominately urea and creatinine) balance and azotemia would occur despite a daily urine output of 1 L.

When oliguria occurs, it starts shortly following the inciting event and lasts an average of 10 to 14 days. However, the oliguric phase may be as short as a few hours or as long as 6 to 8 weeks in the elderly patient with underlying vascular disease. If oliguria persists for longer than 4 weeks, the diagnosis of acute tubular necrosis should be reconsidered; diffuse cortical necrosis, rapidly progressive glomerulonephritis, renal artery occlusion, renal vasculitis, renal emboli, and superimposed volume depletion may be present. Anuria is not characteristic of acute tubular necrosis, but severe oliguria with urine volume less than 100 mL per day may last for several days.

Urinary elimination of nitrogenous wastes, water, electrolytes, and acid is impaired in the initiating and maintenance phases of acute renal failure. The magnitude of resultant abnormalities in blood chemistry depends on whether the patient is oliguric or nonoliguric and on the patient's catabolic state. Nonoliguric patients have higher levels of glomerular filtration than do oliguric patients and thus excrete more nitrogenous waste, water, and electrolytes in their urine. Hence, abnormalities in blood chemistry are generally milder in nonoliguric than oliguric patients with acute renal failure. The complications, need for dialysis, and mortality are also less in nonoliguric patients.

In the afebrile, noncatabolic, oliguric patient with acute renal failure, the daily increments in blood urea nitrogen (BUN) and serum creatinine average 4 to 8 mmol/L (10 to 20 mg/dL) and 40 to 80 μmol/L (0.5 to 1.0 mg/dL), respectively. In catabolic patients with fever, sepsis, or extensive trauma, daily increments in BUN and serum creatinine may be much higher. In patients with acute renal failure due to rhabdomyolysis, the daily increment in serum creatinine may be disproportionately higher than the BUN. This is due to the release from muscle of creatine, which is converted by nonenzymatic hydrolysis to creatinine.

Salt and water overload with resultant hyponatremia, edema, and pulmonary congestion are ever-present dangers in patients with acute renal failure, particularly oliguric patients. Hyponatremia results from excessive water intake, and edema is due to excessive sodium and water intake. In contrast, if urinary losses are not replaced, the nonoliguric patient with a relatively high rate of urine flow and high concentration of urine sodium may develop intravascular volume depletion which can retard recovery of renal function.

Hyperkalemia due to decreased renal elimination of potassium and continued tissue potassium release is a frequent accompaniment of acute tubular necrosis. The usual rate of increase in serum potassium in the noncatabolic, oliguric patient is 0.3 to 0.5 mmol per day. Higher rates of rise in serum potassium concentration suggest the possibility of an endogenous (tissue destruction, hemolysis) or exogenous (medication, diet, blood transfusion) potassium load or of cellular shift of potassium due to acidemia. Generally, hyperkalemia is asymptomatic until serum potassium increases to values above 6.0 to 6.5 mmol/L. Then electrocardiographic abnormalities (bradycardia, recent appearance of left axis deviation, peaked T waves, prolonged QRS complexes, prolonged PR interval, and decreased amplitude of the P waves) and ultimately cardiac arrest can occur. Hyperkalemia can also cause muscle weakness and flaccid quadriparesis.

Hyperphosphatemia, hypocalcemia, and mild *hypermagnesemia* are usually present in acute tubular necrosis. Hyperphosphatemia results from decreased renal phosphorus elimination in the presence of continued release of phosphorus from tissues. The serum phosphorus is usually in the range of 2 to 2.3 mmol/L, but higher values may occur in the traumatized, catabolic patient or in the patient with rhabdomyolysis. Hypocalcemia often develops during acute renal failure. The reason is not clear, but resistance to parathyroid hormone may play a role. Increases in serum magnesium are mild (to levels of 0.8 to 1.2 mmol/L), unless magnesium-containing compounds such as antacids are ingested.

Metabolic acidosis is a regular accompaniment of acute tubular necrosis. The usual daily production of approximately 1 mmol per kilogram of body weight of nonvolatile acid from endogenous metabolic sources can no longer be eliminated by the damaged kidney. The retention of organic acids is sufficient to produce a daily decrease of 1 to 2 mmol/L in plasma bicarbonate and metabolic acidosis with an anion gap.

Mild hyperuricemia is due to decreased renal uric acid excretion. In catabolic patients with extensive tissue damage, higher values of serum uric acid may be observed. Elevation of serum amylase due to impaired renal amylase excretion may occur in the absence of evidence of pancreatitis. The elevations of amylase are usually less than twice the upper limit of normal.

Hematologic abnormalities are usually present in acute tubular necrosis. A normocytic normochromic anemia occurs shortly following the onset of significant azotemia. This anemia is due to impaired erythropoiesis as well as to a mild and variable shortened red blood cell survival. Additional factors that may contribute to anemia include hemodilution, gastrointestinal blood loss, and suppressed erythropoiesis due to infections or drug administration. White blood cell production is not severely disturbed in acute renal failure. However, mild leukocytosis is usually present. Leukocytosis persisting after the initial week of acute renal failure should suggest the possibility of infection. Mild degrees of thrombocytopenia due to reduction of bone marrow platelet production may be observed early in the course. Qualitative defects in platelet function occur and, in association with additional poorly defined coagulation disturbances, contribute to the bleeding tendency of acute renal failure. Acute renal failure may follow intravascular hemolysis and may also be a complication of several primary hematologic or vascular disorders that have major hematologic manifestations such as disseminated intravascular coagulation, thrombotic thrombocytopenic purpura, hemolytic uremic syndrome, and systemic lupus erythematosus.

Infections complicate 30 to 70 percent of all cases of acute tubular necrosis and are a leading cause of morbidity and mortality. The sites of infection include the respiratory tract, operative sites, and urinary tract. Resultant septicemia is frequent, and both gram-positive and gram-negative organisms are encountered. Operative site abscesses (especially intraabdominal) are associated with a poor prognosis if not recognized and treated promptly. Although the exact factors responsible for the high rate of infection remain to be determined, disruption of normal anatomic barriers with intravenous infusions and indwelling catheters may play a role. Host defenses including leukocyte function may be impaired in the setting of uremia. Minimization of use of catheters and intravenous lines, careful daily examination, and prompt thorough evaluation of fever are important. It is also important to emphasize that uremia may obscure fever associated with infections.

Cardiovascular complications include volume overload, hypertension, arrhythmias, and pericarditis. Volume overload is usually due to excessive sodium and water administration. Mild hypertension is seen in 15 to 25 percent of cases and usually appears in the second week of oliguria. This hypertension is usually also a manifestation of extracellular fluid volume overload; however, increased activity of the renin-angiotensin system may also be involved in some instances. Supraventricular arrhythmias may complicate 20 to 30 percent of cases of acute renal failure. Known causes for these arrhythmias include congestive heart failure, electrolyte abnormalities, digitalis intoxication, pericarditis, and anemia. Pericarditis currently occurs infrequently, probably because of prompt dialysis.

Neurologic abnormalities are common in acute renal failure. In undialyzed patients, lethargy, somnolence, confusion, disorientation, asterixis, agitation, myoclonic muscle twitching, and generalized seizures may be observed. These neurologic abnormalities are most often encountered in the elderly patient and generally respond well to dialysis. In addition to uremia per se, drug administration, metabolic and electrolyte abnormalities, and primary neurologic disease may cause neurologic disturbances in the patient with acute renal failure.

Gastrointestinal complications include anorexia, nausea, vomiting, ileus, and poorly defined abdominal complaints. The combination of stress of acute illness and bleeding disorders can lead to gastrointestinal hemorrhage in 10 to 30 percent of patients. Fortunately, the gastrointestinal hemorrhage is usually mild and easily controlled with conservative therapy. Intravenous desmopressin (0.4 μg/kg intravenously) lowers the bleeding time and improves hemostasis in some patients with acute renal failure. Cryoprecipitate can also be used especially in cases refractory to desmopressin.

The recovery phase of acute renal failure commences when the glomerular filtration rate increases so that the BUN and serum creatinine concentrations no longer continue to increase. In oliguric acute renal failure, the recovery phase is heralded by a progressive increase in urine volume. Generally, in the first days the urine volume may double daily, and in some cases a daily urine volume may be greater than 2 L for a few days. In nonoliguric patients, a marked diuretic phase is usually not observed. The duration of the recovery phase in patients with serum creatinine concentrations greater than 440 μmol/L (5 mg/dL) averages 10 to 25 days in oliguric patients and 5 to 10 days in nonoliguric patients. The major complications of acute renal failure, such as infections, gastrointestinal hemorrhage, fluid and electrolyte disturbances, and cardiovascular dysfunction, may persist or first appear during the recovery phase. In addition, persistent abnormalities in glomerular and tubular function during the recovery phase can lead to over- or underhydration or electrolyte disturbances unless careful daily weight, intake and output, biochemical, and clinical monitoring are continued. Hypercalcemia may occur during the recovery phase, especially in patients with rhabdomyolysis. The cause of this complication remains obscure, but mobilization of calcium from damaged muscle into extracellular fluid has been suggested.

Although the major improvement in renal function occurs within the first 1 to 2 weeks of the recovery phase, renal function continues to improve for up to a year following acute renal failure. Sensitive tests of glomerular and tubular function also suggest that some mild defects in renal function may persist indefinitely following acute tubular necrosis. However, the majority of patients achieve clinically normal renal function, and there is no evidence of late progression of renal dysfunction or of complications such as hypertension.

Mortality rates in large series of patients with acute renal failure vary from 20 to 90 percent. Mortality rates are highest in postoperative or traumatized patients, intermediate in patients with acute renal failure encountered in a medical setting, and lowest in acute renal failure observed in an obstetric setting. Advanced age, the presence of serious underlying illness, a catabolic state, and the development of multiple medical complications (especially concomitant acute respiratory failure) during the course are associated with higher mortality rates. Another determinant of outcome is the severity of

TABLE 223-3 General therapeutic approach to patient with acute renal failure

1 Exclude all specifically treatable causes of decreasing renal function including correction of prerenal and postrenal factors.
2 Attempt to establish a urine output.
3 Conservative therapy:
   a Decrease intake of nitrogen, water, and electrolytes to match output.
   b Provide adequate nutrition.
   c Alter medication therapy.
   d Maintain clinical monitoring (frequency of vital signs determined by patient status; intake and output, body weight, inspection of wound and intravenous sites, and physical examination required daily).
   e Maintain biochemical monitoring (frequency of BUN, creatinine, electrolytes, and blood counts will be dictated by patient status; in catabolic oliguric patients, daily determination will be needed; calcium, phosphorus, magnesium, and uric acid can often be determined less often).
4 Provide dialytic therapy.

the renal failure. As stated above, oliguric acute renal failure requiring dialysis is associated with three- to fivefold increases in mortality when compared with nonoliguric acute renal failure that usually does not require dialysis. Infections, complications resulting from fluid and electrolyte disturbances, gastrointestinal hemorrhage, and progression of the primary underlying disease are the major causes of mortality in acute renal failure.

MANAGEMENT (Table 223-3) The first principle of therapy is to exclude causes of deterioration in renal function that are potentially remedial. A search for prerenal factors, obstructive uropathy, glomerulonephritis, renal vascular and interstitial disease, and intrarenal crystal precipitation should be performed. Once the diagnosis of acute tubular necrosis is made by exclusion, little specific therapy is available. Dialysis for the removal of nephrotoxins, such as carbon tetrachloride, ethylene glycol, and heavy metals following chelation therapy, may be indicated. Even in the presence of acute tubular necrosis, any prerenal abnormalities should be corrected both to improve the circulation and to avoid delay in the onset of the recovery phase. In the oliguric patient in whom prerenal factors have been corrected, it has become common clinical practice to administer either a potent loop diuretic or mannitol in an attempt to enhance urine flow. In patients who remain oliguric despite potent diuretics, low-dose infusions of dopamine (1 to 3 mg per kilogram body weight per minute) may increase renal blood flow and allow a diuretic response to potent diuretics. The rationale for such therapy is based on the thought that there is an early phase of renal failure during which the correction of prerenal factors and establishment of urine flow can prevent an oliguric state. Prospective studies have demonstrated lower morbidity and mortality rates in nonoliguric as compared with oliguric acute renal failure. However, a prospective controlled study of the utility of potent diuretics and dopamine in early acute renal failure to convert oliguric to nonoliguric renal failure is needed.

Conservative therapy is capable of controlling many of the manifestations of acute renal failure. After any defects in intravascular volume have been corrected, fluid intake should equal measured output plus estimated insensible losses. Sodium and potassium administration should not exceed measured losses. Daily monitoring of fluid balance and body weight allow assessment of the volume status. A daily weight loss of 0.2 to 0.3 kg occurs in the well-managed patient with acute renal failure. Greater weight loss suggests hypercatabolism or volume depletion, and lesser weight loss suggests excessive salt and water administration. Since most pharmacologic agents are eliminated at least in part by the kidney, careful attention to medication usage and dosage adjustment is needed. The serum sodium concentration provides a guideline for water administration. A decrease in serum sodium indicates a relative excess of total-body water, while an abnormally high concentration indicates a relative deficiency of body water as compared to total-body sodium.

To minimize catabolism, daily intake should include at least 100 g of carbohydrate. Some studies suggest in addition that intravenous administration of a mixture of amino acids and hypertonic glucose improves morbidity and mortality in patients with acute renal failure following surgical procedures or trauma (see Chap. 75). Since parenteral hyperalimentation may be associated with significant complications, this form of nutrition should be reserved for catabolic patients in whom the enteral routine of alimentation does not prove to be satisfactory. Additional means of minimizing catabolism include early removal or debridement of necrotic tissue, control of pyrexia, and early, specific antimicrobial therapy.

The mild metabolic acidosis associated with acute tubular necrosis is generally not treated unless serum bicarbonate falls to below 10 mmol/L. Rapid correction of acidemia by acute alkali administration may decrease ionized calcium concentrations and precipitate tetany. Hypocalcemia is usually asymptomatic and rarely requires specific therapy. Hyperphosphatemia should be controlled with 30 to 60 mL aluminum hydroxide administered orally four to six times per day, since a high calcium-phosphorus product may cause soft tissue calcification. For the occasional patient with profound hyperphosphatemia, early dialysis therapy may be warranted. Unless acute uric acid nephropathy is a diagnostic consideration, the secondary hyperuricemia of acute renal failure is usually not treated with allopurinol. Because of the decreased glomerular filtration rate, the filtered load of uric acid, and thus intratubular deposition, is low. Also, for unknown reasons, clinical gout rarely complicates acute renal failure, despite hyperuricemia. Careful observation of the hematocrit and stool for occult blood is important for the early detection of gastrointestinal blood loss. If a rapid decrease in hematocrit appears to be out of proportion to the degree of renal failure, alternative causes of anemia should be sought.

Congestive heart failure and hypertension indicate volume overload and should be treated accordingly, recognizing, of course, that many drugs such as digoxin are largely excreted by the kidneys. Continuous arteriovenous hemofiltration can remove large amounts of extracellular fluid in the setting of acute renal failure. This therapy is often utilized in patients with oliguric acute tubular necrosis who require large amounts of hyperalimentation fluid to maintain caloric and nitrogen balance. As suggested earlier, hypertension occasionally may persist in the absence of volume overload; thus factors such as hyperreninemia may contribute to the hypertension. Selective histamine-2-receptor blockade (cimetidine, ranitidine) therapy has been of benefit in preventing gastrointestinal bleeding in some seriously ill patients but has not yet been studied in acute renal failure. Avoidance and early detection of infection require minimization of interruption of normal anatomic barriers, including avoidance of long-term catheterization of the urinary bladder, provision of mouth and skin care, promotion of early mobilization, utilization of aseptic techniques for intravenous and tracheostomy sites, and close clinical monitoring. Fever and suspected infection should be promptly evaluated with careful inspection of lung, wounds, urinary tract, and intravenous sites.

Hyperkalemia is an ever-present threat in acute renal failure. Mild elevations of serum potassium (<6.0 mmol/L) can best be treated by withdrawal of all sources of potassium and by continued close laboratory observation. If serum potassium increases to values greater than 6.5 mmol/L and particularly if any electrocardiographic changes appear, active therapy should be instituted. Therapy of such hyperkalemia can be divided into emergent and nonemergent forms. Emergent therapy includes intravenous administration of calcium (5 to 10 mL of 10% calcium chloride solution intravenously over 2 min with electrocardiographic monitoring), bicarbonate (44 mmol intravenously over 5 min), and insulin and glucose (200 to 300 mL of 20% glucose with 20 to 30 units regular insulin given intravenously over 30 min). Nonemergent therapy includes administration of potassium-binding ion exchange resins such as sodium polystyrene sulfonate. This can be administered orally every 3 to 4 h in 25- to 50-g doses with 100 mL 20% sorbitol to avoid constipation. Alternatively, in the patient who cannot take oral medications, 50 g sodium polystyrene sulfonate and 50 g sorbitol in 200 mL water can be given as a retention enema at 1- to 2-h intervals. With refractory hyperkalemia, hemodialysis may be necessary.

Some patients with acute tubular necrosis, particularly those who are nonoliguric and noncatabolic, can be successfully managed with minimal or no dialytic therapy. There has been an increasing tendency to use dialysis therapy early in acute renal failure in an attempt to minimize the development of complications. Early (prophylactic) use of dialysis frequently simplifies management, allowing more liberal fluid and potassium intake and improvement of the general well-being of the patient. Absolute indications for dialysis include symptomatic uremia (usually manifested by central nervous system and/or gastrointestinal symptoms), development of resistant hyperkalemia, severe acidemia or fluid overload not responsive to medical therapy, and pericarditis. In addition, many centers attempt to keep predialysis levels of serum creatinine less than 700 to 900 μmol/L (8 to 10 mg/dL). Adequate prevention of uremic symptoms may require no or infrequent dialysis in the noncatabolic, nonoliguric patient or daily dialysis in the catabolic, traumatized patient. Often, peritoneal dialysis is an acceptable alternative to hemodialysis. Peritoneal dialysis may be especially useful in the patient with noncatabolic acute tubular necrosis when the need for infrequent dialysis is anticipated. Slow, continuous arteriovenous filtration using highly permeable filters has been advocated as a means of controlling extracellular volume. Currently available filters connected via an arteriovenous shunt allow for removal of 5 to 12 L of plasma ultrafiltrate per day without use of a pump. Thus, these devices appear particularly useful in the oliguric volume-overloaded patient with hemodynamic instability.

PREVENTION Because of the high mortality and morbidity of acute renal failure, prophylactic therapy deserves special mention. The first principle of prevention is aggressive resuscitation of the traumatized patient. A fivefold reduction in deaths secondary to acute renal failure occurred from the Korean War to the Vietnamese conflict. This reduction in mortality was probably due to earlier evacuation from the field and more rapid restoration of extracellular fluid volume. A second factor in prevention of acute renal failure is minimization of the use of potential nephrotoxins, particularly in high-risk patients. Finally, maintenance of normal extracellular fluid volume and high urinary flow and solute excretion rates may prevent and/or attenuate the development of acute renal failure in selected situations, such as open-heart surgery, following severe trauma, when rhabdomyolysis and/or intravascular hemolysis is present, and in association with some nephrotoxins including cisplatin, radiographic contrast agents, and amphotericin B. Maintenance of high urine flow and solute excretion rates also can preserve renal function in the setting of high renal loads of potentially insoluble crystalline material such as uric acid and methotrexate.

ACUTE RENAL FAILURE IN PREGNANCY When acute renal failure occurs during pregnancy, it is usually in either the earlier or later stages of gestation. During the first trimester, acute renal failure usually occurs in the setting of nontherapeutic, nonsterile abortion. In these cases, volume depletion, sepsis, and nephrotoxins contribute to the acute renal failure. This form of acute renal failure has markedly declined with the widespread availability of sterile abortion.

Acute renal failure late in pregnancy can occur from either excessive postpartum hemorrhage or preeclampsia. Most such patients generally recover total renal function, but for those who do not histologic evidence of diffuse cortical necrosis is found, which usually complicates the severe hemorrhage of abruptio placentae and is associated with clinical and laboratory evidence of intravascular coagulation.

A rare form of acute renal failure occurring 1 to 12 weeks following uncomplicated pregnancy has been described and termed postpartum glomerulosclerosis. This disorder is usually characterized by irreversible, rapidly progressive renal failure, although milder cases have been described. These patients have an associated microangiopathic hemolytic anemia. The renal histopathologic changes are indistinguishable from those associated with malignant hypertension or scleroderma. The pathophysiology of this disorder has not been defined. No therapy is consistently successful, although heparin therapy has been advocated.

HEPATORENAL SYNDROME The hepatorenal syndrome is a complication of advanced liver disease in which renal failure occurs in the absence of clinical, laboratory, or anatomic evidence of other causes of renal dysfunction. The renal failure is usually associated with oliguria, an unremarkable urinary sediment, and low urinary sodium concentrations (<10 mmol/L). Generally, the renal failure occurs in the setting of advanced hepatic cirrhosis complicated by jaundice, ascites, and hepatic encephalopathy. Occasionally, this syndrome may complicate fulminant hepatitis. The mechanism of the renal failure is not known. The lack of consistent histopathologic alterations in kidneys and the restoration of normal renal function when kidneys from donors with hepatorenal syndrome are transplanted into recipients without liver disease suggest a functional defect. The administration of nonsteroidal anti-inflammatory agents to patients with decompensated cirrhosis may cause a clinical picture identical to that seen with hepatorenal syndrome. With cessation of these drugs, renal function often improves.

Treatment of the hepatorenal syndrome is usually unsuccessful. Care should be taken in the cirrhotic patient not to induce major changes in intravascular volume by large paracentesis or aggressive diuresis, maneuvers that may precipitate hepatorenal syndrome. Since this syndrome mimics prerenal azotemia, a cautious trial of expansion of intravascular volume is warranted. In a few cases, recovery has followed portacaval shunting, insertion of an abdominal-venous (Leveen) shunt, or prolonged hemodialysis. These treatments have not been subjected to controlled trials. The abdominal-venous shunt may be associated with peritonitis, intravascular coagulation, and pulmonary congestion. Improvement in hepatic function often results in parallel improvement in renal function. Every effort should be made to ensure that more specifically treatable causes of concomitant liver and renal dysfunction, such as infections (leptospirosis, hepatitis with immune-complex disease), toxins (aminoglycosides, carbon tetrachloride), and circulatory disorders (severe heart failure, shock), are not present. It should also be recalled that jaundiced patients with liver disease may be particularly susceptible to acute tubular necrosis.

REFERENCES

Anderson RJ, Schrier RW: Acute tubular necrosis, in *Diseases of the Kidney*, RW Schrier, CW Gottschalk (eds). Boston, Little, Brown, 1988, p 1413

Badr KF, Ichikawa I: Prerenal failure: A deleterious shift from renal compensation to decompensation. N Engl J Med 319:623, 1988

Brenner BM, Lazarus JM (eds): *Acute Renal Failure*. Philadelphia, Saunders, 1987

Meyers BD, Moran SM: Hemodynamically mediated acute renal failure. N Engl J Med 314:97, 1986

Shusterman N et al: Risk factors and outcome of hospital-acquired acute renal failure. Am J Med 83:65, 1987

224 CHRONIC RENAL FAILURE

BARRY M. BRENNER / J. MICHAEL LAZARUS

In contrast to the remarkable capacity of the kidney to regain function following the various forms of acute renal injury discussed in the preceding chapter, renal injury of a more sustained nature is often not reversible but leads instead to progressive destruction of nephron mass. Despite successful treatment of hypertension, urinary tract obstruction and infection, and systemic disease, many forms of renal injury associated with permanent nephron loss progress inexorably to chronic renal failure (CRF). Reduction of renal mass causes structural and functional hypertrophy of remaining nephrons. This "compensatory" hypertrophy is due to adaptive hyperfiltration mediated by increases in glomerular capillary pressures and flows. Eventually these adaptations prove "maladaptive" in that they predispose to glomerular sclerosis, an enhanced functional burden on less affected glomeruli, leading in turn to their ultimate destruction.

Glomerulonephritis, in its several forms, was the most common initiating cause of chronic renal failure in the past. In recent years, possibly because of more aggressive treatment of glomerulonephritis and because of changing practices in patient acceptance of end-stage renal disease programs, diabetes mellitus and hypertension have become the leading causes of chronic renal failure (see Table 224-1). These and other progressive forms of renal disease are considered in detail in the remaining chapters of this section. Irrespective of cause, the eventual impact of severe reduction in nephron mass is an alteration in function of virtually every organ system in the body. *Uremia* is the term generally applied to the clinical syndrome in patients suffering from profound loss of renal function. Although the cause(s) of the syndrome remain unknown, the term *uremia* was adopted originally because of the presumption that the abnormalities seen in patients with CRF resulted from retention in the blood of urea and other end products of metabolism normally excreted in the urine. But the term *uremia* represents more than renal excretory failure alone. A host of metabolic and endocrine functions normally subserved by the kidney are also impaired in CRF, and the inexorable course to renal failure is often accompanied by severe malnutrition, impaired metabolism of carbohydrates, fats, and proteins, and defective utilization of energy. Therefore, the *uremia* no longer carries pathophysiologic meaning but instead refers generally to the constellation of signs and symptoms associated with CRF, regardless of cause.

The presentation and severity of signs and symptoms of uremia often vary greatly from patient to patient, depending, at least in part, on the magnitude of the reduction in functioning renal mass as well as the rapidity with which renal function is lost. As discussed in Chap. 222, in the relatively early stage of CRF [i.e., when total glomerular filtration rate (GFR) is reduced but not to levels below about 35 to 50 percent of normal], overall renal function is sufficient to maintain the patient symptom-free, although renal reserve may be diminished. At this stage of renal impairment baseline excretory, biosynthetic, and other regulatory functions of the kidney are generally well maintained. At a somewhat later stage in the course of CRF (GFR about 20 to 35 percent of normal), *azotemia* occurs, and initial manifestations of renal insufficiency usually appear. Although patients are relatively asymptomatic at this stage, renal reserve is diminished sufficiently that any sudden stress, such as intercurrent infection, urinary tract obstruction, dehydration, or administration of a nephrotoxic drug, may compromise renal function still further, often leading to signs and symptoms of overt uremia. With further loss of nephron mass (GFR below 20 to 25 percent of normal), the patient develops *overt renal failure*. Uremia may be viewed as the final stage in this inexorable process, when many of or all the untoward manifestations of CRF become evident clinically. In this chapter the causes and clinical characteristics of the disturbances of the various organ systems seen in patients with CRF will be considered.

TABLE 224-1 Primary Diagnoses—Medicare End-Stage Renal Disease Program*

Diabetic nephropathy	27.7%
Hypertension	24.5%
Glomerulonephritis	21.2%
Polycystic kidney disease	3.9%
Other/unknown	22.7%

* Number of new patients in 1985, 28,944.

SOURCE: Health Care Financing Administration, Bureau of Data Management and Strategy.

PATHOPHYSIOLOGY AND BIOCHEMISTRY OF UREMIA

ROLE OF RETAINED TOXIC METABOLITES The finding that sera from patients with uremia exert toxic effects in a variety of biologic test systems has motivated a diligent search to identify the responsible toxin(s). The most likely candidates thought to qualify as toxins in uremia are the *by-products of protein and amino acid metabolism*. Unlike fats and carbohydrates, which are eventually metabolized to carbon dioxide and water, substances that are easily excreted even in uremic subjects via lungs and skin, the products of protein and amino acid metabolism depend largely on the kidneys for excretion. A vast number of such products have been identified, with urea being quantitatively the most important. *Urea* represents some 80 percent or more of the total nitrogen excreted into the urine in patients with CRF maintained on diets containing 40 or more grams of protein per day. The *guanidino compounds* are the next most abundant of the nitrogenous end products of protein metabolism and include substances such as guanidine, methyl- and dimethylguanidine, creatinine, creatine, and guanidinosuccinic acid. As with urea, guanidines are derived, at least in part, from urea cycle amino acids. Other metabolic products of amino acid and protein catabolism that have been implicated as possible uremic toxins include *urates and other end products of nucleic acid metabolism, aliphatic amines,* a variety of *peptides,* and, finally, several *derivatives of the aromatic amino acids tryptophan, tyrosine, and phenylalanine*. The role of these substances in the pathogenesis of the clinical and biochemical abnormalities seen in CRF is unclear. It is generally believed that uremic symptoms correlate only in a rough and inconsistent way with concentrations of urea in blood. Nevertheless, although urea is probably not a major cause of overt uremic toxicity, it may account for some of the clinical abnormalities, including anorexia, malaise, vomiting, and headache. On the other hand, elevated levels of plasma *guanidinosuccinic acid,* by interfering with activation of platelet factor III by adenosine diphosphate (ADP), contribute to the impaired platelet function seen in CRF. *Creatinine,* generally regarded as a nontoxic substance, may cause adverse effects following conversion to more toxic metabolites such as sarcosine and methylguanidine. Whether these substances, as well as *creatine,* a metabolic precursor of creatinine, and the other compounds cited above, are of clinical importance in the pathogenesis of uremic toxicity remains to be established.

Nitrogenous compounds of larger molecular weight are also retained in CRF. A toxic role for these substances has been suggested because of the impression that patients treated with intermittent peritoneal dialysis are less troubled with neuropathy than patients maintained on chronic hemodialysis, despite higher levels of urea and creatinine in blood in the former group. Since the clearance of small molecules depends mainly upon blood and dialysate flow rates, which are higher with hemodialysis, whereas clearance of larger molecules depends more on membrane surface area and time, which are greater with peritoneal dialysis, this latter form of therapy may be a more effective means of removing these substances of larger molecular weight. A multicenter study examining clearance of small vs. middle-sized molecular substances, dialysis time, and morbidity indicated that urea or other small-molecular-weight substances play a more important role. Evidence that removal of "middle" molecules is associated with objective improvement in clinical well-being is unsubstantiated. The role of middle molecules in the uremic syndrome remains speculative.

Not all these middle-sized molecules accumulate in uremic plasma because of decreased renal excretion alone. The kidney normally *catabolizes* a number of circulating plasma proteins and polypeptides; with reduced renal mass, this capacity may be impaired greatly. Furthermore, plasma levels of many polypeptide hormones [including parathyroid hormone (PTH), insulin, glucagon, growth hormone, luteinizing hormone, and prolactin] rise with advancing renal failure, often markedly so, not only because of impaired renal catabolism but also because of enhanced secretion. Of these, excessive parathyroid hormone (PTH) may be an important uremic "toxin" because of its adverse effect on several organ systems. The consequences of high circulating levels of PTH and other hormones in chronic renal failure are considered below and in Chap. 222.

EFFECTS OF UREMIA ON CELLULAR FUNCTIONS

Alterations in the composition of intracellular and extracellular fluids in CRF have long been recognized. Such abnormalities are believed to be a consequence, at least in part, of *defective ion transport* across cell membranes generally, with retained uremic toxins possibly mediating these alterations in transmembrane ion transport. Integrity of cellular volume and composition depends to a large extent on the active outward transport of Na^+ from cell interior to exterior, the resulting intracellular fluid being relatively low in Na^+ and high in K^+, whereas the reverse is true for extracellular fluid. Active Na^+ transport is a metabolically costly process, accounting for a major fraction of basal energy utilization and oxygen consumption. The consequences of this efflux of Na^+ from cells are many and include, most notably, (1) the generation of a resting electrical potential difference across the cell membrane (with this transcellular voltage oriented so that cell interior is electronegative to cell exterior), and (2) a mechanism for enhancing the influx of K^+ into cells.

In experimental animals, partial inhibition of this active efflux mechanism for Na^+ across cell membranes leads to alterations in body composition and cell functions similar to those demonstrable in erythrocytes, leukocytes, skeletal muscle, and other tissues obtained from uremic subjects. These include increased and decreased intracellular concentrations of Na^+ and K^+, respectively, and reduction in magnitude of the transcellular voltage. These alterations have been shown to be largely reversed by efficient hemodialysis and, for erythrocytes at least, to be recreated when cells from normal subjects are incubated in uremic serum. Other derangements in cellular function have also been implicated as causes for altered body composition in uremia. For example, *Na^+- and K^+-stimulated ATPase activity* is decreased in erythrocytes and brain from uremic patients and animals, respectively. Whether the "uremic toxins" that account for these derangements in cellular function represent abnormally retained products of metabolism which fail to be excreted or normal substances present in increased quantities in response to reduced renal mass remains unknown. *Parathyroid and natriuretic hormones,* examples of this category of substances, are discussed in this context in Chap. 222.

EFFECTS OF UREMIA ON WHOLE-BODY COMPOSITION

What is the impact of these disturbances in active transcellular Na^+ transport on the uremic organism as a whole? From the pathophysiologic considerations already discussed, CRF is likely to lead to abnormally high intracellular Na^+ concentrations, and hence to osmotically induced overhydration of cells generally, whereas these same cells are thought to be relatively deficient in K^+. With the inevitable onset of malaise, anorexia, nausea, vomiting, and diarrhea, patients with CRF may eventually develop protein-calorie malnutrition and negative nitrogen balance, often with profound losses of lean body mass and fat deposits. Owing to the concomitant tendency for salt and water retention, these losses often go unnoticed until the late stages of CRF. Whereas a large fraction of the increase in total-body water in uremia is the result of expansion of intracellular volume, extracellular volume expansion also is observed commonly. With initiation of intermittent hemodialysis or renal transplantation, there is often an immediate and substantial loss of body weight, due primarily to correction of this overhydration. With successful transplantation, the initial diuresis is followed by a period of weight gain, due to restoration of lean body mass and fat deposits to preillness levels. For patients on chronic dialysis, the anabolic response is less dramatic, even when therapy is regarded as optimal, involving mainly reaccumulation of fat deposits. The failure to restore lean body mass to normal with chronic dialysis may reflect insufficient intake of protein, which, in adequately dialyzed patients, should be maintained at levels of 0.8 to 1.4 g per kilogram of body weight per day.

Deficits in intracellular K^+ concentration in CRF have already been mentioned and may result from inadequate intake (poor diet or overzealous K^+ restriction by the physician), excessive losses (vomiting, diarrhea, diuretics), reduction of Na^+- and K^+-stimulated ATPase, or a combination of these. In addition to promoting losses of K^+ into urine (which may be substantial if urine volume remains relatively normal in uremic subjects), the high levels of plasma aldosterone often seen in CRF may also augment net secretion of K^+ into the colon, thereby contributing to marked K^+ losses in stool or diarrheal fluids. Despite deficits in intracellular K^+ concentration, serum K^+ is usually normal or high in CRF, owing most often to metabolic acidosis, which induces an efflux of K^+ from cells. Additionally, uremic patients are relatively resistant to the action of insulin (see below), which normally enhances K^+ uptake by skeletal muscle.

EFFECTS OF UREMIA ON METABOLISM

HYPOTHERMIA In animals injections of urine, urea, or other retained toxic metabolites can induce hypothermia, and basal heat production diminishes soon after nephrectomy. Since active Na^+ transport across cell membranes accounts for a major proportion of basal energy production, the inverse relationship between body temperature and degree of azotemia is due, probably in part, to inhibition of the sodium pump by some retained toxin(s). Dialysis usually returns body temperature to normal.

CARBOHYDRATE METABOLISM The ability to metabolize glucose is impaired in most patients with CRF. The defect largely involves a slowing of the rate at which blood glucose concentration declines to the normal range after administration of a glucose load. Fasting blood sugar levels are usually normal or only slightly elevated; severe hyperglycemia and/or ketosis is uncommon. Consequently, the *glucose intolerance of CRF* usually does not require specific therapy (hence the term *azotemic pseudodiabetes*). Because insulin depends to a large extent on the kidney for its removal from plasma and degradation, circulating insulin levels tend to be increased in uremia. Whereas insulin levels in plasma are only slightly to moderately increased in most fasting uremic subjects, levels in excess of normal are usually found in response to a glucose load. The response to intravenous insulin in patients with CRF is also abnormal, and the rate of utilization of glucose by peripheral tissues often is diminished. The glucose intolerance of uremia results largely from this peripheral resistance to the action of insulin. Other possible factors contributing to glucose intolerance include intracellular deficits of potassium, metabolic acidosis, increased levels of glucagon and other hormones including catecholamines, growth hormone, and prolactin, as well as the myriad of potentially toxic metabolites retained in CRF. In true insulin-dependent diabetics, there is often a decrease in insulin requirement with progressive azotemia, a phenomenon not related solely to decreased caloric intake.

NITROGEN AND LIPID METABOLISM Since the capacity to eliminate the nitrogenous end products of protein catabolism is reduced, CRF may be regarded as a state of *protein intolerance.* As discussed above, retention of the end products of nitrogen metabolism is a dominant cause of the signs and symptoms of uremic toxicity.

Hypertriglyceridemia and decreased high-density lipoprotein cholesterol are common in uremia, whereas cholesterol levels in plasma are usually normal. Whether uremia accelerates triglyceride production by the liver and intestine is unknown. The well-known lipogenic effect of hyperinsulinism may contribute to increased triglyceride synthesis. The rate of removal of triglycerides from the circulation, which depends in large part on the enzyme *lipoprotein lipase,* is depressed in uremia, an effect not corrected appreciably by hemodialysis. The high incidence of premature atherosclerosis in patients on chronic dialysis (see "Cardiovascular and Pulmonary Abnormalities" below) may be related in part to these abnormalities in lipid metabolism.

CLINICAL ABNORMALITIES IN UREMIA

The diagnosis of chronic renal failure is based on recognition of a constellation of signs and symptoms with or without reduced urine output but always with elevation in serum urea nitrogen and creatinine concentrations. As pointed out in Chap. 222, elevation of serum urea nitrogen and creatinine occur late in the course of renal failure. Differentiation between acute and chronic renal failure can be difficult. The history is often most helpful, particularly if normal renal function existed prior to a sudden recent insult. The laboratory findings and physical examination may not be helpful in the differentiation. The hallmark of chronic renal failure is the presence of reduced kidney size on either ultrasound, abdominal scout film, or pyelogram. In the absence of small kidneys, renal biopsy may be necessary for diagnosis.

As noted earlier, CRF leads ultimately to disturbances in function of every organ system. With the application of chronic dialysis in the past three decades, the incidence and severity of these disturbances have been modified, so that where modern medicine is practiced, the overt and florid manifestations of uremia have largely disappeared. Unfortunately, however, even optimal dialysis therapy is not a panacea for the patient with CRF, because, as indicated in Table 224-2, some disturbances resulting from impaired renal function fail to respond fully, while others progress despite dialysis treatment. Furthermore, as with many complex therapeutic modalities, intermittent dialysis may be responsible for the appearance of unique abnormalities not seen prior to initiation of therapy; these abnormalities should be viewed as complications of dialysis.

FLUID, ELECTROLYTE, AND ACID-BASE DISORDERS (See also Chaps. 50 and 51) **Sodium and volume homeostasis** In most patients with stable CRF, modest increases in total body Na^+ and water content can be documented, although objective signs of extracellular fluid (ECF) volume expansion may not be apparent. With ingestion of excessive amounts of salt and water, however, control of excess volume becomes an important clinical and therapeutic consideration. In general, excessive *salt* ingestion contributes to, or aggravates, congestive heart failure, hypertension, ascites, and edema. On the other hand, hyponatremia and weight gain are the consequence of excessive ingestion of *water,* abnormalities which in most patients are relatively mild or asymptomatic. In most patients, daily intake of fluid equal in volume to urine volume per day plus about 500 mL usually maintains the serum Na^+ concentration at normal levels. Hypernatremia is relatively infrequent in CRF. In the edematous patient with CRF not on dialysis, diuretics and modest restriction of salt and water intake are the mainstays of therapy. In volume-expanded dialysis patients, management should include ultrafiltration and restriction of salt and water intake between dialyses.

Patients with CRF have impaired renal mechanisms for conserving Na^+ and water (see Chap. 222). When an *extrarenal* cause for increased fluid loss is present (e.g., vomiting, diarrhea, fever), these patients are prone to develop ECF volume depletion, with signs and symptoms of dry mouth and other mucous membranes, dizziness, syncope, tachycardia, decreased filling of jugular veins, orthostatic hypotension, and vascular collapse. Depletion of extracellular fluid volume typically results in deterioration of residual renal function and, in the previously stable and asymptomatic patient with mild CRF, signs and symptoms of overt uremia. Cautious fluid repletion usually restores extracellular and intravascular volumes to normal and often, but not always, returns renal function to previously stable levels.

Potassium homeostasis Derangements in K^+ balance (see Chaps. 50 and 222) are occasionally documented by laboratory analysis in patients with CRF but are rarely responsible for clinical symptoms unless GFR is below 5 mL/min or an endogenous (hemolysis, trauma, infection) or exogenous (stored blood, K^+-containing medications) K^+ load is administered. Despite progression of renal failure, most patients maintain normal serum K^+ concentrations until the final stages of uremia. This ability to sustain K^+ balance with

TABLE 224-2 Clinical abnormalities in uremia*

FLUID AND ELECTROLYTE DISTURBANCES
Volume expansion and contraction (I)
Hypernatremia and hyponatremia (I)
Hyperkalemia and hypokalemia (I)
Metabolic acidosis (I)
Hyperphosphatemia and hypophosphatemia (I)
Hypocalcemia (I)
ENDOCRINE-METABOLIC DISTURBANCES
Renal osteodystrophy (I or P)
Osteomalacia (D)
Secondary hyperparathyroidism (I or P)
Carbohydrate intolerance (I)
Hyperuricemia (I or P)
Hypothermia (I)
Hypertriglyceridemia (P)
Protein-calorie malnutrition (I or P)
Impaired growth and development (P)
Infertility and sexual dysfunction (P)
Amenorrhea (P)
Dialysis (amyloid, $beta_2$ microglobulin) arthropathy (D)
NEUROMUSCULAR DISTURBANCES
Fatigue (I)
Sleep disorders (P)
Headache (I or P)
Impaired mentation (I)
Lethargy (I)
Asterixis (I)
Muscular irritability (I)
Peripheral neuropathy (I or P)
Restless legs syndrome (I or P)
Paralysis (I or P)
Myoclonus (I)
Seizures (I or P)
Coma (I)
Muscle cramps (D)
Dialysis disequilibrium syndrome (D)
Dialysis dementia (D)
Myopathy (P or D)
CARDIOVASCULAR AND PULMONARY DISTURBANCES
Arterial hypertension (I or P)
Congestive heart failure or pulmonary edema (I)
Pericarditis (I)
Cardiomyopathy (I or P)
Uremic lung (I)
Accelerated atherosclerosis (P or D)
Hypotension and arrhythmias (D)
DERMATOLOGIC DISTURBANCES
Pallor (I or P)
Hyperpigmentation (I, P, or D)
Pruritus (P)
Ecchymoses (I or P)
Uremic frost (I)
GASTROINTESTINAL DISTURBANCES
Anorexia (I)
Nausea and vomiting (I)
Uremic fetor (I)
Gastroenteritis (I)
Peptic ulcer (I or P)
Gastrointestinal bleeding (I, P, or D)
Hepatitis (D)
Refractory ascites on hemodialysis (D)
Peritonitis (D)
HEMATOLOGIC AND IMMUNOLOGIC DISTURBANCES
Normocytic, normochromic anemia (P)
Microcytic (aluminum-induced) anemia (D)
Lymphocytopenia (P)
Bleeding diathesis (I or D)
Increased susceptibility to infection (I or P)
Splenomegaly and hypersplenism (P)
Leukopenia (D)
Hypocomplementemia (D)

* Virtually all the abnormalities contained in this table are completely reversed in time by successful renal transplantation. The response of these abnormalities to hemo- or peritoneal dialysis therapy is more variable. (I) denotes an abnormality that usually improves with an optimal program of dialysis and related therapy. (P) denotes an abnormality that tends to persist or even progress, despite an optimal program. (D) denotes an abnormality that develops only after initiation of dialysis therapy.

advancing renal failure is due to adaptations in the renal distal tubules and colon, sites where aldosterone and other factors serve to enhance K^+ secretion (see Chap. 222). Not surprisingly, oliguria, or disruption of key adaptive mechanisms, can lead to *hyperkalemia* and its potentially ominous effects on cardiac function. Antikaliuretic drugs such as spironolactone, triamterene, or amiloride should be used with extreme caution in chronic renal failure. Likewise, angiotensin-converting enzyme inhibitors and beta blockers may be a cause of hyperkalemia. In the transplanted patient, cyclosporin A is another common cause of increased serum potassium. Hyperkalemia in CRF may also be induced by abrupt lowering of arterial blood pH, since acidosis is associated with efflux of K^+ from intracellular to extracellular fluids. A useful index of the magnitude of this hydrogen-potassium exchange is that for every 0.1-unit change in blood pH, there will be a reciprocal change in serum K^+ concentration of approximately 0.6 mmol/L. Correction of acidosis-induced hyperkalemia with sodium bicarbonate is the treatment of choice. Intravenous insulin and dextrose are useful in lowering serum potassium acutely, while the ion exchange resin sodium polystyrene sulfonate is useful in longer-term control of hyperkalemia. When hyperkalemia persists in the absence of excessive K^+ intake, oliguria, or acute acidosis, the possibility of *hyporeninemic hypoaldosteronism* should be considered. Patients with this syndrome have reduced circulating levels of renin and aldosterone in the plasma and often also have diabetes mellitus.

Hypokalemia due to diminished ability of the kidneys to conserve K^+ is uncommon in most forms of CRF. When hypokalemia occurs in these patients, poor dietary K^+ intake, usually in association with excessive diuretic therapy or gastrointestinal losses, is likely to be the underlying cause. When hypokalemia occurs as a result of primary K^+ wasting in urine, it may represent a solitary renal reabsorptive defect or, more commonly, may be associated with other solute transport abnormalities, as in Fanconi's syndrome, renal tubular acidosis, or other forms of hereditary or acquired tubulointerstitial diseases (see Chaps. 229 and 231). A discussion of the clinical consequences and management of hypokalemia and hyperkalemia is given in Chap. 50.

Metabolic acidosis With advancing renal failure, total daily acid excretion and buffer production fall below the level needed to maintain external balance of hydrogen ions. Metabolic acidosis is the inevitable result, and the mechanisms involved are considered in Chap. 222. In most patients with stable renal insufficiency, administration of 20 to 30 mmol sodium bicarbonate or sodium citrate per day usually corrects the acidosis. In response to a sudden acid challenge (whether from an endogenous or exogenous source), however, patients with CRF are susceptible to acidosis, which requires more substantial quantities of alkali for correction. Administration of sodium must be carried out with careful attention to the patient's volume status.

Phosphate, calcium, and bone As discussed in detail in Chap. 222, hypocalcemia in chronic renal failure results from the impaired ability of the diseased kidney to synthesize 1,25-dihydroxyvitamin D [$1,25(OH_2)D$], the active metabolite of vitamin D (Fig. 224-1). Reabsorption of calcium in the gut is impaired when circulating levels of this active metabolite are low. Also serum phosphate concentration begins to rise when GFR falls below about 25 percent of normal. Calcium deposition in bone is dependent on the availability of phosphate; retention of phosphate in plasma, therefore, facilitates calcium entry into bone and contributes to the hypocalcemia and elevation of plasma PTH levels in CRF. Finally, in advanced CRF, the ability of PTH to mobilize calcium salts from bone may be altered. Despite these various causes of hypocalcemia, symptoms of tetany are rare unless patients are treated with large amounts of alkali.

Overproduction of parathyroid hormone, disordered vitamin D metabolism, chronic metabolic acidosis, and excessive fecal losses of calcium all contribute to the bone diseases in uremia (Fig. 224-1). *Renal* and *metabolic osteodystrophy* are imprecise terms that encompass a number of skeletal abnormalities, including osteomalacia, osteitis fibrosa cystica, osteosclerosis, and, in children especially, impaired bone growth. Although clinical symptoms of bone disease are uncommon, occurring in less than 10 percent of predialysis patients with advanced renal failure, radiologic and histologic abnormalities are observed in, respectively, about 35 and 90 percent. In patients treated by dialysis for several years, symptoms of bone disease are a major cause of morbidity. Renal osteodystrophy is more common in children than in adults, and especially in patients with congenital renal anomalies associated with slowly progressive renal insufficiency. On radiologic examination, three types of lesions can be identified: (1) changes analogous to those in children with nutritional rickets, namely, widened osteoid seams at the growth margin of

FIGURE 224-1 Pathogenesis of bone diseases in chronic renal failure.

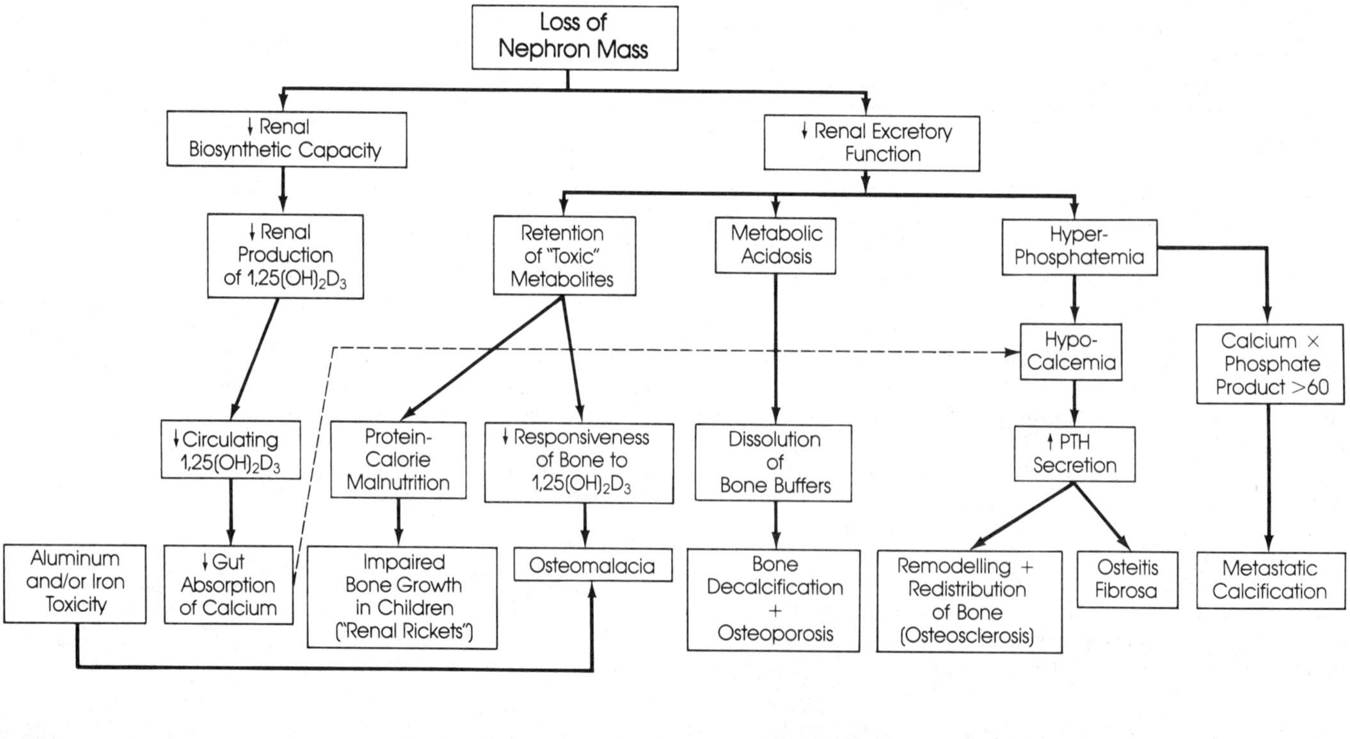

bones (so-called renal rickets); (2) the bone changes of *secondary hyperparathyroidism* (*osteitis fibrosa cystica*), characterized by osteoclastic bone resorption and manifested by subperiosteal erosions, especially of the phalanges, long bones, and distal ends of the clavicles; and (3) *osteosclerosis,* often best evidenced by enhanced bone density in the upper and lower margins of vertebrae, producing the so-called rugger jersey spine.

Osteomalacia was initially thought to be secondary to decreased availability of 1,25(OH_2)D. There is now evidence that osteomalacia is also due to deposition of aluminum in the calcification fronts. The sources are aluminum in dialysate as well as aluminum-containing phosphate-binding agents. In aluminum-induced osteomalacia, the serum level of parathyroid hormone is usually low and that of calcium is often high. With osteitis fibrosa cystica and osteomalacia there is a tendency to spontaneous fractures which are often slow to heal. The ribs are most commonly involved. Painful joints may occur due to calcium deposition in bursa and other periarticular structures. Bone pain may be seen in the absence of fractures. When bone pain is severe, a proximal *myopathy* often coexists, giving rise to gait abnormalities and even leading to cessation of ambulation. The incidence of *aseptic necrosis of the hip* is increased in renal transplant recipients, probably related to chronic glucocorticoid therapy, secondary hyperparathyroidism, and altered vitamin D metabolism. In CRF there is often a tendency to *extraosseous,* or *metastatic, calcification,* especially when the calcium-phosphate product is very high. Medium-sized blood vessels; subcutaneous, articular, and periarticular tissues; myocardium; eyes; and lungs are common sites of metastatic calcification. An arthropathy in chronic dialysis patients is associated with deposition of amyloid or beta$_2$ microglobulin. The cause is unknown but may be related to chronic exposure of blood to certain dialysis membranes.

Management of renal osteodystrophy includes reduction in dietary phosphate available for absorption through the use of a restricted phosphate diet as well as phosphate-binding agents. Calcium carbonate is the preferred phosphate-binding agent, but in some circumstances a combination of aluminum hydroxide and calcium carbonate is necessary. Dialysate calcium, oral calcium, aluminum hydroxide, and calcitriol or dihydrotachysterol must be properly balanced to maintain the serum phosporus at approximately 1.4 mmol/L (4.5 mg/dL) and the serum calcium at approximately 2.5 mmol/L (10 mg/dL) in an attempt to improve osteitis fibrosa cystica, osteomalacia, and myopathy. Treatment should be initiated early in chronic renal failure so that secondary hyperparathyroidism and bone disease may be prevented. It is particularly important to keep the calcium-phosphorous product in the normal range to avoid metastatic calcification or any possible role of these substances in progressive renal insufficiency.

Other solutes Other derangements in CRF include *hyperuricemia* and *hypermagnesemia*. Uric acid retention is a common feature of CRF but rarely leads to symptomatic gout. Hypophosphatemia is usually a consequence of overzealous oral administration of phosphate-binding gels. Because serum magnesium levels tend to rise in CRF, magnesium-containing antacids and cathartics should be avoided.

CARDIOVASCULAR AND PULMONARY ABNORMALITIES Fluid retention in uremic patients often results in congestive heart failure and/or pulmonary edema. A unique form of pulmonary congestion and edema may occur even in the absence of volume overload and is associated with normal or mildly elevated intracardiac and pulmonary wedge pressures. This entity, characterized radiologically by perihilar vascular congestion giving rise to a "butterfly wing" distribution, is due to increased permeability of the alveolar capillary membrane. This low-pressure pulmonary edema, as well as cardiopulmonary abnormalities associated with circulatory overload, usually responds promptly to vigorous dialysis.

Arterial hypertension is the most common complication of end-stage renal disease. When it is not present, the patient either has a salt-wasting form of renal disease (e.g., polycystic or medullary cystic disease or chronic pyelonephritis), is receiving antihypertensive therapy, or is volume-depleted, the last condition usually being due to excessive gastrointestinal fluid losses or overzealous diuretic therapy. Since fluid overload is the major cause of hypertension in uremic subjects, the normotensive state can usually be restored by dialysis. Nevertheless, some patients remain hypertensive, despite rigorous salt and water restriction and ultrafiltration, because of hyperreninemia. In most cases, routine antihypertensive drug therapy is effective. A small minority of these patients develop *accelerated or malignant hypertension,* manifested by markedly elevated systolic and diastolic pressures, severe hyperreninemia, encephalopathy, seizures, retinal changes, and papilledema. Use of drugs such as diazoxide, minoxidil, captopril, enalapril and nitroprusside, along with control of extracellular volume, generally controls such hypertension.

Pericarditis, once a common complication of CRF, is now infrequent because of early initiation of dialysis. Retained metabolic toxins are thought to be the cause of *pericarditis.* The unusual occurrence of pericarditis in the well-dialyzed patient is usually due to viral infection or systemic disease.

The clinical presentation of pericarditis in uremic subjects is generally similar to that of other etiologies (Chap. 193), except that pericardiocentesis for effusions usually yields hemorrhagic fluid. Treatment with intensive dialysis is recommended, and systemic anticoagulation should be avoided to minimize the occurrence of hemorrhagic tamponade. In some patients, pericardiocentesis with intrapericardial instillation of air or glucocorticoids is effective for pericardial tamponade. Pericardiectomy should be considered only after more conservative treatment has failed.

Chronically dialyzed patients have a disturbingly high incidence of *accelerated atherosclerosis,* leading to development of significant coronary, cerebral, and peripheral vascular manifestations. There are ample causes for these complications, including hypertension, hyperlipidemia, glucose intolerance, chronic high cardiac output, and metastatic vascular and myocardial calcification.

HEMATOLOGIC ABNORMALITIES *Normochromic, normocytic anemia* occurs regularly in CRF and contributes to fatigability and listlessness in these patients. Erythropoiesis is depressed in CRF, due both to the effects of retained toxins on bone marrow and to diminished biosynthesis of erythropoietin by the diseased kidney or to the presence of erythropoietin inhibitors. The use of recombinant human erythropoietin results in a dramatic increase in hematocrit and hemoglobin suggesting that reduced serum erythropoietin is perhaps the more important of these factors. The anemia of chronic uremia may also be due in part to aluminum intoxication, which causes a microcytic anemia, fibrosis of the bone marrow due to hyperparathyroidism, and, occasionally, inadequate replacement of folic acid. *Hemolysis* also occurs and involves an extracorpuscular defect since survival of erythrocytes from normal subjects is reduced when these cells are transfused into uremic patients, and erythrocytes from patients with CRF have relatively normal survival times when transfused into normal individuals. Gastrointestinal and chronic dialyzer *blood loss* contributes to anemia, as does *hypersplenism* in the occasional patient. Blood loss is exaggerated in hemodialysis patients because of the need for heparin during dialysis. Transfusions may contribute to suppression of erythropoiesis in CRF and, due to increased risk of hepatitis and hemosiderosis, should be avoided unless anemia aggravates other underlying disorders (for example, coronary or cerebrovascular disease). Androgen therapy has been shown to improve erythropoiesis in some dialysis patients not previously subjected to nephrectomy. Parenteral or oral iron therapy is indicated only in patients with documented iron deficiency due to chronic blood loss. In those patients in whom multiple blood transfusions have been administered, one should consider the possibility of hemachromatosis. Folic and ascorbic acids and the soluble B vitamins should be given to offset chronic losses of these substances via dialysis. As indicated above, clinical trials with recombinant human erythropoietin show this agent to be extremely effective in correcting anemia. Commercial availability of erythropoietin is expected in the near future.

Abnormal hemostasis is another common derangement in CRF, characterized by a tendency to abnormal bleeding and bruising. Bleeding from the surgical wounds or spontaneously into the gastrointestinal tract, pericardial sac, and intracranial vault, in the form of subdural hematoma or intracerebral hemorrhage, is of greatest concern. Prolongation of bleeding time, decreased platelet factor III activity, abnormal platelet aggregation and adhesiveness, and impaired prothrombin consumption contribute to the clotting defects. The abnormality in factor III correlates with increased plasma levels of guanidinosuccinic acid and can largely be corrected by dialysis. Prolongation of the bleeding time is common even in the well-dialyzed patient. Abnormal bleeding times and coagulopathy in renal failure may be reversed with desmopressin, cryoprecipitate, conjugated estrogens, and blood transfusions, and possibly by use of recombinant human erythropoietin.

A wide variety of changes in leukocyte formation and function also occur in uremia leading to *enhanced susceptibility to infection.* Lymphocytopenia and atrophy of lymphoid structures occur in CRF, whereas neutrophil production is relatively unimpaired. Nevertheless, all leukocyte cell types may be affected adversely by uremic serum. Decreased chemotaxis is among the best documented of the defects occurring in uremic leukocytes, with resulting impairment of acute inflammatory response and decreased delayed hypersensitivity. There is a tendency for uremic patients to have less fever in response to infection. For these reasons, infections may be difficult to recognize in uremia. Leukocyte function may also be impaired in patients with CRF because of coexisting acidosis, hyperglycemia, protein-calorie malnutrition, and serum and tissue hyperosmolarity (due to azotemia). Mucosal barriers to infection may also be defective, and, in dialysis patients, vascular access devices are also common portals of entry for pathogens, particularly staphylococci. Glucocorticoids and immunosuppressive drugs add further to the risk of serious infection in many of these patients. Leukopenia is a common transient finding in patients exposed to cellophane-derived membranes during dialysis (Chap. 225).

NEUROMUSCULAR ABNORMALITIES Subtle disturbances of central nervous system function, including inability to concentrate, drowsiness, and insomnia, are among the earliest symptoms of uremia. Mild behavioral changes, loss of memory, and errors in judgment soon follow and often are associated with signs of neuromuscular irritability, including hiccups, cramps, and fasciculations and twitching of large muscle groups. Asterixis, myoclonus, and chorea are common in terminal uremia, as are stupor, seizures, and coma. Many of these neuromuscular complications of severe uremia resolve with dialysis, although nonspecific EEG abnormalities may persist.

Peripheral neuropathy is a common complication of advanced CRF. Initially, sensory nerve involvement exceeds motor, lower extremities are involved more than the upper, and the distal portions of the extremities more than proximal. The "restless legs syndrome," characterized by ill-defined sensations of discomfort in the feet and lower legs and frequent leg movement, is a disturbing complication. If dialysis is not instituted soon after onset of sensory abnormalities, motor involvement follows, often leading to loss of deep tendon reflexes, weakness, peroneal nerve palsy (foot drop), and, eventually, flaccid quadriplegia. Accordingly, early evidence of peripheral neuropathy is generally taken as a firm indication to initiate dialysis or transplantation.

Two types of neurologic disturbances appear to be unique to patients on chronic dialysis. One is the syndrome of *dialysis dementia,* seen in patients who have been on dialysis for a number of years. This syndrome is characterized by speech dyspraxia, myoclonus, dementia, and eventually seizures and death. Aluminum intoxication is probably a major contributor to this syndrome. Other factors (viral infection?) also likely play a role since only a small percent of patients with increased aluminum exposure develop the syndrome. The other disturbance, dialysis disequilibrium, occurs during the first few dialyses, in association with rapid reduction of blood urea levels. Nausea, vomiting, drowsiness, headache, and even grand mal seizures have been attributed to the more rapid (dialysis-induced) pH change and reduction in osmolality of extracellular than intracellular fluids within the cranium, leading to cerebral edema and raised intracranial pressure.

GASTROINTESTINAL ABNORMALITIES Anorexia, hiccups, nausea, and vomiting are common and early manifestations of uremia. The use of carefully monitored protein restriction in the diet may be useful to slow progression of renal insufficiency if initiated early. Protein restriction is also useful in diminishing nausea and vomiting late in the course. Protein restriction should not, of course, be implemented in those patients with severe protein-calorie malnutrition. *Uremic fetor,* a uriniferous odor to the breath, derives from the breakdown of urea in saliva to ammonia and is often associated with unpleasant taste sensation. Mucosal ulcerations leading to blood loss can occur at any level of the gastrointestinal tract in very late stages of CRF—so-called uremic gastroenteritis. Peptic ulcer disease is particularly common, occurring in as many as one-fourth of uremic subjects. Whether this high incidence is related to increased gastric acidity, hypersecretion of gastrin, or secondary hyperparathyroidism is unknown. Most of the gastrointestinal symptoms, except those related to peptic ulcer disease, usually improve with dialysis. A syndrome of idiopathic ascites is seen rarely in patients on chronic dialysis, presumably secondary to fluid overload and/or chronic passive hepatic congestion. Patients with chronic renal failure, particularly those with polycystic kidney disease, have an increased incidence of diverticulosis. Hbs Ag hepatitis is more common in patients on chronic dialysis and is discussed in detail in Chap. 225.

ENDOCRINE-METABOLIC DISTURBANCES The common disturbances in parathyroid function, glucose, and insulin metabolism, as well as the lipid, protein-calorie, and other nutritional abnormalities of uremia have already been considered. In general, pituitary, thyroid, and adrenal gland functions are relatively normal, often despite abnormalities in circulating thyroxine, growth hormone, aldosterone, and cortisol levels. In women, estrogen levels are low, and amenorrhea and inability to carry pregnancies to term are early manifestations of uremia. While menses frequently reappear after chronic dialysis is initiated, successful pregnancies remain rare. In men with CRF, including those on chronic dialysis, impotence, oligospermia, and germinal cell dysplasia are common, as are reduced plasma testosterone levels. As with growth, sexual maturation is often impaired in adolescent children, even among those on chronic dialysis.

DERMATOLOGIC ABNORMALITIES The skin shows many abnormalities. This is not surprising in view of anemia (pallor), defective hemostasis (ecchymoses and hematomas), calcium deposition and secondary hyperparathyroidism (pruritus, excoriations), dehydration (poor skin turgor, dry mucous membranes), and the general cutaneous consequences of protein-calorie malnutrition. A sallow, yellow cast may reflect the combined influences of anemia and retention of a variety of pigmented metabolites, or *urochromes.* In advanced uremia urea concentrations in sweat may reach sufficiently high levels that, after evaporation, a fine white powder can be found on the skin surface—so-called uremic (urea) frost. Although many of these cutaneous abnormalities improve with dialysis, *uremic pruritus* is usually resistant to most systemic and topical therapies. Hemochromatosis causes a slate-gray–bronze discoloration of the skin and is common in the dialysis patient who has received multiple transfusions.

REFERENCES

Acchiardo SR et al: Malnutrition as the main factor in morbidity and mortality of hemodialysis patients. Kidney Int 24:S199, 1983

Anderson S, Brenner BM: Effects of aging on the renal glomerulus. Am J Med 80:435, 1986

Andrassy K, Ritz E: Uremia as a cause of bleeding. Am J Nephrol 5:313, 1985

Deykin D: Uremic bleeding. Kidney Int 24:698, 1983

Dumbauld S et al: Carbohydrate metabolism during fasting in chronic hemodialysis patients. Kidney Int 24:222, 1983

Eschbach JW et al: Correction of the anemia of end-stage renal disease with recombinant human erythropoietin: Results of a combined phase I and II clinical trial. N Engl J Med 316:73, 1987
Gokal R et al: Iron metabolism in hemodialysis patients: A study of the management of iron therapy and overload. Q J Med 48:369, 1979
Goldblum SE, Reed WP: Host defenses and immunologic alterations associated with chronic hemodialysis. Ann Intern Med 93:597, 1980
Jubelirer SJ: Hemostatic abnormalities in renal disease. Am J Kidney Dis 5:219, 1985
Klahr S et al: Factors that may retard the progression of renal disease. Kidney Int 32:S35, 1987
Kopple JD, Massry SG: Uremic toxins: What are they? How are they identified? Semin Nephrol 3:263, 1983
Lim VS: Reproductive function in patients with renal insufficiency. Am J Kidney Dis 9:363, 1987
Livio M et al: Conjugated estrogens for the management of bleeding associated with renal failure. N Engl J Med 315:731, 1986
Luger A et al: Abnormalities in the hypothalamic-pituitary-adrenocortical axis in patients with chronic renal failure. Am J Kidney Dis 9:51, 1987
Mahoney C et al: Central and peripheral nervous system effects of chronic renal failure. Kidney Int 24:170, 1983
Massry SG: Neurotoxicity of parathyroid hormone in uremia. Kidney Int 28:S17, 1985
——— et al: Current status of the use of 1,25(OH)$_2$D$_3$ in the management of renal osteodystrophy. Kidney Int 18:409, 1980
Sherrard DJ: Renal osteodystrophy. Semin Nephrol 6:56, 1986
Slatopolsky E: The interaction of parathyroid hormone and aluminum in renal osteodystrophy. Kidney Int 31:842, 1987

225 DIALYSIS AND TRANSPLANTATION IN THE TREATMENT OF RENAL FAILURE

CHARLES B. CARPENTER / J. MICHAEL LAZARUS

Over the past four decades, dialysis and transplantation have become effective in prolonging the lives of patients with renal insufficiency. The approach to treatment in acute renal failure is different than in chronic renal failure because of the irreversible nature of the latter. Conservative medical management and dialysis are the mainstays of therapy for acute renal failure. Obviously, transplantation is not a treatment for this group of patients. Options for treatment of patients with *chronic* or *irreversible* renal failure are outlined in Fig. 225-1.

Initially patients are managed with conservative therapy, but eventually they require hemodialysis, peritoneal dialysis, or cadaver or related donor transplantation. Because of limited success with each of these treatment modalities, chronic renal failure should be approached with the concept of moving from one form of therapy to another as indicated by the degree of success and incidence of complications with each.

Therapy for renal failure should be initiated at a time when complications will be moderate, but not when the patient is completely asymptomatic. The advanced complications of uremia, as noted in Chaps. 222 and 224, should be avoided by early treatment. Early dialysis is especially applicable to patients with acute renal failure in whom resumption of renal function can be expected and to patients with chronic renal failure who have a good immunologic match with a related donor. In the latter group, early transplantation will likely

FIGURE 225-1 Options for patients with chronic or irreversible renal failure.

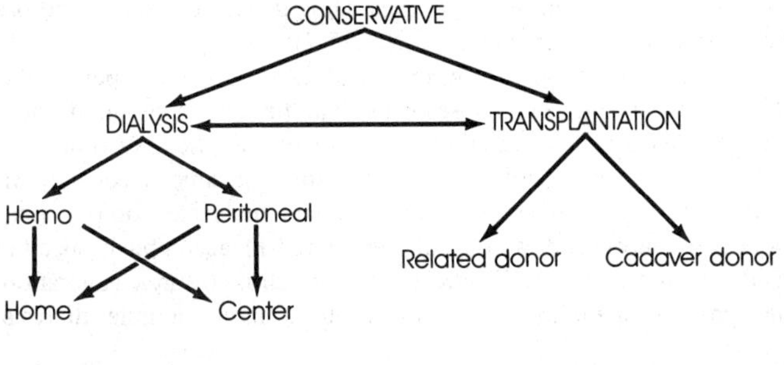

TABLE 225-1 Contraindications to kidney transplantation

1 Absolute contraindications
- *a* Reversible renal involvement
- *b* Ability of conservative measures to maintain useful life
- *c* Advanced forms of major extrarenal complications (cerebrovascular or coronary disease, neoplasia)
- *d* Active infection
- *e* Active glomerulonephritis
- *f* Previous sensitization to donor tissue

2 Relative contraindications (see text)
- *a* Age
- *b* Presence of vesical or urethral abnormalities
- *c* Iliofemoral occlusive disease
- *d* Psychiatric problems
- *e* Oxalosis

lead to resumption of normal renal function. In the remainder of patients, the clinical judgment to move from conservative treatment to dialysis or transplantation is determined by the patient's quality of life and whether or not the benefits of treatment outweigh the risks. Treatment with dietary protein restriction and aggressive control of hypertension, as described in Chap. 224, may prolong the time before dialysis and/or transplantation are required, but should be carried out only if complications of such therapy do not worsen long-term morbidity and mortality.

Selection of patients to receive dialysis and/or transplantation is a matter of some debate. Because of the reversible nature of acute renal failure, *all* patients with this diagnosis should be supported with dialysis, at least for some period of time, to allow return of renal function. In patients with irreversible or chronic renal failure, criteria for selection for transplantation are generally more stringent than those for dialysis and are guided by the possibility of complications related to immunosuppressive therapy. Table 225-1 lists practical considerations in the selection of a recipient for a human renal allograft. Such a procedure should be undertaken only when conservative treatment has failed, when there are no reversible elements in the patient's renal failure, and when the patient is too ill to be maintained comfortably with the usual methods of treatment. However, morbidity is less if transplantation is performed before the patient is critically ill. Transplantation should not be utilized in an attempt to salvage patients from failure to thrive on dialysis.

The recipient should be free of life-threatening extrarenal complications such as cancer, severe coronary artery disease, and cerebrovascular disease. Provided that diffuse vascular involvement is not present, diabetes mellitus is not a contraindication. Oxalosis may recur in relatively short order in a transplanted kidney and is generally a contraindication for this procedure. Although age may be a limiting factor, it is advanced "physiologic" rather than chronologic age which contraindicates transplantation. In general, patients reach a "physiologic" limit at approximately age 60 to 65 years when the incidence of complications due to glucocorticoids becomes much higher than in younger patients. Although abnormalities of the bladder and urethra present additional hazards, successful renal allografts have been placed in individuals with these abnormalities by prior constitution of an artificial bladder (i.e., ileal conduit) into which the donor ureter is placed. Patients with any disease process that may be aggravated by glucocorticoids, cyclosporine, azathioprine, or other immunosuppressive agents, or any patient with medical complications so severe that the risks of operation and drug therapy are high, should not be offered transplantation. In evaluating potential exclusionary diseases, it should be kept in mind that quality of life and long-term results are superior in the *successful* renal transplantation.

Criteria for treatment with hemodialysis or peritoneal dialysis are more liberal since dialysis has less morbidity than transplantation in older patients and those with the aforementioned medical complications. Because of the cost of these programs, some have suggested that entry be restricted in those of advanced age. Such decisions based on moral, social, and economic issues continue to generate debate. In general, nearly all patients are accepted if they or their families desire prolongation of life. In most areas of the world, the cost of medical care for chronic renal failure is borne by government.

CONSERVATIVE TREATMENT

As discussed in Chap. 224, conservative (nondialytic, nontransplant) therapy should be instituted early to control symptoms, minimize complications, prevent long-term sequelae of uremia, and slow the progression of renal insufficiency. Every effort should be made to correct any of the reversible components which aggravate renal impairment. In patients with acute renal failure, prerenal factors, such as volume depletion, decreased cardiac output, or renal artery stenosis, or postrenal components, such as urethral or ureteral obstruction, must be sought and corrected. Such pre- and postrenal components may exacerbate underlying parenchymal disease in patients with chronic renal insufficiency and must be treated in this group as well. Most important is treatment of the underlying disease or complications of renal insufficiency which further hasten the loss of nephrons. Hypertension, urinary tract infections, nephrolithiasis, structural abnormalities of the urinary tract, or those forms of glomerulonephritis which may respond to therapy should be treated aggressively. Preventive aspects include avoidance of nephrotoxic drugs and radiopaque agents in the patient with already compromised renal insufficiency.

Modification of diet is an important aspect of conservative therapy. Early restriction of sodium and fluid may be important in the treatment of hypertension. As renal insufficiency progresses, restriction of foods high in phosphate and potassium is necessary. Reduction of protein content reduces anorexia, nausea, and vomiting and, if initiated early, may retard progression of the disease. Adult patients should receive no less than 0.6 g of protein per kilogram of body weight per day to avoid negative nitrogen balance. Supplementation of low-protein diets with essential ketoamino acid therapy may be useful in prolonging the period of conservative therapy by allowing utilization of urea as a source of nonessential nitrogen. Preliminary results from a study by the multicenter National Institutes of Health/Health Care Financing Administration suggest that control of hypertension may be as important as protein content of the diet. Correction of electrolyte imbalance, e.g., use of sodium bicarbonate or calcium carbonate to correct mild acidosis, or bicarbonate, dextrose and insulin, and potassium exchange resins for treatment of hyperkalemia, is necessary in more advanced states of uremia. Some chemical abnormalities of renal failure do not require or are not amenable to treatment; hypermagnesemia, hyperamylasemia, hypertriglyceridemia, or mild carbohydrate intolerance generally do not require therapy. Treatment of hyperuricemia may be in order if the patient suffers from gout. However, hyperuricemia alone may not be detrimental. Secondary hyperparathyroidism may accentuate progression of renal failure. Whether this is due to hyperphosphatemia, an elevated calcium-phosphorus product, or parathyroid hormone itself is not clear. Nonetheless, vigorous efforts using phosphate-binding agents and calcium supplements and vitamin D products (dihydrotachysterol or calcitriol) to maintain the serum calcium are effective in suppressing parathyroid stimulation, perhaps in slowing renal insufficiency, and likely avoiding severe bone disease later (see Chap. 340). To avoid visceral and vascular calcification, it is important to maintain the calcium-phosphorus product in the physiologic range. Fluid, sodium, potassium, phosphate, and protein restrictions offer the patient a very restricted and often unacceptable diet. This, coupled with the administration of multiple medications, often occurs at a time when the complications of uremia appear and consideration for dialysis and/or transplantation is in order.

While conservative measures are being carried out, it is necessary to prepare the patient with an intensive educational program to explain the possibilities of eventual renal failure and the various forms of therapy available. The more knowledgeable patients are concerning hemodialysis, peritoneal dialysis, and transplantation, the easier and more appropriate will be their decisions at a later time. With hemodialysis, the major method of obtaining blood for treatment is from an arteriovenous fistula. Since these devices often take several months to develop, prophylactic placement of a fistula in a patient planning for hemodialysis is important in minimizing future complications of circulatory access. For those patients who select peritoneal dialysis (continuous ambulatory peritoneal dialysis—CAPD; or continuous cyclic peritoneal dialysis—CCPD), placement of the peritoneal catheter does not require preparation, and therapy can be instituted as soon as uremic signs and symptoms develop. In those patients who may perform home dialysis or undergo transplantation, early education of family members for selection and preparation as a home dialysis helper or a related donor for transplantation should occur well before the onset of symptomatic renal failure. In those patients who may have a good antigenic match with a willing donor, transplantation without intervening hemodialysis or peritoneal dialysis should be considered. In considering related donor transplantation, the risk of unilateral nephrectomy, including development of proteinuria and hypertension, should be considered. As discussed below, the success rate of cadaver donor transplantation has improved sufficiently that this form of therapy should be carefully considered both with the patient and with family members who are potential donors.

DIALYSIS

HEMODIALYSIS Hemodialysis employs the process of diffusion across a semipermeable membrane (cellulose acetate, Cupraphane, polyacrilonitrile, polymethylmethacrylate, polysulfone) to remove unwanted substances from the blood while adding desirable components. A constant flow of blood on one side of the membrane and a cleansing solution–dialysate on the other allows removal of waste products in a fashion grossly similar to that of glomerular filtration. By altering the composition of the dialysate, the method of exposure of blood and dialysate (geometry of the dialyzer), the type and surface area of dialysis membrane, and the frequency and duration of exposure, patients without renal function can be maintained in a relatively healthy state. Hemodialysis equipment consists of three components—the blood delivery system, the composition and delivery system of the dialysate, and the dialyzer itself. Blood is pumped to the dialyzer by a roller pump through lines with appropriate equipment to measure flow and pressures within the system; blood flow should be approximately 300 to 350 mL/min. Hydrostatic pressure within the system can be manipulated to achieve desirable fluid removal, so-called ultrafiltration. The dialysate is delivered to the dialyzer from a storage tank or proportioning system which manufactures dialysate on line. In most systems dialysate passes once across the membrane, countercurrent to blood flow at a rate of 500 mL/min, or it may be recirculated multiple times at higher flow rates. The composition of the dialysate is similar to plasma water, but may be altered depending upon the patient's needs. The dialysate potassium is most often varied, but the sodium, calcium, and acetate or bicarbonate may be varied depending upon the situation. The principal type of dialyzer now in use in most dialysis units in the United States is the hollow fiber or capillary dialyzer, in which membrane material is spun into fine capillaries, thousands of which are packed into bundles with blood flowing through the capillaries while dialysate is circulated on the outside of the fiber bundle (Fig. 225-2).

Most patients require between 9 and 12 h of dialysis per week, equally divided into several sessions. The time depends upon body size, residual renal function, dietary intake, complicating illnesses, and the degree of anabolism or catabolism. The time, frequency of treatments, type and size of dialyzer, and dialysate composition, blood, or dialysate flow may all be altered to accomplish specific needs. In recent years, kinetic modeling, utilizing urea generation and protein catabolic rates, has led to a more definite dialysis

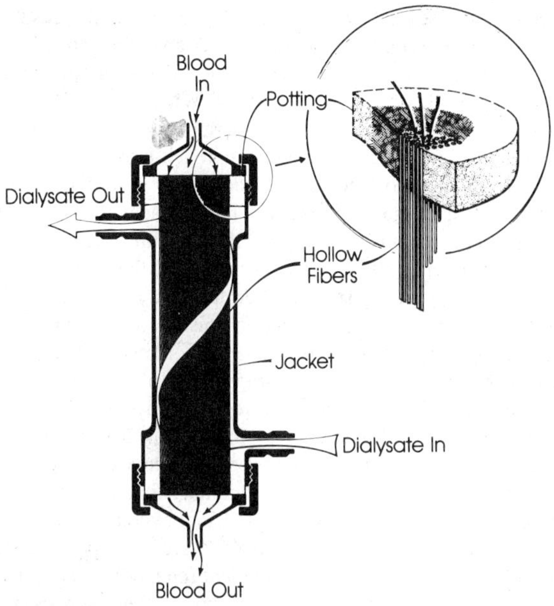

FIGURE 225-2 Hollow fiber or capillary dialyzer; the most commonly used artificial kidney.

prescription. The development of bicarbonate dialysis, variable sodium delivery, high flux or ultraefficient membranes, and urea kinetic modeling has allowed for significant reductions in dialysis time. Clinical trials of this so-called high flux, short-time dialysis are underway. Forms of treatment for the patient with acute renal failure include slow continuous ultrafiltration (SCUF) or continuous arteriovenous hemodialysis (CAVHD)—techniques that employ high efficiency dialyzers with very slow blood and/or dialysate flow rates. This therapy is useful in the unstable, acute renal failure patient and has essentially replaced acute peritoneal dialysis in the ICU and is often preferable to intermittent hemodialysis.

Many complications in the chronic dialysis patient are related to underlying disease or those uremic conditions not reversed by dialytic therapy. These and other related problems of hemodialysis are discussed in Chap. 224. The Achilles' heel of hemodialysis is access to the circulation. The development of the arteriovenous shunt made chronic dialysis possible. This device has had a high failure rate because of infection and thrombosis and led in 1966 to the development of the arteriovenous (AV) fistula. The fistula is preferably created from a native vein, but if not available, a prosthetic conduit (extended polytetrafluoroethylene) subcutaneously placed between an artery and a nearby vein may be utilized. Cannulation of arteriovenous fistulas with 15- to 16-gauge needles allows blood flow sufficient to carry out hemodialysis. Unfortunately, infection, thrombosis, and aneurysm formation also occur in the arteriovenous fistula, particularly in prosthetic devices. There is a relatively high incidence of septicemia and septic embolization associated with shunt and fistula infection; the most common infecting agent is *Staphylococcus aureus*.

In addition, failure of the AV fistula has a significant psychological impact. Depression and altered self-image are common psychiatric problems. The rapid flux in osmolality may cause a disequilibrium syndrome, while rapid changes in electrolytes (particularly potassium) may lead to arrhythmia during dialysis. Hypotension is a common phenomenon during hemodialysis and is due to many factors—the size of the extracorporeal circulation, degree of ultrafiltration, change in serum osmolality, presence of autonomic neuropathy, concomitant use of antihypertensive agents, removal of catecholamines, or infusion of acetate (used as the dialysate buffer) which is a cardiac depressant and vasodilator. Syndromes of dialysis dementia and osteomalacia may be secondary to aluminum contamination of dialysate water or from oral intake of aluminum hydroxide. An increased incidence of HBsAG (hepatitis B surface) antigenemia is related to decreased immunologic integrity. Patients with chronic antigenemia are usually asymptomatic and have little derangement of liver function. There is a higher rate of non-A, non-B hepatitis and cytomegalovirus infection, but these, too, are usually of mild degree. Patients with AIDS often have renal failure terminally and have poor prognosis with or without dialysis. Because of the high incidence of AIDS in IV drug abusers who also have heroin nephropathy, the presence of HIV-positive patients is now common in dialysis units. There is little to suggest that multiple blood transfusions in dialysis patients have played a role in this incidence. Based on clinical experience and recommendations from the Centers for Disease Control, these patients are treated in dialysis units as are other patients with no special precautions. All patients should receive universal precautions for infection control. Mechanical and/or iatrogenic complications such as hemolysis, air embolus, blood leaks, and contaminated dialysate are less common with improved equipment. Membrane-induced adverse reactions may occur, as exemplified by complement-mediated leukopenia and hypoxemia. More prominent symptoms such as back and chest pain, bronchospasm, and anaphylaxis may rarely occur in this reaction. Heparin, necessary during the hemodialysis procedure, may lead to complications such as subdural hematoma and retroperitoneal, gastrointestinal, pericardial, and pleural hemorrhage. One of the major concerns in long-term dialysis patients is the high incidence of mortality related to myocardial infarction and cerebral vascular accidents. These are likely due to the preexistence and continuation of common risk factors in the uremic patient such as hypertension, hyperlipidemia, vascular calcification due to hyperparathyroidism, and high cardiac output due to anemia or other factors. The potential for complications should cause the physician to evaluate the risk/benefit ratio with dialysis treatment before proceeding in the individual patient. Advantages of hemodialysis are the relatively short treatment time and minimal interruption of life-style between treatments. It is more efficient than peritoneal dialysis, allowing rapid changes in abnormal serum values. Hemodialysis can be performed in the home, but the patient requires an assistant during treatment. It is the most widely utilized form of dialysis.

PERITONEAL DIALYSIS Peritoneal dialysis, like hemodialysis, may be performed in various settings and with a number of different techniques. In patients with acute renal failure, intermittent peritoneal dialysis has largely been displaced by intermittent hemodialysis or CAVHD. Chronic peritoneal dialysis was attempted in the late 1940s but was relatively unsuccessful until development of a permanent peritoneal catheter in 1968—the Tenckhoff catheter. Use of this indwelling catheter and closed continuous-cycle dialysate delivery equipment led to treatment protocols with which patients were treated 2 to 3 times per week for a total of 30 to 40 h (intermittent peritoneal dialysis—IPD) to achieve clearances and fluid removal similar to those of hemodialysis. In 1978, the concept of constant peritoneal lavage with prolonged dwell times led to the development of CAPD, which differs from intermittent peritoneal dialysis in that patients instill fluid into the peritoneal cavity, seal the catheter, continue in an ambulatory mode, and every 4 to 6 h empty the peritoneal cavity and replace the dialysate. This technique utilizes 2-L containers of dialysate and obviates the need for dialysis equipment. Modification of the technique using a cyclic dialysate delivery device to exchange dialysate during the night and chronic dwelling of fluid during the waking hours (CCPD) is more acceptable to some patients.

IPD or CCPD may be performed in a center or at home (usually overnight), while CAPD can be performed anywhere. As with hemodialysis, the composition of the dialysate can be modified for ultrafiltration and clearance needs. The major difference in peritoneal dialysate formulas is in the amount of dextrose used as an osmotic agent. Advantages of peritoneal dialysis are avoidance of heparinization and vascular surgery and a slower clearance rate (helpful for some cardiovascular patients). It is more amenable to total self-treatment. Disadvantages include the longer treatment time (intermittently or continuous involvement). It should not be used in patients with extensive abdominal surgery or pulmonary compromise. Inadequate clearance may occur in patients with scleroderma, vasculitis, malignant hypertension, or peritoneal disease. Complications include catheter tunnel infection, peritonitis, moderate protein loss, hypertriglyceridemia, hypercholesterolemia, obesity, and inguinal and abdominal hernias. CAPD is the predominant peritoneal dialysis but requires greater patient compliance and has a higher rate of peritonitis than IPD because of multiple entries into the system.

RESULTS At the end of 1987, approximately 98,400 patients were on chronic dialysis in the United States. Approximately 85 percent of patients are on hemodialysis, and 15 percent perform peritoneal dialysis. Over the past 20 years nearly 87,000 patients have undergone renal transplantation in this country. Approximately 1800 living related and 7000 cadaver renal transplants are performed in the United States per year. Of new patients with end-stage renal disease, approximately 35 to 50 percent are physically and psychologically suitable for transplantation. Many of these patients are on hemodialysis and peritoneal dialysis awaiting availability of a cadaver kidney. An acutely ill or medically complicated patient will likely undergo dialysis in a hospital dialysis unit or intensive care unit, while stable patients may be dialyzed as outpatients in the hospital dialysis unit, in an out-of-hospital dialysis center, or at home. Most centers attempt to have patients participate in their own care, so-called self-dialysis. Approximately 18,000 patients were performing home dialysis, either hemodialysis or peritoneal dialysis (CAPD or CCPD) at the end of 1987, this number representing 19 percent of all patients on dialysis. Home dialysis (either hemodialysis or peritoneal) is preferable for many because of self-reliance and freedom from hospital or center dialysis schedules. Patient motivation is the primary factor in selection of home or in-center self-dialysis. Dialysis performed in the hospital setting is most expensive, while home dialysis with a nonpaid family assistant or alone (peritoneal dialysis only) is somewhat less expensive than in-center dialysis. Despite absence of equipment, peritoneal dialysis is as expensive as home hemodialysis because of the cost of dialysate and of hospitalization related to an increased incidence of peritonitis. The total amount of Medicare payments for end-stage renal disease (covering hemodialysis, peritoneal dialysis, and transplantation) in the year 1987 was 2.5 billion dollars, substantially greater than anticipated at the initiation of the end-stage renal disease program in 1973. This cost reflects an increasing number of recipients and not an increasing cost per patient.

The mean age for patients on dialysis is the late fifties, partly because nephrosclerosis and eventual renal failure from other parenchymal diseases occur in older patients, but more likely because the selection process favors transplantation in younger patients.

Approximately 10 to 20 percent of patients with chronic renal failure are totally rehabilitated by dialysis, and another 30 to 40 percent of nondiabetic patients may be expected to be rehabilitated to a functional status even if not employed. Twenty percent of patients will be returned to a level of function not considered rehabilitated but able to care for themselves. The remainder (approximately 20 percent) are fully dependent on support from others. Diabetics, who have a rehabilitation rate and survival rate significantly lower than that of nondiabetic patients, make up much of the latter two groups. Determination of mortality rates is variable, related to the age of the patient and the disease process(es) involved. Mean mortality for the entire ESRD program is approximately 18 percent per year. This number has substantially increased over the past 10 years, probably in relation to the increased age and co-morbid complications of this population. In patients less than 45 years of age and with no complicating medical illnesses, mortality with hemodialysis, peritoneal dialysis, or transplantation is below 5 percent per year.

TRANSPLANTATION

Transplantation of the human kidney is frequently appropriate for the treatment of advanced chronic renal failure. Worldwide, tens of thousands of such procedures have been performed. When azathioprine and prednisone are used as immunosuppressive drugs, the results with properly matched familial donors are superior to those obtained with organs from cadaveric donors, with 75 to 90 percent compared to 50 to 60 percent graft survival rates at 1 year. When antilymphocyte globulins (ALG) have been added to the treatment regimens in some centers, the results with cadaveric donors approach those with living related donors, at least for the first 2 years after transplantation. Cyclosporine has significantly improved 1-year cadaveric survival rates to the 80 percent range, when used along with prednisone in place of azathioprine and ALG. With all therapies, the rate of graft loss from rejection is much slower after the first year, although occasionally an acute irreversible rejection episode may occur after many months of good function. This is especially likely if the patient neglects to take the immunosuppressive drugs. Clinical renal transplant results in recent years have improved in regard to patient morbidity and mortality rates, the latter declining to less than 5 percent in a number of centers. These findings represent an increasing tendency on the part of transplant teams to decrease immunosuppressive therapy so that in the case of severe rejection the kidney rather than the patient is lost. Second and even third transplants are being performed, and the overall results show a 10 to 20 percent reduction in expected survival compared to first transplants; cyclosporine therapy does not erase the increased risk of rejecting subsequent transplants, however. Overall, transplantation returns the majority of patients to a near-normal life-style.

DONOR SELECTION Donor sources are cadavers or volunteer blood-related living donors. Living volunteer donors should be normal on physical examination and of the same major ABO blood group, because there is good evidence that crossing major blood group barriers prejudices survival of the allograft. It is, however, possible to transplant a kidney of a type O donor into an A, B, or AB recipient. Selective renal arteriography should be performed on volunteer donors to rule out the presence of multiple or abnormal renal arteries, because the surgical procedure is difficult and the ischemic time of the transplanted kidney long when vascular abnormalities exist. Cadaveric donors should be free of malignant neoplastic disease because of the possible transmission of cancer to the recipient.

In the United States, a coordinated national system (United Network for Organ Sharing) of computerized information sharing and logistical support for the transportation of cadaver kidneys to suitable recipients is under development. It is now possible to remove cadaver kidneys and to maintain them for over 48 h on cold pulsatile perfusion or simple flushing and cooling. This permits adequate time for various typing, cross matching, transportation, and selection problems to be solved.

TISSUE TYPING AND CLINICAL IMMUNOGENETICS Matching for antigens of the HLA major histocompatibility gene complex (Chap. 14) is the ideal criterion for selection of donors for renal allografts. Each mammalian species has a single chromosomal region that encodes the strong, or major, transplantation antigens, and the analogous sixth chromosomal region is called *HLA* in human beings. Other antigens, called "minor," may nevertheless play crucial roles, especially the ABH(O) blood groups and an endothelial antigen which is shared with blood monocytes, but not lymphocytes. Evidence for designation of HLA as the genetic region encoding strong transplantation antigens comes from the success rate in living related donor renal and bone marrow transplantation, with superior results in HLA-identical sibling pairs. Nevertheless, 5 to 10 percent of HLA-identical renal allografts are rejected, often within the first weeks after transplantation. It is likely, though not proved, that these failures represent states of prior sensitization to non-HLA antigens. Non-HLA antigens are relatively weak and therefore suppressible by conventional immunosuppressive therapy. Once priming has occurred, however, secondary responses are much more refractory to treatment. In fact, ABH incompatibilities are hazardous because of the presence of natural anti-A and anti-B antibodies in recipients and the normal expression of A and B blood group substances on endothelium.

Living related donors From 1962 to 1982 when azathioprine was the main immunosuppressive drug, living related donors provided superior graft survivals. Among first-degree relatives, the general level of expected graft success was in direct proportion to matching for 2,1, or no HLA haplotypes, as defined by HLA serologic typing and the presence or absence of a proliferative response in the mixed lymphocyte response (MLR) (Chap. 14). HLA-incompatible siblings did slightly better than the overall average with cadaveric donors (50 to 60 percent at 1 year), while HLA semi-identicals (haploidentical) were in the 70 to 75 percent range. Intrafamilial MLRs among haploidenticals were found to be a measure of responsiveness. Low responder donor-recipient pairs had a 1-year graft survival rate of 90 percent, while vigorous responders were at the level of 55 percent unless donor-specific blood transfusions were given to eliminate this disadvantage. The MLR is a relatively imprecise technique, but it has been repeatedly shown that for both living related and cadaveric donors, MLR reactivity with a specific donor is more predictive of graft outcome than serologic typing for HLA-A, -B, -C, or -DR antigens.

Cyclosporine has had a major impact upon the assumption that living related donors are generally superior to cadaveric donors, because in most recent series the improvement in cadaveric results rivals the 80 percent 1-year result previously attained only with haploidentical relatives. One must now weigh the choices in light of the availability of organs and waiting times on dialysis, rather than on the initial rate of graft success. Long-term survival rates, comparing the various donor types and treatment protocols, are not improved in the cyclosporine era, if one assesses graft survival over a decade in terms of half-lives. With azathioprine or cyclosporine, the half-life measured after the first year is 30 to 34 years with HLA-identical donors, 11 to 12 years with haploidentical donors, and 7 to 9 years with cadaveric donors. The major advantage of cyclosporine over azathioprine, therefore, is in the superior level of initial results at 1 to 2 years for cadaveric transplantation and not in the rate of graft loss thereafter.

There has been concern expressed regarding the potential risk to a volunteer kidney donor of premature renal failure after several years of increased blood flow and hyperfiltration per nephron in the remaining kidney. There are a few reports of development of hypertension, proteinuria, and even lesions of focal segmental sclerosis in donors under long-term followup. Documentation of difficulties in significant numbers of donors followed for 15 or more years is unusual, however, and it may be that having a single kidney becomes significant only when another condition, such as hypertension, is superimposed. In this regard, it is desirable to consider the risk of development of type I diabetes mellitus in a family member who is a potential donor to a diabetic renal failure patient. Measurements of anti-insulin and anti-islet antibodies should be made and glucose tolerance tests should be performed in such cases to rule out a prediabetic state. The acceptance of living unrelated donors (spouses, distant relatives, close friends) has been debated as a means to improve the supply of organs and to shorten the waiting period on dialysis. Since volunteer donors who are not matched for one or both HLA haplotypes present as strong a tissue barrier as randomly matched cadaveric donors, they cannot be expected to provide, on average, as reliable a source for long-functioning grafts as a well-matched cadaveric organ. It is illegal in the United States to purchase organs for transplantation.

HLA matching and cadaveric donors The question of whether matching of HLA antigens in unrelated donor-recipient pairs would approximate the high initial success rates and slow rates of subsequent graft loss found with HLA-identical sib pairs could not be answered until the 1980s when reliable class II histocompatibility (DR) typing became widely available. With the 1-year success rate now at 80 to 85 percent for first cadaveric grafts, it is difficult to see an early improvement related to matching when small series of cases are compiled, especially, as is often the case, when the reporting centers have a very small fraction of well-matched cases. Now that pooled data on several thousands of cadaveric renal transplants from all over the world are available, the HLA-matching effect can be clearly seen, especially in the long-term survival figures. Figure 225-3 shows data for 3 years and projections to 10 years, based on the exponential nature of the actuarial plot. Well-matched cases, compatible for HLA-A, -B, and -DR antigens show results comparable to those with HLA-identical sibs. Poorly matched cases, though starting off well at 1 to 2 years, are projected to lose 70 percent of grafts by the end of the first decade. Other analyses show that HLA-DR compatibility alone is the most powerful influence, followed by HLA-B, and to a lesser extent HLA-A. Repeat transplants, following rejection of first grafts, do less well by about 15 to 20 percent, and in these cases the benefits of HLA matching are even more striking, while cyclosporine adds relatively little. These results indicate that HLA antigens of various loci are not of equal strength in the immunosuppressed patient and that only 2 or 3 of them need to be matched to produce improved results. The likelihood of obtaining compatibility for HLA-B and -DR in a given case depends upon the relative frequencies of the recipient's antigens in the general population and upon the pool size of donors available. In addition, the chances depend upon how many

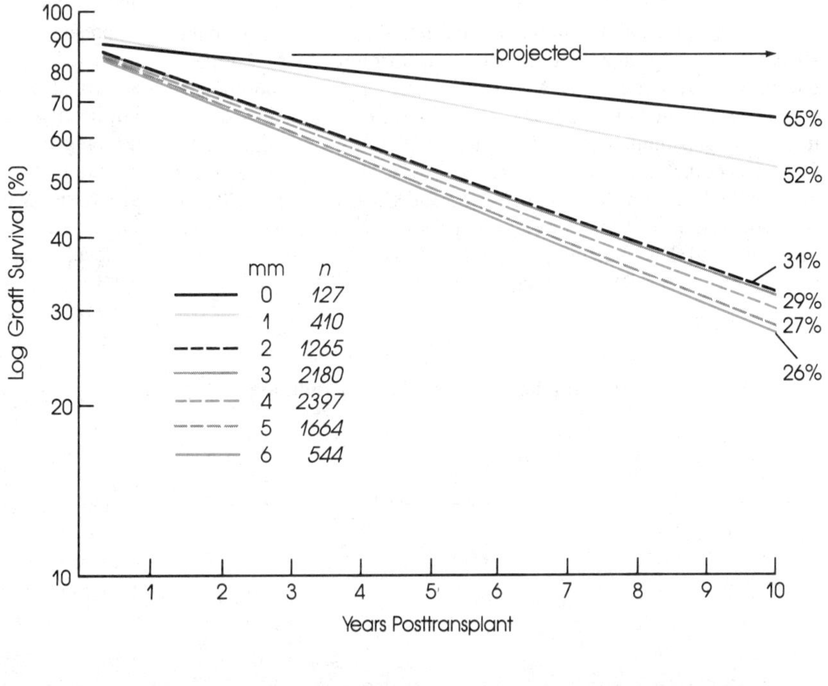

FIGURE 225-3 Survival of first cadaveric renal grafts in the cyclosporine era. The effects of mismatches (mm) for HLA-A, -B, -DR antigens (zero to 6) are shown through 3 years and projected to 10 years. *(From PI Terasaki.)*

other potential recipients are waiting and upon the willingness of transplant centers to share organs on this basis. A 20 to 30 percent rate of DR-compatible cadaveric transplants has been achieved by some organ sharing systems. With the United Network for Organ Sharing waiting list of over 12,000 potential recipients and 8000 or more donors per year, levels approaching these rates and higher are possible.

Presensitization A positive cross match of recipient serum with donor T lymphocytes representing anti-HLA class I is usually predictive of an acute vasculitic event termed *hyperacute* rejection. A few years ago it was thought that patients making such antibodies, tested against a surrogate panel of normal lymphocytes, were at high risk for accelerated, if not hyperacute, rejection, even when the donor-specific cross match was negative. That this is no longer so can be attributed to the greater efforts being made in monitoring patients on dialysis, defining not only the presence or absence of antibodies but also the HLA antigens to which they are directed. Patients with anti-HLA antibodies can be safely transplanted if careful cross matching is performed. Patients sustained by hemodialysis often show fluctuating antibody titers and specificity patterns, sometimes, but not always, temporally related to receipt of blood transfusions. At the time of assignment of a cadaveric kidney, cross matches are performed with more than one highly reactive serum, and the previously analyzed antibody specificities are also taken into account. Anti-HLA antibody responses do not necessarily recur several months later when the incompatible antigen is given in a blood product transfusion. Indeed, it seems relatively safe to ignore positive cross matches with sera kept in storage for several months as long as recent sera are negative. Data on this point are conflicting, showing either no risk or a 15 percent increased risk of early graft loss if only the stored serum samples older than 6 months are reactive with donor cells. The loss of anamnesis to HLA by chronic dialysis patients may result from development of specific unresponsiveness due to suppressor cell activation, or from anti-idiotypic immunity. Presensitization to antigens expressed on B lymphocytes, but not T lymphocytes, is not a contraindication to transplantation. Some of these antibodies are anti-DR, while others are non-HLA IgM antibodies active in the cold and at room temperature, but apparently not relevant to graft survival.

Endothelial-monocyte system In some cases of unexpected accelerated rejection, antibodies with reactivity to renal endothelium and blood monocytes have been found, both in the circulation and in eluates from rejected grafts. Practical aspects of typing and cross matching for this non-HLA system are difficult. Second transplants following rapid loss of the first graft seem to be particularly at risk.

Overview of transplantation immunogenetics In addition to the ABH(O) blood groups, the important histocompatibility antigens presently known are HLA-A, -B, -C, -DR, and the endothelial-monocyte system (Table 225-2). The best current data suggest that major primary immunogenicity lies in the DR antigens, while A, B, C, and endothelial-monocyte antigens provide the major targets for effector IgG, and in the case of A, B, and C, at least, for killer T lymphocytes. Hence the current emphasis is on A, B, and C cross matching and DR matching, although HLA-B compatibility adds significantly to the DR-matching effect.

TABLE 225-2 Histocompatibility in renal transplantation

RELATIVE IMPORTANCE OF TYPING AND CROSS MATCHING FOR SEROLOGICALLY DEFINED ANTIGENS

Antigens	Typing (antigen matching)	Cross matching
Class I (HLA-A, -B, -C)	+ +	+ + +
Class II (HLA-DR)	+ + +	−
Endothelial-monocyte (non-HLA)	? −	+ + +

Blood transfusions At a time when it appeared that transfusion-induced sensitization against a random lymphocyte panel was predictive of a high graft failure rate, a number of transplantation units undertook a policy of withholding blood from as many dialysis patients as possible. The clinical need for blood was found to be less than originally thought, especially in nonnephrectomized patients, and avoidance of possible exposure to hepatitis was also a consideration. The overall experience with the nontransfused patients was a dramatic one, confirmed many times over: such patients were at the *highest risk* for graft failure. Since the early 1980s, however, there has been a progressive loss of the transfusion effect, with little or no detriment now remaining in the nontransfused patients. The loss of the transfusion effect cannot be directly attributed to the introduction of cyclosporine, as the transfusion effect had declined before large numbers of patients received this agent. It seems unlikely that worldwide changes in blood bank processing practices are involved. It is most likely that the overall level of clinical management, particularly in recognition and prompt treatment of rejection, has played a role. Indeed, when looked at carefully, some centers withholding transfusions have noted increased rejection activity in their nontransfused patients but have not had difficulty in treating them. One study shows, however, that graft survival is still decreased in that subset of nontransfused patients who also have an early clinically apparent rejection episode. The current practice to use little or no blood in preparation for transplantation comes at a propitious time because of concerns regarding HIV transmission. The efficacy of recombinant erythropoietin in sustaining red blood cell mass in chronic renal failure patients will further reduce the clinical need for blood transfusions.

IMMUNOLOGY OF REJECTION Knowledge of the immunology of tissue transplantation stems largely from animal experimentation. However, enough evidence has accumulated in humans, particularly in kidney transplantation, to indicate that the evidence is similar though not identical for the different species. The immunologic mechanisms are not qualitatively different from those found in other areas of immunology (Chap. 13). The evidence is that early rejection is associated with T lymphocytes having direct specificity against donor antigens. These may be cytotoxic cells (CD8+ or CD4+) or cells which mediate DTH (CD4+); however, significant numbers of B lymphocytes, null cells, natural killer (NK) cells, and macrophages appear in the early infiltrate, and cells capable of mediating antibody-dependent cell-mediated cytotoxicity (ADCC) are also present (Fig. 225-4). Many of the B lymphocytes produce immunoglobulins. The spectrum of cellular and humoral response and graft injury is quite varied, depending upon specific genetic differences between donor and recipient and states of presensitization. The greater the degree of presensitization, the more likely it is that one will find antibody-mediated vascular lesions. All of the processes shown in Fig. 225-4 are possible, but their relative contribution varies from case to case. Further dissection of the heterogeneity of the human allograft response, utilizing newer techniques for identification of lymphocyte subsets, is adding to the value of graft biopsy as a guide to therapy and prognosis. Monitoring of peripheral blood lymphocyte subsets, utilizing monoclonal antibodies (Chap. 13) to functionally related surface molecules, such as CD4 (T-helper cells) and CD8 (T-suppressor/cytotoxic cells), has been related to the degree of rejection activity in some surveys, but the CD4/CD8 ratio has not always been clinically meaningful. Part of the problem may lie in the fact that these subsets are not as uniquely related to function as originally believed. Indeed, the principal role of the CD4 molecule appears to be the promotion of interaction of T cells with class II HLA molecules on antigen-presenting cells, and, similarly, CD8 interacts with class I HLA (Chaps. 13, 14). Finally, the cytokine mediators of the cellular immune response (IL-1, IL-2, IL-3, IL-4, IL-6, IFNγ) (Chap. 13) are involved in the control and expression of the alloimmune rejection response. For example, T-cell production of IFNγ causes increased expression of HLA antigens upon endothelial cells. In normal immunobiology this effect may be to promote more efficient pre-

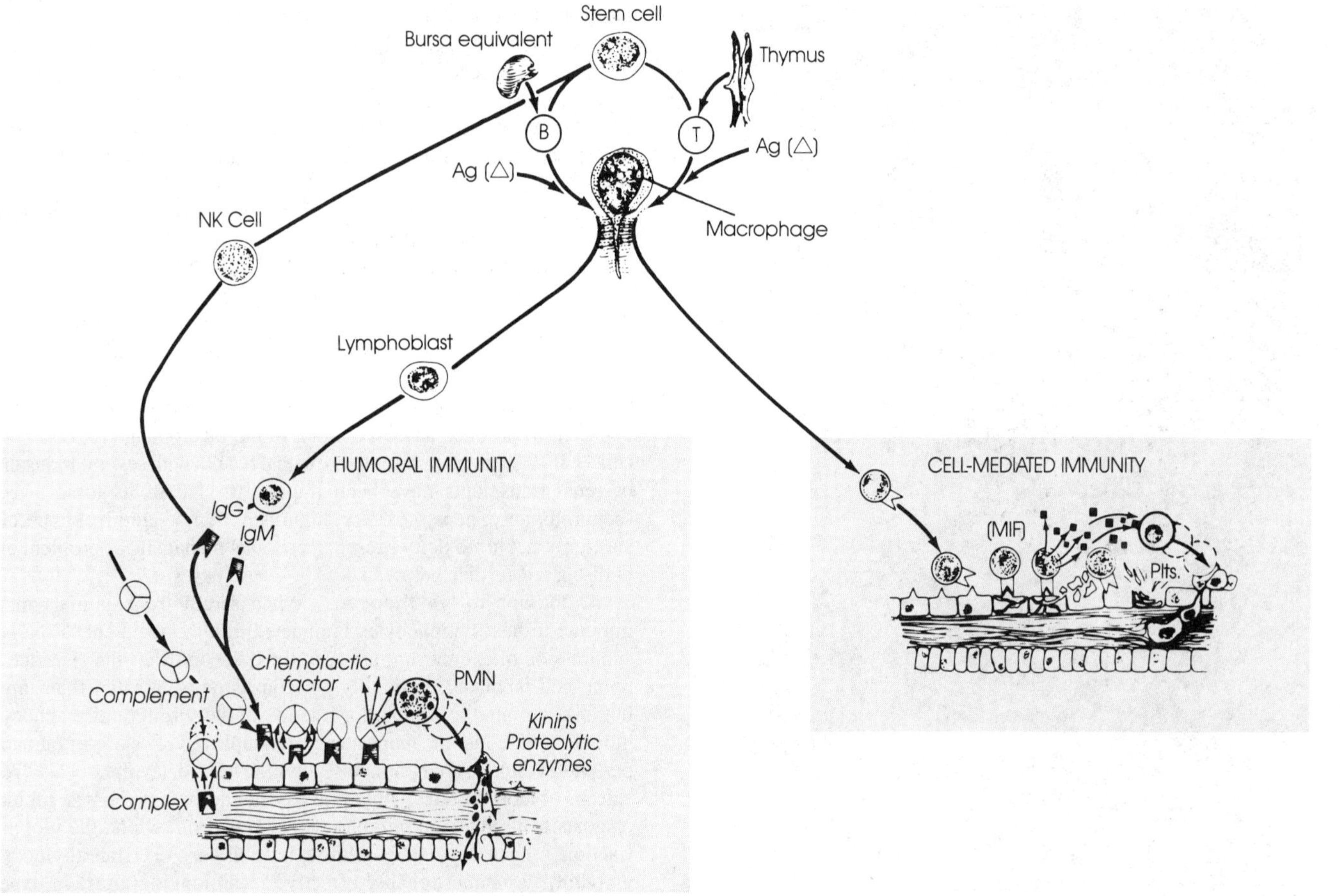

FIGURE 225-4 Overall scheme of the development of effector mechanisms in graft rejection. Bone marrow stem cells differentiate under the influence of the thymus gland into mature thymus-derived (T) lymphocytes, or under the influence of an equivalent to the avian bursa of Fabricius into mature bone marrow–derived (B) lymphocytes. Exposure to antigen (Δ) results in an interaction between T cells and B cells, and often involves macrophages. The sensitized B cells, after mitoses, develop into immunoglobulin-secreting cells (e.g., plasma cells), illustrated here by IgG and IgM. Such immunoglobulins may form immune complexes with antigen in the circulation which activate the complement sequence, or they may react directly with antigens on the blood vessel surface. Elaboration of secondary mediators, including the products of complement activation, results in vascular damage as illustrated. Sensitized T lymphocytes are the primary effector cells in cell-mediated immunity and may react directly with antigens in the graft to exert a cytotoxic effect. In addition, T cells release factors, such as macrophage migration inhibition factor (MIF), which may accelerate the rate of mononuclear cell infiltration. This process is similar to delayed-type hypersensitivity (DTH). It has also been shown that unsensitized non-T cells (NK cells) can be activated to exert cytotoxic effects by the fixation of IgG to target cells, followed by interaction of the IgG (Fc portion) with an Fc receptor on the NK cell. Finally, platelet aggregation and thrombosis can occur following the endothelial damage induced by any of these mechanisms. (See Fig. 13-1.)

sentation of foreign antigen, while in transplantation it enhances the immunogenicity of the vascularized transplant. Also, IL-2 is the major growth factor for expansion of effector T cells. It is the product of a major subset of CD4 cells, while other CD4 cells produce B-cell growth factors, such as IL-4.

The failure of transplanted kidneys after several years of adequate function is due to a form of ''chronic rejection.'' In such kidneys the development of nephrosclerosis, with proliferation of the vascular intima of renal vessels, and intimal fibrosis, with marked decrease in the lumen of the vessels, takes place (Fig. 225-5). The result is renal ischemia, hypertension, widespread tubular atrophy, interstitial fibrosis, and glomerular atrophy with eventual renal failure. It is not established, however, whether slow deterioration of graft function over years is due to the same mechanisms in all cases. Except for the established influence of HLA incompatibility, little is known about the pathogenesis of progressive renal failure in the transplanted population.

IMMUNOSUPPRESSIVE TREATMENT When histocompatibility differences exist between donor and recipient, it is necessary to modify or suppress the immune response in order to enable the recipient to accept a graft. Immunosuppressive therapy, in general, suppresses all immune responses, including those to bacteria, fungi, and even malignant tumors. In the 1950s when clinical renal transplantation began, sublethal total-body irradiation was employed. Currently, immunosuppression is more safely induced pharmacologically. Agents used in humans to suppress the immune response are discussed in the following paragraphs.

Drugs *Azathioprine*, an analogue of mercaptopurine, is the keystone to immunosuppressive therapy in humans. This agent can inhibit synthesis of DNA, RNA, or both. Because cell division and proliferation are a necessary part of the immune response to antigenic stimulation, suppression by this agent may be mediated by the inhibition of mitosis of immunologically competent lymphoid cells, interfering with synthesis of DNA. Alternatively, immunosuppression may be brought about by blocking the synthesis of RNA (possibly messenger RNA), inhibiting processing of antigens prior to lymphocyte stimulation. This drug has little effect in suppressing a secondary immune response, however. Therapy with azathioprine is generally instituted 2 days prior to transplantation in the recipient of a living donor kidney and on the day of transplantation in the case of a cadaveric donor kidney recipient at a level of 4 mg/kg per day. The drug is later tapered to levels of 1.5 to 3 mg/kg per day, as long as the allograft functions. Because the drug is rapidly metabolized by the liver, its dosage need not be varied directly in relation to renal

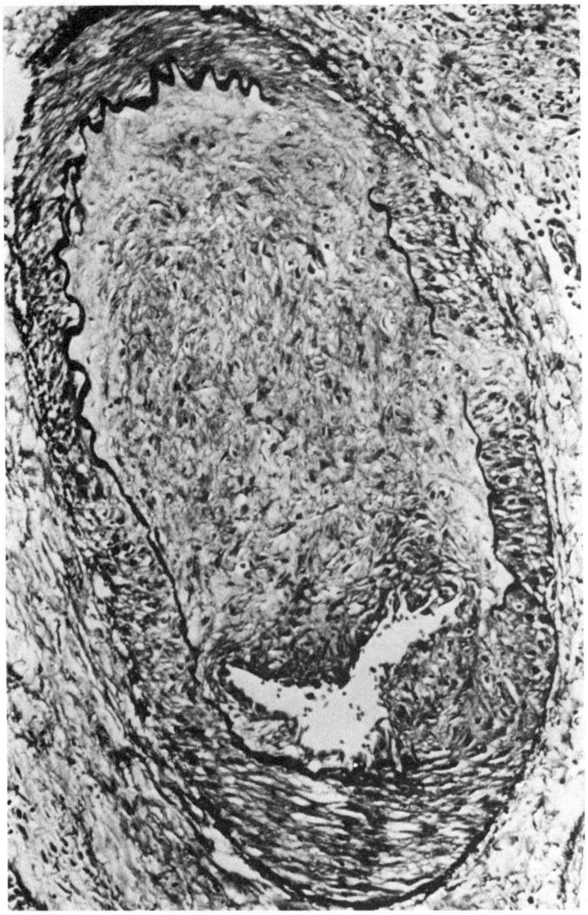

FIGURE 225-5 Biopsy of the renal cadaveric allograft illustrating obliterative endarteritis. Loss of the media is associated with intimal thickening. The elastic tissue shows dissolution of the elastica. The evidence for arteritis with subsequent thrombosis is typically the gaps in the elastica and media. The intimal thickening probably represents organization of a thrombus formed in response to the arteritis. *[From GJ Dammin, JP Merrill, in Structural Basis for Renal Disease, EL Becker (ed), New York, Hoeber-Harper, 1968.]*

function, even though renal failure results in retention of the metabolites of azathioprine. Some patients are unusually sensitive to this drug, particularly when renal function is compromised, and reduction in dosage is required because of leukopenia and occasionally thrombocytopenia. Excessive amounts of azathioprine may also cause jaundice, anemia, and alopecia. If it is essential to administer allopurinol concurrently, the azathioprine dose must be drastically reduced, since inhibition of xanthine oxidase delays degradation. This combination is best avoided.

The *glucocorticoids* are important adjuncts to immunosuppressive therapy. Of all the agents employed, prednisone has effects that are easiest to assess, and in large doses it is the most effective agent for the reversal of rejection. In general, 30 to 40 mg prednisone is given immediately prior to or at the time of transplantation, and the dosage is gradually reduced. The well-known side effects of the glucocorticoids, particularly impairment of wound healing and predisposition to infection, make it desirable to taper the dose as rapidly as possible in the immediate postoperative period. Customarily methylprednisolone, 0.5 to 1.0 g intravenously, is administered immediately upon diagnosis of beginning rejection and continued once daily for 3 days. When the drug is effective, the results are usually apparent within 96 h. Such "pulse" doses are less effective in the chronic rejection process. Most patients whose renal function is stable after 6 months or a year do not require large doses of prednisone; maintenance doses of 15 or 20 mg per day are the rule. Many patients tolerate an alternate-day course of steroids better than daily doses without an increased risk of rejection.

A major effect of steroids is upon the monocyte-macrophage system, preventing the release of IL-6 and IL-1. Although lymphopenia results from large doses of glucocorticoids, this is primarily due to sequestration of recirculating blood lymphocytes to lymphoid tissue.

Cyclosporine A is a fungal peptide with potent immunosuppressive activity in animals and in in vitro systems. It appears to have a preferential effect upon early activation of helper-inducer T lymphocytes, thereby sparing suppressor T-cell responses. Assessment of this agent in human renal transplantation has generally shown that although it works alone, it is more effective in conjunction with glucocorticoids. Since cyclosporine blocks production of IL-2 by helper-inducer (CD4+) T cells, its combination with steroids is expected to produce a double block in the macrophage → IL-1 → T cell → IL-2 sequence. As noted, clinical results with several thousands of renal transplants have been impressive. Of all its toxic effects (nephrotoxicity, hepatotoxicity, hirsutism, tremor, gingival hyperplasia), only nephrotoxicity presents a serious management problem and is discussed further below.

Antibodies to lymphocytes When serum from animals made immune to host lymphocytes is injected into the recipient, a marked suppression of cellular immunity to the tissue graft results. The action upon cell-mediated immunity is considerably greater than upon humoral immunity. A globulin fraction of the serum (antilymphocyte globulin, ALG) is the agent generally employed. For use in humans, peripheral human lymphocytes, thymocytes, or lymphocytes from spleens or thoracic duct fistulas have been injected into horses, rabbits, or goats to produce antilymphocyte serum, from which the globulin fraction is then separated. Although ALG, or ATG (antithymocyte globulin), is unquestionably effective in prolonging grafts in experimental animals, its efficacy in the transplantation of human tissue is less clear, as it varies from source to source. Heterologous antibody against defined T-lymphocyte subsets, in the form of mouse antihuman monoclonal antibody, may offer a more precise approach to this form of therapy. OKT3, in common clinical use, is such an antibody. It is directed to the CD3 molecules which form a portion of the T-cell antigen–receptor complex; hence, CD3 is expressed on all mature T cells. CD4 or CD8 molecules also form part of the fully activated cluster of molecules, and monoclonal antibodies to these offer the potential for more selective targeting of T-cell subsets. Another approach to more selective therapy already under clinical trial is to target the 55-kDa beta chain of the IL-2 receptor, expressed only on T cells that have been recently activated. When the antibody is administered during the first 10 days after transplantation, a powerful immunosuppression results, allowing marked reduction or elimination of cyclosporine during the first few days after graft placement.

Other techniques Among other techniques of immunosuppression, thymectomy and splenectomy have not been widely accepted. Local irradiation of the transplanted kidney in two or three doses of 3500 mGy (350 rad) has also been utilized. This technique may result in fewer early rejection episodes in cadaveric transplants than in nonirradiated controls. Fractional total-lymph-node irradiation (TLI), as employed in the therapy of Hodgkin's disease, is continuing under investigation.

CLINICAL COURSE AND MANAGEMENT OF THE RECIPIENT Bilateral nephrectomy at some point prior to transplantation is performed for a specific cause but not as a routine. Hypertension which is difficult to control or infection involving the end-stage kidneys are the two most common indications. Nephrectomized patients maintain a much lower hematocrit level, but this is no longer considered a disadvantage per se, because blood transfusions need not be avoided in preparation for transplantation. Difficulties do arise when these multiply transfused patients become sensitized and must remain on dialysis. Nephrectomy per se does not appear to affect the survival of subsequent renal allografts.

Adequate hemodialysis should be performed within 48 h of surgery, and care should be taken that the serum potassium level is not markedly elevated so that intraoperative cardiac arrhythmias can be averted. The diuresis that commonly occurs postoperatively must be carefully monitored; in many instances it may be massive, reflecting the inability of ischemic tubules to regulate sodium and water excretion. Massive potassium losses may occur and occasionally be symptomatic. Most chronically uremic patients have some excess of extracellular fluid, and some degree of negative balance should be accomplished, provided hemodynamics remain stable. Acute tubular necrosis (ATN) may cause immediate oliguria or may follow an initial short period of graft function. ATN is most likely to occur when cadaveric donors have been hypotensive, or if the interval between cessation of blood flow and organ harvest (warm ischemic time) has been more than a few minutes. Recovery usually occurs within 3 weeks, although periods as long as 6 weeks have been reported. Superimposition of rejection upon ATN is common, and the differential diagnosis may be difficult. Cyclosporine therapy prolongs ATN, and some patients do not diurese until they are switched to azathioprine. Many centers avoid starting cyclosporine for the first several days, using ALG or a monoclonal antibody along with azathioprine and prednisone until renal function is established.

The rejection episode Early diagnosis of rejection allows prompt institution of therapy to preserve renal function and prevent irreversible damage due to fibrosis. Clinical evidence of rejection may be characterized by fever, swelling, and tenderness over the allograft, and by significant reduction in urine volume. In patients whose renal function is good initially, oliguria may be accompanied by decreased urinary sodium concentration and increased osmolarity. These changes may not be present in the more chronic stages of rejection or when renal function is impaired at the onset of rejection.

Arteriography and radioactive iodohippurate sodium renograms of the transplanted kidney may be useful in ascertaining changes in the renal vasculature and in renal blood flow, even in the absence of urinary flow. Diagnostic ultrasound is the procedure of choice to rule out urinary obstruction or to confirm the presence of perirenal collections of urine, blood, or lymph. When renal function has been good initially, a rise in the serum creatinine level and a decrease in the creatinine clearance is the most sensitive and reliable indicator of possible rejection.

Cyclosporine may cause deterioration in renal function in a manner similar to a rejection episode. In fact, rejection processes tend to be more indolent with cyclosporine, and the only way to make a diagnosis may be by renal biopsy. Cyclosporine has an afferent arteriolar constrictor effect upon the kidney and, in addition, may produce permanent vascular and interstitial injury after sustained high-dose therapy. There is no universally accepted lesion(s) which makes a diagnosis of cyclosporine toxicity, although interstitial fibrosis and thickening of arteriolar walls have been noted by some. Basically, if the biopsy does not reveal moderate and active cellular rejection activity, the serum creatinine will most likely respond to a reduction in cyclosporine dose. Blood levels of drug can be useful if very high or very low but precise correlation with renal function does not exist. If rejection activity is present in the biopsy, appropriate therapy is indicated.

OKT3 monoclonal antibody, given intravenously for 10 to 14 days, is effective in more than 90 percent of first rejections, although it is less effective if methylprednisolone pulses have failed and in cases of severe recurrent rejection activity. A major problem with OKT3 is that severe systemic reactions may be produced during the first day or two of therapy. Chills, fever, hypotension, and headache are the direct result of the antibody effects upon the targeted T cells, most likely related to the known potential of OKT3 to activate T cells nonspecifically. If the antibody is administered to overhydrated oliguric patients, pulmonary edema may be induced. These reactions are not characteristic of other monoclonal antibodies, such as those to the IL-2 receptor. Recurrent or rebound rejection activity may require additional therapy. In such circumstances methylprednisolone may be effective even though it failed initially. Second courses of OKT3 may be given in spite of anti-mouse antibodies generated in response to the first course, if the titers are low and the human antibodies are not directed to the combining site region (idiotype) of the OKT3.

Management problems Modification of the usual clinical manifestations of infection by immunosuppressive therapy is a major problem in the posttransplant period. The major toxic effect of azathioprine is bone marrow suppression, while cyclosporine has no marrow effects. They both may predispose to unusual opportunistic infections, however. The signs and symptoms of infection may be masked and distorted, and fever without obvious cause is common. Only after days or weeks will it become apparent that it has a viral or fungal origin. Bacterial infections are most common during the first month after transplantation. The importance of blood cultures in such patients cannot be overemphasized, because systemic infection without obvious foci is frequent, although wound infections with or without urinary fistulas are most common. Particularly ominous are rapidly occurring pulmonary lesions, which may result in death within 5 days of onset. When these become apparent, immunosuppressive agents should be discontinued except for maintenance doses of prednisone. Aggressive diagnostic procedures, including transbronchial and open lung biopsy, are freqently indicated. In the case of *Pneumocystis carinii* (Chap. 163) trimethoprim-sulfamethoxazole is the treatment of choice; amphotericin B has been used effectively in systemic fungal infections. Prophylaxis against *P. carinii* with daily low-dose trimethoprim-sulfamethoxazole is very effective. Involvement of the oropharynx with *Candida* (Chap. 151) may be treated with local nystatin. Small doses (a total of 300 mg) of amphotericin given over a period of 2 weeks may be effective in refractory oral candidiasis. *Aspergillus* (Chap. 151), *Nocardia* (Chap. 152), and cytomegalovirus (CMV) (Chap. 138) infections also occur. CMV is a common and dangerous infection in transplant recipients. It does not generally appear until the end of the first posttransplant month. Active CMV infection is sometimes associated, or occasionally confused, with rejection episodes. Patients at highest risk for severe CMV disease are those without anti-CMV antibodies who receive a graft from a CMV antibody–positive donor (15 percent mortality). Serial intravenous administration of high titer CMV immune globulin is effective in reducing this risk. Prophylactic use of acyclovir and other antiviral agents is under study. The complications of glucocorticoid therapy are well known and include gastrointestinal bleeding, impairment of wound healing, osteoporosis, diabetes, cataract formation, and hemorrhagic pancreatitis. The treatment of jaundice in transplant patients should include cessation of azathioprine or cyclosporine therapy, if hepatitis or drug toxicity is suspected. It is surprising that total cessation of azathioprine or cyclosporine therapy often does not result in rejection of a graft. Antiplatelet agents and anticoagulants, although effective in theory, have not been successful in the prevention of the chronic vascular lesion. Persistent elevation of serum creatinine levels above 220 μmol/L (2.5 mg/dL) in patients maintained on cyclosporine is an indication for dose reduction, but if rejection activity develops, addition of azathioprine is indicated. Some centers convert patients from cyclosporine to azathioprine after 6 to 12 months. Our own experience with such conversions between 4 and 8 months after transplantation has been satisfactory; however, 30 percent of patients had temporally related rejection episodes requiring additional steroid therapy. Subsequent follow-up showed improved renal function in most cases. The alternative to conversion is to use lower doses of cyclosporine. Since the question of long-term cumulative toxicity to the kidney remains open, lower doses are recommended for the long term. Reduction of cyclosporine is best accomplished by routine use of "triple therapy" in which the following dose levels are common for maintenance after 6 to 8 months: cyclosporine, 3 to 5 mg per kilogram of body weight per day; azathioprine, 1.0 to 1.5 mg/kg per day; prednisone, 0.15 to 0.20 mg/kg per day.

In spite of the potential teratogenic effects of immunosuppressive agents, both women and men have become parents after transplantation. The incidence of congenital abnormalities in the offspring is not unusual.

Glomerular lesions Even identical twins who do not require immunosuppression may develop glomerular lesions after transplantation. These represent recurrence of a glomerulonephritic process. Glomerular lesions may occur in 10 to 15 percent of allografts, even when the original disease was accidental removal of a solitary kidney. The pathogenesis is related to a chronic rejection process. In other cases the lesions resemble those of the patient's own original disease. The recurrence of the nephrotic syndrome with "nil disease" in transplanted kidneys whose recipient's original nil disease had progressed to renal failure with focal sclerosis, and the recurrence in renal allografts of the classic lesions of IgA nephropathy and of membranoproliferative glomerulonephritis with electron-dense deposit disease are classic examples. In the last of these, the incidence of recurrence has been reported to be as high as 30 to 40 percent. In most instances, however, the recurrence of the original renal lesions represents no threat to the patient's immediate prognosis, and a primary diagnosis of glomerulonephritis is rarely taken as a contraindication to transplantation.

Malignancy The incidence of tumors arising in patients on immunosuppressive therapy is 5 to 6 percent, or approximately 100 times greater than that observed in the general population in the same age range. The most common lesions are cancer of the skin and lips and carcinoma in situ of the cervix, as well as lymphomas, particularly reticulum cell sarcoma in the central nervous system and gastrointestinal tract.

Other complications *Hypercalcemia* after transplantation may indicate failure of hyperplastic parathyroid glands to regress. Aseptic necrosis of the head of the femur is probably due to preexisting hyperparathyroidism. With improved management of calcium and phosphorus metabolism during chronic dialysis, the incidence of parathyroid-related complications has fallen dramatically.

Hypertension may be caused by (1) native kidneys, (2) rejection activity in the transplant, (3) renal artery stenosis, if an end-to-end anastomosis was constructed with an iliac artery branch, and (4) renal vasoconstriction from cyclosporine toxicity. The latter may improve with reduction in cyclosporine dose. Whereas angiotensin-converting enzyme inhibitors may be useful, calcium channel blockers are frequently more effective in cyclosporine-treated patients.

Chronic hepatitis, particularly when due to hepatitis B virus, can be a progressive fatal disease over a decade or so. Patients who are persistently HBsAg positive are at higher risk, according to some studies, but the presence of non-A non-B disease is also a concern when one embarks upon a course of deliberate immunosuppression in a transplant recipient.

Both chronic dialysis and renal transplant patients have a higher incidence of death from myocardial infarction and stroke than in the population at large, and this is particularly true in diabetics. Contributing factors are hypertension and hypertriglyceridemia. Increased low density lipoprotein cholesterol and depressed high-density lipoprotein cholesterol concentrations may be exaggerated after transplantation and require treatment.

REFERENCES

CARPENTER CB, MILFORD EL: Renal transplantation: Immunobiology, in *The Kidney*, 3d ed, B Brenner, F Rector (eds). Philadelphia, Saunders, 1986, p 1907

———, ———: HLA matching in cadaveric renal transplantation, in *Transplantation Immunology*, PF Halloran (ed). Philadelphia, Saunders, Immunol Aller Clin North Am 9:1, 1989

COLLINS AJ, KESHAVIAH PR: Are there limitations to shortening dialysis treatment? Trans Am Soc Artif Intern Organs 34:1, 1988

GOTCH FA, SARGENT JA: A mechanistic analysis of the National Cooperative Dialysis Study (NCDS). Kidney Intern 28:526, 1985

HAKIM RM, LAZARUS JM: Medical aspects of hemodialysis, in *The Kidney*, 3d ed, B Brenner, F Rector (eds). Philadelphia, Saunders, 1986, p 1791

———, ———: Hemodialysis in acute renal failure, in *Acute Renal Failure*, B Brenner, JM Lazarus (eds). Philadelphia, Saunders, 1986, p 643

LOERTSCHER R et al: Postoperative management of the renal transplant recipient and long-term complications, in *Renal Transplantation, Contemporary Issues in Nephrology*, Vol 19, EL Milford, BM Brenner, JH Stein (eds). New York, Churchill Livingstone, 1989, p 197

NOLPH KD et al: Continuous ambulatory peritoneal dialysis in the United States: A three year study. Kidney Intern 28:198, 1985

RUBIN RH: Infection in the renal transplant recipient, in *Renal Transplantation, Contemporary Issues in Nephrology*, Vol 19, EL Milford, BM Brenner, JH Stein (eds). New York, Churchill Livingstone, 1989, p 147

SIGLER MH et al: Solute transport in continuous hemodialysis: A new treatment for acute renal failure. Kidney Intern 32:562, 1987

TERASAKI PI (ED): *Clinical Transplants 1987*. Los Angeles, UCLA Tissue Typing Laboratory, 1987

226 IMMUNOPATHOGENIC MECHANISMS OF RENAL INJURY

RICHARD J. GLASSOCK / BARRY M. BRENNER

Recognition of the important role played by immunologic processes in many forms of renal injury, especially those involving the glomerular circulation, constitutes one of the significant advances in the understanding of renal diseases. Through investigation of experimental models of disease in animals, the details of the immune processes responsible for renal injury have been evaluated; yet large gaps in our knowledge still exist regarding etiologic factors and pathogenetic events.

IMMUNOPATHOLOGY Immune renal injury may be divided into the initiating pathogenetic events and the processes that mediate the actual tissue injury. The general concepts of immunopathogenesis are presented in Chap. 13. One mechanism of injury involves the reaction of a circulating antibody with its respective renal antigen in situ. Thus, an immune complex is formed at the site of tissue injury rather than at a distant location. The antigen may either be an intrinsic, or native, constituent of the kidney or one that has been bound to the renal tissue by a particular biochemical or immunologic reaction. This mechanism is often referred to as *anti-tissue antibody-mediated disease*. The intrinsic antigens may be insoluble and slowly renewable components of the extracellular matrix (e.g., basement membrane or mesangial matrix glycoproteins) or soluble components of cells or cell membranes (e.g., epithelial, mesangial, or endothelial cells) associated with the matrix components. Bound or extrinsic antigens can be derived from a variety of sources. The mechanisms of binding of extrinsic antigens to the constituents of renal tissue can be quite diverse. The reactions of circulating antibody to the intrinsic or bound (planted) tissue antigens can give rise to distinctive structural alterations and immunohistochemical appearances, as discussed below.

Another pathogenetic category involves the localization of circulating macromolecular aggregates composed of antigens and antibodies (i.e., circulating immune complexes) within renal structures, principally glomeruli. This mechanism is referred to as *immune-complex-induced disease*. The immune complexes need not bear any special immunochemical relationships with renal structures, and the kidney is a passive participant, damaged by processes that originate elsewhere. The source of the antigen in immune-complex-induced disease may be either *endogenous* (autologous) or *exogenous* (environmental). Further, exogenous antigens may either be biologically inert or derived from an organism capable of self-replication (e.g., bacteria, viruses). Under special circumstances environmental agents may combine with autologous substances to result in new antigenic compounds (hapten-protein conjugates) that act in concert with antibodies to form immune complexes.

In contrast to the above mechanisms, which involve antibody, cell-mediated immune processes may also result in injury to glomerular, vascular, and tubulointerstitial regions of the kidney. A precise role for the cell-mediated immune processes in human renal disease is less well established than for certain experimental models.

Finally, certain human glomerular diseases are prominently associated with an abnormal activation of the alternative pathway of the complement cascade (see also Chap. 13), although such activation need not be directly involved in the pathogenesis of tissue injury.

ANTIBODY REACTION WITH INTRINSIC OR PLANTED RENAL ANTIGENS **Anti-basement membrane antibody disease** This form of renal injury is relatively uncommon in humans. By mechanisms that remain obscure, autoantibodies (usually of the IgG isotype) directed to epitopes on the noncollagen domains of type IV (basement membrane) collagen arise in the circulation. These autoantibodies deposit in the kidney glomerular basement membrane (GBM) and/or tubular basement membrane (TBM) and, on occasion, elsewhere (alveolar basement membrane, choroid plexus basement membrane). Since the epitope is part of a repeating subunit uniformly expressed in basement membranes, the deposits of IgG appear linear by immunofluorescent microscopy (Fig. 226-1*A*). Electron-dense lattices of antigen-antibody complexes are not seen by electron microscopy. The local interaction of the autoantibody with the fixed and native basement membrane antigen leads to a perturbation in the structural components and also to the local activation of mediator systems to be described below. Although activation of the complement cascade facilitates injury by virtue of chemotactic and cytolytic effects, glomerular injury may also occur independent of complement activation. Because the antigen-antibody interaction occurs within the lamina rara interna or on the capillary luminal side of the lamina densa, circulating polymorphonuclear leukocytes, monocytes, and platelets are frequently involved in the mediation of glomerular injury.

Proteinuria results from the loss of glomerular anionic residues (see Chap. 49) and by structural defects in the capillary wall brought about by the local release of cationic lysosomal enzymes within infiltrating inflammatory cells. The glomerular filtration rate may decline if the loss of filtering surface area is sufficient to overcome adaptive increases in capillary flows and pressures in remaining capillary channels or nephron units. Obstruction of individual capillary channels may be the consequence of local coagulation, infiltration by inflammatory cells, or endothelial disruption. Leakage of macromolecules and cells such as fibrinogen and monocytes into Bowman's space through gaps in the capillary wall may provoke extracapillary proliferation as fibrinogen is polymerized to fibrin and monocytes release monokines locally.

Renal disease due to anti-basement membrane antibody production is seen primarily in three circumstances: in connection with glomerulonephritis and pulmonary hemorrhage due to anti-GBM autoantibodies (Goodpasture's syndrome), in idiopathic glomerulonephritis due to anti-GBM antibodies without pulmonary hemorrhage, and in idiopathic tubulointerstitial nephritis due to anti-TBM antibody production. In all instances, characteristic findings serve to identify the pathogenetic mechanism: (1) circulating autoantibodies react with basement membrane antigens in vitro; (2) linear deposits of IgG are found in the involved tissue; and (3) eluates of disease tissue contain immunoglobulin reactive with normal, native basement membrane antigens in vivo and in vitro.

Antibodies reactive with non-GBM-related antigens The glomerular capillary wall and mesangium are composed of a number of potentially immunogenic glycoproteins in addition to the GBM glycoprotein mentioned above. These antigens are distributed throughout the basement membrane, mesangial matrix, and cell surfaces.

Binding in situ of passively administered heterologous antibody or actively induced antibody to these antigens produces differing patterns of immunoglobulin localization and functional and structural alteration of the capillary wall. If the antigen is localized in clusters in relationship to the epithelial aspect of the capillary wall, the reaction with antibody in situ may give rise to granular or beadlike deposits of IgG detected by immunofluorescence and to electron-dense subepithelial deposits (Fig. 226-1*B*).

While the number of possible antigen-antibody interactions in this category is large, few have been documented to be responsible for human glomerular or tubulointerstitial disease. Thus far, animal

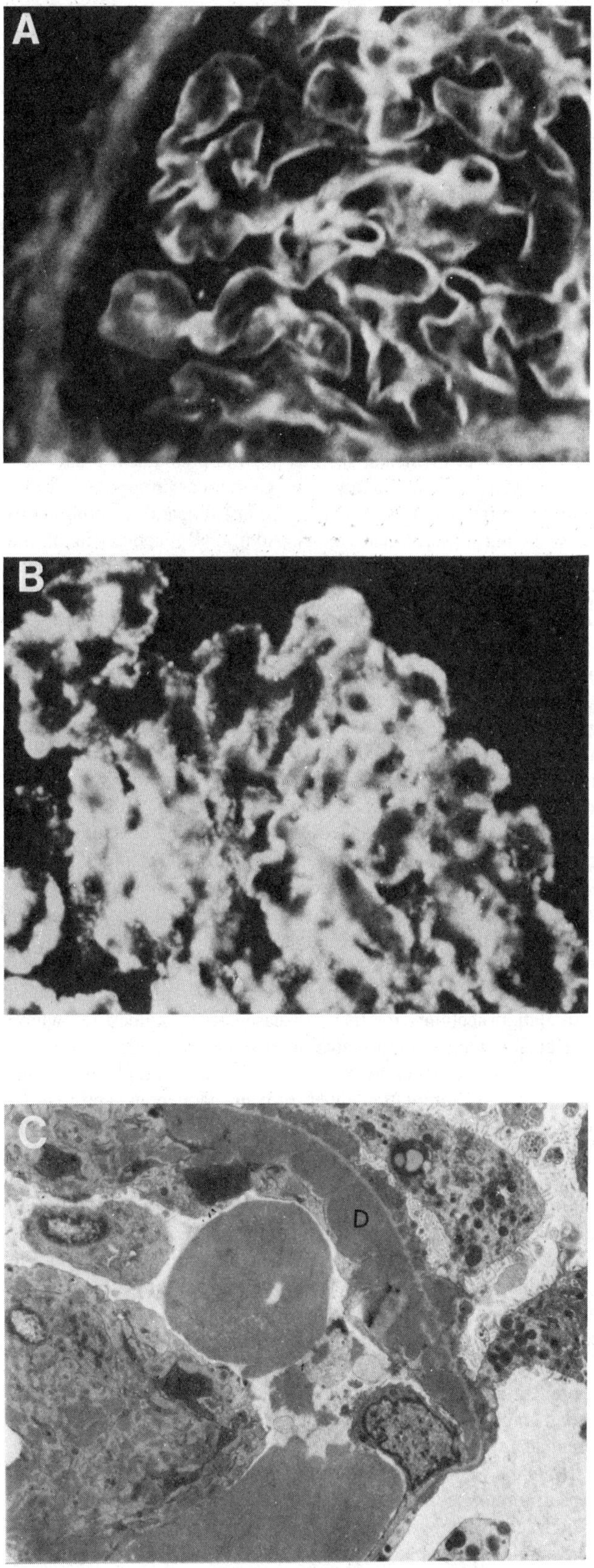

FIGURE 226-1 *A*. Immunofluorescence photomicrograph of a portion of a glomerulus from a patient with anti-glomerular basement membrane antibody–mediated glomerular injury. Note the linear deposits (fluorescein-labeled antihuman IgG). *B*. Immunofluorescence photomicrograph of a portion of a glomerulus from a patient with immune-complex-mediated (in situ or circulating) glomerular injury. Note the irregular, granular deposits (fluorescein-labeled antihuman IgG). *C*. Electron micrograph of a portion of a glomerular capillary from a patient with immune-complex-mediated glomerular injury. Note the electron-dense deposits, *D*.

experimentation has proceeded at a greater pace than understanding of human analogues of this mechanism. The best studied animal model is Heymann's nephritis, which is induced in rats by passive administration of a heterologous antibody to a particular glomerular capillary wall antigen or by active immunization with the antigen in complete Freund's adjuvant. The antigen-antibody interaction occurs in the subepithelial space in the glomerulus and at the brush border of the proximal tubule, where the antigen is synthesized as a component of endocytotic clathrin-coated pits on the surface of the glomerular visceral and proximal tubular epithelial cells. A granular pattern of IgG deposits and subepithelial electron-dense deposits are seen by immunofluorescence and electron microscopy, respectively. Localized activation of the complement cascade, including assembly of the membrane attack complex, may be responsible for altered glomerular permeability, but local variations in the basement membrane may also account for the changes in permselectivity. Since the antigen-antibody reactions occur on the epithelial side of the capillary wall, circulating cellular elements, such as polymorphonuclear leukocytes and monocytes, are not involved in glomerular injury. A similar mechanism might also be active in some idiopathic membranous glomerulonephritis in human beings. Additional reactions involving the binding of circulating antibody to intrinsic structural or self-surface antigens have been described in animals.

Antibodies reacting with planted glomerular antigens Circulating endogenous or environmental substances with special affinity for glomerular structures, including the glomerular capillary wall or mesangium, may deposit in these structures and thus act as a "planted" antigen. An antibody or cellular response to these planted nonglomerular or extrinsic antigens could result in disease as a result of the formation of antigen-antibody complexes in situ. The pattern of disease produced depends upon the sites of the planted antigen and the nature of the immune response. Examples of such planted antigens thus far described include certain drugs, plant lectins, cationized plasma proteins, aggregated immunoglobulins, and deoxyribonucleic acid. Experimental models of this sequence have been described, but there is little definitive information.

CIRCULATING IMMUNE-COMPLEX DISEASE (See Chap. 268) The deposition in the kidney of immune complexes formed in the circulation accounts for many diseases of the kidney for which there is clear evidence of participation of some immunologic process. In this category an immunogenic replicating or nonreplicating substance arises in the circulation either from an endogenous (autologous) or exogenous (environmental) source. Antibody response to the antigen while the antigen remains in the circulation leads to the formation of an aggregate of antigen and antibody known as a *circulating immune complex*. The complement system plays an important role in the transport and removal of circulating immune complexes, and defects in the complement system may predispose to the deposition and accumulation of immune complexes at various tissue sites, including the glomerulus. Activated complement components, particularly C1q and C3b, interfere with the precipitation of immune complexes or solubilize preformed immune complexes, thus preventing their deposition as insoluble aggregates. Circulating immune complexes containing bound C3b are transported to the mononuclear phagocyte system (liver, spleen) via the erythrocyte CR1 receptor. Such transport and delivery favors uptake and degradation of immune complexes by the mononuclear phagocyte system. A small fraction of circulating immune complexes may escape removal by the mononuclear phagocyte system and instead be trapped by vascular structures including the glomeruli. Circulating immune complexes trapped in these sites have the capability of evoking inflammation utilizing many of the mediator systems described above. One of the best-studied examples of this circulating immune-complex disease involving a nonreplicating antigen is serum sickness, which results from the acute or chronic administration of an immunogenic, soluble, heterologous, foreign serum protein (see Fig. 268-1). A small portion of the immune complexes localize within the glomerular mesangium; in the walls of peripheral capillaries; and in joints, heart valves, choroid plexus, splenic sinusoids, and larger blood vessels, particularly at sites of turbulent flow. Once deposited, these complexes evoke an inflammatory response at the site of deposition.

Although this formulation presupposes that immune complexes form within the circulation and then are deposited in vascular structures, immune complexes may form in the extravascular (interstitial) compartment by virtue of diffusion into this fluid compartment of cell-derived antigens and circulating antibody. Such a phenomenon may explain the deposition of immune complexes in the interstitial areas of the kidney, with relative sparing of the glomerular circulation. Regardless of the nature of the antibody or antigen or the particular circumstances surrounding the immunologic events, a valuable clue to the presence of immune-complex deposition or in situ formation is the morphologic pattern found when tissues are examined by immunofluorescence or electron-microscopic techniques. Granular, discontinuous, and irregular deposits of Ig, often in conjunction with complement components, are found by immunofluorescence (Fig. 226-1*B*), whereas electron-dense deposits are seen by electron microscopy (Fig. 226-1*C*). Sometimes these deposits acquire a definite substructure, but for the most part they are rather homogeneous. The deposits may develop in several locations within the glomerulus: beneath the epithelial cells (subepithelial), within the basement membrane (intramembranous), beneath the endothelium (subendothelial), and within the mesangial matrix. Immune complexes may also localize in the peritubular capillary network. The reason for localization at these differing sites may involve factors such as size or charge of the complexes, receptors for the Fc or complement components within glomerular structures, or local hemodynamic events. The deposits appear to increase in size by aggregation, and glomerular cells may participate in their removal. The persistence of deposits is related to the rate of formation balanced by the activity of removal systems. Ig itself in a circulating immune complex trapped in the glomerular circulation may behave as a planted antigen, either via the idiotypic determinants in the antigen-binding sites of antibody or via the Fc portions evoking an anti-immunoglobulin (rheumatoid factor) response. The roles played by anti-idiotype antibody or rheumatoid factor in the evolution of glomerular lesions in immune-complex-mediated disease is not clear. Once deposited in glomeruli, circulating immune complexes evoke local inflammatory and functional changes, which at least for the glomerular circulation may be relatively independent of complement or polymorphonuclear leukocytes. In situ formation of an immune complex in the subepithelial space may not be associated with the accumulation of inflammatory cells. Infiltrating monocytes may play a critical role in mediating glomerular injury. The morphologic lesions which result from immune-complex deposition may vary considerably, from diffuse proliferative to nonproliferative membranous or sclerosing lesions. Coagulation, platelet aggregation, activation of the complement cascade, and release of vasoactive amines may participate in determining the pattern of morphologic response.

The *exogenous* antigens involved in circulating immune-complex-mediated disease are derived chiefly from infectious agents such as bacteria, viruses, or parasites. Replication of the organism provides a continuing source of antigen. The best-studied examples of these in humans are *infective endocarditis, leprosy, syphilis, hepatitis B,* and *malaria*. The *endogenous* antigens involved in human disease vary considerably and include *DNA, thyroglobulin, autologous immunoglobulins, erythrocyte stroma, renal tubule antigens,* and *tumor-specific* or *tumor-associated* antigens.

CELL-MEDIATED IMMUNITY IN GLOMERULAR AND TUBULOINTERSTITIAL DISEASES The roles of specifically sensitized cells acting independently of antibody (T cytotoxic cells), "armed" macrophages, and antibody-dependent cell-mediated cytotoxicity in the pathogenesis of glomerular and tubulointerstitial diseases have been difficult to establish. The glomerulus and probably the cortical interstitium possess the necessary elements to support a cell-mediated response to an autologous or heterologous antigen. Mononuclear cells capable of processing antigen and activating T helper-inducer cells in a major histocompatibility complex–restricted fashion are present in the glomerular mesangium and interstitium. A number of experimental diseases of the kidney, most notably tubulointerstitial nephritis, are the consequence of a cell-mediated immune response. However, relatively few human diseases can be ascribed to cell-mediated immune processes exclusively. The rejection of renal allografts in nonsensitized recipients is clearly a cell-mediated process (see Chap. 225).

By utilizing a variety of in vitro techniques cell-mediated hypersensitivity to both environmental and endogenous antigens is demonstrable in diseases of the kidney, including glomerulonephritis. The precise role such "sensitized" cells play in the actual tissue injury is unclear. It is likely that diseases that do not fit into an antibody- or immune-complex-mediated category will be explained as reactions of the cell-mediated variety. One likely candidate for this category is so-called minimal change disease, one of the subsets of idiopathic nephrotic syndrome. Furthermore, because of the prominence of lymphoid cell infiltration, various forms of chronic tubulointerstitial nephritis may also be cell-mediated reactions (see Chap. 229).

COMPLEMENT-ASSOCIATED GLOMERULAR INJURY Although there is little evidence that complement activation, independent of antitissue antibody or circulating immune complexes, can bring about glomerular injury, there are certain associations between complement and renal disease. The clinicopathologic entity known as *idiopathic mesangiocapillary glomerulonephritis* (see also Chap. 227) may be associated with serum complement deposition within glomeruli suggestive of involvement of the alternative pathway of complement activation, perhaps independent of immune-complex deposition. These patterns are not necessarily unique to this group of disorders since they may also be observed in postinfectious glomerulonephritides and in certain collagen-vascular diseases.

The activation of the complement cascade and the assembly of active cleaving enzymes is discussed more fully in Chap. 13. Briefly, the classical pathway of complement activation is initiated when antibodies (usually IgG or IgM) bind to their respective antigens and expose a C1q binding site on the Fc portion of the Ig molecule. Bound C1q activates C1r and C1s to form active C1qrs, which results in cleavage of C4 and C2 and leads to the assembly of the classical C3 and C5 convertases, C4b2a and C4b2a3b, respectively. The alternative pathway of complement is initiated when an active form of C3 in the fluid phase ($C3H_2O$) reacts with factors B, D, and properdin, forming a C3 convertase, C3Bb. IgA immune complexes, polysaccharides, or lipopolysaccharides have the potential of activating C3 via the alternative pathway. The resultant conversion of native C3 to C3b autocatalytically generates additional C3Bb. The amplification of C3Bb formation contributes to the generation of the C5 convertases, C42Bb3Bb from the classical pathway and C3bBGP from the alternative pathway. These C5 convertases cleave native C5 to C5a and C5b. The two pathways of complement activation thus converge upon C5, and with the interaction of the terminal complement components (C6, C7, C8, and C9) a lytic polymer of C5b6, 7, 8, 9 (n) is formed on the cell surface (the membrane attack complex). Several cleaved molecules (C3a, C5a) have potent proinflammatory and chemotactic properties. Inhibitor proteins control the activation of complement, including C1 inhibitor, factor H (β_1H), and factor I. As discussed previously, C1q and C3b have important functions relating to the aggregation and solubilization of immune complexes, and C3b participates in the transport of immune complexes to the removal sites in the mononuclear phagocyte system.

In *idiopathic mesangiocapillary glomerulonephritis,* particularly the subset known as *dense deposit disease,* serum C3 levels are depressed; C4, C1, and C2 levels tend to be normal; and C3 may be deposited in glomeruli without Ig (see also Chap. 227). In addition, an autoantibody (an immunoconglutinin) to alternative pathway C3 convertase is frequently found in the circulation. This autoantibody reacts with a conformational neoantigen of the alternative pathway C3 convertase and stabilizes this enzyme from the influence of C3b inactivator and β_1H in a fashion similar to properdin. As a result sera containing this autoantibody are capable of inducing C3 cleavage in vitro by permitting the assembly of a stable fluid phase C3 convertase. This antibody is also known as C3 nephritic factor (C3NeF) and was first described in patients with glomerulonephritis and persistent depression of C3 levels.

The relationship between these aberrations in the complement pathway and glomerular injury is uncertain. No experimental models of persistent activation of the alternative pathway are associated with glomerulonephritis; thus, glomerular injury may be a closely associated but unrelated phenomenon, perhaps genetically determined. The recognition that certain structural genes for complement components (C2, C4) are closely associated with the major histocompatibility complex provides a potential explanation for the association of disease susceptibility with defects in biosynthesis of complement proteins. On the other hand, persistent hypocomplementemia may interfere with the normal removal processes for environmental antigens such as viruses. Such a defect might favor the persistence of these antigens in the circulation and enhance the likelihood of formation of circulating immune complexes. The discovery that C3 and its degradation product (primarily C3b) are able to solubilize aggregates of antigen and antibody may provide an additional explanation for the occurrence of immune-complex disease in association with defects of complement synthesis or activation.

Once initiated, immune injury is mediated by the interaction of humoral and cellular factors. Activation of the complement (C) cascade may lead to the cytolysis of the cellular constituents of the glomerulus or to the production of biologically active fragments capable of enhancing vascular permeability or attracting polymorphonuclear leukocytes and other cellular constituents. Coagulation may be initiated by alterations in the endothelial surface and exposure of collagen matrix, followed by localized platelet aggregation. Interactions between the complement cascade and the coagulation process are numerous and complex. Complement activation may trigger coagulation and vice versa. Activation of the Hageman factor can initiate the kallikrein-kinin system. Potent vasoactive peptides, prostaglandins, and leukotrienes may thus be released and play a role in alterations in local and systemic hemodynamics observed in conjunction with immunologically induced renal diseases. Polymorphonuclear leukocytes, eosinophils, monocytes (macrophages), and platelets can be called forth to participate in immune-mediated injury to varying degrees. Polymorphonuclear leukocytes and monocytes appear to participate in glomerular injury by virtue of their ability to release factors that degrade basement membrane glycoproteins and by facilitating the local production of toxic oxygen species (hydroxyl radical and superoxide anion). Activated monocytes may also express a membrane-bound procoagulant, thus fostering local fibrin deposition. Platelet deposition may be involved in the proliferation of glomerular cells via the release of a platelet-derived growth factor or may alter the anionic charge of the capillary wall by local release of cationic proteins, thus facilitating altered glomerular permselectivity. The composite result of these events is to alter the structural and functional integrity of the glomerular capillary and/or peritubular capillary wall, leading to reduced filtration capacity, enhanced permeability to plasma proteins, and migration of cellular elements (i.e., erythrocytes and leukocytes) outside the intravascular compartment.

REFERENCES

COUSER WG et al: Complement and the direct mediation of glomerular injury. A new perspective. Kidney Int 29:879, 1985

FRIES JWV et al: Determinants of immune complex–mediated glomerulonephritis. Kidney Int 34:333, 1988

SCHIFFERLI JA et al: The role of complement and its receptors in the elimination of immune complexes. N Engl J Med 315:488, 1986

SCHREINER GF JR et al: Macrophages and cellular immunity in experimental glomerulonephritis. Springer Semin Immunopathol 5:251, 1982

WILSON CB (guest ed): Immunopathology of renal disease, in *Contemporary Issues in Nephrology,* vol 18, BM Brenner, JH Stein (eds). New York, Churchill Livingstone, 1988

227 THE MAJOR GLOMERULOPATHIES

RICHARD J. GLASSOCK / BARRY M. BRENNER

Alterations of the structural and functional integrity of the glomerular capillary circulation are often associated with the findings, either singly or in combination, of hematuria, proteinuria, reduced glomerular filtration rate (GFR), and hypertension. Five major glomerulopathic syndromes are recognized: *acute glomerulonephritis, rapidly progressive glomerulonephritis, chronic glomerulonephritis,* the *nephrotic syndrome,* and *asymptomatic urinary abnormalities.* This chapter deals with diseases in which the kidney is either the sole or the predominant organ involved (i.e., the primary glomerulopathies) or is involved as a complication of infection or drug exposure. Glomerular injury associated with multisystem disorders or heredofamilial conditions is discussed in Chap. 228.

ACUTE GLOMERULONEPHRITIS

The causes of acute glomerulonephritis (AGN) are given in Table 227-1. The "acute nephritic syndrome" consists of the abrupt onset of *hematuria* and *proteinuria,* accompanied by evidence of *azotemia* (i.e., reduced GFR) and renal *salt and water retention.* If GFR is reduced markedly, oligoanuria may be present (see also Chap. 223). Salt and water retention leads to circulatory congestion, hypertension, and edema. Hematuria is most likely the consequence of migration of erythrocytes across damaged glomerular and/or peritubular capillary walls leading to the presence of erythrocytes in tubule fluid in the early part of the nephron. Proteinuria is the consequence of either a loss of anionic charges of the capillary wall (charge-selective defect) or the appearance of glomerular capillaries with larger-than-normal pore radius, permitting large plasma protein molecules to traverse the glomerular filter. Glomerular filtration rate is reduced presumably because of infiltration of the capillaries by inflammatory cells, which thereby reduce filtering surface area. Alternatively, the filtering surface area could be functionally decreased due to the local elaboration of vasoactive compounds capable of reversibly contracting mesangial cells (e.g., angiotensin II, leukotrienes), thereby leading to a reduction in the number of perfused glomerular capillaries. Extensive crescentic disease may obliterate Bowman's space, further impeding filtration. Fluid retention is due in part to decreased glomerular filtration rate but probably also to persistence of avid distal nephron salt and water reabsorption. Extracellular and intravascular fluid volumes are expanded by salt and fluid retention.

The edema of acute glomerulonephritis tends to appear initially in areas of low tissue pressure, such as the *periorbital* areas, but may subsequently progress to involve dependent portions of the body and lead to *ascites* and/or *pleural effusions. Circulatory congestion* is manifested by an increase in systemic and pulmonary vascular pressures, normal or increased cardiac output, and a shortened circulation time. In the absence of underlying valvular, myocardial, or coronary artery disease or severe diastolic hypertension there is little likelihood that true left ventricular congestive heart failure will develop. If pulmonary capillary pressure rises above the opposing plasma oncotic pressure, however, pulmonary edema may ensue. *Arterial diastolic hypertension* is the consequence of several factors, including extracellular fluid volume expansion, enhanced cardiac output, and modest increases in peripheral vascular resistance. Plasma renin activity, aldosterone, and the sympathetic nervous system are relatively suppressed. Hypertension may at times be accompanied by encephalopathy, particularly in young children.

TABLE 227-1 Causes of acute glomerulonephritis

I Infectious diseases
  A Poststreptococcal glomerulonephritis*
  B Nonstreptococcal postinfectious glomerulonephritis
    1 Bacterial: infective endocarditis,* "shunt nephritis," sepsis,* pneumococcal pneumonia, typhoid fever, secondary syphilis, meningococcemia
    2 Viral: hepatitis B, infectious mononucleosis, mumps, measles, varicella, vaccinia, echovirus, and coxsackievirus
    3 Parasitic: malaria, toxoplasmosis
II Multisystem diseases: systemic lupus erythematosus,* vasculitis,* Henoch-Schönlein purpura,* Goodpasture's syndrome
III Primary glomerular diseases: mesangiocapillary glomerulonephritis, Berger's disease (IgA nephropathy),* "pure" mesangial proliferative glomerulonephritis
IV Miscellaneous: Guillain-Barré syndrome, irradiation of Wilms's tumor, self-administered diphtheria-pertussis-tetanus vaccine, serum sickness

* Most common causes.

The extent and severity of urinary abnormalities in AGN vary considerably. Gross (macroscopic) *hematuria* is the most common, and is often described by the patient as smoky-, coffee-, or cola-colored urine. Lesser degrees of hematuria may go unrecognized by the patient or parent; for this reason, the features of fluid retention and hypertension may be ascribed erroneously to other illnesses if examination of the urine sediment is omitted from the initial evaluation. Hematuria is often, but not invariably, accompanied by the excretion of *red cell casts.* The erythrocytes in the urinary sediment are characteristically small, distorted, fragmented, and hypochromic (dysmorphic hematuria). Leukocyturia and leukocyte casts may indicate the presence of inflammation in the glomerulus and interstitium. The degree of *proteinuria* varies according to the nature and severity of the underlying glomerular lesions. Rarely, protein excretion rates are within the normal range, but generally they are between 0.2 and 3 g/d. If proteinuria is marked and sustained, the nephrotic syndrome may appear (see below).

The short-term evolution of acute glomerulonephritis generally depends upon the nature of the underlying glomerular lesions and their treatment. For example, in infective endocarditis resolution of urinary findings and improved renal function may occur rapidly after control of the bacteremia by antimicrobials. Within a week or so of onset, most patients with poststreptococcal acute glomerulonephritis begin to experience spontaneous resolution of fluid retention and hypertension. Urinary abnormalities often take longer to resolve. A few patients with the acute nephritic syndrome in the ensuing weeks will develop a rapidly progressive form of renal failure (i.e., rapidly progressive glomerulonephritis, discussed below). The long-term outlook for patients with AGN is considered below in the context of treatment of specific lesions. Renal biopsy is useful in characterizing the nature of the underlying lesion but need not be done in every case.

ACUTE POSTSTREPTOCOCCAL GLOMERULONEPHRITIS

Clinical features and diagnosis This disorder can be viewed as the archetype of AGN. Poststreptococcal glomerulonephritis (PSGN) follows in the wake of *pharyngeal or cutaneous infection* with one of a limited number of strains of *group A β-hemolytic streptococci.* These potentially "nephritogenic" streptococci may be identified by serotyping of a cell wall antigen (M protein). Among outbreaks of infection with proved "nephritogenic" strains of streptococci the PSGN attack rate is relatively uniform, but because of variation in the nephritogenicity among group A streptococci, attack rates with outbreaks of infection vary considerably. Among families, asymptomatic episodes of PSGN exceed symptomatic episodes by a factor of 3 or 4 to 1. Immunity to M protein is type-specific, long-lasting, and protective. Repeated episodes of PSGN are therefore unusual. Outbreaks of pharyngeal infection–associated PSGN are commonest in children aged 6 to 10. AGN following cutaneous streptococcal infection is more commonly associated with poor personal hygiene, overcrowding, and concomitant cutaneous disease, such as scabies infestation. Seasonal and geographic variations in prevalence of PSGN are more marked for pharyngeal- than for cutaneous-associated disease.

An important feature of PSGN is the existence of a *latent period* between the earliest manifestations of infection and the onset of recognizable signs and symptoms of nephritis. Following pharyngeal infections the latent period usually is 6 to 10 days in duration. Cutaneous infections are associated with longer latent periods, averaging about 2 weeks. Definitive signs of glomerular inflammation occurring at the same time as, or shortly after, infection usually indicate an *exacerbation* of a preexisting chronic glomerular disease such as Berger's disease (IgA nephropathy) (see below).

The diagnosis of PSGN rests upon the demonstration of at least two of the following three features: (1) A group A β-hemolytic streptococcus of a potentially nephritogenic M-protein type is found in a throat or skin lesion. (2) An immune response to one or more of the streptococcal *exoenzymes,* including antistreptolysin O (ASO), antistreptokinase (ASK), anti-deoxyribonuclease B (ADNAase B), anti-nicotinyl adenine dinucleotidase (ANADase), or antihyaluronidase (AH), can be demonstrated. ASO responses are typically brisk in pharyngeal infections, but often absent in cutaneous infection, whereas AH, ADNAase, and ANADase responses occur after the latter. Testing for multiple antibody responses and serial determinations are necessary to achieve a diagnostic accuracy of 90 percent. Early antimicrobial therapy may prevent the antibody response to exoenzymes and render throat cultures negative but may not prevent the development of PSGN; this makes accurate serologic diagnosis difficult or impossible. (3) A transient decline in the serum concentration of the C3 component of complement, with a return to normal within 8 weeks after the first signs of renal disease, can be demonstrated. Other complement components (i.e., C1q and C4) are frequently less depressed. In addition to these laboratory features it is desirable to document a latent period appropriate to the nature of the infection. Furthermore, the patient should not have any known preexisting renal disease.

Other laboratory features commonly observed in PSGN include transient cryoimmunoglobulinemia and positive tests for circulating immune complexes. The erythrocyte sedimentation rate is usually elevated, while C-reactive protein and rheumatoid factor are generally normal or undetectable. Mild anemia and hypoalbuminemia, both largely dilutional in origin, may be present. Severe hypoalbuminemia may be encountered if heavy proteinuria is present and prolonged. Excretion rates of urinary protein in excess of 3.5 g/d occur in less than 20 percent of hospitalized patients. Proteinuria is usually of a nonselective character and frequently contains high concentrations of fibrin-degradation products and C3 protein, particularly during the diuretic phase. Hyponatremia, hyperchloremia, hyperkalemia, and metabolic acidosis may be seen in azotemic or oliguric patients, especially those with free access to water or potassium. Plasma renin activity and aldosterone secretion rates are low, reflecting suppression secondary to expanded plasma volume. Urinary sodium concentration is usually low, reflecting avid salt reabsorption in the distal nephron. Abdominal films reveal normal or enlarged kidneys. The chest x-ray may be normal or reveal a slightly enlarged heart, often accompanied by signs of pulmonary congestion. The electrocardiogram may reveal nonspecific T-wave abnormalities. Rheumatic fever rarely coexists with acute PSGN.

The differential diagnosis of PSGN includes other infectious or primary renal diseases which may produce an identical acute nephritic syndrome (Table 227-1). Multisystem diseases such as systemic lupus erythematosus, Henoch-Schönlein purpura, and vasculitis may present initially as acute nephritis (Chap. 228). Predominantly nonglomerular diseases, including thrombotic thrombocytopenic purpura, hemolytic-uremic syndrome, atheroembolic renal disease, and acute hypersensitivity interstitial nephritis may also present the features of the acute nephritic syndrome (Chaps. 229 and 230).

Pathology and pathogenesis Renal biopsies performed early in the course reveal *diffuse, endocapillary proliferative glomerulonephritis.* Infiltration of glomeruli with polymorphonuclear leukocytes and monocytes is common. The glomerular capillary walls are usually thin and delicate and free of necrosis. Occasional discrete proteinaceous deposits projecting from the outer aspects of the capillary wall toward the urinary space (humps) may be recognized by light microscopy and coincide with the electron-dense deposits seen by electron microscopy. Segmental extracapillary proliferation (crescents) may involve a few glomeruli, but diffuse and extensive circumferential crescent formation is uncommon except among a subset of patients presenting with severe and rapidly progressive acute renal failure (see section below on rapidly progressive glomerulonephritis). Extraglomerular vessels and tubulointerstitial areas are usually normal. Red blood cells are frequently seen in the lumens of distal tubules, where they form red blood cell casts and dysmorphic erythrocytes.

By immunofluorescence microscopy, granular deposits of IgG are seen in peripheral capillary loops and mesangium, nearly always accompanied by C3 and properdin and less commonly by C1q and C4 (Chap. 226). Several patterns of Ig and/or C3 deposition have been described. Extensive involvement of the peripheral capillary loops with deposits may be associated with a poorer prognosis, while deposits exclusively involving the mesangium usually indicate a more benign outcome. The precise nature of the antigen-antibody systems involved remains unknown. Most likely the antigen is derived from the streptococcal organism itself, but this has been difficult to verify. The profile of altered serum complement components described above, and the prominent C3 and properdin deposition in glomeruli, are suggestive of involvement of the alternative pathway of complement activation (Chap. 226).

Course and treatment The ultimate *prognosis* for PSGN differs between sporadic and epidemic forms and between adults and children. *Epidemic* forms of the disease in *children* have a uniformly favorable short- and long-term prognosis. Few patients die of complications of renal failure (fewer than 1 percent), and nearly all experience a spontaneous resolution of clinical signs within a week after the onset of illness. Abnormalities in the urinary sediment and protein excretion subside slowly in the ensuing months; in a few cases, several years elapse before the urinary sediment is consistently normal. Among children with PSGN during epidemics of streptococcal infection, and in whom some form of preexisting chronic glomerular disease was absent, long-term follow-up has revealed little or no evidence of progression to chronic renal disease. A small percentage may develop extensive crescentic glomerulonephritis with its relentlessly progressive course. The site of the streptococcal infection, the type of M protein, the severity of abnormalities of complement or urinary sediment, or the extent of the rise in antibody response to exoenzymes have little or no bearing on the ultimate prognosis. Prolonged and persistent heavy proteinuria and/or abnormal GFR imply a more unfavorable outcome. *Sporadic* cases of PSGN among *children* may have more serious long-term consequences, although this remains controversial. After the subsidence of the acute disease, some children develop slowly progressive glomerular capillary obliteration (glomerulosclerosis), reduced GFR, and hypertension; after several decades, end-stage renal failure from chronic glomerulonephritis may result. The persistence of proteinuria is the rule in such cases.

The prognosis for *adults* with PSGN is less favorable than for children. The reason for this apparent difference is poorly understood. Although the overall prognosis for PSGN in *epidemics* seems good, *sporadic* PSGN in adults is associated with lasting and/or progressive deterioration in renal function in as many as one-third to one-half of cases. This may take the form of persistent proteinuria and/or hematuria or of slowly progressive glomerulosclerosis and renal failure, often accompanied by hypertension. This evolution seems more likely to occur when the initial disease is unusually severe. Whether milder forms of sporadic PSGN can lead to chronic disease is an unresolved issue (see "Chronic Glomerulonephritis" below).

The *treatment* of acute PSGN is supportive. It is reasonable to recommend bed rest until the signs of glomerular inflammation and circulatory congestion (primarily hypertension) subside, but prolonged periods of inactivity are of no demonstrable benefit in the healing process. Fluid retention, circulatory congestion, and edema may be treated with sodium and fluid restriction or loop diuretics. Diuresis alone often ameliorates mild to moderate hypertension. If severe hypertension is present, vasodilator drugs such as nitroprusside, nifedipine, hydralazine, or diazoxide may be useful. Encephalopathy and pulmonary congestion generally improve with lowering of blood pressure and the relief of circulatory overload. Digitalis should be avoided except in instances of well-documented organic heart disease with congestive failure. Treatment with ion exchange resins and/or dialysis may be required for cases of severe oliguria, fluid overload, and hyperkalemia. Mild protein restriction is desirable for azotemic patients. A 7- to 10-day course of antimicrobials (e.g., penicillin or erythromycin) should be given if streptococcal infection is documented. Long-term chemoprophylaxis is not indicated. Steroids and cytotoxic drugs are not of value.

NONSTREPTOCOCCAL ACUTE POSTINFECTIOUS GLOMERULONEPHRITIS Clinical features and diagnosis A wide variety of infectious illnesses other than those caused by group A β-hemolytic streptococci may also be associated with AGN (Table 227-1). These include *bacteremic states* and various *viral* and *parasitic* diseases. Ordinarily these diseases can be diagnosed by the presence of typical extrarenal clinical features or by bacteriologic or serologic findings. Infective endocarditis, sepsis of other types, typhoid fever, infectious mononucleosis, acute viral hepatitis (hepatitis B), falciparum malaria, and toxoplasmosis are examples of infectious diseases capable of evoking AGN. Circulating immune complexes play an important role in the pathogenesis of AGN in these diseases. Chronic or subacute bacteremic states are frequently associated with persistent depression of serum complement components C1q, C4, and C3, elevated levels of rheumatoid factor, circulating cryoimmunoglobulins, and strongly positive tests for circulating immune complexes. Control of infection usually results in the resolution of glomerular inflammation, although, in occasional instances, rapidly progressive or chronic glomerulonephritis may ensue.

TABLE 227-2 Causes of rapidly progressive glomerulonephritis

I Infectious diseases
- *A* Poststreptococcal glomerulonephritis*
- *B* Infective endocarditis*
- *C* Occult visceral sepsis
- *D* Hepatitis B infection (with vasculitis and/or cryoimmunoglobulinemia)
- *E* Human immunodeficiency virus infection (?)

II Multisystem diseases
- *A* Systemic lupus erythematosus*
- *B* Henoch-Schönlein purpura*
- *C* Systemic necrotizing vasculitis (including Wegener's granulomatosis)*
- *D* Goodpasture's syndrome*
- *E* Essential mixed (IgG/IgM) cryoimmunoglobulinemia
- *F* Malignancy
- *G* Relapsing polychondritis
- *H* Rheumatoid arthritis (with vasculitis)

III Drugs
- *A* Penicillamine*
- *B* Hydralazine
- *C* Allopurinol (with vasculitis)
- *D* Rifampin

IV Idiopathic or primary glomerular disease
- *A* Idiopathic crescentic glomerulonephritis*
  - *1* Type I—with linear deposits of Ig (anti-glomerular basement membrane antibody–mediated)
  - *2* Type II—with granular deposits of Ig (immune-complex–mediated)
  - *3* Type III—with few or no immune deposits of Ig ("pauci-immune")
  - *4* Anti-neutrophil cytoplasmic antibody–induced, ? "forme fruste" of vasculitis
- *B* Superimposed on another primary glomerular disease
  - *1* Mesangiocapillary (membranoproliferative glomerulonephritis)* (especially type II)
  - *2* Membranous glomerulonephritis*
    Berger's disease (IgA nephropathy)*

* Most common.

RAPIDLY PROGRESSIVE GLOMERULONEPHRITIS

Transient azotemia, often associated with a brief period of oliguria, is common in AGN. A diuresis usually follows within days or a few weeks, and GFR returns to normal. On the other hand, some cases of AGN are characterized by a rapidly progressive form of renal failure, which often develops abruptly and displays little tendency for spontaneous or complete recovery. The clinical term *rapidly progressive glomerulonephritis* (*RPGN*) is often applied to this group to connote the development of renal failure in a period of weeks to months, rather than years or decades, as is typical of chronic glomerulonephritis (see below). Usually, but not invariably, extensive *extracapillary* (*crescentic*) *glomerulonephritis* is the pathologic lesion underlying the syndrome of RPGN, and the two terms are often used interchangeably.

RPGN can arise in four clinical settings (Table 227-2): (1) as a renal complication of an acute or subacute infectious disease, (2) as a renal complication of many multisystem diseases, (3) in association with the use of certain drugs, and (4) as a primary or idiopathic glomerular disease. In the latter circumstance the RPGN can arise de novo or be superimposed on another primary glomerular disease process. RPGN occurring as a primary glomerular disease will be discussed here, while that arising secondary to infectious diseases, multisystem diseases, or drugs will be considered in Chap. 228.

IDIOPATHIC RAPIDLY PROGRESSIVE GLOMERULONEPHRITIS Clinical features and diagnosis This disorder affects individuals in a broad age distribution and has a predilection for males. Wide geographic differences in the prevalence of the disease have been noted, and outbreaks ("miniepidemics") may occur. Some patients have had recent heavy exposure to volatile hydrocarbons, but there is little evidence to support a cause-and-effect relationship. While a flulike or viral prodrome may occur, frank arthritis, sinusitis, otitis, skin rash, neuritis, or encephalopathy are uncommon and are more in keeping with a multisystem disease. Symptoms of weakness, nausea, and vomiting (indicative of azotemia) usually dominate the clinical picture. Oliguria, abdominal or flank pain, and hemoptysis may also be present (see "Goodpasture's Syndrome," Chap. 228). The blood pressure is normal or modestly elevated. Urinalysis typically reveals dysmorphic hematuria and red cell casts, but relatively benign urine sediments may be present. Proteinuria is always present and may be massive. Other biochemical features of the nephrotic syndrome are uncommon, probably because of the concomitant reduction in GFR. Proteinuria is typically nonselective, and high concentrations of fibrin degradation products are found in urine. Azotemia develops early and tends to progress at a rapid rate. Other clinical and laboratory features relate to the underlying pathology and pathogenesis.

Pathology and pathogenesis Idiopathic RPGN is not a homogeneous disease. By light microscopy the characteristic abnormality in the kidneys is *extensive extracapillary proliferation,* i.e., *crescents.* The extent and degree of glomerular involvement varies; however, among patients with rapid deterioration of renal function it is usual for more than 70 percent of glomeruli to be involved with circumferential crescents. Endocapillary proliferation, if prominent, suggests the presence of infection. Segmental or diffuse endocapillary necrosis suggests underlying systemic necrotizing vasculitis. Fibrin-related antigens are nearly always demonstrable within the crescents by special stains or by immunofluorescence. Gaps or focal discontinuities in the glomerular basement membrane (GBM) and/or Bowman's capsule are observed in association with crescents.

Variations in the underlying pathogenetic mechanisms responsible for RPGN are illustrated by immunofluorescence studies of renal biopsies (Chap. 226). In approximately 5 to 20 percent of cases, *linear deposits* of IgG indicate involvement of *anti-GBM antibodies.* Circulating anti-GBM antibodies can be demonstrated by indirect immunofluorescence, hemagglutination, or radioimmunoassay techniques. Patients in this subgroup tend to have normal serum complement levels and a marked tendency to develop hemoptysis (see also "Goodpasture's Syndrome," Chap. 228). These patients frequently are HLA-DR2 antigen–positive. About 30 to 40 percent of cases will have findings of *immune-complex–mediated disease,* namely, *granular deposits* of immunoglobulin by immunofluorescence microscopy and electron-dense deposits by electron microscopy. This mechanism of RPGN tends to occur in older individuals, to produce more constitutional symptoms, and to result in more disturbances of the complement pathways than does anti-GBM antibody–mediated disease. Hemoptysis may also occur, but circulating anti-GBM antibodies are absent. C3 levels may be decreased. The remainder of cases of RPGN reveal scanty or no immunoglobulins or complement by immunofluorescence (''pauci-immune''); their pathogenesis is unknown. This group also tends to include older individuals, in whom serum complement concentrations are normal and anti-GBM antibodies are absent. Occasionally, mild hemoptysis may occur. This latter variation may represent a ''forme fruste'' of systemic necrotizing vasculitis with isolated renal involvement. Such patients often have detectable anti-neutrophil cytoplasmic antibody characteristic of systemic necrotizing vasculitis and Wegener's granulomatosis (see Chap. 228).

Lung hemorrhage may be observed in a variety of circumstances associated with RPGN. This subject is covered in greater detail in the section on Goodpasture's syndrome in Chap. 228. Uncommonly, other idiopathic (primary) glomerular diseases may be complicated by a superimposed rapidly progressive glomerulonephritis accompanied by extensive crescent formation. These primary glomerular diseases include mesangiocapillary (membranoproliferative) glomerulonephritis, Berger's disease (IgA nephropathy), and membranous glomerulonephritis (Table 227-2). The pathogenetic mechanisms underlying this complication vary.

Course and treatment The prognosis for preservation of renal function in RPGN is poor. Patients with crescent formation in 70 percent or more of glomeruli or oliguria or severe reduction in GFR (less than 5 mL/min) at the time of presentation and those with an anti-GBM antibody–mediated process have the worst prognosis. Although advances in treatment are changing the outlook for patients with RPGN, as many as one-half require maintenance hemodialysis within 6 months of discovery of the illness. Exceptional patients with crescentic glomerulonephritis have a more protracted illness. Spontaneous resolution is uncommon, except among patients with infection as the basis for formation of antigen-antibody complexes, where removal of antigen can take place.

Glucocorticoids, in the form of ''pulses'' of parenteral methylprednisolone in high doses, and daily oral prednisone, often combined with *cytotoxic agents* (azathioprine or cyclophosphamide), have yielded varying degrees of success, particularly in the patients with granular or minimal Ig deposits in glomeruli, especially in association with vasculitis. Since no controlled studies have yet been conducted, however, it is difficult to ascertain the value of these regimens. Nonetheless, more than two-thirds of patients treated with several ''pulses'' of intravenous methylprednisolone have experienced improvement in renal function often sufficient to avoid the necessity of dialysis. The addition of *anticoagulants* (heparin or warfarin sodium) and antithrombotic agents (dipyridamole, sulfinpyrazone) seems rational on the basis of evidence for involvement of the coagulation process in the genesis of crescent formation. However, evidence of benefit from such therapies in animals with experimentally induced crescentic glomerulonephritis is inconsistent, in part because of variations in the severity of the disease models, the timing of treatment, and the nature of the anticoagulant or antithrombotic agent used. Anticoagulants may be hazardous in patients with advanced renal failure. *Ancrod,* a fibrinogenolytic agent not yet released in the United States, may also be an effective agent. *Intensive plasma exchange* (plasmapheresis—2 to 4 L of plasma daily or three times weekly), combined with steroids and cytotoxic agents, has been employed in patients with RPGN with very encouraging preliminary results, especially in patients revealing linear Ig deposits in glomeruli (anti-GBM antibody–mediated disease). A beneficial effect of intensive plasma exchange combined with immunosuppressive agents has also been claimed in patients with RPGN who do not demonstrate evidence of anti-GBM antibody production. Such benefit has been observed even when the patients have progressed to dialysis-dependent renal failure. Some of these latter patients may have a forme fruste of systemic necrotizing vasculitis. Since few prospective studies comparing the efficacy of glucocorticoids plus immunosuppressive agents versus combined intensive plasma exchange, glucocorticoids, and immunosuppressive agents have been performed, the contribution of intensive plasma exchange to the observed improvements has not been established.

Beneficial effects appear to be greatest when such combined therapy is instituted early in the course of disease, before glomerular abnormalities are advanced. Renal biopsy assessment of the nature, severity, and potential reversibility of disease is a vital aspect of evaluation of patients suspected of having rapidly progressive glomerulonephritis. Such biopsies should be performed early in the course of disease. Despite aggressive therapy, many patients with oliguria do poorly. Treatment must be individualized, and because regular dialysis therapy and/or transplantation are available to most patients with RPGN, one should probably err on the side of a conservative approach, unless compelling evidence in support of potential reversibility is present.

RPGN may recur after renal transplant. It is difficult to be certain of the precise risk in individual cases. At present it seems prudent to recommend that, after initiating dialysis, a period of 3 to 6 months be allowed to elapse before undertaking renal transplantation in patients who have circulating anti-GBM antibodies. There is no convincing evidence that bilateral nephrectomy in advance of transplantation reduces the risk of recurrent disease in the transplant.

THE NEPHROTIC SYNDROME

In its overt form, the nephrotic syndrome (NS) is characterized by *albuminuria, hypoalbuminemia, hyperlipidemia,* and *edema.* These abnormalities are direct or indirect consequences of excessive glomerular leakage of plasma proteins into the urine (see also Chaps. 38 and 49). The defects in the charge- or size-selective barriers of the glomerular capillary wall that underline the excessive filtration of plasma proteins can arise as a consequence of a wide variety of disease processes, including immunologic disorders, toxic injuries, metabolic abnormalities, biochemical defects, and vascular disorders. Thus, nephrotic syndrome is a common end point of a variety of disease processes damaging the permeability properties of the glomerular capillary wall. *Heavy proteinuria* is the hallmark of the nephrotic state. Arbitrarily, protein excretion rates in excess of 3.5 g per 1.73 m^2 surface area per day [or urinary protein concentration of greater than 0.4 mg/mmol (3.5 mg/dL) creatinine] are considered to be in the nephrotic range, primarily because proteinuria of this magnitude is seldom observed in tubulointerstitial and vascular diseases of the kidney. Sustained heavy proteinuria is often, but not invariably, accompanied by *hypoalbuminemia.* Excessive urinary losses, increased renal catabolism, and inadequate hepatic synthesis of albumin all contribute to this depression of plasma albumin. The resulting decrease in plasma oncotic pressure leads to a disturbance in the Starling forces acting across peripheral capillaries. Intravascular fluid migrates into the interstitial tissue (i.e., *edema*), particularly in areas of low tissue pressure. These disturbances initiate a series of homeostatic adjustments designed to correct the resulting deficit in effective plasma volume. These include activation of the renin-angiotensin-aldosterone system, enhanced vasopressin secretion, stimulation of the sympathetic nervous system, and perhaps an alteration in the secretion or renal response to atrial natriuretic peptide. These and other poorly understood adjustments lead to renal sodium and water retention, primarily because of avid reabsorption in distal nephron segments, resulting in unrelenting edema. The severity of edema correlates with the level of serum albumin and with the extent of urinary protein losses. The extent and severity of edema are conditioned by factors such as heart disease or peripheral vascular disease. Profound hypoalbuminemia may occasionally be associated with severe plasma volume reduction, postural hypotension, syncope, and shock. Occasionally acute renal failure may occur. Although this formulation indicates that nephrotic syndrome is invariably accompanied by a significant deficit in intravascular volume and homeostatically appropriate renal salt and water retention, this pattern is not always observed. In fact, measurements of plasma volume, renin, and aldosterone, and determination of the events underlying renal salt and water reabsorption have documented heterogeneity in the pathophysiology of fluid volume homeostasis. Some have expanded intravascular fluid volume and suppressed renin-aldosterone axis, presumably mediated by primary, non-aldosterone-dependent renal salt and fluid retention, resembling the pathophysiology of acute nephritis (see above). These patients often, but not invariably, have some decrease in GFR and structural glomerular lesions. At the other end of the spectrum are patients with overt hypovolemia, hyperreninemia, and avid secondary renal salt retention. Serum albumin levels are low, extracellular fluid volume is expanded, and edema is usually present in both groups.

The diminished plasma oncotic pressure also appears to stimulate hepatic lipoprotein synthesis, and *hyperlipidemia* is a frequent accompaniment of the nephrotic state. Low-density lipoproteins and cholesterol are elevated most frequently, but as the plasma oncotic pressure falls further, very low density lipoproteins and triglycerides also increase. Excessive urinary losses of plasma protein factors regulating lipoprotein synthesis or disposal may also contribute to the hyperlipidemic state. Whether these lipid abnormalities contribute to accelerated atherosclerosis remains controversial. Lipid bodies (fatty casts, oval fat bodies) commonly appear in the urine.

Urine losses of plasma proteins other than albumin are also of importance. Loss of thyroxine-binding globulin may produce abnormalities in thyroid function tests, including a low thyroxine and an enhanced resin triiodothyronine uptake. Loss of cholecalciferol-binding protein may lead to a vitamin D deficiency state and secondary hyperparathyroidism and may contribute to the hypocalcemia and hypocalciuria seen commonly. Enhanced urinary excretion of transferrin may produce an iron-resistant microcytic, hypochromic anemia. Zinc and copper deficiency may result from urinary losses of metal-binding proteins. A hypercoagulable state frequently accompanies severe nephrotic syndrome [serum albumin less than 20 g/L (2 g/dL)]. A variety of factors contribute to the enhanced tendency to thrombosis in nephrotic patients including deficiencies in antithrombin III (due to urine losses), reduced levels or activity of protein C or protein S, hyperfibrinogenemia, enhanced platelet aggregation, and hyperlipidemia.

Some patients develop severe IgG deficiency, in part due to urinary losses and hypercatabolism. Low-molecular-weight complement components may also be lost in the urine and contribute to defects in the opsonization of bacteria. Various drug-binding proteins (chiefly albumin) may be decreased, altering the pharmacokinetics and toxicity of many drugs. Cellulose acetate electrophoresis of serum reveals, in addition to diminished albumin levels, increases of alpha and beta globulins.

COMPLICATIONS AND MANAGEMENT OF THE NEPHROTIC SYNDROME *Edema* should be managed cautiously and conservatively. Overly vigorous diuresis with potent loop diuretics (furosemide or ethacrynic acid) may result in an abrupt decline in effective plasma volume as the deficit in plasma oncotic pressure may preclude mobilization of the extracellular fluid into the intravascular compartment. This is more likely to occur if plasma volume is diminished and may lead to further reduction in GFR, worsening azotemia, and postural hypotension. Severe extracellular volume depletion may predispose to the development of acute renal failure. The temptation to administer concentrated salt-poor albumin should be resisted, as nearly all the administered protein will be excreted in 24 to 48 h, so that any beneficial effect on plasma oncotic pressure will be transient. However, such treatment may be necessary in severely hypoalbuminemic patients suffering from profound postural symptoms or very refractory anasarca.

The treatment of *hyperlipidemia* is frequently unsuccessful, and its influence on morbidity and mortality is uncertain. Colestipol, probucol, and lovastatin can all result in modest decrements in plasma total cholesterol in patients with nephrotic hyperlipidemia. Whether such treatment will be associated with a reduction in risk for atherosclerosis and ischemic heart or cerebral disease is not proven.

The *thromboembolic complications* of NS are reasonably common, including spontaneous peripheral venous and/or arterial, pulmonary arterial, and renal venous occlusions. *Renal vein thrombosis* (RVT), either unilateral or bilateral, is a particularly distressing complication. In the past, this was regarded as a cause rather than a consequence of NS, a conclusion no longer held. Certain glomerular lesions are more likely than others to be associated with RVT. These include membranous glomerulonephritis, mesangiocapillary glomerulonephritis, and amyloidosis. Features suggestive of *acute* RVT include unilateral or bilateral flank or loin pain, gross hematuria, left-sided varicocele, widely fluctuating GFR and urinary protein excretion rates, and asymmetry of renal size and/or function. Scalloping of the ureters (due to collateral circulation) and evidence of pulmonary emboli and/or infarction (Chap. 230) may occur in chronic RVT.

Chronic forms of RVT are commonly asymptomatic. Some advocate an aggressive approach in patients with nephrotic syndrome due to lesions associated with inherently high prevalence of RVT (e.g., membranous glomerulonephritis), routinely employing selective renal venous angiography. If RVT is detected, long-term (optimal duration unknown) anticoagulants are prescribed. Such an approach might prevent later development of serious embolic complications, but since the true risk of pulmonary embolism in this group of patients is not known, although probably low, the benefits-risk relationship of this approach cannot be determined. A more conservative approach has also been advocated in which renal venous angiography is performed only in those patients who have a pulmonary embolism (e.g., symptoms, compatible laboratory findings, and a high-probability ventilation-perfusion scan or pulmonary angiogram) and who have negative noninvasive studies directed toward detecting deep venous thrombosis in the lower extremities. Since such patients would receive anticoagulant therapy in any case, the value of localizing the site of thrombosis is not established. Positive ventilation-perfusion scans in asymptomatic nephrotic patients are likely to have limited value, since subsegmental defects in perfusion may be observed in nephrotic patients even in the absence of renal vein or lower extremity deep venous thrombosis. These changes could conceivably be due to in situ pulmonary arterial thrombosis. The risk of renal vein thrombosis or deep venous thrombosis is increased primarily in patients with nephrotic syndrome and a very low serum albumin level [e.g., less than 20 g/L (2 g/dL)]. The presence of a documented thromboembolic complication is usually regarded as a clear indication for long-term oral anticoagulation. The effectiveness of heparin may be impaired by concomitant antithrombin III deficiency, a factor required for the full expression of the heparin-induced antithrombin effect.

High-protein diets are frequently prescribed; however, the beneficial effect of this approach can be challenged since the main effect of increasing dietary protein is to increase urinary protein excretion rate and the effect on serum albumin levels is modest. Furthermore, such diets are difficult to manage with concomitant salt restriction and, at least theoretically, could aggravate the progression of an underlying structural glomerular lesion. An alternative approach is to prescribe modest protein restriction (e.g., 0.6 g/kg body weight per day), particularly in azotemic patients; some also advocate adding a supplementary amount of dietary protein equal to urinary protein losses. Dietary protein should be of high biologic value and can be supplemented with amino acids. Plasma albumin and transferrin concentrations as well as urinary protein excretion rates should be monitored to evaluate the effect of diet on overall nutritional status. Correction of transport protein deficiencies is not feasible. Supplemental vitamin D might be desirable if deficiency is present, but this has not been fully evaluated clinically. In rare circumstances, profound protein malnutrition or other complications of massive proteinuria may justify ablation of renal function by medical or surgical means.

TABLE 227-3 Causes of the nephrotic syndrome

I Primary glomerular diseases*
A Minimal change disease*
B Mesangial proliferative glomerulonephritis†
C Focal and segmental glomerulosclerosis*
D Membranous glomerulonephritis*
E Mesangiocapillary glomerulonephritis*
1 Type I
2 Type II
3 Other variants
F Other uncommon lesions
1 Crescentic glomerulonephritis
2 Focal and segmental proliferative glomerulonephritis†
3 Unclassifiable lesions
II Secondary to other diseases
A Infections: poststreptococcal glomerulonephritis,* endocarditis, "shunt nephritis," secondary syphilis, leprosy, hepatitis B,* acquired immunodeficiency syndrome (AIDS), infectious mononucleosis, malaria, schistosomiasis, filariasis
B Drugs: organic gold; inorganic, organic, and elemental mercury; penicillamine; "street" heroin,* probenecid; captopril; Tridione; mesantoin; perchlorate; antivenom; antitoxins; contrast media
C Neoplasia: Hodgkin's disease, lymphomas, leukemia, carcinomas, melanoma, Wilms's tumor
D Multisystem: systemic lupus erythematosus,* Henoch-Schönlein purpura,* vasculitis, Goodpasture's syndrome, dermatomyositis, dermatitis herpetiformis, amyloidosis,* sarcoidosis, Sjögren's syndrome, rheumatoid arthritis
E Heredofamilial: diabetes mellitus,* Alport's syndrome, sickle cell disease, Fabry's disease, nail-patella syndrome, lipodystrophy, congenital nephrotic syndrome
F Miscellaneous: preeclamptic toxemia, thyroiditis, myxedema, malignant obesity, renovascular hypertension, chronic interstitial nephritis with vesicoureteric reflux, chronic allograft rejection, bee stings

* Most common.
† Includes Berger's disease (IgA nephropathy).

A classification of the causes of nephrotic syndrome is provided in Table 227-3. The multisystemic, heredofamilial, neoplastic, and metabolic causes are discussed in Chap. 228. The primary (idiopathic) glomerular diseases associated with nephrotic syndrome, as well as the diseases secondary to infectious or drug etiologies, are considered below.

IDIOPATHIC NEPHROTIC SYNDROME This diagnosis is arrived at by exclusion of known causes of NS, such as infections, drug exposure, malignancy, multisystem disease, or hereditary disorders. The idiopathic forms of NS are further classified according to the morphologic features found on renal biopsy (Table 227-4). Performance of a renal biopsy, at least among adults, is required for the accurate diagnosis of idiopathic NS and for the formulation of a rational plan of treatment. Children need not always be subjected to renal biopsy since careful clinical study can often lead to accurate diagnosis.

Minimal change disease This is often referred to as *lipoid nephrosis, nil lesion,* or *foot process disease*. In this form of idiopathic NS, although little or no alterations of the glomerular capillaries are demonstrable by light microscopy (hence the designation "minimal change"), *diffuse epithelial foot process effacement*[1] is evident by electron microscopy. Immunofluorescence microscopy reveals absent or irregular and nonspecific deposits of immunoglobulin and complement components (chiefly IgM and C3). Minimal change disease is the most frequently encountered form of idiopathic NS in children, accounting for more than 70 to 80 percent of cases diagnosed before

[1] The term "fusion" is often used to describe these changes in foot processes, although true fusion of cell membranes does not occur.

TABLE 227-4 Idiopathic nephrotic syndrome

SELECTED FEATURES OF UNDERLYING PRIMARY GLOMERULAR LESIONS

Lesion	Morphology* LM	IFM	EM	Approximate prevalence in children/adults, %	Common clinical/lab features	Response to therapy†	Likelihood of maintaining renal function‡
Minimal change	Normal or very mild proliferation	Negative–trace IgM	Foot process fusion, no deposits	70+/15–20	Highly selective proteinuria,§ *normal* C3, decreased IgG, increased IgM	Steroids++ Cytotoxic drugs+ (cyclophosphamide, chlorambucil) Frequent relapses	95+
Mesangial proliferative	Diffuse proliferation	Negative or variable mesangial IgM, IgG, C3¶	Mesangial deposits	15–20/5–10	Hematuria, *normal* C3	Steroids± Cytotoxic drugs (?)	80 (?)
Focal sclerosis	Focal and segmental sclerosis	Focal and segmental IgM, C3	Foot process fusion, sclerosis, hyaline	10/10–20	Hematuria, leukocyturia, poorly selective proteinuria, *normal* C3	Steroids + Cytotoxic drugs –	45–50
Membranous glomerulonephritis	Thick capillary wall, spikes of BM material	Diffuse granular capillary wall IgG	Subepithelial deposits	<5/30–40	Variable protein selectivity, *normal* C3, renal vein thrombosis	Steroids± Cytotoxic drugs +	70+
Mesangial proliferative glomerulonephritis							
Type I	Mesangial interposition, lobular change	Diffuse C3; variable IgG, IgM	Subendothelial deposits	8/<5	Hematuria, *reduced* C3 (intermittent)	Steroids (?) Anticoagulants (?) Cytotoxic drugs (?) Antithrombotics +	60
Type II	Mesangial interposition	C3 capillary wall and mesangial nodules	Intramembranous deposits	3/<5	Hematuria, *reduced* C3 (persistent), +C3NF	Steroids – Cytotoxic drugs –	45

* LM = light microscopy, IFM = immunofluorescence microscopy, EM = electron microscopy, BM = basement membrane.
† Response to therapy: ++ = highly responsive, + = variably responsive, ± = occasionally responsive, – = unresponsive.
‡ Percent of patients maintaining sufficient renal function to obviate need for chronic dialysis or transplantation within 5 years.
§ Protein selectivity = differential protein clearance, e.g., IgG/transferrin clearance ratio. Highly selective = <0.1, moderately selective = 0.11 to 0.20, poorly selective = >0.20.
¶ Ig deposits are seen in Berger's disease.
NOTE: C3NF = C3 nephritic factor.

the age of 8. This lesion is not rare in adults, representing 15 to 20 percent of cases of idiopathic NS in patients over the age of 16. There is a slight predilection for males. Typically patients present with overt NS, normal blood pressure, normal or slightly reduced GFR, and a "benign" urinary sediment. Varying degrees of microscopic hematuria are found in up to 20 percent of cases. Urinary protein is typically highly selective in children (e.g., it contains principally albumin and minimal amounts of high-molecular-weight plasma proteins such as IgG, $alpha_2$ macroglobulin, or C3) but is variable in adults. The pattern of protein excretion indicates a major "charge-selective" defect in permselectivity. Fibrin split products and C3 are absent in the urine. Serum levels of complement components are normal, except for a slight reduction in C1q. IgG concentrations are often quite depressed during relapse, whereas IgM levels are modestly increased, both during remission and relapse. Some cases may have associated allergic diathesis (e.g., to milk, pollens, etc.), a history of recent immunization, or upper respiratory infection. Circulating immune complexes may be found in some patients using certain assays. The histocompatibility antigen HLA-B12 is more prevalent when minimal change disease is associated with atopy, indicating a possible genetically based predisposition to this disease. Thromboembolic manifestations occur, but renal vein thrombosis is uncommon.

Spontaneous remissions and relapses of heavy proteinuria may occur. Interestingly, an identical lesion is encountered in patients with Hodgkin's disease in whom NS develops, suggesting a role for lymphocytes in its pathogenesis. Except for patients who develop focal and segmental sclerosing lesions (see below), a progressive decline in GFR does not occur. Acute renal failure is rare. In the preantibiotic era infection with encapsulated organisms (e.g., pneumococci) was a leading cause of death, but now the mortality rate is low, and most deaths are associated with complications of treatment rather than the disease itself. Rarely, acute renal failure may occur even without profound hypovolemia. The mechanism is obscure but could relate to tubular obstruction from heavy proteinuria or interstitial edema or severe glomerular epithelial cell effacement. The renal failure is often responsive to steroids and diuretics.

Since the etiology and pathogenesis are unknown, treatment is empirical and symptomatic. Glucocorticoids markedly enhance the natural tendency for this disease to undergo spontaneous remission. Daily or alternate-day oral steroid therapy seems to be equally effective; the latter is associated with fewer steroid-related complications. Daily prednisone (60 mg/m^2 surface area in children, 1 to 1.5 mg/kg body weight in adults) for 4 weeks, followed by alternate-day prednisone (35 to 40 mg/m^2 in children, 1 mg/kg in adults) for 4 additional weeks is a regimen often recommended for initial treatment of this disorder.

Over 95 percent of children (less than age 16) with minimal change disease respond with a complete disappearance of proteinuria within 8 weeks of the institution of prednisone therapy. Because of the high probability of minimal change disease in children, many pediatricians prefer to treat without an initial renal biopsy. A complete steroid response in such circumstances is highly indicative of underlying minimal change disease in children.

On the other hand, only about 30 to 70 percent of adults with minimal change disease respond within 8 weeks of instituting prednisone therapy, with a maximum response often not attained until 20 to 24 weeks from initiation of treatment. Patients over the age of 40 seem to be less responsive to steroids than those under the age of 40 when the disease is discovered. Ultimately the overall response rate in adults is only slightly less than that observed in children. The delayed response to glucocorticoids in adults could be due, in part, to the lower doses of prednisone relative to the doses used in children. Because of the likelihood of a lesion other than minimal change disease and the fact that some of these other lesions (e.g., focal sclerosis) may also sometimes respond to glucocorticoids, a steroid-responsive adult patient with idiopathic nephrotic syndrome cannot be assumed to have minimal change disease.

Among both adults and children, 50 to 60 percent of patients with minimal change disease relapse during the tapering phase of steroid withdrawal or at varying intervals after the cessation of therapy. Such relapses generally indicate a steroid-dependent patient. Frequent relapses (more than three per year) may require repetitive treatment with steroids and may be associated with exogenous Cushing's syndrome. Such patients can ordinarily be identified within 12 to 18 months after steroid treatment. Relapses may be treated with the initial regimen but with more gradual withdrawal of prednisone and with low maintenance doses of 5 to 10 mg daily or on alternate days for 3 to 6 months.

A steroid-dependent patient or one with multiple relapses may benefit by a brief course of cyclophosphamide 2 to 3 mg/kg body weight per day or chlorambucil 0.1 to 0.2 mg/kg body weight per day for 8 to 10 weeks. The steroid-dependent frequently relapsing patient has a lower likelihood of having a prolonged relapse-free interval after such therapy. Overall, only about half of frequently relapsing patients with minimal change disease treated with cyclophosphamide or chlorambucil remain free of disease after 5 years. Among children with minimal change disease the frequency of relapses declines with age. However, cytoxic agents have adverse effects on bone marrow and, in the case of cyclophosphamide, the gonads and urinary bladder. Careful monitoring of hematologic and urinary findings is mandatory. They may also be oncogenic. Azathioprine, previously believed to be ineffective in minimal change disease, will require reevaluation because of anecdotal reports of slow but eventual disappearance of proteinuria in patients with minimal change disease and steroid-sensitive or steroid-dependent nephrotic syndrome treated for 6 months to 1 year with azathioprine 2 to 2.5 mg/kg body weight per day. Cyclosporine in doses of 4 to 6 mg/kg body weight per day induces lasting remissions of nephrotic syndrome in as many as 50 percent of patients treated for 8 to 10 weeks. Further controlled trials are needed before this nephrotoxic agent can be recommended for routine use. Cyclosporine may yet prove to be valuable for steroid-dependent patients who continue to relapse despite cyclophosphamide or chlorambucil therapy or who become steroid unresponsive.

The use of cytotoxic agents should be reserved for patients who develop serious complications of multiple courses of steroid therapy. The long-term prognosis of patients with the minimal change lesion is excellent; a 10-year survival is in excess of 90 percent, but a few develop renal failure as a consequence of development of focal sclerosing glomerular lesions (see below) in association with acquired resistance to glucocorticoid therapy.

Mesangial proliferative glomerulonephritis The lesion is characterized by a mild to moderate diffuse, but distinct, increase in the cellularity of the glomerular capillary bed. The peripheral glomerular capillary walls are thin and delicate, and extracapillary proliferation is not seen. The precise nature of the proliferating cells is not clearly understood but may represent combinations of proliferating mesangial cells, endothelial cells, and infiltrating mononuclear cells. Glomerular involvement is usually reasonably uniform, although there may be segmental accentuation of hypercellularity. Necrosis of glomerular tufts is absent. Deposits of proteinaceous material, if seen, are confined to the mesangial areas. Interposition of mesangial cells and cytoplasm into the periphery of the glomerular capillary wall is not seen. By immunofluorescence, a variety of patterns are observed. If granular IgA deposits in the mesangium predominate, accompanied by C3 and fibrin-reactive antigens but not the early acting components of the complement cascade, then the lesion is categorized as IgA nephropathy, or Berger's disease (see below). Other patterns of immunofluorescence include a predominance of IgM deposits in a granular pattern diffusely throughout the mesangium, isolated mesangial C3 deposits, scattered mesangial IgG deposits, and no immunoglobulin or complement deposits. Thus, mesangial proliferative glomerulonephritis represents a heterogeneous group of glomerular diseases. Some patients with this morphologic lesion may in fact represent instances of resolving postinfectious glomerulonephritis, hereditary nephritis, or other multisystem diseases such as Henoch-

Schönlein purpura, vasculitis, or systemic lupus erythematosus. Electron-microscopic findings are nonspecific. Occasionally small electron-dense paramesangial deposits may be observed.

The findings of large electron-dense deposits in the mesangium in association with the morphologic appearance of mesangial proliferative glomerulonephritis should heighten the suspicion of a multisystem disease or Berger's IgA nephropathy. This lesion accounts for approximately 10 percent of idiopathic nephrotic syndrome in adults and 15 percent in children. It is more common in older children and young adults. Males are affected slightly more often than females. Hematuria, either gross or microscopic, is common. Loin pain, bilateral or unilateral, may be seen in the idiopathic disorder but is more frequently observed in patients who have underlying IgA nephropathy. Laboratory features are not distinctive. Renal function may be modestly decreased or normal at the time of diagnosis. Complement component levels are most often normal. IgG levels may be modestly reduced, and IgA levels may be increased. Antistreptolysin O titers are usually normal. Proteinuria is most often nonselective. The pathogenesis of this lesion is unknown and almost certainly the result of diverse pathogenetic processes. The presence of mesangial immunoglobulin deposits and circulating immune complexes in some, but not all, patients suggests an immune-complex pathogenesis, although the antigen(s) is unknown.

Among adult patients with well-developed nephrotic syndrome and moderate to severe diffuse mesangial proliferation, there is a tendency for persistence of proteinuria and progression to renal insufficiency. This is particularly true if focal and segmental glomerular sclerosis are superimposed on the mesangial proliferative lesion at the time of the initial biopsy. Patients with milder forms of mesangial proliferative glomerulonephritis, particularly when unassociated with mesangial immunoglobulin deposition, may follow a more benign course. Some patients, particularly children, behave in a fashion similar to those with the minimal change lesion. Since renal biopsies from patients with the minimal change lesion may display mild degrees of glomerular hypercellularity, the benign course followed by these patients may indicate that they have the minimal change lesion with more prominent mesangial proliferation rather than a separate disorder under the heading of mesangial proliferative glomerulonephritis. Well-developed mesangial proliferative lesions, particularly in association with mesangial IgM deposits, tend to be unresponsive to glucocorticoid therapy and to evolve into focal and segmental glomerular sclerosis. Indeed, mesangial proliferative glomerulonephritis may be a predecessor of the lesion of focal and segmental glomerulosclerosis. Patients with mesangial proliferative glomerulonephritis who have complete remission of proteinuria following treatment with glucocorticoids similar to that for the minimal change lesion tend to do well, with little inclination toward progressive renal insufficiency. Exacerbations and remissions of proteinuria may occur. Steroid-unresponsive patients with persistent nephrotic syndrome progress at variable rates to renal insufficiency. The role of adjunctive cytotoxic therapy (cyclophosphamide, chlorambucil, or azathioprine) has not yet been established in this disorder.

Because of the variable pathogenesis and the relative rarity of this disorder, long-term prospective studies of natural history and therapy have not been conducted. Many patients, particularly those with mild degrees of proliferation and a remitting course following glucocorticoids, have a very benign prognosis. Other patients, particularly those with steroid unresponsiveness and superimposed focal and segmental glomerulosclerosis on the initial biopsy, have a poor prognosis, often developing end-stage renal failure 5 to 10 years after the diagnosis.

Focal and segmental glomerulosclerosis (focal sclerosis) This lesion is characterized by sclerosis and hyalinization of some, but not all, glomeruli (hence the term *focal*). Among affected glomeruli, only a portion of the glomerular tuft is abnormal (hence, *segmental*). There is a predilection for these lesions initially to affect the *juxtamedullary glomeruli* and to be associated with progressive tubulointerstitial damage. By immunofluorescence, granular and nodular deposits of IgM and C3 are found in the segmental sclerosing lesion. By electron microscopy, focal basement membrane collapse and denudation of epithelial surfaces are noted. All glomeruli reveal diffuse epithelial foot process effacement. This lesion accounts for 10 to 15 percent of cases of idiopathic NS among children and adults. Males are affected more often than females. Focal sclerosis may represent a stage in the evolution of a subgroup of patients with minimal change disease or "pure" mesangial proliferative glomerulonephritis (see above). In more than two-thirds of cases of focal sclerosis overt NS is present at diagnosis; the remainder have proteinuria in the nonnephrotic range. Hypertension, reduced GFR, abnormal tubule function, and abnormal urinary sediment occur commonly. Focal sclerosis may have features indistinguishable from either minimal change disease, mesangial proliferative glomerulonephritis, or membranous glomerulopathy (see below). Proteinuria is nearly always nonselective or becomes so on follow-up. Fibrin degradation products and C3 may be present in the urine. Serum levels of C3 are normal and IgG levels are reduced, but not as severely as in minimal change disease. Similar lesions may be seen in association with heroin abuse, vesicoureteral reflux, acquired immunodeficiency syndrome, solitary kidney, and renal allograft rejection and may complicate other primary glomerular diseases in the late stages. The occurrence of focal and segmental glomerulosclerosis in remnant glomeruli after extensive renal ablation has led to the suggestion that hyperfiltration (or some hemodynamic determinant thereof) may play a causative role in pathogenesis. The attendant lipid abnormalities (e.g., hypercholesterolemia) may also contribute to the progressive nature of the underlying lesion. Abnormalities in the prevalence of HLA antigens have not been consistently described. Renal vein thrombosis is uncommon.

There is little tendency for spontaneous remission, except among children. GFR declines, albeit at variable rates. A subset of patients with focal sclerosis, heavy proteinuria (i.e., greater than 15 to 20 g/d), and profound hypoalbuminemia progress quite rapidly to end-stage renal failure, occasionally in a period of only a few months.

The etiology and pathogenesis of focal sclerosis are unknown. Immune-complex–mediated disease has been postulated, primarily on the basis of immunofluorescence findings, and circulating immune complexes have been found in some cases.

Although few prospective trials have been conducted, a decline in the level of proteinuria concomitant with glucocorticoid therapy and a lowered risk of progressive renal failure among patients with complete or partial remission of proteinuria suggest that steroids exert a beneficial effect on the natural history of the disorder. Indeed, between 20 and 40 percent of patients treated with either alternate-day prednisone (100 to 200 mg) or daily prednisone in a fashion similar to that described for minimal change disease experience complete or partial remissions of proteinuria. If such remissions persist following reduction of steroid dosage, significant protection from progressive renal failure may be provided. The effect of cytotoxic drugs and anticoagulants requires further study. At least half of patients with persistent heavy proteinuria develop end-stage renal failure or die of intercurrent illnesses within 10 years of diagnosis. The rate at which renal failure develops is inversely related to the magnitude of proteinuria. Patients who consistently excrete more than 10 g/d develop end-stage renal failure in a median of approximately 3 years. The prognosis is worse for those patients with azotemia or hypertension at diagnosis. This lesion recurs in renal allografts, occasionally within a few hours of transplantation, suggesting as its cause a circulating glomerular permeability "toxin."

Membranous glomerulonephritis This lesion is characterized by irregular, discontinuous proteinaceous deposits along the outer (or subepithelial) aspect of the glomerular capillary wall. These deposits contain IgG and appear dense by electron microscopy. Unlike focal sclerosis, *all glomeruli are involved uniformly*. At an early stage all glomeruli may appear normal by light microscopy, but as the disease progresses, immune deposits coalesce, and new basement membrane-like material is produced, causing the capillary wall to thicken.

Eventually, increased amounts of basement membrane material project toward the urinary space, giving the appearance of "spikes." There is little proliferation of capillary endothelial or mesangial cells, although mesangial sclerosis may occur in advanced cases. Tubulointerstitial atrophy and vascular lesions are other late manifestations.

This disorder accounts for 30 to 40 percent of cases of idiopathic NS in adults but is rare in children. In over 80 percent of cases the nephrotic syndrome is overt. In the remainder only isolated proteinuria is found. Men are affected more often than women. Blood pressure, GFR, and urinary sediment tend to be normal early in the course, making it difficult to distinguish membranous glomerulopathy from minimal change disease on clinical grounds. Urinary protein selectivity is quite variable. Serum complement components are normal, but IgG levels are modestly depressed. Membranous glomerulonephritis may develop in association with systemic lupus erythematosus (Chap. 228), certain chronic infections (e.g., malaria, hepatitis B), solid tumors (e.g., melanoma and cancer of the lung and colon), or exposure to heavy metals (gold, mercury) or drugs (penicillamine, captopril). A careful search for these causes is warranted in every case of membranous glomerulonephritis. Renal vein thrombosis is frequent in affected patients (see above).

Spontaneous complete remissions of NS are common in children and occur in 20 to 40 percent of adults. Steroid treatment does not greatly influence the development of lasting complete remissions, but may reduce proteinuria to nonnephrotic levels. A long-term beneficial effect of steroids is still a source of controversy. There is no agreement as to the optimal management. Retrospective surveys have often demonstrated no apparent difference in overall mortality or progression to renal failure. Prospective clinical trials have reported efficacy for short-term, high-dose, alternate-day prednisone and for combinations of intravenous methylprednisolone, oral prednisone, and chlorambucil and combinations of prednisone and cyclophosphamide, particularly in the subgroup with progressive renal failure and persistent heavy proteinuria.

Since the long-term prognosis for patients with idiopathic membranous glomerulonephritis is favorable, a conservative approach to treatment is generally recommended. Parameters to identify patients likely to develop progressive renal insufficiency include male sex, older age at onset, presence of hypertension, presence of elevated serum creatinine at discovery, presence of hypertension, and, possibly, severe hyperlipidemia and proteinuria greater than 10 g/d. Renal biopsy findings do not greatly aid in the determination of prognosis, but very advanced glomerular capillary wall alterations, segmental sclerosis, interstitial fibrosis, and tubular atrophy all augur a poor prognosis. Patients with several features associated with a poor prognosis may be candidates for a more aggressive therapeutic approach. Delay of such an aggressive approach to therapy (e.g., combined cytotoxic agents and glucocorticoids) until *after* renal impairment is progressive is advocated by some investigators. Nevertheless, many physicians treat patients with idiopathic membranous glomerulonephritis with a course of alternate-day prednisone as described above for 8 weeks followed by a week of tapering dosage. Such a regimen is seldom associated with adverse consequences unless some contraindication to steroid administration is present. Whether such treatment will prevent end-stage renal failure in patients so treated remains to be established. As indicated above, slowly progressive renal functional impairment occurs almost exclusively in those patients with persistent proteinuria in the nephrotic range. Such renal failure seldom develops within 3 to 4 years of diagnosis. However, on occasion patients may have a more rapidly progressive course. The rapid decline of renal function in a patient with membranous glomerulonephritis suggests a complicating drug-induced interstitial nephritis, acute renal vein thrombosis, or superimposed crescentic glomerulonephritis. Within 10 years of the time of the diagnosis, however, 20 to 30 percent of patients die of intercurrent illness or develop end-stage renal failure. The majority of survivors have complete or partial remission of proteinuria. A few patients have developed superimposed RPGN.

Mesangiocapillary glomerulonephritis This disorder is characterized by proliferation of mesangial cells, often with segmental or diffuse interposition of these cells or their cytoplasm into peripheral capillary loops. Mesangial matrix synthesis is increased as well. The glomerular capillary wall is irregularly thickened, by virtue of the mesangial extensions and the attendant synthesis of basement membrane–like material. This group of disorders is also known as *membranoproliferative* or *lobular glomerulonephritis*. Several immunofluorescence and electron-microscopic patterns are present and reflect heterogeneous mechanisms of pathogenesis. In the *type I* lesion, subendothelial electron-dense deposits are present, C3 is deposited in a granular pattern indicative of immune-complex pathogenesis, and IgG and the early components of complement may or may not be present. In the *type II* lesion the lamina densa of the GBM is transformed into an electron-dense character, giving rise to the term *dense deposit disease*. Basement membranes in Bowman's capsules and in tubules are similarly affected. C3 is found irregularly in the GBM and in granules or rings in the mesangium. Small amounts of Ig (typically IgM) are present, but the early acting complement components are absent from the deposits. Properdin deposition is variable. Additional ultrastructural variants, based upon location of deposit and basement membrane changes, have also been described.

Mesangiocapillary glomerulonephritis, types I and II, is found in 5 to 10 percent of idiopathic NS in children, particularly between the ages of 8 to 16 years, and somewhat less commonly in adults. Type I accounts for at least two-thirds of cases. Males and females are affected equally. In 50 to 75 percent of patients, a full-blown NS is present, often with features of AGN. In the remainder, proteinuria in the nonnephrotic range is nearly always accompanied by microscopic hematuria. Blood pressure and GFR are frequently abnormal, and the urinary sediment is active. Functional abnormalities of the renal tubules are common. Urinary protein selectivity is usually poor; fibrin degradation products and C3 are found in the urine. Serum C3 levels are reduced in the majority of cases. The early acting complement components C1q, C4, and C2 are often normal, especially in type II disease. This pattern may be indicative of activation of the alternate complement pathway (see Chap. 226). C3 nephritic factor (C3NF) is often found in the serum of patients with type II, especially if the C3 level is quite low. Circulating immune complexes are found in type I. Lesions similar to type I membranoproliferative glomerulonephritis may also be found in SLE, hemolytic-uremic syndrome, transplant rejection, chronic hepatitis B antigenemia, and "shunt" nephritis. Renal vein thrombosis may occur. Type II nephritis may be associated with partial lipodystrophy.

Spontaneous remissions are uncommon. Long-term, alternate-day prednisone therapy (0.3 to 0.5 mg/kg body weight every other day) may delay the progression of the disease. Treatment regimens that combine steroids and cytotoxic agents are not of proven value. Anticoagulants and inhibitors of platelet aggregation (acetylsalicylic acid plus dipyridamole) may have a beneficial effect. The course is progressive, and approximately half of patients die or develop end-stage renal failure within 10 years of the diagnosis. The prognosis for type II lesions seems somewhat worse than for type I. Type II disease almost invariably recurs in the transplanted kidney but does not always result in the premature loss of the allograft.

Other forms of idiopathic nephrotic syndrome In a small percentage of adults and children with idiopathic NS (i.e., 5 to 10 percent) other lesions are encountered on renal biopsy. These include *crescentic glomerulonephritis* and *focal* and *segmental proliferative glomerulonephritis*. The pathogenetic mechanisms for these lesions vary. For example, some cases of focal and segmental glomerulonephritis may have extensive mesangial IgA deposits and fit into the category of Berger's disease (see below). Serum C3 levels are usually normal. The clinical characteristics, natural history, and response to treatment of these lesions are not well defined. Hematuria is common and may be recurrent. Proteinuria tends to be nonselective. Spontaneous remissions of NS are uncommon. Since no controlled studies have been conducted, it is not possible to evaluate the effectiveness of treatment. Crescentic glomerulonephritis is likely to have a poor prognosis, whereas mesangial and focal and segmental proliferative glomerulonephritis have a more favorable long-term outlook.

NEPHROTIC SYNDROME CAUSED BY INFECTIOUS AGENTS, DRUGS, OR CHEMICALS Table 227-3 lists the common infectious and drug-related etiologies of NS. In many instances, NS abates following cure of the infection or withdrawal of the offending medication. In patients receiving gold therapy for rheumatoid arthritis or in those exposed to inorganic, organic, or elemental mercury or to penicillamine, membranous glomerulonephritis is usually the lesion responsible for NS. NS is known to follow immunization and antiserum treatment of tetanus or snakebite and to occur in situations associated with atopy.

ASYMPTOMATIC URINARY ABNORMALITIES

This group of patients has *proteinuria in the nonnephrotic range and/or hematuria,* unaccompanied by edema, reduced GFR, or hypertension. Abnormalities are often discovered incidentally and may be persistent or recurrent. In some this syndrome is a phase in the natural history of other glomerulopathic syndromes, especially nephrotic syndrome or chronic glomerulonephritis. Common glomerular disorders that present as asymptomatic proteinuria and/or hematuria are listed in Table 227-5. The heredofamilial and multisystem diseases are discussed in Chap. 228. The presence of dysmorphic erythrocytes and/or red cell casts indicates a glomerular cause for the hematuria.

IDIOPATHIC RENAL HEMATURIA (See also Chap. 49) **Berger's disease (IgA nephropathy)** This disorder was first described by Berger and Hinglais in 1968 and is characterized by recurrent episodes of gross or microscopic hematuria. The diagnosis depends on the finding of prominent IgA deposits in the mesangium by immunofluorescence microscopy. Berger's disease is the most common cause of recurrent hematuria of glomerular origin. It most commonly affects young adults, mostly men. Typically, episodes of macroscopic hematuria are associated with minor flulike illnesses or vigorous exercise. Vague constitutional symptoms may be present, but skin rash, arthritis, and abdominal pain are absent. Urine protein excretion rates are usually less than 3.5 g/d; protein excretion is normal or only mildly increased. The nephrotic syndrome develops occasionally. In some patients a self-limited and reversible form of acute renal failure may occur. Such episodes are frequently preceded by an upper respiratory infection and accompanied by bouts of macroscopic hematuria. Thus, these patients resemble those with acute poststreptococcal glomerulonephritis. Renal biopsy may reveal scattered noncircumferential crescentic glomerulonephritis, usually involving less than half of glomeruli, accompanied by marked tubular abnormalities, interstitial nephritis, and erythrocytes in tubular lumina. On rare occasions, patients present with the syndrome of malignant hypertension. Blood pressure, GFR, and serum albumin are usually normal early in the disease. Serum IgA levels are increased in about 50 percent of cases, while serum complement component levels remain normal. Biopsy of the skin of the volar surface of the forearm sometimes reveals dermal capillary deposits of IgA, C3, and fibrin but not early acting complement components or IgA secretory fragments. Similar skin biopsy findings are encountered in Henoch-Schönlein purpura (Chap. 228). Indeed, Berger's disease may be a monosymptomatic form of Henoch-Schönlein purpura.

TABLE 227-5 Glomerular causes of asymptomatic urinary abnormalities

I Hematuria with or without proteinuria
- *A* Primary glomerular diseases
  - *1* Berger's disease (IgA nephropathy)*
  - *2* Mesangiocapillary glomerulonephritis
  - *3* Other primary glomerular hematurias accompanied by "pure" mesangial proliferation, focal and segmental proliferative glomerulonephritis, or other lesions
  - *4* "Thin basement membrane" disease (? forme fruste of Alport's syndrome)
- *B* Associated with multisystem or heredofamilial diseases
  - *1* Alport's syndrome and other "benign" familial hematurias*
  - *2* Fabry's disease
  - *3* Sickle cell disease
- *C* Associated with infections
  - *1* Resolving poststreptococcal glomerulonephritis*
  - *2* Other postinfectious glomerulonephritides*

II Isolated nonnephrotic proteinuria
- *A* Primary glomerular diseases
  - *1* "Orthostatic" proteinuria*
  - *2* Focal and segmental glomerulosclerosis*
  - *3* Membranous glomerulonephritis*
- *B* Associated with multisystem or heredofamilial diseases
  - *1* Diabetes mellitus*
  - *2* Amyloidosis*
  - *3* Nail-patella syndrome

* Most common.

Renal biopsy reveals a spectrum of changes, but diffuse mesangial proliferative or focal and segmental proliferative glomerulonephritis is found most often. In some cases glomerular morphology may be normal by light microscopy; uncommonly, crescents may be found (see above). The distinguishing feature is the finding by immunofluorescence microscopy of *diffuse mesangial deposition of IgA,* often accompanied by lesser amounts of IgG and nearly always by C3 and properdin, but not by C1q or C4. Fibrin reactive antigens are also common in the mesangium or in association with crescents if the latter are present. The pathogenesis of IgA nephropathy is unknown, but the systemic character of the IgA deposits (skin and glomerular capillaries), the presence of circulating IgG and IgA complexes in the majority of cases, and its similarity to Henoch-Schönlein purpura suggest that it is an immune-complex–mediated disease. The nature and source of the antigen are unknown.

The prognosis is variable, but the disease tends to progress slowly. Approximately 50 percent of patients develop end-stage renal failure within 25 years of the time of diagnosis. Azotemia, hypertension, or proteinuria in the nephrotic range at diagnosis are associated with a poor prognosis. At present, there is no evidence that therapy influences the natural history, although intermittent steroid therapy or broad-spectrum antibiotics may reduce the frequency of episodes of gross hematuria. Glucocorticoids may also result in remissions of proteinuria in those patients with nephrotic syndrome and mild glomerular abnormalities by light microscopy. IgA nephropathy recurs in the transplanted kidney in approximately 30 to 40 percent of cases. Such recurrences seldom result in loss of renal function but may be associated with hematuria.

Other primary renal hematurias Some cases of recurrent hematuria do not reveal the typical immunofluorescence findings seen in Berger's disease. This group of patients is poorly defined, and the etiology and pathogenesis are varied. Some may represent resolving episodes of acute glomerulonephritis or early examples of mesangiocapillary or hereditary glomerulonephritis (Alport's syndrome, see Chap. 228). The common morphologic lesions are focal and segmental or diffuse mesangial proliferative glomerulonephritis, although mild and nonspecific glomerular changes may also be observed. Immunofluorescence studies reveal varying degrees of immunoglobulin and/or complement component deposition (principally IgM and/or C3) in the mesangium. Some cases show linear deposits of IgG, suggesting a possible anti-GBM antibody pathogenesis. Electron microscopy may reveal dense deposits in the mesangium or thin and attenuated glomerular basement membranes. Overall, these patients have an excellent prognosis, with frequent spontaneous permanent remissions of recurrent hematuria. Progressive renal insufficiency is unusual. Because of the benign prognosis no treatment is indicated.

ISOLATED NONNEPHROTIC PROTEINURIA OF GLOMERULAR ORIGIN (See also Chap. 49) Mild to moderate degrees of proteinuria (i.e., greater than 150 mg but less than 2.0 g/d), unaccompanied by abnormalities in the urinary sediment or evidence of hypertension or reduced renal function, are common. Such patients may display other features of heredofamilial or multisystem diseases, including diabetes mellitus, amyloidosis, rheumatoid arthritis, or cancer. The abnormality may either be persistent or evanescent. Proteinuria may occur primarily in the upright posture (*orthostatic proteinuria*) or be present both in recumbent and erect positions (*constant proteinuria*). Fixed and reproducible orthostatic proteinuria has a benign prognosis and frequently disappears on long-term follow-up. Renal biopsies reveal normal glomeruli or trivial alterations of dubious significance. On the other hand, persistent and constant proteinuria may be indicative of a more serious disease, and renal biopsies often reveal definite evidence of a structural lesion. Some of the lesions have been discussed in the context of idiopathic nephrotic syndrome. Other patients have an unsuspected disease such as amyloidosis or diabetes mellitus. In the remainder, the lesions are usually trivial and nonspecific, and the long-term significance is uncertain. In primary glomerular diseases, so long as urinary protein excretion remains modest, the prognosis is excellent, and deterioration of renal function is uncommon. Renal biopsy is not commonly undertaken in patients with persistent and isolated nonnephrotic proteinuria, as determining underlying morphology seldom leads to specific therapy and adds information chiefly of a prognostic nature. Since patients with proteinuria more than 2.0 g/d are more likely to have lesions that will progress, many nephrologists limit renal biopsies to this latter group of patients.

CHRONIC GLOMERULONEPHRITIS

The syndrome of chronic glomerulonephritis (CGN) is characterized chiefly by *persistent urinary abnormalities* (e.g., proteinuria and/or hematuria) and by *slowly progressive impairment of renal function,* eventuating in hypertension, contracted, granular kidneys, and end-stage renal failure. With the possible exception of the minimal change lesion associated with idiopathic nephrotic syndrome (see above) all the disorders described in this chapter and in Chap. 228 can lead eventually to CGN. The pathophysiology of CGN in the context of renal failure is described in Chaps. 222 and 224.

The structural alterations in this syndrome may be categorized as *proliferative* (including mesangial, endo- and/or extracapillary proliferative glomerulonephritis, and focal and segmental proliferative glomerulonephritis), *sclerosing* (including focal and diffuse glomerular sclerosis), and *membranous*. Such lesions are found in most patients with CGN. In the remainder, the underlying lesions are not readily categorized morphologically, and they are often referred to as *chronic "nonspecific" glomerulonephritis.*

The clinical characteristics of the specific lesions are described in other sections of this chapter. The etiologic and pathogenetic origins of chronic nonspecific glomerulonephritis are undoubtedly heterogeneous. Complicating vascular disease contributes to the glomerular obliteration. Some of the patients categorized as having chronic nonspecific glomerulonephritis may have had an earlier unrecognized or undiagnosed episode of acute PSGN.

The detection of CGN usually occurs in one of several ways: (1) the incidental finding of abnormal urine, impaired renal function, or hypertension during multiphasic screening of asymptomatic individuals or evaluation of such individuals for an unrelated illness; (2) the result of the insidious onset of progressive symptoms or signs of advanced renal disease, especially anemia and hypertension; or (3) after an exacerbation of glomerulonephritis, usually during the course of a nonspecific viral or bacterial illness. In advanced stages, the clinical separation of CGN from other causes of renal failure may be difficult; however, the presence of symmetrically contracted kidneys, moderate to heavy proteinuria, abnormal urinary sediment (especially red blood cell casts), and x-ray evidence of normal pyelocalyceal systems are all suggestive of CGN.

The evolution of CGN varies, depending upon the nature of the underlying disease and the presence or absence of complications, especially hypertension. Ten, fifteen, twenty, or more years may elapse from the first discovery of an abnormal urine sediment until the development of end-stage renal failure. Renal biopsy is necessary to define the precise nature of the underlying glomerular lesion. The principal advantage of a morphologic evaluation among patients presenting with the syndrome of CGN is to determine prognosis rather than therapy.

Treatment is supportive and symptomatic. Despite many years of controlled and uncontrolled trials, unequivocal evidence of a favorable effect of treatment with steroids, cytotoxic agents, nonsteroidal anti-inflammatory agents, and anticoagulants has yet to be provided. The management of specific lesions is discussed in greater detail in the relevant sections of this chapter. Hypertension and symptomatic urinary tract infections should be treated vigorously, taking care to avoid nephrotoxic agents. Diuretics should generally be employed only as adjuncts to antihypertensive management or to deal with debilitating degrees of edema. Rigorous salt restriction is usually unnecessary and may be hazardous. In the absence of congestive heart failure or marked hypoalbuminemia, severe edema is rare until the terminal phases of the illness. Potassium restriction is usually unnecessary. Protein and phosphate restriction may slow the rate of progression of renal failure.

REFERENCES

Cameron JS, Glassock RJ (eds): *The Nephrotic Syndrome*. New York, Dekker, 1988

Emancipator S, Schena FP (eds): Immunoglobulin A nephropathy. Semin Nephrol 7:275, 1987

Glassock RJ et al: Primary glomerular diseases, in *The Kidney*, 3d ed, BM Brenner, FC Rector Jr (eds). Philadelphia, Saunders, 1986, p 929

Korbet SM et al: Minimal-change glomerulopathy of adulthood. Am J Nephrol 8:291, 1988

Rodriguez-Iturbe B: Epidemic post-streptococcal glomerulonephritis. Kidney Int 25:129, 1984

Short CD, Mallick N: Membranous glomerulopathy, in *Textbook of Nephrology*, 2d ed, S Massry, R Glassock (eds). Baltimore, Williams and Wilkins (in press)

228 GLOMERULOPATHIES ASSOCIATED WITH MULTISYSTEM DISEASES

RICHARD J. GLASSOCK / BARRY M. BRENNER

Glomerular injury may be a prominent feature of diseases that affect multiple organs and systems. By and large the etiologies of these diseases are unknown, but aberrant immunologic processes, neoplasia, metabolic disturbances, and biochemical abnormalities are believed to be dominant factors in their pathogenesis. These processes lead to alterations in glomerular structure and function. Some of the glomerular lesions are specific for the underlying disease (e.g., amyloidosis, nodular diabetic glomerulosclerosis); however, the majority are nonspecific. Proteinuria results from defects in the charge- and/or size-selective glomerular permeability barriers. Reductions in glomerular filtration rate develop because of loss of filtration surface area. Although the extrarenal manifestations are useful in establishing a diagnosis, some may present with predominant or exclusive renal involvement and only covert extrarenal manifestations.

IMMUNOLOGICALLY MEDIATED MULTISYSTEM DISEASES

SYSTEMIC LUPUS ERYTHEMATOSUS (See also Chap. 269) Systemic lupus erythematosus (SLE) is the archetype of an immunologically mediated disease and is representative of the multisystem diseases in which renal involvement is common. The etiology of SLE is unknown; however, viral infection, genetic factors, and abnormal immune responsiveness probably interact to produce the disease. The principal mechanism for tissue injury in SLE appears to be the deposition of circulating immune complexes, although other mechanisms may also play a role, including antitissue antibody and in situ immune-complex formation (see Chap. 226). The circulating immune complexes may be composed of a variety of endogenous antigens combined with autoantibodies. DNA (single-stranded and double-stranded) is a major antigenic component of immune complexes. The prevalence of clinical renal involvement in SLE ranges from as low as 35 percent to more than 90 percent in different series. Manifestations of renal disease range from mild abnormalities of the urinary sediment (predominantly hematuria) to massive proteinuria, and from chronic indolent glomerulonephritis to a fulminant inflammatory process leading to rapidly progressive renal failure.

The diagnosis and extrarenal manifestations of SLE are described in Chap. 269. This section will deal with the renal involvement. Although extrarenal features usually dominate the clinical picture, SLE may present initially with renal manifestations. Morphologic evidence of renal involvement may exist with or without clinical manifestations. If immunofluorescence and electron-microscopic studies of renal tissue are performed, abnormalities are present in virtually every patient with SLE. The abnormal glomerular morphologic lesions in SLE form a spectrum based upon correlative light- and electron-microscopic and immunofluorescence studies of renal biopsies.

Minimal lupus glomerular lesion This pattern is characterized by few or no changes by light microscopy. Immunofluorescence studies reveal moderate immunoglobulin (Ig) and complement deposits exclusively in mesangium. Scattered electron-dense deposits are found in mesangium by electron microscopy. Clinical manifestations may include mild proteinuria and microscopic hematuria. Nephrotic syndrome is uncommon. Glomerular filtration rate (GFR) is almost always normal. Serologic manifestations vary depending upon the activity of extrarenal disease. Antibodies to DNA are usually present in low titer, and levels of C3 and C4 may be decreased, especially if dermatitis is severe. Circulating immune complexes may also be detected in skin lesions.

Mesangial lupus glomerulonephritis This pattern is characterized by mild to moderate diffuse mesangial cell proliferation and/or mesangial sclerosis. Immunofluorescence studies reveal immunoglobulins (IgG, IgM, and IgA) and complement components (C1q, C4, and C3) deposited in a granular pattern principally in the mesangium. By electron microscopy, electron-dense deposits are also found to be confined to the mesangium. This morphologic appearance may be present in the absence of clinical renal disease or may be associated with minor abnormalities in the urinary sediment and modest proteinuria. Nephrotic syndrome and hypertension may occasionally be present. GFR is almost always normal. Mesangial lupus glomerulonephritis may be the initial renal involvement in SLE, from which other patterns evolve. Associated serologic abnormalities depend upon the degree of extrarenal activity. These include increased levels of antibody to denatured, single-stranded DNA (ssDNA) or native, double-stranded DNA (dsDNA); depressed serum levels of C3, C4, and C1q; and detectable levels of circulating immune complexes (CIC) (Table 228-1).

Focal and segmental lupus glomerulonephritis This pattern is characterized by focal and segmental cellular proliferation, often associated with necrosis, superimposed on diffuse mesangial hypercellularity. Granular deposits of immunoglobulins and complement involve both the mesangium and occasional glomerular capillary loops. By electron microscopy, dense subendothelial deposits are found in the mesangium and in a few peripheral capillary loops. Clinical and laboratory evidence of renal injury is more common than in mesangial lupus glomerulonephritis. Nephrotic syndrome may occur in 10 to 20 percent of patients, but in general GFR is well preserved. This lesion may persist, resolve, or progress to diffuse proliferative lupus glomerulonephritis. Serologic features of active disease are often present in untreated patients.

Diffuse proliferative lupus glomerulonephritis This pattern is characterized by diffuse mesangial and endothelial cell proliferation that may include extensive peripheral capillary wall interposition of mesangial cells. In addition focal cellular necrosis, hematoxylinophilic bodies, fibrinoid necrosis, and "wire loops" (capillaries whose basement membranes are thickened markedly owing to subendothelial deposits) may be present. Extensive extracapillary proliferative (crescentic) glomerulonephritis, vasculitis, and interstitial nephritis may also be found. Varying degrees of chronic lesions may also be present. These include focal and segmental glomerulosclerosis, fibrocellular crescents, interstitial fibrosis, tubular atrophy, and nephroangiosclerosis. Granular deposits of immunoglobulins and complement components are extensive and involve the mesangium and nearly every capillary loop. Electron microscopy reveals extensive subendothelial and mesangial electron-dense deposits as well as occasional intramembranous or subepithelial deposits. Most patients have an active urinary sediment, heavy proteinuria, and progressive impairment of renal function; occasionally, clinical evidence of renal involvement is lacking. In the untreated patient evidence of serologic activity is usually present, including depressed serum C3 and C4 concentrations, high levels of precipitating and nonprecipitating complement-fixing antibody to dsDNA, cryoimmunoglobulinemia, and circulating immune complexes. This lesion is associated with an ominous prognosis, although vigorous treatment may modify the course (see below).

Membranous lupus glomerulonephritis This pattern is nearly identical with that described for idiopathic membranous glomerulonephritis (Chap. 227), except that mesangial deposits and mesangial proliferation are more frequent. There is thickening of the glomerular capillary wall due to the presence of immunoglobulin and complement-

TABLE 228-1 Serologic findings in selected multisystem diseases

Disease	C3	Ig	FANA	Anti-dsDNA	Anti-GBM	Cryo-Ig	CIC	ANCA
Systemic lupus erythematosus	↓ ↓	↑ IgG	+ + +	+ +	−	+ +	+ + +	±
Goodpasture's syndrome	−	−	−	−	+ + +	−	±	−
Henoch-Schönlein purpura	−	↑ IgA	−	−	−	±	+ +	−
Polyarteritis	↓ ↑	↑ IgG	+	±	−	+ +	+ + +	+ + +
Wegener's granulomatosis	↓ ↑	↑ IgA, IgE	−	−	−	±	+ +	+ + +
Cryoimmunoglobulinemia	↓	±	−	−	−	+ + +	+ +	−
Multiple myeloma	−	↓ ↑ IgG, IgA, IgD, IgE	−	−	−	+	±	−
Waldenström's macroglobulinemia	−	↑ IgM	−	−	−	−	−	−
Amyloidosis	−	± Ig	−	−	−	−	−	−

NOTE: C3 = C3 component of complement; Ig = immunoglobulin levels; FANA = fluorescent antinuclear antibody assay; anti-dsDNA = antibody to double-stranded (native) DNA; anti-GBM = antibody to glomerular basement membrane antigens; cryo-Ig = cryoimmunoglobulin; CIC = circulating immune complexes; ANCA = anti-neutrophil cytoplasmic antibody; − = normal; + = occasionally slightly abnormal; + + = often abnormal; + + + = severely abnormal.

containing electron-dense deposits in the subepithelial space, often associated with a spike-like basement membrane reaction. Nearly all patients have heavy proteinuria and the nephrotic syndrome. Although GFR may be normal initially, most patients ultimately develop progressive renal failure. A proliferative lesion may occasionally evolve, and the prognosis then assumes that of diffuse proliferative glomerulonephritis. Serologic features of SLE may or may not be present at the time of diagnosis of this nephropathy. Antibody to dsDNA tends to be nonprecipitating. Some patients with membranous lupus glomerulonephritis may be erroneously categorized as having idiopathic membranous glomerulopathy (see Chap. 227). Measurements of the level of antibody to dsDNA or ssDNA and circulating immune complexes and biopsies of skin for dermal-epidermal deposits of Ig (''lupus band test'') may be helpful for diagnosis in such cases.

Sclerosing or end-stage lupus glomerulonephritis This pattern is characterized by obliterative and sclerosing lesions of the glomeruli and probably represents a late stage of proliferative lesions. Immunofluorescence studies may be only weakly positive for immunoglobulins; subendothelial deposits are infrequent. Hypertension and impaired renal function are common. Serologic parameters of activity of SLE may or may not be present.

Prognosis and treatment The prognosis and treatment of SLE with renal involvement depends upon the nature of the underlying renal lesion especially with regard to the class and the activity of the morphologic disease and to the extent and severity of associated glomerulosclerosis and interstitial fibrosis. Patients with milder forms of renal disease (e.g., minimal, mesangial, or focal lupus glomerulonephritis) tend to do well if treatment is directed to control of the extrarenal manifestations of the disease. Glucocorticoids in modest doses, salicylates, or antimalarials are usually sufficient. Potent nonsteroidal, anti-inflammatory agents may cause functional depression of GFR and should be used with caution in patients with known renal involvement. Serologic parameters, including anti-dsDNA and complement components (C3, C4), should be followed serially. Fluorescent antinuclear antibody tests have little value in prognosis or in following the effectiveness of treatment. A return to normal values for antibody to dsDNA and/or complement components is a favorable sign; however, persistently abnormal serologic features do not necessarily indicate worsening or progressive renal involvement, especially in patients with active extrarenal manifestations. For patients with mild lesions, 85 percent or more can be expected to survive at least 10 years. Patients with membranous lupus glomerulonephritis who receive treatment directed primarily at the extrarenal features also have favorable long-term prognosis. On the other hand, patients with diffuse proliferative lupus glomerulonephritis do less well and, therefore, warrant a more aggressive approach toward ameliorating the renal disease. High-dose, long-term oral glucocorticoid therapy, although capable of improving extrarenal signs of active disease and reducing the acute inflammatory component of the renal lesions, is not an altogether satisfactory regimen for lupus nephritis. Such treatment is associated with a high prevalence of side effects and may not prevent progression of chronic lesions. High-dose, short-term intravenous methylprednisolone is effective in reducing signs of systemic activity of the disease, especially in patients with recent deterioration. Adjunctive use of cytotoxic agents (azathioprine, cyclophosphamide, or chlorambucil) exerts a steroid-sparing effect and may prevent progression of chronic lesions, particularly among those with mild chronic lesions prior to therapy. The optimal regimen has not yet been established; however, intermittent intravenous cyclophosphamide (500 to 1000 mg/m^2 surface area monthly for 6 to 12 months) plus low-dose oral prednisone (0.5 mg/kg body weight per day) and combinations of azathioprine, cyclophosphamide, and low-dose oral prednisone appear to be relatively safe and more effective. Because prospective randomized trials have involved only small numbers of patients, it is premature to adopt any particular regimen as the treatment of choice. Even combinations of azathioprine and low-dose prednisone may exert an overall beneficial effect in certain patients. Little is gained by using a combined steroid-cytotoxic approach in patients with advanced renal failure due to progressive glomerular capillary obliteration and sclerosis. These patients are best treated with dialysis and/or transplantation. Reports claiming efficacy of combined intensive plasma exchange and immunosuppressive therapy for severe glomerulonephritis have not been substantiated in a randomized prospective trial. Such treatment therefore cannot be recommended for the *routine* management of patients with severe and progressive glomerular disease. However, anecdotal reports of dramatic recovery from extrarenal manifestations (e.g., central nervous system lupus) consequent to the use of intensive plasma exchange plus immunosuppression have appeared. Since, from time to time, patients with systemic lupus erythematosus may develop a syndrome closely resembling thrombotic thrombocytopenic purpura, the beneficial effect of intensive plasma exchange may be the consequence of an alteration in thrombotic microangiopathy rather than control of an active immunologically mediated process.

Serologic studies, especially serial measurements of antibody to dsDNA, complement components, and circulating immune complexes, may be useful in assessing patients under therapy. Return of these parameters to normal usually indicates satisfactory control of disease and indicates that drug dosage can be safely diminished. These measurements can be monitored to guide more aggressive therapy when appropriate. However, too heavy reliance on serologic parameters of activity should be discouraged. The correlation between clinical activity and serologic disturbances is poor, at least among patients receiving therapy with steroids and immunosuppressive agents.

Overall, long-term prognosis for patients with SLE and renal involvement has greatly improved. Whether changes in methods of diagnosis, serologic monitoring, or treatment are responsible is unknown. Progression to end-stage renal disease is now relatively uncommon even for patients with diffuse proliferative glomerulonephritis. Cerebral involvement and infectious complications of therapy are now major causes of morbidity and mortality in SLE. Patients with SLE seem to do well on regular chronic dialysis; moreover, as uremia develops, some patients experience remissions of extrarenal activity. In transplanted patients, recurrence of SLE in the renal allograft is uncommon. Thus, patients with SLE and nephritis are satisfactory candidates for both dialysis and transplantation.

GOODPASTURE'S SYNDROME There is a lack of agreement concerning the use of the term *Goodpasture's syndrome*. Some apply this eponym to clinical states and diseases having in common glomerulonephritis and pulmonary hemorrhage. Others restrict the use of the eponym to patients displaying the triad of *glomerulonephritis*, *pulmonary hemorrhage*, and *antibody to basement membrane antigens*. As was mentioned earlier (Chap. 227), pulmonary hemorrhage, covert or overt, can accompany many forms of glomerular disease including systemic necrotizing vasculitis, Wegener's granulomatosis, systemic lupus erythematosus, cryoimmunoglobulinemia, Henoch-Schönlein purpura, and several nonglomerular diseases associated with renal function abnormalities (e.g., *Legionella* infection, renal vein thrombosis with pulmonary embolus). This section will deal with Goodpasture's syndrome as mediated by antibody to basement membrane antigens. The etiology is unknown. Goodpasture's syndrome may appear at any age and typically affects young men. However, the frequency may be increasing in women.

Pulmonary hemorrhage may be mild and easily overlooked or severe and life-threatening. The initial manifestations of pulmonary involvement are cough, mild shortness of breath, and hemoptysis. Hilar pulmonary infiltrates may be seen by chest x-ray, and hypoxia is frequent. With marked intraalveolar hemorrhage pulmonary carbon monoxide uptake is increased, and the pulmonary clearance of radioactive carbon monoxide is depressed. Pulmonary iron sequestration may be documented by scanning of the lungs with ^{59}Fe. Hemosiderin-laden macrophages may be seen in the sputum, but this is a nonspecific finding. Iron-deficiency anemia may result if pulmonary bleeding is prolonged and severe. A history of recent inhalation of volatile hydrocarbons or of viral influenza may be obtained. Fever, arthralgias, and other systemic symptoms are mild or absent at the time of presentation. Other disorders in which renal disease is associated with pulmonary (alveolar) hemorrhage can ordinarily be differentiated from Goodpasture's syndrome by their extrarenal features and by typical serologic findings (Table 228-1).

The glomeruli in Goodpasture's syndrome range from normal or nearly normal to focal proliferative and necrotizing glomerulonephritis; most often there is extensive extracapillary proliferation (crescents). Rapidly progressive renal failure is the common feature, although patients may initially have normal renal function and mild microscopic abnormalities in the urinary sediment. Immunofluorescence studies of renal biopsy material reveal the typical *linear deposits* of anti-basement membrane antibody, often but not necessarily always accompanied by C3 deposition. Electron-microscopic studies do not reveal electron-dense deposits.

Circulating antibody to glycopeptide antigens related to the noncollagenous domains on type IV (basement membrane) collagen are found in over 90 percent of cases if sera are examined early in the course by immunofluorescence or radioimmunoassay (Table 228-1). The level of circulating antibody does not correlate well with the severity of the renal or pulmonary manifestations. Measurements of circulating antibody are of diagnostic value and have no prognostic significance. Serum complement components are nearly always normal, and circulating immune complexes, anti-neutrophil cytoplasmic antibodies, and cryoimmunoglobulins are absent. About 80 to 85 percent of patients are HLA-DR2 antigen–positive.

The course is variable. Patients surviving an initial bout of severe hemoptysis may undergo long-term remissions or may have repeated bouts of pulmonary hemorrhage. Mild forms of glomerular injury may not progress, and the principal clinical problems may be related to recurrent hemoptysis. The diagnosis in such patients may be confused with idiopathic pulmonary hemosiderosis. More commonly the renal disease is progressive, sometimes fulminant, leading to oliguric renal failure in a matter of a few weeks or months (i.e., rapidly progressive glomerulonephritis).

Life-threatening degrees of pulmonary hemorrhage may respond temporarily to high doses of parenteral methylprednisolone (10 to 15 mg/kg body weight) given over short periods. The effectiveness of such therapy in reversing extensive crescentic glomerular lesions is not established. Anticoagulants are contraindicated in the face of active pulmonary hemorrhage. Intensive plasma exchange (2 to 4 L/d plasma), in combination with cytotoxic drugs and modest doses of glucocorticoids, has been associated with dramatic remissions of pulmonary hemorrhage and improvement of the glomerular lesions. This is particularly true if treatment is initiated early in patients with relatively acute disease in whom oliguria has not yet developed. The duration and frequency of plasma exchanges depend upon the response of the patient and the changes in levels of circulating antibody to glomerular basement membrane antigens. Renal biopsy is helpful in guiding the management, but even in the presence of extensive crescent formation responses may be satisfactory. If irreversible glomerular obliteration, extensive interstitial fibrosis, and tubular atrophy are found, especially in the oliguric patient with long-standing disease, plasma exchange offers little hope for improving the renal lesion. Such patients are best managed by regular hemodialysis and/or transplantation. Although recurrences may occasionally develop, the diagnosis is not a contraindication to transplantation so long as the procedure is delayed until levels of circulating anti-basement membrane antibody decrease to undetectable levels.

HENOCH-SCHÖNLEIN PURPURA (See also Chap. 288) This disorder is characterized by nonthrombocytopenic purpura, arthralgias, abdominal pain, and glomerulonephritis. Renal involvement is common and is manifested chiefly by hematuria and proteinuria. In some instances renal involvement is severe, leading to rapidly progressive glomerulonephritis or nephrotic syndrome. The onset of the disease may resemble acute postinfectious glomerulonephritis. Serum complement component levels are usually normal. Serum IgA levels are increased in about half the patients (Table 228-1). Renal biopsy reveals a spectrum of abnormalities. Mild diffuse mesangial cell proliferation and/or focal and segmental proliferative glomerulonephritis is most common when bouts of macroscopic hematuria and proteinuria are present. More severe and diffuse proliferative glomerulonephritis, sometimes accompanied by extracapillary proliferation (crescents), arises in patients with heavy proteinuria and/or rapidly diminishing GFR. Characteristically, immunofluorescence studies reveal mesangial and peripheral capillary granular deposits of IgA, IgG, C3, and fibrinogen but not C1q, C4, or IgA secretory piece. Similar immunofluorescence findings are present in the dermal capillaries of biopsies of involved and uninvolved skin. Electron microscopy reveals electron-dense deposits principally in the mesangium. These findings suggest that Henoch-Schönlein purpura is due to circulating IgA-containing immune complexes. Circulating cryoimmunoglobulins and immune complexes may be present, but the nature of the antigen and the antibody reactivity of the IgA are unknown. Although food allergies and upper respiratory infections may be present, there is no clear-cut etiologic relationship. *Berger's disease* (IgA nephropathy, Chap. 227) may represent a form of Henoch-Schönlein purpura.

The diagnosis is ordinarily not difficult when the typical clinical features are present. The differential diagnosis includes SLE, polyarteritis, infective endocarditis, postinfectious glomerulonephritis, and essential cryoimmunoglobulinemia.

The course is usually benign; however, progressive renal failure may occur. Renal biopsy is a useful prognostic tool. Patients with persistent urinary abnormalities may experience deterioration of renal function several years after diagnosis. Treatment is symptomatic. There is no convincing evidence that glucocorticoid or immunosuppressive therapy is beneficial for the renal lesion, although these treatments may ameliorate extrarenal features. Patients with rapidly progressive (crescentic) glomerulonephritis benefit from intensive plasma exchange combined with immunosuppressive drugs (see Chap. 227).

SYSTEMIC NECROTIZING VASCULITIS (See also Chap. 276) Glomerular involvement is common in the heterogeneous group of disorders that result from widespread inflammatory and necrotizing lesions of blood vessels. Several variations are recognized, including microscopic polyarteritis (hypersensitivity angiitis), macroscopic polyarteritis (periarteritis nodosa), Wegener's granulomatosis, allergic angiitis and granulomatosis, rheumatoid vasculitis, temporal arteritis, and Takayasu's arteritis. Henoch-Schönlein purpura and SLE can also be considered as examples of vasculitis. Many patients with glomerulonephritis accompanying systemic necrotizing vasculitis have characteristic extrarenal findings such as cutaneous palpable purpura, necrotizing skin lesions, pulmonary infiltrates, upper airway or sinus lesions, mononeuritis multiplex, fever, and wasting. Hypertension is frequent in polyarteritis nodosa but may be absent in hypersensitivity vasculitis and Wegener's granulomatosis. Necrotizing pulmonary infiltrates, upper airway disease, sinusitis, and otitis characterize the Wegener's granulomatosis variant. Laboratory findings, often nonspecific, include anemia, mild leukocytosis, eosinophilia, and markedly elevated erythrocyte sedimentation rate. Autoantibodies to a cytoplasmic antigen present in polymorphonuclear leukocytes have been reported in a high percentage of patients with Wegener's granulomatosis and possibly also systemic necrotizing vasculitis (Table 228-1). The detection of such autoantibodies may be helpful in establishing the nature of the underlying disease in patients suspected of having vasculitis. Renal biopsies are a poor means of establishing the diagnosis, since they frequently reveal segmental or diffuse necrotizing glomerulonephritis with or without crescents in the absence of any extraglomerular vascular involvement. Lung biopsies more frequently reveal the typical granulomatous necrotizing vasculitis characteristic of Wegener's granulomatosis. Sural nerve biopsies may be useful in establishing the diagnosis of vasculitis in patients presenting with mononeuritis multiplex.

The prognosis is generally poor for patients with systemic necrotizing vasculitis, especially in the absence of treatment; however, aggressive management with glucocorticoids combined with cyclophosphamide has been associated with improvement in overall prognosis. Treatment of patients with Wegener's granulomatosis with combined glucocorticoid-cyclophosphamide regimens for 6 to 12 months has resulted in long-term remissions. Some patients with fulminant glomerulonephritis secondary to systemic necrotizing vasculitis in which severe glomerular involvement is accompanied by extensive crescent formation and rapidly progressive renal failure may be benefited by combined therapy involving plasma exchange, glucocorticoids, and intravenous or oral cyclophosphamide. The long-term prognosis for such patients remains uncertain, since extrarenal involvement and/or complications of immunosuppressive treatment may ultimately be fatal.

MISCELLANEOUS IMMUNOLOGICALLY MEDIATED MULTISYSTEM DISEASES **Mixed connective tissue disease (MCTD)** In this disorder (also see Chap. 272) renal disease is uncommon and, if present, mild. Clinical manifestations include hematuria and proteinuria and occasionally nephrotic syndrome. Pathologically, membranous glomerulonephritis or mesangiocapillary glomerulonephritis is seen. The prognosis is generally favorable, and treatment is directed at extrarenal manifestations. Glucocorticoid therapy often results in improvement of the glomerular lesions.

Rheumatoid arthritis Several forms of glomerular injury may occur in rheumatoid arthritis (Chap. 270). Secondary amyloidosis is present in 5 to 10 percent of patients with long-standing arthritis. Nephrotic syndrome may arise as a complication of either gold or penicillamine therapy (see Chap. 227). In addition, the kidney may share in the vasculitis seen occasionally in severe rheumatoid arthritis. Finally, patients with rheumatoid arthritis (untreated with gold or penicillamine) may develop a mild proliferative glomerulitis or membranous glomerulonephritis which resembles lesions seen in SLE. Proteinuria, sometimes with nephrotic syndrome, is the principal clinical feature of such lesions. Prolonged and excessive use of analgesics may lead to renal papillary necrosis.

Other disorders *Sjögren's syndrome* (Chap. 273) may be associated with nephrotic syndrome due to membranous or mesangiocapillary glomerulonephritis (type I) or, more frequently, interstitial nephritis. *Sarcoidosis* is rarely complicated by membranous glomerulonephritis. *Partial or total lipodystrophy* may be associated with mesangiocapillary glomerulonephritis (type II, dense deposit disease) (see Chaps. 227 and 336). Complement abnormalities consist of depressed C3 levels, normal C1q and C4 levels, and circulating C3 nephritic factor.

Chronic liver disease may be complicated by glomerular disease. The nephrotic syndrome may appear in the course of *chronic active hepatitis* associated with persistent hepatitis B surface antigenemia. Glomerular lesions include membranous glomerulonephritis or mesangiocapillary (type I) glomerulonephritis. Immunofluorescence studies in such patients reveal granular deposits of immunoglobulins, complement components, and hepatitis B viral antigens, indicating an immune-complex disease. Serum C3 levels are often reduced, and tests for circulating immune complexes and cryoimmunoglobulins are frequently positive. Occasionally patients with little clinical evidence of liver disease develop distinct glomerular lesions secondary to chronic hepatitis B infection. *Acute viral hepatitis* may be associated with transient hematuria or proteinuria and may resemble other postinfectious glomerulonephritides (see Chap. 227). Severe *chronic liver disease* (cirrhosis) may be associated with diffuse glomerulosclerosis. Few clinical manifestations of glomerular disease are found. Prominent mesangial IgA deposits, of unknown pathogenic significance, have been noted in patients with cirrhosis.

MULTISYSTEM DISEASES ASSOCIATED WITH PARAPROTEINEMIA AND NEOPLASIA

ESSENTIAL (MIXED) CRYOIMMUNOGLOBULINEMIA This disorder is associated with circulating cold precipitable immunoglobulins (cryoimmunoglobulins), usually consisting of IgG and IgM; the latter possesses rheumatoid factor activity. Purpura, necrotizing skin lesions in cold-exposed areas, arthralgias, fever, and hepatosplenomegaly are common. Hepatitis B infection and other occult fungal, bacterial, or viral infections may be the cause of this syndrome. Circulating cryoimmunoglobulins are also found in chronic infections and probably represent circulating immune complexes with unusual physical properties. Glomerular disease results from the precipitation of the cryoimmunoglobulin in the glomerular capillaries and may result in acute renal failure, rapidly progressive (crescentic) glomerulonephritis, or the nephrotic syndrome. Serum complement components are depressed, and circulating immune complexes are present (Table 228-1). Pathologically, a diffuse proliferative glomerulonephritis may be seen with findings consistent with the deposition of the circulating cryoimmunoglobulin. Eradication of the underlying infection, if possible, is of value in treatment. Intensive plasma exchange, accompanied by the administration of glucocorticoids and cytotoxic agents, has been of some success in severe cases.

MONOCLONAL GAMMOPATHIES *Multiple myeloma* (Chap. 265) may be associated with at least three types of glomerular injury. Amyloidosis (Chap. 266) (see below) occurs in 10 to 15 percent of patients with multiple myeloma. Lesions may resemble nodular diabetic glomerular sclerosis, and monoclonal cryoimmunoglobulins may be deposited in glomeruli. Proteinuria and the nephrotic syndrome are common. In addition, a tubulointerstitial lesion (myeloma kidney) consisting of large, laminated intratubular casts, tubule cell atrophy, interstitial fibrosis, and inflammation is common in patients with multiple myeloma and acute or chronic renal failure. *Waldenström's macroglobulinemia* may cause acute renal failure when the IgM paraprotein precipitates in glomerular capillaries as "thrombi." Intensive plasma exchange and therapy with alkylating agents may be beneficial. Hyperviscosity may cause functional alterations in GFR. Renal amyloidosis is uncommon. *Benign monoclonal gammopathies* are seldom associated with glomerular complications, except for mild asymptomatic proteinuria and, rarely, nephrotic syndrome. Excessive production of *light chains of Ig* (especially kappa type) may evoke glomerular alterations (nodular glomerulosclerosis, focal sclerosis) due to deposition of the protein in mesangium or along the subendothelial aspect of the glomerular capillary wall.

AMYLOIDOSIS (See also Chap. 266) This disorder may occur in the absence of systemic disease (primary amyloidosis), may be secondary to chronic inflammatory processes (e.g., rheumatoid arthritis, osteomyelitis, paraplegia), multiple myeloma or other neoplastic diseases, or may occur in a hereditary form. All forms may affect the glomeruli.

Primary amyloidosis commonly affects the kidneys and usually occurs in older age groups. Proteinuria, often of nephrotic proportions, is the most common manifestation of renal involvement. The urine sediment tends to be benign. The degree of proteinuria is not necessarily related to the extent of glomerular deposition of amyloid. Enlarged kidneys may be present in patients with well-preserved renal function, but this is a nonspecific finding. The blood pressure is normal unless advanced uremia is present. Typical pathologic features include hypocellular glomeruli infiltrated with amorphous deposits that stain with Congo red and exhibit green birefringence under polarized light. The fibrillar nature of the amyloid deposits can be demonstrated by electron microscopy. Immunofluorescence studies reveal amorphous deposits of immunoglobulin and complement in glomeruli. Renal vein thrombosis may complicate the course of amyloidosis.

Renal amyloidosis is a progressive disease for which there is no established treatment. Remissions may occur in secondary amyloidosis if the cause can be eliminated. Remissions in primary amyloidosis are exceedingly rare; a few reports describe remissions following the use of cytotoxic agents. Overall the 5-year survival for patients with primary amyloidosis is less than 20 percent. Azotemia, persistent nephrotic syndrome, and myocardial involvement confer an even more ominous prognosis.

NEOPLASTIC DISEASE Glomerular alterations may develop with a variety of neoplastic diseases. *Carcinomas,* especially adenocarcinoma of lung, colon, stomach, and breast, may be accompanied by glomerular lesions resembling idiopathic membranous glomerulonephritis, although, on occasion, crescentic or focal and segmental proliferative glomerulonephritis or amyloidosis may be present. Nephrotic syndrome is the most common clinical renal manifestation, and approximately 3 to 10 percent of patients with idiopathic nephrotic syndrome associated with membranous glomerulonephritis harbor an underlying malignancy. Successful treatment of the tumor, especially by surgical means, may lead to a remission of the renal manifestation. Presumably the glomerular lesions arise because of the deposition of circulating immune complexes that are composed of tumor antigen and antitumor antibody. Amyloidosis may occasionally occur.

Lymphomas and leukemias may also give rise to glomerular abnormalities. Hodgkin's disease is commonly associated with the findings of idiopathic nephrotic syndrome (minimal change disease). Other glomerular lesions may include membranous glomerulonephritis, focal proliferative and sclerosing glomerulonephritis, and amyloidosis. The mechanism of the association of Hodgkin's disease with minimal change disease may involve an underlying T-cell abnormality. Proteinuria may wax and wane with fluctuations in the clinical activity of the Hodgkin's disease. Remissions may be produced by local irradiation of involved lymph nodes or by systemic chemotherapy.

METABOLIC, BIOCHEMICAL, AND HEREDITARY DISORDERS

DIABETIC NEPHROPATHY (See also Chap. 319) Diabetes mellitus affects the structure and function of the kidney in many ways. The term *diabetic nephropathy* encompasses all the lesions occurring in the kidneys of patients with diabetes mellitus. These lesions include *glomerulosclerosis* (diffuse or nodular), *arterionephrosclerosis, chronic interstitial nephritis, papillary necrosis,* and various tubular lesions. Diabetic nephropathy is associated with a variety of clinical syndromes, including mild asymptomatic proteinuria, nephrotic syndrome, progressive renal failure (acute, rapidly progressive, or chronic), and hypertension. Glomerular lesions are particularly common and account for the majority of abnormal clinical findings referable to the kidney. *Diffuse diabetic glomerulosclerosis* (diffuse intercapillary glomerulosclerosis) is the most common lesion and can be identified in the vast majority of diabetic patients regardless of the presence of abnormal clinical findings referable to the kidney. This lesion consists of a mild diffuse increase in mesangial matrix accompanied by an increased width of the glomerular basement membrane. Various exudative lesions, such as capsular drops and fibrin caps, may also be present. Hyaline arteriosclerosis, particularly of the efferent arteriole, is also common. Taken together, these lesions suggest the diagnosis of diabetes mellitus, but individually they are not specific. *Nodular glomerulosclerosis* (Kimmelstiel-Wilson lesion), on the other hand, is reasonably specific for juvenile onset (type I) diabetes mellitus. This lesion consists of PAS-positive, laminated, intercapillary nodules on a background of an increase in mesangial matrix. At the periphery of the nodules open glomerular capillary loops are found. The nodules are relatively acellular, in contrast to the cellular lesions of membranoproliferative glomerulonephritis (often referred to as *lobular glomerulonephritis*). A variable percentage of glomeruli may be affected. The pathogenesis of diffuse or nodular diabetic glomerulosclerosis is poorly understood.

The principal clinical manifestation of diabetic glomerular disease is proteinuria. Initially, only small amounts of albumin (20 to 40 μg/min) are excreted, particularly following exercise (microalbuminuria). This amount of albumin excretion is undetectable by routine screening methods. Under ordinary circumstances, microalbuminuria develops within 10 to 15 years from the onset of hyperglycemia and usually progresses within 3 to 7 years to overt proteinuria and clinical diabetic nephropathy. With ''tight'' control of hyperglycemia and/or rigorous control of elevated blood pressure, the development of microalbuminuria may be prevented or reversed. With time, the quantity of protein excreted usually increases and may progress to an overt nephrotic syndrome. Glomerular filtration rate is initially elevated and subsequently falls towards normal coincident with the onset of overt proteinuria. The urinary sediment is typically benign, although microhematuria and/or pyuria may also be present if a complicating urinary tract infection or papillary necrosis is present. Hypertension develops as GFR falls but is seldom of malignant proportions. When hypertension is severe or abrupt in onset, one should suspect a complicating atherosclerotic renal arterial stenosis. Typically, plasma renin activity is normal or decreased. Acquired hyporeninemic hypoaldosteronism with persistent hyperkalemia and mild hyperchloremic metabolic acidosis is common. Once azotemia develops, the disease progresses at variable rates. End-stage renal failure usually develops within 5 years of the onset of overt proteinuria and clinical nephropathy. Despite poor control of hyperglycemia, only about 50 to 60 percent of insulin-dependent diabetic patients develop clinical nephropathy. The factors that protect the remaining patients from renal failure are unknown. Patients with non-insulin-dependent diabetes mellitus may also develop clinical nephropathy.

Until the cause of diabetes mellitus is established, prevention of the glomerulopathy will not be feasible. If the abnormal diabetic milieu is responsible for the vascular complications (including glomerular disease), as some have suggested, then very precise regulation of blood sugar (e.g., meticulous attention to diet, exercise, and insulin dosage and servofeedback devices for insulin administration) may be effective in reducing the development of nephropathy. Once the nephropathy has reached a clinically recognizable stage, aggressive management of hypertension may slow the rate of loss of renal function, but strict control of blood sugar does not seem to retard the rate of progression once overt nephropathy (proteinuria >500 mg/d) has emerged. Patients with end-stage renal failure due to diabetic nephropathy are not ideal candidates for long-term dialysis because of concomitant multiple organ dysfunction secondary to widespread arteriovascular disease. Mortality rates among diabetics on chronic dialysis are about three times higher than among similarly treated nondiabetics of comparable age. Renal transplantation may be successful in the younger diabetic, especially if a living related donor is available. The success rate is somewhat less than in the nondiabetic population, due to the adverse effects of extrarenal vascular involvement (e.g., coronary artery disease), but transplantation is a viable alternative to dialysis in selected patients. Recurrence of typical diabetic glomerular lesions has been documented in renal allografts, but thus far, progressive loss of GFR secondary to recurrent disease has not been noted.

ALPORT'S SYNDROME This disorder consists of sensorineural deafness associated with hereditary nephritis. Renal disease manifests itself at an early age, principally as recurrent hematuria. Men are more frequently and more severely affected than women. Slowly progressive renal insufficiency in men commonly terminates in end-stage renal disease in the second to third decade. There is no clear-cut relationship between the onset or severity of the hearing abnormality and the extent of renal disease. Other associated abnormalities include two related ophthalmologic complications, spherophakia and lenticonus, as well as thrombopenia, hyperprolinemia, and cerebral dysfunction. Family studies have indicated autosomal dominant or X-linked modes of inheritance with variable expressivity. The pathogenesis may be due to defective synthesis of glycopeptide (noncollagenous) components of glomerular and tubular basement membranes.

The pathologic features detected by light microscopy are nonspecific, and a diagnosis cannot be established by optical microscopy alone. Both glomerular and interstitial lesions are present. Focal and diffuse glomerular proliferation, with segmental sclerosis, is common. Interstitial foam cells are nonspecific findings. Electron microscopy reveals thinning, splitting, and delamination of both glomerular and tubular basement membranes, thought by some to be specific for the syndrome. Immunofluorescence studies fail to reveal deposits of immunoglobulins or complement components. The autoantibody to basement membrane antigens found in patients with Goodpasture's syndrome does not react with the glomeruli of some patients with Alport's syndrome. Treatment is supportive; glucocorticoids and cytotoxic agents are ineffective. The disease is not known to recur following transplantation.

FABRY'S DISEASE (See also Chap. 331) This disorder, angiokeratoma corporus diffusum, is an X-linked inborn error of glycosphingolipid metabolism that leads to the accumulation of neutral glycosphingolipids in many tissues including the kidney. A milder disease may develop in heterozygous females. Manifestations include angiokeratomas involving the lower trunk, scrotum, and buttocks; acroparesthesia; corneal opacities; tortuous retinal veins; and premature coronary and cerebral ischemic disease. Renal manifestations include hematuria and modest proteinuria, often associated with slowly progressive renal failure. Light-microscopic findings include foamy alterations of the epithelial cells of the glomerulus due to the accumulation of lipid. Electron microscopy reveals intracellular rounded laminated bodies (''myelin figures''). The disorder is untreatable unless replacement of the deficient enzyme can be ensured; successful renal transplantation may correct the enzyme deficiency.

NAIL-PATELLA SYNDROME This autosomal dominant disease is characterized by dystrophic nails, absence of one or both patellae, iliac horns, and renal disease. The renal manifestations include isolated proteinuria and hematuria and occasionally the nephrotic syndrome. Progressive renal failure is uncommon. Glomerular lesions are nonspecific by light microscopy, but electron microscopy reveals a characteristic moth-eaten appearance of the glomerular basement membrane associated with intramembranous collagen fibrils. The prognosis is generally favorable. No treatment is known.

CONGENITAL NEPHROTIC SYNDROME This autosomal recessive trait is characterized by the development of nephrotic syndrome at the time of or shortly after birth. It occurs with highest frequency in families of Finnish origin. Affected individuals have very large placentas, low birth weight, anasarca, polycythemia, and initially normal GFRs. Levels of alpha fetoprotein are increased in amniotic fluid and maternal serum. Proteinuria is marked and nonselective. Nephrotic syndrome appearing several months after birth is usually due to other causes, especially minimal change disease or focal glomerular sclerosis (Chap. 227). Congenital syphilis and congenital toxoplasmosis may produce similar syndromes and must be excluded. Pathologically, microcystic transformation of the cortical nephrons results in proximal tubular dilatation. Glomerular changes are nonspecific. The anionic charge density on glomerular basement membrane is reduced. Extensive effacement of the foot processes and sclerosis of the glomerular tufts are seen by electron microscopy. Immunofluorescence findings are nonspecific. The course is progressive, and few patients survive the first year of life. Treatment is ineffective. Death is usually due to inanition, infection, or renal failure. A few patients may survive long enough to be considered for renal transplantation.

SICKLE CELL DISEASE (See also Chap. 295) This disorder is an autosomal trait characterized by an abnormal hemoglobin (hemoglobin S). Glomerular lesions occur occasionally in homozygous disease. The medulla is affected, leading to impairment of concentrating ability and acid excretion and, occasionally, to papillary necrosis. Rarely, patients develop mainly glomerular lesions, either membranous or mesangiocapillary glomerulonephritis, accompanied by proteinuria and a nephrotic syndrome. Immunofluorescence studies demonstrate renal deposition of immunoglobulin and complement in a granular pattern suggesting immune-complex–mediated disease. In a few instances, renal tubuloepithelial antigens are localized in these deposits, suggesting that ischemic damage of the kidney may release autologous antigens to provoke the immune-complex disease. The course in patients with the glomerulopathy of sickle cell disease is often relentless, leading to end-stage renal disease. No treatment is known to be effective. Transplantation is occasionally successful.

TABLE 228-2 Drugs associated with glomerular lesions

Elemental, inorganic, or organic mercury compounds
Organic gold compounds
Penicillamine
Captopril
Heroin
Amphetamines
Probenecid
Oxazoladinedione derivatives (e.g., trimethadione)
Antivenoms and antitoxins
Sulfonamides
Vaccinations
Allopurinol
Hydralazine
Rifampin
Nonsteroidal anti-inflammatory agents

LECITHIN:CHOLESTEROL ACYLTRANSFERASE DEFICIENCY (See also Chap. 326) This autosomal recessive trait leads to absence in plasma of the enzyme that catalyzes the conversion of lecithin and cholesterol to lysolecithin and cholesteryl ester. Multiple lipoprotein abnormalities develop, including absence of α and pre-β lipoproteins, hypertriglyceridemia, accumulation of abnormal lipoproteins, and increased plasma-esterified cholesterol. Corneal opacities, anemia, hyperuricemia, proteinuria, and progressive renal failure are characteristic. Foam cells are present in bone marrow and glomeruli, and a picture resembling focal and segmental glomerulosclerosis may evolve. Treatment is generally ineffective, but plasma or blood transfusions may transiently correct the disorder. Renal failure has been corrected by renal transplantation, but recurrence of disease in allografts may occur.

DRUG-INDUCED GLOMERULAR DISEASE Many drugs have been associated with the development of glomerular disease; however, it is usually difficult to establish a direct cause and effect relationship. In a few situations the association is clear-cut, and reexposure has led to recurrence of disease. A partial listing of these drugs is provided in Table 228-2. Certain *heavy metals* (Hg, Au) and their inorganic salts or organic compounds may produce membranous glomerulonephritis and nephrotic syndrome. Removal of the drug is not invariably associated with resolution. *Sulfhydryl compounds* (penicillamine, captopril) may also cause membranous or proliferative glomerulonephritis. The risk of developing a renal complication following penicillamine or gold therapy for rheumatoid arthritis is influenced by genes in the major histocompatibility complex. *Nonsteroidal anti-inflammatory agents* may produce nephrotic syndrome (minimal change disease), interstitial nephritis, and acute renal failure. *Probenecid, trimethadione,* or *paramethadione* may be associated with nephrotic syndrome and a variety of glomerular lesions, including minimal change disease and membranous glomerulonephritis. *Heroin* abuse may be associated with focal and segmental glomerulosclerosis that may progress to nephrotic syndrome and progressive renal failure. *Intravenous amphetamine abuse* may be associated with systemic necrotizing vasculitis. Chronic hepatitis B infection may be involved in the development of glomerular lesions in association with intravenous drug abuse. Allopurinol, hydralazine, and rifampin may be associated with vasculitis and/or crescentic glomerulonephritis.

REFERENCES

Balow JE: Renal vasculitis. Kidney Int 27:954, 1985
——— et al: Effect of treatment on the evolution of renal abnormalities in lupus nephritis. N Engl J Med 311:491, 1984
Glassock R et al: Secondary glomerular diseases, in *The Kidney*, 3d ed, BM Brenner, FC Rector Jr (eds). Philadelphia, Saunders, 1986, p 1014
Grunfeld JP: The clinical spectrum of hereditary nephritis. Kidney Int 27:83, 1985
Kyle RA, Greipp PR: Amyloidosis (AL): Clinical and laboratory features in 229 cases. Mayo Clin Proc 58:665, 1983
Ponticelli C et al (eds): *Antiglobulins, Cryoglobulins and Glomerulonephritis*. Dodrecht, Martinus Nijhoff, 1986
Salant D: Immunopathogenesis of crescentic glomerulonephritis and lung purpura. Kidney Int 32:408, 1987

229 TUBULOINTERSTITIAL DISEASES OF THE KIDNEY

BARRY M. BRENNER / THOMAS H. HOSTETTER

An etiologically diverse group of bilateral renal diseases can be distinguished from those considered in Chaps. 227 and 228 because the histologic and functional abnormalities involve the tubules and interstitium to a greater degree than the glomeruli and renal vasculature (see Table 229-1). Morphologically, acute forms of these disorders are characterized by interstitial edema, often associated with cortical and medullary infiltration by polymorphonuclear leukocytes and patchy areas of tubule cell necrosis. In more chronic forms, interstitial fibrosis predominates, inflammatory cells are typically mononuclear, and abnormalities of the tubules tend to be more widespread, as evidenced by atrophy, luminal dilatation, and thickening of tubule basement membranes. In the past, the diagnosis of chronic pyelonephritis (see Chap. 95) was almost universally applied when these chronic tubulointerstitial abnormalities were found. It is now apparent that only a small proportion of these lesions result from infection. Nonbacterial factors, including exogenous toxins and metabolic and immunologic derangements, constitute the major pathogenic mechanisms thought to be involved. Because of the nonspecific nature of the histology, particularly in chronic tubulointerstitial diseases, biopsy specimens rarely provide a specific diagnosis. The urine sediment is also unlikely to be diagnostic, except in allergic forms of acute tubulointerstitial disease in which eosinophils may predominate in the urinary sediment.

Defects in tubule function often accompany these alterations of tubule and interstitial structure. Proximal tubule dysfunction may be manifested as selective reabsorptive defects leading to hypokalemia, aminoaciduria, glycosuria, phosphaturia, uricosuria, or bicarbonaturia (proximal or type II renal tubular acidosis, see Chap. 231). In combination these defects constitute the *Fanconi syndrome*. Protein excretion is usually modest, rarely exceeding 2 g/d. The excreted proteins are typically of low molecular weight and include beta$_2$ microglobulin, lysozyme, and immunoglobulin light chains. Defective proximal tubule reabsorption of these readily filtered small proteins accounts for their augmented excretion. Tubule sodium reabsorption may also be deranged in patients with advanced tubulointerstitial diseases, predisposing to salt wasting and hypovolemia. One or more of these reabsorptive defects are commonly encountered with heavy metal poisoning, multiple myeloma, and other diffuse tubulointerstitial processes.

Defects in urinary acidification and concentrating ability often represent the most troublesome of the tubule dysfunctions encountered in patients with tubulointerstitial disease. Hyperchloremic metabolic acidosis often develops at a relatively early stage in the course. Patients with this finding generally elaborate urine of maximal acidity (pH of 5.3 or less). In such patients the defect in acid excretion is usually caused by a reduced capacity to generate and excrete ammonia due to the reduction in renal mass. Preferential damage to the collecting ducts, as in amyloidosis or chronic obstructive uropathy, may also predispose to distal or type I renal tubular acidosis, characterized by high urine pH (>5.5) during spontaneous or NH_4Cl-induced metabolic acidosis. Patients with tubulointerstitial diseases affecting medullary and papillary structures predominantly may also evidence concentrating defects, with resultant nocturia and polyuria. The impairment in maximal concentration is typically unresponsive to the administration of vasopressin, and hence is a form of nephrogenic diabetes insipidus. Analgesic nephropathy and sickle cell disease are prototypes of this form of injury.

Although the major structural defects originate in the tubules and interstitium, progressive reduction in glomerular filtration rate (GFR) is a functional accompaniment of most, if not all, forms of tubulointerstitial damage, reflecting secondary injury to glomeruli and other elements of the renal microcirculation. Indeed oliguric, acute renal failure may be caused by acute forms of tubulointerstitial disease, and about a third of patients with chronic renal insufficiency suffer from a primary chronic tubulointerstitial disease.

TABLE 229-1 Principal causes of tubulointerstitial disease of the kidney

I Toxins
- *A* Exogenous toxins
  - *1* Analgesic nephropathy
  - *2* Lead nephropathy (see Chap. 372)
  - *3* Miscellaneous nephrotoxins (e.g., antibiotics, cyclosporine, radiographic contrast media, heavy metals)
- *B* Metabolic toxins
  - *1* Acute uric acid nephropathy (see Chap. 329)
  - *2* Gouty nephropathy (see Chap. 329)
  - *3* Hypercalcemic nephropathy (see Chap. 340)
  - *4* Hypokalemic nephropathy (see Chap. 50)
  - *5* Miscellaneous metabolic toxins (e.g., hyperoxaluria, cystinosis, Fabry's disease)

II Neoplasia
- *A* Lymphoma (see Chap. 302)
- *B* Leukemia (see Chap. 296)
- *C* Multiple myeloma (see Chap. 265)

III Immune disorders
- *A* Hypersensitivity nephropathy
- *B* Sjögren's syndrome (see Chap. 273)
- *C* Amyloidosis (see Chap. 266)
- *D* Transplant rejection (see Chap. 225)
- *E* Tubulointerstitial abnormalities associated with glomerulonephritis (see Chaps. 227 and 228)
- *F* AIDS (see Chap. 264)

IV Vascular disorders (see Chaps. 223 and 230)
- *A* Arteriolar nephrosclerosis
- *B* Atheroembolic disease
- *C* Sickle cell nephropathy
- *D* Acute tubular necrosis

V Hereditary renal diseases
- *A* Hereditary nephritis (Alport's syndrome) (see Chap. 228)
- *B* Medullary cystic disease (see Chap. 231)
- *C* Medullary sponge kidney (see Chap. 231)
- *D* Polycystic kidney disease (see Chap. 231)

VI Infectious injury (see Chap. 95)
- *A* Acute pyelonephritis
- *B* Chronic pyelonephritis

VII Miscellaneous disorders
- *A* Chronic urinary tract obstruction (see Chap. 233)
- *B* Vesicoureteral reflux
- *C* Radiation nephritis

TOXINS

A number of factors make the renal tubules and interstitium particularly prone to toxic injury. Although the kidneys constitute less than 1 percent of total body mass, they receive approximately 20 percent of the cardiac output, and 90 percent or more of renal blood flow is distributed to the renal cortex. Exposure of tubules and interstitium of the renal cortex to circulating toxins is, therefore, quantitatively greater than is that of most other tissues. Transport processes in renal tubules contribute further to the intrarenal accumulation of toxins, enhancing local concentrations of noxious agents. The urinary concentrating mechanism can also establish high levels of toxins within medullary and papillary portions of the kidney, predisposing these regions to chemical injury. Finally, the relatively acid pH of the fluid within most nephron segments may affect the ionization characteristics of potentially toxic compounds and thereby influence local concentration and solubility. Although these processes render the kidney vulnerable to toxic injury, the role of nephrotoxins in renal damage often goes unrecognized because the manifestations of such injury are usually nonspecific in nature and insidious in onset. Diagnosis largely depends upon a history of exposure to a certain toxin, a difficult matter since exposure may be occult. Particular attention should be paid to the occupational history, as well as to an assessment of exposure—current and remote—to drugs, especially antibiotics and analgesics. The recognition of a potential association between a patient's renal disease and exposure to a nephrotoxin is crucial, because, unlike many other forms of renal disease, progression of the functional and morphologic abnormalities associated with toxin-induced nephropathies may be prevented, and even reversed, by eliminating additional exposure.

EXOGENOUS TOXINS **Analgesic nephropathy** Individuals who ingest large quantities of analgesic drugs are particularly prone to develop tubulointerstitial damage and papillary necrosis. Indeed, in Australia, Switzerland, and Sweden, analgesic abuse is one of the most common causes of chronic renal failure, and it is an important cause of renal insufficiency in the United States as well. In animals *phenacetin* and *aspirin* can induce papillary necrosis when either of these drugs is given in quantities far in excess of usual therapeutic doses. However, these drugs are most likely to cause renal damage when ingested in combination. Epidemiologic studies leave no doubt that the chronic ingestion of mixtures of these analgesics can produce permanent and irreversible renal injury in humans.

Morphologically, analgesic nephropathy is characterized by papillary necrosis and tubulointerstitial inflammation. At an early stage, damage to the vascular supply of the inner medulla (vasa recta) leads to a local interstitial inflammatory reaction and, eventually, to papillary ischemia, necrosis, fibrosis, and calcification. Destruction of papillae usually precedes extension of the tubulointerstitial abnormalities to the renal cortex and, therefore, occurs before renal size and GFR are reduced significantly. Although papillary necrosis is a common finding in patients with the nephropathy of analgesic abuse, necrosis of papillae may also occur in patients with chronic pyelonephritis, diabetes mellitus, sickle cell disease, and obstructive uropathy. The susceptibility of the renal papillae to damage by phenacetin is believed to be related to the establishment of a renal gradient for the phenacetin metabolite *acetaminophen,* resulting in papillary tip concentrations tenfold higher than those in renal cortex. Hydration dissipates this gradient and may explain the protective effect of this maneuver in preventing phenacetin-induced papillary necrosis in animals. Aspirin in these analgesic compounds contributes to renal injury by uncoupling oxidative phosphorylation in renal mitochondria and by inhibiting the synthesis of renal prostaglandins, which are potent endogenous renal vasodilator hormones. Both effects of aspirin favor hypoxia in renal tissues and, therefore, enhance the susceptibility of the inner medulla to nephrotoxic injury.

Analgesic nephropathy occurs some three to five times more commonly in women than men. A direct relationship exists between the total amount of analgesic compounds ingested and the degree of renal impairment. The intake of 1.0 g phenacetin per day for 1 to 3 years or the total ingestion of 2 kg phenacetin in combination with other analgesics appear to represent minimum requirements for the development of analgesic nephropathy. In such patients, renal function usually declines gradually, in association with chronic necrosis of papillae and diffuse tubulointerstitial damage to the renal cortex. Occasionally, papillary necrosis may be associated with hematuria and even renal colic, due to obstruction of a ureter by necrotic tissue. More than half of patients with analgesic nephropathy have pyuria, which, if persistently associated with sterile urine, provides an important clue to the diagnosis. Nonetheless, active pyelonephritis may coexist in patients with analgesic nephropathy. Proteinuria, if present, is typically mild (less than 1 g/d). Patients with analgesic nephropathy are usually unable to generate maximally concentrated urine, reflecting the underlying medullary and papillary damage. An acquired form of distal renal tubular acidosis may contribute to the development of *nephrocalcinosis.* The occurrence of anemia out of proportion to the degree of azotemia may also provide a clue to the diagnosis of analgesic nephropathy. Occult gastrointestinal bleeding (usually secondary to analgesic-induced gastritis) and, in an occasional patient, hemolysis (particularly in those with glucose-6-phosphate dehydrogenase deficiency) contribute to the anemia. Vague abdominal complaints, nonspecific headaches, and arthralgias are common. Moderate hypertension is also common and progresses to a malignant phase in only a small minority. When analgesic nephropathy has progressed to renal insufficiency, the kidneys usually appear bilaterally shrunken on intravenous pyelography, and the calyces are deformed. A "ring sign" on the pyelogram is pathognomonic of papillary necrosis and represents the radiolucent sloughed papilla surrounded by the radiodense contrast material in the calyx. Transitional cell carcinoma may develop in the urinary pelvis or ureters as a late complication of analgesic abuse.

Every effort must be made to convince the patient who ingests excessive analgesics to discontinue this hazardous practice. When renal damage is at an early stage, cessation of abuse usually arrests the progression of the nephrotoxic process; not infrequently, overall renal function improves with time. With continued abuse, however, progressive renal damage leads invariably to chronic renal failure.

Lead nephropathy (See also Chap. 375) Children and adults suffering from lead intoxication often develop a chronic tubulointerstitial renal disease. In children, lead poisoning usually results from ingestion of lead-based paints (pica). The oxide of lead liberated from paint, or present in the vapor arising from the welding of metals covered with lead-based paint, may be inhaled in substantial quantities, thereby constituting an industrial form of exposure in adults. Alcohol, illegally distilled in an apparatus constructed from automobile radiators (so-called moonshine), is another cause of lead poisoning. Tubule transport processes enhance the accumulation of lead within renal cells, particularly in the proximal convoluted tubule, leading to cell degeneration, mitochondrial swelling, and eosinophilic intranuclear inclusion bodies rich in lead. In addition to tubule degeneration and atrophy, lead nephropathy is associated with ischemic changes in the glomeruli, fibrosis of the adventitia of small renal arterioles, and focal areas of cortical scarring. Eventually, the kidneys become atrophic. In addition to progressive azotemia, abnormalities of tubule function may occur, particularly *renal glycosuria* and *aminoaciduria.* Urinary excretion of lead, bile pigments, and porphyrin precursors, such as δ-aminolevulinic acid, coproporphyrin, and urobilinogen, may be increased. Patients with chronic lead nephropathy are characteristically *hyperuricemic,* a consequence of enhanced reabsorption of filtered urate. Acute gouty arthritis (so-called saturnine gout) occurs in about 50 percent of patients with lead nephropathy, in striking contrast to other forms of chronic renal failure in which gout is rare (also see Chap. 329). Hypertension is also a complication. Therefore, in any patient with slowly progressive renal failure, atrophic kidneys, gout, and hypertension, the diagnosis of lead intoxication should be considered. In addition, patients with chronic lead poisoning often complain of abdominal colic and have evidence of anemia, peripheral neuropathy, and encephalopathy. The diagnosis may be suspected by finding elevated serum levels of lead. However, because blood levels may not be elevated even in the presence of a toxic total-body burden of lead, the quantitation of lead excretion following a standardized infusion of the chelating agent calcium disodium edetate is a more reliable indicator of serious lead exposure. Urinary excretion of more than 0.6 mg of lead per day is indicative of overt or potential toxicity. Treatment includes removing the patient from the source of exposure and augmenting lead excretion with a chelating agent such as calcium disodium edetate.

Miscellaneous nephrotoxins Therapeutic use of lithium salts for manic-depressive illness has been associated with tubulointerstitial disease. The most frequent clinical finding is a mild to moderate nephrogenic diabetes insipidus resulting in polyuria and polydipsia. It is unclear whether long-term lithium therapy produces irreversible chronic tubulointerstitial lesions and impairment of glomerular filtration rate. Though present evidence suggests that some patients develop histologic evidence of such injury, there are only rare reports of chronic renal insufficiency attributable to this agent. In any case, renal function should be followed in patients taking this drug, and caution should be exercised if lithium is employed in patients with underlying renal disease.

The immunosuppressant cyclosporine causes both acute and chronic renal injury. The acute injury and the use of cyclosporine in transplantation are discussed in Chap. 225. The chronic injury is a progressive decline in filtration rate with mild proteinuria and arterial hypertension. The histologic changes in renal tissue comprise patchy interstitial fibrosis and tubular atrophy. In addition, the intrarenal vasculature often demonstrates hyalinosis, and focal segmental glomerular sclerosis can be present as well. Indeed, renal vasoconstriction induced by the drug appears to be a major mechanism of the renal injury. In patients receiving this drug for renal transplantation, chronic rejection and recurrence of the primary disease may coincide with chronic cyclosporine injury, and on clinical grounds, distinction among these may be difficult. Whether the chronic injury can be prevented by dose reduction is uncertain. However, use of the lowest doses of cyclosporine consistent with adequate immunosuppression appears to mitigate nephrotoxicity. In addition, treatment of any associated arterial hypertension may lessen renal injury.

Many agents that commonly lead to acute renal failure are also capable of producing tubulointerstitial injury (see Chap. 223). These include antibiotics (e.g., aminoglycosides, amphotericin B), radiographic contrast agents, various hydrocarbons (e.g., carbon tetrachloride), and heavy metals (e.g., mercury, cadmium, and bismuth).

METABOLIC TOXINS **Acute uric acid nephropathy** (See also Chap. 329) Acute overproduction of uric acid and extreme hyperuricemia often lead to a rapidly progressive renal insufficiency, so-called acute uric acid nephropathy. This tubulointerstitial disease is usually seen in patients given cytotoxic drugs for the treatment of lymphoproliferative or myeloproliferative disorders but may also occur in these patients before such treatment is begun. The pathologic changes are largely the result of deposition of uric acid crystals in the kidneys and their collecting systems, leading to partial or complete obstruction of collecting ducts, renal pelvis, or ureter. Since obstruction is often bilateral, patients typically show the clinical course of acute renal failure, characterized by oliguria and rapidly rising serum creatinine concentration. In the early phase uric acid crystals can be found in urine, usually in association with microscopic or gross hematuria. Peak serum uric acid levels vary but are almost always above 1200 μmol/L (20 mg/dL) and may even exceed 3500 μmol/L (60 mg/dL).

Prevention of hyperuricemia in patients at risk by treatment with allopurinol in doses of 200 to 800 mg/d prior to cytotoxic therapy reduces the danger of acute uric acid nephropathy. Once hyperuricemia develops, however, efforts should be directed to preventing deposition of uric acid within the urinary tract. Increasing urine volume with potent diuretics (furosemide or mannitol) effectively lowers intratubular uric acid concentrations, and alkalinization of the urine to pH 7 or greater with sodium bicarbonate and/or a carbonic anhydrase inhibitor (acetazolamide) enhances uric acid solubility. If these efforts, together with allopurinol therapy, are ineffective in preventing acute renal failure, dialysis should be instituted to lower the serum uric acid concentration as well as to treat the acute manifestations of uremia. The combination of conservative therapy and hemodialysis allows most patients with acute uric acid nephropathy to survive acute renal failure and ultimately recover renal function.

Gouty nephropathy (See also Chap. 329) Patients with less severe but prolonged forms of hyperuricemia are predisposed to a more chronic tubulointerstitial disorder, often referred to as *gouty nephropathy*. Since other conditions associated with hyperuricemia, such as hypertension, nephrolithiasis, pyelonephritis, and even lead poisoning, may contribute to renal damage, the effect of chronic hyperuricemia per se on renal function is unclear. Nevertheless, the severity of renal involvement correlates with the duration and magnitude of the elevation of the serum uric acid concentration. Histologically, the distinctive feature of gouty nephropathy is the presence of crystalline deposits of uric acid and monosodium urate salts in kidney parenchyma. These deposits are believed to represent the primary pathogenic process in gouty nephropathy, with intraluminal crystallization of uric acid taking place in distal tubules and collecting ducts where urine pH is generally quite low and where uric acid concentrations are considerably in excess of levels in plasma. These deposits not only cause intrarenal obstruction, but also incite an inflammatory response, leading to lymphocytic infiltration, foreign-body giant cell reaction, and eventual fibrosis, especially of medullary and papillary regions of the kidney. Bacteriuria and pyelonephritis occur in about one-fourth of cases, presumably as complications of intrarenal urinary stasis. Since patients with gout frequently suffer from hypertension and hyperlipidemia, degenerative changes of the renal arterioles may constitute a striking feature of the histologic abnormality, often out of proportion to other morphologic defects. Clinically, gouty nephropathy is an insidious cause of renal insufficiency. Early in its course, GFR may be near normal, often despite focal morphologic changes in medullary and cortical interstitium, proteinuria, and diminished urinary concentrating ability. Whether reducing serum uric acid levels with allopurinol exerts a beneficial effect on the kidney remains to be demonstrated. Although such undesirable consequences of hyperuricemia as gout and uric acid stones respond well to allopurinol, use of this drug in asymptomatic hyperuricemia has not been shown to improve renal function consistently. On the other hand, uricosuric agents such as probenecid, which may increase uric acid stone production, clearly have no role in the treatment of renal disease associated with hyperuricemia.

Hypercalcemic nephropathy (See also Chap. 340) Chronic hypercalcemia, as occurs in primary hyperparathyroidism, sarcoidosis, multiple myeloma, vitamin D intoxication, or metastatic bone disease, can cause tubulointerstitial damage and progressive renal insufficiency. The earliest renal lesion induced by hypercalcemia is a focal degenerative change in renal epithelia, primarily in collecting ducts, distal convoluted tubules, and loops of Henle. Tubule cell necrosis leads to nephron obstruction and stasis of intrarenal urine, favoring local precipitation of calcium salts and infection. Dilatation and atrophy of tubules eventually occur, as do interstitial fibrosis, mononuclear leukocyte infiltration, and interstitial calcium deposition (nephrocalcinosis). Calcium deposition may also occur in glomeruli and the walls of renal arterioles. Clinically, the most striking defect is an inability to concentrate the urine maximally, resulting in polyuria and nocturia. Defective transport of chloride in the ascending limb of Henle's loop is responsible, at least in part, for this concentrating defect. Additionally, reduced collecting duct responsiveness to vasopressin may contribute to this abnormality. Reductions in GFR and renal blood flow also occur, both in states of acute severe hypercalcemia and with prolonged hypercalcemia of lesser severity. Distal renal tubular acidosis and sodium and potassium wasting have also been described in these chronic states. Eventually, uncontrolled hypercalcemia leads to severe tubulointerstitial damage and overt renal failure. Urinalysis is rarely a clue to the presence of hypercalcemic renal failure, but abdominal x-rays may demonstrate nephrocalcinosis as well as nephrolithiasis, the latter due to the hypercalciuria which often accompanies hypercalcemia. Treatment for hypercalcemic nephropathy consists of reducing the serum calcium concentration toward normal and correcting the primary abnormality of calcium metabolism. The management of hypercalcemia is discussed in Chap. 340. Prognosis for recovery of renal function depends upon the severity of the renal lesion at the time hypercalcemia is corrected. Renal dysfunction of recent onset secondary to acute hypercalcemia may be completely reversible. Gradual, progressive renal insufficiency related to chronic hypercalcemia, however, may not improve with correction of the calcium disorder. Nonetheless, every effort should be made to return serum calcium concentration to normal in order to minimize further loss of renal function.

Hypokalemic nephropathy (See also Chap. 50) Disturbances of renal structure and function occur commonly in patients with moderate to severe potassium depletion of at least several weeks' duration. Histologically, renal epithelial cells are often seen to contain numerous vacuoles, most marked in proximal, and to a lesser extent, distal convoluted tubules. These findings usually disappear with potassium repletion. Glomeruli are reduced in size and may become sclerotic while larger blood vessels are usually uninvolved. Whether prolonged or recurrent potassium deficiency results in irreversible tubulointerstitial fibrosis, scarring, and atrophy is unresolved. Loss of urinary concentrating ability is the most commonly encountered functional defect. Studies in animals have shown that this urinary concentrating abnormality is preceded by a period of primary polydipsia. The reduced concentrating capacity which eventually develops is due, at least in part, to defective operation of the countercurrent multiplier system. Elevated rates of intrarenal prostaglandin synthesis may also contribute to this concentrating defect, since prostaglandins antagonize the hydroosmotic action of antidiuretic hormone on collecting-duct epithelium. Symptoms of nocturia, polyuria, and polydipsia are frequently encountered in patients with chronic potassium depletion, although, occasionally, patients with severe hypokalemia have no complaints referable to the urinary tract. Patients with hypokalemic nephropathy may have an enhanced susceptibility to pyelonephritis. The polydipsia is probably due to both the impaired renal concentrating ability and a primary disorder of the thirst mechanism, which is believed to be a common feature of chronic potassium depletion. Urinalysis often reveals no abnormalities except for mild proteinuria. Serum creatinine and urea nitrogen concentrations usually remain within normal limits. Treatment should be directed at repleting body potassium stores and correcting the primary process responsible for potassium loss. With correction of body potassium, functional and histologic abnormalities of the kidneys usually disappear, although maximal urinary concentrating ability may not return to normal for several months.

Miscellaneous metabolic toxins Urinary oxalate, derived from the metabolism of glycine and, to a variable extent, from ingested oxalate, may deposit as insoluble intratubular calcium oxalate crystals and result in chronic tubulointerstitial damage in patients with hereditary or acquired forms of *hyperoxaluria*. *Cystinosis* and *Fabry's disease* are other hereditary depositional disorders affecting the renal tubules and interstitium (see Chaps. 228, 231, and 232).

RENAL PARENCHYMAL DISEASE ASSOCIATED WITH EXTRARENAL NEOPLASM

In addition to being the site of origin of several benign and malignant neoplasms (see Chap. 234), the kidneys are frequently affected by neoplasms arising outside the urinary tract. Except for the glomerulopathies associated with lymphomas and several solid tumors (see Chap. 228), the renal manifestations of primary extrarenal neoplastic processes are confined mainly to the interstitium and tubules. Although metastatic renal involvement by solid tumors is unusual, the kidneys are often invaded by neoplastic cells in various lymphomas and leukemias and in multiple myeloma. In postmortem studies of patients with *lymphoma*, renal involvement is found in approximately half. The involvement may be focal, in the form of multiple discrete nodules, or diffuse, with lymphomatous infiltration throughout the renal parenchyma. Diffuse infiltration is seen most commonly in lymphomas other than Hodgkin's disease. There may be flank pain related to massive renal infiltration, and x-rays may show enlargement of one or both kidneys. Renal insufficiency occurs in a minority of cases, and overt uremia is rare. Treatment of the primary disease may improve renal function in these cases.

The kidneys are also commonly involved in various forms of *leukemia*. At postmortem examination, bilateral renal involvement is present in approximately 50 percent of cases. As with lymphoma, uremia is rarely, if ever, a consequence of leukemic infiltration of the kidneys. The kidneys can also be involved in leukemias because of the associated high incidence of hyperuricemia, hypercalcemia, and lysozymuria. The myelogenous leukemias, particularly of the monocytic type, may be complicated by tubule defects involving potassium and magnesium wasting.

In contrast, infiltration of the kidneys with *myeloma* cells is infrequent (see also Chap. 265). When it occurs, the process is usually focal, so that renal insufficiency from this cause is also uncommon. The more usual lesion is *myeloma kidney*, characterized histologically by atrophic tubules, many with eosinophilic intraluminal casts, and numerous multinucleated giant cells within tubule walls and in the interstitium. The frequent occurrence of myeloma kidney in patients with Bence Jones proteinuria has suggested a causal relation. Bence Jones proteins are thought to cause myeloma kidney through direct toxicity to renal tubule cells. In addition, Bence Jones proteins may precipitate within the distal nephron where the high concentrations of these proteins and the acid composition of the tubule fluid favor intraluminal cast formation and intrarenal obstruction. Indeed, positive immunofluorescence staining for immunoglobulin light chains can often be demonstrated in casts found in myeloma kidneys. Occasionally, acute renal failure occurs after intravenous pyelography in patients with multiple myeloma and is believed to result from the further precipitation of Bence Jones proteins induced by dehydration prior to radiographic study. Dehydration of the patient with myeloma in preparation for intravenous pyelography should, therefore, be avoided. Multiple myeloma may also affect the kidneys indirectly. Hypercalcemia or hyperuricemia may lead to the nephropathies described above. Proximal tubule disorders are also seen occasionally, including type II proximal renal tubular acidosis and the Fanconi syndrome. Additionally, intrarenal deposits of *amyloid* (see below) may contribute to impaired excretory function.

IMMUNE DISORDERS

HYPERSENSITIVITY NEPHROPATHY An acute diffuse tubulointerstitial reaction may result from hypersensitivity to a number of drugs. First reported after the use of sulfonamides, acute tubulointerstitial damage is now seen most often with the antibiotic *methicillin*, although *ampicillin, penicillin, cephalothin, phenindione, thiazides, furosemide*, and nonsteroidal anti-inflammatory drugs have also been implicated. Of note, the tubulointerstitial nephropathy which develops in some patients taking nonsteroidal anti-inflammatory drugs may be associated with nephrotic-range proteinuria and histologic evidence of minimal change glomerulopathy. Grossly, the kidneys are usually enlarged. Histologically, the glomeruli appear normal. The principal pathologic abnormalities are in the interstitium of the kidney, which reveals pronounced edema and infiltration with polymorphonuclear leukocytes, lymphocytes, plasma cells, and, in some cases, large numbers of eosinophils. If the process is severe, tubule cell necrosis and regeneration may also be apparent. Immunofluorescence studies either have been unrevealing or have demonstrated a linear pattern of immunoglobin and complement deposition along tubule basement membranes. In a few cases of methicillin-induced acute tubulointerstitial disease, circulating anti-tubule basement membrane antibodies have also been found, suggesting that autoantibody formation may have been induced by the penicilloyl hapten of methicillin (by conjugation of hapten with tubule basement membrane proteins, thereby altering the native antigenicity of the basement membrane). In cases associated with nonsteroidal anti-inflammatory drugs a role for cell-mediated immunity has been proposed, since renal infiltration by both T and B lymphocytes has been observed with a relative predominance of cytotoxic T cells. Evidence for an immunologic basis for these various drug-related nephropathies also derives from the facts that the onset of nephropathy does not appear to be dose-related, often follows a second exposure to the drug presumed to be responsible for the renal injury, and often is associated with increased levels of serum IgE. In the case of methicillin, the patients usually develop evidence of renal injury after about 2 weeks of drug administration. Hematuria, fever, skin rash, and eosinophilia are prominent. Many patients develop azotemia which typically resolves after withdrawal of the offending drug. Proteinuria and pyuria often accompany the hematuria, and occasionally eosinophils are found in the urine sediment. The clinical picture may be confused with acute glomerulonephritis, but when acute azotemia and hematuria are accompanied by eosinophilia, skin rash, and a history of drug exposure, a hypersensitivity reaction leading to acute tubulointerstitial nephritis should be regarded as the leading diagnostic possibility. Discontinuation of the drug usually results in complete reversal of the renal injury; rarely, renal damage may be irreversible. Glucocorticoids have been used, but their value has not been established.

SJÖGREN'S SYNDROME (See also Chap. 273) Keratoconjunctivitis sicca, or Sjögren's syndrome, is an immunologic disorder characterized by dryness of mucous membranes and mononuclear cell infiltration of salivary and lacrimal glands; it is often seen in patients with rheumatoid arthritis. When the kidneys are involved, the predominant histologic findings are those of chronic tubulointerstitial disease. Interstitial infiltrates are composed primarily of lymphocytes, causing the histology of the renal parenchyma in these patients to resemble that of the salivary and lacrimal glands. Renal functional defects associated with this disorder include diminished urinary concentrating ability and distal (type I) renal tubular acidosis. Urinalysis may show pyuria (predominantly lymphocyturia) and mild proteinuria.

AMYLOIDOSIS (See also Chaps. 228 and 266) Glomerular pathology usually predominates and leads to heavy proteinuria and azotemia. However, tubule function may also be deranged, giving rise to a nephrogenic diabetes insipidus and to distal (type I) renal tubular acidosis. In several cases these functional abnormalities correlated with peritubular deposition of amyloid, particularly in areas surrounding vasa rectae, loops of Henle, and collecting ducts. Bilateral enlargement of the kidneys, especially in a patient with massive proteinuria and tubule dysfunction, should raise the possibility of amyloid renal disease.

AIDS (See also Chap. 264) Tubulointerstitial and glomerular pathology in patients with acquired immunodeficiency syndrome (AIDS) causes proteinuria and renal insufficiency. Some of the abnormalities result from associated nephrotoxic insults including intravenous drug abuse and multiple exposure to nephrotoxic antibiotics. In addition, the accumulated effects of multiple septic episodes, such as infectious granulomatous cytomegalovirus inclusions, and Kaposi's sarcoma obviously are secondary to the compromised immune state and should not be considered AIDS-specific renal disease. However, glomerular sclerosis has been reported as a complication of AIDS without apparent other cause. The prevalence of a specific AIDS-related renal lesion appears to be variable with few if any such cases noted in some areas of the United States. The reason for this disparity is uncertain. Based on the limited available data, black patients with AIDS may be especially at risk for renal complications, and the variations in reported prevalence of renal disease in AIDS may, in part, reflect different racial distributions among the AIDS populations studied.

TUBULOINTERSTITIAL ABNORMALITIES ASSOCIATED WITH GLOMERULONEPHRITIS A number of primary glomerulopathies may also be associated with damage to tubules and interstitium. Pathogenetically, the extraglomerular component in these renal disorders often involves the same mechanisms that are responsible for the more pronounced glomerular injury. For example, in more than half of patients with the nephropathy of systemic lupus erythematosus, deposits of immune complexes can be identified in tubule basement membranes, usually accompanied by an interstitial mononuclear inflammatory reaction. Similarly, in many patients with glomerulonephritis associated with antiglomerular basement membrane antibody, the same antibody can be shown to be reactive against tubule basement membranes as well.

MISCELLANEOUS DISORDERS

VESICOURETERAL REFLUX (See also Chaps. 95 and 227) Normally, the junction of the terminal ureter with the urinary bladder provides a competent sphincter so that during micturition urine leaves the bladder only via the urethra. However, when the function of the ureterovesical junction is impaired, urine may reflux into the ureters due to the high intravesical pressure that develops during voiding. Clinically, reflux is often detected on the voiding and postvoiding films obtained during intravenous pyelography, although voiding cystourethrography may be required for definitive diagnosis. Bladder infection may ascend the urinary tract to the kidneys through incompetent ureterovesical sphincters. Not surprisingly, therefore, reflux is often discovered in patients with acute and/or chronic urinary tract infections. In children particularly, reflux of minor degree may disappear with time and standard therapy of intercurrent urinary infection. With more severe degrees of reflux, characterized by marked dilatation of ureters and renal pelves, progressive renal damage often appears, and although active infection may also be present, uncertainty exists as to the necessity of infection in producing the scarred kidney of reflux nephropathy. In contrast to those with other forms of chronic tubulointerstitial disease, patients with renal insufficiency and scarring due to reflux often demonstrate substantial proteinuria. Indeed, in such cases glomerular lesions similar to those of idiopathic focal glomerulosclerosis (Chap. 227) are often present in addition to the usual changes of chronic tubulointerstitial disease. Surgical correction of reflux is usually necessary only with the more severe degrees of reflux since renal damage correlates with the extent of reflux. Obviously, if extensive glomerulosclerosis already exists, urologic repair may no longer be warranted.

RADIATION NEPHRITIS Renal dysfunction can be expected to occur if 23,000 Gy (2300 rad) or more of x-ray irradiation is administered to both kidneys during a period of 5 weeks or less. Histologic examination of the kidneys reveals hyalinized glomeruli, atrophic tubules, extensive interstitial fibrosis, and hyalinization of the media of renal arterioles. Radiation-induced renal ischemia is believed to be the main pathogenic factor responsible for the tubulointerstitial damage, which may not become evident clinically for months after completion of radiation. The presentation of acute radiation nephritis includes rapidly progressive azotemia, moderate to malignant hypertension, anemia, and proteinuria which may reach the nephrotic range. More than 50 percent of these cases progress to chronic renal failure. A more insidious form of radiation nephritis is characterized by slower development of azotemia, anemia, and nephrotic syndrome. Malignant hypertension may follow unilateral renal irradiation and resolve with ipsilateral nephrectomy. Radiation nephritis in recent years has all but vanished because of heightened awareness of its pathogenesis by radiotherapists.

REFERENCES

ADLER SG et al: Hypersensitivity phenomena and the kidney: Role of drugs and environmental agents. Am J Kidney Dis 5:75, 1985

BATUMEN V et al: The role of lead in gout nephropathy. N Engl J Med 304:520, 1981

BOTON R et al: Prevalence, pathogenesis, and treatment of renal dysfunction associated with chronic lithium therapy. Am J Kidney Dis 10:329, 1987

BUCKALEW VM JR, SCHEY HM: Analgesic nephropathy: A significant cause of morbidity in the United States. Am J Kidney Dis 7:164, 1986

COE FL, BUSHINSKY DA: Clinical and laboratory assessment on patients with renal and urinary tract disease, in *Clinical Nephrology*, BM Brenner et al (eds). Philadelphia, Saunders, 1987, p 1

COTRAN RS: Glomerulosclerosis in reflux nephropathy. Kidney Int 21:528, 1982

——— et al: Tubulointerstitial diseases, in *The Kidney*, 3d ed, BM Brenner, FC Rector Jr (eds). Philadelphia, Saunders, 1986, p 1143

HUMES HD, WEINBERG J: Toxic nephropathies, in *The Kidney*, 3d ed, BM Brenner, FC Rector Jr (eds). Philadelphia, Saunders, 1986, p 1491

HUMPHREYS MH, SCHOENFELD PY: AIDS and renal disease. Kidney 20:7, 1987

MURRAY T, GOLDBERG M: Chronic interstitial nephritis: Etiologic factors. Ann Intern Med 82:453, 1975

MYERS BD: Cyclosporine nephrotoxicity. Kidney Int 30:964, 1986

WILSON CB, DIXON FJ: Renal response to immunological injury, in *The Kidney*, 3d ed, BM Brenner, FC Rector Jr (eds). Philadelphia, Saunders, 1986, p 800

230 VASCULAR INJURY TO THE KIDNEY

KAMAL F. BADR / BARRY M. BRENNER

Adequate delivery of blood to the glomerular capillary network is crucial for glomerular filtration and overall salt and water balance. Thus, in addition to the threat to the viability of renal tissue, vascular injury to the kidney may compromise the maintenance of body fluid volume and composition. Involvement of the renal vessels by atherosclerotic, hypertensive, embolic, inflammatory, and hematologic disorders is usually a manifestation of generalized vascular pathology. The morphologic and clinical responses to these insults and the unique renal vasculopathy associated with the toxemias of pregnancy are considered in this chapter.

THROMBOEMBOLIC DISEASES OF THE RENAL ARTERIES

Thrombosis of the major renal arteries or their branches is an important cause of deterioration of renal function, especially in the elderly. It is often difficult to diagnose and therefore requires a high index of suspicion. Thrombosis may occur as a result of intrinsic pathology in the renal vessels (posttraumatic, atherosclerotic, or inflammatory) or as a result of emboli originating in distant vessels, most commonly fat emboli, emboli originating in the left heart (mural thrombi following myocardial infarction, bacterial endocarditis, or aseptic vegetations), or ''paradoxical'' emboli passing from the right side of the circulation via a patent foramen ovale or atrial septal defect. Emboli are bilateral in 15 to 30 percent of cases.

The clinical presentation is variable, depending on the time course and the extent of the occlusive event. Acute thrombosis and infarction, such as follows embolization, may result in sudden onset of flank pain and tenderness, fever, hematuria, leukocytosis, nausea, and vomiting. If infarction occurs, renal enzymes may be elevated, namely, aspartate transaminase (AST), lactic dehydrogenase (LDH) most reliable, and alkaline phosphatase, which rise and fall in the order listed. Urinary LDH and alkaline phosphatase may also increase after infarction. Renal function deteriorates acutely, leading in bilateral thrombosis to acute oliguric renal failure. More gradual (i.e., atherosclerotic) occlusion of a single renal artery may go undetected. A spectrum of clinical presentations lies between these two extremes (Table 230-1). Hypertension usually follows renal infarction and results from renin release in the peri-infarction zone. Hypertension is usually transient but may be persistent. Diagnosis is established by renal arteriography.

Management of *acute* renal arterial thrombosis includes surgical intervention, anticoagulant therapy, conservative and supportive therapy, and control of hypertension. The choice of treatment depends mainly on: (1) the condition of the patient, in particular the patient's ability to withstand major surgery, and (2) the extent of renovascular occlusion and amount of renal mass at risk of infarction. In general, supportive care and anticoagulant therapy are indicated in unilateral disease. In bilateral thrombosis, medical and surgical therapies yield comparable results. Twenty-five percent of patients die during the acute episode, usually from extrarenal complications. In *chronic* ischemic renal disease, surgical revascularization is more likely to preserve and improve renal function and to control the hypertension (see below).

ATHEROEMBOLIC DISEASE OF THE RENAL ARTERIES

Atheroembolic disease typically results from multiple showers of cholesterol-containing microemboli dislodged from atheromatous plaques in large arteries. Such emboli occlude small (150- to 200-μm diameter) vessels in the kidney and in other organs (retina, brain, pancreas, muscles, skin, and extremities). It usually occurs in an elderly individual with atherosclerotic disease elsewhere and usually follows aortic surgery or renal or coronary arteriography. Spontaneous atheroembolic disease has been reported. Manifestations include deterioration of renal function (sudden or gradual), mild proteinuria, microscopic hematuria, and leukocyturia. Urine volume may remain normal or fall to oliguric levels depending on severity. Renal ischemia can induce or exacerbate preexisting hypertension.

TABLE 230-1 Clinical presentations of ischemic renal disease

1. Acute renal failure
2. Progressive azotemia in a patient with known renovascular hypertension (usually on medical therapy)
3. Unexplained progressive azotemia in an elderly patient with or without refractory hypertension
4. Hypertension and azotemia in a renal transplant patient

Antemortem diagnosis of atherosclerotic renal emboli is difficult. The demonstration of cholesterol emboli in the retina is helpful, but a firm diagnosis is established only by demonstration of cholesterol crystals in the smaller arteries and arterioles in renal biopsy or autopsy specimens. These may also be seen in asymptomatic skeletal muscle or skin. No specific treatment is available.

RENAL VEIN THROMBOSIS Thrombosis of one or both main renal veins (RVT) occurs in a variety of settings (Table 230-2). The pathogenesis is not always clear, particularly when it occurs in so-called hypercoagulable states such as may develop in pregnant women, users of oral contraceptives, subjects with nephrotic syndrome, or dehydrated infants. Nephrotic syndrome accompanying membranous glomerulopathy and certain carcinomas seems to predispose to the development of RVT, which occurs in 10 to 50 percent of patients with these disorders. RVT may exacerbate preexisting proteinuria but is infrequently the cause of the nephrotic syndrome.

The clinical manifestations depend on the severity and abruptness of its occurrence. Acute cases occur typically in children and are characterized by sudden loss of renal function, often accompanied by fever, chills, lumbar tenderness (with kidney enlargement), leukocytosis, and hematuria. Hemorrhagic infarction and renal rupture may lead to hypovolemic shock. In young adults RVT is usually suspected from an unexpected and relatively acute or subacute deterioration of renal function and/or exacerbation of proteinuria and hematuria in the appropriate clinical setting (underlying nephrotic syndrome, trauma, pregnancy, oral contraceptive use). In cases of gradual thrombosis, usually occurring in the elderly, the only manifestation may be recurrent pulmonary emboli or development of hypertension. A Fanconi-like syndrome and proximal renal tubular acidosis have been described.

The definitive diagnosis can only be established through selective renal venography with visualization of the occluding thrombus. Treatment consists of anticoagulation, the main purpose of which is prevention of pulmonary embolization, although some authors have also claimed improvement in renal function and proteinuria. Encouraging reports have appeared concerning the use of streptokinase. Spontaneous recanalization with clinical improvement has also been observed. Anticoagulant therapy is more rewarding in the acute thrombosis seen in younger individuals. Nephrectomy is advocated in infants with life-threatening renal infarction. Thrombectomy is effective in some cases.

RENAL ARTERY STENOSIS Stenosis of the main renal artery and/or its major branches accounts for 2 to 5 percent of hypertension. The common cause in the middle-aged and elderly is an atheromatous plaque at the origin of the renal artery. In younger women, stenosis is due to intrinsic structural abnormalities of the arterial wall caused by a heterogeneous group of lesions termed *fibromuscular dysplasia*.

TABLE 230-2 Conditions associated with renal vein thrombosis

1. Trauma
2. Extrinsic compression (lymph nodes, aortic aneurysm, tumor)
3. Invasion by renal cell carcinoma
4. Dehydration (infants)
5. Nephrotic syndrome
6. Pregnancy or oral contraceptives

Renal artery stenosis should be suspected when hypertension develops in a previously normotensive individual over 50 years of age or in the young (under 30 years) with suggestive features: symptoms of vascular insufficiency to other organs, high-pitched epigastric bruit on physical exam, symptoms of hypokalemia secondary to hyperaldosteronism (muscle weakness, tetany, polyuria), and metabolic alkalosis. If renovascular hypertension is suspected, a positive captopril test, which has a sensitivity and specificity of greater than 95 percent, constitutes an excellent screening procedure to assess the need for more invasive radiographic evaluation. The test relies on the exaggerated increase in plasma renin activity (PRA) following administration of captopril to patients with renovascular hypertension as compared to those with essential hypertension. It is considered positive when all of the following criteria are satisfied: stimulated PRA of 12 (μg/L)/h; absolute increase in PRA of 10 (μg/L)/h or more; and increase in PRA of greater than 150 percent (or 400 percent if baseline PRA is less than 3 (μg/L)/h. In the appropriate clinical setting, particularly in the presence of a positive captopril test, digital subtraction renal arteriography should be performed. This procedure obviates the need for cannulation of the arterial system and has a low incidence of false-positive (5 percent) and false-negative (10 percent) results. The most definitive diagnostic procedure is bilateral arteriography with repeated bilateral renal vein and systemic renin determinations. If renal vein renin measurements from the two kidneys differ by a factor of 1.5:1 or more (higher value from the affected kidney) in a patient with radiographic unilateral renal artery stenosis, the chance of cure of hypertension by surgical reconstruction is almost 90 percent, particularly if renal vein renin from the unaffected kidney is equal to or less than systemic levels (suppressible). A ratio of less than 1.5:1, however, does not exclude the diagnosis of renovascular hypertension, particularly in the presence of bilateral disease.

The aims of treatment are control of the blood pressure and restoration of perfusion to the ischemic kidney. In general, it is now firmly established that interventional therapy (i.e., surgery or angioplasty) is superior to medical therapy, which, while controlling blood pressure, does little to salvage renal mass lost to ischemic injury. Success rates with percutaneous transluminal angioplasty in young patients with fibromuscular dysplasia are 50 percent cure and 30 percent improvement in blood pressure control. Due to its relative noninvasiveness as compared to surgery, therefore, angioplasty is the primary therapeutic option for patients with renal artery stenosis. Angioplasty is best suited for noncalcified segmental short lesions and is also useful in some elderly patients who are poor surgical risks. About half of elderly individuals with reduced renal function as a result of renal arterial stenosis improve following angioplasty or surgery, even when preintervention arteriography shows little evidence of cortical perfusion. If angioplasty fails, surgical reperfusion should be considered.

Renal artery stenosis, particularly if atherosclerotic, is a progressive disease that may lead to gradual and silent loss of renal functional tissue. Compensatory contralateral hypertrophy may maintain renal function until affected by superimposed pathologic processes, at which time azotemia supervenes. Even if angioplasty or surgery fail to return blood pressure to normal, these procedures usually render medical therapy easier.

HEMOLYTIC UREMIC SYNDROME (HUS) AND THROMBOTIC THROMBOCYTOPENIC PURPURA (TTP) HUS and TTP, consumptive coagulopathies characterized by microangiopathic hemolytic anemia and thrombocytopenia, have a particular predilection for the kidney and the central nervous system, the latter especially in TTP. The kidneys of patients with HUS or TTP often exhibit a "flea-bitten" appearance, the result of multiple cortical hemorrhagic infarcts. The major sites of pathology are the small renal arteries and afferent arterioles, which are nearly occluded as a result of marked intimal hyperplasia (particularly in TTP) and fibrin deposits in the subintimal regions. When the vasoocclusive process is extensive, bilateral cortical necrosis may occur. In addition, arteriolar microaneurysms, glomerular infarction, or nonspecific focal changes may be seen. In keeping with the focal nature of the vascular lesions, patchy areas of interstitial edema, tubular necrosis, and, eventually, fibrosis occur. By immunofluorescence staining, complement components and immunoglobulins may be demonstrated in the arterioles, and fibrinogen deposits are present in arteries, arterioles, and glomerular capillary loops.

Several mechanisms have been implicated in the etiology of the intravascular coagulopathy seen in HUS and TTP including induction of a generalized Shwartzman phenomenon by microorganisms or endotoxin, genetic predisposition, and deficiency of platelet antiaggregatory substance(s) (e.g., prostacyclin). Some patients improve following exchange transfusion or plasmapheresis, suggesting accumulation of an as yet unidentified toxin.

Renal failure is common in both HUS and TTP, usually manifested by oligoanuria (more severe in HUS), azotemia, mild proteinuria, microscopic and/or gross hematuria, and cylindruria. Patients with HUS have more severe renal failure, often marked by oligoanuria and hypertension and commonly progressing to chronic renal failure. The prognosis in HUS is better in children than adults. In TTP, the course of which may span days to months, renal failure is usually less severe. The overall prognosis, however, remains poor in view of the severe CNS involvement.

In the management of TTP, high-dose glucocorticoids and plasma exchange often provide complete remission or cure. Plasma exchange should be initiated as early as possible, and the treatment cycles can be repeated if thrombocytopenia recurs. Splenectomy and antiplatelet therapy have also been used with varying degrees of success in TTP patients. The success of plasma exchange in adult HUS is less well established than in TTP.

ARTERIOLAR NEPHROSCLEROSIS Whether hypertension is "essential" or of known etiology, persistent exposure of the renal circulation to elevated intraluminal pressures results in development of intrinsic lesions of the renal arterioles (hyaline arteriolosclerosis) that eventually lead to loss of function (nephrosclerosis). Nephrosclerosis is divided into two distinct entities: "benign" and "malignant" (or accelerated).

Benign arteriolar nephrosclerosis Benign arteriolar nephrosclerosis is seen in patients who are hypertensive for an extended period of time (blood pressure more than 150/90) but whose hypertension has not progressed to a malignant form (described below). Such patients, usually in the older age group, are often discovered to be hypertensive on routine physical examination or as a result of nonspecific symptomatology (e.g., headaches, weakness, palpitations).

Kidney size is normal to reduced, with loss of cortical mass leading to a fine granularity. Although the larger arteries may show atherosclerotic changes, the characteristic pathology is in the afferent arterioles, which have thickened walls due to deposition of homogeneous eosinophilic material (hyaline arteriolosclerosis). This material is composed of plasma proteins and fats that have been deposited in the arteriolar wall due to injury to the endothelium, probably secondary to the elevated intraluminal hydraulic pressure. Narrowing of vascular lumina results, with consequent ischemic injury to glomeruli and tubules.

Nephrosclerosis accompanying long-standing systemic arterial hypertension is only one manifestation of a generalized process affecting the cardiovascular system. Physical examination, therefore, may reveal changes in retinal vessels (arteriolar narrowing and/or flame-shaped hemorrhages), cardiac hypertrophy, and possibly signs of congestive heart failure. Renal disease may manifest as a mild to moderate elevation of serum creatinine concentration, microscopic hematuria, and/or mild proteinuria. In general, clinical evaluation does not reveal significant renal abnormalities. More specialized examination may disclose elevated urinary albumin excretion, tapering and loss of caliber of intrarenal vessels on arteriography, and an exaggerated natriuresis in response to a fluid challenge. Patients with benign nephrosclerosis maintain a near-normal glomerular filtration rate despite a reduction in renal blood flow.

Malignant arteriolar nephrosclerosis Patients with long-standing benign hypertension or patients not known to be hypertensive previously may develop malignant hypertension characterized by a sudden (accelerated) elevation of blood pressure (diastolic often above 130 mmHg) accompanied by papilledema, central nervous system manifestations, cardiac decompensation, and acute progressive deterioration of renal function. The absence of papilledema does not rule out the diagnosis in a patient with markedly elevated blood pressure and rapidly declining renal function. The kidneys are characterized by a flea-bitten appearance resulting from hemorrhages in surface capillaries. Histologically, two distinct vascular lesions can be seen. The first, affecting arterioles, is fibrinoid necrosis, i.e., infiltration of arteriolar walls with eosinophilic material including fibrin. There is thickening of vessel walls and, occasionally, an inflammatory infiltrate (necrotizing arteriolitis). The second lesion, involving the interlobular arteries, is a concentric hyperplastic proliferation of the cellular elements of the vascular wall with deposition of collagen to form a hyperplastic arteriolitis (onion-skin lesion). Fibrinoid necrosis occasionally extends into the glomeruli, which may also undergo proliferative changes or total necrosis. Most glomerular and tubule changes are secondary to ischemia and infarction. The sequence of events leading to the development of malignant hypertension is poorly defined. Two pathophysiologic alterations appear central in its initiation and/or perpetuation: (1) increased permeability of vessel walls to invasion by plasma components, particularly fibrin, which activates clotting mechanisms leading to a microangiopathic hemolytic anemia, thus perpetuating the vascular pathology; and (2) activation of the renin-angiotensin-aldosterone system at some point in the disease process, which contributes to the acceleration and maintenance of blood pressure elevation and, in turn, to vascular injury.

Malignant hypertension is most likely to develop in a previously hypertensive individual, usually in the third or fourth decade of life. There is a higher incidence among men, particularly black men. The presenting symptoms are usually neurologic (dizziness, headache, blurring of vision, altered states of consciousness, and focal or generalized seizures). Cardiac decompensation and renal failure appear thereafter. Renal abnormalities include a rapid rise in serum creatinine, hematuria (at times macroscopic), proteinuria, and red and white blood cell casts in the sediment. Nephrotic syndrome may be present. Elevated plasma aldosterone levels cause hypokalemic metabolic alkalosis in the early phase. Uremic acidosis and hyperkalemia eventually obscure these early findings. Hematologic indices of microangiopathic hemolytic anemia (i.e., schistocytes) are often seen.

Control of hypertension is the principal goal of therapy for both benign and malignant forms. The time of initiation of therapy, its effectiveness, and patient compliance are crucial factors in arresting the progression of benign nephrosclerosis. Untreated, most of these patients succumb to the extrarenal complications of hypertension. In contrast, malignant hypertension is a medical emergency; its natural course includes a death rate of 80 to 90 percent within 1 year of onset, almost always due to uremia. Supportive measures should be instituted to control the neurologic, cardiac, and other complications of acute renal failure, but the mainstay of therapy is prompt and aggressive reduction of blood pressure, which, if successful, can reverse all complications in the majority of patients. Presently, 5-year survival is 50 percent, and some patients have evidence of partial reversal of the vascular lesions and a return of renal function to near-normal levels.

SCLERODERMA (PROGRESSIVE SYSTEMIC SCLEROSIS) Renal vascular involvement in scleroderma is characterized by a distinctive lesion of the small arteries (diameters of 150 to 500 μm) consisting of intimal proliferation, medial thinning, and increased collagen deposition in the adventitial layer. Fibrinoid changes in the walls of afferent arterioles and microinfarcts may occur. Glomerular changes are generally nonspecific and secondary to ischemic damage. Tubules are often atrophic. As part of a generalized increase in vasomotor tone, a vasospastic (Raynaud-like) phenomenon at the level of the renal vasculature contributes to the renal insufficiency. Reduction in renal blood flow is the major mechanism underlying the deterioration in kidney function, being present in 80 percent of patients, even in the absence of other clinical abnormalities. As vascular narrowing progresses, hypertension, azotemia, and proteinuria eventually develop. Plasma renin rises in response to sustained renal ischemia. The resulting hypertension causes further renal injury and may play a role in the intimate destruction of nephrons. As more and more nephrons are lost to the combined insults of ischemia and hypertension, development of azotemia heralds a particularly grim prognosis. Proteinuria, usually mild, is a consequence of ischemic and hypertensive glomerular injury.

Although the majority of patients with scleroderma present with extrarenal manifestations, renal involvement is eventually manifested in half of patients followed for up to 20 years. Renal involvement can present in one of two ways, depending on whether malignant hypertension is superimposed on the renal pathology: (1) *Persistent urinary abnormalities* with or without hypertension tend to follow an indolent course with mild proteinuria, occasional casts, cellular elements in the urinary sediment, and a propensity for development of hypertension. Azotemia is absent initially, but when it develops, dialysis is required within 1 year. (2) *Scleroderma renal crisis* is a rapid deterioration in renal function, usually accompanied by malignant hypertension, oliguria, fluid retention, microangiopathic hemolytic anemia, and central nervous system involvement. It may occur in patients with previously undemonstrable or slowly progressive renal disease. Untreated, it leads to chronic renal failure within days to months.

The prognosis of scleroderma renal disease is generally poor, particularly following the onset of azotemia. Aggressive antihypertensive therapy may be effective in delaying the progression of renal failure. In scleroderma renal crisis, prompt treatment with beta blockers, minoxidil, and particularly angiotensin I converting enzyme (ACE) inhibitors may reverse acute renal failure. The effect of these interventions on renal function over the long term is uncertain.

SICKLE CELL NEPHROPATHY Sickle cell disease causes renal complications that arise mainly as a result of sickling of red blood cells in the microvasculature. The hypertonic and relatively hypoxic environment of the renal medulla, coupled with the slow blood flow in the vasa recta, favors the sickling of red blood cells, with resultant local infarction (papillary necrosis). Functional tubule defects in patients with sickle cell disease are likely the result of partial ischemic injury to the renal tubules.

In addition to the intrarenal microvascular pathology described above, young patients with sickle cell disease are characterized by renal hyperperfusion, glomerular hypertrophy, and hyperfiltration. Many of these individuals eventually develop a glomerulopathy leading to proteinuria (present in as many as 30 percent) and, in some, the nephrotic syndrome. Mild azotemia and hyperuricemia can also develop, but advanced renal failure and uremia are rare. Although an immunologic basis for the glomerulopathy of sickle cell disease has been proposed, hemodynamically mediated renal injury, resulting from intrarenal hyperperfusion and glomerular hyperfiltration, may be the major pathogenetic mechanism. Nephron loss secondary to ischemic injury also contributes to the development of azotemia in these patients.

The renal complications of sickle cell disease include the following: *Cortical infarcts* can cause loss of function, persistent hematuria, and perinephric hematomas. *Papillary infarcts*, demonstrated radiographically in 50 percent of patients with sickle trait, lead to an increased risk of bacterial infection in the scarred renal tissues and functional tubule abnormalities. Painless gross hematuria occurs with a higher frequency in sickle trait than in sickle cell disease and likely results from infarctive episodes in the renal medulla. *Functional tubule abnormalities* such as nephrogenic diabetes insipidus result from marked reduction in vasa recta blood flow, combined with ischemic tubule injury. This concentrating defect places these patients at increased risk of dehydration and, hence, sickling crises. The concentrating defect also occurs in individuals with sickle trait. Other tubule defects involve potassium and hydrogen ion excretion, occasionally leading to hyperkalemic, metabolic acidosis and a defect in uric acid excretion which, combined with increased purine synthesis in the bone marrow, results in hyperuricemia. Glomerulopathy is an established consequence of sickle cell disease and is due to a combination of hemodynamically mediated glomerular injury referred to earlier and an immune-complex glomerulonephritis in which tubule epithelial antigens, released into the circulation during episodes of ischemic injury, provoke an antibody response leading to immune-complex deposition in the glomeruli. Proteinuria is the chief manifestation of sickle cell glomerulopathy and may reach nephrotic proportions.

TOXEMIAS OF PREGNANCY Renal function is ''reset'' at a higher level during normal pregnancy. Renal plasma flow (RPF) and glomerular filtration rate (GFR) both increase by 30 to 50 percent. Therefore, serum creatinine levels above 70 μmol/L (0.8 mg/dL) or blood urea nitrogen (BUN) levels above 4.6 mmol/L (13 mg/dL) are abnormal in pregnant women and should be investigated. Systolic and diastolic blood pressures decrease by an average of 10 to 15 mmHg below pregravid values. A diastolic pressure above 75 mmHg during the second trimester or above 85 mmHg during the third trimester is therefore abnormal. Vasodilation in the uterine, renal, and cutaneous beds, vasodilator prostaglandin release from the uteroplacental unit, and a decrease in arteriolar sensitivity to angiotensin II all play a role in the decline of blood pressure during pregnancy.

Preeclampsia-eclampsia The toxemia syndrome, usually occurring in the third trimester of primigravidas, includes hypertension, proteinuria, edema, consumptive coagulopathy, sodium retention, hyperreflexia (preeclampsia), and, if uncontrolled, convulsions (eclampsia). In pure preeclampsia (i.e., not superimposed on previously existing hypertensive or renal disease) the primary sites of pathology are the glomerular endothelial cells. These cells show marked swelling due to an increase in cytoplasmic volume with vacuolization (endotheliosis) and encroach on the vascular lumen, rendering the enlarged glomeruli ischemic. The glomerular basement membrane and the extraglomerular blood vessels are intact. The pathogenesis is unknown. Coagulation abnormalities, hormonal factors, uteroplacental ischemia, and immune mechanisms have all been implicated. The mechanisms mediating the hypertension are also not understood. Despite sodium retention, intravascular volume is contracted as compared to pregravid values. An increased sensitivity to angiotensin II is the basis for the ''roll-over test'' (an increase in diastolic blood pressure of 20 mmHg or more upon changing the patient's position from lateral recumbent to supine, presumably due to alterations in circulating angiotensin levels). In the supine position, the reduction in venous return due to compression by the gravid uterus increases circulating levels of angiotension II. This results in a hypertensive response in preeclamptic patients, who are hyperresponsive to angiotensin II, but not in normal women, in whom pregnancy leads to a relative resistance to the pressor effects of this hormone.

A diagnosis of preeclampsia-related hypertension can be made when repeated measurements over a 4- to 6- h period show a blood pressure of 140/85 mmHg or more. The rise in blood pressure tends to be more severe at night. When preeclampsia occurs in a previously hypertensive patient, a rapid acceleration of the blood pressure elevation is accompanied by an increase in proteinuria, oliguria, edema, and coagulopathy. This is a life-threatening syndrome and tends to recur with future pregnancies. In addition to proteinuria, which correlates with the severity of the renal lesion, GFR and RPF are depressed. In view of the preexisting high levels, however, GFR in preeclamptic women often remains above nonpregnant levels. Uric acid clearance also falls, resulting in hyperuricemia. In the postpartum period, these patients are particularly susceptible to the development of ''postpartum renal failure,'' which is thought to be a form of adult HUS.

Management consists of bed rest in a quiet environment and control of neurologic manifestations and blood pressure, the former with magnesium sulfate and the latter usually with vasodilators such as hydralazine and methyldopa. Diuretics are avoided. The ultimate ''treatment'' is delivery, which should be induced if fetal maturity is adequate or if life-threatening coagulopathy or renal failure occur. The long-term prognosis is generally favorable.

Bilateral cortical necrosis Acute bilateral cortical necrosis is associated with septic abortions, abruptio placentae, and preeclampsia. Coagulation in cortical vessels and arterioles leads to renal tissue necrosis. Anuria and renal failure ensue, and may be irreversible. In other cases renal function returns partially, but on long-term follow-up most patients slowly progress to uremia.

VASCULITIS The kidney is commonly involved in systemic disorders in which necrotizing inflammatory injury to vessels is a primary feature. Several lines of evidence point toward an immunologic pathogenesis for the vasculitides, the prototype of which is periarteritis nodosa (PAN).

Periarteritis nodosa In PAN, arcuate and intralobular arteries are primarily involved. Acute lesions are characterized by destruction of the internal elastic lamina, segmental fibrinoid necrosis of the intima and/or the entire vessel wall, intense intra- and periarterial leukocytic infiltration, and occasional aneurysmal dilatation of the vessel wall (demonstrable radiographically). Fibroblast proliferation leads eventually to occlusion and obliteration of vessel lumina. These vascular changes typically lead to glomerular ischemia, occasionally associated with proliferative changes in the glomerular tufts and juxtaglomerular apparatus. Progression to acute necrotizing crescentic glomerulonephritis may occur.

Clinically, renal involvement in PAN is often associated with hypertension (renin-mediated) which at times progresses to a severe or malignant form. Hematuria, microscopic or gross, can also occur as a result of ischemia, hypertensive renal injury, or glomerulonephritis. Proteinuria is usually mild, and the urinary sediment contains all of the formed elements (red and white blood cells, renal epithelial cells, and their respective casts). Nephrotic syndrome is uncommon. Acute renal failure occurs in approximately 10 percent of cases and is usually the result of malignant hypertension and/or the development of rapidly progressive, crescentic glomerulonephritis. The diagnosis of PAN can be established by documenting the typical arterial lesions in biopsy material from involved organs (testes, muscle, skin). Renal biopsy seldom shows the arterial lesions but may reveal focal or diffuse crescentic glomerulonephritis. Renal and celiac arteriography, however, frequently demonstrates characteristic aneurysmal dilatation of the involved arteries.

Untreated, PAN is generally progressive, causing death from renal failure, gastrointestinal bleeding, or other extrarenal catastrophes. Encouraging therapeutic results have been obtained with glucocorticoid therapy in combination with cytoxic agents (cyclophosphamide or azathioprine) and plasma exchange. In addition, hypertension should be controlled. Early initiation of antihypertensive therapy prolongs survival in more than 90 percent of patients and causes complete remission in 20 percent. Allergic granulomatosis (Churg-Strauss syndrome), a variant of PAN, is similar in its renal manifestations but also causes immediate-type hypersensitivity reactions, including primary pulmonary involvement, asthma, and eosinophilia.

Hypersensitivity angiitis (microscopic form of PAN) Hypersensitivity angiitis is an acute fulminant form of necrotizing vasculitis in which the characteristic pathologic finding is an intense leukocytic infiltration of the smaller renal vessels (arterioles, venules, capillaries) with or without fibrinoid necrosis. Thus, the pathology is more often limited to the glomerular vessels (including the afferent and postglomerular arterioles). The infiltrating leukocytes fragment as they invade the vessel walls giving rise to the term *leukocytoclastic angiitis*. Endothelial proliferative changes are also seen, and in severe cases the pathologic picture may be indistinguishable from crescentic (rapidly progressive) glomerulonephritis. Immunofluorescence staining may reveal IgG and IgM in the mesangium. In contrast to the subacute or chronic course of PAN, hypersensitivity angiitis is characterized by rapid onset of renal failure. Urinalysis reveals proteinuria (at times reaching nephrotic range), hematuria, and casts. Microangiopathic hemolytic anemia and systemic eosinophilia are often present. Hypertension, however, is characteristically absent or mild. Uremia leads to death in the majority. Treatment regimens are similar to PAN, but the response to glucocorticoids appears to be more favorable in this disease than in PAN.

Other vasculitides in which renal involvement is present include Wegener's granulomatosis (in which the renal lesion is primarily in the form of a necrotizing glomerulitis) and Takayasu's arteritis, which may involve the main renal arteries and their branches (see Chap. 276).

REFERENCES

Barré P et al: Successful treatment with streptokinase of renal vein thrombosis associated with oral contraceptive use. Am J Nephrol 6:316, 1986

Eknoyan G, Riggs SA: Renal involvement in patients with thrombotic thrombocytopenic purpura. Am J Nephrol 6:117, 1986

Hakim RM et al: Successful management of thrombocytopenia, microangiopathic anemia, and acute renal failure by plasmapheresis. Am J Kidney Dis 3:170, 1985

Hollenberg NK: The treatment of renovascular hypertension: Surgery, angioplasty, and medical therapy with converting enzyme inhibitors. Am J Kidney Dis 1(Suppl):52, 1987

Jacobson HR: Ischemic renal disease: An overlooked clinical entity? Kidney Int 34:729, 1988

Kashgarian M: Pathology of small blood vessels in hypertension. Am J Kidney Dis 5:A104, 1985

Lindheimer MD, Baylis C (eds): Renal function and disease in pregnancy: An international symposium. Am J Kidney Dis 9:243, 1987

Llach F: *Renal Vein Thrombosis*. New York, Futura, 1983

Materson BJ: Special uses for captopril. Am J Kidney Dis 1(Suppl):88, 1987

Muller FB et al: The captopril test for identifying renovascular disease in hypertensive patients. Am J Med 80:6333, 1986

Ratliffe N: Renal vascular disease: Pathology of large blood vessel disease. Am J Kidney Dis 5:A93, 1985

Working Group on Renovascular Hypertension: Final Report: Detection, evaluation, and treatment of renovascular hypertension. Arch Intern Med 147:820, 1987

231 HEREDITARY TUBULAR DISORDERS

FREDRIC L. COE / SATISH KATHPALIA

POLYCYSTIC RENAL DISEASE IN ADULTS

ETIOLOGY AND PATHOLOGY This disease is found in 1 in 500 autopsies and 1 in 3000 hospital admissions and accounts for approximately 10 percent of end-stage renal failure. Inheritance is autosomal dominant and is linked in most families to the alpha-hemoglobin gene complex and the phosphoglycerate kinase genes on the short arm of chromosome 16. The cortex and medulla of both kidneys are usually filled with thin-walled, spherical cysts, ranging from millimeters to centimeters in diameter, that enlarge the organs and interfere with their function, presumably by compressing the nephrons and causing localized obstruction. The cysts, which are lined by a low cuboidal epithelium, contain straw-colored fluid that becomes hemorrhagic with trauma or infection. The intervening renal parenchyma may be normal or show changes of nephrosclerosis or interstitial nephritis.

CLINICAL FEATURES Symptoms usually begin in the third or fourth decades. Flank pain is frequent. Other common symptoms include gross and microscopic hematuria, especially after trauma, and nocturia due to impaired concentrating ability. Ten percent of patients pass renal calculi whose composition and pathogenesis have not been well studied. Stones and blood clots both cause renal colic. Usually the kidneys are palpable and asymmetric and have a knobby surface. Hypertension develops in 75 percent of patients, and progression to chronic renal failure usually occurs (Table 231-1).

Proteinuria is common but rarely exceeds 2 g/d. Urinary infection occurs at some time in most patients, especially as a consequence of instrumentation and renal calculi; women are infected more frequently than men. Erythrocytosis may occur because of high erythropoietin levels; in other patients blood loss anemia may result from the hematuria.

Acute renal failure can result from infection, ureteral obstruction due to clots or stone, or sudden angulation of a ureter by a nearby cyst. Azotemia progresses slowly in the absence of these complications. Patients with end-stage chronic renal failure tend to have higher hematocrits than their counterparts with other renal diseases. Fluid overload is infrequent because of a tendency for renal salt wasting.

Hepatic cysts are present in about 30 percent of patients. Hepatic function is usually normal, and the liver cysts can be asymptomatic or cause epigastric discomfort or biliary colic or become infected. Cysts also may occur in the spleen, pancreas, lungs, ovaries, testes, epididymis, thyroid, uterus, broad ligament, and bladder. Subarachnoid hemorrhage from intracranial aneurysm causes death or neurologic injury in about 9 percent of patients, but routine cerebral arteriography is not warranted. Mitral valve prolapse (26 percent) and mitral, aortic, and tricuspid valve incompetence occur more often than in control groups.

DIAGNOSIS Palpable kidneys, hypertension, or abnormalities of urine in asymptomatic individuals are often the only manifestations. Excretory or retrograde urography typically shows large kidneys with elongated pelvises and flat calyces indented by cysts. Ultrasonography and radioisotopic renal scanning can both demonstrate the cysts quite well. Gray scale sonography is preferable to intravenous pyelography for screening individuals at risk, especially when genetic counseling is desired. Computed tomography may be useful.

TREATMENT Superimposed renal damage such as is produced by analgesics, obstruction, urinary infection, nephrotoxic antibiotics, and hypertension must be guarded against. Dehydration and inadequate intake of sodium chloride (less than 100 mmol/d) should be avoided. The management of chronic renal failure is simplified because fluid overload is not a usual problem and the hypertension is usually amenable to treatment, but the cysts can cause special problems, such as pain, bleeding, infection, or ureteral obstruction. Puncture of cysts, and in some instances even nephrectomy, may be necessary.

POLYCYSTIC RENAL DISEASE IN INFANTS AND CHILDREN

CLINICAL FEATURES The *infantile form* manifests itself at birth by diffusely enlarged kidneys, renal failure, and maldevelopment of intrahepatic bile ducts. The *childhood form* consists of medullary ductal ectasia which is usually asymptomatic, in association with congenital hepatic fibrosis and portal hypertension. Both conditions are rare, and both are inherited as autosomal recessive traits. Renal failure develops frequently in both forms, but death in the childhood form usually results as a consequence of hepatic disease.

MORPHOLOGY In the infantile form, the distal tubules and collecting ducts are dilated into elongated cysts that are arranged in a radial fashion, particularly in the cortex, and make the kidneys large and spongy. In the childhood form, cysts are fewer in number, cortical collecting ducts are less involved, and the kidneys are not as large. Small intrahepatic bile ducts are irregularly dilated, and large interconnecting spaces, lined by hyperplastic epithelium, fill the portal areas. There is portal fibrosis rather than dilatation and proliferation of small bile ducts, and portal hypertension is the rule by late childhood.

DIAGNOSIS AND TREATMENT Infantile polycystic kidneys may be large enough to cause dystocia. At birth they do not function and cause oliguric renal failure, respiratory distress, hypertension, and

TABLE 231-1 Renal tubule defects

Disease	Renal morphologic abnormalities	Functional abnormalities	Mode of Inheritance*	Associated abnormalities
Adult polycystic disease	Cortical and medullary cysts	Chronic renal failure	AD	Hepatic cysts, intracranial aneurysms
Infantile polycystic disease	Distal tubule and collecting duct cysts	Renal failure in the newborn	AR	Intrahepatic bile duct abnormalities
Childhood polycystic disease	Medullary ductal ectasia	Variable chronic renal failure	AR	Hepatic fibrosis and portal hypertension
Medullary sponge kidneys	Ectatic ducts of Bellini	Nephrocalcinosis	AD+S	None
Medullary cystic disease, recessive	Distal tubule and collecting duct cysts	Chronic renal failure, <20 yr salt wasting, polyuria	AR	Variable retinal degeneration (renal retinal dysplasia)
Medullary cystic disease, dominant	Same	Chronic renal failure, >20 yr salt wasting, polyuria	AD	None
Bartter's syndrome	Hyperplasia of juxtaglomerular and medullary interstitial cells	Hypokalemia, high renin and aldosterone levels, polyuria	AR	None
Liddle's syndrome	None	Hypokalemia, low aldosterone levels	AR	None
Familial nephrogenic diabetes insipidus	None	Vasopressin-resistant renal concentrating defect	XL	None
Renal tubular acidosis, type 1	Papillary nephrocalcinosis	Inability to lower urine pH normally, reduced acid excretion	AD	Periodic paralysis, hypokalemia, non-anion-gap metabolic acidosis, growth retardation, rickets
Renal tubular acidosis, type 2	None	Reduced bicarbonate reabsorption	AR AD XL	Non-anion-gap metabolic acidosis, growth retardation rickets, Fanconi syndrome
Renal tubular acidosis, type 4	Underlying renal disease	Reduced proton and potassium secretion	ACQ	Azotemia
X-linked vitamin D–resistant rickets	None	Reduced phosphate reabsorption, hypophosphatemia	XL	Rickets, osteomalacia, normal serum 1,25-D
Vitamin D–dependent rickets, type 1	None	Defective renal 1,25-D production	AR	Rickets, osteomalacia, low serum 1,25-D
Vitamin D–dependent rickets, type 2	None	Defective cell, 1,25-D receptors	AR	Rickets, osteomalacia, high serum 1,25-D, variable alopecia
Oncogenic osteomalacia	None	Reduced phosphate reabsorptions, hypophosphatemia	ACQ	Osteomalacia; mesenchymal tumors; cancer of the prostate or lung
Renal glucosuria	None	Reduced glucose reabsorption	AD	None
Isolated hypouricemia	None	Reduced urate reabsorption	AR	Variable hypercalciuria, bone demineralization
Cystinuria	Cystine stones	Reduced reabsorption of dibasic amino acids	AR	Short stature
Hartnup's disease	None	Reduced reabsorption of monoamino and carboxylic amino acids	AR	Pellagra-like rash, ataxia, delirium
Iminoglycinuria	None	Reduced reabsorption of proline, hydroxyproline, and glycine	AR	None
Adult Fanconi syndrome	Swan neck deformity of the proximal tubule	Reduced proximal tubule reabsorption of bicarbonate, glucose, uric acid, phosphate, and amino acids	AR	Rickets, osteomalacia, acidosis, dwarfism, low serum potassium
Lowe's syndrome (oculocerebrorenal syndrome)	Same	Same	XL	Ocular and cerebral malformations

* AR, autosomal recessive; AD, autosomal dominant; XL, X-linked; ACQ, acquired; S, sporadic.

congestive heart failure. Intravenous pyelography may reveal a mottled nephrogram with variable retention of contrast material in cysts that correspond to dilated cortical and medullary collecting ducts. On retrograde urography the calyces are blunted, and pyelotubular reflux may be seen. In the childhood type the intravenous pyelogram may suggest medullary sponge kidney, because medullary tubular ectasia is prominent. Renal failure and chronic infection are common.

MEDULLARY SPONGE KIDNEY

PATHOLOGY The ducts of Bellini, i.e., the terminal collecting ducts that reach the ends of the papillae and drain the urine into the renal pelvis, are dilated to cystic proportions and frequently contain calcium oxalate calculi. The kidneys are asymmetric, and the more abnormal kidney is usually the larger. One or more medullary cysts are found near the tip of each involved papilla, and calculi form in the terminal collecting ducts in, or proximal to, the cysts (Fig. 231-1). Parenchymal alterations are secondary to intrarenal obstruction. The cysts are lined by cuboidal and, sometimes, by pseudostratified and stratified squamous epithelium.

CLINICAL DIAGNOSIS AND TREATMENT Medullary sponge kidney is present in 1 of 200 unselected intravenous pyelograms. Although most cases are sporadic, autosomal dominant inheritance has been described. The disease has a bimodal pattern of appearance, the first in adolescence and the second during the third and fourth

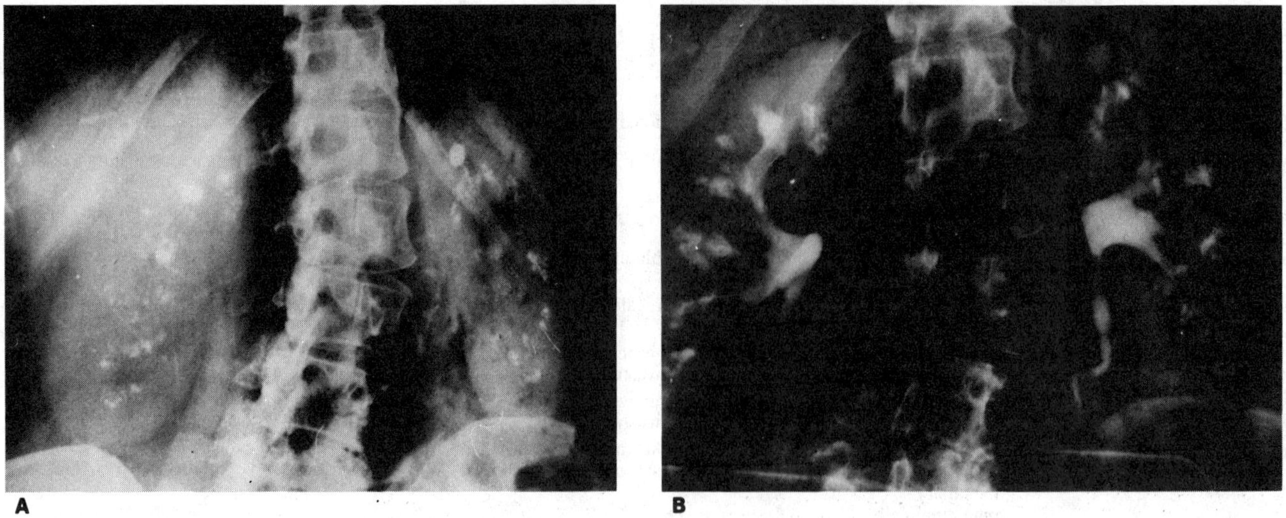

FIGURE 231-1 *A*. Radiographic appearance of medullary sponge kidney. Abdominal flat plate reveals multiple bilateral calcifications. *B*. Radiographic contrast material accumulates in the dilated and cystic terminal collecting ducts and obscures the calcifications.

decades. Calculi, infection, and hematuria occur in 60, 35, and 30 percent of patients, respectively. Papillary nephrocalcinosis due to clusters of stones in cysts is common. Hypercalciuria occurs in nearly half of stone-forming patients but is equally common in other forms of calcium stone disease (Chap. 232). Hypertension is no more common than in the general population. Renal failure is rare, unless nephrolithiasis and/or renal infections are severe.

The diagnosis is made by intravenous urography. The magnitude of pyelotubular backflow varies from a simple papillary blush to tubular ectasia at the tips of the papillae. Small pyramidal cysts and nephrocalcinosis are frequent, and papillary concretions are obscured by the urographic contrast medium. Ectatic collecting ducts are difficult to fill during retrograde pyelography, and the contrast material remains separate from papillary concretions in the cysts.

Asymptomatic patients require no treatment except advice to avoid dehydration and thereby reduce the risk of stone formation. The metabolic etiology of stones should be sought and treated conventionally, while infection and urologic consequences of stones should be treated as described in Chap. 232. Medullary sponge kidneys are vulnerable to infection, and urologic instrumentation should, therefore, be minimized.

MEDULLARY CYSTIC DISEASE (NEPHRONOPHTHISIS COMPLEX)

ETIOLOGY Several hereditary medullary cystic diseases have similar morphology but different patterns of inheritance. The recessive form is associated with renal failure before 20 years of age (early-onset type), whereas the dominant form causes renal failure only after the second decade (adult-onset type). When renal disease is associated with retinal degeneration (renal retinal dysplasia), inheritance is always recessive, but renal failure occurs during adult life.

PATHOLOGY In both forms, most of the cysts are in the medulla and the corticomedullary region and involve the collecting ducts and distal convoluted tubules. Cysts have a low, frequently atrophic, epithelium and range in size from microscopic dimensions to millimeters. The kidneys usually are asymmetrically scarred and shrunken. Both tubular atrophy and periglomerular fibrosis are present, but the former is more severe. In advanced cases, glomeruli become sclerotic and hyalinized, cortical fibrosis and cellular interstitial infiltration appear, and the histology is difficult to differentiate from that of chronic interstitial nephritis.

DIAGNOSIS AND TREATMENT Concentrating ability, acid excretion, and sodium conservation are defective as might be expected from a lesion that damages distal segments of the nephron. The disease is marked by polyuria, progressive renal failure, stunted growth, severe anemia, hyperchloremic metabolic acidosis, and poor sodium conservation. In adults, the inability to conserve sodium may cause a salt-wasting syndrome that resembles adrenal insufficiency but is unresponsive to mineralocorticoids. Hypertension usually is a terminal event. The urinalysis is normal at first, but proteinuria may develop. On intravenous pyelography, the kidneys are small, scarred, and without calcification. The calyces are distorted by numerous cysts in the corticomedullary area.

High sodium and water intake and alkali replacement for acidosis are needed. Treatment of infections, anemia, hypertension, and other aspects of end-stage renal failure are as discussed in Chap. 224. Genetic counseling may be helpful in family planning and in selection of an unaffected related donor for renal transplantation.

BARTTER'S SYNDROME

Bartter's syndrome consists of hypokalemia due to renal potassium wasting, elevated plasma renin activity and aldosterone secretion, normal blood pressure, hyporesponsiveness of blood pressure to infused angiotensin II, and hyperplasia of the granular cells of the juxtaglomerular apparatus of the kidney. Weakness or periodic paralysis and polyuria occur because of chronic potassium depletion. Hypomagnesemia may be present. Hyperplasia of renal medullary interstitial cells, which produce prostaglandins PGE and PGF, has been described, along with elevated PGE_2 production. Inheritance is autosomal recessive, and manifestations commonly begin in childhood.

PATHOGENESIS The main defect seems to be reduced NaCl reabsorption by the thick ascending limb of Henle's loop (TAHL). Volume depletion stimulates aldosterone production and raises serum aldosterone levels, and the combination of high aldosterone levels and increased delivery of NaCl and water to the distal nephron causes kaliuresis and hypokalemia. Magnesuria and hypomagnesemia occur, perhaps because TAHL is a main site for magnesium reabsorption and because hypomagnesemia worsens kaliuresis. Hypokalemia further increases aldosterone production by stimulating release of prostaglandins E_2 and I_2, which promote increased secretion of renin. Both angiotensin II and aldosterone increase renal kallikrein, which increases plasma bradykinin. The normal blood pressure reflects an interaction between the vasodepressor actions of PGE_2 and bradykinin and the elevated angiotensin II. Bartter's syndrome may be mimicked by magnesium deficiency, covert laxative use, or vomiting. Magnesium depletion causes kaliuresis; laxatives cause potassium and volume depletion; vomiting causes renal potassium wasting and volume depletion.

Excessive production of PGE_2 resulting from hypokalemia, a known stimulator of PGE_2 synthesis, may be a secondary consequence of the syndrome. In some cases blockade of PGE_2 production with indomethacin lowers renin levels and restores vascular response to angiotensin II infusion, but does not reduce potassium wasting.

TREATMENT The dietary intake of sodium chloride and potassium should be liberal; potassium supplements may be required. Pharmacologic blockade of aldosterone action on the distal tubules by spironolactone can prevent potassium wasting, though sodium intake must be increased. Inhibition of prostaglandin synthesis with indomethacin, ibuprofen, or aspirin has met with varying success, as indicated above. Beta-adrenergic blockade may lower renin production.

LIDDLE'S SYNDROME (PSEUDOHYPERALDOSTERONISM)

This rare inherited disorder is characterized by hypertension, hypokalemic alkalosis, and negligible aldosterone secretion. It appears to be due to an unusual tendency of distal tubules or collecting ducts to conserve sodium and excrete potassium despite the virtual absence of aldosterone. No other biochemical abnormalities have been described. However, transport rates of sodium in red blood cells are altered. These patients respond to 100 mg per day of triamterene (Chap. 182), a diuretic agent that blocks sodium and potassium exchange in the distal tubule.

FAMILIAL NEPHROGENIC DIABETES INSIPIDUS (DI)

In this disease the distal tubules and collecting ducts are unresponsive to vasopressin because of an X-linked recessive disorder, with variable expressivity in heterozygous females. Affected individuals excrete large volumes of hypotonic urine even when plasma osmolality and vasopressin concentration are both high. Polyuria, polydipsia, and hypertonic dehydration after restriction of fluid intake all result from renal tubular insensitivity to vasopressin (AVP) (also see Chap. 315). Unresponsiveness to vasopressin may be secondary to reduced production of cyclic adenosine 5′-monophosphate (cyclic AMP) in the epithelium of the collecting ducts, to the inability of cyclic AMP to increase the permeability of collecting duct luminal cell membranes to water, or to a combination of the two. Other hereditary tubular defects such as juvenile nephronophthisis, medullary cystic and polycystic diseases, cystinosis, and congenital or acquired chronic urinary tract obstruction can also cause vasopressin-resistant (nephrogenic) DI, but in these syndromes the characteristic features of the underlying disorder are present.

Affected infants easily become dehydrated, hypernatremic, and hyperthermic, and damage of the central nervous system, including mental retardation, may result. In the absence of dehydration, overall renal function is normal. On intravenous pyelography the renal pelvis, ureters, and bladder are dilated, as in any form of DI, because of massive diuresis.

Oral hydration usually is adequate treatment except during early infancy, when hypotonic parenteral fluids may be required. Vasopressin and its synthetic analogues are ineffective, but diuretic agents such as chlorothiazide reduce polyuria. This drug inhibits NaCl reabsorption in the cortical portions of the TAHL, thereby reducing production of free water. In addition, chlorothiazide produces a diuresis that causes contraction of extracellular fluid volume which, in turn, stimulates reabsorption of NaCl and water in the proximal tubule and limits their delivery to the TAHL. Sodium restriction enhances its effect.

RENAL TUBULAR ACIDOSIS (RTA)

In this group of disorders renal excretion of acid is reduced out of proportion to any reduction of glomerular filtration rate. Metabolic acidosis results, but in contrast to renal failure the anions that accompany surplus hydrogen ions in the blood, such as sulfate and phosphate, are excreted normally and are unavailable to balance the fall in serum bicarbonate. Therefore, the kidneys reabsorb chloride in unusually large amounts, and serum chloride rises to preserve electroneutrality in the extracellular fluid. The result is *hyperchloremic acidosis*, and the unmeasured anion gap is normal. There is general agreement that four types of RTA exist (Table 231-2). Types 1 and 2 are often hereditary. Type 3 is a rare mixture of types 1 and 2. Type 4 is acquired and is associated with either hyporeninemic hypoaldosteronism or tubular hyporesponsiveness to circulating mineralocorticoids.

TYPE 1 (DISTAL) RTA Sporadic cases occur, but autosomal dominant inheritance is usual. The kidney does not lower urine pH normally, either because the collecting ducts permit excessive back-diffusion of hydrogen ions from lumen to blood or because they fail to transport hydrogen ions against a steep pH gradient. Since titration of urine buffers and diffusion trapping of NH_4^+ in the tubules both depend upon a low intraluminal pH, excretion of acid is deficient. However, urine ammonium excretion is as high or higher than in normal people whose urine is equally alkaline. Urinary osmotic concentration and potassium conservation also tend to be impaired.

Chronic acidosis lowers tubule reabsorption of calcium, causing renal hypercalciuria and mild secondary hyperparathyroidism. The hypercalciuria, alkaline urine, and low levels of urine citrate—which normally complexes about 40 percent of urine calcium—cause calcium phosphate stones and nephrocalcinosis. Growth is stunted in children because of rickets; this growth defect responds to amelioration of the acidosis with sodium bicarbonate or other alkali. In the adult, bone disease takes the form of osteomalacia. In both children and adults, bone disease may result, in part, from acidosis-induced loss of bone mineral and from inadequate production of 1,25-dihydroxyvitamin D_3 [$1,25(OH)_2D_3$]. Since the kidney does not conserve potassium or concentrate the urine normally, polyuria and hypokalemia occur. Given the stress of an intercurrent illness, acidosis and hypokalemia can be life-threatening.

The diagnosis is suggested by osteomalacia or rickets, hyperchloremic acidosis associated with alkaline urine, and calcium phosphate stones or nephrocalcinosis. To prove that the urine pH cannot be lowered normally, the oral ammonium chloride (NH_4Cl) loading test should be carried out: 0.1 g (1.9 mmol) NH_4Cl per kilogram of body weight is administered, and the blood and urine pH are followed with time. Although systemic acidosis worsens, urine pH does not fall below 5.5. Urinary infection must not be present during this test because bacteria may possess urease, which hydrolyzes urea to ammonia and produces an alkaline urine. When hyperchloremic acidosis is severe and the urine is grossly alkaline, the test is unnecessary.

TABLE 231-2 Comparison of three types of renal tubular acidosis*

Finding	Type 1	Type 2	Type 4
Non-anion-gap acidosis	Yes	Yes	Yes
Minimum urine pH	>5.5	<5.5	<5.5
% filtered HCO_3 excreted	<10	>15	<10
Serum potassium	Low	Low	High
Fanconi syndrome	No	Yes	No
Stones/nephrocalcinosis	Yes	No	No
Daily acid excretion	Low	Normal	Low
Ammonium excretion	High for pH	Normal	Low for pH
Daily HCO_3 replacement needs	<4 mmol/kg	>4 mmol/kg	<4 mmol/kg

* HCO_3, bicarbonate. Type 3 renal tubular acidosis is a rare form of a mixture of types 1 and 2.

A confusing situation may occur when type 1 RTA results from nephrocalcinosis due to hereditary idiopathic hypercalciuria. In this circumstance, stones may be composed of calcium phosphate, but hypokalemia and metabolic acidosis are absent; urine pH is abnormally high and does not fall below 5.5 after NH_4Cl administration. Incomplete RTA is a common term for this circumstance. Other hereditary diseases that cause RTA, such as medullary sponge kidney, galactosemia, Ehler-Danlos syndrome, Fabry's disease, and hereditary elliptocytosis, can be excluded by clinical findings. The relatives of patients with type 1 RTA should be screened for this treatable cause of renal damage.

Treatment Sodium bicarbonate tablets (10 grains = 7.2 mmol base) and Shohl's solution (1 mmol base per milliliter, as Na and K citrate) are both convenient for treatment; the dose should be 0.5 to 2.0 mmol/kg body weight in four or five divided doses daily. The total dose of alkali should be raised until acidosis and hypercalciuria are both eliminated, and the patients should be followed by measurements of serum chloride and CO_2 content and of urine calcium excretion approximately twice yearly. Potassium supplementation is normally not required. Requirements for alkali usually rise during intercurrent illnesses but are usually below 4 mmol/kg body weight per day. Incomplete RTA is best treated using thiazide diuretics as in ordinary idiopathic hypercalcemia (Chap. 232).

TYPE 2 (PROXIMAL) RTA Proximal RTA usually occurs as part of a generalized disorder of proximal tubule function. It can be a transient disorder of infancy which usually disappears in childhood. An isolated form, i.e., without accompanying phosphaturia, aminoaciduria, and uricosuria, has been described in one family. The pathophysiology of proximal RTA is the same whether isolated or part of a generalized disorder. Bicarbonate reabsorption in the proximal tubule is defective, and renal bicarbonate wasting occurs at a normal concentration of plasma bicarbonate. As plasma bicarbonate falls, the filtered load drops to a level that the defective tubule can reabsorb. Then the urine is free of bicarbonate and has a low pH. Potassium wasting and hypokalemia occur, especially when supplementary alkali is given, because bicarbonate is excreted in the urine partly as the potassium salt. Hypercalciuria is moderate, and stone formation is rare. During the NH_4Cl loading test, urine pH falls below 5.5.

Treatment is often not required. When acidosis is severe, bicarbonate must be given in large amounts daily, often above 4 mmol/kg body weight, and even up to 10 mmol/kg per day, because bicarbonate is rapidly excreted in the urine. Another approach is to use a thiazide diuretic and a low-salt diet, which induce mild volume depletion and enhance proximal bicarbonate reabsorption, thereby reducing the required dose. Potassium supplements are needed during treatment because excessive sodium bicarbonate reaches the distal nephron, where much of the sodium is exchanged for potassium, which is then lost in the urine.

TYPE 4 RTA Some patients have a form of renal tubular acidosis that differs from types 1 and 2 and has been called type 4. They have metabolic acidosis without an elevation of the anion gap but differ from type 1 patients in having an acid urine during periods of severe acidosis (Table 231-2), and from type 2 patients in having low urine excretion of bicarbonate and a daily replacement alkali requirement of <4 mmol/kg body weight. They differ from both types 1 and 2 in having a high serum potassium level and a low urine ammonia excretion rate. They have neither Fanconi syndrome nor stone disease. Because potassium and hydrogen excretion are abnormal, they are considered to have generalized distal nephron dysfunction that is due either to intrinsic renal disease or to abnormal aldosterone levels. Hyperkalemia worsens acidosis by suppressing renal production of ammonia, which is the most important urinary buffer, and thereby limiting acid excretion.

The most common patients with type 4 renal tubular acidosis have hyporeninemic hypoaldosteronism; plasma levels of renin and aldosterone are subnormal, even during extracellular volume depletion. Diabetic nephropathy, nephrosclerosis from hypertension, and chronic tubulointerstitial nephropathies are the usual causes. Hyperkalemia and acidosis can be treated with replacement doses of a mineralocorticoid hormone such as fludrocortisone, 0.1 to 0.2 mg/d; some patients may require 0.3 to 0.5 mg/d, suggesting tubule unresponsiveness to the hormone. Furosemide can also improve the hyperkalemia and acidosis, provided salt intake is sufficient to prevent extracellular volume contraction.

A less common condition is *mineralocorticoid-resistant hyperkalemia;* hyperkalemia and acidosis do not improve despite mineralocorticoid hormone treatment. This occurs in occasional patients with underlying renal disease who also have severe salt wasting, as a consequence of distal nephron damage. Plasma renin and aldosterone levels are elevated, and extracellular fluid volume depletion may occur. Treatment requires salt and alkali, but mineralocorticoid supplements are not necessary. Other patients with mild acidosis have no evidence of renal disease and do not waste salt in the urine. Plasma renin and aldosterone levels are low, but hyperkalemia and acidosis do not respond to mineralocorticoid hormone treatment. The cause is thought to be abnormally high distal tubule permeability to chloride ion; sodium chloride reabsorption is elevated, the potential across the distal tubule epithelium is presumed to be below normal, potassium secretion is reduced because it is driven by the transepithelial voltage, hyperkalemia causes acidosis by suppressing ammonia production, and extracellular volume expansion from sodium chloride absorption suppresses renin and aldosterone levels and causes hypertension. The main evidence for this formulation is that infusion of sodium with anions such as bicarbonate or sulfate raises potassium excretion to normal or supranormal levels. Treatment of this rare condition is with thiazide diuretics or low-sodium diet.

Primary mineralocorticoid deficiency from diseases of the adrenals also causes hyperkalemia and acidosis. Evaluation and treatment of adrenal disorders is discussed in Chap. 317.

VITAMIN D DISORDERS

FAMILIAL X-LINKED HYPOPHOSPHATEMIC VITAMIN D–REFRACTORY RICKETS (See also Chap. 341) Reduced tubular reabsorption of phosphate by the proximal tubule and hypophosphatemia occur in this X-linked dominant disease, which is also termed *renal phosphate leak.* Patients may be asymptomatic but are usually short and have rachitic bones; the legs are particularly short and deformed, and osteomalacia develops in adult life. Bone age and dentition are retarded, and the teeth are poorly developed. The skull becomes deformed, and the maxillofacial region may be abnormal. Overgrowth of bone at sites of muscular attachment can limit movement or compress nerves. Bony abnormalities are less common in women. Serum alkaline phosphatase is elevated, serum parathyroid levels are normal or high, serum calcium is usually normal, and urinary calcium excretion is normal or low.

The hypophosphatemia arises in part from decreased tubular reabsorption of phosphate and increased fractional excretion of phosphate. Intestinal absorption of calcium and phosphate may be decreased in untreated patients but increased during treatment with vitamin D. Although glycinuria and mild glucosuria may occur, most patients exhibit only a defect in excretion of phosphate. Absence of hyperchloremic acidosis and a normal serum calcium concentration help to exclude RTA, malabsorption, and nutritional rickets.

Treatment requires oral neutral phosphate, 1 to 4 g daily, in divided doses, and 10,000 to 50,000 units of vitamin D; one must watch for hypercalcemia. Combination of oral phosphate with calcitriol may be more beneficial. Bony deformities require orthopedic management, but corrective surgery, except for genu valgum, should be postponed until active growth is completed.

VITAMIN D–DEPENDENT RICKETS TYPE 1 (See also Chap. 341) Also known as hereditary pseudovitamin D–deficiency rickets, this disease is inherited as an autosomal recessive trait. Defective production of $1,25(OH)_2D_3$ by the kidneys, perhaps because of a genetic defect in 25-hydroxycholecalciferol 1α-hydroxylase, has been proposed as the basis for the disease. However, the dose of calcitriol required to heal rickets is higher than that for vitamin D–deficiency rickets, suggesting an attenuated response to, or excessive degradation of, $1,25(OH)_2D_3$.

Rickets usually begins before 2 years of age. Serum calcium is low, parathyroid hormone concentration and alkaline phosphatase are high, and plasma phosphorus is variable. Urinary calcium is decreased, fecal calcium is increased, and tubular phosphate reabsorption is reduced. Serum levels of $1,25(OH)_2D_3$ are undetectable. Aminoaciduria and hyperchloremic acidosis can occur, but urinary cyclic AMP increases normally in response to PTH infusion.

The 1α-hydroxylated metabolites of vitamin D bypass the enzyme defect and produce a dramatic healing of rickets. Vitamin D_2, 10,000 to 40,000 units per day, is also effective, but oral calcium, 0.5 to 2.0 g/d, is needed as well. The need for vitamin D persists throughout life. Calcitriol, an ideal replacement therapy, is the drug of choice, but one must watch for hypercalcemia.

VITAMIN D–DEPENDENT RICKETS TYPE 2 Like type 1, this disease causes rickets, hypocalcemia, hypophosphatemia, and secondary hyperparathyroidism. Serum levels of $1,25(OH)_2D_3$ are elevated, and treatment with additional $1,25(OH)_2D_3$ does not increase the serum calcium level or heal the bone disease even though it can reduce serum levels of parathyroid hormone. Generalized alopecia is often present and may be either a linked defect or the result of the mineral disorder. The cause appears to be an autosomal recessive defect of the $1,25(OH)_2D_3$ receptor. Treatment with a high dose of calcitriol and mineral supplements may achieve healing of bone, but relapse may occur despite continued treatment.

ONCOGENIC OSTEOMALACIA Mesenchymal tumors, usually benign, can cause renal phosphate wasting similiar to that of X-linked hypophosphatemic rickets, with resulting osteomalacia. Carcinoma of the prostate and oat cell carcinoma of the lung also have caused this syndrome. The disease almost always occurs in adults and develops gradually, over years. The tumors occur mainly in the extremities, head, nose, and mandible, in close association with bone. Their removal cures the phosphate wasting and leads to healing of the osteomalacia.

RENAL GLUCOSURIA

See Chap. 336.

ISOLATED HYPOURICEMIA (See also Chap. 336)

This disorder, in which there is a defect in proximal tubular reabsorption of sodium urate, is inherited as an autosomal recessive trait. Hypouricemia can also occur in the Fanconi syndrome, Hartnup's disease, and Wilson's disease. Uric acid clearance is high, and urine oxypurine levels are normal, excluding hereditary xanthinuria. Patients are asymptomatic except for occasional uric acid nephrolithiasis. No specific treatment is needed except the avoidance of dehydration. Coexistent hypercalciuria and decreased bone density have been described in a few patients, who may have a related disease.

SELECTIVE DISORDERS OF AMINO ACID TRANSPORT

HARTNUP'S DISEASE (See also Chap. 336) In this rare autosomal recessive disorder, renal and intestinal transport of monoamino–monocarboxylic amino acids is defective. An erythematous, scaly, pellagra-like rash appears after exposure to sunlight, and episodic cerebellar ataxia, emotional instability, delirium, and aminoaciduria all occur. The prevalence is 1 in 15,000 newborns.

Dietary monoamino–monocarboxylic amino acids undergo bacterial degradation in the intestinal lumen. At the same time, they are lost in the urine. Inadequate tryptophan availability limits nicotinamide synthesis and leads to secondary pellagra (see Chap. 76). Decreased absorption and urine loss of the other monoamino–monocarboxylic amino acids can cause generalized malnutrition.

The diagnosis is based upon demonstration of massive urine losses of alanine, serine, threonine, asparagine, glutamine, valine, leucine, isoleucine, phenylalanine, tyrosine, tryptophan, histidine, glycine, and citrulline. Hypouricemia may occur. Renal function is otherwise normal. Most patients respond to treatment with oral nicotinamide, 40 to 200 mg/d, and a high-protein diet to compensate for amino acid malabsorption and loss. The ultimate prognosis is good, and the disease often improves with age.

FAMILIAL IMINOGLYCINURIA (See also Chap. 336) This autosomal recessive trait is characterized by excessive urinary excretion of proline, hydroxyproline, and glycine despite normal plasma levels of these amino acids, probably because of deletion or alteration of a membrane transport protein of the renal tubule cells. The patients are asymptomatic. Iminoglycinuria can occur in normal newborn infants up to 3 months of age.

FANCONI SYNDROME

Fanconi syndrome is a constellation of transport defects in the proximal tubule involving amino acids, monosaccharides, sodium, potassium, calcium, phosphate, bicarbonate, uric acid, and proteins. Generalized aminoaciduria, glucosuria, salt wasting, hypercalciuria, hypophosphatemia, proximal renal tubular acidosis, hypouricemia, and tubular proteinuria (Chap. 49) may result. Fanconi syndrome can be acquired secondary to diseases such as cystinosis, tyrosinemia, galactosemia, fructose intolerance, glycogen storage disease (type 1), Wilson's disease, familial nephrosis, and hereditary amyloidosis. Lowe's (or oculocerebrorenal) syndrome is an X-linked recessive form of the Fanconi syndrome associated with ocular and cerebral abnormalities.

An autosomal recessive disease, *adult Fanconi syndrome*, occurs in the absence of any systemic disorder. The term *adult* is misleading since cases are recognized in childhood, but no abnormalities are apparent at birth. Dwarfism and hypophosphatemic rickets occur along with the laboratory abnormalities of Fanconi syndrome. Renal failure is rare, and the prognosis is good when the systemic manifestations are treated. Typically, there is a "swan-neck" deformity and cellular atrophy of the initial portion of the proximal tubule which is probably the anatomic basis of this tubular disorder. The associated defects in the transport of water, sodium, potassium, acid, and phosphate excretion often require treatment. Water, sodium, and potassium intake must be liberal, and phosphate supplements may be needed. Metabolic acidosis can be corrected by the administration of alkali. Vitamin D helps promote bone healing. Glucosuria, uricosuria, and tubular proteinuria do not require treatment.

CYSTINURIA

See Chap. 336.

REFERENCES

Avioli LV: Vitamin D–resistant rickets, in *Diseases of the Kidney*, 3d ed, LE Earley, CW Gottschalk (eds). Boston, Little, Brown, 1979, p 1055

Bernstein J, Kissane JM: Hereditary disorders of the kidney. Part 1: Parenchymal defects and malformations. Perspect Pediatr Pathol 1:117, 1973

Cantani A et al: Familial juvenile nephronophthisis: A review and differential diagnosis. Clin Pediatr 25:90, 1986

Coe FL, Parks JH: Calcium phosphate stones and renal tubular acidosis, in *Nephrolithiasis: Pathogenesis and Treatment*. Chicago, Year Book, 1988, chap 5

DeFronzo FA, Thier SO: Inherited disorders of renal tubule function, in *The Kidney*, 3d ed, BM Brenner, FC Rector Jr (eds). Philadelphia, Saunders, 1986, p 1297

Gabow PA et al: Polycystic kidney disease: Prospective analysis of nonazulemic patients and family members. Ann Intern Med 101:238, 1984

GAMBLIN GT et al: Vitamin D–dependent rickets type 2. J Clin Invest 75:954, 1985
GARRICK R et al: Bartter's syndrome: A unifying hypothesis. Am J Nephrol 5:379, 1985
HUSSACK KF et al: Echocardiographic findings in autosomal dominant polycystic kidney disease. N Engl J Med 319:907, 1988
KIMBERLING WF et al: Linkage heterogeneity of autosomal dominant polycystic kidney disease. N Engl J Med 319:913, 1988
KUPIER JJ: Medullary sponge kidney, in *Cystic Diseases of the Kidney*, KD Gardner Jr (ed). New York, Wiley, 1976, p 151
LEVEY AS et al: Occult intracranial aneurisms in polycystic kidney disease. N Engl J Med 308:986, 1983
LEVY HL: Hartnup disorder, in *The Metabolic Basis of Inherited Disease*, 6th ed, CR Scriver et al (eds). New York, McGraw-Hill, 1989, chap 101, p 2515
LIBBER S et al: Treatment of nephrogenic diabetes insipidus with prostaglandin synthesis inhibitors. J Pediatr 108:35, 1986
LIDDLE GW et al: A familial renal disorder simulating primary aldosteronism but with negligible aldosterone secretion. Trans Assoc Am Phys 76:199, 1963
NARINS RG et al: Metabolic acid-base disorders, in *Fluid, Electrolyte and Acid-Base Disorders*, AI Arieff, RA DeFronzo (eds). NY, Churchill Livingstone, 1985, p 269
RASMUSSEN H, TENENHOUSE HT: Hypophosphatemias, in *The Metabolic Basis of Inherited Disease*, 6th ed, CR Scriver et al (eds). New York, McGraw-Hill, 1989, chap 105, p 2581
REEVES WB, ANDREOLI TE: Nephrogenic diabetes insipidus, in *The Metabolic Basis of Inherited Disease*, 6th ed, CR Scriver et al (eds). New York, McGraw-Hill, 1989, chap 78, p 1985
SCHWAB SJ et al: Renal infections in autosomal dominant polycystic kidney disease. Am J Med 82:714, 1987
SCRIVER CR: Familial renal iminoglycinuria, in *The Metabolic Basis of Inherited Disease*, 6th ed, CR Scriver et al (eds). New York, McGraw-Hill, 1989, chap 102, p 2529
SIRIS ES et al: Tumor-induced osteomalacia. Am J Med 82:307, 1987
TOFUKU Y et al: Hypouricemia due to renal urate wasting: Two types of tubular transport defects. Nephron 30:39, 1982

232 NEPHROLITHIASIS

FREDRIC L. COE / MURRAY J. FAVUS

TYPES OF STONES

Calcium salts, uric acid, cystine, and struvite ($MgNH_4PO_4$) are the basis of most kidney stones in the western hemisphere. Calcium oxalate and calcium phosphate stones make up 75 to 85 percent of the total (Table 232-1) and may be admixed in the same stone. Calcium phosphate in stones is usually hydroxyapatite [$Ca_5(PO_4)_3OH$] or, less commonly, brushite ($CaHPO_4 \cdot H_2O$).

Calcium stones are more common in men; the average age of onset is the third decade. Most persons who form a single calcium stone eventually form another, and the intervals between successive stones shorten or remain constant, suggesting that stone-forming activity usually does not wane with time. The average rate of new stone formation in patients who have previously formed a stone is about one stone every 2 or 3 years. Calcium stone disease is frequently familial.

In the urine, calcium oxalate monohydrate crystals (whewellite) usually grow as biconcave ovals that resemble red blood cells in shape and size but may occur in a larger, "dumbbell" form. In polarized light the crystals appear bright against a dark background with an intensity that is dependent upon orientation, a property known as *birefringence*. Calcium oxalate dihydrate crystals (weddellite) are bipyramidal and only weakly birefringent. Apatite crystals do not exhibit birefringence and appear amorphous, because the actual crystals are too small to be resolved by light microscopy. Brushite produces elongated lathlike (narrow, long, rectangular) crystals.

Uric acid stones (Table 232-1) are radiolucent and are also formed mainly by men. Half of patients with uric acid stones have gout; uric acid lithiasis is usually familial whether or not gout is present. In urine, uric acid crystals are red-orange in color because they adsorb the pigment uricine. Anhydrous uric acid produces small crystals that appear amorphous by light microscopy. They are indistinguishable from apatite crystals, except for their birefringence. Uric acid dihydrate tends to form teardrop-shaped crystals as well as flat, square plates; both are strongly birefringent. Uric acid gravel appears like red dust, and the stones are also orange or red on some occasions. *Cystine stones* are uncommon (Table 232-1), are lemon yellow, and sparkle; they are radiopaque because they contain sulfur. Cystine crystals appear in the urine as flat, hexagonal plates.

Struvite ($MgNH_4PO_4$) *stones* are common (Table 232-1) and potentially dangerous. These stones, formed mainly by women, result from urinary tract infection with urease-producing bacteria, usually *Proteus* species. The stones can grow to a large size and fill the renal pelvis and calyces to produce a "staghorn" appearance. They are radiopaque and have a variable internal density. In urine, struvite crystals are rectangular prisms that have been likened to coffin lids.

MANIFESTATIONS OF STONES

As stones grow upon the surfaces of the renal papillae or within the collecting system, they need not produce symptoms. Accordingly, asymptomatic stones may be discovered during the course of abdominal radiographic studies undertaken for unrelated reasons. Sometimes stones cause gross or microscopic hematuria. In fact, stones rank, along with benign and malignant neoplasms, renal cysts, and genitourinary tuberculosis, as among the common causes of isolated hematuria. Much of the time, however, stones break loose and enter the ureter or occlude the ureteropelvic junction, causing pain and obstruction.

STONE PASSAGE A stone can traverse the ureter without symptoms, but most of the time passage produces pain and bleeding. The pain begins gradually, usually in the flank, but increases over the next 20 to 60 min to become so severe that narcotic drugs are often needed for its control. The pain may remain in the flank or spread downward and anteriorly toward the ipsilateral loin, testicle, or vulva. Pain that migrates downward always indicates that the stone has passed to the lower third of the ureter, but if the pain does not migrate, the position of the stone cannot be predicted. A stone in the portion of the ureter within the bladder wall causes frequency, urgency, and dysuria that may be confused with urinary tract infection. Hematuria is usual with passage of a stone.

OTHER SYNDROMES **Staghorn calculi** Struvite, cystine, and uric acid stones often grow too large to enter the ureter. They gradually fill the renal pelvis and may extend outward through the infundibula to the calyces themselves.

Nephrocalcinosis Calcium stones grow on the renal papillae. Most break loose and cause colic, but sometimes they remain in place so that multiple papillary calcifications are found by x-ray, a condition termed *nephrocalcinosis*. Papillary nephrocalcinosis is very common in hereditary distal renal tubular acidosis and in other states characterized by severe hypercalciuria. In medullary sponge kidney disease (Chap. 231) calcification may occur in dilated distal collecting ducts.

Sludge There can be enough uric acid or cystine in the urine to plug both ureters with precipitate. Calcium oxalate crystals do not do this because less than 100 mg oxalate usually is excreted daily in the urine even in severe hyperoxaluric states, compared with 1000 mg uric acid in patients with ordinary hyperuricosuria and 400 to 800 mg cystine in patients with cystinuria. Calcium phosphate crystals can render the urine milky but do not plug the urinary tract.

INFECTION Although urinary tract infection is not a direct consequence of stone disease, it can occur after instrumentation or surgery of the urinary tract, which are frequent in the treatment of stone disease. Stone disease and urinary infection can enhance the seriousness of one another and interfere with treatment. Obstruction of an infected kidney by a stone may lead to sepsis and extensive damage of renal tissue, since it converts the urinary tract proximal to the obstruction into a closed, or partially closed, space that can become an abscess. On the other hand, some forms of infection, those due to bacteria that possess the enzyme urease, can cause stones composed of struvite.

ACTIVITY OF STONE DISEASE *Active disease* means that new stones are forming or that preformed stones are growing. Sequential

TABLE 232-1 Major causes of renal stones

Stone type and causes	Percent of all stones*	Percent occurrence of specific causes*	Ratio of men to women	Etiology	Diagnosis	Treatment
Calcium stones	75–85		2:1 to 3:1			
Idiopathic hypercalciuria		50–55	2:1	Hereditary (?)	Normocalcemia, unexplained hypercalciuria†	Thiazide diuretic agents
Hyperuricosuria		20	4:1	Diet	Urine uric acid >750 mg per 24 h (women), >800 mg per 24 h (men)	Allopurinol or diet
Primary hyperparathyroidism		5	3:10	Neoplasia	Unexplained hypercalcemia	Surgery
Distal renal tubular acidosis		Rare	1:1	Hereditary	Hyperchloremic acidosis, minimum urine pH >5.5	Alkali replacement
Intestinal hyperoxaluria		~1–2	1:1	Bowel surgery	Urine oxalate >50 mg per 24 h	Cholestyramine or oral calcium loading
Hereditary hyperoxaluria		Rare	1:1	Hereditary	Urine oxalate and glycolic or L-glyceric acid increased	Fluids and pyridoxine
Idiopathic stone disease		20	2:1	Unknown	None of the above present	Oral phosphate, fluids
Uric acid stones	5–8					
Gout		~50	3:1 to 4:1	Hereditary	Clinical diagnosis	Alkali to raise urine pH
Idiopathic		~50	1:1	Hereditary (?)	Uric acid stones, no gout	Allopurinol if daily urine uric acid above 1000 mg
Dehydration		?	1:1	Intestinal, habit	History, intestinal fluid loss	Alkali, fluids, reversal of cause
Lesch-Nyhan syndrome		Rare	Men	Hereditary	Reduced hypoxanthine-guanine phosphoribosyltransferase level	Allopurinol
Malignant tumors		Rare	1:1	Neoplasia	Clinical diagnosis	Allopurinol
Cystine stones	1		1:1	Hereditary	Stone type; elevated cystine excretion	Massive fluids, alkali, D-penicillamine if needed
Struvite stones	10–15		2:10	Infection	Stone type	Antimicrobial agents and judicious surgery

* Values are percent of patients who form a particular type of stone and who display each specific cause of stones.
† Urine calcium above 300 mg per 24 h (men), 250 mg per 24 h (women), or 4 mg/kg per 24 h either sex. Hyperthyroidism, Cushing syndrome, sarcoidosis, malignant tumors, immobilization, vitamin D intoxication, rapidly progressive bone disease, and Paget's disease all cause hypercalciuria and must be excluded in diagnosis of idiopathic hypercalciuria.

radiographs of the renal areas are needed to document the growth or appearance of new stones and to ensure that stones which pass are actually newly formed, not preexistent ones.

PATHOGENESIS OF STONES

Urinary stones usually arise because of the breakdown of a delicate balance. The kidneys must conserve water, but they must also excrete materials that have a low solubility. These two opposing requirements must be balanced during adaptation to a particular combination of diet, climate, and activity. The problem is mitigated to some extent by the fact that urine contains substances that inhibit crystallization of calcium salts and others that bind calcium in soluble complexes. But these protective mechanisms are less than perfect. When the urine becomes supersaturated with insoluble materials, because excretion rates are excessive and/or because water conservation is extreme, crystals form and may grow and aggregate to form a stone.

SUPERSATURATION In a solution in equilibrium with crystals of calcium oxalate, the product of the chemical activities of the calcium and oxalate ions in the solution is termed the *equilibrium solubility product,* because it is the activity product that is unique to the equilibrium condition. If the crystals are removed, and if either calcium or oxalate ions are added to the solution, the activity product will increase, but the solution may remain clear; no new crystals form. Such a solution is considered to be *metastably supersaturated.* If new calcium oxalate seed crystals are now added, they will grow in size. Ultimately, the activity product reaches a critical value at which a solid phase begins to develop spontaneously. This value is called the *upper limit of metastability,* or the *formation product.* Stone growth in the urinary tract requires a urine that, on the average, is above the equilibrium solubility product. Persistence of a stone requires an average activity product at least equal to the solubility product. Excessive supersaturation is common in stone formation.

Calcium, oxalate, and phosphate form many stable soluble complexes among themselves and with other substances in urine, such as citrate. As a result, their free ion activities are considerably below their chemical concentrations and can be measured only by indirect techniques. Reduction in ligands such as citrate can increase ion activity without measurably changing total urinary calcium. Urine supersaturation can be increased by dehydration or by overexcretion of calcium, oxalate, or phosphate. Supersaturation of the urine with cystine or uric acid also occurs when overexcretion or low urine volume is present. Urine pH can also be an important factor; phosphate and uric acid are weak acids that dissociate readily over the physiologic range of urine pH. Alkaline urine contains more urate and dissociated phosphate, favoring deposits of sodium hydrogen urate, brushite, and apatite. Below a urine pH of 5.5, uric acid crystals (pK 5.47) predominate, whereas phosphate crystals are rare. The solubility of calcium oxalate, on the other hand, is not influenced by changes in urine pH. Measurements of supersaturation in a pooled 24-h urine sample are averages that probably underestimate the risk of precipitation. Transient dehydration or postprandial bursts of overexcretion may cause values that are considerably above the average.

NUCLEATION Homogeneous nucleation In urine that is supersaturated with respect to calcium oxalate, these two ions form clusters. The higher the supersaturation, the larger and more numerous the clusters become. Most small clusters eventually disperse because the internal forces that hold them together are too weak to overcome the random tendency of ions to move away. Clusters of over 100 ions can remain stable because attractive forces balance surface losses. Once they are stable, nuclei can grow at levels of supersaturation below that needed for their creation. The formation product marks the point at which stable nuclei become frequent enough to create a permanent solid phase.

Heterogeneous nucleation If a supersaturated urine is seeded with preformed nuclei of a crystal that is similar in structure to calcium oxalate, calcium and oxalate ions in solution will bind to the crystal's surface as they would upon a seed crystal of calcium oxalate itself. The organized growth of one crystal on the surface of another is called *epitaxial growth*, and the seeding of a supersaturated solution by foreign nuclei is called *heterogeneous nucleation*. Sodium hydrogen urate, uric acid, and hydroxyapatite crystals can serve as heterogeneous nuclei that permit calcium oxalate stones to form even though urine calcium oxalate supersaturation never exceeds the metastable limit.

INHIBITORS OF CRYSTAL GROWTH AND AGGREGATION Stable nuclei must grow and aggregate to produce a stone of clinical significance. Urine contains potent inhibitors of both of these processes for calcium oxalate and calcium phosphate but not for uric acid, cystine, or struvite. Inorganic pyrophosphate is a potent inhibitor that appears to affect calcium phosphate more than calcium oxalate crystals. Other urine components that appear to be glycoproteins inhibit the growth of calcium oxalate crystals. Slowing of crystal growth increases the apparent upper limit of metastability, because the critical growth of ion clusters into stable nuclei is hindered. As a consequence of the presence of these inhibitors, crystal growth in urine is slow compared with growth in simple salt solutions, and the upper limit of metastability is higher. Urine citrate may also inhibit crystal growth or nucleation.

EVALUATION AND TREATMENT OF PATIENTS WITH NEPHROLITHIASIS

A majority of patients with nephrolithiasis have remediable metabolic disorders that cause stones and can be detected by chemical analysis of the serum and urine. A practical outpatient evaluation consists of three 24-h urine collections, each with a corresponding blood sample; measurements of serum and urine calcium, uric acid and creatinine, urine oxalate and citrate, and serum electrolytes should be made. When possible, the composition of kidney stones should be determined because treatment depends on stone type (Table 232-1). No matter what disorders are found, every patient should be counseled to avoid dehydration and to drink six to eight glasses of water daily. Since treatment is prolonged, the use of medications must be justified by the activity and severity of stone disease and the importance of protection against new stones.

The management of stones that are already present in the kidneys or urinary tract requires a combined medical and surgical approach. The specific treatment for any individual depends upon the location of the stone, the extent of obstruction, the function of the affected and unaffected kidneys, the presence or absence of urinary tract infection, the progress of stone passage, and the risk of operation or anesthesia, given the overall clinical state of the patient. In general, severe obstruction, infection, intractable pain, or serious bleeding are indications for removal of a stone.

In the past, stones could be removed only by operation or by passing a flexible basket retrograde up the ureter from the bladder during cystoscopy. However, there now are three new alternatives. Extracorporeal lithotripsy causes the in situ fragmentation of stones in the kidney, renal pelvis, or proximal ureter by exposing them to extracorporeal shock waves. The patient is submerged in a water tank, the kidney with the stone is centered at the focal point of parabolic reflectors, and high-intensity shock waves are created by high-voltage discharge. The waves are focused by the reflectors so that they pass through the patient and fracture the stone as they pass. After multiple discharges, most stones are reduced to powder that moves through the ureter into the bladder. Larger fragments are removed by cystoscopy. Percutaneous ultrasonic lithotripsy requires the passage of a rigid cystoscope-like instrument into the renal pelvis through a small incision in the flank. Stones can be disrupted by a small ultrasound transducer, and fragments can be removed directly. The last method is endoscopic passage of an ultrasonic transducer into the ureter via a cystoscope; ureteral stones that are inaccessible to extracorporeal or percutaneous lithotripsy can be fragmented and removed. These various forms of lithotripsy are replacing pyelolithotomy and ureterolithotomy.

CALCIUM STONES **Idiopathic hypercalciuria** (See also Chap. 340) This condition appears to be hereditary, and its diagnosis is straightforward (Table 232-1). In some patients, primary intestinal hyperabsorption of calcium causes transient postprandial hypercalcemia that suppresses secretion of parathyroid hormone. The renal tubules are deprived of the normal potent stimulus to reabsorb calcium at the same time that the filtered load of calcium is increased. In other patients, reabsorption of calcium by the renal tubules appears to be defective, and secondary hyperparathyroidism is evoked by urinary losses of calcium. Renal synthesis of 1,25-dihydroxyvitamin D is increased, producing intestinal hyperabsorption of calcium. In the past, the separation of "absorptive" and "renal" forms of hypercalciuria has been used to guide treatment. However, these may not be distinct entities but the extremes of a continuum of behavior. Hypercalciuria contributes to stone formation by raising urine saturation with respect to calcium oxalate and calcium phosphate.

Thiazide diuretics lower urine calcium in both types of hypercalciuria and are effective in preventing the formation of stones. The drug effect requires slight contraction of the extracellular fluid volume, and massive use of NaCl will reduce its therapeutic effect. Potassium citrate is useful to prevent hypokalemia and raise urine citrate; the latter lowers urine calcium ion levels.

Hyperuricosuria About 20 percent of calcium oxalate stone formers are hyperuricosuric, primarily because of an excessive intake of purine from meat, fish, and poultry. The mechanism of stone formation probably is heterogeneous nucleation of calcium oxalate by crystals of sodium hydrogen urate or uric acid that lodge in the terminal ends of the collecting ducts and produce an anchored site on which calcium oxalate can deposit. A low purine diet is desirable but difficult for many patients to achieve. The alternative is allopurinol, usually 100 mg bid. Some patients eventually alter their diets so that allopurinol can be withdrawn.

Primary hyperparathyroidism (See also Chap. 340) The diagnosis of this condition is established by documenting hypercalcemia that cannot be otherwise explained accompanied by inappropriately elevated serum concentrations of parathyroid hormone. Hypercalciuria, usually present, raises the urine supersaturation of calcium phosphate and/or calcium oxalate (Table 232-1). Prompt diagnosis is important since parathyroidectomy is effective treatment and should be carried out before renal damage has occurred.

Distal renal tubular acidosis (See also Chap. 231) The defect in this condition seems to reside in the distal nephron, which cannot establish a normal pH gradient between urine and blood, leading to hyperchloremic acidosis. The minimum urine pH in response to an oral challenge with NH_4Cl, 1.9 mmol per kilogram of body weight, is above 5.5. Hypercalciuria, an alkaline urine, and a low urine citrate cause supersaturation with respect to calcium phosphate. Calcium phosphate stones form, nephrocalcinosis is common, and osteomalacia or rickets may occur. Renal damage is frequent, and glomerular filtration rate falls gradually. Treatment with supplemental alkali reverses hypercalciuria and limits the production of new stones. The usual dose of sodium bicarbonate is 0.5 to 2.0 mmol per kilogram of body weight per day, in four to six divided doses. An alternative is Shohl's solution, which contains citrate and citric acid. Incomplete renal tubular acidosis (RTA) is a form of the disorder in which systemic acidosis is absent but urine pH cannot be lowered below 5.5 after an exogenous acid load such as ammonium chloride. Incomplete RTA may develop in some patients who form calcium oxalate stones because of idiopathic hypercalciuria; the importance of the RTA in producing stones in this situation is uncertain, and thiazide treatment is a reasonable alternative. Some patients with incomplete RTA form calcium phosphate stones because of low urine citrate and an abnormally alkaline urine and are best treated with alkali as if RTA were complete.

Hyperoxaluria Overabsorption of dietary oxalate and consequent oxaluria, i.e., so-called intestinal oxaluria, is one consequence of fat malabsorption (Chap. 240). The latter can be caused by a variety of conditions, including bacterial overgrowth syndromes, chronic disease of the pancreas and biliary tract, jejunoileal bypass in treatment of obesity, or ileal resection for inflammatory bowel disease. With fat malabsorption, calcium in the bowel lumen is bound by fatty acids instead of oxalate, which is left free for absorption in the colon. Delivery of unabsorbed fatty acids and bile salts to the colon may injure the colonic mucosa and enhance oxalate absorption. Dietary excess of oxalate, ascorbic acid loading, and hereditary hyperoxaluric states are less common causes of hyperoxaluria. Ethylene glycol intoxication and methoxyflurane can also cause oxalate overproduction and hyperoxaluria. Hyperoxaluria from any cause can produce tubulointerstitial nephropathy (Chap. 229) and lead to stone formation.

The oxalate-binding resin cholestyramine, at a dose of 8 to 16 g per day, correction of fat malabsorption, and a low-fat diet are effective treatments for oxaluria secondary to intestinal absorption. Calcium lactate, 8 to 14 g per day, which precipitates oxalate in the gut lumen is an alternative form of therapy. There is no effective treatment for primary hyperoxaluria, the result of an enzymatic defect involving the metabolism of the precursor of oxalate that is inherited as an autosomal recessive (also see Chap. 335). A high fluid intake, phosphate, and pyridoxine (200 mg per day) are recommended, but irreversible renal failure secondary to recurrent stone formation usually occurs before age 20.

Idiopathic calcium lithiasis At least 20 percent of patients have no obvious cause for stones (Table 232-1). The best treatment appears to be a high fluid intake, so that the urine specific gravity remains at 1.005 or below throughout the day and night. Oral phosphate at a dose of 2 g phosphorus daily may lower urine calcium and increase urine pyrophosphate and thereby reduce the rate of recurrence. Orthophosphate causes mild nausea and diarrhea initially, but tolerance may improve with continued intake. Thiazide treatment to reduce calcium excretion and allopurinol to diminish uric acid output may also be helpful. There are no adequate studies to support the use of supplemental magnesium, pyridoxine, or methylene blue.

URIC ACID STONES These stones form because the urine becomes supersaturated with undissociated uric acid, uric acid that is protonated at its N-9 position. In gout, idiopathic uric acid lithiasis, and dehydration, the average pH is abnormally low, usually below 5.4, and often below 5.0. Undissociated uric acid therefore predominates and is soluble in urine only in concentrations of 100 mg per liter. Concentrations above this level represent supersaturation that causes crystals and stones to form. Hyperuricosuria, when present, increases supersaturation, and urine of low pH can be excessively supersaturated with undissociated uric acid even though the daily excretion rate is normal. Myeloproliferative syndromes, chemotherapeutic treatment of malignant tumors, and the Lesch-Nyhan syndrome cause such massive production of uric acid and consequent hyperuricosuria that stones and uric acid sludge occur even at a normal urine pH. The renal collecting tubules can be plugged by uric acid crystals with consequent acute renal failure.

The two goals of treatment are to raise urine pH and to lower excessive urine uric acid excretion to less than 1 g per day. Supplemental alkali, 1 to 3 mmol per kilogram of body weight per day, should be given in three or four evenly spaced, divided doses, one of which should be given at bedtime. The form of the alkali may be important. Potassium citrate may reduce the risk of calcium salts crystallizing when urine pH is increased, whereas sodium citrate or sodium bicarbonate may increase the risk. If the overnight urine pH is below 5.5, the evening dose of bicarbonate may be raised, or 250 mg acetazolamide added at bedtime. With massive overexcretion of uric acid, high doses of allopurinol, exceeding 300 mg daily, may be needed. Treatment with allopurinol should be instituted before chemotherapy of highly cellular tumors, since massive hyperuricosuria can be expected. Alkali treatment must be avoided if hypercalciuria is also present.

CYSTINURIA AND CYSTINE STONES (See also Chap. 336) In this disorder proximal tubular and jejunal transport of cystine and the other dibasic amino acids, lysine, arginine, and ornithine, are defective, and excessive amounts are lost in the urine. Clinical disease is due solely to the insolubility of cystine, which forms stones.

Pathogenesis Cystinuria probably occurs because of defective transport of amino acids by the brush borders of renal tubule and intestinal epithelial cells. Cystine, lysine, arginine, and ornithine appear to share a common renal transport pathway, since infusion of lysine decreases tubular reabsorption of the other three. But cystine is also transported by a separate transport mechanism, because cystinuria and dibasic aminoaciduria can each occur independently. The intestinal defects are not similar in all patients who are homozygous for cystinuria, and the extent of aminoaciduria in those relatives of cystinuric patients who are heterozygous carriers of the defect varies from family to family. Three types of inheritance have been described (see Chap. 336).

Diagnosis and treatment Cystine stones are formed only by patients with cystinuria, but 10 percent of stones formed by cystinuric patients do not contain cystine; therefore, every stone former should be screened for the disease. The sediment from a first morning urine specimen in many patients with homozygous cystinuria reveals typical flat hexagonal platelike cystine crystals. Cystinuria can also be detected using the urine sodium nitroprusside test. The test is positive with 75 to 125 mg cystine per gram of creatinine, a concentration lower than that in the urine of patients with cystinuria but above the levels in normal urine. Because the test is sensitive, it is positive in many asymptomatic heterozygotes for cystinuria. A positive nitroprusside test or the finding of cystine crystals in the urine sediment should be evaluated by measurement of daily cystine excretion. Normal adults excrete 40 to 60 mg cystine per gram of creatinine, heterozygotes usually excrete less than 300 mg/g, and patients with homozygous cystinuria almost always excrete above 250 mg/g.

Treatment consists of a high fluid intake, even at night. Daily urine volume should exceed 3 L. Raising urine pH with alkali is helpful, provided the urine pH exceeds 7.5. Because side effects are frequent, penicillamine, which forms the soluble disulfide cysteine-penicillamine, should be used only when fluid loading and alkali therapy are ineffective. Mercaptopropinylglycine has been used to dissolve renal calculi by perfusion of the renal pelvis and has been given by mouth to prevent stones. Low-methionine diets have not proved to be practical for clinical use.

STRUVITE STONES These stones are a result of urinary infection with bacteria, usually *Proteus* species, which possess urease, an enzyme that degrades urea to NH_3 and CO_2. The NH_3 hydrolyzes to NH_4^+ and raises pH, usually to 8 or 9. The CO_2 hydrates to H_2CO_3 and then dissociates to CO_3^{2-} which precipitates with calcium as $CaCO_3$. The NH_4^+ precipitates PO_4^{3-} and Mg^{2+} to form the triple salt $MgNH_4PO_4$. The result is a stone of calcium carbonate admixed with struvite. Struvite does not form in urine in the absence of infection, because NH_4^+ concentration is low in urine that is alkaline in response to physiologic stimuli. Chronic *Proteus* infection can occur because of impaired urinary drainage, urologic instrumentation or surgery, and especially with chronic antibiotic treatment, which can favor the dominance of *Proteus* in the urinary tract.

Treatment Methenamine mandelate, which lowers urine pH and liberates formaldehyde, is used for chronic suppression of infection when a stone is present. More extreme lowering of urine pH with chronic administration of NH_4Cl may retard stone growth but may also raise urine calcium level and promote the formation of calcium oxalate stones. Antimicrobial treatment is best reserved for dealing with acute infection and for maintenance of a sterile urine after surgery, in the hope of preventing recurrence or minimizing stone growth. Surgery may be appropriate for severe obstruction, pain, bleeding, or intractable urinary infection. Since stones can regrow from any infected fragment which is left behind, recurrences following operation are quite common. In some centers, it is possible to irrigate the renal pelvis and calyces with Renacidin, a solution that dissolves struvite, using a catheter passed through a cutaneous flank incision into the kidney.

REFERENCES

COE FL, PARKS JH: *Nephrolithiasis: Pathogenesis and treatment.* Chicago, Year Book, 1988

——— et al: Effect of low calcium diet on urine calcium excretion, parathyroid function, and serum 1,25(OH)$_2$D$_3$ levels in patients with idiopathic hypercalciuria and in normal subjects. Am J Med 72:25, 1982

FLEISCH H, FAVUS MJ: Disorders of stone formation, in *The Kidney,* 3d ed, BM Brenner, FC Rector Jr (eds). Philadelphia, Saunders, 1986, p 1403

NAKAGAWA Y et al: Purification and characterization of the principal inhibitors of calcium oxalate monohydrate crystal growth in human urine. J Biol Chem 258:12594, 1983

NEWMAN DM et al: Long-term follow-up of 1,900 ESWL treatments, in *Shock Wave Lithotripsy,* JE Lingeman, DM Newman (eds). New York, Plenum, 1988

PAK CYC (ed): Urolithiasis. Kidney Int 13:341, 1978

———: Kidney stones, in *Williams' Textbook of Endocrinology,* 7th ed, JD Wilson, DW Foster (eds). Philadelphia, Saunders, 1985, p 1256

SMITH LH: Urolithiasis, in *Diseases of the Kidney,* 4th ed, RW Schrier, CW Gottschalk (eds). Boston, Little, Brown, 1988, p 785

STRAUSS AL et al: Factors that predict relapse of calcium nephrolithiasis during treatment. Am J Med 72:25, 1982

WEBB DR et al: Extracorporeal shockwave lithotripsy, endourology and open surgery: The management and follow-up of 200 patients with urinary calculi. Ann R Coll Surg Engl 67:337, 1985

233 URINARY TRACT OBSTRUCTION

BARRY M. BRENNER / EDGAR L. MILFORD / JULIAN L. SEIFTER

Obstruction to the flow of urine, with attendant stasis and elevation in urinary tract pressure, impairs renal and urinary conduit functions and represents a common cause of acute and chronic renal failure. With early relief of obstruction, the defects in function usually disappear completely. However, chronic obstruction may produce profound and permanent loss of renal mass (renal atrophy) and excretory capability, as well as enhanced susceptibility to local infection and stone formation. Early and accurate diagnosis and prompt and appropriate therapy are, therefore, essential to minimize the otherwise devastating effects of obstruction on urinary tract structure and function.

ETIOLOGY Obstruction to urine flow can result from *intrinsic* or *extrinsic mechanical blockade* as well as from *functional defects* not associated with fixed occlusion of the urinary drainage system. Lesions causing mechanical obstruction can occur at any level of the urinary tract, from the renal calyces to the external urethral meatus. Normal points of narrowing, such as the ureteropelvic and ureterovesical junctions, bladder neck, and urethral meatus, are common sites of obstruction. When blockage is above the level of the bladder, unilateral dilatation of the ureter (*hydroureter*) and renal pyelocalyceal system (*hydronephrosis*) occur; when the lesion is at or below the level of the bladder, bilateral involvement is the rule.

Common forms of obstruction are listed in Table 233-1. In childhood, *congenital malformations,* including marked narrowing of the ureteropelvic junction, anomalous (retrocaval) location of the ureter, and posterior urethral valves predominate. The latter defect is the most common cause of bilateral hydronephrosis in boys. Children may also have bladder dysfunction secondary to congenital urethral stricture, urethral meatal stenosis, or bladder neck obstruction. In adults, urinary tract obstruction is due mainly to *acquired defects.* Pelvic tumors, calculi, and urethral stricture predominate. Ligation of, or injury to, the ureter during pelvic or colonic surgery can lead to hydronephrosis which, if unilateral, may remain relatively silent and undetected. Obstructive uropathy may also result from extrinsic neoplastic (carcinoma of cervix or colon, retroperitoneal lymphoma) or inflammatory disorders. One such inflammatory disorder is retroperitoneal fibrosis, a process of unknown cause seen most commonly in middle-aged men, which occasionally leads to bilateral ureteral obstruction. Occurring in some patients taking methysergide for relief of migraine, retroperitoneal fibrosis must be distinguished from other retroperitoneal causes of ureteral obstruction, particularly lymphomas and pelvic neoplasms.

TABLE 233-1 Common mechanical causes of urinary tract obstruction

Ureter	Bladder outlet	Urethra
CONGENITAL		
Ureteropelvic junction narrowing or obstruction Ureterovesical junction narrowing or obstruction Ureterocele Retrocaval ureter	Bladder neck obstruction Ureterocele	Posterior urethral valves Anterior urethral valves Stricture Meatal stenosis Phimosis
ACQUIRED INTRINSIC DEFECTS		
Calculi Inflammation Trauma Sloughed papillae Tumor Blood clots Uric acid crystals	Benign prostatic hypertrophy Cancer of prostate Cancer of bladder Calculi Diabetic neuropathy Spinal cord disease	Stricture Tumor Calculi Trauma Phimosis
ACQUIRED EXTRINSIC DEFECTS		
Pregnant uterus Retroperitoneal fibrosis Aortic aneurysm Uterine leiomyomata Carcinoma of uterus, prostate, bladder, colon, rectum Retroperitoneal lymphoma Accidental surgical ligation	Carcinoma of cervix, colon Trauma	Trauma

Functional impairment of urine flow usually results from disorders that involve both the ureter and bladder. Common functional lesions include neurogenic bladder, often with adynamic ureter, and vesicoureteral reflux. Reflux of urine from bladder to ureter(s) is more common in children than adults and may result in severe unilateral or bilateral hydroureter and hydronephrosis. Abnormal insertion of the ureter into the bladder is the most common cause of vesicoureteral reflux in children. Reflux in the absence of urinary tract infection or bladder neck obstruction usually does not lead to renal parenchymal damage and often resolves spontaneously as the child matures. Surgical reinsertion of the ureter into the bladder is indicated if reflux is severe and unlikely to improve spontaneously, if renal function deteriorates, or if urinary tract infections recur despite chronic antimicrobial therapy.

CLINICAL FEATURES The pathophysiology and clinical features of urinary tract obstruction are summarized in Table 233-2. *Pain* is the symptom which most commonly provokes the need for medical attention. The pain of urinary tract obstruction is due to distention of the collecting system or renal capsule. The severity of the pain is influenced more by the rate at which distention develops than by the degree of distention. Acute supravesical obstruction, as from a stone lodged in a ureter (Chap. 232), is associated with excruciatingly severe pain, usually called *renal colic.* This pain is relatively steady and continuous, with little fluctuation in intensity, and often radiates to the lower abdomen, testes, or labia. By contrast, more insidious causes of obstruction, such as chronic narrowing of the ureteropelvic junction, may produce little or no pain yet result in total destruction of the affected kidney. Flank pain which comes on only with micturition is pathognomonic of vesicoureteral reflux.

TABLE 233-2 Pathophysiology of bilateral ureteral obstruction

Hemodynamic effects	Tubule effects	Clinical features
ACUTE		
↑ Renal blood flow ↓ GFR ↓ Medullary blood flow ↑ Vasodilator prostaglandins	↑ Ureteral and tubule pressures ↑ Reabsorption of Na^+, urea, water	Pain (capsule distention) Azotemia Oliguria
CHRONIC		
↓ Renal blood flow ↓ ↓ GFR ↑ Vasoconstrictor prostaglandins ↑ Renin-angiotensin production	↓ Medullary osmolarity ↓ Concentrating ability Structural damage; parenchymal atrophy ↓ Transport functions for Na^+, K^+, H^+	Azotemia Hypertension ADH-insensitive polyuria Natriuresis Hyperkalemic, hyperchloremic acidosis
RELEASE OF OBSTRUCTION		
Slow ↑ in GFR (variable)	↓ Tubule pressure ↑ Solute load per nephron (urea, NaCl) Natriuretic factors present	Postobstructive diuresis Potential for volume depletion and electrolyte imbalance (Na^+, K^+, PO_4^{2-}, Mg^{2+} excretion)

Azotemia develops in urinary tract obstruction when overall excretory function is impaired. This may occur in the setting of bladder outlet obstruction, bilateral renal pelvic or ureteric obstruction, or unilateral disease in a patient with a solitary functioning kidney. Complete bilateral obstruction should be suspected when acute renal failure is accompanied by anuria. Any patient with renal failure otherwise unexplained or with a history of nephrolithiasis, hematuria, prostatic enlargement, pelvic surgery, trauma, or tumor should be evaluated for urinary tract obstruction.

Symptoms of *polyuria* and *nocturia* commonly accompany chronic partial urinary tract obstruction and result from impaired renal concentrating ability. This defect usually does not improve with administration of vasopressin and is therefore a form of acquired nephrogenic diabetes insipidus. Disturbances in sodium chloride transport in the ascending limb of Henle and, in azotemic patients, the osmotic (urea) diuresis per nephron lead to decreased medullary hypertonicity and, hence, a concentrating defect. Partial obstruction, therefore, may be associated with increased rather than decreased urine output. Indeed, wide fluctuations in urinary output in a patient with azotemia should always raise the possibility of intermittent or partial urinary tract obstruction. If fluid intake is inadequate, severe dehydration and hypernatremia may develop. Hesitancy and straining to initiate the urinary stream, postvoid dribbling, urinary frequency, and (overflow) incontinence are common in patients with obstruction at or below the level of the bladder (see Chap. 49).

In addition to loss of urinary concentrating ability and azotemia, partial bilateral urinary tract obstruction often results in other derangements of renal function, including *acquired distal renal tubular acidosis, hyperkalemia,* and *renal salt wasting.* These defects in tubule function are often accompanied by evidence of widespread renal tubulointerstitial damage. Morphologic abnormalities appear early in the course of obstruction; initially the interstitium becomes edematous and infiltrated with mononuclear inflammatory cells. With continued obstruction, the interstitium becomes fibrotic; scarring and atrophy of the papillae and medulla occur and precede these processes in the cortex.

The possibility of urinary tract obstruction must always be considered in patients with urinary tract infections or urolithiasis. Urinary stasis encourages the growth of organisms as well as the formation of crystals, especially magnesium ammonium phosphate (struvite). *Hypertension* is seen frequently in acute and subacute forms of unilateral obstruction and is usually a consequence of increased release of renin by the involved kidney. Chronic unilateral or bilateral hydronephrosis, in the presence of extracellular volume expansion or other forms of renal disease, may result in significant hypertension. *Polycythemia,* an infrequent complication of obstructive uropathy, is probably secondary to increased erythropoietin production by the obstructed kidney.

DIAGNOSIS A history of difficulty in voiding, pain, infection, or changes in urinary volume is common. Evidence for distention of the kidney or urinary bladder often can be obtained by palpation and percussion of the abdomen. A careful rectal examination may reveal enlargement or nodularity of the prostate, abnormal rectal sphincter tone, or a rectal or pelvic mass. The penis should be inspected for evidence of meatal stenosis or phimosis. In the female, vaginal, uterine, and rectal lesions responsible for urinary tract obstruction are usually revealed by inspection and palpation.

Urinalysis and examination of the urine sediment may reveal hematuria, pyuria, and bacteriuria. Often, however, the urine sediment is devoid of abnormal elements, even when obstruction leads to marked azotemia and extensive structural damage. An abdominal scout film should be obtained to evaluate the possibility of nephrocalcinosis or a radiopaque stone at any level of the urinary collecting system. As indicated in Fig. 233-1 if urinary tract obstruction is

FIGURE 233-1 Diagnostic approach for urinary tract obstruction in unexplained renal failure. Circles represent diagnostic procedures, and squares indicate clinical decisions based on available data. CT, computed tomography; IVP, intravenous pyelogram.

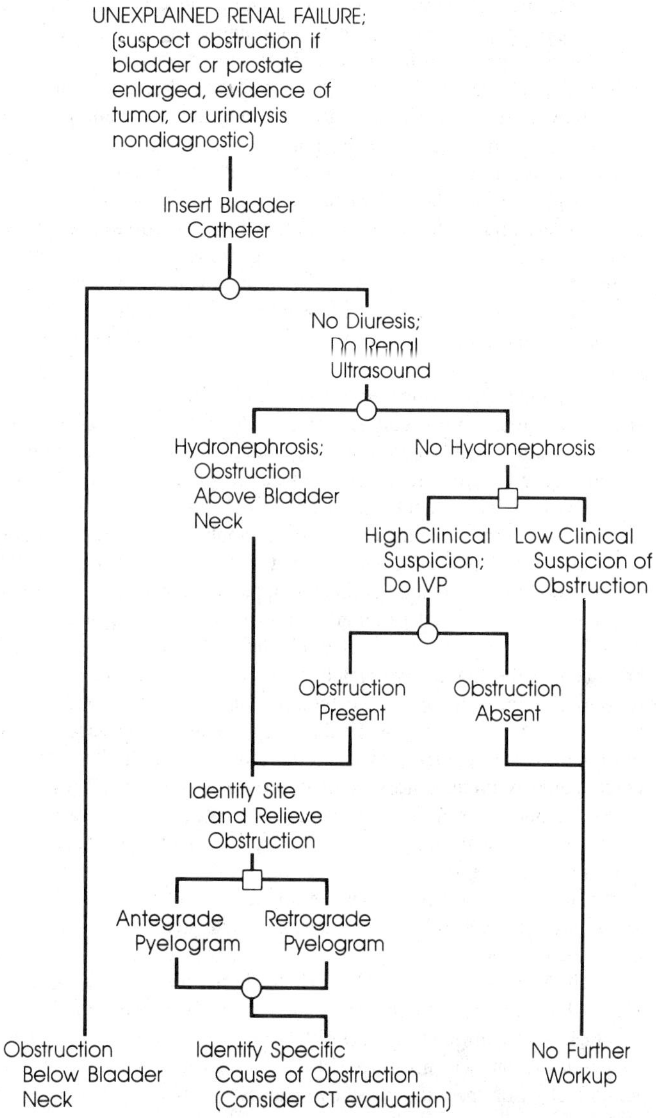

suspected, abdominal ultrasonography should be performed to evaluate renal and bladder size, as well as pyelocalyceal and ureteral contours. If distention of these structures is absent, functionally significant urinary tract obstruction can safely be excluded in differential diagnosis. Abdominal ultrasound may also detect an obstructing pelvic mass.

Intravenous pyelography is indicated if an obstructive abnormality is revealed by ultrasound. If the patient is not azotemic, a standard dose of contrast medium usually provides adequate information. With renal insufficiency, however, high-dose (drip-infusion) pyelography with nephrotomography is usually required for adequate visualization. In the presence of obstruction, the appearance time of the nephrogram is often delayed but eventually becomes more dense than normal because of slow tubular fluid flow rate which results in enhanced water reabsorption by the nephrons and greater concentration of contrast medium within tubules. The kidney involved by an acute obstructive process is usually slightly enlarged, and there is dilatation of the calyces, renal pelvis, and ureter above the obstruction. The ureter, however, is not tortuous, as is the case when the obstruction is chronic. In comparison with the nephrogram, the pyelogram may be extremely faint, especially if the dilated renal pelvis is voluminous, causing dilution of the contrast medium. The radiographic study should be continued until the site of obstruction is determined or the contrast medium is excreted. Delayed films taken as long as 48 h after contrast administration may be necessary to determine the exact site of obstruction. Radionuclide scans define less anatomic detail than intravenous pyelography and, like the pyelogram, are of limited value when renal function is poor. Nonetheless, such scans are sensitive in the detection of obstruction and provide a substitute test in some patients at high risk for reaction to intravenous contrast dyes.

Patients suspected of having intermittent ureteropelvic obstruction (whether functional or mechanical) should have radiologic evaluation while they are in pain, since a normal pyelogram is commonly seen during asymptomatic periods. Hydration or mannitol infusion often helps to provoke a symptomatic attack. Voiding cystourethrography is of great value in the diagnosis of vesicoureteral reflux and bladder neck and urethral obstructions. Patients with obstruction at or below the level of the bladder exhibit thickening, trabeculation, and diverticula of the bladder wall. Postvoiding films reveal residual urine. If these radiographic studies fail to provide adequate information for diagnosis, endoscopic visualization by the urologist often permits precise identification of lesions involving the urethra, prostate, bladder, and ureteral orifices. To facilitate visualization of a suspected lesion in a ureter or renal pelvis, *retrograde* or *antegrade pyelography* should be attempted. These diagnostic studies may be preferable to the intravenous pyelogram in the azotemic patient in whom poor excretory function precludes adequate visualization of the collecting system. Furthermore, intravenous pyelography carries the risk of contrast-induced renal failure in some patients with renal insufficiency, diabetes mellitus, and multiple myeloma, particularly when performed under conditions of dehydration. For these reasons retrograde and antegrade pyelography may offer advantages over the intravenous approach in the diagnostic evaluation of the azotemic patient. The retrograde approach involves catheterization of the involved ureter under cystoscopic control, while the antegrade technique necessitates placement of a catheter into the renal pelvis via a needle inserted percutaneously under ultrasonic or fluoroscopic guidance. While the antegrade approach carries the added advantage of providing immediate and certain decompression of a unilateral obstructing lesion, many urologists initially attempt the retrograde approach and resort to the antegrade method only when attempts at retrograde catheterization are unsuccessful or when cystoscopy or general anesthesia is contraindicated.

Computed tomography (CT) is useful in the diagnosis of specific intraabdominal and retroperitoneal causes of obstruction but is less practical as an initial test to establish the presence of obstruction. Magnetic resonance imaging (MRI) may also be useful in the identification of specific obstructive causes.

TREATMENT AND PROGNOSIS An individual with any form of urinary tract obstruction complicated by infection requires relief of obstruction as soon as possible to prevent development of generalized sepsis and progressive renal damage. On a temporary basis, depending on the site of obstruction, drainage is often satisfactorily achieved by nephrostomy, ureterostomy, or ureteral, urethral, or suprapubic catheterization. The patient with acute urinary tract infection and obstruction should be given appropriate antibiotics based on in vitro bacterial sensitivity and ability of the drug to concentrate in the kidney and urine. Treatment may be required for 3 to 4 weeks. Chronic or recurrent infections in an obstructed kidney with poor intrinsic function may necessitate nephrectomy. When infection is not present, immediate surgery often is not required, even in the presence of complete obstruction and anuria (because of the availability of dialysis), at least until acid-base, fluid and electrolyte, and cardiovascular status are restored to normal. Nevertheless, the site of obstruction should be ascertained as soon as feasible, in part because of the possibility that sepsis may occur and necessitate prompt urologic intervention. Elective relief of obstruction is usually recommended in patients with urinary retention, recurrent urinary tract infections, persistent pain, or progressive loss of renal function. Infrequently, mechanical obstruction can be alleviated by nonsurgical means, as with radiation therapy for retroperitoneal lymphoma. Likewise, functional obstruction secondary to neurogenic bladder may be decreased with the combination of frequent voiding and cholinergic drugs. The approach to obstruction secondary to renal stones is discussed in Chap. 232.

With relief of obstruction, the *prognosis* regarding return of renal function depends largely upon whether irreversible renal damage has occurred. When obstruction is not relieved, the course will depend mainly on whether the obstruction is complete or incomplete, bilateral or unilateral, and whether urinary tract infection is also present. Complete obstruction with infection can lead to total destruction of the kidney within days. Studies in dogs suggest that relief of complete obstruction of 1 and 2 weeks' duration restores glomerular filtration rate to 60 and 30 percent of normal, respectively; after 8 weeks of obstruction, recovery does not occur. Nevertheless, in the absence of definitive evidence of irreversibility, every effort should be made to decompress in the hope of restoring renal function at least partially.

In patients undergoing cystectomy for bladder cancer, the ileal conduit is the currently preferred urinary diversionary procedure. In benign disease a sigmoid conduit may result in less ureteral reflux and secondary chronic renal insufficiency. These approaches are preferable to ureterosigmoidostomy, a procedure complicated by a high incidence of ureteral obstruction, reflux, hypokalemic metabolic acidosis, pyelonephritis, and neoplasms developing at the ureteral anastomotic site.

POSTOBSTRUCTIVE DIURESIS Relief of bilateral, but not unilateral, complete urinary tract obstruction commonly leads to a postobstructive diuresis, characterized by polyuria, which may be massive. The urine is usually hypotonic and may contain a large amount of sodium chloride. The natriuresis is due, at least in part, to the excretion of retained urea, which acts as a poorly reabsorbable solute and diminishes salt and water reabsorption in the tubules (osmotic diuresis). The increase in intratubular pressure very likely also contributes to the impairment in net sodium chloride reabsorption, especially in the terminal nephron segments. Natriuretic factors (other than urea) may also accumulate during uremia induced by obstruction and depress salt and water reabsorption when urine flow is reestablished. In the majority of patients this diuresis is physiologic, resulting in the *appropriate* excretion of the excesses of salt and water retained during the period of obstruction. When extracellular volume and composition return to normal, the diuresis usually abates spontaneously. Therefore, replacement of urinary losses should serve only to prevent hypovolemia, hypotension, or disturbances in serum electrolyte concentrations. Occasionally, iatrogenic expansion of extracellular volume, secondary to administration of excessive quantities of intravenous fluids, is responsible for, or sustains, the diuresis observed in the postobstructive period. Replacement of no more than two-thirds of urinary volume losses per day is usually effective in avoiding this complication. In a rare patient, however, relief of obstruction may be followed by urinary salt and water losses severe enough to provoke profound dehydration and vascular collapse. In these patients, an intrinsic defect in tubule reabsorptive function is probably responsible for the marked diuresis. Appropriate therapy in such patients includes intravenous administration of large quantities of salt-containing solutions to replace sodium and volume deficits.

REFERENCES

HARRIS RH, YARGER WE: The pathogenesis of post-obstructive diuresis. J Clin Invest 56:880, 1975

KAYE AD, POLLACK HM: Diagnostic imaging approach to the patient with obstructive uropathy. Semin Nephrol 2:55, 1982

KLAHR S et al: Urinary tract obstruction, in *The Kidney*, 3d ed, BM Brenner, FC Rector Jr (eds). Philadelphia, Saunders, 1986, p 1443

WILSON DR: Renal function during and following obstruction. Ann Rev Med 28:329, 1977

———: Urinary tract obstruction, in *Diseases of the Kidney*, 4th ed, RW Schrier, SW Gottschalk (eds). Boston, Little, Brown, 1988, p 715

234 TUMORS OF THE URINARY TRACT

MARC B. GARNICK / BARRY M. BRENNER

TUMORS OF THE KIDNEY

RENAL CELL CARCINOMA Renal cell carcinoma (renal adenocarcinoma, formerly "hypernephroma") accounts for 85 percent of all primary renal neoplasms. Approximately 18,000 new cases are diagnosed annually with 8000 deaths in the United States. The peak age incidence is between 55 and 60 years; the male-to-female ratio is 2:1. Environmental risk factors include exposure to cigarette smoke and cadmium. Hereditary forms of renal cell carcinoma, which are commonly multifocal and bilateral, occur in a high proportion of patients with von Hippel–Lindau disease (retinal and central nervous system hemangiomas, autosomal dominant transmission). The genetic defect associated with the disease has been identified. Marker chromosomal translocations between chromosomes 3 and 8 and 3 and 11 have been found in several kindreds with familial renal cancer. Patients with end-stage renal disease on chronic dialysis may develop renal cystic disease and associated renal carcinomas. Renal cell carcinoma arises from the proximal convoluted tubular epithelium. The term "hypernephroma" for renal cell carcinoma (reflecting the previously held notion of cellular origin from adrenal "rests") should be abandoned.

Clinical features Renal cell carcinoma has been called the "internist's tumor" because the lesion is often diagnosed, even in the absence of metastases, by its *systemic* rather than by urologic manifestations. The triad of *gross hematuria, flank pain,* and a *palpable abdominal mass,* although considered classic evidence for the clinical diagnosis, is encountered in less than 10 percent of cases; however, many patients demonstrate at least one of these manifestations. The most common presenting abnormality is *hematuria,* which occurs in 60 percent of cases. Although microscopic hematuria is a consistent abnormality of the urinary sediment, bleeding is not usually evident grossly, allowing the tumor to grow to a large size before clinical manifestations such as flank pain and fullness appear. Contiguous extension to the renal capsule, perirenal fat, lymph nodes, renal vein, inferior vena cava, and ipsilateral adrenal gland is common. The most common sites of distant metastases include lung, mediastinum, bone, central nervous system, thyroid, and liver.

Systemic symptoms of fatigability, weight loss, and cachexia occur in about 50 percent of patients. Intermittent fever, unassociated with infection, occurs occasionally and may be the only presenting sign. Anemia is present at the onset in approximately 50 percent of cases. Erythrocytosis is seen in about 5 percent of patients and has been linked to elaboration of erythropoietin. Eosinophilia, leukemoid reactions, thrombocytosis, and increased erythrocyte sedimentation rate also occur. Renal cell carcinomas may produce hormones or hormone-like substances, including parathyroid hormone and prostaglandins (which may lead to hypercalcemia), prolactin (galactorrhea), renin (hypertension), gonadotropins (feminization and masculinization), and glucocorticoids (Cushing's syndrome). In vascular tumors, intrarenal arteriovenous fistulas may predispose to high-output congestive heart failure. Tumor invasion of the renal vein and inferior vena cava may result in the development of abrupt, symptomatic left varicocele and lower extremity edema, respectively. Hepatic vein occlusion by tumor, with or without vena caval obstruction, may lead to hepatosplenomegaly and ascites. Disturbances in liver function (elevated alkaline phosphatase, hypoalbuminemia, and prolonged prothrombin time) are sometimes found in patients without demonstrable liver metastases and are often reversed following removal of the primary tumor.

Diagnosis (See Fig. 234-1) Although intrarenal calcifications and/or alterations in renal contours seen on the abdominal scout film may suggest the presence of a renal cell carcinoma, *intravenous pyelography* (IVP) with *nephrotomography* is the primary examination by which most renal masses are detected and evaluated. The major task is to differentiate cystic lesions from renal neoplasms. Splaying, distortion or nonvisualization of the collecting system, and distorted renal outlines suggest cancer. Nephrotomography provides clear delineation of renal borders and further aids in distinguishing cystic from solid lesions. *Ultrasonography* has improved the ability to distinguish cysts from renal neoplasms. When combined with nephrotomography, the accuracy of ultrasonography in diagnosing a benign cyst approaches 97 percent. If a cystic lesion on IVP, combined with a benign-appearing sonolucent cystic lesion on ultrasound, is found in an asymptomatic patient without hematuria, cyst puncture is probably unnecessary. Repeat IVP or ultrasound should then be performed periodically, initially every year and then, if no change has occurred during the interval, less often.

If diagnostic accuracy beyond 97 percent is required or if there are changes on repeat IVP or ultrasound, needle aspiration with evaluation of the aspirated fluid for cytology can be performed. The finding of clear yellow fluid or negative cytology usually supports the diagnosis of a simple cyst. Aspiration of cloudy or bloody fluid usually demands a surgical diagnosis, even though the cytology may be negative for cancer. A renal cystogram following aspiration can sometimes provide additional valuable information. Although renal cell carcinoma may coexist within a simple cyst, this is rare.

If the IVP or ultrasound examination demonstrates a lesion which does not satisfy the criteria for a benign, simple cyst, *computed tomography* (CT) is the next modality employed. CT is comparable and possibly superior to selective renal arteriography in both diagnosing and staging renal cell carcinoma. In addition, CT is equivalent to selective renal arteriography in the determination of renal vein involvement and superior to arteriography in determining whether regional nodes are enlarged (representing either tumor or hyperplasia) and/or the liver is involved. CT is the preferred modality for the diagnosis and staging of renal cell carcinoma. Thus, selective renal arteriography is not necessarily needed preoperatively. If, however, the findings on CT are equivocal or additional definition of vascular anatomy is required, renal arteriography should complement CT studies. Magnetic resonance imaging (MRI) has also been used extensively in the evaluation of renal masses. Its role compared to CT scanning is being defined.

OTHER STUDIES Evaluation of urinary cytology is not useful in the diagnosis of renal adenocarcinomas. Retrograde pyelography may be a useful adjunct for opacifying the collecting systems that are not

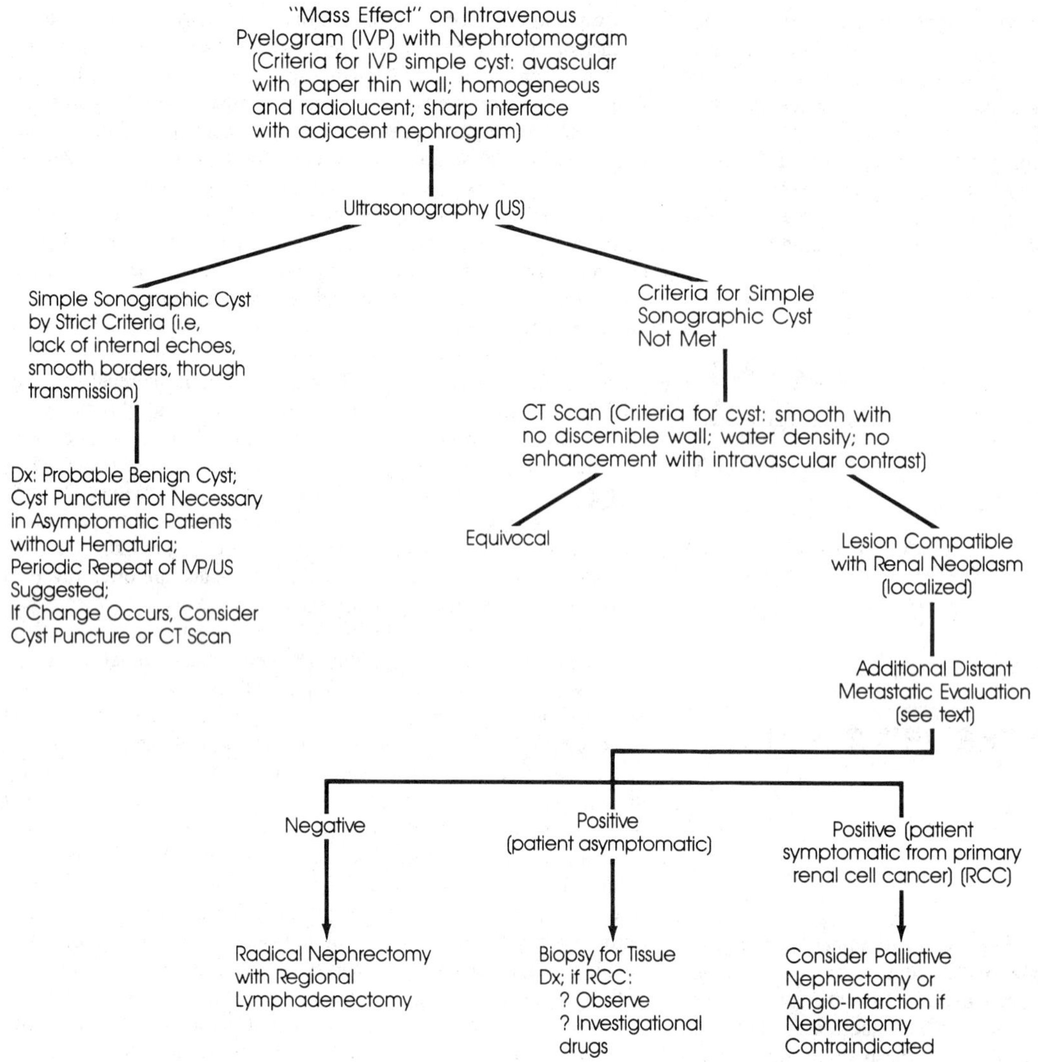

FIGURE 234-1 Diagnostic evaluation for renal mass.

filled by standard IVP and may suggest the diagnosis of transitional cell carcinoma of the renal pelvis. In patients who present with hematuria and a renal mass, cystoscopy is an important adjunct to exclude the coexistence of an unsuspected urothelial tumor, such as carcinoma of the bladder.

If the diagnosis of renal cell carcinoma is considered likely, the patient should then undergo routine chest x-ray, bone scan, and liver function studies, in addition to the abdominal CT, to evaluate other potential sites of tumor spread.

Staging, primary treatment, and prognosis If there is no evidence of metastatic disease following the preoperative evaluation, the treatment of choice for renal cell carcinoma is radical nephrectomy. In addition to en bloc removal of the kidney with the surrounding Gerota's fascia, many urologic surgeons advocate regional lymphadenectomy to help determine prognosis. Preoperative arterial embolization of the main renal artery with a variety of agents may help to simplify the operative approach for large lesions. There is no role for localized pre- or postoperative radiation therapy.

Following surgical and pathologic evaluation, renal cell cancers are staged as follows: stage I, tumor confined within the kidney capsule; stage II, invasion through the renal capsule but confined within Gerota's fascia; stage III, involvement of regional lymph nodes, ipsilateral renal vein, or vena cava; stage IV, distant metastases. Five-year survival rates for stage I range from 60 to 75 percent; for stage II, 47 to 65 percent; for stage III without regional lymph node involvement, 25 to 50 percent; with regional lymph node involvement, 5 to 15 percent; for stage IV, less than 5 percent.

Systemic therapy for metastatic disease There is no standard chemotherapeutic, hormonal, or immunologic program for patients with metastatic renal cancer. Although early reports demonstrated a favorable effect using progestational or androgenic agents, there seems to be very little role for hormonal therapy of renal cell carcinoma. Commonly employed chemotherapy programs include the use of vinblastine sulfate, with or without the use of nitrosoureas. Interferons have been used with limited success. The use of interleukin 2 and lymphokine-activated killer cells (LAK cells) has been reported to be successful in selected patients. The management of patients with renal adenocarcinoma is investigational, and entry of patients into phase II clinical trials is encouraged.

Selected management of patients with metastatic disease There is little wisdom in hoping for spontaneous regression of metastases by removing the kidney of a patient who presents with stage IV renal cell carcinoma who is otherwise asymptomatic. If, however, the primary lesion is associated with pain, bleeding, or other paraneoplastic phenomena, it is sometimes useful to remove the primary tumor or to consider angioinfarction for local therapy despite the presence of metastatic disease. In patients who have had renal cell cancer in the past who then present with an isolated pulmonary or central nervous system metastasis, it is often useful to resect these metastases. Generally, patients selected for surgical nodulectomy have been disease-free for at least 1 year from the original diagnosis to the time of metastatic development and have tumors with a slow doubling time. On occasion, radiation therapy may offer palliation to painful bony lesions and may relieve an obstructed bronchus or ureter.

MISCELLANEOUS TUMORS OF THE KIDNEY In children, Wilms's tumor (nephroblastoma) is the most common cancer of the kidney. These tumors respond well to multimodality therapy including surgery, radiation, and combination chemotherapy, usually with dactinomycin and vincristine. Metastatic lesions to the kidney occur commonly in patients with lung and breast cancer and melanoma. Kidney involvement with malignant lymphoma, too, is common; however, functional renal abnormalities from parenchymal involvement are unusual.

Benign renal tumors are usually recognized as incidental findings at autopsy. However, on occasion, the lesion can cause persistent hematuria and, like the renal oncocytoma, can undergo malignant degeneration. These lesions are usually managed with nephrectomy when detected clinically. In newborns and infants, mesoblastic nephroma (fetal hamartoma) is the most common benign tumor and is successfully treated by simple nephrectomy.

TUMORS OF THE URINARY COLLECTING SYSTEM

The lining of the urinary collecting system from the renal pelvis to the urethra is made up of transitional cell epithelium or "urothelium." This entire lining is subject to carcinogenic influences which may explain the multicentric characteristics of urothelial neoplasms. Numerically, cancer of the bladder is the most common followed by tumors of the renal pelvis. Ureteral and urethral cancers are rare.

BLADDER CARCINOMA Approximately 40,000 new cases of bladder cancer are diagnosed annually with 11,000 deaths in the United States. Men are affected three times as frequently as women, and the disease is unusual in patients under 40 years of age. Epidemiology studies have demonstrated an increased incidence of transitional cell carcinoma following exposure to aromatic amines, particularly 2-naphthylamine. This probably accounts for the high incidence of urothelial cancers among cigarette smokers and workers in the dye, chemical, and certain rubber industries. Individuals with chronic, recurrent nephrolithiasis and recurrent upper urinary tract infections also have an increased incidence of urothelial cancers. Squamous carcinomas occur more frequently in patients with chronic infestation with *Schistosoma haematobium*. Squamous and adenocarcinomas have a worse prognosis compared to transitional cell tumors. Long-term administration of the anticancer alkylating agent cyclophosphamide, which is metabolized to the active compounds acrolein and phosphoramide mustard, is associated with the development of urothelial neoplasms.

Clinical features Gross and microscopic hematuria are the most common presenting complaints (75 percent of patients); other features include dysuria, urinary frequency, and urgency (25 percent of patients), which may be the only manifestations of bladder cancer. Persistence of these symptoms in a previously asymptomatic patient deserves careful attention. Other manifestations, such as ureteral obstruction, pelvic pain, or symptoms from visceral or osseous metastases, occur in a minority of patients at presentation.

Diagnosis and staging Urinary cytology, obtained by examination of bladder washing, catheterized urine or voided urine, IVP, and cystoscopic evaluation with tumor biopsies and selected mucosal biopsies, as well as bimanual examination under anesthesia, are the mainstays for diagnosis of bladder cancer. Findings on IVP that suggest a bladder carcinoma include unilateral or bilateral ureteral obstruction with hydronephrosis, filling defect, or lack of distensibility of the bladder. Additional staging information may be obtained with abdominal or pelvic CT scanning. Following endoscopic resection of a bladder neoplasm, the depth of penetration into the bladder wall is assessed. If additional staging workup, including physical examination, chest x-ray, and routine serum chemistries, are within normal limits, the patient is clinically staged, based upon the cystoscopic biopsy, as having either *superficial* or *invasive* disease. Additional information about perivesical extension or nodal metastases can be obtained at the time of cystectomy and indicates the true pathologic stage of disease. A substantial number of patients who are clinically staged endoscopically as having muscle-invasive disease will have occult lymphatic or distant metastases if surgically staged at the time of cystectomy. Such occult micrometastatic disease indicates systemic involvement and accounts for the high percentage of patients who eventually develop distant metastatic disease despite treatment of the primary bladder lesion.

Treatment Bladder cancer can be subdivided conceptually as being *superficial, invasive,* or *metastatic. Superficial carcinoma* of the bladder includes patients with carcinoma in situ, mucosal involvement (stage 0), or submucosal involvement (stage A). These patients are generally treated with endoscopic resection and selected bladder biopsies with repeat cystoscopic evaluations every 3 to 6 months. Approximately 50 to 70 percent of these patients have a superficial recurrence (limited to the mucosa or submucosa) within a period of 3 years following initial diagnosis. Patients with superficial recurrences are then often treated with intravesical therapies, including thiotepa, doxorubicin mitomycin, bacillus Calmette-Guérin (BCG) or interferons, in addition to cystoscopic resection. The use of intravesical therapy may decrease the number of superficial recurrences, but its effect on the natural history of the disease, in terms of preventing the development of invasive lesions, is unclear.

An additional 12 percent with initial superficial disease eventually develop progressive disease into the bladder muscularis (stage B), perivesical fat (stage C) or metastatic disease to lymph nodes (stage D1), bone, or other viscera (stage D2). Alternatively, patients may present initially with invasive or metastatic disease.

INVASIVE DISEASE These patients generally have extension of tumor into the muscle and/or perivesical fat. Traditional treatments are cystectomy (radical or simple), radiation therapy, or preoperative radiation therapy followed by cystectomy. Five-year survival rates are approximately 45 percent with such treatments. The majority of these patients die of distant metastatic disease despite radical surgery or radiation rather than from local recurrences. In addition, the use of multimodality therapy, including chemotherapy with radiation therapy, may spare individuals with invasive disease radical cystectomy. Surgical techniques, utilizing portions of the small bowel as bladder reservoirs, have enhanced the quality of life in individuals undergoing radical cystectomy. Such procedures allow continent urinary diversion (e.g., Koch pouch), thus eliminating the need for an external ostomy appliance.

METASTATIC DISEASE For patients who have distant metastatic disease in lymph nodes, viscera, or bone, the use of systemic chemotherapy has produced responses from 30 to 70 percent of patients, but usually not lasting more than 6 months. Following the development of metastatic disease, most patients die within 2 years. The most active agents include cisplatin, methotrexate, doxorubicin, cyclophosphamide, and vinblastine, and combinations of these agents have on occasion produced meaningful and durable remissions. One therapeutic strategy for patients with invasive disease consists of initiating chemotherapy followed by definitive local treatment to the bladder (surgery or radiation). The goal of such programs is to eradicate micrometastases that are commonly present in patients with invasive disease.

TRANSITIONAL CELL CANCER OF THE RENAL PELVIS Renal pelvic tumors account for approximately 10 percent of all primary renal cancer. Nearly 90 percent are transitional cell carcinomas. In addition to the etiologic associations implicated for bladder carcinoma, renal pelvic tumors also occur with analgesic abuse nephropathy. These patients are usually middle-aged women with a psychiatric history or chronic headaches who ingest >3 kg of analgesics over years. The exact amount and type of analgesic which induces transitional cell cancer of the renal pelvis is unknown, although aspirin and/or phenacetin can induce the disease experimentally.

Most patients present with painless, gross hematuria. Ureteral obstruction and pain secondary to clots are unusual. The diagnosis is suggested by IVP, which may demonstrate an obstructed, poorly functioning, or nonvisualized kidney or filling defects in a visualized kidney, and a positive urinary cytology. Cystoscopy and retrograde pyelography with brush biopsy generally establish the nature and location of the renal pelvic or ureteral tumor. For low-grade, low-stage tumors, conservative treatment with local excision and preservation of the kidney parenchyma is associated with favorable 5-year survival rates. For high-stage, high-grade lesions, the treatment of choice is radical nephroureterectomy and removal of the cuff of the bladder containing the ipsilateral ureteral orifice. This latter operative approach is dictated by the high likelihood of recurrence in the ureteral stump and orifice if not removed. In addition, routine follow-up with cystoscopies and urinary cytologies are mandatory to help detect the subsequent development of metachronous bladder carcinomas and/or contralateral ureteral and renal pelvic tumors. Five-year survival rates range from 10 to 50 percent. Although chemotherapy programs employed for bladder cancer have been used for patients with metastatic transitional cell carcinoma of the renal pelvis, the overall results are not as successful.

REFERENCES

Brodsky G, Garnick MG: Renal tumors in the adult patient, in *Renal Pathology*, CC Tisher, BM Brenner (eds). Philadelphia, Lippincott, 1989, p 1467

Chisholm GD, Roy RR: The systemic effects of malignant renal tumors. Br J Urol 43:687, 1971

Cronan J, Zeman RK: Renal mass imaging: The internist's role. Am J Med 81:1026, 1986

Cronin RE et al: Renal cell carcinoma: Unusual systemic manifestations. Medicine 55:291, 1976

Garnick MB (ed): Genitourinary cancer, in *Contemporary Issues in Clinical Oncology*, vol 5. New York, Churchill Livingstone, 1985

Hricak H: Detection and staging of renal neoplasms: A reassessment of MR imaging. Radiology 166:643, 1988

Kalish LA et al: A determination of appropriate endpoints in assessing efficacy of intravesical therapies in superficial bladder cancer. J Clin Oncol 5:2004, 1987

Rieselbach RE, Garnick MB (eds): *Cancer and the Kidney*. Philadelphia, Lea & Febiger, 1982

Sternberg CN et al: M-VAC (methotrexate, vinblastine, doxorubicin, and cisplatin) for advanced transitional cell carcinoma of urothelium. J Urol 139:461, 1988

West WH et al: Constant infusion recombinant interleukin-2 in adoptive immunotherapy of advanced cancer. N Engl J Med 316:898, 1987

PART NINE DISORDERS OF THE GASTROINTESTINAL SYSTEM

section 1 Disorders of the alimentary tract

235 APPROACH TO THE PATIENT WITH GASTROINTESTINAL DISEASE

KURT J. ISSELBACHER / DANIEL K. PODOLSKY

BIOLOGIC CONSIDERATIONS The mucosal surface of the gastrointestinal tract comprises a remarkably dynamic population of epithelial cells that are highly developed in their capacity for transmembrane absorption and secretion. These secretory and absorptive abilities facilitate the essential role of the digestive tract in digestion and nutrient uptake, which must be accomplished while maintaining the barrier between the host and potentially harmful pathogens and mutagens in the lumen. The latter is accomplished through both the physical integrity of the intact mucosal surface and the extensive population of resident immune cells.

The intestinal surface itself also contains the distinctive M cells that serve to sample the antigenic milieu of the lumen. The predominance of suppressor lymphocytes within the surface epithelial layer (intraepithelial lymphocytes) suggests that dampening of the body's response to the enormous number of potentially antigenic substances in the lumen is necessary to prevent the constant and unrestrained activation of immune and inflammatory processes. Conversely, the presence of large numbers of helper lymphocytes as well as other cellular effectors of immune response in the lamina propria and submucosa attests to a large armamentarium ready to respond when surface defenses have been breached. No doubt the concentration of so many immume cells capable of attracting and activating inflammatory cells predisposes to the numerous inflammatory conditions to which the gastrointestinal tract is subject.

The mucosal surface of the gastrointestinal tract is also remarkable for the very rapid turnover of the epithelial cell population. It has been suggested that the surface epithelial cell populations turn over in their entirety every 24 to 72 h. This may permit rapid restitution of a functional cell population following an acute insult and may reduce the risk of malignancy through loss of cells affected by the many potential and actual mutagens in the luminal contents. Nevertheless, this proliferative potential must inherently create the setting for neoplastic disorders, which are so common to the gastrointestinal tract. Another fundamental feature of gastrointestinal mucosa is the spatial segregation of the proliferative compartment from the terminally differentiated cells. This is true throughout the gastrointestinal tract but is most apparent in the small intestine where a gradient of differentiation exists from the depths of the crypts of Lieberkühn to the villus tip. This organization is important in understanding the histology and pathophysiology of many mucosal disorders, e.g., nontropical sprue.

In view of the important secretory and absorptive activities of mucosal surface, diseases of the gastrointestinal tract may result in clinical consequences secondary to the physical disruption of the mucosal layer (e.g., blood loss, fluid loss, pathogenic invasion) or nutritional derangements due to impaired digestion and nutrient absorption. In focal or localized disease processes the former predominate, while the latter may be especially prominent in disorders that affect the gastrointestinal tract in a diffuse manner.

While the essential role of the gastrointestinal tract is the absorption of nutrients and excretion of the products is in large part accomplished at the luminal surface, these processes are also dependent on the deeper muscular layers for the coordinated propulsion of food through the lumen. The complexity of both local and distant neural and endocrine factors that contribute to the regulation of intestinal motility is only now becoming fully appreciated. Disruption of normal motility is quite common, with functional bowel complaints affecting as much as 15 percent of adult individuals. Alterations in frequency of bowel movements, abdominal distention, abdominal pain, and nausea, individually or in varying combinations, may result from dysmotility. In addition, structural lesions may also indirectly lead to symptoms through their impact on motility involving some or all regions of the gastrointestinal tract. These range from the *direct* effects of an obstructing lesion to the *indirect* actions of substances released by a primary mucosal disorder (e.g., inflammatory mediators such as arachidonic acid metabolites that also affect smooth-muscle activity).

Although valid unifying generalizations can be made about the gastrointestinal tract in its entirety, the spectrum of diseases affecting this system and their clinical manifestations are significantly related to the constituent organ(s) involved. Thus, esophageal disorders predominantly manifest through their relationship to swallowing, while gastric disorders are dominated by features relating to acid secretion, and disease of the small and large intestine by disruption of nutrition and alterations of bowel movements. Similarly, diseases of the related ancillary organs, the exocrine pancreas and the hepatobiliary system, present characteristic clinical challenges. Finally, it should be remembered that in addition to intrinsic disease, the gastrointestinal tract may be affected by systemic disorders. These include vascular, inflammatory, infectious, and neoplastic conditions leading to focal or diffuse structural lesions. Metabolic and endocrine abnormalities as well as drugs can disrupt normal bowel motility.

CLINICAL CONSIDERATIONS **History** A thorough clinical history is almost uniformly reliable in directing the clinician's attention to appropriate diagnostic considerations in the patient with gastrointestinal symptoms. The most common complaints resulting from disorders involving the gastrointestinal tract include pain, alteration in bowel habit, especially diarrhea and constipation, and indigestion. Among these, abdominal pain is the most frequent and variable and may reflect a broad spectrum of problems from the least threatening to the most urgent. Ascertaining the location (upper or lower, localized or diffuse), character (sharp, burning, cramping), and relationship of the pain to meals will often provide significant insight into the most important diagnostic considerations. If eating produces the symptom, the clinician should determine whether the discomfort occurs while eating (as in esophageal disorders and abdominal angina), shortly after the meal (as often occurs in biliary tract disease), or 30 to 90 min later (as typically seen in peptic disease). Pain that is not affected by eating suggests a process outside of the bowel lumen, such as an abscess, peritonitis, pancreatitis, and some malignancies. Conversely, identification of factors that relieve the symptom is also helpful, e.g., relief with eating or antacids is characteristic of peptic ulcer disease or gastritis. Relationship of the discomfort to bowel movement, especially in association with an altered bowel habit, should focus attention on a disorder of the small or large bowel such as inflammatory bowel disease.

Alterations in bowel habit can result either from disruption of normal intestinal motility or significant structural pathology. A thorough determination of the temporal evolution of the change and the nature of the alteration in conjunction with other constitutional symptoms such as weight loss, fever, or anorexia is important. Temporary variation in bowel habit in association with some life stress and in the absence of signs of systemic illness is suggestive of the common "irritable bowel syndrome," especially when the alteration varies between diarrhea and constipation. Small pellet-like stools are often described by the patient. Associated symptoms of bloating, nausea, and "gas" are also common. This diagnosis can essentially be made only on the basis of a thorough history and physical examination which exclude structural disease. In contrast, the onset of worsening constipation in an adult with previously regular habits, especially when accompanied by systemic symptoms such as weight loss, suggests the possible presence of an underlying obstructing process, particularly malignancy. If diarrhea is present, one should determine the average number of stools, their consistency, their pattern, and if any blood is present. Although *diarrhea* refers to an increased frequency of movements, patients will often use the term to describe loose or watery stools primarily. The occurrence of nocturnal or true bloody diarrhea almost always reflects structural rather than functional bowel disease. A pungent odor or the presence of undigested meat in the movement are suggestive of pancreatic insufficiency. An alteration in color can be seen in cholestasis or steatorrhea (light-colored) or hemorrhage (melenic to maroon or bright red). Mucus in the movement is usually a sign of functional bowel syndrome, while pus is more strongly suggestive of infectious or inflammatory disease. Less common but more dramatic are the symptoms of acute gastrointestinal bleeding, including hemetemesis, melena, and hematochezia, which usually leads to prompt efforts to find medical attention but should always be solicited by the clinician.

In the evaluation of male patients, especially those with diarrhea, a tactful inquiry into sexual activity is essential. Homosexual males are at increased risk for a large variety of gastrointestinal disorders as well as the acquired immunodeficiency syndrome, which may first manifest itself with gastrointestinal symptoms. Finally, careful attention must be given to a general medical history with an emphasis on any medications or nonprescription drugs that may have been used. Thyroid and other metabolic disorders, especially those affecting calcium metabolism, can cause a variety of gastrointestinal symptoms. Unless asked, patients may forget to mention that they take aspirin almost daily for headache, and this may account for occult blood found in the stool. The use of daily laxatives may explain chronic diarrhea.

Physical examination, endoscopy, and radiology All of the cardinal methods of examination are helpful in evaluating the patient with gastrointestinal symptoms. *Inspection* may disclose signs of cholestasis or nutritional deficiencies. An abnormal contour of the abdomen or inspection of the perianal region may manifest signs of a mass or a draining fistula. *Auscultation* is also important. A succussion splash can be elicited in the patients with symptoms of gastric outlet obstruction. The absence of bowel sounds or alteration in pitch can lead to recognition of an evolving ileus or an obstructing process. A bruit may also be appreciated where there are symptoms of ischemic bowel disease. Careful *palpation* of the abdomen is especially important in detecting tenderness and masses, which in the appropriate clinical setting will lead to the recognition of cholecystitis, regional enteritis, periappendiceal abscess, and many other disorders. These findings will often be complemented by *percussion*, which is essential to assessing liver and spleen size. In addition to the examination of the abdomen, a carefully performed digital rectal examination is also essential. In the patient with complaints of incontinence the integrity of the sphincter can be assessed. Most importantly, masses intrinsic to the rectum as well as abnormalities in the pelvis or the pouch of Douglas may only be detected by this examination, and the presence or absence of frank or occult blood in the stool is always important diagnostic information. Sigmoidoscopy should be viewed as a routine extension of the physical examination in the patient with diarrhea or other alteration in bowel habit as well as in the patient with known or suspected blood loss from the lower bowel. This procedure, which can be performed with either the rigid sigmoidoscope or a flexible fiberoptic instrument, allows for direct inspection of the rectosigmoid mucosa permitting detection of cancers and polyps in this segment that may well be missed by barium x-rays. Inflammatory changes of the mucosa can help identify the patient with infectious dysentery or other forms of colitis, most notably ulcerative colitis. The findings of edema, granularity, and diffuse friability (easily induced mucosal bleeding) as well as superficial ulcerations are characteristic in the latter disorder. Fresh stool samples for microbiologic studies and superficial mucosal biopsies obtained at the time of sigmoidoscopy can also yield crucial diagnostic information.

Definitive demonstration or exclusion of structural lesions of the gastrointestinal tract, particularly the great majority of disorders that primarily affect mucosal surface, can often not be accomplished by physical examination alone. Many disorders of the upper or lower gastrointestinal tract are accessible to inspection through fiberoptic instruments. As a result, endoscopic studies are supplanting conventional contrast x-ray studies for many clinical problems, both because of the heightened precision of these diagnostic tools and the opportunity in some instances to accomplish a meaningful therapeutic intervention as an adjunct to the acquisition of diagnostic information. However, it should be emphasized that *no procedure should be considered routine* and used indiscriminately; there must be a rational basis for its use in the individual patient. These techniques are discussed in detail in Chap. 236. Upper gastrointestinal endoscopy permits evaluation of the esophagus, stomach, and duodenum and, with specially designed instruments, the proximal jejunum. When the clinical history warrants a diagnostic examination of the upper gastrointestinal tract for a structural lesion, endoscopic examination is preferable to radiologic study in most patients when the choice is available. Side-viewing scopes permit inspection and cannulation of the ampulla of Vater facilitating retrograde cholangiopancreatography. The colonoscope can be used to visualize the entire colon and often the terminal ileum, resulting in more accurate diagnosis of inflammatory bowel disease. Frequently colonic polyps can be removed at the time of initial colonoscopic identification.

While endoscopic techniques are relatively precise in defining many problems, the limitations of these tools as well as the continued advantages of x-ray studies in some situations should be recognized. Endoscopic tools are not useful in assessing gastrointestinal (GI) motility, which may be more accurately gauged by barium studies. In addition, some areas, notably the small intestine, remain relatively inaccessible to fiberoptic instruments. In hospitals where endoscopy is not feasible, the upper GI series and barium enema remain good diagnostic modalities for the upper and lower GI tract especially when air-contrast techniques are employed. However, they should generally be avoided in the patient with GI bleeding or suspected bowel obstruction. In addition the physician must exercise judgment in preparing the patient for these studies, recognizing that cathartics may markedly worsen the condition of a patient with obstructing lesions or colitis.

Although endoscopy has obviated the role for many conventional GI x-rays, other radiologic imaging modalities are assuming an increasingly crucial role in the approach to the patient with gastrointestinal symptoms. These techniques include ultrasound (US), computed tomography (CT), and magnetic resonance imaging (MRI). The application of these tools to the liver and biliary tract is discussed in Chap. 248. Both US and CT are useful in the delineation of abdominal masses. CT, though more expensive, is often more effective in the evaluation of the lower abdomen, where inflammatory masses in patients with Crohn's disease or complications of diverticular disease may be accurately imaged. MRI may permit exquisitely accurate information on the anatomic extent of invasive rectal cancers and blood flow in patients with vascular disorders, but the full range of its uses in GI disorders remains to be delineated.

Finally, one must emphasize that the optimal use of endoscopic and radiologic imaging techniques also depends on the recognition that each modality has inherent limitations. Only the clinician can determine whether the information is sufficient to establish or exclude a diagnosis in a patient with relevant historical and/or physical findings and a negative or nondiagnostic study. Was the preparation of the patient or the examination of sufficient quality to have detected an abnormality if present? Was the examiner aware of the important diagnostic considerations, and was the study adapted to address those concerns? Conversely only the physician can determine whether irregularities found in diagnostic studies are indeed causally related to the patient's symptoms. This judgment usually relies upon a sound understanding of the biologic basis of gastrointestinal disorders.

DIAGNOSTIC APPROACHES Problems of swallowing The approach should be as follows:

1 *Thorough determination of the nature of dysphagia.* Is the difficulty primarily in swallowing liquids, solids, or both? The location of the difficulty from the patient's perspective and presence or absence of accompanying odynophagia are important to ascertain. These historical clues are complemented by careful visual and neurologic examination of the oropharynx when appropriate.

2 *Routine esophageal x-rays* in the upright and lateral or Trendelenburg position. The horizontal views are essential for demonstration of the swallowing mechanism, unaided by gravity, and of the esophagogastric junction. For details of the pharyngoesophageal area cineradiography is necessary because of the rapidity with which the contrast medium passes through. Hiatus hernia is extremely common (in 15 to 35 percent of persons over 50) and often asymptomatic unless spontaneous reflux of gastric contents can be demonstrated to occur repeatedly. Careful attention is usually needed to detect lower esophageal rings or webs which may be visible as indentations in the barium column only from a limited angle.

3 *Esophagoscopy.* This procedure is desirable to describe lesions suggested by x-ray or, if the lesion is unsuspected, to obtain biopsies from masses or abnormal mucosa and to obtain washings for exfoliative cytologic study. The diagnoses of peptic esophagitis and Barrett's esophagus are made endoscopically. Endoscopy is the most sensitive technique for identifying esophageal or gastric varices, although they are seldom important in the absence of hemorrhage.

4 *Manometric studies* of the upper esophagus, particularly in conjunction with cineradiography. At present, this procedure offers the best differential between disorders primary in the central nervous system, primary pharyngeal muscular disease, and cricopharyngeal dystonia. Manometry of the lower esophagus is useful in the diagnosis of diffuse esophageal spasm, achalasia, and infiltrative diseases that can alter esophageal motility.

Peptic or digestive disorders The approaches to these disorders include:

1 *Insertion of a nasogastric tube.* This is used to establish whether significant gastric retention (more than 75 mL of gastric contents in the fasting state) exists and whether there is acid, bile, blood, or other material in these contents. If pyloric obstruction or gastric atony is present, the tube is used to maintain suction while the patient's electrolyte and fluid balance is restored to normal; the stomach is kept as clean as possible so that reliable diagnostic investigation may be carried out.

2 *Upper intestinal endoscopy.* This procedure is most helpful in identifying the diffuse mucosa in gastritis or, together with biopsy and brushings for cytology, in differentiating between peptic and neoplastic ulcerating lesions. It may identify a specific bleeding site in clinical situations where several potential bleeding sites could exist, such as in the patient with portal hypertension. The significance of the described association of gastritis with *Campylobacter pylori* in patients with nonulcer dyspepsia, particularly the elderly, remains uncertain, but it can be detected by endoscopy and biopsy. Endoscopy can detect a number of potential sources of upper GI bleeding which are often missed by x-ray studies (e.g., erosive gastritis, Mallory-Weiss syndrome). Gastroscopy is also particularly helpful in inspecting the postoperative stomach, especially in detecting stomal ulceration or so-called alkaline reflux gastritis. The first and second portions of the duodenum can also be examined with the fiberoptic gastroscope, and important information about ulcers and other lesions can be obtained by this procedure. Radiologic studies may be useful when endoscopy is not readily available or in the assessment of suspected motility disorders (e.g., gastroparesis). In addition, radiologic examination may be preferred when there are contraindications to safe endoscopy.

3 *Gastric acid secretory studies.* These are useful in the diagnosis of the Zollinger-Ellison syndrome or atrophic gastritis and for determination of completeness of vagotomy. Suspected gastric carcinoma is better diagnosed directly through gastroscopy and biopsy than indirectly through acid secretory studies (achlorhydria). These studies should not be obtained for the routine diagnosis of uncomplicated duodenal ulcer. There is no convincing evidence that acid studies are useful in determining the type of surgery for duodenal ulcer.

Obstructive and vascular disorders of the small intestine When intestinal problems present as obstructive syndromes, the plain x-ray of the abdomen is the most important diagnostic adjunct to careful physical examination. Patterns of dilatation of individual loops of intestine may be characteristic, as in volvulus or acute pancreatitis; erect and decubitus views will often show fluid levels in the affected segments. Motility disorders of the small intestine (temporary ileus or chronic intestinal pseudo-obstruction) may also present with obstructive symptoms and similar x-ray findings but must be managed medically without surgical intervention. Air under the diaphragm is diagnostic of a perforated viscus; air in the portal vein usually results from intestinal necrosis secondary to mesenteric vascular occlusion. The diagnostic accuracy of the plain x-ray in all types of intestinal obstruction is about 75 percent. In patients with symptoms of incomplete obstruction, the radiographic small-bowel series will often be diagnostic in defining the site and degree of obstruction. Infrequently, in this setting, all conventional x-ray studies are unremarkable. In such cases, the radiologist may perform a small-bowel enteroclysis study by passing a special tube into the proximal jejunum; the rapid instillation of barium through the tube will distend the intestine and often reveal subtle lesions missed by other tests.

Vascular diseases of the small intestine are among the most difficult diseases to diagnose. In chronic mesenteric ischemia, radiographic, endoscopic, and laboratory tests are usually normal. Early in the course of acute mesenteric ischemia, the plain film of the abdomen may be unremarkable despite complaints of severe abdominal pain. In these settings, prompt mesenteric angiography is essential in confirming the diagnosis of vascular disease.

Inflammatory and neoplastic diseases of small and large intestine Patients with these conditions are usually identified by history, physical examination, and careful examination of the stools for exudate and blood. Examination of fresh stool samples for common bacterial pathogens and parasites by laboratories skilled in these techniques is important in identifying or excluding infectious causes of diarrhea, particularly in the patient with colitis. Sigmoidoscopy is valuable in identifying mucosal and neoplastic lesions of the lower 25 cm of the colon. The mucosal surface of the entire colon and terminal ileum can be examined directly and biopsied through the fiberoptic sigmoidoscope or colonoscope. The radiologic examination of the small intestine is highly reliable in identifying the prestenotic and stenotic lesions of Crohn's disease. In the colon a single barium enema examination in a well-prepared patient has a diagnostic accuracy of 80 to 85 percent; the addition of air-contrast technique brings the accuracy up over 90 percent, but none of these figures is meaningful if the patient is poorly prepared for the examination, and the cecal area is hard to examine adequately because of its anatomy. Colonoscopy may be preferable, if available, for its greater accuracy and the capability to remove the vast majority of polyps as well as to obtain preoperative tissue confirmation in the patient who probably has cancer. The immunologic assay for the carcinoembryonic antigen has not proved to be specific for colonic cancer; nevertheless, it does contribute to the detection of residual or recurrent disease in postoperative patients.

Peroral biopsy of the small intestine and forceps biopsy of the rectosigmoid are of considerable importance in revealing mucosal disease. Rectal biopsy is an excellent means of demonstrating amyloidosis, schistosomiasis, and amebiasis. Submucosal disease is not seen in these superficial biopsies. Hirschsprung's disease is histologically diagnosed by a deep surgical biopsy of the lower part of the rectum.

Malabsorption syndromes Malabsorption may be suspected on the basis of history and physical examination and is confirmed by examination of the stools. Radiologic examination is of general help in ruling out local lesions and suggesting motor and secretory dysfunction, but it is rarely diagnostic unless an abnormal small-bowel mucosa or fistulas between intestine and stomach are demonstrated.

The tests useful in the diagnosis of malabsorption are discussed in Chap. 240. A simple screening test for excessive fat in the stools can be accomplished by the microscopic examination of a stool specimen stained with Sudan. Chemical analysis of 3-day stool collection for fat, with the patient on a standard diet, is used to establish the diagnosis of steatorrhea. The D-xylose absorption test is about 90 percent accurate in separating mucosal disease from pancreatic insufficiency. Peroral biopsy of the small intestine is of value in the diagnosis of celiac disease, and it may show the less common infiltrations of the mucosa by amyloid or bacterial mucoproteins (Whipple's disease). Leakage of protein into the intestinal lumen may cause hypoproteinemia and can be demonstrated by the recovery in stools of the serum protein alpha$_1$ antitrypsin or intravenously administered markers such as albumin labeled with iodine or chromium isotopes.

Pancreas The pancreas is difficult to study directly because of its anatomic location and relative inaccessibility. Calcification of the pancreas on a plain abdominal film is highly suggestive of chronic pancreatitis and may be associated with fat malabsorption. Pancreatic exocrine insufficiency can be documented by intubation of the duodenum and collection of pancreatic juice after stimulation with secretin or a test meal. Abdominal ultrasound and CT are the best radiographic means of searching for pancreatic enlargement (see Chaps. 259 and 260). Both techniques may also be used to guide needle biopsies of the pancreas and may provide sufficient diagnostic information to obviate the need for exploratory surgery. The pancreatic duct can be cannulated via the fiberoptic duodenoscope and visualized by the injection of radiographic dye. Visualization of the duct may be helpful in the diagnosis of pancreatic pseudocysts, carcinoma, or chronic pancreatitis.

REFERENCES

JOHNSON LR et al: *Physiology of the Gastrointestinal Tract*, 2d ed. New York, Raven, 1987

SLEISENGER MH, FORDTRAN JS: *Gastrointestinal Disease*, 4th ed. Philadelphia, Saunders, 1989

236 GASTROINTESTINAL ENDOSCOPY

MICHAEL B. KIMMEY / FRED E. SILVERSTEIN

Fiberendoscopes have revolutionized the examination of the gastrointestinal tract. Because of the flexibility of the fiberoptic bundles and because of controllability of the instrument tip, the operator can steer the instrument around multiple bends under visual control. A channel permits passage of a variety of endoscopic tools such as biopsy forceps, foreign-body forceps, cytology brushes, wash tubes, and electrocautery snares. The viewing window and the light at the instrument's distal end can be washed free of obscuring material. Fluid can be aspirated from hollow organs, and air can be insufflated as needed to improve visualization. The video endoscope is a modification of the fiberendoscope in which a charged coupled device on the distal tip of the instrument transmits the image onto a TV screen. This system is being increasingly used because it permits storage, analysis, and transmission of the endoscopic images.

The usefulness of fiberendoscopy in diagnosing gastrointestinal disease is well established. Shallow lesions such as erosions or healing ulcers are missed by single-contrast x-ray but not by endoscopy. The brilliant success of polypectomy via the colonoscope has led to the development of other endoscopic therapeutic techniques such as endoscopic sphincterotomy; endoscopic therapy is now a recognized alternative to surgery in many situations.

Although esophagogastroduodenoscopy (EGD) is not a procedure for the occasional operator, it should be available in every general hospital. It is a relatively easy procedure to perform technically, but training and continued experience are necessary for optimal diagnostic accuracy. Complications are most frequent when the operator is inexperienced. Before the procedure the competent endoscopist always takes a history and examines the patient. Particular attention to cardiac, pulmonary, and blood clotting functions is essential.

The more complex procedures such as colonoscopy and endoscopic retrograde cholangiopancreatography (ERCP) require special dexterity, a substantial investment of time for learning, and constant practice to maintain adequate skill; they are probably best accomplished by subspecialists.

UPPER GASTROINTESTINAL ENDOSCOPY Here forward-, oblique-, and side-viewing instruments may be used for EGD. After a careful explanation of the procedure to the patient, pharyngeal topical anesthesia with viscous lidocaine or various anesthetic sprays is followed by intravenous diazepam to the point of mild sedation. With small-caliber instruments less or no diazepam is needed. The tip of the endoscope is placed at the cricopharyngeal sphincter of the esophagus and the patient is encouraged to swallow while gentle pressure is exerted. Small amounts of air are passed through the endoscope to visualize the esophageal lumen. The endoscope is then passed under direct vision into the stomach. The gastric body and antrum are carefully examined. The instrument tip is retroflexed to view the gastric cardia, the fundus, and the whole lesser curvature. The pylorus is traversed, and the first and second portions of the duodenum are visualized. The examination is repeated as the instrument is withdrawn. Visualized lesions can be recorded on photographs or videotape. Biopsies and brush cytologic examinations can be obtained from suspicious areas.

EGD is a relatively safe procedure in experienced hands. Several large surveys suggest a risk of serious complications during diagnostic EGD of approximately 1 in 800 and a risk of death of approximately 1 in 5000. The risks are higher in emergency procedures and in the elderly or seriously ill. In a survey of patients examined by endoscopy during bleeding, 1 in 200 had serious complications and 1 in 700 died from the procedure. The main causes of mortality were cardiopulmonary complications and perforations by the instrument. Endoscopy is preferred over x-ray in the urgent diagnosis of gastrointestinal illness in women who might be pregnant.

Gastroesophageal reflux disease Esophagitis is one of the commonest diseases of the upper gastrointestinal tract (see Chap. 237). Esophageal pain may be confused with cardiac disease, or esophagitis may present as painless blood loss. Because esophagitis usually involves only the superficial mucosa, it cannot be diagnosed by routine single-contrast radiography. At endoscopy, friable mucosa, linear erosions, and ulcerations of erosive esophagitis are clearly visible. Not every patient with heartburn requires esophagoscopy, but the procedure is indicated if the patient complains of dysphagia, if an x-ray shows a stricture, a mass, or an ulcer, if symptoms persist despite therapy, or if antireflux surgery is contemplated.

The squamous mucosa of the esophagus is more vulnerable to peptic digestion than is the columnar epithelium of the stomach. Thus, esophagitis is located on the squamous side of the esophagogastric junction and is most severe in the distal esophagus where the squamous mucosa is most exposed to regurgitated acid and pepsin from the stomach. Discrete peptic ulceration of the esophagus is uncommon.

A short area of esophagitis or a stricture can be seen at levels as high as the arch of the aorta. This is explained by progressive replacement of distal eroded squamous mucosa with metaplastic epithelium, which is more resistant to peptic digestion (Barrett's epithelium). This finding can be documented by biopsy. Such epithelium is more prone to malignant transformation and, therefore, may merit regular surveillance with esophagoscopy and biopsy every 12 to 24 months. If dysplasia is present, more frequent surveillance may be indicated to detect carcinoma.

Esophagitis may progress to scarring and stricture formation. The endoscopic appearance of a benign stricture is characteristic but not diagnostic; a malignancy should be ruled out by biopsy and cytologic brushing before medical treatment is undertaken with dilation and antacids. The whole length of the stricture should be sampled. Endoscopy is also indicated to biopsy the rim of an esophageal ulcer to rule out cancer.

Dilations of difficult strictures are best initiated by passing a flexible-tipped guidewire via the biopsy channel of the endoscope through the stricture under direct vision. The endoscope can then be withdrawn over the wire, which serves as a guide for passage of progressively larger polyvinyl dilators through the stricture under fluoroscopic control. An alternative technique utilizes balloon catheters passed via the endoscope channel or over a guidewire through the stricture. The balloon is inflated under endoscopic and/or fluoroscopic guidance to dilate the stricture.

Peptic ulcer Esophagogastroduodenoscopy is more accurate than upper gastrointestinal x-ray in detecting ulcers. It has been suggested that x-ray be abandoned entirely in favor of endoscopy for detecting ulcers. This makes sense when the source of acute upper gastrointestinal bleeding is sought and urgent surgical intervention is being considered. However, in the workup of the patient with less pressing ulcer complaints, an upper gastrointestinal x-ray is still often used as the initial diagnostic test. As more radiologists routinely use air contrast to obtain better mucosal detail, diagnostic sensitivity for superficial lesions will increase. The greater expense and discomfort of endoscopy are justified if the x-ray is equivocal, or suggests that the ulcer is malignant, if the x-ray is negative but the clinical picture suggests peptic ulceration, or if the patient is about to be operated on for ulcer. Patients with duodenal ulcers shown by x-ray or with classic ulcer deformities of the duodenal bulb do not require endoscopy for diagnosis if the presenting symptoms are characteristic and if the symptomatic response to antiulcer treatment is good. Screening endoscopy using small-diameter endoscopes without sedation is a reasonable alternative to contrast x-rays as the initial diagnostic test in the symptomatic patient.

There are some situations in which x-ray reveals ulcers missed by endoscopy, e.g., ulcers in hourglass constrictions of the stomach or in small, incompletely visualized duodenal bulbs. Fiberendoscopy is especially useful in visualizing postbulbar ulcers, giant duodenal ulcers, and stomal ulceration after partial gastrectomy, all of which can be missed by x-ray. Endoscopy may be of use in determining the cause of gastric outlet obstruction. In most circumstances, patients with duodenal ulcers do not need follow-up endoscopy to see if the ulcer has healed.

In the enthusiasm for fiberendoscopy one must not forget that visual interpretation of gross pathology is subjective—one observer's ulcer is another's erosion. An erosion is confined to the mucosa and heals without a trace, whereas an ulcer is deeper and usually implies a chronic recurrent disease. Endoscopically, erosions are superficial, small, and multiple; ulcers are deeper and larger and tend to be solitary. In the future it is likely that lesions seen endoscopically will be easily recorded for review on videotape or disk, just as currently all lesions seen fluoroscopically are demonstrated in spot films.

Cancer The endoscopic appearance of upper gastrointestinal cancer may seem obvious, especially if there is a mass growing into the lumen. On the other hand, malignant ulcers, infiltrative carcinomas, or small early carcinomas are frequently impossible to diagnose by their gross appearance. Six to eight biopsies should be taken from the rim of a gastric ulcer to exclude malignancy. Experience and skill in choosing the biopsy site improves the accuracy. A cytologic examination of lavage or brush specimen adds to the diagnostic accuracy in all areas of the upper gastrointestinal tract (see Chap. 239).

In most patients gastric ulcers should be assessed for healing by endoscopy after 12 weeks of antiulcer therapy. Persistent ulcers should be biopsied if they were not biopsied at the time of the initial diagnosis. Some patients with a low likelihood of malignancy, for example, a young person taking anti-inflammatory drugs, can be assessed for healing radiographically.

Primary gastric lymphoma can mimic benign gastric ulcer or adenocarcinoma on gastroscopy or x-ray. It can be diagnosed by biopsy or cytology, although the accuracy is not as high as in adenocarcinoma. The 5-year survival for lymphoma is higher than for adenocarcinoma.

If a polypoid lesion of the stomach is covered by mucosa that appears normal by gastroscopy, the likelihood of malignancy is very small. Such lesions are often intramural, extramucosal benign tumors such as leiomyomas or pancreatic rests. Polyps covered by abnormal-appearing mucosa can be benign or malignant. Random biopsy can miss carcinoma within a polyp. If technically feasible, polyps should, therefore, be removed in their entirety by snare cautery for histologic examination. If over 2 cm in diameter, they are more likely to contain cancer (see Chap. 239). Large polyps may require surgical excision.

Ampullary carcinoma may be diagnosed by biopsy during duodenoscopy although a prior endoscopic sphincterotomy may increase diagnostic yield. Other primary duodenal malignancies are very rare. Extensions from pancreatic or biliary tract cancer are difficult to diagnose because the tumor may not have extended into the mucosa and may therefore not be accessible for endoscopic biopsy or cytologic examination. In these secondary tumors, diagnosis must depend upon some combination of echography, hypotonic duodenography, selective pancreatic angiography, and endoscopic retrograde cholangiopancreatography, with cytologic examination of ductal contents.

Upper gastrointestinal bleeding (See also Chap. 46) Endoscopy within the first 12 to 24 h of an upper gastrointestinal hemorrhage can be very helpful in planning rational therapy by visualizing the bleeding source. Shallow lesions not visible by x-ray may be seen (esophagitis, Mallory-Weiss tear, erosive gastritis, shallow stress ulcer, and telangiectasia). Lesions that are visible by x-ray may not be the source of bleeding. Only endoscopy can determine the actual bleeding site. For example, visualization of a spurting artery which is flooding the stomach indicates massive ongoing bleeding requiring prompt therapeutic intervention. Several studies have shown that the demonstration at endoscopy of any bleeding whatsoever or a non-bleeding vessel or sentinel clot in the ulcer base makes rebleeding more likely.

A conservative estimate of the diagnostic accuracy of emergency endoscopy in upper gastrointestinal bleeding is 80 to 85 percent. Endoscopic diagnosis of bleeding erosive gastritis may be made too frequently when blood from another unsuspected source spreads over the gastric mucosa or when trauma from overly vigorous antecedent lavage creates submucosal ecchymoses. To avoid overdiagnosis of erosive gastritis, portions of the gastric wall should be washed free of blood to determine the true appearance of the underlying gastric mucosa.

Every patient having endoscopy for upper gastrointestinal bleeding merits a complete endoscopic examination of the esophagus, stomach, and duodenum. Finding a potential bleeding lesion is not proof that this is the source of hemorrhage unless active bleeding is seen. Up to 50 percent of patients with esophageal varices can be shown endoscopically to be bleeding from another source such as erosive gastritis, duodenal ulcer, or gastric ulcer. Occasionally it is not possible to diagnose the exact lesion that is bleeding, but localizing the area of bleeding can be very helpful; for example, bright red arterial blood may be seen pouring into the stomach from the duodenum when the esophagus and stomach are relatively free of blood.

There are three controversial areas. First, *do all bleeders need endoscopy?* Endoscopy is indicated in all patients who may require surgery because of continual bleeding or rebleeding because selection of the type of operation depends on what lesion is bleeding. Although 85 percent of upper gastrointestinal bleeders stop spontaneously, it is impossible to predict which ones will; therefore, endoscopy is recommended for most bleeders. Second, *how early should endoscopy be performed in the acutely bleeding patient?* Most studies suggest that the diagnostic accuracy of esophagogastroduodenoscopy remains high for the first 12 to 24 h after the bleeding episode. All would agree that it is desirable to delay endoscopy until vital signs have been stabilized after adequate blood replacement. Upper endoscopy is usually performed during waking hours at a time during the first day of bleeding when the patient's vital signs are stable and when the full endoscopic team is available. Emergency endoscopy at night should be reserved for those patients with continued massive bleeding or rebleeding requiring an immediate decision regarding surgery or other treatment. If the patient is exsanguinating, endoscopy can follow induction of anesthesia just preceding surgery. Thus, the patient's airway is protected by an endotracheal tube. Finally, *does endoscopy affect the clinical outcome?* Earlier studies suggest that it does not. Recent studies of the endoscopic treatment of bleeding lesions with heater probes and bipolar probes suggest that these methods are safe and reduce blood requirements, need for surgery, and mortality in some patients with bleeding ulcers.

Injection therapy of bleeding lesions is another therapeutic modality used to stop bleeding. Injection of a dilute solution of epinephrine followed by injection of either alcohol or a sclerosing agent often stops active bleeding from peptic ulcers. Injection of various sclerosing solutions into or next to esophageal varices is currently the treatment of choice for stopping active variceal bleeding. Repeated injection sclerotherapy to achieve variceal eradication produces results comparable to portacaval shunting in terms of mortality, although rebleeding after sclerotherapy may necessitate further sclerotherapy or shunting.

Emergency and therapeutic endoscopy is not for the inexperienced. It requires considerable technical skill and interpretive experience and the best available instruments.

Percutaneous endoscopic gastrostomy The placement of feeding or decompression gastrostomy tubes can be facilitated with the use of an endoscope. Under sedation, the endoscope's light within the stomach is used to identify a suitable location for a gastrostomy in the left upper quadrant of the abdomen. A needle is introduced into the stomach percutaneously and then a snare passed through the endoscope is used to capture a wire or suture placed through the needle. A feeding tube is advanced over the wire into the stomach. Feedings are begun the following day. Hospitalization time and morbidity and mortality associated with operative gastrostomy is reduced.

Patients with transfer dysphagia secondary to strokes and degenerative neurologic disorders benefit the most from this procedure. Other indications for percutaneous endoscopic gastrostomy include dysphagia produced by head and neck neoplasms, and the inability to eat secondary to diffuse cerebral injury. Patients with severe gastroparesis can be fed through a jejunal feeding tube placed through the gastrostomy and then directed through the pylorus. Simultaneous gastric decompression is possible through a separate lumen in the gastrostomy.

Palliation of esophageal carcinoma Patients with dysphagia caused by malignant esophageal strictures usually cannot be cured by esophagectomy. Surgical resection and radiation therapy are often chosen for palliation of dysphagia in this situation. The endoscopist can also help palliate these patients when radiation therapy has failed or when surgical risks are too great.

Dilatation of malignant strictures is usually possible with polyvinyl dilators passed over an endoscopically placed guidewire. Dilatation may improve the patient's swallowing initially, but more definitive therapy is usually needed. This can be in the form of laser ablation or by placement of a prosthesis or stent. Tumor within the esophageal lumen can be destroyed by application of Nd:YAG laser energy using a laser waveguide placed through the biopsy channel of the endoscope. Alternatively, after stricture dilatation large-caliber stents can be placed over a dilator. When the dilator is removed, the stent lumen is available for the passage of food. Stenting is especially useful in the palliation of malignant tracheoesophageal fistulas.

Other indications Upper endoscopy is usually substituted for x-ray in the urgent diagnosis of gastrointestinal illness in *pregnancy*. Patients with *dysphagia* merit esophagoscopy because the cause is frequently organic and may be missed by x-ray. Dysphagia caused by esophageal spasm or dysrhythmia is best diagnosed by manometry or cineradiography in addition to endoscopy. *Painful swallowing* (odynophagia), especially in immunosuppressed or diabetic patients, may merit esophagoscopy because biopsy and brushings of the involved esophageal wall may reveal monilial, herpetic, or cytomegalic virus infections. Soon after ingestion of a corrosive agent, if there is no indication of wall necrosis, limited and gentle esophagoscopy is useful in evaluating the severity of injury. Many impacted foreign bodies can be removed from the esophagus or stomach with a snare or forceps; sharp foreign bodies are usually best removed by pulling them into the lumen of a rigid tubular esophagoscope or by pulling them into a protective overtube around a fiberoptic endoscope. Careful esophagoscopy after removal of an esophageal foreign body is important to determine whether there is an underlying lesion which caused the impaction (e.g., cancer, benign stricture, peptic esophagitis).

In the postoperative stomach, gastroscopy is especially useful in detecting carcinoma, recurrent ulceration, retrograde intussusception, and stomal stricture. Several European studies indicate a definite threat of carcinoma developing in the gastric stump 10 to 20 years after a Billroth II gastrectomy. The diagnosis of such postoperative carcinomas may require many biopsies of seemingly normal mucosa near the anastomosis. Studies of the natural history of this condition in the United States do not suggest a similar high incidence of postoperative carcinoma.

When the duodenal bulb shows reddening or nodularity, many endoscopists diagnose *duodenitis*. There is little evidence to suggest

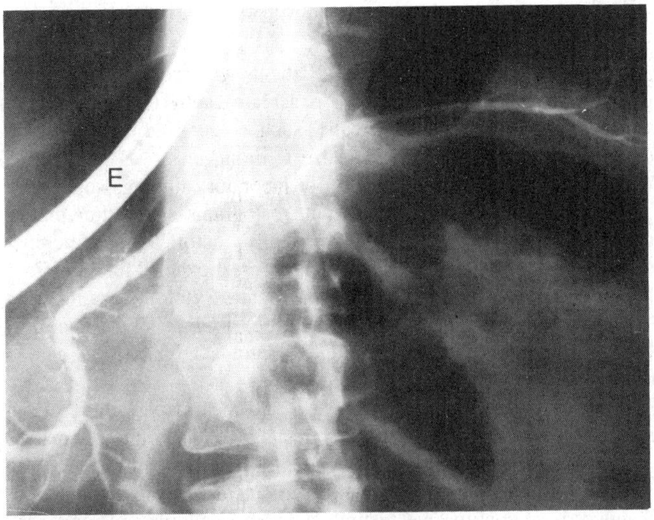

A

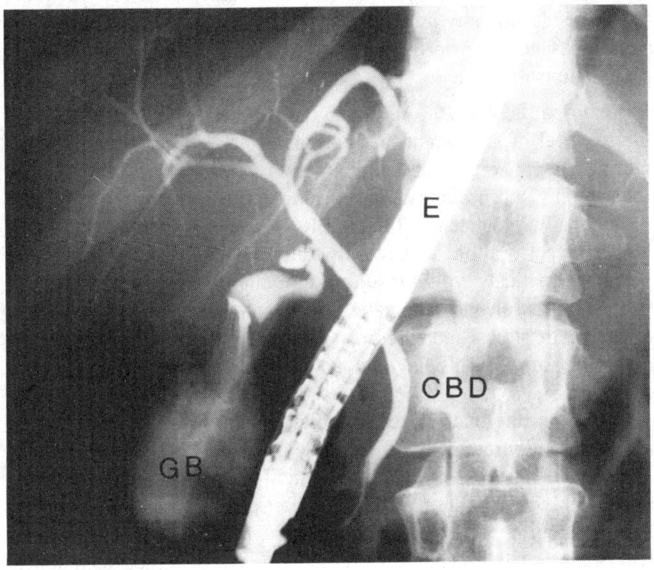

B

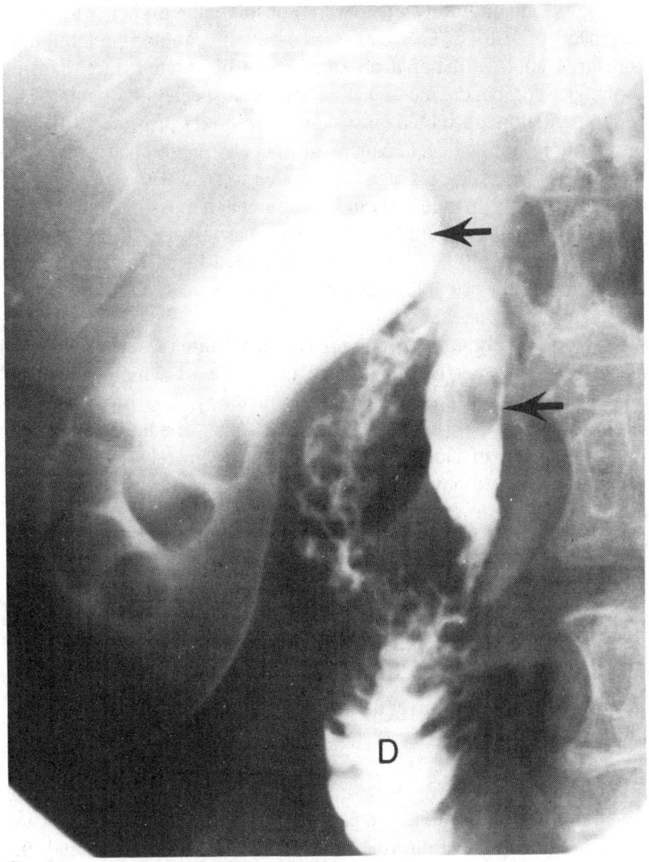

C

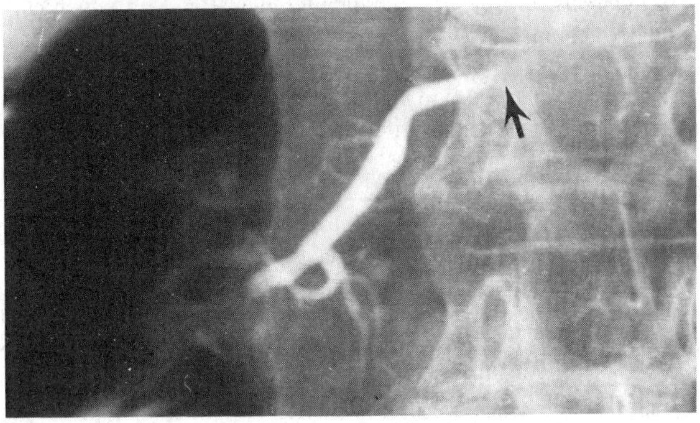

D

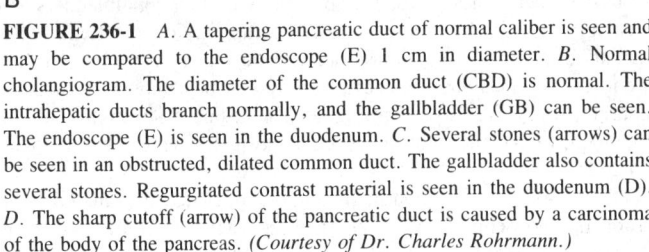

FIGURE 236-1 *A*. A tapering pancreatic duct of normal caliber is seen and may be compared to the endoscope (E) 1 cm in diameter. *B*. Normal cholangiogram. The diameter of the common duct (CBD) is normal. The intrahepatic ducts branch normally, and the gallbladder (GB) can be seen. The endoscope (E) is seen in the duodenum. *C*. Several stones (arrows) can be seen in an obstructed, dilated common duct. The gallbladder also contains several stones. Regurgitated contrast material is seen in the duodenum (D). *D*. The sharp cutoff (arrow) of the pancreatic duct is caused by a carcinoma of the body of the pancreas. *(Courtesy of Dr. Charles Rohrmann.)*

that this picture is of significance. On the other hand, diffuse and bleeding erosions of the duodenal bulb merit a diagnosis of *erosive duodenitis,* especially after ingestion of mucosal irritants such as aspirin. A nodular or narrow duodenum will occasionally yield granulomas on biopsy, indicative of Crohn's disease.

ENDOSCOPIC RETROGRADE CHOLANGIOPANCREATOGRAPHY (ERCP) This endoscopic technique involves placing a side-viewing instrument in the descending duodenum. The papilla of Vater is cannulated, contrast medium is injected, and the pancreatic ducts and hepatobiliary tree are visualized radiographically. Skilled operators can visualize 90 to 95 percent of pancreatic ducts and 90 percent of biliary ducts.

ERCP is performed on an x-ray table. The oropharynx is usually anesthetized with topical lidocaine, and most endoscopists sedate the patient with intravenous diazepam. Atropine and glucagon are given intravenously to induce duodenal hypotonia. The pancreatic duct is usually visualized first and gently filled throughout its entire length with 2 to 5 mL of contrast material with constant fluoroscopic monitoring (Fig. 236-1*A*). Injection is continued until the first side branches are seen or until the patient complains of pain. Overfilling is avoided. By insertion of the cannula at a more acute cephalad angle, the common bile duct and the whole biliary tract including the gallbladder are visualized (Fig. 236-1*B*).

ERCP is a safe procedure when performed by an experienced operator. Asymptomatic amylase elevations occur in 30 to 40 percent of patients after pancreatography and are rarely of clinical significance. Pancreatitis occurs in only 1 percent of patients but is usually benign and self-limited. By monitoring the pancreas during injection using a high-resolution TV screen, the force of injection can be limited to avoid filling of pancreatic acini. This probably minimizes the complication of pancreatitis. In a nationwide survey of complications, the morbidity rate was 3 percent and mortality rate 0.2 percent.

Morbidity and mortality rates were substantially higher with inexperienced operators. The main serious complication is retention of nonsterile contrast material proximal to an obstructed duct, causing cholangitis or pancreatic sepsis. Patients suspected of having bile duct obstruction are started on systemic antibiotics prior to the ERCP. Furthermore, if bile duct or pancreatic duct obstruction is first revealed by ERCP, antibiotic coverage is indicated to reduce the incidence of bacteremia; such patients should be drained if possible either with endoscopic therapy (papillotomy, stents, nasobiliary drains, etc.) or surgically within 36 h. No patient should have ERCP unless advance arrangements for possible operation have been made with the patient and a surgical consultant.

Retrograde cholangiography This procedure is especially useful in patients with persistent jaundice the cause of which cannot be established by conventional diagnostic methods. The important differential diagnosis is between "surgical" and "medical" jaundice. When the cause of jaundice is unclear, approximately 15 percent of patients thought to have "medical" jaundice prove to have extrahepatic biliary obstruction requiring surgery or endoscopic therapy, and, conversely, the same percentage of patients thought to have "surgical" jaundice prove to have an open ductal system by ERCP and can be spared unnecessary intervention.

Remediable causes of obstructive jaundice which can be diagnosed by retrograde cholangiography include common duct stones (Fig. 236-1*C*) and benign and malignant strictures. In jaundiced patients with suspected primary liver disease, such as primary biliary cirrhosis, ERCP can relieve the worry that an operable obstruction is being missed.

In addition to ERCP, there are four other methods of visualizing the biliary tree in the jaundiced patient. Which test to use first depends on the clinical situation, the availability of equipment, and the experience of the specialists using the techniques. The first method is *percutaneous transhepatic cholangiography* (PTC), in which contrast material is injected from the exterior via a "skinny" needle into the intrahepatic bile ducts under fluoroscopic control; success in visualizing the ducts is 90 to 100 percent if the ducts are dilated, but only approximately 70 percent if they are not dilated. PTC is generally safe, but complications do occur (sepsis, bleeding, bile leak, etc.). The morbidity for this procedure is approximately 10 percent; the reported mortality varies from 0.1 to 0.9 percent. The three other methods, which are noninvasive, use *ultrasound, computed tomography* (CT scan), and radionuclide biliary scintigraphy. The first two techniques employ sound waves or x-rays to visualize organs and any stones, cysts, or solid masses within them. They can also be used to determine whether the biliary ducts or gallbladder are enlarged. The radionuclide scans are used to determine patency of the cystic and common ducts and to study gallbladder emptying after administration of cholecystokinin (CCK).

The relative usefulness of these five tests is not established. Many physicians first try ultrasound or CT scan to see whether the biliary ducts are dilated and to seek the cause of the patient's jaundice (stones, pancreatic mass, etc.). The radionuclide scan will determine if the cystic duct and bile ducts are patent. Direct visualization is undertaken if the diagnosis is not established. PTC is often attempted first if an intrahepatic or proximal bile duct obstruction is suggested by imaging tests. ERCP is used first if distal obstruction is suspected. Advantages of the endoscopic approach are that the papilla and the pancreatic duct are seen (in addition to the biliary ducts) and that therapy can be performed with endoscopic sphincterotomy or drainage when appropriate. In the event of a technical failure or incomplete information resulting from either ERCP or PTC, the other technique is tried. This approach detects most lesions requiring surgical intervention.

ERCP or PTC can also be useful in patients with biliary pain, cholangitis, or impaired liver function after previous biliary surgery. Remediable postoperative lesions such as strictures can be discovered and sometimes treated endoscopically. Should endoscopic therapy fail, their precise anatomy is outlined so that reoperation is less difficult.

Retrograde pancreatography Patients with recurrent or chronic pancreatitis may merit retrograde pancreatography to seek a lesion which can be approached surgically, such as localized pancreatitis in the tail or ductal pathology amenable to drainage.

Patients with symptoms, signs, or laboratory findings suggesting pancreatic carcinoma may have pancreatograms suggesting malignancy with a narrowed, encased, or sharply "cutoff" pancreatic duct (Fig. 236-1*D*). Differentiation of such pancreatic ductal findings from benign inflammatory disease can be difficult. Cytologic examination of pancreatic duct contents obtained during ERCP may prove helpful. Unfortunately, most patients with symptomatic pancreatic cancer diagnosed by ERCP are inoperable.

Patients presenting with painless steatorrhea of pancreatic origin may be shown to have a ductal pattern suggesting chronic pancreatitis or pancreatic carcinoma. Pancreatography has not been useful in the study of obscure upper abdominal pain. Pancreatic cysts can be better diagnosed by noninvasive techniques such as ultrasound, and pancreatography should be reserved for those cases where it is desirable to outline the anatomy immediately prior to surgery. Pancreatography alone does not seem promising as a method of screening for early pancreatic carcinoma.

Therapeutic ERCP Access to the pancreatic and biliary tree for the removal of stones and the placement of stents is made possible by endoscopic retrograde sphincterotomy (ERS). The pancreatic or biliary sphincter mechanism is cut using electrosurgical current passed through a wire attached to the ERCP catheter. Complications of bleeding, perforation, pancreatitis, and cholangitis occur in about 8 percent of patients with a resulting mortality rate of approximately 1 percent. The role of pancreatic sphincterotomy in the management of pancreatic stones and strictures is currently controversial; however, biliary sphincterotomy is now an established therapy for several conditions.

Common bile duct stones in patients with prior cholecystectomy are successfully removed from the bile duct after ERS by experienced operators 90 percent of the time. Small stones are pulled into the duodenum with a balloon catheter or after being captured by a basket. Stones larger than 1.5 cm in diameter may be difficult to extract without prior fragmentation by mechanical or other techniques. Common duct stones in younger patients with intact gallbladders are best removed at the time of cholecystectomy. Older patients with increased surgical risks can sometimes be managed with ERS and stone extraction alone; cholecystectomy can be delayed or avoided entirely. ERS is also assuming an increasing role in the initial treatment of patients with acute cholangitis and severe biliary pancreatitis.

Patients with benign and malignant bile duct strictures may benefit from the endoscopic placement of biliary stents after ERS. Benign strictures frequently remain dilated following removal of stents that have been left in place for several months. Patients with either pancreatic carcinoma or cholangiocarcinoma resulting in obstructive jaundice can be effectively palliated by placement of a biliary stent. Stents usually occlude after 3 to 6 months and must be exchanged if recurrent jaundice or cholangitis develops. Strictures involving the hilum of the liver (see Chap. 258) are difficult to palliate endoscopically because stents must be placed into both sides of the liver. These patients may be more effectively palliated with surgical or percutaneous radiologic techniques.

Other diagnostic techniques Critical comparative studies are needed of the various approaches to biliary tree disorders and to pancreatic diseases (ERCP, PTC, angiography, CT scanning, and ultrasound). The role of magnetic resonance imaging in diseases of the pancreas and biliary tree is yet to be defined. Endoscopic ultrasound may also prove to be a valuable technique to image the intestinal wall and adjacent organs.

COLONOSCOPY The interior of the entire length of the colon from anus to cecum can be visualized by the experienced colonoscopist. This is one of the most significant diagnostic and therapeutic applications of fiberoptic endoscopy because it can diagnose potentially curable colonic cancers missed by other techniques and remove potentially precancerous adenomatous polyps.

Approximately 40 percent of colonoscopies are performed because of an abnormal barium enema showing a polyp or a narrowing or filling defect suggesting carcinoma. Approximately 40 percent of colonoscopies are done because of gastrointestinal bleeding. The ability to examine the whole colon is proving valuable in the management of some patients with inflammatory bowel disease.

Patients are prepared for colonoscopy with a liquid diet for 2 days, magnesium citrate laxation the evening before examination, and tap water enemas the morning of the procedure. Another increasingly utilized method of preparing the colon is a total-gut lavage with a nonabsorbable electrolyte solution. This method prepares the patient without laxatives or enemas and only requires a few hours. Immediately before the procedure patients are lightly sedated with intravenous diazepam and meperidine.

The main complications of colonoscopy are hemorrhage and perforation (morbidity rate is 0.5 to 1.3 percent; mortality rate is 0.02 percent). The complication rate for polypectomy is 1 to 2 percent. Diverticular or ischemic disease and prior irradiation make the procedure more difficult and hazardous. The risk of perforation is also increased in the patient with very active colitis, and colonoscopy should be avoided during the acute phase.

Polyps (See also Chap. 243) A polyp seen on barium enema merits colonoscopy for two reasons: it may be an artifact or a cancer, and a second polyp or cancer may have been missed. The polyp can usually be excised, with lower morbidity and mortality rates than with surgery. The best way to rule out cancer within a polyp is to remove it completely for histologic examination. Hyperplastic polyps do not become malignant; colonic polyps that show benign neoplasia histologically may become malignant (tubular and villous adenomas). The risk of neoplastic polyps being cancerous increases with their size. The risk is also higher in villous adenomas. Pedunculated polyps with cancer confined to the mucosa and with an uninvolved stalk can be cured by removal with an electrocautery snare during colonoscopy. Thus, most colonoscopists will remove all polyps more than 0.5 cm in diameter. It is more difficult to know what to do with polyps smaller than 0.5 cm in diameter because more than 50 percent may be adenomatous. A coagulating biopsy technique can be used to both biopsy and destroy even the smallest adenomatous polyp in the hope that the subsequent risk of developing colonic cancer will be reduced. The wisdom of this course of action is suggested by a sigmoidoscopic study in which the removal of all polyps reduced the expected incidence and invasiveness of subsequently developing cancers in the anatomic area screened. Most agree that the patient with adenomatous polyps is more likely to develop another polyp or cancer and therefore merits a regular screening program. The optimal frequency of follow-up examinations after polypectomy is not yet established. The current recommendation is a digital examination and stool test for occult blood yearly. When a polyp is discovered, the entire colon should be examined for synchronous polyps or cancer. This should probably be repeated at 1 year and, if negative, every 3 years thereafter. If stools are positive for occult blood or symptoms develop, immediate evaluation is indicated.

Cancer screening by x-ray All filling defects on barium enema merit evaluation by colonoscopy. If the lesion is a pedunculated polyp, it can be removed for histologic examination; if its appearance suggests a cancer, it can be biopsied and brushed for histologic and cytologic confirmation. When a polyp or a carcinoma is found, the remainder of the colon should be screened for additional polyps and synchronous carcinoma. This avoids multiple colotomies to search for a second lesion and reduces surgical morbidity. Approximately 40 percent of lesions diagnosed as a mass by x-ray are not present on colonoscopy or are found to be due to lesions such as a polyp rather than a cancer.

Narrowing by x-ray An etiologic diagnosis of segmental narrowing may be difficult by x-ray. Colonoscopy often determines the cause of segmental narrowing and differentiates adenocarcinoma from inflammation secondary to ischemia, irradiation, diverticular disease, or Crohn's colitis. Even the most classic "apple-core" lesion indicated by x-ray may be covered by normal mucosa at colonoscopy, suggesting an extrinsic inflammatory lesion. In 10 to 30 percent of patients, narrowed segments present on x-ray are not visualized during colonoscopy, probably because they are areas of temporary spasm. Such findings avoid unnecessary operations.

Chronic bleeding (x-ray and sigmoidoscopy negative) This condition leads to approximately 40 percent of colonoscopies. The x-ray is more likely to miss a lesion when single contrast is used rather than air contrast. The cause of bleeding is found in approximately 40 percent of such patients. The common bleeding sources are adenomatous polyp (20 percent), adenocarcinoma (10 percent), and Crohn's disease (7 percent). Many of these carcinomas are resectable, and this group may benefit most from colonoscopy. If no bleeding source is found, a search may be appropriate for an upper gastrointestinal source with an upper gastrointestinal x-ray and/or upper endoscopy.

Inflammatory bowel disease Colonoscopy is not routinely indicated in patients with inflammatory bowel disease. Colonoscopy may help in the initial diagnosis, especially in differentiating Crohn's colitis from ulcerative colitis. It can aid the surgeon in assessing the activity and extent of the disease before surgery. Colonoscopy can evaluate radiographic abnormalities suggesting cancer, such as strictures, polyps, or masses. Colonoscopy may be indicated in patients with ulcerative colitis of more than 10 years' duration because of the increased risk of carcinoma; it is hoped that repeated colonoscopies will serve to detect these malignancies earlier than x-ray and while the lesions are still curable. The frequency of colonoscopy and/or double-contrast barium enema examination in such patients is not yet established. If an expert gastrointestinal pathologist finds high-grade dysplasia in colonic biopsies in a patient with long-standing ulcerative colitis, most would consider this to be an indication for colectomy. Preparation for colonoscopy must often be modified for patients with inflammatory bowel disease. Colonoscopy is contraindicated in patients with toxic megacolon, very active disease, or a possible intestinal perforation.

Other indications The flexible sigmoidoscope is replacing the rigid 25-cm sigmoidoscope for routine screening because it can be passed to 40 to 60 cm with minimal preparation, less discomfort, and a higher diagnostic yield. After segmental colonic resection for carcinoma, colonoscopy may detect early mucosal recurrence and differentiate it from benign anastomotic strictures or bleeding suture granulomas. These patients must also be periodically screened for the development of polyps or additional carcinomas. Colonoscopy is occasionally used during laparotomy to assist the surgeon in ruling out other lesions. The colonoscope can be advanced to the cecum rapidly with the surgeon's assistance, and additional polyps removed without colotomy. Colonscopy is useful in the management of selected patients with lower gastrointestinal bleeding. Patients with severe active bleeding are best managed with radionuclide-labeled red blood cell scans followed immediately, if active bleeding is present, by selective angiography. Colonoscopic visualization in this setting is difficult because of excessive luminal blood. If the labeled red blood cell scan is negative, colonic lavage with a balanced electrolyte solution followed in several hours by colonoscopy may identify the bleeding site. Bleeding polyps may be removed by snare electrocautery. Endoscopic hemostatic therapy may be useful in other bleeding lesions such as angiodysplasia.

Colonoscopy detects some carriers of the dominant familial polyposis gene before diagnosis by barium enema and sigmoidoscopy. Carcinoma is a great threat in those familial polyposis syndromes which produce many adenomatous polyps (familial polyposis and Gardner's syndrome); in these conditions, polypectomy is useful for diagnosis, but colectomy is the only treatment which prevents development of carcinoma. These patients are also at risk of developing duodenal and periampullary cancer and should probably undergo periodic surveillance with a side-viewing duodenoscope.

CONTRAINDICATIONS All types of fiberoptic endoscopy are contraindicated in certain patients, including those who are uncooperative or combative or who have perforation of the intestine. Patients with acute medical illness such as myocardial infarction have increased risks at endoscopy. The relative benefits and risks of the procedure must be carefully weighed in these situations.

CONSCIOUS LAPAROSCOPY The potentials for laparoscopy in conscious patients have not been as fully appreciated in North America as they have been in other countries, where it has been used widely for over 20 years. This procedure has extremely low mortality and morbidity rates in experienced hands. The instrument usually used for laparoscopy is a stiff tube with a lens system that provides a superb view. Under local anesthesia pneumoperitoneum is gradually induced with air or nitrous oxide.

Much of the exterior of the liver, gallbladder, spleen, peritoneum, diaphragm, and pelvic organs can be clearly visualized. Portions of the colon and small bowel can also be seen. Lesions can be biopsied under direct vision and any resultant bleeding controlled by electrocoagulation. Furthermore, in centers with extensive experience contrast material can be injected into the liver to visualize vascular, lymphatic, and biliary systems.

Laparoscopy may permit one to make a difficult diagnosis without resorting to laparotomy by biopsying localized hepatic disease under direct vision. Laparoscopy can often help differentiate "medical" from "surgical" jaundice and may also enable staging of malignant disease without laparotomy.

REFERENCES

Cello JP et al: Endoscopic sclerotherapy versus portacaval shunt in patients with severe cirrhosis and acute variceal hemorrhage: Long-term follow-up. N Engl J Med 316:11, 1987

Cotton PB: Endoscopic management of bile duct stones (apples and oranges). Gut 25:587, 1984

Fleischer D: Endoscopic therapy of upper gastrointestinal bleeding in humans. Gastroenterology 90:217, 1986

Haggitt RC et al: Prognostic factors in colorectal carcinomas arising in adenomas: Implications for lesions removed by endoscopic polypectomy. Gastroenterology 89:328, 1985

Jensen DM, Machicado GA: Diagnosis and treatment of severe hematochezia: The role of urgent colonoscopy after purge. Gastroenterology 95:1569, 1988

Laine L: Multipolar electrocoagulation in the treatment of active upper gastrointestinal tract hemorrhage. N Engl J Med 316:1613, 1987

Silverstein FE, Tytgat GNJ: *Atlas of Gastrointestinal Endoscopy*. Philadelphia, Saunders, 1987

Sivak MV: *Gastroenterologic Endoscopy*. Philadelphia, Saunders, 1987

237 DISEASES OF THE ESOPHAGUS

RAJ K. GOYAL

The two major functions of the esophagus are the transport of the food bolus from the mouth to the stomach and the prevention of retrograde flow of gastrointestinal contents. The transport function is achieved by peristaltic contractions (see Chap. 42). Retrograde flow is prevented by the two esophageal sphincters, which remain closed between swallows. The upper esophageal sphincter remains closed by the elastic properties of its wall and by tonic contraction of the cricopharyngeus and inferior pharyngeal constrictor muscles due to continuous neural excitation of the lower motor neurons which innervate these muscles via motor end plates. The opening of the upper sphincter is due to inhibition of contraction of the cricopharyngeus and inferior pharyngeal constriction and forward displacement of the larynx by the suprahyoid muscles. In contrast, the lower esophageal sphincter remains closed because of its intrinsic myogenic tone, and a neural pathway, consisting of preganglionic parasympathetic fibers in the vagus nerve and postganglionic myenteric inhibitory neurons, causes its relaxation. A reflex increase in the lower sphincter pressure occurs with an increase in intraabdominal pressure and ingestion of a protein meal. Fatty meals, smoking, and beverages with a high xanthine content (tea, coffee, cola) cause a reduction in sphincter pressure. Many hormones and neurotransmitters can modify lower sphincter pressure. Cholinergic muscarinic (M-2 receptor) agonists, alpha-adrenergic agonists, gastrin, pancreatic polypeptide, substance P, and prostaglandin $F_{2\alpha}$ cause contraction; in contrast, ganglionic stimulants, beta-adrenergic agonists, dopamine, cholecystokinin, secretin, vasoactive intestinal peptide (VIP), calcitonin-gene-related peptide (CGRP), ATP, and adenosine cause relaxation of the sphincter. These effects are mediated by actions on the inhibitory intramural neurons or on the sphincter muscle directly. Effects of many of these agents are pharmacologic rather than physiologic.

SYMPTOMS

DYSPHAGIA See Chap. 42.

ESOPHAGEAL PAIN *Heartburn*, or pyrosis, is characterized by burning retrosternal discomfort that may move up and down the chest like a wave. When severe, it may radiate to the sides of the chest, neck, and angles of the jaw. Heartburn is a characteristic symptom of reflux esophagitis and may be associated with regurgitation or a feeling of warm fluid climbing up the throat. It is aggravated by bending forward, straining, or lying recumbent and is worse after meals. It is relieved by upright posture, by swallowing of saliva or water, or, more reliably, by antacids. Heartburn appears to be produced by heightened mucosal sensitivity and can be reproduced by infusion of dilute (0.1 *N*) hydrochloric acid (Bernstein test) or neutral hyperosmolar solutions into the esophagus.

Odynophagia, or painful swallowing, is characteristic of nonreflux esophagitis, particularly monilial and herpes esophagitis. Odynophagia may also occur with peptic ulcer of the esophagus (Barrett's ulcer), carcinoma with periesophageal involvement, caustic damage of the esophagus, and esophageal perforation. Odynophagia is unusual in uncomplicated reflux esophagitis. Crampy chest pain associated with impaction of the small bowel should be distinguished from odynophagia.

Chest pain other than heartburn and odynophagia occurs when the esophageal muscle contracts with excessive force, for a long duration, and repetitively, as in diffuse esophageal spasm. This may occur spontaneously or during a meal. Chest pain due to periesophageal involvement caused by carcinoma or peptic ulcer may be constant and agonizing. Sometimes different types of esophageal pains exist together in the same patient, and frequently patients are not able to describe the pain accurately enough to allow its classification.

REGURGITATION Regurgitation is the effortless appearance of gastric or esophageal contents in the mouth. In distal esophageal obstruction and stasis, as in achalasia or a large diverticulum, the regurgitated material consists of tasteless mucoid fluid or undigested food. Regurgitation of sour or bitter-tasting material occurs in severe gastroesophageal reflux and is associated with incompetence of both the upper and lower esophageal sphincters. Regurgitation may result in laryngeal aspiration, with spells of coughing and choking that awaken the patient from sleep, and aspiration pneumonia. Water brash is reflex salivary hypersecretion which occurs in response to peptic esophagitis; it should not be confused with regurgitation.

DIAGNOSTIC TESTS

RADIOLOGIC STUDIES Barium swallow with fluoroscopy and esophagogram is the most widely used test for diagnosis of esophageal

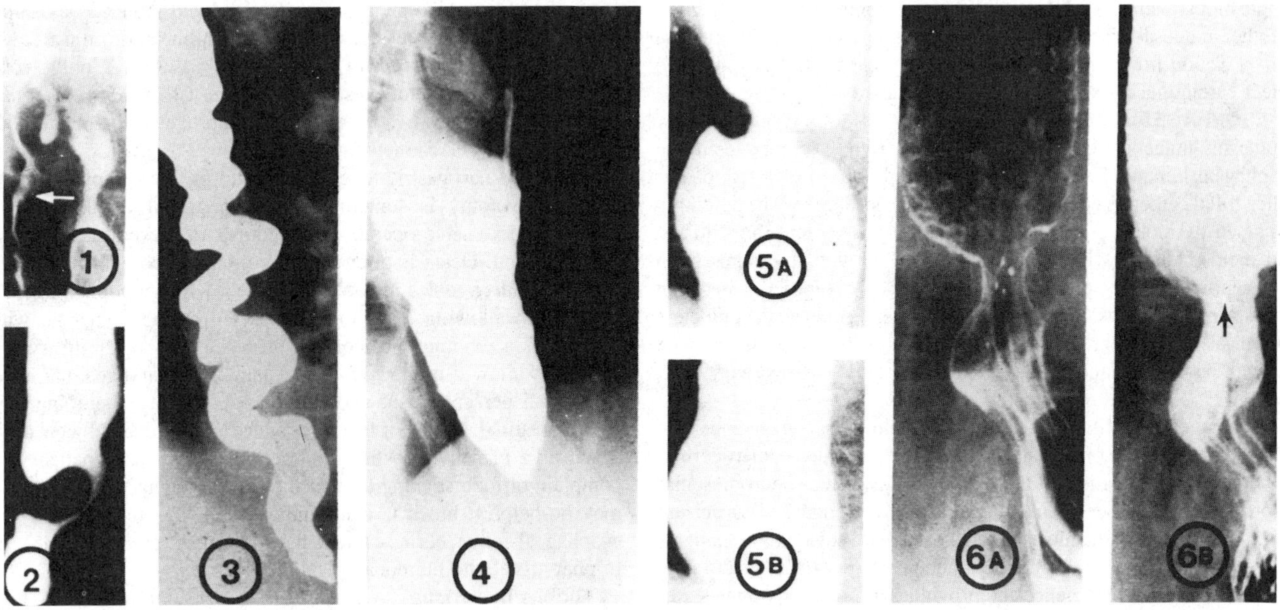

FIGURE 237-1 Radiographic appearance of some motor disorders of the pharynx and esophagus. (1) Pharyngeal paralysis with tracheal aspiration (arrow). (2) Cricopharyngeal achalasia. Note the prominent cricopharyngeus, which is recognized by its smoothness and location in the posterior wall. (3) Diffuse esophageal spasm. Note typical corkscrew appearance of the lower part of the esophagus. (4) Achalasia showing dilation of esophageal body with air-fluid level and closed lower esophageal sphincter. (5) Muscular (contractile) lower esophageal ring. Note a symmetric contraction in *5A* that has disappeared in *5B*, obtained during the same examination. (6) Scleroderma esophagus showing dilated esophagus with a stricture in *6A* and reflux of barium from the stomach into the esophagus in *6B*. *(Courtesy of Dr. Harvey Goldstein.)*

disease and can be used to evaluate both structural and motor disorders. The pharynx is examined to detect stasis of barium in the valleculae and pyriform sinuses and regurgitation of barium into the nose and tracheobronchial tree. Since the pharyngeal phase of swallowing lasts no more than a second, cineradiography may be necessary to permit detection and analysis of abnormalities of pharyngeal function. Spontaneous reflux of barium from the stomach into the esophagus should be sought in patients with suspected reflux esophagitis. Esophageal peristalsis is best studied in the recumbent position since in the upright position the passage of most of the barium occurs by gravity alone. A double-contrast esophagogram, obtained by coating the esophageal mucosa with barium and distending the esophageal lumen with air using effervescent granules, is particularly useful in demonstrating mucosal ulcers and early cancers. Figures 237-1 and 237-2 illustrate the radiographic appearance of some esophageal disorders.

ESOPHAGOSCOPY Fiberoptic esophagogastroduodenoscopy is described in Chap. 236. Esophagoscopy is the direct method of establishing the cause of mechanical dysphagia and of identifying mucosal lesions, such as superficial ulcers and esophagitis, which may not be identified by the usual barium swallow. In the presence of marked luminal narrowing, examination can be achieved by using a smaller caliber endoscope, although on occasion a stricture must be dilated prior to a complete endoscopic examination. Transendo-

FIGURE 237-2 Selected structural lesions of the esophagus. (1) Carcinoma of the esophagus with typical annular narrowing with overhanging margins and destruction of the mucosa. (2) Leiomyoma of the esophagus with smooth filling defect and right angles of origin from the esophageal wall. (3) Esophageal ulcer in columnar-cell-lined esophagus (Barrett's esophagus). (4) Monilial esophagitis with irregular plaquelike filling defects. (5) Long stricture secondary to lye ingestion. (6) Peptic stricture, short and tubular, with associated hiatus hernia. (7) Mucosal lower esophageal mucosal (Schatzki) ring. Thin weblike annular constriction at the esophagogastric junction is associated with a small hiatal hernia. *(Courtesy of Dr. Harvey Goldstein.)*

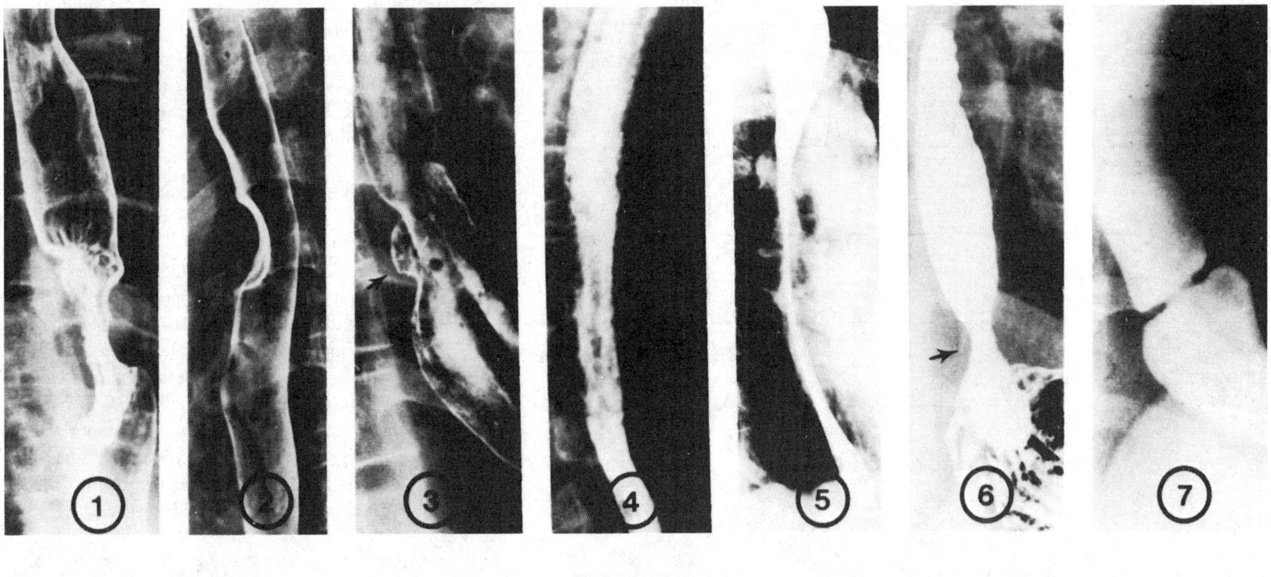

scopic biopsies are useful in diagnosing carcinoma, reflux esophagitis, or other mucosal diseases. Obtaining cells by scraping the mucosa with a Teflon brush during endoscopy may enable the cytologist to detect carcinoma missed by mucosal biopsies.

ESOPHAGEAL MOTILITY The study of esophageal motility entails simultaneous recording of pressures from different sites in the esophageal lumen. This is usually done with a train of three to four water-filled catheters connected to pressure transducers. The assembly is passed by mouth or nose through the esophagus into the stomach and then gradually withdrawn 1 cm at a time until pressures from each centimeter of the esophagus and pharynx are recorded in between and during swallows. The upper and lower esophageal sphincters appear as zones of high pressure that relax on swallowing. The pharynx and esophageal body show peristaltic waves with each swallow.

Esophageal motility studies are very helpful in the diagnosis of achalasia, diffuse esophageal spasm and its variants, scleroderma, and other motor disorders of the esophagus, as well as neuromuscular disorders of the upper esophagus and pharynx (Fig. 237-3) but are of no value in the diagnosis of mechanical dysphagia. In patients with reflux esophagitis, esophageal manometry is useful in quantitating lower esophageal competence and providing information on the status of the esophageal body motor activity. The information obtained by manometry is quantitative and cannot be obtained by barium swallow or endoscopy.

Special tests for the evaluation of reflux esophagitis are described later.

MOTOR DISORDERS

STRIATED MUSCLE Pharyngeal paralysis Pharyngeal paralysis is characterized by dysphagia, nasal regurgitation, and tracheobronchial aspiration during swallowing. It occurs in a variety of neuromuscular disorders (see Table 42-2). Some of these disorders may also involve laryngeal and orofacial muscles. When the suprahyoid muscles are also paralyzed, the upper sphincter does not open with swallowing, leading to paralytic achalasia of the upper esophageal sphincter and severe dysphagia.

Barium swallow, oropharyngography, and cineradiography reveal stasis of barium in the valleculae and pyriform sinuses, nasal and tracheobronchial aspiration, and closed upper sphincter (Fig. 237-1). Pharyngeal motility studies demonstrate reduced amplitude of pharyngeal and upper esophageal contractions and reduced basal upper esophageal sphincter pressure without further relaxation on swallowing (Fig. 237-3). Patients with myasthenia gravis and polymyositis respond to treatment for these diseases (see Chap. 366). Dysphagia in patients with cerebrovascular accident improves with time, although not completely. Treatment in most instances is mainly supportive, consisting of nasogastric tube feeding and physiotherapy. Cricopharyngeal myotomy is sometimes performed, but its usefulness is unproved. Extensive operative procedures to prevent aspiration are rarely needed. Death is often due to pulmonary complications.

Cricopharyngeal achalasia Failure of the cricopharyngeus to relax on swallowing leads to a contracted cricopharyngeus, which appears as a prominent bar on the posterior wall of the pharynx on barium swallow (Fig. 237-1). A transient cricopharyngeal bar is seen in up to 5 percent of subjects without dysphagia undergoing upper gastrointestinal studies; it can be produced in normal subjects during a Valsalva maneuver. When contraction is persistent, patients may complain of food sticking in their throats. Cricopharyngeal myotomy may be helpful, but it is contraindicated in the presence of gastroesophageal reflux because in such patients this procedure may lead to pharyngeal and pulmonary aspiration.

Globus hystericus A sensation of a constant lump in the throat but with no difficulty during swallowing occurs especially in subjects with emotional disorders, particularly in women. Barium studies are normal, but manometry shows a hypertensive upper sphincter. Treatment is primarily one of reassurance.

SMOOTH MUSCLE Achalasia Achalasia is a motor disorder of the esophageal smooth muscle in which the lower esophageal sphincter is hypertensive, does not relax properly with swallowing, and the normal peristalsis of the esophageal body is replaced by abnormal contractions. Based upon the changes in the esophageal body, achalasia can be of two types: in *classic achalasia* simultaneous contractions of small amplitude occur, while in *vigorous achalasia* contractions are simultaneous in onset, large in amplitude, and repetitive, resembling those seen in diffuse esophageal spasm.

PATHOPHYSIOLOGY The underlying abnormality is defective innervation of the smooth-muscle portion of the esophageal body and the lower esophageal sphincter. Pathologically, vigorous achalasia is associated with less severe neural damage than classic achalasia, which shows a marked reduction in myenteric neurons. Primary idiopathic achalasia accounts for most of the patients seen in the United States. Secondary achalasia may be caused by gastric carcinoma infiltrating the esophagus, lymphoma, Chagas' disease, neu-

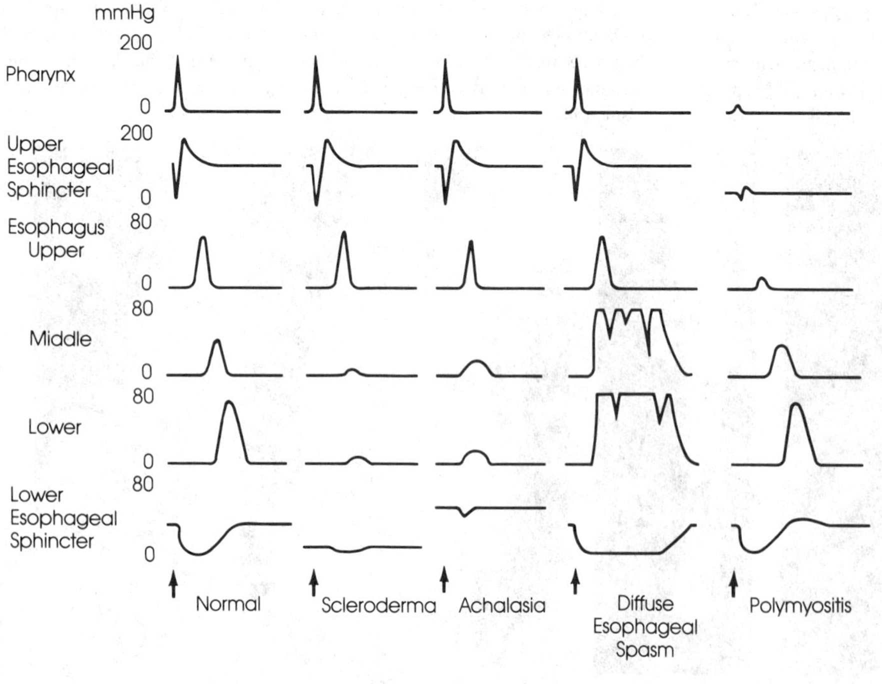

FIGURE 237-3 Motility patterns in selected esophageal and pharyngeal disorders. In normal subjects, the upper and lower esophageal sphincters appear as zones of high pressure. With a swallow (indicated by ↑), pressure in the sphincters falls and a contraction wave starts in the pharynx and progresses down the esophagus. In scleroderma, the lower part of the esophagus (smooth muscle) shows reduced amplitude of contractions, which may be peristaltic or simultaneous in onset, and hypotension of the lower sphincter. In achalasia, the lower part of the esophagus shows reduced amplitude of contractions that are simultaneous in onset. In contrast to scleroderma, the lower esophageal sphincter in achalasia is hypertensive and fails to relax in response to a swallow. In diffuse esophageal spasm, the lower part of the esophagus shows simultaneous onset, large amplitude, long duration, repetitive contractions. In polymyositis, the smooth-muscle part of the esophagus is normal. The skeletal muscle part shows reduced amplitude of contractions. The upper esophageal sphincter is hypotensive and may not relax normally on swallowing due to associated weakness of the suprahyoid muscles.

ropathic chronic intestinal pseudoobstruction syndrome, irradiation, and certain toxins and drugs. Hypertensive or hypercontracting lower esophageal sphincter may be considered as variants of achalasia.

CLINICAL FEATURES Achalasia affects patients of all ages and both sexes. Dysphagia, chest pain, and regurgitation are the main symptoms. Dysphagia occurs early with both liquids and solids and is worsened by emotional stress and hurried eating. Various maneuvers designed to increase intraesophageal pressure, including the Valsalva, may help passage of the bolus into the stomach. Chest pain is more pronounced in vigorous achalasia than in classic achalasia. Regurgitation and pulmonary aspiration occur because of retention of large volumes of saliva and ingested food in the esophagus. The presence of gastroesophageal reflux argues against achalasia, although some of these patients may describe their chest pain as heartburn. The overall course is usually chronic with progressive dysphagia and weight loss over months to years.

DIAGNOSIS Chest x-ray shows absence of the gastric air bubble and sometimes a tubular mediastinal mass beside the aorta. The presence of an air-fluid level in the mediastinum in the upright position represents unpassed food in the esophagus and is characteristic. Barium swallow shows esophageal dilatation, and in advanced cases the esophagus may become sigmoid. On fluoroscopy normal peristalsis is lost in the lower two-thirds of the esophagus. The terminal part of the esophagus shows a persistent beaklike narrowing representing the nonrelaxing lower esophageal sphincter [Fig. 237-1(*2*)]. In patients with vigorous achalasia, there may be pronounced nonperistaltic contractions without a dilated esophagus.

Manometry shows normal or elevated basal lower esophageal sphincter pressure and swallow-induced relaxation which is absent or reduced in degree, duration, and consistency (Fig. 237-3). The esophageal body shows elevated resting pressure. In response to swallows, primary peristaltic waves are replaced by simultaneous-onset contractions. These contractions may be of poor amplitude (classic achalasia) or of large amplitude and long duration (vigorous achalasia). Administration of the cholinergic muscarinic agonist mecholyl causes a marked increase in baseline esophageal pressure, and administration of cholecystokinin (CCK), which normally causes a fall in the sphincter pressure, paradoxically causes contraction of the lower esophageal sphincter. Endoscopy is helpful in excluding the secondary causes of achalasia, particularly gastric carcinoma.

TREATMENT Medical treatment using soft foods, sedatives, nitrates, and anticholinergic drugs is usually unsatisfactory. Calcium channel antagonists such as nifedipine have been used with some success. The best available therapy involves balloon dilation to reduce the basal lower esophageal sphincter pressure by tearing muscle fibers. In experienced hands this technique is effective in about 85 percent of patients. Perforation and bleeding are potential complications. Heller's extramucosal myotomy of the lower sphincter, in which the circular muscle layer is incised, is equally effective. Reflux esophagitis and peptic stricture may follow successful treatment of achalasia. However, this complication is more frequent with myotomy than with balloon dilation.

Diffuse esophageal spasm and related motor disorders Diffuse esophageal spasm is a motor disorder of the esophageal smooth muscle characterized by multiple spontaneous contractions and by swallow-induced contractions that are of simultaneous onset, large amplitude, long duration, and repetitive occurrence. Variants of diffuse esophageal spasm show some but not all of these motor abnormalities.

PATHOPHYSIOLOGY The pathogenesis of the various abnormalities of peristalsis in diffuse esophageal spasm is not known. Histopathologic studies show patchy neural degeneration localized to nerve processes rather than the prominent degeneration of nerve cell bodies seen in achalasia.

Variants of diffuse esophageal spasm, such as large amplitude but peristaltic contractions (sometimes called nutcracker esophagus) or normal amplitude but simultaneous contractions, frequently occur as a primary disease or in association with a variety of diseases as well as emotional stress and aging. Collagen vascular disease, diabetic neuropathy, reflux esophagitis, irradiation esophagitis, esophageal obstruction, and cholinergic and anticholinergic drugs can cause esophageal motor abnormalities. The relationship between reflux esophagitis and motor abnormalities is controversial. Overlapping features of diffuse esophageal spasm and achalasia occur in vigorous achalasia. The variant syndromes are more frequent in clinical practice than classic diffuse esophageal spasm.

CLINICAL FEATURES The symptomatic patient with diffuse spasm or its variants presents with chest pain, dysphagia, or both. Chest pain is particularly marked in patients with esophageal contractions of large amplitude and of long duration. Chest pain usually occurs at rest but may be brought on by swallowing or by emotional stress. The pain is retrosternal; it may radiate to the back, sides of the chest, both arms, or the sides of the jaw and may last for a few seconds to several minutes. It may be acute and severe, mimicking the pain of myocardial ischemia. Dysphagia for solids and liquids may occur with or without chest pain.

Diffuse esophageal spasm must be differentiated from other causes of chest pain, particularly ischemic heart disease with atypical angina. Often a complete cardiac workup is done before the esophageal etiology is seriously considered. The presence of dysphagia in association with pain should point to the esophagus as the site of disease. Symptoms of esophageal spasm should be carefully distinguished from those of reflux esophagitis; sometimes the two may coexist.

DIAGNOSIS Barium swallow shows that normal sequential peristalsis below the aortic arch is replaced by uncoordinated simultaneous contractions that produce the appearance of curling or multiple ripples in the wall, sacculations, and pseudodiverticula—the "corkscrew" esophagus [Fig. 237-1(*3*)]. Sometimes an esophageal contraction obliterates the lumen and barium is pushed away in both directions. The lower esophageal sphincter opens normally.

Manometry reveals the characteristic prolonged large amplitude and repetitive contractions of simultaneous onset in the lower part of the esophagus (Fig. 237-3). Only one or two of these abnormalities may be present in variants of diffuse spasm. Because the abnormalities may be episodic, manometry may be normal at the time of the study; therefore, several techniques are used in attempts to provoke esophageal spasm. Cold swallows produce chest pain but do not produce spasm on manometric studies. Solid boluses and pharmacologic agents, particularly edrophonium, induce both chest pain and motor abnormalities. However, there is a poor correlation between induction of pain and motility changes. Ergonovine may cause coronary artery spasm and should not be used. Overall, the usefulness of pharmacologic provocative tests is limited.

TREATMENT Anticholinergics are usually of limited value because the main nerves that mediate esophageal contractions are noncholinergic. Agents that relax smooth muscle such as sublingual nitroglycerin (0.3 to 0.6 mg) or longer acting agents such as isosorbide dinitrate (2.5 to 10 mg sublingually before meals) and nifedipine (10 to 20 mg before meals) may be helpful in some cases. Esophageal dilation with mercury-filled rubber dilators may produce symptomatic relief as a result of distention of the lower esophagus, but this is largely a placebo effect. Reassurance and tranquilizers are helpful in allaying patients' apprehension. Balloon dilation is sometimes attempted but can be hazardous in inexperienced hands. In severe cases resistant to all therapy, a longitudinal myotomy of esophageal circular muscle is performed; it relieves pain in up to two-thirds of patients.

Scleroderma involving the esophagus The esophageal lesions in systemic sclerosis consist of muscular atrophy of the smooth-muscle portion, with weakness of contraction in the lower two-thirds of the esophageal body and incompetence of the lower esophageal sphincter. The esophageal wall is thin and atrophic with or without areas of patchy fibrosis. Patients present with dysphagia to solids and to liquids in the recumbent position. They may also present with heartburn and regurgitation due to gastroesophageal reflux and esophagitis, which in turn may lead to stricture formation and more pronounced dysphagia. Barium swallow shows dilation and loss of peristaltic contractions in the middle and distal portions of the esophagus. The lower esophageal sphincter is patulous, and gastroesophageal reflux may occur freely (Fig. 237-1). Mucosal changes from esophageal ulceration may be detected, and esophageal stricture may be present. Motility studies show marked reduction in the amplitude of smooth-muscle contractions, which may be peristaltic or nonperistaltic. Lower esophageal sphincter resting pressure is subnormal, but relaxation is normal (Fig. 237-3). Currently, there is no effective treatment for the motor difficulty. Reflux esophagitis and its complications should be treated aggressively as described under reflux esophagitis.

INFLAMMATORY DISORDERS

GASTROESOPHAGEAL REFLUX AND ESOPHAGITIS Reflux esophagitis consists of esophageal mucosal damage resulting from reflux of gastric or intestinal contents into the esophagus. Depending on the causative agent, it is referred to as peptic, bile, or alkaline esophagitis.

Pathophysiology Three considerations involved in the pathophysiology of reflux esophagitis are (1) the pathogenesis of the esophageal reflux episode, (2) the cumulative, or net, esophageal reflux, and (3) the pathogenesis of esophagitis.

Two conditions must be met for a *reflux episode* to occur: the gastrointestinal contents must be "ready" to reflux, and the antireflux mechanism at the lower end of the esophagus must be compromised. Gastrointestinal contents are most likely to reflux (1) when gastric volume is increased (after meals, with pyloric obstruction or gastric stasis syndrome, and in acid hypersecretory states), (2) when the gastric contents are located near the gastroesophageal junction (due to recumbency or bending), and (3) when gastric pressure is increased (with obesity, pregnancy, ascites, or tight binders or girdles).

The normal antireflux mechanisms consist of the lower esophageal sphincter (LES) and the anatomic configuration of the gastroesophageal junction. Reflux occurs only when the LES–gastric pressure gradient is lost. It can be caused by increased intragastric pressure or a transient or sustained decrease in the sphincter tone itself. Most patients with reflux have lower than normal LES pressures. The incompetence of the LES may be primary or secondary. The secondary causes include scleroderma-like diseases, a myopathic type of chronic intestinal pseudoobstruction syndrome, pregnancy, female sex hormones, smoking, smooth-muscle relaxants (such as beta-adrenergics, aminophylline, nitrates, and calcium channel blockers), destruction of the sphincter by surgical resection, myotomy or balloon dilation, and esophagitis. Some patients have normal lower esophageal sphincter pressures but their sphincter relaxes inappropriately, allowing reflux to occur. The importance of the anatomic configuration of the esophagogastric junction is not fully known at present. However, the role of a sliding hiatal hernia in the impairment of the reflux barrier is not felt to be so important as was once thought.

The net or *cumulative esophageal reflux,* i.e., the amount and duration of refluxed material remaining in the esophagus, is dependent on (1) the amount of refluxed material per episode and frequency of episodes, (2) the clearing of the esophagus by gravity and peristaltic contraction, and (3) neutralization by salivary secretion.

Esophagitis is a complication of reflux, and it develops when the mucosal defenses that normally counteract the effect of injurious agents on the esophageal mucosa succumb to the onslaught of the refluxed acid pepsin or bile. *Mild esophagitis* shows microscopic changes of mucosal infiltration with granulocytes or eosinophils, hyperplasia of basal cells, and elongation of dermal pegs. It can occur with or without endoscopic abnormalities. *Erosive esophagitis* shows endoscopically visible damage to the mucosa in the form of marked redness, friability, bleeding, superficial linear ulcers, and exudates. *Peptic stricture* results from fibrosis that causes constriction of the esophageal lumen. The fibrosis is predominantly submucosal, but it may involve the whole wall. Peptic strictures occur in about 10 percent of patients with reflux esophagitis. Short peptic strictures caused by spontaneous reflux are usually 1 to 3 cm long and are present in the distal esophagus near the squamocolumnar junction (Fig. 237-2). Long and tubular peptic strictures are the result of persistent vomiting or prolonged nasogastric intubation. Replacement of the squamous epithelium of the esophagus by columnar epithelium *(Barrett's esophagus)* may also result from reflux esophagitis. Columnar-cell-lined esophagus may be further complicated by peptic ulcer or peptic stricture high up in the lower or midesophagus, and adenocarcinoma in 2 to 5 percent.

Clinical features Heartburn is the characteristic symptom and is produced by the contact of refluxed material with the inflamed esophageal mucosa. Angina-like or atypical chest pain may occur in some patients, while others may experience no heartburn or chest pain. Dysphagia suggests development of peptic stricture. In peptic strictures, the usual history is of several years of heartburn preceding dysphagia. However, in one-third of patients dysphagia may be the presenting symptom. Progressive dysphagia and weight loss may indicate development of adenocarcinoma in Barrett's esophagus. Bleeding occurs due to mucosal erosions or Barrett's ulcer. Reflux in the absence of esophagitis is usually asymptomatic. Severe reflux may reach the pharynx and mouth and result in laryngitis, morning hoarseness, and pulmonary aspiration. Recurrent pulmonary aspiration can cause aspiration pneumonia, pulmonary fibrosis, or chronic asthma.

Diagnosis Evaluation of reflux esophagitis is designed to assess the presence and severity of reflux, nature of refluxant, presence and severity of esophagitis, and pathophysiology of reflux. History, barium swallow, esophagoscopy, mucosal biopsy, esophageal motility, and a variety of special tests are utilized.

The *presence of reflux* is suggested by history. Spontaneous reflux from the stomach into the esophagus on barium examination suggests advanced reflux. Reflux of barium induced by stressful maneuvers is not very helpful, however, because of a high incidence of false-positive and false-negative results. Recently, scintiscan using ^{99m}Tc-sulfur colloid has been used to quantitate gastroesophageal reflux. Several tests that utilize the recording of esophageal luminal pH with a small pH electrode have been proposed to detect and quantitate reflux of gastric acid. In these tests the pH electrode is swallowed, positioned in the stomach, gradually withdrawn across the LES, and then fixed at 5 cm above the sphincter. In the standard acid reflux test, a diagnosis of reflux can be made by failure of the pH to rise as the electrode enters the esophagus and by a decrease in esophageal pH with straining maneuvers. Quantitative information on the acid reflux is obtained by long-term (24-h) esophageal pH recording. The pH recordings are helpful only in the evaluation of acid reflux. The presence of bile or alkaline reflux is suggested by the occurrence of reflux symptoms in the absence of gastric acid and by the demonstration of bile in the aspirate of esophageal reflux.

The *presence and complications of reflux esophagitis* are assessed by barium swallow, esophagoscopy, mucosal biopsy, and the Bernstein test. Barium swallow is usually normal in uncomplicated esophagitis but may reveal the complication of stricture or ulcer formation. A high esophageal peptic stricture, deep ulcer, and adenocarcinoma suggest complications of Barrett's esophagus. Uncomplicated Barrett's esophagus is not diagnosed by barium studies. Esophagoscopy may reveal the presence of erosive esophagitis, distal peptic stricture, or columnar-cell-lined lower esophagus with or without a proximally located peptic stricture, ulcer, or adenocarcinoma. Esophagoscopy may be normal in many patients with esophagitis; in such patients mucosal biopsies and Bernstein tests are helpful. The mucosal biopsies should be obtained 5 cm above the LES because in the distal esophagus mucosal changes are quite frequent in normal subjects. False-positive and false-negative results occur in approximately 10 percent of biopsies. Patients with Barrett's esophagus will show columnar mucosa lining the esophagus which may be of gastric fundic, cardiac, or specialized type. The Bernstein test consists of an infusion of solutions of 0.1 *N* HCl and normal saline into the esophagus. It is useful in diagnosing reflux esophagitis which is not endoscopically obvious. In patients with reflux esophagitis, infusion of acid, but not of saline, reproduces the symptoms of heartburn. Infusion of acid in normal subjects produces no symptoms. Reflux esophagitis should be included in the differential diagnosis of chest pain, esophagitis, upper gastrointestinal bleeding, and dysphagia.

The *causative and predisposing factors* are assessed by history, esophageal motility, and esophageal clearance studies. Esophageal motility studies may provide useful quantitative information on the competence of the LES and of esophageal motor function. Barium swallow and scintiscans can be used to study esophageal clearance. An esophageal acid clearance test using a pH electrode quantifies the number of swallows necessary to clear the esophagus of 10 mL of instilled dilute 0.1 *N* HCl.

Full diagnostic evaluation is not necessary in every patient with reflux esophagitis. In transient and mild cases with a clear-cut history of reflux esophagitis, a therapeutic trial may be sufficient. In persistent cases, and when the diagnosis is not clear, barium swallow, esophagoscopy, and esophageal motility with pH monitoring are indicated.

Patients with angina-like chest pain in whom coronary artery disease has been excluded may be investigated by 24-h ambulatory esophageal pH and motility recording. Most of these patients are found to have reflux esophagitis, while a few have esophageal motor disorders. It should also be remembered that reflux esophagitis may frequently coexist with coronary artery disease.

Treatment The goals of treatment are to decrease gastroesophageal reflux, neutralize refluxate, improve esophageal clearance, and protect the esophageal mucosa. These goals can be achieved by certain general measures and specific drug treatments. The management of uncomplicated cases generally includes weight reduction, sleeping with elevation of the head of the bed, and elimination of factors that increase abdominal pressure. Patients should avoid smoking, fatty foods, coffee, chocolate, alcohol, mint, orange juice, ingestion of large quantities of fluids with meals, and certain medications (such as anticholinergic drugs, calcium channel blockers, and other smooth-muscle relaxants). Antacids (40 to 80 meq, 1 and 3 h after meals) or H-2-blocking agents (cimetidine 300 mg, ranitidine 150 mg, or famotidine 20 mg at bedtime) to neutralize acidity are usually successful.

In moderate to severe cases, the above measures are more strictly enforced. H-2 blockers are used in higher doses (cimetidine, 300 mg qid; ranitidine, 150 mg tid; famotidine, 20 mg tid). A protective agent such as sucralfate (1-g chewable tablet, 1 h before meals) is useful in many cases. If the patient does not respond fully, a prokinetic agent such as metoclopramide, 10 mg qid, domperidone, or cisapride is prescribed to raise sphincter pressure, hasten gastric emptying, and improve esophageal clearance. (Domperidone and cisapride have not yet been approved for use in the United States.) Inhibition of H^+,K^+-ATPase, the pump that is responsible for acid secretion, with omeprazole (currently undergoing clinical trials in the United States) may be very effective in resistant cases. Reflux esophagitis requires prolonged therapy for 3 to 6 months or longer if the disease recurs quickly. Patients with reflux esophagitis with complications such as Barrett's esophagus (with or without a deep ulcer) should be treated vigorously. Patients who have an associated peptic stricture are treated with dilators to relieve dysphagia in addition to vigorous treatment for reflux. Close follow-up with periodic endoscopic biopsies is indicated in patients with Barrett's esophagus to detect and treat high-grade dysplasia and early adenocarcinoma.

Antireflux surgery (Belsey repair, Nissen's fundoplication, and Hill repair), in which the gastric fundus is wrapped around the esophagus, increases the lower sphincter pressure and should be considered in resistant and complicated cases of reflux esophagitis that do not fully respond to medical therapy and when there is persistently inadequate lower sphincter pressure but normal peristaltic contractions in the esophageal body.

Patients with alkaline esophagitis are treated with general measures and neutralization of bile salts with cholestyramine, aluminum hydroxide, or sucralfate. Sucralfate is particularly useful in these cases, as it also serves as a surface protector.

INFECTIOUS ESOPHAGITIS With the recent increase in immunodeficiency states, infectious esophagitis has become increasingly important. Infectious esophagitis can be due to viral, bacterial, fungal, or parasitic organisms. In severely immunocompromised patients, multiple organisms may coexist.

Viral esophagitis (See also Chap. 135) *Herpes simplex virus* (HSV) type I may occasionally cause esophagitis in the immunocompetent person, but either type I or II may afflict patients who are immunosuppressed. These patients complain of the acute onset of chest pain, odynophagia, and dysphagia. Bleeding may occur in severe cases, and systemic manifestations such as nausea, vomiting, fever, chills, and mild leukocytosis may be present. The persistent infection may lead to superinfection of denuded esophageal mucosa with fungi or bacteria, and HSV pneumonia. Herpes blisters on the nose and lips provide a clue to the diagnosis. Barium swallow is inadequate to detect early lesions and cannot reliably distinguish HSV from other types of infections. Endoscopy shows vesicles and small, discrete, punched-out superficial ulcerations with or without fibrinous exudate. In later stages there is diffuse erosive esophagitis caused by enlargement and coalescence of the ulcers. Mucosal cells from biopsy of the edge of an ulcer or cytological smear show ballooning degeneration, ground glass change in the nuclei with eosinophilic intranuclear inclusions (Cowdry type A), and giant cell formation on routine stains. Culture becomes positive within days and is helpful in diagnosis. For prophylaxis in a severely immunocompromised host, acyclovir, 800 mg orally twice daily or 250 mg/m^2 body surface area every 12 h intravenously, is recommended. For treatment of esophagitis, intravenous therapy, 250 mg/m^2 every 8 h is usually initiated. As swallowing improves, the therapy is changed to 200 to 400 mg orally five times daily. Symptoms usually resolve in 1 week, but large ulcerations may take longer to heal. These patients may also have reflux esophagitis which may worsen the symptoms and add to complications.

Varicella-zoster virus (VZV) rarely produces esophagitis in children with chickenpox and adults with herpes zoster. Esophageal VZV can also be the source of disseminated VZV infection in the absence of skin involvement. In an immunocompromised host, VZV esophagitis causes vesicles and confluent ulcers and usually resolves spontaneously, but it may cause necrotizing esophagitis in a severely compromised host. On routine histology of mucosal biopsies or cytology specimens, VZV is difficult to distinguish from HSV, but the distinction can be made immunohistologically or on culture. Acyclovir is effective in prevention and treatment of esophagitis, but much higher doses are needed than those for HSV.

Cytomegalovirus (CMV) infections occur only in the immunocompromised patient. CMV is usually activated from a latent stage or may be acquired from blood product transfusions. CMV lesions initially appear as serpiginous ulcers in an otherwise normal mucosa. These may coalesce to form giant ulcers, particularly in the distal esophagus. The virus involves submucosal fibroblasts and endothelial cells of the blood vessels but not the epithelial cells.

Patients present with painful swallowing, chest pain, hematemesis, nausea, and vomiting. Barium swallow may show nonspecific abnormalities or large esophageal ulcers. Diagnosis requires endoscopy and biopsies of the center of the ulcer. Mucosal brushings are not useful. Routine histology shows intranuclear and small intracytoplasmic inclusions in large fibroblasts and endothelial cells of blood vessels. Immunohistology with monoclonal antibodies to CMV and in situ hybridization of CMV DNA can be performed on centrifugation culture and are useful for early diagnosis. Ganciclovir (DHPG) 5 mg/kg every 12 h intravenously and, more recently, Foscarnet are investigational drugs which are active against CMV. Therapy is continued until healing, which may take weeks to months.

Human immunodeficiency virus (HIV) may be associated with a self-limited syndrome of acute esophageal ulceration associated with oral ulcers and a maculopapular skin rash. This syndrome occurs in homosexual men coincident with both HIV seroconversion and the inversion of the T-lymphocyte helper/suppressor ratio. Electron microscopy of affected tissue reveals retrovirus-like particles that are different from CMV or HSV.

Bacterial esophagitis *Bacterial esophagitis* is unusual, but esophagitis caused by *Lactobacillus* and beta-hemolytic streptococci has been described in the immunocompromised host. In profoundly granulocytopenic patients and in patients with cancer, bacterial esophagitis is often missed because it is commonly present with other organisms including viruses and fungi, and because bacteria are difficult to identify on routine histology. In patients with AIDS, infection with *Cryptosporidium* and *Pneumocystis carinii* may cause nonspecific inflammation of the distal esophagus.

Candida esophagitis Many *Candida* species are normal in the throat but become pathogenic and produce esophagitis in immunodeficiency states. These include HIV; malignant neoplasms (particularly lymphoma and leukemia); treatment with immunosuppressive agents, glucocorticoids, and broad-spectrum antibiotics; diabetes mellitus; hypoparathyroidism; systemic lupus erythematosus; hemoglobinopathy; corrosive esophageal injury; and esophageal stasis. Occasionally, monilial esophagitis occurs in the absence of any of the above predisposing factors. Patients may be asymptomatic or complain of odynophagia and dysphagia. Oral thrush or other evidence of mucocutaneous candidiasis may be absent. Rarely, *Candida* esophagitis may be complicated by esophageal bleeding, perforation, and stricture or by systemic invasion. Barium swallow may be normal or may show multiple nodular filling defects of various sizes (Fig. 237-2). Large nodular defects may resemble clusters of grapes. Endoscopy shows small yellow-white raised plaques with surrounding erythema in mild disease. In extensive disease, confluent linear and nodular plaques are seen. Diagnosis is made by demonstration of yeast or hyphae forms in the smear of plaques and exudate stained with Gram's, periodic acid Schiff, or silver stains. Biopsies are usually not positive. Culture is not useful in diagnosis but may be helpful in confirming the species and, if needed, the drug sensitivities of the yeast (see Chap. 151). In normal or minimally immunocompromised patients, nystatin or clotrimazole is often successful. Nystatin is used as an oral suspension (100,000 units per milliliter) in doses of 10 to 20 mL every 6 h; clotrimazole (10-mg tablet) is to be sucked every 6 h. Ketoconazole (200 to 400 mg in a single oral dose) is considered the treatment of choice; the higher dose is used in the severely immunocompromised host. Poorly responsive patients are treated with amphotericin, 10 to 15 mg as an intravenous infusion for 6 h daily for a total dose of 300 to 500 mg. Miconazole and amphotericin lozenges are currently not available in the United States. The treatment is for 7 to 10 days followed by nystatin, clotrimazole, or ketoconazole for as long as the host resistance remains low.

OTHER TYPES OF ESOPHAGITIS *Radiation esophagitis* is a common occurrence during radiation treatment for lung, mediastinal, or esophageal carcinoma. The frequency and severity of esophagitis increases with the amount of radiation to the area and the concomitant use of certain chemotherapeutic agents such as doxorubicin, bleomycin, cyclophosphamide, and cisplatin. Dysphagia and odynophagia are the main symptoms and may last several weeks to several months after the conclusion of therapy. The esophageal mucosa becomes erythematous, edematous, and friable. Superficial erosions coalesce to form larger superficial ulcers. Submucosal fibrosis and degenerative changes in the blood vessels, muscles, and myenteric neurons may be present. The treatment is relief of pain with viscous lidocaine during the acute phase, while indomethacin may lessen the radiation damage. Esophageal stricture may develop and require dilation. *Corrosive esophagitis* occurs following ingestion of caustic agents, such as strong alkalies or acids. When severe, corrosive injury may lead to esophageal perforation, bleeding, and death. Healing is usually associated with stricture formation. Caustic strictures are usually long and rigid (Fig. 237-2) and generally require dilation with dilators passed over a guide-wire through the stricture. *Pill-induced esophagitis* is associated with the ingestion of certain pills and accounts for many cases of erosive esophagitis. Antibiotics such as doxycycline, tetracycline, and clindamycin account for over half of the cases. Other commonly prescribed pills that cause esophageal injury include aspirin, potassium chloride, ferrous sulfate, quinidine, alprenolol, and various steroidal and nonsteroidal anti-inflammatory agents. *Sclerotherapy* for bleeding esophageal varices usually produces transient retrosternal chest pain and dysphagia due to edema, inflammation, and deranged motility. Esophageal ulcer, stricture, hematoma, or perforation may occur. *Esophagitis associated with mucocutaneous and systemic diseases* is usually associated with blister and bulla formation, epithelial desquamation, and thin, weblike or dense esophageal strictures. Esophageal involvement is indicated by development of odynophagia and dysphagia. Pemphigus vulgaris and bullous pemphigoid form intraepithelial and subepithelial bullae, respectively, and can be distinguished by a specific immunohistology. They are both characterized by sloughing of epithelium or esophageal casts. Glucocorticoid treatment is usually effective. Dystrophic epidermolysis bullosa is an inherited disease that presents in childhood in which local trauma is associated with bulla formation and scarring. Cicatricial pemphigoid, Stevens-Johnson syndrome, and toxic epidermolysis bullosa can produce esophageal bullous lesions and strictures requiring gentle dilation. Graft-versus-host disease occurs in patients who have received allogeneic bone marrow transplants and is associated with generalized desquamation and esophageal strictures. Beçhet's disease may involve the esophagus and may respond to steroid therapy. Crohn's disease, ulcerative colitis, and an erosive lichen planus can also involve the esophagus. Crohn's disease and ulcerative colitis cause aphthous ulcers, and Crohn's disease may cause inflammatory strictures, sinus tract, filiform polyps, and fistulas in the esophagus.

OTHER ESOPHAGEAL DISORDERS

DIVERTICULA Diverticula are outpouchings of the wall of the esophagus. *Zenker's diverticula* appear in the natural weakness in the posterior hypopharyngeal wall and cause halitosis and regurgitation of saliva and food particles consumed several days previously. When they become large and filled with food, they can compress the esophagus and cause dysphagia or complete obstruction. *Midesophageal diverticula* may be caused by traction from old adhesions or by propulsion associated with esophageal motor abnormalities. *Epiphrenic diverticula* may be associated with achalasia. Small or medium-sized diverticula and midesophageal and epiphrenic diverticula are usually asymptomatic. *Diffuse intramural diverticulosis* of the esophagus is due to dilation of the deep esophageal glands. This may lead to chronic candidiasis or a stricture high up in the esophagus. These patients may present with dysphagia. Symptomatic Zenker's diverticula are treated by cricopharyngeal myotomy with or without diverticulectomy. Very large symptomatic esophageal diverticula are removed surgically. When they are associated with motor abnormalities, distal myotomy is performed. Strictures associated with diffuse intramural diverticulosis are treated with rubber dilators.

WEBS AND RINGS Weblike constrictions of the esophagus are usually congenital or inflammatory in origin. Asymptomatic hypopharyngeal webs are demonstrated in up to 10 percent of normal individuals. When concentric, they cause intermittent dysphagia to solids. Symptomatic hypopharyngeal webs with iron-deficiency anemia in middle-aged women constitute Plummer-Vinson syndrome. The clinical importance of this syndrome is uncertain. Midesophageal webs are rare. *Lower esophageal mucosal ring* (Schatzki ring) is a thin, weblike constriction located at the squamocolumnar mucosal junction at or near the border of the lower esophageal sphincter (Fig. 237-2). It invariably produces dysphagia when the diameter is less than 1.3 cm. The dysphagia to solids is the only symptom, and it is usually episodic. Asymptomatic rings may be present in about 10 percent of normal individuals. Lower esophageal ring is one of the common causes of dysphagia. Symptomatic webs and mucosal lower esophageal ring are easily treated by dilation. *Lower esophagitis muscular ring* (contractile ring) is located proximal to the site of mucosal rings and may represent the abnormal uppermost segment of the lower esophageal sphincter. These rings are characterized by a change in size and shape from one time to another (Fig. 237-1). They may also cause dysphagia and should be differentiated from peptic strictures, achalasia, and lower esophageal mucosal ring. They are treated by dilation.

HIATAL HERNIA Hiatal hernia is a herniation of a part of the stomach into the thoracic cavity through the esophageal hiatus in the diaphragm. *Sliding hiatal hernia* is one in which the gastroesophageal junction and fundus of the stomach slide upward. A sliding hernia may result from weakening of the anchors of the gastroesophageal junction to the diaphragm, longitudinal contraction of the esophagus, or increased intraabdominal pressure. Small sliding hernias can be demonstrated commonly during barium studies if intraabdominal pressure is increased. Their incidence increases with age; in the sixth decade of life the prevalence of such hernias is around 60 percent. It is unlikely that a small sliding hiatal hernia by itself produces any clinical symptoms, and its role in the pathogenesis of reflux esophagitis is uncertain. *Paraesophageal hernia* is one in which the esophagogastric junction remains fixed in its normal location and a pouch of stomach is herniated beside the gastroesophageal junction through the esophageal hiatus. A paraesophageal or mixed paraesophageal and sliding hernia may become incarcerated and strangulate. This situation is manifested by acute chest pain, dysphagia, and a mediastinal mass, and requires prompt operative treatment. A herniated gastric pouch may cause dysphagia and may be the site of gastritis and ulceration causing chronic blood loss. A large paraesophageal hernia should be surgically repaired because of a high rate of complications.

MECHANICAL TRAUMA *Esophageal rupture* may be caused by (1) iatrogenic damage from instrumentation of the esophagus or external trauma; (2) increased intraesophageal pressure associated with forceful vomiting or retching (this is also called spontaneous rupture or Boerhaave's syndrome); or (3) diseases of the esophagus such as corrosive esophagitis, esophageal ulcer, and neoplasm. The site of perforation is variable and depends on the cause. Instrumental perforation usually occurs in the pharynx or in the lower esophagus. The esophageal perforation often occurs just above the diaphragm in the posterolateral wall. Esophageal perforation causes severe retrosternal chest pain that may be worsened by swallowing and breathing. Free air enters the mediastinum and spreads to neighboring structures and causes palpable subcutaneous emphysema in the neck, mediastinal crackling sounds on auscultation, and pneumothorax. With time, secondary infection supervenes, and mediastinal abscess and pleuropulmonary suppurative complications may develop. Esophageal perforation associated with vomiting usually deposits gastric contents in the mediastinum and causes severe mediastinal complications. On the other hand, instrumental perforation may be mild and free of severe complications. Spontaneous rupture of the esophagus may mimic myocardial infarction, pancreatitis, or ruptured abdominal viscus. Symptoms of chest pain may be mild, particularly in the elderly. Mediastinal emphysema may develop late. X-ray of the chest shows abnormalities in the majority of patients, and diagnosis is confirmed by swallow of radiopaque contrast material. Treatment includes esophageal and gastric suction and parenteral broad-spectrum antibiotics. Surgical drainage and repair of the laceration should be performed as soon as possible. In patients with terminal carcinoma, surgical repair may not be feasible, and those with minor instrumental perforation can be treated conservatively. Extensive corrosive damage may require esophageal diversion and subsequent excision of the damaged portion of the esophagus.

Mucosal tear (Mallory-Weiss Syndrome) This is usually caused by vomiting and retching, and it usually involves the gastric mucosa near the squamocolumnar mucosal junction but may also involve the esophageal mucosa. Patients present with upper gastrointestinal bleeding that may be severe. Most patients recover with only conservative management, but those with severe arterial bleeding require surgery.

Intramural hematoma Emetogenic injury, particularly in patients with bleeding abnormalities, can cause bleeding between the mucosa and muscle layers of the esophagus. The patients develop sudden dysphagia. Diagnosis is made by barium swallow and computed tomographic scan. Spontaneous resolution usually occurs.

FOREIGN BODIES Foreign bodies may lodge in the cervical esophagus just beyond the upper esophageal sphincter, around the aortic arch, or above the lower esophageal sphincter. Impaction of a bolus of food, particularly a piece of meat or bread, may occur when the esophageal lumen is narrowed due to stricture, carcinoma, or a lower esophageal ring. Acute impaction causes complete inability to swallow and severe chest pain. Both foreign bodies and food boluses may be removed endoscopically. Use of meat tenderizer to facilitate passage of an obstructed meat bolus is to be discouraged because of potential esophageal perforation and aspiration pneumonia.

REFERENCES

AGHA FP et al: Esophageal involvement in epidermolysis bullosa dystrophica: Clinical and roentgenographic manifestations. Gastrointest Radiol 8:111, 1983

BOTT S et al: Medication-induced esophageal injury: Survey of the literature. Am J Gastroenterol 82:758, 1987

CASTELL DO, JOHNSON LF (eds): *Esophageal Function in Health and Disease*. New York, Elsevier, 1983

CLOUSE R: Motor disorders (of the esophagus), in *Gastrointestinal Disease*, MH Sleisenger, JS Fordtran (eds). Philadelphia, Saunders, 1989, pp 559–593

CRIST J et al: Intramural mechanism of esophageal peristalsis: Roles of cholinergic and noncholinergic nerves. Proc Natl Acad Sci USA 81:3595, 1984

DODDS WJ The pathogenesis of gastroesophageal reflux disease. AJR 151:49, 1988

GOYAL RK, CRIST JR: Chest pain of esophageal etiology. Hosp Pract 23:15, 1988

McDONALD GB et al: Esophageal infections in immunosuppressed patients after marrow transplantation. Gastroenterology 88:1111, 1985

MELLOW MH et al: Esophageal acid perfusion in coronary artery disease: Induction of myocardial ischemia. Gastroenterology 85:306, 1983

SHAPIRO J, GOYAL RK: Disorders of the upper esophageal sphincter, in *The Larynx: A Multidisciplinary Approach*, M Fried (ed). Boston, Little, Brown, 1988, pp 293–317

SPECHLER SJ, GOYAL RK: Barrett's esophagus. N Engl J Med 315:362, 1986

SUBRAMANYAM K, PATTERSON M: Chronic esophageal ulceration after endoscopic sclerotherapy. J Clin Gastroenterol 8:58, 1986

WHEELER RR et al: Esophagitis in the immunocompromised host: Role of esophagoscopy in diagnosis. Rev Infect Dis 9:88, 1987

238 PEPTIC ULCER AND GASTRITIS

JAMES E. McGUIGAN

Peptic ulcer is a term used to refer to a group of ulcerative disorders of the upper gastrointestinal tract, involving principally the most proximal portion of the duodenum and the stomach, which have in common participation of acid-pepsin in their pathogenesis. The major forms of common peptic ulcer are duodenal ulcer and gastric ulcer, both of which are chronic diseases. Ulcer associated with the Zollinger-Ellison syndrome, caused by gastrin-releasing tumors (gastrinomas) usually located in the pancreas, is also considered a form of peptic ulcer.

Although our present knowledge of the etiology of peptic ulcer is incomplete, available information supports a crucial role for acid-pepsin. The development of ulcer or the resistance to ulceration is determined by the balance between *aggressive factors* (including secreted gastric acid and pepsin) and those factors that comprise *mucosal defense* or *mucosal resistance* to ulceration. Peptic ulcer results when the aggressive effects of acid-pepsin outweigh the protective effects of gastric or duodenal mucosal resistance. Considering the extraordinary corrosive character of acid-pepsin, why do not all humans develop peptic ulcer? The normal capacity of gastric and proximal duodenal mucosa to resist the corrosive effects of acid and pepsin is unique. This resistance is not shared by other tissues; hence the susceptibility of the esophageal mucosa to injury from refluxed gastric juice, the frequent ulceration of the small intestine when attached surgically to actively secreting gastric mucosa, and corrosion of the skin predictably produced with gastrocutaneous fistulas.

Much has been learned about mechanisms regulating gastric secretion and factors that appear important in development of peptic ulcer. Consideration of gastric physiology provides an understanding of some etiologic elements as well as a rational basis for treatment of peptic ulcer.

GASTRIC PHYSIOLOGY RELATED TO PEPTIC ULCER

AGGRESSIVE FACTORS: ACID AND PEPSINS The gastric mucosa possesses an extraordinary capacity to secrete acid. Parietal cells (oxyntic cells), interspersed along the course of mucosal glands of the body and fundus of the stomach, secrete hydrochloric acid by a process involving oxidative phosphorylation. Parietal cells secrete hydrogen ions at a concentration 3 million times that found in blood. The estimated concentration of HCl secreted directly by parietal cells is approximately 160 m*M*. Each secreted hydrogen ion (H^+) is accompanied by a chloride ion (Cl^-). With each increase in hydrogen ion secretion, there is a reciprocal decrease in sodium ion secretion. For each hydrogen ion secreted into the gastric lumen, one bicarbonate ion (HCO_3^-) is released into the gastric venous circulation, accounting for the *alkaline tide*, a direct reflection of the magnitude of gastric H^+ secretion. Bicarbonate is released from carbonic acid generated from carbon dioxide by parietal cell carbonic anhydrase. The final step in hydrogen ion secretion is accomplished by a proton pump mechanism involving a specific hydrogen-potassium adenosine triphosphatase (H^+,K^+-ATPase) located in the microvillus membrane of the parietal cells' secretory canaliculi. This H^+,K^+-ATPase exchanges hydrogen for potassium across the microvillus membrane. The two-component hypothesis for secretion of acid-containing gastric juice proposes that parietal cells secrete a virtually pure HCl solution, which is mixed (in various proportions) with nonparietal cell alkaline gastric glandular secretions that are similar in ionic composition to extracellular fluid.

Multiple *chemical, neural*, and *hormonal* factors participate in regulation of gastric acid secretion. *Acid secretion is stimulated* by gastrin and by vagal cholinergic postganglionic fibers via muscarinic receptors on parietal cells. Gastrin, the most potent known stimulant of gastric acid secretion, is contained in and released into the circulation from cytoplasmic secretory granules of gastrin cells (or G cells) which are scattered singly or in small clusters among the epithelial lining cells of the mid and deeper portions of the antral pyloric glands. Gastrin is present in tissues and body fluids in multiple molecular forms (Fig. 238-1). The principal form of gastrin in the gastric antral mucosa (or in gastrinoma) is heptadecapeptide gastrin (G-17), which contains 17 amino acid residues, the active site region being the carboxyl-terminal tetrapeptide amide (Try-Met-Asp-Phe-NH_2). Gastrin II is the form of gastrin in which the tyrosyl residue at position 12 is sulfated, and gastrin I is the nonsulfated form. G-17 accounts for more than 90 percent of gastrin in antral mucosa. Approximately two-thirds of serum gastrin consists of a larger molecular species of gastrin, which contains 34 amino acids (G-34). The carboxyl-terminal 17 amino acids of G-34 are identical to those of G-17 and may also be sulfated (G-34 II) or nonsulfated (G-34 I). Although G-17 has a shorter half-life than G-34, circulating G-17 is approximately as potent as G-34 in stimulating gastric acid secretion.

Gastrin is also present in duodenal mucosa, with its highest concentration in the most proximal duodenum (approximately 10 percent of antral concentration). The mucosal concentration of gastrin and the proportion of G-17 decrease with progression down the duodenum. The effects of gastrin and vagal stimulation on gastric acid secretion are intimately interrelated. Vagal stimulation increases gastric acid secretion by cholinergic stimulation of parietal cell secretion, by stimulating release of gastrin into the circulation, and by lowering the parietal cell threshold for response to circulating gastrin concentrations. There is also some evidence suggesting that certain vagal branches or fibers may inhibit gastrin release.

Large amounts of histamine are present in mast cells, and in endocrine cells of some species, in the parietal cell–containing regions of the gastric mucosa. Mast cells are located in close proximity to parietal cells, with a ratio of one mast cell to every two or three parietal cells. For many years views differed on the importance of histamine in stimulating gastric acid secretion; some suggested that histamine was the "final common pathway" for cholinergic and gastrin stimulation of parietal cell acid secretion, while others were skeptical about any role for histamine in the acid secretory process. Interest in the role of histamine in acid secretion was renewed by the discovery of H-2-receptor antagonists which inhibited competitively the action of histamine on H-2 receptors (located on gastric parietal, cardiac atrial, and uterine smooth-muscle cells). These drugs were shown to exert negligible effect on H-1 receptors, which are inhibited readily by conventional antihistamines (H-1-receptor antagonists). H-2-receptor antagonists (e.g., cimetidine, ranitidine, famotidine, nizatidine) inhibit basal acid secretion as well as secretion in response to feeding, gastrin, histamine, hypoglycemia, or vagal stimulation. Most data support the conclusions that (1) histamine plays an important role in stimulating gastric acid secretion and (2) histamine acts in concert with gastrin and cholinergic activity on parietal cells, which bear receptors for histamine, gastrin, and acetylcholine, but that (3) there is still uncertainty as to whether histamine is the final common effector molecule in the stimulation of parietal cell secretion. Histamine stimulates gastric acid secretion by increasing parietal cell cyclic adenosine monophosphate (AMP), thereby activating cyclic AMP–dependent protein kinase(s). Gastrin and cholinergic agents, which do not stimulate cyclic AMP production, stimulate acid secretion by increasing parietal cell cytosolic calcium.

The major physiologic stimulus for gastric acid secretion is ingestion of food. Traditionally, regulation of gastric acid secretion has been classified into three phases—cephalic, gastric, and intestinal. This classification is of some value in analyzing factors that participate in regulation of gastric acid secretion. The *cephalic phase* encompasses the gastric acid secretory response to the sight, smell, taste, and anticipation of food. The *gastric phase* is induced by the presence

Big Gastrin (G34)	⌐Glu-Leu-Gly-Pro-Gln-Gly-Pro-Pro-His-Leu-Val-Ala-Asp-Pro-Ser-Lys-Lys- -Gln-Gly-Pro-Trp-Leu-Glu-Glu-Glu-Glu-Glu-Ala-Tyr*-Gly-Trp-Met-Asp-Phe-NH_2
Heptadecapeptide Gastrin (G 17)	⌐Glu-Gly-Pro-Trp-Leu-Glu-Glu-Glu-Glu-Glu-Ala-Tyr*-Gly-Trp-Met-Asp-Phe-NH_2
Minigastrin (G 14)	Trp-Leu-Glu-Glu-Glu-Glu-Glu-Ala-Tyr*-Gly-Trp-Met-Asp-Phe-NH_2
C-Terminal Pentapeptide	Gly-Trp-Met-Asp-Phe-NH_2

FIGURE 238-1 Amino acid sequences of selected gastrin peptides, all of which contain the common C-terminal pentapeptide amide. (*Tyrosyl is sulfated in gastrin II and nonsulfated in gastrin I molecules.)

of food in the stomach. The *intestinal phase* is due to the entry or presence of food within the lumen of the small intestine. Although these three phases are convenient for considering the diverse contributions to gastric acid secretion, each phase is complex and not necessarily due to a single stimulatory control mechanism.

The cephalic phase, which includes cortical and hypothalamic components, is considered to be mediated primarily by vagal activation, which increases gastric acid secretion principally by effecting stimulation of parietal cells and to lesser extent by promoting gastrin release. The gastric phase results from stimulation of chemical and mechanical receptors in the gastric wall by luminal contents. Mechanical distention of the stomach stimulates gastric acid secretion but results in little, if any, gastrin release; this mechanical effect is inhibited by atropine and appears to be mediated by vagal reflexes. Food in the stomach promotes gastric acid secretion by increasing gastrin release, principally due to the content of *protein* and especially the *products of protein digestion* contained in the meal; oral glucose and fat cause slight increases in serum gastrin but do not stimulate gastric acid secretion. Food in the proximal small intestine stimulates the intestinal phase of gastric acid secretion. A peptone meal (which contains partially hydrolyzed meat protein) introduced into the small intestine stimulates gastric acid secretion but not gastrin release. Food in the small intestine may induce release of an intestinal hormone(s) (distinct from gastrin) that stimulates gastric acid secretion. Increases in circulating amino acids, absorbed from the small intestine, may also contribute to the intestinal phase of gastric acid secretion. *Basal* or *interdigestive gastric acid secretion* can be considered to be a *fourth phase* of acid secretion. This phase is unrelated to feeding, it reaches its peak around midnight and its lowest point about 7 A.M., and neural pathways are probably most important in its regulation.

Ingestion of both caffeine-containing and caffeine-free *coffee* stimulates gastric acid secretion: both forms of coffee stimulate gastrin release. Ingestion of *ethanol* and ethanol-containing beverages stimulates gastric acid secretion. Specifically, ingestion of 5 or 10% ethanol solutions or 10% bourbon whiskey results in prompt gastric acid secretion without increasing gastrin release; however, white wine stimulates gastric acid secretion and gastrin release. Intravenous ethanol stimulates gastric acid secretion, suggesting that both systemic and local mechanisms are involved.

Intravenous *calcium* stimulates gastric acid secretion and produces minimal increases in serum gastrin levels. Oral calcium has been reported to stimulate gastric acid secretion directly, i.e., without an increase in serum calcium or gastrin concentrations. Except in patients who harbor gastrinomas, hypercalcemia is not usually associated with gastric acid hypersecretion or with increases in serum gastrin.

Inhibition of gastric acid secretion can be produced by several mechanisms. Acid secretion may be inhibited by acid in the stomach or duodenum, by hyperglycemia, or by hypertonic fluids or fat in the duodenum. Reduction of the intragastric pH to 3.0 produces partial inhibition of gastrin release; further reduction to pH 1.5 or below blocks completely release of gastrin to almost all stimuli. The precise mechanism by which this pH-dependent feedback control of gastrin release operates has not been defined. Cholinergic and noncholinergic intramural neurons have been proposed as potential mediators. *Somatostatin* appears to play an important role in inhibition of gastrin release produced by acid in the gastric lumen. Somatostatin-containing antral mucosal endocrine cells (D cells) have cytoplasmic processes which extend to neighboring gastrin cells. Somatostatin inhibits gastrin release by its local (paracrine) effects on gastrin cells. In addition, in the acid-secreting portion of the stomach cytoplasmic processes of somatostatin cells extend to intimate contact with parietal cells and other cells. Somatostatin reduces gastric acid secretion by inhibiting gastrin release and by directly inhibiting parietal cell secretion. Acid in the duodenum decreases acid secretion by the stomach, perhaps by promoting release into the circulation of intestinal peptides that then inhibit gastric acid secretion. *Secretin*, which is a linear polypeptide (27 amino acids) related structurally to glucagon, is capable of inhibiting gastric acid secretion. Secretin is released from endocrine cells (S cells) in the mucosa of the small intestine in response to mucosal acidification. Fat in the duodenum also inhibits gastric acid secretion; gastric inhibitory peptide (GIP) has been proposed as a candidate for this enterogastrone action; however, this effect of GIP remains to be proved. The mechanisms by which hyperglycemia or intraduodenal hyperosmolality inhibit gastric acid secretion are not known. Additional peptides residing in the mucosa of the proximal small intestine which possess the capacity to inhibit gastric acid secretion include vasoactive intestinal peptide (VIP), enteroglucagon, neurotensin, peptide YY, and urogastrone. Vasoactive intestinal peptide, a neuropeptide and putative neurotransmitter, is restricted in its location to neurons; it is unlikely to inhibit gastric acid secretion as a circulating hormone since, although released in response to feeding, it is inactivated during its portal passage through the liver. Enteroglucagon is composed of oxyntomodulin (glucagon with an 8-amino acid carboxyl-terminal extension) and glicentin (oxyntomodulin with a 32-amino acid amino-terminal extension). Neurotensin, oxyntomodulin, and peptide YY are released from the small intestine in response to luminal lipid perfusion. Urogastrone is structurally and functionally identical to epidermal growth factor. The extent to which these numerous peptides in the mucosa of the small intestine contribute to the physiologic regulation of gastric acid secretion has not been defined.

The proteolytic effects of *pepsins* in concert with the corrosive properties of secreted gastric acid are integral components in the tissue injury which produces peptide ulceration. Gastric acid catalyzes the cleavage of inactive pepsinogen molecules, converting them to proteolytically active pepsins, and also provides the appropriate low pH required for pepsin activity. Pepsin activity, maximal in the range of pH 1.5 to 2.0, is reduced substantially above pH 4.0, and these enzymes are denatured and irreversibly inactivated at neutral or alkaline pH. A variety of pepsinogens and their respective pepsins are present in gastric juice. Pepsinogens (and their corresponding active pepsins) have been classified by immunochemical techniques as either PG I (pepsinogens 1 through 5) or PG II (pepsinogens 6 and 7). Pepsinogen I is found in chief and mucous cells in the body and fundus of the stomach. Pepsinogen II is located in cells of the pyloric glands, Brunner's glands of the duodenum, mucous cells of the gastric cardiac glands, and the same cells in which PG I is found. Both PG I and PG II are present in plasma, whereas only PG I can be detected in urine. In general, there is a direct correlation between PG I serum concentrations and maximal gastric acid secretion. Most agents which stimulate gastric acid secretion also stimulate pepsinogen secretion. Cholinergic action is particularly potent in promoting pepsinogen secretion. Although it inhibits gastric acid secretion, secretin stimulates pepsinogen secretion.

In addition to secretion of hydrochloric acid parietal cells also secrete *intrinsic factor*. Agents which stimulate gastric acid secretion also lead to secretion of intrinsic factor.

MUCOSAL DEFENSE The precise mechanisms whereby the normal stomach and duodenum resist the corrosive effects of acid-pepsin (i.e., *mucosal resistance* to injury or *mucosal defense*) have not been defined completely. However, a variety of factors have been advanced as potential contributors to mucosal defense. *Gastric mucus* is proposed to play an important role in mucosal defense and thereby in preventing peptic ulceration. Gastric mucus is secreted by gastric mucous cells located on the surface of the gastric mucosal epithelium and in gastric glands. Mucus secretion is enhanced by mechanical or chemical irritation and by cholinergic stimulation. Gastric mucus is present in gastric juice in a soluble phase and as an insoluble mucus gel layer, approximately 0.6 mm in thickness, which coats the mucosal surface of the stomach. Normally the mucus gel is secreted constantly by gastric mucous epithelial cells and is continuously solubilized by pepsins secreted into the gastric lumen. Gastric mucus is a large polymeric glycoprotein (2×10^6 mol wt) containing four subunits connected by disulfide bridges. Depolymerization of the glycoprotein subunits of mucus, by peptic digestion or disruption of disulfide bonds, renders the glycoprotein incapable of forming or maintaining the gel. When intact, this mucus gel serves as an unstirred water layer which slows ionic diffusion but is much more impermeable to penetration by macromolecules such as pepsins (34,000 mol wt). Pepsin molecules secreted into the gastric lumen are denied reentry by the intact mucus gel, thereby potentially protecting mucosal cells from proteolytic injury. *Bicarbonate ions*, secreted by nonparietal gastric epithelial cells, enter the mucus gel, contributing to the development of a microenvironment in the gel with a substantial hydrogen ion gradient between the zone of the gel facing the gastric lumen (more acid, approaching pH of 2) and the zone in contact with the gastric mucosal cells (more alkaline, approaching pH of 7). As an unstirred water layer the mucus gel slows hydrogen ion diffusion back toward the gastric mucosal surface, allowing buffering by bicarbonate within the gel. Gel thickness is increased by administration of prostaglandins of the E series and reduced by nonsteroidal anti-inflammatory drugs, including aspirin. Gastric bicarbonate secretion is stimulated by calcium, certain prostaglandins of the E and F series, cholinergic agents, and dibutyryl cyclic guanosine monophosphate. It is inhibited by NSAIDs including aspirin, and by acetazolamide, alpha-adrenergic agents, and ethanol.

Gastric mucus also contains antigenic determinants used to classify AB(H) blood group substances. Approximately three-fourths of the population secrete gastric juice containing these AB(H) substances, and those individuals are referred to as *secretors*.

Normally the gastric luminal epithelial cell surfaces and intercellular tight junctions provide an almost completely impermeable *gastric mucosal barrier* to back-diffusion of hydrogen ions from the lumen: this barrier may be an important component of mucosal resistance to acid-peptic injury. The barrier can be interrupted by bile acids, salicylates, ethanol, and weak organic acids, thereby permitting back-diffusion of hydrogen ions from lumen to gastric tissues. This may cause cell injury, release of histamine from mast cells, further stimulation of acid secretion, damage to small blood vessels, mucosal hemorrhage, and erosion or ulceration. Interruption of the gastric mucosal barrier appears to contribute to the hemorrhagic erosive gastritis associated with salicylate or ethanol ingestion and to other forms of gastric mucosal injury. Maintenance of normal *mucosal blood flow* is an essential component of mucosal resistance to injury. Decreased mucosal blood flow, accompanied by back-diffusion of luminal hydrogen ions, is important in producing gastric mucosal damage.

Prostaglandins are present in abundant quantities in the gastric mucoas. Various prostaglandins, particularly those of the E series, have been shown to inhibit gastric mucosal injury caused by a wide variety of agents. Endogenous prostaglandins appear to play several important roles in mucosal defense. Prostaglandins stimulate secretion of gastric mucus and gastric and duodenal mucosal bicarbonate. Prostaglandins participate in the maintenance of gastric mucosal blood flow, in the integrity of the gastric mucosal barrier, and in epithelial cell renewal in response to mucosal injury.

MEASUREMENT OF GASTRIC ACID SECRETION Since HCl secretion by the stomach appears to be important in the production of peptic ulcer disease, measurement of basal and stimulated gastric acid secretion may be of value in the assessment of some patients with peptic ulcer. The range of values for normal subjects is extremely broad and overlaps substantially with the values in patients with duodenal ulcer, gastric ulcer, and even the Zollinger-Ellison syndrome. Mean basal acid output (BAO) in normal males without known ulcer disease is about 1.5 to 2.0 mmol/h. In general, basal and stimulated acid outputs in females are approximately two-thirds to three-fourths those found in males. In duodenal ulcer patients mean basal acid output averages from 4 to 6 mmol/h, again, with a wide degree of variation. Patients with gastric ulcer tend to have gastric acid secretory rates that are normal or often slightly less than those for normal subjects.

Measurement of gastric acid output is not helpful in the diagnosis or exclusion of peptic ulcer and is clearly not necessary in most ulcer patients. However, it is of value in selected clinical situations. Detection of gastric acid hypersecretion is important when the Zollinger-Ellison syndrome is suspected. Measurement of gastric acid output is useful to detect achlorhydria, as in patients with pernicious anemia. Since patients with benign gastric ulcer virtually always secrete some acid, pentagastrin-fast achlorhydria in a patient with a gastric ulcer is almost always associated with malignancy. Measurement of gastric acid secretion is indicated in the search for the cause of ulcer recurrence after peptic ulcer surgery; it is also of value in patients in whom hypergastrinemia has been identified, in order to distinguish between clinical conditions characterized by gastric acid hypersecretion or achlorhydria.

In order to measure gastric acid output, a radiopaque gastric tube is passed so that its tip is located in the most dependent portion of the stomach. With the patient reclining or in a semirecumbent position on the left side, the position of the tube is verified by fluoroscopy. Gastric contents are aspirated and discarded. Basal gastric acid secretions are then collected in four consecutive 15-min intervals to determine the 1-h basal acid output. Secretion volume and acid concentration (titrated with sodium hydroxide to pH 7.0 or calculated by formula from the pH of the aspirated gastric juice) are measured, and acid output is expressed in millimoles per hour.

A variety of substances have been used to stimulate maximal acid output (MAO) by the stomach. These have included *histamine*, *betazole* (Histalog)—a structural analogue of histamine, and *pentagastrin* (Peptavlon). Histamine, the first standard stimulant used for gastric acid secretory testing, requires the simultaneous administration of an antihistaminic agent (H-1-receptor antagonist) to inhibit untoward systemic side effects. Betazole possesses fewer undesired side effects than histamine and does not require concomitant administration of an antihistamine. Pentagastrin (*N*-tert-butyloxycarbonyl-β-Ala-Try-Met-Asp-Phe-NH_2) contains the biologically active carboxyl-terminal tetrapeptide amide portion of the gastrin molecule and is currently the preferred and most commonly used agent to induce maximal acid secretion. Following collection of basal acid secretion, gastric juice is collected for four additional consecutive 15-min periods after the subcutaneous injection of pentagastrin (6 μg/kg). MAO is expressed as millimoles of acid aspirated during the 1 h after pentagastrin administration. Peak acid output (PAO) is calculated by combining the two highest consecutive 15-min acid outputs following pentagastrin injection and multiplying by 2.

DUODENAL ULCER

Duodenal ulcer is characteristically a chronic and recurrent disease. Duodenal ulcers are usually deep and sharply demarcated. They tend to penetrate through the submucosa, often into the muscularis propria. This is in contrast to erosions which are limited to the mucosa. The ulcer floor contains no intact epithelium and usually consists of a zone of eosinophilic necrosis resting on a base of granulation tissue surrounded by variable amounts of fibrosis. The ulcer bed may be clear or may contain blood or a proteinaceous exudate with entrapped erythrocytes and acute and chronic inflammatory cells. More than 95 percent of duodenal ulcers occur in the first portion of the duodenum, and approximately 90 percent of those are located within 3 cm of the junction of the pyloric and duodenal mucosa. Duodenal ulcers are usually round or oval, but may be irregular or elliptic. They are usually less than 1 cm in diameter. Rarely, duodenal ulcers may be extremely large (3 to 6 cm in diameter) and may be mistaken radiographically for the entire duodenal bulb. These giant ulcers often escape radiologic detection and are usually identified by endoscopy, or at surgery or postmortem examination.

The absolute prevalence of duodenal ulcer in the population is not known. Estimates have ranged from 6 to 15 percent. This variation in estimates may be explained by differences in the populations examined, study designs, diagnostic methods (e.g., endoscopy vs. radiologic examination) and by actual changes occurring in the frequency of duodenal ulcer. During the past 40 years the frequency of duodenal ulcer (and its complications) has been decreasing in the United States and England, especially in males. The reasons for this reduction are not known. The best current estimates suggest that approximately 10 percent of the population have clinical evidence of duodenal ulcer at some time in their lives. The natural history of duodenal ulcer is spontaneous healing and recurrence: about 60 percent of healed duodenal ulcers recur within 1 year, and 80 to 90 percent recur within 2 years. Duodenal ulcer is slightly more common in males than in females and is approximately three times as frequent as clinically recognized gastric ulcer.

ETIOLOGY AND PATHOGENESIS Although much is now known concerning factors that contribute to the development of duodenal ulcer, we do not completely understand its pathogenesis. It is clear that acid secretion by the stomach is required for production of a duodenal ulcer, but the factors which render the acid-secreting subject susceptible to duodenal ulceration have not been defined completely. Though as a group duodenal ulcer patients secrete more acid than normal, from one-half to two-thirds of them have acid secretory rates (BAO and MAO) within the normal range. Duodenal ulcer patients have approximately 1.9 billion parietal cells, with a maximum capacity of approximately 42 mmol gastric acid secreted per hour; this is in contrast to 1.0 billion parietal cells and a 22 mmol/h secretion rate for nonduodenal ulcer subjects (mean approximate values). However, variations in both groups are so large that most duodenal ulcer patients fall within the normal range. As a group duodenal ulcer patients also have comparable increases in gastric secretion of pepsin and in serum pepsinogen I levels. Peptic ulcer develops when there is an unfavorable balance between acid-pepsin secretion and mucosal resistance: in the pathogenesis of duodenal ulcer, evidence favors the importance of absolute or, in most instances, relative gastric hypersecretion. In contrast, for gastric ulcer defective mucosal resistance appears to be the major contributing factor.

Fasting *serum gastrin* concentrations are normal in duodenal ulcer patients. However, in many duodenal ulcer patients more gastrin is released into the circulation in response to a protein-containing meal than by normal subjects. Duodenal ulcer patients also have greater gastric acid secretory responses to administered gastrin than do nonulcer subjects. In duodenal ulcer patients intragastric acid may be less effective in inhibiting gastrin release and further gastric acid secretion. Therefore, although fasting serum gastrin levels are in the normal range in patients with common duodenal ulcer, gastrin may still play an important role in their frequent, but not invariable, gastric acid hypersecretion. Duodenal ulcer patients tend to empty their stomachs more rapidly than do nonduodenal ulcer patients. This phenomenon, when coupled with gastric acid hypersecretion, may contribute to a greater rate of acid delivery to the first part of the duodenum (the primary location of ulceration) in patients with duodenal ulcer.

Genetic factors appear to be important. Duodenal ulcers are approximately three times as common in first-degree relatives of duodenal ulcer patients as in the general population. Patients with duodenal ulcers have an increased frequency of blood group O and of the nonsecretory status [those who do not secrete AB(H) blood group antigens in their gastric juice], but these associations are weak. An increased incidence of HLA-B5 antigen has been reported in white male subjects with duodenal ulcer. Elevated serum pepsinogen I (PG I) levels, inherited as an autosomal dominant trait, are found in about 50 percent of patients with duodenal ulcer. Individuals with this trait have a frequency of duodenal ulcer which is eight times greater than that of the general population.

Cigarette smoking has been associated with increased duodenal ulcer frequency, decreased response to therapy, and increased duodenal ulcer mortality. Cigarette smoking does not increase gastric acid secretion. It has been suggested that the increased incidence of duodenal ulcer among cigarette smokers may be due to inhibition of pancreatic bicarbonate secretion (an endogenous neutralizer of secreted gastric acid) by nicotine or cigarette smoking and/or by accelerated emptying of gastric acid into the duodenum.

The incidence of duodenal ulcer has also been reported to be increased in patients with chronic renal failure, alcoholic cirrhosis, renal transplantation, hyperparathyroidism, systemic mastocytosis, and chronic obstructive pulmonary disease.

Gastric colonization with *Helicobacter pylori* has been reported in 80 to 100 percent of patients with duodenal ulcer. This has been proposed as a potential contributing factor in the pathogenesis of duodenal ulcer. At present it is uncertain whether *H. pylori* plays a role in producing duodenal ulcer or if its presence reflects a commensal association. Antibodies to herpes simplex have been reported to be higher in titer and more frequent in sera of patients with duodenal ulcer than in normals.

The importance of *psychological factors* in the pathogenesis of duodenal ulcer remains controversial. Contrary to earlier views, there is no single, characteristic duodenal ulcer personality. Chronic anxiety and psychological stress may, however, be factors in exacerbation of ulcer activity. There is some evidence that patients with duodenal ulcer may view stress more negatively than nonulcer subjects. There have been no differences identified in the frequency of duodenal ulcer among different socioeconomic classes or occupation groups.

CLINICAL FEATURES Epigastric pain is by far the most frequent symptom of duodenal ulcer. The pain is often described as sharp, burning, or gnawing. Alternatively, the pain may be ill-defined, boring, or aching, or may be perceived as abdominal pressure or fullness, or as a hunger sensation. In approximately 10 percent of patients the pain is located to the right of the epigastrium. The pain of duodenal ulcer characteristically occurs from 90 min to 3 h after eating. It frequently awakens the patient at night. Pain on awakening before breakfast is sufficiently rare in patients with duodenal ulcer as to challenge the diagnosis. The pain is usually relieved within a few minutes by food or antacids. Symptoms tend to be recurrent and episodic. The severity of pain varies widely from patient to patient. Duodenal ulcers recur often in the absence of pain. Episodes of pain may persist for periods of several days to weeks or months. Periods of remission usually last from weeks to years and are almost always longer than the episodes of pain. In some patients the disease is more aggressive, with frequent and persistent symptoms and/or development of complications. Pain relief with antacids or food is believed to result from acid neutralization. Ingestion of food leads to transient partial neutralization of gastric acid, which is followed by gastrin release and resultant stimulation of acid secretion. With subsequent gastric emptying and increasing gastric acid secretion, a sufficiently low pH is achieved in the stomach and first portion of the duodenum that pain results. Acid-induced pain in patients with duodenal ulcer is believed to be due to (1) acid stimulation of chemical receptors and/or (2) alterations in gastric motility.

Changes in the character of ulcer pain may signal the development of complications. For example, ulcer pain which becomes constant, is longer relieved by food or antacids, or radiates to the back or to either upper quadrant may herald *penetration* of the ulcer (often posteriorly into the pancreas). Pain associated with duodenal ulcer which is accentuated, rather than relieved, by food and/or is accompanied by vomiting often indicates *gastric outlet obstruction*. Abrupt, severe, or generalized abdominal pain is characteristic of free ulcer *perforation* into the peritoneal cavity. Weight loss, in the absence of some degree of gastric outlet obstruction, is unusual. Duodenal ulcer may cause acute gastrointestinal *hemorrhage*, with vomiting of blood or coffee-grounds material, or with the passage of black, tarry stools or even frankly red blood, if the bleeding is massive. More commonly blood loss with duodenal ulcer is more subtle, with occult blood loss detected by stool examination or by variable degrees of anemia which may be accompanied by iron deficiency.

It is important to emphasize that *many patients with active duodenal ulcer have no ulcer symptoms*. This leads to a significant, although not precisely quantifiable, underestimate of duodenal ulcer frequency in the population. Prospective studies using upper gastrointestinal endoscopy suggest that approximately half of duodenal ulcers recur in the absence of symptoms. Endoscopic studies also show a lack of good correlation between ulcer activity, symptom resolution, and ulcer healing. The absence of prior ulcer-type pain does not exclude duodenal ulcer as a potential cause for acute or chronic gastrointestinal hemorrhage, gastric outlet obstruction, or abrupt ulcer perforation.

On *physical examination* epigastric tenderness is by far the most frequent abnormal finding. The area of tenderness is usually in the midline, often midway between the umbilicus and the xiphoid process. In approximately 20 percent of patients the tender area is to the right of the midline. Acute free ulcer perforation into the peritoneal cavity often produces a rigid, boardlike abdomen, usually with generalized rebound tenderness. Initially auscultation of the abdomen may reveal hyperactive bowel sounds which, with clinical progression, may diminish or disappear. Patients with gastric outlet obstruction caused by a duodenal or pyloric channel ulcer may have a ''succussion splash'' produced by fluid and air in the distended stomach. Tachycardia and/or hypotension, in some instances demonstrable only by orthostatic maneuvers, may result from acute duodenal ulcer hemorrhage. Cutaneous and mucosal pallor may reflect anemia from acute or chronic blood loss.

Only about 5 percent of duodenal ulcers are located distal to the duodenal bulb, and most of these are in the immediate postbulbar portion of the first part of the duodenum. Postbulbar ulcer pain may be located in the right upper quadrant or may radiate through the back. Obstruction and hemorrhage are more frequent with postbulbar ulcers than with those in the duodenal bulb. Most immediate postbulbar ulcers, i.e., within 2 cm of the duodenal bulb, are of the common duodenal ulcer variety. Ulceration, located in or beyond the second portion of the duodenum, suggests the Zollinger-Ellison syndrome.

The pyloric channel, which is 1 to 2 cm in length, is the narrowest portion of the gastric outlet. Because of their gastric acid secretory characteristics and clinical features, pyloric channel ulcers are classified with duodenal rather than with gastric ulcers. Ulcers in this location often produce symptoms similar to those of a duodenal ulcer; however, symptoms tend to be less responsive to food and antacids. In patients with pyloric channel ulcers, food may accentuate rather than relieve ulcer pain and may produce vomiting due to partial gastric outlet obstruction. In general, surgery is required more frequently for pyloric channel ulcers than for those in the duodenal bulb.

FIGURE 238-2 Deformed duodenal bulb with ulcer crater.

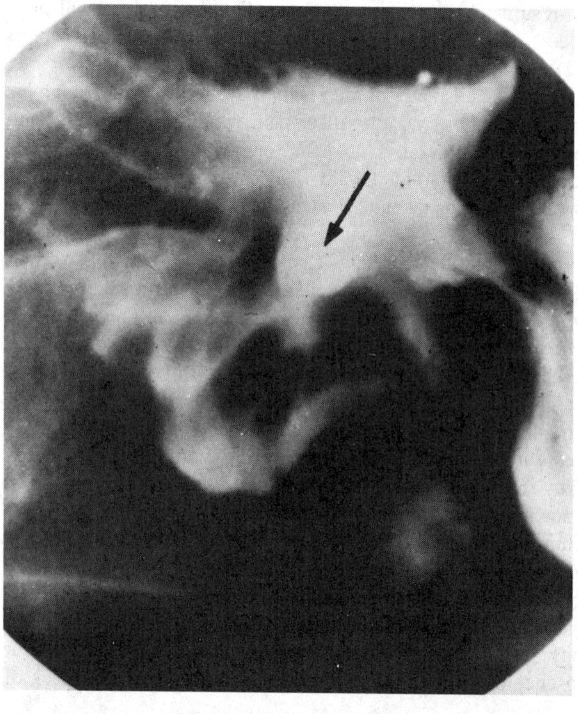

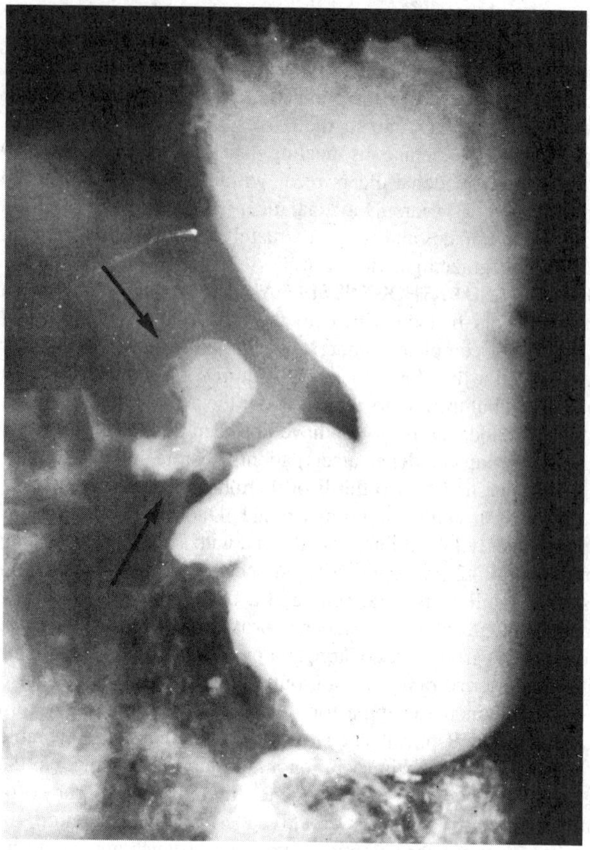

FIGURE 238-3 Distortion of the duodenal bulb with ''cloverleaf'' deformity.

DIAGNOSIS Barium examination of the upper gastrointestinal tract is of value in identifying duodenal ulcer and is still the most common initial method used to establish the diagnosis. The proportion of ulcers identified radiographically depends on the skill, persistence, enthusiasm, and diagnostic criteria of the radiologist. Using conventional single contrast barium techniques, 70 to 80 percent of duodenal ulcers found at endoscopy can be identified by x-ray examination. With double-contrast barium examinations, it is possible to detect about 90 percent of duodenal ulcers. On x-ray the typical duodenal ulcer appears as a discrete crater in the proximal portion of the duodenal bulb. Marked deformity of the duodenal bulb, common in patients with chronic recurrent duodenal ulcer, may make radiographic identification of the ulcer difficult or impossible (Figs. 238-2 and 238-3).

Use of fiberoptic endoscopic examination of the upper gastrointestinal tract has facilitated accurate diagnosis of duodenal ulcer. Duodenoscopy is not required for diagnosis of duodenal ulcer when it has been identified by barium radiographic examination. Endoscopy may be of greatest value, however, (1) in detecting duodenal ulcer suspected in the absence of a radiographically demonstrable ulcer, (2) in patients with radiographic deformity and uncertainty regarding ulcer activity, (3) in identifying ulcers too small or too superficial to be recognized by x-ray, and (4) in identifying (or excluding) an ulcer as the source of active gastrointestinal hemorrhage. Duodensocopy permits direct visualization and photographic documentation of the character of the ulcer—its size, shape, and location—and may provide a reference base for assessment of ulcer healing.

Measurement of gastric acid secretion is not necessary in the assessment of most patients with clinical features of typical duodenal ulcer. Determination of serum gastrin is recommended in those patients in whom surgery is planned or gastrinoma is suspected. Epigastric pain readily relieved by food or antacids strongly suggests duodenal ulcer. However, even after careful radiographic and endoscopic examination many patients with these ulcer-like symptoms have no evidence of ulcer: this has led to the term *nonulcer dyspepsia*. Although symptoms are similar, it is uncertain whether this entity is related to peptic ulcer.

MEDICAL TREATMENT Major objectives of duodenal ulcer therapy are relief of pain and acceleration of ulcer healing. Prevention of ulcer recurrence and complications are additional important objectives. In the past enthusiasm has been expressed for virtually every kind of treatment ever tried for duodenal ulcer. Conclusions regarding the effectiveness of therapy were obscured by spontaneous healing of duodenal ulcer, an intrinsic component of the natural history of the disease, and by imprecise methods used to assess ulcer activity. Specific effective agents currently available and recommended for consideration in treatment of duodenal ulcer are considered below.

Antacids For many decades antacids have been the major form of treatment for duodenal ulcer. Prospective endoscopic studies conducted only relatively recently have verified the effectiveness of antacids in accelerating duodenal ulcer healing. Many types of antacids are available for use in treatment of duodenal ulcer. The ideal antacid should be potent in neutralizing acid, inexpensive, not adsorbed from the gastrointestinal tract, and should contain negligible amounts of sodium. It should be sufficiently palatable to be tolerated with repeated dosage and should be free from side effects. Individual antacids differ substantially in their capacities to neutralize acid, their sodium contents, their absorption properties, and their potential adverse effects. Although the ideal antacid is yet to be developed, a number of preparations are available that can be used effectively in treatment of patients with duodenal ulcer.

The most widely used antacid preparations are mixtures of aluminum hydroxide and magnesium hydroxide, in some instances with additional agents. *Aluminum hydroxide* neutralizes hydrochloric acid with the production of aluminum chloride and water. Use of aluminum hydroxide tends to produce constipation. Aluminum binds phosphate within the gut lumen, thereby facilitating phosphate excretion. As a consequence, prolonged and regular use of aluminum hydroxide may induce systemic phosphate depletion with resultant weakness, malaise, and anorexia. Phosphate depletion is probably restricted to, and should be considered in, those patients with phosphate-poor diets, e.g., dietary deficiency with chronic alcoholism or other states of reduced dietary protein intake.

Magnesium hydroxide is a potent antacid which neutralizes hydrochloric acid, producing magnesium chloride and water. Magnesium hydroxide may produce loose stools. This laxative effect and the constipating effects of aluminum hydroxide can be overcome by using these agents in combination or by alternating their use. From 5 to 10 percent of magnesium in magnesium hydroxide is absorbed by the small intestine. Magnesium is excreted by the kidney, and hypermagnesemia, which is not a problem with normal renal function, does develop in a small number of patients with renal insufficiency who are treated with magnesium-containing antacids. *Magnesium trisilicate*, which is included in various antacid mixtures, is a slow-acting weak antacid.

Calcium carbonate is a potent and inexpensive antacid. In neutralizing acid, it is converted to calcium chloride in the stomach. Approximately 10 percent of calcium ingested as calcium carbonate is absorbed from the proximal small intestine. Calcium carbonate is unique among antacids in that its ingestion is followed by stimulation of gastric acid secretion ("acid rebound"). This is due to the direct action of calcium in stimulating parietal cell acid secretion and, perhaps to a lesser extent, to calcium-mediated stimulation of gastrin release. Chronic calcium carbonate adminstration may be associated with the milk-alkali syndrome, producing elevations of serum calcium, phosphate, urea nitrogen, creatinine, and bicarbonate. These patients may develop renal calcinosis and progressive renal insufficiency. Because of its potential adverse effects, calcium carbonate is not recommended for use as an antacid for treatment of patients with peptic ulcer.

Sodium bicarbonate is a potent, rapidly acting, inexpensive antacid. However, because of its tendency to induce systemic alkalosis and its high sodium content, it should not be used as an antacid in treatment of peptic ulcer.

Acceptance of the crucial role of acid in the pathogenesis of duodenal ulcer has provided a rational basis for the use of antacids in treatment of patients with duodenal ulcer. In a controlled endoscopic study, 4 weeks of treatment with a potent magnesium and aluminum hydroxide antacid mixture increased the rate of duodenal ulcer healing. Ulcer healing occurred in 45 percent of patients receiving placebo and in 78 percent of those treated with 30 mL antacid (144 mmol) given 1 and 3 h after meals and at bedtime. It has been proposed more recently that smaller and less frequent doses may also achieve satisfactory ulcer healing.

H-2-receptor antagonists It has been known for decades that conventional antihistamines, which readily block the actions of histamine on smooth muscle of blood vessels, the gut, or bronchi do not inhibit histamine-stimulated gastric acid secretion. The parietal cell receptor for histamine has been classified as an H-2 receptor and that blocked by classic antihistamines as an H-1 receptor. H-2-receptor antagonists are potent inhibitors of basal (unstimulated) and of stimulated gastric acid secretion. At the present time H-2-receptor antagonists are the therapeutic agents selected most frequently for the management of patients with duodenal ulcer.

Cimetidine was the first H-2-receptor antagonist developed and has been used most extensively in the treatment of duodenal ulcer. Cimetidine is related structurally to histamine (Fig. 238-4), sharing the same imidazole ring, but bearing an extended side chain which

FIGURE 238-4 Chemical structures of histamine and the H-2-receptor antagonists cimetidine, ranitidine, famotidine and nizatidine. Note the imidazole ring shared by histamine and cimetidine but absent in ranitidine, nizatidine, and famotidine.

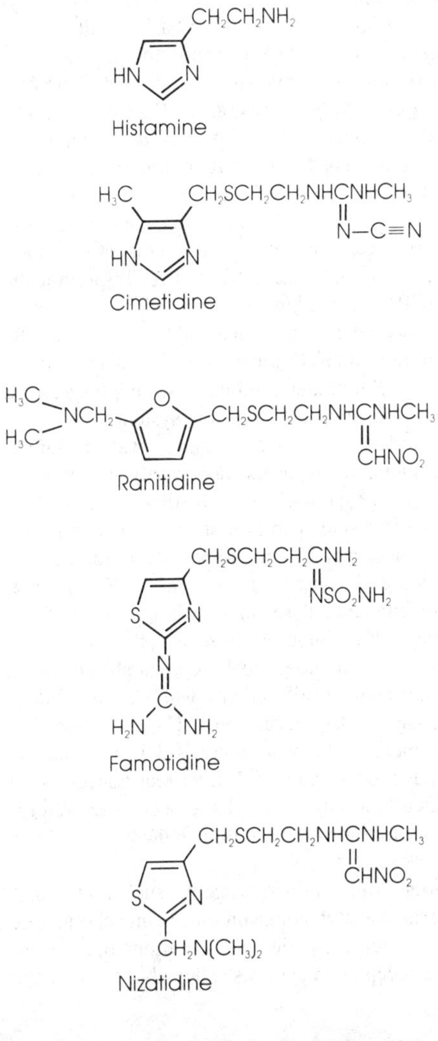

contains a cyanoguanidine group. Much of the information regarding the actions of H-2-receptor antagonist was obtained in the detailed characterization of the actions of cimetidine. Cimetidine (300 mg) was shown to inhibit basal acid secretion by more than 80 percent and meal-stimulated acid secretion by approximately 70 percent. It strikingly reduced acid secretory responses to histamine, caffeine, insulin, hypoglycemia, and gastrin, Cimetidine has been shown to be effective in promoting endoscopically verified duodenal ulcer healing. Initially the oral dose of cimetidine recommended and used in treatment of duodenal ulcer was 300 mg four times daily, with meals and at bedtime. More recently 400 mg cimetidine twice each day or 800 mg once daily has been shown to be equally effective. Treatment of active duodenal ulcer with cimetidine is continued for periods from 4 to 8 weeks. In patients with healed duodenal ulcer prolonged administration of cimetidine (400 mg at bedtime) has been shown to reduce substantially the frequency of duodenal ulcer recurrence.

Considering the enormous number of patients who have been treated with cimetidine, few serious adverse effects have been experienced. Slight and reversible increases in serum transaminase and creatinine levels may occur. Central nervous system abnormalities have been reported in a small number of patients with substantial hepatic-renal functional impairment. Brief increases in serum prolactin have been found after intravenous and oral cimetidine. Cimetidine has been shown to inhibit the cytochrome P_{450} hepatic enzyme system, and therefore may increase blood levels, duration of action, and pharmacologic effects of drugs metabolized by this system. Tender gynecomastia due to the weak antiandrogenic effect of cimetidine may occur in patients with the Zollinger-Ellison syndrome, who require large doses for prolonged periods of time.

Ranitidine, the second H-2-receptor antagonist made available for use, is also prescribed widely in treatment of patients with duodenal ulcer. It is a substituted aminomethylfuran which is structurally unrelated to histamine (Fig. 238-4). On a molar basis, ranitidine is about six times as potent as cimetidine in inhibiting gastric acid secretion. Cimetidine and ranitidine have similar half-lives, approximately 120 min. They appear to be comparably effective in accelerating healing of duodenal ulcer and in reducing duodenal ulcer recurrence. The initial recommended dose of ranitidine for treatment of duodenal ulcer was 150 mg twice each day; 300 mg at bedtime has been found to be equally effective. The maintenance dose for reducing duodenal ulcer recurrence is 150 mg once a day at bedtime. Ranitidine may increase levels of serum AST and ALT (previously designated SGOT and SGPT). There have been occasional reports of reversible hepatitis, hepatocellular, hepatocanalicular, or mixed, with or without jaundice, with ranitidine adminstration. It appears to have no antiandrogen properties. Ranitidine exhibits less inhibitory effect on the cytochrome P_{450} mixed oxygenase enzyme system.

The most recently introduced H-2-receptor antagonists are famotidine and nizatidine. *Famotidine* is an extraordinarily potent H-2-receptor antagonist, being approximately 8 to 10 times as potent as ranitidine in inhibiting gastric acid secretion. It contains a thiazole ring and is not related structurally to cimetidine or ranitidine (Fig. 238-4). The recommended daily dose of famotidine is 40 mg once daily at bedtime. The maintenance dose for prevention of duodenal ulcer recurrence is 20 mg/d at bedtime. *Nizatidine* is the latest H-2-receptor antagonist and has been shown to be comparable to other agents in this class in the treatment of patients with duodenal ulcer and in reduction of duodenal ulcer recurrence. The recommended once daily dose for treatment of duodenal ulcer is 300 mg, and the maintenance dose for reduction of duodenal ulcer recurrence is 150 mg at bedtime. Associated blood dyscrasias have been noted rarely, and hepatotoxicity, similar to that with ranitidine and cimetidine, has also been reported.

Anticholinergic agents Anticholinergic agents, such as atropine, act by inhibiting the effects of acetylcholine on muscarinic cholinergic receptors. These agents decrease gastric acid secretion, but are not nearly as effective as H-2-receptor antagonists. They also delay gastric emptying. Most studies have *not* shown that anticholinergic agents hasten healing or improve symptoms of duodenal ulcer; therefore, they are not recommended as primary agents for treatment for duodenal ulcer. Side effects include dryness of mouth, blurring of vision, cardiac arrhythmias, and urinary retention. They should not be used in patients with glaucoma, impaired gastric emptying, or history or symptoms of urinary retention. There are at least two classes of muscarinic cholinergic receptors (M-1 and M-2). *Pirenzepine* is a relatively selective anticholinergic agent, which is more specific in inhibiting gastric acid secretion, with fewer side effects, than other anticholinergic agents. Pirenzepine, not yet available for prescribing in the United States, has been shown to be effective in treatment of duodenal ulcer. It may prove useful as primary therapy or as adjunctive therapy in duodenal ulcer patients.

Coating agents Several drugs that act neither by neutralization nor by inhibition of gastric acid secretion have been used in treatment of duodenal ulcer. Among these is *sucralfate*, a complex polyaluminum hydroxide salt of sucrose sulfate. Sucralfate becomes highly polar at acid pH and binds to the ulcer bed for up to 12 h, whereas relatively little binds to intact gastric or duodenal mucosa. It is believed that adherence of sucralfate to granulation tissue impedes diffusion of H^+ to the base of the ulcer. In addition sucralfate binds bile acids and pepsins and may, therefore, reduce their injurious effects. Sucralfate may increase endogenous tissue prostaglandins and thereby increase mucosal defense. It is only minimally absorbed, with less than 5 percent appearing in the urine. Sucralfate appears to be similar to antacids and H-2-receptor antagonists in its effectiveness in treatment of duodenal ulcer and in prevention of duodenal ulcer recurrence. The recommended dose of sucralfate is 1 g 1 h before each meal and at bedtime. *Colloidal bismuth* compounds also aid ulcer healing. They form (in an acid medium) a bismuth-protein coagulant which is believed to protect the ulcer from acid-peptic digestion. Bismuth-containing compounds may also be of value in treatment of duodenal ulcer because of their effects on *H. pylori*, a bacterium which appears important in the pathogenesis of some form(s) of gastritis (see below) and, as noted previously, which has been proposed as a potential pathogenetic factor in the etiology of duodenal ulcer. Several duodenal and gastric ulcer trials have shown good healing rates and reduced ulcer recurrence rates in patients treated with colloidal bismuth subcitrate. Colloidal bismuth compounds appear to be the only class of antiulcer drugs that eradicate *H. pylori* and the gastritis associated with its colonization. Some investigators have found lower relapse rates in patients with duodenal ulcer after treatment with colloidal bismuth compared with H-2-receptor antagonists.

Prostaglandins A variety of *prostaglandins*, particularly those of the E series (PGE_1 and PGE_2), have been shown effective in clinical trials in treatment of duodenal ulcer, with healing rates comparable to those achieved with antacid therapy and H-2-receptor antagonists. Their action is believed to be twofold: (1) they reduce basal and stimulated gastric acid secretion, and (2) they enhance mucosal resistance to tissue injury. The principal mechanism by which exogenous prostaglandins enhance mucosal defense has not been clarified completely. However, they exert the following actions which appear important in mucosal defense to injury. PGEs (1) stimulate gastric mucus secretion, (2) stimulate gastric and duodenal bicarbonate secretion, (3) maintain gastric mucosal blood flow, (4) maintain the gastric mucosal barrier to back-diffusion of H^+, and (5) stimulate mucosal cellular renewal and regeneration.

Proton pump inhibition The final phase of hydrogen ion secretion by parietal cells is accomplished by an enzyme (H^+,K^+-ATPase) which serves as a proton pump, exchanging potassium for hydrogen. *Omeprazole*, a specific inhibitor of parietal call H^+,K^+-ATPase, has been shown to be extraordinarily potent in decreasing gastric acid secretion. Omeprazole binds to the H^+,K^+-ATPase, irreversibly inactivating the enzyme. This drug, currently being evaluated in clinical trials, is very effective in accelerating healing of common duodenal ulcers and ulcers in patients with gastrinoma (see below). Omeprazole is not yet approved for prescribing.

Diet With little or no justification, many different diet programs have been used for treatment of patients with duodenal ulcer. There is no evidence that bland diets reduce gastric acid secretion, promote healing, or relieve symptoms of duodenal ulcer. Similarly, soft diets or diets free of spices or fruit juices have not been proven to be of benefit. Although traditionally milk and cream have been prescribed in treatment of ulcer patients, there is no evidence that they benefit ulcer healing. They may contribute to development of the milk-alkali syndrome and may accelerate atherogenesis. Many physicians recommend that patients with duodenal ulcer avoid coffee, with or without caffeine, and other caffeine-containing beverages because of their effects on gastric secretion. It may also be desirable to restrict alcohol intake in these patients. It is reasonable to suggest that if patients experience symptoms after ingestion of certain foods, these foods should be avoided.

General therapeutic considerations How does one integrate the large amount of available information concerning treatment of duodenal ulcer in selecting a therapeutic program for individual patients? There are several reasonable alternatives: effective therapy may be based on neutralization of gastric acid by antacids, on inhibition of gastric acid secretion by antisecretory agents, or on local actions of some other agents. There is no evidence that combinations of these drugs are required in treatment of duodenal ulcer. The various classes of agents appear to be comparably effective in accelerating duodenal ulcer healing and in reducing ulcer recurrence. In general, although side effects differ from group to group, these are all safe and effective drugs. Most duodenal ulcers will heal within 4 or 6 weeks of treatment with each of these groups of agents. It is seldom necessary to continue treatment of active duodenal ulcer for more than 8 weeks.

There is not yet general agreement concerning which patients should receive prolonged maintenance therapy to reduce the frequency of duodenal ulcer recurrence. Most physicians do not initiate maintenance treatment after the first (uncomplicated) episode of duodenal ulcer activity. Maintenance therapy is often recommended in patients with frequent, especially severe, duodenal ulcer recurrences, in those with previous, especially recurrent, duodenal ulcer complications, and perhaps in those with troublesome ulcer disease and other medical conditions which would make ulcer complication or surgery particularly hazardous. Maintenance therapy, when recommended, is usually continued for at least 1 year. Elimination of cigarette smoking, in most studies, appears to facilitate ulcer healing and may reduce duodenal ulcer recurrence. There is no evidence that dietary manipulation plays an important role in duodenal ulcer treatment.

GASTRIC ULCER

The peak incidence for gastric ulcer is in the sixth decade, approximately 10 years later than for duodenal ulcer. Slightly more than half of gastric ulcers occur in males. Gastric ulcers are deep, penetrating beyond the mucosa of the stomach and are similar histologically to duodenal ulcer, but often with more extensive gastritis surrounding the ulcer. Almost all benign gastric ulcers are found immediately distal to the junction of the antral mucosa with the acid-secreting mucosa of the body of the stomach. The location of this junction is variable, especially on the lesser gastric curvature. In general, the antrum extends approximately two-thirds of the way up the lesser curvature and one-third of the way up the greater curvature of the stomach. Benign gastric ulcers are rare in the fundus of the stomach. Benign gastric ulcers are virtually always accompanied by antral gastritis with variable amounts of mucosal atrophy. Gastritis may be present or absent with aspirin-associated gastric ulcers; they are usually located in the antrum, but they are not confined to the junction of the antral and parietal cell mucosa, as are common gastric ulcers.

ETIOLOGY AND PATHOGENESIS Acid-pepsin appears to be important in the pathogenesis of gastric ulcer; however, in contrast to duodenal ulcer, gastric ulcer patients generally have acid secretory rates that are normal or reduced compared with nonulcer subjects. Although many patients with gastric ulcer have reduced rates of acid secretion, true achlorhydria (in response to pentagastrin stimulation) almost never occurs in patients with benign gastric ulcer. Ten to twenty percent of patients with gastric ulcers also have duodenal ulcers. Patients with both duodenal and gastric ulcers tend to have acid secretory patterns that parallel those of duodenal ulcer. Patients with pyloric channel ulcers have acid secretory rates and clinical patterns similar to those found with common duodenal ulcer.

Most evidence supports the primary importance of defective gastric mucosal resistance and/or direct gastric mucosal injury as most important elements in the pathogenesis of gastric ulcer. Unlike duodenal ulcer, serum gastrin levels are increased in a significant proportion of gastric ulcer patients, but increases are limited to those with gastric acid hyposecretion. Gastric emptying has been shown to be delayed in gastric ulcer. It has been suggested that regurgitation of duodenal contents, especially those containing bile, may induce gastric mucosal injury and subsequent gastric ulceration by interruption of the gastric mucosal barrier with resultant back diffusion of secreted hydrogen ions.

CLINICAL FEATURES As with duodenal ulcer, epigastric pain is the most common symptom; however, it is less typical and predictable than in patients with duodenal ulcer. Some gastric ulcer patients experience no relief of pain with eating. Pain may actually be precipitated or accentuated by food, and relief of symptoms with antacids is less consistent than with duodenal ulcers. Gastric ulcers tend to heal, but then recur, often in the same location. Recognizable episodes of recurrent gastric ulcer activity are, in general, less frequent than those of duodenal ulcer. The precise incidence of gastric ulcer is not known, since many gastric ulcer patients are asymptomatic. Although duodenal ulcer is identified clinically more frequently than gastric ulcer, most autopsy studies show an equal or greater proportion of gastric ulcers. This may be due in part to acute preterminal events, but also may reflect the often asymptomatic clinical course of gastric ulcer. Whereas in duodenal ulcer patients nausea and vomiting almost always indicate gastric outlet obstruction, in patients with gastric ulcer they may occur in the absence of mechanical obstruction. Weight loss may occur due to anorexia or aversion to food due to discomfort produced by eating.

Hemorrhage is a common complication, occurring in approximately 25 percent. Mortality is greater in patients with gastric ulcer than with duodenal ulcer. Gastric ulcer perforation occurs less frequently than hemorrhage. Mortality with perforation of gastric ulcers is approximately three times that with duodenal ulcers. Increased mortality is due in part to the increased age of gastric ulcer patients, but also may result from uncertainty and delay in diagnosis and from greater soilage of the peritoneum with gastric ulcer perforation. Gastric outlet obstruction may develop when ulcers are in the pyloric channel or in the most distal antrum but is rare with ulcer in other parts of the stomach.

DIAGNOSIS The history is of value in suspecting gastric ulcer, but it is not as characteristic as in duodenal ulcer. The two major methods for diagnosis are barium examination and endoscopy. Gastric ulcer can usually be identified by standard barium examination with an accuracy that approaches 90 percent. Both benign and malignant gastric ulcers are more common on the lesser than on the greater curvature (Fig. 238-5). Radiation of gastric mucosal folds from the margin of the ulcer crater suggests a benign lesion. Large gastric ulcers, i.e., those greater than 3 cm in diameter, are more often malignant than smaller ones. An ulcer within a mass, as defined radiographically, also suggests malignancy. Approximately 4 percent of gastric ulcers which appear benign radiographically prove to be malignant (by endoscopic biopsy or at surgery). Because of false-positive and false-negative errors, radiographic appearance cannot be used as the sole criterion for the benign or malignant nature of a gastric ulcer.

Endoscopic visualization of the ulcer allows definition of its size,

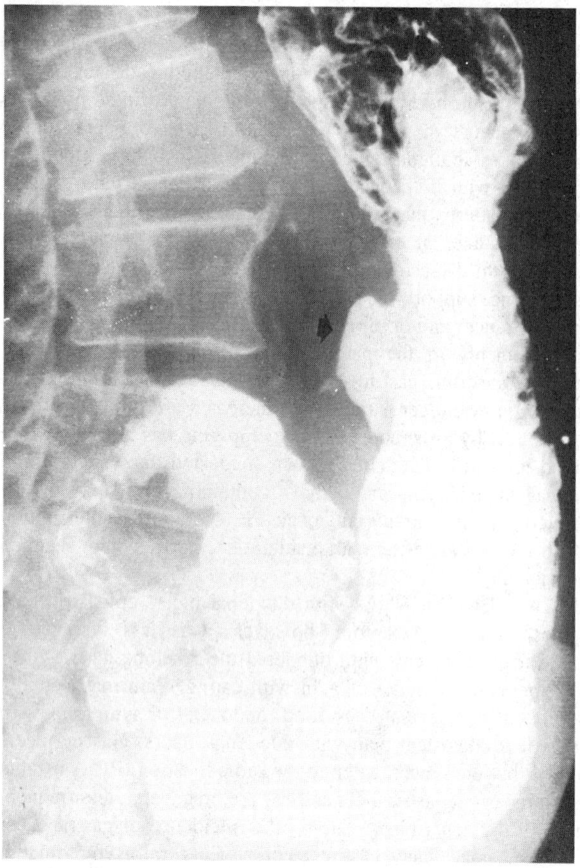

FIGURE 238-5 Benign lesser curvature gastric ulcer. Note ulceration beyond the projected margins of the stomach and the collar of edema.

location, and, by biopsy, its histologic characteristics. At gastroscopy a total of at least six biopsies should be obtained from the inner margin of the ulcer and from the ulcer bed. If accurate cytology is available, brushings of the ulcer should be obtained prior to biopsy. By application of combined radiographic, endoscopic, and histologic techniques, distinguishing a malignant from a benign gastric ulcer should be possible with substantially more than 95 percent confidence.

Gastric ulcer with pentagastrin-fast achlorhydria is rare. When it occurs it almost always indicates gastric carcinoma. However, most patients with gastric carcinoma (about two-thirds to three-fourths) are capable of secreting some gastric acid, although usually less than normal.

MEDICAL TREATMENT In general, with whatever medical treatment modality is selected gastric ulcers tend to heal more slowly than duodenal ulcers, and the healing response rates are somewhat less than those for duodenal ulcer. *Antacids* are effective in gastric ulcer treatment. However, since acid hypersecretion is not characteristic of the disease, smaller doses of antacid may be required than for treatment of duodenal ulcer. *H-2-receptor antagonists* and *sucralfate* are approximately as effective as antacid therapy in the treatment of gastric ulcer. The dosage schedules used for these drugs are similar to those for patients with duodenal ulcer.

Anticholinergic agents have been recommended by some physicians. However, because of substantial side effects of anticholinergic drugs, their tendency to reduce gastric emptying which is already impaired in these patients, the fact that gastric ulcer patients are often older and, therefore, more susceptible to the complications of these agents, and the lack of evidence for their benefit, the use of anticholinergic drugs in gastric ulcer treatment does not appear justified. Some studies have suggested that hospitalization and/or cessation of smoking are of benefit in gastric ulcer healing.

Since salicylates and other nonsteroidal anti-inflammatory drugs (NSAIDs) have been associated with the development of gastric ulcers, patients with gastric ulcer should not ingest these or should be treated with the lowest doses required. Alcohol, because of its injurious effects on the gastric mucosa, should probably also be avoided. Milk and cream, as well as bland or homogenized diets, have not been shown to be of value in treatment. In general, it is probably sufficient to recommend that patients consume a diet of their own choice. Since coffee (caffeine-containing or caffeine-free) and other caffeine-containing liquids stimulate gastric acid secretion, it may be desirable to avoid these beverages.

Carbenoxolone has been used in many countries (though it is not available in the United States) in the treatment of gastric ulcer. This drug is a hydrolytic produce of glycyrrhizic acid (derived from licorice) and has been shown to decrease symptoms and increase the rate of gastric ulcer healing. Carbenoxolone does not decrease gastric acid secretion but increases the life span of gastric mucosal epithelial cells and increases the secretion and viscosity of gastric mucus. Carbenoxolone possesses aldosterone-like effects, so sodium and water retention tend to occur. It is possible to inhibit the aldosterone-like effects of carbenoxolone by use of aldosterone antagonists; however, the latter also abolish the ulcer-healing effect of carbenoxolone. Problems with sodium and water retention and availability of alternative drugs have led to its decreased use worldwide.

Benign gastric ulcers should heal completely within 3 months of vigorous therapy. The failure of gastric ulcer to decrease satisfactorily in size and to heal with medical treatment has been used to suggest gastric malignancy. The following is suggested as one reasonable scheme to monitor gastric ulcer healing. Upper gastrointestinal barium examination or gastroscopy is suggested after 4 weeks of treatment, at which time definite healing of benign gastric ulcers should be demonstrable: the diameter of most ulcers should be reduced by more than 50 percent. If not, malignancy must be suspected and exfoliative cytology and biopsies of the ulcer should be performed. If no malignancy is identified, medical therapy should be continued. If the ulcer has not healed completely at 8 weeks, endoscopic examination should be repeated in another month, at which time most benign gastric ulcers should have healed. In general, large gastric ulcers heal more slowly than smaller ones. It is important to continue treatment to endoscopically verified complete ulcer healing. One must be alert, however, for the occasional "healing" of an ulcerating gastric carcinoma with treatment. Apparently complete healing does not guarantee the benign nature of a gastric ulcer, since approximately 70 percent of gastric ulcers eventually found to be malignant will undergo significant (albeit usually incomplete) healing with medical treatment.

COMPLICATIONS AND SURGERY FOR PEPTIC ULCER

Surgery is reserved for patients with complications of peptic ulcer and for those who do not respond to vigorous and attentive medical treatment. Complications include hemorrhage, obstruction, and perforation.

Hemorrhage occurs in approximately 15 percent of patients with duodenal ulcers; a recurrence of bleeding is estimated to occur in about 40 percent of patients with an initial hemorrhage. In most patients hemorrhage from peptic ulcer responds satisfactorily to medical management, including gastric suction and antacid or H-2-receptor antagonist administration.

Free *perforation* into the peritoneal cavity occurs in approximately 6 percent of patients with duodenal ulcer. Five to ten percent of these patients will have had no recognizable ulcer symptoms prior to perforation. Simultaneous hemorrhage occurs in approximately 10 percent of patients with duodenal ulcer perforation; mortality is greatly increased in this group. Duodenal ulcers, especially those located posteriorly, may penetrate into adjacent structures, most often the pancreas, frequently resulting in increased serum amylase levels. Less commonly, duodenal ulcers may penetrate into the liver, biliary tract, or colon.

Gastric outlet *obstruction* occurs in 2 to 4 percent of patients admitted to the hospital with duodenal or pyloric channel ulcers. Symptoms include abdominal bloating, nausea, vomiting, and weight loss. These patients usually have had ulcer symptoms for many years and often obstructive symptoms for several months.

Failure to respond satisfactorily to medical treatment requires consideration of surgery. The true incidence of lack of ulcer healing with vigorous medical programs is not known. It is clear that, especially with currently available drugs, the vast majority of patients with peptic ulcer can be treated successfully without surgery.

Decisions regarding surgery for patients with complications of peptic ulcer must be individualized. Risks of surgery must be balanced against risks of the disease. The patient's discomfort, costs of medical care and hospitalization, and time lost from work must be examined in relation to the morbidity and possible mortality associated with surgery and anesthesia, risks of recurrent ulcer, and long-term postoperative sequelae. The skill and experience of the surgeon must be weighed as major factors in considering operation.

SURGERY FOR DUODENAL ULCER No single surgical procedure has been accepted universally as the most satisfactory duodenal ulcer operation. At present the most commonly performed surgical procedures are *vagotomy with antrectomy, vagotomy with pyloroplasty, and parietal cell vagotomy* (also referred to as *proximal gastric or superselective vagotomy*) without a gastric drainage procedure.

With conventional (truncal) vagotomy and antrectomy, the vagal trunks are transected, the antrum is removed, and gastrointestinal continuity is reestablished by anastomosis of the remaining stomach with the proximal duodenum (Billroth I anastomosis) or with a loop of the jejunum (Billroth II anastomosis). Vagotomy and antrectomy is an effective procedure with a low recurrence rate (approximately 1 percent). Morbidity and mortality with vagotomy and antrectomy are variable, depending upon patient selection and the skill of the surgeon, but are probably slightly greater than with vagotomy and pyloroplasty.

When the procedure of vagotomy and pyloroplasty is selected, pyloroplasty is performed to facilitate gastric drainage after truncal or selective vagotomy. Vagotomy is performed to inhibit vagal stimulation of gastric acid secretion. Vagotomy does not inhibit gastrin release; in fact, release of gastrin is enhanced after vagal interruption. Three types of vagotomy are now used in the surgical treatment of duodenal or pyloric channel ulcer, namely, *truncal vagotomy, selective vagotomy*, and *parietal call vagotomy*. Pyloroplasty with truncal vagotomy is associated with approximately 1 percent mortality. Ulcer recurrence during the 5 years after surgery is about 5 to 8 percent. With selective vagotomy only the branches of the vagus that supply the stomach are transected, preserving the vagal innervation of the other abdominal viscera. Selective vagotomy has been found by some surgeons to result in a more complete vagotomy, less ulcer recurrence, and fewer postvagotomy complications than truncal vagotomy. Parietal cell vagotomy denervates only the acid-secreting portion of the stomach, sparing the branches of the vagus that innervate the antrum, which makes a gastric drainage procedure (e.g., pyloroplasty) unnecessary. Both immediate and late postoperative complications are less common with parietal cell vagotomy than with truncal vagotomy, and reductions in acid secretion are similar to those achieved with truncal or selective vagotomy. Mortality with parietal cell vagotomy is less than 1 percent. Most studies indicate that with experience, recurrence is comparable to that of other forms of vagotomy with pyloroplasty. This procedure, which is being used with increasing frequency, appears to be a safe and effective surgical therapy.

SURGERY FOR GASTRIC ULCER Surgical treatment is required for gastric ulcer patients who do not respond satisfactorily to medical therapy or who develop complications similar to those described for duodenal ulcer. With the available diagnostic accuracy of careful radiographic examination, endoscopy, biopsy of the ulcer margins, and exfoliative cytology, it should rarely be necessary to operate because of remaining uncertainty regarding the malignant or benign nature of the ulcer. The recommended surgical procedure for the treatment of gastric ulcer is antrectomy with gastroduodenal (Billroth I) anastomosis. It is not necessary to perform a vagotomy when antrectomy is performed by gastric ulcer (not located in the pyloric channel).

CONSEQUENCES AND SYNDROMES AFTER PEPTIC ULCER SURGERY

Modern surgery for peptic ulcer is effective in the treatment of ulcer complications and in the prevention of ulcer recurrence. However, numerous postoperative sequelae and syndromes may occur.

RECURRENT ULCERATION Recurrent ulceration has been reported in approximately 5 percent of all patients after surgery for peptic ulcer. Approximately 95 percent of these recurrences follow surgery for duodenal ulcer disease. The risk of development of recurrent ulcer is 3 to 10 percent after surgery for duodenal ulcer and approximately 2 percent after gastric ulcer surgery. Recurrence is more common after vagotomy and pyloroplasty and after parietal cell vagotomy than after vagotomy and antrectomy. When ulcers occur after partial gastric resection, the ulcer is usually located at the anastomosis (stomal or marginal ulcer) or immediately distal to it in the small intestine. Abdominal pain is the most common symptom in patients with a stomal ulcer. The pain is usually epigastric but is often not characteristic of common duodenal ulcer. It is usually, but not always, relieved by meals or antacids and, in general, tends to be more persistent and progressive than that observed with unoperated duodenal ulcer. Hemorrhage or anemia due to blood loss, nausea and vomiting from obstruction, weight loss, or symptoms from perforation may occur. The development of a stomal ulcer after duodenal ulcer surgery usually indicates that an incomplete vagotomy was performed. Inadequate gastric resection, when performed without vagotomy, may also result in stomal ulceration. Additional causes for the development of recurrent ulcer include an excessively long jejunal afferent loop, and inadvertently performed gastroileal or gastrocolic anastomosis, poor gastric drainage, and ingestion of ulcerogenic drugs. Less commonly, a marginal ulcer may be caused by acid hypersecretion secondary to gastrinoma or a retained antrum.

Radiographic examination with barium is of limited diagnostic value and identifies only from 50 to 65 percent of stomal ulcerations. Surgical deformity at the anastomotic site often may mimic stomal ulcer in its absence or conceal it when present. When suspected, endoscopic examination is required to identify stomal ulceration. Medical treatment with antacids is almost always unsatisfactory in patients with stomal ulcer. H-2-receptor antagonists have been used successfully to induce healing of stomal ulcers. The long-term effectiveness of these agents on stomal ulcers and prevention of their recurrence remain to be established. Surgery is usually necessary for treatment of ulcer recurrence, and it is usually, but not invariably, successful. In patients with recurrent ulcer provocative testing with measurements of serum gastrin should be performed to identify or exclude gastrinoma (see below).

RECURRENT ULCER DUE TO RETAINED ANTRUM Recurrent ulcers have been described in a small number of patients after antrectomy with gastrojejunostomy (Billroth II anastomosis) in which the antral resection was not complete. In these patients the distal antrum, inadvertently not resected, remains in continuity with the duodenum after surgery. These patients usually develop or continue to have gastric acid hypersecretion due to gastrin release by the residual antral mucosa which is no longer in contact with gastric acid, the normal inhibitor of gastrin release. In these patients fasting serum gastrin levels may be normal to moderately increased. Patients with retained antrum can be distinguished from those with gastrinoma by intravenous injection of secretion with measurements of serum gastrin. Gastrinoma patients exhibit substantial increases in serum gastrin, whereas in those with retained antrum, serum gastrin levels

TABLE 238-1 Provocative gastrin tests

Disorder	Serum gastrin response (change from basal levels) After IV secretion injection	After test meal
Zollinger-Ellison (gastrinoma)	Increase (greater than 200 pg/mL)	Little or no increase (increases less than 50%)
Common duodenal ulcer	No change, slight decrease, or small increase	Moderate increase (may be slightly more than normal, but less than in gastrin cell hyperplasia)
Antral gastrin cell hyperplasia	No change, slight decrease, or small increase	Striking increase (greater than 200%)
Achlorhydria (e.g., pernicious anemia, chronic gastritis)	No change, slight decrease, or small increase	Moderate increase

decrease after secretin adminstration (see Table 238-1). These patients can be treated successfully by surgical removal of the remaining antrum.

AFFERENT LOOP SYNDROMES Patients with partial gastric resection with gastrojejunostomy (Billroth II anastomosis) may experience abdominal bloating and pain 20 min to 1 h after eating, frequently followed by nausea and vomiting. The vomitus often contains large amounts of bile. Characteristically, the bloating and abdominal discomfort are relieved by vomiting. This type of afferent loop syndrome, which is uncommon, is believed to be caused by distention of an incompletely draining afferent intestinal loop by pancreatic and biliary secretions which are stimulated by eating. Serum amylase levels may be mildly or moderately increased. Because of partial obstruction it is often difficult to demonstrate the afferent loop by barium meal examination. Treatment is surgical correction of the incomplete afferent loop obstruction, and, in some instances, revision to a gastroduodenal anastomosis.

A second form of afferent loop dysfunction is that due to stasis with bacterial overgrowth within the afferent loop. These patients may exhibit the same characteristics as are found with other forms of small intestinal bacterial overgrowth or blind loop syndromes (see Chap. 240). These include malabsorption, especially of fat and vitamin B_{12}. Correction of the afferent loop bacterial overgrowth syndrome can be accomplished by surgical revision of the afferent loop.

BILE REFLUX GASTRITIS After peptic ulcer surgery a small proportion of patients experience early satiety, abdominal discomfort, and vomiting, which is believed due to reflux of duodenal contents into the stomach. Endoscopic examination usually reveals regurgitated bile in the stomach and diffuse gastritis, often involving the entire gastric remnant. Various terms assigned to this entity include *alkaline reflux gastritis, bile reflux gastritis, duodenogastric reflux*, and *bilious vomiting*. The mechanisms or materials contained in the refluxed intestinal contents accounting for these symptoms have not been defined. Although the term bile reflux gastritis has been used, there is no certainty that regurgitated bile is responsible for the syndrome. Administration of cholestyramine, intended to bind bile acids and facilitate their excretion, has not been of benefit in this disorder. Some surgeons have reported successful treatment of bile reflux gastritis by diversion of duodenal contents from proximity to the stomach with a Roux en Y anastomosis.

DUMPING SYNDROME Following peptic ulcer surgery some patients experience an assortment of vasomotor symptoms after eating. These include palpitation, tachycardia, lightheadedness, diaphoresis, and less frequently, postural hypotension. Abdominal discomfort and vomiting may also occur. The vasomotor symptoms, referred to as the *early dumping syndrome*, are usually experienced within 30 min after eating and are believed to result from rapid emptying of hyperosmolar gastric contents into the proximal small intestine. This leads to a shift of fluid into the gut lumen and produces intestinal distention and contraction of plasma volume. Additional proposed mechanisms for these symptoms include stimulation of autonomic reflexes secondary to small intestinal distention and/or release of hormones from the gut in response to rapid entry of gastric contents into the duodenum or jejunum.

The *late dumping syndrome* refers to a symptom complex comprising dizziness, lightheadedness, palpitation, diaphoresis, confusion, and, in rare instances, syncope, occurring 90 min to 3 h after eating. The symptoms can often be precipitated by meals rich in simple carbohydrates, especially sucrose. The syndrome appears to be caused by hypoglycemia due to insulin release stimulated by abrupt increases in blood glucose secondary to rapid emptying of sugar-containing meals into the proximal small intestine.

Both forms of the dumping syndrome are treated by dietary measures. These include limitation of simple sugar-continuing liquids and solids (sweets), elimination of liquids at mealtime, and frequent small meals. Most patients have not been benefited by surgical procedures such as creation of reversed jejunal loops and isoperistaltic jejunal interposition.

POSTVAGOTOMY DIARRHEA A significant number of patients experience diarrhea after peptic ulcer surgery, especially with a procedure including truncal vagotomy. Diarrhea usually occurs within 2 h of eating. Although the mechanism is not clear, interruption of vagal fibers to the abdominal viscera appears to play an important role in the production of the diarrhea. The surgical drainage procedure, pyloroplasty or antrectomy, which removes the pyloric regulatory emptying mechanism, may also contribute to the diarrhea. Diarrhea has been estimated to occur in 20 to 30 percent of patients after truncal vagotomy with drainage, in 10 to 20 percent with selective vagotomy and drainage, and in only 1 to 8 percent of those with parietal cell vagotomy (without drainage). Rapid emptying of gastric contents into the small intestine, resulting in increased fluid volume within the intestinal lumen, due to the osmotic action of the meal, may also contribute to the diarrhea.

HEMATOLOGIC COMPLICATIONS Intrinsic factor secreted by gastric parietal cells is necessary for active absorption of vitamin B_{12} by the distal ileum. Patients who have had total gastrectomy invariably will develop malabsorption of vitamin B_{12} and should receive monthly intramuscular injections of vitamin B_{12} (50 to 100 μg) indefinitely. Megaloblastic anemia due to vitamin B_{12} deficiency is rare after partial gastric resection; however, reduced serum vitamin B_{12} levels have been observed in about 14 percent of these patients. Even more rarely vitamin B_{12} deficiency may be produced by bacterial overgrowth in a stagnant afferent loop following Billroth II anastomosis. Gastritis in the remaining stomach develops in more than 60 percent of duodenal ulcer patients after vagotomy and antrectomy or vagotomy and pyloroplasty. This may result in decreased vitamin B_{12} absorption. Inasmuch as the stomach secretes intrinsic factor in excess of need by approximately 100 times, peptic ulcer patients treated with partial gastric resection do not develop vitamin B_{12} deficiency secondary to the amount of stomach resected. (In addition, the resected portion of the stomach is almost always principally antrum, which contains few parietal cells.) However, after peptic ulcer surgery patients may develop decreased serum vitamin B_{12} levels due to reduced absorption of food-bound vitamin B_{12}; these patients will often have normal absorption of free vitamin B_{12}, as used in the Schilling test. The precise mechanism of the malabsorption of food-bound vitamin B_{12} is not known. It may be due in part to rapid emptying of gastric contents, with reduced efficiency of intrinsic factor binding of vitamin B_{12}. Anemia after peptic ulcer surgery may also result from deficiency produced by malabsorption of iron or folate. A combined deficiency of vitamin B_{12}, iron, and folate is common in patients with anemia following partial or subtotal gastric resection. Iron deficiency is the most common single hematologic defect after peptic ulcer surgery and may result from either blood loss (e.g., with persistent or recurrent ulcers) or from iron malabsorption. Patients with gastric resection malabsorb dietary iron but have normal absorption of iron salts;

therefore they will respond favorably to treatment with therapeutic oral iron preparations. Folate deficiency may result from either reduced dietary intake or impaired folate absorption. Except for the anemia produced by blood loss in association with early recurrent ulcer disease, the development of anemia after peptic ulcer surgery is gradual, usually occurring several years postoperatively.

The nature of the anemia after ulcer surgery should be clarified by determination of the red blood cell morphology and by measurements of serum iron, folate, and vitamin B_{12}. Iron or folate deficiency may be treated by oral replacement. Vitamin B_{12} deficiency should be treated with monthly intramuscular injections of the vitamin.

OSTEOMALACIA AND OSTEOPOROSIS Osteoporosis and osteomalacia may develop after partial or complete gastrectomy but occur rarely after vagotomy and pyloroplasty. Osteomalacia is extremely frequent following gastrojejunostomy or Billroth II anastomosis. These bone changes are believed to result from malabsorption of calcium and vitamin D. Patients may develop bone pain and have pathologic fractures. The incidence of bone fractures in men following gastric resection has been estimated to be almost twice that of control subjects of similar age. Reduced bone density requires years to develop and can be identified by x-ray. Patients with osteomalacia usually have increased levels of serum alkaline phosphatase and may have reduced serum calcium concentrations. These patients should be treated by supplemental oral vitamin D and calcium. In fact, the frequency of osteoporosis and osteomalacia after partial or complete gastrectomy is sufficiently great that treatment with vitamin D and calcium should probably be instituted and continued indefinitely in these patients, especially females, following gastric resection.

GENERAL MALABSORPTION (See Chap. 240) Mild, chemically demonstrable steatorrhea is common in patients after ulcer surgery. Weight loss is more common after partial gastric resection than with vagotomy without resection and occurs in approximately 60 percent of patients in whom a portion of the stomach has been removed. The major cause of weight loss after peptic ulcer surgery is reduced food intake. On a 100-g fat diet, loss of stool fat seldom exceeds 15 g per day (normal individuals, less than 7 g per day). The causes of maldigestion and malabsorption after peptic ulcer surgery include rapid gastric emptying, reduced dispersion of food in the stomach, reduced bile concentrations in the gut lumen, increased rate of transit of the meal through the small intestine, and reduced or delayed pancreatic secretory responses to feeding. Steatorrhea and weight loss, sometimes accompanied by vitamin B_{12} malabsorption, may develop as a result of bacterial overgrowth, especially in patients with afferent loop bacterial stasis. Overt symptoms and other manifestations of malabsorption appearing after surgery for peptic ulcer may also be due to other preexisting conditions, including latent celiac sprue and chronic pancreatitis.

CARCINOMA AFTER PARTIAL GASTRECTOMY Several studies have documented an increased incidence of adenocarcinoma of the stomach in duodenal ulcer patients following partial gastric resection and after vagotomy and drainage without resection. This usually develops 10 or more years after ulcer surgery. The possibility of carcinoma of the stomach should be considered when abdominal symptoms, which may be similar to or distinct from those due to the original ulcer, appear many years after apparently successful surgery.

ZOLLINGER-ELLISON SYNDROME (GASTRINOMA)

In 1955 Zollinger and Ellison described the syndrome that bears their names, which consists of ulcer disease of the upper gastrointestinal tract, marked increases in gastric acid secretion, and nonbeta islet cell tumors of the pancreas.

ETIOLOGY AND PATHOGENESIS Zollinger and Ellison, in their original description of the syndrome, suggested that the ulcer disease in these patients resulted from release of a secretagogue from these tumors into the circulation which accounted for the often enormously increased rates of gastric acid secretion. Their proposal proved correct when in 1960 extracts of Zollinger-Ellison (Z-E) tumors were shown to stimulate gastric acid secretion. Subsequently, it was found that these pancreatic islet cell tumors contained gastrin and that there were large amounts of this hormone in the circulation producing the pathophysiologic characteristics of the syndrome. These gastrin-containing tumors are therefore now called *gastrinomas*.

Most gastrinomas are found within the pancreas. Pancreatic gastrinomas may vary in size from 2 mm to more than 20 cm in diameter. Multiple, apparently primary tumors are common. In from one-half to two-thirds of patients multiple gastrinomas are in the pancreas; however, more than half are not identified at surgery. Pancreatic gastrinomas are most common in the head of the pancreas. Approximately 13 percent of patients with this syndrome have tumors in the wall of the duodenum, especially in its second portion. Gastrinomas have also been located less commonly in other sites, including the hilum of the spleen and rarely in the stomach. Primary gastrinomas, surrounded by lymphoid tissue, have been found in proximity to the pancreas, proximal duodenum, and spleen. These may be confused with, but are distinct from, metastasis to regional lymph nodes. In rare instances, the Z-E syndrome has resulted from other gastrin-containing tumors, e.g., parathyroid and ovarian adenomas. About two-thirds are histologically or biologically malignant. Malignant gastrinomas usually grow slowly; however, a small portion may be rapidly invasive and may metastasize early and widely. Metastasis is most common to regional lymph nodes and liver; spread may also be to peritoneal surfaces, spleen, bone, skin, or mediastinum. Gastrinomas have light-microscopic similarities to carcinoid tumors and may be mistaken for carcinoid tumors, especially when they arise from the mucosa of the small intestine or stomach. Pancreatic islet cell hyperplasia occurs in approximately 10 percent of patients with the Z-E syndrome. Hyperplasia of the islets, accompanying recognized or unidentified gastrinoma, appears to be an association or a consequence, rather than a cause, of excess gastrin release, since gastrin is not present in the hyperplastic tissue.

In 20 to 25 percent of patients with the Z-E syndrome, the gastrinoma is a component of the multiple endocrine neoplasia type I (MEN I) syndrome, an autosomal dominant disorder with a high degree of penetrance and great variability in expressivity. Patients with MEN I may have hyperplasia, adenomas, or carcinoma involving, in order of frequency, the parathyroid glands, pancreatic islets, and pituitary. Hyperparathyroidism is present in 87 percent of patients with MEN I syndrome, and gastrinoma is present in approximately half of these patients (see Chap. 325).

In most gastrinomas approximately 80 to 95 percent of gastrin is in the form of heptadecapeptide gastrin (G-17), with most of the remainder being G-34. In contrast, approximately two-thirds of circulating gastrin in gastrinoma patients is G-34; most of the remainder is G-17. However, smaller amounts of even larger forms of gastrin and smaller gastrin fragments can be detected in the serum. When sought for, almost all gastrin secreting islet cell tumors are found to contain multiple hormones, which are usually clinically silent. These have included, among others, ACTH, glucagon, melanocyte-stimulating hormone, parathyroid hormone, growth hormone releasing factor (GRF), insulin, pancreatic polypeptide, and vasoactive intestinal peptide. Of these ACTH is the most common; it is found in approximately 30 percent of gastrin-secreting tumors in patients with the Z-E syndrome. Cushing's syndrome with increased serum ACTH levels has been reported in 8 percent of 75 Z-E patients. ACTH-releasing gastrinomas are often aggressively malignant. Alternatively, in patients with gastrinoma associated with MEN I, Cushing's syndrome may result from ACTH release from associated pituitary tumors; the symptoms of Cushing's syndrome are generally mild and the gastrinomas are usually not metastatic. Approximately one-third of patients with gastrinomas have increases in serum concentrations of *pancreatic polypeptide*.

The parietal cell mass is substantially expanded to from three to six times normal, secondary to the tropic effects of circulating gastrin on parietal cells. Small, multicentric, noninvasive carcinoid tumors have been identified in the gastric mucosa of patients with the Z-E syndrome. These tumors and associated focal areas of enterochromatin-like (ECL) cell hyperplasia are believed to represent consequences of substantial and sustained hypergastrinemia. They have also been found in the gastric mucosa of patients with pernicious anemia, in which substantial increases in serum gastrin are found in the absence of gastric acid secretion.

While the true incidence of the Z-E syndrome is not known, estimates are that it accounts for 0.1 to 1 percent of peptic ulcers. The Z-E syndrome may occur at any age, but initial manifestations are most common between ages 30 and 60.

CLINICAL FEATURES From 90 to 95 percent of patients with gastrinomas develop ulceration of the gastrointestinal tract at some point during the course of their disease. Profound gastric acid hypersecretion is found in most, but not all, patients. Especially early in the course of the disease symptoms are usually similar to those of patients with typical peptic ulcer. However, ulcer symptoms may be more fulminant, progressive, and persistent, and, in general, respond poorly to the usual medical and surgical peptic ulcer treatment programs. The anatomic site of the ulcers in patients with gastrinoma is similar, but not identical, to that of patients with common types of peptic ulcer. About 75 percent of gastrinoma patients have ulcers in the first portion of the duodenum or in the stomach; these are usually single, but may be multiple. When multiple ulcers occur, they are frequently located not only in the first portion of the duodenum, the site of common duodenal ulcer, but also in the remainder of the duodenum or even the jejunum. In one large series, 14 percent of the ulcers were in the duodenum beyond its first portion and 11 percent in the jejunum.

Diarrhea occurs in about 40 percent of patients, and about 7 percent of patients with gastrinoma have diarrhea in the absence of ulcer disease. The diarrhea is due to the outpouring of large amounts of hydrochloric acid into the proximal duodenum and can be reduced or eliminated by aspiration of gastric juice. The excessive acid has been shown to reduce the pH of the contents of the proximal and distal jejunum to as low as 1 and 3.6, respectively. Inflammatory changes may be produced in the mucosa of the small intestine, secondary to the injurious effect of large amounts of acid and pepsin. Steatorrhea, which is less common than diarrhea, results from inactivation of pancreatic lipase by large concentrations of acid in the proximal small intestine and from decreases in luminal bile acids. The decrease in intraluminal bile acid concentration is caused by precipitation of the major bile acids at low pH. This then leads to impaired micelle formation, which, in turn, reduces intestinal absorption of fatty acids and monoglycerides (see Chap. 240). Vitamin B_{12} malabsorption, not correctable by addition of intrinsic factor, has been detected in some patients with the Z-E syndrome. Although gastric secretion of intrinsic factor appears normal, the reduced pH within the gut interferes with intrinsic factor–mediated vitamin B_{12} absorption. This can be corrected by neutralization of the intestinal contents. The mechanism by which low pH in the gut interferes with intrinsic factor action is not known.

DIAGNOSIS The presence of gastrinoma should be suspected in patients with a compatible clinical history, especially in those with marked acid hypersecretion. Two-thirds of gastrinoma patients have basal gastric acid outputs (BAO) that exceed 15 mmol/h. In some instances the basal output may be greater than 100 mmol/h. However, there is substantial overlap in rates of gastric acid secretion among patients with gastrinoma and duodenal ulcer and normal subjects. Gastrinoma patients often have BAO rates that are greater than 60 percent of those induced by maximal stimulation (MAO). In most normal subjects and duodenal ulcer patients basal acid secretory rates are less than 60 percent of maximal secretion. However, because of frequent exceptions to these guidelines in patients with gastrinomas and common duodenal ulcers, the use of the BAO/MAO ratio is of no value in the certain identification of patients with gastrinoma.

Some radiographic features may suggest the diagnosis of the Z-E syndrome. Large mucosal folds may be demonstrated most prominently in the stomach, but also in the duodenum, and, in some instances, the jejunum. The lumen of the stomach and small intestine often contains large amounts of fluid. Radiographic features of most ulcers in these patients, except when they are multiple and/or distal in location, are similar to those of common peptic ulcer. Gastrinomas are difficult to localize. In almost half of patients with clinical and laboratory evidence the tumors cannot be identified at surgery. Arteriography is of limited value in identifying gastrinomas; only from 20 to 30 percent of primary tumors or hepatic metastases found at surgery have been identified by arteriography. Computed tomography is of slightly greater value in identifying gastrinomas. Use of both selective arteriography and CT has been reported to identify 44 percent of gastrinomas in Z-E patients and 80 percent of those located at surgery. Endoscopic retrograde pancreaticoduodenography has not proved to be of assistance in the diagnosis or exclusion of pancreatic gastrinomas. A small number of duodenal wall gastrinomas have been identified and confirmed histologically by duodenoscopy.

The diagnosis in a patient with clinical features consistent with the Z-E syndrome depends upon the demonstration of *increased serum gastrin levels* by radioimmunoassay. Fasting serum gastrin levels in normal subjects and patients with typical duodenal ulcer average approximately 20 to 50 pg/mL and usually do not exceed 150 pg/mL. Patients with gastrinoma almost always have fasting serum gastrin levels that are greater than 200 pg/mL and have been found as high as 450,000 pg/mL. Approximately half of these patients have fasting serum gastrin levels that are less than 1000 pg/mL (an approximate mean value for serum gastrin for patients with gastrinoma).

Several provocative tests have been used to evaluate patients with possible gastrinoma, especially those who do not exhibit pronounced hypergastrinemia (i.e., serum gastrin > 1000 pg/mL). These tests utilize measurements of serum gastrin levels in response to intravenous secretin injection, calcium infusion, or ingestion of a standard test meal (see Table 238-1).

In the *secretin injection test,* secretin (Kabi secretin, 2 units per kilogram) is given intravenously over 30 to 60 s. Gastrin is measured in serum samples obtained before injection of secretin and at 5-min intervals thereafter for 30 min. In normal individuals and patients with common duodenal ulcer, secretin produces no change, small reductions, or small increases in serum gastrin levels. In contrast, in gastrinoma patients intravenous secretin induces substantial increases in serum gastrin. The gastrin levels increase promptly by at least 200 pg/mL, usually at 5 min (and virtually always by 10 min), then gradually decrease toward or to preinjection levels by 30 min. In the *calcium infusion test* serum samples for gastrin measurements are obtained before and at 30-min intervals for 4 h after initiation of a constant 3-h intravenous infusion of calcium gluconate (5 mg calcium per kilogram per hour). In gastrinoma patients serum gastrin concentrations usually increase above the basal serum gastrin by more than 400 pg/mL. The third provocative test involves the *feeding of a standard meal:* gastrin is measured in serum samples obtained before the meal and at 15-min intervals after it for 90 min. In gastrinoma patients serum gastrin levels increase little or not at all, seldom reaching values 50 percent greater than fasting levels (see Table 238-1).

The secretin injection test is by far the most valuable provocative test in identifying gastrinoma patients. Positive serum gastrin responses to intravenous secretin are found in more than 95 percent of patients with gastrinoma. Using the criteria suggested, substantial increases in serum gastrin following secretin injection have been detected only rarely in nongastrinoma patients. Reduced gastric acid secretion, achlorhydria or profound hypochlorhydria, is by far the most common cause of hypergastrinemia. For this reason gastric acid secretion should be measured before consideration of the secretin injection test. Exaggerated release of gastrin in response to calcium infusion is found in more than 80 percent of gastrinoma patients; however, this exaggerated response to calcium infusion occurs in some nongastrinoma patients with hypergastrinemia (e.g., with achlorhydria). Enhanced gastrin release with calcium infusion is not observed in gastrinoma patients in the absence of the abnormally large gastrin release in response to secretin. Since the calcium infusion test does not add to the sensitivity or specificity of the secretin injection test and since calcium infusion is potentially more hazardous, it is not now recommended.

In a very small proportion of duodenal ulcer patients (much less than 1 percent), gastric acid hypersecretion may be accompanied by increased serum gastrin levels due to hyperfunction and/or hyperplasia of antral gastrin cells (G cells). These patients can be distinguished from those with gastrinoma by the secretin and meal stimulation tests. In patients with this antral gastrin cell abnormality, intravenous secretin does not produce the large increases in serum gastrin characteristic of gastrinoma, but ingestion of the test meal does lead to generous increases in serum gastrin levels, frequently exceeding the fasting serum gastrin concentration by more than 200 percent (see Table 238-1).

TREATMENT In general, patients with Z-E syndrome are resistant to those medical therapies and surgical procedures designed for and usually effective in treating common peptic ulcer. Antacids may produce transient symptomatic relief but rarely, if ever, induce ulcer healing or sustained relief of symptoms. Incomplete gastric resection (with or without vagotomy) or pyloroplasty with vagotomy is frequently followed by prompt and often fulminant ulcer recurrence. Many patients with gastrinoma have had multiple surgical procedures, particularly in those instances in which the diagnosis was not established initially. Mortality was reported to be lowest in those patients with multiple gastric surgical procedures in whom gastrectomy was the initial gastric surgery for the Z-E syndrome: this led to the conclusion that when gastric surgery was required in gastrinoma patients, total gastrectomy was the surgical procedure of choice.

Recent development of more effective drugs to reduce acid secretion and more precise diagnostic techniques to locate the gastrinomas have increased substantially the therapeutic options. The key to management in these patients is individualization of treatment, since patients with the Z-E syndrome are highly heterogeneous with respect to clinical manifestations and extent of disease. As with many other predominantly malignant tumors, the ideal treatment is removal of the gastrinoma.

H-2-receptor antagonists are effective in reducing gastric acid secretion, producing symptom relief, and inducing ulcer healing in patients with the Z-E syndrome. They are indicated as initial treatment of gastrinoma patients, for prolonged treatment of those patients who are not candidates for tumor resection, and in those in whom total gastrectomy is not anticipated. *Cimetidine* was the first H-2-receptor antagonist used widely and successfully in the treatment of these patients. Improvement in clinical symptoms, decreases in gastric acid output, and ulcer healing were found in 80 to 85 percent. Administration of cimetidine has been required at 4- to 6-h intervals, with total daily doses usually four to eight times those used in the treatment of common duodenal ulcer. More recently, *ranitidine* and *famotidine* have been used effectively in treatment of patients with the Z-E syndrome. These H-2-receptor antagonists require comparable increases in dosage when compared with doses used in treatment of common duodenal ulcer. When instituted, H-2-receptor antagonist therapy must be continued indefinitely, since even temporary discontinuance is usually followed by ulcer recurrence. The dose of H-2-receptor antagonist required to maintain a satisfactory reduction in gastric acid secretion can be assessed by measuring the basal gastric acid output during the hour immediately prior to the next anticipated dose of the drug: the goal is to reduce gastric acid output to less than 10 mmol/h at that time.

The most effective drug in reducing gastric acid secretion and in inducing ulcer healing in patients with the Z-E syndrome is the H^+,K^+-ATPase inhibitor omeprazole. This drug is extremely potent in inhibiting gastric acid secretion, and, as a function of potency and dosage, its effectiveness can be prolonged and sustained. This drug is not yet available for prescribing in the United States. Some Z-E patients, in whom gastrinomas could not be identified or removed surgically, have been treated effectively with parietal cell vagotomy, which has reduced or, in a few instances, eliminated the doses of H-2-receptor antagonists required in these patients.

Treatment for patients with the Z-E syndrome should be individualized. In selecting the best therapy, the biologic behavior of these tumors and the clinical manifestations in each patient must be taken into consideration. Early studies indicated that morbidity and mortality in patients with the Z-E syndrome were due principally to complications of severe ulcer disease. However, with earlier diagnosis, effective antiulcer treatment, and longer follow-up, more frequent consequences of the malignant invasive properties of gastrinoma are now being recognized. Complete *surgical resection of the tumors,* when possible, represented *optimal treatment in patients with gastrinoma.* Complete surgical removal of gastrinoma, with cure, has been achieved in approximately 25 percent of patients with the Z-E syndrome. Successful tumor resection is rarely, if ever, achieved in gastrinoma patients with MEN I because of the overwhelming likelihood that multifocal tumors, often with metastasis though frequently indolent, are present at the time of diagnosis.

Therapeutic doses of H-2-receptor antagonists are indicated in the period during which the diagnosis is being established, while the location and extent of the tumor are being determined, and also as treatment prior to anticipated surgery. At present, H-2-receptor antagonists are certainly indicated for patients who are poor operative candidates, who refuse surgery, and in whom surgical removal of the tumor is not possible. Patients with aggressively invasive gastrinoma have been treated with streptozotocin and 5-fluorouracil, in some instances combined with adriamycin, in attempts to reduce tumor bulk and associated symptoms. Success with chemotherapy is limited, with only an approximate 40 percent initial response and no complete responses. When metastatic and/or otherwise nonresectable gastrinoma is present, control of the ulcer disease may be achieved in most instances by treatment with H-2-receptor antagonists, perhaps with parietal cell vagotomy, or rarely, when required, by total gastric resection. There is no convincing evidence that tumor progression is usually influenced by gastrectomy.

STRESS ULCERS AND EROSIONS

A variety of acute ulcerative lesions of the gastrointestinal tract are distinct clinically from chronic peptic ulcer. Among these are the acute upper gastrointestinal erosions and ulcers often observed in patients with shock, massive burns, sepsis, and severe trauma. These are often referred to as *stress erosions* and *ulcers.* These lesions, which are frequently multiple, are most common in the acid-secreting portion of the stomach, but they may also occur in the antrum and duodenum.

These erosions and superficial ulcers are extremely frequent and occur in about 90 percent of patients with massive injuries and burns. The most common clinical finding in these patients is painless gastrointestinal hemorrhage. Blood loss is usually minimal but may be substantial. Erosions develop most frequently approximately 24 h after trauma. Small amounts of blood loss may be detected in the first 24 to 48 h after trauma. However, when massive hemorrhage occurs, it is usually more than 2 or 3 days after the acute insult. The diagnosis is best established by upper gastrointestinal endoscopy. The erosions are most often too superficial to be recognized by barium examination of the upper gastrointestinal tract. Acute stress ulcers and erosions should be suspected when there is evidence of upper gastrointestinal bleeding in patients with severe injuries, burns, infections, and/or shock.

Many theories have been proposed to explain stress-associated acute mucosal ulceration. Mucosal ischemia and tissue injury from gastric acid appear to be important in the production of these acute stress erosions and ulcers. There is usually no evidence of acid hypersecretion; however, the lesions cannot be produced in experimental animals in the absence of acid. Most evidence supports the conclusion that mucosal ischemia is the most important element in the production of stress erosions and ulceration.

The treatment of acute stress ulcerations and erosions is principally preventive. In high-risk patients the frequency of stress ulcerations can be diminished by vigorous use of antacids to neutralize gastric contents and H-2-receptor antagonists to inhibit gastric acid secretion. When medical therapy fails to arrest bleeding, surgical approaches have included pyloroplasty and vagotomy and total gastrectomy.

The term *Cushing's ulcer* has been applied to acute ulcer of the upper gastrointestinal tract associated with intracranial injury or increases in intracranial pressure, e.g., with brain tumors or subdural hematoma. These ulcers may involve the stomach, proximal duodenum, or esophagus and frequently lead to hemorrhage or perforation. They do not differ histologically from acute stress ulceration. However, unlike stress ulcers, Cushing's ulcers are frequently associated with gastric acid hypersecretion. Treatment includes correction of increased intracranial pressure, when possible, and the usual measures for treatment of acute erosions and ulcerations, including vigorous therapy with antacids or H-2-receptor antagonists.

DRUG-ASSOCIATED ULCERS AND EROSIONS

Gastric and duodenal ulcers have been described following administration of many drugs. Aspirin ingestion has been shown to be associated with an increased incidence of gastric ulcer and, probably to a lesser extent, duodenal ulcer, and is a frequent cause of hemorrhagic erosive gastritis. Gastric mucosal injury, similar to that produced by aspirin, has also been observed in patients treated with a variety of other NSAIDs (e.g., indomethacin, ibuprofen, naproxen, tolmetin, sulindac, piroxicam, diflunisal, fenoprofen). The specific mechanism by which salicylates and other NSAIDs induce, or are associated with, gastric ulcer has not been established. Several mechanisms have been proposed, with most evidence favoring depletion of protective tissue prostaglandins by the well-recognized capacities of these agents to inhibit prostaglandin synthesis (see "Gastritis," below). They may contribute to development of gastric ulcer by interruption of the gastric mucosal barrier, permitting back-diffusion of hydrogen ions that may injure the gastric mucosa. Misoprostol, a prostaglandin E analogue, is effective in prevention of NSAID-induced gastric ulcers at dosage of 200 μg four times daily.

Administration of glucocorticoids has been reported and is commonly assumed to be associated with ulcer disease of the upper gastrointestinal tract. The subject remains controversial, since some data support and other data reject this association.

GASTRITIS

Gastritis is *inflammation of the gastric mucosa*. Gastritis is not a single disease. Rather, it is a group of disorders that have inflammatory changes in the gastric mucosa in common, but that have different clinical features, histologic characteristics, and pathogenesis. Several classifications have been used for consideration of gastritis. In general, these classifications have been based on (1) the acuteness or chronicity of the clinical manifestations, (2) the histologic features characterizing the gastritis, (3) the anatomic distribution of the gastritis, or, in some instances, (4) the proposed pathogenesis of each of the two principal forms of chronic gastritis. Based on the *clinical features* of the gastritis, the two principal forms, which constitute very different clinical entities, are *acute gastritis* and *chronic gastritis*. Different types of chronic gastritis exhibit histologic features which permit their classification according to the presence or absence of mucosal atrophy associated with the gastritis and the anatomic distribution of the gastritis or atrophy in the gastric mucosa.

In this section the major clinical forms of acute gastritis and chronic gastritis will be addressed, including reference to the histologic features of the major forms of gastritis. Attention will also be directed to additional specific forms of gastritis.

ACUTE GASTRITIS The principal, and certainly the most dramatic, form of acute gastritis is *acute hemorrhagic gastritis*, which is also referred to as *acute erosive gastritis*. These terms reflect the bleeding from the gastric mucosa almost invariably found in this form of gastritis and the characteristic loss of integrity of the gastric mucosa (erosion) that accompanies the inflammatory lesion. Gross examination in hemorrhagic gastritis shows edema, mucosal friability, erosions, and sites of bleeding with extravasation of blood into the mucosa and the lumen of the stomach. Gastric erosions and sites of hemorrhage may be distributed diffusely throughout the gastric mucosa or may be localized to the body or antrum of the stomach. They are often placed linearly on the crests of the gastric folds.

Histologic examination of the gastric mucosa reveals infiltration of the lamina propria with mononuclear cells and polymorphonuclear leukocytes with extravasation of blood in the mucosa, distorting the glandular structures. Proteinaceous exudate containing polymorphonuclear leukocytes may be present in gastric glands. Gastric erosions, by definition, are limited to the mucosa and do not extend beneath the muscularis mucosae. Acute erosive gastritis may accompany deeper, more focal lesions, which represent acute ulcers and may extend to and through all layers of the gastric wall.

Etiology and pathogenesis Acute erosive gastritis may develop without apparent explanation but is more likely to occur in several specific clinical circumstances. Erosive gastritis is usually associated with serious illness or with various drugs. Erosive gastritis has been estimated to occur in up to 80 to 90 percent of critically ill hospitalized patients. It is most often found in patients in medical or surgical intensive care units with severe trauma, major surgery, hepatic, renal, or respiratory failure, shock, massive burns, or severe infections with septicemia. Acute erosive gastritis associated with these severe illnesses is often referred to as *stress-induced gastritis*. The contributions of all mechanisms responsible for erosive gastritis in critically ill patients have not been defined completely. However, important participating elements appear to include ischemia of the gastric mucosa, acid diffusion from the gastric lumen into gastric mucosal tissues, and, perhaps in some forms, bile acids and/or other duodenal-pancreatic secretions refluxed into the gastric lumen. Mucosal ischemia and acid in the gastric lumen are clearly crucial elements in the etiopathogenesis of stress-induced gastritis. Septic shock with resulting mucosal ischemia produces gastric erosions in experimental animals. During such experimentally induced shock the intramural pH of the gastric mucosa falls precipitously when the gastric lumen is irrigated with HCl: this produces severe hemorrhagic lesions. The decrease in intramural pH results from diffusion of luminal hydrogen ions, which damage the gastric mucosa. With neutral pH irrigation the fall in intramural pH is much less and gastric lesions are minimal. Counteracting the effects of acid by vigorous and continuous treatment with antacids or by inhibiting secretion with H-2-receptor antagonists has been effective in reducing the incidence and the hemorrhagic complications of acute erosive gastritis in critically ill patients.

Various agents are known to injure the gastric mucosa. These include aspirin and other NSAIDs, bile acids, pancreatic enzymes, and ethanol. These agents disrupt the gastric mucosal barrier, which under normal conditions impedes the back-diffusion of hydrogen ions from the gastric lumen to the mucosa (despite and against an enormous H^+ concentration gradient). The most common and very important cause of drug-associated acute erosive gastritis is ingestion of aspirin or other NSAIDs. These drugs inhibit gastric mucosal cyclooxygenase activity, thereby reducing the synthesis and tissue levels of endogenous mucosal prostaglandins, which appear to play important roles in mucosal defense. This reduction in tissue prostaglandins is thought to be a principal, but perhaps not the exclusive, mechanism by which aspirin and other NSAIDs damage the gastric mucosa. It is possible that aspirin may injure small vessels in the gastric mucosa by inhibition of prostacyclin in the walls of small blood vessels or by inhibition of synthesis of thromboxane by platelets. An additional proposed mechanism for aspirin-induced gastrointestinal mucosal injury is via the effects of sodium salicylate, the product of aspirin metabolism found in the circulation, which is toxic to mitochondrial respiration and oxidative phosphorylation of cells. This may produce endothelial and epithelial cell injury with hemorrhage into the tissues or vascular thrombosis by endothelial cell disruption. Acid in the gastric lumen appears crucial to the production of salicylate-associated injury to the gastric mucosa.

Ethanol damage to the gastric mucosa is associated principally with subepithelial hemorrhages with surrounding edema and only slight to moderate increases in mucosal inflammatory cells. The mechanism by which alcohol injures the gastric mucosa is uncertain. Proposals have included cell injury due to its inherent lipophilic and lipolytic properties and/or interruption of the gastric mucosal barrier or direct damage to small mucosal blood vessels.

Clinical features Bleeding from the gastric mucosa with acute gastritis may range from abrupt and dramatic upper gastrointestinal hemorrhage to the most subtle blood loss, perhaps detected only by the presence of occult blood in the stool or development of mild, asymptomatic, and unexplained anemia. Patients with acute erosive gastritis may have hematemesis and/or melena as well as less apparent forms of gastrointestinal blood loss. Except for possible consequences of blood loss, erosive gastritis is usually asymptomatic. However, less common symptoms may include epigastric or upper abdominal pain, nausea, and vomiting. Pain is much less common with erosive gastritis than with ulcer disease, with painless gastrointestinal hemorrhage more commonly the only clinical manifestation. Physical examination is often normal in patients with acute hemorrhagic gastritis. However, they may have upper abdominal tenderness or evidence of blood loss such as pallor, tachycardia, and hypotension. When they occur, abnormalities of white blood cell count, such as leukocytosis or leukopenia, more often reflect the associated serious illness than the gastritis.

Diagnosis The presence of erosive gastritis is usually first suspected by detection of blood in the stool or in the gastric aspirate. The diagnosis is best established by upper gastrointestinal endoscopic examination, which reveals mucosal hemorrhages, friability and congestion, erosions, and, in some instances, superficial or deep ulcerations which, when present, are usually in the fundus or body of the stomach. Radiographic examination is much less reliable in detecting acute hemorrhagic-erosive gastritis.

Treatment Treatment should be directed to prevention of erosive gastritis, treatment of the associated disease, withdrawal of the offending agent, and general supportive measures, as required, including maintenance of oxygen, blood volume, and fluid and electrolyte requirements. In the past, iced-saline lavage has been used in treatment of patients with hemorrhagic gastritis. However, this has never been shown to be effective in reducing gastrointestinal hemorrhage in these patients. Hourly antacid administration (e.g., 30 mL of an aluminum-magnesium hydroxide liquid preparation) and/or administration of an H-2-receptor antagonist (usually intravenously) have been shown to be effective in reducing the frequency of hemorrhagic gastritis in critically ill patients. These drugs should be used in doses and frequency sufficient to maintain the pH of gastric contents above 4. Although proven of value in prevention, it is less certain that they are effective in treatment of acute hemorrhagic gastritis. However, a similar therapeutic program with antacids or H-2-receptor antagonists does seem reasonable and generally is advised. Sucralfate has also been used in treatment of these patients. Misoprostol is effective in prevention of hemorrhagic gastritis, erosions, or gastric ulceration associated with ingestion of aspirin and other nonsteroidal agents.

Most patients respond favorably during vigorous treatment by the measures indicated. Acute hemorrhagic gastritis tends to improve as the patient's clinical condition improves. Because of the rapid cell renewal and restitutive properties of the gastric mucosa, lesions of acute hemorrhagic gastritis may return to normal, both endoscopically and histologically, within 48 h of an acute event. However, occasionally further measures are required in attempts to arrest persistent life-threatening blood loss. These have included embolization or vasopressin infusion of the left gastric artery. Uncommonly, surgery is required for relentless hemorrhage. Vagotomy and pyloroplasty with oversewing of focal bleeding ulcerations has been used with limited success, and, rarely, total gastrectomy may be required. Morbidity and mortality with surgery in these patients is very great, usually reflecting the severity of their associated illnesses. Surgical treatment should not be performed unless absolutely necessary.

Enteropathic erosive gastritis Enteropathic erosive gastritis is a rare clinical entity with multiple erosions of the gastric mucosa found in the absence of recognized precipitating factors. These patients may have anorexia, nausea, vomiting, or poorly defined upper abdominal discomfort. Less commonly they show evidence of gastrointestinal blood loss or weight loss. Endoscopic examination is usually required to establish the diagnosis. Erosions, which may be few or numerous, are usually located on the crests of the folds, but may be found in any portion of the gastric mucosa. Gastric biopsies are performed primarily to exclude other abnormalities, e.g., gastric lymphoma, carcinoma, and Crohn's disease. Erosions usually heal completely and may or may not return. The etiology is not known, nor are there accepted principles for specific recommendations for therapy.

Acute gastritis associated with *Helicobacter pylori* *Helicobacter pylori* (previously called *Campylobacter pylori*) is a short (0.2 to 0.5 μm in length), spiral-shaped, microaerophilic gram-negative bacillus which has been suggested as a potential cause of certain forms of acute and chronic gastritis. Gastric colonization has also been associated with duodenal and gastric ulcer (see "Peptic Ulcer," above). With gastric colonization *H. pylori* are found in the deep portions of the mucus gel layer that coats the gastric mucosa and between the mucus gel layer and the apical surfaces of the gastric mucosal epithelial cells. They also may be located in the regions of the tight junctions between adjacent mucosal epithelial cells. They do not invade the gastric mucosa. *H. pylori* is associated with inflamed gastric mucosal epithelium in the stomach as well as with metaplastic gastric epithelium found elsewhere, e.g., in the duodenal bulb of most patients with duodenal ulcer.

There is evidence that *H. pylori* is the cause, or at least a principal cause, of a form of gastritis that has been designated *active chronic gastritis*. Active chronic gastritis is characterized by dense infiltration of the lamina propria of the gastric mucosa with invasion of the epithelial cell layer by polymorphonuclear leukocytes. The mucosal surface is usually intact, without erosions or hemorrhagic lesions. When erosions do occur, they are usually small and limited to the superficial epithelial cell layer. There is poor correlation between the histologic abnormalities and the endoscopic appearance of the mucosa: endoscopy may reveal subtle abnormalities, or, more often, the endoscopic appearance is totally normal. Histologic abnormalities are associated with positive culture for *H. pylori*, and the degree of histologic abnormality, in general, parallels the number of organisms that can be identified. In addition, the more active the gastritis, reflected by infiltration of the mucosa with polymorphonuclear leukocytes, the greater the likelihood that *H. pylori* will be found. Healing of the gastritis occurs when cultures become negative. Spontaneous disappearance of *H. pylori* has not been noted. It has been observed to persist in gastric mucosal biopsies of untreated patients for more than 2 years.

H. pylori has been identified in gastric samples by histologic examination, culture, urease activity, and by endonuclease analysis. On stained tissue sections *H. pylori* is Giemsa-positive and faintly hematoxylin-positive. It can be cultured successfully from biopsy material, but usually not from gastric secretions. *H. pylori* produce large amounts of urease. The rapid urease test of gastric biopsy material is a relatively simple and reliable method for presumptive identification of the presence of *H. pylori*. The test is inexpensive with good sensitivity and specificity. A urea breath test using ^{13}C or

^{14}C has also been developed for identifying *H. pylori*. Antibodies (IgG and IgA) to *H. pylori* have been identified in sera of individuals with *H. pylori* colonization. There is a high degree of correlation between these serum antibodies and histologic gastritis.

H. pylori synthesizes a protease that hydrolyzes gastric mucous glycoproteins, which may therefore disrupt the gastric mucus gel layer, contributing to mucosal injury. There is evidence that this form of acute gastritis with *H. pylori* is associated with reductions in gastric acid secretion. By retrospective examination, *H. pylori* were demonstrated in gastric mucosal biopsy specimens described from volunteers participating in gastric secretory studies who developed epidemic gastritis, with concurrent reductions in rates of gastric acid secretion.

When sought for, *H. pylori* has been identified in a large proportion of gastric biopsies of patients with several upper gastrointestinal diseases. It has been cultured from antral biopsy specimens in 90 to 100 percent of patients with duodenal ulcer, 70 percent with gastric ulcer, 80 percent with chronic gastritis involving the antral mucosa, and in 50 percent of patients with nonulcer dyspepsia.

H. pylori is also frequent in asymptomatic individuals considered to be otherwise well. Histologic gastritis has long been recognized as common in healthy asymptomatic individuals; recently it has been shown to be associated strongly with gastric *H. pylori* colonization. *H. pylori* with associated gastritis was found in the gastric biopsy samples of from 20 to 25 percent of healthy volunteer subjects. When these asymptomatic individuals were examined, there was no relationship between the histologic and endoscopic appearances of the gastric mucosa. Endoscopic examination usually appeared normal, in spite of the histologic evidence of gastritis and *H. pylori*.

Colloidal bismuth compounds have been shown to eradicate *H. pylori* from gastric mucosa. It is uncertain by what mechanism. Eradication may be due to antibacterial effects or perhaps to binding or coating of the organism. Amoxicillin (50 mg tid or qid), bismuth subsalicylate (30 mL qid), and metronidazole (500 mg tid) have each been used singly or in combination for periods of from 1 week to 2 months to eradicate *H. pylori*. Eradication of *H. pylori* results in disappearance of inflammatory changes in the gastric mucosa. Recolonization of the organism after treatment, usually with the same bacterial subtype, with recurrence of gastritis is very frequent and usually occurs within 1 month after initial eradication and discontinuance of treatment.

CHRONIC GASTRITIS The inflammatory cell infiltrate in chronic gastritis is composed principally of chronic inflammatory cells, predominantly lymphocytes and plasma cells. Polymorphonuclear leukocytes and eosinophils may be present in small numbers, but do not predominate. Chronic gastritis is often patchy and irregular in distribution.

Histologic classification Chronic gastritis has been classified descriptively on the basis of several characteristic histologic abnormalities. In its evolution chronic gastritis initially involves the superficial and glandular areas of the gastric mucosa and progresses to glandular destruction, which may be followed by a profound reduction in gland number (atrophy) and/or gland metaplasia.

Superficial gastritis is that form of gastritis with inflammatory changes in the lamina propria of the superficial mucosa, with cellular infiltration and edema separating the gastric glands. Superficial gastritis appears to represent the initial stage in the development of chronic gastritis. With superficial gastritis the inflammatory cell infiltrate is limited to the lamina propria of the upper (epithelial) half of the gastric mucosa and the glands are preserved. There may be a decrease in mucus in glandular mucous cells and in mitotic figures in cells of the glands.

Atrophic gastritis is the next stage in the developmental chronology of chronic gastritis. In atrophic gastritis the inflammatory infiltrate extends to the deep portions of the mucosa. There is progressive distortion and destruction of the glands, which become separated by the inflammatory process. Atrophic gastritis is followed by the development of the final stage of chronic gastritis, which is *gastric atrophy*. With gastric atrophy there is a profound loss of the glandular structures, which are now separated widely by connective tissue, with a greatly reduced or absent inflammatory infiltrate. The mucosa is thin, often revealing the prominence of its underlying vessels by endoscopic examination.

As chronic gastritis progresses, there may be changes in the morphology of the gastric glandular elements. *Intestinal metaplasia* is the term used to describe the conversion of gastric glands to the appearance of small-intestinal mucosal glands containing goblet cells. Intestinal metaplasia may be patchy or extensive in the gastric mucosa. With *pseudopyloric gland metaplasia* the glands of the body of the stomach assume the appearance of antral pyloric glands. Pseudopyloric metaplasia may occur with either atrophic gastritis or gastric atrophy.

Chronic gastritis: types A and B The two major forms of chronic gastritis have been classified as types A and B based on their distributions in the gastric mucosa coupled with some implications regarding their pathogenesis. *Type A gastritis* is the less common form of chronic gastritis: it characteristically involves the body and fundus of the stomach with relative sparing of the antrum. This is the form of gastritis that may lead to pernicious anemia. The frequent presence of antibodies to parietal cells and antibodies to intrinsic factor in sera of patients with type A gastritis and pernicious anemia has suggested an immune or autoimmune pathogenesis for this form of gastritis. Antibodies to parietal cells have been shown to be cytotoxic for gastric mucosal cells. Cell-mediated immune mechanisms have also been proposed to participate in gastric mucosal cell injury in pernicious anemia and related forms of type A gastritis. Antibodies to parietal cells have been found in sera of approximately 90 percent of patients with pernicious anemia and in more than half of other patients with type A gastritis. Relatives of patients with pernicious anemia have a higher than normal frequency of serum antibodies to parietal cells, atrophic gastritis, and reduced gastric acid secretion. In control populations parietal cell antibodies may be found in up to 20 percent of individuals over age 60 and in approximately 20 percent of all patients with hypoparathyroidism, Addison's disease, and vitiligo. About 50 percent of patients with pernicious anemia have antibodies to thyroid antigens, and approximately 30 percent of patients with thyroid disease have circulating antibodies to parietal cells. Serum antibodies to intrinsic factor are more specific than parietal cell antibodies and are present in about 40 percent of patients with pernicious anemia.

In patients with pernicious anemia the gastric parietal cell–containing glands are invariably destroyed, accounting for their inability to secrete gastric hydrochloric acid. Since, in human beings, parietal cells also secrete intrinsic factor, there is failure to absorb vitamin B_{12} actively with resulting hematologic and/or neurologic consequences characteristic of pernicious anemia. It has been estimated that the risk of cancer of the stomach in patients with type A gastritis and pernicious anemia is approximately three times that of the general population.

Type B gastritis is much the more common form of chronic gastritis. In younger patients type B gastritis principally involves the antrum, whereas in older patients the entire stomach is affected. This transition is estimated to require about 15 to 20 years. The incidence of chronic gastritis, most of it type B gastritis, increases with age, reaching 78 percent in individuals over age 50 and virtually 100 percent after age 70.

A large number of studies from various parts of the world have shown a strong association of *H. pylori* with type B gastritis. Chronic gastritis with *H. pylori* infection and/or persistence is associated with reduced gastric acid secretion. Eradication of *H. pylori* produces improvement in histologic findings; when treatment is stopped, inflammatory changes recur, and organisms reappear. These observations have favored the proposal that type B gastritis is caused by chronic bacterial infection by *H. pylori*. Chronic reflux of pancreatic-biliary secretions, bile acids and lysolecithin, in particular, has also been proposed as a potential factor in the production of type B chronic gastritis.

Gastric acid secretion is reduced in both type A and type B chronic gastritis. In general, the reduction in gastric acid secretion, which is complete in patients with pernicious anemia, is proportionate to the severity of parietal cell destruction and mucosal atrophy in the body and fundus of the stomach. Serum gastrin levels are usually elevated substantially in patients with pernicious anemia and are in approximately the same range as those of patients with the Z-E syndrome (gastrinoma). Since the antral mucosa is relatively spared, the antral gastrin-containing cells, deprived of feedback control normally exercised by acid in the stomach, release gastrin continuously. Serum gastrin levels are also often similarly elevated in patients with type A gastritis with achlorhydria or profound hypochlorhydria who do not have pernicious anemia. Patients with type B gastritis have serum gastrin levels that are highly variable, not consistently elevated and often in the normal range. A small portion of patients with type B gastritis have serum antibodies to gastrin, leading some to propose an autoimmune mechanism for this form of gastritis. Alternatively, and probably more likely, these antibodies represent responses to the inflammatory process rather than contributing factors.

There is no persuasive evidence that acute gastric mucosal injury associated with stress or with ethanol or aspirin or other NSAIDs progresses to chronic gastritis. Acute gastritis caused by *H. pylori* may be a form of gastritis in which there is sufficient information to suspect progression to a chronic form of gastritis, i.e., type B chronic gastritis.

Diagnosis Biopsy of the gastric mucosa provides the most reliable means of identifying and classifying gastritis. Caution must be exercised in the interpretation of a single gastric mucosal biopsy in a patient with suspected acute or chronic gastritis. The patchy and irregular distribution of the gastritis may lead to substantial sampling error. Therefore, several biopsies of suspected areas, when safe and possible, are recommended.

Treatment No specific treatment is required for type A or type B chronic gastritis with or without mucosal atrophy. The only form of chronic gastritis that requires specific treatment is pernicious anemia, the most complete expression of type A gastritis. Vitamin B_{12} deficiency in these patients, resulting from malabsorption of vitamin B_{12} secondary to destruction of parietal cells in the body and fundus of the stomach, requires indefinite regular parenteral vitamin B_{12} administration.

Ménétrier's disease *Ménétrier's* disease is a clinical entity characterized by large tortuous gastric mucosal folds. The abnormalities in Ménétrier's disease may be localized or diffused throughout the stomach. Prominent mucosal folds are often most conspicuous in the gastric body and fundus. Histologic inflammation is not a component of this disease. Therefore, it is not a form of gastritis. The primary pathologic feature is thickening of the gastric mucosa due to hyperplasia of surface and glandular mucous cells, which replace most of the chief and parietal cells. Pits of the gastric glands elongate and may become extremely tortuous. The lamina propria may contain an increased number of lymphocytes. Intestinal metaplasia may be present.

The most common symptom is epigastric pain. Anorexia, nausea, vomiting, and weight loss are less frequent. Gastric bleeding is unusual and, when present, is due to superficial mucosal erosions. Uncommonly, gastric ulcer or gastric carcinoma may develop in these patients. Patients often develop a protein-losing gastropathy resulting in hypoalbuminemia and edema. Gastric acid secretion is usually reduced or may be absent. Barium examination of the upper gastrointestinal tract reveals the large gastric folds, which are readily confirmed by endoscopic examination. The diagnosis is best established by deep mucosal biopsy (and cytology) to exclude gastric malignancy. The depth of these lesions and the disconcerting prominence of the folds may require a surgical full-thickness biopsy to exclude lymphoma or infiltrating carcinoma.

Anticholinergic agents and H-2-receptor antagonists have been reported to decrease protein loss in patients with Ménétrier's disease. Treatment includes a high-protein diet to replace protein losses. If present, ulcers should be treated as described previously for common gastric ulcer. Severe disease with persistent substantial protein loss may require total gastrectomy.

Gastritis due to corrosive agents Ingestion of a variety of corrosive chemicals can cause severe damage to the gastric mucosa. Because of its anatomic location, the antrum is a frequent site for such injury. Ingested substances which are particularly injurious to the gastric mucosa include strong acids (e.g., hydrochloric acid, sulfuric acid) or strong alkali (e.g., sodium hydroxide). Depending on dose and concentration these agents can cause injury ranging from mild inflammation to extensive tissue necrosis. With alkali ingestion (especially lye) the esophagus is particularly susceptible to severe injury, necrosis, and potential subsequent stricture. The stomach, especially the antrum, is more susceptible to acute injury by ingestion of strong acid. With ingestion of these corrosive substances patients may describe burning of the mouth, throat, and retrosternal area. Epigastric pain and vomiting often signal gastric injury. Hemorrhage and/or perforation may occur. Treatment of strong acid ingestion includes dilution with water, followed by antacids and supportive therapy as required. Neutralization of ingested lye by administrated acid is not recommended.

Infectious gastritis Infectious causes of gastritis, other than gastritis associated with gastric *H. pylori* colonization, are unusual. *Phlegmonous gastritis,* a rare form of bacterial gastritis, is a life-threatening disease with extensive infiltration of the gastric wall, tissue necrosis, and manifestations of generalized sepsis. Responsible infectious agents include, among others, streptococci, staphylococci, *Proteus* species, and *Escherichia coli*. Treatment includes appropriate intravenous antibiotics and necessary supportive care including fluid and electrolyte replacement as required. Lack of response to therapy may require gastrectomy. Additional infectious causes of gastritis may be found in immunocompromised patients. Gastric erosions may be produced by herpes simplex virus. Typical intranuclear inclusions of cytomegalovirus, with positive cultures, have been found by endoscopic gastric biopsy in some immunocompromised patients. This has been interpreted to represent disseminated cytomegalovirus infection.

Eosinophilic gastritis *Eosinophilic gastritis* may occur as isolated involvement of the stomach or as a component of eosinophilic gastroenteritis. Eosinophilic gastritis is characterized by extensive eosinophilic infiltration of the wall of the stomach, usually with circulating eosinophilia. Biopsy reveals extensive eosinophilic infiltration which may involve all coats of the stomach or may be limited to mucosa, submucosa, or muscular regions of the gastric wall. The antrum is involved more frequently than the gastric body or fundus. There may be prominent antral mucosal folds with edema and mucosal thickening, uncommonly leading to gastric outlet obstruction. Epigastric pain, which may be accompanied by nausea and vomiting, is the most frequent symptom. These patients usually respond favorably to treatment with glucocorticoids. Rarely surgery is required to establish the diagnosis or for relief of obstructive symptoms.

Granulomatous gastritis A variety of generalized diseases, some of which are infectious, can involve the stomach, producing *granulomatous gastritis*. Crohn's disease, as in the small intestine, may produce ulceration, granulomatous infiltration, and/or scarring with stricture formation. Its distinction from other gastric lesions requires biopsy at the time of endoscopic examination. Less common infectious causes of granulomatous disease of the stomach include, among others, histoplasmosis, candidiasis, syphilis, and tuberculosis. Rarely, idiopathic granulomatous gastritis and eosinophilic granulomas also involve the stomach. In patients with granulomatous disease of the stomach multiple biopsies and cytology are usually required to establish the diagnosis and to exclude malignancy. If the diagnosis is not established by biopsy at endoscopy, surgical exploration may be required.

Gastritis and prior gastric surgery Variable amounts of gastritis almost always occur in the remaining stomachs of patients treated surgically by partial gastrectomy and, to a somewhat lesser extent, after vagotomy and pyloroplasty. Gastritis is especially common and often severe after gastrojejunal (Billroth II) anastomosis.

Gastric surgery appears to accelerate the development of gastritis, with progressive loss of parietal cells in the gastric remnant after surgery. Most patients are asymptomatic; however, a small proportion develop mild or severe symptoms, most commonly epigastric pain, nausea, and vomiting. This form of gastritis been referred to as *alkaline gastritis* or *bile reflux gastritis*. It has been assumed, but not proven, that gastritis results from reflux of pancreaticobiliary secretions. Endoscopic examination often reveals a beefy red and sometimes friable gastric mucosa. Abnormalities may be limited to mucosa in the region of the anastomosis or may involve all the remaining gastric mucosa. Bile is often seen in the gastric remnant. Biopsies of involved mucosa at endoscopy show variable degrees of acute and/or chronic gastritis. Gastric acid secretion is usually decreased.

Managing patients with severe symptoms is very difficult. Various therapeutic approaches have been used with limited, if any, success. These have included cholestyramine, H-2-receptor antagonists, sucralfate, antacids, and pancreatic enzyme replacement. Surgery, which is sometimes successful, is Roux-en-Y, which diverts pancreaticobiliary secretions away from the gastric remnant. Nonsurgical modalities should be exhausted before proceeding with attempts to treat this disease by surgery.

REFERENCES

Peptic ulcer

BARDHAN KD et al: Double blind comparison of cimetidine and placebo in the maintenance and healing of chronic duodenal ulceration. Gut 20:158, 1979

DOOLEY CP, COHEN H: The clinical significance of *Campylobacter pylori*. Ann Intern Med 108:70, 1988

FRUCHT H et al: Secretin and calcium provocative tests in the Zollinger-Ellison syndrome: A prospective study. Ann Intern Med 111:713, 1989

KLOPPEL G et al: Pancreatic lesions and hormonal profile of pancreatic tumors in multiple endocrine neoplasia type I: An immunocytochemical study of nine patients. Cancer 57:1824, 1986

MATON PN et al: Cushing's syndrome in patients with the Zollinger-Ellison syndrome. N Engl J Med 315:1, 1986

MCARTHUR KE et al: Treatment of acid-peptic diseases by inhibition of gastric H^+,K^+-ATPase. Annu Rev Med 37:97, 1986

MCGUIGAN JE, TRUDEAU WL: Differences in rates of gastrin release in normal persons and patients with duodenal ulcer. N Engl J Med 288:64, 1973

PEURA DA, JOHNSON LF: Cimetidine for prevention and treatment of gastroduodenal lesions in patients in an intensive care unit. Ann Intern Med 103:173, 1985

RATHBONE BJ et al: *Campylobacter pyloridis*—a new factor in peptic ulcer disease? Gut 27:635, 1986

RICHARDSON CT: Sucralfate. Ann Intern Med 97:269, 1982

——— et al: Treatment of Zollinger-Ellison syndrome with exploratory laparotomy, proximal gastric vagotomy, and H_2-receptor antagonists: A prospective study. Gastroenterology 89:357, 1985

TAKEUCHI KD: Role of pH gradient in mucus in protection of gastric mucosa. Gastroenterology 84:331, 1983

VINAYEK R: et al: Famotidine in the therapy of gastric hypersecretory states. Am J Med 81:49, 1986

VON SCHRENK T et al: Prospective study of chemotherapy in patients with metastatic gastrinoma. Gastroenterology 94:1326, 1988

WOLFE MM, SOLL AH: The physiology of gastric acid secretion. N Engl J Med 319:1707, 1988

Gastritis

BARTHEL JS et al: Gastritis and *Campylobacter pylori* in healthy, asymptomatic volunteers. Arch Intern Med 148:1149, 1988

Campylobacter pylori becomes *Helicobacter pylori* (editorial). Lancet 2:1019, 1989

DOOLEY CP, COHEN H: The clinical significance of *Campylobacter pylori*. Ann Intern Med 108:70, 1988

LAINE L, WEINSTEIN WM: Histology of alcoholic hemorrhagic "gastritis": A prospective evaluation. Gastroenterology 94:1254, 1988

PEURA DA, JOHNSON LF: Cimetidine for prevention and treatment of gastroduodenal lesions in patients in an intensive care unit. Ann Intern Med 103:173, 1985

RAUWS EAJ et al: *Campylobacter pyloridis*–associated chronic active antral gastritis: A prospective study of its prevalence and the effects of antibacterial and antiulcer treatment. Gastroenterology 94:33, 1988

ROBERT A: Cytoprotection by prostaglandins. Gastroenterology 77:761, 1979

SEARCY CM, MALAGELADA J-R: Ménétrier's disease and idiopathic hypertrophic gastropathy. Ann Intern Med 100:565, 1984

SLOMIANY BL et al: *Campylobacter pyloridis* degrades mucin and undermines gastric mucosal integrity. Biochem Biophys Res Commun 144:307, 1987

TAKEUCHI KD: Role of pH gradient of mucus in protection of gastric mucosa. Gastroenterology 84:331, 1983

VANE JR: Inhibition of prostaglandin synthesis as a mechanism for aspirin-like drugs. Nature 23:232, 1971

239 NEOPLASMS OF THE ESOPHAGUS AND STOMACH

ROBERT J. MAYER

ESOPHAGEAL CANCER

Incidence and etiology In the United States, cancer of the esophagus is a relatively uncommon but extremely lethal malignant condition. It is estimated that the diagnosis was made in 10,100 Americans in 1989, leading to 9400 deaths. Worldwide, the incidence of esophageal cancer varies strikingly. It occurs frequently within a so-called Asian esophageal cancer belt extending from the southern shore of the Caspian Sea on the west to northern China on the east and encompassing parts of Iran, Soviet Central Asia, Afghanistan, Siberia, and Mongolia. Additionally, high incidence "pockets" of the disease are present in such disparate locations as Finland, Iceland, Curaçao, southeastern Africa, and northwestern France. In North America and western Europe, the disease is far more common in blacks than whites, greater in males than females, appearing most frequently after age 50, and appearing to be an illness associated with lower socioeconomic classes.

A variety of causative factors have been implicated in the development of the disease (Table 239-1). In the United States, 80 to 90 percent of esophageal cancer cases are believed attributable to excess consumption of alcohol and/or a long-standing history of cigarette smoking. The relative risk increases with either the amount of tobacco smoked or alcohol consumed. The consumption of whiskey is seemingly linked to a higher incidence than the consumption of wine or beer. The development of esophageal cancer has also been associated with the ingestion of other carcinogens such as nitrites, smoked opiates, and fungal toxins in pickled vegetables, as well as with mucosal damage caused by such physical insults as long-term exposure to extremely hot tea, the ingestion of lye, radiation-induced strictures, and chronic achalasia. The presence of an esophageal web in association with glossitis and iron deficiency (i.e., Plummer-Vinson or Paterson-Kelly syndrome) and congenital hyperkeratosis and pitting of the palms and soles (i.e., tylosis palmaris et plantaris) have each been linked with esophageal cancer, as have dietary deficiencies of

TABLE 239-1 Some etiologic factors believed to be associated with esophageal cancer

I Excess alcohol consumption
II Cigarette smoking
III Other ingested carcinogens
- *A* Nitrates (converted to nitrites)
- *B* Smoked opiates
- *C* Fungal toxins in pickled vegetables

IV Mucosal damage from physical agents
- *A* Hot tea
- *B* Lye ingestion
- *C* Radiation-induced strictures
- *D* Chronic achalasia

V Host susceptibility
- *A* Esophageal web with glossitis and iron deficiency (i.e., Plummer-Vinson or Paterson-Kelly syndrome)
- *B* Congenital hyperkeratosis and pitting of the palms and soles (i.e., tylosis palmaris et plantaris)

VI ? Dietary deficiencies—molybdenum, zinc, vitamin A
VII ? Celiac sprue
VIII Chronic gastric reflux (i.e., Barrett's esophagus)—for adenocarcinoma

molybdenum, zinc, and vitamin A. The risk for esophageal cancer may be slightly greater in individuals with celiac sprue and is definitely increased in the presence of chronic gastric reflux (i.e., Barrett's esophagus).

Clinical features Approximately 15 percent of esophageal cancers occur in the upper third of the esophagus ("cervical esophagus"), 50 percent in the middle third, and 35 percent in the lower third. More than 85 percent of esophageal tumors are squamous cell carcinomas, arising from the squamous epithelium which lines the lumen of the esophagus. Adenocarcinomas, while far less frequent, develop more commonly from columnar epithelium which may appear in the distal esophagus in association with chronic gastric reflux (i.e., Barrett's esophagus). These malignancies have the biologic behavior of gastric rather than esophageal cancers. Attempts at endoscopic and cytologic screening for carcinoma in patients with Barrett's esophagus have not yet proved successful. It should be noted that squamous cell carcinomas and adenocarcinomas of the esophagus cannot be distinguished radiographically or endoscopically.

Progressive dysphagia and weight loss of short duration are the initial symptoms in the vast majority of patients. Dysphagia initially occurs with solid foods and gradually progresses to include semisolids and liquids. By the time these symptoms develop, the disease is usually incurable since difficulty in swallowing does not occur until 60 percent or more of the esophageal circumference is infiltrated with cancer. Dysphagia may be associated with pain on swallowing (odynophagia), pain radiating to the chest and/or back, regurgitation or vomiting, and aspiration pneumonia. The disease most commonly spreads to adjacent and supraclavicular lymph nodes, liver, lungs, and pleura. Tracheoesophageal fistulas may develop as the disease advances, leading to severe suffering. As with other squamous cell carcinomas, hypercalcemia may occasionally occur in the absence of osseous metastases. This is believed to result from a tumor-secreted protein structurally analogous to a portion of parathyroid hormone.

Diagnosis Routine, contrast radiographs effectively identify esophageal lesions of sufficient size to cause symptoms. In contrast to benign esophageal leiomyomata which result in esophageal narrowing with preservation of a normal mucosal pattern, esophageal carcinomas characteristically cause ragged, ulcerating changes in the mucosa in association with deeper infiltration, producing a picture resembling achalasia. Smaller, potentially resectable tumors are often poorly visualized despite technically adequate esophagograms. Because of this, esophagoscopy should be performed in all patients suspected of having an esophageal abnormality in order to visualize the tumor and to obtain histopathologic confirmation of the diagnosis. Since the same population of patients at risk for esophageal carcinoma (i.e., smokers and drinkers) also has a high rate of cancers of the lung and head and neck region, endoscopic inspection of the larynx, trachea, and bronchi should also be carried out. A thorough examination of the fundus of the stomach (by retroflexing the endoscope) is imperative as well. Endoscopic biopsies of esophageal tumors fail to recover malignant tissue in one-third of cases because the biopsy forceps cannot penetrate deeply enough through normal mucosa pushed in front of the carcinoma. Cytologic examination of tumor brushings frequently complements standard biopsies and should be performed routinely. The extent of tumor spread to the mediastinum and paraaortic lymph nodes should also be assessed by computed tomography (CT) scans of the chest and abdomen.

Treatment The prognosis for patients with esophageal carcinoma is poor. Less than 5 percent of patients are alive 5 years after the initial diagnosis, leading many physicians to focus management efforts solely on symptomatic control. Surgical resection of all gross tumor (i.e., total resection) is feasible in only 40 percent of cases, with residual tumor cells frequently present at the resection margins. Such esophagectomies are associated with a postoperative mortality rate in excess of 20 percent due to anastomotic fistulas, subphrenic abscesses, and respiratory complications. Less than 20 percent of patients who survive a total resection can be expected to be alive after 5 years. The therapeutic outcome following the administration of primary radiation therapy [55 to 60 Gy (5500 to 6000 rad)] is not dissimilar to that of radical surgery, sparing patients perioperative morbidity but often resulting in less satisfactory palliation of obstructive symptoms. The evaluation of chemotherapeutic agents in patients with esophageal carcinoma has been hampered by ambiguity in the definition of "response" (i.e., benefit) and the debilitated physical condition of many treated individuals. Nonetheless, significant reductions in the size of measurable tumor masses have been reported in 15 to 25 percent of patients given single-agent treatment and in 30 to 60 percent of patients treated with drug combinations which include cisplatin. Recent therapeutic efforts have been directed at utilizing combination chemotherapy and radiation therapy as the initial therapeutic approach, either alone or followed by an attempt at operative resection. It remains to be determined whether such an intensive multimodality approach will increase the cure rate.

For the incurable, surgically unresectable patient with esophageal cancer, dysphagia, malnutrition, and the management of tracheoesophageal fistulas loom as major issues. Approaches to palliation of these cancer-related complications include repeated endoscopic dilatation, the surgical placement of a gastrostomy or jejunostomy for hydration and feeding, and the surgical insertion of a polyvinyl prosthesis to bypass the tumor. Endoscopic fulguration of the obstructing tumor with lasers appears to be the most promising of these techniques.

TUMORS OF THE STOMACH

GASTRIC ADENOCARCINOMA **Incidence and epidemiology** For reasons which remain uncertain, the incidence and mortality rates for gastric cancer have decreased markedly during the past 60 years. In 1930, gastric cancer represented the leading cause of cancer-related deaths among American men by a factor of two, while the disease in women ranked just behind tumors of the uterine cervix and breast. During the ensuing years, the mortality rate from gastric cancer in the United States has dropped in men from 28 to 7.8 per 100,000 population, while in women, the rate has decreased from 27 to 3.7 per 100,000. Nonetheless, it was estimated in 1989 that 20,000 new cases of stomach cancer were diagnosed in the United States and that 13,900 Americans died of the disease. The decreased incidence in gastric cancer in the United States is also reflected worldwide. The incidence of gastric cancer varies widely among different countries, being comparatively high in Japan, China, Chile, and Ireland; however, a decrease in both incidence and mortality has occurred in these areas as well.

Epidemiologic surveys have suggested the risk of gastric cancer to be greater among lower socioeconomic classes. Furthermore, migrants from high- to low-incidence nations appear to maintain their susceptibility to gastric cancer while the risk for their offspring more closely approximates that of the new homeland. These findings suggest that an environmental exposure, probably beginning early in life, is related to the development of gastric cancer with dietary carcinogens considered the most likely factor(s).

Pathology Approximately 90 percent of stomach cancers are adenocarcinomas with 10 percent due to non-Hodgkin's lymphomas and leiomyosarcomas. Gastric adenocarcinomas may be subdivided into two categories: a *diffuse type* in which cell cohesion is absent, resulting in individual cells infiltrating and thickening the stomach wall without forming a discrete mass; and an *intestinal type* characterized by cohesive neoplastic cells forming glandlike tubular structures. The diffuse carcinomas occur more often in younger patients, develop throughout the stomach including the cardia, result in a loss of distensibility of the gastric wall (so-called linitis plastica or "leather bottle" appearance), and are associated with a far more ominous prognosis. Intestinal-type lesions are frequently ulcerative, more commonly appear in the antrum and lesser curvature of the stomach, and are often preceded by a prolonged precancerous process. While the incidence of diffuse carcinomas is similar in most populations,

TABLE 239-2 Dietary factors as a cause of gastric carcinoma*

Sources of nitrate-converting bacteria

I Exogenous
 A Bacterially contaminated food
 B Frequent in lower socioeconomic classes who have higher incidence of the disease
 C Diminished by improved food preservation and refrigeration
II Endogenous
 A Decreased gastric acidity
 B Prior gastric surgery (antrectomy)—15 to 20 year latency period
 C Atrophic gastritis and/or pernicious anemia
 D ? Prolonged exposure to histamine-2-receptor antagonists

*HYPOTHESIS: Dietary nitrates are converted to carcinogenic nitrites by bacteria

the intestinal type tends to predominate in the high-risk geographic regions mentioned earlier and is less likely to be found in areas where the frequency of gastric cancer is declining. Thus, different etiologic factor(s) may be involved in these two subtypes. In the United States, the distal stomach is the site of origin of about half of gastric cancers. Approximately 20 percent of these tumors arise in the lesser curvature, 25 percent in the cardia, and only 3 to 5 percent in the greater curvature. More than 10 percent of gastric carcinomas involve the entire stomach.

Etiology The relationship between dietary patterns and the development of gastric carcinoma has been extensively investigated. The long-term ingestion of high concentrations of nitrates in dried, smoked, and salted foods appears to be associated with a higher risk. The nitrates are thought to be converted to carcinogenic nitrites by bacteria (Table 239-2). Such bacteria may be introduced exogenously through the ingestion of the partially decayed foods which are consumed in abundance worldwide by the lower socioeconomic classes. Bacteria may also appear endogenously as a result of a lack or loss of gastric acidity. This may occur when acid-producing cells of the gastric antrum have been surgically removed 15 to 20 years previously at the time of a partial gastrectomy to control benign peptic ulcer disease or when achlorhydria, atrophic gastritis, and even pernicious anemia develop in the elderly. Serial endoscopic examinations of the stomach in patients with atrophic gastritis have documented replacement of the usual gastric mucosa by intestinal-type cells. This process of intestinal metaplasia may lead to cellular atypia and eventual neoplasia. Since the declining incidence of gastric cancer in the United States is primarily a reflection of a decline in distal, ulcerating, intestinal-type lesions, it is conceivable that better food preservation and the availability to all socioeconomic classes of refrigeration for food storage have resulted in a decrease in the dietary ingestion of exogenous bacteria. It remains uncertain whether the iatrogenic achlorhydria induced by the widespread, prolonged use of parietal cell histamine antagonists will result in a future increase in intestinal-type gastric cancer.

Several additional etiologic factors have been associated with gastric carcinoma. Gastric ulcers and adenomatous polyps have occasionally been so linked, but data regarding a cause-and-effect relationship are unconvincing. The inadequate clinical distinction between benign gastric ulcers and small ulcerating carcinomas may, in part, account for this presumed association. The presence of extreme hypertrophy of gastric rugal folds (i.e., Ménétrier's disease), giving the impression of polypoid lesions, has been associated with a striking frequency of malignant transformation; such hypertrophy, however, does not represent the presence of true adenomatous polyps. Individuals with blood group A have been reported to have a higher incidence of gastric cancer than persons with blood group O; it is possible that this observation is related to differences in the mucous secretion of the various ABO blood groups, thereby leading to greater or lesser mucosal protection from carcinogens. No association has been identified between duodenal ulcers and gastric cancer.

Clinical features Gastric cancers, when superficial and surgically curable, usually produce no symptoms. As the tumor becomes more extensive, patients may complain of an insidious upper abdominal discomfort varying in intensity from a vague, postprandial fullness to a severe, steady pain. Anorexia, often with slight nausea, is very common but is not the usual presenting complaint. Weight loss may eventually be observed and nausea and vomiting are particularly prominent with tumors of the pylorus; dysphagia may be the major symptom caused by lesions of the cardia. There are no early physical signs of the disease, and the finding of a palpable abdominal mass generally indicates long-standing growth and, all too often, regional extension.

Gastric carcinomas spread by direct extension through the gastric wall to the perigastric tissues, occasionally adhering to adjacent organs such as the pancreas, colon, or liver. The disease also spreads via lymphatics or by seeding of peritoneal surfaces. Metastases to intraabdominal and supraclavicular lymph nodes may occur frequently as may metastatic nodules to the ovary (Krunkenberg's tumor) or to the peritoneal cul-de-sac (Blumer's shelf); malignant ascites may also develop. The liver is the most common site for hematogenous spread of tumor.

The presence of iron-deficiency anemia in men and occult blood in the stool of both sexes should mandate a search for an occult lesion in the gastrointestinal tract. Such a careful assessment is of particular importance in patients having atrophic gastritis or pernicious anemia. Unusual clinical features associated with gastric adenocarcinomas include migratory thrombophlebitis, microangiopathic hemolytic anemia, and acanthosis nigricans.

Diagnosis A double-contrast radiographic examination is the simplest diagnostic procedure for the evaluation of a patient with epigastric complaints. The use of double-contrast techniques helps to detect small lesions by improving mucosal detail. The stomach should be distended at some time during every radiographic examination since decreased distensibility may be the only indication of a diffuse infiltrative carcinoma. Although gastric ulcers can be detected fairly early, it may be impossible to distinguish benign from malignant lesions. The anatomic location of an ulcer is not in itself an indication of the presence or absence of a cancer.

The x-ray demonstration of a benign-appearing gastric ulcer presents special problems. Some physicians believe that gastroscopy is not mandatory if the radiographic features are typically benign, if complete healing can be visualized by x-ray within 6 weeks, and if a follow-up contrast radiograph several months later is normal. However, many feel that gastroscopic biopsy and brush cytology are required for all patients with a gastric ulcer in order to exclude a malignancy. The identification of malignant gastric ulcers prior to their penetration into surrounding tissues is crucial since the curability of such early lesions when limited to the mucosa or submucosa, even in the United States, is greater than 80 percent. Since gastric carcinomas are difficult to distinguish clinically or radiographically from gastric lymphomas, endoscopic biopsies should be made as deeply as possible due to the submucosal location of lymphoid tumors.

Treatment Surgical removal of the complete tumor with resection of adjacent lymph nodes offers the only chance for cure. However, this is possible in less than one-third of patients. In general, a subtotal gastrectomy represents the treatment of choice for patients with distal carcinomas while total or near-total gastrectomies are required for more proximal tumors. The prognosis following complete surgical resection is adversely influenced by the degree of tumor penetration into the stomach wall, regional lymph node involvement, and vascular invasion, characteristics found in the vast majority of American patients. As a result, the probability of survival after five years for the 25 to 30 percent of patients in the United States able to undergo a complete resection of a gastric cancer is approximately 25 percent for distal tumors and less than 10 percent for proximal tumors, with continued tumor recurrences being observed for at least 8 years following surgery. In the absence of ascites or extensive hepatic or peritoneal metastases, however, even the patient who is believed to be surgically incurable should be offered an attempt at resecting the primary lesion since the reduction of residual tumor offers the best form of palliation and may possibly enhance the probability for subsequent benefit if chemotherapy and/or radiation therapy are administered.

Gastric adenocarcinoma is a relatively radioresistant tumor, requiring doses of external beam irradiation in excess of the tolerance of surrounding structures such as bowel mucosa and spinal cord if adequate control of the primary tumor is to be achieved. As a result, the major role of radiation therapy in patients with gastric cancer has been limited to palliation of pain. Controlled trials have not been conducted to determine whether radiation therapy after a complete resection can prolong survival. In the setting of surgically unresectable disease limited to the epigastrium, comparative studies have shown that patients treated with 35 to 40 Gy (3500 to 4000 rad) did not live longer than similar patients not receiving radiotherapy; however, survival was prolonged slightly when 5-fluorouracil (5-FU) was given concomitantly with radiation therapy. In this clinical setting, the 5-FU may well be functioning as a radiosensitizer.

The administration of combinations of cytotoxic drugs to patients with advanced gastric carcinoma has been associated with reductions of greater than 50 percent in measurable tumor masses ("partial responses") in 30 to 50 percent of cases, providing significant benefit to individuals who respond to treatment. Such drug combinations have generally included 5-FU and doxorubicin together with mitomycin-C, cisplatin, or semustine (methyl-CCNU). Despite this encouraging response rate for a malignant condition once thought untreatable, complete disappearances of tumor masses remain uncommon, the partial responses are transient, and the overall impact of such multidrug therapy on survival has been a source of debate. The use of prophylactic (i.e., adjuvant) chemotherapy following the complete resection of a gastric cancer as a means of eradicating clinically undetectable micrometastases and improving the potential for cure has led to conflicting results; the role of adjuvant treatment remains an unsettled issue and such therapy should continue to be considered investigational.

PRIMARY GASTRIC LYMPHOMA Primary lymphoma of the stomach is relatively uncommon, comprising about 7 percent of gastric malignancies and about 2 percent of all lymphomas. It is, however, the most frequent extranodal location for lymphoma. The disease is difficult to distinguish clinically from gastric adenocarcinoma; both tumors are most often detected during the sixth decade of life, present with epigastric pain, early satiety, and generalized fatigue, and are usually characterized by ulcerations with a ragged, thickened mucosal pattern demonstrated by contrast radiographs. The diagnosis of lymphoma of the stomach may occasionally be made through cytologic brushings of the gastric mucosa, but usually requires a biopsy at the time of gastroscopy or laparotomy. The failure of gastroscopic biopsies to detect lymphoma should not be interpreted as being conclusive since superficial biopsies may miss the more deeply situated lymphoid infiltrate. The macroscopic pathology of gastric lymphoma may also mimic adenocarcinoma, either as a bulky ulcerated lesion localized in the corpus or antrum or as a diffuse process spreading throughout the entire gastric submucosa and even extending into the duodenum. Microscopically, the vast majority of gastric lymphoid tumors are non-Hodgkin's lymphomas of B-cell origin; Hodgkin's disease involving the stomach is extremely uncommon. Gastric lymphomas spread initially to regional lymph nodes (often to Waldeyer's ring) and may then disseminate.

Primary gastric lymphoma is a far more treatable disease than adenocarcinoma of the stomach, underscoring the need for making the correct diagnosis. All detectable tumor can be removed in over two-thirds of patients by some type of a subtotal gastrectomy. The prognosis in such patients is encouraging with 5-year survival rates of 40 to 60 percent having been reported. The best prognosis seems to be associated with those gastric lymphomas having small, single lesions, more differentiated histologies, and absence of spread to adjacent lymph nodes. While postoperative radiation therapy to the abdomen has been employed in the past, even when all obvious disease has been resected, the value of such a practice is open to serious question since the majority of recurrences develop in anatomic sites distant from the epigastrium and outside the fields of radiation treatment. Combination chemotherapy, which has proved to be highly effective in the management of disseminated non-Hodgkin's lymphoma including the diffuse large cell subtype, has recently gained increased favor as an adjunct to surgery, particularly when regional lymph node involvement is present. In the past, such drug therapy was not considered to be a substitute for surgery, even if the lymphoma were localized, since the rapid destruction of lymphoma masses by chemotherapy occasionally led to life-threatening hemorrhage. The results of recent clinical trials, however, have suggested that the probability for such bleeding may be relatively small and that drug treatment alone may be adequate to eradicate the lymphoma. If widespread disease is discovered at the time of laparotomy, combination chemotherapy should be utilized.

GASTRIC (NONLYMPHOID) SARCOMA Leiomyosarcomas are the most common of this group of gastric malignancies and comprise approximately 1 to 3 percent of all gastric neoplasms. They most frequently involve the anterior and posterior walls of the gastric fundus and often ulcerate and bleed. Even those lesions which appear benign on histologic examination may behave in a malignant fashion. Leiomyosarcomas rarely invade adjacent viscera and characteristically do not metastasize to lymph nodes but may spread to the liver and lungs. The treatment of choice is surgical resection. Combination chemotherapy should be reserved for patients with metastatic disease.

REFERENCES

Esophageal cancer

Boyce HW: Palliation of advanced esophageal cancer. Semin Oncol 11:186, 1984

Coia LR et al: Nonsurgical management of esophageal cancer: Report of a study of combined radiotherapy and chemotherapy. J Clin Oncol 5:1783, 1987

Kelsen D: Chemotherapy of esophageal cancer. Semin Oncol 11:159, 1984

Lightdale CJ, Winawer SJ: Screening diagnosis and staging of esophageal cancer. Semin Oncol 11:101, 1984

Poplin E et al: Combined therapies for squamous-cell carcinoma of the esophagus, a Southwest Oncology Group Study (SWOG - 8037). J Clin Oncol 5:622, 1987

Reid BJ et al: Barrett's esophagus. Correlation between flow cytometry and histology in detection of patients at risk for adenocarcinoma. Gastroenterology 93:1, 1987

Schottenfeld D: Epidemiology of cancer of the esophagus. Semin Oncol 11:92, 1984

Skinner DB: Surgical treatment for esophageal carcinoma. Semin Oncol 11:136, 1984

Gastric tumors

Allum WH et al: Adjuvant chemotherapy in operable gastric cancer. Lancet 1:571, 1989

Antonioli DA, Goldman H: Changes in the location and type of gastric adenocarcinoma. Cancer 50:775, 1982

Bedikian AY et al: The natural history of gastric cancer and prognostic factors influencing survival. J Clin Oncol 2:305, 1984

Correa P: Clinical implications of recent developments in gastric cancer pathology and epidemiology. Semin Oncol 12:2, 1985

Douglass HO, Nava HR: Gastric adenocarcinoma—management of the primary disease. Semin Oncol 12:32, 1985

Gohmann JJ, Macdonald JS: Chemotherapy of gastric cancer. Cancer Invest 7:39, 1989

Haber DA, Mayer RJ: Primary gastrointestinal lymphoma. Semin Oncol 15:154, 1988

Kurtz RC, Sherlock P: The diagnosis of gastric cancer. Semin Oncol 12:11, 1985

Langman MJS: Antisecretory drugs and gastric cancer. Br Med J 290:1850, 1985

Licht JD et al: Gastrointestinal sarcomas. Semin Oncol 15:181, 1988

List AF et al: Non-Hodgkin's lymphoma of the gastrointestinal tract: An analysis of clinical and pathologic features affecting outcome. J Clin Oncol 6:1125, 1988

Lundegardh G et al: Stomach cancer after partial gastrectomy for benign ulcer disease. N Engl J Med 319:195, 1988

240 DISORDERS OF ABSORPTION

NORTON J. GREENBERGER / KURT J. ISSELBACHER

MECHANISMS OF ABSORPTION

Diseases of the small intestine are frequently accompanied by alterations in intestinal function, and clinically this impaired function is seen as the malabsorption syndrome. In order to obtain a better appreciation of the derangements which occur in the many disorders of intestinal function, the processes of normal absorption will first be reviewed.

It is important to distinguish between digestion and absorption, since an increased loss of nutrients in the stool may be a reflection of a derangement of either process. Digestion involves the breakdown or hydrolysis of nutrients to smaller molecules in order to prepare the ingested substances for absorption, or transport across the intestinal cell. It will be recalled that most of the digestive process is initiated in the stomach by acid and pepsin and is continued in the upper small intestine primarily by the action of pancreatic enzymes such as lipase, amylase, and trypsin. As a result of these digestive actions carbohydrates are broken down to monosaccharides and disaccharides, proteins to peptides and amino acids, and fats to monoglycerides and fatty acids. In the adult it is in this form that nutrients are, to a large extent, transported across the epithelial surface of the intestinal cell.

ANATOMIC AND PHYSIOLOGIC FACTORS The intestine has an enormous surface area. This can be attributed in large part to its length, which in the adult is more than 4 m, and to the foldings of the surface plicae. At the light microscopic level, the villi of the small intestine provide additional surface area, which is further augmented by the presence of microvilli (approximately 2×10^8 per square centimeter) on the outer, or brush border, region of epithelial cells. Thus the total absorptive area of the small intestine is enormous.

Motility (contractility) of the bowel is an important process which permits nutrients to remain in intimate contact with the intestinal cells and possibly influences the continued movement of the nutrients *into* and along the absorbing channels, such as the lymphatics. Two types of motility aid in this process: the gross motility of the intestine itself and the motility of individual villi. Entrance of the nutrients into the general circulation is achieved via the capillaries into the portal system or via the lacteals into the intestinal lymphatics.

TYPES OF ABSORPTION Four mechanisms have been considered to be important in the transport of substances across the intestinal cell membrane, namely, active transport, passive diffusion, facilitated diffusion, and endocytosis.

Active transport involves the transport of a substance across the cell against an electric or chemical gradient; this process requires energy, is carrier-mediated, and is subject to competitive inhibition. *Passive diffusion* is the opposite of this process; energy is not required, transport is with (rather than against) the electric or chemical gradient, the process is not carrier-mediated, and it does not show properties of competitive inhibition. Thus active transport may be viewed as "uphill" transport, whereas passive diffusion is equivalent to "downhill" transport. *Facilitated diffusion* is similar to passive diffusion except that such a process shows evidence of being carrier-mediated and frequently subject to competitive inhibition.

Endocytosis is a process akin to phagocytosis. By this mechanism nutrients (soluble or particulate) upon entering the cell are surrounded by the components of the outer plasma cell membrane. In the intestinal tract endocytosis occurs in the neonatal period and, contrary to earlier belief, also occurs to a limited extent in the adult organism. While quantitatively limited, it appears to account, for example, for uptake of antigens.

SITES OF ABSORPTION While many substances are absorbed throughout the length of the small intestine, certain nutrients tend to be absorbed more in one region than in others. The proximal intestine is a major area for the absorption of iron, calcium, water-soluble vitamins, and fat (monoglycerides and fatty acids). Sugars are absorbed in the proximal intestine and also the midintestine. While the amino acids appear to be absorbed primarily in the middle of the small intestine, or jejunum, some absorption also occurs in the upper and lower areas. The distal small intestine appears to be the *major* absorptive area for bile salts and vitamin B_{12}. As is emphasized below, this factor is of clinical significance in circumstances where there has been removal or disease of the ileum.

The colon is important for the absorption of water and electrolytes, a process which occurs predominantly in the cecum. Although the rectum is not a usual site for absorption of ingested foodstuffs, drugs introduced by rectum may be absorbed there. Thus drugs introduced by this route, such as salicylates or steroids, may have systemic as well as local effects.

ABSORPTION OF SPECIFIC NUTRIENTS Carbohydrate absorption Much of the carbohydrate we ingest is in the form of starch, a complex polysaccharide consisting of many hexose units (attached either in a 1,4 or 1,6 linkage). By the action of salivary and pancreatic amylase, starch is hydrolyzed to oligosaccharides and then to disaccharides (mostly maltose). While monosaccharides such as glucose are readily absorbed, disaccharides are not. Disaccharides are split enzymatically into their component sugars by disaccharidases (or oligosaccharidases) located on or within the microvilli of intestinal epithelial cells. The two types of disaccharidases are β-galactosidases (lactase) and α-glucosidases (sucrase, maltase). By the action of these enzymes, lactose is split into glucose and galactose, sucrose into glucose and fructose, and maltose into two molecules of glucose. The resultant monosaccharides are then transported through the cell into the portal circulation. Most disaccharides are hydrolyzed so rapidly by brush border enzymes that the capacity of the transport mechanism is exceeded and some monosaccharides diffuse back into the intestinal lumen. Lactose, however, is hydrolyzed at a slower rate, and thus lactose hydrolysis is the rate-limiting step in lactose absorption.

Sugars such as glucose and galactose are absorbed by an active transport mechanism. The transport rate of sugars can be related to the substrate concentration by the expression K_t, where K_t stands for the monosaccharide substrate concentration that produces half the maximal transport rate. Published K_t values for glucose transport have varied widely, partly because of failure to consider the unstirred water layer, which constitutes a diffusion barrier for solutes.

Glucose (and galactose) entry into the cell is largely coupled to sodium ions (so-called symport); both sodium and glucose appear to bind to the hexose carrier in the microvillus membrane. Energy is required for the movement of glucose into the cell, which seems largely to come from the sodium pump and the Na^+,K^+-ATPase of the basolateral membrane (see below).

Protein and amino acid absorption Dietary proteins are initially subject to degradation in the stomach by pepsin. However, complete hydrolysis is largely achieved by the action of the pancreatic enzymes trypsin and chymotrypsin as well as by other endopeptidases and exopeptidases such as carboxypeptidase. By these enzymatic processes oligopeptides, dipeptides, and amino acids are formed. Just as there are disaccharidases in mucosal cells to digest disaccharides, there are also oligopeptidases to split small peptides. Dipeptidases are located in the cytoplasm as well as on the microvilli. Dipeptides are absorbed more rapidly than amino acids, and presumably their uptake involves a separate mechanism. Thus, digestion of proteins to amino acids occurs in three locations: intestinal lumen, brush border, and cytoplasm of mucosal cells. As indicated above, contrary to earlier beliefs proteins can also be absorbed by the adult intestine. Although quantitatively limited, protein absorption probably is immunologically significant.

Most naturally occurring amino acids are L-amino acids, and these are subject to a number of different transport processes. *Neutral* amino acids seem to share a common carrier mechanism; thus amino acids such as tryptophan and alanine show competitive inhibition. Among the *dibasic* amino acids which appear to have a distinct transport mechanism are arginine, ornithine, and lysine. The neutral amino acid cystine shares this mechanism. There is also a separate transport system for *glycine* and the *imino acids* proline and hydroxyproline. There is also a transport system for *dicarboxylic* acids such as glutamic and aspartic acids. Therefore, in genetic disorders, such as cystinuria, one will find impaired absorption not only of cystine but also of arginine, ornithine, and lysine. Similarly in Hartnup disease, a defect in the transport of neutral amino acids (especially of tryptophan, phenylalanine, histidine) is found. In these genetic disorders uptake and absorption of dipeptides is normal.

Absorption of amino acids is rapid in the duodenum and jejunum but slow in the ileum. The actual mechanism of the absorption of amino acids by the intestine has not been elucidated. As in the case of carbohydrates, sodium ions appear to be required for the entry of these acids and the energy needed for their concentration within the cell. Some amino acids have affinity for more than one mechanism. For example, glycine may be transported by both the neutral and imino acid transport systems.

Fat absorption (Fig. 240-1) Most of the ingested dietary fats are in the form of long-chain triglycerides. These triglycerides contain both saturated fatty acids (such as palmitic and stearic) and unsaturated fatty acids (such as oleic and linoleic). The particle size of the fat is decreased largely by the churning action of the stomach. The entry of fat into the duodenum plus the presence of acid causes release of secretin and pancreozymin-cholecystokinin, which in turn leads to a stimulation of the flow of bile and pancreatic juice.

ROLE OF PANCREATIC LIPASE The hydrolysis of triglycerides by pancreatic lipase is a complex process involving lipase, colipase, and bile salts. Pancreatic lipase is an enzyme that binds to the oil-water interface of an emulsified triglyceride substrate. The detergent properties of bile salts permit pancreatic lipase to gain access to water-insoluble lipids. One of the important functions of bile salts is to clear the oil-water interface of dietary fat from proteins of exogenous and endogenous origin, thus making it available for pancreatic lipolysis. Colipase, a protein present in pancreatic juice, is also essential for the action of lipase; its function is to anchor the lipase close to the surface of the triglyceride droplet. All three components, i.e., pancreatic lipase, colipase, and bile salts, form a *ternary complex,* which generates lipolytic products that diffuse away from the complex and are absorbed. With colipase present, lipase remains at the interface and forms 2-monoglycerides and fatty acids, which are the major end products of triglyceride hydrolysis. Less than 5 percent of ingested fat remains in the form of diglycerides and triglycerides. Without colipase, bile acids would actually wash pancreatic lipase away from the interface, and the hydrolytic rate of triglycerides would be reduced.

ROLE OF BILE SALTS (Fig. 240-2) Bile salts play an important role in the digestion and absorption of fat. They are synthesized in the liver (approximately 200 to 600 mg daily) from cholesterol and excreted in the bile in the form of their glycine or taurine conjugates. In humans the principal bile acids excreted are conjugates of cholic and chenodeoxycholic acid. Bile salts are good detergents, because they have both polar (hydrophilic) and nonpolar (hydrophobic) groups. During digestion the concentration of conjugated bile salts in the lumen is in the range of 5 to 15 μmol/mL, and at these concentrations the bile salts aggregate to form *micelles.* Fatty acids and monoglycerides enter these micelles, forming mixed micelles. An emulsion of triglyceride is turbid; mixed micelles containing bile salts, fatty acids, and monoglycerides are clear solutions. The formation of *mixed micelles* and hence the solubilization of fatty acids and monoglycerides is much more effectively achieved with *conjugated bile salts* at the pH which normally exists in the intestinal lumen (Fig. 240-2).

Most conjugated bile salts are absorbed in the ileum and after entering the portal vein are subject to an enterohepatic circulation. By this process about 90 percent of the conjugated bile salts reaching the ileum is reabsorbed. As a consequence only about 200 to 600 mg bile salts is excreted in the feces per day, while, as part of the enterohepatic circulation, the 3- to 4-g bile salt pool circulates many times each day so that actually 20 to 30 g of bile salts may enter the duodenum each day. When the enterohepatic circulation is intact, the size of the bile salt pool is largely determined by the frequency of the enterohepatic circulation, i.e., the number of cycles per day (see also Chap. 258). If the ileum is diseased or removed, absorption of bile salts is impaired, and a significant fecal loss of bile salts will occur. As a consequence of this bile salt depletion, the concentration of bile salts in the intestinal lumen will also decrease, leading to further impairment of fat absorption. A similar result will occur if bile salt reabsorption is prevented by chelating agents, such as cholestyramine (see "Regional Enteritis" below). Diarrhea per se may result in increased fecal excretion of bile salts. This has been demonstrated both in normal subjects in whom diarrhea has been induced and in patients with chronic idiopathic diarrhea.

INTRAMUCOSAL ASPECTS OF FAT ABSORPTION (Fig. 240-1) After the hydrolysis of fatty acids to monoglycerides and their interaction with bile salts to form mixed micelles, the lipids pass through an "unstirred" water layer covering the cell surface. The mixed micelles apparently do not enter the cell, but instead the component fatty acids and monoglycerides are released from the micellar phase and then enter the cell by diffusion. In aqueous duodenal contents, large bile salt mixed micelles saturated with products of lipolysis coexist with larger liquid crystal liposomes of the same lipids saturated with free fatty acids and mixed bile salts. These phases are interconvertible and both may be important in fat digestion and absorption. Upon

FIGURE 240-1 Scheme of intestinal digestion, absorption, esterification, and transport of dietary triglycerides. TG = triglycerides; FA = fatty acids; MG = monoglycerides; BS = bile salts.

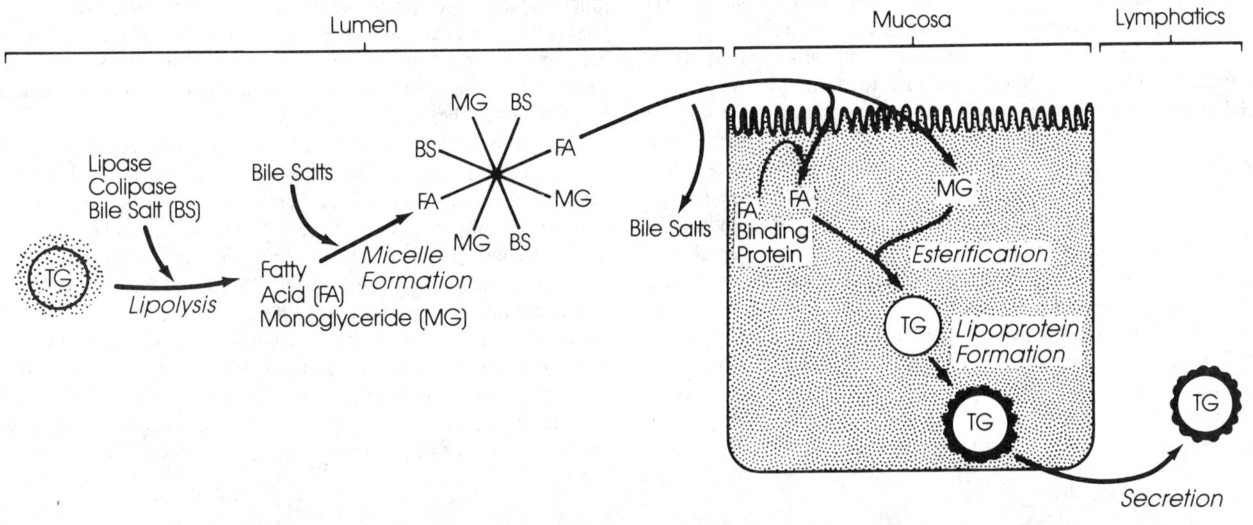

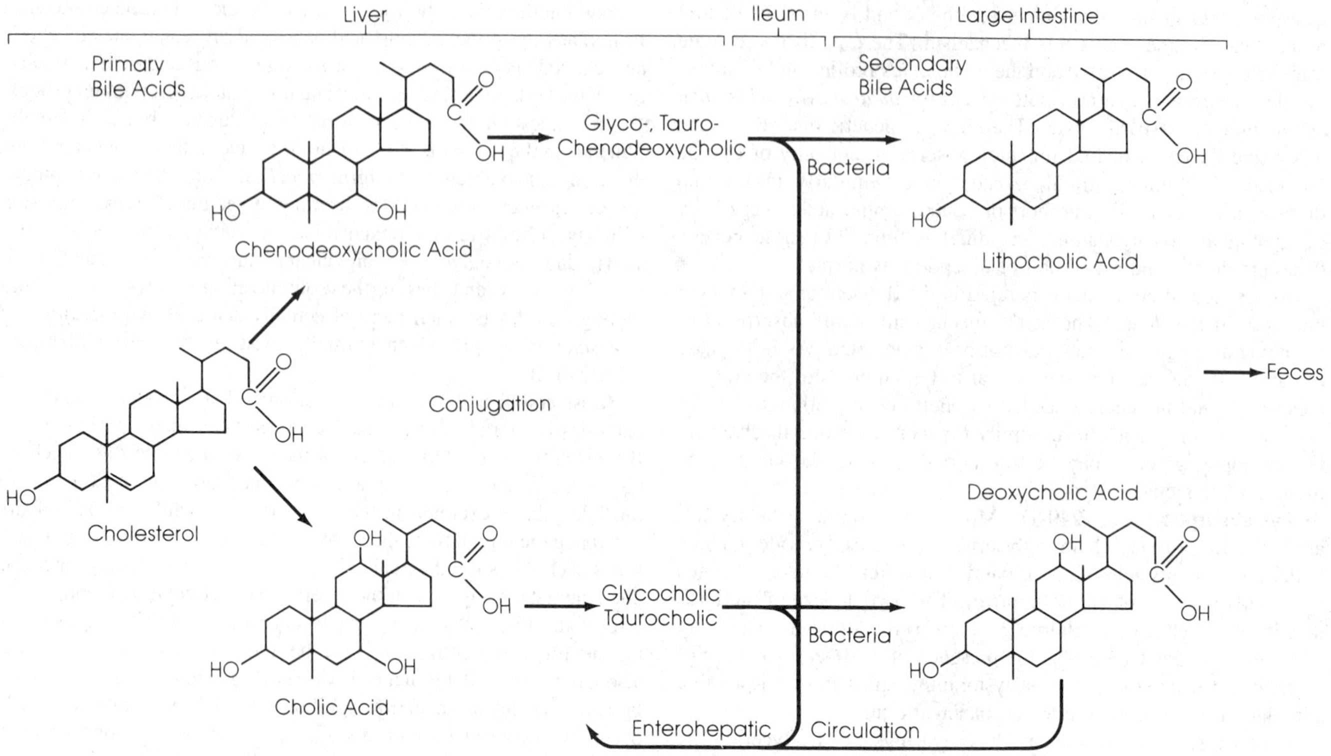

FIGURE 240-2 Scheme of hepatic and intestinal metabolism of bile salts and the enterohepatic circulation (from ileum to liver). Note that bacteria lead to the formation of secondary bile acids; of the latter, only deoxycholic acid is absorbed to any appreciable extent.

entry into the mucosal cell, fatty acids may interact with specific binding proteins. The subsequent fate of the intracellular lipid is strongly influenced by the fatty acid chain length. Fatty acids and monoglycerides derived from long-chain triglycerides (i.e., containing C-16 to C-18 fatty acids) are promptly *reesterified to triglycerides* by enzymes of the endoplasmic reticulum. These triglycerides then interact with specific apolipoproteins plus cholesterol and phospholipid to form chylomicrons and very low density lipoproteins. These initially accumulate in the Golgi region of the cell and then are secreted into the lacteals and the intestinal lymph. There are thus four major steps in the absorption of long-chain fatty acids and monoglycerides: (1) mucosal uptake and interaction with binding proteins, (2) reesterification to triglycerides, (3) lipoprotein formation, and (4) secretion into lymph.

By contrast, fatty acids derived from medium-chain triglycerides (i.e., containing C-8 and C-12 fatty acids) are *not reesterified* to any significant extent within the cell and are not incorporated into lipoproteins. Instead, they rapidly enter the portal venous system, where they are transported as fatty acids bound to albumin. The major aspects of fat absorption are summarized in Fig. 240-1.

Absorption of cholesterol and fat-soluble vitamins (A, D, E, K) In addition to contributing significantly to the total-body synthesis of cholesterol, the intestine also plays an active role in the absorption of cholesterol and its esters. Within the lumen, cholesterol esters from the bile and diet are hydrolyzed by a pancreatic esterase. There is also a separate cholesterol esterase in the intestinal microvilli, which completes this hydrolysis. As a result, only free cholesterol appears to enter the intestinal cell. However, just as in the case of long-chain fatty acids, much of the cholesterol is reesterified and is then secreted primarily into lymph.

The absorption mechanisms of the fat-soluble vitamins A, D, E, and K are not well understood. The intestine is able to convert β-carotene into vitamin A. The vitamin A thus formed or absorbed from the lumen is esterified in the mucosa primarily with palmitic acid, transported in the chylomicrons of the lymph, and stored as retinol palmitate in the liver. The other lipid-soluble vitamins also appear in lymph chylomicrons, but esterification with fatty acids does not appear to be necessary for their transport.

Water and sodium absorption In spite of extensive investigations the main mechanisms of water and electrolyte transport are not well understood. The mechanisms responsible for fluid absorption differ in the jejunum, ileum, and colon. There are two pathways by which water and ions cross the intestinal mucosa: the paracellular and transcellular pathways. Individual intestinal mucosa cells are joined near their apex by a "tight junction," and ions and water traverse this *paracellular* pathway during absorption and secretion. It is believed that the tight junction pathway contains aqueous-filled channels or pores. Such intercellular spaces are closed in the resting state and dilated during absorption. Considerable evidence has accumulated indicating that pumps and carriers are involved in intestinal water and solute transport. For example, in the ileum, Na^+ enters in exchange for H^+, and Cl^- enters in exchange for HCO_3^-. Sodium entry into the cell also occurs coupled with glucose via the glucose-sodium carrier in the microvillus membrane. Inside the cell, the Na^+ pump located in the basolateral membrane actively transports Na^+ out of the mucosal cell and into the intercellular space. *Transcellular* transport requires passage of ions through two membrane barriers, i.e., the apical brush border plasma membrane and the basolateral membrane. After Na^+ and Cl^- are transported across the brush border membrane into the cell, Na^+ is pumped across the basolateral membrane and Cl^- either follows passively or is also pumped into the intercellular space. The Na^+,K^+-ATPase is present in the basolateral but not in the brush border membrane and is the biochemical mediator of this pump. Bulk water movement obviously influences the movement of Na^+, K^+, and Cl^-. This "solvent drag" effect is explained by two mechanisms: (1) solutes may be caught in a moving stream of water and transported across a membrane, and (2) water movement results in increased concentration of solute on the side of the membrane from which water was transported, which causes solute to diffuse through the direction of flow. Diarrhea can

TABLE 240-1 Some mechanisms in the production of diarrhea

I Secretory diarrhea
- *A* Secretory agents associated with adenylate cyclase system
  - *1* Enterotoxin-producing bacteria *(Vibrio cholerae, Escherichia coli)*
  - *2* Methylxanthines (caffeine, theophylline)
  - *3* Prostaglandins
  - *4* Vasoactive intestinal peptide (VIP)
  - *5* Dihydroxy bile acids (affect colon primarily; effects seen after ileal resection)
- *B* Secretory agents *not associated* with adenylate cyclase system
  - *1* Glucagon, secretin, cholecystokinin-pancreozymin, serotonin, calcitonin, gastrin inhibitory polypeptide (GIP)
  - *2* Some laxatives* (ricinoleic acid, bisacodyl, phenolphthalein, dioctyl sodium sulfosuccinate)
  - *3* Bacterial enterotoxins *(Shigella, Staphylococcus aureus, Clostridium perfringens)*
- *C* Mucosal injury, altered cell permeability
  - *1* *Salmonella, Shigella,* invasive *E. coli,* gastroenteritis viruses
  - *2* Celiac sprue
  - *3* Inflammatory bowel disease (ulcerative colitis, regional enteritis)
- *D* Neoplasms with or without hormone production
  - *1* Gastrinoma (gastrin)
  - *2* Carcinoid syndrome (serotonin, prostaglandins)
  - *3* Medullary carcinoma of thyroid (calcitonin, prostaglandins)
  - *4* Pancreatic cholera syndrome (? VIP)
  - *5* Villous adenoma

II Osmotic diarrhea
- *A* Impaired carbohydrate absorption
  - *1* Disaccharidase deficiency (lactose or sucrose-isomaltose intolerance)
  - *2* Glucose-galactose malabsorption
- *B* Laxative ingestion or abuse
  - *1* Nonabsorbable osmotically active agents (lactulose, sorbitol, mannitol)
  - *2* Saline purgatives (magnesium phosphate, magnesium hydroxide–containing antacids)
- *C* Postsurgical disorders
  - *1* Vagotomy and pyloroplasty*
  - *2* Gastrojejunostomy* (Billroth I and II)

III Motility disorders
- *A* Laxative abuse*
- *B* Irritable bowel syndrome
- *C* Diverticular disease of the colon
- *D* Diabetic diarrhea with visceral neuropathy

* Multiple mechanisms involved in production of diarrhea.

be simply defined as impaired net absorption of water and electrolytes by the small intestine or colon. Some mechanisms producing diarrhea are listed in Table 240-1.

Calcium absorption Calcium is actively transported by the small intestine, and this process is intimately linked to the active form of vitamin D_3, namely, 1,25-dihydroxycholecalciferol. The role of two other intestinal cell proteins, calcium-binding protein and calmodulin, in the absorption of calcium remains unclear. Recent studies indicate that calcium is absorbed to the same extent from various calcium salts (carbonate, citrate, gluconate, lactate, and acetate) and from milk in healthy subjects; an average of 32 percent of the ingested calcium was absorbed from the various sources.

Iron absorption The formation of soluble iron complexes is important for maintaining intraluminal iron in an absorbable form. Gastric acid facilitates the chelation of inorganic iron with substances such as ascorbic acid, sugars, amino acids, and bile; these macromolecular complexes then remain soluble in the more alkaline duodenum and jejunum. With the average western diet the iron intake averages 15 to 25 mg per day; iron absorption averages 0.5 to 1.0 mg per day in men and 1.0 to 2.0 mg per day in women during their reproductive years. A regulatory mechanism for the absorption of inorganic iron appears to exist within the small-intestinal mucosal cells. Iron is actively transported by the small intestine, and the duodenum is the principal site of iron absorption. The absorption of elemental iron in humans and animals involves at least two distinct steps: (1) mucosal uptake of iron from the lumen and (2) mucosal transfer of iron to the plasma. Much of the iron entering the mucosal cell is not transferred to the plasma but remains trapped within the cell and is excreted into the lumen when the cell is shed. Iron lost by this mechanism seems to vary inversely with body iron stores. However, this mucosal regulatory mechanism can be overcome when pharmacologic doses of iron are ingested. Hemoglobin iron is also absorbed by human subjects, depending upon body requirements for iron; the heme is split from globin in the lumen and absorbed as an intact metalloporphyrin. Organic iron in the form of hemoglobin is absorbed more effectively than iron from cereals and vegetables. The absorption of inorganic iron is increased by ascorbic acid. Similarly, the presence of anemia, liver injury, pregnancy, idiopathic hemochromatosis, or a portacaval shunt may result in increased iron absorption. Conversely, the prior ingestion of large doses of iron and the presence in the lumen of phosphates, carbonates, and phytates may lead to decreased absorption of inorganic iron. Impaired absorption of iron is frequent in disorders (such as nontropical sprue) which involve the duodenal mucosa.

Water-soluble vitamins *Vitamin B_{12} absorption* is discussed in Chap. 292. In the case of *folic acid absorption,* it should be emphasized that folates exist in food conjugated with glutamyl peptides. These *polyglutamates* must be deconjugated (by folic deconjugase) to monoglutamates for absorption to occur. Certain drugs (such as oral contraceptives, sulfasalazine, diphenylhydantoin, trimethoprim, and pyrimethamine) inhibit the absorption of dietary folate and hence can cause folate deficiency. Sulfasalazine, for example, competitively inhibits three enzymes important in the intestinal metabolism of folate, i.e., dihydrofolate reductase, methylene tetrahydrofolate reductase, and serine transhydroxymethylase. Thiamine and riboflavin appear to be absorbed by passive diffusion.

TESTS USEFUL IN THE DIAGNOSIS OF MALABSORPTION

Most of the tests useful in the diagnosis of malabsorption indicate the presence of abnormal absorptive or digestive function, and only a few tests may suggest a specific diagnosis. Accordingly, it is frequently necessary to employ a combination of tests to establish a diagnosis. To illustrate the use of various tests, the characteristic findings in nontropical sprue, an example of a primary malabsorptive disorder, and pancreatic insufficiency, an example of impaired digestion, are compared in Table 240-2.

Stool fat The qualitative examination of the stool for undigested muscle fibers, neutral fat, and split fat is a simple and reliable screening test for steatorrhea. The finding of an increased number of muscle fibers indicates impaired intraluminal digestion. Properly performed, the qualitative microscopic examination of a stool specimen with the Sudan III stain is of value and correlates well with the quantitative determination of fecal fat by the Van de Kamer method. The latter remains the most reliable measurement of steatorrhea. A normal fecal fat excretion is less than 6 g for 24 h, or greater than 94 percent coefficient of fat absorption.

Oral [^{14}C]triolein can also be used as an effective test for fat absorption. During the digestive process the triolein is hydrolyzed, and the labeled glycerol is absorbed and metabolized by the liver. The $^{14}CO_2$ produced is exhaled and can then be measured hourly (for 6 h) in the expired air. Normally more than 3.5 percent of the administered label [0.185 MBq (5 μCi)] appears in the breath per hour.

Xylose absorption In the most commonly employed test of carbohydrate absorption, the patient ingests 25 g D-xylose. A 5-h urine xylose excretion of 26 mmol (4.0 g) or greater is considered normal. Low values may be obtained in patients with ascites, intestinal bacterial overgrowth, or renal insufficiency, after administration of certain drugs (e.g., aspirin, indomethacin), and most commonly if the urine collection is incomplete. To prevent difficulties in interpreting the test, it is advisable to determine the blood xylose level 2 h after ingestion of xylose. A blood xylose level of 2 mmol/L (30 mg/dL) or greater indicates normal absorption of D-xylose. An abnormal D-xylose absorption test is found most frequently in disorders affecting the mucosa of the proximal small intestine, such as nontropical and tropical sprue.

Gastrointestinal x-ray studies All patients with malabsorption should have radiographic examinations of the small intestine and, in

TABLE 240-2 Tests useful in the diagnosis of malabsorptive disorders

		Typical findings		
Test	Normal values	Malabsorption (nontropical sprue)	Maldigestion (pancreatic insufficiency)	Comment
I Quantitative determination of stool fat	<6 g per 24 h; >95% coefficient of fat absorption	>6 g per 24 h	>6 g per 24 h	Best test for establishing presence of steatorrhea
II Carbohydrate absorption				
A D-Xylose absorption (25-g oral dose)	5-h urinary excretion 26 mmol (>4.5 g); peak blood level >2.0 mmol/L (>30 mg/dL)	↓	Normal	A good screening test for carbohydrate absorption
III Small-intestine x-rays		Malabsorption pattern	Normal or minimal malabsorption pattern; occasionally pancreatic calcification	
IV Blood tests				
A Serum calcium	2.2–2.7 mmol/L (9–11 mg/dL)	Frequently ↓	Usually normal	
B Serum albumin	35–55 g/L (3.5–5.5 g/dL)	Frequently ↓	Usually normal	Decreased levels of both serum albumin and globulins should raise the question of protein-losing enteropathy
C Serum cholesterol	3.90–6.45 mmol/L (150–250 mg/dL)	↓	Frequently ↓	Usually decreased in disorders associated with significant steatorrhea
D Serum iron	14–24 μmol/L (80–150 μg/dL)	Frequently ↓	Normal	Low values may reflect decreased body iron stores
E Serum magnesium	0.6–1.0 mmol/L (1.2–2.0 meq/liter)	Frequently ↓	Usually normal	
F Serum zinc	12–20 μmol/liter	Frequently ↓	Usually normal	Decreased levels common in malnutrition, cirrhosis, and malabsorption
G Serum carotenes	>100 IU/dL	↓	Usually ↓	Fairly satisfactory screening tests for malabsorption
H Serum vitamin A	>100 IU/dL	↓		
I Prothrombin time	70–100%; 12–15 s	Frequently ↓	Frequently ↓	
V Small intestinal mucosal biopsy		Abnormal	Normal	A specific diagnosis can be established in a small number of disorders (see text)
VI Urine tests				
A Vitamin B_{12} absorption	>8% urinary excretion in 48 h	Frequently ↓	Frequently ↓	Useful in determining whether vitamin B_{12} malabsorption is due to gastric or small-intestinal disorders
B Urine 5-hydroxyindoleacetic acid (5-HIAA)	10–47 μmol per 24 h (2–9 mg per 24 h)	↑	Normal	Slightly increased level (12–16 mg per 24 h) characteristically found in nontropical sprue
VII Breath tests				
A Breath H_2 (after 50 g lactose)	Minimal breath H_2	May be ↑	Normal	Secondary to lactase deficiency (see text)
B Breath H_2 (after 10 g lactulose)	Minimal breath H_2	May be normal or ↓	Normal	Early peak in bacterial overgrowth; can be used to determine intestinal transit time
C Breath $^{14}CO_2$ (after ^{14}C xylose)	Minute amounts $^{14}CO_2$	May be ↓	Usually normal	Increased in bacterial overgrowth
D Glycocholic acid metabolism (oral glycine-1-[^{14}C]glycocholate)	<1% of dose excreted $^{14}CO_2$ in 4 h	Normal	Normal	Increased $^{14}CO_2$ excretion with bacterial overgrowth or bile acid malabsorption (due to ileal resection or inflammatory disease)
	<4% of dose excreted in stools	Normal	Normal	Increased fecal excretion of ^{14}C in bile acid malabsorption
E [^{14}C]Triolein absorption (breath test)	>3.5% of dose as breath $^{14}CO_2$ per hour	Decreased	Decreased	Correlates well with chemical stool fat; recently introduced test
VIII Miscellaneous				
A Bacteria (culture)	<10^3 organisms per milliliter	Normal	Normal	>10^5 organisms per milliliter indicates bacterial overgrowth
B Secretin test	Volume >1.8 (mL/kg)/h Bicarbonate concentration >80 mmol/liter	Normal	Abnormal	See discussion of pancreatic insufficiency in Chaps. 259 and 260
C Bentiromide test	Urine excretion arylamines ≥50%	May be abnormal	Abnormal	See discussion of pancreatic disease in Chaps. 259 and 260

many cases, of the esophagus, stomach, and colon as well. Occasionally, the latter two examinations may provide important clues to the presence of such disorders as gastroileostomy, scleroderma, Zollinger-Ellison syndrome, ulcerative colitis, and intestinal fistulas. Traditional radiographic findings suggesting a diagnosis of malabsorption include flocculation of barium within fluid-filled loops causing fragmentation and segmentation of the barium column. However, these patterns are no longer demonstrated reliably in small-bowel series because of widespread use of barium products that contain a nonflocculating suspension of micropulverized barium sulfate. In

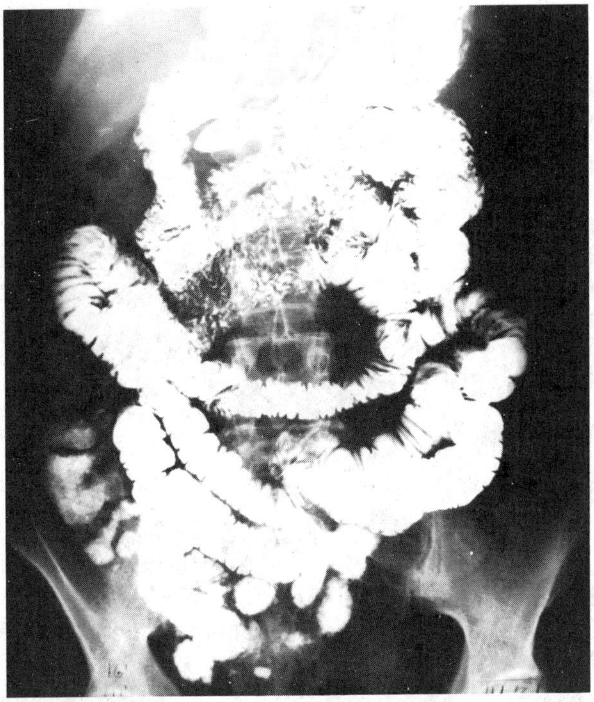

A

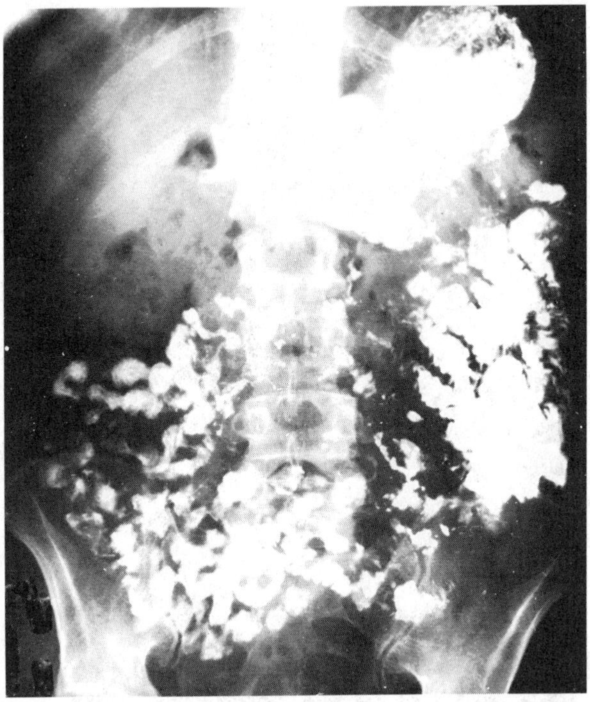

B

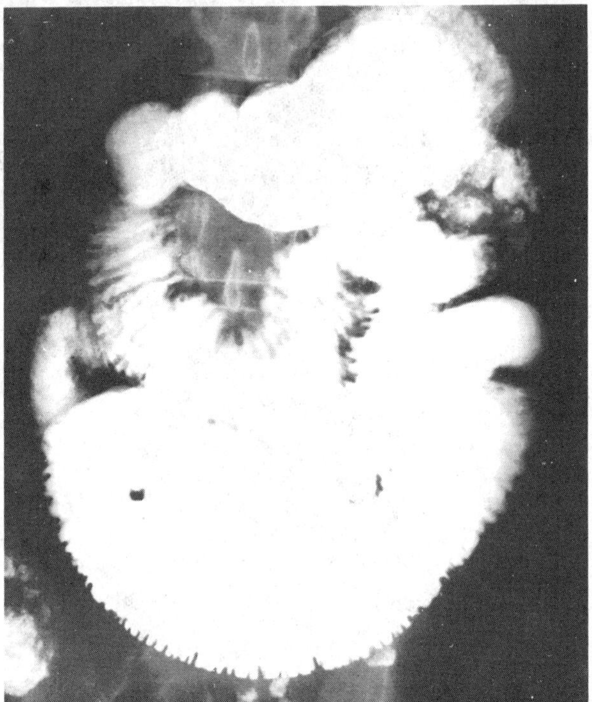

C

FIGURE 240-3 *A*. X-ray of a normal small intestine showing good mucosal pattern. *B*. Intestinal x-ray of a patient with nontropical sprue. Note dilatation of small bowel, lack of mucosal markings, and segmentation and clumping of barium. *C*. Intestinal x-ray of patient with obstructed lymphatics due to Köhlmeier-Degos disease, with "accordion-pleated" pattern (lower edge).

nontropical sprue, the most consistent abnormalities are thickened and nodular duodenal folds and dilatation of the small bowel. However, these findings are nonspecific and may be found in several of the disorders listed in Table 240-3. Some representative examples of abnormal small-bowel radiographs are shown in Fig. 240-3.

Small-intestinal biopsy The most commonly used instruments for obtaining peroral biopsy specimens from the small intestine include the Rubin tube, the Crosby, Carey, and Ross-Moore capsules, and the upper gastrointestinal endoscope. Examination of small-bowel biopsy specimens has proved to be of considerable value in the differential diagnosis of malabsorptive disorders. Table 240-3 lists disorders associated with abnormalities in intestinal biopsies, and Fig. 240-4 depicts some illustrative lesions.

Schilling test for vitamin B_{12} absorption The Schilling test is valuable in the differential diagnosis of malabsorption and is frequently carried out in three stages: (1) without intrinsic factor, (2) with intrinsic factor, and (3) after a course of treatment with antibiotics or anti-inflammatory drugs. Since vitamin B_{12} is absorbed primarily

TABLE 240-3 Disorders associated with abnormalities in small-bowel biopsy specimens

I Disorders in which biopsy is of diagnostic value (diffuse lesions)
- *A* Whipple's disease: Lamina propria infiltrated with macrophages containing PAS-positive glycoproteins
- *B* Abetalipoproteinemia: Villus structure normal; epithelial cells vacuolated due to excess fat
- *C* Agammaglobulinemia: Flattened or absent villi; increased lymphocyte infiltration; absence of plasma cells

II Disorders in which biopsy may be of diagnostic value (patchy lesions)
- *A* Intestinal lymphoma: Infiltration of lamina propria and submucosa with malignant cells
- *B* Intestinal lymphangiectasia: Dilated lacteals and lymphatics in lamina propria; clubbed villi
- *C* Eosinophilic enteritis: Diffuse or patchy eosinophilic infiltration in lamina propria and mucosa
- *D* Amyloidosis: Presence of amyloid confirmed by special stains
- *E* Regional enteritis: Noncaseating granulomas
- *F* Parasitic infestations: Parasitic invasion of mucosa; adherence of trophozoites to mucosal surface, as in giardiasis
- *G* Systemic mastocytosis: Mast cell infiltration of lamina propria

III Disorders in which biopsy is abnormal but not diagnostic
- *A* Celiac sprue: Shortened or absent villi; hypertrophied crypts; damaged surface epithelium; mononuclear infiltrate
- *B* "Collagenous" sprue: Indistinguishable from celiac sprue; extensive subepithelial collagen deposition
- *C* Tropical sprue: Lesion similar to celiac sprue with shortened or absent villi; lymphocyte infiltration
- *D* Folate deficiency: Shortened villi; megalocytosis; decreased mitoses in crypts
- *E* Vitamin B_{12} deficiency: Similar to folate deficiency
- *F* Acute radiation enteritis: Similar to folate deficiency
- *G* Systemic scleroderma: Fibrosis around Brunner's glands
- *H* Bacterial overgrowth syndromes: Patchy damage to villi and increased lymphocyte infiltration

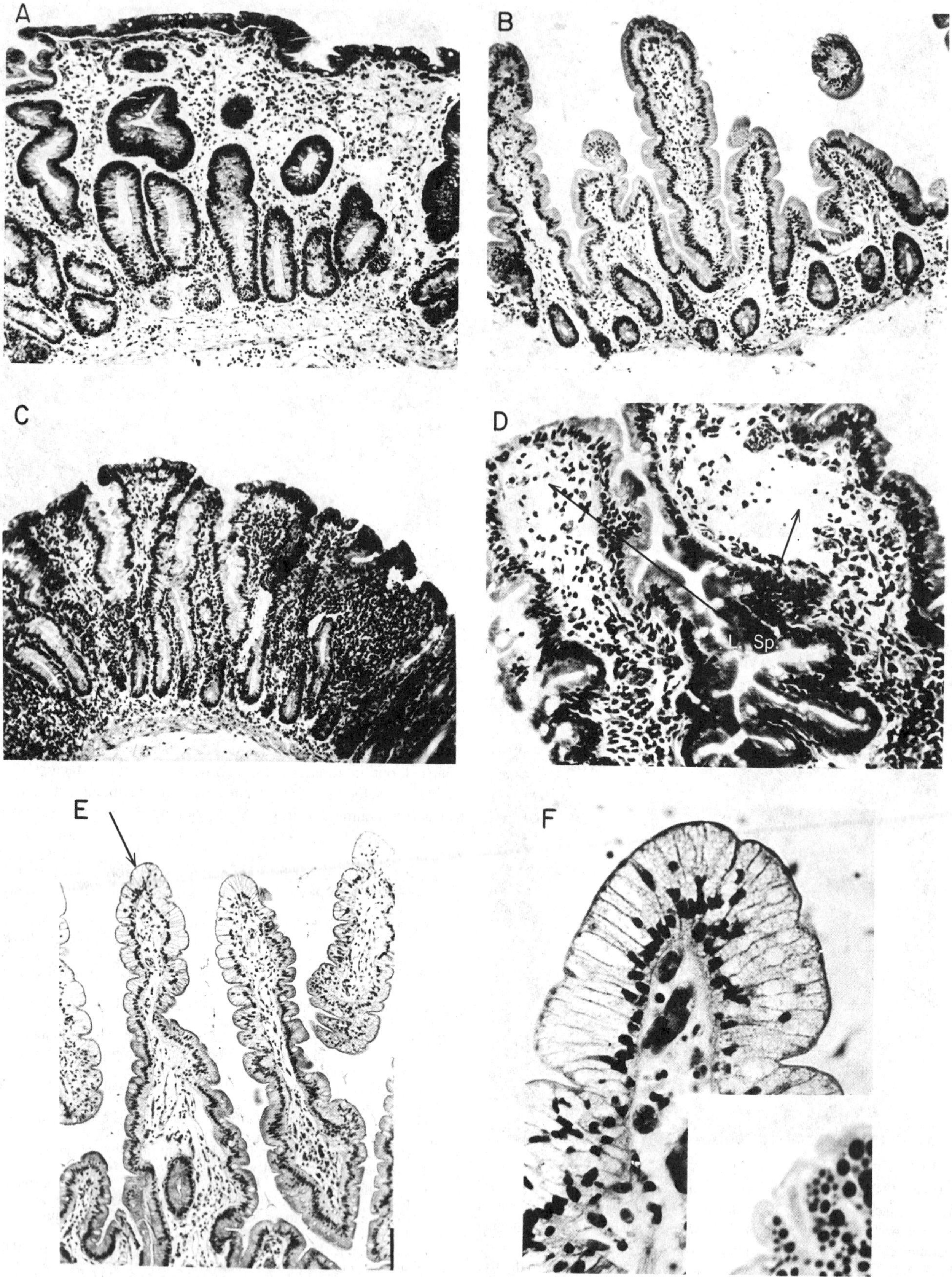

FIGURE 240-4 Typical peroral intestinal biopsies. *A*. Jejunal mucosa of patient with nontropical sprue. Note virtual absence of villi, elongated crypts (some cut in cross section), mononuclear infiltrate, cuboidal instead of columnar epithelium on top of villi (300×). *B*. Biopsy from the same patient as in *A*, after 9 months on a gluten-free diet. Note reappearance of villi with normal-appearing columnar cells and reduction in infiltrate and crypt height (300×). *C*. Biopsy from patient with agammaglobulinemia. The features bear a striking resemblance to those of nontropical sprue. There is a marked mononuclear infiltration, some of it in aggregates (200×). *D*. Close-up of villi of patient with protein-losing enteropathy. Note broadened and dilated tips, and lymphatic spaces (arrows). (450×). *E*. Intestinal biopsy from patient with abetalipoproteinemia. The villus tips have a ''lacy'' appearance (arrow) due to retained fat (300×). *F*. High-power micrograph of villus in *E*. Vacuoles are filled with lipid (750×). Insert shows dark-staining (osmium) lipid droplets in mucosal cells (osmium counterstained with Giemsa; 800×).

in the distal ileum, an abnormal Schilling test may indicate a pathologic condition of the distal small bowel. In disorders affecting the terminal ileum, such as regional enteritis and lymphomas, the first- and second-stage Schilling test are frequently abnormal. The ileal receptor site appears to be damaged in these disorders, and the impaired absorption of B_{12} is not corrected by the addition of intrinsic factor or the use of antibiotics. However, the Schilling test may normalize after treatment with prednisone or sulfasalazine. The Schilling test may also be useful in establishing a diagnosis of abnormal bacterial overgrowth of the small bowel, which may be present in disorders such as blind loop syndrome, scleroderma, and multiple small-bowel diverticula (see below). In the blind loop syndrome, for example, the bacteria can actually take up vitamin B_{12} with resultant impaired absorption of B_{12}. Under these conditions the first-stage Schilling test is frequently abnormal, as is the second stage. After appropriate antibiotic treatment the Schilling test usually returns to normal. Vitamin B_{12} absorption is frequently abnormal in patients with exocrine pancreatic insufficiency (see Chap. 260).

Secretin and other pancreatic tests The secretin test, secretin cholecystokinin test, intraduodenal perfusion with essential amino acids, and bentiromide test, which may be useful in establishing a diagnosis of pancreatic insufficiency, are discussed in detail in Chap. 259.

Serum calcium, albumin, cholesterol, magnesium, and iron Abnormal serum calcium, albumin, cholesterol, magnesium, and iron values may be found in several malabsorptive disorders. The primary value of such tests is to suggest that abnormal intestinal absorptive function may be present. These tests are usually of limited value in the *differential diagnosis* of malabsorption, but if abnormal, may be helpful in supporting this diagnosis.

Serum carotenes, vitamin A, and prothrombin time Absorption of the fat-soluble vitamins A, D, K, and E is frequently impaired in patients with steatorrhea. Measurements of serum carotene and vitamin A levels are useful as screening tests for malabsorption. However, other tests not only are more sensitive but often give more specific information than the serum carotene and vitamin A levels. The blood prothrombin time is an important test, since patients with malabsorption may present with abnormal bleeding due to vitamin K deficiency. If the decreased prothrombin activity is due to malabsorption, it should be readily correctable with parenteral vitamin K.

Breath tests The bile acid breath test utilizing [^{14}C]cholylglycine is a reasonably reliable screening test for bacterial overgrowth syndromes. Approximately two-thirds of patients with a positive small-bowel culture will have an abnormal bile acid breath test. However, in patients with suspected malabsorption of bile acids the test is rather insensitive without the additional determination of fecal bile acid excretion. The excretion of breath hydrogen after ingestion of lactose is a sensitive, specific, and noninvasive test for detecting lactase deficiency. Lactulose and [^{14}C]xylose breath tests for bacterial overgrowth have also been found helpful.

PATHOPHYSIOLOGIC BASIS FOR SYMPTOMS AND SIGNS IN MALABSORPTIVE DISORDERS The common symptoms and signs found in malabsorptive disorders are listed in Table 240-4. The most frequent symptoms are those of malnutrition, weight loss, and diarrhea. However, in each of the clinical settings listed in Table 240-4, it is important to consider the cause of the malabsorption.

TABLE 240-4 Pathophysiologic basis for symptoms and signs in malabsorptive disorders

Symptom or sign	Pathophysiology
GASTROINTESTINAL	
Generalized malnutrition and weight loss	Malabsorption of fat, carbohydrate, and protein → loss of calories
Diarrhea	Impaired absorption or increased secretion of water and electrolytes; unabsorbed dihydroxy bile acids and fatty acids → decreased absorption of water and electrolytes; excess load of fluid and electrolytes presented to the colon may exceed its absorptive capacity
Flatus	Bacterial fermentation of unabsorbed carbohydrate
Glossitis, cheilosis, stomatitis	Deficiency of iron, vitamin B_{12}, folate, and other vitamins
GENITOURINARY	
Nocturia	Delayed absorption of water, hypokalemia
Azotemia, hypotension	Fluid and electrolyte depletion
Amenorrhea, ↓ libido	Protein depletion and "caloric starvation" → secondary hypopituitarism
HEMATOPOIETIC	
Anemia	Impaired absorption of iron, vitamin B_{12}, and folic acid
Hemorrhagic phenomena	Vitamin K malabsorption → hypoprothrombinemia
MUSCULOSKELETAL	
Bone pain	Protein depletion → impaired bone formation → osteoporosis Calcium malabsorption → demineralization of bone → osteomalacia
Osteoarthropathy	Cause uncertain
Tetany, paresthesias	Calcium malabsorption → hypocalcemia; magnesium malabsorption → hypomagnesemia
Weakness	Anemia; electrolyte depletion (hypokalemia)
NERVOUS SYSTEM	
Night blindness	Impaired absorption vitamin A → vitamin A deficiency
Xerophthalmia	Vitamin A deficiency
Peripheral neuropathy	Vitamin B_{12}, thiamine deficiency
SKIN	
Eczema	Cause uncertain
Purpura	Vitamin K deficiency
Follicular hyperkeratosis and dermatitis	Deficiency of vitamin A, zinc, essential fatty acids, and other vitamins

DISORDERS OF MALABSORPTION

(See Table 240-5)

INADEQUATE DIGESTION Liver and biliary tract disease It is not generally appreciated that patients with acute or chronic liver disease may develop malabsorption due to impaired intraluminal digestion. Steatorrhea has been described in acute viral hepatitis, chronic extrahepatic biliary tract obstruction, primary biliary cirrhosis, and postnecrotic and nutritional cirrhosis. Absorption of D-xylose and vitamin B_{12} are usually normal, and small-intestinal mucosal biopsy specimens are generally unremarkable. The steatorrhea associated with liver and biliary tract disease is thought to be due to impaired hepatic synthesis or excretion of conjugated bile salts, resulting in impaired formation of micellar lipid. In addition to steatorrhea, patients with liver disease may have impaired absorption of vitamin D and calcium, resulting in severe metabolic bone disease. This is particularly common in patients with primary biliary cirrhosis. Skeletal roentgenograms may show increased porosity of bone, cortical thinning, vertebral compression, and spontaneous pathologic fractures. Patients with alcohol-induced liver disease may also have exocrine pancreatic insufficiency. Accordingly, pancreatic function should be evaluated in patients with liver disease and malabsorption.

TABLE 240-5 Classification of the malabsorption syndromes

I Inadequate digestion
- *A* Postgastrectomy steatorrhea*
- *B* Deficiency or inactivation of pancreatic lipase
  - *1* Exocrine pancreatic insufficiency
    - *a* Chronic pancreatitis
    - *b* Pancreatic carcinoma
    - *c* Cystic fibrosis
    - *d* Pancreatic resection
  - *2* Ulcerogenic tumor of the pancreas (Zollinger-Ellison syndrome, gastrinoma)*

II Reduced intestinal bile salt concentration (with impaired micelle formation)
- *A* Liver disease
  - *1* Parenchymal liver disease
  - *2* Cholestasis (intrahepatic or extrahepatic)
- *B* Abnormal bacterial proliferation in the small bowel
  - *1* Afferent loop stasis
  - *2* Strictures
  - *3* Fistulas
  - *4* Blind loops
  - *5* Multiple diverticula of the small bowel
  - *6* Hypomotility states (diabetes, scleroderma, intestinal pseudoobstruction)
- *C* Interrupted enterohepatic circulation of bile salts
  - *1* Ileal resection
  - *2* Ileal inflammatory disease (regional ileitis)
- *D* Drugs (by sequestration or precipitation of bile salts)
  - *1* Neomycin
  - *2* Calcium carbonate
  - *3* Cholestyramine

III Inadequate absorptive surface
- *A* Intestinal resection or bypass
  - *1* Mesenteric vascular disease with massive intestinal resection
  - *2* Regional enteritis with multiple bowel resections
  - *3* Jejunoileal bypass
- *B* Gastroileostomy (inadvertent)

IV Lymphatic obstruction
- *A* Intestinal lymphangiectasia
- *B* Whipple's disease*
- *C* Lymphoma

V Cardiovascular disorders
- *A* Constrictive pericarditis
- *B* Congestive heart failure
- *C* Mesenteric vascular insufficiency
- *D* Vasculitis

VI Primary mucosal absorptive defects
- *A* Inflammatory or infiltrative disorders
  - *1* Regional enteritis*
  - *2* Amyloidosis
  - *3* Scleroderma*
  - *4* Lymphoma*
  - *5* Radiation enteritis
  - *6* Eosinophilic enteritis
  - *7* Tropical sprue
  - *8* Infectious enteritis (e.g., salmonellosis)
  - *9* Collagenous sprue
  - *10* Nonspecific ulcerative jejunitis
  - *11* Mastocytosis
  - *12* Dermatologic disorders (e.g., dermatitis herpetiformis)
- *B* Biochemical or genetic abnormalities
  - *1* Nontropical sprue (gluten-induced enteropathy); celiac sprue
  - *2* Disaccharidase deficiency
  - *3* Hypogammaglobulinemia
  - *4* Abetalipoproteinemia
  - *5* Hartnup disease
  - *6* Cystinuria
  - *7* Monosaccharide malabsorption

VII Endocrine and metabolic disorders
- *A* Diabetes mellitus*
- *B* Hypoparathyroidism
- *C* Adrenal insufficiency
- *D* Hyperthyroidism
- *E* Ulcerogenic tumor of the pancreas (Zollinger-Ellison syndrome, gastrinoma)*
- *F* Carcinoid syndrome

* Malabsorption caused by multiple defects.

Postgastrectomy malabsorption The presence of a malabsorption syndrome has been documented frequently in patients after subtotal gastrectomy. Steatorrhea is more common with a Billroth II than a Billroth I type of anastomosis. Usually the fat loss is minimal, ranging from 7 to 10 g per 24 h. Patients with gross steatorrhea usually have impaired intraluminal fat digestion due to several factors: (1) With a Billroth II anastomosis the duodenum is bypassed, and there is a decreased entry of stomach contents into the proximal duodenum (i.e., afferent loop). This leads to a decreased stimulus for the release of *secretin* and *cholecystokinin-pancreozymin* from the duodenum and may result in a depressed pancreatic enzyme response. (2) There may be *inadequate mixing* of the pancreatic enzymes and bile salts secreted into the proximal duodenum with the gastric contents entering the jejunum. (3) There may be *stasis* of intestinal contents in the afferent loop, resulting in abnormal bacterial proliferation in the proximal small bowel. This in turn may lead to abnormalities in bile salt metabolism (see "Malabsorption Due to Bacterial Overgrowth of the Small Bowel, Pathophysiology" below). (4) The presence of maldigestion may lead to *protein depletion*, which in turn may produce further impairment in pancreatic function. (5) The *loss of the reservoir function of the stomach* may result in decreased intestinal transit time. Perhaps the most important factor is rapid gastric emptying, which results in low luminal concentrations of digestive secretions for the first 60 to 80 min after a meal. Such a disorder has been described in patients with subtotal gastrectomy and duodenostomy (Billroth I), gastrojejunostomy (Billroth II), and truncal vagotomy and pyloroplasty (V&P). That gastric emptying rates are somewhat slower in patients with V&P may account for the overall less severe nutritional deficiencies in such patients. In some patients treatment with pancreatic enzymes may lead to significant improvement. Specimens of duodenal or jejunal fluid should be obtained for culture of both aerobic and anaerobic organisms and appropriate antibiotic therapy instituted if there is evidence of abnormal bacterial overgrowth (colony count of greater than 10^7 per milliliter of jejunal fluid). Because the duodenum is the principal site of absorption of iron and calcium, in patients with a Billroth II anastomosis impaired absorption of calcium and iron may also develop. Occult metabolic bone disease occurs frequently in this setting.

INADEQUATE ABSORPTIVE SURFACE (SHORT BOWEL SYNDROME) Extensive intestinal resection often results in the short bowel syndrome. The most common disorders resulting in short bowel syndrome are (1) massive intestinal resection following a vascular insult to the small intestine, (2) regional enteritis with multiple bowel resections, and (3) jejunoileal bypass for morbid obesity. In general, the absorption of nutrients will be influenced by the extent and site of small bowel resected, the presence of the ileocecal valve, and adaptation of the remaining small bowel. Resection of 40 to 50 percent of the small bowel is usually well tolerated, provided the proximal duodenum, the distal half of the ileum, and the ileocecal valve are spared. By contrast, resection of the ileum and the ileocecal valve alone may induce severe diarrhea and malabsorption, even though less than 30 percent of the small intestine is resected.

Several measures are important in the management of short bowel syndrome: (1) The diet should contain at least 2500 kcal and consist primarily of carbohydrate and protein with fat restricted to less than 40 g per day. A fat-restricted diet is effective in reducing diarrhea, presumably because there is decreased production of hydroxy fatty acids from long-chain fats. Such hydroxy fatty acids, in essence, are cathartics and increase net secretion of water and electrolytes by the colon as well as the small bowel. (2) It is often necessary to provide vitamin and mineral supplements, which usually include K^+, Cl^-, Mg^{2+}, Ca^{2+}, trace metals (Zn, Cd, Mn), iron, folate, vitamin B_{12}, other vitamins (A, D, E, K, B_1, B_2, B_6, biotin), and essential fatty acids. (3) Specific drugs (for example, belladonna alkaloids, diphenoxylate, loperamide, and codeine), which decrease intestinal motility and prolong mucosal contact time, are helpful in controlling diarrhea. These agents also decrease ileostomy outputs. (4) A bile salt–sequestering agent such as cholestyramine blunts the effects of bile salts, which stimulate net secretion of water and electrolytes by the colon. (5) Patients with short-bowel syndrome may have gastric acid hypersecretion, which is often transient, and which results in dilution of pancreatic secretions as well as inactivation of pancreatic enzymes. Under these conditions, a histamine H-2 receptor antagonist is useful because it will suppress gastric acid secretion and decrease the volume of fluid entering the proximal small bowel, thus leading to an increased concentration of pancreatic enzymes. In addition, supplemental pancreatic enzyme therapy may be required. (6) A bypassed colon can be used to receive infusions of fluid and electrolytes since a portion of the colon can still absorb 1000 to 1500 mL fluid per day. Finally, (7) total parenteral nutrition is frequently required during the first 6 months after massive intestinal resection until some degree of adaptation has occurred. Such patients may also require long-term parenteral hyperalimentation with a silicone rubber catheter in the superior vena cava, and this can be done at home.

For a discussion of regional enteritis see Chap. 241.

MALABSORPTION DUE TO BACTERIAL OVERGROWTH OF THE SMALL BOWEL The proximal small intestine is usually bacteriologically sterile because of three factors: (1) the acid milieu of the stomach; (2) intestinal peristalsis, which sweeps bacteria to the distal small bowel; and (3) secretion into the lumen of the intestine of immunoglobulins, which may serve as coproantibodies. When bacteria are isolated from the upper small bowel, they are frequently contaminants transported from the mouth and upper respiratory tract, and the colony count rarely exceeds 10^4 per milliliter of jejunal fluid. The major mechanism limiting the growth of bacteria in the small intestine is normal peristalsis. Any disorder leading to impaired intestinal motility may result in abnormal stasis of intestinal contents with ineffective mechanical cleansing of bacteria. This in turn may lead to abnormal bacterial proliferation and malabsorption. Several malabsorptive disorders have been associated with bacterial overgrowth of the small bowel, and these are listed in Table 240-6.

Pathophysiology Bacterial overgrowth may result in changes in bile salt metabolism, and these are believed directly and indirectly to account for the steatorrhea. First, bacteria (especially anaerobic gram-positive bacteria) may lead to the intraluminal deconjugation of bile salts with a consequent production of free bile acids. In contrast to conjugated bile salts, unconjugated bile salts may be absorbed in the proximal small bowel by nonionic diffusion, resulting in decreased intraluminal concentrations of bile salts in the jejunum. Second, the decreased bile salt concentrations, the increase of unconjugated bile salts, and the decrease of the conjugated salts all serve to contribute to impaired intraluminal micelle formation and hence fat malabsorption. In addition to abnormalities in bile salt metabolism, intestinal mucosal lesions have been demonstrated in patients with intestinal stasis. Such lesions are often patchy in distribution, and the histologic appearance ranges in severity from minimal changes in villous architecture to severe lesions with virtual absence of villi. The etiology of these lesions is unclear; possible causes include damage caused by bacterial invasion, bacterial toxins, or metabolic products such as unconjugated bile salts. In this regard, certain bacteria such as *Bacteroides* elaborate proteases which solubilize brush border proteins and destroy disaccharidases such as sucrase and maltase. The impaired absorption of vitamin B_{12} is not related to the disturbed bile salt metabolism but appears to be due to uptake of vitamin B_{12} by microorganisms.

Many of the above abnormalities in bile salt metabolism may be reversed by appropriate antibiotic therapy. When such treatment is instituted, unconjugated bile salts in the jejunal fluid decrease, an increase in the micellar lipid phase will occur, and steatorrhea diminishes or disappears. In addition, significant improvement in the absorption of vitamin B_{12} will occur with broad-spectrum antibiotics such as tetracycline.

Clinical manifestations Breath tests, i.e., tests with [^{14}C]-labeled bile acid, [^{14}C]xylose, and lactulose, are useful screening tests for malabsorption syndrome due to abnormal bacterial overgrowth of the small intestine. A definitive diagnosis is established by demonstrating larger numbers of microorganisms (greater than 10^5 per milliliter) and a polymicrobial flora in cultures of duodenal or jejunal fluid. Other clinical features include the following: (1) steatorrhea of a moderate degree, usually in the range of 15 to 30 g fecal fat per 24 h; (2) macrocytic anemia with a megaloblastic bone marrow; (3) impaired absorption of vitamin B_{12} which is not corrected by intrinsic factor; and (4) correction of steatorrhea and impaired vitamin B_{12} absorption by antibiotic therapy. Absorption of D-xylose, peroral small-intestinal biopsy specimens, and other tests of absorptive function (Table 240-2) may be normal in these patients. A single course or intermittent courses (2 to 3 weeks per month) of therapy with antibiotics such as tetracycline, ampicillin, or trimethoprim-sulfamethoxazole are usually given.

Chronic intestinal pseudoobstruction (See also Chap. 243) Chronic intestinal pseudoobstruction is a heterogeneous syndrome with a variety of causes (Table 240-7). Primary or idiopathic intestinal pseudoobstruction is a chronic illness characterized by recurrent episodes of intestinal obstruction in which all known causes of mechanical obstruction and other illnesses known to produce intestinal pseudoobstruction have been excluded. In addition to abnormalities in small-bowel motility, derangements in esophageal, gastric, and colonic motility have also been described. The primary clinical manifestations are nausea and vomiting, abdominal pain, distention, constipation, diarrhea, and urinary tract symptoms. Patients typically exhibit prolonged transit of chyme along the gastrointestinal tract, especially the small bowel where pressure activity patterns are markedly disordered. Oral cisapride accelerates gastric emptying, normalizes intestinal transit, and improves propulsive small-bowel activity in patients with pseudoobstruction. Malabsorption, secondary to stasis of intestinal contents with resultant abnormal bacterial proliferation in the small bowel, is frequently present.

TABLE 240-6 Causes of intestinal bacterial overgrowth (intestinal colonization)

I Structural abnormalities producing stasis of intestinal contents
  A Multiple small-bowel diverticula
  B Strictures
    1 Regional enteritis*
    2 Radiation enteritis*
    3 Occlusive vascular disease; vasculitis
  C Billroth II subtotal gastrectomy with afferent loop stasis*
  D Multiple laparotomies resulting in adhesions and partial small-bowel obstruction
II Fistulas
  A Gastrocolic, gastroileal, jejunoileal, jejunocolic
III Motor abnormalities resulting in intestinal hypomotility
  A Scleroderma*
  B Amyloidosis*
  C Diabetes mellitus*
  D Hypothyroidism
  E Vagotomy
  F Intestinal pseudoobstruction (see Table 240-7)
IV Miscellaneous
  A Hypogammaglobulinemia*
  B Nodular lymphoid hyperplasia
  C Pernicious anemia
  D Pancreatic insufficiency
V No underlying disorder detected

* Multiple mechanisms may contribute to malabsorption in these disorders

TABLE 240-7 Causes of chronic intestinal pseudoobstruction

I Primary: Idiopathic
II Secondary
  A Collagen vascular disease
    1 Scleroderma
    2 Dermatomyositis/polymyositis
    3 Systemic lupus erythematosus
  B Amyloidosis
  C Endocrine disorders
    1 Myxedema
    2 Diabetes mellitus
  D Neurologic diseases
    1 Chagas' disease
  E Others
    1 Jejunoileal bypass
    2 Jejunal diverticulosis
    3 Drugs (tricyclic antidepressants, clonidine, etc.)

Tropical sprue Tropical sprue is a malabsorptive disorder of unknown cause affecting residents of or visitors to tropical regions. Both epidemic and endemic forms of the disease have been recognized. Tropical sprue may have its onset months or even years after a patient has returned from the tropics. The etiology of the disorder has not been elucidated, but it might well result from one or more of the following: (1) a nutritional deficiency, (2) a transmissible infectious microorganism, and (3) a toxin elaborated by a microorganism or contained in the diet. It is of interest that coliform organisms, shown to produce an enterotoxin causing fluid secretion, have been isolated from the jejunum of tropical sprue patients but not from other patients with bacterial overgrowth of the proximal small bowel. Anorexia, diarrhea, weight loss, symptoms of anemia, sequelae of nutritional deficiency (Table 240-4), and abdominal distention are common findings. Patients are frequently deficient in iron as well as vitamin B_{12} and folate. Laboratory studies usually reveal anemia (megaloblastic in 60 percent of cases) and impaired absorption of fat, xylose, and vitamin B_{12}. Malabsorption of at least two nutrients is considered essential for the diagnosis. Jejunal biopsy classically reveals shortened and thickened villi, increased crypt depth, and increased infiltration of mononuclear cells in the lamina propria and epithelium (Table 240-3). However, these biopsy findings are not specific, and the lesion may be patchy; in addition, interpretation is difficult because "control" biopsies from asymptomatic residents in the same tropical region are often considered abnormal when compared with normal biopsies from patients in temperate zones. Such histologic findings have been termed *tropical jejunitis*. Treatment with vitamin B_{12}, folate, and antibiotics have all been effective in inducing a remission. A short course, i.e., 2 to 4 weeks, of therapy with a sulfonamide or tetracycline is usually given. Occasional patients require more prolonged antibiotic therapy.

Scleroderma Although there are numerous reports of small-intestinal involvement in scleroderma, frank malabsorption has been reported infrequently. It has been suggested that malabsorption may be due to several factors: (1) lymphatic obstruction; (2) reduced arterial blood supply to the gut; (3) impaired intestinal motility leading to relative stasis of intestinal contents and hence bacterial overgrowth; and (4) involvement of the intestinal wall by the disease. At present there is little evidence to support the first two postulated mechanisms. In some cases abnormal bacterial proliferation in the upper small bowel has been documented, and in these patients antibiotic therapy has resulted in decrease in steatorrhea, gain in weight, and increased absorption of vitamin B_{12}. In the intestinal wall there may also be extensive deposition of collagen, especially in the muscular mucosa, submucosa, and muscularis externa, with significant muscle atrophy. Studies of duodenal myoelectric activity in scleroderma revealed normal slow-wave frequency and propagation velocity but decreased excitability of the bowel to mechanical stimuli such as distention and humoral stimuli such as pentagastrin and secretin. This motor dysfunction may be an important factor in the dilatation, atony, and stasis of intestinal contents in scleroderma.

Malabsorption in the acquired immunodeficiency syndrome Diarrhea and weight loss occur frequently in patients with the acquired immunodeficiency syndrome (AIDS). These symptoms are often due to enteric infections or small-intestinal Kaposi's sarcoma. However, such symptoms can be due to malabsorption, which has been well-documented in patients with AIDS in whom identifiable enteric infections and intestinal involvement with Kaposi's sarcoma have been excluded. The presence of malabsorption in these patients has been documented by steatorrhea and abnormal D-xylose absorption tests. Serum zinc levels may be decreased. In addition, small-bowel biopsy specimens have revealed dense infiltration of mononuclear cells and histiocytes. Microorganisms have also been identified in the mucosa.

DISORDERS ASSOCIATED WITH LYMPHATIC OBSTRUCTION

Whipple's disease This is a rare disorder characterized clinically by arthralgia, abdominal pain, diarrhea, progressive weight loss, dilated lacteals in the bowel wall, and impaired intestinal absorption. Wasting, low-grade fever, increased skin pigmentation, and peripheral lymphadenopathy are frequently present. In addition, central nervous system manifestations including confusion, memory loss, focal cranial nerve signs, nystagmus, and ophthalmoplegia may be present. Laboratory examination usually reveals the presence of steatorrhea, impaired xylose absorption, abnormal small-bowel x-rays, hypoalbuminemia, and anemia. Hypoalbuminemia is due to excessive loss of serum albumin into the gastrointestinal tract as well as impaired synthesis of albumin.

The diagnosis is established by demonstrating the presence in the mucosa of macrophages containing large cytoplasmic granules which give a brilliant magenta stain with the periodic acid Schiff reagent (PAS). Such macrophages may also be seen in other tissues such as lymph nodes, spleen, or liver. The finding of PAS-positive macrophages in the lamina propria is not specific for Whipple's disease, but virtual replacement of most cellular elements in the lamina propria by these macrophages has been seen only in this disorder. In addition to the PAS-positive macrophages, jejunal biopsies frequently show dilated lymphatics and some degree of blunting of the intestinal mucosal villi.

Electron-microscopic studies have revealed the presence of rod-shaped structures (or bacilliform bodies) 0.3 by 1.5 to 2.5 μm within and adjacent to the macrophages in the lamina propria as well as within epithelial cells and polymorphonuclear leukocytes. The ultrastructural features of these bacilliform bodies suggest that they are microorganisms. It is of particular interest that after treatment of the patient with antibiotics the bacilliform bodies decrease or disappear together with a decrease in the number of PAS-positive macrophages. In addition, the reappearance of the bacteria often heralds the onset of a clinical relapse after antibiotics have been withdrawn.

Whipple's disease at one time was thought to be invariably fatal. However, it is now clear that therapy with antibiotics will usually induce a clinical remission. In a few cases there has been complete reversal of the histologic abnormalities in the jejunal mucosa, and some of these cases have been followed for 10 years. Patients with Whipple's disease should be treated with antibiotics such as trimethoprim-sulfamethoxazole for at least 1 year. Treatment with tetracycline alone or penicillin alone is not adequate initial therapy; relapse rates with these drugs are approximately 40 percent. The most important parameter for following the disease and predicting its course is the presence or absence of bacilli in sections of small-bowel biopsies.

Intestinal lymphoma Steatorrhea is a manifestation of *primary* intestinal lymphoma. The disease occurs predominantly in men, and the mean age of onset of symptoms is about 50 years. The diagnosis should be suspected in patients with malabsorption with the following findings: (1) a malabsorption syndrome in which clinical and biopsy features resemble those of nontropical sprue but in which there is an incomplete response to a gluten-free diet, (2) the presence of *abdominal pain* and *fever*, and (3) signs and symptoms of intestinal obstruction. The usual stigmata of generalized lymphoma are frequently absent. Hepatomegaly, splenomegaly, palpable abdominal masses, and peripheral adenopathy are usually not found. Lymphangiography and CT scanning may reveal abnormal intraabdominal nodes. The diagnosis can be established by laparotomy and often may be made by thorough examination of multiple mucosal biopsy specimens obtained perorally. There may be a total absence of villi or lesser degrees of blunting and shortening of the villi. In contrast to nontropical sprue, the lamina propria is usually massively infiltrated with lymphoid cells. Malignancy may be diagnosed by demonstrating lymphoid cells with the cytologic features of malignancy, the presence of reticulum cells outside germinal centers, and infiltration and destruction of crypts by pleomorphic lymphoid cells. Some patients elaborate or secrete a fragment of the heavy chain of IgA immunoglobulins (*α-chain disease*). The latter is probably a variant of intestinal lymphoma.

The mechanism of malabsorption in intestinal lymphoma may be related to several factors: (1) diffuse involvement of the small-intestinal mucosa; (2) involvement of the bowel wall with lymphatic obstruction; and (3) localized stenosis with stasis of intestinal contents and bacterial overgrowth. It should be emphasized that it is often difficult, by clinical and morphologic features alone, to distinguish nontropical sprue from intestinal lymphoma. Indeed, there is evidence to suggest that lymphoma may develop as a late complication of nontropical sprue.

The course of intestinal lymphoma has ranged from 4 months to 4 years from the onset of symptoms. Perforation, bleeding, and intestinal obstruction are common terminal complications. There is insufficient evidence to determine whether radiation therapy, chemotherapy, or localized surgical resection modify the natural course of the disease.

CARDIOVASCULAR DISORDERS Steatorrhea has been described in patients with chronic congestive heart failure, superior mesenteric artery insufficiency, and constrictive pericarditis. Abnormal dilated mucosal lymphatics and excessive enteric loss of protein have been demonstrated in patients with constrictive pericarditis. The mechanism of steatorrhea in patients with chronic heart failure remains uncertain. It might be due to congestion and edema of the mucosa, mucosal hypoxia, or abnormalities in pancreatic function. Although pronounced steatorrhea is uncommon in congestive heart failure, these patients are frequently anorectic, and a low fat intake could mask a latent steatorrhea. Steatorrhea is quite infrequent in patients with vasculitis and is thought to be due to segmental infarction of the small bowel in addition to intestinal ischemia.

DEFECTS IN MUCOSAL FUNCTION

INFLAMMATORY OR INFILTRATIVE DISORDERS Regional enteritis The clinical features of regional enteritis are described in Chap. 241. Malabsorption in regional enteritis may result from several factors: (1) interruption of the enterohepatic circulation of bile salts by ileal disease or resection; (2) deconjugation of bile salts due to bacterial overgrowth, in turn related to strictures and/or fistulas; (3) active inflammatory bowel disease causing impaired mucosal cell function; (4) inadequate absorptive surface resulting from intestinal resection or fistulas; and (5) severe protein depletion producing impaired exocrine pancreatic function. Active ileal disease and/or ileal resection resulting in an interrupted enterohepatic circulation of and deficiency of conjugated bile salts appears to be the major factor responsible for steatorrhea as well as impaired absorption of vitamin B_{12}. Small-bowel absorptive function has been correlated with the extent of ileal disease or resection. When the length of ileal dysfunction exceeds 90 to 100 cm, virtually all patients will have steatorrhea and vitamin B_{12} malabsorption. After intestinal resection, the functional capacity of the remaining small bowel will depend on the site and extent of resection as well as the presence of residual inflammatory disease. Massive intestinal resection usually results in impaired absorption of all food constituents. When the malabsorption is due to strictures and blind loops as a result of previous surgical therapy, antibiotic therapy may be helpful, but surgical removal of these areas is usually necessary for long-term improvement. With diffuse inflammatory disease a florid malabsorption syndrome may occur with steatorrhea, hypocalcemia, impaired vitamin B_{12} absorption, and hypoalbuminemia due to increased enteric protein loss. Treatment with sulfasalazine and glucocorticoids drugs may be beneficial (see Chap. 241).

After *ileal resection*, patients frequently have bothersome diarrhea. This appears to be due to *interruption of the enterohepatic circulation* whereby increased amounts of bile salts reach the colon, where they interfere with water and electrolyte absorption and thus have a cathartic effect. The *bile salt–induced diarrhea* after ileal resection may respond to treatment with cholestyramine, an exchange resin which binds bile salts and causes them to lose their biochemical effect on the bowel. Patients with ileal resection of less than 100 cm and fecal fat excretion less than 20 g per day show the best symptomatic response to cholestyramine.

Chronic nongranulomatous ulcerative jejunoileitis This disorder is characterized by abdominal pain, weight loss, fever, diarrhea, steatorrhea, hypoalbuminemia, and protein-losing enteropathy. Clinical features mimic those found in both regional enteritis and celiac sprue. Indeed, the intestinal lesion may be indistinguishable from celiac sprue. However, exclusion of gluten from the diet does not result in any benefit. Glucocorticoid treatment has resulted in transient improvement, but long-term effects are unpredictable.

Amyloidosis This disorder is discussed in detail in Chap. 266.

Radiation injury to the small bowel Extensive morphologic damage of the small-intestinal mucosa often follows normal or excessive abdominal irradiation. These changes include a decrease in crypt mitoses, marked shortening of the villi, megalocytosis of epithelial cells, and inflammatory cell infiltration of the lamina propria. This may be associated with transient diarrhea and impaired intestinal absorption. However, restoration of normal intestinal architecture is usually complete within 2 weeks after cessation of therapy. Persistent diarrhea and malabsorption may develop shortly after x-ray therapy, or there may be a latent period of several years before the onset of diarrhea. Steatorrhea, ranging from 10 to 40 g per day, has been frequently observed, but impaired absorption of calcium, iron, D-xylose, or vitamin B_{12} is less common. In some patients intestinal strictures due to vasculopathy and ischemia may develop following irradiation, and thus stasis of intestinal contents and abnormal bacterial proliferation may occur. In others, intestinal lymphangiectasia, presumably due to lymphatic obstruction, has been documented. Diarrhea and malabsorption may be refractory to all methods of management. Treatment with antibiotics, pancreatic enzymes, gluten-free diet, adrenal glucocorticoids, and opiates has met with but limited success.

Eosinophilic enteritis Eosinophilic gastroenteritis is a disorder of the stomach, small bowel, and colon of unknown etiology characterized by peripheral blood eosinophilia and eosinophilic infiltration of the gut wall but without evidence of vasculitis. The clinical manifestations, usually recurrent, are protean and relate to the site of gastrointestinal tract involvement. Three main patterns have been identified: (1) Predominant mucosal disease manifested by iron-deficiency anemia, hypoalbuminemia due to protein-losing enteropathy, and mild steatorrhea. Patients in this group often present with a malabsorption syndrome and a history of intolerance to specific foods. (2) Predominant muscle layer disease characterized by marked thickening and rigidity of the stomach and proximal small bowel with obstructive symptoms and radiologic features of pyloric narrowing and obstruction. The obstructive form of eosinophilic gastroenteritis accounts for half of the cases reported since 1970. Accordingly, eosinophilic enteritis should be considered in the differential diagnosis of gastric outlet obstruction, diffuse small-bowel disease, and ileocolitis. Indeed, eosinophilic enteritis often mimics regional enteritis. (3) Predominant subserosal disease in which the cardinal manifestation is ascites with marked eosinophilia in the ascitic fluid. Although the above classification based on tissue layer of major involvement is useful in understanding the principal manifestations, it should be emphasized that multiple clinical forms, e.g., ascites (serosal involvement) and obstruction (muscular involvement), also occur.

Previous reports have emphasized food allergy and mucosal features of this disease. However, food sensitivity is related to symptoms in less than 20 percent of patients. In such patients fasting serum IgE levels are often elevated, and challenge with offending foods frequently evokes symptoms of abdominal pain and diarrhea in addition to a marked increase in serum IgE levels. In most patients with eosinophilic enteritis, however, immunologic studies including serum immunoglobulins, serum complement, lymphocyte quantitation, and lymphocyte response to nonspecific mitogens reveal no abnormalities. Thus, both IgE-mediated and IgE-dependent mechanisms may be operative in different patients with eosinophilic gastroenteritis. Several nonreaginic factors influence peripheral blood and tissue eosinophilia. It seems clear that evidence of allergy or food sensitivity is often absent and is not required for the diagnosis of eosinophilic enteritis. In addition, even in patients with food allergies, elimination diets are frequently ineffective and such patients may require prolonged glucocorticoid therapy to remain well. Surgical treatment for relief of obstructive symptoms and glucocorticoids are the mainstays of therapy.

Dermatitis and malabsorption A malabsorption syndrome, usually mild, has been reported in patients with a variety of dermatologic disorders, including psoriasis, eczematoid dermatitis, and dermatitis herpetiformis. Proximal intestinal mucosal abnormalities are almost invariably found in patients with dermatitis herpetiformis. In one study 21 of 22 patients had lesions ranging in severity from a completely "flat" to an almost normal intestinal mucosa. The mucosal lesions were often patchy in distribution. Clinical and laboratory evidence of significant malabsorption was infrequent, possibly due to the limited length of small intestine involved in this skin disorder. While the skin lesions of dermatitis herpetiformis respond to sulfone, the gut lesions do not. By contrast, in some patients with blunted and flattened intestinal mucosal lesions, and steatorrhea, there may be a striking improvement in villous architecture and regression of steatorrhea after withdrawal of gluten from the diet without improvement in the skin lesions. Further, in patients with dermatitis herpetiformis and a morphologically normal small-intestinal mucosa, administration of a high-gluten diet may result in blunted and flattened mucosal lesions indistinguishable from those of nontropical sprue. As in the latter disease, an increased frequency of HLA-A1 and HLA-B8 are also seen. These observations raise the interesting question as to whether certain patients with dermatitis herpetiformis and a malabsorption syndrome have latent nontropical sprue.

BIOCHEMICAL OR GENETIC ABNORMALITIES Nontropical sprue Nontropical sprue is a disorder characterized by malabsorption, abnormal small-bowel structure, and intolerance to gluten, a protein found in wheat and wheat products. It has been appropriately referred to as *gluten-induced enteropathy*. Celiac disease in children and nontropical sprue of the adult are probably one and the same disorder with the same pathogenesis.

There are insufficient data to provide an accurate estimation of the incidence of nontropical sprue in any population. This is largely because the severity of the disease varies greatly and individuals may have typical mucosal change and yet have no overt symptoms. Seventy percent of the cases in most reported series are women. The incidence in siblings appears to be many times higher than that in the general population, and it has been suggested that sprue may be inherited through a dominant gene of incomplete penetrance. Celiac sprue patients have an increased frequency of serum histocompatibility antigens, particularly of the HLA-B8 and HLA-Dw3 types. The HLA-B8 phenotype has been found in 85 to 90 percent of sprue patients as compared with 20 to 25 percent in normal subjects. The HLA-B8 antigen may be linked to immune response genes which may determine the immunologic recognition of certain substances. It has been suggested that such genetic factors may predispose to immunologic tolerance of dietary proteins such as the peptides in gluten or to the production of pathogenic antigluten antibodies which could result in binding of gluten to epithelial cells with subsequent tissue damage.

PATHOPHYSIOLOGY Gluten and the related substance gliadin are high-molecular-weight proteins found especially in wheat. These proteins, as well as the larger peptide hydrolysis products (containing glutamine), are toxic when administered to patients with sprue in remission. The exact mechanism for this effect is not clear, but two theories have been proposed, namely, a "toxic" and an immunologic theory. One possible mechanism is that patients with sprue lack a specific mucosal peptidase, so that gluten or its larger glutamine-containing peptides are not effectively hydrolyzed to smaller peptides (i.e., dipeptides or amino acids). As a consequence "toxic" peptides might accumulate in the mucosa. It has been demonstrated that patients with sprue in remission will develop steatorrhea and typical mucosal changes when they are given gluten. Similar results will occur with the administration of peptide hydrolysates containing at least eight amino acids with a terminal glutamine residue. It has been shown that when gluten is instilled into the *ileum* of sprue patients, histologic changes begin to occur within hours. This does not occur in the *upper jejunum*, suggesting that the effect is immediate and local rather than systemic. After noxious gluten fractions damage surface absorptive cells, the damaged cells are sloughed rapidly from the mucosal surface into the gut lumen. To compensate for this, cell proliferation increases, crypts undergo hypertrophy, and cell migration accelerates to replace the damaged and sloughed epithelial cells. This more rapid than normal epithelial cell renewal can be reversed by a gluten-free diet. The intestinal mucosa of patients with sprue shows many enzyme alterations, including decreased levels of disaccharidases, alkaline phosphatase, and peptide hydrolases, as well as impaired ability to digest gluten peptides. However, these abnormalities usually revert toward normal after successful treatment with a gluten-free diet. There is additional evidence supporting the concept of toxicity of gluten and gluten breakdown products in sprue. First, gliadin, especially the A-gliadin moiety, is toxic to sprue mucosa maintained in organ culture, causing ultrastructural changes and depression of disaccharidase activity. Second, sprue mucosa hydrolyzes a specific fraction of a gliadin digest (i.e., fraction 9) in a defective manner, and fraction 9 is selectively toxic to sprue mucosa. Third, specific fractions of gluten fed to sprue patients cause transient alterations in mucosal histology and depression of disaccharidase activity, but full recovery is observed in 72 h. The rapid onset of these changes and prompt recovery are consistent with a direct toxic effect. Despite intensive study, however, no persistent, specific, or selective peptidase deficiency has been demonstrated.

It has also been suggested that gluten or gluten metabolites may initiate an *immunologic reaction* in the intestinal mucosa. The presence of a mononuclear inflammatory cell infiltrate in the lamina propria of the mucosa, the beneficial response to glucocorticoid drugs, the finding of abnormal antibodies to gliadin in the serum of sprue patients, the synthesis of increased amounts of antigliadin antibody by sprue mucosa maintained in organ culture, and the elaboration of lymphokines such as migration inhibitory factor (MIF) by sprue mucosa incubated with gliadin have all been cited as evidence in support of this hypothesis. However, the evidence indicating that an abnormal (immune) mechanism is important in initiating or perpetuating this disease process remains to be determined.

A possible role for adenovirus serotype 12 (Ad12) in the pathogenesis of celiac sprue has been proposed based on two observations: (1) homology of amino acid sequences between a portion of A-gliadin and a viral-encoded protein (E16) produced by Ad12; and (2) patients with untreated celiac sprue have a much higher frequency of antibodies to Ad12 compared to treated celiac patients and controls. These observations are in accord with the hypothesis that there must be an *environmental* factor as well as a *genetic predisposition* to explain why only certain people develop celiac sprue.

Jejunal biopsy specimens from patients with nontropical sprue usually show a characteristic lesion. There is blunting and flattening of the mucosal surface, with villi either absent or broad and short. The crypts are elongated, and there is generally a dense infiltration of inflammatory cells in the lamina propria. The surface epithelium is altered with a sparse brush border, cuboidal rather than the normal columnar cells, and infiltration of inflammatory cells in the epithelial layer. These changes are usually most severe in the proximal small bowel, presumably because this area of the bowel is exposed to the highest gluten concentration. The typical morphologic changes illustrated in Fig. 240-4 are characteristic of nontropical sprue but are not specific. Similar changes have been described in other conditions, including lymphoma, tropical sprue, and hypogammaglobulinemia associated with malabsorption. Many biochemical abnormalities have been demonstrated in mucosal biopsy specimens from nontropical sprue patients. Impaired esterification of fatty acids to triglycerides, decreased uptake of amino acids, and decreased activity of intestinal disaccharidases (especially lactase) have been well documented. The latter observation may account for the high incidence of milk intolerance in untreated sprue patients or those in relapse. However, the greater abundance of undifferentiated crypt cells may be important, since crypt cells normally have a lower capacity for nutrient uptake than do villus cells.

Since the mucosa is damaged and altered in patients with nontropical sprue, there may be *decreased release of pancreato-tropic hormones* (secretin and cholecystokinin, i.e., CCK). This results in decreased stimulation of the pancreas with lower than normal intraluminal levels of pancreatic enzymes in response to a meal. In addition, the gallbladder appears to be resistant to the action of cholecystokinin, resulting in absent or minimal contractions of the gallbladder, in turn leading to sequestration of bile salts in an inert gallbladder. These two defects may result in impaired intraluminal digestion of fat and protein, which will be superimposed on the defect in intestinal transport caused by a damaged mucosa.

Diarrhea is common in sprue patients and is due to a number of factors, including *impaired absorption* of salt and water by duodenum and jejunum, net *secretion* of water and electrolytes by an abnormally permeable jejunal mucosa, and net colonic secretion of water and electrolytes induced by unabsorbed fatty acids and hydroxy fatty acids. However, the distal small intestine in sprue has the ability to adapt to the damage and loss of absorptive capacity in the proximal small intestine. Indeed, increased ileal absorption of sodium, chloride, and water has been demonstrated in sprue patients.

CLINICAL FEATURES Most patients with nontropical sprue will have a typical malabsorption syndrome characterized by weight loss, abdominal distention and bloating, diarrhea, steatorrhea, and abnormal tests of absorptive function. The characteristic alterations in tests of intestinal absorption are outlined in Table 240-2. It should be emphasized, however, that some sprue patients may present with isolated abnormalities which initially do not suggest the diagnosis of nontropical sprue. Thus, a patient may be admitted for investigation of iron-deficiency anemia without apparent blood loss or of abnormal bleeding due to hypoprothrombinemia but may not have diarrhea or overt steatorrhea. Likewise, sprue patients may present with puzzling metabolic bone disease without diarrhea or steatorrhea. Such patients usually complain of bone pain and tenderness and frequently are found to have extensive demineralization of bone, compression deformities, kyphoscoliosis, and Milkman's fractures. Emotional disturbances are common in these patients, and many individuals with a diagnosis of weight loss initially considered related to severe anxiety and depression are subsequently found to have nontropical sprue. In each of the above clinical settings, the diagnosis of sprue should be considered in the differential diagnosis.

Since there is no specific diagnostic test, three criteria should be met in order to establish a definite diagnosis of nontropical sprue: (1) evidence of malabsorption; (2) an abnormal small-bowel (jejunal) biopsy showing blunting and flattening of the villi along with changes in the surface epithelium; and (3) clinical, biochemical, and histologic improvement after institution of a gluten-free diet. In equivocal cases, the patient can be challenged with 30 to 50 g gluten orally, and if this promptly results in increased diarrhea and steatorrhea, the diagnosis of gluten-induced enteropathy is established. It should be emphasized that tests of intestinal absorption may reveal abnormalities which range from very minimal alterations to severe changes. Abnormalities in absorption tests have been shown to correlate reasonably well with the length of small-bowel involvement and to a lesser extent with the severity of the proximal lesion. A possible variant of celiac sprue is *collagenous* sprue. In this disorder small-bowel biopsy specimens characteristically reveal a blunted and flattened mucosa and large masses of eosinophilic hyalin material in the lamina propria. In one study of 349 jejunal biopsy specimens from 145 patients with celiac sprue, 45 (31 percent) showed basement membrane thickening often associated with collagen deposition, but dense collagen deposition was found in only 11 patients. Fatal, unremitting malabsorption developed in four of the latter patients. These observations suggest that collagenous membrane thickening is a fairly frequent finding in jejunal biopsies from patients with sprue but that dense collagen deposits are an unusual feature and may indicate a poor prognosis.

TREATMENT Despite the uncertainties concerned with the diagnosis of nontropical sprue, approximately 80 percent of the patients improve after institution of a *gluten-free diet*. Symptomatic improvement usually occurs within a few weeks, but improvement in tests of absorptive function and small-bowel histologic characteristics may not occur for months. It has been repeatedly demonstrated that strict adherence to a gluten-free diet more consistently results in improvement than does suboptimal gluten restriction. Nevertheless, even with strict diet adherence some cases show little improvement in intestinal histologic features. Patients with nontropical sprue treated with glucocorticoids but continuing a normal gluten-containing diet have shown symptomatic improvement as well as improvement in intestinal histology and tests of intestinal absorptive function. The mechanism by which glucocorticoids protect the mucosa from the effects of gluten is not clear.

If a patient with nontropical sprue does not respond to a gluten-free diet, other possibilities or complicating factors must be considered: (1) the diagnosis is incorrect; (2) the patient is not adhering strictly to the diet; (3) there may be another concurrent disease, such as pancreatic insufficiency; (4) the patient may have ulceration of the jejunum or ileum; (5) lactase deficiency may be present with resultant milk intolerance; (6) the patient may have collagenous sprue; or (7) he or she may have developed intestinal lymphoma, a disease which appears to occur more frequently in patients with sprue than in the general population. Finally, it should be emphasized that a small number of patients show a markedly delayed response to a gluten-free diet, with significant improvement occurring only after 24 to 36 months of therapy. Approximately 50 percent of patients with refractory sprue respond to glucocorticoids; such patients may also require parenteral hyperalimentation.

Systemic mastocytosis Some evidence of malabsorption occurs in 30 percent of patients with systemic mastocytosis. Malabsorption is usually not severe and is manifested primarily as minimal or moderate steatorrhea and impaired absorption of D-xylose and vitamin B_{12}. Small-bowel biopsy specimens typically show moderate blunting of villi and mast cell infiltration.

Disaccharidase deficiency syndromes As indicated above, the hydrolysis of disaccharides occurs on or within the brush border (microvilli) of intestinal epithelial cells by specific disaccharidases located there. As would be anticipated, both primary (genetic or familial) and secondary (acquired) deficiencies of these disaccharidases have been observed.

LACTASE DEFICIENCY IN THE ADULT Instances of isolated deficiency of mucosal lactase occur; they are associated with symptoms of lactose intolerance. Since lactose is the principal carbohydrate of milk, such individuals show milk intolerance with symptoms of abdominal cramps, bloating or distention, and diarrhea. Similar symptoms will occur following the ingestion of lactose. The symptoms are due to the fact that lactose when not hydrolyzed is not absorbed, and its osmotic effect in the lumen leads to shifts of fluid into the intestinal tract. The pH of the stool will also decrease because of the production of lactic acid and short-chain fatty acids from the fermentation of lactose by colonic bacteria. Although primary intestinal lactase deficiency seems to be hereditary, lactose or milk intolerance may not become clinically evident until puberty or late adolescence. There are significant racial differences in the incidence of this entity. It would appear that about 5 to 15 percent of the adult white population shows intestinal lactase deficiency, but in black Americans, Bantus, and Orientals, the incidence has been reported as high as 80 to 90 percent.

The diagnosis may be suspected when one obtains a history of gastrointestinal symptoms following milk ingestion. It should be emphasized that the ingestion of only moderate amounts of lactose, e.g., 5 to 12 g or the amount contained in 100 to 240 mL milk, often results in symptoms. Bloating, cramps, and flatulence, but not diarrhea, are usually produced with ingestion of small to moderate amounts of lactose. The vast majority of lactose-intolerant patients are aware that they are milk-intolerant and avoid milk. That these symptoms are not due to allergic reactions to the proteins in milk (i.e., milk allergy or hypersensitivity) can be demonstrated by performing a lactose tolerance test. This test consists of administering an oral dose of lactose (usually from 0.75 to 1.5 g per kilogram of body weight) and obtaining serial blood samples for measurements of blood glucose. In a positive test, intestinal symptoms occur, and the blood glucose increases less than 1.1 mmol/L (20 mg/dL) above the fasting level. However, false-positive and false-negative tests occur in 20 percent of normal subjects because the test is influenced by gastric emptying and glucose metabolism. Measurement of breath hydrogen after ingestion of 50 g lactose is a more sensitive and specific test. The rationale for this test is that hydrogen is released from unabsorbed lactose by colonic bacteria and breath hydrogen excretion subsequently rises. The test is noninvasive and is not influenced by gastric emptying or metabolic factors. Approximately 70 percent of patients with primary lactose intolerance will respond to a lactose-restricted diet while the remaining 30 percent will not because of an underlying irritable bowel syndrome.

Acquired lactase deficiency is often seen in association with a variety of gastrointestinal diseases, in many of which there is histologic evidence of mucosal damage. The disorders in which lactose intolerance and lactase deficiency may occur include nontropical and tropical sprue, regional enteritis, viral and bacterial infections of the intestinal tract, giardiasis, abetalipoproteinemia, cystic fibrosis, and ulcerative colitis. Patients with both primary and acquired (secondary) lactase deficiency are often able to tolerate yogurt because the latter contains bacterial-derived lactases.

DEFICIENCY OF OTHER DISACCHARIDASES Damage to the intestinal mucosa may produce decreased levels of other disaccharidases, such as sucrase-isomaltase, but usually these are not as depressed as lactase, and symptoms of specific intolerance, such as sucrose intolerance, are uncommon. There are instances of primary and apparently hereditary sucrose intolerance, but these always occur in association with sucrase-isomaltase deficiency. Sucrase-isomaltase deficiency, while not as frequent as lactase deficiency, is nonetheless an important cause of diarrhea, bloating, and cramping abdominal pain in children. Such patients are often unable to adhere to a low-sucrose diet. Thus, the observation that the symptoms of sucrose malabsorption can be ameliorated by the simple expedient of ingesting viable yeast cells is of considerable practical importance.

Hypogammaglobulinemia Malabsorption may be associated with hypogammaglobulinemia or agammaglobulinemia. The hypogammaglobulinemia may be of the congenital or the acquired type, with the onset either in childhood or adulthood. When malabsorption has been noted, it has included impaired absorption of fat, D-xylose, and vitamin B_{12}. Peroral intestinal biopsy may reveal changes comparable to those seen in nontropical sprue, but often one finds a more striking mononuclear infiltrate giving a nodular appearance to the mucosa both microscopically and macroscopically. Diarrhea and steatorrhea may precede or follow the development of hypogammaglobulinemia, and these may worsen during infections and subside after the infection is controlled with antibiotics. Intestinal infestation with *Giardia lamblia* is common in hypogammaglobulinemic patients. Meticulous collection and culture of intestinal fluids have revealed excessive numbers of anaerobic bacteria in the small bowel of some patients with hypogammaglobulinemia. However, the relationship between such overgrowth with anaerobes and diarrhea and steatorrhea remains to be clarified. Arthritis, resembling rheumatoid arthritis, and thymoma have also been described in patients with this syndrome. In some patients improvement in diarrhea and malabsorption may occur spontaneously, whereas in others improvement may follow treatment with a gluten-free diet, glucocorticoids, antibiotics, injections of gammaglobulin, and cholestyramine. These forms of therapy have not been uniformly successful. Although transient improvement is common, complete cessation of symptoms is distinctly unusual.

The relationship between hypogammaglobulinemia and malabsorption remains obscure. There is no evidence to date indicating that excessive enteric loss of gammaglobulin or alteration of the intestinal microflora occurs, but abnormalities in IgA metabolism may be important in this syndrome. This immunoglobulin is the predominant one in the intestinal mucosa and is found in many exocrine secretions, including tears, saliva, gastric juice, and intestinal juice. A few patients have been described with malabsorption and selective deficiency of IgA.

Abetalipoproteinemia See Chap. 326.

Hartnup disease, cystinuria See Chap. 336.

ENDOCRINE AND METABOLIC DISORDERS Diabetes mellitus The occurrence of diarrhea and steatorrhea in patients with diabetes mellitus has been well documented. When steatorrhea accompanies diabetes, it may be due to the presence of (1) exocrine pancreatic insufficiency, (2) coexistent nontropical sprue, (3) abnormal bacterial proliferation in the proximal small bowel, or (4) severe and uncontrolled diabetes per se (e.g., so-called diabetic diarrhea). Patients falling into the first three categories will usually respond in a satisfactory manner to treatment with pancreatic extracts, a gluten-free diet, and antibiotics, respectively. The pathogenesis of diarrhea and steatorrhea in patients in the fourth category remains poorly understood, and the response to various forms of therapy has been quite variable. It has been demonstrated that patients with diabetic diarrhea and steatorrhea may have involvement of the autonomic nervous system with degenerative changes in the sympathetic and parasympathetic nerves and ganglia. In some patients bacterial overgrowth in the stomach and proximal small bowel may occur and contribute to the diarrhea and steatorrhea.

The clinical features in patients with diarrhea and steatorrhea due to diabetes per se seem to be fairly uniform. Diabetes usually develops at a young age and is often severe and difficult to control. There is a distinct predominance of males. Several signs of autonomic neuropathy are usually present, including postural hypotension, anhydrosis, impotence, and bladder irregularities. Peripheral vascular disease and peripheral neuropathy are also common. Gastrointestinal x-rays may show delayed gastric emptying and disordered transit through the small bowel. Peroral small-bowel biopsy specimens are normal. Tests of intestinal absorptive function are normal except for steatorrhea and azotorrhea. There has been no consistent response to therapy with pancreatic extracts, gluten-free diet, or glucocorticoids. When bacterial overgrowth is present, broad-spectrum antibiotics may be helpful. Clonidine has proved useful in patients with large volume diarrhea not responding to dietary measures and anticholinergics.

Hypoparathyroidism Steatorrhea has been documented in several patients with idiopathic hypoparathyroidism. In addition to hypocalcemia, impaired absorption of D-xylose and vitamin B_{12}, decreased serum iron values, and abnormal small-intestinal roentgenograms have been demonstrated in some cases. In such patients the serum phosphorus level is elevated (due to the hypoparathyroidism) rather than low (as in primary malabsorption). The cause of malabsorption in this disorder is unclear.

Adrenal insufficiency Although there are few studies on fat excretion in adrenal insufficiency in human beings, malabsorption, especially of fat, appears to occur more frequently than has been generally appreciated. Patients with adrenal insufficiency have been found to have steatorrhea which is corrected by therapy with adrenal glucocorticoids.

Hyperthyroidism There are few detailed studies on intestinal absorptive function in patients with hyperthyroidism. Mild to moderate steatorrhea and hypoalbuminemia have been reported, but absorption of D-xylose and vitamin B_{12} is frequently normal. Steatorrhea usually remits after successful treatment of hyperthyroidism. Clinical studies suggest that steatorrhea in hyperthyroidism is not due to any defect of pancreatic, biliary, or small-intestinal mucosal function but is a result of hyperphagia with ingestion of unusually large amounts of fat occurring in association with rapid gastric emptying and intestinal transit.

Ulcerogenic tumor of the pancreas (Zollinger-Ellison syndrome) The clinical features of ulcerogenic tumor of the pancreas are described in Chap. 238. Malabsorption is frequently found in this disease. The acidification and dilution of intestinal contents caused by gastric acid hypersecretion leads to major disturbances in fat digestion and absorption. Impaired formation of micellar lipid due to inactivation of pancreatic lipase is probably the major factor in the production of steatorrhea. Other factors contributing to fat malabsorption in this disorder include (1) precipitation of glycine-conjugated bile salts due to low intraluminal pH, (2) alteration of the intestinal mucosa with ulceration and metaplasia, and (3) impaired fatty acid esterification and chylomicron formation.

Carcinoid syndrome (See Chap. 262) Although diarrhea is common in the carcinoid syndrome, malabsorption with significant steatorrhea is unusual. In many of the cases of carcinoid syndrome with steatorrhea there has been a prior intestinal resection (usually ileal), and in these cases the resection is the important factor in the causation of steatorrhea. However, direct involvement of the bowel wall and mesentery by the carcinoid tumor have been well documented. That abnormalities in serotonin metabolism may also be important is suggested from the decrease in the steatorrhea observed in some of these patients when treated with the antiserotonin drug methysergide. Although side effects may occur, for control of diarrhea and steatorrhea patients may be given a trial of 8 to 12 mg methysergide per day.

PROTEIN-LOSING ENTEROPATHY The gastrointestinal tract has been shown to play a significant role in the metabolism and physiologic degradation of plasma proteins. The exact magnitude of the normal gastrointestinal protein loss in human beings has remained unclear, but studies with labeled albumin have suggested that between 10 and 20 percent of the normal turnover of albumin may be accounted for by enteric protein loss. However, under certain pathologic conditions, excessive gastrointestinal protein loss may develop. An extensive number of disorders have been found to be associated with intestinal protein loss. Some of these are listed in Table 240-8.

Pathophysiology Several mechanisms have been proposed for the passage of plasma proteins across the gastrointestinal mucosa, both normally and in certain disease states. First, plasma proteins may pass into the gastrointestinal tract through an inflamed or ulcerated mucosa and account for the protein loss occasionally seen in regional enteritis and ulcerative colitis. Second, plasma protein loss may occur as a result of disordered mucosal cell structure. For example, patients with nontropical sprue have abnormal villous structure and surface epithelium, and these changes could facilitate the diffusion of plasma protein between the cells. Third, in the presence of increased lymphatic pressure, there may be increased passage of plasma proteins into the lumen via the intercellular spaces of the mucosal epithelium. This might be expected to occur in disorders in which there is granulomatous or neoplastic involvement of lymphatics. Fourth, dilated lymph vessels in the mucosa may rupture through the surface epithelium, discharging their contents into the intestinal lumen. This is thought to be important in the pathogenesis of steatorrhea and hypoproteinemia in patients with idiopathic intestinal lymphangiectasia (see "Intestinal Lymphangiectasia" below).

Several techniques have been developed for the detection and quantitation of gastrointestinal protein loss. In the past these have primarily involved the use of intravenously administered radiolabeled macromolecules such as ^{125}I-labeled serum albumin, $^{51}CrCl_3$, ^{51}Cr-labeled albumin, and indium 111. ^{111}In-labeled transferrin and $^{51}CrCl_3$ (which rapidly become attached to circulating transferrin) are the compounds available commercially for clinical use. After the intravenous administration of 0.93 to 1.11 MBq (25 to 30 μCi) of the labeled compound to normal subjects, between 0.1 and 0.7 percent of the administered radioactivity is recovered in the stool over a 4-day period. Patients with excessive enteric protein loss may excrete from 2 to 40 percent of the injected radioactive label. False-positive results may be obtained if the stool specimen is contaminated with urine. There is also a reliable and sensitive nonisotopic method to measure intestinal protein loss which involves the measurement of α_1-antitrypsin (AT). This serum enzyme, which has the same molecular weight as albumin (50,000), is resistant to proteolysis and when leaked into the intestinal lumen is not degraded. One can easily measure AT in serum and stool by radial immunodiffusion in order to obtain AT loss in stool (normal loss is less than 2.6 mg per gram of stool) or intestinal clearance of AT (normal is less than 13 mL/day). Results using AT as a marker of intestinal protein loss correlate well with the more cumbersome and costly isotopic methods. Random fecal AT assays can also be used as a simple screening method for enteric protein loss.

The rate of albumin synthesis and degradation can be determined using intravenously administered radioiodinated albumin and measuring the decline in radioactivity in the serum. Such studies carried out in patients with protein-losing enteropathies have demonstrated a reduced circulating (intravascular) and total-body pool of albumin, a normal or increased rate of albumin synthesis, markedly shortened albumin survival, and increased fecal protein loss. Whereas normal subjects catabolize 5 to 10 percent of their intravascular albumin pool each day (the fractional catabolic rate), patients with excessive enteric protein loss may have fractional catabolic rates of 50 to 60 percent.

Studies utilizing radioiodinated immunoglobulins have demonstrated a decreased intravascular globulin pool and increased fractional catabolic rate. However, the synthesis of IgG is usually normal, suggesting that a decreased level of IgG and increased enteric protein loss is not a potent stimulus for IgG synthesis. The increase in fractional catabolic rate is comparable for albumin, IgG, and IgM immunoglobulins, further suggesting that there is bulk loss of plasma proteins into the intestinal tract and not a selective loss of certain proteins. The finding of decreased globulins often is an ancillary aid in excluding renal, cardiac, and hepatic cases of hypoalbuminemia.

Abnormalities in albumin and globulin metabolism in patients with a protein-losing enteropathy may be reversed or diminished within a few months after the institution of appropriate therapy. It is obviously important that a specific etiologic diagnosis should be established in all patients with treatable disorders, who may be expected to have a remission induced by the appropriate therapy for the underlying disease. The intestinal protein loss in patients with nontropical sprue, Whipple's disease, constrictive pericarditis, re-

TABLE 240-8 Disorders associated with protein-losing enteropathy

I Stomach
- *A* Gastric carcinoma
- *B* Giant hypertrophy of the gastric mucosa
- *C* Atrophic gastritis
- *D* Postgastrectomy syndrome

II Small intestine
- *A* Intestinal lymphangiectasia
- *B* Nontropical sprue
- *C* Tropical sprue
- *D* Regional enteritis
- *E* Whipple's disease
- *F* Lymphoma
- *G* Intestinal tuberculosis
- *H* Acute infectious enteritis
- *I* Scleroderma
- *J* Jejunal diverticulosis
- *K* Allergic gastroenteropathy

III Colon
- *A* Colonic neoplasm
- *B* Ulcerative colitis
- *C* Granulomatous colitis
- *D* Megacolon

IV Heart
- *A* Congestive heart failure
- *B* Constrictive pericarditis
- *C* Interatrial septal defect
- *D* Primary cardiomyopathy

V Miscellaneous
- *A* Esophageal carcinoma
- *B* Gastrocolic fistula
- *C* Agammaglobulinemia
- *D* Nephrosis

gional enteritis, ulcerative colitis, and Ménétrier's disease has been ameliorated by therapy appropriate to the underlying disorder.

Intestinal lymphangiectasia PATHOPHYSIOLOGY The disorder intestinal lymphangiectasia is characterized by increased enteric loss of protein, hypoproteinemia, edema, lymphocytopenia, malabsorption, and abnormal dilated lymphatic channels in the small intestine. The high incidence of chylous effusions and abnormal peripheral, retroperitoneal, and thoracic lymphatics indicates that intestinal lymphangiectasia is part of a generalized congenital disorder of the lymphatic system. It has been suggested that the hypoplastic visceral lymphatic channels result in obstruction to lymph flow, with the subsequent development of increased intestinal lymphatic pressure. This in turn may lead to dilated lymphatic vessels throughout the small-bowel wall and mesentery. Hypoproteinemia and steatorrhea are thought to be due to rupture of the dilated lymphatic vessels with discharge of lymph into the bowel lumen. In adults approximately 1500 mL lymph, containing 70 g fat and 50 g albumin, passes through the thoracic duct each day. The leakage of a small amount of this lymph might be expected to result in considerable loss of protein and fat into the intestinal lumen. In addition, absorption of dietary long-chain triglycerides stimulates lymph flow, and this may increase further the retrograde leakage of intestinal lymph into the lumen. Three lines of evidence support the concept of intestinal leakage of lymph in intestinal lymphangiectasia: (1) chylous fluid has been recovered from the duodenum in these patients; (2) retrograde passage of contrast material from retroperitoneal lymphatics into the duodenum and jejunum has been documented; and (3) significant steatorrhea may persist in patients after institution of a completely fat-free diet, suggesting an increased enteric loss of endogenous fat present in lymph.

CLINICAL FEATURES The disease affects primarily children and young adults. All patients have edema, which may be asymmetric because of hypoplastic peripheral lymphatics. Chylous effusions and diarrhea are common symptoms. The primary laboratory finding is hypoproteinemia with decreased serum levels of albumin, immunoglobulins IgG, IgA, and IgM, transferrin, and ceruloplasmin. Despite moderate to severe hypogammaglobulinemia there does not appear to be an increased incidence of pyogenic bacterial infections. In addition, circulating antibody response to challenge with *Brucella* and typhoid antigens is normal. Steatorrhea is usually mild, although in some instances fat loss may be as much as 40 g per day. Some patients have hypocalcemia and impaired absorption of vitamin B_{12}. Lymphocytopenia (due to the loss of lymphocytes in lymph) is common, with lymphocyte counts ranging from 400 to 1000 per milliliter (normal: 1500 to 4000 per milliliter). This is associated with abnormal delayed hypersensitivity, as evidenced by prolonged homograft survival and impaired cutaneous responsiveness to antigens such as mumps and monilia.

Small-bowel roentgenograms are frequently abnormal, showing changes of mucosal edema and a malabsorption pattern. Lymphangiograms may demonstrate hypoplastic peripheral and visceral lymphatics with the absence of groups of retroperitoneal lymph nodes. Specimens of jejunal mucosa characteristically reveal dilated and telangiectatic lymphatic vessels in the lamina propria and submucosa. The villi may be club-shaped because of distortion from grossly dilated lymphatics (Fig. 240-4). Such changes in the intestinal mucosa may be reversed after appropriate therapy. The diagnosis of intestinal lymphangiectasia is therefore established by (1) small-intestinal biopsy and (2) demonstration of increased enteric protein loss using radioactive macromolecules.

TREATMENT A low-fat diet, by decreasing lymph flow, usually results in significant improvement with decreased fecal fat excretion, decreased enteric protein loss, increased serum calcium and albumin levels, and an increased half-life of injected ^{125}I-labeled albumin. Similar results may be obtained by the substitution of medium-chain triglycerides (MCT) for dietary long-chain triglycerides, since MCT are transported as medium-chain fatty acids by the portal vein rather than via the lymph.

REFERENCES

CALDWELL JH et al: Eosinophilic gastroenteritis with obstruction. Immunological studies of seven patients. Gastroenterology 74:825, 1978

CHERNER JA et al: Gastrointestinal dysfunction in systemic mastocytosis. A prospective study. Gastroenterology 95:657, 1988

CHUNG YC et al: Protein digestion and absorption in human small intestine. Gastroenterology 76:1415, 1979

COOPER BT et al: Celiac disease and malignancy. Medicine (Baltimore) 59:249, 1980

FLORENT C et al: Intestinal clearance of α_1-antitrypsin: A sensitive method for the detection of protein-losing enteropathy. Gastroenterology 81:777, 1981

GASKIN KJ et al: Colipase and maximally activated pancreatic lipase in normal subjects and patients with steatorrhea. J Clin Invest 69:368, 1982

GILLIN JS et al: Malabsorption and mucosal abnormalities of the small intestine in the acquired immunodeficiency syndrome. Ann Intern Med 102:619, 1985

HARMS HK: Enzyme substitution therapy with the yeast saccharomyces cerevisial in congenital sucrase-isomaltase deficiency. N Engl J Med 316:1306, 1987

HOWDLE PDet al: Cell-mediated immunity to gluten within the small intestinal mucosa in coeliac disease. Gut 23:115, 1982

KAGNOFF M et al: Evidence for the role of human intestinal adenovirus in the pathogenesis of coeliac disease. Gut 28:5, 1987

KEINATH RD et al: Antibiotic treatment and relapse in Whipple's disease. Long term followup of 88 patients. Gastroenterology 88:1867, 1985

KHOURI MR et al: Sudan stain of fecal fat: New insight into an old test. Gastroenterology 96: 421, 1989

KERLID P, WONG L: Breath hydrogen testing in bacterial overgrowth of the small intestine. Gastroenterology 95:982, 1988

KLIPSTEIN FA: Tropical sprue in travelers and expatriates living abroad. Gastroenterology 80:590, 1981

LOUGHRAN TP et al: T-cell intestinal lymphoma associated with celiac sprue. Ann Intern Med 104:44, 1986

LUBY LD et al: Lactulose/mannitol test: An ideal screen for celiac disease. Gastroenterology 96:79, 1989

MACGREGOR I et al: Gastric emptying of liquid meals and pancreatic and biliary secretion after subtotal gastrectomy or truncal vagotomy and pyloroplasty in man. Gastroenterology 72:195, 1977

MARA CS et al: Duodenal manifestations of nontropical sprue. Gastrointest Radiol 11:30, 1986

PETERS TJ, BJARNASON I: Coeliac syndrome: Biochemical mechanisms and the missing peptidase hypothesis revisited. Gut 25:913, 1984

SCHILLER LR et al: Studies on the prevalence and significance of radiolabeled bile acid malabsorption in a group of patients with idiopathic chronic diarrhea. Gastroenterology 92:151, 1987

SLEIKH MS et al: Gastrointestinal absorption of calcium from milk and calcium salts. N Engl J Med 317:532, 1987

STANGHELLINI V: Chronic idiopathic intestinal pseudo-obstruction: Clinical and intestinal manometric findings. Gut 28:5, 1987

241 INFLAMMATORY BOWEL DISEASE
Ulcerative colitis and Crohn's disease

ROBERT M. GLICKMAN

DEFINITION *Inflammatory bowel disease* (IBD) is a general term for a group of chronic inflammatory disorders of unknown etiology involving the gastrointestinal tract. Since there are no pathognomonic features or specific diagnostic tests, in a strict sense, these disorders remain diagnoses of exclusion. Their features are sufficiently characteristic, however, to permit accurate diagnosis in the majority of cases. Chronic IBD may be divided into two major groups, chronic nonspecific *ulcerative colitis* and *Crohn's disease*. The original description of the disease by Crohn, Ginzberg, and Oppenheimer in 1932 localized the disease to segments of ileum. However, the same process may involve the buccal mucosa, esophagus, stomach, and duodenum as well as the jejunum and ileum. Crohn's disease of the small bowel is also known as *regional enteritis*. In addition, a similar inflammatory picture may occur in the colon, either alone or with accompanying small-intestinal involvement. In most instances, this form of colitis can be distinguished clinically and pathologically from ulcerative colitis and is also referred to as *Crohn's disease of the colon*. Granulomatous colitis is a less accurate term since only a portion of cases exhibit granulomas. Clinically these disorders are characterized by recurrent inflammatory involvement of intestinal segments with diverse clinical manifestations often resulting in a chronic, unpredictable course.

EPIDEMIOLOGY The epidemiologic and etiologic considerations in ulcerative colitis and Crohn's disease share many features in common and will be discussed together. These diseases are more common in whites than in blacks and orientals with an increased incidence (three- to sixfold) in Jews compared to non-Jews. Both sexes are equally affected.

The incidence and prevalence of the two diseases differ slightly with most studies showing ulcerative colitis to be more common. When analyzed in western Europe and the United States, ulcerative colitis (including ulcerative proctitis) has an incidence of approximately 6 to 8 cases per 100,000 population and an estimated prevalence of approximately 70 to 150 cases per 100,000 population. Estimates of the incidence of Crohn's disease (colonic plus small bowel) are approximately 2 cases per 100,000 population; the prevalence is estimated at 20 to 40 per 100,000 population. Many believe the incidence of Crohn's disease (especially colonic) to be increasing.

While peak occurrence of both diseases is between ages 15 and 35, it has been reported in every decade of life. A familial incidence of IBD has been recorded with estimates that 2 to 5 percent of persons with Crohn's disease or ulcerative colitis will have one or more relatives affected. There is no specificity, however, for a given form of IBD within a given family. Such epidemiologic clustering of cases could argue for either genetic or common environmental influences on the development of these diseases (see below). It has been suggested that there is a probable hereditary basis for these disorders plus a strong environmental component.

ETIOLOGY AND PATHOGENESIS While the cause of ulcerative colitis and Crohn's disease remains unknown, certain features of these diseases have suggested several areas of possible etiologic importance. These include familial or genetic, infectious, immunologic, and psychological factors.

Inflammatory bowel disease is more common in whites, occurs with an increased frequency in Jews, and exhibits some familial clustering. This suggests that there may be a *genetic* predisposition to the development of the disease. In addition, the disease has been described in monozygotic twins. A search for genetic markers which might be of value in identifying susceptible individuals has not identified any single marker (i.e., histocompatibility antigen) in patients with inflammatory bowel disease.

The chronic inflammatory nature of these diseases has prompted a continuing search for a possible *infectious etiology*. In spite of numerous attempts to find known bacterial, fungal, or viral agents, no etiologic agent has thus far been isolated. Preliminary reports of isolates of cell wall variants of *Pseudomonas* or of transmissible agents producing cytopathic effects in tissue culture have yet to be confirmed. Efforts to produce specific granulomatous tissue reactions with filtrates from Crohn's disease tissue have yielded conflicting and nonreproducible results. As discussed below, many infectious agents can produce *acute* colitis or ileitis; however, there is no evidence that these agents are involved in *chronic* inflammatory bowel disease.

The theory that an *immune* mechanism may be involved is based on the concept that the extraintestinal manifestations which may accompany these disorders (e.g., arthritis, pericholangitis) may represent autoimmune phenomena and that therapeutic agents, such as glucocorticoids and azathioprine, may exert their effects via immunosuppressive mechanisms. Patients with inflammatory bowel disease may have *humoral antibodies* to colon cells, bacterial antigens such as *Escherichia coli*, lipopolysaccharide, and foreign proteins such as cow milk protein. In general, the presence and titer of these antibodies do not correlate with disease activity. It is likely that these antigens gain access to immunocompetent cells secondary to epithelial damage. In addition, IBD has been described in association with agammaglobulinemia as well as IgA deficiency, casting further doubt on the pathogenetic role of humoral antibodies. *Immune complexes* have also been invoked to explain extraintestinal manifestations of IBD. While there are well-defined examples of tissue injury resulting from immune complexes, studies utilizing specific detection techniques have failed to demonstrate an increased frequency of immune complexes in patients with IBD.

Associated abnormalities of *cell-mediated immunity* include cutaneous anergy, diminished responsiveness to various mitogenic stimuli, and decreases in the number of peripheral T cells. Since many of these changes may revert to normal when the disease is quiescent, it is likely that they are secondary phenomena. Experimental colitis has been produced in laboratory animals by prior sensitization with dinitrochlorobenzene, suggesting a T-cell–dependent mechanism of tissue injury. It remains to be determined whether the regulation of immune function (e.g., suppressor T cells) is of pathogenic importance in the etiology of IBD. Thus far, none of the altered immunologic findings have been specific for either ulcerative colitis or Crohn's disease.

The *psychological* features of patients with inflammatory bowel disease have also been stressed. It is not uncommon for these diseases to present initially or to flare in association with major psychological stresses such as the loss of a family member. It has been suggested that patients with IBD have a characteristic personality which renders them susceptible to emotional stresses which in turn may precipitate or exacerbate their symptoms. While there is little evidence directly relating possible emotional factors to the etiology of inflammatory bowel disease, there is little doubt that a chronic disease of unknown etiology affecting individuals in the prime of their life often results in feelings of anger, anxiety, and some degree of depression. These reactions are undoubtedly important factors in modifying the course of these diseases and in the response to therapy.

PATHOLOGY In ulcerative colitis there is an inflammatory reaction primarily involving the colonic mucosa. Grossly, the colon appears ulcerated, hyperemic, and usually hemorrhagic (Fig. 241-1). A striking feature of the inflammation is that it is *uniform* and *continuous* with no intervening areas of normal mucosa. The rectum is usually involved (95 percent of cases) and the inflammation extends proximally in a continuous fashion but for a variable distance. When there is involvement of the entire colon, there may be minimal involvement of a few centimeters of the terminal ileum, referred to as "backwash ileitis." This involvement never leads to the thickening and narrowing characteristic of Crohn's disease. The surface mucosal cells as well as the crypt epithelium and submucosa are involved in an inflammatory reaction with neutrophilic infiltration (Fig. 241-2*A*). This progresses to epithelial damage with loss of surface epithelial cells resulting in multiple ulcerations. Infiltration of the crypts with

FIGURE 241-1 Ulcerative colitis. Resected colon with portion of terminal ileum. The specimen showed uniform inflammation, erythema, and hemorrhage and a normal terminal ileum.

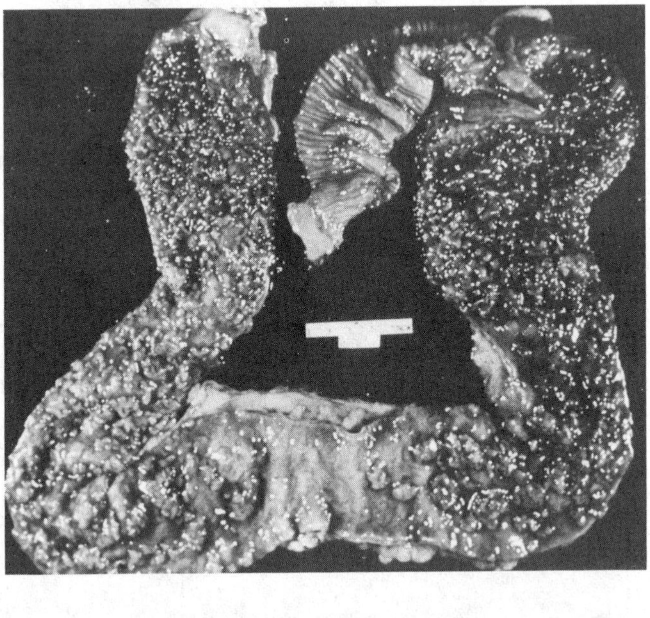

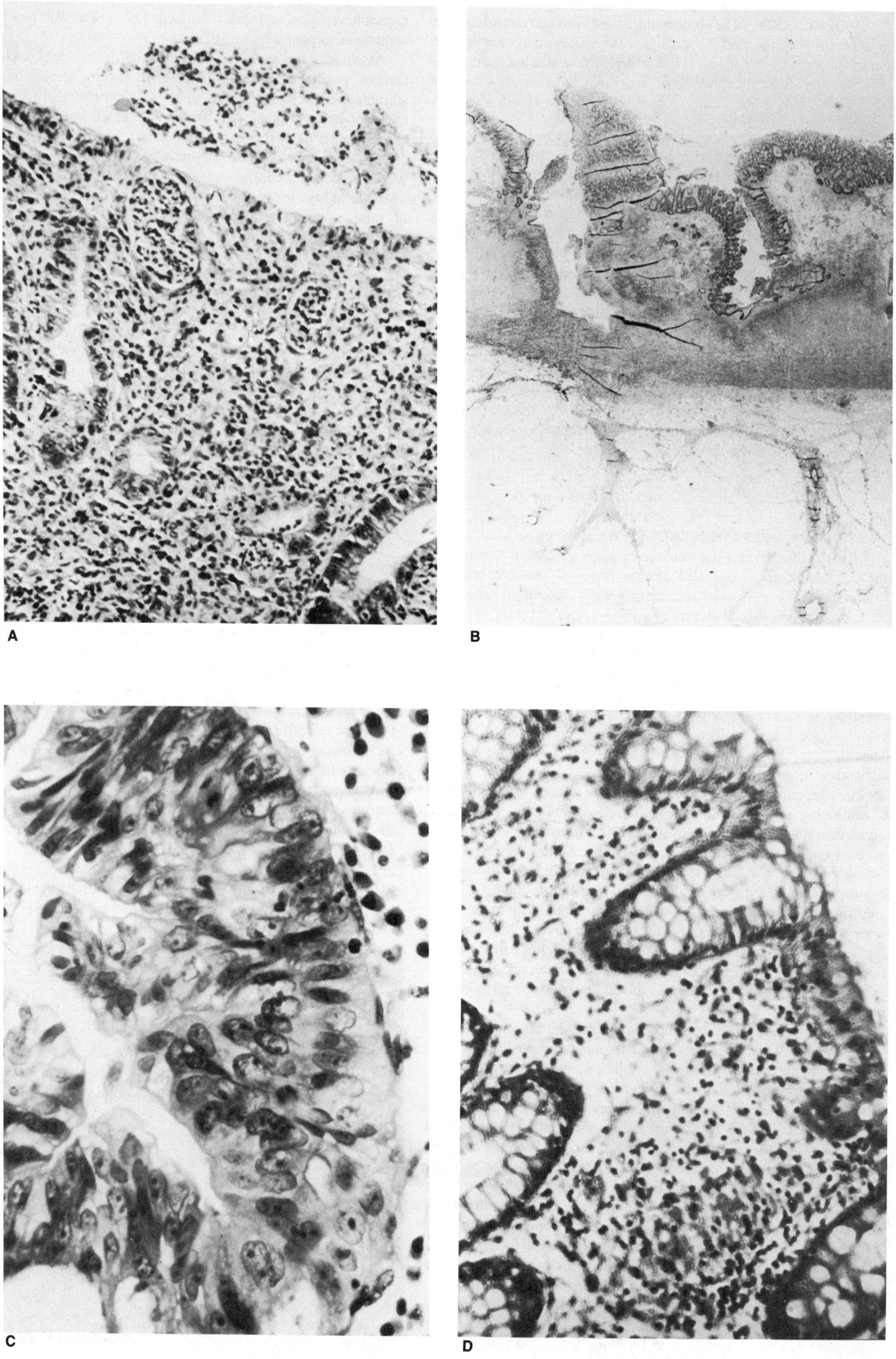
A
B
C
D

neutrophils results in characteristic (but not specific) small crypt abscesses and their eventual destruction. There may also be loss of crypt epithelium with a loss of goblet (mucus-producing) cells and submucosal edema. With repetitive cycles of inflammation, mild submucosal fibrosis develops. Regenerative activity is evidenced by irregular crypt epithelium often showing bifurcation at the base of the crypts. It is important to stress that, unlike Crohn's disease, deeper layers of the bowel beneath the submucosa usually are not involved. In severe ulcerative colitis, as seen with toxic megacolon, the bowel wall may become extremely thin, the mucosa denuded with inflammation extending to the serosa leading to dilatation and subsequent perforation.

Recurrent inflammation may lead to characteristic features of chronicity. Fibrosis and longitudinal retraction result in shortening of the colon. Loss of the normal haustral pattern leads radiologically to a smooth, "lead-pipe" appearance of the colon. Regenerating islands of mucosa surrounded by areas of ulceration and denuded mucosa appear as "polyps" protruding into the lumen of the colon. However, these protrusions are inflammatory in nature and not neoplastic and are therefore called pseudopolyps (Fig. 241-2*B*).

With long-standing ulcerative colitis, the surface epithelium may show features of *dysplasia*. Changes of nuclear and cellular atypia are thought to represent a premalignant change occurring in the setting of long-standing ulcerative colitis. Marked dysplasia in colonic biopsies in the setting of long-standing colitis is associated with a significant risk of a coexistent carcinoma elsewhere in the colon and may influence the decision to advise colectomy.

Crohn's disease, in contrast to ulcerative colitis, is characterized by chronic inflammation extending through *all layers of the intestinal wall* and involving the mesentery as well as regional lymph nodes. Whether or not the small bowel or colon is involved, the basic pathologic process is the same.

The earliest pathologic changes in Crohn's disease are poorly defined since surgery is usually not electively undertaken early in the course of the disease. At laparotomy, the terminal ileum appears hyperemic and boggy, with mesentery and mesenteric lymph nodes swollen and reddened. At this early stage, the bowel wall, although edematous, is usually pliable. While some patients with this initial presentation will subsequently develop typical regional enteritis, a significant number will recover completely. This acute form of ileitis will undoubtedly be shown to have diverse etiologies. Indeed, approximately 80 percent of patients with this presentation have been shown to be infected with *Yersinia enterocolitica,* an organism capable of producing a self-limited, acute inflammatory ileitis.

As the disease progresses, the gross appearance assumes a characteristic picture. The bowel appears greatly thickened and leathery with the lumen narrowed (Fig. 241-3). This characteristic stenosis can occur in any portion of the intestine and may be associated with varying degrees of intestinal obstruction. The mesentery appears greatly thickened, fatty, and often extends over the serosal surface of the bowel in characteristic fingerlike projections. The appearance of the mucosa is variable, depending on the severity and stage of the disease, but may appear relatively normal in sharp contrast to ulcerative colitis. In more advanced cases, the mucosa has a nodular, "cobblestoned" look. This is the result of submucosal thickening and mucosal ulceration, often linear in the long axis of the bowel at the base of mucosal folds. These ulcerations may penetrate into the submucosa

FIGURE 241-2 Colonic biopsies in inflammatory bowel disease. *A*. Ulcerative colitis. The surface mucosa is destroyed and the submucosa is diffusely infiltrated with polymorphonuclear leukocytes. Crypt abscesses are also present. *B*. Pseudopolyp. Regenerating island of mucosa with adjacent area of ulceration. *C*. Ulcerative colitis. Severe dysplasia occurring in long-standing chronic ulcerative colitis. Note atypical changes in the nuclei and marked palisading of nuclei of the crypt epithelium. *D*. Crohn's disease of the colon. Note the relatively intact mucosa with a solitary granuloma in the lamina propria.

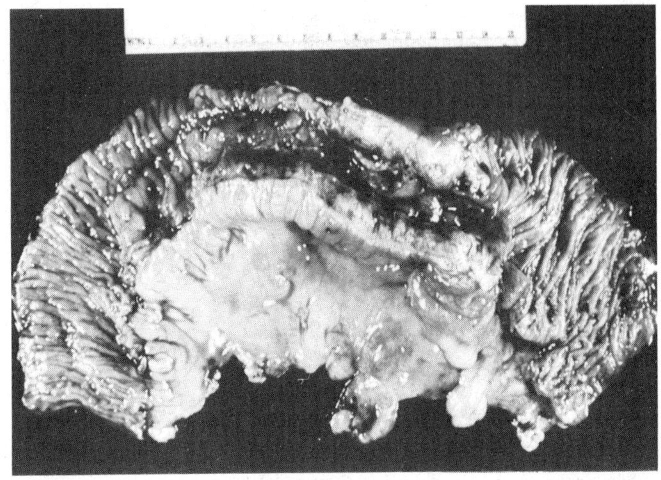

FIGURE 241-3 Regional enteritis. Resected specimen of terminal ileum demonstrates thickened bowel wall and chronically inflamed mucosa. Note the relatively sharp demarcation of the diseased segment with grossly normal mucosa on either side.

and muscularis and coalesce to form intramural channels which become manifested as fistulas and fissures.

There are other morphologic features distinguishing Crohn's disease from ulcerative colitis. In Crohn's disease, the disease is often *discontinuous;* severely involved segments of bowel are separated from each other with intervening segments of apparently normal bowel, producing "skip areas." In approximately 50 percent of Crohn's disease of the colon, the rectum may be spared. In sharp contrast, in ulcerative colitis the involvement is contiguous and the rectum is almost always involved. In addition, in Crohn's disease the transmural inflammatory process, involving serosa and mesentery, also accounts for the characteristic fistula and abscess formation. As a result of serosal inflammation, adjacent loops of small intestine may become adherent and matted together by a fibrinous peritoneal reaction, leading to palpable mass, most often in the right lower quadrant. Fistula formation may occur between adherent loops of intestine, colon, or other adjacent organs such as the bladder or vagina. Fistulous tracts may also lead to the skin or end blindly within the peritoneum or retroperitoneum, surrounded by adherent loops of bowel and inflammatory tissue. Fistula formation is not seen in ulcerative colitis.

Microscopically, granulomas are most helpful in distinguishing Crohn's disease from other forms of inflammatory bowel disease; they do not occur in ulcerative colitis. They may be seen in rectal or colonoscopic biopsies (Fig. 241-2*D*). While granulomas are a helpful finding when present, it is the chronic inflammation involving all layers of the intestinal wall which is most characteristic.

In most series reporting the distribution of Crohn's disease, approximately 30 percent will involve the small intestine (usually the terminal ileum) without colonic disease, 30 percent with only colonic involvement, and 40 percent with ileocolic involvement usually of the ileum and right colon. In a small number of patients (mostly children and adolescents) there may be diffuse and extensive ulceration of the jejunum and ileum.

While there often are sufficient features to permit distinction between ulcerative colitis and Crohn's disease of the colon (Table 241-1), in 10 to 20 percent of cases this distinction may not be possible.

CLINICAL FEATURES

ULCERATIVE COLITIS The major symptoms of ulcerative colitis are bloody diarrhea and abdominal pain, often with fever and weight loss in more severe cases. With mild disease, there may be one or two semiformed stools containing little blood and with no systemic

TABLE 241-1 Pathologic and clinical features of IBD

	Ulcerative colitis	Crohn's disease
PATHOLOGIC		
Segmental	0	+ +
Transmural involvement	+/−	+ +
Granulomas	0	+/+ + (50%)
Fibrosis	+	+ +
Fissuring, fistulas	+/−	+ +
Mesenteric fat, lymph node involvement	0	+ +
CLINICAL		
Diarrhea	+ +	+ +
Rectal bleeding	+ +	+
Abdominal pain	+	+ +
Palpable mass	0	+ +
Fistulas	+/−	+ +
Strictures	+	+ +
Small bowel involvement	+/− ("backwash ileitis")	+ +
Rectal involvement	+ + (95%)	+/+ + (50%)
Extracolonic disease	+	+
Toxic megacolon	+	+/−
Recurrence after colectomy	0	+
Malignancy (with long-standing disease)	+	+/−

NOTE: 0 = never; +/− = rare; + = occasional; + + = frequent, common.

manifestations. In contrast, the patient with severe disease may have frequent liquid stools containing blood and pus, complain of severe cramps, and demonstrate symptoms and signs of dehydration, anemia, fever, and weight loss. With predominantly rectal involvement, constipation rather than diarrhea may be present, and tenesmus may be a major complaint. On occasion, intestinal symptoms may be overshadowed by fever, weight loss, or one of the extracolonic manifestations of the disease (see below).

The physical findings in ulcerative colitis are usually nonspecific; there may be some abdominal distention or tenderness along the course of the colon. In mild cases, the general physical examination will be normal. Extracolonic manifestations include arthritis, skin changes, or evidence of liver disease. Fever, tachycardia, and postural hypotension are usually associated with more severe disease. The laboratory findings are often nonspecific and usually reflect the degree and severity of bleeding and inflammation. There may be anemia which reflects chronic disease as well as iron deficiency from chronic blood loss. Leukocytosis with a left shift and an elevated sedimentation rate are often seen in the severely ill, febrile patient. Electrolyte abnormalities, especially hypokalemia, reflect the degree of diarrhea. Hypoalbuminemia is common with extensive disease and usually represents luminal protein loss through an ulcerated mucosa. An elevated alkaline phosphatase may indicate associated hepatobiliary disease (see below).

The clinical course of ulcerative colitis is variable. The majority of patients will suffer a relapse within 1 year of the first attack, reflecting the recurrent nature of the disease. There may, however, be prolonged periods of remission with only minimal symptoms. In general, the severity of symptoms reflects the extent of colonic involvement and the intensity of the inflammation. At one end of the spectrum are patients who present with limited involvement of the rectum (ulcerative proctitis) or rectum and sigmoid (ulcerative proctosigmoiditis). Consistent with this limited colonic involvement, the disease is usually mild, with minimal systemic or extracolonic manifestations. The major symptoms are rectal bleeding and tenesmus. Most of these patients, especially those with only rectal involvement, will not develop more extensive disease. In the remainder, the disease may extend proximally with variable involvement. Most patients with ulcerative colitis (perhaps 85 percent) will have mild to moderate disease of an intermittent nature and can be managed without hospitalization. In approximately 15 percent of patients, the disease assumes a more fulminant course, involves the entire colon, and presents with severe bloody diarrhea and systemic signs and symptoms. The patients are at risk to develop toxic dilatation and perforation of the colon (described below) and represent a medical emergency.

CROHN'S DISEASE As discussed above, the basic pathologic features of Crohn's disease are the same whether the disease involves the small bowel or colon. The clinical presentation, however, will largely reflect the anatomic location of the disease and to some degree will predict which complications of the disease may develop. The clinical features of ulcerative colitis and Crohn's disease are compared in Table 241-1.

The major clinical features of Crohn's disease are fever, abdominal pain, diarrhea often without blood, and generalized fatigability. There may be associated weight loss. With *colonic involvement* diarrhea and pain are the most frequent symptoms. Rectal bleeding is distinctly less common than with ulcerative colitis and reflects (1) sparing of the rectum in many patients, and (2) the transmural nature of the disease with only irregular mucosal involvement. There may be associated severe anorectal complications such as fistulas, fissures, and perirectal abscess. Such features may antedate the clinical onset of colitis and should always raise the suspicion of associated Crohn's disease. With recurrent perirectal inflammation the anal canal may be thickened, and perianal fistulas or scarring may be present. With extensive colonic involvement, dilatation of the colon may occur. However, since Crohn's disease often results in a thickened colonic wall, this is less common with Crohn's disease than with ulcerative colitis. Extracolonic manifestations (discussed below), particularly arthritis, are seen more commonly with colonic than with small bowel Crohn's disease (regional enteritis).

With involvement of the *small bowel* there may be additional presenting signs and symptoms. Typically, the disease has its onset in a young adult with a history of fatigue, variable weight loss, right lower quadrant discomfort or pain, and diarrhea. Low-grade fever, anorexia, nausea, and vomiting may also be present. The abdominal pain may be steady and localized to the right lower quadrant or may assume a colicky or crampy pattern, reflecting variable degrees of intestinal stenosis. The diarrhea is often moderate, usually without gross blood; if there is no rectal involvement, tenesmus is absent. Physical examination at this time often reveals right lower quadrant tenderness with an associated fullness or mass reflecting adherent loops of bowel. At this time the patient may have mild anemia, mild to moderate leukocytosis, and an elevated sedimentation rate.

Since acute ileitis may have an abrupt onset with fever, leukocytosis, and right lower quadrant pain, the clinical picture may be indistinguishable from acute appendicitis. The diagnosis can be made only at laparotomy, when the characteristic beefy red terminal ileum, boggy mesenteric fat, and succulent mesenteric lymph nodes indicate that appendicitis alone could not produce this picture.

While the symptoms of diarrhea and abdominal pain will usually alert the clinician to the possibility of regional enteritis, other symptoms may dominate the clinical presentation. In children and the aged, fever of undetermined origin and unexplained weight loss may be prominent and initially may cause one to suspect underlying malignancy. In some patients, the first manifestation of the disease may be intestinal obstruction; in others the disease may present with fistula formation in the form of perianal sepsis or urinary tract infection resulting from an enterovesical fistula. Similarly, right ureteral obstruction and hydronephrosis may occur due to external compression of the ureter by a right lower quadrant inflammatory mass. On occasion, often in the setting of extensive small-bowel involvement, features of malabsorption may be prominent. These features, along with anorexia and the catabolic effects of the chronic inflammatory process, may combine to produce striking degrees of weight loss.

The complications of the disease are often local, resulting from intestinal inflammation and involvement of adjacent structures.

Intestinal obstruction is a frequent complication, occurring in 20 to 30 percent of patients during the course of the disease. In the initial stages, the obstruction usually is due to the acute inflammation and edema of the involved intestinal segment, usually the terminal ileum. However, as the disease progresses and fibrosis develops, obstruction may be due to a fixed narrowing of the bowel.

Fistula formation is a frequent complication of chronic regional enteritis as well as Crohn's disease of the colon. Fistulas may occur between contiguous segments of intestine; they may also burrow into the retroperitoneal spaces and present as cutaneous fistulas or indolent abscesses. In a significant number of patients, the first indication of the disease may be the presence of persistent rectal fissures, a perirectal abscess, or a rectal fistula. Although uncommon, pneumaturia should raise the suspicion of enterovesical fistula and is often associated with a persistent urinary tract infection.

Since Crohn's disease is a transmural disease with the bowel wall greatly thickened, free *intestinal perforation* is uncommon. In a small number of cases, however, it may be the presenting feature, and the disease is first discovered at the time of laparotomy for a perforated viscus. The passage per rectum of bright red blood should alert one to the possible coexistence of rectal involvement (i.e., ileocolitis). Crohn's disease may also involve the *stomach* and *duodenum*. The involvement is usually of the antrum and/or the first and second portions of the duodenum. Symptoms may include pain mimicking peptic ulcer disease. Later in the course of the disease, chronic scarring may produce gastric outlet or duodenal obstruction.

There are increasing reports of *small-bowel* and *colonic malignancy* developing in the setting of long-standing Crohn's disease. Although the risk of developing malignancy is statistically increased, the complication is uncommon when compared with the frequency of malignancy in ulcerative colitis (see below). As in other chronic inflammatory diseases, patients with long-standing Crohn's disease may rarely develop secondary *amyloidosis,* which may manifest itself with hepatosplenomegaly or significant proteinuria. The presence of extensive ileal disease, resulting in *bile salt malabsorption,* is associated with a decreased bile salt pool and an increased lithogenicity of bile (see Chap. 240). Up to 30 percent of patients with extensive ileal disease will develop gallstones. Also, in the setting of ileal disease and an intact colon there is increased colonic absorption of dietary oxalate with resultant hyperoxaluria and the development of *urinary oxalate stones.* Dehydration due to diarrhea is an additional predisposing factor in renal stone formation.

DIAGNOSIS

The diagnosis of IBD should be entertained in all patients presenting with diarrhea or bloody diarrhea, persistent perianal sepsis, and abdominal pain. There may be atypical presentations such as fever of unexplained origin in the absence of bowel symptoms or with extracolonic manifestations such as arthritis or liver disease antedating or overshadowing the bowel involvement. Since Crohn's disease may also involve the small intestine, it should be considered in the differential diagnosis of all types of malabsorption syndromes, intermittent intestinal obstruction, and abdominal fistulas.

The laboratory examination is usually nonspecific and reflects the extent and severity of the inflammatory reaction. In addition, when Crohn's disease involves the small bowel, laboratory features of malabsorption may be present. There may be a variable degree of anemia, from occult blood loss or the effect of chronic inflammation on the bone marrow. Folate or vitamin B_{12} malabsorption may also contribute to the anemia. While the Schilling test may be abnormal in patients with extensive ileal disease, frank macrocytic anemia due to vitamin B_{12} malabsorption alone is unusual, attesting to the marked efficiency of ileal absorption of the vitamin. When there is significant diarrhea, electrolyte abnormalities (hypokalemia, hypomagnesemia) may be prominent. Hypocalcemia may reflect extensive mucosal involvement and malabsorption of vitamin D. Hypoalbuminemia may result from amino acid malabsorption as well as from protein-losing enteropathy. Variable degrees of steatorrhea may result from bile salt depletion and mucosal damage. Mild abnormalities of liver function (especially an increased serum alkaline phosphatase) may reflect the development of a fatty liver in the malnourished patient or a coexisting pericholangitis. Significant jaundice is unusual. Proteinuria may reflect secondary amyloidosis, a rare complication.

Sigmoidoscopy and *radiologic* studies of the bowel are most important in establishing the diagnosis of inflammatory bowel disease. Sigmoidoscopy must be performed in all patients presenting with chronic diarrhea and in all instances of rectal bleeding. While meticulous air-contrast barium enema examination of the perfectly prepared colon may disclose the earliest mucosal changes in either ulcerative colitis or Crohn's disease (see below), a conventional barium enema examination is often "normal" in early disease. Direct visualization of the colonic mucosa combined with biopsy is the most sensitive way of determining whether rectal inflammation is present. It can often be performed without prior enema preparation in the patient actively having diarrhea. The goal of sigmoidoscopy is to establish *whether* mucosal inflammation is present and not necessarily to determine its full *extent* at the initial examination. Thus, if sigmoidoscopic changes are encountered within the first 8 to 10 cm, it is not necessary to pass the instrument to its full length which may cause discomfort when the bowel is acutely inflamed. In ulcerative colitis, findings include a loss of mucosal vascularity, diffuse erythema, friability of the mucosa, and often an exudate consisting of mucus, blood, and pus. The most characteristic feature is mucosal friability, best demonstrated by lightly wiping the surface of the mucosa with a cotton swab and observing the mucosa for the appearance of diffuse, small bleeding points. Equally characteristic is the uniformity of involvement. Once diseased mucosa is encountered (usually in the rectum), there are no areas of intervening normal mucosa before the proximal extent of the disease is reached. Ulceration is shallow, may be small or confluent, but invariably occurs in segments of active colitis. Rectal biopsy may corroborate mucosal inflammation. With more chronic disease, the mucosa may show a granular appearance and pseudopolyps may be present.

Endoscopic examination of the colon is also of value in the diagnosis of colonic Crohn's disease. The findings are of ulcerations which may be tiny, aphthous erosions or deep, longitudinal fissures. They usually occur in segments of otherwise normal mucosa. Since the mucosa is not uniformly involved, friability and diffuse granularity, which are hallmarks of ulcerative colitis, are not characteristic of Crohn's colitis. Rather a cobblestone appearance, which is a coarse irregularity of the mucosal surface, reflects submucosal inflammation and is characteristic of Crohn's disease. Pseudopolyps, edema, and strictures may be seen in Crohn's colitis as well as in ulcerative colitis. Colonic mucosal biopsy reveals granulomas in 30 to 50 percent of specimens taken from involved areas. Features such as crypt abscesses, infiltration with inflammatory cells, or ulcerations are nonspecific but compatible features. Since skip areas and rectal sparing are characteristic of Crohn's disease, colonoscopy may be superior to sigmoidoscopy in the evaluation of Crohn's disease. Colonoscopic examination is also indicated when Crohn's disease appears only to involve the small bowel. Ileal biopsy may be feasible, and coexisting colonic involvement occurs in a significant number of cases. Perianal inflammatory lesions as well as areas of rectal disease seen at endoscopy will often show granulomatous inflammation. Rectal biopsy of seemingly "uninvolved" areas may also show microscopic evidence of granulomatous inflammation in only 5 to 15 percent of patients.

The *radiologic evaluation* of the bowel provides essential information in the diagnosis of IBD. Barium enema, in ulcerative colitis, may reveal the extent of the disease and help define associated features such as stricture, pseudopolyposis, or carcinoma. The earliest features seen in ulcerative colitis are irritability and incomplete filling

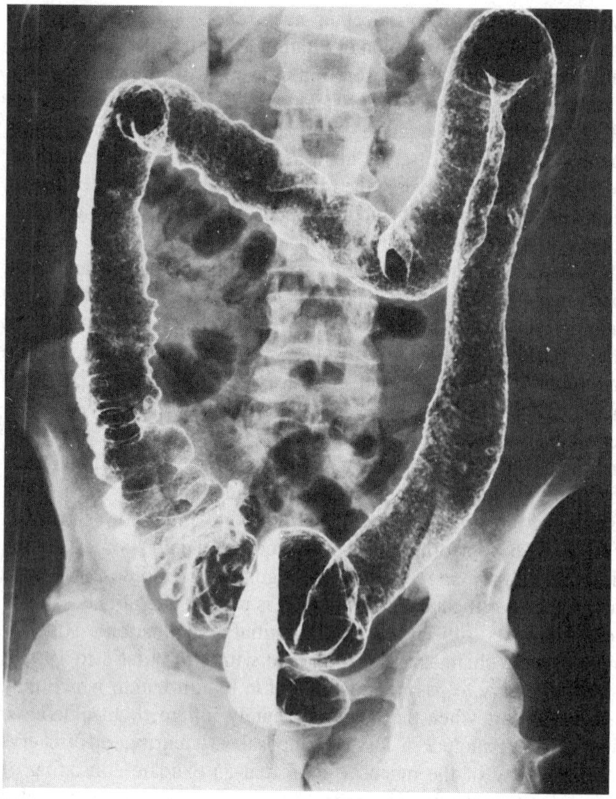

FIGURE 241-4 Acute ulcerative colitis, air-contrast study. Note the diffuse fine ulceration of the entire colon, producing serration along the contour of the bowel. *(Courtesy of R Gold, Columbia Presbyterian Medical Center.)*

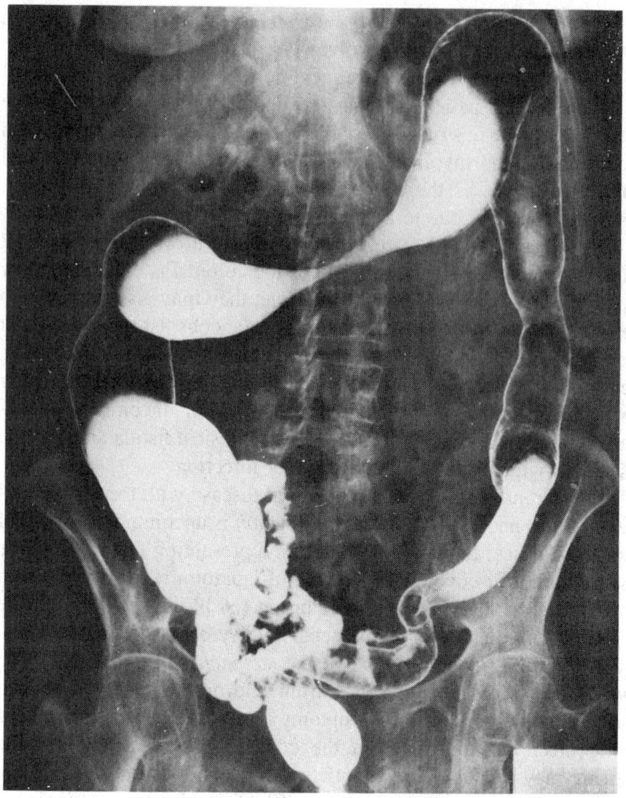

FIGURE 241-5 Chronic ulcerative colitis. Note the loss of haustrations and the fusiform stricture in the transverse colon. *(Courtesy of R Gold, Columbia Presbyterian Medical Center.)*

due to associated inflammation. Fine ulcerations may be seen at this time as serrations along the contour of the bowel producing a hazy margin (Fig. 241-4). The ulcerations may become deeper and with more fulminant disease produce a grossly ragged and irregular contour. Polypoid defects appear as a result of edematous mucosa between ulcerations. The diffuse pattern of ulceration is best seen on the evacuation film or on air-contrast barium enema. In the chronic stage of the disease (Fig. 241-5), the characteristic features are shortening of the bowel, depression of the flexures, narrowing of the bowel lumen, and rigidity. The bowel has a symmetric, ahaustral, tubular appearance with a decreased mucosal pattern. Although strictures are uncommon, when they occur they have a concentric lumen with fusiform tapering margins. Eccentricity should raise the suspicion of an associated carcinoma.

Barium enema examination in Crohn's disease of the colon has features which usually distinguish it from ulcerative colitis. Features characteristic of Crohn's disease include rectal sparing, the presence of skip lesions, and the finding of small ulcerations occurring on small irregular nodules. The small ulcerations often extend to produce longitudinal ulcers (Fig. 241-6) and transverse fissures which in reality are limited sinus tracts. These may extend into adjacent tissues to produce fistulas. Irregular thickening and fibrosis may lead to stricture formation which may be multiple. In 10 to 15 percent of cases the disease may uniformly involve the entire colon, making differentiation from ulcerative colitis more difficult. Reflux of barium into the terminal ileum during barium enema may reveal characteristic ileal changes of regional enteritis.

When Crohn's disease involves the small intestine, the terminal ileum is most characteristically involved with features similar to colonic involvement. Careful x-ray examination of the small bowel may demonstrate loss of mucosal detail and rigidity of involved segments resulting from submucosal edema or stenosis. The submucosal inflammation may lead to the characteristic radiologic cobblestoned appearance of the mucosa (Fig. 241-7), and fistulous tracts may be seen, especially in the ileocecal area (Fig. 241-8). Involvement of the stomach and duodenum usually appears radiologically as stiffening and infiltration of the mucosa and can mimic an infiltrative tumor. If such an appearance is due to regional enteritis, there is almost always coexistent involvement of either the jejunum or ileum. In Crohn's disease computed tomography (CT) imaging of the abdomen may be of value in the evaluation of thickened, separated bowel loops and to help distinguish thickened, matted loops (phlegmon) from intraabdominal abscess.

While barium studies often provide information on the pattern and extent of inflammatory bowel disease, caution must be exercised in obtaining these studies in the acutely ill patient with severe colitis in whom barium study and the bowel cleansing which precedes it may result in a worsening of the disease and can precipitate toxic dilatation of the colon.

Fiberoptic colonoscopy has added greatly to the diagnosis of colonic inflammatory bowel disease. Areas formerly beyond the reach of the sigmoidoscope can now be directly visualized and biopsy material obtained. Early in the course of colonic inflammation, endoscopic examination and biopsy are the most sensitive techniques to demonstrate mucosal involvement. Polypoid lesions, strictures, and unclear x-ray features can usually be fully defined. Periodic colonoscopic examination and biopsy are being increasingly used in cancer surveillance in patients with long-standing inflammatory bowel disease (see below).

DIFFERENTIAL DIAGNOSIS

Many entities must be considered in the differential diagnosis in IBD. The focus of the differential diagnosis will in large measure be determined by the presenting features of the disease. When *rectal bleeding* is the presenting complaint, a colonic source should be considered. While *hemorrhoids* are commonly found, they must be

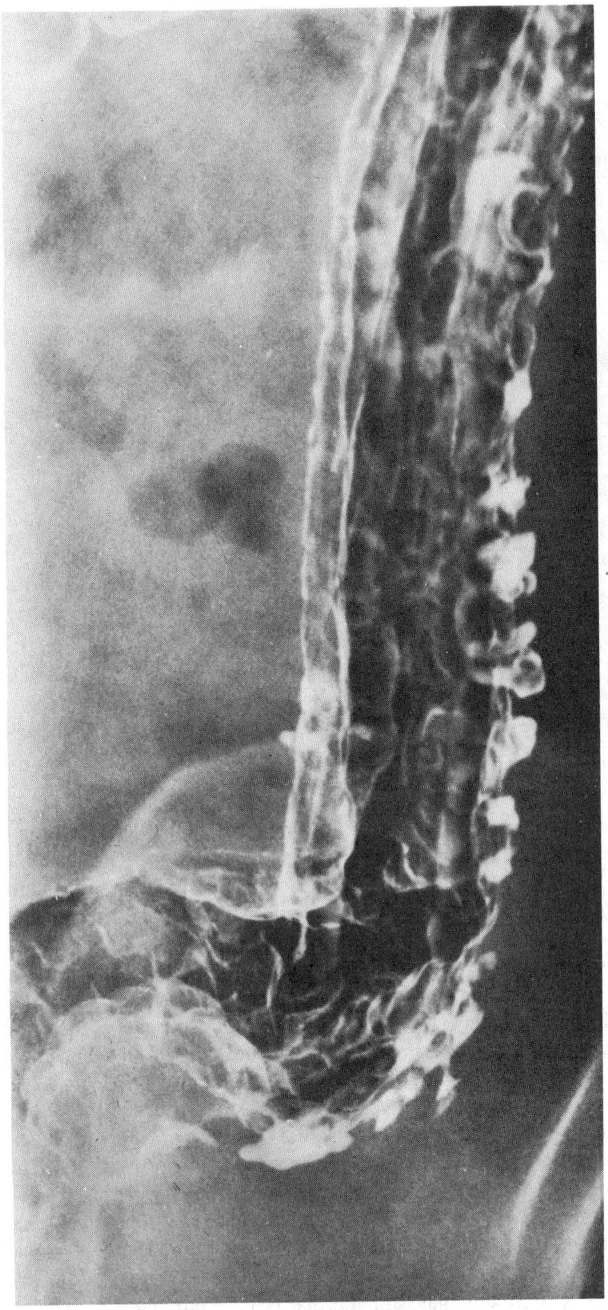

FIGURE 241-6 Crohn's colitis. Air-contrast study.

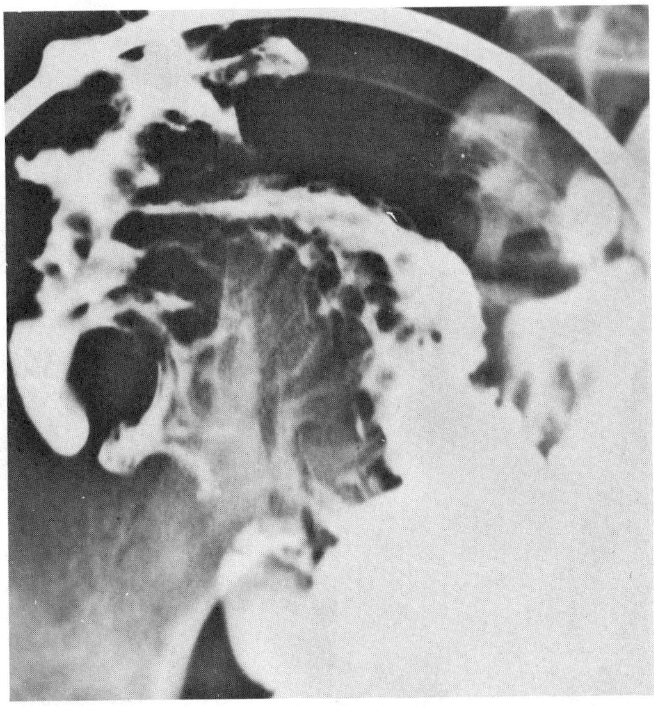

FIGURE 241-7 Crohn's ileocolitis. Note the nodularity and ulceration of the terminal ileum and the deformity of the cecum.

considered a tentative source of bleeding until sigmoidoscopy and barium enema have eliminated other colonic lesions. Colonic *neoplasms* (carcinoma, adenomatous polyps) may also present with rectal bleeding and can usually be diagnosed by barium enema with subsequent sigmoidoscopic or colonoscopic biopsy. It should be remembered that carcinoma may complicate long-standing colitis. Rectal bleeding from *colonic diverticula* or *arteriovenous malformations* usually present no problem in differential diagnosis since radiologic and endoscopic features of inflammatory bowel disease are absent. *Radiation proctitis,* which may present as a localized area of colitis, is usually found in the setting of pelvic irradiation. The onset may, however, occur at variable (months to years) periods of time after irradiation. Characteristic features on sigmoidoscopy include mucosal atrophy and telangiectasia along with friability and small ulcerations. A colitis sometimes indistinguishable from ulcerative colitis may occur in Behçet's syndrome and is associated with aphthous oral ulceration, uveitis, and urethritis.

Acute colitis may be caused by a variety of *infectious* agents (Chap. 92). Often presenting with bloody diarrhea, infectious colitis may be difficult to distinguish from IBD at initial presentation. Rectal biopsy in infectious colitis shows marked polymorphonuclear infiltration with pronounced edema and relative sparing of the crypts, features which may distinguish it from idiopathic inflammatory bowel disease. A listing of these agents is given in Table 241-2.

Amebiasis may present with bloody diarrhea and at sigmoidoscopy be indistinguishable from idiopathic ulcerative colitis. A history of recent foreign travel or homosexual exposure should always be sought. Since specific amebicidal therapy is necessary to eradicate this infection and corticosteroids may be detrimental, every effort should be made to exclude this diagnosis in appropriate individuals. Acute *bacillary dysentery* may be caused by *Shigella* and *Salmonella* or *Campylobacter,* all easily diagnosed by stool culture. *Yersinia enterocolitis,* which often presents as acute ileitis, can also produce a self-limited colitis, sometimes with granulomatous reaction. Infectious agents may cause acute proctitis indistinguishable from idiopathic ulcerative proctitis. Such infections, often seen in homosexuals, may be due to herpes simplex virus, *gonorrhea,* or *lymphogranuloma venereum* (LGV) as well as *amebiasis.* Recently, in homosexual men, non-LGV strains of *Chlamydia* have been shown to produce a granulomatous proctitis closely resembling Crohn's disease of the rectum.

Pseudomembranous colitis (antibiotic-associated colitis) is caused by a necrolytic toxin elaborated by *Clostridium difficile,* which under certain circumstances proliferates within the bowel. Most often the

TABLE 241-2 Microbiologic causes of colitis

Shigella
Salmonella
Amebiasis
Yersinia
Campylobacter
Lymphogranuloma venereum (LGV)
"Non-LGV" *Chlamydia*
Gonorrhea
Pseudomembranous colitis (*Clostridium difficile* toxin)
Tuberculosis

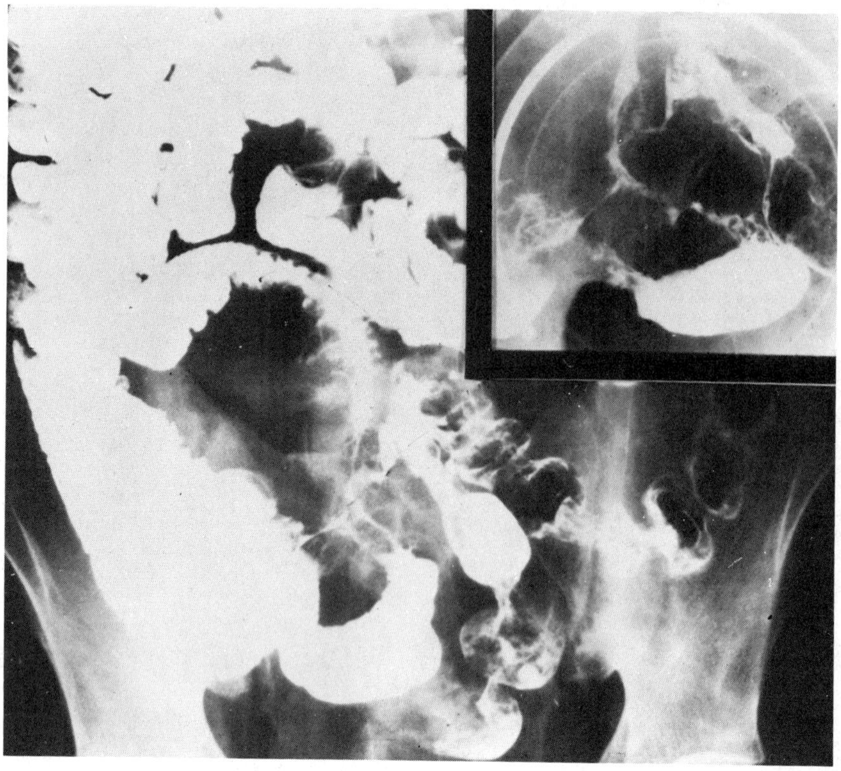

FIGURE 241-8 Regional enteritis. X-ray showing fistulas between loops of bowel. Insert is a compression film of this area; note fistulas between adjacent loops of bowel.

disease is a result of antibiotic therapy which presumably upsets the normal ecologic balance of the bowel flora permitting *C. difficile* to proliferate. Almost every antibiotic has been implicated, although cases related to the use of vancomycin or aminoglycosides are rare. Most often diarrhea is profuse and watery, although bloody diarrhea occurs in 5 percent of cases. Characteristic lesions are seen on sigmoidoscopy and appear as multiple, discrete yellowish plaques which on biopsy show features of acute inflammation and ulceration with a pseudomembrane of fibrin and necrotic material. On occasion lesions may be beyond reach of the sigmoidoscope and require colonoscopy. Diagnosis is best made by detecting *C. difficile* toxin in the stool. Treatment is either directed at binding the toxin or at eradicating the *C. difficile* organisms. Anion exchange resins such as cholestyramine (4 g PO qid for 5 days) will bind the toxin and may be used in mild cases. Vancomycin (250 mg PO qid for 7 to 14 days) is the treatment of choice for more severely ill patients and should produce clinical improvement within 5 days. Since vancomycin therapy is expensive, alternative therapies have been proposed. Metronidazole (500 mg PO tid) or bacitracin (25,000 units PO qid) have been suggested as alternative therapies. With all forms of therapy, relapse rates (15 to 30 percent) have been observed and may require a subsequent course of therapy to eradicate the organism. On occasion, infectious causes of colitis will be superimposed on ulcerative colitis or Crohn's disease. In this case, once the acute infection has subsided, symptoms and inflammatory mucosal changes may persist, raising the possibility of associated idiopathic IBD. Similar considerations apply to the patient with IBD who uncommonly may develop associated *pseudomembranous* colitis. The finding of *C. difficile* toxin in the stool and subsequent treatment will serve to clarify this presentation.

Abdominal pain in association with rectal bleeding, especially in the older age group, may be due to *ischemic colitis*. Because of an excellent collateral circulation, the rectum is usually spared. Radiologic features are often characteristic.

Inflammatory bowel disease may be difficult to distinguish from functional diarrhea early in the course of disease. The presence of constitutional symptoms such as fatigue, fever, and weight loss, coupled with laboratory features of anemia, elevated erythrocyte sedimentation rate, or occult blood in the stool should alert the clinician to the possibility of IBD. Similarly, finding leukocytes in a stained stool specimen points to an inflammatory basis for the diarrhea. In all cases, stool cultures and parasitologic examination of the stool are required to rule out enteric bacterial pathogens or amebiasis. In the *irritable bowel syndrome* sigmoidoscopy, rectal biopsy, and barium enema examination are all normal.

Once the diagnosis of idiopathic IBD has been established, the distinction between ulcerative colitis and Crohn's disease of the colon is usually possible. Differential diagnostic features are shown in Table 241-1.

With small-intestinal involvement (regional enteritis) the differential diagnosis should include disorders presenting with intraabdominal abscesses, fistulas, intestinal obstruction, and malabsorption. The finding of associated colonic involvement in patients with ileal disease will often serve to distinguish Crohn's disease from other ileal disorders. With diffuse involvement of the jejunum and ileum, regional enteritis must be distinguished from *nongranulomatous ulcerative jejunoileitis*. Abdominal pain and diarrhea are prominent features of this disorder, and weight loss, malabsorption, and hypoproteinemia tend to be more prominent than in regional enteritis. Small-bowel biopsy shows a more diffuse lesion with flattened villi (similar to celiac sprue), infiltration of the lamina propria, and mucosal ulceration. *Abdominal lymphoma* may likewise present with clinical and radiologic features difficult to distinguish from regional enteritis. Hepatosplenomegaly and peripheral adenopathy, when present, are helpful clues, but often disease is confined to the intestine. In such cases, laparotomy is usually required to make the definitive histologic diagnosis.

The advanced presentation of regional enteritis with areas of stenosis and draining fistulas may also be confused with *chronic fungal infection of the bowel,* including actinomycosis, aspergillosis, and blastomycosis. These infections often are seen in debilitated patients with impaired host defenses. Fungal skin tests and examination of fistula drainage and biopsy material for characteristic granules and fungi are helpful in making the diagnosis.

Intestinal tuberculosis characteristically produces stenotic lesions, usually in the terminal ileum, also often involving the contiguous cecum and ascending colon. Unlike regional enteritis, "skip areas" are unusual. Histologically, the granulomatous inflammation seen with *Mycobacterium* tuberculosis may be indistinguishable from regional enteritis; acid-fast stains and cultures are required. Fortunately in western countries primary intestinal tuberculosis is now rare; when intestinal involvement does occur, it invariably is associated with pulmonary tuberculosis.

COMPLICATIONS OF INFLAMMATORY BOWEL DISEASE

The complications of IBD may be classified as local, which are a direct reflection of mucosal inflammation and its extension, or systemic complications (Table 241-3). Local complications of IBD such as fistulas, abscesses, and strictures have been described above. In addition, perforation, toxic dilatation, and the development of carcinoma may complicate both ulcerative colitis and Crohn's disease.

PERFORATION Intestinal perforation can occur in severe ulcerative colitis since with extensive ulceration the bowel wall may become extremely thin. The clinical features are those of acute peritonitis with signs of peritoneal inflammation and the demonstration of free air under the diaphragm on upright film of the abdomen. These are an indication for immediate colectomy.

Toxic dilatation of the colon may occur in Crohn's colitis but is more common in ulcerative colitis. This complication can best be considered as a severe form of ulcerative colitis with the additional feature of colonic dilatation. It is thought that the neuromuscular tone of the bowel is affected by the severe inflammation resulting in dilatation. Injudicious use of hypomotility agents (codeine, diphenoxylate, loperamide, paregoric, anticholinergic agents) to treat diarrhea in the setting of acute colitis can precipitate this complication. Similarly, cathartic preparation and barium enema examination as well as superimposed hypokalemia may be contributing factors. Clinically, features of severe colitis are present with high fever, tachycardia, volume depletion, electrolyte imbalance, and abdominal pain. On examination, the patient appears toxic, and colonic dilatation may be evident. There is abdominal tenderness and if perforation has already occurred, peritoneal signs are present. Diarrhea may actually decrease markedly due to colonic atony, creating the false impression that the colitis is clinically improved. Plain film of the abdomen will show colonic dilatation with the colonic diameter more than 6 cm.

TABLE 241-3 Some systemic complications of inflammatory bowel disease

1 Nutritional and metabolic
- *a* Weight loss, ↓ muscle mass, growth retardation (children)
- *b* Electrolyte deficiency (K^+, Ca^{2+}, Mg^{2+})
- *c* Hypoalbuminemia (↓ nutrition, protein-losing enteropathy)
- *d* Anemia (chronic disease, iron deficiency; rarely folate or vitamin B_{12} deficiency in Crohn's disease)
- *e* Bile salt deficiency with ileal disease (steatorrhea and fat-soluble vitamin deficiency; ↑ colonic oxalate absorption → renal stones; ↑ lithogenicity of bile → gallstones)

2 Musculoskeletal
- *a* Peripheral arthralgia, arthritis
- *b* Ankylosing spondylitis, sacroileitis
- *c* Granulomatous myositis (rare)

3 Hepatobiliary disease
- *a* Fatty liver
- *b* Cholelithiasis
- *c* Pericholangitis, biliary cirrhosis (rare)
- *d* Sclerosing cholangitis
- *e* Bile duct carcinoma
- *f* Chronic active hepatitis and cirrhosis

4 Skin and mucous membrane
- *a* Erythema nodosum
- *b* Pyoderma gangrenosum
- *c* Aphthous stomatitis
- *d* Crohn's disease of buccal mucosa, gingiva, vagina

5 Eye
- Iritis, uveitis, episcleritis

6 Venous thrombosis and thromboembolism (hypercoagulability, dehydration, stasis)

There may be air in the wall of the colon, and irregular, ulcerated islands of mucosa may be silhouetted against the air shadow. While the transverse colon is the most common site of dilatation, this is probably largely positional, since with the patient supine, this is the highest portion of the colon. This presentation of colitis represents a true medical emergency and is associated with a mortality of greater than 30 percent if perforation has occurred. Appropriate therapy is discussed below.

CARCINOMA AND INFLAMMATORY BOWEL DISEASE There is an increased incidence of carcinoma in patients with chronic IBD when compared to the general population, especially in patients who have more extensive mucosal involvement (i.e., pancolitis) and those who have had their disease for extended periods of time. Cumulative risk of cancer rises steadily with the duration of disease. It has been estimated that with pancolitis there is a risk of cancer of 12 percent at 15 years, 23 percent at 20 years, and 42 percent at 24 years, although estimates in community-based practices have been lower. In children, the risk of cancer appears to rise more sharply after the first 10 years of disease, perhaps reflecting the higher incidence of pancolitis in children. Limited involvement of the colon (i.e., proctitis) has a low risk of malignant degeneration. Malignancy developing in Crohn's disease of the colon or small bowel is less well documented, but the incidences of both small- and large-bowel malignancies are increased compared to the general population. The incidence, however, is less than in ulcerative colitis.

The development of colon carcinoma arising in the setting of IBD demonstrates important differences when compared to carcinoma arising in a noncolitic population. Clinically, many of the earlier warning signs of a colonic neoplasm (i.e., rectal bleeding, change in bowel habits) will be difficult to interpret in the setting of colitis. In colitic patients the distribution of carcinomas is more uniform throughout the colon than in noncolitic patients; in the latter the majority of carcinomas are in the rectosigmoid within reach of the sigmoidoscope. In colitis patients the tumors are more often multiple, flat, and infiltrating and appear to have a higher grade of malignancy. There is some evidence to suggest that these features may reflect the younger age at which they occur rather than the associated colitis. Further adding to the difficulty in diagnosis is the frequent occurrence of mucosal irregularities, ulcerations, and pseudopolyps, making a small carcinoma difficult to diagnose radiologically or endoscopically.

Efforts have been directed to devise effective screening procedures to detect carcinoma developing in the setting of IBD. Carcinoembryonic antigen (CEA) may be elevated nonspecifically in ulcerative colitis and therefore is of limited value. Periodic barium enemas and/or sigmoidoscopy or colonoscopy have been suggested, but interpretation is sometimes hampered by abnormalities related to the colitis itself. The addition of colonic mucosal biopsy may add a significant dimension. It was originally suggested that a generalized precancerous lesion may be present in high-risk patients with colitis who either harbor an occult malignancy or who will develop cancer. Subsequent studies of rectal biopsies in patients with long-standing colitis showed that if dysplasia was present, there was approximately a 50-percent chance that an associated malignancy was present in those patients who subsequently came to colectomy. Complicating these findings was the fact that dysplastic changes were only found in rectal biopsies 60 percent of the time, making colonoscopy with multiple biopsies desirable. In addition, in some patients not undergoing colectomy, dysplasia was not a consistent finding on subsequent biopsies. While more information is needed on the prognostic significance and reproducibility of finding dysplastic changes on mucosal biopsy, it seems prudent to examine patients with colonic IBD of greater than 8 to 10 years' duration with colonoscopy and multiple mucosal biopsies at regular intervals. The frequency of such examinations has not been established, with recommendations varying from 6 months to 2 years. If severe dysplasia is found, then confirmation at less than 6-month intervals seems prudent. While most authorities would not advise "prophylactic" colectomy in the patient with long-standing colitis, the finding of severe dysplasia may well identify a subgroup who already harbor an occult carcinoma or who are at high risk of its development. There can be no uniform recommendation for this small group of patients, but many physicians will advise colectomy in this setting.

EXTRAINTESTINAL MANIFESTATIONS OF INFLAMMATORY BOWEL DISEASE

There are a variety of nonintestinal symptoms and signs which may be associated with IBD and occur in both ulcerative colitis and Crohn's disease (Table 241-3). Since some of these manifestations may not coincide with, or may overshadow, the underlying bowel disease, they may on occasion pose difficult diagnostic problems. Their etiology is currently unknown.

Joint manifestations are common in patients with IBD (~25 percent incidence). These may range from arthralgia only to an acute arthritis with painful, swollen joints.

The nondeforming arthritis is mono- or polyarticular and often migratory. Knees, ankles, and wrists are most commonly involved, but any joint may be affected. Joint fluid, if aspirated, reveals findings of an acute arthritis without crystals or evidence of infection. Tests for specific forms of arthritis (rheumatoid factor, antinuclear antibody, and LE factor) are negative. Typically, the arthritis correlates with activity of the underlying bowel disease. Rarely, peripheral arthritis may truly antecede clinical bowel symptoms. Arthritis is more commonly found in patients with colonic than with small-bowel involvement alone (regional enteritis).

In contrast, the central arthritis or ankylosing spondylitis associated with IBD is unrelated to the activity of the underlying bowel disease. It may antedate the bowel disease by years and persist after surgical or medical remission of the disease has been achieved. Symptoms are of low backache and stiffness with eventual limitation of motion. This may be associated with sacroileitis as well. X-rays usually reveal characteristic changes. In contrast to the peripheral arthritis, there is a strong association of HLA-B27 with ankylosing spondylitis, whether or not IBD is present.

Like the peripheral arthritis *skin manifestations* are more common with colonic disease. They occur in about 15 percent of patients, and when present the severity correlates with activity of the bowel disease. *Erythema nodosum* may be seen and heals without scarring. *Pyoderma gangrenosum,* an ulcerating lesion often occurring on the trunk, is relatively painless and may heal with scarring. In the rare patient, the lesion may persist even after colectomy for ulcerative colitis. *Aphthous ulcers* resemble "canker sores" of the mouth, and in approximately 5 to 10 percent of patients they are present during periods of active disease and then resolve. Their etiology is unknown and they are treated symptomatically. *Ocular manifestations* such as episcleritis, recurrent iritis, and uveitis occur in approximately 5 percent of patients and may represent a severe manifestation of the disease. In general, their activity parallels the course of the bowel disease, and the lesions may respond dramatically when colectomy is done for other indications.

Abnormalities of *liver function* are common in IBD. In the severely ill, malnourished patient, mild abnormalities of serum aminotransferases and alkaline phosphatase are often seen and represent nonspecific focal hepatitis or fatty infiltration. Factors favoring fatty infiltration of the liver in the severely ill patient are poor nutrition and often concomitant steroid therapy. The lesion is not progressive and resolves with disease remission. *Pericholangitis* is characterized histologically by portal tract inflammation, some bile ductular proliferation, and concentric fibrosis around bile ductules. Some authorities feel that this lesion represents the intrahepatic form of sclerosing cholangitis. Most often, the lesion is clinically insignificant, and its sole manifestation is an elevated serum alkaline phosphatase. It is usually nonprogressive and requires no therapy. Rarely, there may be an apparent progression to cirrhosis of either the postnecrotic or biliary type. Uncommonly, patients with IBD may develop *sclerosing cholangitis* (Chap. 258), a chronic inflammation of unknown etiology involving the extrahepatic and intrahepatic bile ducts which may produce varying degrees of extrahepatic biliary obstruction. Corticosteroids and immunosuppressive therapy are not beneficial. Reversal of the disease after colectomy is an inconsistent result and should not form the sole indication for colectomy. Cholangiocarcinoma, arising in the extrahepatic biliary tree, has an increased incidence in patients with chronic ulcerative colitis. Such patients will present with extrahepatic biliary obstruction which must be distinguished from sclerosing cholangitis. Finally, *chronic active hepatitis* which may progress to *cirrhosis* may be seen in IBD, although the exact relationship between these disorders is unknown. The evaluation and therapy are similar to the disease occurring in noncolitic patients. There is no clear evidence that colectomy influences the course of this form of liver disease.

TREATMENT

In general, the treatment of ulcerative colitis and Crohn's disease shares certain common principles. Initial treatment of all forms of uncomplicated IBD is primarily medical, and the principles of medical therapy are similar. Surgery is reserved for (1) specific complications and (2) intractability of disease. There are certain important differences, however, between ulcerative colitis and Crohn's disease; namely, the response to drug therapy may differ, complications often differ, and the prognosis after surgical therapy is not the same.

ULCERATIVE COLITIS Medical therapy Once the diagnosis is established, the severity of the disease must be assessed. Mild ulcerative colitis, including ulcerative proctitis, can usually be treated on an ambulatory basis. More severe disease, especially at initial presentation, is best treated in a hospital setting. The disease can rapidly worsen, and the course of a given attack cannot be predicted at the outset. The aims of therapy are to control the inflammatory process and replace nutritional losses. A certain degree of improvement usually follows intravenous correction of fluid and electrolyte disturbances. Blood transfusions may be required in severe anemia, especially when there is continued active bleeding. Agents to control diarrhea (diphenoxylate, loperamide, codeine, anticholinergics) should be used with extreme caution for fear of precipitating colonic dilatation and toxic megacolon. The decision to institute specific nutritional replacement therapy will be determined by the nutritional status of the patient and whether a protracted clinical course can be anticipated. In the severely ill patient, even clear liquids orally may stimulate colonic activity, and it is often wise to give the patients nothing by mouth. In this setting, intravenous alimentation, either peripheral or central, has been used as interim nutritional replacement therapy (see Chap. 75). While there is no evidence that intravenous alimentation is effective as primary therapy, it is an important component of a treatment program. In the less severely ill patients able to tolerate fluids by mouth, the use of elemental oral diets may be beneficial providing supplemental nutrition with low fecal volume. While milk is not contraindicated in ulcerative colitis, diarrhea will be exacerbated if there is an associated lactase deficiency.

The principal drugs used in the therapy of ulcerative colitis are the *anti-inflammatory agents, sulfasalazine* (Azulfidine) and *adrenal glucocorticoids* or ACTH. Sulfasalazine consists of a sulfonamide (sulfapyridine) moiety chemically bound to a salicylate (5-aminosalicylate); it undergoes bacterial cleavage in the colon. The liberated sulfapyridine is efficiently absorbed and largely excreted in the urine; the liberated 5-aminosalicylate believed to be the active component remains largely in the colon and is excreted in the stool. The salicylate moiety is thought to exert its action through inhibition of prostaglandin synthesis. While most physicians are familiar with the use of sulfasalazine to prevent recurrences of ulcerative colitis, it is less well appreciated that this agent is effective in the therapy of acute ulcerative colitis of mild to moderate severity. Therapeutic doses of 4 to 6 g daily are required. The drug is usually started at a dose of

500 mg bid and then increased daily or every other day by 1 g until the therapeutic dose is achieved.

In the severely ill patient who may not tolerate oral medication and for whom a more rapid time frame of therapy is often desired, initial therapy is begun with glucocorticoids or ACTH. While some physicians still prefer ACTH to corticosteroids, these agents appear equally effective when given in equivalent dosages and by comparable routes of administration. The choice is one of individual preference; however, oral prednisone (45 to 60 mg daily) is often employed initially. Alternatively, intravenous ACTH may be given (40 to 60 units) over an 8-h drip infusion. In the severely ill patient, parenteral administration of corticosteroids (i.e., intravenous hydrocortisone 300 to 400 ng daily) is preferable to avoid the uncertainty of adequate oral absorption. Improvement is usually noted after 7 to 10 days of such therapy by a reduction in fever, decreased bloody diarrhea, and an improvement in appetite.

After initial improvement low-roughage oral feedings can be resumed. At this point the dose of steroids can be tapered, or if ACTH was used initially, oral prednisone at reduced dosage can be started. There is no specific schedule for tapering glucocorticoids. The guiding principle, however, is that once clinical remission is achieved, there is no evidence that chronic steroid administration favorably influences the long-term outlook of the disease or that recurrences can be prevented by chronic steroid therapy. In practice, steroid therapy can be tapered and discontinued over a 2- to 3-month period after discharge. In some patients (10 to 15 percent) efforts to completely eliminate steroids may be associated with a flare of the disease, and low to moderate steroids (10 to 15 mg of prednisone daily) may be required to suppress disease activity. This should not be confused with the prophylactic administration of steroids to patients in remission, but rather represents incompletely responsive disease. Once the acutely ill patient is taking oral feedings, sulfasalazine should be added as described above in a daily dose of 2 g. Controlled trials have shown that this dose of sulfasalazine, when administered chronically to patients with ulcerative colitis, is effective in decreasing the frequency of relapses and should be continued chronically after glucocorticoids have been discontinued. Patients with glucose phosphate dehydrogenase deficiency or those exhibiting severe allergic reactions to the drug unfortunately cannot be maintained on it. Patients who exhibit intolerance for the drug (headache, nausea) or mild skin allergic reactions can be "desensitized" by gradually reintroducing the drug in small doses. Sulfasalazine is discontinued for 1 to 2 weeks and then is restarted at a dose of 0.125 to 0.25 g per day for 1 week with a gradual increase by 0.125 g per week to a maintenance dose of 2 g per day. The knowledge that the 5-aminosalicylate portion of the molecule is therapeutically efficacious has led to formulations of this compound without the sulfa moiety responsible for allergic reactions. 5-Aminosalicylate incorporated into enemas, enteric coated 5-ASA, or oral azodisalicylate (consisting of two molecules of 5-aminosalicylate joined by an azo bond) have shown encouraging results in the treatment of mild to moderate ulcerative colitis.

The use of immunosuppressive therapy with drugs such as azathioprine is less well established in ulcerative colitis. As a single agent in the therapy of acute ulcerative colitis, the drug is ineffective. However, the drug may be added to the regimen at a dose of 1.5 to 2.0 mg/kg when glucocorticoids fail or when the steroid dose needed to reduce inflammation is too high. It is desirable to monitor the blood count and observe the patient carefully for infection. Azathioprine may also have a limited role as a "steroid-sparing agent" in the patient with chronic ulcerative colitis who must be maintained on corticosteroids to control disease activity.

Toxic megacolon is a major complication of severe ulcerative colitis which requires rapid, intensive management best carried out jointly by the internist or gastroenterologist and surgeon. Once the diagnosis is established, prompt and vigorous use of intravenous fluids, electrolyte replacement therapy, and blood transfusions are indicated. Because of the fear of perforation and high likelihood that bacteremia and occult perforation have occurred, many physicians will institute broad-spectrum antibiotic coverage after appropriate cultures have been obtained. The patient is given nothing by mouth, and nasogastric suction is often instituted. Full intravenous corticosteroid therapy is also begun. Majority opinion favors an initial period of medical stabilization for the first 24 to 48 h. If significant objective improvement has not occurred and if perforation seems imminent, emergency colectomy should be carried out. While it is certainly true that some patients, under maximal medical therapy, may slowly improve and thus avoid colectomy, the risk of this course of action must be carefully considered. If perforation occurs, mortality rates rise sharply, approaching 50 percent in those who subsequently go on to colectomy.

At the other end of the spectrum is the patient with mild ulcerative colitis, limited to the rectum or rectosigmoid, who is managed on an ambulatory basis. Therapy is started with sulfasalazine, 0.5 to 1.0 g four times a day with meals. If rectal symptoms such as tenesmus are prominent, topical steroids in the form of small enemas may produce marked improvement. The equivalent of 100 mg hydrocortisone (20 mg prednisone) in 60 to 100 mL saline is used as a bedtime enema. On occasion the use of steroid foam preparations may be better tolerated in the patient with severe tenesmus. Retention enemas have been shown to deliver medication as far as the descending colon, and absorption of steroid is small (~10 to 20 percent). If large doses of rectal steroids are required for control, it is preferable to use oral prednisone at a moderate dosage (20 mg daily).

Psychotherapy The elements of trust and mutual understanding combined with the compassion and expertise of the physician are essential in the therapy of any chronic disease and are particularly important in the long-term management of patients with inflammatory bowel disease. Often these patients are intelligent young adults who are frequently resentful of a disease affecting them during the most productive years. Through the vigorous participation of the physician many patients are able to lead reasonably stable and productive lives. More formal psychiatric assistance may be required in the chronically ill patient, in particular children or adolescents, or in the elderly where severe depressive reactions are common. This is particularly true when colectomy is being advised and in the emotional adjustment which must be made after colectomy.

Pregnancy and ulcerative colitis While many physicians are apprehensive about the management and prognosis of ulcerative colitis in the pregnant patient, the outcome for the patient and the fetus is excellent. In general, the pregnancy is not threatened by coexistent colitis, with no increase in stillbirths or premature deliveries when compared to the general population. When patients with inactive colitis become pregnant, approximately 50 percent may have an exacerbation of their disease with some clustering of these flares during the first trimester and in the postpartum period. The therapy of ulcerative colitis during pregnancy is largely the same as in the nonpregnant patient. Sulfasalazine is used to treat mild to moderate disease since there is no evidence that the drug is harmful to the fetus or leads to increased incidence of fetal malformations. Women with inactive colitis who enter a pregnancy on maintenance sulfasalazine should be continued on the drug. Since sulfapyridine appears in breast milk, in the newborn with unconjugated hyperbilirubinemia from other causes, breast feeding should be discontinued or the drug stopped if the colitis is inactive. In most situations, however, the drug should be continued to protect the mother during the postpartum period from a relapse of disease. Corticosteroids should be used in the same dosage and for the same indications as in the nonpregnant patient.

Thus, it is clear that the patient with colitis can realistically plan to have a family. It is prudent, however, to bring active disease under control before pregnancy is undertaken to ensure the most optimal physical and emotional setting for the pregnancy. Similar conclusions apply to the management of Crohn's disease during pregnancy.

Surgical therapy Approximately 20 to 25 percent of patients with ulcerative colitis will require colectomy during the course of their disease. A major indication for colectomy is failure to respond to intensive medical management. Such patients, although not showing colonic dilatation, may fail to improve after 7 to 10 days of optimal medical therapy. Fever, persistent bloody diarrhea, and severe fatigue may persist, and consideration should be given to semielective colectomy. Elective colectomy may be performed in patients whose disease remains chronically active and who require continuous corticosteroid administration. Such patients are at risk of developing the complications of chronic steroid therapy. After colectomy these patients often feel more energetic and usually gain back weight to their preillness level. As discussed above, the patient with long-standing colitis is at high risk for colonic cancer. While most authorities do not advise ''prophylactic'' colectomy in the patient with quiescent disease, the finding of marked dysplasia on colonoscopic biopsies done as a part of a surveillance program should make the physician think seriously about advising colectomy.

The decision to advise colectomy in other than emergency circumstances is difficult for both patient and physician. Many patients have an understandable reluctance to undergo colectomy and have difficulty in conceptualizing life with an ileostomy. In most metropolitan centers there are ileostomy groups who visit patients preoperatively and can provide answers to many practical questions. It is also desirable for the patient to be visited by a nurse familiar with stoma care to instruct the patient on the practical aspects of handling the ileostomy.

While total proctocolectomy with permanent ileostomy is the procedure of choice for almost all patients undergoing colectomy, several alternative approaches have been suggested. The *continent ileostomy* is an ileal loop reservoir fashioned under the skin with a nipple valve to prevent spilling of ileal contents. Ileal effluent collects in this reservoir which must be emptied with a soft rubber catheter. Only a small stoma is externally visible, thus eliminating an external ileostomy appliance. Problems with this procedure include a failure of continence, irritation of the mucosa of the ileal reservoir from stasis (''pouchitis''), and bacterial overgrowth which may lead to mild malabsorption. Repeat operations are common, and this procedure should only be done by skilled surgeons familiar with the technique. *Ileorectal anastomosis* with *mucosal stripping* of the rectal segment is sometimes done in children who require colectomy. Newer forms of surgical therapy include ileoanal anastomosis with internal reservoirs thus preserving sphincteric function. These approaches are recent and not generally available.

CROHN'S DISEASE The medical management of colonic Crohn's disease is similar in most respects to that of ulcerative colitis. In a multicenter study (National Cooperative Crohn's Disease Study), sulfasalazine was shown to be effective in the therapy of active colonic disease. Glucocorticoids also were efficacious but less so than with small-bowel involvement. The indications and dosages of these medications are similar to those for ulcerative colitis. Since in Crohn's disease, intraabdominal sepsis can result from fistula or abscess formation, corticosteroids must be used with caution and constant attention is required to detect evidence of sepsis, which can be masked by these agents. In general, the disease is less explosive in onset, and although toxic dilatation and perforation can occur, they are less common than in ulcerative colitis. The principles of management are the same. Because of the indolent nature of the disease, the response to therapy is often less complete than in ulcerative colitis, and the disease tends to progress despite apparent clinical inactivity. It may be more difficult to achieve a clinical remission and to withdraw steroids completely. As in ulcerative colitis, controlled studies have shown no benefit to continuing steroids after remission since the frequency of recurrence is not altered by prophylactic steroid therapy. Disappointingly, sulfasalazine did not decrease recurrence rates in Crohn's disease.

While response to therapy of the initial attack of Crohn's colitis may be satisfactory, many patients continue to have persistently active disease. This may express itself as progressive weight loss, diarrhea, and deterioration of general health. Perianal disease with predominantly left-sided colonic involvement (fistula formation and perirectal abscesses) may constitute a recurrent problem. In one controlled study, *metronidazole* (20 mg/kg per day in divided dosage) resulted in marked improvement in 10 of 18 patients with chronic perineal fistulas associated with Crohn's disease. It is not clear whether the drug is active because of its antibacterial properties or through another mechanism. It is possible that this drug may prove to be of value in the therapy of the perineal complications of Crohn's disease before surgical therapy is attempted. The role of immunosuppressive therapy such as azathioprine has been controversial in Crohn's disease. The multicenter United States study (National Cooperative Study) found azathioprine to be ineffective as a single agent in the therapy of active Crohn's disease. Yet there have been reports of dramatic improvement in a small percentage of patients when azathioprine (1.5 to 2 mg/kg) is added to a maximal program in the nonresponding patient. Some investigators have found 6-mercaptopurine (the active metabolite of azathioprine) effective in controlling disease activity when added to corticosteroids and sulfasalazine. However, a beneficial response may take 6 to 8 months in some patients.

The management of Crohn's disease of the small intestine (regional enteritis) is similar to that for colonic Crohn's disease, and as noted many patients have concomitant small- and large-bowel disease. Several additional considerations are pertinent, however. *Intestinal obstruction* is not uncommonly a presenting feature with ileal involvement. Initially, this may be secondary to acute inflammation and will respond to corticosteroids. With recurrent involvement and the development of fibrosis, steroid therapy is less effective and surgical decompression is required. *Nutritional problems* often are more severe with involvement of the small intestine than with colonic involvement alone. Added to the general catabolic nature of the disease may be loss of absorptive surface which may result from progressive involvement or because of surgical resection. Refinements in the technique of parenteral alimentation have made it possible to provide a patient's total daily caloric intake intravenously for a period of weeks or even months (see Chap. 75). Parenteral alimentation has been employed with increasing frequency in the severely ill patient as a means of placing the gastrointestinal tract ''at rest'' and in preparing the malnourished patient for surgery. With this approach the disease may become quiescent, and the drainage from fistulas may decrease. However, disease activity frequently recurs when oral feedings are resumed. On occasion, prolonged intravenous alimentation, administered at home, may be required when oral feedings are not effective or in children exhibiting severe growth failure associated with Crohn's disease. Most often it is possible to design a dietary program of oral supplementation to nourish the patient adequately.

In patients with extensive small-bowel involvement or in those with a short bowel resulting from extensive intestinal resection, supplementation of electrolytes, minerals, and vitamins will be required. Extensive ileal disease or resection often results in diarrhea induced by bile salts and in malabsorption; cholestyramine may be needed to control the diarrhea and medium-chain triglycerides added to reduce fat malabsorption (see Chap. 240). In patients with stenotic segments of intestine, a low-residue (low-fiber) diet should be recommended. A lactose-free diet should be instituted if there is an associated lactase deficiency. Other dietary modifications have not been shown to have any beneficial effect on the primary disease process. Patients should be encouraged to eat a nutritious, appealing diet of their own choosing. *Surgical therapy* is generally reserved for the complications of Crohn's disease rather than as a primary form of therapy. In contrast to ulcerative colitis, more patients with Crohn's disease will require surgery in the chronic management of the disease. Approximately 70 percent of patients will require at least one operation during the course of their disease. Although each case and situation must be individualized, in general, surgery may be required (1) for persistent or fixed bowel narrowing or obstruction; (2) for symptomatic fistula formation to the bladder, vagina, or skin; (3) for persistent anal fistulas or abscesses; and (4) for intraabdominal abscesses, toxic dilatation of the colon, or perforation. In contrast to ulcerative colitis, where colectomy is curative, in Crohn's disease surgical resection of the small or large intestine is followed by a high rate of recurrence. With resection of segments of small bowel or ileum and reanastomosis a recurrence rate of 50 to 75 percent over a 5-year period is not unusual. Recurrence of disease is invariably proximal to the created anastomosis. When total colectomy and ileostomy are performed for Crohn's disease of the colon without significant small-intestinal involvement, recurrence rates are lower, varying from 10 to 30 percent. Despite these recurrences, most patients do not develop a short-bowel syndrome and usually can expect significant improvement. Faced with the possibility of recurrent disease many physicians are reluctant to advise surgery in Crohn's disease, except for the type of clear-cut complications described above. Alternatively, patients with persistently active disease may require chronic maintenance on unacceptably high levels of corticosteroids and with the appreciable risk of steroid side effects. Just as a failure of medical therapy should lead to colectomy in ulcerative colitis, it should be the conclusion in the patient with Crohn's colitis without major small-bowel involvement. While in this setting there is also a definite rate of recurrence, such recurrences are often not disabling. When extensive small-bowel disease is present, surgical therapy is often not feasible and should only be reserved for specific disease complications.

The therapy of Crohn's disease in children presents special problems since normal growth and development may be retarded in the presence of active disease. In addition to conventional drug therapy, intensive nutritional therapy or the judicious use of surgery may be required.

PROGNOSIS

The overall prognosis of IBD has been favorably affected by the use of corticosteroids and sulfasalazine, as well as by supportive techniques such as intravenous alimentation. In *acute* ulcerative colitis these therapeutic modalities can result in a remission in almost 90 percent of patients. The mortality of an initial acute attack is approximately 5 percent. Poor prognostic factors and an increased mortality rate are likely when there is total colonic involvement, when the onset occurs over age 60, and when toxic megacolon develops.

The long-term prognosis of *chronic* ulcerative colitis is more difficult to assess due to the variable and intermittent nature of the disease and improvements in therapy. Left-sided colitis and ulcerative proctitis have a very favorable prognosis and probably no increase in mortality; similarly the long-term prognosis for extensive colitis has improved greatly. Older studies suggested a poor prognosis for extensive colitis, with less than 50 percent of patients surviving 15 years after onset. More recent observations (longest follow-up 11 years) show a 10-year mortality rate of between 5 and 10 percent for severe first attacks (excluding toxic megacolon). Approximately 75 percent of patients will experience relapses, and 20 to 25 percent will require colectomy. The problem of carcinoma developing in the setting of long-standing chronic ulcerative colitis is an important factor in determining the long-term prognosis of ulcerative colitis. As discussed above, periodic surveillance with colonoscopy and multiple biopsies to detect dysplastic changes is indicated to detect a high-risk group for which to advise colectomy.

The prognosis for Crohn's disease is not as favorable as for ulcerative colitis. An exception is *acute regional enteritis*, often discovered during laparotomy for suspected appendicitis; this has an excellent prognosis. More than two-thirds of such patients may show no subsequent evidence of regional enteritis, and this form of acute ileitis may well be due to *Yersinia* infection (see above). Prevailing surgical opinion favors a conservative approach in this situation, and in most instances operative resection is not advised.

In the majority of patients with Crohn's disease the course is chronic and intermittent regardless of the site of involvement. The disease responds less well to medical therapy with time, and over two-thirds of patients develop complications requiring surgery at some point in their disease. In contrast to ulcerative colitis, where mortality appears greatest early in the disease, in Crohn's disease the mortality rate increases with the duration of the disease, and probably ranges from 5 to 10 percent. Most deaths occur from peritonitis and sepsis. As indicated above, following surgery patients with Crohn's disease often have recurrence and relapses. Nevertheless, the therapy of Crohn's disease will result in reasonably stable and productive lives for most Crohn's disease patients.

REFERENCES

General

KIRSNER JB, SHORTER RG (eds): *Inflammatory Bowel Disease*, 2d ed. Philadelphia, Lea & Febiger, 1980

———, ———: Recent developments in "nonspecific" inflammatory bowel disease. N Engl J Med 306:775, 837, 1982

SLEISENGER MH, FORDTRAN JS (eds): *Gastrointestinal Diseases*, 4th ed. Philadelphia, Saunders, 1989

Etiology and diagnostic aspects

BLASER MJ, RELLER LB: *Campylobacter* enteritis. N Engl J Med 305:1444, 1981

CHAPMAN RW et al: Serum antibodies, ulcerative colitis, and sclerosing cholangitis. Gut 27:86, 1986

GOLDBERG HI et al: Computed tomography in the evaluation of Crohn's disease. Am J Roent 140:277, 1983

GREENSTEIN AJ et al: The extraintestinal complications of ulcerative colitis and Crohn's disease: A study of 700 patients. Medicine 55:401, 1976

JESS P: Acute terminal ileitis: A review of recent literature on the relationship to Crohn's disease. Scand J Gastroenterol 16:321, 1981

QUINN TC et al: *Chlamydia trachomatis* proctitis. N Engl J Med 305:195, 1981

SURAWICZ CM, BELIC L: Rectal biopsy helps to distinguish acute self limited colitis from idiopathic inflammatory bowel disease. Gastroenterology 86:104, 1984

TRNKA YM, LAMONT JT: Association of *Clostridium difficile* toxin with symptomatic relapse of chronic inflammatory bowel disease. Gastroenterology 80:693, 1981

VAN TRAPPEN G et al: *Yersinia* enteritis and enterocolitis: Gastroenterological aspects. Gastroenterology 72:220, 1977

Therapy of inflammatory bowel disease

AZAD KHAN AK et al: Optimum dose of sulphasalazine for maintenance treatment in ulcerative colitis. Gut 12:232, 1980

BERNSTEIN LH et al: Healing of perineal Crohn's disease with metronidazole. Gastroenterology 79:357, 1980

FARMER RG et al: Long-term follow-up of patients with Crohn's disease. Relationship between clinical pattern and prognosis. Gastroenterology 88:1818, 1985

KELTS DG et al: Nutritional basis of growth failure in children and adolescents with Crohn's disease. Gastroenterology 76:720, 1979

LENNARD JONES JE et al: Cancer in colitis: Assessment of the individual risk by clinical and histological criteria. Gastroenterology 73:1280, 1977

PEPPERCORN MA: Sulfasalazine. Ann Intern Med 3:377, 1984

PRESENT DH et al: 6-Mercaptopurine in the management of inflammatory bowel disease: short- and long-term toxicity. Ann Intern Med 111:641, 1989

RIDDELL RH et al: Dysplasia in inflammatory bowel disease. Hum Pathol 14:931, 1983

SCHROEDER KW et al: Coated oral 5-aminosalicylate acid therapy for mild to moderately active ulcerative colitis. A randomized study. N Engl J Med 317:1625, 1987

SUMMERS RW et al: National cooperative Crohn's disease study: Results of drug treatment. Gastroenterology 77:849, 1979

URSING B et al: A comparative study of metronidazole and sulfasalazine for active Crohn's disease. The Cooperative Crohn's Disease Study in Sweden. Gastroenterology 83:550, 1982

242 DISEASES OF THE SMALL AND LARGE INTESTINE

J. THOMAS LaMONT / KURT J. ISSELBACHER

SYMPTOMS OF INTESTINAL DISEASE

SYMPTOMS OF DISEASES OF THE SMALL INTESTINE The major clinical manifestations of small-bowel disease are *motility disturbances*, abdominal *pain* and *distention*, gastrointestinal *bleeding*, and *malabsorption*.

Altered intestinal peristalsis is a common manifestation of a variety of diseases. The presentation may be one of decreased motility, such as paralytic ileus resulting from metabolic disturbance or peritonitis, or intestinal obstruction caused by tumors, adhesions, volvulus, or intussusception (Chap. 244). Diarrhea frequently accompanies small-bowel disease (Chap. 44) resulting from direct mucosal involvement by inflammatory or infiltrative lesions (sprue, regional enteritis). The associated malabsorption of fat and bile salts is an important factor in the pathogenesis of diarrhea in these conditions (Chaps. 44 and 240).

Abdominal pain due to small-intestinal disease is usually periumbilical or supraumbilical and often poorly localized. With obstruction, pain is classically described as intermittent or colicky. Visceral pain arises from distention or stretching of the intestinal wall, or from inflammation of the overlying parietal peritoneum. As the intestine becomes progressively dilated with loss of muscular tone, the colicky nature of the pain may become less apparent. Acute inflammation of the small intestine which involves the visceral or parietal peritoneum is associated with steady, aching pain, usually located directly over the inflamed area, and may be accompanied by guarding and rebound tenderness if the parietal peritoneum is involved. *Gastrointestinal bleeding* due to small-bowel disease may be detected as occult bleeding or, less commonly, brisk hemorrhage. In general, bleeding from the stomach or small intestine causes black or tarry stool (melena), while bleeding from the colon causes passage of red blood or clots. Obviously, the appearance of blood in the stool depends not only on site of bleeding but also on the rate of the hemorrhage and the rapidity of transit; thus localization of the bleeding site by stool appearance alone may be misleading.

An important clue to the presence of small-bowel disease is the demonstration of malabsorption of fat. With extensive mucosal damage or lymphatic obstruction, the presenting symptoms may relate to any of the features of a malabsorption syndrome or protein-losing enteropathy (Chap. 240) and should direct attention to the small intestine.

SYMPTOMS OF COLONIC DISEASE The major symptoms of colonic disease are *alteration in bowel habit, rectal bleeding,* and *pain.* Alteration in bowel habit implies a change from previous patterns of defecation; hence a detailed history is important. Most normal individuals have one to three movements of well-formed stools each day. *Diarrhea* means the passage of watery or loose stools usually with increased frequency, while *constipation* implies infrequent passage of hard, dry stools; *obstipation* is the absence of spontaneous bowel movements. A persistent change in bowel habit, particularly in older individuals with no previous irregularity, is usually an important early symptom of organic disease of the colon and should never be labeled *functional* unless a thorough diagnostic evaluation is negative. The appearance of the stool may also provide important diagnostic clues. Blood coating the exterior of a formed stool implies a lesion in the anal canal or rectum, while blood admixed with the feces indicates a bleeding source higher in the colon. Brisk hemorrhage from the colon or distal small intestine results in passage of fresh blood, called *hematochezia.* This may appear as fresh blood and clots if the lesion is in the left colon, or darker maroon-colored blood if the bleeding source is in the right colon.

Pain resulting from colonic disease is usually localized to either of the lower abdominal quadrants, as opposed to pain of small-intestinal origin, which is localized to the periumbilical area or higher. Rectal pain is often felt deep in the pelvis, while pain in the anal canal is accurately localized to the perineum. The mechanisms of colonic pain are similar to those in other intestinal viscera (see Chap. 17). Distention from gas or fluid causes crampy or colicky pain from stretching of the muscle layers and resulting contraction or spasm. Pain of this type is often relieved by passage of flatus or stool. Pain may also result if the colonic wall is inflamed or infiltrated by tumor. Acute colonic inflammation which involves the visceral or parietal peritoneum produces sharply localized pain, which may be accompanied by abdominal guarding and rebound tenderness. An important symptom of rectal disease is *tenesmus,* or painful straining at stool, with a sensation of incomplete emptying after defecation. This symptom can be caused by retention of stool in the rectum, by tumors of the rectum which simulate retained stools, or by colonic inflammation.

DIAGNOSTIC PROCEDURES

PHYSICAL EXAMINATION Careful *examination* of the abdomen may disclose a mass or fistula associated with inflammatory or neoplastic disease, localized tenderness, or abdominal distention resulting from ileus or intestinal obstruction. The physical examination and findings in the patient with acute abdominal pain are discussed in Chap. 17.

Thorough examination may also reveal extraintestinal findings associated with small-intestinal diseases. Thus buccal pigmentation or telangiectasia may indicate coexistent small-bowel polyposis or intestinal telangiectasia and may clarify episodes of abdominal pain or chronic bleeding. Similarly, evidence of iritis, arthritis, or erythema nodosum may suggest the presence of inflammatory bowel disease.

Perhaps the most important part of the physical examination in the diagnosis of colonic diseases is the *digital rectal examination.* This procedure should never be omitted for reasons of modesty or fear of embarrassment because it is essential in the diagnosis of perianal, sphincteric, and ampullary lesions; prostatic and uterine abnormalities; and even small rectal masses. A metastatic tumor may be felt in the perirectal tissues as a shelf-like deformity (Blumer's shelf), especially anteriorly above the prostate. The fecal material on the glove should be immediately tested with guaiac-impregnated cards for occult blood. Approximately one-half of all rectal carcinomas lie within reach of the index finger, and omission of the rectal examination may delay diagnosis and worsen the prognosis.

STOOL EXAMINATION Abnormal stools constitute important objective evidence of colonic disease. Stools should be examined by the physician as soon as possible after defecation for the presence of visible blood on the surface or within the specimen. A small sample should be tested for occult blood. Microscopic examination of fresh stool is important in the diagnosis of parasitic diseases, particularly in amebic colitis when motile trophozoites can be seen in fresh, warm stool suspensions. Stool suspensions can also be stained with a drop of methylene blue for polymorphonuclear leukocytes, which indicate the presence of an acute inflammatory exudate as occurs in ulcerative colitis, amebic colitis, and bacillary dysentery. Fixed and stained slides of stool may also reveal amebas and other parasites, while stool culture is essential for the diagnosis of bacillary dysentery. Sudan III stain of stool is a useful screening test for steatorrhea.

BARIUM STUDIES The considerable length of the small intestine (some 4 to 7 m in the adult) makes *radiologic studies* of the small bowel of prime importance and usually forms the basis for the diagnosis of small-bowel diseases. *Small-bowel x-rays* are not usually part of a routine upper gastrointestinal series and must be specifically requested. In view of the length of the small bowel and wide variations in transit time, it is essential to provide the radiologist with as much information as possible, since the precise nature of the problem may determine various technical aspects of the examination. Enteroclysis is a specialized small-bowel barium study during which barium is infused rapidly via a nasogastric tube into the jejunum. This technique allows distention of bowel loops and rapid filling of the entire small intestine, thus avoiding the problems of inadequate distention and poor transit sometimes encountered in routine small-bowel barium studies. Enteroclysis is indicated in patients with suspected small-bowel lesions not visualized by ordinary barium studies.

Barium enema is a useful diagnostic tool for the identification of certain colonic diseases, including diverticulosis and its complications, motility disturbances, and displacement of the colon by extrinsic lesions. Barium enema is also useful for detection of loss of haustral markings in chronic ulcerative colitis, and for diagnosis of intestinal fistulas. Fiberoptic colonoscopy is more accurate for the diagnosis of early changes of inflammatory bowel disease, or for detection of colonic neoplasms. Colonoscopy offers the additional advantage of allowing biopsy of suspicious lesions, and removal of most polyps.

SIGMOIDOSCOPY The technique of fiberoptic sigmoidoscopy is not difficult to master, and with practice the discomfort to the patient is minimal. The availability of flexible fiberoptic sigmoidoscopes now makes it possible to examine the lower 40 to 60 cm of the colon, compared to the 25-cm limit of the rigid sigmoidoscope. Flexible sigmoidoscopy is generally less painful than rigid sigmoidoscopy. Because approximately half of all colorectal neoplasms lie in the distal 50 cm of the bowel, sigmoidoscopy is an important diagnostic tool. It should be stressed that a rectal carcinoma can be missed on routine barium enema yet easily visualized and biopsied through the sigmoidoscope. Furthermore, the earliest changes of ulcerative colitis may not be demonstrated radiographically but may be obvious through the sigmoidoscope. Rectal biopsy is easily and painlessly accomplished through the instrument and is associated with minimal morbidity except in the presence of bleeding disorders.

COLONOSCOPY See Chap. 236.

MESENTERIC ANGIOGRAPHY Angiography is helpful in the diagnosis of two conditions: intestinal ischemia and gastrointestinal hemorrhage. Patients suspected of having acute intestinal ischemia from arterial embolus as well as chronic ischemia (intestinal angina) should undergo angiography to locate the site of blockage. Angiography may be diagnostic in some patients with acute gastrointestinal blood loss, especially when bleeding exceeds 0.5 mL/min.

RADIONUCLIDE BLEEDING SCAN Bleeding from the small or large bowel can be localized in certain circumstances by radionuclide scanning of the abdomen after intravenous injection of technetium 99m sulfur colloid or autologous red cells labeled with the same agent (Fig. 242-1). If the patient is bleeding at a rate of 0.1 to 0.5 mL/min or greater, the location of radioactivity in the abdomen may indicate the source of bleeding. This diagnostic approach usually requires confirmation by another diagnostic modality such as angiography or endoscopy. The radionuclide bleeding scan is noninvasive, a particular advantage in older patients with bleeding from the small bowel or colon. The bleeding scan is not recommended in patients with suspected bleeding from the esophagus, stomach, or duodenum, who are best studied by upper endoscopy.

FIGURE 242-1 Radionuclide bleeding scan using intravenous injection of technetium-labeled autologous red cells. Ten minutes after injection, a blush appears in the right abdomen over the cecum (arrow). Thirty minutes after injection, the blush has increased in intensity. The cardiac blood pool is noted at the top. Surgery revealed a bleeding diverticulum in the cecum.

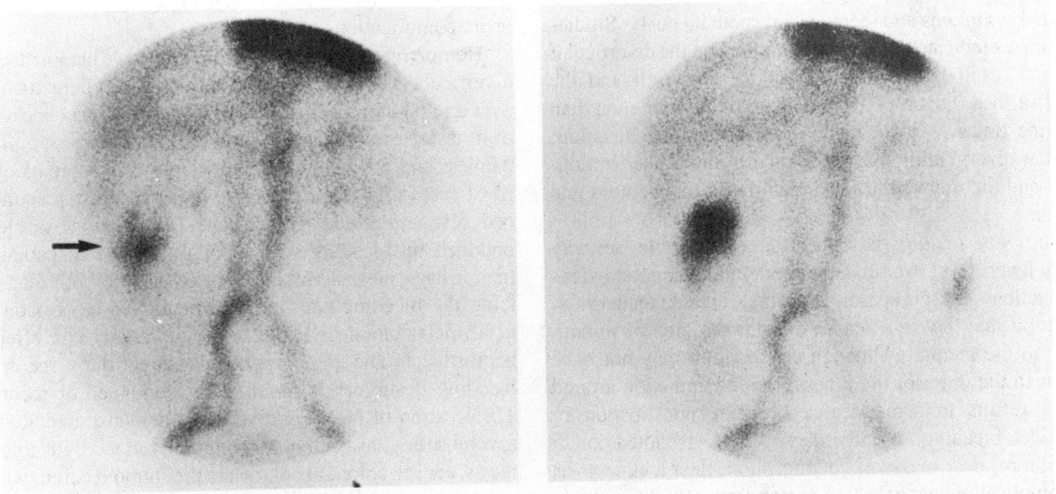

DISORDERS OF INTESTINAL MOTILITY

A major function of the intestinal tract is to propel the intestinal contents (food, secretions, chyme, feces) from stomach toward anus. Abnormalities of motility comprise the most common intestinal diseases: diverticulosis, megacolon, constipation, and irritable bowel syndrome. Although these conditions share a common abnormality, i.e., dysmotility, their clinical features are quite diverse.

DIVERTICULOSIS Diverticula may be either congenital or acquired and may affect either the small or large intestine. Congenital diverticula are herniations of the entire thickness of intestinal wall, while the more common acquired diverticula consist of herniations of the mucosa through the muscularis, generally at the site of a nutrient artery.

Small-intestinal diverticula Diverticula may occur in any portion of the small intestine; however, with the exception of Meckel's diverticulum, the most common locations are in the duodenum and jejunum. Most often diverticula are asymptomatic and discovered incidentally on upper gastrointestinal x-rays. On occasion, however, they may cause symptoms either because of their anatomic proximity to other structures or rarely from inflammation or bleeding.

Duodenal diverticula arise singly from the medial surface of the second portion of the duodenum. In most patients, they cause no symptoms. Rarely, they may present as acute diverticulitis with abdominal pain, fever, gastrointestinal bleeding or, most rarely, perforation. Adjacent structures, such as the bile or pancreatic ducts, may become involved; cases of common-duct obstruction and pancreatitis have been reported. Jejunal diverticula, while less common, may also be the site of acute inflammation, bleeding, or perforation with resulting abscess or peritonitis.

Multiple jejunal diverticula may be associated with a malabsorption syndrome related to bacterial overgrowth within the diverticula, similar to other situations where intestinal stasis (i.e., blind loops) permits bacterial proliferation. The consequences of bacterial proliferation with resultant mucosal damage, deconjugation of bile salts, and vitamin B_{12} malabsorption are discussed in Chap. 240.

Meckel's diverticulum, a persistent omphalomesenteric duct, is the most frequent congenital anomaly of the digestive tract, occurring in approximately 2 percent of autopsied adults. The diverticulum is wide-mouthed, about 5 cm long, and arises from the antimesenteric border of the ileum, usually within 100 cm of the ileocecal valve. The sac may be lined with normal ileal mucosa (approximately 50 percent) or contain gastric, duodenal, pancreatic, or colonic mucosa. While rarely symptomatic after age 5, Meckel's diverticulum may produce hemorrhage, inflammation, and obstruction in children and teenagers.

Hemorrhage occurs almost exclusively before age 10 and invariably results from peptic ulceration of ileal mucosa adjacent to a Meckel's diverticulum lined with gastric mucosa. The diagnosis may be established by isotope scanning of the abdomen after injection of technetium, which is taken up by the ectopic gastric mucosa in the diverticulum. False-negative and false-positive Meckel's scans are not uncommon; thus other clinical and laboratory features must be carefully assessed before recommending surgery. In older children and young adults inflammation of the diverticulum may mimic acute appendicitis. Mechanical obstruction may also occur if the diverticulum intussuscepts into the lumen of the bowel or twists on a fibrous remnant of the omphalomesenteric duct which extends from the diverticulum to the abdominal wall. The treatment of any of these complications of Meckel's diverticulum is surgical excision.

Colonic diverticula Diverticula of the colon are herniations or saclike protrusions of the mucosa through the muscularis, at the point where a nutrient artery penetrates the muscularis. Diverticula occur most commonly in the sigmoid colon and decrease in frequency in the proximal colon. They increase with age, and the incidence ranges between 20 and 50 percent in western populations over age 50. The exact mechanism for their formation is unknown but may be related to an increase in intraluminal pressure. Thickening of the muscle coat of the colon in most patients with diverticula suggests that herniations of mucosa are caused by increased pressure produced by colonic muscle contractions. The rarity of colonic diverticula in underdeveloped nations in contrast to their frequent occurrence in western countries has led to the speculation that diverticula result from the highly refined western diet, which is deficient in dietary fiber or roughage. It is proposed that such diets result in decreased fecal bulk, narrowing of the colon, and an increase in intraluminal pressure in order to move the smaller fecal mass. The role of dietary fiber in the etiology and treatment of diverticular disease remains to be determined.

Colonic diverticula are usually asymptomatic and are an incidental finding on barium enema performed for other reasons. The major complications of inflammation, both acute and chronic, and hemorrhage occur in only a small percentage of individuals with diverticulosis. Since diverticulosis is quite common in older patients, one must avoid the temptation of attributing symptoms to the diverticula unless other conditions, especially colonic neoplasm, have been excluded.

Diverticulitis Inflammation can occur in or around the diverticular sac. The cause of diverticulitis is probably mechanical, related to retention in the diverticula of undigested food residues and bacteria, which may form a hard mass called a *fecalith*. This compromises the blood supply to the thin-walled sac (made up solely of mucosa and serosa) and renders it susceptible to invasion by colonic bacteria. The inflammatory process may vary from a small intramural or pericolic abscess to generalized peritonitis. Some attacks are accompanied by minimal symptoms and seem to heal spontaneously. Studies of resected specimens indicate that most perforations of the diverticular sac are small and result in inflammation of the sac itself and the adjacent serosal surface. Diverticulitis occurs more often in men than women, and three times as often in the left as in the right colon. This suggests that diverticulitis may be related to the higher intraluminal pressures and the more solid fecal material in the sigmoid and descending colon.

Acute colonic diverticulitis is a disease of variable severity characterized by fever, left lower quadrant abdominal pain, and signs of peritoneal irritation—muscle spasm, guarding, rebound tenderness. Rectal examination may reveal a tender mass if the area of inflammation is close to the rectum. Although constipation may not have been noted prior to the onset of the illness, the inflammation around the colon often results in some degree of acute constipation or obstipation. Rectal bleeding, usually microscopic, is noted in 25 percent of cases; it is rarely massive. Polymorphonuclear leukocytosis is common. Complications include free perforation, which results in acute peritonitis, sepsis, and shock, particularly in the elderly. The perforation may be walled off by adherent omentum or neighboring structures such as the bladder or small bowel. Abscess formation or fistulas then occur as the inflammatory mass burrows into other organs. Severe pericolitis may cause a dense, fibrous reaction or stricture around the bowel which can be associated with colonic obstruction.

DIFFERENTIAL DIAGNOSIS In the less acute situation differential diagnosis is principally that of a neoplasm in the area of the diverticulosis. During the acute phase of diverticulitis, barium enema and sigmoidoscopy may be hazardous, since contrast material or air under pressure may lead to rupture of an inflamed diverticulum and convert a walled-off inflammatory lesion to a free perforation. These examinations are usually safe after adequate treatment and healing of the diverticulitis. The radiologic findings on barium enema suggestive of diverticulitis are leakage of barium from a diverticular sac, stricture formation, and the presence of a pericolic inflammatory mass. In many patients, the distortion caused by inflammation prevents a clear distinction between cancer and diverticulitis. In these cases colonoscopy or surgical excision may be required for accurate diagnosis.

TREATMENT For the mild case without signs of perforation, treatment consists of bed rest, stool softeners, liquid diet, and a wide-spectrum antibiotic such as tetracycline or ampicillin. Repeated attacks of diverticulitis in the same area generally require surgical resection. Severe attacks with acute peritoneal signs, suspected abscess, or perforation require intravenous antibiotics directed against gram-negative anaerobic bacteria, followed by surgical drainage or resection. The usual procedure is a diverting colostomy with resection of the involved colon; reanastomosis is then performed at a second operation.

Painful diverticular disease without diverticulitis Some patients with diverticulosis develop recurrent left lower quadrant colicky pain without clinical or pathologic evidence of acute diverticulitis. They often have bouts of alternating constipation and diarrhea, and the pain may be relieved by defecation or passage of flatus. These features suggest the coexistence of the irritable bowel syndrome (see below). Examination during a bout of pain reveals tenderness of the sigmoid colon, but signs of peritoneal inflammation such as rebound tenderness, muscle guarding, fever, and leukocytosis are absent. Barium enema shows typical diverticula without evidence of inflammation and stricture, plus a "sawtooth" irregularity of the lumen reflecting muscle hypertrophy and spasm. In some patients the pain is severe enough to warrant observation in a hospital and restriction of food since feeding aggravates the pain by causing colonic contraction. Anticholinergics, which reduce sigmoid contractions, and mild sedation are usually all that is required. After recovery the patient should be started on a high-residue diet or given a bulk laxative such as hemicellulose, unprocessed bran, or psyllium extract. Surgical excision is usually not indicated unless acute diverticulitis or its complications occur.

Hemorrhage from diverticula Massive hemorrhage from colonic diverticula is one of the commonest causes of hematochezia in patients over age 60. This complication of diverticulosis is caused by erosion of a vessel by a fecalith within the diverticular sac. The bleeding is painless and not accompanied by signs or symptoms of diverticulitis. Most cases of mild or moderate hemorrhage stop spontaneously with bed rest and blood transfusion. Localization of bleeding can be obtained by bleeding scan or angiography. In patients with severe hemorrhage mesenteric angiography can be both diagnostic in localizing the bleeding site and therapeutic since vasoconstrictive drugs or artificial blood clot infused intraarterially can effectively control hemorrhage. The angiographer can direct the surgeon to the area of bleeding if surgery is required for continued or recurrent bleeding. The location of bleeding diverticula demonstrated at angiography on several series has been more commonly in the right colon, particularly the ascending colon, in contrast to the sigmoid colon, where diverticula are more numerous.

MEGACOLON Megacolon, or giant colon, is characterized by massive distention of the colon usually accompanied by severe constipation or obstipation. This condition can be either congenital or acquired and is seen in all age groups. Acute toxic megacolon is a severe complication of chronic ulcerative colitis (see Chap. 241).

Aganglionic megacolon (Hirschsprung's disease) This is a congenital disorder which becomes manifest in early infancy, occurring more frequently in males, and is often familial. These infants have massive abdominal distention, absent bowel movements, and impaired nutrition due to chronic obstruction of the colon. In some individuals with less severe symptoms the disease may not be diagnosed until adolescence or early adulthood. The inability to defecate is caused by the absence of ganglion cells (Meissner's and Auerbach's plexuses) in a small segment of the distal colon, usually near the anus. This aganglionic segment is unable to relax to permit passage of stool, causing the normal colon proximal to it to become greatly dilated. On rectal examination the ampulla is empty of feces and the anal sphincter is normal. Barium enema reveals a narrowed segment in the rectosigmoid area, with massive dilatation above. Diagnosis is made by full-thickness surgical biopsy under anesthesia and demonstration of absent ganglion cells in the diseased segment. In most patients the aganglionic segment is in the rectosigmoid colon; in rare instances the lesion may involve more proximal bowel or even the entire colon. The treatment of choice is surgery which restores normal defecation. The most effective operation is a pull-through procedure in which normally innervated colon is anastomosed to the distal rectum just above the internal sphincter, thus bypassing the contracted aganglionic segment.

Chronic idiopathic megacolon This condition, also called *psychogenic megacolon,* has its onset later in childhood, usually at the time toilet training begins. It is characterized by severe chronic constipation and distention and, in contrast to Hirschsprung's disease, digital examination reveals the rectal ampulla to be invariably distended with feces. Barium enema shows the entire colon to be distended with stools, no narrowed segment is seen, and rectal biopsy discloses the normal complement of ganglion cells in Auerbach's plexus. Treatment is based on education in normal bowel habits, but a long course of enemas or large doses of mineral oil may be required until the patient acquires more normal bowel movements.

Acquired megacolon In Central and South America infection with *Trypanosoma cruzi* (Chagas' disease) can result in destruction of the ganglion cells of the colon, producing a clinical picture similar to congenital megacolon, except that the onset is in adult life rather than childhood. A number of other diseases are associated with megacolon in adults. Patients with schizophrenia or depression, particularly institutionalized patients, may have obstipation and massive colonic dilatation. Severe neurologic disorders including cerebral atrophy, spinal cord injury, and parkinsonism may also cause megacolon. Myxedema, infiltrative diseases such as amyloidosis, and scleroderma can also reduce colonic motility and produce marked colonic distention. Narcotic drugs, particularly morphine and codeine, can cause severe constipation, especially when administered to bedridden patients. Digital rectal examination of adults with acquired megacolon reveals a rectum distended with feces, as opposed to the empty rectum in aganglionic megacolon. Treatment is aimed at the underlying disease as well as the careful use of enemas and cathartics.

INTESTINAL PSEUDOOBSTRUCTION Intestinal pseudoobstruction is an acute or chronic motility disorder characterized by distention or dilatation of the small and large intestine. Abdominal pain, nausea, and vomiting may lead to diagnostic confusion with mechanical obstruction, but as the name of this condition implies, the underlying cause is not obstruction but rather a severe dysmotility resulting in distention. Pseudoobstruction may be primary or secondary and acute or chronic. In primary or idiopathic pseudoobstruction no other contributing condition can be identified, and the motility disorder is attributed to abnormalities of sympathetic innervation or of the muscle layers of the intestine. Secondary pseudoobstruction may result from scleroderma, diabetes, amyloidosis, neurologic diseases, drugs, or sepsis.

Chronic or intermittent secondary pseudoobstruction Numerous medical conditions can cause chronic dilatation of the large and small bowel. Some of these may involve the intestinal smooth muscle such as scleroderma, dermatomyositis, amyloidosis, or muscular dystrophy. Endocrine disorders, including myxedema and diabetes mellitus, may result in chronic distention which in the diabetic results from autonomic visceral neuropathy. Chronic neurologic diseases including Parkinson's disease and stroke may be complicated by chronic pseudoobstruction; in these patients drugs and relative immobility are contributing features. Finally, psychotic patients (especially those who are institutionalized) may suffer from prolonged megacolon.

The symptoms of chronic secondary pseudoobstruction are chronic or intermittent constipation, crampy abdominal pain, anorexia, and bloating. Gastric distention and disordered swallowing may be present. Abdominal x-rays reveal gaseous distention of the large and small bowel, and occasionally of the stomach. Air fluid levels are unusual and should raise the possibility of mechanical obstruction. Upper gastrointestinal series and barium enema do not reveal specific abnormalities of the intestine such as tumor, stricture, or volvulus. The presence of an autoimmune disorder or endocrinopathy may require confirmation by serologic or blood tests; biopsy may be needed as in amyloidosis or muscular dystrophy.

The treatment of chronic intestinal pseudoobstruction is made difficult due to the complexity and chronicity of the underlying systemic disease. Patients with scleroderma may respond to broad-spectrum antibiotics if intestinal bacterial overgrowth is suspected. Metoclopramide may benefit gastric dysmotility in the diabetic. Discontinuation of psychotropic or anti-Parkinson drugs may occasionally result in improvement. Cathartics and enemas may be required to relieve fecal impaction, and the regular use of stool softeners and a high-fiber diet may help prevent recurrences.

Idiopathic intestinal pseudoobstruction This term encompasses patients with signs and symptoms of pseudoobstruction in whom no systemic disease can be identified. The typical patient has recurrent attacks of abdominal pain and distention with nausea and vomiting. The small intestine is primarily involved, and chronic constipation is much less frequent than in secondary pseudoobstruction. Steatorrhea secondary to bacterial overgrowth of the small intestine is common and may lead to chronic diarrhea and malnutrition. Many patients exhibit abnormalities of motility in the esophagus and urinary bladder, in addition to the small and large intestine. Various defects have been described in patients with this syndrome, including abnormalities of the mesenteric plexus and myopathy of the intestinal and urinary bladder smooth muscle (so-called hollow visceral myopathy). Elevated prostaglandin E levels have been reported in some patients. Treatment of idiopathic pseudoobstruction is unsatisfactory. Surgery to relieve "obstruction" is to be avoided, since the condition is often worsened by abdominal surgery. Medical therapy with metoclopramide and cholinergic agents has been unsuccessful. Nutritional support in the form of low-residue elemental diets or parenteral hyperalimentation may be helpful. Unfortunately the lack of effective therapy and the progressive nature of the illness make the prognosis of idiopathic pseudoobstruction rather unfavorable. Death from malnutrition and steatorrhea are common. The long-term impact of total parenteral nutrition on this disease is not yet clear.

Acute intestinal pseudoobstruction This entity, sometimes referred to as Ogilvie's syndrome, is characterized by acute intestinal dilatation, involving primarily the colon but occasionally also the small intestine. As in other forms of pseudoobstruction, the clinical features are difficult to distinguish from mechanical obstruction. The patient may complain of colicky lower abdominal pain and acute constipation. Examination reveals a distended, tympanitic abdomen, with reduced or absent bowel sounds. Localized tenderness over the distended colon is common, but diffuse abdominal tenderness, rigidity, or rebound tenderness are unusual. Abdominal films reveal massive dilatation of the colon and small intestine, occasionally with the presence of air fluid levels. The cecum, being the most capacious part of the colon, is often massively dilated and tender. The onset of these symptoms usually occurs in patients who have recently undergone severe surgical or medical stress such as major surgery, myocardial infarction, sepsis, or respiratory failure. Patients with acute pseudoobstruction are frequently on respirators, have received narcotics or sedatives, and have metabolic and electrolyte disturbances.

Management of acute pseudoobstruction requires careful correction of fluid and electrolyte abnormalities, intubation of the stomach or small intestine for decompression, and avoidance of drugs which depress intestinal motility. Barium enema may be hazardous because of the risk of perforating the already dilated bowel. Some authorities recommend cecostomy when the diameter of the colon exceeds 8 cm to avoid ischemic necrosis and perforation. Decompressive colonoscopy is beneficial in some patients. The outcome depends in large part on the prognosis of the associated medical or surgical conditions. Patients who recover from the underlying medical or surgical conditions usually have a return of normal colonic function.

IRRITABLE BOWEL SYNDROME The irritable bowel syndrome (IBS) is the most common gastrointestinal disease in clinical practice, and although not a life-threatening illness, it causes great distress to those afflicted and feelings of helplessness and frustration for the physician attempting to treat it. The patient with irritable bowel syndrome may present with one of *three clinical variants.* Patients with so-called spastic colitis complain primarily of chronic abdominal pain and constipation. A second group has chronic intermittent diarrhea, often without pain. Some patients have both features and complain of alternating constipation and diarrhea.

The basic pathophysiologic abnormality in the irritable bowel syndrome is an alteration of intestinal motility. Patients with the spastic colon variant (pain and constipation) have *increased* resting colonic motility; in contrast, those presenting primarily with diarrhea have *decreased* resting colonic motility. Both groups have an increase in colonic motility after injection of cholinergic drugs or cholecystokinin; motility may also be increased in association with psychological stress. It has been suggested that cholecystokinin may be a normal stimulus of intestinal motility and that the spastic colon may result from an exaggerated response to the normal release of cholecystokinin after eating.

Patients with the irritable bowel syndrome also exhibit an abnormal basic electrical rhythm in the colon, characterized by an increase in 3-cycle-per-minute slow-wave activity. It is not certain, however, whether these abnormalities of smooth-muscle contraction are primary or secondary to another underlying abnormality of intestinal neuromuscular function.

Evidence of significant psychological disturbances may be seen in some patients with irritable bowel syndrome. Depression, hysteria, and obsessive-compulsive traits are common, and psychological stress frequently triggers an exacerbation of symptoms. It should be noted, however, that increased intracolonic pressure has been observed in normal volunteers during acute stress. This suggests that psychological stress may be a nonspecific trigger of symptoms in the irritable bowel syndrome, as is the case in many other illnesses of diverse etiology.

Clinical features The irritable bowel syndrome is a disease of young or middle-aged adults; female/male ratio is 2:1. The predominant feature is a history of chronic constipation, diarrhea, or both. The typical patient describes watery diarrhea occurring *intermittently* for months or years. The diarrhea is usually worse in the morning upon arising or after breakfast. After the passage of three or four loose stools with excessive mucus the patient may feel well for the remainder of the day. Diarrhea throughout the day or especially nocturnal diarrhea is most unusual. The diarrhea may last for weeks or months and then disappear spontaneously for variable periods of time. Some patients describe "pencil-like" pasty stools rather than diarrhea.

Another typical presentation is that of chronic abdominal pain with constipation, or with alternating constipation and diarrhea. These patients describe intermittent crampy lower abdominal pain, often over the sigmoid colon, which is usually relieved by passage of flatus or stool. The patient may describe excessive bloating which is not discernible to the physician. A variety of other complaints, such as heartburn, excessive bloating, back pain, weakness, faintness, and palpitations, are frequent in patients with irritable bowel syndrome. The pain may occasionally be in the right upper quadrant or midepigastrium, leading to diagnostic confusion with biliary tract or peptic ulcer disease.

Physical examination reveals these patients to be anxious but otherwise normal. During intense pain, the abdomen may be distended, but no visible peristalsis is noted; the abdominal musculature is relaxed, and a tender sigmoid full of feces may be palpated in the left lower quadrant. Characteristically, the rectal ampulla is empty of feces. Sigmoidoscopy may reveal a prominent vascular pattern, muscle spasm, or excess mucus. The mucosa itself is normal.

The *diagnosis* of the irritable colon syndrome is suggested by the chronic intermittent nature of symptoms without obvious signs of physical deterioration, the relation of symptoms to environment or emotional stress, and the exclusion of other conditions. The evaluation should include a careful history, complete physical examination, and stool examination for occult blood, parasites, and pathogenic bacteria. In some patients colonoscopy will be necessary to exclude inflammation or neoplasia. Barium enema may reveal spasticity of the sigmoid, accentuated haustra, and a tubular appearance to the descending colon. Lactase deficiency may masquerade as irritable colon syndrome and should be excluded by a trial of milk restriction, a lactose tolerance test, or a lactose breath hydrogen test (see Chap. 240). Thyrotoxicosis is easily confused with irritable bowel syndrome and should be excluded by appropriate laboratory studies.

Treatment of the irritable colon syndrome requires both skill and patience. It is important that the patient be reassured that this condition normally does not lead to the development of chronic inflammatory bowel disease (i.e., ulcerative colitis) or colonic malignancy. It is also important for both the patient and the physician to realize that the condition is chronic, and while it may be alleviated, it cannot be cured. The patient should be encouraged to adapt to the symptoms so as to minimize their impact on life-style. The physician should not imply that the symptoms are largely emotional or psychological in origin, since this is usually rejected by the patient. It is appropriate, however, to emphasize the relationship between psychological stress and the onset of severity of symptoms, as this may allow the patient to better deal with the disease. After the diagnosis is established, frequent x-rays and endoscopies are not necessary; general physical examinations, hemograms, and stool examinations for occult blood, however, should be carried out at regular intervals.

Drug treatment is aimed at altering the abnormal colonic motility in this disease. Patients with constipation may respond to an increase in dietary bulk in the form of unprocessed bran or psyllium bulk laxatives. Mild sedation with phenobarbital or tranquilizers may be indicated, and anticholinergic drugs are useful in some patients. Troublesome diarrhea may respond to diphenoxylate (Lomotil) or paregoric. Unfortunately, no specific drug or dietary regimen affords good relief in all patients, and thus a number of therapeutic maneuvers need to be tried.

CHRONIC CONSTIPATION In Chap. 44 the mechanism of defecation is discussed. Disorders involving the sensory or motor components of this mechanism may arise from destruction of the nerves subserving these functions, from invasion or inflammation of the rectosigmoid itself, or from central nervous system lesions. Most cases of chronic constipation arise from habitual neglect of afferent impulses, failure to initiate defecation, and accumulation of large, dry fecal masses in the rectum. This voluntary suppression of the call to stool may arise during the period of toilet training in childhood, or later in life because of a sense of social impropriety, unaccustomed surroundings, uncomfortable toilet facilities, or illnesses which require confinement to bed. Chronic constipation is much more common in women, with onset typically in late adolescence or early adulthood. As constant distention of the rectum with feces becomes chronic, the patient grows less aware of rectal fullness. Bowel movements become progressively more difficult, and painful hemorrhoids or anal fissures reinforce suppression of the urge to defecate. To avoid these problems, the patient begins the chronic use of laxatives or enemas, without which defecation becomes impossible.

Treatment The physician should make every attempt to educate the patient about the chain of events which has led to chronic constipation. Attempts should be made to alter patterns of many years' duration, and the patient must recognize the importance of responding to, rather than suppressing, the urge to defecate. It is helpful to initiate a routine whereby defecation is attempted at a given time each day. In most individuals the call to stool occurs in the morning after breakfast. Physical exercise such as a brisk walk just before attempts at defecation may be helpful. Patients are instructed to increase dietary bulk with foods rich in fiber, such as green vegetables and unprocessed cereal grains, or by the regular use of bulk laxatives, such as hemicellulose, psyllium extract, and powdered unprocessed bran. The success of such a regimen depends to some extent on the duration of symptoms. Elderly patients with long-standing constipation and reliance on enemas or laxatives are more resistant to these measures than younger patients whose bowel patterns are less established. Moreover, poor muscle tone, reduced physical activity, and increased incidence of other medical conditions make the problem more difficult in the older age group. Bedridden elderly patients often develop severe constipation and even fecal impaction unless preventive measures are taken. This applies not only to patients with previous constipation but also to those with regular bowel movements prior to their confining illness. Regular administration of stool softeners, bulk laxatives, or mild cathartics is necessary until full ambulation and a normal diet are resumed. The onset of fecal impaction in bedridden patients is heralded by a feeling of rectal distention, urgency of defecation, or tenesmus. Occasionally the fecal impaction will result in low-grade chronic obstruction with dilatation and increased fluid content proximal to the impaction; "paradoxical diarrhea" may thus occur as fluid moves past the obstructing fecal mass. This situation will be aggravated if antidiarrheal drugs are given because the underlying constipation will be worsened. The appropriate maneuver is to disimpact the rectum manually or to administer gentle enemas if the impaction is beyond the reach of the finger.

VASCULAR DISORDERS OF THE INTESTINE

Ischemia is the end result of interruption or reduction of the blood supply of the intestine. However, the clinical manifestations of intestinal ischemia range from mild chronic symptoms to catastrophic episodes, depending on the segment involved, the degree of involvement, and the rapidity of the process, and the clinician should be aware of this spectrum of manifestations (Table 242-1). The gut derives its arterial blood supply from the celiac axis and the superior and inferior mesenteric arteries. The small intestine is supplied by the celiac and superior mesenteric arteries; the colon is supplied by branches of the superior and inferior mesenteric arteries. A rich network of anastomotic vessels and the possible development of collateral circulation determine the clinical picture of acute or chronic intestinal arterial insufficiency.

TABLE 242-1 Patterns of intestinal ischemia

Condition	Etiology	Clinical features	Management
Mesenteric artery embolus	Arterial embolus associated with atrial fibrillation or rheumatic heart disease	Acute central abdominal pain, shock, peritonitis	Immediate angiography and embolectomy if possible
Abdominal angina	Atherosclerosis of celiac and superior mesenteric arteries	Chronic postprandial pain, weight loss	Angiography and surgery in selected cases
Ischemia colitis	Low-flow state	Acute lower abdominal pain, rectal bleeding	Sigmoidoscopy; surgery only for peritonitis

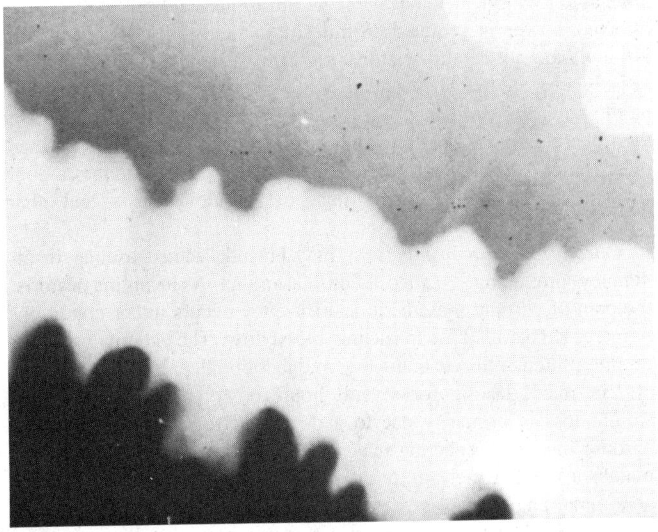

FIGURE 242-2 Barium enema showing "thumbprinting" or submucosal edema of the inferior margin of the transverse colon, in a patient with acute ischemic colitis.

MESENTERIC ISCHEMIA AND INFARCTION Acute small-intestinal ischemia may be classified as *occlusive* or *nonocclusive*. Occlusion may result from arterial thrombus or embolus of the celiac or superior mesenteric arteries, or from venous occlusion in the same distribution. Arterial embolus occurs most commonly in patients with chronic or recurrent atrial fibrillation, artificial heart valves, or valvular heart disease, while arterial thrombosis is associated with extensive atherosclerosis or low cardiac output. Venous occlusion is quite rare and is occasionally seen in women taking oral contraceptives. Approximately one-half of patients with mesenteric ischemia do not have a definite occlusion of a major vessel, a condition referred to as *nonocclusive* ischemia. The exact cause of nonocclusive disease is obscure; systemic arterial hypotension, cardiac arrhythmias, prolonged heart failure, digitalis therapy, dehydration, and endotoxemia have been suggested as contributing factors.

The outstanding clinical feature of acute mesenteric ischemia is severe abdominal pain, often colicky and periumbilical at the onset, later becoming diffuse and constant. Vomiting, anorexia, diarrhea, and constipation are also frequent but of little diagnostic help. Examination of the abdomen may reveal tenderness and distention. Bowel sounds are often normal even in the face of severe infarction. Some patients have a surprisingly normal abdominal examination in spite of severe pain. Mild gastrointestinal bleeding is often detected by guaiac examination of stool, but gross hemorrhage is unusual except in ischemic colitis (see below). A typical laboratory finding is a pronounced polymorphonuclear leukocytosis. Late in the course of the disease (24 to 72 h) gangrene of the bowel occurs with diffuse peritonitis, sepsis, and shock. Abdominal plain films in patients with mesenteric ischemia may reveal air fluid levels and distention. Barium study of the small intestine reveal nonspecific dilatation, poor motility, and evidence of thick mucosal folds ("thumbprinting") (Fig. 242-2).

Acute mesenteric ischemia is a grave condition with a high morbidity and mortality. Patients suspected of having acute arterial embolus should undergo immediate celiac and mesenteric angiography to localize the embolus, followed by embolectomy. Restoration of normal circulation may allow complete recovery if performed before irreversible necrosis or gangrene has occurred. Unfortunately infarction and transmural necrosis are frequently found at surgery, necessitating resection. Arterial or venous thrombosis is not generally amenable to surgical removal of the thrombus, and resection of the affected bowel is required. Similarly, patients with nonocclusive ischemia are not candidates for corrective vascular surgery (as major vessels are patent). These individuals often have extensive necrosis of the small or large intestine because of the widespread nature of the ischemic event. The decision to operate on patients with suspected mesenteric ischemia is a difficult one as the typical patient is a poor surgical risk owing to advanced age, dehydration, sepsis, and other serious medical conditions.

Chronic arterial insufficiency may precede acute vascular insufficiency, producing so-called abdominal angina. As in angina pectoris, the pain of chronic mesenteric insufficiency occurs under conditions of increased demand for splanchnic blood flow. The patient complains of intermittent dull or cramping midabdominal pain 15 to 30 min after a meal, lasting for several hours postprandially. Significant weight loss is primarily due to a decreased food intake; however, chronic intestinal ischemia may also produce mucosal damage and malabsorption, which in turn aggravates the weight loss. Since abdominal angina may progress to bowel infarction, serious consideration should be given to performing arteriographic studies to confirm the diagnosis in those patients who are candidates for abdominal vascular surgery. The only definitive treatment is surgical removal of the arterial obstruction or the construction of bypass arterial grafts to the ischemic bowel.

A variety of systemic conditions are associated with *vasculitis* of the large and small arteries supplying the intestine. Most often, these disorders can be recognized by the associated extraintestinal manifestations as in polyarteritis nodosa, lupus erythematosus, dermatomyositis, Henoch-Schönlein purpura (allergic vasculitis), and rheumatoid vasculitis. When larger arteries are involved, as in polyarteritis nodosa, the picture of acute intestinal infarction is similar to embolic or atherosclerotic vascular occlusion. Often the involvement of smaller vessels leads to areas of intramural hemorrhage and edema leading to abdominal pain, variable degrees of intestinal obstruction, and bleeding. Barium enema may show "thumbprinting" and "spiculation" due to localized edema, hemorrhage, and ulceration. In many instances, treatment of the underlying disorder may lead to regression of symptoms. If signs of an acute abdomen develop, surgical exploration is usually indicated.

Intramural small-intestinal hemorrhage may occur with vasculitis, trauma, or impaired coagulation, especially in patients receiving anticoagulants. The clinical and radiologic features resemble those seen with vasculitis and local mucosal hemorrhage.

ISCHEMIC COLITIS Ischemia of the colon most often affects the elderly population because of the greater frequency of vascular disease in that group. Ischemic colitis is almost always a nonocclusive disease, that is, obstruction of major arteries is not seen. Shunting of blood away from the mucosa may contribute to this condition, but the mechanism of ischemia is not known.

The clinical picture depends upon the degree of ischemia and the rate of its development. In *acute fulminant ischemic* colitis the major manifestations are severe lower abdominal pain, rectal bleeding, and hypotension. Dilatation of the colon and physical signs of peritonitis are seen in severe cases. Plain abdominal films may reveal thumbprinting from submucosal hemorrhage and edema. Barium enema is hazardous in the acute situation because of the risk of perforation. Sigmoidoscopy or colonoscopy may detect ulcerations, friability, and bulging folds from submucosal hemorrhage. Angiography is not helpful in the management of patients with presumed ischemic colitis since a remedial occlusive lesion is very rarely found. Surgical resection may be required in some patients with fulminant ischemic colitis to remove gangrenous bowel; others with lesser degrees of ischemia may respond to conservative medical management.

Subacute ischemic colitis, the most common clinical variant of ischemic colonic disease, produces lesser degrees of pain and bleeding, often occurring over several days or weeks. The left colon may be involved, but the rectum is usually spared because of collateral blood flow, a distinguishing feature from acute ulcerative colitis. Barium enema reveals edema, cobblestoning, thumbprinting, and occasionally superficial ulceration. Angiography is not indicated as almost all cases are nonocclusive. Occasionally *stricture formation* may follow a bout of ischemic colitis or may present de novo without a history of antecedent pain or bloody diarrhea. Most cases of nonocclusive ischemic colitis resolve in 2 to 4 weeks and do not recur. Surgery is not required except for obstruction secondary to postischemic stricture.

ANGIODYSPLASIA OF THE COLON These are vascular ectasias (not neoplasms) which occur in the right colon of many older individuals and may cause bleeding (see Chap. 46). Angiodysplasia is a degenerative lesion consisting of dilated, distorted, thin-walled vessels lined by vascular endothelium. Angiodysplasia may result from partial obstruction of the submucosal venous plexus by the tension generated in the cecal wall during muscular contraction. Aortic stenosis occurs in some patients, and may cause chronic ischemia of the colon that leads to angiodysplasia. Grossly angiodysplasias look similar to spider angiomas of the skin and appear as star-shaped branching vessels in the submucosa measuring from 2 mm to 1 cm in diameter. The lesions are usually multiple and are found primarily in the cecum and ascending colon.

Cecal angiodysplasia is important because of the likelihood of bleeding, either massively or chronically. In patients over 60 approximately one-quarter of colonic bleeding episodes are secondary to angiodysplasia. The diagnosis requires careful angiography showing extravasation of contrast material into the lumen, or colonoscopy with visualization of bleeding lesions. Hemorrhage from angiodysplasia may be controlled by embolization during arteriography or by electrocautery through the colonoscope. Some patients with massive uncontrolled bleeding or multiple sites of angiodysplasia may require right hemicolectomy.

ANORECTAL PROBLEMS

HEMORRHOIDS The internal hemorrhoidal plexus of veins is located in the submucosal space above the valves of Morgagni. The anal canal separates it from the external hemorrhoidal venous plexus, but the two spaces communicate under the anal canal, the submucosa of which is attached to underlying tissue to form the interhemorrhoidal depression. Whenever the internal hemorrhoidal plexus is enlarged, there is associated increase in supporting tissue mass, and the resultant venous swelling is called an *internal hemorrhoid.* When veins in the external hemorrhoidal plexus become enlarged or thrombosed, the resultant bluish mass is called an *external hemorrhoid.*

Both types of hemorrhoids are very common and are associated with increased hydrostatic pressure in the portal venous system, such as during pregnancy, straining at stool, or with cirrhosis. When internal hemorrhoids enlarge, pain is not a usual feature until the situation is complicated by thrombosis, infection, or erosion of the overlying mucosal surface. Most persons complain of bright red blood on the toilet tissue or coating the stool, with a feeling of vague anal discomfort. The discomfort is increased when the hemorrhoid enlarges or prolapses through the anus; prolapse is often accompanied by edema and sphincteric spasm. Prolapse, if not treated, usually becomes chronic as the muscularis stays stretched, and the patient complains of constant soiling of underclothing with very little pain. Prolapsed hemorrhoids may become infected or thrombosed; the overlying mucous membrane may bleed profusely as the result of the trauma of defecation.

External hemorrhoids, because they lie under the skin, are quite often painful, particularly if there is a sudden increase in their mass. These episodes result in a tender blue swelling at the anal verge due to thrombosis of a vein in the external plexus and need not be associated with enlargement of the internal veins. Since the thrombus usually lies at the level of the sphincteric muscles, anal spasm often occurs.

The diagnosis of internal and external hemorrhoids is made by inspection, digital examination, and direct vision through the anoscope and proctoscope. Since such lesions are very common, they must not be regarded as the cause of rectal bleeding or chronic hypochromic anemia until a thorough investigation has been made of the more proximal gastrointestinal tract. Acute blood loss can occasionally be attributed to internal hemorrhoids. Chronic anemia in the presence of large but not definitely bleeding hemorrhoids should provoke a search for a polyp, cancer, or ulcer.

Most hemorrhoids respond to conservative therapy such as sitz baths or other forms of moist heat, suppositories, stool softeners, and bed rest. Internal hemorrhoids which remain permanently prolapsed are best treated surgically; milder degrees of prolapse or enlargement with pruritus ani or intermittent bleeding can be successfully handled by banding or injection of sclerosing solutions. External hemorrhoids which become acutely thrombosed are treated by incision, extraction of the clot, and compression of the incised area following clot removal. No surgical procedure should be carried out in the presence of acute inflammation of the anus, ulcerative proctitis, or ulcerative colitis. Both proctoscopy and barium enema should always be performed before a patient is subjected to hemorrhoidectomy.

ANAL INFLAMMATION Perianal inflammatory lesions may be primary or may be associated with inflammatory bowel disease or diverticular disease as mentioned above. Anal *fissures* are superficial erosions of the anal canal which usually heal rapidly with conservative therapy. Anal *ulcers* are more chronic and deep and give symptoms largely as the result of painful spasm of the external anal sphincter during and after defecation. Bleeding may occur with either fissure or ulcer; healing of the ulcer often is associated with a hypertrophied anal papilla and some degrees of anal contracture. *Fistula in ano,* a tract leading from the rectal lumen to the perianal skin, usually results from local crypt abscesses; fewer than 5 percent of such lesions found in medical practice in the United States are due to tuberculosis or cancer. The fistula is a chronically inflamed canal made up of fibrous tissue surrounding granulation tissue, the lumen of which may be difficult to demonstrate. Perirectal *abscesses* often represent the tracking down into the anal area of purulent material escaping from the rectosigmoid; diverticulitis, Crohn's disease, ulcerative colitis, or previous surgery may be the underlying cause. Fistulas between the rectum and vagina or the rectum and bladder represent serious complications of granulomatous, septic, or malignant disorders and require the patient to be hospitalized for definitive diagnostic and therapeutic procedures.

REFERENCES

Disorders of motility

BODE WE et al: Colonoscopic decompression for acute dilatation of the colon. Am J Surg 147:243, 1984

SCHUFFLER MD et al: Chronic intestinal pseudo-obstruction. Medicine 60:173, 1981

TROTMAN IF, MISEWICZ JJ: Sigmoid motility in diverticular disease and the irritable bowel syndrome. Gut 29:218, 1988

Diverticular diseases

BRIAN JE, STAIR JM: Non-colonic diverticular disease. Surg Gynecol Obstet 161:189, 1985

THOMPSON WG, PATEL DG: Clinical picture of diverticular disease of the colon. Clinics Gastrol 15:903, 1986

Intestinal ischemia and angiodysplasia

SANTOS JC et al: Angiodysplasia of the colon: Endoscopic diagnosis and treatment. Br J Surg 75:256, 1988

WILLIAMS L: Mesenteric ischemia. Surg Clin North Am 68:331, 1988

243 TUMORS OF THE LARGE AND SMALL INTESTINE

ROBERT J. MAYER

COLORECTAL CANCER

INCIDENCE Cancer of the large bowel is second only to lung cancer as a cause of cancer death in the United States. Approximately 151,000 new cases were anticipated in 1989, resulting in 61,300 deaths. The incidence and mortality rates for this extremely common malignant condition have not changed substantially in males during the past 40 years, although, for some reason, a slight decrease in the mortality rate has appeared in females. Colorectal cancer generally occurs in individuals 50 years of age or older.

ETIOLOGY AND RISK FACTORS (Table 243-1) **Diet** The etiology for most cases of large-bowel cancer appears to be related to environmental factors. The disease occurs more often in upper socioeconomic populations who live in urban areas. Epidemiologic studies in various countries have documented a direct correlation between mortality from colorectal cancer and per capita consumption of calories, meat protein, and dietary fat and oil as well as elevations in the serum cholesterol concentration and mortality from coronary artery disease. Any geographic variations in incidence do not appear to be related to genetic differences, since migrant groups tend to assume the large-bowel cancer incidence rates of their adopted countries. Furthermore, population groups such as Mormons and Seventh Day Adventists, whose lifestyle and dietary habits differ somewhat from those of their neighbors, have significantly lower-than-expected incidence and mortality rates for colorectal cancer, while the appearance of colorectal cancer has increased in Japan since that nation has adopted a more "western" diet. It is therefore assumed that dietary patterns influence the development of colorectal cancer. At least two hypotheses have been proposed to explain this relationship, neither of which is fully satisfactory.

ANIMAL FATS Based on the association of colorectal cancer with hypercholesterolemia and coronary artery disease as well as the increased incidence of large-bowel tumors in geographic areas where meat is a dietary staple, it has been suggested that the ingestion of animal fats leads to an increased proportion of anaerobes in the gut microflora, resulting in the conversion of normal bile acids into carcinogens. This provocative hypothesis is supported by several reports of increased amounts of fecal anaerobes in the stools of patients with colorectal cancer. However, there are conflicting data from population studies relating fat intake to the risk for colon cancer and from unsuccessful attempts at altering the profile of fecal microflora through short-term alterations in diet. Any definitive assessment of the animal fat concept must await a prospective survey of a defined population, correlating carefully obtained and periodically updated dietary histories with quantitative cultures of stool microflora, and determining the incidence of colorectal cancer in these individuals over a 10 to 20 year period of time.

FIBER The observation that South African Bantus ingest a diet far higher in roughage, produce more frequent, bulkier stools, and

TABLE 243-1 Risk factors for the development of colorectal cancer

Diet
- ? Animal fat
- ? Fiber

Hereditary syndromes (autosomal dominant inheritance)
- Polyposis coli
- Non-polyposis syndrome

Inflammatory bowel disease
Streptococcus bovis bacteremia
Ureterosigmoidostomy

have a lower incidence of large-bowel cancer than their American and European counterparts led to the proposal that the higher rate of colorectal cancer in western society is in large part the result of a low intake of dietary fiber. This theory suggests that dietary fiber accelerates intestinal transit time, thereby reducing the exposure of colonic mucosa to potential carcinogens and diluting these carcinogens because of enhanced fecal bulk. Such a proposition appears somewhat simplistic when subjected to careful scrutiny. Although an enhanced fiber intake increases fecal bulk, there has been no consistent evidence that a high fiber intake actually shortens the transit time of stool. Additionally, despite the generally higher fiber intake in low-incidence countries, the environmental differences between developing and industrialized nations are myriad and include such other important dietary variables as meat and fat consumption. Finally, a diet low in fiber may lead to chronic constipation and such associated conditions as diverticulosis. If a low fiber diet were a significant factor in the etiology of colorectal cancer, individuals having diverticulosis should be at higher risk for the development of large-bowel tumors; this does not appear to be the case.

OTHER Emerging data suggest that the risk for the development of colorectal cancer may be diminished by the addition of calcium supplements to the diet. It is thought that such dietary calcium may inactivate bowel carcinogens through the formation of insoluble soaps. In support of this concept are (1) the finding that supplementary dietary calcium reduced the proliferation of colonic epithelial cells in familial colon cancer kindreds and (2) the results of a survey of the dietary habits of a cohort of about 2000 men over a 19-year period, suggesting that the risk of colonic cancer decreased with increased oral intake of calcium.

Thus, while the weight of epidemiologic evidence implicates diet as being the major etiologic factor for colorectal cancer, no single foodstuff has been sufficiently identified as being a causative or protective agent to justify specific recommendations for widespread changes in eating habits.

Hereditary factors and syndromes As many as 25 percent of patients with colorectal cancer may have a family history of the disease, suggesting a hereditary predisposition. Such inherited large-bowel cancers can be divided into two main groups: the well-studied but uncommon polyposis syndromes and the less well defined non-polyposis syndromes (Table 243-2).

Polyposis coli (i.e., familial polyposis of the colon) is a rare condition characterized by the appearance of thousands of adenomatous polyps throughout the large bowel. The condition is transmitted in an autosomal dominant manner, although occasional patients with no family history are thought to have developed the polyposis due to a spontaneous mutation. Molecular studies have recently associated polyposis coli with a deletion in the long arm of chromosome 5. It has been hypothesized that the loss of this genetic material (i.e., allelic loss) results in the absence of tumor-suppressor genes whose protein products would normally inhibit neoplastic growth. The presence of soft tissue and bony tumors in addition to the colonic polyps characterizes a subset of polyposis coli known as *Gardner's syndrome,* while the appearance of malignant tumors of the central nervous system accompanying polyposis coli defines *Turcot's syndrome*. The colonic polyps in all these conditions are rarely present prior to puberty but are generally evident in affected individuals by age 25. If left surgically untreated, colorectal cancer will develop in almost all patients prior to age 40. Polyposis coli has been studied intensively and appears to result from a defect in the colonic mucosa leading to an abnormal proliferative pattern and an impaired ability for cellular repair following exposure to radiation or ultraviolet light. Once the multiple polyps that constitute polyposis coli are detected, patients should have a total colectomy. It remains unclear whether the optimal operative approach in such a clinical setting is to resect the entire colon and rectum, requiring the young patient to have a permanent ileostomy, or to perform an ileoproctostomy. While the latter procedure retains the distal rectum and anal sphincter, it places the patient at continued risk for the development of cancer in the rectal remnant and necessitates semiannual or annual proctoscopic surveillance. The offspring of patients with polyposis coli, who are often prepubertal when the diagnosis is made in the parent, have a 50 percent risk for the eventual development of this premalignant disorder and should be carefully screened on a periodic basis until age 35. Such screening should include endoscopic and/or contrast radiographic examinations. Testing for occult blood in the stool is an inadequate screening maneuver. Unfortunately, no disease-specific screening technique is generally available for the children of polyposis coli patients, although radioautographic measurements of colonic mucosal proliferation have been utilized with apparent efficacy in a small number of patients at highly specialized medical centers. Conceivably, molecular probes for the chromosome 5 deletion will prove to be useful in this regard in the future.

The hereditary predisposition for colorectal cancer in families having no history of polyposis coli has received increased attention since the identification of several kindreds who displayed risks as high as 50 percent for the development of a colonic malignancy. These colorectal lesions involve the proximal large bowel in an unusually high frequency. Such families frequently include patients having multiple primary cancers, with the association of colorectal and endometrial adenocarcinomas being especially prominent in women. The trait for cancer appears to be transmitted in an autosomal dominant manner and the median age for the appearance of an adenocarcinoma is under age 50, 10 to 15 years below the usual age for the general population. The offspring of such predisposed patients should undergo intensive screening beginning by age 25, and the screening should include triannual colonoscopies or double-contrast barium enemas.

Inflammatory bowel disease (See also Chap. 241) Large-bowel cancer represents a not infrequent complication in patients with long-standing inflammatory bowel disease. The development of a neoplasm appears to occur more commonly in patients with ulcerative colitis than in those with granulomatous colitis, but such an impression may result in part from the occasional difficulty in differentiating these two conditions. The risk of colorectal cancer in a patient with inflammatory bowel disease is relatively small during the initial 10 years following the onset of the disease, but then appears to increase at a rate of approximately 0.5 to 1.0 percent per year. Actuarially derived cumulative cancer rates in such symptomatic patients have ranged from 8 to 30 percent after 25 years. The risk is generally considered to be higher in younger patients with pancolitis.

TABLE 243-2 Hereditable (autosomal dominant) gastrointestinal polyp syndromes

Syndrome	Distribution of polyps	Histologic type	Malignant potential	Associated lesions
Familial colonic polyposis	Large intestine	Adenoma	Common	None
Gardner's syndrome	Large and small intestines	Adenoma	Common	Osteomas, fibromas, lipomas, epidermoid cysts
Turcot's syndrome	Large intestine	Adenoma	Common	Brain tumors
Non-polyposis syndrome	Large intestine	Adenoma	Common	Endometrial tumors
Peutz-Jeghers syndrome	Small and large intestines, stomach	Hamartoma	Rare	Mucocutaneous pigmentation; tumors of the ovary, breast, pancreas, endometrium
Juvenile polyposis	Large and small intestines, stomach	Hamartoma rarely progressing to adenoma	Rare	Various congenital abnormalities

Cancer surveillance in patients with inflammatory bowel disease is unsatisfactory. Symptoms such as bloody diarrhea, abdominal cramping, and obstruction, which may signal the appearance of a tumor, are similar to the complaints of patients whose underlying disease is flaring. In patients with a history of inflammatory bowel disease lasting 15 years or more who continue to experience exacerbations, the surgical removal of the colon can significantly reduce the risk for cancer and also eliminate the target organ for the underlying chronic gastrointestinal disorder. The value of such surveillance techniques as colonoscopy with mucosal biopsies and brushings for less symptomatic individuals with chronic inflammatory bowel disease is uncertain. The purpose of such procedures has been the identification of premalignant mucosal dysplasia, thereby justifying surgical intervention. The lack of uniformity regarding the pathologic criteria that characterize dysplasia and the absence of data that such surveillance reduces the development of lethal cancers, however, has made this costly practice an area of controversy.

Other high-risk conditions *STREPTOCOCCUS BOVIS* BACTEREMIA For unknown reasons, individuals who develop endocarditis or septicemia from this fecal bacteria seem to have a high incidence of occult colorectal tumors. Endoscopic or radiographic screening for such patients appears advisable.

URETEROSIGMOIDOSTOMY There is a 5 to 10 percent incidence of colon cancer 15 to 30 years after ureterosigmoidostomy to correct congenital extrophy of the bladder. Neoplasms characteristically are found at a site distal to the ureteral implant where colonic mucosa is chronically exposed to both urine and feces.

POLYPS The majority of colorectal cancers, regardless of etiology, are believed to arise from adenomatous polyps. A polyp is a grossly visible protrusion from the mucosal surface and may be classified pathologically as a nonneoplastic hamartoma *(juvenile polyp)*, a hyperplastic mucosal proliferation *(hyperplastic polyp)*, or an adenomatous polyp. Only adenomas are clearly premalignant and only a minority of such lesions ever develop into cancer. Population-screening studies and autopsy surveys have revealed that adenomatous polyps may be found in the colons of about 30 percent of middle-aged or elderly people. Based on this prevalence and the known incidence of colorectal cancers, it appears that less than 1 percent of polyps ever become malignant. Most polyps produce no symptoms and remain clinically undetected. Occult blood in the stool may be found in less than 5 percent of patients with such lesions.

A number of molecular changes have been described in the DNA obtained from adenomatous polyps, dysplastic lesions, and polyps containing microscopic foci of tumor cells (i.e., *carcinoma in situ*). Consistent with the multistep process leading to cancer, a series of alterations has been observed, often beginning with a specific mutation in the *ras* proto-oncogene followed by deletions in chromosomes 5, 18, and 17. The loss of genetic material on the short arm of chromosome 17 appears to be associated with activation of a gene leading to the production of transformation-associated protein p53. Thus, the altered proliferative pattern of the colonic mucosa (which results in the progression to a polyp and then to a carcinoma) may involve the mutational activation of an oncogene followed by and coupled with the loss of genes which normally suppress tumorigenesis. Based on this model, it is believed that neoplasia develops only in those polyps in which all of these mutational events take place.

Clinically, the probability of an adenomatous polyp becoming a cancer is dependent upon the gross appearance of the lesion and its histologic features. Adenomatous polyps may be pedunculated (i.e., extending from adjacent bowel on a stalk) or sessile (i.e., flat). Cancers develop more frequently in sessile polyps, with the probability being directly related to the size of the lesion. Histologically, adenomatous polyps may be tubular, villous (i.e., papillary), or tubulovillous. Villous adenomas, which are predominantly sessile in appearance, become malignant more than three times as often as tubular adenomas.

Following the detection of an adenomatous polyp, the entire large bowel should be visualized endoscopically or radiographically since synchronous lesions are present in approximately one-third of cases. Colonoscopy should then be repeated periodically, even in the absence of a previously documented malignancy, since such patients have a 30 to 50 percent probability of developing another adenoma and are at a higher-than-average risk for developing a colorectal carcinoma. Adenomatous polyps are thought to require more than 5 years of growth before becoming clinically significant; therefore, colonoscopy need not be carried out more frequently than every 3 years.

SCREENING The rationale for colorectal cancer screening programs is that the earlier detection of localized, superficial neoplasms in asymptomatic individuals will increase the surgical cure rate. Screening strategies have been based on the assumption that more than 60 percent of such early lesions are located in the rectosigmoid, making them accessible to rigid proctosigmoidoscopy. For unexplained reasons, however, there has been a consistent decrease during the past several decades in the proportion of large-bowel cancers arising in the rectum with a corresponding increase in the more proximal descending colon. As such, the potential for rigid proctosigmoidoscopy to detect a sufficient number of occult neoplasms to make the procedure cost-effective has been questioned. The availability of flexible, fiberoptic sigmoidoscopes, permitting trained operators to visualize the colon for up to 60 cm, should enhance cancer detection. Whether this added detection justifies the expenses of the device and the examination remains to be determined.

Most programs directed at the early detection of colorectal cancers have focused on digital rectal examinations and testing stool for the presence of occult blood. The digital examination should be part of any routine physical evaluation in adults older than age 40, serving as the best screening test for prostate cancer in men, a component of the pelvic examination in women, and as an inexpensive maneuver for the detection of masses in the rectum. The development of the Hemoccult test has greatly facilitated the potential to detect occult fecal blood. Unfortunately, even when performed optimally, the Hemoccult test has major limitations as a screening technique. Between 35 to 50 percent of patients with documented colorectal cancers have a negative fecal Hemoccult test, consistent with the intermittent bleeding pattern of these tumors. When random cohorts of asymptomatic persons have been tested, 3 to 6 percent have Hemoccult-positive stools. Colorectal cancers have been found in only 5 to 10 percent of these "test-positive" cases, with benign polyps being detected in an additional 20 to 30 percent. Consequently, a colorectal neoplasm will *not* be found in the majority of asymptomatic individuals with occult blood in their stool. Nonetheless, persons found to have Hemoccult-positive stool routinely undergo further medical evaluation that includes sigmoidoscopy, barium enema, and/or colonoscopy—procedures that not only are uncomfortable and expensive, but also are associated with a low but finite risk for significant complications. The added cost of these studies would appear justifiable, if the minority of patients found to have occult neoplasms because of Hemoccult screening could be shown to have an improved prognosis and prolonged survival. Prospectively controlled trials addressing this issue are ongoing.

Therefore, screening techniques for large-bowel cancer in asymptomatic persons remain unsatisfactory. Thus far, no controlled clinical study has demonstrated any screening maneuver that enhances the likelihood for cure. As a result, recommendations from governmental and private agencies are conflicting, and the issue remains unresolved.

CLINICAL FEATURES Presenting symptoms Symptoms vary with the anatomic location of the tumor.

Since stool is relatively liquid as it passes through the ileocecal valve into the right colon, neoplasms arising in the cecum and ascending colon may become quite large, significantly narrowing the bowel lumen, without resulting in any obstructive symptoms or noticeable alterations in bowel habits. Lesions of the right colon commonly ulcerate, leading to chronic, insidious blood loss without a change in the appearance of the stool. Consequently, patients with tumors of the ascending colon often present with symptoms such as fatigue, palpitations, and even angina pectoris and are found to have

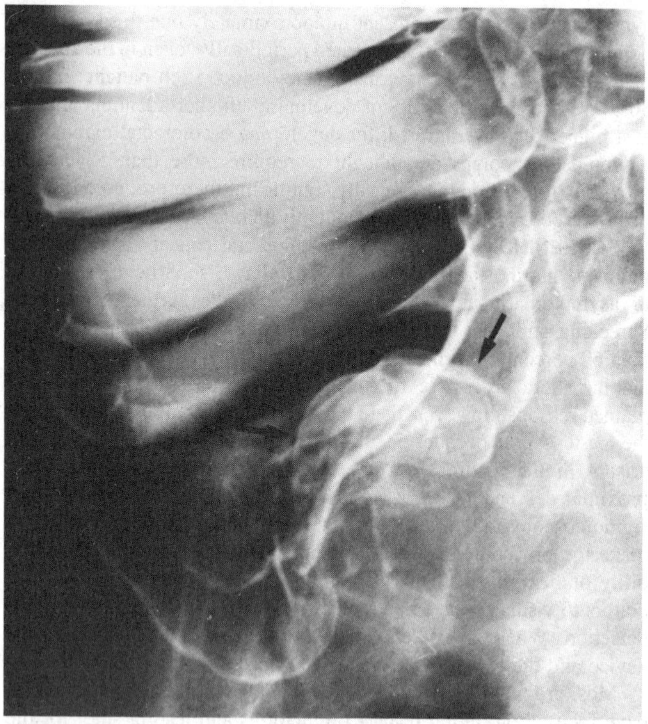

FIGURE 243-1 Double-contrast air-barium enema revealing a sessile tumor of the cecum in a patient with iron-deficiency anemia and guaiac-positive stool. The lesion at surgery was a stage B adenocarcinoma.

FIGURE 243-2 Annular, constricting adenocarcinoma of the descending colon. This radiographic appearance is referred to as an ''apple-core'' lesion and is always highly suggestive of malignancy.

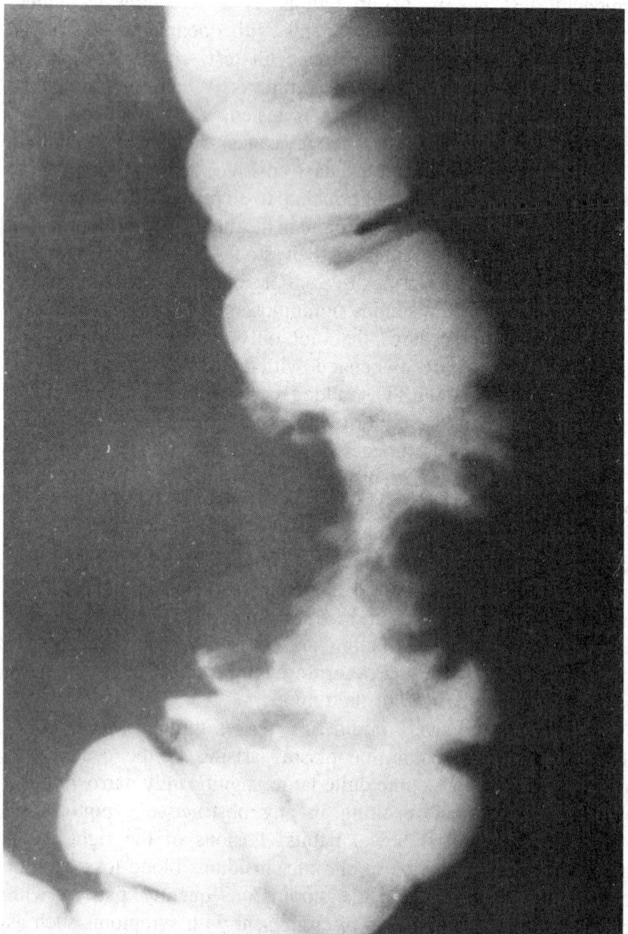

a hypochromic, microcytic anemia indicative of iron deficiency. Since the cancer may bleed intermittently, however, a random test for the presence of occult blood in the stool may be negative. As a result, the unexplained presence of iron-deficiency anemia in any adult (with the possible exception of a premenopausal, multiparous woman) mandates a thorough endoscopic and/or radiographic visualization of the entire large bowel (Fig. 243-1).

Since stool becomes more concentrated as it passes into the transverse and descending colon, tumors arising there tend to impede the passage of stool, resulting in the development of abdominal cramping, occasional obstruction, and even perforation. Radiographs of the abdomen often reveal characteristic annular, constricting lesions (''apple-core'' or ''napkin-ring'') (Fig. 243-2).

Neoplasms arising in the rectosigmoid often are associated with hematochezia, tenesmus, and narrowing in the caliber of stool; nonetheless, anemia is an infrequent finding. While these symptoms may lead patients and their physicians to suspect the presence of hemorrhoids, the development of rectal bleeding and/or altered bowel habits demands a prompt digital rectal examination and proctosigmoidoscopy.

Staging, prognostic factors, patterns of spread The prognosis for individuals having colorectal cancer is closely related to the depth of tumor penetration into the bowel wall and the presence of both regional lymph node involvement and distant metastases. These variables are incorporated into the staging system introduced by Dukes (Table 243-3). Patients with superficial lesions not penetrating into the muscularis or involving regional lymph nodes are designated as having *stage A* disease; those individuals whose tumors penetrate more deeply but without spread to lymph nodes are termed as having *stage B* disease; regional lymph node involvement defines *stage C* disease; and metastatic spread to sites such as liver, lung, or bone indicates *stage D* disease. Unless gross evidence of metastatic disease is present, it is impossible to accurately determine disease stage prior to surgical resection and pathologic analysis of the operative specimens.

Most recurrences after a surgical resection of a large-bowel cancer occur within the first 4 postoperative years, making the 5-year mark a fairly reliable indicator of cure. The likelihood for 5-year survival in patients with colorectal cancer is closely associated with their Dukes' stage (Table 243-3). That likelihood has appeared to improve during the past several decades when similar surgical stages have been compared. The most plausible explanation for this improvement appears to be more thorough intraoperative and pathologic staging. In particular, more exacting attention to pathologic detail has revealed that the prognosis following the resection of a colorectal cancer is not related merely to the presence or absence of regional lymph node involvement but may be more precisely assessed by the number of involved lymph nodes (i.e., 1 to 4 lymph nodes versus >5 lymph nodes). Other predictors of a poor prognosis after a total surgical resection include tumor penetration through the bowel wall into pericolic fat, poorly differentiated histology, perforation and/or tumor adherence to adjacent organs (increasing the risk for an anatomically adjacent recurrence), and venous invasion by tumor (Table 243-4). Regardless of the clinicopathologic stage, a preoperative elevation of the plasma carcinoembryonic antigen (CEA) titer is suggestive of eventual tumor recurrence. The presence of abnormal DNA content

TABLE 243-3 Dukes' classification of colorectal cancer

Stage	Pathologic description	Approximate 5-year survival, %
A	Cancer limited to mucosa and submucosa	>90
B	Cancer extends into muscularis or serosa	70–85
C	Cancer involves regional lymph nodes	30–60
D	Distant metastases (i.e., liver, lung, etc.)	5

TABLE 243-4 Poor prognostic predictors following total surgical resection

Tumor spread to regional lymph nodes
Number of regional lymph nodes involved
Tumor penetration through the bowel wall
Poorly differentiated histology
Perforation
Tumor adherence to adjacent organs
Venous invasion
Preoperative elevation of CEA titer (>5.0 ng/mL)
? Aneuploidy
? Specific chromosomal deletion (allelic loss)

(i.e., aneuploidy) and specific chromosomal deletions (i.e., so-called allelic loss) in tumor cells, as determined by flow cytometry and restriction fragment length polymorphism analysis respectively, appears to predict a higher risk for metastatic spread. In contrast to most other carcinomas and sarcomas, the prognosis in individuals with colorectal cancer is *not* influenced by the size of the primary lesion when adjusted for nodal involvement and histologic differentiation.

Cancers of the large bowel generally spread to regional lymph nodes or to the liver via the portal venous circulation. The liver represents the most frequent visceral site of metastatic dissemination; it is the initial site of distant spread in one-third of recurring colorectal cancers and eventually becomes involved in greater than two-thirds of such patients at the time of death. In general, colorectal cancer rarely metastasizes to the lungs, supraclavicular lymph nodes, bone, or brain without prior spread to the liver. A major exception to this rule occurs in patients having primary tumors in the distal rectum, from where tumor cells may spread through the paravertebral venous plexus, escaping the portal venous system and thereby reaching the lungs or supraclavicular lymph nodes without hepatic involvement. The median survival after the detection of distant metastases may range from 6 to 9 months (hepatomegaly, liver abnormalities) to 20 to 24 months (small liver nodule initially identified by elevated CEA level and subsequent CT scan).

TREATMENT Total resection of tumor represents optimal management when a malignant lesion is endoscopically or radiographically detected in the large bowel. An evaluation for the presence of metastatic disease, including a thorough physical examination, a chest x-ray, biochemical assessment of liver function, and a plasma CEA level, should be performed prior to surgery. When possible, a colonoscopy of the entire large bowel should be performed to identify synchronous neoplasms and/or polyps. The detection of metastases should not preclude surgery in patients with tumor-related symptoms such as gastrointestinal bleeding or obstruction, but may often result in a less radical operative procedure being carried out. At the time of laparotomy, the entire peritoneal cavity should be examined with the liver, pelvis, and hemidiaphragm being thoroughly inspected and the full length of the large bowel being carefully palpated. Following recovery from a complete resection, patients should be carefully observed for 5 years by semiannual physical examinations and yearly blood chemistries. If a complete colonoscopy was not performed preoperatively, this should be carried out within the first several postoperative months. Some authorities favor obtaining plasma CEA levels at 3-month intervals because of the sensitivity of this test as a marker for otherwise undetectable tumor recurrence. Subsequent endoscopic or radiographic surveillance of the large bowel, probably at triannual intervals, is indicated, since patients who have been cured of one colorectal cancer have a 3 to 5 percent probability of developing an additional bowel cancer during their lifetime and a risk in excess of 15 percent for the development of adenomatous polyps. Anastomotic (i.e., ''suture-line'') recurrences are infrequent in colorectal cancer patients, if the surgical resection margins were adequate and free of tumor.

Radiation therapy to the pelvis is generally recommended for patients with rectal cancer because of the 30 to 40 percent probability of regional recurrences following complete surgical resection of stages B and C tumors, especially if they have penetrated through the serosa. This alarmingly high rate of local disease recurrence is believed to be due to the fact that the contained anatomic space within the pelvis limits the extent of the resection and because the rich lymphatic network of the pelvic side wall immediately adjacent to the rectum facilitates the early spread of malignant cells into surgically inaccessible tissue. Prospectively randomized trials have indicated that the prophylactic use of radiation therapy, either pre- or postoperatively, reduces the likelihood of pelvic recurrences but does not appear to prolong survival. Preoperative radiotherapy is clearly indicated for patients with large, potentially unresectable rectal cancers, since such anatomically fixed lesions may shrink sufficiently to permit subsequent surgical removal.

Chemotherapy in patients with advanced colorectal cancer has proven to be of only marginal benefit. Since its introduction into clinical trials more than 25 years ago, 5-fluorouracil (5-FU) remains the most effective treatment for this disease. It is as useful when given alone as when combined with other drugs, but is associated with only a 15 to 20 percent likelihood of reducing measurable tumor masses by 50 percent or more (i.e., partial response). While the probability for tumor response appears to be somewhat greater for patients with liver metastases when such chemotherapy is infused directly into the hepatic artery as compared to a peripheral vein, intraarterial treatment is costly and toxic and does not appear to prolong survival. The results of recent studies have suggested that the concomitant administration of folinic acid (also known as leucovorin or citrovorum factor) will improve the efficacy of 5-FU in patients with advanced colorectal cancer, presumably by enhancing the binding of 5-FU to its target enzyme, thymidylate synthetase, thereby increasing the suppression of DNA synthesis and accompanying cytotoxicity. The majority of randomized trials have indicated a threefold improvement in the likelihood of partial response when folinic acid is combined with 5-FU; however, the effect on survival is uncertain and the optimal dose-schedule remains to be defined.

The value of postoperative chemotherapy and/or radiation therapy has been assessed in patients with stages B and C cancers as a means of eradicating clinically undetectable micrometastases and thereby increasing the probability for cure. The weight of evidence from more than 12 prospectively randomized trials in patients who have undergone the resection of a colon cancer suggests that the use of such prophylactic chemotherapy (i.e., including 5-FU given alone or in combination with other cytotoxic drugs) does not reduce the recurrence rate or prolong survival. However, the results of two clinical studies have indicated that the administration of adjuvant 5-FU with an anthelmintic agent, levamisole, to patients with stage C cancers leads to a decrease in the likelihood of recurrence and a modest improvement in survival. The levamisole is thought to act in this therapeutic setting as a nonspecific immunomodulator. In contrast, in patients who have undergone the resection of a rectal cancer, data from controlled studies indicate that postoperative radiation therapy when combined with chemotherapy appears to reduce the likelihood of regional recurrences and increase the potential for cure. It has been postulated that the chemotherapy, ineffective when given prophylactically for patients with colon lesions, acts as a radiation sensitizer when given to individuals who have been operated upon for rectal cancer, thereby enhancing the biologic effect of the radiotherapy.

TUMORS OF THE SMALL INTESTINE

Small-bowel tumors comprise only 3 to 6 percent of gastrointestinal neoplasms. Because of their rarity, a correct diagnosis is often delayed. Abdominal symptoms are usually vague and poorly defined, and conventional radiographic studies of the upper and lower intestinal tract are often normal. Small-bowel tumors should be considered in the following situations: (1) recurrent, unexplained episodes of crampy abdominal pain; (2) intermittent bouts of intestinal obstruction, especially in the absence of inflammatory bowel disease or prior abdominal surgery; (3) intussuception in the adult; and (4) evidence of chronic intestinal bleeding in the presence of negative conventional radiographs. A careful small-bowel barium study is the diagnostic procedure of choice; the diagnostic accuracy may be improved by infusing barium through a nasogastric tube placed into the duodenum (enteroclysis).

BENIGN TUMORS In general, the histology of benign small-bowel tumors is difficult to predict on clinical and radiologic grounds alone. The symptomatology of benign tumors is not distinctive, with pain, obstruction, and hemorrhage being the most frequent symptoms. These tumors are usually discovered during the fifth and sixth decades of life, more often in the distal rather than the proximal small intestine. The most common benign tumors are adenomas, leiomyomas, lipomas, and angiomas.

Adenomas These tumors include those of the islet cells and Brunner's glands as well as polypoid adenomas. *Islet cell adenomas* are occasionally located outside the pancreas, and the associated syndromes are discussed in Chap. 320. *Brunner's gland adenomas* are not truly neoplastic but represent a hypertrophy or hyperplasia of submucosal duodenal glands. These appear as small nodules in the duodenal mucosa that secrete a highly viscous alkaline mucus. Most often this is an incidental radiographic finding not associated with any specific clinical disorder.

Polypoid adenomas (See Table 243-2) Approximately 25 percent of benign small-bowel tumors are polypoid adenomas. They may present as single polypoid lesions or, less commonly, as papillary villous adenomas. As in the colon, the sessile or papillary form of the tumor is sometimes associated with a coexistent carcinoma. Occasionally, patients with Gardner's syndrome (a variant of polyposis coli) may develop premalignant adenomas in the small bowel; such lesions are generally in the duodenum. Multiple polypoid tumors may occur throughout the small bowel (and occasionally the stomach and colorectum) in the Peutz-Jeghers syndrome. The polyps are usually hamartomas (juvenile polyps) having a low potential for malignant degeneration. Mucocutaneous melanin deposits as well as tumors of the ovary, breast, pancreas, and endometrium are also associated with this autosomal dominant condition.

Leiomyomas These neoplasms arise from smooth-muscle components of the intestine and are usually intramural, affecting the overlying mucosa. Ulceration of the mucosa may cause gastrointestinal hemorrhage of varying severity.

Lipomas These tumors occur with greatest frequency in the distal ileum and at the ileocecal valve. They have a characteristic radiolucent appearance, are usually intramural and asymptomatic, but may on occasion be associated with bleeding.

Angiomas While not true neoplasms, these lesions are important because they frequently cause intestinal bleeding. They may take the form of telangiectasia or hemangiomas. Multiple intestinal telangiectasia occur in a nonhereditary form confined to the gastrointestinal tract or as part of the hereditary Osler-Rendu-Weber syndrome. Vascular tumors may also take the form of isolated hemangiomas, most commonly in the jejunum. Angiography, especially during bleeding, is the procedure of choice in evaluating these lesions.

MALIGNANT TUMORS While infrequent in appearance, small-bowel malignancies occur in patients with long-standing regional enteritis and celiac sprue as well as in individuals with the acquired immunodeficiency syndrome (AIDS). In contrast to benign tumors, malignant tumors of the small bowel are frequently associated with fever, weight loss, anorexia, bleeding, and a palpable abdominal mass. After ampullary carcinomas (many of which arise from biliary or pancreatic ducts), the most frequently occurring small-bowel malignancies are adenocarcinomas, lymphomas, carcinoid tumors, and leiomyosarcomas.

Adenocarcinomas The most common primary cancers of the small bowel are adenocarcinomas, which account for about 50 percent of the malignant tumors. These neoplasms occur with highest frequency in the distal duodenum and proximal jejunum, where they tend to ulcerate and cause hemorrhage or obstruction. Radiologically, they may be confused with chronic duodenal ulcer disease or with Crohn's disease if the patient has long-standing regional enteritis. The diagnosis is best made by endoscopy and biopsy under direct vision. Surgical resection is the treatment of choice.

Lymphomas Lymphomatous involvement of the small bowel may be primary or secondary. A diagnosis of a primary intestinal lymphoma requires histologic confirmation of a lymphoproliferative neoplasm in a clinical setting in which palpable adenopathy and hepatosplenomegaly are absent and there is no evidence of lymphoma on a chest radiograph, CT scan, peripheral blood smear, or on bone marrow aspiration and biopsy. In general, symptoms referable to the small bowel are present, usually accompanied by an anatomically discernible lesion. Secondary lymphoma of the small bowel refers to involvement of the intestine by a lymphoid malignancy extending from involved retroperitoneal lymph nodes and hence is a manifestation of a generalized systemic neoplasm (see Chap. 300).

Primary intestinal lymphoma comprises 25 percent of malignancies of the small bowel. Essentially all these neoplasms are non-Hodgkin's lymphomas, most frequently having a diffuse, large-cell (i.e., "high-grade") histology. Intestinal lymphoma involves the ileum more frequently than the jejunum, which, in turn, is more commonly affected than the duodenum, a pattern which mirrors the relative amount of normal lymphoid cells in these anatomic areas. The risk of small-bowel lymphoma is increased in patients with a prior history of malabsorptive conditions (e.g., celiac sprue), regional enteritis, and depressed immunologic function due to congenital immunodeficiency syndromes, prior organ transplantation, autoimmune disorders, or AIDS.

The development of localized or nodular masses that narrow the lumen results in periumbilical pain (made worse by eating) as well as weight loss, vomiting, and occasional intestinal obstruction. The diagnosis of small-bowel lymphoma may be suspected by the appearance on contrast radiographs of patterns such as infiltration and thickening of mucosal folds, mucosal nodules, areas of irregular ulceration, or stasis of contrast material. The diagnosis can be confirmed by surgical exploration and resection of involved segments. Intestinal lymphoma may occasionally be diagnosed by peroral intestinal mucosal biopsy, but since the disease mainly involves the lamina propria, full-thickness surgical biopsies are usually required.

Resection of the tumor constitutes the initial treatment modality. While postoperative radiation therapy has been offered to some patients following such a total resection, most authorities favor short-term systemic treatment with combination chemotherapy. The frequent presence of widespread intraabdominal disease at the time of diagnosis and the occasional multicentricity of the tumor often make a total resection impossible. Combination chemotherapy would appear to be appropriate management for these patients as well. The probability of sustained remission or cure is approximately 75 percent in patients with localized disease, but 25 percent or less in individuals with unresectable lymphoma.

A unique form of small-bowel lymphoma, diffusely involving the entire intestine, was first described in oriental Jews and Arabs and is referred to as immunoproliferative small intestinal disease (IPSID), Mediterranean lymphoma, or alpha-heavy chain disease. The typical presentation includes chronic diarrhea and steatorrhea associated with vomiting and abdominal cramps; clubbing of the digits may be observed as well. A curious feature in many patients with IPSID is the presence in the blood and intestinal secretions of an abnormal IgA which contains a shortened alpha-heavy chain and is devoid of light chains. It is suspected that the abnormal alpha chains are produced by plasma cells infiltrating the small bowel. The clinical course of patients with IPSID is generally one of exacerbations and remissions, with death frequently resulting from either progressive malnutrition and wasting or the development of an aggressive lymphoma. Chemotherapy and radiation therapy have been ineffective.

Carcinoid tumors Among the more common epithelial tumors of the small intestine are carcinoid tumors. They arise from argentaffin cells of the crypts of Lieberkühn and are found from the distal duodenum to the ascending colon, areas embryologically derived from the midgut. More than 50 percent of intestinal carcinoids are found in the distal ileum, with the majority congregating in close proximity to the ileocecal valve. Most intestinal carcinoids are asymptomatic and of low malignant potential, but invasion and metastases may occur, leading to the carcinoid syndrome (Chap. 262).

Leiomyosarcomas Large, bulky tumors, leiomyosarcomas often are greater than 5 cm in diameter and may be palpable on abdominal examination. Bleeding, obstruction, and perforation are common.

CANCERS OF THE ANUS

Cancers of the anus account for 1 to 2 percent of the malignant tumors of the large bowel. The majority of such lesions arise in the anal canal which is defined as the anatomic area extending from the anorectal ring to a zone approximately halfway between the pectinate (or dentate) line and the anal verge. Carcinomas arising proximal to the pectinate line (i.e., in the transitional zone between the glandular mucosa of the rectum and the squamous epithelium of the distal anus) are known as basaloid, cuboidal, or cloacogenic tumors; approximately one-third of anal cancers have this histologic pattern. Malignancies arising distal to the pectinate line have a squamous cell histology, ulcerate more frequently, and represent approximately 55 percent of anal cancers. The prognosis for patients with basaloid and squamous cell cancers of the anus is identical when corrected for tumor size and the presence or absence of nodal spread.

Anal cancers occur most commonly in individuals with a prior history of chronic anal irritation. Such irritation may result from condylomata accuminata (i.e., viral lesions thought to be caused by papilloma virus infection), perianal fissures and/or fistulas, chronic hemorrhoids, and leukoplakia. The risk for anal cancer appears to be increased among homosexual males, presumably due to trauma related to anal intercourse. There presently are no data to indicate that anal cancers are AIDS-related tumors associated with infection by the human immunodeficiency virus. Anal cancers occur most commonly in middle-aged individuals, develop more frequently in women than men, and are most often associated with bleeding, pain, the sensation of a perianal mass, and perianal pruritus at the time of diagnosis.

Until recently, radical surgery (abdominal-perineal resection with lymph node sampling and a permanent colostomy) was the treatment of choice for this tumor type. The probability of survival 5 years following such a procedure ranged from 55 to 70 percent in the absence of spread to regional lymph nodes and decreased to less than 20 percent if nodal involvement was present. However, an alternative therapeutic approach combining external beam radiation with concomitant chemotherapy has resulted in biopsy-proven disappearance of all tumor in more than 80 percent of patients whose initial lesion was less than 5 cm in size. Tumor recurrences have occurred in less than 10 percent of these patients. Thus, it appears that more than 80 percent of patients with anal cancers can be cured with nonoperative treatment and that disfiguring surgery should be reserved for the minority of individuals who are found to have residual tumor after being managed initially with radiation combined with chemotherapy.

REFERENCES

Colorectal cancer

Etiology and risk factors

COLLINS RH JR et al: Colon cancer, dysplasia, and surveillance in patients with ulcerative colitis. N Engl J Med 316:1654, 1987

HAGGITT RC, REID BJ: Hereditary gastrointestinal polyposis syndromes. Am J Surg Path 10:871, 1986

LIPKIN M, NEWMARK H: Effect of added dietary calcium on colonic epithelial cell proliferation in subjects at high risk for familial colonic cancer. N Engl J Med 313:1381, 1985

VOGELSTEIN B et al: Genetic alterations during colorectal-tumor development. N Engl J Med 319:595, 1988

ZARIDZE DG: Environmental etiology of large bowel cancer. J Natl Cancer Inst 70:389, 1982

Polyps

CANNON-ALBRIGHT LA et al: Common inheritance of susceptibility to colonic adenomatous polyps and associated colorectal cancers. N Engl J Med 319:533, 1988

FENOGLIO-PREISER CM, HUTTER RVP: Colorectal polyps: Pathologic diagnosis and clinical significance. Cancer 35:322, 1985

Screening

GROSSMAN S et al: Colonoscopic screening of persons with suspected risk factors for colon cancer: II Past history of colorectal neoplasms. Gastroenterology 96:299, 1989

KNIGHT KK et al: Occult blood screening for colorectal cancer. JAMA 261:586, 1989

NEUGUT AI, PITA S: Role of sigmoidoscopy in screening for colorectal cancer: A critical review. Gastroenterology 95:492, 1988

SELBY JV, FRIEDMAN GD: Sigmoidoscopy in the periodic health examination of asymptomatic adults. JAMA 261:594, 1989

SIMON JB: Occult blood screening for colorectal carcinoma: A critical review. Gastroenterology 88:820, 1985

Clinical features

GASTROINTESTINAL TUMOR STUDY GROUP: Adjuvant therapy of colon cancer—results of a postoperatively randomized trial. N Engl J Med 310:737, 1984

KERN SE et al: Allelic loss in colorectal carcinoma. JAMA 261:3099, 1989

WANEBO JH et al: Preoperative carcinoembryonic antigen level as a prognostic indicator in colorectal cancer. N Engl J Med 229:448, 1978

Treatment

GASTROINTESTINAL TUMOR STUDY GROUP: Prolongation of the disease-free interval in surgically treated rectal carcinoma. N Engl J Med 312:1465, 1985

MAYER RJ et al: The status of adjuvant therapy for colorectal cancer. J Natl Cancer Inst 81:1359, 1989

MOERTEL CG et al: Levamisole and fluorouracil for adjuvant therapy of resected colon carcinoma. N Engl J Med 322:352, 1990

Tumors of the small intestine

HABER DA, MAYER RJ: Primary gastrointestinal lymphoma. Semin Oncol 15:154, 1988

LEVIN B: Neoplasms of the small bowel, in *Medical Oncology. Basic Principles and Clinical Management of Cancer,* P Calabresi et al (eds). New York, Macmillan, 1985, pp 875–883

Anal cancer

DALING JR et al: Sexual practices, sexually transmitted diseases, and the incidence of anal cancer. N Engl J Med 317:973, 1987

LEICHMAN L et al: Cancer of the anal canal: Model for preoperative adjuvant combined modality therapy. Am J Med 78:211, 1985

244 ACUTE INTESTINAL OBSTRUCTION

WILLIAM SILEN

ETIOLOGY AND CLASSIFICATION Intestinal obstruction may be *mechanical* or *nonmechanical* (resulting from neuromuscular disturbances which produce either *adynamic* or *dynamic ileus*). The causes of mechanical obstruction of the lumen are conveniently divided into (1) lesions *extrinsic* to the intestine, e.g., adhesive bands, internal and external hernias; (2) lesions *intrinsic* to the wall of the intestine, e.g., diverticulitis, carcinoma, regional enteritis; and (3) obturation of the lumen, e.g., gallstone obstruction, intussusception. From the clinical standpoint, however, it is most useful to consider whether the obstructive mechanism involves the small or large intestine, because the causes, symptoms, and treatment are different (see below). Adhesions and external hernias are the most common causes of obstruction of the small intestine, constituting 70 to 75 percent of cases of this type. Adhesions, however, almost never produce obstruction of the colon, while carcinoma, sigmoid diverticulitis, and volvulus, in that order, are the most common etiologies and together account for about 90 percent of the cases.

Adynamic ileus is probably the most common overall cause of obstruction. Recent studies indicate that the development of this condition is mediated via the hormonal component of the sympathoadrenal system. Adynamic ileus will occur after any peritoneal insult, and its severity and duration will be dependent to some degree on the type of peritoneal injury. Hydrochloric acid, colonic contents, and pancreatic enzymes are among the most irritating substances, whereas blood and urine are less so. Adynamic ileus occurs to some degree after any abdominal operation, and its severity varies directly with the amount of intestinal handling and the length of the operation; it usually lasts 2 to 3 days after most operative procedures. Retroperitoneal hematomas, particularly associated with vertebral fracture, commonly cause severe adynamic ileus, and the latter may occur with other retroperitoneal conditions such as ureteral calculus or severe pyelonephritis. Thoracic diseases including lower-lobe pneumonia, fractured ribs, and myocardial infarction frequently produce adynamic ileus, as do electrolyte disturbances, particularly potassium depletion. Finally intestinal ischemia, whether the result of vascular occlusion or intestinal distention itself, may perpetuate an adynamic ileus. Spastic or dynamic ileus is very uncommon and results from extreme and prolonged contraction of the intestine. It has been observed in heavy metal poisoning, uremia, porphyria, and extensive intestinal ulcerations.

PATHOPHYSIOLOGY Distention of the intestine is caused by the accumulation of gas and fluid proximal to and within the obstructed segment. Seventy to eighty percent of intestinal gas consists of swallowed air, and because this is composed mainly of nitrogen, which is poorly absorbed from the intestinal lumen, removal of air by continuous gastric suction is a useful adjunct in the treatment of intestinal distention. The accumulation of fluid proximal to the obstructing mechanism results not only from ingested fluid, swallowed saliva, gastric juice, and biliary and pancreatic secretions but also from interference with normal sodium and water transport. During the first 12 to 24 h of obstruction there is a marked depression of flux from lumen to blood of sodium and consequently water in the distended proximal intestine. After 24 h, there is also movement of sodium and water into the lumen, contributing further to the distention and fluid losses. Intraluminal pressure rises from a normal of 2 to 4 cmH_2O to 8 to 10 cmH_2O. During peristalsis, when simple obstruction or a "closed loop" is present, pressures reach 30 to 60 cmH_2O. Closed-loop obstruction of the small intestine results when the lumen is occluded at two points by a single mechanism such as a hernial ring or adhesive band, thus producing a closed loop whose blood supply is often obstructed at the same time. Strangulation of the loop itself is thus common in association with marked distention proximal to the involved loop. A form of closed-loop obstruction is encountered when complete obstruction of the colon exists in the presence of a competent ileocecal valve (85 percent of individuals). Although the blood supply of the colon is not entrapped within the obstructing mechanism, distention of the cecum is extreme because of its greater diameter (LaPlace's law), and impairment of the intramural blood supply is considerable with consequent gangrene of the cecal wall, usually anteriorly. Necrosis of the small intestine may occur by the same mechanism of interference with intramural blood flow when distention is extreme, but this sequence is uncommon in the small intestine. Once impairment of blood supply occurs, bacterial invasion supervenes and peritonitis develops. The systemic effects of extreme distention include elevation of the diaphragm with restricted ventilation and subsequent atelectasis. Venous return via the inferior vena cava may also be impaired.

The loss of fluids and electrolytes may be extreme, and unless replacement is prompt, leads to hemoconcentration, hypovolemia, renal insufficiency, shock, and death. Vomiting, accumulation of fluids within the lumen by the mechanisms described above, and the sequestration of fluid into the edematous intestinal wall and peritoneal cavity as a result of impairment of venous return from the intestine all contribute to massive loss of fluid and electrolytes. As soon as significant impedance to venous return is present, the intestine becomes severely congested, and blood begins to seep into the intestinal lumen. Blood loss may reach significant levels when long segments of intestine are involved.

SYMPTOMS *Mechanical small-intestinal obstruction* is characterized by cramping midabdominal pain which tends to be more severe the higher the obstruction. The pain occurs in paroxysms, and the patient is relatively comfortable in the intervals between the pains. Audible borborygmi are often noted by the patient simultaneously with the paroxysms of pain. The pain may become less severe as distention progresses, probably because motility is impaired in the edematous intestine. When strangulation is present, the pain is usually more localized and may be steady and severe without a colicky component, a fact which often causes delay in diagnosis of obstruction. Vomiting is almost invariable, and it is earlier and more profuse the higher the obstruction. The vomitus initially contains bile and mucus and remains as such if the obstruction is high in the intestine. With low ileal obstruction, the vomitus becomes feculent, i.e., orange-brown in color with a foul odor, which results from the overgrowth of bacteria proximal to the obstruction. Singultus is common. Obstipation and failure to pass gas by rectum are invariably present when the obstruction is complete, although some stool and gas may be passed spontaneously or after an enema shortly after onset of the complete obstruction. Diarrhea is occasionally observed in partial obstruction. Blood in the stool is rare, even in the completely obstructed patient, but does occur in cases of intussusception. Other than some minor but inconsistent differences in pain patterns noted above, the symptoms of strangulating obstructions cannot be distinguished from those of nonstrangulating obstructions.

Mechanical colonic obstruction produces colicky abdominal pain similar in quality to that of small-intestinal obstruction but of much lower intensity. Complaints of pain are occasionally absent in stoic elderly patients. Vomiting occurs late, if at all, particularly if the ileocecal valve is competent. Paradoxically, feculent vomitus is very rare. A history of recent alterations in bowel habits and blood in the stool is common because carcinoma and diverticulitis are the most frequent causes. Constipation becomes progressive, and obstipation with failure to pass gas ensues. Acute symptoms may develop over a period of a week.

In *adynamic ileus,* colicky pain is absent, and only discomfort from distention is evident. Vomiting may be frequent but is rarely profuse. It usually consists of gastric contents and bile and is almost never feculent. Complete obstipation may or may not occur. Singultus is very common.

PHYSICAL FINDINGS *Abdominal distention* is the hallmark of all forms of intestinal obstruction. It is least marked in cases of obstruction high in the small intestine and most marked in colonic obstruction. Early in the course of the disease, especially in closed-loop strangulating small-bowel obstruction, distention may be barely perceptible or absent. Tenderness and rigidity are usually minimal; the temperature is rarely above 37.8°C (100°F) in nonstrangulating obstruction of the small and large intestine. Contrary to popular belief the same is true of strangulating obstruction until very late in the course of the disease, a fact which has often resulted in unfortunate delay in treatment. Signs and symptoms of shock also occur *very late* in strangulating obstruction. The appearance of shock, tenderness, rigidity, and fever often means that there has been contamination of the peritoneum with infected intestinal content. The presence of a palpable abdominal mass usually signifies a closed-loop strangulating small-bowel obstruction because the tense fluid-filled loop is the palpable lesion. Auscultation may reveal loud high-pitched borborygmi coincident with the colicky pain, but this classic finding is often not present late in strangulating or nonstrangulating obstruction. A quiet abdomen does not eliminate the possibility of obstruction, nor does it necessarily establish the diagnosis of adynamic ileus.

LABORATORY AND X-RAY FINDINGS Leukocytosis, with shift to the left, usually occurs when strangulation is present, but a normal white blood cell count does not exclude strangulation. Elevation of the serum amylase is encountered occasionally in all forms of intestinal obstruction, especially the strangulating variety.

The x-ray is extremely valuable but under certain circumstances may also be misleading. In nonstrangulating complete small-bowel obstruction, x-rays are almost completely reliable. Distention of fluid- and gas-filled loops of small intestine usually arranged in a "step-

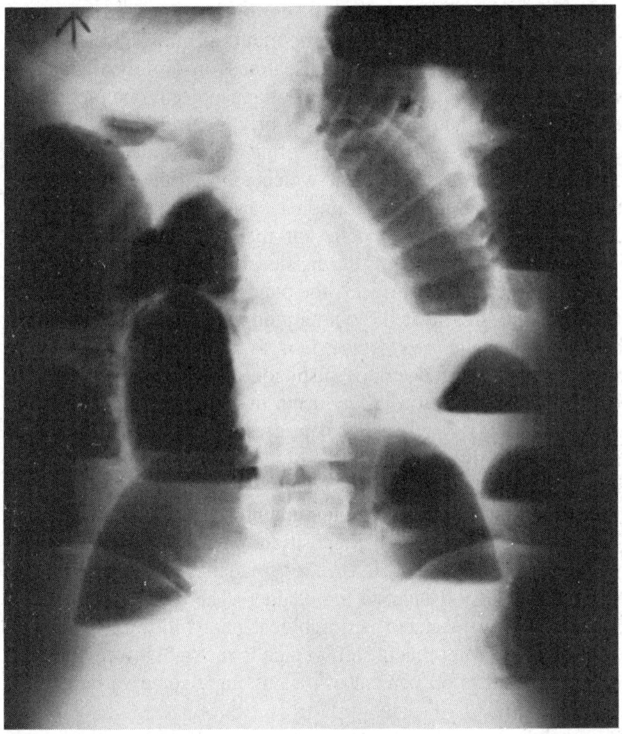

FIGURE 244-1 Acute mechanical obstruction of small intestine (upright film). Note air-fluid levels, marked distention of bowel loops, and absence of colonic gas.

ladder'' pattern with air-fluid levels and an absence or paucity of colonic gas are pathognomonic (Fig. 244-1). These findings, however, are absent in slightly over half the cases of strangulating small-bowel obstruction, especially early in the disease. A general haze due to peritoneal fluid and sometimes a ''coffee-bean''-shaped mass are seen in strangulating obstruction. Occasionally the films are normal, but when symptoms are consistent with obstruction of the small intestine, a normal film should suggest strangulation. Roentgenographic differentiation of partial mechanical small-bowel obstruction from adynamic ileus may be impossible since gas is present in both small and large intestine; however, colonic distention is usually more prominent in adynamic ileus. A radiopaque dye given by mouth is useful in making this distinction.

Colonic obstruction with a competent ileocecal valve is easily recognized because distention with gas is mainly confined to the colon. Barium enema, sigmoidoscopy, or colonoscopy, depending upon the suspected site of obstruction, are usually advisable to determine the nature of the lesion except when concomitant perforation is suspected, a rare occurrence. Sigmoidoscopy may be therapeutic in cases of sigmoid volvulus. When the ileocecal valve is incompetent, the films resemble those of partial small-bowel obstruction or adynamic ileus, and barium enema or colonoscopy is necessary to establish the correct diagnosis. Barium given by mouth is perfectly safe when obstruction is in the small intestine since the barium sulfate does not become inspissated in this location. *Barium should never be given by mouth to a patient with possible colonic obstruction* until that possibility has been excluded by barium enema.

PROGNOSIS AND TREATMENT **Small-intestinal obstruction** The overall mortality rate for obstruction of the small intestine is about 10 percent, even under the most optimal conditions. While the mortality rate for nonstrangulating obstruction is as low as 5 to 8 percent, that for strangulating obstruction has been reported to be between 20 and 75 percent. Well over half of the deaths from small-bowel obstruction occur in those with strangulation; however, the latter constitute only one-fourth to one-third of the cases. Careful studies indicate that the clinical, laboratory, and x-ray findings are not reliable in distinguishing strangulating from nonstrangulating obstruction when obstruction is complete. Complete obstruction is suggested when there has been a total cessation in the passage of gas or stool per rectum and when gas is absent in the distal intestine by x-ray. Since strangulating small-bowel obstruction is always complete, operation should always be undertaken in such patients after suitable preparation. Prior to operation, fluid and electrolyte balance should be restored, and decompression instituted by means of a nasogastric tube. Six to eight hours of preparation may be necessary. During this period broad-spectrum antibiotics are indicated if strangulation is felt to be likely, but operation should not be delayed unless there is unequivocal clinical and roentgenographic evidence of resolution of the obstruction during the period of preparation. Attempts to pass a long tube into the small intestine usually fail while putting the patient through uncomfortable unproductive manipulations which delay appropriate fluid replacement and decompression. *There are probably few if any indications for the use of a long intestinal tube.* Procrastination of operation because of improvement in well-being of the patient during resuscitation and gastric decompression usually leads to unnecessary and hazardous delay in proper treatment. Purely nonoperative therapy is safe only in the presence of incomplete obstruction and is best utilized in patients with (1) repeated episodes of partial obstruction, (2) recent postoperative partial obstruction, and (3) partial obstruction following a recent episode of diffuse peritonitis.

Colonic obstruction The mortality rate for colonic obstruction is about 20 percent. As in small-bowel obstruction, nonoperative treatment is contraindicated unless the obstruction is incomplete. Occasionally, but not always, when the obstruction is incomplete, nonoperative therapy may result in sufficient decompression that a definitive operative procedure can be undertaken at a later date. This can usually be accomplished by discontinuation of all oral intake and perhaps by nasogastric suction, although attempts to decompress a *completely* obstructed colon by intubation are almost invariably futile. A long intestinal tube will not decompress an obstructed colon with a competent ileocecal valve. When obstruction is complete, early operation is mandatory, especially when the ileocecal valve is competent; cecal gangrene is likely if the cecal diameter exceeds 10 cm on plain abdominal film. For obstruction on the left side of the colon, the most common site, preliminary operative decompression by cecostomy or transverse colostomy followed by definitive resection of the primary lesion is the treatment of choice. For a lesion of the right or transverse colon, primary resection and anastomosis can safely be performed because distention of the ileum with consequent discrepancy in size and hazard in suture are not present.

Adynamic ileus This type of ileus usually responds to nonoperative continuous decompression and adequate treatment of the primary disease. The prognosis is usually good. Recently, successful decompression of severe colonic ileus has been accomplished by colonoscopy, but this should be avoided if tenderness in the right lower quadrant suggests possible cecal gangrene. Rarely, adynamic colonic distention may become so great that cecostomy is required if cecal gangrene is feared. Spastic ileus usually responds to treatment of the primary disease.

REFERENCES

Becker WF: Acute adhesive ileus: A study of 412 cases with particular reference to the abuse of tube decompression in treatment. Surg Gynecol Obstet 95:472, 1952

Bulkley GB et al: Intraoperative determination of small intestinal viability following ischemic injury: Prospective controlled trial of two adjuvant methods (Doppler and fluorescein) compared with standard clinical judgement. Ann Surg 193:628, 1981

Cohn I, Atik M: Strangulation obstruction: Closed loop studies. Ann Surg 153:94, 1961

Dubois A et al: Postoperative ileus: Physiopathology, etiology and treatment. Ann Surg 178:781, 1973

Gough IR: Strangulating adhesive small bowel radiographs. Br J Surg 65:431, 1978

Hofsetter SR: Acute adhesive obstruction of the small intestine. Surg Gynecol Obstet 152:141, 1981

Jackson BR: The diagnosis of colonic obstruction. Dis Colon Rectum 25:603, 1982

Nolan DJ: Barium examination of the small intestine. Gut 22:682, 1981

SHIELDS R: The absorption and secretion of fluid and electrolytes by the obstructed bowel. Br J Surg 52:774, 1965

SILEN W: *Cope's Early Diagnosis of the Acute Abdomen*, 17th ed. London, Oxford, 1987

245 ACUTE APPENDICITIS

WILLIAM SILEN

INCIDENCE AND EPIDEMIOLOGY The maximum incidence of acute appendicitis occurs in the second and third decades of life. While the disease may be encountered at any time of life, it is relatively rare at the extremes of age. Males and females are equally affected except between puberty and age 25, when males predominate in a 3:2 ratio. Perforation is relatively much more common in infancy and in the aged, during which periods mortality rates are highest. The mortality rate has decreased steadily in Europe and the United States from 8.1 per 100,000 of the population in 1941 to less than 1 per 100,000 in 1970 and subsequently. The absolute incidence of the disease also decreased by about 40 percent between 1940 and 1960 but since then has remained unchanged. Although various factors such as changing dietary habits, altered intestinal flora, and better nutrition and intake of vitamins have been suggested to explain the reduced incidence, the exact reasons have not been elucidated. Of interest is that the overall incidence of appendicitis is much lower in underdeveloped countries, especially parts of Africa, and in lower socioeconomic groups.

PATHOGENESIS The primary pathogenetic hallmark has always been thought to be luminal obstruction. While obstruction can be identified by careful examination in 30 to 40 percent of cases, recent studies have shown that ulceration of the mucosa is the initial event in the majority. The causation of the ulceration is unknown, although a viral etiology has been postulated. Recently, it has been suggested that infection with *Yersinia* organisms may cause the disease since careful study has shown that high complement fixation titers have been found in as many as 30 percent of cases of proven appendicitis 1 week after operation. Whether the inflammatory reaction attendant with ulceration is sufficient to obstruct the tiny appendiceal lumen even transiently is also not clear. Obstruction, when present, is most commonly caused by a fecalith, which results from accumulation and inspissation of fecal matter around vegetable fibers. Enlarged lymphoid follicles associated with viral infections (e.g., measles), inspissated barium, worms (e.g., pinworms, *Ascaris*, and *Taenia*), and tumors (e.g., carcinoid or carcinoma) may also obstruct the lumen. Secretion of mucus distends the organ, which has a capacity of only 0.1 to 0.2 mL, and luminal pressures rise as high as 60 cmH_2O. Luminal bacteria multiply and invade the appendiceal wall as venous engorgement and subsequent arterial compromise result from the high intraluminal pressures. Finally, gangrene and perforation occur. If the process evolves slowly, adjacent organs such as the terminal ileum, cecum, and omentum may wall off the appendiceal area so that a localized abscess will develop, whereas rapid progression of vascular impairment may cause perforation with free access to the peritoneal cavity. Subsequent rupture of primary appendiceal abscesses may produce fistulas between the appendix and bladder, small intestine, sigmoid, or cecum. Occasionally, acute appendicitis may be the first manifestation of Crohn's disease. While chronic infection of the appendix with tuberculosis, amebiasis, and actinomycosis may occur, a useful clinical aphorism states that *chronic appendiceal inflammation is not usually the cause of prolonged abdominal pain of weeks' or months' duration*. In contrast, it is clear that recurrent acute appendicitis does occur, often with complete resolution of inflammation and symptoms between attacks. Recurrent acute appendicitis may become more frequent as antibiotics are dispensed more freely.

CLINICAL MANIFESTATIONS The history and sequence of symptoms are among the most important diagnostic features of appendicitis. The initial symptom is almost invariably *abdominal pain* of the visceral type, resulting from appendiceal contractions or distention of the lumen. It is usually poorly localized in the periumbilical or epigastric regions. There is often an accompanying urge to defecate or pass flatus, neither of which relieves the distress. This visceral pain is mild, often cramping, and rarely catastrophic in nature, usually lasting 4 to 6 h, but may not be noted by stoic individuals or by some patients during sleep. As inflammation spreads to the parietal peritoneal surfaces, the pain becomes somatic, steady, and more severe, aggravated by motion or cough and usually located in the *right lower quadrant*. *Anorexia* is so frequent that the presence of hunger should arouse serious suspicion of the diagnosis of acute appendicitis. *Nausea* and *vomiting* occur in 50 to 60 percent of cases, but vomiting is rarely profuse and protracted. The development of nausea and vomiting before the onset of pain is extremely rare. Change in bowel habit is of little diagnostic value since any or no alteration may be observed, although the presence of diarrhea caused by an inflamed appendix in juxtaposition to the sigmoid may cause serious diagnostic difficulties. Urinary frequency and dysuria occur if the appendix lies adjacent to the bladder. The typical sequence of symptoms (poorly localized periumbilical pain followed by nausea and vomiting with subsequent shift of pain to the right lower quadrant) occurs in only 50 to 60 percent of patients, and some variations are considered below.

Physical findings vary with time after onset of the illness and according to the location of the appendix, which may be situated deep in the pelvic cul-de-sac, in the right lower quadrant in any relation to the peritoneum, cecum, and small intestine, in the right upper quadrant, or even in the left lower quadrant. *The diagnosis cannot be established unless tenderness can be elicited.* While tenderness is sometimes absent in the early visceral stage of the disease, it ultimately always develops and is found in any location corresponding to the position of the appendix. Abdominal tenderness may be completely absent if a retrocecal or pelvic appendix is present, in which case the sole physical finding may be tenderness in the flank or on rectal or pelvic examination. Percussion, rebound tenderness, and referred rebound tenderness are often, but not invariably, present; they are most likely to be absent early in the illness. Flexion of the right hip and guarded movement by the patient are due to parietal peritoneal involvement. Hyperesthesia of the skin of the right lower quadrant and a positive psoas or obturator sign are often late findings and are rarely of diagnostic value. When the inflamed appendix is in close proximity to the anterior parietal peritoneum, muscular rigidity is present, yet is often minimal early. The temperature is usually normal or slightly elevated [37.2 to 38°C (99 to 100.5°F)], but a temperature above 38.3°C (101°F) should always suggest the presence of perforation. Tachycardia is commensurate with the elevation of the temperature. Rigidity and tenderness become more marked as the disease progresses to perforation and localized or diffuse peritonitis. Distention is rare unless severe diffuse peritonitis has developed. The alleged disappearance of pain and tenderness just prior to perforation is extremely unusual. A mass may develop if localized perforation has occurred but usually will not be detectable before 3 days after onset of the disease. Earlier presence of a mass suggests carcinoma of the cecum or Crohn's disease. Perforation is rare before 24 h after onset of symptoms, but the rate may be as high as 80 percent after 48 h.

Laboratory examination does not establish the diagnosis since the latter is based primarily on clinical grounds. Although moderate leukocytosis of 10,000 to 18,000 cells per microliter is frequent (with a concomitant shift to immature cells), the absence of leukocytosis does not eliminate the possibility of acute appendicitis. Leukocytosis of greater than 20,000 cells per microliter should alert the clinician to the probability of perforation. Anemia and blood in the stool suggest a primary diagnosis of carcinoma of the cecum, especially in elderly individuals. The urine may contain a few white or red blood cells without bacteria if the appendix lies close to the right ureter or bladder.

Urinalysis is most useful, however, in excluding genitourinary conditions which may mimic acute appendicitis. X-rays are rarely of value except when an opaque fecalith (5 percent of patients) is observed in the right lower quadrant (especially in children) together with other clinical findings consistent with appendicitis. Consequently there is no routine need to obtain films of the abdomen unless there is a possibility of other conditions such as intestinal obstruction or ureteral calculus. In some cases in which symptoms are either recurrent or more prolonged, a careful barium enema may disclose an extrinsic defect on the medial wall of the cecum or a calcified fecalith. The diagnosis may also be established by the ultrasonic demonstration of an enlarged and thick-walled appendix, but if the appendix cannot be seen, the diagnosis cannot be excluded.

While the typical historical sequence and physical findings are present in 50 to 60 percent of cases, it is obvious that a wide variety of atypical patterns of disease are encountered, especially at the age extremes and during pregnancy. The 70 to 80 percent incidence of perforation and generalized peritonitis in infants under 2 years of age is dramatic testimony to the importance of the history in the early detection of the disease. Any infant or child with diarrhea, vomiting, and abdominal pain is highly suspect. Fever is much more common in this age group, and abdominal distention is often the only physical finding. In the elderly, pain and tenderness are often obtunded, and thus the diagnosis is frequently delayed. A 30 percent incidence of perforation in patients over 70 attests to the importance of this delay. Elderly patients often present themselves initially with a slightly painful mass (a primary appendiceal abscess), or sometimes appear with adhesive intestinal obstruction 5 or 6 days after a previously undetected perforated appendix. Appendicitis occurs about once in every 1000 pregnancies and is the most common extrauterine condition requiring abdominal operation. The diagnosis may be missed or delayed because of the frequent occurrence of mild abdominal discomfort and nausea and vomiting during pregnancy. During the last trimester when the mortality rate from appendicitis is highest, uterine displacement of the appendix to the right upper quadrant and laterally leads to confusion in diagnosis.

DIFFERENTIAL DIAGNOSIS A listing of the differential diagnoses of acute appendicitis would produce an encyclopedic compendium of all conditions which cause abdominal pain since appendicitis may simulate any of these diseases. Diagnostic accuracy is about 75 to 80 percent for experienced clinicians and must be based solely on the clinical criteria outlined above. It is probably better to err slightly in the direction of overdiagnosis since delay is associated with perforation and increased morbidity and mortality. In unperforated appendicitis the mortality rate is 0.1 percent, little more than that associated with general anesthesia; for perforated appendicitis there is an overall mortality of 3 percent, a figure which increases to 15 percent in the elderly. In doubtful cases 4 to 6 h of observation is always more beneficial than harmful, however. The most common conditions discovered at operation when acute appendicitis is erroneously diagnosed are, in rough order of frequency, mesenteric lymphadenitis, no organic disease, acute pelvic inflammatory disease, ruptured graafian follicle or corpus luteum cyst, and acute gastroenteritis. In addition, acute cholecystitis, perforated ulcer, acute pancreatitis, acute diverticulitis, strangulating intestinal obstruction, ureteral calculus, and pyelonephritis frequently present diagnostic difficulties.

It is useful to consider separately some of the more common and difficult diagnostic possibilities, especially in the female. Differentiation of *pelvic inflammatory disease* from acute appendicitis may be virtually impossible. Gram-negative intracellular diplococci on cervical smear are not pathognomonic unless *Neisseria gonorrhea* can be cultured. Pain on movement of the cervix is not specific and may occur in appendicitis if perforation has occurred or if the appendix lies adjacent to the uterus or adnexa. *Rupture of a graafian follicle* (mittelschmerz) occurs at midcycle with spill of blood and fluid to produce pain and tenderness more diffuse and usually of a less severe degree than in appendicitis. Fever and leukocytosis are usually absent. *Rupture of a corpus luteum cyst* is identical clinically to rupture of a graafian follicle but develops about the time of menstruation. The presence of an adnexal mass and evidence of blood loss help differentiate *ruptured tubal pregnancy*. *Twisted ovarian cyst* and *endometriosis* occasionally are difficult to distinguish from appendicitis. In all of these female conditions, ultrasonic examination of the pelvis and laparoscopy may be of great value.

Acute mesenteric lymphadenitis is the appellation usually given when enlarged, slightly reddened lymph nodes at the root of the mesentery and a normal appendix are encountered at operation in a patient who usually has right lower quadrant tenderness and a somewhat higher temperature than most patients with acute appendicitis. Whether this is a single, discrete entity is unclear since the causative factor is not known. It has been recognized recently that some of these patients have infection with *Yersinia pseudotuberculosis* or *Y. enterocolytica* in which case the diagnosis can be established by culture of the mesenteric nodes or by serologic titers (Chap. 121). The diagnosis is essentially impossible clinically, although retrospectively there often appears to have been more diffuse pain and tenderness. Children seem to be affected more frequently than adults. Operation should be undertaken unless there is rapid resolution of all symptoms and findings. *Acute gastroenteritis* usually causes profuse watery diarrhea, often with nausea and vomiting but without localized findings. Between cramps, the abdomen is completely relaxed. In salmonella gastroenteritis the abdominal findings are similar, although the pain may be more severe and more localized, and fever and chills are common. The occurrence of similar symptoms among other members of the family may be helpful. When the diagnosis of acute pelvic appendicitis with perforation has been missed, gastroenteritis is the most common previous working diagnosis. Persistent abdominal or rectal tenderness should eliminate the diagnosis of gastroenteritis. *Regional enteritis* (Crohn's disease) is usually associated with a more prolonged history, often with previous exacerbations regarded by the patient or physician as episodes of gastroenteritis unless the diagnosis has been established previously. *Meckel's diverticulitis* usually cannot be distinguished from acute appendicitis but is very rare.

TREATMENT Cathartics and frequent enemas should be avoided if appendicitis is under consideration, and antibiotics should not be administered when the diagnosis is in question, as they will only mask the presence or development of perforation. The treatment is early operation and appendectomy as soon as the patient can be prepared. Preparation rarely takes more than 1 to 2 h in early appendicitis but may require 6 to 8 h in cases of severe sepsis and dehydration associated with late perforation. The *only* circumstance in which operation is *not* indicated is the presence of a palpable mass 3 to 5 days after the onset of symptoms. Should operation be undertaken at that time, a phlegmon rather than a definitive abscess will be found, and complications from dissection of such a phlegmon are frequent. Such patients treated with broad-spectrum antibiotics, parenteral fluids, and rest usually show resolution of the mass and symptoms within 1 week. *Interval appendectomy* can and should be done safely 3 months later. Should the mass enlarge or the patient become more toxic, drainage of the abscess is necessary. The complications of subphrenic, pelvic, or other intraabdominal abscesses usually follow perforation with generalized peritonitis and can be avoided by early diagnosis of the disease.

REFERENCES

BOLTON JP: Assessment of the value of the white cell count in management of suspected acute appendicitis. Br J Surg 62:906, 1975

BUSUTTIL RW et al: Effect of prophylactic antibiotics in acute nonperforated appendicitis: A prospective, randomized double-blind clinical study. Ann Surg 194:502, 1981

BUTLER C: Surgical pathology of acute appendicitis. Hum Pathol 12:870, 1981

JULIEN BCM et al: A prospective study of ultrasonography in the diagnosis of appendicitis. N Engl J Med 317:666, 1987

KOEPSELL TD et al: Factors affecting perforation in acute appendicitis. Surg Gynecol Obstet 153:508, 1981

RAVAL B et al: Use of computed tomography in appendicitis: Technique, findings, and pitfalls. J Comput Tomogr 11:17, 1987

SCHWERK WB et al: Ultrasonography in the diagnosis of acute appendicitis: A retrospective study. Gastroenterology 97:630, 1989

VANTRAPPEN G et al.: *Yersinia* enteritis and enterocolitis: Gastroenterological aspects. Gastroenterology 72:220, 1977

246 DISEASES OF THE PERITONEUM AND MESENTERY

KURT J. ISSELBACHER / J. THOMAS LaMONT

ACUTE PERITONITIS Peritonitis is a localized or generalized inflammatory process of the peritoneum that may appear in both acute and chronic forms. In the acute form the motor activity of the intestine is decreased, and the intestinal lumen becomes distended with gas and fluid. Fluid accumulates as a result of failure to reabsorb the 7 or 8 liters normally secreted daily into the lumen and absorbed from the distal small bowel and colon. There is also accumulation of fluid in the peritoneal cavity as well as decreased oral intake. These combined losses can lead to rapid depletion of the plasma volume with impaired cardiac and renal function.

Etiology Peritonitis may be due to entry of bacteria into the peritoneal cavity from a perforation in the gastrointestinal tract or from an external penetrating wound. It may be secondary to severe chemical reactions from the release of pancreatic enzymes, the digestive juices of the upper gastrointestinal tract, or bile as a result of injury or perforation of the intestine or biliary tract. Patients with systemic lupus erythematosus may have bouts of sterile peritonitis during attacks of their disease.

The most common causes of bacterial peritonitis are appendicitis, perforations associated with diverticulitis, peptic ulcer, gangrenous gallbladder, and gangrenous obstruction of the small bowel from adhesive bands, incarcerated hernia, or volvulus. Any lesion leading to the escape of intestinal bacteria may be a source, including a perforating carcinoma, foreign body, and ulcerative colitis. The peritoneal cavity is remarkably resistant to contamination, and unless continuing contamination occurs, the disease process becomes localized. Patients with alcoholic cirrhosis and ascites have an increased susceptibility to spontaneous bacterial peritonitis, usually from enteric pathogens. This complication occurs in the absence of recognizable perforation of a viscus, and may be due to leakage of bacteria through the intestinal wall.

Clinical features These usually consist of increasing abdominal pain, distention, nausea and vomiting, inability to pass feces or flatus, fever, hypotension, tachycardia, thirst, and oliguria. On physical examination the patient appears acutely ill and febrile and has a variable degree of abdominal distention. The abdomen is usually acutely tender and tympanitic, often with rebound tenderness. The location of the pain and tenderness depends on the underlying cause and whether the inflammation is localized or generalized. In *localized* peritonitis, as seen in uncomplicated appendicitis or diverticulitis, the physical findings are limited to the area of inflammation. With widespread peritoneal inflammation there is *generalized* peritonitis with diffuse abdominal tenderness and rebound. Rigidity of the abdominal wall is a common finding in peritonitis and may be localized or generalized.

Peristalsis may be present initially but usually disappears as the illness progresses. Hypotension is common, as is leukocytosis, which often is greater than 20,000 cells per microliter. Plain abdominal films may reveal dilatation of the large and small bowel with edema of the small-bowel wall as evidenced by the distance between adjacent loops of gas-filled small intestine. Diagnostic paracentesis is sometimes valuable in determining the nature of the exudate as well as whether bacteria can be demonstrated or cultured. Diabetic ketoacidosis, lead colic, gastric crises of syphilis, and acute porphyria may cause severe abdominal symptoms that resemble the picture of acute peritonitis.

GONOCOCCAL PERITONITIS This usually involves an extension of gonococcal infection from a primary focus in the female reproductive tract. The signs of inflammation usually are limited to the pelvis, but there may be findings of a mild generalized peritonitis. Occasionally the patient has right upper quadrant pain and tenderness caused by gonococcal perihepatitis involving the liver capsule and adjacent peritoneum (Fitz-Hugh–Curtis syndrome; see also Chap. 110).

STARCH PERITONITIS An acute granulomatous peritonitis can develop in some patients as a foreign-body reaction to cornstarch used to powder surgical gloves. The clinical picture is that of acute abdominal pain and fever 10 to 30 days after an abdominal operation. The diagnosis can be made by paracentesis and demonstration of starch granules in monocytes. However, most patients are reexplored because of the fear of abscess or bacterial peritonitis, with the finding of foreign-body granuloma studding the peritoneum.

PSEUDOMYXOMA PERITONEI This is a rare condition resulting from rupture of a mucocele of the appendix or of a mucinous ovarian cyst. The abdomen becomes filled with masses of jelly-like material. Occasionally, with removal of the mucocele or the ovarian cyst and most of the myxomatous material, a cure may ensue. In other cases, however, the mucoid material recurs, leading to progressive wasting and eventual death. Colloid carcinoma arising from the stomach or colon with peritoneal implants may resemble pseudomyxoma at laparotomy. The course of this type of highly malignant tumor is one of rapid cachexia and early death. The diagnosis can usually be made by the appearance of many highly malignant cells in the peritoneal implants.

CANCER OF THE PERITONEUM Aside from mesothelioma, which in most patients is caused by previous exposure to asbestos, cancer of the peritoneum is usually secondary to a neoplasm within the abdomen, most commonly of the stomach and ovary. This type of metastatic malignancy is invariably associated with progressive ascites with a high specific gravity and high protein content, often with large numbers of red blood cells or even gross blood. The diagnosis is established by demonstrating malignant cells in the fluid. The clinical progress of this malignant spread can sometimes be arrested by installations of radioactive gold, nitrogen mustard, or chloroquine.

FAMILIAL MEDITERRANEAN FEVER See Chap. 278.

PNEUMATOSIS CYSTOIDES INTESTINALIS This is a condition in which multiple gas-filled blebs or cysts accumulate in the intestinal wall beneath the serosal surface of the bowel. The exact source of the gas has not been explained satisfactorily. In some instances, this disease is associated with specific ulceration of the intestinal mucosa, in particular peptic ulcer with outlet obstruction. Cysts in the wall of the small bowel are seen as an occasional complication of mesenteric vascular occlusion. In the large bowel, these cysts are usually benign, may be seen with a variety of other disorders, and usually disappear in time.

There are no specific physical findings secondary to the pneumatosis, and the diagnosis is made either by x-ray or at laparotomy. Occasionally the subserosal cysts may rupture, resulting in pneumoperitoneum.

CHYLOUS ASCITES This term refers to the accumulation of chyle (intestinal lymph) in the peritoneal cavity. The condition is sometimes associated with chylothorax. The fluid in the peritoneal cavity appears milky or creamy because of the presence of chylomicrons. This fat may be demonstrated microscopically by staining with Sudan III and may be removed by acidification of the fluid followed by extraction with ether. The chyle (lipid) will then go into the ether phase. Many conditions may be associated with the cloudy or milky-appearing peritoneal fluid, so-called pseudochylous ascites. The milky or turbid appearance is usually due to the presence of protein and desquamated cells. The turbidity of this fluid will not be removed with the ether but will clear with addition of alkali.

The causes of chylous ascites include (1) penetrating or nonpenetrating trauma that damages the main duct in the lymphatic system within the abdomen, (2) intestinal obstruction if it is associated with rupture of a major lymphatic channel, (3) congenital lymphangiectasia, (4) malignant disease or tuberculous infection that obstructs the intestinal lymphatics, (5) filariasis, or (6) cirrhosis.

The sudden accumulation of chyle in the peritoneal cavity often results in abdominal pain, signs of peritoneal irritation, and leukocytosis. These symptoms gradually subside, leaving the patient with a distended but nontender, fluid-filled abdomen. Lymphangiography is of value in determining the location of the leak or site of obstruction to the lymphatic channels. The course depends upon the underlying etiologic factors.

MESENTERIC LIPODYSTROPHY This is a rare disorder usually affecting middle-aged women and characterized pathologically by infiltration of the mesentery with lipid-laden macrophages and fibrous tissue. These patients present with ill-defined abdominal pain and occasionally an abdominal mass. The diagnosis is made at laparotomy by demonstration of thick fibrofatty masses at the root of the mesentery with retraction and distortion of the bowel loops.

REFERENCES

KIPFER RE et al: Mesenteric lipodystrophy. Ann Intern Med 80:582, 1974
LIMBER GK et al: Pseudomyxoma peritonei. Ann Surg 1978:587, 1973
PRESS OW et al: Evaluation and management of chylous ascites. Ann Intern Med 96:358, 1982
SCHWARTZ SI et al: *Principles of Surgery*, 5th ed. New York, McGraw-Hill, 1989
TITO L et al: Spontaneous bacterial peritonitis. Hepatology 8:27, 1988
WARSHAW AL: Diagnosis of starch peritonitis by paracentesis. Lancet 2:1054, 1972

section 2 Liver and biliary tract disease

247 BIOLOGIC AND CLINICAL APPROACHES TO LIVER DISEASE

KURT J. ISSELBACHER / DANIEL K. PODOLSKY

BIOLOGIC CONSIDERATIONS An understanding of diseases of the liver and their clinical manifestations can be derived from an understanding of fundamental hepatic structure and function. An appreciation of anatomic aspects of the liver and biliary tree from the gross level to that of the individual hepatocyte and other cellular constituents is needed to understand the spectrum of clinical manifestations of liver disease. The dual blood supply, unique to the liver and including the portal venous system, makes the liver an intermediate filter for most of the venous drainage of the abdominal viscera. This often leads to secondary hepatic involvement in a number of extrahepatic diseases and makes the liver a relatively common site of solid tumor metastases. Furthermore, an appreciation of the relevant anatomy, especially that of the portal venous system, is important in understanding clinically important manifestations of portal hypertension, a common complication of chronic liver disease when scarring and regeneration lead to distortion of the intrahepatic microvasculature. These anatomic considerations lead the clinician to look for evidence of splenic enlargement and hypersplenism, gastrointestinal bleeding, accumulation of ascites, and signs of portal-systemic encephalopathy. Certainly an understanding of the anatomy of the biliary tract from canaliculus to common bile duct is integral to understanding the basis and sequelae of obstructive jaundice. While inflammation of the gallbladder may lead to fever and pain, choledocholithiasis will cause biliary colic as well as jaundice. Diffuse processes affecting the intrahepatic ducts, such as primary sclerosing cholangitis, will lead to cholestasis and its attendant symptoms while a focal process affecting a single branch of the biliary tree, such as a neoplasm, usually will not.

The structural organization at a level intermediate between the gross anatomic and the cellular also contributes to the clinical patterns seen with disorders of the liver. While various concepts have been offered, most useful is that of the traditional liver lobule. Blood emanates from the portal venules at the periphery and passes through the hepatic sinusoids to the central vein. The portal venules, terminal bile ductules, and hepatic arterioles are arranged in a *triad*. Appreciation of this organization and the presence of concentric zones of function within the lobule explain distinct patterns of injury such as the centrilobular injury resulting from ischemia. These structural features no doubt also provide the basis for the relative preservation of hepatocellular function in many disorders that can lead to significant portal hypertension, such as schistosomiasis and biliary cirrhosis.

As important as the anatomic features are in understanding liver disease, many liver disorders and their manifestations can only be appreciated in the context of the functional complexity of the liver at the cellular level. As detailed in Chap. 250, the hepatocyte plays an important role in diverse general metabolic processes that may be deranged as a consequence of liver disease. In addition this metabolic diversity leads to hepatic involvement in many inborn errors of metabolism, including a wide variety of storage diseases, and less well-understood disorders of iron metabolism (hemosiderosis and hemochromatosis) and copper homeostasis (Wilson's disease).

Some other functional aspects should also be emphasized. The hepatocyte modifies numerous endogenous (e.g., bilirubin) and exogenous (e.g., alcohol, acetaminophen) potentially toxic compounds through oxidation, reduction, and conjugation carried out by several enzymes of the endoplasmic reticulum. Conjugation of substrates generally facilitates their hepatic excretion, converting water-insoluble substances to water-soluble derivatives. It is therefore not surprising that parenchymal liver disease may lead to either conjugated or unconjugated hyperbilirubinemia and jaundice. Metabolic modifications may significantly alter the pharmacologic activity of drugs through formation of derivatives with either decreased or enhanced activity. These metabolic processes may create intermediates which are toxic to the liver itself. This explains the selective susceptibility of the liver to the toxicity of carbon tetrachloride, acetaminophen, and, most importantly, alcohol, which is converted to acetaldehyde.

Additional functions of the hepatocyte that may have significant clinical ramifications include the production of a variety of soluble proteins for secretion into the circulation and the presence of receptors specific for various circulating ligands. The latter is a property shared with the Kupffer cell which fulfills much of its function as a constituent of the reticuloendothelial system by clearing a number of serum glycoproteins through asialoglycoprotein receptor–mediated endocytosis. There is evidence to suggest that some of the substances taken up by this endocytotic mechanism may subsequently pass to and through the hepatocyte to complete an enterohepatic circulation. Carcinoembryonic antigen (CEA) is a glycoprotein and putative tumor marker which is handled in this manner, leading to artifactual elevations in hepatobiliary disease. In contrast to the Kupffer cell, the spectrum of ligands taken up by hepatocytes via specific receptors is much broader. In addition to ligands targeted for lysosomal degradation, the hepatocyte possesses receptors for ligands which are metabolically active after their uptake and dissociation from their receptors. These include transferrin-bound iron and, most important, low-density lipoprotein (LDL) which contributes to regulation of overall body cholesterol metabolism. Disruption of lysosomal degradation of specific ligands in hereditary storage disease leads to hepatomegaly and to a variety of infiltrative disorders. Disruption of the nonlysosomal endocytotic pathway ligands can lead to systemic disorders. It is not clear whether specific receptors or other hepatocyte membrane components play a role in the relative or absolute tropism of infectious agents (particularly the hepatitis viruses) which account for a large proportion of both acute and chronic liver disease. However, the relative selectivity of the hepatitis viruses (A, B, non-A, non-B, and indirectly D) for the hepatocyte is essential in understanding the clinical features, which derive from the extent of hepatocyte destruction, of the illnesses caused by these agents. At the same time the hepatocyte may be infected by less strictly organotropic agents including other viruses (e.g., Epstein-Barr virus) and a wide variety of bacterial and parasitic organisms. The vascular supply of the liver leads to its frequent involvement in disseminated infections.

A final feature of hepatocyte cell biology that contributes to the expression of liver disease is the potential for proliferation and regeneration. Although few mitotic figures are seen in normal hepatic parenchyma, rapid regeneration involving both proliferation and cellular hypertrophy occurs following hepatic resection in experimental animals and humans. The capacity for hepatocellular regeneration is evident in the complete recovery which usually occurs following fulminant hepatitis (due either to viral or toxic agents) if the patient can be sustained through the period of acute injury. Architecturally disordered regeneration in concert with fibrosis is an essential factor in the development of cirrhosis and leads both to disruption of blood flow through the hepatic parenchyma and to uneven hepatocellular function due to distortion of normal lobular structure. Although the mechanisms which control hepatocyte proliferation after hepatocellular loss are incompletely understood, evidence suggests that a complex balance of various peptide growth factors plays an important role.

CLINICAL CONSIDERATIONS In approaching the patient with known or suspected liver disease, consideration of the patient's problem in the context of a few salient questions permits the clinician to focus on the most important diagnostic possibilities and the severity of the illness. Is the problem primarily hepatocellular or cholestatic? Was the onset of the illness abrupt or gradual? Has the problem led to clinically significant impairment of normal hepatocellular function such as signs of altered mentation or coagulopathy? Are there signs or symptoms of portal hypertension? Important and reliable clues which address these questions may often be obtained from a careful history and physical examination.

Clinical History A number of historic features may distinguish cholestatic and hepatocellular disease processes. A history of marked right upper quadrant pain or previous indigestion suggests cholelithiasis, cholecystitis, or choledocholithiasis, whereas vague nagging discomfort suggests hepatocellular or infiltrative disease with hepatomegaly causing pain due to distention of Glisson's capsule. Additional important symptoms which should be elicited include pruritus, jaundice, anorexia, weight loss, and fever. Complaints of easy bruising or mental confusion by the patient (or family) should be regarded as ominous signs of either fulminant acute or advanced chronic liver disease.

Family history is important with respect to jaundice, anemia, splenectomy, or cholecystectomy; a positive history may be helpful in diagnosing hemolytic anemia, congenital or familial hyperbilirubinemia, or gallstones. In Wilson's disease (hepatolenticular degeneration), there may be a family history of tremor or neurologic abnormalities. *Occupation* should be reviewed in detail, and *environmental factors* need to be examined. Note should be made of the use of any medications or exposure to known or putative toxins such as carbon tetrachloride, beryllium, or vinyl chloride. The patient should be asked about travel to other countries, especially to areas where hepatitis may be endemic. Careful questioning regarding alcohol intake is important in most cases. Since the alcoholic often denies or understates the amounts consumed, it may be desirable to check the validity of the history with relatives or close friends.

Contact with jaundiced patients (especially intimate or sexual relations) should be noted. If the patient has had any *injections*, hepatitis B or non-A, non-B infection may be the underlying disease. Injections include blood tests, blood or plasma transfusions, tattooing, and dental treatment. Postoperative jaundice may be due to the anesthetic, especially after multiple uses of halothane, or to impaired hepatic excretory function resulting from relative hypoxemia of liver cells during the operative or postoperative period.

As suggested, the *onset of the illness* should be noted. The relatively abrupt onset of nausea, anorexia, and aversion to smoking followed by progressive jaundice suggests viral hepatitis. A gradual development of jaundice associated with pruritus suggests cholestasis. Intermittent right upper quadrant abdominal pain followed by cholestatic jaundice points to gallstone disease, while the gradual onset of painless jaundice with weight loss is suggestive of tumor, such as carcinoma of the head of the pancreas. Jaundice associated with fever and chills makes cholangitis and extrahepatic biliary obstruction likely possibilities. The awareness of progressive abdominal swelling, perhaps first noticed because of tightness of clothing, suggests ascites which may be due to malignancy or an insidious first manifestation of cirrhosis. The patient with hepatitis generally feels ill, and dark urine and light stools occur before the appearance of scleral or skin icterus. In cholestatic hepatitis, the patient may feel relatively well and complain only of symptoms due to the obstruction, such as pruritus.

Physical examination Jaundice is looked for in the sclera as well as the skin. Pallor indicative of anemia may be a reflection of hemolysis, cirrhosis, or neoplasm. Significant cachexia, especially of the extremities, may be associated with cancer or cirrhosis. In the cirrhotic patient, one should look for stigmas of alcohol abuse such as parotid and lacrimal gland enlargement and Dupuytren's contracture, as well as other features of cirrhosis such as gynecomastia, testicular atrophy, and diminished axillary or pubic hair.

The *skin examination* may reveal ecchymoses due to prothrombin deficiency, or purpura due to thrombocytopenia. *Palmar erythema* or *spider angiomas* may reflect acute or chronic liver disease. Spider angiomas are usually found above the umbilicus and especially on the face, neck, shoulders, forearms, and dorsum of the hands. The presence of a few spider angiomas is not abnormal in women, especially during pregnancy. However, their appearance in men is always abnormal and should be carefully searched for. In chronic cholestasis, *scratch marks, finger clubbing,* and *xanthoma* of the eyelids and extensor surfaces of the tendons of the wrists and ankles may be found. A *slate color* to the skin due to increased melanin should suggest the presence of hemochromatosis.

Evaluation of the *mental state* and *neurologic function* is important. Slight deterioration of the intellect and minimal personality changes may suggest hepatocellular disease or the presence of portal-systemic venous shunts, but care must be taken to exclude other causes such as neurologic disease. The presence of flapping tremor of the hands (asterixis) may be found in association with portal-systemic encephalopathy or impending hepatic coma.

Abdominal examination may reveal ascites, which, together with dilated periumbilical veins, suggests cirrhosis and extensive portal collateral circulation. If additional features of liver disease are lacking, malignancy must be more seriously considered. A very large nodular and rock-hard liver suggests the presence of hepatoma or hepatic metastases. Careful percussion is necessary to evaluate the size of a nonpalpable liver. A small liver may indicate cirrhosis (especially postnecrotic); a small liver which diminishes in size suggests severe hepatitis or massive hepatic necrosis. In the alcoholic, fatty infiltration and cirrhosis often produce a uniform enlargement of the liver. The liver edge is tender in hepatitis, in congestive heart failure, and occasionally in malignant disease and with alcoholism (especially "alcoholic hepatitis").

A palpable and sometimes visibly enlarged gallbladder (Courvoisier's sign) suggests extrahepatic biliary obstruction often due to pancreatic cancer. A tender gallbladder and positive Murphy's sign suggest cholelithiasis or choledocholithiasis. A palpable spleen may indicate hepatitis or cirrhosis; significant splenomegaly may be a reflection of portal hypertension.

Abdominal auscultation may reveal the presence of a venous hum over dilated collateral veins radiating from the umbilicus, the so-called caput medusae. In advanced cirrhosis this venous hum is virtually diagnostic of significant portal hypertension. A bruit may sometimes be heard over large regenerating nodules in cirrhosis and occasionally over hepatomas and metastatic nodules in the liver. A friction rub may occasionally be heard over hepatomas and metastatic liver nodules.

Serum assays for biochemical markers of liver disease are an integral part of the proper evaluation of liver and biliary tract disease. In general, the serum bilirubin is measured to confirm the presence and severity of jaundice and determine the extent of bilirubin conjugation. Aminotransferase (transaminase) elevations reflect the severity of active hepatocellular damage, while alkaline phosphatase elevations are found with cholestasis and hepatic infiltrates. Serum albumin and the prothrombin time are used as indexes of hepatic synthetic function. These and other tests are reviewed in Chaps. 47 and 249.

The further evaluation of patients with hepatobiliary disease should be individualized depending on the history, physical findings, and initial screening laboratory tests. Hepatocellular disease such as hepatitis is often sufficiently clear so that only serologic tests are needed. Nonetheless in many patients, computed tomography (CT), ultrasound, scintiscans, or liver biopsy may be needed to determine the nature of the liver disease. When hepatic tumors are suspected, CT, ultrasound, or scintiscan may be performed followed by liver biopsy or laparoscopy for a more specific diagnosis. When biliary obstruction is suspected, the first examination is usually an ultrasound study to determine the size of the bile ducts, whether gallstones are present, or whether there is the suggestion of a mass in the head of the pancreas. Frequently more information is needed and thus a cholangiogram, performed through the endoscope or through percutaneous puncture under ultrasound or CT guidance, should be obtained.

CLASSIFICATION OF LIVER DISEASE No single classification of the various types of liver disease is entirely satisfactory because in many instances the etiology and pathogenetic mechanism are obscure. As a consequence, one finds an abundance of labels and names applied to hepatic disorders. Some individuals use the term *hepatitis* to imply viral infection, others simply to connote evidence of hepatic inflammation. The often used words *acute, subacute,* and *chronic* are ambiguous. *Chronicity* should refer to continuing or recurrent disease (i.e., duration). *Activity* should refer to evidence of the presence of perpetuation of liver cell injury; this is most readily identified by serum transaminase elevations and by the degree of hepatocellular necrosis on biopsy.

Because of the difficulties involved in defining the etiology of many types of liver disease, in most instances the process is best defined and described by an examination of the morphologic character of the lesion. Therefore, a *morphologic classification* of liver disease, as outlined in Table 247-1, appears at present more practical than one based on etiology.

TABLE 247-1 Classification of liver disease

I Parenchymal
- *A* Hepatitis (viral, drug-induced, toxic)
  - *1* Acute
  - *2* Chronic (persistent or active)
- *B* Cirrhosis
  - *1* Alcoholic (portal, nutritional, Laennec's cirrhosis)
  - *2* Postnecrotic
  - *3* Biliary
  - *4* Hemochromatosis
  - *5* Rare types (e.g., Wilson's disease, galactosemia, cystic fibrosis of pancreas, alpha$_1$-antitrypsin deficiency)
- *C* Infiltrations
  - *1* Glycogen
  - *2* Fat (neutral fat, cholesterol, gangliosides, cerebrosides)
  - *3* Amyloid
  - *4* Lymphoma, leukemia
  - *5* Granuloma (e.g., sarcoidosis, tuberculosis, idiopathic)
- *D* Space-occupying lesions
  - *1* Hepatoma, metastatic tumor
  - *2* Abscess (pyogenic, amoebic)
  - *3* Cysts (polycystic disease, *Echinococcus*)
  - *4* Gummas
- *E* Functional disorders associated with jaundice
  - *1* Gilbert's syndrome
  - *2* Crigler-Najjar syndrome
  - *3* Dubin-Johnson and Rotor syndromes
  - *4* Cholestasis of pregnancy and benign recurrent cholestasis

II Hepatobiliary
- *A* Extrahepatic biliary obstruction (by stone, stricture, or tumor)
- *B* Cholangitis

III Vascular
- *A* Chronic passive congestion and cardiac cirrhosis
- *B* Hepatic vein thrombosis (Budd-Chiari syndrome)
- *C* Portal vein thrombosis
- *D* Pylephlebitis
- *E* Arteriovenous malformations

REFERENCES

SCHIFF L, SCHIFF ER: *Diseases of the Liver,* 6th ed. Philadelphia, Lippincott, 1987

SHERLOCK S: *Diseases of the Liver and Biliary System,* 8th ed. Oxford, Blackwell, 1989

WRIGHT R et al: *Liver and Biliary Disease,* 2d ed. Philadelphia, Saunders, 1985

248 HEPATOBILIARY IMAGING

LAWRENCE S. FRIEDMAN / LAURENCE NEEDLEMAN

Selection of appropriate imaging techniques for the liver and biliary tract in a given patient depends on the particular clinical problem and on an understanding of the uses and limitations of each technique; in many situations, two or more imaging methods may provide complementary and useful information. In determining the optimal studies, communication between the clinician and the radiologist is essential.

PLAIN ABDOMINAL RADIOGRAPHS AND BARIUM STUDIES OF THE GASTROINTESTINAL TRACT Standard plain films of the abdomen provide little diagnostic information about the hepatobiliary system. They may permit a rough estimation of hepatic size and detection of splenic enlargement or gross ascites. Their major value is in demonstrating *calcified lesions,* including gallstones (about 15 percent are radiopaque) and intrahepatic lesions such as echinococcal cysts, calcified granulomas due to previous tuberculosis or histoplasmosis, or, rarely, tumors or vascular lesions. Plain abdominal x-rays may also demonstrate *air in the biliary tract,* as may occur after endoscopic papillotomy or with a biliary-enteric fistula, either surgical or as a result of inflammation or erosion of a stone from the gallbladder into the intestine. Emphysematous cholecystitis is associated with air in the wall of the gallbladder as a result of severe inflammation. Air seen in a branching pattern extending to the periphery of the liver is usually within portal venous branches and associated with serious inflammatory processes in the intestine.

A barium swallow may demonstrate large esophageal varices in patients with portal hypertension, although endoscopy is more sensitive for the detection of varices.

ULTRASONOGRAPHY Ultrasonography has the advantages of relatively low cost, potential portability, and safety, as ionizing radiation is not required. Ultrasound imaging depends on small differences in the acoustic properties of soft tissue. Short pulses (1 μs) of high-frequency sound (3 to 10 million Hz) are transmitted into the patient; at each interface between tissues of different acoustic properties, a small portion of the energy is reflected back to the transducer, which also acts as a receiver. With *B-mode,* or *gray-scale,* ultrasound scanning, ultrasound reflections are displayed as shades of gray; cross-sectional, transverse, longitudinal, or oblique images of organs can be produced depending on the orientation of the transducer. With *real-time* ultrasonography, scanning is so rapid that a continuously changing ("real time") image is displayed, thus permitting a survey of the abdominal anatomy in a short period of time and demonstration of physiologic tissue movements, such as arterial pulsations. The major limitation of ultrasonography is its inability to penetrate bone or air, including bowel gas, which may limit complete examination of abdominal organs. In general, tissue penetration of ultrasound decreases as resolution increases.

Ultrasonography is the preferred initial method for imaging the gallbladder and biliary tree (Fig. 248-1). It is sensitive and specific (>95 percent) for the detection of *cholelithiasis,* and, unlike oral cholecystography, is not limited by the presence of jaundice or dye allergy in the patient. Ultrasonography is also highly sensitive for detecting a *dilated biliary tract* in patients with cholestasis and may indicate whether the site of obstruction is in the intra- or extrahepatic ducts. The cause of biliary obstruction, such as a mass lesion in the head of the pancreas or porta hepatis, may also be detected by ultrasonography, although the area around the distal common bile duct may be obscured by bowel gas.

FIGURE 248-1 Sonogram showing dilated bile ducts due to pancreatic carcinoma. The diameter of the extrahepatic bile ducts is 1.2 cm measured anterior to the portal vein (between asterisks). The site of maximal dilatation is 2.0 cm in the distal common bile duct (between arrows).

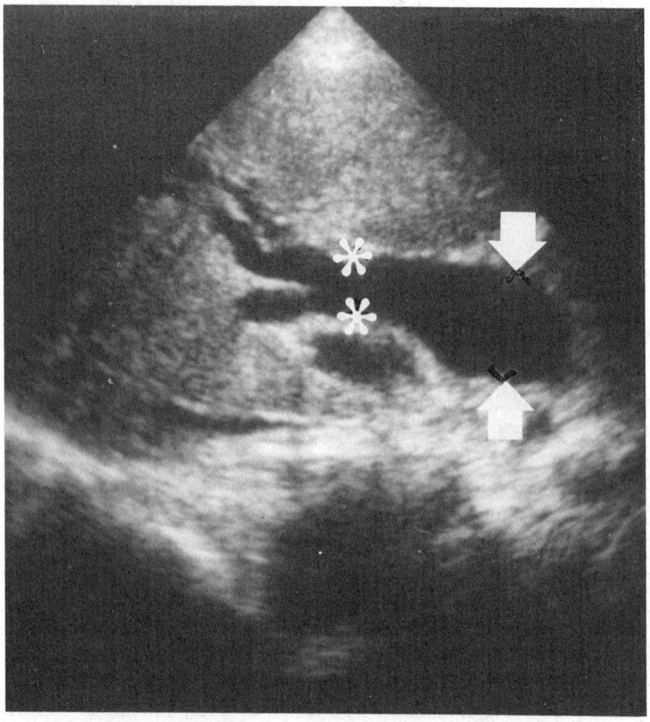

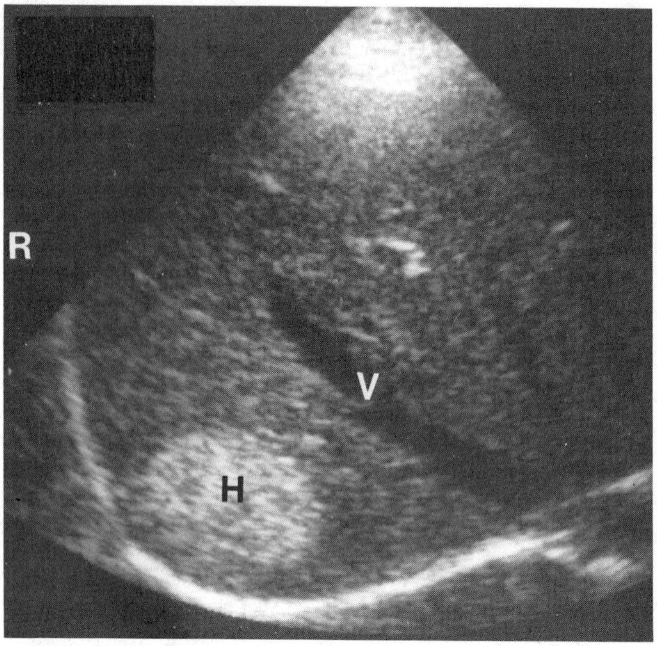

FIGURE 248-2 Sonogram showing an echogenic mass which represents a hemangioma (H) in the posterior right lobe of the liver lateral to the right hepatic vein (V). R = right side of the patient.

Ultrasonography is also a primary screening examination for hepatic disease, which may be suspected because of symptoms, hepatomegaly, abnormal liver function tests, jaundice, or the suspicion of a mass lesion (Fig. 248-2). In general, *focal hepatic lesions* are better visualized than diffuse parenchymal disease such as fatty liver, hepatitis, or cirrhosis. Hepatic masses as small as 1 cm may be detected, and cystic lesions or abscesses can be distinguished from solid lesions, although the nature of a solid hepatic mass (adenoma, hepatocellular carcinoma, metastasis, hemangioma, etc.) may not be identified. Nevertheless, a specific diagnosis may be facilitated by percutaneous "thin"-needle biopsy of hepatic lesions under ultrasound guidance, and insertion of a catheter under ultrasound guidance may permit nonoperative drainage of an abscess. Other uses of ultrasonography include detection of ascites when the physical examination is equivocal, demonstration of portal vein thrombosis in patients with bleeding gastroesophageal varices, and evaluation of patency of portosystemic shunts in patients with recurrent variceal bleeding after shunt surgery. Ultrasonography is usually the first imaging study performed in patients with hepatic dysfunction after liver transplantation to look for a biliary leak or vascular occlusion.

Doppler ultrasonography allows detection of the presence and direction of blood flow based on changes in the frequency of backscattered ultrasound waves caused by the movement of blood. *Intraoperative ultrasonography* involves the application of the ultrasound transducer to the exposed liver at surgery, thereby increasing the sensitivity of detecting occult hepatic metastases. *Endosonography* involves the attachment of an ultrasound transducer to the tip of an endoscope to permit ultrasonographic imaging from within the bowel lumen, thereby minimizing the obscuring effects of bowel gas. Compared to conventional imaging techniques, endosonography permits more precise determination of the depth of tumor invasion through the bowel wall and improved detection of early pancreatic lesions.

COMPUTED TOMOGRAPHY Because computed tomographic (CT) scans can detect very small differences in the attenuation of x-rays, structures not visible on conventional radiographs can be identified. With current CT scanning techniques, the radiation dose received by the patient is similar to that of diagnostic procedures such as barium enema. The identification of anatomic structures can be facilitated by the administration of an oral contrast agent to define

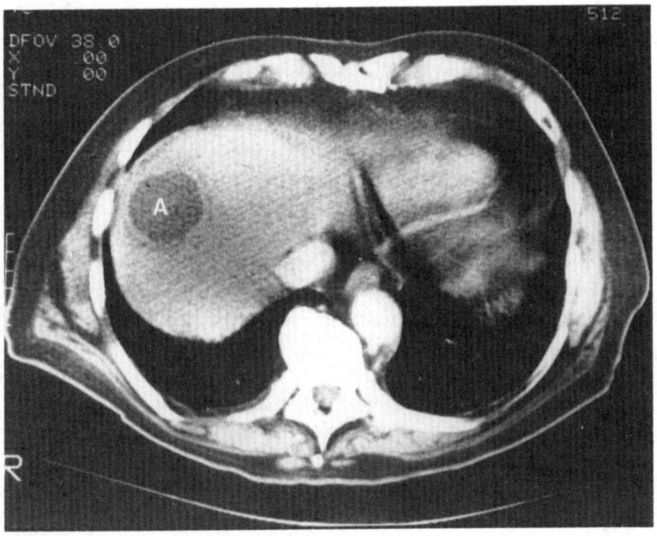

FIGURE 248-3 CT scan with contrast showing a low attenuation mass (*A*) in the dome of the liver, which represents an amebic abscess. R = right side of the patient.

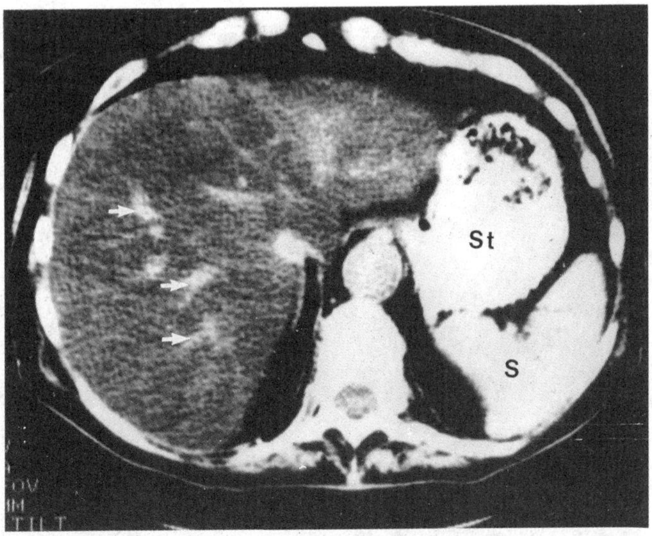

FIGURE 248-4 CT scan showing fatty infiltration of the liver. Note that the attenuation of the liver is lower than that of the spleen (S). The more highly attenuated linear structures of the liver (arrows) are the intrahepatic vessels. St = stomach filled with orally administered barium contrast agent.

the bowel lumen or an intravenous contrast agent to enhance blood vessels and tissues. In general, anatomic definition is more complete with CT scanning than with ultrasonography, and CT scanning has the additional advantage that obesity and intestinal gas do not reduce the quality of the examination. However, a paucity of fat in malnourished patients or children may limit the resolution of the CT image. The disadvantages of CT scanning are radiation exposure and cost. In many instances, CT scanning is reserved for patients in whom ultrasonography is technically difficult or inconclusive.

CT scanning before and after intravenous administration of a contrast agent is an excellent method of evaluating *hepatic masses*. Cystic lesions are readily identified, and abscesses can usually be distinguished from tumors (Fig. 248-3). Masses as small as 1 cm can usually be identified by CT scanning, and, as with ultrasonography, the lesions can be biopsied under CT guidance. Intravenous administration of a contrast agent may result in enhancement of a primary or secondary tumor relative to the surrounding liver, and certain lesions, such as a cavernous hemangioma, may show a pattern of enhancement that is characteristic enough to confirm the diagnosis. Invasion of blood vessels by tumor may also be demonstrated in this way. CT scanning has a more limited role in the evaluation of diffuse liver disease, such as cirrhosis, in which the density of the liver remains in the normal range. However, characteristic CT findings may be associated with *fatty infiltration* of the liver, in which the density of the liver is significantly reduced (Fig. 248-4), and *hemochromatosis*, or *secondary iron overload*, in which the density of the liver is increased, and an estimate of hepatic iron concentration may be made.

Although CT scanning is nearly as accurate as ultrasonography in detecting cholelithiasis or dilated bile ducts, ultrasonography is usually the preferred initial test because of its availability, lack of risk, and lower cost. However, CT scanning is more accurate than ultrasonography in identifying the level and cause of biliary obstruction. CT scanning may be used to define the extent of carcinoma of the gallbladder.

MAGNETIC RESONANCE IMAGING Magnetic resonance (MR) imaging detects the density of protons in tissue water and lipids and their relaxation times. Since hydrogen nuclei (protons) have an odd number of particles, they behave like magnets when placed in a strong magnetic field. In MR imaging, protons aligned in a magnetic field are subjected to a brief pulse of weak radio waves, the frequency of which (termed the *resonant frequency*) is related mathematically to the externally applied magnetic field. The pulse of radio waves causes the protons to change their direction of spin and alignment. After the radio wave pulse, the protons return to their original orientation and emit energy with the same radio frequency as that absorbed. Imaging may be accomplished by the detection and analysis of proton density, the T1 relaxation time (a measure of the rate at which the nuclei realign themselves in the magnetic field), or the T2 relaxation time (a measure of the rate at which the emitted radio frequency energy decays). Each method produces a slightly different type of image. The choice of imaging technique depends on the contrast resolution needed for a particular organ. In general, because the magnetic environments of protons in fat, intracellular water, and extracellular water differ, MR imaging provides sharp contrast differentiation of tissues containing varying amounts of water or fat.

In addition to excellent contrast resolution between normal and abnormal tissues, advantages of MR imaging include the lack of ionizing radiation and the ability to image in transverse, longitudinal, coronal, or even oblique planes. Its disadvantages include cost, slow imaging time that results in blurred images due to respiration and peristalsis, and limitations imposed by a strong magnetic field, such as the inability to study patients with pacemakers and other metallic devices.

The range of applications of MR imaging and its role relative to other imaging modalities are under evaluation. MR imaging of *mass lesions* of the liver appears to have greater sensitivity than CT scanning; however, like CT scanning, MR imaging cannot reliably distinguish primary from metastatic tumors (Fig. 248-5). Hepatic abscesses can be detected readily, although on occasion, it may be difficult to distinguish abscesses from tumors with necrotic centers. MR imaging is sensitive in the detection of hemangiomas, which often have an appearance sufficiently characteristic to permit differentiation from hepatic malignancy. Whereas its value in diffuse parenchymal liver disease such as hepatitis or cirrhosis is uncertain, MR imaging can serve as a useful noninvasive method for the diagnosis and monitoring of iron and copper deposition in hemochromatosis, secondary iron overload, or Wilson's disease. Similarly, a modification of MR imaging (*proton spectroscopic imaging*), in which the image of fat is subtracted from the image of water, shows promise in identifying fatty liver and quantifying hepatic fat content. Since rapidly flowing blood is often signal-free on MR imaging, blood vessels can be distinguished without the need for a contrast agent in most cases; thus, MR imaging may be useful in assessing the surgical resectability of vascular tumors.

The gallbladder and bile ducts can be demonstrated by MR

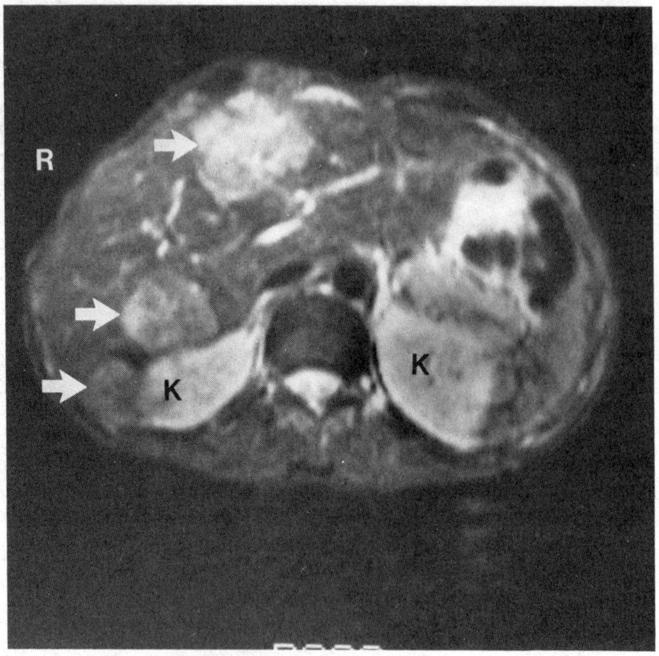

FIGURE 248-5 Magnetic resonance (MR) image of the liver showing three hepatic metastases (arrows) with higher signal than the surrounding liver. R = right side of the patient, K = kidney.

imaging, and cholelithiasis and cholecystitis can be detected; however, MR imaging currently offers no advantages over other imaging techniques. Although gallstones in the common bile duct are not detected by MR imaging, other causes of bile duct obstruction, such as pancreatitis or pancreatic carcinoma, may be identified.

Currently, MR imaging is based on hydrogen, which is the most abundant nucleus in the body and very sensitive to MR. *MR spectroscopy* also permits imaging based on other isotopes, such as phosphorus 31, with the ability to permit study of the metabolic state of normal and diseased organs.

RADIOISOTOPE SCANNING A variety of radioisotopes can be used to study the anatomy and function of the liver and biliary system. After injection into a peripheral vein, the radioisotope is extracted by the liver and excreted in the bile. A scintillation (gamma) camera produces an image by detecting the radiation emitted during the decay of the radioisotope. Depending on the information desired, radioisotopes can be chosen that are taken up by hepatic parenchymal cells, Kupffer cells, or neoplastic and inflammatory cells or that are rapidly excreted in bile. Because radioisotope scanning of the liver seldom provides a precise diagnosis, it has largely been replaced by ultrasonography and CT scanning for first-line imaging. However, radioisotope scanning of the biliary tract is an important tool in the investigation of acute cholecystitis.

Technetium 99m–labeled sulfur colloid scanning The most commonly used radiopharmaceutical for anatomic evaluation of the liver is ^{99m}Tc-labeled sulfur colloid, which is taken up by reticuloendothelial (Kupffer) cells in the liver. Such scanning can be used to assess the size and shape of the liver. Any disease process that results in replacement of Kupffer cells, including *primary and metastatic tumors, cysts,* and *abscesses,* produces a "cold" area in the hepatic scintigram. Lesions greater than 2 to 3 cm in diameter can be reliably detected. The resolution of ^{99m}Tc-sulfur colloid scanning is nearly equivalent to that of ultrasonography, CT scanning, and MR imaging, but it is not as specific as these techniques in determining the nature of the lesion. Because of impaired blood flow and reticuloendothelial function, *diffuse hepatic disease,* such as hepatitis and cirrhosis, may result in decreased or patchy uptake of radiocolloid with preferential uptake by the bone marrow and spleen, particularly when portal hypertension is present. Occasionally, the irregular uptake of radiocolloid in cirrhosis results in the falsely positive appearance of hepatic filling defects. *Obstruction of the hepatic veins* (Budd-Chiari syndrome) may result in preferential uptake of radiocolloid by the caudate lobe of the liver.

Gold (^{198}Au)- and indium (^{111}In)-labeled colloids are also taken up by Kupffer cells and may be used to image the liver but are more expensive than ^{99m}Tc-sulfur colloid and expose the patient to a greater radiation dose. Newer scintigraphic techniques designed to improve the sensitivity of liver imaging include *single photon emission computed tomography* (SPECT), which permits visualization of the cross-sectional distribution of a radioisotope, and *positron emission tomography* (PET), which utilizes isotopes that decay by positron emission and provides information about regional blood flow and alterations in tissue metabolism.

Gallium scanning ^{67}Gallium citrate accumulates in tissues actively synthesizing protein and is taken up by *tumors and abscesses;* ^{75}selenomethionine has similar properties. On scanning, the lesion appears as an area of increased activity, or "hot spot." Imaging with this agent may be useful in detecting hepatocellular carcinomas, Hodgkin's disease, some non-Hodgkin's lymphomas, and melanomas, although nonspecific uptake of gallium by the liver, bone marrow, and gastrointestinal tract limit the reliability of gallium scanning.

Tagged blood cell scanning Intravenous injection of *autologous white blood cells* labeled with ^{111}In increases the specificity of radioisotope scanning for the detection of hepatic (and abdominal) *abscesses*. Similarly, *autologous red blood cells* or circulating proteins such as albumin or transferrin labeled with ^{111}In or ^{99m}Tc provide a sensitive method of identifying *hemangiomas* that are detected as mass lesions by ultrasonography or CT scanning (Fig. 248-6).

Biliary scanning A variety of radiopharmaceuticals are rapidly cleared by hepatocytes and excreted in the bile, thus permitting scintigraphic evaluation of the biliary tract. The earliest agent used for this purpose was ^{131}I-rose bengal, which, because of its high radiation dose, has been replaced by agents that can be labeled with ^{99m}Tc. The most widely used agents are *N*-substituted iminoacetic acids (HIDA, PIPIDA, DISIDA), which concentrate in the bile even when serum bilirubin levels are elevated. Biliary scanning is used most often in evaluating patients with suspected *acute cholecystitis,* in whom visualization of the gallbladder excludes obstruction of the cystic duct and hence acute cholecystitis (Fig. 248-7). Persistent nonvisualization of the gallbladder over several hours with normal visualization of the liver, bile ducts, and intestine indicates a diagnosis of acute cholecystitis with 95 percent accuracy. False-positive results may occur in patients receiving parenteral nutrition or narcotics and those with hepatitis. Biliary scanning is less accurate in patients with chronic cholecystitis, in whom delayed visualization of the gallbladder is frequent. However, biliary scanning may be useful in identifying

FIGURE 248-6 ^{99m}Tc-labeled autologous red blood cell scan of the hemangioma shown in Fig. 248-2. S = spleen, K = kidney.

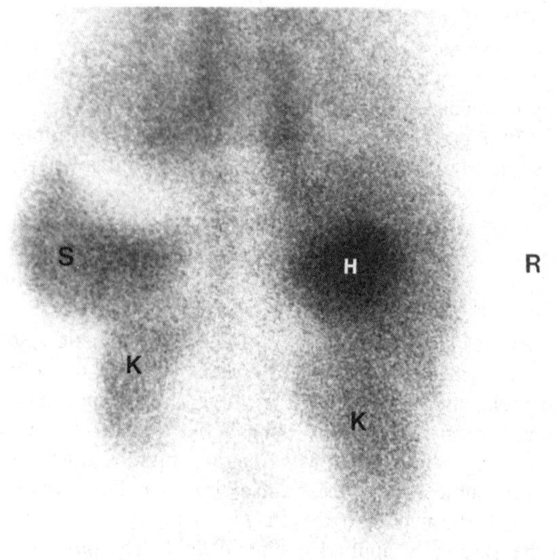

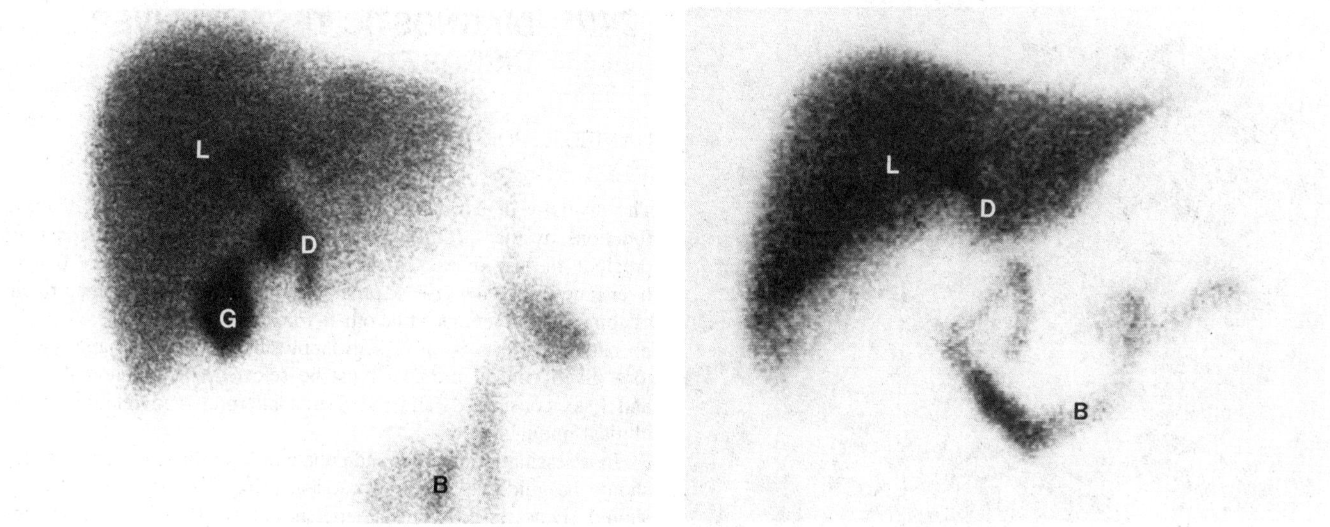

FIGURE 248-7 *A*. Hepatobiliary scan using ^{99m}Tc-DISIDA in a normal person showing uptake in the liver (L), gallbladder (G), bile ducts (D), and bowel (B) with patency of the cystic duct and biliary system. *B*. Abnormal hepatobiliary scan showing radioisotope in the liver (L), bile ducts (D), and bowel (B) but not in the gallbladder. This is due to an obstructed cystic duct (with a patent common bile duct) due to acute cholecystitis.

cholestasis, acute and chronic biliary obstruction, bile leaks, biliary-enteric fistulas, and *choledochal cysts.*

ORAL CHOLECYSTOGRAPHY Although the use of oral cholecystography declined markedly with the advent of ultrasonography, the recent development of nonsurgical approaches to the treatment of cholelithiasis (e.g., extracorporeal shock wave lithotripsy and oral dissolution therapy with chenodeoxycholic or ursodeoxycholic acid) had led to a resurgence of interest in oral cholecystography. The test is simple and inexpensive. It involves radiographic assessment of gallbladder opacification 14 to 16 h after oral administration of iopanoic acid or 10 to 12 h after oral administration of sodium tyropanoate, both of which are concentrated in the gallbladder after intestinal absorption and hepatic excretion. A second dose of dye may need to be administered to as many as 15 to 25 percent of persons in whom gallbladder opacification is not achieved after a single dose.

Nonvisualization of the gallbladder indicates *gallbladder disease* with nearly 95 percent certainty, whereas normal visualization excludes gallbladder disease with 97 percent certainty. Failure of the gallbladder to opacify may also result from patient noncompliance, intestinal malabsorption, and liver disease; the gallbladder will not visualize when the serum direct bilirubin level is greater than 34 μmol/L (2 mg/dL). Oral cholecystography is as sensitive as ultrasonography in the overall detection of gallbladder disease (stones, polyps, adenomyomatosis, cholesterolosis, cholecystitis), although ultrasonography is more sensitive in detecting stones per se. However, oral cholecystography is more accurate in determining the *number and size of stones* and, unlike ultrasonography, can demonstrate *cystic duct patency,* factors that are important in determining a patient's suitability for nonoperative gallstone therapy.

CHOLANGIOGRAPHY In the past, *intravenous cholangiography,* in which contrast dye is administered as a bolus by peripheral vein, was the principal radiographic technique to visualize the bile ducts. Because of a high rate of serious reactions to the dye, the lack of bile duct visualization when the serum bilirubin level was above 42 μmol/L (2.5 mg/dL), and the development of more effective radiologic techniques to visualize the bile ducts, intravenous cholangiography has become obsolete.

Percutaneous transhepatic cholangiography (THC) This technique involves the direct percutaneous injection, via a "thin" (22-gauge) needle, of contrast dye into bile ducts in the liver under fluoroscopic guidance. When intrahepatic ducts are dilated, the success rate of duct opacification approaches 100 percent, but when the intrahepatic ducts are not dilated, as in primary sclerosing cholangitis, the success rate is around 90 percent and multiple attempts may be required. Serious complications occur in no more than 3 percent of cases and include hemorrhage, bile peritonitis, and sepsis.

THC may be used to determine the cause of *biliary obstruction* or *cholestasis* and is of particular value in evaluating the potential surgical resectability of proximal cholangiocarcinomas. In addition, biliary biopsies and cytologic brushings may be obtained and strictures may be balloon-dilated via a catheter inserted through the THC tract. In patients with biliary obstruction who are poor operative risks, an external drain may be left in place to permit biliary decompression or an internal stent (endoprosthesis) may be placed to relieve obstruction.

Endoscopic retrograde cholangiopancreatography (ERCP) (See Chap. 236) This technique uses fiberoptic endoscopy to visualize the ampulla of Vater and guide the insertion of a catheter through the ampulla for the selective injection of contrast material into the common bile and pancreatric ducts, which are then imaged radiologically (see Chap. 236). The success rate for cannulation depends on the experience of the endoscopist and can approach 95 percent or more; unlike THC, successful biliary cannulation does not depend on a dilated bile duct. Serious complications may occur in about 5 percent of cases and include pancreatitis and cholangitis.

Using THC, ERCP, or both, the biliary system can be visualized in nearly all patients. ERCP is preferable when the bile ducts are not dilated and when an *ampullary, pancreatic, or distal bile duct lesion* is suspected. In patients with *choledocholithiasis,* ERCP permits sphincterotomy and stone extraction. Additionally, ERCP may permit ampullary biopsy, pancreatic or biliary ductal brushings for cytologic examination, balloon dilation of a stricture, placement of a nasobiliary drain to decompress an obstructed biliary system, and insertion of a stent to relieve biliary obstruction caused by tumors. ERCP can also be used for *manometric measurements of the sphincter of Oddi,* a potentially valuable technique in the diagnosis of papillary stenosis and ampullary spasm.

ANGIOGRAPHY Angiography is required less often now than in the past for evaluating the hepatobiliary system. Nevertheless, newer contrast agents, improved techniques of vascular catheterization, and the development of therapeutic applications make angiography of value in certain situations. Selective cannulation of the hepatic artery or one of its branches may be helpful in distinguishing certain *vascular lesions* of the liver, including hemangiomas, adenomas, focal nodular hyperplasia, hemangioendotheliomas, and hepatocellular carcinomas (Fig. 248-8). Angiography may be particularly valuable in assessing the *surgical resectability* of an isolated hepatic lesion or in identifying

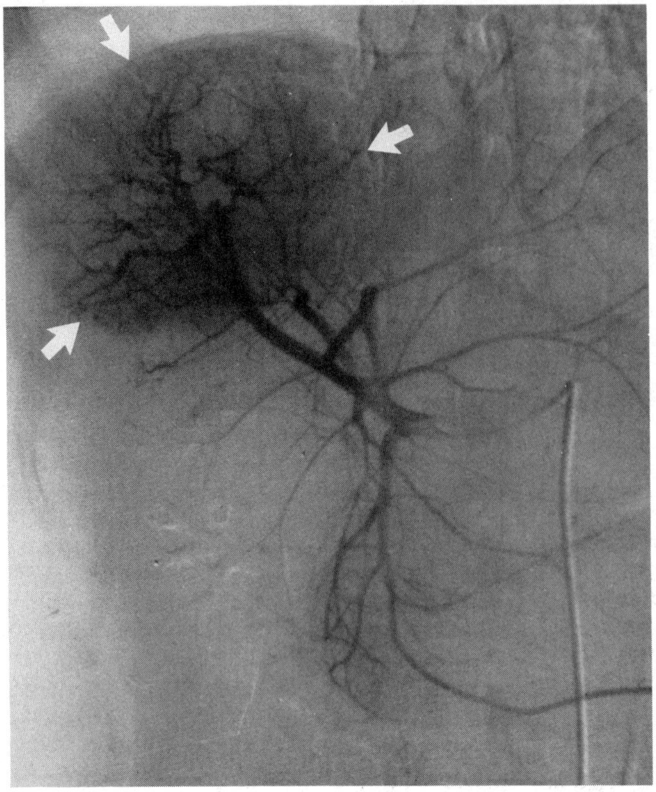

FIGURE 248-8 Arterial phase of a selective hepatic angiogram showing a hepatocellular carcinoma as a hypervascular mass (outlined by arrows) with many irregular and corkscrew-shaped tumor vessels in the right lobe of the liver.

a vascular occlusion after liver transplantation. In planning portosystemic shunt surgery, angiography is the best imaging technique to define portal venous anatomy and assess the patency of the vessels to be used. The portal venous system may be examined on the venous phase of celiac and superior mesenteric arteriography or after direct injection of contrast into the portal venous system via a splenic or transhepatic route. Hepatic venography and hemodynamic measurements, including wedged hepatic venous pressures, can be obtained concurrently (see Chap. 254). Therapeutic applications of angiography include *embolization* of bleeding vessels, arteriovenous fistulas, and certain highly vascular or inoperable tumors.

REFERENCES

COOPERBERG PL, GIBNEY RG: Imaging of the gallbladder, 1987. Radiology 163:605, 1987

COUNCIL ON SCIENTIFIC AFFAIRS, AMERICAN MEDICAL ASSOCIATION: Magnetic resonance imaging of the abdomen and pelvis. JAMA 261:420, 1989

FERRUCCI JT et al: Advances in hepatobiliary radiology. Radiology 168:3198, 1988

MARTON KI, DOUBILET P: How to image the gallbladder in suspected cholecystitis. Ann Intern Med 109:722, 1988

ROTHSCHILD MA, ORATZ M: Hepatic imaging. Semin Liv Dis 9:1, 1989

SHERLOCK S: *Diseases of the Liver and Biliary System*, 8th ed. Oxford, Blackwell, 1989

TAYLOR KJW et al: Noninvasive imaging of the hepatobiliary system, in *Diseases of the Liver*, 6th ed, L Schiff, ER Schiff (eds). Philadelphia, Lippincott, 1987, pp 261–309

WRIGHT R et al: *Liver and Biliary Disease: Pathophysiology, Diagnosis, Management*, 2d ed. London, Saunders, 1985

249 DIAGNOSTIC TESTS IN LIVER DISEASE

DANIEL K. PODOLSKY / KURT J. ISSELBACHER

The diversity of normal liver functions and the disruption of these functions by the spectrum of disorders which may affect the liver preclude the use of any single test as a reliable measure of overall liver function. Many disease processes may lead to severe impairment of some liver functions while others remain entirely unaffected. Since no battery of tests is universally applicable, those most appropriate to a given clinical problem must be selected, their potential value and risks considered, and the results interpreted in relation to the clinical findings.

In assessing the severity and course of liver disease, the physician should be guided by several practical principles. The tests selected should (1) assess different parameters of liver function, (2) be used *serially* in order to evaluate the evolution or course of the disease, and (3) be interpreted within the total clinical context, with recognition that any single laboratory test may be fallible.

BLOOD TESTS OF LIVER FUNCTION (See Table 249-1)

BILIRUBIN Bilirubin metabolism and its assessment are discussed in detail in Chaps. 47 and 251. Spectrophotometric determinations of serum bilirubin in the clinical laboratory measure two pigment fractions: (1) the water-soluble conjugated fraction that gives a *direct reaction* with the diazo reagent and consists largely of conjugated bilirubin (as the mono- and diglucuronide), and (2) the lipid-soluble *indirect-reaction* fraction (total minus direct) that represents primarily unconjugated bilirubin. The serum of normal adults (when measured by the van den Bergh reaction) contains less than 4.2 μmol/L (0.25 mg/dL) direct-reacting bilirubin and 17 μmol/L (1 mg/dL) or less of total bilirubin. Studies with high-performance liquid chromatography (HPLC) suggest that even these levels may be artifactually high in normal persons (see Chap. 47).

Conjugated hyperbilirubinemia with elevated direct- and indirect-reacting material indicates impairment of secretion into the bile, while unconjugated hyperbilirubinemia reflects impaired conjugation. The latter is found in a limited number of processes including such nonhepatic conditions as hemolytic anemia and ineffective erythropoiesis (increased pigment load) and a few hepatic disorders, principally Gilbert's syndrome or the relatively rare Crigler-Najjar syndrome. Although measurement of both the direct and total serum bilirubin will determine whether the patient has predominantly unconjugated or conjugated hyperbilirubinemia, this distinction is of limited usefulness since the majority of hepatobiliary disorders lead to conjugated hyperbilirubinemia. In most instances, fractionation of serum bilirubin does not distinguish cholestasis due to parenchymal disease from that arising from biliary tract processes.

TABLE 249-1 Abnormalities shown by tests of liver function

Test	Type of liver disease: Obstructive	Parenchymal
AST and ALT (SGOT and SGPT)	↑	↑–↑↑↑
Alkaline phosphatase	↑↑↑	↑
Albumin	N	↓–↓↓↓
Prothrombin time	N–↑*	↑–↑↑↑
Bilirubin	N–↑↑↑	N–↑↑↑
γ-Glutamyl transpeptidase (GGT)	↑↑↑	N–↑↑↑
5′-Nucleotidase	↑–↑↑↑	N–↑

* Correctable with parenteral vitamin K if elevated.
NOTE: N, normal: ↑, elevated; ↓, decreased.

Bilirubin appears in the urine only after it is converted to a water-soluble form; generally this involves conjugation with polar glucuronide groups which enhance water solubility. Rapid assessment of bilirubinuria is possible using commercially available dipsticks and may be helpful as an initial screening measure. Bilirubinuria occurs with even minimal degrees of jaundice and may be detected before jaundice is evident. Its usefulness is otherwise quite limited. Urobilinogen, a product of luminal bacterial metabolism of bilirubin, is reabsorbed from the bowel and secreted in the urine. Complete bile duct obstruction blocks excretion of bilirubin into the gut and results in disappearance of urobilinogen from the urine. Assessment of urobilinogen in a freshly collected 2-h urine specimen by the Watson method (normal values 0.2 to 1.2 units) may distinguish biliary tract obstruction from parenchymal dysfunction, but this test has been largely superseded by newer methods.

SERUM ENZYME ASSAYS A number of serum enzymes have been used to distinguish and assess hepatocellular injury and biliary tract dysfunction or obstruction. All have inherent limitations in sensitivity and specificity, and none truly distinguish these processes definitively. Elevations in enzyme activities may also be seen in association with nonhepatic disorders. Nevertheless, with proper and careful interpretation, a number of serum enzymes provide important clinical tools.

Aminotransferases (transaminases) Assays of many serum enzymes have been proposed as indicators of hepatocellular damage. Of these, aspartate aminotransferase (AST,SGOT) and alanine aminotransferase (ALT,SGPT) activities have proven most useful. These enzymes catalyze the transfer of the γ-amino groups of aspartate and alanine, respectively, to the γ-keto group of ketoglutarate, leading to the formation of oxaloacetic acid and pyruvic acid. In contrast to ALT, which is found primarily in the liver, AST is present in many tissues including heart, skeletal muscle, kidney, and brain and is thus somewhat less specific as an indicator of liver function. The source of serum AST and ALT in the normal person [less than 0.58 μkat/L (35 U/L)] is unclear, and the mechanism responsible for clearance of these enzymes is uncertain. In the hepatocyte, ALT is found exclusively in the cytosol, while different isoenzymes of AST exist in mitochondria and the cytosol. Although elevated serum levels of AST or ALT may be observed in a variety of nonhepatic diseases, notably in myocardial infarction and skeletal muscle disorders, these disorders can usually be clinically distinguished from liver disease. Conversely, uremia may lead to spuriously low aminotransferase values.

Serum AST and ALT are elevated to some extent in nearly all liver disorders. Highest levels are found in association with conditions causing extensive hepatic necrosis, such as severe viral hepatitis, toxin-induced liver injury, or prolonged circulatory collapse. Lesser elevations are encountered in mild acute viral hepatitis as well as in both diffuse and focal chronic liver diseases (e.g., chronic active hepatitis, cirrhosis, and hepatic metastases). However, the absolute levels of aminotransferases correlate poorly with severity of liver injury or prognosis, and serial determinations are usually most helpful. Thus in the patient with massive hepatic necrosis, there may be marked elevations in the early phase (i.e., 24 to 48 h), but by the time the patient is tested 3 to 5 days later the levels may be in the range of 3.34 to 5.8 μkat/L (200 to 350 U/L). It is noteworthy that in severe alcoholic hepatitis one commonly finds only modest increases in these enzymes (generally less than 5.0 μkat/L). Minimal elevations of AST and ALT (less than 1.67 μkat/L) may also be found in association with biliary tract obstruction; higher levels suggest the development of cholangitis with resultant hepatic cell necrosis.

In general AST and ALT levels parallel each other, with one exception. In alcoholic hepatitis the AST/ALT ratio may be greater than 2; this appears to result from a reduction in hepatic ALT content due to a deficiency in the cofactor pyridoxine-5-phosphate.

Alkaline phosphatase Human serum contains several forms of alkaline phosphatase, a plasma membrane–derived enzyme of uncertain physiologic function which hydrolyzes synthetic phosphate esters at pH 9. These activities arise from bone, intestine, liver, and placenta. A number of different assays have been developed which utilize different substrates.

In the absence of bone disease or pregnancy, elevated levels of alkaline phosphatase activity usually reflect impaired biliary tract function. The increased levels reflect increased synthesis of the enzyme by hepatocytes and biliary tract epithelium rather than regurgitation of enzyme due to obstruction. Bile acids may play a role both by inducing synthesis and by promoting solubilization of the membrane-associated enzyme activity.

Slight to moderate increases in alkaline phosphatase (1 to 2 times normal) occur in many patients with parenchymal liver disorders such as hepatitis and cirrhosis; transient increases may occur in all types of liver disease. However, the most striking increases in alkaline phosphatase (3 to 10 times normal) occur with extrahepatic biliary tract (mechanical) obstruction or with intrahepatic (functional) cholestasis, as in drug-induced cholestasis or primary biliary cirrhosis. Conversely, it is unusual for the serum alkaline phosphatase to remain normal when there is obstructive jaundice, and a normal enzyme level argues strongly against the presence of cholestasis. The alkaline phosphatase is usually mildly elevated in metastatic or infiltrative liver disease (e.g., leukemia, lymphoma, and sarcoid). The enzyme may be elevated in the presence of incomplete biliary obstruction or when there is obstruction of only one hepatic duct, conditions in which the serum bilirubin is often normal or only slightly elevated. Serum alkaline phosphatase is also elevated in nonhepatic disorders, most notably in some bone disorders (e.g., Paget's disease, osteomalacia, and metastases to bone) and sometimes with malignancy. Occasionally tumors produce an alkaline phosphatase which is identical or similar to the placental form, the so-called Regan isoenzyme.

Although one can usually make a reasonable assessment as to whether an elevation of the alkaline phosphatase is of hepatic or nonhepatic origin, several methods can distinguish the different isoenzymes facilitating resolution of any uncertainty. In contrast to that derived from bone, the hepatic isozyme is stable to treatment with heat (56°C for 15 min) or urea. These enzymes can also be separated by electrophoresis, but this is usually impractical. Parallel determination of serum 5′-nucleotidase activity is also helpful; an increase of both 5′-nucleotidase and alkaline phosphatase is consistent with an hepatobiliary source of the enzyme elevation. Even after correction for age and sex (higher levels being found in the young and in older women), isolated elevations in alkaline phosphatase may occasionally be encountered in adults with no apparent disease.

5′-Nucleotidase, leucine aminopeptidase, and γ-glutamyltranspeptidase *5′-Nucleotidase* catalyzes the hydrolysis of phosphate from the 5′ position of the pentose component of the nucleotide. Although tissue distribution is widespread, elevations are generally associated with hepatobiliary disease. The principal value of the 5′-nucleotidase measurement is to confirm the hepatic origin of an elevated alkaline phosphatase level in children, pregnant women, or in those settings where coincident bone disease may be present. However, 5′-nucleotidase levels do not always parallel alkaline phosphatase in liver disease, and lack of elevation does not exclude an hepatic source of elevated serum alkaline phosphatase.

Despite a widespread tissue distribution, *leucine aminopeptidase,* a protease which cleaves amino-terminal amino acids from peptides, is significantly elevated only in diseases of the pancreas and hepatobiliary system. There is considerable overlap in values of the peptidase levels found in patients with hepatocellular disease and in those with cholestatic jaundice; thus, in general, its measurement is of little clinical value.

γ-Glutamyltranspeptidase GGT catalyzes the transfer of the γ-glutamyl group from peptides such as glutathione to other amino acids and may play a role in amino acid transport. It is found throughout the hepatobiliary system as well as in other tissues. In liver disease, GGT correlates with alkaline phosphatase levels and is the most sensitive indicator of biliary tract disease. However, elevations of GGT are nonspecific and may be associated with pancreatic, cardiac, renal, and pulmonary disorders as well as with diabetes and alcoholism. This enzyme may be increased by agents which induce microsomal enzymes, and it has been suggested as a potential marker of alcoholism. However, overall lack of specificity has limited its clinical usefulness.

Other enzymes Measurement of total serum lactic dehydrogenase (LDH) or its isoenzymes is usually not helpful in diagnosis of liver disease because of this enzyme's nearly ubiquitous body distribution. Moderate LDH elevations are common in acute viral hepatitis, cirrhosis, and metastatic carcinoma to the liver. Biliary tract disease may also produce slight elevations. Numerous other dehydrogenases (e.g., isocitrate dehydrogenase, sorbitol dehydrogenase, and glutamate dehydrogenase) have been used or proposed as markers of liver disease, but none appear to offer significant diagnostic improvement over standard aminotransferase determinations. Elevation of serum ornithine carbamyl transferase (OCT), a urea cycle enzyme present only in liver and intestine, occurs primarily in liver disease, but its lack of association with any specific type of liver disease has limited its diagnostic usefulness also.

SERUM PROTEINS Extensive liver injury may lead to *decreased* blood levels of albumin, prothrombin, fibrinogen, and other proteins synthesized exclusively by hepatocytes. In contrast to measurements of serum enzymes, serum protein levels reflect liver synthetic function rather than just cell injury. Three important caveats should be remembered regarding interpretation of serum protein levels: (1) they are neither early nor sensitive indicators of liver disease (because of the extent of hepatic reserve and their half-life, see below), (2) they are of little value in the differential diagnosis of liver disease, and (3) decreases in their serum levels are not specific for liver disease.

Albumin and globulin Albumin is quantitatively the most important serum protein synthesized by the liver; the normal serum value ranges from 35 to 55 g/L (see Chap. 250). Albumin has a fairly long half-life (14 to 20 days) with less than 5 percent turnover daily; it is therefore not a good indicator of acute or mild liver injury. Furthermore, there is a substantial reserve of hepatic albumin synthesis; thus, adequate synthesis may continue until there is extensive hepatocellular injury. Serum levels are influenced by a variety of nonhepatic factors, most notably nutritional status, hormonal factors, and plasma oncotic pressure. Routes of degradation in health remain undefined, but nonhepatic conditions may lead to depressed serum albumin levels mainly due to excessive loss despite adequate synthetic function (e.g., nephrotic syndrome or protein-losing enteropathy). Nonetheless, reduction in the serum albumin levels provides an excellent indication of the severity of chronic liver disease. In the patient with ascites, an increased volume of distribution as well as an absolute reduction in protein synthesis may contribute to hypoalbuminemia.

Serum globulins are a heterogeneous group of proteins whose production in a variety of tissues is influenced by a number of factors. Serum globulins (normal: 20 to 35 g/L) include alpha and beta globulins as well as serum immunoglobulins, the latter largely accounting for the gamma fraction. Serum globulins are often diffusely elevated in association with chronic liver disease and in other nonhepatic disorders. In cirrhosis varying degrees of hyperglobulinemia may occur; this may reflect increased stimulation of the peripheral reticuloendothelial compartment due to shunting of antigens past the liver and impaired clearance by hepatic Kupffer cells. Although some have suggested that elevations in different globulin fractions as assessed by electrophoretic or other means may have a differential diagnostic value, this remains a largely unfulfilled promise. Similarly, the albumin/globulin ratio has no physiologic significance.

Clotting factors The liver synthesizes six coagulation factors: fibrinogen (factor I), prothrombin (factor II), and factors V, VII, IX, and X. With the exception of factor V, production of functional proteins requires the presence of the cofactor, vitamin K. Because most of these factors are normally present in excess, impaired coagulation is usually seen only in severe liver disease. Abnormalities of these factors can be most efficiently determined by the one-stage *prothrombin time,* which measures the rate of prothrombin conversion to thrombin in the presence of thromboplastin and calcium and requires the integrity of most of the vitamin K–dependent clotting factors (see Chap. 62). Factor VII is the rate-limiting factor in this pathway and thus has the greatest influence on the prothrombin levels. The prothrombin time is dependent on normal hepatic synthesis of clotting factors and sufficient intestinal uptake of vitamin K. Absorption of this fat-soluble vitamin itself requires adequate dietary intake and normal function of intestinal mucosa and biliary secretion. Severe acute or chronic parenchymal liver injury may lead to prolongation of the prothrombin time due to impaired synthesis of the clotting proteins. Because these proteins have a shorter half-life than that of albumin, the prothrombin time may be an earlier indicator than serum albumin of severe liver injury. In both acute and chronic hepatocellular injury, an increase in the prothrombin time serves as an ominous prognostic sign. Because it is a fat-soluble vitamin, prolongation of the prothrombin time may result from vitamin K malabsorption which may occur with cholestasis due to biliary tract disease or due to fat malabsorption (steatorrhea) of any cause (e.g., pancreatic insufficiency). Poor dietary intake, antibiotic therapy, or use of warfarin-type anticoagulants are additional causes of a prolonged prothrombin time, owing to deficiencies of active vitamin K. These processes can be distinguished from hepatic synthetic failure by demonstrating normalization of the prothrombin time (within 24 to 48 h) after parenteral injections of vitamin K. The *partial thromboplastin time,* which reflects the activities of fibrinogen, prothrombin, and factors V, VIII, IX, X, XI, and XII, may also be prolonged in severe liver disease. Clotting functions should be assessed in all patients with liver disease prior to any surgical procedure, including liver biopsy (see Chaps. 62 and 288).

BLOOD AMMONIA Ammonia is elevated in the blood of some patients with either acute or chronic liver disease. Although influenced by a number of factors (summarized in Chap. 250), elevations in blood ammonia reflect disruption of the pathways of urea synthesis by which the liver detoxifies amine groups. A markedly elevated blood ammonia usually reflects severe hepatocellular necrosis. Cirrhotic patients, especially those with endogenous or surgically created portal-systemic shunting, often have varying degrees of hyperammonemia and hepatic encephalopathy. However, there is only a rough correlation between blood ammonia levels and the degree of hepatic encephalopathy; some patients will function normally with a twofold elevation, while others will be stuporous at the same concentration. Ammonia levels may increase before the onset of coma; similarly, they may return to normal some 48 to 72 h before improvement of the neurologic status.

SERUM LIPIDS AND LIPOPROTEINS AND BILE ACIDS Abnormalities in serum lipids and lipoproteins are sensitive but nonspecific indicators of liver diseases. Acute parenchymal liver disease is commonly associated with increased plasma triglycerides, decreased cholesterol esters, and abnormal lipoproteins. The absence of alpha and prebeta bands with a concomitant increase in the beta fraction is typical of acute viral hepatitis. Less marked but more persistent abnormalities are found in patients with chronic parenchymal disease reflecting deficiencies in lecithin:cholesterol acyltransferase (LCAT) and hepatic triglyceride lipase. Either intra- or extrahepatic cholestasis may lead to an increase in unesterified cholesterol and in serum phospholipids. Lipoprotein X, a distinctive lipoprotein encountered in cholestasis, consists of equimolar amounts of unesterified cholesterol and lecithin which is regurgitated from the biliary tract. Although characteristically seen in patients with extrahepatic biliary obstruction, lipoprotein X may be found in any cholestatic condition.

Removal of bile acids from portal blood is impaired in liver disease because of parenchymal damage and portal-systemic shunts; there may also be reentry of bile acids into blood from injured hepatocytes or an obstructed biliary tract. Although there are a variety of techniques for measuring serum bile acids, these determinations are not yet of proven value for routine clinical use.

IMMUNOLOGIC AND OTHER TESTS

A number of immunologic derangements may be seen in liver disease. Antimitochondrial antibodies are found in 85 to 90 percent of patients with primary biliary cirrhosis. In this test, serum is incubated with rabbit hepatocytes. The presence of antimitochondrial antibodies can then be assessed after subsequent staining with a fluorescein-tagged second antibody. However, this marker is not entirely specific and is occasionally found in patients with chronic active hepatitis and drug-induced hepatitis. Its primary value is in helping to distinguish primary biliary cirrhosis from extrahepatic biliary obstruction. In chronic active hepatitis the *lupus erythematosus–cell test* (LE-cell test) may be positive, and *antinuclear antibodies* as well as *anti-smooth-muscle antibodies* may be present (see Chap. 269). Alpha fetoprotein is of value in the diagnosis of hepatocellular carcinoma (see Chap. 255). Measurements of serum alpha$_1$-antitrypsin and ceruloplasmin should be performed in infants with cirrhosis or hepatitis since they may reflect alpha$_1$-antitrypsin deficiency or Wilson's disease, respectively (see Chaps 256 and 330).

OTHER DIAGNOSTIC PROCEDURES

PERCUTANEOUS NEEDLE BIOPSY OF THE LIVER Percutaneous needle biopsy is a safe, simple, and valuable method for the diagnostic evaluation of liver disease. *Diffuse parenchymal disorders* such as cirrhosis, hepatitis, and drug reactions may be diagnosed with remarkable accuracy. In *disseminated focal diseases* (such as granulomas or tumor infiltrates) serial sections may demonstrate characteristic lesions.

Biopsy is performed under local anesthesia, usually with the Menghini (aspiration), Klatskin, or Vim-Silverman (cutting) needle, by either a transpleural or subcostal approach. If the operator is skillful and patients carefully selected, morbidity should be quite low and limited to occasional postbiopsy pain or vasovagal reactions.

Some of the most frequent indications for needle biopsy are (1) unexplained hepatomegaly or hepatosplenomegaly; (2) cholestasis of uncertain cause; (3) persistently abnormal liver function tests; (4) suspected systemic or infiltrative diseases such as sarcoidosis, miliary tuberculosis, or fever of unknown origin; and (5) suspected primary or metastatic liver tumor. Percutaneous liver biopsy may be performed either for diagnostic purposes or to evaluate the extent and severity of a known disease process. However, other new and improved noninvasive diagnostic methods have obviated the need for biopsy in many circumstances, and thus biopsy should be performed only when information from these other techniques is inadequate.

Needle biopsy should not be performed if (1) the patient is unable to cooperate; (2) clinical or laboratory evidence indicates impaired hemostasis (prothrombin time prolonged by 3 s or more over control, thrombocytopenia less than 80 to 100 $\times$ 10^9 platelets per liter, or partial thromboplastin time or bleeding time prolonged); (3) there is infection of the right pleural space or septic cholangitis; (4) tense ascites is present, with risk of continued leakage of ascitic fluid; (5) compatible blood is not available for transfusion in case of hemorrhage; or (6) high-grade biliary obstruction is suspected and there is an increased risk of bile peritonitis. With the increasing use of CT scan and ultrasonography, it is possible to perform "directed" aspiration biopsies of isolated lesions with very thin needles. Aspirated material can be used for cytology (tumors) and culture (abscesses) but is often inadequate for assessment of liver architecture.

LAPAROSCOPY AND LAPAROTOMY (PERITONEOSCOPY) See Chap. 236.

REFERENCES

Brensilver HL, Kaplan MM: Significance of elevated liver alkaline phosphatase in serum. Gastroenterology 68:1556, 1975

Ferrucci JT Jr et al (eds): *Interventional Radiology of the Abdomen*, 2d ed. Baltimore, Williams and Wilkins, 1985

Kemeny MM et al: A projected analysis of laboratory tests and imaging studies to detect hepatic lesions. Ann Surg 195:163, 1982

Moss, AA et al Hepatic tumors: Magnetic resonance and CT appearance. Radiology 150:191, 1984

Rothschild MA et al: Serum albumin. Hepatology 8:385, 1988

Sabesin SM: Cholestatic lipoproteins—Their pathogenesis and significance. Gastroenterology 83:704, 1982

250 DERANGEMENTS OF HEPATIC METABOLISM

DANIEL K. PODOLSKY / KURT J. ISSELBACHER

The liver plays a central role in the maintenance of metabolic homeostasis. It is therefore not surprising that the development of clinically important liver disease is accompanied by diverse systemic manifestations of disordered metabolism. The liver has considerable reserve capacity, so minimal or even moderate cell injury may not be reflected by measurable changes in its metabolic function. However, some functions of the liver are more sensitive than others, and a variety of defects may be seen, depending on the nature and extent of the initial insult.

The biochemical functions in which the liver plays a major role include (1) the intermediate metabolism of amino acids and carbohydrates, (2) synthesis and degradation of proteins and glycoproteins, (3) metabolism and degradation of drugs and hormones, and (4) regulation of lipid and cholesterol metabolism. The derangements of these functions are discussed in connection with their occurrence in various forms of parenchymal liver disease. Alterations of bilirubin, bile salt, and porphyrin metabolism are discussed elsewhere (Chaps. 46, 240, 328).

Metabolic derangements are most evident in the patient with advanced liver disease, and the manifestations are similar regardless of the initial etiologic insult. To a varying degree similar abnormalities are observed in patients with severe chronic hepatitis, micronodular cirrhosis, and postnecrotic cirrhosis. Since the many functions of the liver may be affected to varying degrees in individual patients, no single test effectively measures the overall state of liver function. The proper interpretation of liver function tests is discussed in Chap. 249.

CARBOHYDRATE METABOLISM The liver functions to maintain normal levels of blood sugar by a combination of glycogenesis, glycogenolysis, glycolysis, and gluconeogenesis. These pathways are regulated by a number of hormones including insulin, glucagon, growth hormone, and certain catecholamines. Although it has been presumed that exquisite sensitivity of the hepatocytes to insulin is responsible for the uptake of an oral glucose load by the liver, there are also data that have challenged the importance of insulin-mediated glucose uptake by the hepatocyte. In the fasting state, the liver contributes to glucose homeostasis by glycogenolysis and gluconeogenesis in response to hypoinsulinemia and hyperglucagonemia. Maintenance of normal blood glucose levels through gluconeogenesis is ultimately related to catabolism of muscle protein, which provides the necessary amino acid precursors, especially alanine. In a complementary fashion, in the postprandial state, the liver directs alanine and branched-chain amino acids to the peripheral tissues, where they are then incorporated into muscle protein. These reciprocal pathways form a glucose-alanine shuttle which is modulated by ambient changes in the hormones mentioned above (Fig. 250-1). While it has been presumed that synthesis of glycogen and fatty acid in the postprandial state arises from direct conversion of glucose, there are data to suggest that, in fact, these pathways are *indirect* with products deriving from 3-carbon metabolites of glucose or other gluconeogenic compounds such as lactate, fructose, and alanine.

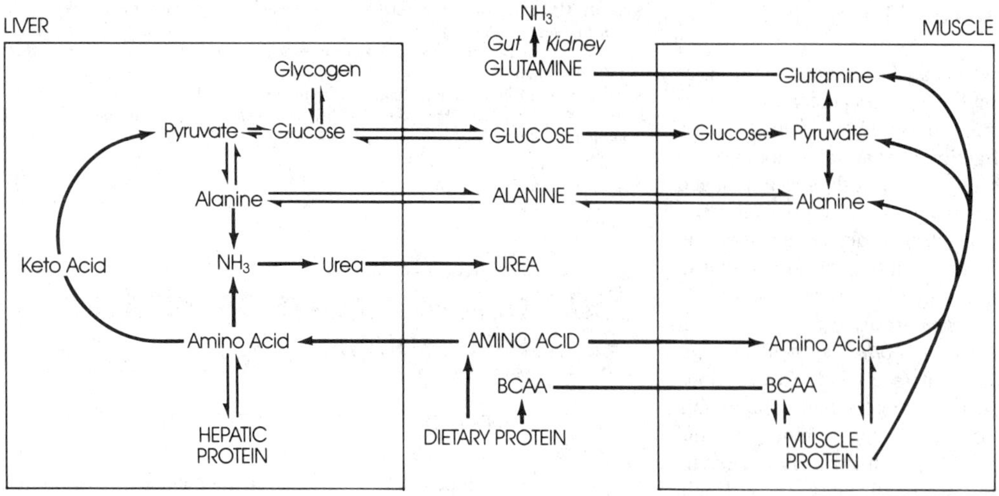

FIGURE 250-1 Carbohydrate-protein exchange between muscle and liver. After an overnight fast there is net release of amino acids by muscle (predominantly alanine and glutamine). These are derived from transamination of pyruvate, degraded amino acids, and glucose. Branched-chain amino acids (BCAA) are particularly important as a source of nitrogen for alanine synthesis. Alanine is utilized for gluconeogenesis by the liver, and urea is formed as a by-product. The main sites of glutamine uptake are the kidney and gut, where it is used for ammonia production and as a possible source of energy, respectively. Following ingestion of dietary protein, skeletal muscle goes into an anabolic phase; there is selective hepatic escape and muscle uptake of dietary BCAA, reduced muscle output of alanine and glutamine, and a reduced rate of hepatic gluconeogenesis. Hepatic tissue protein also goes into an anabolic phase following protein ingestion. (*Modified with permission from AS Tavill in Wright et al.*)

Abnormalities of glucose homeostasis are common in cirrhosis (Table 250-1). Most frequently hyperglycemia and glucose intolerance are observed. Glucose intolerance is associated with normal or increased levels of plasma insulin (except in patients with hemochromatosis), suggesting that insulin resistance rather than insulin deficiency may be responsible. One of the factors that may play a role in the apparent insulin resistance is an absolute decrease in the liver's ability to metabolize a glucose load because of a decrease in functioning hepatocellular mass. There is also evidence that response to insulin is diminished due to both receptor and postreceptor defects in hepatocytes of patients with cirrhosis. In addition, both hyperinsulinemia and hyperglucagonemia may be present due to decreased hepatic clearance of this hormone resulting from portal-systemic shunting. In patients with hemochromatosis, insulin levels, however, may indeed be low due to pancreatic iron deposition and sometimes concomitant genetic diabetes mellitus. Patients with cirrhosis may also have elevated serum lactate levels reflecting the decreased capacity of the liver to utilize lactate for gluconeogenesis.

Hypoglycemia, although more common in acute fulminant hepatitis, may also be seen with end-stage cirrhosis. Glycogen in the liver accounts for 5 to 7 percent of the normal tissue weight. Because the capacity of the liver to store glycogen is limited (approximately 70 g) and glucose consumption continues at a constant rate (approximately 150 g per day), hepatic glycogen stores are depleted after 1 day of fasting. Hypoglycemia in end-stage cirrhosis may be due to decreased hepatic glycogen stores, diminished glucagon responsiveness, or decreased capacity to synthesize glycogen due to extensive parenchymal destruction.

TABLE 250-1 Alteration of glucose metabolism in cirrhosis

Factors leading to hyperglycemia:
Decreased hepatic glucose uptake
Decreased hepatic glycogen synthesis
Hepatic resistance to insulin
Portal-systemic glucose shunting
Peripheral insulin resistance
Hormonal abnormalities (serum)
↑ Glucagon
↓ Cortisol
↑ Insulin (↓ in hemochromatosis)
Factors leading to hypoglycemia:
Decreased gluconeogenesis
Decreased hepatic glycogen content
Hepatic resistance to glucagon
Poor oral intake
Hyperinsulinemia secondary to portal-systemic shunting

AMINO ACID AND AMMONIA METABOLISM Through a variety of anabolic and catabolic processes, the liver is the major site of amino acid interconversion. Amino acids utilized for hepatic protein synthesis are derived from dietary protein, metabolic turnover of endogenous protein (primarily from muscle), and direct synthesis in the liver. Most of the amino acids entering the liver via the portal vein are catabolized to urea (except for the branched-chain amino acids leucine, isoleucine, and valine). A lesser amount is released into the general circulation as free amino acids, and these may play an important role in the glucose-alanine cycle mentioned above. In addition, amino acids are utilized for the synthesis of liver intracellular proteins, plasma proteins, and special compounds such as glutathione, glutamine, taurine, carnosine, and creatine. Disruption of normal amino acid metabolism may be reflected in altered plasma amino acid concentrations. In general, levels of aromatic amino acids normally metabolized by the liver (as well as methionine) are elevated, while those of the branched-chain amino acids, largely utilized by skeletal muscle, tend to be normal or depressed. It has been suggested that an alteration in the ratio of these two types of amino acids plays a role in the development of hepatic encephalopathy (see below), but there is not agreement on this concept.

Hepatic catabolism or degradation of amino acids involves two major reactions: transamination and oxidative deamination. In transamination an amino group of an amino acid is transferred to a keto acid. This process is catalyzed by aminotransferases which are found in very high amounts in liver but are also present in other tissues, such as kidney, muscle, heart, lung, and brain. Glutamic-oxaloacetic acid transaminase (aspartate aminotransferase, AST) has been studied most extensively, and increased levels are found in the serum secondary to various types of liver injury (e.g., acute viral and drug-induced hepatitis). As a result of transamination, amino acids can enter the citric acid cycle and then function in the intermediary metabolism of carbohydrates and lipids. Most of the nonessential amino acids are also synthesized in the liver by transamination. Oxidative deamination, which results in conversion of amino acids to keto acids (and ammonia), is catalyzed by L-amino-acid oxidase with two exceptions: glycine oxidation is catalyzed by glycine oxidase, and glutamic oxidation is catalyzed by glutamic dehydrogenase. With severe liver damage (e.g., massive hepatic necrosis), utilization of amino acids is impaired, free amino acids in the bloodstream increase, and an "overflow" type of aminoaciduria may occur.

Urea production is intimately related to the metabolic pathways outlined above, providing a means for disposal of ammonia, the toxic product of nitrogen metabolism. Disruption of this process is of particular clinical importance in the patient with severe acute and chronic liver disease. The fixation of amino acid–derived NH_3 in the form of urea is carried out via the Krebs-Henseleit cycle. The final step of this cycle, the formation of urea by arginase, is irreversible. In advanced liver disease urea synthesis is often depressed, leading to an accumulation of NH_3, usually with a significant reduction in blood urea nitrogen (BUN), an ominous sign of liver failure. This finding may be obscured by superimposed renal impairment, which often develops in patients with severe hepatic failure. Urea is mostly excreted by the kidney, but approximately 25 percent will diffuse into the intestine where it is converted to NH_3 by bacterial urease. The intestinal production of ammonia also occurs from the bacterial deamination of unabsorbed amino acids and of protein derived from the diet, exfoliated cells, or blood in the gastrointestinal tract.

Gut NH_3 is absorbed and transported to the liver via the portal vein, where it is again converted to urea. The kidney also produces varying amounts of NH_3, largely by the deamination of glutamine. The contributions of the gut and kidney to ammonia synthesis have important implications for the management of the hyperammonemic state frequently seen in patients with advanced liver disease usually in association with portal-systemic shunting of blood.

While the exact chemical mediators of hepatic encephalopathy remain unknown, elevated levels of blood NH_3 generally correlate with the degree of encephalopathy, although approximately 10 percent of such patients have normal levels of blood ammonia. In addition, therapeutic measures that reduce serum NH_3 levels also usually lead to clinical improvement. The several mechanisms known to lead to increased blood NH_3 levels in patients with cirrhosis are illustrated in Fig. 250-2 and include the following: (1) If there is excessive nitrogenous material in the intestine (from bleeding or dietary protein), excessive amounts of NH_3 will be formed by bacterial deamination of amino acids. (2) If renal function declines (as in the hepatorenal syndrome), blood urea nitrogen rises, leading to increased diffusion of urea into the intestinal lumen, where bacterial urease converts it to NH_3. (3) If hepatic function is significantly depressed, diminished

FIGURE 250-2 Major factors (steps 1 to 4) influencing the level of blood ammonia. In cirrhosis with portal hypertension, venous collaterals allow ammonia to bypass the liver (step 5), permitting the entry of ammonia into the systemic circulation (portal-systemic shunting).

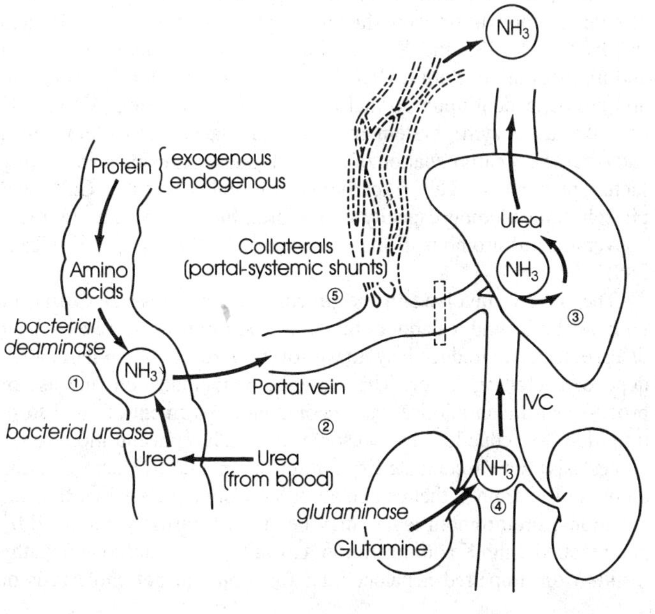

urea synthesis may occur with a resultant decrease in the removal of NH_3. (4) If alkalosis (often due to central hyperventilation) and hypokalemia accompany hepatic decompensation, there may be a decrease in the renal availability of H^+ ions; as a result, the NH_3 produced from glutamine by the action of renal glutaminase is permitted to enter the renal vein (rather than being excreted as NH_4^+) leading to increased peripheral blood NH_3 levels. In addition hypokalemia itself leads to increased NH_3 production. (5) If portal hypertension is present and anastomoses exist between the portal vein and systemic venous channels, these portal-systemic shunts will allow NH_3 from the gut to bypass hepatic detoxification, leading to elevated blood NH_3 levels. Thus, with portal-systemic shunting of blood, elevated NH_3 levels may develop even with relatively little hepatocellular dysfunction. It is unclear what effects these same factors may have on other compounds which may play a role in the development of hepatic encephalopathy.

An additional factor important in determining whether a given NH_3 level in the blood will be detrimental to the central nervous system is the blood pH. The more alkaline the pH, the more toxic a given level of NH_3 is likely to be. At 37°C the p*K* of NH_3 is 8.9; this is close enough to the pH of blood that minor changes in pH can affect the NH_4^+/NH_3 ratio. Because un-ionized NH_3 crosses membranes more readily than NH_4^+ ions, alkalosis favors the entry of ammonia into the brain (with subsequent changes in cell metabolism) by shifting the equilibrium of the following reaction to the right

$$NH_4^+ + OH^- \rightleftharpoons NH_3 + HOH$$

As a result, alkalosis not only increases peripheral blood NH_3 levels by renal mechanisms but also increases tissue levels by influencing the diffusion of NH_3 across membranes.

PROTEIN SYNTHESIS AND DEGRADATION The liver is an important site of protein synthesis and degradation. Although the body muscle mass produces the greatest total amount of protein, the liver has the highest rate of synthesis per gram of tissue. The liver synthesizes not only the proteins it needs, but also and perhaps more importantly it produces numerous export proteins. Among the latter, albumin is the most important; *it is produced at a rate of approximately 12 g per day,* representing 25 percent of total hepatic protein synthesis and half of all exported protein. The average normal half-life of serum albumin is 17 to 20 days. The proportion of hepatocytes carrying out active albumin synthesis varies from 10 to 60 percent depending on the body's requirements. Approximately 60 percent of albumin is found in the extravascular spaces, but plasma albumin is still the most abundant circulating protein.

Albumin contributes significantly to the plasma oncotic pressure. In addition, it is the principal binding and transport protein for numerous substances including some hormones, fatty acids, trace metals, tryptophan, bilirubin, and other organic anions of both endogenous and exogenous origin. Despite the many important functions of albumin, rare individuals with congenital analbuminemia appear to have no major physiologic derangements other than the excessive accumulation of extravascular fluid. While many of the less hydrophobic ligands may be transported in the unbound form, this suggests that other serum proteins may also play a role in binding and transport.

Much has been learned about the mechanisms involved in the synthesis of secretory proteins, especially of albumin (see Fig. 250-3). Polyribosomes bound to the rough endoplasmic reticulum (RER) of the hepatocyte are the principal site of translation of messenger ribonucleic acid (mRNA) coding for export proteins; in contrast proteins destined for intracellular use, such as ferritin, are synthesized on free rather than bound polyribosomes in the cytoplasm. After a short-term fast, there is a decrease in the amount of albumin mRNA associated with the RER; instead more mRNA is found in the cytosol and in a state dissociated from polyribosomes. Albumin, like secretory proteins produced by other organs, appears to be synthesized initially as a larger precursor, preproalbumin. This precursor molecule contains an additional 24 extra amino acid residues

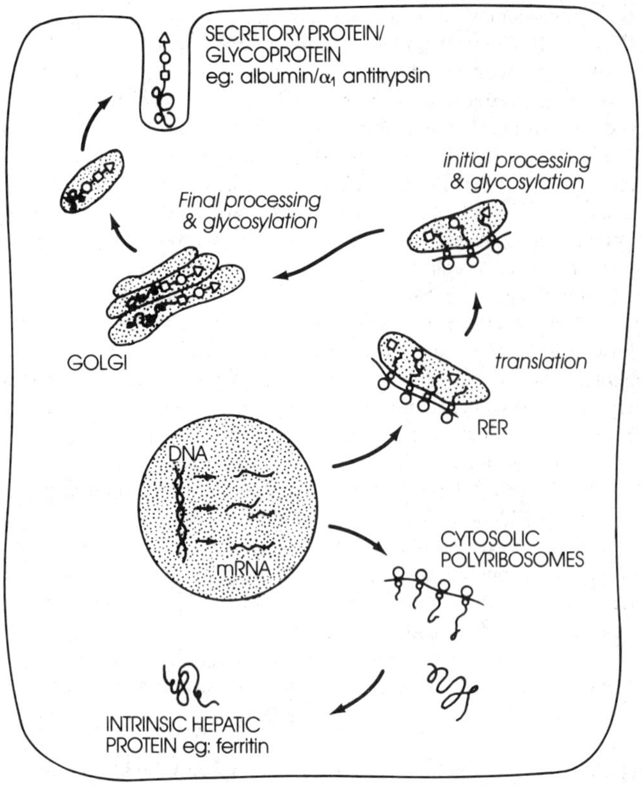

FIGURE 250-3 Schematic diagram illustrating major steps in synthesis, processing, and secretion of proteins and glycoproteins by the liver. Ribosomal subunits and mRNA form polysome complexes to initiate protein synthesis. Polyribosomes synthesizing proteins destined for export (e.g., albumin) associate with membranes to form membrane-bound polysomes [i.e., the rough endoplasmic reticulum (RER)]. Synthesis of precursor molecule (e.g., "preproalbumin") occurs and is followed by stepwise proteolytic cleavage and secretion from the cell. Other export proteins (e.g., α_1-antitrypsin) are first glycosylated in the RER and Golgi prior to secretion. Proteins produced for intracellular use (e.g., ferritin) are synthesized on non-membrane-bound cytosolic polyribosomes and processed by stepwise proteolytic cleavage and secretion from the cell.

on the *N* terminus, referred to as a "signal peptide," which undergoes two sequential cleavages (or "processing"); the molecule is then transported to the Golgi apparatus prior to secretion. The "pre" portion of preproalbumin is cleaved within the RER even before protein synthesis is completed; the "pro" segment is removed within the lumen of the ER. Once synthesis and processing are completed, albumin is transported from the Golgi vesicles to the hepatocyte surface by mechanisms which are unclear but almost certainly involve the microfilaments and microtubule apparatus of the cell. Although the hepatic lymph space of Disse provides a potential avenue for the newly released albumin, most secreted proteins enter the plasma.

Albumin synthesis is subject to a number of regulatory influences. These include the rate of transcription of specific mRNAs and the availability of the substrate tRNA (transfer RNA). At the translational level, the integrity of polyribosomes and their synthetic abilities is modified by factors affecting initiation, elongation, and release of peptides and proteins as well as by the availability of ATP, GTP, and magnesium ions. The rate of albumin synthesis is also influenced by the availability of amino acid precursors, especially tryptophan, the scarcest of the essential amino acids. Indeed in patients with large carcinoid tumors albumin synthesis may decrease precipitously when tryptophan is consumed by carcinoid cells in the production of 5-hydroxytryptophan (serotonin) (see Chap. 262). The rate of albumin synthesis is also affected by colloid oncotic pressure with increased production occurring in response to falling oncotic pressure. Finally, influences of hormones such as insulin and glucagon on hepatic protein metabolism are closely integrated with the nutritional factors discussed above.

The liver also produces a wide variety of other secretory proteins, most of which have a synthetic pathway and processing procedure similar to that of albumin (Fig. 250-3). The presence of a *signal peptide,* such as the "prepro" segment of albumin, which is subsequently removed during protein maturation appears to be a general mechanism for orienting proteins in the membranes of the endoplasmic reticulum and directing them for export rather than for intracellular use or degradation. Most proteins undergo even further modification in the form of sequential *glycosylation* in the RER and Golgi apparatus. The carbohydrate moieties of these glycoproteins appear to be important in determining their site of action and their rate of tissue uptake after secretion. Some of the clinically important secretory glycoproteins include ceruloplasmin, α_1-antitrypsin, and most other alpha and beta globulins. While the site of albumin catabolism is uncertain, the removal of terminal sialic acid residues after secretion and the resultant exposure of penultimate galactose or *N*-acetylglucosamine residues appears to result in receptor-mediated uptake of "aged" proteins by hepatocytes and Kupffer cells, followed by their subsequent degradation. Reduced amounts of the hepatic receptor for asialoglycoproteins appear to result in elevated serum concentrations of these glycoproteins in patients with severe and chronic liver disease.

One of the clinically most important derangements in protein metabolism is the development of hypoalbuminemia, which results largely from reduced synthetic activity. Decreased synthesis may be caused by a decrease in the number as well as the function of hepatocytes. A decrease in the dietary supply of amino acids can also contribute to deficient synthesis. To some extent the body attempts to compensate for decreased albumin synthesis by reducing the rate of degradation. Attempts to raise the serum albumin level by intravenous infusions are often futile because this compensatory mechanism can be blunted and the decrease in albumin degradation may not occur. The reduced degradation of albumin is not a general phenomenon in chronic liver disease because other proteins such as fibrinogen are degraded more rapidly than normal. The degree of hypoalbuminemia is also augmented in the patient with ascites, in which large amounts of the body's albumin are present in the ascitic fluid. When there is increased hepatic venous pressure (as in postsinusoidal or hepatic vein outflow block), there may be increased hepatic lymph production with extravasation into the peritoneal cavity. In contrast to intestinal lymph, the protein content of hepatic lymph appears to be relatively uninfluenced by ascitic oncotic pressure, most likely reflecting the lack of tight junctions between sinusoidal endothelial cells.

Other proteins produced by the liver include many of the blood-clotting factors: fibrinogen (factor I), prothrombin (factor II), and factors V, VII, IX, and X as well as inhibitors of both coagulation and fibrinolysis. Factors II, VII, IX, and X are vitamin K–responsive and are dependent upon normal intestinal fat absorption. Vitamin K activates an enzyme system in liver endoplasmic reticulum which catalyzes the γ carboxylation of selected glutamyl residues in clotting factor precursors. The γ carboxylation enhances the Ca^{2+} and phospholipid binding capacity of prothrombin and permits its rapid conversion to thrombin in the presence of factors V and X (Chap. 288).

The liver is involved in the process of hemostasis by virtue of both anabolic and catabolic functions. As expected, severe liver disease leads to reduced synthesis of prothrombin, a vitamin K–dependent clotting factor. The presence of malnutrition, the use of broad-spectrum antibiotics, or concomitant impairment of fat absorption due to reduction in intestinal bile salt concentration (e.g., cholestasis) may accentuate hypoprothrombinemia by decreasing the amount of vitamin K that can be absorbed from the intestine. In these situations, prothrombin levels may be at least partially corrected by parenteral vitamin K administration. However, when the coagulopathy results from impaired hepatocellular function and not cholestasis or intestinal factors, exogenous vitamin K is unlikely to correct or improve prothrombin synthesis. The vitamin K–dependent clotting proteins have a substantially shorter serum half-life than albumin; therefore, hypoprothrombinemia usually precedes the development of hypoalbuminemia, especially in the patient with acute hepatocellular disease. In cirrhosis, coagulopathy may be further aggravated by the thrombocytopenia resulting from hypersplenism.

Since the liver is also the site of production of non-vitamin K–dependent clotting factors, severe liver disease injury may lead to decreased plasma concentrations of factor V in addition to factors II, VII, IX, and X. It is unusual for fibrinogen to be reduced significantly, unless there is an associated disseminated intravascular coagulation (DIC). For unclear reasons, the damaged liver may actually produce increased amounts of fibrinogen as well as other proteins collectively designated acute-phase reactants (C-reactive proteins, haptoglobin, ceruloplasmin, and transferrin). The latter are produced both in response to liver injury (e.g., severe chronic active hepatitis) and in association with systemic illnesses such as cancer, rheumatoid arthritis, bacterial infections, burns, and myocardial infarctions. However, while the diseased liver may produce normal or increased amounts of fibrinogen, the molecules themselves may be qualitatively abnormal (i.e., structurally and functionally), reflecting more subtle derangements in protein synthesis. These functionally abnormal fibrinogen molecules may contribute to the altered hemostasis frequently found in patients with chronic liver disease.

DETOXIFICATION MECHANISMS Water-soluble drugs and endogenous substances usually are excreted unchanged in the urine or bile. However, lipid-soluble compounds tend to accumulate in the body and affect cellular processes, unless they are converted to less active compounds or to more water-soluble metabolites which are more easily excreted. Hepatic blood flow, protein binding, and the intrinsic capacity of the liver to eliminate a drug are all primary determinants of hepatic drug clearance. The liver has an important role in the metabolism of many exogenous drugs and endogenous hormones by virtue of several enzyme systems involved in biochemical transformation. The relative importance of these various factors differs depending on how well a drug is extracted by the liver. There are two major types of reactions. The first, *phase I reactions,* result in chemical modification of reactive groups by oxidation, reduction, hydroxylation, sulfoxidation, deamination, dealkylation, or methylation. Such modifications usually involve one of several enzymatic systems, including the mixed-function oxidases, cytochromes b_5 and P_{450} (microsomal), and the glutathione *S*-acyltransferases (cytoplasmic). These biochemical reactions usually lead to *inactivation* of drugs such as barbiturates and benzodiazepines. However, *activation* may also occur. For example, cortisone is activated to cortisol and prednisone to prednisolone (both products being more potent than the parent compounds); imipramine, a depressant, is converted to desmethylimipramine, an antidepressant. In the same manner, phase I reactions may even convert a nontoxic compound to a toxic one as in the metabolism of isoniazid and acetaminophen. Similarly, some carcinogens may be activated by formation of highly reactive epoxide intermediates in the liver, while other carcinogens may be detoxified.

The enzymes responsible for phase I reactions, especially those involving the cytochrome P_{450} system, can be induced by drugs such as ethanol, barbiturates, haloperidol, and glutethimide. Conversely, hepatic microsomal enzymes may be inhibited by agents such as chloramphenicol, cimetidine, disulfiram, dextropropoxyphene, allopurinol, and, paradoxically, by ethanol. The concomitant administration of two drugs metabolized by the same microsomal enzyme may result in modification, potentiation, or diminution of the pharmacologic efficacy of either or both drugs. Activity of phase I reactions may also change with aging.

Phase II reactions may follow phase I reactions or proceed independently; these involve the conversion of substances to their glucuronide, sulfate, acetyl, taurine, or glycine derivatives, thereby converting lipophilic substances to water-soluble derivatives and permitting their excretion in bile or urine. Conjugation catalyzed by microsomal UDP (uridine diphosphate)-glucuronyltransferases to form glucuronide derivatives is one of the most common phase II reactions. In general, the conjugates are more soluble than the parent compound and are pharmacologically inactive.

An awareness that there may be varying degrees of impairment in the hepatic uptake, detoxification, and excretion of certain drugs is important in the clinical management of patients with chronic liver disease. Portal-systemic shunting of blood may decrease the "first-pass effect" of drugs absorbed from the gut. In cirrhosis, altered intrahepatic hemodynamics due to a disordered liver architecture may also reduce the rates of hepatic drug clearance. Hypoalbuminemia will permit drugs usually bound to albumin to be present in increased concentrations of their unbound form in the circulation and extracellular spaces; this may result in an increased activity of such drugs. Most importantly, a decrease in the amount of function of microsomal enzymes responsible for phase I and phase II reactions will result in slower rates of drug inactivation and elimination. Drugs for which there may be a decreased clearance in patients with liver disease include anticonvulsants (e.g., phenytoin, phenobarbital), anti-inflammatory agents (e.g., acetaminophen, phenylbutazone, glucocorticoids), minor tranquilizers, cardioactive drugs (e.g., lidocaine, quinidine, propranolol), and antibiotics (e.g., nafcillin, chloramphenicol, tetracyclines, clindamycin, trimethoprim, rifampin, pyrazinamide). This will lead to decreased dosage requirements and a narrowing of the range between therapeutic and toxic drug levels. Finally, the patient with chronic liver disease may demonstrate alterations in the pharmacologic effects of drugs in addition to or independent of changes in their pharmacokinetics such as an increased central nervous system sensitivity to opiates and other sedatives.

The difficulties in safely administering pharmacologic agents to patients with both acute and chronic liver disease are underscored by the frequency with which administration of benzodiazepines is cited as precipitating hepatic coma. It may be very difficult clinically to determine whether agitation, confusion, and irrational behavior are due to early hepatic encephalopathy or are related to the concurrent use of benzodiazepines, opiates, barbiturates, and other depressants. It should be recognized that there is great variation of drug clearance in patients with liver disease; although data on average clearances may provide a reasonable estimate for initial dosages, subsequent adjustments in dose need to be individualized in order to attain the desired plasma drug concentration.

The mechanism by which some agents exert a hepatotoxic effect may involve the same metabolic pathways responsible for normal drug detoxification. The mechanism of acetaminophen toxicity is particularly illustrative. Acetaminophen is metabolized and detoxified by the hepatic mixed-function oxygenase system, but one of the intermediate products is a potent free radical (postulated metabolite *N*-acetylimidoquinone) which can inactivate many enzymes and proteins by binding irreversibly to their sulfhydryl groups. Normally this interaction can be prevented by reduced glutathione. In the presence of excessive amounts of the acetaminophen free radical (e.g., from overdosage or underlying liver disease), the glutathione levels of the hepatocytes are readily exhausted and the excess free radicals can lead to inactivation of cellular proteins and produce widespread hepatocellular necrosis. In the case of acetaminophen overdosage, the very early administration of sulfhydryl groups in the form of *N*-acetylcysteine can often prevent this drug-induced liver injury.

HORMONE METABOLISM In addition to its role in the metabolism of diverse pharmacologic agents, the liver is also responsible for inactivation or modification of several endogenous hormones; therefore, chronic liver disease may be accompanied by signs of apparent hormonal imbalance. Some hormones (e.g., insulin and glucagon) are inactivated in the liver by proteolysis or deamination. Thyroxine and triiodothyronine are metabolized in the liver by reactions involving deiodination. Steroid hormones, such as glucocorticoids and aldosterone, are first inactivated to their tetrahydro derivative (by reduction of the Δ^4 double bond and the 3-keto group), followed by conjugation, mostly with glucuronic acid. Testosterone is metabolized to the isomeric 17-ketosteroids androsterone and etiocholanolone and excreted in the urine mostly as sulfate conjugates. Estrogens, such as estradiol, may be converted to estriol and estrone and then conjugated with glucuronic acid or sulfate. Abnormalities in estrogen (and testosterone) metabolism are believed to be involved in the development of the spider angiomas, loss of axillary or pubic hair, and testicular atrophy frequently seen in patients with chronic liver disease. In addition, increased portal-systemic shunting of testosterone and androstenedione secondary to portal hypertension may lead to the development of gynecomastia in cirrhotic males due to increased peripheral conversion to estradiol and estrone, especially in patients with alcoholic cirrhosis. In patients with alcoholic liver disease, feminization may also be related to the direct toxic effects of alcohol on the gonadal-pituitary-hypothalamic axis which lead to the overall reduction in serum testosterone found in patients with cirrhosis. Similar effects are also seen in patients with hemochromatosis due to deposition of iron in these sites. However, gynecomastia is often lacking in the latter, apparently due to a coincident reduction in plasma concentration of androstenedione, a major precursor for estrogen synthesis.

Estrogens also act directly on the liver to impair hepatic secretory activity. Estradiol and related estrogens, such as those present in contraceptive pills, interfere with sodium sulfobromophthalein and bile salt excretion and worsen the preexisting defect in secretion of conjugated bilirubin in patients with Dubin-Johnson syndrome; they may also elevate plasma alkaline phosphatase levels (see Chap. 249). Related steroids such as etiocholanolone and pregnanediol have been shown to stimulate δ-aminolevulinic acid (ALA) synthetase activity leading to increased porphobilinogen excretion. Since these steroids exert these effects only in their unconjugated form, the increased hepatic levels of δ-aminolevulinic acid synthetase in patients with alcoholic cirrhosis may be secondary to the action of gonadal steroids.

LIPID METABOLISM: FATTY ACIDS AND TRIGLYCERIDES Under normal conditions, most of the fatty acids taken up by the liver and esterified to triglyceride are derived from adipose tissue or the diet. Some fatty acids (especially saturated ones) are synthesized in the liver from acetate. The fatty acids may then be converted enzymatically to triglyceride, esterified with cholesterol, incorporated into phospholipids, or oxidized to CO_2 or ketone bodies. Most of the triglyceride is produced for export, but in order to be secreted it must be converted to lipoproteins by combining with relatively specific apoprotein moieties. This emphasizes the importance of protein synthesis for the release and secretion of triglyceride from the liver. It should be noted that the liver plays a major role in regulating lipoprotein levels by virtue of both its degradative and synthetic functions. Thus, the liver is quantitatively the major site of low-density lipoprotein (LDL) catabolism with dual high- and low-affinity receptor-mediated pathways playing a role. In addition chylomicron remnants are removed and degraded by the liver, where their constituents have a number of metabolic effects. The liver is not only the primary site of very low density lipoprotein (VLDL) secretion but also accounts for a major portion of its subsequent degradation by mechanisms similar to that of chylomicron remnant degradation and conversion to LDL via the action of hepatic lipase. The liver may also play a role in high-density lipoprotein (HDL) catabolism. It is noteworthy that with the exception of cholestatic disease (see below), clinically significant alterations in lipoprotein and cholesterol metabolism are usually not found in patients with chronic liver disease.

Studies on the production of fatty liver have shown that singly or in combination, one or more of the steps depicted in Fig. 250-4 may be involved. An increased influx of fatty acids mobilized from adipose tissue due to drugs (e.g., ethanol or glucocorticoids) or secondary to diabetic ketosis may lead to a fatty liver. Similarly, increased levels of fatty acids in the liver, either from enhanced fatty acid synthesis or from decreased fatty acid oxidation, may lead to increased triglyceride formation. In some instances (e.g., ethanol excess) there

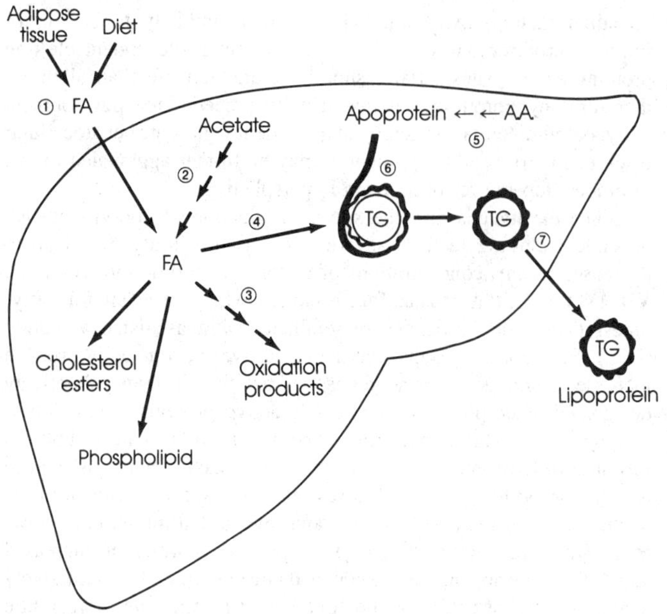

FIGURE 250-4 Factors in the uptake and esterification of fatty acids to triglyceride by the liver, including the formation and release of triglyceride as lipoprotein. The numbers refer to steps, which, if altered, may result in increased liver triglyceride (i.e., fatty liver).

may also be increases in the carbohydrate backbone, α-glycerophosphate, involved in fatty acid esterification to triglyceride. Since release of triglyceride involves the formation of lipoproteins, lipid accumulation may occur because of decreased apoprotein synthesis. This appears to be the case in fatty livers seen in patients with protein-calorie malnutrition (kwashiorkor) and due to toxins such as carbon tetrachloride, phosphorus, or ethionine, as well as following excessive doses of antibiotics like tetracycline that can inhibit protein synthesis. Finally, there may be impaired lipoprotein secretion from the liver. Alcohol is perhaps the most common agent leading to a fatty liver, but the mechanism(s) whereby alcohol leads to increased liver triglyceride is not clear. Depending on factors such as dose or duration, alcohol ingestion may affect any of the seven steps shown in Fig. 250-4; however, the primary factor for the production of the alcohol-induced fatty liver remains to be determined. The alterations in the redox state due to excessive accumulation of NADH resulting from oxidation of alcohol may also contribute.

In addition to the changes leading to fatty liver, there are many metabolic alterations which may be found in the blood of patients following the ingestion of large amounts of alcohol. These include, among others, *increased* plasma levels of lactate, proline, urate, and triglycerides and *decreased* plasma levels of glucose, magnesium, phosphate, and triiodothyronine (T_3).

CHOLESTEROL Cholesterol and bile acid synthesis is carried out primarily by the liver. Cholesterol synthesis is subject to a number of metabolic controls, most of them mediated via the rate-limiting biosynthetic enzyme 3-hydroxy-3-methylglutaryl coenzyme A reductase (HMG-CoA reductase). Cholesterol exists either free or combined with fatty acids in the form of cholesterol esters; in the plasma both are found primarily in association with β-lipoproteins. The plasma and liver also contain lecithin–cholesterol acyltransferase (LCAT), an enzyme involved in the conversion of free cholesterol to its esterified form. Since there is exchange of free cholesterol between tissues, changes in plasma cholesterol levels reflect changes in total body cholesterol. However, decreases in plasma cholesterol esters may reflect hepatic damage and impaired hepatic cholesterol esterification.

Severe liver injury often leads to a decrease in *total* serum cholesterol levels, including both free and esterified fractions. This may be due to decreased synthesis of cholesterol and cholesterol esters, decreased apoprotein synthesis, or both. In cholestasis (either intra- or extrahepatic) total serum cholesterol often increases strikingly. Disorders of cholestasis are associated with marked abnormalities of lipoprotein metabolism. In primary biliary cirrhosis there are pronounced elevations in serum free cholesterol and LDL; conversely, serum HDL is reduced and may disappear from the serum in patients with long-standing disease. Similar but less marked changes are seen in other cholestatic conditions.

The increase in serum free cholesterol (and phospholipid) and the concomitant decrease in esterified cholesterol in cholestasis may be related to a decrease in the hepatic production of LCAT. Reduced levels of LCAT are also correlated with the appearance of an abnormal LDL, referred to as lipoprotein X (LP-X). Although LP-X, which has a high content of free cholesterol and triglyceride, was originally thought to be a specific indicator of biliary tract obstruction, it is evident that it appears in any cholestatic condition. While the depressed hepatic production of LCAT may be responsible for altered lipid content and composition of lipoproteins, the factors leading to the overall increase in total serum cholesterol are not clear. In experimental animals, bile duct ligation results in a net increase in hepatic cholesterol synthesis, and in ''regurgitation'' of bile salts, cholesterol, and LP-X into venous radicals. However, it is difficult to translate these experimental findings to the patient with primary biliary cirrhosis unless any insult to cells lining the biliary canaliculi and ductules can impair the delicate balance of lipid synthesis and removal.

Most of the derangements of hepatic metabolism discussed above are evident only in patients with severe or long-standing liver disease. Indeed, in all but the most severe cases of acute viral hepatitis, hepatic metabolic functions are remarkably well preserved, and in most cases of mild to moderate acute viral hepatitis, it is uncommon to observe clinically important alterations in carbohydrate, protein, and lipid metabolism. However, in the patients with severe or fulminant hepatitis, whether from a viral or toxic agent, the metabolic derangements may be similar to those seen in more chronic disease. For example, in fulminant hepatitis there may be pronounced hypoprothrombinemia and impaired coagulation, hypoalbuminemia, and the relatively acute development of ascites, as well as hyperammonemia and encephalopathy. However, in contrast to patients with cirrhosis, abnormalities in carbohydrate metabolism are more likely to lead to profound hypoglycemia than to hyperglycemia. This hypoglycemia appears to reflect both a marked decrease in hepatic glycogen stores and a diminished glucagon responsiveness. There may also be poor oral intake due to nausea and anorexia together with increased glucose utilization secondary to hyperinsulinemia (due to portal-systemic shunting and decreased insulin degradation).

REFERENCES

Arias IM et al: *The Liver: Biology and Pathophysiology,* 2d ed. New York, Raven, 1988

Cavallo-Perin P et al: Mechanism of insulin resistance in human liver cirrhosis. Evidence of a combined receptor and post-receptor defect. J Clin Invest 75:1659, 1985

Cooper AD: Role of the liver in the degradation of lipoproteins. Gastroenterology 88:192, 1984

Flannery DB et al: Current status of hyperammonemic syndromes. Hepatology 2:495, 1982

Hoyumpa AM et al: Hepatic encephalopathy. Gastroenterology 77:803, 1979

Kleg HK et al: Conversion of androgens to estrogens in idiopathic hemochromatosis: Comparison with alcoholic liver disease. J Clin Endocrin Metab 61:1, 1985

Owen OE et al: Hepatic, gut and renal substrate flux rates in patients with hepatic cirrhosis. J Clin Invest 68:240, 1981

Rothschild MA et al: Serum albumin. Hepatology 8:355, 1988

Sherlock S: *Diseases of the Liver and Biliary System,* 8th ed. Oxford, Blackwell, 1989

Smith AR et al: Alteration in plasma and CSF amino acids, amines and metabolites in hepatic coma. Ann Surg 187:343, 1978

Williams RC: Drug administration in hepatic disease. N Engl J Med 309:1616, 1983

Wright R et al: *Liver and Biliary Disease,* 2d ed. Philadelphia, Saunders, 1985

251 BILIRUBIN METABOLISM AND HYPERBILIRUBINEMIA

KURT J. ISSELBACHER

The normal metabolism of bilirubin and the approach to the patient with jaundice have been presented in Chap. 47. With a consideration of these pathways, the disorders of bilirubin metabolism can be divided into four major categories, namely, those due to (1) increased pigment production, (2) reduced hepatic uptake of bilirubin, (3) impaired hepatic conjugation, and (4) decreased excretion of the conjugated pigment from the liver into bile. The first three of these disorders are associated with predominantly unconjugated hyperbilirubinemia. The fourth group, defective excretion, is associated with predominantly conjugated hyperbilirubinemia and bilirubinuria.

DISORDERS CAUSING PREDOMINANTLY UNCONJUGATED HYPERBILIRUBINEMIA

The plasma concentration of unconjugated bilirubin is determined by (1) the rate at which newly synthesized bilirubin enters the plasma (bilirubin turnover) and (2) the rate of removal of bilirubin by the liver (hepatic bilirubin clearance). Disturbances of the latter can result from derangements of hepatic bilirubin uptake, conjugation, or both. Measurements of these variables, although not routinely available, permit a classification of patients into those with *increased bilirubin turnover* (e.g., hemolysis), those with *decreased bilirubin clearance* (e.g., Gilbert's syndrome), and those in whom both mechanisms operate.

OVERPRODUCTION OF BILIRUBIN (INCREASED TURNOVER)

Increased destruction of circulating erythrocytes (intravascular and extravascular hemolysis) In disorders associated with hemolysis, most commonly the hemolytic anemias, the rate of bilirubin production is increased and may even exceed the amount that can be removed by a normal liver. The resulting jaundice is primarily an unconjugated hyperbilirubinemia. There is often also a small increase in the serum conjugated bilirubin (see Chap. 47). If significant anemia or other adverse factors are present (e.g., fever, sepsis, hypoxemia, or vascular collapse), the ability of the liver to handle the pigment load will be compromised, and the degree of jaundice will be greater.

The clinical and diagnostic features of the various hemolytic anemias are described in Chap. 294. The presence of reticulocytosis, shortened red blood cell survival, and increased fecal urobilinogen, in the absence of clinical and laboratory evidence of liver disease, strongly suggest hemolysis and overproduction of bilirubin as the cause of the jaundice. It is obvious, however, that in some cases (e.g., cirrhosis, tumors, and sepsis), hemolysis *plus* deranged liver function may be present. In most cases of uncomplicated hemolytic states, the mean serum bilirubin level will be in the range of 51 to 86 μmol/L (3 to 5 mg/dL); rarely, higher levels may be seen.

Jaundice due to increased pigment production may also be seen as a consequence of *tissue infarction* (e.g., pulmonary infarcts) and large *collections of blood in tissues* (e.g., leakage from blood vessels after catheterization studies, rupture of an aortic aneurysm). If hypotension and hypoxemia also supervene, jaundice is usually more pronounced, and the resulting impairment of liver function may also lead to a significant increase in the serum conjugated bilirubin level (see ''Postoperative Jaundice'' below).

Except in early infancy, elevations of serum unconjugated bilirubin levels are not generally harmful per se, and the prognosis is that of the hemolytic process itself. However, in the neonatal state and infancy, unconjugated bilirubin levels above 340 μmol/L (20 mg/dL) may lead to *kernicterus* due to bilirubin deposition in the lipid-rich basal ganglia (see Chap. 358). Chronic overproduction of bilirubin may result in the formation of gallstones composed predominantly of bilirubin ("pigment stones"). In this situation, all the potential complications of calculus disease of the biliary tract (Chap. 258) may be superimposed on the chronic hemolytic state which produced it.

Increased production of bilirubin from sources other than circulating erythrocytes As indicated in Chap. 47, about 15 to 20 percent of the circulating bilirubin is normally derived from sources other than the destruction of circulating red blood cells. This represents the so-called early-labeled fraction; it includes the synthesis of bilirubin from nonhemoglobin heme in the liver and from hemoglobin heme in the marrow.

In some conditions, jaundice results from an increased destruction of red blood cells or their precursors in the marrow—a process referred to as *ineffective erythropoiesis* (see Chaps. 47 and 61). In patients with thalassemia, pernicious anemia, and congenital erythropoietic porphyria, such an increased rate of formation of the early-labeled bilirubin fraction has been demonstrated. It is possible that some cases of unexplained unconjugated hyperbilirubinemia may be caused by an increased hepatic production of bilirubin from nonhemoglobin heme, but this phenomenon has not yet been demonstrated clinically.

IMPAIRED HEPATIC UPTAKE OF BILIRUBIN **Drugs** Only a few drugs have been definitely shown to influence the uptake of bilirubin by the liver. Flavaspidic acid, used in the treatment of tapeworm infestation, may cause unconjugated hyperbilirubinemia, as well as impairment of sodium sulfobromophthalein (BSP) clearance, during its administration. The jaundice readily subsides following treatment. Flavaspidic acid competes with bilirubin for binding to ligandin, leading thereby to unconjugated hyperbilirubinemia. The jaundice which may occur with novobiocin and some cholecystographic dyes is also apparently due to an interference in bilirubin uptake.

Gilbert's syndrome Some cases of this syndrome of chronic unconjugated hyperbilirubinemia may be due to a defect in hepatic uptake (as reflected by alteration in BSP kinetics). In most cases, however, a deficiency of bilirubin glucuronyl transferase can be demonstrated. Hence this syndrome is best considered as a defect in bilirubin conjugation (see below).

IMPAIRED BILIRUBIN CONJUGATION (DECREASED ACTIVITY OF BILIRUBIN GLUCURONYL TRANSFERASE) **Neonatal jaundice (physiologic jaundice of the newborn)** Almost every infant exhibits some transient unconjugated hyperbilirubinemia between the second and fifth days of life. While during gestation the placenta serves to clear bilirubin from the fetus, after birth infants must detoxify the pigments themselves. However, at this stage the hepatic enzyme glucuronyl transferase is still "immature" and inadequate for the task. As a result, unconjugated bilirubinemia develops, usually not exceeding 86 μmol/L (5 mg/dL). The activity of glucuronyl transferase increases within several days to 2 weeks after birth, and concomitantly the serum bilirubin returns to normal. In the premature infant the glucuronyl transferase activity is less, and the neonatal jaundice may be more pronounced. The "maturation" of the fetal and neonatal liver may be enhanced by treatment of the pregnant mother or the newborn infant with phenobarbital or related drugs. This results in a clear-cut reduction of the degree and duration of unconjugated hyperbilirubinemia in the newborn. In infants with a superimposed hemolytic process (e.g., erythroblastosis), the excessive pigment load leads to more pronounced jaundice, and bilirubin levels may exceed 340 μmol/L (20 mg/dL). It should be emphasized that neonatal jaundice is not present at the time of delivery; if jaundice is present at birth, other causes must be considered.

The cytoplasmic liver cell protein ligandin binds bilirubin in the hepatocyte and may assist in the transfer of bilirubin to the endoplasmic reticulum for conjugation (Chap. 47). It has been proposed that deficiency of ligandin may contribute to neonatal jaundice.

An additional facet of the "immature" liver is a concomitant defect in the excretion of *conjugated* bilirubin. Rarely this defect persists beyond the time needed for the development of adequate glucuronide conjugation and may explain the occasional presence of conjugated hyperbilirubinemia in infants with erythroblastosis (*inspissated bile syndrome*).

When in the neonatal state unconjugated bilirubin levels approach or exceed 340 μmol/L (20 mg/dL), the infants may develop and die of *kernicterus* (bilirubin encephalopathy). This condition results from unconjugated bilirubin deposition in the lipid-rich basal ganglia. In the past treatment consisted of exchange transfusions, and albumin infusions were used to increase binding of bilirubin in the circulation and diminish its entry into the brain. The current approach is *phototherapy;* intense illumination of these patients with strong white or blue light leads to the photoisomerization of bilirubin to water-soluble isomers that are rapidly excreted in the bile without the prior need of conjugation. However, another novel approach involves decreasing bilirubin production from heme by inhibitors of the enzyme, heme oxygenase. Synthetic protoporphyrins, such as tin protoporphyrin, have been successfully administered to patients with neonatal hyperbilirubinemia with marked reduction in the serum bilirubin and with no major side effects.

Hereditary glucuronyl transferase deficiency There are currently three syndromes that fall into this category. As indicated in Table 251-1, they reflect progressive decreases in the activity of glucuronyl transferase and thus may be part of a spectrum, i.e., from minimal deficiency to complete absence of bilirubin glucuronyl transferase.

GILBERT'S SYNDROME Since the original report by Gilbert in 1907, there has been an increased recognition of this benign but chronic disorder characterized by mild, persistent, unconjugated hyperbilirubinemia. The patient usually does not manifest this disorder until after the second decade and is often unaware of the jaundice until it is detected by physical examination or routine laboratory testing. The total serum bilirubin level usually ranges and fluctuates from 21 to 51 μmol/L (1.2 to 3 mg/dL) and rarely exceeds 86 μmol/L (5 mg/dL). With the van den Bergh diazo reaction, less than 20 percent of the bilirubin gives a direct reaction; however, studies using more accurate methods (such as high-pressure liquid chromatography) show that the serum bilirubin in patients with Gilbert's syndrome is almost all unconjugated. Typically the jaundice fluctuates and is exacerbated following prolonged fasting (see below), surgery, fever or infection, and excessive exertion or alcohol ingestion. Liver function tests are normal, and the liver cells usually appear normal by light microscopy.

With the exception of hemolytic anemias, this disorder is probably the most common cause of mild unconjugated hyperbilirubinemia. Detailed studies show these patients to have a partial deficiency of bilirubin glucuronyl transferase. Some patients also manifest decreased bilirubin uptake and increased hemolysis. Decreased glucuronyl transferase alone or together with a decrease in bilirubin uptake

TABLE 251-1 Hereditary unconjugated hyperbilirubinemias with deficiency of glucuronyl transferase

Features	Mild (Gilbert's syndrome)	Moderate (Crigler-Najjar syndrome type II)	Severe (Crigler-Najjar syndrome type I)
Inheritance	Unclear*	Dominant†	Recessive
Serum bilirubin, μmol/L (mg/dL)	17–102 (1–6)	102–340 (6–20)	340–770 (20–45)
Kernicterus	No	Rare	Yes
Conjugated bilirubin in bile	Yes (↑ monoconjugates)	Yes (↑↑ monoconjugates)	No
Response to phenobarbital	Yes	Yes	No
Bilirubin conjugation	↓‡	↓↓	Absent

* Many cases are without familial incidence.
† Variable expressivity.
‡ Other defects such as occult hemolysis and ↓ bilirubin uptake may coexist.

appears to account for the observed *decrease in hepatic bilirubin clearance*. A decreased clearance and hepatic uptake of bile salts has also been shown.

Previously Gilbert's syndrome was traditionally defined as mild, chronic, unconjugated hyperbilirubinemia occurring in the absence of hemolysis. However, with the use of radiobilirubin kinetics and erythrocyte half-life studies, at least two forms of Gilbert's syndrome have been described. One group includes patients with decreased bilirubin clearance and *no hemolysis*. A second group includes those who also have *evidence of hemolysis* (often occult) and hence increased bilirubin turnover. The simultaneous presence of both derangements appears to be a chance occurrence of two not uncommon disorders in the same patient and does not imply a causal relationship. There is additional evidence of the heterogeneity of patients with Gilbert's syndrome. Some patients have an increase in hepatocyte lipofuscin and an increase in the smooth endoplasmic reticulum (SER); others show an increase in hepatic lysosomal enzymes.

A feature of Gilbert's syndrome which can be useful diagnostically is the increase in serum bilirubin following prolonged fasting or calorie deprivation. Patients with this disorder, when placed on 1255 kJ (300 kcal) per day for 2 days, will increase their serum bilirubin by 26 μmol/L (1.5 mg/dL) or more, the major increase being in the unconjugated fraction. It appears that a decrease in glucuronyl transferase activity is needed in order to obtain this effect. Patients with hemolysis do not show an increase in serum bilirubin with fasting. As a reflection of the mild decrease in glucuronyl transferase in Gilbert's syndrome (1) serum bilirubin levels will decrease when the enzyme activity is enhanced following phenobarbital administration, and (2) the bile shows a modest increase in monoconjugates of bilirubin (see Table 251-1).

In general, the diagnosis of this benign but not uncommon disorder is made by exclusion. The syndrome is suspected in a patient with low-grade unconjugated hyperbilirubinemia with (1) no systemic symptoms, (2) *no overt* or clinically recognizable hemolysis, (3) normal tests of routine liver function, and (4) a liver biopsy (although usually not necessary) that is normal by light microscopy.

CRIGLER-NAJJAR SYNDROME (TYPES I AND II) This disorder is known to exist in two forms. Type I is the clinically *severe* form (originally described by Crigler and Najjar) and is due to *absence of glucuronyl transferase*. Type II has more *moderate* clinical findings due to *partial deficiency of glucuronyl transferase*. The major differences between the two variants are summarized in Table 251-1.

Type I (Crigler-Najjar) is a rare disorder. Infants develop high unconjugated bilirubin levels in the serum [340 to 770 μmol/L (20 to 45 mg/dL)]. Absence of the enzyme can be demonstrated in the liver. Routine liver function tests are normal, as is liver histology. Because of the absence of glucuronyl transferase no conjugated bilirubin is formed by the liver; hence no bilirubin is secreted by the liver, and the bile is colorless.

Phototherapy may temporarily and transiently reduce the unconjugated bilirubin level. Phenobarbital has no effect since the enzyme defect is complete and no drug "induction" is therefore possible. Affected infants usually die within the first year of life, although some patients have survived to the second or third decade of life. Death is usually from kernicterus. A strain of rats (Gunn rat) with the type I defect exists and is widely used as an animal model of the Crigler-Najjar syndrome (type I).

Type II patients have a *partial deficiency* of glucuronyl transferase, and their disorder is less severe. Serum unconjugated bilirubin levels are lower [103 to 340 μmol/L (6 to 20 mg/dL)], jaundice may not appear until adolescence, and neurologic complications are uncommon. The bile contains variable amounts of conjugated bilirubin with a significant increase in monoconjugates. Phenobarbital is effective in lowering the serum bilirubin level in type II patients. However, the disorder is relatively benign in those patients whose bilirubin is less than 308 to 340 μmol/L (18 to 20 mg/dL).

Acquired deficiency of glucuronyl transferase As with any enzyme, glucuronyl transferase is susceptible to inhibition by a variety of agents, and because of the decreased activity of the enzyme in the neonatal state, such inhibition may be more evident at that time. Neonatal jaundice may be aggravated or prolonged in infants treated with *drugs* such as chloramphenicol or novobiocin, or with *vitamin K*. In some breast-fed infants jaundice has been ascribed to the presence in *breast milk* of pregnane-3β,20α-diol, an inhibitor of glucuronyl transferase. When the infant is removed from the breast, the "breast-milk jaundice" subsides.

Hypothyroidism delays the normal "maturation" of glucuronyl transferase. In cretins, neonatal jaundice may be prolonged for weeks or months. In fact, the presence of prolonged unconjugated hyperbilirubinemia after birth may be a clue to an underlying hypothyroidism.

In the infant, as well as in the adult, *liver cell damage* leads to impairment in glucuronide conjugation as a result of decreased transferase activity. However, since excretion is probably the rate-limiting step in bilirubin metabolism and since this step is always interfered with to a greater extent than conjugation in parenchymal liver disease, the pigment which accumulates in the blood is predominantly conjugated bilirubin.

DISORDERS CAUSING COMBINED CONJUGATED AND UNCONJUGATED HYPERBILIRUBINEMIA

In jaundice due to primary liver disease, the plasma usually exhibits elevated levels of both conjugated and unconjugated bilirubin, and *urine contains bilirubin*. The relative proportions of the two pigments are highly variable. In many familial hepatic abnormalities (described below) and in some forms of liver injury, the jaundice is largely due to increases in conjugated bilirubin. Such a serum pigment pattern is also seen with extrahepatic biliary obstruction. One *cannot differentiate* intrahepatic and extrahepatic causes of jaundice from either the levels or proportions of unconjugated and conjugated bilirubin in serum. Thus the main purpose of the initial fractionation of the serum bilirubin is to distinguish hepatic parenchymal and biliary obstructive disease from the disorders associated with predominantly unconjugated hyperbilirubinemia.

FAMILIAL DEFECTS IN HEPATIC EXCRETORY FUNCTION

Dubin-Johnson syndrome This disorder, also called *chronic idiopathic jaundice*, is a benign, autosomally inherited hyperbilirubinemia characterized by the presence of a dark pigment in the centrilobular region of the liver cells. Functionally there exists a *defect in biliary excretion* of bilirubin, cholephilic dyes, and porphyrins. Using the diazo method for measuring bilirubin, the serum pigment in these patients typically has been observed to be in the range of 51 to 257 μmol/L (3 to 15 mg/dL) and predominantly of the conjugated type. However, with the newer and more accurate method (alkaline methanolysis and high-pressure liquid chromatography), homozygous patients with the Dubin-Johnson syndrome have been shown to have significant levels of serum *unconjugated bilirubin*. This finding may in part reflect pigment which, after conjugation by the liver, is deconjugated in the hepatobiliary system and refluxed into the plasma. Moreover, the serum contains more diconjugated than monoconjugated bilirubin, just the reverse of what is seen in acquired hepatobiliary disease and Rotor syndrome. This reversed ratio is believed to be characteristic and diagnostic for homozygous patients.

Patients with Dubin-Johnson syndrome may be asymptomatic or have vague constitutional or gastrointestinal symptoms. Not infrequently the liver is slightly enlarged; in about one-fourth of the cases there is mild hepatic tenderness. Oral and intravenous cholangiography fails to visualize the biliary tract. There is typically and characteristically a late rise in the plasma BSP elimination curve at *90 min*. This is caused by the reflux from the liver of the conjugated dye and reflects the defect in the hepatic excretory transport maximum (T_m). It is noteworthy that there is no such secondary rise in plasma when dyes which are not conjugated by the liver are given, such as indocyanine green. When bile salts such as ursodeoxycholic acid are given, these patients show a decreased hepatic uptake and clearance. In the liver the striking feature is the presence of a brown or black pigment in the hepatocytes. Some findings suggest that this unique pigment is "melanin-like"; others indicate it to be a polymer of epinephrine metabolites.

These patients also show an abnormality in coproporphyrin excretion. Normal urine contains mostly coproporphyrin III and small amounts of coproporphyrin I; Dubin-Johnson patients show a reversal of this pattern, i.e., they excrete predominantly coproporphyrin I. Heterozygotes show an intermediate excretory pattern.

There is impaired excretion of many metabolites, including conjugated bilirubin, BSP, and iodinated dyes. Excretion of bile acids, however, is normal. Oral contraceptive agents may accentuate hyperbilirubinemia or may produce jaundice for the first time. Features of cholestasis such as pruritus or steatorrhea are usually lacking, and, specifically, serum alkaline phosphatase levels are *not* elevated. The overall prognosis of the disorder is excellent.

Rotor syndrome This is similar in many respects to the Dubin-Johnson syndrome. However, *there is no pigment in the liver cells,* and the serum conjugated bilirubin has more monoconjugates than diglucuronide conjugates. The gallbladder is usually visualized on cholecystography, and there is an increase in the *total* urinary coproporphyrins but *not* an increased percentage in excretion of coproporphyrin I. The BSP excretion pattern does *not* show a secondary rise at 90 min. The impairment in excretion which is typical of Dubin-Johnson syndrome is not present; instead in most cases of the Rotor syndrome there is impairment of *hepatic storage capacity* (*S*). This rare syndrome is inherited as an autosomal recessive trait and is genetically distinct from Dubin-Johnson syndrome.

Benign familial recurrent cholestasis This is a relatively rare syndrome characterized by recurrent attacks of pruritus and jaundice. During an attack the serum alkaline phosphatase and bile acid levels are markedly elevated, and liver biopsy shows the morphologic features of cholestasis. However, there is no mechanical biliary obstruction, with cholangiography revealing a patent biliary tree. Remissions are the rule, and at such times hepatic function tests and liver morphologic features are usually normal. The cause of the disorder is unknown; cirrhosis does not develop, and the disorder is benign. A congenital origin has been postulated on the basis of the early age of onset and familial incidence.

Recurrent jaundice of pregnancy This form of jaundice is also known as *intrahepatic cholestasis of pregnancy*. During a normal pregnancy some derangements in liver function occur, especially during the last trimester. Usually these consist of slight increases in BSP retention and in serum alkaline phosphatase. This mild increase in alkaline phosphatase during pregnancy is normally of placental rather than of hepatic origin. With a normal pregnancy elevations of serum bilirubin either do not occur or are less than 34 μmol/L (2 mg/dL).

In a small number of pregnant women an intrahepatic cholestasis may appear. This usually occurs in the third trimester but may develop any time after the seventh week of gestation. The clinical features consist primarily of pruritus and jaundice. Serum bilirubin levels are usually less than 103 μmol/L (6 mg/dL). The serum alkaline phosphatase and cholesterol levels are elevated significantly, while other liver function tests are only mildly deranged. Histologically the liver shows varying degrees of cholestasis but only a few parenchymal cell changes. The clinical and laboratory abnormalities subside promptly after delivery and are usually normal within 7 to 14 days.

This condition has been seen more frequently in Scandinavia and Europe than in the United States. Since steroid hormones and specifically estrogens can induce changes in hepatic excretory function in normal individuals (see Chap. 250), these patients probably have an increased susceptibility or sensitivity to the hepatic effects of estrogenic and progestational hormones. The intrahepatic cholestasis is usually termed *recurrent*, since the syndrome often (but not always) reappears in subsequent pregnancies. The process is benign and self-limited, and treatment is usually not needed, but cholestyramine administration will diminish the pruritus. This disorder must be distinguished from the many other causes of jaundice not unique to pregnancy, such as viral hepatitis. It must also be distinguished from the idiopathic *acute fatty liver of pregnancy* and the *tetracycline-induced* fatty liver. The latter two conditions are rare, occur in the last trimester, and have a high fatality rate; however, in these disorders there is evidence of diffuse parenchymal damage and not just cholestasis.

ACQUIRED DEFECTS OF HEPATIC EXCRETORY FUNCTION

Drug-induced cholestasis A condition entirely analogous to the intrahepatic cholestasis of pregnancy may occur in some women following the use of oral contraceptive agents. In some, mild cholestatic jaundice may occur, liver function returns to normal when the drugs are withdrawn, and chronic liver disease does not appear to result. It is relevant that one-third of the reported patients with jaundice due to oral contraceptives also have a history of recurrent intrahepatic cholestasis of pregnancy.

The nature of these changes produced by the natural and synthetic female sex hormones is very similar to those resulting from the administration of certain testosterone analogues, especially those with α substitutions at the 17 position of the steroid nucleus. These agents (such as methyltestosterone and norethandrolone) commonly cause BSP retention and less commonly cause jaundice or significant changes in other liver functions. However, unlike the female hormones, these agents have been implicated as a cause of chronic liver disease, especially biliary cirrhosis.

Because of these phenomena, synthetic steroid sex hormones should not be used in patients with liver disease. Conversely, in individuals using these agents the appearance of jaundice or elevations in serum aminotransferase (transaminase) levels or alkaline phosphatase contraindicates their further use. However, mild to moderate increases in BSP retention alone are probably not of clinical significance, although liver function tests should be carried out periodically.

As is discussed in detail in Chap. 252, there are many drugs which may produce not only cholestasis but liver injury resembling acute hepatitis or cholestatic hepatitis. In contrast to the jaundice produced by the steroid hormones, the clinical features are those of fever, rash, arthralgia, and eosinophilia, with the liver showing a pronounced inflammatory reaction. These features suggest that such reactions are *allergic* or *toxic* in nature and therefore differ from the effects caused by the steroid hormones, which probably represent an exaggerated response by the liver to the normal action of these hormones.

Postoperative jaundice The occurrence of postoperative jaundice is a problem of increasing importance. It is perhaps seen more frequently now than in earlier years, because patients are able to undergo more major surgical procedures (i.e., cardiac surgery, repair of ruptured aneurysms) and survive. In approaching this problem the possible pathogenic mechanisms listed in Table 251-2 need to be considered. The patient may have *pigment overload,* especially from blood transfusions (with hemolysis of stored blood), from resorption of blood in extravascular spaces, and less commonly from hemolytic anemia. *Hepatocellular damage* and decreased liver cell function may occur due to concurrent use of hepatotoxic drugs (Chap. 252) or anesthetics such as halothane. Hepatocellular necrosis may follow profound shock; with lesser degrees of hypotension or hypoxemia, morphologic damage may be slight, but significant impairment of function may occur. Hence, prior shock or hypotension plus pigment overload may produce significant jaundice. Extensive sepsis can also produce jaundice, often of a cholestatic type. Concurrent renal impairment due to hypotension and hypoxemia may enhance the degree of jaundice because the renal excretion of conjugated bilirubin is decreased. *Extrahepatic obstruction* due to surgical damage or stones needs to be considered, and may be excluded by ultrasound studies.

A form of jaundice referred to as *benign postoperative intrahepatic*

TABLE 251-2 Conditions causing or contributing to postoperative jaundice

I Increased pigment load
  A Hemolytic anemia
  B Transfusions (especially of stored blood)
  C Resorption of hematomas, blood in extravascular spaces
II Impaired hepatocellular function
  A Hepatitis-like picture
    1 Halothane anesthesia
    2 Drugs
    3 Shock
    4 Infection with hepatitis viruses
  B Cholestatic picture
    1 Hypotension, hypoxemia
    2 Drugs
    3 Sepsis
III Extrahepatic obstruction
  A Bile duct injury
  B Choledocholithiasis

cholestasis may be seen. In the typical case the patient has had major and prolonged surgery for a catastrophic event such as a ruptured aortic aneurysm complicated by hypotension and hypoxemia, extensive blood loss into tissues, and massive blood replacement. Jaundice may be noted on the second or third postoperative day, and the serum bilirubin, predominantly conjugated, may reach 340 to 680 μmol/L (20 to 40 mg/dL) by the eighth to tenth day. Serum alkaline phosphatase levels may be elevated three- to tenfold. Typically the serum aspartate aminotransferase (AST, SGOT) is only mildly elevated. The liver morphology is striking in that necrosis is not seen, only cholestasis and erythrophagocytosis.

The cause of this type of postoperative cholestatic jaundice is uncertain. However, it probably reflects (1) increased pigment load, (2) decreased liver function due to hypoxemia and hypotension, and (3) decreased renal bilirubin excretion due to varying degrees of tubular necrosis as a result of shock. This diagnostic possibility must be considered in the postoperative patient with marked cholestatic jaundice. The course of the jaundice is self-limited and will subside if the other systemic complications do not predominate and lead to death.

Hepatitis and cirrhosis These disorders, discussed in detail in Chaps. 252 to 254, constitute the *most common disorders associated with jaundice*. As has been stated previously, when the liver cell is damaged, as in viral hepatitis, there is often impairment in all three major hepatic phases of bilirubin metabolism, namely, uptake, conjugation, and excretion. Since the excretory step is the one which is rate-limiting and most readily affected by injury, significant amounts of conjugated bilirubin reenter the systemic circulation. There are also usually lesser increases in the serum unconjugated bilirubin. This phenomenon is probably a reflection of the impaired uptake and conjugation, and is due in part to the shortened life span of red blood cells often found in liver disease. In most patients with hepatitis and cirrhosis, the total serum bilirubin levels tend not to exceed 860 μmol/L (50 mg/dL). (For a summary of laboratory features in icteric states, see Table 251-3.)

EXTRAHEPATIC BILIARY OBSTRUCTION Anatomic or mechanical obstruction of the bile ducts is most commonly due to stones, tumors, or strictures. The clinical picture is quite similar to that of intrahepatic cholestasis with pronounced elevations of the serum conjugated bilirubin and alkaline phosphatase levels. Usually, but not always, fever, pain, and chills may be present. In contrast to hepatitis and cirrhosis, the serum bilirubin level often tends to plateau and rarely exceeds levels of 600 μmol/L (35 mg/dL). The reason for this plateau is not clear but may be related to renal excretion of

TABLE 251-3 Laboratory features in icteric states

	Serum bilirubin			
Bilirubin disorder	Unconjugated	Conjugated	Urine bilirubin	Comments
I Overproduction				
A Hemolysis (intra- and extravascular)	↑	N	0	↑ Bilirubin turnover; serum bilirubin rarely exceeds 68 μmol/L (4 mg/dL)
B Ineffective erythropoiesis	↑	N	0	Splenomegaly; normal RBC survival; normoblasts in marrow
II Defective hepatic uptake				
A Some drugs (e.g., flavaspidic acid, novobiocin)	↑	N	0	Normal liver biopsy
B Gilbert's syndrome (some cases)				
III Defective conjugation				
A Neonatal jaundice	↑	Low	0	↓ Glucuronyl transferase; ? ↓ ligandin
B Gilbert's syndrome	↑	Low	0	↓ Glucuronyl transferase and ↓ bilirubin uptake; some may have ↑ hemolysis; bile contains ↑ monoconjugates
C Crigler-Najjar syndrome (types I and II)	↑	Low	0	Type I = absence of transferase Type II = deficiency of transferase; bile contains ↑ ↑ monoconjugates
IV Defective excretion				
A Intrahepatic obstruction				
1 Familial syndromes				
a Dubin-Johnson	↑	↑	+	Abnormal BSP curve, hepatic lipochrome pigment; ↑ urinary coproporphyrin type I
b Rotor	↑	↑		No liver pigment; ↑ total urinary coproporphyrin
2 Drugs (e.g., chloramphenicol, methyltestosterone)	↑	↑	+	↑ Alkaline phosphatase but other function tests usually normal
3 Benign recurrent cholestasis	↑	↑	+	↑ Alkaline phosphatase
4 Recurrent jaundice of pregnancy (third trimester)	↑	↑	+	↑ Alkaline phosphatase; may be reproduced in afflicted subjects by estrogens or progesterone
B Extrahepatic obstruction (tumors, stone, stricture of bile duct)				↑ ↑ Alkaline phosphatase (often > fourfold)
1 Partial	↑	↑	+	
2 Complete	↑	↑	+	
V Hepatocellular disease*				
A Hepatitis	↑	↑	+	Conjugated/total serum bilirubin >50–70%; liver biopsy important for diagnosis
B Cirrhosis: Same as hepatitis	↑	↑		

* Note that in hepatocellular disease there is generally an interference in all pathways of bilirubin metabolism (i.e., impaired uptake, conjugation, and excretion).

conjugated bilirubin or alternative pathways of bilirubin catabolism in obstructive jaundice.

REFERENCES

Benign familial recurrent cholestasis

DEPAGTER AGF et al: Familial benign intrahepatic cholestasis. Gastroenterology 71:202, 1976

ENDO T et al: Bile acid metabolism in benign recurrent intrahepatic cholestasis. Gastroenterology 76:1002, 1979

Dubin-Johnson and Rotor syndromes

BERK PD et al: Inborn errors of bilirubin metabolism. Med Clin North Am 59:803, 1975

ROSENTHAL P et al: Homozygous Dubin-Johnson syndrome exhibits a characteristic serum bilirubin pattern. Hepatology 1:540, 1981

SWARTZ HM et al: On the nature and excretion of the hepatic pigment in the Dubin-Johnson syndrome. Gastroenterology 76:958, 1979

WOLKOFF AW et al: Hereditary jaundice and disorders of bilirubin metabolism, in *The Metabolic Basis of Inherited Disease*, 6th ed. CR Scriver et al (eds). New York, McGraw, 1989, pp 1367–1408

WOLPERT E et al: Abnormal sulfobromophthalein metabolism in Rotor's syndrome and obligate heterozygotes. N Engl J Med 206:1099, 1977

Glucuronyl transferase deficiency states

BERTHELOT P, DHUMEAUS D: New insights into the classification and mechanisms of hereditary, chronic, non-hemolytic hyperbilirubinemia. Gut 19:474, 1978

DAWSON J et al: Gilbert's syndrome: Evidence of morphologic heterogeneity. Gut 20:848, 1979

FELSHER BF, CARPIO NM: Caloric intake and unconjugated hyperbilirubinemia. Gastroenterology 69:42, 1975

FEVERY J et al: Unconjugated bilirubin and an increased proportion of bilirubin monoconjugates in the bile of patients with Gilbert's syndrome and Crigler-Najjar disease. J Clin Invest 60:970, 1977

OHKUBO H et al: Ursodeoxycholic acid oral tolerance test in patients with constitutional hyperbilirubinemias and effect of phenobarbital. Gastroenterology 81:126, 1981

——— et al: Effects of corticosteroids on bilirubin metabolism in patients with Gilbert's syndrome. Hepatology 1:168, 1981

OLSSON R et al: Gilbert's syndrome: does it exist? A study of the prevalence of symptoms in Gilbert's syndrome. Acta Med Scand 224:485, 1988

Postoperative jaundice

HOOTEGEM PV et al: Serum bilirubins in hepatobiliary disease: Comparison with other liver function tests and changes in the postobstructive period. Hepatology 5:112, 1985

KOFF RS: Postoperative jaundice. Med Clin North Am 59:823, 1975

LAMONT JT, ISSELBACHER KJ: Postoperative jaundice, in *Liver and Biliary Disease*, 2d ed, R Wright et al (eds). Philadelphia, Saunders, 1985

252 ACUTE HEPATITIS

JULES L. DIENSTAG / JACK R. WANDS / KURT J. ISSELBACHER

ACUTE VIRAL HEPATITIS

Acute viral hepatitis is a systemic infection affecting the liver predominantly. Five categories of viral agents have been implicated: hepatitis A virus (HAV), hepatitis B virus (HBV), two types of non-A, non-B hepatitis agents, one bloodborne, the other enterically transmitted, and the HBV-associated delta agent. Although these agents can be distinguished by their antigenic properties, all five types produce clinically similar illnesses. These range from asymptomatic and inapparent to fulminant and fatal acute infections common to all five types, on the one hand, and from subclinical persistent infections to rapidly progressive chronic liver disease with cirrhosis and even hepatocellular carcinoma, common to the bloodborne types (HBV, delta, and bloodborne non-A, non-B), on the other.

VIROLOGY AND ETIOLOGY **Hepatitis A** Hepatitis A virus (HAV) is a nonenveloped 27-nm, heat-, acid-, and ether-resistant RNA virus in the picornavirus family; it has been classified as enterovirus type 72 (Fig. 252-1). Its virion is composed of four polypeptides designated VP1 to VP4. Inactivation of viral activity can be achieved by boiling for 1 min, by contact with formaldehyde and chlorine, or by ultraviolet irradiation. All strains of this virus identified to date are immunologically indistinguishable and belong to one serotype. Hepatitis A has an incubation period of approximately 4 weeks. The virus is present in the liver, bile, stools, and blood during the late incubation period and acute preicteric phase of illness. Despite persistence of virus in the liver, viral shedding in feces, viremia, and infectivity diminish rapidly once jaundice becomes apparent. Unlike other hepatitis viruses, hepatitis A virus can be grown readily in tissue culture. In addition, its 7500-nucleotide genome has been cloned and characterized.

Antibodies to HAV (anti-HAV) can be detected during acute illness when serum aminotransferase activity is elevated and fecal HAV shedding is still occurring. This early antibody response is predominantly of the IgM class and persists for several months. During convalescence, however, anti-HAV of the IgG class becomes the predominant antibody (Fig. 252-2). Therefore, the diagnosis of hepatitis A is made during acute illness by demonstrating high-titer anti-HAV of the IgM class. Following acute illness, anti-HAV of the IgG class remains detectable indefinitely, and patients with serum anti-HAV are immune to reinfection. Indeed, the IgG anti-HAV present in immune globulin accounts for the protection it affords against HAV infection.

Hepatitis B This viral infection is unique in that concentrations of viral antigen and viral particles in the blood may reach 500 μg/mL and 10 trillion particles per milliliter, respectively. Electron-microscopic studies have demonstrated three particulate forms (Table 252-1) of HBV (see Fig. 252-1). The most numerous are the 22-nm particles which appear as spherical or long filamentous forms; these are antigenically identical with the outer surface or coat of HBV, and they are thought to represent excess viral coat protein. Outnumbered in serum by a factor of 100 or 1000 to 1 compared to the spheres and tubules are large 42-nm spherical particles, which represent the intact hepatitis B virion. These large particles consist of an outer coat and an inner icosahedral nucleocapsid core measuring 27 nm in diameter. Previous studies have shown that antiserum obtained from hemophiliacs, who had presumably been exposed repeatedly to hepatitis viruses through multiple blood transfusions, would form a precipitin line by diffusion in agar gel with an antigen present in hepatitis serum. This antigen, identified in the serum of an Australian aborigine, was originally called Australia antigen or hepatitis-associated antigen and is now referred to as hepatitis B surface antigen (HBsAg). The discovery of this antigen provided the first serologic test to distinguish hepatitis B from other types of hepatitis. HBsAg consists primarily of two major polypeptides, one of 24,000 mol wt and its glycosylated counterpart of 28,000 mol wt. A number of different HBsAg subdeterminants have been identified. There is a common group-reactive antigen, *a*, shared by all HBsAg isolates. In addition, HBsAg may contain one of several subtype-specific antigens, namely, *d* or *y*, *w* or *r*, as well as other more recently characterized specificities. These HBsAg subtypes provide additional epidemiologic markers in evaluating the transmission of hepatitis B infection in that subtypes "breed true." For example, studies of hepatitis outbreaks have shown that index cases and their contacts have identical HBsAg subtypes. Clinical course and outcome, however, are independent of subtype.

The intact 42-nm virion can be disrupted by mild detergents and the 27-nm nucleocapsid core particle isolated. Naked core particles do not circulate in serum. The antigen expressed on the surface of the nucleocapsid core is referred to as hepatitis B core antigen (HBcAg), and the corresponding antibody is anti-HBc. HBcAg does not cross-react with HBsAg. A third antigen associated with hepatitis B is hepatitis B e antigen (HBeAg). HBeAg is a soluble, nonparticulate antigen which is found only in HBsAg-positive serum and is immunologically and biochemically distinct from HBsAg and intact HBcAg but appears to be an internal component or degradation

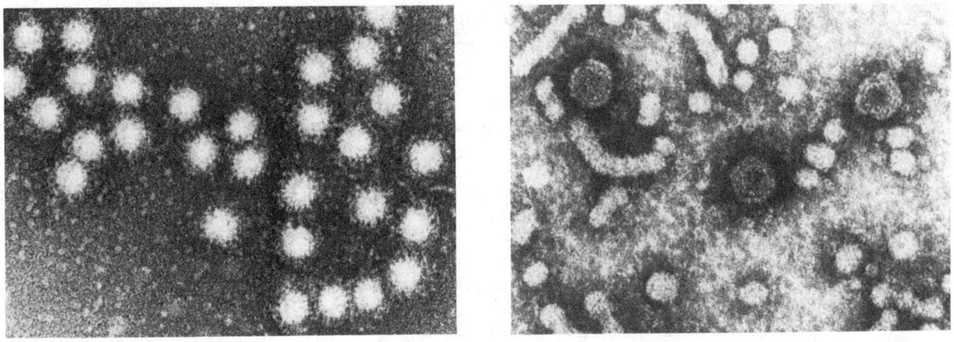

FIGURE 252-1 *A*. Electron micrograph of 27-nm hepatitis A virus particles purified from stool of a patient with acute hepatitis A virus infection and aggregated by hepatitis A antibody. *B*. Electron micrograph of concentrated serum from a patient with acute hepatitis B infection, demonstrating the 42-nm virions, tubular forms, and spherical 22-nm particles of hepatitis B surface antigen. 132,000×.

product of the core of HBV. HBsAg-positive serum containing HBeAg is more likely to be highly infectious and to be associated with the presence of hepatitis B virions (and DNA polymerase and HBV DNA, see below) than HBeAg-negative or anti-HBe-positive serum. For example, HBsAg carrier mothers who are HBeAg-positive almost invariably transmit hepatitis B infection to their offspring, while HBsAg carrier mothers with anti-HBe rarely infect their offspring.

In every individual with acute hepatitis B infection, HBeAg develops transiently, early in the course of illness, but persistent HBeAg positivity correlates with ongoing viral replication and may be associated with continuing disease actvity in chronic hepatitis; its disappearance may be a harbinger of biochemical improvement and potential resolution of infection. Unfortunately HBeAg is not a sufficiently discriminating marker to support prognostic predictions or to substitute for morphologic evaluation of severity in patients with chronic hepatitis.

Within the nucleocapsid core, in addition to HBeAg, is a predominantly double-stranded, but partially single-stranded, DNA genome measuring 3200 nucleotides as well as a DNA polymerase, which directs replication and repair of HBV DNA. In vitro, the polymerase can repair the single-stranded gap and render it double-stranded. Once thought to be unique among viruses, HBV is now recognized as one of a family of animal viruses, hepadnaviruses (hepatotropic DNA viruses), and is classified as hepadnavirus type 1. Viruses similar to HBV infect certain species of woodchucks, ground squirrels, and Pekin ducks, to mention the most carefully characterized. Like HBV, all have the same distinctive three morphologic forms, have counterparts to the virus antigens of HBV, replicate within the liver, contain their own, endogenous DNA polymerase, have partially double-stranded, partially single-stranded genomes, and, for the most part, are associated with acute and chronic hepatitis and hepatocellular carcinoma. Evidence suggests that hepadnaviruses rely on replicative strategies typical of retroviruses. Instead of DNA replication directly from a DNA template, hepadnaviruses rely on reverse transcription (effected by the DNA polymerase) of minus-strand DNA from an RNA intermediate. Although HBV has not been cultivated in vitro, its genome has been cloned in bacterial, yeast, and mammalian cell vectors and has been completely characterized. Four segments of the genome have been characterized: (1) the pre-S and S gene, which code for HBsAg and several other poorly characterized pre-S gene products, including receptors on the HBV surface for polymerized human serum albumin and hepatocyte receptors; (2) the C gene, which codes for HBcAg and HBeAg; (3) the P gene, which codes for DNA polymerase; and (4) the X gene, which codes for a recently identified protein seen more frequently in patients with chronic hepatitis and hepatocellular carcinoma but which remains to be further characterized. The pre-S region consists of both pre-S1 and pre-S2. The protein product of the S gene is HBsAg (''major protein''); the product of the pre-S2 plus S gene region is the ''middle protein''; and the product of the pre-S1 plus pre-S2 plus S regions is the ''large protein.'' Compared to the smaller spherical and tubular particles of HBV, complete virions are enriched in ''large protein.'' Both pre-S proteins and their respective antibodies can be detected during HBV infection. Not only has the HBV genome been cloned but its gene products have been expressed by recombinant vectors. In addition, the delineation of the gene and amino acid maps of HBV has led to the production in the laboratory of synthetic HBsAg polypeptides. Although HBV cannot be cultivated from clinical material in in vitro systems, several cell lines have been transfected with HBV DNA. Such transfected cells support in vitro replication of the intact virus and its component proteins.

FIGURE 252-2 Scheme of typical clinical and laboratory features of viral hepatitis type A.

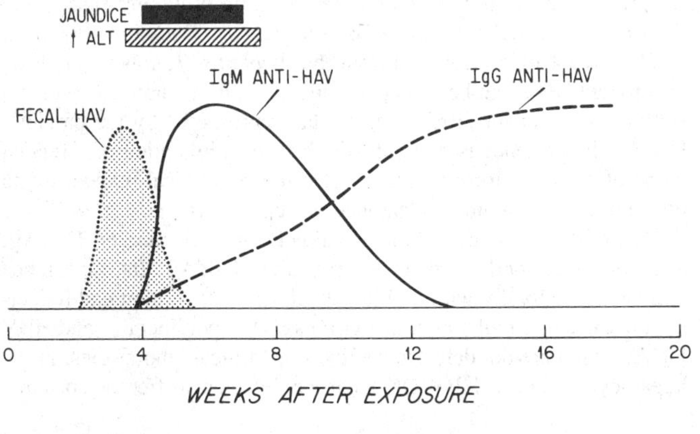

After infection with HBV, the first virologic marker detectable in serum is HBsAg (Fig. 252-3). Circulating HBsAg precedes elevations of serum aminotransferase activity and clinical symptoms and remains detectable during the entire icteric or symptomatic phase of acute hepatitis B and beyond. In typical cases, HBsAg becomes undetectable 1 to 2 months following the onset of jaundice and rarely persists beyond 6 months. After HBsAg disappears, antibody to HBsAg (anti-HBs) becomes detectable in serum and remains detectable indefinitely thereafter. Because HBcAg is sequestered within an HBsAg coat, HBcAg is not detectable routinely in the serum of patients with HBV infection. On the other hand, antibody to HBcAg (anti-HBc) is readily demonstrable in serum, beginning within the first 1 to 2 weeks after the appearance of HBsAg and preceding detectable levels of anti-HBs by weeks to months. Because variability exists in the time of appearance of anti-HBs following HBV infection, occasionally a gap of several weeks or longer may separate the disappearance of HBsAg and the appearance of anti-HBs. During this ''gap'' or ''window'' period, anti-HBc may represent serologic evidence of current or recent HBV infection, and blood containing anti-HBc in the absence of HBsAg and anti-HBs has been implicated in the development of transfusion-associated hepatitis B. In part because the sensitivity of immunoassays for HBsAg and anti-HBs has increased, however, this window period is rarely encountered. In some persons, years after HBV infection, anti-HBc may persist in the circulation longer than anti-HBs. Therefore, isolated anti-HBc does not necessarily indicate

TABLE 252-1 Nomenclature and features of hepatitis antigens and antibodies

Hepatitis type	Particle diameter, nm	Description	Antigen	Corresponding antibody	Remarks
A	27	Icosahedral virus particle	Hepatitis A virus (HAV)	Hepatitis A antibody (anti-HAV)	RNA virus; present in stool and serum early in course of hepatitis A
B	42	Intact virion (surface and core); spherical	Hepatitis B surface antigen (HBsAg) Hepatitis B core antigen (HBcAg)	Hepatitis B surface antibody (anti-HBs) Hepatitis B core antibody (anti-HBc)	DNA virus; found in serum
	27	Nucleocapsid core of virion, icosahedral	HBcAg	Anti-HBc	Core contains DNA and DNA polymerase; present in hepatocyte nuclei but not in serum Anti-HBc detected in serum during and after acute infection
	22	Appear as spherical and filamentous forms; both have same antigenic properties as surface of virion; represent excess viral coat material	HBsAg	Anti-HBs	HBsAg detectable in > 90% of patients with acute hepatitis B; found in serum, body fluids, and hepatocyte cytoplasm Anti-HBs appears following B infection; protective antibody
	Nonparticulate	Soluble protein, internal component of nucleocapsid	Hepatitis B e antigen (HBeAg)	Hepatitis B e antibody (anti-HBe)	HBeAg found in HBsAg-positive serum only, correlates with infectivity and presence of intact virus particles
C	(presumed 30–60 nm)	Particle not identified	HCAg	Anti-HCV	10,000 nucleotide single-stranded RNA virus; cause of bloodborne non-A, non-B hepatitis; antibody appears after 1 to 3 months
D	35–37	Hybrid particle with HBsAg coat and delta nucleocapsid core	Hepatitis delta antigen (HDAg)	Hepatitis delta antibody (anti-HD)	Defective RNA virus, requires helper function of HBV
E	27–32 nm	Icosahedral virus particle	HEAg	Anti-HEV	RNA virus present in stool; cause of enteric non-A, non-B hepatitis

active virus replication; most instances of isolated anti-HBc represent hepatitis B infection in the remote past. Distinction between recent and remote HBV infection can be accomplished by determination of the immunoglobulin class of anti-HBc. Anti-HBc of the IgM class (IgM anti-HBc) predominates during the first approximately 6 months after acute infection, whereas IgG anti-HBc is the predominant class of anti-HBc beyond 6 months. Therefore, patients with current or recent acute hepatitis B, including those in the anti-HBc window, have IgM anti-HBc in their serum. In patients who have recovered from hepatitis B in the remote past as well as those with chronic HBV infection, anti-HBc is predominantly of the IgG class. Infrequently, in no more than 1 to 5 percent of patients with acute HBV infection, levels of HBsAg are too low to be detected; in such cases, the presence of IgM anti-HBc establishes the diagnosis of acute hepatitis B. Similarly, isolated anti-HBc may occur in the rare patient with chronic hepatitis B whose HBsAg level is below the sensitivity threshold of contemporary immunoassays (a low-level carrier); in such cases, the anti-HBc is of the IgG class. Generally, in persons who have recovered from hepatitis B, anti-HBs and anti-HBc persist indefinitely.

FIGURE 252-3 Scheme of typical clinical and laboratory features of acute viral hepatitis type B.

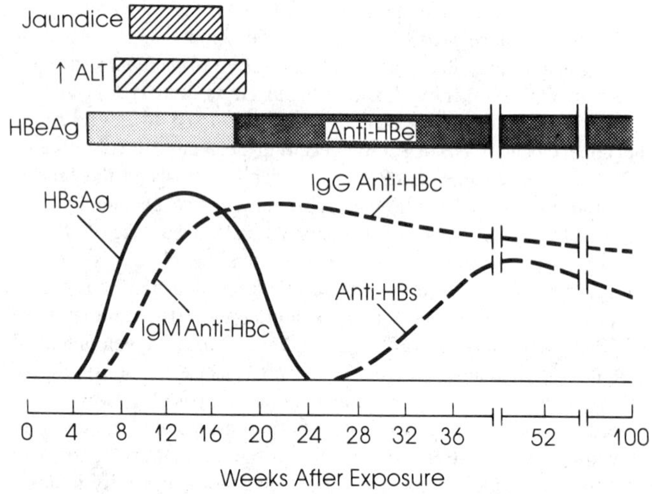

The temporal association between the appearance of anti-HBs and resolution of HBV infection as well as the observation that persons with anti-HBs in serum are protected against reinfection with HBV suggest that *anti-HBs is the protective antibody*. Therefore, strategies for prevention of HBV infection are based on providing susceptible persons with circulating anti-HBs (see below). Occasionally, in 10 to 20 percent of patients with chronic hepatitis B, low-level, low-affinity anti-HBs can be detected. This antibody is directed against a subtype determinant different from that represented by the patient's HBsAg; its presence is thought to reflect the stimulation of a related clone of antibody forming cells, but it has no clinical relevance and does not signal imminent clearance of hepatitis B.

The other readily detectable hepatitis B virologic marker, HBeAg, appears concurrently with or shortly after HBsAg. Its appearance coincides temporally with high levels of virus replication and reflects the presence of circulating intact virions, DNA polymerase, and HBV DNA, which are not detected routinely in clinical laboratories; in the hepatocyte nucleus, HBV DNA can be detected in free or episomal form. This *replicative* stage of HBV infection is the time of maximal infectivity. In self-limited HBV infections, HBeAg becomes undetectable shortly after peak elevations in aminotransferase activity, before the disappearance of HBsAg, and anti-HBe then becomes detectable, coinciding with a period of relatively lower infectivity (Fig. 252-3). In protracted HBV infection, HBeAg may remain detectable, indicating persistent replicative infection. When HBeAg is absent and anti-HBe present in chronic hepatitis B, infection is usually *nonreplicative*. In this phase of chronic infection, when HBV DNA is demonstrable in hepatocyte nuclei, it tends to be integrated into the host genome. In the nonreplicative phase, only spherical and tubular forms of HBV, *not intact virions,* circulate. Occasionally, nonreplicative HBV infection converts back to replicative infection. Such spontaneous reactivations are accompanied by reexpression of HBeAg and HBV DNA as well as by exacerbations of liver injury.

Hepatitis B antigens and DNA have been identified in extrahepatic tissues, such as lymph nodes, bone marrow, circulating lymphocytes, spleen, and pancreas. The clinical relevance of these findings remains obscure.

Delta hepatitis The delta hepatitis agent, hepatitis D virus (HDV), is a defective RNA virus which coinfects with and requires the helper function of HBV for its replication and expression. Slightly smaller than HBV, delta is a formalin-sensitive, 35- to 37-nm virus with a hybrid structure. Its nucleocapsid expresses delta antigen, which bears no antigenic homology with any of the HBV antigens, and contains a small, 1700-nucleotide RNA genome that is nonhomologous with HBV DNA but that has features of plant satellite viruses or viroids. This delta core is ''encapsidated'' by an outer coat of HBsAg. Thus, delta can either infect a person simultaneously with HBV (''coinfection'') or superinfect a person already infected with HBV (''superinfection''); when delta infection is transmitted from a donor with one HBsAg subtype to an HBsAg-positive recipient with a different subtype, the delta agent assumes the HBsAg subtype of the recipient, rather than the donor. Because delta relies absolutely on HBV, the duration of delta infection is determined by the duration of and cannot outlast HBV infection. Delta antigen is expressed primarily in hepatocyte nuclei and is occasionally detectable in serum. During acute delta infection, anti-delta of the IgM class predominates; in self-limited infection, anti-delta is low-titer and transient, rarely remaining detectable beyond the clearance of HBsAg and delta antigen. In chronic delta infection, anti-delta circulates in high titer, and both IgM and IgG anti-delta can be detected. Delta antigen in the liver and delta RNA in serum and liver can be detected during HDV replication.

Non-A, non-B hepatitis Sensitive serologic tests for identifying both types A and B hepatitis have led to the identification of hepatitis cases with incubation periods and modes of transmission consistent with an infectious disease but without serologic evidence of hepatitis A or B infection. Identified initially among recipients of transfused blood, these cases of so-called non-A, non-B hepatitis have not been associated serologically with Epstein-Barr virus or cytomegalovirus (except in rare instances) or with other viruses known to involve the liver. Long before a non-A, non-B hepatitis virus had been identified definitively, cross-challenge studies in chimpanzees suggested that there are at least two different bloodborne non-A, non-B hepatitis agents. One has been isolated from clotting factor VIII concentrates, is chloroform-sensitive, and induces ultrastructural cytoplasmic tubular changes in hepatocytes. The other has been isolated from clotting factor IX concentrates, is chloroform-resistant, and does not induce cytoplasmic tubular changes in hepatocytes. The former type appears to be the most frequently encountered after blood transfusion.

An almost 15-year quest to identify an agent of non-A, non-B viral hepatitis ended in 1988 with the identification of an RNA virus with immunologic specificity for transfusion-associated non-A, non-B hepatitis. Among complementary DNA (cDNA) fragments cloned in *Escherichia coli* from the pellet of a chimpanzee plasma with unusually high infectivity, one clone expressed a protein that reacted with antibody in convalescent serum but not preillness serum from chimpanzees with experimentally induced non-A, non-B hepatitis. This viral antigen was found as well in the livers of infected, but not uninfected-control, chimpanzees. Most chimpanzees and humans studied with well-pedigreed transfusion-related non-A, non-B hepatitis acquire antibody to this virus between 1 and 3 months after the onset of acute illness. Validation of an immunoassay for antibody to this agent came most convincingly from its ability to distinguish, in panels of coded serum samples, between pedigreed non-A, non-B hepatitis cases and pedigreed negative, noninfectious samples as well as other-disease controls. The virus appears to be a single-stranded RNA virus with a genome of approximately 10,000 nucleotides. It has *no homology with HBV,* retroviruses, or other hepatitis viruses; however, its genome, size, and stability are consistent with its inclusion in the togavirus family of lipid-enveloped agents that includes the arboviruses (such as yellow fever and dengue viruses) and rubella virus. Only one continuous open reading frame (gene) has been identified. This agent has been named *hepatitis C virus (HCV).* The question remains whether this is the only agent of ''bloodborne'' non-A, non-B hepatitis or whether another agent will be identified, as suggested by the chimpanzee cross-challenge studies cited above. Because the titer of this agent in serum is so low, practical diagnostic tests for virus antigen remain to be developed.

In addition, a distinct type of waterborne non-A, non-B hepatitis has been identified in India, Asia, and Central America (so-called epidemic or enteric non-A, non-B hepatitis), which, because of its epidemiologic resemblance to hepatitis A, has been labeled by some ''non-A hepatitis'' and has been classified provisionally as ''hepatitis E'' (for enteric) virus (HEV). Enteric non-A, non-B hepatitis is caused by a 27- to 32-nm HAV-like virus; however, there is no genomic or antigenic homology between the enteric non-A, non-B agent and HAV or other picornaviruses. This virus has been detected in stools from patients with epidemic non-A, non-B hepatitis and has been transmitted serially in chimpanzees. Fecal excretion of the virus and immune responses to it have been documented in experimentally infected chimpanzees. Routine tests for clinical purposes, however, have not yet been developed. Details of virologic events and humoral immune responses remain to be described.

PATHOGENESIS While data on the pathogenesis of hepatitis A, non-A, non-B hepatitis, and delta hepatitis are very limited, evidence suggests that the clinical manifestations of and outcomes following acute liver injury associated with HBV infection are determined by the immunologic responses of the host. The existence of asymptomatic hepatitis B carriers with normal liver histology and function suggests that the virus is not directly cytopathic. The facts that lymphoid cells are juxtaposed with necrotic hepatocytes in the livers of patients with liver injury and that patients with defects in cellular immune competence are more likely to remain chronically infected rather than to clear the virus are cited to support the role of cellular immune responses in the pathogenesis of hepatitis B–related liver injury. To date, however, because adequate animal and laboratory models are lacking, support for this hypothesis remains circumstantial. Still, the model that has the most experimental support involves cytolytic T cells sensitized specifically to recognize host and hepatitis B viral antigens on the liver cell surface. Although HBsAg was initially thought to be the most likely viral target antigen on the hepatocyte surface, recent laboratory observations suggest that HBcAg, present on the cell membrane in minute quantities, is the viral target antigen that, with host antigens, invites cytolytic T cells to destroy HBV-infected hepatocytes. Debate does continue, however, over the relative importance of viral and host factors in the pathogenesis of liver injury associated with hepatitis B and its outcome.

Although the mechanism of HBV-induced liver injury remains uncertain, immune complex–mediated tissue damage appears to play a major pathogenetic role in the extrahepatic manifestations of acute hepatitis B. The occasional prodromal serum sickness–like syndrome observed in acute hepatitis B appears to be related to the deposition in tissue blood vessel walls of circulating immune complexes leading to activation of the complement system. The clinical consequences are urticarial rash, angioedema, fever, and arthritis. During the early prodrome of hepatitis B in these patients, HBsAg in high titer in association with small amounts of anti-HBs leads to the formation of soluble, circulating immune complexes (in antigen excess). Complement components in the serum are depressed during the arthritic phase of the illness and are also detectable in the circulating immune complexes. In addition to complement components, these complexes contain HBsAg, anti-HBs, IgG, IgM, IgA, and fibrin. After the patient recovers from the serum sickness–like syndrome, these immune complexes disappear.

In patients who become carriers of HBsAg following acute hepatitis, other types of immune-complex disease may be seen. Glomerulonephritis with the nephrotic syndrome is occasionally observed; HBsAg, immunoglobulin, and C3 deposition has been found in the glomerular basement membrane. While polyarteritis nodosa develops in considerably fewer than 1 percent of patients with hepatitis B, 20 to 30 percent of patients with polyarteritis nodosa have HBsAg in serum. In these patients, the affected small and medium-sized arterioles have been shown to contain HBsAg, immunoglobulins, and complement components.

PATHOLOGY The typical morphologic lesions of hepatitis A, B, delta, and non-A, non-B are often similar and consist of panlobular infiltration with mononuclear cells, hepatic cell necrosis, hyperplasia of Kupffer cells, and variable degrees of cholestasis. Hepatic cell regeneration is present, as evidenced by numerous mitotic figures, multinucleated cells, and "rosette" or "pseudoacinar" formation. The mononuclear infiltration consists primarily of small lymphocytes, although plasma cells and eosinophils are occasionally seen. Liver cell damage consists of hepatic cell degeneration and necrosis, cell dropout, ballooning of cells, and acidophilic degeneration of hepatocytes (forming so-called Councilman-like bodies). Large hepatocytes with a ground glass appearance of the cytoplasm may be seen in chronic but not in acute hepatitis B; these cells have been shown to contain HBsAg and can be identified histochemically with orcein or aldehyde fuchsin. In uncomplicated viral hepatitis, the reticulin framework is preserved.

In bloodborne non-A, non-B hepatitis, the histologic lesion is often remarkable for a relative paucity of inflammation, a marked increase in activation of sinusoidal lining cells, the presence of fat, and occasionally bile duct lesions in which biliary epithelial cells appear to be piled up without interruption of the basement membrane.

In enteric non-A, non-B hepatitis, a common histologic feature is marked cholestasis.

A more severe histologic lesion, *bridging hepatic necrosis,* also termed *subacute* or *confluent necrosis,* is occasionally observed in some patients with acute hepatitis. "Bridging" between lobules results from large areas of hepatic cell dropout, with collapse of the reticulin framework. Characteristically, the bridge consists of condensed reticulum, inflammatory debris, and degenerating liver cells that span adjacent portal areas, portal to central veins, or central vein to central vein. This lesion has been thought to have prognostic significance; in many of the originally described patients with this lesion, a subacute course terminated in death within several weeks to months, or chronic active hepatitis and postnecrotic cirrhosis developed. More recent investigations have failed to uphold the association between bridging necrosis and such a poor prognosis in patients with acute hepatitis. Although the frequency of bridging may be higher among hospitalized patients with severe acute hepatitis, and although cirrhosis, chronic hepatitis, and even death have been observed in this group, the frequency of bridging necrosis in uncomplicated acute viral hepatitis is probably on the order of 1 to 5 percent. Prospective studies have failed to demonstrate a difference in prognosis between patients with acute hepatitis who have bridging necrosis and those who do not. Therefore, although demonstration of this lesion in patients with chronic hepatitis has prognostic significance (see Chap. 253), its demonstration during acute hepatitis is less meaningful, and liver biopsies to identify this lesion are no longer undertaken routinely in patients with acute hepatitis. In *massive hepatic necrosis* (fulminant hepatitis, acute yellow atrophy), the striking feature at postmortem examination is the finding of a small, shrunken, and soft liver. Histologic examination reveals massive necrosis and dropout of liver cells of most lobules with extensive collapse and condensation of the reticulin framework.

Immunofluorescence and immunoperoxidase antibody studies have been instrumental in localizing HBsAg to the cytoplasm and plasma membrane of infected liver cells. In contrast, HBcAg predominates in the nucleus, but, occasionally, scant amounts are also seen in the cytoplasm and on the cell membrane. Electron-microscopic studies of liver biopsy material have demonstrated the presence of HBsAg particles in the cytoplasm and HBcAg particles in the nucleus of liver cells during hepatitis B infection. These morphologic observations suggest that DNA is synthesized and packaged within core particles in the nucleus, while the surface coat is assembled in the cytoplasm, resulting in the formation of intact hepatitis B virus. Delta antigen is localized to the hepatocyte nucleus, while HAV antigen is localized to the cytoplasm.

EPIDEMIOLOGY Prior to the availability of serologic tests for hepatitis viruses, all viral hepatitis cases were labeled either as "infectious" or "serum" hepatitis. Modes of transmission overlap, however, and *a clear distinction among the different types of viral hepatitis cannot be made solely on the basis of clinical or epidemiologic features* (Table 252-2). The most accurate means to distinguish the various types of viral hepatitis involves specific serologic testing.

Hepatitis A *This agent is transmitted almost exclusively by the fecal-oral route*. Spread of HAV is enhanced by poor personal hygiene and overcrowding, and large outbreaks as well as sporadic cases have been traced to contaminated food, water, milk, and shellfish. Intrafamily and intrainstitutional spread are also common. Early epidemiologic observations suggested that there is a predilection for hepatitis A to occur in late fall and early winter. In temperate zones, epidemic waves have been recorded every 5 to 20 years as new segments of nonimmune population appeared; however, in developed countries, the incidence of type A hepatitis has been declining, presumably as a function of improved sanitation, and these cyclic patterns are no longer being observed. No HAV carrier state has been identified after acute type A hepatitis; perpetuation of the virus in nature depends presumably on nonepidemic, inapparent subclinical infection.

In the general population, anti-HAV, an excellent marker for previous HAV infection, increases in prevalence as a function of increasing age and of decreasing socioeconomic status. Serologic evidence of prior hepatitis A infection occurs in about 40 percent of urban populations in the United States, fewer than 5 percent of whom recall having had a symptomatic case of hepatitis. In developing countries, exposure, infection, and subsequent immunity are almost universal in childhood. As the frequency of subclinical childhood infections declines in developed countries, a susceptible cohort of adults emerges. Hepatitis A tends to be more symptomatic in adults; therefore, paradoxically, as the frequency of HAV infection declines, the likelihood of clinically apparent, even severe, HAV illnesses increases in the susceptible adult population. Travel to endemic areas is a common source of infection for adults from nonendemic areas.

Hepatitis B It has long been recognized that a major route of hepatitis B transmission is percutaneous, but the outmoded designation "serum hepatitis" is an inaccurate label for the epidemiologic spectrum of HBV infection recognized today. As detailed below, most of the hepatitis transmitted by blood transfusion is not caused by HBV; moreover, in approximately half of patients with acute type B hepatitis, there is no history of an identifiable percutaneous exposure. We now recognize that many cases of type B hepatitis result from less obvious modes of nonpercutaneous or covert percutaneous transmission. HBsAg has been identified in almost every body fluid from infected persons—saliva, tears, seminal fluid, cerebrospinal fluid, ascites, breast milk, synovial fluid, gastric juice, pleural fluid and urine and even rarely in feces. Although there is abundant evidence to suggest that feces are not infectious, at least some of these body fluids—most notably semen and saliva—have been shown

TABLE 252-2 Comparisons of type A, type B, and non-A, non-B hepatitis

Feature	Hepatitis A	Hepatitis B*	Non-A, non-B hepatitis: Bloodborne (hepatitis C)	Non-A, non-B hepatitis: Enteric (hepatitis E)
Incubation	15–45 days (mean 30)	30–180 days (mean 60–90)	15–160 (mean 50)	14–60 (mean 40)
Onset	Acute	Often insidious	Insidious	Acute
Age preference	Children, young adults	Any age	Any age but more common in adults	Young adults (20–40 years)
Transmission route:				
Fecal-oral	+ + +	−	Unknown	+ + +
Other nonpercutaneous†	+/−	+ +	+ +	+/−
Percutaneous	Unusual	+ + +	+ + +	−
Severity	Mild	Often severe	Moderate	Mild
Prognosis	Generally good	Worse with age, debility	Moderate	Good
Progression to chronicity	None	Occasional (5–10%)	Occasional (10–50%)	None
Prophylaxis	IG	Standard IG (not documented) HBIG, hepatitis B vaccine	?	?
Carrier	None	0.1–30%‡	Approximately 1%	None

* Concomitant delta hepatitis is similar in these features to hepatitis B, but more severe outcomes are favored.
† For example, sexual or maternal-neonatal contact.
‡ Varies considerably throughout the world, see text.

to be infectious, albeit less so than serum, when administered percutaneously or nonpercutaneously to experimental animals. Among the nonpercutaneous modes of HBV transmission, oral ingestion has been documented as a potential route of exposure but one whose efficiency is quite low. On the other hand, the two nonpercutaneous routes considered to have the greatest impact are intimate (especially sexual) contact and perinatal transmission.

In sub-Saharan Africa, intimate contact among toddlers is considered instrumental in contributing to the maintenance of the high frequency of HBsAg in the population. Perinatal transmission occurs primarily in infants born to HBsAg carrier mothers or mothers with acute hepatitis B during the third trimester of pregnancy or during the early postpartum period. Perinatal transmission is uncommon in North America and western Europe but occurs with great frequency and is the most important mode of HBV perpetuation in the Far East and developing countries. Although the precise mode of perinatal transmission is unknown, and although approximately 10 percent of infections may be acquired in utero, epidemiologic evidence suggests that most infections occur approximately at the time of delivery and are not related to breast feeding. Likelihood of perinatal transmission of HBV correlates with the presence of HBeAg; 90 percent of HBeAg-positive mothers but only 10 to 15 percent of anti-HBe-positive mothers transmit HBV infection to their offspring. In most cases, acute infection in the neonate is clinically asymptomatic, but the child is very likely to become an HBsAg carrier.

The more than 200 million HBsAg carriers in the world constitute the main reservoir of hepatitis B in human beings. Serum HBsAg is infrequent (0.1 to 0.5 percent) in normal populations in the United States and western Europe; however, a prevalence of up to 5 to 20 percent has been found in the far east and in some tropical countries, and as high as 30 percent in persons with Down's syndrome, lepromatous leprosy, leukemia, Hodgkin's disease, polyarteritis nodosa, patients with chronic renal disease on hemodialysis, and needle-using drug addicts.

Other groups with high rates of HBV infection include spouses of acutely infected persons, sexually promiscuous persons (especially promiscuous homosexual men), health care workers exposed to blood, persons who require repeated transfusions especially with pooled blood product concentrates (e.g., hemophiliacs), residents and staff of custodial institutions for the mentally retarded, prisoners, and, to a lesser extent, family members of chronically infected patients. In volunteer blood donors, the prevalence of anti-HBs, a reflection of previous HBV infection, ranges from 5 to 10 percent, but the prevalence is higher in lower socioeconomic strata, older age groups, and persons—including those mentioned above—exposed to blood products.

Prevalence of infection, modes of transmission, and human behavior conspire to mold geographically different epidemiologic patterns of HBV infection. In the Far East and Africa, hepatitis B, a disease of the newborn and young children, is perpetuated by a cycle of maternal-neonatal spread. In North America and western Europe, hepatitis B is primarily a disease of adolescence and early adulthood, the time of life when intimate sexual contact as well as recreational and occupational percutaneous exposures tend to occur.

Delta hepatitis Infection with the delta agent has a worldwide distribution, but two epidemiologic patterns exist. In Mediterranean countries (northern Africa, southern Europe, the Middle East), delta infection is endemic among those with hepatitis B, and the disease is transmitted predominantly by nonpercutaneous means, especially close personal contact. In nonendemic areas, such as the United States and northern Europe, delta infection is confined to persons exposed frequently to blood and blood products, primarily drug addicts and hemophiliacs. Delta hepatitis can be introduced into a population through drug addicts or by migration of persons from endemic to nonendemic areas. Thus, patterns of population migration and human behavior facilitating percutaneous contact play important roles in the introduction and amplification of delta infection. Occasionally, the migrating epidemiology of delta hepatitis is expressed in explosive outbreaks of severe hepatitis, such as those that have occurred in remote South American villages as well as in urban centers in the United States. Ultimately, such outbreaks of delta hepatitis—either of coinfections with acute hepatitis B or of superinfections in those already infected with HBV—may blur the distinctions between endemic and nonendemic areas.

Non-A, non-B hepatitis (hepatitis C) Routine screening of blood donors for HBsAg and the elimination of commercial blood sources have markedly decreased the frequency of hepatitis B after transfusion, but posttransfusion hepatitis still remains an important medical problem. The likelihood of posttransfusion hepatitis has been reported to be from 0.3 to 9 cases per 1000 units transfused, and the risk of anicteric hepatitis following transfusion is much greater than that of clinical hepatitis with jaundice. The risk of viral hepatitis after transfusion of blood derivatives is dependent on the methods by which these products are processed. The *greatest risk* follows the use of multiple pooled donor products such as concentrates of factors II, VII, VIII, IX, and X. Hepatitis has developed in 20 to 30 percent of individuals receiving these pooled products for the first time. Blood products associated with an *average risk* include whole blood, packed red blood cells, single donor platelets, and plasma. Products such as albumin and immune and hyperimmune globulin, because of prior treatment of these substances by heating to 60°C or by cold ethanol extraction, involve *no risk*. It had been suggested that frozen, glycerol-treated, washed red blood cells may carry a reduced risk of hepatitis, but this has been disproved.

Currently, hepatitis B accounts for only 5 to 10 percent of posttransfusion hepatitis. More of a problem is the occurrence of non-A, non-B hepatitis, which, prior to the development of a virus-specific screening test, accounted for approximately 90 to 95 percent or more of posttransfusion hepatitis cases following transfusion of voluntarily donated blood prescreened for HBsAg. The fact that non-A, non-B hepatitis is transmitted by transfused blood from asymptomatic donors (Table 252-2) and that it can be transmitted to chimpanzees by blood from patients with chronic hepatitis suggests that there is a carrier state for it. The frequency of posttransfusion non-A, non-B hepatitis approaches 5 to 10 percent of blood recipients, especially recipients of multiple units of blood products. Now that there is a serologic screening test to identify the major agent of this hepatitis, reduction and even elimination of infection due to transfusion may be possible.

In addition to being transmitted by transfusion, non-A, non-B hepatitis cases have been observed in other settings of percutaneous and nonpercutaneous exposure, e.g., intrafamily contact, intravenous drug abuse, occupational contact, nosocomial infection, use of hemodialysis units, and intrainstitutional contact. Special attention is merited by non-A, non-B hepatitis in hemophiliacs, in whom the incubation period may be as brief as 1 to 4 weeks, and in renal transplant recipients, up to 20 percent of whom have chronic liver disease. In the early years after transplantation, the death rate in patients with hepatitis is higher, as a result not of liver failure but of severe infections outside the hepatobiliary tree. However, 5 to 10 years after transplantation complications of chronic liver disease account for increased morbidity and mortality.

In western countries, non-A, non-B hepatitis accounts for approximately 15 to 30 percent of sporadic cases of viral hepatitis presenting for medical evaluation. Occurrence of multiple bouts of among drug abusers and hemophiliacs reinforces cross-challenge studies in chimpanzees that suggest that there is more than one such bloodborne agent. Eight percent of patients with transfusion-associated non-A, non-B hepatitis and 50 to 60 percent with the sporadic form have detectable anti-HCV; whether a more sensitive test for anti-HCV will raise these frequencies, or whether another non-A, non-B virus accounts for the residual cases, remains to be seen.

Non-A, non-B hepatitis (hepatitis E) Enteric non-A, non-B hepatitis identified in India, Asia, Africa, and Central America resembles hepatitis A in its primarily enteric mode of spread. The commonly recognized cases occur after contamination of water supplies as after monsoon flooding, but sporadic, isolated cases occur. Infections arise in populations that are immune to HAV, and favor young adults. It is not known if the E form occurs outside of recognized endemic areas, for example, in the United States, or if it accounts for any of the sporadic non-A, non-B cases in nonendemic areas. Cases imported from endemic areas have been found in the United States.

CLINICAL AND LABORATORY FEATURES Symptoms and signs The *prodromal symptoms* of acute viral hepatitis are systemic and quite variable. Constitutional symptoms of anorexia, nausea and vomiting, fatigue, malaise, arthralgias, myalgias, headache, photophobia, pharyngitis, cough, and coryza may precede the onset of jaundice by 1 to 2 weeks. The nausea, vomiting, and anorexia are frequently associated wth alterations in olfaction and taste. A low-grade fever between 38 and 39°C/(100 to 102°F) is more often present in hepatitis A than in non-A, non-B or B, except when hepatitis B is heralded by a serum sickness–like syndrome; rarely, a fever of 39.5 to 40°C/(103 to 104°F) may accompany the constitutional symptoms. Dark urine and clay-colored stools may be noticed by the patient from 1 to 5 days prior to the onset of clinical jaundice.

With the onset of *clinical jaundice* the constitutional prodromal symptoms usually diminish, but in some patients mild weight loss (2.5 to 5 kg) is common and may continue during the entire icteric phase. The liver becomes enlarged and tender and may be associated with right upper quadrant pain and discomfort. Infrequently, patients present with a cholestatic picture, suggesting extrahepatic biliary obstruction. Splenomegaly and cervical adenopathy are present in 10 to 20 percent of patients with acute hepatitis. Rarely, a few spider angiomas appear during the icteric phase and disappear during convalescence. During the *recovery phase,* constitutional symptoms disappear, but usually some liver enlargement and abnormalities in biochemical tests of hepatic function are still evident. The duration of the posticteric phase is variable, ranging from 2 to 12 weeks, and usually is more prolonged in acute hepatitis B and in non-A, non-B hepatitis. Complete clinical and biochemical recovery is to be expected 1 to 2 months after all cases of hepatitis A and E and 3 to 4 months after the onset of jaundice in three-quarters of uncomplicated cases of hepatitis B and C. In the remainder biochemical recovery may be delayed. A substantial proportion of patients with viral hepatitis never become icteric.

Infection with the delta agent (HDV) can occur in the presence of acute or chronic HBV infection; the duration of HBV infection determines the duration of delta infection. When acute delta and HBV infection occur simultaneously, clinical and biochemical features may be indistinguishable from those of HBV infection alone. As opposed to patients with *acute* HBV infection, patients with *chronic* HBV infection can support HDV replication indefinitely. This can happen when acute HDV infection occurs in the presence of a nonresolving acute HBV infection. More commonly, acute HDV infection becomes chronic when it is superimposed on an underlying chronic HBV infection. In such cases, the delta superinfection appears as a clinical exacerbation or an episode resembling acute viral hepatitis in someone already chronically infected with HBV. In the past, events resembling acute hepatitis in a HBV carrier or a patient with chronic hepatitis B were attributed to superimposed non-A, non-B hepatitis or to the natural history of the disease. A proportion of such episodes, however, represent acute superinfection with HDV. Delta superinfection in a patient with chronic hepatitis B often leads to clinical deterioration (see below).

In addition to superinfections with other hepatitis agents, acute hepatitis-like clinical events in persons with chronic hepatitis B may accompany spontaneous HBeAg–to–anti-HBe seroconversion or spontaneous reactivation, i.e., reversion from nonreplicative to replicative infection. Such reactivations can occur as well in therapeutically immunosuppressed patients with chronic HBV infection when cytotoxic-immunosuppressive drugs are withdrawn; in these cases, restoration of immune competence is thought to allow resumption of previously checked cell-mediated cytolysis of HBV-infected hepatocytes.

Laboratory features The serum aminotransferases AST and ALT (previously designated SGOT and SGPT) show a variable increase during the prodromal phase of acute viral hepatitis and precede the rise in bilirubin level (see Figs. 252-2 and 252-3). The acute level of these enzymes, however, does not correlate well with the degree of liver cell damage. Peak levels vary from 400 to 4000 IU or more; these levels are usually reached at the time the patient is clinically icteric and diminish progressively during the recovery phase of acute hepatitis. The diagnosis of anicteric hepatitis is difficult and requires a high index of suspicion; it is based on clinical features and on aminotransferase elevations, although mild increases in conjugated bilirubin may also be found.

Jaundice is usually visible in the sclera or skin when the serum bilirubin value exceeds 43 μmol/L (2.5 mg/dL). When jaundice appears, the serum bilirubin typically rises to levels ranging from 85 to 340 μmol/L (5 to 20 mg/dL). The serum bilirubin may continue to rise despite falling serum aminotransferase levels. In most instances the total bilirubin is equally divided between the conjugated and unconjugated fractions. Bilirubin levels above 340 μmol/L (20 mg/dL) extending and persisting late into the course of viral hepatitis are more likely to be associated with severe disease. In certain patients with underlying hemolytic anemia, however, such as glucose-6-phosphate dehydrogenase deficiency and sickle cell anemia, high serum bilirubin is common, resulting from superimposed hemolysis. In such patients bilirubin levels greater than 513 μmol/L (30 mg/dL) have been observed and are not necessarily associated with a poor prognosis.

Neutropenia and lymphopenia are transient and are followed by a relative lymphocytosis. Atypical lymphocytes (varying between 2 and 20 percent) are common during the acute phase. These atypical lymphocytes are indistinguishable from those seen in infectious mononucleosis. Measurement of the prothrombin time (PT) is important in patients with acute viral hepatitis, for a prolonged value may reflect a severe synthetic defect, signify extensive hepatocellular necrosis, and indicate a worse prognosis. Occasionally a prolonged PT may occur with only mild increases in the serum bilirubin and aminotransferase levels. Prolonged nausea and vomiting, inadequate carbohydrate intake, and poor hepatic glycogen reserves may contribute to hypoglycemia noted occasionally in patients with severe viral hepatitis. Serum alkaline phosphatase may be normal or only mildly elevated, while a fall in serum albumin is uncommon in uncomplicated acute viral hepatitis. In some patients mild and transient steatorrhea has been noted as well as slight microscopic hematuria and minimal proteinuria.

A diffuse but mild elevation of the gamma globulin fraction is common during acute viral hepatitis. Serum IgG and IgM are elevated in about one-third of patients during the acute phase of viral hepatitis, but serum IgM elevation is seen more characteristically during acute hepatitis A. During the acute phase of viral hepatitis, antibodies to smooth muscle and other cell constituents may be present, and low titers of rheumatoid factor, antinuclear antibody, and heterophil antibody can also be found occasionally. These antibodies are nonspecific and can also be associated with other viral and systemic diseases. In contrast, virus-specific antibodies, which appear during and after hepatitis virus infection, are serologic markers of diagnostic importance.

As described above, serologic tests are available with which to establish a diagnosis of hepatitis A, B, delta, and C. Tests for fecal or serum HAV are not routinely available. Therefore, a diagnosis of type A hepatitis is based on detection of IgM anti-HAV during acute illness (Fig. 252-2). Rheumatoid factor can give rise to false-positive results in this test.

A diagnosis of HBV infection can usually be made by detection of HBsAg in serum. Infrequently, levels of HBsAg are too low to be detected during acute HBV infection even with the current generation of highly sensitive immunoassays. In such cases, the diagnosis can be established by the presence of IgM anti-HBc. Alternatively, de novo appearance of anti-HBc and anti-HBs during illness and convalescence may support the diagnostic impression.

The titer of HBsAg bears little relation to the severity of clinical disease. Indeed, there may be an inverse correlation between the serum concentration of HBsAg and the degree of liver cell damage. For example, titers are highest in immunosuppressed patients, lower in chronic liver disease (but higher in chronic persistent than in chronic active hepatitis), and very low in acute fulminant hepatitis. These observations suggest that in hepatitis B the degree of liver cell damage and the clinical course are probably related to variations in the patient's immune response to HBV rather than to the amount of circulating HBsAg. In immunocompetent persons, however, there is a correlation between markers of HBV *replication* and liver injury (see below).

Another serologic marker which may be of value in patients with hepatitis B is HBeAg. Its principal clinical usefulness is as an indicator of relative infectivity. Because HBeAg is invariably present during early acute hepatitis B, HBeAg testing is indicated primarily during follow-up of chronic infection.

In patients with hepatitis B surface antigenemia of unknown duration, e.g., blood donors whose blood is found to be HBsAg-positive and who are referred to a physician for evaluation, testing for IgM anti-HBc may be useful to distinguish between acute or recent infection (IgM anti-HBc-positive) and chronic HBV infection (IgM anti-HBc-negative, IgG anti-HBc-positive). A false-positive test for IgM anti-HBc may be encountered in patients with high-titer rheumatoid factor.

Anti-HBs is rarely detectable in the presence of HBsAg in patients with *acute* hepatitis B, but 10 to 20 percent of persons with *chronic* HBV infection may harbor low-level anti-HBs. This antibody is directed not against the common group determinant, *a*, but against the heterotypic subtype determinant (e.g., HBsAg of subtype *ad* with anti-HBs of subtype *y*). In most cases, this serologic pattern cannot be attributed to infection with two different HBV subtypes, and the presence of this antibody is not a harbinger of imminent HBsAg clearance. When such antibody is detected, its presence is of no recognized clinical significance.

After immunization with hepatitis B vaccine, which consists of HBsAg alone, anti-HBs is the only serologic marker to appear. A summary of the commonly encountered serologic patterns of hepatitis B and their interpretations appears in Table 252-3. Tests for the detection of HBV DNA in liver and serum or DNA polymerase in serum are available in a limited number of research laboratories. Like HBeAg, serum HBV DNA and DNA polymerase are indicators of HBV replication, but they are more sensitive. These markers are useful in following the course of HBV replication in patients with chronic hepatitis B receiving experimental antiviral chemotherapy, with interferon for example. In immunocompetent persons a general correlation does appear to exist between the level of HBV replication, as reflected by the level of HBV DNA in serum, and the degree of liver injury. High serum HBV DNA levels, increased expression of viral antigens, and necroinflammatory activity in the liver go hand

TABLE 252-3 Commonly encountered serologic patterns of hepatitis B infection

HBsAg	Anti-HBs	Anti-HBc	HBeAg	Anti-HBe	Interpretation
+	–	IgM	+	–	Acute HBV infection, high infectivity
+	–	IgG	+	–	Chronic HBV infection, high infectivity
+	–	IgG	–	+	Late-acute or chronic HBV infection, low infectivity
+	+	+	+/–	+/–	*1* HBsAg of one subtype and heterotypic anti-HBs (common) *2* Process of seroconversion from HBsAg to anti-HBs (rare)
–	–	IgM	+/–	+/–	*1* Acute HBV infection *2* Anti-HBc window
–	–	IgG	–	+/–	*1* Low-level HBsAg carrier *2* Remote past infection
–	+	IgG	–	+/–	Recovery from HBV infection
–	+	–	–	–	*1* Immunization with HBsAg (after vaccination) *2* Remote past infection (?) *3* False-positive

in hand unless immunosuppression interferes with cytolytic T-cell responses to virus-infected cells; reduction of HBV replication with antiviral drugs, such as interferon, tends to be accompanied by an improvement in liver histology.

Before the availability of reliable serologic tests for hepatitis C, a diagnosis of non-A, non-B hepatitis was made by serologic exclusion of HAV and HBV infection in the setting of a compatible history. Now that a specific antibody test is available, the potential exists for making a specific serologic diagnosis; however, delays of 1 to 3 months before the appearance of detectable antibody may interfere with serodiagnosis during acute illness. Furthermore, the level of antibody appears to be quite low. A helpful clinical clue is the episodic pattern of aminotransferase elevation seen frequently in non-A, non-B hepatitis. A diagnosis of acute non-A, non-B hepatitis can be entertained if tests for HBsAg, IgM anti-HBc, and IgM anti-HAV are negative. If follow-up samples are obtained 1 or more months after the onset of acute illness, a specific serologic diagnosis of bloodborne non-A, non-B hepatitis (''hepatitis C'') may be made. If the specific antibody test remains negative, infection with a second bloodborne or an enteric non-A, non-B hepatitis agent (''hepatitis E'') should be considered. A diagnosis of non-A, non-B hepatitis may be more difficult to establish in patients with chronic hepatitis who have anti-HBc in their blood. The anti-HBc in such cases will almost invariably be of the IgG class; it represents either HBV infection in the remote past or current HBV infection with low-level virus carriage.

The presence of HDV infection can be identified by demonstrating intrahepatic delta antigen or, more practically, an antidelta seroconversion (a rise in titer of anti-HD or de novo appearance of IgM anti-HD). Circulating HDAg, also diagnostic of acute infection, is detectable only briefly, if at all. Because IgM anti-HD is transient and IgG anti-HD is often undetectable once HBsAg disappears, retrospective serodiagnosis of acute self-limited, simultaneous HBV and HDV infection is difficult.

When a patient presents with acute hepatitis and has HBsAg and anti-HD in the serum, determination of the class of anti-HBc is helpful in establishing the relationship between infection with HBV and HDV. Although IgM anti-HBc does not distinguish *absolutely* between acute and chronic HBV infection, its presence is a reliable indicator of recent infection and its absence a reliable indicator of infection in the remote past. In simultaneous acute HBV and HDV infections, IgM anti-HBc will be detectable, while in acute HDV infection superimposed upon chronic HBV infection, anti-HBc will be of the IgG class.

In the future, tests for the presence of HDV-associated RNA will be useful for determining the presence of ongoing HDV replication and relative infectivity. Currently, probes for this marker are restricted to a limited number of research laboratories. Similarly, diagnostic tests for the enteric non-A, non-B hepatitis agent are cumbersome and remain limited to a small number of research laboratories.

Liver biopsy is rarely necessary or indicated in acute viral hepatitis, except when there is a question about the diagnosis or when there is clinical evidence suggesting a diagnosis of chronic active hepatitis.

Little agreement exists over routine diagnostic algorithms to be applied in the evaluation of cases of acute viral hepatitis. One potential approach is to test every patient with three serologic tests, HBsAg, IgM anti-HAV, and IgM anti-HBc (Table 252-4). The presence of HBsAg, with or without IgM anti-HBc, represents HBV infection. If IgM anti-HBc is present, the HBV infection is considered acute; if IgM anti-HBc is absent, the HBV infection is considered chronic. A diagnosis of acute hepatitis B can be made in the absence of HBsAg when IgM anti-HBc is detectable. A diagnosis of acute hepatitis A is based on the presence of IgM anti-HAV. If IgM anti-HAV coexists with HBsAg, a diagnosis of simultaneous HAV and HBV infections can be made; if IgM anti-HBc (with or without HBsAg) is detectable, the patient has simultaneous acute hepatitis A and B, and if IgM anti-HBc is undetectable, the patient has acute hepatitis A superimposed on chronic HBV infection. Absence of all serologic markers is consistent with a diagnosis of non-A, non-B hepatitis. A follow-up test for antibody to hepatitis C can be done to confirm the diagnosis serologically.

TABLE 252-4 Simplified diagnostic approach in patients presenting with acute hepatitis

Test patient's serum for			
HBsAg	IgM anti-HAV	IgM anti-HBc	Diagnostic conclusion
+	−	+	Acute hepatitis B
+	−	−	Chronic hepatitis B
+	+	−	Acute hepatitis A superimposed on chronic hepatitis B
+	+	+	Acute hepatitis A and B
−	+	−	Acute hepatitis A
−	+	+	Acute hepatitis A and B (HBsAg below detectable level)
−	−	+	Acute hepatitis B (HBsAg below detectable level)
−	−	−	Compatible with non-A, non-B hepatitis*

* Confirm with follow-up test for antibody to non-A, non-B hepatitis agent.

If a serologic diagnosis of chronic hepatitis B is made, testing for HBeAg and anti-HBe is indicated to evaluate relative infectivity. Testing for HBV DNA in such patients provides a more quantitative and sensitive test for the level of virus replication and, therefore, is very helpful during antiviral therapy (see Chap. 253). In patients with hepatitis B, testing for anti-HD is useful under the following circumstances: severe and fulminant cases, severe chronic cases, cases of acute hepatitis-like exacerbations in patients with chronic hepatitis B, persons with frequent percutaneous exposures, and persons from areas where delta infection is endemic.

PROGNOSIS Virtually all previously healthy patients with hepatitis A recover completely from their illness with no clinical sequelae. Similarly in acute hepatitis B, 90 percent of patients have a favorable course and recover completely. There are, however, certain clinical and laboratory features which suggest a more complicated and protracted course. Patients of advanced age and with serious underlying medical disorders such as congestive heart failure, severe anemia, and diabetes mellitus may have a prolonged course and are more likely to experience severe hepatitis. Initial presenting features such as ascites, peripheral edema, and symptoms of hepatic encephalopathy suggest a poorer prognosis. In addition, a prolonged prothrombin time, low serum albumin, hypoglycemia, and very high serum bilirubin values suggest severe hepatocellular disease. Patients with these clinical and laboratory features deserve prompt hospital admission. The case fatality rate in hepatitis A and B is very low (approximately 0.1 percent) but is increased by advanced age and underlying debilitating disorders. Among patients ill enough to be hospitalized for acute hepatitis B, the fatality rate is 1 percent. Non-A, non-B hepatitis occurring after transfusion is less severe during the acute phase than type B hepatitis and is more likely to be anicteric; fatalities are rare, but the precise case fatality rate is not known. In outbreaks of the waterborne type of non-A, non-B hepatitis (hepatitis E) in India and Asia, the case fatality rate is 1 to 2 percent, and up to 10 percent in pregnant women. Patients with simultaneous acute hepatitis B and delta hepatitis do not necessarily experience a higher mortality rate than do patients with acute hepatitis B alone; however, in several recent outbreaks of acute simultaneous HBV and HDV infection among drug addicts, the case fatality rate has approximated 5 percent. In the case of delta superinfection of a person with chronic hepatitis B, the likelihood of fulminant hepatitis and death is increased substantially. Although the case fatality rate for delta hepatitis has not been defined adequately, in outbreaks of severe delta superinfection in isolated populations with a high hepatitis B carrier rate, the mortality rate has been recorded as in excess of 20 percent.

COMPLICATIONS AND SEQUELAE A small proportion of patients with hepatitis A experience *relapsing hepatitis* weeks to months after apparent recovery from acute hepatitis. Relapses are characterized by recurrence of symptoms, aminotransferase elevations, occasionally jaundice, and fecal excretion of HAV. Another unusual variant of acute hepatitis A is *cholestatic hepatitis,* characterized by protracted cholestatic jaundice and pruritus. Even when these complications occur, hepatitis A remains self-limited and does not progress to chronic liver disease. During the prodromal phase of acute hepatitis B, a serum sickness–like syndrome characterized by arthralgia or arthritis, rash, angioedema, and rarely hematuria and proteinuria may develop in some patients. This syndrome occurs prior to the onset of clinical jaundice, and these patients are often erroneously diagnosed as having rheumatoid arthritis or other rheumatologic diseases such as systemic lupus erythematosus. This syndrome occurs in about 5 to 10 percent of patients with acute hepatitis B. The diagnosis can be established by measuring serum aminotransferase levels, which are almost invariably elevated, and serum HBsAg.

The most feared complication of viral hepatitis is *fulminant hepatitis* (massive hepatic necrosis); fortunately this is a rare event. This is primarily seen in hepatitis B and delta hepatitis as well as enteric non-A, non-B hepatitis. Hepatitis B accounts for more than 50 percent of fulminant hepatitis cases, a sizeable proportion of which are associated with delta infection. Participation of the delta agent can be documented in approximately one-third of patients with acute fulminant hepatitis B and two-thirds of patients with fulminant hepatitis superimposed on chronic hepatitis B. Fulminant hepatitis is seen less frequently in bloodborne non-A, non-B hepatitis, and only occasionally in hepatitis A. Patients usually present with signs and symptoms of encephalopathy that may evolve to deep coma. The liver is usually small, and the prothrombin time excessively prolonged. The combination of rapidly shrinking liver size, rapidly rising bilirubin level, and marked prolongation of the prothrombin time, together with clinical signs of confusion, disorientation, somnolence, ascites, and edema, indicates that the patient has hepatic failure with encephalopathy. Cerebral edema is common; brainstem compression, gastrointestinal bleeding, sepsis, respiratory failure, cardiovascular collapse, and renal failure are terminal events. The mortality is exceedingly high (greater than 80 percent in patients with deep coma), but patients who survive may have a complete biochemical and histologic recovery.

It is particularly important to document the disappearance of HBsAg following apparent clinical recovery from acute hepatitis B. Before laboratory methods were available to distinguish between acute and acute hepatitis–like exacerbations (''spontaneous reactivations'') of chronic hepatitis B, observations suggested that approximately 10 percent of patients remained HBsAg-positive for longer than 6 months after the onset of clinically apparent acute hepatitis B. Half of these persons were found to clear the antigen from their circulations during the next several years, but the other 5 percent remained chronically HBsAg-positive. More recent observations suggest that the true rate of chronic infection after clinically apparent acute hepatitis B is as low as 1 to 2 percent in normal, immunocompetent, young adults. Earlier, higher estimates may have been biased by inadvertent inclusion of acute exacerbations in chronically infected patients; these patients, chronically HBsAg-positive before exacerbation, were unlikely to seroconvert to HBsAg-negative thereafter. Whether the rate of chronicity is 10 or 1 percent, such patients have anti-HBc in serum; anti-HBs is either undetected or detected at low titer against the opposite subtype specificity of the antigen (see ''Laboratory Features'' above). These patients may (1) be asymptomatic carriers, (2) have low-grade chronic persistent hepatitis, or (3) have chronic active hepatitis with or without cirrhosis. The likelihood of becoming an HBsAg carrier after acute HBV infection is especially high among neonates, persons with Down's syndrome, chronically hemodialyzed patients, and immunosuppressed patients, including persons with human immunodeficiency virus infection.

Chronic active hepatitis is a major late complication of acute hepatitis B occurring in a small proportion of acute cases but more common in those with chronic infection (see Chap. 253). Certain clinical and laboratory features suggest progression of acute hepatitis to chronic active hepatitis: (1) lack of complete resolution of clinical symptoms of anorexia, weight loss, and fatigue and the persistence of hepatomegaly; (2) the presence of bridging or multilobular hepatic necrosis on liver biopsy during protracted, severe acute viral hepatitis; (3) failure of the serum aminotransferase, bilirubin, and globulin levels to return to normal within 6 to 12 months following the acute illness; and (4) the continued presence of HBsAg 6 months or more after acute hepatitis, suggesting chronic viral infection of the liver.

Although acute delta hepatitis infection does not increase the likelihood of chronicity of simultaneous acute hepatitis B, delta hepatitis has the potential for contributing to the severity of chronic hepatitis B. Delta hepatitis superinfection can transform asymptomatic or mild chronic hepatitis B into severe, progressive chronic active hepatitis and cirrhosis; it can also accelerate the course of chronic active hepatitis B. Some delta superinfections in patients with chronic hepatitis B lead to fulminant hepatitis. After transfusion-associated acute non-A, non-B hepatitis, as many as 50 percent of patients have abnormal biochemical liver tests for more than a year. In a majority of such patients, liver histology is consistent with chronic active hepatitis. Although many of these patients have no symptoms and a nonprogressive course, ultimately, cirrhosis develops in as many as 20 percent of those with *chronic* posttransfusion non-A, non-B hepatitis within 10 years of acute illness. The likelihood of chronic hepatitis is also approximately 50 percent after sporadic non-A, non-B hepatitis occurring in the absence of identifiable percutaneous inoculation with blood products or contaminated needles. In contrast, neither HAV nor enteric non-A, non-B hepatitis causes chronic liver disease.

Rare complications of viral hepatitis include pancreatitis, myocarditis, atypical pneumonia, aplastic anemia, transverse myelitis, and peripheral neuropathy. *Carriers* of HBsAg, particularly those infected in infancy or early childhood, have an enhanced risk of hepatocellular carcinoma (see Chap. 255). In children, hepatitis B may present rarely with anicteric hepatitis, a nonpruritic papular rash of the face, buttocks, and limbs, and lymphadenopathy (papular acrodermatitis of childhood or Gianotti-Crosti syndrome).

DIFFERENTIAL DIAGNOSIS Viral diseases such as infectious mononucleosis; those due to cytomegalovirus, herpes simplex, and coxsackieviruses; and toxoplasmosis may share certain clinical features with viral hepatitis and cause elevation in serum aminotransferase and less commonly in serum bilirubin levels. Tests such as the differential heterophil and serologic tests for these agents may be helpful in the differential diagnosis if HBsAg, anti-HBc, and IgM anti-HAV determinations are negative. A complete drug history is particularly important, for many drugs and certain anesthetic agents can produce a picture of either acute hepatitis or cholestasis (see below). Equally important is a past history of unexplained ''repeated episodes'' of acute hepatitis. This should alert the physician to the possibility that the underlying disorder is chronic active hepatitis. Alcoholic hepatitis must also be considered, but usually the serum aminotransferase levels are not as markedly elevated and other stigmata of alcoholism may be present. The finding on liver biopsy of fatty infiltration, a neutrophilic inflammatory reaction, and ''alcoholic hyaline'' would be consistent with alcohol-induced rather than viral liver injury. Because acute hepatitis may present with right upper quadrant abdominal pain, nausea and vomiting, fever, and icterus, it is often confused with acute cholecystitis, common duct stone, or ascending cholangitis. Patients with acute viral hepatitis may tolerate surgery poorly; therefore, it is important to exclude this diagnosis, and in confusing cases, a percutaneous liver biopsy may be necessary prior to laparotomy. Viral hepatitis in the elderly is often misdiagnosed as obstructive jaundice resulting from a common duct stone or carcinoma of the pancreas. Because acute hepatitis in the elderly may be quite severe and the operative mortality high, a thorough evaluation including biochemical tests, radiographic studies of the biliary tree, and even liver biopsy may be necessary to exclude primary parenchymal liver disease. Another clinical constellation that may mimic acute hepatitis is right ventricular failure with passive hepatic congestion or hypoperfusion syndromes, such as those associated with shock, severe hypotension, and severe left ventricular failure. Clinical features are usually sufficient to distinguish between the two entities. Very rarely, malignancies metastatic to the liver can mimic acute or even fulminant viral hepatitis. Occasionally, genetic or metabolic liver disorders (e.g., Wilson's disease, $alpha_1$ antitrypsin deficiency) are confused with viral hepatitis.

MANAGEMENT Treatment of acute attack There is no specific treatment for *typical acute viral hepatitis.* Although hospitalization may be required for clinically severe illness, most patients do not require hospital care. Forced and prolonged bed rest is not essential for full recovery, but many patients will feel better with restricted physical activity. A high-calorie diet is desirable, and because many patients may experience nausea late in the day, the major caloric intake is best tolerated in the morning. Intravenous feeding is necessary in the acute stage if the patient has persistent vomiting and cannot maintain oral intake. Drugs capable of producing adverse reactions such as cholestasis and drugs metabolized by the liver should be avoided. If severe pruritus is present, the use of the bile salt–sequestering resin cholestyramine will usually alleviate this symptom. Glucocorticoid therapy has no value in acute viral hepatitis. Even in severe cases associated with *bridging necrosis,* controlled trials have failed to demonstrate the efficacy of steroids. In fact, such therapy may be hazardous.

Physical isolation of patients with hepatitis to a single room and bathroom is rarely necessary except in the case of fecal incontinence for hepatitis A and E or uncontrolled, voluminous bleeding for hepatitis types B (with or without concomitant delta hepatitis) and bloodborne non-A, non-B. Because most patients hospitalized with hepatitis A excrete little if any HAV, the likelihood of HAV transmission from these patients during their hospitalization is low. Therefore, burdensome *enteric precautions are no longer recommended.* Although gloves should be worn when the bedpans or fecal material of patients with hepatitis A are handled, these precautions do not represent a departure from sensible procedure for all hospitalized patients. For patients with types B and bloodborne non-A, non-B hepatitis, emphasis should be placed on blood precautions, i.e., avoiding direct, ungloved hand contact with blood and other body fluids. Enteric precautions are unnecessary. The importance of simple hygienic precautions, such as hand washing, cannot be overemphasized.

Hospitalized patients may be discharged when there is substantial symptomatic improvement, a significant downward trend in the serum aminotransferase and bilirubin values, and a return to normal of the prothrombin time. Mild aminotransferase elevations should not be considered contraindications to the gradual resumption of normal activity.

In *fulminant hepatitis,* the goal of therapy is to support the patient by maintenance of fluid balance, support of circulation and respiration, control of bleeding, correction of hypoglycemia, and treatment of other complications of the comatose state in anticipation of liver regeneration and repair. Protein intake should be restricted and oral lactulose or neomycin administered. Massive doses of glucocorticoids have been administered, but such therapy has been shown in controlled trials to be ineffective. Likewise, exchange transfusion, plasmapheresis, human cross-circulation, porcine liver cross-perfusion, and hemoperfusion have not been proven to enhance survival. Meticulous intensive care is the one factor that does appear to improve survival. Orthotopic liver transplantation is resorted to with increasing frequency, with excellent results, in patients with fulminant hepatitis (see Chap. 257).

HAZARDS TO MEDICAL AND PARAMEDICAL PERSONNEL Health care workers exposed frequently to blood, body tissues, and fluids have an increased risk of viral hepatitis, primarily hepatitis B. Approximately 15 percent of health workers have one or more serologic markers of HBV infection, and 1 percent are HBsAg-positive. The risk is higher in surgeons, pathologists, laboratory technologists who process blood specimens, technologists who draw blood and insert intravenous cannulas, hemodialysis staff, and others who perform invasive procedures. Transmission of HBV infection in health care settings, however, appears to be unidirectional, from patients to staff. With rare exceptions, HBsAg-positive health personnel do not increase the risk of HBV infection for their patients. Asymptomatic HBsAg carriers represent the greater risk to health personnel, because there are no readily identifiable clinical features that allow their recognition. Approximately 1 percent of all patients admitted to large metropolitan hospitals are HBsAg-positive, but 90 percent of these are not identified routinely. Patients with a past history of hepatitis or multiple transfusions, patients from countries where hepatitis B is endemic, sexually active homosexual men, intravenous drug abusers, and patients with chronic liver disease, chronic renal failure, polyarteritis nodosa, and Down's syndrome should have routine HBsAg determinations because of the high frequency of HBsAg positivity in these groups. If positive, they are potentially infectious, and appropriate precautions should be taken during operative or other acute-care procedures. In hemodialysis units, introduction of patient and staff education, routine periodic screening for HBsAg and aminotransferase elevations, and segregation of HBsAg-positive patients from susceptible patients have reduced dramatically the incidence of new HBV infections in both patients and medical personnel. Immunization with hepatitis B vaccine is another important measure in limiting the spread of hepatitis B to health workers (see below).

PROPHYLAXIS Because therapy for viral hepatitis is limited, emphasis is placed on prevention through immunization. The prophylactic approach differs for each of the types of viral hepatitis. In the past, immunoprophylaxis relied exclusively on passive immunization with antibody-containing globulin preparations purified by cold ethanol fractionation from the plasma of hundreds of normal donors. Currently, for hepatitis B, active immunization with a vaccine is available as well.

Hepatitis A All preparations of immune globulin (IG) contain anti-HAV. Although the titers may vary, all IG preparations appear to have an antibody concentration sufficient to be protective. When administered before exposure or during the early incubation period, IG is effective in preventing clinically apparent type A hepatitis. In some cases, IG does not abort infection but, by attenuating it, renders it inapparent. As a result long-lasting "passive-active" immunity occurs; however, this is now considered to be the exception rather than the rule. For intimate contacts (household, institutional) of persons with hepatitis A, administration of 0.02 mL/kg is recommended as early after exposure as possible; it may be effective even when administered as late as 2 weeks after exposure. Prophylaxis is not necessary for casual contacts (office, factory, school, or hospital), for most elderly persons, who are very likely to be immune, or for those known to have anti-HAV in their serum. In day-care centers, recognition of hepatitis A cases in children or staff should provide a stimulus for immunoprophylaxis in the center and in the children's family members. By the time most common-source outbreaks of type A hepatitis are recognized, it is usually too late in the incubation period for IG to be effective; however, prophylaxis may limit the frequency of secondary cases. For travelers to tropical countries, developing countries, and other areas outside of standard tourist routes, IG prophylaxis is recommended. When such travel lasts less than 3 months, 0.02 mL/kg is given; for longer travel or residence in these areas, a dose of 0.06 mL/kg every 4 to 6 months is recommended. Administration of plasma-derived globulin is safe; it has not been associated with transmission of AIDS to recipients, and the AIDS virus (human immunodeficiency virus, HIV) is inactivated by 25 percent alcohol, to which plasma is subjected during the cold ethanol fractionation process. Killed, live attenuated, and genetically engineered hepatitis A vaccines are being developed.

Hepatitis B Until recently, prevention of hepatitis B was based on *passive* immunoprophylaxis either with standard IG, containing modest levels of anti-HBs, or hepatitis B immune globulin (HBIG), containing high-titer anti-HBs. The efficacy of standard IG has never been established and remains questionable; even the efficacy of HBIG, demonstrated in several clinical trials, has been challenged, and its contribution appears to be in reducing the frequency of clinical *illness*, not in preventing *infection*. Although HBV cannot be cultivated in vitro in the classical sense, a vaccine for *active* immunization has been prepared from purified, noninfectious 22-nm spherical forms of HBsAg derived from the plasma of healthy HBsAg carriers. The vaccine is subjected to three different chemical inactivation steps which, cumulatively, destroy the infectivity of every known virus, including HIV. In controlled clinical trials among high-risk persons, this plasma-derived vaccine was shown to be immunogenic, highly effective in preventing HBV infection, and, despite its unconventional source, very safe. In addition, a genetically engineered vaccine derived from recombinant yeast has been introduced. The latter vaccine consists of HBsAg particles that are nonglycosylated but are otherwise indistinguishable from natural HBsAg; this second-generation vaccine is comparable in immunogenicity, protective efficacy, and safety to the first-generation, plasma-derived vaccine. Current recommendations can be divided into those for preexposure and postexposure prophylaxis.

For *preexposure* prophylaxis against hepatitis B in settings of frequent exposure (health workers exposed to blood, hemodialysis patients and staff, residents and staff of custodial institutions for the developmentally handicapped, intravenous drug abusers, promiscuous homosexual men as well as promiscuous heterosexuals, persons such as hemophiliacs who require long-term, high-volume therapy with blood derivatives, household and sexual contacts of HBsAg carriers, and persons living in or traveling extensively in endemic areas), three intramuscular (deltoid, not gluteal) injections of hepatitis B vaccine are recommended at 0, 1, and 6 months. Pregnancy is *not* a contraindication to vaccination. The recommended dose for each injection of plasma-derived vaccine is 20 μg for immunocompetent adults, 40 μg for immunosuppressed patients (hemodialysis patients, transplant recipients, and oncology patients receiving chemotherapy), and 10 μg for infants and children under the age of 10. One of the available recombinant vaccines is formulated to contain 10 μg for normal adults and 5 μg for children; another contains 20 μg and 10 μg for adults and children, respectively.

For unvaccinated persons sustaining an exposure to HBV, *post-exposure* prophylaxis with a combination of HBIG (for rapid achievement of high-titer circulating anti-HBs) and hepatitis B vaccine (for achievement of long-lasting immunity as well as its apparent efficacy in attenuating clinical illness after exposure) is recommended. For *perinatal* exposure of infants born to HBsAg-positive mothers, a single dose of HBIG, 0.5 mL, should be administered intramuscularly in the thigh *immediately after birth,* followed by a complete course of three 10-μg injections of plasma-derived hepatitis B vaccine (or 5 μg of recombinant vaccine) to be started within the first 12 h to 1 week of life. For those experiencing a direct percutaneous inoculation or transmucosal exposure to HBsAg-positive blood or body fluids (e.g., accidental *needle stick,* other mucosal penetration, or ingestion), a single intramuscular dose of HBIG, 0.06 mL/kg, administered as soon after exposure as possible, is followed by a complete course of hepatitis B vaccine to begin within the first week. For those exposed by *sexual* contact to a patient with acute hepatitis B, the Immunization Practices Advisory Committee of the United States Public Health Service recommends a single intramuscular dose of HBIG, 0.06 mL/kg, within 14 days of exposure, to be followed by either a second HBIG injection or, only when HBsAg positivity in the index case persists beyond 3 months, a complete course of hepatitis B vaccine. Other authorities, however, recommend a combination of HBIG followed by a complete course of hepatitis B vaccine injections for all sexual contacts of patients with acute hepatitis B, regardless of the duration of HBsAg positivity in the index case. When both HBIG and hepatitis B vaccine are recommended, they may be given at the same time but at separate sites.

The precise duration of protection afforded by hepatitis B vaccine is unknown; however, approximately 80 to 90 percent of immunocompetent vaccinees retain protective levels of anti-HBs for at least 5 years. Thereafter and even after anti-HBs becomes undetectable, protection persists against clinical hepatitis B, hepatitis B surface antigenemia, and chronic HBV infection. Currently *booster* immunizations are not recommended routinely, except in immunosuppressed persons who have lost detectable anti-HBs or immunocompetent persons who sustain percutaneous HBsAg-positive inoculations after losing detectable antibody.

Delta hepatitis Infection with the delta hepatitis agent can be prevented by vaccinating susceptible persons with hepatitis B vaccine. No product is available for immunoprophylaxis to prevent delta superinfection in HBsAg carriers; for them, avoidance of percutaneous exposures and limitation of intimate contact with persons who have delta infection are recommended.

Non-A, non-B hepatitis For transfusion-associated non-A, non-B hepatitis, the effectiveness of IG prophylaxis has not been demonstrated consistently and is not recommended. The most effective measure for reducing the frequency of posttransfusion non-A, non-B hepatitis is the elimination of commercially obtained donor blood and reliance exclusively on volunteer blood donors. The presence of elevated ALT and/or anti-HBc in donor blood was found to correlate with the risk of non-A, non-B hepatitis in recipients. Both of these markers appear to identify segments of the blood donor population with an increased risk of bloodborne viral infections. In the late 1980s, screening of donor blood for these surrogate markers was introduced. At the same time, exclusion of blood donors in high-risk groups for AIDS and screening of blood donors for anti-HIV were introduced. These measures, introduced to limit transfusion-associated AIDS, have the potential to lower the risk of infection with other bloodborne agents, like non-A, non-B hepatitis virus, as well. Finally, the recent introduction of blood donor screening for antibody to hepatitis C is expected to reduce further the risk of non-A, non-B hepatitis after transfusion. Another approach, chemical treatment of blood products and concentrates to inactivate non-A, non-B hepatitis virus infectivity, is also being pursued. Studies to test the efficacy of standard IG after needle stick, sexual, or perinatal exposure to non-A, non-B hepatitis have not been done. Because the inoculum is considerably smaller in these settings than that associated with transfusion, and because of its safety and low cost, some authorities do recommend postexposure prophylaxis with a single dose of IG, 0.06 mL/kg (or 0.5 mL for neonatal exposure), in these situations. The efficacy of IG for prevention of enteric non-A, non-B hepatitis remains to be evaluated.

TOXIC AND DRUG-INDUCED HEPATITIS

Liver injury may follow the inhalation, ingestion, or parenteral administration of a number of pharmacologic and chemical agents. These include industrial toxins (e.g., carbon tetrachloride, trichloroethylene, and yellow phosphorus), the heat-stable toxic bicyclic octapeptides of certain species of *Amanita* and *Galerina* (hepatotoxic mushroom poisoning), and more commonly, pharmacologic agents used in medical therapy. It is essential that any patient presenting with jaundice or impaired liver function be questioned carefully about exposure to chemicals used in work or at home and drugs taken by prescription or bought "over the counter." In general, two major types of chemical hepatotoxicity have been recognized: (1) direct toxic type and (2) idiosyncratic type.

As shown in Table 252-5, direct toxic hepatitis occurs with predictable regularity in individuals exposed to the offending agent and is dose-dependent. The latent period between exposure and liver injury is usually short (often several hours), although clinical manifestations may be delayed for 24 to 48 h. Agents producing toxic hepatitis are generally systemic poisons or are converted in the liver to toxic metabolites. The direct hepatotoxins result in morphologic abnormalities which are reasonably characteristic and reproducible

TABLE 252-5 Some features of toxic and drug-induced hepatic injury

	Direct toxic effect		Idiosyncratic			Other
Features	(Carbon tetrachloride, e.g.)	(Acetaminophen, e.g.)	(Halothane, e.g.)	(Isoniazid, e.g.)	(Chlorpromazine, e.g.)	(Oral contraceptive agents, e.g.)
Predictable and dose-related toxicity	+	+	0	0	0	+
Latent period	Short	Short	Variable	Variable	Variable	Variable
Arthralgia, fever, rash, eosinophilia	0	0	+	0	+	0
Liver morphology	Necrosis, fatty infiltration	Centrilobular necrosis	Similar to viral hepatitis	Similar to viral hepatitis	Cholestasis *with* portal inflammation	Cholestasis *without* portal inflammation, vascular lesions

for each toxin. For example, carbon tetrachloride and trichloroethylene characteristically produce a centrilobular zonal necrosis, whereas yellow phosphorus poisoning typically results in periportal injury. The hepatotoxic octapeptides of *Amanita phalloides* usually produce massive hepatic necrosis. The lethal dose of the toxin is about 10 mg, the amount found in a single deathcap mushroom. Tetracycline, when administered in intravenous doses greater than 1.5 g daily, leads to microvesicular fat deposits in the liver. Liver injury, which is often only one facet of the toxicity produced by the direct hepatotoxins, may go unrecognized until jaundice appears.

In idiosyncratic drug reactions the occurrence of hepatitis is usually infrequent and unpredictable, the response is not dose-dependent, and it may occur at any time during or shortly after exposure to the drug. Extrahepatic manifestations of hypersensitivity, such as rash, arthralgias, fever, leukocytosis, and eosinophilia occur in about one-quarter of patients with idiosyncratic hepatotoxic drug reactions; this observation and the unpredictability of idiosyncratic drug hepatotoxicity contributed to the hypothesis that this category of drug reactions is immunologically mediated. More recent evidence, however, suggests that even idiosyncratic reactions represent direct hepatotoxity but are caused by drug metabolites rather than by the intact compound. Even the prototype of idiosyncratic hepatoxicity reactions, halothane hepatitis, and isoniazid hepatotoxicity, associated frequently with hypersensitivity manifestations, are now recognized to be mediated by toxic metabolites which damage liver cells directly. Currently, idiosyncratic reactions are thought to result from differences in metabolic reactivity to specific agents; host susceptibility is mediated by the kinetics of toxic metabolite generation, which differs among individuals. Idiosyncratic reactions lead to a morphologic pattern that is more variable than those produced by direct toxins; a single agent is often capable of causing a variety of lesions, although certain patterns tend to predominate. Depending on the agent involved, idiosyncratic hepatitis may result in a clinical and morphologic picture indistinguishable from viral hepatitis (e.g., halothane) or may simulate extrahepatic bile duct obstruction clinically with morphologic evidence of cholestasis and minimal hepatocellular damage (e.g., chlorpromazine). Morphologic alterations may also include bridging hepatic necrosis (e.g., methyldopa), or, infrequently, hepatic granulomas (e.g., sulfonamides).

Not all adverse hepatic drug reactions can be classified as either toxic or idiosyncratic in type. For example, oral contraceptives, which combine estrogenic and progestational compounds, may result in impairment of hepatic function and occasionally in jaundice. However, they do not produce necrosis or fatty change, manifestations of hypersensitivity are generally absent, and susceptibility to the development of oral contraceptive–induced cholestasis appears to be genetically determined.

Because drug-induced hepatitis is often a presumptive diagnosis and many other disorders produce a similar clinicopathologic picture, evidence of a causal relationship between the use of a drug and subsequent liver injury may be difficult to establish. The relationship is most convincing for the direct hepatotoxins, which lead to a high frequency of hepatic impairment after a short latent period. Idiosyncratic reactions may be reproduced, in some instances, when rechallenge, after an asymptomatic period, results in a recurrence of signs, symptoms, and morphologic and biochemical abnormalities. Rechallenge, however, is often ethically unfeasible, because severe reactions may occur.

Treatment of toxic and drug-induced hepatic disease is largely supportive, as in acute viral hepatitis. Withdrawal of the suspected agent is indicated at the first sign of an adverse reaction. In the case of the direct toxins, liver involvement should not divert attention from renal or other organ involvement which may also threaten survival.

In Table 252-6 several classes of chemical agents are listed, together with examples of the pattern of liver injury produced by them. Certain drugs appear to be responsible for the development of chronic as well as acute hepatic injury. For example, oxphenisatin, alpha methyldopa, and isoniazid have been associated with chronic active hepatitis, and halothane and methotrexate have been implicated in the development of cirrhosis. A syndrome resembling primary biliary cirrhosis has been described following treatment with chlorpromazine, methyl testosterone, tolbutamide, and other drugs. Portal hypertension in the absence of cirrhosis may result from alterations in hepatic architecture produced by vitamin A or arsenic intoxication, industrial exposure to vinyl chloride, or administration of thorium dioxide. The latter three agents have also been associated with

TABLE 252-6 Principal alterations of hepatic morphology produced by some commonly used drugs and chemicals

Principal morphologic change	Class of agent	Example
Cholestasis	Anabolic steroid	Methyl testosterone*
	Antithyroid	Methimazole
	Chemotherapeutic	Erythromycin estolate
	Oral contraceptive	Norethynodrel with mestranol
	Oral hypoglycemic	Chlorpropamide
	Tranquilizer	Chlorpromazine*
Fatty liver	Chemotherapeutic	Tetracycline
	Anticonvulsant	Sodium valproate
	Antiarrhythmic	Amiodarone
Hepatitis	Anesthetic	Halothane†
	Anticonvulsant	Phenytoin
	Antihypertensive	Methyldopa†
	Chemotherapeutic	Isoniazid†
	Diuretic	Chlorothiazide
	Laxative	Oxyphenisatin†
Toxic (necrosis)	Hydrocarbon	Carbon tetrachloride
	Metal	Yellow phosphorus
	Mushroom	*Amanita phalloides*
	Analgesic	Acetaminophen
	Solvent	Dimethylformamide
Granulomas	Anti-inflammatory	Phenylbutazone
	Chemotherapeutic	Sulfonamides
	Xanthine oxidase inhibitor	Allopurinol

* Rarely associated with primary biliary cirrhosis-like lesion.
† Occasionally associated with chronic active hepatitis or bridging hepatic necrosis or cirrhosis.

angiosarcoma of the liver. Oral contraceptives have been implicated in the development of hepatic adenoma and, rarely, hepatocellular carcinoma and occlusion of the hepatic vein (Budd-Chiari syndrome). Another unusual lesion, peliosis hepatis (blood cysts of the liver), has been observed in some patients treated with oral contraceptives or anabolic steroids. The existence of these hepatic disorders expands the spectrum of liver injury induced by chemical agents and emphasizes the need for a thorough drug history in all patients with liver dysfunction.

The following are the patterns of adverse hepatic reactions for some prototypic agents.

ACETAMINOPHEN HEPATOTOXICITY (DIRECT TOXIN) Acetaminophen, an analgesic and antipyretic that is available without a prescription, has caused severe centrolobular hepatic necrosis when ingested in large amounts in suicide attempts or accidentally by children. A single dose of 10 to 15 g, occasionally less, may produce clinical evidence of liver injury. Fatal fulminant disease is usually (although not invariably) associated with ingestion of 25 g or more. Blood levels of acetaminophen correlate with the severity of hepatic injury (levels above 300 μg/mL 4 h after ingestion are predictive of the development of severe damage, while levels below 150 μg/mL suggest that hepatic injury is highly unlikely). Nausea, vomiting, diarrhea, abdominal pain, and shock are early manifestations occurring 4 to 12 h after ingestion. Then 24 to 48 h later, when these features are abating, hepatic injury becomes apparent. Maximal abnormalities and hepatic failure may not be evident until 4 to 6 days after ingestion. Renal failure and myocardial injury may be present.

Acetaminophen hepatotoxicity is mediated by a toxic reactive metabolite formed from the parent compound by the cytochrome P_{450} mixed-function oxidase system of the hepatocyte. This metabolite is detoxified by binding to glutathione. When excessive amounts of the metabolite are formed, glutathione levels in liver fall, and the metabolite is covalently bound to nucleophilic hepatocyte macromolecules. This process is believed to lead to hepatocyte necrosis; the precise sequence and mechanism are unknown. Hepatic injury may be potentiated by prior administration of alcohol or other drugs, by conditions which stimulate the mixed-function oxidase system, or by conditions such as starvation which reduce hepatic glutathione levels. In chronic alcoholics, the toxic dose of acetaminophen may be as low as 2 g.

Treatment of acetaminophen overdosage includes gastric lavage, supportive measures, and oral administration of activated charcoal or cholestyramine to prevent absorption of residual drug. Neither of the latter agents appears to be effective if given more than 30 min after acetaminophen ingestion; if they are used, the stomach lavage should be done before other agents are administered orally. In patients with high acetaminophen blood levels (>200 μg/mL measured at 4 h or >100 μg/mL at 8 h after ingestion) the administration of sulfhydryl compounds (e.g., cysteamine, cysteine, or *N*-acetylcysteine) appears to reduce the severity of hepatic necrosis. These agents appear to act by providing a reservoir of sulfhydryl groups to bind the toxic metabolites or by stimulating synthesis and repletion of hepatic glutathione. Therapy should be begun within 8 h of ingestion but may be effective even if given as late as 24 h after overdose. Later administration of sulfhydryl compounds is of uncertain value.

Survivors of acute acetaminophen overdose usually have no evidence of hepatic sequelae. In a few patients prolonged or repeated administration of acetaminophen in therapeutic doses appears to have led to the development of chronic active hepatitis and cirrhosis.

HALOTHANE HEPATOTOXICITY (IDIOSYNCRATIC REACTION) Halothane, a nonexplosive fluorinated hydrocarbon anesthetic agent that is structurally similar to chloroform, has been reported to result in severe hepatic necrosis in a small number of individuals, many of whom have previously been exposed to this agent. The failure to produce similar hepatic lesions reliably in animals, the rarity of hepatic impairment in human beings, and the delayed appearance of hepatic injury suggest that halothane is not a direct hepatotoxin but may be a sensitizing agent. However, manifestations of hypersensitivity are seen in fewer than 25 percent of cases. A genetic predisposition leading to an idiosyncratic metabolic reactivity has been postulated and appears to be the most likely mechanism of halothane hepatotoxicity. Supporting this postulate is the demonstration in patients with halothane hepatitis and their family members of increased lymphocyte susceptibility to damage in vitro by electrophilic drug metabolites. Adults (rather than children), obese people, and women appear to be particularly susceptible. Fever, moderate leukocytosis, and eosinophilia may occur in the first week following halothane administration. Jaundice usually is noted 7 to 10 days after exposure but may occur earlier in previously exposed patients. Nausea and vomiting may precede the onset of jaundice. Hepatomegaly is often mild, but liver tenderness is common. The serum aminotransferase levels are elevated. The pathologic changes at autopsy are indistinguishable from massive hepatic necrosis resulting from viral hepatitis. The case fatality rate of halothane hepatitis is not known but may vary from 20 to 40 percent in cases with severe liver involvement. In rare instances cirrhosis has been observed following repeated bouts of halothane hepatitis; however, in most patients who recover, the liver returns to normal. It is strongly suggested that patients in whom unexplained spiking fever, especially delayed fever, or jaundice develops after halothane anesthesia not receive this agent again. Because cross-reactions between halothane and methoxyfluorane have been reported, the latter agent should not be used after halothane reactions. Later-generation halogenated hydrocarbon anesthetics are felt to be associated with a lower risk of hepatotoxicity; however, rare cases have been observed.

METHYLDOPA HEPATOTOXICITY (TOXIC AND IDIOSYNCRATIC REACTION) Minor alterations in liver tests are reported in about 5 percent of patients treated with this antihypertensive agent. These trivial abnormalities typically resolve despite continued drug administration. In less than 1 percent of patients, acute liver injury resembling viral hepatitis, or chronic active hepatitis, or rarely a cholestatic reaction is seen 1 to 20 weeks after methyldopa is started. In 50 percent of cases the interval is shorter than 4 weeks. A prodrome of fever, anorexia, and malaise may be noted for a few days before the onset of jaundice. Rash, lymphadenopathy, arthralgia, and eosinophilia are rare. Serologic markers of autoimmunity are infrequently detected, and fewer than 5 percent of patients have a Coombs-positive hemolytic anemia. In about 15 percent of patients with methyldopa hepatotoxicity the clinical, biochemical, and histologic features are those of chronic active hepatitis with or without bridging necrosis and macronodular cirrhosis. With discontinuation of the drug, the disorder usually resolves, although progression has been seen in a few patients.

ISONIAZID HEPATOTOXICITY (TOXIC AND IDIOSYNCRATIC REACTION) In approximately 10 percent of adults treated with the antituberculosis agent isoniazid, elevated serum aminotransferase levels develop during the first few weeks of therapy; this appears to represent an adaptive response to a toxic metabolite of the drug. Whether or not isoniazid is continued, these values (usually below 200 units) return to normal in a few weeks. In about 1 percent of treated patients, an illness develops which is indistinguishable from viral hepatitis; approximately half of these cases occur within the first 2 months of treatment, while in the remainder, clinical disease may be delayed for many months. Liver biopsy reveals morphologic changes similar to those of viral hepatitis or bridging hepatic necrosis. The disease may be severe, with a case fatality rate of 10 percent. Important liver injury appears to be age-related, increasing substantially in frequency after age 35; the highest frequency is in patients over age 50, the lowest under the age of 20. Fever, rash, eosinophilia, and other manifestations of drug allergy are distinctly unusual. A reactive metabolite of acetylhydrazine, a metabolite of isoniazid, may be responsible for liver injury. A picture resembling chronic active hepatitis has been observed in a few patients.

SODIUM VALPROATE HEPATOTOXICITY (TOXIC AND IDIOSYNCRATIC REACTION) Sodium valproate, an anticonvulsant useful in the treatment of petit mal and other seizure disorders, has been associated with the development of severe hepatic toxicity and, rarely, fatalities in both children and adults. Asymptomatic elevations of serum aminotransferase levels have been recognized in as many as 45 percent of treated patients. These "adaptive" changes, however, appear to have no clinical importance, for major hepatotoxicity is not seen in the majority of patients despite continuation of drug therapy. In those rare patients in whom jaundice, encephalopathy, and evidence of hepatic failure are found, examination of liver tissue reveals microvesicular fat and bridging hepatic necrosis predominantly in the centrolobular zone. Bile duct injury may also be apparent. It seems likely that sodium valproate is not directly hepatotoxic but that its metabolite, 4-pentenoic acid, may be responsible for hepatic injury.

PHENYTOIN HEPATOTOXICITY (IDIOSYNCRATIC REACTION) Phenytoin, diphenylhydantoin, a mainstay in the treatment of seizure disorders, has been associated in rare instances with the development of severe hepatitis-like liver injury leading to fulminant hepatic failure in some instances. In many patients the hepatitis is associated with striking fever, lymphadenopathy, rash (Stevens-Johnson syndrome or exfoliative dermatitis), leukocytosis, and eosinophilia, suggesting an immunologically mediated hypersensitivity mechanism. Despite these observations, there is also evidence that metabolic idiosyncrasy may be responsible for hepatic injury. In the liver, phenytoin is converted by the cytochrome P_{450} system to metabolites which include the highly reactive electrophilic arene oxides. These metabolites are normally metabolized further by epoxide hydrolases. A defect (genetic or acquired) in epoxide hydrolase activity would permit covalent binding of arene oxides to hepatic macromolecules, thereby leading to hepatic injury. Regardless of the mechanism, hepatic injury is usually manifest within the first 2 months after beginning phenytoin therapy. With the exception of an abundance of eosinophils in the liver, the clinical, biochemical, and histologic picture resembles that of viral hepatitis. In rare instances, bile duct injury may be the salient feature of phenytoin hepatotoxicity with striking features of intrahepatic cholestasis. Asymptomatic elevations of aminotransferase and alkaline phosphatase levels have been observed in a sizeable proportion of patients receiving long-term phenytoin therapy. These liver changes are believed by some authorities to represent the potent hepatic enzyme–inducing properties of phenytoin and are accompanied histologically by swelling of hepatocytes in the absence of necroinflammatory activity or evidence of chronic liver disease.

CHLORPROMAZINE HEPATOTOXICITY (CHOLESTATIC IDIOSYNCRATIC REACTION) In about 1 percent of patients receiving chlorpromazine, intrahepatic cholestasis with jaundice develops after 1 to 4 weeks of treatment. In rare instances, jaundice has been reported after a single exposure. Anicteric reactions are frequent. The onset may be abrupt with fever, rash, arthralgias, lymphadenopathy, nausea, vomiting, and epigastric or right upper quadrant pain. Pruritus may precede the appearance of jaundice, dark urine, and light stools. Eosinophilia with or without mild leukocytosis may be present, and conjugated hyperbilirubinemia, moderately elevated serum alkaline phosphatase, and mildly elevated serum aminotransferase levels (100 to 200 units) are noted. Liver biopsy reveals cholestasis, bile plugs in dilated bile canaliculi, and a dense portal infiltrate of polymorphonuclear, eosinophilic, and mononuclear leukocytes. Occasionally, scattered foci of hepatic parenchymal necrosis may be evident. Jaundice and pruritus usually subside within 4 to 8 weeks following cessation of therapy, without sequelae, and fatalities are rare. Cholestyramine may be of value in relieving severe pruritus. In a small number of patients, jaundice is prolonged for several months to years; rarely, a disorder resembling but distinct from primary biliary cirrhosis may develop.

AMIODARONE HEPATOTOXICITY (TOXIC AND IDIOSYNCRATIC REACTION) Therapy with this potent antiarrhythmic drug is accompanied in 15 to 50 percent of patients by modest elevation of serum aminotransferase levels that may remain stable or diminish despite continuation of the drug. Such abnormalities may appear days to many months after beginning therapy. A proportion of those with elevated aminotransferase levels have detectable hepatomegaly, and clinically important liver disease develops in fewer than 5 percent of patients. Features that represent a direct effect of the drug on the liver and that are common to the majority of long-term recipients are ultrastructural phospholipidosis, unaccompanied by clinical liver disease, and interference with hepatic mixed-function oxidase metabolism of other drugs. The relatively common elevations in aminotransferase levels are also considered a predictable, dose-dependent, direct hepatotoxic effect. On the other hand, in the rare patient with clinically apparent, symptomatic liver disease, liver injury resembling that seen in alcoholic liver disease is observed. The so-called pseudoalcoholic liver injury can range from steatosis, to alcoholic hepatitis–like neutrophilic infiltration and Mallory's hyaline, to cirrhosis. Electron-microscopic demonstration of phospholipid-laden lysosomal lamellar bodies can help to distinguish amiodarone hepatotoxicity from typical alcoholic hepatitis. This category of liver injury appears to be a metabolic idiosyncracy which allows hepatotoxic metabolites to be generated. Rarely, an acute idiosyncratic hepatocellular injury, resembling viral hepatitis or cholestatic hepatitis, occurs. Hepatic granulomas have occasionally been observed. Because amiodarone has a long half-life, liver injury may persist for months after the drug is stopped.

ERYTHROMYCIN HEPATOTOXICITY (CHOLESTATIC IDIOSYNCRATIC REACTION) The most important adverse effect associated with erythromycin is the infrequent occurrence of a cholestatic reaction. Although most of these reactions have been associated with erythromycin estolate, other erythromycins may also be responsible. The reaction usually begins during the first 2 or 3 weeks of therapy and includes nausea, vomiting, fever, right upper quadrant abdominal pain, jaundice, leukocytosis, and moderately elevated aminotransferase levels. The clinical picture can resemble acute cholecystitis or bacterial cholangitis. Liver biopsy reveals variable cholestasis, portal inflammation comprising lymphocytes, polymorphonuclear leukocytes, and eosinophils, and scattered foci of hepatocyte necrosis. Symptoms and laboratory findings usually subside within a few days of drug withdrawal, and evidence of chronic liver disease has not been found on follow-up. The precise mechanism remains ill-defined.

ORAL CONTRACEPTIVE HEPATOTOXICITY (CHOLESTATIC REACTION) The administration of oral contraceptive combinations of estrogenic and progestational steroids results in significant bromsulphthalein (BSP) retention in a high proportion of patients, and, to a far lesser extent, elevation of serum alkaline phosphatase. Weeks to months after taking these agents, intrahepatic cholestasis with pruritus and jaundice is noted in a small number of patients. Especially susceptible seem to be patients with recurrent idiopathic jaundice of pregnancy, severe pruritus of pregnancy, or a family history of these disorders. Laboratory studies, with the exception of liver biochemical tests, are normal, and extrahepatic manifestations of hypersensitivity are absent. Liver biopsy reveals cholestasis with bile plugs in dilated canaliculi and striking bilirubin staining of liver cells. In contrast to chlorpromazine-induced cholestasis, portal inflammation is absent. The lesion is reversible on withdrawal of the agent, and sequelae have not been reported. The two steroid components appear to act synergistically on hepatic function, although the estrogen may be primarily responsible. Oral contraceptives are contraindicated in patients with a history of recurrent jaundice of pregnancy. Primarily benign but, rarely, malignant neoplasms of the liver, hepatic vein occlusion, peliosis hepatis, and peripheral sinusoidal dilatation have also been associated with oral contraceptive therapy.

17,α-ALKYL-SUBSTITUTED ANABOLIC STEROIDS (CHOLESTATIC REACTION) In the majority of patients receiving these agents, used therapeutically mainly in the treatment of bone marrow failure but used surreptitiously and without medical indication by athletes to improve their performance, mild hepatic dysfunction develops. Impaired excretory function is the predominant defect, but the precise mechanism is uncertain. Jaundice, which appears to be dose-related, develops in only a minority of patients and may be the sole clinical manifestation of hepatotoxicity, although anorexia, nausea, and malaise are described in some patients. Pruritus is not a prominent feature. Serum aminotransferase levels are usually under 100 units, and serum alkaline phosphatase levels are normal, mildly elevated, or, in less than 5 percent of patients, three or more times the upper limit of normal. Examination of liver tissue reveals cholestasis without inflammation or necrosis. Hepatic sinusoidal dilatation and peliosis hepatis have been found in a few patients. The cholestatic disorder is usually reversible on cessation of treatment, although fatalities have been linked to peliosis. An association with hepatic adenoma and hepatocellular carcinoma has been reported.

TRIMETHOPRIM-SULFAMETHOXAZOLE HEPATOTOXICITY (IDIOSYNCRATIC REACTION) This antibiotic is used routinely for urinary tract infections in immunocompetent persons and for prophylaxis against and therapy of *Pneumocystis carinii* pneumonia in immunosuppressed persons (transplant recipients, patients with AIDS). With its increasing use, its occasional hepatotoxicity is being recognized with growing frequency. Its likelihood is unpredictable, but, when it occurs, trimethoprim-sulfamethoxazole hepatotoxicity follows a relatively uniform latency period of several weeks and is often accompanied by eosinophilia, rash, and other features of a hypersensitivity reaction. Biochemically and histologically, acute hepatocellular necrosis predominates, but cholestatic features are quite frequent. Occasionally, cholestasis without necrosis occurs, and, very rarely, a severe cholangiolytic pattern of liver injury is observed. In most cases, liver injury is self-limited, but rare fatalities have been recorded. The hepatotoxicity is attributable to the sulfamethoxazole component of the drug and is similar in features to that seen with other sulfonamides; tissue eosinophilia and granulomas may be seen.

REFERENCES

Viral hepatitis

ALTER HJ et al: Detection of antibody to hepatitis C virus in prospectively followed transfusion recipients with acute and chronic non-A, non-B hepatitis. N Engl J Med 321:1494, 1989

——— (ed): Viral hepatitis. Semin Liver Dis 6:1, 1986

BRADLEY DW et al: Enterically transmitted non-A, non-B hepatitis: Serial passage of disease in cynomolgus macaques and tamarins and recovery of disease-associated 27- to 34-nm viruslike particles. Proc Natl Acad Sci USA 84:6277, 1987

DAVIS GL, HOOFNAGLE, JH: Reactivation of chronic type B hepatitis presenting as acute viral hepatitis. Ann Intern Med 102:762, 1985

DIENSTAG JL, ISSELBACHER KJ: Therapy of acute and chronic hepatitis. Arch Intern Med 141:1419, 1981

———: Non-A, non-B hepatitis. I. Recognition, epidemiology, and clinical features. II. Experimental transmission, putative virus agents and markers, and prevention. Gastroenterology 85:439 and 743, 1983

GERETY RJ (ed): *Non-A, Non-B Hepatitis*. New York, Academic 1981

——— (ed): *Hepatitis A*. Orlando, Academic, 1984

——— (ed): *Hepatitis B*. Orlando, Academic, 1985

IMMUNIZATION PRACTICES ADVISORY COMMITTEE: Recommendations for protection against viral hepatitis. Ann Intern Med 103:391, 1985

———: Update on hepatitis B prevention. Ann Intern Med 107:353, 1987

JACOBSON IM, DIENSTAG JL: Viral hepatitis vaccines. Annu Rev Med 36:241, 1985

KUO G et al: An assay for circulating antibodies to a major etiologic virus of human non-A, non-B hepatitis. Science 244:362, 1989

LEMON SM: Type A viral hepatitis: New developments in an old disease. N Engl J Med 313:1059, 1985

RIZZETTO M: The delta agent. Hepatology 3:729, 1983

——— et al (eds): *The Hepatitis Delta Virus and Its Infection*. New York, Alan R Liss, 1987

——— et al: Hepatitis delta virus infection of the liver: Progress in virology, pathobiology, and diagnosis. Semin Liver Dis 8:350, 1988

SEEFF LB, HOOFNAGLE JH: Immunoprophylaxis of viral hepatitis. Gastroenterology 77:161, 1979

———, KOFF R: Passive and active immunoprophylaxis of hepatitis B. Gastroenterology 86:958, 1984

——— et al: A serologic follow-up of the 1942 epidemic of post-vaccination hepatitis in the United States Army. N Engl J Med 316:765, 1987

SEEGER C et al: Biochemical and genetic evidence for the hepatitis B virus replication strategy. Science 232:477, 1986

SZMUNESS W et al: Hepatitis B vaccine: Demonstration of efficacy in a controlled clinical trial in a high-risk population in the United States. N Engl J Med 303:833, 1980

——— et al (eds): Viral Hepatitis: 1981 International Symposium. Philadelphia, Franklin Institute Press, 1982

THEILMANN L et al: Detection of pre-SI proteins in serum and liver of HBsAg-positive patients: A new marker for hepatitis B virus infection, Hepatology 6:186, 1986

VERME G et al (eds): *Viral Hepatitis and Delta Infection*. New York, Alan R. Liss, 1983

VYAS GN et al (eds): *Viral Hepatitis and Liver Disease*. Orlando, Grune & Stratton, 1984

ZUCKERMAN AJ (ed): *Viral Hepatitis and Liver Disease*. New York, Alan R Liss, 1988

Drug-induced hepatitis

BLACK M et al: Isoniazid-associated hepatitis in 114 patients. Gastroenterology 69:389, 1975

ISHAK KG, IREY NS: Hepatic injury associated with the phenothiazines: Clinicopathologic and follow-up study of 36 patients. Arch Pathol 93:283, 1972

LUDWIG J, AXELSEN R: Drug effects on the liver: An updated tabular compilation of drugs and drug-related hepatic diseases. Dig Dis Sci 28:651, 1983

MITCHELL JR, JOLLOW DJ: Metabolic activation of drugs to toxic substances. Gastroenterology 68:392, 1975

RIGAS B et al: Amiodarone hepatotoxicity. Ann Intern Med 104:348, 1986

SHERLOCK S: Hepatic reactions to drugs. Gut 20:634, 1979

SMILKSTEIN MJ et al: Efficacy of *N*-acetylcysteine in the treatment of acetaminophen overdose. N Engl J Med 319:1557, 1988

ZAFRANI ES et al: Cholestatic and hepatocellular injury associated with erythromycin esters: Report of nine cases. Am J Dig Dis 24:38, 1979

ZIMMERMAN HJ: *Hepatotoxicity*. New York, Appleton-Century-Crofts, 1978

——— (ed): Drug-induced liver disease. Semin Liver Dis 1:91, 1981

———, ISHAK KG: Valproate-induced hepatic injury: Analysis of 23 fatal cases. Hepatology 2:591, 1982

253 CHRONIC HEPATITIS

JACK R. WANDS / KURT J. ISSELBACHER

Chronic hepatitis refers to three related disorders—chronic persistent hepatitis, chronic lobular hepatitis, and chronic active hepatitis. These are characterized by a combination of hepatocyte necrosis and inflammation of varying severity persisting for more than 6 months. The clinically most important disorder, chronic active hepatitis, may lead to hepatic failure and death or result in the development of cirrhosis and its sequelae. While all three forms of chronic hepatitis share some common histopathologic features and appear to be incited by similar etiologic factors, their pathogeneses, clinical presentations, natural histories, prognoses, and therapies are different.

CHRONIC PERSISTENT AND CHRONIC LOBULAR HEPATITIS

Definition and etiology Chronic persistent and chronic lobular hepatitis result from infections with hepatitis B virus (HBV) and non-A, non B hepatitis viruses. Other etiologies may exist but are poorly defined. In general, these are both nonprogressive disorders; hepatic failure is not seen and evolution into cirrhosis is exceedingly rare. Occasionally, however, patients with chronic active hepatitis may be seen during spontaneous remission, at which time the histopathologic findings may suggest chronic persistent or chronic lobular hepatitis. Under these circumstances relapses and progression to the more serious underlying chronic active hepatitis may occur. Another exception to the nonprogression of chronic persistent and lobular hepatitis occurs in patients positive to hepatitis B surface antigen (HBsAg), in whom superinfection with delta agent (HDV) may lead to the development of chronic active hepatitis (see Chap. 252). Indeed, the clinical presentation of rapidly progressive liver injury in a known chronic HBsAg carrier should suggest infection with HDV.

Pathology In typical chronic persistent hepatitis there is infiltration of the portal areas with mononuclear cells, but there is no erosion of the limiting plate (so-called piecemeal necrosis) or extension of the inflammation into the liver lobule. A "cobblestone" arrangement of liver cells, indicative of hepatic regenerative activity, is a common feature. Minimal fibrosis may be observed, but *cirrhosis is characteristically absent*. In chronic lobular hepatitis, in addition to the portal inflammatory changes, lobular inflammation and focal hepatocellular necrosis are prominent features during clinically active phases. The morphologic features of chronic persistent, lobular, and active hepatitis are compared in Table 253-1.

Clinical and laboratory features Most patients with chronic persistent and/or lobular hepatitis are asymptomatic, although some may complain of anorexia, fatigue, and occasionally of nausea and

TABLE 253-1 Some distinguishing features of chronic persistent, chronic lobular, and chronic active hepatitis

Features	Chronic persistent hepatitis	Chronic lobular hepatitis	Chronic active hepatitis
CLINICAL			
Onset like acute hepatitis	≈70%	≈90%	≈30%
Recurrent acute episodes	Infrequent	Common	Common
Extrahepatic involvement	Rare	Rare	Common
Prognosis	Good	Good	Variable
LIVER HISTOLOGY			
Piecemeal necrosis	Inconstant	Inconstant	Typical
Site of inflammation	Portal	Portal/lobular in active phase	Portal, extending into lobule
Lobular architecture	Preserved	Preserved	Distorted
Fibrosis	Slight	Slight	Common
Progression to cirrhosis	Rare	Rare	Common

vomiting. Physical findings are usually normal, but the liver may be slightly enlarged and tender. Laboratory data show mild elevations of aminotransferase and alkaline phosphatase levels and these abnormalities may persist for months to years. During active phases of chronic lobular hepatitis, aminotransferase levels may resemble those seen in acute viral hepatitis.

Management Once the diagnosis of chronic persistent or lobular hepatitis has been established by liver biopsy, no specific therapy is required since such patients generally do not develop fibrosis and cirrhosis. Follow-up examination is recommended every 6 to 12 months until aminotransferase values have returned to normal and to identify the rare patient who may progress to chronic active hepatitis.

CHRONIC ACTIVE HEPATITIS Definition Chronic active hepatitis is a disorder of diverse etiologies characterized by continuing hepatic necrosis, active inflammation, and fibrosis which may lead to or be accompanied by liver failure, cirrhosis, and death. The prominence of extrahepatic features and seroimmunologic abnormalities has led to the use of a variety of terms to describe this disorder. These terms include autoimmune hepatitis, lupoid hepatitis, subacute hepatitis, and chronic active liver disease. *Chronic active hepatitis* seems to be the most appropriate designation for this clinicopathologic entity, regardless of the etiology and the clinical variations.

Pathology Although chronic active hepatitis may be suspected from the clinical history and the physical findings, *liver biopsy is necessary to establish the diagnosis*. The cardinal histopathologic features observed in the liver include (1) a dense mononuclear and plasma cell infiltration of the portal zones which greatly expands into the liver lobule; (2) destruction of the hepatocytes at the periphery of the lobule (piecemeal necrosis) with erosion of the limiting plate surrounding the portal triads; (3) connective tissue septa extending from the portal zones into the lobule, isolating parenchymal cells into clusters and enveloping bile ducts; and (4) evidence of hepatic regeneration with "rosette" formation, thickened liver cell plates, and regenerative "pseudolobules." This process may be patchy, and individual liver lobules may remain uninvolved. Councilman-like bodies, which represent necrosis of single liver cells, may be seen in the periportal areas. The lesion of bridging hepatic necrosis may be seen in some patients with chronic active hepatitis. This lesion or its more extensive variant, multilobular bridging hepatic necrosis, suggests the presence of severe disease.

There is substantial morphologic evidence that in some instances chronic active hepatitis will progress to or is accompanied by the development of cirrhosis. On liver biopsy, cirrhosis can be demonstrated in 20 to 50 percent of patients, even early in the course of the disease, and at autopsy postnecrotic cirrhosis may be found. It is also possible that many cases of so-called cryptogenic cirrhosis are the result of chronic active hepatitis after inflammation and necrosis have subsided. In other patients fibrosis is not progressive and morphologic evidence of cirrhosis cannot be found.

Etiology Multiple etiologic agents may initiate chronic active hepatitis. Probably the most important and common triggering factors are infection with hepatitis B virus or the non-A, non-B hepatitis viruses. In about one-third of patients the disease begins abruptly following an illness typical of acute viral hepatitis. Persistence of HBsAg in the serum is found in 20 to 30 percent of patients with chronic active hepatitis, suggesting that persistent hepatitis B virus infection may be related to the development of this disease. Many of these HBsAg-positive patients also have positive tests for the hepatitis B e antigen (HBeAg) and have high levels of HBV-DNA in serum, indicating active viral replication (see Chap. 252). Superinfection with delta hepatitis agent in HBsAg-positive individuals may lead to the development of chronic active hepatitis and in general leads to a more serious clinical course than HBV infection alone. Similarly, persistent non-A, non-B hepatitis virus infections may be responsible for cases of chronic active hepatitis following transfusion-associated and sporadic non-A, non-B hepatitis. Drugs are involved in the pathogenesis of some cases. For example, features typical of chronic active hepatitis have been found in some patients in association with the administration of methyldopa. In these patients challenge with methyldopa has led to increased activity of the disease, while discontinuance has resulted in clinical, biochemical, and histologic improvement. Oxyphenisatin, isoniazid, nitrofurantoin, and other drugs have also been incriminated as etiologic agents in patients with chronic active hepatitis. Thus, chemical as well as viral agents may play a role in the production of chronic active hepatitis. The existence of other triggering factors seems likely, but their nature and mechanisms of action remain to be determined.

Immunopathogenesis There is increasing evidence that the progressive parenchymal cell destruction in patients with chronic active hepatitis involves an interaction with the immune system conditioned or controlled by genetic factors. Evidence to support this concept includes the following facts: (1) In the liver the histopathologic lesions are composed predominantly of thymus-derived or T lymphocytes and plasma cells in association with progressive liver cell destruction and replacement by fibrous tissue. (2) A variety of circulating "autoantibodies" are frequently detected, such as anti-smooth-muscle, antimitochondrial, and antithyroid antibodies. (3) The persistence of HBsAg in the serum and the hepatitis B core antigen (HBcAg) in the liver cell following an attack of acute hepatitis B is frequently associated with the development of chronic active or chronic persistent hepatitis. (4) Other "autoimmune" diseases such as thyroiditis, diabetes mellitus, ulcerative colitis, Coombs-positive hemolytic anemia, proliferative glomerulonephritis, and Sjögren's syndrome may be associated with chronic active hepatitis or may occur in relatives of affected patients. (5) Histocompatibility antigens HLA-B1 or -B8 and -DRw3 and -DRw4 are more prevalent than expected in patients with chronic active hepatitis without HBsAg. (6) Finally, the use of glucocorticoids, believed to be effective in a variety of immunologic and autoimmune disorders, is often beneficial in the treatment of severe chronic active hepatitis.

There is increasing evidence that cellular immune reactions may be important in the pathogenesis of chronic active hepatitis. It has been suggested that lymphocytes become sensitized to altered or new antigens present on the surface membranes of hepatocytes. This hypothesis is supported in part by studies demonstrating that circulating and liver-derived lymphocytes may have the capability of causing liver cell damage in vitro.

Humoral immune mechanisms may be responsible for some of the clinical manifestations of chronic active hepatitis. In particular, extrahepatic features such as arthralgias, arthritis, rash, and glomerulonephritis appear to be mediated by the deposition of circulating immune complexes. Furthermore, complement activation, as demonstrated by low serum complement levels, and the presence of complement components in immune complexes suggest that circulating immune complexes may be involved in mediating extrahepatic inflammation and tissue damage.

Clinical features The clinical spectrum of chronic active hepatitis ranges from asymptomatic illness at one end to fatal hepatic failure at the other. All age groups are affected. In approximately two-thirds of patients the disease has an *insidious onset* over a period of several weeks to months, or the disease is discovered incidentally, and the duration of the illness is uncertain. In the remainder an abrupt onset similar to that in acute viral hepatitis is seen, but features of chronic active hepatitis usually develop during the ensuing 12 to 24 months. The clinical and laboratory features suggesting progression from acute hepatitis to chronic active hepatitis are discussed in Chap. 252. *Fatigue* is a common symptom. Persistent or recurrent *jaundice* is a common feature in severe disease. Intermittent deepening of jaundice and recurrent symptoms of *malaise, anorexia,* and *low-grade fever,* suggestive of a superimposed acute hepatitis, are common throughout the course of the illness. In some patients complications of cirrhosis, such as ascites, variceal bleeding, encephalopathy, coagulopathy, or hypersplenism, may first bring the patient to medical attention. In others the extrahepatic features dominate the clinical picture, and liver disease is entirely unsuspected. Extrahepatic presenting features may include amenorrhea, bloody diarrhea (due to associated ulcerative colitis), abdominal pain, arthralgia or arthritis, macular or papular eruptions, acne, erythema nodosum, pleurisy, pericarditis, anemia, azotemia, and sicca syndrome (of keratoconjunctivitis and xerostomia). These extrahepatic features and abnormal serologic reactions tend to be more frequent in women than men and in patients without serologic evidence of preceding hepatitis B.

The *course* of chronic active hepatitis is variable, and the disease may persist for long periods without clinically overt liver disease. This appears to be particularly true of chronic active hepatitis associated with hepatitis B virus or non-A, non-B hepatitis viruses. The condition may on occasion spontaneously remit into a clinically inactive phase, although continuing hepatocellular necrosis or progression to cirrhosis is usually the rule. The histologic lesion may reverse itself completely before the development of cirrhosis in some HBsAg-positive patients after their antigenemia has spontaneously cleared or following the loss of viral replication as measured by disappearance of HBV-DNA from serum and seroconversion of HBeAg from positive to negative and the development of anti-HBe. If untreated, the case fatality rate may be high during the first few years of illness, especially in patients with clinically and histologically severe disease. Death usually occurs as a result of liver failure and hepatic coma. Later death is often due to a complication of cirrhosis—variceal hemorrhage or intercurrent infection. Primary hepatocellular carcinoma is an uncommon complication of HBsAg-negative chronic active hepatitis even when the disease has progressed to postnecrotic cirrhosis. This finding is in contrast to long-term HBsAg carriers with chronic active hepatitis and/or cirrhosis in whom the incidence of liver carcinoma is high (see Chap. 252).

Laboratory findings Liver function tests are invariably abnormal but may not correlate with the clinical severity or histopathologic findings in the individual case. Many patients have normal serum bilirubin, alkaline phosphatase, and globulin levels with only minimal aminotransferase elevations or HBsAg positivity and yet have a liver biopsy consistent with severe chronic active hepatitis. Serum aspartate aminotransferase (SGOT) and alanine aminotransferase (SGPT) levels are increased and fluctuate in the range of 100 to 1000 units in most cases. In severe cases the serum bilirubin is moderately elevated [51.3 to 171 μmol/L (3 to 10 mg/dL)]. Mild hypoalbuminemia occurs in patients with active disease or in those with advanced cirrhosis. Serum alkaline phosphatase levels may be moderately elevated or near normal. The prothrombin time is often prolonged, particularly late in the disease or during active phases.

Hypergammaglobulinemia (greater than 2.5 g/dL) is common, particularly in patients with extensive plasma cell infiltration of the liver. A variety of abnormal serologic reactions and circulating autoantibodies are found in chronic active hepatitis. Some of these serologic reactions are nonspecific and may be seen in other viral diseases. Circulating autoantibodies against DNA, IgG, smooth muscle, and mitochrondria support the concept that chronic active hepatitis is indeed a systemic disease. HBsAg may be found in 20 to 30 percent of patients with chronic active hepatitis, more commonly in men than women.

Differential diagnosis Early in the course of chronic active hepatitis the disease may resemble typical *acute viral hepatitis.* However, the persistence of symptoms, including biochemical abnormalities such as elevated serum aminotransferase and bilirubin levels or circulating HBsAg over the ensuing months indicates that a chronic liver disorder is present. The major entities which must be distinguished from chronic active hepatitis are *chronic persistent and lobular hepatitis.* As indicated in Table 253-1, in chronic persistent and lobular hepatitis the onset of the illness frequently resembles acute hepatitis. The aminotransferase enzyme values are variably elevated, and HBsAg may be present in serum. Fatigue, anorexia, malaise, right upper quadrant discomfort, and hepatomegaly may be associated with all three forms of chronic hepatitis. Thus, a definitive diagnosis can only be established by liver biopsy since a *differentiation between chronic active, chronic persistent, and lobular hepatitis cannot be made by clinical and biochemical criteria.* This distinction is important because chronic persistent and lobular hepatitis are not progressive disorders, rarely if ever result in cirrhosis, and require no therapy.

The presence of extrahepatic manifestations in chronic active hepatitis such as pleuritis, arthritis, and arthralgias may cause confusion with *connective tissue disorders* such as rheumatoid arthritis and systemic lupus erythematosus. The existence of clinical and biochemical features suggestive of progressive liver disease clearly distinguishes chronic active hepatitis from these disorders. In adolescence, *Wilson's disease* may present with features of chronic active hepatitis before the neurologic manifestations become apparent; serum ceruloplasmin, serum and urinary copper determination, and measurement of the liver copper levels will establish the diagnosis. Late in the course of chronic active hepatitis some patients may present with *postnecrotic cirrhosis* without evidence of active hepatitis. This lesion, termed cryptogenic cirrhosis, may also represent an end stage of other destructive liver diseases (e.g., primary biliary cirrhosis) *Primary biliary cirrhosis* may share histologic similarities with chronic active hepatitis, particularly early in the disease. However, in primary biliary cirrhosis the prominence of pruritus plus markedly elevated serum alkaline phosphatase and cholesterol levels, the presence of high titers of antimitochondrial antibodies (in contrast to the low levels seen in chronic active hepatitis), and the pattern of histologic progression will usually permit differentiation from chronic active hepatitis.

Management In chronic active hepatitis *not* associated with hepatitis B virus or non-A, non-B viruses glucocorticoid therapy is the treatment of choice. Glucocorticoids have been shown to be effective in prolonging survival of these patients during the first few years of illness when the mortality rate is high. A therapeutic response characterized by a complete clinical, biochemical, and histologic remission is to be expected in 60 to 80 percent of patients. Either prednisone or prednisolone therapy should be initiated at a dose of 20 to 40 mg daily. This dose can usually be gradually tapered within 2 to 3 months to 10 to 20 mg daily. The beneficial effects of glucocorticoid treatment on the course and prognosis of patients with mild or asymptomatic chronic active hepatitis has not been established.

Improvement of fatigue and anorexia is usually noted within days to several weeks. Biochemical improvement is to be expected over several weeks to months, with a fall in serum bilirubin and globulin levels and a rise in serum albumin. The serum aminotransferase level usually drops promptly, but the absolute value of the aminotransferase *alone* does not appear to be a useful marker of recovery in the individual patient. Histologic improvement, characterized by a decrease in mononuclear infiltration and subsequent improvement in the extent of hepatocellular necrosis, may be delayed for 6 to 24 months. After a favorable clinical and biochemical response, repeat liver biopsy may show features consistent with chronic persistent hepatitis. Despite this histologic improvement, relapses are common when glucocorticoids are discontinued.

Reduction of the suppressive glucocorticoid doses should be performed cautiously, particularly at lower prednisone levels, since even small decrements in therapy may be associated with clinical worsening, and increasing dosage may be needed for control of spontaneous exacerbation. Unless major complications require discontinuation of glucocorticoids, they should be prescribed for at least 12 months or longer in order to reduce the risk of relapse.

Other therapeutic approaches have been used in the treatment of severe chronic active hepatitis, particularly in the elderly and in patients with major side effects from glucocorticoids. An initial prednisone dosage of 30 mg, tapered down to 10 to 20 mg, in combination with 50 to 75 mg azathioprine has been demonstrated to be effective; this treatment avoids the adverse effects of high dosage of glucocorticoids. However, *azathioprine alone is not effective* in the treatment of chronic active hepatitis. Alternate-day prednisone therapy diminishes steroid side effects but usually does not provide adequate therapy.

Glucocorticoids have little if any beneficial effect on the natural course of HBsAg-positive chronic active hepatitis. Treatment of *asymptomatic* HBsAg carriers who only have evidence of chronic active hepatitis on liver biopsy is not justified. In *symptomatic* HBsAg-positive patients with severe chronic active hepatitis, glucocorticoids have not been shown to be of value either in short- or long-term therapy. Similarly, in chronic active hepatitis caused by non-A, non-B viruses long-term glucocorticoid therapy is not beneficial and may be detrimental. Other therapeutic modalities have been used in the treatment of chronic active hepatitis associated with hepatitis B virus or non-A, non-B viruses including azathioprine, D-penicillamine, cyclophosphamide, interleukin 2, acyclovir, adenine arabinoside, and adenine arabinoside monophosphate. These agents have not yet been shown to be effective in the majority of patients. Randomized controlled studies on a limited number of patients with chronic active hepatitis caused by hepatitis B virus or non-A, non-B viruses using alpha interferon showed some promise in reducing or eliminating viral replication. In those patients who responded, improvement in serum alanine aminotransferase values and liver histopathology has been observed. These and other therapeutic strategies (e.g., combination of different interferons, glucocorticoid therapy and withdrawal followed by interferon, and others) are currently undergoing controlled clinical trials. While none of these therapeutic strategies can be recommended for general use at present, patients with chronic active viral hepatitis may benefit from referral to medical centers participating in therapeutic trials.

REFERENCES

CASELMANN WH et al: β and γ interferon in chronic active hepatitis: A pilot trial of short term combination therapy. Gastroenterology 96:449, 1989

CZAJA AJ et al: Laboratory assessment of severe chronic active liver disease during and after corticosteroid therapy. Correlation of serum transaminase and gamma globulin levels with histologic features. Gastroenterology 80:667, 1981

HODGES JR et al: Chronic active hepatitis: The spectrum of disease. Lancet 1:550, 1982

HOOFNAGEL JH et al: Randomized, control trial of recombinant alpha interferon in patients with chronic active hepatitis B. Gastroenterology 95:1318, 1988

JACYNA MR et al: Randomized controlled trial of interferon alpha (lymphoblastoid interferon) in chronic non-A, non-B hepatitis. Br Med J 298:80, 1989

LAM KC et al: Deleterious effect of prednisolone in HBsAg-positive chronic active hepatitis. N Engl J Med 304:380, 1981

MACKAY IR, TAIT BD: HLA associations with autoimmune-type chronic active hepatitis: Identification of B8-DRw3 haplotypes by family studies. Gastroenterology 79:95, 1980

SEEF LB, KOFF RS: Therapy for chronic active hepatitis. Adv Intern Med 29:109, 1984

WEISSBERG JI et al: Survival in chronic hepatitis B. An analysis of 379 patients. Ann Intern Med 101:613, 1984

WELLER IVD et al: Effects of prednisone/azathioprine in chronic hepatitis B viral infection. Gut 23:650, 1982

254 CIRRHOSIS OF THE LIVER

DANIEL K. PODOLSKY / KURT J. ISSELBACHER

Cirrhosis is a pathologically defined entity which is associated with a spectrum of characteristic clinical manifestations. The cardinal pathologic features reflect irreversible chronic injury of the hepatic parenchyma and include extensive fibrosis in association with the formation of regenerative nodules. These features result from hepatocyte necrosis, collapse of the supporting reticulin network with subsequent connective tissue deposition, distortion of the vascular bed, and nodular regeneration of remaining liver parenchyma. The pathologic process should be viewed as a final common pathway of many types of chronic liver injury. Clinical features of cirrhosis derive from the morphologic alterations and often reflect the severity of hepatic damage rather than the etiology of the underlying liver disease. Loss of functioning hepatocellular mass may lead to jaundice, edema, coagulopathy, and a variety of metabolic abnormalities; fibrosis and distorted vasculature lead to portal hypertension and its sequelae, including gastroesophageal varices and splenomegaly. Ascites and hepatic encephalopathy result from both hepatocellular insufficiency and portal hypertension.

Classification of the various types of cirrhosis based solely on etiology or morphology is unsatisfactory. A single pathologic pattern may result from a variety of insults, while the same insult may produce several morphologic patterns. Nevertheless most types of cirrhosis may be usefully classified by a mixture of etiologically and morphologically defined entities as follows: (1) alcoholic; (2) cryptogenic and postviral or postnecrotic; (3) biliary; (4) cardiac; (5) metabolic, inherited, and drug-related; and (6) miscellaneous. This chapter considers first the various types of cirrhosis and then the major clinical complications of chronic liver disease and cirrhosis.

ALCOHOLIC LIVER DISEASE AND CIRRHOSIS

Definition Alcoholic cirrhosis, historically referred to as Laennec's cirrhosis, is the most common type of cirrhosis encountered in North America and many parts of western Europe and South America. It is usually characterized by diffuse fine scarring, fairly uniform loss of liver cells, and small regenerative nodules, and therefore, it is sometimes referred to as micronodular cirrhosis. However, micronodular cirrhosis may also result from other types of liver injury (e.g., following jejunoileal bypass), and thus alcoholic cirrhosis and micronodular cirrhosis are not necessarily synonymous. Conversely alcoholic cirrhosis may progress to macronodular cirrhosis with time.

Alcoholic cirrhosis is only one of many consequences resulting from chronic alcoholic ingestion, and it often accompanies other forms of alcohol-induced liver injury. The three principal alcohol-induced hepatic lesions are designated: (1) alcoholic fatty liver, (2) alcoholic hepatitis, and (3) alcoholic cirrhosis. These morphologic categories are rarely found in a pure form, and features of each may be present to varying degrees in an individual patient.

Etiology Although chronic alcoholism is the most common cause of cirrhosis, the quantity and duration of drinking necessary to cause cirrhosis remain unclear. The typical alcoholic patient with cirrhosis has had a daily consumption of a pint or more of whiskey, several quarts of wine, or an equivalent amount of beer for at least 10 years. The amount and duration of ethanol ingestion, rather than the type of alcoholic beverage or the pattern of ingestion, appear to be the important determinants of liver injury. In general, the latent period preceding the development of cirrhosis is inversely related to the level of daily alcohol intake. Rates of ethanol metabolism are under genetic control, but no metabolic defect has been identified in cirrhotic patients or their families to suggest a unique "susceptibility" to ethanol or its toxic effects. Although malnutrition per se does not appear to lead to cirrhosis, it is possible that nutritional factors may augment the detrimental effects of chronic alcohol ingestion on the liver. The finding that only 10 to 15 percent of alcoholics develop cirrhosis suggests that other factors may affect the impact of alcohol on the liver. Women, on average, appear to develop alcohol-induced liver injury at lesser levels of consumption than men, suggesting that hormonal factors may play a role in susceptibility.

Alcoholic fatty liver occurs in most heavy drinkers but is reversible on cessation of alcohol consumption and is not thought to be an inevitable precursor of alcoholic hepatitis or cirrhosis. In contrast, alcoholic hepatitis, an inflammatory lesion characterized by infiltration of the liver with leukocytes, liver cell necrosis, and alcoholic hyaline, is thought to be the major precursor of cirrhosis. Subsequent healing accompanied by fibrosis distorts the normal lobular architecture. Indeed, *deposition of collagen in perivenular spaces* may be the earliest manifestation of the process which ultimately leads to cirrhosis.

Pathology and pathogenesis ALCOHOLIC FATTY LIVER The liver is enlarged, yellow, greasy, and firm. Hepatocytes are distended by large cytoplasmic fat vacuoles which push the hepatocyte nucleus against the cell membrane. Accumulation of fat in the liver of the alcoholic results from the combination of impaired fatty acid oxidation, increased uptake and esterification of fatty acids to form triglycerides, and diminished lipoprotein biosynthesis and secretion.

ALCOHOLIC HEPATITIS Morphologic features include hepatocyte degeneration and necrosis, often with ballooned cells, and an infiltrate of polymorphonuclear leukocytes and lymphocytes. The polymorphonuclear cells may encircle damaged hepatocytes which contain *Mallory bodies,* or *alcoholic hyaline*. These are clumps of perinuclear, deeply eosinophilic material believed to represent aggregated intermediate filaments. Mallory bodies are highly suggestive of, but *not specific* for, alcoholic hepatitis, since morphologically similar material has been seen in association with morbid obesity, jejunoileal bypass surgery, poorly controlled diabetes mellitus, and a variety of other disorders including Wilson's disease and Indian childhood cirrhosis. Deposition of collagen around the central vein and in perisinusoidal areas, often termed central hyaline sclerosis, may be associated with an increased likelihood of progression to cirrhosis.

ALCOHOLIC CIRRHOSIS With continued alcohol intake and destruction of hepatocytes, fibroblasts (including myofibroblasts with contractile properties) appear at the site of injury and stimulate collagen formation. Weblike septa of connective tissue appear in periportal and pericentral zones and eventually connect portal triads and central veins. This fine connective tissue network surrounds small masses of remaining liver cells which regenerate and form nodules. Although regeneration occurs within the small remnants of parenchyma, cell loss generally exceeds replacement. With continuing hepatocyte destruction and collagen deposition, the liver shrinks in size, acquires a nodular appearance, and becomes hard as "end-stage" cirrhosis develops. Although alcoholic cirrhosis is usually a progressive disease, appropriate therapy and strict avoidance of alcohol may arrest the disease at most stages and permit functional improvement.

Clinical features SIGNS AND SYMPTOMS Clinical manifestations of *alcoholic fatty liver* are often minimal or entirely absent, and the disorder may not be recognized unless another illness (frequently alcohol-related) brings the patient to medical attention. Hepatomegaly, at times accompanied by tenderness, may be the only finding. Jaundice, ascites, and edema are only seen with more serious liver injury.

The clinical severity of *alcoholic hepatitis* varies enormously, ranging from asymptomatic or mild illness to fatal hepatic insufficiency. Typically, the clinical features of alcoholic hepatitis resemble those of viral or toxic liver injury. Patients often experience anorexia, nausea and vomiting, malaise, weight loss, abdominal distress, and jaundice. Fever as high as 39.4°C (103°F) may be seen in about half of cases. On physical examination, tender hepatomegaly is common, and splenomegaly is found in about one-third of patients. The patient may have cutaneous arterial "spider" angiomas and jaundice. More severe cases may be complicated by ascites, edema, bleeding, and encephalopathy. At the time of initial presentation, the central nervous system findings may be difficult to distinguish from manifestations of concurrent alcohol intoxication or withdrawal (see below).

Although jaundice, ascites, and encephalopathy may subside with abstinence, continued alcohol excess and poor dietary habits usually lead to repeated acute episodes of hepatic decompensation. Some patients die during these acute exacerbations, but most recover after several weeks or months. Even after complete abstinence, clinical recovery may be protracted, and histologic abnormalities can persist up to 6 months or longer. Cholestatic jaundice mimicking biliary tract obstruction may also develop in some cases of acute alcoholic hepatitis.

Alcoholic cirrhosis may also be clinically silent; in fact 10 percent of cases are discovered incidentally at laparotomy or autopsy. In many cases symptoms are insidious in onset, occurring usually after 10 or more years of excessive alcohol use and progressing slowly over subsequent weeks and months. Anorexia and malnutrition lead to weight loss and a reduction in skeletal muscle mass. The patient may experience easy bruising, increasing weakness, and fatigue. Eventually the clinical manifestations of hepatocellular dysfunction and portal hypertension ensue, including progressive jaundice, bleeding from gastroesophageal varices, ascites, and encephalopathy. The abrupt onset of one of these complications may be the first event prompting the patient to seek medical attention. In other cases, cirrhosis first becomes evident when the patient requires treatment of symptoms related to alcoholic hepatitis.

A firm, nodular liver may be an early sign of disease; the liver may be either enlarged, normal, or decreased in size. Other frequent findings include jaundice, palmar erythema, spider angiomas, parotid and lacrimal gland enlargement, clubbing of fingers, splenomegaly, muscle wasting, and ascites with or without peripheral edema. Men may have decreased body hair and/or gynecomastia and testicular atrophy, which, like the cutaneous findings, result from disturbances in hormonal metabolism, including increased peripheral formation of estrogren due to diminished hepatic clearance of the precursor androstenedione. Testicular atrophy may reflect hormonal abnormalities or the toxic effect of alcohol on the testes. In women, signs of virilization or menstrual irregularities may occasionally be encountered. Dupuytren's contractures resulting from fibrosis of the palmar fascia with resulting flexion contracture of the digits are associated with alcoholism but are not specifically related to cirrhosis.

Over a period of 3 to 5 years, the cirrhotic patient typically becomes emaciated, weak, and chronically jaundiced. Ascites and other signs of portal hypertension become increasingly prominent. Most patients with advanced cirrhosis die in hepatic coma, commonly precipitated by hemorrhage from esophageal varices or intercurrent infection. Progressive renal dysfunction often complicates the terminal phase of the illness.

LABORATORY FINDINGS Routine hematologic and biochemical blood tests are usually normal in patients with alcoholic fatty liver, except for minimal elevations of the serum AST (aspartate aminotransferase, SGOT); occasionally alkaline phosphatase and bilirubin levels are also elevated. In more advanced alcoholic liver disease, abnormalities of laboratory tests are more common. Anemia may result from acute and chronic gastrointestinal blood loss, coexistent nutritional deficiency (notably of folic acid and vitamin B_{12}), hypersplenism, and a direct suppressive effect of alcohol on the bone marrow. Hemolytic anemia presumably due to effects of hypercholesterolemia on erythrocyte membranes resulting in unusual spurlike projections (acanthocytosis) has been described in some alcoholics with cirrhosis. Leukocytosis is often present in severe alcoholic hepatitis; however, some patients with this disorder may have leukopenia and thrombocytopenia due to hypersplenism or an inhibitory effect of alcohol on the bone marrow. Mild or pronounced hyperbilirubinemia may be found, usually in association with varying elevations of serum alkaline phosphatase levels. Frequently elevated are levels of serum AST, but levels greater than 5 μkat (300 units) are unusual and should prompt one to look for other coincident or complicating factors. In contrast to viral hepatitis, the serum AST is usually disproportionately elevated relative to alanine aminotransferase (AST/ALT ratio > 2).* This discrepancy may result from the proportionally greater inhibition of ALT synthesis by ethanol, which may be partially reversed by pyridoxal phosphate.

The serum prothrombin time is frequently prolonged, reflecting reduced synthesis of clotting proteins, most notably the vitamin K–dependent factors (see "Coagulopathy" below). The serum albumin level is usually depressed, while serum globulins are increased. Hypoalbuminemia reflects in part overall impairment in hepatic protein synthesis, while hyperglobulinemia is thought to result from nonspecific stimulation of the reticuloendothelial system. Elevated blood ammonia levels in patients with hepatic encephalopathy reflect diminished hepatic clearance because of impaired liver function and shunting of portal venous blood around the cirrhotic liver into the systemic circulation (see below and Chap. 250).

A variety of metabolic disturbances may be detected. Glucose intolerance due to endogenous insulin resistance may be present; however, clinical diabetes is uncommon. Central hyperventilation may lead to respiratory alkalosis in patients with cirrhosis. *Dietary deficiency* and *increased urinary losses* lead to hypomagnesemia and *hypophosphatemia*. In patients with ascites and dilutional hyponatremia, hypokalemia may occur from increased urinary potassium losses due in part to hyperaldosteronism. Prerenal azotemia is also observed in such patients.

Diagnosis *Alcoholic fatty liver* should be suspected in alcoholic patients with hepatomegaly and normal or minimally deranged liver function tests. Alcoholic fatty liver may be seen in combination with alcoholic hepatitis or established cirrhosis. *Alcoholic hepatitis* should be considered in an alcoholic who has been drinking heavily and demonstrates jaundice, fever, an enlarged, tender liver, or ascites. The clinical impression is often supported by the deranged results of tests of liver function and other laboratory abnormalities described above. Alcoholic hepatitis or fatty liver may be present in association with alcoholic cirrhosis.

Alcoholic cirrhosis should be strongly suspected in patients with a history of prolonged or excessive alcohol intake and physical signs of chronic liver disease. The clinical features and laboratory findings are usually sufficient to provide reasonable indication of the presence and extent of hepatic injury. Although a percutaneous needle biopsy of the liver is not usually necessary to confirm the typical findings of alcoholic hepatitis or cirrhosis, it may be helpful in distinguishing patients with less advanced liver disease from those with cirrhosis and in excluding other forms of liver injury such as viral hepatitis. Biopsy may also be helpful as a diagnostic tool in evaluating patients with clinical findings suggestive of alcoholic liver disease who deny alcohol intake. In patients with features of cholestasis, ultrasonography may be appropriate to exclude the presence of extrahepatic biliary obstruction. When the clinical status of an otherwise stable cirrhotic patient deteriorates without an obvious explanation, complicating conditions, such as infection, portal vein thrombosis, and hepatocellular carcinoma, should be sought.

Prognosis The patient with an alcoholic fatty liver and no complications has a good prognosis; rapid and complete resolution usually follows cessation of alcohol intake. In patients with alcoholic hepatitis, the presence of marked hyperbilirubinemia, rising serum creatinine, marked prolongation of the prothrombin time (> 1.5 times control), ascites, and encephalopathy are associated with a poor short-term prognosis; the in-hospital mortality in these patients may exceed 50 percent. In milder cases, clinical recovery may be complete, but repeated bouts of alcoholic hepatitis usually lead to irreversible and progressive chronic liver injury. Abstinence from alcohol as well as early and appropriate medical care can decrease long-term morbidity and mortality, and delay or prevent the appearance of further complications. Patients who have had a major complication of cirrhosis and who continue to drink, have a 5-year survival of less than 50 percent. However, those patients who remain abstinent have a substantially better prognosis. In general, overall outlook in patients with advanced liver disease remains poor; most of these patients eventually die as a result of massive variceal hemorrhage and/or profound hepatic encephalopathy.

Treatment Alcoholic hepatitis and cirrhosis are serious illnesses that require long-term medical supervision and careful management. Therapy of the underlying liver disease is largely supportive. Specific treatment is directed at particular complications such as variceal bleeding and ascites (see below). Some studies suggest that administration of prednisone or prednisolone in moderately large doses may be helpful in patients with severe alcoholic hepatitis and encephalopathy. However, the use of glucocorticoids in acute alcoholic hepatitis remains controversial and is not recommended. Although a number of studies have supported the use of propylthiouracil in the management of acute alcoholic hepatitis, the way it works is as yet undefined, and its efficacy has not been unequivocally established. More recently maintenance therapy with colchicine (0.6 mg PO bid) in the patient has been shown to slow progression and increase longevity of alcoholic liver disease in one long-term study. Other agents, such as penicillamine and intravenous infusion of insulin and glucagon, have been used experimentally, but their therapeutic efficacy and safety remain to be demonstrated.

In the absence of signs of impending hepatic coma, the patient should be placed on a diet containing at least 1 g protein per kilogram of body weight and 8500 to 12,500 kJ (2000 to 3000 kcal) per day. Use of diets enriched in branched-chain amino acids has been advocated in patients predisposed to hepatic encephalopathy, but the value of these diets in patients with compensated cirrhosis is unproven. Daily multivitamin supplements should be prescribed, with the addition of large parenteral doses of thiamine in patients with Wernicke-Korsakoff disease (see Chap. 357). The patient should be made to realize that there is no medication that will protect the liver against the effects of further alcohol ingestion. Therefore, alcohol should be absolutely forbidden. An important component of the complete care of such patients is encouragement to become involved in an appropriate alcohol counseling program.

All medicines must be administered with caution in the patient with cirrhosis, especially those eliminated or modified through hepatic metabolism or biliary pathways. In particular, care must be taken to avoid overzealous use of drugs that may directly or indirectly precipitate complications of cirrhosis. For example, vigorous treatment of ascites with diuretics may result in electrolyte abnormalities or hypovolemia which can lead to coma. Similarly, even modest doses of sedative can lead to deepening encephalopathy.

POSTNECROTIC CIRRHOSIS, POSTVIRAL CIRRHOSIS

Definition Postnecrotic cirrhosis represents the final common pathway of many types of advanced liver injury. *Coarsely nodular, posthepatitic,* and *multilobular cirrhosis* are terms synonymous with postnecrotic cirrhosis. The term *cryptogenic cirrhosis* has been used interchangeably with postnecrotic cirrhosis, but this designation should be reserved for those cases in which the etiology of cirrhosis is unknown (approximately 10 percent of all patients with cirrhosis).

Postnecrotic cirrhosis is characterized morphologically by (1) extensive confluent loss of liver cells, (2) stromal collapse and fibrosis resulting in broad bands of connective tissue containing the remains of many portal triads, and (3) irregular nodules of regenerating hepatocytes, varying in size from microscopic to several centimeters in diameter.

Etiology Postnecrotic cirrhosis is a morphologic term referring to a defined stage of advanced chronic liver injury of both specific and unknown (cryptogenic) causes. Epidemiologic and serologic evidence suggests that viral hepatitis (hepatitis B or non-A, non-B) may be an antecedent factor in at least one-fourth of cases of

* ALT = alanine aminotransferase, SGPT.

apparently cryptogenic postnecrotic cirrhosis. In areas where hepatitis B virus infection is endemic (e.g., southeast Asia, sub-Saharan Africa), up to 15 percent of the population may acquire the infection in early childhood, and cirrhosis may ultimately develop in one-fourth of these chronic carriers. Although hepatitis B infection is much less prevalent in the United States, it is relatively common among certain high-risk groups (e.g., promiscuous homosexual men, intravenous drug abusers), and contributes to an increased incidence of cirrhosis. In the United States non-A, non-B hepatitis agents appear to account for many cases of cirrhosis following blood transfusions. It is estimated that non-A, non-B hepatitis occurs in up to 10 percent of blood recipients, of whom as many as 5 to 10 percent may ultimately develop postnecrotic cirrhosis. Because reliable serologic markers for non-A, non-B hepatitis are not yet available, the number of cases of postnecrotic cirrhosis attributable to this agent (or agents) is difficult to determine but may be substantial (see Chap. 252). Postnecrotic cirrhosis may also develop in patients with chronic active hepatitis of the autoimmune type (see Chaps. 252 and 253).

Other probable causes of postnecrotic cirrhosis, including drugs and toxins, are listed in Table 254-1. In some instances, advanced alcoholic liver disease and primary biliary cirrhosis may lead to postnecrotic cirrhosis.

Pathology The postnecrotic liver is typically shrunken in size, distorted in shape, and composed of nodules of liver cells separated by dense and broad bands of fibrosis. The microscopic picture is consistent with the gross impression: nodules are highly variable in size with large amounts of connective tissue separating the disorganized islands of regenerating parenchyma.

Clinical features In patients with cirrhosis of known etiology in whom there is progression to a postnecrotic stage, the clinical manifestations are an extension of those resulting from the initial disease process. Usually clinical symptoms are related to portal hypertension and its sequelae, such as ascites, splenomegaly, hypersplenism, encephalopathy, and bleeding esophageal varices. The hematologic and liver function abnormalities resemble those seen with other types of cirrhosis. In a few patients with postnecrotic cirrhosis the diagnosis may be made incidentally at operation, at postmortem, or by a needle biopsy of the liver performed to investigate asymptomatic hepatosplenomegaly.

Diagnosis and prognosis Postnecrotic cirrhosis should be suspected in patients with signs and symptoms of cirrhosis or portal hypertension. Needle or operative liver biopsies confirm the diagnosis, although nonuniformity of the pathologic process may result in sampling errors. The diagnosis of cryptogenic cirrhosis is reserved for those patients in whom no known etiology can be demonstrated. About 75 percent of patients have progressive disease despite supportive therapy and die within 1 to 5 years from complications including exsanguinating variceal hemorrhage, hepatic encephalopathy, or superimposed hepatocellular carcinoma.

Treatment Management is usually limited to treatment of the complications of portal hypertension, including control of ascites, avoidance of drugs or excessive protein intake that may induce hepatic coma, and prompt treatment of infections (see below). In patients with asymptomatic cirrhosis, expectant management alone is appropriate. In those patients in whom postnecrotic cirrhosis has developed as a result of a treatable condition, therapy directed at the primary disorder may limit further progression (e.g., Wilson's disease, hemochromatosis).

TABLE 254-1 Cirrhosis and/or liver disease associated with infectious, metabolic, hereditary, drug-related, and other types of disorders

1 Infectious diseases
- *a* Viral hepatitis [hepatitis B, non-A, non-B, hepatitis D, cytomegalovirus (Chaps. 138, 326, and 333)]
- *b* Toxoplasmosis (Chap 162)
- *c* Schistosomiasis (Chap. 170)
- *d* Ecchinococcus (Chap. 171)
- *e* Brucellosis (Chap. 119)

2 Inherited and metabolic disorders (see also Chap. 256)
- *a* Hemochromatosis (Chap. 327)
- *b* Wilson's disease (Chap. 330)
- *c* Alpha$_1$-antitrypsin deficiency (Chap. 208)
- *d* Galactosemia (Chap. 337)
- *e* Glycogen storage disease (Chap. 332)
- *f* Gaucher's disease (Chap. 331)
- *g* Hereditary fructose intolerance (Chap. 337)
- *h* Hereditary tyrosinemia (Chap. 334)
- *i* Fanconi's syndrome (Chap. 331)

3 Drugs and toxins (Chap. 252)
- *a* Methyldopa
- *b* Methotrexate
- *c* Isoniazid
- *d* Perhexilene maleate
- *e* Oxyphenisatin
- *f* Arsenicals
- *g* Pyrrolidizine alkaloids (venoocclusive disease)
- *h* Oral contraceptives (Budd-Chiari)

4 Other or unproven causes
- *a* Sarcoidosis (Chap. 252)
- *b* Graft-versus-host disease
- *c* Chronic inflammatory bowel disease (Chap. 241)
- *d* Cystic fibrosis (Chap. 209)
- *e* Jejunoileal bypass (Chap. 45)
- *f* Diabetes mellitus (Chap. 319)

BILIARY CIRRHOSIS

Biliary cirrhosis results from injury to or prolonged obstruction of either the intrahepatic or extrahepatic biliary system. It is associated with impaired biliary excretion, destruction of hepatic parenchyma, and progressive fibrosis. Primary biliary cirrhosis is characterized by chronic inflammation and fibrous obliteration of intrahepatic bile ductules. Secondary biliary cirrhosis is the result of long-standing obstruction of the larger extrahepatic ducts. Although primary and secondary biliary cirrhosis are separate pathophysiologic entities with respect to the initial insult, many clinical features are similar.

PRIMARY BILIARY CIRRHOSIS Etiology and pathogenesis The cause of primary biliary cirrhosis remains unknown. Several observations suggest that a disordered immune response may be involved. Primary biliary cirrhosis is frequently associated with a variety of disorders presumed to be autoimmune in nature, such as the CRST syndrome (calcinosis, Raynaud's phenomenon, sclerodactyly, telangiectasia), the sicca syndrome (dry eyes and dry mouth), autoimmune thyroiditis, and renal tubular acidosis. Most importantly, a circulating IgG antimitochondrial antibody is detected in more than 95 percent of patients with primary biliary cirrhosis and only rarely in other forms of liver disease. In addition, elevated serum levels of IgM and cryoproteins consisting of immune complexes capable of activating the alternate complement pathway are found in 80 to 90 percent of patients. Lymphocytes are prominent in the portal regions and surround damaged bile ducts. These histologic findings resemble those noted in graft-versus-host disease following liver and bone marrow transplantation and suggest that damage to bile ducts may be immunologically mediated, perhaps reflecting a defect in a suppressor cell population.

Pathology Primary biliary cirrhosis is often divided into four stages based on morphologic findings. The earliest recognizable lesion (stage I), termed *chronic nonsuppurative destructive cholangitis*, is a necrotizing inflammatory process of the portal triads. It is characterized by destruction of medium and small bile ducts, a dense infiltrate of acute and chronic inflammatory cells, mild fibrosis, and occasionally bile stasis. At times, periductal granulomas and lymph follicles are found adjacent to affected bile ducts. Subsequently, the inflammatory infiltrate becomes less prominent, the number of bile ducts is reduced, and smaller bile ductules proliferate (stage II). Progression over a period of months to years leads to a decrease in interlobular ducts, loss of liver cells, and expansion of periportal fibrosis into a network of connective tissue scars (stage III). Ultimately, cirrhosis, which may be micronodular or macronodular, develops (stage IV).

Clinical features SIGNS AND SYMPTOMS Many patients with primary biliary cirrhosis are asymptomatic, and the disease is initially detected on the basis of elevated serum alkaline phosphatase levels during routine screening. The majority of such patients remain asymptomatic and do not develop progressive liver injury.

Among patients with symptomatic disease 90 percent are women ages 35 to 60. The earliest symptom is usually pruritus, which may be either generalized or limited initially to the palms and soles. After several months or years, jaundice and gradual darkening of the exposed areas of the skin (melanosis) may ensue. Other early clinical manifestations of primary biliary cirrhosis reflect impaired bile excretion. These include steatorrhea and the malabsorption of lipid-soluble vitamins often resulting in easy bruising (vitamin K deficiency), bone pain due to osteomalacia (vitamin D deficiency), occasionally night blindness (vitamin A deficiency), and dermatitis (possibly vitamin E and/or essential fatty acid deficiency). Protracted elevation of serum lipids, especially cholesterol, leads to subcutaneous lipid deposition around the eyes (xanthelasmas) and over joints and tendons (xanthomas). Over a period of months to years, the itching, jaundice, and hyperpigmentation slowly worsen. Eventually signs of hepatocellular failure and portal hypertension develop and ascites appears. Death due to hepatic insufficiency usually occurs within 5 to 10 years after the first signs of the illness and is often precipitated by uncontrolled variceal hemorrhage or infection.

Physical examination may be entirely normal in the early phase of the disease, when patients are asymptomatic or pruritus is the sole complaint. Later there may be jaundice of varying intensity, hyperpigmentation of the exposed skin areas, xanthelasmas and tendinous and planar xanthomas, moderate to striking hepatomegaly, splenomegaly, and clubbing of the fingers. Bone tenderness, signs of vertebral compression, ecchymoses, glossitis, and dermatitis may all be noted. Clinical evidence of the sicca syndrome can be found in as many as 75 percent of patients, and serologic evidence of autoimmune thyroid disease in 25 percent. Other conditions encountered with increased frequency include rheumatoid arthritis, CRST syndrome, scleroderma, pernicious anemia, and renal tubular acidosis.

LABORATORY FINDINGS Primary biliary cirrhosis is increasingly diagnosed at a presymptomatic stage, prompted by the finding of a two- to fivefold elevation of the serum alkaline phosphatase during routine screening. Serum 5′-nucleotidase activity is also elevated. In this setting, serum bilirubin and aminotransferase levels are usually normal, but the diagnosis is supported by a positive antimitochondrial antibody test (titer > 1:40). The latter is both *relatively* specific and sensitive; a positive test is found in over 90 percent of symptomatic patients. As the disease evolves, the serum bilirubin level rises progressively and may reach 510 μmol/L (30 mg/dL) or more in the final stages. Serum aminotransferase values rarely exceed 2.5 to 3.3 μkat (150 to 200 units). Hyperlipidemia is common, and a striking increase of the serum unesterified cholesterol is often noted. An abnormal serum lipoprotein (lipoprotein X) may be present in primary biliary cirrhosis but is not specific and appears in other cholestatic conditions. A deficiency of bile salts in the intestine leads to moderate steatorrhea and impaired absorption of the fat-soluble vitamins and hypoprothrombinemia. Patients with primary biliary cirrhosis have elevated liver copper levels, but this finding is not specific and is found in all disorders in which there is prolonged cholestasis.

Diagnosis Primary biliary cirrhosis should be considered in middle-aged women with unexplained pruritus or an elevated serum alkaline phosphatase and in whom there may be other clinical or laboratory features of protracted impairment in biliary excretion. Although a positive serum antimitochondrial antibody determination provides important diagnostic evidence, false-positive results do occur, and therefore liver biopsy should be performed to confirm the diagnosis. In most cases the biliary tract should be evaluated to exclude remediable extrahepatic biliary tract obstruction especially in view of the frequent presence of coexisting cholelithiasis.

Treatment There is no specific therapy for primary biliary cirrhosis. Corticosteroids are ineffective and may actually worsen the bone disease. D-Penicillamine has been tried because of its ability to chelate copper and because of its possible antifibrotic and immunomodulating activities. However, the drug appears to be ineffective and has a high incidence of unacceptable side effects. While some have suggested that azathioprine may be helpful in slowing the progression of disease, this has not been established. Colchicine has been shown to have some effect in slowing the progression of disease in symptomatic patients and should be tried (0.6 mg PO bid) unless gastrointestinal intolerance is limiting. Although not yet confirmed, treatment with low-dose methotrexate has been reported to halt or reverse progression of primary biliary cirrhosis.

Treatment is generally directed toward the relief of symptoms. Although the mechanism of the protracted pruritus is not entirely clear, cholestyramine, an oral bile salt–sequestering resin, may be helpful in doses of 8 to 12 g per day to decrease both the pruritus and the hypercholesterolemia. Steatorrhea can be reduced by a low-fat diet and substituting medium-chain triglycerides for dietary long-chain triglycerides. Fat-soluble vitamins A and K should be given by parenteral injection at regular intervals to prevent or correct night blindness and hypoprothrombinemia, respectively. Zinc supplementation may be necessary if night blindness is refractory to vitamin A therapy. Osteomalacia may be ameliorated by dietary calcium supplements in conjunction with oral vitamin D. In advanced disease, $25(OH)D_3$ or $1,25(OH_2)D_3$ may be preferred to vitamin D since poor hepatic function may limit conversion of vitamin D to the active metabolites. The management of ascites, variceal hemorrhage, and encephalopathy is described below. The role of hepatic transplantation for patients with primary biliary cirrhosis is under study; this may offer the best, and only, hope for survival in patients with end-stage disease.

SECONDARY BILIARY CIRRHOSIS Etiology Secondary biliary cirrhosis results from prolonged partial or total obstruction of the common bile duct or its major branches. In adults, obstruction is most frequently caused by postoperative strictures or gallstones, usually with superimposed infectious cholangitis. Chronic pancreatitis may lead to biliary stricture and secondary cirrhosis. Secondary biliary cirrhosis may also develop in patients with pericholangitis or idiopathic sclerosing cholangitis. Patients with malignant tumors of the common bile duct or pancreas rarely survive long enough to develop secondary biliary cirrhosis. In children, congenital biliary atresia and cystic fibrosis are common causes of secondary biliary cirrhosis. Choledochal cysts if unrecognized may also be a rare cause of secondary biliary cirrhosis.

Pathology and pathogenesis Unrelieved obstruction of the extrahepatic bile ducts leads to (1) bile stasis and focal areas of centrilobular necrosis followed by periportal necrosis, (2) proliferation and dilatation of the portal bile ducts and ductules, (3) sterile or infected cholangitis with accumulation of polymorphonuclear infiltrates around bile ducts, and (4) progressive expansion of portal tracts by edema and fibrosis. Extravasation of bile from ruptured interlobular bile ducts into areas of periportal necrosis leads to the formation of "bile lakes" surrounded by cholesterol-rich pseudoxanthomatous cells. As in other forms of cirrhosis injury is accompanied by regeneration in residual parenchyma. These changes gradually lead to a finely nodular cirrhosis. In general, at least 3 to 12 months is required for biliary obstruction to result in cirrhosis. Relief of the obstruction is frequently accompanied by biochemical and morphologic improvement.

Clinical features SIGNS AND SYMPTOMS The signs and symptoms of secondary biliary cirrhosis are similar to those of primary biliary cirrhosis. Jaundice and pruritus are usually the most prominent features. In addition, fever and/or right upper quadrant pain, reflecting bouts of cholangitis or biliary colic, are typical. The manifestations of portal hypertension are found only in advanced cases.

LABORATORY TESTS Elevation in serum alkaline phosphatase and conjugated hyperbilirubinemia are nearly always present. There is a moderate increase in serum aminotransferases. When the disease is complicated by cholangitis, elevations in aminotransferase levels and leukocytosis are more pronounced. As in primary biliary cirrhosis, there are abnormalities in serum lipids (including the presence of lipoprotein X) and laboratory findings consistent with steatorrhea. However, the antimitochondrial antibody test is usually negative.

Diagnosis Secondary biliary cirrhosis should be considered in any patient with clinical and laboratory evidence of prolonged obstruction to bile flow, especially when there is a history of previous biliary tract surgery or gallstones, bouts of ascending cholangitis, or right upper quadrant pain. Cholangiography (either percutaneous or endoscopic) usually demonstrates the underlying pathologic process. Liver biopsy, although not always necessary from a clinical standpoint, can document the development of cirrhosis.

Treatment Relief of obstruction to bile flow, by either surgical or endoscopic means, is the most important step in the prevention and therapy of secondary biliary cirrhosis. Effective decompression of the biliary tract results in a significant improvement in both symptoms and survival, even in patients with established cirrhosis. When obstruction cannot be relieved, as in sclerosing cholangitis, antibiotics may be helpful acutely in controlling superimposed infection or, when administered on a chronic basis, as prophylactic therapy in suppressing recurring episodes of ascending cholangitis. Without relief of obstruction, there is a steady progression to end-stage cirrhosis and its terminal manifestations.

CARDIAC CIRRHOSIS

Definition Prolonged, severe right-sided congestive heart failure may lead to chronic liver injury and cardiac cirrhosis. The characteristic pathologic features of fibrosis and regenerative nodules distinguish cardiac cirrhosis from both reversible passive congestion of the liver due to acute heart failure and acute hepatocellular necrosis (''ischemic hepatitis'' or ''shock liver'') resulting from systemic hypotension and hypoperfusion of the liver.

Etiology and pathology In right-sided heart failure, retrograde transmission of elevated venous pressure via the inferior vena cava and hepatic veins leads to congestion of the liver. Hepatic sinusoids become dilated and engorged with blood, and the liver becomes tensely swollen. With prolonged passive congestion and ischemia from poor perfusion secondary to reduced cardiac output, necrosis of centrilobular hepatocytes ensues and leads to fibrosis in these central areas. Ultimately centrilobular fibrosis develops with collagen extending outward in a characteristic stellate pattern from the central vein. Gross examination of the liver shows alternating red (congested) and pale (fibrotic) areas, a pattern often referred to as ''nutmeg liver.'' Improvement in management of cardiac disorders, particularly advances in surgical treatment, has reduced the frequency of cardiac cirrhosis.

Clinical features In acute passive congestion, the liver becomes enlarged and tender, and the patient may complain of severe right upper quadrant pain due to stretching of Glisson's capsule. The serum bilirubin is usually only mildly increased and may be predominantly either conjugated or unconjugated. The AST level is mildly elevated but may be transiently very high following a period of marked systemic hypotension (shock liver), when the clinical picture can mimic acute viral or drug-induced hepatitis. The serum albumin and prothrombin are usually normal, but may become abnormal in shock liver or with the development of cirrhosis. In cases of tricuspid insufficiency the liver may be pulsatile, but this finding disappears as cirrhosis develops. With prolonged right-sided heart failure the liver is enlarged, firm, and usually nontender. The signs and symptoms of heart failure usually overshadow the liver disease. Bleeding from esophageal varices is rare, but chronic encephalopathy may be prominent with a waxing and waning course reflecting variations in the severity of right-sided heart failure. Ascites and peripheral edema, often primarily related to the underlying cardiac dysfunction, may be worsened by the superimposed liver disease.

Diagnosis The presence of a firm, enlarged liver with signs of chronic liver disease in a patient with valvular heart disease, constrictive pericarditis, or cor pulmonale of long duration (>10 years) should suggest cardiac cirrhosis. Liver biopsy can confirm the diagnosis but is usually contraindicated because of coagulopathy or ascites. Coexistent chronic heart and liver disease should also raise the possibility of hemochromatosis, amyloidosis, or other infiltrative diseases.

Budd-Chiari syndrome resulting from the occlusion of the hepatic veins or inferior vena cava may be confused with acute congestive hepatomegaly. In this condition the liver is grossly enlarged and tender, and severe intractable ascites is present. However, signs and symptoms of heart failure are notably absent. The most common cause is thrombosis of the hepatic veins, often in the setting of polycythemia rubra vera, myeloproliferative syndromes, paroxysmal nocturnal hemoglobinuria, or other hypercoagulable states; it may also result from invasion of the inferior vena cava by tumor, such as renal cell or primary hepatocellular carcinoma. Idiopathic membranous obstruction of the inferior vena cava is the most common cause of this syndrome in Japan. Hepatic venography or liver biopsy showing centrilobular congestion and sinusoidal dilatation in the absence of right-sided heart failure establishes the diagnosis of Budd-Chiari syndrome. Venoocclusive disease affecting the sublobular branches of the hepatic veins and the hepatic venules may result from hepatic irradiation, treatment with some antineoplastic agents, use of oral contraceptives, or ingestion of pyrrolidizine alkaloids present in some herbal teas (''bush tea disease'') and can mimic congestive hepatomegaly.

Treatment Prevention or treatment of cardiac cirrhosis depends on the diagnosis and therapy of the underlying cardiovascular disorder. Improvement in cardiac function frequently results in improvement of liver function and stabilization of the liver disease.

METABOLIC, HEREDITARY, DRUG-RELATED, AND OTHER TYPES OF CIRRHOSIS (See Table 254-1). Cirrhosis or hepatitis may result from a wide variety of other processes encompassing the spectrum of etiologic factors listed in Table 254-2. Although some of these disorders have distinctive clinical or morphologic features, the manifestations of cirrhosis are largely independent of the underlying pathogenic mechanism.

NONCIRRHOTIC FIBROSIS OF THE LIVER Several diseases, either congenital or acquired, may be associated with localized or generalized hepatic fibrosis. They are distinguished from cirrhosis by the absence of hepatocellular damage and the lack of nodular regenerative activity. The clinical manifestations in such cases are largely secondary to portal hypertension. The different types of these disorders are indicated in Table 254-2; with the exception of schistosomiasis, all these conditions are relatively rare.

TABLE 254-2 Some causes of noncirrhotic hepatic fibrosis

1 Idiopathic portal hypertension (noncirrhotic portal fibrosis, Banti's syndrome); three variants:
- *a* Intrahepatic phlebosclerosis and fibrosis
- *b* Portal and splenic vein sclerosis
- *c* Portal and splenic vein thrombosis

2 Schistosomiasis (''pipe-stem'' fibrosis with presinusoidal portal hypertension)

3 Congenital hepatic fibrosis (may be associated with polycystic disease of liver and kidneys)

MAJOR SEQUELAE OF CIRRHOSIS

The clinical course of patients with advanced cirrhosis is usually complicated by a number of important sequelae which are independent of the etiology of the underlying liver disease. These include portal hypertension and its consequences (i.e., gastroesophageal varices and splenomegaly), ascites, hepatic encephalopathy, spontaneous bacterial peritonitis, hepatorenal syndrome, and hepatocellular carcinoma.

PORTAL HYPERTENSION Definition and pathogenesis Normal pressure in the portal vein is low (10 to 15 cm saline; 7 to 10 mmHg) because vascular resistance in the hepatic sinusoids is minimal. Portal hypertension (>30 cm saline) most commonly results from increased resistance to portal blood flow. Because the portal venous system lacks valves, resistance at any level between the heart and splanchnic vessels results in retrograde transmission of an elevated pressure. Increased resistance can occur at three levels relative to the hepatic sinusoids: (1) presinusoidal, (2) sinusoidal, and (3) postsinusoidal. Obstruction in the *presinusoidal* venous compartment may be anatomically outside of the liver (e.g., portal vein thrombosis) or within the liver itself but at a functional level proximal to the hepatic sinusoids so that the liver parenchyma is not exposed to the elevated venous pressure (e.g., schistosomiasis). *Postsinusoidal* obstruction may also occur outside the liver at the level of the hepatic veins (e.g., Budd-Chiari syndrome), the inferior vena cava, or, less commonly, within the liver (e.g., venoocclusive disease in which the central hepatic venules are the primary site of injury). When cirrhosis is complicated by portal hypertension, the increased resistance is usually sinusoidal. While distinctions between pre-, post-, and sinusoidal processes are conceptually appealing, functional resistance to portal flow in a given patient may occur at more than one level. Portal hypertension may also arise from increased blood flow (e.g., massive splenomegaly or arteriovenous fistulas), but the low-outflow resistance of the normal liver makes this a rare clinical problem.

Cirrhosis is the most common cause of portal hypertension in the United States. Clinically significant portal hypertension is present in greater than 60 percent of patients with cirrhosis. *Portal vein obstruction* is the second most common cause; it may be idiopathic or occur in association with cirrhosis, infection, pancreatitis, or abdominal trauma. *Hepatic vein thrombosis* (Budd-Chiari syndrome) and hepatic venoocclusive disease are relatively infrequent causes of portal hypertension (see above). Portal vein occlusion may result in massive hematemesis from gastroesophageal varices, but ascites is usually found only with cirrhosis. Noncirrhotic portal fibrosis accounts for only a few patients with portal hypertension.

Clinical features The major clinical manifestations of portal hypertension include hemorrhage from gastroesophageal varices, splenomegaly with hypersplenism, ascites, and acute and chronic hepatic encephalopathy. All of these features are related, at least in part, to the development of portal-systemic collateral channels. The absence of valves in the portal venous system facilitates retrograde (hepatofugal) blood flow from the high pressure portal venous system to the lower-pressure systemic venous circulation. Major sites of collateral flow involve the veins around the rectum (hemorrhoids), cardioesophageal junction (esophagogastric varices), retroperitoneal space, and the falciform ligament of the liver (periumbilical or abdominal wall collaterals). Abdominal wall collaterals appear as tortuous epigastric vessels that radiate from the umbilicus toward the xiphoid and rib margins (caput medusae).

Diagnosis In patients with known liver disease, the development of portal hypertension usually becomes evident by the appearance of splenomegaly, ascites, encephalopathy, and/or esophageal varices. Conversely, the finding of any of these features should lead one to evaluate the patient for the presence of underlying portal hypertension and liver disease. Varices may be documented by either barium swallow or fiberoptic esophagoscopy and lend indirect support to the diagnosis of portal hypertension. Although rarely necessary, portal venous pressure may be measured directly by percutaneous transhepatic "skinny needle" catheterization or indirectly through transjugular cannulation of the hepatic veins. Both free and wedged hepatic vein pressure (WHVP) should be measured. While WHVP is elevated in sinusoidal and postsinusoidal portal hypertension including cirrhosis, this measurement is usually normal in presinusoidal portal hypertension. In patients in whom additional information is necessary (e.g., preoperative evaluation before portal-systemic shunt surgery) or percutaneous catheterization is not feasible, mesenteric and hepatic angiography may be helpful. Particular attention should be directed to the venous phase to assess the patency of the portal vein and the direction of portal blood flow.

Treatment Although treatment is usually directed toward a specific complication of portal hypertension, attempts are sometimes made to reduce the pressure in the portal venous system. Surgical decompression procedures have been used for many years to lower portal pressure in patients with bleeding esophageal varices (see below). However, portal-systemic shunt surgery does not result in improved survival rates in patients with cirrhosis. There are also reports that beta-adrenergic receptor blockers, such as propranolol, may reduce portal venous pressure. Treatment of patients with clinically significant sequelae of portal hypertension, especially variceal bleeding, with doses of propranolol titrated to reduce the resting pulse by 25 percent is reasonable if no contraindications exist.

Vigorous treatment of patients with alcoholic hepatitis and cirrhosis, chronic active hepatitis, and other liver diseases may lead to a fall in portal pressure and to a reduction in variceal size. In general, however, portal hypertension due to cirrhosis is not reversible. In selected patients hepatic transplantation may be beneficial (e.g., end-stage primary biliary cirrhosis).

VARICEAL BLEEDING Pathogenesis While vigorous hemorrhage may arise from any portal-systemic venous collaterals, bleeding is most common from varices in the region of the gastroesophageal junction. The factors contributing to bleeding from gastroesophageal varices are not entirely understood but include the degree of portal hypertension and the size of the varices. Esophagitis with erosion of underlying varices does not appear to play an important role.

Clinical features and diagnosis Variceal bleeding often occurs without obvious precipitating factors and usually presents with painless but massive hematemesis with or without melena. Associated signs range from mild postural tachycardia to profound shock, depending on the extent of blood loss and degree of hypovolemia. Because patients with varices may bleed from other gastrointestinal lesions (e.g., peptic ulcer, gastritis), exclusion of other bleeding sources is important even in patients with prior variceal hemorrhage. Fiberoptic endoscopy is the best choice for evaluating upper gastrointestinal hemorrhage in patients with known or suspected portal hypertension.

Treatment Variceal bleeding is a life-threatening emergency. Prompt estimation and vigorous replacement of blood losses to maintain intravascular volume are essential and take precedence over diagnostic studies and more specific intervention to stop the bleeding. Replacement of clotting factors with fresh frozen plasma is important in patients with coagulopathy. Patients are best managed in an intensive care unit and often require close monitoring of central venous or pulmonary capillary wedge pressures, urine output, and mental status. Only when the patient is hemodynamically stable should attention be directed toward specific diagnostic studies (especially endoscopy) and other therapeutic modalities to prevent further or recurrent bleeding.

About half of all episodes of variceal hemorrhage cease without intervention, although the risk of rebleeding is very high. The medical management of acute variceal hemorrhage includes the use of vasoconstrictors (vasopressin), balloon tamponade, and endoscopic sclerosis of varices (sclerotherapy). Intravenous infusion of *vasopressin* at a rate of 0.1 to 0.9 units per minute results in generalized vasoconstriction leading to diminished blood flow in the portal venous system. Intravenous infusion of vasopressin has been shown to be as effective as selective intraarterial administration. Control of bleeding can be achieved in up to 80 percent of cases, but bleeding recurs in more than half after the vasopressin is tapered and discontinued. Furthermore, a number of serious side effects, including cardiac and gastrointestinal tract ischemia, acute renal failure, and hyponatremia, may be associated with vasopressin therapy. If bleeding is too vigorous or endoscopy is not available, *balloon tamponade* of the bleeding varices may be accomplished with a triple-lumen (Sengstaken-Blakemore) or four-lumen (Minnesota) tube with esophageal and gastric balloons. After the tube is introduced into the stomach, the gastric balloon is inflated and pulled back into the cardia of the stomach. If bleeding does not stop, the esophageal balloon is inflated for additional tamponade. Careful monitoring for complications such as esophageal rupture is essential. Where available, *endoscopic sclerosis* of esophageal varices should be employed to control bleeding acutely. In this procedure, the varices are injected with one of several sclerosing agents (e.g., sodium morrhuate) via a needle-tipped catheter passed through the endoscope. After initial endoscopic identification of varices as the presumed source of bleeding, such "sclerotherapy" controls acute bleeding in up to 90 percent of cases. In addition, repeated sclerotherapy until obliteration of all varices is accomplished should be performed in an effort to prevent recurrent bleeding. While available data support the efficacy of sclerotherapy in controlling bleeding acutely, further studies are needed to define the technique and the overall role of sclerotherapy in the management of variceal bleeding. Prophylactic sclerosis of esophageal varices in the absence of proven bleeding is not indicated. Although beta-adrenergic blocking agents (e.g., propranolol) have no role in the management of acute variceal bleeding, a number of studies suggest they may be of value in reducing the risk of recurrent upper gastrointestinal hemorrhage in the patient with portal hypertension.

Surgical therapy of portal hypertension and variceal bleeding involves the creation of a portal-systemic shunt to permit decompression of the portal system. Two types of portal systemic shunts have been used: *nonselective shunts* to decompress the entire portal system and *selective shunts* intended to decompress only the varices while maintaining blood flow to the liver itself. Nonselective shunts include end-to-side or side-to-side portacaval and proximal splenorenal anastomoses; selective shunts include the distal splenorenal shunt. Nonselective shunts are more likely to be complicated by encephalopathy than selective shunts. Emergency portal-systemic nonselective shunts may control acute hemorrhage, but such surgery is usually used only as a last resort because early operative mortality is greater than 30 percent. The role of portal-systemic shunt surgery after initial control of bleeding by nonoperative means is also uncertain. Surgically created shunts effectively reduce the risk of recurrent hemorrhage, but the overall mortality of patients undergoing such surgery is comparable to that of unoperated patients. Although patients who have undergone portal-system surgery succumb to recurrent bleeding less commonly than unoperated patients, this improvement is counterbalanced by increased morbidity from encephalopathy and death from progressive liver failure. Prophylactic shunt surgery should not be performed in patients with nonbleeding varices. Increasingly, therapeutic portal-systemic shunt has been reserved for patients who experience further bleeding despite serial endoscopic sclerotherapy. Other surgical procedures (e.g., esophageal transection) have also been advocated for the management of acute variceal bleeding although their efficacy remains unproven.

SPLENOMEGALY Definition and pathogenesis Congestive splenomegaly is common in patients with severe portal hypertension. Rarely, massive splenomegaly from nonhepatic disease leads to portal hypertension due to increased blood flow in the splenic vein.

Clinical features Although usually asymptomatic, splenomegaly may be massive and contribute to the thrombocytopenia or pancytopenia of cirrhosis. In the absence of cirrhosis, splenomegaly in association with variceal hemorrhage should suggest the possibility of splenic vein thrombosis.

Treatment Splenomegaly usually requires no specific treatment, although massive enlargement of the spleen may occasionally necessitate splenectomy at the time of shunt surgery. Splenectomy may also be indicated if splenomegaly is the cause rather than the result of portal hypertension. Thrombocytopenia alone is rarely severe enough to necessitate removal of the spleen.

ASCITES Definition Ascites is the accumulation of excess fluid within the peritoneal cavity. It is most frequently encountered in patients with cirrhosis and other forms of severe liver disease, but a number of other disorders may lead to either transudative or exudative ascites (see Chap. 48).

Pathogenesis The accumulation of ascitic fluid represents a state of total-body sodium and water excess, but the event that initiates this imbalance is unclear. Two theories have been proposed (see Fig. 254-1). The "underfilling" theory suggests that the primary abnormality is inappropriate sequestration of fluid within the splanchnic vascular bed due to portal hypertension and a consequent decrease in effective circulating blood volume. According to this theory, an apparent decrease in intravascular volume (underfilling) is sensed by the kidney, which responds by retaining salt and water. The "overflow" theory suggests that the primary abnormality is inappropriate renal retention of salt and water in the absence of volume depletion.

Regardless of the initiating event, a number of factors contribute to accumulation of fluid in the abdominal cavity (see Fig. 254-1). *Portal hypertension* plays an important role in the formation of ascites by raising hydrostatic pressure within the splanchnic capillary bed. *Hypoalbuminemia* and *reduced plasma oncotic pressure* also favor the extravasation of fluid from plasma to peritoneal cavity, and thus ascites is infrequent in patients with cirrhosis unless both portal hypertension and hypoalbuminemia are present. *Hepatic lymph* may weep freely from the surface of the cirrhotic liver due to distortion and obstruction of hepatic sinusoids and lymphatics and contribute to ascites formation. In contrast to the contribution of transudative fluid from the portal vascular bed, hepatic lymph may weep into the peritoneal cavity even in the absence of marked hypoproteinemia because the endothelial lining of the hepatic sinusoids is discontinuous. This mechanism may account for the high protein concentration present in the ascitic fluid of some patients with the Budd-Chiari syndrome.

Renal factors also play an important role in perpetuating ascites. Patients with ascites fail to excrete a water load in a normal fashion. They have increased renal sodium reabsorption by both proximal and distal tubules, the latter due largely to secondary hyperaldosteronism and increased plasma renin activity. Renal vasoconstriction, perhaps

FIGURE 254-1 Multiple factors involved in development of ascites. Current concepts suggest that initiating factor may be either primary sodium retention ("overflow") or diminished effective intravascular volume ("underfilling").

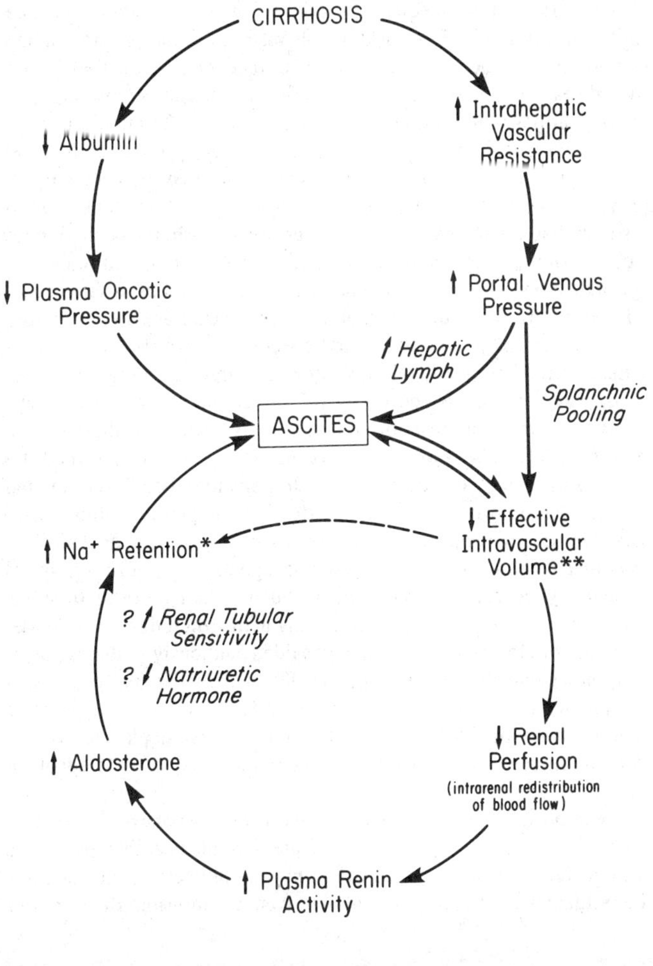

resulting from increased serum prostaglandin or catecholamine levels, may also contribute to sodium retention.

Clinical features and diagnosis Usually ascites is first noticed by the patient because of increasing abdominal girth. More pronounced accumulation of fluid may cause shortness of breath because of elevation of the diaphragm. When peritoneal fluid accumulation exceeds 500 mL, ascites may be demonstrated on physical examination by the presence of shifting dullness, a fluid wave, or bulging flanks. Ultrasound examination can detect smaller quantities of ascites and should be performed when physical examination is equivocal. Paracentesis should usually be performed with a small-gauge needle at the time of initial evaluation or at the time of any clinical deterioration of a cirrhotic patient. A small amount of fluid (less than 200 mL) should be obtained and examined for evidence of infection, tumor, or other possible causes and complications of ascites.

Treatment When ascites develops in the setting of severe, acute liver disease, resolution of ascites is likely to follow improvement in liver function. More commonly, ascites develops in patients with stable or steadily worsening liver function. Therapeutic intervention is indicated both to prevent potential complications and to control progressive increase in ascites, which may become pronounced enough to cause physical discomfort. However, overzealous attempts to reduce ascites may deplete the intravascular volume faster than fluid can be mobilized from the ascitic compartment and may precipitate renal failure. Thus, therapy aimed at reducing ascites should be gentle and incremental (see below). The goal is the loss of no more than 1.0 kg daily if both ascites and peripheral edema are present and no more than 0.5 kg daily in patients with ascites alone. To initiate therapy it may be desirable to hospitalize the patient so that daily weights and frequent serum electrolyte levels can be monitored and compliance ensured. Although abdominal girth measurements are frequently used as an index of fluid loss, they tend to be unreliable.

Strict bed rest is often recommended because of improved renal clearance in the supine position. However, salt restriction is the most important cornerstone of therapy. A diet containing 800 mg sodium (2 g NaCl) is often adequate to induce a negative sodium balance and permit diuresis. Response to salt restriction and bed rest alone is more likely to occur if the ascites is of recent onset, the underlying liver disease is reversible, a precipitating factor can be corrected, or the patient has a high urinary sodium excretion (~25 mmol per day) and normal renal function. Fluid restriction of approximately 1500 mL per day does little to enhance diuresis but may be necessary to prevent or correct hyponatremia. If sodium restriction alone fails to result in diuresis and weight loss, diuretic therapy should be instituted. Because of the role of hyperaldosteronism in sustaining salt retention, spironolactone or other distal tubule–acting diuretics (triamterene, amiloride) are the drugs of choice. These agents are also preferred because of their gentle action and specific potassium-sparing properties. Spironolactone is initially given in a dose of 25 mg four times a day and increased as needed by 100 mg per day every several days up to a maximum dose of 400 mg daily. An indication of the minimum effective dose of spironolactone may be obtained by monitoring urinary electrolyte concentrations for a rise in sodium and fall in potassium levels reflecting effective competitive inhibition of aldosterone. In some patients, diuresis cannot be initiated despite maximal doses of distal tubule–acting agents (e.g., 400 mg spironolactone) because of avid proximal tubular sodium absorption. When this occurs, more potent and proximally acting diuretics (furosemide, thiazide, or ethacrynic acid) may be added cautiously to the regimen. Spironolactone plus furosemide, 40 or 80 mg daily, is usually sufficient to initiate a diuresis in most patients. However, such aggressive therapy must be used with great caution to avoid plasma volume depletion, azotemia, and hypokalemia which may lead to encephalopathy.

A minority of patients with advanced cirrhosis have "refractory ascites" and fail to respond, despite intensive medical therapy. When this occurs in patients with marked hypoalbuminemia, diuresis may be initiated following cautious intravenous infusion of *salt-poor albumin*. Because of the short half-life of infused albumin, this approach is of short-term benefit and may, in fact, precipitate variceal hemorrhage due to expansion of the intravascular volume. In some patients a side-to-side *portacaval shunt* may result in improvement in ascites although generally these patients are extremely poor surgical risks. Intractable ascites can also be treated with the surgical implantation of a plastic *peritoneovenous shunt* which has a pressure-sensitive, one-way valve allowing ascitic fluid to flow from the abdominal cavity to the superior vena cava. However, the usefulness of this technique is limited by a high rate of complications such as infection, disseminated intravascular coagulation, and thrombosis of the shunt. Although clinical experience has long led to caution in removing large volumes of ascites by paracentesis for fear of precipitating progressive renal failure, recent studies have demonstrated the safety of this approach when combined with concomitant intravenous infusion of albumin in amounts proportional to those removed. Removal of up to 5 L of fluid using this approach has been found to speed reduction of ascites safely in the patient with tense ascites.

SPONTANEOUS BACTERIAL PERITONITIS Patients with ascites and cirrhosis may develop acute bacterial peritonitis without an obvious primary source of infection. Typical features include abrupt onset of fever, chills, generalized abdominal pain, and rebound abdominal tenderness accompanied by cloudy ascitic fluid with a high white cell count and usually positive bacterial cultures. However, the clinical symptoms *may be minimal,* and some patients manifest only worsening jaundice or encephalopathy in the absence of localizing abdominal complaints. The diagnosis is based on careful examination of the ascitic fluid. An ascitic fluid leukocyte count of greater than 500 cells per cubic millimeter or more than 250 polymorphonuclear leukocytes should suggest the possibility of bacterial peritonitis while results of bacterial cultures of ascitic fluid are pending. Empiric therapy with ampicillin and an aminoglycoside or cefotaximene should be initiated when the diagnosis is first suspected because enteric gram-negative bacilli are found in the majority of cases; less frequently the infection is caused by pneumococci and other gram-positive bacteria. Specific antibiotic therapy can be selected once the specific organism is identified. Therapy is usually administered for 10 to 14 days.

HEPATORENAL SYNDROME Definition and pathogenesis Hepatorenal syndrome is a serious complication in the patient with cirrhosis and ascites, and is characterized by worsening azotemia with avid sodium retention and oliguria in the absence of identifiable specific causes of renal dysfunction. The exact basis for this syndrome is not clear, but altered renal hemodynamics appear to be involved. The kidneys are structurally intact; urinalysis and pyelography are usually normal. Renal biopsy although rarely needed is also normal, and in fact kidneys from such patients have been successfully used for renal transplantation. There are indications that an imbalance in certain metabolites of arachidonic acid (prostaglandins and thromboxane) may play a pathogenetic role.

Clinical features and diagnosis Worsening azotemia, hyponatremia, progressive oliguria, and hypotension are the hallmarks of the hepatorenal syndrome. This syndrome, which is distinct from prerenal azotemia, may be precipitated by severe gastrointestinal bleeding, sepsis, or overly vigorous attempts at diuresis or paracentesis; it may also occur without an obvious cause. The diagnosis is supported by the demonstration of avid urinary sodium retention. Typically the urine sodium concentration is less than 5 mmol per liter, a concentration lower than that generally found in uncomplicated prerenal azotemia. The urinary sediment is unremarkable.

Treatment Treatment is usually unsuccessful. Although some patients with hypotension and decreased plasma volume may respond to infusions of salt-poor albumin, volume expansion must be undertaken with caution to avoid precipitating variceal bleeding. Vasodilator therapy, including intravenous infusion of dopamine, is not effective.

HEPATIC ENCEPHALOPATHY Definition Hepatic (portal-systemic) encephalopathy is a complex neuropsychiatric syndrome characterized by disturbances in consciousness and behavior, personality changes, fluctuating neurologic signs, asterixis or "flapping tremor," and distinctive electroencephalographic changes. Encephalopathy may be *acute* and reversible or *chronic* and progressive. In severe cases, irreversible coma and death may occur. Acute episodes may recur with variable frequency.

Pathogenesis The specific cause of hepatic encephalopathy is unknown. The most important factors in the pathogenesis are severe hepatocellular dysfunction and/or intrahepatic and extrahepatic shunting of portal venous blood into the systemic circulation, so that the liver is largely bypassed. As a result of these processes, various toxic substances absorbed from the intestine are not detoxified by the liver and lead to metabolic abnormalities in the central nervous system. Ammonia is the substance most often incriminated in the pathogenesis of encephalopathy. Many, but not all, patients with hepatic encephalopathy have elevated blood ammonia levels, and recovery from encephalopathy is often accompanied by declining blood ammonia levels. Other compounds and metabolites which may contribute to the development of encephalopathy include mercaptans (derived from intestinal metabolism of methionine), short-chain fatty acids, and phenol. Several observations suggest that excessive concentrations of gamma-aminobutyric acid (GABA), an inhibitory neurotransmitter, in the CNS are important in the reduced levels of consciousness seen in hepatic encephalopathy. Increased CNS GABA may reflect failure of the liver to efficiently extract precursor amino acids. False neurochemical transmitters (e.g., octopamine), resulting in part from alterations in plasma levels of aromatic and branched-chain amino acids, may also play a role. An increase in the permeability of the blood-brain barrier to some of these substances may be an additional factor involved in the pathogenesis of hepatic encephalopathy.

In the patient with otherwise stable cirrhosis, hepatic encephalopathy often follows a clearly identifiable precipitating event (see Table 254-3). Perhaps the most common predisposing factor is *gastrointestinal bleeding,* which leads to an increase in the production of ammonia and other nitrogenous substances which are then absorbed. Similarly, *increased dietary protein* may precipitate encephalopathy as a result of increased production of nitrogenous substances by colonic bacteria. *Electrolyte disturbances,* particularly hypokalemic alkalosis secondary to overzealous use of diuretics, vigorous paracentesis, or vomiting, may precipitate hepatic encephalopathy. Systemic alkalosis causes an increase in the amount of nonionic ammonia (NH_3) relative to ammonium ions (NH_4^+). Only nonionic (uncharged) ammonia readily crosses the blood-brain barrier and accumulates in the central nervous system. Hypokalemia also directly stimulates renal ammonia production. Hypoxia, injudicious use of central nervous system–depressing drugs (e.g., barbiturates, benzodiazepines), and acute infection may trigger or aggravate hepatic encephalopathy, although the mechanisms involved are not clear. Other potential precipitating factors include superimposed acute viral hepatitis, alcoholic hepatitis, extrahepatic bile duct obstruction, surgery, and other coincidental medical complications.

Clinical features and diagnosis Hepatic encephalopathy has protean manifestations, and any neurologic abnormality, including focal deficits, may be encountered. In patients with acute encephalopathy, neurologic deficits are completely reversible upon correction of underlying precipitating factors and/or improvement in liver function, but in patients with chronic encephalopathy the deficits may be irreversible and progressive. Cerebral edema is frequently present and contributes to the clinical picture and overall mortality in patients with both acute and chronic encephalopathy.

The diagnosis of hepatic encephalopathy should be considered when four major factors are present: (1) acute or chronic hepatocellular disease and/or extensive portal-systemic collateral shunts (the latter may be either spontaneous, e.g., secondary to portal hypertension, or surgically created, e.g., portacaval anastomosis); (2) disturbances of awareness and mentation which may progress from forgetfulness and confusion to stupor and finally coma; (3) shifting combinations of neurologic signs, including asterixis, rigidity, hyperreflexia, extensor plantar signs, and rarely, seizures; and (4) a characteristic (but nonspecific) symmetric, high-voltage, slow-wave (2 to 5 per second) pattern on the electroencephalogram. Asterixis ("liver flap," "flapping tremor") is a nonrhythmic asymmetric lapse in voluntary sustained position of the extremities, head, and trunk. It is best demonstrated by having the patient extend the arms and dorsiflex the hands. Because elicitation of asterixis depends on sustained voluntary muscle contraction, it is not present in the comatose patient. Asterixis is nonspecific and also occurs in patients with other forms of metabolic brain disease. Alterations in personality, mood disturbances, confusion, deterioration in self-care and handwriting, and daytime somnolence are additional clinical features of encephalopathy. *Fetor hepaticus,* a unique musty odor of the breath and urine believed to be due to mercaptans, may be noted in patients with varying stages of hepatic encephalopathy. Some patients may develop spastic paraparesis or *chronic progressive hepatocerebral degeneration,* the latter a clinical variant of hepatic encephalopathy characterized by a slow decline in intellectual function, tremor, cerebellar ataxia, choreoathetosis, and psychiatric symptoms.

Grading or classifying the stages of hepatic encephalopathy is often helpful in following the course of the illness and assessing response to therapy. One useful classification is shown in Table 254-4.

The diagnosis of hepatic encephalopathy is usually one of exclusion. There are no diagnostic liver function test abnormalities, although an elevated serum ammonia level in the appropriate clinical setting is highly suggestive of the diagnosis. Examination of the cerebrospinal fluid is unremarkable, and computed tomography of the brain shows no characteristic abnormalities. A number of conditions, particularly disorders related to acute and chronic alcoholism, can mimic the clinical features of hepatic encephalopathy. These include acute alcohol intoxication, sedative overdose, delirium tremens, Wernicke's encephalopathy, and Korsakoff's psychosis (see Chap. 357). Subdural hematoma, meningitis, and hypoglycemia or other metabolic encephalopathies must also be considered, especially in patients with

TABLE 254-3 Common precipitants of hepatic encephalopathy

1 Increased nitrogen load
- *a* Gastrointestinal bleeding
- *b* Excess dietary protein
- *c* Azotemia
- *d* Constipation

2 Electrolyte imbalance
- *a* Hypokalemia
- *b* Alkalosis
- *c* Hypoxia
- *d* Hypovolemia

3 Drugs
- *a* Narcotics, tranquilizers, sedatives
- *b* Diuretics (see *2*)

4 Miscellaneous
- *a* Infection
- *b* Surgery
- *c* Superimposed acute liver disease
- *d* Progressive liver disease

TABLE 254-4 Clinical stages of hepatic encephalopathy

Stage	Mental status	Asterixis	EEG
I	Euphoria or depression, mild confusion, slurred speech, disordered sleep	+/−	Usually normal
II	Lethargy, moderate confusion	+	Abnormal
III	Marked confusion, incoherent speech, sleeping but arousable	+	Abnormal
IV	Coma; initially responsive to noxious stimuli, later unresponsive	−	Abnormal

alcoholic cirrhosis. In young patients with liver disease and neurologic abnormalities, Wilson's disease should be excluded.

Treatment Early recognition and prompt treatment of hepatic encephalopathy are essential. Patients with acute, severe hepatic encephalopathy (stage IV) require the usual supportive measures for the comatose patient. Specific treatment of hepatic encephalopathy is aimed at (1) elimination or treatment of precipitating factors and (2) lowering of blood ammonia (and other toxin) levels by decreasing the absorption of protein and nitrogenous products from the intestine. In the setting of acute gastrointestinal bleeding, blood in the bowel should be promptly evacuated with enemas and laxatives in order to reduce the nitrogen load. Protein should be excluded from the diet, and constipation should be avoided. Ammonia absorption can be decreased by the administration of lactulose, a nonabsorbable disaccharide that acts as an osmotic laxative. Metabolism of lactulose by colonic bacteria may also result in an acid pH that favors conversion of ammonia to the poorly absorbed ammonium ion. In addition lactulose may actually diminish ammonia production through its direct effects on bacterial metabolism. Lactulose syrup can be administered in a dose of 30 to 50 mL every hour until diarrhea occurs; thereafter the dose is adjusted (usually 15 to 30 mL three times daily) so that the patient has two to four soft stools daily. Intestinal ammonia production by bacteria can also be decreased by oral administration of the antibiotic neomycin, at a dose of 0.5 to 1.0 g every 6 h. Although poorly absorbed, neomycin may reach sufficient concentrations in the bloodstream to cause renal toxicity. The use of agents such as levodopa, bromocriptine, keto-analogues of essential amino acids, and intravenous amino acid formulations rich in branched-chain amino acids in the treatment of acute hepatic encephalopathy remain of unproven benefit. Hemoperfusion to remove toxic substances and therapy directed primarily toward coincident cerebral edema in acute encephalopathy are also of unproven value.

Chronic encephalopathy may be effectively controlled by administration of lactulose. Management of patients with chronic encephalopathy should include dietary protein restriction, sometimes to levels as low as 40 g daily, in combination with low doses of lactulose or neomycin. Nephrotoxicity or ototoxicity may be limiting in prolonged usage of neomycin. There are suggestions that vegetable protein may be preferable to animal protein.

OTHER SEQUELAE OF CIRRHOSIS Coagulopathy Patients with cirrhosis often demonstrate a variety of abnormalities in both cellular and humoral clotting function. Thrombocytopenia may result from hypersplenism. In the alcoholic patient, there may be direct bone marrow suppression by ethanol. Diminished protein synthesis may lead to reduced production of fibrinogen (factor I), prothrombin (factor II), and factors V, VII, IX, and X. Reduction in levels of all factors except factor V may be worsened by the coincident malabsorption of the fat-soluble cofactor vitamin K due to cholestasis (see Chap. 240). Recent reports have documented the appearance of normal factor VIII levels following liver transplantation in patients with classical hemophilia probably as a result of production by nonhepatocellular components of the donor organ.

Hepatocellular carcinoma (See Chap. 255.)

REFERENCES

Alcoholic and postnecrotic cirrhosis

BARRY RE, MCGIVAN JD: Acetaldehyde alone may initiate hepatocellular damage in acute alcoholic liver disease. Gut 26:1065, 1985

BASKIN B et al: Ethanol and liver regeneration. Hepatology 8: 408, 1988

CARITHERS RL et al: Methylprednisolone therapy in patients with severe alcoholic hepatitis: A randomized multicenter trial. Ann Intern Med 110:685, 1989

GLUUD C et al: Prognostic indicators in alcoholic cirrhotic men. Hepatology 8:222, 1988

ORREGO H et al: Long-term treatment of alcoholic liver disease with propylthiouracil. N Engl J Med 317: 1421, 1987

SATO S et al: Liver fibrosis in alcoholics: Detection by FAB radioimmunoassay of serum procollagen III peptides. JAMA 256: 1471, 1986

SØRENSEN TIA et al: Prospective evaluation of alcohol abuse and alcoholic liver injury in man as predictors of development of cirrhosis. Lancet 2:241, 1984

Biliary cirrhosis

BABB C et al: Type III procollagen peptide: A marker of disease activity and prognosis in primary biliary cirrhosis. Lancet 1,1021, 1988

BESWICK DR et al: Asymptomatic primary biliary cirrhosis: A progress report on long-term follow-up and natural history. Gastroenterology 89:267, 1985

BODENHEIMER H JR et al: Evaluation of colchicine therapy in primary biliary cirrhosis. Gastroenterology 95:124, 1988

CHRISTENSEN E et al: Beneficial effects of azathioprine and predictor of prognosis in primary biliary cirrhosis: Final results of an international trial. Gastroenterology 89:1084, 1985

ESQUIVEL CO et al: Transplantation for primary biliary cirrhosis. Gastroenterology 94: 1207, 1988

KAPLAN MM et al: Primary biliary cirrhosis treated with low dose oral pulse methotrexate. Ann Int 109:429, 1988

NEUBERGER J et al: Double-blind controlled trial of D-penicillamine in patients with primary biliary cirrhosis. Gut 26:114, 1985

YEAMAN SJ et al: Primary biliary cirrhosis: Identification of two major M2 mitochondrial autoantigens. Lancet 1:1067, 1988

Hepatic encephalopathy

BASSETT ML et al: Amelioration of hepatic encephalopathy by pharmacologic antagonism of the GABA-Benzodiazepene receptor complex in a rabbit model of fulminant hepatic failure. Gastroenterology 93:1069, 1987

DUDLEY FJ et al: Hepatorenal syndrome without avid sodium retention. Hepatology 6:248, 1986

FRASER CL, ARIEFF AI: Hepatic encephalopathy. N Engl J Med 313:865, 1985

JONES EA et al: The neurobiology of hepatic encephalopathy. Hepatology 4:1235, 1984

MORGAN MY, HAWLEY KE: Lactitol vs. lactulose in the treatment of acute hepatic encephalopathy in cirrhotic patients: A double blind randomized study. Hepatology 7:1278.

SCHAFER DF: Hepatic coma: Studies on the target organ. Gastroenterology 93: 1131, 1987

SKOLNICK P: The γ-aminobutyric acid A ($GABA_A$)-benzodiazepine receptor complex, pp 534–536, in: Jones EA, moderator. The γ-aminobutyric A ($GABA_A$) receptor complex and hepatic encephalopathy: some recent advances. Ann Intern Med 110:532, 1989

Portal hypertension and ascites

CELLO JP et al: Endoscopic sclerotherapy versus portacaval shunt in patients with severe cirrhosis and variceal hemorrhage. N Engl J Med 311:1589, 1984

CROSSLEY JR, WILLIAMS R: Spontaneous bacterial peritonitis. Gut 26:325, 1985

EPSTEIN M: The sodium retention of cirrhosis: A reappraisal. Hepatology 6:312, 1986

GINÉS P et al: Comparison of paracentesis and diuretics in the treatment of cirrhotics with tense ascites: Results of a randomized study. Gastroenterology 93:234, 1987

MILLIKAN WJ et al: The Emory prospective randomized trial: Selective versus nonselective shunt to control variceal bleeding. Ann Surg 201:712, 1985

NICHOLLS KM et al: Sodium excretion in advanced cirrhosis: Effect of expansion of central blood volume and suppression of plasma aldosterone. Hepatology 6:235, 1986

PASTA L et al: Propranolol for prophylaxis of bleeding in cirrhotic patients with large varices: A multicenter randomized clinical trial. Hepatology 8:1, 1988

PINTO PC et al: Large-volume paracentesis in nonedematous patients with tense ascites: Its affect on intravascular volume. Hepatology 8: 207, 1988

PINZANI M et al: Altered furosemide pharmacokinetics in chronic alcoholic liver disease with ascites contributes to diuretic resistance. Gastroenterology 92:294, 1987

TERBLANCHE J et al: Controversies in the management of bleeding esophageal varices. N Engl J Med 320:1394, 1469, 1989

255 NEOPLASMS OF THE LIVER

KURT J. ISSELBACHER / JACK R. WANDS

PRIMARY CARCINOMA Tumors of hepatocytes or hepatocellular carcinomas account for 80 to 90 percent of liver carcinomas; but there are also bile duct cell carcinomas (cholangiocarcinomas) or those of mixed origin. There is, however, little practical purpose in distinguishing between the two types, since both may be found in different parts of the same tumor and the clinical courses are similar.

Epidemiology and etiology In North and South America and Europe primary liver cancers account for only 1 to 2 percent of malignant tumors found at autopsy. However, in parts of Africa and Asia they may account for up to 20 to 30 percent of all types of malignancy. Liver cell carcinoma is up to four times more common in men than in women. The peak incidence occurs in the fifth and sixth decades of life in western countries, but one to two decades earlier in Africa and Asia, areas with a high prevalence of liver carcinoma. Cirrhosis, usually macronodular or postnecrotic, is found in 60 to 75 percent of autopsied patients with primary liver cell carcinoma in all parts of the world. In view of the wide geographic variation in the incidence of hepatocellular carcinoma, different etiologic factors appear to be involved.

1 *Chronic liver disease* of any type predisposes to the development of carcinoma. A variety of metabolic, alcoholic, viral, or idiopathic chronic liver diseases can lead to liver cell carcinoma. Thus, α_1-*antitrypsin deficiency* and hereditary tyrosinosis, with active liver disease since birth, has a high incidence of developing into carcinoma. In the adult age group, *hemochromatosis* has the highest risk of malignant degeneration, presumably owing to the long duration of the chronic liver inflammation and cirrhosis. Alcoholic and postnecrotic cirrhosis are the most common forms of underlying liver disease in patients with liver carcinoma in western countries.
2 *Hepatitis B (HBV)* is endemic in many areas of Africa and Asia. The prevalence of HBV antigenemia in the normal population is up to 10 to 15 percent in some parts of Africa and the Far East. In these areas, most patients with hepatocellular carcinoma (90 to 95 percent) will have serologic evidence of recent or past HBV infection (see Chap. 252). Approximately 60 to 70 percent of these patients will have chronic hepatitis and/or cirrhosis at the time of clinical presentation. In most instances HBV-DNA integration has been found in the genome of tumor cells as well as in the adjacent uninvolved hepatocytes. HBV-DNA integration appears to occur most commonly in long-term chronic carriers and in those individuals who acquire infection at birth. The relative risk of developing a primary hepatocellular carcinoma in an HBV chronic carrier as compared to an uninfected individual is approximately 100:1. It is recommended that known chronic HBV carriers have biannual alpha fetoprotein (AFP) determinations to screen for subclinical hepatocellular carcinoma (see below).
3 *Mycotoxins,* metabolites of saprophytic fungi, including certain known hepatic carcinogens (e.g., aflatoxins), are continuously ingested in foodstuffs in small amounts and are found in high concentrations in foods in parts of Africa and Asia, where liver cell carcinoma is found more frequently. Ingested mycotoxins and viral inflammation and cirrhosis as the result of HBV infection may act synergistically to increase the risk of liver cell cancer.
4 *Hormonal factors* may be important in view of the male predominance in liver cancer and the effect of sex hormones on experimental carcinogenesis. Hepatocellular carcinoma has been reported in some patients on long-term androgenic therapy. Long-term use of *oral contraceptives* rarely leads to development of hepatic cell adenoma, a benign neoplasm, but malignant transformation into carcinoma has been reported.

Clinical features Cancers of the liver may escape clinical recognition during life because they often occur in patients with underlying cirrhosis, and the symptoms and signs may initially suggest a progression of the underlying liver disease. *Hepatomegaly,* with *pain* or *tenderness,* usually moderate in degree and localized to the upper abdomen or the right upper quadrant, is often the major complaint. Other important clinical features which should alert the clinician to the diagnosis include a *mass* in the liver, particularly if tender; the presence of a *friction rub* or *bruit* over the liver; and *blood-tinged ascites* (hemoperitoneum) which occurs in about 20 percent of cases. However, all such signs and symptoms reflect far advanced and usually inoperable disease and this underscores the value of early detection by AFP screening or ultrasound determinations. Jaundice is characteristic of cholangiocarcinoma but is relatively uncommon in hepatocellular carcinoma in the absence of active liver disease.

Anemia and *elevated alkaline phosphatase* and *AFP* levels are common laboratory findings. In a patient with cirrhosis, a disproportionately high serum alkaline phosphatase in relation to other abnormal liver function tests is often a clue to an infiltrating or partially obstructing liver carcinoma.

Diagnosis The clinical features outlined above should suggest the possibility of primary liver carcinoma. A number of imaging procedures are used to detect liver tumors including ultrasound, CT scanning, MRI, or hepatic artery angiography (see Chap. 248). Ultrasound is frequently used to screen high-risk populations and should be the first procedure used when hepatocellular carcinoma is suspected; it is relatively sensitive and can detect most tumors greater than 3 cm. MRI is also being used with increasing frequency. Celiac axis angiography is sensitive and indispensable before surgery.

AFP, a unique fetal α_1-globulin, is found in the serum of many patients with hepatocellular carcinoma. Very high levels, greater than 500 μg/L, occur in about 70 percent of patients. The serum AFP may be *slightly elevated* in about 5 to 10 percent of patients with large hepatic metastases from gastrointestinal tumors, and in about one-third of patients with acute or chronic viral hepatitis; only rarely do levels over 500 μg/L occur in these conditions. Minimally elevated levels of AFP may persist in some patients with chronic hepatitis. AFP is also elevated up to 500 μg/L in maternal sera during normal pregnancy. The detection and persistence of *high levels* of serum AFP (over 500 or 1000 μg/L) in an adult with liver disease and without an obvious gastrointestinal tract tumor strongly suggest the presence of primary liver carcinoma. However, gradually increasing AFP levels even when starting at a low (<50 μg/L) serum level may signal the development of a small (<3 cm) subclinical hepatocellular carcinoma, particularly in the high-risk HBV carrier group with and without chronic hepatitis and cirrhosis.

Percutaneous *liver biopsy* can be diagnostic, especially if the biopsy is taken in the area of a palpable nodule or mass localized by ultrasound or CT scans. False negatives may occur in as many as one-fourth of patients if the biopsy is performed in a routine, blind manner with the intercostal approach, and well-differentiated hepatocellular carcinoma may be difficult to diagnose by aspiration cytology or even needle biopsy. Cytologic examination of ascitic fluid is invariably negative for tumor cells. *Laparoscopy* or *laparotomy* with open liver biopsy may be required for diagnosis. This direct approach has the additional advantage of identifying the occasional patient with localized resectable tumor who may be suitable for partial hepatectomy.

Course and management The course of the disease is fatal and usually rapid. Most patients die within 3 to 6 months from gastrointestinal hemorrhage, progressive cachexia, or hepatic failure.

Surgical resection offers the only chance of cure but the 5-year survival is low and only a few patients have resectable tumors at presentation. However, with AFP and ultrasound screening programs to identify subclinical hepatocellular carcinoma in high-risk populations, it is likely that 5-year survival rates will be substantially improved.

If the patient is young, in good general health, and has no obvious extrahepatic involvement, solitary hepatic lesions may be excised with *partial hepatectomy,* but the 5-year survival rate is low. Persistently high or rising levels of AFP after excision of the tumor are suggestive of residual or recurrent tumor. Hepatocellular carcinoma may respond for brief periods to systemic or intraarterial chemotherapy. However, the results are still poor, and further trials of combined drug therapy are in progress. Liver transplantation can now be considered a therapeutic option, but recurrence of tumor and frequent appearance of metastases after transplantation have limited the usefulness of this procedure (see Chap. 257). Aggressive surgery or transplantation may prove to be of value in the treatment of small, localized tumors if diagnosed early or in the slower-growing fibrolamellar type of liver cell carcinoma. Other approaches which are of limited usefulness include hepatic artery embolization and hepatic artery perfusion (via implanted pumps) with fluorouracil and doxorubicin. Monoclonal antibodies tagged with radioactive or cytotoxic agents are also being investigated as potentially effective approaches.

OTHER BENIGN AND MALIGNANT TUMORS These tumors are very rare. Hepatoblastomas are histologically distinct primary malignant tumors of the liver occurring only in infancy and early childhood and characteristically have very high levels of serum AFP. They are usually solitary masses, may be resectable and have a higher 5-year survival rate than hepatocellular carcinoma. *Hemangiomas,* the most common benign tumors, are usually single and small, but may present as a large hepatic nodule. Percutaneous needle liver biopsy is contraindicated if the diagnosis is suspected because of the danger of hemorrhage. The diagnosis can be made by angiography. Surgical excision is usually not indicated unless the tumors are large and symptomatic or a malignant lesion cannot be excluded. *Hemangioendotheliomas* or *angiosarcomas* are rare malignant vascular tumors. They can be caused by chronic *vinyl chloride* exposure and may appear 15 to 20 years after the administration of thorium dioxide.

Hepatic adenomas, although rare, are particularly prone to occur in women taking oral contraceptives for long periods. These benign neoplasms may regress when the pill is discontinued. Focal nodular hyperplasia, a nonneoplastic hamartoma, may also become more vascular with long-term use of oral contraceptives leading to increased risk of pain or hemorrhage. Other rare tumors include benign cholangiomas, rhabdomyomas, rhabdomyosarcomas, and a number of other benign and malignant tumors arising from various mesenchymal elements. These tumors usually present as a palpable mass in the liver or with intraabdominal hemorrhage. They can be visualized and their extent defined by angiography. Surgical exploration and open biopsy or resection are usually required for definitive diagnosis.

METASTATIC TUMORS Metastatic malignant tumors of the liver are common in clinical practice, ranking second only to cirrhosis as a cause of fatal liver disease. In the United States the incidence of clinically significant metastatic carcinoma is at least 20 times greater than that of primary carcinoma. Hepatic metastases have been reported at autopsy in 30 to 50 percent of patients dying from malignant disease.

Pathogenesis The liver is uniquely vulnerable to invasion by tumor cells. Its size, high rate of blood flow, and double perfusion by hepatic artery and portal vein combine to make it the most common site of metastases except for the lymph nodes. In addition, local tissue factors or endothelial membrane characteristics appear to enhance metastatic implants. Virtually all types of neoplasms except those primary in the brain may metastasize to the liver. The most common primary tumors are those of the gastrointestinal tract, lung, breast, and melanomas. Less common are metastases from tumors of the thyroid, prostate, and skin.

Clinical features Most patients with metastatic malignancy of the liver present with (1) symptoms referable only to the primary tumor, with asymptomatic hepatic involvement discovered in the course of clinical evaluation; (2) nonspecific symptoms of weakness, weight loss, fever, sweating, and loss of appetite; or rarely, with (3) features indicating active hepatic disease, especially abdominal pain, hepatomegaly, or ascites.

Patients with widespread metastatic liver involvement usually have suggestive clinical signs of cancer and hepatic enlargement. Some have localized induration or tenderness, and occasionally a friction rub may be found over tender areas of the liver.

Abnormal liver function tests are frequent but often mild and nonspecific. They reflect the effects of fever and wasting, as well as the infiltrating neoplastic process itself. An increase in serum alkaline phosphatase is the most common and frequently the only abnormality noted. Hypoalbuminemia, anemia, and occasional mild elevation of transaminase levels may also be found with more widespread disease. Greatly elevated serum levels of carcinoembryonic antigen (CEA) are usually found when the metastases are from primary malignancies in the gastrointestinal tract, breast, or lung.

Diagnosis Evidence of metastatic invasion of the liver should be sought actively in any patient with a primary malignancy, especially of the lung, gastrointestinal tract, or breast, before resection of the primary lesion is undertaken. Abnormal liver function tests, particularly an elevated alkaline phosphatase, or demonstration of a mass by liver scintiscan, ultrasound, or CT may provide a presumptive diagnosis. Blind percutaneous needle biopsy of the liver will result in a positive diagnosis of metastatic disease in only 60 to 80 percent of cases with hepatomegaly and elevated alkaline phosphatase levels. Serial sectioning of specimens, two or three repeat biopsies, or cytologic examination of biopsy smears may increase the diagnostic yield by 10 to 15 percent. The yield is greatly increased when biopsies are directed by ultrasound or CT or obtained by laparoscopy.

Treatment Most metastatic carcinomas respond poorly to all forms of treatment, which is usually only palliative. Surgical removal of a single large metastasis is rarely feasible. Systemic chemotherapy with combinations of different chemotherapeutic agents briefly may slow tumor growth and reduce symptoms in some patients but does not significantly alter the prognosis. It remains to be determined whether newer drugs or combination chemotherapy eventually will prove to be more effective.

REFERENCES

BEASLEY RP et al: Hepatocellular carcinoma and hepatitis B virus. Lancet 2:1129, 1981

BRECHOT C et al: Evidence that hepatitis B virus has a role in liver cell carcinoma in alcoholic liver disease. N Engl J Med 306:1384, 1982

DIBICEGLIE AM: Hepatocellular carcinoma. Ann Intern Med 108:390, 1988

LIAW Y-F et al: Early detection of hepatocellular carcinoma in patients with chronic type B hepatitis. A prospective study. Gastroenterology 90:263, 1986

LOTZE MT: Surgical management of hepatocellular carcinomas. Gastroenterology Clin North Am 16:613, 1987

MALT RA: Surgery for hepatic neoplasms. N Engl J Med 313:1591, 1985

OKUDA K et al: Natural history of hepatocellular carcinoma and prognosis in relation to treatment. Study of 850 patients. Cancer 56:918, 1985

OMATA M et al: Hepatocellular carcinoma in the USA: Etiologic considerations. Localization of hepatitis B antigens. Gastroenterology 76:279, 1979

ORDER SE et al: Iodine 131 antiferritin, a new treatment modality in hepatoma. A radiation therapy oncology group study. J Clin Onc 3:1573, 1985

POPPER H et al: Relationship of the hepatitis B virus carrier state to hepatocellular carcinoma. Hepatology 7:764, 1987

SHAFRITZ DA et al: Integration of hepatitis B virus DNA into the genome of liver cells in chronic liver disease and hepatocellular carcinoma. N Engl J Med 305:1067, 1981

TANG ZHAO-YON: *Subclinical Hepatocellular Carcinoma*. New York, Springer, 1985

ZAMAN SN et al: Risk factors in development of carcinoma in cirrhosis: Prospective study of 613 patients. Lancet 1:1357, 1985

256 INFILTRATIVE AND METABOLIC DISEASES AFFECTING THE LIVER

KURT J. ISSELBACHER / DANIEL K. PODOLSKY

Many disseminated, systemic, or metabolic diseases involve the liver in a diffuse manner by the infiltration of abnormal cells or the accumulation of chemical substances or metabolites. Chemical accumulation may be extracellular or intracellular and may involve hepatocytes, Kupffer cells, or other elements of the reticuloendothelial system. Although infiltrative diseases may vary widely in their etiology and extrahepatic manifestations, the findings in the liver may be quite similar. Generalized enlargement and firmness of the liver, gradual and nonspecific deterioration of liver function, and, less often, signs of portal hypertension or ascites are typical features of this group of diseases. Differential diagnosis by clinical means may be difficult on occasion, but in patients in whom ancillary clinical findings do not establish the diagnosis, the diffusely infiltrated liver provides an excellent source of tissue for diagnostic purposes.

As discussed in Chap. 6, the tools of molecular biology, especially recombinant DNA probes and restriction fragment length polymorphism will undoubtedly play a significant role in arriving at the molecular basis for many of these disorders. Some diseases will reflect the manifestation of mutant structural genes causing absent or reduced amounts of a gene product (e.g., phenylalanine hydroxylase deficiency leading to classic phenylketonuria), or a structurally *altered* gene which is functionally inactive (e.g., $alpha_1$ antitrypsin). In other instances the mutation may affect *gene regulation* as in Menke's syndrome, a rare disorder of zinc metabolism that affects the liver, which appears to result from faulty regulation of metallothionein gene expression.

LIPID INFILTRATIONS

FATTY LIVER Slight to moderate enlargement of the liver due to diffuse infiltration of liver cells by neutral fat (triglyceride) is a common clinical and pathologic finding. Although minimal fatty changes are often transient and have no clinical significance, persistent or extensive fatty infiltration may produce dysfunction and symptoms that require careful evaluation.

Etiology The major causes of fatty liver encountered in clinical practice depend on the age, geographic location, and metabolic-nutritional status of the patient population. *Chronic alcoholism* is the most common cause of fatty liver in this country and in other countries with a high alcohol intake. The severity of fatty involvement is roughly proportional to the duration and degree of alcoholic excess. *Protein malnutrition,* especially in infancy and early childhood, accounts for most cases of severe fatty liver in the tropical zones of Africa, South America, and Asia. The hepatic changes may be associated with other clinical and pathologic features of kwashiorkor. Patients with adult-onset *diabetes mellitus,* especially those who are overweight and are poorly controlled, often have fatty livers. *Obesity* is commonly associated with fatty infiltration of the liver; this recedes as weight reduction occurs. However, *jejunoileal bypass* for surgical treatment of morbid obesity is sometimes associated with severe fatty liver and hepatic failure that may be fatal. In patients with Cushing's syndrome and in those receiving large doses of corticosteroids, fatty infiltration of the liver may occur. In many *chronic illnesses,* especially those complicated by impaired nutrition or malabsorption, increased fat is found in liver cells. For example, patients with ulcerative colitis, chronic pancreatitis, or protracted heart failure frequently have moderately fatty livers at the time of death. Patients maintained on prolonged *intravenous hyperalimentation* may also develop fatty livers.

Acute fatty liver is caused by a number of hepatotoxins and is frequently accompanied by signs and symptoms of liver failure. Carbon tetrachloride intoxication, DDT poisoning, and ingestion of substances containing yellow phosphorus result in severe fatty liver. Acute and prolonged alcohol ingestion may also be considered in this category and may be associated with a rapidly enlarging and fat-laden liver. *Acute fatty liver of pregnancy* is a rare but often fatal condition seen during the third trimester of pregnancy which is characterized by nausea, vomiting, abdominal pain, renal failure, and coma. It should be distinguished from the benign cholestasis more frequently encountered during the third trimester of pregnancy. *Massive tetracycline therapy,* in amounts of 3 to 12 g intravenous, is a rare cause of acute fatty liver and fatal hepatic coma. Other drugs (e.g., valproic acid) have also been associated with the development of a fatty liver.

Pathogenesis The hepatic lipid deposits, which consist largely of triglycerides and lesser amounts of phospholipid and cholesterol, appear as vacuoles of varying size within the cytoplasm of liver cells. In extreme cases, every liver cell is involved, and lipids comprise up to 30 to 40 percent of the total liver weight.

The biochemical mechanisms leading to hepatic triglyceride accumulation are described in Chap. 250. Fatty infiltration has been produced in experimental animals by a variety of toxic agents and drugs, such as alcohol, carbon tetrachloride, and orotic acid. Deficiencies, such as choline deficiency, readily lead to increased fat in the liver in the rat. Many of these factors appear to disrupt synthesis of proteins, including the apoproteins needed for transport of triglycerides out of the liver as lipoproteins. However, with few exceptions experimental studies do not explain the pathogenesis of fatty liver in clinical disease. Moderate doses of ethanol may produce both acute and chronic fatty changes in human subjects, probably by its direct effects on hepatic triglyceride and fatty acid metabolism (Chap. 250). Protein deficiency seems to account for the fatty liver of kwashiorkor, and impaired protein synthesis for the fat accumulation following tetracycline and carbon tetrachloride administration. In diabetes mellitus and in starvation, increased mobilization of fatty acids from adipose tissue may be involved. Fatty infiltration during hyperalimentation appears to be derived from the high concentration of dextrose rather than from any lipid infusions.

Clinical features The signs and symptoms of fatty liver are related to the degree of fat infiltration, the time course of its accumulation, and the underlying cause. The obese or diabetic patient with chronic fatty liver is usually asymptomatic and has only mild tenderness over the enlarged liver. The liver function tests are normal or show mild elevations of alkaline phosphatase, transaminases, or aminotransferases. In contrast, the rapid accumulation of fat seen in the setting of hyperalimentation may lead to marked tenderness, presumably resulting from stretching of Glisson's capsule. Similarly, alcoholic patients with acute fatty liver following a bout of heavy drinking may have right upper quadrant pain and tenderness often with laboratory evidence of cholestasis. The clinical presentation of acute fatty liver of pregnancy or fatty liver from hepatotoxins is similar to that of fulminant hepatic failure arising from any cause, with evidence of hepatic encephalopathy, marked elevations of prothrombin time and transaminases, and variable degrees of jaundice.

Diagnosis The findings of a firm, nontender, and generally enlarged liver with minimal hepatic dysfunction in a patient with chronic alcoholism, malnutrition, poorly controlled diabetes mellitus, or obesity should suggest a fatty liver. When diagnostic uncertainty exists, needle biopsy of the liver will demonstrate the increased fatty content and possibly the underlying primary disorder. In acute fatty liver of pregnancy and in most cases of Reye's syndrome (see below), fat accumulates in small vacuoles (microvesicular fat) rather than in the large cytoplasmic droplets encountered in other disorders. The reason for the morphologic appearance of the fat in these two disorders is unclear.

Treatment Adequate nutritional intake, removal of alcohol or offending toxins, and correction of any associated metabolic disorders usually result in recovery. There is no clinical rationale for the use of lipotropic agents such as choline. When indicated, attention should be directed to abstinence from alcohol, careful control of diabetes, weight loss, or correction of intestinal absorptive defects. In the alcoholic fatty liver there is gradual disappearance of fat from the liver after 4 to 8 weeks of adequate diet and abstinence from alcohol. Similarly, fatty infiltration usually resolves within 2 weeks after discontinuation of parenteral hyperalimentation. However, restitution of intestinal continuity may not prevent progression of disease in patients who have had extensive intestinal bypass surgery.

REYE'S SYNDROME (FATTY LIVER WITH ENCEPHALOPATHY) This acute illness is encountered exclusively in children below 15 years of age. It is characterized clinically by vomiting, and signs of progressive central nervous system damage, signs of hepatic injury, and hypoglycemia. Morphologically there is extensive fatty vacuolization of the liver and renal tubules. The cause is unknown, although viral and toxic agents, especially salicylates, have been implicated. Increased aspirin use and much higher serum salicylate levels in children with this illness than in the general population have been described during outbreaks of Reye's syndrome. However, it seems clear that this illness may also occur in the absence of exposure to salicylates. In fatal cases, the liver is enlarged and yellow with striking diffuse fatty microvacuolization of cells. Peripheral zonal hepatic necrosis has also been present in some cases. Fatty changes of the renal tubular cells, cerebral edema, and neuronal degeneration of the brain are the major extrahepatic changes. Electron microscopic studies show structural alterations of mitochondria in liver, brain, and muscle.

The onset usually follows an upper respiratory tract infection, especially influenza or chickenpox. Within 1 to 3 days persistent vomiting occurs, together with stupor, which usually progresses rapidly to generalized convulsions and coma. The liver is enlarged, but *jaundice is characteristically absent or minimal.* Elevations in serum aminotransferases and prothrombin time, hypoglycemia, metabolic acidosis, and elevated serum ammonia levels are the major laboratory findings. The mortality rate in Reye's syndrome is approximately 50 percent. Therapy consists of infusions of glucose and fresh frozen plasma, as well as intravenous mannitol to reduce the cerebral edema. Chronic liver disease has not been reported in survivors.

NIEMANN-PICK DISEASE (See Chap. 331) This rare heritable disorder, of which there are five types, is found mainly in Jewish infants and is characterized by the accumulation of sphingomyelin and cholesterol in reticuloendothelial cells of the liver, spleen, bone marrow, and brain due to deficiency of sphingomyelinase. Hepatomegaly and splenomegaly are present, together with elevations in serum aminotransferase and alkaline phosphatase levels, but jaundice and other evidence of hepatic dysfunction are rare. The liver, which is typically large, yellow, and fatty, shows clusters of lipid-filled, foamy Kupffer cells. Diagnosis is made by lipid analysis of the tissue obtained from bone marrow aspiration.

GAUCHER'S DISEASE (See Chap. 331) Accumulations of large reticuloendothelial cells containing the cerebroside glucosylceramide (Gaucher's cells) in the liver and spleen account for the characteristic moderate to massive hepatosplenomegaly found in patients with the juvenile and adult forms of this disorder. Rarely, ascites or portal hypertension is produced by compression of the intrahepatic vasculature. The diagnosis may be made readily by liver biopsy and demonstration of the Gaucher's cells but should be confirmed by demonstration of a deficiency of the enzyme glucosylceramide β-glucosidase in peripheral leukocytes.

WOLMAN'S AND CHOLESTEROL ESTER STORAGE DISEASES Wolman's disease is a rare and fatal familial lipidosis of infancy producing hepatosplenomegaly and stippled calcification of the adrenal glands. Liver biopsy shows clusters of foam cells (reticuloendothelial cells filled with cholesterol ester and triglycerides), hepatocytes containing fat, and patchy fibrosis. A related but less severe genetic disorder is cholesterol ester storage disease. In this condition there is hypercholesterolemia and accumulation of both cholesterol esters and triglycerides in hepatic lysosomes. Both of these storage disorders are associated with hepatic deficiencies of cholesterol ester hydrolase and triglyceride lipase.

Other rare lipid disorders associated with hepatomegaly and increased fat in the liver include abetalipoproteinemia, Tangier disease, Fabry's disease, and types I and V hyperlipoproteinemia. (See Chap. 326 for details.)

HEPATIC GLYCOGEN ACCUMULATION

DIABETIC GLYCOGENOSIS Hepatic enlargement caused by distention of liver cells with glycogen is present in some poorly controlled diabetic patients and often in juvenile diabetic patients (see Chap 319). More often, however, hepatomegaly is related to fatty infiltration (see above). Ketoacidosis and vigorous insulin therapy may further enhance hepatic enlargement and glycogen deposition. In the absence of cirrhosis, hepatomegaly usually decreases with careful control of the diabetes.

GLYCOGEN STORAGE DISEASE (See Chap. 332) The normal liver contains 1 to 5 percent glycogen (by weight). Except for types V and VII, the liver is involved in all genetically determined glycogen storage diseases. There is disruption of glucose homeostasis due to an inability to mobilize hepatic glycogen stores. In types I, II, and VI hereditary glycogen storage diseases, increased amounts of glycogen (and fat) are found. Types III and IV are associated with derangements of glycogen structure, and cirrhosis may be present. Fasting hypoglycemia is present in all these diseases. Enzymatic and chemical analysis of liver tissue is usually needed for diagnosis.

Hepatic changes are common in patients with unrecognized or untreated galactosemia. In early weeks of life fatty infiltration and cholestasis may be noted in acutely ill infants. If the disease goes unrecognized for months or years, cirrhosis may develop. (See also Chap. 337.)

HEPATIC MINERAL ACCUMULATION

WILSON'S DISEASE (See Chap. 330) This rare disease, predominantly of young people, is characterized by cirrhosis, softening and degeneration of the basal ganglia, and pigmentation of the cornea (Kayser-Fleischer rings). Increased copper deposition in the tissues seems to be responsible for the liver and basal ganglia changes. Liver cells are ballooned and show increased glycogen with glycogen vacuolization in the nuclei. The liver shows all grades of changes, from minimal to severe periportal or macronodular cirrhosis.

HEMOCHROMATOSIS (See Chap. 327) This relatively common genetically determined disorder involves accumulation of abnormal amounts of iron due to inappropriate absorption in the intestine. The liver, as a primary site of iron storage, is most directly affected. There is diffuse deposition of excess iron in hepatocytes, in contrast to the characteristic accumulation of iron in the reticuloendothelial compartment typical of secondary iron overload and hemosiderosis. Hepatic iron overload commonly results in hepatomegaly. Although liver function is initially well preserved, if the disease is untreated, progressive impairment is followed by the development of cirrhosis.

OTHER INFILTRATIVE DISEASES

HURLER'S SYNDROME (See Chap. 333) This is an uncommon hereditary disease that is characterized by the widespread tissue deposition of mucopolysaccharide (chondroitin sulfate B and heparin sulfate) in many tissues. The liver is frequently enlarged and firm. Microscopically, Kupffer cells and other macrophages are enlarged and filled with metachromatic granular material. Cirrhosis may be a late complication.

ALPHA$_1$ ANTITRYPSIN DEFICIENCY (See also Chap. 210) Patients with homozygous deficiency of serum alpha$_1$ antitrypsin (α1AT) are prone to develop emphysema in adult life. The disease is suggested by the absence of alpha$_1$ globulin on serum electrophoresis (α1AT makes up 90 percent of this fraction normally) and confirmed by direct measurement of α1AT. The exact phenotype can then be determined by starch electrophoresis. Although there are 16 recognized alleles, only PiZ and PiS are associated with clinical disease. The molecular bases of these altered products have been related to single nucleic acid substitutions, e.g., PiZ is caused by a G (guanine) to A (adenine) transposition which results in a substitution of a glutamic acid for lysine at residue 292 in the α1AT protein. Hepatocytes of some patients with this deficiency contain globules positive to the periodic acid Schiff (PAS) reaction. Approximately 10 percent of children with homozygous deficiency (PiZZ phenotype) of α1AT will develop significant liver disease including neonatal hepatitis and progressive cirrhosis. It has been suggested that 15 to 20 percent of all chronic liver disease in infancy may be attributed to α1AT deficiency. In adults, the most common manifestation of α1AT deficiency is asymptomatic cirrhosis, which may progress from a micronodular to a macronodular state and may be complicated by the development of hepatocellular carcinoma. The occurrence of liver disease in these patients is not dependent upon the development of lung disease.

RETICULOENDOTHELIAL DISORDERS (See also Chaps. 63 and 302)

Moderate to massive hepatomegaly and splenomegaly occur frequently in the various types of leukemia and lymphoma. Jaundice, when present, is usually slight and results from hemolysis. Deep and protracted jaundice is distinctly rare and is caused by obstruction of the intrahepatic or extrahepatic bile ducts by tumor. Liver biopsy specimens reveal portal and sinusoidal infiltrates in most cases of leukemia, but the cellular pattern may be mixed and nonspecific. Liver biopsy is diagnostic in only 5 percent of patients with Hodgkin's disease. This percentage is increased in those with advanced disease or splenomegaly. Directed biopsy at laparoscopy or laparotomy is more likely to be positive than "blind" needle biopsy. Nonspecific histologic changes in the liver have been described in patients with lymphoma and may contribute to the abnormal liver function tests.

Myeloid metaplasia and other myeloproliferative disorders associated with extramedullary hematopoiesis produce hepatomegaly which may reach huge proportions, especially following splenectomy. Serum alkaline phosphatase elevations are often found. Ascites and portal hypertension, resulting from diffuse involvement of portal venules and lymphatics, are rare complications.

GRANULOMATOUS INFILTRATIONS

Perhaps as a result of the large population of mononuclear phagocytes, a number of systemic granulomatous diseases involve the liver, including sarcoidosis, miliary tuberculosis, histoplasmosis, brucellosis, schistosomiasis, berylliosis, and drug reactions. In addition, isolated granulomas of no diagnostic importance may be found occasionally in patients with various forms of cirrhosis and hepatitis. The liver infiltrated by granulomas may be slightly enlarged and firm, but hepatic dysfunction is usually limited and manifested only by mild increases in serum alkaline phosphatase and occasionally aminotransferase levels. In a few patients with sarcoidosis or brucellosis, portal hypertension may develop, and extensive postnecrotic scarring or postnecrotic cirrhosis may follow healing of the granulomatous lesions as in schistosomiasis.

Needle biopsy of the liver reveals granulomas and often provides the first definite evidence of a systemic or disseminated granulomatous disease. In patients with sarcoidosis who have neither clinical nor laboratory evidence of hepatic involvement, needle biopsy is positive in about 80 percent of cases. In cases of suspected miliary tuberculosis a portion of the biopsy should be cultured and stained for mycobacteria. The organism can be detected in the majority of cases, particularly when caseating granulomas are present. Serial sections of the biopsy specimen should be examined if granulomas are not apparent. Individual granulomas are rarely specific in their microscopic appearance, and final diagnosis usually requires other clinical, laboratory, or histologic data.

In approximately 20 percent of patients it is not possible to identify a cause for the granulomatous infiltration. When these infiltrates are accompanied by fever of unknown etiology, the diagnosis of granulomatous hepatitis should be considered. This is an uncommon disorder of unknown etiology and is diagnosed by exclusion. While granulomatous hepatitis invariably responds to moderate doses of corticosteroids, relapses are frequent, and such therapy should never be undertaken unless tuberculous disease or other causes of granulomatous infiltration have been excluded. This may include an initial empiric trial of antituberculous therapy.

AMYLOIDOSIS (See also Chap. 266)

Systemic amyloidosis, whether primary and idiopathic, familial, or secondary to chronic inflammatory or neoplastic diseases, often involves the liver. Grossly, the liver infiltrated with amyloid is enlarged and pale and rubbery in consistency. Microscopically, the birefringent amyloid deposits appear as homogeneous waxy material within the space of Disse, often being concentrated in the periportal areas and associated with atrophy of adjacent liver cell plates. Selective involvement of the walls of blood vessels, especially of the hepatic arterioles, may be a striking feature of primary amyloidosis. With this possible exception, however, the hepatic lesions are the same in all forms of amyloidosis and are present in 60 to 90 percent of cases.

An enlarged and firm liver is found in about 60 percent of patients, and ascites occurs in advanced stages of the disease in about 20 percent. Jaundice, portal hypertension, and other signs of chronic liver disease are usually absent. Liver function changes, although frequent, correlate poorly with the extent of liver infiltration. Hypoalbuminemia and elevated serum alkaline phosphatase are common. Hypoalbuminemia, however, may be related to the nephrotic syndrome owing to renal involvement; the prothrombin time is usually normal. The diagnosis is established by biopsy of rectum, skin, liver, or other involved organs and demonstration of the characteristic Congo red–staining deposits by polarizing microscopy.

REFERENCES

BOVE KE: Reye's syndrome, in *Hepatology, A Textbook of Liver Disease*, D Zakim, TD Boyer (eds). Philadelphia, Saunders, 1982, pp 1212–1220

GISHAN FK, GREENE HL: Liver disease in children with PIZZ α_1-antitrypsin deficiency. Hepatology 8:307, 1988

GLENNER GG: Amyloid deposits and amyloidosis. The β-fibrilloses. N Engl J Med 302:1283, 1980

HEUBI JE et al: Grade I Reye's syndrome: Outcome and predictors of progression to deeper coma grades. N Engl J Med 311:1539, 1984

HURWITZ ES et al: Public Health Service Study on Reye's syndrome and medications. N Engl J Med 313:842, 1985

KIDD VJ, WOO SLC: Recombinant DNA probes used to detail genetic disorders of the liver. Hepatology 4:731, 1984

REYNOLDS TB et al: Hepatic granulomas, in *Hepatology, A Textbook of Liver Disease*, D Zakim, TD Boyer (eds). Philadelphia, Saunders, 1982, pp 995–1009

RILEY C et al: Acute fatty liver of pregnancy: A reassessment based on observations in nine patients. Ann Intern Med 106:703, 1987

SCHIFF L, SCHIFF ER: *Diseases of the Liver*, 6th ed. Philadelphia, Lippincott, 1987

SPECHLER SJ, KOFF RS: Wilson's disease: Diagnostic difficulties in the patient with chronic hepatitis and hyperceruloplasminemia. Gastroenterology 78:103, 1980

SCRIVER CR et al (eds): *The Metabolic Basis of Inherited Disease*, 6th ed. New York, McGraw-Hill, 1989

257 LIVER TRANSPLANTATION

RUDI SCHMID

Orthotopic liver transplantation, i.e., replacement of a diseased liver by a healthy organ recovered from a recently brain-dead individual, is surgically difficult, requires a full array of supporting services usually available only in large tertiary medical centers, and carries a considerable operative and postoperative mortality. However, the risk-versus-benefit ratio has improved to an extent where liver transplantation has become a promising approach for selected patients whose liver disease is progressive, life-threatening, and beyond the reach of traditional therapy.

The first orthotopic liver transplantation in a human was performed by Starzl and associates in 1963 at the University of Colorado in Denver, but the survival of this patient and several subsequently transplanted patients was less than 1 month. The following years brought refinements in both surgical technique and postoperative management that improved survival rates, but by 1976 only 24 percent of adults and 33 percent of children who underwent liver transplantation survived for more than 1 year. Until the 1970s, performance of the operation remained almost entirely limited to the Denver center and to another liver transplantation facility established by Calne in 1968 in Cambridge, England. Since 1980, however, the prospect for prolonged survival with good quality of life has improved owing largely to development of better techniques for organ preservation, improvements in surgical techniques including the development of a pump-driven venovenous bypass system, and advances in immunosuppression, particularly the use of cyclosporine in combination with steroids. As a result, an increasing number of transplant centers are being established, and the total number of successful liver transplants exceeded 3,000 by the end of 1986. Over 1200 liver transplantations were performed in the United States in 1988.

INDICATIONS FOR LIVER TRANSPLANTATION In the absence of absolute or relative contraindications (see below), potential candidates for liver transplantation are children and adults who suffer from severe, irreversible liver disease for which alternative medical or surgical treatments have been exhausted. Timing of the operation is of critical importance; the disease should be in a late enough stage to allow the patient all opportunity for spontaneous stabilization or recovery but early enough to give the surgical procedure a fair chance of success. As a general rule, transplantation should be considered in patients with end-stage liver disease who are experiencing or have experienced life-threatening complications of hepatic failure, whose quality of life has deteriorated to unacceptable levels, or whose liver disease predictably will result in irreversible damage to the central nervous system. The decision to transplant requires the combined judgment of an experienced team of hepatologists, transplant surgeons, anesthesiologists, and specialists in supporting services; the well-informed consent of the patient or the patient's family or authorized representative must also be obtained.

TRANSPLANTATION IN CHILDREN **Biliary atresia** The most common indication for transplantation in children is biliary atresia, which results in progressive distortion of intrahepatic bile ducts and cirrhosis, leading to hepatic insufficiency and death. Hepatoportoenterostomy (Kasai procedure) performed in the first two months of life may provide substantial, albeit usually transient, improvement, but in a small percentage of patients this procedure has been reported to result in prolonged stabilization obviating further surgery. In the majority of patients, however, progressive liver disease eventually requires transplantation, but the operation preferably should be delayed as long as possible to permit the child optimal development.

Metabolic disorders Genetically transmitted diseases associated with progressive liver failure constitute another major indication in children and adolescents. In progressive cirrhosis due to α_1-antitrypsin deficiency, transplantation results in appearance of the donor α_1-antitrypsin phenotype and return of the plasma enzyme level toward normal. In Wilson's disease presenting with acute hepatic failure or with progressive neurologic deficiency that is unresponsive to chelation therapy, liver transplantation is the treatment of choice. Improvement in neurologic function and return of plasma ceruloplasmin concentration to normal have been reported. Liver failure in Byler's, Alagille's, and Wolman's disease and in protoporphyria, tyrosinemia, and some types of glycogenosis have been indications for transplantation. In Crigler-Najjar disease type I and in certain hereditary disorders of the urea cycle and of amino acid or lactate-pyruvate metabolism, transplantation may be the only way to prevent impending deterioration of central nervous system function, despite the fact that the replaced liver is structurally normal. Combined heart and liver transplantation have yielded dramatic improvement in cardiac function and plasma cholesterol level in children with homozygous familial hypercholesterolemia. In hereditary oxalosis, improvement has been reported after combined liver and kidney transplantation.

TRANSPLANTATION IN ADULTS **Nonalcoholic cirrhosis** Chronic active hepatitis due to presumed autoimmunity and cirrhosis of nonviral etiology with liver failure are important indications for transplantation. From the mid-1970s to 1985, the actuarial 1-year survival of 275 patients transplanted for these conditions progressively rose from 31 percent to approximately 70 percent.

Primary biliary cirrhosis Because primary biliary cirrhosis has an indolent and often fluctuating course, liver transplantation is indicated only in patients who have progressed to an end stage of the disease or whose quality of life has deteriorated to an unacceptable level. Survival is similar to that in nonalcoholic cirrhosis. In the posttransplantation period, it may be difficult to distinguish between homograft rejection and potential recurrence of the original disease because the clinical, laboratory, and histologic features of the two conditions are similar.

Sclerosing cholangitis Transplantation has been successful in patients with primary sclerosing cholangitis or with Caroli's disease in whom surgical drainage procedures failed to prevent progressive deterioration of hepatic function. Recurrent infections with sepsis are frequent indications for transplantations in these patients.

Hepatic vein thrombosis Transplantation has been reported in 17 patients with Budd-Chiari syndrome with an actuarial 3-year survival of 60 percent. Because spontaneous recannulation of the obstructed hepatic veins occasionally occurs, the operation should be reserved for patients with progressive hepatic decompensation or irreversible hepatorenal syndrome. Postoperative anticoagulation is essential in these patients. Although many patients with Budd-Chiari syndrome have underlying polycythemia vera or a covert myeloproliferative disorder, this usually is no contraindication for liver transplantation.

Hepatobiliary cancer Overall survival of patients who undergo transplantation for primary hepatocellular carcinoma or cholangiocarcinoma is significantly less than that for other categories of liver disease because the majority of patients succumb to disseminated carcinomatosis. Moreover, because the results have improved only slightly in recent years, the proportion of transplanted patients who received homografts for primary liver cancer has progressively decreased since 1980. The most promising approach to primary liver cancer clearly is early detection when the tumor is small and amenable to total resection. Several experimental protocols including lethal irradiation of the cancer-containing liver followed by resection and orthotopic transplantation are currently being evaluated.

CONTRAINDICATIONS FOR TRANSPLANTATION Absolute contraindications for transplantation include life-threatening systemic diseases, infections, preexisting cardiovascular or pulmonary disease, metastatic malignancies, and therapy-resistant arterial hypotension. Preexisting renal disease is a relative contraindication; successful concomitant renal transplantation has been reported. Portal vein thrombosis is another relative contraindication; successful thrombectomy or construction of a venous bypass with subsequent liver transplantation have been performed. In alcohol-related liver disease, the outcome of transplantation generally has been disappointing; only 27 out of 819 patients reported up to August 1984 were transplanted for this condition. In patients with advanced alcohol-related cirrhosis who, despite abstinence for at least 6 months and adequate nutritional state, develop hepatic decompensation, transplantation may be contemplated when all other means of therapy have failed; relatively few patients, however, fulfill these qualifications. Patients with chronic viral hepatitis B, particularly those positive for HBsAg and HBeAg and those with non-A, non-B hepatitis, although the infection usually recurs in the homograft, increasingly are transplanted with acceptable survival results. Information is inadequate to determine whether recurrent infection also occurs in chronic hepatitis B without evidence of active viral replication. Patients with delta hepatitis are poor risks for transplantation. In fulminant hepatitis of all etiologies associated with encephalopathy and/or hepatorenal syndrome, results of transplantation generally have been discouraging. Interpretation of available results is difficult because most reports fail to distinguish between hepatic coma stages III and IV, which have strikingly different prognoses with conservative management.

RESULTS OF TRANSPLANTATION **Survival** Since 1983, the survival rate of patients undergoing liver transplantation has steadily improved. In 1985, the overall prospect for 1-year survival was about

70 percent, with children faring slightly better than adults. Of 152 patients who underwent liver transplantation at various centers between January 1980 and April 1983 and who survived the initial three postoperative months, the 3-year survival rate was 79 percent in adults with nonalcoholic cirrhosis and 92 percent in children with biliary atresia; in 102 patients transplanted after April 1983 who survived the initial three postoperative months, 1-year survival rates reached 89 percent in adults and 96 percent in children.

Posttransplantation quality of life In patients who have undergone transplantation for life-threatening chronic liver disease, objective evaluation of the quality of life after surgery is inherently difficult, and reliable information is sparse. Nonetheless, full rehabilitation seems to have been achieved in the majority of those who survived the first three postoperative months and escaped chronic rejection or unmanageable infection. Immunosuppressive medication in reduced doses is continued indefinitely. Several women who underwent transplantation and received immunosuppressive therapy have conceived and carried the pregnancy to term without demonstrable damage to the infants.

TECHNICAL AND MANAGEMENT ASPECTS Surgical techniques Liver donors commonly are procured from accident victims 2 months to 45 years of age who are brain-dead and without detectable hepatic dysfunction. Cardiovascular and respiratory functions are sustained artificially until the liver can be removed. Prolonged periods of hypotension or hypoxia preclude donation, and compatibility of ABO blood type and organ size are important considerations in donor selection, although successful ABO-incompatible or reduced donor organ transplants have been performed successfully. A recent report suggests that implantation of a female liver into a male recipient results in reduced homograft survival. Multiple-organ procurement (including the liver, heart, and kidneys, but not the pancreas) is technically feasible. Following perfusion with cold electrolyte solution the donor liver is packed in ice; a new perfusion solution recently developed by Belzer at the University of Wisconsin allows for at least 20 h of preservation without significant impairment of graft viability.

Removal of the recipient's liver is technically difficult, particularly in the presence of varices or scarring from previous abdominal operations. After the portal vein and inferior vena cava are dissected, a pump-driven bypass system is applied that reroutes blood from the portal vein and inferior vena cava to the superior vena cava, thereby preventing congestion of visceral organs. In implanting the new liver, meticulous attention must be directed to reestablishment of the portal venous and hepatic arterial circulations and to reconstruction of biliary drainage. The latter usually is achieved by anastomosis of the common bile ducts or by choledochojejunostomy to a Roux en Y limb, if the common bile duct of the recipient cannot be used for reconstruction.

A transplant operation requires 8 to 12 h. Because of excessive bleeding associated with portal hypertension and liver failure, large volumes of blood, blood products, and volume expanders may be required during surgery.

POSTOPERATIVE COURSE AND MANAGEMENT Postoperative complications Patients who undergo liver transplantation are frequently malnourished, so that attention to multiple organ failure is of primary importance. Because of the fluids administered during surgery, patients may become overloaded during the immediate postoperative period, necessitating continuous monitoring of cardiovascular and pulmonary function. Cardiovascular instability also may result from electrolyte imbalance during reperfusion of the donor liver. Pulmonary function may be further compromised by paralysis of the right hemidiaphragm caused by phrenic nerve injury. The hyperdynamic state with increased cardiac output frequently occurring in patients with liver failure rapidly reverses after successful liver transplantation. Postoperative jaundice is almost invariable and reflects the large administered pigment load and variable degrees of ischemic or mechanical injury sustained by the liver during harvesting, preservation, and implantation. Prerenal azotemia, acute kidney injury due to hypotension, or renal toxicity caused by antibiotics or cyclosporine are frequently encountered in the postoperative period and sometimes require dialysis. Other postoperative complications related to technical difficulties include stenosis or leakage of the anastomosed common bile duct, intraperitoneal hemorrhage, and thrombosis of the reconstructed hepatic artery or of the portal or hepatic vein. Acute upper gastrointestinal hemorrhage or unexplained transient hemolytic anemia, with or without thrombocytopenia, may occur.

Bacterial, viral, or fungal infections related to the required immunosuppressive therapy may be life-threatening in the postoperative period. These infections may involve the biliary tree, liver, upper gastrointestinal tract, or lungs, and they demand early recognition and prompt management. *Candida, Nocardia, Pneumocystis carinii*, and cytomegalovirus are frequent infective agents, but viruses of the herpes group, other mycoses, or gram-negative bacteria may also be pathogens. In most transplant centers, patients routinely are given antibiotic and antifungal therapy prophylactically. Routine use of sulfamethoxazole with trimethoprim decreases the incidence of postoperative *P. carinii* infection.

Immunosuppression The introduction in 1980 of cyclosporine as an immunosuppressive agent contributed substantially to the improvement in transplant survival. The drug depresses both humoral and cell-mediated immunity via inhibition of interleukin 2 production without affecting rapidly dividing cells in the bone marrow, which may account for the reduced incidence of systemic posttransplantation infection. Unfortunately, cyclosporine causes dose-related renal tubular injury and direct renal artery vasospasm, which usually can be managed by reducing the dose. Other adverse effects of long-term cyclosporine use are hypertension, hyperkalemia, tremor, hirsutism, and hyperplasia of the gums. Because of these side effects, combinations of cyclosporine and prednisone or cyclosporine, prednisone, and azathioprine are preferable regimens for immunosuppressive treatment during the initial postoperative months. For long-term management, renal toxicity may make it necessary to reduce cyclosporine to very low doses. In many centers, cyclosporine treatment is initiated prior to or on the day of surgery and is continued by intravenous route through the operation and the immediate postoperative period until oral administration can be resumed.

Transplant rejection Despite the use of cyclosporine in various combinations, homograft rejection still occurs in the majority of patients 1 to 6 weeks after surgery. To date no clinically documented "hyperacute" rejections have been observed in humans although a reproducible animal model has now been developed. Early signs suggesting liver rejection are leukocytosis, increase in serum bilirubin level, and rise in aminotransferase and alkaline phosphatase activity; these may be followed by fever, tenderness in the right upper abdomen, diarrhea, ascites, and progressive deterioration of hepatic function. Because of the lack of specificity of these manifestations, differential diagnosis between homograft rejection, biliary obstruction, viral hepatitis, and recurrence of the original liver disease frequently is difficult. Radiographic visualization of the biliary tree and/or percutaneous liver biopsy often are helpful in establishing the correct diagnosis. Early morphologic features of rejection characteristically include portal infiltration with small lymphocytes and variable numbers of polymorphonuclear leukocytes, centrolobular bile stasis, selective injury to bile duct epithelium associated with polymorphonuclear infiltration, and, at times, endothelial inflammation of portal or central veins and occasionally of hepatic arterioles. These findings are similar to those in graft-versus-host disease and may be indistinguishable from those of primary biliary cirrhosis. As soon as transplant rejection is suspected, it is treated with intravenous methylprednisolone in repeated boluses; if this fails to reverse the rejection processes, many centers are also using antilymphocyte antibodies, either as polyclonal antilymphocyte globulin or the monoclonal agent OKT-3.

Chronic rejection is a relatively rare event that appears to be unrelated to the occurrence of preceding acute rejection episodes. It is associated with progressive cholestasis, bile duct proliferation, focal parenchymal necrosis, mononuclear infiltration, and fibrosis. These morphologic findings may be so similar to those of chronic viral hepatitis that differentiation between the two may be difficult. In some patients with therapy-resistant chronic rejection, retransplantation has yielded encouraging results.

REFERENCES

Busuttil RW, Moderator: Liver transplantation today. Ann Intern Med 104:377, 1986

Demetris AJ et al: Pathologic analysis of liver transplantation for primary biliary cirrhosis. Hepatology 8:939, 1988

Maddrey WC (ed): *Transplantation of the Liver*. New York, Elsevier, 1988

O'Grady TG, Williams R: Present position of liver transplantation and its impact on hepatologic practice. Gut 29:566, 1988

Polson RJ et al: Evidence for disease recurrence after liver transplantation for primary biliary cirrhosis. Clinical and histologic follow-up studies. Gastroenterology 97:7P5,1989

Scharschmidt BF: Human liver transplantation: An analysis of 819 patients from 8 centers, in *Recent Advances in Hepatology*, HC Thomas, EA Jones (eds). London, Churchill-Livingstone, 1985, vol 2

Starzl TE et al: Liver transplantation. N Engl J Med 321:1014, 1092, 1989

258 DISEASES OF THE GALLBLADDER AND BILE DUCTS

NORTON J. GREENBERGER / KURT J. ISSELBACHER

PHYSIOLOGY OF BILE PRODUCTION AND FLOW **Bile secretion and composition** Bile formed in the hepatic lobules is secreted into a complex network of canaliculi, small bile ductules, and larger bile ducts which run with lymphatics and branches of the portal vein and hepatic artery in portal tracts situated between hepatic lobules. These interlobular bile ducts coalesce to form larger septal bile ducts that join to form the right and left hepatic ducts, which in turn unite to form the common hepatic duct. The common hepatic duct is joined by the cystic duct of the gallbladder to form the common bile duct which enters the duodenum (often after joining the main pancreatic duct) through the ampulla of Vater.

Hepatic bile is a pigmented isotonic fluid with an electrolyte composition resembling blood plasma. The electrolyte composition of gallbladder bile differs from that of hepatic bile since most of the inorganic anions, chloride and bicarbonate, have been removed by reabsorption across the basement membrane.

Major components of bile by weight include water (82 percent), bile acids (12 percent), lecithin and other phospholipids (4 percent), and unesterified cholesterol (0.7 percent). Other constituents include conjugated bilirubin, proteins (IgA, by-products of hormones, and other proteins metabolized in the liver), electrolytes, mucus, and, often, drugs and their metabolic by-products.

The total daily basal secretion of hepatic bile is approximately 500 to 600 mL. The metabolic products of hepatocyte uptake and synthesis are secreted into the bile canaliculi, which are lined by microvillus membrane components associated with microfilaments of actin, microtubules, and other contractile elements. Within the hepatocyte, conjugation of many of the bile constituents may occur, while other components of bile such as primary bile acids, lecithin, and some cholesterol are synthesized de novo. Three mechanisms are important in regulating bile flow: (1) active transport of bile acids from hepatocytes into the canaliculi, (2) bile acid–independent ATPase-mediated transport of sodium, and (3) ductular secretion. The last is a secretin-mediated and cyclic AMP–dependent phenomenon which appears to result from the active transport of sodium and bicarbonate into the ductule with resulting passive movement of water across the cell membrane.

The bile acids The primary bile acids, cholic and chenodeoxycholic acids, are synthesized from cholesterol in the liver, conjugated with glycine or taurine, and excreted into the bile. Secondary bile acids, including deoxycholate and lithocholate, are formed in the colon as bacterial metabolites of the primary bile acids. However, lithocholic acid is much less efficiently absorbed from the colon than deoxycholic acid. Other secondary bile acids, found in trace amounts, which include ursodeoxycholic acid (a stereoisomer of chenodeoxycholate) and a variety of other unusual or "aberrant" bile acids, may be produced in increased amounts in patients with chronic cholestatic syndromes. In normal bile, the ratio of glycine to taurine conjugates is about 3:1, while in patients with cholestasis, increased concentrations of sulfate and glucuronide conjugates of bile acids are often found.

Bile acids are detergents which in aqueous solutions and above a critical concentration of about 2 m*M* form molecular aggregates called *micelles*. Cholesterol alone is poorly soluble in aqueous environments, and its solubility in bile depends upon both the lipid concentration and the relative molar percentages of bile acids and lecithin. Normal ratios of these constituents favor the formation of solubilizing "mixed micelles," while abnormal ratios promote the precipitation of cholesterol crystals in bile.

In addition to facilitating the biliary excretion of cholesterol, bile acids are necessary for the normal intestinal absorption of dietary fats via a micellar transport mechanism (see Chap. 240). Bile acids also serve as a major physiologic driving force for hepatic bile flow and aid in water and electrolyte transport in the small bowel and colon.

Enterohepatic circulation Bile acids are efficiently conserved under normal conditions. Conjugated and unconjugated bile acids are absorbed by *passive diffusion* along the entire gut. Quantitatively much more important for bile salt recirculation, however, is the *active transport* mechanism for conjugated bile acids in the distal ileum (see Chap. 240). The reabsorbed bile acids enter the portal bloodstream and are taken up rapidly by hepatocytes, reconjugated, and resecreted into bile (enterohepatic circulation).

The normal bile acid pool size is approximately 2 to 4 g. During digestion of a meal, the bile acid pool undergoes at least one or more enterohepatic cycles depending upon the size and composition of the meal. Normally the bile acid pool circulates approximately 5 to 10 times daily. Intestinal absorption of the pool is about 95 percent efficient, so that fecal loss of bile acids is in the range of 0.3 to 0.6 g/d. This fecal loss is compensated by an equal daily synthesis of bile acids by the liver, and thus the size of the bile salt pool is maintained. Bile acids returning to the liver suppress de novo hepatic synthesis of primary bile acids from cholesterol by inhibiting the rate-limiting enzyme 7α-hydroxylase. While the loss of bile salts in stool is usually matched by increased hepatic synthesis, the maximum rate of synthesis is approximately 5 g/d, which may be insufficient to replete the bile acid pool size when there is pronounced impairment of intestinal bile salt reabsorption.

Gallbladder and sphincteric functions In the fasting state, the sphincter of Oddi offers a high-pressure zone of resistance to bile flow from the common bile duct into the duodenum. This tonic contraction serves to (1) prevent reflux of duodenal contents into the pancreatic and bile ducts, and (2) promote bile filling of the gallbladder. The major factor controlling the evacuation of the gallbladder is the peptide hormone cholecystokinin, which is released from the duodenal mucosa in response to the ingestion of fats and amino acids. Cholecystokinin produces (1) powerful contraction of the gallbladder, (2) decreased resistance of the sphincter of Oddi, (3) increased hepatic secretion of bile, and thus (4) enhanced flow of biliary contents into the duodenum.

Hepatic bile is "concentrated" within the gallbladder by energy-dependent transmucosal absorption of water and electrolytes. Almost the entire bile acid pool may be sequestered in the gallbladder following an overnight fast for delivery into the duodenum with the first meal of the day. The normal capacity of the gallbladder is 30 to 75 mL of bile.

DISEASES OF THE GALLBLADDER

CONGENITAL ANOMALIES Anomalies of the biliary tract may be found in 10 to 20 percent of the population, including abnormalities in number, size, and shape (e.g., agenesis of the gallbladder, duplications, rudimentary or oversized ''giant'' gallbladders, and diverticula). Phrygian cap is a clinically innocuous entity in which a partial or complete septum (or fold) separates the fundus from the body. Anomalies of position or suspension are not uncommon and include left-sided gallbladder, intrahepatic gallbladder, retrodisplacement of the gallbladder, and ''floating'' gallbladder. The latter condition predisposes to acute torsion, volvulus, or herniation of the gallbladder.

GALLSTONES **Pathogenesis of gallstones** Gallstones are quite prevalent in most western countries. In the United States, autopsy series have shown gallstones in at least 20 percent of women and in 8 percent of men over the age of 40. It is estimated that 16 to 20 million persons in the United States have gallstones and that approximately 1 million new cases of cholelithiasis develop each year.

Gallstones are crystalline structures formed by concretion or accretion of normal or abnormal bile constituents. These stones are divided into three major types; cholesterol and mixed stones account for 80 percent of the total, with pigment stones comprising the remaining 20 percent. Mixed and cholesterol gallstones usually contain more than 70 percent cholesterol monohydrate plus an admixture of calcium salts, bile acids and bile pigments, proteins, fatty acids, and phospholipids. Pigment stones are primarily composed of calcium bilirubinate; they contain less than 10 percent cholesterol.

CHOLESTEROL AND MIXED STONES AND BILIARY SLUDGE Cholesterol is relatively water insoluble and requires aqueous dispersion into either micelles or vesicles, both of which require the presence of a second lipid to ''liquify'' the cholesterol. When the cholesterol content of bile exceeds the amount which can be solubilized by bile salt and bile salt–lecithin micelles, the excess is dispersed in larger lipid vesicles (Fig. 258-1). Vesicles are spherical particles composed of lecithin and cholesterol and contain only traces of bile salts. Vesicles and micelles are important cholesterol-solubilizing and -transport agents in bile supersaturated with cholesterol.

There are several important mechanisms in the formation of lithogenic (stone-forming) bile. The most important is increased biliary secretion of cholesterol. This may occur in association with obesity, high-caloric diets, or drugs (e.g., clofibrate) and may result from increased activity of hydroxymethylglutaryl-coenzyme A (HMG-CoA) reductase, the rate-limiting enzyme of hepatic cholesterol synthesis. In some patients, impaired hepatic conversion of cholesterol to bile acids may also occur, resulting in an increase of the lithogenic cholesterol/bile acid ratio. Lithogenic bile also results from decreased hepatic secretion of bile salts and phospholipids which may follow impaired hepatic synthesis (e.g., rare inborn errors of metabolism such as cerebrotendinous xanthomatosis) or conditions affecting the enterohepatic circulation of these constituents (e.g., prolonged parenteral alimentation or ileal disease or resection). In addition, most patients with gallstones appear to have reduced activity of hepatic cholesterol 7α-hydroxylase, the rate-limiting enzyme for primary bile acid synthesis.

A second important abnormality is defective vesicle formation because the vesicles have too little phospholipid and an excess of cholesterol. While cholesterol saturation of bile is an important prerequisite for gallstone formation, it is not sufficient by itself to produce cholesterol precipitation in vivo.

A third important mechanism is *nucleation* of cholesterol monohydrate crystals, which is greatly accelerated in human lithogenic bile; it is this feature rather than the degree of cholesterol supersaturation that distinguishes lithogenic from normal gallbladder bile. Accelerated nucleation of cholesterol monohydrate in bile may be due to either an *excess* of *pronucleating factors* or a *deficiency* of *antinucleating* factors. Nonmucin and mucin glycoproteins and lysine

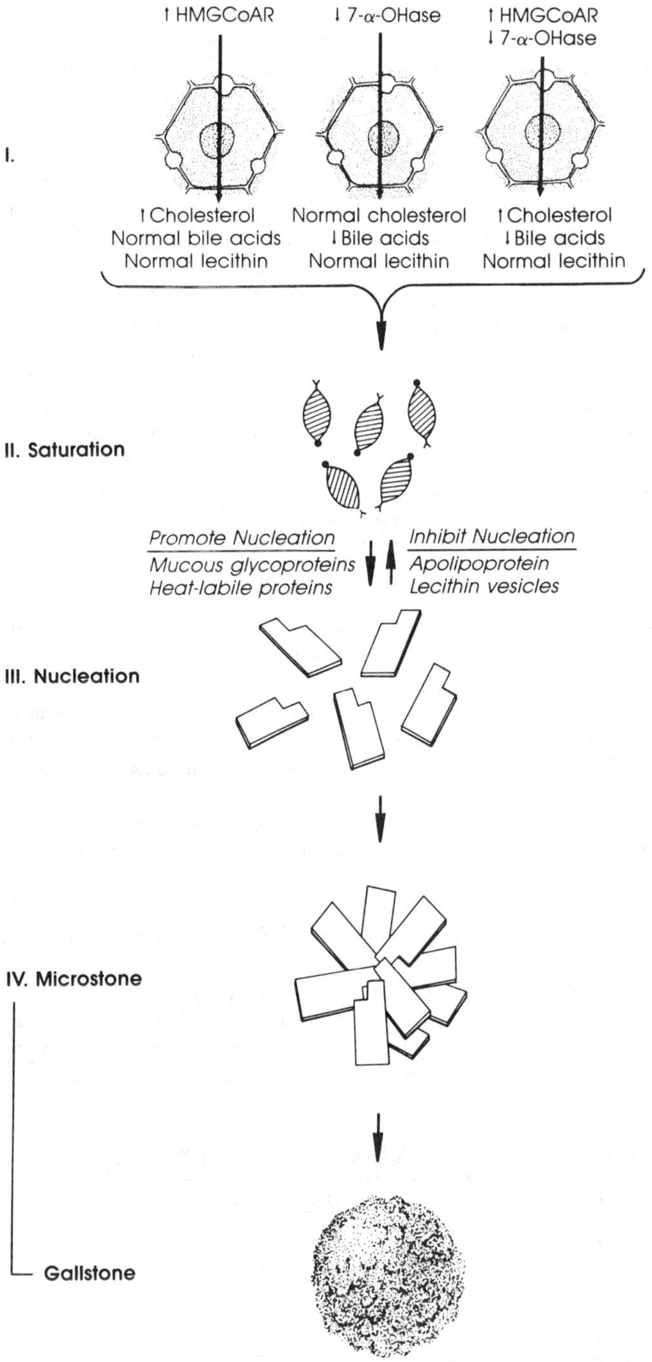

FIGURE 258-1 Scheme showing pathogenesis of gallstone formation. Conditions or factors that increase the ratio of cholesterol to bile acids and lecithin favor gallstone formation. (HMG CoAR = hydroxymethylglutaryl-coenzyme A reductase; 7-α-OHase = 7α-hydroxylase.)

phosphatidylcholine appear to be pronucleating factors while apolipoproteins AI and AII appear to be antinucleating factors. However, the characterization of additional pronucleating and antinucleating factors remains incomplete. Cholesterol monohydrate crystal nucleation and crystal growth probably occur within the mucin gel layer. Vesicle fusion leads to liquid crystals which in turn nucleate into solid cholesterol monohydrate crystals. Continued growth of the crystals occurs by direct nucleation of cholesterol molecules from supersaturated unilamellar biliary vesicles.

A fourth important mechanism in cholesterol gallstone formation concerns *biliary sludge*. Biliary sludge is a thick mucous material which upon microscopic examination reveals lecithin-cholesterol crystals, cholesterol monohydrate crystals, calcium bilirubinate, and mucin thread or mucous gels. Biliary sludge typically forms a crescentlike layer in the most dependent portion of the gallbladder and is recognized by characteristic echoes on ultrasonography (see below). In vitro, cholesterol monohydrate crystals (>50 μm) mixed with mucus produce echoes that are indistinguishable from gallbladder sludge observed in patients. The presence of biliary sludge implies two abnormalities: (1) the normal balance between gallbladder mucin secretion and elimination has become deranged; and (2) nucleation from biliary solutes has occurred. That biliary sludge is a precursor form of gallstone disease is evident from several observations. In one study, 96 patients with gallbladder sludge were followed prospectively by several ultrasound studies. In 17 patients (18 percent), biliary sludge disappeared and did not recur for at least two years. In 58 patients (60 percent), biliary sludge disappeared and reappeared. Importantly, gallstones developed in 14 patients in 8 of whom the gallstones were "silent." In 12 patients, cholecystectomies were performed, 6 for gallstone-associated biliary pain and 3 in symptomatic patients with sludge but without gallstones who had prior attacks of pancreatitis; the latter did not recur after cholecystectomy. It should be emphasized that biliary sludge can develop with disorders that cause gallbladder hypomotility, i.e., surgery, burns, total parenteral nutrition, pregnancy, and oral contraceptives—all of which are associated with gallstone formation. Finally, biliary sludge can account for the observation that most cholesterol gallstones have a pigmented center.

To summarize briefly, cholesterol gallstone disease occurs because of several defects which include: (1) bile supersaturation with cholesterol; (2) nucleation of cholesterol monohydrate with subsequent crystal retention and stone growth; and (3) abnormal gallbladder motor function with delayed emptying and stasis. Other important factors known to predispose to cholesterol stone formation are summarized in Table 258-1.

PIGMENT STONES Gallstones composed largely of calcium bilirubinate are much more common in the orient than in western countries. The presence of increased amounts of unconjugated, insoluble bilirubin in bile results in the precipitation of bilirubin which may aggregate to form pigment stones or may fuse to form the nidus for growth of mixed cholesterol gallstones. In western countries, chronic hemolytic states (with increased conjugated bilirubin in bile) or alcoholic liver disease are associated with an increased incidence of pigment stones. Deconjugation of soluble bilirubin mono- and diglucuronide may be mediated by the enzyme β-glucuronidase, which is sometimes produced when bile is chronically infected by bacteria. Pigment stone formation is especially prominent in Asians and is often associated with infections in the biliary tree (see Table 258-1).

TABLE 258-1 Predisposing factors for cholesterol and pigment gallstone formation

1 Cholesterol and mixed stones
 a Demography: northern Europe and North and South America greater than orient; probable familial, hereditary aspects
 b Obesity, high-calorie diet (↑ cholesterol output)
 c Clofibrate therapy (↑ cholesterol output)
 d Malabsorption of bile acids (e.g., ileal disease or resection) (↓ bile salt secretion)
 e Female sex hormones: women > men after puberty; oral contraceptives and other estrogens (↓ bile salt secretion)
 f Age, especially among males
 g Other factors: pregnancy, diabetes mellitus, dietary polyunsaturated fats (↑ cholesterol output)
 h Prolonged parenteral alimentation
2 Pigment stones
 a Demographic/genetic factors: orient, rural setting
 b Chronic hemolysis
 c Alcoholic cirrhosis
 d Chronic biliary tract infection, parasite infestation
 e Increasing age

Diagnosis of gallstones Procedures of potential use in the diagnosis of cholelithiasis and other diseases of the gallbladder are detailed in Table 258-2. The plain abdominal film may detect gallstones containing sufficient calcium to be radiopaque (10 to 15 percent of cholesterol and mixed stones and approximately 50 percent of pigment stones). Plain radiography may also be of use in the diagnosis of emphysematous cholecystitis, porcelain gallbladder, limey bile, and gallstone ileus.

Ultrasonography of the gallbladder is very accurate in the identification of cholelithiasis and has several advantages over oral cholecystography (see Fig. 258-2*A*). The gallbladder is easily visualized with the technique, and, in fact, failure to image the gallbladder

TABLE 258-2 Diagnostic evaluation of the gallbladder

Procedure	Diagnostic advantages	Diagnostic limitations	Comment
Plain abdominal x-ray	Low cost Readily available	Relatively low yield ?Contraindicated in pregnancy	Pathognomonic findings in: Calcified gallstones Limey bile, porcelain GB Emphysematous cholecystitis Gallstone ileus
Oral cholecystogram (OCG)	Low cost Readily available Accurate identification of gallstones (90–95%) Identification of GB anomalies, hyperplastic cholecystoses Identification of chronic GB disease after nonvisualization on double dose	?Contraindicated in pregnancy ?Contraindicated with history of reaction to iodinated contrast Nonvisualization with: Serum bilirubin >34–68 μmol/L (2–4 mg/dL) Failure to ingest or absorb tablets Impaired hepatic excretion Very small stones may be undetected More time-consuming than GBUS	A useful procedure in identification of gallstones if diagnostic limitations prevent GBUS
Gallbladder ultrasound (GBUS)	Rapid Accurate identification of gallstones (>95%) Simultaneous scanning of GB, liver, bile ducts, pancreas "Real-time" scanning allows assessment of GB volume, contractility Not limited by jaundice, pregnancy May detect very small stones	Bowel gas Massive obesity Ascites Recent barium study	Procedure of choice for detection of stones
Radioisotope scans (HIDA, DISIDA, etc.)	Accurate identification of cystic duct obstruction Simultaneous assessment of bile ducts	?Contraindicated in pregnancy Serum bilirubin >103–205 μmol/L (6–12 mg/dL) Cholecystogram of low resolution	Indicated for confirmation of suspected cholecystitis

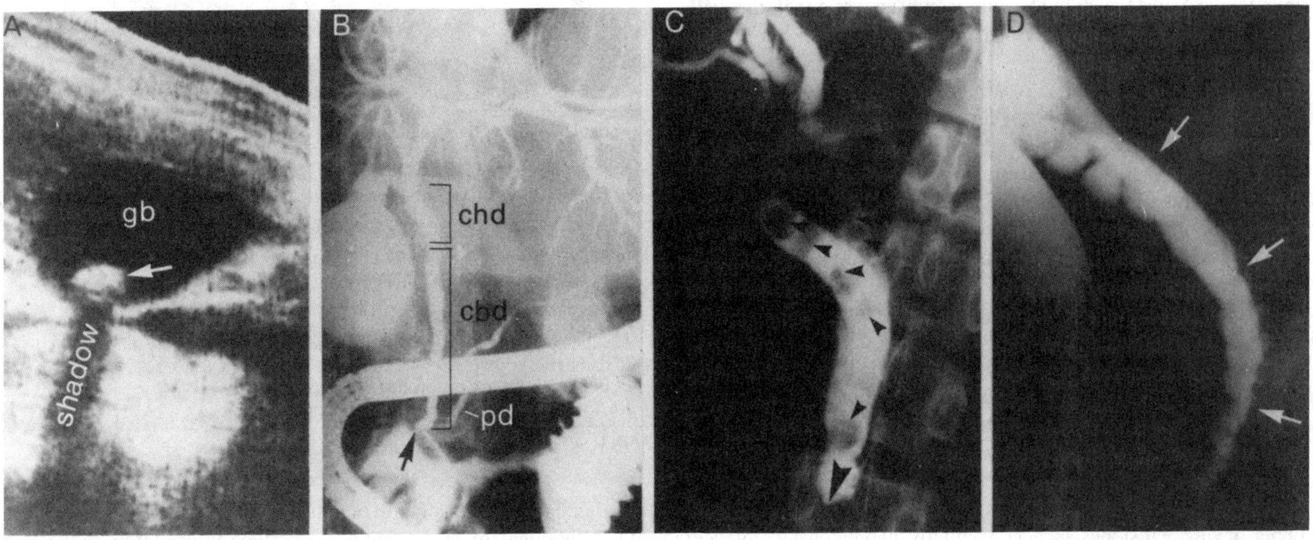

FIGURE 258-2 Examples of ultrasound and radiologic studies of the biliary tract. *A*. An ultrasound study showing a distended gallbladder containing a single large stone (arrow) which casts an acoustic shadow. *B*. Endoscopic retrograde cholangiopancreatogram (ERCP) showing normal biliary tract anatomy. In addition to the endoscope and large vertical gallbladder filled with contrast dye, the common hepatic duct (chd), common bile duct (cbd), and pancreatic duct (pd) are shown. The arrow points to the ampulla of Vater. *C*. Percutaneous transhepatic cholangiogram (PTHC) showing choledocholithiasis. The biliary tract is dilatated and contains multiple radiolucent calculi (small arrows). The dilatation is due to obstruction by a large stone in the distal portion of the duct (large arrow). *D*. ERCP showing sclerosing cholangitis. The common bile duct is to the right of the endoscope. Following retrograde cholangiography, the common bile duct shows thickening of the wall with a narrow, beaded lumen typical of sclerosing cholangitis.

successfully in a fasting patient correlates well with the presence of underlying gallbladder disease. Stones as small as 2 mm in diameter may be confidently identified provided that firm criteria are used [e.g., acoustic ''shadowing'' of opacities that are within the gallbladder lumen and that change with the patient's position (by gravity)]. In major medical centers the false-negative and false-positive rates for ultrasound in gallstone patients are about 2 to 4 percent. Biliary sludge is material of low echogenic activity that typically forms a layer in the most dependent position of the gallbladder. This layer shifts with postural changes but fails to produce acoustic shadowing; these two characteristics distinguish sludges from gallstones.

Oral cholecystography (OCG) is a useful procedure for the diagnosis of gallstones but has been largely replaced by ultrasound. False-positive results are rare, but the oral cholecystogram may be falsely negative (when good opacification is achieved) in approximately 5 to 10 percent of patients with gallstones. Factors which may produce nonvisualization of the OCG are summarized in Table 258-2. When these can be excluded, nonvisualization of the gallbladder following a second dose of oral contrast agent is highly correlated with underlying cystic duct obstruction or chronic inflammation of the gallbladder.

Radiopharmaceuticals such as ^{99m}Tc-labeled *N*-substituted iminodiacetic acids (HIDA, DIDA, DISIDA, etc.) are rapidly extracted from the blood and are excreted into the biliary tree in high concentration even in the presence of mild to moderate serum bilirubin elevations. Failure to image the gallbladder in the presence of biliary ductal visualization may indicate cystic duct obstruction, acute or chronic cholecystitis, or surgical absence of the organ. Such scans have their greatest application in the diagnosis of acute cholecystitis.

Symptoms of gallstone disease Gallstones usually produce symptoms by causing inflammation or obstruction following their migration into the cystic duct or common bile duct. The most specific and characteristic symptom of gallstone disease is biliary colic. Obstruction of the cystic duct or common bile duct by a stone produces increased intraluminal pressure and distention of the viscus which cannot be relieved by repetitive biliary contractions. The resultant visceral pain is characteristically a severe, steady aching or pressure in the epigastrium or right upper quadrant of the abdomen with frequent radiation to the interscapular area, right scapula, or shoulder.

Biliary colic begins quite suddenly and may persist with severe intensity for 1 to 4 h, subsiding gradually or rapidly. An episode of biliary pain is sometimes followed by a residual mild ache or soreness in the right upper quadrant which may persist for 24 h or so. Nausea and vomiting frequently accompany episodes of biliary colic, and mild elevations of serum bilirubin [not exceeding 85.5 μmol/L (5 mg/dL)] occur in 25 percent of patients. Persistence of a high serum bilirubin level suggests common duct stones. Fever or chills (rigors) with biliary colic usually imply an underlying complication, i.e., cholecystitis, pancreatitis, or cholangitis. Complaints of vague epigastric fullness, dyspepsia, eructation, or flatulence, especially following a fatty meal, should not be confused with biliary colic. Such symptoms are frequently elicited from patients with gallstone disease but are not specific for biliary calculi. Biliary colic may be precipitated by eating a fatty meal, by consumption of a large meal following a period of prolonged fasting, or by eating a normal meal.

Natural history of gallstones Gallstone disease discovered in an asymptomatic patient or in a patient whose symptoms are not referable to cholelithiasis is a common clinical problem. The natural history of ''silent'' or asymptomatic gallstones has occasioned much debate. In contrast to previous reports, a study of predominantly male silent gallstone patients suggests that the cumulative risk for the development of symptoms or complications requiring surgery is relatively low—10 percent at 5 years, 15 percent at 10 years, and 18 percent at 15 years. Patients remaining asymptomatic for 15 years were found to be unlikely to develop symptoms during further follow-up, and most patients who did develop complications from their gallstones experienced *prior* warning symptoms. Similar conclusions apply to diabetics with silent gallstones. Decision analysis has suggested that (1) the cumulative risk of death due to gallstone disease while on expectant management is small; and (2) prophylactic cholecystectomy is not warranted.

Complications requiring cholecystectomy appear to be much more common in gallstone patients who have developed symptoms of biliary colic. Patients found to have gallstones at a young age are more likely to develop symptoms from cholelithiasis than are patients older than 60 years at the time of initial diagnosis. Patients with diabetes mellitus and gallstones may be somewhat more susceptible to septic complications, but the magnitude of risk of septic biliary complications in diabetic patients is incompletely defined. In addition, asymptomatic gallstone patients with nonvisualization of the gallbladder on OCG appear to have an increased tendency to develop symptoms and complications.

Treatment of gallstones SURGICAL THERAPY Although the management of silent gallstones remains controversial, the risk of developing symptoms or complications requiring surgery is quite small (in the range of 1 to 2 percent per year) in most asymptomatic gallstone patients. Thus, a recommendation for prophylactic cholecystectomy in a patient with gallstones should probably be based on assessment of three factors: (1) the presence of symptoms which are frequent enough or severe enough to interfere with the patient's general routine; (2) the presence of a prior complication of gallstone disease, i.e., history of acute cholecystitis, pancreatitis, gallstone fistula, etc.; or (3) the presence of an underlying condition predisposing the patient to increased risk of gallstone complications (e.g., calcified or porcelain gallbladder, cholesterolosis, adenomyomatosis, nonvisualizing gallbladder on oral cholecystography, and/or a previous attack of acute cholecystitis regardless of current symptomatic status). Patients with very large gallstones (over 2 cm in diameter) and patients having gallstones in a congenitally anomalous gallbladder might also be considered for prophylactic cholecystectomy. Although age under 50 years is a worrisome factor in asymptomatic gallstone patients, few authorities would now recommend routine cholecystectomy in all young patients with silent stones.

MEDICAL THERAPY—GALLSTONE DISSOLUTION Treatment with oral chenodeoxycholic acid (CDCA, chenic acid) or its 7β-epimer, ursodeoxycholic acid (UDCA), to dissolve cholesterol or mixed gallstones has resulted in complete or partial dissolution of such stones in approximately 50 to 60 percent of patients with radiolucent gallstones. Biliary secretion of these agents following oral bile acid administration alters the bile acid/cholesterol/lecithin ratio in bile (the lithogenic index). The major therapeutic effect of CDCA, however, is thought to be secondary to a decrease in HMG-CoA reductase activity, which in turn results in decreased hepatic cholesterol synthesis. UDCA administration appears to produce a lamellar liquid crystalline phase in bile which allows dispersion of cholesterol from stones by physical-chemical means.

Oral bile acid therapy is essentially ineffective in dissolving (1) pigment gallstones, which represent approximately 20 percent of radiolucent stones; (2) radiopaque or calcified gallstones; (3) gallstones greater than approximately 1.5 cm in diameter; and (4) gallstones in gallbladders poorly opacified following oral cholecystography. In patients with multiple, small, radiolucent gallstones in a functioning gallbladder, success rates for CDCA therapy of up to 80 percent have been reported if daily doses of 10 to 15 mg/kg of CDCA are used over a 1- to 3-year treatment period. However, lower daily doses of CDCA, i.e., 5 to 10 mg/kg, have resulted in much lower complete dissolution (5 to 15 percent) as well as lower partial dissolution rates (40 percent). Further, some massively obese patients may require doses as high as 20 to 25 mg/kg per day of CDCA to achieve cholesterol desaturation of bile. Ultrasound appears to be more sensitive than oral cholecystography in following patients during and after stone dissolution therapy (Table 258-3).

Chenodeoxycholic acid therapy is usually associated with self-limited diarrhea in most patients given an optimal therapeutic dose. In addition, approximately 25 percent of patients treated with CDCA acid develop mild (two- to threefold) and transient (less than 6 months) elevations of serum aminotransferase levels. Although hepatic injury has been described, biopsy and liver function studies in humans have shown serious CDCA-related hepatotoxicity in less than 1 to 2 percent of patients.

Ursodeoxycholic acid is therapeutically effective at lower doses (5 to 10 mg/kg per day) than chenodeoxycholic acid and has not been associated with the relatively high incidence of diarrhea and serum aminotransferase elevations seen in CDCA-treated patients. On the other hand, UDCA treatment has been associated with calcification of previously uncalcified gallstones in more than 10 percent of patients.

TABLE 258-3 Chenodeoxycholic acid (CDCA) and gallstone dissolution

RESULTS OF U.S. NATIONAL COOPERATIVE GALLSTONE STUDY

1 Patients—916 with radiolucent stones, treated 24 months
- *a* Placebo
- *b* Low-dose CDCA; 375 mg per day
- *c* High-dose CDCA; 750 mg per day

2 Results—best with high dose
- *a* Complete dissolution, 13.5%
- *b* Partial dissolution, 27.3%; complete plus partial, 40.8%
- *c* Best results—women, thin patients, small stones

3 Side effects
- *a* Mild diarrhea
- *b* Changes in hepatic structure, function; 3% clinically significant liver damage
- *c* Elevation (10%) of serum LDL cholesterol

4 Recurrence—likely when CDCA stopped

SOURCE: *Schoenfield et al.*

After complete dissolution of gallstones by either CDCA or UDCA and withdrawal of such treatment, current information suggests a recurrence rate of 30 to 55 percent over 3 to 12 years of follow-up. There appears to be an approximately linear increase in gallstone recurrence of 10 to 15 percent per annum over the first 3 to 5 years after which there may be a plateau with no further recurrence. The recurrence rate is lower in patients who had a single gallstone compared to those with multiple stones. In clinical trials designed to prevent recurrences, UDCA in doses of 3 mg/kg or 200 to 300 mg/d may delay and/or reduce recurrence.

Direct dissolution of gallstones within a period of hours using methyl tertiary butyl ether or other solvents through percutaneously placed biliary catheters has also been reported. Such solvent dissolution of gallbladder or ductal stones by continuous perfusion appears promising.

GALLSTONE LITHOTRIPSY Electrohydraulic extracorporeal shock wave lithotripsy, combined with medical litholytic therapy, is a safe and effective treatment in selected patients with radiolucent gallbladder calculi. The usual criteria for selection of patients include: (1) history of biliary colic; (2) radiolucent stones; (3) gallbladder visualization by oral cholecystography; (4) 1 to 4 stones with the diameter of the largest <30 mm; and (5) absence of acute cholecystitis, cholangitis, biliary obstruction, acute pancreatitis, and pregnancy. Approximately 30 percent of patients referred for lithotripsy meet the selection criteria. In one study of 175 patients, gallstones disintegrated in all but one patient; with concurrent litholytic therapy (oral CDCA and UDCA) gallstones completely disappeared in 30 percent of the patients at 2 months, 48 percent at 2 to 4 months, 63 percent at 4 to 8 months, 78 percent at 8 to 12 months, and 91 percent at 12 to 18 months. Side effects include biliary colic (35 percent), cutaneous petechiae (14 percent), transient hematuria (37 percent), and pancreatitis (1.5 percent). Important issues to be addressed with future studies are: (1) What is the recurrence rate after complete disappearance of stones? (2) Is lithotripsy effective in patients with calcified stones? (3) What is the efficacy of other types of lithotripters i.e., ultrasound waves generated by piezoelectric devices?

ACUTE AND CHRONIC CHOLECYSTITIS Acute cholecystitis Acute inflammation of the gallbladder wall usually follows obstruction of the cystic duct by a stone. Inflammatory response can be evoked by three factors: (1) *mechanical inflammation* produced by increased intraluminal pressure and distention with resulting ischemia of the gallbladder mucosa and wall; (2) *chemical inflammation* caused by the release of lysolecithin (due to the action of phospholipase on lecithin in bile) and other local tissue factors; and (3) *bacterial inflammation,* which may play a role in 50 to 85 percent of patients with acute cholecystitis. The organisms most frequently isolated by culture of gallbladder bile in these patients include *Escherichia coli, Klebsiella* species, group D *Streptococcus, Staphylococcus* species, and *Clostridium* species.

Acute cholecystitis often begins as an attack of biliary colic which progressively worsens. Approximately 60 to 70 percent of patients report having experienced prior attacks which resolved spontaneously. As the episode progresses, however, the pain of acute cholecystitis becomes more generalized in the right upper abdomen. As with biliary colic, the pain of cholecystitis may radiate to the interscapular area, right scapula, or shoulder. Peritoneal signs of inflammation such as increased pain with jarring or on deep respiration may be apparent. The patient is anorectic and often nauseated. Vomiting is relatively common and may produce symptoms and signs of vascular and extracellular volume depletion. Jaundice is unusual early in the course of acute cholecystitis but may occur when edematous inflammatory changes involve the bile ducts and surrounding lymph nodes.

A low-grade fever is characteristically present, but shaking chills or rigors are not uncommon. The right upper quadrant of the abdomen is almost invariably tender to palpation. An enlarged, tense gallbladder is palpable in one-quarter to one-half of patients. Deep inspiration or cough during subcostal palpation of the right upper quadrant usually produces increased pain and inspiratory arrest (Murphy's sign). A light blow delivered to the right subcostal area may elicit a marked increase in pain. Localized rebound tenderness in the right upper quadrant is common, as are abdominal distention and hypoactive bowel sounds from paralytic ileus, but generalized peritoneal signs and abdominal rigidity are usually lacking, absent perforation.

The diagnosis of acute cholecystitis is usually made on the basis of a characteristic history and physical examination. The triad of sudden onset of right upper quadrant tenderness, fever, and leukocytosis is highly suggestive. Typically, leukocytosis in the range of 10,000 to 15,000 cells per microliter with a left shift on differential count is found. The serum bilirubin is mildly elevated [(less than 85.5 μmol/L (5 mg/dL)] in 45 percent of patients, while 25 percent have modest elevations in serum aminotransferases (usually less than a fivefold elevation). The radionuclide (e.g., HIDA) biliary scan may be confirmatory if bile duct imaging is seen without visualization of the gallbladder. Ultrasound will demonstrate calculi in 90 to 95 percent of cases.

Approximately 75 percent of patients treated medically have remission of acute symptoms within 2 to 7 days following hospitalization. In 25 percent, however, a complication of acute cholecystitis will occur despite conservative treatment (see below). In this setting, prompt surgical intervention is required. Of the 75 percent of patients with acute cholecystitis who undergo remission of symptoms, approximately one-quarter will experience a recurrence of cholecystitis within 1 year, and 60 percent will have at least one recurrent bout within 6 years. In view of the natural history of the disease, acute cholecystitis is best treated by early surgery whenever possible.

ACALCULOUS CHOLECYSTITIS In 5 to 10 percent of patients with acute cholecystitis, calculi obstructing the cystic duct are not found at surgery. In over 50 percent of such cases an underlying explanation for acalculous inflammation is not found. An increased risk for the development of acalculous cholecystitis is especially associated with serious trauma or burns, with the postpartum period following prolonged labor, and with orthopedic and other nonbiliary major surgical operations in the postoperative period. Other precipitating factors include vasculitis, obstructing adenocarcinoma of the gallbladder, diabetes mellitus, torsion of the gallbladder, "unusual" bacterial infections of the gallbladder (e.g., *Leptospira, Streptococcus, Salmonella,* or *Vibrio cholerae*), and parasitic infestation of the gallbladder. Acalculous cholecystitis may also be seen with a variety of other systemic disease processes (sarcoidosis, cardiovascular disease, tuberculosis, syphilis, actinomycosis, etc.) and may possibly complicate periods of prolonged parenteral hyperalimentation.

Although the clinical manifestations of acalculous cholecystitis are indistinguishable from those of calculous cholecystitis, the setting of acute gallbladder inflammation complicating severe underlying illness is characteristic of acalculous disease. Ultrasound, CT scanning, or radionuclide examinations demonstrating a large, tense, static gallbladder without stones and with evidence of poor emptying over a prolonged period may be diagnostically useful in some cases. The complication rate for acalculous cholecystitis exceeds that for calculous cholecystitis. Successful management of acute acalculous cholecystitis appears to depend primarily upon early diagnosis and surgical intervention with meticulous attention to postoperative care.

EMPHYSEMATOUS CHOLECYSTITIS So-called emphysematous cholecystitis is thought to begin with acute cholecystitis (calculous or acalculous) followed by ischemia or gangrene of the gallbladder wall and infection by gas-producing organisms. Bacteria most frequently cultured in this setting include anaerobes such as *Clostridium welchii,* or *perfringens,* and aerobes such as *E. coli.* This condition occurs most frequently in elderly men and in patients with diabetes mellitus. The clinical manifestations are essentially indistinguishable from those of nongaseous cholecystitis. The diagnosis is usually made on plain abdominal film by the finding of gas within the gallbladder lumen, dissecting within the gallbladder wall to form a gaseous ring, or in the pericholecystic tissues. The morbidity and mortality rates with emphysematous cholecystitis are considerable. Prompt surgical intervention coupled with appropriate antibiotics is mandatory.

Chronic cholecystitis Chronic inflammation of the gallbladder wall is almost always associated with the presence of gallstones and is thought to result from repeated bouts of subacute or acute cholecystitis or from persistent mechanical irritation of the gallbladder wall. The presence of bacteria in the bile occurs in more than one-quarter of patients with chronic cholecystitis. Although the presence of infected bile in a patient with *chronic* cholecystitis undergoing elective cholecystectomy probably adds little to the operative risk, intraoperative Gram's staining and routine culturing of bile has been advocated to identify those patients whose gallbladder is colonized with *Clostridium* species. Appropriate antibiotics intra- and postoperatively are recommended in such patients because colonization with these organisms may be associated with devastating septic complications following surgery. Chronic cholecystitis may be asymptomatic for years, may progress to symptomatic gallbladder disease or to acute cholecystitis, or may present with complications (see below).

Complications of cholecystitis EMPYEMA AND HYDROPS Empyema of the gallbladder usually results from progression of acute cholecystitis with persistent cystic duct obstruction to superinfection of the stagnant bile with a pus-forming bacterial organism. The clinical picture resembles that of cholangitis with high fever, severe right upper quadrant pain, marked leukocytosis, and, often, prostration. Empyema of the gallbladder carries a high risk of gram-negative sepsis and/or perforation. Emergency surgical intervention with proper antibiotic coverage is required as soon as the diagnosis is suspected.

Hydrops or mucocele of the gallbladder may also result from prolonged obstruction of the cystic duct, usually by a large solitary calculus. In this instance, the obstructed gallbladder lumen is progressively distended, over a period of time, by mucus (mucocele) or by a clear transudate (hydrops) produced by mucosal epithelial cells. A visible, easily palpable, nontender mass often extending from the right upper quadrant into the right iliac fossa may be found on physical examination. The patient with hydrops of the gallbladder frequently remains asymptomatic, although chronic right upper quadrant pain also may occur. Cholecystectomy is indicated since empyema, perforation, or gangrene may complicate the condition.

GANGRENE AND PERFORATION Gangrene of the gallbladder results from ischemia of the wall and patchy or complete tissue necrosis. Underlying conditions often include marked distention of the gallbladder, vasculitis, diabetes mellitus, empyema, or torsion resulting in arterial occlusion. Gangrene usually predisposes to perforation of the gallbladder, but perforation may also occur in chronic cholecystitis without premonitory warning symptoms. *Localized perforations* are usually contained by the omentum or by adhesions produced by recurrent inflammation of the gallbladder. Bacterial superinfection of the walled-off gallbladder contents results in abscess formation. Most patients are best treated with cholecystectomy, but some seriously ill patients may be managed with cholecystostomy and drainage of the abscess. *Free perforation* is less common but is associated with a mortality rate of approximately 30 percent. Such patients may experience a sudden transient relief of right upper quadrant pain as the distended gallbladder decompresses; this is followed by signs of generalized peritonitis.

FISTULA FORMATION AND GALLSTONE ILEUS *Fistulization* into an adjacent organ adherent to the gallbladder wall may result from inflammation and adhesion formation. Fistulas into the duodenum are most common, followed in frequency by those involving the hepatic flexure of the colon, stomach or jejunum, abdominal wall, and renal pelvis. Clinically "silent" biliary-enteric fistulas occurring as a complication of chronic cholecystitis have been found in up to 5 percent of patients undergoing cholecystectomy. Asymptomatic cholecystoenteric fistulas may sometimes be diagnosed by finding gas in the biliary tree on plain abdominal films. Barium contrast studies or endoscopy of the upper gastrointestinal tract or colon may demonstrate the fistula, but oral cholecystography will almost never result in opacification of either the gallbladder or the fistulous tract. Treatment in the symptomatic patient usually consists of cholecystectomy, common bile duct exploration, and closure of the fistulous tract.

Gallstone ileus refers to mechanical intestinal obstruction resulting from the passage of a large gallstone into the bowel lumen. The stone customarily enters the duodenum through a cholecystoenteric fistula at that level. The site of obstruction by the impacted gallstone is usually at the ileocecal valve, provided that the more proximal small bowel is of normal caliber. The majority of patients do not give a history of either prior biliary tract symptoms or complaints suggestive of acute cholecystitis or fistulization. Large stones over 2.5 cm in diameter are thought to predispose to fistula formation by gradual erosion through the gallbladder fundus. Diagnostic confirmation may occasionally be found on the plain abdominal film (e.g., small-intestinal obstruction with gas in the biliary tree and a calcified, ectopic gallstone) or following an upper gastrointestinal series (cholecystoduodenal fistula with small-bowel obstruction at the ileocecal valve). Early laparotomy is indicated with enterolithotomy and careful palpation of the more proximal small bowel and gallbladder to exclude other stones.

LIMEY (MILK OF CALCIUM) BILE AND PORCELAIN GALLBLADDER Calcium salts may be secreted into the lumen of the gallbladder in sufficient concentration to produce calcium precipitation and diffuse, hazy opacification of bile or a layering effect on plain abdominal roentgenography. This so-called limey bile or milk of calcium bile is usually clinically innocuous, but cholecystectomy is recommended since limey bile most often occurs in an hydropic gallbladder. In the entity called porcelain gallbladder, calcium salt deposition within the wall of a chronically inflamed gallbladder may be detected on the plain abdominal film. Cholecystectomy is advised in all patients with porcelain gallbladder since in a high percentage of cases this finding appears to be associated with the development of carcinoma of the gallbladder.

Treatment of cholecystitis MEDICAL THERAPY Although surgical intervention remains the mainstay of therapy for acute cholecystitis and its complications, a period of in-hospital stabilization may be required before cholecystectomy. Oral intake is eliminated, nasogastric suction is initiated, and extracellular volume depletion and electrolyte abnormalities are repaired. Meperidine or pentazocine are usually employed for analgesia since they may produce less spasm of the sphincter of Oddi than drugs such as morphine. Intravenous antibiotic therapy is usually indicated in patients with severe acute cholecystitis even though bacterial superinfection of bile may not have occurred in the early stages of the inflammatory process. Postoperative complications of wound infection, abscess formation, or sepsis are reduced in antibiotic-treated patients. Effective single-agent antibiotics include ampicillin, cephalosporins, chloramphenicol, or aminoglycosides, but in diabetic or debilitated patients and in those with signs of gram-negative sepsis, combination antibiotic treatment may be preferable (see also Chap. 83).

SURGICAL THERAPY The optimal timing of surgical intervention in patients with acute cholecystitis remains controversial. Urgent (emergency) cholecystectomy or cholecystostomy is probably appropriate in most patients in whom a complication of acute cholecystitis such as empyema, emphysematous cholecystitis, or perforation is suspected or confirmed. In uncomplicated cases of acute cholecystitis up to 30 percent of patients fail to resolve their symptoms on appropriate medical therapy, and progression of the attack or a supervening complication leads to the performance of early operation (within 24 to 72 h). The technical complications of surgery are not increased in patients undergoing early as opposed to delayed cholecystectomy. Delayed surgical intervention is probably best reserved for (1) patients in whom the overall medical condition imposes an unacceptable risk for early surgery, and (2) cases in which the diagnosis of acute cholecystitis is in doubt. Early cholecystectomy is the treatment of choice for most patients with acute cholecystitis. Mortality figures for emergency cholecystectomy in most centers approach 3 percent, while the mortality risk for elective or early cholecystectomy approximates 0.5 percent in patients under age 60. Of course, the operative risks increase with age-related diseases of other organ systems and with the presence of long-term or short-term complications of gallbladder disease. Seriously ill or debilitated patients with cholecystitis may be managed with cholecystostomy and tube drainage of the gallbladder. Elective cholecystectomy may then be done at a later date.

Postcholecystectomy complications Early complications following cholecystectomy include atelectasis and other pulmonary disorders, abscess formation (often subphrenic), external or internal hemorrhage, biliary-enteric fistula, and bile leaks. Jaundice may indicate absorption of bile from an intraabdominal collection following a biliary leak, or mechanical obstruction of the common bile duct by retained calculi, intraductal blood clots, or extrinsic compression. Routine performance of intraoperative cholangiography during cholecystectomy has helped to reduce the incidence of these early complications.

Overall, cholecystectomy is a very successful operation which provides total or near-total relief of presurgical symptoms in 75 to 90 percent of patients. The most common cause of persistent postcholecystectomy symptoms is an overlooked extrabiliary disorder (e.g., reflux esophagitis, peptic ulceration, postgastrectomy syndrome, pancreatitis, or irritable bowel syndrome). In a small percentage of patients, however, a disorder of the extrahepatic bile ducts may result in persistent symptomatology. These so-called postcholecystectomy syndromes may be due to (1) biliary strictures, (2) retained biliary calculi, (3) cystic duct stump syndrome, (4) stenosis or dyskinesia of the sphincter of Oddi, or (5) bile salt–induced diarrhea or gastritis.

CYSTIC DUCT STUMP SYNDROME In the absence of cholangiographically demonstrable retained stones, symptoms resembling biliary colic or cholecystitis in the postcholecystectomy patient have frequently been attributed to disease in a long (>1 cm) cystic duct remnant (cystic duct stump syndrome). Careful analysis, however, reveals that postcholecystectomy complaints are attributable to other causes in almost all patients in whom the symptom complex was originally thought to result from the existence of a long cystic duct stump. Accordingly, considerable care should be taken to investigate the possible role of other factors in the production of postcholecystectomy symptoms before attributing them to cystic duct stump syndrome.

PAPILLARY DYSFUNCTION, PAPILLARY STENOSIS, SPASM OF THE SPHINCTER OF ODDI, AND BILIARY DYSKINESIA Symptoms of biliary colic accompanied by signs of recurrent, intermittent biliary obstruction may be produced by papillary stenosis, papillary dysfunction, spasm of the sphincter of Oddi, and biliary dyskinesia. Papillary stenosis is thought to result from acute or chronic inflammation of the papilla of Vater or from glandular hyperplasia of the papillary segment. Five criteria have been used to define papillary stenosis: (1) upper abdominal pain, usually right upper quadrant or epigastric; (2) abnormal liver tests; (3) dilatation of the common bile duct upon endoscopic retrograde cholangiopancreatogram (ERCP) examination;

(4) delayed (longer than 45 min) drainage of contrast material from the duct; and (5) increased basal pressure of the sphincter of Oddi, a finding that may be of only minor significance. A useful alternative to ERCP is hepatobiliary scintigraphy using ^{99m}Tc-diisopropyl iminodiacetic acid, especially if ERCP and/or biliary manometry are either unavailable or not feasible. In patients with papillary stenosis, quantitative hepatobiliary scintigraphy has revealed delayed transit from the common bile duct to the bowel, ductal dilatation, and abnormal time-activity dynamics. This technique can also be used before and after sphincterotomy to document improvement in biliary emptying. Treatment consists of endoscopic or surgical sphincteroplasty to ensure wide patency of the distal portions of both the bile and pancreatic ducts. The greater the number of the above criteria present, the greater the likelihood that a patient does have a degree of papillary stenosis sufficient to justify correction. The factors usually considered as indications for sphincterotomy include: (1) prolonged duration of symptoms; (2) lack of response to symptomatic treatment; (3) presence of severe disability; and (4) the patient's choice of sphincterotomy over surgery (given a clear understanding on his or her part of the risks involved in both procedures).

Criteria for diagnosing dyskinesia of the sphincter of Oddi are even more controversial than those for papillary stenosis. Proposed mechanisms include spasm of the sphincter, denervation sensitivity resulting in hypertonicity, and abnormalities of the sequencing or frequency rates of sphincteric contraction waves. When thorough evaluation has failed to demonstrate another cause for the pain, and when cholangiographic and manometric criteria suggest a diagnosis of biliary dyskinesia, medical treatment with nitrites or anticholinergics to attempt pharmacologic relaxation of the sphincter has been proposed. Endoscopic sphincterotomy or surgical sphincteroplasty may be indicated in patients who fail to respond to a 2 to 3 month trial of medical therapy, especially if basal sphincter of Oddi pressures are elevated.

BILE SALT–INDUCED CATHARSIS AND GASTRITIS Postcholecystectomy patients may develop symptoms and signs of gastritis, which has been attributed to duodenogastric reflux of bile. However, firm data linking an increased incidence of bile gastritis with surgical removal of the gallbladder are lacking. Similarly, the occurrence of cholestyramine-responsive diarrhea in a small number of patients following cholecystectomy has been attributed to an alteration of the enterohepatic circulation of bile acids induced or unmasked by removal of the gallbladder.

THE HYPERPLASTIC CHOLECYSTOSES The term *hyperplastic cholecystoses* is used to denote a group of disorders of the gallbladder characterized by excessive proliferation of normal tissue components.

Adenomyomatosis is characterized by a benign proliferation of gallbladder surface epithelium with gland-like formations, extramural sinuses, transverse strictures, and/or fundal nodule (''adenoma'' or ''adenomyoma'') formation. Outpouchings of mucosa termed Rokitansky-Aschoff sinuses may be seen on oral cholecystography in conjunction with hyperconcentration of contrast medium. Characteristic dimpled filling defects may also be seen.

Cholesterolosis is characterized by abnormal deposition of lipid, especially cholesterol esters, in the lamina propria of the gallbladder wall. In its diffuse form (''strawberry gallbladder''), the gallbladder mucosa is brick red and speckled with bright yellow flecks of lipid. The localized form shows solitary or multiple ''cholesterol polyps'' studding the gallbladder wall. Cholesterol stones of the gallbladder are found in nearly half the cases. Cholecystectomy is indicated in both adenomyomatosis and cholesterolosis when symptomatic or when cholelithiasis is present.

CANCER OF THE GALLBLADDER Most cancers of the gallbladder develop in conjunction with stones rather than polyps. In patients with gallstones, the risk for developing gallbladder cancer, while increased, is still quite low. In one study, gallbladder cancer developed in only 5 of 2583 patients with gallstones followed for a median of 13 years. In the United States, adenocarcinomas comprise the vast majority of the estimated 6500 new cases of gallbladder cancer diagnosed each year. The female/male ratio is 4:1 and the mean age at diagnosis is approximately 70 years. The clinical presentation is most often one of unremitting right upper quadrant pain associated with weight loss, jaundice, and a palpable right upper quadrant mass. Cholangitis may supervene. The gallbladder is rarely visualized on OCG, and preoperative diagnosis of the condition is rare. Once symptoms have appeared, spread of the tumor outside the gallbladder by direct extension or by lymphatic or hematogenous routes is almost invariable. Over 75 percent of gallbladder carcinomas are unresectable at the time of surgery, the exceptions being tumors discovered incidentally at laparotomy. The 1-year mortality rate for unresectable disease is approximately 95 percent, and only 5 percent of patients survive 5 years or more from the time of diagnosis. Radical operative resection does not appear to improve survival. Results of trials with radiation and chemotherapy of primary gallbladder cancer have also been disappointing.

DISEASES OF THE BILE DUCTS

CONGENITAL ANOMALIES Biliary atresia and hypoplasia Atretic and hypoplastic lesions of the extrahepatic and major intrahepatic bile ducts are the most common biliary anomalies of clinical relevance encountered in infancy. The clinical picture is one of severe obstructive jaundice during the first month of life, with pale stools. The diagnosis is confirmed by surgical exploration with operative cholangiography. Approximately 10 percent of cases of biliary atresia are treatable with Roux en Y choledochojejunostomy, with the Kasai procedure (hepatic portoenterostomy) being attempted in the remainder in an effort to restore some bile flow. Most patients, even those having successful biliary-enteric anastomoses, eventually develop chronic cholangitis, extensive hepatic fibrosis, and portal hypertension.

Choledochal cysts Cystic dilatation may involve the free portion of the common bile duct, i.e., choledochal cyst, or may present as diverticulum formation in the intraduodenal segment. In the latter situation chronic reflux of pancreatic juice into the biliary tree can produce inflammation and stenosis of the extrahepatic bile ducts leading to cholangitis or biliary obstruction. Because the process may be gradual, approximately 50 percent of patients present with onset of symptoms after age 10. The diagnosis may be made by ultrasound, abdominal computed tomography (CT), or cholangiography. Surgical treatment involves excision of the ''cyst'' and biliary-enteric anastomosis. Patients with choledochal cysts are at increased risk for the subsequent development of cholangiocarcinoma.

Congenital biliary ectasia Cystic dilatation of the intrahepatic bile ducts may involve either the major intrahepatic radicles (Caroli's disease) or the inter- and intralobular ducts (congenital hepatic fibrosis) or both. In Caroli's disease, clinical manifestations include recurrent cholangitis, abscess formation in and around the affected ducts, and, sometimes, gallstone formation within portions of ectatic intrahepatic biliary radicles. The CT scan and cholangiographic patterns are usually diagnostic, and treatment with ongoing antibiotic therapy is usually undertaken in an effort to limit the frequency and severity of recurrent bouts of cholangitis. Progression to secondary biliary cirrhosis with portal hypertension, amyloidosis, extrahepatic biliary obstruction, cholangiocarcinoma, or recurrent episodes of sepsis with hepatic abscess formation is common.

CHOLEDOCHOLITHIASIS Pathophysiology and clinical manifestations Passage of gallstones into the common bile duct occurs in approximately 10 to 15 percent of patients with cholelithiasis. The incidence of common duct stones increases with increasing age of the patient, so that up to 25 percent of elderly patients may have calculi in the common duct at the time of cholecystectomy. Undetected duct stones are left behind in approximately 1 to 5 percent of cholecystectomy patients. The overwhelming majority of bile duct stones are cholesterol or mixed stones formed in the gallbladder which then migrate into the extrahepatic biliary tree through the cystic duct. Primary calculi arising de novo in the ducts are usually pigment stones developing in patients with (1) chronic hemolytic diseases; (2) hepatobiliary parasitism or chronic, recurrent cholangitis; (3) congenital anomalies of the bile ducts (especially Caroli's disease); or (4) dilated, sclerosed, or strictured ducts. Common duct stones may remain asymptomatic for years, may pass spontaneously into the duodenum, or (most often) may present with biliary colic or a complication.

Complications CHOLANGITIS Cholangitis may be acute or chronic, and symptoms result from inflammation which usually requires at least partial obstruction to the flow of bile. Bacteria are present on bile culture in approximately 75 percent of patients with acute cholangitis early in the symptomatic course. The characteristic presentation of acute cholangitis involves biliary colic, jaundice, and spiking fevers with chills (Charcot's triad). Blood cultures are frequently positive and leukocytosis is typical. *Nonsuppurative* acute cholangitis is most common and may respond relatively rapidly to supportive measures and to treatment with antibiotics (see Chap. 83). In *suppurative* acute cholangitis, however, the presence of pus under pressure in a completely obstructed ductal system leads to symptoms of severe toxicity—mental confusion, bacteremia, and septic shock. Response to antibiotics alone in this setting is relatively poor, multiple hepatic abscesses are often present, and the mortality rate approaches 100 percent unless prompt surgical correction of the obstructing lesion and drainage of infected bile is carried out.

OBSTRUCTIVE JAUNDICE Gradual obstruction of the common bile duct over a period of weeks or months usually leads to initial manifestations of jaundice or pruritus without associated symptoms of biliary colic or cholangitis. Painless jaundice may occur in patients with choledocholithiasis, but this manifestation is much more characteristic of biliary obstruction secondary to malignancy of the head of pancreas, bile ducts, or ampulla of Vater.

In patients whose obstruction is secondary to choledocholithiasis, associated chronic calculous cholecystitis is very common and the gallbladder in this setting may be relatively indistensible. The absence of a palpable gallbladder in most patients with biliary obstruction from duct stones is the basis for *Courvoisier's law,* i.e., that the presence of a palpably enlarged gallbladder suggests that the biliary obstruction is secondary to an underlying malignancy rather than to calculous disease. Biliary obstruction causes progressive dilatation of the intrahepatic bile ducts as intrabiliary pressures rise. Hepatic bile flow is suppressed, and regurgitation of conjugated bilirubin into the bloodstream leads to jaundice accompanied by dark urine (bilirubinuria) and light-colored (acholic) stools.

Common bile duct stones should be suspected in any patient with cholecystitis whose serum bilirubin level exceeds 85.5 μmol/L (5 mg/dL). The maximum bilirubin level is seldom over 256.5 μmol/L (15.0 mg/dL) in patients with choledocholithiasis unless concomitant hepatic disease or another factor leading to marked hyperbilirubinemia exists. Serum bilirubin levels of 342.0 μmol/L (20mg/dL) or more should suggest the possibility of neoplastic obstruction. The serum alkaline phosphatase level is almost always elevated in biliary obstruction. A rise in alkaline phosphatase often precedes clinical jaundice and may be the only abnormality in routine liver function tests. There may be a two- to tenfold elevation of serum aminotransferases, especially in association with acute obstruction. Following relief of the obstructing process, serum aminotransferase elevations usually return rapidly to normal, while the serum bilirubin level may take 1 to 2 weeks to return to normal. The alkaline phosphatase usually falls slowly, lagging behind the decrease in serum bilirubin.

PANCREATITIS The most common associated entity discovered in patients with nonalcoholic acute pancreatitis is biliary tract disease. Biochemical evidence of pancreatic inflammation complicates acute cholecystitis in 15 percent of cases and choledocholithiasis in over 30 percent, and the common factor appears to be the passage of gallstones through the common duct. Coexisting pancreatitis should be suspected in patients with symptoms of cholecystitis who develop (1) back pain or pain to the left of the abdominal midline, (2) prolonged vomiting with paralytic ileus, or (3) a pleural effusion, especially on the left side. Surgical treatment of gallstone disease is usually associated with resolution of the pancreatitis.

SECONDARY BILIARY CIRRHOSIS Secondary biliary cirrhosis may complicate prolonged or intermittent duct obstruction with or without recurrent cholangitis. Although this complication may be seen in patients with choledocholithiasis, it is more common in cases of prolonged obstruction from stricture or neoplasm. Once established, secondary biliary cirrhosis may be progressive even after correction of the obstructing process, and increasingly severe hepatic cirrhosis may lead to portal hypertension or to hepatic failure and death. Prolonged biliary obstruction may also be associated with clinically relevant deficiencies of the fat-soluble vitamins A, D, and K.

Diagnosis and treatment The diagnosis of choledocholithiasis is usually made by cholangiography (see Table 258-4), either preoperatively or intraoperatively at the time of cholecystectomy. The incidence of coexisting common duct stones in patients with cholelithiasis is relatively high. Operative cholangiography should be performed routinely during surgical procedures on the biliary tract. Preoperative indications for common duct exploration include (1) cholangiographic demonstration of ductal stones, (2) jaundice or cholangitis preceding operation, (3) a history of gallstone-related pancreatitis, and (4) cholangiographic evidence of a markedly enlarged common bile duct. Operative indications for exploration of the duct include (1) manual palpation of stones in the common bile duct, (2) positive intraoperative cholangiogram, (3) enlargement of the common bile duct or cystic duct at operation, (4) multiple small stones or "sand" in the gallbladder, and (5) a gallbladder empty of stones at surgery in a patient with previously documented gallstones.

In most cases of choledocholithiasis, the treatment of choice is cholecystectomy with choledocholithotomy and T-tube drainage of the bile ducts. A T-tube cholangiogram is usually performed prior to T-tube removal on or before the tenth postoperative day. Retained calculi seen on T-tube cholangiography may be removed percutaneously by placement of a steerable basket catheter under radiographic guidance through the matured T-tube sinus tract. Endoscopic sphincterotomy followed by spontaneous or basket stone extraction is an additional nonsurgical alternative in the management of patients with common duct stones, especially in elderly or poor-risk patients.

TRAUMA, STRICTURES, AND HEMOBILIA Benign strictures of the extrahepatic bile ducts result from surgical trauma in approximately 95 percent of cases and occur in about 1 in 500 cholecystectomies. Strictures may present with bile leak or abscess formation in the immediate postoperative period or with biliary obstruction or cholangitis as long as 2 years or more following the inciting trauma. The diagnosis is established by percutaneous or endoscopic cholangiography. Successful operative correction by a skillful surgeon with duct-to-bowel anastomosis is usually possible, although mortality rates from surgical complications, recurrent cholangitis, or secondary biliary cirrhosis are high.

Hemobilia may follow traumatic or operative injury to the liver or bile ducts, intraductal rupture of a hepatic abscess or aneurysm of the hepatic artery, biliary or hepatic tumor hemorrhage, or mechanical complications of choledocholithiasis or hepatobiliary parasitism. Diagnostic procedures such as liver biopsy, percutaneous transhepatic cholangiography (PTHC), and transhepatic biliary drainage catheter placement may also be complicated by hemobilia. Patients often present with a classic triad of biliary colic, obstructive jaundice, and melena or occult blood in the stools. The diagnosis is sometimes made by cholangiographic evidence of blood clot in the biliary tree, but selective angiographic verification may be required. Although minor episodes of hemobilia may resolve without operative intervention, surgical ligation of the bleeding vessel is frequently required.

EXTRINSIC COMPRESSION OF THE BILE DUCTS Partial or complete biliary obstruction may sometimes be produced by extrinsic compression of the ducts. The most common cause of this form of obstructive jaundice is carcinoma of the head of the pancreas. Biliary obstruction may also occur as a complication of either acute or

TABLE 258-4 Diagnostic evaluation of the bile ducts

Procedure	Diagnostic advantages	Diagnostic limitations	Contraindications	Complications	Comment
Hepatobiliary ultrasound (HBUS)	Rapid Simultaneous scanning of GB, liver, bile ducts, pancreas Accurate identification of dilated bile ducts Not limited by jaundice, pregnancy Guidance for fine-needle biopsy	Bowel gas Massive obesity Ascites Barium Partial bile duct obstruction Poor visualization of distal CBD	None	None	Initial procedure of choice in investigating possible biliary obstruction
Computed body tomography (CT)	Simultaneous scanning of GB, liver, bile ducts, pancreas Accurate identification of dilated bile ducts, masses Not limited by jaundice, gas, obesity, ascites High-resolution image Guidance for fine-needle biopsy	Extreme cachexia Movement artifact Ileus Partial bile duct obstruction High cost May not be readily available	Pregnancy	Reaction to iodinated contrast, if used	Indicated for evaluation of hepatic or pancreatic masses Procedure of choice in investigating possible biliary obstruction if diagnostic limitations prevent HBUS
Percutaneous transhepatic cholangiogram (PTHC)	Extremely successful when bile ducts dilated Best visualization of proximal biliary tract Possible separate visualization of obstructed left ductal system Bile cytology/culture Percutaneous transhepatic drainage	Nondilated or sclerosed ducts	Pregnancy Uncorrectable coagulopathy Massive ascites ? Hepatic abscess	Bleeding Hemobilia Bile peritonitis Bacteremia, sepsis	Usually, initial cholangiogram of choice when bile ducts are dilated
Endoscopic retrograde cholangiopancreatogram (ERCP)	Simultaneous pancreatography Visualization/biopsy of ampulla and duodenum Best visualization of distal biliary tract Bile or pancreatic cytology Endoscopic sphincterotomy and stone removal ? Biliary manometry Not limited by ascites, coagulopathy, abscess	Gastroduodenal obstruction ? Roux en Y biliary-enteric anastomosis	Pregnancy ? Acute pancreatitis ? Severe cardiopulmonary disease	Pancreatitis Cholangitis, sepsis Infected pancreatic pseudocyst Perforation (rare) Hypoxemia, aspiration	Cholangiogram of choice in: Absence of dilated ducts ? Pancreatic, ampullary or gastroduodenal disease Prior biliary surgery PTHC contraindicated or failed Endoscopic sphincterotomy a treatment possibility

NOTE: Intravenous cholangiography (IVC) is an obsolete technique because 40% of common duct stones are missed and there is poor resolution even with tomography. There are few indications for its use especially since other cholangiographic techniques are usually available.

chronic pancreatitis or involvement of lymph nodes in the porta hepatis by lymphoma or metastatic carcinoma. The latter should be distinguished from cholestasis resulting from massive replacement of the liver by tumor.

HEPATOBILIARY PARASITISM Infestation of the biliary tract by adult helminths or their ova may produce a chronic, recurrent pyogenic cholangitis with or without multiple hepatic abscesses, ductal stones, or biliary obstruction. This condition is relatively rare but does occur in inhabitants of southern China and elsewhere in southeast Asia. The organisms most commonly involved are trematodes or flukes, including *Clonorchis sinensis*, *Opisthorchis viverrini* or *felineus*, and *Fasciola hepatica*. The biliary tract may also be involved by intraductal migration of adult *Ascaris lumbricoides* from the duodenum or by intrabiliary rupture of hydatid cysts of the liver produced by *Echinococcus* species. The diagnosis is made by cholangiography and the presence of characteristic ova on stool examination. When obstruction is present, the treatment of choice is laparotomy under antibiotic coverage, with common duct exploration and a biliary drainage procedure. It should be emphasized that in the orient, one also sees cholangiohepatitis associated with pigment lithiasis, which may, in fact, be more common than cholangitis due to parasites.

SCLEROSING CHOLANGITIS Primary or idiopathic sclerosing cholangitis is a disorder characterized by a progressive, inflammatory, sclerosing and obliterative process affecting the extrahepatic and, often, the intrahepatic bile ducts. The lesion may appear as an isolated entity or may occur in association with inflammatory bowel disease, especially ulcerative colitis, or with multifocal fibrosclerosis syndromes such as retroperitoneal, mediastinal, and/or periureteral fibrosis, Riedel's struma, or pseudotumor of the orbit. Papillary stenosis and sclerosing cholangitis are also important complications of the acquired immunodeficiency syndrome (AIDS); cytomegalovirus and cryptosporidia infections have been observed frequently in such patients, raising the question whether these microbes may be a pathogenetic factor in primary sclerosing cholangitis. Secondary sclerosing cholangitis may occur as a long-term complication of choledocholithiasis, cholangiocarcinoma, operative or traumatic biliary injury, or contiguous inflammatory processes.

Patients with sclerosing cholangitis often present with signs and symptoms of chronic or intermittent biliary obstruction: jaundice, pruritus, right upper quadrant abdominal pain, or acute cholangitis. Late in the course, complete biliary obstruction, secondary biliary cirrhosis, hepatic failure, or portal hypertension with bleeding varices may occur. The diagnosis is usually established by finding thickened ducts with narrow, beaded lumina on cholangiography (see Fig. 258-2*D*). The cholangiographic technique of choice in suspected cases is probably ERCP since intrahepatic ductal involvement may make PTHC difficult or impossible. When a diagnosis of sclerosing cholangitis has been established, a search for associated diseases, especially for chronic inflammatory bowel disease, should be carried out.

Therapy with cholestyramine may help control symptoms of

pruritus, and antibiotics are useful when cholangitis complicates the clinical picture. Vitamin D and calcium supplementation may help prevent the loss of bone mass frequently seen in patients with chronic cholestasis. Glucocorticoids have not been shown to be efficacious. In cases where complete or high-grade biliary obstruction has occurred, surgical intervention may be appropriate. Efforts at biliary-enteric anastomosis or stent placement may, however, be complicated by recurrent cholangitis and further progression of the stenosing process. The role of colectomy in patients with sclerosing cholangitis complicating chronic ulcerative colitis is uncertain. The prognosis is unfavorable, with a mean survival of 4 to 10 years following the diagnosis, regardless of therapy. Primary sclerosing cholangitis is one of the most common indications for liver transplantation. In one study, the mean follow-up time from the diagnosis of primary sclerosing cholangitis to the time of liver transplantation was 5.8 years.

CHOLANGIOCARCINOMA Benign tumors of the extrahepatic bile ducts are extremely rare causes of mechanical biliary obstruction. The majority of these are papillomas, adenomas, or cystadenomas which present with obstructive jaundice or hemobilia. Adenocarcinoma of the extrahepatic ducts is relatively more common. There is a slight male preponderance (60 percent), and the peak age incidence is in the fifth to seventh decades. Apparent predisposing factors include (1) some chronic hepatobiliary parasitic infestations, (2) congential anomalies with ectactic ducts, (3) sclerosing cholangitis and chronic ulcerative colitis, and (4) occupational exposure to possible biliary tract carcinogens (workers in rubber or automotive plants). Cholelithiasis is not clearly associated with cholangiocarcinoma as a predisposing factor. The lesions may be diffuse or nodular; the latter often arise at the confluence of the hepatic ducts (Klatskin tumors). This tumor is usually associated with a *collapsed* gallbladder and such a finding mandates that the proximal hepatic ducts be optimally visualized by cholangiography.

Patients with cholangiocarcinoma usually present with biliary obstruction, painless jaundice, pruritus, weight loss, and acholic stools. A deep-seated, vaguely localized right upper quadrant pain may be an associated complaint. Hepatomegaly and a palpable, distended gallbladder are frequent accompanying signs. Fever is unusual unless associated with ascending cholangitis. Because the obstructing process is gradual, the cholangiocarcinoma is often far advanced by the time it presents clinically. The diagnosis is most frequently made by cholangiography following ultrasound demonstration of dilated intrahepatic bile ducts. Any focal strictures of the bile ducts should probably be considered malignant until proved otherwise. Long-term palliation of the tumor is possible in some cases when radiation and/or chemotherapy are combined with palliative drainage of the biliary tree.

CARCINOMA OF THE PAPILLA OF VATER The ampulla of Vater may be involved by extension of tumor arising elsewhere in the duodenum or may itself be the primary site of origin of sarcomas, carcinoid tumors, or adenocarcinomas. Papillary adenocarcinomas are associated with slow growth and a more favorable clinical prognosis than diffuse, infiltrative cancers of the ampulla, which are more frequently widely invasive. The presenting clinical manifestation is usually obstructive jaundice. ERCP is probably the preferred diagnostic technique when ampullary carcinoma is suspected, because it allows for direct endoscopic inspection and biopsy of the ampulla as well as for performance of pancreatography to exclude a diagnosis of pancreatic malignancy. Cancer of the papilla is usually treated by wide, often radical, surgical excision. Lymph node or other metastases are present at the time of surgery in approximately 20 percent of cases, and the 5-year survival rate following surgical therapy in this group is only 5 to 10 percent. In the absence of metastases, however, radical pancreaticoduodenectomy (Whipple procedure) is associated with 5-year survival rates as high as 40 percent, and several long-term survivors have been reported.

REFERENCES

Bismuth H, Malt RA: Carcinoma of the biliary tract. N Engl J Med 301:704, 1979

Carey MC et al: Whither biliary sludge? Gastroenterology 95:508, 1988

Dowling RH et al: Gallstone recurrence and post dissolution management, in *Enterohepatic circulation of Bile Acids and Sterol Metabolism*, G Paumgartren, A Stichl, W Gersk (eds). Lancaster, PA, MTP Press, 1985, pp 361–369

Ferrucci JT Jr, Mueller PR: Interventional radiology of the biliary tract. Gastroenterology 82:974, 1982

Gracie WA, Ransohoff DF: The natural history of silent gallstones. The innocent gallstone is not a myth. N Engl J Med 307:798, 1982

Holzbach RT et al: Biliary proteins: Unique inhibitors of cholesterol crystal nucleation in human gallbladder bile. J Clin Invest 72:35, 1984

Hood K et al: Prevention of gallstone recurrence by non-steroidal antiinflammatory drugs. Lancet 2:1223, 1988

Lee SP et al: Origin and fate of biliary sludge. Gastroenterology 94:170, 1988

Levy PF et al: Human gallbladder mucin accelerates nucleation of cholesterol in artifical bile. Gastroenterology 87:270, 1984

Maringhini A et al: Gallstones, gallbladder cancer, and other gastrointestinal malignancies: An epidemiologic study in Rochester, Minnesota. Ann Intern Med 107:30, 1987

Maton PN et al: Outcome of chenodeoxycholic acid (CDCA) treatment in 125 patients with radiolucent gallstones. Medicine 61:86, 1982

Messin B et al: Does total parenteral nutrition induce gallbladder sludge formation and lithiasis? Gastroenterology 84:1012, 1983

Palme KR, Hofmann AF: Intraductal monooctanoin for the direct dissolution of bile duct stones: Experience in 343 patients. Gut 27:196, 1986

Podda M et al: Efficacy and safety of a combination of dienodeoxycholic acid and ursodeoxycholic acid for gallstone dissolution. Gastroenterology 96:222, 1989

Ransohoff DF: Assessment of prophylactic cholecystectomy and medical therapy for diabetics with silent gallstones. Gastroenterology 92:1588, 1987

Sackman M et al: Shock wave lithotripsy of gallbladder stones. The first 175 patients. N Engl J Med 318:393, 1988

Sauerbruch T et al: Fragmentation of bile duct stones by extracorporeal shock waves. Gastroenterology 96:222, 1989

Schneidermon D et al: Papillary stenosis and sclerosing cholangitis in the acquired immunodeficiency syndrome. Ann Intern Med 106:546, 1987

Shaffer EA et al: Cholescintigraphic detection of functional obstruction of the sphincter of Oddi: Effect of papillotomy. Gastroenterology 90:728, 1986

Silvis SE et al: What is the post-cholecystectomy pain syndrome? Gastrointestinal Endoscopy 31:401, 1985

Smith BF, Lamont JT: The central issue of cholesterol gallstones. Hepatology 6:529, 1986

Thistle JL et al: Dissolution of cholesterol gallbladder stones by methyl-tert-butyl ether administered by percutaneous transhepatic catheter. N Engl J Med 320:633, 1989

Wiesner RH et al: Comparison of clinicopathologic features of primary sclerosing cholangitis and primary biliary cirrhosis. Gastroenterology 88:108, 1985

section 3 Disorders of the pancreas

259 APPROACH TO THE PATIENT WITH PANCREATIC DISEASE

NORTON J. GREENBERGER / PHILLIP P. TOSKES

GENERAL CONSIDERATIONS

Inflammatory disease of the pancreas may be acute or chronic. Although good data exist concerning the frequency of acute pancreatitis (about 5000 new cases per year in the United States with a mortality rate of about 10 percent), the number of patients who suffer with relapsing pancreatitis or chronic pancreatitis is largely undefined. The relative inaccessibility of the pancreas to direct examination and the nonspecificity of the abdominal pain associated with pancreatitis make the diagnosis of pancreatitis difficult and usually dependent on elevation of blood amylase levels. Many patients with chronic pancreatitis do not have elevated blood amylase levels. Some patients with chronic pancreatitis develop signs and symptoms of pancreatic exocrine insufficiency, and thus objective evidence for pancreatic disease can be demonstrated. However, greater than 90 percent of the pancreas must be damaged before maldigestion of fat and protein is manifested. Obviously there is a very large reservoir of pancreatic exocrine function, and the signs and symptoms usually associated with exocrine insufficiency are late manifestations, depending on virtually complete destruction of the gland. Even the secretin stimulation test, which is the most sensitive method of assessing pancreatic exocrine function, is probably abnormal only when greater than 70 percent of exocrine function has been lost. Thus, the number of patients who have subclinical exocrine dysfunction (i.e., less than 90 percent loss of function) is unknown.

The clinical manifestations of acute and chronic pancreatitis and pancreatic insufficiency are protean. Thus, patients may present with hyperlipidemia, vitamin B_{12} malabsorption, hypercalcemia, hypocalcemia, hyperglycemia, ascites, pleural effusions, and chronic abdominal pain with normal amylase levels. Indeed, if the clinician considers pancreatitis as a possible diagnosis only when presented with a patient having classic symptoms (i.e., severe, constant epigastric pain that radiates through to the back, along with an elevated blood amylase level), only a minority of the patients with pancreatitis will be correctly diagnosed.

As emphasized in Chap. 260, the etiologies as well as the clinical manifestations are quite varied. Although it is well appreciated that *pancreatitis* is frequently secondary to alcohol abuse and biliary tract disease, pancreatitis is also caused by drugs, trauma, and viral infections, and is associated with metabolic and connective tissue disorders. In addition, in approximately 15 percent of patients with acute pancreatitis and 25 percent of patients with chronic pancreatitis, the etiology is obscure.

TESTS USEFUL IN THE DIAGNOSIS OF PANCREATIC DISEASE

Several tests have proved of value in the evaluation of pancreatic exocrine function. Examples of specific tests and usefulness in the diagnosis of acute and chronic pancreatitis are summarized in Table 259-1.

PANCREATIC ENZYMES IN BODY FLUIDS The serum amylase is widely used as a screening test for acute pancreatitis in the patient with acute abdominal or back pain. A value greater than 150 Somogyi units per deciliter should raise the question of acute pancreatitis. Levels greater than 300 units make the diagnosis more likely, and values greater than three times normal virtually clinch the diagnosis if gut perforation or infarction is excluded. In acute pancreatitis the serum amylase is usually elevated within 24 h and remains so for 1 to 3 days. Levels return to normal within 3 to 5 days unless there is extensive pancreatic necrosis, incomplete ductal obstruction, or pseudocyst formation. Approximately 70 to 75 percent of patients with acute pancreatitis will have an elevated serum amylase. Normal values, however, may occur if (1) there is a delay (2 to 5 days) in obtaining blood samples, (2) the underlying disorder is chronic pancreatitis rather than acute pancreatitis, and (3) hypertriglyceridemia is present. Patients with hypertriglyceridemia and proven pancreatitis have been found to have spuriously low levels of amylase activity. Importantly, serum lipase and urinary amylase levels may be abnormal in this setting, thus facilitating the diagnosis of acute pancreatitis.

The serum amylase is often elevated in other conditions (Table 259-2), in part because the enzyme is found in many organs in addition to the pancreas (salivary glands, liver, small intestine, kidney, fallopian tube) and can be produced by various tumors (carcinoma of the lung, esophagus, breast, and ovary). Isoenzymes of amylase fall into two general categories, those arising from the pancreas (P isoamylases) and those from nonpancreatic sources (S isoamylases). The measurement of serum isoamylases is of clinical importance. Isoamylase analysis of normal serum shows that about 35 to 45 percent of the amylase is of pancreatic origin. For example, in patients with acute pancreatitis, the total serum amylase returns to normal more rapidly than pancreatic isoamylase. Thus, in patients seen after the first day, the pancreatic isoamylase is a more sensitive indicator of pancreatitis than the total serum amylase. In addition, in certain conditions, such as the postoperative state, acute alcohol intoxication, and diabetic ketoacidosis, it had been assumed that elevations in serum amylase indicated acute pancreatitis. However, the elevation of serum amylase in such conditions has been shown to actually be of the S type. The general availability of a simple assay that employs a protein which selectively inhibits nonpancreatic amylase has led to more widespread use of isoamylase determinations.

Urine amylase is increased in acute pancreatitis and may be elevated after serum values have returned to normal. The finding that the renal clearance of amylase is increased in acute pancreatitis has led to the suggestion that the amylase/creatinine clearance ratio (C_{am}/C_{cr}) may be a more sensitive and specific test for the diagnosis of acute pancreatitis.

However, experience with the C_{am}/C_{cr} has demonstrated that it is no more sensitive than the serum amylase. In addition, the specificity of the C_{am}/C_{cr} has been seriously questioned because the ratio is also increased in a number of other disorders, e.g., diabetic ketoacidosis, burns, pancreatic neoplasms, renal failure, and the postoperative state. The mechanism of increased renal amylase clearance in acute pancreatitis is secondary to a reversible renal tubular defect which results in decreased amylase reabsorption.

Elevation of ascitic fluid amylase occurs in acute pancreatitis as well as (1) in pancreatogenous ascites due to disruption of the main pancreatic duct of a leaking pseudocyst and (2) in other abdominal disorders which simulate pancreatitis (e.g., intestinal obstruction, intestinal infarction, and perforated peptic ulcer). Elevation of pleural

TABLE 259-1 Tests useful in the diagnosis of acute and chronic pancreatitis and pancreatic tumors

Test	Principle	Comment
I Pancreatic enzymes in body fluids		
A Amylase		
1 Serum	Pancreatic inflammation leads to increased enzyme levels	Simple; 20–40% false-negatives and -positives; reliable if test results are two to three times the upper limit of normal
2 Urine	Renal clearance of amylase is increased in acute pancreatitis	May be abnormal when serum levels normal; false-negatives and -positives
3 Amylase/creatinine clearance ratio (C_{am}/C_{cr})	Renal clearance of amylase greater than clearance of creatinine	No more sensitive than the serum amylase; many false-positives
4 Ascitic fluid	Disruption of gland or main pancreatic duct leads to increased amylase concentration	Can establish diagnosis of pancreatitis; false-positives with intestinal obstruction and perforated ulcer
5 Pleural fluid	Exudative pleural effusion with pancreatitis	False-positives with carcinoma of the lung and esophageal perforation
6 Isoenzymes	P isoamylases arise from the pancreas; S isoamylases are from other sources	More sensitive than total serum amylase in diagnosis of acute pancreatitis; useful in identifying nonpancreatic causes of hyperamylasemia
B Serum lipase	Pancreatic inflammation leads to increased enzyme levels	New methods of determination greatly simplified; positive in 70–85% of cases; excellent specificity; normal in nonpancreatic hyperamylasemic conditions
C Serum trypsin-like immunoreactivity (TLI)	Pancreatic inflammation leads to increased levels	*Elevated* in acute pancreatitis and renal failure; *decreased* in chronic pancreatitis *with* steatorrhea; normal in chronic pancreatitis *without* steatorrhea and steatorrhea with normal pancreatic function
D Pancreatic polypeptide (PP)	PP confined almost totally to the pancreas; release stimulated by nutrients and hormones; such release parallels pancreatic enzyme secretion	Basal, meal-simulated, and hormone (secretin CCK)-stimulated PP levels *decreased* in chronic pancreatitis; fasting PP levels >125 pg/mL argues against chronic pancreatitis and pancreatic cancer
II Studies pertaining to pancreatic structure		
A Radiologic and radionuclide tests		
1 Plain film of the abdomen	Abnormal in acute and chronic pancreatitis	Simple; normal in >50% of both acute and chronic pancreatitis
2 Upper gastrointestinal x-rays	Abnormally thickened duodenal folds; displacement of stomach or widening of duodenal loop suggests a pancreatic mass (inflammatory, neoplastic, cystic)	Simple; frequently normal; largely superseded by US and CT scanning
3 Ultrasonography (US)	Can provide information on edema, inflammation, calcification, pseudocysts, and mass lesions	Simple, noninvasive; sequential studies quite feasible; useful in diagnosis of pseudocyst
4 CT scan	Permits detailed visualization of pancreas and surrounding structures	Useful in the diagnosis of pancreatic calcification, dilated pancreatic ducts, and pancreatic tumors; may not be able to distinguish between inflammatory and neoplastic mass lesions
5 Selective angiography	Can identify pancreatic neoplasms (1) by sheathing of celiac or superior mesenteric branches by tumor or (2) by tumor staining; displacement of vessels by tumor	Indicated (1) in suspected islet cell tumors and (2) prior to pancreatic or duodenal resection; most reliable features reflect nonresectable pancreatic cancer
6 Endoscopic retrograde cholangiopancreatography (ERCP)	Cannulation of pancreatic and common bile duct permits visualization of pancreatic-biliary ductal system	Provides diagnostic data in 60–85% of cases; differentiation of chronic pancreatitis from pancreatic carcinoma may be difficult
B Pancreatic biopsy with US or CT guidance	Percutaneous biopsy with skinny needle and localization of lesion by US	High diagnostic yield; laparotomy avoided; requires special technical skills
III Tests of exocrine pancreatic function		
A Direct stimulation of the pancreas with analysis of duodenal contents		
1 Secretin-pancreozymin (CCK) test	Secretin leads to increased output of pancreatic juice and HCO_3^-; CCK leads to increased output of pancreatic enzymes; pancreatic secretory response related to functional mass of pancreatic tissue	Sensitive enough to detect occult disease; involves duodenal intubation and fluoroscopy; poorly defined normal enzyme response; overlap in chronic pancreatitis; large secretory reserve capacity of the pancreas
B Indirect stimulation of pancreas with measurement of pancreatic enzymes		
1 Lundh test meal	Test meal (fat, carbohydrate, and protein) causes increased release of CCK, which causes increased enzyme output; trypsin concentration measured	Useful in pancreatic exocrine insufficiency; false-negatives with delayed gastric emptying; false-positives in primary mucosal disease of the gut and choledocholithiasis; does not measure secretory capacity
2 Benzoyl-tyrosyl-*p*-aminobenzoic (Bz-Ty-PABA, bentiromide) test	Synthetic peptide (Bz-Ty-PABA) specifically cleaved by chymotrypsin, liberating PABA which is absorbed and PABA metabolite excreted in the urine	Simple and reliable test of pancreatic exocrine function
C Measurement of intraluminal digestion products		
1 Microscopic examination of stool for undigested meat fibers and fat	Lack of proteolytic and lipolytic enzymes causes decreased digestion of meat fibers and triglycerides	Simple, reliable; not sensitive enough to detect milder cases of pancreatic insufficiency
2 Quantitative stool fat determination	Lack of lipolytic enzymes brings about impaired fat digestion	Reliable, reference standard for defining severity of malabsorption; does not distinguish between maldigestion and malabsorption

TABLE 259-1 Tests useful in the diagnosis of acute and chronic pancreatitis and pancreatic tumors *(continued)*

Test	Principle	Comment
3 Fecal nitrogen	Lack of proteolytic enzymes leads to imparied protein digestion, causing increase in stool nitrogen	Does not distinguish between maldigestion and malabsorption; low sensitivity
D Measurement of pancreatic enzymes in feces		
1 Chymotrypsin	Pancreatic secretion of proteolytic enzymes	May be useful in cystic fibrosis; tedious; 10% false-positives and false-negatives

fluid amylase occurs in acute pancreatitis, chronic pancreatitis, carcinoma of the lung, and esophageal perforation.

In the past, serum lipase levels were not frequently performed because of methodological problems. However, newer methods are now available and development of automated lipase assays should lead to their routine use and obviate present reliance on total amylase measurements in the diagnosis of acute pancreatitis. In two representative studies, lipase determinations exhibited good *sensitivity* and excellent *specificity;* lipase levels were elevated in 70 to 85 percent of patients with acute pancreatitis, and the specificity was 99 percent. An obvious advantage of the lipase assay is that this enzyme is normal in several disorders associated with hyperamylasemia (e.g., macroamylasemia, diabetic ketoacidosis, renal failure, salivary gland lesions).

Assay for trypsinogen (or trypsin-like immunoreactivity) has a theoretical advantage over amylase and lipase determinations in that the pancreas is the only organ that contains this enzyme. The test appears to be useful in the diagnosis of both acute and chronic pancreatitis. Sensitivity and specificity are comparable to amylase and lipase determinations. Since trypsinogen is also excreted by the kidney, elevated values are found in renal failure.

A recent study evaluated the sensitivity and specificity of five assays used to diagnose acute pancreatitis: two amylase assays, one lipase, one trypsinlike immunoreactivity (TLI), and one pancreatic isoamylase. The data obtained show that (1) if the best cutoff level is used, all assays have similar specificities and suggest that (2) total serum amylase is as good an indicator of acute pancreatitis as any of the others. However, inherent in many such studies is the problem that the recognition and diagnosis of acute pancreatitis hinges upon the finding of an elevated serum amylase. The question arises as to whether any diagnostic test result can be proved superior to the total serum amylase level if hyperamylasemia is required for the diagnosis. In other studies, when "objective" confirmation of the clinical diagnosis of pancreatitis was required (ultrasonography, CT, laparotomy), the sensitivity of the serum amylase has been as low as 68 percent. With these limitations in mind, the recommended screening tests for acute pancreatitis are *total serum amylase and serum lipase activities*. Serum amylase values greater than three times normal are highly specific.

TABLE 259-2 Causes of hyperamylasemia and hyperamylasuria

I Pancreatic disease
- *A* Pancreatitis
  - *1* Acute
  - *2* Chronic: ductal obstruction
  - *3* Complications of pancreatitis
    - *a* Pancreatic pseudocyst
    - *b* Pancreatogenous ascites
    - *c* Pancreatic abscess
- *B* Pancreatic trauma
- *C* Pancreatic carcinoma

II Nonpancreatic disorders
- *A* Renal insufficiency
- *B* Salivary gland lesions
  - *1* Mumps
  - *2* Calculus
  - *3* Irradiation sialadenitis
  - *4* Maxillofacial surgery
- *C* "Tumor" hyperamylasemia
  - *1* Carcinoma of the lung
  - *2* Carcinoma of the esophagus
  - *3* Breast carcinoma, ovarian carcinoma
- *D* Macroamylasemia
- *E* Burns
- *F* Diabetic ketoacidosis
- *G* Pregnancy
- *H* Renal transplantation
- *I* Cerebral trauma
- *J* Drugs: morphine

III Other abdominal disorders
- *A* Biliary tract disease: cholecystitis, choledocholithiasis
- *B* Intraabdominal disease
  - *1* Perforated or penetrating peptic ulcer
  - *2* Intestinal obstruction or infarction
  - *3* Ruptured ectopic pregnancy
  - *4* Peritonitis
  - *5* Aortic aneurysm
  - *6* Chronic liver disease
  - *7* Postoperative hyperamylasemia

SOURCE: After WB Salt II, S Schenker, Medicine 55:269, 1976.

STUDIES PERTAINING TO PANCREATIC STRUCTURE **Radiologic tests** Plain films of the abdomen provide useful information in 30 to 50 percent of patients with acute pancreatitis. The most frequent abnormalities include (1) a localized ileus usually involving the jejunum ("sentinel loop"); (2) a generalized ileus with air-fluid levels; (3) the "colon cutoff sign," which results from isolated distention of the transverse colon; (4) duodenal distention with air-fluid levels; and (5) a mass, which is frequently a pseudocyst. In chronic pancreatitis, an important radiographic finding is pancreatic calcification, which characteristically is localized adjacent to and superimposed on the second lumbar vertebra (see Fig. 260-1).

Upper gastrointestinal x-rays may reveal displacement of the stomach by the retroperitoneal mass (see Fig. 260-2A) or widening and effacement of the duodenal C loop, which also suggests the presence of a pancreatic mass that could be an inflammatory, cystic, or neoplastic process. However, their use has been largely superceded by ultrasound.

Ultrasonography (echography) can provide important information in patients with acute pancreatitis, chronic pancreatitis, pancreatic calcification, pseudocyst, and pancreatic carcinoma. It is a useful procedure in the evaluation of the patient with acute pancreatitis. Echographic appearances can indicate the presence of edema, inflammation, and calcification (not obvious on plain films of the abdomen), as well as pseudocysts, mass lesions, and gallstones (see Figs. 260-1 to 260-3). In acute pancreatitis the pancreas is characteristically enlarged. In pancreatic pseudocyst the usual appearance is that of an echo-free, smooth, round fluid collection. Pancreatic carcinoma distorts the usual landmarks, and mass lesions greater than 3.0 cm are usually detected as localized, echo-free solid lesions. Ultrasound is often the initial investigation for most patients with suspected pancreatic disease. However, obesity, excess small- and large-bowel gas, and recently performed barium-contrast examinations can interfere with ultrasound studies, which are often technically unsatisfactory.

Computed tomography is the best imaging study for initial evaluation of a suspected chronic pancreatic disorder. It is especially useful in the detection of pancreatic tumors, fluid-containing lesions such as pseudocysts and abscesses, and calcium deposits. Most lesions are characterized by (1) enlargement of the pancreatic outline, (2) distortion of the pancreatic contour, or (3) fluid-containing lesions that have different attenuation coefficients than normal pancreas. However, it is occasionally difficult to distinguish between inflammatory and neoplastic lesions. Oral water-soluble contrast agents may be used to opacify the stomach and duodenum during CT scans; this permits more precise delineation of various organs as well as mass lesions.

Selective catheterization of the celiac and superior mesenteric arteries combined with superselective catheterization of others such as the hepatic, splenic, and gastroduodenal arteries permits visualization of the pancreas and detection of pancreatic neoplasms and pseudocysts. Pancreatic neoplasms can be identified by the sheathing of blood vessels by a mass lesion (see Fig. 260-3). Hormone-producing pancreatic tumors are especially likely to exhibit increased vascularity and tumor staining. Angiographic abnormalities are noted in many patients with pancreatic carcinoma but are uncommon in patients without pancreatic disease. Angiography complements ultrasonography and endoscopic retrograde cholangiopancreatography (ERCP) in the study of a patient with a suspected pancreatic lesion and may be carried out if ERCP is either unsuccessful or nondiagnostic.

Endoscopic retrograde cholangiopancreatography ERCP may provide useful information on the status of the pancreatic ductal system and thus aid in the differential diagnosis of pancreatic disease (see Figs. 260-2 and 260-3). Pancreatic carcinoma is characterized by stenosis or obstruction of either the pancreatic duct or common bile duct; both ductal systems are often abnormal. In chronic pancreatitis ERCP abnormalities include (1) luminal narrowing; (2) irregularities in the ductal system with stenosis, dilatation, sacculation, and ectasia; and (3) blockage of the pancreatic duct by calcium deposits. Differentiation from carcinoma may be difficult because of similar overlapping features, i.e., ductal stenosis and irregularity. Elevated serum and/or urine amylase levels following ERCP have been reported in 25 to 75 percent of patients, but clinical pancreatitis is uncommon. In a series of 300 patients pancreatitis occurred in only five patients following ERCP. If no lesion is found within the biliary and/or pancreatic ducts in a patient with repeated attacks of acute pancreatitis, manometric studies of the sphincter of Oddi may be indicated.

Pancreatic biopsy with radiologic guidance Percutaneous aspiration biopsy of a pancreatic mass often distinguishes between a pancreatic inflammatory mass and a pancreatic neoplasm.

TESTS OF EXOCRINE PANCREATIC FUNCTION

Pancreatic function tests (Table 259-1) can be divided into the following:

1 *Direct stimulation of the pancreas* by intravenous infusion of secretin or secretin plus cholecystokinin (CCK) followed by collection and measurement of duodenal contents
2 *Indirect stimulation of the pancreas* utilizing nutrients or amino acids, fatty acids, and synthetic peptides followed by assay of proteolytic, lipolytic, and amylolytic enzymes
3 Study of *intraluminal digestion products* such as undigested meat fibers, stool fat, and fecal nitrogen
4 *Measurement of fecal pancreatic enzymes* such as chymotrypsin

The secretin test, used to detect diffuse pancreatic disease, is based on the physiologic principle that the pancreatic secretory response is directly related to the functional mass of pancreatic tissue. In the standard assay, secretin is given intravenously in a dose of 1 clinical unit (CU) per kilogram, either as a bolus or continuous infusion. Obviously, results will vary with the secretin preparation used, dose, mode of administration, and completeness of collection of duodenal contents. Normal values for the standard secretin test are (1) volume output >2.0 mL/kg per hour, (2) bicarbonate (HCO_3^-) concentration >80 meq/L, and (3) HCO_3^- output >10 meq in 1 h. The most reproducible measurement having the highest level of discrimination between normal subjects and patients with chronic pancreatitis appears to be the maximal bicarbonate concentration.

The *combined secretin-CCK test* permits measurement of pancreatic amylase, lipase, trypsin, and chymotrypsin. Although there is overlap in the distribution of enzyme output in normal subjects and patients with pancreatitis, markedly decreased enzyme outputs suggest advanced damage and destruction of acinar cells. With frank exocrine pancreatic insufficiency there is usually an overall reduction in both HCO_3^- concentration and output of several enzymes. However, with lesser degrees of pancreatic damage there may be a dissociation between HCO_3^- concentration and enzyme output. There may also be a dissociation between the results of the secretin test and other tests of absorptive function. For example, patients with chronic pancreatitis often have abnormally low outputs of HCO_3^- after secretin but have normal fecal fat excretion. Thus, the secretin test measures the secretory capacity of ductular epithelium, while fecal fat excretion indirectly reflects intraluminal lipolytic activity. Steatorrhea does not occur until intraluminal levels of lipase are markedly reduced, underscoring the fact that only small amounts of enzymes are necessary for intraluminal digestive activities. An abnormal secretin test should suggest only that chronic pancreatic damage is present; it will not consistently distinguish between chronic pancreatitis and pancreatic carcinoma.

Another test of exocrine pancreatic function, which indirectly reflects intraluminal chymotrypsin activity, has been evaluated in patients with pancreatic disease. This test (the *tripeptide hydrolysis* or *bentiromide* test) utilizes a synthetic peptide, *N*-benzoyl-L-tyrosyl-*p*-aminobenzoic acid (Bz-Ty-PABA), that is specifically cleaved by chymotrypsin to Bz-Ty and PABA. Normally, after oral administration, the peptide reaches the small intestine, where it is hydrolyzed by chymotrypsin with the liberation of PABA, which is rapidly absorbed and excreted in the urine. Results in several hundred patients with chronic pancreatitis and other disorders indicate that PABA excretion is significantly lower in chronic pancreatitis compared with controls. Depending on the severity of pancreatic exocrine impairment, the overall sensitivity is 60 percent (range 46 to 74 percent), and the specificity if coupled with a D-xylose test approximates 90 percent.

Measurement of *intraluminal digestion products,* i.e., undigested muscle fibers, stool fat, and fecal nitrogen, is discussed in Chap. 240. Measurement of chymotrypsin in stool reflects pancreatic output of this proteolytic enzyme. Decreased chymotrypsin activity in stool has been reported in patients with chronic pancreatitis and cystic fibrosis. However, normal values may occur in patients with pancreatic insufficiency, and false-positive results have been reported in up to 10 percent of normal individuals.

Tests useful in the diagnosis of exocrine pancreatic insufficiency and the differential diagnosis of malabsorption are also discussed in Chaps. 240 and 260.

260 ACUTE AND CHRONIC PANCREATITIS

NORTON J. GREENBERGER / PHILLIP P. TOSKES / KURT J. ISSELBACHER

BIOCHEMISTRY AND PHYSIOLOGY OF PANCREATIC EXOCRINE SECRETION

GENERAL CONSIDERATIONS The pancreas secretes 1500 to 3000 mL isosmotic alkaline (pH > 8.0) fluid per day containing about 20 enzymes and zymogens. The pancreatic secretions provide the enzymes needed to effect the major digestive activity of the gastrointestinal tract and provide an optimum pH for the function of these enzymes.

REGULATION OF PANCREATIC SECRETION **Hormonal and neural mechanisms** The exocrine pancreas is under both hormonal and neural control, with hormonal control being of primary importance. *Gastric acid* is the stimulus for the release of secretin, a peptide with 27 amino acids. Sensitive radioimmunoassay studies for secretin suggest that the pH threshold for the release of secretin from the duodenum and jejunum is 4.5. Secretin stimulates the secretion of pancreatic juice rich in *water and electrolytes*. Release of cholecystokinin (CCK) from duodenum and jejunum is largely produced by long-chain fatty acids, certain essential amino acids (tryptophan, phenylalanine, valine, methionine), and gastric acid itself. CCK evokes an *enzyme-rich secretion from the pancreas*. Gastrin, although it shares an identical terminal tetrapeptide with CCK, is a weak stimulus for pancreatic enzyme output. The *parasympathetic nervous system* (via the vagus) exerts some control over pancreatic secretion. Part of this is mediated by the release of gastrin, and part is secondary to a direct effect of acetylcholine on the pancreatic acinar cell. Also, vagal stimulation effects release of vasoactive intestinal peptide (VIP), a secretin agonist. Vagal control of pancreatic secretion seems to be most important following a truncal vagotomy, but even in such patients severe maldigestion does not ensue. Bile salts also stimulate pancreatic secretion, thereby integrating the functions of the biliary tract, pancreas, and small intestine.

Pancreatic secretion at the cellular level There appear to be two functionally distinct pathways by which secretagogues can stimulate pancreatic secretion. Studies with isolated pancreatic acinar cells indicate that secretin, VIP, and cholera toxin interact with receptors on the acinar cell, leading to an increase in cellular cyclic adenosine monophosphate (cyclic AMP). CCK, acetylcholine, gastrin, and various other peptides (e.g., bombesin, caerulein) react with other receptors on the acinar cell to cause an increased turnover of phosphatidylinositol and the release of membrane calcium and induce changes in the electrical properties of the pancreatic acinar cell surface and junctional membranes. When a secretagogue that increases cyclic AMP is added to a secretagogue that increases calcium outflux, potentiation of enzyme secretion occurs.

WATER AND ELECTROLYTE SECRETION Although sodium, potassium, chloride, calcium, zinc, phosphate, and sulfate are found within pancreatic secretion, *bicarbonate is the ion of primary physiologic importance*. In the acini and in the ducts, secretin causes the cells to add water and bicarbonate to the fluid. In the ducts an exchange occurs between bicarbonate and chloride. There is a good correlation between the maximal bicarbonate output after stimulation with secretin and the pancreatic mass. The bicarbonate output of 120 to 300 mmol/d helps neutralize gastric acid production and creates the appropriate pH for the activity of the pancreatic enzymes.

ENZYME SECRETION The pancreas secretes amylolytic, lipolytic, and proteolytic enzymes. Amylolytic enzymes such as amylase hydrolyze starch to oligosaccharides and to the disaccharide maltose. The *lipolytic enzymes* include lipase, phospholipase A, and cholesterol esterase. Bile salts *inhibit* lipase, but colipase, another constituent of pancreatic secretion, binds to lipase and prevents this inhibition. Bile salts *activate* phospholipase A and cholesterol esterase. *Proteolytic enzymes* include *endopeptidases* (trypsin, chymotrypsin), which act on the internal peptide bonds of proteins and polypeptides; exopeptidases (carboxypeptidases, aminopeptidases), which act on the free carboxyl-terminal end and free amino-terminal end of peptides, respectively; and elastase. The proteolytic enzymes are secreted as inactive precursors (zymogens). Ribonucleases (deoxyribonucleases, ribonuclease) are also secreted. While parallel secretion of pancreatic enzymes usually occurs, nonparallel secretion can occur as a result of exocytosis from heterogeneous sources within the pancreas. *Enterokinase*, an enzyme found within the duodenal mucosa, cleaves the lysine-isoleucine bond of trypsinogen to form trypsin. Trypsin then activates the other proteolytic zymogens in a cascade phenomenon. All pancreatic enzymes have pH optima in the alkaline range.

AUTOPROTECTION OF THE PANCREAS Autodigestion of the pancreas is prevented by the packaging of proteases in precursor form and by the synthesis of protease inhibitors. These protease inhibitors are found within the acinar cell, the pancreatic secretions, and the alpha$_1$- and alpha$_2$-globulin fractions of plasma.

EXOCRINE-ENDOCRINE RELATIONSHIPS Pancreatic glucagon (29 amino acid residues) has a high degree of structural similarity to secretin. It decreases volume and enzyme secretion by the pancreas but not bicarbonate secretion. Glucose, in large concentrations, may also inhibit pancreatic exocrine secretion. The choleretic and insulinotropic effects of secretin are shared by glucagon.

ENTEROPANCREATIC AXIS AND FEEDBACK INHIBITION Pancreatic enzyme secretion in human beings is controlled, at least in part, by a negative feedback mechanism induced by the presence of active serine proteases in the duodenum. To illustrate, intraduodenal perfusion with phenylalanine causes a prompt increase in plasma CCK levels as well as increased secretion of chymotrypsin. However, simultaneous perfusion with trypsin blunts both responses. Conversely, duodenal perfusion with protease inhibitors actually leads to enzyme hypersecretion. It appears that serine proteases inhibit pancreatic secretion by acting upon a CCK-releasing peptide found within the lumen of the small intestine.

ACUTE PANCREATITIS

GENERAL CONSIDERATIONS Pancreatic inflammatory disease may be classified as follows: (1) acute pancreatitis and (2) chronic pancreatitis. This classification is based primarily on clinical criteria with the obvious difference between the acute and chronic varieties being restoration of normal function in the former and permanent residual damage in the latter. The pathologic spectrum of acute pancreatitis varies from *edematous pancreatitis*, which is usually a mild and self-limited disorder, to *necrotizing pancreatitis*, in which the degree of pancreatic necrosis correlates with the severity of the attack and its systemic manifestations. The term *hemorrhagic pancreatitis* is less meaningful in a clinical sense because variable amounts of interstitial hemorrhage can be found in pancreatitis as well as in other disorders such as pancreatic trauma, pancreatic carcinoma, and severe congestive heart failure.

The incidence of pancreatitis varies in different countries and depends upon etiologic factors, e.g., alcohol, gallstones, metabolic factors, and drugs (Table 260-1). In the United States, for example, acute pancreatitis is related to alcohol ingestion more commonly than to gallstones; in England the opposite obtains. Epidemiologic data based on autopsy data indicate that in the United States the overall prevalence of acute pancreatitis is approximately 0.5 percent. An upward trend has been noted in the crude death rate from 1.0 per 100,000 in 1955 to 1.3 in 1965.

ETIOLOGY AND PATHOGENESIS There are many causative factors in the pathogenesis of acute pancreatitis (Table 260-1), but the mechanisms by which these conditions trigger pancreatic inflammation have not been identified. Alcoholic patients with pancreatitis may represent a special subset, since most alcoholics do not develop pancreatitis. The list of identifiable causes is growing, and it is likely that pancreatitis related to viral infections, drugs, and as yet undefined factors is more common than heretofore recognized.

Autodigestion is one pathogenetic theory which proposes that proteolytic enzymes (e.g., trypsinogen, chymotrypsinogen, proelastase, and phospholipase A) are activated within the pancreas rather than in the intestinal lumen. A variety of factors (such as endotoxins, exotoxins, viral infections, ischemia, anoxia, and direct trauma) are believed to activate these proenzymes. Activated proteolytic enzymes, especially trypsin, not only digest pancreatic and peripancreatic tissues but also can activate other enzymes such as elastase and phospholipase. The active enzymes then digest cellular membranes and cause proteolysis, edema, interstitial hemorrhage, vascular damage, coagulation necrosis, fat necrosis, and parenchymal cell necrosis. Cellular injury and death result in the liberation of activated enzymes. In addition, activation and release of bradykinin peptides and vasoactive substances (e.g., histamine) are believed to produce vasodilatation,

TABLE 260-1 Causes of acute pancreatitis

I Alcohol ingestion (acute and chronic alcoholism)
II Biliary tract disease (gallstones)
III Postoperative (abdominal, nonabdominal)
IV Postendoscopic retrograde cholangiopancreatography (ERCP)
V Trauma (especially blunt abdominal type)
VI Metabolic
  A Hypertriglyceridemia
  B Apolipoprotein CII deficiency syndrome
  C Hypercalcemia, e.g., hyperparathyroidism
  D Renal failure
  E After renal transplantation*
  F Acute fatty liver of pregnancy†
VII Hereditary pancreatitis
VIII Infections
  A Mumps
  B Viral hepatitis
  C Other viral infections (coxsackievirus, echovirus)
  D Ascariasis
  E Mycoplasma
IX Drug-associated
  A Definite association
    1 Azathioprine
    2 Sulfonamides
    3 Thiazide diuretics
    4 Furosemide
    5 Estrogens (oral contraceptives)
    6 Tetracycline
    7 Valproic acid
    8 Pentamidine
  B Probable association
    1 Chlorthalidone
    2 Ethacrynic acid
    3 Procainamide
    4 Iatrogenic hypercalcemia
    5 L-Asparaginase
X Connective tissue disorders with vasculitis
  A Systemic lupus erythematosus
  B Necrotizing angiitis
  C Thrombotic thrombocytopenic purpura
XI Penetrating peptic ulcer
XII Obstruction of the ampulla of Vater
  A Regional enteritis
  B Duodenal diverticulum
XIII Pancreas divisum
XIV Recurrent bouts of acute pancreatitis without obvious cause
  A Consider
    1 Occult disease of the biliary tree or pancreatic ducts
    2 Drugs
    3 Hypertriglyceridemia
    4 Pancreas divisum
XV Other

* Pancreatitis occurs in 3 percent of renal transplant patients and is due to many factors including surgery, hypercalcemia, drugs (corticosteroids, azathioprine, L-asparaginase, diuretics), and viral infections.
† Pancreatitis also occurs in otherwise uncomplicated pregnancy and is most often associated with cholelithiasis.

increased vascular permeability, and edema. There is thus a cascade of events culminating in the development of acute necrotizing pancreatitis.

The autodigestion theory has largely eclipsed two older theories. First, the "common channel" theory holds that such an anatomic arrangement facilitates reflux of bile into the pancreatic duct, and this results in activation of pancreatic enzymes. (Actually, a common channel with free communication between the common bile duct and main pancreatic duct is infrequently encountered.) The second theory is that obstruction and hypersecretion are pivotal in the development of pancreatitis. Obstruction of the main pancreatic duct, however, produces pancreatic edema but not pancreatitis.

A recent hypothesis to explain the intrapancreatic activation of zymogens is that they become activated by *lysosomal hydrolases* within the pancreatic acinar cell itself. In two different types of experimental pancreatitis, it has been demonstrated that digestive enzymes and lysosomal hydrolases become admixed; as a result the former can be activated within the acinar cell by the latter. *In vitro,* lysosomal enzymes such as cathepsin B can activate trypsinogen, and trypsin can activate the other protease precursors.

CLINICAL FEATURES *Abdominal pain* is the major symptom of acute pancreatitis. Pain may vary from a mild and tolerable discomfort to severe, constant, and incapacitating distress. Characteristically, the pain, which is steady and boring in character, is located in the epigastrium and periumbilical region and often radiates to the back as well as to the chest, flanks, and lower abdomen. The pain is frequently more intense when the patient is supine, and patients often obtain relief by sitting with the trunk flexed and knees drawn up. Nausea, vomiting, and abdominal distention due to gastric and intestinal hypomotility and chemical peritonitis are also frequent complaints.

Physical examination frequently reveals a distressed and anxious patient. Low-grade fever, tachycardia, and hypotension are fairly common. Shock is not unusual and may result from (1) hypovolemia secondary to exudation of blood and plasma proteins into the retroperitoneal space, i.e., a "retroperitoneal burn"; (2) increased formation and release of kinin peptides which cause vasodilatation and increased vascular permeability; and (3) systemic effects of proteolytic and lipolytic enzymes released into the circulation. Jaundice occurs infrequently; when present it usually is due to edema of the head of the pancreas with compression of the intrapancreatic portion of the common bile duct. Erythematous skin nodules due to subcutaneous fat necrosis may occur. In 10 to 20 percent of patients there are pulmonary findings, including basilar rales, atelectasis, and pleural effusion, the latter most frequently left-sided. Abdominal tenderness and muscle rigidity are present to a variable degree, but compared with the intense pain, these signs may be unimpressive. Bowel sounds are usually diminished or absent. A pancreatic pseudocyst may be palpable in the upper abdomen. A faint blue discoloration around the umbilicus (Cullen's sign) may occur as the result of hemoperitoneum, and a blue-red-purple or green-brown discoloration of the flanks (Turner's sign) reflects tissue catabolism of hemoglobin. The latter two findings, which are uncommon, indicate the presence of a severe necrotizing pancreatitis.

LABORATORY DATA The diagnosis of acute pancreatitis is usually established by the presence of an increased serum amylase. Values elevated threefold above normal virtually clinch the diagnosis if overt salivary gland disease and gut perforation or infarction are excluded. However, there appears to be no definite correlation between the severity of pancreatitis and the degree of serum amylase elevation. After 48 to 72 h, even with continuing evidence of pancreatitis, total serum amylase values tend to return to normal. However, pancreatic isoamylase and lipase levels may remain elevated for 7 to 14 days. It will be recalled that amylase elevations in serum and urine occur in many conditions other than pancreatitis (see Table 259-2). Importantly, patients with *acidemia* (arterial pH $\leq$7.32) may have spurious elevations in serum amylase. In one study, 12 of 33 acidemic patients had an elevated serum amylase but only one had an elevated lipase value; 9 had salivary-type amylase as the predominant serum isoamylase. This explains why patients with diabetic ketoacidosis may have marked elevations in serum amylase without any other evidence to support a diagnosis of acute pancreatitis. The urine amylase C_{am}/C_{cr} ratio is usually elevated in patients with severe pancreatitis; this ratio usually is not increased in patients with normal serum amylase. Serum lipase activity increases in parallel with amylase activity, and measurement of both enzymes increases the diagnostic yield. An elevated serum lipase or trypsin value is usually diagnostic of acute pancreatitis; these tests are especially helpful in patients with nonpancreatic causes of hyperamylasemia (see Table 259-4). Markedly increased levels of peritoneal or pleural fluid amylase [>1500 nmol/L (>5000 units per deciliter)] are also helpful, if present, in establishing the diagnosis.

Leukocytosis (15,000 to 20,000 leukocytes per microliter) occurs frequently. More severe cases may show hemoconcentration with hematocrit values exceeding 50 percent because of loss of plasma into the retroperitoneal space and peritoneal cavity. *Hyperglycemia* is common and is due to multiple factors that include decreased insulin release, increased glucagon release, and increased output of adrenal glucocorticoids and catecholamines. *Hypocalcemia* occurs in approximately 25 percent of cases, and its pathogenesis is incompletely understood. While earlier studies suggested that the parathyroid gland response to a decrease in serum calcium is impaired, subsequent observations have failed to confirm this. Intraperitoneal saponification of calcium by fatty acids in areas of fat necrosis occurs occasionally with large amounts (up to 6.0 g) dissolved or suspended in ascitic fluid. Such "soap formation" also may be significant in patients with pancreatitis, mild hypocalcemia, and little or no obvious ascites. *Hyperbilirubinemia* [serum bilirubin >68 μmol/L (>4.0 mg/dL)] occurs in approximately 10 percent of patients. However, jaundice is transient and serum bilirubin levels return to normal in 4 to 7 days. Serum alkaline phosphatase and aspartate aminotransferase (AST) levels are also transiently elevated and parallel serum bilirubin values. When markedly elevated [i.e., >8.5 μmol/L (>500 units per deciliter)], serum lactic dehydrogenase (LDH) levels suggest a poor prognosis. Serum albumin is decreased to ≤30 g/L (≤3.0 g/dL) in about 10 percent of cases and is associated with more severe pancreatitis and an increased mortality rate (Table 260-2). Methemalbumin, a circulating heme metabolite attached to albumin, has been considered as a useful index of severe necrotizing pancreatitis. Its usefulness, however, has been limited by its nonspecificity for pancreatitis (it occurs, for example, in abdominal trauma, bone fractures, soft-tissue trauma, and retroperitoneal hematoma) and its absence in the majority of cases of severe necrotizing pancreatitis. *Hypertriglyceridemia* occurs in 15 to 20 percent of cases, and serum amylase levels in such patients are often spuriously normal (see Chap. 259). Most patients with hypertriglyceridemia and pancreatitis, when subsequently examined, show evidence of an underlying derangement in lipid metabolism which probably antedated the pancreatitis. Approximately 25 percent of patients have *hypoxemia* (arterial $P_{O_2} \leq$ 60 mmHg), which may herald the onset of adult respiratory distress syndrome. Finally, the electrocardiogram is occasionally abnormal in acute pancreatitis with ST-segment and T-wave abnormalities simulating myocardial ischemia.

Radiologic studies useful in the diagnosis of acute pancreatitis are listed in Table 259-1 and discussed in Chap. 259. Although one or more of the abnormalities are found in over 50 percent of patients, the findings are inconstant and nonspecific. The chief value of conventional x-rays [chest; kidney, ureter, and bladder (KUB)] in acute pancreatitis is to help exclude other diagnoses, especially a perforated viscus. Upper gastrointestinal tract x-rays have been superseded by ultrasonography and CT scanning. A CT scan may confirm the clinical impression of acute pancreatitis even in the face of normal serum amylase levels. Importantly, CT is quite helpful in indicating the severity of acute pancreatitis and its expected morbidity and mortality. Sonography and radionuclide scanning (PIPIDA, HIDA) are useful in acute pancreatitis to evaluate the gallbladder and biliary tree.

DIAGNOSIS Any severe acute pain in the abdomen or back should suggest acute pancreatitis. The diagnosis is usually entertained when a patient with a possible predisposition to pancreatitis presents with severe and constant abdominal pain, nausea, emesis, fever, tachycardia, and abnormal findings on abdominal examination. Laboratory studies frequently reveal leukocytosis, abnormal x-rays of the abdomen and chest, hypocalcemia, and hyperglycemia. The diagnosis is usually confirmed by finding an elevated serum amylase and/or lipase. Obviously, not all the above features have to be present for the diagnosis to be established.

The *differential diagnosis* should include consideration of the following disorders: (1) perforated viscus, especially peptic ulcer; (2) acute cholecystitis and biliary colic; (3) acute intestinal obstruction; (4) mesenteric vascular occlusion; (5) renal colic; (6) myocardial infarction; (7) dissecting aortic aneurysm; (8) connective tissue disorders with vasculitis; (9) pneumonia; and (10) diabetic ketoacidosis. A penetrating duodenal ulcer can usually be identified by upper gastrointestinal x-rays and/or endoscopy. A perforated duodenal ulcer is readily diagnosed by the presence of free intraperitoneal air. It may be difficult to differentiate acute cholecystitis from acute pancreatitis since an elevated serum amylase may be found in both disorders. Pain of biliary tract origin is more right-sided and gradual in onset, and ileus is usually absent; sonography and radionuclide scanning are helpful in establishing the diagnosis of cholelithiasis and cholecystitis. Intestinal obstruction due to mechanical factors can be differentiated from pancreatitis by the history of colicky pain, findings on abdominal examination, and x-rays of the abdomen showing characteristic changes of mechanical obstruction. Acute mesenteric vascular occlusion is usually evident in elderly debilitated patients with brisk leukocytosis, abdominal distention, and bloody diarrhea, in whom paracentesis shows sanguinous fluid and arteriography shows vascular occlusion. Serum as well as peritoneal fluid amylase levels are increased, however, in patients with intestinal infarction. Systemic lupus erythematosus and polyarteritis nodosa may be confused with pancreatitis, especially since pancreatitis may develop as a complication of those diseases. Diabetic ketoacidosis is often accompanied by abdominal pain and elevated total serum amylase levels, thus closely mimicking acute pancreatitis. However, the serum lipase and pancreatic isoamylase are not elevated in diabetic ketoacidosis.

COURSE OF THE DISEASE AND COMPLICATIONS There is an increased mortality rate with three or more risk factors identifiable either at the time of admission to hospital or during the initial 48 h of hospitalization (see Table 260-2). It is important to identify the patient with acute pancreatitis with an increased risk of dying. This subgroup is characterized by the following features: (1) respiratory failure with an arterial P_{O_2} <60 mmHg; (2) shock; (3) massive colloid replacement; (4) serum calcium <2.0 mmol/L (<8 mg/dL); and (5) the presence of "toxic broth" or dark (hemorrhagic) fluid on abdominal paracentesis. The presence of any one factor constitutes a severe attack. In one large series characterized by at least three of the first four features, the survival rate was only 29 percent in the patients treated with medical measures but increased to 64 percent with operative treatment. In another series, the mortality rate was 0.9 percent in patients with zero to two factors (Table 260-2), 16 percent in patients with three to four factors, and 40 percent with five to six factors present. The high mortality rate of such severely ill patients is due in large part to infection and warrants intensive radiologic intervention and monitoring and/or a combination of radiologic and surgical means as discussed in detail below.

The local and systemic complications of acute pancreatitis are listed in Table 260-3. Patients frequently develop an inflammatory mass in the first 2 to 3 weeks after pancreatitis. These may be phlegmons, abscesses, or pseudocysts (see below). Systemic complications include pulmonary, cardiovascular, hematologic, renal, metabolic, and central nervous system abnormalities. Pancreatitis, hypertriglyceridemia, and alcoholism constitute a triad in which cause and effect remain incompletely understood. However, several reasonable conclusions can be drawn. First, hypertriglyceridemia can precede and apparently cause the development of pancreatitis. Second,

TABLE 260-2 Factors adversely influencing survival in acute pancreatitis*

I Risk factors identifiable upon admission to hospital
- *A* Increasing age
- *B* Hypotension
- *C* Abnormal pulmonary findings
- *D* Abdominal mass
- *E* Hemorrhagic or discolored peritoneal fluid
- *F* Increased serum LDH levels
- *G* Leukocytosis
- *H* Hyperglycemia
- *I* First attack of pancreatitis

II Risk factors identifiable during initial 48 h of hospitalization
- *A* Fall in hematocrit > 10 percent with hydration and/or hematocrit < 30 percent
- *B* Necessity for massive fluid and colloid replacement
- *C* Hypocalcemia
- *D* Hypoxemia with or without adult respiratory distress syndrome
- *E* Hemorrhagic brown peritoneal fluid, i.e., "toxic broth"
- *F* Hypoalbuminemia
- *G* Azotemia

* Increased mortality with three or more risk factors.

TABLE 260-3 Complications of acute pancreatitis

I Local
- *A* Pancreatic phlegmon
- *B* Pancreatic abscess
- *C* Pancreatic pseudocyst
  - *1* Pain
  - *2* Rupture
  - *3* Hemorrhage
  - *4* Infection
  - *5* Obstruction of gastrointestinal tract (stomach, duodenum, colon)
- *D* Pancreatic ascites
  - *1* Disruption of main pancreatic duct
  - *2* Leaking pseudocyst
- *E* Involvement of contiguous organs by necrotizing pancreatitis
  - *1* Massive intraperitoneal hemorrhage
  - *2* Thrombosis of blood vessels
  - *3* Bowel infarction
- *F* Obstructive jaundice

II Systemic
- *A* Pulmonary
  - *1* Pleural effusion
  - *2* Atelectasis
  - *3* Mediastinal abscess
  - *4* Pneumonitis
  - *5* Adult respiratory distress syndrome
- *B* Cardiovascular
  - *1* Hypotension
    - *a* Hypovolemia
    - *b* Hypoalbuminemia
  - *2* Sudden death
  - *3* Nonspecific ST-T changes in electrocardiogram simulating myocardial infarction
  - *4* Pericardial effusion
- *C* Hematologic
  - *1* Disseminated intravascular coagulation (DIC)
- *D* Gastrointestinal hemorrhage*
  - *1* Peptic ulcer disease
  - *2* Erosive gastritis
  - *3* Hemorrhagic pancreatic necrosis with erosion into major blood vessels
  - *4* Portal vein thrombosis, variceal hemorrhage
- *E* Renal
  - *1* Oliguria
  - *2* Azotemia
  - *3* Renal artery and/or renal vein thrombosis
- *F* Metabolic
  - *1* Hyperglycemia
  - *2* Hypertriglyceridemia
  - *3* Hypocalcemia
  - *4* Encephalopathy
  - *5* Sudden blindness (Purtscher's retinopathy)
- *G* Central nervous system
  - *1* Psychosis
  - *2* Fat emboli
- *H* Fat necrosis
  - *1* Subcutaneous tissues (erythematous nodules)
  - *2* Bone
  - *3* Miscellaneous (mediastinum, pleura, nervous system)

* Aggravated by coagulation abnormalities (DIC).

the vast majority (>80 percent) of patients with acute pancreatitis do not have hypertriglyceridemia. Third, almost all patients with pancreatitis and hypertriglyceridemia are *either* alcoholics who have been drinking shortly before the onset of pancreatitis *or* patients with preexistent hypertriglyceridemia. Fourth, many of the patients with this triad have persistent hypertriglyceridemia after recovery from pancreatitis and abstention from alcohol. Finally, patients with a deficiency of apolipoprotein CII have an increased incidence of pancreatitis; apolipoprotein CII activates lipoprotein lipase, which is important in clearing chylomicrons from the bloodstream.

Purtscher's retinopathy, a relatively unusual complication, refers to the sudden and severe loss of vision in patients with acute pancreatitis. It is characterized by a peculiar funduscopic appearance with cotton-wool spots and hemorrhages confined to an area limited by the optic disk and macula; it is believed to be due to posterior retinal artery occlusion with aggregated granulocytes.

TREATMENT In most patients (approximately 85 to 90 percent) with acute pancreatitis, the disease is self-limited and subsides spontaneously, usually within 3 to 7 days after treatment is instituted. Medical therapy is aimed at reducing pancreatic secretion and, in essence, "putting the pancreas at rest." Conventional measures include (1) analgesics for pain, (2) intravenous fluids and colloids to maintain normal intravascular volume, (3) no oral alimentation, and (4) nasogastric suction to decrease gastrin release from the stomach and prevent gastric contents from entering the duodenum. Recent controlled trials, however, have shown that nasogastric suction offers no clear-cut advantages in the treatment of mild to moderately severe acute pancreatitis. Its use, therefore, must be considered elective rather than mandatory.

It has been demonstrated that CCK-stimulated pancreatic secretion is almost abolished in four different experimental models of acute pancreatitis. This probably explains why drugs to block pancreatic secretion in acute pancreatitis have failed to have any therapeutic benefit. For this and other reasons, anticholinergic drugs are not indicated in acute pancreatitis. Although antibiotics have been used in the treatment of acute pancreatitis, three recent randomized prospective trials have shown no benefit from the use of antibiotics in acute pancreatitis of mild to moderate severity. However, because secondary infection of necrotic pancreatic tissue (phlegmon, abscess, pseudocyst) or obstructed biliary passages (ascending cholangitis, complicating choledocholithiasis) contributes to much of the late mortality, appropriate *antibiotic therapy of established infection* is obviously quite important. Previous reports suggested that glucagon was useful in acute pancreatitis, but controlled trials have not provided convincing evidence of effectiveness. Similarly, a protease inhibitor such as aprotinin (Trasylol) and cimetidine have not proved effective.

A CT scan provides valuable information on the severity and prognosis of acute pancreatitis (Fig. 260-1). The following classification is in widespread use: grade A, normal; grade B, focal or diffuse pancreatic edema; grade C, extension of inflammatory changes to the peripancreatic fat; grade D, phlegmon or a single ill-defined fluid collection in or around the pancreas and often extending to the lesser sac and/or pararenal space; grade E, two or more fluid collections *or* presence of gas in or adjacent to the pancreas. Recent studies suggest that the likelihood of prolonged pancreatitis or serious complications is negligible when CT scans are either grade A or B; possible although unlikely with a grade of C; and most likely to occur with grades D and E. The patient with mild to moderate pancreatitis usually requires treatment with intravenous fluids, fasting, and possibly nasogastric suction for 2 to 4 days. A clear liquid diet is frequently started on the third to sixth day and a regular diet by the fifth to seventh day. The patient with unremitting *fulminant pancreatitis* usually requires inordinate amounts of fluid and close attention to complications such as cardiovascular collapse, respiratory insufficiency, and pancreatic infection. The latter should be managed by a combination of radiologic and surgical means (see below). While earlier uncontrolled studies suggested that *peritoneal lavage* via a percutaneous dialysis catheter is helpful in severe pancreatitis, recent studies indicate that such treatment does not influence the outcome of such attacks. Laparotomy with adequate drainage and removal of necrotic tissue should be considered if conventional therapy does not halt the patient's deterioration. The use of parenteral nutrition makes it possible to give nutritional support to patients with severe, acute, or protracted pancreatitis who are unable to eat normally. Finally, patients with severe gallstone-induced pancreatitis may improve dramatically if papillotomy is carried out within the first 36 to 72 h of the attack.

PANCREATIC PHLEGMON, ABSCESS, AND PSEUDOCYST The *phlegmon* is a solid mass of swollen, inflamed pancreas often containing patchy areas of necrosis; it may be present for 1 to 2 weeks. This prolonged inflammatory process should not be confused with a pseudocyst, a differentiation which is usually accomplished by sonography. A phlegmon should be suspected if abdominal pain, fever, leukocytosis, and hyperamylasemia persist for more than 5 days and especially if an abdominal mass is also present. Differentiation from an abscess may be difficult even with a CT scan. Occasionally, extensive areas of pancreatic necrosis develop in phlegmons and require incision and drainage. Phlegmons may also

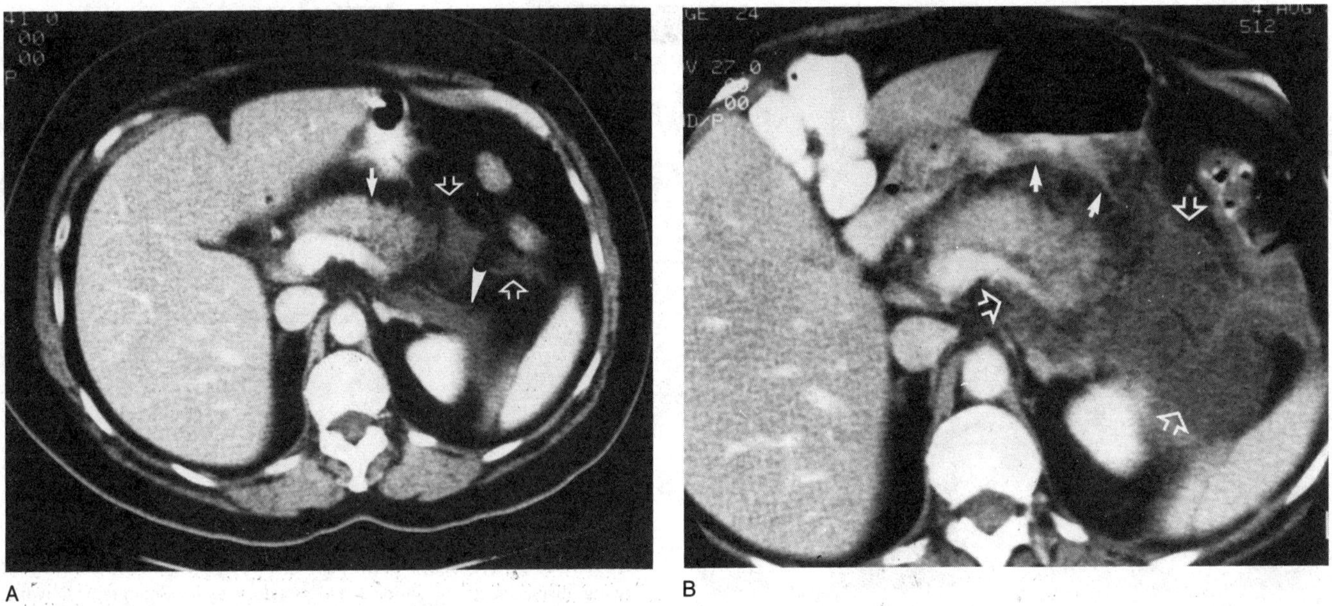

FIGURE 260-1 Acute pancreatitis: CT evolution. *A*. This contrast-enhanced CT scan of the abdomen was performed on the day of admission on a patient with clinical evidence of acute pancreatitis. Note the mildly decreased density of the body of the pancreas to the left of the midline (arrow). There are a few linear strands in the peripancreatic fat, suggesting inflammation (open arrows). A small amount of fluid is seen in the anterior pararenal space (arrowhead). *B*. Nine days after admission, there is a marked worsening with severe inflammation of the pancreas evidenced by anterior displacement of the posterior gastric wall (arrows), increased inflammation of the peripancreatic fat, and increased pancreatic effusion in the anterior perirenal space and around the splenic vein (open arrows). *(Courtesy of Dr. P.R. Ros, University of Florida College of Medicine.)*

be secondarily infected, resulting in abscess formation. The latter occurs in 10 percent of patients with acute pancreatitis. The early diagnosis of pancreatic infection can be accomplished by CT-guided needle aspiration. In one study, 60 patients, representing 5 percent of all admissions for acute pancreatitis, were suspected of harboring a pancreatic infection on the basis of fever, leukocytosis, and an abnormal CT scan (phlegmon, pseudocyst, or extrapancreatic fluid collection). Importantly, 36 of 60 patients (60 percent) had a pancreatic infection with 20 of the 36 (55 percent) developing infection within the first 2 weeks. This study suggests that only guided aspiration can reliably distinguish sterile from infected pancreatitis. The following are guidelines for patients meeting the above selection criteria: (1) pseudocysts and phlegmons should be aspirated promptly because more than half could be infected; (2) extrapancreatic fluid collections need not be aspirated promptly as most are sterile; (3) if a phlegmon is found initially to be sterile but fever and leukocytosis persist, allow several days of observation before considering reaspiration, as clinical improvement frequently occurs; and (4) if fever and leukocytosis recur after an interval of well-being, consider reaspiration.

Severe pancreatitis with the presence of three or more risk factors, postoperative pancreatitis, early oral feeding, early laparotomy, and perhaps injudicious use of antibiotics predispose to the development of pancreatic abscess. Pancreatic abscess may also develop because of communication of a pseudocyst with the colon, after inadequate surgical drainage of a pseudocyst, or after needling of a pseudocyst. The characteristic signs of abscess are fever, leukocytosis, ileus, and rapid deterioration in a patient initially recovering from pancreatitis. However, the only manifestations may be persistent fever and signs of continuing pancreatic inflammation. Drainage of pancreatic abscesses by nonsurgical percutaneous catheter techniques, using CT guidance, has been only moderately successful (resolution in 50 to 60 percent of patients). Accordingly, laparotomy with radical sump drainage and possibly resection of necrotic tissue is usually required because the mortality rate for undrained pancreatic abscess approaches 100 percent. Multiple abscesses are common and reoperation is frequently required.

Pseudocysts of the pancreas are collections of tissue, fluid, debris, pancreatic enzymes, and blood, which develop over a period of 1 to 4 weeks after the onset of acute pancreatitis in approximately 15 percent of patients. In contrast to true cysts, pseudocysts do not have epithelial lining and the walls consist of necrotic tissue, granulation tissue, and fibrous tissue. Disruption of the pancreatic ductal system is common. However, the subsequent course of this disruption varies widely, namely, from spontaneous healing to continuous leakage of pancreatic juice causing tense ascites. Pseudocysts are preceded by pancreatitis in 90 percent of cases and by trauma in 10 percent. Approximately 85 percent are located in the body or tail of the pancreas and 15 percent in the head. Some patients have two or more pseudocysts. Abdominal pain, with or without radiation to the back, is the usual presenting complaint. A palpable, tender mass may be found in the middle or left upper abdomen. The serum amylase is elevated in 75 percent of patients some time during their illness and may fluctuate markedly.

Pseudocysts often displace some portion of the gastrointestinal tract on x-ray examination in 75 percent of cases (Fig. 260-2). Sonography, however, is reliable in detecting pseudocysts. Sonography also permits differentiation between an edematous and an inflamed pancreas (pancreatic phlegmon), which can give rise to a palpable mass and an actual pseudocyst. Furthermore, serial ultrasound studies will indicate whether a pseudocyst has resolved. CT scanning complements the use of ultrasound in the diagnosis of pancreatic pseudocyst (Fig. 260-2), especially when it is infected.

The management of pseudocysts is compromised by incomplete knowledge of the natural history of this disorder. In studies utilizing sonography, pseudocysts resolved in 25 to 40 percent of patients. However, pseudocysts that are greater than 5 cm and that persist for greater than 6 weeks rarely disappear. In others, serious complications may occur such as (1) pain caused by expansion of the lesion and pressure on other viscera, (2) rupture, (3) hemorrhage, and (4) abscess. Rupture of a pancreatic pseudocyst is a particularly serious complication. Shock almost always supervenes and mortality rates range from 14 percent if the rupture is not associated with hemorrhage to over 60 percent if hemorrhage has occurred. Rupture and hemorrhage are the prime causes of mortality in pancreatic pseudocyst. A triad of findings, e.g., increase in size of the mass, localized bruit over the mass, and a sudden decrease in hemoglobin and hematocrit levels without obvious signs of external blood loss, should alert one to the diagnosis of hemorrhage from a pseudocyst. Thus, in pseudocyst

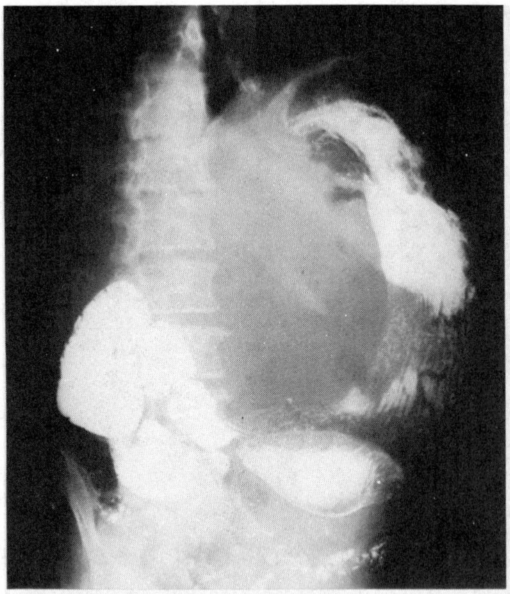

A

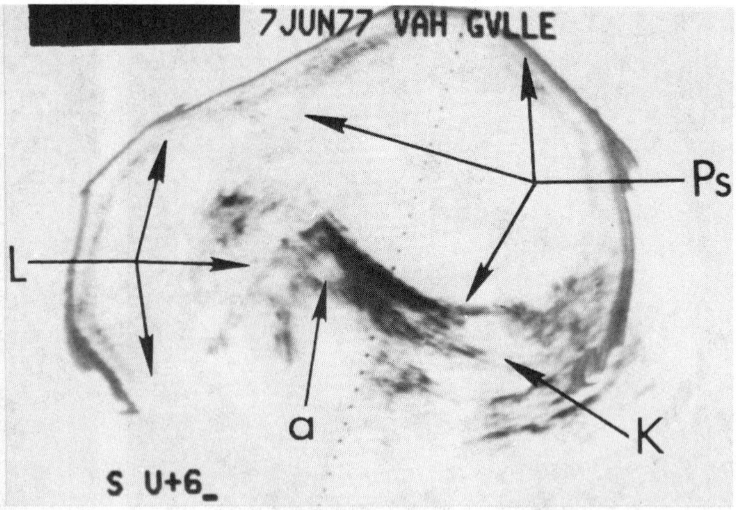

B

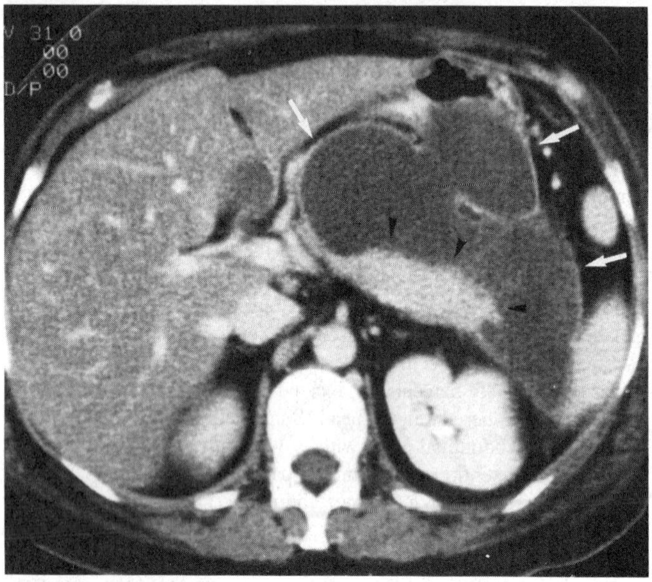

C

FIGURE 260-2 Pseudocyst of the pancreas. *A*. Upper gastrointestinal x-ray showing displacement of stomach by pseudocyst. *B*. Sonogram showing pseudocyst (Ps). K = kidney; a = aorta; L = liver. *C*. CT scan showing pseudocyst. Note a large lobulated fluid collection (arrows) surrounding the tail of the pancreas (arrowheads). Note the dense, thin rim in the periphery representing the fibrous capsule of the pseudocyst. (*Courtesy of Dr. P. R. Ros, University of Florida College of Medicine.*)

patients who are stable and uncomplicated and in whom serial ultrasound studies show a decreasing pseudocyst, conservative therapy is indicated. Conversely, patients with a pseudocyst which is expanding and which is complicated by rupture, hemorrhage, and abscess should be operated on. Using ultrasound or CT guidance, sterile chronic pseudocysts can be treated safely with single or repeated needle aspiration or more prolonged catheter drainage with an expected success rate of 45 to 75 percent. The success rate with infected pseudocysts is considerably less, i.e., 40 to 50 percent. Patients not responding to drainage require surgical therapy. Therapy consists of internal or external drainage of the cyst. Prolonged observation of a nonresolving pancreatic pseudocyst exposes the patient to increased risks which exceed those of elective surgery.

PANCREATIC ASCITES AND PANCREATIC PLEURAL EFFUSIONS Pancreatic ascites is usually due to disruption of the main pancreatic duct, often associated with an internal fistula between the duct and the peritoneal cavity or a leaking pseudocyst (see also Chap. 48). The diagnosis of pancreatic ascites is suggested in a patient with an elevated serum amylase who also has increased levels of albumin [>30 g/L (>3.0 g/dL)] and amylase in the ascitic fluid. In addition, endoscopic retrograde cholangiopancreatography (ERCP) will often demonstrate passage of contrast material from a major pancreatic duct or a pseudocyst into the peritoneal cavity. As many as 15 percent of patients with pseudocysts have concurrent pancreatic ascites. The differential diagnosis should include intraperitoneal carcinomatosis, tuberculous peritonitis, constrictive pericarditis, and Budd-Chiari syndrome.

If the pancreatic duct disruption is posterior, an internal fistula may develop between the pancreatic duct and pleural space producing a pleural effusion, which is usually left-sided and often massive. This often requires thoracentesis or chest tube drainage.

Treatment usually involves placing the patient on nasogastric suction and parenteral alimentation to decrease pancreatic secretion. In addition, paracentesis is performed to keep the peritoneal cavity free of fluid and, it is hoped, effect sealing of the leak. If ascites continues to recur after 2 to 3 weeks of medical management, the patient should be operated on following pancreatography to define the anatomy of the abnormal duct.

CHRONIC PANCREATITIS AND PANCREATIC EXOCRINE INSUFFICIENCY

GENERAL AND ETIOLOGIC CONSIDERATIONS Chronic inflammatory disease of the pancreas may present as episodes of acute inflammation superimposed upon a previously injured pancreas or as chronic damage with persistent pain or malabsorption. The causes of relapsing chronic pancreatitis are similar to those of acute pancreatitis (Table 260-2), except that frequently there is an appreciable incidence of cases of undetermined origin. In addition, the pancreatitis associated with gallstones is predominantly acute or relapsing acute in nature. A cholecystectomy is almost always performed in patients after the first or second attack of gallstone-associated pancreatitis. Patients with chronic pancreatitis may present with persistent abdominal pain, with or without steatorrhea, and some may present with steatorrhea and no pain.

Patients with chronic pancreatitis who develop extensive destruction of the pancreas (i.e., less than 10 percent of exocrine function remaining) will demonstrate steatorrhea and azotorrhea. In the adult in the United States, alcoholism is the most common cause of clinically apparent pancreatic exocrine insufficiency, while cystic

TABLE 260-4 Causes of pancreatic exocrine insufficiency

I Alcohol, chronic alcoholism
II Cystic fibrosis
III Severe protein calorie malnutrition with hypoalbuminemia
IV Pancreatic and duodenal neoplasms
V Pancreatic resection
VI Gastric surgery
  A Subtotal gastrectomy with Billroth II anastomosis
  B Subtotal gastrectomy with Billroth I anastomosis
  C Truncal vagotomy and pyloroplasty
VII Gastrinoma (Zollinger-Ellison syndrome)
VIII Hereditary pancreatitis
IX Traumatic pancreatitis
X Hemochromatosis
XI Shwachman's syndrome (pancreatic insufficiency and bone marrow dysfunction)
XII Trypsinogen deficiency
XIII Enterokinase deficiency
XIV Isolated deficiencies of amylase, lipase, or proteases
XV Alpha$_1$-antitrypsin deficiency
XVI Idiopathic pancreatitis

fibrosis is the most frequent cause in children. In up to 25 percent of adults in the United States with chronic pancreatitis, the cause is not known, i.e., they have idiopathic chronic pancreatitis. In other parts of the world, severe protein calorie malnutrition is a common etiology. Table 260-4 lists other causes of pancreatic exocrine insufficiency, but they are relatively uncommon.

PATHOPHYSIOLOGY Unfortunately, the events that initiate an inflammatory process within the pancreas are still not well understood, and the many hypotheses will not be reviewed. In the case of alcohol-induced pancreatitis, however, it has been suggested that the primary defect may be the precipitation of protein (inspissated enzymes) within the ducts. The resulting ductal obstruction can lead to duct dilatation, diffuse atrophy of the acinar cells, fibrosis, and eventual calcification of some of the protein plugs. While patients with alcohol-induced pancreatitis generally consume large amounts of alcohol, some consume very little (i.e., 50 g or less per day). Thus, prolonged consumption of "socially acceptable" amounts of alcohol is compatible with the development of pancreatitis. In addition, the finding of extensive pancreatic fibrosis in patients who have expired during their first attack of clinical acute alcohol-induced pancreatitis supports the concept that such patients already have chronic pancreatitis.

CLINICAL FEATURES Patients with relapsing chronic pancreatitis may present with symptoms identical with those found in acute pancreatitis, but their pain may be continuous or intermittent, or pain may be absent. The pathogenesis of this pain is poorly understood. Although the classic description is that of epigastric pain radiating through the back, the pain pattern is often atypical. The pain may be maximal in the right or left upper quadrants in the back or diffuse throughout the upper abdomen; it may even be referred to the anterior chest or flank. Characteristically, the pain is persistent, deep-seated, and unresponsive to antacids. It often is increased by alcohol and ingestion of heavy meals (especially foods rich in fat). Often the pain is so severe as to require the frequent use of narcotics.

Weight loss, abnormal stools, and other signs of symptoms suggestive of malabsorption (see Table 240-5) are common in chronic pancreatitis. However, clinically apparent deficiencies of fat-soluble vitamins are surprisingly rare. The physical findings in these patients are usually not impressive such that there is a disparity between the severity of the abdominal pain and the paucity of physical signs (save some abdominal tenderness and mild temperature elevation).

DIAGNOSTIC EVALUATION (See Chap. 259) In contrast to patients with relapsing acute pancreatitis, the serum amylase and lipase levels are usually not elevated. Elevations of the serum bilirubin and alkaline phosphatase may indicate cholestasis secondary to chronic inflammation around the common bile duct (Fig. 260-3). Many patients demonstrate impaired glucose tolerance, and some may have an elevated fasting blood glucose level.

The classic triad of pancreatic calcification, steatorrhea, and diabetes mellitus usually establishes the diagnosis of chronic pancreatitis and exocrine pancreatic insufficiency but is found in less than one-third of chronic pancreatitis patients. Accordingly, it is often necessary to perform an intubation test such as the *secretin stimulation test,* which usually becomes abnormal when 70 percent or more of pancreatic exocrine function has been lost. Approximately 40 percent of patients with chronic pancreatitis have *cobalamin (vitamin B_{12}) malabsorption* which is corrected by the administration of oral pancreatic enzymes. There is usually a marked excretion of fecal fat (see Chap. 240), which can be reduced with the administration of oral pancreatic enzymes. A fecal fat concentration $\geq$9.5 percent is characteristic of pancreatogenous steatorrhea (see Table 259-1). The bentiromide test (Chap. 259) and D-xylose urinary excretion test are useful in patients with "pancreatic steatorrhea," since the bentiromide test will be abnormal and the D-xylose excretion usually normal. A decreased serum trypsinogen strongly suggests pancreatic exocrine insufficiency.

The radiographic hallmark of chronic pancreatitis is the presence of scattered calcification throughout the pancreas (Fig. 260-3). Diffuse pancreatic calcification indicates that significant damage has occurred and obviates the need for a secretin test. Alcohol is by far the most common cause of pancreatic calcification, but it may also be seen in severe protein-calorie malnutrition, hereditary pancreatitis, posttraumatic pancreatitis, hyperparathyroidism, islet cell tumors, and idiopathic chronic pancreatitis. An ongoing prospective study of 107 patients has shown convincingly that pancreatic calcification may decrease or even disappear either following ductal decompression or spontaneously in one-third of patients with severe chronic pancreatitis. Pancreatic calcification is a dynamic process that is incompletely understood.

Special techniques such as sonography, CT scanning, and ERCP have added new dimensions to the diagnosis of pancreatic disease. In addition to excluding pseudocysts and pancreatic cancer, sonography may show calcification or dilated ducts associated with chronic pancreatitis (Fig. 260-4). Similar benefits can be derived from CT scans. ERCP is the only nonoperative technique which provides a direct view of the pancreatic duct. In patients with alcohol-induced pancreatitis, ERCP may reveal a pseudocyst missed by sonography or CT scan.

COMPLICATIONS OF CHRONIC PANCREATITIS The complications of chronic pancreatitis are protean. *Cobalamin (vitamin B_{12}) malabsorption* occurs in 40 percent of patients with alcohol-induced chronic pancreatitis and in virtually all with cystic fibrosis. The cobalamin malabsorption is consistently corrected by the administration of pancreatic enzymes (containing proteases). The cobalamin malabsorption may be due to excessive binding of cobalamin by nonintrinsic factor cobalamin-binding proteins. The latter are ordinarily destroyed by pancreatic proteases, but with pancreatic insufficiency the nonspecific binding proteins escape degradation and compete with intrinsic factor for cobalamin binding. Although the majority of patients show *impaired glucose tolerance,* the development of diabetic ketoacidosis and coma is uncommon. Similarly, end organ damage (retinopathy, neuropathy, nephropathy) is also uncommon, and the appearance of these complications should raise the question of concomitant genetic diabetes mellitus. A nondiabetic retinopathy, peripheral in location and secondary to vitamin A and/or zinc deficiency, is common in these patients. High-amylase-containing *effusions* occur within the pleura, pericardium, or peritoneum. *Gastrointestinal bleeding* may occur from a peptic ulcer, gastritis, a pseudocyst eroding into the duodenum, or from ruptured varices secondary to splenic vein thrombosis due to inflammation of the tail of the pancreas. *Icterus* may occur, owing to either edema of the head of the pancreas compressing the common bile duct or chronic cholestasis secondary to chronic inflammatory reaction around the intrapancreatic portion of the common bile duct (Fig. 260-3). This chronic obstruction may lead to cholangitis and ultimately biliary cirrhosis. *Subcutaneous fat necrosis* may appear as tender red nodules on the lower extremities. *Bone pain* may be secondary to intramedullary fat necrosis. Inflammation of the large and small joints of the

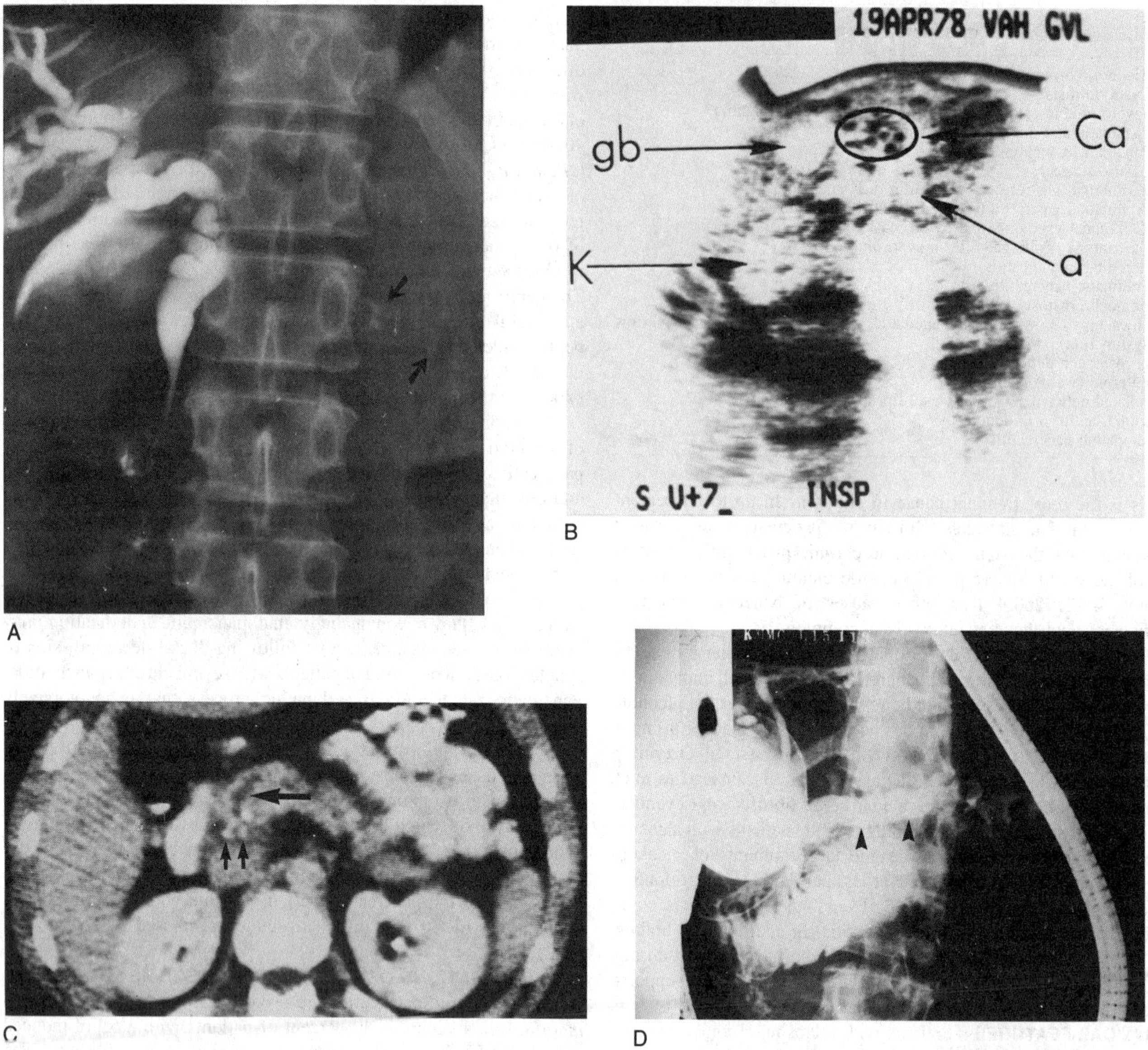

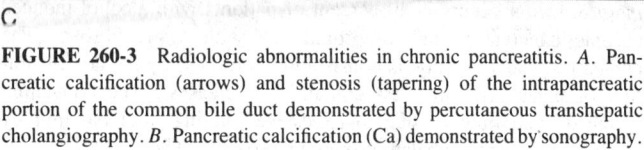

FIGURE 260-3 Radiologic abnormalities in chronic pancreatitis. *A*. Pancreatic calcification (arrows) and stenosis (tapering) of the intrapancreatic portion of the common bile duct demonstrated by percutaneous transhepatic cholangiography. *B*. Pancreatic calcification (Ca) demonstrated by sonography. gb = gallbladder; K = kidney; a = aorta. *C*. Pancreatic calcification (vertical arrows) and dilated pancreatic duct (horizontal arrow) demonstrated by CT scan. D. Endoscopic retrograde cholangiopancreatogram shows grossly dilated pancreatic ducts (arrows) in a patient with long-standing pancreatitis.

upper and lower extremities may occur. The incidence of pancreatic carcinoma is probably increased in patients with diffuse calcification. Perhaps the most common and troublesome complication is addiction to narcotics.

TREATMENT AND APPROACH TO MANAGEMENT Therapy for patients with chronic pancreatitis is directed to two major problems, namely, pain and malabsorption. Patients with intermittent attacks of pain are essentially treated like those with acute pancreatitis (see above). Patients with severe and persistent pain should avoid alcohol completely and avoid large meals rich in fat. Since the pain is often severe enough to require frequent use of narcotics (and hence addiction), a number of surgical procedures have been developed for pain relief. ERCP allows the surgeon to plan the operative approach. If there is a stricture of the pancreatic duct, then a *local resection* may ameliorate the pain. Unfortunately isolated localized strictures are not common. In most patients with alcohol-induced disease, the pancreas is diffusely involved and surgically correctible localized ductal disease is rare. When there is primary ductal obstruction and dilatation, ductal decompression may provide effective pain palliation. Short-term pain relief may be achieved in up to 80 percent of patients, while long-term pain relief occurs in approximately 50 percent. In some of these patients, however, pain relief can be achieved only by resecting 50 to 95 percent of the gland. Although pain relief is achieved in three-quarters of these patients, they tend to develop pancreatic endocrine and exocrine insufficiency and must be on pancreatic enzyme replacement therapy. It is important to screen the patients carefully, for such radical surgery is contraindicated in those who are severely depressed or suicidal or continue to drink. Procedures such as sphincteroplasty, splanchnicectomy and celiac ganglionectomy, and nerve blocks usually bring only temporary relief and are not recommended.

Two double-blind controlled trials have demonstrated that large doses of conventional pancreatic enzymes (eight tablets with each meal and at bedtime) decrease the abdominal pain in patients with chronic pancreatitis. The patients most likely to respond to such therapy with amelioration of pain are those with mild to moderate exocrine pancreatic dysfunction as evidenced by an abnormal secretin test, normal fat absorption, and minimal abnormalities upon ERCP examination. These clinical observations seem to fit in with data in human beings and experimental animals which demonstrate a negative

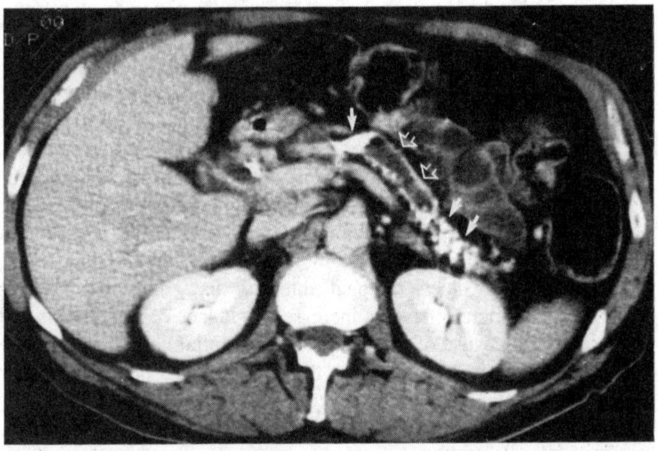
A

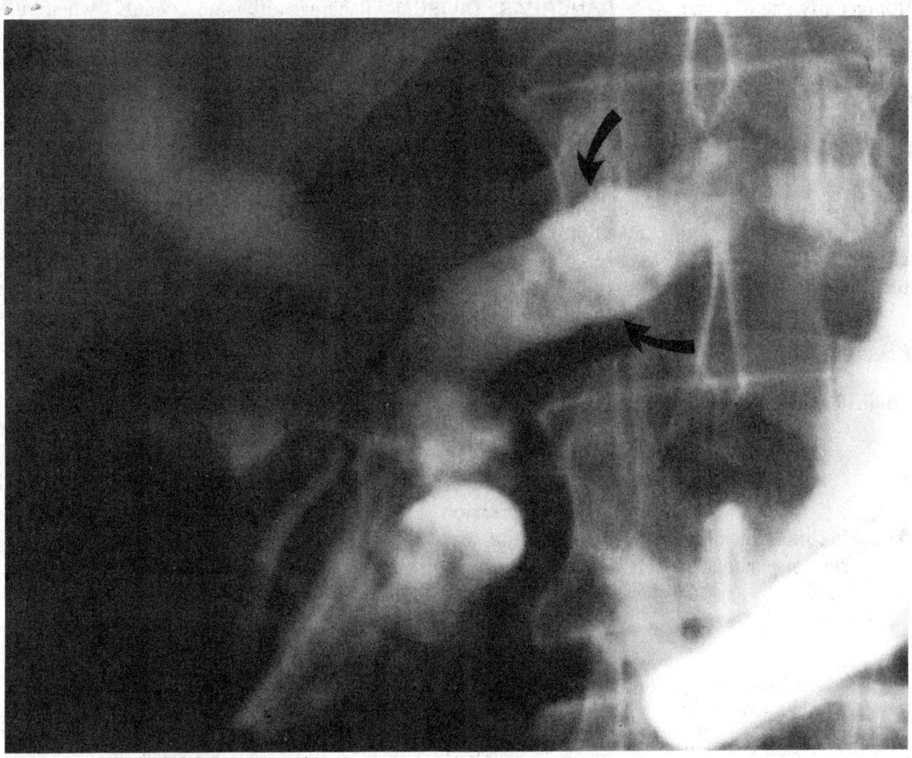
B

FIGURE 260-4 Chronic pancreatitis and pancreatic calculi: CT scan and ERCP appearance. *A*. In this contrast-enhanced CT scan of the abdomen, there is evidence of an atrophic pancreas with multiple calcifications (arrows). Note a markedly dilated pancreatic duct seen in this section through the body and tail (open arrows). *B*. ERCP in the same patient demonstrates the dilated pancreatic duct as well as an intrapancreatic duct calculus (arrows). These findings correlate nicely with the CT scan appearance.

feedback regulation for pancreatic exocrine secretion controlled by the amount of proteases within the lumen of the proximal small intestine. It seems reasonable to approach the patient with severe persistent or continuous abdominal pain thought to be secondary to chronic pancreatitis in the following manner. After other causes of abdominal pain (peptic ulcer, gallstones, etc.) have been appropriately excluded, a pancreatic *sonogram* should be done. If no mass is found, a *secretin test* may be performed, since with chronic pancreatitis and pain this test usually will be abnormal. If the secretin test is abnormal (i.e., decreased bicarbonate concentration or volume output), a 3- to 4-week *trial of pancreatic enzymes* is appropriate. Eight conventional tablets or three enteric-coated capsules are taken at meals and at bedtime. If no relief is obtained, and especially if the volume secreted during the secretin test is very low, ERCP should be performed. If a pseudocyst or a localized ductal obstruction is found, appropriate surgery should be considered. A provocative study from South Africa questions the significance of the relationship of dilated ducts and/or strictures to pain. The finding of an appreciable obstruction or stricture in 65 percent of the patients who were pain-free more than 1 year, compared with 79 percent of the group with pain, suggests that factors other than duct obstruction or narrowing may be important in the pathogenesis of pain. It may be that the most important factors in the relief of pain are abstinence from alcohol and progressive pancreatic dysfunction rather than the surgical procedure per se. If no surgically remedial lesion is found and severe pain continues despite abstinence from alcohol, subtotal pancreatic resection may be necessary.

The treatment of malabsorption rests upon the use of pancreatic enzyme replacement therapy. Although diarrhea and steatorrhea are usually improved, the results are frequently less than satisfactory. The major problem is delivery of enough active enzyme into the duodenum. Steatorrhea can be abolished if 10 percent of the normal amount of lipase could be delivered into the duodenum at the proper time. This concentration of lipase cannot be achieved with the presently available preparations of pancreatic enzymes, even if the latter are given in large doses. These poor results may be due to inactivation of lipase by gastric acid, food emptying from the stomach more rapidly than the exogenously administered pancreatic enzymes, and variation in the enzyme activity of various batches of commercially available pancreatic extracts.

For the usual patient three to eight tablets or capsules of a potent enzyme preparation should be administered with meals. Some patients on conventional tablets require adjuvant therapy to improve enzyme replacement treatment. Although initially cimetidine was considered an effective adjuvant, studies have failed to confirm this. Sodium bicarbonate (1.3 g with meals) is effective and inexpensive. Antacids containing calcium carbonate or magnesium hydroxide are not effective and may actually result in increased steatorrhea. Adjuvant therapy should not be given with enteric-coated microsphere preparations because such therapy may increase the gastric pH such that these preparations would release their enzymes into the stomach rather than the small intestine.

Patients with severe exocrine pancreatic insufficiency secondary to alcohol who continue to drink have a high mortality (in one series 50 percent were dead when followed for 5 to 12 years) and significant morbidity (weight loss, lassitude, vitamin deficiency, and narcotic addiction). Pain may abate if progressive severe exocrine insufficiency continues. If abstinence is pursued and vigorous replacement therapy is utilized for the maldigestion-malabsorption, the patients do reasonably well.

HEREDITARY PANCREATITIS Hereditary pancreatitis is a rare disease similar to chronic pancreatitis except for an early age of onset and evidence of hereditary factors (involving an autosomal dominant gene with incomplete penetrance). These patients have recurring attacks of severe abdominal pain which may last from a few days to a few weeks. The serum amylase and lipase levels may be elevated during acute attacks but are usually normal. Patients frequently develop pancreatic calcification, diabetes mellitus, and steatorrhea, and in addition, they have an increased incidence of pancreatic carcinoma. Such patients often require ductal decompression to obtain pain relief. Abdominal complaints in relatives of patients with hereditary pancreatitis should raise the question of pancreatic disease.

PANCREATIC ENDOCRINE TUMORS

Pancreatic endocrine tumors are summarized in Table 260-5 and discussed in Chap. 262.

OTHER CONDITIONS

ANNULAR PANCREAS When there is a failure in communication of the ventral and dorsal anlage of the pancreas, a ring of pancreatic tissue encircles the duodenum. Such an annular pancreas may cause intestinal obstruction in the neonate or the adult. Symptoms of postprandial fullness, epigastric pain, nausea, and vomiting may be present for years before the diagnosis is entertained. The radiographic findings are symmetric dilatation of the proximal duodenum with bulging of the recesses on either side of the annular band, effacement of the duodenal mucosa without destruction of the mucosa, accentuation of the findings in the right anterior oblique position, and the lack of change on repeated examinations. The differential diagnosis should include duodenal webs, tumors of the pancreas or duodenum, postbulbar peptic ulcer, regional enteritis, and adhesions. Patients with annular pancreas have an increased incidence of pancreatitis and peptic ulcer. Because of these and other potential complications, the treatment is surgical even though the condition has been present for years. Retrocolic duodenojejunostomy is the procedure of choice, although some surgeons advocate Billroth II gastrectomy, gastroenterostomy, and vagotomy.

PANCREAS DIVISUM Pancreas divisum occurs when the embryologic ventral and dorsal parts of the pancreas fail to fuse so that pancreatic drainage is accomplished mainly through the accessory papilla. Pancreas divisum is the most common congenital anatomic variant of the human pancreas. Current evidence indicates that this anomaly is not a predisposing factor to the development of pancreatitis in the great majority of patients with this anomaly. However, the combination of pancreas divisum and a small accessory orifice could result in dorsal duct obstruction. The challenge is to identify this subset of patients with dorsal duct pathology. Cannulation of the dorsal duct by ERCP is not as easily done as is cannulation of the ventral duct (Fig. 260-5). Patients with pancreatitis and pancreas divisum demonstrated by ERCP should be treated with conservative measures including pancreatic enzyme therapy. Many of these patients have idiopathic pancreatitis unrelated to the pancreas divisum and will respond well to pancreatic enzyme therapy. Endoscopic or surgical intervention is indicated only when the above methods fail. If marked dilation of the dorsal duct can be demonstrated, surgical ductal decompression should be performed. The appropriate therapy for those patients without dilation of the dorsal duct is not yet defined. It should be stressed that the ERCP appearance of pancreas divisum,

TABLE 260-5 Pancreatic endocrine tumors

Syndrome	Hormone(s) produced	Primary hormone effects	Pathologic features	Clinical features
Zollinger-Ellison	Gastrin	Gastric acid hypersecretion with basal acid outputs usually >15 mmol/h (>15 meq/h)	Delta cell islet tumors; 10% aberrant (duodenal); 60% malignant	Severe peptic ulcer disease often refractory to therapy; ectopic ulcers; diarrhea; multiple endocrine adenomas (parathyroid, pituitary, adrenal, thyroid)
Insulinoma	Insulin	Hypoglycemia with inappropriately increased serum insulin levels	Beta cell islet tumors; 80–90% benign	Hypoglycemic symptoms
Glucagonoma	Glucagon; pancreatic polypeptide	Hyperglucagonemia →glucose intolerance	Alpha cell islet tumors; 60% malignant	Slow-growing pancreatic tumor; hyperglycemia; bullous and eczematoid dermatitis, weight loss; anemia; gastric and intestinal motor abnormalities
Somatostatinoma	Somatostatin; pancreatic polypeptide	Somatostatin inhibits insulin, gastrin and pancreatic enzyme secretion; decreased bile flow	Delta cell islet tumor	Pancreatic tumor; diarrhea; steatorrhea; gallstones; diabetes mellitus; anemia
Pancreatic cholera	Vasoactive intestinal peptide (VIP) ? Gastric inhibitory polypeptide ? Prostaglandin E ? Pancreatic peptide	Net secretion of salt and water by gut	? Delta cell tumor; >50% malignant	Pancreatic tumor with severe watery diarrhea; flushing; weight loss; hypokalemia; hypercalcemia; hypochlorhydria; hyperglycemia; inordinate fecal water and electrolyte losses
Carcinoid	Serotonin; prostaglandins	Altered gut motility; diarrhea	Enterochromaffin cells; nonbeta cell islet tumors	Carcinoid syndrome with flushing; wheezing; diarrhea; alcohol intolerance; hepatomegaly

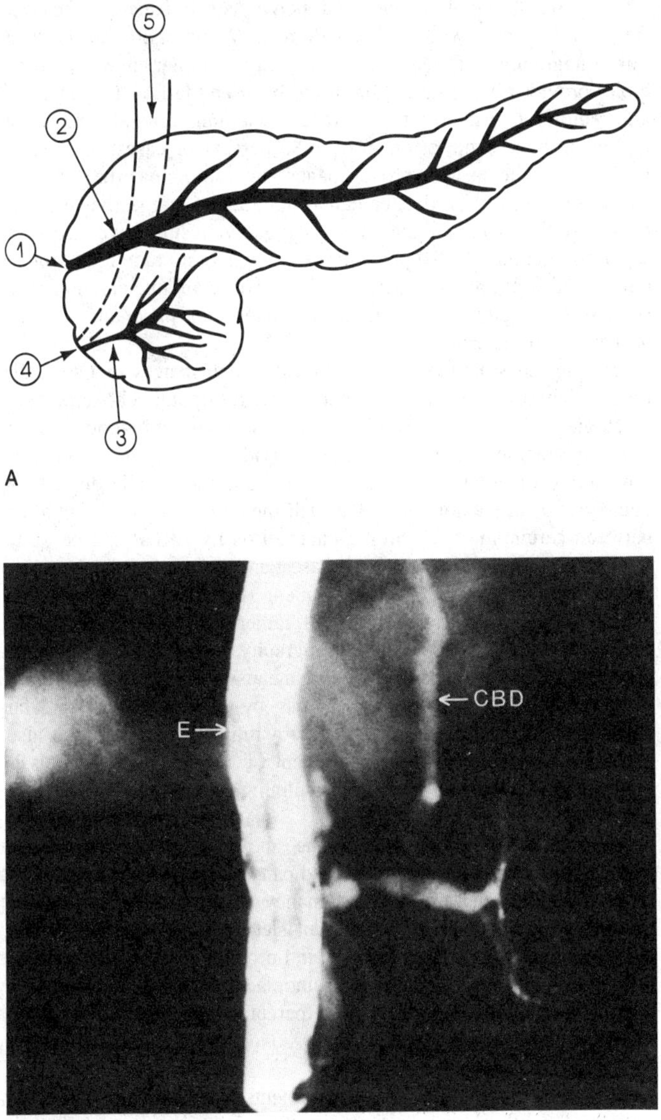

FIGURE 260-5 Illustration of the pancreatic ducts and typical ERCP of pancreas divisum. *A*. Diagram of the ventral and dorsal structures of the pancreas: (1) duct of Santorini; (2) pancreatic duct from the dorsal anlage; (3) pancreatic duct from the ventral anlage; (4) duct of Wirsung; and (5) common bile duct. *B*. ERCP showing filling only of the ventral component of the pancreatic duct and the common bile duct (CBD) from cannulization of the duct of Wirsung. Failure to fill the pancreatic duct of the body and tail of the pancreas is diagnostic of ventral pancreas or pancreas divisum. E = endoscope.

i.e., a small-caliber ventral duct with an arborizing pattern, may be confused with an obstructed main pancreatic duct secondary to a mass lesion.

MACROAMYLASEMIA Macroamylasemia is a condition whereby amylase is circulating in the blood in a polymer form too large to be easily excreted by the kidney. The patient with this condition will demonstrate an elevated serum amylase value, a low urinary amylase, and a C_{am}/C_{cr} of less than 1 percent. The presence of macroamylase can be documented by chromatography of the serum. The prevalence of macroamylasemia is 1.5 percent of the nonalcoholic general adult hospital population. Usually macroamylasemia is an incidental finding and is not related to disease of the pancreas or other organs. It is important to be aware of this condition so that patients with macroamylasemia will not be needlessly evaluated and treated for pancreatic disease.

REFERENCES

AMMANN RW et al: Evolution and regression of pancreatic calcification in chronic pancreatitis. A prospective long-term study of 107 patients. Gastroenterology 95:1018, 1988

BALTHAZAR EJ et al: Acute pancreatitis: Prognostic value of CT. Radiology 156:767, 1985

BLOCK H et al: Identification of pancreas necrosis in severe acute pancreatitis: Imaging procedures versus clinical staging. Gut 227:1035, 1986

CERZOF SG et al: Early diagnosis of pancreatic infection by computed tomography guided aspiration. Gastroenterology 93:1315, 1987

CHOI TK et al: Somatostatin in the treatment of acute pancreatitis: A prospective randomized trial. Gut 30:223, 1989

COTTON PB: Pancreas divisum. Pancreas 3:245, 1988

ECKFELDT JH et al: High prevalence of hyperamylasemia in patients with acidemia. Ann Intern Med 104:362, 1986

GARDNER JD, JENSEN RT: Gastrointestinal peptides: The basis of action at the cellular level, in *Recent Progress in Hormone Research*, vol 39. New York, Academic, 1983

GULLO L et al: Effect of cessation of alcohol use on the course of pancreatic dysfunction in alcoholic pancreatitis. Gastroenterology 95:1063, 1988

JACOBSON DG et al: Trypsin-like immunoreactivity as a test for pancreatic insufficiency. N Engl J Med 310:1307, 1984

KOLARS JC et al: Comparison of serum amylase, pancreatic isoamylase and lipase in patients with hyperamylasemia. Dig Dis Sci 29:289, 1984

LIENER IE et al: Effect of trypsin inhibitor from soybeans (Bowman-Birk) on the secretory activity of the human pancreas. Gastroenterology 94:419, 1988

MOOSSA AR: Surgical treatment of chronic pancreatitis: An overview. Br J Surg 74:661, 1987

NEOPTOLEMOS JP et al: Control trial of urgent endoscopic retrograde cholangiopancreatography and endoscopic sphincterotomy versus conservative treatment for acute pancreatitis due to gallstones. Lancet 2:979, 1988

NIEDERAU C, GRENDELL JH: Diagnosis of chronic pancreatitis. Gastroenterology 88:1973, 1985

RANSON JH-C: Risk factors in acute pancreatitis. Hosp Pract 20:69, 1985

SLAFF J et al: Protease specific suppression of pancreatic exocrine secretion. Gastroenterology 87:44, 1984

STEER ML et al: Pancreatitis. The role of lysosomes. Dig Dis Sci 29:934, 1984

STEWART AF et al: Hypocalcemia associated with calcium soap formation in a patient with a pancreatic fistula. N Engl J Med 315:496, 1986

TOSKES PP, GREENBERGER NJ: Acute and chronic pancreatitis. DM, vol 24, 1983

VAN DYKE JA et al: Pancreatic imaging. Ann Intern Med 102:212, 1985

VENTRUCCI M et al: Role of serum pancreatic assays in the diagnosis of pancreatic disease. Dig Dis Sci 34:39, 1989

261 PANCREATIC CANCER

ROBERT J. MAYER

INCIDENCE AND ETIOLOGY The incidence of pancreatic carcinoma in the United States has increased significantly as the median life expectancy of the American population has been prolonged. The tumor results in the death of more than 95 percent of afflicted patients. Approximately 25,000 individuals died of pancreatic cancer in 1989, making it the fifth most common cause of cancer-related mortality. The disease appears to occur somewhat more frequently in males than in females and in blacks than in whites. It rarely develops prior to the age of 50.

Little is known about the causes of pancreatic cancer. Cigarette smoking represents the most consistently observed risk factor for the development of the tumor, with the disease being two to three times more common in heavy smokers than in nonsmokers. It is uncertain whether this apparent association reflects a direct carcinogenic effect of metabolites of cigarette smoke on the pancreas or whether an as yet undefined exposure occurring more frequently in cigarette smokers is responsible for the enhanced risk. There are no convincing data to link such epidemiologic factors as alcohol abuse, chronic pancreatitis, cholelithiasis, or preexisting diabetes mellitus with the development of pancreatic cancer. Furthermore, the weight of clinical data has failed to support any association between coffee consumption and pancreatic cancer.

CLINICAL FEATURES More than 90 percent of pancreatic cancers are ductal adenocarcinomas, with islet cell tumors constituting

TABLE 261-1 Presenting signs and symptoms of pancreatic carcinoma

Frequent:
- Abdominal pain
- Weight loss
- Jaundice (lesions of pancreatic head only)

Infrequent:
- Glucose intolerance
- Palpable gallbladder
- Migratory thrombophlebitis
- Gastrointestinal hemorrhage
- Splenomegaly

the remaining 5 to 10 percent. Pancreatic cancers occur twice as frequently in the pancreatic head (about 70 percent of cases) as in the body (about 20 percent) or tail (about 10 percent) of the gland.

With the exception of jaundice, the initial symptoms associated with pancreatic cancer are often insidious in nature and are usually present for longer than 2 months prior to the time the cancer is diagnosed (Table 261-1). Pain and weight loss are present in more than 75 percent of patients. The pain typically has a gnawing, visceral quality, occasionally radiating from the epigastrium to the back, and generally representing a more severe problem in lesions arising in the body or tail since such tumors may become quite large prior to being detected. Characteristically, the pain improves somewhat on bending forward. The development of significant pain is suggestive of retroperitoneal invasion and infiltration of the splanchnic nerves, indicating the primary lesion to be far advanced and surgically unresectable. The weight loss observed in the majority of patients having pancreatic carcinoma is primarily the result of anorexia, although in the initial period of the disease, subclinical malabsorption may also be a contributing factor.

Jaundice due to biliary obstruction is found in more than 80 percent of patients having tumors in the pancreatic head and is typically accompanied by darkening of urine, a claylike appearance of stool, and pruritus. In contrast to the "painless jaundice" sometimes observed in patients having carcinomas of the bile ducts, duodenum, or periampullary regions, the majority of icteric individuals having ductal carcinomas of the pancreatic head will complain of significant abdominal discomfort. Although the gallbladder is usually enlarged in patients with carcinoma of the head of the pancreas, it is palpable in less than 50 percent of cases (Courvoisier's sign). The presence, however, of an enlarged gallbladder in a jaundiced patient without biliary colic should suggest malignant obstruction of the extrahepatic biliary tree.

The vast majority of patients with pancreatic cancer do not develop clinical diabetes mellitus; in one study, glucose intolerance was found in only 6 percent of a group of 924 patients whose presenting symptoms were carefully analyzed. Other uncommon initial manifestations include venous thrombosis and migratory thrombophlebitis, gastrointestinal hemorrhage resulting from varices due to tumor compression of the portal venous system, and splenomegaly caused by cancerous encasement of the splenic vein.

DIAGNOSTIC PROCEDURES (Fig. 261-1) Despite the availability of serologic tests for tumor-associated antigens such as the carcinoembryonic antigen (CEA) and CA 19-9 and noninvasive imaging techniques such as CT scanning and ultrasonography, the early diagnosis of a potentially resectable pancreatic carcinoma remains extremely difficult. The nonspecificity of the initial symptoms and the poor sensitivity of both serologic assays and noninvasive techniques have frustrated the development of effective screening procedures. When the disease is clinically suspected in a patient having vague, persistent abdominal complaints, an ultrasound to visualize the gallbladder as well as the pancreas should be performed as well as upper GI contrast radiographs to rule out the presence of a hiatal hernia or a peptic ulcer. If these studies fail to provide an explanation for the symptoms, a CT scan should be considered. Such a scan should encompass not only the pancreas but also the liver, retroperitoneal lymph nodes, and pelvis, since pancreatic cancer frequently spreads within the abdomen. While more costly than ultrasonography, CT scanning is technically simpler, more reproducible, provides better definition of the body and tail of the pancreas, and requires less interpretive skill. CT scanning generally detects a malignant pancreatic lesion in over 80 percent of cases; in 5 to 15 percent of patients with proven pancreatic carcinoma, the CT scan shows only generalized pancreatic enlargement suggestive of pancreatitis rather than malignancy. False-positive results have also been reported in about 5 to 10 percent of cases where no tumor was found when a laparotomy was performed. The role of nuclear magnetic resonance imaging (MRI) in the evaluation of pancreatic lesions remains to be determined.

In selected situations where clinical circumstances dictate additional diagnostic evaluation, endoscopic retrograde cholangiopancreatography (ERCP) may clarify the cause of ambiguous CT or ultrasonographic findings. The characteristic findings are stenosis or obstruction of either the pancreatic or the common bile duct; both duct systems are abnormal in over half the cases. The differentiation between carcinoma and chronic pancreatitis by ERCP can be quite difficult, particularly if both diseases are present. False-negative results with ERCP are quite infrequent (less than 5 percent) and usually occur in the setting of islet cell, rather than ductal, carcinomas.

Selective and superselective angiography may be of value in some patients. Angiography is an effective means of detecting carcinomas in the body and tail of the pancreas by demonstrating vascular narrowing, displacement, or occlusion by tumor. Angiography is also useful in assessing whether encasement of peripancreatic vessels is present; this is of importance in determining the potential for surgical resection.

Regardless of the results of the above diagnostic studies, a histologic confirmation of a presumed pancreatic cancer is mandatory to be absolutely certain that malignancy exists and to rule out the presence of such other neoplasms as an islet cell tumor or a lymphoma, for which the therapeutic approach and prognosis differ significantly from those for the usual ductal carcinoma. Such tissue confirmation may often be obtained through a percutaneous needle aspiration biopsy of the pancreas with CT or ultrasonographic guidance, thereby obviating surgical exploration.

It should be emphasized that patients with carcinoma of the pancreas may undergo several months of investigation before a diagnosis is established. In the past, this period of diagnostic delay and accompanying emotional uncertainty erroneously led to an impression that the pain and weight loss might not have had an organic cause, resulting in an association of pancreatic cancer and depression. The availability of CT scans has resulted in a prompter diagnosis and dispelled this incorrect notion. Unfortunately, however, even laparotomy may not provide a definitive diagnosis, because chronic pancreatitis may also produce a hard mass in the head of the pancreas, making it indistinguishable from carcinoma by palpation. Furthermore, a superficial biopsy of such a mass may not show neoplastic tissue, revealing only evidence of pancreatitis since the cancer itself is often surrounded by edematous, inflamed, and fibrotic tissue (i.e., changes associated with chronic pancreatitis).

TREATMENT Complete surgical resection of pancreatic tumors offers the only effective treatment for this disease. Unfortunately, such "curative" operations are only possible in 10 to 15 percent of patients with pancreatic cancer and are limited, for all practical purposes, to those individuals having tumors in the pancreatic head in whom jaundice was the initial symptom. Patients considered for such a procedure should have no evidence of metastatic spread on a chest radiogram and abdominal-pelvic CT scan, should undergo preoperative celiac angiography (to exclude evidence of surgical unresectability such as vascular invasion by tumor), and should involve care by an experienced surgeon, since mortality rates of greater than 15 percent have been associated with this procedure. Although the potential for cure in patients with pancreatic cancer is restricted to those few who are able to undergo a complete surgical

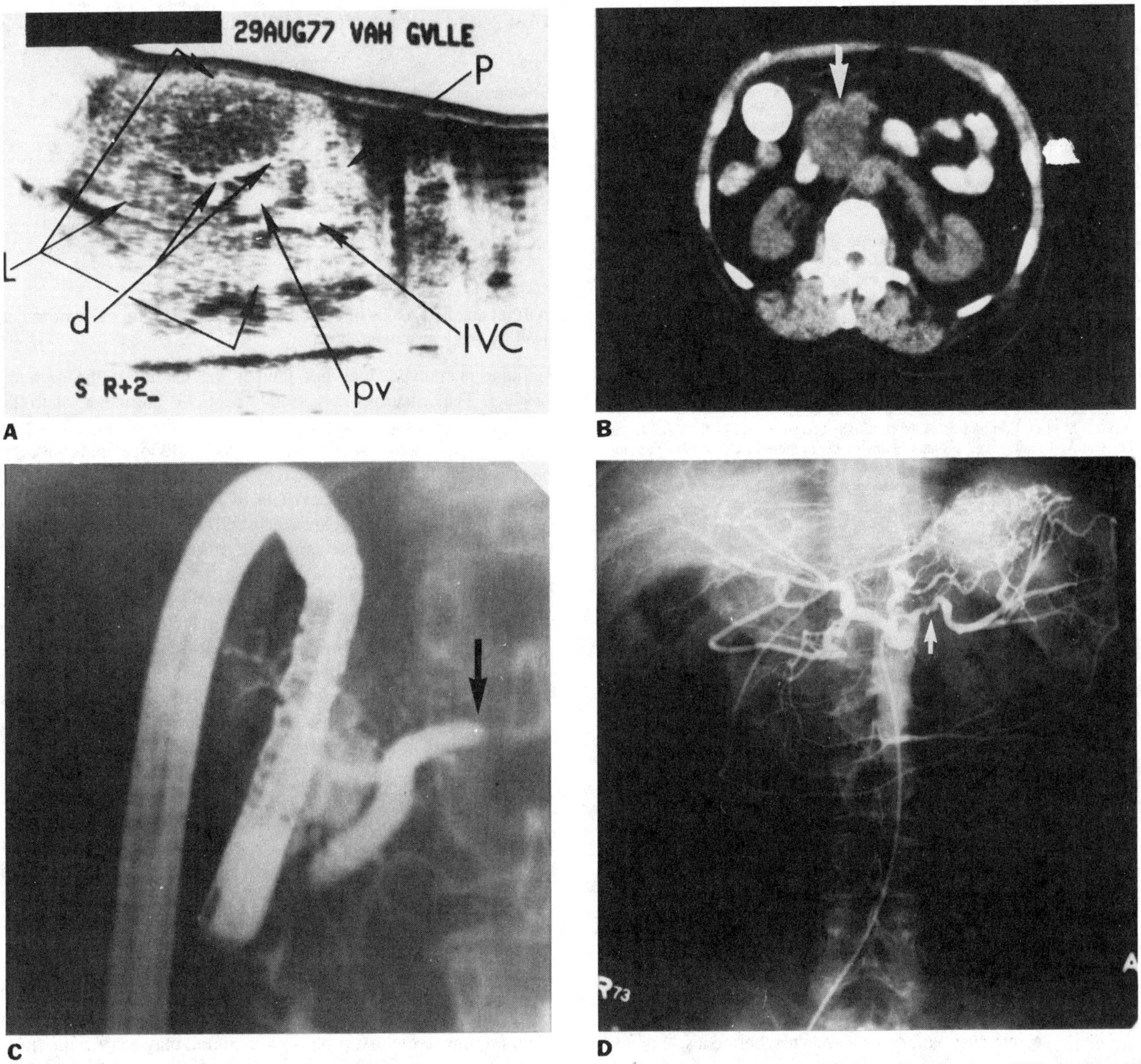

FIGURE 261-1 Carcinoma of the pancreas. *A*. Sonogram showing pancreatic carcinoma (P), dilated intrahepatic bile ducts (d), dilated portal vein (pv), and inferior vena cava (IVC). *B*. CT scan showing pancreatic carcinoma (arrow). *C*. ERCP showing abrupt cut off of the duct of Wirsung (arrow). *D*. Arteriogram showing sheathing of splenic artery by tumor encasement (arrow).

resection, the 5-year survival rate following such operations is only 10 percent. Nonetheless, an attempt at the procedure merits strong consideration, particularly for lesions in the pancreatic head, since ductal carcinomas often cannot be distinguished preoperatively from ampullary, duodenal, and distal bile duct tumors or pancreatic cyst adenocarcinomas, all of which have far higher resectability and cure rates. Furthermore, survival is prolonged three- to fourfold in those patients who eventually experience disease recurrence following pancreatic resection than in those whose tumor is not excised, indicating that such operations have a palliative as well as curative potential. The risk for tumor recurrence is unaffected by the type of operative procedure [i.e., total pancreatectomy versus pancreaticoduodenectomy (''Whipple resection'')] but is increased by the presence of lymph node metastases or tumor invasion into adjacent viscera.

The median survival for patients whose pancreatic cancers are surgically unresectable is approximately 5 months. Management of such individuals should be directed at symptomatic palliation. Ambulatory patients having tumors in the pancreatic head should be considered for surgical diversion of the biliary system. If jaundice has already developed, therapeutic options include either nonoperative biliary decompression by endoscopic or percutaneous, transhepatic biliary drainage or surgical biliary bypass. External beam radiation in patients with unresectable tumors which have not spread beyond the pancreas does not appear to prolong survival, although a sufficient reduction in tumor size may lead to palliation of pain. However, the addition of 5-fluorouracil (5-FU) chemotherapy to external beam irradiation has increased the survival time for these patients, perhaps by acting as a radiosensitizing agent. A similar combination of radiation therapy and 5-FU appears to have prolonged the survival and increased the cure rate when compared to a prospectively randomized nontreatment control group of patients who had a complete surgical resection of their pancreatic cancer. This observation has been made in a small patient population and thus demands confirmation prior to the general acceptance of the efficacy of postoperative (''adjuvant'') treatment.

The experience utilizing chemotherapy in the management of patients with widely metastatic pancreatic cancer has been disappointing. No presently available drug regimen can be considered as being ''standard.'' Newer forms of therapy must be developed and should constitute the initial treatment for consenting, ambulatory patients.

Pancreatic endocrine tumors are discussed in Chap. 262.

REFERENCES

BERG RJ, CONNELLY RR: Updating the epidemiologic data on pancreatic cancer. Semin Oncol 6:275, 1979

CANCER OF THE PANCREAS TASK FORCE: Staging of cancer of the pancreas. Cancer 47:1631, 1981

CONNOLLY MM et al: Survival in 1001 patients with carcinoma of the pancreas. Ann Surg 206:366, 1987

GASTROINTESTINAL TUMOR STUDY GROUP: Pancreatic cancer. Adjuvant combined radiation and chemotherapy following curative resection. Arch Surg 120:899, 1985

GUDJONSSON B et al: Cancer of the pancreas. Diagnostic accuracy and survival statistics. Cancer 42:2494, 1978

MOERTEL CT et al: Therapy of locally unresectable pancreatic adenocarcinoma: A randomized comparison of high dose (6,000 rads) radiation alone, moderate dose radiation (4,000 rads) + 5-fluorouracil, and high dose radiation + 5-fluorouracil. The Gastrointestinal Tumor Study Group. Cancer 48:1705, 1981

MOOSA AR, LEVIN B: The diagnosis of "early" pancreatic cancer: The University of Chicago experience. Cancer 47:1688, 1981

O'CONNELL MJ: Current status of chemotherapy for advanced pancreatic and gastric cancer. J Clin Oncol 3:1031, 1985

SPEER AG et al: Randomized trial of endoscopic versus percutaneous stent insertion in malignant obstructive jaundice. Lancet 2:57, 1987

STEINBERG WM et al: Comparison of the sensitivity and specificity of the CA 19-9 and carcinoembryonic antigen assays in detecting cancer of the pancreas. Gastroenterology 90:343, 1986

WARSHAW AL, SWANSON RS: Pancreatic cancer in 1988: Possibilities and probabilities. Ann Surg 208:541, 1988

262 ENDOCRINE TUMORS OF THE GASTROINTESTINAL TRACT AND PANCREAS

LEE M. KAPLAN

Tumors arising from neuroendocrine cells of the gastrointestinal tract and pancreas present special challenges in diagnosis and therapy. Unlike other gastrointestinal neoplasms, these tumors may cause symptoms from excess hormone secretion rather than from growth, invasion, or local anatomic effects. Frequently slow growing, they may nonetheless be life-threatening because of uncontrolled release of specific hormones and neurotransmitters. These neoplasms arise from within the gastrointestinal mucosa and pancreatic islets in cells that normally secrete monoamines and peptide hormones. For example, gastrin-secreting G cells within the gastric and duodenal mucosa regulate gastric acid secretion, and insulin-secreting β cells within the pancreatic islets serve a crucial role in the homeostatic control of glucose metabolism. Overall, more than 30 distinct secretory products have been identified within neuroendocrine cells of the gut.

BIOLOGIC CONSIDERATIONS

A striking feature of neuroendocrine tumors is the preservation of highly differentiated cell function. Tumor cells contain secretory granules and maintain the capacity for *a*mine *p*recursor *u*ptake and *d*ecarboxylation (APUD), a process essential for the production of monoamine neurotransmitters such as serotonin, dopamine, and histamine. This characteristic has fostered the term *APUDomas* for neoplasms derived from these cells, which can be located in the thyroid (C cells), adrenal medulla, lung (neuroendocrine cells), skin (melanocytes), and nervous system (glial cells and neuroblasts), as well as the gastrointestinal tract and pancreas. These cells also synthesize and secrete peptide hormones by a separate mechanism. Several of the known APUDomas are listed in Table 262-1. It was postulated that this specialized capability implies a common embryologic origin for these diverse cells, but in fact cells of *varied* heritage can acquire the APUD phenotype during differentiation.

Studies of neuroendocrine cell physiology have revealed several important characteristics of secretory cells and the clinical syndromes caused by their products:

TABLE 262-1 Distribution of APUD tumors

Origin	Tumors
Gastrointestinal tract	Carcinoid tumor
Pancreas	Islet cell carcinoma
Central nervous system	Ganglioneuroblastoma, neuroblastoma, chemodactoma, paraganglionoma
Thyroid	Medullary thyroid carcinoma
Skin	Melanoma
Adrenal medulla	Pheochromocytoma
Lung	Carcinoid tumor, small cell carcinoma

1 Cellular phenotype does not predict the nature of the secreted product. Thus, neurons may secrete peptide "hormones" into the synaptic cleft, and endocrine cells may secrete monoamines previously classified as "neurotransmitters." Individual cells have the capacity to synthesize and secrete both peptide and monoamine transmitters, which may coexist in individual secretory granules. Many symptoms of enterochromaffin cell tumors (carcinoid tumors) appear to arise from the combined actions of monoamine and peptide products.

2 Transmitter secretion by neuroendocrine cells is frequently episodic or pulsatile. Although the regulation of secretion is poorly understood, the temporal pattern of hormone release may vary depending on the hormonal milieu, physiologic state, or stage of development. Thus, symptoms produced by abnormal secretion of hormones from neuroendocrine tumors may be intermittent, especially in early stages when tumor cells may behave more like their normal counterparts.

3 Individual cells have the *potential* to secrete a wide array of transmitters. This feature is particularly evident for the peptide hormones. Depending on the stage of development, cellular environment, and other as-yet-unidentified factors, neuroendocrine cells can change secretory profiles dramatically. For example, in cell culture, clonal populations may suddenly change from the secretion of insulin to cholecystokinin, gastrin, or even glucagon. Endocrine tumors may contain heterogeneous populations of cells so that within individual tumors a single cell type may predominate, or there may be multiple cell types in varying proportions. In addition, the secretory profile of a tumor may vary with time, producing a dramatic alteration of symptoms. Individual metastatic implants can also display different phenotypes from the primary tumor and from each other.

4 Individual hormones and transmitters secreted by neuroendocrine cells may regulate physiologic activity (e.g., secretion, absorption, or contractility), stimulate or inhibit growth, or affect the development of target cells. Thus, the humoral activity of gut neuroendocrine tumors can cause a wide variety of effects, including gastric acid hypersecretion, abnormal intestinal motility, gastric epithelial hyperplasia, gallstone formation, mesenteric and cardiac fibrosis, and necrosis of the skin.

5 Hormone production by neuroendocrine cells is tightly regulated at many levels, including RNA transcription, precursor peptide processing, and secretion. These cells in addition may be subject to control by neighboring secretory cells (*paracrine regulation*). Thus, multiple cell types may act in concert to control the growth, secretory characteristics, and thus the clinical manifestations of individual tumors. Abnormal secretion by the tumors themselves may disrupt the normal regulated function of neighboring neuroendocrine cells, and neoplastic transformation may disturb hormone secretion by these cells. Cells may secrete partially processed hormone precursors, leading to unpredictable effects, or display altered susceptibility to regulation by exogenous stimuli. Occasionally, such characteristics can be exploited to permit specific diagnostic tests for individual tumors.

TABLE 262-2 Gastrointestinal endocrine tumor syndromes

Syndrome	Cell type	Clinical features	Percentage malignant	Major products
Carcinoid syndrome	Enterochromaffin, enterochromaffin-like	Flushing, diarrhea, wheezing, hypotension	~100	Serotonin, histamine, miscellaneous peptides
Zollinger-Ellison, gastrinoma	Non-β islet cell, duodenal G cell	Peptic ulcers, diarrhea	~70	Gastrin
Insulinoma	Islet β cell	Hypoglycemia	~10	Insulin
Verner-Morrison, WDHA, VIPoma, pancreatic cholera	Islet D_1 cell	Diarrhea, hypokalemia, hypochlorhydria	~60	Vasoactive intestinal peptide
Glucagonoma	Islet A cell	Mild diabetes mellitus, erythema necrolytica migrans, glossitis	>75	Glucagon
Somatostatinoma	Islet D cell	Diabetes mellitus, diarrhea, steatorrhea, gallstones	~70	Somatostatin
GRFoma	Non-β islet cell	Acromegaly	—	Growth hormone–releasing hormone (GRF)
CRFoma	Non-β islet cell	Cushing's syndrome	—	Corticotropin-releasing hormone (CRF)
PPoma	Islet PP cell	Rare necrolytic erythema	—	Pancreatic polypeptide (PP)
Neurotensinoma	Non-β islet cell	None	—	Neurotensin
Miscellaneous tumors	Non-β islet cell	Hypercalcemia	—	Parathyroid hormone
		Inappropriate ADH	—	Vasopressin
		Hyperpigmentation	—	Melanocyte-stimulating hormone

Neuroendocrine tumors of the gastrointestinal tract can be classified by cell type, major hormone secreted, and site of origin. These characteristics, alone or in combination, correlate well with the observed clinical syndromes. Table 262-2 lists the important tumors in this category, along with their clinical presentations, major secreted products, cells of origin, and biologic behavior.

DIAGNOSTIC CONSIDERATIONS

Several distinct syndromes of hormone excess have been described in which symptoms may suggest the presence of an endocrine tumor of the gastrointestinal tract or pancreas. Moreover, these tumors may present as part of the type I multiple endocrine neoplasia (MEN I) syndrome (see Chap. 325). MEN I patients frequently develop parathyroid and pituitary adenomas that may produce symptoms of hypercalcemia, hyperprolactinemia, hyperthyroidism, or growth hormone excess. Diagnosis is suggested by history, physical findings, elevated blood levels of the relevant peptide hormone(s), or elevated urinary levels of the major metabolites of monoamine transmitters. Further confirmation of hormone-producing tumors may be provided by provocative tests that reveal abnormalities in the regulation of hormone secretion. For example, tolbutamide may enhance somatostatin secretion from somatostatinoma cells. Normal somatostatin-secreting D cells do not show this effect. Other examples of *abnormal* regulation in tumor cells include enhancement by secretin of gastrin secretion in gastrinomas, and pentagastrin stimulation of calcitonin secretion in medullary thyroid (C cell) tumors.

Anatomic definition for pancreatic tumors should be sought by computed tomography (CT), and endoscopic visualization or barium contrast studies should be obtained for suspected mucosal and submucosal tumors. In cases where tumors are too small to be visualized by these noninvasive methods, angiography or selective venous sampling for hormone determination may provide anatomic localization. CT and magnetic resonance imaging are the preferred means of assessing metastatic spread, since the liver and lymph nodes are the initial sites of tumor metastasis.

THERAPEUTIC CONSIDERATIONS

Therapy of endocrine tumors has two goals: (1) to decrease or reverse the growth and spread of the tumor, and (2) to relieve the symptoms of hormone overproduction. When the tumor is localized, both goals may be accomplished by surgical excision. However, most of these tumors are malignant and have spread by the time of diagnosis, and control of growth in such malignant tumors has proven difficult. Thus far, the greatest benefit has been seen with chemotherapeutic regimens that include streptozocin, alone or in combination with fluorouracil or doxorubicin. Control of hepatic metastases has been achieved with hepatic artery embolization, although this approach is palliative rather than curative.

Several approaches are used to control the effects of excess hormone production by these tumors. The most common is to block the function of the target tissue. For example, gastric acid hypersecretion induced by gastrin-producing tumors may be reversed by medications that inhibit acid secretion (e.g., H-2-receptor blockers or proton pump blockers) or by surgical resection of the stomach. Diazoxide is used to help reverse the effects of hyperinsulinemia, and hypomotility agents may ameliorate the diarrhea caused by hypersecretion of vasoactive intestinal peptide (VIP), gastrin, somatostatin, neurotensin, or serotonin.

A second approach is to block release of the transmitter from the tumor cells. The success of this approach depends upon the continued ability of the tumor cells to respond to such physiologic or pharmacologic stimuli. Initial trials used somatostatin, a peptide hormone that inhibits the release of numerous hormones and amine transmitters. While somatostatin controls the symptoms of many of these tumors, it has a short half-life and must be given intravenously. These limitations have been largely overcome by the use of octreotide, a longer-acting analogue of somatostatin with similar actions that can be administered subcutaneously. The chemical structures of somatostatin and octreotide are shown in Fig. 262-1 (see also Chap. 313). Octreotide frequently relieves the symptoms of several endocrine tumors that are inadequately controlled by tumor resection or ablation. In addition, tumor regression occurs in occasional patients, suggesting that the hormone agonist may have some growth-inhibiting effects. The major known side effects of octreotide are dose-dependent and are similar to symptoms of somatostatin excess, including steatorrhea, mild hyperglycemia, nausea, and abdominal pain. The clinical disorders that respond to therapy with octreotide are summarized in Table 262-3.

CARCINOID TUMORS

Carcinoid tumors are the most protean and the most common gastrointestinal endocrine tumors, accounting for approximately 55

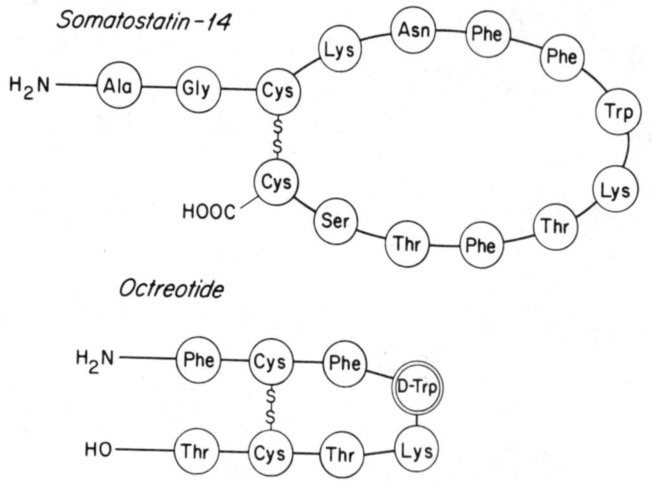

FIGURE 262-1 Structures of somatostatin-14 and octreotide. The double circle denotes the substitution of D-tryptophan for the naturally occurring L-tryptophan. This substitution inhibits peptide degradation and prolongs serum half-life.

percent of such neoplasms. They may present with gastrointestinal bleeding, abdominal pain, obstruction from tumor growth or tumor-induced mesenteric fibrosis, or symptoms arising from tumor-secreted hormones. The name *carcinoid* was applied to these tumors because slow growth and the homogeneous appearance of tumor cells led early investigators to underestimate their malignant potential. They pursue an indolent course and the interval between onset of symptoms and diagnosis averages 4.5 years. Carcinoid tumors arise from neuroendocrine cells throughout the body but are most prevalent in the gastrointestinal tract, pancreas, and pulmonary bronchi. Ninety percent of these tumors arise in the enterochromaffin or Kulchitsky cells within the gastrointestinal tract. The tumors can be found anywhere from the stomach to the rectum and are most common in the appendix, rectum, and ileum. Gastrointestinal carcinoids frequently cause abdominal pain, bleeding, or intestinal obstruction. Although they are rarely large, the tumors may become the leading point for intussusception. In addition, mesenteric spread stimulates a local fibrous reaction, causing intestinal kinking, obstruction, and vascular compromise. Rare sites of carcinoid tumors include the thymus, esophagus, biliary duct, Meckel's diverticulum, breast, and ovary. No risk factors have been clearly defined for these tumors, although the incidence of gastric carcinoids may be increased in patients with pernicious anemia, achlorhydria, and Hashimoto's thyroiditis. Carcinoids of the bronchus and small intestine may occur in association with MEN I. Thymic carcinoids may be associated with hyperparathyroidism or Cushing's syndrome.

TABLE 262-3 Clinical uses of octreotide in gastrointestinal disease

Hormone-secreting tumors	
Carcinoid tumor	Inhibits cutaneous flushing, controls diarrhea, reverses hypotension, aids perioperative management, ?inhibits growth
VIPoma	Controls diarrhea
Insulinoma	Controls hypoglycemia acutely, aids perioperative management
Gastrinoma	Perioperative management, ?controls diarrhea
Glucagonoma	Controls necrolytic erythema
Dumping syndrome	Controls diarrhea, vasomotor symptoms
Diarrhea	Inhibits intestinal secretion, motility
Short-bowel syndrome	
Ileostomy	
Diabetic neuropathy	
Acquired immunodeficiency syndrome	
Fistulas	Inhibits fluid and enzyme secretion, promotes healing
Pancreatic	
Enteric	
Crohn's disease	
Gastrointestinal bleeding	
Portal hypertensive gastropathy	Reduces portal pressure, splanchnic blood flow
Esophageal and gastric varices	Reduces portal pressure, splanchnic blood flow

Appendiceal tumors comprise nearly half of all carcinoid tumors and are incidental findings in 0.3 to 0.7 percent of routine appendectomy specimens. They are usually small, solitary, and benign. Local invasion is common but metastatic spread is rare, and the presence of tumor does not necessarily confer appreciable morbidity or mortality. Colorectal carcinoids have a similarly benign course and are usually asymptomatic. In contrast, small-bowel and bronchial carcinoids have a more malignant course. Local transmural invasion, early metastasis to lymph nodes and liver, and symptoms from hormone secretion are common. Other sites of metastatic spread include bone, and less commonly, heart, breast, and eye. The risk of metastatic spread is dependent on tumor size. Metastases are found in fewer than 2 percent of tumors less than 1 cm in diameter, but in nearly 100 percent of tumors greater than 2 cm. Additional primary tumor implants within the gastrointestinal tract are found in 40 percent of patients.

CARCINOID SYNDROME Enterochromaffin cells secrete a variety of hormones and are embryologically related to thyroid C cells, adrenal medullary cells, and melanocytes. Tumors of each of these cell types may produce syndromes of hormone excess. Hormone secretion by carcinoid cells can cause distinctive and debilitating effects (carcinoid syndrome) long before local growth or metastastic spread is apparent. Manifestations of the carcinoid syndrome include the triad of cutaneous flushing, diarrhea, and valvular heart disease and, less commonly, telangiectasias, wheezing, and paroxysmal *hypo*tension. Early in the course, symptoms are usually episodic and may be provoked by stress, catecholamines, and ingestion of food or alcohol. During acute paroxysms, systolic blood pressure typically falls 20 to 30 mmHg. Diarrhea may result from several mechanisms. The most common type is mixed secretory and hypermotility-induced, producing watery stools unresponsive to fasting. Other causes include partial mechanical obstruction from tumor or fibrosis, and mesenteric vascular insufficiency from local fibrosis. Endocardial fibrosis can cause valvular heart disease, usually affecting the proximal side of the tricuspid and pulmonary valves and leading to tricuspid insufficiency, pulmonary stenosis, and secondary right-sided heart failure. Left-sided valvular disease may occur in association with bronchial carcinoids, presumably because venous effluent from these tumors passes directly into the pulmonary veins, avoiding inactivation of the hormone mediators in the lung.

Approximately 5 percent of all patients with carcinoid tumors experience one or more symptoms of the carcinoid syndrome. The likelihood of developing symptoms is strongly dependent on the origin and behavior of the tumor. While 30 to 60 percent of small-bowel carcinoids are associated with systemic manifestations, only 3.5 percent of lung, 1 percent of appendix, and virtually no rectal carcinoids produce the syndrome. In patients with intestinal carcinoids, the humoral symptoms only develop in the setting of metastatic disease to the liver. Bronchial and other extraintestinal carcinoids, whose hormone products are not immediately cleared by the liver, may produce the carcinoid syndrome in the absence of metastasis.

Carcinoid tumors may be classified on the basis of embryonic origin (Table 262-4). Clinical features, secreted hormones, diagnostic evaluation, and prognosis vary according to whether a carcinoid arises in foregut, midgut, or hindgut structures. For example, carcinoid syndrome is less common in patients with foregut carcinoids than midgut tumors, but the syndrome, when it occurs, is more likely to include wheezing. Patients with foregut carcinoid syndrome more often have dramatic cutaneous flushing involving the whole body than those with tumors of midgut or hindgut organs. The flush of bronchial carcinoids may be prolonged (lasting hours to days);

TABLE 262-4 Characteristics of carcinoid tumors

			Carcinoid syndrome	
Embryonic origin	Site of primary tumor	Frequency, %	Characteristics	Monoamines
Foregut	Bronchus	3.5	Intense flush, lasting up to several hours; associated lacrimation, salivation, facial edema; wheezing; diarrhea; left- and right-sided cardiac lesions	5-HT, ± Histamine
	Stomach	~5	Intense, patchy, whole body flush, with defined borders, wheals, usually lasting several minutes; pruritus; wheezing; diarrhea	5-HTP, Histamine, ± 5-HT
	Duodenum, jejunum	~40	Diarrhea	5-HT
	Pancreas, gallbladder	Rare	Occasional necrolytic erythema	
Midgut	Ileum Appendix	~40 ~1	Facial flush, usually lasting seconds to minutes; telangiectasias; cardiac lesions; peritoneal fibrosis; diarrhea	5-HT, ± Histamine
Hindgut	Colon	Rare	Mild facial flush	5-HT
	Rectum	0	Diarrhea	

NOTE: 5-HT = 5-hydroxytryptamine (serotonin); 5-HTP = 5-hydroxytryptophan.

associated with excessive lacrimation, salivation, and facial edema; and occasionally producing significant hypotension. The cutaneous manifestations of gastric carcinoids, though lasting only minutes, are frequently well-circumscribed and associated with wheals, pruritus, and high levels of histamine secretion. Midgut carcinoids commonly cause the carcinoid syndrome. Acute episodes of flushing tend to be less severe than those associated with foregut tumors, but facial telangiectasias may develop late in the course. Midgut tumors are more frequently associated with cardiac manifestations and peritoneal fibrosis. Hindgut tumors rarely cause the carcinoid syndrome. A rare variant syndrome associated with ovarian carcinoids causes severe peritoneal fibrosis.

Serotonin (5-hydroxytryptamine, 5-HT) is the most common secretory product of carcinoid tumors. As shown in Fig. 262-2,

FIGURE 262-2 Metabolic pathway of serotonin in the carcinoid syndrome.

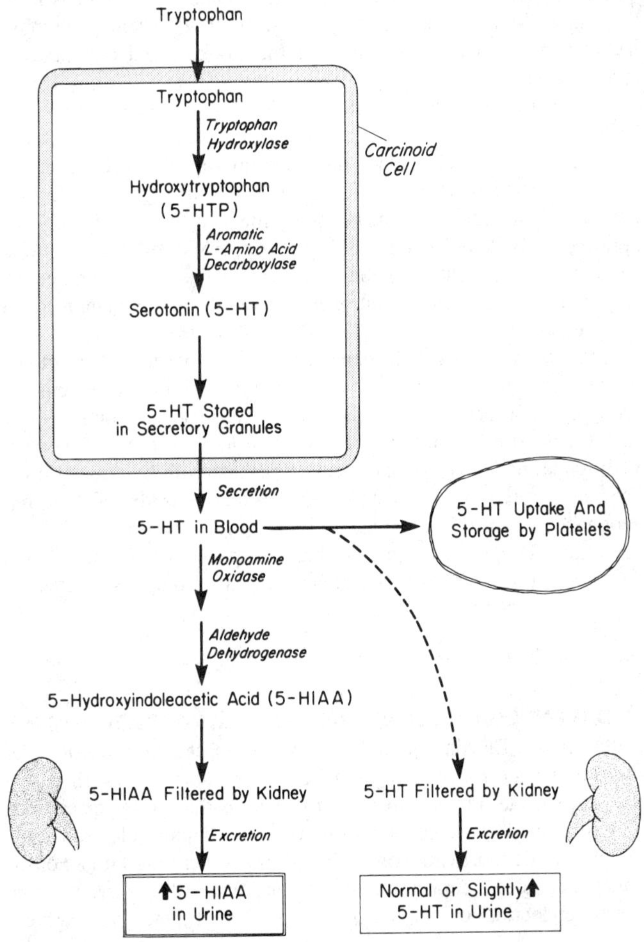

carcinoid tumors synthesize serotonin by enzymatic modification of circulating tryptophan. Up to 50 percent of the dietary intake of tryptophan can be converted to serotonin by these cells, which may leave inadequate substrate for incorporation into proteins and conversion to niacin. As a result, patients with widely metastatic carcinoid tumors may suffer symptoms of protein malnutrition (see Chap. 71) or mild pellagra (see Chap. 76). Serotonin induces intestinal secretion, inhibits intestinal absorption, and stimulates intestinal motility. High serotonin levels are likely the cause of diarrhea in most cases of carcinoid syndrome. Serotonin also stimulates fibroblast growth and fibrogenesis and thus may mediate or accelerate the peritoneal and cardiac valvular fibrosis in this disease. Excess serotonin secretion alone does not account for cutaneous flushing. Multiple monoamine and peptide factors contribute to the vasomotor changes; the relative contributions of each mediator may vary from patient to patient.

Carcinoid tumors elaborate multiple monoamines and peptide hormones, including histamine, catecholamines, bradykinins, tachykinins, enkephalins and endorphins, vasopressin, gastrin, adrenocorticotrophin, and prostaglandins (Table 262-5). Many secrete somatostatin, neurotensin, substance P, neurokinin A, and motilin. The elevated circulating levels of these substances mediate many of the pathophysiologic changes of carcinoid syndrome, although the relative contributions of each remain to be identified.

DIAGNOSIS The diagnosis of carcinoid tumors is influenced by the presenting features of the tumor. Patients with nonfunctional tumors (i.e., without the carcinoid syndrome) usually present with symptoms due to the direct effects of the tumor in the gastrointestinal tract, including abdominal pain or tenderness, nausea, malaise, weight loss, intestinal or biliary obstruction, or gastrointestinal bleeding. Depending on the location of the tumor and whether metastases are

TABLE 262-5 Hormone mediators of carcinoid syndrome

Clinical feature	Frequency, %	Candidate mediators
Diarrhea	78	5-HT, histamine, prostaglandins, VIP, glucagon, gastrin, calcitonin
Cutaneous flushing	94	5-HT, 5-HTP, kallikrein, NKA, histamine, SK, SP, prostaglandins
Telangiectasia	25	Unknown
Wheezing	18	5-HT, histamine
Abdominal pain	51	Tumor, hepatic enlargement, bowel ischemia (fibrosis)
Heart disease		5-HT
Right-sided	40	
Left-sided	13	
Pellagra dermatosis	7	Tryptophan depletion (5-HT synthesis)

NOTE: 5-HT = 5-hydroxytryptamine (serotonin); 5-HTP = 5-hydroxytryptophan; NKA = neurokinin A; SK = substance K; SP = substance P; VIP = vasoactive intestinal peptide.

SOURCE: After W Creutzfeldt and F Stockmann, Am J Med 82:4, 1987.

present, endoscopy, barium studies, or CT may allow anatomic localization. Radiographic studies should include small-bowel follow-through or direct instillation of radiographic contrast material into the small bowel (enteroclysis) to identify tumors in the jejunum and ileum. Despite the improved detection of tumors, however, their pathologic identity is usually not suspected before resection or liver biopsy.

Evaluation of patients with clinical features of carcinoid syndrome is based on the observation that serotonin is secreted by the large majority of functional carcinoid tumors. As shown in Fig. 262-2, serotonin is metabolized in the blood to 5-hydroxyindoleacetic acid (5-HIAA), which is cleared by the kidneys. Plasma and platelet serotonin and urinary 5-HIAA levels are usually elevated in the setting of carcinoid syndrome. Measurement of urinary 5-HIAA excretion is the most useful diagnostic test, and approximately 75 percent of patients excrete more than 80 μmol/d (15 mg/d). Specificity of this test approaches 100 percent after exclusion of ingested substances known to elevate 5-HIAA levels; these include bananas, plantain, pineapple, kiwi fruit, walnuts, plums, pecans, avocados, guaifenesin, and acetaminophen. Conversely, aspirin and levodopa ingestion can cause a falsely depressed 5-HIAA level. In some patients with carcinoid syndrome and normal urinary 5-HIAA, documentation of elevated plasma or platelet serotonin concentrations may establish the diagnosis. However, many gastric carcinoid tumors lack the aromatic L-amino acid decarboxylase and convert 5-hydroxytryptophan (5-HTP) serotonin with low efficiency. Since 5-HTP is not metabolized to 5-HIAA, urinary studies may be misleading. These patients may have elevated urinary serotonin levels, since renal cells contain aromatic L-amino acid decarboxylase. Diagnosis in these cases may be confirmed by demonstrating elevated plasma 5-HTP, histamine, or peptide hormone levels, although it frequently rests on the anatomic detection of the tumor itself. Attempts to provoke cutaneous flushing are helpful for documenting flushing in cases when the clinical history is equivocal. Ethanol, pentagastrin, or *micro*gram quantities of epinephrine can be used for this purpose. Abdominal ultrasonography, CT, and selective angiography are the most sensitive tests for detecting metastatic disease in the liver. Since most patients with the humoral syndrome have metastases, liver biopsy is the most common access to histologic diagnosis. Additional information about bone metastases and cardiac sequelae may be obtained with bone scans and echocardiography, respectively. In patients in whom a tumor cannot be detected, imaging with radiolabeled metaiodobenzyl guanidine may be helpful. This agent is concentrated by neuroendocrine cells and accumulates in many carcinoid tumors.

TREATMENT Effective treatment of the carcinoid syndrome may require more than one approach. Therapy should be selected according to the severity of symptoms. Since nearly all patients with carcinoid syndrome have metastatic disease, resection is rarely curative. Mild diarrhea may be controlled with hypomotility agents such as loperamide or diphenoxylate/atropine. In patients who have undergone ileal resection, diarrhea can be exacerbated by bile salt malabsorption and frequently responds to cholestyramine. Flushing, if rare and mild, may not require therapy. Combination therapy with histamine H-1- and H-2-receptor antagonists (e.g., diphenhydramine and ranitidine) can inhibit the cutaneous flush associated with foregut carcinoids. Phenoxybenzamine may provide additional benefit by inhibiting the release of bradykinin. Methyl xanthine bronchodilators and glucocorticoids are helpful in relieving the dyspnea and wheezing associated with bronchial carcinoids. β-Adrenergic agonists should be avoided since they may provoke acute exacerbations. Serotonin antagonists, including cyproheptadine and methysergide, have been used to provide relief of diarrhea. Unfortunately, these agents have little effect on flushing and other vasomotor symptoms and methysergide can induce fibrosis similar to that caused by the carcinoid itself. ICS 205-930, an investigational agent that selectively blocks the 5-HT_3 subset of neuronal serotonin receptors, inhibits diarrhea in the carcinoid syndrome.

Octreotide is a potent inhibitor of hormone secretion by carcinoid cells. Indeed, this agent provides effective control of diarrhea, flushing, and wheezing in more than 75 percent of cases. Octreotide is effective in the management of acute manifestations of the carcinoid syndrome such as hypotension or resulting angina, as well as the transient exacerbation caused by hepatic artery embolization or the induction of general anesthesia. However, octreotide must be administered in two or three subcutaneous injections each day. It is not yet known whether octreotide can prevent the observed cardiac (or mesenteric) fibrosis. Established valvular heart disease is not reversed by any form of medical therapy.

Surgery, hepatic artery embolization, and chemotherapy have been used to reduce the burden of tumor tissue. Surgery is the treatment of choice for small (<2-cm diameter) carcinoid tumors of the appendix or large bowel. Patients with carcinoid syndrome from isolated bronchial or other extraintestinal carcinoids may also be amenable to curative resection. Most patients with carcinoid syndrome, however, have gross metastatic disease. Hepatic resection generally provides only transient amelioration of symptoms and no improvement in survival. In isolated cases, however, long-term palliation has been achieved by resection of a *single* hepatic metastasis after removal of the primary tumor. Several less-invasive approaches have been tried to limit the hepatic tumor burden and control humoral symptoms, including selective hepatic artery infusion of chemotherapy, local irradiation, and hepatic arterial occlusion. Unfortunately, carcinoid tumors are generally radioresistant and respond weakly to chemotherapy. Arterial occlusion by gel foam embolization provides transient relief of symptoms in approximately 90 percent of patients. Its success derives in part from the fact that the hepatic artery supplies less than half of the blood supply of normal liver tissue but nearly all the blood supply of the tumor. Side effects of therapy include pain, fever, and occasional synthetic liver dysfunction. Effectiveness of therapy can be monitored with serum transaminase levels, which should rise substantially over the first 24 to 48 h after embolization. Patients undergoing embolization may experience acute exacerbation of carcinoid symptoms provoked by the sudden release of hormones from the tumor. Although such effects are rarely life-threatening, prophylactic treatment with histamine-receptor blockers and octreotide is recommended.

Several systemic chemotherapeutic protocols have been evaluated. Various combinations of streptozocin, fluorouracil, cyclophosphamide, and doxorubicin induce objective responses in approximately one-third of patients with metastatic disease, although the effect on survival is minimal. Leukocyte interferon decreases tumor size in approximately 20 percent and decreases urinary 5-HIAA excretion in about half of patients. Although octreotide has induced objective responses in a few cases, controlled trials have not yet demonstrated a significant effect.

The prognosis is highly dependent on the site and stage of the disease at diagnosis. As noted above, appendiceal and rectal carcinoids rarely affect survival. For other gastrointestinal carcinoids, 5-year survival is approximately 95 percent with local disease, 65 percent with lymph node involvement, and 18 percent with liver metastases. Median survival is $2\frac{1}{2}$ years after the first episode of flushing. Prognosis is inversely correlated with the degree of urinary 5-HIAA elevation. Despite attempts at therapy, patients excreting >800 μmol/d (>150 mg/d) have a median survival of only 13 months.

PANCREATIC ISLET-CELL TUMORS

GASTRINOMA (ZOLLINGER-ELLISON SYNDROME) In 1955, Zollinger and Ellison reported the association of severe peptic ulcer disease and gastrin-secreting tumors of the pancreas. These gastrinomas generate high serum gastrin levels, leading to hypersecretion of gastric acid and consequent duodenal and jejunal ulcers. Gastrinomas are the most common of the hormone-secreting tumors of the pancreatic islets, comprising nearly one-tenth of gastroenteropancreatic endocrine tumors and occurring with a frequency of approximately 4×10^{-7} in an unselected population in Ireland. Zollinger-Ellison syndrome may account for up to 0.1 percent of patients with duodenal ulcer disease in the United States. Ulcer disease develops in almost all patients with gastrinoma and is the presenting problem in approximately 70 percent. More than half of patients experience diarrhea (either watery stools or steatorrhea), and approximately 30 percent present with diarrhea alone. Radiologic and endoscopic examinations frequently reveal increased gastric fluid and thickened rugal folds. The age distribution of patients with gastrinoma is similar to that in ordinary acid peptic disease, with a broad peak in the fifth to eighth decades. Gastrinoma should be considered in all patients with recurrent or refractory ulcer disease, ulcers associated with gastric hypertrophy, ulcers in the distal duodenum or jejunum, ulcers in patients with diarrhea, kidney stones, hypercalcemia, or pituitary disease, or a strong family history of duodenal ulcer disease or endocrine tumors.

In patients with ulcer disease or diarrhea, serum fasting gastrin levels of greater than 200 ng/L (200 pg/mL) suggest the diagnosis. However, since gastric acid exerts a negative feedback on the *normal* G-cell secretion of gastrin, inhibition of acid secretion can also lead to elevated gastrin levels in this range. Thus, the serum gastrin level does not reliably predict gastrinoma in the presence of atrophic gastritis, partial gastric resection, histamine-receptor blockers such as cimetidine or ranitidine, or proton pump blockers such as omeprazole. The *sine qua non* of Zollinger-Ellison syndrome is hypergastrinemia in the presence of gastric acid hypersecretion. More than 90 percent of patients have a basal acid output (BAO) greater than 15 mmol/h. In the setting of ulcer disease without gastric outlet obstruction, this level of hyperchlorhydria is diagnostic of gastrinoma. In patients who have previously undergone gastric surgery, BAO >5 mmol/h is diagnostic. Secretin infusion provides a second means of distinguishing gastrinoma from other causes of hypergastrinemia. Secretin has little effect on gastrin secretion from normal G cells (causing a modest increase or decrease in serum gastrin levels) but usually stimulates gastrin secretion by gastrinoma cells. This provocative test is particularly useful in the 50 percent of gastrinoma patients with modest elevations in serum gastrin. Zollinger-Ellison syndrome is predicted by an *increase* in serum gastrin of at least 200 ng/L (200 pg/mL) within 15 min of a single intravenous injection of secretin (2 units per kg body weight). Approximately 90 percent of patients with gastrinoma will demonstrate a diagnostic rise in serum gastrin at 2, 5, 10, or 15 min after secretin injection.

Between one-fourth and one-half of gastrinomas occur in association with the MEN I syndrome (see Chap. 325). Hyperparathyroidism is the most common component of MEN I and occurs in about 80 percent of patients with this form of Zollinger-Ellison syndrome. All gastrinoma patients should be screened for possible MEN I by measurement of serum calcium, phosphorus, cortisol, and prolactin levels and imaging of the sella turcica. First-degree relatives of patients with MEN I also should be similarly screened.

Approximately 80 percent of gastrin-secreting tumors arise in pancreatic islets, including nearly all of those associated with MEN I, and most are located in the pancreatic head. Another 10 to 15 percent arise from G cells in the duodenum, and the remainder are scattered in the distal small bowel, stomach, spleen, liver, lymph nodes, and ovary (mucinous cystadenoma). The tumors are usually small and are frequently multifocal, especially when associated with MEN I. The biologic behavior may be variable. In most reported series, one-half to two-thirds of these tumors are malignant, with metastases in lymph nodes and liver and less frequently in bone. However, the prevalence of metastatic disease at the time of diagnosis appears to have decreased, perhaps owing to the more widespread consideration and earlier detection of these tumors. Such observations have important therapeutic implications since isolated tumors are more likely to be cured by resection. Gastrinomas, like most other islet-cell tumors, are generally slow-growing, but growth patterns vary widely and metastases may be more aggressive than the primary tumor itself.

Treatment of Zollinger-Ellison syndrome is directed at the sequelae of excess gastrin secretion and at the tumor itself. The availability of potent inhibitors of gastric acid secretion has reduced the need for gastric surgery in these patients. Reduction of BAO to <10 mmol/h is usually sufficient to control symptoms. H-2-receptor blockers, including cimetidine, ranitidine, famotidine, and nizatidine, are effective, although optimal therapy may require two to three times the standard daily dose for ordinary peptic ulcer disease and more frequent administration for control of acid output and symptoms. Omeprazole, which inactivates the parietal cell H^+,K^+-ATPase, is a more potent inhibitor of gastric acid secretion and controls symptoms of Zollinger-Ellison syndrome in nearly all patients. With each of these medical regimens, control of symptoms and acid secretion frequently requires increasing doses over time. Basal acid output or gastric pH should be measured yearly to evaluate the continued efficacy of therapy, and the rare patient who fails to respond to medical therapy should be treated surgically. However, patients with coexistent hyperparathyroidism should undergo parathyroid resection before a decision is made about gastric surgery, since resolution of hypercalcemia may permit better medical control of gastric acid secretion. In most cases, parietal cell vagotomy reduces acid secretion sufficiently to permit effective medical therapy. In rare cases, uncontrollable gastric acid secretion or complications of the ulcer disease mandate total gastrectomy.

Because of the effective control of hormone-mediated symptoms, morbidity and mortality from gastrinoma is increasingly related to the growth and spread of tumor itself. Curative resection of the gastrinoma is possible in 15 to 20 percent of cases and is favored by extrapancreatic location and inability to detect the tumor mass preoperatively. Gastrinomas in association with MEN I syndrome are not amenable to surgical cure, although these tumors generally have a benign natural history. Preoperative evaluation with CT and selective angiography is used to exclude multiple primary tumors and metastases. Treatment of unresectable gastrinoma includes chemotherapy, hormonal therapy, and hepatic artery embolization. Chemotherapeutic regimens including streptozocin and fluorouracil, with or without doxorubicin, commonly induce partial responses. Leukocyte interferon may also cause objective response, but octreotide does not appear to be effective. Hepatic artery embolization may decrease hepatic tumor burden and ameliorate pain. Unfortunately, none of these approaches prolongs survival of patients with metastatic disease, which approximates 25 percent at 10 years.

INSULINOMA (β CELL TUMOR) The hallmark of pancreatic β cell tumors is the development of symptomatic hypoglycemia from unregulated insulin hypersecretion (see also Chap. 320). Insulinomas are the second most common functioning islet cell tumors and have a reported prevalence of approximately 8×10^{-7} in an unselected Irish population. They arise most frequently in the fifth to seventh decades although cases have been reported at all ages. In infants and children, insulinoma must be distinguished from diffuse β cell adenomatosis or nesidioblastosis. Whipple's triad describes the classic presentation of insulinoma and includes fasting hypoglycemia, *symptoms* of hypoglycemia, and immediate relief after intravenous glucose administration. Weight gain may result from increased food ingested to combat symptoms of hypoglycemia. In the current era, the diagnosis of insulinoma is made by demonstrating fasting hypoglycemia in the presence of normal or elevated plasma insulin levels. Symptoms related to the hypoglycemia include headache, slurred speech, psychologic alterations, visual disturbances, confusion, and, ultimately, coma and death. Hypoglycemia also induces the secondary release of catecholamines, leading to tremulousness, diaphoresis, pallor, palpitations, cardiac arrhythmias, and behavioral irritability. Because of the episodic release of insulin, symptoms early in the course may be intermittent or occur only after somewhat prolonged periods of fasting. However, symptoms do develop early so that tumors are usually small and solitary at the time of diagnosis. Multiple primary tumors are found in approximately 10 percent of patients. An additional 10 percent are malignant, with spread to the local lymph nodes and the liver. As with gastrinomas, insulinomas are frequently associated with MEN I (see Chap. 325) and such tumors are more likely to be multifocal. Extrapancreatic insulin-secreting tumors are rare and usually arise in ectopic pancreatic tissue.

Diagnosis is made by demonstrating fasting hypoglycemia and an inadequate response of insulin to the hypoglycemia. Patients are fasted under close supervision for up to 72 h, followed, if necessary, by an exercise tolerance test. Serum glucose, insulin, and cortisol levels are determined every 1 to 2 h or at any time that symptoms appear. Approximately 75 percent of patients with insulinoma develop hypoglycemia within 24 h, as evidenced by a serum glucose less than 2.8 mmol/L (50 mg/dL) in men or 2.5 mmol/L (45 mg/dL) in women. However, there is no absolute glucose level which defines hypoglycemia, so the diagnosis of insulinoma depends on demonstrating inadequate insulin suppression in the face of falling glucose levels. Because hypoglycemia inhibits insulin secretion from normal β cells, the ratio of plasma insulin (in μU/mL) to serum glucose (in mg/dL) is maintained at less than 0.3. In patients with insulinoma, the ratio is usually >0.4 and increases with fasting. Documentation of rising cortisol levels excludes hypoglycemia secondary to hypothalamic-pituitary-adrenal dysfunction. It is also necessary to exclude other causes of fasting hypoglycemia, including administration of exogenous insulin, sulfonylurea ingestion, severe liver failure, and tumors that secrete insulinlike growth factors (e.g., fibrosarcoma, mesothelioma, and hemangiopericytoma). Exogenous insulin administration can be excluded by measuring levels of the C peptide of proinsulin, which normally vary in parallel with the plasma insulin concentrations. Since insulin administration suppresses endogenous insulin secretion, detection of normal or elevated C-peptide levels is inconsistent with insulin abuse. In addition, because insulinoma cells often process proinsulin incompletely, the serum often has an increased ratio of proinsulin to insulin. A ratio greater than 20 percent in the appropriate clinical setting is suggestive of insulinoma. Serum levels of sulfonylureas should be elevated if hyperinsulinemic hypoglycemia is caused by these agents. Normal glucose/insulin ratios exclude liver failure and tumors which secrete insulinlike growth factors. (Refer to Chap. 320 for a more complete discussion of hypoglycemia syndromes.)

Once a diagnosis of insulinoma is established, acute treatment is supportive with intravenous glucose infusion as required to maintain plasma levels within the normal range. Hyperglycemic agents, including diazoxide, beta-adrenergic-receptor blockers, and phenytoin can be used to support serum glucose levels but their effects are variable and may last only a short time. Octreotide is a potent inhibitor of insulin secretion by these tumors and may be the most effective agent for acute management. Definitive therapy is accomplished by surgical resection. Because insulinomas are usually small (90 percent are <2 cm in diameter), only half are detected by CT. Angiography with selective venous sampling for insulin levels is about 80 percent sensitive and palpation at laparotomy detects 80 to 90 percent of tumors. At surgery, detectable tumors should be resected. The effectiveness of intervention is monitored by determination of intraoperative blood glucose levels. If no detectable tumors are found, stepwise distal pancreatectomy is performed until frozen sections of resected specimens and/or blood glucose measurements indicate that all tumor has been removed. If no tumor is found, or if multiple tumors are present, pancreatectomy is limited to 70 to 80 percent to preserve digestive and endocrine pancreatic function.

Patients with metastatic disease and those whose insulinomas are not removed by partial pancreatectomy can frequently be managed with hyperglycemic agents such as diazoxide or octreotide. In one study, all of the seven patients with metastatic insulinoma showed a response to octreotide, although the degree of response was variable. However, hypoglycemia may be worsened by octreotide administration, perhaps owing to inhibition of glucagon or growth hormone by this agent. Diazoxide, though frequently effective, can cause troubling side effects, including salt and fluid retention, hypertrichosis, and gastrointestinal upset. The combination of streptozocin and fluorouracil is the mainstay of chemotherapy for metastatic disease. These agents induce objective remission in approximately half of patients and are associated with a modest but significant increase in survival. Patients with residual tumor should be followed carefully for changes in secretory profile which may affect therapy. Such changes may include development of hyperglycemia as a result of glucagon-secreting metastases.

VIPOMA [VERNER-MORRISON SYNDROME; WATERY DIARRHEA HYPOKALEMIA ACHLORHYDRIA (WDHA) SYNDROME; PANCREATIC CHOLERA] Verner and Morrison described a syndrome of watery diarrhea, hypokalemia, and renal failure in association with non-β cell tumors of the pancreatic islets. The clinical features of this syndrome are caused by the high levels of vasoactive intestinal peptide (VIP) secreted by the tumors. VIPomas comprise approximately 2 percent of gastroenteropancreatic tumors and have a prevalence of approximately 1×10^{-7} in the Irish population studied. The manifestations of VIPoma include secretory diarrhea, profound weakness, hypokalemia, and hypochlorhydria. Stool volume is greater than 3 L/d in 80 percent of patients, and nonanion gap acidosis usually occurs as a result of bicarbonate losses in the stool. Other electrolyte abnormalities include hypercalcemia in approximately two-thirds of patients and hypophosphatemia. Approximately half of patients develop hyperglycemia, which results from hypokalemia- and VIP-induced glycogenolysis in the liver, and a fifth of patients experience cutaneous flushing. Although most symptoms can be reproduced by infusion of exogenous VIP, these tumors also contain other peptide hormones, including the VIP-related peptide histidine-methionine (PHM), somatostatin, helodermin, and neurotensin, each of which may contribute to clinical features exhibited by individual patients. Diagnosis rests on the demonstration of high plasma VIP levels in the setting of a stool volume of at least 1 L/d. Lesser increases in VIP levels occur in patients with hepatic failure and intestinal ischemia.

VIPomas are most commonly pancreatic tumors. Unlike gastrinomas and insulinomas, however, VIPomas frequently grow to a large size before becoming clinically apparent. On average, the size of these tumors at the time of diagnosis is second only to the nonfunctioning pancreatic islet cell tumors. Although they are slow-growing, these tumors are usually malignant. Approximately three-fifths are metastatic at the time of diagnosis. Eighty percent of VIPomas are located in the body or tail of the pancreas. A few cases have been seen in association with MEN I. However, there is no constant relation between the two syndromes. Between 10 and 15 percent of VIP-secreting tumors arise from neuroendocrine cells in the intestinal mucosa, and a few are ganglioneuroblastomas, mastocytomas, pheochromocytomas, or small cell carcinomas of the lung.

Treatment is surgical extirpation whenever possible. However, metastases may preclude this approach. Preoperative evaluation should include CT to localize the tumor and any metastases that may be present. In addition to supportive therapy with fluids and electrolytes, prednisone is frequently effective in reducing the volume of diarrhea, despite its inability to alter serum VIP levels. Octreotide inhibits the secretion of VIP and ameliorates symptoms in approximately 80 percent of patients. VIPomas often produce symptoms related to the large size of the tumor itself. Surgery may be indicated to relieve local effects or to remove a single large primary tumor. For patients with symptomatic metastatic disease, chemotherapy and hepatic artery embolization have the greatest benefit on tumor burden. Regimens containing streptozocin and fluorouracil are the most effective chemotherapy, inducing objective partial remission in up to 90 percent of cases.

GLUCAGONOMA In 1966, McGovern described a rare syndrome of diabetes mellitus and necrolytic migratory erythema in association with a pancreatic islet cell tumor. To date, fewer than 200 cases have been reported, most presenting in middle age. The observation that these tumors secrete high levels of glucagon suggested a cause for the diabetes and that the peptide may have a role in the other clinical features. Although these tumors frequently synthesize and secrete additional peptides, including pancreatic polypeptide, somatostatin, insulin, and gastrin, the common link is hyperglucagonemia. Glucagonomas are characteristically single, large, and slow-growing. More than 75 percent have metastasized at the time of diagnosis, most commonly to the liver and bones. Glucagonoma has been reported in association with MEN I. A fasting plasma glucagon of >1000 ng/L (>1000 pg/mL) establishes the diagnosis. More modest elevations of plasma glucagon levels may occur in diabetic ketoacidosis, renal failure, hepatic failure, sepsis, prolonged fasting, and gluten-sensitive enteropathy. Hypocholesterolemia and hypoaminoacidemia are common, with alanine, glycine, and serine levels usually less than 25 percent of normal. Glucagonoma may be distinguished from other hyperglucagonemic syndromes by the failure of glucose to suppress and the failure of arginine to enhance serum glucagon concentrations.

The characteristic glucagonoma skin rash is erythematous, raised, scaly, sometimes bullous, sometimes psoriatic, and ultimately crusted. It is located primarily on the face, abdomen, perineum, and distal extremities. After resolution, the regions of the acute eruption usually remain indurated and hyperpigmented. Patients may also experience glossitis, stomatitis, angular cheilitis, dystrophic nails, and hair-thinning. The diabetes is usually mild or asymptomatic and may manifest only as an abnormality on an oral glucose tolerance test. Ketoacidosis has not been reported. Weight loss, hypoaminoacidemia, anemia, and thromboembolic disease also occur in association with this syndrome. A causal association between hyperglucagonemia and skin disease has been difficult to prove, leading to speculation that the rash may result from nutritional deficiency. In some patients, the rash responds to oral zinc or intravenous amino acid therapy. Octreotide therapy has also yielded good results. However, dermatologic symptoms frequently recur after each of these therapies.

Because the tumor is usually large and found only in the pancreas, it is easily identified by CT, ultrasound, or angiography. Surgical therapy is curative in approximately 30 percent of patients. Resection is more frequently aimed at decreasing tumor burden. Despite occasional objective responses, attempts at chemotherapy with combinations of streptozocin, fluorouracil, doxorubicin, and dacarbazine have little impact. Fortunately, the slow-growing nature of the tumor allows for prolonged survival even in many cases of metastatic disease.

SOMATOSTATINOMA Somatostatin-secreting tumors are the most recent group to be identified with a defined clinical syndrome. The classic triad of somatostatinoma includes diabetes mellitus, steatorrhea, and cholelithiasis. These symptoms derive from the widespread inhibitory actions of somatostatin, including inhibition of insulin release, pancreatic enzyme and bicarbonate secretion, and gallbladder motility, respectively. The diabetes is usually mild, and in a few cases, *hypo*glycemia has been seen, perhaps from the cosecretion of other peptides. Individual somatostatinomas have been shown to secrete insulin, calcitonin, gastrin, VIP, adrenocorticotrophin, prostaglandins, substance P, motilin, and glucagon. Patients with somatostatinomas may also develop hypochlorhydria, weight loss, and paroxysmal hypertension.

Approximately 60 percent of reported somatostatinomas are located in the pancreas. The second most common site is in the small intestine, although intestinal tumors are associated with lower plasma somatostatin levels and are more commonly asymptomatic. Like glucagonomas and VIPomas, these tumors are usually single, large, and metastatic at the time of diagnosis. Somatostatinomas have not been reported in association with MEN I. Curiously, the occasional coincidence of pheochromocytoma, café au lait spots, and neurofibromatosis suggests a possible association with MEN type IIb (see Chap. 325). Small cell lung carcinomas, medullary thyroid carcinomas, pheochromocytomas, and paragangliomas that secrete somatostatin have also been described.

MISCELLANEOUS FUNCTIONAL ISLET CELL TUMORS In addition to the diseases described above, islet cell tumors have been associated with several other syndromes of hormone excess, including acromegaly (growth hormone or growth hormone–releasing hormone), hypercalcemia (parathormone-like peptide), diarrhea and diabetes mellitus (neurotensin), and Cushing's syndrome (corticotropin-releasing factor or adrenocorticotropin).

NONFUNCTIONING ISLET CELL TUMORS (See also Chap. 261) More than 15 percent of pancreatic islet cell tumors are not associated with any definable hormone-mediated syndrome. Nonetheless, many of these nonfunctioning islet cell tumors synthesize and secrete one or more regulatory peptides, including pancreatic polypeptide, substance P, and motilin. With increasing availability of radioimmunoassay and immunohistochemical reagents, protein products will probably be defined for more and more of these tumors. Nonetheless, most of these tumors behave in a similar fashion. They arise most commonly in the head and tail of the pancreas and are frequently large (5 to 10 cm in diameter) at the time of diagnosis. The most common clinical manifestations are abdominal pain, jaundice, a palpable mass, malaise, and bleeding esophageal or gastric varices (from splenic vein compression). Though slow-growing, at least half of these tumors present with metastases to the liver or lymph nodes. Surgical cure is achieved in approximately 20 percent. The remainder are poorly responsive to chemotherapy. Streptozocin with or without fluorouracil induces objective responses in approximately 60 percent of patients. Five-year survival for patients with these tumors is approximately 40 percent, with many long-term survivors despite known metastatic disease.

REFERENCES

Carcinoid tumors and syndrome

FELDMAN JM: Carcinoid tumors and syndrome. Semin Oncol 14:237, 1987

FELDMAN JM, O'DORISIO TM: Role of neuropeptides and serotonin in the diagnosis of carcinoid tumors. Am J Med 81 (Suppl 6B):41, 1986

GODWIN JD: Carcinoid tumors: An analysis of 2837 cases. Cancer 36:560, 1975

KVOLS LK et al: Treatment of the malignant carcinoid syndrome: Evaluation of a long-acting somatostatin analogue. N Engl J Med 315:663, 1986

MARTENSSON H et al: Bronchial carcinoids: An analysis of 91 cases. World J Surg 11:356, 1987

MOERTEL CG et al: Carcinoid tumor of the appendix: Treatment and prognosis. N Engl J Med 317:1699, 1987

NORHEIM I et al: Malignant carcinoid tumors: An analysis of 103 patients with regard to tumor localization, hormone production, and survival. Ann Surg 206:115, 1987

OBERG K et al: Treatment of malignant carcinoid tumors with human leukocyte interferon: Long-term results. Cancer Treatment Rep 70:1297, 1986

THORSON A et al: Malignant carcinoid of the small intestine with metastases to the liver, valvular disease of the right side of the heart, peripheral vasomotor symptoms, bronchoconstriction, and an unusual type of cyanosis: A clinical and pathologic syndrome. Am Heart J 47:795, 1954

Islet cell tumors

BLOOM SR, POLAK JM: Glucagonoma syndrome. Amer J Med 82 (Suppl 5B):25, 1987

BOSTWICK DG et al: Expression of opioid peptides in tumors. N Engl J Med 317:1439, 1987

BRANDI ML et al: Familial multiple endocrine neoplasia type I: A new look at pathophysiology. Endocrine Rev 8:391, 1987

GORDEN P et al: Somatostatin and somatostatin analogue (SMS 201-995) in treatment of hormone-secreting tumors of the pituitary and gastrointestinal tract and non-neoplastic diseases of the gut. Ann Intern Med 110:35, 1989

KENT RB et al: Nonfunctioning islet cell tumors. Ann Surg 193:185, 1981

KREJS GJ: VIPoma syndrome. Amer J Med 82 (Suppl 5B):37, 1987

KVOLS LK et al: Treatment of metastatic islet cell carcinomas with a somatostatin analogue (SMS 201-995). Ann Intern Med 107:162, 1987

VINIK AI et al: Somatostatinomas, PPomas, neurotensinomas. Semin Oncol 14:263, 1987

WOLFE MM, JENSEN RT: Zollinger-Ellison syndrome. N Engl J Med 317:1200, 1987

WYNICK D et al: Symptomatic secondary hormone syndromes in patients with established malignant pancreatic endocrine tumors. N Engl J Med 319:605, 1988

PART TEN DISORDERS OF THE IMMUNE SYSTEM, CONNECTIVE TISSUE, AND JOINTS

section 1 Disorders of the immune system

263 PRIMARY IMMUNE DEFICIENCY DISEASES

MAX D. COOPER / ALEXANDER R. LAWTON III

INTRODUCTION Immunologic functions are mediated by two developmentally independent, but functionally interacting, families of lymphocytes. The activities of B and T lymphocytes, and their products, in host defense are closely integrated with the functions of other cells of the reticuloendothelial system. Macrophages, dendritic cells, and the Langerhans' cells in the skin play an important role in the trapping and presentation of antigens to T and B cells to initiate the immune response. Macrophages also become effector cells, especially when activated by products of lymphocytes. The scavenger activity of polymorphonuclear leukocytes is directed and made specific by antibodies in concert with products of the complement system (see Chap. 13). Natural killer (NK) cells, a population of granular lymphocytes, may spontaneously kill tumor and virus-infected cells, activities that are enhanced by the interferon products of immune and inflammatory cells. Killing by NK cells can also be targeted by IgG antibodies for which NK cells have cell-surface receptors. The interaction of basophils and tissue mast cells with IgE antibodies in causation of immediate-type hypersensitivity is discussed in Chap. 267. Consideration of these interrelationships is an important part of the analysis of patients with suspected immune deficiency.

CLINICAL DISEASE FEATURES COMMON TO IMMUNE DEFICIENCY Immunodeficiency syndromes, whether congenital, spontaneously acquired, or iatrogenic, are characterized by unusual susceptibility to infection and not infrequently to autoimmune disease and lymphoreticular malignancies. The types of infection often provide the first clue to the nature of the immunologic defect.

Patients with *defects in humoral immunity* have recurrent or chronic sinopulmonary infection, meningitis, and bacteremia, most commonly caused by pyogenic bacteria such as *Haemophilus influenzae, Streptococcus pneumoniae,* and staphylococci. These and other pyogenic organisms also cause frequent infections in individuals who have either neutropenia or a deficiency of the pivotal third component of complement (C3). The tripartite collaboration of antibody, complement, and phagocytes in host defense against pyogenic organisms makes it important to assess all three systems in individuals with unusual susceptibility to bacterial infections.

Antibody-deficient patients in whom cell-mediated immunity is intact have an interesting response to viral infections. The clinical course of primary infection with viruses such as varicella zoster or rubeola, unless complicated by bacterial infection, does not differ significantly from that of the normal host. However, long-lasting immunity may not develop, and as a result multiple bouts of chickenpox and measles may occur. Such observations suggest that intact T cells may be sufficient for control of established viral infections, while antibodies play an important role in limiting the initial dissemination of virus and in providing long-lasting protection. Exceptions to this generalization are becoming more widely recognized. Agammaglobulinemic patients fail to clear hepatitis B virus from their circulation and have a progressive, and often fatal, course. Poliomyelitis has occurred following live-virus vaccination in some patients. Chronic encephalitis, which may progress over a period of months to years, is being observed with apparently increasing frequency. Echoviruses and adenoviruses have been isolated from brain, spinal fluid, or other sites in such patients; in others no agent has been detected.

The occurrence of an unusually serious infection, for example, *H. influenzae* meningitis in an older child or adult, warrants consideration of humoral immune deficiency. Bacterial infections in certain sites may also suggest this possibility. Chronic otitis media occurs frequently in patients with hypogammaglobulinemia, and is significant because of its relative rarity in normal adults. Pansinusitis, although almost invariably present in immunoglobulin deficiency, is a less helpful finding because it is not rare in apparently normal people. Bacterial infections of the skin or urinary tract are less frequent problems in hypogammaglobulinemic patients.

Infestation with the intestinal parasite *Giardia lamblia* is a frequent enough cause of diarrhea in antibody-deficient patients to warrant diagnostic duodenal aspiration and intestinal biopsy when the organism cannot be demonstrated in the stool.

Abnormalities of cell-mediated immunity predispose to disseminated virus infections, particularly with latent viruses such as herpes simplex (see Chap. 135), varicella zoster (see Chap. 136), and cytomegalovirus (see Chap. 138). In addition, patients so affected almost invariably develop mucocutaneous candidiasis and frequently acquire widely disseminated fungal infections. Pneumonia caused by the protozoan *Pneumocystis carinii* is also common (see Chap. 163).

T-cell deficiency is probably always accompanied by some abnormality of antibody responses (see Fig. 263-1), although this may not be reflected by hypogammaglobulinemia. This may explain in part why patients with primary T-cell defects are also subject to overwhelming bacterial infection.

The most severe form of immune deficiency occurs in individuals, often infants, who lack both cell-mediated and humoral immune functions. Individuals with severe combined immunodeficiency are susceptible to the whole range of infectious agents including organisms not ordinarily considered pathogenic. Multiple infections with viruses, bacteria, and fungi occur, often simultaneously. Because donor

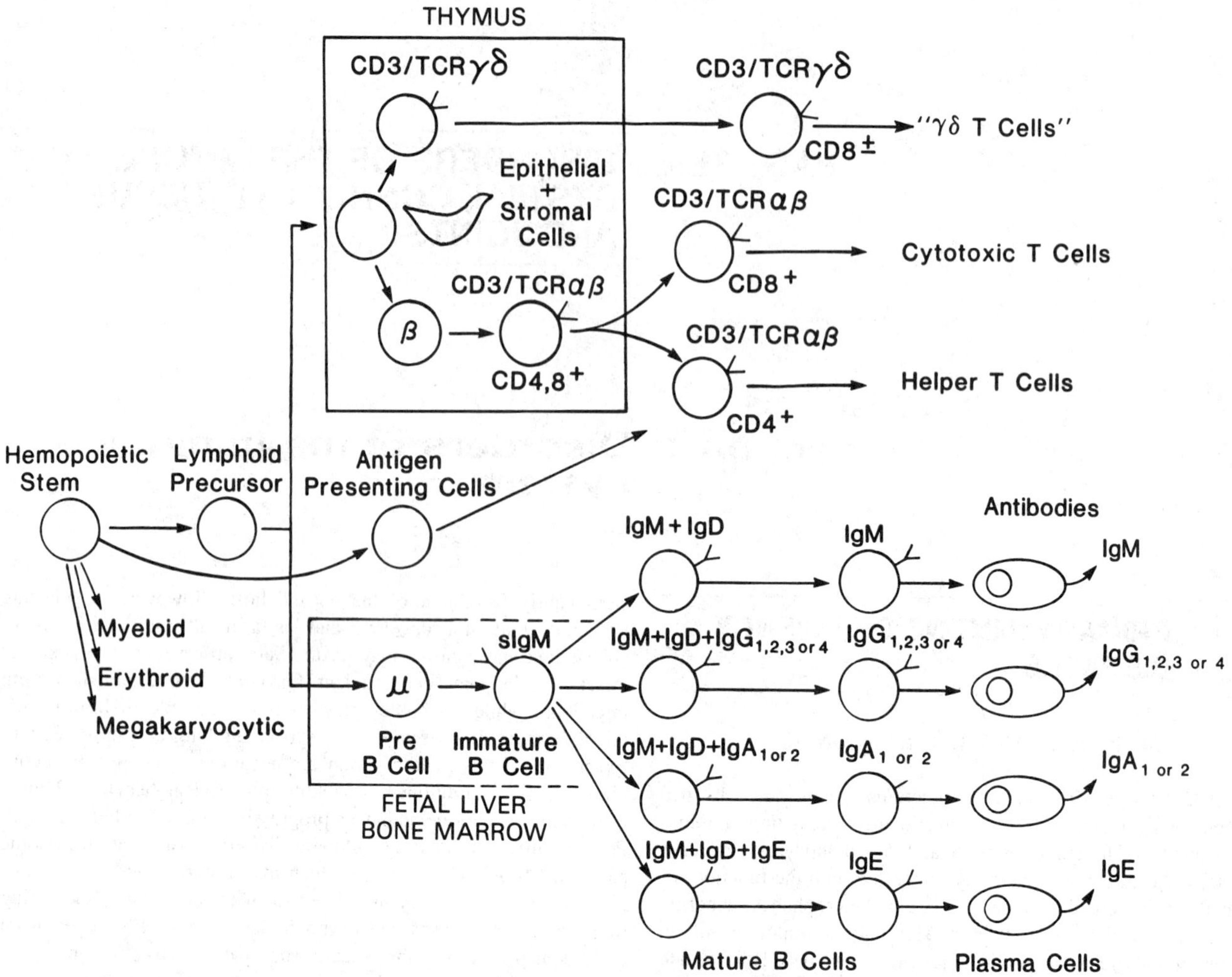

FIGURE 263-1 Hypothetical model outlining the differentiation of hemopoietic stem cells along T- and B-cell lineages. Failure to develop T and B cells may result from defective stem cells or from inborn metabolic errors affecting both cell types. Rarely, other hematopoietic cell lines are also absent. Absence of either T or B cells suggests malfunction of central lymphoid tissues, including the thymus and the fetal liver–bone marrow complex. B-cell deficiency may result from failure to generate pre-B cells from their stem cell precursors or from failure of pre-B cells to give rise to their B-lymphocyte progeny. Similarly, differentiation may be arrested at several levels within the T-cell lineage; arrests at the thymocyte level and failure to develop the helper subset have been observed in immunodeficient patients. Agammaglobulinemia and deficiencies of some T-cell functions may occur despite the presence of normal numbers of B or T cells in the circulation. Failure of B lymphocytes to differentiate to plasma cells can be due to intrinsic cellular abnormalities or to faulty T-cell regulation.

lymphocytes cannot be rejected by the recipients, blood transfusions can produce fatal graft-versus-host disease.

DIFFERENTIATION OF T AND B CELLS The functional deficits which occur in both congenital and acquired immunodeficiencies are usefully viewed as being caused by defects at various points along the differentiation pathways of immunocompetent cells. For this reason certain features of the development and differentiation of T and B cells that are especially relevant to the analysis of immunodeficiency are briefly presented here; Chap. 13 provides a general account of their roles in cellular and humoral immunity.

A subpopulation of hematopoietic stem cells may become restricted to lymphoid differentiation prior to migration to the thymus, where T cells are generated, or to the fetal liver and adult bone marrow, where B-cell development begins (Fig. 263-1). A major function of central lymphoid tissues is to generate the clonal diversity characteristic of the immune system. Each T or B lymphocyte is induced to express surface receptor molecules of a unique specificity for antigen. The receptors of B lymphocytes are immunoglobulin molecules which are formed by paired heavy and light chains of either κ or λ type. The heavy chain gene loci are on the long arm of chromosome 14; the 5′-3′ order of these is V_H (variable), D (diversity), and J_H (joining) minigene families followed by the C_H (constant region) genes, C_μ, C_δ, $C_{\gamma 3}$, $C_{\gamma 1}$, $C_{\alpha 1}$, $C_{\gamma 2}$, $C_{\gamma 4}$, C_ϵ, and $C_{\alpha 2}$. The κ gene family, consisting of V_κ, J_κ, and C_κ genes, is located on chromosome 2, and the homologous λ gene loci on chromosome 22.

The T-cell receptors are related cell surface molecules with antigen-binding specificity. The receptor on most T cells is composed of two polypeptide chains, called α and β. The β-chain family is located on chromosome 7, and consists of V_β, D_β, J_β, and C_β minigene loci. The α-chain family on chromosome 14 similarly consists of a series of V_α, D_α, J_α, and C_α genes. A smaller subpopulation of T cells express a T-cell receptor composed of γ and δ polypeptide chains. The γ-chain gene family is located on chromosome 7, and the δ-chain family is located in the midst of the α gene locus on chromosome 14.

The genetic strategy for creating functional gene complexes encoding antigen receptors is similar for T and B cells. For example, a functional V region gene of the immunoglobulin heavy chain is formed by productive rearrangement of one each of the V_H, D, and J_H genes and deletion of the intervening DNA to generate a contiguous coding structure which is then transcribed together with the nearest C_H gene. Functional light chain genes are formed by a V-J rearrangement in either the κ or λ gene loci. The V_β gene is similarly composed of a rearranged set of V_β, D_β, and J_β genes forming a contiguous coding structure, which the T cell then transcribes along with the nearest C_β gene. Because there are many different V, D, and J genes, they can be put together in various combinations to encode a large number of receptor molecules having different antigen-binding specificities.

Generation of clonal diversity requires cellular proliferation, such that each of the different receptor specificities encoded in the genome comes to be uniquely expressed by individual cells. A clone consists of all cells that express the identical antigen-binding receptors. Estimates for the total number of B-cell clones usually vary between 10 and 100 million. T-cell clonal diversity may be equally extensive. The initial step in clonal development is independent of antigen and reflects a genetically programmed sequence of differentiation analogous to that of primary erythropoiesis or myelopoiesis. This phase, termed *primary differentiation,* begins early in human fetal development and may continue into adult life.

The most primitive morphologically identifiable cell in the B lineage is called a pre-B cell. These cells have undergone a productive V_HDJ_H rearrangement and express cytoplasmic μ chains (the heavy chain of IgM). Since light chain gene rearrangement and expression occurs later, pre-B cells lack the membrane-bound immunoglobulin receptors which characterize B lymphocytes. Pre-B cells are generated in fetal liver and in the bone marrow of adults. Pre-B cells proliferate in response to growth factors made by neighboring stromal cells and, after undergoing a productive rearrangement of light chain VJ genes, become immature B lymphocytes that express surface IgM receptors. These B lymphocytes differ from their more mature counterparts in an important physiologic characteristic; they are highly susceptible to inactivation when their receptors bind antigen. Consequently, immature B cells encountering self-antigens may be eliminated or rendered anergic.

The developmental sequence for expression of diverse immunoglobulin classes by human B lymphocytes begins with expression of IgM. The expression of IgD on IgM-bearing cells occurs later. Lymphocytes committed to synthesis of IgG, IgA, and IgE are derived from IgM-bearing precursors through a genetic switch mechanism. Each of the heavy chain constant region genes except C_δ is preceded by a switch region composed of repetitive nucleotide sequences. The heavy chain class switch is accomplished by splicing of the switch region of μ with the switch region in front of the downstream heavy chain gene to be expressed next.

T-lineage cells also undergo sequential rearrangements of the minigene families encoding their antigen receptors. On entering the epithelial thymus, lymphoid precursor cells may follow one of two T-cell pathways. The first involves rearrangement of V_γ and J_γ genes to express γ chains and rearrangement of V_δ, D_δ, and J_δ genes to express δ chains. These associate with the CD3 proteins to form the CD3/γδ T-cell receptor (TCR) complex of γδ T cells. Pre-T cells beginning development along the second differentiation pathway in the thymus rearrange one each of the V_β, D_β, and J_β genes prior to the expression of a complete β chain. At a later differentiation stage, similar rearrangements of V_α and J_α genes occur in the α-chain family, and then the completed antigen receptor molecule of one α chain and one β chain is expressed together with the CD3 protein complex on the cell surface of an immature αβ T cell. Initially the αβ T cells express both the CD4 and CD8 accessory molecules on their surface. Later, as these cells mature under the influence of a self-antigen selection process, they either down-regulate the CD8 molecule to become CD4+ T cells with helper cell potential or they cease to express the CD4 molecule to become CD8+ T cells with cytotoxic potential. The CD4+ αβ T cells leaving the thymus have been selected to recognize peptide fragments presented in the groove of class II major histocompatibility (MHC) molecules of antigen-presenting cells. The CD8+ αβ T cells migrating from the thymus have been selected to recognize peptide fragments in the cleft of class I MHC molecules expressed by virtually all types of nucleated cells. The CD4 and CD8 molecules are called accessory molecules because they have binding affinity for class II or class I MHC molecules, respectively. While the γδ T cells express neither CD4 nor CD8 molecules during their intrathymic development, they may express CD8 molecules as mature T cells in peripheral lymphoid tissues. The expression of these cell surface molecules, called differentiation antigens, can be defined by their reactivity with monoclonal antibodies. This provides a powerful tool for elucidating the developmental relationships of both T and B lymphocytes (Fig. 263-1).

The γδ T cells constitute a minor population of peripheral T cells and their function is presently unknown. The αβ T cells bearing the CD4 markers constitute approximately 70 percent of circulating T cells and function as helper-inducer cells, necessary for expression of effector functions of both T and B cells. The αβ T cells expressing CD8 molecules constitute 20 to 30 percent of circulating T cells, mediate cytotoxic reactions, and may be responsible for suppression of immune responses. Developmental arrests or failure of function of one or more of these T-cell subsets may be responsible for immunodeficiency or autoimmune diseases.

The events designated *secondary differentiation* follow stimulation of specific clones of lymphocytes by antigen. These processes are synonymous with the immune response (see Chap. 13). Particularly important in consideration of immunodeficiencies are the collaborative interactions among macrophages, T cells, and B cells. While B lymphocytes may differentiate to IgM-secreting plasma cells when stimulated by thymus-independent antigens, such as lipopolysaccharides, most antibody responses, particularly those of the IgA and IgG classes, require intimate collaboration between T and B cells. Antigens bound to the antibody receptors on B cells are internalized, partially digested, and recycled to the cell surface, where they are presented on class II molecules to the T cell. The activated T cell in turn produces soluble factors that promote growth and differentiation of the B cell. These factors include the interleukins IL-2, IL-4, IL-5, IL-6, and γ interferon.

Differentiation of T or B cells may be arrested at either the primary or secondary stages. Reflecting the complex cellular interactions involved in immune responses and the pivotal role played by T lymphocytes, immune deficiencies primarily involving T cells are usually also associated with abnormal B-cell function. Conversely, immunodeficiencies manifested primarily by inability to produce antibodies may be caused by T-cell defects not associated with abnormal cell-mediated immunity.

EVALUATION OF IMMUNODEFICIENT PATIENTS A careful history and physical examination will usually indicate whether the major problem involves the antibody-complement-phagocyte system or cell-mediated immunity. A history of a normal response to smallpox vaccination or of contact dermatitis due to poison ivy suggests intact cellular immunity. Persistent mucocutaneous candidiasis suggests deficient cell-mediated immunity. Lymphopenia and the absence of palpable lymph nodes may be important findings. However, patients with profound immunodeficiency may have diffuse lymphoid hyperplasia. Most immunodeficiencies may be diagnosed by thoughtful use of tests available in local or regional clinical laboratories. More precise evaluation of immunologic functions and treatment may require referral to specialized centers. Table 263-1 presents a résumé of widely available laboratory investigations.

Humoral immunity With rare exceptions, deficiency of humoral immunity is accompanied by diminished serum concentration of one or more classes of immunoglobulin. Normal values vary with age, and adult concentrations of IgM (0.8 g/L) are reached at about 1 year, of IgG (8.0 g/L) at 5 to 6 years, and of IgA (1.0 g/L) at puberty (see Chap. 13). Also, the wide range of values among normal adults creates difficulty in defining the lower limits of normal. Reasonable estimates for low normal values are 0.4 g/L for IgM, 5 g/L for IgG, and 0.5 g/L for IgA. In the presence of borderline hypogammaglobulinemia, assessing the patient's capacity to produce specific antibodies becomes particularly important. Most hospital laboratories can measure isohemagglutinins, anti-streptolysin O, and "febrile agglutinins." Typhoid H and O agglutinins can be measured before and after immunization with standard typhoid vaccine. State public health laboratories and private specialty laboratories can perform titrations

TABLE 263-1 Laboratory evaluation of host defense status

I Initial screening assays*
  A Complete blood count with differential smear
  B Serum immunoglobulin levels: IgM, IgG, IgA, IgD, IgE
II Other readily available assays
  A Quantification of blood mononuclear cell populations by immunofluorescence assays employing monoclonal antibody markers†
    T cells: CD2, CD3, CD4, CD8
    B cells: CD20, CD21, μ, δ, γ, α, κ, λ immunoglobulin determinants
    NK cells: CD16
    Monocytes: CD15
    Activation markers: HLA-DR, CD25
  B T-cell functional evaluation
    1 Delayed hypersensitivity skin tests (PPD, Candida histoplasmin, tetanus toxoid)
    2 Proliferative response to mitogens (phytohemagglutinin, concanavalin A) and allogeneic cells (mixed lymphocyte response)
  C B-cell functional evaluation
    1 Natural or commonly acquired antibodies: isohemagglutinins; antibodies to common viruses (influenza, rubella, rubeola) and bacterial toxins (diphtheria, tetanus)
    2 Response to immunization with protein (tetanus toxoid) and carbohydrate (pneumococcal vaccine, *H. influenza B* vaccine) antigens
    3 Quantitative IgG subclass determinations
  D Complement
    1 CH_{50}
    2 C3, C4
  E Phagocyte function
    1 Reduction of nitroblue tetrazolium
    2 Chemotaxis assays
    3 Bactericidal activity

* Together with a history and physical examination, these tests will identify more than 95 percent of patients with primary immunodeficiencies.
† The menu of monoclonal antibody markers may be expanded or contracted to focus on particular clinical questions.

for antibodies to common viral agents and bacterial toxins, such as diphtheria and tetanus.

Since antibody deficiency may be mimicked clinically by deficiency of complement components, measurement of total hemolytic complement (CH_{50}) should be a part of the evaluation of host defense. Measurement of C3 alone is inadequate for screening, since deficiencies of both early and late complement components may predispose to bacterial infection (see Chap. 13). Estimation of numbers of circulating B lymphocytes has been of great value in determining the pathogenesis of certain types of immune deficiency. B lymphocytes are identified by the presence of membrane-bound immunoglobulins; additional markers include HLA-DR antigens, receptors for aggregated IgG (Fc receptor), and receptors for the d fragment of the third complement component (CR2) which also binds the Epstein-Barr virus. Following activation, B cells express increased levels of several cell surface antigens, some of which serve as receptors for soluble growth and differentiation-promoting factors that are made by T cells. Most of these molecules on the B-cell surface can be identified and enumerated by specific monoclonal antibodies.

Pokeweed mitogen (PWM), an extract of the plant *Phytolacca americana*, has the capacity to induce primed B lymphocytes to proliferate and differentiate to plasma cells. This activity requires the presence of T lymphocytes, which also proliferate in response to PWM. Thus, this in vitro assay can measure not only the capacity of B lymphocytes to differentiate but also the "helper" function of patients' T lymphocytes.

Cellular immunity Human T lymphocytes may be enumerated by their expression of the TCR/CD3 complex of surface molecules. The CD2 antigenic molecule is also expressed by almost all of the T cells, and a few non-T-lineage lymphocytes. This molecule can bind to the LFA-3 molecule present on sheep erythrocytes and on antigen-presenting cells. The CD4 molecule serves as a marker for helper T cells, but macrophages also express this molecule in relatively low levels. Conversely, the CD8 molecule is expressed by cytotoxic T cells. This cell surface molecule may also be expressed by subpopulations of γδ T cells and non-T-lineage lymphocytes with natural killer activity.

Normal levels of serum immunoglobulins and antibody responsiveness are reliable indices of intact helper T-cell function. T-lymphocyte function can be measured directly by delayed hypersensitivity skin testing, using a variety of antigens to which the majority of older children and adults have been sensitized. The most generally useful skin test antigen is a 1:5 dilution of tetanus toxoid injected intradermally, since almost all individuals will have been sensitized. Purified protein derivative (PPD), histoplasmin, mumps antigen, and extracts of *Candida* or *Trichophyton* may also be used.

T-lymphocyte function may be estimated in vitro by the capacity of cells to proliferate in response to antigens to which the patient has been sensitized, to lymphocytes from an unrelated donor, to antibodies that cross-link the CD3/TCR complex, or to the T-cell mitogens, which include phytohemagglutinin, concanavalin A, and pokeweed mitogen. The response is usually quantified by measurement of incorporation of radioactive thymidine into newly synthesized DNA. It is also possible to measure the production of lymphokines (or interleukins) by activated T cells. Finally, the ability of T cells activated in mixed lymphocyte culture to lyse target cells can be measured.

The capacity of T lymphocytes from immunologically normal persons to be activated in vitro with antigens or mitogens may be markedly diminished by acute febrile illness, treatment with corticosteroids, or stress. Caution should be exercised in interpreting abnormal results in these circumstances.

CLASSIFICATION Primary immunodeficiencies may be either congenital or acquired, and are currently classified according to mode of inheritance and whether the defect involves T cells, B cells, or both (Table 263-2). In general, this classification will be followed in the following discussion, which emphasizes three related concepts; first, that immunodeficiencies are most logically viewed as defects of cellular differentiation; second, that these defects may involve either primary development of T or B cells or the antigen-dependent phase of their differentiation; and third, that defects of secondary B-cell differentiation may in some instances reflect T-cell abnormalities resulting from faulty T-B collaboration.

Secondary immunodeficiencies are those not caused by intrinsic abnormalities in development or function of T and B cells. The best known of these is the acquired immunodeficiency syndrome (AIDS) which may follow infection with the human immunodeficiency virus (HIV) (see Chap. 264). Other examples are immune deficiency associated with malnutrition, protein-losing enteropathy, and intestinal lymphangiectasia. Also considered secondary are immunodeficiencies resulting from hypercatabolic states such as occur in myotonic dystrophy, immunodeficiency associated with lymphoreticular malignancy, and immunodeficiency resulting from treatment with x-rays, antilymphocyte serum, or cytotoxic drugs.

Incidence As a group, the primary immunodeficiencies are relatively common. Isolated IgA deficiency may occur in approximately 1 in 600 individuals. While no other specific category approaches this frequency, the cumulative total is approximately 1 in 400 individuals in North America.

The more severe forms of primary immunodeficiency have their onset early in life and all too frequently result in death during childhood. Immunodeficiencies may become apparent at any age, however, and a substantial number of patients with congenital hypogammaglobulinemia survive to middle age or beyond. In a referral center for patients with immunodeficiency diseases, approximately two-thirds of the immunodeficient patients will be adults. Improved methods of diagnosis and treatment may increase this ratio in the future.

Severe combined immunodeficiency (SCID) This syndrome is characterized by gross functional impairment of both humoral and cell-mediated immunity and by susceptibility to devastating fungal, bacterial, and viral infections. It is usually congenital, may be inherited either as an X-linked or autosomal recessive defect, or may occur sporadically. Affected infants rarely survive beyond 1 year without treatment. This syndrome has been associated with a diversity

TABLE 263-2 WHO classification of primary immunodeficiencies

A Combined immunodeficiencies
- *1* Severe combined immunodeficiency (SCID):
  - *a* X-linked
  - *b* Autosomal recessive ("Swiss-type agammaglobulinemia")
- *2* Adenosine deaminase (ADA) deficiency
- *3* Purine nucleoside phosphorylase (PNP) deficiency
- *4* MHC class II deficiency
- *5* Reticular dysgenesis

B Predominantly antibody deficiencies
- *1* X-linked agammaglobulinemia
- *2* X-linked hypogammaglobulinemia with growth hormone deficiency
- *3* Ig deficiency with increased IgM ("Hyper-IgM syndrome")
- *4* Ig heavy chain–gene deletions
- *5* κ-chain deficiency
- *6* IgA deficiency
- *7* Selective deficiency of IgG subclasses (with or without IgA deficiency)
- *8* Common variable immunodeficiency (CVID)
- *9* Transient hypogammaglobulinemia of infancy

C Other well-defined immunodeficiency syndromes
- *1* Wiskott-Aldrich syndrome
- *2* Ataxia telangiectasia
- *3* 3d and 4th pouch/arch syndrome (DiGeorge)

D Syndromes associated with immunodeficiency
- *1* Chromosome abnormalities:
  - *a* Bloom syndrome
  - *b* Fanconi anemia
  - *c* Down syndrome
- *2* Multiple organ system abnormalities:
  - *a* Partial albinism
  - *b* Short-limbed dwarfism
  - *c* Cartilage hair hypoplasia
  - *d* Agenesis of the corpus callosum
- *3* Hereditary metabolic defects:
  - *a* Transcobalamin II deficiency
  - *b* Acrodermatitis enteropathica (zinc deficiency)
  - *c* Type I orotic aciduria
  - *d* Biotin-dependent carboxylase deficiency
- *4* Hypercatabolism of Ig:
  - *a* Familial hypercatabolism of Ig
  - *b* Myotonic dystrophy
  - *c* Intestinal lymphagiectasia
- *5* Other:
  - *a* Hyper-IgE syndrome
  - *b* Chronic mucocutaneous candidiasis
  - *c* Thymoma
  - *d* Immunodeficiency following hereditarily-determined susceptibility to Epstein-Barr virus

of defects in development of immunocompetent cells, some of which may be related to specific enzymatic abnormalities.

The classic example of SCID, *Swiss-type agammaglobulinemia*, is characterized by severe lymphopenia involving both T and B cells, and is inherited with an autosomal recessive pattern. Rarely, other hematopoietic cell lines fail to develop in a variant form of SCID called *reticular dysgenesia*. About half of patients with autosomal recessive SCID are deficient in an enzyme involved in purine metabolism, adenosine deaminase (ADA). Studies of the pathophysiologic relationship of ADA deficiency to abortive lymphoid differentiation suggest that intracellular accumulation of adenosine and deoxyadenosine triphosphate, by inhibiting ribonucleotide reductase enzymes, interferes with DNA synthesis. Improvement of both clinical status and immunologic function has occurred in patients treated with a source of exogenous ADA. The cellular defect in the lymphopenic forms of SCID logically rests with the precursor cells for both T and B lineages. The immunologic defects in all of these types of SCID patients have been repaired following transplantation of bone marrow or fetal liver as a source of stem cells, confirming the hypothesis that the stromal microenvironments of the thymus and bone marrow of these patients are capable of supporting T- and B-cell differentiation of normal stem cells.

SCID may also occur with an X-linked inheritance pattern. Affected boys may not have severe lymphopenia; most have normal numbers of B lymphocytes with few or no circulating T lymphocytes. This developmental disorder can also be repaired by transplantation of bone marrow stem cells from a histocompatible sibling. Transplants of haploidentical bone marrow, depleted of donor T cells to prevent graft-versus-host disease, may also correct the T-cell deficit, but the antibody deficiency may persist for years in this instance.

Treatment of SCID patients should probably be attempted only in centers with a strong research interest in this problem. It is crucial that these patients be recognized early and not be given blood transfusions which may cause fatal graft-versus-host disease.

T-cell immunodeficiency Reflecting the diversity of T-cell functions, abnormalities of T-cell development may be responsible for a wide spectrum of immune deficiencies including severe combined immunodeficiency, selective defects in cell-mediated immunity, and syndromes presenting as antibody deficiency with apparently normal cell-mediated immunity. These defects may be acquired (see Chap. 264) as well as congenital. Until recently, laboratory assays of T-lymphocyte function were limited to correlates of cell-mediated immunity; no means were available for studying T-cell regulatory functions. Quantification of T-cell subsets and of their growth factor receptors using monoclonal antibodies, accompanied by functional measurements of helper and cytotoxic activity, are expanding the spectrum of immunodeficiencies primarily related to T-cell abnormalities. The genes for the T-cell receptors, the CD3 protein complex, other surface molecules involved in signal reception and transduction, and T-cell-derived interleukins have all been cloned. Assays for their products are also becoming available. The availability of these assays and DNA probes will also allow more precise definition of T-cell disorders, the numbers of which will increase with the use of these sophisticated tools for T-cell analysis.

DI GEORGE'S SYNDROME This is the classic example of isolated T-cell deficiency which results from maldevelopment of thymic epithelial elements derived from the third and fourth pharyngeal pouches. Defective development of other organs formed in part by cells of embryonic neural crest origin is also seen in these patients. Affected infants usually present with congenital cardiac defects, particularly those involving the great vessels, hypocalcemic tetany due to failure of parathyroid development, and absence of a normal thymus. Associated abnormalities may include abnormal ears, shortened philtrum, micrognathia, and hypertelorism. Serum immunoglobulin concentrations are frequently normal, but antibody responses, particularly of IgG and IgA isotypes, are usually impaired. Lymphocyte counts may be near normal, but most of the lymphocytes are B cells. Carefully performed autopsies have often revealed a tiny, histologically normal thymus, usually in an ectopic location. With time, most patients develop functional T cells. A few patients with Di George's syndrome transplanted with fetal thymus have rapidly developed immunocompetent T cells of host origin. However, it is difficult to be certain whether long-term improvement is the result of a small thymus gland in an ectopic location or due to grafted thymus epithelium.

Children lacking the congenital anomalies associated with Di George's syndrome may present with severe impairment of cell-mediated immunity. Some have normal or even increased immunoglobulin levels, while others have selective deficiencies of one or more immunoglobulin classes. Specific antibody responses are usually impaired even in patients with normal concentrations of immunoglobulins. This ill-defined entity has been called the *Nezelof's syndrome*.

Inherited deficiency of the enzyme purine nucleoside phosphorylase (PNP) is associated with an often severe and selective deficiency of T-lymphocyte function. This enzyme functions in the same purine salvage pathway as ADA; toxic effects of the *PNP deficiency* may be related to intracellular accumulation of deoxyguanosine triphosphate (GTP).

ATAXIA-TELANGIECTASIA This is an autosomal recessive genetic disorder characterized by cerebellar ataxia, oculocutaneous telangiectasia, and immunodeficiency. The responsible gene appears to be closely linked to the thy-1 gene on chromosome 11. Onset of truncal ataxia usually occurs in infancy and is progressive. Immunodeficiency may be clinically manifest by recurrent and chronic sinopulmonary infection leading to bronchiectasis. However, not all patients have immunodeficiency. The two most frequent causes of death are chronic pulmonary disease and malignancy. Lymphomas are most common, although carcinomas have also occurred.

The immunologic abnormalities seem to be related to maldevelopment of the thymus. The thymus is markedly hypoplastic and similar in appearance to an embryonic thymus. The peripheral T cell pool is frequently reduced in size, especially in lymphoid tissue compartments. Cutaneous anergy and delayed rejection of skin grafts are common. Although the number and class distribution of B lymphocytes are usually normal, most patients are deficient in serum IgE and IgA, and a smaller number have reduced serum levels of IgG, particularly of the IgG2, IgG4 subclasses. IgM and IgD are usually normal.

There is circumstantial evidence that ataxia-telangiectasia may involve a generalized defect in cellular differentiation related to the defects in DNA repair mechanisms which have been identified in these patients. Cultured cells from these patients are highly susceptible to radiation-induced chromosomal damage. Defective DNA repair mechanisms may account for the high incidence of malignancies in these patients. Ovarian agenesis also occurs frequently. Persistence of very high serum levels of oncofetal proteins, including alpha-fetoprotein and carcinoembryonic antigen, may be of diagnostic value.

Only symptomatic treatment is available. Unless a severe IgG deficiency is present, therapy with gamma globulin is not indicated. Unusual sensitivity to x-irradiation should be kept in mind in planning therapy for patients who develop cancer.

Immunoglobulin deficiency syndromes X-LINKED AGAMMAGLOBULINEMIA Males with this syndrome often begin to have recurrent bacterial infections late in the first year of life, when maternally derived immunoglobulins have disappeared. Affected individuals have very few immunoglobulin-bearing B lymphocytes in their circulation and lack primary and secondary lymphoid follicles. However, pre-B cells are found in normal frequency in their bone marrow. This developmental block at the pre-B to B cell level contrasts with earlier and later arrests in B-cell differentiation characterizing other immunodeficiencies (see below and Fig. 263-1). The gene defect has been mapped to the Xq 21.3–22 region. B cells from obligate carriers utilize the normal X chromosome exclusively, while T cells and myeloid cells express either X chromosome. *X-linked agammaglobulinemia with growth hormone deficiency* is a rare disorder that maps to a different region of the X chromosome.

Agammaglobulinemia is a misnomer, as most patients with this and other forms of severe panhypogammaglobulinemia synthesize some immunoglobulins. Within the same family some affected males have had substantial levels of IgM, IgG, and IgA, while others have been nearly agammaglobulinemic. All these patients were markedly deficient in circulating B lymphocytes. This observation suggests that the few B lymphocytes which escape the block in differentiation are fully capable of plasma cell maturation and immunoglobulin synthesis. However, antibody replacement therapy is needed in all of these patients because of the limited number of B-cell clones that are generated.

A form of arthritis with some of the features of rheumatoid disease occurs in some of these patients. *Mycoplasma* organisms are sometimes the cause of the arthritis. Chronic encephalitis of viral etiology appears to be an increasingly frequent terminal complication. Some of these patients have also had an associated dermatomyositis. The frequency with which these complications occur is reduced by adequate treatment with gamma globulin.

TRANSIENT HYPOGAMMAGLOBULINEMIA OF INFANCY This is a reversible syndrome in which normal physiologic hypogammaglobulinemia of infancy is unusually prolonged and severe. IgG levels of normal-term infants commonly drop to levels of 3.0 to 4.0 g/L between 3 and 6 months of age as maternally derived IgG is catabolized; levels subsequently rise reflecting the infants' increased synthetic capacity. Periodic immunologic assessment is needed to differentiate transient hypogammaglobulinemia from other forms of antibody deficiency. Antibody replacement therapy is recommended only in rare instances of severe or recurrent infections.

ISOLATED DEFICIENCY OF IgA This immunodeficiency occurs with a frequency of approximately 1 in 600 individuals of European origin. IgA deficiency is much less common in people of Asian and African origin. In Japan, for example, the incidence is approximately 1 in 18,500. While the precise genetic basis for this difference in incidence is unknown, IgA deficiency is frequently associated with certain MHC haplotypes in caucasians. The defective gene(s) predisposing to IgA deficiency may be in the class III region of the MHC genes on chromosome 6.

With rare exceptions, IgA1 and IgA2 subclasses are both deficient in serum and in mucous secretions. Many adults with isolated IgA deficiency do not seem to have unusual problems with infection. Nevertheless, this condition is not benign. As a group, individuals with IgA deficiency have an increased number of respiratory infections of varying severity, and a few have had severe pulmonary disease such as bronchiectasis. Chronic diarrheal disease also occurs. The incidence of asthma and other atopic diseases among IgA-deficient patients is high, and, conversely, the incidence of IgA deficiency among atopic children has been found to be 20 to 40 times that in the normal population. IgA deficiency is also significantly associated with autoimmune diseases such as rheumatoid arthritis and systemic lupus erythematosus. Selective reductions in the IgG2 and IgG4 subclasses have been associated with the increased infections seen in some IgA-deficient individuals. Finally, some IgA-deficient patients develop significant levels of antibodies to IgA. These patients may have severe anaphylactic reactions when transfused with normal blood or blood products.

IgA deficiency is often familial, but can also occur in association with congenital intrauterine infections, such as toxoplasmosis, rubella, and cytomegalovirus infection. IgA deficiency sometimes follows treatment with phenytoin or penicillamine. Most commonly, the syndrome appears as a sporadic defect.

The pathogenesis of IgA deficiency, whether genetic or induced by environmental insult, involves a block in terminal differentiation of B lymphocytes. Virtually all patients have detectable IgA-bearing B lymphocytes, although their numbers may be reduced. In normal children and adults, most of the B lymphocytes bearing IgA have only that immunoglobulin class on their surface, while in IgA-deficient patients and normal neonates, IgA-bearing lymphocytes also bear surface IgM. This immature phenotype is associated in most patients with failure of their cultured lymphocytes to secrete IgA when stimulated by pokeweed mitogen. While there is as yet no generally accepted pathogenic mechanism, suspicion remains high that many of these patients have a primary defect in essential regulatory interactions between T and B cells.

Treatment of IgA deficiency is essentially symptomatic. IgA cannot be effectively replaced by exogenous gamma globulin or plasma, and use of either can increase the risk of development of antibodies to IgA. IgA-deficient patients in need of transfusion should be screened for the presence of antibodies to IgA, and ideally should be given blood only from IgA-deficient donors. Treatment with immune globulin may benefit the exceptional IgA-deficient person in whom IgG2 and IgG4 subclass deficiencies are associated with severe infections. The risk of anaphylactic reactions to contaminating IgA must always be considered in treating IgA-deficient patients.

X-LINKED IMMUNODEFICIENCY WITH INCREASED LEVELS OF IgM This is a specific syndrome only because of its inheritance pattern. IgG and IgA levels are usually very low or undetectable, while IgD levels may be high. The number and distribution of B lymphocytes bearing IgM and IgD have been normal, while IgG and IgA B lymphocytes are often undetectable, suggesting a defect in isotype switching. The clinical patterns of infection are similar to those occurring with other hypogammaglobulinemic states. Neutropenia often occurs in affected males and can increase their vulnerability to infections. Adequate antibody replacement by immune globulin administration may both reverse the neutropenia and reduce the frequency of infections

ISOLATED DEFICIENCY OF IgM This syndrome has been reported rarely in this country but was detected frequently in a British population. Approximately 20 percent of these patients were asymptomatic while 60 percent had severe recurrent infections, often with bacteremia. Pneumococcal pneumonia and meningococcal meningitis have been noted in IgM-deficient patients. Other associated conditions included gastrointestinal disease, atopy, splenomegaly, and development of malignancy. The condition was frequently familial, and was four times more common in males than females. The number of circulating B lymphocytes has varied from very low to normal.

IgG SUBCLASS DEFICIENCIES Selective deficiencies in one or more of the four IgG subclasses are seen in some patients with repeated infections. The IgG subclass deficiency may easily go undetected when the total serum IgG level is measured, because IgG2, IgG3, and IgG4 together account for only 30 to 40 percent of the IgG antibodies, and even a deficiency in IgG1 may be masked by increases in the remaining IgG isotypes. However, the current availability of subclass-specific monoclonal antibodies allows precise measurement of IgG subclass levels.

Homozygous deletions of genes encoding the constant region of the different γ chains is the basis for the IgG subclass deficiency in some individuals. For example, deletion of the $C_{\alpha 1}$, $C_{\gamma 2}$, $C_{\gamma 4}$, and C_{ϵ} was responsible for one individual's inability to make IgA1, IgG2, IgG4, and IgE. Interestingly, individuals with this and other patterns of C_H-gene deletions often do not have unusual infections.

Most of the IgG subclass–deficient individuals with repeated infections appear to have regulatory defects which prevent normal B-cell differentiation. The defect may extend to other isotypes. IgA deficiency may accompany IgG2 and IgG4 subclass deficiencies (see the section on IgA deficiency, above), and an inability to produce IgM antibodies to polysaccharide antigens often reflects a broader defect in antibody responsiveness. This subgroup of patients may benefit from administration of gamma globulin. However, a thorough immunologic assessment is needed to identify the relatively few patients with IgG subclass deficiency who need this therapy.

COMMON VARIABLE IMMUNODEFICIENCY This represents a heterogeneous group of syndromes which may be congenital or acquired, sporadic or familial, and which occur in both males and females. These patients have in common the clinical manifestations of antibody deficiency associated with panhypogammaglobulinemia. The majority of these patients have normal numbers of B lymphocytes. These are clonally diverse, but have an immature phenotype. In the few patients studied, B lymphocytes capable of binding specific antigens were present, and these increased in frequency following immunization. Consistent with the evidence that B lymphocytes in these patients are able to recognize antigens and proliferate but fail to differentiate to plasma cells is the frequent occurrence of nodular lymphoid hyperplasia, including splenomegaly and intestinal lymphoid hyperplasia.

By use of assays capable of measuring B-lymphocyte differentiation to plasma cells in vitro, three major types of defects have been tentatively identified. First, and most common, is an intrinsic abnormality of B lymphocytes. B lymphocytes from these patients can be activated via their immunoglobulin receptors to express functional receptors for T cell–derived growth factors, but they fail to differentiate into immunoglobulin-secreting plasma cells even when provided with differentiation factors from normal T cells. Second, there is evidence that in some patients the T cells, or their products, may actively suppress terminal differentiation of autologous or normal B lymphocytes. The increase in suppressor activity could be either a primary or secondary abnormality. Finally, quantitative deficiency of helper T-cell function has been observed in some patients, usually also in association with defective B-cell function. This functional defect may or may not be associated with reduced numbers of CD4+ T cells.

It is important to consider the diagnosis of common variable immunodeficiency in adults with chronic pulmonary infections, some of whom will present with unexplained bronchiectasis. Intestinal diseases, including chronic giardiasis, intestinal malabsorption, and atrophic gastritis with pernicious anemia, are common in this group of patients. Patients with common variable immunodeficiency may also present with signs and symptoms highly suggestive of lymphoid malignancy, including fever, weight loss, splenomegaly, generalized lymphadenopathy, and lymphocytosis. Routine histologic examination of lymphoid tissues usually reveals germinal center hyperplasia which may be difficult to distinguish from nodular lymphoma (see Chap. 302). Demonstration of a normal distribution of immunoglobulin isotypes and light chain classes on circulating and tissue B lymphocytes can serve to distinguish these patients from those having a monoclonal B-cell malignancy with secondary hypogammaglobulinemia. The monthly administration of immune gamma globulin in adequate doses (see below) is an essential part of the treatment of all of these complications.

IMMUNODEFICIENCY WITH THYMOMA The association of hypogammaglobulinemia with spindle cell thymoma usually occurs relatively late in adult life. Bacterial infections and severe diarrhea often reflect the antibody deficiency, whereas fungal and viral infections are infrequent complications. T-cell numbers and cell-mediated immunity are usually intact, but these patients are very deficient in circulating B lymphocytes and pre-B cells in the bone marrow. They also frequently have eosinopenia, and may develop erythroid aplasia. Complete bone marrow failure has occurred in a few immunodeficient patients with thymoma. The relationship between the thymoma and apparent abnormalities of hematopoietic stem cells remains conjectural.

WISKOTT-ALDRICH SYNDROME This is an X-linked genetic disease characterized by eczema, thrombocytopenia, and repeated infections. Affected boys often present with bleeding in infancy. Most do not survive childhood, dying of complications of bleeding, infection, or lymphoreticular malignancy. The immunologic defects in this disease are well characterized but poorly understood. Serum concentrations of IgM are usually decreased, while IgA and IgG are normal and IgE is frequently increased. However, synthetic rates for all three classes may be elevated, indicating a significant element of hypercatabolism. The number and class distribution of B lymphocytes are usually normal. Functionally, these boys are consistently unable to make antibodies to polysaccharide antigens normally; responses to protein antigens are often not impaired early in the course of the disease. While most patients acquire a diminished number of T cells, serial appraisal of affected males suggests that the T-cell defects are secondary. They frequently become anergic, and their T cells do not respond normally to challenge with ubiquitous antigens. The nature of the primary defect is still unknown.

Transplantation of histocompatible bone marrow from a sibling donor has corrected both hematologic and immunologic abnormalities in several patients. In patients lacking a suitable donor, splenectomy may improve platelet counts and reduce the risk of serious hemorrhage. Because of the increased risk of pneumococcal bacteremia, splenectomized patients should probably receive prophylactic penicillin.

Miscellaneous immunodeficiency syndromes Infection with *Candida albicans* is the almost universal accompaniment of severe deficiencies in cell-mediated immunity. The syndrome of *chronic mucocutaneous candidiasis* is different because superficial candidiasis is usually the only major manifestation of immunodeficiency. These patients rarely develop systemic infection with *Candida* or other fungal agents and are not unusually susceptible to virus or bacterial disease. The syndrome is often congenital and may be associated with single or multiple endocrinopathies as well as iron deficiency. Treatment of associated conditions may lead to improvement or even cure of *Candida* infection.

No uniformity of immunologic defects has been identified in these patients, although defects of antibody formation have been detected occasionally. Humoral immunity, including ability to make specific anti-*Candida* antibodies, is usually normal. Many patients are anergic, some to a variety of antigens and some only to *Candida;* anergy in some patients has been related to inability of their lymphocytes to produce migration inhibition factor.

Results of treatment with antifungal agents, such as amphotericin B, have been variable. In some patients, intensive treatment with amphotericin B coupled with surgical removal of infected nails has led to sustained improvement. Ketoconazole, an oral antifungal agent, is reported to be quite effective.

X-LINKED LYMPHOPROLIFERATIVE SYNDROME This is an X-linked recessive disease in which there appears to be a selective impairment in immune elimination of Epstein-Barr virus (EBV). Infectious mononucleosis in affected males may have a fulminant and fatal outcome, may be associated with development of B-cell malignancies, or may result in acquired hypogammaglobulinemia, aplastic anemia, or agranulocytosis. Antibodies to EBV have been detected in some patients but are often absent in the face of infection. Generation of cytotoxic T cells appears to be the primary mechanism of control of EBV infection in normal persons, and natural killer cells may also play a role in eliminating EBV-infected B cells. While the gene defect has been mapped to the Xq 24–27 region, the nature of the cellular defect which prevents a normal response to EBV in patients with the X-linked lymphoproliferative syndrome has not been defined.

Metabolic abnormalities associated with immunodeficiency The relation of deficiencies of the purine salvage enzymes, adenosine deaminase and purine nucleoside phosphorylase, to immunodeficiency was discussed earlier. Other inherited metabolic defects should be briefly mentioned because of their potential importance in understanding the molecular basis of immunologic function. Inherited *deficiency of transcobalamin II,* the serum carrier molecule responsible for transport of vitamin B_{12} to tissues, is associated with failure of immunoglobulin production as well as megaloblastic anemia, leukopenia, thrombocytopenia, and severe malabsorption. All abnormalities are reversed by administration of pharmacologic doses of vitamin B_{12}. The syndrome of *acrodermatitis enteropathica* includes severe desquamating skin lesions, intractable diarrhea, bizarre neurologic symptoms, variable combined immunodeficiency, and an often fatal outcome. This disease is apparently caused by an inborn error of metabolism resulting in malabsorption of dietary zinc, and can be effectively treated by parenteral or large oral doses of zinc. Zinc deficiency might in part account for the immunodeficiency which accompanies severe malnutrition.

TREATMENT OF IMMUNODEFICIENCIES Most immunodeficiency diseases involving severe abnormalities of T-cell function, with or without hypogammaglobulinemia, are treated with bone marrow transplants. Histocompatible marrow from a sibling donor is preferred but haploidentical marrow may be used after removal of T cells. This therapy is complex and is best done by experienced research teams.

The increasing availability of purified gamma interferon, lymphocyte growth factors, and other biologically active cytokines promises to be important in the therapy of certain immunologic disorders. Genetic engineering also holds promise for future therapy of certain genetic defects of the immune system.

Replacement therapy with human gamma globulin should be used in patients who have recurrent bacterial infections and are deficient in IgG. Maintenance of serum IgG levels between 3.0 and 5.0 g/L is sufficient to prevent most serious infections, although chronic sinusitis, otitis media, and bronchitis may persist. These serum levels usually can be achieved by intravenous administration of IgG, 300 to 400 mg/kg, at monthly intervals. Alternatively, intramuscular injections of 100 mg/kg, at two- to four-week intervals, may suffice in some hypogammaglobulinemic patients.

The advantage of intravenous immune globulin is that higher amounts of antibodies can be given with less discomfort. Since higher levels of serum antibodies afford better protection from infections, intravenous antibody replacement is currently considered the treatment of choice for hypogammaglobulinemia. In patients with mild to moderate IgG deficiency (3.0 to 4.0 g/L), the decision to treat should be based on clinical symptoms and response to antigenic challenge.

Gamma globulin treatment is of no value in patients with deficiencies of immunoglobulins other than IgG. This form of treatment is not benign. Some patients develop symptoms of diaphoresis, tachycardia, flank pain, and hypotension during or immediately following injections. This reaction may be mediated by aggregates of IgG in the intramuscular preparations of gamma globulin but also may occur as a consequence of antibodies produced by the patient against donor immunoglobulins, particularly IgA.

Infusion of fresh plasma, 10 to 20 mL/kg at intervals of 3 to 4 weeks, has the advantage of replacing IgM and IgA as well as IgG. However, both IgM and IgA have a half-life of only a few days, and this source of antibodies can be recommended only in rare cases in which IgM antibodies may be needed to control an unusually resistant infection. The major disadvantage of plasma is the risk of transmitting hepatitis virus or other viruses, which can be particularly devastating in immunodeficient patients. This risk can be minimized by use of selected donors, usually family members, carefully screened for the absence of HIV and hepatitis virus infections.

Use of plasma or immune globulin selected on the basis of a high titer of antibodies to a particular agent may be indicated in certain situations. For example, antibodies to the causative echovirus may dramatically improve encephalitis in immunodeficient patients.

Therapy with exogenous IgG may not suffice to eliminate the chronic sinopulmonary inflammation and its progression to pulmonary fibrosis and bronchiectasis. Therefore, maintenance of good pulmonary toilet with regular postural drainage can be an especially important part of patient management. The principles of antibiotic therapy are not different in these than other patients, except that the index of suspicion of bacterial infection should remain very high.

REFERENCES

BURKS WA, STEEL RW: Selection IgA deficiency. Ann Allergy 57:3, 1986

COOPER MD: B lymphocytes: Normal development and function. N Engl J Med 317:1452, 1987

EIBL M et al: Primary immunodeficiency diseases—Report of a WHO Scientific Group. Immunodeficiency Rev 2:1, 1989

GOOD RA: Bone marrow transplantation for immunodeficiency diseases. Am J Med Sci 294:68, 1987

HANSON LA et al: Immunoglobulin subclass deficiency. Pediatr Infect Dis J 7:S17, 1988

PAUL WE: *Fundamental Immunology*, 2d ed. New York, Raven, 1989

ROIFMAN CM, GELFAND EW: Replacement therapy with high dose intravenous gammaglobulin improves sinopulmonary disease in patients with hypogammaglobulinemia. Pediatr Infect Dis J 7:S92, 1988

ROSEN FS et al: The primary immunodeficiencies. N Engl J Med 311:235, 300, 1984

ROYER HD, REINHERZ EL: T lymphocytes: Ontogeny, function, and relevance to clinical disorders. N Engl J Med 274:1171, 1987

264 THE ACQUIRED IMMUNODEFICIENCY SYNDROME (AIDS)

ANTHONY S. FAUCI / H. CLIFFORD LANE

DEFINITION The acquired immunodeficiency syndrome was originally defined for surveillance purposes by the Centers for Disease Control (CDC) as the presence of a reliably diagnosed "opportunistic" disease that is at least moderately indicative of an underlying defect in cell-mediated immunity in the absence of known causes of underlying immune defects such as iatrogenic immunosuppression or malignant neoplasms. Following the demonstration in 1984 that the human immunodeficiency virus (HIV) is the etiologic agent of AIDS, reliable tests for HIV antibody as well as for the virus itself became available. Since that time the case definition of AIDS has undergone several revisions with regard to inclusion and exclusion criteria. Despite this complexity the simple common denominator of AIDS is infection with HIV and subsequent development of persistent constitutional symptoms and/or AIDS-defining diseases such as secondary infections, neoplasms, and neurologic disease (see below). It is appropriate to think in terms of the spectrum of HIV-related disease rather than the presence or absence of AIDS according to a strict definition. This concept has been reinforced by prospective, natural history studies of HIV-infected individuals. In those studies, the risk for developing a typical AIDS-defining opportunistic infection (*Pneumocystis carinii* pneumonia) within 1 year was 15 percent in individuals with less than 0.200×10^9 CD4+ T lymphocytes per liter (200 cells per microliter) in the absence of prior symptoms of HIV infection, and as high as 47 percent in individuals with two or more symptoms of HIV infection. Thus, the risk of serious outcome of HIV infection, particularly with regard to opportunistic infections, is predictable on the basis of the degree of immunosuppression as measured by the level of circulating CD4+ T cells. Since, in the absence of therapy (see below), most HIV-infected individuals experience progressive diminution of circulating CD4+ T cells, HIV infection itself is part of the spectrum of HIV-related disease.

ETIOLOGY AIDS is caused by HIV, a human retrovirus of the lentivirus group. The four recognized human retroviruses belong to two distinct groups: the human T lymphotropic (or leukemia) retroviruses, HTLV-I and HTLV-II, and the human immunodeficiency viruses, HIV-1 and HIV-2. The former are transforming viruses, and the latter are cytopathic viruses (see Chap. 134). The most common cause of AIDS throughout the world is HIV-1. HIV-2 has about 40 percent sequence homology with HIV-1 and is more closely related to some members of a group of simian immunodeficiency viruses (SIV). It has been identified predominantly in western African countries, is much less common, and is felt to be less pathogenic than HIV-1. HIV has the usual retroviral genes (*env, gag,* and *pol*) and six extra genes involved in the replication and other biologic activities of the virus (see Chap. 134). Various isolates of HIV-1 manifest heterogeneity, particularly in the region of the envelope gene.

INCIDENCE AND PREVALENCE AIDS was first recognized in the United States in the summer of 1981 when the CDC reported the unexplained occurrence of *Pneumocystis carinii* pneumonia in 5 previously healthy homosexual men in Los Angeles and Kaposi's sarcoma in 26 previously healthy homosexual men in New York and Los Angeles. By mid-1990, approximately 120,000 cases among adults and adolescents and approximately 2000 cases among children less than 13 years old had been reported in the United States. It is estimated that between 1 and 1.5 million people are infected in the United States, and in the absence of effective therapy (see below) it is projected that by 1992 there will have been 365,000 reported cases.

AIDS is a global epidemic with virtually every country in the world reporting cases. In addition to the United States, areas of the world with the highest incidence include western Europe, central Africa, South America (particularly Brazil), and Canada.

Sexual contact is the major mode of transmission of HIV worldwide. The virus can also be transmitted by blood or blood products both in individuals who share contaminated needles for intravenous drug use and in those who receive tranfusions of blood or blood products. Infected mothers efficiently (30 to 40 percent) transmit the virus to their infants perinatally and as early as the first and second trimesters of pregnancy. Virus can also be transmitted from mother to infant via breast feeding. There is absolutely no evidence that HIV can be transmitted by casual contact or that the virus can be spread by insects such as by a mosquito bite.

Among the adult cases reported in the United States, approximately 60 percent are in homosexual or bisexual men who do not use intravenous drugs. The next largest number of cases (20 percent) is seen among heterosexual men and women intravenous drug users and is related to the sharing of needles and other drug paraphernalia. Seven percent of cases are in men who are homosexual or bisexual and who also use intravenous drugs. Approximately 1 percent of cases are in hemophiliacs with no history of other risk factors. These individuals were exposed to HIV because of the large quantities of factor VIII and/or plasma concentrates that they received intravenously as replacement for deficient clotting factors. An additional 2 percent of cases are in nonhemophiliacs who have received transfusions of blood or blood products. Five percent of cases are in persons who have had heterosexual contact with an individual known to be infected or one belonging to a known risk category for HIV infection. Approximately half of these individuals with heterosexually acquired AIDS were infected by having sex with an intravenous drug user, and an additional 30 percent of such patients have had heterosexual contact with a person born in a country (such as certain central African countries) with a high incidence of heterosexually acquired HIV infection. Despite the fact that the majority of cases of AIDS have occurred among homosexual or bisexual men, the rate of new cases of AIDS is now higher among intravenous drug users than among homosexual men in cities, such as New York, where there are high concentrations of intravenous drug users. This has led to a progressive increase in the proportion of heterosexually acquired AIDS since intravenous drug users can infect their sexual partners. Furthermore, this pattern has also led to a dramatic increase in HIV-infected infants and new cases of pediatric AIDS. Approximately 80 percent of all pediatric (<13 years of age) AIDS cases have infection from their mothers, and of these the vast majority of infants were born of mothers who were either intravenous drug users themselves or the sexual partners of intravenous drug users. The remainder of pediatric cases have occurred among blood transfusion recipients (11 percent) and hemophiliacs (5 percent).

The epidemic of HIV infection and the epidemic of HIV disease in the United States are somewhat discordant. Although the figures vary widely from city to city, the prevalence of HIV infection among homosexual men is extremely high; approximately 50 to 60 percent of homosexual men attending sexually transmitted diseases clinics in high-incidence cities, such as San Francisco and New York, are HIV seropositive. However, a saturational effect and, more importantly, behavior modification together have brought the epidemic of new infection among homosexual men in the United States to a peak. This is indicated by the fact that the rate of new infection among homosexual men in San Francisco in 1982 to 1983 was approximately 19 percent per year, while it is now less than 1 percent per year. Nonetheless, the epidemic of disease among homosexual men has far from peaked. In the absence of effective therapy that can prevent disease in infected individuals (see below), the majority of new cases within the next few years will still be among homosexual men. Likewise, despite the fact that over 70 percent of persons with hemophilia A are HIV seropositive, screening of blood donors and heat treatment of factor VIII concentrates has resulted in a virtual halt in the new infections among hemophiliacs. Yet those infected will continue to develop disease. The same holds true for infections acquired via blood transfusions among nonhemophiliacs. Rare infections will continue to occur by transfusion of contaminated blood, since a very small percentage of individuals who are infected may escape detection by screening tests conducted among blood donors (see below). The chance of a single unit of donated blood containing HIV is estimated to range from 1 in 40,000 to 1 in 250,000.

The situation is somewhat different among intravenous drug users. The prevalence of HIV infection among intravenous drug users is high, especially among inner-city minority populations in the United States; in New York City the HIV seroprevalence in this group approximates 55 to 60 percent. Furthermore, there is no evidence that the epidemic of new infections has peaked among this group. Seroprevalence studies of emergency room patients in a hospital in inner-city Baltimore indicated that approximately 5 percent of all emergency room admissions were HIV-seropositive, a reflection of the high incidence of intravenous drug use of that population and of spread to heterosexual partners of intravenous drug users. Likewise, studies of approximately 5000 patients attending two inner-city sexually transmitted disease clinics in Baltimore indicated that approximately 5 percent of patients were infected with HIV. Of HIV-infected patients 25 years of age or younger, 46 percent of men and 72 percent of women denied high-risk behavior other than heterosexual activity, adding further credence to the concept that substantial secondary spread of HIV is occurring through heterosexual contact, predominantly with infected intravenous drug users. In this regard, there is a significant association of HIV infection with syphilis (see Chap. 128) in accord with the correlation of genital ulcers and heterosexual transmission of HIV noted in other studies (see below).

Although the precise prevalence of HIV infection in the general population in the United States is unknown, it is felt to be quite low. This belief is based on data collected from millions of blood donors that indicate that among this group, which voluntarily excludes individuals who knowingly practice high-risk behavior, less than 0.04 percent of people are HIV-seropositive. This is in contrast to the central African country of Zaire in which as many as 3 to 5 percent of the general population may be positive. Surveys of new military recruits in the United States have shown that approximately 0.15 percent are HIV-seropositive. The discrepancy between this group and the blood donor population likely reflects the fact that military recruits are younger, are more sexually active, and contain a higher proportion of inner-city minorities (see above). Broad seroprevalence studies designed to be representative of the entire population of the United States are currently being undertaken by the CDC.

There is a small but real occupational risk of HIV infection among health care workers who are exposed to the virus through penetrating injuries and, to a much lesser extent, through mucosal splash incidents involving large amounts of blood. Of the several hundred health care workers who have sustained penetrating injuries with instruments contaminated with HIV-infected blood, less than 0.5 percent have become infected.

PATHOPHYSIOLOGY AND IMMUNOPATHOGENESIS The common denominator of AIDS is a profound immunosuppression, predominantly of cell-mediated immunity, that leads to a variety of opportunistic diseases, particularly certain infections and neoplasms. Other features of AIDS, such as Kaposi's sarcoma and neurologic abnormalities, cannot be explained directly by the immunosuppressive effects of HIV since these complications may occur prior to the development of severe immunologic impairment.

The main cause of the immune defect in AIDS is a quantitative and qualitative deficiency in the subset of thymus-derived (T) lymphocytes termed the *T4 population*. This subset of cells is defined phenotypically by the presence of the CD4 surface molecule, which is the cellular receptor for HIV. Although the T4 cell is the major cell type infected with HIV, virtually any human cell that expresses the CD4 molecule on its surface is capable of binding to and being infected with HIV. Of particular importance are cells of the monocyte-macrophage lineage.

HIV binds specifically and with high affinity, via a stretch of amino acids in the viral envelope (gp 120), to a portion of the V1 region of the CD4 molecule located near its *N*-terminus. Following binding, the virus fuses with the target cell membrane and is internalized. It then utilizes the enzyme reverse transcriptase to transcribe its genomic RNA to DNA, which is integrated into the cellular DNA where it exists for the life of the cell as a "provirus" (see Chap. 134). The provirus may remain latent or be activated to transcribe mRNA and genomic RNA, leading to protein synthesis, assembly, new virion formation, and budding of virus from the cell surface. Although the precise mechanism by which the virus induces cell death has not been established, it is felt that the major mechanism is massive viral budding from the cell surface, which leads to disruption of the plasma membrane and resulting osmotic disequilibrium. Other mechanisms that might contribute to the diminution of T4 cells are: infection of a T4-cell precursor leading ultimately to reduction by attrition of T4 cells; selective depletion of CD4+ lymphoid or nonlymphoid cells that serve T4 cells, such as by supplying an essential cytokine; formation of syncytia between uninfected cells and infected cells expressing viral envelope proteins on their surface, leading to the "innocent bystander" death of uninfected cells from fusion with infected cells; autoimmune phenomena whereby virus-specific cellular or humoral immune responses eliminate infected cells expressing viral proteins or uninfected cells that have bound or expressed viral proteins on their surface; and secretion of substances toxic to T4 cells by HIV-infected cells.

Functional abnormalities of uninfected T4 cells have been well documented in HIV-infected individuals. This is particularly true of the antigen-responsive T4-cell subset, which is defective early in the course of HIV infection. The precise mechanism of this defect is unclear. However, it may be related to a variety of factors including the selective infection of the memory subset of T4 cells, which leads to their early elimination and results in defective responses to recall antigens in the remaining cells. In addition, HIV proteins can interfere in vitro with the interaction between the CD4 molecule and its natural ligand, the major histocompatibility (MHC) class II molecule, which is critical to the monocyte-T4 cell interactions essential for specific immune responses to soluble antigen. Furthermore, antibodies to the HIV envelope protein may cross-react with class II MHC molecules and interfere with immune function.

Following initial infection with HIV, there is generally an abrupt, slight-to-moderate decrease in circulating T4 lymphocytes, which usually levels off with counts remaining stable for years. This sequence may reflect containment of the virus by immune responses. After variable periods, the T4 cells usually insidiously and progressively decrease in number, likely reflecting a gradual escape from immune containment. However, the course of infection in certain individuals may be punctuated by abrupt and dramatic decreases in T4 counts. Once the T4-lymphocyte count drops to 0.200×10^9 per liter (200 cells per microliter) or less, the chances of developing an opportunistic infection such as *Pneumocystis carinii* pneumonia are high, and this level of T4 cells is prognostic of a serious clinical complication.

In the early phases of HIV infection, the suppressor-cytotoxic subset of T cells, phenotypically defined by the CD8 surface molecule, is sometimes initially elevated. The T8 subset is believed to be responsible for the containment of HIV infection in T4 cells. As infection progresses, T8-cell numbers may be normal or, in many cases, become decreased late in the course of infection.

Although only 1 in 10,000 to 1 in 1000 T4 cells in the peripheral blood of AIDS patients actively expresses virus at any given time (the figure is lower during the asymptomatic phase), the number of cells that harbor latent HIV provirus is as high as 1 in 100 to 1 in 10. The viral burden per constant number of T4 cells increases as the T4-cell number is depleted and as disease progresses. Factors that induce the conversion of latent infection to actively replicating virus are potentially important in the pathogenesis of HIV disease. Mitogens, antigens, and transfected heterologous viral genes have been demonstrated to induce virus expression in vitro. Furthermore, cytokines such as tumor necrosis factor alpha (TNF-α), IL-6, and granulocyte-macrophage colony stimulating factor (GM-CSF) can also induce virus expression in infected cells. Since TNF-α is secreted in response to a number of infections, many of which occur as opportunistic infections in HIV-infected individuals, a cycle of progressive induction of HIV from latently infected cells may occur as disease progression occurs, and more secondary infections ensue. Thus, certain cytokines involved in the regulation of the normal immune response may serve as cofactors (see below) in the in vitro induction of virus expression in cells already infected with HIV.

The relationship between the depletion of T4 lymphocytes and profound immunosuppression is clear. Since the T4-lymphocyte subset is responsible for the induction and/or regulation of virtually the entire immune system, the selective defect in this subset results in global impairment of components of immunity that depend, at least in part, on inductive signals from the T4 cell. These include defects in natural killer cells, virus-specific cytotoxic T cells, B cells, and monocytes. Some of these defects can be corrected in vitro by supplying inductive signals in the form of lymphokines derived from T4 cells.

B lymphocytes from AIDS patients are polyclonally activated, resulting in hypergammaglobulinemia and circulating immune complexes. The consequences of B-cell abnormalities are most obvious in children with AIDS, in whom there is an increase in bacterial infections with organisms against which an intact humoral immune response is required for protection. It is felt that the nonspecific polyclonal activation of B cells interferes with the ability to mount an adequate de novo humoral immune response. The mechanism of the polyclonal hyperactivity of B cells in HIV-infected individuals is unclear, but may relate to activation of Epstein-Barr virus (EBV) in the absence of the normal regulatory T-cell influences, the elaboration of factors derived from T cells and monocytes that can trigger B cells, or the possible direct triggering of B cells by HIV itself. There is no evidence that HIV can infect B cells in vivo.

Circulating monocytes are normal in number in HIV-infected individuals; however, a number of monocyte functional abnormalities have been reported including defects in chemotaxis, secretion of interleukin 1, certain cytotoxic functions, and the ability to present antigen to T cells. Infection of circulating monocytes cannot explain these functional abnormalities, since in vivo infection of circulating monocytes occurs rarely and in very low frequency, whereas infection of tissue macrophages and of macrophage lineage cells in the brain (see below) and other organs is easily demonstrable. The reported abnormalities of circulating monocytes are likely related in part to the activation of these cells in vivo by cytokines. Infection of monocyte precursors in bone marrow with HIV may directly or indirectly be responsible for certain of the hematologic abnormalities in HIV-infected individuals. Given the fact that HIV can persist in macrophages without causing a cytopathic effect, macrophages may serve as reservoirs of HIV and may contribute to the dissemination of virus in the body.

HIV has been demonstrated in the brains of infected individuals with neuropsychiatric abnormalities (see below). In addition, the virus can be isolated from the cerebrospinal fluid (CSF) of a high percentage of infected individuals without detectable neuropsychiatric findings. The predominant brain cells infected with HIV are of the monocyte-macrophage lineage such as microglial cells. There is no convincing evidence that neurons can be infected with HIV. Although the mechanisms of nervous system tissue damage by HIV are unknown, it is felt that release of toxic cytokines from HIV-infected monocyte-macrophage lineage cells may play a role. In addition, products of HIV may impair neuron function.

HIV-infected individuals have an increased incidence of neoplasms such as Kaposi's sarcoma, some B-cell lymphomas, Hodgkin's disease, and certain carcinomas. The mechanism of this diathesis is unknown, and immunosuppression is not the only factor involved. For example, EBV has been implicated in some of the B-cell lymphomas that occur with HIV infection. HIV does not cause these tumors directly since viral sequences have not been demonstrated in the DNA from the tumor cells. HIV may contribute to the development of Kaposi's sarcoma by inducing the secretion of a growth factor from infected CD4+ cells which in turn induces endothelial cells to secrete a number of cytokines that cause the proliferation of the mixed cell types characteristic of Kaposi's sarcoma (see Chap. 134).

The pathogenesis of the hypercatabolic wasting syndrome seen in many HIV-infected individuals is unclear, but may be due in part to increased levels of cytokines such as TNF-α, also termed *cachetin*, which causes cachexia in animals (see Chap. 20).

A variety of potential cofactors may play a role in the transmission of and susceptibility to HIV infection and in the development of disease in infected individuals. For example, there is a strong association between genital ulcerations and susceptibility to HIV infection through sexual contact. In addition, cytokines such as TNF-α may be important cofactors in the induction of expression of virus in already infected cells (see above). Furthermore, coinfection with HTLV-I or human herpesvirus 6 enhances the expression of HIV in vitro.

The precise role of the immune system in the prevention or slowing of progression of disease in HIV-infected individuals is unclear. Such individuals make antibodies directed against a number of viral proteins, and neutralizing antibodies can be demonstrated in most infected persons. However, studies of the relationship between the presence and level of neutralizing antibodies and clinical outcome have produced conflicting results. Likewise, HIV-specific, MHC-restricted, cytotoxic T cells have been demonstrated in HIV-infected persons, but their relationship to protection is also unclear. Other immune mechanisms, such as antibody-dependent cellular cytotoxicity and natural killer cell activity, have been demonstrated in vitro against the virus; their role, if any, in protection remains to be determined.

CLINICAL MANIFESTATIONS The clinical consequences of HIV infection form a spectrum ranging from the asymptomatic state to severe disease (Table 264-1). The majority of individuals experience no recognizable symptoms or signs at the time of initial infection, but some patients develop an *acute illness* (group I) approximately 3 to 6 weeks following primary infection. It is characterized by nonspecific signs and symptoms including fevers, rigors, arthralgias, myalgias, maculopapular rash, urticaria, abdominal cramps, diarrhea, and aseptic meningitis. The syndrome lasts 2 to 3 weeks and resolves spontaneously. Seroconversion usually occurs 8 to 12 weeks after presumed exposure.

Although the length of time from initial infection to the development of clinical disease varies greatly, the mean period is estimated to be between 8 and 10 years. During that period of time, individuals are classified as having *asymptomatic infection* (group II). Approximately 75 percent of individuals will develop some degree of symptoms, including full-blown AIDS (36 percent), within 7 years of initial infection, and up to 80 to 90 percent of infected persons develop some degree of deterioration of immune function within 3 years of infection, usually in the absence of symptoms.

Certain patients, otherwise asymptomatic, develop *persistent generalized lymphadenopathy* (group III). This syndrome is defined as palpable lymphadenopathy (lymph node enlargement of $\geq$ 1 cm) at two or more extrainguinal sites that persists for more than 3 months in the absence of a concurrent illness or condition, other than HIV infection, to explain the findings. It has been postulated that this phenomenon in the absence of other symptoms represents a state of immunologic containment of the virus and is a favorable sign. However, patients at this stage frequently go on to disease progression, and so any viral containment that occurs is only transient.

The stage of HIV infection that has defied precise clinical classification is that of nonspecific signs or symptoms with or without a substantial decrease in T4 cells (<200 T4 cells per microliter). This has generally been referred to empirically as early *AIDS-related complex* (ARC) if individuals manifest one or two signs or symptoms such as fatigue, fever, weight loss, persistent skin rash, oral hairy leukoplakia, herpes simplex, and oral thrush, and advanced ARC if more than two of these manifestations are present. The line between advanced ARC and full-blown AIDS is not clear, and a certain level of *constitutional disease* (group IV, subgroup A) should be considered as AIDS. This latter group is defined as consisting of one or more of the following: fever persisting for more than 1 month, involuntary weight loss of greater than 10 percent of baseline, or diarrhea persisting for more than 1 month in the absence of another cause to explain the findings. Patients may develop a hypercatabolic wasting syndrome in the absence of any other signs or symptoms of HIV infection and may be categorized as group IV, subgroup A patients,

TABLE 264-1 Classification system for HIV infection

Group I	Acute infection
Group II	Asymptomatic infection
Group III	Persistent generalized lymphadenopathy
Group IV	Other disease:
Subgroup A	Constitutional disease
Subgroup B	Neurologic disease
Subgroup C	Secondary infectious diseases
Subgroup D	Secondary neoplasms
Subgroup E	Other conditions

SOURCE: Modified from Centers for Disease Control, 1986 and 1987.

or more frequently this syndrome may occur in patients who already have developed another AIDS-defining condition such as opportunistic infections or neoplasms (see below). In any case, in the majority of patients no underlying direct cause of the wasting syndrome is identified.

Neurologic disease is common in HIV-infected individuals; 40 to 60 percent of patients with AIDS manifest neurologic dysfunction and 80 to 90 percent manifest neuropathologic abnormalities at autopsy. The most common neurologic disorder is HIV encephalopathy, also referred to as the AIDS dementia complex. If this syndrome or myelopathy or peripheral neuropathy occur in the absence of a concurrent condition or illness other than HIV infection, it constitutes in itself an AIDS-defining illness (group IV, subgroup B). Other neurologic complications of AIDS include cryptococcal meningitis, central nervous system (CNS) toxoplasmosis, primary CNS lymphoma, progressive multifocal leukoencephalopathy, cytomegalovirus (CMV) infection, peripheral neuropathies, vacuolar myelopathy, and aseptic meningitis. CNS mass lesions in an HIV-infected individual should be considered either toxoplasmosis or primary CNS lymphoma until proven otherwise. The former gives a typical "ring-enhancing" appearance on computed tomography (CT) with contrast (see Chap. 162).

The most common clinical manifestation of AIDS is opportunistic infection (group IV, subgroup C). It is not unusual for an AIDS patient to have more than one opportunistic infection simultaneously (Table 264-2). *Pneumocystis carinii* pneumonia (see Chap. 163) is the most common opportunistic infection, occurring in approximately 80 percent of patients at some point during the course of their illness.

TABLE 264-2 Commonly encountered opportunistic infections in AIDS and their treatments

Infecting agent	Reference chapters*	Manifestations	Treatment	Toxicities of treatment	Comment
Pneumocystis carinii	163	Pneumonia (usually interstitial); rarely dissemination	Trimethoprim/sulfamethoxazole, 15–20/75–100 mg/kg per day PO or IV in 3–4 divided doses for 2–3 weeks	Skin rash, neutropenia, megaloblastosis, thrombocytopenia	Trimethoprim (5 mg/kg q 6 h) and dapsone 100 mg/d may be as effective as trimethoprim/sulfamethoxazole.
			or Pentamidine isethionate, 3–4 mg/kg per day by slow IV; 2–3 weeks duration of therapy	Hypoglycemia, hyperglycemia, hypocalcemia, azotemia, hepatic dysfunction, hypotension	After episode of *P. carinii* pneumonia or in patients with CD4+ lymphocytes <0.200 × 10^9/L (<200 cells/μL) prophylaxis is recommended with aerosolized pentamidine isethionate, 300 mg monthly, or trimethoprim/sulfamethoxazole 320/1600 mg bid.
Cytomegalovirus	138	Retinitis, enteritis, cerebritis, pneumonitis, esophagitis, adrenalitis	Ganciclovir [9-(1,3-dihydroxy-2 propoxymethyl) guanine (DHPG)] 5 mg/kg IV bid for 2–3 weeks, then 5 mg/kg IV qd maintenance	Bone marrow suppression	Bone marrow toxicity of ganciclovir may be additive with that of zidovudine. Maintenance therapy should be continued indefinitely; reinductions required often with both drugs. Foscarnet still in clinical trials.
			or Foscarnet (phosphonoformate) 60 mg/kg tid for 2–3 weeks, then 90 mg/kg qd maintenance, IV	Azotemia, seizures, hypomagnesemia	
Candida albicans	151,87	Oral thrush	Clotrimazole troches, 5 times daily	Generally free of toxicity	
			or Nystatin suspension 5 mL swish and swallow, qid	Generally free of toxicity	
			or Ketoconazole, 200–400 mg/d PO	Hepatitis, adrenal insufficiency	
		Esophagitis	Mild: Swallow nystatin suspension, sucking clotrimazole troches		
			or Ketoconazole 200–400 mg/d PO	Hepatitis, adrenal insufficiency	
			Severe: Amphotericin B, 0.3 mg/kg per day IV for 5–10 d	Fever, chills, nausea, vomiting, thrombophlebitis, azotemia, hypokalemia, anemia, hypomagnesemia	
		Rarely disseminated	Amphotericin B, 0.4–0.5 mg/kg per day or as a double dose on alternate days for several weeks		
Mycobacterium avium-intracellulare	127,85	Disseminated, particularly in bone marrow, lung, lymph node, liver	No recognized therapy; 3 to 5 drugs chosen from among isoniazid, ethambutal, rifampin, ethionamide, pyrazinamide, cycloserine, streptomycin, amikacin, clofazimine, ansamycin	See Chaps. 85 and 127	No regimen yet shown to be reliably effective.

TABLE 264-2 Commonly encountered opportunistic infections in AIDS and their treatments *(continued)*

Infecting agent	Reference chapters*	Manifestations	Treatment	Toxicities of treatment	Comment
Mycobacterium tuberculosis	125,85	Pulmonary; disseminated (frequent)	2 or 3 drugs chosen from among isoniazid, rifampin, ethambutol, pyrazinamide, streptomycin and others (see Chap. 125)	See Chaps. 85 and 125	Short-course regimens not recommended. Initial response to therapy generally good. Role for long-term maintenance therapy remains unclear.
Cryptococcus neoformans	151	Meningitis; pulmonary; disseminated	Amphotericin 8, 0.5–0.6 mg/kg per day IV when used alone or 0.3 mg/kg per day when used in combination with 5-fluorocytosine (5FC, flucytosine) *or in combination with* 5-Fluorocytosine, 150 mg/kg per day in 4 divided doses q 6 h PO	See above for *Candida albicans* treatment Rash, myelosuppression, hepatitis	Requires indefinite maintenance therapy; ketoconazole or fluconazole may be effective. Fluconazole (still in clinical trials) may also be effective as initial therapy.
Toxoplasma gondii	162	Encephalitis; intracerebral mass; ocular disease (rare)	Pyrimethamine loading dose of 100–200 mg PO in 2 divided doses for 2 days; maintenance dose of 25 mg/d in single dose *plus* Sulfadiazine loading dose of 50–75 mg/kg PO; thereafter maintenance dose of 75–100 mg/kg per day in 4 divided doses q 6 h PO *plus* Folinic acid, 10 mg/d PO in single dose	Anemia, neutropenia, thrombocytopenia, rash Usual for sulfonamides (see Chap. 85), especially crystalluria, hematuria, rash	Initial response in patients who recover usually occurs within 2 to 3 weeks. Requires indefinite maintenance therapy.
Herpes simplex	135,86	Severe mucocutaneous disease including perianal skin Esophagitis; pneumonia; disseminated (rare)	Acyclovir, 250 mg/m^2 q 8 h for 7 d IV; *or* 200 mg PO, 5 times daily for 10 d Acyclovir, 10 mg/kg q 8 h for 10 d IV	Generally free of toxicity Azotemia, CNS changes, rash, mild hepatitis	May recur, but maintenance therapy usually not indicated
Herpes zoster	136,86	Severe cutaneous disease; dissemination (rare)	Acyclovir, 500 mg/m^2 q 8 h IV for 7 d	Azotemia, CNS changes, rash, mild hepatitis	
Cryptosporidium	166	Prolonged, severe diarrhea; malnutrition, wasting	None proven; spiramycin in clinical trials Supportive care including antimotility agents.		Protracted diarrhea, unresponsive to therapy, may lead to inanition
Isospora belli	166	Severe diarrhea; may be indistinguishable from cryptosporidiosis	Trimethoprim/sulfamethoxazole, 160/800 mg qid PO for 10 d, then bid for 3 weeks	See above for *Pneumocystis carinii*	Prophylaxis using trimethoprim/sulfamethoxazole 160/800 mg 3 times weekly or sulfadoxine/pyramethamine 500/25 mg once per week has been effective.
Salmonella sp.	113	Septicemia, diarrhea	Ampicillin, trimethoprin/sulfamethoxazole, quinolones, or chloramphenicol depending on microbial sensitivities; see Chap. 85 for details	See Chap. 85	Ciprafloxacin may also be effective.

* The reader is referred to the indicated chapter for detailed discussion of infection, treatment, and treatment toxicities.

Patients may present with typical findings such as fever, dyspnea, and hypoxia. However, in contrast to the presentation in immunosuppressed patients without AIDS in whom the onset is usually abrupt and explosive, patients with AIDS often have an indolent presentation with symptoms gradually accelerating over weeks prior to the establishment of the diagnosis. The chest x-ray may be normal, show an interstitial infiltrate or, in the case of patients receiving aerosolized pentamidine, reveal upper lobe cavitary disease. Because of the large number of microorganisms in AIDS patients, the diagnosis can usually be made by histochemical staining of induced sputum, or if that fails by bronchoscopy with staining of material from transbronchial biopsy or bronchial lavage. It is unusual to have to resort to thoracotomy and lung biopsy to establish the diagnosis. Extrapulmonary disseminated *P. carinii* may occur more frequently in individuals receiving aerosolized pentamidine isethionate as prophylaxis against pulmonary infection (see below).

Cytomegalovirus infections (see Chap. 138) are common in AIDS patients and appear as fever and disseminated organ system involvement. CMV chorioretinitis can result in serious visual impairment and even blindness. CMV can cause enteritis with intractable diarrhea, interstitial pneumonitis, and adrenalitis. CMV infection of the CNS is an uncommon cause of neurologic complications.

Candida albicans (see Chap. 151) is an extremely common infection in AIDS patients and is usually manifested as oral thrush or esophagitis. Detectable candidemia and disseminated candidiasis are unusual. Oral candidiasis in an HIV-infected individual without other opportunistic infections indicates ARC and is prognostic of progression to AIDS.

Mycobacterium avium-intracellulare (see Chap. 127) is uncommon in individuals without HIV infection but can exist as a localized or disseminated infection in AIDS patients and is readily isolated from bone marrow, lymph nodes, liver biopsies, and blood of infected individuals. It generally occurs as a smoldering infection, is rarely the primary cause of death, but is associated with wasting syndromes. Active infection with *M. tuberculosis* (see Chap. 125) occurs in as many as 10 percent of AIDS patients. The risk of active tuberculosis is particularly high among HIV-infected nonwhites and intravenous drug users and has led to a resurgence of tuberculosis in some cities. Although the prevalence and incidence of *M. tuberculosis* infection are similar in HIV-infected and non-HIV-infected intravenous drug users, the risk of active tuberculosis is elevated only for HIV-seropositive subjects. As in non-AIDS patients, the lungs are the most frequent site of disease, but more than half of AIDS patients with tuberculosis have at least one extrapulmonary site. As a consequence, the CDC includes extrapulmonary tuberculosis as an AIDS-defining diagnosis in HIV-infected individuals.

Cryptococcus neoformans infection (see Chap. 151) occurs in approximately 10 percent of AIDS patients as meningitis (approximately 75 percent of infections) or as disseminated disease with the lungs being the predominant organ involved. In patients with meningitis, CSF leukocyte count and protein and glucose levels may be normal. Diagnosis is established on the basis of CSF cultures and CSF cryptococcal antigen levels, with the latter usually reaching extremely high titers. Serum crytococcal antigen may be positive in these patients.

Toxoplasma gondii (see Chap. 162) is one of the most common CNS infections in AIDS patients. It occurs as an encephalitis or as an intracerebral mass lesion. Manifestations include focal neurologic changes or diffuse signs and symptoms such as mental status abnormalities and seizures. CT scans with contrast usually show multiple lesions with ring enhancement. Ocular disease occurs rarely. Serologic studies that suggest recrudescence rather than primary infection are not reliable for diagnosis, and microbiologic confirmation is often required on tissue obtained by stereotactic needle biopsy or at craniotomy. If these latter approaches are not feasible because of the location of lesions deep in the cerebral cortex, empiric treatment may be indicated in some patients in the absence of a confirmed diagnosis.

Herpes simplex virus infection (see Chap. 135) in patients with AIDS or ARC may be manifest as severe mucocutaneous disease, including perianal involvement and esophagitis; pneumonitis has been reported. Herpes zoster infection (see Chap. 136) can involve a single or several dermatomes and rarely disseminates beyond the skin.

Persistent diarrhea is frequent in AIDS patients, and in fact diarrhea that persists for longer than 1 month without an obvious cause in an HIV-infected individual establishes the diagnosis of AIDS (Table 264-1; group IV, subgroup A). The enteric pathogen *Cryptosporidium* (see Chap. 166) is an important cause of prolonged or recurrent diarrhea and may lead to malabsorption and wasting. In an immunocompetent host cryptosporidia usually cause an explosive, profuse, watery diarrhea accompanied by abdominal cramping that lasts for 5 to 11 days and abates spontaneously. In AIDS patients cryptosporidiosis is usually indolent in onset and prolonged in duration with abdominal cramping and systemic manifestations similar to those seen in normal hosts. However, prolonged and often intractable diarrhea may lead to inanition. *Isospora belli* (see Chap. 167) also causes a severe diarrhea in AIDS patients and may be indistinguishable clinically from that caused by cryptosporidia. Diarrheal syndromes can also occur secondary to CMV enteritis, Kaposi's sarcoma in the gastrointestinal tract, or other intestinal parasites and microbes.

Bacterial infections, in particular infections with encapsulated organisms, occur more commonly in children with AIDS. Even among adults, *Salmonella* infections (see Chap. 113) are a relatively common cause of diarrhea and bacteremia. Other pyogenic bacterial infections include *Haemophilus influenza* (see Chap. 115) and *Streptococcus pneumoniae* (see Chap. 99). Because of the frequent use of indwelling venous catheters in AIDS patients, infections around these devices and septicemia with *Staphylococcus aureus* and *Staph. epidermidis* (see Chap. 100) are common.

Less common infections in AIDS patients include *coccidioidomycosis* (see Chap. 151), *aspergillosis* (Chap. 151), *histoplasmosis* (Chap. 151), and *nocardiosis* (Chap. 152), and disseminated cat-scratch disease (Chap. 98).

Kaposi's sarcoma (group IV, subgroup D) is characterized histopathologically by proliferation of a mixed cell population including endothelial cells. It is often the presenting clinical manifestation of AIDS. HIV is not the direct cause of Kaposi's sarcoma, and there is no evidence of malignant transformation of cells. Furthermore, the presence and extent of Kaposi's sarcoma is not necessarily related to the degree of HIV-induced immunosuppression. The role of HIV in Kaposi's sarcoma may be the induction of growth factors that cause proliferation of the cells composing the tumor (see Chap. 134). Kaposi's sarcoma occurs in approximately 34 percent of male homosexuals with AIDS and in less than 10 percent of heterosexual AIDS patients. The reason for this discrepancy is unclear; there has been speculation that one or more cofactors present in the homosexual population accounts for the relatively higher prevalence of Kaposi's sarcoma among this group. However, such cofactors have not been identified.

Kaposi's sarcoma presents clinically as multifocal vascular nodules in the skin and viscera. The course ranges from indolent, with only skin manifestations, to fulminant, with extensive visceral involvement. The pattern of Kaposi's sarcoma in AIDS patients differs significantly from that of non-HIV-infected patients. In elderly men in the United States and Europe and in organ transplant recipients who are pharmacologically immunosuppressed, the disease is generally indolent, and extracutaneous involvement occurs in only 10 percent of patients. In non-HIV-infected children and young adults with Kaposi's sarcoma in central Africa, there is a 20 percent incidence of extracutaneous spread of disease. In contrast, extracutaneous involvement occurs in over 70 percent of AIDS patients with Kaposi's sarcoma.

The skin lesions of Kaposi's sarcoma generally present as papules or plaques that ultimately evolve into nodules. Lesions can occur in any location, but the face is a common site, especially the tip of the nose and pinnae of the ears. In advanced cases, involvement of lymphatics can cause facial edema. Oral mucous membranes are also involved frequently as are the lower extremities, particularly the soles of the feet. In the early stages, the lesions are usually painless, but some patients experience considerable pain, especially in lower extremities. Significant edema can occur with lower extremity disease. The skin and mucous membrane lesions are red or purple, do not blanch on pressure, and turn a brownish color if they resolve on therapy.

Although any organ system can be involved in the disseminated form of Kaposi's sarcoma, lymph nodes, gastrointestinal tract, and lungs are most commonly involved. Kaposi's sarcoma in the lungs often leads to extensive interstitial disease with severe impairment of diffusing capacity and may result in massive pulmonary hemorrhage. Pulmonary Kaposi's sarcoma must be differentiated from *P. carinii* pneumonia since both can present with fever and interstitial patterns on chest x-ray. Pleural effusions and bilateral lower lobe infiltrates are much more common in Kaposi's sarcoma.

Certain *lymphoid neoplasms* (see Chap. 302) are associated with HIV infection. There is an increased incidence of high-grade non-Hodgkin's lymphoma of a B-cell type, including primary B-cell lymphoma of the brain. In fact, non-Hodgkin's lymphoma occurring in an HIV-infected individual constitutes a diagnosis of AIDS (group IV, subgroup D, Table 264-1). In addition to the brain, common extranodal sites of lymphoma include bone marrow, gastrointestinal tract, liver, skin, and mucous membranes. The lymphomas are particularly aggressive, and mortality rates are high. Hodgkin's disease in HIV-infected individuals usually follows an atypically aggressive clinical course with involvement of multiple extranodal sites. The histopathologic types are usually nodular sclerosing and of mixed cellularity. The relationship between the lymphomas and HIV infection is unclear; there is no evidence that HIV directly transforms the tumor cells (see Chap. 134).

Thrombocytopenia may occur as the initial presenting sign of HIV infection. Various mechanisms of thrombocytopenia have been reported including the nonspecific deposition of complement and immune complexes on platelets, resulting in their clearance from the circulation, as well as the presence of an antibody against a 25-kD platelet protein. Platelet counts are usually 20 to 50 × 10^9 per liter (20,000 to 50,000 per microliter), but may be much lower; severe purpura has been reported. In some patients the thrombocytopenia has resolved spontaneously, but most require therapy such as glucocorticoid administration, which generally results in temporary remissions but further suppresses the immune system; splenectomy has also induced remissions (see Chap. 287). Treatment of HIV infection with zidovudine (see below) has resulted in remissions of HIV-associated thrombocytopenia.

Nonspecific interstitial pneumonitis accounts for approximately 30 percent of all episodes of clinical pneumonitis in AIDS patients. It must be distinguished from pulmonary Kaposi's sarcoma and microbial pneumonitis, particularly that caused by *P. carinii* (see above). Nonspecific interstitial pneumonitis should be suspected in patients with a clinical pneumonitis whose CD4+ lymphocyte count is >0.200 × 10^9 per liter (>200 cells per microliter). *Lymphocytic interstitial pneumonia* occurs rarely in adults with AIDS, but is found in 30 to 50 percent of children. It is felt to be an EBV-associated lymphoproliferative disease of the lungs.

DIAGNOSIS The diagnosis of AIDS is made in an HIV-infected individual who falls within the classification level of group IV disease in Table 264-1 (see above). However, it is more appropriate to think of HIV infection as a continuous spectrum of disease rather than a strict AIDS versus non-AIDS type of categorization (see Table 264-1).

Laboratory detection of HIV infection is accomplished by a number of diagnostic tests. The most widely used is a test for HIV antibody employing the enzyme-linked immunosorbent assay (ELISA). This extremely sensitive technique has been useful in screening large numbers of individuals for HIV infection. Its major disadvantage is a relatively high incidence of false-positive reactions when used to screen people at low risk of infection. The rate of false-positive reactions with first-generation ELISAs, which employ lysates from HIV-infected cells as a source of antigen, has been reduced with second-generation tests, which use recombinant DNA proteins or synthetic peptides of the virus as antigens. All positive ELISA reactions should be repeated, and if the repeat determination is also reactive, the results should be confirmed by a more specific test for antibody. The most commonly employed confirmatory test is a western blot test that identifies antibodies to specific viral proteins. Other confirmatory tests are the immunofluorescence assay (IFA) and the radioimmunoprecipitation assay (RIPA).

Detectable antibodies to HIV usually do not appear for weeks or months following infection. Ninety-five percent of infected individuals develop detectable antibodies within 5 months of infection. However, patients may rarely be infected for 3 to 4 years before antibody is detectable. Under these circumstances, demonstration of the virus is necessary to make the diagnosis of HIV infection. Virus can be detected by assays for circulating viral protein (antigenemia), particularly the p24 core antigen. The disadvantage of this test is that although p24 antigenemia may be present prior to the development of antibodies, the antigen may not be detectable in a substantial proportion of healthy HIV-infected antibody-positive patients. In experienced laboratories, virus can be isolated in a high proportion of cases by coculture of infected patient cells with mitogen-activated peripheral blood blast cells from normal subjects. A research tool that may ultimately be a highly sensitive clinical test for detecting virus is the polymerase chain reaction (Chap. 6), which selectively amplifies viral genes allowing detection of HIV DNA present at very low frequencies in infected cells.

TREATMENT AND PROGNOSIS The period between infection and development of symptoms is long, but variable. Mathematical models suggest that the mean incubation period for adults is approximately 8 to 10 years, whereas children under 5 years of age generally develop symptoms within 2 years. Prospective studies of a large cohort of homosexual and bisexual men indicated that after approximately 7 years of infection, 36 percent had progressed to AIDS and another 40 percent had other manifestations of infection; only 20 percent remained symptom-free. It is currently believed that virtually all infected individuals will ultimately develop progressive disease. Consequently, the therapeutic approach is to treat the HIV infection with antiretroviral drugs when indicated (see below), to treat prophylactically to prevent certain opportunistic infections when appropriate (see below), and to treat opportunistic infections and neoplasms as they occur.

Patients with AIDS or ARC should be treated with the nucleoside analogue zidovudine (3′-azido-3′-deoxythymidine; AZT) at a dose of 200 mg, orally every 4 h. If this dose cannot be tolerated, it should be reduced to 100 mg every 4 h. One report indicates that the lower dose is as effective as the higher dose and is accompanied by considerably less toxic side effects. HIV-infected individuals who have one or two symptoms and levels of CD4+ lymphocytes <0.500 × 10^9 per liter (<500 cells per microliter) benefit from zidovudine, 200 mg every 4 h, as evidenced by delay of progression to advanced ARC or AIDS. In addition, asymptomatic individuals with similar CD4+ cell counts have benefited from zidovudine, 100 mg every 4 h while awake for a total daily dose of 500 mg, because the progression to advanced ARC or AIDS is likewise delayed. Dramatic improvements in HIV-related neurologic manifestations have also been reported after administration of zidovudine. The most common toxic side effects are bone marrow suppression, resulting in anemia (often requiring transfusions) and neutropenia, and gastrointestinal intolerance. These toxicities are dose-dependent and often resolve upon reduction of the dose. Other nucleoside analogues such as dideoxyinosine (ddI) are currently being evaluated.

Treatments of the most common opportunistic infections encountered in AIDS patients are listed in Table 264-2 and in the individual chapters dealing with each infection. All of these infections have high rates of recurrence to varying degrees. For example, infections causes by CMV, *Toxoplasma gondii,* and *Cryptococcus neoformans* require maintenance treatment for life. In addition, continuous treatment or prophylaxis for other infections may be required. It is recommended that *aerosolized pentamidine isethionate,* 300 mg once per month, or trimethoprim/sulfamethoxazole, 320/1600 mg twice daily, be given to individuals who have had a previous bout of *P. carinii* pneumonia or whose CD4+ lymphocyte level is ≤0.200 × 10^9 per liter (≤200 cells per microliter).

Kaposi's sarcoma that is cosmetically acceptable to the patient, does not interfere with function, and is without significant symptoms should not be treated. When indicated, radiation therapy in the form of superficial photon or electron beam [200 cGy (200 rad) for 10 treatments] to the involved cutaneous areas or high-energy megavoltage irradiation [1500 to 3500 cGy (1500 to 3500 rad) depending on the tissue involved] may palliate localized cutaneous and extracutaneous disease. Alternatively, in patients with Kaposi's sarcoma and CD4+-lymphocyte levels >0.150 × 10^9 per liter (>150 cells per microliter) interferon alpha (5 to 35 × 10^6 units per day adjusted for toxicity) may induce complete or partial responses in tumors in 30 to 40 percent of patients. In addition, inferferon alpha has a significant antiretroviral effect that may be helpful in combination with other antiretroviral agents. Other single agents, such as vinblastine or doxorubicin, and combinations of drugs, including etoposide (VP-16), doxorubicin, vinblastine, and bleomycin (see Chap. 301), have resulted in transient improvement in advanced disease. A major difficulty with chemotherapy is the compounding of the immunosuppressed state and the increase in risk of opportunistic infections.

Treatment of the lymphoid neoplasms should follow guidelines of therapy for non-AIDS patients (see Chap. 302). Since these tumors generally follow a more aggressive course in AIDS patients, response rates and duration of responses are less favorable than in a non-AIDS population.

A number of attempts at immune reconstitution have been undertaken. These have included bone marrow transplantation, especially between identical twins when one of the pair has AIDS; infusion of histocompatible lymphocytes; and administration of soluble mediators such as interleukin 2 and interferon gamma. Temporary partial reconstitution of the immune response has been noted in some cases.

There is no cure for AIDS, and no antiretroviral regimen is capable of eliminating HIV completely from infected individuals. As a consequence, the prognosis for infected individuals, particularly those that have advanced to symptomatic disease, is grave. Nonetheless, at least one drug (zidovudine) causes limited prolongation of survival in AIDS patients and a delay in the progression of disease in infected individuals. It is generally felt that the ultimate chemotherapeutic regimen for HIV infection, which it is hoped will lead to it becoming a chronic manageable disease, will be a combination of several antiretroviral agents acting at different phases of the HIV life cycle together with an immunoenhancing agent.

PREVENTION Education, counseling, and behavior modification are the cornerstones of prevention of HIV infection. Widespread voluntary testing for HIV infection together with counseling of infected individuals should prove helpful in behavioral modification programs among infected individuals who would otherwise be unaware of their HIV status and who could potentially infect sexual partners. In addition, infected individuals may benefit from early therapeutic intervention even if they are asymptomatic. The incidence of new infections per year among homosexual and bisexual men in certain high-prevalence cities such as San Francisco has decreased dramatically from the early years of the epidemic. This has resulted, at least in part, from behavioral modifications regarding the number of sex partners and safe sexual practices. Several studies indicate that condom use decreases the risk of HIV transmission.

Screening of the blood supply for antibodies to HIV has almost eliminated infections among transfusion recipients and hemophiliacs who require replacement of plasma components. Continuing high rates of new infections among intravenous drug users, their heterosexual partners, and children born to intravenous drug users or to the female sexual partners of intravenous drug users will require intensive efforts aimed at treatment of drug abuse together with behavioral modification.

Health care workers should practice universal precautions when handling blood and body fluids and follow all guidelines for the prevention of transmission of HIV and hepatitis B virus that have been issued by the Centers for Disease Control (see Chap. 83).

The development of a vaccine to prevent infection and/or disease with HIV will be an important tool in the strategy for world-wide containment of the AIDS epidemic. Several candidate vaccines are undergoing early phase I testing in humans. In the monkey model of simian immunodeficiency virus (SIV), immunization with whole killed SIV is effective in protecting animals from challenge with live virus by preventing either infection or the development of disease following infection. These studies lend optimism to the feasibility of developing a safe and effective vaccine for HIV in the future.

REFERENCES

CENTERS FOR DISEASE CONTROL: Classification system for human T-lymphotropic virus type III/lymphadenopathy-associated infections. Morb Mort Week Rep 35:334, 1986

———: Revision of the CDC surveillance case definition for acquired immunodeficiency syndrome. Morb Mort Week Rep 36:1S, 1987

———: Guidelines for prevention of transmission of human immunodeficiency virus and hepatitis B virus to health-care and public safety workers. Morb Mort Week Rep 38:S-6, 1989

CURRAN JW et al: Epidemiology of HIV infection and AIDS in the United States. Science 239:610, 1988

FAUCI AS: The human immunodeficiency virus: Infectivity and mechanisms of pathogenesis. Science 239:617, 1988

FISCHL MA et al: The efficacy of azidothymidine (AZT) in the treatment of patients with AIDS and AIDS-related complex. A double-blind, placebo-controlled trial. N Engl J Med 317:185, 1987

GALLO RC, MONTAGNIER L: AIDS in 1988. Sci Am 259:41, 1988

HO DD et al: The acquired immunodeficiency syndrome (AIDS) dementia complex. Ann Intern Med 111:400, 1989

KNOWLES DM et al: Lymphoid neoplasia associated with the acquired immunodeficiency syndrome (AIDS). Ann Intern Med 108:744, 1988

LANE HC et al: Anti-retroviral effects of interferon-α in AIDS-associated Kaposi's sarcoma. Lancet 2:1218, 1988

PHAIR J et al: The risk of *Pneumocystis carinii* pneumonia among men infected with human immunodeficiency virus type 1. N Engl J Med 322:161, 1990

PIZZO PA et al: Acquired immune deficiency syndrome in children. Current problems and therapeutic considerations. Am J Med 85:(Suppl 2A) 195, 1988

PRICE RW et al: The brain in AIDS: Central nervous system HIV-1 infection and AIDS dementia complex. Science 239:586, 1988

ROSENBERG ZF, FAUCI AS: The immunopathogenesis of HIV infection. Adv Immunol 46:377, 1989

SELWYN PA et al: A prospective study of the risk of tuberculosis among intravenous drug users with human immunodeficiency virus infection. N Engl J Med 320:545, 1989

265 PLASMA CELL DISORDERS

DAN L. LONGO

GENERAL PRINCIPLES The plasma cell disorders are monoclonal neoplasms related to each other by virtue of their development from common progenitors in the B-lymphocyte lineage. Multiple myeloma, Waldenström's macroglobulinemia, primary amyloidosis (see Chap. 266), and the heavy chain diseases comprise this group and may be designated by a variety of synonyms such as monoclonal gammopathies, paraproteinemias, plasma cell dyscrasias, and dysproteinemias. A schema for the normal development of B lymphocytes is depicted in Fig. 265-1. Mature B lymphocytes destined to produce IgG, bear surface immunoglobulin molecules of both M and G heavy chain isotypes with both isotypes having identical idiotypes (variable regions). Under normal circumstances, maturation to antibody-secreting plasma cells is stimulated by exposure to the antigen for which the surface immunoglobulin is specific; however, in the plasma cell disorders the control over this process is lost. The clinical manifestations of all the plasma cell disorders relate to the expansion of the neoplastic cells, to the secretion of cell products (immunoglobulin molecules or subunits, lymphokines), and to some extent to the host's response to the tumor.

There are three categories of structural variation among immunoglobulin molecules that form antigenic determinants, and these are used to classify immunoglobulins (Chap. 13). *Isotypes* are those determinants that distinguish among the main classes of antibodies of a given species and are the same in all normal individuals of that species. Therefore, isotypic determinants are by definition recognized by antibodies from a distinct species (heterologous sera) but not by antibodies from the same species (homologous sera). There are five heavy chain isotypes (M, G, A, D, E) and two light chain isotypes (kappa, lambda). *Allotypes* are distinct determinants that reflect regular small differences between individuals of the same species in the amino acid sequences of otherwise similar immunoglobulins. These differences are determined by allelic genes, and by definition they are detected by antibodies made in the same species. *Idiotypes* are the third category of antigenic determinants. They are unique to the molecules produced by a given clone of antibody-producing cells. Idiotypes are formed by the unique structure of the antigen binding portion of the molecule.

Antibody molecules (see Fig. 265-2) are composed of two heavy chains (mol wt ~ 50,000) and two light chains (mol wt ~ 25,000). Each chain has a constant portion (limited amino acid sequence variability) and a variable region (extensive sequence variability).

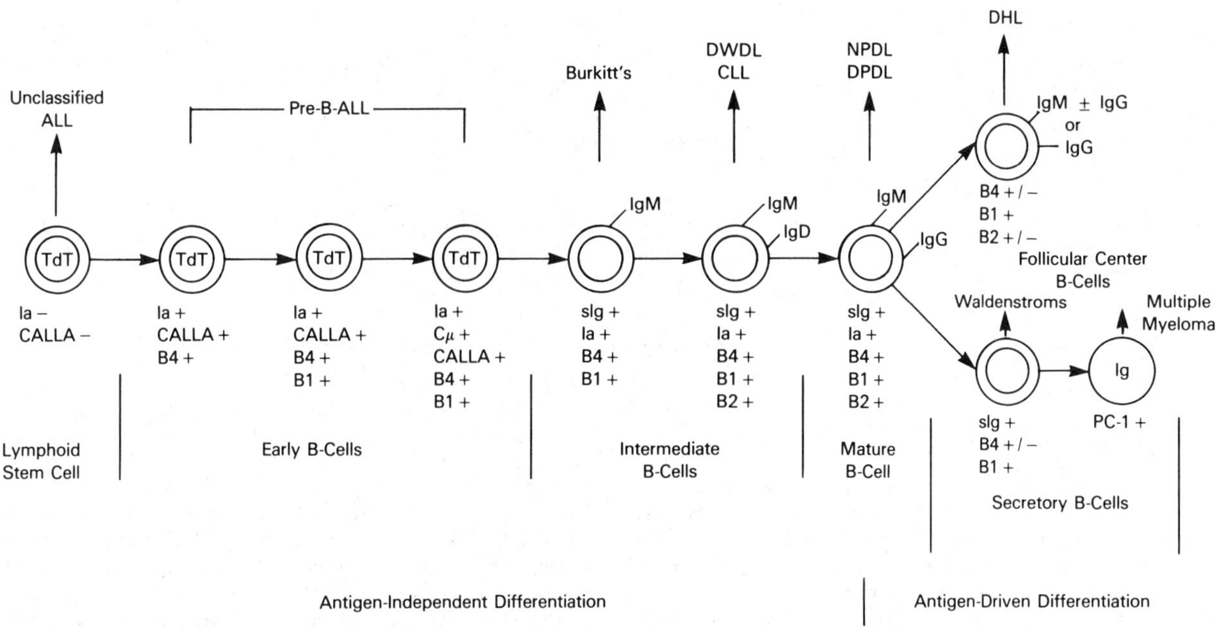

FIGURE 265-1 Schematic representation of the pathway of differentiation of normal B cells. CALLA, B1, B2, B4, Ia, PC-1, and sIg (surface immunoglobulin) are cell markers used to distinguish discrete stages of development. Terminal transferase (TdT) is a cellular enzyme. The stage of differentiation arrest for each lymphoproliferative disorder is shown. The following abbreviations are used: ALL, acute lymphoblastic leukemia; DWDL, diffuse well-differentiated lymphocytic lymphoma; CLL, chronic lymphocytic leukemia; NPDL, nodular poorly differentiated lymphocytic lymphoma; DPDL, diffuse poorly differentiated lymphocytic lymphoma; DHL, diffuse histiocytic or large-cell lymphoma.

The light and heavy chains are linked by disulfide bonds and are aligned so their variable regions are adjacent to one another. This variable region forms the antigen recognition site of the antibody molecule; its unique structural features form a particular set of determinants called idiotypes that are reliable markers for a particular clone of cells because each antibody is formed and secreted by a single clone. Each chain is specified by distinct genes, synthesized separately, and assembled into an intact antibody molecule after translation (see Fig. 265-3). Because of the mechanics of the gene rearrangements necessary to specify the immunoglobulin variable regions (VDJ joining for the heavy chain, VJ joining for the light chain; see Fig. 265-3), a particular clone rearranges only one of the two chromosomes to produce an immunoglobulin molecule of only one light chain isotype and only one allotype (allelic exclusion). After exposure to antigen, the variable region may become associated with a new heavy chain isotype (class switch). Each clone of cells performs these sequential gene arrangements in a unique way. This results in each clone producing a unique immunoglobulin molecule. In most cells, light chains are synthesized in slight excess, are secreted as free light chains by plasma cells, and are cleared by the kidney, but less than 10 mg of such light chains is excreted per day.

Electrophoretic analysis of components of the serum proteins permits determination of the amount of immunoglobulin in the serum (Fig. 265-4). The variety of immunoglobulins move heterogeneously in an electric field and form a broad peak in the gamma region. The gamma globulin region of the electrophoretic pattern is usually increased in the serum of patients and animals with plasma cell tumors. There is a sharp spike in this region called an M component

FIGURE 265-2 Schematic depiction of an IgG molecule. Each molecule consists of two heavy and two light chains linked by disulfide bonds. There are two types of light chains, kappa (genes on chromosome 2) and lambda (chromosome 22), each containing two domains. There are 10 types of heavy chains: 4 types of G (G1 to G4), 2 of A (A1, A2), 2 of M (M1, M2), and 1 each of D and E (all on chromosome 14), each with four domains. A domain is 100 to 110 amino acids in length. Within each domain is an intrachain disulfide bond that produces a loop. V_H (variable domain of the heavy chain) and V_L (variable domain of the light chain) form an antigen binding site whose unique determinants form an idiotype. Immunoglobulins of the same isotype (e.g., IgG1κ) differ between individuals. The determinants that distinguish them are called allotypic determinants and are located on C_L (constant domain of the light chain) and C_{H2} (second constant domain of the heavy chain). C_{H2} is also the main site of glycosylation (CHO) and complement binding. Papain cleaves the molecule into antigen-binding (Fab) and crystallizable (Fc) components. The portion of the heavy chain in an Fab fragment is called the Fd piece. Fc receptors on cells bind to the C_{H3} domain. IgM and IgA occur as polymers and each unit of two heavy and two light chains is connected by a J (joining) chain. The heavy chain isotypes determine the function of the antibody.

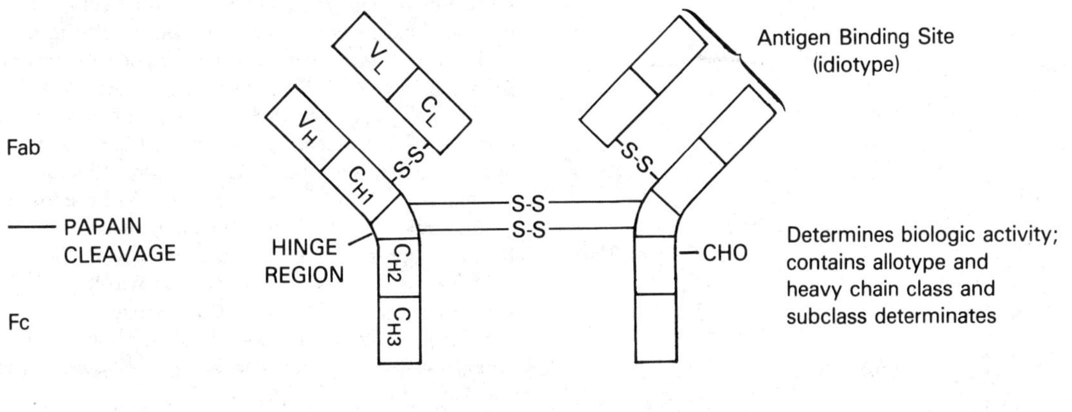

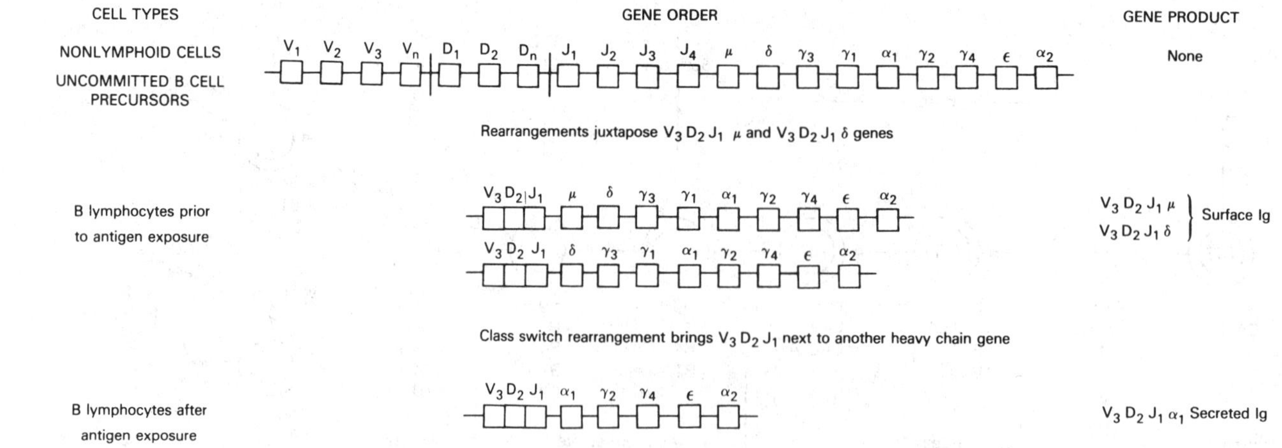

FIGURE 265-3 Schematic diagram of the organization and translocation of immunoglobulin genes. Immunoglobulin heavy chains are encoded by four distinct genetic elements, variable (Igh-V), diversity (Igh-D), joining (Igh-J), and constant (Igh-C) genes. The variable region of the immunoglobulin heavy chain is encoded by the V, D, and J genes. The same variable region may be associated with any of the 10 heavy chain constant region genes. In the germline genome (all cells except B cells) the V, D, and J genes are widely separated and there are numerous forms of each. Once a cell becomes committed to B-cell differentiation, a single V gene and a single D gene translocate to a single J gene, and the intervening genetic material is excised. This is called VDJ joining. The newly formed VDJ gene is transcribed into a single message along with either an M or D isotype C gene. Upon exposure to antigen, another rearrangement may occur so that the VDJ gene may be associated with a G, A or E isotype C gene. In light chain genes, there appear to be no D genes, and thus, light chain variable regions are formed by VJ joining.

(M for monoclonal). Less commonly the M component may appear in the beta$_2$ or alpha$_2$ globulin region. The antibody must be present at a concentration of at least 5g/L (0.5 g/dL) to be detectable by this method. This corresponds to approximately 10^9 cells producing the antibody. Confirmation that such an M component is truly monoclonal relies on the use of immunoelectrophoresis that shows a single light and heavy chain type. Hence, immunoelectrophoresis and electrophoresis provide qualitative and quantitative assessment of the M component, respectively. Once the presence of an M component has been confirmed, electrophoresis provides the more practical information for managing patients with monoclonal gammopathies. In a given patient, the amount of M component in the serum is a reliable measure of the tumor burden. This makes the M component an excellent tumor marker; yet it is not specific enough to be used to screen asymptomatic patients. In addition to the plasma cell disorders, M components may be detected in other lymphoid neoplasms such as chronic lymphocytic leukemia and lymphomas of B- or T-cell origin; nonlymphoid neoplasms such as chronic myelogenous leukemia, breast and colon cancer; a variety of nonneoplastic conditions such as cirrhosis, sarcoidosis, parasitic diseases, Gaucher's disease, and pyoderma gangrenosum; and a number of autoimmune conditions, including rheumatoid arthritis, myasthenia gravis, and cold agglutinin disease. A very rare skin disease known as lichen myxedematosus or papular mucinosis is associated with a monoclonal gammopathy. Highly cationic IgGλ is deposited in the dermis of patients with this disease. It is unclear whether this organ specificity reflects the specificity of the antibody for some antigenic component of the dermis. The nature of the M component is variable. It may be an intact antibody molecule of any heavy chain subclass, or it may be an altered antibody or fragment. Isolated light or heavy chains may be produced. In some plasma cell tumors such as extramedullary or solitary bone plasmacytomas, less than a third of patients will have an M component. In about 20 percent of myelomas, only light chains are produced and in most cases are secreted in the urine as Bence Jones proteins. The frequency of myelomas of a particular heavy chain class is roughly proportional to the serum concentration, so that IgG myelomas are more common than IgA and IgD myelomas. In some cases, the antigen specificity of the monoclonal antibody is known.

FIGURE 265-4 Representative electrophoretic patterns of serum and urine. The upper panel illustrates the normal pattern of serum and urine protein on electrophoresis. Since there are many different immunoglobulins in the serum, their differing mobilities in an electric field produce a broad peak. The lower panel illustrates the patterns of serum and urine proteins in a patient with myeloma. The predominance of a product of a single cell is reflected by a "church spire" sharp peak. The presence of free light chains in the urine is reflected in a peak, as well.

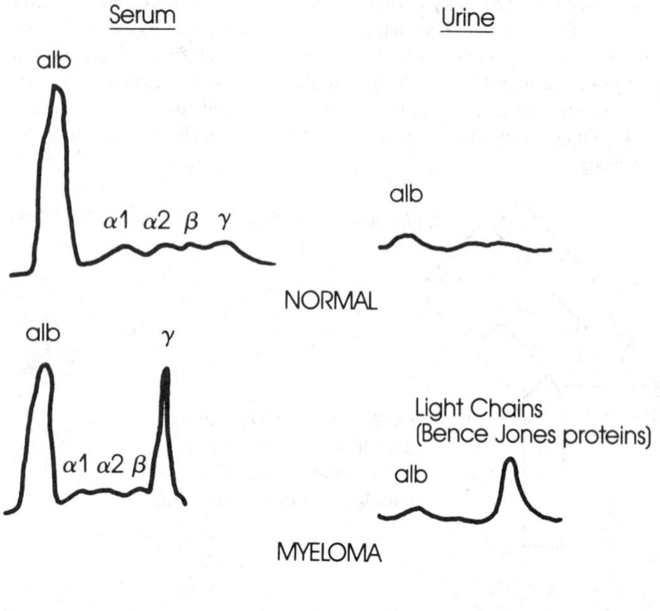

MULTIPLE MYELOMA Definition Multiple myeloma represents a malignant proliferation of plasma cells. The terms multiple myeloma and myeloma may be used interchangeably. The disease results from the uncontrolled proliferation of plasma cells derived from a single clone. The tumor, its products, and the host response to it result in a number of organ dysfunctions and symptoms of bone pain or fracture, renal failure, susceptibility to infection, anemia, hypercalcemia, and occasionally clotting abnormalities, neurologic symptoms, and vascular manifestations of hyperviscosity.

Etiology The etiology of myeloma is not known. Myeloma was found to occur with increased frequency in those exposed to the radiation of nuclear warheads in World War II after a 20-year latency. Although there is no direct evidence implicating oncogenes in human myeloma, the observations of c-*myc* and b-*lym* oncogenes in Burkitt's lymphoma, the high incidence of chromosomal translocations in human B-cell tumors, and the role of type C RNA viruses in murine plasmacytoma formation suggest that cells of the B-cell lineage may be susceptible to growth deregulation by such stimuli. The murine plasmacytoma models are particularly interesting in that there is evidence that the induction of plasmacytomas may require exposure to foreign antigens as well as a cellular event. This suggests that chronic antigenic stimulation may play a role in the transformation of a particular B-cell clone. There is also some evidence for a genetic predisposition to myeloma in humans. Patients with myeloma have a significantly higher incidence of expressing the Glm(x) heavy chain allotype marker, and there is a weak but significant linkage disequilibrium that shows the HLA-B5 determinant being expressed more commonly than expected in myeloma patients. There is the possibility that the neoplastic event in myeloma may involve cells earlier in B-cell differentiation than the plasma cell. Circulating B cells bearing surface immunoglobulin that share the idiotype of the M component are present in myeloma patients. It is possible that the malignant clone escapes normal control mechanisms at a pre-plasma cell stage of differentiation and the chronic exposure to a particular antigenic stimulus drives the cell to terminal differentiation. It remains difficult to distinguish benign from malignant plasma cells on the basis of morphologic criteria in all but a few cases.

Incidence and prevalence Myeloma is primarily a disease of the elderly and increases in incidence with age. The median age at diagnosis is 64 years. The disease is rare under age 40. The yearly incidence is around 3 per 100,000 and remarkably similar in a variety of countries throughout the world. Males are slightly more commonly affected than females and blacks have nearly twice the incidence of whites. In the age group over 25 years of age the incidence is 30 per 100,000.

Pathogenesis and clinical manifestations (Table 265-1) Bone pain is the most common symptom in myeloma and is present in nearly 70 percent of patients. The pain usually involves the back and ribs, and unlike the pain of metastatic carcinoma which often is worse at night, the pain of myeloma is precipitated by movement. Persistent localized pain in a patient with myeloma usually signifies a pathologic fracture. The bone lesions of myeloma are caused by the proliferation of the tumor cells and the activation of osteoclasts which destroy the bone. The osteoclasts respond to osteoclast activating factors (OAF) made by the myeloma cells (OAF activity can be mediated by several cytokines including interleukin 1, lymphotoxin, and tumor necrosis factor). However, production of these factors stops following administration of corticosteroids or interferon-gamma. The bone lesions are lytic in nature and are rarely associated with osteoblastic new bone formation; therefore, radioisotopic bone scanning is less useful in diagnosis than plain radiography. The bony lysis results in substantial mobilization of calcium from bone, and serious acute and chronic complications of hypercalcemia may dominate the clinical picture (see below). Localized bone lesions may expand to the point that mass lesions may be palpated, especially on the skull (Fig. 265-5), clavicles, and sternum, and the collapse of vertebrae may lead to symptoms of spinal cord compression.

TABLE 265-1 Pathogenesis and clinical manifestations of multiple myeloma

Clinical finding	Underlying cause	Pathogenic mechanism
Hypercalcemia, pathologic fractures, cord compression, lytic bone lesions, osteoporosis, bone pain	Skeletal destruction	Tumor expansion; production of osteoclast activating factors (OAF) by tumor cells
Renal failure	Light chain proteinuria, hypercalcemia, urate nephropathy, amyloid glomerulopathy (rare)	Toxic effects of tumor products; light chains, OAF, DNA breakdown products:
	Pyelonephritis	Hypogammaglobulinemia
Anemia	Myelophthisis, decreased production, increased destruction	Tumor expansion; production of inhibitory factors and autoantibodies by tumor cells
Infection	Hypogammaglobulinemia, decreased neutrophil migration	Decreased production due to tumor-induced suppression; increased IgG catabolism
Neurologic symptoms	Hyperviscosity, cryoglobulins, amyloid deposits	Products of tumor; properties of M component; light chains
	Hypercalcemia, cord compression	OAF
Bleeding	Interference with clotting factors, amyloid damage of endothelium, platelet dysfunction	Products of tumor; antibodies to clotting factors; light chains; antibody coating of platelets
Mass lesions		Tumor expansion

The next most common clinical problem in patients with myeloma is susceptibility to bacterial infections. The most common infections are pneumonias and pyelonephritis, and the most frequent pathogens are *Streptococcus pneumoniae*, *Staphylococcus aureus*, and *Klebsiella pneumoniae* in the lungs and *Escherichia coli* and other gram-negative organisms in the urinary tract (Chap. 82). In about 25 percent of patients recurrent infections are the presenting features, and over 75 percent of patients will have a serious infection at some time in their course. The susceptibility to infection has several contributing causes. First, patients with myeloma have diffuse hypogammaglobulinemia if the M component is excluded. The hypogammaglobulinemia is related to both decreased production and increased destruction of normal antibodies. Moreover, some patients generate a population of circulating regulatory cells in response to their myeloma that can suppress normal antibody synthesis. In the case of IgG myeloma, normal IgG antibodies are broken down more rapidly than normal because the catabolic rate for IgG antibodies varies directly with the serum concentration. The large M component results in fractional catabolic rates of 8 to 16 percent instead of the normal 2 percent. These patients have very poor antibody responses, especially to polysaccharide antigens such as those on bacterial cell walls. Such responses are normally T-cell-independent. Most measures of T-cell function in myeloma are normal but a subset of CD4+ cells may be decreased. Granulocyte lysozyme content is low and granulocyte migration is not as rapid as normal in patients with myeloma, probably

FIGURE 265-5 Bony lesions in multiple myeloma. The skull demonstrates the typical "punched out" lesions characteristic of multiple myeloma. The lesion represents a purely osteolytic lesion with little or no osteoblastic activity. *(Courtesy of Dr. Geraldine Schechter.)*

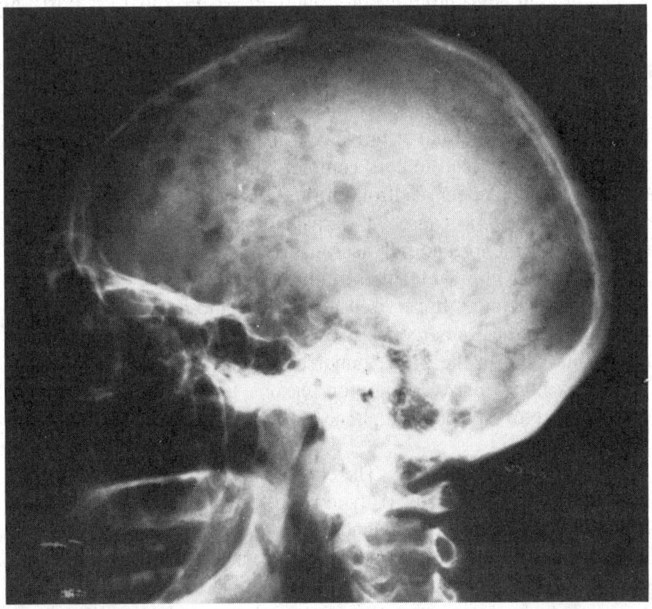

the result of a product of the tumor. There are also a variety of abnormalities in complement functions in myeloma patients. All of these factors contribute to the immune deficiency of these patients.

Renal failure occurs in nearly 25 percent of myeloma patients, and some renal pathology is noted in over half. There are many contributing factors. Hypercalcemia is the most common cause of renal failure. Glomerular deposits of amyloid, hyperuricemia, recurrent infections, and occasional infiltration of the kidney by myeloma cells all may contribute to renal dysfunction. However, tubular damage associated with the excretion of light chains is almost always present. Normally, light chains are filtered, reabsorbed in the tubules and catabolized. With the increase in amount of light chains presented to the tubule, the tubular cells become overloaded with these proteins, and tubular damage results either directly from light chain toxic effects or indirectly from the release of intracellular lysosomal enzymes. The earliest manifestation of this tubular damage is the adult Fanconi syndrome (a type 2 proximal renal tubular acidosis) with increased loss of glucose, amino acids, and defects in the ability of the kidney to acidify and concentrate the urine. The proteinuria is not accompanied by hypertension, and the protein is nearly all light chains. Generally, there is very little albumin in the urine because glomerular function is usually normal. When the glomeruli are involved, the proteinuria is nonselective. Patients with myeloma also have a decreased anion gap [i.e., sodium minus (chloride plus bicarbonate)] because the M component is cationic, resulting in retention of chloride. This is often accompanied by hyponatremia that is felt to be artificial (pseudohyponatremia) because each volume of serum has less water as a result of the increased protein.

Anemia occurs in about 80 percent of myeloma patients. It is usually normocytic and normochromic and related both to the replacement of normal marrow by expanding tumor cells and to the inhibition of hematopoiesis by factors made by the tumor. In addition, mild hemolysis may contribute to the anemia. A larger than expected fraction of patients may have megaloblastic anemia due to either folate or vitamin B_{12} deficiency. Granulocytopenia and thrombocytopenia are very rare. Clotting abnormalities may be seen due to the failure of antibody-coated platelets to function properly or to the interaction of the M component with clotting factors I, II, V, VII, or VIII. Raynaud's phenomenon and impaired circulation may result if the M component forms cryoglobulins, and hyperviscosity syndromes may develop depending on the physical properties of the M component (most common with IgM, IgG3, and IgA paraproteins). Hyperviscosity is defined on the basis of the relative viscosity of serum as compared to water. Normal relative serum viscosity is 1.8 (i.e., serum is normally almost twice as viscous as water). Symptoms of hyperviscosity occur at a level of 5 to 6, a level usually reached at paraprotein concentrations of around 40 g/L (4 g/dL) for IgM, 50 g/L (5 g/dL) for IgG3, and 70 g/L (7 g/dL) for IgA.

Although neurologic symptoms occur in a minority of patients, they may have many causes. Hypercalcemia may produce lethargy, weakness, depression, and confusion. Hyperviscosity may lead to headache, fatigue, visual disturbances, and retinopathy. Bony damage and collapse may lead to cord compression, radicular pain, and loss of bowel and bladder control. Infiltration of peripheral nerves by amyloid can be a cause of carpal tunnel syndrome and other sensorimotor mono- and polyneuropathies.

Many of the clinical features of myeloma, e.g., cord compression, pathologic fractures, hyperviscosity, sepsis, and hypercalcemia, can present as medical emergencies. Despite the widespread distribution of plasma cells in the body, tumor expansion is dominantly within bone and bone marrow and, for reasons unknown, rarely causes enlargement of spleen, lymph nodes, or gut-associated lymphatic tissue.

Diagnosis and staging The classic triad of myeloma is marrow plasmacytosis (>10 percent), lytic bone lesions, and a serum and/or urine M component. The diagnosis may be made in the absence of bone lesions if the plasmacytosis is associated with a progressive increase in the M component over time or if extramedullary mass lesions develop. There are two important variants of myeloma, solitary bone plasmacytoma and extramedullary plasmacytoma. These lesions are associated with an M component in less than 30 percent of the cases, they may affect younger individuals, and both are associated with median survivals of 10 or more years. Solitary bone plasmacytoma is a single lytic bone lesion without marrow plasmacytosis. Extramedullary plasmacytomas usually involve the submucosal lymphoid tissue of the nasopharynx or paranasal sinuses without marrow plasmacytosis. Both tumors are highly responsive to local radiation therapy. If an M component is present, it should disappear after treatment. Solitary bone plasmacytomas may recur in other bony sites or evolve into myeloma. Extramedullary plasmacytomas rarely recur or progress.

The most difficult differential diagnosis in patients with myeloma involves their separation from people with benign monoclonal gammopathies or monoclonal gammopathies of uncertain significance (MGUS). MGUS is vastly more common than myeloma, occurring in 1 percent of the population over age 50 and in up to 10 percent over age 75. Patients with MGUS usually have fewer than 20 g/L (2 g/dL) of M components, no urinary Bence Jones protein, less than 5 percent marrow plasmacytosis, and no anemia, renal failure, lytic bone lesions, or hypercalcemia. When bone marrow cells are exposed to radioactive thymidine in order to quantitate dividing cells, patients with MGUS always have a labeling index less than 1 percent and patients with myeloma always have a labeling index greater than 1 percent. Other discriminators include plasma cell acid phosphatase and β-glucuronidase, both of which are low in MGUS patients, and the salmon calcitonin stimulation test, which is positive only in patients with active ongoing bone destruction. Only about 11 percent of patients with MGUS go on to develop myeloma. Typically, patients with MGUS require no therapy.

The clinical evaluation of patients with myeloma includes a careful physical examination searching for tender bones and masses. It is paradoxic that only a small minority of patients have an enlargement of the spleen and lymph nodes, the physiologic sites of antibody production. Chest and bone radiographs may reveal lytic lesions or diffuse osteopenia. A complete blood count with differential may reveal anemia. Erythrocyte sedimentation rate is elevated. Very rare patients (~2 percent) may have plasma cell leukemia with more than 2000 plasma cells per microliter. This may be seen in disproportionate frequency in IgD (~12 percent) and IgE (~25 percent) myelomas. Serum calcium, urea nitrogen, creatinine, and uric acid may be elevated. Protein electrophoresis and measurement of serum immunoglobulins are useful for detecting and characterizing M spikes, supplemented by immunoelectrophoresis, which is especially sensitive for identifying low concentrations of M components not detectable by protein electrophoresis. A 24-h urine specimen is necessary to quantitate protein excretion and a concentrated aliquot is used for electrophoresis and immunological typing of any M component. Serum alkaline phosphatase is usually normal even with extensive bone involvement because of the absence of osteoblastic activity. It is also important to quantitate serum $beta_2$ microglobulin (see below).

The serum M component will be IgG in 53 percent of patients, IgA in 25 percent, IgD in 1 percent, and 20 percent of patients will have only light chains in serum and urine. Dipsticks for detecting proteinuria are not reliable at identifying light chains, and the heat test for detecting Bence Jones protein is falsely negative in about 50 percent of patients with light chain myeloma. Fewer than 1 percent of patients have no identifiable M component, and these are usually light chain myelomas in which renal catabolism has made them undetectable in the urine. About two-thirds of patients with serum M components also have urinary light chains. The light chain isotype may have an impact on survival. Patients secreting lambda light chains have a significantly shorter overall survival than those secreting kappa light chains. It is not clear whether this is due to some genetically important determinant of cell proliferation or because lambda light chains are more likely to cause renal damage and form amyloid than are kappa light chains. The heavy chain isotype may have an impact on patient management as well. About half of patients with IgM paraproteins develop hyperviscosity compared to only 2 to 4 percent of patients with IgA and IgG M components. Among IgG myelomas, it is the IgG3 subclass that has the highest tendency to form both concentration- and temperature-dependent aggregates, leading to hyperviscosity and cold agglutination at lower serum concentrations.

The staging system for patients with myeloma is a functional system for predicting survival and is based on a variety of clinical and laboratory tests, unlike the anatomic staging systems for solid tumors. Details of the staging system are given in Table 265-2. Based upon the hemoglobin, calcium, M component, and degree of skeletal involvement, the total-body tumor burden is estimated to be low (stage I, <0.6 × 10^{12} cells per square meter), intermediate (stage II, 0.6 to 1.2 × 10^{12} cells per square meter), or high (stage III, >1.2 × 10^{12} cells per square meter), and the stages are further subdivided on the basis of renal function (A if serum creatinine <2 mg/dL, B if >2). Patients in stage IA have a median survival of more than 5 years and those in stage IIIB about 15 months. Beta$_2$ microglobulin is a protein of 11,000 mol wt with homologies with the constant region of immunoglobulins that is the light chain of the class I major histocompatibility antigens (HLA-A, -B, -C) on the surface of every cell. Serum beta$_2$ microglobulin is the single most powerful predictor of survival and can substitute for staging. Patients with beta$_2$ microglobulin levels less than 0.004 g/L have a median survival of 43 months and those with levels higher than 0.004 g/L only 12 months. It is also felt that once the diagnosis of myeloma is firm, histologic features of atypia may also exert an influence on prognosis.

Treatment and course About 10 percent of patients with myeloma will have an indolent course demonstrating only very slow progression of disease over many years. Such patients only require antitumor therapy when the serum myeloma protein rises above 50 g/L (5 g/dL) or progressive bone lesions develop. Patients with solitary bone plasmacytomas and extramedullary plasmacytomas may be expected to enjoy prolonged, disease-free survival after local radiation therapy to a dose of around 40 Gy. There is a low incidence of occult marrow involvement in patients with solitary bone plasmacytoma. Such patients are usually detected because their serum M component falls slowly or disappears initially only to return after a few months. These patients respond well to systemic chemotherapy.

The vast majority of patients with myeloma require therapeutic intervention. In general, such therapy is of two sorts: systemic chemotherapy to control the progression of myeloma and symptomatic supportive care to prevent serious morbidity from the complications of the disease. All patients with stage II or III disease and stage I patients exhibiting Bence Jones proteinuria, progressive lytic bone lesions, vertebral compression fractures, recurrent infections, or rising serum M component should be treated with systemic combination chemotherapy. Although there are no reported cases of long-term disease-free survival (i.e., cured patients), there is no doubt that therapy can prolong and improve the quality of life for myeloma patients.

The standard treatment has consisted of intermittent pulses of an alkylating agent [L-phenylalanine mustard (L-PAM, melphalan), cyclophosphamide, or chlorambucil] and prednisone administered for 4 to 7 days every 4 to 6 weeks. The alkylating agents appear to be roughly equally active, but resistance to one agent is often accompanied by resistance to the others. The usual doses are as follows: melphalan, 8 mg/m^2 body surface area per day; cyclophosphamide, 200 mg/m^2 per day; chlorambucil, 8 mg/m^2 per day; prednisone, 25 to 60 mg/m^2 per day. Because of their near equivalence in antitumor efficacy, we favor cyclophosphamide as the alkylating agent because it is less toxic to the marrow stem cell compartment and results in a lower incidence of acute myelodysplastic syndromes than do the other alkylating agents. Doses may need adjustment based on marrow tolerance. However, there are few constraints on the dose of the steroid pulse and it appears that more is better. Recent evidence suggests that higher dose-intensity of the steroid (i.e., mg/m^2 per week) is associated with significantly longer survival. Patients responding to therapy generally have a prompt and gratifying reduction in bone pain, hypercalcemia, and anemia, and often have fewer infections. The serum M component lags substantially behind the symptomatic improvement, often taking 4 to 6 weeks to fall. This fall depends upon the rate of tumor kill and the fractional catabolic rate of immunoglobulin, which in turn depends upon the serum concentration (for IgG). Light chain excretion, with a functional half-life of approximately 6 h, may fall within the first week of treatment. However, since urine light chain levels may relate to renal tubular function, they are not a reliable measure of tumor cell kill. Calculations of tumor cell kill are made by extrapolation of the serum M-component level and rely heavily on the assumption that every tumor cell produces immunoglobulin at a constant rate. The data on which this assumption is based are reasonable, but recently it has been possible to alter the rate of immunoglobulin production of a myeloma in vitro with calcium channel blockers, a finding that may have clinical utility, for example, in patients with hyperviscosity. Thus, it is possible that a treatment might affect immunoglobulin production without killing the tumor cell, a situation that would result in an overestimation of the antitumor effects of the treatment if current criteria for response were applied. About 60 percent of patients will achieve at least a 75 percent reduction in serum M-component level and tumor cell mass in response to an alkylating agent and prednisone. Although this is a tumor reduction of less than one log, clinical responses may last many months. Efforts to improve the fraction of patients responding and the degree of response have involved adding other active chemotherapeutic agents to the treatment program. Patients with more advanced disease may benefit most from such an approach, but 3- to 5-drug therapy is experimental at this time.

The ideal duration of therapy has not been determined. Most physicians treat every 4 to 6 weeks for 1 or 2 years. Cessation of therapy is followed by relapse, usually within a year. Retreatment may be associated with a second response in up to 80 percent of

TABLE 265-2 Myeloma staging system

Stage	Criteria	Estimated tumor burden (× 10^{12} cells/m^2)
I	All of the following: *1* Hemoglobin >100 g/L (10 g/dL) *2* Serum calcium <12 mg/dL *3* Normal bone x-ray or solitary lesion *4* Low M-component production *a* IgG level <50 g/L (<5 g/dL) *b* IgA level <30 g/L (<3 g/dL) *c* Urine light chain <4 g/24 h	<0.6 (low)
II	Fitting neither I nor III	0.6–1.20 (intermediate)
III	One or more of the following: *1* Hemoglobin <85 g/L (<8.5 g/dL) 2 Serum calcium (>12 mg/dL) *3* Advanced lytic bone lesions *4* High M-component production *a* IgG level >70 g/L (>7 g/dL) *b* IgA level >50 g/L (>5 g/dL) *c* Urine light chains >12 g/24 h	>1.20 (high)

SUBCLASSIFICATION BASED ON SERUM CREATININE LEVELS

Level	Stage	Median survival, months
A <2 mg/dL	IA	61
B >2 mg/dL	IIA,B	55
	IIIA	30
	IIIB	15

ALTERNATIVE STAGING BASED ON SERUM BETA$_2$ MICROGLOBULIN LEVELS

Level	Stage	Median survival, months
<4 μg/mL	I	43
>4 μg/mL	II	12

patients. Maintenance therapy may prolong the duration of response, but no study has demonstrated this to result in prolonged survival. The regrowth rate of the tumor during relapse accelerates with each relapse. Patients primarily resistant to initial therapy have a median survival of less than a year. High-dose pulsed steroids used alone (200 mg prednisone every other day or 1 g/m^2 per day methylprednisolone for 5 days) or VAD combination chemotherapy (vincristine, 0.4 mg per day 4-day continuous infusion; doxorubicin, 9 mg/m^2 per day in a 4-day continuous infusion; dexamethasone, 40 mg per day for 4 days per week for 3 weeks) may offer useful palliation in patients resistant to primary therapy.

About 15 percent of patients die within the first 3 months after diagnosis, and subsequently the death rate is about 15 percent per year. The disease usually follows a chronic course for 2 to 5 years before developing an acute terminal phase usually marked by the development of pancytopenia with a cellular marrow that is refractory to treatment. Widespread organ infiltration by myeloma cells occurs and survival is less than 6 months. About 46 percent of patients die in the chronic phase of disease from progressive myeloma (16 percent) and renal failure (10 percent), sepsis (14 percent), or both (6 percent). Death in the acute terminal phase (26 percent) is chiefly from progressive myeloma (13 percent) and sepsis (9 percent). Five percent of patients die of acute leukemia, myeloblastic or monocytic, and although it has been debated that this is related to the primary disease, it appears more likely to be the result of chronic therapy with alkylating agents. Nearly 23 percent of patients die of myocardial infarction, chronic lung disease, diabetes, or strokes, all intercurrent illnesses related more to the age of the patient group than the tumor.

Supportive care directed at the anticipated complications of the disease may be as important as primary antitumor therapy. The hypercalcemia generally responds well to corticosteroid therapy, hydration, and natriuresis. Calcitonin may add to the inhibitory effects of steroids on bone resorption. Dichloromethane diphosphonate has also been shown to reduce osteoclastic bone resorption. Treatments aimed at strengthening the skeleton, like fluorides, calcium, and vitamin D with or without androgens, have been suggested but are not of proven efficacy. Iatrogenic worsening of renal function may be prevented by the use of allopurinol during chemotherapy to avoid urate nephropathy and by maintaining a high fluid intake to help excrete light chains and calcium. In the event of acute renal failure, plasmapheresis is approximately 10 times more effective at clearing light chains than peritoneal dialysis, and acutely reducing the protein load may result in functional improvement. Urinary tract infections should be watched for and treated early. Chronic dialysis probably should not be initiated in patients who have failed to respond to antitumor therapy. Plasmapheresis may be the treatment of choice for hyperviscosity syndromes. Although the pneumococcus is a dreaded pathogen in myeloma patients, they do not respond to pneumococcal polysaccharide vaccines. The advent of intravenous gamma globulin preparations raises some hope that prophylactic administration may prevent some serious infections, but this has not been tested. Chronic oral antibiotic prophylaxis is probably not warranted. Patients developing neurologic symptoms in the lower extremities, severe localized back pain, or problems with bowel and bladder control may need emergency myelography and radiation therapy for palliation. Most bone lesions respond to analgesics and chemotherapy, but certain painful lesions may respond most promptly to localized radiation. The chronic anemia may respond to hematinics (iron, folate, cobalamin) and some have responded to androgens. The pathogenesis of the anemia should be established and specific therapy instituted, where possible.

WALDENSTRÖM'S MACROGLOBULINEMIA In 1948, Waldenström described a malignancy of lymphoplasmacytoid cells that secreted IgM. In contrast to myeloma, the disease was associated with lymphadenopathy and hepatosplenomegaly, but the major clinical manifestation was the hyperviscosity syndrome. The disease resembles the related diseases chronic lymphocytic leukemia, myeloma, and lymphocytic lymphoma. Waldenström's macroglobulinemia and IgM myeloma both follow a similar clinical course. The diagnosis of IgM myeloma is usually reserved for patients with lytic bone lesions and is important only because of the hazard of pathologic fractures.

The etiology of macroglobulinemia is unknown. The disease is similar to myeloma in being slightly more common in men and occurring with increased incidence with age (median, 64 years). There have been reports that the IgM in some patients with macroglobulinemia may have specificity for myelin-associated glycoprotein (MAG), a protein that has been associated with demyelinating disease of the peripheral nervous system and may be lost earlier and to a greater extent than the better known myelin basic protein in patients with multiple sclerosis. There is a surface antigen on natural killer cells that is cross-reactive with the MAG, and coincidentally, natural killer cells are decreased in multiple sclerosis. Sometimes patients with macroglobulinemia develop a peripheral neuropathy before the appearance of the neoplasm. There is speculation that the whole process begins with a viral infection that may elicit an antibody response that cross-reacts with a normal tissue component.

Like myeloma, the disease involves the bone marrow, but unlike myeloma, it does not cause bone lesions or hypercalcemia. Like myeloma, a serum M component is present in the serum in excess of 30 g/L (3 g/dL), but unlike myeloma, the size of the IgM paraprotein results in little renal excretion and only around 20 percent of patients excrete light chains. Therefore, renal disease is not common. The light chain isotype is kappa in 80 percent of the cases. Patients present with weakness, fatigue, and recurrent infections, similar to myeloma patients, but epistaxis, visual disturbances, and neurologic symptoms like peripheral neuropathy, dizziness, headache, and transient paresis are much more common in macroglobulinemia. Physical examination reveals adenopathy and hepatosplenomegaly, and ophthalmoscopic examination may reveal vascular segmentation and dilatation of the retinal veins characteristic of hyperviscosity states. Patients may have a normocytic, normochromic anemia, but rouleaux formation and a positive Coombs' test are much more common than in myeloma. Malignant lymphocytes are usually present in the peripheral blood. About 10 percent of macroglobulins are cryoglobulins. These are pure M components and are not the mixed cryoglobulins seen in rheumatoid arthritis and other autoimmune diseases. Mixed cryoglobulins are composed of IgM or IgA complexed with IgG, for which they are specific. In both cases, Raynaud's phenomenon and serious vascular symptoms precipitated by the cold may occur, but mixed cryoglobulins are not commonly associated with malignancy. Patients suspected of having a cryoglobulin based on history and physical examination should have their blood drawn into a warm syringe and delivered to the laboratory in a container of warm water to avoid errors in quantitating the cryoglobulin.

Control of serious hyperviscosity symptoms like an altered state of consciousness or paresis can be achieved acutely by plasmapheresis because 80 percent of the IgM paraprotein is intravascular. Aside from this, management is identical to that of myeloma. About 80 percent of patients respond to chemotherapy and their median survival is over 3 years. The absence of other serious organ toxicities results in a longer life span of patients with macroglobulinemia compared to those with myeloma.

HEAVY CHAIN DISEASES The heavy chain diseases are rare lymphoplasmacytic malignancies. Their clinical manifestations vary with the heavy chain isotype. They secrete a defective heavy chain that usually has an intact Fc fragment and a deletion in the Fd region. Gamma, alpha, and mu heavy chain diseases have been described, but no reports of delta or epsilon heavy chain diseases have appeared. Molecular biologic analysis of these tumors has revealed structural genetic defects that may account for the aberrant chain secreted.

Gamma heavy chain disease (Franklin's disease) This disease affects people of widely different age groups and countries of origin. It is characterized by lymphadenopathy, fever, anemia, malaise, hepatosplenomegaly, and weakness. Its most distinctive symptom is palatal edema, resulting from node involvement of Waldeyer's ring, and this may progress to produce respiratory compromise. The diagnosis depends upon the demonstration of an anomalous serum M component [often <20 g/L (<2 g/dL)] that reacts with anti-IgG but not anti-light chain reagents. The M component is typically present in *both serum* and *urine*. Most of the paraproteins have been of the gamma$_1$ subclass, but other subclasses have been seen. The patients may have thrombocytopenia, eosinophilia, and nondiagnostic bone marrow. Patients usually have a rapid downhill course and die of infection; however, some patients have survived 5 years with chemotherapy.

Alpha heavy chain disease (Seligmann's disease) This is the commonest of the heavy chain diseases. It is closely related to a malignancy known as Mediterranean lymphoma, a disease that affects young people in parts of the world such as the Mediterranean, Asia, and South America in which intestinal parasites are common. The disease is characterized by an infiltration of the lamina propria of the small intestine with lymphoplasmacytoid cells that secrete truncated alpha chains. Demonstrating alpha heavy chains is difficult because the alpha chains tend to polymerize and appear as a smear instead of a sharp peak on electrophoretic profiles. Despite the polymerization, hyperviscosity is not a common problem in alpha heavy chain disease. Without J-chain–facilitated dimerization, viscosity does not increase dramatically. Light chains are absent from serum and urine. The patients present with chronic diarrhea, weight loss, and malabsorption and have extensive mesenteric and paraaortic adenopathy. Respiratory tract involvement occurs rarely. Patients may vary widely in their clinical course. Some may develop diffuse aggressive histologies of malignant lymphoma. Chemotherapy may produce long-term remissions. Rare patients appear to have responded to antibiotic therapy, raising the question of the etiologic role of antigenic stimulation perhaps by some chronic intestinal infection.

Mu heavy chain disease The secretion of isolated mu heavy chains into the serum appears to occur in a very rare subset of patients with chronic lymphocytic leukemia. The only features that may distinguish patients with mu heavy chain disease are the presence of vacuoles in the malignant lymphocytes and the excretion of kappa light chains in the urine. The diagnosis requires ultracentrifugation or gel filtration to confirm the nonreactivity of the paraprotein with the light chain reagents because some intact macroglobulins fail to interact with these serums. The tumor cells seem to have a defect in the assembly of light and heavy chains because they appear to contain both in their cytoplasm. There is no evidence that such patients should be treated differently from other patients with chronic lymphocytic leukemia.

REFERENCES

ALEXANIAN R et al: Prognosis of asymptomatic multiple myeloma. Arch Intern Med 148: 1963, 1988

BELCH A et al: A randomized trial of maintenance versus no maintenance melphalan and prednisone in responding multiple myeloma patients. Br J Cancer 57:94, 1988

CHAK LY et al: Solitary plasmacytoma of bone: Treatment, progression and survival. J Clin Oncol 5:1811, 1987

DURIE BGM et al: Pretreatment tumor mass, cell kinetics and prognosis in multiple myeloma. Blood 55:364, 1980

FARHANGI M (ed): Plasma cell myeloma and the myeloma proteins. Semin Oncol 13:259, 1986

GRIEPP PR et al: Value of beta-2-microglobulin level and plasma cell labeling indices as prognostic factors in patients with newly diagnosed myeloma. Blood 72:219, 1988

KYLE RA: Monoclonal gammopathy of undetermined significance. Natural history in 241 cases. Am J Med 64:814, 1978

KYLE RA (ed): Myeloma and related disorders, in *Neoplastic Diseases of the Blood*, New York, Churchill Livingstone, 1985, pp 385–676

PALMER M et al: Dose-intensity analysis of melphalan and prednisone in multiple myeloma. J Natl Cancer Inst 80:414, 1988

PILARSKI LM et al: Pre-B cells in peripheral blood of multiple myeloma patients. Blood 66:416, 1985

SALMON SE et al: Alternating combination chemotherapy and levamisole improves survival in multiple myeloma: A Southwest Oncology Group study. J Clin Oncol 1:453, 1983

SHEEHAN T et al. The efficacy and toxicity of VAD in the treatment of myeloma and related disorders. Scand J Haematol 37:426, 1986

266 AMYLOIDOSIS

ALAN S. COHEN

DEFINITION AND CLASSIFICATION Amyloidosis may be defined as the extracellular deposition of the fibrous protein amyloid in one or more sites of the body. It was named by Virchow in 1854 on the basis of its color after staining with iodine and sulfuric acid. This protein has unique ultrastructural, x-ray diffraction, and biochemical characteristics. It can be deposited locally where it has no clinical consequences or may involve virtually any organ system of the body leading to severe pathophysiologic changes, or the disease may fall between these two extremes. The natural history of amyloidosis is poorly understood, and the clinical diagnosis is often not made until the disease is far advanced. It is now clear that there are multiple clinically and biochemically different forms of amyloid, that are so classified because of the unique fibrous structure that they all possess. The following classification is clinically the most useful: (1) primary (AL type) amyloidosis (no evidence for preexisting or coexisting disease); (2) amyloid associated with multiple myeloma (also AL type); (3) secondary or reactive (AA type) amyloidosis associated with chronic infectious diseases (e.g., osteomyelitis, tuberculosis, leprosy) or chronic inflammatory diseases (e.g., rheumatoid arthritis); (4) heredofamilial amyloidosis, a variety of neuropathic [AF transthyretin (prealbumin) type], renal, cardiovascular, and other syndromes, plus the amyloidosis associated with familial Mediterranean fever (AA type); (5) local amyloidosis (focal, often tumorlike, deposits which occur in isolated organs, often endocrine, without evidence of systemic involvement); (6) amyloidosis associated with aging, especially in the heart and in the brain, and (7) amyloid associated with long-term hemodialysis. These clinical forms and their current biochemical classification are listed in Table 266-1.

PATHOLOGY AND STRUCTURE Amyloid is amorphous, eosinophilic, extracellular, and ubiquitous in distribution. The involved organs may have a rubbery consistency and a waxy, pink or gray appearance. Organ enlargement, especially of the liver, kidney, spleen, and heart, may be prominent.

Microscopically, amyloid stains pink with the hematoxylin-eosin stain and shows metachromasia with crystal violet. The Congo red stain imparts a unique green birefringence when sections are viewed in the polarizing microscope. This is the single most useful procedure for establishing the presence of amyloid. Amyloid deposits may be focal in almost any area of the body but are most often perivascular.

The heart may show focal or diffuse interstitial deposits in the myocardium, endocardium, or pericardium. In the aged heart, the atrium is usually focally involved or there may occur more diffuse lesions of the atria and ventricles. In the kidney, the glomerulus is primarily affected, although interstitial, peritubular, and vascular amyloid occur. In early lesions, small nodular or diffuse deposits appear near the basement membrane and, as the disease progresses, the glomerulus may be massively laden with amyloid, and its capillary bed will be occluded. In the gastrointestinal tract, there may be perivascular deposits only, or irregular or diffuse deposits may be found in the submucosa, in the muscularis mucosa, or subserosa. The amyloid may appear at any level or portion of the gastrointestinal tract including the gallbladder and pancreas. In the nervous system, amyloid has been described along peripheral nerves, in autonomic ganglia, and in senile plaques, in neurofibrillary tangles, as well as blood vessels ("congophilic angiopathy") of the central nervous system. It may be found in any portion of the orbit including the vitreous humor and cornea. In summary, there is virtually no area of the body that is spared. This ubiquitous distribution elicits a wide variety of clinical symptoms and signs.

All types of human amyloid consist of fine, nonbranching rigid fibrils that in tissue sections measure approximately 10×10^9 m (100 Å) in diameter. Isolated amyloid fibrils have a delicate, thin,

TABLE 266-1 Biochemical and clinical classification of amyloid

Biochemical type	Clinical form	Comment
AL	*1* Primary	Homologous to *N*-terminal residue of variable region of kappa or lambda light chain (or rarely whole chain). Varied molecular weight.
	2 Multiple myeloma-associated	
AA	*3* Secondary (reactive)	Serum protein SAA is putative precursor; Arg-Ser-Phe-Phe-Ser sequence to 76 amino acids.
$AF_{transthyretin}$	*4* Heredofamilial* especially familial amyloid polyneuropathy (Portuguese, Japanese, Swedish, Greek, Italian)	Many with single amino substitution of methionine for valine at position 30; multiple other variants exist.
AE	*5* Local Focal skin, lung, etc. amyloid Focal endocrine-related amyloid i.e., thyroid (medullary carcinoma)	Calcitonin precursor; other endocrine-related forms of amyloid exist.
AS	*6* Senile (aging) Heart	Two types: (1) transthyretin; (2) atrial natriuretic peptide.
	Brain	Beta protein (A4) of Alzheimer's disease
AH	*7* Chronic hemodialysis-related amyloid	$Beta_2$ microglobulin

* The sole hereditary recessive amyloid is that associated with familial Mediterranean fever. This amyloid is biochemically of the AA type.

nonbranching fibrous character. The individual fibril (or filament) has a diameter of about 7 × 10^9 m (70 Å) and tends to aggregate laterally. Each fibril (filament) has subunit protofibrils of 3 to 3.5 × 10^9 m (30 to 35 Å) diameter. X-ray diffraction of isolated amyloid fibrils reveals a cross beta pattern, the "pleated sheet" of Pauling and Corey, indicating that the polypeptide chain runs transversely to the long axis of the fibril specimen.

A second component, the plasma component or pentagonal unit (P component or AP) with a different ultrastructure, x-ray diffraction pattern, and chemical characteristics, has also been isolated from amyloid and is identical with a serum alpha globulin (SAP). It has many similarities to C-reactive protein, but it does not behave in humans as a classic acute phase protein. It is not responsible for the characteristic tinctorial properties or ultrastructure of amyloid.

BIOCHEMISTRY OF AMYLOID FIBRILS The bulk of amyloid deposits consists of fibrils. Purified amyloid derived from the fibril is a protein. The chemical composition of the different clinical forms of amyloid are distinct and allow for more precise diagnosis (Table 266-1). The homology of the fibril of primary and myeloma amyloid to the *N*-terminal region of the variable fragment of an immunoglobulin light chain and subsequently, in a limited number of cases, to a homogeneous light polypeptide chain, has been demonstrated. These light chain–related proteins range in size from about 5000 to 25,000 Da and are now termed amyloid light chain (AL) or AL_κ or AL_λ (Table 266-1). Amino acid sequence analysis indicates that most primary amyloid proteins contain the *N*-terminal amino acid residue identical to the variable regions of the light chain (Asp-Ile-Gln-Ser-Pro-Ser-Ser-Leu- . . .).

Another protein that is unrelated to any known immunoglobulin has been described in the secondary amyloid deposits. This protein, amyloid A (AA) protein, can be isolated from the amyloid of patients with secondary amyloidosis and from that associated with familial Mediterranean fever. It is a unique protein with a molecular weight of about 8500 Da made up of 76 amino acid residues arranged in a single chain, and an amino acid sequence beginning with Arg-Ser-Phe. . . . Some heterogeneity has been demonstrated (i.e., AAs of different molecular weights).

Antisera to alkali-degraded amyloid fibrils of the AA protein have detected an antigenically related serum component, SAA. Amino acid analysis, peptide maps, and sequence studies suggest that AA protein is an amino terminal fragment of SAA and is derived from it by proteolysis. SAA behaves as an acute phase reactant and is elevated in infection and inflammation. In addition, SAA is elevated in amyloid-resistant animals suggesting that the appearance of amyloid is not solely determined by the level of SAA. SAA associates with the HDL_3 subclass of serum lipoproteins and is often referred to as apoSAA. It is likely that humans have a three-gene family for SAA. Human SAA_1 and SAA_2 are similar by restriction mapping and SAA_3 is different in the region of exon 3. An SAA inducing factor (now known to be interleukin 1) is released from stimulated macrophages and causes the release of SAA from hepatocytes, the site of SAA synthesis. The precise regulation of the conversion of SAA to the insoluble AA protein of amyloidosis is not understood.

Familial amyloid polyneuropathy (FAP) is a dominant hereditary disease affecting kinships originating in Portugal, Japan, Sweden, and elsewhere. A 14,000-Da protein has been isolated from the tissues of patients from each of the above-noted geographically distributed kinships. Immunologic and amino acid sequence analysis has identified it as transthyretin (prealbumin), the first association of this molecule with a disease. It has also been shown that in many kinships there is a single amino acid substitution, methionine for valine at position 30 in the transthyretin isolated from the amyloid. Multiple other variants have also been shown to exist (Table 266-2).

A number of other amyloid proteins have been isolated and characterized. These include several from focal endocrine-related amyloid lesions such as precalcitonin from the amyloid of medullary carcinoma of the thyroid and insulinoma amyloid polypeptide (IAPP) of the pancreas that is related to calcitonin gene-related peptide. Transthyretin has also been isolated from senile cardiac amyloid and atrial natriuretic peptide has been isolated as a distinct and separate

TABLE 266-2 Amino acid variations in hereditary amyloidoses

Clinical geography	Mutant position	Normal amino acid	Mutant amino acid
Familial amyloid polyneuropathy: amyloid protein = transthyretin			
1 Portugal; Sweden; Japan; Greece; Italy	30	Val	Met
2 Poland (Israel)	33	Phe	Ile
3 U.S.A.—West Virginia (Appalachia)	60	Thr	Ala
4 U.S.A.—Illinois (German)	77	Ser	Tyr
5 U.S.A.—Indiana (Swiss)	84	Ile	Ser
Familial amyloid cardiopathy: amyloid protein = transthyretin			
1 Denmark	111	Leu	Met
Familial amyloid cerebral hemorrhage			
1 Iceland: abnormal protein = cystatin C (gamma trace)	?58	?Gln	NK*
2 Netherlands: abnormal protein = ?beta protein			

* NK = Not known

protein from these lesions. $Beta_2$ microglobulin has been identified as the protein from the amyloid associated with chronic hemodialysis.

Of great interest is confirmation that the lesions known as senile plaques (which contain amyloid) and the meningeal vascular amyloid of Alzheimer's disease consist of a newly described protein, beta protein (or A4 protein).

P component of amyloid In addition to the characteristic fibrils described above, a second component, the P component, has been noted in most amyloid deposits. P component (AP) has been recognized by electron microscopy as a pentagonal-shaped structured unit having an outside diameter of about 9×10^9 m (90 Å) and an inside diameter of about 4×10^9 m (40 Å). On immunoelectrophoresis it migrates as an alpha globulin, and it possesses antigenic identity with a constituent of normal human plasma (SAP). The amino acid sequence is distinct from that of the amyloid fibrils. Its pentagonal ultrastructure is similar to C-reactive protein (CRP), but the latter is one-half the molecular weight of AP and has other well-defined differences despite a 50 to 60 percent homology on amino acid sequence. AP binds to amyloid fibrils in a calcium-dependent fashion almost universally and has been used as a marker of amyloid.

IMMUNOBIOLOGY OF AMYLOID The precise etiology and pathogenesis of amyloidosis are unknown. Experimentally, the induction of AA amyloidosis has been shown to be a multifactorial process that is contributed to by the type of inflammatory stimulation, the nature of the SAA isotype, and the genetic background of the host. During inflammation, the mediator, interleukin 1, stimulates hepatic cells to produce increased SAA. SAA is partially degraded by monocyte or leukocyte surface enzymes to form AA. It is likely that macrophages play a role in the SAA degradation. Related abnormalities such as altered connective tissue glycosaminoglycans, altered macrophage enzymes, or enzyme inhibitors have all been postulated.

In AL amyloid, a monoclonal population of bone marrow plasma cells appears to be present and either consistently produces small lambda or kappa fragments or clones of immunoglobulins that are processed (cleaved) in an abnormal fashion by macrophage enzymes to produce the partially degraded light chains responsible for AL amyloidosis.

The formation of amyloid may also be determined in part by the intrinsic beta configuration of at least a portion of the polypeptide chain such as in transthyretin, $beta_2$ microglobulin, and other amyloidogenic proteins. Clearly in the hereditary amyloidoses the substitution of a single amino acid variant contributes to the overall pathogenesis.

It has also been demonstrated that a new substance known as amyloid enhancing factor (AEF), possibly a cytokine, contributes at least to the accelerated formation of secondary and probably other forms of amyloid.

CLINICAL MANIFESTATIONS The clinical manifestations of amyloidosis are varied and depend entirely on the area of the body which is involved.

Kidney Renal involvement may consist of mild proteinuria or frank nephrosis. In some cases, the urinary sediment may show only a few red blood cells. The renal lesion is usually not reversible and in time leads to progressive azotemia and death. The prognosis does not appear to be related to the degree of the proteinuria; when azotemia finally develops, the prognosis is grave. In one series the mean survival of patients with renal amyloid from the time of biopsy was 29 months, but in a few cases there was presumptive evidence of regression of the renal amyloid. The utilization of chronic hemodialysis and of kidney transplantation will clearly improve the prognosis of renal amyloid. Hypertension is rare except in long-standing amyloidosis. Renal tubular acidosis or renal vein thrombosis may occur. Localized accumulation of amyloid may be noted in the ureter, bladder, or other parts of the genitourinary tract.

Liver While hepatic involvement is common, liver function abnormalities are minimal and occur late in the disease. The two tests most useful in indicating hepatic amyloid are the Bromsulphalein (BSP) extraction and serum alkaline phosphatase activity; however, no liver function tests are truly specific or sensitive for amyloid. Liver scans produce variable and nonspecific results. Portal hypertension occurs but is uncommon. Intrahepatic cholestasis has been noted in about 5 percent of patients with AL (primary) amyloidosis. In a series of 38 patients in whom liver tissue was available for examination, all 38 had some amyloid present, irrespective of the type of amyloidosis (primary or secondary), and contrary to previous notions, parenchymal amyloid was more extensive in the AL cases. Hepatomegaly is common, and AL hepatic amyloid is usually accompanied by the nephrotic syndrome and by congestive heart failure. Prognosis is poor, and one group of 80 patients with proven AL hepatic amyloid had a median survival of 9 months. Amyloidosis of the spleen characteristically is not associated with leukopenia and anemia.

Heart Cardiac manifestations consist primarily of congestive failure and cardiomegaly (with or without murmurs) and a variety of arrhythmias. Although the cardiac manifestations predominantly reflect diffuse myocardial amyloid, the endocardium, valves, and pericardium may be involved as well. Pericarditis with effusion is rare, although the differential diagnosis of constrictive pericarditis versus restrictive cardiomyopathy frequently arises. Echocardiography has demonstrated symmetric thickening of the left ventricular wall, hypokinesia and decreased systolic contraction and thickening of the interventricular septum and left ventricular posterior wall, and left ventricular cavities of small to normal size. Two-dimensional echocardiography produces the characteristic findings of thickened right and left ventricles, a normal left ventricular cavity, and especially a diffuse hyperrefractile ''granular sparkling'' appearance. Hearts which are heavily infiltrated with amyloid may or may not show an enlarged silhouette. Fluoroscopy usually shows decreased mobility of the ventricular wall; angiographic studies usually demonstrate thickened ventricular wall, decreased ventricular mobility, and absence of rapid ventricular filling in early diastole. Cardiac amyloidosis can present as intractable heart failure. Electrocardiographic abnormalities include a low-voltage QRS complex and abnormalities in atrioventricular and intraventricular conduction, often resulting in varying degrees of heart block. Owing to their propensity to develop conduction defects and arrhythmias, patients with cardiac amyloidosis appear to be especially sensitive to digitalis, and this drug should be used with caution. Radionuclide techniques utilizing technetium 99 pyrophosphate for cardiac scanning are often positive, especially in patients with amyloid related congestive heart failure.

Skin Involvement of the skin is one of the most characteristic manifestations of primary amyloidosis. The lesions may consist of slightly raised, waxy papules or plaques which usually are clustered in the folds of the axillae, anal, or inguinal regions, the face and neck, or mucosal areas such as ear or tongue. Periorbital ecchymoses (''black eye syndrome'') have been reported. The lesions are seldom pruritic. Involvement of the skin or mucosa may not be apparent clinically but may be demonstrated by biopsy. Gentle rubbing of the skin may induce bleeding into the skin, leading to purpura. Cutaneous involvement also can occur in secondary amyloidosis; in one series it was found in 42 percent of such patients, in 55 percent of a group of patients with primary disease, and in all 11 patients with hereditary amyloid neuropathy.

Gastrointestinal tract Gastrointestinal symptoms are common in amyloidosis. They may result from direct involvement of the gastrointestinal tract at any level or from infiltration of the autonomic nervous system with amyloid. The symptoms include those of obstruction, ulceration, malabsorption, hemorrhage, protein loss, and diarrhea. Infiltration of the tongue occasionally leads to macroglossia. When not enlarged, the tongue may become stiffened and firm to palpation. While infiltration of the tongue is characteristic of primary amyloidosis or amyloidosis accompanying multiple myeloma, it is occasionally seen in the secondary form of the disease.

Gastrointestinal bleeding may occur from any of a number of sites, notably the esophagus, stomach, or large intestine, and may be severe. Amyloid infiltration of the esophagus may lead to an incompetent or nonrelaxing lower esophageal sphincter, nonspecific motility disorders of the esophageal body, or rarely achalasia. Small-bowel lesions may lead to clinical and x-ray changes of obstruction. A malabsorption syndrome is seen at times. Amyloidosis may develop in association with other entities involving the gastrointestinal tract, especially tuberculosis, granulomatous enteritis, lymphoma, and Whipple's disease; differentiation of these conditions, which give rise to secondary amyloidosis, from diffuse primary amyloidosis of the small bowel may be difficult. Similarly, amyloidosis of the stomach may closely mimic gastric carcinoma, with obstruction, achlorhydria, and the radiologic appearance of tumor masses.

Nervous system Neurologic manifestations may include peripheral neuropathy, postural hypotension, inability to sweat, Adie's pupil, hoarseness, and sphincter incompetence. These manifestations are especially prominent in the heredofamilial amyloidoses. The cranial nerves are generally spared except for those involving the pupillary reflexes. Carpal tunnel syndrome may be caused by several amyloidoses, especially primary (AL) and chronic hemodialysis (B_2M) amyloid. Peripheral neuropathy is frequent in the former type. Amyloid occurs in the central nervous system as a component of senile plaques, neurofibrillary tangles, and in blood vessels ("congophilic angiopathy"). The protein concentration in the cerebral spinal fluid may be increased. Infiltrates of the cornea or vitreous body may be present in hereditary amyloid syndromes. Certain of these syndromes are characterized by a bilateral scalloping appearance of the pupil.

Endocrine Amyloid may infiltrate the thyroid or other endocrine glands but rarely causes endocrine dysfunction. Local amyloid deposits almost invariably accompany medullary carcinoma of the thyroid. Amyloid is often found in the adrenal gland, pituitary gland, and pancreas. Little if any clinical dysfunction is present unless there is massive replacement of the gland by amyloid.

Joints Amyloid can directly involve articular structures by its presence in the synovial membrane and synovial fluid or in the articular cartilage. Amyloid arthritis can mimic a number of rheumatic diseases because it can present as a symmetric arthritis of small joints with nodules, morning stiffness, and fatigue. Most patients with amyloid arthropathy eventually are found to have multiple myeloma. The synovial fluid usually has a low white blood cell count, a good to fair mucin clot, a predominance of mononuclear cells, and no crystals. Studies of surgical specimens suggest a significant incidence of amyloid in cartilage, capsule, and synovium in osteoarthritis. Amyloid infiltration of muscle may lead to a pseudomyopathy.

Respiratory system The nasal sinuses, larynx, and trachea may be involved by accumulations of amyloid which block the ducts, in the case of the sinuses, or the air passages. Amyloidosis of the lung involves the bronchi and alveolar septa diffusely. The lower respiratory tract is affected most frequently in primary amyloidosis and in the disease associated with dysproteinemia. Pulmonary symptoms attributable to amyloid are present in about 30 percent of these patients and in some are the most serious manifestations of the disease. In secondary amyloidosis, pulmonary disease is a frequent histopathologic accompaniment but seldom gives rise to clinically significant symptoms. Amyloid may also be localized in the bronchi or pulmonary parenchyma and may resemble a neoplasm. In these cases, local excision should be attempted and, when successful, may be followed by prolonged remissions.

Hematopoietic system Hematologic changes may include fibrinogenopenia, increased fibrinolysis, and selective deficiency of clotting factors. Deficient factor X seems to be due to nonspecific calcium-dependent binding to the polyanionic amyloid fibrils. Splenectomy in the patient with such a factor-X deficiency can relieve the deficiency and the associated bleeding disorder, since factor X has been shown to bind to the large masses of splenic amyloid.

HEREDOFAMILIAL AMYLOIDOSIS There is no generally accepted nosology for the heredofamilial amyloid syndromes. Some reports emphasize the site of predominant organ involvement as neuropathic, nephropathic, or cardiopathic amyloidosis, while others stress the genetic aspects. To date, virtually all analyses of pedigrees have shown that, with one major exception, the mode of inheritance is autosomal dominant. The exception is amyloidosis of familial Mediterranean fever (FMF), which is inherited as an autosomal recessive disorder and is an AA type of amyloid. Even in FMF amyloid, however, several kinships with autosomal dominant inheritance have been reported. The recognizable clinical patterns still form the basis for classification, although serum abnormalities (decreased serum prealbumin in several types of familial amyloid polyneuropathy) have been reported. Table 266-3 proposes a tentative classification and is based largely on the major site of organ involvement, in addition to genetic data and ethnic background. Specific single amino acid mutations have already been listed in Table 266-2.

The heredofamilial amyloidoses include a group primarily involving the nervous system. Among these are lower limb neuropathy [familial amyloid polyneuropathy (FAP)], first described in Portugal, which has a poor prognosis and is characterized by progressively severe neuropathy including marked autonomic nervous system involvement. This variety also has been described in Japan, Sweden, and in families of Greek, of Swedish and of Italian origin. In some of these individuals, bilateral "scalloped" pupils are pathognomonic of the disease. The second type of neuropathy has been found in families of Swiss origin in Indiana and of German origin in Maryland. It is a milder disease and is often associated with a carpal tunnel syndrome and vitreous opacities. A more severe variety of generalized neuropathy associated with renal amyloidosis has been described in Iowa in a family of English-Irish-Scottish ancestry.

Several types of severe familial renal disease in association with amyloid have been described. Possibly the most remarkable is FMF, a disorder subdivided into phenotype I, with irregularly occurring fever and abdominal, chest, or joint pain, preceding or accompanying renal amyloid, and phenotype II, in which renal amyloidosis is the first or only manifestation of the disease. Colchicine treatment prevents attacks of FMF and appears to prevent subsequent deposition of amyloid as well. Sporadically, other hereditary forms of renal amyloidosis have been described, including the curious association of urticaria, deafness, and renal amyloid.

Severe familial amyloid heart disease has been described in a Danish family, and familial persistent atrial standstill with amyloid in a family of Mexican-American origin. Hereditary cerebral amyloid with hemorrhage in an Icelandic family appears to be due to gamma trace protein (cystatin C) deposits and is associated with a decrease of these proteins in the cerebrospinal fluid. A similar disorder has been reported from the Netherlands. Miscellaneous hereditary amyloid syndromes include hereditary multiple endocrine neoplasms type II (including medullary carcinoma of the thyroid with amyloid) as well as others listed in Table 266-3.

DIAGNOSIS The specific diagnosis of amyloidosis depends upon obtaining a tissue specimen by biopsy and the demonstration of amyloid with appropriate stains. First, of course, the disease must be suspected. When a patient with a chronic disorder predisposing to amyloid such as rheumatoid arthritis, tuberculosis, paraplegia, multiple myeloma, bronchiectasis, or leprosy develops hepatomegaly, splenomegaly, malabsorption, cardiac disease, or, most importantly, proteinuria, amyloid should come to mind. In addition, in any heredofamilial syndromes, especially those which have a dominant autosomal mode of inheritance and are characterized by peripheral neuropathy, nephropathy, or cardiopathy, the diagnosis of amyloid should be considered. Finally, primary systemic amyloid should be considered in any individual with a diffuse noninflammatory infiltrative disease involving either mesenchymal tissues—blood vessels, heart, gastrointestinal tract—or parenchymal tissues—kidney, liver, spleen, adrenal.

When the diagnosis is suspected, it is good practice to perform an abdominal subcutaneous fat pad aspirate or a rectal biopsy. If there is a specific reason for not carrying out these procedures, other sites including skin, gums, or the suspected organ—kidney, liver—

TABLE 266-3 Classification of heredofamilial amyloidoses

Types	Forms
Familial amyloid polyneuropathy	
Type I Portuguese (Andrade)	*1* Portuguese
	2 Swedish
	3 Japanese
	4 Greek
	5 English
	6 German
	7 Italian
Type II Indiana (Rukavina)	*1* Swiss
	2 German
Type III Iowa (Van Allen) (possibly same as type I)	*1* Scottish-English-Irish
Type IV Cranial neuropathy and corneal lattice dystrophy (Meretoja)	*1* Finnish
	2 Danish
	3 Dutch
Familial oculoleptomeningeal amyloid	*1* German
	2 Dutch
	3 Japanese
Hereditary cerebral amyloid with hemorrhage	*1* Icelandic
	2 Dutch
Familial nephropathy	
Type I Familial Mediterranean fever (Heller)(recessive)	*1* Sephardic Jewish
	2 Armenian
	3 Turkish
Type II Fever and abdominal pain	*1* Swedish
	2 Sicilian
Type III Urticaria, deafness, renal disease	
Familial cardiopathy	
Type I Progressive heart failure	*1* Danish
Type II Hereditary atrial standstill	*1* Mexican-American

may be biopsied. All tissues obtained must be stained with Congo red and examined in the polarizing microscope for green birefringence. A modified potassium permanganate stain will allow reasonably accurate differentiation of the AA type from AL amyloid. In the former, pretreatment with permanganate, followed by the standard Congo red stain, abolishes the green birefringence (i.e., the tissue is permanganate-sensitive). Beta$_2$ microglobulin amyloid is also permanganate-sensitive. The AL and AF prealbumin types are permanganate-resistant.

In order to establish the relationship of immunoglobulin-related amyloid to multiple myeloma, electrophoretic and immunoelectrophoretic studies on serum or urine should be performed when the biopsy reveals amyloid deposition. Most of these patients will have only relatively small paraprotein components and only a few will have frank multiple myeloma.

PROGNOSIS AND TREATMENT The course of amyloidosis is difficult to document since dating the time of origin of the disease is rarely possible. When amyloidosis develops in patients with rheumatoid arthritis, it seldom becomes evident when the arthritis is less than 2 years in duration. The mean duration of arthritis before amyloidosis was detected was 16 years in one series. When amyloidosis develops in patients with multiple myeloma, manifestations leading to initial hospitalization are more apt to be related to amyloid disease than to myeloma. In these cases prognosis is very poor, and life expectancy is usually less than 6 months.

Instances have been reported of amyloidosis accompanying treatable infections, such as osteomyelitis, in which at least partial remission has occurred following treatment of the primary disease. There have been similar experiences following successful treatment of tuberculosis or drainage of chronic empyema. However, many such reports are not substantiated by biopsy proof of resorption.

Generalized amyloidosis is usually a slowly progressive disease and leads to death in several years, but it may have a better prognosis than was suspected in the past. The average survival in most large series is 1 to 4 years, but a number of individuals with amyloid have been followed 5 to 10 years and longer.

The major cause of death is renal failure. Sudden death, presumably due to arrhythmias, is also quite common. Occasionally, gastrointestinal hemorrhage, respiratory failure, intractable heart failure, and superimposed infections are the terminal events.

There is no specific therapy for any variety of amyloidosis. Rational therapy should be directed at (1) decreasing chronic antigenic stimuli that produce amyloid, (2) inhibition of the synthesis and extracellular deposition of amyloid fibrils, and (3) promoting lysis or mobilization of existing amyloid deposits.

A variety of agents have been used to treat amyloidosis. Proof of their efficacy is not available. The finding that a portion of the immunoglobulin light chain is incorporated in the amyloid of patients with primary amyloidosis and its presumed synthesis by plasma cells has led to the use of alkylating agents. However, these agents cause bone marrow depression, and there are reports of acute leukemia developing in amyloidosis patients receiving melphalan. Moreover, there is experimental evidence that immunosuppressive agents may enhance the deposition of preexisting amyloid. Hence, conservative and supportive measures have been the mainstay of management. Recent trials have indicated that a prednisone/melphalan regimen or a prednisone/melphalan/colchicine program prolongs life. Studies in several centers are underway to compare these programs to each other and to colchicine alone (see below).

Patients with severe renal amyloidosis and azotemia have been subjected to bilateral nephrectomy and renal transplantation followed by immune therapy. One of two patients died of infection 5 months after surgery. The donor kidney showed no evidence of amyloidosis. The second patient achieved a 10-year clinical remission after receiving a transplanted kidney. Notwithstanding the hazards of operating upon patients with systemic amyloidosis who may have cardiac involvement, carefully selected azotemic patients clearly benefit from transplantation.

Colchicine has been shown to be effective in preventing acute attacks in patients with FMF, and two groups of investigators independently have reported the inhibition of amyloid deposition in the mouse model by colchicine. It is conceivable, therefore, that colchicine is effective in blocking amyloid deposition. One large study has shown it to be effective in prolonging life in primary (AL) amyloidosis using a life-table survivorship analysis. However, the exact mechanism of its action is unknown. The use of dimethylsulfoxide (DMSO) in the treatment of amyloid has had variable results.

REFERENCES

COHEN AS: Amyloidosis. N Engl J Med 277:522, 1967

———, SKINNER M: Diagnosis of amyloidosis, in *Laboratory Diagnostic Procedures in the Rheumatic Diseases*, 3d ed, AS Cohen (ed). Orlando, Fla, Grune & Stratton, 1985

——— et al: Amyloid proteins, precursors, mediator, and enhancer. Lab Invest 48:1, 1983

GLENNER GG et al: Amyloid fibril proteins: Proof of homology with immunoglobulin light chains. Science 172:1150, 1971

——— et al: *Amyloid and Amyloidosis*. New York, Excerpta Medica, 1980

HUSBY G, SLETTEN K: Chemical and clinical classification of amyloidosis, 1985. Scand J Immunol 23:253, 1986

KISILEVSKY R: From arthritis to Alzheimer's disease: Current concepts on the pathogenesis of amyloidosis. Can J Physiol Pharm 65:1805, 1987

KYLE RA, GREIPP PR: Amyloidosis (AL): Clinical and laboratory features in 229 cases. Mayo Clin Proc 58:665, 1983

section 2 Disorders of immune-mediated injury

267 DISEASES OF IMMEDIATE TYPE HYPERSENSITIVITY

K. FRANK AUSTEN

The term *atopic allergy* implies a familial tendency to manifest alone or in combination such conditions as asthma, rhinitis, urticaria, and eczematous dermatitis (atopic dermatitis). However, individuals without an atopic background may also develop hypersensitivity reactions, particularly urticaria and anaphylaxis, associated with the same class of antibody, IgE, found in atopic individuals. The designation *diseases of immediate type hypersensitivity* presents a more suitable framework than the broad term *allergy* or the restrictive definition of atopy.

The fixation of IgE to human basophils has been demonstrated by radioautography and electron microscopy and to intraepithelial and perivenular mast cells in tonsils, adenoids, and nasal polyps of humans by immunofluorescence. IgE-dependent mediator generation and release also occur in the mast cells of human lung slices, nasal polyps, or skin and have been observed in those tissues most involved in diseases of immediate type hypersensitivity.

Studies with purified rat peritoneal mast cells have indicated that the IgE receptor is transmembrane-linked and that stereospecific receptor perturbation activates a polyphosphatidyl inositol–selective phospholipase C to elaborate 1,2-diacylglycerols (1,2-DAG) and inositol-1,4,5-*bis*-phosphate (IP_3), which in turn activate protein kinase C and mobilize intracellular calcium ions, respectively. These events may be augmented by the formation of calcium ion channels and attenuated by the activation of adenylate cyclase with formation of cyclic 3′,5′-adenosine monophosphate (cyclic AMP) and activation of cyclic AMP–dependent protein kinase. The calcium ion-dependent activation of phospholipases cleaves membrane phospholipids to generate lysophospholipids, which like 1,2-DAG, are fusogenic and may facilitate the fusion of the secretory granule perigranular membrane with the cell membrane, a step which releases the membrane-free granule containing the preformed or primary mediators of mast cell effects. The arachidonic acid generated simultaneously by phospholipase action is processed oxidatively into secondary mediators of the prostaglandin and leukotriene (Fig. 267-1) classes. The lysophospholipid formed from release of arachidonic acid from 1-*0*-alkyl-2-acyl-*sn*-glyceryl-3-phosphorylcholine can be acetylated in the second position to form platelet activating factor (PAF) (Fig. 267-2). The secretory granule of the human mast cell has a crystalline structure, unlike mast cells of lower species, and IgE-dependent cell activation can be characterized morphologically by solubilization and swelling of the granule contents within the first minute of receptor perturbation; this reaction is followed by the ordering of intermediate filaments about the swollen granule, movement toward the cell surface, and fusion of the perigranular membrane with that of other granules and with the plasmalemma to form extracellular channels for mediator release while maintaining cell viability.

Important insight into the diversity of mast cells within a species has been gained from studies of serosal mast cells considered to be connective tissue mast cell (CTMC) and mucosal mast cell (MMC) populations from rats infected with *Nippostrongylus brasiliensis*. The CTMC secretory granules stain with alcian blue and counterstain with safranin, contain large amounts of histamine, heparin proteoglycan, chymotryptic protease termed neutral protease I, and carboxypeptidase A, generate prostaglandin D_2 upon IgE-Fc–dependent activation, and remain viable ex vivo in coculture with fibroblasts in the absence of added T-cell factors. The MMC secretory granules stain with alcian blue but not safranin, contain small amounts of histamine and a distinct chymotryptic protease termed neutral protease II, generate leukotriene C_4 in preference to prostaglandin D_2 (PGD_2) during activation-secretion, and are T-cell factor–dependent for appearance in vivo or generation from progenitors in vitro. Upon stimulus-specific activation in vitro, the membrane-derived lipid mediators such as leukotrienes, PGD_2, and PAF along with histamine and selected secretory granule–associated acid hydrolases are solubilized, whereas the neutral proteases, which are cationic, remain largely complexed to the anionic proteoglycans. It is speculated that the macromolecular complex serves to deliver the neutral proteases so that the endo- and exoproteases can function in concert at the substrate site.

Histamine and the various lipid mediators alter venular permeability, and the cysteinyl leukotrienes constrict both vascular and nonvascular smooth muscle. Leukotrienes C_4 and D_4 (LTC_4 and

FIGURE 267-1 Metabolism of phospholipids to arachidonic acid and cyclooxygenase-derived products. Cleavage of arachidonic acid from membrane phospholipids during cellular activation proceeds either by the action of phospholipase A_2 (PLase A_2) or by the sequential action of phospholipase C (PLase C) and diacylglycerol lipase (DAG lipase). Biosynthesis of prostaglandins is depicted with the structure of PGD_2, which is the predominant product from mast cells via the terminal action of a PGD_2 synthetase. The η-lipoxygenase family of monolipoxygenases; includes 5-lipoxygenase, which initiates the pathway to leukotriene generation. Abbreviations: PGG_2, PGH_2, PGI_2, PGE_2, $PGF_{2\alpha}$, PGD_2, prostaglandins G_2, H_2, I_2, E_2, $F_{2\alpha}$, and D_2, respectively; TxA_2, TxB_2, thromboxane A_2 and B_2, respectively; 6-k-$PGF_{1\alpha}$, 6-keto-prostaglandin $F_{1\alpha}$; HHT, 12-hydroxy-heptadecatrienoic acid. *(Modified from Schwartz and Austen, Immunological Diseases, 4th ed.)*

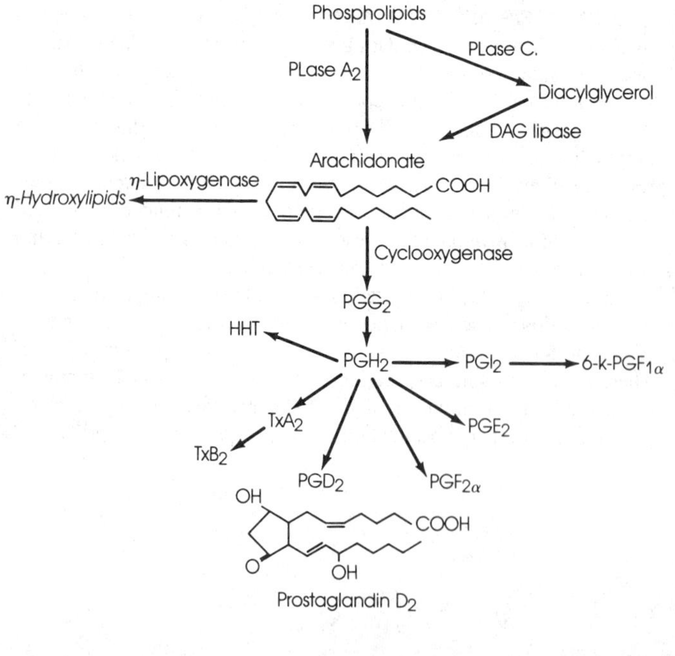

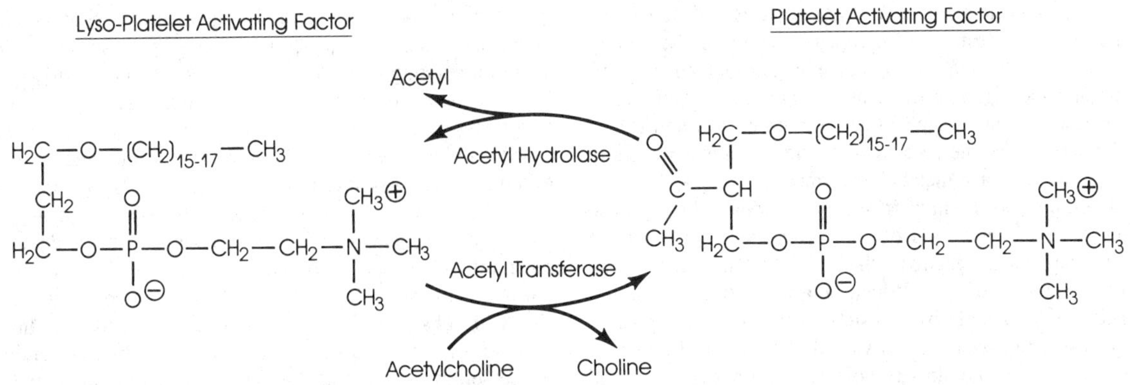

FIGURE 267-2 Synthesis and degradation of platelet activating factor. *(From Schwartz and Austen, Immunological Diseases, 4th ed.)*

LTD_4) are logs more potent than histamine in constricting human airway smooth muscle when administered by aerosol, and leukotriene E_4 (LTE_4), the most stable member of the family, is also somewhat more potent than histamine. The 5-lipoxygenation of arachidonic acid to 5*S*-hydroperoxy-6-*trans*-8,11,14-*cis*-eicosatetraenoic acid (5-HPETE) and then to 5,6-*trans*-oxido-7,9-*trans*-11,14-*cis*-eicosatetraenoic acid (LTA_4) is followed by the adduction of glutathione via a microsomal LTC_4 synthase to yield 5*S*-hydroxy-6*R*-*S*-glutathionyl-7,9-*trans*-11,14-*cis*-eicosatetraenoic acid (LTC_4); upon transport across the membrane to the extracellular environment LTC_4 undergoes sequential cleavage of the glutathione portion to yield the cysteinyl-glycyl (LTD_4) and cysteinyl (LTE_4) derivatives. Alternatively, a cytosolic LTA_4 epoxide hydrolase converts LTA_4 into 5*S*-12*R*-dihydroxy-6,14-*cis*-8,10-*trans*-eicosatetraenoic acid (LTB_4), which mediates leukocyte margination and directed (chemotactic) migration in human sites.

The evidence for diversity of mast cells within the human is more subtle than in the rat, but nonetheless is sufficient to suggest possible functional implications. Mast cells of human lung, intestine, and skin each stain with alcian blue but not safranin and have a similar histamine content. Dispersed partially purified human lung and intestinal mast cells respond to activation by IgE-Fc–dependent mechanisms with generation of LTC_4 and PGD_2; are not activated by various peptide agonists; are enriched for the secretory granule neutral protease tryptase; and exhibit secretory granules with a scroll and crystalline ultrastructure. In the lung they synthesize heparin proteoglycan in a 2:1 ratio to chondroitin sulfate E proteoglycan, and in the intestine they are T-cell-dependent, as revealed by their absence from mucosal sites in patients with T-cell deficiencies. The skin mast cells are readily stimulated for exocytosis by diverse peptides such as C5a anaphylatoxin, substance P, and f-Met-Leu-Phe; elaborate PGD_2 with IgE-Fc receptor–dependent activation; are much enriched for the secretory granule neutral proteases—tryptase, chymase, and carboxypeptidase A—and for heparin proteoglycan; exhibit secretory granules with a lattice and crystalline ultrastructure; and are present in the intestinal submucosa of patients with T-cell deficiencies. Whether mast cell diversity is determined entirely by the microenvironment or is dictated in part by different progenitors derived from a common marrow precursor is not established.

In any event, mast cells bearing specific recognition units are distributed at cutaneous and mucosal surfaces and in deeper tissues about venules, are an expansile population during T-cell stimulation, and could regulate the entry of foreign substances by their rapid response capability. A local increase in venular permeability via the action of histamine and membrane-derived lipid mediators could introduce critical plasma proteins such as complement and immunoglobulin. Phagocytic cells such as eosinophils would be elicited by PAF and specific peptides, while LTB_4 would recruit neutrophils and, in time, monocyte-macrophages. The secretory granule exo- and endoproteases might function to clear damaged connective tissue elements and facilitate tissue repair. There is even evolving evidence that mast cells via their constituents can regulate fibroblast proliferation and/or angiogenesis. Local and subclinical regulation of the tissue microenvironment would represent an initial and homeostatic physiologic response, while an intense or continuous stimulus would result in inflammation and tissue injury which could be either beneficial or detrimental (hypersensitivity) depending upon the appropriateness of the immunologic specificity.

Consideration of the mechanism of immediate type hypersensitivity diseases in the human has focused largely on the IgE-dependent recognition of otherwise nontoxic substances. Support for this thesis has come from the finding that clinical atopic allergy is associated with elevated total levels of IgE and in some instances with an immune response that is specifically linked to the histocompatibility locus. Populations of allergic whites have a significantly higher total serum level of IgE than nonallergic individuals, and highly atopic persons with asthma have significantly higher serum levels of IgE than those with fewer allergic manifestations. IgE distribution in normal families is consistent with the dominant inheritance of the low-IgE phenotype. As a result of the action of a single IgE regulator gene, the majority of family members would have elevated IgE levels as a possible basis for their atopic state. The association between HLA histocompatibility type and the immediate hypersensitivity response has been noted in persons of the low-IgE phenotype who were studied with highly purified allergens, generally of small size. Such presumptive evidence of immune response (Ir) genes by linkage disequilibrium, that is, the association of the hypersensitivity response with a particular histocompatibility haplotype, represents an additional element in the polygenic atopic allergic state. Nonetheless, all the studies taken together, both of families and of populations, seem to indicate that the genetically determined elevated IgE levels found in about three-fourths of atopic allergic subjects exert the predominant influence on most specific IgE responses. It is also likely that diseases of immediate type hypersensitivity may occur because of deficient intracellular controls of mediator generation or release, or both, or that the extracellular controls directed against mediator inactivation may be impaired.

ANAPHYLAXIS Definition The life-threatening anaphylactic response of a sensitized human appears within minutes after administration of specific antigen and is manifested by respiratory distress often followed by vascular collapse or by shock without antecedent respiratory difficulty. Cutaneous manifestations exemplified by pruritus and urticaria with or without angioedema are characteristic of such systemic anaphylactic reactions. Gastrointestinal manifestations include nausea, vomiting, crampy abdominal pain, and diarrhea.

Predisposing factors and etiology There is no convincing evidence that age, sex, race, occupation, or geographic location predisposes a human to anaphylaxis except through exposure to some immunogen. According to most studies, atopy does not predispose individuals to penicillin anaphylaxis.

The materials capable of eliciting the systemic anaphylactic reaction in the human include the following: heterologous proteins in the form of antiserum, hormones, enzymes, Hymenoptera venom, pollen extracts, and foods; polysaccharides such as iron dextran; and most commonly diagnostic agents and drugs such as antibiotics and even vitamins. The diagnostic and therapeutic agents are generally of low molecular weight and, other than nonsteroidal anti-inflammatory agents and radiographic dyes, are considered to function as haptens which form immunogenic conjugates with host proteins. The conjugating hapten may be the parent compound, a nonenzymatically derived storage product, or a metabolite formed in the host.

Pathophysiology and manifestations Individuals differ in the time of appearance of perception of symptoms and signs, but the hallmark of the anaphylactic reaction is the onset of some manifestation within seconds to minutes after introduction of the antigen, generally by injection or less commonly by ingestion. There may be upper or lower airway obstruction or both. Laryngeal edema may be experienced as a ''lump'' in the throat, hoarseness, or stridor, while bronchial obstruction is associated with a feeling of tightness in the chest or audible wheezing. A particularly characteristic feature is the eruption of well-circumscribed, discrete cutaneous wheals with erythematous, raised, serpiginous borders and blanched centers. These urticarial eruptions are intensely pruritic and may be localized or distributed. They may coalesce to form giant hives, and seldom persist beyond 48 h. A localized, nonpitting, deeper edematous cutaneous process, angioedema, may also be present. It may be asymptomatic or cause a burning or stinging sensation.

In fatal cases with clinical bronchial obstruction, the lungs show marked hyperinflation on gross and microscopic examination. The microscopic findings in the bronchi, however, are limited to luminal secretions, peribronchial congestion, submucosal edema, and eosinophilic infiltration, and the acute emphysema is attributed to intractable bronchospasm which subsides with death. The angioedema resulting in death by mechanical obstruction occurs in the epiglottis and larynx, but the process is also evident in the hypopharynx and to some extent the trachea; on microscopic examination there is wide separation of the collagen fibers and the glandular elements; vascular congestion and eosinophilic infiltration are also present. Patients dying of vascular collapse without antecedent hypoxia from respiratory insufficiency have visceral congestion but no major shift in the distribution of blood volume. The associated electrocardiographic abnormalities, with or without infarction, noted in some patients could reflect a primary cardiac event or be secondary to a critical reduction in plasma volume.

The angioedematous and urticarial manifestations of the anaphylactic syndrome have been attributed to release of endogenous histamine. A role for the cysteinyl leukotrienes in altering pulmonary mechanics by causing marked bronchiolar constriction seems likely. Vascular collapse without respiratory distress in response to experimental challenge with the sting of a hymenopteran was associated not only with marked and prolonged elevations in blood histamine but also with evidence of intravascular coagulation and kinin generation. Based upon the findings that patients with systemic mastocytosis and episodic hypotension proceeding to vascular collapse excrete large amounts of PGD_2 in addition to histamine and are controlled by administration of a nonsteroidal agent but not by antihistamines alone, it may be that PGD_2 is also of importance in the hypotensive anaphylactic reactions. Because of the marked coronary arterial constrictor action of the cysteinyl leukotrienes upon administration to experimental animals, these substances may be involved in the disease process of patients with myocardial ischemia without or with infarction.

Diagnosis The diagnosis of an anaphylactic reaction depends largely upon an accurate history revealing the onset of the appropriate symptoms and signs within minutes after the responsible material is encountered. When only a portion of the full syndrome is present, such as isolated urticaria, sudden bronchospasm in an asthmatic patient, or vascular collapse after intravenous administration of an agent, it is difficult to exclude a nonimmunologic, toxicologic or idiosyncratic response. For example, intravenous administration of a chemical mast cell–degranulating agent may elicit generalized urticaria, angioedema, and a sensation of retrosternal oppression with or without clinically detectable bronchoconstriction or hypotension. Furthermore, nonsteroidal anti-inflammatory agents such as indomethacin, aminopyrine, mefenamic acid, and aspirin may precipitate a life-threatening episode of obstruction of upper or lower airways in asthmatic subjects that is clinically reminiscent of anaphylaxis but is not associated with a detectable IgE response. This syndrome may reflect a unique reactivity to an imbalance in the ratio of prostaglandin to leukotriene biosynthesis when cyclooxygenase is inhibited.

The presence of a labile reagin (IgE) in the heart blood of a patient dying of systemic anaphylaxis has been demonstrated at postmortem by passive transfer of the serum intradermally into a normal recipient, followed in 24 h by antigen challenge into the same site, with subsequent development of a wheal and flare, the Prausnitz-Küstner reaction. Indeed, such a reagin can be transiently identified in the serum of most patients who develop systemic anaphylaxis to a variety of different agents. In order to avoid the hazards of transferring hepatitis to the recipient in the Prausnitz-Küstner reaction, it is preferable to employ the less sensitive monkey recipient or a human leukocyte suspension enriched with basophils for subsequent antigen challenge. It is presumed that the activity responsible for most cases of systemic anaphylaxis resides with the IgE class, since the Prausnitz-Küstner activity in the serums of patients with systemic reactions to Hymenoptera venom or human seminal plasma protein can be removed by IgE immunosorbent columns. Furthermore, radioimmunoassays have demonstrated specific IgE antibodies in patients with anaphylactic reactions to insulin and to parathormone, but such approaches require purified antigens. In the transfusion anaphylactic reaction that occurs in patients with IgA deficiency, the responsible specificity resides in IgG anti-IgA rather than in IgE; the mechanism of the reaction is presumed to be complement activation with secondary mast cell participation.

Treatment and prevention Early recognition of an anaphylactic reaction is mandatory, since death occurs within minutes to hours after the first symptoms. Mild symptoms such as pruritus and urticaria can be controlled by administration of 0.2 to 0.5 mL of 1:1000 epinephrine subcutaneously, with repeated doses as required at 3-min intervals for a severe reaction. If the antigenic material was injected into an extremity, the rate of absorption may be reduced by prompt application of a tourniquet proximal to the reaction site, administration of 0.2 mL of 1:1000 epinephrine into the site, and removal without compression of an insect stinger, if present. An intravenous infusion should be initiated to provide a route for administration of epinephrine, diluted 1:50,000, volume expanders, and vasopressor agents if intractable hypotension occurs. Epinephrine most likely acts to reverse the action of mediators on target tissues, and its early administration appears critical. When epinephrine fails to control the situation, hypoxia due to airway obstruction or related to a cardiac arrhythmia, or both, must be considered. Oxygen via a nasal catheter or intermittent positive pressure breathing of oxygen with 0.5 mL isoproterenol diluted 1:200 in saline may be helpful, but either endotracheal intubation or a tracheostomy is mandatory if progressive hypoxia exists. Ancillary agents such as the antihistamine diphenhydramine, 50 to 80 mg intramuscularly or intravenously, and aminophylline, 0.25 to 0.5 g intravenously, are appropriate for urticaria-angioedema and bronchospasm, respectively. Intravenous corticosteroids are not effective for the acute event but may be considered for persistent bronchospasm and hypotension.

Prevention of anaphylaxis must take into account the sensitivity of the recipient, the dose and character of the diagnostic or therapeutic agent, and the effect of the route of administration on the rate of absorption. If there is a definite history of a past anaphylactic reaction, even though mild, it is advisable to select another agent or procedure. A skin test should be performed before the administration of certain materials producing a high incidence of anaphylactic reactions, such as horse serum or allergenic extracts, or when the nature of the past adverse reaction is unknown. Since even a skin or conjunctival test can produce a serious reaction, a scratch test should precede these tests in a high-risk situation. With regard to penicillin, two-thirds of patients with a positive reaction history and positive intradermal skin tests to benzylpenicilloyl-polylysine (BPL) and/or the minor determinant mixture (MDM) of benzylpenicillin products experience allergic reactions with treatment, and these are almost uniformly of the anaphylactic type in those patients with minor determinant reactivity. Even patients without a history of previous clinical reactions have a 6 percent incidence of positive skin tests to the two test materials, and about 3 per 1000 with a negative history experience anaphylaxis with therapy with a mortality of about 1 per 100,000. The value of skin testing is both to permit therapy with the agent in question when the risk does not exist and to emphasize the hazards where the sensitivity is confirmed. In the event that an agent must be used despite a positive history, a positive skin test, or both, the following precautionary measures should be taken: An intravenous infusion should be started, with intubation equipment and a tracheostomy set at hand; the material should be given intradermally, then subcutaneously, and then intramuscularly in increasing doses at 20- to 30-min intervals so that the initial dose by the next route does not exceed the final dose by the previous route. It is difficult to be certain that the mediator-containing cells have been exhausted, and therapeutic use of the agent may be accompanied by untoward consequences. It may be critical to give the therapeutic agent at regular intervals to prevent the reestablishment of a sensitized cell pool of large size. A different form of protection involves the development of blocking antibody of the IgG class which is protective against Hymenoptera venom–induced anaphylaxis by interacting with antigen so that less reaches the sensitized tissue mast cells; to be effective this immunotherapy requires the use of specific or cross-reacting Hymenoptera venom rather than whole-insect-body extracts.

URTICARIA AND ANGIOEDEMA **Definition** Urticaria and angioedema may appear separately or together as cutaneous manifestations of localized nonpitting edema; a similar process may occur at mucosal surfaces of the upper respiratory or gastrointestinal tract. *Urticaria* involves only the superficial portion of the dermis presenting as well-circumscribed wheals with erythematous raised serpiginous borders with blanched centers which may coalesce to become giant wheals. *Angioedema* is a well-demarcated localized edema involving the deeper layers of the skin including the subcutaneous tissue. Recurrent episodes of urticaria and/or angioedema of less than 6 weeks' duration are considered acute, while attacks persisting beyond this period are designated chronic.

Predisposing factors and etiology The occurrence of urticaria and angioedema is probably more frequent than usually described because of the evanescent, self-limited nature of such eruptions, which seldom require medical attention when limited to the skin. Although persons in any age group may experience acute or chronic urticaria and/or angioedema, these lesions increase in frequency after adolescence, with the highest incidence occurring in persons in the third decade of life; indeed, one survey of college students indicated that some 15 to 20 percent had experienced a pruritic wheal reaction.

The classification of urticaria-angioedema presented in Table 267-1 focuses on the different mechanisms for eliciting clinical disease. Only the IgE-dependent and the IgG-mediated reactions in IgA-deficient persons should be considered immediate hypersensitivity. However, the other mechanisms are important for differential diagnosis, and most cases of chronic urticaria are idiopathic. The appearance of urticaria and angioedema in atopic persons in the absence of a specific exposure is attributed to the atopic diathesis and implies an IgE mechanism. Urticaria and/or angioedema occurring during the appropriate season in patients with seasonal respiratory allergy or as a result of exposure to animals or molds is attributed to inhalation of pollens, animal dander, and mold spores, respectively. However, urticaria and angioedema secondary to inhalation are relatively uncommon compared with ingestion of fresh fruits, shellfish, chocolate, nuts, tomatoes, and various drugs, including penicillin-contaminated milk products, which may elicit not only the anaphylactic syndrome with prominent gastrointestinal complaints but also chronic urticaria. Additional etiologies include physical stimuli such as cold, solar rays, exercise, and mechanical irritation (dermographism).

TABLE 267-1 Classification of urticaria with angioedema

1 IgE-dependent
- *a* Atopic diathesis
- *b* Specific antigen sensitivity (pollens, foods, drugs, fungi, molds, Hymenoptera venom, helminths)
- *c* Physical: dermographism; cold; light; cholinergic; vibratory; exercise-related

2 Complement-mediated
- *a* Hereditary angioedema: type 1; type 2
- *b* Acquired angioedema: type 1; type 2
- *c* Necrotizing vasculitis
- *d* Serum sickness
- *e* Reactions to blood products

3 Nonimmunologic
- *a* Direct mast cell–releasing agents: opiates; antibiotics; curare, D-tubocurarine; radiocontrast media
- *b* Agents which presumably alter arachidonic acid metabolism: aspirin and nonsteroidal anti-inflammatory agents; azo dyes and benzoates

4 Idiopathic

Angioedema without urticaria occurs with $C\bar{1}$ inhibitor ($C\bar{1}INH$) deficiency that can be inborn as an autosomal dominant characteristic or can be acquired in association with lymphoproliferative disorders. The urticaria and angioedema associated with classical serum sickness or with idiopathic cutaneous necrotizing angiitis is believed to be an immune-complex disease when hypocomplementemia is a concomitant. The idiosyncratic drug reactions to mast cell granule-releasing agents and to nonsteroidal anti-inflammatory drugs can be systemic, resembling anaphylaxis, or limited to cutaneous sites.

Pathophysiology and manifestations Urticarial eruptions are distinctly pruritic, involve any area of the body from the scalp to the soles of the feet, and appear in crops of 24- to 72-h duration with old lesions fading as new ones appear. The most common sites are the extremities, external genitalia, and face, particularly the region of the eyes and lips. Although self-limited in duration, angioedema of the upper respiratory tract may be life-threatening due to laryngeal obstruction, while gastrointestinal involvement may present with abdominal colic, with or without nausea and vomiting, and may precipitate unnecessary surgical intervention. No residual discoloration occurs with either urticaria or angioedema unless there is an underlying process leading to superimposed extravasation of erythrocytes.

The pathology of urticaria and angioedema is usually characterized by massive edema of the dermis in urticaria, and of the subcutaneous tissue as well as the dermis in angioedema. Collagen bundles in affected areas are widely separated, and the venules are sometimes dilated. The perivenular infiltrate may consist of lymphocytes, eosinophils, and neutrophils that are present in varying combination and number throughout the dermis. Allergen-induced wheal-and-flare reactions are characterized by mast cell degranulation and an accumulation of eosinophils over hours to days. The elicitation of a wheal-and-flare response upon injection of the relevant allergen into a patient with urticaria and/or angioedema, or into a site in a normal recipient prepared with serum from the patient, the Prausnitz-Küstner reaction, indicates an IgE-dependent, mast cell–mediated reaction.

Perhaps the best-studied example of mast cell–mediated urticaria and angioedema is *cold urticaria*. Acquired cold urticaria is a disorder in which patients exposed to cold experience an urticarial eruption that may evolve into angioedema and be associated with syncope. Cryoglobulins, cryofibrinogens, cold agglutinins, or hemolysins may be recognized, but not in the majority of patients. The finding in a number of patients of a serum factor, characterized as being of the IgE class, that is capable of transferring the cold urticaria reaction to a skin site of a normal recipient has focused attention upon the mast cell in this condition. Immersion of an extremity in an ice bath precipitates angioedema of the distal portion with urticaria at the air interface within minutes of the challenge. Histologic studies reveal marked mast cell degranulation with associated edema of the dermis and subcutaneous tissues. The venous effluent of the cold-challenged and angioedematous extremity reveals a marked rise in plasma content of histamine, low-molecular-weight eosinophilotactic activity, and high-molecular-weight neutrophil chemotactic activity, which are presumably of mast cell origin, whereas the venous effluent of the contralateral normal extremity contains none of these mediators. Elevations of plasma histamine with biopsy-proven mast cell degranulation have also been demonstrated with systemic attacks of *cholinergic urticaria* and *exercise-induced erythema-angioedema* precipitated experimentally by exercise on a treadmill while wearing a wet suit.

Diagnosis The rapid onset and self-limited nature of urticarial and angioedematous eruptions are distinguishing features. Additional characteristics are the occurrence of the urticarial crops in various stages of evolution and the asymmetric distribution of the angioedema. Urticaria and/or angioedema involving IgE-dependent mechanisms are often appreciated by historical considerations implicating specific allergens, by seasonal incidence, by exposure to certain environments, or by physical stimuli such as cold, exercise, sunlight (solar urticaria), or trauma (dermographism). Direct reproduction of the lesion with physical stimuli is particularly valuable because it so often establishes the cause of the lesion. The diagnosis can be confirmed by careful testing with the putative foreign substance to determine if a local wheal and flare results, and by passive transfer of such a reaction with serum of the patient to a skin site in a normal recipient, the Prausnitz-Küstner phenomenon. Passive transfer to the skin of a nonhuman primate or in vitro to human basophils may also be attempted. IgE-mediated urticaria and/or angioedema may or may not be associated with an elevation of total IgE or with peripheral eosinophilia. Fever, leukocytosis, or an elevated sedimentation rate are characteristically absent.

The classification of urticarial and angioedematous states noted in Table 267-1 in terms of possible mechanisms necessarily includes some differential diagnostic points. Hypocomplementemia is not observed in IgE-mediated mast cell disease and can reflect either an acquired abnormality generally attributed to the formation of immune complexes or a genetic deficiency of C$\bar{1}$INH. Chronic recurrent urticaria, generally in females, associated with arthralgias, an elevated sedimentation rate, and normo- or hypocomplementemia suggests an underlying cutaneous necrotizing angiitis. Confirmation depends upon a biopsy which reveals cellular infiltration, nuclear debris, and fibrinoid necrosis of the venules.

Hereditary angioedema is an autosomal dominant state associated with the absence of functional C$\bar{1}$INH. The diagnosis is suggested not only by family history but also by the lack of urticarial lesions, the prominence of recurrent gastrointestinal attacks of colic, and episodes of laryngeal edema. Laboratory diagnosis depends upon demonstrating the antigenic lack of C$\bar{1}$INH (type 1) in most kindreds, but some kindreds have an antigenically intact nonfunctional protein (type 2) and require a functional assay to establish the diagnosis. The natural substrates of uninhibited C$\bar{1}$, C4, and C2 are chronically depleted but fall further during attacks due to the activation of additional C1 to C$\bar{1}$. An acquired form of C$\bar{1}$INH deficiency, associated with lymphoproliferative disorders, has the same clinical manifestations and differs in the lack of a familial element; in the reduction of C1/C$\bar{1}$ as well as C$\bar{1}$INH, C4, and C2; and in the presence of an anti-idiotypic antibody to the monoclonal immunoglobulin expressed on the B cells (type 1). In a second acquired form of C$\bar{1}$INH deficiency with angioedema due to appearance of IgG anti-C$\bar{1}$INH (type 2) B cell malignancy has not been prominent.

Urticaria and angioedema must be differentiated from contact sensitivity, an acute vesicular eruption that progresses to chronic thickening of the skin with continued allergenic exposure. They must also be differentiated from atopic dermatitis, a condition that may present as erythema, edema, papules, vesiculation, and oozing proceeding to a subacute and chronic stage in which vesiculation is less marked or absent, and in which scaling, fissuring, and lichenification predominate in a distribution that characteristically involves the flexor surfaces. In cutaneous mastocytosis the reddish-brown macules and papules, characteristic of urticaria pigmentosa, urticate with pruritus upon trauma, and in systemic mastocytosis, without or with urticaria pigmentosa, there is an episodic systemic flushing with or without urticaria but no angioedema.

Prevention and treatment Identification of the etiologic factor(s) and their elimination provide the most satisfactory therapeutic program; this approach is feasible to varying degrees with IgE-mediated reactions to allergens or physical stimuli. Topically applied steroids are of no benefit in the management of urticaria and/or angioedema, and while systemic steroids have no general value, they are helpful in an occasional patient with necrotizing cutaneous angiitis, pressure urticaria, or even ordinary urticaria and angioedema. Antihistamines of the H1 class and sympathomimetic agents often provide symptomatic relief; cyproheptadine, hydroxyzine, and a combination of H1 and H2 antihistamines are held to be even more beneficial. The therapy of inborn C$\bar{1}$INH deficiency has been simplified by the finding that attenuated androgens correct the biochemical defect and afford prophylactic protection. Since the affected individuals are heterozygous, with the depletion of C$\bar{1}$INH being due to a combination of deficient synthesis and excessive utilization of the normal gene product, the efficacy of the attenuated androgens is attributed to production by the normal gene of an amount of functional C$\bar{1}$INH sufficient to control the spontaneous activation of C1 to C$\bar{1}$. Since the use of such agents for children and pregnant women is not yet accepted, the antifibrinolytic agent ϵ-aminocaproic acid may be used occasionally to control spontaneous attacks or for preoperative prophylaxis in some patients.

ALLERGIC RHINITIS Definition Allergic rhinitis is characterized by sneezing, rhinorrhea, obstruction of the nasal passages, conjunctival and pharyngeal itching, and lacrimation. Although commonly seasonal because of its relation to airborne pollens, other patterns and etiologies occur. The use of the term "hay fever" to describe seasonal allergic rhinitis is a common convention but is literally inappropriate because the symptom complex is neither produced by hay nor associated with fever.

Predisposing factors and etiology Allergic rhinitis generally presents in atopic individuals, that is, in persons with a family history of a similar or related symptom complex and a personal history of collateral allergy expressed as eczematous dermatitis, urticaria, and/or asthma (see Chap. 204). Symptoms generally appear before the fourth decade of life and tend to diminish gradually with aging, although complete spontaneous remissions are uncommon. A relatively small number of weeds which depend upon wind rather than insects for cross-pollination, as well as certain grasses and trees, produce sufficient quantities of pollen suitable for wide distribution by air currents to elicit seasonal allergic rhinitis. The dates of pollination of these species generally vary little from year to year in a particular locale but may be quite different in another climate. Molds, which are widespread in nature because they occur in soil or decaying organic matter, may propagate spores in a pattern dependent upon climatic conditions. Perennial allergic rhinitis occurs in response to allergens that are present throughout the year such as in desquamating epithelium in animal dander, the processed materials or chemicals utilized in an industrial setting, or the dust accumulating at work or at home. Dust has a diverse content including mites, and many patients with perennial rhinitis are sensitive only to house dust. Moreover, in many patients with perennial rhinitis, no clear-cut allergen can be demonstrated. The ability of allergens to cause rhinitis rather than lower respiratory symptoms may be attributed to their size, 10 to 100 μm, and retention within the nose. However, even when the allergen penetrates to the lower respiratory tract, whether it elicits a bronchoconstrictor response resulting from mediator release depends on the presence of chronically hyperirritable airways.

Pathophysiology and manifestations Episodic rhinorrhea, sneezing, and obstruction of the nasal passages with lacrimation and pruritus of the conjunctiva, nasal mucosa, and oropharynx are the hallmarks of allergic rhinitis. The nasal mucosa is pale and boggy, but the nares are not reddened or excoriated. The conjunctiva may be congested and edematous; the pharynx is generally unremarkable but may appear injected. Swelling of the turbinates and mucous membranes with obstruction of the sinus ostia and eustachian tubes precipitates secondary infections of the sinuses and middle ear, respectively, commonly in perennial but rarely in seasonal disease. Nasal polyps often arise concurrently with edema and/or infection within the sinuses and increase obstructive symptoms.

The nose presents a large mucosal surface area through the folds of the turbinates and serves to adjust the temperature and moisture content of inhaled air and to filter out particulate materials. The convoluted nasal passages readily filter out particles above 10 μm in size by impingement in a mucous blanket at bends in their course; ciliary action then moves the entrapped particles toward the pharynx. Entrapment of pollen and digestion of the outer coat by mucosal enzymes such as lysozymes release protein allergens generally of 10,000 to 40,000 molecular weight. Although the initial interaction occurs between the allergen and intraepithelial mast cells sensitized with specific IgE, the bulk of the mast cells are located beneath the mucosal surface and are recruited secondarily. During the symptomatic season when the mucosa are already swollen and hyperemic, there is enhanced adverse reactivity to the seasonal pollen as well as to antigenically unrelated pollens for which there is underlying hypersensitivity. This priming effect is attributed to improved penetration of the allergens to the deeper perivenular mast cells. Biopsy specimens of nasal mucosa during an episodic allergic reaction show profound submucosal edema with infiltration predominantly by eosinophils, although some neutrophil polymorphonuclear leukocytes are present. Polyps, a feature in perennial rhinitis, are mucosal protrusions containing chiefly edema fluid with variable degrees of eosinophilic infiltration.

The mucosal surface fluid contains not only IgA that is present preferentially because of its secretory piece, but also IgE, which apparently arrives by diffusion from plasma cells distributed in proximity to mucosal surfaces. IgE fixes to mucosal and submucosal mast cells, and the intensity of the clinical response to inhaled allergens is quantitatively related to the naturally occurring or experimentally defined pollen dose. Specific IgE is distributed not only to tissue mast cells but also to circulating basophilic leukocytes; patients with more severe clinical disease have basophils which release histamine in response to lesser concentrations of allergen in vitro than do cells from patients with milder disease. Human nasal polyps from ragweed-sensitive patients release histamine, eosinophilotactic peptides, and spasmogenic leukotrienes upon challenge with ragweed allergen in vitro. In sensitive individuals, the introduction of allergen into the nose is associated with sneezing, "stuffiness," and discharge, and the fluid contains histamine, PGD_2, and leukotrienes. Thus, the mast cells of nasal polyp tissue, and of the nasal mucosa and submucosa, generate and release mediators through IgE-dependent reactions which are capable of producing tissue edema and eosinophilic infiltration.

Diagnosis The diagnosis of seasonal allergic rhinitis depends largely upon an accurate history of occurrence coincident with the pollination of the offending weeds, grasses, or trees. The continuous character of perennial allergic rhinitis due to contamination of the home or place of work makes historical analysis difficult, but there may be a variability in symptoms that can be related to animal exposure or work habits. Patients with perennial rhinitis commonly develop the problem in adult life, are more often women than men, and manifest nasal polyps and thickening of the sinus membranes by x-ray. The term *vasomotor rhinitis* designates a symptom complex resembling perennial allergic rhinitis without an established allergic basis. Other entities to be excluded are exposure to irritants, upper respiratory infection, pregnancy with prominent nasal mucosal edema, prolonged topical use of alpha-adrenergic agents in the form of nose drops, and the use of certain therapeutic agents such as rauwolfia. Nasal polyps are a characteristic of perennial allergic rhinitis and are often associated with sinus infection.

The nasal secretions of allergic patients are rich in eosinophils, and peripheral eosinophilia with elevations in relation to clinical exacerbations is a common feature. Local or systemic neutrophilia implies infection. Total serum IgE is frequently elevated, but the demonstration of immunologic specificity for IgE is critical to an etiologic diagnosis. Some normal individuals will exhibit a wheal-and-flare skin response to intracutaneous inoculation of high concentrations of common airborne allergens. The diagnosis rests not only on the skin test alone, but also on the correlation of the clinical history with skin reactivity to concentrations of allergen selected by controlled testing. This provides the best balance of selectivity with specificity. Scratch tests with food allergens are unreliable, while intracutaneous testing may be dangerous, and elimination diets are the best approach to the diagnosis. Regardless of method of testing, food allergy is uncommon as a significant cause of allergic rhinitis.

Although standard radioimmunodiffusion techniques can be used to screen for patients with markedly elevated levels of IgE, their sensitivity of less than 1000 ng/mL is insufficient to detect the elevations in most atopic allergic patients. A commonly employed technique, sensitive to about 50 ng/mL, is known as the competitive radioimmunosorbent test (RIST). In this procedure, the IgE of the serum competes with radiolabeled IgE for solid-phase-bound anti-IgE; the displacement of radiolabeled IgE is compared to a standard curve to yield the IgE concentration of the serum. Other assays, such as the noncompetitive RIST, in which the anti-IgE immunosorbent is exposed to a series of standard IgE preparations before introducing the unknown, and double-antibody radioimmunoprecipitin test (RIP), have greater sensitivity and reproducibility, respectively, and, like the competitive RIST, establish a normal geometric mean serum IgE for nonallergic whites of less than 120 ng/mL. Even more useful is the measurement of specific anti-IgE in serum by its binding to a solid-phase allergen and quantitation by the subsequent uptake of radiolabeled anti-IgE. This radioallergosorbent technique (RAST) correlates satisfactorily with the bioassay of specific IgE by skin test or histamine release from peripheral blood leukocytes and is convenient for the patients; however, it requires defined allergens and full standardization. Further, neither the immunochemical nor bioassay detection of a previous immune response to a foreign material mandates a therapeutic intervention, unless there is relevant concomitant evidence of a significant clinical problem.

Prevention and treatment Avoidance of exposure to the offending allergen is the most effective means of controlling allergic diseases; removal of pets from the home to avoid animal danders, utilization of air filtration devices to minimize the concentrations of airborne pollens, travel to nonpollinating areas during the critical periods, and even a change of domicile to eliminate a mold spore problem may be necessary. *Immunotherapy,* often termed *hyposensitization,* consists of repeated subcutaneous injections of gradually increasing concentrations of the allergen(s) considered to be specifically responsible for the symptom complex. Controlled studies in ragweed and grass allergic rhinitis have established that patients are partially relieved of their symptoms by such treatments applied over a period of years. Improvement appears to be dose-related, and the end point is based either on severe adverse local or systemic reactions to the allergen injection or on satisfactory relief of symptoms. The immunologic characteristics of a response include a rise in antibodies of the IgG class, a small increase in specific IgE early in the treatment course followed by a plateau or decline, and a decline in the percentage of histamine released from peripheral blood basophilic leukocytes challenged with a fixed concentration of the allergen. The antibodies of the IgG class might well reduce or neutralize the quantity of allergen available for interaction with the tissue mast cells but, more importantly, could modify the seasonal booster response in specific IgE synthesis. None of the individual parameters of the response to immunotherapy correlates well with the assessments of clinical efficacy, suggesting that benefit is derived from a complex of effects. Immunotherapy should be reserved for clearly documented seasonal diseases that cannot be managed with drugs because of their side effects.

Management with pharmacologic agents offers a diverse approach. Antihistamines are the only specific end-organ antagonists available for control of a mast cell–derived reaction and are limited to competition with but one mediator. Nonetheless, antihistamines are very effective for some patients, and the side effects such as drowsiness and gastrointestinal distress, which limit the dosage of a particular preparation, can sometimes be circumvented by use of an agent of different structure. An orally active agent with alpha-adrenergic activity is often employed for its decongestant effects and to partially counteract the drowsiness produced by antihistamines. Topical administration of alpha-adrenergic agents may be helpful but has the immediate disadvantage of rebound vasodilatation, and prolonged usage may produce a chronic rhinitis. The topically active steroids of the beclomethasone class ameliorate symptoms of both seasonal and perennial rhinitis without detectable adrenal suppression and represent a major advance in therapy. Cromolyn sodium inhaled nasally has also given encouraging prophylactic results and is of particular merit because it acts to prevent mast cell activation.

REFERENCES

Austen KF: Biologic implications of the structural and functional characteristics of the chemical mediators of immediate-type hypersensitivity. The Harvey Lectures, Series 73, 1977–1978, p 93

Caulfield JP et al: Secretion in dissociated human pulmonary mast cells. Evidence for solubilization of granule contents before discharge. J Cell Biol 85:299, 1980

Creticos PS et al: Peptide leukotriene release after antigen challenge in patients sensitive to ragweed. N Engl J Med 310:1626, 1984

Green GR et al: Evaluation of penicillin hypersensitivity: Value of clinical history and skin testing with penicilloyl-polylysine and penicillin G. J Allerg Clin Immunol 60:339, 1977

Ishizaka T, Ishizaka K: Activation of mast cells for mediator release through IgE receptors. Progr Allergy 34:188, 1984

Lewis RA, Austen KF: The biologically active leukotrienes: Biosynthesis, metabolism, receptors, functions, and pharmacology. J Clin Invest 73:889, 1984

Marsh DG et al: Genetics of the human immune response to allergens. J Allerg Clin Immunol 65:322, 1980

Schwartz LB, Austen KF: The mast cells and mediators of immediate hypersensitivity, in *Immunological Diseases*, 4th ed, M Samter et al (eds). Boston, Little, Brown, 1988, p 157

Soter NA et al: Urticaria and arthralgias as manifestations of necrotizing angiitis (vasculitis). J Invest Dermatol 63:485, 1974

———: Release of mast cell mediators and alterations in lung function in patients with cholinergic urticaria. N Engl J Med 302:604, 1980

268 IMMUNE-COMPLEX DISEASES

THOMAS J. LAWLEY / MICHAEL M. FRANK

DEFINITION The term *immune-complex disease* refers to a group of diseases thought to be mediated by the deposition of immune complexes in specific organ or tissue sites including the glomerulus of the kidney and blood vessel walls. In general these immune deposits are thought to arise from antigen-antibody complexes formed in the circulation. Once deposited in tissues, the complexes activate a variety of potent soluble mediators of inflammation, such as the complement proteins, causing an influx of polymorphonuclear neutrophils and monocytes. These activated cells release toxic products of oxygen metabolism as well as various proteases and other enzymes, ultimately causing tissue damage. While the specific etiology of these diseases is variable, they share a common pathophysiology. The clinical features of these diseases are quite diverse, ranging from mild cutaneous eruptions to severe organ involvement with pericarditis, glomerulonephritis, and vasculitis.

PATHOPHYSIOLOGY The introduction of foreign or noxious materials into an individual is often followed by an immune response. Specific antibody produced in the course of this response binds to antigen, forming immune complexes. In general, these complexes are phagocytosed and destroyed by macrophages of the reticuloendothelial system. However, at times these complexes are deposited in tissues, causing inflammation and tissue damage. In recent years, there has been a concerted effort to understand the mechanisms underlying this damage.

The biologic activity of the complexes has been studied in detail. It has been shown that the isotype of antibody affects biologic activity. Thus IgG- and IgM-containing complexes activate the classic complement pathway, and IgA-containing complexes may activate the alternative complement pathway. In contrast, cell surface IgE complexes are capable of mediating the degranulation of mast cells by a noncytotoxic, complement-independent mechanism.

The size of the immune complexes in the circulation is an important parameter of toxicity. In general the larger (>19 S) complexes cause more tissue damage than the smaller complexes. The size is related to the concentration and molar ratio of antibody and antigen, as well as to the avidity of the antibody for the antigen. The ratio of antigen to antibody may range from antibody excess through antigen-antibody equivalence to antigen excess. In marked antibody excess, antigen valences are saturated and in general the complexes are small. Under conditions of marked antigen excess, antibody-combining sites are saturated, chances for lattice formation are limited, and, again, the complexes are small. At equivalence or mild antigen excess, lattice formation is facilitated, and large complexes can form. Immune complexes formed at moderate antigen excess are thought to be most pathogenic, perhaps because they are most efficient at activating the various mediator systems like the complement cascade.

Net charge of antigen and antibody also appears to be important in determining the pathophysiologic effect of the complexes. It has been shown that positively charged immune complexes tend to deposit in renal glomeruli, while complexes containing similar antigen with neutral charge tend to penetrate glomeruli slowly. This is presumably due to the fact that the glomerulus presents a negatively charged surface to the circulation. Similarly, there is a relationship between the degree of binding of immune complexes to the basement membrane of skin, which is also negatively charged, and the degree of positive charge of the complexes.

The first human disease in which circulating immune complexes were thought to play a pathogenic role was serum sickness. In their classic monograph, "Die Serumkrankheit," Clemens von Pirquet and Bela Schick described in great detail their experiences with the use of horse antidiphtheria toxin in children. They found that a reproducible reaction pattern occurred 8 to 13 days following the subcutaneous injection of horse serum protein. The patients developed fever, malaise, cutaneous eruptions, arthralgias, leukopenia, lymphadenopathy, and albuminuria. The authors suggested that this reaction pattern was caused by the interaction of host antibody, formed in the 8 days following the injection of the horse serum, with horse serum protein. They believed that this interaction led to the deposition of antigen-antibody complexes in tissue with resulting tissue damage, but the technology necessary to pursue this hypothesis was not available.

Numerous large retrospective studies of human serum sickness confirmed the observations of von Pirquet and Schick, but it was not until the studies of Germuth and Dixon that evidence for the role of circulating immune complexes in serum sickness was obtained. These investigators utilized rabbit models of serum sickness.

In the acute serum sickness model, the injection of antigen is followed by a period of intravascular equilibration and then by intravascular-extravascular equilibration lasting several days. The equilibration period is followed by a progressive decline in the level of antigen in the circulation, representing the normal degradation of the injected serum protein. Following this period of decay, there is a sudden acceleration in the clearance of the antigen from the circulation, usually beginning at about 7 to 8 days. The period of rapid decline in the level of antigen in the circulation is due to the development of an immune response in the recipient animal. This

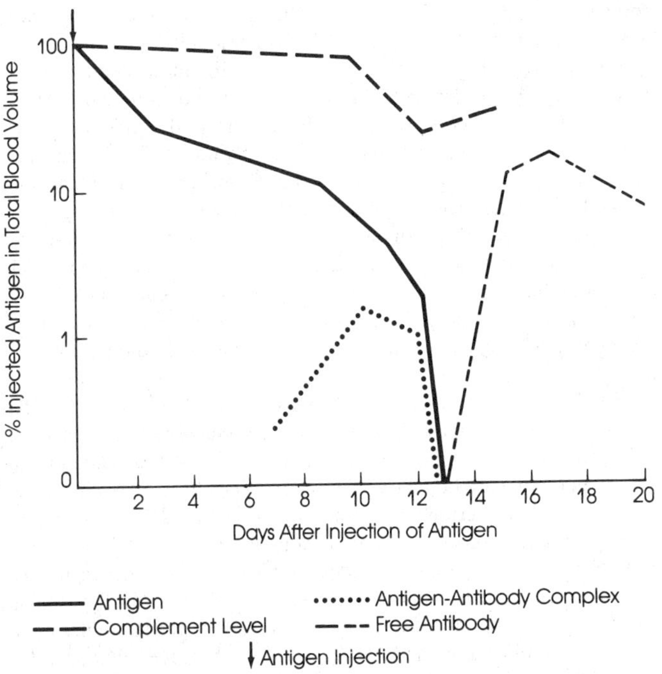

FIGURE 268-1 The rabbit model of acute serum sickness. Radiolabeled antigen is injected at day 0. After a period of equilibration of antigen between the intravascular and extravascular space, there is progressive elimination of antigen from the circulation. With the onset of the animal's immune response there is rapid elimination of antigen from the circulation. Coincident with the phase of rapid elimination is the appearance of antigen-antibody complexes in the circulation and a fall in serum complement. Complete antigen clearance is associated with the appearance of free antibody in the circulation. At the time when antigen-antibody complexes are seen in the circulation, immunopathologic findings are maximal.

results in the formation of antigen-antibody complexes and subsequent clearance of the complexes from the circulation by the cells of the reticuloendothelial system (RES) (Fig. 268-1). During the period in which the complexes are being formed in the circulation, there is a fall in the animal's serum complement levels. At this time pathologic changes occur in large arteries, renal glomeruli, joints, and cardiac vessels. The glomerulonephritis noted during this period has been studied extensively. It is characterized by swelling of the endothelial cells and marked proteinuria with little hematuria; an infiltrate of monocytes but very few granulocytes is found in the renal glomeruli. Immunofluorescence studies have shown that antigen, host immunoglobulin, and C3 are deposited along the glomerular basement membrane in a typical granular pattern. On electron-microscopic examination of kidney sections, few abnormalities are seen except swelling of endothelial cells. Late in the reaction subepithelial deposits of electron-dense material are noted in some animals; however, at this time fluorescent antibody examination is negative for immunoglobulin and complement in the glomeruli. The deposits may represent immunologically altered immunoglobulin or complement.

There is also a very high incidence of arteritis in the coronary artery outflow tract and at branching points of the aorta in the acute serum sickness model. The arteritis is characterized by marked intimal proliferation of endothelium. This is followed by degradation of the internal elastic lamina and adventitia with resulting fibrinoid necrosis of the vessel. On immunofluorescence microscopy, host immunoglobulin, antigen, and C3 are found roughly in the region of the internal elastic lamina, but these immunoreactive materials are rapidly removed and are gone in several days. It has been suggested that the polymorphonuclear neutrophils present in the lesions phagocytize these complexes. In contrast to the findings in glomerulonephritis, materials which decrease complement activity or inhibit the polymorphonuclear leukocytic response diminish or block the development of arteritis.

At the time of the development of serum sickness in this animal model, there are high-molecular-weight immune complexes in the circulation; the animals that become sick regularly have complexes that are greater than 19 S in their sedimentation characteristics. Acute serum sickness is present only as long as these circulating immune complexes persist and resolves rapidly once the antigen is cleared from the circulation and the immune complexes are gone.

It is possible to induce chronic glomerulonephritis in animals by the repeated intravenous injection of the antigen. The dose of antigen injected is critical to the development of the disease. Antigen excess must be produced after each antigen administration, and immune complexes must circulate in the animals. These animals develop glomerulonephritis but not the arteritis characteristic of acute serum sickness.

Other animal models of immune-complex disease closely resemble systemic lupus erythematosus. The most widely studied and best characterized is the disease that occurs spontaneously in the F_1 hybrid of New Zealand black (NZB) and New Zealand white (NZW) mice. These animals develop antibodies to nucleic acids including double-stranded DNA and have decreased numbers of suppressor T cells. They also develop circulating immune complexes and an immune-complex-mediated glomerulonephritis that eventuates in renal insufficiency and death. Direct immunofluorescence microscopy of the kidneys in these animals reveals deposits of DNA, antibodies to DNA, and C3 in the glomerular basement membrane. The female NZB-NZW mice develop these changes before the males, and this sex difference may be related to a switch in the class of antibodies to DNA from IgM to IgG that occurs much earlier in the females than in the males.

Over the years a great deal of attention has been paid to the fate of immune complexes in animal models. Injection of antigens into immunized animals is followed by the deposition of the antigen in the liver, spleen, and lung, all elements of the RES. Detailed studies have examined the fate of preformed immune complexes of carefully determined size in a variety of animals. In general, the findings of these studies have paralleled those reported in the animal models of serum sickness. The very large insoluble complexes are rapidly removed from the circulation. Soluble complexes that are greater than 19 S in their sedimentation characteristics are removed by the liver and persist in the circulation for only a matter of minutes. The major factor appearing to govern the rate of clearance of these large, preformed complexes from the circulation is the rate of hepatic blood flow. In some studies complement activation by complexes is also important in their metabolism, and injected complexes go through a complex series of processing steps. Large-lattice-size complexes appear to be dissociated by complement into smaller entities. Following injection, complexes containing complement components become associated with cells with complement receptors. Human erythrocytes have complement receptors, and these cells appear to be particularly important in the processing of complexes. It is believed that complement-coated complexes associate with complement receptors on red cell surfaces and that the complexes are stripped from these cells as they course through the sinusoids of the liver. They are then metabolized. Fc receptors for IgG also play a prominent role in the removal of IgG-containing immune complexes from the circulation, and any manipulation that affects the interaction of Fc receptors and the Fc fragment of IgG in the complexes predisposes to failure to clear the complexes and to tissue deposition. It is possible to measure RES Fc-receptor functional activity in patients and normal individuals by intravenously injecting IgG-sensitized autologous radiolabeled erythrocytes and then monitoring the rate of disappearance of these immune particles from the bloodstream. In those diseases with tissue deposition of immune complexes there tends to be an associated RES Fc-receptor defect and delayed clearance of the antibody-sensitized cells from the circulation. Another form of immune-complex-mediated tissue damage follows local formation of immune complexes in tissues such as the kidney. Glomerular subepithelial immune-complex deposits are thought to form often on an in-site basis. This may occur as a result of antibody binding to fixed glomerular antigens or antibody binding to "planted" nonglomerular antigens. In the latter instance it is believed that certain cationic antigens can bind to the laminae rarae of the capillary wall in a glomerulus through charge-dependent mechanisms. This "planted" antigen is then recognized by antibody, and local tissue damage results.

DETECTION OF CIRCULATING IMMUNE COMPLEXES Many different assays are available for the detection of soluble immune complexes in various biologic fluids. Although these assays vary in their sensitivity and reproducibility, they have expanded our understanding of circulating immune complexes and their role in various disease states. In general, early tests for the detection of circulating immune complexes relied on physical characteristics of the immune complexes, such as their high molecular weight or cold insolubility. These rather insensitive techniques have been replaced by assays for immunologic components or biologic activities of immune complexes. Although there are now sensitive radioimmunoassays for the detection of circulating immune complexes containing IgG, IgM, and IgA, these tests are not antigen-specific. In fact, in most cases in which circulating immune complexes are demonstrable, the component antigen(s) is (are) unknown. As with most laboratory tests, immune-complex assays may be influenced by other factors. Anticoagulants, endotoxin, and free DNA as well as immunoglobulin aggregates formed after the sample is obtained may result in false-positive results. The impact of these factors can be reduced by the selection of immune-complex assays that are unaffected by these variables and by the use of two or more different assays in situations in which critical evaluation of circulating immune complexes is desired. Several of the most sensitive and commonly used immune-complex assays will be described briefly: (1)C1q binding, or solid-phase radioassays, (2)Raji cell assays, and (3)conglutinin assays. *C1q* is a subcomponent of the first component of complement and will bind to immune complexes containing IgG subclasses 1 to 3 or IgM via noncovalent attachment to a specific site on the Fc portion of immunoglobulin. *Raji cells* are a lymphoblastoid cell line with cell surface receptors for complement, especially C3. The assays are based on the ability of circulating immune complexes that contain bound complement components in their lattices to bind to the surface of the Raji cells via the complement receptors. The bound complexes are easily detected. *Conglutinin* is a 750-kDa nonimmunoglobulin protein found in certain bovine sera that will bind to a cleavage fragment of human C3 known as iC3b. Immune complexes containing iC3b will bind to conglutinin attached to a solid-phase substrate and can be detected.

SERUM SICKNESS Drug hypersensitivity reactions are the most common cause of serum sickness today. It is hypothesized that the drug acting as a hapten binds to a plasma protein. The drug-protein complex is seen as foreign and induces typical serum sickness. Commonly occurring signs and symptoms of serum sickness include fever, cutaneous eruptions (morbilliform and/or urticarial), arthralgias, lymphadenopathy, and albuminuria. Less common manifestations are arthritis, nephritis, neuropathy, and vasculitis. The time required for primary sensitization to an offending agent is approximately 1 to 3 weeks. However, clinical manifestations may develop within 12 to 36 h if there is a history of a previous immunizing exposure. Drug-induced serum sickness usually abates within days after withdrawal of the causative agent. Reactions may persist for longer intervals, particularly if repository or long-acting agents are responsible for the problem. Drugs responsible for serum sickness include penicillin, sulfonamides, thiouracils, hydantoins, *p*-aminosalicylic acid, phenylbutazone, thiazides, and streptomycin. Foreign antisera and blood products may also induce serum sickness reactions.

Recent studies of patients receiving intravenous infusions of horse antithymocyte globulin (ATG) as therapy for bone marrow failure have confirmed and expanded the immunologic findings in animal models of serum sickness in humans. The patients develop signs and symptoms of serum sickness 8 to 13 days after beginning therapy with ATG (Fig. 268-2). These include fever; malaise; cutaneous eruptions; arthralgias and arthritis, mainly of the large joints; gastrointestinal distress with nausea, vomiting, and melena; lymphadenopathy; and proteinuria. Clinical disease coincides with the development of very high levels of circulating immune complexes as measured by the ^{125}I-labeled C1q binding assay and marked decreases in serum C3, C4, and CH_{50} levels. Interestingly, the first cutaneous manifestation of serum sickness is a previously undescribed cutaneous sign, namely, a serpiginous band of erythema occurring along the sides of the hands, feet, fingers, and toes at the junction of palmar or plantar skin with the dorsolateral surface. Direct immunofluorescence of involved skin during serum sickness reveals deposits of immunoglobulins and C3 in the walls of small cutaneous blood vessels in most patients. These studies provide strong support for a pathogenic role for circulating immune complexes in the pathophysiology of human serum sickness.

SYSTEMIC LUPUS ERYTHEMATOSUS Systemic lupus erythematosus (SLE) is a multisystem disease associated with a number of immunologic abnormalities including the production of autoantibodies, hypergammaglobulinemia, suppressor-T-cell abnormalities, decreased levels of serum complement, and increased levels of circulating immune complexes. Immune complexes are thought to play a critical role in the pathophysiology of SLE. Early evidence for the role of circulating immune complexes in SLE included the finding by direct immunofluorescence of glomerular deposits of immunoglobulin, complement, and DNA in kidney biopsies. Mixed IgM-IgG cryoglobulins were found in the sera of a substantial number of SLE patients, and when the antibody specificity of these cryoprecipitates was examined, reactivity was found against single- and double-stranded DNA as well as ribonucleoprotein. Utilizing the newer, more sensitive assays, circulating immune complexes have been found in a high percentage of patients with SLE. An explanation for the continued circulation of immune complexes in patients with SLE has been provided by the demonstration of defective function of the reticuloendothelial system (RES) in these patients. Patients with SLE have been shown to have delayed clearance of autologous red blood cells coated with IgG from the circulation, suggesting an impaired function of RES Fc-IgG receptors. The prolonged RES clearance in these patients was found to be correlated with increased levels of circulating immune complexes as measured by the C1q binding assay and with clinical disease activity. Studies in the same patients after their disease improved with treatment revealed a significant correlation between clinical improvement, improvement of Fc-mediated clearance, and decreased levels of circulating immune complexes. Individuals with SLE also have decreased numbers of C3b receptors on their erythrocytes. Whether the decreased number of receptors is primary or secondary remains to be established. Nonetheless, abnormalities of both Fc-IgG and C3b receptors which are responsible for phagocytosis of circulating immune complexes are present in patients with SLE.

VASCULITIS There is strong circumstantial evidence for the role of circulating immune complexes in the various forms of hypersensitivity or necrotizing vasculitis. Features of the classic "palpable purpura" of cutaneous necrotizing vasculitis closely resemble the clinical, histopathologic and immunopathologic features of the Arthus reaction. The Arthus reaction is a model for immune-complex-mediated vascular damage in which antigen is injected intradermally into an animal which possesses circulating antibody against that antigen. In both vasculitis and the Arthus reaction, deposits of immunoglobulin and complement are found in the walls of blood vessels in early lesions. The histopathology of both consists of infiltrates of polymorphonuclear neutrophils, leukocytoclasis, endothelial cell damage and necrosis, hemorrhage, and perivascular deposits of fibrin. Electron microscopy of lesions of cutaneous necrotizing vasculitis reveals subendothelial electron-dense deposits compatible with immune complexes. The available evidence indicates the presence of immune complexes at the site of tissue damage in necrotizing vasculitis. In accord with these findings is the demonstration of circulating immune complexes in a high percentage of patients with this disease.

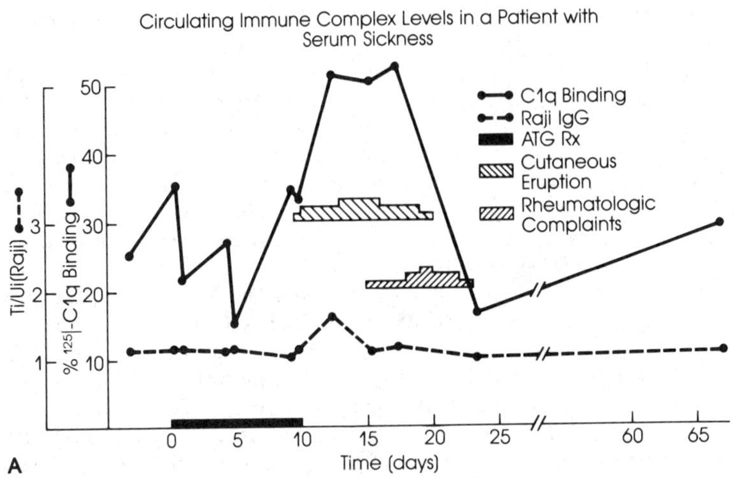

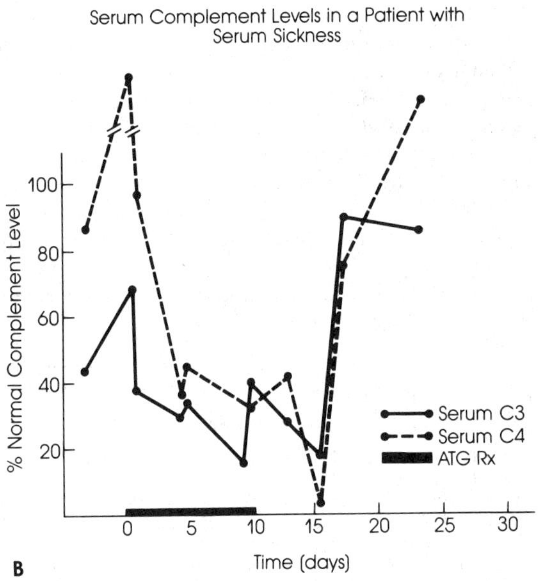

FIGURE 268-2 Serum sickness in human beings. Horse antithymocyte globulin was injected into patients with aplastic anemia daily for 10 days. After the fifth day of injection, C1q binding activity begins to rise (*A*). At the same time there is a dramatic fall in plasma levels of C3 and C4 and onset of clinical symptoms (*B*).

LABORATORY FINDINGS In theory the essential feature of immune-complex disease would be the finding of circulating immune complexes. In practice there is great variability from disease to disease in the frequency of positive immune-complex assays. In some diseases, such as SLE, there is a high frequency of positive immune-complex assays. In others, like membranoproliferative glomerulonephritis, the frequency of positive assays is much lower. Part of the reason for this has to do with the stage of disease under study. In some cases immunologic phenomena are responsible for the initiation of the disease and the initial tissue insult. However, subsequent injury is caused by scarring, inflammation, and repair mechanisms that result in more extensive tissue damage. Thus, progression of disease may occur at a time when immunologic injury is no longer occurring. A second reason for the failure to detect circulating immune complexes in diseases thought to be mediated by them has to do with technical difficulties in the measurement of such complexes. There are many types of assays for immune complexes. Most are indirect and rely on a biologic or biochemical property of the complexes such as the binding of complement components. The pattern of positive reaction clearly varies from disease to disease. Clearly each assay recognizes a different type of complex with maximal efficiency. Since multiple assays are rarely performed on one specimen, complexes, although present, may not be detected. Finally, although a disease is classified as immune-complex-related because of the finding of immune deposits in affected tissues or because of the similarity of its pathologic findings to those of animal models of immune-complex disease, the disease may not be actually caused by circulating immune complexes. For example, antibody may be formed to a tissue component, bind to it in a tissue site, and induce damage. Such is thought to be the case in Goodpasture's disease. For all of these reasons, assays for the detection of circulating immune complex, while often useful, are rarely critical for diagnosis or patient management.

Examination of tissues using immunofluorescent techniques to detect immune deposits is also of great interest in establishing the diagnosis of immune-complex disease. Immune complexes deposited in tissues may be evanescent. For example, in cutaneous vasculitis, lesions must be biopsied within 12 h of their appearance. Although helpful in diagnosis and in establishing pathogenesis, testing for immune deposits in tissue is rarely required for diagnosis.

Another test commonly used to infer the presence of immune complexes is the measurement of serum complement. Decreased levels are taken to indicate the presence of complexes. In fact, it has been suggested that the levels of serum C4 and C3 are the most sensitive indexes of disease activity in SLE. However, the correlation between disease activity and complement levels is rough at best, and some patients with active SLE may have relatively normal complement levels for several reasons. The normal range of complement component levels is wide, and a given patient may have depressed levels with serum concentrations falling from high-normal levels to low-normal levels. In general complement components act as acute phase reactants, and the lowering of serum complement may be masked by increased synthesis. Moreover, under many circumstances activation of complement may mediate profound pathophysiologic effects, although few molecules of complement are actually involved. For example, complement binding to red cells may be responsible for much of the red cell destruction that occurs with ABO-mismatched transfusions; yet serum complement levels may be unchanged because too few molecules are used in erythyrocyte destruction to detect a fall in titer. Finally, all types of complexes do not activate complement in the same way. Massive antigen release from red cells occurring during the course of vivax malaria infection leads to the rapid formation of antigen-antibody complexes in the circulation. For unknown reasons these complexes only interact with the early components of the classic complement pathway, while C3 and the later complement components are not recruited. Thus, if one measures levels of C3, no fall in titer is noted, although complexes are present and massive complement activation has taken place. The complexes formed in SLE activate optimally the classic pathway; presumably those involved in IgA glomerulonephritis activate the alternative pathway. Therefore, the complement test chosen for examination may be important.

Other tests may suggest indirectly the presence of immune-complex disease. For example, a finding of mixed IgG-IgM cryoprecipitates suggests the presence of immune complexes. The presence of antinuclear antibodies suggests autoimmunity, as does the presence of a number of tissue-component-specific antibodies. Similarly, the presence of specific antigen such as hepatitis B surface antigen in the circulation together with appropriate clinical symptoms may suggest an immune-complex disease. Most patients with active immune-complex-mediated disease have an elevated erythrocyte sedimentation rate, although this is not invariably the case. Patients with Takayasu's arteritis may have a normal erythrocyte sedimentation rate during the later phases of the evolution of lesions when most pathology is caused by scarring, fibrosis, and repair within vessel walls. Finally, specific laboratory test findings such as red cell casts in the urine in glomerulonephritis or mild cerebrospinal fluid pleocytosis in the presence of cerebritis are discussed in the chapters concerning those diseases.

TREATMENT The therapy of immune-complex-mediated disease relies upon removal of the offending antigen and interruption of the inflammatory response. In general serum sickness is a self-limited disease that is seldom life-threatening. In the case of drug-induced serum sickness it is most important to discontinue the offending agent. In many instances, supportive care combined with antihistamines for urticaria and acetaminophen for fever, myalgias, and arthralgias is adequate. If serious renal, vascular, or central nervous system involvement occurs, the use of systemic glucocorticoid therapy is indicated.

The therapy of SLE is discussed in Chap. 269 and the therapy of vasculitis is discussed in Chap. 276.

REFERENCES

Cochrane CB, Koffler D: Immune complex disease in experimental animals and man. Adv Immunol 16:185, 1963

Dixon F: The role of antigen-antibody complexes in disease. Harvey Lect 52:21, 1963

Frank MM et al: Immunoglobulin G–Fc receptor mediated clearance in autoimmune diseases. Ann Intern Med 98:206, 1983

Germuth FC Jr.: A comparative histologic and immunologic study in rabbits of induced hypersensitivity of the serum sickness type. J Exp Med 97:257, 1953

Lawley TJ et al: A prospective clinical and immunologic analysis of patients with serum sickness. N Engl J Med 311:1407, 1984

Mannik M, Arend WP: Fate of preformed immune complexes in rabbits and rhesus monkeys. J Exp Med 134:19s, 1971

Von Pirquet C, Schick B: *Serum Sickness*. Baltimore, Williams & Wilkins, 1951

Theofilopoulos AN, Dixon FJ: The biology and detection of immune complexes. Adv Immunol 28:89, 1979

269 SYSTEMIC LUPUS ERYTHEMATOSUS

BEVRA HANNAHS HAHN

DEFINITION AND PREVALENCE Systemic lupus erythematosus (SLE) is a disease of unknown etiology in which tissues and cells are damaged by deposition of pathogenic autoantibodies and immune complexes. Ninety percent of cases are in women, usually of child-bearing age, but children, men, and the elderly can be affected. In the United States, the prevalence of SLE in urban areas varies from 15 to 50 per 100,000; it is more common and more severe in blacks than in whites. Hispanic and Asian populations are also susceptible.

PATHOGENESIS AND ETIOLOGY Production of pathogenic antibodies and immune complexes, coupled with failure to suppress them, are the basic abnormalities underlying SLE. These antibodies are listed in Table 269-1. Not all antibodies or immune complexes are pathogenic. Some antibodies cause disease because of their antigen specificity. Examples are antibodies to erythrocyte surface antigens or to coagulation factors. Others cause disease because of their immunoglobulin (Ig) isotype, ability to fix complement (C′), avidity, and/or electrical charge. For example, complement-fixing cationic antibodies bind to the polyanions in glomerular basement membrane, bind antigen, and cause damage.

The pathogenesis of SLE includes genetic, environmental, and sex hormonal factors. These result in abnormal humoral and cellular immune responses and inadequate clearing of antibodies and immune complexes. Genetic predisposition is indicated by higher concordance for clinical disease in monozygotic than in dizygotic twins, a 10 percent frequency of patients with more than one affected individual in the family; and the fact that 6 percent of SLE patients have inherited deficiencies of complement components. Several genes in the HLA class II and III regions increase the relative risk (RR) for SLE as follows: DR2 (RR3), DR3 (RR3), and null alleles for C4, as in C4A.Q0 (RR3), and C4A.Q0.Q0 (RR17). Combinations of these genes increase RR even further: DR2, C4A.Q0 confers a RR of 25. There are probably additional genes, independent of HLA I, II, and III, which confer susceptibility. Viruses have been suspected as etiologic agents but not yet proven to be. Phospholipids in cell walls of enteric bacteria may act as polyclonal B-cell activators or antigens to elicit antibodies cross-reactive with the ribose phosphate backbone in DNA. In some patients, exposure to ultraviolet light causes disease flares, probably by altering the antigenicity of DNA or the composition of dermal-epidermal junctions. Sex hormone influences contribute to the pathogenesis of SLE. In general, estrogen enhances and testosterone reduces antibody responses. Men and women with SLE have increased hydroxylation of estrogen and estrone to 16 α-hydroxyestrone, producing prolonged estrogenic stimulation. The ultimate outcome of all of these factors is B-cell hyperactivity, accompanied by multiple abnormalities in immunoregulation. For example, quantities of T helper-inducer and T suppressor-cytotoxic cells are diminished during periods of disease activity, and many functions are abnormal. Helper activity is increased, while the ability of suppressors to reduce anti-DNA synthesis is impaired. Direct and antibody-mediated cytotoxicity are also abnormal. Ability of T cells to secrete interleukin 2 is suppressed, and abnormal interferons are produced. Failure to suppress antibody production also results from abnormalities in the humoral idiotype–anti-idiotype network. Finally, immune complexes are cleared more slowly than normal, related in part to both inherited and acquired deficiencies of complement (CR1) receptors on cell surfaces.

Clinical manifestations of the disease are determined by which antibody subpopulations and immune complexes are present in the patient's repertoire; which organs, cells, or cell products are their targets; and the ability of the patient to correct the abnormalities.

CLINICAL MANIFESTATIONS At onset, SLE may involve only one organ system (with additional manifestations occurring later) or may be multisystemic. Clinical manifestations are listed in Table 269-2. Autoantibodies are usually detectable on the patient's initial visit. Disease severity varies from mild and intermittent to persistent and ultimately fatal. Most patients experience exacerbations interspersed with periods of relative quiescence. Fewer than 10 percent have long-lasting, symptom-free remissions. *Systemic symptoms* are usually prominent and include fatigue, malaise, fever, anorexia, weight loss, and nausea.

Musculoskeletal Almost all SLE patients experience arthralgias and myalgias; most develop arthritis. Pain is often out of proportion to physical findings, which include symmetric fusiform swelling of joints [most frequently proximal interphalangeal (PIP) and metacarpophalangeal (MCP) joints of the hands, wrists, and knees], diffuse puffiness of hands and feet, and tenosynovitis. Joint deformities are unusual, although 10 percent of patients develop swan-neck deformities and ulnar drift at the MCP joints. Erosions are rare, but subcutaneous nodules over elbows and fingers occur. Myopathy can be inflammatory and related to active disease or iatrogenic, secondary to hypokalemia or to glucocorticoids or hydroxychloroquine. Ischemic necrosis of bone also causes ''joint'' pain and is a common cause of hip, knee, and shoulder pain in these patients.

Cutaneous The *malar (''butterfly'') rash* is a fixed erythematous rash, flat or raised, over the cheeks and bridge of the nose, often involving the chin and ears. It is usually exacerbated by ultraviolet light. Scarring is absent, but telangiectases may develop. A more diffuse maculopapular rash, predominant in sun-exposed areas, is also common. Its presence usually indicates disease flare. Loss of scalp hair (which often heralds a flare) is usually patchy but can be extensive; the hair will regrow except in discoid lupus erythematosus (DLE). *Vasculitic skin lesions* include subcutaneous nodules, ulcers (usually on the legs), purpura, and infarcts of skin or digits. *DLE lesions* occur in some patients with SLE and can be disfiguring. They are circular with an erythematous rim, raised, and scaly with follicular plugging and telangiectasia. Central scarring produces depigmentation and permanent loss of appendages. They occur over the scalp, ears, face, and sun-exposed areas of the arms, back, and chest. Only 5

TABLE 269-1 Autoantibodies in patients with SLE

	Incidence, %	Antigen detected	Clinical importance
Antinuclear antibodies	95	Multiple nuclear and cytoplasmic antigens	Human cell line substrates are more sensitive than standard murine tissues. A repeatedly negative test on both makes SLE diagnosis unlikely. Multiple antibodies are detected.
Anti-DNA	70	DNA	Anti-dsDNA is relatively disease specific; anti-ssDNA is not. Associated with nephritis and clinical activity.
Anti-Sm	30	Protein complexed to 6 species of small nuclear RNA	Specific for SLE.
Anti-RNP	40	Protein complexed to U1RNA	High titer seen in syndromes with features of polymyositis, scleroderma, lupus, and mixed connective tissue disease. If present in SLE without anti-DNA, risk for nephritis is low.
Anti-Ro (SSA)	30	Protein complexed to Y_1–Y_5 RNA	Associated with Sjögren's syndrome, DR3 haplotype, subacute cutaneous lupus, inherited complement deficiencies, ANA-negative lupus, lupus in the elderly, neonatal lupus, congenital heart block in infants. Can cause nephritis.
Anti-La (SSB)	10	Phosphoprotein complexed with RNA pol III transcripts	Always associated with anti-Ro; risk for nephritis is low if present in SLE. Associated with Sjögren's syndrome.
Antihistone	70	Histones	More frequent in drug-induced LE (95%) than in spontaneous SLE.
Anticardiolipin	50	Phospholipid	Increases risk for venous or arterial thrombosis, thrombocytopenia, and spontaneous abortion. Associated with prolonged PTT (lupus anticoagulant) and false-positive VDRL.
Antierythrocyte	60	Erythrocyte surface antigens	A small proportion of these patients develop overt hemolysis.
Antiplatelet	—	Platelet surface	Associated with thrombocytopenia.
Antilymphocyte	70	Lymphocyte surface antigens	Probably associated with leukopenia and abnormal T-cell function.
Antineuronal	60	Neuronal and lymphocyte surface antigens	In CSF, high IgG titers correlate with diffuse CNS lupus.

percent of individuals with DLE progress to SLE; however, 20 percent of SLE patients have DLE lesions. Less frequent SLE skin lesions include urticaria, periorbital edema, bullae, erythema multiforme, lichen planus–like lesions, and panniculitis (''lupus profundus'').

Patients with *subacute cutaneous lupus* (SCLE) are a distinct subset with recurring extensive skin lesions. Arthritis and fatigue are frequent; central nervous system and renal involvement are not. Some patients are antinuclear antibody (ANA)–negative. The majority have antibodies to Ro (SS-A) or to single-stranded (ss) DNA and carry the HLA-DR3 phenotype. The skin lesions are photosensitive polycyclic annular or papulosquamous psoriasiform lesions over the arms, trunk, and face; they become hypopigmented but not scarred.

Mucous membrane lesions are usually small, shallow, painless ulcers in the mouth and nose.

Renal manifestations Although almost all patients with SLE have deposits of immunoglobulin in glomeruli, only one-half have clinical nephritis, defined by persistent proteinuria. At presentation, most patients are asymptomatic (unless already uremic), except those with edema of the nephrotic syndrome. Urinalysis shows hematuria, cylindruria, and proteinuria. As discussed under ''Pathology'' (see below), most patients with mesangial or mild focal glomerulonephritis do not develop deterioration of renal function. In patients with more severe active or chronic lesions, renal failure is a major cause of death. Since mild lesions may not require aggressive therapy with glucocorticoids and/or cytotoxic drugs whereas severe lesions do, renal biopsy may provide information that will affect therapeutic decisions over the subsequent several months. Patients with deteriorating renal function and active urine sediment also require prompt, aggressive therapy; biopsy is not necessary unless they fail to respond. However, patients with a high proportion of sclerotic glomeruli on biopsy, usually with a serum creatinine of >265 μmol/L (>3 mg/dL), are unlikely to respond to immunosuppressive therapy. In these cases, dialysis or transplantation should be planned. Patients with persistently abnormal urinalyses associated with high titers of antibodies to double-stranded (ds) DNA and hypocomplementemia are also at risk for severe nephritis; kidney biopsy is useful in these cases if the results are likely to have an impact on therapeutic decisions.

Nervous system Any region of the brain can be involved in SLE, as can the meninges, spinal cord, and cranial and peripheral nerves. Central nervous system (CNS) events may be isolated, single or multiple, but they usually occur in the setting of active disease in other systems. Mild mental dysfunction is the most frequent manifestation. Seizures are frequent and may be grand mal, petit mal, or focal. Other manifestations include psychosis, organic brain syndromes, headache (including migraine), focal infarcts with resultant deficits, extrapyramidal disorders, cerebellar dysfunction, hypothalamic dysfunction with inappropriate antidiuretic hormone (ADH) secretion, pseudotumor cerebri, subarachnoid hemorrhage, aseptic meningitis, transverse myelitis with paraplegia or quadriplegia, optic neuritis, cranial nerve palsies, and peripheral sensorimotor neuropathy resulting either in mononeuritis multiplex or glove-and-stocking deficits. Depression and anxiety are frequent.

Laboratory diagnosis of CNS disease can be difficult. Abnormal electroencephalograms are found in about 70 percent of patients and usually show diffuse slowing or focal abnormalities. The cerebrospinal fluid (CSF) shows elevated protein levels in 50 percent and an elevated number of mononuclear cells in 30 percent of patients. Lumbar puncture should be performed whenever CNS symptoms could result from infection, especially in patients receiving immunosuppressive therapy. Brain scans (including CT) and angiograms are most likely to be positive when focal neurologic deficits are present and are less helpful in cases with diffuse, nonfocal manifestations. Magnetic resonance imaging is the most sensitive radiographic technique to

TABLE 269-2 Clinical manifestations of SLE

	Percent of patients positive during course of disease	
Systemic		95
Fatigue, malaise, fever, anorexia, nausea, weight loss		
Musculoskeletal		95
Arthralgias/myalgias	95	
Nonerosive polyarthritis*	60	
Hand deformities	10	
Myopathy/myositis	40/5	
Ischemic necrosis of bone	15	
Cutaneous		80
Malar rash*	50	
Discoid rash*	15	
Photosensitivity*	40	
Oral ulcers*	40	
Other rashes—maculopapular, urticarial, bullous, subacute cutaneous lupus	40	
Alopecia	40	
Vasculitis	20	
Panniculitis	5	
Hematologic	85	
Anemia (of chronic disease) } *	70	
Hemolytic anemia } *	10	
Leukopenia (<4000/mm³) } *	65	
Lymphopenia (<1500/mm³) } *	50	
Thrombocytopenia (<100,000/mm³) } *		
Circulating anticoagulant	15	
Splenomegaly	10–20	
Lymphadenopathy	15	
	20	
Neurologic		60
Organic brain syndromes	35	
Psychosis } *	10	
Seizures } *	20	
Other CNS (see text)	15	
Peripheral neuropathy	15	
Cardiopulmonary		60
Pleurisy } *	50	
Pericarditis } *	30	
Myocarditis } *	10	
Endocarditis (Libman-Sachs)	10	
Pleural effusions	30	
Lupus pneumonitis	10	
Interstitial fibrosis	5	
Pulmonary hypertension	<5	
ARDS/hemorrhage	<5	
Renal		50
Proteinuria >500 mg/24 h } *	50	
Cellular casts } *	50	
Nephrotic syndrome } *	25	
Renal failure } *	5–10	
Gastrointestinal		45
Nonspecific (anorexia, nausea, mild pain, diarrhea)	30	
Vasculitis with bleeding or perforation	5	
Ascites	<5	
Abnormal liver enzymes	40	
Thrombosis		15
Venous	10	
Arterial	5	
Fetal loss		30 (of pregnancies)
Ocular		15
Retinal vasculitis	5	
Conjunctivitis/episcleritis	10	
Sicca syndrome	15	

* In addition to two positive laboratory tests [positive ANA plus one or more of (1) positive LE cells, (2) anti-dsDNA, (3) anti-Sm, or (4) false-positive VDRL], a combination of these clinical and laboratory manifestations totalling four meet American Rheumatism Association criteria for classifying patients as SLE. Bracketed features count as one, even if more than one are present, e.g., leukopenia plus thrombocytopenia = one criterion.

TABLE 269-3 Laboratory manifestations of SLE

Tests that help *confirm the clinical diagnosis and predict severity*	Tests that may be helpful in *following the clinical course**
Relatively specific for SLE:	Titer of anti-dsDNA
anti-dsDNA	Serum complement levels
anti-Sm	Westergren erythrocyte sedimentation rate
Not specific:	Hematocrit
ANA (most sensitive)	Leukocyte count
THC, C3, C4	Platelet count
Anti-Ro	Urinalysis
Direct Coombs' test	Serum creatinine
VDRL	
PTT	
Anticardiolipin	
Hematocrit	
Leukocyte count	
Platelet count	
Urinalysis	
Serum creatinine	

* For each patient, the pattern of laboratory abnormalities (if any) associated with a disease flare should be established and only those tests used subsequently as adjuncts to clinical assessment.

detect structural abnormalities; however, it may be normal in certain SLE patients with CNS disease. Standard laboratory measures of disease activity (Table 269-3) often do not correlate with neurologic manifestations. Neurologic problems usually improve (with the exception of deficits related to infarcts) with therapy and/or time; recurrences are common.

Vascular Thrombosis in capillaries, small vessels, and medium-sized veins and arteries can be a major problem. Although vasculitis may play a role in the thrombotic process, there is increasing evidence that antibodies against phospholipids (anticardiolipin) are associated with clotting. These antibodies may be the ''lupus anticoagulant.'' In addition, degenerative vascular changes associated with years of immune-complex deposition in vessel walls may predispose to symptomatic coronary artery disease in relatively young individuals with SLE. Anticoagulation with warfarin sodium is usually effective in reducing recurrences of venous clots; it is unclear whether any therapies reduce the incidence of arterial clotting.

Hematologic abnormalities The lupus anticoagulant usually binds to phospholipids in the prothrombin activator complex. It prolongs the partial thromboplastin time, an abnormality not corrected by addition of normal plasma. Three clinical sequelae may be associated with it. First, some patients experience repeated episodes of either venous or arterial clotting; these are often serious, especially if associated with pulmonary emboli, strokes, or occlusion of major arteries. Second, if the anticoagulant is associated with thrombocytopenia or hypoprothrombinemia, significant bleeding can occur. Third, in the absence of clotting or bleeding disorders, it may be a benign laboratory abnormality; biopsies and surgery can be performed without increased risk of bleeding. Antibodies to clotting factors (VIII, IX) are often associated with bleeding. Bleeding syndromes usually respond to glucocorticoids.

Anemia of chronic disease occurs in most patients during periods of disease activity. Frank hemolysis occurs in a small proportion of those with positive Coombs' tests; that syndrome is usually responsive to high-dose glucocorticoids. Splenectomy is often effective in steroid-resistant patients.

Leukopenia is common and usually reflects lymphopenia. In general, it is not associated with recurrent infections and does not require treatment.

Mild thrombocytopenia is common. Severe thrombocytopenia with bleeding and purpura occurs in 5 percent of patients and should be treated with high-dose glucocorticoids. If the platelet count has not risen to a safe range in 5 to 14 days, splenectomy should be considered.

Cardiopulmonary Pericardial pain is the most frequent symptom of cardiac lupus; effusions can occur. Tamponade has been reported and constrictive pericarditis occurs, but is rare. Myocarditis can cause arrhythmias and/or cardiac failure. Endocarditis of the Libman-Sachs verrucous type, a diagnosis made at autopsy, is usually not clinically significant; however, it can cause aortic or mitral regurgitation. Rarely, myocardial infarcts result from vasculitis of coronary arteries; more often they are associated with degenerative arterial disease.

Pleurisy and pleural effusions are common manifestations of SLE. Lupus pneumonitis causes recurrent episodes of fever, dyspnea, and cough; x-rays show infiltrates which come and go over a period of days or weeks, and/or areas of platelike atelectasis; this syndrome responds to glucocorticoids. However, *the most common cause of pulmonary infiltrates in patients with SLE is infection.* Interstitial pneumonitis leading to fibrosis occurs in a small proportion of patients; the inflammatory phase may respond to treatment, while the fibrosis does not. Occasionally, patients develop pulmonary hypertension. Infrequent but often fatal pulmonary manifestations include adult respiratory distress syndrome (ARDS) and massive intraalveolar hemorrhage.

Gastrointestinal Nonspecific gastrointestinal symptoms are common, but vasculitis of the intestine is the most dangerous manifestation. It causes acute or subacute crampy pain, vomiting, and diarrhea and can lead to intestinal perforation and death. Vasculitis is usually present simultaneously in other systems. Another gastrointestinal manifestation of SLE is a pseudoobstruction in which patients present with acute crampy abdominal pain; x-rays show dilated loops of small bowel which may be edematous. Surgery should be avoided unless true obstruction is present. Patients generally respond to glucocorticoid therapy. Acute pancreatitis occurs and can be severe; it may result from active SLE or from glucocorticoid therapy. Elevated serum levels of liver enzymes, especially transaminases, are common in patients with active SLE but are not associated with significant hepatic damage; they return to normal as the disease is treated.

Ocular The most important ocular manifestation of SLE is retinal vasculitis with infarcts; blindness can develop over a period of days. Examination of the retina shows areas of sheathed, narrow arterioles, and cytoid bodies (white exudates) adjacent to vessels. Other ocular abnormalities include conjunctivitis, episcleritis, and optic neuritis. The sicca syndrome is frequent.

PATHOLOGY **Cutaneous lesions** Acute systemic discoid (DLE) and subacute cutaneous LE skin lesions show similar histopathology. Characteristic changes include degeneration of the basal layer of the epidermis with disruption of the dermal-epidermal junction (DEJ) and scattered mononuclear cell infiltrates around vessels and appendages in the upper dermis. In DLE follicular plugging and hyperkeratosis are prominent. Deposits of immunoglobulin (Ig) and C′ are seen in the DEJ in 80 to 100 percent of lesional and 50 percent of nonlesional skin in patients with active SLE; the proportions are lower during remissions. Active subacute cutaneous lesions are positive for deposits of Ig and C′ only 50 percent of the time. Ig deposition in the DEJ *is not specific* for *LE*. Vasculitic lesions usually show leukocytoclastic angiitis.

Renal lesions Most renal lesions are caused by in situ immune-complex formation or deposition of circulating complexes in glomeruli. In mild nephritis, histology shows either no changes or proliferation confined to the mesangium. When Ig deposits are found solely in the mesangium, prognosis is good and renal failure is rare. If Ig and C′ extend outside the mesangium into capillary loops, the prognosis worsens. Associated glomerular histologic changes in ascending order of severity are (1) focal proliferative, (2) membranoproliferative, and (3) diffuse proliferative (see Chap. 228). Membranous changes without proliferation occur. In addition to those histologic categories, *active disease* and *increased risk of progression to renal failure* are associated with glomerular necrosis, cellular epithelial crescents, hyaline thrombi, leukocytic or mononuclear cell infiltrates in the tubular interstitium, and necrotizing vasculitis. In addition, measures of *chronicity* are important, as they are associated with a *high incidence of renal failure*. They include glomerular sclerosis, fibrous crescents, interstitial fibrosis, and tubular atrophy. Focal proliferative and membranous changes are associated with 85 percent 5-year survival; diffuse proliferative glomerulonephritis is associated with 70 percent 5-year survival. Progression from focal to diffuse lesions can occur.

LABORATORY MANIFESTATIONS The presence of characteristic antibodies (Table 269-1) confirms the diagnosis of SLE. Antinuclear antibodies are the best screening test. If the test substrate is living human nuclei, as in WIL-2 or HEP-2 cells, more than 95 percent of lupus patients will have positive tests. Rodent liver or kidney substrates do not detect as wide a range of ANA or anticytoplasmic antibodies; approximately 85 percent of SLE serums are positive on those substrates. A positive ANA is not specific for SLE; ANA occur (usually in low titer) in some normal individuals; the frequency increases with aging. Furthermore, other autoimmune diseases, acute viral infections, chronic inflammatory processes, and several drugs may cause ANA positivity. Therefore, a positive ANA supports a diagnosis of SLE but *is not specific*; a negative ANA makes the diagnosis unlikely but not impossible. Antibodies to dsDNA and to Sm are relatively specific for SLE; other autoantibodies listed in Table 269-1 are not. High serum levels of ANA and anti-DNA and low levels of complement usually reflect disease activity, especially in patients with nephritis. Serum levels of cryoglobulins or other immune complexes occasionally correlate with disease activity. Total functional hemolytic complement (CH_{50}) levels are the most sensitive measure of complement activation but are also most subject to laboratory error. Quantitative levels of C3 and C4 are widely available. Very low levels of CH_{50} with normal levels of C3 suggest inherited deficiency of a complement component.

Hematologic abnormalities are common and include anemia (usually normochromic, normocytic but occasionally hemolytic), leukopenia, lymphopenia, and thrombocytopenia. In some patients the Westergren erythrocyte sedimentation rate correlates with disease activity.

Urinalysis and serum creatinine should be measured periodically in patients with SLE. When active nephritis is present, the urinalysis usually shows proteinuria, microscopic hematuria, and cellular or granular casts. Renal biopsy is indicated when results would influence therapeutic decisions. (See discussion under "Clinical Manifestations.")

Other tests that may be abnormal in SLE include false-positive tests for syphilis and abnormal coagulation tests, especially a prolonged partial thromboplastin time. Both are related to antibodies to cardiolipin, discussed under "Clinical Manifestations." Rheumatoid factors are present in 30 to 50 percent of patients.

The tests which are useful for diagnosis and for following the clinical course of patients with SLE are listed in Table 269-3.

PREGNANCY Since SLE is a disease of young women, pregnancy is a frequent occurrence. Fertility rates are normal in patients with SLE, but the rate of spontaneous abortion and stillbirths is high (30 to 50 percent), especially in women with lupus anticoagulant and/or antibodies to cardiolipin. A debate has arisen regarding treatment of pregnant women with SLE and these antibodies who have experienced fetal loss. Some authorities recommend no intervention; others have reported high rates of successful births if mothers are treated with high daily doses of glucocorticoids plus low doses of aspirin or with anticoagulating doses of subcutaneous heparin.

There may be increased flares of SLE during the first trimester (SLE may begin during pregnancy) and especially during the first 6 weeks postpartum. If severe renal or cardiac disease is absent and SLE is controlled, the majority of patients complete pregnancy safely and deliver normal infants. Glucocorticoids (except dexamethasone and betamethasone) are inactivated by placental enzymes and do not cause fetal abnormalities except for low birth weights. Neonatal lupus (related to the presence of anti-Ro in maternal serum) occurs in infants but is rare. A transient DLE-like rash, congenital heart block, and thombocytopenia can occur.

DIFFERENTIAL DIAGNOSIS The American Rheumatism Association has developed diagnostic criteria for SLE. Manifestations included are indicated by asterisks in Table 269-2. Any four of those, or a total of four when combined with certain autoantibodies, establish a diagnosis of definite SLE. Disease confined to one or two systems may be more difficult to classify. The disorders with which SLE can be confused include rheumatoid arthritis; skin disorders such as urticaria, erythema multiforme, rosacea, lichen planus; neurologic disorders such as idiopathic epilepsy or multiple sclerosis; hematologic disorders such as idiopathic thrombocytopenic purpura; and psychiatric disorders. It may also be difficult to distinguish SLE from other autoimmune disorders such as dermatomyositis and overlap syndromes. Some authorities classify patients with features of SLE, rheumatoid arthritis, polymyositis, and scleroderma, accompanied by high titers of anti-RNP, under the rubric "mixed connective tissue disease" (Chap. 272) and report a low incidence of nephritis and CNS disease and a high incidence of pulmonary disease and evolution into scleroderma. It is impossible to put some patients into a definite category; therapy should be directed toward the dominant manifestations. The possibility of drug-induced lupus should always be considered.

DRUG-INDUCED LUPUS Several drugs can cause a syndrome resembling SLE in individuals without any obvious predisposition to the disease. The most common offender is procainamide, which induces ANA in 50 to 75 percent of individuals within a few months; 20 percent of patients receiving the drug develop clinical drug-induced LE. Hydralazine induces ANA in 25 to 30 percent of individuals, and lupus-like symptoms in 10 percent. Both procainamide and hydralazine-induced lupus are more likely to occur in individuals who acetylate the drug slowly. The clinical syndrome consists of polyarthralgias and systemic symptoms in most patients. Polyarthritis occurs in 25 to 50 percent and pleuropericarditis occurs in 30 percent of patients with hydralazine-induced lupus and in 50 percent of patients with procainamide-induced lupus. Other manifestations typical of idiopathic SLE are unusual, including nephritis and CNS involvement. All patients with drug-induced lupus are ANA-positive; most have antibodies to histones. Antibodies to dsDNA and hypocomplementemia are rarely present—a helpful point in distinguishing drug-induced from idiopathic lupus. Anemia, leukopenia, lupus anticoagulant, thrombocytopenia, cryoglobulins, rheumatoid factors, false-positive VDRL, and positive direct Coombs' tests can occur. The initial therapeutic approach should be discontinuation of the suspect drug; most patients improve in days or a few weeks. In patients with severe symptoms, a short course (2 to 10 weeks) of glucocorticoids is indicated. Clinical symptoms rarely persist more than 6 months; ANA may remain positive for years. Other drugs which infrequently induce lupus-like illness include isoniazid, chlorpromazine, *d*-penicillamine, practolol, methyldopa, oral contraceptives, and possibly hydantoins and ethosuximide. Most lupus-inducing drugs can be used safely in patients with idiopathic lupus if there are limited alternatives.

PROGNOSIS The overall survival in patients with SLE is approximately 71 percent over 10 years. Patients with severe involvement of brain, lungs, heart, or kidney have the worst outcomes in terms of survival and disability. Infections and renal failure are the leading causes of death.

TREATMENT There is no cure for SLE. Complete remissions occur but are rare; therefore, patient and physician should plan, first, to control acute, severe flares and, second, to develop maintenance therapies in which symptoms are suppressed to an acceptable level, usually at the cost of some drug side effects. From 20 to 30 percent of SLE patients have mild disease with no life-threatening manifestations. However, their disease may be disabling because of pain and fatigue. These patients should be managed without glucocorticoids. Arthralgias, arthritis, myalgias, fever, and mild serositis may improve on nonsteroidal anti-inflammatory drugs (NSAIDs) including salicylates. However, some NSAID toxicities such as hepatitis, aseptic meningitis, and renal impairment are especially frequent in SLE patients. The dermatitides of SLE (including DLE) and, occasionally, lupus arthritis may respond to antimalarials. Doses of 400 mg hydroxychloroquine daily may be associated with improvement of skin lesions in a few weeks. Side effects include retinal toxicity, rash, myopathy, and neuropathy. Regular ophthalmologic examinations should be performed at least every 6 months, since retinal toxicity is related to cumulative dose. Other therapies for skin rash include use of sunscreens (an SPF rating of 15 or higher is recommended) to prevent rashes and topical or intralesional glucocorticoids if rashes develop. Systemic glucocorticoids should be reserved for patients with disabling, severe lesions.

Life-threatening and severely disabling manifestations of SLE are treated with high doses of *glucocorticoids* (1 to 2 mg/kg per day). When the disease is active, glucocorticoids should be given in divided doses every 8 to 12 h. After the disease has been controlled for several days, doses should be consolidated to one morning dose; thereafter, the daily dose should be tapered as rapidly as clinical disease permits. Ideally, patients should be slowly converted to alternate-day therapy with a single morning dose of short-acting glucocorticoid (prednisone, prednisolone, methylprednisolone) to minimize side effects. However, the disease may flare on alternate days, in which case the lowest single daily dose that suppresses symptoms and major organ damage should be used. Undesirable side effects of chronic glucocorticoid therapy include cushingoid habitus, weight gain, hypertension, infection, capillary fragility, acne, hirsutism, accelerated osteoporosis, ischemic necrosis of bone, cataracts, glaucoma, diabetes mellitus, myopathy, hypokalemia, irregular menses, irritability, insomnia, and psychosis. Prednisone doses of 15 mg daily (or less) given before the hour of noon usually do not significantly suppress the hypothalamic pituitary axis. Some side effects can be minimized if one is alert for them; hyperglycemia, hypertension, edema, and hypokalemia should be treated. The physician should identify infections early and treat promptly. Immunizations with influenza and pneumococcal vaccines are safe and generally effective in patients with stable disease. Supplemental calcium (1000 to 1500 mg daily) with vitamin D (50,000 U weekly) in carefully selected patients (with normal 24-h urine calcium and normal serum calcium; ambulatory) receiving stable doses of glucocorticoids may help maintain bone mass. Some acutely ill lupus patients, including those with diffuse nephritis, have been treated with 3 to 5 days of 1000-mg intravenous "pulses" of methylprednisolone, followed by maintenance daily or alternate-day glucocorticoids. It is unclear whether there are any special advantages or toxicities to this regimen.

The use of *cytotoxic agents* (azathioprine, chlorambucil, cyclophosphamide) in SLE is somewhat controversial. Their use in lupus nephritis is probably associated with a lower rate of renal failure and fewer disease flares, and it permits faster tapering and lower maintenance doses of glucocorticoids. Undesirable side effects include bone marrow suppression, irreversible ovarian failure, hepatotoxicity (azathioprine), bladder toxicity (cyclophosphamide), and an increased risk for malignancies. If a lupus patient has life-threatening disease unresponsive to glucocorticoids or requires an unacceptably high maintenance dose of glucocorticoids, it is appropriate to consider cytotoxic drugs. Azathioprine is the least toxic; it may be given in a dose of 2 to 3 mg/kg per day orally. Cyclophosphamide is probably the most effective and the most toxic. Intravenous pulse doses (10 to 15 mg/kg) given once every 4 weeks have less urinary bladder toxicity and more rapid onset of action (5 to 15 days) than daily oral doses, but bone marrow suppression can be severe. Cyclophosphamide can also be used in daily oral doses (1.5 to 2.5 mg/kg per day) or in combination with low doses of azathioprine (0.5 to 1 mg/kg per day of each). After disease activity has been controlled for several months, tapering of cytotoxic agents and attempts to discontinue them are appropriate.

Several experimental therapies are being studied, including plasmapheresis, total-lymph-node irradiation, cyclosporine, sex hormone therapy, and intravenous gamma globulin.

Patients with nephrotic syndrome often maintain stable renal function in spite of persistent edema and hypoalbuminemia; hypertension is usually a concomitant problem. Such patients should be treated with 3 to 6 months of high-dose glucocorticoid therapy; if proteinuria does not diminish, the drug should be tapered and discontinued and treatment directed toward control of hypertension and hyperlipidemia.

It is appropriate in patients with end-stage nephritis to plan for dialysis or transplantation; their survival is similar to that of patients with other immune nephritides.

In the subsets of patients with SLE who do not have progressive, severe disease, patients should be informed that although SLE is a chronic, potentially serious disease, some patients can lead relatively normal lives if their disease is appropriately managed.

REFERENCES

AUSTIN HA III et al: Prognostic factors in lupus nephritis. Am J Med 75:382, 1983

BALOW JE et al: NIH conference: Lupus nephritis (includes treatment). Ann Intern Med 106:79, 1987

EBLING FM, HAHN BH: Pathogenic subsets of antibodies to DNA, in *International Reviews in Immunology*, H Kohler and C Bona (eds) 5:7995, 1989

GINZLER E et al: A multi-center study of outcome in systemic lupus erythematosus. I. Entry variables as predictors of prognosis. Arthritis Rheum 25:601, 1982

HARRIS EN et al: Thrombosis, recurrent fetal loss, thrombocytopenia: Predictive value of the anticardiolipin test. Arch Intern Med 146:2153, 1986

HOWARD PF et al: Relationship between C4 null genes, HLA-D region antigens and genetic susceptibility to systemic lupus erythematosus in Caucasian and Black Americans. Am J Med 81:187, 1986

LEAKER B et al: Lupus nephritis: Clinical and pathological correlation. Q J Med 62:163, 1987

REICHLIN M: *Antibodies to Cytoplasmic Antigens in Systemic Lupus Erythematosus*, R G Lahita (ed). New York, Wiley, 1987, chap 8, pp 257–269

ROTHFIELD N: Systemic lupus erythematosus: Clinical aspects and treatment, in *Arthritis and Allied Conditions*, 11th ed, DJ McCarty (ed). Philadelphia, Lea & Febiger, 1989, chap 67, pp 1022–1048

TAN EM: Systemic lupus erythematosus: Immunological aspects, in *Arthritis and Allied Conditions*, 11th ed, DJ McCarty (ed). Philadelphia, Lea & Febiger, 1989, chap 68, pp 1049–1054

——— et al: The 1982 revised criteria for the classification of systemic lupus erythematosus. Arthritis Rheum 25:1271, 1982

270 RHEUMATOID ARTHRITIS

PETER E. LIPSKY

Rheumatoid arthritis (RA) is a chronic, multisystem disease of unknown etiology. Although there are a variety of systemic manifestations, the characteristic feature of RA is persistent inflammatory synovitis, usually involving peripheral joints in a symmetric distribution. The potential of the synovial inflammation to cause cartilage destruction and bone erosions and subsequently joint deformities is the hallmark of the disease. Despite its destructive potential, the course of RA can be quite variable. Some patients may experience only a mild oligoarticular illness of brief duration with minimal joint damage, while others will have a relentless progressive polyarthritis with marked joint deformity. Most patients will experience an intermediate course.

EPIDEMIOLOGY AND GENETICS The prevalence of RA is approximately 1 percent of the population (range 0.3 to 2.1 percent); women are affected approximately three times more often than men. The prevalence increases with age, and sex differences diminish in the older age group. RA is seen throughout the world and affects all races. The onset is most frequent during the fourth and fifth decade of life, with 80 percent of all patients developing the disease between the ages of 35 and 50.

Family studies indicate a genetic predisposition. For example, severe RA is found at approximately four times the expected rate in first-degree relatives of individuals with seropositive disease. Moreover, 30 percent of monozygous twins are concordant for RA, whereas only 5 percent of dizygous twins are concordant. The role of genetic influences in the etiology of RA was established by the demonstration of an association with the class II major histocompatibility complex gene product, HLA-DR4. As many as 70 percent of whites or Japanese with classic or definite RA express HLA-DR4 compared with 28 percent of control individuals. An association with HLA-DR4 has also been noted in blacks, Latin Americans, and Chippewa Indians, although the incidence of HLA-DR4 positivity in individuals with RA in these groups is not as great as in whites. In a number of groups, including Israeli Jews and Asian Indians, however, there is no association between the development of RA and HLA-DR4. In these individuals, there is an association between RA and HLA-DR1. Molecular analysis of HLA-DR antigens has provided insight into these apparently disparate findings. Thus, HLA-DR4 consists of a family of closely related antigens, including HLA-Dw4, Dw10, Dw13, Dw14, and Dw15, that differ structurally in the amino acids that surround position 70 of the third hypervariable region of the β chain of the molecule. Different members of the HLA-DR4 family of molecules are found to predominate in different ethnic groups. Thus, for example, in HLA-DR–positive North American whites, HLA-Dw4 and Dw14 are the most frequent subtypes, whereas HLA-Dw15 is most frequent in Japanese, and HLA-Dw10 is most common in Israeli Jews. Moreover, only some HLA-DR4 subtypes are associated with the development of RA. Thus, HLA-Dw4, Dw14, and Dw15, but not Dw10 or Dw13, are associated with the development of RA. The amino acids surrounding position 70 of the third hypervariable region of the HLA-DR β chain are very similar in HLA-Dw4, Dw14, and Dw15, whereas there are significant differences in HLA-Dw10 and Dw13. Of note, the amino acid sequence of the third hypervariable region of HLA-DR1 is identical to that of Dw14. These results suggest that this particular amino acid sequence in this region of the HLA-DR molecule may be a major genetic element conveying susceptibility to RA, regardless of whether it occurs in HLA-DR4 or HLA-DR1. Since this region of the HLA-DR molecule is involved in binding foreign peptides and thereby facilitating their presentation to specific T lymphocytes, it is possible that the association between particular HLA-DR molecules and RA may be explained by the capacity of individuals expressing these HLA-DR determinants to recognize an antigen that initiates the disease process.

Additional genes in the HLA-D complex may also convey susceptibility to RA. The haplotype HLA-DR4, DQw3.1 appears to be associated with more severe manifestations of RA, including Felty's syndrome, whereas pulmonary involvement in RA is associated with HLA-DR4. Finally, genes outside the HLA complex, such as those controlling the expression of the antigen receptor on T cells have also been associated with the development of RA.

To date, genetic risk factors cannot fully account for the incidence of RA, suggesting that environmental factors also play a role in the etiology of the disease. This is emphasized by epidemiologic studies in Africa that have indicated that climate and urbanization have a major impact on the incidence and severity of RA in groups of similar genetic background.

Besides an association between the development of RA and genes of the major histocompatibility complex, there appears to be a genetic predisposition for the development of certain toxic reactions induced by drugs used to treat RA. For example, the presence of the HLA-DR3 allele is highly associated with the development of side effects to gold therapy, including proteinuria, thrombocytopenia, and perhaps skin rash. Similarly, the presence of this allele appears to predispose to the development of proteinuria following therapy with D-penicillamine. In general, no association has been noted between HLA type and the response to therapy.

CLINICAL MANIFESTATIONS Onset Characteristically, RA is a chronic polyarthritis. In approximately two-thirds of patients, it begins insidiously with fatigue, anorexia, generalized weakness, and vague musculoskeletal symptoms until the appearance of synovitis becomes apparent. This prodrome may persist for weeks or months and defy diagnosis. Specific symptoms usually appear gradually as several joints, especially those of the hands, wrists, knees, and feet, become affected in a symmetric fashion. In approximately 10 percent of individuals, the onset is more acute with a rapid development of polyarthritis often accompanied by constitutional symptoms including fever, lymphadenopathy, and splenomegaly. In approximately one-third of patients, symptoms may initially be confined to one or a few joints. Although the pattern of joint involvement may remain asymmetric in a few patients, a symmetric pattern is more typical.

Signs and symptoms of articular disease Pain, swelling, and tenderness may initially be poorly localized to the joints. Pain in affected joints, aggravated by movement, is the most common manifestation of established RA. It corresponds in pattern to the joint involvement but does not always correlate with the degree of apparent inflammation. Generalized stiffness is frequent and is usually greatest after periods of inactivity. Morning stiffness of greater than 1-h duration is an almost invariable feature of inflammatory arthritis and serves to distinguish it from various noninflammatory joint disorders. The length and intensity of the stiffness can be used as a crude assessment of disease activity. The majority of patients will experience constitutional symptoms such as weakness, easy fatigability, anorexia, and weight loss. Although fever to 40°C occurs on occasion, temperature elevation in excess of 38°C is unusual and suggests the presence of an intercurrent problem such as infection.

Clinically, synovial inflammation causes swelling, tenderness, and limitation of motion. Warmth is usually evident on examination, especially of large joints such as the knee, but erythema is infrequent. Pain originates predominantly from the joint capsule, which is abundantly supplied with pain fibers and is markedly sensitive to stretching or distention. Joint swelling results from accumulation of synovial fluid, hypertrophy of the synovium, and thickening of the joint capsule. Initially, motion is limited by pain. The inflamed joint is usually held in flexion to maximize joint volume and minimize distention of the capsule. Later, fibrous or bony ankylosis, or soft tissue contractures lead to fixed deformities.

Although inflammation can affect any diarthrodial joint, RA most often causes symmetric arthritis with characteristic involvement of certain specific joints such as the proximal interphalangeal and metacarpophalangeal joints. The distal interphalangeal joints are rarely involved. Synovitis of the wrist joints is a nearly uniform feature of RA and may lead to limitation of motion, deformity, and median nerve entrapment (carpal tunnel syndrome). Synovitis of the elbow joint often leads to flexion contractures that may develop early in the disease. The knee joint is commonly involved with synovial hypertrophy, chronic effusion, and frequently ligamentous laxity. Pain and swelling behind the knee may be caused by extension of inflamed synovium into the popliteal space (Baker's cyst). Arthritis in the forefoot, ankles, and subtalar joints can produce severe pain with ambulation as well as a number of deformities. Axial involvement is usually limited to the upper cervical spine. Involvement of the lumbar spine is not seen, and lower back pain cannot be ascribed to rheumatoid inflammation. On occasion, inflammation from the synovial joints and bursae of the upper cervical spine leads to atlantoaxial subluxation. This usually presents as pain in the occiput but on rare occasions may lead to compression of the spinal cord.

With persistent inflammation, a variety of characteristic deformities develop. These can be attributed to a number of pathologic events including laxity of supporting soft tissue structures; destruction or weakening of ligaments, tendons, and the joint capsule; cartilage destruction; muscle imbalance; and unopposed physical forces associated with the use of affected joints. Characteristic deformities of the hand include (1) radial deviation at the wrist with ulnar deviation of the digits often with palmar subluxation of the proximal phalanges ("Z" deformity); (2) hyperextension of the proximal interphalangeal joints, with compensatory flexion of the distal interphalangeal joints (swan-neck deformity); (3) flexion deformity of the proximal interphalangeal joints and extension of the distal interphalangeal joints (boutonnière deformity); and (4) hyperextension of the first interphalangeal joint and flexion of the first metacarpophalangeal joint with a consequent loss of thumb mobility and pinch. Typical deformities may also develop in the feet, including eversion at the hindfoot (subtalar joint), plantar subluxation of the metatarsal heads, widening of the forefoot, hallux valgus, and lateral deviation and dorsal subluxation of the toes.

Extraarticular manifestations RA is a systemic disease with a variety of extraarticular manifestations. Although these occur frequently, not all of them have clinical significance. However, on occasion, they may be the major evidence of disease activity and source of morbidity and require management per se. As a rule, these manifestations take place in individuals with high titers of autoantibodies to the Fc component of immunoglobulin G (rheumatoid factors).

Rheumatoid nodules develop in 20 to 30 percent of persons with RA. They are usually found on periarticular structures, extensor surfaces, or other areas subjected to mechanical pressure, but they can develop elsewhere including the pleura and meninges. Common locations include the olecranon bursa, the proximal ulna, the Achilles tendon, and the occiput. Nodules vary in size and consistency and are rarely symptomatic, but on occasion they break down as a result of trauma or become infected. They are found almost invariably in individuals with circulating rheumatoid factor. Histologically, rheumatoid nodules consist of a central zone of necrotic material including collagen fibrils, noncollagenous filaments, and cellular debris, a midzone of palisading macrophages that express HLA-DR antigens, and an outer zone of granulation tissue. Examination of early nodules has suggested that the initial event may be a focal vasculitis.

Clinical weakness and atrophy of skeletal muscle are common. Muscle atrophy may be evident within weeks of the onset of RA and usually is most apparent in musculature approximating affected joints. Muscle biopsy may show type II fiber atrophy and muscle fiber necrosis with or without a mononuclear cell infiltrate.

Rheumatoid vasculitis which can affect nearly any organ system is seen in patients with severe RA and high titers of circulating rheumatoid factor. Rheumatoid vasculitis is very uncommon in blacks. In its most aggressive form, rheumatoid vasculitis can cause polyneuropathy and mononeuritis multiplex, cutaneous ulceration and dermal necrosis, digital gangrene, and visceral infarction. While such widespread vasculitis is very rare, more limited forms are not uncommon, especially in white patients with high titers of rheumatoid factor. Neurovascular disease presenting either as a mild distal sensory neuropathy or as mononeuritis multiplex may be the only signs of vasculitis. Cutaneous vasculitis usually presents as crops of small brown spots in the nail beds, nail folds, and digital pulp. Larger ischemic ulcers, especially in the lower extremity, may also develop. Myocardial infarction secondary to rheumatoid vasculitis has been reported as has vasculitic involvement of lungs, bowel, liver, spleen, pancreas, lymph nodes, and testes. Renal vasculitis is rare.

Pleuropulmonary manifestations, which are more commonly observed in men, include pleural disease, interstitial fibrosis, pleuropulmonary nodules, pneumonitis, and arteritis. Evidence of pleuritis is found commonly at autopsy, but symptomatic disease during life is infrequent. Typically, the pleural fluid contains very low levels of glucose in the absence of infection. Pleural fluid complement is also low compared with the serum level when these are related to the total protein concentration. Pulmonary fibrosis can produce impairment of the diffusing capacity of the lung. Pulmonary nodules may appear singly or in clusters. When they appear in individuals with pneumoconiosis, a diffuse nodular fibrotic process (Caplan's syndrome) may develop. On occasion, pulmonary nodules may cavitate and produce a pneumothorax or bronchopleural fistula. Rarely pulmonary hypertension secondary to obliteration of the pulmonary vasculature occurs. In addition to pleuropulmonary disease, upper airway obstruction from cricoarytenoid arthritis or laryngeal nodules may develop.

Clinically apparent heart disease attributed to the rheumatoid process is rare, but evidence of asymptomatic pericarditis is found at autopsy in 50 percent of cases. Pericardial fluid has a low glucose level and is frequently associated with the occurrence of pleural effusion. Although pericarditis is usually asymptomatic, on rare occasions death has occurred from tamponade. Chronic constrictive pericarditis may also occur.

RA tends to spare the central nervous system directly, although vasculitis can cause peripheral neuropathy. *Neurologic manifestations* may also result from atlantoaxial or midcervical spine subluxations. Nerve entrapment secondary to proliferative synovitis or joint deformities may produce neuropathies of median, ulnar, radial (interosseous branch), or anterior tibial nerves.

The rheumatoid process involves the *eye* in less than 1 percent of patients. Affected individuals usually have long-standing disease and nodules. The two principal manifestations are episcleritis, which is usually mild and transient, and scleritis, which involves the deeper coats of the eye and is a more serious inflammatory condition. Histologically, the lesion is similar to a rheumatoid nodule and may result in thinning and perforation of the globe (scleromalacia perforans). Fifteen to twenty percent of persons with RA may develop Sjögren's syndrome with attendant keratoconjunctivitis sicca.

Felty's syndrome consists of chronic RA, splenomegaly, neutropenia, and on occasion anemia and thrombocytopenia. It is most common in individuals with long-standing disease. These patients frequently have high titers of rheumatoid factor, subcutaneous nodules, and other manifestations of systemic rheumatoid disease. Felty's syndrome is very uncommon in blacks. It may develop after joint inflammation has regressed. Circulating immune complexes are often present, and evidence of complement consumption may be seen. The leukopenia is a selective neutropenia with polymorphonuclear leukocyte counts of less than 1500 per microliter, and sometimes less than 1000 per microliter. Bone marrow examination usually reveals moderate hypercellularity with a paucity of mature neutrophils. However, the bone marrow may be normal, hyperactive, or hypoactive; maturation arrest may be seen. Hypersplenism has been proposed as one of the causes of leukopenia, but splenomegaly is not invariably found and splenectomy does not always correct the abnormality. Excessive margination of granulocytes caused by antibodies to these cells, complement activation, or binding of immune complexes may contribute to granulocytopenia. Patients with Felty's syndrome have increased frequency of infections usually associated with neutropenia. The cause of the increased susceptibility to infection is related to the defective function of polymorphonuclear leukocytes as well as the decreased number of cells.

Osteoporosis secondary to rheumatoid involvement is common and may be aggravated by corticosteroid therapy and immobilization. Osteopenia involves both juxtaarticular bone and long bones distant from involved joints.

LABORATORY FINDINGS No tests are specific for diagnosing RA. However, rheumatoid factors, which are autoantibodies reactive with the Fc portion of IgG, are found in more than two-thirds of adults with the disease. Widely utilized tests largely detect IgM rheumatoid factors. The presence of rheumatoid factor is not specific for RA. Rheumatoid factors are found in 5 percent of healthy persons. The frequency of rheumatoid factor in the general population increases with age, and 10 to 20 percent of individuals over 65 years old have a positive test. In addition, a number of conditions besides RA are associated with the presence of rheumatoid factor. These include systemic lupus erythematosus, Sjögren's syndrome, chronic liver disease, sarcoidosis, interstitial pulmonary fibrosis, infectious mononucleosis, hepatitis B, tuberculosis, leprosy, syphilis, subacute bacterial endocarditis, visceral leishmaniasis, schistosomiasis, and malaria. In addition, rheumatoid factor may appear transiently in normal individuals after vaccination or transfusion and may also be found in relatives of individuals with RA.

The presence of rheumatoid factor does not establish the diagnosis of RA but can be of prognostic significance because patients with high titers tend to have more severe and progressive disease with extraarticular manifestations. Rheumatoid factor is uniformly found in patients with nodules or vasculitis. The predictive value of the presence of rheumatoid factor in determining a diagnosis of RA is poor. Thus, less than one-third of unselected patients with a positive test for rheumatoid factor will be found to have RA. The test is not useful as a screening procedure but can be employed to confirm a diagnosis in individuals with a suggestive clinical presentation and, if present in high titer, to designate patients at risk for severe systemic disease.

Normochromic, normocytic anemia is frequently present in active RA. It is thought to reflect ineffective erythropoiesis; large stores of iron are found in the bone marrow. In general, anemia and thrombocytosis correlate with disease activity. The white blood cell count is usually normal, but a mild leukocytosis may be present. Leukopenia may also exist without the full-blown picture of Felty's syndrome. Eosinophilia, when present, usually reflects severe systemic disease.

The erythrocyte sedimentation rate is increased in nearly all patients with active RA. A variety of other acute phase reactants including ceruloplasmin and C-reactive protein are also elevated, and generally such elevations correlate with disease activity and the likelihood of progressive joint damage.

Synovial fluid analysis confirms the presence of inflammatory arthritis, although none of the findings is specific. The fluid is usually turbid, with reduced viscosity, increased protein content, and a slightly decreased or normal glucose concentration. The white cell count varies between 5 and 50,000 per microliter; polymorphonuclear leukocytes predominate. Total hemolytic complement, C3, and C4 are markedly diminished in synovial fluid relative to total protein concentration as a result of activation of the classic complement pathway by locally produced immune complexes.

When monoclonal antibodies specific for T-lymphocyte subsets are used to examine peripheral blood mononuclear cells of patients with RA, no specific changes in the numbers of circulating CD4+ (helper-inducer) or CD8+ (suppressor-cytotoxic) T cells are noted. However, an increased number of circulating T cells expressing HLA-DR, an indication of T-cell activation, can be observed. This finding is most frequent in patients with active joint disease.

RADIOGRAPHIC EVALUATION Early in the disease, roentgenograms of the affected joints are usually not helpful in establishing a diagnosis. They reveal only that which is apparent from physical examination, namely, evidence of soft tissue swelling and joint effusion. As the disease progresses, abnormalities become more pronounced, but none of the radiographic findings is diagnostic of RA. The diagnosis, however, is supported by a characteristic pattern of abnormalities including the tendency toward symmetric involvement. Juxtaarticular osteopenia may become apparent within weeks of onset. Loss of articular cartilage and bone erosions develop after months of sustained activity. The primary value of radiography is to determine the extent of cartilage destruction and bone erosion produced by the disease, particularly when one is considering therapy with disease-modifying drugs or surgical intervention.

CLINICAL COURSE AND PROGNOSIS The course of RA is quite variable and difficult to predict in an individual patient. Most patients experience persistent but fluctuating disease activity, accompanied by a variable degree of joint deformity. After 10 to 12 years, fewer than 20 percent of patients will have no evidence of disability or deformity. Features of patients that predict the development of disability include older age, female sex, more severe radiographic involvement, and the presence of rheumatoid nodules or elevated titers of rheumatoid factor. Neither pattern of disease onset nor currently available therapies appear to have an impact on the development of disabilities. Approximately 15 percent of patients with RA will have a short-lived inflammatory process that remits without major deformity.

Several features of patients with RA appear to have prognostic significance. Remissions of disease activity are most likely to occur during the first year. White females tend to have more persistent synovitis and progressively erosive disease than males. Persons who present with high titers of rheumatoid factor, C-reactive protein, and haptoglobin also have a worse prognosis, as do individuals with subcutaneous nodules or radiographic evidence of erosions at the time of initial evaluation. Although sustained disease activity of more than 1 year's duration portends a poor outcome, the rate of progression of joint abnormalities is not constant; the greatest progression takes place during the first 6 years of disease and at a much slower rate thereafter.

The median life expectancy of persons with RA is shortened by 3 to 7 years. Of the 2.5-fold increase in mortality rate, RA itself is a contributing feature in 15 to 25 percent. The increased mortality rate seems to be limited to patients with more severe articular disease and can be attributed largely to infection and gastrointestinal bleeding. Drug therapy may also play a role in the increased mortality rate seen in these individuals.

DIAGNOSIS The diagnosis of RA is easily made in persons with typical established disease. In a majority of patients, the disease assumes its characteristic clinical features within 1 to 2 years of onset. The typical picture of bilateral symmetric inflammatory polyarthritis involving small and large joints in both the upper and lower extremities with sparing of the axial skeleton except the cervical spine suggests the diagnosis. Constitutional features indicative of the inflammatory nature of the disease, such as morning stiffness, support the diagnosis. Demonstration of subcutaneous nodules is a helpful diagnostic feature. Additionally, the presence of rheumatoid factor, inflammatory synovial fluid with increased numbers of polymorphonuclear leukocytes, and radiographic findings of juxtaarticular bone demineralization and erosions of the affected joints substantiate the diagnosis.

The diagnosis is somewhat more difficult early in the course when only constitutional symptoms or intermittent arthralgias or arthritis in an asymmetric distribution may be present. A period of observation may be necessary before the diagnosis can be established. A definitive diagnosis of RA depends predominantly on characteristic clinical features and the exclusion of other inflammatory processes. The isolated finding of a positive test for rheumatoid factor or an elevated erythrocyte sedimentation rate, especially in an older person with joint pains, should not itself be used as evidence of RA.

Recently, the American Rheumatism Association has developed revised criteria for the classification of rheumatoid arthritis (Table 270-1). The newer criteria are simpler to apply than the previous ones and demonstrate a sensitivity of 91 to 94 percent and a specificity of 89 percent when used to classify patients with RA compared with control subjects with rheumatic diseases other than RA. The major differences between the new and old criteria are that results of invasive procedures such as biopsies are not included, the classifications of probable, definite, and classic RA have been eliminated, and patients with more than a single diagnosis are not eliminated by exclusion criteria. Although these criteria were developed as a means of disease classification for epidemiologic purposes, they are useful as guidelines for establishing the diagnosis. Failure to meet these criteria, however, especially during the early stages of the disease, does not exclude the diagnosis.

TABLE 270-1 The 1987 revised criteria for the classification of rheumatoid arthritis

1 Guidelines for classification
- *a* Four of seven criteria are required to classify a patient as having rheumatoid arthritis.
- *b* Patients with two or more clinical diagnoses are not excluded.

2 Criteria*
- *a* Morning stiffness: Stiffness in and around the joints lasting 1 h before maximal improvement.
- *b* Arthritis of 3 or more joint areas: At least 3 joint areas, observed by a physician simultaneously, have soft tissue swelling or joint effusions, not just bony overgrowth. The 14 possible joint areas involved are right or left proximal interphalangeal, metacarpophalangeal, wrist, elbow, knee, ankle, and metatarsophalangeal joints.
- *c* Arthritis of hand joints: Arthritis of wrist, metacarpophalangeal joint, or proximal interphalangeal joint.
- *d* Symmetric arthritis: Simultaneous involvement of the same joint areas on both sides of the body.
- *e* Rheumatoid nodules: Subcutaneous nodules over bony prominences, extensor surfaces, or juxtaarticular regions observed by a physician.
- *f* Serum rheumatoid factor: Demonstration of abnormal amounts of serum rheumatoid factor by any method for which the result has been positive in less than 5% of normal control subjects.
- *g* Radiographic changes: Typical changes of RA on posteroanterior hand and wrist radiographs which must include erosions or unequivocal bony decalcification localized in or most marked adjacent to the involved joints.

* Criteria *a–d* must be present for at least 6 weeks. Criteria *b–e* must be observed by a physician.

PATHOLOGY AND PATHOGENESIS Microvascular injury and an increase in the number of synovial lining cells appear to be the earliest lesions in rheumatoid synovitis. The nature of the insult causing this response is not known. Subsequently, an increased number of synovial lining cells is seen along with perivascular infiltration with mononuclear cells. As the process continues, the synovium becomes edematous and protrudes into the joint cavity as villous projections.

Light-microscopic examination discloses a characteristic constellation of features which include hyperplasia and hypertrophy of the synovial lining cells, focal or segmental vascular changes, including microvascular injury, thrombosis and neovascularization, edema, and infiltration with mononuclear cells often collected into aggregates around small blood vessels. Although this pathologic picture is typical of RA, it can also be seen in a variety of other chronic inflammatory arthritides. The mononuclear cell collections are variable in composition and size. The predominant infiltrating cell is the T lymphocyte. T4 (helper-inducer) cells predominate over T8 (suppressor-cytotoxic) cells and are frequently found in close proximity to HLA-DR+ macrophages and dendritic cells. Analysis of T cells in synovial fluid has documented an enrichment in CD29-expressing memory T4 cells and a marked reduction in the number of CD45R-expressing naive T4 cells. In addition, the T8 cells are largely of the cytotoxic and not the suppressive phenotype.

Although the etiologic stimuli have not been identified, established rheumatoid synovitis is characterized by persistent immunologic activity. The infiltrating T cells appear to be activated, since they express activation antigens such as HLA-DR. In addition, they express an increased density of molecules, such as leukocyte function associated antigen 1 (LFA-1, CD11a/CD18) that have been implicated in a variety of cell-to-cell interactions, including binding of circulating cells to postcapillary venules just prior to entry into sites of tissue inflammation. Finally, the T cells appear to have proliferated locally in the synovial tissue, perhaps in response to sequestered antigen, since they express determinants such as very late antigen (VLA-1) that appears on T cells only after prolonged proliferation. Evidence of B-cell activation can also be found in the inflamed synovium, and plasma cells producing immunoglobulin and rheumatoid factor are characteristic features of rheumatoid synovitis. Large numbers of macrophages with an activated phenotype are also found in rheumatoid synovium.

The rheumatoid synovium is characterized by the presence of a number of secreted products of activated lymphocytes, macrophages, and other cell types. The local production of these cytokines appears to account for many of the pathologic and clinical manifestations of RA. Table 270-2 lists cytokines that have been identified in rheumatoid synovial fluid and indicates their putative role in the rheumatoid inflammatory process. These cytokines include those that are derived from T lymphocytes such as interleukin 2 (IL-2), IL-6, granulocyte-macrophage colony stimulating factor (GM-CSF), tumor necrosis factor α, and transforming growth factor β; those originating from activated macrophages, including IL-1, tumor necrosis factor α, IL-6, GM-CSF, macrophage CSF, platelet-derived growth factor, insulin-like growth factor, and transforming growth factor β; as well

TABLE 270-2 Cytokines in rheumatoid inflammation

Manifestation	Cytokine involved
1 Synovial tissue inflammation	
a Increased adherence of postcapillary venules	IL-1, TNFα, IFN-γ
b T-cell activation and proliferation	IL-1, TNFα, IL-6, IL-2
c B-cell differentiation and antibody formation	IL-1, TNFα, IL-6, IL-2, IFN-γ
d Increased expression of HLA antigens	IFN-γ, TNFα
e Macrophage activation	IFN-γ, GM-CSF, M-CSF, IL-2
2 Synovial fluid inflammation	
a Increased adherence of postcapillary venules	IL-1, TNFα, IFN-γ
b Chemotactic for PMN	TNFα
c Activation of PMN	TNFα, GM-CSF
3 Synovial proliferation	
a Fibroblast growth	PDGF, IL-1, IGF, FGF, TGFβ, EGF
b Neovascularization	TNFα, FGF, TGFβ
4 Cartilage and bone damage	
a Activation of chondrocytes	IL-1, TNFα
b Activation of fibroblasts	IL-1, TNFα
c Activation of osteoblasts-osteoclasts	IL-1, TNFα
5 Systemic manifestations	
a Fever, constitutional symptoms	IL-1, TNFα
b Acute phase reactants	IL-1, TNFα, IL-6

NOTE: IL-1, interleukin 1; IL-2, interleukin 2, IL-6, interleukin 6, TNFα, tumor necrosis factor α; IFN-γ, interferon γ; GM-CSF, granulocyte-macrophage colony stimulating factor; M-CSF, macrophage colony stimulating factor; PDGF, platelet-derived growth factor; PMN, polymorphonuclear cells; IGF, insulin-like factor; FGF, fibroblast growth factor; TGFβ, transforming growth factor β; EGF, epidermal growth factor.

as those secreted by other cell types in the synovium, such as fibroblasts and endothelial cells, including IL-1, IL-6, GM-CSF, and macrophage CSF. The activity of these cytokines appears to account for many of the features of rheumatoid synovitis including the synovial tissue inflammation, synovial fluid inflammation, synovial proliferation, and cartilage and bone damage as well as the systemic manifestations of RA. In addition to the production of cytokines that propagate the inflammatory process, local factors are produced that tend to slow the inflammation including specific inhibitors of cytokine action and additional cytokines, such as transforming growth factor β, which inhibits many of the features of rheumatoid synovitis including T-cell activation and proliferation, B-cell differentiation, and migration of cells into the inflammatory site.

These findings have suggested that the propagation of RA is an immunologically mediated event, although the original initiating stimulus has not been characterized. One view is that the inflammatory process in the tissue is driven by the T4 helper-inducer cells infiltrating the synovium. Evidence for this includes (1) the predominance of T4 cells in the synovium; (2) the increase in soluble IL-2 receptors, a product of activated T cells, in blood and synovial fluid of patients with active RA; and (3) amelioration of the disease by removal of T cells by thoracic duct drainage or suppression of their function by total lymphoid irradiation. T lymphocytes produce a number of cytokines, including gamma interferon and GM-CSF, that can lead to activation of macrophages and also increased expression of HLA molecules. Moreover, T lymphocytes produce a variety of cytokines that promote B-cell proliferation and differentiation into antibody-forming cells and, therefore, may also promote local B-cell stimulation. The resultant production of immunoglobulin and rheumatoid factor can lead to immune-complex formation with consequent complement activation and exacerbation of the inflammatory process by the production of the anaphylatoxins, C3a and C5a, and the chemotactic factor, C5a. The tissue inflammation is reminiscent of delayed-type hypersensitivity reactions occurring in response to soluble antigens or microorganisms. It is, however, unclear whether this represents a response to a persistent exogenous antigen or to altered autoantigens such as collagen, or immunoglobulin. Alternatively, it could represent persistent responsiveness to activated autologous cells such as might occur as a result of Epstein-Barr virus infection. Also, the persistent inflammation could result from deranged immunoregulatory mechanisms that are either primary abnormalities or develop as a result of the local inflammatory response.

Overriding the chronic inflammation in the synovial tissue is an acute inflammatory process in the synovial fluid. The exudative synovial fluid contains a large number of polymorphonuclear leukocytes and relatively few mononuclear cells. A number of mechanisms play a role in stimulating the exudation of synovial fluid. Locally produced immune complexes can activate complement and generate anaphylatoxins and chemotactic factors. Local production by mononuclear phagocytes of factors such as IL-1, tumor necrosis factor α, and leukotriene B_4 can stimulate the endothelial cells of postcapillary venules to become more efficient at binding circulating cells, whereas tumor necrosis factor α and leukotriene B_4 stimulate the migration of polymorphonuclear leukocytes into the synovial site. In addition, vasoactive mediators such as histamine produced by the mast cells that infiltrate the rheumatoid synovium may also facilitate the exudation of inflammatory cells into the synovial fluid. Finally, the vasodilatory effects of locally produced prostaglandin E_2 may also facilitate entry of inflammatory cells into the inflammatory site. Once in the synovial fluid, the polymorphonuclear leukocytes can ingest immune complexes, with the resultant production of reactive oxygen metabolites and other inflammatory mediators, further adding to the inflammatory milieu. Locally produced cytokines such as tumor necrosis factor α and GM-CSF can additionally stimulate polymorphonuclear leukocytes. The production of large amounts of cyclooxygenase and lipoxygenase pathway products of arachidonic acid metabolism by cells in the synovial fluid and tissue further accentuates the signs and symptoms of inflammation.

The precise mechanism by which bone and cartilage destruction occurs has not been completely resolved. Although the synovial fluid contains a number of enzymes potentially able to degrade cartilage, the majority of destruction occurs in juxtaposition to the inflamed synovium, or pannus, that spreads to cover the articular cartilage. This vascular granulation tissue is composed of proliferating fibroblasts, small blood vessels, and a variable number of mononuclear cells. The cytokines IL-1 and tumor necrosis factor α play an important role by stimulating the cells of the pannus to release collagenase and other neutral proteases. These same two cytokines also activate chondrocytes in situ, stimulating them to produce proteolytic enzymes that can degrade cartilage locally. Finally, these two cytokines may contribute to the local demineralization of bone by activating osteoclasts. Prostaglandin E_2 produced by fibroblasts and macrophages may also contribute to bone demineralization.

TREATMENT General principles The goals of therapy of RA are: (1) relief of pain; (2) reduction of inflammation; (3) preservation of functional capacity; (4) resolution of the pathologic process; and (5) facilitation of healing. Currently available medications are capable of providing pain relief and some reduction in inflammation. Since the etiology of RA is unknown and the pathogenesis speculative, therapy remains empirical. None of the therapeutic interventions are curative, and, therefore, all must be viewed as palliative, aimed at relieving the signs and symptoms of the disease. The various therapies employed are directed at nonspecific suppression of the inflammatory process in the hope of ameliorating symptoms and preventing progressive damage to articular structures.

Management of patients with RA involves an interdisciplinary approach which attempts to deal with the various problems that these individuals have with functional as well as psychosocial interactions. A variety of physical therapies may be useful in decreasing the symptoms of RA. Rest ameliorates symptoms and can be an important component of the total therapeutic program. In addition, splinting to reduce unwanted motion of inflamed joints may be useful. Exercise directed at maintaining muscle strength and joint mobility without exacerbating joint inflammation is also an important aspect of the therapeutic regimen. A variety of orthotic devices can be helpful in supporting and aligning deformed joints to reduce pain and improve function.

Medical management of RA involves three general approaches. The first is the use of aspirin and other nonsteroidal anti-inflammatory drugs, simple analgesics, and if necessary, low-dose glucocorticoids to control the symptoms and signs of the local inflammatory process. These agents are rapidly effective at mitigating signs and symptoms, but they appear to exert little effect on the progression of the disease. A second group of drugs includes a variety of agents that have been classified as the disease-modifying drugs. These agents appear to have the capacity to decrease elevated levels of acute phase reactants in treated patients and, therefore, are thought to modify the destructive capacity of the disease. A third class of agents includes the immunosuppressive and cytotoxic drugs that have been shown to ameliorate the disease process in some patients.

A number of experimental approaches such as total-lymphoid irradiation, lymphoplasmapheresis, and the administration of the immunosuppressive agent cyclosporin have also been used to treat RA. Although some show potential for ameliorating disease, none has been shown to be a safe and cost-effective way to treat patients on a long-term basis. Recently, substitution of dietary omega-6 essential fatty acids with omega-3 fatty acids such as eicosapentaenoic acid found in certain fish oils has also been shown to provide symptomatic improvement in patients with RA. A variety of nontraditional approaches have also been claimed to be effective in treating RA, including diets, plant and animal extracts, vaccines, hormones, and topical preparations of various sorts. Many of these are costly, and none has been shown to be effective. However, belief in their efficacy ensures their continued use by some patients.

Nonsteroidal anti-inflammatory drugs Besides aspirin, there are now several additional nonsteroidal anti-inflammatory drugs (NSAIDs) available to treat RA. These include fenoprofen, ibuprofen, indomethacin, naproxen, meclofenamate, piroxicam, sulindac, tolmetin, dicloferac, and flurbiprofen. As a result of the capacity of these agents to block the activity of the enzyme cyclooxygenase and therefore the production of prostaglandins, prostacyclin, and thromboxanes, they have analgesic, anti-inflammatory, and antipyretic properties. These agents are all associated with a wide spectrum of toxic side effects. Some, such as gastric irritation, azotemia, platelet dysfunction, and exacerbation of allergic rhinitis and asthma, are related to the inhibition of cyclooxygenase activity, while a variety of others, such as rash, liver function abnormalities, and bone marrow depression, may not be. Elderly patients on diuretics may be at higher risk for certain toxic effects. None of the NSAIDs has been shown to be more effective than aspirin in the treatment of RA. However, these nonaspirin drugs are associated with a lower incidence of gastrointestinal intolerance. None of the newer NSAIDs appears to show significant therapeutic advantages over the other available agents. In addition, there is no consistent advantage of any of these newer agents over the others with respect to the incidence or severity of toxic manifestations.

Disease-modifying drugs Clinical experience has delineated a number of agents that appear to have the capacity to alter the course of RA. This group of agents includes gold compounds, D-penicillamine, the antimalarials, and sulfasalazine. In practice, these agents share a number of characteristics. They exert minimal direct nonspecific anti-inflammatory or analgesic effects, and therefore NSAIDs must be continued during their administration, except in a few cases when true remissions are induced with them. The appearance of benefit from disease-modifying drug therapy is usually delayed for weeks or months. As many as two-thirds of patients develop some clinical improvement as a result of therapy with any of these agents, although the induction of true remissions is unusual. In addition to clinical improvement, there is frequently an improvement in serologic evidence of disease activity, and titers of rheumatoid factor and the erythrocyte sedimentation rate frequently decline. Despite this, there is minimal evidence that disease-modifying drugs actually retard the development of bone erosions or facilitate their healing.

Each of these drugs is associated with considerable toxicity, and therefore, careful patient monitoring is necessary. Which disease-modifying drug should be the drug of first choice remains controversial, and trials have failed to demonstrate a consistent advantage of one over the other. Toxicity of the various agents thus becomes important in determining the drug of first choice. Failure to respond or development of toxicity to one agent does not preclude responsiveness to another. For example, a similar percentage of RA patients who have failed to respond to gold will respond to D-pencillamine when it is given as the second disease-modifying drug. No characteristic features of patients have emerged that predict responsiveness to a disease-modifying drug. Moreover, the indications for the initiation of therapy with one of these agents are not well defined.

Glucocorticoid therapy Although systemic glucocorticoid therapy can provide effective symptomatic therapy in patients with RA, these drugs should be avoided if possible because they do not alter the course of the disease and the potential toxicity of long-term therapy is substantial. Low-dose (less than 7.5 mg per day) prednisone has been advocated as useful additive therapy to control symptoms, but trials have not provided convincing evidence of efficacy and even low-dose therapy may promote osteoporosis.

Immunosuppressive therapy The immunosuppressive drugs azathioprine and cyclophosphamide have been shown to be effective in the treatment of RA and to exert therapeutic effects similar to those of the disease-modifying drugs. However, these agents are no more effective than the disease-modifying drugs. Moreover, they cause a variety of toxic side effects, and cyclophosphamide appears to predispose the patient to the development of malignant neoplasms. Therefore, these drugs have been reserved for patients who have clearly failed therapy with disease-modifying drugs. On occasion, extraarticular disease such as rheumatoid vasculitis may require cytotoxic immunosuppressive therapy.

The folic acid antagonist methotrexate, given in an intermittent low-dose (7.5 to 15 mg once weekly), also may be useful in the treatment of RA. Recent trials have documented the efficacy of methotrexate and have indicated that its onset of action is more rapid than that of disease-modifying drugs. Long-term trials have indicated that methotrexate does not induce remission, but rather suppresses symptoms while it is being administered. Maximal improvement is observed after 6 months of therapy with little additional improvement thereafter. Major toxicity includes gastrointestinal upset and liver function abnormalities that appear to be dose-related and hepatic fibrosis that can be quite insidious, requiring liver biopsy for detection in its early stages.

Surgery Surgery plays a role in the management of patients with severely damaged joints. Although arthroplasties and total joint replacements can be done on a number of joints, the most successful procedures are carried out on hips and knees. Realistic goals of these procedures are relief of pain, correction of deformity, and modest functional improvement. Reconstructive hand surgery may lead to cosmetic improvement and some functional benefit. Open or arthroscopic synovectomy may be useful in some patients with persistent monarthritis, especially of the knee. In addition, early tenosynovectomy of the wrist may prevent tendon rupture.

Approach to the patient with RA At the onset of disease it is difficult to predict the natural history of an individual patient's illness. Therefore, the usual approach is to attempt to alleviate the patient's symptoms with nonsteroidal anti-inflammatory drugs. Some patients may have mild disease that requires no additional therapy. Since the disease-modifying drugs are potentially toxic and not universally effective, their use is usually delayed until it is apparent that symptoms cannot be controlled adequately with nonsteroidal anti-inflammatory drugs.

At some time during most patients' course, the possibility of initiating disease-modifying drug therapy is entertained. With aggressive disease this might occur sooner, often within 3 to 6 months of disease onset, whereas in patients with more indolent disease, smoldering activity may not require such therapy for many years.

The development of bone erosions or radiographic evidence of cartilage loss is clear-cut evidence of the destructive potential of the inflammatory process and indicates the need for disease-modifying drug therapy. The other indications such as persistent pain, joint swelling, or functional impairment are much more subjective, however. The decision to begin use of a disease-modifying drug requires careful monitoring of joint swelling and functional activity, as well as an understanding of the patient's pain tolerance and expectation of therapy. In this setting, the fully informed patient must play an active role in the decision to begin disease-modifying drug therapy, after careful review of the therapeutic and toxic potential of the various drugs.

If a patient responds to a disease-modifying drug, therapy is continued with careful monitoring to avoid toxicity. All disease-modifying drugs provide a suppressive effect and therefore require prolonged administration. Even with successful therapy, local injection of glucocorticoids may be necessary to diminish inflammation that may persist in a limited number of joints. In addition, nonsteroidal anti-inflammatory drugs may be necessary to mitigate symptoms. Even after inflammation has totally resolved, symptoms from loss of cartilage and supervening degenerative joint disease or deformities may require additional treatment. Surgery may also be necessary to relieve pain or diminish the functional impairment secondary to deformity. Only when patients have persistent inflammatory disease or severe extraarticular manifestations is the use of cytotoxic immunosuppressive drugs or experimental procedures justified.

REFERENCES

ARNETT FC et al: The American Rheumatism Association 1987 revised criteria for the classification of rheumatoid arthritis. Arthritis Rheum 31:315, 1988

ATHANASON NA et al: Immunohistology of rheumatoid nodules and rheumatoid synovium. Ann Rheum Dis 47:398, 1988

CLELAND LG et al: Clinical and biochemical effects of dietary fish oil supplements in rheumatoid arthritis. J Rheum 15:10, 1988

CUSH JJ, LIPSKY PE: Phenotypic analysis of synovial tissue and peripheral blood lymphocytes isolated from patients with rheumatoid arthritis. Arthritis Rheum 31:1230, 1988

EMERY P et al: Deficiency of the suppressor-inducer subset of T lymphocytes in rheumatoid arthritis. Arthritis Rheum 30:849, 1987

FEIGENBAUM SL et al. Prognosis in rheumatoid arthritis: A longitudinal study of newly diagnosed younger adult patients. Am J Med 66:377, 1979

FIRESTEIN G, ZVAIFLER N: The pathogenesis of rheumatoid arthritis, in *Immunology of Rheumatic Diseases,* DS Pisetsky et al (eds). Rheumatic Dis Clin North Am 13:447, 1987

GOTO M et al: T cytotoxic and helper cells are markedly increased and T suppressor and inducer cells are markedly decreased in rheumatoid synovial fluids. Arthritis Rheum 30:737, 1987

HOCHBERG MC: Adult and juvenile rheumatoid arthritis: Current epidemiologic concepts. Epidemiol Rev 3:27, 1981

KEYSTONE EC et al: Elevated soluble interleukin-2 receptor levels in the sera and synovial fluids of patients with rheumatoid arthritis. Arthritis Rheum 31:844, 1988

KREMER JM, LEE JK: A long-term prospective study of the use of methotrexate in rheumatoid arthritis. Update after a mean of fifty-three months. Arthritis Rheum 31:577, 1988

LIPSKY PE: Gold, penicillamine and antimalarials, in *Inflammation: Basic Principles and Clinical Correlates,* JI Gallin et al (eds). New York, Raven Press, 1988, pp 897–910

MITCHELL DM et al: Survival, prognosis and causes of death in rheumatoid arthritis. Arthritis Rheum 29:706, 1986

NEPOM GT et al: The molecular basis for HLA class II associations with rheumatoid arthritis. J Clin Immunol 7:1, 1987

PINALS RS: Sulfasalazine in the rheumatic diseases. Semin Arthritis Rheum 17:246, 1988

PINCUS T et al: Severe functional declines, work disability, and increased mortality in seventy-five rheumatoid arthritis patients studied over nine years. Arthritis Rheum 27:864, 1984

SCHNEIDER HA et al: Rheumatoid vasculitis: Experience with 13 patients and review of the literature. Semin Arthritis Rheum 14:280, 1985

SCOTT TE et al: HLA-DR4 and pulmonary dysfunction in rheumatoid arthritis. Am J Med 82: 765, 1987

SHERRER YS et al: The development of disability in rheumatoid arthritis. Arthritis Rheum 29:494, 1986

UTSINGER DD et al (eds): *Rheumatoid Arthritis.* Philadelphia, Lippincott, 1985

271 SYSTEMIC SCLEROSIS (SCLERODERMA)

BRUCE C. GILLILAND

DEFINITION Systemic sclerosis (SSc) is a multisystem disorder of unknown etiology characterized by fibrosis of the skin, blood vessels, and visceral organs including the gastrointestinal tract, lungs, heart, and kidneys. The degree and rate of skin and internal organ involvement vary among patients. Two subsets, however, can be identified, even though there is some overlap. One subset is referred to as *diffuse cutaneous scleroderma* and is characterized by the rapid development of symmetric skin thickening of proximal and distal extremity, face, and trunk. These patients are at greater risk for developing kidney and other visceral disease early in their course. The other subset is *limited cutaneous scleroderma,* which is defined by symmetric skin thickening limited to fingers or distal extremity and to the face. This subset frequently has features of CREST syndrome, an acronym standing for calcinosis, Raynaud's phenomenon, esophageal dysmotility, sclerodactyly, and telangiectasia. The prognosis in limited cutaneous scleroderma is better except for the occasional patient who, after many years, develops pulmonary arterial hypertension or biliary cirrhosis. Systemic sclerosis of visceral organs also may occur in the absence of any skin involvement. Survival is determined by the severity of visceral disease, especially involving the heart, lungs, and/or kidneys.

Scleroderma can also occur in a localized form limited to the skin, subcutaneous tissue, and muscle, and without systemic involvement. The two localized forms are morphea, which occurs as single or multiple plaques of skin induration, and linear scleroderma, which involves an extremity or face.

SSc also occurs in association with features of other connective tissue diseases. The term *overlap syndrome* has been used to describe such patients. *Undifferentiated connective tissue disease* has been suggested as a designation for patients who do not have diagnostic criteria for any one connective tissue disease. *Mixed connective tissue disease* is a syndrome involving features of systemic lupus erythematosus, systemic sclerosis, polymyositis, and rheumatoid arthritis and very high titers of circulating antibody to nuclear ribonucleoprotein antigen (see Chap. 272). *Eosinophilic fasciitis* is a scleroderma-like illness and will be discussed in this chapter.

EPIDEMIOLOGY SSc has a worldwide distribution and affects all races. The onset of disease is usually in the third to fifth decade, and the incidence increases with age. Women are affected approximately three times as often as men, and even more often during the childbearing years. The onset of scleroderma in childhood is unusual. The annual incidence has been estimated to be 14.1 cases per million population based on a 20-year study performed in Allegheny County, Pennsylvania. The role of heredity has not been clarified. Several examples of familial SSc have been reported, and the finding of other connective tissue diseases and autoantibodies in relatives of involved patients suggests a hereditary predisposition.

Several environmental factors have been associated with the development of SSc and scleroderma-like illnesses. SSc appears to be more common in coal and gold miners, especially in those with more extensive exposure, suggesting that silica dust may be a predisposing factor. Workers exposed to polyvinyl chloride may develop Raynaud's phenomenon, acroosteolysis, scleroderma-like skin lesions, and nailfold capillary abnormalities similar to those observed in SSc. These workers may also develop hepatic fibrosis and angiosarcoma. The development of scleroderma has been associated with exposure to vinyl chloride, epoxy resins, and aromatic hydrocarbons such as benzine and toluene. In 1981, in Spain, a multisystem disease resembling scleroderma occurred following the ingestion of adulterated cooking oil (rapeseed oil). Approximately 20,000 people were affected. The patients initially develop interstitial pneumonitis, eosinophilia, arthralgias, arthritis, and myositis, followed subsequently by joint contractures, skin thickening, Raynaud's phenomenon, pulmonary hypertension, sicca syndrome, and resorption of the distal fingertips. Extensive sclerosis of the dermis and subcutaneous tissue has been noted in patients receiving pentazocine, a nonnarcotic analgesic agent. Bleomycin, an anticancer agent, produces fibrotic skin nodules, linear hyperpigmentation, alopecia, gangrene of fingers, and pulmonary fibrosis affecting mainly the lower lobes. In Japan, the use of paraffin or silicone for breast augmentation has been associated with the development of SSc.

PATHOGENESIS The outstanding feature of SSc is the overproduction of collagen that is qualitatively normal. The increased collagen production is thought to be due to aberrant regulation of fibroblast cell growth and/or to increased biosynthesis of connective tissue. While etiology for this abnormal production is unknown, immunologic and vascular mechanisms are thought to play a role in the development of fibrosis and other features of SSc.

Numerous immunologic abnormalities have been noted in patients with SSc. Antinuclear antibodies are found in approximately 95 percent of patients and hypergammaglobulinemia in at least one-third of patients. Systemic sclerosis is also found in association with other connective tissue diseases suspected to be of autoimmune origin. Abnormalities of T-cell population have been noted, and include decreased CD8-suppressor-cell activity and increased CD4-helper-cell activity. The CD4/CD8 ratio is increased in peripheral blood and in early skin lesions of SSc due to decreased number of CD8 lymphocytes. CD4 cells have been shown to produce more interleukin 2 than cells from normal subjects. Natural killer (NK) cell activity is also reduced in the peripheral blood of patients, particularly in those with diffuse cutaneous disease early in their course. NK cells are a subpopulation of lymphocytes which participate in surveillance against certain microbes and neoplasms as well as in the control of the immune system. They have been shown to produce a number of immunomodulary proteins that inhibit B-cell differentiation, suppress immunoglobulin production, and lyse antigen-processing cells. The number of NK cells is normal in SSc patients, suggesting that the loss of function represents an intrinsic cellular defect.

Lymphocytes and monocytes are found in close proximity to fibroblasts in active skin disease of patients with SSc, which suggests a role for cell-mediated immunity in stimulating increased collagen production. These lymphocytes are mostly T cells. Studies have shown the number of circulating T cells in SSc patients to be normal or decreased; the latter finding may indicate attraction of T cells to sites of active disease in skin and other organs. Supernatants from activated normal peripheral lymphocytes contain lymphokines that can stimulate cultured fibroblasts to produce collagen. Crude extracts from skin of SSc patients or normals have been observed to stimulate patients' lymphocytes as measured by the macrophage migration inhibition test. Interleukin 1, a product of activated monocytes, also can stimulate fibroblast proliferation, but its importance in SSc is uncertain since studies have shown increased as well as decreased interleukin 1 production. Additional support for involvement of cell-mediated immunity in the pathogenesis of SSc is the appearance of scleroderma-like lesions in patients with graft-versus-host disease (GVHD) after bone marrow transplantation and in a murine model of chronic GVHD, conditions known to be associated with activated T cells. More recently, mast cells have been implicated in the development of fibrosis. Increased numbers of mast cells are found in the deeper layer of dermis in the early phase of disease. On interaction with T lymphocytes, mast cells release products that stimulate fibroblasts to secrete increased amounts of collagen. Further studies are required to better understand the role of altered immunity in the pathogenesis of SSc.

Vascular damage is also involved in the pathogenesis of SSc. Vascular abnormalities are noted before the appearance of fibrosis. Fibrosis is initially often perivascular, suggesting that vascular inflammatory events may subsequently affect the surrounding connective tissue. The initial event is postulated to be endothelial cell injury, which subsequently leads to intimal thickening, narrowing of the lumen, decreased distensibility, and eventual obliteration of blood vessels. The cause of endothelial damage is not known. The finding of a serum nonimmunoglobulin cytotoxic factor for endothelial cells in some patients has not been confirmed in other studies. The sera of some patients mediate antibody-dependent cellular cytotoxicity (ADCC) directed against human microvascular endothelial cells. Endothelial cell damage is reflected by elevated plasma levels of von Willebrand factor in SSc patients. The binding of von Willebrand factor to exposed subendothelium permits adhesion and activation of platelets. Activated platelets release platelet derived growth factor (PDGF), which has been demonstrated to be chemotactic and mitogenic for both smooth-muscle cells and fibroblasts. PDGF may be one of several factors stimulating intimal fibrosis and with its passage through the injured endothelium could also account for adventitial and perivascular fibrosis. Intravascular fibrin deposits appear in small arteries and arterioles and may cause the microangiopathic hemolytic anemia observed in some patients. The number of small arteries, arterioles, and capillaries in skin and other organs is eventually reduced. The remaining capillaries in skin dilate and proliferate to become visible telangiectatic lesions.

Chromosomal abnormalities have been noted in greater than 90 percent of SSc patients. These acquired abnormalities include chromatid breaks, acentric fragments, and ring chromosomes and are found in approximately 30 percent of mitotic cells. A chromosomal breakage factor has been found in the serum of SSc patients. The significance of these chromosomal abnormalities is unknown.

PATHOLOGY In the skin, a thin epidermis overlies compact bundles of collagen which lie parallel to the epidermis. Fingerlike projections of collagen extend from the dermis into the subcutaneous tissue and bind the skin to the underlying tissue. Dermal appendages are atrophied, and rete pegs are lost. In early stages of disease, increased numbers of T cells, monocytes, plasma cells, and mast cells are found, particularly in the lower dermis of involved skin.

In the lower two-thirds of the esophagus, the histologic findings consist of a thin mucosa and increased collagen in the lamina propria, submucosa, and serosa. The degree of fibrosis is less than in the skin. Atrophy of the muscularis in the esophagus and throughout the involved portions of the gastrointestinal tract is more prominent than the amount of fibrotic replacement of muscle. Ulceration of the mucosa is often present and may be due to either SSc or superimposed peptic esophagitis. Striated muscles in the upper one-third of the esophagus are relatively spared. Similar changes may be found throughout the gastrointestinal tract, especially in the second and third portions of the duodenum, jejunum, and large intestine. Atrophy of the muscularis of the large intestine may lead to the development of large-mouth diverticula. In the later stages of the disease, the involved portions of the gastrointestinal tract become dilated. Infiltration of lymphocytes and plasma cells in the lamina propria is also present.

With pulmonary involvement, diffuse interstitial fibrosis, thickening of the alveolar membrane, and peribronchial fibrosis are observed. Bronchiolar epithelial proliferation accompanies the pulmonary fibrosis. Rupture of septa produces small cysts and areas of bullous emphysema. Small pulmonary arteries and arterioles show intimal thickening, fragmentation of the elastica, and muscular hypertrophy; this may occur without interstitial pulmonary fibrosis and produce pulmonary hypertension.

The synovium in patients with arthritis is similar to that seen in early rheumatoid arthritis and shows edema with infiltration of lymphocytes and plasma cells. A characteristic finding is a thick layer of fibrin overlying and within the synovium. Later in the disease the synovium may become fibrotic. Fibrinous deposits appear on the surfaces of tendon sheaths and in the overlying fascia and may lead to audible creaking over moving tendons.

Histologic features of primary myopathy consist of interstitial and perivascular lymphocytic infiltrations, degeneration of muscle fibers, and interstitial fibrosis. Arterioles may be thickened, and capillaries may be decreased in number. Pathologic and electrophysiologic findings of polymyositis in proximal muscles are present in the few patients who are considered to have the overlap syndrome of SSc and polymyositis.

Cardiac involvement consists of degeneration of myocardial fibers and irregular areas of interstitial fibrosis that is most prominent around blood vessels. Fibrosis also involves the conduction system, leading to atrioventricular conduction defects and arrhythmias. The wall of smaller coronary arteries may be thickened. Fibrinous pericarditis and pericardial effusions are found in some patients.

Renal involvement is found in over half the patients and consists of intimal hyperplasia of the interlobular arteries, fibrinoid necrosis of the afferent arterioles, including the glomerular tuft, and thickening of the glomerular basement membrane. Small cortical infarctions and glomerulosclerosis may be present. The renal pathologic change is often indistinguishable from that observed in malignant hypertension. Renal vascular lesions, however, may be present in the absence of hypertension. Immunofluorescence studies of kidney have shown IgM, complement components, and fibrinogen in the walls of affected vessels. Angiographic renal studies in patients with SSc may show constriction of the intralobular arteries, a finding that simulates the vasospasm of the digital arteries observed in Raynaud's phenomenon. Cold-induced Raynaud's phenomenon has been shown to decrease renal blood flow.

Primary liver involvement is not common. Primary biliary cirrhosis occurs in some patients, particularly in those with the limited cutaneous form of SSc. Fibrosis of the thyroid gland may develop in the presence or absence of autoimmune thyroiditis.

Thickening of the periodontal membrane with replacement of the lamina dura is demonstrated radiographically as widening of the periodontal space and rarely causes loosening of the teeth.

Pathologic changes in small arteries and arterioles consist of concentric subintimal proliferation and periadventitial fibrosis, with narrowing or occlusion of the lumen. These vascular abnormalities have been described in digits, skin, muscle, lung, kidney, and other viscera. Arteritis with fibrinoid necrosis is occasionally observed.

CLINICAL MANIFESTATIONS Systemic sclerosis usually begins insidiously; the first symptoms are frequently Raynaud's phenomenon and puffy fingers. Ninety-five percent of patients will experience Raynaud's phenomenon, which is defined as episodic vasoconstriction of small arteries and arterioles of fingers, toes, and sometimes the tip of the nose and the earlobes. Episodes are brought on by cold exposure, vibration, or emotional stress. Patients experience pallor and/or cyanosis followed by rubor on rewarming. Pallor and/or cyanosis are usually associated with coldness and numbness of fingers and/or toes, and rubor with pain and tingling. Raynaud's phenomenon may precede skin changes by several months or even years in those patients who subsequently develop the limited cutaneous form of SSc. After 2 or more years of Raynaud's phenomenon, few patients who have this as their only symptom will subsequently develop SSc.

In early disease, fingers and hands are swollen. Swelling may also involve forearms, feet, lower legs, and face. However, lower extremities are relatively spared. This edematous phase may last for a few weeks, months, or even longer. The edema may be pitting or nonpitting. The skin gradually becomes firm, thickened, and eventually tightly bound to underlying subcutaneous tissue (indurative phase). In patients with diffuse cutaneous scleroderma, skin changes will become generalized and involve the extremities, face, and trunk. Rapid progression of these changes over a 2- to 3-year period is associated with a greater risk of visceral disease, particularly of the lungs, heart, or kidneys. On the other hand, patients with limited cutaneous scleroderma will usually have a more gradual progression of skin changes which are restricted to fingers or distal extremity and face. After many years of disease, the skin may soften and return to normal thickness or become thin and atrophic.

In the extremity, the taut skin over fingers gradually limits full extension, and flexion contractures develop. Ulcers may appear on the volar pads of the fingertips and over bony prominences such as elbows, malleoli, and the extensor surface of the proximal interphalangeal joints of the hands. These ulcers may become secondarily infected. The soft tissue of fingertips is lost. In some instances, resorption of the terminal phalanges occurs. Skin over the extremities, face, and trunk may become darkly pigmented, even without exposure to the sun. Pigmentation of the skin may occur over superficial blood vessels and tendons. The skin loses hair, oil, and sweat glands and so becomes dry and coarse.

In some patients, particularly those with the limited cutaneous form of disease, calcific deposits develop in intracutaneous and subcutaneous tissue. The sites commonly involved are periarticular tissue, digital pads, olecranon and prepatellar bursae, and skin along the extensor surface of the forearms. The overlying skin may break down, with drainage of calcific material. Involvement of the face results in loss of skin wrinkles and facial expression, as well as microstomia, which may make eating and dental hygiene difficult. The capillary bed of nailfolds of the fingers may show enlargement of capillaries with little or no capillary loss, usually indicative of limited cutaneous scleroderma. In diffuse cutaneous scleroderma, there is disorganization of the capillary bed and decreased numbers of capillaries. These capillary changes, which are observed by wide angle microscopy or with an ophthalmoscope used as a magnifier, are not found in patients who have only Raynaud's phenomenon.

More than half the patients with SSc complain of pain, swelling, and stiffness of the fingers and knees. A symmetric polyarthritis, resembling rheumatoid arthritis, may be seen. In more advanced stages of the disease, leathery crepitation can be palpated over moving joints, especially the knee. Extensive fibrotic thickening of the tendon sheaths in the wrist can produce a carpal tunnel syndrome. Muscle weakness usually is present in patients with severe skin involvement and, in most cases, is due to disuse atrophy. There is a distinctive histologic myopathy that accompanies SSc which is not associated with muscle enzyme abnormalities. A few patients develop a myositis characterized by proximal muscle weakness and muscle enzyme elevations that are identical to polymyositis (overlap syndrome). In addition to terminal phalanges, resorption of bone may involve ribs, clavicle, and angle of mandible.

Symptoms attributable to esophageal involvement are present in more than 50 percent of patients and include epigastric fullness, burning pain in the epigastric or retrosternal regions, and regurgitation of gastric contents. These symptoms, most noticeable when the patient is lying flat or bending over, are due to the reduced tone of the gastroesophageal sphincter and to dilatation of the distal esophagus. Peptic esophagitis frequently occurs and may lead to strictures and narrowing of the lower esophagus. However, it seldom results in bleeding. Dysphagia, particularly of solid foods, may occur independent of other esophageal symptoms and is caused by the loss of esophageal motility due to neuromuscular dysfunction. Manometry or cineradiography reveals decreased amplitude or disappearance of peristaltic waves in the lower two-thirds of the esophagus. Raynaud's phenomenon in the absence of a connective tissue disease is also associated with esophageal dysmotility. Later in the course of the illness, dilatation and atony of the lower portion of the esophagus as well as reflux are seen. With gastric involvement, barium studies show dilatation, atony, and delayed gastric emptying.

Hypomotility of the small intestine produces symptoms of bloating and abdominal pain, and may suggest an intestinal obstruction or paralytic ileus (pseudoobstruction). Malabsorption syndrome with weight loss, diarrhea, and anemia is due to bacterial overgrowth in the atonic intestine or possibly to obliteration of lymphatics by fibrosis. Roentgenographic features of the second and third portions of the duodenum and of the jejunum include dilatation, loss of the usual feathery pattern, and delayed disappearance of barium. Pneumatosis intestinalis occasionally occurs and appears as radiolucent cysts or linear streaks within the wall of the small intestine. Benign pneumoperitoneum may result from the rupture of these cysts. Involvement of the large intestine may cause chronic constipation and fecal impaction with episodes of bowel obstruction. Barium studies of the large intestine may show dilatation, atony, and large-mouth diverticula. Some patients may have gastrointestinal features of SSc with little or no cutaneous or other organ involvement.

The lungs are affected in SSc in at least two-thirds of the patients. The most common symptom is exertional dyspnea, often accompanied by a dry, nonproductive cough. Symptoms may occur in the absence of pulmonary fibrosis, and patients with pulmonary fibrosis can be relatively asymptomatic. Bilateral basilar rales may be present. Restriction of chest movement caused by extensive skin involvement of the thorax rarely occurs. Aspiration pneumonia may result from gastric reflux due to lower esophageal atony. Superimposed bacterial or viral pneumonia can be a serious complication in patients with pulmonary fibrosis. There is an increased frequency of alveolar cell and bronchogenic carcinoma in patients with pulmonary fibrosis. Pulmonary function tests are frequently abnormal and show a reduction in vital capacity and decreased lung compliance. Impairment of gas exchange is reflected by a low diffusing capacity and low P_{O_2} with exercise. These abnormalities may be present even when the chest radiograph is normal. Chest film may show a pattern of linear densities, mottling, and honeycombing involving most prominently the lower two-thirds of the lung. In the absence of significant interstitial fibrosis, a severe form of pulmonary arterial hypertension develops after many years of disease in patients with limited cutaneous scleroderma. Less than 10 percent of patients will develop this complication, which is caused by narrowing and obliteration of pulmonary arteries and arterioles by intimal fibrosis and medial hypertrophy. Pulmonary hypertension is manifested by progressive worsening of dyspnea and eventually by appearance of right-sided heart failure. Electrocardiographic evidence of pulmonary hypertension is usually present. The prognosis is extremely poor with the development of pulmonary hypertension; the mean duration of survival is approximately 2 years.

Primary cardiac involvement in SSc includes pericarditis with or without effusions, heart failure, and varying degrees of heart block or arrhythmias. Cardiomyopathy attributable to myocardial fibrosis appears in fewer than 10 percent of patients, and involves primarily those patients with diffuse cutaneous scleroderma. Radionuclide studies have shown abnormalities of left ventricular function due to myocardial fibrosis. Cold-induced vasospasm of the hands produces defects in myocardial thallium perfusion. The characteristic pathologic feature of contraction band necrosis results from cardiac muscle damage caused by intermittent vasospasm of coronary vessels. Patients may experience angina pectoris even though coronary angiograms are normal. Patients can also develop left ventricular failure secondary to systemic hypertension or cor pulmonale secondary to pulmonary arterial hypertension.

Renal failure is the leading cause of death in SSc, accounting for almost half of the deaths. Significant renal disease occurs mostly in those patients with diffuse cutaneous scleroderma. A high risk of renal crisis is present in those patients who have rapidly progressive widespread skin thickening early in their course. Renal crisis is characterized by malignant hypertension, which can rapidly progress to renal failure. These patients manifest hypertensive encephalopathy, severe headache, retinopathy, seizures, and left ventricular failure. Hematuria and proteinuria are followed by oliguria and renal failure. The mechanism for the hypertensive crisis is activation of the renin-angiotensin system. Before the advent of effective antihypertensive drugs, the majority of these patients died within 6 months. Renal failure can also develop insidiously later in the course of disease in the setting of mild to moderate hypertension and proteinuria. In these patients or those with clinically unrecognized renal disease, reduction of renal plasma flow secondary to heart failure or volume depletion resulting from overdiuresis may precipitate renal crisis. An indicator of impending renal failure is microangiopathic anemia, which may occur in a normotensive patient. The presence of a chronic pericardial effusion may also herald subsequent renal failure.

Symptoms of dry eyes and/or dry mouth are frequently present in patients with SSc. Lip biopsy may show lymphocytic infiltration of minor salivary glands characteristic of Sjögren's syndrome or intraglandular or periglandular fibrosis. Antibodies to SS-A (Ro) and/or SS-B (La) are found in those patients with lip biopsies consistent with Sjögren's syndrome and not in those with salivary gland fibrosis.

Hypothyroidism occurs in a significant number of patients and may be associated with high levels of antithyroid antibodies. Fibrosis of the thyroid gland may be present, but also occurs in the absence of autoimmune thyroiditis. Other manifestations of SSc include trigeminal neuralgia and male impotence secondary to decreased penile tumescence. These men have normal serum levels of testosterone and gonadotropins. Pathogenesis of this abnormality has been considered to be due either to vascular and/or autonomic nervous system abnormalities.

LABORATORY FINDINGS The erythrocyte sedimentation rate may be elevated. Hypoproliferative anemia related to chronic inflammation is the most common cause of anemia in SSc. Anemia may also be caused by iron deficiency secondary to gastrointestinal bleeding. Bacterial overgrowth due to atony of the small bowel may lead to vitamin B_{12} and/or folic acid–deficiency anemia. Microangiopathic hemolytic anemia is most often associated with renal involvement and is caused by the presence of intravascular fibrin in renal arterioles. Hypergammaglobulinemia, consisting mostly of IgG, is found in approximately half the patients. Rheumatoid factor, in low titer, is present in 25 percent of patients. Antinuclear antibodies detected by using a cultured human laryngeal carcinoma cell line (HEp-2) substrate are present in 95 percent of patients. Antinuclear antibodies that have a high specificity for SSc are antitopoisomerase 1 (Scl-70), antinucleolar, and anticentromere. Antitopoisomerase 1, originally called anti-Scl-70, recognizes the nuclear enzyme DNA topoisomerase 1. These antibodies are found in about 20 percent of patients, and are associated with diffuse cutaneous involvement and interstitial pulmonary disease. They are seldom present in other disorders or in conjunction with anticentromere antibodies. Antinucleolar antibodies are relatively specific for SSc and are present in approximately 20 to 30 percent of patients. Anticentromere antibodies react with protein antigens located in the kinetochore region of chromosomes and are strongly associated with limited cutaneous scleroderma or CREST syndrome. Anticentromere antibodies are found in only about 10 percent of patients with diffuse cutaneous scleroderma and rarely in other connective tissue diseases. They are occasionally found in patients with only Raynaud's phenomenon and may indicate subsequent development of limited cutaneous disease. High titers of anti-RNP are present in those patients with features of mixed connective tissue disease. Anti-PM-Scl, formerly referred to as anti-PMl, may be found in SSc patients with polymyositis and renal involvement. Anti-SS-A and/or anti-SS-B are present in those patients with overlap syndrome of SSc and Sjögren's syndrome.

DIAGNOSIS The diagnosis of SSc presents no difficulty in the presence of Raynaud's phenomenon, with typical skin lesions and visceral involvement. Although Raynaud's phenomenon may be the first symptom of SSc, most patients with Raynaud's phenomenon alone do not develop a connective tissue disease. Other causes of Raynaud's phenomenon include thoracic outlet (scalenus anticus and cervical rib) syndromes, shoulder-hand syndrome, trauma (jackhammer or vibratory machine operators), previous cold injury, vinyl chloride exposure, and circulating cryoglobulins or cold agglutinins. Linear scleroderma and morphea are localized forms of scleroderma that can usually be distinguished clinically. In early disease, SSc may initially be confused with rheumatoid arthritis, systemic lupus erythematosus, or polymyositis when articular or muscle involvement is prominent. SSc without cutaneous involvement should be considered in patients with unexplained pulmonary fibrosis, pulmonary hypertension, cardiomyopathies, heart block, dysphagia, or malabsorption syndrome. Several conditions have scleroderma-like features but lack the visceral involvement. Scleredema (scleredema adultorum of Buschke) occurs predominantly in children and is characterized by painless edematous induration involving the face, scalp, neck, trunk, and proximal portions of the extremities. Involvement of the hands and feet usually does not occur. Scleredema may be associated with previous streptococcal infection and is usually self-limited, resolving in 6 to 12 months. Histology reveals accumulation of mucopolysaccharides in the dermis and skeletal muscle. A rare entity, scleromyxedema (lichen myxedematosus), is manifested by yellowish or pale red papules in association with diffuse skin thickening which may involve the face and hands. Acid mucopolysaccharide deposits are found in the dermis. Monoclonal IgG may be detected in some of these patients. Primary amyloidosis may involve the skin of the extremities and face diffusely to give the appearance of scleroderma. Biopsy will clearly differentiate these entities.

COURSE AND PROGNOSIS The course of SSc is quite variable. Until disease differentiates into recognizable subsets, prognosis in early disease is difficult to predict. Patients with limited cutaneous scleroderma, especially those with anticentromere antibodies, have a good prognosis, with the notable exception of those few patients, less than 10 percent, who after 10 to 20 years or longer develop pulmonary arterial hypertension. Malabsorption syndrome and primary biliary cirrhosis are the causes of morbidity and mortality in some patients with limited cutaneous disease. On the other hand, the prognosis is generally worse in patients with diffuse cutaneous disease, particularly when the onset occurs at an older age. In addition, males have a worse prognosis. Renal and other visceral organ disease may develop early in the course of those patients with rapidly progressive generalized skin thickening. Death occurs most often from cardiac, renal, or pulmonary involvement. In one study the 10-year cumulative survival of patients with only renal involvement was 30 percent and of patients with only lung involvement, 50 percent. In patients without heart, lung, or kidney involvement, survival was 71 percent.

Skin may spontaneously soften after years of disease. Softening occurs in the reverse order of original skin involvement beginning with the trunk and followed by the proximal and then the distal extremities. Sclerodactyly may persist. Skin thickness may eventually approach normal.

TREATMENT Even though SSc cannot be cured, treatment of involved organ systems can relieve symptoms and improve function. The doctor-patient relationship is extremely important in caring for patients with this chronic debilitating illness. Once the diagnosis of SSc has been made, the patient and family should be instructed about this disorder. The patient will need repeated explanations and reassurances throughout his or her illness. Depending on the severity of illness, the patient will require monitoring of blood pressure, blood counts, urinalysis, and renal and pulmonary function on a regular basis.

Effectiveness of drug therapy in SSc is difficult to evaluate because of the variable course and severity of the disease. Many drugs have been used in the treatment of SSc without any consistent or prolonged benefit. In uncontrolled studies D-penicillamine has been reported to reduce skin thickening and prevent development of significant organ involvement. This drug interferes with inter- and intramolecular cross-linking of collagen and is also immunosuppressive. Its immunosuppressive activity may also lead to decrease of collagen production. Penicillamine is better tolerated when started at a low dose, usually 250 mg per day, and then increased at 1- to 3-month intervals up to 1.5 g per day as tolerated. Although a few patients can tolerate higher doses, most patients are maintained on a dose between 0.5 and 1 g per day. For optimal absorption, it is important to give this drug 1 h before or 2 h after a meal. This drug can be quite toxic; its more serious complications include glomerulonephritis with nephrotic syndrome, aplastic anemia, leukopenia, thrombocytopenia, and myasthenia gravis. Other side effects are fever, rash, anorexia, nausea, and loss of taste. Patients should have monthly complete blood counts (including platelet count) and urinalysis. Azathioprine and other immunosuppressives have also been used in SSc, and should be reserved for those patients with rapidly progressive and life-threatening disease. Control studies are lacking. A trial of treatment with recombinant γ-interferon is currently in progress. This agent has been shown to inhibit collagen production.

Antiplatelet therapy may play a role in the treatment of SSc since the biologic products of platelets affect blood vessels. Low doses of aspirin block the formation of thromboxane A_2, a powerful vasoconstrictor and platelet aggregator. In addition, dipyridamole 200 to 400 mg in divided daily doses also decreases platelet adhesion to damaged vessel walls. While these drugs have a reasonable therapeutic rationale, a 2-year double-blind study did not show any benefit from their use. Reports of beneficial effects of colchicine or chlorambucil have not been documented in controlled studies.

Glucocorticoids are indicated in those patients with inflammatory myositis or pericarditis. The initial dose is 40 to 60 mg per day and is tapered based on clinical improvement. Prednisone 10 mg per day or less may be beneficial in treating arthritis refractory to nonsteroidal anti-inflammatory drugs and in reducing edema associated with the edematous phase of early skin involvement. Glucocorticoids are not otherwise indicated in the long-term treatment of SSc. High doses of glucocorticoids may play a role in precipitating acute renal failure. However, this association remains unclear.

The management of Raynaud's phenomenon is directed at control of vasospasm. Patients should be advised to dress warmly and wear mittens and socks, not to smoke, to remove causes of external stress, and to avoid drugs such as amphetamine and ergotamine. Beta blocking drugs may make Raynaud's phenomenon worse. Warmth of the central body induces peripheral vasodilatation. Drugs that block sympathetic vasoconstriction, such as reserpine, α-methyldopa, phenoxybenzamine, and prazosin may be useful in the treatment of Raynaud's phenomenon, but their side effects often curtail extended use. Calcium channel blockers, nifedipine and diltiazam, can be effective in alleviating Raynaud's phenomenon, but side effects of light-headedness and palpitations may limit their use. The dose of nifedipine is 10 to 20 mg tid. Ketanserin, an oral serotonin antagonist, has also been shown to be effective. Techniques of biofeedback have also been used with variable success for teaching patients to control the temperature of their hands. Surgical sympathectomy usually provides only temporary improvement, and it, along with other forms of therapy, does not prevent progression of the vascular lesion. The response to any therapy for Raynaud's phenomenon is limited by the degree of existing structural narrowing of digital arteries. Gangrene of distal digits may occur and require surgical amputation.

Numerous drugs have been claimed to soften the hidebound skin, but documentation in controlled studies is lacking. These drugs include D-penicillamine, colchicine, *p*-aminobenzoic acid, and vitamin E. Dryness of the skin may be reduced by avoiding frequent use of detergent soaps and by applying regularly hydrophilic ointments and bath oils. Regular exercise helps to maintain flexibility of extremities and pliability of skin. Massaging the skin several times a day may also be beneficial. Fingertip ulcerations can be protected by applying a guard or cage over the end of the finger. The use of an occlusive dressing over a noninfected ulcer may promote healing and protect the finger. Skin ulcers should be kept clean by soaking or by surgical or chemical debridement. Sympatholytic drugs or local nitroglycerine paste applied to the ulcer may be beneficial in promoting healing. Infected ulcers can usually be treated with topical antibiotics but may require systemic antibiotics especially when there is a question of underlying osteomyelitis.

Patients with reflux esophagitis are treated with small frequent meals, antacids between meals, and elevation of the head of the bed. Patients should be advised not to lie down for a few hours after a meal, and to avoid coffee, tea, and chocolate, which reduce the pressure of the lower esophageal sphincter. Cimetidine or ranitidine may be beneficial in some patients. Metoclopramide can also be of help in some patients. Patients with dysphagia should be instructed to chew their food thoroughly and wash it down with fluids. Malabsorption syndrome due to duodenal hypomotility and bacterial overgrowth may improve with intermittent use of appropriate antibiotics. Patients with severe debilitating malabsorption may benefit from parenteral hyperalimentation. Stool softeners and mild laxatives are usually adequate for treating constipation due to hypomotility of the colon.

Acute myositis is usually responsive to glucocorticoids; these drugs should not be used for the indolent primary form of muscle disease of SSc. Articular symptoms are treated with aspirin or other nonsteroidal anti-inflammatory agents.

Pulmonary fibrosis is not reversible, and therefore treatment is directed at symptoms or complications. Pulmonary infection requires prompt treatment with antibiotics. Hypoxia necessitates giving low concentrations of oxygen. The role of glucocorticoids in preventing progression of interstitial lung disease is not clear. Patients should receive Pneumovax and yearly influenza immunizations.

Recognition of early renal failure is important in order to preserve remaining function. Renal involvement is often accompanied by hypertension and mild to moderate proteinuria. An occasional patient may be normotensive. Antihypertensive agents are often effective in lowering blood pressure and stabilizing or reversing renal failure. These drugs include propranolol, clonidine, and minoxidil. Particularly effective are the angiotensin-converting enzyme inhibitors, which include captopril and enalapril. Dialysis may be required in patients with progressive renal failure. Some patients, however, have a slow return of renal function after several months and may no longer require dialysis.

Patients with cardiac failure require careful monitoring of digitalis and diuretic administration. Pericardial effusions may also improve with diuretics. Care should be taken to avoid overdiuresis which may lead to decreased renal blood flow, decreased cardiac output, and renal failure.

EOSINOPHILIC FASCIITIS Eosinophilic fasciitis is a scleroderma-like syndrome characterized by inflammation followed later by sclerosis of the dermis, subcutis, and deep fascia. The disease affects adults, and often occurs after strenuous physical activity. Patients do not have Raynaud's phenomenon or internal organ involvement. Several immunologic abnormalities have been associated with eosinophilic fasciitis and include aplastic anemia, myelodysplastic syndrome, and thrombocytopenia. Patients usually have the abrupt onset of symmetric tenderness and swelling of the extremities which is rapidly followed by induration of the skin and subcutaneous tissue. The skin takes on a cobblestone or puckered appearance. Carpal tunnel syndrome appears early in the course, and flexion contractures develop later. A marked eosinophilia is found in the early stage of disease and subsequently decreases. Increased levels of polyclonal IgG and immune complexes are often present in the serum. A full-thickness biopsy consisting of skin, fascia, and superficial muscle shows perivascular infiltration of histiocytes, eosinophils, lymphocytes, and plasma cells. Biopsies later in the course show sclerosis. Spontaneous improvement and occasionally complete remission may occur after 2 to 5 years of disease. Some patients have persistent disease while others are left with flexion contractures. Administration of glucocorticoids may provide symptomatic improvement and will decrease the eosinophilia. Improvement has been reported with the use of the H-2 blocker cimetidine.

REFERENCES

EARNSHAW W et al: Three human chromosomal autoantigens are recognized by sera from patients with anti-centromere antibodies. J Clin Invest 77:426, 1986

HAWKINS RA et al: Increased dermal mast cell populations in progressive systemic sclerosis: A link in chronic fibrosis? Ann Intern Med 102:182, 1985

MARICQ HR et al: Microvascular abnormalities as possible predictors of disease subsets in Raynaud phenomenon and early connective tissue disease. Clin Exp Rheumatol 1:195, 1983

MEDSGER TA: Systemic sclerosis (scleroderma), localized scleroderma, eosinophilic fasciitis, and calcinosis, in *Arthritis and Allied Conditions*, 11th ed, McCarty DJ (ed). Philadelphia, Lea & Febiger, 1989, p 1118

MILLER EB et al: Reduced natural killer cell activity in patients with systemic sclerosis: Correlation with clinical disease type. Arthritis Rheum 31:1515, 1988

SEIBOLD JR: Scleroderma (systemic sclerosis), in *Textbook of Rheumatology*, 3d ed, WN Kelly et al (eds). Philadelphia, Saunders, 1989

SHULMAN LE: Diffuse fasciitis with eosinophilia: A new syndrome. Arthritis Rheum 20:S205, 1977

SILVER RM, LEROY EC: Systemic sclerosis (scleroderma), in *Immunological Diseases*, 4th ed, Samter M et al (eds). Boston, Little, Brown, 1988, p 1459

STEEN VD et al: D-Penicillamine therapy in progressive systemic sclerosis (scleroderma). Ann Intern Med 97:652, 1982

WEINER ES et al: Clinical associations of anti-centromere antibodies and antibodies to topoisomerase I. Arthritis Rheum 31:378, 1988

WHITESIDE TL et al: Soluble mediators from mononuclear cells increase the synthesis of glycosaminoglycan by dermal fibroblast cultures derived from normal subjects and progressive systemic sclerosis patients. Arthritis Rheum 28:188, 1985

272 MIXED CONNECTIVE TISSUE DISEASE

GORDON C. SHARP

DEFINITION Mixed connective tissue disease (MCTD) is a syndrome characterized by a combination of clinical features similar to those of systemic lupus erythematosus (SLE), scleroderma, polymyositis, and rheumatoid arthritis and unusually high titers of circulating antibody to a nuclear ribonucleoprotein (RNP) antigen.

ETIOLOGY, PATHOGENESIS, AND PATHOLOGY The etiologic and pathogenic mechanisms of MCTD remain unknown, but a number of clues point to the involvement of immune aberrations: (1) persistence of extremely high titers of antibody to nuclear RNP and a marked polyclonal hypergammaglobulinemia indicative of B-cell hyperactivity; (2) a suppressor T-cell defect; (3) circulating immune complexes during active disease; (4) deposition of IgG, IgM, and complement within vascular walls and along sarcolemmal and glomerular basement membranes; and (5) widespread lymphocytic and plasma cell infiltration of numerous tissues. One of the chief underlying pathologic findings in some adults and children with MCTD is a proliferative intimal and/or medial vascular lesion resulting in narrowing of the lumen of large vessels (e.g., pulmonary, renal, and coronary vessels and aorta) and of small arterioles of many organs. Such lesions in the lungs may contribute to pulmonary hypertension and abnormalities of pulmonary function.

CLINICAL MANIFESTATIONS The age range in published reports of MCTD is from 4 to 80 years, with a mean of 37 years. Approximately 80 percent of patients have been female. Typical clinical features include Raynaud's phenomenon, polyarthritis, swollen hands or sclerodactyly, esophageal dysfunction, pulmonary involvement, and inflammatory myopathy. Malar rash, alopecia, lymphadenopathy, and cardiac and renal disease are less frequent manifestations.

Cutaneous manifestations of MCTD include the swollen, sausage-like appearance of the fingers, nonscarring alopecia, lupus-like rashes, heliotrope eyelids, erythematous patches over the knuckles, periungual telangiectasia, and "squared" telangiectasia over the hands and face. Scleroderma-like changes may be present but only occasionally become extensive.

Musculoskeletal abnormalities occur in most patients. Arthritis is usually nondeforming but may resemble rheumatoid arthritis. Proximal muscle weakness is frequent and may be severe. Serum levels of creatine phosphokinase and aldolase are often markedly elevated, electromyograms are typical of inflammatory myopathy, and biopsies show degeneration of muscle fibers and interstitial and perivascular infiltrates of lymphocytes and plasma cells.

Esophageal dysfunction has been demonstrated in 80 percent of all patients, including 70 percent of asymptomatic patients. Characteristic abnormalities include reduced upper and lower esophageal sphincter pressures and decreased amplitude of peristalsis in the distal two-thirds of the esophagus.

Pulmonary involvement occurs in 85 percent of patients with MCTD but may be clinically silent until far advanced. The most common clinical finding is exertional dyspnea, followed by pleuritic pain and bibasilar rales. Reduced diffusing capacity for carbon monoxide is the most frequent functional abnormality.

Cardiac disease is less common than pulmonary involvement in adults with MCTD but may be more frequent in children. Pericarditis is the most common cardiac finding; other findings have included mitral valve prolapse, myocarditis, congestive heart failure, and aortic insufficiency.

Renal disease in children and adults with MCTD has a combined prevalence of about 28 percent. Progressive renal failure is uncommon, and clinical and histologic findings suggest that vascular lesions may represent a more serious problem than immune complex nephritis in MCTD.

Other less frequent clinical manifestations include fever, lymphadenopathy, neurologic abnormalities, Sjögren's syndrome, hepatosplenomegaly, and intestinal involvement similar to that seen in scleroderma.

LABORATORY FINDINGS Almost all patients have positive fluorescent antinuclear antibody tests at high titers (usually greater than 1:1000) with a speckled pattern and very high titers of antibodies directed against the ribonuclease-sensitive nuclear RNP component of extractable nuclear antigen (ENA). Elevated anti–native DNA antibody titers and antibodies to the ribonuclease-resistant Sm component of ENA are uncommon in MCTD; their presence is usually associated with a severe flare-up of lupus-like features. High titers of circulating RNP antibodies usually persist for years, but antibody levels may decline significantly or become undetectable in patients who are in prolonged remission.

Recent studies have further elucidated the nature of the RNP and Sm antigens. Antibodies to RNP immunoprecipitate U1 snRNA-protein complexes and react with proteins designated 68K, A, and C, whereas Sm antibodies immunoprecipitate snRNA-protein complexes containing U1, U2, U4, U5, and U6 snRNAs and react with proteins designated B/B′ and D. Furthermore, these antigenic complexes have been shown to have important biologic roles in the processing of messenger RNA. Several reports indicate that antibodies to the 68K protein are associated with anti-U1 RNP antibodies in MCTD, but rarely occur in SLE. Other preliminary studies have revealed that U1 68K-positive MCTD patients have disease associated with HLA-DR4 but not with HLA-DR3 as is found in patients with SLE.

Rheumatoid factor is found, often at very high titers, in over half of the patients with MCTD. Diffuse hypergammaglobulinemia is frequently noted and may be elevated to a level of 50 g per liter. A mild to moderate reduction in serum complement levels occurs in about 30 percent of patients. Other less frequent laboratory findings include leukopenia, anemia, and thrombocytopenia (mainly in children).

DIAGNOSIS The diagnosis of MCTD is based on a combination of typical overlapping clinical findings and high titers of circulating antibody to nuclear RNP antigen. In some patients, all the clinical manifestations may be present on initial evaluation. However, as clinicians have become more aware of the syndrome and tests for RNP antibody are being performed more frequently, MCTD is being recognized in an earlier phase in patients presenting with minimal symptoms (e.g., Raynaud's phenomenon, arthralgias, myalgias, and swollen hands). In some this mild "undifferentiated connective tissue disease" syndrome may persist for years, but a recent prospective, long-term study showed that the majority of patients with high titers of RNP antibodies and limited clinical manifestations ultimately developed signs and symptoms consistent with a diagnosis of MCTD.

TREATMENT AND PROGNOSIS Lacking controlled studies, specific treatment recommendations for MCTD are based on anecdotal information. Salicylates, other nonsteroidal anti-inflammatory agents, hydroxychloroquine, vasodilators, and/or low doses of glucocorticoids are used to treat mild disease. In general, mild disease is quite responsive to low-dose glucocorticoids. If the disease is more severe and significantly involves major organ systems, higher doses of glucocorticoids (e.g., 1 mg/kg per day of prednisone) are usually required. As with SLE, a cytotoxic agent may be added in steroid-resistant or -dependent cases. However, the efficacy of this latter therapeutic regimen has not been substantiated by controlled clinical trials. The prognosis for MCTD is generally similar to that of SLE and somewhat better than for scleroderma.

REFERENCES

PETTERSSON I et al: The use of immunoblotting and immunoprecipitation of (U) small nuclear ribonucleoproteins in the analysis of sera of patients with mixed connective tissue disease and systemic lupus erythematosus. Arthritis Rheum 29:986, 1986

SHARP GC, SINGSEN BH: Mixed connective tissue disease, in *Arthritis and Allied Conditions*, 11th ed, DJ McCarty (ed). Philadelphia, Lea & Febiger, 1988, p 1080

SULLIVAN WD et al: A prospective evaluation emphasizing pulmonary involvement in patients with mixed connective tissue disease. Medicine 63:92, 1984

TAKEDA Y et al: Enzyme-linked immunosorbent assay using isolated (U) small nuclear ribonucleoprotein polypeptides as antigens to investigate the clinical significance of autoantibodies to these polypeptides. Clin Immunol Immunopathol 50:213, 1989

273 SJÖGREN'S SYNDROME

H. CLIFFORD LANE / ANTHONY S. FAUCI

DEFINITION Sjögren's syndrome is an immunologic disorder characterized by progressive destruction of the exocrine glands leading to mucosal and conjunctival dryness (sicca syndrome) accompanied by a variety of autoimmune phenomena. The disease can occur either by itself, in which case it is referred to as primary Sjögren's syndrome, or in association with other autoimmune diseases (see Chaps. 269 and 270), in which case it is referred to as secondary Sjögren's syndrome. In addition, some authors have divided the disease into two forms: glandular, when the only clinical manifestations are within the exocrine system, and extraglandular, when other tissues are involved as well.

INCIDENCE AND PREVALENCE The disease predominantly affects women in the third or fourth decades of life. Although precise incidence figures are not known, it has been suggested that Sjögren's syndrome is the second most common rheumatologic disease in the United States. Up to 30 percent of patients with rheumatoid arthritis, 10 percent of patients with systemic lupus erythematosus, and 1 percent of patients with scleroderma have been reported as having secondary Sjögren's syndrome. Immunogenetic predisposition appears to play an important role in the incidence of Sjögren's syndrome. The frequency of the HLA-B8, the HLA-DRw3, and the MT-2 histocompatibility antigens is significantly increased in patients with primary Sjögren's syndrome.

PATHOPHYSIOLOGY AND IMMUNOPATHOGENESIS The two main mechanisms of tissue destruction in Sjögren's syndrome are lymphocytic infiltration and immune-complex deposition. In addition, approximately 10 percent of these patients develop a lymphoproliferative process known as *pseudolymphoma*. This disorder has many histologic features of lymphoma but is associated clinically with a benign course.

Virtually any organ system of the body may be affected in the patient with Sjögren's syndrome. The disease process is most striking in the salivary and lacrimal glands, where there is a progressive mononuclear cell infiltrate which generally leads to complete scarring. Renal disease may result from a lymphocytic interstitial nephritis or an immune-complex glomerulonephritis. Pulmonary involvement is most frequently due to interstitial pneumonitis caused by an infiltration of mononuclear cells, although discrete mass lesions due to pseudolymphoma may occur. Patients with Sjögren's syndrome may also develop an immune-complex vasculitis, at times associated with cryoglobulinemia. Thromboangiitis obliterans has also been seen, usually in patients with preexisting Raynaud's phenomena. Both the peripheral and the central nervous system manifestations of this disease are felt to be due to blood vessel inflammation.

Patients with Sjögren's syndrome exhibit two main types of immunoregulatory defects. The first of these is an abnormally active cellular immune system. This is evident by the intense inflammatory mononuclear cell infiltrates seen in the salivary glands of these patients. These infiltrates are made up predominantly of activated T cells; however, activated B lymphocytes can be detected as well. These mononuclear cell infiltrates are responsible for many of the clinical manifestations of Sjögren's syndrome, including the profound dryness of conjunctival and mucosal surfaces, interstitial nephritis, interstitial pneumonitis, and meningoencephalitis. The second immunoregulatory defect seen in patients with Sjögren's syndrome is oligoclonal B-cell activation. This results in hypergammaglobulinemia, oligoclonal spikes on protein electrophoresis, elevated levels of circulating immune complexes, and the production of autoantibodies. Among the autoantibodies seen are rheumatoid factor, SSA (anti-Ro), and SSB (anti-La). While the precise clinical significance of these and other serologic markers is unclear, it does appear that most patients with the more serious systemic manifestations of Sjögren's syndrome are SSA-positive.

CLINICAL MANIFESTATIONS AND LABORATORY ABNORMALITIES The most common clinical manifestations of Sjögren's syndrome are keratoconjunctivitis sicca and xerostomia. Patients often complain initially of a gritty sensation in the eyes or severe dryness of the mouth. The lack of saliva may be associated with an increased rate of dental caries. Mucosal dryness may extend into the upper airway, in which case patients may complain of a persistent cough or hoarseness that is worse in cold weather. Corneal dryness may be so severe as to result in corneal ulcerations.

Renal involvement is seen in approximately 40 percent of patients with primary Sjögren's syndrome. This generally presents clinically as a mild interstitial nephritis that may result in renal tubular acidosis. This form of kidney disease rarely leads to chronic renal failure; however, it may be associated with a 50 percent reduction in creatinine clearance. A minority of patients with renal disease demonstrate an immune-complex glomerulonephritis. This is seen usually in the context of systemic vasculitis.

Twenty-five percent of patients with primary Sjögren's syndrome develop vasculitis (Chap. 276). This usually takes the form of a cutaneous palpable purpura or hypersensitivity vasculitis of the lower extremities. Patients with Sjögren's syndrome may also develop a severe, systemic vasculitis. This is often seen in the setting of cryoglobulinemia and may result in fever, skin rash, and bowel infarction. The vasculitic syndromes seen in patients with Sjögren's syndrome are generally episodic rather than chronic.

A variety of neurologic conditions have been described in patients with Sjögren's syndrome. The most common nervous system presentation is that of a sensory polyneuropathy and/or mononeuritis multiplex. Central nervous system involvement has been reported in this illness and may be focal or diffuse in its presentation. Patients have also been noted to develop a diffuse proximal myositis.

Pulmonary involvement generally takes the form of an interstitial pneumonitis which is usually of little clinical significance. Pulmonary mass lesions may occur that may be infectious, inflammatory, or neoplastic.

Approximately 10 percent of patients with Sjögren's syndrome develop pseudolymphoma. This unusual lymphoproliferative disorder may present as lymphadenopathy, parotid gland enlargement, or pulmonary nodules. Approximately 10 percent of the Sjögren's syndrome patients with pseudolymphoma may go on to develop a lymphocytic (non-Hodgkin's) lymphoma.

Autoimmune thyroid disease resembling Hashimoto's thyroiditis is a common accompaniment of Sjögren's syndrome. Approximately 50 percent of patients with Sjögren's syndrome have some evidence of biochemical hypothyroidism, and 10 percent of patients require thyroid supplement.

Pregnant women with anti-Ro (SSA) antibodies are at an increased risk of delivering infants with cardiac conduction defects. Thus, pregnancies need to be carefully monitored in this group of patients.

A variety of laboratory abnormalities may be seen in patients with Sjögren's syndrome. Among the serologic and hematologic abnormalities are elevated levels of circulating immune complexes, autoantibodies, leukopenia, thrombocytosis, and an elevation in the erythrocyte sedimentation rate. In addition, patients often have a high urine pH.

While the presence of these abnormalities may increase one's level of suspicion of a diagnosis of Sjögren's syndrome, they are not diagnostic by themselves.

DIAGNOSIS A diagnosis of Sjögren's syndrome is made when the triad of keratoconjunctivitis sicca, xerostomia, and mononuclear cell infiltration of the salivary gland is noted. This latter finding is made by a lower lip biopsy. The differential diagnosis of Sjögren's syndrome includes sarcoidosis, lymphoma, primary amyloidosis, HIV infection, and graft-versus-host disease.

TREATMENT AND PROGNOSIS Treatment is geared toward symptomatic relief of mucosal dryness and meticulous oral hygiene, and includes artificial tears, ophthalmologic lubricating ointments, nasal sprays of normal saline, moisturizing skin lotions, frequent sips of water, and oral fluoride treatments. There is currently no effective treatment for the ongoing exocrine gland destruction. Glucocorticoids have been used with varying degrees of success in the management of glomerulonephritis, interstitial pneumonitis, and pseudolymphoma. They have not proved to be effective in the management of the cutaneous vasculitis. Patients with systemic vasculitis associated with cryoglobulinemia may benefit from brief courses of immunosupressive therapy (Chap. 276). It should be stressed that this form of systemic vasculitis is episodic, and therefore, in contrast to most forms of systemic necrotizing vasculitis, does not require chronic immunosuppressive therapy. Therapy of pseudolymphoma should be reserved for those cases in which vital organ function is threatened. Because cytotoxic therapy may predispose to the transition from pseudolymphoma to true lymphoma, this form of immunosuppressive therapy should be reserved for potentially life-threatening situations.

The overall prognosis for patients with Sjögren's syndrome is quite good. Patients with secondary Sjögren's syndrome generally have less severe manifestations of Sjögren's than those with the primary form. Patients with primary disease are best managed with ocular and mucosal lubricants, attention to oral hygiene, frequent monitoring of thyroid function, and the reassurance that their disease, while a substantial source of morbidity, generally does not shorten life.

REFERENCES

Fox RI et al: Primary Sjögren's syndrome: Clinical and immunopathologic features. Semin Arthritis Rheum 14:77, 1984

Malinoiv KL et al: Neuropsychiatric dysfunction in primary Sjögren's syndrome. Ann Intern Med 103:344, 1985

Talal N et al (eds): *Sjögren's Syndrome: Clinical and Immunological Aspects*. New York, Springer-Verlag, 1987, p 299

Tsokos M et al: Vasculitis in primary Sjögren's syndrome. Histologic classification and clinical presentation. Am J Clin Pathol 88:26, 1987

274 ANKYLOSING SPONDYLITIS AND REACTIVE ARTHRITIS

JOEL D. TAUROG / PETER E. LIPSKY

ANKYLOSING SPONDYLITIS

Ankylosing spondylitis (AS) is an inflammatory disorder of unknown etiology that primarily affects the axial skeleton; peripheral joints and extraarticular structures may also be involved. The disease usually begins in the second or third decade; the prevalence in men is approximately three times that in women. It is considered the prototype of the group of disorders collectively referred to as the *spondyloarthropathies,* which includes ankylosing spondylitis, reactive arthritis, psoriatic arthritis and spondylitis, and enteropathic arthritis and spondylitis. In Europe, ankylosing spondylitis is often referred to by the eponyms Marie-Strümpell disease or Bekhterev's disease.

EPIDEMIOLOGY Ankylosing spondylitis shows a striking correlation with the presence of the histocompatibility antigen HLA-B27. The disease occurs throughout the human populations of the world in proportion to the prevalence of this antigen. In North American Caucasians, the prevalence of HLA-B27 in the general population is 7 percent, whereas over 90 percent of patients with AS have inherited this antigen. The association with HLA-B27 is independent of disease severity.

In large population surveys, 1 to 2 percent of adults inheriting HLA-B27 have been found to have AS. In contrast, in families of patients with AS, 10 to 20 percent of adult first-degree relatives inheriting HLA-B27 have been found to have the disease. The concordance rate in identical twins is estimated to be 60 percent or less. These epidemiologic findings indicate that both genetic and environmental factors play a role in the pathogenesis of the disease and that the genetic factors may include allelic genes in addition to HLA-B27.

PATHOLOGY Sacroiliitis is usually, but not invariably, one of the earliest manifestations of AS. The early lesion consists of subchondral granulation tissue containing lymphocytes, plasma cells, mast cells, macrophages, and chondrocytes. Usually, the thinner iliac cartilage is eroded first, then the thicker sacral cartilage. The irregularly eroded, sclerotic margins of the joint are gradually replaced by fibrocartilage regeneration and ultimately by ossification, so that in the end stage the joint may be totally obliterated. Radiographically, this progression is evident as erosion of the cortical margins of the joint with subchondral bony sclerosis, followed by apparent widening of the joint space caused by extensive erosion of the cortical margins, bony bridging, then fusion.

In the spine, the initial lesion consists of inflammatory granulation tissue at the junction of the annulus fibrosus of the disk cartilage and the margin of vertebral bone. The outer annular fibers are eroded and eventually replaced by bone, forming the beginning of a bony excrescence called a *syndesmophyte,* which then grows by continued enchondral ossification, ultimately bridging the adjacent vertebral bodies. Ascending progression of this process leads to the ''bamboo spine'' observed radiographically. Other lesions in the spine include diffuse osteoporosis, erosion of vertebral bodies at the disc margin (Romanus lesion), ''squaring'' of vertebrae, and inflammation and destruction of the disc-bone border. Inflammatory arthritis of the apophyseal joints is common; early, there is pannus eroding cartilage, often followed by bony ankylosis.

The pathology of arthritis in peripheral joints in AS can show synovial hyperplasia, lymphoid infiltration, and pannus formation, but the process lacks the exuberant synovial villi, fibrin deposits, ulcers, and plaques of plasma cells seen in rheumatoid arthritis. Furthermore, central cartilaginous erosions due to proliferation of subchondral granulation tissue are common in AS but rarely found in rheumatoid arthritis.

The enthesis, the site of tendinous or ligamentous attachment to bone, is another common site of pathology in AS, especially at sites localized around the spine and pelvis. Enthesitis is characterized by erosive, inflammatory lesions that may eventually undergo ossification.

Approximately 20 percent of patients with AS are affected by acute anterior uveitis. Few cases have been studied histologically, and none at an early stage. After recurrent attacks, the iris shows nonspecific inflammatory changes, scarring, increased vascularity, and many macrophages laden with pigment.

Aortic insufficiency develops in a small percentage of cases. There is thickening of the aortic valve cusps and the aorta near the sinuses of Valsalva, with dense adventitial scar tissue and intimal fibrous proliferation, the scar tissue often extending into the ventricular septum with resultant heart block.

Recently, microscopic inflammatory lesions of the colon and ileocolonic valve were reported in patients with AS lacking any clinical evidence of inflammatory bowel disease.

PATHOGENESIS The pathogenesis of AS is poorly understood. A number of features of the disease implicate immune-mediated mechanisms, including elevated serum levels of IgA and acute phase reactants, inflammatory histology, and close association with HLA-B27. No specific event or exogenous agent that triggers the onset of the disease has been identified, although overlapping features with reactive arthritis and inflammatory bowel disease suggest that enteric bacteria may play a role. Evidence has been obtained suggesting antigenic interrelatedness between HLA-B27 and certain enteric bacteria, but it is not yet known whether this contributes to the pathogenesis of AS. There is also some evidence both in AS patients and in animal models for an association between spondylitis and immunity to cartilage proteoglycan.

CLINICAL MANIFESTATIONS The symptoms of the disease are usually first noticed in late adolescence or early adulthood; onset after age 40 is unusual. In the majority of patients, the initial symptom is dull pain, insidious in onset, felt deep in the lower lumbar or gluteal region. Characteristically, this is accompanied by low-back morning stiffness of up to a few hours' duration that improves with activity. The stiffness may return following prolonged periods of inactivity. Within a few months of onset, the pain usually has become persistent and bilateral, and nocturnal exacerbation of the pain that forces the patient to get up and move around may be frequent.

In some patients, bony tenderness may accompany back pain or stiffness, while in others, it may be the predominant complaint. Common sites include the costosternal junctions, spinous processes, iliac crests, greater trochanters, ischial tuberosities, tibial tubercles, and heels. Occasionally, chest pain is the presenting complaint, because of involvement of the thoracic spine and chest wall articulations. Arthritis in the hips and shoulders occurs at some stage in 25 to 35 percent of all patients, and can lead to early symptoms. Arthritis of peripheral joints other than the hips and shoulders has been reported in up to 30 percent of patients and can occur at any stage of the disease. Peripheral arthritis is usually asymmetric. Neck pain and stiffness, indicating involvement of the cervical spine, is usually a relatively late manifestation. Occasional patients, especially those with a juvenile onset, present with predominantly constitutional symptoms such as fatigue, anorexia, fever, weight loss, or night sweats.

The most common extraarticular manifestation is acute anterior uveitis, which can antedate the onset of the joint disease. Attacks are typically unilateral and tend to recur, causing pain, photophobia, and increased lacrimation. Aortic insufficiency, sometimes producing the symptoms of congestive heart failure, occurs in a few percent of patients and occasionally occurs early in the course of the spinal disease.

Initially, the physical findings reflect the manifestations of the inflammatory process. The most specific findings involve loss of spinal mobility, with limitation of anterior flexion, lateral flexion, and extension of the lumbar spine, and limitation of chest expansion.

Limitation of motion is usually out of proportion to the degree of bony ankylosis, reflecting spasm secondary to pain and inflammation. Pain in the sacroiliac joints may be elicited either with direct pressure or with maneuvers that stress the joints. In addition, there is commonly tenderness upon palpation at the sites of symptomatic bony tenderness mentioned above, and paraspinous muscle spasm is often present.

The Schober test is a useful measure of forward flexion of the lumbar spine. The patient stands erect, with heels together, and marks are made directly over the spine 5 cm below and 10 cm above the lumbosacral junction (identified by a horizontal line between the posterior superior iliac spines). The patient then bends forward maximally, while not bending the knees, and the distance between the two marks is measured. The distance between the two marks increases 5 cm or more in the case of normal lumbar mobility and less than 4 cm in the case of decreased lumbar mobility. Chest expansion is measured as the difference between maximal inspiration and maximal forced expiration in the fourth intercostal space in males, or just below the breasts in females. Normal chest expansion is 5 cm or greater.

Limitation or pain with motion of the hips or shoulders is usually present if either of these joints is involved. Careful examination is also necessary to detect inflammatory disease of peripheral joints. It should be emphasized that early in the course of mild cases, symptoms may be mild and nonspecific, and the physical examination may be completely normal.

The course of the disease is extremely variable, ranging from the individual on one end of the spectrum with mild stiffness and radiographically evident disease confined to the sacroiliac joints to the patient on the other end of the spectrum with a totally fused spine, severe bilateral hip arthritis and ankylosis, possibly accompanied by severe peripheral arthritis and extraarticular manifestations. Pain tends to be persistent early in the disease and then to become intermittent, with alternating exacerbations and quiescent periods. In a typical severe case with progression of the spondylitis to syndesmophyte formation, the patient's posture undergoes characteristic changes. The lumbar lordosis is obliterated with accompanying atrophy of the buttocks. The thoracic kyphosis is accentuated. If the cervical spine is involved, there may be a forward stoop of the neck. Hip involvement with ankylosis may lead to flexion contractures, compensated by flexion at the knees. The progression of the disease may be followed by measuring the patient's height, chest expansion, Schober test, and the distance between the occiput and the wall when the patient stands erect with the heels and back flat against the wall (occiput-to-wall test).

Onset of the disease in adolescence correlates with both a worse prognosis and more severe hip involvement. The disease in women tends to be milder than in men, with less frequent progression to total spinal ankylosis, although there is some evidence for an increased prevalence of isolated cervical ankylosis and of peripheral arthritis in women with AS.

The most serious complication of the spinal disease is spinal fracture, which can occur with even minor trauma to the rigid, osteoporotic spine. Most commonly, the cervical spine is involved, often leading to quadriplegia. Cauda equina syndrome is another infrequent complication of long-standing spinal disease in AS. Pulmonary involvement, characterized by slowly progressive upper lobe fibrosis, is a rare complication of long-standing AS; eventually the lesions can cavitate and become colonized by *Aspergillus*. Although cardiovascular involvement can occur early in the course of the disease, the prevalence of aortic insufficiency and of cardiac conduction disturbances, including third-degree heart block, increases with prolonged disease. Amyloidosis, especially involving the kidney, was found in 6 percent of one autopsy series, but the true prevalence appears to be considerably lower. Prostatitis has been reported to have an increased prevalence in men with AS.

Despite the persistence of the disease, most patients with AS do not experience disabling symptoms and are able to remain gainfully employed. Only in uncommon instances does the disease appear to shorten life, these being due largely to spinal trauma, aortic insufficiency, respiratory failure, amyloid nephropathy, or complications of therapy such as upper gastrointestinal hemorrhage. An excess mortality from leukemia was noted in patients treated with deep x-ray therapy to the spine, a common mode of therapy for AS until effective anti-inflammatory medications became available in the mid-1950s.

LABORATORY FINDINGS There is no laboratory test that is diagnostic of AS. In most ethnic groups, the HLA-B27 gene is present in approximately 90 percent of patients with AS; American blacks appear to represent an exception, since the prevalence of B27 in this group has been reported to be only 50 percent. Most patients with active disease have an elevated erythrocyte sedimentation rate and an elevated C-reactive protein. A mild normochromic normocytic anemia may be present. Patients with severe disease may show an elevated alkaline phosphatase. Elevated serum IgA levels are common. Rheumatoid factor and antinuclear antibodies are uniformly absent unless caused by a coexistent process unrelated to AS. Synovial fluid from inflamed peripheral joints in AS is not distinctly different from that of other inflammatory joint diseases. In cases with restriction of chest wall motion, pulmonary function tests may demonstrate decreased vital capacity and increased functional residual capacity, but airflow measurements are normal and ventilatory function is usually well maintained.

RADIOGRAPHIC FINDINGS Radiographically demonstrable sacroiliitis is usually present in AS. The earliest changes in the sacroiliac joints demonstrable by plain x-ray radiography show blurring of the cortical margins of the subchondral bone, followed by erosions and sclerosis. Progression of the erosions leads to "pseudowidening" of the joint space; as fibrous and then bony ankylosis supervene, the joints may become obliterated radiographically. The changes and progression of the lesions are usually symmetric.

In mild cases, years may elapse before unequivocal sacroiliac abnormalities are evident on plain radiographs. Although computed tomography and magnetic resonance imaging have been shown to detect abnormalities reliably at an earlier stage than plain radiography, these techniques are not generally used for routine diagnostic purposes.

Roentgenographic abnormalities generally appear in the sacroiliac joints before appearing elsewhere in the spine. In the lumbar spine, progression of the disease leads to straightening caused by loss of lordosis and reactive sclerosis caused by osteitis of the anterior corners of the vertebral bodies with subsequent erosion, leading to "squaring" of the vertebral bodies. Progressive ossification of the superficial layers of the annulus fibrosus leads to eventual formation of marginal syndesmophytes, visible on plain films as bony bridges connecting successive vertebral bodies on the anterior and lateral sides.

DIAGNOSIS The diagnosis of early AS before the development of irreversible deformity can be difficult to establish. Criteria for the diagnosis of AS were formulated in 1961 (Rome criteria) and revised in 1966 (New York criteria). For definite AS, the New York criteria require the presence of advanced radiographic sacroiliitis and at least one of three clinical findings (limitation of motion of the lumbar spine in all three planes, pain at the thoracolumbar junction or in the lumbar spine, or chest expansion limited to $\leq$2.5 cm).

In 1984, modifications to the New York criteria were proposed, which, although not yet formally adopted, have been shown to be comparably specific but more sensitive than the original New York criteria, especially in diagnosing the disease at an earlier stage. The modified criteria consist of the following: (1) a history of inflammatory back pain (see below); (2) limitation of motion of the lumbar spine in both the sagittal and frontal planes; (3) limited chest expansion, relative to standard values for age and sex; and (4) definite radiographic sacroiliitis. Under the proposed modified New York criteria, the presence of radiographic sacroiliitis plus any one of the other three criteria is sufficient for a diagnosis of definite AS. The increased sensitivity of these modified criteria is largely the result of the inclusion of earlier stages of radiographic sacroiliitis than are permitted under the original New York criteria.

Several studies have identified a sizeable population of B27-positive individuals with symptoms typical of AS who lack definite radiographic sacroiliitis. However, when followed over time, most of these patients eventually develop radiographic changes. These studies indicate that diagnostic criteria based on radiographic findings may in some cases be too insensitive for the diagnosis of early AS. The B27 test is useful only as a diagnostic adjunct, since the presence of B27 is neither necessary nor sufficient for the diagnosis.

AS must be differentiated from numerous other causes of low back pain. The inflammatory back pain of AS is usually distinguished by the following five features: (1) age of onset below 40; (2) insidious onset; (3) duration greater than 3 months before medical attention is sought; (4) morning stiffness; and (5) improvement with exercise or activity. The most common causes of back pain other than AS are primarily mechanical or degenerative rather than inflammatory and do not show these features. Less common metabolic, infectious, and malignant causes of back pain must also be differentiated from AS.

TREATMENT There is no definitive treatment for AS. The principal goal of management is the conscientious participation of the patient in an exercise program designed to maintain functional posture and to preserve range of motion. Most patients require anti-inflammatory agents to achieve sufficient symptomatic relief to be able to remain functional and carry out the exercise program. It is not known whether drug treatment alone can alter the progression of the disease.

Worldwide, the most commonly used drug therapy for AS is indomethacin, although several other nonsteroidal anti-inflammatory drugs (NSAIDs) have also been proven to be effective in reducing pain and stiffness and are commonly used. Indomethacin is particularly effective as a 75-mg slow-release preparation taken once or twice daily. Although phenylbutazone at doses of 200 to 400 mg/d has been considered by several authorities to be the most effective agent in AS, because of its greater potential for serious side effects such as aplastic anemia and agranulocytosis, its use in the United States is confined to patients with severe disease whose symptoms do not respond well to other agents. Recent controlled trials suggest that sulfasalazine[1] in doses of 2 to 3 g/d may be useful in reducing axial and peripheral joint symptoms as well as in reversing laboratory evidence of inflammation. No therapeutic role for gold, penicillamine, immunosuppressive drugs, or systemic corticosteroids has been documented in AS. Occasionally, intralesional or intraarticular corticosteroid injections may be beneficial in patients with persistent enthesopathy or synovitis unresponsive to anti-inflammatory agents.

The most common indication for surgery in patients with AS is severe hip joint arthritis, the pain and stiffness of which are often dramatically relieved by total hip arthroplasty. A smaller number of patients may benefit from surgical correction of extreme flexion deformities of the spine or of atlantoaxial subluxation.

Attacks of acute anterior uveitis are usually effectively managed with local corticosteroid administration in conjunction with mydriatic agents. Coexistent cardiac disease may require pacemaker implantation or aortic valve replacement.

REACTIVE ARTHRITIS

Reactive arthritis refers to acute nonpurulent arthritis complicating an infection elsewhere in the body. In recent years, the term has been used primarily to refer to spondyloarthropathies following enteric or urogenital infections and occurring predominantly in individuals with the histocompatibility antigen HLA-B27. Included in this category is the constellation of clinical findings often referred to as *Reiter's syndrome*. Other forms of reactive arthritis not associated with HLA-B27 and showing a different spectrum of clinical features, such as rheumatic fever, are discussed elsewhere in this volume.

[1]This drug has not been approved for this purpose by the Food and Drug Administration at the time of publication.

HISTORICAL BACKGROUND In 1916, Reiter described a patient who, following an episode of bloody diarrhea, developed a systemic illness with polyarthritis, conjunctivitis, and nongonococcal urethritis. Although similar cases had previously been described, this report served to focus attention on the triad of arthritis, urethritis, and conjunctivitis which subsequently was referred to as Reiter's syndrome. Additional clinical featues, particularly mucocutaneous lesions, were later recognized to be frequent accompaniments of the syndrome.

In recent years, the identification of several bacterial species capable of triggering the clinical syndrome, as well as the finding that three-fourths of the patients possess the HLA-B27 antigen, have led to the unifying concept of reactive arthritis as a clinical syndrome triggered by a specific etiologic agent in a genetically susceptible host. It is now recognized that a similar spectrum of clinical manifestations can be triggered by enteric infection with any of several *Shigella, Salmonella, Yersinia,* and *Campylobacter* species or with *Clostridium difficile,* by genital infection with *Chlamydia trachomatis,* and possibly by other agents as well. Although Reiter's syndrome can be said to represent one part of the spectrum of the clinical manifestations of reactive arthritis, it can be reasonably argued that the term is now largely of historical interest.

EPIDEMIOLOGY Like ankylosing spondylitis, reactive arthritis occurs predominantly in individuals who have inherited the HLA-B27 gene; in most series, 60 to 85 percent of the patients are B27-positive. In epidemics of arthritogenic bacterial infection, e.g., *Shigella flexneri,* it has been estimated that reactive arthritis develops in ~20 percent of the B27-positive individuals at risk. Some studies of families with multiple cases of AS or reactive arthritis have suggested that the two conditions tend to "breed true"; whether this is caused by genetic or environmental factors is not known. The disease is most common in individuals 18 to 40 years of age, but it is well-recognized both in children over 5 years of age and in older adults.

Although Reiter's syndrome has long been described as a disease predominantly of men, this conclusion is probably overstated and related to the ascertainment of cases. The sex ratio in reactive arthritis following enteric infection is nearly 1:1, whereas venereally acquired reactive arthritis is predominantly a male disease. The overall prevalence and incidence of reactive arthritis are difficult to assess because of the variable prevalence of the triggering infections and genetic susceptibility factors in different populations. Certain populations, such as the Navajo Indians of the southwestern United States and the Inuit Eskimos of Greenland, show a very high occurrence of reactive arthritis, whereas the disease is quite uncommon in certain other populations, such as the Haida Indians, with an equally high prevalence of HLA-B27. The reasons for these differences are not clear.

A particularly severe form of reactive arthritis has been described in patients with the acquired immunodeficiency syndrome. Most of these patients are HLA-B27-positive. From the incidence figures it can be inferred that B27-positive individuals with human immunodeficiency virus infection develop reactive arthritis at a higher than expected frequency.

PATHOLOGY Synovial histology is similar to that of other inflammatory arthropathies, including rheumatoid arthritis. Enthesitis is a common clinical finding in reactive arthritis; the histology of this lesion resembles that of ankylosing spondylitis. Microscopic histopathologic evidence of inflammation has been noted in the colon and ileum of patients with postvenereal as well as postenteritic reactive arthritis. The skin lesions of keratoderma blennorrhagica are histologically indistinguishable from psoriatic lesions.

ETIOLOGY AND PATHOGENESIS The first bacterial infection to be causally related to reactive arthritis was *Shigella flexneri*. An outbreak of shigellosis among Finnish troops in 1944 resulted in numerous cases of reactive arthritis. Of the four species of *Shigella, sonnei, boydii, flexneri,* and *dysenteriae, S. flexneri* has most often been implicated in cases of reactive arthritis, both sporadic and epidemic. *S. sonnei*, although responsible for the majority of cases of shigellosis in the United States, has only rarely been implicated in cases of reactive arthritis.

Other bacteria that have been definitively identified as triggers of reactive arthritis include several *Salmonella* species, *Yersinia enterocolitica*, and *Campylobacter jejuni*. There is suggestive evidence implicating several other microorganisms, including *Brucella*, *Yersinia pseudotuberculosis*, *Clostridium difficile*; the genitourinary pathogens *Chlamydia trachomatis*, *Neisseria gonorrhoeae*, and *Ureaplasma urealyticum*; and *Streptococcus pyogenes*. There are also numerous isolated reports of acute arthritis preceded by other bacterial, viral, or parasitic infections, but whether the microorganisms involved are actual triggers of reactive arthritis remains to be determined.

It has not been determined whether reactive arthritis occurs by the same pathogenetic mechanism following infection with each of these microorganisms, nor has the mechanism been fully elucidated in the case of any one of the known bacterial triggers. The immune response is presumed to play a principal role, but there is not yet general agreement on the relative importance of humoral versus cellular mechanisms. Most, if not all, of the triggering organisms share a capacity to invade host cells and survive intracellularly.

The largest body of data regarding the immune response in reactive arthritis has been generated by studies of *Y. enterocolitica*, particularly serotypes O:3 and O:9 in Finland, where these organisms frequently cause enteric infection in a population in which the prevalence of HLA-B27 is 14 percent. In comparison with individuals who fail to develop reactive arthritis following enteric infection with *Yersinia*, patients with *Yersinia*-triggered reactive arthritis show far fewer gastrointestinal symptoms attributable to the infection, a smaller initial IgM response, stronger and more persistent IgA and IgG responses, higher levels of IgA anti-*Yersinia* antibodies with a secretory component, and reduced T-cell proliferative responses to *Yersinia* antigens. These findings suggest an unusual persistence of the immune response to the infecting organism in those individuals in whom reactive arthritis develops. Circulating immune complexes containing *Yersinia* antigens have been found in a higher proportion of arthritic than nonarthritic individuals, and occasionally in the inflamed joints, but the significance of these findings is not clear.

It is not known to what extent reactive arthritis represents an autoimmune response against host tissues, as opposed to an immune response against antigens of the triggering organism that have disseminated to the target tissues. Both mechanisms appear to operate in animal models. Chlamydial antigens have been demonstrated in the synovium of a few patients with venereally acquired reactive arthritis, but it is not known whether they are the inciting antigenic stimulus. Similarly, *Yersinia enterocolitica* antigen has been detected in synovial fluid cells in patients with *Y. enterocolitica*–induced reactive arthritis, but the significance of this is unclear.

The role of HLA-B27 in reactive arthritis has yet to be fully elucidated. At present, the evidence favors some form of molecular mimicry, or the sharing of antigenic determinants between the HLA-B27 molecule and molecules encoded by the inciting microbial agent. Several reports have documented antigenic cross-reactivity between the B27 molecule and envelope glycoproteins of arthritogenic bacteria, including *Shigella flexneri* and *Yersinia pseudotuberculosis*, but the pathogenetic significance of this is not known. Many but not all B27-negative individuals with reactive arthritis possess HLA-B alleles that are antigenically cross-reactive with HLA-B27, notably HLA-B7.

CLINICAL FEATURES The clinical manifestations of reactive arthritis constitute a spectrum that ranges from an isolated, transient monarthritis to a more severe multisystem disease. In the majority of cases, a careful history will elicit some evidence of an antecedent infection 1 to 4 weeks before the onset of symptoms of the reactive disease. However, in a sizeable minority, particularly in cases of relapse, no clinical or laboratory evidence of an antecedent infection can be found. In many cases of presumed venereally acquired reactive disease, there is a history of a recent new sexual partner, even in the absence of laboratory evidence of infection.

Constitutional symptoms are common, including fatigue, malaise, fever, and weight loss. The musculoskeletal symptoms are usually acute in onset. Arthritis is usually asymmetric and additive, with involvement of new joints occurring over a period of a few days to 1 or 2 weeks. The joints of the lower extremities, especially the knee, ankle, and subtalar, metatarsophalangeal, and toe interphalangeal joints, are the most common sites of involvement, but the wrist and fingers can be involved as well. The arthritis is usually quite painful, and tense joint effusions are not uncommon, especially in the knee. Dactylitis, or "sausage digit," a diffuse swelling of a solitary finger or toe, is a distinctive feature of both reactive arthritis and psoriatic arthritis. Tendinitis and fasciitis are particularly characteristic lesions, producing pain at multiple insertion sites, especially the Achilles insertion, the plantar fascia, and sites along the axial skeleton. Spinal and low back pain are quite common, and may be caused by insertional inflammation, muscle spasm, acute sacroiliitis, or presumably, arthritis in intervertebral articulations.

Urogenital lesions may occur throughout the course of the disease. In males, urethritis may be marked or relatively asymptomatic, and may be either an accompaniment of the triggering infection or a result of the reactive phase of the disease. Prostatitis is also common. Similarly, in females cervicitis or salpingitis may be caused either by the infectious trigger or the sterile reactive process.

Ocular disease is common, ranging from transient, asymptomatic conjunctivitis to an aggressive anterior uveitis that occasionally proves refractory to treatment and results in blindness.

Mucocutaneous lesions are frequent. Oral ulcers tend to be superficial, transient, and often asymptomatic. The characteristic skin lesion, keratoderma blennorrhagica, consists of vesicles that become hyperkeratotic, ultimately forming a crust before disappearing. It is most common on the palms and soles, but may occur elsewhere as well. In patients with HIV infection, these lesions are often extremely severe and extensive, dominating the clinical picture. Lesions on the glans penis (*circinate balanitis*) are common; these consist of vesicles that quickly rupture to form painless superficial erosions, which in circumcised individuals can form crusts similar to those of keratoderma blennorrhagica. Nail changes are common and consist of onycholysis, distal yellowish discoloration, and/or heaped up hyperkeratosis.

Less frequent or rare manifestations of reactive arthritis include cardiac conduction defects, aortic insufficiency, central or peripheral nervous system lesions, and pleuropulmonary infiltrates.

Long-term follow-up studies suggest that some joint symptoms persist in many, if not most, patients with reactive arthritis. Recurrences of the acute syndrome are common, and as many as 25 percent of patients either become unable to work or are forced to change occupations because of persistent joint symptoms. Chronic heel pain is often a particularly distressing symptom. Ankylosing spondylitis is also a common sequela. In most studies, HLA-B27-positive patients have a worse outcome than B27-negative patients. The extent to which the long-term prognosis varies with different inciting agents is not known. However, patients with *Yersinia*-induced arthritis appear to have less chronic disease than those whose initial episode follows epidemic shigellosis.

LABORATORY AND RADIOGRAPHIC FINDINGS The erythrocyte sedimentation rate is elevated during the acute phase of the disease. Mild anemia may be present, and acute phase reactants tend to be increased. Synovial fluid is nonspecifically inflammatory, showing an elevated white cell count with a predominance of neutrophils. In most ethnic groups, three-fourths of the patients possess the HLA-B27 antigen. Although it is unusual for the triggering infection to persist through the time of onset of the reactive disease, it may occasionally be possible to culture the organism, for example, in the case of *Shigella*- or *Chlamydia*-induced disease. Serologic evidence of a recent infection may be present, such as a marked elevation of antibodies to *Yersinia* or *Chlamydia*.

In early or mild disease, radiographic changes may be absent or confined to juxtaarticular osteoporosis. With long-standing persistent disease, marginal erosions and loss of joint space can be seen in affected joints. Periostitis with reactive new bone formation is characteristic of the disease, as it is with all of the spondyloarthropathies. Spurs at the insertion of the plantar fascia are common.

Sacroiliitis and spondylitis similar to those described for ankylosing spondylitis may be seen as late sequelae. However, sacroiliitis is more commonly asymmetric than in AS, and the spondylitis, rather than ascending symmetrically from the lower lumbar segments, can begin anywhere along the lumbar spine. The syndesmophytes may be coarse and nonmarginal, arising from the middle of a vertebral body, a pattern rarely seen in primary AS.

DIAGNOSIS Reactive arthritis is a clinical diagnosis, there being no definitively diagnostic laboratory test or radiographic finding. The diagnosis should be entertained in any patient with an acute inflammatory, asymmetric, additive arthritis or tendinitis. The evaluation of such a patient should include careful questioning regarding possible antecedent triggering events such as an episode of diarrhea or dysuria. On physical examination, careful attention must be paid to the distribution of the joint and tendon involvement and to possible sites of extraarticular involvement, such as the eyes, mucous membranes, skin, nails, and genitalia. Synovial fluid aspiration and analysis may be helpful in excluding septic or crystal-induced arthritis.

Although typing for B27 is not needed to secure the diagnosis in clear-cut cases, it has prognostic significance in terms of severity, chronicity, and the propensity for spondylitis and uveitis. Furthermore, it can be helpful diagnostically in atypical cases, a positive test increasing and a negative test decreasing the probability that the diagnosis of reactive arthritis is correct.

It is particularly important to differentiate reactive arthritis from disseminated gonococcal disease, both of which can be venereally acquired and associated with urethritis. Gonococcal arthritis and tenosynovitis tend to involve both upper and lower extremities equally, whereas in reactive arthritis the symptoms usually predominate in the lower extremities. Back pain is common in reactive arthritis but is not a feature of gonococcal disease, whereas the vesicular skin lesions characteristic of disseminated gonococcal disease are not found in reactive arthritis. A positive gonococcal culture from the urethra or cervix does not exclude a diagnosis of reactive arthritis; however, culturing gonococci from blood, skin lesion, or synovium establishes the diagnosis of disseminated gonococcal disease. Occasionally, the only definitive way to distinguish the two is through a therapeutic trial of antibiotics.

Reactive arthritis shares many features with psoriatic arthropathy, including the asymmetry of the arthritis, a propensity for sausage digits and nail involvement, an association with uveitis, and skin lesions of similar histology. However, psoriatic arthritis is usually gradual in onset, the arthritis tends to affect primarily the upper extremities, and there is far less associated periarthritis. Psoriatic arthritis is not associated with mouth ulcers, urethritis, or bowel symptoms; and there is a female predominance. Although psoriatic arthropathy shows some distinctive radiographic features that are not found in reactive arthritis, these only occur late in the disease and are of little help diagnostically. Only psoriatic spondylitis, not the peripheral arthritis, is associated with HLA-B27, about 50 percent of the patients being positive. Occasional patients, usually B27-positive, following what appears to be a typical episode of reactive arthritis, will develop typical psoriasis and persistent arthritis, such that the two entities become indistinguishable.

TREATMENT Most patients with reactive arthritis are benefitted to some degree by nonsteroidal anti-inflammatory drugs, although rarely are symptoms of the acute arthritis completely ameliorated and some patients fail to respond at all. Indomethacin, 75 to 150 mg/d in divided doses, is the initial treatment of choice, with phenylbutazone, 100 mg tid or qid, being the NSAID of last resort because of its potentially serious side effects.

Patients with debilitating symptoms refractory to NSAID therapy may respond to cytotoxic agents such as azathioprine, 1 to 2 mg/kg per day, or methotrexate, 7.5 to 15 mg per week. Recent studies have suggested that sulfasalazine, up to 3 g/d in divided doses, also may be beneficial to patients with persistent reactive arthritis.[2] There appears to be no place for systemic corticosteroids, antimalarials, gold, or penicillamine in the treatment of reactive arthritis. Although many clinicians routinely administer courses of antibiotics to patients with reactive arthritis, there is little evidence that this is beneficial.

Tendinitis and other enthesitic lesions occasionally may benefit from intralesional corticosteroids. Uveitis may require aggressive treatment with corticosteroids to prevent serious sequelae. Skin lesions ordinarily require only symptomatic treatment. In patients with HIV infection and reactive arthritis, many of whom have severe skin lesions, the skin lesions in particular appear to respond dramatically to systemic treatment with azidothymidine. Cardiac complications are managed conventionally; management of neurologic complications is symptomatic.

Patients need to be educated with regard to the nature of the disease and the factors that predispose to its recurrence. Comprehensive management includes counseling of patients in the use of condoms, avoidance of sexual promiscuity, and exposure to enteropathogens. Appropriate use of physical therapy, vocational counseling, and continued surveillance for long-term complications such as ankylosing spondylitis are also part of comprehensive care.

REFERENCES

CALABRO JJ, DICK C (eds): *Ankylosing Spondylitis—New Clinical Applications in Rheumatology*. Lancaster, UK, MTP Press, 1987

CALIN A (ed): *Spondylarthropathies*. Orlando, Grune & Stratton, 1984

GRANFORS K et al: *Yersinia* antigens in synovial fluid cells from patients with reactive arthritis. N Engl J Med 320:216, 1989

KEAT A: Reiter's syndrome and reactive arthritis in perspective. N Engl J Med 309:1606, 1983

KHAN MA et al: Spondylitic disease without radiographic evidence of sacroiliitis in relatives of HLA-B27-positive ankylosing spondylitis patients. Arthritis Rheum 28:40, 1985

LEIRISALO M et al: Ten-year follow-up study of patients with *Yersinia* arthritis. Arthritis Rheum 31:533, 1988

MIELANTS H et al: HLA antigens in seronegative spondylarthropathies. Reactive arthritis and arthritis in ankylosing spondylitis: Relation to gut inflammation. J Rheumatol 14:466, 1987

NISSILA M et al: Sulfasalazine in the treatment of ankylosing spondylitis: A twenty-six week, placebo-controlled clinical trial. Arthritis Rheum 31:1111, 1988

TOIVANEN A, TOIVANEN P (eds): *Reactive Arthritis*. Boca Raton, CRC Press, 1988

VAN DER LINDEN SM et al: Evaluation of diagnostic criteria for ankylosing spondylitis: A proposal for modification of the New York criteria. Arthritis Rheum 27:361, 1984

WINCHESTER R et al: The co-occurrence of Reiter's syndrome and acquired immunodeficiency. Ann Intern Med 106:19, 1987

275 BEHÇET'S SYNDROME

HARALAMPOS M. MOUTSOPOULOS

BEHÇET'S SYNDROME Behçet's syndrome is a multisystem disorder presenting with recurrent oral and genital ulcerations as well as uveitis often leading to blindness.

PREVALENCE, PATHOGENESIS, AND PATHOLOGY The disease has a worldwide distribution. The prevalence of Behçet's syndrome ranges from 1:1000 in Japan to 1:500,000 in North America and Europe. In the Mediterranean countries the prevalence might be higher. It affects mainly young adults, with men having more severe disease than females.

The etiology and pathogenesis of this syndrome remain obscure. Bacteria and viruses have been suggested as the causative agents, but there is no convincing proof. Today, Behçet's syndrome is considered an autoimmune disease because of the common denominator of vasculitis in most patients. Circulating autoantibodies to human oral mucous membrane and immune complexes are found in

[2]Azathioprine, methotrexate, and sulfasalazine have not been approved for this purpose by the Food and Drug Administration at the time of publication.

approximately 50 percent of the cases. Familial occurrence has been reported, and in patients from eastern Mediterranean countries and Japan, the disease appears to be linked to HLA-B5 and HLA-DR5 alloantigens.

CLINICAL FEATURES The recurrent aphthous ulcerations are a sine qua non for the diagnosis. The ulcers are usually painful with a diameter ranging from 2 to 10 mm. They can be shallow or deep with a central yellowish necrotic base; appear singly or in crops; and are located on the lips, gums, buccal mucosa, and tongue. The palate, tonsils, and larynx are rarely involved. The ulcers persist for 1 to 2 weeks and subside without leaving scars. The genital ulcers resemble the oral ones in both appearance and course. Vaginal ulcers are usually painless and may be detected during routine pelvic examination. Painful genital ulcers may occur on the external genitalia.

Skin involvement includes folliculitis, erythema nodosum, and an acne-like exanthem. Severe dermal vasculitis is an infrequent event. Nonspecific skin inflammatory reactivity to any scratches, needle pricks, and intradermal saline injection (pathergy test) is a common and specific manifestation in Japanese and eastern Mediterranean patients.

Eye involvement is the most dreaded complication, as it occasionally progresses rapidly to blindness. The eye disease is usually present at the onset but also may develop within the first few years. In addition to iritis, posterior uveitis, retinal vessel occlusions, and optic neuritis can be seen in some cases of the syndrome. Hypopyon uveitis, which is considered the hallmark of Behçet's syndrome, is in fact a rare manifestation.

The arthritis of Behçet's syndrome is not deforming and affects the knees and ankles.

Superficial or deep peripheral vein thrombosis is seen in one-fourth of the patients. Pulmonary emboli, however, appear to be an exceptionally rare complication. The superior vena cava is obstructed occasionally, producing a dramatic clinical picture. Arterial involvement occurs infrequently and presents with aortitis or peripheral arterial aneurysm and arterial thrombosis.

The prevalence of central nervous system involvement differs geographically. High figures are quoted from northern Europe and the United States. The most common lesions are benign intracranial hypertension, a multiple sclerosis-like picture, and pyramidal involvement. Psychiatric disturbances are frequent.

Gastrointestinal involvement is reported in patients from Japan and include mucosal ulcerations of the gut.

Laboratory findings are mainly nonspecific indices of inflammation such as leukocytosis and elevated erythrocyte sedimentation rate as well as C-reactive protein levels; antibodies to human oral mucosa are also found.

PROGNOSIS AND TREATMENT The severity of the syndrome usually abates with time; male sex and younger age at onset seem to predispose for severe illness. Apart from the cases with neurologic complications, the life expectancy seems to be normal, and the only serious complication is blindness.

Treatment of Behçet's syndrome is symptomatic and empirical. Mucous membrane involvement may respond to topical corticosteroids in the form of mouthwash or paste. The arthritis responds to rest and analgesics. Thrombophlebitis is treated with aspirin, 500 mg/d, and dipyridamole, 250 mg/d. Colchicine can be beneficial in the mild forms of the syndrome. The serious manifestations of Behçet's syndrome, i.e., uveitis and central nervous system involvement, require systemic corticosteroid therapy (prednisone, 1 mg/kg per day) and/or cytotoxic agents (chlorambucil, 0.1 mg/kg per day; azathioprine, 1 to 2 mg/kg per day; or cyclophosphamide, 1 to 2 mg/kg per day). There are early reports of the beneficial use of cyclosporin A in the uveitis of Behçet's syndrome.

REFERENCES

NUSSENBLATT RB et al: Effectiveness of cyclosporin therapy for Behçet's disease. Arthritis Rheum 28:671, 1985

O'DUFFY JD et al: Summary of the Third International Conference on Behçet's disease. J Rheumatol 10:154, 1983

SHIMIZU T et al: Behçet's disease (Behçet's syndrome). Semin Arthritis Rheum 8:223, 1979

YAZICI H, MOUTSOPOULOS HM: Behçet's disease, in *Current Therapy in Allergy and Immunology*, LM Lichtenstein, AS Fauci (eds). Philadelphia, Decker, 1985

276 THE VASCULITIS SYNDROMES

ANTHONY S. FAUCI

DEFINITION Vasculitis is a clinicopathologic process characterized by inflammation of and damage to blood vessels. The vessel lumen is usually compromised, and this is associated with ischemia of the tissues supplied by the involved vessel. A broad and heterogeneous group of syndromes may result from this process since any type, size, and location of blood vessel may be involved. Vasculitis and its consequences may be the primary or sole manifestation of a disease; alternatively, vasculitis may be a secondary component of another primary disease. Vasculitis may be confined to a single organ such as the skin, or it may simultaneously involve several organ systems.

PATHOPHYSIOLOGY AND PATHOGENESIS Generally, most of the vasculitic syndromes are assumed to be mediated at least in part by immunopathogenic mechanisms. However, evidence to this effect is for the most part indirect. Deposition of immune complexes in tissues (see Chap. 268) is the most widely accepted pathogenic mechanism of vasculitis. Nonetheless, the causal role of immune complexes has not been clearly established in most of the vasculitic syndromes. Circulating immune complexes need not result in deposition of the complexes in blood vessels with ensuing vasculitis, and many patients with active vasculitis do not have demonstrable circulating or deposited immune complexes. This situation may result from an inadequacy of the techniques for detecting certain types of immune complexes or from the rapidity with which complexes may be cleared from the circulation. The actual antigen contained in the immune complex has only rarely been identified in vasculitic syndromes. In this regard, hepatitis B antigen has been identified in both the circulating and deposited immune complexes in a subset of patients with systemic vasculitis, most notably within the polyarteritis nodosa group (see below).

The mechanisms of tissue damage in immune-complex–mediated vasculitis resemble those described for serum sickness (Chap. 268). In this model, antigen-antibody complexes are formed in antigen excess and are deposited in vessel walls whose permeability has been increased by vasoactive amines such as histamine, bradykinin, and leukotrienes released from platelets or from mast cells as a result of IgE-triggered mechanisms. The deposition of complexes results in activation of complement components, particularly C5a, which is strongly chemotactic for neutrophils. These cells then infiltrate the vessel wall, phagocytose the immune complexes, and regurgitate their intracytoplasmic enzymes, which damage the vessel wall. As the process becomes subacute or chronic, mononuclear cells infiltrate the vessel wall. The common denominator of the resulting syndrome is compromise of the vessel lumen with ischemic changes in the tissues supplied by the involved vessel.

In addition to the classic immune-complex–mediated mechanisms of vasculitis, other immunopathogenic mechanisms may be involved in damage to vessels. The most prominent of these is cell-mediated immune injury as reflected in the histopathologic feature of granulomatous vasculitis. However, immune complexes themselves may induce granulomatous responses, and the presence of granulomas in or around blood vessels may be indicative of immune-complex mechanisms, delayed hypersensitivity or cell-mediated immune responses, or both. Vascular endothelial cells can express HLA class

II molecules following activation by cytokines such as interferon gamma. This allows these cells to participate in immunologic reactions such as interaction with T4 lymphocytes in a manner similar to antigen-presenting macrophages. In addition, endothelial cells can secrete interleukin 1 which may activate T lymphocytes and initiate or propagate in situ immunologic processes within the blood vessel. Other mechanisms such as direct cellular cytotoxicity or antibody directed against vessel components or antibody-dependent cellular cytotoxicity have been suggested in certain types of vessel damage. However, there is no convincing evidence to support their contribution to the pathogenesis of any of the recognized vasculitic syndromes.

It is unclear why certain individuals develop vasculitis in response to certain antigenic stimuli whereas others do not. However, it is likely that a number of factors are involved in the ultimate expression of a vasculitic syndrome. These include the genetic predisposition, the regulatory mechanisms associated with immune response to certain antigens, and the ability of the reticuloendothelial system to clear circulating complexes from the blood. The size and physicochemical properties of immune complexes, the relative degree of turbulence of blood flow, the intravascular hydrostatic pressure in different vessels, and the preexisting integrity of the vessel endothelium likely explain why only certain types of immune complexes cause vasculitis and why the vasculitic process is selective for only certain vessels in individual patients.

CLASSIFICATION OF VASCULITIC SYNDROMES A major feature of the vasculitic syndromes as a group is the fact that there is a great deal of heterogeneity at the same time as there is considerable overlap among them. This has led to both difficulty and confusion with regard to the categorization of these diseases. The classification scheme listed in Table 276-1 takes into account this heterogeneity and overlap, and will serve as a matrix to emphasize the fact that certain syndromes are predominantly systemic in nature and almost invariably lead to irreversible organ system dysfunction and even death if untreated, while others are usually localized to the skin and rarely result in irreversible dysfunction of vital organs. The distinguishing and overlapping features of the diseases listed in Table 276-1, which justify this classification scheme, will be discussed below.

SYSTEMIC NECROTIZING VASCULITIS

CLASSIC POLYARTERITIS NODOSA Definition Polyarteritis nodosa (PAN) in its classic form was described in 1866 by Kussmaul and Maier. It is a multisystem, necrotizing vasculitis of small- and medium-sized muscular arteries in which involvement of the renal and visceral arteries is characteristic. Classic PAN does not involve pulmonary arteries, although bronchial vessels may be involved; granulomas, significant eosinophilia, and an allergic diathesis are not part of the classic syndrome.

Incidence and prevalence It is difficult to establish an accurate incidence of this disease because of the fact that many reports of PAN actually have included diseases other than the classic syndrome. It is clearly an uncommon, but not a rare, disease. The mean age at onset is 45 years and the male to female ratio is 2.5:1.

Pathophysiology and pathogenesis The vascular lesion in classic PAN is a necrotizing inflammation of small- and medium-sized muscular arteries. The lesions are segmental and tend to involve bifurcations and branchings of arteries. They may spread circumferentially to involve adjacent veins. However, involvement of venules is not seen in classic PAN, and if present, suggests the polyangiitis overlap syndrome (see below). In the acute stages of disease, polymorphonuclear neutrophils infiltrate all layers of the vessel wall and perivascular areas, which results in intimal proliferation and degeneration of the vessel wall. Mononuclear cells infiltrate the area as the lesions progress to the subacute and chronic stages. Fibrinoid necrosis of the vessels ensues with compromise of the lumen, thrombosis, infarction of the tissues supplied by the involved vessel, and, in some cases, hemorrhage. As the lesions heal, there is collagen deposition, which may lead to further occlusion of the vessel lumen. Aneurysmal dilatations up to 1 cm in size along the involved arteries are characteristic of classic PAN. Granulomas and substantial eosinophilia with eosinophilic tissue infiltrations are not characteristically found and suggest allergic angiitis and granulomatosis (see below).

Multiple organ systems are involved, and the clinicopathologic findings reflect the degree and location of vessel involvement and the resulting ischemic changes (Table 276-2). As mentioned above, pulmonary arteries are not involved in classic PAN, and bronchial artery involvement is uncommon. The pathology in the kidney is predominantly that of arteritis; however, glomerulitis occurs in up to 30 percent of patients. In patients with significant hypertension, typical pathologic features of glomerulosclerosis may be seen alone or superimposed on lesions of glomerulonephritis. In addition, pathologic sequelae of hypertension may be found elsewhere in the body.

The presence of hepatitis B antigenemia in approximately 30 percent of patients with systemic vasculitis, particularly of the classic PAN type, together with the isolation of circulating immune complexes composed of hepatitis B antigen and immunoglobulin, as well as the demonstration by immunofluorescence of hepatitis B antigen, IgM, and complement in the blood vessel walls, strongly suggest the role of immunologic phenomena in the pathogenesis of this disease.

TABLE 276-1 Classification of the vasculitic syndromes

- Systemic necrotizing vasculitis
  - Classic polyarteritis nodosa
  - Allergic angiitis and granulomatosis of Churg-Strauss
  - Polyangiitis overlap syndrome
- Hypersensitivity vasculitis:
  - Exogenous stimuli proved or suspected
    - Henoch-Schönlein purpura
    - Serum sickness and serum sickness–like reactions
    - Other drug-induced vasculitides
    - Vasculitis associated with infectious diseases
  - Endogenous antigens likely involved
    - Vasculitis associated with neoplasms
    - Vasculitis associated with connective tissue diseases
    - Vasculitis associated with other underlying diseases
    - Vasculitis associated with congenital deficiencies of the complement system
- Wegener's granulomatosis
- Giant cell arteritis
  - Temporal arteritis
  - Takayasu's arteritis
- Other vasculitic syndromes
  - Mucocutaneous lymph node syndrome (Kawasaki's disease)
  - Isolated central nervous system vasculitis
  - Thromboangiitis obliterans (Buerger's disease)
  - Miscellaneous vasculitides

TABLE 276-2 Classic PAN: Organ system involvement at autopsy

Organ system	Percent
Kidney	85
Heart	76
Liver	62
Gastrointestinal tract:	51
Jejunum	37
Ileum	27
Mesentery	24
Colon	20
Duodenum	10
Gallbladder	10
Rectosigmoid	10
Appendix	7
Muscle	39
Pancreas	35
Testes	33
Peripheral nerves	32
Central nervous system	27
Skin	20

SOURCE: Cupps and Fauci, 1981, p 32.

TABLE 276-3 Clinical manifestations related to organ system involvement in classic PAN

Organ system	Percent incidence	Clinical manifestations
Renal	60	Renal failure, hypertension
Musculoskeletal	64	Arthritis, arthralgia, myalgia
Peripheral nervous system	51	Peripheral neuropathy, mononeuritis multiplex
Gastrointestinal tract	44	Abdominal pain, nausea and vomiting, bleeding, bowel infarction and perforation, cholecystitis, hepatic infarction, pancreatic infarction
Skin	43	Rash, purpura, nodules, cutaneous infarcts, livedo reticularis, Raynaud's phenomenon
Cardiac	36	Congestive heart failure, myocardial infarction, pericarditis
Genitourinary	25	Testicular, ovarian, or epididymal pain
Central nervous system	23	Cerebral vascular accident, altered mental status, seizure

SOURCE: Cupps and Fauci, 1981, p 29.

Clinical and laboratory manifestations Nonspecific signs and symptoms are the hallmarks of classic PAN. Fever, weight loss, and malaise are present in over one-half of cases. Patients usually present with vague symptoms such as weakness, malaise, headache, abdominal pain, and myalgias. Specific complaints related to the vascular involvement within a particular organ system may also dominate the presenting clinical picture as well as the entire course of the illness (Table 276-3). Renal involvement most commonly manifests as ischemic changes in the glomeruli; however, glomerulonephritis is seen in approximately 30 percent of patients. Hypertension may be related to both the renal polyarteritis as well as the glomerulitis and may dominate the clinical picture. Classic PAN may involve any organ system; the clinical manifestations related to specific organ system involvement are listed in Table 276-3.

There are no diagnostic serologic tests for classic PAN. In over 75 percent of patients the leukocyte count is elevated with a predominance of neutrophils. Eosinophilia is only rarely seen and, when present at high levels, suggests the diagnosis of allergic angiitis and granulomatosis. The anemia of chronic disease may be seen, and an elevated erythrocyte sedimentation rate (ESR) is invariably present. Other common laboratory findings reflect the particular organ involved. Hypergammaglobulinemia may be present, and up to 30 percent of patients have a positive test for hepatitis B surface antigen. Arteriograms may demonstrate characteristic abnormalities such as aneurysms in the small- and medium-sized muscular arteries of the kidneys and abdominal viscera.

Diagnosis The diagnosis of classic PAN is based on the demonstration of characteristic findings of vasculitis on biopsy material of involved organs. In the absence of easily accessible tissue for biopsy, the angiographic demonstration of involved vessels, particularly in the form of aneurysms of small- and medium-sized arteries in the renal, hepatic, and visceral vasculature, is sufficient to make the diagnosis. Aneurysms of vessels are not pathognomonic of classic PAN; furthermore, aneurysms need not always be present, and angiographic findings may be limited to stenotic segments and obliteration of vessels. Biopsy of symptomatic organs such as nodular skin lesions, painful testes, and muscle groups provides the highest diagnostic yields, while blind biopsy of asymptomatic organs is frequently negative. In cases associated with hepatitis B antigenemia, the demonstration of circulating hepatitis B antigen serves as important circumstantial evidence in support of the diagnosis.

Treatment and prognosis The prognosis of untreated classic PAN is extremely poor. The usual clinical course is characterized either by fulminant deterioration or by relentless progression associated with intermittent acute flare-ups. Death usually results from renal failure; from gastrointestinal complications, particularly bowel infarcts and perforation; and from cardiovascular causes. Intractable hypertension often compounds dysfunction in other organ systems such as the kidneys, heart, and central nervous system leading to additional late morbidity and mortality. The 5-year survival rate of untreated patients has been reported to be 13 percent, while glucocorticoid treatment may increase this figure to over 40 percent. Extremely favorable therapeutic results have been reported in classic PAN with the combination of prednisone, 1 mg/kg per day, and cyclophosphamide, 2 mg/kg per day (see section on "Wegener's Granulomatosis" for a detailed description of this therapeutic regimen). This regimen has been reported to result in up to a 90 percent long-term remission rate even following the discontinuation of therapy. Isolated reports have indicated favorable therapeutic responses in classic PAN using plasmapheresis together with corticosteroids and cytotoxic agents.

ALLERGIC ANGIITIS AND GRANULOMATOSIS (CHURG-STRAUSS DISEASE) Definition Allergic angiitis and granulomatosis was described in 1951 by Churg and Strauss and is a disease characterized by granulomatous vasculitis of multiple organ systems, particularly the lung. It is similar in many respects to classic PAN except that the former has a high frequency of lung involvement, vasculitis of blood vessels of various types or sizes including veins and venules, intra- and extravascular granuloma formation together with eosinophilic tissue infiltration, and a strong association with severe asthma and peripheral eosinophilia.

Incidence and prevalence Allergic angiitis and granulomatosis is an uncommon disease whose exact incidence, similar to classic PAN, is difficult to determine due to the grouping of multiple types of vasculitic syndromes in many reported series. The disease can occur at any age with the possible exception of infants. The mean age of onset is 44 years with a male to female ratio of 1.3:1.

Pathophysiology and pathogenesis The vasculitis which is characteristic of allergic angiitis and granulomatosis is similar to that of classic PAN (see above) with certain notable exceptions. In addition to small- and medium-sized muscular arteries, capillaries, veins, and venules can be involved in the former disease. The characteristic histopathologic features of allergic angiitis and granulomatosis are granulomatous reactions that may be present in the tissues or even within the walls of the vessels themselves. These are usually associated with infiltration of the tissues with eosinophils. This process can occur in any organ in the body; however, in sharp contrast to classic PAN, lung involvement is predominant, with skin, cardiovascular system, kidney, peripheral nervous system, and gastrointestinal tract also commonly involved. Although the precise pathogenesis of this disease is uncertain, its strong association with asthma, its clinicopathologic manifestations which strongly suggest hypersensitivity phenomena, and its close similarity to classic PAN point to aberrant immunologic phenomena.

Clinical and laboratory manifestations Patients with allergic angiitis and granulomatosis exhibit nonspecific manifestations such as fever, malaise, anorexia, and weight loss similar to patients with classic PAN. In contrast to the latter disease, the pulmonary findings in allergic angiitis and granulomatosis clearly dominate the clinical picture with severe asthmatic attacks and the presence of pulmonary infiltrates. Skin lesions occur in approximately 70 percent of patients and include purpura in addition to cutaneous and subcutaneous nodules. Apart from the characteristic pulmonary findings, the multisystem involvement in this disease is quite similar to that of classic PAN (see above); an important exception is the fact that the renal disease in allergic angiitis and granulomatosis is less common and generally less severe than that of classic PAN.

The characteristic laboratory finding in virtually all patients with allergic angiitis and granulomatosis is a striking eosinophilia which reaches levels greater than 1000 cells per microliter in more than 80 percent of patients. The other laboratory findings are similar to those of classic PAN and reflect the organ systems involved.

Diagnosis Similar to classic PAN, the diagnosis of allergic angiitis and granulomatosis is made by biopsy, demonstrating vasculitis in a patient with the characteristic clinical manifestations. The biopsy findings are distinctive in the latter disease in that granulomatous vasculitis with eosinophilic tissue involvement together with peripheral eosinophilia are typical. Furthermore, pulmonary involvement is extremely common and is usually manifested by severe asthma associated with pulmonary infiltrates that may be fleeting in nature.

Treatment and prognosis The prognosis of untreated allergic angiitis and granulomatosis is poor with a reported 5-year survival of 25 percent. Unlike classic PAN, the cause of death is more likely to be related to pulmonary and cardiac disease as opposed to renal or gastrointestinal involvement. Glucocorticoid therapy has been reported to increase the 5-year survival to more than 50 percent. In glucocorticoid failures or in patients who present with fulminant multisystem disease, the treatment of choice is a combined regimen of cyclophosphamide and alternate-day prednisone which has resulted in a high rate of complete remission similar to the experience with classic PAN (see above).

POLYANGIITIS OVERLAP SYNDROME Many patients with systemic vasculitis manifest clinicopathologic characteristics which do not fit precisely into any classification, but which have overlapping features of classic PAN, allergic angiitis and granulomatosis, Wegener's granulomatosis, Takayasu's arteritis, or the hypersensitivity group of vasculitides. This subgroup has been referred to as the "polyangiitis overlap syndrome" and is part of the major grouping of systemic necrotizing vasculitis. It is clear that this entity does exist, and it has been designated with a distinct classification in order to avoid confusion in attempting to fit such overlap syndromes into one or other of the more classic vasculitic syndromes. This subgroup is truly a systemic vasculitis with the same potential for resulting in irreversible organ system dysfunction as the other systemic necrotizing vasculitides. The diagnostic and therapeutic considerations as well as the prognosis for this subgroup are the same as those for classic PAN and allergic angiitis and granulomatosis.

HYPERSENSITIVITY VASCULITIS

DEFINITION The term hypersensitivity vasculitis has been used to designate a heterogeneous group of disorders which are characterized by a vasculitic syndrome presumed to be associated with a hypersensitivity reaction following exposure to an antigen such as an infectious agent, a drug, or other foreign or endogenous substances. The common denominator of this group of diseases is the involvement of small vessels. Although any organ can be involved with this type of vasculitis, skin involvement generally dominates the clinical picture and the extracutaneous involvement is usually much less severe than that of the systemic vasculitides. There are multiple subgroups within the larger category of hypersensitivity vasculitis.

INCIDENCE AND PREVALENCE Although the exact incidence of this group of vasculitic syndromes is uncertain, it is clearly more common than the systemic necrotizing vasculitis group. The disease can occur at any age and in both sexes; however, different subgroups have a higher incidence in certain age groups and some are more common in males than females, or vice versa.

PATHOPHYSIOLOGY AND PATHOGENESIS The typical histopathologic feature of the hypersensitivity vasculitides is the presence of vasculitis of small vessels. Postcapillary venules are the most commonly involved vessels; capillaries and arterioles may be involved less frequently. This vasculitis is characterized by a leukocytoclasis which refers to the nuclear debris remaining from the neutrophils which have infiltrated in and around the vessels during the acute stages. In the subacute or chronic stages, mononuclear cells predominate; in certain subgroups, eosinophilic infiltration is seen. Erythrocytes often extravasate from the involved vessels, leading to palpable purpura.

Immune-complex deposition is generally considered to be the immunopathogenic mechanism of this type of vasculitis; however, formal proof that this is the case has not been established for all subgroups (see above). The hypersensitivity vasculitides can be broken down into two major categories depending on the type of putative antigen involved in the hypersensitivity reaction. In the originally described group, the antigen was foreign to the host, i.e., a drug, microbe, or foreign protein. In the second category, the antigen is felt to be endogenous to the host. Examples of these are the "self" proteins such as DNA or immunoglobulin which form immune complexes with their respective antibodies and lead to vasculitic complications in systemic lupus erythematosus and rheumatoid arthritis, respectively; other examples are the tumor antigens which form immune complexes with antibody and lead to vasculitis associated with certain neoplasms.

CLINICAL AND LABORATORY MANIFESTATIONS The hallmark of the broad group of hypersensitivity vasculitides is the predominance of skin involvement. Skin lesions may appear typically as palpable purpura; however, other cutaneous manifestations of the vasculitis may occur, including macules, papules, vesicles, bullae, subcutaneous nodules, ulcers, as well as recurrent or chronic urticaria. Despite the fact that skin lesions predominate, other organ systems may be involved to varying degrees and the extent to which this occurs may define a relatively distinct subgroup. Even in patients with isolated cutaneous involvement, the disease may be characterized by systemic signs and symptoms such as fever, malaise, myalgia, and anorexia. The skin lesions may be pruritic or even quite painful with a burning or stinging sensation. Lesions most commonly occur in the lower extremities in ambulatory patients or in the sacral area in bedridden patients due to the effects of hydrostatic forces on the postcapillary venules. Edema may accompany certain lesions, and hyperpigmentation often occurs in areas of recurrent or chronic lesions.

There are no specific laboratory tests which are diagnostic of hypersensitivity vasculitis. A mild leukocytosis with or without eosinophilia is characteristic as is an elevated ESR. Cryoglobulins and rheumatoid factor may be seen in certain cases, and serum complement levels follow no definite pattern. Laboratory abnormalities related to specific organ dysfunction reflect the involvement of these organs in the particular syndrome in question.

Henoch-Schönlein purpura The most distinctive subgroup of the hypersensitivity vasculitides is Henoch-Schönlein purpura, also referred to as anaphylactoid purpura, which is characterized by palpable purpura, most commonly distributed over the buttocks and lower extremities; arthralgias; gastrointestinal signs and symptoms; and glomerulonephritis. The disease is usually seen in children; however, individuals of any age may be affected. It has a remarkable tendency to resolve and recur several times over a period of weeks or months, usually ending in spontaneous resolution. A small percentage of patients progress to chronic disease. A number of antigens have been implicated in the immunopathogenesis of this disease, including infectious agents, drugs, certain foods, insect bites, and immunizations. IgA is the antibody class most often seen in the immune complexes of these patients. The typical palpable purpura is seen in virtually all patients; most patients develop polyarthralgias in the absence of frank arthritis. Gastrointestinal involvement, which is seen in almost 70 percent of pediatric patients, is characterized by colicky abdominal pain usually associated with nausea, vomiting, diarrhea, or constipation, which is frequently accompanied by the passage of blood and mucus per rectum; bowel intussusception may occur rarely. The renal involvement is usually characterized by a mild glomerulitis leading to hematuria with red blood cell casts (see also Chap. 228). Most patients recover completely and some do not require therapy. When glucocorticoid therapy is required, it is usually administered as 1 mg/kg per day of prednisone and tapered according to the clinical response.

Serum sickness and serum sickness–like reactions These reactions are characterized by the occurrence of fever, urticaria, polyarthralgias, and lymphadenopathy 7 to 10 days after primary exposure and 2 to 4 days after secondary exposure to a heterologous protein (classic serum sickness) or a nonprotein drug such as penicillin or sulfa (serum sickness–like reaction). Most of the manifestations are not due to a vasculitis; however, occasional patients will have typical cutaneous venulitis which may progress rarely to a systemic vasculitis. This disorder is discussed in detail in Chap. 268.

Vasculitis associated with other underlying primary diseases A number of diseases have vasculitis as a secondary manifestation of the underlying primary process. Foremost among these are the connective tissue diseases, particularly systemic lupus erythematosus (Chap. 269), rheumatoid arthritis (Chap. 270), and Sjögren's syndrome (Chap. 273). The most common form of vasculitis in these conditions is the small vessel venulitis isolated to the skin and clinically indistinguishable from the hypersensitivity vasculitides noted in response to an exogenous antigen. However, certain patients may develop a fulminant systemic necrotizing vasculitis indistinguishable from the polyarteritis nodosa group. Cryoglobulinemia may be seen in a number of the diverse vasculitic syndromes. Essential mixed cryoglobulinemia may present as a typical hypersensitivity vasculitis confined to the skin. However, typically it is associated with glomerulonephritis, arthralgias, hepatosplenomegaly, and lymphadenopathy in addition to skin involvement. The cryoglobulins usually consist of cryoprecipitable IgM rheumatoid factor directed against normal endogenous IgG.

Vasculitis can be associated with certain malignancies, particularly lymphoid or reticuloendothelial neoplasms. Leukocytoclastic venulitis confined to the skin is the most common finding; however, widespread systemic vasculitis may occur. Of particular note is the association of hairy-cell leukemia (Chap. 296) with classic PAN.

A leukocytoclastic vasculitis predominantly involving the skin with occasional involvement of other organ systems may be a minor component of many other diseases. These include subacute bacterial endocarditis, Epstein-Barr virus infection, chronic active hepatitis, ulcerative colitis, congenital deficiencies of various complement components, retroperitoneal fibrosis, and primary biliary cirrhosis. Association of hypersensitivity vasculitis with $alpha_1$ antitrypsin deficiency, intestinal bypass surgery, and relapsing polychondritis have been reported.

DIAGNOSIS The diagnosis of hypersensitivity vasculitis is made by the demonstration of vasculitis on biopsy. Given the predominance of cutaneous involvement, biopsy material is generally readily available. Patients who present with what appears to be isolated cutaneous vasculitis should undergo a systemic (usually noninvasive) workup of other organ systems since skin involvement is often the presenting feature of systemic vasculitis.

TREATMENT AND PROGNOSIS Most cases of hypersensitivity vasculitis resolve spontaneously, and others, such as Henoch-Schönlein purpura, remit and relapse before finally remitting completely. In those patients in whom persistent cutaneous disease evolves or in whom extracutaneous organ system involvement occurs, a variety of therapeutic regimens have been tried with variable results. In general, the treatment of this type of vasculitis has not been satisfactory. This is in contrast to the systemic necrotizing vasculitis group (see above) and Wegener's granulomatosis (see below) which generally are much more serious diseases than hypersensitivity vasculitis, but usually respond dramatically to the combination of prednisone and cyclophosphamide. Fortunately, since the disease is generally limited to the skin, this lack of consistent response to therapy usually does not lead to a life-threatening situation. When an antigenic stimulus is recognized as the precipitating factor in the vasculitis, it should be removed; if this is a microbe, appropriate antimicrobial therapy should be instituted. If the vasculitis is associated with another underlying disease, treatment of the latter often results in resolution of the former. In situations where disease is apparently self-limited, no therapy, except possibly symptomatic therapy, is indicated. When disease persists or results in progressive organ system dysfunction such as renal failure in Henoch-Schönlein purpura, glucocorticoid therapy should be instituted, usually as prednisone, 1 mg/kg per day, in a regimen aimed at rapid tapering where possible, either directly to discontinuation or by conversion to an alternate-day regimen followed by ultimate discontinuation. In cases that prove refractory to glucocorticoids in which irreversible organ system dysfunction is likely, a trial of a cytotoxic agent such as cyclophosphamide in the regimen described above for systemic vasculitis is warranted. Patients with chronic vasculitis isolated to cutaneous venules rarely respond dramatically to any therapeutic regimen, and cytotoxic agents should be used only as a last resort in these patients. Plasmapheresis has been used with some success in fulminant cases. Dapsone has been tried in a number of patients with isolated cutaneous vasculitis with rare anecdotal reports of success. However, this drug has been consistently beneficial as therapy for cutaneous vasculitis only in patients with erythema elevatum diutinum (see below).

WEGENER'S GRANULOMATOSIS

DEFINITION Wegener's granulomatosis is a distinct clinicopathologic entity characterized by granulomatous vasculitis of the upper and lower respiratory tracts together with glomerulonephritis. In addition, variable degrees of disseminated vasculitis involving both small arteries and veins may occur.

INCIDENCE AND PREVALENCE Wegener's granulomatosis is an uncommon disease whose true incidence is difficult to determine. It is extremely rare in blacks compared to whites; the male to female ratio is 1.3:1. The disease can be seen at any age but is infrequent among preadolescents; the mean age of onset is approximately 40 years.

PATHOPHYSIOLOGY AND PATHOGENESIS The histopathologic hallmarks of Wegener's granulomatosis are necrotizing vasculitis of small arteries and veins together with granuloma formation which may be either intravascular or extravascular. Lung involvement typically appears as multiple, bilateral, nodular cavity infiltrates which on biopsy almost invariably reveal the typical necrotizing granulomatous vasculitis. Endobronchial disease either in its active form or as a result of fibrous scarring may lead to obstruction with atelectasis. Upper airway lesions, particularly those in the sinuses and nasopharynx, typically reveal inflammation, necrosis, and granuloma formation with or without vasculitis.

It its earliest form, renal involvement is characterized by a focal and segmental glomerulitis which may evolve into a rapidly progressive crescentic glomerulonephritis. Granuloma formation is only rarely seen on renal biopsy. In addition to the classic triad of upper and lower respiratory tracts and kidney disease, virtually any organ can be involved with vasculitis, granuloma, or both.

The immunopathogenesis of this disease is unclear, although the involvement of upper airways and lung suggests an aberrant hypersensitivity response to an exogenous or even endogenous antigen that enters through or resides in the upper airway. The demonstration of circulating and deposited immune complexes in certain patients together with granulomatous reactivity suggests either an overlap of delayed hypersensitivity and immune-complex–mediated mechanisms or a granulomatous response to the immune complexes themselves. Antibodies to a protein contained in the intracytoplasmic azurophil granules of neutrophils have been demonstrated in a high percentage of patients with active Wegener's granulomatosis. The pathophysiologic significance of these findings is unclear at present.

CLINICAL AND LABORATORY MANIFESTATIONS A typical patient presents with severe upper respiratory tract findings such as paranasal sinus pain and drainage, and purulent or bloody nasal discharge with or without nasal mucosal ulceration. Nasal septal perforation may follow, leading to saddle nose deformity. Serous otitis media may occur as a result of eustachian tube blockage.

Pulmonary involvement may be manifested as asymptomatic infiltrates or may be clinically expressed as cough, hemoptysis, dyspnea, and chest discomfort. It is present in approximately 95 percent of patients. Subglottic stenosis resulting from active disease or scarring may result in severe airway obstruction.

Eye involvement (60 percent of patients) may range from a mild conjunctivitis to episcleritis, scleritis, granulomatous sclerouveitis, ciliary vessel vasculitis, and retroorbital mass lesions leading to proptosis.

Skin lesions (45 percent of patients) appear as papules, vesicles, palpable purpura, ulcers, or subcutaneous nodules; biopsy reveals vasculitis, granuloma, or both. Cardiac involvement (12 percent of patients) manifests as pericarditis, coronary vasculitis, or, rarely, cardiomyopathy. Nervous system manifestations (22 percent of patients) include cranial neuritis, mononeuritis multiplex, or, rarely, cerebral vasculitis and/or granuloma.

Renal disease (85 percent of patients) generally dominates the clinical picture and, if left untreated, accounts directly or indirectly for most of the mortality in this disease. Although it may smolder in some cases as a mild glomerulitis with proteinuria, hematuria, and red blood cell casts, it is clear that once clinically detectable renal functional impairment occurs, rapidly progressive renal failure usually ensues unless appropriate treatment is instituted.

While the disease is active, most patients have nonspecific symptoms and signs such as malaise, weakness, arthralgias, anorexia, and weight loss. Fever may indicate activity of the underlying disease, but more often reflects secondary infection, usually of the upper airway.

Characteristic laboratory findings include a markedly elevated ESR, mild anemia and leukocytosis, mild hypergammaglobulinemia, particularly of the IgA class, and mildly elevated rheumatoid factor. Thrombocytosis may be seen as an acute phase reactant; hypocomplementemia is not seen despite the presence of circulating immune complexes in some patients. Antineutrophil cytoplasmic autoantibodies are seen in the majority of patients with active disease (see above).

DIAGNOSIS The diagnosis of Wegener's granulomatosis is a clinicopathologic one made by the demonstration of necrotizing granulomatous vasculitis on biopsy of appropriate tissue in a patient with the clinical findings of upper and lower respiratory tract disease together with evidence of glomerulonephritis. Pulmonary tissue, preferably obtained by open thoracotomy, offers the highest diagnostic yield, almost invariably revealing granulomatous vasculitis. Biopsy of upper airway tissue usually reveals granulomatous inflammation with necrosis but may not show vasculitis. Renal biopsy confirms the presence of glomerulonephritis

In its typical presentation, the classic clinicopathologic complex of Wegener's granulomatosis usually provides ready differentiation from other disorders. However, if all of the typical features are not present at once, it needs to be differentiated from the other vasculitides, particularly allergic angiitis and granulomatosis, Goodpasture's syndrome (Chap. 228), tumors of the upper airway or lung, and infectious or noninfectious granulomatous diseases. Of particular note is the differentiation from idiopathic midline granuloma (see Chap. 279) which frequently erodes through the skin of the face, a feature never seen in Wegener's granulomatosis.

Of particular importance in the differential diagnosis is a disease called *lymphomatoid granulomatosis*. It is characterized by lung, skin, central nervous system, and kidney involvement in which atypical lymphocytoid and plasmacytoid cells infiltrate tissue in an angioinvasive manner. In this regard, it clearly differs from Wegener's granulomatosis in that it is not an inflammatory vasculitis in the classic sense, but an infiltration of vessels with atypical mononuclear cells; granuloma may be present in involved tissues. Approximately 50 percent of patients develop a true malignant lymphoma.

TREATMENT AND PROGNOSIS Wegener's granulomatosis was formerly universally fatal, usually within a few months after the onset of clinically apparent renal disease. Glucocorticoids alone led to some symptomatic improvement with little effect on the ultimate course of the disease. It has been well established that the treatment of choice in this disease is cyclophosphamide given in doses of 2 mg/kg per day orally. The leukocyte count should be closely monitored during therapy and the dosage adjusted in order to maintain the count above 3000 per cubic millimeter, which generally maintains the neutrophil count at approximately 1500 per microliter. With this approach, clinical remission can usually be induced and maintained without causing severe leukopenia with its associated risk of infection. Cyclophosphamide should be continued for 1 year following the induction of complete remission and gradually tapered and discontinued thereafter. Patients who cannot tolerate cyclophosphamide or who develop serious toxicity such as severe cystitis may be treated with azathioprine in similar doses.

At the initiation of therapy, glucocorticoids should be administered together with cyclophosphamide. This can be given as prednisone, 1 mg/kg per day initially (for the first month of therapy) as a daily regimen with gradual conversion to an alternate-day schedule followed by tapering and discontinuation after approximately 6 months.

Using the above regimen, the prognosis of this disease is excellent and long-term remission is achieved in over 90 percent of patients. A number of patients who developed irreversible renal failure, but who achieved subsequent remission on appropriate therapy, have undergone successful renal transplantation.

Because of anecdotal reports of some success with an intermittent, intravenous bolus of cyclophosphamide (1 gm/m^2 per month) in the treatment of Wegener's granulomatosis and other systemic vasculitides, prospective studies using this regimen are currently underway. In addition, recent reports have indicated a potential role for trimethoprim/sulfamethoxazole in the treatment of Wegener's granulomatosis. However, controlled prospective clinical trials are needed to substantiate these claims. Chronically administered cyclophosphamide in the regimen indicated above is still clearly the treatment of choice for Wegener's granulomatosis.

TEMPORAL ARTERITIS

DEFINITION Temporal arteritis, also referred to as cranial or giant cell arteritis, is an inflammation of medium- and large-sized arteries. It characteristically involves one or more branches of the carotid artery, particularly the temporal artery, hence the name cranial or temporal arteritis. However, it is a systemic disease and can involve arteries in multiple locations.

INCIDENCE AND PREVALENCE Temporal arteritis is an uncommon disease estimated to occur in 24 per 100,000 people. It is a disease of the elderly, occurring almost exclusively in individuals older than 55 years; however, well-documented cases have occurred in patients 40 years old or younger. It is more common in women than in men and is rare in blacks. Familial aggregation of this disease has been reported.

PATHOPHYSIOLOGY AND PATHOGENESIS Although the temporal artery is most frequently involved in this disease, patients often have a systemic vasculitis of multiple medium- and large-sized arteries which may go undetected. Histopathologically, the disease is a panarteritis with inflammatory mononuclear cell infiltrates within the vessel wall with frequent giant cell formation. There is proliferation of the intima and fragmentation of the internal elastic lamina. Pathophysiologic findings in organs result from the ischemia related to the involved vessels. Immunopathogenic mechanisms, particularly cell-mediated immunity, are felt to be involved in this disease, although the etiology is entirely unknown.

CLINICAL AND LABORATORY MANIFESTATIONS The disease is characterized clinically by the classic complex of fever, anemia, high ESR, and headaches in an elderly patient. Other manifestations include malaise, fatigue, anorexia, weight loss, sweats, and arthralgias. Temporal arteritis is closely associated with the polymyalgia rheumatica syndrome, which is characterized by stiffness, aching, and pain in the muscles of the neck, shoulders, lower back, hips, and thighs.

In patients with involvement of the temporal artery, headache is the predominant symptom and may be associated with a tender, thickened, or nodular artery which may pulsate early in the disease but may become occluded later. Scalp pain and claudication of the jaw and tongue may occur. A well-recognized and dreaded complication of temporal arteritis, particularly in untreated patients, is ocular involvement due primarily to ischemic optic neuritis, which may lead to serious visual symptoms, even sudden blindness in some patients. However, most patients have complaints relating to the head or eyes for months before objective eye involvement. Claudication of the extremities, strokes, myocardial infarctions, aortic aneurysms and dissections, and infarctions of visceral organs have been reported.

Characteristic laboratory findings in addition to the elevated ESR include a normochromic or slightly hypochromic anemia. Liver function abnormalities are common, particularly increased alkaline phosphatase levels. Increased levels of IgG and complement have been reported as have increased levels of circulating immune complexes.

DIAGNOSIS The diagnosis of temporal arteritis and its associated clinicopathologic syndrome can often be made clinically by the demonstration of the classic picture of fever, anemia, and high ESR with or without symptoms of polymyalgia rheumatica in an elderly patient. The diagnosis is confirmed by biopsy of the temporal artery. Since involvement of the vessel may be segmental, the diagnosis may be missed on routine biopsy. Dramatic response to a trial of glucocorticoid therapy can confirm the diagnosis.

TREATMENT AND PROGNOSIS Temporal arteritis and its associated symptoms are exquisitely sensitive to glucocorticoid therapy. Treatment should begin with prednisone, 40 to 60 mg per day followed by a gradual tapering to a maintenance dose of 7.5 to 10 mg per day. When ocular signs and symptoms occur, it is important that therapy be initiated or adjusted to control them. Because of the possibility of relapse, therapy should be continued for at least 1 to 2 years. The prognosis is generally good, and most patients achieve complete remission that is often maintained after withdrawal of therapy.

TAKAYASU'S ARTERITIS

DEFINITION Takayasu's arteritis is an inflammatory and stenotic disease of medium- and large-sized arteries characterized by a strong predilection for the aortic arch and its branches. For this reason, it is often referred to as the aortic arch syndrome.

INCIDENCE AND PREVALENCE Takayasu's arteritis is an uncommon disease, much less common than temporal arteritis. It is most prevalent in adolescent girls and young women. Although it is more common in the Orient, it is neither racially nor geographically restricted. An association of the disease has been described with HLA-DR2, MB1 in Japan and HLA-DR4, MB3 in the United States.

PATHOPHYSIOLOGY AND PATHOGENESIS The disease involves medium- and large-sized arteries with a strong predilection for the aortic arch and its branches; the pulmonary artery may also be involved. The most commonly affected arteries seen by angiography are the subclavians, followed by the aortic arch, ascending aorta, carotids, and femorals. The involvement of the major branches of the aorta is much more marked at their origin than distally. Partial renal artery occlusion with resulting hypertension is common. The disease is a panarteritis with inflammatory mononuclear cell infiltrates and occasionally giant cells. There is marked intimal proliferation and fibrosis, scarring and vascularization of the media, and disruption and degeneration of the elastic lamina. Narrowing of the lumen occurs with or without thrombosis. The vasa vasorum are frequently involved. Pathologic changes in various organs reflect the compromise of blood flow through the involved vessels.

Immunopathogenic mechanisms, the precise nature of which is uncertain, are suspected in this disease.

CLINICAL AND LABORATORY MANIFESTATIONS Takayasu's arteritis is a systemic disease with generalized as well as local symptoms. The generalized symptoms include malaise, fever, night sweats, arthralgias, anorexia, and weight loss which may occur months before vessel involvement is apparent. These symptoms may merge into those related to pain over the involved vessels followed by symptoms of ischemia in organs supplied by the compromised vessels. Pulses are commonly absent in the involved vessels, particularly the subclavian artery. Aortic regurgitation may occur; hypertension is seen in almost 50 percent of cases. Cardiomegaly and cardiac failure secondary to aortic or pulmonary hypertension occur commonly; the coronary arteries themselves are rarely involved. Carotid artery involvement leads to a variety of central nervous system signs and symptoms with over one-half of patients experiencing syncopal episodes; stroke, which occurs in 15 percent of patients, may represent the first sign of disease; ocular signs and symptoms are present in 60 percent of patients.

The clinical course may be fulminant, may progress gradually, or may stabilize. Complications are related to the distribution of the involved vessels. Death usually occurs from congestive heart failure or cerebrovascular accidents.

Characteristic laboratory findings include an elevated ESR, mild anemia, leukocytosis, and elevated immunoglobulin levels.

DIAGNOSIS The diagnosis of Takayasu's arteritis should be suspected strongly in a young woman who develops a decrease or absence of peripheral pulses, discrepancies in blood pressure, and arterial bruits. The diagnosis is confirmed by the characteristic pattern on arteriography which includes irregular vessel walls, stenosis, poststenotic dilatation, aneurysm formation, occlusion, and evidence of increased collateral circulation. Histopathologic demonstration of inflamed vessels adds confirmatory data; however, tissue is rarely readily available for examination.

TREATMENT AND PROGNOSIS The course of the disease is variable, and spontaneous remissions may occur. Reported mortality statistics range from less than 10 percent to 75 percent, likely reflecting duration of follow-up. Although glucocorticoid therapy in doses of 40 to 60 mg prednisone per day alleviates symptoms, there are no convincing studies which indicate that they alone increase survival. However, recent studies suggest that glucocorticoid therapy can induce remissions in a high percentage of individuals. In addition, surgery and/or angioplasty may remarkably improve survival by decreasing the risk of stroke and correcting hypertension due to renal artery stenosis. A few patients who were refractory to glucocorticoid therapy responded favorably to cyclophosphamide, 2 mg/kg per day. However, long-term studies will be needed to confirm this.

MUCOCUTANEOUS LYMPH NODE SYNDROME (KAWASAKI'S DISEASE)

Mucocutaneous lymph node syndrome is an acute, febrile, multisystem disease of children. It is characterized by unresponsiveness to antibiotics; nonsuppurative cervical adenitis; and changes in the skin and mucous membranes such as edema, congested conjunctivae, erythema of the oral cavity, lips, and palms, and desquamation of the skin of the fingertips. Although the disease is generally benign and self-limited, it is associated with coronary artery aneurysms in 17 to 31 percent of cases, with an overall case fatality rate of 0.5 to 2.8 percent. These complications usually occur between the third and fourth week of illness during the convalescent stage. Vasculitis of the coronary arteries is seen in almost all of the fatal cases which have been autopsied. There is typical intimal proliferation and infiltration of the vessel wall with mononuclear cells. Beadlike aneurysms and thromboses may be seen along the artery. Most investigators agree that many of the cases of PAN formerly reported in children were actually arteritic complications of unrecognized mucocutaneous lymph node syndrome. Other manifestations include pericarditis, myocarditis, myocardial ischemia and infarction, and cardiomegaly.

Apart from the up to 2.8 percent of patients who develop fatal complications, the prognosis of this disease for uneventful recovery is excellent. High-dose intravenous gamma globulin (400 mg/kg per day for 4 consecutive days) together with aspirin (100 mg/kg per day for 14 days followed by 3 to 5 mg/kg per day for several weeks) have been shown to be effective in reducing the prevalence of coronary artery abnormalities when administered early in the course of the disease.

ISOLATED VASCULITIS OF THE CENTRAL NERVOUS SYSTEM

Isolated vasculitis of the central nervous system is an uncommon clinicopathologic entity characterized by vasculitis restricted to the vessels of the central nervous system without other apparent systemic vasculitis. Although the arteriole is most commonly affected, vessels of any size can be involved. The inflammatory process is usually composed of mononuclear cell infiltrates with or without granuloma formation. Cases have been associated with cytomegalovirus, syphilis, pyogenic bacterial and varicella-zoster infections, as well as with Hodgkin's disease and amphetamine abuse; however, in several cases no underlying disease process has been identified.

Patients may present with severe headaches, altered mental function, and focal neurologic defects. Systemic symptoms are generally absent. Devastating neurologic abnormalities may occur depending on the extent of vessel involvement. The diagnosis is generally made by demonstration of characteristic vessel abnormalities on arteriography and confirmed by biopsy of the brain parenchyma and leptomeninges. The prognosis of this disease is poor; however, some reports indicate that glucocorticoid therapy alone or together with cyclophosphamide in steroid-resistant patients administered as described above for the systemic vasculitides has induced sustained clinical remissions in a small number of patients.

THROMBOANGIITIS OBLITERANS (BUERGER'S DISEASE)

Thromboangiitis obliterans is an inflammatory occlusive peripheral vascular disease of unknown etiology which affects arteries and veins. Thrombosis of the vessels is likely the primary event, and so this disease is not a classic vasculitis. However, it is considered among the vasculitides because of the intense inflammatory response within the thrombus and the fact that there is often a vasculitis of the vasa vasorum in the arterial wall. The disease is discussed in detail in Chap. 198.

MISCELLANEOUS VASCULITIDES

A variety of disorders, many of which are uncommon, are characterized by varying degrees of inflammatory responses involving blood vessels. *Behçet's syndrome* is a clinicopathologic entity characterized by recurrent episodes of oral and genital ulcers, iritis, and cutaneous lesions. The underlying pathologic lesion is a leukocytoclastic venulitis, although vessels of any size and in any organ can be involved. This disorder is described in detail in Chap. 275.

Cogan's syndrome is a disease characterized by nonsyphilitic interstitial keratitis together with vestibuloauditory symptoms. It may be associated with a systemic vasculitis involving vessels of different sizes as well as the aortic valve.

Erythema nodosum is a common disease which is recognized as a hypersensitivity manifestation of a number of other disorders. It is a painful nodular process of the dermis and subcutaneous tissues. However, histopathologically, there is a vasculitis of small venules (see Chap. 56).

Erythema elevatum diutinum is a rare, chronic skin disorder of unknown etiology characterized by persistent red, purple, and yellowish papules, plaques, and nodules usually distributed symmetrically over the extensor surface of the limbs which on biopsy demonstrate a leukocytoclastic venulitis together with a marked dermal inflammatory infiltrate. The disease responds dramatically to dapsone therapy.

Eales' disease is a retinal vasculitis which predominantly affects males in the second and third decade of life and which produces a syndrome of recurrent hemorrhages into the retina and vitreous.

REFERENCES

ALARCON-SEGOVIA D: The necrotizing vasculitides. Med Clin North Am 61:240, 1977

CUPPS TR, FAUCI AS: *The Vasculitides*. Philadelphia, Saunders, 1981

——— et al: Chronic, recurrent small-vessel cutaneous vasculitis. Clinical experience in 13 patients. JAMA 247:1994, 1982

——— et al: Isolated angiitis of the central nervous system. Prospective diagnostic and therapeutic experience. Am J Med 74:97, 1983

FAUCI AS: Vasculitis, in *Clinical Immunology*, CW Parker (ed). Philadelphia, Saunders, 1980, pp 475–519

———: Vasculitis. J Allergy Clin Immunol 72:211, 1983

——— et al: The spectrum of vasculitis. Clinical, pathologic, immunologic, and therapeutic considerations. Ann Intern Med 89:660, 1978

——— et al: Wegener's granulomatosis: Prospective clinical and therapeutic experience with 85 patients for 21 years. Ann Intern Med 98:76, 1983

FAUCI AS, LEAVITT RY: Vasculitis, in *Arthritis and Allied Conditions: A Textbook of Rheumatology*, 11th ed, DJ McCarty (ed). Philadelphia, Lea & Febiger, 1989, pp 1166–118

KADISON P, HAYNES BF: Vasculitis: Mechanisms of vessel damage, in *Inflammation: Basic Principles and Clinical Correlates*. JI Gallin et al. New York, Raven, 1988, pp 703–717

LEAVITT RY, FAUCI AS: Polyangiitis overlap syndrome. Am J Med, 1986

SHELHAMER JH et al: Takayasu's arteritis and its therapy. Ann Intern Med 103:121, 1985

277 SARCOIDOSIS

RONALD G. CRYSTAL

DEFINITION Sarcoidosis is a chronic, multisystem disorder of unknown etiology characterized in affected organs by an accumulation of T lymphocytes and mononuclear phagocytes, noncaseating epithelioid granulomas, and derangements of the normal tissue architecture. Although there are usually skin anergy and depressed cellular immune processes in the blood, sarcoidosis is characterized at the sites of disease by exaggerated helper-T-lymphocyte immune processes. All parts of the body can be affected, but the organ most frequently affected is the lung. Involvement of the skin, eye, and lymph nodes is also common. The disease is often acute or subacute and self-limiting, but in many individuals it is chronic, waxing and waning over many years.

ETIOLOGY The etiology of sarcoidosis is unknown. A variety of infectious and noninfectious agents have been implicated, but there is no proof that any specific agent is responsible. However, all available evidence is consistent with the concept that the disease results from an exaggerated cellular immune response (acquired, inherited, or both) to a limited class of antigens or self-antigens.

INCIDENCE AND PREVALENCE Sarcoidosis is a relatively common disease affecting individuals of both sexes and almost all ages, races, and geographic locations. Females appear to be slightly more susceptible than males. Cases of sarcoid have been described in all of the major races, and the disease is found throughout the world. It has been suggested that sarcoid is more common in certain geographic areas such as the southeastern part of the United States, but when case-matched controls have been used, these geographic differences are less convincing. There is a remarkable diversity of the prevalence of sarcoidosis among certain ethnic and racial groups. The prevalence of sarcoidosis is from 10 to 40 per 100,000 in the United States and Europe. In the United States, the majority of patients are black, with a ratio of blacks to whites ranging from 10:1 to 17:1. In Europe, however, the disease affects mostly whites. Furthermore, while the prevalence per 100,000 in Sweden is 64, in France it is 10, in Poland 3, yet for Irish females living in London it is 200. In contrast, the disease is very rare among Eskimos, Canadian Indians, New Zealand Maoris, and southeast Asians.

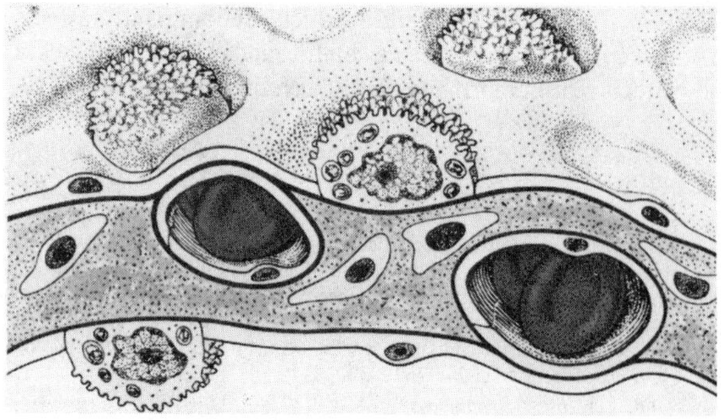

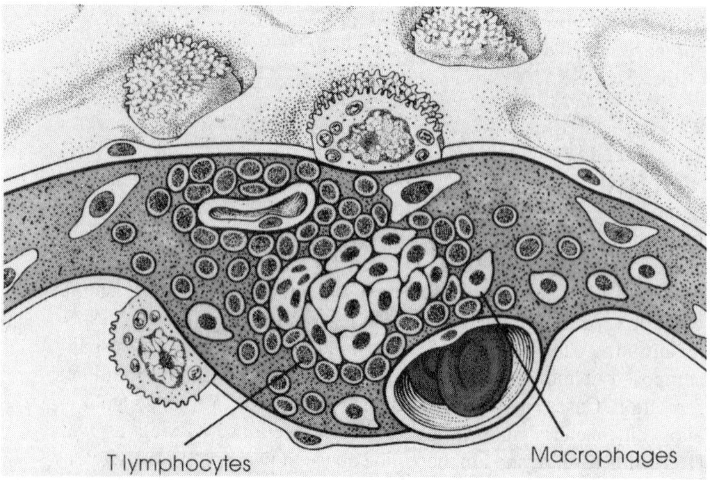

A

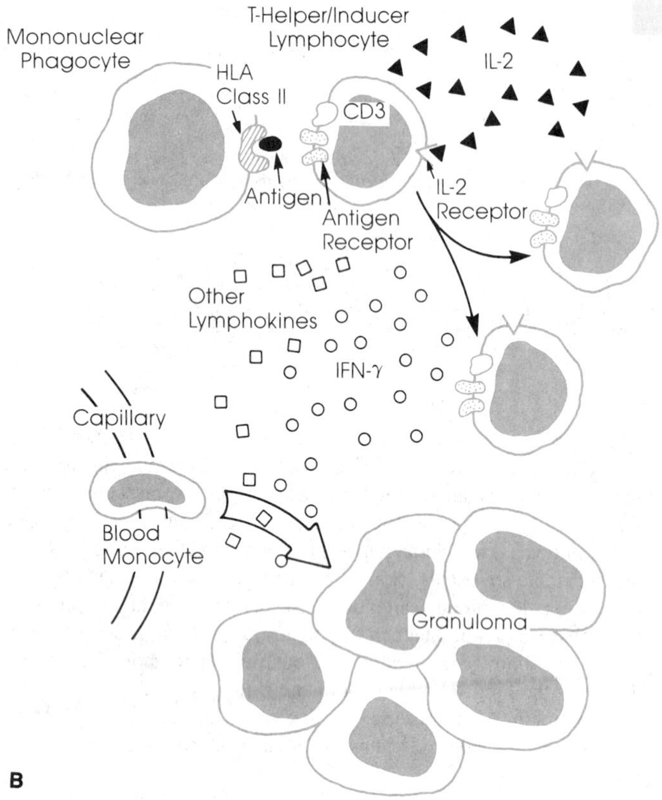

B

FIGURE 277-1 Pathogenesis of sarcoidosis. *A.* Histologic abnormalities. Normal alveoli *(left)* and alveoli in active sarcoidosis *(right)*. The latter are distorted by the accumulated T helper-inducer lymphocytes, alveolar macrophages, and macrophages aggregated into granulomas. There is mild damage to alveolar epithelial and endothelial cells. *B.* The exaggerated processes of T helper-inducer lymphocytes in affected organs result in the accumulation of these cells along with macrophages and macrophages aggregated into granulomas. The trigger for the T helper-inducer cells is unknown. It may be a limited class of antigens or self-antigens presented in the context of class II HLA surface molecules by mononuclear phagocytes to the T helper-inducer lymphocyte. The antigen class II HLA complex is identified by the T-cell antigen receptor, the CD3 signal transducing complex is triggered, and the T cell is activated. Consequent to this process the immune response is exaggerated and skewed to produce activated T helper-inducer cells that release interleukin 2, which drives the accumulation of more T helper cells. The activated T helper-inducer cells also release γ-interferon (IFN-γ) and other lymphokines, mediators that contribute to the recruitment and activation of blood monocytes and hence to granuloma formation.

Most patients present with sarcoidosis between the ages of 20 and 40, but it can occur in children and in the elderly. Several hundred kindred groups with familial sarcoidosis have been described, and the disease has been observed in twins, more commonly in monozygotic than in dizygotic pairs. There have also been several instances of husband-wife pairs identified, and geographic foci of sarcoid among unrelated individuals living closely within a community, arguing for some environmental factors in the pathogenesis of the disease. Although the histocompatibility locus HLA-B8 has been suggested to confer certain responses to sarcoidosis, no clear patterns in any HLA locus have emerged. Unlike many diseases in which the lung is involved, sarcoidosis favors nonsmokers.

PATHOPHYSIOLOGY AND IMMUNOPATHOGENESIS The first manifestation of the disease is an accumulation of mononuclear inflammatory cells, mostly T helper lymphocytes and mononuclear phagocytes, in affected organs. This inflammatory process is followed by the formation of granulomas, aggregates of macrophages and their progeny, epithelioid cells, and multinucleated giant cells. The typical sarcoid granuloma is a compact structure composed of an aggregate of mononuclear phagocytes surrounded by a rim of T helper-inducer lymphocytes and, to a far lesser extent, B lymphocytes. The overall structure is relatively discrete and is interspersed with fine collagen fibrils, presumably remnants of the underlying connective tissue matrix. The giant cells within the granuloma can be of the Langhans' or foreign-body variety and often contain inclusions such as Schaumann bodies (conch-like structures), asteroid bodies (stellate-like structures), and residual bodies (refractile calcium-containing inclusions).

Together, the accumulated T cells, mononuclear phagocytes, and granulomas represent the active disease. Other than the fact that they take up space and thus their bulk modifies the local architecture, there is no evidence that the mononuclear inflammatory cells either alone or in the granuloma injure the affected organ by releasing mediators that damage the normal parenchymal cells or the extracellular matrix. Rather, organ dysfunction in sarcoid results from the accumulated inflammatory cells distorting the architecture of the affected tissue; if a sufficient number of structures vital to the function of the tissue are involved, the disease becomes clinically apparent in that organ. Thus, while autopsy series show that, to some extent, sarcoidosis involves most organs in the majority of patients, the disease manifests clinically only in organs where it affects function (such as the lung and eye) or in organs where it is readily observed (such as the skin or, by x-ray, the hilar nodes). For example, in the lung the inflammatory cells and granulomas distort the walls of the alveoli, bronchi, and blood vessels (Fig. 277-1*A*), thus altering the intimate relationships between air and blood necessary for normal gas exchange. When a sufficient amount of pulmonary tissue is involved, it is sensed by the individual as dyspnea. In contrast, most individuals with sarcoidosis have granulomatous mononuclear cell inflammation in the liver but usually do not have symptoms or functional derangements referable to that organ, likely because the disease process does not modify the local structures sufficiently to affect function.

If the disease is suppressed, either spontaneously or with therapy, the mononuclear inflammation is reduced in intensity and the number of granulomas is reduced. The granulomas resolve either by dispersion of the cells or by centripetal proliferation of fibroblasts from the periphery of the granuloma inward, to form a small scar. In chronic cases, the mononuclear cell inflammation persists for years. If the intensity of the inflammation is sufficiently high for a sufficiently long period, the derangements to the affected tissues result in extensive damage, the development of fibrosis, and permanent loss of organ function.

All available evidence suggests that active sarcoidosis results from an exaggerated cellular immune response to a variety of antigens or self-antigens, in which the process of T-lymphocyte triggering, proliferation, and activation is skewed in the direction of helper-inducer-T-lymphocyte processes (Fig. 277-1*B*). The result is an exaggerated helper-inducer-T-cell response, and thus the accumulation of large numbers of activated T cells in the affected organs. Since the activated helper-inducer T lymphocyte releases mediators that attract and activate mononuclear phagocytes, it is likely that the process of granuloma formation is a secondary phenomenon which is a consequence of the exaggerated helper-inducer-T-cell process. In this context, the current hypotheses of the cause of sarcoidosis, not mutually exclusive, include: (1) the disease is caused by a class of antigens, nonself or self, that trigger only the helper-inducer-T-cell arm of the immune response; (2) the disease results from an inadequate suppressor arm of the immune response, such that helper-inducer-T-cell processes cannot be shut down in a normal fashion; or (3) the disease results from inherited (and/or acquired) differences in immune response genes, such that the response to a variety of antigens is an exaggerated, helper-inducer-T-cell process.

Independent of the inciting agent(s) or the reason why there is an exaggerated helper-inducer-T-cell response, there is a general understanding of the processes responsible for the maintenance of the inflammation and the development of the granuloma. The T helper-inducer lymphocytes accumulate at the sites of disease, at least in part, because they proliferate in these sites at an exaggerated rate. This T-cell proliferation is maintained by the spontaneous release of interleukin 2 (IL-2), the T-cell growth factor, by activated T helper-inducer cells in the local milieu. In this regard, sarcoidosis is a remarkable example of compartmentalization of the immune system and a dramatic illustration of why disease activity of sarcoidosis cannot be assessed by evaluating the immune system only in the blood. Whereas the T helper-inducer cells in the involved organs are releasing IL-2 and proliferating at an enhanced rate, the T cells in other sites, such as blood, are quiescent. Furthermore, while there is a marked enhancement of the number of T helper-inducer cells at the sites of disease, the numbers of T helper-inducer cells in the blood are normal or slightly reduced. In the involved organs, the ratio of helper-inducer to suppressor-cytotoxic T cells may be as high as 10:1 compared to the ratio of 2:1 found in normal tissues or in the blood of affected individuals.

In addition to driving other T helper-inducer cells in the affected organs to proliferate, the T helper-inducer cells at the sites of disease are activated and release mediators that both recruit and activate mononuclear phagocytes. The T helper-inducer cells accomplish this by releasing a variety of mediators (lymphokines) including proteins capable of recruiting blood monocytes to the local milieu of the activated T cells and γ-interferon, a protein that, among its many actions, activates mononuclear phagocytes. Together, these mediators recruit blood monocytes to the affected organs and activate them, providing the building blocks for the formation of the granuloma.

In addition to these exaggerated cellular immune processes, active sarcoid is also characterized by hyperglobulinemia. Included among the immunoglobulins are antibodies against a variety of infectious agents as well as IgM anti-T-cell antibodies. However, there is no evidence that any of these antibodies plays a role in the pathogenesis of the disease, and they are thought to result from the nonspecific polyclonal stimulation of B cells by the activated T cells at the site of disease.

If the damage in the affected organs is sufficiently extensive so that the remaining parenchymal cells cannot reestablish the normal tissue architecture, the usual result is fibrosis, the proliferation of mesenchymal cells and deposition of their connective tissue products. There is convincing evidence that the fibroblast proliferation is directed by tissue macrophages spontaneously releasing growth signals for fibroblasts, including platelet-derived growth factor, fibronectin, and insulin-like growth factor 1. It is not known, however, why this fibrotic process occurs only in a relatively small proportion of individuals with sarcoidosis.

CLINICAL MANIFESTATIONS Sarcoidosis is a systemic disease, and thus the clinical manifestations may be generalized or focused on one or more organs. However, because the lung is almost always involved, most patients have symptoms referable to the respiratory system. Independent of the site, the clinical manifestations of the disease relate directly to the exaggerated helper-inducer T cell–mononuclear phagocyte granulomatous inflammatory process itself, or to the sequela resulting from the permanent damage caused by this process.

Sarcoidosis is occasionally discovered in a completely asymptomatic individual, but more commonly it presents abruptly over 1 to 2 weeks or the affected individual develops symptoms insidiously over several months. Independent of the mode of presentation, about 75 percent of all cases present when the individual is less than 40 years of age.

The asymptomatic form is usually detected by a routine examination, such as a chest film. In the United States, this represents about 10 to 20 percent of all cases, but in countries where chest films are mandatory in preemployment screening programs, the proportion of asymptomatic patients is higher.

So-called acute or subacute sarcoidosis develops abruptly over a period of a few weeks and represents 20 to 40 percent of all cases. These individuals usually have constitutional symptoms such as fever, fatigue, malaise, anorexia, or weight loss. These symptoms are usually mild, but in approximately 25 percent of the acute cases, the constitutional complaints are extensive. Many patients have respiratory symptoms, including cough, dyspnea, or a vague retrosternal chest discomfort. Two syndromes have been identified in the acute group. Löfgren's syndrome, frequent in Scandinavian, Irish, and Puerto Rican females, includes the complex of erythema nodosum and x-ray findings of bilateral hilar adenopathy, often accompanied by joint symptoms. The Heerfordt-Waldenstrom syndrome describes individuals with fever, parotid enlargement, anterior uveitis, and facial nerve palsy.

The insidious form of sarcoidosis develops over months and is associated usually with respiratory complaints without constitutional symptoms. In the United States, 40 to 70 percent of all sarcoid patients are in this category. About 10 percent of these individuals have symptoms referable to organs other than the lung. It is the individuals who present with the insidious form of sarcoidosis who most commonly go on to develop chronic sarcoidosis, with permanent damage to the lung and other organs.

Despite the fact that sarcoidosis is a systemic disease and some evidence of inflammation can be detected in most organs in the majority of patients, sarcoidosis is important clinically because of the pulmonary abnormalities and, to a lesser extent, lymph node, skin, and eye involvement. Far less commonly, other organs are involved significantly.

Lung Of individuals with sarcoidosis, 90 percent have an abnormal chest x-ray at some time during their course. Overall, approximately 50 percent develop permanent pulmonary abnormalities and 5 to 15 percent have progressive fibrosis of the lung parenchyma. Sarcoidosis of the lung is primarily an interstitial lung disease (see Chap. 211) in which the inflammatory process involves the alveoli, small bronchi, and small blood vessels. These individuals typically have symptoms of dyspnea, particularly with exercise, and a dry cough. In acute and subacute cases, physical examination usually reveals dry rales. Hemoptysis is rare, as is production of sputum.

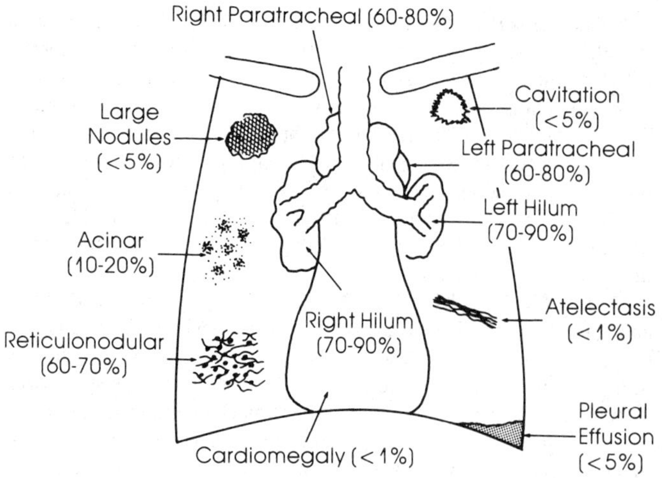

A

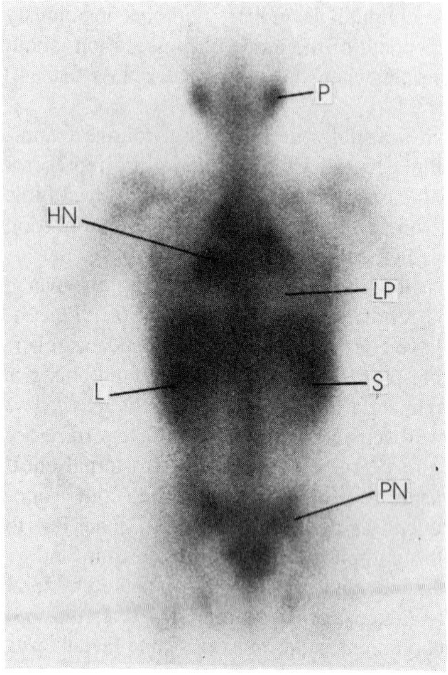

B

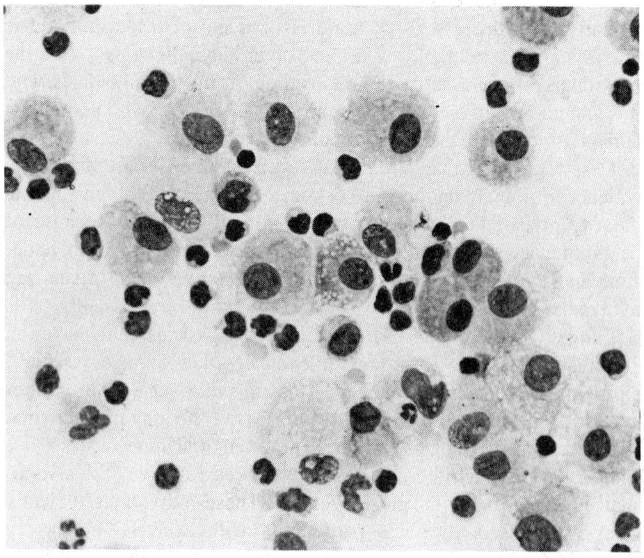

C

Occasionally, the large airways are involved to a degree sufficient to cause dysfunction. Distal atelectasis can result from endobronchial sarcoidosis or from external compression from enlarged intrathoracic nodes. Rarely, wheezing is heard, incorrectly suggesting asthma. Large-vessel pulmonary granulomatous arteritis is common, but it rarely causes major problems. If it dominates the pulmonary lesions, it is sometimes called "necrotizing sarcoidal granulomatosis." The pleura is involved in 1 to 5 percent of cases, almost always manifesting as a unilateral pleural effusion with characteristics of an exudate containing lymphocytes. The effusions usually clear within a few weeks, but chronic pleural thickening can result. Pneumothorax is very rare.

Lymph nodes Lymphadenopathy is very common in sarcoidosis. Intrathoracic nodes are enlarged in 75 to 90 percent of all patients; usually this involves the hilar nodes, but the paratracheal nodes are commonly involved (Fig. 277-2*A*). Less frequently, there is enlargement of subcarinal, anterior mediastinal, or posterior mediastinal nodes. Peripheral lymphadenopathy is very common, particularly involving the cervical, axillary, epitrochlear, and inguinal nodes. The nodes in the retroperitoneal area and in the mesenteric chain can also enlarge. All of these nodes are nonadherent, with a firm, rubbery texture. Palpation causes no pain. Unlike nodes in tuberculosis, the nodes do not ulcerate. The lymphadenopathy rarely causes a problem for the affected individual; however, if it is massive, it can be disfiguring and can impinge on other organs and lead to functional impairment.

Skin Sarcoidosis involves the skin in about 25 percent of cases. The most common lesions are erythema nodosum, plaques, maculopapular eruptions, subcutaneous nodules, and lupus pernio. Erythema nodosum, comprising bilateral, tender red nodules on the anterior surface of the legs, is not specific for sarcoidosis but is common, particularly in acute sarcoidosis, in combination with systemic symptoms and polyarthralgias. Treatment is not required since the lesions resolve spontaneously in 2 to 4 weeks. Erythema nodosum is much more common among sarcoid patients in Europe than in the United States. Skin plaques associated with sarcoid are purple, indolent lesions, often raised, and usually occur on the face, buttocks, and extremities. The maculopapular eruptions occur on the face around the eyes and nose, on the back, and on the extremities. These are elevated lesions less than 1 cm in diameter with a flat, waxy top. Subcutaneous nodules are most common on the trunk and extremities. Lupus pernio is characterized by indurated blue-purple, swollen, shiny lesions on the nose, cheeks, lips, ears, fingers, and knees. The lesions on the tip of the nose cause a bulbous appearance, sometimes associated with varicosities. The nasal mucosa is usually involved, and underlying bone can be destroyed. Sarcoidosis can also involve old surgical scars and tattoos. Although it may be disfiguring, cutaneous sarcoidosis rarely causes major problems. Clubbing of the fingers is occasionally observed in sarcoidosis if there is extensive pulmonary fibrosis.

Eye Eye involvement occurs in approximately 25 percent of patients with sarcoidosis, and it can cause blindness. The usual lesions involve the uveal tract, iris, ciliary body, and choroid. Of those cases with eye involvement, approximately 75 percent have anterior uveitis and 25 to 35 percent have posterior uveitis. There is blurred vision, tearing, and photophobia. The uveitis can develop

FIGURE 277-2 Common laboratory findings of sarcoidosis. *A*. Schematic view of the abnormal findings on the chest x-ray. Shown are changes observed with the average frequency of occurrence. *B*. Typical gallium 67 scan of an individual with active sarcoidosis. The isotope has accumulated in the lung parenchyma (LP), liver (L), spleen (S), parotid (P), hilar nodes (HN), and pelvic nodes (PN). *C*. Cells recovered by bronchoalveolar lavage of an individual with active pulmonary sarcoidosis. The lavage analysis reflects the inflammation in the tissue. Shown are alveolar macrophages (large cells) and lymphocytes (small cells). The cell population is dominated by lymphocytes, in contrast to normals, in whom lymphocytes represent <20 percent of the cell population.

rapidly and may clear spontaneously over a 6- to 12-month period. It can also develop insidiously and be chronic. Conjunctival involvement is also common, usually with small, yellow nodules. When the lacrimal gland is involved, a keratoconjunctivitis sicca syndrome, with dry, sore eyes, can result.

Upper respiratory tract The nasal mucosa is involved in up to 20 percent of patients, usually presenting with nasal stuffiness. Any of the structures of the mouth can be involved, particularly the tonsils. Sarcoidosis involves the larynx in about 5 percent of cases. The epiglottis and areas around the true vocal cords are usually involved, but the cords themselves are not. These individuals are usually hoarse and they have dyspnea, wheezing, and stridor; complete obstruction can occur.

Bone marrow and spleen Sarcoidosis of the marrow is reported in 15 to 40 percent of cases, but it rarely causes hematologic abnormalities other than a mild anemia, neutropenia, and eosinophilia, and occasionally thrombocytopenia. Although splenomegaly occurs in only 5 to 10 percent of patients, celiac angiography or splenic biopsy reveals involvement in 50 to 60 percent of cases. The presentation and complications of splenomegaly in sarcoidosis are similar to those of splenomegaly in general.

Liver Although liver biopsy reveals liver involvement in 60 to 90 percent of cases, usually it is not important clinically. Sarcoidosis involves generally the periportal areas. Approximately 20 to 30 percent have hepatomegaly and/or biochemical evidence of liver involvement. Usually these changes reflect a cholestatic pattern and include an elevated alkaline phosphatase level; the bilirubin and aminotransferases are only mildly elevated, and jaundice is rare. Rarely, portal hypertension can occur, as can intrahepatic cholestasis with cirrhosis.

Kidney Clinically apparent primary renal involvement in sarcoidosis is rare, although tubular, glomerular, and renal artery disease have been reported. More commonly, but still in only 1 to 2 percent of all cases, there is a disorder of calcium metabolism with hypercalcinuria, with or without hypercalcemia. If chronic, nephrocalcinosis and nephrolithiasis can result. It is believed that the calcium abnormalities are associated with enhanced calcium absorption in the gut, which is related to an abnormally high level of circulating 1,25-dihydroxyvitamin D produced by mononuclear phagocytes in the granulomas.

Nervous system All components of the nervous system can be involved in sarcoidosis. Neurologic findings are observed in about 5 percent of patients. Seventh nerve involvement with unilateral facial paralysis is most common. It occurs suddenly and is usually transient. Other common manifestations of neurosarcoid include optic nerve dysfunction, papilledema, palate dysfunction, hearing abnormalities, hypothalamic and pituitary abnormalities, chronic meningitis, and occasionally, space-occupying lesions. Psychiatric disturbances have been described, and seizures can occur. Rarely, multiple lesions which mimic multiple sclerosis, spinal cord abnormalities, and peripheral neuropathy can occur.

Musculoskeletal system The bones, joints, and/or muscles can be involved in sarcoidosis. Bone lesions are observed in 5 percent of patients and include variable-sized cysts in areas of expanded bone, well-defined round punched-out lesions, or lattice-like changes. Hand and foot bones are the common sites, but most bones can be involved. Occasionally, the bone lesions are tender and painful. Joint involvement is more common, with an incidence of 25 to 50 percent in known cases of sarcoidosis. Arthralgias and frank arthritis occur mostly in large joints; they can be migratory and are usually transient, but can be chronic and result in deformities. Although muscle biopsy frequently demonstrates granulomatous inflammation, muscle dysfunction is rare. However, nodules, polymyositis, and chronic myopathy have been described.

Heart Approximately 5 percent of patients have significant heart involvement, with clinical evidence of cardiac dysfunction. Left ventricular wall involvement is common. Arrhythmias are frequent, and serious conduction disturbances, including complete heart block, can occur. Papillary muscle dysfunction, pericarditis, and congestive heart failure are also observed. Cor pulmonale secondary to chronic pulmonary fibrosis may occur but is uncommon.

Endocrine and reproductive system The hypothalamic-pituitary axis is the part of the endocrine system most commonly involved; this usually presents as diabetes insipidus. Anterior pituitary dysfunction is also seen, manifesting as a deficiency in one or more pituitary hormones. Complete hypopituitarism is rare. Much less frequently, sarcoidosis can cause primary dysfunction of other endocrine glands. Adrenal cortical involvement resulting in Addison's syndrome has been described. Involvement of the reproductive organs occurs, but infertility is rare. Pregnancy is not affected by sarcoidosis, and patients with sarcoidosis who become pregnant usually improve during pregnancy. However, the disease may flare post partum; presumably this variation results from fluctuations in endogenous glucocorticoid production.

Exocrine glands Parotid enlargement is a classic feature of sarcoidosis, but clinically apparent parotid involvement occurs in less than 10 percent of patients. Bilateral involvement is the rule. The gland is usually nontender, firm, and smooth. Xerostomia can occur; other exocrine glands are affected only rarely.

Gastrointestinal tract Although sarcoidosis involvement of the gastrointestinal tract is found occasionally at autopsy, it rarely has clinical importance. Occasionally, patients have esophageal or gastric symptoms.

COMPLICATIONS The respiratory tract abnormalities cause most of the morbidity and mortality associated with sarcoidosis. The major problems are those characteristic of interstitial lung disease (see Chap. 211), particularly dyspnea and insufficient oxygen delivery to vital organs. Respiratory failure with carbon dioxide retention is rare. In some patients, lung destruction results in formation of bullae that may harbor mycetomas, which are usually aspergillomas; erosion into the parenchyma can result in massive bleeding. The most common complications apart from the lung are associated with the eye; however, with therapy blindness is rare. Complications of other organs include a gamut of abnormalities. The most serious are central nervous system lesions or cardiac involvement leading to congestive heart failure or sudden death.

LABORATORY ABNORMALITIES Common abnormalities in the blood include lymphocytopenia, an occasional mild eosinophilia, an increased erythrocyte sedimentation rate, hyperglobulinemia, and an elevated level of angiotensin-converting enzyme. Hypercalcemia is rare. Other serum abnormalities relate to involvement of specific organs such as liver, kidney, or endocrine glands.

Because the lung is involved so commonly, the routine chest film is almost always abnormal (Fig. 277-2*A*). The three classic x-ray patterns of pulmonary sarcoidosis are type I—bilateral hilar adenopathy with no parenchymal abnormalities; type II—bilateral hilar adenopathy with diffuse parenchymal changes; and type III—diffuse parenchymal changes without hilar adenopathy. The type III pattern is sometimes split into two categories with films that show fibrosis and upper lobe retraction classified separately. Although patients with type I x-rays tend to have the acute or subacute, reversible form of the disease while those with types II and III often have the chronic, progressive disease, these patterns do not represent the "stages" of sarcoidosis. Thus, except for epidemiologic purposes, this x-ray categorization is mostly of historic interest. The hilar adenopathy is almost always bilateral, but unilateral node enlargement can be seen. Nodes are also common in the paratracheal region. The diffuse parenchymal changes are typically reticulonodular infiltrates, but an acinar pattern is observed occasionally. Large nodules, similar to those of metastatic disease, are unusual but can occur. When there is massive fibrosis, the hila are pulled upward and there are conglomerate masses in the midlung zones. Some of the unusual chest x-ray findings in sarcoidosis include "egg shell" calcification of hilar nodes, pleural effusions, cavitation, atelectasis, pulmonary hypertension, pneumothorax, and cardiomegaly.

The lung function abnormalities of sarcoidosis are typical for interstitial lung disease (see Chap. 211) and include decreased lung volumes and diffusing capacity with a normal or supernormal ratio of the forced expiratory volume in 1 s to the forced vital capacity. Occasionally there is evidence of airflow limitation. There is usually mild hypoxemia and a mild, compensated hypocarbia.

The gallium 67 lung scan is usually abnormal, showing a pattern of diffuse uptake. If present, enlarged nodes are detected in these scans, as is inflammation in a variety of extrathoracic sites that usually have no clinical importance (Fig. 277-2*B*). Bronchoalveolar lavage demonstrates typically an increased proportion of lymphocytes, most of which are activated helper-inducer T lymphocytes (Fig. 277-2*C*). The remainder of the cells are mostly alveolar macrophages. In patients with significant fibrosis, a small number of neutrophils are also found. Eosinophils are rare.

The other laboratory features of sarcoidosis depend on the specific organ involved.

DIAGNOSIS For a typical case, the diagnosis of sarcoidosis is made by a combination of clinical, radiographic, and histologic findings. In a young adult with constitutional complaints, respiratory symptoms, erythema nodosum, blurred vision, and bilateral hilar adenopathy, the diagnosis is almost always sarcoidosis. Commonly, however, the findings are more subtle. Furthermore, because sarcoidosis can occur in almost any place in the body, like tuberculosis or syphilis, it can be confused with many other disorders. In this context, the differential diagnosis of sarcoidosis must cover a wide range. However, it is confused most commonly with neoplastic diseases such as lymphoma or with disorders characterized also by a mononuclear cell granulomatous inflammatory process, such as the mycobacterial and fungal disorders.

The presence of skin anergy is typical but not diagnostic of sarcoidosis. The Kveim-Siltzbach skin test, the intradermal injection of a heat-treated suspension of a sarcoidosis spleen extract which is biopsied 4 to 6 weeks later, yields sarcoidosis-like lesions in 70 to 80 percent of individuals with sarcoidosis with less than 5 percent false-positives. However, the material is not widely available, and with the use of the transbronchial biopsy to obtain lung parenchyma for diagnostic purposes, the Kveim-Siltzbach test is not in general use.

No blood findings are diagnostic of the disease. Angiotensin-converting enzyme is elevated in the serum in approximately two-thirds of patients with sarcoidosis, but false-positives and false-negatives are common. An elevated 24-h urine calcium level is consistent with the diagnosis, but is not specific.

The chest x-ray cannot be used as the sole criterion for the diagnosis of sarcoidosis. While the finding of bilateral hilar adenopathy is the hallmark of this disease, a similar pattern is occasionally observed in lymphoma, tuberculosis, coccidioidomycosis, brucellosis, and bronchogenic carcinoma.

The pattern of the gallium 67 scan is not diagnostic for sarcoidosis nor is the finding of an increased proportion of lymphocytes among the cells recovered by bronchoalveolar lavage. However, the typical patterns of these tests (Fig. 277-2*B* and *C*) put the diagnosis in the general category of granulomatous lung disorders.

Whether or not the presentation is "classic," biopsy evidence of a mononuclear cell granulomatous inflammatory process is mandatory in order to make a definitive diagnosis of sarcoidosis. Because the lung is involved so frequently, it is the most common site to be biopsied, usually through a fiberoptic bronchoscope. Less common, but acceptable, sites for biopsy are the hilar nodes (by mediastinoscopy), the skin, conjunctiva, or lip. Rarely, the spleen, intraabdominal nodes, muscle, parotid or other salivary glands, upper respiratory tract, or the heart are biopsied for diagnostic purposes. At any of these sites, the findings must include the typical noncaseating granulomas. However, although histologic evidence is mandatory for a definitive diagnosis of sarcoidosis, the histologic findings are not sufficiently specific to make the diagnosis by themselves, as noncaseating granulomas are found in a number of other diseases, including infections and malignancy. Furthermore, although the liver or scalene nodes often reveal "positive" biopsies in cases of sarcoidosis, noncaseating granulomas from other causes are so frequent in these sites that they are not considered acceptable sites for establishing the diagnosis. Thus, the definitive diagnosis of sarcoidosis is based on the biopsy in the context of the history, physical examination, blood tests, x-ray, lung function, and, if available, gallium 67 scan and bronchoalveolar lavage. Patients with immunodeficiency virus (HIV) infection commonly have lymphocytopenia, chest x-ray abnormalities, positive gallium 67 chest scans, increased proportions of lavage lymphocytes (early in the course of the disease), and can have lung granulomas, and thus serologic testing for HIV infection should always be done in individuals suspected of having sarcoidosis.

PROGNOSIS Overall, the prognosis in sarcoidosis is good. Most individuals who present with the acute disease are left with no significant sequela. Approximately half of all patients have some permanent organ dysfunction, but for most, this is mild, stable, and progresses rarely. In approximately 15 to 20 percent of cases, the disease remains active or recurs intermittently. Death is attributable directly to the disease in about 10 percent of all those affected.

TREATMENT The therapy of choice for sarcoidosis is glucocorticoids. A variety of other drugs have been tried, including indomethacin, oxyphenbutazone, chloroquine, methotrexate, *p*-aminobenzoate, allopurinol, levamisole, and cyclophosphamide, but there is no evidence, apart from anecdotal, uncontrolled reports, to support their efficacy. Cyclosporine is ineffective for the pulmonary manifestations of the disease; anecdotal reports suggest it may be useful in extrathoracic sarcoid not responding to glucocorticoids.

The major problem in treating sarcoidosis is in deciding when to treat. Because the disease clears spontaneously in about 50 percent of patients, and because the permanent organ derangements often do not improve with glucocorticoids, there is controversy among clinicians as to the criteria for treatment. However, there is no question that glucocorticoids suppress effectively the activated T-helper-inducer-cell processes occurring at the sites of disease. Thus the major problem in making decisions concerning therapy in sarcoidosis is to determine the extent and activity of the inflammatory process in the organs at greatest risk, such as the lung, eye, heart, and central nervous system.

For the lung, this is based on a combination of history, physical findings, chest x-ray, and pulmonary function tests. Centers that see large numbers of these individuals also use criteria based on gallium 67 lung scans and bronchoalveolar lavage findings. The serum level of the angiotensin-converting enzyme has been suggested as a criterion for disease activity, but it is not specific for the lung. Unless the respiratory impairment is devastating, active pulmonary sarcoidosis is observed usually without therapy for 2 to 3 months; if the inflammation does not subside spontaneously, therapy is instituted. For the eye, decisions concerning therapy are based on slit-lamp examination and tests for visual acuity. For the heart and central nervous system, decisions are based on an estimate of the severity of the involvement; patients with minor dysfunction are usually observed, while patients with significant cardiac or neurologic abnormalities are treated. Usually, it is not necessary to treat the systemic symptoms, but occasionally the extent of the fevers, fatigue, and/or weight loss will necessitate therapy.

The usual therapy for sarcoidosis is prednisone, 1 mg/kg, for 4 to 6 weeks followed by a slow taper over 2 to 3 months. This is repeated if the disease again becomes active. Alternate-day therapy is used by some clinicians, but there is no evidence that it is as effective. High-dose bolus intravenous glucocorticoids are used occasionally, but are probably not as effective as oral therapy. Inhaled glucocorticoids are not efficacious. Mild ocular disease responds usually to local therapy but suppression of the uveitis often requires systemic glucocorticoids.

REFERENCES

CRYSTAL RG Interstitial lung disease of unknown etiology: Disorders characterized by chronic inflammation of the lower respiratory tract. N Engl J Med 310:154, 235, 1984

FANBURG BL, PITT EA: Sarcoidosis, in *Textbook of Respiratory Medicine*, JF Murray, JA Nadel (eds). Philadelphia, Saunders, 1988, pp 1486–1500
GRASSI C et al: *Sarcoidosis and Other Granulomatous Disorders, Proceedings of the XI World Congress*. Amsterdam, Excerpta Medica, 1988
HUNNINGHAKE GW et al: Maintenance of granuloma formation in pulmonary sarcoidosis by T-lymphocytes within the lung. N Engl J Med 302:594, 1980
JOHNS CJ: Sarcoidosis, in *Pulmonary Diseases and Disorders*, AP Fishman (ed). New York, McGraw-Hill, 1988, pp 645–666
MOLLER DR et al: Bias toward use of a specific T-cell receptor β-chain variable region in a subgroup of individuals with sarcoidosis. J Clin Invest 82:1183, 1988
PINKSTON P et al: Spontaneous release of interleukin-2 by lung T-lymphocytes in active pulmonary sarcoidosis. N Engl J Med 208:793, 1983
ROBINSON BWS et al: Gamma interferon is spontaneously released by alveolar macrophages and lung T-lymphocytes in patients with pulmonary sarcoidosis. J Clin Invest 75:1488, 1985
SALTINI C et al: Spontaneous release of interleukin-2 by lung T-lymphocytes in active pulmonary sarcoidosis is primarily from the Leu3 + DR + T-cell subset. J Clin Invest 77:1962, 1986
SHARMA OP: *Sarcoidosis: Clinical Management*. London, Butterworth, 1984
VENET A et al: Enhanced alveolar macrophage-mediated antigen-induced T-lymphocyte proliferation in sarcoidosis. J Clin Invest 75:293, 1985

278 FAMILIAL MEDITERRANEAN FEVER (FAMILIAL PAROXYSMAL POLYSEROSITIS)

SHELDON M. WOLFF

DEFINITION Familial Mediterranean fever (FMF) is an inherited disorder of unknown etiology, characterized by recurrent episodes of fever, peritonitis, and/or pleuritis. Arthritis, skin lesions, and amyloidosis are seen in some patients.

TERMINOLOGY The variety of names given to FMF has led to confusion concerning its clinical features. None of the names, including FMF, is completely satisfactory. Such terms as *periodic disease* and *periodic peritonitis* are inaccurate because the disease usually is not cyclical. *Benign paroxysmal peritonitis* is inappropriate because many of the patients have involvement of serosal surfaces other than the peritoneum, and some die of amyloidosis. *Familial paroxysmal polyserositis* is an acceptable alternative for the term *familial Mediterranean fever*.

ETHNOLOGY AND GENETICS FMF occurs predominantly in patients of non-Ashkenazi (Sephardic) Jewish, Armenian, and Arabic ancestry. However, the disease is not restricted to these groups, and has been seen in patients of Italian, Ashkenazi Jewish, and Anglo-Saxon descent as well as others.

The best studies of the genetics of FMF have been done in Israel, where the disease appears to be inherited as an autosomal recessive. Nevertheless, approximately 50 percent of patients give no family history of the disease. Consanguinity among the parents of FMF patients is as high as 20 percent, a figure which may be an underestimate. Approximately 60 percent of patients are male.

ETIOLOGY Although numerous pathogenetic mechanisms have been suggested, the etiology of FMF is unknown. Fever and inflammation are such prominent signs that frequent attempts have been made to implicate infectious agents and/or their products. However, extensive studies have failed to implicate these or any other specific infectious agents. Recently it has been suggested that FMF is caused by an abnormality of catecholamine metabolism. Others have suggested defects in complement, thus implicating alterations in the immune system. Substantiation of such potential pathogenic mechanisms is awaited.

It has been suggested that FMF may be a pathologic exaggeration of normal periodic temperature rhythmicity. However, extensive studies of temperature and other circadian rhythms in FMF patients have failed to demonstrate alterations from normal.

Because many FMF patients note that certain emotional or environmental changes may have profound effects on the frequency with which episodes of their disease occur, a psychosomatic basis has been suggested for the illness. There is no question that most patients eventually have transient or even permanent psychological alterations, which probably reflect their reaction to a chronic recurring illness that is forever threatening their social, economic, and personal well-being, but there is no evidence for a functional etiology for FMF.

The demonstration that FMF is inherited as an autosomal recessive disorder has led to the thesis that it is another inborn error of metabolism. Despite extensive studies, no such error has been found. Reported instances of excessive urinary excretion of porphyrins in FMF are probably examples of true porphyria and not FMF.

It has been reported that blood levels of unconjugated etiocholanolone were elevated during fever in six patients with FMF. Subsequent studies, however, showed no correlation between levels of etiocholanolone and fever.

PATHOLOGY Despite the striking clinical manifestations during an acute attack of FMF, no specific pathologic alterations have been found. At laparotomy, only acute peritoneal inflammation in which the exudate contains a predominance of polymorphonuclear leukocytes is found to be present. A disproportionately large number of male patients develop gallbladder disease with and without cholelithiasis, but extensive histopathologic examination has failed to reveal any specific pathologic changes. Pleural and joint inflammation are also nonspecific.

In the amyloidosis which accompanies FMF, amyloid is deposited in the intima and media of the arterioles, the subendothelial region of venules, the glomeruli, and the spleen. Aside from their vessels, the heart and liver are uninvolved.

MANIFESTATIONS In the majority of patients, the symptoms of FMF begin between the ages of 5 and 15, although attacks sometimes commence during infancy, and onset has occurred as late as age 52. The duration and frequency of attacks vary greatly in the same patient, and there is no set rhythm or periodicity to their occurrence. The usual acute episode lasts 24 to 48 h, but some may be prolonged for 7 to 10 days. The attacks range in frequency from twice weekly to once a year, but 2 to 4 weeks is the commonest interval. Spontaneous remissions lasting years have been seen. In the majority of cases, pregnancy is associated with an absence of acute episodes, and many patients note less frequent attacks in the summer than in the winter. There may be a decrease in the severity and frequency of the attacks with age or with development of amyloidosis.

Fever Fever is a cardinal manifestation of FMF and is present during most but not all attacks. Rarely, fever may be present without serositis. The temperature may be preceded by a chill and will peak in 12 to 24 h. Defervescence is often accompanied by diaphoresis. The fever ranges from 38.5 to 40°C but is quite variable.

Abdominal pain Abdominal pain occurs in more than 95 percent of patients, and may vary in severity in the same patient. Minor premonitory discomfort may precede an acute episode by 24 to 48 h. The pain usually starts in one quadrant and then spreads to involve the whole abdomen. The initial site is usually very tender. Tenderness may remain localized with referred pain in other areas, and there may be radiation to the back. There may be splinting of the chest and pain in one or both shoulders, typical of diaphragmatic irritation. Nausea and vomiting sometimes occur. The abdomen is usually distended, and may become rigid with decreased or absent bowel sounds. On x-ray, the wall of the small intestine may appear edematous, transit of barium is slowed, and fluid levels may be seen. An abdominal operation may precipitate an acute attack of FMF which may be confused with other postoperative complications.

Chest pain Most patients with abdominal attacks have referred chest pain at one time or another, and 75 percent also develop acute pleuritic pain with or without abdominal symptoms. In 30 percent, the attacks of pleuritis precede the onset of abdominal attacks by varying periods of time, and a small number of patients never develop abdominal attacks. Chest pain is usually unilateral and is associated with diminished breath sounds, a friction rub, or a transient pleural effusion.

Joint pain In Israel, 75 percent of patients report at least one episode of acute arthritis. Arthritis can be distinct from abdominal or pleural attacks, can be acute or, rarely, chronic, and may involve one or several joints. Effusions are common and the large joints are involved most frequently. Radiologic findings are nonspecific. Despite careful search, frank arthritis rarely has been seen in the United States. Some patients have a history of rheumatic fever–like illness in childhood, but in a large series of patients, including 30 from the Middle East, acute arthritis was not observed. Mild arthralgia is common during acute attacks but is nonspecific.

Skin manifestations Skin involvement is reported by 25 to 35 percent of patients. These lesions consist of painful, erythematous areas of swelling from 5 to 20 cm in diameter, usually located on the lower legs, the medial malleolus, or the dorsum of the foot. They may occur without abdominal or pleural pain and subside within 24 to 48 h.

Other signs and symptoms Involvement of other serosal membranes has been reported, but pericarditis and meningitis are rare. Hematuria, splenomegaly, and small white dots called *colloid bodies* in the ocular fundus are among the findings of questionable significance. Rarely migraine-like headaches accompany acute abdominal attacks, and some patients have become somewhat irrational or show extreme emotional lability during attacks. Whether these are primary manifestations of FMF or secondary effects of pain and fever is not known.

Complications A serious, but increasingly uncommon, complication of FMF is drug addiction or habituation. Obviously, efforts should be made to avoid use of narcotics. Depression and lack of motivation are common, and patients with FMF require considerable encouragement and support. A striking number of patients in one American series have developed gallbladder disease.

Amyloidosis has been reported in Israel, North Africa, and elsewhere in the Middle East, but there have been only rare reported instances of amyloidosis complicating FMF in the United States. These findings are even more striking because there are probably as many known FMF patients in the United States as in Israel. These differences are unexplained and suggest that environmental or nutritional, as well as genetic, factors may play a role in the development of amyloidosis in FMF.

LABORATORY FINDINGS Polymorphonuclear leukocytosis ranging from 10,000 to 30,000 cells per microliter is almost invariable during acute attacks. The erythrocyte sedimentation rate is elevated during attacks but returns to normal between attacks. Plasma fibrinogen, serum haptoglobin, ceruloplasmin, and C-reactive protein increase during the episodes. Increased levels of plasma dopamine beta-hydroxylase activity have been reported in FMF patients (see below). Plasma lipids are normal, and there are no consistent abnormalities of hepatic or renal function. When amyloidosis is present, laboratory findings are typical of a nephrotic syndrome followed by renal insufficiency. Electrocardiographic and electroencephalographic changes are inconstant and nonspecific.

DIAGNOSIS When the typical acute attacks of FMF occur in an individual of appropriate ethnic background who has a family history of FMF, the diagnosis is easy. When a patient is seen for the first time, a variety of other febrile illnesses must be excluded by appropriate study or observation. These include acute appendicitis, acute pancreatitis, porphyria, cholecystitis, intestinal obstruction, and other major abdominal catastrophes.

Some of the inherited forms of the hyperlipidemias may mimic the clinical picture of FMF, but lipid analysis will eliminate them from consideration. The patient with FMF is not immune to other diseases, and when an attack differs from the usual pattern or is more prolonged, consideration should be given to other diagnostic possibilities. The pleural form of the disease is sometimes difficult to differentiate from acute pulmonary infection or infarction, but the rapid disappearance of signs and symptoms resolves the problem. The joint manifestations may be more prolonged than other forms of FMF, and differentiation from septic arthritis, gout, and acute rheumatoid disease may be necessary. The erythema is sometimes difficult to differentiate from superficial thrombophlebitis or cellulitis.

Whether or not the patient is of the appropriate ethnic group, the most difficult diagnostic problem in FMF is the patient who presents with fever alone. In this situation, an extensive diagnostic workup for fever of unknown origin may be required. Fortunately, such patients are rare, and all eventually develop serosal involvement. Until specific diagnostic tests for FMF are available, patients with recurrent fever but without signs of inflammation of one of the serosal membranes should not be categorized as having FMF.

Recently it has been reported that FMF patients have increased levels of plasma dopamine beta-hydroxylase (RHP) activity and that these levels returned to normal during colchicine treatment. Confirmation of these findings should provide the basis for the first diagnostic test for FMF.

PROGNOSIS Despite the severity of the symptoms during some acute attacks, most patients are remarkably free of any debilitation during the intervals between attacks. With encouragement and an understanding of their disease, most FMF patients lead fairly normal lives. The greatest hazard to patients is prolonged periods of hospitalization due to erroneous diagnoses or failure to understand the disease. In the United States, the prognosis of patients with FMF does not seem to be different from that of patients with other chronic nonfatal illnesses. Death usually results from causes unrelated to the underlying disease.

The complication of amyloidosis in Israel, parts of North Africa, Turkey, and other parts of the Middle East makes the prognosis quite different from that in America. In the past, approximately 25 percent of FMF patients in Israel were known to have amyloidosis, and this complication usually led to death. However, the widespread use of colchicine has resulted in dramatically decreasing the incidence of amyloidosis.

TREATMENT Among the therapies tried have been antibiotics, hormones (including estrogens and adrenal corticosteroids), antipyretic drugs, immunotherapy, psychotherapy, elimination and low-fat diets, chloroquine, and phenylbutazone. When carefully studied and followed up, none of these therapies proved effective.

During the past 15 years, the outlook of patients with FMF has been altered dramatically. Goldfinger reported in 1972 that the prophylactic use of colchicine in five patients dramatically reduced the number of attacks. Subsequently, controlled trials in the United States and Israel have shown that chronic administration of colchicine will greatly reduce the number of acute attacks of FMF. It is recommended that 0.6 mg colchicine be taken by mouth three times a day. Patients often develop gastrointestinal side effects with this dose, however, in which case the dose should be reduced to 0.6 mg taken twice a day. Although an occasional patient will respond to 0.6 mg taken only once a day, this amount is less likely to be beneficial. Most FMF patients will respond favorably to colchicine prophylaxis.

In some patients, intermittent therapy may be beneficial. The patient should take 0.6 mg colchicine by mouth every hour for 4 h, then every 2 h for 4 h, and every 12 h thereafter for 48 h. The colchicine should be given at the first premonitory sign of an attack. If both acute and prophylactic colchicine therapy fail, supportive therapy is all that can be offered. Except for unusual circumstances, narcotics should not be given to FMF patients.

REFERENCES

BARAKAT MH et al: Plasma dopamine beta-hydroxylase: Rapid diagnostic test for recurrent hereditary polyserositis. Lancet 2:1280, 1988

DINARELLO CA et al: Colchicine therapy for familial Mediterranean fever. A double-blind trial. N Engl J Med 291:934, 1974

MATZNER Y et al: C5a-Inhibitor deficiency in peritoneal fluids from patients with familial Mediterranean Fever. N Engl J Med 314:1001, 1986

MEYERHOFF J: Familial Mediterranean fever: Report of a large family, review of the literature, and discussion of the frequency of amyloidosis. Medicine 59:66, 1980

ZEMER D et al: Colchicine in the prevention and treatment of the amyloidosis of familial Mediterranean fever. N Engl J Med 314:1001, 1986

279 MIDLINE GRANULOMA

SHELDON M. WOLFF

DEFINITION Midline granuloma is an uncommon disease characterized by localized inflammation, destruction, and often mutilation of the tissues of the upper respiratory tract and face. This condition has also been referred to as *lethal midline granuloma, malignant granuloma,* and *granuloma gangrenescens,* none of which is an appropriate term.

ETIOLOGY The etiology of midline granuloma is unknown. In view of the intense granulomatous inflammation, the disease is thought to represent a localized hypersensitivity reaction which leads to tissue destruction and mutilation. However, the responsible antigen(s) is unknown, and there is no immunologic evidence supporting this hypothesis. A variety of microorganisms have been considered as possible causative agents, but detailed microbiologic investigations have failed to detect the consistent presence of pathogenic organisms. In view of the clinical and pathologic features of the illness as well as the fact that some tumors, such as malignant reticulosis (or polymorphic reticulosis), can elicit a similar intense inflammatory response, some authors have suggested a neoplastic basis for midline granuloma. However, when malignant tissue is found in the lesions, the diagnosis of midline granuloma is no longer tenable.

It is possible that midline granuloma is part of the spectrum of what has been recently termed *angiocentric immunoproliferative lesions*. The latter are considered to represent a spectrum of postthymic T-cell proliferative lesions. In fact, the association of malignant reticulosis and also of lymphomatoid granulomatosis with this group seems justified. Whether "idiopathic" midline granuloma is an early or arrested form of angiocentric immunoproliferative lesions awaits the kind of sophisticated immunocytologic studies that have been performed in patients with T-cell lymphoproliferative diseases.

PATHOLOGY The most characteristic pathologic finding is acute or chronic inflammation with necrosis. Superimposed pyogenic infection of the involved tissues, including the sinuses, may contribute to nonspecific histologic findings. The pathologic hallmark, noncaseating granulomas, with or without giant cells, may be obscured by the inflammatory reaction, but when present this is strong evidence in favor of the diagnosis. Primary vasculitis is seen rarely; when it occurs, a search for other causes, most notably Wegener's granulomatosis, should be made (see Chap. 276). The presence of malignant cells makes the diagnosis of midline granuloma unacceptable. Until an etiology is established, the diagnosis of midline granuloma will rest on the characteristic clinical features outlined below.

CLINICAL FEATURES The disease may occur at any age, but the majority of patients are in the fifth and sixth decades. It is more common in women than men and has been reported in all races. Many patients report recurrent "sinus" problems, and some have histories of allergic rhinitis, although the significance of these features is unknown.

The major symptoms are usually related to the nose. Patients frequently complain of nasal stuffiness and occasionally of discharge. The first symptom in a smaller percentage of patients relates to ulceration of the mucosa of the nose, the buccal mucosa, or the gums. This has led to loosening of the teeth, and dentists are often consulted first by these patients. Rarely, patients will present first with eye findings related to conjunctival inflammation or even ulceration. Although the progression of symptoms in some patients may be slow, all too often the disease steadily, and sometimes rapidly, progresses. The characteristic symptoms of nasal discharge, difficulty in breathing through the nose, and pain over the sinuses, nose, or eye become more prominent with time. Once ulceration begins, the disease often progresses rapidly. The ulcers frequently involve the nasal septum and will lead to the characteristic septal perforation and a saddlenose deformity. The majority of patients develop ulceration and eventually perforations of the soft and hard palates. Untreated, the disease can lead to massive destruction and mutilation of the tissues involved, including the skin of the face and the eyes. Frequently, the necrotic tissue becomes infected, and systemic symptoms such as fever and anorexia appear. The destructive lesions can become very malodorous. The disease extends to involve local tissues and does not progress below the neck; if this happens, other diseases should be considered. As the necrotic process progresses and involves vital organs, patients may lose sight in the affected eye, experience dysphagia, and have difficulty in speech. Although spontaneous temporary remissions have been reported, untreated midline granuloma is fatal. The progression of the disease can be rapidly accelerated by surgical procedures in the affected areas. The patient usually dies from secondary infection, although erosion by the process into a major blood vessel or penetration into the central nervous system with superimposed meningitis can also cause death.

Aside from the granulomatous inflammation, necrosis, and destruction, no other specific clinical or pathologic findings are associated with midline granuloma. Occasionally, with superimposed infection, local lymphadenopathy may be noted, but it is not characteristic of the disease per se.

LABORATORY FINDINGS With progression of the disease, a variety of nonspecific abnormalities may be noted. These changes are characteristic of inflammatory processes in general or of secondary infections. For example, mild anemia, leukocytosis, elevated sedimentation rate, and hyperglobulinemia are common in these patients. Radiographic examination reveals pansinusitis, and as the disease advances, destruction of bone in the involved areas is characteristic.

DIFFERENTIAL DIAGNOSIS The diagnosis of midline granuloma is made by finding the characteristic histologic lesions in biopsies of the affected tissues. When the specimens show only inflammatory tissue, a presumptive diagnosis of midline granuloma can be made only when the characteristic clinical picture is present and other diseases with similar presentation have been excluded. The diagnosis of Wegener's granulomatosis is ruled out by the absence of vasculitis in the biopsy specimens and the localized nature of midline granuloma (i.e., no pulmonary or renal involvement). In addition, Wegener's granulomatosis rarely, if ever, causes erosion through facial tissues. It is often difficult to differentiate true midline granuloma from neoplasms of the upper airways such as malignant reticulosis and certain lymphomas. These may be clinically similar to midline granuloma and are often associated with granulomatous inflammation. Careful examination of generous biopsy material as well as concomitant workup for disseminated neoplasm often provides the clinicopathologic distinction. Other diseases to be excluded by appropriate laboratory techniques are histoplasmosis, blastomycosis, coccidioidomycosis, leprosy, tuberculosis, syphilis, mucocutaneous leishmaniasis, rhinoscleroma, and pseudotumor of the orbit. Occasional patients who inhale cocaine develop septal perforations with inflammation that may be difficult to differentiate from midline granuloma (if the patients deny cocaine abuse).

TREATMENT The complications of midline granuloma such as superimposed infections can be treated specifically. Although adrenal glucocorticoids are often used in the therapy of midline granuloma, they are of no value and probably are contraindicated if infection is present. Sporadic reports of therapy with cytotoxic agents are difficult to interpret, since some of the patients reported clearly had lymphoma or Wegener's granulomatosis, diseases where such agents are of definite value. However, some patients appear to respond to cytotoxic chemotherapy. Surgical removal of the involved tissue has been attempted but is useless and may, in fact, cause rapid progression of the disease.

The treatment of choice is radiotherapy to the local lesion. Although low dosages [10,000 mGy (1000 rad) and below] have been reported to be effective, many patients relapse after such therapy. Radiotherapy should be given in a dose of 50,000 mGy (5000 rad) to the involved areas. Where such a regimen is employed, long-lasting remissions (more than 20 years) and probable cures have been achieved. Following irradiation and after an appropriate period to allow for tissue healing (usually 1 year), reconstructive and plastic surgery, which may be of enormous cosmetic and functional value, can be undertaken.

REFERENCES

FAUCI AS et al: Radiation therapy of midline granuloma. Ann Intern Med 84:140, 1976

FECHNER RE, LAMPPIN DW: Midline malignant reticulosis. Arch Otolaryngol 95:467, 1972

LIPFORD EH JR: Angiocentric immunoproliferative lesions: A clinicopathologic spectrum of post-thymic T-cell proliferation. Blood 72:1674, 1988

section 3 Disorders of the joints

280 APPROACH TO ARTICULAR AND MUSCULOSKELETAL DISORDERS

JOHN J. CUSH / PETER E. LIPSKY

Musculoskeletal complaints account for nearly 10 percent of all outpatient evaluations in general medical practice. Many of the musculoskeletal complaints that cause patients to seek medical attention are related to self-limited conditions requiring minimal evaluation and only symptomatic therapy and reassurance. However, some patients with similar symptoms may require additional laboratory testing to confirm a suspected diagnosis or document the extent and nature of the pathologic process. The initial goal of the clinician is to diagnose accurately and provide timely therapy while avoiding excessive diagnostic testing and unnecessary treatment.

Individuals with musculoskeletal complaints should be evaluated in a uniform, logical manner with a thorough history, a comprehensive physical examination, and appropriate laboratory testing. With such an approach and an understanding of the pathophysiologic processes underlying musculoskeletal complaints, an adequate diagnosis can be made in the vast majority of individuals. However, some patients will not fit immediately into an established diagnostic category. Many musculoskeletal disorders resemble each other at the outset and may take months or even years to evolve fully into a specific, recognizable syndrome. Such knowledge should temper the desire to establish a definitive diagnosis at the first encounter.

A paramount objective during the initial encounter is to determine whether the condition requires additional evaluation or immediate therapy. To make this decision, a knowledge of the particular anatomic sites of involvement (articular, periarticular, or extraarticular) and the nature of the pathologic processes (inflammatory or noninflammatory) is important (Table 280-1). Information derived from the patient's symptoms and signs allows the clinician to narrow the diagnostic considerations and assess the need for immediate diagnostic testing, therapeutic intervention, or continued observation over a period of time.

CLINICAL HISTORY Historic features of the disorder are important in establishing the nature and extent of the pathologic process and may also provide important clues to the diagnosis. Aspects of the patient profile including age, sex, race, and family history can provide important information. Certain diagnoses are more frequent in different age groups. Systemic lupus erythematosus and Reiter's syndrome occur more frequently in the young, whereas fibrositis is most frequent in middle age and osteoarthritis and polymyalgia rheumatica are more prevalent among the elderly. Diagnostic clustering is also evident when *sex* and *race* are considered. Gout and the spondyloarthropathies are more common in men, whereas rheumatoid arthritis and fibrositis are more frequent in women. Racial predilections are noted with disorders such as polymyalgia rheumatica and giant cell arteritis (whites) and sarcoidosis (blacks). *Familial aggregation* may be seen in disorders such as ankylosing spondylitis, gout, rheumatoid arthritis, and Heberden's nodes of osteoarthritis.

The type of clinical presentation also provides important diagnostic clues. The *mode of onset* is characteristically acute in septic arthritis or gout, whereas osteoarthritis and fibrositis may have more indolent presentations.

Precipitating events such as trauma, drug administration, or antecedent illnesses should be sought. The *number and pattern* of involved structures often provide useful information. Disorders such as trauma and gout are typically focal, whereas others, such as polymyositis and fibrositis, are more diffuse in their involvement. Rheumatoid arthritis tends to be symmetric, whereas the spondyloarthropathies are asymmetric. The upper extremities are frequently involved in rheumatoid arthritis, whereas lower extremity arthritis is characteristic of Reiter's syndrome and gout at their onsets. Involvement of the axial skeleton is common in ankylosing spondylitis but is infrequent in rheumatoid arthritis with the notable exception of the

TABLE 280-1 Musculoskeletal disorders

I Anatomic sites of involvement	*II* Pathologic processes
A Articular	*A* Inflammatory
1 Synovium	*1* Infectious
2 Articular cartilage	*2* Crystal-induced
3 Juxtaarticular bone	*3* Immunologic
4 Other—menisci, capsule	*4* Reactive
B Periarticular	*5* Idiopathic
1 Ligaments	*B* Noninflammatory
2 Tendons	*1* Traumatic
3 Bursae	*2* Mechanical or degenerative
C Extraarticular	*3* Neoplastic
1 Muscle	*4* Functional
2 Fascia	*5* Other
3 Bone	
4 Nerve	
5 Skin and subcutaneous tissue	

cervical spine. The *chronology and evolution* of the patient's complaints may also be useful in suggesting diagnostic possibilities. Chronic (osteoarthritis), intermittent (gout), migratory (rheumatic fever), and additive (Reiter's syndrome) patterns are suggestive of certain disease processes. The duration of signs and symptoms alters the diagnostic considerations. Thus, the musculoskeletal signs and symptoms of hepatitis B virus infection may be identical with those of early rheumatoid arthritis, but rarely persist beyond 2 to 3 weeks.

Associated features outside the musculoskeletal system may also provide useful diagnostic information. A variety of musculoskeletal disorders may be associated with systemic features such as fever (systemic lupus erythematosus, infection), rash (systemic lupus erythematosus, Reiter's syndrome, rheumatic fever), or morning stiffness (inflammatory arthritis). In addition, some are associated with involvement of other organs including the eyes (Behçet's disease, sarcoid, Reiter's syndrome), the organs of the gastrointestinal tract (scleroderma, inflammatory bowel disease), the genitourinary tract (Reiter's syndrome, gonococcemia), or the nervous system (rheumatoid arthritis, vasculitis).

PHYSICAL EXAMINATION The goal of the physical examination is to ascertain the structures involved, the nature of the disorder, the extent and functional consequences of the process, and the presence of systemic manifestations. A knowledge of topographic anatomy is necessary to identify the primary site(s) of involvement and differentiate between articular, periarticular, and extraarticular disease. The musculoskeletal evaluation is largely dependent on careful inspection, palpation, and a variety of specific physical maneuvers to elicit diagnostic signs.

Examination of involved and uninvolved joints will determine the absence or presence of *warmth, erythema,* or *swelling*. The examination should distinguish true articular swelling caused by synovial effusion or synovial proliferation from periarticular involvement which usually extends beyond the normal joint margins. Synovial effusion can be distinguished from synovial hypertrophy or bony hypertrophy by palpation. Bursal effusions (i.e., olecranon, prepatellar) overlie bony prominences and are fluctuant with sharply defined borders. Joint *stability* can be assessed by palpation and by the application of manual stress. Subluxation or dislocation, which may be secondary to traumatic, mechanical, or inflammatory causes, can be assessed by inspection and palpation. Joint *volume* can be assessed by palpation. Distention of the articular capsule by various processes causes pain. The patient will attempt to minimize the pain by maintaining the joint in the position of greatest volume and least intraarticular pressure, usually partial flexion. Clinically, this may be reflected as obvious swelling, voluntary or eventually fixed flexion deformities, or diminished range of motion, especially on extension when joint volumes are decreased. Active and passive *range of motion* should be assessed in all planes and is best quantified by a goniometer with contralateral comparison. Joint *crepitus* may be felt during these maneuvers and may be prominent in degenerative disorders. Limitation of motion is frequently caused by effusion, pain, deformity, or contracture. Contractures may be an indication of antecedent synovial inflammation. Joint *deformity* usually indicates a long-standing pathologic process. Deformities may result from ligament destruction, soft tissue contracture, bony enlargement, ankylosis, erosive disease, or subluxation. Examination of the musculature will document strength and the presence of atrophy, and also will elicit pain or spasm. The examiner should assess carefully for periarticular involvement, especially when articular complaints are not supported by objective findings referable to the joint capsule. The identification of musculoskeletal pain of soft tissue origin (periarticular or extraarticular) will prevent unwarranted and often expensive further evaluations.

ADDITIONAL INVESTIGATIONS The vast majority of musculoskeletal disorders can be easily diagnosed by a complete history and physical examination. However, in a number of circumstances, additional investigations may be required to establish the diagnosis or confirm a suspected etiology. A number of features indicate the need for additional evaluation. Patients with *acute monarticular* conditions require additional evaluation, as do those who present with *traumatic* or *inflammatory* conditions or those with *neurologic changes* or *systemic manifestations* of serious disease. Finally individuals with *chronic (>6 weeks)* symptoms, even of minor severity, are candidates for additional evaluation. The extent and nature of the additional investigation should be dictated by the pattern of the involvement and suspected pathologic process. Broad batteries of diagnostic tests and radiographic procedures are rarely a useful or cost-effective means to establish a diagnosis.

Besides a complete blood count, including a white blood cell and differential count, the routine evaluation should include a determination of the erythrocyte sedimentation rate, and C-reactive protein, which can be useful in discriminating inflammatory from noninflammatory musculoskeletal disorders.

Synovial fluid aspiration and analysis is always indicated in acute monarthritis or when a septic or crystal-induced arthropathy is suspected. Synovial fluid can be classified according to its appearance, cell count, glucose level, and viscosity. Noninflammatory synovial fluid is clear, amber-colored, with a white blood cell count of <3000 cells per microliter and a mononuclear cell predominance. The glucose concentration is normal and is usually within 0.55 to 0.83 mmol/L (10 to 15 mg/dL) of serum values. Synovial fluid viscosity is assessed by expressing fluid from the syringe one drop at a time. Normally there is a stringing effect, with a long tail behind each synovial drop. Such effusions are typical of osteoarthritis and trauma. Inflammatory fluid is turbid and yellow with an increased white cell count (3000 to 50,000 cells per microliter) and a polymorphonuclear leukocyte predominance. The protein is elevated, the glucose is normal or low, and the viscosity is poor, reflected by a short or nonexistent tail following each drop of synovial fluid. Such effusions are found in rheumatoid arthritis, gout, other inflammatory arthritides, and occasionally septic arthritis. Infectious fluid is turbid and opaque, with a white cell count >50,000 cells per microliter, and a polymorphonuclear leukocyte predominance. The protein is elevated, the glucose is low, and viscosity is poor. Such effusions are typical of septic arthritis but may rarely occur with sterile inflammatory arthritides such as rheumatoid arthritis or gout. Additionally, hemorrhagic synovial fluid may be seen with hemarthrosis or trauma. Synovial fluid should be analyzed immediately for crystals using a polarizing microscope. Monosodium urate, seen in gouty effusions, appears as long, needle-shaped, negatively birefringent, usually intracellular crystals, whereas calcium pyrophosphate dihydrate found in chondrocalcinosis and pseudogout is usually seen as short, rhomboid-shaped, positively birefringent crystals. When infection is suspected, synovial fluid should be Gram-stained and cultured appropriately. Whenever gonococcal arthritis is suspected, immediate plating of the fluid on appropriate culture medium is indicated. It should be noted that on occasion both crystal-induced arthritis and infection may occur in the same joint.

Serologic tests for rheumatoid factor (antibodies to IgG), antinuclear antibodies, complement levels, or antistreptolysin O titers should only be carried out when there is clinical evidence to suggest a specific diagnosis, as these have poor predictive value as screening tests.

DIAGNOSTIC IMAGING IN JOINT DISEASES Historically, *conventional radiography* has played an integral part in the diagnosis and staging of articular disorders. Plain films are most appropriate when there is a history of prior trauma, suspected chronic infection, progressive disability, monarticular involvement, when therapeutic alterations are considered, or as a baseline assessment for what appears to be a chronic process. However, in most inflammatory disorders, early radiography is rarely helpful in establishing a diagnosis and often reveals only soft tissue swelling and juxtaarticular demineralization. As the disease progresses, calcification (soft tissue, cartilage, or bone), joint space narrowing, erosions, bony ankylosis, new bone formation (sclerosis, osteophytes, or periostitis), or subchondral cysts may develop and provide diagnostic information. The

TABLE 280-2 Application of diagnostic imaging techniques to musculoskeletal disorders

Method	Cost	Conditions evaluated	Indications
Ultrasound	+*	Focal	Synovial (Baker's) cyst Rotator cuff tears Tendon injury
Radionuclide scintigraphy			
^{99m}Tc	++	Diffuse	Metastatic bone survey Evaluation of Paget's disease Quantitative joint assessments Early polymyalgia rheumatica
^{111}In-WBC	++	Diffuse	Acute infections Prosthetic infections Osteomyelitis
^{67}Ga	++	Diffuse	Acute and chronic infections Osteomyelitis
Computed tomography	+++	Focal	Herniated intervertebral disks Sacroiliitis Spinal stenosis Osteoid osteoma Spinal trauma
Magnetic resonance imaging	++++	Focal	Avascular necrosis Osteomyelitis Derangements of axial skeleton and spinal cord

* +, Arbitrary cost of ultrasound compared to other modalities.

use of high-quality films and proper positioning can eliminate the need for further studies.

The advent of additional imaging techniques has enhanced diagnostic sensitivity and can facilitate the early diagnosis of certain articular disorders. In selected circumstances, the appropriate use of these modalities is indicated when conventional radiography cannot provide adequate information (Table 280-2). *Ultrasonography* is useful in the detection of soft tissue abnormalities that cannot be fully appreciated by clinical eximination. There are a limited number of circumstances wherein ultrasound is the preferred method of evaluation. These include the assessment of synovial (Baker's) cysts, rotator cuff tears, and various tendon injuries. *Radionuclide scintigraphy* of the musculoskeletal disorders is useful to provide information regarding the metabolic status of bone and, along with radiography, is well suited for total-body assessment of the extent and distribution of musculoskeletal involvement. Scintigraphy, using ^{99m}Tc, ^{67}Ga, and ^{111}In-labeled white blood cells (In-WBC), has been applied to a variety of articular disorders with variable success. The proper application of these radioisotope techniques is dependent upon knowledge of their distribution and uptake about the joint under normal and diseased states. *[^{99m}Tc] pertechnate* is bound to albumin and accumulates in areas of increased vascularity; hence, the increased uptake observed with synovitis, infection, or neoplasia and the decreased uptake seen in early osteonecrosis. By contrast, *[^{99m}Tc] phosphate* is utilized as a bone-seeking radionuclide, whose distribution is dependent upon blood flow and uptake during new bone formation. Increased uptake is seen with inflammation, increased blood flow, bone remodeling, and heterotopic bone formation (Fig. 280-1). The nonspecificity of ^{99m}Tc scanning has limited its use to investigational and serial assessments of joint/bone involvement or metastatic bone surveys. *Gallium 67* binds to serum and cellular transferrin and lactoferrin and is preferentially taken up by neutrophils and tumor tissue (lymphoma) and is thus useful in the identification of infection and malignancies. Scanning with *^{111}In-WBC* has been used to detect both infectious and inflammatory arthritis. Although both have been used with success, ^{111}In-WBC scanning is more sensitive than use of ^{67}Ga in the early diagnosis of osteomyelitis and infected arthroplasties. Prior treatment with antibiotics reduces the diagnostic sensitivities of both ^{67}Ga and ^{111}In-WBC scintigraphy.

Computed tomography (CT) provides the physician with rapid reconstruction of sagittal, coronal, and axial images and spatial relationships among anatomic structures. It has proved to be most useful in the assessment of the axial skeleton because of its ability to visualize in the axial plane. Articulations previously considered difficult to visualize using conventional radiography, such as the zygoapophyseal, sacroiliac, sternoclavicular, and hip joints, can be effectively evaluated using CT. CT has been demonstrated to be

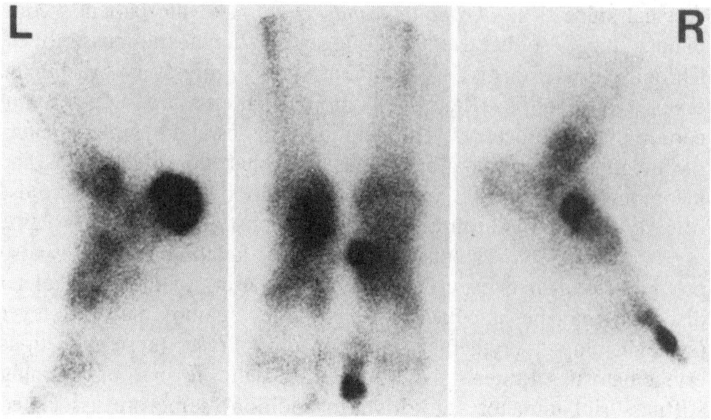

FIGURE 280-1 [^{99m}Tc] phosphate scintigraphy of the feet of a 33-year-old black male with Reiter's syndrome, manifested by sacroiliitis, urethritis, uveitis, asymmetric oligoarthritis, and enthesitis. This bone scan demonstrates increased uptake indicative of enthesitis involving the insertions of the left Achilles tendon and plantar aponeurosis and the right tibialis posterior tendon and arthritis of the right first interphalangeal joint.

FIGURE 280-2 Superior sensitivity of magnetic resonance imaging in the diagnosis of osteonecrosis of the femoral head. A 25-year-old white male taking high-dose glucocorticoids for idiopathic thrombocytopenic purpura developed bilateral hip pain. Conventional x-ray films (*A*) demonstrated abnormalities only in the right hip consistent with stage II osteonecrosis (arrow). A bone scan (*B*) revealed increased uptake in the right hip only (arrow). MRI using spin echo proton density images (*C* and *D*) demonstrated low-density signals from both femoral heads (arrows), indicative of bilateral osteonecrosis.

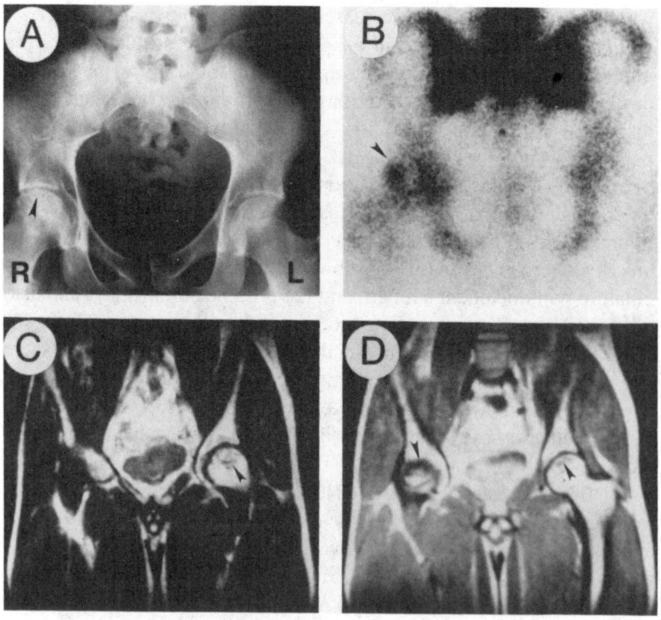

TABLE 280-3 Common musculoskeletal disorders in the elderly

I	Inflammatory
	Polymyalgia rheumatica
	Temporal (giant cell) arteritis
	Gout
	Calcium pyrophosphate dihydrate deposition disease
II	Mechanical
	Degenerative joint disease
	Spinal stenosis
III	Metabolic
	Osteoporosis
	Myxedema
	Paget's disease
IV	Associated with neoplastic disease
	Carcinomatous arthropathy or neuromyopathy
	Dermatomyositis
	Hypertrophic osteoarthropathy
V	Drug-induced
	Diuretics (gout)
	Drug-induced lupus
	Corticosteroids (osteopenia, myopathy)

useful in the diagnosis of low back pain syndromes, sacroiliitis, avascular necrosis, osteoid osteoma, tarsal coalition, osteomyelitis, and intraarticular osteochondral fragments.

In recent years, *magnetic resonance imaging* (MRI) has emerged as a useful method of musculoskeletal imaging. MRI has the advantages of providing greater anatomic detail and contrast resolution (Fig. 280-2). However, the cost and limited availability of MRI have thus far constrained its application to the evaluation of musculoskeletal disorders. MRI is capable of imaging muscle, cartilage, ligaments, tendons, pannus, synovial effusions, and bone. MRI has been shown to be a sensitive and effective means to detect soft tissue injuries (meniscal and rotator cuff tears), ischemic osteonecrosis of bone, and osteomyelitis and to assess the cervical spinal cord following cervical injury, subluxation, and/or arthritis.

EVALUATION OF THE ELDERLY FOR RHEUMATIC DISEASES Musculoskeletal disorders in geriatric patients are often not diagnosed since complaints in the elderly may be insidious in onset and chronic in nature. In addition, older individuals frequently possess multiple interactive variables, including other medical conditions and therapies that may obscure the nature of the problem. This is compounded by the diminished reliability of laboratory testing in the elderly, owing to the wider range of nonpathologic serologic variability, including elevated erythrocyte sedimentation rates and low titers of rheumatoid factor or antinuclear antibodies. Although nearly all rheumatic disorders can afflict the elderly, certain diseases and drug-induced disorders are more common in this age group (Table 280-3). The elderly should be approached in the same manner used for all patients with musculoskeletal complaints, with additional inquiry to exclude common geriatric musculoskeletal disorders. An emphasis on identifying intercurrent medical conditions and therapies is extremely important. Drug-induced lupus erythematosus, gout, and chronic salicylate toxicity are all more common in the elderly. The physical examination should emphasize coexistent disease that may influence subsequent diagnosis and treatment.

REFERENCES

BELTRAN J et al: Rheumatoid arthritis: MR imaging manifestations. Radiology 165:153, 1987

BROWER AC: Imaging techniques and modalities, in *Arthritis in Black and White*, AC Brower (ed). Philadelphia, Saunders, 1988, p 1

ETTINGER WH: Approach to the diagnosis and management of musculoskeletal disease. Clin Geriatr Med 4:269, 1988

FRIES JF, MITCHELL DM: Joint pain or arthritis. JAMA 235:199, 1976

GATTER RA: *Practical Handbook of Joint Fluid Analysis*. Philadelphia, Lea & Febiger, 1984

GAYLIS NB: Initial evaluation of the arthritic patient: Piecing together the diagnostic clues. Postgrad Med 80(5):65, 1986

HALL H: Examination of the patient with low back pain. Bull Rheum Dis 33:1, 1983

HUGHES GRV: Autoantibodies in lupus and its variants: Experience in 1000 patients. Br Med J 289:339, 1984

KEAN W: Arthritis in the elderly. Clin Rheum Dis 12:1, 1986

NAMEY TC: Nuclear medicine and special radiologic imaging and technique in the diagnosis of rheumatic disease, in *Textbook of Rheumatology*, WN Kelley et al (eds). Philadelphia, Saunders, 1985, p 608

POLLEY HF, HUNDER GG: *Rheumatologic Interviewing and Physical Examination of the Joints*. Philadelphia, Saunders, 1978

TAN EM: Antinuclear antibodies in diagnosis and management. Hosp Pract 18:79, 1983

WILSON FC: Principles of diagnosis and treatment of musculoskeletal trauma, in *The Musculoskeletal System: Basic Processes and Disorders*, FC Wilson (ed). Philadelphia, Lippincott, 1983, p 270

281 OSTEOARTHRITIS

KENNETH D. BRANDT / KAREN KOVALOV–ST. JOHN

Osteoarthritis (OA), also termed degenerative joint disease (DJD), represents failure of the diarthrodial (movable, synovial-lined) joint. In idiopathic (primary) OA, the most common form of the disease, no predisposing factor is apparent. Secondary OA appears pathologically indistinguishable from idiopathic OA but is attributable to an obvious underlying cause (Table 281-1).

EPIDEMIOLOGY OA is the most common joint disease of human beings and the leading cause of disability in the elderly; it has been estimated that 100,000 people in this country are unable to walk independently from bed to bathroom because of OA. A progressive increase in prevalence of OA is seen with increasing age. In a radiographic survey of women less than 45 years of age, only 2 percent had OA; between the ages of 45 to 64 years, however, the prevalence was 30 percent while for those older than 65 years it was 68 percent. The figures were similar in males but somewhat lower in the older age groups. OA is rare in children and young adults.

Under the age of 55 years the joint distribution of OA in men and women is similar; in older individuals hip OA is more common in men, while OA of interphalangeal joints and the thumb base is more common in women. The pattern of joint involvement is markedly influenced by prior vocational or avocational overload. Thus, OA is common in ankles of ballet dancers and metacarpophalangeal joints of prize fighters, although it is uncommon in those sites in the general population.

There are racial differences in both the prevalence of OA and the pattern of joint involvement. The Chinese in Hong Kong have a lower incidence of OA of the hip than do whites; OA is more frequent in Native Americans than in whites. Whether these differences are genetic or relate to cultural differences in joint usage is unknown.

Hereditary factors also underlie development of OA. For example, the mother of a woman with OA in distal interphalangeal joints (Heberden's nodes) is twice as likely to exhibit OA in these joints, and her sister three times as likely, as the mother and sister of an unaffected woman.

PATHOLOGY The earliest gross pathologic finding in OA is softening of the articular cartilage in habitually loaded areas of the joint surface (Fig. 281-1). With progression of OA the integrity of the surface is lost and the articular cartilage thins. Vertical clefts (fibrillation) extend into the depth of the cartilage. With joint motion, shards of fibrillated cartilage are shed, unmasking bone, which undergoes eburnation (sclerosis into a substance resembling ivory) with wear. Subchondral cysts develop. Some are filled with fibromyxomatous tissue; others communicate with the surface and contain synovial fluid. The fluid, under pressure during joint loading, may expand the cysts into large geodes. Beneath the damaged articular cartilage and at the joint margins osteophytes (bone spurs) form. Some may severely restrict joint movement. Blood vessels, arising from the subchondral marrow, infiltrate the calcified cartilage, leading to fragmentation and duplication of the tidemark. Endochondral ossification results in new bone at these sites.

TABLE 281-1 Classification of OA

I Idiopathic
- *A* Localized
  - *1* Hands: Heberden's and Bouchard's nodes (nodal), erosive interphalangeal arthritis (nonnodal), carpal–1st metacarpal
  - *2* Feet: hallux valgus, hallux rigidus, contracted toes (hammer/cock-up toes), talonavicular
  - *3* Knee:
    - (*a*) Medial compartment
    - (*b*) Lateral compartment
    - (*c*) Patellofemoral compartment
  - *4* Hip:
    - (*a*) Eccentric (superior)
    - (*b*) Concentric (axial, medial)
    - (*c*) Diffuse (coxae senilis)
  - *5* Spine:
    - (*a*) Apophyseal joints
    - (*b*) Intervertebral joints (disk)
    - (*c*) Spondylosis (osteophytes)
    - (*d*) Ligamentous (hyperostosis, Forestier's disease, diffuse idiopathic skeletal hyperostosis
  - *6* Other single sites, e.g., glenohumoral, acromioclavicular, tibiotalar, sacroiliac, temporomandibular
- *B* Generalized OA includes 3 or more of the areas listed above (Kellgren-Moore)

II Secondary
- *A* Trauma
  - *1* Acute
  - *2* Chronic (occupational, sports)
- *B* Congenital or developmental
  - *1* Localized diseases: Legg-Calvé-Perthes, congenital hip dislocation, slipped epiphysis
  - *2* Mechanical factors: unequal lower extremity length, valgus/varus deformity, hypermobility syndromes
  - *3* Bone dysplasias: epiphyseal dysplasia, spondyloapophyseal dysplasia, osteonychodystrophy
- *C* Metabolic
  - *1* Ochronosis (alkaptonuria)
  - *2* Hemochromatosis
  - *3* Wilson's disease
  - *4* Gaucher's disease
- *D* Endocrine
  - *1* Acromegaly
  - *2* Hyperparathyroidism
  - *3* Diabetes mellitus
  - *4* Obesity
  - *5* Hypothyroidism
- *E* Calcium deposition diseases
  - *1* Calcium pyrophosphate dihydrate deposition
  - *2* Apatite arthropathy
- *F* Other bone and joint diseases
  - *1* Localized: fracture, avascular necrosis, infection, gout
  - *2* Diffuse: rheumatoid (inflammatory) arthritis, Paget's disease, osteopetrosis, osteochondritis
- *G* Neuropathic (Charcot joints)
- *H* Endemic
  - *1* Kashin-Beck
  - *2* Mseleni
- *I* Miscellaneous
  - *1* Frostbite
  - *2* Caisson's disease
  - *3* Hemoglobinopathies

SOURCE: From Mankin et al, 1986.

In the face of this breakdown of the extracellular matrix, the chondrocytes undergo mitotic division. Clones of new cells appear. Later in the disease, however, the cartilage becomes hypocellular. In many areas fibrocartilage replaces hyaline cartilage. The synovium shows foci of mononuclear cell infiltration, although pannus does not develop. Shards of cartilage which have broken off the articular surface may become embedded in the synovium, where they incite an inflammatory reaction. Marked fibrosis of the joint capsule may develop, further restricting joint motion.

PATHOGENESIS In normal joints articular cartilage serves two essential mechanical functions: First, it provides a smooth weight-bearing surface, so that one bone is able to glide effortlessly over the other within the joint. Secondly, it transmits load from one bone to the next so that the bones do not shatter with loading of the joint. Articular cartilage is made up of two major macromolecules, proteoglycans and collagen. Proteoglycans (PGs) provide elasticity and stiffness on compression; collagen provides tensile strength.

In OA, the earliest physicochemical change in the cartilage is an increase in water content, due to disruption of the collagen network which normally constrains the densely packed PGs and maintains them in an underhydrated state. Although no biochemical abnormalities have been detected in the type II collagen fiber itself, an abnormality in cross-linking of adjacent fibers may exist. Type IX collagen, a minor collagen of articular cartilage which is covalently linked to type II and present on the surface of the type II fiber, may function as a "cross-linker." With the increase in cartilage water the PG concentration falls. The cartilage softens (chondromalacia) and offers diminished resistance to compression.

Levels of matrix-degrading enzymes, e.g., collagenase and proteoglycanases (PGases), are increased in OA cartilage. These enzymes are not derived from the synovial membrane or joint fluid but are secreted by the chondrocytes themselves in a latent form, which is converted to active enzyme by physiologic activator(s) (e.g., plasminogen activator/plasmin or other proteases). Normal articular cartilage contains inhibitors of matrix-degrading enzymes. In OA cartilage a stoichiometric imbalance appears to exist between the levels of degradative enzymes and of inhibitors.

The basis for the increased synthesis and secretion of matrix-degrading enzymes by the OA chondrocyte is unclear. Interleukin 1 and tumor necrosis factor, which are released by mononuclear cells in the OA synovium, may stimulate chondrocytes to synthesize and release degradative enzymes. Whether mechanical factors may directly stimulate enzyme release from the chondrocyte is unclear.

In addition to the increase in matrix degradation in OA, evidence exists of a marked synthetic response by the chondrocyte. Rates of synthesis of PGs, collagen, noncollagenous proteins, DNA, and RNA all are severalfold greater than normal, reflecting a very active "repair" effort by the OA chondrocyte. In some cases this may maintain a biomechanically adequate matrix. With progression of OA, however, the chondrocyte "fails," the rate of PG synthesis falls, and the articular surface is lost.

Not only the articular cartilage but also the subchondral bone is metabolically active in OA. Appositional growth results in the subchondral sclerosis seen radiographically. Stiffening of the subchondral bone, which reduces its ability to absorb the energy of joint loading, may lead to mechanical breakdown of the overlying cartilage.

The pathogenesis of OA can be related to an abnormality in the geometry of the involved joint, in the material properties of the cartilage or bone, or in the supporting structures (e.g., ligaments or neuromuscular apparatus). Idiopathic primary OA of the hip appears to be related in most cases to incongruity of joint surfaces due, for example, to subtle degrees of acetabular dysplasia or slipped femoral capital epiphysis.

Ochronosis may be cited as an example of a condition in which OA is caused by an abnormality in the biomaterials of the joint. Congenital deficiency of the enzyme homogentisic acid oxidase leads to accumulation of homogentisic acid polymers in articular cartilage, where they bind to type II collagen and stiffen the tissue. The shock-absorbing properties of cartilage become compromised, and the risk of cartilage fibrillation is increased. Clinically, most patients with ochronosis develop severe generalized OA by the age of 40. Osteopetrosis, which leads to stiffening of the bone, is similarily associated with generalized OA in most patients who survive to middle age. In contrast, osteoporosis, which results in an abnormal softening of bone, bears an inverse relationship to OA.

That abnormalities in the ligamentous support of joints may be important in the pathogenesis of OA is suggested by the increased frequency of OA in Ehlers-Danlos syndrome. Neuropathic joint disease (Charcot arthropathy) is a severe form of degenerative joint disease seen in patients with a severe neurosensory disorder.

CLINICAL FEATURES OA usually affects a single joint or only a few joints. While the early stages are painless, joint pain eventually leads the patient to seek medical attention. This is often described as a deep ache, localized to the involved joint. Typically, the pain is aggravated by use and relieved by rest. As the disease progresses,

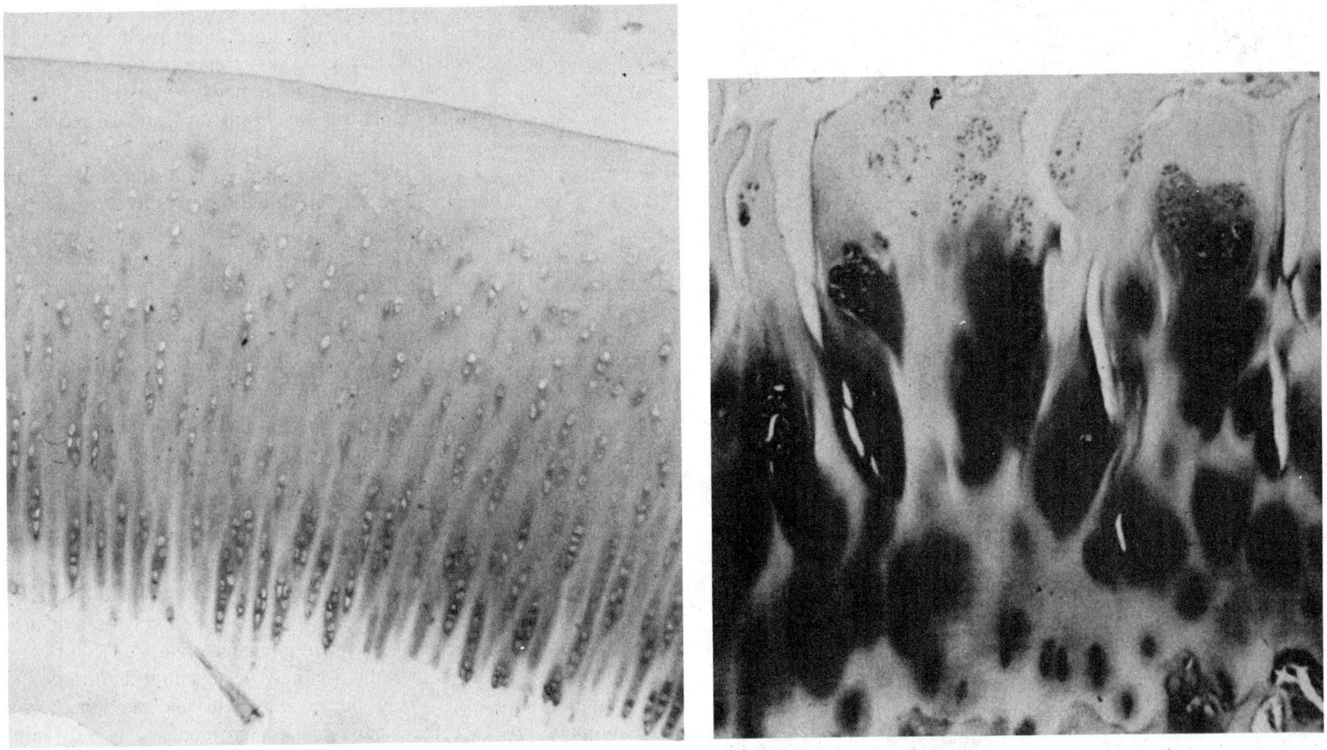

FIGURE 281-1 *A.* Normal articular cartilage. Note the intact surface and even distribution of chondrocytes. Mitotic figures are not present in normal adult articular cartilage. *B.* Osteoarthritic cartilage. Note the disruption of surface integrity, with vertical fissues (fibrillation) and irregular distribution of cells. Many of the chondrocytes have replicated and exist in clusters. Stained with Safranin-O, which binds to the sulfated glycosaminoglycan chains of proteoglycans. Note areas of diminished staining (pale extracellular matrix) due to patchy proteoglycan depletion.

the pain may become persistent. Stiffness of the involved joint upon arising in the morning or after immobility (e.g., following an automobile ride or an evening in a theater seat) may be prominent, but usually lasts less than 20 min. Systemic manifestations are not associated with primary OA.

Although the most striking structural changes in OA occur in the cartilage, joint pain in OA must arise from other structures since cartilage is aneural. In some patients pain may be due to stretching of nerve endings in the periosteum covering osteophytes. In others it may arise from microfractures in subchondral bone or from medullary hypertension caused by distortion of blood flow by hypertrophic subchondral trabeculae. Indeed, OA pain may be relieved temporarily by medullary core decompression, emphasizing the importance of hydraulic factors in some cases. Muscle spasm and joint instability leading to capsular stretching also may cause pain in OA.

In some patients with OA, joint pain may be due to synovitis. In patients with advanced OA marked synovial inflammation may be present. This may be due to phagocytosis of pieces of cartilage and bone derived from the abraded joint surface or to release from the cartilage of soluble matrix macromolecules, e.g., glycosaminoglycans or PGs. Synovitis may be due also to crystals of calcium pyrophosphate or calcium hydroxyapatite, which have been demonstrated in most synovial effusions from patients with OA. In other cases immune complexes, containing antigens derived from cartilage matrix, may be sequestered in collagenous tissue of the joint, leading to low-grade chronic immune synovitis. In the earlier stages of OA synovial inflammation may be absent. However, even in the absence of synovitis joint pain may be relieved by a nonsteroidal anti-inflammatory drug (NSAID) suggesting that these drugs have analgesic actions independent of their anti-inflammatory effects.

Physical examination of the OA joint may reveal localized tenderness and bony or soft tissue swelling. Bony crepitus (the sensation of bone rubbing against bone, evoked by joint movement) is characteristic. Synovial effusions are relatively uncommon and, when present, usually small in volume. Palpation may reveal some warmth over the joint. Disuse, secondary to pain, can lead to periarticular muscle atrophy, suggesting even greater bony enlargement than actually exists. In advanced stages, gross deformity, bony hypertrophy, subluxation, and marked loss of joint motion may be striking. Although it is a common impression that OA is inevitably progressive, in many patients the disease stabilizes. In some, regression of symptoms, and even of radiographic changes, occurs.

Interphalangeal joints *Heberden's nodes,* bony enlargements of the distal interphalangeal joints, represent the most common form of idiopathic OA (Fig. 281-2). A similar process at the proximal interphalangeal joints leads to *Bouchard's nodes.* Often Heberden's nodes develop gradually, with little discomfort. However, they may present acutely with pain, redness, and swelling, sometimes triggered by minor trauma. Gelatinous dorsal cysts, filled with hyaluronic acid, may develop at the insertion of the digital extensor tendon into the base of the distal phalanx.

The second most frequent area of involvement in OA is the thumb base. Swelling, tenderness, and marked crepitus on movement of the joint are typical. Osteophytes may lead to a ''squared'' appearance of the thumb base.

The hip Congenital or developmental defects (e.g., acetabular dysplasia, Legg-Calvé-Perthes disease, slipped capital epiphysis) may be implicated in as many as 80 percent of cases of hip OA. Twenty percent of patients will develop bilateral involvement. Pain from hip OA is generally referred to the inguinal area but may be referred to the buttock or proximal thigh. Less commonly, hip OA presents as knee pain. Pain can be evoked by putting the involved hip through its range of motion; initially, flexion may be painless but internal rotation will exacerbate pain. Loss of internal rotation occurs early, followed by loss of extension, adduction, and flexion due to capsular fibrosis and/or buttressing osteophytes.

The knee OA of the knee may involve medial or lateral femorotibial compartments and/or the patellofemoral compartment. Palpation may reveal bony hypertrophy (osteophytes) and tenderness.

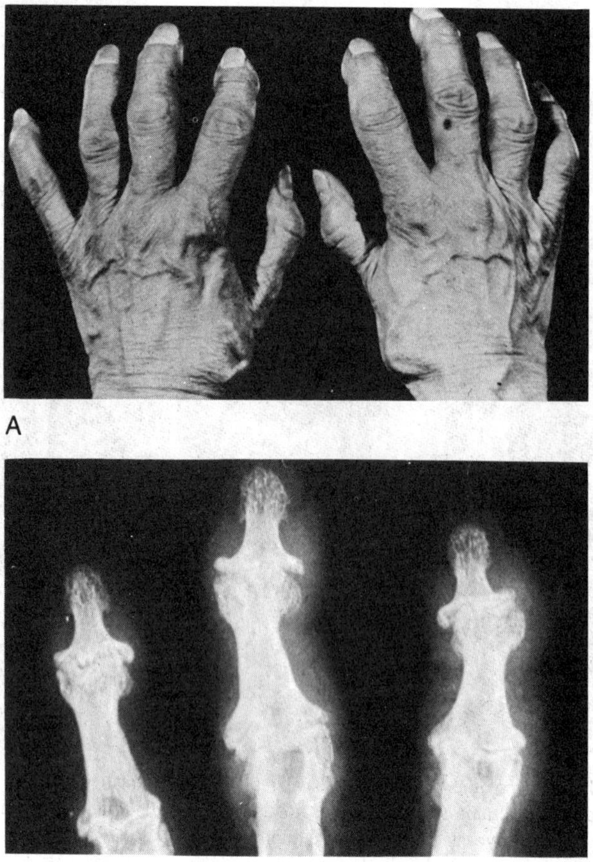

A

B

FIGURE 281-2 Osteoarthritis. *A.* Heberden's nodes of the distal interphalangeal joints and Bouchard's nodes of the proximal interphalangeal joints are present. The carpometacarpal joint is radially subluxed giving the hand a squared appearance. There is also angulation of the distal and proximal interphalangeal joints. *B.* Radiograph of the second, third, and fourth proximal and distal interphalangeal joints. Loss of joint space, osteophytes, and subchondral sclerosis and cysts are evident.

Effusions, if present, are generally small. Joint movement commonly elicits bony crepitus. OA in the medial compartment may result in a varus (bow-legged) deformity; in the lateral compartment it produces a valgus (knock-knee) deformity. A "shrug" sign (pain when the patella is compressed manually against the femur during quadriceps contraction) may be a sign of OA in the patellofemoral joint.

Chondromalacia patellae, which also is characterized by knee pain and a positive shrug sign, is a syndrome of patellofemoral pain, often bilateral, occurring in teenagers and young adults. It is more common in females than in males. It may be caused by a variety of factors (e.g., abnormal quadriceps angle, patella alta, trauma). Although exploration of the knee may reveal softening and fibrillation of cartilage on the posterior aspect of the patella, this is usually not progressive. In most cases chondromalacia patellae is not a precursor of OA. Usually, analgesics or NSAIDs and physical therapy are effective. In other cases, pain may be relieved by correction of patellar malalignment.

The spine Degenerative disease of the spine can involve the apophyseal joint, intervertebral disks, and/or paraspinous ligaments. *Spondylosis* refers to degenerative *disk* disease. The term *OA of the spine* should be reserved for degeneration of the apophyseal joints (true diarthrodial joints). Symptoms of spinal OA include localized pain and stiffness. Nerve root compression by an osteophyte blocking a neural foramen, prolapse of a degenerated disk, or subluxation of an apophyseal joint may cause radicular pain and motor weakness.

Marked calcification and ossification of paraspinous ligaments occur in *diffuse idiopathic skeletal hyperostosis* (DISH). Although DISH is often categorized as a variant of OA, diarthrodial joints are not involved. Ligamentous calcification and ossification are usually most prominent in the anterior spinal ligaments and give the appearance of "flowing wax" on the anterior bodies of the vertebrae. However, a radiolucency may be seen between the newly deposited bone and the vertebral body, differentiating DISH from the marginal osteophytes in spondylosis. Intervertebral disk spaces are preserved, and sacroiliac and apophyseal joints appear normal, helping to differentiate DISH from spondylosis and ankylosing spondylitis, respectively.

DISH occurs in middle age and in the elderly and is more common in men than in women. Patients are frequently asymptomatic, but may have musculoskeletal stiffness. Radiographic changes are generally much more severe than might be predicted from the mild symptoms caused by DISH.

Generalized OA Generalized OA is characterized by involvement of three or more joints or groups of joints (distal interphalangeal and proximal interphalangeal joints are counted as one group each). Heberden's and Bouchard's nodes are prominent. Symptoms may be episodic, with "flare-ups" of inflammation marked by soft tissue swelling, redness, and warmth. The erythrocyte sedimentation rate may be elevated, but serum rheumatoid factor tests are negative.

Erosive OA In erosive OA distal and/or proximal interphalangeal joints of the hands are most prominently affected. Erosive OA tends to be more destructive than typical OA, and radiographic evidence of collapse of the subchondral plate is characteristic. In contrast to other forms of OA, bony ankylosis may occur. Joint deformity and functional impairment may be severe. Pain and tenderness are commonly episodic. The synovium is much more extensively infiltrated with mononuclear cells than in other forms of OA.

LABORATORY AND RADIOGRAPHIC FEATURES The diagnosis of OA is usually based on clinical and radiographic features. In the early stages radiographs may be normal, but joint space narrowing becomes evident as articular cartilage is lost. Other characteristic radiographic findings include subchondral bone sclerosis, subchondral cysts, and marginal osteophytes. A change in joint contours, due to bony remodeling, and subluxation may be seen. In OA, great disparity often exists between the severity of radiographic findings, severity of symptoms, and functional ability. Thus, while more than 90 percent of people over the age of 40 have some radiographic changes of OA in weight-bearing joints, only 30 percent of these will have symptoms.

No laboratory studies are diagnostic of OA, but specific laboratory testing may help in identifying one of the underlying causes of secondary OA. Since primary OA is not systemic, the erythrocyte sedimentation rate, serum chemistry determinations, blood counts, and urinalysis are normal. Analysis of synovial fluid reveals mild leukocytosis (<2000 white blood cells per microliter), with a predominance of mononuclear cells.

Prior to the appearance of radiographic changes clinical diagnosis of OA without an invasive procedure (e.g., arthroscopy, arthrotomy) is limited. Approaches such as magnetic resonance imaging (MRI) and ultrasonography are expensive and not widely available, and the limits of resolution do not justify their routine clinical use for diagnosis of OA or for monitoring disease progression. Much effort is currently being devoted to evaluation of serologic tests for these purposes. The approach depends upon detection in synovial fluid and/or serum of macromolecules (e.g., PGs, glycosaminoglycans) released from degenerating cartilage or bone. None of these tests has yet proved suitable for clinical use.

TREATMENT No cure exists for OA. Treatment is aimed at reducing pain, maintaining mobility, and minimizing disability. The vigor of the therapeutic intervention should be dictated by the condition in the individual patient. For those with only mild disease, reassurance, instruction in joint protection, and an occasional analgesic may be all that is required.

Drug therapy Drug therapy in OA today is symptomatic. Often the joint pain can be controlled with only a simple analgesic (e.g., acetaminophen). For more severe pain dextrapropoxyphene hydrochloride may be used. Narcotics are rarely indicated in OA.

NSAIDs often decrease pain and improve mobility in OA. However, it is unclear whether this is due to their anti-inflammatory effect or to an analgesic action independent of their effect on inflammation. As indicated above, patients with OA may obtain symptomatic benefit from an NSAID even when evidence of synovitis is lacking. The superiority of NSAIDs over compounds providing comparable analgesia but without anti-inflammatory effect has not yet been adequately demonstrated in OA. Nonetheless, if signs of joint inflammation are present or simple analgesics are inadequate, it is reasonable to prescribe an NSAID for the patient with OA.

Claims have been made that some agents, such as polysulfated glycosaminoglycans, retard the progression of OA in human beings; it has been suggested that some NSAIDs also may have a "chondro-protective" effect. However, adequately controlled long-term clinical trials in human beings to support such claims have not been performed.

Systemic glucocorticoids have no place in the treatment of OA. However, intra- or periarticular injection of a depot glucocorticoid preparation may provide marked symptomatic relief. The injection should not be repeated in a given joint more often than every 4 to 6 months, since too frequent injections may accelerate cartilage break-down. Temporary reduction of usage of the joint after the steroid injection may prolong the therapeutic response.

Reduction of joint loading OA may be caused or aggravated by poor body mechanics. Correction of poor posture and a support for excessive lumbar lordosis can be helpful. Excessive loading of the involved joint should be avoided. Overloading of the knee due to pronated feet or varus or valgus knee deformities may be corrected by orthotics or osteotomy. Running shoes may be helpful in cushioning load.

Patients with OA of the knee or hip should seek alternatives to prolonged standing, kneeling, and squatting. Obese patients should be counseled to lose weight, but this may be difficult to accomplish since caloric expenditure may be reduced due to the inactivity imposed by the painful joint.

Rest periods during the day may be of benefit, but complete immobilization of the painful joint is rarely indicated. For unilateral OA of the hip or knee a cane, held in the contralateral hand, is often useful. Bilateral disease may necessitate the use of crutches or a walker.

Physical therapy Heat applied to joints prior to exercise reduces pain and stiffness. A variety of modalities are available. Often the least expensive and most convenient is a hot shower or bath. Occasionally, better analgesia may be obtained with ice than with heat. Transcutaneous electrical nerve stimulation (TENS) may be helpful, especially for low back pain due to OA of the lumbar spine.

Disuse of the OA joint because of pain leads to muscle atrophy. Since muscles play a major role in protecting articular cartilage from stress, strengthening periarticular muscles is important. The atrophy of joint cartilage and bone which develops with disuse of a limb is due chiefly to reduction in loading of the joint by contraction of periarticular muscles (e.g., hamstrings and quadriceps for the knee). Exercises should be designed to maintain range of motion and strengthen muscles surrounding the joint. Isometric exercises are generally preferable to isotonic exercises, since they minimize joint stress.

Orthopedic surgery Joint replacement surgery should be re-served for patients with advanced OA in whom aggressive medical management has been unsuccessful. Arthroplasty may relieve pain and increase mobility. Osteotomy, which is surgically more conserva-tive, may eliminate abnormal dynamic loading by correcting mala-lignment. In patients with hip or knee OA it may provide effective pain relief; it is of greatest benefit when the disease is only moderately advanced. Arthroscopic removal of loose cartilage fragments can prevent locking and also may relieve pain. Lavage of the joint with large quantities of Ringer's lactate, to flush out fibrin, cartilage shards, and other debris, may provide several months of comfort for patients whose joint pain has been refractory to analgesics and NSAIDs, but controlled studies that support the efficacy of this procedure have not been published.

Chondroplasty (abrasion arthroplasty) has gained some popularity as treatment for OA. Well-controlled studies of its efficacy are lacking, however, and the fibrocartilaginous tissue which resurfaces the abraded bone is inferior to normal hyaline cartilage in its ability to withstand compressive and shear stresses.

REFERENCES

BRANDT KD: Osteoarthritis: Clinical patterns and pathology, in *Textbook of Rheumatology*, 2d ed, WN Kelley et al (eds). Philadelphia, Saunders, 1985, pp 1432–1448

———: Osteoarthritis. Clin Geriatr Med 4:279, 1988

———: Management of osteoarthritis, in *Textbook of Rheumatology*, 3d ed, WN Kelley et al (eds). Philadelphia, Saunders, 1989, pp 1501–1512

———, RADIN E: The physiology of articular stress: Osteoarthrosis. Hosp Practice 22:103, 1987

CIOMS: The epidemiology of chronic rheumatism, in *Atlas of Standard Radiographs of Arthritis*. Oxford, Blackwell, 1963

LAWRENCE JS et al: Osteoarthritis prevalence in the population and relationship between symptoms and x-ray changes. Ann Rheum Dis 25:1, 1966

MANKIN HJ, BRANDT KD: Pathogenesis of osteoarthritis, in *Textbook of Rheumatology*, WN Kelley et al (eds). Philadelphia, Saunders, 1989, pp 1469–1479

——— et al: Workshop on etiopathogenesis of osteoarthritis. J Rheumatol 13:1127, 1986

282 ARTHRITIS DUE TO DEPOSITION OF CALCIUM CRYSTALS

GARY S. HOFFMAN

CRYSTALLOGRAPHY AND ARTHRITIS The use of polarizing microscopy to identify sodium urate crystals in synovial fluid of patients with gout was described in 1961. Since then, application of this relatively simple technique and research tools such as electron microscopy, energy-dispersive elemental analysis, and x-ray diffrac-tion have established the role of additional types of microcrystals, including calcium pyrophosphate dihydrate (CPPD), calcium hydroxy-apatite (HA), and calcium oxalate (CaOx), in other forms of arthritis. Each of these materials may cause acute or chronic arthritis or periarthritis. In spite of differences in crystal morphology, chemistry, and physical properties, the clinical events that result from deposition and release of sodium urate, CPPD, HA, and CaOx may be indistinguishable. Prior to the use of crystallographic techniques in rheumatology, much of what was considered to be gouty arthritis, in fact, was not. The great frequency (at least 60 percent) with which either HA or CPPD are found in chronic effusions from osteoarthritic joints has raised many questions about their role in causing or enhancing arthritis in the elderly. Patients with the most severe osteoarthritis appear to have the highest incidence of concurrent HA and/or CPPD synovitis, implying an additive or synergistic relation-ship. The occasional coexistence of sodium urate, CPPD, HA, or CaOx in the same joint further emphasizes the importance of crystallographic analysis for these potentially difficult diagnostic problems. In the setting of acute articular or periarticular inflammation, aspiration and analysis of effusions are most important to assess the possibility of infection. Polarization microscopy, alone, may identify most typical crystals and allow diagnosis. HA, however, represents an exception. Because these crystals are not birefringent and may be extremely small, more sophisticated techniques would be required to confirm their presence. Apart from the identification of specific microcrystalline materials or organisms, synovial fluid characteristics are not pathognomonic. Chronic monarticular or pauciarticular ef-fusions of uncertain etiology should be approached with an inquisi-tiveness similar to that given to the acute effusion. Although chronicity makes septic arthritis far less likely, it remains part of the differential diagnosis, as does microcrystalline arthropathy.

CALCIUM PYROPHOSPHATE DIHYDRATE (CPPD) DEPOSITION DISEASE **Pathogenesis** CPPD crystal deposition in articular cartilage, synovium, and periarticular ligaments and tendons is most common in the elderly, affecting 10 to 15 percent of persons 65 to 75 years old and 30 to 60 percent of those more than 85 years old. In most cases this process is asymptomatic and the cause of CPPD deposition is uncertain. Because over 80 percent of patients are more than 60 years old, and 70 percent have preexisting joint damage from other conditions, it is likely that physical and chemical changes in aging cartilage favor crystal nucleation. Examples of such chemical alterations include the following: (1) Increased production of inorganic pyrophosphate and decreased levels of pyrophosphatases in cartilage extracts from patients with CPPD arthritis. The increase in pyrophosphate appears related to enhanced activity of ATP pyrophosphohydrolase, which catalyzes the reaction of ATP to AMP and pyrophosphate. (2) Diminution of cartilage glycoproteins that normally inhibit and regulate crystal nucleation and impair the ability of crystals to trigger the release of enzymes from neutrophils. Such inhibitors are probably chemically unique for different types of crystals. Inhibitor deficiencies may thus lead to increased crystal deposition, and at a later time, crystal shedding may be associated with an inadequately inhibited inflammatory response. The release of CPPD crystals in the joint space is followed by neutrophil phagocytosis of crystals and the release of inflammatory substances. In addition, neutrophils release a glycopeptide that is chemotactic for other neutrophils, thus augmenting inflammatory events. The same substance is present in gout. In both gout and CPPD arthritis, production of this glycopeptide can be suppressed by colchicine.

A minority of patients with CPPD arthropathy have an increased incidence of metabolic abnormalities or hereditary CPPD disease. These associations suggest that a variety of different metabolic products may enhance CPPD deposition. Included among these conditions are hyperparathyroidism, hemochromatosis, gout, hypophosphatasia, hypomagnesemia, hypothyroidism, ochronosis, Wilson's disease, and amyloid. Hemochromatosis is a good example. Ferrous ions may either directly alter cartilage or inhibit inorganic pyrophosphatases, leading to enhanced susceptibility to CPPD deposition. The presence of CPPD arthritis in individuals less than 50 years old should lead to consideration of these metabolic disorders and evaluation of serum calcium, phosphorus, alkaline phosphatase, iron, iron-binding capacity, magnesium, thyroxine, and thyroid-stimulating hormone. However, the likelihood of discovering these diseases, as occult conditions, in older persons with CPPD deposition is very small.

Clinical manifestations CPPD arthropathy may be asymptomatic, acute, subacute, or chronic or cause acute synovitis superimposed upon chronically involved joints. Acute CPPD arthritis was originally termed "pseudogout" by McCarty and coworkers because of its striking similarity to gout. He and others have since recognized that the clinical sequelae of CPPD deposition include: (1) induction or enhancement of some forms of osteoarthritis; (2) induction of severe resorptive disease that may radiographically mimic neuropathic arthritis; and (3) production of symmetric proliferative synovitis, clinically similar to rheumatoid arthritis.

The knee is the most frequently affected joint in CPPD arthropathy. Other sites include the wrist, shoulder, ankle, elbow, and hands. Rarely the temporomandibular joint and ligamentum flavum of the spinal canal may be involved. Clinical and radiographic evidence indicates that CPPD deposition is polyarticular in at least two-thirds of patients. When acute synovitis occurs, diagnosis is made by identification of rod- or rhomboid-shaped weakly positively birefringent crystals (Fig. 282-1) that stain with alizarin red S in synovial fluid. When the clinical picture resembles that of slowly progressive osteoarthritis, diagnosis may be more difficult. Joint distribution may provide important clues, suggesting a nonosteoarthritic process. For example, primary osteoarthritis almost never involves the metacarpophalangeal, wrist, elbow, shoulder, or ankle joint. If radiographs reveal punctate and/or linear radiodense deposits in fibrocartilaginous joint menisci or articular hyaline cartilage (chondrocalcinosis), the diagnostic certainty of CPPD is further enhanced. *Definitive diagnosis* requires demonstration of typical crystals in synovial fluid or articular tissue. In the absence of joint effusion or indications to obtain a synovial biopsy, chondrocalcinosis is presumptive of CPPD deposition. One exception is chondrocalcinosis due to CaOx in some patients with chronic renal failure.

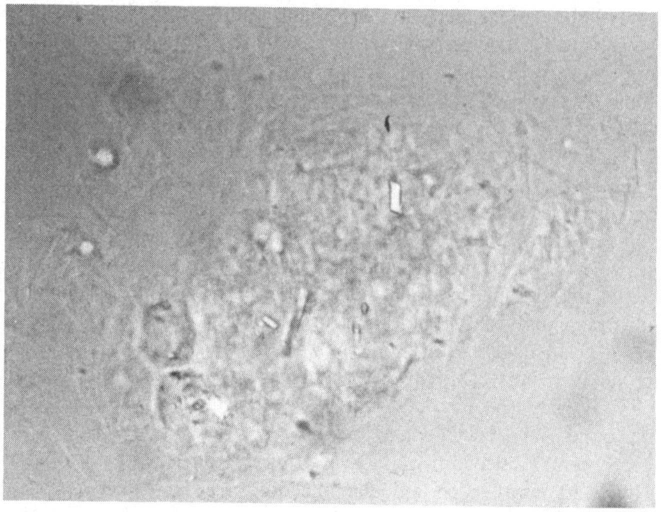

FIGURE 282-1 Calcium pyrophosphate dihydrate crystals, in a fragment of connective tissue, illustrate positive birefringence of rods and rhomboids (compensated polarized light microscopy). ×400. (*Courtesy of Ralph Schumacher.*)

Acute attacks of CPPD arthritis may be precipitated by trauma, such as physical injury to an extremity, joint surgery, a sprain, or even a long walk. These events are believed to cause cartilaginous abrasion and microcrystal shedding into the joint space. Rapid diminution of serum calcium concentration, as may occur in severe medical illness or after surgery (especially parathyroidectomy), can also lead to pseudogout. How transient calcium disequilibrium may facilitate CPPD release is unclear.

In as many as 50 percent of cases, CPPD pseudogout may be associated with low-grade fever and on occasion temperature as high as 40°C. Whether or not radiographic proof of chondrocalcinosis is evident in the involved joint(s), synovial analysis with microbial stains and cultures is essential to rule out the possibility of infection. In fact, infection in a joint with any microcrystalline deposition process can lead to crystal shedding and subsequent synovitis from both crystals and microorganisms. Synovial fluid in uncomplicated pseudogout has inflammatory qualities. The WBC count can range from several thousand cells to 100,000 per milliliter, the mean being about 24,000 per milliliter and the predominant cell being the neutrophil. Polarization microscopy usually reveals weakly positively birefringent crystals in the extracellular fluid and within neutrophils.

Untreated, acute attacks may last a few days to as long as a month. *Treatment* by joint aspiration (to decrease intraarticular pressure) and nonsteroidal anti-inflammatory agents or intraarticular glucocorticoid injection may result in return to prior status within 10 days or less. For patients with frequent recurrent attacks of pseudogout, daily prophylactic treatment with low doses of colchicine may be helpful. Unfortunately, effective treatment does not exist to remove CPPD deposits from cartilage and the joint capsule. As a result, CPPD tends to cause progressive forms of arthritis.

CALCIUM HYDROXYAPATITE DEPOSITION DISEASE **Pathogenesis** Calcium hydroxyapatite is the primary mineral of bone and teeth. Abnormal accumulation can occur in areas of tissue damage (dystrophic calcification), in hypercalcemic or hyperparathyroid states (metastatic calcification), and in certain conditions of unknown cause, such as tumoral calcinosis and periarticular calcification leading to acute and chronic tendinitis and/or bursitis. HA-induced tendinitis and bursitis are most common in the setting of overuse of an extremity. In chronic renal failure, hyperphosphatemia enhances HA deposits within as well as around joints. It was not until 1976 that HA was clearly established as a cause of arthritis.

HA and other basic calcium phosphates may be released from exposed bone and cause the acute synovitis occasionally seen in chronic stable osteoarthritis (e.g., the "hot" Heberden's node). HA deposition is also an important factor in an extremely destructive chronic arthropathy of the elderly that occurs most often in knees and shoulders. Joint destruction is associated with attenuation or rupture of supporting structures, leading to instability and deformity. Progression tends to be indolent, and synovial fluid WBC counts are usually less than 1000 cells per milliliter. Symptoms range from minimal to severe pain and disability that may lead to joint replacement surgery. Whether severely affected patients merely represent an extreme synovial tissue response to HA crystals that are so common in osteoarthritis is uncertain. Observations that favor articular HA deposition and joint destruction being a unique entity, rather than just a sequel of osteoarthritis, include the following: (1) Primary osteoarthritis of the shoulders is infrequent. (2) High levels of activated collagenase and neutral protease, as well as fragments of collagen, have been found in the noninflammatory synovial fluids of patients with severe HA arthropathy; the concentration of these enzymes exceeded those for rheumatoid arthritis and uncomplicated osteoarthritis. (3) Synovial membrane tissue cultures, exposed to HA crystals (or CPPD), markedly increased release of these enzymes, underscoring the destructive potential of abnormally stimulated synovial lining cells. (4) Although rare, HA crystals have been isolated from individuals less than 30 years old who have no evidence of osteoarthritis.

Clinical manifestations Periarticular and articular deposits may coexist and be associated with acute and/or chronic damage to the joint capsule, tendons, bursa, or articular surfaces. The most common sites of HA deposition include those in and/or around the knees, shoulders, hips, and fingers. Clinical manifestations include asymptomatic radiographic abnormalities, acute synovitis or tendinitis, and chronic destructive arthropathy. Most patients with HA arthropathy are elderly. Although the true incidence of HA arthritis is not known, 30 to 50 percent of patients with osteoarthritis have HA microcrystals in their synovial fluid. Such crystals can frequently be identified in clinically stable osteoarthritic joints, but are more likely to come to attention in persons experiencing acute or subacute worsening of joint pain and swelling. The synovial fluid WBC count in HA arthritis is usually low (<2000 per milliliter), but may at times have as many as 50,000 per milliliter. Most synovial fluid analyses reveal a predominance of mononuclear cells. Occasionally neutrophils may dominate.

Diagnosis Radiographic findings in HA arthropathy are not diagnostic. Intra- and/or periarticular calcifications with or without erosive, destructive, or hypertrophic changes may be present. X-ray films may also be normal.

Definitive diagnosis of HA arthropathy depends on identification of crystals from synovial fluid or tissue (Fig. 282-2). Individual crystals are very small, non-birefringent, and can only be seen by electron microscopy. Clumps of crystals may appear as 1- to 20-μm shiny intra- or extracellular globules that stain purplish on Wright's stain and bright red with alizarin red S. Absolute identification depends on electron microscopy with energy dispersive elemental analysis, x-ray diffraction, or infrared spectroscopy.

Treatment of HA arthritis is nonspecific. Acute attacks of synovitis may be selflimiting within days to several weeks. Aspiration of effusions, plus the use of nonsteroidal anti-inflammatory agents for 2 weeks or intraarticular injection of glucocorticoid salts appear to shorten the duration and intensity of symptoms. In patients with underlying severe destructive articular changes, response to medical therapy is usually less rewarding.

CALCIUM OXALATE (CaOx) DEPOSITION DISEASE Pathogenesis *Primary oxalosis* is a rare hereditary metabolic disorder (Chap. 335). Enhanced production of oxalic acid may result from at least two different enzyme defects, leading to hyperoxalemia and deposition of calcium oxalate crystals in tissues. Nephrocalcinosis, renal failure, and death usually occur prior to 20 years of age. Acute and/or chronic CaOx arthritis and periarthritis may complicate primary oxalosis during later years of illness.

Secondary oxalosis is more common than the primary disorder. It is one of the many metabolic abnormalities that complicate end-stage renal disease (ESRD). In ESRD calcium oxalate deposits have long been recognized in visceral organs, blood vessels, bones, and even cartilage. However, it was not until 1982 that such deposits were demonstrated to be one of the causes of arthritis in chronic renal failure. Thus far, reported patients have been dependent on long-term hemodialysis or peritoneal dialysis (see also Chap. 225), and many had received vitamin C (ascorbic acid) supplements. Ascorbic acid is metabolized to oxalate, which is inadequately cleared in uremia and by dialysis. Such supplements are now usually avoided in dialysis programs because of the risk of enhancing hyperoxalosis and its sequelae.

Clinical manifestations and diagnosis As was noted for the other calcium salts, CaOx aggregates can be found in articular cartilage, synovium, and periarticular tissues. From these sites,

FIGURE 282-2 *A.* Apatite rods from synovial fluid (electron microscopy). ×105,000. *B.* An electron micrograph demonstrates a cluster of dark apatite crystals within a synovial fluid mononuclear cell. (*Courtesy of Ralph Schumacher.*)

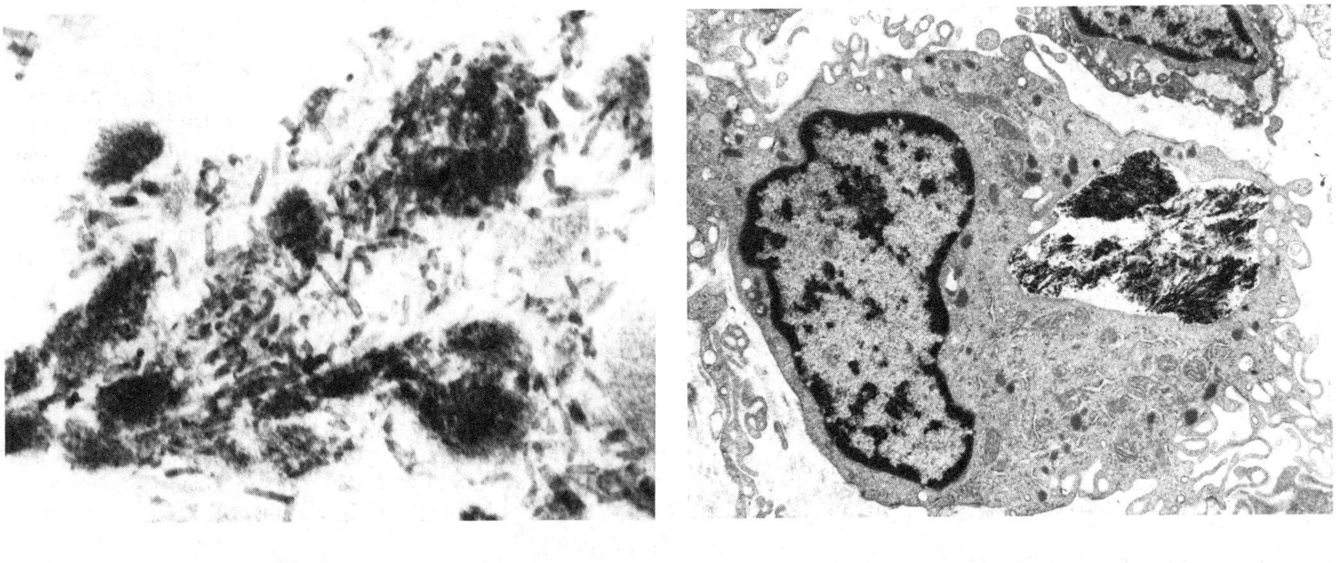

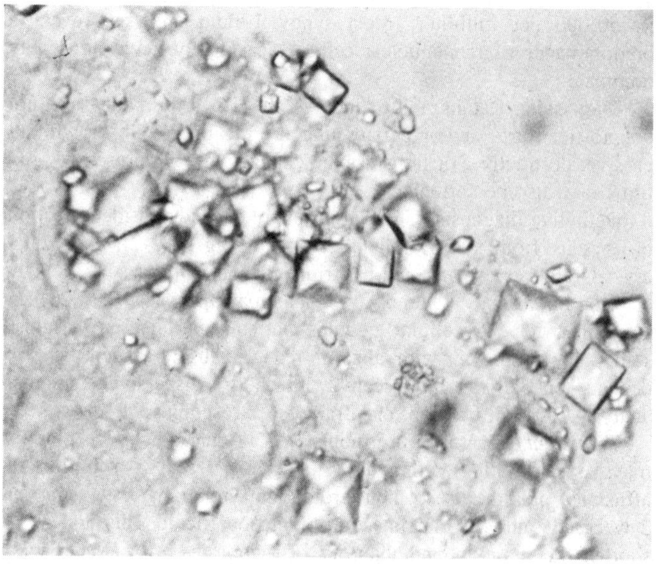

FIGURE 282-3 Calcium oxalate crystals demonstrate typical bipyramidal morphology (regular light microscopy). ×400. (*Courtesy of Ralph Schumacher.*)

crystals may be shed, causing acute synovitis. Persistent aggregates of CaOx may, like HA and CPPD, stimulate synovial proliferation and enzyme release, resulting in progressive articular destruction. Few well-studied cases have been reported. Deposits have been documented in fingers, wrists, elbows, knees, ankles, and feet. Any articular site could potentially be involved.

Each of the known microcrystalline arthropathies may be a complication of ESRD, and rare patients may have more than one type of crystal present in a joint effusion. The advent of crystallographic techniques has made it clear that most arthritic problems in ESRD are not, as was once believed, due to gout. Clinical features of acute CaOx arthritis may not be distinguishable from those due to sodium urate, CPPD, or HA. Radiographs may reveal chondrocalcinosis, a feature of either CPPD or CaOx deposition. CaOx-induced synovial effusions are usually noninflammatory, with less than 2000 leukocytes per milliliter. Predominant cell types have varied from being either neutrophils or mononuclear cells. In most instances, crystals are extracellular, although CaOx has been identified within neutrophils. Synovial membranes show modest signs of inflammation. CaOx has a variable shape and variable birefringence to polarized light. The most easily recognized forms are bipyramidal and strongly positively birefringent (Fig. 282-3).

Treatment of CaOx arthropathy with nonsteroidal anti-inflammatory agents, colchicine, intraarticular glucocorticoids, and increased frequency of dialysis has produced only slight improvement.

REFERENCES

ALVARELLOS A, SPILBERG I: Colchicine prophylaxis in pseudogout. J Rheumatol 13:804, 1986

DIEPPE PA et al: Apatite deposition disease. A new arthropathy. Lancet 1:266, 1976

———: Pyrophosphate arthropathy: A clinical and radiological study of 105 cases. Ann Rheum Dis 41:371, 1982

DOHERTY M, DIEPPE P: Crystal deposition disease in the elderly. Clin Rheum Dis 12:97, 1986

HALVERSON PB et al: Milwaukee shoulder syndrome: Eleven additional cases with involvement of the knee in seven (basic calcium phosphate crystal deposition disease). Semin Arthritis Rheum 14:36, 1984

HOFFMAN GS et al: Calcium oxalate microcrystalline-associated arthritis in end-stage renal disease. Ann Intern Med 97:36, 1982

MASUDA I, ISHIKAWA K: Clinical features of pseudogout attack. A survey of 50 cases. Clin Orthop 229:173, 1988

MCCARTY DJ et al: The significance of calcium phosphate crystals in the synovial fluid of arthritic patients: The "pseudogout syndrome." Ann Intern Med 56:711, 1962

———: "Milwaukee shoulder"—association of microspheroids containing hydroxyapatite crystals, active collagenase, and neutral protease with rotator cuff defects. I. Clinical aspects. Arthritis Rheum 24:464, 1981

MOSKOWITZ R: Diseases associated with the deposition of calcium pyrophosphate or hydroxyapatitie, in *Textbook of Rheumatology*, 3d ed, WN Kelly et al (eds). Philadelphia, Saunders, 1989, chap 79

REGINATO AJ et al: Arthropathy and cutaneous calcinosis in hemodialysis oxalosis. Arthritis Rheum 29:1387, 1986

SCHUMACHER HR JR: Crystals, inflammation, and osteoarthritis. Am J Med 83 (Suppl 5A):11, 1987

TERKELTAUB RA et al: Serum and plasma inhibit neutrophil stimulation by hydroxyapatite crystals. Arthritis Rheum 31:1081, 1988

283 PSORIATIC ARTHRITIS AND ARTHRITIS ASSOCIATED WITH GASTROINTESTINAL DISEASES

PETER H. SCHUR

PSORIATIC ARTHRITIS Psoriatic arthritis is an inflammatory arthritis that occurs in patients with psoriasis. While psoriasis occurs in about 1 to 2 percent of the general population, psoriatic arthritis occurs in about 0.1 percent. Between 2.6 and 7 percent of people with arthritis have psoriasis; 0.5 to 40 percent of people with psoriasis have some form of arthritis (5 to 7 percent have "psoriatic arthritis").

Etiology and pathogenesis The etiology and pathogenesis are unknown. Indirect evidence has suggested that (viral) infections, trauma, increased cellular immunity to streptococci, decreased suppressor cell activation, immune complexes, and abnormal polymorphonuclear leukocyte (PMN) function may each play a role. Familial aggregation suggests the influence of genetic factors. Although HLA-B13, B17, CW6, and perhaps DR7 are increased in frequency in patients with psoriasis, most studies have observed an increased frequency of HLA-B17 and B27 in patients with psoriatic arthritis. The increase in HLA-B27 is noted especially in those with psoriatic spondylitis, while B27, B38, B39, and DR7 have been noted in association with peripheral arthritis in different studies.

Clinical manifestations Three major types of psoriatic arthritis have been recognized. A mean of 47 percent of patients (range 16 to 70 percent) have an asymmetric inflammatory arthritis. The psoriasis tends to precede the arthritis by many years. Disease appears equally in men and women. The proximal and distal interphalangeal (PIP, DIP) joints are most frequently involved (with characteristic sausage-shaped digits) and knees, hips, ankles, and wrists less frequently involved. Many have morning stiffness. Most patients have onychodystrophy (onycholysis, ridging, pitting), whose course does not parallel that of the synovitis. The prognosis is good, with only one-fourth of the patients developing progressive destructive disease; one-third develop inflammatory occular complications (conjunctivitis, iritis, episcleritis).

A mean of 25 percent of patients (range 15 to 39 percent) develop symmetric arthritis. Psoriasis and inflammatory arthritis usually develop simultaneously, and occur twice as frequently in women. The DIP, PIP, MCP, MTP, and, in particular, large peripheral joints are involved. Most patients experience morning stiffness. Practically all have onychodystrophy, which helps distinguish these patients from those with rheumatoid arthritis. Over half of this group go on to develop destructive arthritis, including arthritis mutilans. Eye complications are uncommon. None have subcutaneous nodules, but one-fourth have rheumatoid factors.

A mean of 23 percent of the patients (range 5 to 33 percent) have psoriatic "spondylitis," with or without peripheral joint involvement. Psoriasis tends to precede the arthritis by a few years and is twice as common in men. About half of this group have ankylosing spondylitis and the other sacroiliitis. Low back pain with morning stiffness is common. Many have onychodystrophy. The back disease is usually slowly progressive with little clinical deterioration; as compared to ankylosing spondylitis, the peripheral disease also tends not to be destructive except for the occasional patient with arthritis mutilans. Few patients have inflammatory ocular complications.

Some authors have described additional subsets of psoriatic arthritis: predominant DIP joint involvement (6 percent of cases), arthritis mutilans (5 percent), and juvenile psoriatic arthritis (2 percent).

The pathology is quite similar to that seen in rheumatoid arthritis: synoviocytic hyperplasia, early PMN infiltration and later mononuclear cell infiltration, cartilage erosion, and pannus formation. Fibrosis of the joint capsule and marrow is prominent in many.

Laboratory findings There are few laboratory abnormalities. Elevated erythrocyte sedimentation rates and complement levels reflect inflammation. Rheumatoid factors are uncommon and are more likely to be observed in those with symmetric arthritis. Immunoglobulin levels are normal. Uric acid levels are often elevated and parallel the extent and severity of the psoriasis. Sodium urate crystals in joint fluids suggest gout.

Radiologic investigation reveals findings quite similar to those of rheumatoid arthritis: soft tissue swelling, loss of the cartilage space, erosions, bony ankylosis, subluxations, subchondral cysts, but less demineralization. More unique, and suggestive of psoriatic arthritis are: erosions at DIP joints; expansion of the base of the terminal phalanx; whittling of the distal middle phalanx; cuplike erosions of the proximal terminal phalanx—"pencil-in-cup" appearance; proliferation of bone about osseous erosions; sacroiliitis, spondylitis; terminal phalangeal osteolysis; bone proliferation and periostitis (especially of phalanges); and telescoping of one bone into its neighbor, leading to the "opera-glass" deformity.

Diagnosis The diagnosis of psoriatic arthritis should be considered in individuals with arthritis and psoriasis. Psoriasis should be distinguished from seborrheic dermatitis and eczema. Psoriatic lesions may be quite small peripherally, or often hidden in the scalp, umbilicus, and gluteal folds. Fungal infection of nails can be distinguished from psoriasis, for the latter will demonstrate pitting and onycholysis. Furthermore, onychodystrophy is uncommon (20 percent) in uncomplicated psoriasis. It is often difficult to distinguish Reiter's syndrome from psoriatic arthritis since both manifest sausage toes. Reiter's syndrome usually presents in younger individuals, especially males; is less frequently progressive or destructive; and more likely associated with characteristic skin lesions (keratoderma blenorrhagica), urethritis, and conjunctivitis. Gout can be distinguished by the presence of intraarticular sodium urate crystals. Psoriasis in association with Heberden's nodes or Bouchard's nodes of the DIP and PIP joints, respectively, does not suggest psoriatic arthritis. Psoriatic arthritis differs from rheumatoid arthritis by the relevant lack of rheumatoid factors, the tendency to asymmetry, the frequent presence of nail lesions (onychodystrophy), and the high frequency of HLA-B27, especially in patients with axial skeletal involvement.

Treatment The treatment of psoriatic arthritis begins with patient education and physical and occupational therapy to maintain muscle strength and joint and muscle function. Orthotics and occasional intraarticular glucocorticoids for isolated acutely and severely inflamed joints may be added as needed. The mainstay, however, is the use of nonsteroidal anti-inflammatory drugs (NSAIDs) including salicylates. They will reduce inflammation and alleviate pain in the majority of patients. Aspirin and indomethacin are particularly useful. Oral colchicine has been reported to be of benefit. For those patients with more severe involvement, a disease-modifying antirheumatic drug should be utilized. While hydroxychloroquin is often successful in either causing amelioration or remission it carries a significant risk of exacerbation of psoriasis. Oral and intramuscular gold salts have caused remission in over 50 percent of patients, with few side effects. For the more severe cases, especially with extensive skin involvement, methotrexate is recommended. A total of three doses of 2.5 to 5 mg given 12 h apart once a week is recommended. Most patients respond well with respect to both skin lesions and arthritis. Patients who are resistant to oral therapy may respond to intravenous therapy. Renal and liver function and a CBC should be monitored frequently, and abnormalities should prompt withholding of the drug until tests normalize. Liver biopsies are recommended after a total of 1.5 g of methotrexate and then every 2 years to identify patients with fibrosis and cirrhosis, which necessitates withdrawal of the drug. This is rare. However, patients are advised to avoid nephrotoxic and hepatotoxic (viz., ethanol) drugs. If methotrexate cannot be tolerated, 6-mercaptopurine and azathioprine have been proven successful. The arthritis of few patients responds to the psoriasis therapy known as PUVA (psoralen with UV-A radiation). Advanced forms of therapy should be provided only in consultation with, or by, persons expert in their use.

ARTHRITIS ASSOCIATED WITH GASTROINTESTINAL DISEASE

Inflammatory bowel disease (IBD) Arthritis has been observed to be associated with inflammatory bowel disease. Peripheral arthritis occurs in 9 to 20 percent of patients with IBD (e.g., ulcerative colitis, Crohn's disease). Arthritis is somewhat more likely to occur in patients with large-bowel disease and in those patients with complicatons such as abscesses, pseudomembranous polyposis, perianal disease, massive hemorrhage, erythema nodosum, stomatitis, uveitis, and pyoderma gangrenosum. Males and females are affected equally. The arthritis tends to be acute, is associated with flares of the bowel disease, occurs early in the course of the bowel disease, is self-limiting (90 percent under 6 months), and does not result in destruction. Involved joints are swollen, erythematous, warm, and painful. The majority of patients (90 percent) have polyarticular disease with knees, ankles, elbows, and wrists more commonly affected than PIP, MCP, and MTP joints. Half of patients have migratory arthritis. Granulomas, associated with Crohn's disease, can cause an erosive arthritis. Rarely a psoas abscess can result from bowel perforation, even resulting in (septic) hip arthritis. Rheumatoid factor tests are negative. In those persons who have only peripheral arthritis, there is no increase in frequency in HLA-B27. Synovial fluids have 5000 to 12,000 white blood cells per microliter, mostly PMNs. Radiographs demonstrate soft-tissue swelling and effusions without erosions or destruction. Pathologic examination of synovial biopsies reveals only nonspecific inflammation. The arthritis responds to successful treatment of the bowel disease such as colectomy (for ulcerative colitis), glucocorticoids, or sulfasalazine. NSAIDs are useful to relieve pain and inflammation, but should be used with caution because of possible gastrointestinal side effects.

Spondylitis occurs in 1.1 to 26 percent of patients with Crohn's disease or ulcerative colitis. Males and females are equally affected. Patients will typically complain of stiffness in the back and/or buttocks in the morning or after rest. Stiffness and associated pain are often relieved by exercise. Back symptoms are unrelated to those of the gastrointestinal disease. Physical examination reveals limited spinal flexion and reduced chest expansion. Some patients may have peripheral arthritis, especially of the hips and/or shoulders. Iritis is a frequent complication. Radiographs of the back show the typical findings of ankylosing spondylitis and bilateral sacroiliitis. HLA-B27 is found in 53 to 75 percent of these patients. Treatment includes NSAIDs, gluococorticoids for the bowel disease, and physical therapy. The axial disease progresses in a slow manner akin to ankylosing spondylitis.

Asymptomatic sacroiliitis detected by radiography occurs in 4 to 25 percent of patients with Crohn's disease or ulcerative colitis. By contrast, 52 percent of patients with IBD have abnormal technetium pyrophosphate bone scans of the sacroiliac joint. There is no increased frequency of HLA-B27. This "disease" does not necessarily progress to spondylitis.

Other complications of chronic IBD include: (1) finger clubbing (observed in 4 to 13 percent of patients with Crohn's disease, especially those with small bowel involvement) that may regress after surgery; (2) development of amyloid, especially in association with Crohn's disease; and (3) osteoporosis resulting from inactivity, malabsorption, and/or treatment with glucocorticoids. Osteomalacia can result from malabsorption. In this setting, acutely increased back pain should make compression fracture suspect.

Intestinal bypass arthritis Intestinal bypass surgery was developed for the treatment of obesity in 1952; 11 years later arthritis was recognized as a postoperative complication. Polyarthralgia and sometimes arthritis may occur weeks, even years following surgery in 8 to 36 percent of patients. Pain and tenderness exceed objective findings in most; others have noted episodes of abrupt onset of pain and inflammation. Tenosynovitis is common. Episodes may last for days and even months; tend to affect the knee, wrist, ankle, shoulder, and finger joints; and cause pain in the neck and back. The syndrome occurs more likely after jejunocolic than after jejunoileal surgery and more in females than males. There is often an associated urticarial, vesicular, pustular, macular, or nodular eruption. Raynaud's symptoms appear in one-third of the patients. X-rays generally show no joint damage, except marginal erosions in patients with persistent arthritis. Synovial fluids generally have white blood cell counts of 500 to 27,000 per microliter of mostly PMNs. Synovial biopsies show chronic synovitis with lymphocytes but without lymphoid follicles. Tests for rheumatoid factors, antinuclear antibodies, and HLA-B27 are usually negative, while immune complexes (and cryoglobulins) are often present. They contain bacterial antigens, their antibodies, IgA secretory component, and various complement components. These observations suggest that the syndrome has the following pathogenesis: bacteria proliferate in intestinal blind loops; bacterial antigens are absorbed; antibodies to these antigens develop and combine with them to form immune complexes which deposit in synovial tissue to cause arthritis. NSAIDs and glucocorticoids can relieve the joint symptoms but more lasting results can be achieved by tetracycline therapy to decrease bacteria; even better is reanastomosis of the bowel.

Whipple's disease (intestinal lipodystrophy) Whipple's disease is rare and occurs mostly in middle-aged Caucasian males who develop arthritis, prolonged diarrhea, malabsorption, and weight loss. Up to 90 percent of patients develop arthritis, usually prior to other symptoms. Knees and ankles and, to a lesser extent, fingers, hips, shoulders, elbows, and wrists are involved. The arthritis is acute in onset and is characterized by tender, red swollen joints. Symptoms are migratory, usually lasting just a few days, and are rarely chronic or cause permanent joint damage. Associated symptoms may include fever (54 percent), edema, serositis (pleurisy, pericarditis, endocarditis), pneumonia, hypotension, lymphadenopathy (54 percent), hyperpigmentation (54 percent), subcutaneous nodules, clubbing, and uveitis. Central nervous system (43 percent) involvement may develop with loss of memory, confusion, depression, headache, diplopia, and papilledema. Laboratory abnormalities include anemia (75 percent), low serum carotene (95 percent) and albumin levels (93 percent), and HLA-B27 (30 percent) in those patients with axial arthritis. Synovial fluids have been reported to contain 450 to 36,000 white blood cells per microliter (30 to 95 percent neutrophils) or a mild monocytosis. Joint x-rays rarely show erosions but may show a sacroiliitis in those occasional patients who have axial skeletal symptoms; abdominal x-rays, or CT scans, may reveal lymphadenopathy. The diagnosis is generally established by the detection of PAS-staining bacilliform structures in the lamina propria and/or in foamy macrophages in the small intestine. These inclusion-containing foamy macrophages have also been detected in the synovium, synovial fluid, abdominal and peripheral lymph nodes, pericardium, myocardium, liver, spleen, kidney, brain, and other tissues. Electron microscopy reveals rod-shaped organisms in the lamina propria of the small intestine. Although bacteria have not been isolated or cultured from these patients, the syndrome responds well to long-term antibiotic therapy: viz., penicillin, tetracycline, or erythromycin 0.5 g qid for one year. Some have recommended an initial 2-week course of penicillin and streptomycin. Trimethoprim-sulfamethoxazole benefits in the event of CNS involvement.

Reactive arthritis A Reiter's-like syndrome of arthritis 2 to 3 weeks following diarrhea caused by either *Shigella, Salmonella, Yersinia*, or *Campylobacter* organisms has been described (see Chap. 274). The term *Reiter's syndrome* applies if patients also have ocular, mucocutaneous, and/or urethral lesions. Synovial fluid cultures are typically negative. Most (90 percent) of these individuals are HLA-B27 positive. One group of investigators has demonstrated that an anti-*Klebsiella* antiserum reacted with cells from B27-positive spondylitic patients, but not from normal B27-positive individuals; the reaction could be inhibited by extracts of the above organisms as well as certain *Klebsiella*. These observations have suggested that a plasmid in these bacteria affect certain B27-positive individuals and may be involved in the pathogenesis of Reiter's syndrome and related spondyloarthropathies.

REFERENCES

FLEMING JL et al: Whipple's disease: Clinical, biochemical, and histopathologic features and assessment of treatment in 29 patients. Mayo Clin Proc 63:539, 1988

GRAVALLESE EM, KANTROWITZ GF: Arthritic manifestations of inflammatory bowel disease. Am J Gastroenterol 83:703, 1988

KAMMER GM et al: Psoriatic arthritis: A clinical, immunologic and HLA study of 100 patients. Semin Arthritis Rheum 9:75, 1979

KERR R, RESNICK D: Radiology of the seronegative spondyloarthropathies. Clin Rheum Dis 11:113, 1985

LAURENT MR: Psoriatic arthritis. Clin Rheum Dis 11:61, 1985

WOLHEIM FA: Enteropathic arthritis, in *Textbook of Rheumatology*, 3d ed, WN Kelley et al (eds). Philadelphia, Saunders, 1989, 62, pp 1064–1073

WOODROW JC: Genetic aspects of the spondyloarthropathies. Clin Rheum Dis 11:1, 1985

284 RELAPSING POLYCHONDRITIS AND MISCELLANEOUS ARTHRITIDES

BRUCE C. GILLILAND

RELAPSING POLYCHONDRITIS

Relapsing polychondritis is an episodic and often progressive inflammatory disorder affecting predominately the cartilage of the ears, nose, and tracheobronchial tree, as well as internal structures of the eyes and ears. Other manifestations include polyarthritis and aortic insufficiency. It is most common between the ages of 40 to 60 years but may affect children and the elderly. Relapsing polychondritis is an uncommon disorder which has been found in all races. Both sexes are equally affected, and no familial tendency is apparent. The etiology is unknown.

PATHOLOGY AND PATHOPHYSIOLOGY The earliest abnormality of cartilage noted histologically is a focal or diffuse loss of basophilic staining indicating depletion of acid mucopolysaccharides from the cartilage matrix. Inflammatory infiltrates are found adjacent to involved cartilage and consist of predominantly mononuclear cells and occasional plasma cells. In acute disease, polymorphonuclear white cells may also be present. Destruction of cartilage begins at the outer edges and advances centrally. There is lacunar breakdown and loss of chondrocytes. Degenerating cartilage is replaced by granulation tissue and later by fibrosis and focal areas of calcification. Small sites of cartilage regeneration may be present. Immunofluorescence studies have shown immunoglobulins and complement at sites of involvement. Fine granular material observed in the degenerating cartilage matrix by electron microscopy has been interpreted to be enzymes or immunoglobulins.

In the eye, lymphocytes and plasma cells have been found around episcleral vessels, as well as in the corneal stroma and iris. In the proximal aorta, mononuclear cells have been noted in the media along with loss of elastic and muscle tissue.

Immunologic mechanisms play a role in the pathogenesis of relapsing polychondritis. Immunoglobulin and complement deposits are found at sites of inflammation. In addition, antibodies to type II collagen and immune complexes are detected in the sera of some patients. The possibility that an immune response to type II collagen may be important in the pathogenesis is supported experimentally by the occurrence of auricular chondritis in rats immunized with type II collagen. Antibodies to type II collagen are found in the sera of these animals, and immune deposits are detected at sites of ear inflammation. Cell-mediated immunity may also be operative in causing tissue injury since lymphocyte transformation can be demonstrated when lymphocytes of patients are exposed to cartilage extracts.

Dissolution of cartilage matrix can be induced by the intravenous injection of crude papain, a proteolytic enzyme, into young rabbits, which results in collapse of their normally rigid ears within 4 h. Reconstitution of the matrix occurs in about 7 days. In relapsing polychondritis, loss of cartilage matrix also most likely results from action of proteolytic enzymes released from chondrocytes and monocytes that have been activated by inflammatory mediators.

CLINICAL MANIFESTATIONS Auricular chondritis is the most frequent presenting manifestation of relapsing polychondritis and eventually affects about 90 percent of patients. Usually both ears are involved. Patients experience the sudden onset of pain, tenderness, and swelling of the cartilaginous portion of the ear. Earlobes are spared since they do not contain cartilage. The overlying skin has a beefy red or violaceous color. Prolonged or recurrent episodes result in a flabby or droopy ear. Swelling may close off the external auditory meatus or the eustachian tube to cause otitis media, either of which can impair hearing. Inflammation of the internal auditory artery or its cochlear branch produces hearing loss, vertigo, ataxia, nausea, and vomiting. The cartilage of the nose becomes inflamed during the first or subsequent attacks. Approximately 80 percent of patients will eventually have nose involvement. The bridge of the nose becomes red, swollen, and tender, and may collapse, producing a saddle deformity. In some patients, the saddle deformity develops insidiously without overt inflammation.

Arthritis is the presenting manifestation in relapsing polychondritis in approximately one-third of patients and may be present for several months before other features appear. The arthritis is usually asymmetric, oligo- or polyarticular, and involves both large and small peripheral joints. An episode of arthritis lasts from a few days to several weeks and resolves spontaneously without residual joint deformity. Attacks of arthritis may not be temporally related to other manifestations of relapsing polychondritis. The joints are warm, tender, and swollen. Joint fluid has been reported to be noninflammatory. In addition to peripheral joints, inflammation may involve the costochondral and sternoclavicular cartilages. Destruction of these cartilages may result in a flail anterior chest wall.

Eye manifestations occur in greater than half of the patients and include conjunctivitis, episcleritis, iritis, and keratitis. Ulceration and perforation of the cornea may occur and cause blindness. Other manifestations include cataracts, proptosis, optic neuritis, and extraocular muscle palsies.

Laryngotracheal involvement occurs in approximately 70 percent of patients. Symptoms include hoarseness, a nonproductive cough, and tenderness over the larynx and proximal trachea. Mucosal edema, strictures, and/or collapse of laryngeal or tracheal cartilage may cause stridor and life-threatening airway obstruction necessitating tracheostomy. Collapse of cartilage in bronchi leads to pneumonia and, when extensive, to respiratory insufficiency.

Aortic regurgitation occurs in about 15 percent of patients and is due to progressive dilatation of the aortic ring or to destruction of the valve cusps. Other heart values can be affected. Aneurysmal dilatation of the proximal aorta as well as other medium to large vessels may also occur. Segmental necrotizing glomerulonephritis and renal vasculitis have been noted in some patients.

The course of disease is highly variable, with episodes lasting from a few days to several weeks and then subsiding spontaneously. In other patients, disease may have a chronic, smoldering course. In one study the 5-year estimated survival rate was 74 percent and the 10-year survival rate 55 percent. In contrast to earlier series, only about half of the deaths could be attributed to relapsing polychondritis or complications of treatment. Pulmonary complications accounted for only 10 percent of all fatalities. In general, patients with more widespread disease have a worse prognosis.

LABORATORY FINDINGS Mild leukocytosis and normocytic normochromic anemia are often present. The erythrocyte sedimentation rate is usually elevated. Rheumatoid factor and antinuclear antibody tests are occasionally positive in low titer. Circulating immune complexes may be detected, especially in patients with early active disease. Elevated levels of gamma globulin may be present. Tracheal stenosis can be demonstrated by regular tomograms or computed tomography of the neck. Bronchography is performed for demonstrating bronchial narrowing. On a chest film, narrowing of main bronchi and, when aortic insufficiency is present, cardiomegaly can be observed. Radiographs may show calcification at previous sites of cartilage damage involving ear, nose, larynx, or trachea.

DIAGNOSIS Diagnosis is based on the recognition of the typical clinical features. Biopsies of the involved cartilage from the ear, nose, or respiratory tract will confirm the diagnosis but are only necessary when clinical features are not typical. Patients with Wegener's granulomatosis may have a saddle nose and pulmonary involvement but can be distinguished by the absence of auricular involvement and the presence of granulomatous lesions in the tracheobronchial tree. Patients with Cogan's syndrome have interstitial keratitis and vestibular and auditory abnormalities, but this syndrome does not involve the respiratory tract or ears. Reiter's syndrome may initially resemble relapsing polychondritis because of oligoarticular arthritis and eye involvement, but it is distinguished in time by the appearance of urethritis and typical mucocutaneous lesions and the absence of nose or ear cartilage involvement. Rheumatoid arthritis may initially suggest relapsing polychondritis because of arthritis and eye inflammation. The arthritis in rheumatoid arthritis, however, is erosive and symmetric. In addition, rheumatoid factor titers are usually high compared to relapsing polychondritis. Bacterial infection of the pinna may be mistaken for relapsing polychondritis, but differs by usually involving only one ear including the earlobe. Auricular cartilage may also be damaged by trauma or frostbite.

Relapsing polychondritis may develop in patients with a variety of autoimmune disorders including systemic lupus erythematosus, rheumatoid arthritis, Sjögren's syndrome, and vasculitis. In most cases, these disorders antedate the appearance of polychondritis usually by months or years. It is likely that these patients have an immunologic abnormality that predisposes them to development of this group of autoimmune disorders.

TREATMENT Prednisone, 40 to 60 mg/d, is often effective in suppressing disease activity and is tapered gradually once disease is controlled. In some patients, prednisone can be stopped, while in others low doses in the range of 10 to 15 mg/d are required for continued suppression of disease. Immunosuppressive drugs such as cyclophosphamide or azathioprine should be reserved for patients who fail to respond to prednisone.

MISCELLANEOUS ARTHRITIDES

NEUROPATHIC JOINT DISEASE Neuropathic joint disease (Charcot's joint) is a severe form of osteoarthritis associated with loss of pain sensation, proprioception, or both. In addition, normal muscular reflexes that modulate joint movement are decreased. Without these protective mechanisms, joints are subjected to repeated trauma, resulting in progressive cartilage damage. The distribution of joint involvement depends on the underlying neurologic disorder. In tabes dorsalis, knees, hips, and ankles are most commonly affected; in syringomyelia, the glenohumeral joint, elbow, and wrist; and in diabetes mellitus, the tarsal and tarsometatarsal joints. Resorption of metatarsals and phalanges is also seen in diabetic patients. In children, neuropathic joint disease is caused by congenital indifference to pain or meningomyelocele. Neuropathic joint disease is also observed in patients with amyloidosis and leprosy or following repeated intraarticular glucocorticoid injections. The mechanism of injury in the latter situation is thought to be an analgesic effect of steroids leading to overuse of a previously damaged joint which results in accelerated cartilage deterioration.

Neuropathic joint disease usually begins in a single joint and then progresses to involve other joints, depending on the underlying neurologic disorder. The involved joint progressively becomes enlarged from bony overgrowth and synovial effusion. Loose bodies may be palpated in the joint cavity. Joint instability, subluxation, and crepitus occur as the disease progresses. Charcot's joints may develop rapidly, and a totally disorganized joint with multiple bony fragments may evolve in a patient within weeks or months. The amount of pain experienced by the patient is less than would be anticipated based on the degree of joint involvement. Patients may experience sudden joint pain from intraarticular fractures of osteophytes or condyles. Initially, radiographs show early features of osteoarthritis followed subsequently by marked destructive and hypertrophic changes. Large, bizarre-shaped osteophytes and intraarticular bone fragments are observed. The radiographic findings of the diabetic Charcot's foot may be difficult to distinguish from those of osteomyelitis. Osteomyelitis is often suspected when the diabetic patient has an infected cutaneous ulcer on the foot. The Charcot's joint radiographically shows osteopenia, sharp cortical margins, and severe disruption and disorganization of the midtarsal and tarsometatarsal joints. In osteomyelitis, the bone margins are indistinct. The synovial fluid from a neuropathic joint is usually noninflammatory, may be bloody or xanthochromic, and may contain fragments of synovium, cartilage, and/or bone.

The primary focus of treatment is to provide stabilization of the joint. Treatment of the underlying disorder, even if successful, usually does not alter the joint disease. Braces and splints are helpful. Their use requires close surveillance since patients may be unable to appreciate pressure from a poorly adjusted brace. Fusion of a very unstable joint may improve function, but nonunion is frequent especially when immobilization of the joint is inadequate.

HYPERTROPHIC OSTEOARTHROPATHY Hypertrophic osteoarthropathy (HOA) is characterized by clubbing of digits, periosteal new bone formation, and arthritis. HOA occurs in a primary or familial form beginning usually in childhood. The secondary form of HOA is associated with intrathoracic malignancies, suppurative lung disease, congenital heart disease, and a variety of other disorders, and is more common in adults. Clubbing is almost always a feature of HOA but can occur as an isolated manifestation. It is unclear whether clubbing alone represents a partial expression of HOA or is a separate entity. The presence of only clubbing in a patient usually has the same clinical significance as HOA.

Pathology and pathophysiology In HOA, the periosteum becomes elevated and new bone is deposited beneath the periosteum while endosteal bone is resorbed. These changes occur primarily at the distal ends of metacarpals, metatarsals and long bones of the extremities. Occasionally, scapulae, clavicles, ribs, and pelvic bones are also affected. Mononuclear cell infiltration may be present in the adjacent soft tissue. Proliferation of connective tissue occurs in the nail bed and volar pad of digits, giving the distal phalanges a clubbed appearance. Small blood vessels in the clubbed digits are dilated and have thickened walls. In addition, the number of arteriovenous anastomoses is increased. The synovium of involved joints is edematous and may have an infiltration of lymphocytes and plasma cells.

The pathogenesis of HOA is not known. Both neurogenic and humoral theories have been proposed. In support of a neurogenic mechanism is the observation that the disorders most often associated with HOA involve sites innervated by the vagus nerve. Also, vagotomy may result in resolution of symptoms. A neural reflex initiated by vagal stimulation from the site of disease is thought to lead to vasodilatation and other features of HOA. The humoral theory postulates that a substance produced by the underlying disease and normally inactivated or removed by its passage through the lung reaches the systemic circulation in an active form and induces the changes of HOA. Several humoral substances, including immunoreactive growth hormone, estrogens, prostaglandins, and ferritin, have been suggested as but not proven to be mediators of HOA.

Clinical manifestations Primary HOA, also referred to as *pachydermoperiostitis* or *Touraine-Solente-Golé syndrome*, usually begins insidiously at puberty. It is inherited as an autosomal dominant with variable expression and is more common in boys than in girls. The skin of the face and scalp thickens, producing deep nasolabial folds, furrowed forehead and corrugated scalp which give the face a leonine appearance. The skin of the face and scalp is usually greasy, and there is excessive sweating, particularly of the palms and soles. The distal extremities are thickened due to proliferation of new bone and soft tissue, and when the process is extensive, they may resemble elephant feet. Marked clubbing of hands and feet produces a spade-like deformity and clumsiness. Acrolysis of the terminal phalanges of feet and hands may occur. Symptoms of bone and joint pain are usually seen only in those who have had their disease for two decades or longer.

HOA secondary to an underlying disease occurs more frequently than primary HOA. It accompanies a variety of disorders and may precede clinical features of the associated disorder by months. The progression of HOA tends to be more rapid when associated with malignancies, most notably bronchogenic carcinoma. Patients experience a burning or deep-seated aching pain in the distal extremities due to periostitis. The pain can be quite incapacitating, and is aggravated by dependency and relieved by elevation of the affected limbs. Joint manifestations vary from arthralgias to very painful arthritis, most often affecting the metacarpal-phalangeal and metatarsal-phalangeal joints, wrists, ankles, and knees. The involved joints are warm, tender, and swollen. Joint effusions are usually small, and the fluid is noninflammatory, containing only a few white cells. The distal extremities may be swollen and the overlying skin warm and erythematous. Pressure applied over the distal end of the forearms and lower legs may be quite painful. Clubbing is usually asymptomatic except for occasional warmth or burning of the fingertips. Clubbing usually evolves over months and often is first noted by the physician and not the patient. Patients, especially those with lung tumor, may experience severe skeletal pain prior to the appearance of clubbing. Clubbing is characterized by widening of the fingertips, enlargement of the distal volar pad, convexity of the nail contour, and the loss of the normal 15° angle between the proximal nail and cuticle. The thickness of the digit at the base of the nail is greater than the thickness at the distal interphalangeal joint. The base of the nail feels spongy when compressed and the nail can be easily rocked on its bed. Marked periungual erythema is usually present. When clubbing is advanced, the finger may have a drumstick appearance. Excessive sweating, oiliness of the skin, and thickening of the facial skin are uncommon in secondary HOA.

HOA occurs in 5 to 10 percent of patients with intrathoracic malignancies, the most common being bronchogenic carcinoma and pleural tumors. Lung metastases infrequently cause HOA. HOA is also seen in patients with intrathoracic infections including lung abscesses, empyema, bronchiectasis, chronic obstructive lung disease, and pulmonary tuberculosis. HOA may also accompany chronic interstitial pneumonitis, sarcoidosis, and cystic fibrosis. In the latter, clubbing is more common than the full syndrome of HOA. Other cases of clubbing include congenital heart disease with right-to-left shunts, Crohn's disease, ulcerative colitis, sprue, and neoplasms of the esophagus, liver, small and large bowel. In patients with congenital heart disease with right-to-left shunts, clubbing alone occurs more often than the full syndrome of HOA.

Unilateral clubbing has been found in association with aneurysms of the aorta, subclavian, or innominate artery and with arteriovenous fistula of brachial vessels. Clubbing of the toes but not fingers has been associated with an infected abdominal aortic aneurysm. Clubbing of a single digit may follow trauma, and has been reported in tophaceous gout and sarcoidosis.

Hyperthyroidism (Graves' disease), treated or untreated, may occasionally be associated with clubbing and periostitis of the bones of the hands and feet. This condition is referred to as *thyroid acropachy*. Periostitis is asymptomatic and occurs in the midshaft and diaphyseal portion of the metacarpal and phalangeal bones. The long bones of the extremities are seldom affected. Elevated levels of long-acting thyroid stimulator (LATS) are found in the serum of these patients.

Laboratory The laboratory abnormalities reflect the underlying disorder. The synovial fluid of involved joints has less than 500 white cells per microliter, and they are predominantly mononuclear. Radiographs show a faint radiolucent line beneath the new periosteal bone along the shaft of long bones at their distal end. These changes are most frequently observed at the ankles, wrists, and knees. The ends of the distal phalanges may show osseous resorption. Radionuclide studies show pricortical linear uptake along the cortical margins of long bones that may be present before any radiographic changes.

Treatment The treatment of hypertrophic osteoarthropathy is to identify the associated disorder and treat it appropriately. The symptoms and signs of hypertrophic osteoarthropathy may disappear completely with removal or effective chemotherapy of a tumor or with antibiotic therapy and drainage of a chronic pulmonary infection. Vagotomy or percutaneous block may lead to symptomatic relief in some patients. Aspirin, other nonsteroidal anti-inflammatory drugs, or analgesics may help control symptoms of hypertrophic osteoarthropathy.

FIBROSITIS Fibrositis, also termed *fibromyalgia*, is a commonly encountered disorder characterized by musculoskeletal pain, stiffness, and easy fatigability which affects predominantly women between the ages of 25 and 45 years. The term *fibrositis* is a misnomer, since this is not an inflammatory disorder of connective tissue. The etiology and pathogenesis of fibrositis are not known. A disturbance of normal stage 4 (non-REM) sleep has been suggested as playing a role in the development of fibrositis. Symptoms of fibrositis were produced in normal subjects by disturbing stage 4 sleep with a buzzer without wakening them. Sleep studies in patients with fibrositis have shown an alpha intrusion pattern superimposed on slow wave sleep. Muscle abnormalities have been found at sites of tenderness in some patients. Psychological abnormalities may also contribute to symptoms. A better understanding of fibrositis awaits further studies.

Symptoms are generalized aching and stiffness of the trunk, hip, and shoulder girdles. Other patients complain of generalized aching and muscle weakness. Patients perceive that their joints are swollen; however, joint examination is normal. Stiffness is usually present on arising in the morning and improves during the day, but may last all day in some patients. Patients complain of exhaustion and wake up tired. They also awake frequently at night and have trouble falling back asleep. Symptoms are made worse by stress or anxiety, cold, damp weather, and overexertion. Patients often feel better during warmer weather and vacations. Disorders commonly associated with fibrositis include irritable bowel syndrome, irritable bladder, headaches, and dysmenorrhea. Symptoms of fibrositis also occur in patients who carry the diagnosis of chronic fatigue syndrome.

The characteristic physical feature is the demonstration of specific tender sites which are exquisitely more tender than adjacent areas. Tender sites should be distinguished from the trigger points found in myofascial pain syndromes. Pressure over trigger points causes pain to be referred to a nearby site, while pressure over tender sites causes pain only at that site. The patient may suddenly jump or withdraw when the tender site is palpated. The sites of tenderness are remarkably constant in location. Common sites of tenderness are over the midpoint of the upper border of the trapezius, lateral epicondyles, supraspinatus, lower cervical spine, lumbar spine, posterior iliac spine, costochondral junctions, especially the second, gluteus maximus, and medial fat pad of the knee. Skinfold tenderness may be present, particularly over the upper scapular region. Subcutaneous nodules may be felt at sites of tenderness. Nodules in similar locations are present in normal persons but are not tender.

The diagnosis of fibrositis is made by recognizing the clinical manifestations. The joint and muscle examination is normal, and there are no laboratory abnormalties. Symptoms suggesting fibrositis are seen in patients with rheumatoid arthritis or other connective tissue diseases, and tender sites may be present. It is not clear whether this is part of the connective tissue disease or should be considered as fibrositis complicating the connective tissue disease.

Patients should be informed that they have a treatable condition which is not a crippling, deforming, or degenerative process. Salicylates or other nonsteroidal anti-inflammatory drugs only partially improve symptoms. Glucocorticoids have been of little benefit and should not be used in these patients. Local measures such as heat, massage, injection of tender sites with steroids or lidocaine, and acupuncture provide only temporary relief of symptoms. The use of tricyclics such as amitriptyline, 10 to 25 mg, doxepin, 10 to 25 mg, and cyclobenzaprine, 10 to 20 mg, at bedtime will give the patient restorative sleep resulting in clinical improvement. Higher doses of these medications may be necessary. Patients should improve their physical fitness by regular exercise and decrease the stress in their lives.

PSYCHOGENIC RHEUMATISM Patients may experience severe joint pain involving a few to several joints without physical findings of arthritis. These patients are often convinced that they have rheumatoid arthritis, systemic lupus erythematosus, or another connective tissue disease. This disorder is recognized by the inconsistencies, exaggerations, and emotional lability of the patient during the history and physical examination. Laboratory studies are normal. Organic disease needs to be excluded, which requires seeing the patient at regular intervals. This condition also needs to be distinguished from fibrositis. Anti-inflammatory or other drugs are not helpful.

CARPAL TUNNEL SYNDROME Carpal tunnel syndrome is an entrapment neuropathy of the median nerve at the wrist producing paresthesias and weakness of the hands. The syndrome is caused by pressure on the median nerve where it passes in company with the flexor tendons of the fingers through the tunnel formed by carpal bones and the transverse carpal ligament.

Compression of the median nerve is produced by any process that encroaches on the carpal tunnel. Localized tenosynovitis of the flexor tendons of the fingers is a frequent cause of carpal tunnel syndrome, particularly in middle-aged women. Premenstrual edema or edema occurring in pregnancy may also cause these symptoms. Symptoms can be precipitated by activities which require repeated flexion, pronation, and supination of the wrist, for example, sewing, driving, and operating computers. Other causes of carpal tunnel syndrome, often bilateral, are rheumatoid arthritis, acromegaly, hypothyroidism, and amyloidosis. Unilateral carpal tunnel syndrome is more likely due to trauma, physical activities involving one wrist, tuberculosis, gout, or calcium pyrophosphate deposition disease.

Patients experience numbness or paresthesias of the palmar surface of the thumb, index and middle fingers, and radial half of the ring finger. Numbness or paresthesias of the whole hand may occur. Pain may be referred to the forearm and less commonly to the shoulder and neck regions. Pain or tingling of the fingers often occurs at night and is relieved by shaking or exercising the hand. Weakness and atrophy of the thenar muscles usually appear later and can occur without significant sensory symptoms.

Thenar muscle weakness is manifested by decreased strength of abduction, opposition, and flexion of the thumb. On examination, symptoms of paresthesia or pain in the fingers may be reproduced by percussion over the volar surface of the wrist (Tinel's sign) or by full flexion of the wrist for 1 min (Phalen's maneuver). Decreased touch or hyperpathia to pinprick may be demonstrated over the fingers supplied by the median nerve. Nerve conduction studies of the median nerve show delayed latency across the wrist, confirming the diagnosis.

Treatment of patients with only sensory symptoms and minor

nerve conduction abnormalities consist of a wrist splint to be worn mainly at night, anti-inflammatory drugs, and local injection with steroids. If symptoms persist or motor abnormalities are present, surgical decompression of the carpal tunnel with release of the transverse carpal ligament and debridement is indicated.

TARSAL TUNNEL SYNDROME Tarsal tunnel syndrome is an entrapment neuropathy of the posterior tibial nerve at the ankle producing aching, burning, tingling, and numbness of the plantar surface of the foot and toes. The syndrome is caused by compression of the posterior tibial nerve and its branches as they pass through the tunnel beneath the flexor retinaculum on the medial side of the ankle inferior and posterior to the medial malleolus. Also passing through this tunnel are the flexor tendons of the toes, vascular bundle, and the medial and lateral plantar branches of the posterior tibial nerve. Compression of the nerve in the tunnel may be caused by tenosynovitis resulting from overuse or trauma and by inflammatory arthritis such as rheumatoid arthritis. Other causes include pregnancy, myxedema, and amyloidosis.

Patients experience paresthesias of the plantar surface of the foot and toes which may radiate up the calf. Symptoms often occur at night and after standing, and may be relieved by movement of the foot and ankle. On examination, there may be loss of sensation over the plantar surface of the foot, but this is variable. Symptoms may be reproduced by percussion over the flexor retinaculum (Tinel's sign) or by applying firm pressure to this area. Diagnosis is confirmed by nerve conduction studies that show prolonged latency across the tunnel. Treatment consists of anti-inflammatory drugs and local injection of steroids. If symptoms persist, surgical decompression is indicated.

REFLEX SYMPATHETIC DYSTROPHY SYNDROME The reflex sympathetic dystrophy syndrome (RSDS) is characterized by pain and tenderness usually of a distal extremity accompanied by signs and symptoms of vasomotor instability, trophic skin changes, and the rapid development of bony demineralization. A precipitating event can be identified in two-thirds of the cases. These include local trauma, myocardial infarction, strokes, and peripheral nerve injuries. RSDS is observed most often in individuals over the age of 50, reflecting the frequency of the accompanying disorder. The sex distribution is equal. An entire hand or foot is usually affected. Occasionally, RSDS will involve an isolated site such as the patella, hip, or one or two rays of a foot or hand. The contralateral side may be affected in up to 50 percent of patients, and subclinical disease may be present in virtually all patients. The pathogenesis of RSDS is poorly understood. The vasomotor manifestations are thought to be caused by abnormal stimulation of the sympathetic nervous system.

RSDS evolves through three clinical phases. The clinical manifestations of the first phase are pain and swelling of a distal extremity, which develop weeks to months following the precipitating event. The pain has an intense, burning quality. The involved extremity is warm, edematous, and tender especially around joints. Increased sweating and hair growth occur. In 3 to 6 months, the skin gradually becomes thin, shiny, and cool (second phase). Clinical features of the first two phases overlap. In another 3 to 6 months, the skin and subcutaneous tissue become atrophic, and irreversible flexion contractures of the hand or foot develop (third phase). Motion of the shoulder on the affected side is frequently painful and greatly restricted, a condition referred to as shoulder-hand syndrome (see "Adhesive Capsulities," below).

The laboratory abnormalities are those of the associated disorder. Radiographs of the involved distal extremity demonstrate mottled osteopenia referred to as Sudeck's atrophy. Later in the course, diffuse osteopenia develops. Similar changes, however, are observed in an immobilized limb following a fracture or paralysis. Bone scan in the early phase shows asymmetric and increased blood flow followed subsequently by increased radionuclide uptake in the periarticular bone of the involved side. Uptake may also be increased on the contralateral side indicating subclinical involvement.

Early recognition and treatment are important to prevent permanent disability. RSDS may be reversible in its early phases. Appropriate mobilization of the patient following a myocardial infarction, stroke, or injury may help to prevent this syndrome. Pain should be properly controlled. Application of heat or cold along with exercises are useful. Sympathetic nerve block may be effective and, if it is, can be followed by surgical sympathectomy. The response, however, may not be sustained. A short course of high-dose prednisone in conjunction with physical therapy has been beneficial in some patients. Prednisone is started at 60 mg/d for 4 days and gradually tapered over a 3-week period.

TSIETZE'S SYNDROME AND COSTOCHONDRITIS Tsietze's syndrome is manifested by painful swelling of one or more costochondral articulations. Age of onset is usually before 40, and both sexes are equally affected. Most patients have only one joint involved, usually the second or third costochondral joint. The onset of anterior chest pain may be sudden or gradual. The pain may radiate to the arms or shoulder and is aggravated by sneezing, coughing, deep inspirations, or twisting motions of the chest. The term *costochondritis* is often used interchangeably with Tsietze's syndrome, but some restrict the former term to pain of the costochondral articulations without swelling. Costochondritis is observed in patients over age 40, tends to affect the third, fourth, and fifth costochondral joints, and occurs more often in women. Both syndromes may mimic cardiac or upper abdominal causes of pain. Rheumatoid arthritis, ankylosing spondylitis, or Reiter's syndrome may involve costochondral joints but are distinguished easily by their other clinical features. Other skeletal causes of anterior chest wall pain are xiphoidalgia and the slipping rib syndome, which usually involves the tenth rib. Analgesics, anti-inflammatory drugs, or local steroid injections usually relieve symptoms.

MUSCULOSKELETAL DISORDERS ASSOCIATED WITH HYPERLIPIDEMIA Musculoskeletal manifestations may be the first indication of a hereditary disorder of lipoprotein metabolism. Patients with type II hyperlipoproteinemia may have recurrent migratory polyarthritis involving knees and other large peripheral joints and, to a lesser degree, peripheral small joints. The involved joints can be warm, erythematous, and swollen. Arthritis usually has a sudden onset, lasts from a few days to 2 weeks, and does not cause joint damage. Several attacks occur a year. Synovial fluid from involved joints is not inflammatory, and contains few white cells and no crystals. Joint involvement may actually represent inflammatory periarthritis or peritendinitis and not intraarticular disease. The recurrent transient nature of the arthritis may suggest rheumatic fever, especially since patients with lipoproteinemia have an elevated erythrocyte sedimentation rate and a falsely elevated antistreptolysin O titer. Furthermore, patients may have aortic valvular disease secondary to atherosclerosis. Patients with type II hyperlipoproteinemia also have tendinous xanthomas in the Achilles, patellar, and extensor tendons of the hands and feet. These are located within tendon fibers and appear in childhood in homozygous patients and after the age of 30 in heterozygous patients. Tuberous xanthomas appear only in patients homozygous for type II hyperlipoproteinemia. They are located over the extensor surfaces of the elbows, knees and hands, and also on the buttocks. Patients with type IV hyperlipoproteinemia may also have a mild inflammatory arthritis affecting large and small peripheral joints, usually in an asymmetric pattern with only a few joints involved at a time. Arthritis may be persistent or recurrent with episodes lasting a few days. Joint fluid is noninflammatory. Periarticular hyperesthesia may be present. Large juxtaarticular bone cysts have been noted in a few patients. The pathogenesis of arthritis in both types of hyperlipoproteinemia is not well understood. Salicylates, other NSAIDs, or analgesics usually provide relief of symptoms.

PERIARTICULAR DISORDERS **Bursitis** Bursitis is inflammation of a bursa, which is a thin-walled sac lined with synovial tissue. The function of the bursa is to facilitate movement of tendons and muscles over bony prominences. Excessive frictional forces, trauma, systemic disease (e.g., rheumatoid arthritis, gout), or infection may cause bursitis. Subacromial bursitis (subdeltoid bursitis) is the most common form of bursitis. Another is trochanteric bursitis, which involves the bursa around the insertion of the gluteus medius to the greater trochanter of the femur. Patients experience pain over the lateral aspect of the hip and upper thigh and are tender over the posterior aspect of the greater trochanter. External rotation and resisted abduction of the hip elicit pain. Olecranon bursitis occurs over the posterior elbow, and when the area is acutely inflamed, infection should be excluded by aspirating and culturing fluid from the bursa. Achilles bursitis involves the bursa located above the insertion of the tendon to the calcaneus and results from overuse and wearing tight shoes. Retrocalcaneal bursitis involves the bursa which is located between the calcaneus and posterior surface of the Achilles tendon. The pain is experienced at the back of the heel, and swelling appears on the medial and/or lateral side of the tendon. It occurs in association with spondyloarthropathies, rheumatoid arthritis, gout and trauma. Ischial bursitis (weaver's bottom) affects the bursa separating the gluteus medius from the ischial tuberosity and develops from prolonged sitting on hard surfaces. Iliopsoas bursitis affects the bursa that lies between the iliopsoas muscle and hip joint and is lateral to the femoral vessels. Pain is experienced over this area and made worse by hip extension and flexion. Bursitis results from trauma or overuse and can be seen in patients with rheumatoid arthritis. Anserine bursitis is an inflammation of the sartorius bursa located over the medial side of the tibia just below the knee and is manifested by pain on climbing stairs. Tenderness is present over the insertion of the conjoint tendon of the sartorius, gracilis, and semitendinosus. Prepatellar bursitis (housemaid's knee) occurs in the bursa situated between the patella and overlying skin and is caused by kneeling on hard surfaces. Treatment of bursitis consists of prevention of the aggravating condition, rest of the involved part, a nonsteroidal anti-inflammatory drug, and local steroid injection.

Rotator cuff tendinitis Tendinitis of the rotator cuff is the major cause of a painful shoulder. Of the tendons forming the rotator cuff, the supraspinatus tendon is most often affected, probably because of its repeated impingement between the acromion and humeral head as well as its reduced blood supply occurring with abduction of the arm. The process evolves through inflammation, fibrosis, and tears of the tendon. Subacromial bursitis may also be present. Symptoms usually occur after injury or overuse, particularly in individuals over age 40. Patients complain of a dull aching in the shoulder that may interfere with sleep. Severe pain is experienced when the arm is actively abducted into an overhead position. Tenderness is present over the lateral aspect of the humeral head just below the acromion. Nonsteroidal anti-inflammatory drugs, local steroid injection, and physical therapy may relieve symptoms.

Patients may tear the supraspinatus tendon acutely by falling on an outstretched arm or lifting a heavy object. Symptoms are pain, along with weakness of abduction and external rotation of the shoulder. Atrophy of the supraspinatus muscles develops. The diagnosis is established by arthrogram. Surgical repair may be necessary in patients who fail to respond to conservative measures.

Calcific tendinitis This is characterized by deposition of calcium salts, primarily hydroxyapatite, within a tendon. The exact mechanism for calcification is not known but may be due to ischemia or degeneration of the tendon. The supraspinatus tendon is most often affected because of its frequent impingement and reduced blood supply when the arm is abducted. It usually develops after age 40. Calcification within the tendon may evoke acute inflammation, producing sudden and severe pain in the shoulder. Tendon calcification, however, may be asymptomatic or not related to the patient's symptoms.

Bicipital tendinitis and rupture Bicipital tendinitis, or tenosynovitis, is produced by friction on the tendon of the long head of the biceps as it passes through the bicipital groove. When the inflammation is acute, patients experience anterior shoulder pain which radiates down the biceps into the forearm. Abduction and external rotation of the arm are painful and limited. The bicipital groove is very tender to palpation. Pain may be elicited along the course of the tendon by resisting supination of the forearm with the elbow at 90° (Yergason's supination sign). Acute rupture of the tendon may occur with vigorous exercise of the arm and is often painful. In a young patient, it should be repaired surgically. Rupture of the tendon in an older person may be associated with little or no pain and is recognized by the presence of persistent swelling of the biceps ("Popeye" muscle). Surgery is usually not necessary in this setting.

Adhesive capsulitis Often referred to as "frozen shoulder," adhesive capsulitis is characterized by pain and restricted movement of the shoulder usually in the absence of intrinsic shoulder disease. Adhesive capsulitis, however, may follow bursitis or tendinitis of the shoulder or be associated with systemic disorders such as chronic pulmonary disease, myocardial infarction, and diabetes mellitus. Prolonged immobility of the arm contributes to the development of adhesive capsulitis, and reflex sympathetic dystrophy is thought to be a pathogenic factor. The capsule of the shoulder is thickened, and a mild chronic inflammatory infiltrate and fibrosis may be present.

Adhesive capsulitis occurs more commonly in women after age 50. Pain and stiffness usually develop gradually over several months to a year, but may progress rapidly in some patients. Pain may interfere with sleep. The shoulder is tender to palpation, and both active and passive movement are restricted. Radiograph of the shoulder shows osteopenia. The diagnosis is confirmed by arthrogram, in that only a limited amount of contrast material, usually less than 15 mL, can be injected under pressure into the shoulder joint.

The majority of patients improve spontaneously 12 to 18 months after the onset of disease, but some may have permanent restriction of movement. Early mobilization of the arm following an injury to the shoulder may prevent the development of this disease. Slow but forceful injection of contrast material into the joint may lyse adhesions and stretch the capsule, resulting in improvement of shoulder motion. Manipulation under anesthesia may be helpful in some patients. Once established, therapy may have little effect on the natural course of the disease. Local injections of corticosteroids, nonsteroidal anti-inflammatory drugs, and physical therapy may provide relief of symptoms.

TUMORS OF JOINTS Primary tumors and tumorlike disorders of synovium are uncommon but should be considered in the differential diagnosis of monarticular joint disease. In addition, metastases to bone and primary bone tumors adjacent to a joint may produce joint symptoms.

Pigmented villonodular synovitis is characterized by exuberant proliferation of synovial cells usually involving a single joint. It occurs most often in young adults and affects both sexes equally. The etiology of this disorder is unknown.

The synovium is a brownish color and has numerous large, fingerlike villi which fuse to form pedunculated nodules. There is marked hyperplasia of synovial cells within the stroma of the villi. Hemosiderin granules and lipids are found in the cytoplasm of macrophages and in the interstitial tissue. Multinucleated giant cells may be present. The proliferative synovium grows into the subsynovial tissue and invades adjacent cartilage and bone.

The clinical picture of pigmented villonodular synovitis is characterized by the insidious onset of swelling and pain in one joint, most commonly the knee. Other joints affected include the hips, ankles, calcaneocuboid joints, elbows, and small joints of the fingers or toes. The disease may also involve the common flexor sheath of the hand. Symptoms may be mild, intermittent, and present for years before the patient seeks medical attention. Radiographs may show joint space narrowing, erosions, and subchondral cysts. The joint fluid contains blood and is dark-red or almost black in color. Lipid containing macrophages may be present in the fluid. The joint fluid may be clear if hemorrhages have not occurred.

The treatment of pigmented villonodular synovitis is complete synovectomy. With incomplete synovectomy, the villonodular synovitis recurs, and the rate of tissue growth may be faster than occurred originally. Irradiation of the involved joint has been successful in some patients.

Synovial chondromatosis is a disorder characterized by multiple focal metaplastic growths of normal-appearing cartilage in the synovium or tendon sheath. Segments of cartilage break loose and continue to grow as loose bodies. When calcification and ossification of loose bodies occur, the disorder is referred to as synovial osteochondromatosis. The disorder is usually monarticular and affects young to middle-aged individuals. The knee is most often involved, followed by hip, elbow, and shoulder. Symptoms are pain, swelling, and decreased motion of the joint. Radiographs may show several rounded calcifications within the joint cavity. Treatment is synovectomy; however, the tumor may recur.

Hemangiomas occur in synovium and in tendon sheaths. The knee is affected most commonly. Recurrent episodes of joint swelling and pain usually begin in childhood. The joint fluid is bloody. Treatment is excision of the lesion. *Lipomas* occur most often in the knee, originating in the subsynovial fat on either side of the patellar tendon. Lipomas also appear in tendon sheaths of the hands, wrists, feet, and ankles.

Synovial sarcoma (malignant synovioma) is a neoplasm of connective origin arising from tissue adjacent to large joints and seldom from the joint itself. It occurs most often in young adults and is more common in men. The tumor presents as a slowly growing mass near a joint, without much pain. The tumor spreads along tissue planes. The most common site of visceral metastasis is lung. The diagnosis is made by biopsy. Treatment is wide resection of the tumor including adjacent muscle and regional lymph nodes. Amputation of the involved distal extremity may be required. Chemotherapy may be beneficial in some patients with metastatic disease.

Synovial chondrosarcoma may arise in the synovium, tendon sheath, or bursa and is very rare. Treatment is radical excision or amputation.

REFERENCES

ALTMAN RD, TENENBAUM J: Hypertrophic osteoarthropathy, in *Textbook of Rheumatology*, WN Kelley et al (eds). Philadelphia, Saunders, 1989, chap 95, pp 1666–1673

BENNETT RM, GOLDENBERG DL (eds): *Rheumatic Disease Clinics of North America: The Fibromyalgia Syndrome*. Philadelphia, Saunders, 1989

ELLMAN MH: Neuropathic joint disease (Charcot joints), in *Arthritis and Allied Conditions*, DJ McCarty (ed). Philadelphia, Lea & Febiger, 1989, chap 81, pp 1255–1272

HERMAN JH: Polychondritis, in *Textbook of Rheumatology*, WN Kelley et al (eds). Philadelphia, Saunders, 1989, chap 83, pp 1513–1522

KOZIN F: Painful shoulder and the reflex sympathetic dystrophy syndrome, in *Arthritis and Allied Conditions*, DJ McCarty (ed). Philadelphia, Lea & Febiger, 1989, chap 97, pp 1509–1544

MICHET CJ JR et al: Relapsing polychondritis: Survival and predictive role of early disease manifestations. *Ann Intern Med* 104:74–78, 1986

NEER CS II: Impingement lesions. *Clin Orthop* 173:70–77, 1983

SCHILLER AL: Tumors and tumor-like lesions involving joints, in *Textbook of Rheumatology*, WN Kelly et al (eds). Philadelphia, Saunders, 1989, chap 100, pp 1775–1797

WEISMAN MH: Arthritis associated with hematologic disorders, storage diseases, disorders of lipid metabolism, and dysproteinemias, in *Arthritis and Allied Conditions*, DJ McCarty (ed). Philadelphia, Lea & Febiger, 1989, chap 84, pp 1312–1315

PART ELEVEN HEMATOLOGY AND ONCOLOGY

285 IMPACT OF MOLECULAR BIOLOGY ON HEMATOLOGY

STUART H. ORKIN

Phenotypic variation is the essence of genetics, whether reflected as normal polymorphism or as inherited disease. Differences between individuals are encoded in cellular DNA (the genome), the reservoir of genetic information for the individual as well as the species. Until recently the precise relationship between a given phenotype (a trait or a disease) and a specific alteration in cellular DNA could only be inferred. For example, where a specific protein was known to be structurally abnormal in a clinical condition, demonstration of an amino acid replacement in the mutant product allowed one to predict a substitution in the DNA on the basis of the genetic code. Thus, the substitution of glutamic acid by valine at the sixth amino acid of the β chain of sickle hemoglobin could be accounted for by a change in a single nucleotide in cellular DNA (Chap. 5).

The past decade has witnessed a revolution in biomedical sciences with the introduction of the extraordinarily powerful methods of recombinant DNA that permit isolation of genes in pure form and their precise characterization. In many spheres of medicine recombinant DNA technology offers great promise, only one tangible consequence of which is the commercial production of new proteins such as growth factors, hormones, and enzymes. Nowhere has the impact of recombinant DNA been more immediate than in the understanding, diagnosis, and potential treatment of hematologic diseases.

RECOMBINANT DNA TECHNOLOGY AND THE NEW GENETICS (See also Chap. 6) With the tools of recombinant DNA, the relationship between a specific gene, an alteration in that gene, and a phenotype (or disease) can be established with certainty. This new capability rests on relatively simple procedures to isolate genes, determine their nucleotide sequences, and put genes back into cells to assess their function. Isolating a pure gene among the approximately 10^5 other genes in a cell is impossible by traditional biochemical means. Recombinant DNA methods, however, permit doing so by molecular cloning. In this context, cloning refers to the process by which one DNA molecule is joined to another (termed a *vector*) that can replicate autonomously in a specially chosen host, usually a bacterium or yeast. A common feature of cloning methods is the use of *restriction enzymes,* reagents that recognize specific sequences in double-stranded DNA and generate cleavages at or near those sites. As cloning methods were devised, techniques also were developed to permit rapid determination of the nucleotide sequence of cloned DNA and assessment of its function in cells. Ultimately direct correlations can be made between gene structure and gene function.

In parallel with the introduction of techniques to examine individual genes, methods were developed that utilize naturally occurring variation in DNA sequence as markers for the inheritance of disease genes and for the mapping of genes to specific chromosomes and subchromosomal regions. These methods are restriction enzyme digestion, electrophoresis, and molecular hybridization (the Southern blot procedure). The variations in DNA sequence they detect are commonly referred to as *restriction fragment length polymorphisms* (RFLPs). RFLPs may be used as markers for specific genes or gene regions in families affected with a disorder (see below). More broadly, RFLPs help determine the relative distance of one marker from another or of a marker from a disease locus to which it is linked (linkage analysis). While linkage analysis is beyond the scope of this chapter (see Chap. 6), it should be noted that sufficient RFLPs have been identified to permit construction of a low-resolution map of the human genome. With such a map, study of the correlation of RFLPs and disease phenotypes in families can be employed to position genes for inherited phenotypes on specific chromosomes. As noted below, the genes involved in inherited disorders can now be located and cloned by such approaches without prior knowledge of the protein product of the normal gene or even its cellular origin ("reverse genetics").

Until very recently cloning methods were the only means by which suitable amounts of pure gene DNA could be obtained for laboratory study. Now, a method termed the *polymerase chain reaction* (PCR) provides a simple technique for the acquisition of sufficient quantities of specific gene regions, if nucleotide sequence information exists regarding the gene itself. The use of specific synthetic DNA primers on either side of a target DNA region and repetitive enzymatic extension and denaturation on the template DNA allow for the in vitro synthesis of pure gene regions. Although PCR may seem unduly specialized or technical, it is remarkably efficient and convenient even for clinical laboratories. As such, its widespread use will probably revolutionize genetic diagnosis.

IMMEDIATE IMPACT OF THE NEW GENETICS ON HEMATOLOGIC DISEASE The application of recombinant DNA technology to the analysis of disease has expanded greatly since its introduction in about 1978; therefore discussion of its impact on hematologic disease must of necessity be selective. In forging an understanding of the molecular basis of disease and testing new approaches to diagnosis based on genetic criteria, consideration of the hemoglobinopathies, particularly thalassemia syndromes, is particularly instructive.

Determining the molecular basis of disease For nearly three decades it has been appreciated that thalassemia syndromes result from unbalanced synthesis of globin chains (Chap. 295). Prior to recombinant DNA methods, reduced (or absent) synthesis of specific globin polypeptides in various thalassemia syndromes was established, as was deficiency of specific messenger RNAs. Whether deficiency was secondary to mutations in globin genes per se or in genes that regulate their expression, and how specific mutations led to reduced mRNA synthesis or function, were largely unknown. This changed with the advent of procedures that permitted isolation of globin genes from patients with thalassemias, determination of their nucleotide sequences, and analysis of expression of the cloned genes upon reintroduction into cells. It became possible to elucidate the precise molecular basis of these syndromes. Rather than representing a single type of mutation, thalassemia syndromes reflected the entire spectrum of molecular defects that might be predicted to interfere with gene expression. Lesions included gross gene deletions, but more commonly consisted of *single base substitutions* in globin genes that adversely affected gene transcription, proper removal of intervening sequences during RNA splicing, mRNA polyadenylation, translatability, or stability. Taken together, the thalassemia syndromes were the first genetic disorders to be described in detail at the molecular level.

The comprehensive dissection of the thalassemia syndromes relied on combining gene cloning with RFLP haplotype analysis. The latter method takes advantage of RFLPs to characterize the chromosome vicinity of the globin genes. In a given chromosomal region, the pattern of restriction site differences constitutes an RFLP haplotype, much as differences at the histocompatibility loci form a haplotype. It was reasoned that haplotype differences surrounding the human β-globin gene might provide a signature for different chromosomal backgrounds upon which mutations in the β-globin gene producing thalassemia might have arisen. It thus became possible to group potentially identical mutant alleles together and focus attention on those among them that differ from the others. Therefore, examination of cloned β-globin genes (representing different chromosome haplotypes) revealed a comprehensive picture of mutations in thalassemia with high efficiency and speed.

Impact on diagnosis At the clinical level, the new genetic methods have had their greatest impact on diagnosis. This has resulted from the development of techniques for the detection of specific gene defects in uncloned DNA samples. The feasibility of assigning specific defects in small DNA samples permits examination of the distribution of mutations in populations, carrier detection in families at risk (or those possibly at risk), and prenatal diagnosis as early as the first trimester by chorionic villus biopsy sampling and later by amniocentesis.

Although extensive DNA deletion, insertion, or rearrangement may often be the molecular basis of an inherited disorder, most gene mutations in inherited disorders are single nucleotide changes that cannot be detected by gross examination of gene structure. To diagnose such defects, highly sensitive assays are required that distinguish mutant from normal DNA sequences in a specific region of a gene. With a catalog of clinically relevant gene mutations for which individuals may be surveyed (as is available for the thalassemia syndromes), these procedures may be applied with great precision. The detection of the sickle cell mutation is already a classic demonstration of the application of recombinant DNA methods to diagnosis. A substitution of T for A in the sixth codon of the β-globin gene, which directs the replacement of valine for glutamic acid, is the underlying basis for sickle cell anemia. Quite fortuitously, this single change abolishes a recognition site in the gene for a restriction enzyme (Mst II) and, thereby, alters the fragments of the gene generated upon digestion of total DNA by this enzyme. With the procedure of Southern, in which DNA fragments are electrophoretically separated in gels and then probed for specific sequences by molecular hybridization (see Fig. 6-2, p. 34), the relevant β-globin gene fragments may be visualized. In this manner a molecular diagnosis of normal, sickle trait, or sickle cell anemia can be achieved accurately and reliably with a small DNA sample from blood cells or fetal material. This approach has been used in the prenatal diagnosis of sickle cell anemia with considerable success (Chap. 295).

Applications of polymerase chain reaction The newer and simpler PCR method was also first applied in the analysis of the sickle cell mutation. With synthetic DNA primers flanking the sickle mutation, the critical DNA segment can be amplified in vitro more than a millionfold to provide material sufficient for analysis by restriction enzyme digestion, molecular hybridization, or even direct DNA sequencing (see Fig. 6-3, p. 34). Since the method requires only minute samples, takes a matter of hours rather than days, and is readily adapted for automated handling, PCR is very rapidly finding its way into clinical as well as research laboratories.

The extraordinary power of PCR methodology is perhaps best exemplified by its application to the analysis of minimal residual disease in hematologic malignancies. In many forms of cancer very specific cytogenetic alterations occur (Chap. 300). Often these involve breakage and union of ordinarily separate chromosomal regions; typical examples are the translocations found in chronic myelogenous leukemia (Chap. 296). To the extent that such translocations are found within a limited target region, these chromosomal abnormalities may be detected with PCR primers flanking the breakpoints. An especially informative example is follicular lymphoma, in which there is frequently a chromosome 14;18 translocation. The 14;18 breakpoints connect one of six immunoglobin heavy chain joining (J_h) regions on chromosome 14 to a small breakpoint region on the BCL2 gene on chromosome 18. With PCR (using primers flanking the junctures), a single abnormal cell among more than 10^6 normal cells is detectable. Therefore, PCR presents the means to identify the subclinical presence of residual neoplastic cells. Although the precise clinical significance of small numbers of residual leukemic cells in patients in apparent remission remains to be determined, it is highly likely that correlations of the residual neoplastic cell burden with clinical outcome and treatment will be important for management of hematologic malignancies.

Detection of clonality in cell populations A related application of recombinant DNA methods to hematologic malignancies is the detection of *clonality in cell populations*. The clonal expansion of lymphoid cells is generally taken to reflect proliferation of malignant cells, whereas polyclonal expansion is not. Rearrangements of immunoglobulin genes and T-cell receptor loci normally accompany differentiation of B- and T-cells, respectively. In light of this, Southern blot analysis of lymphoid cell DNA with appropriate molecular probes can provide evidence regarding the clonality of cell populations. Taken together with other findings, such information can make clinical diagnoses more precise.

Using DNA probes that detect RFLPs, the cellular DNAs of virtually any two (or more) individuals can be distinguished, particularly if highly polymorphic probes (called *fingerprinting probes*) are employed. The capability of distinguishing the genotypes of cells has also found an application in the management of patients following bone marrow transplantation. Analysis of RFLPs following allogeneic transplantation enables assessing the relative contribution of host and donor hematopoietic cells. Engraftment of donor marrow, reemergence of host elements, and mixed cell chimerism can be evaluated with RFLP analysis.

Selected applications of recombinant DNA methods in clinical diagnosis are summarized in Table 285-1.

IMPACT ON THE UNDERSTANDING OF DISEASE AND NORMAL BIOLOGY Some diseases reflect a disturbance of normal cellular physiology. An understanding of their biochemical basis can often provide novel insights into normal biology. Until very recently, the analysis of inherited human disorders required identification and characterization of specific proteins and their corresponding genes. Many conditions, however, including those affecting the hematopoietic system, display phenotypes for which adequate biochemical explanations are lacking. In general, animal models that faithfully mimic human disorders are not available. However, using an approach that combines classical genetics and recombinant DNA methods, the gene affected in a disorder can now be identified without specific

TABLE 285-1 Recombinant DNA analysis in clinical diagnosis

Application	Examples
Detection of specific mutations in populations and families at risk	Carrier detection of sickle cell anemia Estimation of specific β-thalassemia mutations in populations
Prenatal diagnosis of disease	β Thalassemia, sickle cell anemia
Detection of minimal residual disease in malignancy	Chromosome 14;18 translocation in follicular lymphoma
Detection of clonality in cell populations	Rearrangement of Ig and T-cell receptor gene loci in lymphomas
Distinguishing genotypes of hematopoietic cells	Assessment of host/donor cell contributions following allogeneic bone marrow transplantation

knowledge of the protein product. With DNA probes that recognize RFLPs within families at risk for an inherited condition, markers that are very closely linked to a particular disease locus may be identified. By a variety of methods, the region of the relevant gene may be further delimited by additional linkage mapping or by use of patient samples bearing DNA deletions or chromosomal translocations. Ultimately, a region of DNA that gives rise to an mRNA that is structurally or quantitatively deranged in the disease defines the gene itself. This approach to the identification and characterization of the affected gene and its product is often termed *reverse genetics*.

Impact of reverse genetics Examples of the impact of this approach to disease are just emerging. One of the first involved the analysis of an inherited hematologic disorder, the X-linked variety of chronic granulomatous disease (X-CGD). In this disease activated phagocytic white blood cells of affected males fail to produce superoxide anion, an important chemical component of the host defense system against microorganisms. The cellular biochemistry of superoxide generation and its derangement in X-CGD had been actively studied since the first description of the rare disorder more than thirty years ago. Nonetheless, considerable controversy existed regarding the nature of the essential cellular proteins and the X-chromosome–encoded locus in the disease. Although the details are beyond the scope of this chapter, the molecular cloning of the gene involved in X-CGD rapidly demonstrated the requirement for a usual cytochrome molecule in white blood cell superoxide production. In addition, further work has provided useful biochemical and molecular reagents with which to pursue dissection of superoxide production in greater depth. Reverse genetics has also elucidated the genetic defects in Duchenne muscular dystrophy and in retinoblastoma.

The tremendous promise of the reverse-genetics approach to the understanding of inherited disorders relates to the extraordinary power of recombinant DNA methods, where in rapid succession (1) the protein product of a gene can be determined from a DNA sequence; (2) specific reagents to that protein can be generated either by immunization with synthetic peptides deduced from the sequence or with material manufactured in bacteria; and (3) the normal versions of the involved genes can be introduced into mammalian cells to analyze protein function. This approach will facilitate understanding of normal cellular physiology as well as efforts to correct disease phenotypes.

IMPACT OF THE NEW GENETICS ON TREATMENT OF HEMATOLOGIC DISORDERS In at least four areas recombinant DNA technology has had a major impact on clinical hematology. First, as noted above, identification of the specific gene mutations leading to thalassemia syndromes has led to effective and efficient prenatal diagnosis of disease. In geographic areas where these conditions are prevalent, programs for prenatal diagnosis, coupled with routine hematologic screening and genetic counseling, have already reduced the incidence of births of newly affected individuals. This is a significant achievement in public health management of a genetic disorder. Second, as also noted above, the development of new methods for the detection of specific DNA abnormalities in only a few cells among many allows better assessment of residual disease in hematologic malignancies. Correlation of clinical outcome with residual disease status and treatment is likely to lead to improved therapy. Third, the availability of new hematopoietic growth factors through molecular cloning and gene expression is beginning to change the clinical management of several conditions. For example, the use of erythropoietin constitutes a major new approach to the treatment of the anemia of chronic renal disease. Abnormalities of white blood cell production, particularly the transient neutropenia accompanying cancer chemotherapy, may be more effectively managed by administration of growth factors (colony stimulating factors) for myelomonocytic cells. Fourth, production of blood clotting factors by recombinant DNA methods provide a promising approach to the treatment of hemophilias.

Other applications of recombinant DNA technology in clinical hematology are more speculative, but two warrant discussion.

Since the production of fetal hemoglobin generally reduces the consequences of sickle cell anemia or thalassemia, studies have focused on the pharmacologic stimulation of fetal hemoglobin production in adults. Based on the observation that the modification of cellular DNA by methylation is often associated with gene inactivity, 5-azacytidine, a drug that causes widespread demethylation, has been tested for its effects on fetal hemoglobin production in patients with thalassemia or sickle cell anemia. While an augmentation in production has been observed, the molecular basis for the effect remains controversial. Nonetheless, this research has led to the testing of a variety of cytotoxic agents, such as hydroxyurea, that appear to exert a similar effect on fetal hemoglobin production. Although the precise mechanisms by which such drugs exert their effect is unclear, increases in fetal hemoglobin production are often in the range believed to be of clinical benefit.

Another attempt to modulate expression of genes in the treatment of an inherited disorder is the recent administration of the lymphokine *γ-interferon* to patients with chronic granulomatous disease. This lymphokine, previously known as macrophage activating factor, augments cellular killing of microbes by phagocytic cells. In part, this phenomenon may relate to the capacity of the γ-interferon to up-regulate expression of genes encoding some of the essential components of the superoxide-generating system of phagocytes. Limited clinical trials suggest that administration of γ-interferon may significantly enhance cellular function in selected patients with chronic granulomatous disease. From these two examples, it is already apparent that knowledge of the molecular biology of specific gene systems will generate novel therapies for the management of severe inherited hematologic disorders.

Somatic gene therapy A potential application of recombinant DNA technology to clinical hematology yet to be explored is *somatic genetic therapy*. The ability to clone genes and reintroduce them into cells offers prospects for correcting inherited disease by genetic means. The intent of such an approach would be to treat only somatic cells of the affected individual (somatic gene therapy), rather than attempting to correct the germline. At present, somatic gene therapy is being contemplated only for severe, life-threatening disorders for which conventional medical management is unsatisfactory. Many methods for the introduction of the normal version of a gene into a cell bearing defective versions have been considered. At present, the most promising avenue would appear to be the use of modified, recombinant RNA viruses (retroviruses) to achieve efficient transfer of new genetic material into hematopoietic stem cells.

In principle, the hematopoietic system is an attractive target for gene therapy as pluripotent stem cells self-renew and also give rise to cell progenitors and mature blood cells. Furthermore, extensive experience in bone marrow transplantation provides a strong base for management of the host, the handling of marrow cells, and the reconstitution of the hematopoietic system by infusion of donor cells. In somatic therapy, genetically modified cells of the affected patient, rather than stem cells from another individual, would be used for cellular reconstitution. The inherited disorders that seem most appropriate for this approach include immunodeficiencies, such as severe combined immunodeficiency due to lack of adenosine deaminase (Chap. 263), hemoglobinopathies (thalassemia and sickle cell anemia), storage disorders (such as Gaucher's disease), and coagulation factor deficiencies (such as hemophilia A). Although considerable progress in the methodologies required for somatic gene therapy has been made, efficient infection of sufficient numbers of stem cells by recombinant retroviruses and adequate expression of the introduced gene in hematopoietic stem cells and their progeny remain formidable problems preventing clinical use. Because correction of a mutant gene in the chromosome (rather than introduction of a normal gene copy randomly into the host cell genome) would be preferable since regulated expression would be guaranteed, attention is also being directed to the use of targeted gene insertion.

Current and potential applications of recombinant DNA methods

TABLE 285-2 Recombinant DNA and management of hematologic disease

Application	Examples
Current	
Prenatal diagnosis of inherited disorders	β Thalassemia and sickle cell anemia
Detection of minimal residual disease in malignancy	Translocation in follicular lymphoma Ig or T-cell receptor gene rearrangements
Administration of hematopoietic growth factors	Erythropoietin for anemia of chronic renal disease
Administration of clotting factors	Factor VIII for hemophilia A
Under study	
Modulation of gene expression to ameliorate severity of clinical disease	Stimulation of fetal hemoglobin production in sickle cell anemia Use of γ-interferon in chronic granulomatous disease
Possible for future	
Somatic therapy for the correction of inherited disease	Candidates Hemoglobinopathies Adenosine deaminase deficiency Storage disorders Coagulation deficiencies

in the management of hematologic disease are summarized in Table 285-2.

Disorders of the hematopoietic system have proved to be a fruitful arena for the application of recombinant DNA methods to clinical medicine. Progressively greater impact of these methods on diagnosis and on the understanding of pathophysiology is virtually assured. Sensitive diagnostic approaches to clonality and minimal residual disease are likely to guide future management of malignant disease. Finally, we can be cautiously optimistic about the potential of recombinant DNA technology to provide novel approaches to treatment, including pharmacologic manipulation of gene expression and somatic genetic therapy.

REFERENCES

Erlich HA (ed): *PCR Technology: Principles and Applications for DNA Amplification.* New York, Stockton Press, 1989

Nichols EK: *Human Gene Therapy.* Cambridge, MA, Harvard, 1989

Orkin SH: Reverse genetics in human disease. Cell 47:845, 1986

———: Molecular genetics and inherited human disease, in *The Metabolic Basis of Inherited Disease,* 6th ed, CR Scriver et al (eds). New York, McGraw-Hill, 1989, vol 1

———, Kazazian HH Jr: Mutation and polymorphism of the human beta-globin gene and its surrounding DNA. Ann Rev Genet 18:131, 1984

286 BLOOD GROUPS AND BLOOD TRANSFUSION

ELOISE R. GIBLETT

BLOOD GROUP ANTIGENS AND ANTIBODIES

Human red blood cell membranes contain over 300 different antigenic determinants, the molecular structure of which is dictated by genes at an unknown number of chromosomal loci. The term *blood group* is applied to any well-defined system of red blood cell antigens controlled by a locus having a variable number of allelic genes, such as *A*, *B*, and *O* in the ABO system. Over twenty blood group systems are currently recognized. The term *blood type* refers to the antigen phenotype, which is the serologic expression of the inherited blood group genes.

Alloantibodies specific for the blood group antigens may occur "naturally" (i.e., in the absence of known stimulus by foreign red blood cells) or in response to transfusion or pregnancy. Naturally occurring antibodies tend to be IgM molecules, and many of them (notably excepting anti-A and anti-B) react poorly at body temperature but readily agglutinate red blood cells at 5 to 20°C. Antibodies formed in response to exposure to another person's red blood cells or soluble blood group substances initially belong to the IgM class but usually change to the IgG class within a few weeks or months. In general, these "immune" antibodies react best at body temperature, and special laboratory procedures are required for their detection.

BLOOD GROUP SYSTEMS ABO system: Genes and antigens There are four major allelic genes in this system: A^1, A^2, *B*, and *O*. The locus for these alleles is on the long arm of chromosome 9. The actual products of the first three genes are glycosyltransferases which select specific sugars, *N*-acetyl-D-galactosamine (GalNAc) by the A^1 and A^2 transferases and D-galactose (Gal) by the *B* transferase, attaching them by alpha-linkage to short (oligo) saccharide chains. These chains comprise the carbohydrate moiety of glycolipid and glycoprotein molecules on the red blood cells or in other tissues and fluids. Although the A^1 and A^2 transferases perform the same function, they have different rate constants, so people who inherit an A^1 gene have more A-reactive sites than those with an A^2 gene. The *O* gene product is a protein which cross-reacts immunologically with the *A* and *B* transferase molecules but has no detectable enzyme activity; thus it is functionally "silent."

Nearly all individuals produce "naturally occurring" antibodies against the A or B antigens not present on their own red blood cells, as shown in Table 286-1. This fact is used as the basis for confirming the red blood cell type. Most of the major phenotypes represent more than one genotype. In the absence of family studies, it is possible to infer the genotype from only three phenotypes: A_1B, A_2B, and O. In routine practice, the ABO type is determined by testing the red blood cells with anti-A and anti-B and by testing the serum against A, B, and O red blood cells. Under special circumstances, a further distinction between A and AB types is made by using anti-A_1, an antiserum prepared by absorbing anti-A typing serum with A_2 red blood cells. The remaining unabsorbed antibodies have A_1 specificity, reacting with A_1 and A_1B, but not with A_2 and A_2B cells. (Alternatively, anti-A_1 is prepared as a lectin from extracts of certain seeds.) The frequencies of the various phenotypes in two American blood donor populations are also given in Table 286-1.

Red blood cells of types O and A_2 have large amounts of another antigen, called H, which is the immediate precursor to A and B. H specificity depends on the presence of a fucose (Fuc) residue attached to the oligosaccharides by a transferase that is the product of a very common gene called *H*. (The H and ABO loci are not genetically linked.) In very rare individuals who fail to inherit an *H* gene from either parent (i.e., they are homozygous for its allele, *h*), the *H* transferase is not made, and the H-determining fucose is not attached. This prevents the addition of specific sugars by the *A* and *B* transferases. As a result, even if an *A* or *B* gene has been inherited, the red blood cells are not agglutinated by anti-A, anti-B, or anti-H, while the serum contains all three antibodies. When a patient requiring transfusion has this so-called O_h (or Bombay) phenotype, special arrangements are necessary to obtain blood of the same rare type from a source such as the Red Cross.

About 80 percent of people are either homozygous or heterozygous for the "secretor," or *Se,* gene, which has no effect on the formation of antigens intrinsic to red blood cells but which governs the production of a fucosyltransferase in secretory tissues. Homozygotes for the apparently inactive allele *se* are called *nonsecretors* because their secretory cells produce a very weakly reactive fucosyl transferase, so their body fluids virtually lack H, A, and B antigen activities.

Antibodies in ABO system Red blood cells of newborn infants have a decreased number of H, A, and B reactive sites, and their

TABLE 286-1 Blood types of the ABO system (including Hh)

Genotype*	Phenotype	Antigens on red blood cells†	Antibodies in serum‡	Phenotype frequencies in Americans, %: Western European descent	African descent
A^1A^1, A^1A^2, A^1O	A_1	A_1, (H)	Anti-B (anti-H)	35	23
A^2A^2, A^2O	A_2	A_2, H	Anti-B (anti-A_1)	10	6
BB, *BO*	B	B, (H)	Anti-A, -A_1	8	17
A^1B	A_1B	A, A_1, B	(Anti-H)	3	3
A^2B	A_2B	A, B, H	(Anti-A_1)	1	1
OO	O	H	Anti-A, -A_1 Anti-B	43	50
hh	O_h	None	Anti-A, -A_1 Anti-B Anti-H	Very rare	Very rare

* In all types except the last, the *H* allele is present as *HH* or *Hh*.
† (H) indicates occasional presence of weakly reacting H antigen.
‡ Antibodies in parentheses are, if present, weak cold agglutinins.
SOURCE: Race and Sanger.

plasma normally contains very little anti-A or anti-B. This finding is due to the fact that fetal immunoglobulin production is minimal, while most of the anti-A and anti-B produced in the mother are IgM molecules which cannot cross the placenta. However, in some type O adults, much of the anti-A, anti-B, and anti-AB (a cross-reacting antibody sometimes called anti-C) are of the IgG class and reach the infant's bloodstream. For this reason, ABO hemolytic disease of the newborn usually occurs in A (or B) infants of O mothers.

It is not acceptable medical practice to transfuse A, B, or AB blood into patients whose red blood cells lack the corresponding antigens, since their plasma contains incompatible antibodies. However, it is acceptable to give A or B blood (preferably as packed red blood cells) to AB recipients, or to give O packed red blood cells (*not* whole blood, except in severe emergencies) to patients of type A, B, or AB when the transfusion requirement exceeds the supply of type-specific blood. Although antibodies with A_1 specificity frequently occur in the plasma of A_2 and A_2B subjects, they are almost always weak cold agglutinins. Therefore, if anti-A_1 has been identified in a transfusion patient, it can be ignored unless it reacts in vitro with A_1 red blood cells at 37°C.

Lewis system Antigens in the Lewis system are not produced by red blood cells but are taken up as glycosphingolipid molecules from the surrounding plasma. There are two well-defined Lewis antigenic determinants, Le^a and Le^b, both of which are structurally related to the H, A, and B antigens.

Anti-Le^a and anti-Le^b are fairly common naturally occurring antibodies, produced mainly by subjects of phenotype O, Le(a − b −). Nearly all examples of these antibodies are of the IgM class, so they rarely, if ever, can cross the placenta during pregnancy. Were they to do so, destruction of the infant's red blood cells would be highly unlikely, since the Lewis glycosphingolipids are very poorly developed during fetal life.

Lewis antibodies (particularly anti-Le^a) are complement-binders; anti-Le^a in very rare instances causes transfusion reactions with intravascular hemolysis. However, the plasma of Le(a +) donors usually contains enough soluble Le^a antigen to neutralize the patient's anti-Le^a before it can attack the vulnerable red blood cells. Nevertheless, patients whose plasma contains anti-Le^a that strongly hemolyzes Le(a +) red blood cells or agglutinates them at temperatures above 30°C should be given blood from either Le(a − b +) or Le(a − b −) donors. Anti-Le^b is virtually never a transfusion hazard.

P system Several structurally related antigens are considered together under the heading of a single system called P. As in the ABO and Lewis systems, the gene products are glycosyltransferases, attaching either D-galactose, *N*-acetyl-D-galactosamine, or *N*-acetyl-D-glucosamine to glycosphingolipids on the red blood cell membrane. P_1 and P, the major antigenic determinants, were previously thought to represent the expression of two allelic genes at the same locus, analogous to A^1 and A^2 in the ABO system. However, these two antigens represent quite different sugar sequences, and the genetic interpretation is complex.

Anti-P_1, which occurs frequently, almost never causes red blood cell destruction—the exceptions being those rare examples which react strongly with P_1 red blood cells in vitro at 37°C. In patients with paroxysmal cold hemoglobinuria, the so-called Donath-Landsteiner autoantibodies frequently react with globoside, a very common red blood cell glycosphingolipid with P specificity.

I system The I and i antigenic determinants are structurally heterogeneous, biochemically related to the H, A, B, Le, and P antigens. Most people inherit a gene associated with I antigen production, but the red blood cells of newborn infants react very weakly with anti-I and strongly with anti-i. A gradual reversal occurs during the first year or two, representing the development of I antigen in association with branching of carbohydrate chains on the cell membrane. In patients with certain kinds of "marrow stress," particularly thalassemia and hypoplastic anemia, red blood cell i activity is increased.

Anti-I is a common antibody, frequently found as a weak cold agglutinin of no clinical concern. In patients with the cold type of autoimmune hemolytic anemia, autoantibodies usually have anti-I or anti-I plus i specificity, and most of them belong to the IgM class (see Chap. 294). Anti-i production is associated mainly with lymphoid cell diseases, especially infectious mononucleosis and lymphosarcoma. A patient already having a "marrow-stressing" disorder such as thalassemia may develop an intense autoimmune hemolytic anemia due to anti-i. When transfusions are required, finding compatible blood poses no problem, since the red blood cells of most adults are i-negative. Even patients with strong cold-reacting anti-I antibodies are usually not difficult to transfuse safely if they are kept warm during the infusion. However, since anti-I often fixes complement, washed red cells may be preferable for transfusion to prevent exposure to additional complement components.

MNS system Closely linked genes on chromosome 4 determine the MN and Ss antigens, respectively. There are four inherited haplotypes: MS, Ms, NS, and Ns. Glycophorin A carries M and N specificity, while S and s are on glycophorin B. Absence of these sialoglycoproteins is associated with rare phenotypes such as En(a-), S^u, and M^k, but there are no accompanying hematologic abnormalities.

Anti-M and anti-N are usually naturally occurring IgM agglutinins with little capability of destroying red blood cells. Patients on long-term renal dialysis tend to form anti-N as either an auto- or alloantibody. These N-specific autoantibodies have no hemolytic potential, but they are alleged to cause rejection of kidneys kept refrigerated before transplantation.

Formation of anti-S or anti-s usually requires the stimulus of transfusion or pregnancy, and accordingly these antibodies often belong to the IgG class. A third antibody, anti-U, behaves serologically somewhat like anti-S plus anti-s, being formed in sensitized black subjects whose red blood cells have the S^u phenotype lacking S and s antigens. All three of these antibodies can hemolyze incompatible red blood cells in vivo, but they are readily detectable by adequate compatibility testing.

Rh system The Rh locus is on chromosome 1. Rh antigenic determinants appear to be dependent on interaction between red blood cell membrane protein and phospholipid molecules. Many Rh phenotypes have been described serologically. While the underlying biochemical genetics is not well defined, recent evidence indicates that there are probably at least three tandem Rh loci, somewhat analogous to the complex HLA and immunoglobulin loci. The Rh alleles dictate the structure of a set of epitopes that are usually antithetical: C or c, E or e, and D or d (the latter having no corresponding antibody and therefore being simply the absence of D). These sets are inherited from each parent as a haplotype, such as CDe, cde, cDE, and so forth.

The D(Rh_o) antigen is by far the most immunogenic of this or any other blood group system (except for those previously described systems in which the formation of antibodies does not depend on exposure to foreign red blood cells). About 15 percent of Caucasians lack the D(Rh_o) antigen and are Rh-negative. When transfused only once with Rh-positive blood, these Rh-negative persons have about a 50 percent chance of forming anti-D(Rh_o) antibodies, which could cause destruction of any subsequently transfused Rh-positive red blood cells. For this reason, Rh-negative patients are always given Rh-negative blood except when the transfusion requirements of a male or postmenopausal female exceed the available supply. Giving Rh-positive blood to Rh-negative premenopausal females is a very serious matter, because, unless adequate amounts of Rh immunoglobulin are given to prevent immunization, any subsequent pregnancy with an Rh-positive infant will almost always stimulate a secondary immune response, resulting in hemolytic disease of the newborn.

The Rh antigens C, c, E, and e are considerably less immunogenic than D, and it is impractical to match these antigens in donors and recipients. Of course, when previously sensitized patients form the corresponding antibodies, it is necessary to find donor blood lacking the specific antigens. The difficulty of this search varies. For example, about 20 percent of the population lack the c antigen and thus are compatible donors for a patient whose plasma contains anti-c. However, only 2 percent lack the e antigen, so patients with anti-e pose serious problems, especially when large amounts of blood are required. Blood banks often maintain donor calling lists or frozen red blood cells for use in such cases, and autologous transfusion is especially desirable for nonemergency procedures.

A large proportion of patients with acquired hemolytic anemia of the warm type have IgG autoantibodies which react with one or more Rh-associated antigens. In some instances, the specificity is clear-cut (for example, anti-e), but more often the antibodies react with all red blood cells except those of the rare type known as Rh_{null}. These cells lack all known Rh antigens, and the cell membrane is defective, reinforcing the belief that in normal red blood cells, molecules bearing the Rh determinants are an intrinsic part of the membrane protein structure.

Kidd, Kell, Duffy, and Lutheran systems In the Kell and Duffy systems, anti-K and anti-Fy^a are frequently encountered antibodies capable of marked alloimmune red blood cell destruction. Even more dangerous are the antibodies in the Kidd system, anti-Jk^a and anti-Jk^b, which are notoriously difficult to detect. Whenever a patient has a hemolytic transfusion reaction after transfusion of blood found to be compatible by the usual laboratory tests, the most likely cause is anti-Jk^a. Antibodies in the Lutheran system have only rarely been reported to cause red blood cell destruction.

Other blood group antigens Many other red blood cell antigens have been described. The Xg^a antigen is of considerable scientific importance, since its locus is on the X chromosome. Other antigens are of clinical interest because they occur on the red blood cells of 95 percent or more of most populations, making it difficult to find compatible blood when their antibodies are present in patients requiring transfusion. Fortunately many of these antibodies have little ability to destroy red blood cells, even though they consist of IgG molecules and react in vitro at 37°C. Included in this category are most examples of anti-Sd^a (Sid), anti-Yt^a (Cartwright), anti-Yk^a (York), and many others. Nevertheless, both caution and experience are necessary when considering the transfusion of serologically incompatible blood, particularly when the antibodies react in vitro at body temperature. Antibodies with Chido (Ch^a) and Rodgers (Rg^a) specificity are incapable of causing hemolysis. Their respective antigenic determinants are located on the C4d fragment of the fourth component of complement and are thereby taken up from the plasma by red cells.

BIOLOGIC SIGNIFICANCE OF BLOOD GROUPS Immune reactions The relationship of blood group antigens and antibodies to alloimmune red blood cell destruction has been briefly discussed in the previous sections. Because antigens in the ABO system are present in other tissues, they play a role in determining histocompatibility, so that transplantation of ABO-incompatible kidneys and other organs carries a risk of rejection (see Chap. 225). However, successful grafting of ABO-incompatible bone marrow is possible when the patient is immunosuppressed and either given exchange transfusions of plasma compatible with the donor's red blood cells or the patient's own plasma is passed over a column containing oligosaccharides with A and/or B specificity.

Infertility and early fetal loss Both of these effects have been ascribed to ABO incompatibility, although in some instances the data are of marginal significance. Nevertheless, many population geneticists believe that this factor plays a significant role in the processes of natural selection.

Disease-related phenotype changes A and, to a lesser extent, B determinants are subject to certain biochemical changes, such as those caused by bacterial glycosidases, acetylases, and other enzymes. As a result, the red blood cells may develop new specificities, becoming either "polyagglutinable" or having "pseudo-B" characteristics. Another acquired alteration in ABO type occurs in some patients with acute myelocytic leukemia whose original type is A_1 or B. This change in phenotype, with partial or complete loss of agglutinability by anti-A or anti-B, can occasionally be a diagnostic aid in the early hypoplastic phase of leukemia. The changes in Ii specificity associated with "marrow stress" are described above (see "I System").

Other disease relationships The incidence of certain diseases is related to blood type. For example, type O "nonsecretors" have about twice the incidence of duodenal ulcer than do secretors of types A or B. On the other hand, type A carries a higher incidence of tumors of salivary glands, stomach, and pancreas than does type O. Persons with the rare Rh_{null} type, whose red cells lack all the Rh antigens, have some degree of increased hemolysis, as do people with the McLeod phenotype. McLeod red blood cells react only weakly with antibodies against antigens of the autosomally controlled Kell system because they lack Kx, a very common X-linked Kell precursor antigen. Some boys with the X-linked form of chronic granulomatous disease also have the McLeod phenotype due to deletion of both genes, which are closely linked on the X chromosome. Individuals (mainly of African origin) who lack both Fy^a and Fy^b—the major antigens in the Duffy system—are protected against infestation by the malarial parasite, *Plasmodium vivax*, presumably because Fy^a and Fy^b act as specific recognition or acceptor sites for the merozoites.

Chromosome mapping Blood genetic markers, including the red and white blood cell allotypes as well as the plasma and blood cell enzyme phenotypes, are very useful for mapping the human chromosomes. Some of these markers are genetically linked to loci for genes causing metabolic diseases, and it is possible to predict the development of inherited malfunctions from specimens obtained in utero or from newborn infants. For example, the secretor gene locus is closely linked to the locus of the gene causing myotonic dystrophy, and a determination of the secretor status of a baby at risk can be used to predict the likelihood of its developing this disease, since both characters are inherited as autosomal dominants. In addition, tests for the restriction fragment length polymorphisms (RFLPs) can be performed on any tissue containing cellular DNA, including blood and amniotic fluid. The very large number of these genetic markers adds greatly to our potential ability to predict the occurrence of inherited diseases.

Medicolegal applications When the red blood cell antigens are combined with HLA, RFLPs, and the other genetic markers in blood, the probability of distinguishing one person from another is over 1 billion to 1. This high degree of individuality promotes the usefulness of genetic markers for ruling out paternity, maternity, and monozygosity in nearly all cases where those relationships do not exist.

BLOOD TRANSFUSION

INTRODUCTION Considerable morbidity and, to a lesser extent, mortality are associated with blood transfusion therapy. Responsible medical practice dictates that physicians have sufficient background information to make soundly reasoned judgments concerning the risks as well as the benefits of this procedure. They must decide not only what blood components (if any) are indicated but also what quantities are needed.

WHOLE BLOOD A unit of whole blood consists of approximately 450 mL blood collected into a plastic bag containing 63 mL of either citrate-phosphate-dextrose (CPD) or citrate-phosphate-dextrose–adenine (CPD-A) solution as anticoagulant and preservative. Blood collected in CPD has a refrigerated storage life of only 3 weeks, while CPD-A blood may be kept 5 weeks. At the end of these periods, about 70 to 80 percent of red blood cells are still viable, white blood cells and platelets are nonviable, and clotting factors V and VIII have low levels of activity. The storage time for packed red blood cells harvested from blood collected in CPD or CPD-A can be increased to 49 days by the addition of preservative solutions that contain mannitol.

Virtually the only reason to transfuse whole blood is to restore blood volume lost through recent hemorrhage, as with gastrointestinal bleeding, major surgery, or trauma. For assessing blood loss, routine laboratory tests are misleading for several hours after hemorrhage. Both hemoglobin and hematocrit measurements reflect the ratio of red blood cell mass to blood volume, rather than indicating the total circulating red blood cells. Since the compensatory vasoconstriction evoked by hemorrhage initially prevents extravascular fluids from replacing intravascular fluid loss, both laboratory measurements may be falsely high. Clinically, postural hypotension provides a warning that blood transfusion may be required. Pallor, syncope, tachycardia, thirst, and air hunger are useful indicators of massive blood loss (i.e., 1500 mL or more in adults), sometimes requiring immediate transfusion of type O red blood cells that have not been cross-matched. In less severe cases, maintaining the blood volume with saline or plasma expanders provides time for accurate blood typing and compatibility testing.

During surgery, blood loss can be measured quite accurately, and there is a tendency to "keep up" or even to "stay ahead" of lost volume by transfusion. Such practices lead to unwarranted use of blood with its attendant hazards. In most adult subjects, blood loss of 500 mL is easily tolerated, being equivalent to the amount given by a blood donor. Judicious use of crystalloid infusions is frequently all that is required to circumvent blood transfusion, even with blood losses up to a liter. In modern medicine, ordering "fresh" blood at any time is not acceptable practice, since proper component therapy is both safer and more scientifically based.

PACKED RED BLOOD CELLS The preparation of packed red blood cells from whole blood involves sedimentation or centrifugation followed by removal of plasma into a satellite bag, all in a closed system. Such packed cells have the same storage periods as whole blood. Removal of the plasma provides protection against circulatory overload as well as against excessive loads of sodium, potassium, citrate, ammonia, and antibodies (particularly anti-A) which might be harmful to the patient. Furthermore, the removed plasma can be used for preparing such products as cryoprecipitate, albumin, and immunoglobulins.

In the absence of recent blood loss, most transfusions are given to patients who need replacement of oxygen-carrying capacity. Packed red blood cells are much preferred to whole blood for this purpose, since the plasma serves no useful purpose and may be detrimental, especially in hypervolemic subjects. Diagnoses most frequently associated with the need for packed red blood cells fall into two major categories of anemia, hypoplastic and hemolytic.

Red blood cell hypoplasia Chronic bone marrow depression not responding to medical therapy may, under favorable circumstances, be treated by bone marrow transplantation (see Chap. 299). However, some patients are either unsuitable candidates or have no access to a marrow donor (although the increasing use of unrelated donors is shrinking the number of such subjects). The red blood cell mass of these patients can be maintained at functional levels for long periods, provided they do not develop multiple antibodies against red blood cell antigens. These patients are in general more liable to become immunologically refractory to platelets and white blood cells than to red blood cells. Patients whose red blood cell hypoplasia is secondary to marrow invasion by malignancy and/or to various chemo- or radiotherapeutic agents also require red blood cell transfusions. Again, sensitization to transfused platelets and white blood cells creates a greater problem than red blood cell immunization.

Hemolytic anemia In severe cases of inherited nonimmune hemolysis due to intrinsic red blood cell defects (e.g., sickle cell anemia, thalassemia, or severe deficiencies of glucose-6-phosphate dehydrogenase), the only hope of maintaining oxygen-carrying capacity through a crisis is the careful use of red blood cell transfusion. Patients with other forms of nonimmune hemolysis or ineffective erythropoiesis (e.g., vitamin B_{12}, folate, or iron deficiencies) are candidates for transfusion only if they are severely anemic and if the cause cannot be corrected by specific replacement therapy. Whenever any infusion is given to a patient with severe anemia, the possibility of precipitating heart failure must be recognized and circumvented by careful monitoring.

Patients with autoimmune hemolytic anemia are not good candidates for red blood cell transfusion. Not only are they liable to develop new alloantibodies, but they may have already formed such antibodies as the result of earlier transfusion or pregnancy. In the presence of circulating *auto*antibodies, alloantibodies are often difficult to detect, and transfused red blood cells may be rapidly destroyed. Consultation with a blood transfusion expert is desirable in cases where severe anemia with hypoxemia or cardiac failure poses an immediate threat to life.

PLATELETS Platelet concentrates are prepared by centrifugation of platelet-rich plasma to yield at least 5×10^{10} platelets from each donor unit. More porous plastic bags and gentle agitation facilitate gas transport across the container walls during storage at room temperature. A continuous supply of oxygen maintains aerobic platelet metabolism and prevents harmful drops in pH due to lactic acid production and CO_2 retention. These factors permit platelet storage for up to 5 days with posttransfusion survivals of 6 to 7 days. In adult thrombocytopenic patients without consumptive coagulopathy or platelet-specific antibodies, 1 unit of platelet concentrate raises the platelet count by about 10,000 per microliter.

Patients with idiopathic thrombocytopenic purpura produce autoantibodies which react with all human platelets (see Chap. 287), and therefore derive little or no benefit from platelet transfusion. Similarly, in patients with thrombocytopenia due to a consumptive coagulopathy (as in infection or metastatic malignancy) the usefulness of platelet therapy is limited, unless its purpose is to keep the patient from bleeding while the primary cause is being treated.

The most rational use of platelets is to control bleeding in patients either with a temporary loss of platelets not due to immunity (e.g., massive blood replacement, prolonged surgery) or with suppressed platelet production (leukemia, lymphoma, treatment with radio- or chemotherapy). Since platelets are very immunogenic, and typing and cross-matching techniques are not yet practical, this blood component should not be given in the absence of clear indication. Most nonbleeding patients with platelet counts above 10,000 per microliter can maintain adequate hemostasis. However, patients in the immediate postoperative period may need to have their platelet counts elevated to as high as 100,000 per microliter. In other bleeding situations, a platelet count of 50,000 per microliter or more suggests other causes for hemorrhage, especially if there is no recent history of ingestion of aspirin or other drugs that interfere with platelet function, which would be reflected by a prolonged bleeding time. The effectiveness of platelet transfusion is assessed by comparing the platelet count before the infusion with counts obtained about 1 and 24 h later.

Choice of blood type Ideally, donors of platelets should have the same ABO and Rh types as the patient, since it is impossible to remove all red blood cells and plasma from the platelet concentrate. When it is necessary to use O donors for A, B, or AB recipients, the plasma may contain sufficient anti-A (or anti-B) to destroy some of the patient's red blood cells. Although this possibility is small, it deserves consideration in children or in adults receiving large numbers of platelet concentrates. When platelets of A, B, or AB donors are given to patients of unlike ABO type, the posttransfusion platelet increment may be somewhat diminished, although this is rarely a major problem. However, it is important that the number of red blood cells in such ABO-incompatible preparations be kept as small as possible.

Since some red blood cells are inevitably present in platelet concentrates, Rh-negative patients should receive platelets from Rh-negative donors whenever feasible, particularly if there is a possibility of subsequent pregnancy. However, lack of platelets from Rh-negative donors should not preclude transfusing Rh-positive donor platelets in a life-threatening situation. Patients who have the potential of becoming mothers can be protected against Rh alloimmunization by an injection of Rh immunoglobulin, about 20 μg for each milliliter of Rh-positive red blood cells present in the infusion. In other Rh-negative patients given platelets from Rh-positive donors, Rh-antibody formation can be expected to occur with a high frequency, but these antibodies do not interfere with the survival of subsequently transfused Rh-positive donor platelets, since they do not themselves contain Rh antigens.

Refractory state Patients who receive random donor platelets on more than one or two occasions frequently develop alloantibodies with either HLA or platelet antigen specificities. Such refractory patients can often be maintained with concentrates prepared by plateletpheresis from family members or HLA-compatible community pheresis donors. Failure to achieve a good response to histocompatible platelets suggests the presence of platelet-specific alloantibodies, nonimmune causes of platelet refractoriness, or hypersplenism.

PREVENTION OF PLATELET ALLOIMMUNIZATION Several approaches to preventing platelet alloimmunization have been tested in limited trials. Platelets express only class I, and not class II, HLA antigens, and may therefore not stimulate antibody production. It is thus possible that removal of white blood cells from platelet and red cell preparations can minimize antibody formation. Unfortunately, conflicting results have been reported from the use of leukocyte-poor preparations, probably reflecting the presence of variable numbers of contaminating white blood cells as well as nonstandard criteria for diagnosing alloimmunization. Efforts to settle this important question are in progress. An alternative method of preventing immunization is to reduce antigen exposure by using single-donor platelets obtained by pheresis rather than by using pooled platelet concentrates. This strategy probably delays but usually does not prevent eventual immunization.

WHITE BLOOD CELL TRANSFUSIONS Since it is now possible with platelet transfusions to control bleeding in many patients with hematologic malignancies, hemorrhage has been supplanted by infection as the most frequent cause of death. In general, neutrophil transfusion therapy should be considered in patients with severe neutropenia who have documented bacterial infections not responsive to appropriate antibiotic therapy. A course of neutrophil support usually consists of daily transfusion of 10 to 30 $\times$ 10^9 neutrophils, obtained from normal donors by leukapheresis. Problems of maintaining patients for long periods in this way are even more difficult than those associated with platelets. Neutrophils have a very short life span in the bloodstream, and many questions remain unanswered about the best dosage schedules, the feasibility of neutrophil storage, the efficacy of neutrophils for fungal infections, and the recognition and management of alloimmunization. Hazards include alloimmunization to HLA and other antigens, pulmonary damage and other transfusion reactions, as well as graft-versus-host reactions and transmission of infection, particularly cytomegalovirus (CMV), to immunosuppressed recipients, including immunoincompetent infants. Irradiated and leukocyte-poor preparations reduce these risks, and are routinely used in patients undergoing marrow transplantation. The possibility of CMV infection is further reduced by selecting CMV-negative donors for these patients and those receiving transfusions of white blood cells if they are CMV negative.

PLASMA COMPONENT THERAPY Fresh frozen plasma and cryoprecipitate are major blood component preparations because they are necessary for the care of patients with coagulation disorders (see Chap. 288). Plasma can be used for expanding intravascular volume, but it carries the risk of viral transmission. Commercially prepared albumin solutions are preferable as volume expanders, as they have been heated to inactivate viruses. They are useful in special cases, such as nephrosis, certain gastroenteropathies, and severe malnutrition. Immunoglobulin preparations are also commercially made, including specific hyperimmune globulin for preventing the development of certain infectious diseases and for blocking the immune response to Rh antigen. Special clotting factor concentrates for the treatment of bleeding disorders and antithrombin III for coronary artery occlusion are discussed in appropriate chapters of this book.

PLASMAPHERESIS The introduction of cell separators has made plasmapheresis a simple procedure wherein as much as one to two plasma volumes may be exchanged in 1 to 3 h. The procedure has generally been used to reduce the plasma concentration of proteins, lipids, protein-bound hormones or toxins, antibodies, antigens, or immune complexes. While the number of different diseases that have been managed by this procedure is considerable, there are only a few in which the role of plasmapheresis is generally accepted. Even then, there is controversy regarding the frequency and volume of exchange as well as the nature of replacement fluids.

The most established indication is symptomatic hyperviscosity syndrome; plasmapheresis in this setting reproducibly results in clinical improvement. Plasmapheresis can also be used successfully in selected patients with myasthenia gravis, Goodpasture's syndrome, thrombotic thrombocytopenic purpura, and immune-complex-mediated vasculitis.

COMPLICATIONS OF BLOOD TRANSFUSION Transfusion reactions are classified as immune or nonimmune. The immunologically mediated reactions may be directed against red or white blood cells, platelets, or at least one of the immunoglobulins, IgA. Other less well defined hypersensitivity reactions also occur. The major nonimmune reactions are due to circulatory overload, massive transfusion, or transmission of an infectious agent.

Reactions due to red blood cells Hemolysis due to red blood cell alloantibodies may occur within the circulation or extravascularly. The very rapid cell destruction associated with *intravascular hemolysis* is usually due to incompatibility within the ABO system, since both anti-A and anti-B fix complement, regardless of whether they are IgM or IgG molecules. Other possibilities to consider are anti-Jk^a, anti-Fy^a, and rarely anti-Le^a. Rh antibodies are usually not associated with hemoglobinemia. Symptoms include restlessness, anxiety, flushing, chest or lumbar pain, tachypnea, tachycardia, and nausea, followed by the typical findings of shock and renal failure. In comatose or anesthetized patients, the first sign of danger is often oozing of blood from the mucous membranes or operative site, due to intravascular coagulation.

Extravascular hemolysis is most commonly caused by antibodies of the Rh system, but several other antibodies, especially of the Kell, Duffy, and Kidd systems, are among the offenders. The clinical manifestations are usually milder, consisting of malaise and fever. Shock and renal complications rarely occur. Some patients have delayed reactions in which the transfused red blood cells have normal survival initially, but about a week later they are rapidly destroyed in the reticuloendothelial system. Such delayed reactions are commonly due to an anamnestic rise in antibodies previously stimulated by transfusion or pregnancy. Rarely, patients are found to have destroyed all the transfused cells in the absence of demonstrable antibodies.

LABORATORY INVESTIGATION Of first importance in the investigation of a hemolytic transfusion reaction is a careful check on the identity of both the donor and the recipient, since clerical errors, especially mistakes in identity, are most frequently involved. Then the necessary steps include demonstrating that red blood cell destruction has occurred, investigating its cause, and determining the status of the patient's renal and coagulation mechanisms.

With recent *intravascular* lysis, the hemoglobin level is elevated in both plasma and urine (blood must be drawn cautiously to avoid red blood cell rupture). Also, depending on the number of red blood cells destroyed, there may be methemalbuminemia accompanied by marked reduction of serum haptoglobin and hemopexin. (Measuring the latter two substances is rarely necessary, and to be meaningful, both tests require knowledge of the pretransfusion levels for comparison.) The best indicator of *extravascular* lysis is a rise in unconjugated bilirubin, accompanied by failure of the hematocrit to reach the expected posttransfusion level.

Having a *pretransfusion* specimen of the patient's blood is very helpful, so that determination of both donor and recipient blood types can be repeated, along with the compatibility test. If antibodies are detected, this pretransfusion specimen is also valuable for determining specificity, aided by knowledge of the full antigen composition, since alloantibodies are formed only against antigens not present on the patient's own cells. The *posttransfusion* specimen may not contain the offending antibodies, since they could have been completely absorbed by the donor's incompatible red blood cells. However, it is desirable to examine the red blood cells in the posttransfusion sample, both microscopically for agglutinates and by the direct antiglobulin (Coombs) test. A positive result usually means that some of the donor's red blood cells, coated by the patient's antibodies, were still present when the blood was drawn. But it is also possible that the *donor's* plasma contained antibodies, missed during the donor screening procedure, which reacted with the red blood cells of the patient. Thus, if the direct antiglobulin test on the posttransfusion specimen is positive, the plasma of both donor and recipient should be examined for the responsible antibodies. In the absence of ABO incompatibility, significant destruction of a patient's red blood cells by a donor's alloantibodies is distinctly rare. More typically, the antibody-coated red blood cells survive well in vivo, but their presence can lead to a misdiagnosis of acquired hemolytic anemia.

TREATMENT The care of patients with extravascular hemolysis should be conservative, avoiding additional transfusion unless the patient's life is otherwise threatened. Intravascular hemolysis is a far greater hazard, since shock and renal failure can occur. Immediate treatment with an osmotic diuretic is indicated unless acute tubular necrosis has already occurred. Renal blood flow can be increased with appropriate agents, shock controlled symptomatically, and disseminated intravascular coagulation treated appropriately. Management of the coagulopathy is discussed in Chap. 289, and treatment of renal shutdown in Chap. 223.

Other immunologically related reactions In the absence of red blood cell destruction, most febrile reactions can be ascribed to immunity against white blood cell, platelet, or plasma antigens. Further laboratory workup is required only when the reaction is unusually severe. For example, patients with antibodies against IgA molecules sometimes undergo severe shock upon exposure to the blood of other human subjects. Such individuals must be transfused only with blood that lacks IgA or with repeatedly washed red blood cells. Patients with antibodies against white blood cells or platelets can usually be given packed red blood cells from which leukocytes have been removed after centrifugation or by filtration. Some centers use frozen and thawed red blood cells for transfusing patients sensitized to white blood cells, or to retard the occurrence of such sensitization in candidates for bone marrow transplantation. However, in patients who are candidates for renal transplantation, prior transfusions with white cell–containing products are often associated with improved prognosis—especially if the blood donor is subsequently used as the kidney donor.

Nonimmune transfusion reactions Included in this category are circulatory overload, adverse effects of massive transfusion, infections, metabolic shock, air and fat embolisms, thrombophlebitis, and siderosis. The first three are by far the most common.

CIRCULATORY OVERLOAD Patients with renal or cardiac insufficiency are liable to develop circulatory failure and pulmonary edema with even modest amounts of intravenous infusion. Infants are also vulnerable, since their vasculature does not accommodate rapidly to infusions. The onset may be immediate or delayed for up to 24 h after transfusion, with dyspnea and chest pain progressing to the full-blown picture of pulmonary edema. Susceptible patients should be transfused in a sitting position, with the rate of red blood cell flow not exceeding 2 mL/min, depending on body size and degree of impairment. A rise in central venous pressure heralds the danger of administering more red blood cells unless they are exchanged with whole blood removed from the patient.

MASSIVE TRANSFUSION When the amount of stored blood transfused to bleeding patients greatly exceeds their normal blood volume, dilutional thrombocytopenia can occur, requiring infusion of platelet concentrates. Fresh frozen plasma is only rarely useful, but if the factor 8 level or fibrinogen content is low, infusing an appropriate amount of cryoprecipitate should be considered.

INFECTION Many diseases, such as hepatitis, cytomegalovirus infection, syphilis, malaria, toxoplasmosis, brucellosis, and the acquired immunodeficiency syndrome (AIDS) can be transmitted by transfusion. In addition, blood that becomes infected during handling and storage can cause very severe shock, owing to toxic bacterial metabolites. Testing donated blood for evidence of transmissible infection is increasingly important to reduce transfusion risks. Tests for hepatitis B virus antigen and syphilis, as well as for the antibody to HIV (the AIDS-associated virus), are routinely performed on all donor units. In addition, many laboratories are now including "surrogate" tests for the hepatitis B core antibody and measurements of the plasma level of alanine–amino transferase. The current risk of hepatitis transmission by transfusion is not known, because these tests have only recently been introduced, and a test for non-A, non-B hepatitis will soon be available.

As mentioned earlier, CMV-negative immunocompromised patients, including low birthweight neonates, are candidates to receive blood products found negative for the CMV antibody. To reduce the risk of AIDS transmission, patients at high risk for the disease are instructed not to serve as donors. In addition, all blood is tested for the HIV antibody using an ELISA technique. Confirmatory tests, such as the Western blot technique, are performed before the donor is informed of a positive result, but blood found positive by the ELISA test is discarded. Transmission of AIDS by transfusion is now very rare, although sporadic cases may still occur when high-risk donors fail to be detected, especially during the early period after their exposure to the virus. The popularity of autologous transfusion has increased considerably in recent years and is a good procedure to consider, especially in patients who are candidates for elective surgery.

REFERENCES

ANSTEE DJ: Blood group active components of the human red cell membrane, in *Red Cell Antigens and Antibodies*, G Garratty (ed). Arlington, VA, American Association of Blood Banks, 1986, p 1

BARNES DM: HTLV-I: To test or not to test. Science 242:372, 1988

BEAL RW, ISBISTER JB: *Blood Component Therapy in Clinical Practice*. New York, Blackwell, 1988

BLOY C et al: Determination of the N-terminal sequence of human red cell Rh(D) polypeptide and demonstration that the Rh(D), (c), and (E) antigens are carried by distinct polypeptide chains. Blood 72:661, 1988

BOVE JR: Transfusion-transmitted diseases: Current problems and challenges, in *Progress in Hematology XIV*, EB Brown (ed). New York, Grune and Stratton, 1986, p 123

DAHR W: Immunochemistry of sialoglycoproteins in human red blood cell membranes, in *Recent Advances in Blood Group Biochemistry*, V Vengelen-Tyler and WJ Judd (eds). Arlington, VA, American Association of Blood Banks, 1986, p 23

GIBLETT ER: Blood group alloantibodies: An assessment of some laboratory practices. Transfusion 17:299, 1977

GIBLETT ER: Erythrocyte antigens and antibodies, in *Hematology*, 3d ed, WJ Williams et al (eds). New York, McGraw-Hill, in press, 1989

HAKOMORI S: Blood group ABH and Ii antigens of human erythrocytes: Chemistry, polymorphism and their developmental change. Semin Hematol 18:39, 1981

ISSITT PD: *Applied Blood Group Serology*, 3d ed. Miami, Montgomery Scientific Publications, 1985

KORETZ RL et al: Non-A, non-B transfusion hepatitis—a decade later. Gastroenterology 88:1251, 1985

MARSH WL, REDMAN CM: Recent developments in the Kell blood group system. Transf Med Rev 1:4, 1987

MOLLISON PL et al: *Blood Transfusion in Clinical Medicine*, 8th ed. Oxford, Blackwell, 1987

PITTIGLIO DH: Genetics and biochemistry of A, B, H and Lewis antigens, in *Blood Group Systems: ABH and Lewis*. Arlington, VA, American Association of Blood Banks, 1986, p 1

PETZ LD, SWISHER SN (eds): *Clinical Practice of Blood Transfusion*. New York, Churchill Livingston, 1981

RACE RR, SANGER R: *Blood Groups in Man*, 6th ed. Oxford, Blackwell, 1975

SLICHTER SJ: Transfusion and bone marrow transplantation. Transf Med Rev 2:1, 1988

WATKINS WM: Biochemistry and genetics of the ABO, Lewis, and P blood group systems, in *Advances in Human Genetics*, H Harris, K Hirschhorn (eds). New York, Plenum, 1980, vol 10, pp 1–136, 379–385

section 1 Clotting disorders

287 DISORDERS OF THE PLATELET AND VESSEL WALL

ROBERT I. HANDIN

Patients with platelet or vessel wall disorders usually bleed into superficial sites such as the skin, mucous membranes, genitourinary or gastrointestinal tract. Bleeding begins immediately after trauma and either responds to simple measures like pressure and packing, or requires systemic therapy with glucocorticoids, plasma fractions, or platelet concentrates. The most common platelet/vessel wall disorders are (1) various forms of thrombocytopenia, (2) von Willebrand's disease, and (3) drug-induced platelet dysfunction. This chapter reviews the diagnosis and treatment of quantitative and qualitative platelet disorders as well as vessel wall defects which cause bleeding. The physiology of normal hemostasis and the cardinal manifestations of bleeding arising from hemostatic disorders have been reviewed in Chap. 62.

PLATELET PRODUCTION AND KINETICS Platelets arise from the fragmentation of megakaryocytes, which are very large, polyploid bone marrow cells produced by several cycles of chromosomal duplication without cytoplasmic division. After leaving the marrow space, approximately one-third of the platelets are sequestered in the spleen, while the other two-thirds circulate for 7 to 10 days. Normally, only a small fraction of the platelet mass is consumed in the process of hemostasis, so that most platelets circulate until they become senescent and are removed by phagocytic cells. The normal blood platelet count is maintained between 150,000 and 450,000 per microliter. Although the regulatory signals are not well-defined, a decrease in platelet mass stimulates an increase in the number, size, and ploidy of megakaryocytes releasing additional platelets into the circulation.

The platelet count varies during the menstrual cycle, rising following ovulation and falling at the onset of menses. It is also influenced by the patient's nutritional state and can be decreased in severe iron, folic acid, or vitamin B_{12} deficiency. Platelets are *acute phase reactants* and patients with systemic inflammation, tumors, bleeding, and mild iron deficiency may have an increased platelet count, a benign condition called *secondary or reactive thrombocytosis*. In contrast, the increase in platelet count that is characteristic of the myeloproliferative disorders such as polycythemia vera, chronic myelogenous leukemia, myeloid metaplasia, and essential thrombocytosis can cause either severe bleeding or thrombosis.

MECHANISM OF THROMBOCYTOPENIA Thrombocytopenia is caused by one of three mechanisms—decreased bone marrow production, increased splenic sequestration, or accelerated destruction of platelets. In order to determine the etiology of thrombocytopenia, each patient should have a careful examination of the peripheral blood film, an assessment of marrow morphology by examination of an aspirate or biopsy, and an estimate of splenic size by bedside palpation. A scheme for classifying patients with thrombocytopenia based on these clinical observations and laboratory tests is outlined in Fig. 287-1.

Impaired production Disorders that injure stem cells or prevent their proliferation in marrow frequently cause thrombocytopenia. They usually affect multiple hematopoietic cell lines so that thrombocytopenia is accompanied by varying degrees of anemia and leukopenia. Diagnosis of a platelet production defect is readily established by examination of a bone marrow aspirate or biopsy, which should show a reduced number of megakaryocytes. The most common causes of decreased platelet production are marrow aplasia, fibrosis, or infiltration with malignant cells, all of which produce highly characteristic marrow abnormalities. Occasionally, thrombocytopenia is the presenting laboratory abnormality in these disorders. Cytotoxic drugs, which are frequently used in cancer chemotherapy, impair megakaryocyte proliferation and maturation and frequently cause thrombocytopenia. There are also rare marrow disorders like congenital amegakaryocytic hypoplasia and thrombocytopenia with absent radii (TAR syndrome), which selectively decrease megakaryocyte production.

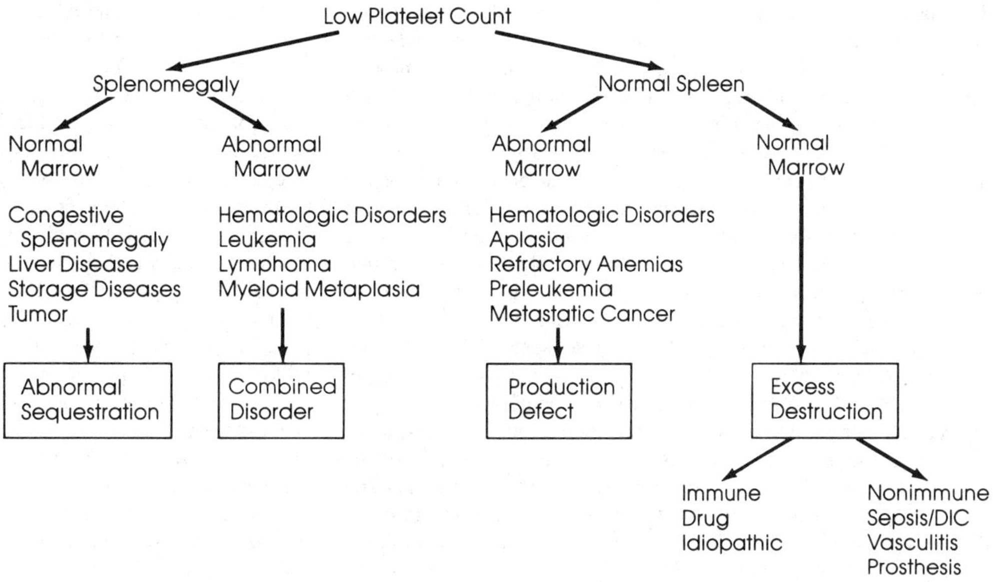

FIGURE 287-1 The clinical evaluation of patients with thrombocytopenia [*Modified from RI Handin, in W Beck (ed). Hematology, 4th ed, MIT Press, Cambridge, MA, 1985.*]

Splenic sequestration Since one-third of the platelet mass is normally sequestered in the spleen, splenectomy will increase the platelet count by 30 percent. In contrast, when the spleen enlarges, the fraction of sequestered platelets increases, lowering the platelet count. The most common causes of splenomegaly are portal hypertension secondary to liver disease, splenic infiltration with tumor cells in myeloproliferative or lymphoproliferative disorders, or with macrophages in storage disorders like Gaucher's disease. Isolated splenomegaly is rare and, in most patients, splenomegaly is accompanied by other clinical manifestations of the underlying disease. Many patients with leukemia, lymphoma, or a myeloproliferative syndrome have both marrow infiltration and splenomegaly and develop thrombocytopenia from a combination of impaired marrow production and splenic sequestration of platelets.

Accelerated destruction Abnormal vessels, fibrin thrombi, or intravascular prostheses can all shorten platelet survival and cause *nonimmunologic thrombocytopenia*. For example, thrombocytopenia is common in patients with vasculitis, the hemolytic uremic syndrome, thrombotic thrombocytopenic purpura (TTP), as one manifestation of disseminated intravascular coagulation (DIC), and in patients with prosthetic cardiac valves. In addition, platelets coated with antibody, immune complexes, or complement are rapidly cleared by mononuclear phagocytes in the spleen or other tissues inducing *immunologic thrombocytopenia*. The most common causes of immunologic thrombocytopenia are viral or bacterial infections, drugs, and a chronic autoimmune disorder referred to as idiopathic thrombocytopenic purpura (ITP). Patients with immunologic thrombocytopenia do not usually have splenomegaly and have an active bone marrow with an increased number of megakaryocytes.

DRUG-INDUCED THROMBOCYTOPENIA Many common drugs can cause thrombocytopenia (see Table 287-1). As previously mentioned, many chemotherapeutic agents are cytotoxic and depress megakaryocyte production. Ingestion of large quantities of alcohol has a similar marrow-depressing effect leading to transient thrombocytopenia. The syndrome is particularly common in binge drinkers. Thiazide diuretics, which are commonly used to treat hypertension or congestive heart failure, impair megakaryocyte production and can produce mild thrombocytopenia (50,000 to 100,000 per microliter), which may persist for several months after the drug is discontinued.

Most drugs induce thrombocytopenia by eliciting an immune response in which the platelet is an innocent bystander. The platelet is damaged by complement activation following the formation of drug-antibody complexes. Current laboratory tests can identify the causative agent in 10 percent of patients with clinical evidence of drug-induced thrombocytopenia. The best proof of a drug-induced etiology is a prompt rise in the platelet count when the suspected drug is discontinued. Patients with drug-induced platelet destruction may also have a secondary increase in megakaryocyte number without other marrow abnormalities.

Although most patients recover within 7 to 10 days and do not require therapy, occasional patients with platelet counts below 10,000 to 20,000 per microliter have severe hemorrhage and may require temporary support with glucocorticoids, plasmapheresis, or platelet transfusions while waiting for the platelet count to rise. A patient who has recovered from drug-induced immunologic thrombocytopenia should be instructed to avoid the offending drug in the future since only minute amounts of drug are needed to set up subsequent immune reactions. Certain drugs like phenytoin and gold salts may induce prolonged thrombocytopenia, since the drugs are cleared from body storage depots quite slowly. Heparin deserves special mention as it is a common cause of thrombocytopenia in hospitalized patients. It is estimated that 10 percent of patients receiving therapeutic doses of heparin develop thrombocytopenia and, occasionally, may have severe bleeding or intravascular platelet aggregation and paradoxical

TABLE 287-1 Drugs implicated in thrombocytopenia

I Suppression of platelet production
- *A* Myelosuppressive drugs
  - *1* Severe: cytosine arabinoside, daunorubicin
  - *2* Moderate: cyclophosphamide, busulfan, methotrexate, 6-mercaptopurine
  - *3* Mild: vinca alkaloids
- *B* Thiazide diuretics
- *C* Ethanol
- *D* Estrogens

II Immunologic platelet destruction
- *A* Clinical suspicion plus convincing experimental evidence
  - *1* Antibiotics: sulfathiazole, novobiocin, *p*-aminosalicylate
  - *2* Cinchona alkaloids: quinidine, quinine
  - *3* Foods: beans
  - *4* Sedatives, hypnotics, anticonvulsants: apronalide, carbamazepine
  - *5* Arsenical drugs used to treat syphilis
  - *6* Digitoxin
  - *7* Methyldopa
  - *8* Stibophen
- *B* Clinical suspicion (major drugs implicated)
  - *1* Aspirin
  - *2* Chlorpropamide
  - *3* Chloroquine
  - *4* Chlorothiazide and hydrochlorothiazide
  - *5* Gold salts
  - *6* Insecticides
  - *7* Sulfadiazine, sulfisoxazole, sulfamerazine, sulfamethazine, sulfamethoxypyridazine, sulfamethoxazole, sulfatolamide

thrombosis. Although many cases of heparin thrombocytopenia are due to drug-antibody binding to platelets, some may be secondary to direct platelet agglutination by heparin. In either case, prompt cessation of heparin will reverse the thrombocytopenia. The syndrome is more common with heparin derived from beef lung.

IDIOPATHIC THROMBOCYTOPENIC PURPURA (ITP) The immunologic thrombocytopenias can be classified on the basis of the pathologic mechanism, the inciting agent, or the duration of the illness. The explosive onset of severe thrombocytopenia following recovery from a viral exanthem or upper respiratory illness is common in children and accounts for 90 percent of the pediatric cases of immunologic thrombocytopenia. This syndrome is usually called *acute idiopathic thrombocytopenic purpura* (acute ITP). Of these patients, 60 percent recover in 4 to 6 weeks and over 90 percent recover within 3 to 6 months. Transient immunologic thrombocytopenia also complicates some cases of infectious mononucleosis, acute toxoplasmosis, or cytomegalovirus infection and can be part of the prodromal phase of viral hepatitis. Acute ITP is rare in adults and accounts for less than 10 percent of postpubertal patients with immune thrombocytopenia. Acute ITP is caused by immune complexes containing viral antigens which bind to platelet Fc receptors or by antibodies produced against viral antigens which cross react with the platelet. In addition to the viral disorders described above, the differential diagnosis should include atypical presentations of aplastic anemia, acute leukemias, or metastatic tumor. A bone marrow examination is essential to exclude these disorders, which can occasionally mimic acute ITP.

Most adults present with a more indolent form of thrombocytopenia which may persist for many years and is referred to as *chronic ITP*. Women aged 20 to 40 are most commonly afflicted and outnumber men by a ratio of 3:1. They may present with an abrupt fall in platelet count and bleeding similar to patients with acute ITP. More often they have a prior history of easy bruising or menometrorrhagia. These patients have an autoimmune disorder with antibodies directed against target antigens on the glycoprotein IIb-IIIa complex or glycoprotein Ib (see Fig. 62-2). Although most antibodies function as opsonins and accelerate platelet clearance by phagocytic cells, occasional antibodies bind to epitopes on critical regions of these glycoproteins and impair platelet function.

Since a low platelet count may be the initial manifestation of systemic lupus erythematosus (SLE) or the first sign of a primary hematologic disorder, all patients with chronic ITP should have a bone marrow examination and an antinuclear antibody determination. In addition, patients with hepatic or splenic enlargement, lymphadenopathy, or atypical lymphocytes should have serologic studies for hepatitis, cytomegalovirus, Epstein-Barr virus, toxoplasma, and HIV. HIV infection has rapidly become a common cause of immunologic thrombocytopenia and should be considered in the differential diagnosis of thrombocytopenia in high-risk groups—homosexuals, hemophiliacs, and intravenous drug abusers. Thrombocytopenia can be (1) the initial symptom of HIV infection, (2) a manifestation of the AIDS-related complex (ARC), or (3) a complication of fully developed AIDS.

Treatment of patients with ITP must take into account the age of the patient, the severity of the illness, and the anticipated natural history. Although adults have a higher incidence of intracranial bleeding than children, specific therapy may not be necessary unless the platelet count is under 20,000 per microliter or there is extensive bleeding. Hemorrhage in patients with either acute or chronic ITP can usually be controlled with glucocorticoids but, in rare cases, may require plasmapheresis to reduce the antibody or immune complex level, or temporary phagocytic blockade with intravenous gamma globulin. Emergency splenectomy is usually reserved for patients with acute or chronic ITP who are desperately ill and have not responded to any medical measures designed to improve hemostasis. The treatment of symptomatic thrombocytopenia in patients with HIV infection presents a special problem because the administration of glucocorticoids or splenectomy may increase susceptibility to the opportunistic infections which threaten these patients. Splenectomy has been effective in the course of HIV infection prior to the onset of symptomatic AIDS.

Symptomatic patients with chronic ITP are usually placed on glucocorticoids. In one standard regimen, 60 mg of prednisone is administered for 2 to 4 weeks and rapidly decreased over another week. Approximately 50 percent of patients with chronic ITP will normalize their platelet count on these high doses of prednisone. However, the majority will have a fall in platelet count following steroid withdrawal. Patients with chronic ITP who fail to maintain a normal platelet count after 2 to 3 weeks of steroids are eligible for elective splenectomy. These steroid-responsive but steroid-dependent patients are very likely to respond to splenectomy, and 70 percent will have a normal platelet count within 1 week after surgery. Some patients who do not respond to glucocorticoids may still respond to splenectomy.

Patients who are still thrombocytopenic after steroid therapy or splenectomy or who relapse months to years after initial therapy have received a variety of immunosuppressive drugs including azathioprine, cyclophosphamide, vincristine, and vinblastine. More recently danazol, an impeded androgen, has been used with some success. Although each of these drugs may be beneficial, it is important to use some restraint as they have serious side effects. If a patient is not bleeding and maintains a platelet count over 20,000 per microliter, consideration should be given to withholding therapy, since there are many patients with severe chronic thrombocytopenia who have lived with their disease for two or three decades.

VON WILLEBRAND'S DISEASE Von Willebrand's disease (vWD) is the most common inherited bleeding disorder and may occur in as many as 1 in 800 to 1000 individuals. The von Willebrand factor (vWF) is a heterogeneous multimeric plasma glycoprotein with two major functions. It facilitates platelet adhesion under conditions of high shear stress by linking platelet membrane receptors to vascular subendothelium; it also serves as the plasma carrier for factor VIII, the antihemophilic factor, a critical blood coagulation protein. The normal plasma vWF level is 10 mg/L. The vWF activity is distributed among a series of plasma multimers with estimated molecular weights ranging from 400,000 to over 20 million. A single large vWF precursor subunit is synthesized in endothelial cells and megakaryocytes, where it is cleaved and assembled into the disulfide-linked multimers present in plasma, platelets, and vascular subendothelium. A modest reduction in plasma vWF concentration, or a selective loss in the high-molecular-weight multimers, decreases platelet adhesion and causes clinical bleeding.

Although vWD is heterogeneous, there are certain clinical features which are common to all the syndromes. With one exception (type III disease), all forms are inherited as autosomal dominant traits and affected patients are heterozygous with one normal and one abnormal vWF allele. In mild cases, bleeding occurs only after surgery or trauma. More severely affected patients have spontaneous epistaxis or oral mucosal, gastrointestinal, or genitourinary bleeding. The laboratory findings are variable. The most diagnostic pattern is the combination of (1) a prolonged bleeding time, (2) a reduction in plasma vWF concentration, (3) a parallel reduction in ristocetin cofactor activity, and (4) reduced factor VIII activity. The variability in laboratory tests is related both to the heterogeneous nature of the defects in vWD and the fact that vWF synthesis or release is increased by ABO blood group type, central nervous disorders, systemic inflammation, or pregnancy. Since vWD is an autosomal dominant disorder, some vWF is produced by the remaining normal allele. Thus, patients with mild defects may have laboratory values that fluctuate over time and may occasionally be within the normal range.

The cDNA for vWF has been cloned and the gene localized to chromosome 12. Information is now appearing regarding the molecular genetics of the von Willebrand syndromes. There are three major types of vWD. Patients with *type I disease*, the most common abnormality, have a mild to moderate decrease in plasma vWF. In the milder cases, although hemostasis is clearly impaired, the vWF level is just below the lower limit of normal (50 percent activity, or 5 mg/L). In type I disease there is a parallel decrease in vWF antigen, factor VIII activity, and ristocetin cofactor activity, with a normal spectrum of multimers detected by sodium dodecyl sulfate–agarose (SDS-agarose) gel electrophoresis. Cultured endothelial cells derived from the umbilical cords of patients with vWD synthesize and secrete reduced quantities of vWF multimer and have a two- to fourfold reduction in vWF mRNA.

The variant forms of vWD (*type II disease*), which are much less common, are characterized by normal or near-normal levels of a dysfunctional protein. Patients with the *type IIa variant* of vWD have a deficiency in the high- and medium-molecular-weight forms of vWF multimer detected by SDS-agarose electrophoresis. This is due either to an inability to assemble the high-molecular-weight multimers or to premature catabolism after they leave the endothelial cell and enter the circulation. vWF protein derived from type IIa endothelial cells is unusually susceptible to proteolysis, in keeping with the observations of in vivo proteolytic degradation and rapid catabolism. The quantity of vWF antigen and the amount of associated factor VIII are usually normal. In the *type IIb variant,* there is also a loss in high-molecular-weight multimers. However, in type IIb cases, it is due to the inappropriate binding of vWF to platelets. This forms intravascular platelet aggregates which are rapidly cleared from the circulation causing mild, cyclic thrombocytopenia. Levels of total vWF antigen and factor VIII usually remain normal.

Approximately 1 in 1 million individuals have a very severe form of vWD that is phenotypically recessive (*type III disease*). Type III patients are usually the offspring of two parents with mild type I disease. However, in many cases, the parents are very mildly affected or are asymptomatic. Type III patients may inherit a different abnormality from each parent (a doubly heterozygous state) or be homozygous for a single defect. Type III patients have severe mucosal bleeding, no detectable vWF antigen or activity, and may have sufficiently low factor VIII levels to have occasional hemarthroses like mild hemophiliacs. Several type III families have been described with major deletions in the vWF gene that were detected by Southern blotting with vWF cDNA.

Appropriate therapy of vWD depends on the symptoms and the underlying type of disease. There are two therapeutic options. One involves the use of cryoprecipitate, which is a plasma fraction enriched in vWF and is appropriate treatment for all the inherited forms of vWD. During surgery, or after major trauma, patients should receive ten bags of cryoprecipitate twice daily. This regimen should be continued twice daily for 48 to 72 h to ensure optimal hemostasis. Minor bleeding episodes such as prolonged epistaxis or severe menorrhagia may respond to a single transfusion of cryoprecipitate. Recurrent menorrhagia, a major problem for women with severe vWD, can be effectively treated with oral contraceptive agents that suppress menses.

A second therapeutic option, which avoids the use of plasma and its attendant risk of serious viral infections, is the use of 1-desamino-8-D-arginine vasopressin (DDAVP), a vasopressin analogue which has minimal blood pressure–elevating and fluid-retaining properties and raises the plasma vWF level in normal individuals and patients with mild vWD. Patients with type I disease are the best candidates for DDAVP therapy. However, they must be tested for an adequate response prior to anticipated surgery, and vWF levels must be closely monitored during therapy since the patient may develop tachyphylaxis when therapy is continued for more than 48 h. DDAVP should not be given to patients with variant forms of vWD without prior testing, since it may not improve multimer pattern or hemostasis in type IIa patients, and it may actually worsen the defect or cause thrombotic complications in type IIb patients, since it increases the number of platelet-vWF aggregates and the degree of thrombocytopenia. It is also ineffective therapy for most patients with the severe form (type III) of vWD.

Although most cases of vWD are inherited, there are also acquired forms of vWD caused by antibodies which inhibit vWF function or by lymphoid or other tumors which selectively adsorb vWF multimers onto their surfaces. Anti-vWF antibodies have developed in patients with severe vWD following multiple transfusions, as well as in patients with autoimmune and lymphoproliferative disorders. Adsorption of vWF to tumor surfaces has been documented in patients with Waldenstrom's macroglobulinemia and Wilm's tumor and inferred in other patients with lymphoma. Treatment of acquired vWD should focus on controlling the underlying disease, since cryoprecipitate and DDAVP are usually not effective and the disorder can be fatal.

PLATELET MEMBRANE DEFECTS Receptors which modulate platelet adhesion and aggregation are located on the two major platelet surface glycoproteins. As previously discussed (see Chap. 62), vWF facilitates platelet adhesion by binding to glycoprotein Ib, while fibrinogen links platelets into aggregates via sites on the glycoprotein IIb-IIIa complex. There are two rare but well-defined platelet defects characterized by the loss of these glycoprotein receptors. Patients with the *Bernard-Soulier syndrome* have markedly reduced platelet adhesion and cannot bind vWF to their platelets owing to a deficiency in glycoprotein Ib complex. They also have reduced levels of several other membrane proteins, mild thrombocytopenia, and extremely large, lymphocytoid platelets. Platelets from patients with *Glanzmann's disease* or *thrombasthenia* are missing or markedly deficient in the glycoprotein IIb-IIIa complex. Their platelets do not bind fibrinogen and cannot form aggregates. The platelets undergo shape change and secretion and are of normal size.

Both of these disorders are inherited as autosomal recessive traits and are characterized by markedly impaired hemostasis and recurrent episodes of severe mucosal hemorrhage. In keeping with the selective nature of the defects, Bernard-Soulier platelets react normally to all stimuli except ristocetin. In contrast, thrombasthenic platelets adhere normally and will agglutinate with ristocetin but will not aggregate with any of the agonists which require fibrinogen binding, such as adenosine diphosphate (ADP), thrombin, or epinephrine.

The only effective therapy for hemorrhagic episodes in these two disorders is transfusion with normal platelets. This is usually effective, although alloimmunization will eventually limit the lifespan of infused platelets. In addition, a few patients have developed inhibitor antibodies with specificity for the missing protein. These antibodies bind to the protein which is expressed on the transfused normal platelets and impair their function.

PLATELET RELEASE DEFECTS The most common mild bleeding disorders arise from the ingestion of aspirin and other nonsteroidal anti-inflammatory drugs (NSAIDs) which inhibit platelet production of thromboxane A_2, an important mediator of platelet secretion and aggregation (see Figs. 62-3, 62-4). These drugs inhibit platelet cyclooxygenase, which converts arachidonic acid to a labile endoperoxide intermediate that is critical for thromboxane formation. Aspirin is the most potent agent, since it irreversibly acetylates the platelet enzyme so that a single dose impairs hemostasis for 5 to 7 days. The other agents are competitive and reversible inhibitors with more transient effects. Blocking thromboxane A_2 synthesis partially inhibits platelet release and aggregation with weak agonists such as ADP and epinephrine and produces a mild hemostatic defect. The administration of high doses of certain antibiotics, particularly penicillin, can coat the platelet surface, block platelet release, and impair hemostasis.

Patients generally have minimal symptoms such as easy bruising, and bleeding is usually confined to the skin. Occasional patients will have prolonged oozing after surgery, particularly with procedures involving mucous membranes such as periodontal, oral, or reconstructive plastic surgery. Not surprisingly, the antiplatelet effect of drugs like aspirin is more dramatic when they are administered to patients with underlying defects like vWD or hemophilia. Patients with drug-induced cyclooxygenase deficiency have a prolonged bleeding time, and their platelets fail to aggregate when incubated with arachidonic acid, epinephrine, or low doses of ADP. Platelet responses to collagen and thrombin are impaired at low doses, but normal at higher doses. Symptomatic patients should be encouraged to use drugs like acetaminophen which do not impair platelet function. Although most cases of cyclooxygenase deficiency are drug-induced, occasional patients have inherited disorders in platelet cyclooxygenase activity which impair thromboxane production or receptor level defects which prevent platelets from responding to thromboxane A_2. Although a number of metabolic disorders can perturb hemostasis, uremic platelet dysfunction is clinically the most important. The mechanism by which uremia impairs platelet function is not well understood, and retention of phenolic and guanidinosuccinic acids, excess prostacyclin production, or impaired vWF-platelet interactions have all been implicated. There is a good correlation between the degree of uremia and bleeding symptoms, and bleeding can usually be reversed by dialysis. In addition, the administration of cryoprecipitate or DDAVP, which raise plasma vWF levels, can also improve hemostasis.

STORAGE POOL DEFECTS Platelet granules have considerable amounts of adenine nucleotides, calcium, and adhesive glycoproteins like thrombospondin, fibronectin, and vWF, all of which promote platelet adhesion and aggregation. Thus, it is not surprising that patients with defective platelet granules have a mild bleeding disorder. Platelet storage pool defects may be inherited as an isolated disorder or be part of systemic granule packaging defects such as oculocutaneous albinism, the Hermansky-Pudlak, or the Chediak-Higashi syndromes. Clinically, these patients cannot be distinguished from those with other functional platelet disorders since they all have easy bruising, mucosal bleeding, and a prolonged bleeding time. They can be differentiated from patients with the cyclooxygenase defects since their platelets will usually aggregate in response to arachidonic acid. In addition, their platelets have decreased levels of specific granule constituents like ADP and serotonin and abnormalities in granule morphology that are best visualized by electron microscopy.

Occasionally, patients with acute and chronic leukemia or one of the myeloproliferative disorders develop an acquired storage pool disorder due to dysplastic megakaryocyte development. In addition, patients with liver disease and some patients with systemic lupus or other immune complex–mediated disorders may have circulating platelets which have degranulated prematurely. Platelet degranulation and a transient storage pool disorder have also been described following prolonged cardiopulmonary bypass.

VESSEL WALL DISORDERS Bleeding from vascular disorders (nonthrombocytopenic purpura) is usually mild and confined to the skin and mucous membranes. The pathogenesis of bleeding is poorly defined in many of the syndromes, and classical tests of hemostasis, including the bleeding time and tests of platelet function, are usually normal. Vascular purpura arise from damage to capillary endothelium, abnormalities in the vascular subendothelial matrix or extravascular connective tissues which support blood vessels, or from the formation of abnormal blood vessels. There are also several idiopathic disorders which involve the vessel wall and which can cause more severe bleeding and organ dysfunction.

Thrombotic thrombocytopenic purpura Thrombotic thrombocytopenic purpura (TTP) is a fulminant, often lethal disorder that may be initiated by endothelial injury and subsequent release of vWF and other procoagulant materials from the endothelial cell. In addition, some patients with TTP may have a unique circulating protein which induces platelet aggregation. Characteristic findings include the microvascular deposition of hyaline thrombi which stain for fibrin, thrombocytopenia, microangiopathic hemolytic anemia, fever, renal failure, fluctuating levels of consciousness, and evanescent focal neurologic deficits. The presence of hyaline thrombi in arterioles, capillaries, and venules without any inflammatory changes in the vessel wall is diagnostic. Gingival biopsies are positive in 30 to 40 percent of patients, and marrow biopsies are occasionally helpful. The presence of a severe Coombs negative hemolytic anemia with schistocytes or fragmented red blood cells in the peripheral blood smear, coupled with thrombocytopenia, and minimal activation of the coagulation system help to confirm the clinical suspicion of TTP. This disorder should be distinguished from vasculitis and systemic lupus erythematosus, which can predispose patients to TTP and ITP. Levels of platelet-associated IgG and complement are usually normal in TTP.

The treatment of acute TTP has changed radically in the past few years. Steroids and heparin or emergency splenectomy have been abandoned, and the enthusiasm for antiplatelet therapy has diminished. Increasingly, treatment has focused on the use of exchange transfusion or intensive plasmapheresis coupled with infusion of fresh frozen plasma. With this therapeutic approach, the overall mortality has been markedly reduced, and over half the patients with TTP are recovering from this formerly fatal disorder. Most patients surviving the acute illness recover completely with no residual renal or neurologic disease. Occasional patients with a chronic relapsing form of TTP require maintenance plasmapheresis and plasma infusion, and a few patients are only controlled with glucocorticoids.

Hemolytic-uremic syndrome Hemolytic-uremic syndrome (HUS) is a disease of infancy and early childhood which closely resembles TTP. Patients present with fever, thrombocytopenia, microangiopathic hemolytic anemia, hypertension, and varying degrees of acute renal failure. In many cases, onset is preceded by a minor febrile or viral illness, and an infectious or immune complex–mediated etiology has been proposed. As in TTP, there is no evidence of disseminated intravascular coagulation. In contrast to TTP, the disorder remains localized to the kidney where hyaline thrombi are seen in the afferent aterioles and glomerular capillaries. Such thrombi are not present in other vessels, and neurologic symptoms, other than those associated with uremia, are uncommon. There is no effective therapy; however, with dialysis for acute renal failure, the initial mortality is only 5 percent. Between 10 and 50 percent of patients are left with some chronic renal impairment.

Henoch-Schönlein purpura Henoch-Schönlein or anaphylactoid purpura is a distinct, self-limited type of vasculitis which occurs in children and young adults. Patients have an acute inflammatory reaction in capillaries, mesangial tissues, and small arterioles which leads to increased vascular permeability, exudation, and hemorrhage. Vessel lesions contain IgA and complement components. The syndrome may be preceded by an upper respiratory infection or streptococcal pharyngitis or be associated with food or drug allergies. Patients develop a purpuric or urticarial rash on the extensor surface of the arms and legs and on the buttocks; they also have polyarthralgias or arthritis, colicky abdominal pain, and hematuria from focal glomerulonephritis. Despite the hemorrhagic features, all coagulation tests are normal. A small number of patients may develop fatal acute renal failure, and 5 to 10 percent develop chronic nephritis. Glucocorticoids provide symptomatic relief of the joint and abdominal pains but do not alter the course of the illness.

Metabolic and inflammatory disorders A number of acute febrile illnesses cause capillary fragility and skin bleeding. Immune complexes containing viral antigens, or the viruses themselves, may damage endothelial cells. In addition, certain pathogens such as the rickettsiae which cause Rocky Mountain spotted fever replicate in endothelial cells and damage them. Thrombocytopenia is also a frequent finding in acute infectious disorders and may contribute to skin bleeding. In addition, whenever the platelet count falls below 10,000 per microliter, gaps which develop between endothelial cells allow the diapedesis of red cells into the dermis leading to the formation of petechiae. Drugs such as the sulfonamides, penicillin, and allopurinol may cause vascular inflammation resulting in maculopapular or urticarial rashes. Some of these mechanisms are additive, and drug reactions in thrombocytopenic individuals cause an intensely hemorrhagic rash.

Occasionally, patients with diffuse polyclonal hyperglobulinemia will develop purpuric lesions on the lower limbs—a benign condition referred to as *hyperglobulinemic purpura*. Vascular purpura may occur in patients with various monoclonal plasma protein abnormalities including Waldenström's macroglobulinemia, multiple myeloma, and cryoglobulinemia. These proteins markedly increase serum viscosity and may impair blood flow through capillaries. Thus, retinal hemorrhage, central nervous system dysfunction, and skin necrosis have all been described in these syndromes due to the marked elevation in viscosity. In addition, the globulins may impair platelet aggregation and adhesion and interfere with fibrin polymerization. Patients with mixed cryoglobulinemia develop a more extensive maculopapular lesion due to immune complex–mediated damage to the vessel wall. The mixed cryoglobulinemia (usually IgG and anti-IgG) may be associated with arthralgias, diffuse weakness, and unexplained nephritis. Plasmapheresis will temporarily lower the level of globulins, remove immune complexes, and improve symptoms in these patients. However, long-term management must include control of the underlying disease which produces the abnormal globulins or immune complexes.

Patients with *scurvy* (vitamin C deficiency) develop painful episodes of perifollicular skin bleeding as well as bleeding into muscles and, occasionally, into the gastrointestinal and genitourinary tracts. The diagnosis is confirmed by the presence of hyperkeratosis of skin, gum swelling, and low levels of the vitamin in leukocytes. Vitamin C–deficient patients have markedly defective collagen synthesis, since ascorbic acid is needed to synthesize hydroxyproline, an essential constituent of collagen. Patients with *Cushing's syndrome,* which is characterized by excess production of glucocorticoids, or patients on large doses of glucocorticoids develop generalized protein wasting and may show skin bleeding or easy bruising due to atrophy of the supporting connective tissue around blood vessels. Aging causes a similar atrophy of perivascular connective tissue on the extensor surface of the hands and arms, leading to "senile purpura." These patients develop dark purple, irregularly shaped hemorrhagic areas due to abnormal skin mobility which tears small blood vessels.

Patients with inherited disorders of the connective tissue matrix such as *Marfan's syndrome, Ehlers-Danlos syndrome,* and *pseudoxanthoma elasticum* also have easy bruising. In addition to having fragile skin vessels and easy bruising, patients with Ehlers-Danlos syndrome may develop aneurysms in intraabdominal vessels and apoplectic rupture and hemorrhage due to defects in the vascular collagen network. Primary vascular abnormalities can also lead to bleeding. Patients with *Osler-Weber-Rendu disease* (hereditary hemorrhagic telangiectasia), an inherited autosomal dominant disorder, have frequent episodes of nasal and gastrointestinal bleeding from abnormal telangiectatic capillaries; patients with *angiodysplasia* of the colon have increased incidence of gastrointestinal bleeding. In the *Kasabach-Merritt syndrome* patients may have very extensive and progressively enlarging vascular malformations which may involve large portions of their extremities. Bleeding is secondary to disseminated intravascular coagulation triggered by stagnant blood flow through the tortuous abnormal vessels.

REFERENCES

HANDIN RI, WAGNER DD: Molecular and cellular biology of von Willebrand factor, in *Progress in Hemostasis and Thrombosis,* vol 9, BS Coller (ed). Philadelphia, Saunders, 1989, pp 233–259

MAJERUS P: Platelets, in *The Molecular Basis of Blood Diseases,* G Stamatoyanopoulis et al (eds). Philadelphia, Saunders, 1987, pp 689–722

SADLER JE, DAVIE EW: Hemophilia A, hemophilia B, and von Willebrand's disease, in *The Molecular Basis of Blood Diseases,* G Stamatoyanopoulis et al (eds). Philadelphia, Saunders, 1987, pp 575–630

STUART MJ, KELTON JG: The platelet: Quantitative and qualitative abnormalities, in *Hematology of Infancy and Childhood,* 3d ed, DG Nathan, FA Oski (eds). Philadelphia, Saunders, 1987, p 1343–1479

WILLIAMS WJ: et al (eds): *Hematology,* 4th ed. New York, McGraw-Hill, 1990

288 DISORDERS OF COAGULATION AND THROMBOSIS

ROBERT I. HANDIN

Patients with congenital plasma coagulation defects characteristically bleed into muscles, joints, and body cavities, hours or days after an injury. Most of the *inherited* plasma coagulation disorders are due to defects in single coagulation proteins, with the two X-linked disorders, factors VIII and IX deficiency, accounting for the majority of the congenital coagulation disorders. These patients merit special attention since they may have severe bleeding and chronic disability and require specialized medical therapy. With the exception of factor XIII deficiency, each of the known disorders prolongs either the prothrombin time (PT), partial thromboplastin time (PTT), or both of these important laboratory screening tests. If they are abnormal, quantitative assays of specific coagulation proteins are then carried out using the PT or PTT tests and plasma from congenitally deficient individuals as substrate. The corrective effect of varying concentrations of patient plasma is measured and expressed as a percentage of a normal pooled plasma standard. The interval range for most coagulation factors is from 50 to 150 percent of this average value, and the minimal level of most individual factors needed for adequate hemostasis is 25 percent.

Acquired coagulation disorders are both more frequent and more complex, arising from deficiencies of multiple coagulation proteins, and simultaneously affecting both primary and secondary hemostasis. The most common acquired hemorrhagic disorders are (1) disseminated intravascular coagulation, (2) the hemorrhagic diathesis of liver disease, and (3) vitamin K deficiency and complications of anticoagulant therapy.

Although congenital and acquired bleeding disorders are relatively rare, venous and arterial thrombosis and embolism are common medical disorders which have been recognized for over a hundred years. Although risk factors such as atherosclerotic vascular disease, congestive heart failure, malignancy, and immobility predispose patients to thrombosis, specific coagulation defects have not yet been identified in most patients with thromboembolism. Several inherited coagulation abnormalities have now been described which induce a hypercoagulable or prethrombotic state and predispose patients to thrombosis. These disorders merit special attention since they affect young people, cause recurrent episodes of thromboembolism, and may involve multiple members of a single family. An understanding of the biochemical basis of thromboembolism is also important since anticoagulant and antithrombotic regimes are based on the premise that modifying critical coagulation reactions will reduce the incidence of thrombosis. This chapter will review the diagnosis, natural history, and therapy of congenital and acquired plasma coagulation disorders, as well as the inherited prethrombotic disorders. The physiology of normal hemostasis and the cardinal manifestations of the hemorrhagic and thrombotic disorders are described in Chap. 62.

FACTOR VIII DEFICIENCY—HEMOPHILIA A Pathogenesis and clinical manifestations The antihemophilic factor (AHF) or factor VIII coagulant protein is a large (265,000-Da), single-chain protein which regulates the activation of factor X by proteases generated in the intrinsic coagulation pathway (see Figs. 62-4, 62-6). It is synthesized in liver parenchymal cells and circulates complexed to the von Willebrand protein (vWF). Previous efforts to purify and characterize the factor VIII molecule were limited by its low concentration (10 μg/L) and susceptibility to proteolysis. However, the cloning and sequencing of complementary DNA (cDNA) encoding the factor VIII molecule and the mapping of the factor VIII gene on the X chromosome have provided the first detailed picture of its structure and have resulted in improved methods for carrier detection and prenatal diagnosis.

One in 10,000 males is born with deficiency or dysfunction of the factor VIII molecule. The resulting disorder, hemophilia A, is characterized by bleeding into soft tissues, muscles, and weight-bearing joints. Although normal hemostasis requires 25 percent factor VIII activity, symptomatic patients usually have factor VIII levels below 5 percent, with a close correlation between the clinical severity of hemophilia and plasma AHF level. Patients with <1 percent factor VIII activity have *severe* disease; they bleed frequently even without discernible trauma. Patients with levels between 1 and 5 percent have *moderate* disease with less frequent bleeding episodes. Those with levels over 5 percent have *mild* disease with infrequent bleeding that is usually secondary to trauma. Occasional patients with factor VIII levels as high as 25 percent are discovered when they bleed after major trauma or surgery, although the vast majority of patients with hemophilia A have factor VIII levels below 5 percent.

Hemophilic bleeding occurs hours or days after injury, can involve any organ, and, if untreated, may continue for days or weeks. This can result in large collections of partially clotted blood putting pressure on adjacent normal tissues and can cause necrosis of muscle (compartment syndromes), venous congestion (pseudophlebitis), or ischemic damage to nerves. For example, hemophiliacs often develop femoral neuropathy due to pressure from an unsuspected retroperitoneal hematoma. They can also develop large calcified masses of blood and inflammatory tissue that are mistaken for soft tissue sarcomas (pseudotumor syndrome).

Patients with severe hemophilia are usually diagnosed shortly after birth because of an extensive cephalhematoma or profuse bleeding at circumcision. However, patients with moderate disease may not bleed until they begin to walk or crawl, and mild hemophiliacs may not be diagnosed until they are adolescents or young adults. Typically, a hemophiliac patient presents with pain followed by swelling in a weight-bearing joint, like the hip, knee, or ankle. The presence of blood in the joint (hemarthrosis) causes synovial inflammation, and repetitive bleeding erodes articular cartilage and causes osteoarthritis, articular fibrosis, joint ankylosis, and eventually muscle atrophy. Although bleeding may occur into any joint, after a joint has been damaged it may become a site for subsequent bleeding episodes.

Hematuria, in the absence of any genitourinary pathology, is also common. It is usually self-limited and may not require specific therapy. The most feared complications of hemophilia are oropharyngeal and central nervous system bleeding. Patients with oropharyngeal bleeding may require emergency intubation to maintain an adequate airway. Central nervous system bleeding can occur without antecedent trauma or without evidence of a specific lesion.

Patients suspected of having hemophilia should have screening tests of hemostasis including a platelet count, bleeding time, PT, and PTT. Typically, the patient will have a prolonged PTT with all other tests normal. Because of the similarity clinically of factors VIII and IX deficiency, any male with an appropriate bleeding history and a prolonged PTT should have specific assays for factor VIII and factor IX.

Therapy There are several tenets regarding the treatment of bleeding in hemophiliac patients: (1) Symptoms often precede objective evidence of bleeding. (2) Signs of bleeding may not appear until several days after well-documented trauma. Physicians caring for these patients have learned to rely on their patients to inform them of early symptoms, usually pain, and to begin treatment at that time. Early treatment is more effective, less costly, and can be lifesaving. (3) It is critical to avoid the use of aspirin or aspirin-containing drugs which impair platelet function and may cause severe hemorrhage.

Plasma products enriched in factor VIII have revolutionized the care of hemophilia patients, reduced the degree of orthopedic deformity, and permitted virtually any form of elective and emergency surgery. The widespread use of factor VIII concentrates has also produced serious complications including viral hepatitis, chronic liver disease, and the acquired immunodeficiency syndrome (AIDS). The standard therapeutic products are cryoprecipitate and factor VIII concentrate. *Cryoprecipitate,* which contains about half the factor VIII activity of fresh frozen plasma in one-tenth the original volume, is simple to prepare and is produced in hospital or regional blood banks. It must be stored frozen and is thawed and pooled prior to administration. However, most patients utilize partially purified *factor VIII concentrate* which is prepared from multiple donors and supplied as a lyophilized powder. It can be refrigerated and reconstituted just prior to use.

There are three recent developments which have increased the safety of factor VIII therapy. First, heating of lyophilized factor VIII concentrates under carefully controlled conditions can inactivate human immunodeficiency virus (HIV) without destroying factor VIII coagulant activity. Second, highly purified factor VIII can be produced by adsorbing and eluting factor VIII from monoclonal antibody columns. Third, recombinant factor VIII is now undergoing clinical trials and may soon be marketed. All patients with hemophilia should receive either heat-treated or monoclonal purified factor VIII, and newly diagnosed hemophiliacs should only receive the monoclonal preparations to minimize viral infections and exposure to irrelevant proteins.

Each unit of factor VIII, which is the amount present in 1 mL of normal plasma, will raise the plasma level of the recipient by 2 percent per kilogram of body weight. Factor VIII has a half-life of 8 to 12 h, making it necessary to infuse it continuously or at least twice daily to sustain a chosen factor VIII level. In patients with mild hemophilia an alternative to the use of plasma products is desmopressin, which transiently increases the factor VIII level.

An uncomplicated episode of soft tissue bleeding, or an early hemarthrosis, can be treated with one infusion of cryoprecipitate or factor VIII concentrate sufficient to raise the factor VIII level to 15 or 20 percent. A more extensive hemarthrosis or retroperitoneal bleeding requires twice-daily or continuous infusions in order to keep the factor VIII level between 25 and 50 percent for at least 72 h. Life-threatening bleeding into the central nervous system, or major surgery, may require therapy for 2 weeks with levels kept at a minimum of 50 percent of normal. In addition to the prompt infusion of factor VIII–enriched plasma products, patients need skilled orthopedic care with immobilization of inflamed joints to promote healing and to prevent contractures, and physical therapy to strengthen muscles and maintain joint mobility. Prior to surgery every patient should be screened for the presence of an inhibitor to factor VIII.

Patients with hemophilia who do not have an inhibitor should receive factor VIII infusions just prior to surgery and will require daily monitoring so that the factor VIII level is maintained above 50 percent for 10 to 14 days after surgery. When patients undergo joint replacement or other major orthopedic surgery, therapy should be continued for 3 weeks. This permits adequate wound healing and the institution of necessary joint mobilization and physical therapy.

Hemophiliacs also require treatment prior to dental procedures. Filling of a carious tooth can be managed by a single infusion of cryoprecipitate or factor VIII concentrate coupled with the administration of 4 to 6 g of ϵ-aminocaproic acid (EACA) four times daily for 72 to 96 h after the dental procedure. EACA is a potent antifibrinolytic agent which will inhibit plasminogen activators present in oral secretions and stabilize clot formation in oral tissue. For major oral and periodontal surgery and extractions of permanent teeth, patients should be hospitalized and treated with factor VIII. Therapy should begin just prior to surgery and be continued for a minimum of 48 to 72 h.

Many centers have organized home care programs so that patients can administer their own factor VIII infusions with the onset of symptoms. Occasional patients with very frequent bleeding receive regularly scheduled infusions. However, the expense and inconvenience usually limit the use of "prophylactic" infusions. Concern regarding transmission of AIDS has complicated therapy of hemophilia, and some patients are reluctant to treat themselves.

Complications Most hemophiliacs have had multiple episodes of hepatitis, and a majority have elevated hepatocellular enzyme levels and abnormalities on liver biopsy. Ten to twenty percent of hemophiliacs also have hepatosplenomegaly, and a small number develop chronic active or persistent hepatitis or cirrhosis. Recently, a few patients with hemophilia and end-stage liver disease have received liver transplants with cure of both diseases. Along with homosexuals and intravenous drug abusers, hemophiliacs are at high risk for AIDS since they frequently receive blood products. Hemophiliacs can also present with the full range of AIDS-related syndromes including diffuse lymphadenopathy and immune thrombocytopenia. Although as many as 80 percent of multiply transfused hemophiliacs are HIV-positive and some have progressed to AIDS-related complex (ARC) or AIDS, recent advances in factor VIII concentrate preparation should prevent future HIV infection.

Despite frequent bleeding, severe iron-deficiency anemia is uncommon since most of the bleeding is internal and iron is effectively recycled. Mild iron deficiency from chronic epistaxis or gastrointestinal bleeding has been noted in some hemophiliacs. In addition, after receiving large doses of factor VIII concentrate, some patients develop a mild Coombs'-positive hemolytic anemia due to small amounts of anti-A and anti-B antibody present in commercial concentrates which bind to red cells and cause hemolysis.

Following multiple transfusions, between 10 and 20 percent of patients with severe hemophilia develop inhibitors to factor VIII. Inhibitors are, generally, IgG antibodies which rapidly neutralize factor VIII activity and prevent effective transfusion therapy. There are two types of inhibitors which have different biologic characteristics and lead to different clinical presentations. Patients with type I inhibitors have a typical anamnestic response and raise their antibody titer following exposure to factor VIII. Patients with a type II inhibitor have a low antibody titer which cannot be stimulated by factor VIII infusion. Patients with the type I inhibitor should not receive factor VIII. In an emergency, control of bleeding may require intensive plasmapheresis, or infusion of prothrombin complex concentrates which contain trace quantities of activated coagulation factors and can bypass the block in coagulation produced by the inhibitor. Patients with low-titer type II antibodies may respond to higher than normal doses of factor VIII.

Genetic counseling and carrier detection Until recently, carrier detection required biologic and immunologic assays which compared the ratio of factor VIII to vWF (von Willebrand factor) protein and were predictive in only 70 to 80 percent of cases. It is now possible to trace the most defective allele in some families by examining the inheritance of restriction fragment length polymorphisms (RFLPs) linked to the factor VIII gene. In addition, certain families have been identified with specific mutations and deletions in the factor VIII gene that can be detected by restriction enzyme digestion of their DNA. Previously, prenatal diagnosis required sampling fetal blood for coagulant activity. Now, in families with an identifiable RFLP linked to the gene or a gene deletion or rearrangement, precise diagnosis is possible early in pregnancy from either chorionic villus biopsy or amniocentesis. The amount of material required has decreased, and the rapidity of diagnosis has increased with the introduction of the polymerase chain reaction to amplify desired segments of genomic DNA.

Most women carriers of hemophilia produce sufficient factor VIII for normal hemostasis from the factor VIII allele on their normal X chromosome. However, occasional hemophilia carriers will have factor VIII levels far below 50 percent due to random inactivation of normal X chromosomes in tissue producing factor VIII. These symptomatic carriers may bleed with major surgery or bleed occasionally with menses. Rarely, true female hemophiliacs arise from consanguinity within families with hemophilia, or from concomitant Turner's syndrome or XO mosaicism in a carrier female.

FACTOR IX DEFICIENCY—HEMOPHILIA B Factor IX is a single-chain, 55,000-Da proenzyme which is converted to an active protease (IXa) by factor XIa or by the tissue factor–VIIa complex. Factor IXa then activates factor X in conjunction with activated factor VIII. Factor IX is one of a group of six proteins, synthesized in the liver, which require vitamin K for biologic activity. As previously discussed (see Chap. 62), vitamin K is a cofactor for a unique posttranslational modification which inserts a second carboxyl group onto certain glutamic acid residues on factor IX. This modification permits calcium binding and adsorption onto phospholipid surfaces. Factor IX cDNA has been cloned, the gene mapped on the X chromosome, linked RFLPs identified, and patients with deletions and mutations in the IX gene have been discovered.

Factor IX deficiency or dysfunction (hemophilia B, Christmas disease) occurs in 1 in 100,000 male births. Accurate laboratory diagnosis is critical, since it is clinically indistinguishable from factor VIII deficiency (hemophilia A) but requires treatment with a different plasma fraction. Either fresh frozen plasma or a plasma fraction enriched in the prothrombin complex proteins is used. In addition to the expected complications of hepatitis, chronic liver disease, and AIDS, the therapy of factor IX deficiency has a special hazard. Trace quantities of activated coagulation factors in prothrombin complex concentrates may activate the coagulation system and cause thrombosis and embolism. This is particularly common in immobilized surgical patients and patients with liver disease. As a result, some centers have returned to fresh frozen plasma for factor-IX–deficient surgical patients while others have recommended the addition of small doses of heparin to the concentrate to activate antithrombin III during the infusion and reduce hypercoagulability.

FACTOR XI DEFICIENCY Factor XI is a 160,000-Da, dimeric protein which is activated via the intrinsic coagulation pathway. It is converted to an active protease (XIa) by factor XIIa, in conjunction with high-molecular-weight kininogen and kallikrein (see Figs. 62-4 and 62-5). Factor XI deficiency is inherited as an autosomal recessive trait and is especially common in Ashkenazi Jews. In contrast to factors VIII and IX deficiency, the correlation between factor level and propensity to bleed is not as precise, there is less spontaneous bleeding, and hemarthroses are rare. Many patients with factor XI deficiency present with posttraumatic bleeding or with bleeding in the perioperative period, and occasional factor XI–deficient women have menorrhagia. Daily infusions of fresh frozen plasma are sufficient since the half-life of factor XI is approximately 24 h.

OTHER FACTOR DEFICIENCIES Deficiencies in factors V, VII, X, and prothrombin (factor II) are all exceedingly rare autosomal recessive disorders. Although spontaneous or posttraumatic musculoskeletal bleeding or menorrhagia can occur with these deficiencies, hemarthroses are uncommon. Fresh frozen plasma is the appropriate therapy, although prothrombin concentrates may be employed for patients with severe prothrombin or factors VII and X deficiency as long as the risks of hepatitis and thrombosis are recognized.

Defects in the contact activation pathway involving Hageman Factor (factor XII), high-molecular-weight kininogen, and prekallikrein cause laboratory abnormalities but no clinical bleeding. Despite dramatic prolongation of the PTT, which is often greater than 100 s, deficient individuals have normal hemostasis and can undergo major surgery without plasma replacement therapy. It is important to recognize and diagnose these disorders since the patients should neither be inappropriately treated with plasma nor denied indicated surgery on the basis of these laboratory abnormalities. As discussed in Chap. 62, there may be as yet undefined alternative pathways to activate factor XI in vivo which bypass this apparent defect in coagulation.

AFIBRINOGENEMIA AND DYSFIBRINOGENEMIA Fibrinogen is a 340,000-Da dimeric molecule made up of two sets of three covalently linked polypeptide chains. Thrombin sequentially cleaves fibrinopeptides A and B from the Aα and Bβ chains of fibrinogen to produce fibrin monomer, which then polymerizes to form a fibrin clot. Although fibrinogen is needed for platelet aggregation and fibrin formation, severe fibrinogen deficiency, paradoxically, does not usually cause serious bleeding except after surgery. Patients with afibrinogenemia, who have no detectable fibrinogen in plasma or platelets, may have infrequent, mild bleeding episodes. Preliminary genetic analyses do not show any deletion or structural changes in the genes encoding the α, β, and γ chains of fibrinogen despite the total absence of plasma fibrinogen.

Fibrinogen is an abundant plasma protein (2.5 g/L) that has been purified and completely sequenced. Mutations have been identified which alter the release of fibrinopeptides from the Aα and Bβ chains of fibrinogen, the rate of polymerization of fibrin monomers, and the sites for fibrin cross-linking. These dysfibrinogenemias are almost always inherited as autosomal dominant traits, so that patients have approximately equal concentrations of normal and mutant fibrinogen in their plasma. Patients with dysfibrinogenemia have a slightly prolonged PT and PTT, a prolonged thrombin time, and a disparity between the quantity of fibrinogen measured with functional and immunologic assays. Despite these abnormalities most patients have no symptoms while other patients have moderate bleeding. A few dysfibrinogenemias induce a hypercoagulable state and increase the risk of thrombosis, and others have been associated with an increased incidence of abortion (see Chap. 289).

FACTOR XIII DEFICIENCY AND DEFECTIVE FIBRIN CROSS-LINKING Factor XIII is a transglutaminase which stabilizes fibrin clots by forming ϵ-amino-γ-glutamyl cross-links between adjacent α and γ chains of fibrin. Factor XIII deficiency is an extremely rare inherited syndrome with only a few hundred documented cases. Patients usually bleed in the neonatal period from their umbilical stump or circumcision. In addition to hemorrhage, these patients may have poor wound healing, a high incidence of infertility among males, abortion among affected females, and a high incidence of intracerebral hemorrhage. These observations suggest that the enzyme may be important in other physiologic and pathologic processes beyond hemostasis, including placental implantation, spermatogenesis, and wound healing. Several drugs, including isoniazid, may bind to cross-linking sites on fibrinogen and mimic factor XIII deficiency by blocking enzyme activity. Normal hemostasis requires only 1 percent of normal enzyme activity, which can be achieved with small amounts of fresh frozen plasma.

VITAMIN K DEFICIENCY Vitamin K is a fat-soluble vitamin which plays a critical role in hemostasis. Dietary vitamin K is absorbed in the small intestine and stored in the liver. The vitamin is also synthesized by endogenous bacterial flora resident in the small intestine and colon; however, there is controversy regarding the quantity of endogenous vitamin K that is absorbed from the large intestine. Following absorption and transport, vitamin K is converted to an active epoxide in liver microsomes, and serves as a cofactor in the enzymatic carboxylation of glutamic acid residues on prothrombin complex proteins (Fig. 288-1).

There are three major causes of vitamin K deficiency—inadequate dietary intake, intestinal malabsorption, and loss of storage sites due to hepatocellular disease. Neonatal vitamin K deficiency, which causes hemorrhagic disease of the newborn, has disappeared from western countries with the routine administration of vitamin K to all newborn infants. Although there is, theoretically, a 30-day store of vitamin K in the normal liver, acutely ill patients can become deficient within 7 to 10 days. Acute vitamin K deficiency is particularly common in patients recovering from biliary tract surgery who have no dietary intake of vitamin K, have T-tube drainage of bile, and are on broad-spectrum antibiotics. Vitamin K deficiency is also seen in chronic liver disease, particularly primary biliary cirrhosis, and in some malabsorption states (see Chaps. 240 and 254).

With the onset of vitamin K deficiency, plasma levels of all the prothrombin complex proteins (factors II, VII, IX, X; protein C and protein S) decrease. Factor VII and protein C, which have the shortest half-lives, decrease first. Because of the rapid fall in factor VII, patients with mild vitamin K deficiency may have a prolonged PT and a normal PTT. Later, as the levels of the other factors fall, the PTT will also become prolonged. Parenteral administration of 10 mg of vitamin K rapidly restores vitamin K levels in the liver and permits normal production of prothrombin complex proteins within 8 to 10 h. Severe hemorrhage can be treated with fresh frozen plasma, which immediately corrects the hemostatic defect. If the cause of vitamin K deficiency cannot be eliminated, patients may need monthly injections. Purified prothrombin complex concentrates should be avoided as they contain trace quantities of activated forms of the prothrombin complex proteins and can cause thrombosis in patients with liver disease. They will also expose patients to an increased risk of hepatitis.

DISSEMINATED INTRAVASCULAR COAGULATION Disseminated intravascular coagulation (DIC) may be an explosive and life-threatening bleeding disorder. Although there is a long list of diseases complicated by DIC, it is most frequently associated with obstetrical catastrophes, metastatic malignancy, massive trauma, and bacterial sepsis (Table 288-1). In each case, a tentative triggering mechanism has been identified. For example, tumors and traumatized or necrotic tissue release materials resembling tissue factor into the circulation, while endotoxin from gram-negative bacteria activates several steps in the coagulation cascade. In addition to a direct effect on the activation of Hageman factor (factor XII), endotoxin induces the expression of tissue factor activity on the surface of monocytes and endothelial cells. These cell surfaces then accelerate coagulation reactions. This combination of potent thrombogenic stimuli causes the deposition of small thrombi and emboli throughout the microvasculature. This early thrombotic phase of DIC is then followed by a phase of procoagulant consumption and secondary fibrinolysis. Continued fibrin formation and fibrinolysis lead to hemorrhage from the depletion of coagulation proteins and platelets and the antihemostatic effects of fibrin degradation products (see Fig. 288-2).

The clinical presentation varies with the stage and severity of the syndrome. Most patients have extensive skin and mucous membrane bleeding and hemorrhage from multiple sites—usually surgical inci-

FIGURE 288-1 The mechanism of action of vitamin K, which is a cofactor in the formation of di-γ-carboxyglutamic acid residues on coagulation proteins, is depicted. Vitamin K is converted to an epoxide in liver microsomes. The epoxide is the active form and is reduced back to vitamin K by a liver membrane reductase. Warfarin blocks the action of the reductase and competitively inhibits the effects of vitamin K.

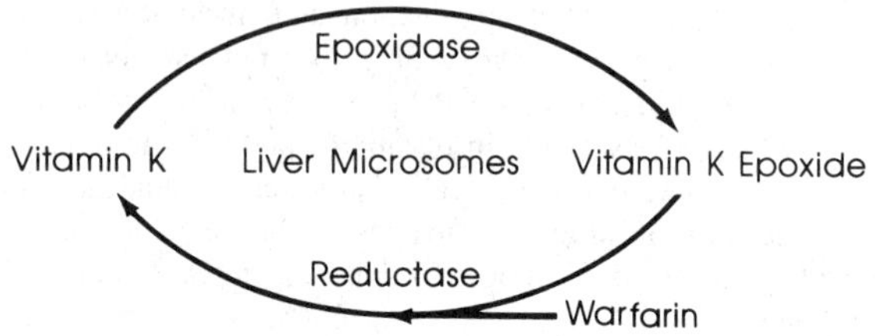

TABLE 288-1 Etiologic factors and disorders causing disseminated intravascular coagulation

Liberation of tissue factors	Obstetrical syndromes—abruptio placentae, amniotic fluid embolism, retained dead fetus, second trimester abortion
	Hemolysis
	Neoplasms, particularly mucinous adenocarcinomas, acute promyelocytic leukemia
	Intravascular hemolysis
	Fat embolism
	Tissue damage—burns, frostbite, head injury, gunshot wounds
Endothelial damage	Aortic aneurysm
	Hemolytic uremic syndrome
	Acute glomerulonephritis
	Rocky Mountain spotted fever
Vascular malformation and decreased blood flow	Kasabach-Merritt syndrome
Infections	Bacterial: staphylococci, streptococci, pneumococci, meningococci, gram-negative bacilli
	Viral: arboviruses, varicella, variola, rubella
	Parasitic: malaria, kala-azar
	Rickettsial: Rocky Mountain spotted fever
	Mycotic: acute histoplasmosis

SOURCE: Modified from RI Handin, RD Rosenberg, in Hematology, 4th ed, WS Beck (ed), Cambridge, MA, MIT Press, 1985.

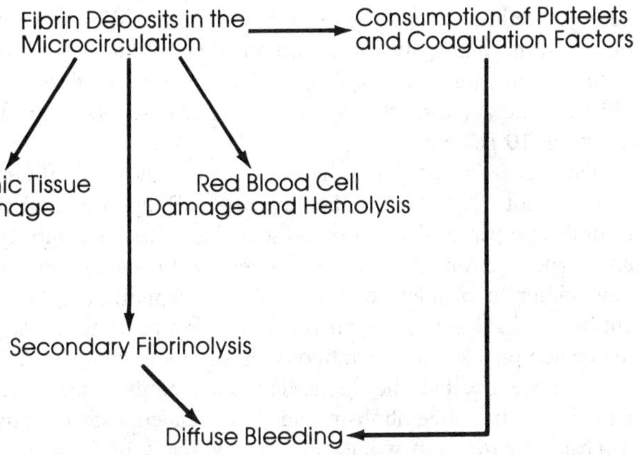

FIGURE 288-2 The pathophysiology of disseminated intravascular coagulation (DIC). Shown are the interactions between coagulation and fibrinolytic pathways which result in bleeding in patients with DIC.

sions, venipuncture, or catheter sites. Less often, patients present with peripheral acrocyanosis, thrombosis, and pregangrenous changes in digits, genitalia, and nose—areas where blood flow is markedly reduced by vasospasm or microthrombi. Occasional patients, particularly those with chronic DIC secondary to malignancy, have laboratory abnormalities without any evidence of thrombosis or hemorrhage.

The laboratory manifestations include thrombocytopenia, and the presence of schistocytes or fragmented red blood cells which arise from cell trapping and damage within fibrin thrombi; prolonged PT and PTT and thrombin time, and a reduced fibrinogen level from depletion of coagulation proteins; and elevated fibrin degradation products (FDPs) from intense secondary fibrinolysis. The cardinal manifestation of DIC, which correlates most closely with bleeding, is the plasma fibrinogen level.

Treatment DIC can cause life-threatening hemorrhage and requires prompt treatment. This should include: (1) an attempt to correct any reversible cause of DIC; (2) measures to control the major symptom, either bleeding or thrombosis; and (3) a prophylactic regimen to prevent recurrence in cases of chronic DIC. Treatment will vary with the clinical presentation. In patients with an obstetric complication like abruptio placentae or acute bacterial sepsis, the underlying disorder is easy to correct, and prompt delivery of the fetus and placenta or treatment with appropriate antibiotics will reverse the DIC syndrome. In patients with metastatic tumor causing DIC, control of the primary disease may not be possible and long-term prophylaxis may be necessary.

Patients with bleeding as a major symptom should receive fresh frozen plasma to replace depleted clotting factors, and platelet concentrates to correct thrombocytopenia. Those with acrocyanosis and incipient gangrene or thrombosis need immediate anticoagulation with intravenous heparin. The use of heparin in the treatment of bleeding is still controversial, although it is a logical way to reduce thrombin generation and prevent further consumption of clotting proteins. It should be reserved for patients with thrombosis or those who continue to bleed despite vigorous treatment with plasma and platelets.

Patients with mild DIC, who may not be symptomatic, may begin to bleed following stresses like surgery or chemotherapy. For example, mild DIC, without clinical bleeding, has been documented during saline- or prostaglandin-induced midtrimester abortions. Prophylactic treatment of patients with heparin may prevent progression of the DIC syndrome and has been used in the treatment of patients with acute promyelocytic leukemia and in some patients with a retained dead fetus who require surgical extraction. However, most patients with low-grade DIC can be managed simply with plasma and platelet replacement and do not require heparin. Chronic DIC does not respond to oral warfarin anticoagulants, but it can be controlled with long-term heparin infusion. Occasional patients with indolent tumors and severe DIC have been maintained on heparin administered by intermittent subcutaneous injection or continuous infusion with portable pumps.

Despite our detailed understanding of the pathophysiology of DIC and a vigorous approach to therapy, there is little evidence that its treatment will change the natural history of the underlying disorder. Therapy will only stabilize the patient, prevent exsanguination or massive thrombosis, and permit institution of definitive therapy.

COAGULATION DISORDERS IN LIVER DISEASE Since the liver plays a central role in the synthesis and metabolism of coagulation proteins, liver dysfunction is frequently accompanied by a hemostatic defect. The major causes of hemorrhage in patients with liver disease are outlined in Table 288-2. It is important to recognize that bleeding is usually due to an anatomic lesion, which is then exacerbated by the hemostatic defects. Most patients bleed from complications of portal hypertension such as esophageal varices, or from gastritis and peptic ulceration of the gastrointestinal tract. Portal hypertension also causes splenomegaly, with splenic sequestration of platelets and thrombocytopenia, which contributes to the hemostatic defect (see Chap. 254).

Patients with hepatocellular liver disease cannot store vitamin K optimally and may have some degree of vitamin K deficiency. Cholestasis, which is a frequent feature of liver disease, impairs vitamin K absorption and further decreases liver vitamin K stores. They may also have decreased production of other coagulation proteins including fibrinogen and factor V. The liver also produces inhibitors of coagulation such as antithrombin III and proteins C and S and is the clearance site for activated coagulation factors and fibrinolytic enzymes. Thus, patients with liver disease are ''hypercoagulable'' and predisposed to developing DIC and may develop systemic fibrinolysis. For these reasons, coagulation defects in advanced liver failure are often difficult to distinguish from those of DIC.

Each patient with hemorrhage and liver disease should have a PT, PTT, platelet count, and fibrinogen determination, although it is not always possible to determine the major hemostatic abnormality from a single set of laboratory values. It is helpful to have previous laboratory data available for patients with chronic liver disease who develop an acute complication. Most patients present with moderate prolongation of the PT and PTT, mild thrombocytopenia, and a normal fibrinogen level. However, they may present with a more complex defect combining defective synthesis, abnormal clearance, and active consumption of coagulation proteins. Since vitamin K deficiency is so common, it is advisable to administer a single parenteral dose of vitamin K after initial laboratory studies have been obtained, even though this may only partially correct the laboratory abnormalities. The presence of severe thrombocytopenia or a low

TABLE 288-2 Causes of bleeding in liver disease

I Anatomic factors
- *A* Portal hypertension
  - *1* Varices
  - *2* Splenomegaly and secondary thrombocytopenia
- *B* Peptic ulceration
- *C* Gastritis

II Hepatic function abnormalities
- *A* Decreased synthesis of procoagulant proteins: fibrinogen, prothrombin, factors V, VII, IX, X, XI
- *B* Decreased synthesis of coagulation inhibitors: protein C, protein S, antithrombin III
- *C* Impaired absorption and metabolism of vitamin K
- *D* Failure to clear activated coagulation proteins leading to
  - *1* Disseminated intravascular coagulation
  - *2* Systemic fibrinolysis

III Complications of therapy
- *A* Dilution of platelets and coagulation proteins from massive transfusions
- *B* Infusion of activated coagulation proteins in prothrombin complex concentrates
- *C* Bleeding from heparin; thrombosis from ε-aminocaproic acid (EACA)

fibrinogen level suggests the additional complication of DIC and may require further studies and therapy.

The safest replacement therapy for a patient with liver disease is fresh frozen plasma since it supplies all known coagulation factors. However, even this form of therapy has drawbacks since large quantities of plasma may precipitate hepatic encephalopathy and cause fluid and sodium overload. Prothrombin complex concentrates should be avoided since they only replace the vitamin K–dependent factors, may be contaminated with hepatitis and AIDS virus, and contain trace quantities of activated coagulation proteins. Similarly, fibrinogen concentrates, or cryoprecipitate, which are rich in factor VIII and fibrinogen should not be used without additional fresh frozen plasma. Anticoagulation with heparin has been advocated to control DIC, but this is particularly hazardous and not recommended in cirrhosis since heparin is metabolized erratically and may thus lead to severe bleeding.

FIBRINOLYTIC DEFECTS Bleeding can also occur from defects in the fibrinolytic system. Patients with $alpha_2$ plasmin inhibitor deficiency have excess fibrinolysis following fibrin deposition after trauma or surgery and so may experience recurrent hemorrhage. Similarly, patients with cirrhosis have an impaired clearance of tissue plasminogen activator and systemic fibrinolysis which may contribute to their hemorrhagic defect. Rarely, patients with tumors such as metastatic prostatic carcinoma may develop diffuse bleeding from primary fibrinolysis rather than DIC. Clues to the diagnosis include a disproportionately low fibrinogen with a relatively normal PT and PTT and the presence of a normal or nearly normal platelet count. However, at times it is difficult or impossible to differentiate primary fibrinolysis from the secondary fibrinolysis accompanying DIC. Patients with clearly established primary fibrinolysis should not receive heparin; they do require plasma therapy and, occasionally, fibrinolytic inhibitors like EACA. However, EACA should not be given to patients suspected of having DIC unless they are also receiving heparin, since EACA can cause massive, often fatal, thrombosis in a patient with DIC.

CIRCULATING ANTICOAGULANTS Circulating anticoagulants, or inhibitors, are usually IgG antibodies which interfere with coagulation reactions. Specific inhibitors inactivate individual coagulation proteins and may cause severe hemorrhage. As discussed above, they arise in 15 to 20 percent of patients with factors VIII or IX deficiency who have received plasma infusions. *Specific* inhibitors also occur in previously normal individuals. Although the most common target protein is factor VIII, inhibitors have been described with a specificity for each of the coagulation proteins. Anti-factor VIII antibodies in nonhemophiliacs are seen in postpartum females, in patients on various drugs, as part of the spectrum of autoantibodies in systemic lupus erythematosus patients, and in normal elderly individuals. *Nonspecific* (lupus-like) inhibitors prolong coagulation tests by binding to phospholipids; they do not perturb hemostasis in vivo, unless associated with thrombocytopenia or prothrombin deficiency. While they are most often encountered in patients with systemic lupus erythematosus, nonspecific inhibitors have also been noted in patients with many other disorders and also in otherwise normal individuals.

The critical laboratory feature, which identifies the presence of either type of inhibitor, is the failure of normal plasma to correct a prolonged PT, PTT, or both. Plasma from patients with a specific inhibitor will progressively inactivate a coagulation protein and thus prolong whichever of these screening tests requires the participation of that clotting factor. This effect persists after dilution. Nonspecific inhibitors immediately prolong the PT and PTT and, at low dilution, block multiple coagulation reactions. However, these effects can be overcome by altering the quantity or type of phospholipid or by diluting the plasma.

Hemorrhage in patients with specific inhibitors may require treatment with massive plasma or concentrate infusion, the use of activated prothrombin complex concentrates to bypass the antibodies against factors VIII or IX, and plasmapheresis or exchange transfusion to lower antibody titer. Chronic immunosuppressive regimens have been sometimes employed and have been particularly useful in otherwise normal individuals with an acquired factor VIII antibody. Many patients lose their antibody and recover within 6 to 12 months, although the acute mortality rate from uncontrollable bleeding may approach 10 percent.

Patients with nonspecific anticoagulants have normal hemostasis and do not require any therapy unless they are concomitantly thrombocytopenic or prothrombin-deficient. Both thrombocytopenia and hypoprothrombinemia are secondary to autoantibodies which bind either to platelets or the prothrombin molecule. While these antibodies have no effect on function, they accelerate clearance of the coated platelets or the antibody-prothrombin complexes. There is some evidence that the lupus-like anticoagulant may predispose patients to thromboembolism and is associated with recurrent mid-trimester abortions in women. However, many of these women can successfully carry their fetuses to term following therapy with glucocorticoids.

INHERITED PRETHROMBOTIC DISORDERS As previously discussed (see Chap. 62), coagulation is carefully regulated by a series of inhibitors which limit thrombin generation and fibrin formation and by the fibrinolytic system which effectively removes fibrin thrombi (see Figs. 62-5 and 62-7). Inherited defects in the natural coagulation inhibitors (i.e., antithrombin, protein C, and protein S), abnormalities in the fibrinolytic system, and certain dysfibrinogenemias predispose patients to thrombosis (see Table 288-3). Although they are an important and rapidly expanding group of disorders, they account for less than 10 percent of patients with recurrent thromboembolism. The known disorders are all inherited as autosomal dominant traits, so that heterozygous individuals, who have a 50 percent reduction in protein concentration or a mixture of mutant and normal molecules, will have an increased risk of thrombosis. The patients all have similar clinical presentations with a strong family history of thrombosis, episodes of recurrent venous thromboembolism, and symptoms by their early twenties. Any patient with this distinctive history should be tested for the molecular abnormalities described below.

ANTITHROMBIN DEFICIENCY Antithrombin complexes with activated coagulation proteins and blocks their biologic activity (see Fig. 62-5). The rate of this reaction is enhanced by heparin-like molecules within the vessel wall or on endothelial cells. Plasma antithrombin III content varies from 5 to 15 mg/L (50 to 150 percent), with values only slightly below normal increasing the risk of thrombosis. For optimal screening, it is important to assess both the antithrombin III concentration by immunoassay and the plasma antithrombin and heparin cofactor activity with functional assays. The most common defect is mild (heterozygous) antithrombin defi-

TABLE 288-3 Prethrombotic disorders

INHERITED FORMS
Antithrombin III deficiency
Protein C deficiency
Protein S deficiency
Dysplasminogenemia
Dysfibrinogenemia
Defective release of plasminogen activator
Diminished venous content of plasminogen activator
Excessive release of plasminogen activator inhibitor
Heparin cofactor II deficiency
Homocystinuria
ACQUIRED DISORDERS
Chronic congestive heart failure
Metastatic tumor
Metastatic malignancy
Extensive trauma or major surgery
Myeloproliferative disorders
Behçet's syndrome
Kawasaki's disease
Ingestion of oral contraceptives or L-asparaginase

ciency, which occurs in 1 out of 2000 individuals. In addition, dysfunctional antithrombin molecules, with mutations affectng either the serine protease–binding site or the heparin-binding site, or activation of inhibitor by heparin have been described. Some investigators have suggested that another molecule called heparin cofactor II may also be a clinically important thrombin inhibitor. Some patients with thrombosis have been described who are heparin cofactor II–deficient.

Patients with antithrombin deficiency who develop acute thrombosis or embolism can be treated with intravenous heparin, since there is usually sufficient normal antithrombin to act as a heparin cofactor. Following their first episode of thromboembolism, patients should be placed on oral anticoagulants for life to prevent recurrent thrombosis. Family studies should be conducted when an antithrombin-deficient individual is discovered, since up to half the members of a kindred may be affected. Asymptomatic individuals with antithrombin deficiency should receive prophylactic anticoagulation with heparin or plasma infusions to raise their antithrombin level prior to medical or surgical procedures which may increase their risk of thrombosis. Chronic oral anticoagulation is not recommended until individuals at risk have a clinical thrombotic episode.

DEFICIENCIES OF PROTEINS C AND S Protein C is a vitamin K–dependent hepatic protein which binds to the endothelial cell surface protein thrombomodulin and is converted to an active protease by thrombin (Fig. 62-5). Activated protein C, in conjunction with protein S, proteolyzes factors Va and VIIIa, which shuts off fibrin formation. Activated protein C may also stimulate fibrinolysis and accelerate clot lysis. Deficiencies of proteins C and S are autosomal dominant disorders which may be more common than antithrombin deficiency and cause identical problems—recurrent venous thrombosis and pulmonary embolism. Dysfunctional molecules have also been definitely identified in patients with thrombosis. In addition, protein S activity may be reduced when there is an excess of C4b binding protein.

Heterozygous patients with acute thrombosis and moderate proteins C or S deficiency should be heparinized and then placed on oral anticoagulants. There are, however, two potential problems with the use of coumarin anticoagulants in these patients. First, these vitamin K antagonists (see Fig. 288-1 and Fig. 62-5), which lower the level of the procoagulant factors II, VII, IX, and X, may also reduce the concentration of proteins C and S and nullify the desired antithrombotic effect. In addition, there are patients with coumarin-induced skin necrosis who have protein C deficiency, suggesting that this defect may predispose patients to a rare but serious complication of oral anticoagulants.

Homozygous protein C deficiency, which is very rare, can cause fulminant intravascular coagulation in the neonatal period. Patients with homozygous protein C deficiency may require periodic plasma infusions rather than oral anticoagulants to prevent recurrent intravascular coagulation and thrombosis.

DYSFIBRINOGENEMIAS AND FIBRINOLYTIC DEFECTS Several families have now been described with recurrent venous thrombosis and embolism due to defects in fibrinogen or plasminogen or with decreased synthesis or release of tissue plasminogen activator. While the majority of dysfibrinogenemias cause bleeding, one variant, fibrinogen New York, is characterized by excessively rapid release of fibrinopeptides and recurrent thromboembolism. Patients with this disorder as well as those with an abnormal plasminogen which resists activation by streptokinase and urokinase have been successfully treated with heparin and oral anticoagulants. Defects in tissue plasminogen activator content or release have not been completely characterized. One group of patients with recurrent venous thrombosis and embolism failed to increase venous blood fibrinolytic activity when challenged with local ischemia or physical exercise. The other group had impaired fibrinolytic activity in extracts prepared from biopsied veins. The recent cloning of cDNA for tissue plasminogen activator (tPA) and the availability of immunoassays for tPA should facilitate more detailed studies of this class of defects. There is also recent evidence that young patients with acute myocardial infarction may have impaired fibrinolysis due to increased plasma levels of plasminogen activator inhibitor (PAI), a serine protease inhibitor which binds to tPA and is derived from endothelial cells.

In addition to the inherited disorders which predispose patients to thromboembolism, many common illnesses are associated with an increased risk of thrombosis (see Table 288-3). These patients are said to have a "hypercoagulable" or "prethrombotic" state. This increased risk is seen in patients with chronic congestive heart failure and metastatic malignancy and in patients undergoing major surgery. In these patients, the generation of tissue factor activity in damaged or ischemic tissue or metastatic tumor, coupled with venous stasis and endothelial injury, induce the formation of venous and, more rarely, arterial thrombi. There are also several hematologic disorders including paroxysmal nocturnal hemoglobinuria, essential thrombocythemia, and polycythemia vera in which poorly defined abnormalities in circulating leukocytes and platelets, or changes in blood flow and viscosity, predispose patients to venous and arterial thrombosis. Diseases which affect the endothelial cell, such as Behçet's syndrome, Kawasaki's disease, and homocystinuria, or the administration of drugs like the oral contraceptives, which lower antithrombin III levels, or L-asparaginase, which inhibits production of multiple coagulation factors, may also predispose patients to thrombosis.

REFERENCES

ANTONARAKIS SE: The molecular genetics of hemophilia A and B in man. Factor III and factor IX deficiency. Adv Hum Genet 17:17, 1988

GIDDINGS JC, PEAKE IR: Laboratory support in the diagnosis of coagulation disorders. Clin Haematol 14:571, 1985

KANE WH, DAVIE EW: Blood coagulation factors V and VIII: Structural and functional similarities and their relationship to hemorrhagic and thrombotic disorders. Blood 71:539, 1988

KASPER CK, DIETRICH SL: Comprehensive management of haemophilia. Clin Haematol 14:489, 1985

LAWN R: The molecular genetics of hemophilia. Sci Am 254:48, 1986

MAMMEN E: Congenital coagulation disorders. Semin Thromb Hemost 9:1, 1983

PIERCE GF et al: The use of purified clotting factor concentrates in hemophilia. Influence of viral safety, cost and supply on therapy. JAMA 261:3434, 1989

WHITE GC, SHOEMAKER CB: Factor VIII gene and hemophilia A. Blood 73:1, 1989

289 ANTICOAGULANT, FIBRINOLYTIC, AND ANTIPLATELET THERAPY

ROBERT I. HANDIN

ANTICOAGULANT AND FIBRINOLYTIC THERAPY

Anticoagulation with heparin, followed by treatment with oral vitamin K antagonists, is the standard treatment for acute venous thrombosis and pulmonary embolism. In addition, chronic oral anticoagulation is used to prevent cerebral arterial embolism from cardiac sources such as ventricular mural thrombi, atrial thrombi, or from an atherosclerotic, partially stenosed carotid or vertebral artery. Anticoagulants are also used, less successfully, to treat peripheral or mesenteric arterial thrombosis. These agents retard fibrin deposition on established thrombi and prevent the formation of new thrombi. The induction of a fibrinolytic state by the infusion of recombinant tissue plasminogen activator (rtPA) or pharmacologic agents such as streptokinase (SK) and urokinase (UK) has become an accepted mode of therapy for some thromboembolic disorders. This approach has been advocated for some patients with massive pulmonary embolism and systemic hypotension and to restore the patency of acutely occluded peripheral and coronary arteries. Prompt fibrinolytic therapy may reduce myocardial damage following acute coronary occlusion (see Chap. 189).

TABLE 289-1 Anticoagulant therapy with heparin

Clinical indication	Dose, U.S.P. units	Route
Prophylaxis in general surgery	5000 q 12 h	SC
Prophylaxis in medical patients with congestive heart failure, cardiomyopathy, or myocardial infarction	10,000 q 12 h	SC
Venous thromboembolism (acute)	5000 (bolus) 1000 qh	IV
Venous thromboembolism (prophylaxis in pregnancy, warfarin failures, or chronic DIC)	1000 qh	SQ (pump)

ACUTE ANTICOAGULATION WITH HEPARIN Heparin is a naturally occurring mucopolysaccharide polymer with tetrasaccharide sequences that bind to and activate antithrombin III. It is an extremely potent anticoagulant that can reduce thrombin generation and fibrin formation in patients with acute venous and arterial thrombosis or embolism (Table 289-1). Heparin is administered to patients with acute thrombosis or embolism by continuous intravenous infusion at a rate sufficient to raise the activated partial thromboplastin time (APTT) to 1.5 to 2 times the control value. This usually requires 1000 U.S.P. units per hour and is continued while patients are begun on oral anticoagulants and achieve appropriate prolongation of the prothrombin time. The usual duration of combined heparin-warfarin therapy is 5 to 7 days. Heparin is then discontinued, and the patient is maintained on warfarin. Alternatives include the administration of 5000 U.S.P. units of heparin four times a day either subcutaneously or intravenously. Long-term heparin administration via portable external or implantable pumps is occasionally needed for recurrent thromboembolism that is refractory to oral anticoagulants, for pregnant women with thromboembolism, and for patients with chronic disseminated intravascular coagulation (DIC). Lower doses of heparin (5000 U.S.P. units every 12 h) have also been used to prevent deep venous thrombosis in high-risk surgical and medical patients. Patients with congestive heart failure, myocardial infarction, or cardiomyopathy may require 10,000 U.S.P. units every 12 h for similar protection.

The major complication of heparin therapy is bleeding—especially from surgical sites and into the retroperitoneum. Aspirin or aspirin-containing drugs impair platelet function, and intramuscular injections in these patients may cause significant bleeding. Heparin's anticoagulant effect can be rapidly reversed by the administration of protamine sulfate. However, this is usually not necessary, and reduction or omission of heparin improves hemostasis and stops bleeding. Thrombocytopenia occurs in about 10 percent of heparin recipients, can be severe, and may be accompanied by intravascular platelet agglutination and arterial thrombosis. Recognition of this rare complication—thrombocytopenia and paradoxical thrombosis—is critical, since discontinuing heparin can reverse the syndrome and may be lifesaving. Heparin administration for longer than 2 months also carries a risk of osteoporosis. Commercial heparin preparations are heterogeneous and only about 20 percent of the infused material has anticoagulant activity. Low molecular weight heparin fractions, which retain anticoagulant activity, are the treatment of choice for patients with heparin-dependent thrombocytopenia who require additional heparin therapy. These fractions do not interact with platelets and may not cause thrombocytopenia.

CHRONIC ORAL ANTICOAGULATION The coumarin anticoagulants, which include warfarin and dicumarol (dicoumarol), prevent the reduction of vitamin K epoxides in the liver microsomes and induce a state analogous to vitamin K deficiency (see Fig. 288-1). They slow thrombin generation and clot formation by impairing the biologic activity of the prothrombin complex proteins and are used to prevent the recurrence of venous thrombosis and pulmonary embolism. Although regimens employing loading doses of drug have been advocated, the simplest way to induce anticoagulation is to administer a single dose of a coumarin compound and monitor the prothrombin time (PT) until the desired prolongation is achieved. For example, treatment can be initiated with 5 to 10 mg/d of warfarin or equivalent, with the goal of prolonging the PT to 1.5 to 2 times the control value. Although the PT may reach this value after a few days of therapy, effective anticoagulation, with stable reduction of all the prothrombin complex proteins, requires at least 1 week of warfarin administration. Most patients require a daily maintenance dose of 2.5 to 7.5 mg of warfarin to remain anticoagulated. As discussed above, patients should remain on heparin until the appropriate dose of a coumarin anticoagulant like warfarin is established.

Although warfarin anticoagulants reduce the recurrence of deep venous thrombosis and pulmonary or cerebral embolism, they may also cause bleeding. Any patient who takes oral anticoagulants requires frequent monitoring of the PT. Despite the most careful management, fluctuations in PT can occur. Various drugs that alter liver microsomal metabolism of coumarins or compete for albumin binding sites can increase or decrease the potency of warfarin (Table 289-2).

There is a direct relation between the duration of anticoagulation and the risk of recurrent thrombosis. Although recommendations vary somewhat, most patients with a single uncomplicated thromboembolic event have maximal benefit after 3 to 6 months of anticoagulation. About 10 percent of patients on an oral anticoagulant for 1 year have a serious complication requiring medical supervision, and 0.5 to 1 percent have a fatal hemorrhagic event despite careful medical management. The anticoagulant effects of coumarins can be reversed by infusion of fresh frozen plasma or by the administration of vitamin K. In many cases, reduction or omission of several doses improves hemostasis and stops hemorrhage. Despite the risk of bleeding, patients with prosthetic heart valves, severe mitral stenosis, cardiomyopathy, chronic congestive heart failure, recurrent or persistent atrial fibrillation, or an inherited "prethrombotic" disorder may require lifelong anticoagulation.

One devastating complication of oral anticoagulation is hemorrhagic skin necrosis. Some patients with this complication are deficient in protein C, a natural anticoagulant protein whose activity is reduced by vitamin K antagonists. Patients with suspected protein C deficiency should not begin oral anticoagulant therapy unless they simultaneously receive heparin or plasma infusions to restore protein C levels to normal. Patients with an inherited trait that causes coumarin resistance may require extremely high doses to get an anticoagulant effect. Psychologically disturbed patients may surreptitiously ingest coumarin and present with unexplained bleeding and a prolonged PT. Plasma coumarin levels can be measured to confirm such ingestion.

TABLE 289-2 Effect of drugs and metabolic changes on oral anticoagulant potency

I Factors leading to enhanced potency and increased prothrombin time
- *A* Reduced coumarin clearance
  - 1 Disulfiram (Antabuse)
  - 2 Metronidazole (Flagyl)
  - 3 Trimethoprim-sulfamethoxazole (Bactrim, Septra)
- *B* Reduced albumin binding
  - 1 Phenylbutazone
- *C* Additive hemostatic effect of certain drugs or disorders
  - 1 Aspirin
  - 2 Heparin
  - 3 Liver disease
  - 4 Thrombocytopenia
  - 5 Vitamin K deficiency
- *D* Increased turnover of vitamin K
  - 1 Clofibrate
  - 2 Hypermetabolism (e.g., hyperthyroidism)

II Factors leading to diminished potency and decreased prothrombin time
- *A* Accelerated coumarin clearance—induction of hepatic metabolizing enzymes
  - 1 Barbiturates
  - 2 Rifampin
- *B* Reduced absorption
  - 1 Cholestyramine
- *C* Impaired metabolism
  - 1 Genetic coumarin resistance

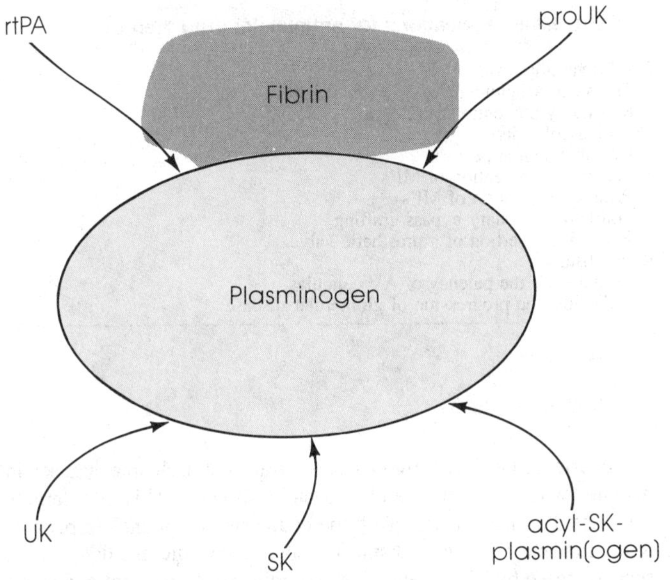

FIGURE 289-1 The mechanism of action of various plasminogen activators used for thrombolytic therapy. Recombinant tissue plasminogen activator (rtPA) and pro-urokinase (proUK) preferentially activate plasminogen bound to fibrin and are called "fibrin-specific" activators. Urokinase (UK), streptokinase (SK), and acylated streptokinase-plasminogen conjugates activate both free and fibrin-bound plasminogen.

FIBRINOLYTIC THERAPY Fibrinolysis, an important part of the normal hemostatic process, is initiated by the release of either tPA or pro-urokinase (proUK) from endothelial cells. These agents preferentially activate plasminogen, which is adsorbed onto fibrin clots. This serves to direct and localize the lytic process to sites that contain fibrin thrombi. Although fibrinolysis begins immediately after vascular injury, clot lysis and vessel recanalization may not be complete for 7 to 10 days. As previously discussed (see Chap. 62), the fibrinolytic pathway is important in normal hemostasis, as defects can predispose patients to either hemorrhage or recurrent thrombosis (see Chap. 288). In addition, activators of the fibrinolytic system are frequently employed to accelerate clot lysis in patients with thromboembolism (see Fig. 289-1, Table 289-3).

Several pharmacologic agents can accelerate clot lysis. These drugs are either naturally occurring products or chemically modified derivatives and differ with respite to fibrin specificity and complications (see Table 289-3). The cloning of the cDNA encoding tPA permitted the large-scale production of rtPA. This and proUK are relatively "fibrin-specific" agents that activate plasminogen more effectively in the presence of fibrin thrombi. This makes it theoretically possible to achieve more selective clot lysis without inducing the systemic lytic state that accompanies the infusion of urokinase (UK) or streptokinase (SK). In practice, some systemic fibrinolysis always

TABLE 289-3 Fibrinolytic activators

Product	Source	MW	Fibrin	Complications
Recombinant tissue plasminogen activator (rtPA)	Recombinant	70,000	+	Bleeding
Pro-urokinase (proUK)	Melanoma cell cultures	55,000	+	Bleeding
Urokinase (UK)	Renal tubular cell cultures	33,000	+	Bleeding
Streptokinase (SK)	β-Hemolytic streptococci	47,000	−	Immune reactions Bleeding
Acyl-SK-plasmin(ogen)	Chemical synthesis	139,00	+/−	Immune reactions Bleeding

TABLE 289-4 Indications for fibrinolytic therapy

Acute coronary occlusion/infarction
Acute peripheral arterial occlusion
Massive pulmonary embolism
Axillary vein thrombosis
Massive iliofemoral vein thrombosis

accompanies the infusion of effective doses of the fibrin-specific agents. In addition, all fibrinolytic agents can cause hemorrhage by attacking essential hemostatic plugs as well as pathologic thrombi. Thus, lytic therapy is not recommended for patients with recent surgery, indwelling cannulas, or a history of neurologic lesions, gastrointestinal bleeding, or hypertension.

Current indications for fibrinolytic therapy are listed in Table 289-4. Fibrinolytic therapy is now recommended for patients with acute myocardial infarction and with massive pulmonary embolism complicated by hypotension, severe hypoxemia, and right heart strain or failure. In addition, fibrinolytic agents have been successfully administered to patients with acute peripheral arterial embolism or occlusion and to patients with extensive iliofemoral thrombophlebitis. While such therapy may hasten lysis of venous thrombi, the long-term benefit remains unproven. There is no firm evidence that lytic therapy reduces postphlebitic complications. In contrast, fibrinolytic therapy may be of distinct benefit for thrombosis of the axillary vein, which does not respond well to conventional anticoagulation.

SK and UK are the oldest and most extensively studied fibrinolytic agents. SK is a bacterial enzyme, and UK is a product of renal tubular epithelial cells. These agents cannot discriminate between free and fibrin-bound plasminogen. When administered systemically for clot lysis, they also cause hypofibrinogenemia and a systemic lytic state. SK is an indirect plasminogen activator that interacts with circulating plasminogen to form an equimolar complex with proteolytic activity. The SK-plasminogen complex then activates additional plasminogen molecules that initiate fibrinolysis. In contrast, UK has intrinsic proteolytic activity and can activate plasminogen directly.

In the case of SK, one usually administers a loading dose of 250,000 units irrespective of body weight. Since patients may have antistreptococcal antibodies, the loading dose may need to be repeated. In addition, patients may develop acute allergic symptoms including urticaria and, occasionally, serum sickness reactions. With UK, a loading dose of 4400 units per kg body weight is administered over 10 to 30 min. Both regimens induce an intense lytic state as evidenced by a drop in fibrinogen, prolongation of the thrombin time, and a prolongation of the euglobulin lysis time—an in vitro measure of fibrinolytic activity, predominantly plasminogen activated. After the initial loading dose, 100,000 units of SK or 4400 units of UK per kg body weight are administered hourly for 24 to 72 h. At the desired time, the lytic state is reversed by discontinuing UK or SK and by administering heparin for 7 to 10 days. Heparin can be started 6 h after the fibrinolytic agent has been stopped. To enhance the likelihood of success, fibrinolytic therapy should be initiated as soon as possible after the onset of thrombosis or embolism.

The majority of myocardial infarcts are due to acute coronary occlusion, and fibrinolytic therapy has been tried extensively for acute coronary events. Initially, the nonspecific agents SK or UK were administered via a catheter placed in the diseased coronary artery in an attempt to achieve localized clot lysis. Fibrin-specific agents such as rtPA or proUK are now being administered intravenously; the former has been studied most extensively. Systemic infusion of 100 mg rtPA over 6 h restores vessel patency in approximately 75 percent of patients. Patients are then maintained on heparin for several days. ProUK given in a similar manner has almost identical effects. As discussed in Chap. 189, it is imperative to begin the therapy within a few hours of the onset of symptoms. Systemic fibrinogen levels fall 25 percent with this regimen. Bleeding is a major complication as rtPA cannot discriminate between pathologic intracoronary thrombi, which are undesirable, and vitally important hemostatic plugs; both contain fibrin and may coexist in the same patient. The most serious complication of fibrinolytic therapy, intracranial hemorrhage, is relatively rare but has devastating and sometimes fatal consequences. Thus, the same stringent contraindications discussed for systemic lytic therapy should be employed with fibrin-specific agents.

ANTIPLATELET DRUG THERAPY

Antiplatelet drugs have a role to play in the management of patients with arterial vascular disease and thromboembolism (see Table 289-5). Aspirin is the most widely studied of these drugs because of its unique pharmacology. A single dose of aspirin irreversibly acetylates and inactivates the enzyme cyclooxygenase and thereby inhibits platelet production of thromboxane A_2. Although aspirin may also inactivate cyclooxygenase in some tissues, including endothelial cells, such cells recover rapidly by synthesizing new enzyme. Platelets, which are anucleate, cannot synthesize new enzyme and remain inactive for the rest of their lifespan. As little as one 160 mg tablet of aspirin daily or a 325 mg tablet every other day inhibits platelet thromboxane production and aggregation.

Many antithrombotic regimens have employed dipyridamole, which inhibits phosphodiesterase and raises intracellular cyclic AMP in vitro. The usual dose of 50 to 100 mg four times daily has no discernible effect on platelet function. Dipyridamole has usually been administered in combination with aspirin; it is not clear that dipyridamole adds benefits when added to aspirin.

Patients with coronary artery disease who have unstable angina are at high risk for myocardial infarction (Chap. 189). In two large clinical trials, the prompt administration of aspirin dramatically reduced the progression to myocardial infarction in this group, although aspirin had no effect on the frequency, intensity, or duration of chronic angina. Aspirin also reduces the incidence of second infarction by 25 percent when administered to men who have had a myocardial infarct. In a large study of asymptomatic physicians, daily aspirin therapy also reduced the incidence of first infarcts and is now widely used for prevention of myocardial infarction. The combination of aspirin and dipyridamole, when begun prior to surgery, may also increase the patency of coronary bypass grafts, and the same combination reduces the incidence of cerebral emboli in patients on warfarin who have prosthetic intracardiac valves.

TABLE 289-5 Indications for antiplatelet drug therapy

Cerebrovascular disease
Transient ischemic attacks
Secondary prevention of CVA's
Cardiovascular disease
Unstable angina pectoris
Secondary prevention of MI's
Primary prevention of MI's
Following coronary bypass grafting
Following insertion of a prosthetic valve
Renal disease
To maintain the patency of AV cannulas
? To slow the progression of glomerular disease

Aspirin reduces the frequency of transient ischemic attacks in patients with occlusive cerebrovascular disease. This has largely supplanted anticoagulation with the coumarin compounds in patients with transient ischemia. Aspirin also reduces the incidence of a second stroke by 25 percent when administered to men following the first cerebrovascular accident. Aspirin is also effective in maintaining the patency of arteriovenous cannulas inserted into patients with renal failure who require hemodialysis. Aspirin plus dipyridamole may also slow the progression of some forms of glomerulonephritis, although these drugs are not widely used in the treatment of renal disease. However, aspirin appears not to be effective in maintaining the patency of vessels following percutaneous angioplasty.

REFERENCES

Clouse LJ, Comp PC: The regulation of hemostasis: The protein C system. N Engl J Med 314:1298, 1986

Goller BS: Platelets and thrombolytic therapy. N Engl J Med 322:33, 1990

Lee TH et al: Candidates for thrombolysis among Emergency Room patients with acute chest pain: Potential true- and false-positive rates. Ann Intern Med 110:957, 1989

Levine MN, Hirsh J: Hemorrhagic complications of anticoagulation therapy. Semin Thromb Hemost 12L:39, 1986

Loscalzo J, Braunwald E: Tissue plasminogen activator. N Engl J Med 319:925, 1988

Saour JN et al: Trial of different intensities of anticoagulation in patients with prosthetic heart valves. N Engl J Med 322:428, 1990

section 2 Disorders of the hematopoietic system

290 PATHOPHYSIOLOGY OF THE ANEMIAS

H. FRANKLIN BUNN

There is a large and coherent body of information on the birth, life, and death of red cells. A thorough familiarity with erythropoiesis and erythrocyte structure and function is necessary to understand the pathogenesis of the various anemias as well as to develop an orderly approach to diagnosis and management. Conversely, investigation of specific red cell disorders has provided unique insights into normal erythroid physiology.

RED CELL PRODUCTION Red cells are derived from an undifferentiated progenitor cell in the bone marrow called the *pluripotent stem cell* (Fig. 290-1). A stem cell is one which is capable of both self-renewal and differentiation. *Pluripotent* implies that granulocytes, monocytes, and platelets also evolve from this ancestor cell. The pluripotent stem cell has the morphologic characteristics of a mature lymphocyte. The control of proliferation into differentiated cell lines is beginning to be understood owing in part to the isolation and characterization of hematopoietic stem cells and growth factors. As Fig. 290-1 shows, the most primitive erythroid progenitor which has been cultured from both bone marrow and peripheral blood is called the *erythroid burst-forming unit* (BFU_e). After 10 to 15 days in tissue culture it produces a large colony of recognizable red cell precursors. The BFU_e is responsive to high doses of the erythroid-promoting hormone erythropoietin, which acts synergistically with other growth

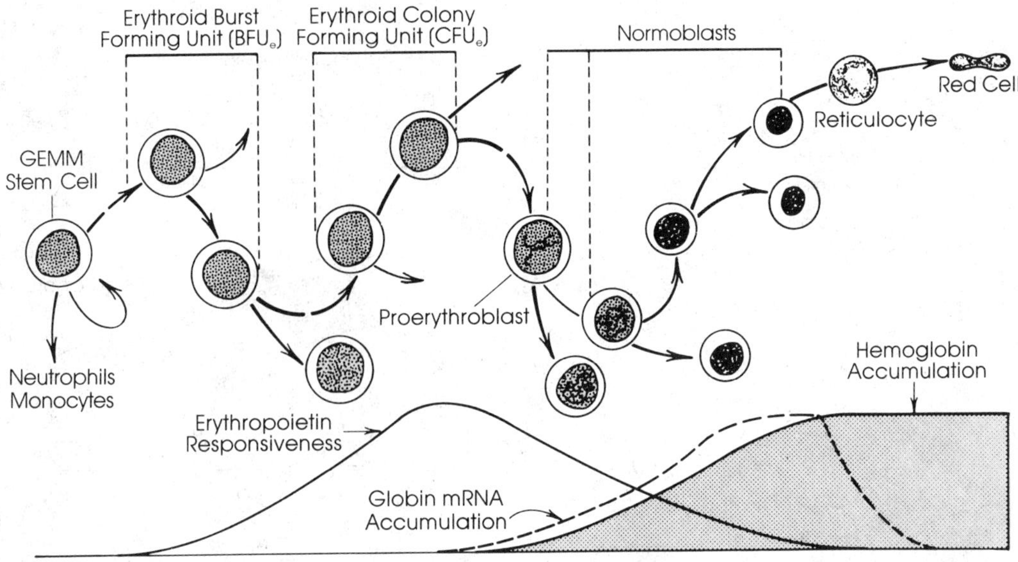

FIGURE 290-1 Differentiation and morphologic maturation of erythroid cells. Erythroid cells are derived from GEMM stem cells (shown on left) which are also capable of differentiating into neutrophils, monocytes (macrophages), and megakaryocytes. Under the influence of erythropoietin, erythroid precursor cells ($BFU_e \rightarrow CFU_e$) differentiate into proerythroblasts, the earliest recognizable erythroid cells in the bone marrow. During further maturation, globin mRNA accumulates, directing the cell to synthesize hemoglobin.

factors derived from lymphocytes, monocytes, and cells of the marrow stroma (fibroblasts, adipocytes, endothelial cells, etc.). A more mature cell, the *erythroid colony-forming unit* (CFU_e), produces a smaller clone of erythroid cells after 4 to 7 days in culture and is very sensitive to erythropoietin. Well-designed experiments involving incubation of uniform hematopoietic and stromal cell populations with purified growth factors should provide considerably more information about the mechanisms underlying the differentiation and maturation of erythroid cells in vivo, as well as insights into certain disorders of erythropoiesis.

Erythropoietin, a glycoprotein having a molecular weight of 34,000, has been purified to homogeneity. The cloning of the erythropoietin gene has made possible the synthesis of large amounts of biologically active hormone. Erythropoietin is produced, primarily by the kidneys, in response to hypoxia and is secreted into the plasma. Levels of this hormone are increased in direct proportion to the degree of hypoxia.

Erythropoietin interacts with a specific receptor on the surfaces of committed erythroid stem cells, inducing them to differentiate into proerythroblasts, the earliest red cell precursor that can be recognized on examination of the bone marrow. Normally the transition from the proerythroblast to the most mature normoblast involves three or four cell divisions over a 4-day period (Fig. 290-1). During this time, the nucleus becomes smaller, and an increasing amount of hemoglobin is produced in the cytoplasm. Following the last division, the pyknotic nucleus is removed from the normoblast, forming the reticulocyte which stays in the bone marrow for 2.5 to 3 days. The reticulocyte is then released into the general circulation, where it remains for another 24 h before it loses its mitochondria and ribosomes and assumes the morphologic appearance of a mature red cell.

Erythroid precursor cells ranging from the pronormoblast to the reticulocyte possess a specific surface receptor for the iron-transferrin complex, enabling them to incorporate sufficient iron for hemoglobin production (Fig. 290-2). The use of a radioactive iron label such as

FIGURE 290-2 Erythrocyte production, circulation, and destruction. Circulating iron-bound transferrin (TF) is bound to specific receptors on the surface of red blood cell precursors in the marrow. Most of this iron is incorporated into hemoglobin; the remainder is stored as ferritin. Following maturation of the erythroid precursor, the nucleus is shed and the red blood cell emerges from the marrow into the plasma where it circulates for approximately 120 days. The senescent red blood cell is taken up by the mononuclear phagocyte system and is destroyed. The heme iron is initially incorporated into ferritin. This storage iron is available for transport to the marrow via transferrin.

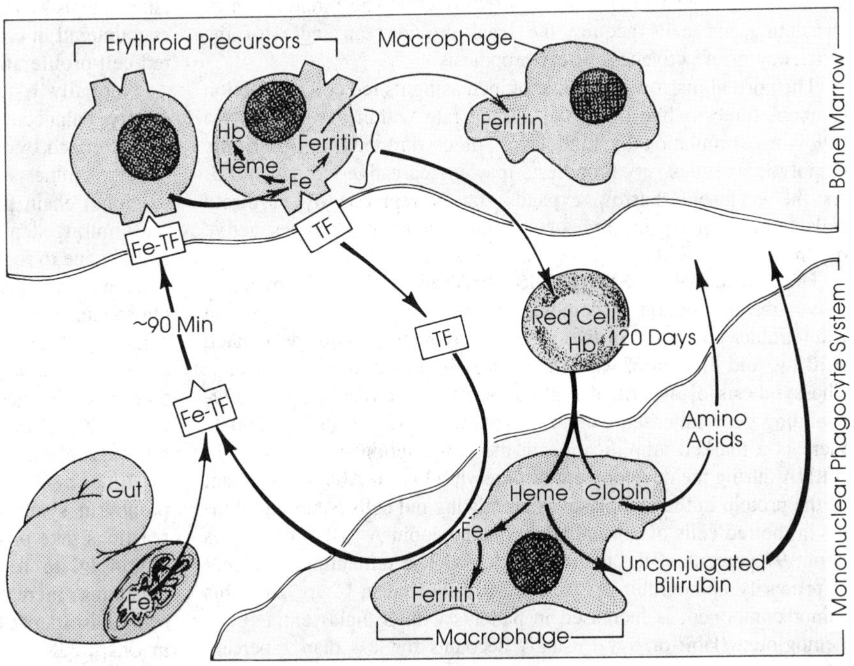

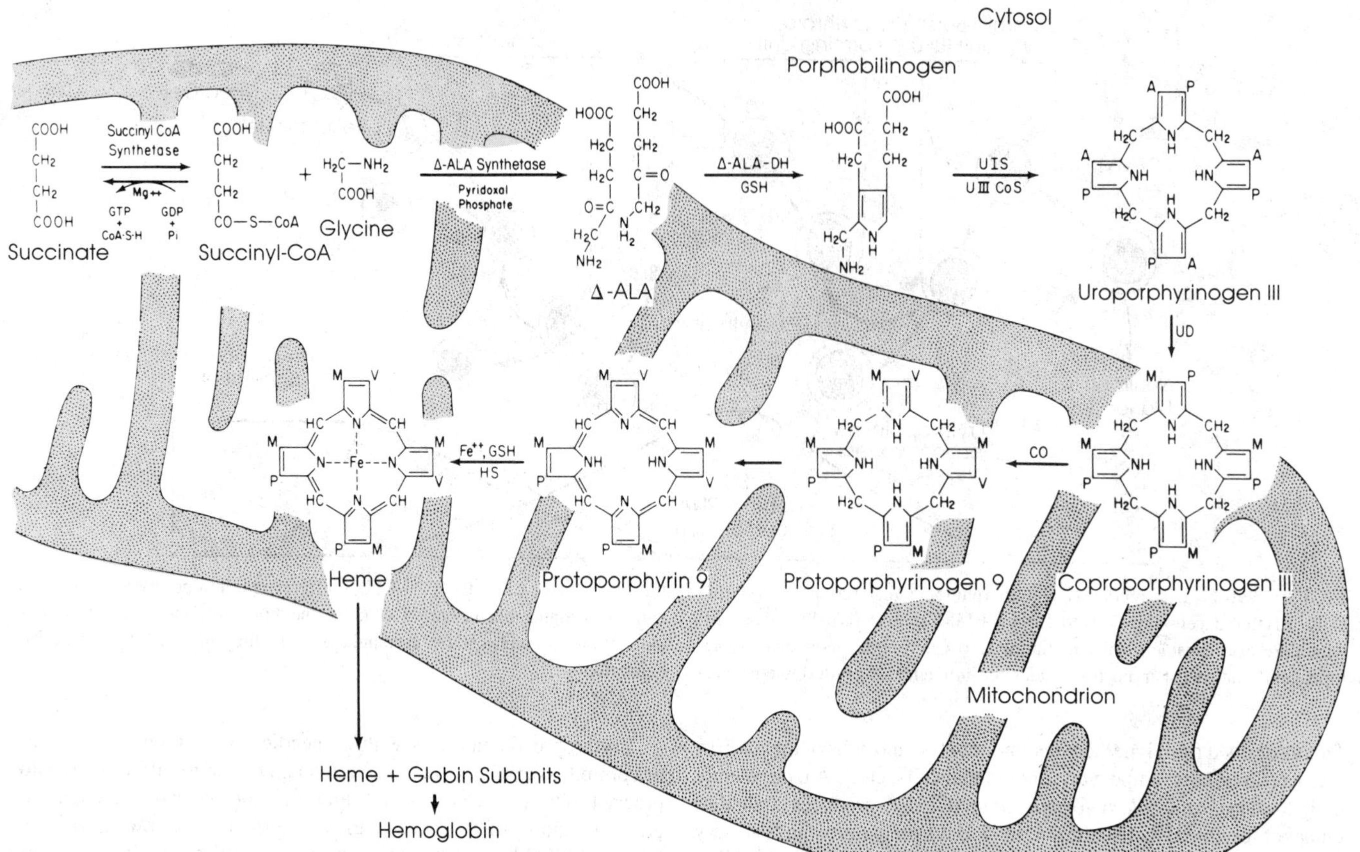

FIGURE 290-3 The biosynthesis of heme. The following abbreviations are used: CoA, coenzyme A; GTP, guanosine triphosphate; GDP, guanosine diphosphate; Pi, inorganic phosphorus; GSH, glutathione; δ-ALA-DH, δ-aminolevulinate dehydrase; UIS, uroporphyrinogen I synthetase; UIII CoS, uroporphyrinogen III cosynthetase; UD, uroporphyrinogen decarboxylase; CO, coproporphyrinogen oxidase; HS, heme synthetase; A, acetate; P, proprionate; M, methyl; V, vinyl. Enzymatic steps that occur in mitochondria are shown.

^{59}Fe permits a quantitative assessment of erythropoiesis. From the rate at which injected ^{59}Fe-labeled transferrin disappears from the plasma, plasma iron turnover can be calculated. This parameter is generally proportional to the total developing erythroid cell mass. Normally, about 80 percent of ^{59}Fe bound to plasma transferrin goes to erythroid cells in the marrow (Fig. 290-3*B*). After 4 to 6 days the labeled iron reappears in circulating erythrocytes. The extent to which circulating red cells acquire the label provides an index of the efficiency or effectiveness of erythropoiesis.

The normal marrow is capable of increasing its red cell production to about three to five times the normal rate within a week or two following stimulation by high levels of erythropoietin. In chronic hemolytic anemias, erythropoiesis may increase five- to sevenfold. As the erythroid marrow expands, fat is replaced by erythroid cells, and formerly inactive or "yellow" marrow becomes active or "red."

HEMOGLOBIN BIOSYNTHESIS Erythroid cell development involves the production of hemoglobin-containing cells. Hemoglobin is a tetramer composed of two pairs of polypeptide chains designated α, β, γ, and δ, each of which is covalently linked to a heme group. The synthesis of a particular globin subunit is directed by a corresponding gene inherited from each parent. As shown in Fig. 290-1, there is a marked amplification in the transcription of globin chain mRNA during the development of proerythroblasts. About 98 percent of the protein in the cytoplasm of circulating red cells is hemoglobin.

In the red cells of normal adults, hemoglobin A ($\alpha_2\beta_2$) composes about 97 percent of the total hemoglobin. The remaining 3 percent is primarily hemoglobin A_2 ($\alpha_2\delta_2$). As discussed in Chap. 295, this minor component is increased in patients with β thalassemia. Fetal hemoglobin (HbF or $\alpha_2\gamma_2$) usually accounts for less than 1 percent of total hemoglobin in normal adult red cells. HbF is localized to 1 to 7 percent of red cells. In contrast, it is the main hemoglobin component of fetal red cells. During the last 3 months of gestation, γ-chain synthesis switches to β-chain synthesis. However, in certain types of congenital hemolytic anemias such as the β thalassemias and sickle cell anemia, the production of γ chains (and therefore of HbF) persists. In addition, increased levels of HbF may also be encountered in certain acquired anemias in which there is disordered red cell proliferation.

Normally α- and β-chain synthesis in erythroid precursors is evenly balanced. In contrast, the thalassemias (Chap. 295) are characterized by imbalance in globin chain synthesis.

The synthesis of *heme* in red cell precursors is closely matched to globin chain production. As shown in Fig. 290-3 the initial and rate-limiting step is the condensation of succinyl coenzyme A (CoA) and glycine to form δ-aminolevulinic acid. This reaction, which takes place in mitochondria, requires that glycine be activated by pyridoxal phosphate. Accordingly, patients with sideroblastic anemia in whom heme synthesis is usually defective may sometimes respond to pyridoxine therapy (Chap. 291). The next steps of heme synthesis take place in the cytosol. Two molecules of δ-aminolevulinic acid condense to form a ring structure, prophobilinogen. This colorless pyrrole is elevated in acute intermittent porphyria and can be detected in urine by the Watson-Schwartz test. The subsequent steps in prophyrin synthesis are also shown in Fig. 290-3. The last three reactions take place in mitochondria. Iron is inserted into protoporphyrin IX to form heme. In iron deficiency, as well as in lead poisoning, increased levels of protoporphyrin can be detected in red cells. Disorders of porphyrin synthesis and metabolism are discussed in Chap. 328.

HEMOGLOBIN STRUCTURE AND FUNCTION The primary role of red cells is to transport oxygen from lungs to tissues and to transport carbon dioxide in the reverse direction. Both of these functions are assumed by hemoglobin. The three-dimensional structure of human hemoglobin has been determined from x-ray crystallographic analysis. The important functional properties of hemoglobin such as heme-heme interaction, the pH dependency of oxygen affinity (the Bohr effect), and the interaction with 2,3-diphosphoglycerate can now be understood in stereochemical terms. This structural information has also been useful in explaining the abnormal functional properties of a number of human hemoglobin variants which are associated with clinical and hematalogic manifestations (see Chap. 295).

During the circulation through the lungs, hemoglobin becomes almost fully saturated with oxygen (1.34 mL O_2 per gram of hemoglobin). As red cells perfuse the capillary beds, oxygen is extracted. Efficient unloading of oxygen at relatively high oxygen tensions is possible because of the sigmoid shape of the oxygen dissociation curve (heme-heme interaction) (see Fig. 290-4). The affinity of hemoglobin for oxygen is modified by three intracellular cofactors: hydrogen ion, carbon dioxide, and 2,3-diphosphoglycerate (2,3-DPG). Increasing the concentrations of each of these three effectors results in a "shift to the right" in the oxygen dissociation curve. In human red cells, 2,3-DPG appears to be an important regulator of hemoglobin function. One molecule of 2,3-DPG binds to the β chains of deoxyhemoglobin, thereby decreasing oxygen affinity. Elevated levels of 2,3-DPG have been noted in various states of hypoxia. The resulting decrease in oxygen affinity permits enhanced oxygen release. The oxygenation of a particular organ or tissue depends on three main factors (depicted in Fig. 290-5): blood flow, oxygen-carrying capacity of the blood (hemoglobin concentration), and the affinity of the hemoglobin for oxygen. Patients with a primary abnormality of one of these three factors depend on adjustments in one or both of the other two in order to maintain optimal tissue oxygenation. For example, patients with anemia have two available modes of compensation: enhanced blood flow and decreased oxygen affinity, mediated by increased levels of 2,3-DPG. Conversely, individuals with a hemoglobin variant having increased oxygen affinity have a primary defect in oxygen unloading. As discussed in Chap. 295, such patients compensate by developing secondary erythrocytosis.

FIGURE 290-4 The oxyhemoglobin dissociation curve of normal blood. The major factors influencing the position of the curve are pH, temperature, and the intracellular concentration of 2,3-DPG. An increase in plasma pH or a decrease in temperature and 2,3-DPG causes an increase in oxygen affinity (shift to the left) and a relative decrease in oxygen unloading when going from an arterial P_{O_2} of 12.7 kPa (95 mmHg) to a venous P_{O_2} of 5.3 kPa (40 mmHg). Conversely, a decrease in pH or an increase in temperature and 2,3-DPG causes a decrease in oxygen affinity (shift to the right) and a relative increase in oxygen unloading.

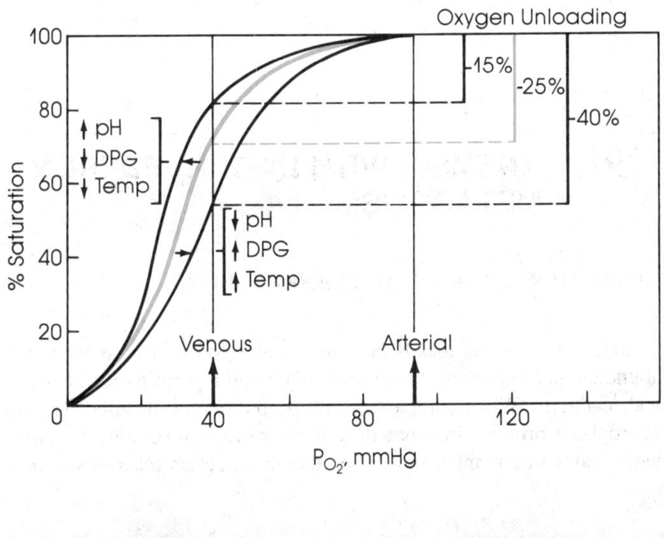

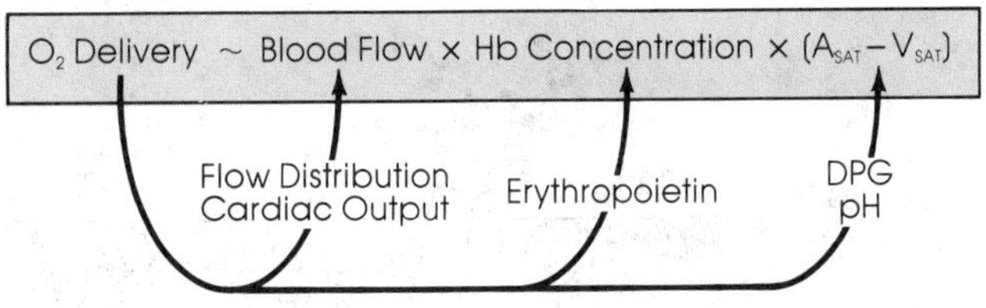

FIGURE 290-5 Oxygen delivered to an organ or tissue is directly proportional to (1) blood flow, (2) hemoglobin concentration, and (3) the difference in oxygen saturation of the arterial and venous blood. Patients with various types of hypoxia may compensate in the following ways: (1) The distribution of blood flow is altered to maintain oxygenation of vital organs; total cardiac output increases when hypoxia is severe. (2) Increased erythropoietin production stimulates erythropoiesis. (3) Oxygen unloading is enhanced by a shift to the right in the oxygen dissociation curve, mediated by an increase in red cell 2,3-DPG.

RED BLOOD CELL METABOLISM As the red cell emerges from the bone marrow, it loses its nucleus, ribosomes, and mitochondria and therefore all capability for cell division, protein synthesis, and oxidative phosphorylation. Compared with other cells, the erythrocyte has a rather simple scheme of intermediary metabolism. Glucose is virtually the only fuel utilized by the red cell. It readily enters the red cell by facilitated diffusion and is then converted to glucose-6-phosphate. There are two major pathways available for glucose-6-phosphate (Fig. 294-2). About 80 to 90 percent of this intermediate is converted to lactate by means of the glycolytic (or Embden-Meyerhof) pathway. Two moles of adenosine triphosphate (ATP) are generated for every mole of glucose that is metabolized. The intracellular mediator of hemoglobin function, 2,3-diphosphoglycerate, is synthesized in a side reaction shown in Fig. 294-2. About 10 percent of intracellular glucose-6-phosphate undergoes oxidation by means of the hexose-monophosphate shunt. This pathway maintains glutathione in the reduced form, thereby protecting sulfhydryl groups in hemoglobin and the red cell membrane from oxidation by peroxides and superoxide as well as by certain drugs and toxins. Such oxidant stress can compromise red cell function and viability in patients with a deficiency in glucose-6-phosphate dehydrogenase, the first enzymatic step in the hexose-monophosphate shunt (see Chap. 294). Less commonly, individuals may have a deficiency in one of the enzymes of the glycolytic pathway or in one of the other enzymes of the hexose-monophosphate shunt.

The red cell has rather modest metabolic obligations in keeping with its simplified structure. A significant portion of the ATP generated by glycolysis is spent in operating the sodium-potassium pump, necessary to preserve the ionic milieu in the cytoplasm and prevent colloid osmotic lysis. In addition, some metabolic energy is expended on maintenance and repair of the red cell membrane. Certain proteins in the membrane become phosphorylated by means of ATP and protein kinases, but the physiologic significance of this process is not yet understood. Finally, a small amount of metabolic currency is spent on maintaining hemoglobin iron atoms in the reduced form (Fe^{2+}).

The 120-day survival of the circulating red cell is dependent on preservation of the pliability of its membrane. The red cell membrane is composed of 50 percent protein, 40 percent lipid, and 10 percent carbohydrate. It is a bilayer consisting of molecules of phospholipid and cholesterol in a 1.2:1 molar ratio oriented in a stacked array so that the hydrophobic portions of the molecules are oriented toward the interior while the polar side groups are either on the external surface of the cell (the plasma membrane) or on the inner cytoplasmic surface (see Fig. 290-6). The distribution of phospholipids differs significantly in the two portions of the bilayer. The outer surface is relatively rich in lecithin and sphingomyelin while the inner surface has relatively more phosphatidyl serine and phosphatidyl ethanolamine. The lipids on the outer surface exchange freely with plasma lipids.

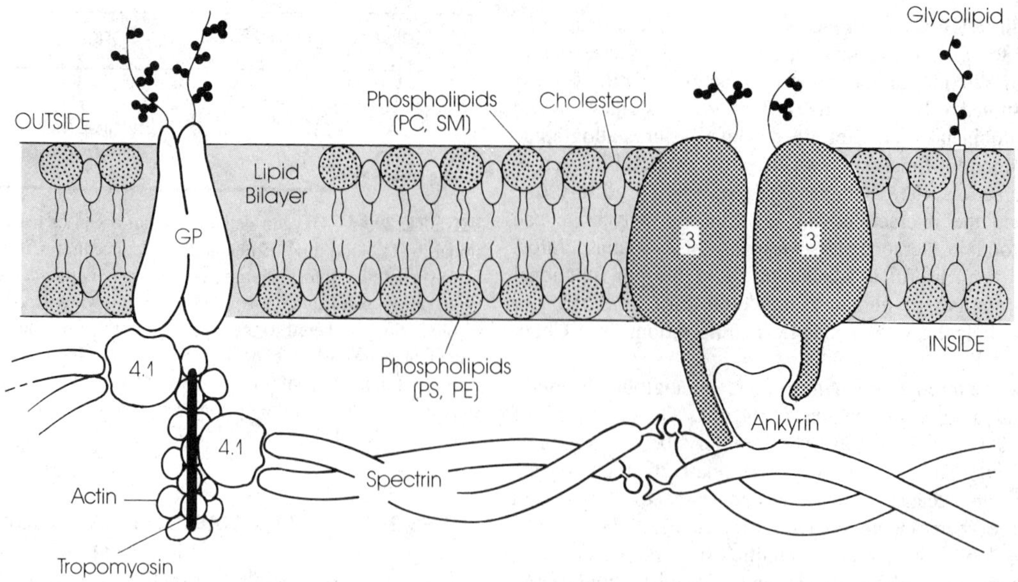

FIGURE 290-6 Diagram of a cross section of the red blood cell membrane. Spectrin, actin, tropomyosin, and protein 4.1 form a meshwork which laminates the inner surface of the membrane. In contrast, other proteins such as the glycophorins (GP) and protein 3 (the anion transport channel) traverse the lipid bilayer. Long polysaccharide chains are covalently attached to these proteins on the outer surface of the cell and also to glycolipid. The protein ankyrin forms a bridge between spectrin and a fraction of the anion transport proteins. Protein 4.1 binds to GP. Phospholipids in the lipid bilayer include phosphatidylcholine (PC) and sphingomyelin (SM), which are located primarily on the outer surface of the membrane, and phosphatidyl serine (PS) and phosphatidyl ethanolamine (PE), which are located primarily on the inner surface of the membrane.

The red cell membrane contains about eight major proteins depicted in Fig. 290-6 and a large number of minor components. These proteins can be divided into two groups. A few span the lipid bilayer so that one end of the polypeptide is on the external cell surface and the other is on the inner surface. Examples include glycophorin, which contains a number of polysaccharide blood group antigens, and band 3, which serves as a channel for the passage of anions in and out of the red cell. Other proteins bind only to the inner surface of the red cell membrane. These include several enzymes as well as structural proteins such as spectrin and actin, which interact to form a meshwork that laminates the cytoplasmic surface of the membrane.

It is likely that the physiologic demise of 120-day-old red cells is due to a loss of membrane flexibility preventing them from negotiating the narrow-bore channels of the microcirculation, including the sinusoids of the spleen. The factors responsible for red cell senescence are poorly understood. Experimental evidence indicates that deterioration of the red cell's metabolic machinery, sufficient to deplete it of ATP, can cause the cell to become spiculated (ecchinocytic) and lose its normal pliability. Depletion of ATP disrupts the spectrin and actin meshwork lining the inner membrane surface, resulting in aggregation of these proteins. Other factors such as enhanced rigidity and, perhaps, coating with immunoglobulin may also contribute to the recognition of the senescent red cell by the mononuclear phagocyte system. In contrast to normal red cells, there is a large and well-documented body of information on the mechanisms responsible for red cell destruction in various hemolytic anemias. These are discussed in Chap. 294.

Once the senescent red cell is sequestered (Fig. 290-2), hemoglobin is readily catabolized. Amino acids are released by proteolytic digestion and subsequently metabolized. The heme group is catabolized by a microsomal oxidizing system. The porphyrin ring is converted to bile pigments which are excreted almost quantitatively by the liver. One mole of carbon monoxide is formed per mole of heme that is broken down. Endogenous carbon monoxide production correlates directly with erythroid cell destruction. As Fig. 290-2 shows, the iron that is released during heme catabolism is initially incorporated into the storage protein ferritin, but it is eventually transported to marrow erythroid precursors by transferrin, the plasma iron–binding protein.

If red cell production is disordered, there may be significant destruction of erythroid cells within the bone marrow. A number of anemias are characterized by *ineffective erythropoiesis,* particularly those in which erythroid maturation is morphologically abnormal and the circulating red cells are abnormal in size. Examples discussed in detail elsewhere include megaloblastic anemias, sideroblastic anemias, and β thalassemia major. Such disorders are characterized by erythroid hyperplasia in the bone marrow and rapid uptake of labeled iron into the marrow but a low recovery of the labeled iron in circulating red cells. Endogenous carbon monoxide production and plasma levels of unconjugated bilirubin are generally elevated in ineffective erythropoiesis.

REFERENCES

Babior BM, Stossel TP: *Hematology: A Pathophysiological Approach.* New York, Churchill Livingston, 1984

Beck WS (ed): *Hematology,* 5th ed. Boston, MIT Press, 1990

Bennett V: The membrane skeleton of human erythrocytes and its implications for more complex cells. Ann Rev Biochem 54:273, 1985

Bunn HF, Forget BG: *Hemoglobin: Molecular, Genetic and Clinical Aspects.* Philadelphia, Saunders, 1986

Erslev AJ, Gabuzda TG: *Pathophysiology of Blood,* 3 ed. Philadelphia, Saunders, 1985

Jandl JH: *Blood, Textbook of Hematology.* Boston, Little, Brown, 1987

Spivak JL: Erythropoietin: A brief review. Nephron 52:289, 1989

291 ANEMIAS WITH DISTURBED IRON METABOLISM

KENNETH R. BRIDGES / H. FRANKLIN BUNN

Among the transition metals that are essential to life, iron is the most abundant and important, being used in a broad repertoire of biochemical reactions. When complexed with porphyrin and inserted into an appropriate protein, iron not only binds oxygen reversibly but also participates in a number of vital oxidation-reduction reactions. Since inorganic iron is highly toxic, specific processes have evolved for its assimilation, transport, and storage. Under normal circumstances, iron homeostasis is precisely maintained but can go awry in a variety of clinical settings, leading either to iron deficiency or iron overload.

PHYSIOLOGY OF IRON

IRON ABSORPTION This occurs predominantly in the duodenum and upper jejunum. Inorganic iron salts exist in either of two valence states, Fe^{2+} (ferrous) or Fe^{3+} (ferric). Most dietary iron consists of ferric salts, which form insoluble ferric hydroxide precipitates at physiologic pH. Absorption is aided by stomach acidity which maintains ferric iron in a soluble form. Normally about 10 percent of the 10 to 20 mg of iron ingested per day in an average diet is absorbed. Heme is much more readily absorbed than inorganic iron. Unfortunately, a dearth of meat in the diets of many people throughout the world limits the availability of this excellent iron source.

The absorption of inorganic iron is greatly influenced by dietary compounds which may chelate the element. Citrate and ascorbate, for example, increase iron absorption by forming soluble complexes which readily enter the epithelial cells lining the upper gastrointestinal tract. Other compounds such as tannates, which are found in teas, plant phytates, and phosphates form very tight complexes with iron and significantly inhibit absorption. The metabolic machinery involved in iron absorption is shared with several heavy metals, including lead, cadmium, and strontium. Increased iron absorption as occurs, for instance in iron deficiency, enhances the uptake of these elements.

TRANSPORT AND STORAGE The precise mechanism by which iron is translocated across the epithelial barrier in the intestine is unknown. Once this task is accomplished, however, the element is coupled to transferrin, an 80-kDa serum glycoprotein which delivers iron to tissues throughout the body (Fig. 291-1). Each transferrin molecule can bind two iron atoms. The aggregate binding sites of all the transferrin in the circulation comprise the total iron-binding capacity (TIBC) of plasma. Normally, 20 to 45 percent of the iron-binding sites are filled. Specific receptors on the plasma membranes of cells recognize transferrin, leading to the internalization of the protein and the release of iron into the cell cytoplasm. As might be expected, erythroid precursor cells in the bone marrow, which have a high requirement for iron, have a correspondingly high density of transferrin receptors.

Excess iron is stored in the body as ferritin or as hemosiderin. The iron in ferritin is enclosed within a protein shell, apoferritin, which can take up Fe^{2+} and oxidize it so that Fe^{3+} is deposited within the iron core. The synthesis of apoferritin is stimulated by iron. Small quantities of ferritin can be measured in serum. Under normal conditions there is a close correlation between serum ferritin concentration and body iron stores, with 1 μg/L serum ferritin equivalent to approximately 10 mg of storage iron. With time, ferritin is engulfed by lysosomes and catabolized to hemosiderin, a nonspecific mixture of partially degraded protein, lipid, and iron. Iron enters and leaves the ferritin molecule in a metabolically controlled fashion, making it available for the normal physiologic functions of the cell. In contrast, iron which is trapped in the hemosiderin meshwork is returned to the metabolic mainstream of the cell in a slow and unregulated fashion.

FIGURE 291-1 The distribution of iron in normal adults and internal iron kinetics. Bold arrows indicate major pathways of iron movement.

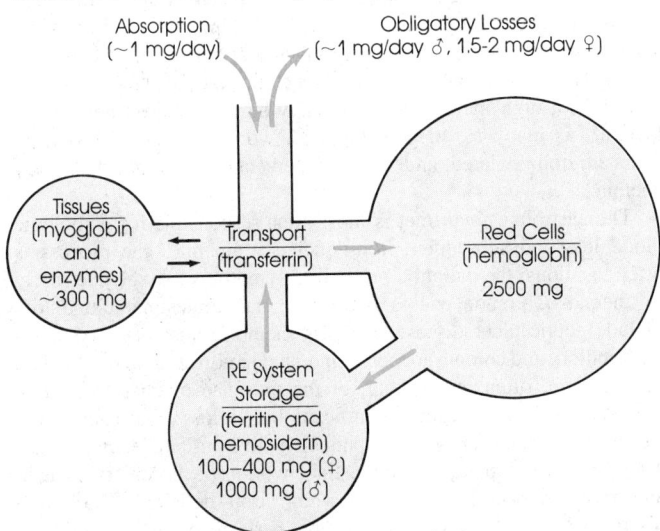

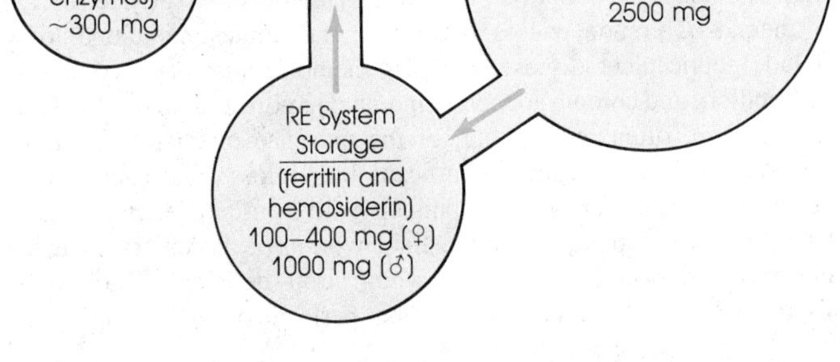

Body iron stores are assiduously conserved. In fact, no physiologic pathway of iron removal exists. A small daily loss of 1 to 2 mg of the element results from the shedding of senescent cells along the gastrointestinal and genitourinary tracts and from desquamation of skin (Fig. 291-1). Normally, this loss closely balances daily absorption. When the demand for iron is increased by depletion of body reserves due to growth spurts, pregnancy, or menstrual and pathologic hemorrhage, the efficiency of iron absorption can increase up to about 20 percent. With iron deficiency, absorption of the element can increase to between 30 and 40 percent of the amount ingested. In contrast, with iron overload no effective counterbalancing mechanism exists.

Iron kinetics Between 80 and 90 percent of absorbed iron is delivered to the bone marrow for erythropoiesis. The dynamics of iron utilization by the peripheral tissues can be monitored by loading plasma transferrin with the radioisotope ^{59}Fe and injecting the labeled protein back into the circulation. Such ferrokinetic studies reveal an exponential loss of label from the plasma, with a half-life of about 75 min. The plasma iron turnover (PIT) is the absolute amount of iron released from transferrin per unit of time, and is determined largely by the rate of erythropoiesis. Effective erythropoiesis results in the incorporation of 80 to 90 percent of iron into hemoglobin in circulating erythrocytes. With some anemias, such as the thalassemias, the megaloblastic anemias, and sideroblastic anemia, there is intramedullary destruction of nascent red cells. The result is a high PIT reflecting the increase in erythropoietic activity, but a diminished incorporation of the labeled iron into circulating erythrocytes. This combination is termed ineffective erythropoiesis. When erythropoiesis is diminished because of marrow hypoplasia, the PIT is correspondingly reduced.

LABORATORY INVESTIGATION OF IRON STORES *Direct assays* for evaluating iron stores require biopsy specimens. Most storage iron is found in the reticuloendothelial cells of the bone marrow, liver, and spleen or in hepatic parenchymal cells. The liver is a homogeneous tissue and therefore an excellent source by which to gauge iron stores. Prussian blue staining of liver biopsies, a commonly used technique, provides only a semiquantitative estimation of iron stores whereas atomic absorption spectroscopy furnishes accurate quantitative data. Formalin-fixed samples can be evaluated by this technique, allowing for transport and later testing. Liver biopsy with atomic absorption spectroscopic measurements is the gold standard for quantitative evaluation of iron overload. Bone marrow specimens do not provide a reliable estimation of iron excess but are useful in the evaluation of iron deficiency. Because of the cellular heterogeneity of bone marrow, histologic evaluation of iron deposits must focus on storage in macrophages. An absence of Prussian blue staining reliably reflects a deficiency in iron stores.

The simplest *indirect assay* of iron stores is the measurement of the ratio of serum iron to TIBC (Fig. 291-2). Iron deficiency depresses serum iron levels and boosts the TIBC. Therefore the transferrin is generally less than 10 percent saturated. Iron loading increases the serum iron with little effect on the TIBC, leading to greater than 80 percent saturation of transferrin. The ratio of iron to TIBC must be viewed with the patient's total clinical picture in mind. For example, serum iron and transferrin levels are depressed by conditions such as inflammation, cancer, and liver disease, leading at times to skewed ratios.

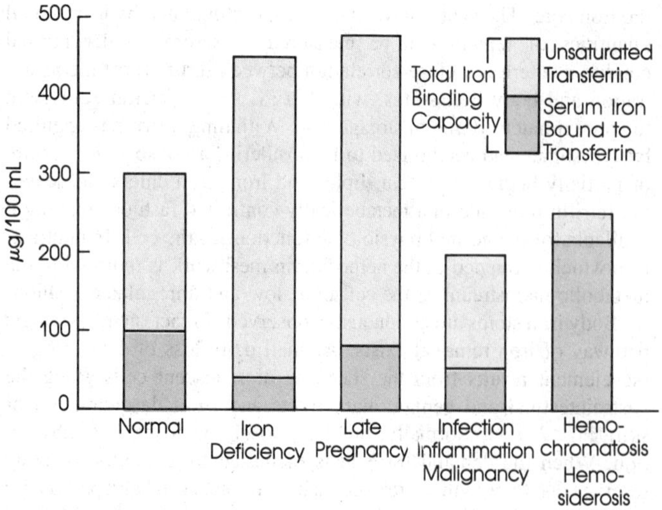

FIGURE 291-2 Serum iron and total iron-binding capacity in various disorders.

Iron stores are also reflected by *serum ferritin* levels. Ferritin in the circulation is a secretory form of the protein which is glycosylated and differs in subunit composition from the storage form found in cells. The physiologic function of serum ferritin is presently unknown. The protein normally contains very little iron. The concentration of serum ferritin rises with iron loading and declines with depletion of tissue iron stores. The serum ferritin level also increases with inflammation, cancer, and liver disease. In addition, the normal ranges for serum ferritin vary with age and sex. Therefore corrections for these factors should be made when values on a specific patient are interpreted.

In patients with iron deficiency, protoporphyrin IX accumulates in the red cell because there is insufficient iron to convert it to heme (see Fig. 290-3). The fluorometric assay of free erythrocyte protoporphyrin (FEP) is a reliable and cost-effective way of screening large groups of individuals such as schoolchildren for iron deficiency.

Computed tomography (CT) of the liver provides an excellent assessment of body iron stores, particularly with iron overload. The iron content of liver biopsy samples correlates well with determination by dual energy CT scanning. Another sensitive noninvasive technique for evaluating liver iron deposition is magnetic resonance imaging. Both instruments permit longitudinal evaluation and are valuable adjuncts in monitoring and treating patients with iron overload.

IRON-DEFICIENCY ANEMIA

ETIOLOGY Iron deficiency occurs when the rate of loss or utilization of the element exceeds its rate of assimilation. The stages of iron deficiency are shown in Table 291-1. Utilization is greatest during the rapid growth spurts of infancy and adolescence (Table 291-2). Depleted iron stores, if not frank anemia, are commonly seen in children in these two age groups. Neonates born to iron-deficient women are rarely anemic, but do have low body iron stores. These infants lack the reserves needed for the swift growth which occurs after birth. The iron content of breast milk is comparable to that of cow's milk, but the bioavailability of iron is greater in breast milk. Iron deficiency during childhood has a number of deleterious consequences, including impaired cognition. Therefore, infants should receive iron supplementation.

TABLE 291-1 Stages in the development of iron deficiency

	Normal	Mild	Moderate	Severe
Hemoglobin:	150 g/L	130 g/L	100 g/L	50 g/L
MCV	N	↓	↓	↓↓
MCHC	N	N	↓	↓↓
Marrow Fe stores	Present	Absent	Absent	Absent
Serum Fe/TIBC, μg/L	1000/3000	~750/3000	~500/4500	~250/6000

NOTE: MCV = mean corpuscular volume; MCHC = mean corpuscular hemoglobin concentration; TIBC = total iron-binding capacity; N = normal; ↓ = decreased.

TABLE 291-2 Causes of iron deficiency

I Increased iron utilization
- *A* Postnatal growth spurt
- *B* Adolescent growth spurt

II Physiologic iron loss
- *A* Menstruation
- *B* Pregnancy

III Pathologic iron loss
- *A* Gastrointestinal bleeding
- *B* Genitourinary bleeding
- *C* Pulmonary hemosiderosis
- *D* Intravascular hemolysis

IV Decreased iron intake
- *A* Cereal-rich, meat-poor diets
- *B* Food faddists
- *C* Elderly and indigent
- *D* Malabsorption

In western countries, the increased demand for iron during adolescence is often accompanied by voluntary consumption of foods with low iron content. Among the elderly and the poor, financial constraints often produce a similar pattern of inadequate iron intake. Large numbers of people throughout the world have become inured to diets consisting largely of grains or cereals, which are inadequate sources of iron. The added burden of blood loss due to parasites such as hookworm makes iron deficiency a problem of staggering proportions.

Decreased absorption of iron This can occur in many clinical settings. After partial or total gastrectomy, the assimilation of dietary iron is impaired, owing primarily to increased motility and bypass of the proximal intestine, which is the primary site of iron absorption. Achlorhydria also contributes to decreased iron absorption. Patients with chronic diarrhea or intestinal malabsorption may also develop iron deficiency, particularly if the duodenum and proximal jejunum are involved. Sometimes iron-deficiency anemia is a harbinger of nontropical (celiac) sprue.

Iron loss This loss may be physiologic or pathologic. Examples of physiologic iron loss include menstruation and pregnancy. Menstrual blood loss doubles the daily iron requirement. With a term pregnancy, about 500 mg of iron are transferred from the mother to the fetus. Some of this iron is derived from increased gastrointestinal absorption of the element by the mother. In the absence of supplemental iron, however, her stores will be depleted to meet the needs of the fetus. Currently, the vast majority of pregnant women who seek medical attention are routinely given prophylactic treatment with iron salts. Pregnant women who do not receive adequate antenatal care have a high incidence of clinically significant iron deficiency. Overall, as many as 40 percent of all women in the childbearing years are iron-depleted, and nearly 20 percent develop iron-deficiency anemia.

The gastrointestinal tract is most often responsible for pathologic blood loss and subsequent iron-deficiency anemia. The process is often insidious; the patient's presenting symptoms may be due solely to anemia. Common causes of chronic gastrointestinal blood loss include peptic ulcer disease, gastritis, hemorrhoids, angiodysplasia of the colon, and colonic adenocarcinoma. Hemorrhoids and salicylate ingestion are often responsible for the presence of occult blood in the stool but rarely cause significant blood loss. Gastrointestinal cancer is a specter haunting all patients with iron-deficiency anemia. Therefore, a complete gastrointestinal workup is necessary in men and postmenopausal women in whom iron deficiency has been discovered. Stool guaiacs should be performed on six different occasions along with a digital rectal examination. Radiologic examination of the gastrointestinal tract and/or endoscopic procedures are obligatory. The patient must be assumed to have a gastrointestinal malignancy until proven otherwise.

In about 15 percent of patients with documented gastrointestinal bleeding, no source can be determined, even after extensive radiologic and endoscopic investigation. In tropical areas, parasitic infestations, particularly hookworm, are a major cause of blood loss. Occasionally, as in patients with hereditary telangiectasia or in those with a bleeding diathesis, gastrointestinal bleeding arises from multiple sites. Thrombocytopenia, qualitative platelet disorders, and von Willebrand's disease are more apt to cause gastrointestinal bleeding than are deficiencies of the soluble coagulation factors.

Blood loss from other sources rarely produces iron-deficiency anemia. Bleeding in the genitourinary tract usually is sufficiently alarming that medical attention is sought early in the process. Intravascular hemolysis with hemoglobin loss in the urine, e.g., paroxysmal nocturnal hemoglobinuria, is very unusual. Pulmonary hemorrhage, secondary to bronchiectasis or idiopathic pulmonary hemosiderosis, may also cause iron-deficiency anemia.

CLINICAL CONSEQUENCES OF IRON DEFICIENCY Cell growth and proliferation are impaired by iron deficiency. The production of red blood cells is in particular jeopardy owing to their high requirement for iron. Many aspects of the presentation of iron-deficiency anemia including weakness, lassitude, palpitations, and sometimes exertional dyspnea are common to all forms of chronic anemia. No definite link between these symptoms and tissue depletion of iron-dependent enzymes and cofactors has been established.

After the cells of the bone marrow, those of the gastrointestinal tract have the highest level of proliferative activity. Consequently many of the signs and symptoms of iron deficiency are localized to this organ system. Glossitis characterized by a reddened, swollen, smooth, shiny, and tender tongue occurs sporadically. Angular stomatitis involves erosion, tenderness, and swelling at the corners of the mouth. Gastric atrophy with achlorhydria occurs occasionally. A postcrycoid web (Plummer-Vinson syndrome) may develop with long-standing iron deficiency. Koilonychia, or spoon-shaped nails, result from slowing in the rate of growth of the nail plate. Menorrhagia is a common symptom in iron-deficient women. Both menorrhagia and gastric atrophy (mentioned above) may be a consequence as well as a cause of iron deficiency.

One peculiar symptom which is quite characteristic of iron deficiency is pica. Patients develop cravings for substances such as starch (amylophagia), ice (pagophagia), and clay (geophagia). Some of these materials, such as starch and clay, bind iron in the gastrointestinal tract, worsening the deficiency. The basis of this bizarre behavior is unknown. A particularly invidious consequence of iron deficiency is increased intestinal absorption of lead. Children from impoverished families, who often have both iron deficiency and pica, are at greatest risk of developing lead poisoning. The toxicity of lead is due at least in part to a disruption of heme synthesis in neural tissues, a process abetted by iron deficiency. These unfortunate children are thereby placed in double jeopardy.

Laboratory findings A variety of laboratory tests can be used to assess varying degrees of iron deficiency. The development of iron deficiency progresses in stages (Table 291-1), each of which correlates with clinical laboratory abnormalities. *Storage iron depletion* occurs first, during which iron reserves are lost without compromise of the iron supply for erythropoiesis. At this stage, a bone marrow aspirate stained with Prussian blue will show markedly reduced or absent deposits of iron in macrophages. This finding is accompanied by a decrease in the level of serum ferritin. The next stage is *iron-deficient erythropoiesis,* during which the erythroid iron supply is reduced without the development of anemia. The iron-binding capacity of the serum (TIBC) first rises, followed by a drop in serum iron. As a result, the fractional saturation of transferrin falls markedly. The circulating red cells become microcytic and hypochromic. This is accompanied by an increase in FEP. The final stage is the development of frank *iron deficiency anemia,* wherein the red cells become more severely hypochromic and microcytic (Fig. A5-4). Often, only a thin rim of cytoplasm appears on the periphery of the red cell. Small fragments and bizarre poikilocytes are also seen. Such misshapen red cells have shortened survival in the circulation. The percentage of reticulocytes is usually normal but may increase temporarily following an acute episode of blood loss. The white count is usually normal, while the platelet count is normal or increased. The bone marrow displays moderate erythroid hyperplasia. Many of the late normoblasts appear to have scanty cytoplasm.

TABLE 291-3 Differential diagnosis of microcytic, hypochromic anemia

	Iron-deficiency anemia	β-Thalassemia trait	Anemia of chronic disease	Sideroblastic anemia
Serum iron	↓	N	↓	↑
TIBC	↑	N	↓	N
Serum ferritin	↓	N	↑	↑
Red cell protoprophyrin	↑	N	↑	↑ or N
Hb A_2	↓	↑	N	↓

NOTE: ↑ = increased; ↓ = decreased, N = normal; TIBC = total iron-binding capacity.

Differential diagnosis In a patient with hypochromic microcytic anemia, the major diagnostic possibilities are iron deficiency, thalassemia, anemia of chronic inflammation, and sideroblastic anemia. Several laboratory tests (shown in Table 291-3) are useful in the differential diagnosis. Mild iron deficiency may be readily confused with β-thalassemia trait or with the two-deletion forms of α thalassemia (α –/α – or – –/αα) (Chap. 295). In these mild forms of thalassemia, microcytosis is much more marked than hypochromia; accordingly the mean corpuscular hemoglobin concentration (MCHC) is usually normal. The red cell size distribution is more uniform than that in iron deficiency. Target cells and basophilic stippling are usually more prominent in thalassemia than in iron deficiency. Hemoglobin A_2 is elevated in β-thalassemia trait and decreased in iron deficiency and α thalassemia. If a patient with β-thalassemia trait develops iron deficiency, the level of Hb A_2 may fall to normal. The serum iron is normal or elevated in the thalassemias and decreased in both iron deficiency and in the anemia of chronic disease. However, as Fig. 291-2 shows, the transferrin level is also decreased in the latter. The laboratory tests shown in Table 291-3 are not very helpful in determining whether a patient with a chronic inflammatory disease, such as rheumatoid arthritis, has become iron-deficient. The finding of a low serum ferritin level or absent iron stores in a bone marrow aspirate would be diagnostic of iron deficiency. A trial of iron therapy may be necessary to settle the issue. The diagnosis of *sideroblastic anemia* (see below) rests on the demonstration of ringed sideroblasts in the bone marrow. These patients often have a population of hypochromic microcytic red cells, even though the red cell indexes are usually normal.

THERAPY Iron deficiency responds very effectively to the administration of oral iron salts such as ferrous sulfate. One 325-mg tablet (60 mg of elemental iron) should be administered three times daily. Iron is best absorbed when taken between meals. The most common side effect is abdominal discomfort, characterized by bloating, fullness, and, on occasion, pain. Switching to ferrous gluconate or ferrous lactate may bring relief. Moreover, iron salts may be better tolerated if taken at mealtime. Iron-containing vitamin cocktails generally should be avoided since these preparations are costly and contain suboptimal amounts of iron.

A reticulocytosis occurs 3 to 4 days after the initiation of iron therapy, with a peak at about 10 days. Patients may not respond to iron replacement due to (1) an incorrect diagnosis; (2) noncompliance; (3) blood loss exceeding the rate of replacement; (4) bone marrow suppression by tumor, chronic inflammation, etc.; or (5) malabsorption. Malabsorption of iron is an infrequent problem, but requires parenteral iron replacement when it occurs. Iron-dextran complex may be administered as intramuscular injections following a 50-mg dose to test for allergic reactions. A total of about 2 g of iron-dextran may be administered in this fashion. A Z-tract should be used for the injections to prevent oozing of the compound into the dermis, which can produce intractable skin discoloration. In occasional patients so emaciated that they cannot tolerate intramuscular injections, iron-dextran can be given intravenously. The most convenient approach is to dilute 500 mg of the compound into 50 mL of sterile water and to infuse a test dose of 1 mL. If no adverse reaction is noted, the remainder of the solution can be delivered over several hours. The intravenous administration of up to 2 g of iron at a single sitting is generally well-tolerated. Occasionally patients experience arthralgias, chills, and fever which may persist for several days after the infusion. Long-term deleterious consequences are rare. The amount of iron required for replacement can be calculated from the deficit in the red cell mass, with an additional 1000 mg to replace the body stores. Blood transfusions are rarely necessary except for patients in whom severe iron-deficiency anemia threatens cardiovascular or cerebrovascular function.

ANEMIAS WITH SECONDARY IRON LOADING

Iron overload in individuals with chronic anemias may result either from multiple transfusions or from increased gastrointestinal absorption of the element owing to ineffective erythropoiesis.

SIDEROBLASTIC ANEMIAS These comprise a group of disorders of diverse cause (Table 291-4) characterized by ringed sideroblasts in the nucleated erythroid percursors in the bone marrow. Greater than 10 percent of the normoblasts contain iron-laden mitochondria which surround the nucleus and appear as pathognomonic "rings" with Prussian blue staining. A number of metabolic abnormalities have been noted in the sideroblastic anemias, including defects in one or more steps in heme synthesis. Since the initial and final steps of heme synthesis are located in the mitochondria (Fig. 290-3), it is difficult to know whether such abnormalities are the cause or the result of iron loading. In addition to the presence of ringed sideroblasts, these disorders share certain other features: bone marrow erythroid hyperplasia with decreased red cell production (ineffective erythropoiesis); a population of hypochromic, microcytic red cells reflecting defective heme synthesis; a marked increased in serum iron and transferrin saturation, sometimes accompanied by generalized iron overload.

Hereditary sideroblastic anemia is a rare X-linked disorder associated with defective activity of δ-aminolevulinic acid synthetase, the initial and rate-limiting enzyme in heme biosynthesis. Affected males have anemia of variable severity that often responds to treatment with large doses of pyridoxine.

Acquired sideroblastic anemias may be caused by a variety of insults including ethanol and isoniazid, which produce abnormalities in pyridoxine metabolism, and lead, which inhibits several steps in the heme synthetic pathway (Table 294-4). Ringed sideroblasts are found in about 30 percent of patients hospitalized for alcohol abuse, particularly in the setting of coexistent folate deficiency and malnutrition. This morphologic abnormality disappears within several days following cessation of alcohol ingestion. Secondary sideroblastic anemia has also been observed in a variety of inflammatory and neoplastic states. A particularly intractable form of the disorder sometimes occurs following treatment of malignancy, especially multiple myeloma, with alkylating chemotherapeutic agents.

TABLE 291-4 The sideroblastic anemias

I Hereditary or congenital sideroblastic anemias
II Acquired sideroblastic anemias
- *A* Associated with drugs and toxins (e.g., alcohol, lead, isoniazid, chloramphenicol)
- *B* Associated with neoplastic and inflammatory disease (e.g., carcinoma, leukemia, lymphoma, rheumatoid arthritis)
- *C* Alkylating agent chemotherapy (e.g., cyclophosphamide)

Most commonly, however, acquired sideroblastic anemia is idiopathic, appearing spontaneously in older individuals. Disturbed growth and maturation occurs in all the lines which emanate from the hematopoietic stem cells. Chromosomal abnormalities are commonly observed in bone marrow cells. Neutropenia develops in a significant number of patients, as does thrombocytopenia. Some individuals have normal numbers of platelets which are, however, dysfunctional. A bleeding diathesis often results. About 10 percent of individuals with sideroblastic anemia will develop acute myelogenous leukemia. This proportion appears to be higher in cases arising from therapy with alkylating agents.

The treatment of secondary sideroblastic anemia focuses primarily on withdrawal of the offending agent. No specific treatment is presently available for idiopathic cases. Since pyridoxine is innocuous and inexpensive, all patients should be given a trial of the vitamin at 200 mg per day for 2 to 3 months, despite the low probability of response in the acquired disorder. Occasionally, an improvement in hematocrit occurs with androgen therapy. This therapy should be used cautiously in patients with liver disease, diabetes, or benign prostatic hypertrophy. Ongoing clinical trials are attempting to define the role of recombinant cytokines such as erythropoietin, granulocyte-monocyte colony stimulating factor (GM-CSF) and interleukin 3 in the treatment of sideroblastic anemia. Supportive therapy, sometimes including blood transfusions, is indicated in all patients.

TRANSFUSIONAL HEMOCHROMATOSIS Repeated blood transfusion is the most common cause of iron overload in patients with anemia. One unit of blood contains 200 to 250 mg iron. Therefore a patient who requires 3 units of blood per month will accumulate about 8 g of iron over the course of a year, enough to cause early clinical sequelae of iron loading. In order for the consequences of iron loading to play a major clinical role, a requirement for chronic transfusions must be coupled with a relatively long survival. The disorders which fulfill these criteria at present include (1) thalassemia major, (2) myeloproliferative and myelodysplastic syndromes (including sideroblastic anemia), and (3) aplastic anemia of moderate severity. Patients with chronic renal failure who are on dialysis also fall under this rubric at present. However, this last indication will be obviated by the recent availability of recombinant erythropoietin.

Transfusional iron overload produces a spectrum of problems similar to those seen with idiopathic hemochromatosis (Chap. 327). Of these, the most serious result from myocardial and hepatic iron deposition. Cardiac siderosis leads to arrhythmias, conduction defects, and congestive failure. The radionuclide ventriculogram is a reliable means of detecting early myocardial dysfunction. Iron deposition in the liver injures hepatocytes, leading to necrosis, fibrosis, and ultimately, cirrhosis. Serum transaminase levels are usually only modestly elevated, even in patients with heavy hepatic iron deposition. Disturbed glucose metabolism occurs commonly, although an oral glucose tolerance test is sometimes needed to demonstrate the defect. Gonadal dysfunction and ACTH deficiency are much less frequent. Hyperpigmentation reflects increased melanin production due to dermal iron deposition, but may not occur in fair-skinned patients. In the assessment of these patients, liver biopsy provides the greatest yield of information since iron content as well as the pathologic state of the organ can be determined. Liver CT scanning or magnetic resonance imaging are the most reliable noninvasive methods of estimating iron deposition. The iron/TIBC ratio and serum ferritin level are both elevated with transfusional hemochromatosis, but do not accurately establish the degree of iron overload in an individual.

The only treatment presently available for transfusional hemochromatosis is chelation therapy. Deferoxamine (deferrox) is the only agent which has been extensively evaluated and shown to prevent or reverse the complications of iron overload. The drug must be given parenterally over a period of 12 to 16 h. Generally, deferoxamine is delivered by subcutaneous infusion with a portable syringe pump. Considerable effort is being devoted to the development of a safe and effective oral iron chelating agent. Oral ascorbic acid supplementation markedly enhances iron excretion in patients on deferoxamine therapy. The vitamin increases the availability of storage iron to the chelator, by slowing the degradation of ferritin to hemosiderin. Cardiac toxicity has occurred in patients with hemochromatosis who consumed excessive amounts of ascorbic acid. The generation of injurious free radicals by iron released from storage sites is the probable mechanism of this effect. Further investigation into the basis of cellular injury in patients with hemochromatosis treated with ascorbic acid is needed to clarify the possible therapeutic utility of this vitamin.

REFERENCES

BRIDGES KR: Transfusion hemochromatosis, in *Transfusion Medicine*, WH Churchill, S Kurtz (eds). Cambridge, MA, Blackwell, 1988, pp 129–144

GIBSON RS, MACDONALD AC: Serum ferritin and dietary iron parameters in a sample of Canadian preschool children. J Can Dietetic Assoc 49:23, 1988

HUEBERS HA, FINCH CA: The physiology of transferrin and transferrin receptors. Physiol Rev 67:520, 1987

JACOBS A, CLARK RE: Pathogenesis and clinical variations in the myelodysplastic syndromes. Clin Haematol 15:925, 1986

KONTOGHIORGHES GJ et al: Effective chelation of iron in β-thalassemia with the oral chelator 1,2-dimethyl-3-hydropyrid-4-one. Br Med J 295:1509, 1987

LANZKOWSKY P: Problems in diagnosis of iron deficiency anemia. Pediatr Ann 14:618, 1985

PIOMELLI S et al: Lead-induced abnormalities of porphyrin metabolism. The relationship with iron deficiency. Ann NY Acad Sci 514:278, 1987

WOLFE LC et al: Prevention of cardiac disease by subcutaneous deferoxamine in patients with thalassemia major. N Engl J Med 312:1600, 1985

292 MEGALOBLASTIC ANEMIAS

BERNARD M. BABIOR / H. FRANKLIN BUNN

The megaloblastic anemias are disorders caused by impaired DNA synthesis. Cells primarily affected are those having a relatively rapid turnover, especially hematopoietic precursors and gastrointestinal epithelial cells. Cell division is sluggish, but cytoplasmic development progresses normally, so megaloblastic cells tend to be large, with an increased ratio of RNA to DNA. Megaloblastic erythroid cells tend to be destroyed in the marrow in excessive numbers, an abnormality termed *ineffective erythropoiesis* (Chaps. 61 and 290).

Most megaloblastic anemias are due to a deficiency of cobalamin (vitamin B_{12}) and/or folic acid. The various clinical entities associated with megaloblastic anemia are listed in Table 292-1. This classification is easier to comprehend if the physiologic and biochemical principles discussed below are kept in mind.

TABLE 292-1 Classification of the megaloblastic anemias

I Cobalamin deficiency
- *A* Inadequate intake: vegetarians (rare)
- *B* Malabsorption
  - *1* Inadequate production of intrinsic factor (IF)
    - *a* Pernicious anemia
    - *b* Gastrectomy
    - *c* Congenital absence or functional abnormality of IF (rare)
  - *2* Disorders of terminal ileum
    - *a* Tropical sprue
    - *b* Nontropical sprue
    - *c* Regional enteritis
    - *d* Intestinal resection
    - *e* Neoplasms and granulomatous disorders (rare)
    - *f* Selective cobalamin malabsorption (Imerslund's syndrome) (rare)
  - *3* Competition for cobalamin
    - *a* Fish tapeworm
    - *b* Bacteria: blind loop syndrome
  - *4* Drugs: *p*-aminosalicylic acid, colchicine, neomycin
- *C* Other
  - *1* Nitrous oxide
  - *2* Transcobalamin II deficiency (rare)

II Folic acid deficiency
- *A* Inadequate intake: unbalanced diet (common in alcoholics, teenagers, some infants)
- *B* Increased requirements
  - *1* Pregnancy
  - *2* Infancy
  - *3* Malignancy
  - *4* Increased hematopoiesis (chronic hemolytic anemias)
  - *5* Chronic exfoliative skin disorders
  - *6* Hemodialysis
- *C* Malabsorption
  - *1* Tropical sprue
  - *2* Nontropical sprue
  - *3* Drugs: Phenytoin, barbiturates, (?) ethanol
- *D* Impaired metabolism
  - *1* Inhibitors of dihydrofolate reductase: methotrexate, pyrimethamine, triamterene, pentamidine, etc.
  - *2* Alcohol
  - *3* Rare enzyme deficiencies: dihydrofolate reductase, others

III Other causes
- *A* Drugs which impair DNA metabolism
  - *1* Purine antagonists: 6-mercaptopurine, azathioprine, etc.
  - *2* Pyrimidine antagonists: 5-fluorouracil, cytosine arabinoside, etc.
  - *3* Others: procarbazine, hydroxyurea, acyclovir, zidovudine
- *B* Metabolic disorders (rare)
  - *1* Hereditary orotic aciduria
  - *2* Others
- *C* Megaloblastic anemia of unknown etiology
  - *1* Refractory megaloblastic anemia
  - *2* Di Guglielmo's syndrome*
  - *3* Congenital dyserythropoietic anemia

* A form of acute nonlymphocytic leukemia with atypical, dysplastic changes in erythroid series.

PHYSIOLOGIC CONSIDERATIONS

FOLIC ACID Folic acid is the common name for pteroylmonoglutamic acid. It is synthesized by many different plants and bacteria. Fruits and vegetables constitute the primary dietary source of the vitamin. Some forms of dietary folic acid are labile and may be destroyed by cooking. The minimum daily requirement is normally about 50 μg but may be increased severalfold during periods of enhanced metabolic demand such as pregnancy.

The assimilation of adequate amounts of folic acid is dependent on the nature of the diet and its means of preparation. Folates in various foodstuffs are largely conjugated to polyglutamic acid. This highly polar side chain impairs the intestinal absorption of the vitamin. However, conjugases (γ-glutamyl carboxypeptidases) in the lumen of the gut convert polyglutamates to mono- and diglutamates, which are readily absorbed in the proximal jejunum.

There are binding proteins in plasma for folates, but their physiologic significance is unclear. Plasma folate is primarily in the form of N^5-methyltetrahydrofolate, a monoglutamate. N^5-Methyltetrahydrofolate is transported into cells by a carrier which is specific for the tetrahydro forms of the vitamin. Once in the cell, the folate is reconverted to the polyglutamate form, after removal of the N^5-methyl group in a cobalamin-requiring reaction (see below). The polyglutamate form may be useful for retention of folate by the cell.

Normal individuals have about 5 to 20 mg folic acid in various body stores, half in the liver. In light of the minimum daily requirement, it is not surprising that a deficiency will occur within months if dietary intake or intestinal absorption is curtailed.

COBALAMIN This vitamin is a complex organometallic compound in which a cobalt atom is situated within a corrin ring, a structure similar to the porphyrin from which heme is formed (Fig. 290-3). Unlike heme, however, cobalamin cannot be synthesized in the human body and must be supplied in the diet. The only dietary source of cobalamin are animal products: meat and dairy foods. The minimum daily requirement for cobalamin is about 2.5 μg.

During gastric digestion, cobalamin in food is released and forms

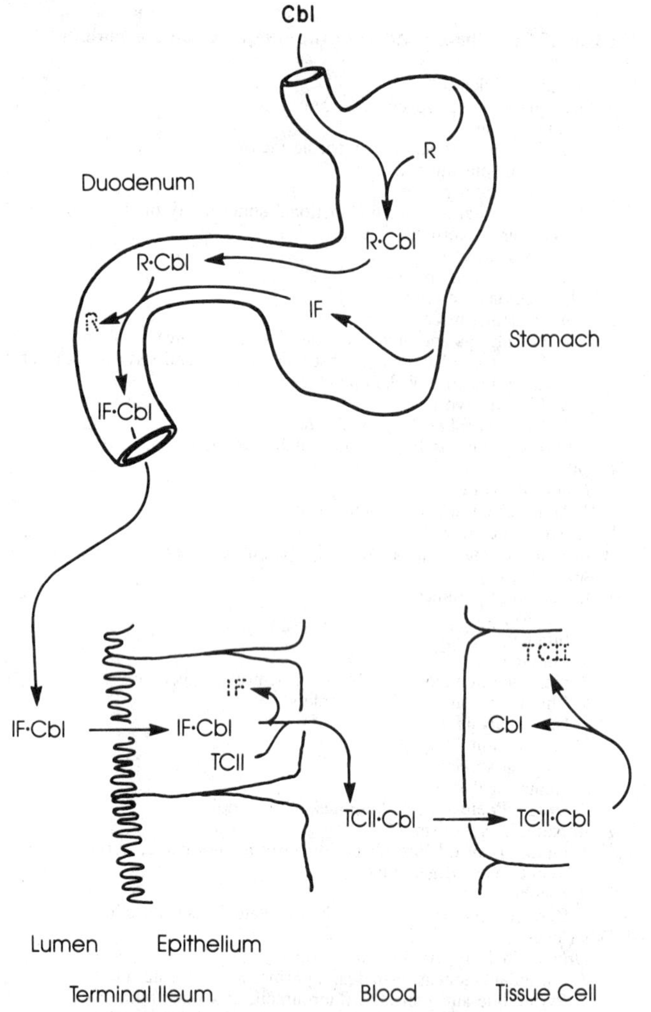

FIGURE 292-1 The assimilation of cobalamin. On entering the stomach dietary cobalamin (Cbl) forms a complex with R binding protein. As this protein is digested, cobalamin is transferred to intrinsic factor (IF). This complex passes through the intestine until it reaches specific receptors on the mucosa of the distal ileum. The internalized Cbl is then transferred to transcobalamin II (TCII) which circulates in the plasma until it is binds to receptors on cells throughout the body and is internalized.

a stable complex with gastric R binder, one of a group of closely related glycoproteins of unknown function which are found in secretions (e.g., saliva, milk, gastric juice, bile), phagocytes, and plasma. On entering the duodenum, the cobalamin–R binder complex is digested, releasing the cobalamin, which then binds to intrinsic factor (IF). This glycoprotein of molecular weight 50,000 is produced by the parietal cells of the stomach. The secretion of intrinsic factor generally parallels that of hydrochloric acid. The cobalamin-IF complex is resistant to proteolytic digestion and travels to the distal ileum, where specific receptors on the mucosal brush border bind the cobalamin-IF complex, thereby enabling the vitamin to be absorbed. Thus, intrinsic factor like transferrin (see Chap. 291) serves as a cell-directed carrier protein. The receptor-bound cobalamin-IF complex is taken into the ileal mucosal cell, where over the course of several hours the IF is destroyed and the cobalamin is transferred to another transport protein, transcobalamin II (TC II). The cobalamin–TC II complex is then secreted into the circulation, from which it is rapidly taken up by the liver, the bone marrow, and other cells. The pathway of cobalamin absorption is shown in Fig. 292-1. Normally, about 2 mg cobalamin is stored in the liver, and another 2 mg is stored elsewhere in the body. In view of the minimum daily requirement, about 3 to 6 years would be required for a normal individual to become deficient in cobalamin if absorption were to cease abruptly.

Although TC II is the acceptor for newly absorbed cobalamin, most circulating cobalamin is bound to transcobalamin I (TC I), a glycoprotein closely related to gastric R binder. TC I appears to be derived in part from leukocytes. The paradox that most circulating cobalamin is bound to TC I rather than TC II, even though TC II initially carries all the cobalamin that is absorbed by the intestine, is explained by the fact that cobalamin bound to TC II is rapidly cleared from the blood ($t_{1/2}$ about 1 h), while clearance of cobalamin bound to TC I requires many days. The function of TC I is unknown.

BIOCHEMICAL CONSIDERATIONS

FOLATE The *prime function* of this vitamin is to transfer 1-carbon moieties such as methyl and formyl groups to various organic compounds (see Fig. 292-2). The source of these 1-carbon moieties is usually serine, which reacts with tetrahydrofolate to produce glycine and $N^{5,10}$-methylenetetrahydrofolate. An alternative source is formiminoglutamic acid, an intermediate in histidine catabolism, which gives up its formimino group to tetrahydrofolate to yield N^5-formiminotetrahydrofolate and glutamic acid. These derivatives provide entry into an interconvertible donor pool consisting of tetrahydrofolate derivatives carrying various 1-carbon moieties (see Fig. 292-2). The constituents of this pool can donate their 1-carbon moieties to appropriate acceptor compounds to form metabolic intermediates which are ultimately converted to building blocks used in the synthesis of biologic macromolecules. The most important building blocks are (1) purines, in which the C-2 and C-8 atoms are introduced in folate-dependent reactions; (2) deoxythymidylate monophosphate (dTMP), synthesized from $N^{5,10}$-methylenetetrahydrofolate and deoxyuridylate monophosphate (dUMP); and (3) methionine, formed by the transfer of a methyl group from N^5-methyltetrahydrofolate to homocysteine. Cobalamin is also required for the formation of methionine from homocysteine (see below).

In all but one of the 1-carbon transfer reactions, tetrahydrofolate is produced. It can immediately accept a 1-carbon moiety and reenter the donor pool. The single exception is the thymidylate synthetase reaction (dUMP → dTMP), in which dihydrofolate is the product (Fig. 292-2). This must be reduced to tetrahydrofolate by the enzyme dihydrofolate reductase before it can reenter the donor pool. A number of drugs are able to inhibit dihydrofolate reductase, thereby diverting folate from the donor pool and producing what amounts to a state of folate deficiency in the face of normal tissue folate concentrations.

COBALAMIN In humans there are two metabolically active forms of cobalamin, identified by the alkyl group attached to the sixth coordination position of the cobalt atom: methylcobalamin and adenosylcobalamin. The vitamin preparation which is used therapeutically is cyanocobalamin (also called vitamin B_{12}). Cyanocobalamin

FIGURE 292-2 Scheme of folate metabolism.

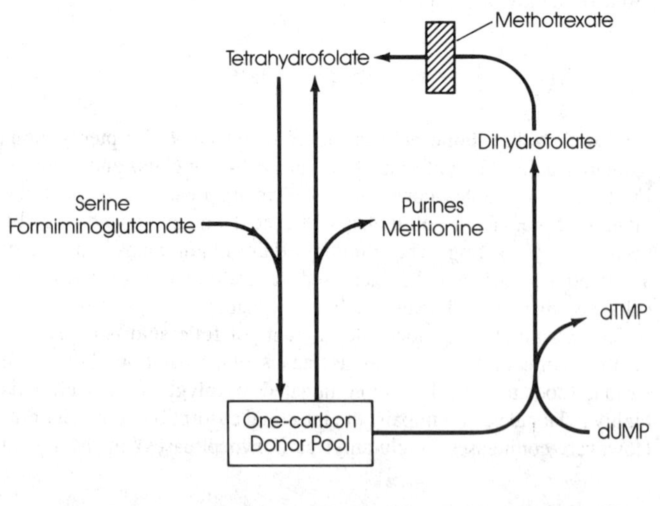

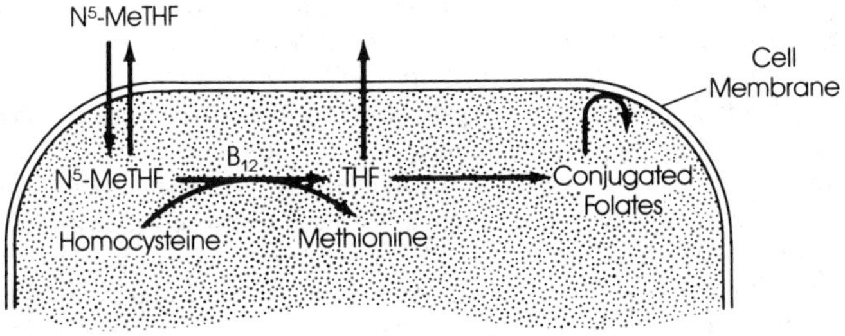

FIGURE 292-3 Diagram showing the interrelationship between cobalamin (methylcobalamin) and folate metabolism within the cell.

has no known physiologic role and must be converted to a biologically active form before it can be used by tissues.

Methylcobalamin is an essential cofactor in the conversion of homocysteine to methionine (Fig. 292-3). When this reaction is impaired, folate metabolism is deranged, and it is this derangement which is thought to underlie the defect in DNA synthesis and the megaloblastic maturation pattern in patients who are deficient in cobalamin (see Fig. 292-3). What appears to happen in cobalamin deficiency is that the unconjugated N^5-methyltetrahydrofolate newly taken from the bloodstream cannot be converted to other forms of tetrahydrofolate by methyl transfer. This is the so-called folate trap hypothesis. Since N^5-methyltetrahydrofolate is a poor substrate for the conjugating enzyme (this has been shown in rats and pigs but has not yet been demonstrated in humans), it largely remains in the unconjugated form and slowly leaks from the cell. Tissue folate deficiency therefore develops, and this results in megaloblastic hematopoiesis. This hypothesis explains the fact that tissue folate stores in cobalamin deficiency are substantially reduced, with a disproportionate reduction in conjugated as compared with unconjugated folates, despite normal or supranormal serum folate levels. It also explains why large doses of folate can produce a partial hematologic remission in patients with cobalamin deficiency.

Impairment in the conversion of homocysteine to methionine may also be partly responsible for the neurologic complications of cobalamin deficiency (see below). The methionine formed in this reaction is needed for the production of choline and choline-containing phospholipids as well as for the methylation of myelin basic protein. Nervous system damage is thought to result from interference with these processes due to decreased methionine production in cobalamin deficiency.

Adenosylcobalamin is required for the conversion of methylmalonyl coenzyme A (CoA) to succinyl CoA. Lack of this cofactor leads to large increases in the tissue levels of methylmalonyl CoA and its precursor, propionyl CoA. As a consequence, nonphysiologic fatty acids containing an odd number of carbon atoms are synthesized and incorporated into neuronal lipids. This biochemical abnormality may also contribute to the neurologic complications of cobalamin deficiency (see below).

CLINICAL DISORDERS

CLASSIFICATION OF MEGALOBLASTIC ANEMIAS (Table 292-1) The etiology of megaloblastic anemia varies in different parts of the world. In temperate zones, folate deficiency in alcoholics and pernicious anemia are the common types of megaloblastic anemias. In certain areas close to the equator, tropical sprue is endemic and an important cause. In Scandinavia, megaloblastic anemia is sometimes secondary to infestation by the fish tapeworm *Diphyllobothrium latum*.

The dietary intake of cobalamin is more than adequate for the body's requirements, except in true vegetarians (individuals who live on a purely vegetable diet) and their breast-fed infants. Thus, deficiency of cobalamin is almost always due to malabsorption. As explained in the section above, the absorption of cobalamin depends upon a specific binding protein produced in the stomach and uptake by a specific receptor in the mucosa of the distal ileum. Accordingly, several steps in this process can go awry and lead to malabsorption. In contrast, the dietary intake of folic acid is marginal in many parts of the world. Furthermore, since the body's stores of folate are relatively low, folic acid deficiency can arise rather suddenly during periods of decreased dietary intake or increased metabolic demand. Finally, folic acid deficiency may be due to malabsorption. Often two or more of these factors coexist in a given patient.

Combined deficiencies of cobalamin and folic acid are not uncommon. Patients with tropical sprue are often deficient in both vitamins. The biochemical lesion that results in megaloblastic maturation of bone marrow cells also causes structural and functional abnormalities of the rapidly proliferating epithelial cells of the intestinal mucosa. Thus, severe deficiency of one vitamin can lead to malabsorption of the other. Furthermore, as discussed above, a deficiency of cobalamin causes a secondary reduction in cellular folic acid.

Finally, megaloblastic anemias may occasionally be induced by factors unrelated to a vitamin deficiency. Most such cases are caused by one or more of the many drugs which interfere with DNA synthesis. Less commonly, megaloblastic maturation is encountered in certain acquired defects of hematopoietic stem cells. Rarest of all are specific congenital enzyme deficiencies in which megaloblastic anemia is characteristically encountered.

COBALAMIN DEFICIENCY There are many conditions in which cobalamin deficiency may develop. Although each has its own characteristic manifestations, certain clinical features are common to all. These clinical features involve the blood, the gastrointestinal tract, and the nervous system.

The hematologic manifestations are almost entirely the result of anemia although very rarely purpura may appear, due to thrombocytopenia. Symptoms of anemia may include weakness, lightheadedness, vertigo, and tinnitus, as well as palpitations, angina, and the symptoms of congestive failure. On physical examination, the patient with florid cobalamin deficiency is pale, with slightly icteric skin and eyes. The pulse is rapid, and the heart may be enlarged; auscultation will reveal a systolic flow murmur. The spleen and liver may be somewhat enlarged. There may be a slight fever.

The gastrointestinal manifestations reflect the effect of cobalamin deficiency on the rapidly proliferating gastrointestinal epithelium. The patient sometimes complains of a sore tongue, which on inspection will be smooth and beefy red. Anorexia with moderate weight loss may also be evident, possibly accompanied by diarrhea and other gastrointestinal symptoms. These latter manifestations may be in part caused by megaloblastosis of the small-intestinal epithelium, which results in malabsorption.

The neurologic manifestations are the most worrisome of all, because they often fail to remit fully on treatment. They begin pathologically with demyelination, followed by axonal degeneration and eventual neuronal death; the final stage, of course, is irreversible. Sites of involvement include peripheral nerves, the spinal cord, where the posterior and lateral columns undergo demyelination, and the cerebrum itself. Signs and symptoms include numbness and paresthesias in the extremities (the earliest neurologic manifestations), weakness, ataxia, and poor finger coordination. There may be sphincter disturbances. Reflexes may be diminished or increased. The Romberg and Babinski signs may be positive, and position sense and vibration sense are usually diminished. Disturbances of mentation will vary from mild irritability and forgetfulness to severe dementia or frank psychosis. It should be emphasized that occasionally *neurologic disease may occur in a patient with a normal hematocrit* and normal red blood cell indexes.

In the usual patient, in whom hematologic problems predominate, the blood and bone marrow show characteristic megaloblastic changes which are described under "Diagnosis" below. The anemia may be very severe—hematocrits of 15 to 20 are not infrequent—but is surprisingly well tolerated by the patient because it develops so slowly.

Pernicious anemia The most common cause of cobalamin deficiency in temperate climates is pernicious anemia, in which intrinsic factor secretion ceases owing to atrophy of the gastric mucosa. It is most frequently seen in individuals of northern European descent and American blacks and is much less common in southern Europeans and Orientals. Men and women are equally affected. It is a disease of the elderly, the average patient presenting near age 60; it is rare under 30, although typical pernicious anemia can be seen in children under 10 (juvenile pernicious anemia). Inherited conditions in which a histologically normal stomach secretes either an abnormal intrinsic factor or none at all will induce cobalamin deficiency in infancy or early childhood.

On the basis of incomplete evidence, pernicious anemia is currently thought to be caused by an autoimmune reaction against gastric parietal cells. There is considerable evidence for immunologic abnormalities in pernicious anemia. The incidence of pernicious anemia is substantially increased in patients with other diseases thought to be of immunologic origin, including Graves' disease, myxedema, thyroiditis, idiopathic adrenocortical insufficiency, vitiligo, and hypoparathyroidism. Patients with pernicious anemia also have abnormal circulating antibodies related to their disease: 90 percent have antiparietal cell antibody while 60 percent have anti-intrinsic factor antibody. Antiparietal cell antibody is also found in 50 percent of patients with gastric atrophy without pernicious anemia as well as in 10 to 15 percent of an unselected patient population, but anti-intrinsic factor antibody is usually absent from these patients. Relatives of patients with pernicious anemia have an increased incidence of the disease, and even clinically unaffected relatives may have anti-intrinsic factor antibody in their serum. A final point supporting an immunologic basis for pernicious anemia is the fact that corticosteroids have been reported to reverse the disease both pathologically and clinically.

The destruction of parietal cells in pernicious anemia is thought to be mediated by complement-fixing antibodies against the parietal cell surface. The observation that pernicious anemia is unusually common in patients with agammaglobulinemia, however, suggests that the cellular immune system may also play a role in its pathogenesis.

Pathologically, the most characteristic finding in pernicious anemia is gastric atrophy affecting the acid- and pepsin-secreting portion of the stomach; the antrum is spared. Other pathologic changes are secondary to the deficiency of cobalamin; these include megaloblastoid alterations in the gastric and intestinal epithelium and the neurologic changes described above. The abnormalities in the gastric epithelium appear as cellular atypia in gastric cytology specimens, a finding which must be carefully distinguished from the cytologic abnormalities seen in gastric malignancy.

The *clinical manifestations* are primarily those of cobalamin deficiency, as described above. The disease is of insidious onset and progresses slowly. Laboratory examination will reveal hypergastrinemia and pentagastrin-fast achlorhydria as well as the hematologic and other laboratory abnormalities discussed below in "Diagnosis."

Through appropriate replacement therapy, patients with pernicious anemia should experience complete and lifelong correction of all abnormalities which are due to cobalamin deficiency, except to the extent that irreversible changes in the nervous system may have occurred prior to treatment. These patients, however, are unusually subject to gastric polyps and have about twice the normal incidence of cancer of the stomach. In view of the latter complication, patients should be followed with frequent stool guaiac examinations together with further diagnostic studies when indicated.

Postgastrectomy Following total gastrectomy or extensive damage to gastric mucosa as, for example, by ingestion of corrosive agents, megaloblastic anemia may develop because the source of intrinsic factor has been removed. In such patients the absorption of orally administered cobalamin is impaired. Megaloblastic anemia may also follow partial gastrectomy, but the incidence is lower than after total gastrectomy, in which cobalamin malabsorption occurs in 100 percent of patients. The cause of cobalamin deficiency after partial gastrectomy may be intestinal overgrowth of bacteria, but it does not always respond to antibiotics.

Intestinal organisms Megaloblastic anemia may occur with intestinal stasis due to anatomic lesions (strictures, diverticula, anastomoses, "blind loops") or pseudoobstruction (diabetes mellitus, scleroderma, amyloid). This anemia is caused by colonization of the small intestine by large masses of bacteria which divert cobalamin from the host. Steatorrhea may also be seen under these circumstances, because bile salt metabolism is disturbed when the intestine is heavily colonized with bacteria. Hematologic responses have been observed after administration of oral antibiotics such as tetracycline and ampicillin.

Megaloblastic anemia is seen, in Scandinavia especially, in persons harboring the fish tapeworm *D. latum*. The anemia has been attributed to competition by the worm for cobalamin. Destruction of the worm eliminates the problem.

Ileal abnormalities Cobalamin deficiency is commonly found in tropical sprue, while it is an unusual complication of nontropical sprue (gluten-sensitive enteropathy; see Chap. 240). Virtually any disorder which compromises the absorptive capacity of the distal ileum can result in cobalamin deficiency. Specific entities include regional enteritis, Whipple's disease, and tuberculosis. Segmental involvement of the distal ileum by disease can cause megaloblastic anemia without any other manifestations of intestinal malabsorption such as steatorrhea. Cobalamin malabsorption is also seen after ileal resection. The Zollinger-Ellison syndrome (intense gastric hyperacidity due to a gastrin-secreting tumor) may cause cobalamin malabsorption by acidifying the small intestine. This will retard the transfer of the vitamin from R binder to intrinsic factor and will impair the binding of the cobalamin–IF complex to the ileal receptors. Chronic pancreatitis may also cause cobalamin malabsorption by impairing the transfer of the vitamin from R binder to intrinsic factor. This abnormality can be detected by tests of cobalamin absorption (see below, Schilling test), but it is invariably mild and never causes clinical cobalamin deficiency. Finally, there is a rare congenital disorder, Imerslund-Gräsbeck disease, in which a selective defect in cobalamin absorption is accompanied by proteinuria.

FOLIC ACID DEFICIENCY Patients with folic acid deficiency are more apt to be malnourished than those with cobalamin deficiency. Accordingly, they are likely to appear wasted. The gastrointestinal manifestations are similar to, but may be more widespread and more severe than those of, pernicious anemia. Diarrhea is often present, and cheilosis and glossitis are also encountered. However, in contrast to cobalamin deficiency, neurologic abnormalities do not occur.

The hematologic manifestations of folic acid deficiency are the same as those of cobalamin deficiency. Folic acid deficiency can generally be attributed to one or more of the following factors: increased demand for folate, inadequate intake, and malabsorption.

Inadequate intake Folic acid malnutrition is commonly encountered among a number of groups. Alcoholics frequently become folate-deficient because their main source of caloric intake is alcoholic beverages. Distilled spirits are virtually devoid of folic acid, while beer and wine do not contain enough of the vitamin to satisfy the daily requirement. In addition, alcohol may interfere with folate metabolism. Narcotic addicts are also prone to become folate-deficient because of malnutrition. Many indigent and elderly individuals who subsist primarily on canned foods or "tea and toast" and occasional teenagers whose diet consists of "junk food" develop folate deficiency.

Increased demand Tissues with a relatively high rate of cell division such as the bone marrow or gut mucosa have a large requirement for folate. Therefore, patients with chronic hemolytic anemias or other causes of very active erythropoiesis may become deficient if their high folate requirement is not met by dietary intake. Likewise, a pregnant woman may become deficient in folic acid because of the high demand of the developing fetus. Folate deficiency may also occur during the growth spurts of infancy and adolescence.

Malabsorption Folic acid deficiency is a common accompaniment of tropical sprue. Both the gastrointestinal symptoms and malabsorption are improved by the administration of either folic acid or antibiotics by mouth. Patients with nontropical sprue (gluten-sensitive enteropathy) may also develop significant folic acid deficiency which parallels other parameters of malabsorption. Similarly, alcohol-related folate deficiency may be due in part to malabsorption. In addition, other primary small-bowel disorders are sometimes associated with vitamin deficiency. These entities are all discussed in Chap. 240.

DRUGS Next to deficiency of folate or cobalamin, the most common cause of megaloblastic anemia is drug ingestion. Drugs which cause megaloblastic anemia do so by interfering with DNA synthesis, either directly or by antagonizing the action of folate. They can be classified as follows:

1 *Direct inhibitors of DNA synthesis.* The drugs in this category are used in the treatment of malignancy. Their efficacy depends on their ability to disrupt DNA synthesis. They include purine analogues (6-thioguanine, azathioprine, 6-mercaptopurine), pyrimidine analogues (5-fluorouracil, cytosine arabinoside), and other drugs which interfere with DNA synthesis by a variety of mechanisms (hydroxyurea, procarbazine).

The antiviral agents acyclovir, used in herpes simplex and herpes zoster infections, and zidovudine (AZT), used against the human immunodeficiency virus (HIV), can cause megaloblastic anemia. Megaloblastic anemia is only rarely seen with acyclovir, but it occurs regularly with zidovudine, representing the major toxicity of this drug.

2 *Folate antagonists.* The most toxic of these is methotrexate, an exceedingly powerful inhibitor of dihydrofolate reductase which is used in the treatment of certain malignancies. Much less toxic, but still capable of inducing a megaloblastic anemia, are several weak dihydrofolate reductase inhibitors that are used to treat a variety of nonmalignant conditions. These include pentamidine, trimethoprim, triamterene, and pyrimethamine.

The megaloblastic changes in methotrexate poisoning appear to result from the following sequence of events. In methotrexate-poisoned cells, the methylation of dUMP to dTMP is grossly impaired. As a consequence, the phosphorylation of dUMP to dUTP, normally a very minor reaction, becomes a major route of dUMP metabolism. The capacity of a highly specific dUTP pyrophosphatase to degrade dUTP back to dUMP is overwhelmed under these conditions, and dUTP accumulates in the cell. This dUTP is incorporated into newly synthesized DNA, because DNA polymerase cannot distinguish between dUTP and the closely related normal substrate, dTTP. As a result, defective strands of DNA are produced in which T is partly replaced by U. The U-containing regions of these defective strands are recognized by a specific repair system, which excises them and attempts to replace them with normal DNA. In methotrexate-poisoned cells, however, there is so much dUTP and so little dTTP that the new DNA is also likely to be defective. It is this futile cycle of faulty replication, error excision, faulty repair, etc., which explains the megaloblastic pattern of DNA synthesis in methotrexate-poisoned cells.

3 *Nitrous oxide.* Nitrous oxide inhalation causes the destruction of endogenous cobalamin. As ordinarily used, this anesthetic does not destroy enough cobalamin to cause clinical manifestations. Repeated or protracted exposure, however, may lead to a megaloblastic anemia. Fatal megaloblastic anemia has been reported in patients with tetanus who were given nitrous oxide continuously for weeks.

4 *Others.* A number of drugs antagonize folate by mechanisms which are poorly understood but are thought to involve an effect on absorption of the vitamin by the intestine. In this category are the anticonvulsants phenytoin (Dilantin) and primidone (Mysoline) and phenobarbital (Luminal). Megaloblastic anemia induced by these agents is mild.

ACUTE MEGALOBLASTIC ANEMIA Occasionally, a full-blown megaloblastic state can develop over the course of just a few days. This is usually seen following nitrous oxide anesthesia, but may occur in any patient with a serious illness requiring intensive care, especially a patient receiving multiple transfusions, dialysis, or total parenteral nutrition. An acute megaloblastic state can also be precipitated by the administration of a weak antifolate (e.g., trimethoprim) to a patient with marginal tissue folate stores.

The condition resembles an immune cytopenia, with a rapidly developing thrombocytopenia and/or leukopenia in the absence of anemia. The blood smear may be completely normal, but the marrow is always floridly megaloblastic. Acute megaloblastic anemia responds rapidly to treatment with folate plus cobalamin in the usual therapeutic doses.

OTHER Hereditary Megaloblastic anemia may be seen in several hereditary disorders. It is a regular feature of orotic aciduria, a deficiency of orotidylic decarboxylase and phosphorylase, leading to a defect in pyrimidine metabolism and characterized by retarded growth and development as well as by the excretion of large amounts of orotic acid. Megaloblastic anemia has been reported in a single case of the Lesch-Nyhan syndrome, a condition resulting from a deficiency of hypoxanthine-guanine phosphoribosyltransferase whose clinical manifestations include gout, mental retardation, and self-mutilation. It has also been described in methylmalonic aciduria due to a defect in the biosynthesis of the two metabolically active alkyl cobalamins, though it is not seen in methylmalonic aciduria due to methylmalonyl CoA mutase deficiency. Congenital folate malabsorption causes megaloblastic anemia, accompanied by ataxia and mental retardation. Megaloblastic anemia has been reported to accompany the congenital deficiency of two other folate-metabolizing enzymes: dihydrofolate reductase and N^5-methyltetrahydrofolate:homocysteine methyltransferase. These deficiencies are less well documented than is congenital folate malabsorption. A thiamine-responsive megaloblastic anemia accompanied by nerve deafness and diabetes mellitus has been reported in several children. Megaloblastic changes as well as multinuclearity of red blood cell precursors are seen in the marrow of certain patients with congenital dyserythropoietic anemia, a group of inherited disorders characterized by mild to moderate anemia presenting at any age and pursuing a benign course.

Transcobalamin II deficiency, like the congenital abnormalities in cobalamin absorption described previously, causes pronounced deficiency in cobalamin in infancy or early childhood, with all the accompanying manifestations. Megaloblastic anemia is not seen in hereditary transcobalamin I deficiency.

Refractory megaloblastic anemia This is a form of myelodysplasia in which megaloblastic erythropoiesis may sometimes be seen. Megaloblastic changes are restricted to the red blood cell series; large granulocyte precursors and giant metamyelocytes are not seen (see below). Like other forms of myelodysplasia, acquired sideroblastic anemia is associated with an increased incidence of acute leukemia.

Megaloblastic changes are seen in erythremic myelosis and acute erythroleukemia (di Guglielmo) where red blood cell precursors are prominently involved. Here, the marrow is characterized by bizarre erythroid maturation, with multinuclearity and multipolar mitotic figures in the red blood cell precursors. Erythremic myelosis is discussed further in Chap. 296.

DIAGNOSIS The finding of significant macrocytosis [mean corpuscular volume (MCV) $>$ 100 fL] suggests the presence of a megaloblastic anemia. Other causes of macrocytosis include hemolysis, liver disease, alcoholism, hypothyroidism, and aplastic anemia. If the macrocytosis is marked (MCV $>$ 110 fL), the patient is much more likely to have a megaloblastic anemia. The reticulocyte count is low, and the leukocyte and platelet count may also be decreased, particularly in severely anemic patients. The blood smear (Fig. A5-2) demonstrates marked anisocytosis and poikilocytosis, together with macroovalocytes, which are large, oval, fully hemoglobinized erythrocytes typical of megaloblastic anemias. There is some basophilic stippling, and an occasional nucleated red blood cell may be seen.

In the white blood cell series, the neutrophils show hypersegmentation of the nucleus. This is such a characteristic finding that a single cell with a nucleus of six lobes or more should raise the immediate suspicion of a megaloblastic anemia. A rare myelocyte may also be seen. Bizarre, misshapen platelets are also observed. The bone marrow examination is very helpful in the diagnosis of megaloblastic anemia. The marrow is hypercellular with a decreased myeloid/erythroid ratio and abundant stainable iron. Red blood cell precursors are abnormally large and have nuclei that appear much less mature than would be expected from the development of the cytoplasm (nuclear-cytoplasmic asynchrony). The nuclear chromatin is more dispersed than it should be and consequently stains less intensely than normal. To the extent that it is aggregated, it condenses in a peculiar fenestrated pattern which is very characteristic of megaloblastic erythropoiesis. Abnormal mitoses may be seen. Granulocyte precursors are also affected, many being larger than normal, including giant bands and metamyelocytes. Megakaryocytes are decreased and show abnormal morphology.

Megaloblastic anemias are characterized by ineffective erythropoiesis (Chap. 290). In a severely megaloblastic patient as many as 90 percent of the red blood cell precursors may be destroyed before they are released into the bloodstream, compared with 10 to 15 percent in the normal subject. Enhanced intramedullary destruction of erythroblasts results in an increase in unconjugated bilirubin and lactic acid dehydrogenase (isoenzyme 1) in plasma. Abnormalities in iron kinetics also attest to the presence of ineffective erythropoiesis, with increased iron turnover but low incorporation of labeled iron into circulating red blood cells.

In evaluating a patient with megaloblastic anemia, it is important to determine whether there is a specific vitamin deficiency by measuring serum cobalamin and folate levels. The normal range of cobalamin in serum is 200 to 900 pg/mL; values less than 100 pg/mL indicate clinically significant deficiency. The normal serum concentration of folic acid ranges from 6 to 20 ng/mL; values of 4 ng/mL or less are generally considered to be diagnostic of folate deficiency. Unlike serum cobalamin, serum folate levels may reflect recent alterations in dietary intake. Measurement of red blood cell folate occasionally provides useful information since it is not subject to short-term fluctuations in folate intake and is, therefore, a better index of tissue folate stores than serum folate.

Once cobalamin deficiency has been established, its pathogenesis can be delineated by means of a Schilling test. A patient is given radioactive cobalamin by mouth followed shortly thereafter by an intramuscular injection of unlabeled cobalamin. The proportion of the administered radioactivity excreted in the urine during the next 24 h provides an accurate measure of absorption of cobalamin, assuming that a complete urine sample has been collected. Since cobalamin deficiency is almost always due to malabsorption (Table 292-1), this first stage of the Schilling test should be abnormal. The patient is then given labeled cobalamin bound to intrinsic factor. Absorption of the vitamin will now approach normal if the patient has pernicious anemia or some other type of intrinsic factor deficiency. If cobalamin absorption is still decreased, the patient may have bacterial overgrowth (blind loop syndrome) or ileal disease (including an ileal absorptive defect secondary to the cobalamin deficiency itself). Cobalamin malabsorption due to bacterial overgrowth can frequently be corrected by the administration of antibiotics. The Schilling test can provide equally reliable information after the patient has had adequate therapy with parenteral cobalamin.

Low serum cobalamin levels are sometimes found in patients who are hematologically normal and have normal Schilling tests. Many of these patients absorb cobalamin poorly when the vitamin is mixed with food. The question has been raised whether the neurologic and psychiatric abnormalities often seen in these patients may be due to a chronic state of cobalamin deficiency. If so—and this question is far from answered—symptomatic cobalamin deficiency in the absence of anemia may be far more widespread than is currently recognized.

TREATMENT

COBALAMIN DEFICIENCY Apart from specific therapy related to the underlying disorder (e.g., antibiotics for intestinal overgrowth with bacteria), the mainstay of treatment for cobalamin deficiency is replacement therapy. Since the defect is one of absorption, replacement should be administered parenterally, specifically in the form of intramuscular cyanocobalamin. (If intramuscular administration is contraindicated or refused, cobalamin deficiency can be managed by oral replacement therapy, but at doses of 300 to 1000 μg daily, it is an expensive mode of treatment which requires very close medical supervision to avoid relapse.) Treatment should be started with 100 μg cobalamin per day for a week. The frequency of administration of the vitamin may then be decreased, the goal being to give a total of 2000 μg during the first 6 weeks. The patient may then be placed on 100 μg cyanocobalamin intramuscularly every month, a regimen that must be maintained for the rest of the patient's life. If necessary, larger doses may be given at less frequent intervals (e.g., 1 mg every 2 to 4 months), but the risk of relapse is substantially greater than if the vitamin is given monthly.

The response to treatment is gratifying. Shortly after treatment is begun, and several days before a hematologic response is evident in the peripheral blood, the patient will experience an increase in strength and an improved sense of well-being. Marrow morphology begins to revert toward normal within a few hours after treatment is initiated. Reticulocytosis begins 4 to 5 days after therapy is started and peaks at about day 7 (Fig. 292-4), with subsequent remission of the anemia over the next several weeks. If a reticulocytosis does not occur, or if it is less brisk than expected from the level of the hematocrit, a search should be made for other factors contributing to the anemia (e.g., infection, coexisting folate deficiency, or hypothyroidism). Hypokalemia and salt retention may occur early in the course of therapy; usually these developments are of no consequence, but occasionally they may lead to severe illness or even death.

In most cases, replacement therapy is all that is needed for the treatment of cobalamin deficiency. Occasionally, however, a patient with a severe anemia will have such a precarious cardiovascular status that emergency transfusion is necessary. This must be done with great care, since it is very easy to precipitate florid congestive failure in such patients by fluid overload. Blood must be administered slowly in the form of packed cells, with very close observation, giving as an initial dose no more than 100 mL. This small volume will frequently be enough to ameliorate the cardiovascular problems sufficiently that further therapy can be restricted to cobalamin replacement. If necessary, blood may be administered by exchanging patient blood (mostly plasma) for packed cells.

With lifelong treatment, patients should experience no further manifestations of cobalamin deficiency. As previously stated, neu-

FIGURE 292-4 Hematologic response of a patient with pernicious anemia to an intramuscular injection of 100 μg cobalamin on day 0. *(From A Erslev, TG Gabuzda, Pathophysiology of Blood, Philadelphia, Saunders, 1975.)*

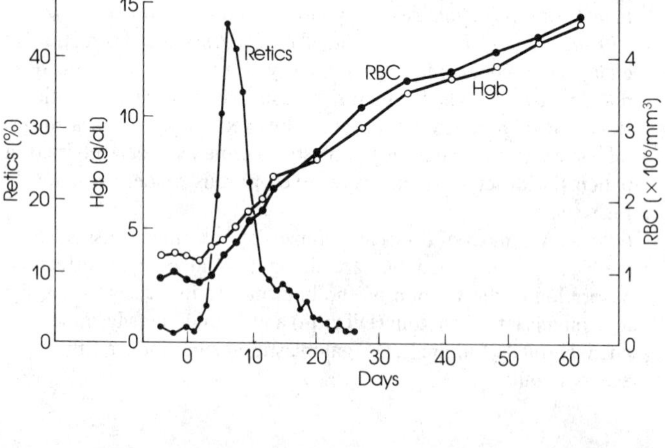

rologic symptoms may not be fully corrected even by optimal therapy. The potential for late development of gastric carcinoma in pernicious anemia necessitates careful follow-up of the patient.

FOLATE DEFICIENCY Like cobalamin deficiency, folate deficiency is treated by replacement therapy. The usual dose of folate is 1 mg per day, by mouth, but higher doses (up to 5 mg per day) may be required for folate deficiency due to malabsorption. Parenteral folate is rarely necessary. The hematologic response is similar to that seen after replacement therapy for cobalamin deficiency—that is, a brisk reticulocytosis after about 4 days, followed by correction of the anemia over the next 1 to 2 months. The duration of therapy depends on the basis of the deficiency state. Patients with a continuously increased requirement (such as patients with hemolytic anemia) or those with malabsorption or chronic malnutrition should continue to receive oral folic acid indefinitely. In addition, the patient should be encouraged to maintain an optimal diet containing adequate amounts of folate.

Folate, particularly in large doses, can correct the megaloblastic anemia of cobalamin deficiency without altering the neurologic abnormalities. The neurologic manifestations may even be aggravated by folate therapy. Cobalamin deficiency can thus be masked in patients who for one reason or another are taking large doses of folate. For this reason, a hematologic response to folate must never be used to rule out cobalamin deficiency in a given patient; cobalamin deficiency can be excluded only by appropriate laboratory evaluation.

OTHER CAUSES OF MEGALOBLASTIC ANEMIA Megaloblastic anemia due to drugs can be treated, if necessary, by reducing the dose of the drug or eliminating it altogether. The effects of folate antagonists which inhibit dihydrofolate reductase can be counteracted by folinic acid (citrovorum factor) in a dose of 100 to 200 mg per day. Since folinic acid is a derivative of tetrahydrofolate, it circumvents the block in folate metabolism imposed by dihydrofolate reductase inhibitors, replenishing the tissues with a form of folate which can directly enter the one-carbon donor pool. Certain of the congenital megaloblastic anemia–producing enzyme deficiencies can be treated by appropriate specific therapeutic regimens. For the megaloblastic forms of sideroblastic anemia, pyridoxine in pharmacologic doses (as high as 300 mg per day) should be tried. A few patients will respond to this therapy. Simple supportive measures are all that appear to be in order for treatment of refractory megaloblastic anemia. Acute erythroleukemia (di Guglielmo's disease) is usually treated like other types of acute nonlymphocytic leukemia (see Chap. 296).

REFERENCES

ALLEN RH: The plasma transport of vitamin B_{12}. Br J Haematol 36:153, 1976

BABIOR BM: The megaloblastic anemias, in *Hematology*, 4th ed, WJ Williams et al (eds). New York, McGraw-Hill, 1990

BORCH K: Epidemiologic, clinicopathologic, and economic aspects of gastroscopic screening of patients with pernicious anemia. Scand J Gastroenterol 21:21, 1986

COOPER BA, ROSENBLATT DS: Inherited defects of vitamin B_{12} metabolism. Annu Rev Nutr 7:291, 1987

ERIKSSON S et al: Pernicious anemia as a risk factor in gastric cancer: The extent of the problem. Acta Med Scand 210:481, 1981

HERBERT V: Megaloblastic anemias. Lab Invest 52:3, 1985

———: Don't ignore low serum cobalamin (vitamin B_{12}) levels. Arch Intern Med 148:1705, 1988

KAPADIA CR, DONALDSON RM: Disorders of cobalamin (vitamin B_{12}) absorption and transport. Ann Rev Med 36:93, 1985

LAWSON DH et al: Early mortality in the megaloblastic anemias. Q J Med 41:1, 1972

LINDENBAUM J: Status of laboratory testing in the diagnosis of megaloblastic anemia. Blood 61:624, 1983

——— et al: Neuropsychiatric disorders caused by cobalamin deficiency in the absence of anemia or macrocytosis. N Engl J Med 318:1720, 1988

SAVAGE D, LINDENBAUM J: Anemia in alcoholics. Medicine 65:322, 1986

SHANE B, STOKSTAD EL: Vitamin B_{12}–folate interrelationships. Annu Rev Nutr 5:115, 1985

SCOTT JM, WEIR DG: Drug induced megaloblastic change. Clin Haematol 9:587, 1980

293 ANEMIA ASSOCIATED WITH CHRONIC DISORDERS

H. FRANKLIN BUNN

Among the most commonly encountered anemias are those that accompany a variety of chronic underlying diseases. They can be corrected only if the primary condition is reversible. As shown in Table 293-1, these anemias can be subdivided into several groups.

ANEMIA OF CHRONIC INFLAMMATION

CLINICAL FEATURES Patients who have a chronic systemic inflammatory disorder persisting more than a month usually develop a mild or moderate anemia. The extent of the anemia is roughly proportional to the duration and severity of the inflammatory process. These disorders include chronic infections such as subacute infective endocarditis, osteomyelitis, lung abscess, tuberculosis, and pyelonephritis. Among noninfectious causes of anemia of chronic inflammation, the most common is rheumatoid arthritis. Other noninfectious inflammatory disorders often associated with chronic anemia include systemic lupus erythematosus, vasculitides (such as temporal arteritis), sarcoidosis, regional enteritis, and tissue injury such as fracture.

This kind of anemia is also commonly encountered in neoplastic disorders, including Hodgkin's disease and a variety of solid tumors such as carcinoma of the lung and breast. Other factors may contribute to the development of more severe anemia in cancer patients. In those with gastrointestinal or uterine cancer, blood loss can be the predominant factor. Chronic bleeding will lead to iron deficiency. Furthermore, cancer patients may develop progressive anemia if the bone marrow is invaded with tumor cells. Myelophthisic anemia is discussed in Chap. 298. Cancer patients are often malnourished and may develop folate deficiency. Rarely, patients with disseminated malignancy develop severe traumatic hemolytic anemia (Chap. 294). Finally, suppression of hematopoiesis by chemotherapeutic agents or radiation therapy may aggravate anemia.

HEMATOLOGIC FEATURES Hemoglobin values generally range between 90 and 110 g/L. A hemoglobin level less than 80 g/L indicates the presence of one or more of the aggravating factors mentioned above. Although this group of anemias is generally classified as normocytic-normochromic, red blood cells are often slightly microcytic. The mean corpuscular hemoglobin concentration is about 320 g/L (normal ≅ 340 g/L). Examination of the bone marrow reveals normal erythroid maturation. However, the red blood cell precursors have less stainable iron than normal (i.e., fewer sideroblasts), while the macrophages in the marrow usually contain increased amounts of iron. Myeloid hyperplasia and an increase in plasma cells are often seen in chronic infections.

The corrected reticulocyte count is low. Careful measurement of red blood cell survival generally reveals moderately shortened erythrocyte life span. Cross-transfusion studies point to an extracorpuscular mechanism, probably hyperplasia of the mononuclear-phagocyte system. There is seldom any other evidence of significant hemolysis. However, in certain chronic infections such as subacute infective

TABLE 293-1 Anemias secondary to chronic systemic diseases

1 Anemia of chronic inflammation
- *a* Infection
- *b* Connective tissue disorders, etc.
- *c* Malignancy

2 Anemia of uremia
3 Anemia due to endocrine failure
4 Anemia of liver disease

endocarditis and miliary tuberculosis, splenomegaly can contribute to further shortening of the red blood cell life span, thereby increasing the severity of the anemia. In this setting spherocytes are often seen on the blood smear.

Serum iron is characteristically subnormal in this group of anemias, but in contrast to iron deficiency, the total transferrin level is also reduced (see Fig. 291-2). The fractional saturation of transferrin is lower than normal. The serum iron falls within hours or days following the onset of the inflammation, whereas several weeks elapse before the transferrin level falls. Serum ferritin is increased in patients with inflammatory disorders. Certain other plasma proteins are characteristically elevated in chronic inflammation, probably under the stimulus of interleukin 1, a protein hormone released by activated macrophages. These "phase reactants" include gamma globulin, the third component of complement, haptoglobin, $alpha_1$ antitrypsin, orosomucoid, and fibrinogen. The latter is usually not measured since protein electrophoresis is routinely done on serum rather than plasma. Elevation of these proteins is responsible for the increased rate of red blood cell sedimentation which is so commonly observed.

It is often difficult to detect iron deficiency in a patient with chronic inflammation. The serum iron is low, and red blood cell protoporphyrin is increased in both conditions. When iron deficiency is superimposed on a chronic inflammatory state, the serum ferritin falls and transferrin level rises, usually to within normal limits. Under such circumstances, the amount of storage iron in the bone marrow is unpredictable. This problem is commonly encountered in patients with rheumatoid arthritis who may have developed iron deficiency owing to gastrointestinal blood loss. Because of this diagnostic uncertainty, it is often prudent to give such a patient a trial of iron and ascertain whether the hemoglobin level increases. However, it is important to avoid prolonged administration of iron unless a true deficiency state persists.

PATHOGENESIS The anemia of chronic inflammation is primarily due to defective red blood cell production and failure to compensate for the slightly decreased red blood cell life span. The subnormal amounts of iron in erythroblasts, in spite of an abundance of storage iron, suggest a defect in the transfer of iron to the developing erythroid cells. The cells that are formed are somewhat "iron deficient," and therefore tend to be small and pale. As in true iron deficiency, increased red blood cell protoporphyrin reflects the reduced availability of iron for heme synthesis. This defect can be quantitated by iron kinetic studies. If radioactive iron bound to transferrin is administered, there is normal uptake into erythroblasts and incorporation into circulating red cells. In contrast, if hemoglobin labeled with radioactive iron is injected, the incorporation of label into circulating red cells is only half normal. The hyperplastic mononuclear phagocyte system which is responsible for decreased survival of circulating red cells probably traps the hemoglobin iron and prevents its transfer to the bone marrow. The macrophages' increased avidity for iron may be due to one of the actions of interleukin 1, i.e., release of lactoferrin from neutrophils. The iron-binding protein lactoferrin captures free iron and rapidly transfers it to macrophages.

The modest suppression of red blood cell production is caused in part by decreased availability of iron. In addition, erythropoietin levels tend to be lower than expected for the degree of anemia. However, erythropoietin levels are not as low as in the anemia of renal failure (see below) and probably do not play a significant role in the pathogenesis of the anemia.

MANAGEMENT The anemia of chronic inflammation is not responsive to hematinic agents such as iron, folic acid, or vitamin B_{12}. Since the anemia is seldom severe, blood transfusion is rarely indicated. Efforts should be directed toward correcting the underlying disorder. In addition, if the anemia is more severe than expected, it is essential to search for other factors such as blood loss or drug-induced myelosuppression that could contribute to the reduction of red blood cell mass.

ANEMIA OF UREMIA

Anemia almost always accompanies the uremic syndrome (Chap. 224). Although the hemoglobin level is highly variable among uremic patients, the severity of the anemia is roughly proportional to the degree of azotemia. The etiology of the renal failure usually has little bearing on the extent of anemia. However, for any level of serum creatinine patients with polycystic disease tend to be less anemic than those with other types of renal disease. In contrast to anemias associated with other chronic disorders discussed in this chapter, the anemia of uremia can be very severe, with hemoglobin levels as low as 40 g/L. However, patients often tolerate such marked anemia fairly well. This is largely due to compensatory adjustments such as redistribution of blood flow and a decrease in the oxygen affinity of the blood (see Chap. 61).

The anemia of uremia is normochromic and normocytic. Examination of the bone marrow seldom reveals any abnormalities. Red blood cell morphology is usually normal. In about one-third of patients, so-called burr cells are seen in the peripheral blood smear. These red blood cells have a characteristic evenly scalloped border (see Fig. A5-9). Neither the degree of anemia nor the red blood cell life span is influenced by the presence of burr cells. In most patients the corrected reticulocyte count is low and the red blood cell survival is only modestly decreased. Thus the low red blood cell mass is due to decreased red blood cell production. The primary basis for this defect is that the diseased kidneys are unable to secrete adequate amounts of erythropoietin. Plasma erythropoietin levels are lower than those of nonuremic patients with a comparable degree of anemia. Erythropoiesis is further impaired but not abolished in patients who have undergone bilateral nephrectomy. In addition, red blood cell production may be suppressed by the accumulation of substances that are normally cleared by the kidneys. Iron kinetic measurements reveal impaired incorporation of iron into circulating red blood cells. Thus, it is likely that the anemia is due in part to ineffective erythropoiesis (see Chap. 290). Improvement in the rate of utilization of iron by the bone marrow has been noted following hemodialysis.

A small minority of uremic patients, particularly those with advanced disease, have brisk hemolysis. Red blood cell survival studies indicate that the hemolysis is due to extracorpuscular factors. Either metabolic or mechanical factors may contribute to the hemolysis. Some patients may acquire a defect in the hexose monophosphate shunt which renders the red blood cell vulnerable to the formation of Heinz bodies (see Chap. 294). The hemolysis can be aggravated by oxidant drugs or oxidant compounds such as chloramine in the dialysis bath. If the renal failure is due to thrombotic thrombocytopenic purpura or hemolytic-uremic syndrome, patients will have a severe form of microangiopathic hemolytic anemia, with characteristic abnormalities of red blood cell morphology (see Chap. 294).

In some patients aluminum salts that contaminate the tap water used in hemodialysis cause a worsening of anemia and the emergence of microcytosis and hypochromia.

Treatment of the anemia of uremia should focus on an attempt to reverse the renal failure. The anemia may be modestly improved following hemodialysis. A prompt and dramatic correction of the anemia follows successful renal transplantation. Occasionally, polycythemia may be encountered following the renal engraftment, and may be a harbinger of impending rejection. In those patients who are not candidates for renal transplantation the administration of androgens provides a modest stimulation of erythropoiesis, particularly in patients who have not undergone bilateral nephrectomy.

The treatment of the anemia of uremia has been revolutionized by the development of recombinant human erythropoietin. Administration of this genetically engineered product thrice weekly by intravenous infusion results in correction of anemia and gratifying symptomatic improvement. The agent is identical in structure to native erythropoietin and therefore safe and virtually free of side effects. However, overtreatment should be avoided since it can aggravate hypertension and increase the likelihood of thromboses. Accordingly, sufficient recombinant erythropoietin should be given to maintain the patient's hematocrit between 0.33 and 0.38.

It is important to be aware of other factors that may aggravate the anemia of renal disease. Uremic patients have a propensity to hemorrhage, owing to a qualitative defect in platelet function. Thus, gastrointestinal blood loss is commonly encountered. Furthermore a small but significant amount of blood loss occurs during hemodialysis. For these reasons some uremic patients become iron deficient. Folic acid deficiency may also occur, owing to the poor nutrition of many patients or to the loss of this vitamin during dialysis.

ANEMIA SECONDARY TO ENDOCRINE FAILURE

A number of hormones, including thyroxine, glucocorticoids, testosterone, and growth hormone are known to affect proliferation of human erythroid cells in vitro. Therefore it is not surprising that a mild to moderate normochromic-normocytic anemia generally accompanies a number of endocrine deficiency states, including hypothyroidism, Addison's disease, hypogonadism, and panhypopituitarism. It is possible that the anemias associated with hypothyroidism and hypopituitarism are related to the decreased need for oxygen transport, since oxygen consumption is reduced when thyroid hormone or growth hormone is lacking.

The anemia of *myxedema* is usually normocytic. Red blood cell life span is normal and erythropoiesis is effective. A minority of patients have macrocytic red blood cells which can usually be attributed to either folic acid or B_{12} deficiency. Patients with myxedema have an increased incidence of pernicious anemia. Hypothyroid patients, particularly females with menorrhagia, often develop iron deficiency and a microcytic anemia. Because the plasma volume may be reduced along with the red blood cell mass, the anemia of hypothyroidism may be masked. Since the signs and symptoms of myxedema are sometimes elusive, this diagnosis should be considered in the evaluation of any patient with unexplained anemia.

The anemia of *Addison's disease* is also masked by a decrease in plasma volume. Untreated patients have an average hemoglobin level of about 130 g/L. Upon hormone replacement, the plasma volume is rapidly reconstituted and the hemoglobin level falls to 80 percent of its pretreatment value. With continued therapy, the red blood cell mass returns to normal.

Testosterone has a physiologic influence on red blood cell mass. During passage through adolescence the mean hemoglobin level of males increases from 130 to 150 g/L. Eunuchoid males generally have a mean hemoglobin level averaging 130 g/L. Pituitary dysfunction or ablation is associated with a mild normochromic normocytic anemia as well as occasional leukopenia.

The anemias secondary to endocrine failure are all readily corrected when adequate hormone replacement is given.

ANEMIA OF LIVER DISEASE

Patients with chronic liver disease, regardless of etiology, usually have a mild to moderate anemia which is normocytic or slightly macrocytic. An increased plasma volume may artificially lower the hematocrit and make the anemia seem worse than it is. Red blood cell morphology is normal, except for the presence of target cells (see Fig. A5-3) and occasional stomatocytes, which have increased membrane surface area owing to increased deposits of cholesterol and phospholipid. The bone marrow is usually normal. Erythropoiesis fails to compensate for a moderate shortening of red blood cell life span. The anemia persists as long as hepatic function is defective, but it may be corrected if normal hepatic function can be restored.

The situation is much more complex in patients with *alcoholic liver disease*. Many factors can contribute to the development of anemia. Alcohol is a direct suppressor of erythropoiesis. In alcoholics who have continued to drink up to the time of clinical evaluation, the bone marrow often reveals vacuoles in the cytoplasm of red and white blood cell precursors. In addition, ringed sideroblasts may be observed, particularly in patients who are malnourished. In alcoholics there is often suboptimal intake of dietary folic acid and impairment of folate utilization. Furthermore, alcoholics commonly develop significant hemorrhage from gastritis, esophageal varices, or duodenal ulcer, which contributes to the anemia. The risk of gastrointestinal blood loss is further increased by the presence of thrombocytopenia or deficiencies in soluble clotting factors. Although alcoholics usually have increased iron stores, they may become iron-deficient after prolonged gastrointestinal bleeding. Rarely patients with alcoholic cirrhosis develop a severe hemolytic anemia accompanied by the appearance of rigid red blood cells with irregular borders called acanthocytes or "spur" cells (see Fig. A5-8). This entity is discussed in detail in Chap. 294. In addition, alcoholics may acquire a defect in the erythrocyte hexose monophosphate shunt, similar to that encountered in patients with uremia.

REFERENCES

BUDMAN DR, STEINBERG AD: Hematologic aspects of systemic lupus erythematosus. Ann Intern Med 86:220, 1977

ESCHBACH JW, ADAMSON J: Anemia of end-stage renal disease. Kideny Int 28:1, 1985

——— et al: Correction of the anemia of end-stage renal disease with recombinant human erythropoietin. N Engl J Med 316:73, 1987

LEE GR: The anemia of chronic disease. Semin Hematol 20:61, 1983

MOWAT AG: Hematologic abnormalities in rheumatoid arthritis. Semin Arthritis Rheum 1:195, 1972

NEFF MS et al: Anemia in chronic renal failure. Acta Endocrinol 271(Suppl):80, 1985

SAVAGE D, LINDENBAUM J: Anemia in alcoholics. Medicine 65:322, 1986

294 HEMOLYTIC ANEMIAS

RICHARD A. COOPER / H. FRANKLIN BUNN

Red blood cells undergo premature destruction by two general mechanisms. First, red blood cells may lyse in the circulation and release their contents directly into the plasma. Intravascular hemolysis may be caused by trauma to the red blood cell, by fixation of complement to the red blood cell, or by exogenous toxins. Second, and more commonly, red blood cells are taken up by macrophages in the spleen and liver (mononuclear-phagocyte system), where they are destroyed and digested (extravascular lysis). The mononuclear-phagocyte system clears the cells from the circulation under two general conditions: first, the presence of surface abnormalities such as bound immunoglobulin for which macrophages have specific receptors; second, the presence of physical characteristics that limit the deformability of red blood cells, thereby impeding their ability to traverse the fine filtering system of the spleen.

The discoid shape of red blood cells favors deformability, providing a surface area that is 60 to 70 percent in excess of the minimum that is necessary to encompass the content of the cell. Deformability is determined by three independent variables: (1) the viscoelastic properties of the red blood cell membrane, (2) the ratio of surface area to volume, and (3) the intracellular concentration of hemoglobin or the aggregation of hemoglobin into polymers or precipitates.

One or more of these factors play a role in the pathogenesis of the various hemolytic anemias that are described in this chapter. A classification of these anemias is shown in Table 294-1. A number of clinical and laboratory features are shared by various types of hemolytic anemia. Patients with congenital hemolysis often have

TABLE 294-1 Hemolytic anemias: Classification based on mechanism of hemolysis

Extracorpuscular	*1* Extrinsic factors	Acquired
	a Splenomegaly	
	b Antibody: immunohemolytic anemias	
	c Mechanical trauma: microangiopathic hemolytic anemia	
	d Direct toxic effect: malaria, clostridial infection, etc.	
	2 Membrane abnormalities	
	a Spur cell anemia	
Intracorpuscular	*b* Paroxysmal nocturnal hemoglobinuria	
	c Hereditary spherocytosis (rare: elliptocytosis, stomatocytosis)	Hereditary
	3 Abnormalities of red blood cell interior	
	a Enzyme defects	
	b Defects in the hexose monophosphate shunt	
	c Hemoglobinopathies	
	d Thalassemias	

lifelong anemia and may have a positive family history. Splenomegaly is seen in most chronic hemolytic anemias, both congenital and acquired. Patients with significant red blood cell turnover may be icteric, owing to an increase in unconjugated bilirubin.

LABORATORY EVALUATION OF HEMOLYSIS

The reticulocyte count is the single most useful test in the initial evaluation (Table 294-2). Patients with hemolytic anemia generally have a brisk reticulocytosis. The bone marrow predictably reveals erythroid hyperplasia. Since it seldom provides useful additional information, a bone marrow examination is generally not indicated in the evaluation of a patient with hemolytic anemia, unless an associated disorder such as lymphoma is suspected.

A number of serum tests are useful in establishing the presence of hemolysis (see Table 294-2), most importantly, the measurement of bilirubin, a tetrapyrrole formed from the oxidative catabolism of heme. *Unconjugated* or *"indirect" bilirubin* circulates in the plasma in transit from the mononuclear-phagocyte system to the liver where it is conjugated. When measured accurately, unconjugated bilirubin is a reliable guide to the presence of increased heme catabolism and is usually elevated in patients with hemolysis. The serum level of conjugated or "direct" bilirubin is normal unless the patient has associated hepatic or biliary dysfunction. Unconjugated bilirubin is also increased in patients with ineffective erythropoiesis, a condition in which there is enhanced destruction of red cell precursors within the bone marrow. Since circulating unconjugated bilirubin is tightly bound to albumin, it does not pass through renal glomeruli. Thus, patients with hemolytic anemia have acholuric jaundice, whereas the hyperbilirubinemia of liver disease is associated with bilirubin in the urine.

TABLE 294-2 Laboratory evaluation of hemolysis

	Moderate hemolysis (RBC life span 20–40 days)	Severe hemolysis (RBC life span 5–20 days)
HEMATOLOGIC		
Routine blood film	Polychromatophilia	Polychromatophilia
Reticulocyte count	↑	↑ ↑
Bone marrow examination	Erythroid hyperplasia	Erythroid hyperplasia
PLASMA OR SERUM		
Bilirubin	↑ Unconjugated	↑ Unconjugated
Haptoglobin	↓, absent	Absent
Hemopexin	Normal, ↓	↓, absent
Plasma hemoglobin	↑	↑ ↑
Lactate dehydrogenase	↑ (variable)	↑ ↑ (variable)
Methemalbumin	0	+ *
URINE		
Bilirubin	0	0
Urobilinogen	Variable	Variable
Hemosiderin	0, +	+
Hemoglobin	0	+ *

* *Intravascular hemolysis.*

Other serum tests are also useful in the assessment of hemolysis. *Haptoglobin* is an alpha globulin which is present in high concentration (~1.0 g/L) in the plasma (and serum). It binds specifically and tightly to the protein (globin) in hemoglobin. The hemoglobin-haptoglobin complex is cleared within minutes by the mononuclear-phagocyte system, while free haptoglobin has a long circulation time ($t_{1/2}$ = 4 days). Thus, patients with significant hemolysis, either intravascular or extravascular, have low or absent levels of serum haptoglobin. Haptoglobin synthesis is decreased in patients with hepatocellular disease. Conversely, synthesis is enhanced in inflammatory states. Haptoglobin, like $alpha_1$ antitrypsin, orosomucoid, and the third component of complement are acute phase reactants. These facts must be considered in the interpretation of serum haptoglobin. *Hemopexin* is a plasma beta globulin which binds specifically to heme. It becomes depleted in patients with moderate and severe hemolysis. In addition to that bound by hemopexin, some of the heme from circulating free hemoglobin is transferred to albumin, resulting in the formation of *methemalbumin.* This complex is encountered only in severe intravascular hemolysis. Plasma hemoglobin is increased in proportion to the degree of hemolysis, but may be falsely elevated owing to lysis of red cells in vitro.

Once the haptoglobin binding capacity of the plasma is exceeded, free hemoglobin permeates renal glomeruli, primarily as $\alpha\beta$ dimers with a molecular weight of 32,000. This filtered hemoglobin is reabsorbed by the proximal tubule, where it is catabolized in situ, and the heme iron is incorporated into storage proteins (ferritin and hemosiderin). The presence of hemosiderin in the urine, detected by staining the sediment with Prussian blue, indicates that a significant amount of circulating free hemoglobin has been filtered by the kidneys. When the absorptive capacity of the tubular cells is exceeded, hemoglobinuria ensues. The presence of hemoglobinuria indicates severe intravascular hemolysis. Sometimes the clinician is faced with the dilemma of whether benzidine-positive heme pigment in the urine is hemoglobin or myoglobin. The easiest way to distinguish between these alternatives is to examine an anticoagulated blood specimen after centrifugation. The plasma of patients with hemoglobinuria has a reddish-brown color. Conversely, patients with myoglobinuria have normal-appearing plasma. Because of its higher molecular weight, hemoglobin has lower glomerular permeability than myoglobin and is less rapidly cleared by the kidneys.

Tagging red cells with an appropriate isotopic label provides the most direct and precise measure of cell survival. The most commonly used label is sodium [^{51}Cr]chromate. Since it does not bind irreversibly to red cells, the measured survival of normal red cells ($t_{1/2}$ = 26 to 32 days) is shorter than the true red cell survival ($t_{1/2} \simeq$ 60 days). Such studies are not necessary or indicated in the diagnostic workup of the majority of patients with hemolytic anemia. However, scanning with a collimated detector can be employed to monitor the sequestration of ^{51}Cr-tagged red cells in the liver and spleen. This approach is sometimes useful in evaluating patients for possible splenectomy.

RED CELL MORPHOLOGY AS A CLUE TO DIAGNOSIS Most hemolytic disorders are associated with a change in the morphologic appearance of red blood cells. Some of these are depicted in Atlas 5. Spherocytes are the most common morphologic abnormality in hemolytic diseases. Small numbers occur in many disorders. They are most striking in patients with hereditary spherocytosis and in patients with warm antibody-induced immunohemolytic disease (Figs. A5-10 and A5-11). Spherocytes are the hallmark of splenic conditioning. Fragmented red blood cells suggest traumatic injury of the red cell including valve hemolysis, one of the microangiopathic hemolytic anemias [thrombotic thrombocytopenic purpura (Fig. A5-7), hemolytic uremic syndrome], or disseminated intravascular coagulation. Target-shaped red blood cells which are well filled with hemoglobin occur in patients with hemoglobin C. They are prevalent in sickle cell anemia, where they were first described, and they are found in patients with the underhydrated form of hereditary stomatocytosis. The most common cause of target cells is liver disease (Fig. A5-3). Target cells which are deficient in hemoglobin (hypochromic) are the hallmark of the thalassemia syndromes (Fig. A5-5).

Spiculated red blood cells often cause confusion because of the frequency with which they are induced as an artifact during the preparation of a blood smear. Under these conditions, they are particularly frequent at the edges of the smear. When surrounded by otherwise normal-appearing red blood cells, spiculated red blood cells can be a clue to diagnosis. They occur, usually in small numbers, in conjunction with uremia or following splenectomy even in the absence of an underlying red blood cell disorder. Bizarrely spiculated red blood cells (acanthocytes) occur in the rare condition abetalipoproteinemia (Chap. 326) and in anorexia nervosa; however, in each of these instances minimal hemolysis is present. As discussed below, acanthocytes are a striking feature of spur cell anemia (Fig. A5-8).

Permanently sickled, crescent-shaped red blood cells (Fig. A5-6) are the hallmark of sickle cell anemia. Boat-shaped red cells are a clue to the double heterozygous state, hemoglobin SC disease. The presence of both crescent-shaped cells and hypochromic target cells on the same smear is suggestive of the doubly heterozygous state, sickle cell–β thalassemia (see Chap. 295).

While in no case can the peripheral blood smear be totally diagnostic, in many it is a low-cost, important clue to the diagnosis. In addition to red blood cell morphology, a large battery of specific diagnostic tests are available for determining the etiology of the various hemolytic anemias. These are discussed in broad outline in Chap. 61 (Table 61-1) and in detail in this chapter.

EXTRINSIC CAUSES OF HEMOLYSIS

SPLENOMEGALY The spleen is particularly efficient in trapping and destroying red blood cells which have minimal defects, often so mild as to be undetectable by in vitro techniques. This unique ability of the spleen to filter mildly damaged red blood cells results from its unusual vascular anatomy. Almost all the blood circulating through the spleen flows rapidly from arterioles in the white pulp to sinuses in the spleen's red pulp, and then on into the venous system. In contrast, a small portion of splenic blood flow (normally 1 to 2 percent) leaves the arterioles of the white pulp to enter a nonendothelialized portion of the spleen. In this sense, it is extravascular, although the entire spleen may be considered as a specialized part of the vascular system. This blood passes into the ''marginal zone'' of the lymphatic white pulp. Although the cells which occupy this zone are not phagocytic, they serve as a mechanical filter hindering the progress of severely damaged red blood cells. As red blood cells leave this zone and enter the red pulp, they flow into narrow cords which end blindly but which communicate with sinuses through small openings between the lining cells of the sinuses. These openings, averaging 3 μm in diameter, test the ability of red blood cells to undergo a deformation of shape. Red blood cells which do not pass the stringent test imposed upon them by the spleen filter are engulfed by phagocytic cells and destroyed.

The normal spleen poses no threat to normal red blood cells. However, splenomegaly exaggerates the adverse conditions to which red blood cells are exposed. Splenic enlargement may be considered in three broad categories. In the first are infiltrative disease (such as myeloproliferative disorders, Chap. 297), lymphomas (Chap. 302), and storage diseases (such as Gaucher's disease, Chap. 331). In the second are systemic inflammatory diseases leading to splenic hypertrophy. In the third are diseases which cause congestive splenomegaly. Hemolysis may occur whenever the spleen is enlarged. Its occurrence is least predictable in infiltrative diseases of the spleen where substantial splenomegaly may exist with no apparent hemolysis. Inflammatory and congestive splenomegaly are commonly associated with mild to moderate shortening of red blood cell survival.

TABLE 294-3 Hemolysis due to antibodies

I Warm-antibody immunohemolytic anemia
A Idiopathic
B Lymphomas: Chronic lymphocytic leukemia, non-Hodgkin's lymphomas, Hodgkin's disease (infrequent)
C Systemic lupus erythematosus
D Tumors (rare)
E Drugs
1 α-Methyldopa type
2 Penicillin type (hapten)
3 Quinidine type (innocent bystander)
II Cold-antibody immunohemolytic anemia
A Cold agglutinin disease
1 Acute: Mycoplasma infection, infectious mononucleosis
2 Chronic: Idiopathic, lymphoma
B Paroxysmal cold hemoglobinuria

RED CELL ANTIBODIES Immune hemolysis in the adult may be induced by three general types of antibodies:

1 Alloantibodies acquired by blood transfusions or pregnancies and directed against transfused red blood cells (Chap. 286).
2 Antibodies reactive at body temperature and directed against the patient's own red blood cells (Table 294-3).
3 Antibodies reactive in the cold and directed against the patient's own red blood cells (Table 294-3).

Coombs' antiglobulin test is the major tool for diagnosing these disorders. This test relies on the ability of antibodies prepared in animals and directed against specific human serum proteins to agglutinate red blood cells if these human serum proteins are present on the red blood cell surface. The serum proteins of particular interest are IgG and C3. The ability of anti-IgG or anti-C3 antiserums to agglutinate the patient's red blood cells is referred to as the *direct Coombs test.* At times it is advantageous to know whether there is antibody in the serum of patients which is reactive against other human red blood cells, e.g., in cross matching prior to blood transfusion (Chap. 286). To determine this, an *indirect Coombs test* is performed by incubating normal ABO- and Rh-compatible red blood cells with the patient's serum and subsequently performing a direct Coombs test on these incubated red cells.

"Warm" antibodies Antibodies which react at body temperature are usually of the IgG class, although occasionally they are IgA. They induce a pattern of hemolysis which affects both the patient's own cells and normal transfused cells. This acquired syndrome is frequently designated *autoimmune hemolytic anemia.* In recent years, as a number of drugs which induce this clinical syndrome have become recognized, attention has focused on the exogenous factors which may underlie the formation of these red blood cell antibodies, and the expression *immunohemolytic anemia* is preferred.

CLINICAL MANIFESTATIONS Warm-antibody immunohemolytic anemia occurs at all ages but is more common in adults, particularly women and older individuals. In approximately one-fourth of patients this disorder occurs as a complication of an underlying disease affecting the immune system, especially chronic lymphocytic leukemia, non-Hodgkin's lymphoma, and systemic lupus erythematosus (SLE). Occasionally, immunohemolytic anemia is seen in patients with advanced, active Hodgkin's disease. Case reports link it to a variety of nonlymphoid neoplasms.

The presentation and course of immunohemolytic anemia are quite variable. In its mildest form, the only manifestation is a positive direct Coombs test. In this instance, insufficient antibody is present on the red blood cell surface to permit the reticuloendothelial system to recognize the cell as abnormal. This is particularly common in SLE. A large fraction of patients with immunohemolytic anemia have a chronic mild anemia and splenomegaly. The direct Coombs test is positive for IgG but seldom for C3, and the indirect Coombs test is negative. In other cases this disorder may be more severe, with hemoglobin levels less than 70 g/L and reticulocyte counts of 30 percent and higher. Spherocytosis is usually marked (Fig. A5-11). Coombs' test is positive for IgG and frequently for C3 as well. Large quantities of antibody are present not only on the patient's red blood cells but also in the patient's serum as demonstrated by the indirect Coombs test. Thrombocytopenia may also be present. The coexistence of immune destruction of red blood cells and platelets is referred to as *Evans' syndrome,* a disorder in which separate antibodies are directed against platelets and red blood cells. In its most severe form, immunohemolytic anemia presents with fulminant, overwhelming hemolysis associated with hemoglobinemia, hemoglobinuria, and shock, a syndrome which may be fatal.

Associated findings include hyperbilirubinemia, decreased or absent haptoglobin levels, and occasionally hepatomegaly. Fever and abdominal pain occur in some patients. Venous thrombosis occurs occasionally, the most frequent site being the deep veins of the legs, but thrombosis of mesenteric and portal veins has also been reported. Arterial thromboses occur as well.

PATHOGENESIS Little is known about the origin of red blood cell antibodies in the immunohemolytic anemias. Much more information exists concerning the mechanism of destruction of red blood cells coated with IgG antibodies. Although spherocytosis is often a prominent feature of hemolysis in vivo, the simple exposure of normal red blood cells to IgG antibodies does not lead to spherocytosis in vitro. However, human red blood cells coated with IgG antibodies are bound to the surface of monocytes or splenic macrophages and undergo a spherical transformation. The ability to cause this red blood cell–leukocyte interaction is greatest with IgG of subclasses 1 and 3 (the most common subclasses). It is not shared by IgM or IgA. However, C3 on the red blood cell surface also promotes this cell-cell interaction, but binding may be more transient because of the ability of the plasma C3 inactivator to release bound cells. Indeed, IgG and C3 behave in a synergistic fashion in this regard, accounting for the more severe hemolytic disease in patients in whom both IgG and C3 are present on the red blood cell surface. Since the slow flow compartment of the spleen is particularly efficient in trapping red blood cells which are coated with IgG antibodies, the spleen is the major site of red blood cell destruction in this disorder.

THERAPY AND PROGNOSIS In the initial evaluation of the patient, it is important to rule out drugs which are known to cause immunohemolytic anemia. This topic is discussed below.

Patients having a mild degree of hemolysis usually do not require therapy. In those with clinically significant hemolysis, initial therapy consists of glucocorticoids (e.g., prednisone, 1.0 mg/kg per day). A rise in hemoglobin is frequently noted within 3 or 4 days and occurs in most patients within 1 week. Prednisone is continued until the hemoglobin level has risen to normal values, and thereafter it is tapered slowly over the course of several months. More than 75 percent of patients will achieve a significant and sustained reduction in hemolysis; however, in half of these patients the disease will relapse either during the period of steroid tapering or following the cessation of steroid therapy. Steroids appear to have two modes of action: an immediate effect due to inhibition of the clearance of IgG-coated red blood cells by the mononuclear phagocyte system, and a later effect due to steroid-induced inhibition of antibody synthesis.

Patients with severe anemia may require blood transfusions. Because the antibody in this disease is a "panagglutinin," reacting with all normal donor cells, the usual cross matching is impossible. The goal in selecting blood for transfusion is to avoid administering red cells with antigens to which patients have previously been sensitized and which are known to be associated with complement lysis and intravascular hemolysis. In addition to A and B, Kell, Kidd (Jk^a), and Duffy (Fy) account for almost all examples of this type of hemolysis. A common procedure is to adsorb the panagglutinin present in patient's serum using the patient's own red cells from which antibody has previously been eluted. Serum freed of autoantibody in this way can then be tested for the presence of alloantibody to specific donor blood groups. ABO-compatible red cells matched in this fashion are administered slowly with attention paid to the possibility of an immediate-type transfusion reaction.

Splenectomy is the second line of therapy in this disorder. It is recommended for patients who cannot tolerate steroid therapy, in whom steroid therapy has been insufficient to control the disease process, or in whom a normal hematologic status can be maintained only with excessive doses of steroids. To provide prophylaxis against pneumococcal infection, a risk in splenectomized individuals, patients should be immunized with polyvalent pneumococcal antiserum.

Patients who have been refractory to steroid therapy and to splenectomy have been treated with immunosuppressive drugs. The greatest experience is with azathioprine and cyclophosphamide. A variable success rate has been reported with each. Recently, intravenous gamma globulin has been administered to rare patients who have failed to respond to the therapies mentioned above. There is insufficient experience to date to assess its efficacy.

In the majority of patients, this disease is controlled by steroid therapy alone, by splenectomy, or by a combination. In most of the remaining patients, a partial degree of control is achieved. Fatalities occur among three categories: first, rare patients with overwhelming hemolysis in whom death is directly attributable to anemia; second, those with major thrombotic events coincident with active hemolysis; third, those whose host defenses are impaired by glucocorticoids, splenectomy, and/or immunosuppressives. In patients in whom immunohemolysis develops as a complication of an underlying disorder, the prognosis is dominated by that of the primary disease.

Immunohemolytic anemia secondary to drugs Drugs which have been directly related to immunohemolytic anemia are of three kinds, as distinguished by their three mechanisms of actions: (1) Drugs, such as α-methyldopa (Chap. 196), which induce a disorder identical almost in every respect to the warm-antibody immunohemolytic anemia described above. (2) Drugs of the penicillin type which can become associated with the red blood cell surface and induce the formation of an antibody directed against the red blood cell–drug complex. (3) Drugs, such as quinidine, that form a complex with plasma proteins to which an antibody forms; this drug–plasma protein–antibody complex settles out on red blood cells or platelets, inducing destruction on an "innocent bystander" basis.

α-METHYLDOPA-TYPE ANTIBODIES A positive direct Coombs test is observed in up to 10 percent of patients receiving α-methyldopa therapy in a dose of 2.0 g daily. A small minority of these patients develop spherocytosis and hemolysis, often of severe degree. This "autoimmune" disorder may be triggered by a deficiency of suppressor T lymphocytes. Two distinctive features are that the indirect Coombs test is positive in almost all patients with hemolysis and that the red cells are coated with IgG but not C3. The IgG antibody is directed against the Rh complex as it is in most patients with idiopathic immunohemolytic anemia due to IgG. Hemolysis decreases over the course of several weeks after cessation of drug therapy, although the direct Coombs test may remain positive for more than 1 year.

PENICILLIN (HAPTEN)-INDUCED IMMUNOHEMOLYSIS An antibody directed against "penicillinized" red blood cells induces hemolysis in patients receiving large, intravenous doses of penicillin and penicillin-type antibiotics (e.g., 15 to 20 million units of penicillin per day, or 12 to 15 g oxacillin per day). Hemolysis usually begins 7 to 14 days after the start of penicillin therapy and is associated with spherocytosis and hyperbilirubinemia. The patient's red blood cells are Coombs-positive for IgG during the period of penicillin therapy. An indirect Coombs test can be demonstrated with the patient's serum using normal red blood cells "penicillinized" in vitro. Hemolysis ceases abruptly when penicillin therapy is stopped, although the serum antibody can be demonstrated for many weeks.

INNOCENT BYSTANDER IMMUNOHEMOLYSIS Innocent bystander antibodies may be of either the IgG or IgM class, and the antigen-antibody complexes which adhere to the red blood cell surface are capable of fixing complement. The drug-antibody complex dissociates from the red blood cell, leaving only C3 to be detected by Coombs' test. The pattern of hemolysis may be primarily extravascular red blood cell destruction, or it may be intravascular hemolysis due to complement lysis with hemoglobinemia, hemoglobinuria, and acute renal failure. This is an uncommon form of hemolysis despite the fact that the drugs associated with it are in very common usage. They include quinine and quinidine, isoniazid, sulfonamides, phenacetin, stibophen, *p*-aminosalicylic acid, dipyrone, and various insecticides.

Immune hemolysis due to cold-reactive antibodies Antibodies which are reactive in the cold induce hemolysis under two general conditions. First, in cold agglutinin disease IgM antibodies, usually reactive with the I antigen, occur spontaneously, in the course of a lymphoproliferative disease or as a complication of infectious mononucleosis or mycoplasma pneumonia. Second, in paroxysmal cold hemoglobinuria, antibodies of the IgG class (Donath-Landsteiner) occur spontaneously or as a complication of certain viral diseases or of syphilis.

COLD AGGLUTININ DISEASE *Clinical manifestations* Agglutination of red blood cells by IgM cold agglutinins is most profound at very low temperatures, and disagglutination occurs quickly upon warming. In most patients agglutination ceases at 32°C. The fixation of complement is a warm-reactive process. Therefore, patients may have very high titers of cold agglutinins as measured at low temperatures, but these antibodies may be inefficient in fixing complement to the cell surface and totally unable to induce agglutination at temperatures achieved in the bloodstream. Most cold agglutinins cause little or no shortening of red blood cell survival.

In mycoplasma pneumonia, cold agglutinins are very common, whereas only the occasional patient will have significant hemolysis about 5 to 10 days after recovery from the infection. Spherocytes may be seen occasionally, but the red blood cell morphology is usually normal. The antibody is directed against the I antigen, and the entire process is self-limited.

The cold agglutinin in infectious mononucleosis is most frequently directed against the i antigen, an antigen accessible on the surface of fetal red blood cells but not adult red blood cells. Therefore, this cold agglutinin is of serologic interest, but rarely induces hemolysis in humans. Antibody directed against the I antigen and complex antibodies involving both antigens have also been reported, with hemolysis.

A chronic form of cold-induced hemolysis occurs in patients de novo or in association with lymphoid neoplasms. It most commonly affects individuals in their seventh or eighth decades. The clinical manifestations relate to hemolysis and less commonly to agglutination of red blood cells in capillaries in those portions of the body exposed to low temperature, causing acrocyanosis. Gangrene is uncommon. Hemoglobin levels are usually above 100 g/L and rarely below 70 g/L. Reticulocytes are fewer in number than might be anticipated, presumably because of the selective destruction of young cells (including reticulocytes) in this disorder.

In most patients with cold agglutinin disease, the antibody titer is very high (e.g., 1:10,000) at 4°C and very low (e.g., 1:16) at 37°C. In some patients the antibody shows a flatter thermal spectrum with a moderately high titer at 4°C (e.g., 1:320) and a readily demonstrable titer at 37°C (e.g., 1:64). Hemolysis tends to be more severe in this latter group. The Coombs test demonstrates the presence of C3 on the red blood cell surface, but IgM (which is responsible for the C3 coating of red cells) is not found.

Pathogenesis The etiology of the antibody is unknown. It appears to exert its hemolytic effect not through agglutination per se but rather by the fixation of C3 to the red blood cell surface. The liver is particularly efficient at detecting red blood cells coated with C3 in the form of C3b and clearing them from the circulation. A plasma enzyme, C3 inactivator, is capable of cleaving C3b into a small fragment (C3c) which leaves the cell surface and reenters the plasma, and C3d, which adheres to the red blood cell surface where it is recognized as C3 in Coombs' test but not as C3 by the mononuclear phagocyte system. The presence of C3d on the red blood cell surface decreases the ability of IgM anti-I to begin anew the complement sequence and thereby reestablish C3b on the red cell surface. Because of this, red blood cells that have survived in the circulation for a period of time have become "protected," while the younger red blood cells are in greater jeopardy.

Therapy The cutaneous manifestations of this disorder are best treated by maintaining the patient in a warm environment. Because transfusion of normal blood presents to the patient a large number of red blood cells which have not previously been exposed to the cold agglutinin and are therefore not "protected," transfusion may be associated with an acceleration of the hemolytic process. Splenectomy is usually not of value in this disorder. Glucocorticoids are of limited value, although patients with the panthermal variety of cold agglutinin disease may respond favorably to this therapy. Chlorambucil and cyclophosphamide are the most commonly employed agents in those patients in whom therapy is indicated. Although some patients have experienced a dramatic improvement, the effectiveness of this therapy is usually marginal.

Cold agglutinin disease tends to be chronic and unremitting. The overall prognosis is dominated by the underlying lymphoproliferative disease, if present. In those patients in whom cold agglutinin disease appears to arise spontaneously, lymphoproliferative disease may become apparent after several years.

PAROXYSMAL COLD HEMOGLOBINURIA (PCH) Now a rare disorder, PCH was more frequent at a time when tertiary syphilis was more prevalent. It results from the formation of the Donath-Landsteiner antibody, an IgG antibody which is directed against the P antigen complex and which can induce complement-mediated lysis. Attacks are precipitated by exposure to cold and are associated with hemoglobinemia and hemoglobinuria, chills and fever, back, leg, and abdominal pain, headache, and malaise. Recovery from the acute episode is prompt, and between episodes patients are asymptomatic. When this syndrome accompanies acute viral infections (e.g., measles and mumps), it is self-limited. When secondary to syphilis, it responds favorably to specific therapy for this disorder. No specific therapy exists for idiopathic cases. Despite the severity of individual episodes, the natural history of this disease extends over many years.

TRAUMA IN THE CIRCULATION Mechanical trauma can cause hemolysis in three ways: (1) when red blood cells flow through small vessels over the surface of bony prominences and are subject to external impact during various physical activities; (2) when they flow across a pressure gradient created by an abnormal heart valve or valve prosthesis and are disrupted by a shear stress; and (3) when the deposition of fibrin in the microvasculature exposes them to a physical impediment that fragments them (Table 294-4).

External impact Hemoglobinemia and hemoglobinuria have been observed in individuals who have undergone a prolonged march or a

TABLE 294-4 Disturbances of the formed elements of blood secondary to intravascular trauma

Etiology	Fragments	Hemolysis	Thrombocytopenia
Impact: march hemoglobinuria, etc.	0	+	0
Cardiac (turbulence):			
Aortic valve prosthesis	+ + + +	+ + + +	0
Mitral valve prosthesis	+ +	+ +	0
Calcific aortic stenoses	+	±	0
Vessel disease:			
Malignant hypertension; Eclampsia; Renal graft rejection; Hemangiomas; Immune disease (scleroderma)	+ + +	+	+
Thrombotic thrombocytopenic purpura	+ + + +	+ + + +	+ + + +
Hemolytic uremic syndrome	+ + + +	+ + + +	+ + + +
Disseminated intravascular coagulation	+ +	±	+ + + +

prolonged jog, most typically on a hard surface and while wearing thin-soled shoes. The role of direct external trauma in this process has been demonstrated by the fact that hemolysis can be prevented by the insertion of a soft inner sole in the runner's shoes. Similar types of hemolysis have been described following karate and the playing of bongo drums. No abnormality of red blood cell morphology has been demonstrated, even during the acute episode, and no underlying red blood cell abnormality has been uncovered. A large percentage of individuals will develop hemoglobinemia and hemoglobinuria when exposed to the conditions described above. As a result of muscle damage during some of these activities, myoglobinuria may also occur, but renal function is preserved. No specific therapy is required.

Cardiac hemolysis Hemolysis associated with fragmented red blood cells (Fig. A5-7) occurs in approximately 10 percent of patients with artificial aortic valve prostheses. This incidence is somewhat greater with valves having stellite rather than silastic occluders, greater with small valves as compared with larger valves, and greater when valves are cloth-covered or when there is a paravalvular leak. Traumatic hemolysis is much less common in recipients of porcine valves. Severe hemolysis may occur after repair of ostium primum or endocardial cushion defects with a prosthetic patch. Mitral valve prostheses have also been associated with hemolysis, but since the pressure gradient across these is lower than across aortic prostheses, the incidence is lower. A moderately shortened red blood cell survival with little or no anemia occurs in some patients with severe calcific aortic stenosis. Indeed, almost any intracardiac lesion which alters hemodynamics may lead to some shortening of red blood cell survival. In addition, traumatic hemolysis has been observed in patients who have undergone aortofemoral bypass.

CLINICAL MANIFESTATIONS In severe cases hemoglobin levels fall to 50 to 70 g/L with reticulocytosis, fragmented red blood cells in the peripheral blood, depressed haptoglobin, elevated serum lactic dehydrogenase, and hemoglobinemia and hemoglobinuria. Iron loss (as hemoglobin or hemosiderin) in the urine may lead to iron deficiency. Direct Coombs test may rarely become positive.

PATHOGENESIS A number of factors combine to cause the fragmentation and destruction of red blood cells in this disorder. Direct mechanical trauma of red blood cells at the time of seating of the occluder of the prosthetic valve, the deposition of fibrin across disrupted attachment points, but probably most important, the shear stress resulting from turbulent blood flow may all result in the fragmentation of red blood cells. The last explains the higher incidence of hemolysis in patients who have a paravalvular leak and therefore greater velocity of blood flow across the aortic orifice during systole.

THERAPY AND PROGNOSIS Iron deficiency should be corrected by the administration of oral iron. The elevated hemoglobin which results may permit a decrease in the cardiac output and a slowing of the hemolytic rate. Limitation in physical activity also lessens the hemolytic rate. When these measures fail, any paravalvular leak must be repaired or the prosthetic valve replaced.

Deposition of fibrin in the microvasculature Fibrin deposition in the microvasculature fragments red blood cells and traps platelets under three general conditions: (1) abnormalities of the vessel wall in recognized disorders, such as malignant hypertension, eclampsia, rejection of a renal allograft, disseminated cancer, and hemangiomas; (2) two potentially fatal syndromes of unknown etiology, thrombotic thrombocytopenic purpura and the hemolytic uremic syndrome; and (3) disseminated intravascular coagulation.

ABNORMALITIES OF THE VESSEL WALL The degree of hemolysis induced by this family of disorders is usually quite mild, although the number of fragments in the peripheral blood may be striking. In occasional patients, thrombocytopenia may be severe. In each case, therapy is best directed at the primary disease. Thus, reversal of renal graft rejection, treatment of malignant hypertension and eclampsia, control of cancer, etc., lead to a cessation of the hemolytic process. The relative importance of the primary vascular abnormality and of the deposition of fibrin in causing hemolysis is unclear.

Thrombotic thrombocytopenic purpura (TTP) This disease of unknown etiology affects individuals of all ages but primarily young adults, more often women.

CLINICAL MANIFESTATIONS Hemolysis is a striking feature of this disease. Anemia occurs in association with fragmented red blood cells, nucleated red cells in the peripheral blood, an elevated reticulocyte count, and thrombocytopenia of varying degree. Platelet counts range from 5000 to 100,000 per cubic millimeter. Jaundice is common, and petechiae may be present, although usually to a less striking degree than in idiopathic thrombocytopenic purpura (ITP). Tests of coagulation, such as the prothrombin time, partial thromboplastin time, fibrinogen concentration, and the level of fibrinogen split products, are usually normal or only mildly abnormal. If the coagulation tests indicate disseminated intravascular coagulation, the diagnosis of TTP is doubtful. Erythroid hyperplasia and an increased number of megakaryocytes are present in the bone marrow. The life span of platelets is decreased to hours, and no site of organ localization of destroyed platelets is observed. A positive antinuclear antibody (ANA) is obtained in approximately 20 percent of patients. Some patients experience significant, although not severe, bleeding of uterine, gastrointestinal, or other origin. Fever is present in almost all patients, and many experience nonspecific constitutional symptoms such as nausea, abdominal pain, and arthralgias. The spleen and liver may be palpable.

The course of TTP spans days to weeks in most patients, but occasionally continues for months. As the disease progresses, the brain and kidneys become progressively involved, and their dysfunction is the ultimate cause of death in the majority of patients. Proteinuria and a moderate elevation of blood urea nitrogen may be found on initial presentation, and there is a continued rise in blood urea nitrogen and a fall in urine output as the disease progresses. Neurologic symptoms evolve in more than 90 percent of patients whose disease terminates in death. Initially, there may be changes in mental status such as confusion, delirium, or altered states of consciousness. Focal findings include seizures, hemiparesis, aphasia, and visual field defects. These neurologic symptoms may fluctuate and terminate in coma. Involvement of myocardial blood vessels may be a cause of sudden death in some patients.

PATHOGENESIS The etiology of TTP is unknown. Arterioles are filled with hyalin material, presumably fibrin and platelets, and similar material may be seen beneath the endothelium of otherwise uninvolved vessels. Immunofluorescence studies have shown the presence of immunoglobulin and complement in arterioles. Microaneurysms of arterioles are often present. Controversy exists concerning the specificity of these changes, some authorities noting them in the hemolytic uremic syndrome (particularly in the kidney) and in disseminated intravascular coagulation. An association with systemic lupus erythematosus (SLE), scleroderma, and Sjögren's syndrome suggests an immunologic etiology. A high-molecular-weight form of von Wilebrand's protein, as well as a platelet-aggregating protein, have been identified in the plasma of TTP patients and may contribute significantly to the pathogenesis of the microvascular defect.

DIAGNOSIS The combination of hemolytic anemia with fragmented and nucleated red blood cells, thrombocytopenia, fever, neurologic disorders, and renal dysfunction is virtually pathognomonic of TTP. The diagnosis is further supported by the finding of normal coagulation tests, although occasional patients have an isolated abnormality of coagulation. Although they are not usually required for diagnosis, biopsies of skin and muscle, gingiva, lymph node, or bone marrow will frequently reveal the pathologic abnormalities described above. TTP should be considered in every patient in whom the diagnosis of ITP or Evans' syndrome (ITP plus immunohemolytic anemia) is made. The finding of fragmented red blood cells in the peripheral blood is particularly helpful in this regard. Because the clinical course can fluctuate widely, therapy is difficult to evaluate.

THERAPY AND PROGNOSIS Until recently, this disease was almost universally fatal. A large number of therapeutic modalities have been attempted with variable success. These include glucocorticoids, plasma exchange, splenectomy, and antiplatelet drugs. Patients are initially treated with high doses of glucocorticoids (100 to 1000 mg prednisone per day). However, additional therapy is indicated. The most consistent improvement (60 to 75 percent) has been noted with exchange transfusion or plasmapheresis. In most patients plasmapheresis is as effective as exchange transfusion. In others the response may depend upon the infusion of plasma. Splenectomy is also effective, but with a lower frequency of response and with additional risk in these critically ill patients. The benefit of antiplatelet drugs (dipyridamole, sulfinpyrazone, dextran, aspirin) is unclear, but they are commonly used together with the therapeutic measures described above. Aspirin may increase the risk of bleeding and should be employed with caution. Vincristine may be effective in otherwise refractory patients. Because of the ever-present risk of sudden death, therapy should be instituted promptly. Even deep coma is not a contraindication to therapy since full neurologic recovery is the rule in patients responding to therapy. If treatment is instituted early in the disease, remission occurs in approximately two-thirds of patients. Relapses have been noted in approximately 10 percent of patients but are usually responsive to therapeutic intervention.

Hemolytic uremic syndrome The hemolytic uremic syndrome is a disorder usually encountered in young children and has laboratory features similar to those of TTP. Often the patient has a prodrome of a viral-like illness. Less commonly, the disorder appears to be familial. Patients present with acute hemolytic anemia, thrombocytopenic purpura, and acute oliguric renal failure. Most patients have either hemoglobinuria or anuria. Unlike TTP, neurologic manifestations are uncommon. The peripheral blood findings and coagulation tests are usually indistinguishable from those of TTP. Pathologic changes are similar but restricted to the kidney. Patients are treated with dialysis and transfusions. The efficacy of glucocorticoids, dextran, and heparin is uncertain. The mortality in children ranges from 5 to 20 percent, but is considerably higher in adults. A disorder resembling the hemolytic-uremic syndrome has recently been described in adults treated with the antineoplastic drug mitomycin C, usually in combination with other drugs.

Disseminated intravascular coagulation (DIC) Red blood cell fragmentation in the microvasculature (microangiopathic hemolytic anemia) is seen in about one-fourth of patients with DIC (Chap. 289). The degree of hemolysis is much less in DIC than in either TTP or the hemolytic uremic syndrome, and anemia with reticulocytosis and nucleated red blood cells is distinctly rare.

DIRECT TOXIC EFFECTS A variety of infections may be associated with severe hemolysis. The microorganisms in bartonellosis (Chap. 123) and malaria (Chap. 159) directly parasitize red blood cells. Babesiosis (Chap. 164) also may cause a mild to moderate hemolytic anemia by direct parasitization of red blood cells.

Other infectious organisms exert their damaging effects on red blood cells indirectly. The most striking is that resulting from septicemia with *Clostridium welchii* (Chap. 107). The phospholipase produced by this organism is capable of cleaving the phosphoryl bond of lecithin thereby lysing human red blood cells. A mild, transient hemolysis frequently accompanies bacteremia with diverse organisms such as pneumococci, staphylococci, and *Escherichia coli*.

Hemolysis may result from the direct action of snake and spider venoms on the red blood cell. Although cobra venom is directly lytic in vitro, the clinical disease induced by the bite of the cobra is one of moderate hemolysis associated with spherocytosis. Spider bites are known to induce acute intravascular hemolysis associated with spherocytosis. It is thought that the brown recluse spider which inhabits the central and southern portions of the United States and portions of South America is responsible. The hemolytic disease continues for several days up to 1 week.

Copper has a direct hemolytic effect on red blood cells. Hemolysis has been observed following exposure of individuals to copper salts (such as during hemodialysis). In addition, the transient episodes of hemolysis observed in patients with Wilson's disease are probably due to copper toxicity.

The red blood cell membrane is unstable at temperatures above 49°C due to denaturation of the cytoskeletal protein, spectrin. When studied in vitro, the red blood cell undergoes a process of budding, cleavage, and resealing above this temperature. The same process is observed in individuals who have suffered extensive burns. These patients have prominent spherocytosis as well as hemoglobinemia and sometimes hemoglobinuria.

MEMBRANE ABNORMALITIES

ACQUIRED DISORDERS OF THE MEMBRANE There are two well-defined acquired disorders of the red blood cell membrane: spur cell anemia and paroxysmal nocturnal hemoglobinuria (PNH).

Spur cell anemia Hemolytic anemia with bizarre-shaped red blood cells occurs in some patients with severe hepatocellular disease. Most patients with spur cell anemia have advanced Laennec's cirrhosis. This hemolytic disorder is observed in approximately 5 percent of patients with manifestations of severe cirrhosis, such as ascites, jaundice, and hepatic encephalopathy. Spur cell anemia has also been reported in neonatal hepatitis.

CLINICAL MANIFESTATIONS Anemia is moderate to severe, with hematocrit levels ranging from 0.16 to 0.30. Thus, the anemia is more severe than is observed in otherwise uncomplicated cirrhosis, in which hematocrit levels are rarely below 0.28, unless there is accompanying folic acid deficiency, blood loss, iron deficiency, etc. (Chap. 293). Splenomegaly is a constant feature, and the spleen is generally more prominent than in patients who have cirrhosis but who do not have spur cell anemia. Jaundice is also a constant feature, and hepatic encephalopathy is common. Other tests of liver function are similar to values obtained in most patients with severe cirrhosis, although there is a tendency to longer prothrombin times. Chromium half-survival times of red blood cells are decreased to as short as 6 days (normal being 26 to 32 days), and red cell destruction is localized to the spleen. Normal transfused red blood cells have a survival similar to that of the patient's own red blood cells. Red blood cells are irregularly shaped with multiple spicules, and a small number of bizarre-shaped fragments are commonly seen on peripheral blood smears (see Fig. A5-8). Reticulocytes range from 5 to 15 percent.

PATHOGENESIS The surface membrane of spur cells contains 50 to 70 percent excess cholesterol, but its total phospholipid content is normal. In this way, spur cells are distinct from the more usual target red blood cells in liver disease, which possess an excess of both cholesterol and phospholipid. Cholesterol out of proportion to phospholipid decreases the fluidity of the spur cell membrane, and cell deformability is also decreased. Normal red blood cells acquire the spur abnormality when incubated in serum from affected patients. This results from the presence in serum of an abnormal low-density lipoprotein with an increased mole ratio of free (unesterified) cholesterol to phospholipid. Thus, red blood cells in spur cell anemia may be considered to be "innocent bystanders." These rigid, cholesterol-laden red blood cells are detected by the filtering system of the spleen, aided by congestive splenomegaly in cirrhosis. In contrast to circulating spur cells, normal red blood cells which have acquired cholesterol in vitro have an increased surface area and a decreased osmotic fragility, and they have a regular pattern of spicule deformity. This is also true in vivo for normal red blood cells during their initial 24 h in the patient's circulation. However, during continued circulation in vivo in the presence of the spleen, cholesterol-rich spur cells lose surface area and transform to the irregular pattern of spiculation associated with acanthocytes (see "Red Blood Cell Morphology" above). This process of membrane "conditioning" by the spleen continues, and the cell is destroyed in the spleen.

DIAGNOSIS Increasing anemia in a patient with chronic cirrhosis most commonly results from blood loss, folic acid deficiency, or iron deficiency. The hemolytic rate may increase transiently during periods of acute fatty liver. The combination of an elevated reticulocyte count and elevated bilirubin in the presence of the characteristic morphologic abnormality on peripheral blood smear is diagnostic. Red blood cells of similar morphologic appearance are seen in patients with abetalipoproteinemia. However, these individuals have a minimal amount of hemolysis.

Spur cells and acanthocytes must be distinguished from regularly scalloped, crenated red blood cells (echinocytes). These are a frequent artifact on blood smears, and they are present in some patients with uremia ("burr cells") (Fig. A5-9). Small, dense crenated spheres (spheroechinocytes) are sometimes seen in congenital nonspherocytic hemolytic anemia due to enzyme deficiencies in the Embden-Meyerhof pathway (see below).

TREATMENT Since normal red blood cells acquire the spur abnormality when transfused into patients with this form of anemia, transfusion therapy is of limited benefit. Attempts to influence red blood cell cholesterol by the use of various lipid-lowering agents have been unsuccessful. Splenectomy has been reported to prevent both the conditioning of red blood cells in the spleen and their premature destruction. However, splenectomy carries a high risk in patients with severe liver disease complicated by portal hypertension and coagulation defects, and it must be reserved for selected patients in whom hemolysis is a major clinical problem and who appear to be relatively good surgical risks.

PROGNOSIS In most patients spur cell anemia occurs during the late stages of cirrhosis, and more than 90 percent of patients succumb to their underlying liver disease within 1 year of the diagnosis of spur cell anemia.

Paroxysmal nocturnal hemoglobinuria (PNH) This condition is distinctive among hemolytic disorders in humans because it is an intracorpuscular defect acquired at the stem cell level. It occurs primarily in young adults.

CLINICAL MANIFESTATIONS Anemia is of exceedingly variable degree with hematocrit values of 0.20 and lower in occasional patients and normal values in others. Mild granulocytopenia and thrombocytopenia are commonly present. Although regarded as a classic feature of this disease, gross hemoglobinuria is present only intermittently in most patients, and never occurs in some. Hemosiderinuria is usually present. Other features of diagnostic significance are a low leukocyte alkaline phosphatase and a low red blood cell acetylcholinesterase. Red blood cells are normochromic and normocytic unless iron deficiency has occurred from the chronic loss of iron in the urine. The diagnosis is established by a positive acid hemolysis test or sucrose lysis test, both of which demonstrate the enhanced sensitivity of PNH red blood cells to complement (see below). Venous thrombosis is a common complication of this disorder, and has been reported in peripheral veins as well as in mesenteric, hepatic, portal, and cerebral veins. Thrombosis is a common cause of death in patients severely affected with PNH. A second manifestation, possibly related to thromboses in small veins, is the occurrence of back and abdominal pain similar in character to that which occurs in sickle cell anemia. Headache has also been reported. Since the widespread use of the sucrose lysis test, many patients have been discovered with mild, chronic disease.

PATHOGENESIS The underlying abnormality which affects red blood cells, granulocytes, and platelets in PNH is an inordinate sensitivity to complement. This may be demonstrated in vitro using a complement-fixing antibody. PNH red blood cells fix more C1 than normal red cells per unit of antibody present, and this C1 promotes more C3 fixation per molecule of C1 than is seen with normal red cells. However, antibody is not necessary for the lysis of red blood cells in PNH. Rather, C3 is readily fixed to the red blood cell surface by means of the alternate (properdin) pathway. Careful analytic procedures have demonstrated two and in some cases three separate populations of red blood cells [type 1 (normal), type 2, type 3] with varying sensitivities to complement in patients with PNH. The clinical manifestations relate directly to the proportion of the red blood cells produced that are most sensitive to complement. Although platelets share with red blood cells this sensitivity to complement, platelet survival is normal in PNH. However, a functional modification of platelets induced by complement may underlie the thrombotic complications of this disease. The increased sensitivity of red blood cells to complement has been demonstrated to result from the lack of a red cell membrane regulatory protein, decay-accelerating factor (DAF), which inhibits activation of C3 at the membrane and, in type 3 PNH cells, a deficiency of C8 binding protein which inhibits activation of C8 and C9. It is surely of pathophysiologic relevance that these two proteins, along with leukocyte alkaline phosphatase and erythrocyte acetylcholinesterase, share a common glycan-phosphatidyl membrane anchor.

Since it affects granulocytes, platelets, and red blood cells but not lymphocytes, this defect is thought to occur because of an acquired change in the pluripotent stem cell which generates these cells. In this respect it is similar to both acute myelogenous leukemia and the myeloproliferative syndromes, disorders which appear to affect the stem cells responsible for platelet, granulocyte, and red blood cell production. A number of patients with PNH have subsequently developed acute myelogenous leukemia. The red blood cell abnormality characteristic of PNH (complement sensitivity) occurs to a mild degree in some patients with aplastic anemia and in some with myelofibrosis, further linking this series of bone marrow disorders. It appears likely that PNH results from a somatic mutation in the marrow stem cell pool.

DIAGNOSIS As indicated above, PNH is commonly undiagnosed for a period of months to years. The classic manifestation of gross hemoglobinuria may be present only intermittently, and an awareness of its presence may be obtained only by repeated questioning of the patient. In some patients, a chronic hemolytic process occurs without gross hemoglobinuria. Therefore, diagnoses such as refractory anemia, hemolytic anemia of unknown etiology, and pancytopenia are common in patients subsequently proven to have PNH. A decreased leukocyte alkaline phosphatase is a clue to the diagnosis, and the presence of hemosiderin in the urine sediment is strongly suggestive. Hemosiderinuria may occur with intravascular hemolysis of any etiology. However, only a few disorders in humans result in intravascular hemolysis. These are PNH, paroxysmal cold hemoglobinuria, hemolytic transfusion reaction, traumatic hemolysis, and hemolysis due to lysins (snake venom, *C. welchii* bacteremia) or to extensive acute burns. The acid hemolysis test is also positive in the rare congenital disorder hereditary erythrocytic multinuclearity with positive acidified-serum test (HEMPAS). In this latter disorder, complement sensitivity results from an inordinate fixation of C4 molecules per molecule of C1. Since this sensitivity exists in the classic (antibody-mediated) pathway but not in the alternate (properdin) pathway, spontaneous fixation of complement with lysis in vivo is not a feature of the HEMPAS disorder.

It should be noted that in PNH chromium survival studies often produce confusing information. This results from the bi- or trimodal population of red blood cells. The cells most sensitive to complement have a very short survival, and they account for a minority of circulating red blood cells, whereas the cells less sensitive to complement have a more normal survival and account for the majority of circulating cells. Thus, the chromium survival is longer than might be anticipated from other measures of hemoglobin turnover.

TREATMENT Transfusion therapy is useful in PNH not only for raising the hemoglobin level but also for suppressing the marrow production of red blood cells during episodes of sustained hemoglobinuria or of sustained painful crisis. The transfusion of blood prior to surgery may reduce the incidence of postoperative thrombotic complications. For reasons that are still unclear, whole blood transfusions frequently cause an exacerbation of the hemolytic process. This can be prevented by using washed red blood cells rather than whole blood.

Therapy with androgens frequently results in a rise of hemoglobin level. Adrenocortical steroids may also be effective in reducing the rate of hemolysis.

Because of iron loss in the urine, iron deficiency is common. An exacerbation of hemolysis often follows the administration of iron

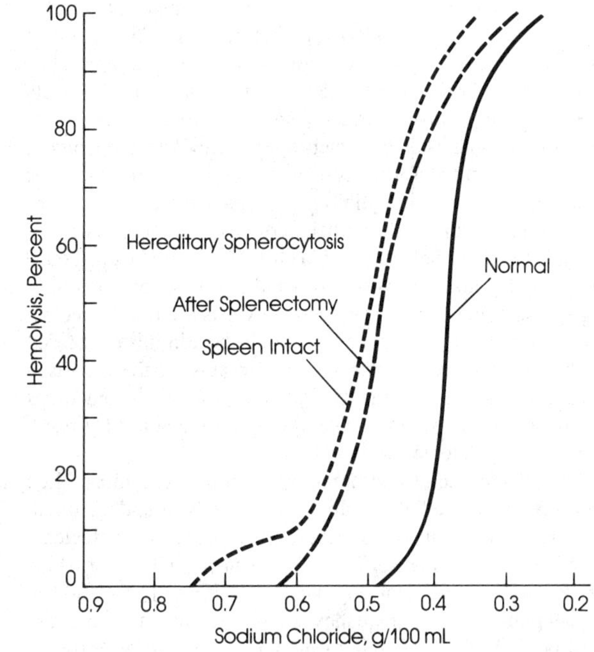

FIGURE 294-1 Osmotic fragility of red blood cells in hereditary spherocytosis. When the spleen is present, a small subpopulation of cells which are "conditioned" in the spleen form the fragile "tail" of the osmotic fragility curve. After splenectomy a single population exists which is more osmotically fragile than normal.

because of the formation of a large number of young red blood cells, many of which are sensitive to complement. This may be minimized by suppressing the bone marrow with transfusions.

Splenectomy has been undertaken in some patients with the hope of decreasing the hemolytic rate and the transfusion requirement. However, because of the limited therapeutic benefit and the increased surgical risk in patients with PNH, splenectomy cannot be recommended.

Anticoagulation with coumarin-type drugs may have some benefit in preventing thromboses, particularly in the postsurgical patient. On the other hand, therapy with heparin has been noted to cause an increased amount of hemolysis in some patients with PNH, and caution must be exercised when using this drug.

PROGNOSIS Most patients with classic PNH have a life expectancy of less than 10 years, although some survive for much longer. A series of 17 patients surviving more than 20 years has been compiled by questioning hematologists nationally. In more than one-third of these patients, there had been an amelioration of disease symptoms, and in two patients PNH was totally quiescent. The major morbidity relates to venous thromboses. Despite the marked degree of iron deposition in the kidney, death from renal failure is rare. The prognosis is uncertain in patients in whom the manifestations of PNH are more subtle and in whom the diagnosis was made because of the widespread use of the sucrose lysis test. Some patients may lead a normal life.

CONGENITAL ABNORMALITIES OF THE RED CELL MEMBRANE There are four types of inherited abnormalities of the red cell membrane: hereditary spherocytosis, hereditary elliptocytosis, hereditary pyropoikilocytosis, and hereditary stomatocytosis. Each syndrome may represent a group of disorders with differing structural defects. The molecular pathogenesis of these disorders has not been completely defined.

Hereditary spherocytosis This is a disease of autosomal dominant inheritance in which intrinsically abnormal red blood cells are destroyed in the presence of an otherwise normal spleen. Its incidence is approximately 1:4500. In 20 percent of patients the absence of hematologic abnormalities in family members suggests that a spontaneous mutation has occurred. The disorder is sometimes clinically apparent in early infancy, but often escapes detection until adult life.

CLINICAL MANIFESTATIONS The major clinical features of hereditary spherocytosis are anemia, splenomegaly, and jaundice. The prominence of the latter finding accounts for its prior designation "congenital hemolytic jaundice" and is due to an increased concentration of unconjugated (indirect-reacting) bilirubin in plasma. Jaundice may be intermittent and tends to be less pronounced in early childhood. Because of the increased bile pigment production, gallstones of pigment type are common, even in childhood. Compensatory normoblastic hyperplasia of the bone marrow occurs with the extension of red marrow into the midshafts of long bones and occasionally with extramedullary erythropoiesis, at times leading to the formation of paravertebral masses visible on chest x-ray. Because the bone marrow's capacity to increase erythropoiesis by six- to tenfold exceeds the usual rate of hemolysis in this disease, anemia is usually mild or moderate and may even be absent in an otherwise healthy individual. Compensation may be temporarily interrupted by episodes of erythroid hypoplasia precipitated by infections, often of a minor nature. Splenomegaly is a constant feature of hereditary spherocytosis. The hemolytic rate may increase transiently during systemic infections which induce further splenic enlargement. Chronic leg ulcers, similar to those observed in sickle cell anemia, occasionally occur.

The characteristic erythrocyte abnormality is the spherocyte (Fig. A5-10). The mean corpuscular volume (MCV) is usually normal or slightly decreased, and the mean corpuscular hemoglobin concentration (MCHC) is increased to 350 to 380 g/L. Spheroidicity may be quantitatively assessed in terms of osmotic fragility (Fig. 294-1). Because spherocytes have a decreased surface area per unit volume, they lyse more readily when exposed to solutions of low salt concentration. On microscopic examination spherocytes are usually detected even when present in very small numbers. However, they will ordinarily not influence the osmotic fragility test unless they constitute more than 1 or 2 percent of the total cell population. A prominent increase in the osmotic fragility of red blood cells following sterile incubation of whole blood for 24 h at 37°C is also characteristic of hereditary spherocytosis. The autohemolysis test is an extension of this latter procedure and measures the amount of spontaneous hemolysis occurring after 48 h of sterile incubation. In hereditary spherocytosis about 10 to 50 percent of the red blood cells are lysed (versus less than 4 percent of normal red blood cells). Autohemolysis of these red blood cells is largely prevented by the addition of glucose prior to incubation.

PATHOGENESIS The molecular abnormality in hereditary spherocytosis involves the proteins of the cytoskeleton. Nearly all patients have a significant deficiency of spectrin which correlates with the severity of the anemia. Some (perhaps most) patients have a decrease and/or a structural abnormality of ankyrin, the protein that links spectrin to protein 3 (see Fig. 290-6). The spheroidal contour and rigid structure of the red blood cells impede their passage through the spleen. There, the red blood cells are exposed to an environment in which their increased metabolic rate cannot be sustained. The first injury imposed upon them by the spleen is a further loss of surface membrane. This "conditioning" produces a subpopulation of hyperspheroidal red blood cells in the peripheral blood. These are subsequently destroyed in the spleen. The intracorpuscular nature of the red blood cell defect in hereditary spherocytosis is demonstrated by a diminished life span of the patient's red cells in normal subjects when the spleen is present and a normal survival of normal cells transfused into patients with hereditary spherocytosis.

DIAGNOSIS Hereditary spherocytosis must be distinguished from the spherocytic hemolytic anemias associated with red blood cell antibodies. The family history is helpful, when present. The diagnosis of immune spherocytosis is usually readily established by a positive direct Coombs test. Spherocytes, often in considerable numbers, are seen in association with hemolysis induced by splenomegaly in patients with cirrhosis or chronic infections, and a few spherocytes are seen in the course of a wide variety of hemolytic disorders, particularly glucose-6-phosphate dehydrogenase (G6PD) deficiency.

TREATMENT AND PROGNOSIS Splenectomy reliably corrects the anemia, although the red blood cell defect persists. The operative risk is low. Red blood cell survival after splenectomy is normal or nearly so. Rare relapses have been reported and are probably attributable to postoperative growth of splenic autotransplants or to hyperplasia of secondary spleens which were overlooked at operation. Because of the potential for gallstones and for episodes of bone marrow hypoplasia or hemolytic crises, splenectomy should be performed in most individuals with hereditary spherocytosis, even those with mild anemia. Splenectomy in children should be postponed until the age of 4 years, if possible. Beyond age 3, severe infections following splenectomy in hereditary spherocytosis are rare. Nonetheless, polyvalent pneumococcal vaccine should be administered to all patients who are to undergo splenectomy. Because of the increased requirement for folic acid in patients with hemolysis, they sometimes become deficient in this vitamin. Therapy with folic acid may result in an increased hemoglobin level.

Hereditary elliptocytosis and hereditary pyropoikilocytosis Red blood cells of oval or elliptic shape are normally found in birds, reptiles, camels, and llamas; however, they occur in appreciable numbers in humans only in *hereditary elliptocytosis,* a disorder which is transmitted as an autosomal dominant and affects 1 per 4000 to 5000 of the population, a frequency similar to that of hereditary spherocytosis. It is also referred to as *hereditary ovalocytosis.* In most affected individuals, a structural abnormality of erythrocyte spectrin leads to impaired assembly. Others often have a deficiency of erythrocyte membrane protein 4.1, which is important in stabilizing the interaction of spectrin and actin in the cytoskeleton (see Fig. 290-6). Homozygotes with total absence of this protein have more marked hemolysis.

The great majority of patients manifest only mild hemolysis, with hemoglobin levels above 120 g/L, reticulocytes less than 4 percent, depressed haptoglobin levels, and red blood cell survivals within or just under the normal range. In 10 to 15 percent of patients the rate of hemolysis is substantially increased with chromium half-survival times of red blood cells as short as 5 days and reticulocytes ranging to 20 percent. Hemoglobin levels rarely fall below 90 to 100 g/L. Red blood cell destruction occurs predominantly in the spleen, which is enlarged in patients with overt hemolysis, and hemolysis is corrected by splenectomy.

In both the anemic and nonanemic varieties of this disorder the red blood cells are normochromic and normocytic. At least 25 percent and, more commonly, greater than 75 percent of red blood cells are elliptic, with an axial ratio (width/length) of less than 0.78. Patients with hemolysis frequently have microovalocytes, bizarre-shaped red blood cells, and red cell fragments, all of which increase in number following splenectomy. The degree of hemolysis does not correlate with the percentage of elliptocytes. Osmotic fragility is usually normal but may be increased in patients with overt hemolysis.

Hereditary pyropoikilocytosis (HPP) is thought to be related to hereditary elliptocytosis, since both have been reported in the same family. HPP is a rare disorder characterized by bizarre-shaped, microcytic red cells which undergo disruption at temperatures of 44 to 45°C (in contrast to the normal thermal instability at 49°C). This results from an abnormality of spectrin structure. Hemolysis, which is usually severe, is recognized in childhood and is partially responsive to splenectomy.

Hereditary stomatocytosis Stomatocytes are red blood cells having a slit-like central zone of pallor on dried smears. The syndrome of hereditary hemolytic anemia and stomatocytic red blood cells is inherited in an autosomal dominant pattern. It may represent a number of discrete entities. Two major red blood cell defects have been delineated in this syndrome. First, the red blood cells have an increased permeability to sodium and potassium, which is compensated for by an increased active transport of these cations. Second, red cells have an increased surface area associated with an increase in membrane lipid content, particularly phosphatidylcholine. In some patients, the red blood cell is swollen with an excess of ions and water and a decreased mean corpuscular hemoglobin concentration (overhydrated stomatocytes, ''hydrocytosis''); in other patients the red cell is shrunken with a decreased ion and water content and an increased mean corpuscular hemoglobin concentration (dehydrated stomatocytes, ''desiccytosis''). Those patients in whom the red blood cells are overhydrated have true stomatocytes on dried smears. Dehydrated stomatocytes assume the morphology of target cells on dried smears. In both instances, red blood cells are cup- or bowl-shaped when examined in wet preparation. Osmotic fragility is increased in overhydrated stomatocytes and decreased in underhydrated stomatocytes. Autohemolysis is increased and is corrected by glucose.

Most patients have splenomegaly and mild anemia. Splenectomy decreases but does not totally correct the hemolytic process. Its indications are similar to those for hereditary spherocytosis.

DISORDERS OF THE INTERIOR OF THE RED CELL

RED CELL ENZYME DEFECTS During its maturation, the red blood cell loses its nucleus, ribosomes, and mitochondria and thus its capability for protein synthesis and oxidative phosphorylation. The mature circulating red blood cell has a relatively simple pattern of intermediary metabolism (Fig. 294-2) in keeping with its modest metabolic obligations. As discussed in Chap. 290, some ATP must be generated from the Embden-Meyerhof pathway to drive the cation pump which maintains the ionic milieu within the red blood cell. Smaller amounts of energy are needed for the preservation of hemoglobin iron in the ferrous (Fe^{2+}) state, and perhaps for the renewal of the lipids in the red blood cell membrane. About 10 percent of the glucose consumed by the red blood cell is metabolized via the hexose-monophosphate shunt (Fig. 294-2). This pathway protects both hemoglobin and the membrane from exogenous oxidants including certain drugs.

Studies of red blood cell enzyme defects have provided valuable information on the metabolic control of normal erythrocytes. Figure 294-2 shows a large number of recognized specific enzyme deficiency states affecting the glycolytic pathway or the hexose-monophosphate shunt. Many of these enzyme abnormalities appear to be restricted to red blood cells. The long life span of the red blood cell and its inability to synthesize proteins pose a challenge to the stability of its enzymes. Therefore, a mutation resulting in decreased stability will be expressed more readily in the red blood cell compared with other tissues.

Defects in the Embden-Meyerhof pathway Deficiencies of most of the enzymes of the Embden-Meyerhof (or glycolytic) pathway have been reported. In general, all these enzymopathies have similar pathophysiologic and clinical features. Patients present with a congenital nonspherocytic hemolytic anemia of variable severity. The red blood cells are often relatively deficient in ATP, considering their young age. As a result, there is an increased leak of potassium ion from inside these cells. Abnormalities in red blood cell morphology (see below) indicate that the red cell membrane is secondarily affected by the enzyme defect. These red blood cells are apt to be rigid and thus more readily sequestered by the mononuclear-phagocyte system.

Some of these glycolytic enzyme deficiencies such as pyruvate kinase (PK) deficiency and hexokinase deficiency are localized to the red blood cell, with no apparent metabolic abnormality in leukocytes or other cells that have been studied. In other disorders, the enzyme deficiency is more widespread. Glucose phosphate isomerase deficiency and phosphoglycerate kinase deficiency also involve leukocytes, although affected individuals have no apparent abnormalities of white blood cell function. Individuals with deficiency of triose phosphate isomerase have decreased levels of enzyme in leukocytes, muscle cells, and central nervous system fluid. Furthermore, they have a progressive neurologic disorder. Some patients with phosphofructokinase deficiency have a myopathy.

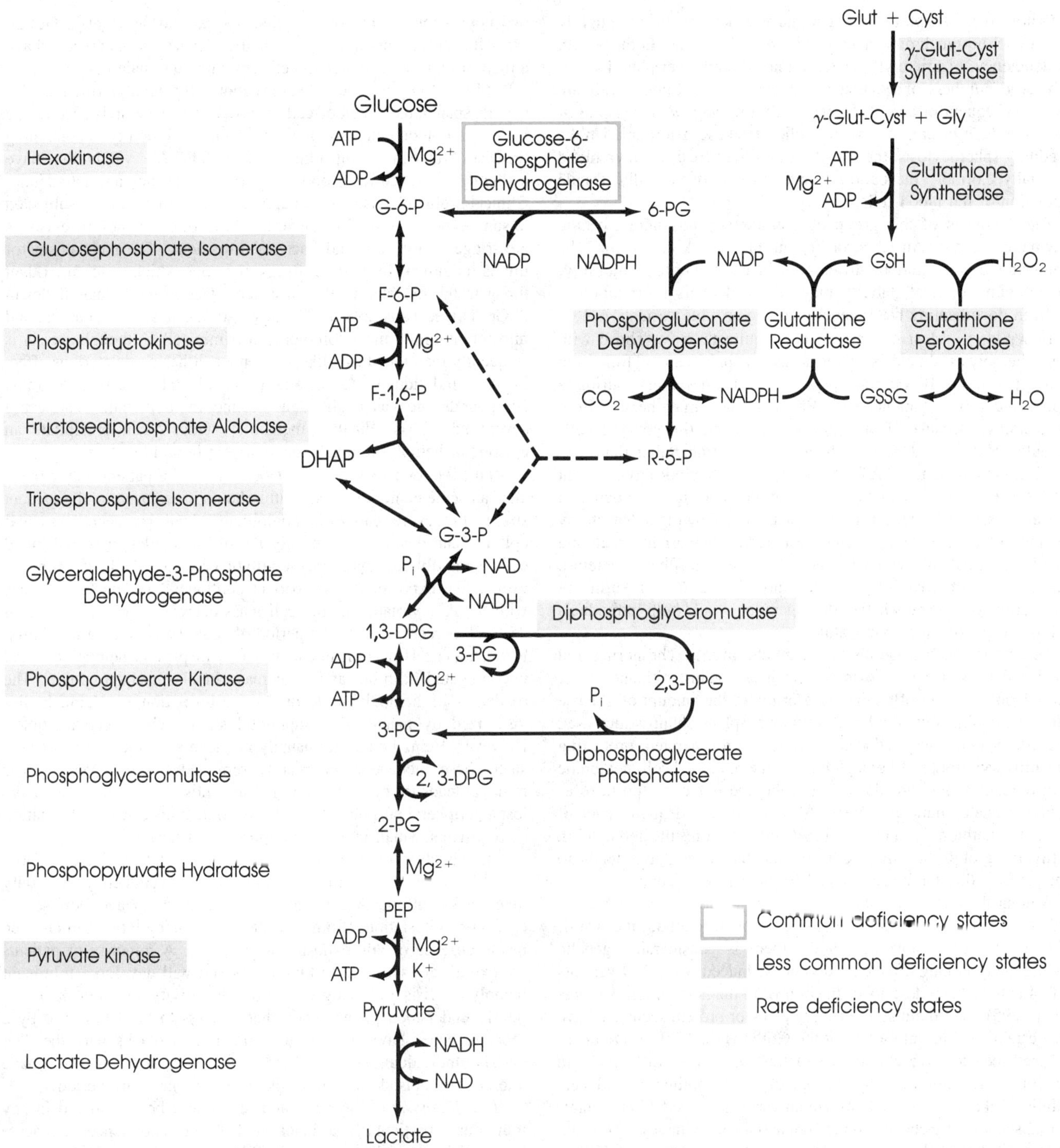

FIGURE 294-2 Metabolic pathways in the red blood cell. The glycolytic pathway is outlined vertically from glucose to lactate. The pentose phosphate pathway is shown on the right. Known enzyme deficiency states are shown. Bold solid lines denote common states, light solid lines less common ones, and dotted lines rare ones. *(From WN Valentine, Semin Hematol 8:309, 1971.)*

Among the reported defects of glycolytic enzymes, about 95 percent are due to PK deficiency and about 4 percent are due to glucose phosphate isomerase deficiency. The remainder shown in Fig. 294-2 are extremely rare. Most have been encountered in isolated families. There is considerable variability in the clinical manifestations and laboratory findings among reported cases of PK deficiency. This is probably due to the fact that a number of different PK variants have been reported. This heterogeneity probably also applies to the other less common glycolytic enzyme defects. Accordingly, the clinical manifestations of these disorders are quite variable.

GENETICS Most of the glycolytic enzyme defects are inherited in an autosomal recessive pattern. Thus, the parents of affected patients are heterozygotes. Heterozygotes generally possess half-normal levels of enzyme activity which are more than adequate for normal metabolic function. Thus, these individuals are entirely asymptomatic. Since the gene frequency for this group of enzymopathies is low, it is not surprising that true homozygotes are often the offspring of a consanguineous mating. Alternatively, affected individuals may be double heterozygotes, inheriting an abnormal allele from each parent. Phosphoglycerate kinase deficiency is inherited as a sex-linked disorder. Affected males have a severe hemolytic anemia while female carriers may have a mild hemolytic process.

CLINICAL MANIFESTATIONS Patients with severe hemolysis usually present during early childhood with anemia, icterus, and splenomegaly. Other stigmata of chronic hemolysis are occasionally seen. Occasionally, siblings are similarly affected.

LABORATORY FINDINGS Patients have a normocytic (or slightly macrocytic) normochromic anemia with reticulocytosis. In those with PK deficiency, bizarre erythrocytes are noted on the peripheral smear with large numbers of spiculated red blood cells. Spherocytes are usually infrequent or absent. Hence, the term *congenital nonspherocytic hemolytic anemia* has been applied to these disorders. Unlike hereditary spherocytosis, the osmotic fragility of freshly drawn blood is usually normal. Incubation brings out an osmotically fragile population of red blood cells.

The diagnosis of this group of anemias depends upon specific enzymatic assays. An abnormality in enzyme kinetics may be demonstrated. In addition, differences in electrophoretic mobility, pH optimum, or heat stability may be noted. This information is useful in documenting heterogeneity among enzyme variants.

TREATMENT Most patients do not require therapy. Those with severe hemolysis should be given a daily supplement of folic acid (1 mg per day). Blood transfusions may be necessary during a hypoplastic crisis. Patients with PK deficiency may benefit from splenectomy. Because of their enzymatic defect, the younger cells (reticulocytes) depend on mitochondrial respiration rather than glycolysis for maintenance of ATP. However, in the hypoxic environment of the spleen, aerobic metabolism is curtailed and the ATP-depleted cells are destroyed in situ. It is of interest that following splenectomy patients with PK deficiency often have a marked increase in circulating reticulocytes. Patients with deficiency of glucose phosphate isomerase may also be improved by splenectomy. There is not sufficient information to indicate whether this operation would help individuals with other glycolytic enzymopathies.

Defects in the hexose-monophosphate shunt The normal red blood cell is well endowed to protect itself against oxidant stress. Upon exposure to an offending drug or toxin, the amount of glucose that is metabolized via the hexose-monophosphate shunt is increased severalfold. In this way reduced glutathione is regenerated, protecting the sulfhydryl groups of hemoglobin and the red blood cell membrane from oxidation. Individuals with an inherited defect in the hexose-monophosphate shunt are unable to maintain an adequate level of reduced glutathione in their red blood cells. As a result, hemoglobin sulfhydryl groups become oxidized, and the hemoglobin tends to precipitate within the red blood cell forming Heinz bodies.

Among the congenital shunt defects, by far the most common is *G6PD deficiency*. It affects millions of people throughout the world. Like the glycolytic enzymopathies, there is considerable genetic heterogeneity among affected individuals. Indeed, over 250 variants of G6PD have been described. In contrast to the hemoglobin variants (Chap. 295) abnormalities in primary DNA or protein sequence have been established in only a few of the G6PD variants. The remainder are presumed to have abnormal structure because of differences in electrophoretic mobility, enzyme kinetics, pH optimum, and heat stability. Like many of the hemoglobin variants, some G6PD mutants were discovered by chance and are not associated with any significant functional abnormalities. The normal or "wild" form of G6PD is designated by type B. About 20 percent of blacks have a G6PD (designated A+) which differs electrophoretically but is functionally normal. Among the clinically significant G6PD variants, the most common is the so-called A− type encountered primarily in blacks who originated from central Africa. The A− G6PD has the same electrophoretic mobility as the A+ type, but it is unstable and has abnormal kinetic properties. Like the HbS gene, the A− type of G6PD may confer protection against malaria. This variant is found in about 15 percent of black males in the United States. A second relatively common G6PD variant is encountered among peoples of the eastern Mediterranean area, particularly Sephardic Jews. A third relatively common variant occurs in the Chinese.

The G6PD gene is located on the X chromosome. Thus the deficiency state is a sex-linked trait. Affected males (hemizygotes) inherit the abnormal gene from their mothers who are usually carriers (heterozygotes). Because of inactivation of one of the two X chromosomes (Lyon hypothesis, see Chap. 5), the heterozygote has two populations of red blood cells: normal and deficient in G6PD. Most female carriers are asymptomatic. Those who happen to have a high proportion of deficient cells resemble the male hemizygotes.

G6PD activity normally declines about 50 percent during the 120-day life span of the red blood cell. This decay is moderately accelerated in A− red blood cells and markedly so in red blood cells containing the Mediterranean variant. Individuals with the A− variant may have a slightly shortened red blood cell survival, but they are not anemic. Clinical problems arise only when the affected individual is subjected to some type of environmental stress. Most often, hemolytic episodes are triggered by viral and bacterial infections. The mechanism for this is unknown. In addition drugs or toxins which pose an oxidant threat to the red blood cell cause hemolysis in individuals deficient in G6PD (see Table 294-5). Of these, sulfa drugs, antimalarials, and nitrofurantoin are most commonly incriminated. Although aspirin is frequently mentioned as a likely offender, it has no deleterious effect in A− individuals. Occasionally, accidental ingestion of toxic compounds such as naphthalene (found in moth balls) can cause severe hemolysis. Finally, metabolic acidosis can precipitate an episode of hemolysis in subjects deficient in G6PD.

CLINICAL AND LABORATORY FEATURES The patient may experience an acute hemolytic crisis within hours of exposure to the oxidant stress. In severe cases, hemoglobinuria and peripheral vascular collapse can develop. Since only the older population of red blood cells is rapidly destroyed, the hemolytic crisis is usually self-limited, even if the exposure to the oxidant continues. Among black males with the A− variant, the red cell mass decreases by a maximum of 25 to 30 percent. During the period of acute hemolysis, a rapid drop in hematocrit is accompanied by a rise in plasma hemoglobin and unconjugated bilirubin and a decrease in plasma haptoglobin. The oxidation of hemoglobin leads to the formation of Heinz bodies visualized by means of a supravital stain such as crystal violet. However, Heinz bodies are usually not seen after the first day or so, since these inclusions are readily removed by the spleen. Their removal leads to the formation of "bite cells," red cells which have lost a peripheral portion of the cell. Multiple bites cause the formation of fragments. Small numbers of spherocytes may also be present.

Individuals with the *Mediterranean type G6PD* have a more unstable enzyme and, therefore, a much lower overall enzyme activity than blacks with the A− variant. As a result, they have more severe clinical manifestations. Some have a chronic hemolytic anemia, even in the absence of any exposure to oxidants. A minority of patients are exquisitely sensitive to fava beans and will develop a fulminant hemolytic crisis following exposure. Sensitivity to *Vicia fava* is a poorly understood phenomenon that appears to be determined by a separate gene. Favism is not encountered in blacks with the A− variant. Individuals with the Mediterranean variant sometimes have a temporary episode of hemolysis during the newborn period.

The *diagnosis* of G6PD deficiency should be considered in any individual, particularly a black male, who experiences an acute hemolytic episode. The patient should be thoroughly questioned about possible exposure to oxidant agents. A number of screening tests are available to establish the diagnosis. However, since the deficiency occurs primarily in older red blood cells, a false-negative test may be seen during a hemolytic episode when there is a high proportion of young red blood cells. It may be necessary to repeat these diagnostic tests after the patient has recovered. Unusual features in

TABLE 294-5 Drugs causing hemolysis in subjects deficient in G6PD

Antimalarials: Primaquine, pamaquine, chloroquine, dapsone
Sulfonamides: Sulfanilamide, sulfasoxazole, etc.
Nitrofurantoin
Analgesics: Phenacetin, acetanilid
Miscellaneous: Vitamin K (water-soluble form), probenecid, methylene blue, *p*-aminosalicylic acid, nalidixic acid, quinine,* quinidine,* chloramphenicol*

* Not known to cause hemolysis in blacks with A− type G6PD.

the case should prompt further investigation including a more complete and specific characterization of the enzyme.

TREATMENT Since hemolysis in patients deficient in A − G6PD is usually self-limited, no specific treatment is necessary. Splenectomy does not appear to be of benefit to Mediterranean patients with chronic hemolysis. Blood transfusions are rarely indicated. If a patient develops a severe hemolytic episode with hemoglobinuria, maintaining adequate urine output is important.

Attention should be directed toward the *prevention* of hemolytic episodes. Infections ought to be treated promptly. Subjects deficient in G6PD should be warned about risks posed by oxidant drugs and fava beans. Any black patient about to be given an oxidant drug should be screened for G6PD deficiency.

OTHER DEFECTS OF THE HEXOSE-MONOPHOSPHATE SHUNT A few kindreds have been found to have congenital deficiency in red blood cell glutathione due to a defect in either of the two enzymes responsible for the synthesis of this tripeptide. Affected individuals have a hemolytic anemia with Heinz bodies that is aggravated by oxidant drugs. Deficiency of glutathione reductase has been reported, but its relationship to clinically significant hemolysis is not well established. Sometimes the deficiency state can be corrected by the administration of riboflavin (5 mg per day). There are also isolated reports of deficiencies of glutathione peroxidase and 6-phosphogluconate dehydrogenase, but, again, their association with hemolysis is uncertain.

Other enzyme defects Hemolytic anemia may sometimes be caused by abnormalities in enzymes of nucleotide metabolism. A growing number of individuals with pyrimidine 5′-nucleotidase deficiency have been encountered. Their red cells have marked basophilic stippling. Hemolytic anemia has also been noted in individuals whose red blood cells have supranormal levels of adenosine deaminase and relatively low levels of ATP.

HEMOGLOBINOPATHIES The sickling disorders constitute an important form of congenital hemolytic anemia. Less commonly, hemolysis may be due to the inheritance of an unstable hemoglobin variant. These disorders of hemoglobin are discussed in Chap. 295.

REFERENCES

ANTMAN KH et al: Microangiopathic hemolytic anemia and cancer: A review. Medicine 58:377, 1979

BYRNE JJ, MOAKE JL: Thrombotic thrombocytopenic purpura and haemolytic-uremic syndrome: Evolving concepts of pathogenesis and therapy. Clin Haematol 15:413, 1986

COOPER RA: Abnormalities of cell-membrane fluidity in the pathogenesis of disease. N Engl J Med 297:371, 1977

———: Hemolytic syndromes and red cell membrane abnormalities in liver disease. Semin Hematol 17:103, 1980

HIRONO A et al: Enzymatic diagnosis in non-spherocytic hemolytic anemia. Medicine 67:110, 1988

LUX SE: Disorders of the red cell membrane, in *Hematology of Infancy and Childhood*, DG Nathan, FA Oski (eds). Philadelphia, Saunders, 1987

PANGBURN et al: Paroxysmal nocturnal hemoglobinuria: Deficiency in factor H–like functions of the abnormal erythrocytes. J Exp Med 157:1971, 1983

PISCIOTTA AV: Thrombotic thrombocytopenic purpura. Ann Intern Med 92:249, 1980

ROSSE WF: Autoimmune hemolytic anemia. Hosp Prac 20:105, 1985

———: *Clinical Immunohematology*. Cambridge, Blackwell Scientific, 1989

———, PARKER CG: Paroxysmal nocturnal hemoglobinuria. Clin Haematol 14:105, 1985

SCHRIER SL (ed): The red blood cell membrane. Clin Haematol 14:1, 1985

VALENTINE WN et al: Hemolytic anemias and erythrocyte enzymopathies. Ann Intern Med 103:245, 1985

295 DISORDERS OF HEMOGLOBIN

H. FRANKLIN BUNN

In 1910, Herrick described a medical student from Jamaica who had a hemolytic anemia in conjunction with elongated "sickled" red blood cells. Subsequently, it was shown that all the red blood cells of such patients assume a classic holly leaf or sickle shape following deoxygenation of the blood. In 1949, Itano and Pauling discovered the association of sickle cell anemia with an electrophoretically abnormal hemoglobin. Eight years later, Ingram demonstrated that this hemoglobin (designated Hb S) differed from normal Hb A by the substitution of valine for glutamic acid at the sixth position of the β chain. Since then, over 400 structurally different human hemoglobin variants have been discovered in widely scattered parts of the world. Generally, a new hemoglobin is named after the place where it is first encountered. No more than a third of these mutant hemoglobins are associated with significant clinical manifestations. The remainder have been discovered by serendipity or as a result of large population surveys. All told, the hemoglobinopathies have taught us many valuable lessons in such diverse areas as the mechanisms of hemolysis, the pathophysiology of oxygen transport, the stereochemistry of hemoglobin function, and the genetic bases of protein synthesis.

This chapter focuses on the clinically significant variants. In addition, disorders of the biosynthesis of globin (the thalassemias) and methemoglobinemia are discussed.

GENETIC CONSIDERATIONS The synthesis of each of the subunits of hemoglobin (α, β, γ, δ, ε, ζ) is governed by separate genes. The ε and ζ subunits are found only in embryonic hemoglobin. Normal individuals inherit two β-chain genes (one from each parent), four α-chain genes, and four γ-chain genes. The ε-, γ-, δ-, and β-chain genes occupy adjacent loci on chromosome 11 (see Fig. 295-1). The ζ and α genes are located on chromosome 16. The structure and function of normal hemoglobin ($\alpha_2\beta_2$) are discussed in Chap. 290. The inheritance of abnormal hemoglobins follows classic mendelian genetics. If two parents are heterozygous for a hemoglobin variant such as Hb S, statistically one-quarter of the offspring will be SS homozygotes, another quarter will be normal (AA genotype), and half will have sickle trait (AS). The commonly encountered hemoglobinopathies such as S, C, and E are β-chain variants. Occasionally, an individual inherits two different β-chain variants, one from each parent. Hemoglobin SC disease is an example of such a double heterozygous state. Genes for β thalassemia are located on the β-chain structural gene. Accordingly, an individual can inherit from one parent (and pass on to a child) either β thalassemia or a β-chain variant, but not both. Among the hemoglobinopathies associated with sickling (described below), only the homozygous state (Hb SS) or double heterozygous state (Sβ thalassemia or SC) has important clinical manifestations. In contrast, the unstable variants and those having abnormal oxygen-binding properties are encountered only in heterozygotes. In some cases, the homozygous state would be incompatible with life.

About 90 percent of these abnormal hemoglobins are single amino acid replacements, due to a single base substitution in the corresponding triplet codon. The structural information accumulated on human mutant hemoglobins has provided ample verification of the fidelity of the genetic code. Other genetic mechanisms must be invoked to explain the structure of a few interesting hemoglobin variants. The Lepore hemoglobins have arisen because of nonhomologous crossover between the adjacent δ- and β-chain genes, giving rise to a fusion subunit in which the *N*-terminal end has the amino acid sequence of the δ chain and the *C*-terminal end has the sequence of the β chain (see Fig. 295-1). Some of the unstable hemoglobins have deletions of one or more residues in sequence within a subunit. Finally there are a few variants which have elongated subunits (e.g., Hb Constant

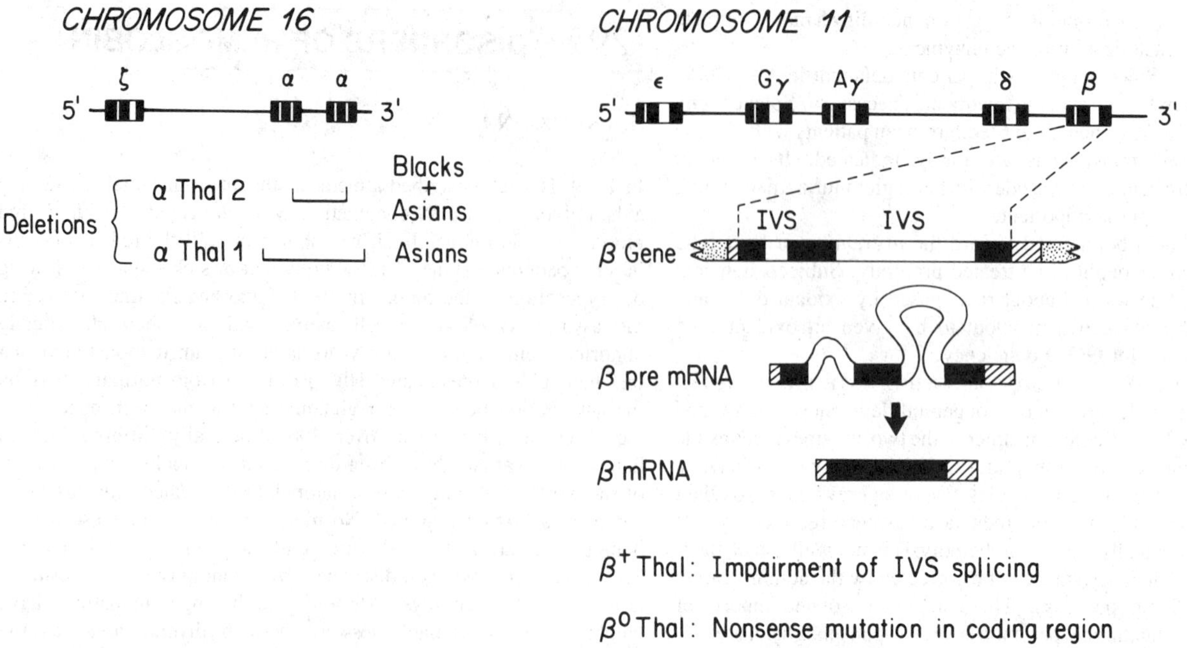

FIGURE 295-1 Diagram of human globin genes. *Left:* The α-globin gene complex includes the embryonic ζ gene as well as two α genes. In the vast majority of individuals with α thalassemia 2 (α −) one α gene is deleted owing to a nonhomologous crossover between adjacent α genes. In α thalassemia 1 (− −) both α genes are deleted. *Right:* The β-globin gene complex includes the embryonic ϵ gene, two fetal genes ($^G\gamma$ and $^A\gamma$), the δ gene, and the β gene. Below is a diagram of the β gene showing the coding regions (■), the intervening segments (IVS) and the flanking regions (▨) that are transcribed into mRNA below. Most cases of β^+ thalassemia in Mediterranean individuals involve a base substitution causing partial impairment of splicing of an IVS. Most cases of β^0 thalassemia in Mediterraneans involve a base substitution that creates either a stop codon or a frame shift.

Spring). These have arisen either because of a base substitution in the termination codon or because of a frame shift which puts the termination codon out of phase.

CLINICAL CLASSIFICATION The clinically significant hemoglobin variants are classified in Table 295-1. By far the most important and prevalent type of hemoglobinopathy is due to the presence of sickle hemoglobin, either in the homozygous state or in conjunction with another type of hemoglobin abnormality. The inheritance of an unstable hemoglobin variant may give rise to congenital hemolytic anemia associated with the presence of inclusions of precipitated hemoglobin within the red blood cells (Heinz bodies). Finally, hemoglobin variants may have abnormal functional or spectral properties, resulting in familial erythrocytosis or familial cyanosis.

SICKLE SYNDROMES

SICKLE CELL TRAIT About 8 percent of black Americans are heterozygous for Hb S. The gene frequency is highest in central Africa, particularly in regions where malaria is endemic. In some parts of Nigeria, over 30 percent of the population has sickle trait. The gene has persisted because heterozygotes gain slight protection against falciparum malaria. This is an example of balanced polymorphism.

The diagnosis of sickle trait or any of the other sickle syndromes depends upon the demonstration of sickling under reduced oxygen tension. In the widely used sickle preparation, sickled cells can be visualized microscopically after the addition of an oxygen-consuming reagent such as metabisulfite. Many clinical laboratories prefer a solubility test which depends on the fact that deoxyhemoglobin S has a low solubility at high ionic strength. These tests are reasonably specific for Hb S although some of the unstable variants may give a false-positive solubility test. Therefore, if one of these screening tests is positive, hemoglobin electrophoresis should be performed. Individuals with sickle trait usually have about 35 to 40 percent Hb S and 55 to 60 percent Hb A.

Hemoglobin S heterozygotes have minimal clinical problems. Their overall life expectancy and frequency of hospitalization are no different from those of a comparable group of individuals with hemoglobin A. AS red blood cells require a much lower oxygen tension for sickling than SS red cells. Accordingly, individuals with sickle trait may develop sickle cell crises only if they become severely hypoxic. They may occasionally sustain a splenic infarct. As discussed below, the renal medulla is particularly susceptible to sickling. Many AS individuals have impaired ability to form concentrated urine, and a few have recurrent episodes of painless hematuria as a result of medullary infarction. Infarction due to sickling has been encountered in other organs in sickle trait but is extremely rare. For these reasons, AS individuals should not be placed in any high-risk group for employment or insurance considerations.

SICKLE CELL ANEMIA Sickle cell anemia is a significant cause of morbidity and mortality among black individuals. About 0.15 percent of black children in the United States have the disease. The prevalence is lower among adults because patients with sickle cell anemia have a decreased life expectancy. The protean clinical manifestations of this disorder can all be attributed to a specific molecular lesion: the substitution of valine for glutamic acid at the sixth residue of the β chain.

Molecular pathogenesis Upon deoxygenation, a red blood cell containing Hb S changes from a biconcave disk to an elongated crescent-shaped or "sickle"-shaped cell (see Fig. 295-2). Electron micrographs reveal the presence of fibers having a diameter of about 20 nm. Each sickle fiber consists of a helical polymer with 14 strands. The polymer is stabilized by hydrophobic bonding between β6 valine and a complementary site on another portion of the β chain on an adjacent strand (Fig. 295-2). In addition, there are many other

TABLE 295-1 Clinically important hemoglobin variants

I Sickle syndromes
- *A* Sickle cell trait (AS)
- *B* Sickle cell anemia (SS)
- *C* Double heterozygous states: Sickle β thalassemia, sickle C disease (SC), sickle D disease (SD)

II Unstable hemoglobin variants: congenital Heinz body hemolytic anemia
III Variants with high oxygen affinity: familial erythrocytosis
IV M hemoglobins: familial cyanosis (see Table 295-3)

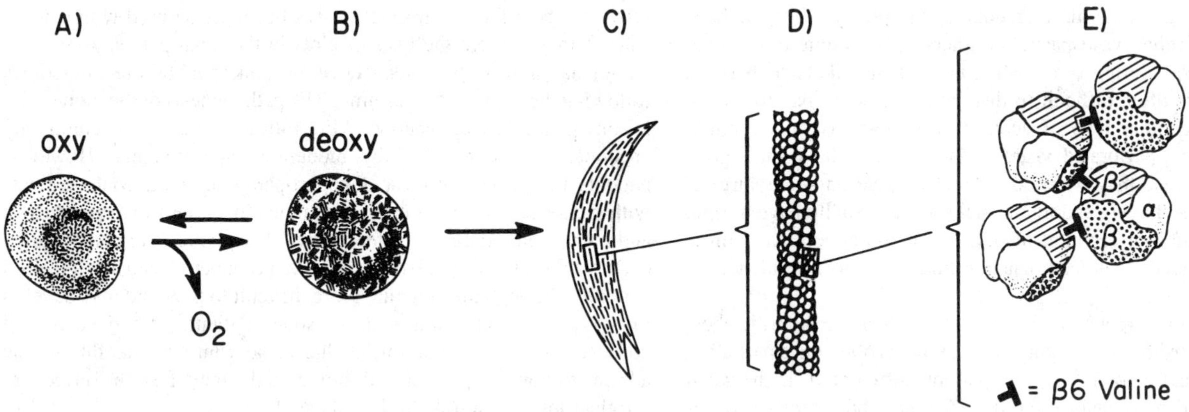

FIGURE 295-2 Polymerization of sickle hemoglobin. When the red cell (*A*) is deoxygenated, deoxyhemoglobin S aggregates to form domains of elongated rodlike polymers (*B*). In most cells these fibers align and distort the cell into the classic sickle shape (*C*). The individual Hb S molecules form a closely packed polymer consisting of 14 strands having a helical configuration (*D*). A close-up of the contacts between a pair of aligned strands (*E*) shows the abnormal β6 valine forming a hydrophobic contact with an acceptor site on the β chain of a molecule on the adjacent strand.

interactions between neighboring molecules. Sickling, both within the intact red blood cell and in free solution, is greatly affected by the presence of non-S hemoglobin. Hb A participates more readily than Hb F in copolymerization with Hb S.

Cellular pathogenesis As discussed in Chap. 290, the ability of red blood cells to traverse the microcirculation depends in large part on their pliability. As sickle polymers are formed during deoxygenation, the red blood cell becomes rigid, and, as a result, may obstruct capillary blood flow. The rate at which polymerization occurs depends primarily on the intracellular concentration of HbS and the extent of deoxygenation. If polymerization occurs before the red cell escapes the narrow-bore capillary, obstruction may occur, resulting in local tissue hypoxia, further deoxygenation, and further sickling. This vicious cycle may result in the amplification of microscopic obstruction into a larger area of infarction. The oxygen-dependent sickle cycle is ordinarily reversible. However, the membrane of SS red blood cells may become sufficiently damaged so that the cells lose potassium and water, leading to the formation of irreversibly sickled forms. In these cells, the characteristic sickle shape persists even after they are exposed to ambient oxygen tension at room temperature and can readily be seen on examination of Wright-stained blood films (see Fig. A5-6). The proportion of irreversibly sickled cells varies considerably among homozygous sicklers and is not correlated with clinical severity. Hemoglobin F is distributed unevenly among red blood cells of SS patients, and composes between 2 and 20 percent of the total hemoglobin (the remainder is almost entirely Hb S). Since Hb F inhibits the polymerization of Hb S, those cells that contain Hb F are protected from sickling, whereas those cells that lack Hb F are likely to become irreversibly sickled. It is not surprising that these rigid cells are readily culled from the circulation and destroyed. The continuous formation and destruction of irreversibly sickled cells contributes significantly to the severe hemolytic anemia shared by all patients with sickle cell anemia. Furthermore, these rigid cells may initiate small-vessel occlusions.

Factors such as acidosis or increased erythrocyte 2,3-diphosphoglycerate, which lower the oxygen affinity of red blood cells, will enhance the formation of deoxyhemoglobin and, therefore, promote intracellular polymerization and eventual sickling. In addition, sickling is highly dependent on hemoglobin concentration. Any pathophysiologic process which tends to pull water out of sickle red blood cells will greatly increase their tendency to sickle. Thus, the hypertonic environment of the renal medulla can cause local sickling and the formation of papillary infarcts, even in individuals with sickle trait.

Clinical manifestations Patients with homozygous sickle cell anemia have a variety of clinical problems broadly outlined in Table 295-2. Signs and symptoms usually do not appear until after the sixth month of life, at which time most of the Hb F has been replaced by Hb S. Among the *constitutional* manifestations of sickle cell anemia are delay of growth and development and a general failure to thrive. In addition, these patients have an increased tendency to develop serious infections, particularly due to pneumococcus. SS patients have marked impairment of splenic function, preventing effective clearance of circulating bacteria. With the passage of time, the organ sustains recurrent infarcts and eventually becomes a nubbin of fibrous tissue.

ANEMIA SS homozygotes have a severe hemolytic anemia with hematocrit values between 18 and 30 percent. The destruction of red blood cells is independent of cell age. The mean red blood cell survival is about 10 to 15 days. Those cells having relatively low levels of Hb F have a shorter life span, in part due to a greater chance of becoming irreversibly sickled. As a result of accelerated red blood cell breakdown, patients with sickle cell disease have characteristic clinical and laboratory findings discussed in Chap. 290. Even though hemolysis is primarily extravascular, plasma haptoglobin is generally low or absent, and plasma hemoglobin levels are moderately elevated.

The anemia becomes increasingly severe if erythropoiesis is suppressed. There are two main causes of "aplastic crises"—infection and folic acid deficiency. As discussed in Chap. 293, infection brings about a transient reduction in red blood cell production. In particular, parvovirus causes an abrupt suppression of erythropoiesis. In SS patients with severe ongoing hemolysis, this usually results in a rapid drop in hematocrit (Table 295-2).

VASOOCCLUSIVE PHENOMENA The morbidity and mortality of sickle cell disease are due primarily to recurrent vasoocclusive phenomena. As shown in Table 295-2, these can be divided into two groups. Throughout their lives, SS patients are plagued by recurrent *painful crises*. These episodes may appear with explosive suddenness and attack various parts of the body, particularly the abdomen, chest, back, and joints. About a third of painful crises are preceded by a viral or bacterial infection. The frequency of painful crises is highly variable. A given patient may have months or even years without a crisis and then have a cluster of frequent severe attacks. In some

TABLE 295-2 Clinical manifestations of sickle cell anemia

I Constitutional
  A Impaired growth and development
  B Increased susceptibility to infection
II Vasoocclusive
  A Microinfarcts → Painful crises
  B Macroinfarcts → Organ damage
III Anemia
  A Severe hemolysis
  B Aplastic crises

individuals, crises occur more frequently in cold weather, perhaps precipitated by reflex vasospasm. In others, crises come more often in warm weather, during times when patients are likely to become dehydrated. It is often difficult to distinguish between painful sickle crisis and some other type of acute process such as biliary colic, appendicitis, or a perforated viscus. Many patients have undergone exploration because they were considered to have an acute surgical problem. Patients having abdominal sickle crises usually have normal bowel sounds and no rebound tenderness. If the abdominal pain is due to sickling, the surgeon usually finds no gross evidence of infarction or ischemia.

SS homozygotes frequently develop attacks of acute pleuritic chest pain with fever. Although the initial chest x-ray is often unremarkable, an infiltrate may evolve. The important differential is between pneumonitis and pulmonary infarction. Culture and Gram's stain of the sputum will be helpful in establishing the presence of pneumonia. In these patients, pulmonary infarctions are much more likely due to thrombosis in situ than to emboli. Occasionally, pulmonary infarcts become secondarily infected.

When a sickle crisis is localized in the extremities, it may mimic osteomyelitis or an acute arthritis such as gout or rheumatoid arthritis. Patients commonly develop acute synovitis with joint effusion. Examination of the joint fluid is helpful in this differential diagnosis. If the effusion is due to sickling, the fluid will be clear and yellow, with a low white blood cell count (100 to 1000 mononuclear cells per cubic millimeter) and an absence of crystals or bacteria.

Sickle crises may occasionally involve the central nervous system. Patients can present with a seizure, stroke, or coma. Although such crises are frequently reversible, they may be fatal.

CHRONIC ORGAN DAMAGE By the time that patients reach adulthood, there is often objective evidence of anatomic or functional damage to various tissues, due to the cumulative effect of recurrent vasoocclusive episodes. Almost any organ may be involved, but the most common are the lungs, kidneys, liver, skeleton, and skin.

Cardiopulmonary Impairment of pulmonary function is a common complication of sickle cell disease. Resting arterial P_{O_2} is usually reduced in part because of intrapulmonary arterial-venous shunting. Since SS red blood cells have decreased oxygen affinity, arterial blood will be significantly undersaturated, leading to an increased tendency for red cells to sickle when they reach the peripheral circulation. SS homozygotes frequently develop congestive heart failure. The chronic severe anemia and hypoxemia impose a sustained burden on the heart. Most patients have a systolic ejection murmur as a result of their hyperdynamic circulation. Even though more oxygen is extracted by the myocardium than any other tissue, SS patients rarely develop myocardial infarction, probably because of rapid transit through the myocardial microcirculation.

Hepatobiliary Like other patients with congenital hemolytic anemia, those with sickle cell anemia have icterus and an increased tendency to form gallstones. It is often difficult to distinguish between the abdominal pain of acute cholecystitis and that due to a sickle crisis. Jaundice deepens markedly if a patient develops choledocholithiasis, and bilirubin levels as high as 855 μmol/L (50 mg/dL) have been reported. As a rule, cholecystectomy is not recommended unless gallstones cause symptoms. In addition, patients with sickle cell anemia may develop hepatic infarcts which occasionally become infected, resulting in abscess formation. If a significant portion of hepatic parenchyma becomes infarcted, fibrosis and deterioration of liver function may result, with deepening of jaundice.

Genitourinary (see also Chaps. 228 and 230) The hypertonic and acidic environment of the renal medulla promotes sickling, resulting in microinfarcts. Virtually all patients have isosthenuria. The inability to form concentrated urine increases the risk of significant dehydration. In addition, like those with sickle trait or SC disease, SS homozygotes may develop significant and prolonged painless hematuria as a result of papillary infarcts. Hematuria may be so extensive that iron deficiency develops. ε-Aminocaproic acid has proved to be effective in severe cases but must be used with caution since it may prevent the lysis of clots in the renal pelvis.

A small number of patients develop frank renal failure, sometimes following the nephrotic syndrome. The pathogenesis of the glomerular lesions is not well understood. Mild nitrogen retention is commonly encountered, accompanied by moderate hyperuricemia. However, patients rarely have uric acid nephropathy or gout. Male patients with sickle cell anemia occasionally develop priapism (spontaneous and painful engorgement of the penis). This distressing complication occurs with about equal frequency in prepubertal and postpubertal patients, although the latter are more difficult to treat and may develop impotence following the acute episode. Patients should be treated conservatively with sedation, analgesia, and intravenous fluids. The administration of packed red blood cells may also be effective. Surgical intervention is rarely indicated.

Skeletal Like other patients with congenital hemolytic anemia, patients with sickle cell anemia demonstrate radiologic abnormalities due to the expansion of red marrow. However, the development of bony infarcts results in more characteristic x-ray abnormalities. The biconcave or "fishmouth" vertebrae are pathognomonic of sickle cell disease. Skeletal infarction generally leads to increased bony trabeculation and sclerosis. Aseptic necrosis of the head of the femur is particularly common in patients with sickle cell disease and can lead to considerable disability. Like infarcts in other organs, bony infarctions are more likely to become infected. In patients who develop osteomyelitis, salmonella is a frequent pathogen.

Ocular A variety of ocular abnormalities are encountered in patients with SS and SC disease. These include retinal infarcts, peripheral vessel disease, arteriovenous anomalies, vitreous hemorrhage, retinitis proliferans, and retinal detachment. In addition, when viewed with a strong magnifying lens, angulated and "corkscrew" vessels can be seen in the bulbar conjunctiva. The major ocular complications are more commonly encountered in SC and sickle β thalassemia patients than in SS patients. The early diagnosis of retinal lesions in sickle disease is important since retinal detachment may be prevented by appropriate therapy.

Skin Chronic skin ulcers often occur in the distal lower extremities. The lesions appear to be commoner in patients with more severe anemia. Ankle ulcers have also been encountered in rare patients with other types of congenital hemolytic anemia. This complication is more commonly seen in tropical areas. Ankle ulcers generally respond to conservative management, such as elevation of the leg, maintenance of strict cleanliness, and application of a mild chemical debriding agent such as Dakin's solution. The weekly application of Unna boots has been effective. In patients with refractory ulcers, a hypertransfusion regimen is probably indicated. Skin grafting should be undertaken only after all other measures have failed.

Neurologic A variety of central nervous system manifestations may be encountered in sickle cell anemia. Although cerebral thrombosis is the principal neurologic complication, SS patients also have an increased incidence of subarachnoid hemorrhage. A patient has about a 25 percent chance of developing some type of neurologic complication during a lifetime. Hemiplegia is encountered more frequently than coma, convulsions, or visual disturbances. Patients generally make a full recovery, particularly from their first cerebral vascular accident. Preliminary studies in children indicate that a hypertransfusion program is beneficial to those who have sustained a major neurologic complication.

Diagnosis The diagnosis of sickle cell anemia should be considered in any black patient with a hemolytic anemia. The history of painful crises, arthropathy, ankle ulcers, etc., can be very helpful. If a patient has a relatively mild form of the disease, the diagnosis may not have been made during childhood. A number of laboratory tests are useful in distinguishing sickle cell anemia from other hemoglobinopathies. Examination of the peripheral blood smear reveals normochromic normocytic red blood cells, many of which appear as targets. The presence of irreversibly sickled forms is very helpful (see Fig. A5-6). In addition, the presence of Howell-Jolly bodies, siderocytes, and occasional normoblasts suggests the absence of effective splenic function. A positive test for sickling, such as the metabisulfite preparation or the solubility test, indicates the presence of Hb S but does not distinguish between SS, AS, and double heterozygotes (SβThal, SC). Hemoglobin electrophoresis is necessary to establish the diagnosis. Patients with homozygous sickle cell anemia have about 2 to 20 percent Hb F and 2 to 4 percent Hb A_2. The remainder is Hb S. No Hb A is detected unless the patient has been transfused within the past 4 months. Patients with sickle β thalassemia will have hypochromic microcytic red blood cells, fewer irreversibly sickled forms, and a variable proportion of Hb A (0 to 30 percent). SC diseases can be readily diagnosed by hemoglobin electrophoresis. In hemoglobin SD disease, the two hemoglobin variants comigrate during conventional electrophoresis at pH 8.6 but can be separated by agar gel electrophoresis at pH 6.0.

Treatment Understanding the molecular pathogenesis of sickling has not yet led to an effective form of therapy. A large array of antisickling regimens has been proposed, but thus far none has stood the test of time. Recent investigation has focused on stimulating the production of Hb F by agents such as hydroxyurea and perhaps recombinant erythropoietin. Currently accepted management of sickle cell anemia is primarily supportive and conservative. Since patients with sickle cell anemia are at increased risk of developing infections, many of which trigger painful and aplastic crises, it is very important to detect infection early and give appropriate antibiotics promptly. Malaria prophylaxis should be administered in endemic areas. The development of pneumococcal sepsis in children may be prevented by the administration of the polyvalent vaccine and prophylactic penicillin.

The anemia of sickle cell disease increases markedly if the patient becomes deficient in folic acid. Since these patients have a continuous increased requirement for folic acid, it is reasonable to maintain them on a daily oral supplement.

Painful crises should be treated promptly with adequate analgesia and hydration. Some patients feel that their crises can be aborted if treated early. Therefore, it is expedient to give these patients a supply of an analgesic such as codeine which can be taken at home. However, these patients are at risk of becoming addicted to opiates. Oxygen should be administered during acute pain crisis if the patient has arterial hypoxemia.

Blood transfusions play a limited role in the management of sickle cell anemia. Between crises, patients tolerate anemia quite well and do not derive much subjective benefit from transfusions. However, partial replacement of the patients' red blood cells by transfused red cells (hypertransfusion) may be an effective way of preventing vasoocclusive crises. In order to lower the viscosity of the patient's blood significantly, it is necessary that over 50 percent of the patient's red blood cells be of donor origin. Hypertransfusion is a reasonable approach to getting a patient through a limited period of risk such as surgery. However, the problems of isoimmunization, iron overload, and hepatitis dictate against its widespread use.

Prevention Genetic counseling can play an important role in the prevention of sickle cell anemia. Parents who are both AS heterozygotes should be informed that there is a 25 percent chance that their offspring will be homozygous. The antenatal diagnosis of sickle cell anemia can be made in the first trimester of pregnancy by obtaining fetal cells from a chorionic villus and analyzing the DNA following digestion with a restriction endonuclease that recognizes the codon involved in the β6 valine mutation. If it is established that the fetus is an SS homozygote, the parents may decide to terminate the pregnancy.

Prognosis The clinical course of patients with sickle cell anemia is highly variable. Many assessments of prognosis that have appeared in the literature have been unduly pessimistic. During the past 30 years there has been considerable improvement in the care of patients with sickle cell anemia. An increasing number of patients are surviving into adulthood and bearing offspring. There has also been a decline in the mortality of SS mothers during pregnancy and childbirth. However, in underdeveloped nations, the mortality in sickle cell anemia remains very high.

No single clinical or laboratory finding is a consistent predictor of prognosis in sickle cell disease. Although those patients who have relatively high amounts of Hb F tend to have milder clinical manifestations, this relationship is of no prognostic value in any given patient. Considerable variation in the severity of sickle cell disease has been reported among different ethnic and geographical groups. A group of Shi Arabs from Saudi Arabia has been found to have a benign form of sickle cell anemia with very high levels of Hb F (15 to 30 percent). A mild type of sickle cell anemia has also been encountered in central India. SS patients with coexisting α thalassemia have less severe hemolysis but do not have a significant reduction in vasoocclusive phenomena.

SICKLE β THALASSEMIA This disease is highly variable in its clinical severity and complications. It is commonly encountered in people from the Mediterranean countries as well as those from central Africa. Sickle β thalassemia tends to be milder in blacks, just as homozygous β thalassemia is much less severe in blacks than in the Mediterranean populations. Patients have a congenital hemolytic anemia of variable severity, accompanied by splenomegaly in about 70 percent of cases. Individuals who produce no normal β chains (sickle β^0 thalassemia) have vasoocclusive manifestations comparable to those encountered in homozygous SS disease. In contrast, patients who are able to produce some normal β chains (sickle β^+ thalassemia) have less severe anemia, fewer pain crises, and less organ damage.

Examination of the blood film reveals hypochromic microcytic red blood cells, with polychromatophilia, target cells, stippling, and rare fixed sickle forms. The electrophoretic pattern shows from 60 to 90 percent Hb S and 10 to 30 percent Hb F. Hemoglobin A will be about 10 to 30 percent if the β-thalassemia gene is capable of producing some β^A chains (β^+ thalassemia, see below). In patients who have sickle β^0 thalassemia, no Hb A will be present, and therefore the disorder may be difficult to distinguish from homozygous sickle cell anemia. Hemoglobin A_2 is moderately elevated in sickle β thalassemia, but it is difficult to measure this minor component accurately in the presence of Hb S. Occasional patients may derive benefit from splenectomy if the spleen is sequestering a significant amount of red blood cells.

SICKLE C DISEASE Although the gene frequency among blacks in the United States for Hb C (β6 Glu→Lys) is only one-fourth that for Hb S, the prevalence of SC disease among adults is almost as high as SS disease since the former group of patients has a nearly normal life expectancy. These individuals have a mild to moderate hemolytic anemia, usually accompanied by splenomegaly. On peripheral blood smears, target cells and occasional plump sickled forms are seen. Hemoglobin electrophoresis reveals 50 percent Hb S, 50 percent Hb C. Hemoglobin S copolymerizes with Hb C to the same extent as with Hb A. The increased tendency of SC red cells to sickle, compared with sickle trait cells, can be explained by two phenomena: increased intracellular hemoglobin concentration and significantly higher percent Hb S. Patients with SC disease may occasionally have painful crises or organ infarcts. They are at particular risk of developing ocular complications described above, including proliferative retinopathy and retinal detachment. In addition, patients with SC disease are at relatively high risk of developing hematuria from renal medullary infarcts and avascular necrosis of the femoral head. Pregnant women with SC disease have a high rate of complications during pregnancy. Individuals with an electrophoretic pattern suggestive of Hb SC disease but with more severe clinical manifestations may be double heterozygotes for Hb S and Hb O Arab (β121 Glu→Lys).

SICKLE D DISEASE A number of hemoglobins comigrate with Hb S on routine electrophoresis. The most commonly encountered variant is Hb D Los Angeles (β121 Glu→Gln). Hemoglobins S and

D can be separated by special electrophoretic methods. The diagnosis of Hb SD disease is suggested by the demonstration of a positive sickle cell preparation in only one of the patient's two parents. SD double heterozygotes have moderately severe anemia.

HOMOZYGOUS Hb C DISEASE Patients have a mild congenital hemolytic anemia accompanied by splenomegaly. Hemoglobin C has a tendency to form intracellular crystals, particularly if red blood cells are suspended in a hypertonic medium. The intracellular hemoglobin concentration is markedly increased owing to loss of potassium and water from the cytoplasm. As a result, the blood film reveals striking target cells. Red blood cell osmotic fragility is decreased. Patients rarely develop significant complications. No specific therapy is indicated.

UNSTABLE HEMOGLOBIN VARIANTS

In the early 1950s several patients in England were found to have congenital nonspherocytic hemolytic anemia associated with inclusions of precipitated hemoglobin (Heinz bodies) within red blood cells. The presence of an abnormal hemoglobin was suspected by the formation of a precipitate when the patients' hemolysates were gently heated. Currently, over 90 different unstable hemoglobin variants have been identified. The great majority are single amino acid substitutions in the β chain. A few are due to deletion of one or more amino acids within the β chain. Patients present with a hemolytic anemia of variable degree. Severe cases are usually detected in late infancy or early childhood and have jaundice, splenomegaly, and dark-colored urine. An autosomal dominant mode of inheritance can usually be established, although about a fifth of the cases appear to be spontaneous mutants.

Pathogenesis These hemoglobin variants have structural alterations at sites in the molecule that drastically affect its stability and solubility. Many involve an amino acid substitution in the portion of the subunit where heme is inserted. In such instances, the heme may be displaced from the heme pocket. As a result, the abnormal hemoglobin has decreased solubility and forms an intracellular precipitate (Heinz body). Red blood cells which contain this type of inclusion are recognized by the mononuclear phagocyte system and are either cleansed of their intracellular debris (pitting) or destroyed. The displaced heme moiety is aberrantly catabolized, forming dipyrroles, such as mesobilifuscin, instead of bilirubin. Pigmenturia is probably due to the excretion of these dipyrroles. The degree of instability of these hemoglobin variants and, therefore, the extent of hemolysis vary considerably. In some, such as Hb Zürich, an additional oxidant stress, such as the ingestion of certain drugs, is required for significant hemolysis. In contrast, patients with Hb Hammersmith have continuous and marked red blood cell breakdown. The degree of anemia is influenced not only by the severity of the hemolysis but also by the ability of the blood to unload oxygen. Thus, patients having unstable variants with increased oxygen affinity, such as Hb Köln, may have a near-normal hemoglobin level, i.e., compensated hemolysis.

Diagnosis The red blood cell morphology is somewhat variable. Often, patients with a functioning spleen have normal-appearing red blood cells. Slight hypochromia and basophilic stippling are not uncommon. The blood may have to be incubated in order to bring out Heinz bodies. In some cases, red blood cells appear as if a bite had been taken from a margin. It is tempting to speculate that at this site a Heinz body had been pitted. Following splenectomy, red blood cells appear much more abnormal, and Heinz bodies are larger and more numerous.

The diagnosis of a congenital Heinz body hemolytic anemia is established by the following laboratory tests and results:

1 *Hemoglobin electrophoresis* will often reveal an abnormal component, usually composing less than 30 percent of the total.
2 *Heinz bodies* can be demonstrated by incubating a freshly drawn sample of blood with a supravital stain.
3 A significant *precipitate* is formed when the hemolysate is incubated at 50°C, or in the presence of 17% isopropanol.
4 The unstable hemoglobins often have an abnormal *oxygen dissociation curve*.

If these tests are negative in a patient with congenital nonspherocytic hemolytic anemia, a defect of the membrane or one of the red blood cell enzymes is likely (Chap. 294).

Treatment The treatment of congenital Heinz body hemolytic anemia is primarily supportive. Anemia is rarely severe enough to warrant blood transfusion. Oxidant drugs should be avoided. Like others with chronic hemolysis, these patients have an increased requirement for folic acid. Those with severe hemolysis often benefit from prophylactic folate therapy. The red blood cell mass may fall during a period of bone marrow suppression, such as that resulting from folate deficiency or acute infection. Although patients with severe hemolysis may benefit from splenectomy, this operation is not curative. Because of the risk of bacterial sepsis in infants and young children who have been splenectomized, this treatment should be postponed until the child is over 4 years old. The diagnostic tests cited above become more abnormal following splenectomy. For this reason, in some cases the diagnosis may not be definitely established until after the operation.

STABLE VARIANTS HAVING ABNORMAL OXYGEN AFFINITY

In 1966 certain members of a large family were discovered to have erythrocytosis in association with an electrophoretically abnormal hemoglobin, Hb Chesapeake, which had a very high affinity for oxygen. Since then, more than 40 other stable high-affinity hemoglobin variants have been encountered in families with erythrocytosis. Their structural alterations tend to be at sites which influence hemoglobin's functional behavior. As a result of the hemoglobin's increased oxygen affinity, oxygen unloading to tissues is decreased, and there is an erythropoietin-mediated stimulus to erythropoiesis. This disorder is manifested in the heterozygous state and follows an autosomal codominant pattern of inheritance. Hematocrit levels are rarely high enough to cause a significant increase in blood viscosity. Thus, affected individuals are generally asymptomatic and lack any pertinent physical findings other than a ruddy complexion. The diagnosis should be suspected in all patients with unexplained erythrocytosis, particularly when other family members are similarly affected, and can be established by the demonstration of increased oxygen affinity of the whole blood. About two-thirds of the high-affinity variants can be readily separated from Hb A by electrophoresis. No treatment is indicated. The patient should be reassured that the disorder is benign.

Hemoglobin variants having a marked decrease in oxygen affinity cause one form of familial cyanosis (Table 295-3). Because of the abnormality of hemoglobin function, arterial blood is partially unsaturated despite normal oxygen tension. Thus, the cyanosis is due

TABLE 295-3 Differential diagnosis of cyanosis

I Decreased oxygenation of hemoglobin (↑ deoxyhemoglobin)
- *A* Reduced arterial oxygen tension (common)
  - *1* Pulmonary disease
  - *2* Cardiac right-to-left shunt
- *B* Hemoglobin variant having decreased oxygen affinity (rare)

II Methemoglobinemia (rare)
- *A* Hereditary
  - *1* M hemoglobins
  - *2* Cytochrome b_5 reductase deficiency
- *B* Acquired
  - *1* Nitrites and nitrates: sodium nitrite, amyl nitrite, nitroglycerin, nitroprusside, silver nitrate
  - *2* Aniline dyes
  - *3* Acetanilid and phenacetin
  - *4* Sulfonamides
  - *5* Other: lidocaine, chlorate, phenazopyridine

to increased levels of deoxyhemoglobin in the blood. Except for this cosmetic problem, affected individuals have no other clinical manifestations. Blood values are otherwise normal.

METHEMOGLOBINEMIA

Oxygen transport depends on the maintenance of intracellular hemoglobin in the reduced (Fe^{2+}) state. When hemoglobin is oxidized to methemoglobin, the heme iron becomes Fe^{3+} and is incapable of binding oxygen. Normal red cells contain less than 1 percent methemoglobin. A small amount of hemoglobin autooxidizes as red cells circulate. This process probably occurs by the dissociation of the superoxide anion from oxyhemoglobin:

$$Hb^{2+}O_2 \rightarrow Hb^{3+} + O_2^-$$

Normally, the methemoglobin that is formed is reduced by the following reaction:

$$Hb^{3+} + \text{RedCyt } b_5 \rightarrow Hb^{2+} + \text{OxCyt } b_5$$

Reduced cytochrome b_5 (RedCyt b_5) is regenerated by the enzyme cytochrome b_5 reductase (methemoglobin reductase):

$$\text{OxCyt } b_5 + \text{NADH} \xrightarrow[\text{reductase}]{\text{Cytochrome } b_5} \text{RedCyt } b_5 + \text{NAD}$$

Hereditary methemoglobinemia is due either to the presence of one of the M hemoglobins or to the deficiency of the enzyme cytochrome b_5 reductase (Table 295-3). These inherited disorders are clinically mild, while the induction of methemoglobinemia by drugs or toxins can be life-threatening.

If methemoglobin exceeds 15 g/L (1.5 g/dL) (10 percent of the total hemoglobin), affected individuals will have clinically obvious cyanosis. The color of the skin is indistinguishable from the much commoner cyanosis due to impairment of oxygen saturation that may occur in pulmonary and cardiac disorders (Table 295-3). With higher amounts of methemoglobin, patients become symptomatic. At a methemoglobin level of about 35 percent, the affected individual experiences headache, weakness, and breathlessness. Levels in excess of 80 percent are usually incompatible with life.

The toxicity of methemoglobinemia can be readily explained in terms of hemoglobin function. The fact that a certain proportion of the heme moieties is no longer able to bind oxygen is not a serious physiologic handicap per se. A proportion of 30 percent methemoglobin is much more deleterious than a 30 percent decrement in red cell mass, because the oxidized hemes have a profound effect on the remaining functional hemes in the hemoglobin tetramer. The conformation of methemoglobin (like that of carboxyhemoglobin) is very similar to that of oxyhemoglobin. Thus, a partially oxidized hemoglobin tetramer has the same tertiary and quaternary structure as a molecule which is comparably oxygenated. In each case, the affinity of the remaining hemes for oxygen is increased. For this reason, methemoglobinemia [as well as carbon monoxide (Chap. 374)] causes a "shift to the left" of the oxyhemoglobin dissociation curve and, consequently, impaired unloading of oxygen to tissues.

CYTOCHROME b_5 REDUCTASE (METHEMOGLOBIN REDUCTASE) DEFICIENCY This condition is inherited in an autosomal recessive pattern. The enzyme is a flavoprotein having properties similar to those of liver microsomal cytochrome b_5 reductase. The soluble erythrocyte enzyme is formed by cleavage of a hydrophobic tail from the microsomal enzyme.

Individuals with cytochrome b_5 reductase deficiency have lifelong cyanosis of variable degree, depending on the level of methemoglobin, but usually have no associated symptoms or other physical findings. Some may have mild polycythemia owing to increased oxygen affinity. Others have been noted to be mentally retarded. Untreated individuals usually have 15 to 30 percent methemoglobin. Methemoglobin levels are higher in the older population of red cells because the activity of the abnormal enzyme declines markedly with red cell age. There appears to be considerable heterogeneity in the variant enzymes from different families, as shown by differences in their electrophoretic mobility and kinetic parameters. In these ways, cytochrome b_5 reductase deficiency resembles glucose-6-phosphate dehydrogenase deficiency (Chap. 294).

ACQUIRED METHEMOGLOBINEMIA This disorder is generally due to exposure to certain drugs or toxins. Compounds which can cause clinically significant methemoglobinemia are listed in Table 295-3. Some agents such as nitrite and chlorate oxidize the heme iron directly. Others such as sulfa drugs and aniline must undergo biochemical transformation before they cause methemoglobinemia. Few drugs currently in use cause significant methemoglobinemia, unless the individual is unusually susceptible. Exposure to local anesthetics such as procaine and to nitroprusside occasionally causes severe methemoglobinemia. As might be expected, individuals heterozygous for methemoglobin reductase deficiency are much more likely than normal individuals to develop clinically apparent methemoglobinemia after exposure to an oxidant stress. Thus, the extent of methemoglobinemia depends not only on the dose of the toxic agent but also on the susceptibility of the exposed individual.

M HEMOGLOBINS Five hemoglobin variants have abnormal absorbance spectra, owing to the oxidation of the heme iron in the affected subunit. They involve amino acid substitutions of residues responsible for the binding of the heme iron to the globin. These so-called M hemoglobins (Table 295-3) result in a rare form of congenital and familial cyanosis. Individuals with the α-chain variants Hb M Boston and Hb M Iwate are cyanotic at birth, while cyanosis does not appear in those with the β-chain variants (Hb M Saskatoon, Hb M Hyde Park, and Hb M Milwaukee) until about 4 to 6 months of age, when fetal hemoglobin has been replaced by adult hemoglobin. As with the unstable and high-affinity variants, an autosomal codominant inheritance pattern is found. Except for cyanosis, patients are asymptomatic.

DIAGNOSIS Methemoglobinemia should be considered in any cyanotic patient with no evidence of heart or lung disease. If the cyanosis is due to decreased oxygen saturation, a blood specimen will change from a purple to a red color upon mixing with air. In contrast, a blood specimen from a methemoglobinemic individual remains a chocolate brown color irrespective of exposure to air. Methemoglobinemia can be documented by spectroscopic examination of the hemolysate. Individuals with hereditary methemoglobinemia will have lower levels than patients symptomatic from acquired methemoglobinemia. Patients who have ingested an oxidant drug may have an additional hemoglobin derivative called sulfhemoglobin in which the protoporphyrin has been chemically modified. Sulfhemoglobinemia tends to cause cyanosis even more readily than methemoglobinemia. Unlike methemoglobin, the absorbance of sulfhemoglobin at 620 to 630 nm is not decreased by the addition of cyanide. The M hemoglobins have characteristic spectral abnormalities which differ from those obtained when normal Hb A is partially oxidized. Furthermore, these hemoglobin variants can be detected by hemoglobin electrophoresis.

Treatment In individuals with methemoglobin reductase deficiency, the oral administration of methylene blue (100 to 300 mg/d) or ascorbic acid (300 to 500 mg/d) will result in a marked reduction in the level of methemoglobin. The purpose of treatment is primarily cosmetic. Severe toxic methemoglobinemia is treated by the intravenous administration of methylene blue (2 mg/kg, repeat if needed). Within an hour, the methemoglobin level is usually reduced by at least 50 percent. Treatment is neither necessary nor possible in individuals having Hb M.

THALASSEMIAS

The thalassemias are a diverse group of congenital disorders in which there is a defect in the synthesis of one (or more) of the subunits of hemoglobin. As a result of decreased production of hemoglobin, the

TABLE 295-4 Classification of the thalassemias

Diagnosis	Globin chain synthesis in reticulocytes	RBC morphology	Hb electrophoresis	Clinical severity
α Thalassemia:	α/β*			
Silent carrier $(\alpha-/\alpha\alpha)$	0.9	Normal	Normal, $\downarrow$ Hb A_2	0
α-thalassemia trait $[(\alpha-/\alpha-)$ or $(--/\alpha\alpha)]$	0.7	$\downarrow$ MCV†	Normal, $\downarrow$ Hb A_2	0
Hb H disease $(--/\alpha-)$	0.3	$\downarrow$ MCV Heinz bodies, targets	$\uparrow$ Hb H (β_4) (10–15%)	2+
Hydrops fetalis $(--/--)$	0	$\uparrow\uparrow$ Nucleated RBC	$\uparrow\uparrow$ Hb Barts (γ_4)	4+
β Thalassemia:	β/α*			
Heterozygous	0.5	$\downarrow$ MCV, stippling	$\uparrow$ Hb A_2 ($\pm$ $\uparrow$ Hb F)	0 to +
Homozygous (or double heterozygous)	0–0.3	$\downarrow$ MCV, hypochromic Nucleated RBC, targets bizarre shapes	$\uparrow\uparrow$ Hb F	4+ (major) 2–3+ (intermedia)

* Normal = 1.
† MCV = mean corpuscular volume.

red blood cells are microcytic and hypochromic (Table 61-2). The thalassemias involve a spectrum ranging from subtle morphologic abnormalities to life-threatening disease. In contrast to the qualitative hemoglobin abnormalities listed in Table 295-1, the thalassemias are quantitative abnormalities of subunit synthesis. Thus, the β chains of patients with β thalassemia have normal structure but are produced in reduced and sometimes undetectable amounts. Conversely, patients with α thalassemia have impaired production of α chains. The reduction in globin chain synthesis can be demonstrated in vitro by incubating reticulocytes with labeled amino acids and determining the incorporation of radioactivity into globin subunits (Table 295-4). Most forms of thalassemia can be identified from the information summarized in Table 295-4. Occasionally, establishing a definitive diagnosis requires measurement of globin chain synthesis or analysis of globin gene structure.

α THALASSEMIA As mentioned at the beginning of this chapter, normal individuals inherit two α-chain genes from each parent. The great majority of cases of α thalassemia can be explained by deletions of α-chain genes, owing to nonhomologous crossover (Fig. 295-1). Specific gene deletions can be identified by analysis of patients' DNA following digestion by restriction endonucleases. The clinical manifestations of α thalassemia depend upon the number of genes deleted (Table 295-4). In the silent carrier state, heterozygous α thalassemia 2 $(\alpha-/\alpha\alpha)$, one of the four genes is deleted. Affected individuals have no hematologic abnormalities. Individuals with deletion of two of the four α-chain genes (α-thalassemia trait) have either homozygous α thalassemia 2 $(\alpha-/\alpha-)$ or heterozygous α thalassemia 1 $(--/\alpha\alpha)$. They have microcytic and slightly hypochromic red blood cells but no significant hemolysis or anemia. Hemoglobin electrophoresis is normal except for a decreased amount of Hb A_2. Deletion of three α-chain genes $(--/\alpha-)$ produces a well-compensated hemolytic state with microcytic hypochromic red blood cells including many target cells. Intracellular inclusions or Heinz bodies are formed by the precipitation of Hb H, a tetramer composed of β chains which accumulates because of the marked impairment of α-chain synthesis. The most severe form of α thalassemia, hydrops fetalis, is usually due to deletion of all four α-chain genes. The affected fetus has red blood cells containing only Hb Barts, a tetramer composed of γ chains. This condition is incompatible with life, since oxygen transport depends upon the presence of heterotetramers such as $\alpha_2\beta_2$ and $\alpha_2\gamma_2$. In orientals both the α− and the −− haplotypes are relatively common; thus both Hb H disease and hydrops fetalis are frequently encountered. In contrast, blacks commonly have the α− haplotype (gene frequency ≅ 0.15) but rarely have the −− haploptype. Therefore Hb H disease is very rare in blacks and hydrops fetalis has not been reported. Homozygous α thalassemia 2 is encountered in about 2 percent of blacks and is therefore a relatively common cause of microcytosis in an individual who is otherwise healthy and not iron-deficient.

The elongated α-chain variant Hb Constant Spring, commonly encountered among southeast Asians, also has an α-thalassemia phenotype, and when inherited with the −− haplotype can cause Hb H disease.

β THALASSEMIA Since individuals inherit only one β-chain gene from each parent, affected individuals are either heterozygotes, homozygotes, or double heterozygotes. The gene frequency for β thalassemia approaches 0.1 in southern Italy and certain Mediterranean islands. β Thalassemia is also encountered quite commonly in central Africa, Asia, the south Pacific, and certain parts of India. Statistically, one-quarter of the offspring of two heterozygotes (β-thalassemia trait) will have the homozygous state: β thalassemia major or Cooley's anemia. An individual may inherit a β-thalassemia gene from one parent and a β-chain structural variant from the other Sickle β thalassemia (discussed above) is a commonly encountered example of such a double heterozygous state.

The molecular pathogenesis of the β thalassemias is more complex and heterogeneous than that of α thalassemia. In contrast to α thalassemia, gene deletion is an uncommon cause of β thalassemia. Among the recognized types of β-gene deletion, an entity known as "pancellular hereditary persistence of fetal hemoglobin" has minimal clinical manifestations owing to efficient synthesis of γ chains on the chromosome in which the β and δ genes are deleted. Hemoglobin Lepore is a fusion protein formed from a nonhomologous crossover between the δ and β genes resulting in the absence of normal β-chain synthesis and therefore a β-thalassemia phenotype (Fig. 295-1). In the great majority of cases of β thalassemia, restriction endonuclease maps reveal no gross abnormalities of the β-globin gene complex. Nevertheless, there are several steps in β-globin synthesis that could go awry and lead to a thalassemic phenotype. A number of cases involve mutations in or near one of the intervening sequences of the β-globin gene, leading to errors in the splicing of mRNA. Often β^A chains are made but in reduced amounts (β^+ thalassemia) (see Fig. 295-1). Other cases have nonsense mutations in the coding region, causing premature termination of β-globin chains. This is the most common cause of β^0 thalassemia (Fig. 295-1).

Cellular pathogenesis As a result of imbalance in globin chain synthesis, the β thalassemias have varying degrees of ineffective erythropoiesis (Chap. 290) and hemolysis. In β thalassemia major there is a marked relative excess of α-chain production. Free α chains have decreased solubility and will form insoluble aggregates or inclusions within red blood cell precursors in the bone marrow. Like congenital Heinz body hemolytic anemia due to unstable hemoglobin variants, the inclusion bodies in thalassemia bring about abnormalities in membrane permeability as well as entrapment and destruction of red blood cells by the macrophages in the mononuclear phagoycte system. As a result, β thalassemia is characterized by both intramedullary erythroid destruction and also a shortening of the life span of circulating red blood cells that emerge from the bone marrow. Thus, these patients have the characteristic parameters of both ineffective erythropoiesis (increased plasma iron turnover, decreased incorporation of iron into red blood cells) and peripheral hemolysis. Because these red blood cells are under double jeopardy, there is an enormous compensatory stimulus to erythropoiesis, resulting both in expansion of the red marrow and in extramedullary hematopoiesis in the liver and spleen. Chain imbalance in β thalassemia is attenuated to a variable degree by the "compensatory" synthesis of γ chains which are able to combine with excess free α chains and form a stable tetramer (Hb F). Patients with Cooley's anemia who have a relatively high rate of γ-chain production have a less severe clinical course. Individuals with β thalassemia minor have absent or very mild ineffective erythropoiesis and hemolysis, detectable in some patients by a slight elevation in fecal urobilinogen and a modest shortening of the red blood cell life span.

In the α thalassemias a relative excess production of non-α chains can be detected, leading to the formation of Hb Barts (γ_4) in the newborn and young infant. Children and adults with deletion of 3 α-globin genes usually have Hb H (β_4). In contrast to the α-chain inclusions found in β thalassemia, the Heinz bodies due to Hb H are more stable and develop in mature circulating red blood cells. As a result, Hb H disease is primarily a hemolytic disorder without a significant amount of ineffective erythropoiesis.

β thalassemia minor This common entity, also referred to as β-*thalassemia trait,* is rarely associated with significant clinical manifestations. The diagnosis is generally made in patients being evaluated for mild anemia or in follow-up of abnormalities found on routine blood studies. Most individuals with β-thalassemia trait escape diagnosis. About one-fifth of affected individuals have splenomegaly. Icterus is occasionally noted, particularly in those individuals who also have Gilbert's disease, another common and benign congenital disorder (Chap. 251).

In otherwise healthy individuals with β-thalassemia trait, the mean hemoglobin level is about 15 percent lower than in normal persons of the same age and sex; the red blood cell count is usually elevated, and the cells are microcytic. Indeed, at any level of hematocrit, patients with β thalassemia minor have more marked microcytosis than those with iron deficiency. In contrast, the mean corpuscular hemoglobin concentration is normal. In addition to microcytosis, examination of the blood film reveals occasional target cells, cigar-shaped cells, and a moderate amount of basophilic stippling; the reticulocyte count is normal. Special isotope techniques are required to demonstrate a slightly reduced red blood cell life span. The red blood cells have decreased osmotic fragility. Serum iron is normal unless the patient also happens to be iron-deficient. Hemoglobin electrophoresis is very useful in establishing the diagnosis of β thalassemia minor. Most affected individuals will have a twofold increase in Hb A_2 (5 percent versus normal of 2.5 percent). In contrast, Hb A_2 is subnormal in α thalassemia, iron deficiency, and sideroblastic anemias. Patients with β-thalassemia trait who become iron-deficient usually have a "normal" level of Hb A_2 which increases to above normal after correction of the deficiency. Approximately half of individuals with β thalassemia minor also have a modest elevation of Hb F (2 to 3 percent). In the less common state, δβ thalassemia, in which there is a deletion of the adjacent δ and β chain genes, Hb A_2 levels will be normal or decreased, but Hb F is increased (5 to 15 percent).

No treatment is indicated for individuals with β-thalassemia trait. They should be reassured that they do not have a serious hematologic problem. The genetic implications of thalassemia should be explained, particularly to those of childbearing age. Many individuals have been given long-term iron treatment on the mistaken impression that they had iron-deficiency anemia. These patients may gradually develop clinically significant siderosis. Establishing the diagnosis of β thalassemia minor should prevent such inappropriate therapy.

β thalassemia major Also termed Cooley's anemia, this is probably the most severe form of congenital hemolytic anemia. Clinical manifestations generally appear after the first 4 to 6 months of life when the switch from γ-chain to β-chain production usually occurs. Patients develop a severe anemia with a hematocrit of less than 20 unless they are supported by transfusions. Accordingly, patients have all the signs and symptoms associated with severe anemia. In addition, they have findings related to severe intramedullary and peripheral hemolysis as well as to iron overload. Patients with β thalassemia major often have marked wasting and appear malnourished. Children have slow rates of growth and development. In adolescents, the onset and development of secondary sex characteristics are delayed. Patients have a peculiar skin color due to a combination of icterus, pallor, and increased melanin deposition. They usually have skeletal abnormalities, secondary to expansion of the erythroid marrow. Enlargement of the malar bones may give the characteristic "chipmunk" facies or cause malocclusion of the jaw. Patients invariably have cardiomegaly which may be accompanied by signs of congestive heart failure. Marked hepatomegaly and splenomegaly are always found in these patients.

The *diagnosis* of β thalassemia major should be considered in any patient with a severe hemolytic anemia and hypochromic microcytic red blood cells. Examination of the peripheral blood smear reveals marked variations in the size and shape of red blood cells, including many target and stippled cells as well as teardrop and cigar-shaped cells (see Fig. A5-5). Normoblasts are usually seen, particularly if the patient has undergone splenectomy. Hemoglobin electrophoresis shows the presence of increased amounts of Hb F and variable amounts of Hb A. In patients who are homozygous for β^0 thalassemia, no Hb A can be detected. Hemoglobin A_2 is usually increased about twofold, although it can be normal in β thalassemia major.

Patients with β thalassemia major have a short life expectancy. It is unusual for a patient with the most severe form of the disease to survive into adulthood. Most patients have such severe anemia that they are dependent upon transfusions. The chronic administration of large amounts of blood along with an inappropriate increase in iron absorption from the gastrointestinal tract inevitably leads to clinically significant hemosiderosis. As a result of iron overload, these patients develop abnormalities in cardiac, endocrine, and hepatic function. The combination of chronic hypoxia and myocardial siderosis leads to cardiac arrhythmias, congestive failure, and ultimately death.

Homozygotes who survive into adulthood are likely to have a less severe form of the disease, designated as β *thalassemia intermedia.* There are several genetic subtypes which are associated with less severe clinical manifestations: (1) β thalassemia with unusually high levels of Hb F synthesis, (2) δβ thalassemia in which there is absence of δ-chain as well as β-chain synthesis, and (3) the presence of α thalassemia in combination with homozygous β thalassemia, leading to more balanced subunit synthesis. A milder clinical course is also seen in individuals who are doubly heterozygous for β thalassemia and hereditary persistence of Hb F. Patients with the above genotypes usually have moderately severe anemia, but do not require transfusions.

Treatment of β thalassemia major is primarily supportive. The obvious benefits of transfusion therapy are partially offset by the risk of iron overload, hepatitis, and alloimmunization. Despite these problems, children with Cooley's anemia fare better if their hemoglobin is maintained at greater than 90 g/L (9 g/dL). In view of the increased demands of the hyperplastic marrow, it is reasonable to maintain these patients on a daily supplement of folic acid. Since splenic sequestration contributes to shortened red blood cell survival, many patients derive some benefit from splenectomy. The prevention and treatment of iron overload is a continuing concern in these patients. Continuous subcutaneous injection of desferrioxamine permits the mobilization and excretion of significant amounts of iron and, when administered over a prolonged period, can prevent or retard the development of chronic iron toxicity.

Considerations of genetic counseling and antenatal diagnosis are as relevant in the *prevention* of β thalassemia major as they are for sickle cell anemia (see above). Because of linkages between β thalassemias and restriction enzyme polymorphisms, prenatal diagnosis can often be made by DNA analysis of amniotic fluid cells.

However, in some cases it is necessary to take the risk of obtaining fetal red blood cells for globin chain synthesis measurements.

REFERENCES

ADAMS JG, HONIG GR: *Human Hemoglobin Genetics*. New York, Springer Verlag, 1986

BUNN HF, FORGET BG: *Hemoglobin: Molecular, Genetic and Clinical Aspects*. Philadelphia, Saunders, 1986

CASTLE WB: From man to molecule and back to mankind. Semin Hematol 13:159, 1976

CHARACHE S: Advances in the understanding of sickle cell anemia. Hosp Pract 21:173, 182, 1986

EATON WA, HOFRICHTER J: Hemoglobin S gelation and sickle cell disease. Blood 70:1245, 1987

EMBURY S: The clinical pathophysiology of sickle cell disease. Ann Rev Med 37:36, 1986

KAN YW: Thalassemia: Molecular mechanism and detection. Am J Hum Genet 38:4, 1986

NIENHUIS AW et al: Advances in thalassemia research. Blood 63:738, 1984

OLD JM et al: First trimester fetal diagnosis for haemoglobinopathies. Lancet 2:763, 1986

SCHECHTER AN, BUNN HF: What determines severity in sickle cell disease. N Engl J Med 306:295, 1982

SERJEANT GR: *The Clinical Features of Sickle Cell Disease*. New York, American Elsevier, 1986

WEATHERALL DJ, CLEGG JB: *The Thalassemia Syndromes*. Oxford, Blackwell, 1982

296 THE LEUKEMIAS

RICHARD CHAMPLIN / DAVID W. GOLDE

The leukemias are a heterogeneous group of neoplasms arising from the malignant transformation of hematopoietic (blood-forming) cells. Leukemic cells proliferate primarily in the bone marrow and lymphoid tissues where they interfere with normal hematopoiesis and immunity. Ultimately they emigrate into the peripheral blood and infiltrate other tissues.

Leukemias are classified according to the cell types primarily involved (*myeloid* or *lymphoid*) and as *acute* or *chronic* based upon the natural history of the disease. Acute leukemias have a rapid clinical course, resulting in death within a matter of months without effective treatment, whereas chronic leukemias have a more prolonged natural history. This chapter will cover acute lymphocytic leukemia (ALL), acute myelogenous leukemia (AML), chronic lymphocytic leukemia (CLL), and hairy cell leukemia. Chronic myelogenous leukemia (CML) is discussed in Chap. 297.

ETIOLOGY The cause of leukemia is not known in most patients, although both genetic and environmental factors may be important. There is a high concordance rate among identical twins if acute leukemia develops in the first year of life, and families with an excessive incidence of leukemia have been identified. Acute leukemia occurs with an increased frequency in a variety of congenital disorders, including Down's, Bloom's, Klinefelter's, Fanconi's, and the Wiskott-Aldrich syndromes.

Environmental factors are also known to play a role in the etiology of leukemia. Ionizing radiation causes leukemia in experimental animals, and there is a clear relationship between such exposure and the development of leukemia in humans. For example, individuals with occupational radiation exposure, patients receiving radiation therapy, or Japanese survivors of the atomic bomb explosions have a predictable and dose-related increased incidence of leukemia. Radiation exposure increases the risk of developing CML, AML, and possibly ALL, but there is no known relationship to CLL or to hairy cell leukemia. Chemicals such as benzene and other aromatic hydrocarbons have also been associated with the development of AML. Treatment with alkylating agents and other chemotherapeutic drugs also leads to an increased incidence of AML.

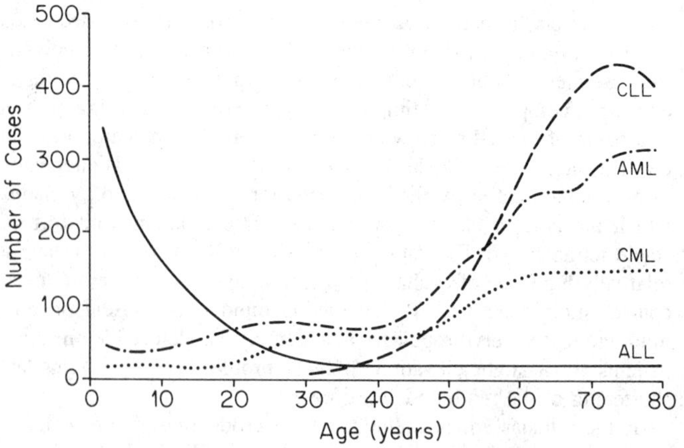

FIGURE 296-1 Age-related incidence of various forms of leukemia: ALL = acute lymphoblastic leukemia, AML = acute myelogenous leukemia, CLL = chronic lymphocytic leukemia, CML = chronic myelogenous leukemia. *(From Surveillance and Mortality Data 1973–1977, U.S. Department of Health and Human Resources.)*

While leukemias induced by retroviruses (RNA viruses) have been studied in laboratory animals for many years, it was not until recently that a viral etiology was established for a form of human leukemia. A unique human retrovirus, referred to as human T-cell leukemia virus I (HTLV-I) (see Chap. 134) has recently been identified as causing adult T-cell leukemia (ATL), an aggressive malignancy composed of mature T-lymphoid cells. A related virus, HTLV-II, has been isolated from cells of patients with rare and poorly defined chronic T-cell leukemias. Adult T-cell leukemia is endemic in southwestern Japan and parts of the Caribbean and central Africa. Except for the HTLV family, no virus has been causally associated with the more common human acute and chronic leukemias.

INCIDENCE AND PREVALENCE The incidence of all leukemias is approximately 13 per 100,000 people per year, and the age-related incidence of the various forms of leukemia is shown in Fig. 296-1. The incidence of both acute and chronic leukemias is somewhat higher in men than in women. ALL is primarily a disease of children and young adults, whereas AML occurs at all ages. CLL and hairy cell leukemia tend to occur in the elderly.

There have been several epidemiologic reports of case clustering of leukemias within communities and even in successive occupants of the same house. The bulk of evidence, however, indicates that the common forms of acute and chronic leukemias are not contagious and the incidence of leukemia is not increased among close contacts, such as marital partners or in the offspring of women who develop leukemia during pregnancy. The clear exception is ATL caused by HTLV-I. The virus may be passed in blood products and from infected to uninfected individuals.

PATHOPHYSIOLOGY Acute leukemia is characterized by proliferation of immature myeloid or lymphoid cells. The leukemia arises following malignant transformation of a single hematopoietic or lymphoid progenitor, followed by cellular replication and expansion of the transformed clone. The most prominent characteristic of the neoplastic cells in acute leukemia is a defect in maturation beyond the myeloblast or promyelocyte level in AML and the lymphoblast level in ALL. Leukemic cells accumulate in the bone marrow due both to excessive proliferation and to a defect in terminal maturation. The failure to mature to nonreplicating end cells is the major factor leading to the accumulation of leukemic cells in AML. The leukemic cells proliferate primarily in the bone marrow, circulate in the blood, and may infiltrate into other tissues such as lymph nodes, liver, spleen, skin, viscera, and the central nervous system.

The cellular blood elements are derived from pluripotent and committed hematopoietic stem cells which reside in the bone marrow.

Leukemic transformation may occur in cells at several levels of differentiation. In some patients with AML who are heterozygous for glucose-6-phosphate dehydrogenase (G6PD) isoenzymes, the granulocytes, macrophages, erythrocytes, and megakaryocytes all contain the single G6PD isoenzyme present in the leukemic cells, suggesting that these cells are derived from the malignant clone and that leukemic transformation involved a pluripotent stem cell. In other AML patients, only granulocytes and/or macrophages appear monoclonal, and in these patients, transformation may have occurred at the level of the committed granulocytic-macrophage progenitor.

The mechanism of neoplastic transformation producing leukemia is poorly understood but involves a fundamental alteration of DNA conferring hereditable malignant characteristics to the transformed cell and its progeny. A neoplastic phenotype can be induced in nonmalignant cells in vitro by transfer (transfection) of DNA from the leukemic cells. In animals, leukemias can be induced by retroviruses which either carry a transforming gene (viral oncogene) or integrate into specific sites in DNA causing activation of cellular proto-oncogenes (insertional mutagenesis). The role of oncogenes in the pathogenesis of neoplasia is discussed in Chap. 10. With sensitive techniques, clonal cytogenetic abnormalities can be detected in most patients with acute and chronic leukemias. A wide range of cytogenetic abnormalities is associated with the various forms of leukemias, and distinctive nonrandom chromosomal abnormalities are associated with AML, ALL, and CLL, as shown in Table 296-1. Chromosomal rearrangements in leukemic cells may alter the structure or regulation of cellular oncogenes, producing quantitative or qualitative changes in their gene products, which may play a role in initiating or maintaining the leukemic state. Most data suggest the development of leukemia is a multistep process. In many cases, acute leukemia develops in patients with a preexisting myelodysplastic or myeloproliferative disorder.

The pathophysiology of bone marrow failure in leukemia is complex. Pancytopenia is typically present and results at least in part from physical replacement of the normal precursor cells by leukemic cells. Some patients with acute leukemia and pancytopenia have a hypocellular bone marrow indicating that marrow failure is not simply due to overcrowding by leukemic cells. Leukemic cells may directly inhibit normal hematopoiesis via cell-mediated or humoral mechanisms. Alternatively, leukemic cells may occupy critical niches in the bone marrow (stromal) microenvironment and interfere with normal cellular interactions. Normal hematopoietic stem cells do remain in the bone marrow and are capable of proliferating and restoring hematopoiesis following effective antileukemic treatment.

Some patients develop AML after a preleukemic syndrome. The preleukemic and myelodysplastic syndromes are a heterogeneous group of disorders, and the nomenclature describing them is confusing. These syndromes generally occur in middle-aged or elderly patients. Included under the heading of myelodysplastic syndromes are refractory anemia with excess blasts, chronic myelomonocytic leukemia, and acquired idiopathic sideroblastic anemia. The term *preleukemia* should be reserved for a recognizable syndrome of hematopoietic dysfunction that typically precedes the classic findings of AML. This syndrome is usually characterized by a picture of ineffective hematopoiesis with anemia, thrombocytopenia, and sometimes granulocytopenia associated with a hypercellular, dysplastic bone marrow. In preleukemia, the leukemic clone is already established, and usually there is progressive impairment of hematopoiesis and accumulation of blasts. Megaloblastic hematopoiesis is common, and folate or vitamin B_{12} deficiency must be ruled out. Cytogenetic abnormalities are frequent; the most common chromosomal abnormalities are 5q−, −5, −7, and trisomy 8. When 5q− exists as the sole abnormality, the patient usually presents with refractory anemia associated with mild thrombocytosis. This disorder, referred to as the 5q− syndrome, usually does not progress to acute leukemia. Many patients with preleukemic or myelodysplastic syndromes never develop overt AML but die from complications of bone marrow failure. Smoldering AML refers to a syndrome in which the diagnostic features of acute leukemia are present, but the disease follows an indolent or subacute course. This disorder also tends to occur in elderly patients.

TABLE 296-1 Chromosomal abnormalities associated with acute leukemias

Abnormalities	Leukemia subtype	Relative prognosis
AML		
t(8;21)	M2 (myelocytic)	Good
+8	M1, M2, M4, M5	—
t(15;17)	M3 (promyelocytic)	Good if remission is achieved
t(9;11)	M5(monocytic)	Poor
inv 16	AML usually M4 with eosinophilia	Good
t(6;9)	AML with basophilia	—
5q−, −5, −7	AML following preleukemic syndrome or treatment-related leukemia	Poor
Ph[1], t(9;22)	Occasionally present in M1, M2, M4, M5, M6; must distinguish from CML blast crisis	Poor
ALL		
Hyperdiploidy	L1, L2	Good
6 q−	L1, L2	Good
14q+	L1, L2	—
t(8;14)	L3 (B-cell)	Poor
Ph[1], t(9;22)	L1, L2	Poor
t(4;11)	L2 (or M4 form AML)	Poor
CLL		
+12	B-cell type	Good
+12, 14 q+	B-cell type	Poor
+12, + other abnormalities	B-cell type	Poor
t(11;14)	B-cell type	Poor

ACUTE LEUKEMIAS: ACUTE LYMPHOCYTIC LEUKEMIA (ALL) AND ACUTE MYELOGENOUS LEUKEMIA (AML)

PATHOLOGY AND CLASSIFICATION The diagnosis of acute leukemia requires the demonstration of leukemic cells in the bone marrow, peripheral blood, or extramedullary tissues. The bone marrow is typically hypercellular with a monomorphic infiltration of leukemic blasts and a marked reduction in normal bone marrow elements. It is critical to distinguish ALL from AML since these two diseases differ in natural history, prognosis, and response to various therapeutic agents.

Acute lymphocytic leukemia can be identified and classified on the basis of morphology and immunologic phenotype related to the stage of lymphoid differentiation. The leukemic lymphoblasts in ALL are generally smaller than myeloblasts (10 to 15 μm in diameter) and typically have only a thin rim of agranular cytoplasm. The nucleus may be round or convoluted (see Fig. A5-24). Three morphologic subtypes are included in the French-American-British classification: L1 cells are small and homogeneous with a regular nuclear membrane and a small nucleolus. L2 cells are larger and have a lower nuclear-cytoplasmic ratio with more pleomorphic size and shape. L2 cells typically have one or more prominent nucleoli. The L3 form of ALL is uncommon, occurring in less than 5 percent of cases; the leukemic cells in this variant contain large vesicular nuclei with basophilic, often vacuolated cytoplasm. L3 cells have a high mitotic index and represent the leukemic form of Burkitt's lymphoma.

Leukemic lymphoblasts in more than 90 percent of patients with

ALL contain a nuclear enzyme *terminal deoxynucleotidyl transferase* (Tdt) which is only rarely present in AML cells. An exception is the L3 subtype, which is Tdt-negative. The functional role of this enzyme is not known. Tdt is normally found in 1 percent of normal bone marrow cells and is present in immature T and B lymphocytes; it is absent in mature lymphocytes, hairy cell leukemia, and CLL. The leukemic cells from approximately half of patients with ALL react with the periodic acid Schiff stain showing blocklike inclusions of glycogen. Lymphoblasts do not contain granulocytic or monocytic lysosomal enzymes and therefore do not react with cytochemical stains for peroxidase, Sudan black, and nonspecific esterase.

Several forms of ALL can be defined based upon immunologic phenotype. Approximately 60 percent of cases are termed *common ALL;* the cells are Tdt-positive and have the common ALL antigen (CALLA) but do not express surface membrane immunoglobulin or T-cell antigens. These cells are usually derived from precursors of the B-cell lineage, as they may express immature B-cell antigens and have immunoglobulin gene rearrangements. CALLA is not a leukemia-specific antigen, since it is present on immature lymphoid cells including approximately 1 percent of cells in the normal bone marrow. About 20 percent of cases of ALL are of the *T-cell type,* where the T lymphoblasts express the E-rosette receptor or other T-lymphocyte-related antigens; these cells are Tdt-positive, usually CALLA-negative, and stain positively for acid phosphatase. T-cell ALL typically occurs in adolescent males and is frequently associated with a high leukocyte count and an anterior mediastinal mass. Less than 5 percent of cases of ALL are *B-cell type.* The cells in this variant produce a monoclonal immunoglobulin which is bound to the surface membrane and have L3 morphology. In B-cell ALL, the cells typically contain the t(8;14) chromosomal abnormality characteristic of Burkitt's lymphoma. Approximately 15 percent of cases of ALL are termed *null cell type* because the cells do not elaborate CALLA or T- or B-cell antigens.

The leukemic cells in AML are 12 to 20 μm in diameter, larger than lymphoblasts, and have a lower nuclear-cytoplasmic ratio. The leukemic myeloblasts usually have discrete nuclear chromatin and multiple nucleoli. The presence of Auer rods, abnormal primary granules, in the cytoplasm of leukemic cells is diagnostic of AML; these inclusions are present in 10 to 20 percent of patients with AML (see Fig. A5-22). Dysplastic morphologic abnormalities may be prominent in residual granulocytic, erythroid, and megakaryocytic cells. Cytochemical stains are often helpful in distinguishing AML from ALL and in classifying the pathologic subtypes of AML. Myeloperoxidase, α-naphthyl-AS-D-chloracetate esterase, and Sudan black are primarily present in cells undergoing granulocytic differentiation. Nonspecific esterase (α-naphthyl butyrate esterase) stains cells of the monocyte-macrophage lineage. A number of cell surface antigens present in AML cells have also been described. These stains and markers, however, may be negative in leukemias of undifferentiated cells.

A collaborative French-American-British group has divided AML into seven pathologic subtypes based upon the degree of differentiation and maturation of the predominant cells toward granulocytes, monocytes, erythrocytes, or megakaryocytes. The characteristics of each subtype are summarized in Table 296-2. There are only subtle differences in the clinical features of each subtype. The acute promyelocytic subtype (M3) is frequently associated with disseminated intravascular coagulation (DIC) induced by thromboplastic material released by the leukemic cells; DIC is usually present at the time of diagnosis and may be markedly exacerbated during chemotherapy. Acute myelomonocytic leukemia (M4) and acute monocytic leukemia (M5) are more likely than other subtypes to have extramedullary involvement of the skin, gingiva, central nervous system, and other tissues.

It is often difficult to distinguish the acute myelogenous leukemia without maturation (M1) from the L2 form of ALL by morphology alone. In these cases additional studies including cytochemical stains and analysis of myeloid and lymphoid antigens are required. Electron microscopy may be helpful in some cases to demonstrate small numbers of promyelocytic granules in cells that appear undifferentiated by light microscopy. Some patients appear to have a *biphenotypic acute leukemia.* In these patients, subpopulations of malignant cells contain both myeloid and lymphoid markers. These cells may represent leukemias of primitive pluripotent stem cells, or more likely they result from aberrant gene expression in a transformed myeloid or lymphoid progenitor.

CLINICAL AND LABORATORY FEATURES ALL and AML share many clinical features. In the majority of patients, the initial symptoms of acute leukemia are present for less than 3 months. A preleukemic syndrome can be identified in approximately 25 percent

TABLE 296-2 Morphologic subtypes of AML

			Reactivity with special stains		
Subtype	% of AML	Morphology	Peroxidase Sudan black	Nonspecific esterase	Periodic acid Schiff
M1 AML without maturation	20	Few if any azurophilic granules	+/−	+/−	−
M2 AML with maturation	30	Blasts with promyelocytic granules, Auer rods may be present	+ + +	+/−	+
M3 Promyelocytic leukemia	5	Hypergranular promyelocytes often with multiple Auer rods per cell	+ + +	+	+
M4 Acute myelomonocytic leukemia	30	Monocytoid-appearing cells in peripheral blood associated with serum lysozyme	+ +	+ + +	+ +/+
M5 Acute monocytic leukemia	10	Two subtypes identified: (a) undifferentiated; (b) differentiated associated with serum lysozyme	+/−	+ + +	+ +/+
M6 Acute erythroleukemia	5	Predominance of erythroblasts and markedly dysplastic erythroid precursors	−	−	+ +
M7 Acute megakaryocytic leukemia	5	Undifferentiated blasts react with antiplatelet antibodies and contain platelet peroxidase	−	+/−	+

of patients with AML; in these patients, anemia and other cytopenias are usually present for months to years preceding the development of overt leukemia.

Patients with ALL and AML may present with pancytopenia without circulating blasts, with a normal leukocyte count, or with marked leukocytosis. Leukostasis due to occlusion of the microcirculation by leukemic blast cells can lead to hypoperfusion of vital tissues, most commonly lung and brain. Leukostasis becomes increasingly common when the number of circulating blasts exceeds 100×10^9 per liter and is seen more often with the larger blast cells in AML than in ALL. Patients may complain of manifestations of anemia such as pallor, easy fatigability, and dyspnea on mild exertion. The metabolic activity of large numbers of blasts can lead to artifactual results in laboratory tests, especially glucose and potassium concentrations and arterial blood gas analysis.

Bleeding is a major problem in patients with acute leukemia and is primarily related to thrombocytopenia. Coagulation defects may also be present. In some patients, megakaryocytes are derived from the leukemic clone and produce platelets with abnormal function. Petechiae and easy bruisability are common. Hemorrhage becomes increasingly common when the platelet count is less than 20×10^9 per liter, typically occurring from oral (particularly gingiva) and gastrointestinal mucous membranes. Spontaneous bleeding involving the central nervous system, lungs, or other viscera may also occur.

Infection is a frequent complication of acute leukemia. The incidence of infection is inversely related to the number of circulating neutrophils and becomes a major risk in patients with granulocyte counts less than 0.5×10^9 per liter. Neutrophils derived from leukemic progenitors may also function abnormally, further compromising host defenses. The leukemia and its treatment cause a breakdown of mucosal barriers, and systemic infections usually develop from organisms colonizing the skin, throat, and gastrointestinal tract. Common sites of infections in patients with acute leukemia include the skin, gingiva, perirectal tissues, lung, and urinary tract. Septicemia often occurs without an apparent source. Gram-negative bacteria, gram-positive cocci, and *Candida* species are frequent pathogens.

Hepatomegaly and splenomegaly due to leukemic infiltration are present in approximately one-half to three-fourths of patients with ALL and a minority of patients with AML. This visceral involvement can produce symptoms of nausea, abdominal fullness, or early satiety. Lymphadenopathy is more common in ALL than in AML. An anterior mediastinal mass is usually present in patients with the T-cell variant of ALL, and rarely occurs in other forms of ALL or in AML. Acute leukemia may infiltrate into extramedullary tissues such as the skin, lung, eye, nasopharynx, or kidneys. Testicular involvement is particularly common in males with ALL. Soft tissue masses of leukemic cells, "chloromas," can develop in any location. Occasionally, extramedullary leukemia can precede detectable involvement in the bone marrow.

Symptoms related to the expanding malignant cell mass, such as bone pain and sternal tenderness, occur in approximately half of patients with acute leukemia; osteolytic lesions are rare. Renal abnormalities can develop as a result of leukemic infiltration, ureteral obstruction by uric acid stones or enlarged lymph nodes, urate nephropathy, or from infectious or hemorrhagic complications. Gastrointestinal symptoms of early satiety, distention, and constipation may result from organomegaly or from leukemic infiltration or bleeding into the bowel and other viscera.

In acute leukemia, the neoplastic cells may infiltrate into the subarachnoid space, causing leukemic meningitis or direct involvement of the brain or spinal cord parenchyma. Neurologic involvement is unusual at the time of diagnosis, but the central nervous system is a frequent site of relapse, particularly in patients with ALL. The first symptoms of leukemic meningitis are usually headache and nausea. Papilledema, cranial nerve palsies, seizures, and altered mentation develop with disease progression. Cytocentrifuge preparations of cerebrospinal fluid (CSF) characteristically reveal leukemic blast cells, an elevated CSF protein, and reduced glucose concentrations.

Patients with acute leukemia often develop metabolic abnormalities. Hyponatremia and hypokalemia are common due to renal tubular abnormalities induced by lysozyme or other products of the leukemic cells. The serum lactic acid dehydrogenase (LDH) level may be increased. Hyperuricemia may be present due to accelerated turnover of cells with increased purine release, and lactic acidosis rarely occurs in patients with a large burden of leukemic cells.

TREATMENT OF ACUTE LEUKEMIA: GENERAL CONSIDERATIONS The growth of leukemic cells follows a Gompertzian growth curve with near exponential growth at a lower cell mass and progressive slowing of the growth rate at higher leukemic cell burdens. The leukemic mass is usually between 10^{11} to 10^{12} cells at the time of diagnosis. Chemotherapeutic agents produce a fractional cell kill, that is, a percentage of tumor cells (not an absolute number) is killed with each course of treatment. Most chemotherapeutic regimens employed for acute leukemias are probably capable of a 3 to 5 log kill, resulting in the elimination of 99.9 to 99.999 percent of the leukemia cells. Another potential effect of some chemotherapeutic drugs is to induce maturation of the leukemic cells to mature nonproliferating cells. When the leukemia cell mass is reduced below approximately 10^9 cells, leukemia can no longer be detected in the blood or bone marrow, and the patient appears to be in complete remission. The clinical criteria for complete remission include (1) less than 5 percent blasts in the bone marrow and absence of leukemic cells in the peripheral blood, (2) the restoration of normal peripheral blood counts, and (3) the absence of physical findings attributable to extramedullary involvement of the leukemia. If no further treatment is given, however, the residual leukemic cells will proliferate, leading to relapse.

The treatment of acute leukemia is divided into distinct phases. *Remission induction chemotherapy* is the most critical phase. Intensive systemic chemotherapy is administered with the goal of reducing the leukemic cell mass below the level of detection. After remission is achieved, additional systemic chemotherapy must be given to further reduce the leukemic cell mass and, ideally, eradicate the leukemia. Intensive chemotherapy administered immediately following remission induction is referred to as *consolidation* or *early intensification* treatment. Lower dose chemotherapy that is generally continued over several years is referred to as *maintenance treatment*. Intensive chemotherapy administered more than 6 months after remission induction is termed *late intensification*. Another aspect of treatment involves local chemotherapy or radiation to frequent sites of relapse which are considered to be sanctuary sites, such as the central nervous system where systemic treatment may fail to eradicate the disease. The value of these forms of treatment for ALL and AML will be discussed separately.

Supportive care The supportive care of patients with pancytopenia is a critical aspect of the treatment of acute leukemia. This primarily involves the appropriate administration of blood products and management of infections.

Adequate levels of hemoglobin can usually be maintained with transfusions of packed red blood cells. An adequate number of circulating platelets can initially be attained by transfusions of platelets from unselected donors, but some transfused patients eventually develop antiplatelet antibodies which shorten platelet survival and render the patient unresponsive to further platelet transfusions. Patients who fail to respond to transfusions of platelets from unselected donors may respond to platelets from an HLA-identical donor. The risk of spontaneous hemorrhage is directly related to the degree of thrombocytopenia. It is generally advisable to transfuse platelets to maintain the platelet count above 20×10^9 per liter. Also, uterine bleeding should be minimized in menstruating women with thrombocytopenia by administering an anovulatory agent.

The potential therapeutic benefit of granulocyte transfusions has been extensively studied in patients receiving treatment for acute leukemia. Most data indicate that survival is not improved by granulocyte transfusions either to prevent infections or to treat documented infections, and that their routine use cannot be recommended. The major limitations in the use of granulocyte transfusions are the current technical difficulty in collecting sufficient numbers of granulocytes from normal donors and the adverse effects associated with their transfusion such as fever, leukoagglutination, pulmonary infiltrates, and transmission of cytomegalovirus (CMV) and other infections.

The prevention and treatment of infections is of critical importance in the management of patients with acute leukemia. Since most infections are caused by organisms colonizing the skin and gastrointestinal tract, a variety of approaches have been evaluated to suppress the endogenous flora in these sites. Most centers recommend the use of face masks, careful hand washing, oral nonabsorbable antibiotics, and reverse isolation for granulocytopenic patients. The development of bacterial and fungal infections may be delayed or avoided by these measures.

Granulocytopenic patients who develop fever or other signs of infection require prompt evaluation and treatment. Fever is usually due to a bacterial, fungal, or viral infection. Gram-negative sepsis is common in this setting and may be rapidly fatal. Granulocytopenic patients with unexplained fever or overt infections should be evaluated and receive empiric treatment for a presumed bacterial infection until a definitive diagnosis can be established. A combination of broad-spectrum antibiotics, such as an aminoglycoside or a third-generation cephalosporin in combination with a semisynthetic penicillin, should be employed and modified when the results of bacterial and fungal cultures are available. Systemic fungal infections are also common in granulocytopenic patients with leukemia and should be suspected in patients who fail to respond to antibiotic or who respond and develop recurrent fever. Definitive diagnosis of fungal infections may be difficult, and a therapeutic trial of amphotericin B is often indicated. The problem of infections in the immunocompromised host is discussed in Chap. 82.

TREATMENT OF ACUTE LYMPHOBLASTIC LEUKEMIA The treatment of ALL is one of the major successes in modern oncology. Forty years ago the disease was uniformly fatal and had a median survival of only 3 months. With current therapy, more than 50 percent of children with ALL achieve long-term remissions and probable cure. Adults and high-risk subgroups of children with ALL have a poorer prognosis, and long-term remissions are only achieved in a minority of patients. Therapy for ALL consists of three phases: (1) remission induction chemotherapy, (2) central nervous system prophylaxis, and (3) continuation (maintenance) chemotherapy.

The goal of remission induction chemotherapy is to eliminate all clinical signs and morphologic evidence of leukemia, as well as to restore normal bone marrow function. The intensity of treatment is important, because the duration of remission is prolonged by reducing the leukemic cell burden to the smallest possible fraction.

The combination of vincristine and prednisone plus either L-asparaginase or daunorubicin induces complete remissions in over 90 percent of children with ALL within 4 weeks. Some patients with persistent leukemia may achieve remission with 2 to 4 additional weeks of treatment with the same or alternate drugs. Failure to achieve remission can be attributed primarily to the development of drug resistance, severe infections, or central nervous system (CNS) leukemia.

In patients who achieve remission, prophylactic treatment to the CNS is required to prevent leukemic meningitis. The rationale for this treatment is based on the hypothesis that circulating leukemic cells infiltrate into the CNS and cerebrospinal fluid early in the course of the disease. Since the drugs used in remission induction in ALL generally penetrate poorly into the cerebrospinal fluid, these leukemic cells are sheltered from the effects of systemic chemotherapy. Over the ensuing months these cells may proliferate, producing overt leukemic meningitis. Leukemic meningitis is the initial site of relapse in up to two-thirds of patients with ALL who do not receive prophylactic therapy. Prophylactic treatment to the CNS, instituted immediately after remission induction, has been successful in dramatically reducing the incidence of CNS relapse. Most centers employ 18- to 24-Gy whole-brain radiation in combination with intrathecal methotrexate. Cranial irradiation does produce subtle abnormalities in neurologic function, particularly in young children, and there is considerable interest in evaluating lower-dose radiotherapy regimens or alternative methods of CNS treatment. Preliminary data suggest that the combination of intrathecal and high-dose systemic methotrexate may provide adequate prophylactic treatment to the CNS.

Since patients in remission still harbor leukemia cells, further systemic treatment is required to prevent or delay leukemic relapse. The optimal approach to continuation therapy involves the administration of combination chemotherapy given in doses approaching maximal tolerance. As a rule, the drugs that are effective in inducing remission in ALL have not been useful in maintenance chemotherapy. The combination of 6-mercaptopurine and methotrexate is the most frequently employed maintenance regimen, but more intensive consolidation and maintenance regimens are required for adult patients and children with poor prognostic features.

The optimal duration of maintenance chemotherapy is unknown. Many patients can discontinue chemotherapy after 2 to 3 years and remain in long-term remission. Up to one-quarter of patients will relapse, however, after maintenance therapy is discontinued. It is not known whether maintenace therapy given for more than 3 years will further reduce the likelihood of relapse. Since there is currently no method to reliably detect small numbers of residual leukemic cells, there is no objective means to determine when therapy can be safely discontinued.

Complications of therapy for ALL Chemotherapy-induced myelosuppression and immunosuppression are inevitable side effects of the treatment for ALL. The chemotherapy directed toward the leukemic lymphoblasts also affects normal T and B lymphocytes, resulting in lymphocytopenia and immunodeficiency. Peripheral blood B cells generally recover to normal levels within several months after treatment is discontinued, but T-cell numbers and function may remain depressed for up to 1 year. *Pneumocystis carinii* pneumonia can occur while patients are in remission; trimethoprim-sulfamethoxazole prophylaxis is effective in preventing this complication. Growth in children is somewhat retarded during the administration of chemotherapy. Catch-up growth generally occurs once therapy is discontinued, and most children ultimately attain near normal height and weight. Sterility may result from treatment with most chemotherapeutic agents and irradiation. Gonadal function may recover after a prolonged interval. The gonads in prepubertal patients are relatively resistant to the effects of chemotherapy, and most patients undergo normal puberty after therapy is discontinued.

Prognosis in ALL The factors most affecting prognosis are age, the leukocyte count at the time of diagnosis, and cytogenetic abnormalities. Children between the ages of 3 and 9 years with white blood counts less than 10×10^9 per liter have the best prognosis; 50 to 70 percent achieve long-term survival and probable cure with current treatment. Older patients and those with higher leukocyte counts have a poorer prognosis. Fewer than 30 percent of adults with ALL are long-term survivors in most series, and it is uncertain whether the maintenance therapy which is effective in children is of benefit for adults. Males have a worse prognosis than females, due in part to the problem of testicular relapse. Children with the L1 morphologic subtype have a better prognosis than those with the L2 form, but this is probably not true in adults. Patients with T-cell ALL tend to have a poorer prognosis than the CALLA subgroup. These patients are generally older and present with a high white blood count, and it is uncertain if T-cell type, per se, is an independent poor prognostic factor. The B-cell (L3) variant of ALL has the worst prognosis.

Chromosomal abnormalities provide independent prognostic information. Approximately one-half of the patients with ALL have detectable cytogenetic abnormalities, including hypodiploidy, pseudodiploidy, or hyperdiploidy. A number of nonrandom chromosomal abnormalities are associated with ALL. Approximately 10 percent of patients with ALL have the Philadelphia (Ph^1) chromosome, an abnormality typical of chronic myelogenous leukemia. Associated with ALL, and possibly with hybrid (biphenotypic) leukemias, is t(4;11). Patients with pseudodiploidy, particularly t(4;11) and t(9;22), have a poor prognosis, while patients with hyperdiploidy have a better prognosis.

Remission and survival rates in adult patients with ALL (those over 15 years of age) are significantly lower than for children with the same disease. Remission induction rates in adults and high-risk children are generally between 50 to 70 percent following treatment with vincristine, prednisone, and daunorubicin; the median duration of remission is 10 to 12 months, and the 5-year survival rate is 10 to 30 percent with standard maintenance chemotherapy. Several centers have reported improved results in high-risk children and in adults with more intensive, multiple-drug consolidation and maintenance programs, but the optimal therapy for high-risk forms of ALL is uncertain.

Treatment of recurrent ALL Leukemia may recur either in the bone marrow or in extramedullary sites. Patients who relapse while receiving maintenance therapy have a very poor prognosis with little possibility of a long-term second remission. Combination chemotherapy with a three- or four-drug regimen including vincristine, prednisone, L-asparaginase, and/or daunorubicin results in a second remission in 50 to 70 percent of these patients. Remission duration, however, is usually brief, and subsequent relapse is inevitable. Patients who relapse after discontinuation of maintenance therapy have a better prognosis. Second remissions can be induced in about 90 percent of these patients. Although most will relapse again, some have achieved long-term survival. These patients should probably have CNS prophylaxis repeated to prevent recurrent disease in this extramedullary site.

Meningeal leukemia is the most common site of extramedullary relapse in patients with ALL. Cranial irradiation plus intrathecal methotrexate alone or in combination with cytarabine is the standard therapy for CNS leukemia. Testicular relapse is common in male patients with ALL and may occur during or after cessation of maintenance therapy. The treatment of choice is irradiation of the affected testicle. Patients with extramedullary relapse involving the CNS, testes, or other tissues are at very high risk for subsequent relapse in the bone marrow. Systemic reinduction therapy is indicated and may prevent generalized relapse of ALL.

TREATMENT OF ACUTE MYELOGENOUS LEUKEMIA The initial goal in the treatment of AML is to induce a complete hematologic remission. The drugs active in AML have little selectivity for leukemic cells over their normal bone marrow counterparts. Induction of severe myelosuppression is necessary in order to achieve a complete remission. The two most active drugs are cytarabine and daunorubicin. The combination of these agents with or without 6-thioguanine results in a complete remission rate of 60 to 80 percent. Mitoxantrone or amsacrine may be substituted for daunorubicin. If residual leukemia is present 2 to 4 weeks after chemotherapy, the treatment is repeated. Patients who fail to enter remission with this approach have a poor prognosis.

Patients with AML who achieve complete remission still have a substantial number of residual leukemic cells. Further therapy is required to reduce and hopefully to eradicate these occult leukemia cells. The benefits of available forms of consolidation and maintenance treatment are controversial. The best results have been achieved in patients receiving one to three intensive cycles of consolidation chemotherapy. Median remission duration varies from 9 months to 2 years in most series. Ten to thirty percent of patients survive over 5 years free of disease, and most of these patients are probably cured. Better results have been reported in preliminary studies using very intensive consolidation regimens, including high-dose cytarabine alone or in combination with other drugs. The results of these studies suggest a benefit for patients receiving consolidation treatment when compared to historical controls, but these observations remain to be confirmed in prospectively controlled clinical trials.

Although some uncontrolled studies suggested that maintenance therapy with lower doses of these same agents or late intensification treatment improved remission duration, recent prospective controlled studies reported no benefit for patients receiving these forms of treatment. Current data suggest that the major benefit in therapy is achieved with intensive induction and consolidation treatment.

Most patients who achieve complete remission will ultimately relapse. At that point, the disease is usually much less responsive to therapy; only a minority of patients achieve a brief second remission, and median survival is 3 to 6 months.

Central nervous system leukemia in AML occurs in 10 to 20 percent of patients at some point in their disease, and most commonly develops in patients with monocytic (M5) or myelomonocytic (M4) subtypes. Unlike ALL, the CNS is rarely an isolated site of relapse in AML; CNS involvement usually occurs in the setting of systemic relapse. This may not be a biologically important leukemic sanctuary in patients with AML, and prophylactic treatment to the CNS has not improved remission duration or survival. Patients who develop meningeal leukemia are treated with cranial irradiation and intrathecal chemotherapy with cytarabine and/or methotrexate.

Prognostic factors in AML Chromosomal abnormalities in AML are of prognostic value; patients with abnormalities such as t(8;21), t(15;17), or inv 16 tend to have a relatively good prognosis, while −5, −7, t(9;22), and complex chromosomal abnormalities are associated with a poor prognosis.

Age is a major prognostic factor in many series; patients over 60 years of age are less likely to achieve complete remission. This group also tolerates intensive therapy poorly and is more difficult to support through the complications of pancytopenia. In addition, elderly patients are more likely to have leukemic cells with poor-risk chromosomal abnormalities such as −7, −5 and are more likely to have a defined preleukemic syndrome. However, elderly patients who do achieve remission have a similar remission duration and survival as younger patients. Since the major factor influencing survival is the achievement of complete remission, intensive chemotherapy should be administered to most elderly patients. Two controlled trials have shown that attenuated doses of daunorubicin in combination with full-dose cytarabine is less toxic and is as effective as higher dose regimens in elderly patients.

The leukemic subtype is of limited prognostic significance. Acute promyelocytic leukemia (M3) is typically associated with disseminated intravascular coagulation, and fatal CNS hemorrhage may complicate remission induction chemotherapy for this type of leukemia. Prophylactic heparin therapy is generally indicated during induction treatment to suppress DIC and prevent hemorrhagic complications. Heparin plus ϵ-aminocaproic acid is indicated in patients with excessive fibrinolysis. Patients with promyelocytic leukemia who do achieve remission appear to have a greater chance of long-term survival than other subgroups. Patients with monocytic or myelomonocytic leukemia may have a poorer prognosis than the M1 to M3 subgroups.

Patients with preleukemia evolving into AML or smoldering leukemia respond poorly to chemotherapy; less than half of these patients achieve complete remission. Such patients also tend to have prolonged bone marrow aplasia following treatment and often succumb to complications of pancytopenia. Patients who do achieve remission have a similar remission duration as patients with de novo AML, and intensive induction therapy is usually indicated. No treatment has been consistently effective during the preleukemic phase, and chemotherapy should be withheld until progressive overt leukemia develops. Low-dose cytarabine has been reported to be successful in occasional patients with preleukemia or smoldering AML; this therapy worsens cytopenias, and rare responses tend to be brief. An innovative approach to therapy for preleukemia involves agents such as retinoic acid which induce cellular maturation. A small number of patients with preleukemia (and progranulocytic leukemias) have had improvement in peripheral blood counts with retinoic acid therapy, but most patients fail to respond, and there is no evidence that survival is improved. Limited studies with hematopoietic hormones such as granulocyte-macrophage colony-stimulating factor (GM-CSF) suggest utility for this class of agents to improve hematopoiesis in preleukemia. Patients who develop acute leukemia after a preexisting myeloproliferative disorder or paroxysmal nocturnal hemoglobinuria usually have a poor prognosis.

Patients who receive cytotoxic chemotherapy with or without concomitant extensive radiation therapy have an increased risk of developing AML. Secondary or treatment-related leukemia is most commonly associated with prolonged therapy with alkylating agents, nitrosoureas, or procarbazine, and has been seen primarily in patients with Hodgkin's disease, multiple myeloma, and ovarian carcinoma. Almost all of the patients with treatment-related AML have chromosomal abnormalities, usually hypodiploidy with −5 and/or −7. These patients typically develop a preleukemic syndrome with pancytopenia several months before overt AML is recognized. They respond poorly to chemotherapy, and despite treatment, median survival is only 3 months after development of AML.

Other factors such as white blood and platelet counts, LDH level, and the presence of fever and hemorrhage have been reported to have prognostic importance. The impact of each of these variables is uncertain.

IMMUNOTHERAPY FOR ACUTE LEUKEMIAS Immunotherapy has been reported to be capable of suppressing small numbers of tumor cells in experimental animals. As such, immunotherapy has been evaluated to prevent leukemic relapse from the residual leukemic cells remaining after induction treatment in patients with ALL and AML. Unfortunately, clinical trials with nonspecific immune potentiating agents such as bacillus Calmette-Guérin (BCG), *Corynebacterium parvum*, or levamisole have not shown any benefit in prolonging the duration of remission. There are no convincing data to support the use of currently available immunotherapy in patients with either ALL or AML.

BONE MARROW TRANSPLANTATION FOR ACUTE LEUKEMIAS Bone marrow transplantation from an identical twin or an HLA-identical sibling donor is effective treatment for both ALL and AML. The objective of this approach is to administer very high doses of chemotherapy alone or with total-body irradiation, and then to rescue the patient from severe myelosuppression by the transplantation of bone marrow from a normal donor. In addition, the transplantation of allogeneic bone marrow may confer an immune-mediated graft-versus-leukemia effect. The current results with bone marrow transplantation are summarized in Table 296-3. Bone marrow transplantation is discussed in detail in Chap. 299.

Allogeneic bone marrow transplantation is associated with substantial risks. Approximately one-third of patients transplanted for leukemia will die from transplant-related complications including graft-versus-host disease, interstitial pneumonitis, and opportunistic infections. Most centers limit the use of bone marrow transplantation to patients under 45 years of age, since older patients generally have a poor outcome. Reports from several centers indicate that 10 to 15 percent of otherwise end-stage patients with refractory leukemia have achieved long-term disease-free survival and probable cure following bone marrow transplantation. Although only a small proportion of patients in this category benefit, the results compare favorably to those obtained with other forms of treatment.

These survival figures are substantially improved when bone marrow transplantation is performed during remission, the burden of leukemic cells is low, and the patients are in relatively good general condition. Because many children with ALL can achieve a prolonged initial remission with chemotherapy, bone marrow transplantation has generally been reserved for patients in second remission; in this group 30 to 60 percent have achieved prolonged survival with marrow transplantation. It is uncertain whether adults or children with high-risk forms of ALL should receive marrow transplants in first complete remission.

Approximately 30 percent of patients with AML transplanted in early relapse or second remission have achieved long-term survival. There is controversy as to whether patients with AML should receive allogeneic bone marrow transplantation or postremission chemotherapy while in first complete remission. Over 500 marrow transplants have been reported in this setting. It is clear that the risk of recurrent leukemia is lower following bone marrow transplantation than with postremission chemotherapy; however, bone marrow transplantation is more likely to be associated with fatal treatment complications. Overall 3- to 5-year survival is 40 to 60 percent with bone marrow transplantation compared with 10 to 50 percent survival achieved with optimal chemotherapy. Patient age is a major prognostic factor with bone marrow transplantation; the best results have been reported in children and young adults. Although young patients probably have better results with bone marrow transplantation than with chemotherapy, it is uncertain whether this is true for patients over 30 years of age. One major limitation of bone marrow transplantation as a general therapeutic approach is that only a minority of patients are currently eligible; most patients are either too old to be considered or lack an HLA-identical related donor. Recently several large registries of potential unrelated donors have been formed and bone marrow transplants from unrelated histocompatible donors are under active evaluation.

Autologous bone marrow transplantation has also been evaluated in patients with acute leukemia. With this approach, remission bone marrow is collected and cryopreserved. The patient may then receive intensive chemoradiotherapy followed by reinfusion of the cryopreserved bone marrow. Since remission bone marrow is likely to contain small numbers of residual leukemic cells, many centers have treated the collected marrow with antileukemic monoclonal antibodies or chemotherapy prior to cryopreservation. Selected patients with ALL and AML transplanted in first or second remission have achieved prolonged survival, but further studies are required to critically assess the efficacy of autologous marrow transplantation for acute leukemia. Furthermore the efficacy of ex vivo treatment of the collected bone marrow to eradicate contaminating malignant cells has not been conclusively demonstrated.

SUMMARY AND FUTURE DIRECTIONS IN ACUTE LEUKEMIA Effective induction chemotherapy capable of inducing remission in most patients with ALL and AML is now available, but long-term survival has been achieved in only a minority of patients. In the next decade, the focus of clinical research should be toward measures to prolong the duration of remission. Innovative methods of consolidation treatment with intensive chemotherapy or high-dose chemoradiotherapy and bone marrow transplantation must be evaluated for their effect on remission duration and survival. It will also be important to develop effective but less toxic approaches for favorable prognostic groups such as children with low-risk forms of ALL to improve the quality of life in long-term survivors. Innovative

TABLE 296-3 Representative results of bone marrow transplantation (BMT) compared with conventional chemotherapy for AML and ALL

	Survival >3 years, %	
	BMT	Chemotherapy
ALL		
First remission	30–60	20–70*
Second remission	30–50	<10
Third remission or relapse	10–20	0
AML		
First remission	40–60	10–50
Second remission or early relapse	30	<10
Third remission or relapse	10–20	0

* Best results in children with low white blood count.

new therapies are required for poor-risk groups, particularly the elderly and patients with preleukemic syndromes.

Sensitive techniques to detect residual leukemia during morphologic complete remission must also be developed to help guide the intensity and duration of treatment. Most importantly, new and effective drugs are required with selectivity toward leukemic cells which would spare the host from morbidity and mortality attendant to the currently available agents.

CHRONIC LYMPHOCYTIC LEUKEMIA

Chronic lymphocytic leukemia (CLL) is a hematologic neoplasm characterized by the accumulation of mature-appearing lymphocytes in the peripheral blood associated with infiltration of the bone marrow, spleen, and lymph nodes. The disease is uncommon before the fourth decade of life and is usually seen in patients over 50 years of age. It is the most common form of chronic leukemia in the United States but is rare in Orientals. CLL is more frequent in males than females.

CLL represents a clonal expansion of neoplastic B lymphocytes in more than 95 percent of cases. These cells commonly have trisomy 12 alone or with additional chromosomal abnormalities. Clonality has also been demonstrated by expression of a single light chain (κ or λ) or immunoglobulin idiotype specificity. In less than 5 percent of cases, CLL may be due to an expansion of T lymphocytes. An unusual type of T-cell CLL is seen in patients with ataxia-telangiectasia and is often associated with a translocation of genetic material between the number 14 chromosomes (t14;14). Other cytogenetic abnormalities occurring in CLL are listed in Table 296-1.

The diagnosis of CLL can usually be made on the basis of physical examination and a review of the peripheral blood smear. Leukocytosis is present, and the malignant cells characteristically appear as morphologically normal small lymphocytes (see Fig. A5-23). They have markers of B lymphocytes. In most cases a monoclonal immunoglobulin can be demonstrated on the cell surface, although immunofluorescent staining is usually weak. Monoclonal surface IgM with or without IgD is characteristically present, and a small amount of this IgM paraprotein can often be detected in the serum with sensitive techniques. The CLL cells also have receptors for the Fc portion of IgG, and complement receptors may or may not be present. Most patients develop some degree of hypogammaglobulinemia. Approximately 5 percent of patients have the T-cell form of CLL. The neoplastic cells form rosettes with sheep erythrocytes and contain other T-cell surface markers. T-cell CLL cannot usually be distinguished from B-cell CLL morphologically.

It is important to distinguish early CLL from reactive lymphocytosis in asymptomatic patients. In reactive lymphocytosis, the cells are polyclonal and predominantly T lymphocytes, whereas in CLL they are usually B cells. The demonstration of monoclonal surface membrane immunoglobulin unambiguously defines a B-cell lymphocytosis as neoplastic. T-cell CLL must be distinguished from Sézary syndrome where the cells have a characteristic lobulated nucleus and there is extensive skin involvement. T-cell CLL also must be distinguished from adult T-cell leukemia (ATL). Prolymphocytic leukemia is a CLL variant seen in older people and is characterized by massive splenomegaly, usually in the absence of lymphadenopathy. The neoplastic cell in prolymphocytic leukemia usually is of B-cell origin. It is larger than that seen in CLL and has a prominent nucleolus. Prolymphocytic leukemia is typically associated with very high white counts (in excess of 200 × 10^9 per liter) and a poor response to therapy. Lymphosarcoma cell leukemia represents a leukemic phase of lymphocytic lymphoma and is generally an aggressive disease (Chap. 302). The cellular morphology is suggestive of an acute rather than a chronic leukemia. Monoclonal immunoglobulin is usually easily detected on these cells, and the fluorescent staining is bright, often with spontaneous capping. Hairy cell leukemia is distinguished on the basis of the typical cellular morphology and the presence of tartrate-resistant acid phosphatase in the hairy cells. Waldenström's macroglobulinemia is differentiated from CLL on the basis of bone marrow morphology and lower white blood cell counts, and the secretion of a large amount of a monoclonal IgM paraprotein.

CLINICAL FEATURES The clinical features of CLL are very different from acute leukemia. In more than 25 percent of patients with CLL, the disorder is discovered as an incidental finding. The common practice of ordering routine complete blood counts in adults has led to an earlier diagnosis of CLL in asymptomatic patients. The signs and symptoms of CLL usually relate to tissue infiltration, peripheral blood cytopenias, or immunosuppression. Patients may present with symptoms of anemia, lymph node enlargement, or intercurrent infection. Splenomegaly seldom leads to symptoms, and the liver is minimally enlarged in only about half of patients.

The white cell count ranges between 15 × 10^9 and 200 × 10^9 per liter, with a preponderance of mature-appearing lymphocytes. There is little correlation between the leukocyte count and symptomatology. Patients with advanced disease may present with anemia, granulocytopenia, and thrombocytopenia resulting from bone marrow infiltration by the leukemic cells. About 20 percent of patients develop a Coombs-positive autoimmune hemolytic anemia during the course of their disease. Occasionally, autoimmune thrombocytopenia may occur. Rarely, CLL evolves into an aggressive lymphocytic lymphoma referred to as *Richter's syndrome,* which is believed to be due to a clonal evolution of the original leukemia.

TREATMENT The therapeutic objectives in CLL differ sharply from those for the acute leukemias. The available drugs and radiation therapies are incapable of eradicating the leukemia and producing true complete remissions. Current therapy is effective to reduce the lymphocyte count and lymphadenopathy and to palliate symptoms produced by the leukemia. There is little evidence, however, that survival is substantially affected.

Although a number of prognostic classifications of CLL have been suggested, the new international classification appears most useful (Table 296-4). Prognosis correlates well with stage of disease; however, the rate of progression of patients from one stage to another is highly variable. Patients with stage A disease, in which the disease is limited to lymphocytosis alone or lymphocytosis plus limited lymphadenopathy, have a good prognosis. Median survival exceeds 7 years; these patients usually require no treatment. Patients with more substantial lymphadenopathy and hepatosplenomegaly (stage B) have an intermediate prognosis with a median survival of approximately 5 years. Patients with anemia or thrombocytopenia (stage C) have a worse prognosis with a median survival of less than 2 years.

The indications for therapy in CLL include hemolytic anemia, important cytopenias, disfiguring lymphadenopathy, symptomatic organomegaly, or marked systemic symptoms. When treatment is required, the cornerstone of therapy is usually an alkylating agent. Chlorambucil is the most frequently prescribed drug for CLL at a recommended daily dose of 0.1 to 0.2 mg/kg per day. The chlorambucil dose is generally reduced, and the drug is eventually stopped when the lymphocyte count falls below 20 × 10^9 per liter. The drug may also be given in pulses every 3 to 6 weeks, or continuously in low daily doses. Cyclophosphamide appears to be as effective as

TABLE 296-4 International workshop on CLL staging classification

Stage	Description	Median survival, years
A	Lymphocytosis with clinical involvement of fewer than 3 lymph node groups*; no anemia or thrombocytopenia	>10
B	More than 3 lymph node groups* involved	5
C	Anemia or thrombocytopenia regardless of number of lymph node groups involved	2

* Lymph node groups—cervical, axillary, inguinal, liver, spleen.

chlorambucil in the treatment of CLL. Maintenance therapy has no definite value, and continuing alkylating agent therapy may increase the risk of future development of AML.

Glucocorticosteroids are useful for CLL in special circumstances. These drugs do not have a prominent lympholytic effect in CLL and are therefore not effective as primary therapy. Glucocorticosteroids are useful, however, in the treatment of associated Coombs-positive hemolytic anemia or immune thrombocytopenia, and may be transiently effective in treating patients with pancytopenia and the "packed marrow" syndrome. Glucocorticosteroids have important side effects, including a predisposition to opportunistic infection. In more advanced CLL, combination chemotherapy may be useful. Regimens that include an alkylating agent, vincristine, and prednisone are often employed, and in advanced disease low-dose doxorubicin (Adriamycin) is often added. Pentostatin has been effective in selected patients. Splenectomy may be indicated in patients with hypersplenism, refractory hemolytic anemia, or thrombocytopenia. Radiation therapy may occasionally be useful for control of localized disease, and total-body radiation has rarely been useful in palliating end-stage disease. In preliminary trials, interferon does not appear to be effective in this disease, although agents such as deoxycoformycin, an adenosine deaminase inhibitor, are promising.

Hypogammaglobulinemia is common in patients with CLL, and life-threatening infectious complications may occur. Intramuscular injections of gamma globulin have not been effective, but recently developed intravenous immunoglobulin preparations may be useful in preventing infections in these patients.

HAIRY CELL LEUKEMIA

Hairy cell leukemia is a lymphoid neoplasm characterized by peripheral blood cytopenias, splenomegaly, and morphologically typical malignant cells in the blood and bone marrow. The disease superficially resembles CLL but has distinct clinical features and requires different therapy. Hairy cell leukemia is usually seen in patients over 40 years of age, and there is a very definite male preponderance. Originally, this disorder was thought to account for about 2 percent of all leukemias; however, the disease is now recognized with increased frequency, and many large series have been reported. Hairy cell leukemia has been reported to occur worldwide.

The disease was originally referred to as leukemic reticuloendotheliosis; however, the term *hairy cell leukemia* is now widely accepted because it is descriptive of the characteristic cytoplasmic projections seen on the leukemic cell. The disorder is due to expansion of neoplastic B lymphocytes which often produce monoclonal immunoglobulin; however, rare T-cell variants have been reported. The etiology of hairy cell leukemia is unknown; a single case of T-cell hairy cell leukemia has been reported, from which a unique species of human T-cell leukemia virus (HTLV-II) was recovered.

CLINICAL FEATURES AND PATHOLOGY Patients with hairy cell leukemia usually present with symptoms due to splenomegaly, infection caused by impaired host defense, or vasculitis. Many asymptomatic patients are detected on routine complete blood counts. More than three-quarters of patients will have palpable splenomegaly, and in some cases splenic involvement is massive. Lymphadenopathy is rare, and substantial hepatomegaly is uncommon at the time of diagnosis, although infiltration of the portal triads by hairy cells is often seen microscopically. Occasionally bone lesions may cause symptoms of hip pain. Approximately 30 percent of patients with hairy cell leukemia have an associated vasculitis-like disorder. Common manifestations include erythema nodosum and cutaneous nodules due to perivasculitis. Visceral involvement similar to polyarteritis nodosa may occur.

Moderate pancytopenia is usually present at diagnosis. The leukocyte count is normal or low, and characteristic hairy cells are seen in the peripheral blood. These cells are about 15 to 20 μm in diameter and have an eccentrically placed nucleus with characteristic foamy cytoplasm. Cytoplasmic projections may be seen on smear, but they are best appreciated by phase microscopy. These cells stain positively for tartrate-resistant acid phosphatase (TRAP), which is a cytochemical stain for the isoenzyme 5 of acid phosphatase. Bone marrow aspiration is seldom successful because of reticulin fibrosis. The biopsy typically shows replacement of the normal architecture by mononuclear cells that are not packed together but maintain spaces between the intercellular contacts. Splenic histology is typical, consisting of mononuclear cell infiltration of the red pulp and engorgement of the sinuses.

Hairy cell leukemia must be distinguished from chronic lymphocytic leukemia, Waldenström's macroglobulinemia, and acute leukemia. Some patients with hairy cell leukemia present with a hypocellular bone marrow which may be misdiagnosed as aplastic anemia. The diagnosis depends on identifying the characteristic cells in the bone marrow and peripheral blood.

TREATMENT OF HAIRY CELL LEUKEMIA The course of hairy cell leukemia can be quite indolent; however, there is a wide spectrum of severity and rate of progression of the disease among patients. Approximately one-quarter of patients present without significant cytopenias and without other complications of the disease; these patients require no immediate treatment. They should be followed at intervals and closely observed for infections. Infection is the primary cause of death in patients with hairy cell leukemia. Common infections include *Legionella* pneumonitis, toxoplasmosis, tuberculosis, and atypical mycobacterial disease, nocardiosis, and pyogenic infections. Patients probably benefit from pneumococcal vaccination. Any significant fever should be thoroughly evaluated and aggressively treated with antibiotics. Since *Legionella* pneumonitis is relatively common in these patients, high-dose erythromycin should usually be administered to patients with pulmonary infiltrates.

Therapy directed at the leukemia is indicated in patients presenting with marked pancytopenia, a history of infections, massive splenomegaly, or a rapid rate of disease progression. The cornerstone of therapy has been splenectomy, which appears to ameliorate the disease in a majority of patients. The role of splenectomy, however, in patients with no splenic enlargement is uncertain. Patients with progressive disease following splenectomy or those who do not elect surgery should be treated with α-interferon. Interferon is now an approved drug highly effective in hairy cell leukemia. Virtually all treated patients respond to α-interferon with about 70 percent achieving major hematologic benefit. Complete remissions are rare, but retreatment of recurrent disease is often successful. Pentostatin is an experimental drug that is highly active in hairy cell leukemia and may become the treament of choice since it often induces complete remissions. Glucocorticosteroids are not effective in hairy cell leukemia, and they are potentially dangerous because they further predispose these patients to infections. Short courses of glucocorticosteroids may be useful, however, in controlling the vasculitis or autoimmune manifestations that are often associated with the disease. Chemotherapy with alkylating agents or other myelotoxic drugs is contraindicated in patients with hairy cell leukemia because of poor bone marrow reserve.

The prognosis in hairy cell leukemia is variable, and published series are outdated because of the recent improvements in diagnosis and treatment. At least 50 percent of patients survive more than 8 years from diagnosis, and this prognosis has improved considerably with the application of interferon, pentostatin, and better supportive care.

REFERENCES

General

Gale RP (ed): *Leukemia Treatment*. Boston, Blackwell, 1986

———, Golde DW (eds): *Recent Advances in Leukemia and Lymphoma*. New York, Alan R Liss Inc., 1987

Golde DW, Takaku E (eds): *Hematopoietic Stem Cells*. New York, Marcel Dekker Inc, 1985

Gunz FW, Henderson ES (eds): *Leukemia*, 4th ed. New York, Grune & Stratton, 1983

Rowley JD: Biological implications of consistent chromosome rearrangements in leukemia and lymphoma. Cancer Res 44:3159, 1984
Wong-Staal F, Gallo RC: The family of human T-lymphotropic leukemia viruses: HTLV-I as the cause of adult T cell leukemia and HTLV-III as the cause of acquired immunodeficiency syndrome. Blood 65:253, 1985
Yunis JJ: The chromosomal basis of human neoplasia. Science 221:227, 1983

Acute leukemias

Bennett JM et al: Criteria for the diagnosis of acute leukemia of megakaryocytic lineage. Ann Intern Med 103:460, 1985
Champlin R, Gale RP: Acute lymphoblastic leukemia: Recent advances in biology and therapy. Blood 73:2051, 1989
———: Bone marrow transplantation for leukemia: Recent advances and comparisons with alternative therapies. Semin Hematol 24:55, 1987

ALL

Gaynor J et al: A cause-specific hazard rate analysis of prognostic factors among 199 adults with acute lymphoblastic leukemia: The Memorial Hospital experience. J Clin Oncol 6:1014, 1988
Hoelzer D et al: Prognostic factors in a multicenter study for treatment of acute lymphoblastic leukemia in adults. Blood 71:123, 1988
Jacobs AD, Gale RP: Recent advances in the biology and treatment of acute lymphoblastic leukemia in adults. N Engl J Med 311:1219, 1984
Johnson FL et al: A comparison of marrow transplantation with chemotherapy for children with acute lymphoblastic leukemia in second or subsequent remission. N Engl J Med 305:846, 1981
Mauer AM: Therapy of acute lymphoblastic leukemia in childhood. Blood 56:1, 1980
Ritz J et al: Autologous bone marrow transplantation in CALLA-positive acute lymphoblastic leukemia after in vitro treatment with J5 monoclonal antibody and complement. Lancet 2:60, 1982
Rivera GK, Mauer AM: Controversies in the management of childhood acute lymphoblastic leukemia: Treatment intensification, CNS leukaemia, and prognostic factors. Semin Hematol 24:12, 1987

AML

Appelbaum FR et al: Bone marrow transplantation or chemotherapy after remission induction for adults with acute nonlymphoblastic leukemia. Ann Intern Med 101:581, 1984
Bagby GC: The preleukemic syndrome (hematopoietic dysplasia). Blood Rev 2:194, 1988
Champlin RE et al: Treatment of acute myelogenous leukemia: A prospective controlled trial of bone marrow transplantation versus consolidation chemotherapy. Ann Intern Med 102:285, 1985
———, Gale RP: Acute myelogenous leukemia: Recent advances in therapy. Blood 69:1551, 1987
——— et al: Prolonged survival in acute myelogenous leukaemia without maintenance chemotherapy. Lancet 1:894, 1984
Fialkow PJ et al: Acute nonlymphocytic leukemia: Heterogeneity of stem cell origin. Blood 57:1068, 1981
Foon KA et al: The role of immunotherapy in acute myelogenous leukemia. Arch Intern Med 143:1726, 1983
Gale RP, Champlin RE: How does bone marrow transplantation cure leukaemia? Lancet 2:28, 1984
Greenberg PL: The smoldering myeloid leukemic states: Clinical and biologic features. Blood 61:1035, 1983
Herzig RH et al: High-dose cytosine arabinoside therapy for refractory leukemia. Blood 62:361, 1983
Koeffler HP: Induction of differentiation of human acute myelogenous leukemia cells: Therapeutic implications. Blood 62:709, 1983
Preisler HD: The treatment of acute nonlymphocytic leukemia. Blood Rev 1:97, 1987
Weinstein HJ et al: Chemotherapy for acute myelogenous leukemia in children and adults: VAPA update. Blood 62:315, 1983

CLL

Binet J-L et al: Chronic lymphocytic leukaemia: Proposals for a revised prognostic staging system. Br J Haematol 48:365, 1981
Caligaris-Cappio F, Janossy G: Surface markers in chronic lymphoid leukemias of B cell type. Semin Hematol 22:1, 1985
Foon K, Gale RP: Staging and therapy of chronic lymphocytic leukemia. Semin Hematol 24:264, 1987
Han T et al: Prognostic importance of cytogenetic abnormalities in patients with chronic lymphocytic leukemia. N Engl J Med 310:288, 1984

Hairy cell leukemia

Cheson BD, Martin A: Clinical trials in hairy cell leukemia. Current status and future directions. Ann Intern Med 106:871, 1987
Genot E et al: Effect of interferon-alpha on the expression and release of the CD23 molecule in hairy cell leukemia. Blood 74:2455, 1989
Glaspy JA et al: Evolving therapy of hairy cell leukemia. Cancer 59:652, 1987
Golomb HM: The treatment of hairy cell leukemia. Blood 69:979, 1987
——— et al: Sequential evaluation of alpha-2b-interferon treatment in 128 patients with hairy cell leukemia. Semin Oncol 14(Suppl 2):13, 1987
Jacobs AD et al: Recombinant alpha-2 interferon for hairy cell leukemia. Blood 65:1017, 1985
Spiers ASD et al: Remissions in hairy-cell leukemia with pentostatin (2′-deoxycoformycin). N Engl J Med 316:825, 1987

297 THE MYELOPROLIFERATIVE DISEASES

JOHN W. ADAMSON

DEFINITION The myeloproliferative diseases are neoplasms of the multipotent hematopoietic stem cell. They include chronic myelogenous leukemia (CML), polycythemia vera (PV), agnogenic myeloid metaplasia with myelofibrosis (AMM/MF), and essential thrombocytosis (ET). In addition to their common stem cell origin, other features are shared which occasionally lead to a blurring between the various disorders. However, apparent transitions from one disorder to another are uncommon. With the exception of CML, the diseases tend to run a chronic course over many years.

The stem cell origin and clonal nature of these diseases have been shown through cytogenetic analyses and through studies in female patients who are heterozygous for glucose-6-phosphate dehydrogenase (G6PD). Consistent with the stem cell origin and neoplastic nature of these diseases a single G6PD enzyme is found in peripheral blood granulocytes, platelets, red cells, and monocytes in patients who have been shown to be G6PD heterozygotes by analysis of skin fibroblasts. In at least some patients, the level of stem cell involvement includes a progenitor capable of giving rise to lymphocytes, as well. In patients with characteristic cytogenetic abnormalities, abnormal metaphases may be found in precursors of platelets, red cells, and granulocytes. These findings indicate that the diseases arise as clonal expansions of single transformed stem cells. At the time of diagnosis, virtually all of the myeloid cells of the blood are derived from the neoplastic clone.

CHRONIC MYELOGENOUS LEUKEMIA

DEFINITION AND ETIOLOGY CML is characterized by marked splenomegaly and the production of increased numbers of granulocytes, particularly neutrophils. The disorder is associated with a characteristic chromosomal abnormality (see below) and runs a generally mild course until it transforms to a frankly leukemic (blastic) phase. Usually no specific etiologic agent can be identified; however, an increased incidence of CML in atomic bomb survivors has been noted. CML occurs at any age, but the peak incidence occurs in the third and fourth decades. The sexes are affected equally.

PATHOPHYSIOLOGY AND SYMPTOMATOLOGY The natural course of CML can be divided into a chronic and a blastic or acute phase. The chronic phase of CML is characterized by an excessive proliferation and accumulation of granulocytes and their precursors in the marrow and blood. Typically, the white blood cell count is markedly elevated, often exceeding 200,000 per microliter. At this stage, myeloblasts are less than 5 percent of the cells in the marrow and blood. The diagnosis often is made because of incidental laboratory tests which reveal an elevated white blood count, or because a patient complains of left upper quadrant discomfort due to an enlarged spleen. About 20 percent of cases are diagnosed on the basis of an elevated blood count in the absence of symptoms. In the majority, however, the signs and symptoms of the disease are related to the expanded myeloid mass in the marrow and spleen. Presenting symptoms are related to splenomegaly, anemia, or hypermetabolism manifested by weight loss and fever. Arthralgias may be severe. Lymphadenopathy is rare in this phase. Thrombohemorrhagic complications such as excessive bleeding, either spontaneously or with surgical or dental procedures, are occasionally found. Ninety percent of patients have palpable splenomegaly.

During the course of the chronic phase of CML the disease transforms to the more malignant blastic phase. After the first 6 to 12 months following diagnosis, the rate of transformation to the blastic phase is about 25 percent of the remaining patients per year and over 85 percent of patients with CML will eventually die in this phase. Occasionally, patients may present in the blastic phase of the disease. The chronic phase may be restored if such patients respond successfully to chemotherapy. There is no single test which predicts precisely when a patient's disease will transform to the blastic phase, but certain features associated with early transformation include the degree of leukocytosis, the presence of an excessively large liver and spleen, the percentage of immature cells in the marrow, and the presence of large numbers of eosinophils or basophils. Overall survival for patients from the time of diagnosis averages 3½ years.

The blastic phase of CML represents an evolution in the disease from hyperplasia of mature elements of the marrow to increased numbers of blasts and promyelocytes. Half of the patients progress to blast crisis through an "accelerated" phase characterized by progressively increasing leukocytosis, thrombocytosis or thrombocytopenia, and splenomegaly, which are refractory to previously effective drugs. In some patients, the transition to a state resembling acute myelogenous leukemia may take only a few weeks. A minority of patients will present with or develop extramedullary tumors, usually in lymph nodes or skin, or osteolytic bone lesions. Meningeal leukemia is rare.

The blastic phase may be lymphoid or myeloid in origin. One-third of cases have characteristics of lymphoblasts including the enzyme terminal deoxynucleotidyl transferase (Tdt), a DNA-synthesizing enzyme associated with acute lymphoblastic leukemia and normal thymic lymphocytes, as well as the common acute lymphoblastic leukemia antigen (CALLA). This is consistent with the known level of stem cell involvement in the original disease. Lymphoid blast crisis in some patients is associated with arrested rearrangements of the immunoglobulin genes, typical of pre-B cells. Myeloid blast crisis resembles acute myelogenous leukemia, but a few patients will have a basophilic or erythroleukemic conversion from the chronic phase of the disease. The latter, and the fact that the blasts may react positively with monoclonal antibodies to erythroid- or megakaryocyte-associated antigens, emphasize the diversity of this phase and the stem cell nature of the disease. Auer rods are virtually never seen in the myeloblasts of CML in blastic phase.

LABORATORY FINDINGS Table 297-1 summarizes the distinguishing laboratory features of the various myeloproliferative diseases. The most prominent laboratory finding in CML is the leukocytosis. Unlike the finding in leukemoid reactions, there is generally a bimodal distribution of neutrophils in the blood with a peak of mature polymorphonuclear neutrophils (PMNs) and a second peak of myelocytes or metamyelocytes. Platelet morphology is more normal than in the other myeloproliferative disorders, and in vitro platelet function, as marked by aggregation in the presence of agents such as epinephrine, is also generally normal. Basophilia, typical of all of the myeloproliferative disorders, may be prominent. A number of unique biochemical abnormalities are also found. Accompanying the leukocytosis of CML is a marked elevation of serum vitamin B_{12} levels, as well as an increased serum vitamin B_{12}–binding capacity. This is due to excessive serum levels of transcobalamin I, a glycoprotein of alpha globulin electrophoretic mobility. A vitamin B_{12}–binding protein with similar properties has been shown to be produced by mature normal and leukemic granulocytes in vitro. Elevated levels in the serum of patients with CML are probably derived from the turnover of the increased granulocytic mass. The high levels of vitamin B_{12}, as well as the increased serum binding capacity, return toward normal with treatment of the disease. Leukocyte alkaline phosphatase, an enzyme in granulocytes, is markedly reduced in the granulocytes of nearly all patients with CML. However, with infection or glucocorticoid administration, the level of the enzyme in granulocytes may rise to the normal range. The levels of the enzyme may also return toward normal with successful therapy of the disease and reduction of the white cell count. The only other hematologic disorders with low or absent leukocyte alkaline phosphatase are paroxysmal nocturnal hemoglobinuria and occasional cases of myelodysplasia. The marrow as well as the spleen of patients with CML may contain glycolipid-laden phagocytes which resemble Gaucher cells. Hyperuricemia related to the increased cell turnover may occur in all the myeloproliferative diseases prior to therapy and can be exacerbated by treatment. The mature granulocyte in CML is a cell that is functionally normal with respect to phagocytosis and bactericidal activity. Granulocyte kinetics in CML have been studied with isotope-labeling techniques, and there is clear evidence for increased production of mature granulocytes. The numbers of primitive myeloid progenitors (colony-forming cells) in the marrow and blood of patients with CML are also increased. This includes both committed erythroid as well as granulocytic progenitors, and their numbers in the blood may be 10,000 times the normal number.

CYTOGENETICS More than 95 percent of patients with CML have a unique and characteristic chromosome marker in metaphases of marrow—the Philadelphia chromosome (Ph). This chromosomal abnormality represents a reciprocal translocation of genetic material between the long arms of chromosome 22 and chromosome 9. This particularly interesting chromosomal rearrangement involves break points near two cellular proto-oncogenes, c-*abl* on chromosome 9 and c-*sis* on chromosome 22. The proto-oncogene c-*sis* is the cellular homologue of the simian sarcoma virus oncogene and encodes sequences for platelet-derived growth factor (PDGF). The proto-oncogene c-*abl* is translocated to a specific region of chromosome 22, the breakpoint cluster region (*bcr*). As a result, a fusion gene product of *bcr/abl* is formed which has tyrosine kinase activity and may have a role in the development and persistence or progression of the disease. This chromosome abnormality persists throughout the course of the disease, in remission and relapse, and is unaffected by the usual therapies. It is present in virtually all metaphases of granulocytic, megakaryocytic, and erythroid precursors but not in traditionally prepared lymphocyte preparations or skin fibroblasts. Some patients with CML, who do not have the Ph chromosome abnormality by routine cytogenetic techniques, can be shown to have the *bcr/abl* rearrangement by molecular analysis. In addition to the Ph chromosome, the blastic phase of CML is often associated with the acquisition of other chromosomal abnormalities, such as aneuploidy, which reflect the more malignant character of this phase of the disease. Double Ph chromosomes also may be seen. Less than 5 percent of patients with clinically typical CML lack the Ph chromosome. These patients are generally younger and have a more rapidly progressive clinical course. Although considered with CML, this disease is probably a distinct myeloproliferative disorder.

While the Ph chromosome is a consistent feature of CML, there is evidence, using other cell markers such as G6PD, that the appearance of the chromosomal abnormality is not the primary event in the acquisition of the disease. Thus, some lymphocyte populations which appear by G6PD analysis to be clonally derived lack the Ph chromosome. These and other results suggest a multistep pathogenesis in

TABLE 297-1 The myeloproliferative diseases

Disease	Hematocrit	White blood cell count	Platelet count	Splenomegaly	Leukocyte alkaline phosphatase	Marrow fibrosis	Ph chromosome
CML	Normal or ↓	↑ ↑ ↑	↑ to ↓	+ + +	↓ to 0	±	+
PV	↑ ↑	↑	↑	+	↑ ↑	±	0
AMM/MF	↓	↑ to ↓	↑ to ↓	+ + +	↑ or normal	+ + +	0
ET	Normal	Normal	↑ ↑ ↑	+	↑ or normal	±	0

CML with the acquisition of the Ph chromosome as a secondary event.

DIAGNOSIS CML which presents with splenomegaly, a markedly elevated white cell count, a low leukocyte alkaline phosphatase, and the Ph chromosome is an easy diagnosis. Atypical presentations must be differentiated from leukemoid reactions associated with infections or neoplasms. In the latter, the leukocyte alkaline phosphatase is usually elevated and the Ph chromosome is absent. A closely related myeloproliferative disorder is agnogenic myeloid metaplasia (AMM/MF) (see below). This disease usually presents with marked myelofibrosis and splenomegaly. The white blood cell count and platelet count may be elevated, but leukocyte alkaline phosphatase is normal or increased and the Ph chromosome is absent. Among the myeloproliferative diseases, the serum vitamin B_{12} level cannot be used as a differential diagnostic test in patients with elevated white cell counts.

THERAPY Chronic phase CML can be controlled by a number of alkylating agents such as busulfan, cyclophosphamide, or melphalan, as well as hydroxyurea, a cell cycle–specific drug. Splenic irradiation is not as effective as chemotherapy for control of the disease. The most commonly used drug is busulfan. It may be administered on an intermittent schedule or on a continuous daily basis with approximately the same results. The most serious complication of busulfan therapy is prolonged myelosuppression. Occasionally, remission of the disease for periods in excess of 1 year may follow a single course of treatment. The principal side effects include increased skin pigmentation resembling that seen with adrenal insufficiency and, rarely, pulmonary or retroperitoneal fibrosis. An initial daily oral dose of 4 to 8 mg will reduce the white cell count to less than 20,000 per microliter in 2 to 3 weeks. The dose of busulfan should be reduced progressively, roughly in proportion to the reduction in white blood cell count. Patients achieve an excellent hematologic remission, with return of blood counts to normal and reduction in organomegaly. The Ph chromosome remains, however. A true remission of the disease does not occur; rather, the proliferating granulocyte mass is reduced to the point where immature cells disappear from the peripheral blood. Furthermore, neither conventional therapy nor high-dose combination chemotherapy designed to eradicate the Ph-positive clone significantly prolongs survival. Encouraging results with interferon, both in terms of reduction of the white cell count and the percent of Ph-positive metaphases in the marrow, have been reported, but the results of randomized trials with this or similar agents are not available.

Splenectomy has little place in the primary management of CML but may be reserved for those patients with evidence of hypersplenism or repeated painful splenic infarctions or for the rare instance in which prolonged thrombocytopenia follows busulfan therapy. Splenectomy in the chronic phase of CML does not prolong survival or delay the onset of blastic transformation.

Acceleration of the disease is reflected by progressive refractoriness to chemotherapy, increased leukocytosis with a larger proportion of immature forms, thrombocytosis, and increasing splenomegaly. Prior to blastic transformation, the drug hydroxyurea can effectively control the proliferative aspects of the disease. The dose ranges from 1 to 3 g/d by mouth. The blastic phase of CML is refractory to most drug regimens, but short-lived remissions in about 20 percent of cases have been obtained with the use of vincristine and prednisone or other intensive combination chemotherapy programs useful in the treatment of acute leukemia (see Chap. 296). There is a correlation between the appearance of Tdt in the blast cells and the response to vincristine and prednisone, drugs commonly used for acute lymphoblastic leukemia in childhood. However, the correlation is not perfect, and therapy for the blastic phase should begin with vincristine and prednisone, regardless of the presence or absence of Tdt or the morphology of the blasts. Hydroxyurea may be used here, as well, to suppress the proliferation of blasts; however, meaningful remissions are rarely, if ever, obtained and patients die of infection or bleeding. Symptomatic extramedullary myeloblastic tumors can be controlled with local radiation therapy.

It has been demonstrated that eradication of Ph-positive cells can be achieved in the majority of chronic phase patients treated with intensive chemotherapy and radiation and transplanted with bone marrow from an identical twin or sibling compatible for human histocompatibility leukocyte antigens (HLA). Analysis of patients receiving bone marrow transplantation suggests that the best results are obtained in patients transplanted in chronic phase within the first year of diagnosis. Busulfan or other alkylating agents should be avoided if marrow transplantation remains an option. Long-term disease-free survival in good-risk transplant patients is approximately 70 percent, although late relapses occur with reappearance of the Ph chromosome. Progressively poorer results with higher relapse rates are obtained if patients are transplanted in the accelerated or blastic phase of the disease.

POLYCYTHEMIA VERA

DEFINITION AND ETIOLOGY Polycythemia vera (PV) is characterized by splenomegaly and an increased production of all myeloid elements; however, the disease is generally dominated by an elevated hemoglobin concentration. PV is gradual in onset and runs a chronic but usually slowly progressive course.

The disease generally begins in late middle life and is slightly more common in males. Only rarely is PV found in children or multiple members of a single family. The disease is relatively uncommon in blacks and occurs with increased frequency in Jews of European ancestry.

PATHOPHYSIOLOGY AND SYMPTOMATOLOGY None of the recognized physiologic mechanisms of increased red blood cell production is present in PV. The disease must be distinguished from secondary forms of polycythemia, in which an elevated hemoglobin concentration results from increased erythropoietin production. Secondary polycythemia may arise through hypoxia or occasionally may be found with certain neoplasms. PV is also distinct from spurious (relative) polycythemia, which results from a decrease in the plasma volume rather than a true increase in red blood cell mass. Also, secondary causes of polycythemia are not associated with splenic enlargement or increased leukocytes and platelets, which are typical of PV.

In PV there is a unique relationship of erythropoietin to red blood cell production. As opposed to the findings in secondary forms of polycythemia, urine and serum levels of erythropoietin in patients with PV are reduced. Presumably, erythropoietin production is suppressed by the elevated hemoglobin concentration, since phlebotomy results in a rise in both erythropoietin levels and red blood cell production (provided that there is no deficiency in iron). This demonstrates the marrow's ability to respond to humoral regulation.

In cell culture, marrow from patients with PV forms colonies of hemoglobin-synthesizing cells in the absence of added erythropoietin. This is rarely the case with marrow cells from normal persons or from patients with secondary polycythemia. A reduced production of erythropoietin, the appearance of "endogenous" erythroid colonies in marrow cultures, and the clonal origin from the pluripotent hematopoietic stem cell indicate that hematopoiesis in PV is not regulated by the usual mechanisms.

PV produces symptoms associated with increased blood volume and blood viscosity. The hemoglobin concentration, hematocrit, and total blood volume may become markedly elevated, a consequence of the sharply increased red blood cell mass. The plasma volume is usually normal but may be increased. Associated with the expanded blood volume is a consistently elevated increase in cardiac output and a less uniform, but significant, increase in cardiac index. Reduction of the hematocrit and blood volume by phlebotomy leads to a reduction in the stroke volume and cardiac output in these patients and generally to an improvement in exercise tolerance. The increased cardiac output occurs in association with an increase in blood viscosity and, presumably, in vascular resistance associated with the elevated hematocrit.

Complaints related to the increased viscosity and/or decreased cerebral perfusion include headache, dizziness, vertigo, a sense of fullness of the head, rushing in the ears, visual alterations (scotomas, double vision, or blurred vision), tinnitus, syncope, and even chorea. Peripheral vascular symptoms of both arterial and venous insufficiency are common; in one large series, more than 35 percent of patients gave a history of some thrombotic or hemorrhagic event during the course of their disease. The risk of thrombosis may be increased by the accelerated atherosclerosis in this disease. Bleeding is common and comes most often from the nose or from peptic ulcer disease. Intramuscular hemorrhages and bruising also are seen. The tendency to increased bleeding may be due to the distended vasculature resulting from the increased blood volume. However, intrinsic platelet dysfunction also may contribute to bleeding, particularly from the gastrointestinal tract. The incidence of peptic ulcer disease is estimated to be four to five times higher in patients with PV than it is in the general population, although the reasons are unclear.

Late in the disease, the spleen may become greatly enlarged, producing symptoms of early satiety, a sense of abdominal fullness, and pleuritic chest or left upper quadrant pain secondary to capsular stretching or infarction. Pruritus, particularly after bathing, is reported frequently and may be disabling. Occasionally, urticaria is seen.

The increased cellular proliferation seen with PV results in hyperuricemia in 25 to 30 percent of patients and may be associated with formation of urate stones and uric acid nephropathy.

LABORATORY FINDINGS The most prominent laboratory feature is the elevated hemoglobin concentration. Unless altered by iron deficiency, the red blood cells are normochromic and normocytic. Polychromasia is frequently seen, and nucleated red blood cells may be found in the later stages of the disease. These findings represent cells released from extramedullary sites of hematopoiesis or reflect damage to marrow stroma due to fibrosis.

The white cell count is elevated in two-thirds of patients and is usually in the range of 15,000 to 25,000 per microliter but may be as high as 60,000 per microliter. An increase in the absolute basophil count (to more than 100 per microliter) is found in about 70 percent of patients. The leukocyte alkaline phosphatase is increased in more than 80 percent of cases. Serum vitamin B_{12} levels vary and are increased in about one-third of the patients; however, the binding capacity is increased in as many as 75 percent. In addition to increased transcobalamin I, transcobalamin III is also increased.

Thrombocytosis is seen in over half of all patients with PV. In vitro studies of platelet function demonstrate defective platelet adhesiveness and impaired secondary release of adenosine diphosphate (ADP) in response to epinephrine. These are poorly correlated with the bleeding time, and the contribution of these functional abnormalities to the thrombotic and hemorrhagic events in patients with PV is uncertain. Abnormal liver function studies, including an elevated alkaline phosphatase, may occur if there is massive hepatomegaly.

Splenomegaly occurs in 75 percent of patients but is usually not as marked as in CML or AMM/MF. Splenomegaly persists even when the elevated hemoglobin concentration has been reduced by repeated phlebotomies. Microscopic examination of the spleen reveals multiple foci of extramedullary hematopoiesis and fibrosis. The follicular pattern of the organ is retained, unlike the loss of normal architectural structure observed in CML. Foci of extramedullary hematopoiesis also may be found in the liver.

Bone marrow examination shows either erythroid hyperplasia or panhyperplasia without distinctive morphologic features. There is increased megakaryocyte nuclear ploidy in the face of thrombocytosis. This pattern of platelet regulation is different from that observed in the reactive thrombocytosis associated with inflammation or neoplasia, where megakaryocyte nuclear ploidy is inversely related to the peripheral platelet count. As PV progresses, fibrosis may appear in central areas of the marrow, and scanning techniques will demonstrate expansion of hematopoietic tissue to more peripheral skeletal sites.

Cytogenetic abnormalities, including trisomy 1, 8, or 9 and 20q−, have been reported in about 10 percent of untreated patients. Prior treatment with myelosuppressive agents or radioactive phosphorus (^{32}P) appears to increase the incidence of such abnormalities.

DIAGNOSIS The plethoric patient with pancytosis and splenomegaly, and without evidence of chronic cardiac or pulmonary disease, presents few diagnostic problems. However, it is more common to see patients with PV who have less than the full clinical disease or in whom an elevated hemoglobin or hematocrit has been discovered at the time of routine laboratory evaluation. Under these circumstances, it is important that the diagnosis of PV be made with certainty in order to direct therapeutic efforts appropriately.

First, there is little statistical likelihood that hematocrits consistently near or greater than 60 percent represent a simple decrease in plasma volume. When hematocrit levels are in the range of 50 to 55 percent, however, the likelihood of true erythrocytosis is reduced to about 50 percent and the red blood cell mass should be determined directly by isotope dilution using ^{51}Cr-labeled autologous red blood cells. While the plasma volume may be calculated indirectly from the red blood cell mass, it is preferable to measure this compartment independently using a second label. The results for red blood cell mass are best expressed as a function of the lean body mass, which may be estimated from the patient's height and weight. If the results of such a study are equivocal, the clinical findings must establish whether the patient has a true increase in red blood cell production or else the patient should be restudied at a later time.

The patient who presents with a hematocrit or hemoglobin in the high normal range, microcytosis, leukocytosis, and iron deficiency should be considered as possibly having PV. Evaluation of red and white blood cell morphology, basophil count, and platelet morphology should be carried out to make certain that this is not a patient with PV who has bled.

While measurements of red blood cell mass distinguish spurious from true erythrocytosis, the results do not distinguish between the various forms of polycythemia. If the diagnosis is uncertain, additional indexes which may be helpful include the absolute basophil count, the leukocyte alkaline phosphatase score, and results of radioisotope scanning to quantitate spleen size. This last is particularly useful in obese individuals or patients in whom the spleen is enlarged but not palpable.

If the diagnosis of PV remains obscure, an intravenous pyelogram or abdominal CT scan should be obtained to exclude hypernephroma or other renal pathology which might result in increased erythropoietin production. Arterial blood gas measurements should be obtained, including carboxyhemoglobin levels if the patient is a smoker. Perhaps 20 percent of patients with PV may have a hemoglobin oxygen saturation below 92 percent, but almost all will have a saturation equal to or greater than 88 percent. This modest impairment of oxygen loading may be due to decreased diffusing capacity of the lung, possibly triggered by repeated episodes of thromboembolism or thrombosis in situ.

When the diagnosis is not clear following routine investigation, measurement of serum erythropoietin levels by radioimmunoassay may be helpful. Patients with PV generally have lower plasma erythropoietin levels than do patients with secondary forms of polycythemia. In vitro growth characteristics of bone marrow cells from patients with PV also may be useful in diagnosis.

COURSE AND PROGNOSIS The course of PV has been a subject of disagreement, some observers believing that later complications are hastened by myelosuppressive therapy. About 15 to 20 percent of patients will progress to marrow fibrosis, marked splenomegaly, and anemia; one view holds that if patients live long enough, all will enter this so-called spent phase of the disease. However, the majority of patients die of vascular complications of their disease or of unrelated causes. Although the incidence is low, there is a statistically significant association of second hematologic neoplasms in patients with PV; these include non-Hodgkin's lymphomas and multiple myeloma. Of patients with PV, 1 to 2 percent experience transformation into acute leukemia even without prior radiation or chemotherapy.

THERAPY Optimal therapy of PV remains unsettled. The median survival has been extended to 10 to 12 years with phlebotomy alone, while patients receiving no therapy at all survive only 2 years. However, neither myelosuppressive therapy nor phlebotomy holds a clear advantage for survival. For many years after its introduction in 1940, ^{32}P was the therapy of choice. However, a retrospective analysis of a large number of cases suggested that ^{32}P increased the incidence of acute leukemia (to over 10 percent) while not clearly enhancing survival over other forms of therapy. In order to resolve the major questions regarding the most effective therapy, the incidence of complicating factors, and the prognostic implication of certain features such as thrombocytosis or cytogenetic abnormalities, the International Polycythemia Vera Study Group was established. This group prospectively assigned patients who met strict diagnostic criteria into three treatment programs at random: ^{32}P therapy augmented by phlebotomy, myelosuppressive therapy plus phlebotomy, and phlebotomy alone. Analysis of the survival curves demonstrated similar survivals for the various treatment groups until the seventh year after randomization. At that point, patients treated with alkylating agents had poorer survival. The findings indicated that those patients in the phlebotomy-only group suffered from increased risk of death due to hemorrhage or thrombosis within the first four years, while leukemia and other neoplasms were more prevalent later in the course of the patients treated with chemotherapy or ^{32}P. However, a simultaneous European cooperative therapy trial did not demonstrate increased leukemia in patients treated with chemotherapy, and the survival in those patients was superior to that of patients treated with phlebotomy alone.

Despite the controversy, certain therapeutic tenets meet with agreement. Phlebotomy is safe, can be done repeatedly, and is preferred in individuals with mild disease, young patients, or those with polycythemia of uncertain etiology. Myelosuppression is best in patients with extreme symptomatic thrombocytosis, rapidly enlarging spleen, or symptoms of hypermetabolism. It may also spare elderly patients the rigors of phlebotomy. Regardless of eventual decisions involving therapy, phlebotomy should be used initially to reduce the red blood cell mass and blood volume. The end point of phlebotomy therapy should be a hematocrit or hemoglobin value in the low-normal range. This form of treatment may lead to prolonged clinical remission. Iron should not be given if phlebotomy is the primary mode of therapy. Phlebotomy is especially important if a patient with PV must undergo emergency surgery, since intra- and postoperative morbidity and mortality are four to five times greater in uncontrolled as opposed to controlled (phlebotomized) patients. Under these circumstances, the red blood cell mass should be reduced acutely by exchange phlebotomies and the blood replaced with a suitable plasma expander. This will prevent the vascular instability associated with too rapid a reduction in total blood volume.

Marrow suppression may be achieved by radiation or chemotherapy. The administration of ^{32}P is easy, provides long, trouble-free remissions in most cases, and successfully reduces the morbidity associated with the disease. The regimen recommended by the International Polycythemia Vera Study Group consists of the intravenous administration initially of 85.2 MBq of $^{32}P/m^2$ body surface area. The patient is then followed for a period of 3 months and retreated at that time, as needed, with a dose 25 percent greater than that given originally. This program may be repeated 3 months later but is rarely required. Remissions may last 6 to 24 months, during which time the patient is often symptom-free. This ^{32}P therapy may be repeated if relapse occurs. Exposure to ^{32}P increases the incidence of leukemia in patients with PV, and the risk of leukemic transformation may be related to the cumulative dose of isotope.

Suppression of marrow function with chemotherapy has been common during the last 15 years. Effective drugs include hydroxyurea, melphalan, busulfan, and chlorambucil. Busulfan, in doses of 4 to 6 mg/d orally, reduces the white blood cell and platelet counts, but suppression may be unpredictable and prolonged and the drug is relatively less effective in suppressing erythropoiesis. Moreover, continued use of this drug may lead to pulmonary fibrosis and a syndrome resembling adrenal insufficiency. Chlorambucil, originally employed in the prospective treatment trial by the International Polycythemia Vera Study Group, resulted in a high incidence (over 10 percent) of acute leukemia, and the study group has recommended against the routine use of this or other alkylating agents in this disease. Currently, no form of treatment is clearly better than any other in terms of patient survival, but management with ^{32}P may be simpler and particularly appropriate in elderly patients. Hydroxyurea, a drug active in the DNA synthetic phase of the cell cycle and not known to be leukemogenic, is effective. Hydroxyurea given orally in doses of 1 to 3 g/d may control symptoms of hypermetabolism and the elevated leukocyte and platelet counts, but phlebotomy is generally required for adequate control of the red cell mass. Small clinical trials of aspirin to control thrombotic complications have not shown benefit.

Other symptoms associated with PV may be managed conservatively. In the case of pruritus, cyproheptadine, 12 to 16 mg/d, may be effective. Allopurinol in doses of 300 mg/d will reduce serum uric acid. Symptomatic splenomegaly is usually improved with treatment, although splenectomy may be indicated in rare instances.

AGNOGENIC MYELOID METAPLASIA/MYELOFIBROSIS

DEFINITION AND ETIOLOGY AMM/MF is characterized by the tendency of the neoplastic stem cells to lodge and grow in multiple sites outside the marrow. Typically, there is progressive splenomegaly, the gradual replacement of marrow elements by fibrosis, progressive anemia, and variable changes in the number of granulocytes and platelets. The disease begins in late middle life and is gradual in onset, chronic, and progressive. Males and females are equally involved, and there is only rare familial occurrence.

While erythrocytes, granulocytes, and platelets are members of a single neoplastic clone, the fibrosis is reactive and not part of the abnormal clone. AMM is an integral part of the disease and is seen early in its course. There is no evidence that AMM arises in compensation for replacement of the marrow by fibrous tissue.

PATHOPHYSIOLOGY AND SYMPTOMATOLOGY AMM/MF presents most commonly with vague constitutional symptoms associated with anemia, such as fatigue, weakness, and anorexia, or with splenomegaly. An enlarged spleen is seen in virtually all patients; however, the disease progresses slowly and splenomegaly may be present for years prior to diagnosis. The enlargement may become so extensive as to produce symptoms of pain, abdominal fullness, and dyspnea. Hepatomegaly occurs in more than 50 percent of patients and also may become massive, but enlargement of the liver due to AMM does not occur in the absence of splenomegaly. Petechiae are found in 20 percent of patients as a result of thrombocytopenia, and a history of bleeding is obtained in 10 percent. Less common findings include lymphadenopathy, jaundice, ascites, and bone pain. Weight loss, fever, sweating, and extremity pain may occur occasionally and are associated with a hypermetabolic state. The increased cellular turnover results in hyperuricemia in 25 to 30 percent of patients.

LABORATORY FINDINGS The blood counts of patients with AMM/MF are variable. Mild anemia is observed in over one-half of the patients at the time of diagnosis and progresses during the course of the disease. Eventually, almost all patients become anemic. The recognized mechanisms leading to anemia include ineffective erythropoiesis, increased splenic pooling of red cells, and a decrease in red blood cell survival. Low serum folate and megaloblastic maturation may contribute. The peripheral blood smear usually shows dramatic changes in red cell and platelet morphology. Basophilic stippling is prominent and bizarre red cell shapes, including teardrop poikilocytes, fragmented cells, and nucleated red cells, are common, as are giant platelet forms.

An elevation in the white blood cell count is found in about 50 percent of patients, and values as high as 50,000 per microliter may be seen. However, 20 percent of patients are leukopenic, with white blood cell counts less than 4000 per microliter. Generally, there is a shift toward immature forms in granulocyte maturation, and circulating blast forms may be found. The appearance of these cells does not imply a bad prognosis. An increase in the absolute basophil count is observed in 25 percent of patients. The leukocyte alkaline phosphatase activity is elevated in about half the patients, the remainder being equally distributed between having normal or low values. Serum vitamin B_{12} levels are normal or slightly elevated, as are vitamin B_{12}-binding proteins. These values usually do not approach those seen with CML.

A normal or elevated platelet count is frequently found early in the course of the disease, but thrombocytopenia eventually develops in most patients, owing to ineffective production and splenic pooling. The circulating platelets vary considerably in size and shape, and megakaryocyte nuclei may be found on the peripheral blood smear. In vitro studies of platelet function reflect defective platelet adhesiveness and impaired secondary release of ADP in response to epinephrine. Abnormal liver function tests, including elevated bilirubin and alkaline phosphatase, may be associated with massive hepatomegaly.

The spleen may become massive. There are multiple foci of extramedullary hematopoiesis on pathologic examination, but the normal follicular architecture of the spleen is maintained. Other organs which may be involved include the kidneys, lymph nodes, adrenal glands, and lungs. Bone marrow examination early in the course of the disease reveals a hypercellular marrow in about 20 percent of patients and may be difficult to distinguish from PV. Special stains of the marrow reveal increased reticulin deposition. However, a minority of patients develops obvious patchy collagen fibrosis separating areas of hyperplastic marrow, or diffuse fibrosis with osteosclerosis. Megakaryocytes may be preserved remarkably well in the areas of fibrosis. One hypothesis to account for the marrow fibrosis is that neoplastic megakaryoblasts and megakaryocytes release growth factors, such as PDGF, which stimulate fibroblasts or other connective tissue cells to synthesize collagen or reticulin. This is also consistent with the fact that successful bone marrow transplantation leads to the reversal of established fibrosis.

The fibrosis and osteosclerosis of the marrow generally correlate with one another and also with the degree of splenomegaly. However, there is no clear relationship between the histopathology of the marrow and the peripheral blood counts. In 40 to 50 percent of patients, the appearance of marrow sclerosis is reflected on x-ray examination by increased bone density involving particularly the axial skeleton and proximal long bones. These x-ray changes result from thickened cortical bone and the loss of medullary spaces due to increased and thickened bony trabeculae.

No unique cytogenetic abnormalities have been described in AMM/MF; however, certain nonrandom abnormalities, including monosomy 7 and trisomy 9, have been found. Reports of the Ph chromosome in this disorder probably reflect examples of atypical CML.

DIAGNOSIS A bone marrow biopsy is essential to the evaluation of this disease, and without it the diagnosis cannot be made with certainty. This disorder may be difficult to distinguish from other myeloproliferative diseases.

In CML the white blood cell count is usually greater than 20,000 per microliter, while in AMM/MF it is generally 10,000 to 20,000 per microliter. Leukocyte alkaline phosphatase is usually lower in CML, and this determination may be useful in distinguishing between the two disorders. Fibrosis of the marrow is found in only 10 to 15 percent of patients with CML and is usually present only as a preterminal event; osteosclerosis is almost never seen. In the absence of the Ph chromosome, however, the distinction between these diseases is occasionally difficult.

The separation of PV and essential thrombocytosis (ET) from AMM/MF occasionally is troublesome because all may present with thrombocytosis, splenomegaly, leukocytosis, and anemia. However, ET generally is not associated with advanced fibrosis. The most difficult distinction is between AMM/MF and the late stages of PV, and attempts to separate them are probably unwarranted. Approximately 15 to 25 percent of patients with PV progress to advanced marrow fibrosis and marked splenomegaly. It is impossible to be certain that a patient with typical AMM/MF did not initially have PV. Postpolycythemia myeloid metaplasia with myelofibrosis has a poorer prognosis.

Secondary causes of myelofibrosis include metastatic carcinoma, leukemia and lymphomas, tuberculosis, Gaucher's disease, Paget's disease, and exposure to toxins such as benzene or to x-rays. These associations are usually not difficult to distinguish from AMM/MF.

THERAPY There is no definitive therapy for this disorder, and no treatment has been shown to affect life span favorably. Anemia is treated with transfusions as required. Androgens may be administered to improve the anemia, although they are helpful in less than half of the cases. Oxymetholone (2 to 4 mg/kg per day) or fluoxymesterone may be given, particularly if there is marked ineffective erythropoiesis. Glucocorticoids may enhance the response to androgens but alone are not helpful. Myelosuppressive therapy is only occasionally indicated, but it may be used to control painful splenomegaly or marked thrombocytosis. Chlorambucil or melphalan may be employed, but other blood elements may be depressed and the period of remission is relatively short (4 to 5 months). External radiation to the spleen will reduce its size, but the effects are transient and therapy may lead to severe pancytopenia. Allopurinol may be given to reduce a high uric acid level.

The role of splenectomy in the treatment of AMM/MF is controversial. Late in the course of the disease the hazards of removing a massively enlarged organ are considerable, and intraoperative mortality and postoperative complications, particularly thrombosis and infection, are frequent. Early removal of the spleen, as soon as the diagnosis is made, does not clearly reduce later complications or make management easier. The only clear indications for splenectomy are hemolysis, severe thrombocytopenia, and intractable symptoms related to spleen size.

COURSE AND PROGNOSIS AMM/MF generally follows a prolonged course, with a median survival of 4 to 5 years from the time of diagnosis; 25 percent of patients may live 15 years. Anemia occurs eventually in most patients, and many will require transfusions. Complicating features of the disease include gout or other problems related to hyperuricemia and symptoms related to the enlarging spleen. Portal hypertension may be seen due to hepatic fibrosis, hepatic vein thrombosis, or the markedly increased blood flow through the spleen. Clinically evident bleeding occurs in about 25 percent, and it is important for thrombocytopenic patients to avoid drugs such as aspirin or nonsteroidal anti-inflammatory agents which further impair platelet function. While the degree of splenomegaly appears to be of no prognostic importance, a platelet count of less than 100,000 per microliter, hemoglobin of less than 100 g/L (10 g/dL), and hepatomegaly are associated with poorer survival.

The major causes of death include infection, congestive heart failure, renal failure, portal hypertension, and hemorrhage. Transformation to acute leukemia occurs in 5 to 10 percent of patients and may be related to radiation or chemotherapy. A particularly fulminant variant of AMM/MF, known as acute myelofibrosis, is characterized by rapid progression of fibrosis and pancytopenia without splenic enlargement. Death due to marrow failure usually occurs within 1 year of diagnosis. This disorder is now more correctly recognized as acute megakaryoblastic leukemia.

ESSENTIAL THROMBOCYTOSIS

DEFINITION AND ETIOLOGY Essential thrombocytosis (ET) is dominated clinically by a markedly elevated platelet count which is invariably above 400,000 per microliter and which may reach levels of 3 to 4 million per microliter. The disease closely resembles PV and AMM/MF. Although an elevated platelet count is the dominant laboratory feature, all cell lines are involved in the expansion of the neoplastic clone.

As opposed to secondary forms of thrombocytosis, which arise in response to inflammation, acute bleeding, iron deficiency, or neoplasms, ET represents the overproduction of platelets in the absence of a recognizable stimulus. In cultures of bone marrow cells from patients with ET, colonies of megakaryocytes from megakaryocytic progenitors often form in the absence of added stimulus. Endogenous erythroid colonies may also form. This does not happen with marrow cell cultures from normal individuals or patients with secondary thrombocytosis.

PATHOPHYSIOLOGY AND SYMPTOMATOLOGY Symptoms associated with ET are linked to the platelet dysfunction and perhaps to platelet aggregation in the microvasculature of the central nervous system. Patients with ET may present with erythromelalgia, venous or arterial thromboses, or spontaneous bleeding. This may be seen as easy bruisability, unusual bleeding following minor dental procedures or other surgery, or large-vessel bleeding into soft tissues or muscles in the absence of a history of trauma. The first clue may be such a hemorrhagic or thrombotic episode. Transient ischemic attacks or even frank strokes may occur in patients with markedly elevated platelet counts. In general, there is a correlation between symptomatology and platelet counts in patients with this disease. However, the correlation is imperfect and individual patients will manifest symptoms at different platelet levels. Young patients, particularly females, are generally asymptomatic, regardless of platelet count.

LABORATORY FINDINGS The most prominent laboratory feature is the elevated platelet count. Examination of the peripheral blood smear reveals platelets of markedly different morphology with many large forms and forms which appear hypogranular. In vitro platelet function tests typically reveal an abnormality in platelet aggregation in response to epinephrine, collagen, or ADP. The epinephrine defect is the most characteristic. These in vitro aggregation abnormalities do not correlate with the history of bleeding or thrombosis or with a prolonged bleeding time. Splenomegaly is seen in two-thirds of patients with this disease but is generally modest, and the spleen does not achieve the size observed in CML or AMM/MF. Bone marrow examination reveals large numbers of hyperploid megakaryocytes and, with disease progression, there may be evidence of fibrosis. This is rarely as marked as in AMM/MF.

DIAGNOSIS A markedly elevated platelet count with typical platelet morphology in the absence of a cause for secondary thrombocytosis is generally sufficient to make the diagnosis. Confirmation may be obtained by in vitro platelet function tests, measurement of bleeding time, or the association of splenomegaly. Cytogenetic abnormalities are uncommon with this disease. A useful feature is the matching of megakaryocyte size to platelet number on examination of a marrow aspirate and biopsy. Secondary thrombocytosis is associated with increased numbers of megakaryocytes which are of generally small diameter and lower ploidy. In ET, the elevated platelet number is associated with increased numbers of large, hyperploid megakaryocytes.

COURSE AND PROGNOSIS The median survival of patients with ET is not well-defined. A prospective study evaluating therapy in this disease is being conducted by the Polycythemia Vera Study Group. It is anticipated that survival will be at least as good as for those patients with PV. Complications of the disease, such as hemorrhage or fatal thrombosis, represent the terminal event in the majority of cases. In 1 or 2 percent of cases the disease transforms to a more aggressive or frankly leukemic phase. If this does occur, aggressive chemotherapy is rarely effective.

THERAPY The indications for therapy in ET are unsettled, particularly in young, asymptomatic patients, and the effect of therapy in prolonging survival has not been quantitated. However, there is agreement that patients with symptomatic thrombocytosis who have had bleeding or thrombotic episodes should be treated. Previous therapy has employed alkylating agents such as busulfan or chlorambucil. However, because of the concern that these drugs may result in or enhance the likelihood of leukemic transformation, therapy with hydroxyurea is being evaluated. The available data suggest good control of the disease, but the overall effect on survival cannot be judged as yet. If patients are symptomatic at a particular platelet count, their counts should be maintained well below that level through the use of myelosuppression. Alkylating agents or ^{32}P may be used if hydroxyurea becomes ineffective. Treatment of acute events such as thrombosis or hemorrhage in an uncontrolled or previously undiagnosed patient with ET should be by emergent plateletpheresis. Aspirin and dipyridamole may prove useful in preventing thrombotic or ischemic symptoms in some patients with ET.

REFERENCES

ADAMSON JW, FIALKOW PJ: Pathogenesis of the myeloproliferative syndromes. Br J Haematol 38:299, 1978

ALLAN HC: Therapeutic options in chronic myeloid leukemia. Blood Rev 3:45, 1989

BERK PD et al: Increased incidence of acute leukemia in polycythemia vera associated with chlorambucil therapy. N Engl J Med 304:441, 1981

CHAMPLIN RE, GOLDE DW: Chronic myelogenous leukemia (CML): Recent advances. Blood 65:1039, 1985

HOCKIN WG, GOLDE DW: Polycythemia: Evaluation and management. Blood Rev 3:57, 1989

Polycythemia vera: An update I and II. In *Seminars in Hematology*, vol 23, PA Miescher, ER Jaffe (eds). Orlando, Grune & Stratton, Nos 2 (April) and 3 (July), 1986

SILVERSTEIN MK: Primary thrombocythemia, in *Hematology*, WJ Williams et al (eds). New York, McGraw-Hill, 1983, pp 218–222

STAM K et al: Evidence of a new chimeric *bcr/abl* mRNA in patients with chronic myelocytic leukemia and the Philadelphia chromosome. N Engl J Med 313:1429, 1985

TALPAZ M et al: Hematologic remission and cytogenetic improvement induced by recombinant human interferon alpha-a in chronic myelogenous leukemia. N Engl J Med 314:1065, 1986

THOMAS ED et al: Marrow transplantation for the treatment of chronic myelogenous leukemia. Ann Intern Med 104:155, 1986

298 BONE MARROW FAILURE: APLASTIC ANEMIA AND OTHER PRIMARY BONE MARROW DISORDERS

JOEL M. RAPPEPORT / H. FRANKLIN BUNN

An important group of anemias is caused by primary disorders of the bone marrow which impair the formation of erythropoietic precursors. The term *aplastic anemia* should be restricted to conditions in which an acellular or markedly hypocellular bone marrow results in pancytopenia (anemia, neutropenia, and thrombocytopenia). Rare patients develop selective aplasia of only erythroid cells (*pure red blood cell aplasia*). Alternatively, in *myelophthisic anemia,* erythropoiesis is suppressed because the marrow is infiltrated with tumor, granulomas, or fibrosis. The dysmyelopoietic or myelodysplastic anemias are associated with variable neutropenia and thrombocytopenia resulting from an acquired disorder of the hematopoietic pluripotent stem cell.

APLASTIC ANEMIA

ETIOLOGY Aplastic anemia is thought to be due to injury or destruction of a common pluripotential stem cell affecting all subsequent cell populations. The diverse factors associated with the development of aplastic anemia are listed in Table 298-1. In approximately half of the cases of aplastic anemia in the United States, no etiologic agent is identifiable. In areas of the world where a larger

TABLE 298-1 Causes of pancytopenia

I Aplastic anemia
  A Idiopathic anemias
  B Constitutional anemias (Fanconi's anemia)
  C Chemical and physical agents
    1 Dose-related: benzene, ionizing irradiation, alkylating agents, antimetabolites (folic acid antagonists, purine and pyrimidine analogues), mitotic inhibitors, anthracyclines, inorganic arsenicals
    2 Idiosyncratic: chloramphenicol, phenylbutazone, sulfa drugs, methylphenylethylhydantoin, gold compounds, organic arsenicals, insecticides
  D Immunologically mediated aplasia
  E Other associations: hepatitis, other viral infections, systemic lupus erythematosus, diffuse eosinophilic faciitis
II Pancytopenia with normal or increased bone marrow cellularity
  A Myelodysplastic syndromes
  B Hypersplenism (Chap. 63)
  C Vitamin B_{12} and folate deficiencies (Chap. 292)
III Paroxysmal nocturnal hemoglobinuria (Chap. 294)
IV Bone marrow replacement
  A Hematologic malignancies (Chaps. 134, 296, 302)
  B Nonhematologic metastatic tumor
  C Storage cell disorders (Chap. 331)
  D Osteopetrosis (Chap. 345)
  E Myelofibrosis (Chap. 297)

percentage of the population may be exposed to toxins such as insecticides and benzenes in uncontrolled dose, the percentage of idiopathic cases is smaller. In some cases, a damaged marrow microenvironment may contribute to marrow failure. The role of lymphokines in aplasia is currently under intense study.

Congenital causes Fanconi's anemia, the most common type of constitutional aplastic anemia, is an autosomal recessively inherited disease usually appearing in childhood. This disorder is often associated with multiple congenital somatic anomalies, including renal and cardiac malformations, hyperpigmentation of the skin, and bony abnormalities, particularly hypoplastic or absent thumbs or radii. Most patients have chromosomal abnormalities owing to a defect in DNA repair. Patients who survive the complications of progressive marrow failure are at high risk of developing leukemia or other malignancies. Other genetic syndromes have been associated with bone marrow failure including dyskeratosis congenita.

Immune causes A number of clinical observations have led to the concept that a significant proportion of cases of aplastic anemia may be mediated by immunologic mechanisms. These include autologous recovery following immunosuppressive preparation for marrow grafting and failure of hematopoietic reconstitution in some patients following marrow transplantation from identical twin donors in the absence of immunosuppression. A variety of in vitro culture techniques have also supported the concept of an antibody or a cellular autoimmune process in some patients with aplasia. However, in any given case the identification of an immune process may be difficult.

Drugs and toxins Multiple and seemingly unrelated drugs and chemical agents have been incriminated as etiologic agents in aplastic anemia. The association varies from a predictable dose-related aplasia to idiosyncratic reactions unrelated to dose.

The agents which in an adequate dose will predictably produce bone marrow depression are the antineoplastic and immunosuppressive drugs along with ionizing radiation. These drugs include folic acid antagonists, alkylating agents, the anthracyclines, and the nitrosoureas, as well as purine and pyrimidine analogues. The degree of aplasia is dose related but may vary from individual to individual. The effects of combination chemotherapy may be additive. Withdrawal of the drug usually permits recovery of the marrow elements, although irreversible aplasia is occasionally noted. Marrow aplasia may also be induced by therapeutic x-rays or, less commonly, by acute exposure from a laboratory or industrial accident. The severity of aplasia is dependent upon the dose and rate of the exposure as well as the extent of marrow irradiated.

Benzene derivatives have been associated with multiple hematologic abnormalities including aplastic anemia. Benzene-induced aplasia may result from both industrial and domestic use of benzene-containing products. This aplasia may be reversible, although mild abnormalities such as macrocytosis may persist.

Chloramphenicol, a commonly used broad-spectrum antibiotic, is associated with two forms of bone marrow toxicity. The more common effect upon the bone marrow is a reversible dose-related suppression of erythroid and, on occasion, granulocytic and megakaryocytic precursors. This condition is characterized by a transient anemia, associated with a drop in reticulocytes and elevation of serum iron. This bone marrow suppression is related to the dose and duration of administration of chloramphenicol. The bone marrow reveals vacuoles in the cytoplasm of early erythroid and granulocytic precursors. Similar morphologic features are seen much more commonly in some patients who have ingested large amounts of alcohol.

The more serious form of bone marrow failure associated with chloramphenicol is an "idiosyncratic" reaction. This nitrobenzene compound has been the single most commonly incriminated drug in cases of aplastic anemia. These patients develop severe pancytopenia and often irreversible, fatal marrow aplasia. This complication occurs in approximately 1 in 50,000 patients who take the drug. The development of aplastic anemia seems to be unrelated to dose or duration of administration. Marrow aplasia cannot be anticipated or prevented by hematologic monitoring, since it may appear after cessation of the drug. Unfortunately, many cases of fatal aplastic anemia have occurred in patients who received chloramphenicol for trivial or dubious reasons. Therefore, this antibiotic should not be used when there are reasonable alternatives.

Other unrelated chemicals and drugs may be responsible for the development of aplastic anemia. These agents can be placed into two classes: those in which a number of associations have been reported and, therefore, a definite toxic potential has been established, and those in which only a few reported cases exist and, therefore, only a possibility of toxic potential exists at present. The establishment of these relationships is often further confused by the fact that many of the patients have taken multiple drugs. Agents in which a definite potential toxicity exists are shown in Table 298-1.

Infections A number of cases of aplastic anemia have been reported following infectious hepatitis. The antecedent hepatitis is not distinguished by its severity, and the aplastic anemia commonly appears as the hepatitis resolves. Aplasia has usually followed non-A, non-B hepatitis but on occasion has been associated with types A and B. The aplasia tends to be severe and frequently has a fatal outcome. Other viruses, including Epstein-Barr virus, have been implicated in aplastic anemia. Many cases of so-called "idiopathic aplastic anemia" are preceded by a benign-appearing viral respiratory illness. Parvovirus selectively infects erythroblasts and therefore acutely aggravates anemia in patients with hemolysis (Chap. 294).

Some patients infected with human immunodeficiency virus will develop pancytopenia and a hypoplastic bone marrow. Contributing factors include direct suppression of hematopoietic cells by the virus, opportunistic infections such as cytomegalovirus or *Mycobacterium avium intracellulare,* and myelotoxic drugs such as trimethoprim-sulfamethoxazole and azidothymidine.

Aplastic anemia has also been reported in association with a number of other illnesses (Table 298-1). The clinical and laboratory findings associated with paroxysmal nocturnal hemoglobinuria may accompany or precede the development of aplasia. Aplastic anemia that develops during pregnancy may remit following delivery of the fetus.

CLINICAL MANIFESTATIONS The onset of aplastic anemia is usually insidious. Initial presenting symptoms include mild progressive weakness and fatigue attributable to the anemia and/or hemorrhage from the skin, nose, gums, vagina, or gastrointestinal tract due to the thrombocytopenia. The bleeding is usually mild, but occasionally retinal or central nervous system hemorrhage may be the initial mode of presentation. Although the patient may be severely neutropenic, it is less common for the initial presentation to be a bacterial infection.

Physical examination generally reveals pallor. Petechiae or ecchymoses may be noted in the skin, mucous membranes, the conjunctivae, and fundi. Lymphadenopathy and hepatosplenomegaly are notably absent. Fever may be present, but despite the presence of an infection, the usual signs of inflammation may be absent because of neutropenia.

The *course* of the disease is generally determined by the severity of the aplasia, rather than by the etiology. Mild disease can progress to a more severe disorder. Conversely, complete recovery or partial recovery of one or more cell lines may develop. It is important to obtain an accurate assessment of the degree of aplasia. Severe aplasia is defined as marked pancytopenia with at least two of the following criteria: granulocytes fewer than 500 per microliter, platelets fewer than 20,000 per microliter, or anemia with corrected reticulocyte count less than 1 percent. The bone marrow is markedly hypoplastic and depleted of hematopoietic cells. Patients with severe disease have a high risk of dying from bleeding and/or infections in a matter of months, while patients with a milder form of the disease may live for years. The clinical course of the disease is affected primarily by infections and by the nature and location of bleeding. Although infections may not dominate the clinical picture initially, they assume greater importance with the passage of time. Because of the need for multiple red blood cell and platelet transfusions, over a period of time one may encounter the sequelae of hemosiderosis and/or hepatitis. Even those patients who recover may have mild thrombocytopenia and persistent macrocytosis for many years. Long-term survivors are at increased risk of developing either acute leukemia or the myelodysplastic syndrome.

LABORATORY DIAGNOSIS The diagnosis of aplastic anemia and the assessment of its relative severity depend upon a thorough laboratory evaluation. The peripheral blood usually shows pancytopenia. The absolute granulocyte count is low, or becomes progressively depressed during the illness. The red blood cells are normochromic and normocytic or mildly macrocytic reflecting stress erythropoiesis, and the corrected reticulocyte count is very low or zero. Since the incidence of serious bleeding and/or infection correlates with the degree of thrombocytopenia or neutropenia, these values must be determined initially and followed serially. A bone marrow aspirate may yield a "dry tap," but a bone marrow biopsy will reveal a severely hypocellular or aplastic marrow with replacement by fat. There is usually a severe depression of megakaryocytes and myeloid cells and a marked but relatively less severe depression of the erythroid precursors.

Elevated serum iron coupled with a normal level of transferrin results in elevated transferrin saturation. Because of the reduction in erythroid precursors, plasma iron clearance is prolonged, and incorporation of iron into red blood cells is markedly decreased. There is no evidence of increased red blood cell destruction.

DIFFERENTIAL DIAGNOSIS The diagnosis of aplastic anemia implies the exclusion of the other causes of pancytopenia that are listed in Table 298-1. Splenomegaly and/or lymphadenopathy argue strongly against aplastic anemia. Malignant and nonmalignant invasion of the bone marrow must be excluded by microscopic examination of the marrow. Paroxysmal nocturnal hemoglobinuria and systemic lupus erythematosus should be ruled out by appropriate tests including the sugar water and acid hemolysis tests. Vitamin B_{12} and folate deficiencies can be excluded by serum assays and morphologic changes. Pancytopenia rarely may be secondary to various infections. Before aplastic anemia can be classified as idiopathic, a careful history must exclude exposure to all known and suspected agents. In our complex society, all patients are exposed to potentially toxic agents in their environment. Nevertheless this difficulty should not discourage a careful and extensive search for a cause.

TREATMENT The management of aplastic anemia has become one of the most challenging aspects of modern medicine, requiring a diligent multidisciplinary team of care givers in a well-equipped tertiary care center. For patients with mild aplasia, every effort should be made to do as little as possible except to remove possible etiologic agents in expectation of spontaneous recovery. As noted below, androgens may be of value in mild aplasia. Patients with severe aplasia should be considered for a bone marrow transplantation, if a suitable donor is available. The efficacy of this treatment with complete correction of the hematopoietic defect has been most clearly demonstrated in younger patients (Chap. 299).

Supportive care Regardless of the therapy chosen, the mainstay of treatment is good supportive care. The first and most immediate step is the removal of any suspected etiologic agent. If the disease is mild at presentation, no further supportive care need be instituted, unless there is subsequent deterioration. If a severe neutropenia exists (polymorphonuclear leukocytes fewer than 500 per microliter), the patient should be shielded from potential infections. Prophylactic systemic antibiotics should not be utilized. Intramuscular injections should be minimized and, if necessary, should be administered with care. Established infections should be treated vigorously with specific antibiotics, and fever of undetermined etiology may, after appropriate evaluation, call for broad-spectrum antibiotic coverage until a specific diagnosis is established. Menstruating females should be placed on suppressive doses of birth control pills.

TRANSFUSIONS These should be used *judiciously* and restricted to appropriate component therapy, since future therapy and ultimate survival may be affected by transfusions. Red blood cells should be administered to maintain the well-being of the patient rather than to establish a certain hemoglobin level. Transfusions pose significant risks such as development of hepatitis or hemosiderosis, as well as sensitization to both red blood cell antigens and transplantation antigens. Platelet transfusions should be administered in the face of serious hemorrhage. Some groups employ prophylactic transfusions when the platelet count is lower than 20,000 per microliter. Others, fearful of the development of resistance to future transfusions, administer platelets only when faced with hemorrhage. Responses to platelet transfusions may be blunted by the presence of infection. If a patient develops immune resistance to platelet transfusions, HLA-compatible platelet transfusions may be useful (Chap. 286). Should a bone marrow transplant be considered, family members should be avoided as a source of blood products since the patient may develop antibodies to minor transplantation antigens. Leukocyte transfusions are not administered prophylactically. However, white blood cell infusions may be of value in patients with documented gram-negative infections and severe neutropenia who have failed to respond to antimicrobial therapy.

Marrow-stimulating agents Although patients with mild aplasia sometimes respond to androgens, and a few appear to be androgen-dependent, those with severe aplasia are usually unresponsive. Patients with mild aplasia should be treated with adequate doses of androgens as the initial mode of therapy. The most widely used drugs at present are oxymetholone, fluoxymesterone, and nandrolone decanoate. Responses may occur as long as 3 to 6 months after the initiation of therapy. The administration of recombinant granulocyte-macrophage colony stimulating factor is effective in treating pancytopenia associated with AIDS, myelodysplasia, or myelotoxic drugs. It is less effective in the treatment of aplastic anemia.

Immunosuppressive agents Increasing clinical and laboratory evidence suggests that 40 to 50 percent of patients will have a complete or, more likely, partial response to immunosuppressive therapy. The specificity and mechanism of this therapy is as yet undefined. The most commonly administered therapy is animal antisera directed against human lymphocytes and thymocytes. The effectiveness as well as the dose and duration of administration of these heterogeneous sera is variable from batch to batch. Serious side effects may accompany the administration of these heteroantisera. Very high doses of glucocorticoids or the immunosuppressive agent cyclosporine may yield similar responses.

In general, splenectomy has no role in the management of aplastic anemia.

Bone marrow transplantation (See Chap. 299)

OTHER PRIMARY BONE MARROW DISORDERS

PURE RED CELL APLASIA Pure red cell aplasia involves a selective failure in the production of erythroid elements in the bone marrow. Granulopoiesis and megakaryocytopoiesis remain normal. Patients have a normochromic normocytic anemia with normal granulocyte count and platelet count. Severe reticulocytopenia exists, and the bone marrow is characterized by a virtual absence of any erythroid precursors in the face of otherwise normal cellular elements. An increase in lymphocytes may be seen in the marrow.

Constitutional red cell aplasia Blackfan-Diamond syndrome, a rare chronic constitutional red blood cell aplasia, may appear in infants from the time of birth to the age of 2 years. Twenty-five percent of patients have minor congenital anomalies. The disorder is of unknown etiology, but has been corrected by both glucocorticoids and marrow transplantation.

Acquired red cell aplasia The rare acquired form of pure red blood cell aplasia is seen predominantly in middle-aged adults. About one-third of patients have thymomas. Five percent of all patients with thymomas have pure red blood cell aplasia. The association between thymoma and myasthenia gravis is somewhat stronger. In many patients both with and without thymomas, erythropoiesis is inhibited by a complement-fixing IgG immunoglobulin which has selective cytotoxicity for marrow erythroblasts. A much smaller group of patients has been noted to have an inhibitor against erythropoietin. Occasionally, pure red cell aplasia is encountered in patients with T-cell chronic lymphatic leukemia. The circulating T cells are distinguished by the presence of receptors for the Fc portion of IgG.

TREATMENT Since these patients have virtually no endogenous red blood cell production, they are totally dependent on red blood cell transfusion. If thymic enlargement is noted, a thymectomy may induce a remission in approximately 50 percent of patients. If the thymus is normal, thymectomy is of no benefit. Patients without thymoma or those with an unsuccessful thymectomy should receive glucocorticoids, alone or in combination with an immunosuppressive agent such as cyclophosphamide. Treatment often results in both prolonged clinical remission and disappearance of the inhibitor.

MYELODYSPLASTIC SYNDROMES Also known as the refractory dysmyelopoietic anemias are a heterogeneous group of normocytic anemias often associated with neutropenia, thrombocytopenia, and/or monocytosis. The bone marrow varies in cellularity and usually reveals disordered maturation of erythroid, myeloid, and megakaryocytic cells. In some patients, erythroid cells accumulate large amounts of iron in mitochondria (ringed sideroblasts) (Chap. 291). The FAB (French, American, British) classification of the myelodysplastic syndrome includes five categories: refractory anemia (RA); refractory anemia with ringed sideroblasts (RARS); refractory anemia with excess of blasts (RAEB); chronic myelomonocytic leukemia (CMML); and refractory anemia with excess blasts in transformation (RAEB-T). This intrinsic disorder of the hematopoietic pluripotential stem cell is most frequently noted in older people. Although the etiology of these disorders is unclear, some patients appear to develop the syndrome secondary to chemotherapy, particularly alkylating agents with or without accompanying radiation therapy. The most common cytogenetic abnormalities noted include the deletion of the long arm of chromosome 5 (5q −), deletion of chromosome 7 or 5 (−7, −5), or trisomy 8. Over time, a variety of additional cytogenetic changes may be observed. Survival is variable among the subtypes with longer median survivals of 76 months noted in RARS and short median survivals of 3 to 6 months noted in RAEB-T. Patients may succumb to infections and hemorrhage because of the associated neutropenia and thrombocytopenia. These clonal disorders are frequently preleukemic with further evolution to a frank leukemic clone noted in 5 to 20 percent of patients with RARS and greater than 50 percent of patients with RAEB-T.

The mainstay of treatment is supportive: appropriate transfusion therapy and antibiotics for febrile episodes. Occasional long-term survivors may require therapy for iron overload. Rarely, patients with sideroblastic anemia will respond to pyridoxine or pyridoxal phosphate. Although differentiation agents such as vitamin D, retinoic acid, and low-dose cytosine arabinoside are effective in vitro, their therapeutic efficacy has been disappointing. Bone marrow transplantation in the appropriate setting has been curative for the myelodysplastic syndromes, as it has for de novo leukemias. Stimulation of the bone marrow by a variety of agents has been studied. Androgen therapy has in some cases resulted in moderate improvement. Hematopoietic growth factors, in particular recombinant granulocyte-macrophage colony stimulating factor (rGM-CSF), are currently under investigation and offer the potential for stimulating blood cell production. Both their long-term therapeutic effect and the possibility of accelerating the development of leukemia are still to be determined. The treatment of leukemia evolving from the myelodysplastic syndrome is discussed in Chap. 296.

MYELOPHTHISIC ANEMIA Infiltration of the bone marrow with tumor, fibrosis, or granulomas can result in the development of a severe anemia. Tumor may be derived from cell lines indigenous to the bone marrow, as in leukemia, lymphoma, or myeloma, or the marrow may be invaded by metastatic deposits of solid tumor, usually carcinoma. Among the solid tumors most frequently associated with myelophthisic anemia are carcinoma of the breast, stomach, prostate, lung, and thyroid. Hepatomegaly and splenomegaly may develop in this setting, along with marrow fibrosis.

Fibrosis in the bone marrow, usually in association with myeloid metaplasia (see Chap. 297), can cause myelophthisic anemia. Granulomatous involvement of the bone marrow is usually due to advanced tuberculosis. Primary lipid storage disorders, such as Gaucher's disease and Niemann-Pick disease, occasionally produce a myelophthisic anemia, and the rare disorder osteopetrosis, or marble bone disease, may also give a similar hematologic picture.

The invasion of the bone marrow by tumor or granulomas impairs both erythropoiesis and thrombopoiesis. In contrast, neutrophil production is generally normal or increased. It is unlikely that the anemia and thrombocytopenia are due merely to "crowding" of the bone marrow space by extrinsic cells. Myelophthisis also causes a distortion of the microcirculation of the marrow, with premature release of immature cells.

Myelophthisis usually results in a severe normochromic normocytic anemia. A variety of misshapen erythrocytes are noted, particularly teardrop cells and fragmented cells with some basophilic stippling. In addition, normoblasts are usually seen in the peripheral blood. The reticulocyte percentage is often slightly increased (4 to 7 percent). However, when corrected for the anemia and the premature release from the bone marrow, the absolute reticulocyte count is actually reduced and reflects a decrease in red blood cell production. While thrombocytopenia is usually present, the white blood cell count is often elevated, with a marked shift to the left in the differential count. The combination of immature myeloid cells and normoblasts in the peripheral blood constitutes the "leukoerythroblastic" morphology so characteristic of myelophthisic anemia. Striking abnormalities are usually seen on examination of the bone marrow. Often an aspirate yields a "dry tap" owing to the infiltration of the marrow with abnormal tissue. Marrow biopsy is more likely to be diagnostic, revealing leukemia, lymphoma, or foci of metastatic tumors or granulomas. However, marrow involvement is often segmental, so that the primary pathologic process may be missed on a single biopsy.

Treatment Treatment consists of attempts to reverse the primary pathologic process. It is particularly important to search for the presence of tuberculosis, since this disease is readily treatable. More often, however, the underlying disease is not amenable to therapy, and supportive measures, such as blood transfusions, must be employed.

REFERENCES

ANASETTI C et al: Marrow transplantation for severe aplastic anemia. Long-term outcome in fifty "untransfused" patients. Ann Intern Med 104:461, 1986

CAMITTA BM et al: Aplastic anemia: Pathogenesis, diagnosis, treatment and prognosis. N Engl J Med 306:645, 1982
CHIKKAPPA G et al: Pure red cell aplasia with chronic lymphatic leukemia. Medicine 65:339, 1986
CLARK DA et al: Studies on pure red cell aplasia. XI. Results of immunosuppressive treatment of 37 patients. Blood 63:277, 1984
GRIFFIN JD (ed): Myelodysplastic syndromes. Clin Haematol 15:909, 1986
HUMPHRIES RK, YOUNG N: Aplastic anemia and stem cell biology, in *Aplastic Anemia*. New York, AR Liss, 1984
KRANTZ SB, DESSYPRIS EN: Pure red cell aplasia, in *Hematopoietic Stem Cells*, DW Golde and F Takaka (eds). New York, Dekker, 1985
RAPPEPORT JM, NATHAN DG: Acquired aplastic anemia: Pathophysiology and treatment. Adv Intern Med 27:547, 1982
SPECK B et al: Treatment of severe aplastic anemia. Exp Hematol 14:126, 1986
VADHAN-RAJ S et al: Effects of recombinant human granulocyte-macrophage colony-stimulating factor in patients with myelodysplastic syndromes. N Engl J Med 317:1545, 1987

299 BONE MARROW TRANSPLANTATION

E. DONNALL THOMAS

SELECTION OF THE PATIENT Marrow transplantation is a rational therapeutic option only if the patient's disease involves the marrow or if hazard to the normal marrow is the limiting factor in aggressive treatment of a disease. A marrow transplant involves a transplant not only of the donor myeloid, erythroid, and megakaryocytic systems but also of the donor lymphoid and macrophage-monocyte systems. The rationale is illustrated by the three types of disease for which marrow transplantation has been widely utilized:

1 *Genetic disease*. For immunologic deficiency diseases, the objective is to replace the recipient's genetically defective lymphoid system with the normal lymphoid system of the donor. For genetic diseases such as thalassemia major, the abnormal marrow must be destroyed and replaced by normal marrow.
2 *Aplastic anemia*. Regardless of etiology, the disease process results in loss of the marrow, and the objective is to replace the defective organ with a normal functioning organ.
3 *Malignant disease*. For leukemia and other hematologic malignancies the objective is the complete destruction of the malignant cell population and, unavoidably, normal marrow cells by intensive chemoradiotherapy with restoration of normal marrow function by the transplanted marrow.

TYPES OF TRANSPLANTS A *syngeneic* graft describes a graft in which donor and recipient are genetically identical, i.e., identical twins. An *allogeneic* graft is one in which donor and recipient are of different genetic origins. A *chimera* is an individual whose body contains living, proliferating cells of different genetic origin. An *autologous* marrow graft refers to the removal of a patient's marrow, administration of chemo- and/or radiotherapy, and then return of the patient's own marrow.

SELECTION OF THE DONOR The donor must be in good health, and the donor, or an appropriate advocate, must be capable of giving informed consent. The principal risk is the anesthesia. Beyond these considerations, selection of the donor is largely determined by histocompatibility testing. Red blood cell incompatibility is not a barrier to marrow transplantation.

Histocompatibility typing (See Chap. 14) The HLA region is composed of a series of closely linked genes on chromosome 6. The array of genes encoded on a single chromosome is known as a *haplotype*. Each individual has two haplotypes, one inherited from each parent. The antigens encoded at HLA-A, -B, -C, -DR, and -DQ are detected on lymphocytes by serologic techniques in a microcytotoxicity assay and those of the D region are also detected by the mixed leukocyte culture reaction. Loci within the D region can now be recognized serologically by typing of B lymphocytes. These closely linked genetic loci, each with a large number of known alleles, make the HLA region the most complex genetic polymorphism yet described. Despite this complexity, within a family there can be only four haplotypes. Therefore, for a given patient, each sibling has one chance in four of being HLA-identical with the patient. The most widely used transplants are those between HLA-identical siblings. There is now an increasing use of other family members and volunteer unrelated donors who match the patient or differ by only one HLA antigen.

PREPARATION OF THE PATIENT Infants with severe combined immunologic deficiency are conditioned to accept a transplant by the nature of their disease. All other patients are immunologically competent, to a greater or lesser degree, and are able to reject the marrow graft unless prepared with some form of immunosuppressive therapy. An immunosuppressive regimen commonly used for patients with aplastic anemia uses large doses of cyclophosphamide. Preparation of the patient with leukemia involves high-dose chemoradiotherapy for immunosuppression and to kill leukemic cells. A commonly used regimen involves cyclophosphamide followed by total-body irradiation (TBI). Approximately 10 gray (Gy) must be used for immunosuppression sufficient to permit consistent engraftment of marrow even though only 4 to 5 Gy will cause lethal marrow injury. Patients with genetic disease of the marrow may be prepared with busulfan or dimethyl busulfan to destroy the abnormal marrow along with cyclophosphamide for immunosuppression.

Marrow aspiration and infusion The pelvic bones are the most readily accessible sites for procurement, although marrow may be obtained from the sternum, ribs, or, in the case of children, the tibia. In the operating room and under general or spinal anesthesia multiple marrow aspirations are performed on the iliac crests. For adult donors, the volume of the mixture of blood and marrow cells is from 500 to 800 mL. As each aspiration is performed, the marrow is mixed with heparin and tissue culture medium. When the collection is completed, the marrow is passed through stainless steel screens to break up particles. It is then given to the recipient by intravenous infusion. The marrow stem cells pass through the lungs and subsequent growth and reconstitution of the marrow is confined almost exclusively to the medullary cavities.

Support for the patient without marrow function Usually 2 to 4 weeks are required before the transplanted marrow starts to produce the critical formed elements of the peripheral blood. Supportive care is crucial for survival. The patient should be cared for using the most effective available isolation facilities. Platelet transfusions are usually unnecessary at levels above 20,000 per microliter (see Chap. 287). Below that level, they should be used until values above 20,000 are sustained, especially if there is any evidence of bleeding. If the patient becomes refractory to random donor platelets, the use of platelets from HLA-matched family members or unrelated donors may be necessary. Aspirin and other drugs that depress platelet function should be avoided. Granulocyte transfusions (see Chaps. 81 and 82) may be indicated for therapy of refractory infection in a granulocytopenic patient. Packed red blood cells should be given as needed to control symptoms of anemia, usually to keep the hematocrit above 25 percent. All blood products should be irradiated with 1.5 Gy to inactivate lymphocytes that might cause a graft-versus-host reaction.

Since infection is an ever-present danger, bacteriologic cultures should be obtained frequently. Onset of significant fever (38.5°C) should arouse a strong suspicion of infection in the granulocytopenic patient. Fever with clinical signs of bacteremia or fever sustained more than 24 h is an indication for starting systemic antibacterial therapy even if cultures are negative. Initial therapy usually includes an aminoglycoside active against *Pseudomonas* (gentamicin, tobramycin, amikacin) and carbenicillin or ticarcillin with additional antibiotics added as indicated by culture results (see Chaps. 82 and 85). Subsequently, if cultures are negative but fever persists, therapy with a combination of trimethoprim and sulfamethoxazole or with amphotericin may be considered. Once broad-spectrum antibiotic therapy has been initiated, it should be continued until the granulocyte count rises above 200 per microliter even if clinical signs of infection disappear.

Many patients coming to marrow transplantation have had inadequate nutrition because of their disease or the efforts to treat it. The preparation for marrow grafting results in nausea, vomiting, and mucositis which results in poor oral intake for at least several weeks. A Hickman modification of the Broviac catheter is installed routinely. The catheter makes it possible to administer hyperalimentation, medications, and blood products and is also used for drawing blood samples. Although some catheters are removed because of infection or suspected infection, about 90 percent of the patients have the catheter in place for approximately 3 months, the period of time when it is needed.

ENGRAFTMENT AND PROOF OF ENGRAFTMENT Engraftment is signaled by a rise in granulocytes and platelets and the reappearance of reticulocytes. The median time required to reach a granulocyte count of 1000 per microliter is 26 days. The rise in platelet count usually occurs a week or two later.

Proof of engraftment depends upon use of cytogenetics, blood genetic markers, and/or restriction enzyme fragment length polymorphisms to distinguish donor from host cells. The regenerating marrow is usually entirely of donor type. Occasional patients show persistence of some host cells for a few weeks. Rare patients have an increasing number of host cells, and eventually the marrow is repopulated by host cells as the graft is lost.

COMPLICATIONS FOLLOWING ENGRAFTMENT The complications that may follow successful marrow engraftment are (1) graft rejection, a problem primarily occurring in patients with aplastic anemia; (2) infection, including early bacterial infections or later opportunistic infections such as cytomegalovirus interstitial pneumonia; (3) acute graft-versus-host disease (GVHD), the result of the immunologic reaction of the engrafted lymphoid elements against tissues of the recipient; (4) chronic GVHD; (5) recurrence of leukemia; and (6) miscellaneous complications such as hemorrhagic cystitis, cardiomyopathy, cataract formation, venocclusive liver disease, leukoencephalopathy, and sterility.

CLINICAL RESULTS OF MARROW TRANSPLANTATION Immunodeficiency diseases Despite the rarity of these disorders, these patients are unique in that immunosuppressive therapy is not necessary to condition the patient to accept a graft, and because some myeloid function is usually present, rapid marrow engraftment is not essential. One such patient was the first to be transplanted from an HLA-identical sibling, and more than 100 similar patients have been successfully reconstituted since then.

Genetically determined hematologic diseases Marrow grafts have now been reported for Kostmann's syndrome, chronic granulomatous disease, Chédiak-Higashi syndrome, Blackfan-Diamond syndrome, congenital aplastic anemia, and sickle cell disease (one patient, transplanted because of leukemia). Of particular interest is marrow transplantation for thalassemia major. Thalassemia major is a significant cause of death in children in many parts of the world. In developed countries, therapy with transfusions and chelating agents can prolong life for one to three decades but at great expense. In 1981, a patient with thalassemia major was prepared with dimethyl busulfan and cyclophosphamide and given a marrow graft from an HLA-identical older sister who did not have the thalassemia trait. There was prompt resolution of laboratory and clinical evidence of thalassemia, and the patient's growth and development are normal. Now more than 200 marrow transplants for thalassemia major have been done. Approximately 10 percent of the children died of complications of marrow grafting, and 10 percent have regenerated their own marrow and again have thalassemia major. Eighty percent of the patients appear to be cured of the disease although some 5 percent of the cured patients are under treatment for chronic GVHD. Results are better for patients less than 8 years of age, but good results are now being reported for older, multiply transfused patients. Marrow grafting can cure genetically determined hematopoietic disorders which, at present, cannot be cured in any other way. Gene transfer for therapy of these diseases is an exciting possibility currently under investigation in many laboratories.

Transplantation for severe aplastic anemia (See Chap. 298) Because of the poor prognosis on conventional therapy, patients with severe aplastic anemia are logical candidates for marrow transplantation.

HLA-IDENTICAL SIBLING DONORS Patients with severe aplastic anemia must be prepared for engraftment with immunosuppressive therapy. The most widely used regimen is cyclophosphamide 50 mg/kg on each of 4 days followed 36 h later by donor marrow. The first two successful transplants were reported in 1972, and these recipients are alive and well.

For ethical reasons the initial marrow transplants were carried out in patients who had failed to benefit from conventional therapy. As a consequence these end-stage patients had already received multiple transfusions, and many were severely infected at the time of transplantation. One-third of the patients rejected the graft, and the long-term survival of these end-stage patients was 40 to 50 percent.

Since blood transfusions can sensitize an intended marrow transplant recipient, resulting in rejection of the marrow graft, patients with severe aplastic anemia were identified early in the course of the disease so that marrow transplantation could be carried out before blood transfusions were given. The long-term survival of these patients is more than 80 percent. Therefore, patients with severe aplastic anemia and their families should have tissue typing performed immediately upon diagnosis. If a suitable donor can be identified, marrow transplantation should be carried out promptly before transfusions become necessary.

However, many patients with severe aplastic anemia present to the physician with bleeding and/or infection, and transfusions must be given as an urgent medical necessity. Therefore, marrow transplant teams are investigating other preparative regimens designed to prevent graft rejection and to improve survival. These include regimens using various combinations of antithymocyte globulin, cyclophosphamide, and total-nodal irradiation. Another regimen is based on the fact that patients given a smaller number of marrow cells have had an increased probability of graft rejection. Since it was not practical to get more marrow cells from the donor, peripheral blood mononuclear cells have been used as an added source of donor cells. The standard cyclophosphamide regimen was administered followed by the marrow transplant. Then, on each of 3 to 5 days following marrow transplantation, buffy coat white blood cells were collected from 4 units of donor blood by a leukapheresis technique and administered intravenously to the recipient without in vitro irradiation. For patients who have been transfused, these modified regimens have largely solved the problem of graft rejection. Long-term survival is approximately 75 percent.

IDENTICAL TWIN DONORS Aplastic anemia is not a common disease, and to find a patient with it who has an identical twin is even more uncommon. Nevertheless, a number of transplants have been carried out for severe aplastic anemia using an identical twin as the marrow donor. In some patients the simple intravenous infusion of marrow without any immunosuppressive treatment resulted in recovery. These results reinforce the concept that aplastic anemia is due to an acquired abnormality of the stem cell which can be corrected by transplantation of normal syngeneic stem cells. However, some patients did not recover after simple intravenous marrow infusion. These patients were then treated with the cyclophosphamide regimen and given a second infusion of marrow from the twin which resulted in complete hematopoietic reconstitution. The results suggest that some cases may be due to an immune mechanism or abnormal regulators of cell growth. Whatever the mechanism, the rare patient with aplastic anemia who has a genetically identical twin has a 90 percent chance of being cured with marrow transplantation.

Transplantation for acute leukemia Acute leukemia (see Chap. 296) has served as a prototype malignant disease of the marrow for treatment by intensive chemoradiotherapy and marrow transplantation. Almost all regimens used for preparing leukemic patients for marrow transplantation have employed supralethal TBI. This has been done for several reasons: (1) irradiation is an effective means of eradicating leukemic cells; (2) irradiation penetrates to the so-called privileged sites where leukemic cells may be inaccessible to chemotherapeutic agents; and (3) irradiation is a powerful immunosuppressive agent. Cyclophosphamide or other antileukemic drugs are given with TBI. Regimens using busulfan and cyclophosphamide (without TBI) are also being explored.

ACUTE LEUKEMIA IN RELAPSE USING HLA-IDENTICAL SIBLING DONORS For ethical reasons, marrow transplantation was initially attempted only in patients with acute leukemia in relapse after combination chemotherapy. These end-stage patients were poor candidates for any therapeutic procedure because they usually presented with a heavy body burden of leukemic cells, were usually granulocytopenic and thrombocytopenic, and often already infected with antibiotic-resistant bacteria and fungi. In early studies 10-Gy TBI was given in preparation for grafting. Then an attempt was made to kill more leukemic cells by giving cyclophosphamide a few days before administration of TBI and the marrow transplant. For these end-stage patients there were many deaths related to advanced illness at the time of transplantation, graft-versus-host disease, opportunistic infections, or recurrence of leukemia. An analysis of survival shows that 10 percent of these patients are long-term survivors with the leading patients now 18 years postgrafting. It appears that these patients, on no maintenance chemotherapy, are cured of their disease. Marrow transplant teams have utilized several different chemoradiotherapy preparative regimens for end-stage patients, but the long-term survival rate remains at 5 to 15 percent.

ACUTE LYMPHOBLASTIC LEUKEMIA (ALL) IN REMISSION USING HLA-IDENTICAL SIBLING DONORS The fact that some patients in the end stages of acute leukemia could apparently be cured led to transplantation earlier in the course of disease. Many patients with ALL, particularly children in the "good-risk" category, can be cured by combination chemotherapy, but once marrow relapse has occurred, long-term survival is rare. Therefore, the decision was made to transplant patients in the second or subsequent remission. It was recognized that some of these patients would be lost early to transplant complications, but this risk seemed acceptable if some patients could, in fact, be cured. Most marrow transplant teams are reporting long term survival and apparent cure of 25 to 50 percent of these patients. Recurrent leukemia is a major problem. These recurrences, in host-type cells, show that the preparative regimen was often ineffective in eradicating the residual leukemic cell population.

ACUTE NONLYMPHOBLASTIC LEUKEMIA (ANL) IN REMISSION USING HLA-IDENTICAL SIBLING DONORS In contrast to patients with ALL, patients with ANL in first remission are known to have a poor prognosis. With combination chemotherapy the median duration of the first remission in most reported series is approximately 12 to 15 months, and only 20 to 25 percent of the patients are alive at 5 years after initial chemotherapy. Therefore, a study of marrow transplantation in these patients in first remission was considered to be ethically acceptable. Several hundred such transplants have now been carried out with various marrow transplant teams reporting 45 to 70 percent long-term disease-free survival.

PATIENTS WITH CHRONIC MYELOGENOUS LEUKEMIA (CML) The term *chronic* is inappropriate in describing the clinical course of patients with CML. The conversion to blast crisis and death occurs at a fairly constant rate, and the median survival in most series of patients is approximately 30 to 40 months (see Chap. 297). Although a small fraction of patients may live for a long time in the chronic phase, in general, the outlook for most patients with CML is quite grim. When blast crisis appears, therapy is usually ineffective. A subset of patients whose blasts appear to be more like lymphoblasts (terminal transferase-positive) and with a hypodiploid number of chromosomes may respond for a period of a few months to treatment with vincristine and prednisone.

Marrow transplantation from HLA-identical donors has been carried out in patients with CML in blast crisis. As expected from the experience with acute leukemia in relapse, there were many deaths. However, 10 to 20 percent of these patients are long-term survivors without the Philadelphia (Ph) chromosome and appear to be cured.

A study of marrow transplantation during the chronic phase of the disease for patients with an identical twin to serve as marrow donor was initiated. The twin donors were clinically and hematologically normal. Preparation was with cyclophosphamide and TBI. Nine of 14 such patients are alive and well without the Ph chromosome 7 to 12 years later. These results of syngeneic marrow transplantation indicated that the Ph chromosome–positive leukemic cell clone can be eliminated and suggested that marrow transplantation could be carried out in the chronic phase of CML utilizing allogeneic donors. HLA-identical grafts have been performed for more than 600 patients in the chronic phase of CML. Long-term survival ranges from 50 to 80 percent and the absence of the Ph chromosome indicates cure for the majority of these patients.

PATIENTS WITH ACUTE LEUKEMIA USING DONORS OTHER THAN HLA-IDENTICAL SIBLINGS The general experience in the United States has been that only one-third of the patients with acute leukemia will have an HLA-identical sibling. The majority of patients will not have an HLA-identical sibling. Marrow transplantation has been carried out in family member donor-recipient pairs in which one of the HLA haplotypes was genetically identical and the other haplotype phenotypically identical for one or more of the HLA loci. The results of these transplants when donor and recipient are phenotypically matched or mismatched at only one locus are quite similar to the results using an HLA-identical sibling donor. The outcome is largely a function of the stage of the disease in which the transplant was carried out. There are too few patients to permit an analysis according to the family relationship of the donor or according to the HLA locus involved in the mismatch.

Serologic HLA typing makes it technically possible to find a suitably matched unrelated donor, at least for patients with the more common HLA haplotypes, given a large panel of potential donors whose HLA types have been determined. The National Marrow Donor Program has recruited more than 20,000 HLA-typed donors, and more than 100 transplants from unrelated donors have been carried out.

Autologous marrow transplantation The technique for procuring and cryopreserving marrow has been established for more than 20 years. The patient's own marrow can be cryopreserved during intensive chemoradiotherapy and then returned to the patient in order to avoid subsequent lethal marrow aplasia. The concept is attractive because use of the patient's own marrow avoids the risk of GVHD. The following points are pertinent in considering autologous marrow transplantation: (1) The patient's marrow should not be contaminated with malignant cells. (2) Autologous marrow is of value only in protecting the patient against lethal hematopoietic toxicity. If the regimen of chemoradiotherapy involves lethal toxicity to other organ systems, autologous marrow will not be of benefit. (3) The tumor being treated must show a dose-response curve such that supralethal chemoradiotherapy can be expected to result in a significantly enhanced antitumor response. Unfortunately, with currently available agents, only a few tumors appear to fall into this category. (4) The protocol must be designed so that the role of autologous marrow can be demonstrated. In animals it is feasible to administer "supralethal" therapy and to demonstrate that animals given syngeneic marrow will survive while those not given marrow will die. For obvious reasons, this kind of controlled experiment cannot be done in humans. Failure to recognize these four principles accounts for much of the current uncertainty about the value of autologous marrow transplantation in the treatment of patients with malignant disease.

Nevertheless, the potential use of autologous marrow is the subject of a new wave of interest, and some results are encouraging. The tumors that might be expected to show a significant improvement in response to high-dose chemoradiotherapy include the leukemias, Hodgkin's disease, non-Hodgkin's lymphoma, small cell cancer of the lung, breast cancer, testicular tumors, and ovarian tumors. Techniques being explored for removal of tumor cells from the marrow include physical separation, destruction by chemotherapeutic agents, and destruction by monoclonal antibodies. Several transplant centers are conducting studies of the utility of cryopreserved autologous marrow, and all have reported successful hematopoietic reconstitution in most patients. Most also describe the high complete remission rate and good disease-free survival over initial periods of 1 to 3 years. It is too early to evaluate fully the impact of these studies on the course of the several diseases.

IMMUNOLOGIC ASPECTS OF MARROW TRANSPLANTATION

Marrow graft rejection "Marrow graft rejection" describes a phenomenon in which the transplanted marrow graft begins to function, but after a few days or weeks, the peripheral blood counts suddenly drop and marrow biopsy shows the marrow to be devoid of myeloid elements. Immunologically mediated marrow graft rejection is usually a consequence of sensitization by transfusions. In addition, inadequate immunosuppressive therapy before grafting may facilitate marrow graft rejection. Marrow graft rejection is a common problem in patients with aplastic anemia, but is very uncommon in patients with leukemia, which may be due to several factors: (1) Transfusions are usually given to leukemic patients while they are receiving antileukemic chemotherapy which is also immunosuppressive. This chemotherapy may prevent sensitization to transplantation antigens contained in blood products. (2) Leukemia may damage the lymphoid system so that the disease process itself interferes with sensitization. (3) Leukemic patients receive a more intensive immunosuppressive regimen before grafting.

Marrow graft failure may be due to causes other than immunologic mechanisms. With a solid organ, such as the kidney, histologic proof of graft rejection is easily obtained, but such proof usually cannot be obtained with a marrow graft since the myeloid marrow simply disappears. Other possible mechanisms of graft failure include (1) defective or inadequate numbers of "stem cells" in the donor marrow; (2) defective microenvironment in the marrow recipient; (3) allogeneic resistance not associated with HLA; and (4) susceptibility of the donor marrow to the same etiologic mechanism(s) responsible for the original disease process.

Acute graft-versus-host disease (GVHD) A "wasting disease" or "runt disease" was described many years ago in newborn mice or in rodents exposed to lethal TBI and given infusions of allogeneic hematopoietic cells. These observations were later confirmed for other species, including humans, and were recognized to be due to an immunologic reaction of engrafted lymphoid cells, presumably T cells, against the tissues of the host. This graft-versus-host reaction is one of the major complications of marrow transplantation in humans. In patients given a marrow graft from an HLA-identical sibling and postgrafting immunosuppression, approximately one-half develop moderate to severe GVHD.

Acute GVHD in humans usually involves the skin, gastrointestinal tract, and/or the liver. A skin rash is usually the first sign of GVHD. Intestinal involvement results in diarrhea and may progress to abdominal pain and ileus. Liver disease is characterized by rises of bilirubin, serum glutamic oxaloacetic transaminase, and alkaline phosphatase. Severe immunologic deficiency accompanies GVHD, and death from infection is frequent.

Since GVHD is immunologically mediated, efforts to prevent its development have involved the use of immunosuppressive therapy. Of the many agents studied, methotrexate, glucocorticoids, and cyclosporine were found to be useful. One regimen consists of methotrexate, 15 mg/m^2 on day 1 postgrafting and 10 mg/m^2 on days 3, 6, 11, and 18, and weekly thereafter through day 102. Cyclosporine is a potent immunosuppressive agent. It is particularly valuable in organ grafts such as kidney, heart, and liver. Cyclosporine given after a marrow graft is useful because it does not cause mucositis as methotrexate does, and it does not suppress the marrow graft so that effective marrow function is evident earlier. Cyclosporine is nephrotoxic, and marrow graft recipients often receive other nephrotoxic agents such as amphotericin for suspected fungal infection. Creatinine level and serum cyclosporine level must be monitored carefully with prompt reduction of dosage if renal function is threatened. A regimen using a short course of methotrexate along with cyclosporine has proved highly effective in reducing the incidence and severity of acute GVHD.

A number of studies have been carried out in an effort to treat acute GVHD once it becomes established. Recipients of HLA-identical marrow have been treated with rabbit, goat, or horse antithymocyte globulin, high-dose methyl prednisolone, cyclosporine, and/or anti-T-cell monoclonal antibodies. About two-thirds of patients will respond to one or another of these agents. However, about one-third of the patients who develop moderate to severe GVHD will die of it or its infectious complications. It is clear that the treatment of acute GVHD is unsatisfactory and that new approaches in preventing or treating GVHD must be found.

Experiments are underway designed to eliminate from the marrow inoculum the T cells believed to be responsible for GVHD while retaining hematopoietic stem cells. One approach involves treatment of the donor marrow with lectins for agglutination and separation of the T cells. Monoclonal antibodies that react with human T cells or subsets of T cells are being used in conjunction with complement, or are bound to toxins, such as the A chain of ricin, to create an immunotoxin. The preliminary results of these studies indicate a reduction in the incidence and severity of GVHD. However, the incidence of graft failure and of recurrence of leukemia is significantly increased. The explanation for these problems is unknown at present.

Chronic GVHD Chronic GVHD occurs in approximately one-fourth of those recipients of marrow from an HLA-identical sibling who survive beyond 100 days. The manifestations include skin disease, keratoconjunctivitis, buccal mucositis, esophageal strictures, small- and large-intestinal involvement, pulmonary insufficiency, chronic liver disease, and generalized wasting. Histologically, the disease resembles the systemic collagen vascular diseases, especially morphea and lupus erythematosus profundus. Chronic GVHD may be associated with recurrent and occasionally fatal bacterial infections.

Initial efforts to treat chronic GVHD with short courses of antithymocyte globulin or prolonged treatment with prednisone were ineffective. Recently, treatment with prednisone with or without azathioprine has resulted in recovery of about 80 percent of the patients, although treatment may be required for 1 or 2 years. Twenty percent continue to have problems which may be disabling, and cyclosporine, intermittent steroids, or monoclonal antibodies alone or bound to a toxin are being tried for the refractory patients.

Recovery of immunologic function Most patients given a marrow transplant from an HLA-identical sibling develop a functional graft with adequate levels of circulating granulocytes and platelets. Nevertheless, particularly in the first 3 months after grafting, these patients are susceptible to a wide variety of opportunistic infections. Approximately one-fifth of patients develop an interstitial pneumonia, and cytomegalovirus can be demonstrated in more than one-half of these pneumonias. The mortality rate is approximately 80 percent. Use of blood products from donors who are serologically negative for CMV for those donor-recipient pairs also serologically negative has almost eliminated CMV infection and pneumonia in this subset of patients. The high incidence of infection is the result of a very slow return of immunologic function, which may be made worse by GVHD and by efforts to prevent or treat GVHD. Fortunately, by the end of the first year after grafting, most patients have recovered immunologically and are able to lead normal lives without an increased incidence of infection.

Tolerance The long-term healthy human recipients of allogeneic marrow transplants are true chimeras. Their myeloid, lymphoid, and monocyte-macrophage systems are entirely made up of cells of donor origin. Clearly, these donor cells in the recipient are "tolerant" of the hosts' tissues. Studies of tolerance constitute a fascinating story in immunobiology, but a clear understanding of the state of tolerance has not emerged. At least three mechanisms may be operative, including classical central tolerance, tolerance maintained by "blocking factors," and tolerance related to the presence of "suppressor" cells.

The effect of age The success of allogeneic marrow grafting is inversely proportional to the age of the recipient. For example, for patients transplanted in first remission of ANL, long-term survival for those under age 20 is approximately 75 percent and for patients aged 30 to 50, 40 percent. The most apparent explanation for this difference is the increased incidence and severity of GVHD in older patients. Most marrow transplant centers do not transplant patients over the age of 50. These age restrictions do not apply to syngeneic transplants since these patients do not have GVHD, although patients over the age of 50 do not tolerate intensive treatment as well as younger patients.

RECURRENT LEUKEMIA AFTER GRAFTING **Frequency of recurrence of leukemia** For patients with leukemia transplanted in relapse or in second remission, an actuarial analysis shows a rather constant rate of recurrence of leukemia in the first year, a decreasing rate in the second year, and few recurrences thereafter. If there were no other causes of death, approximately 35 percent of the patients would be cured, while 65 percent would be destined to relapse. However, the risk of relapse is only about 20 percent for patients with ANL transplanted in first remission or CML transplanted in chronic phase. It is evident that recurrent leukemia after grafting is a major problem for patients transplanted in relapse or in second or subsequent remission.

Nature of recurrent leukemia Blood genetic makers, cytogenetic techniques, and restriction enzyme fragment length polymorphisms can be used to identify the donor or host origin of the leukemic cells in patients who relapse after marrow transplantation. In the vast majority of patients the recurrent leukemia is in host-type cells, indicating that the preparative regimen and the graft did not eliminate all the leukemic cells. However, several cases have now been reported in which the recurrent leukemic cells were shown to be of donor origin. The mechanism of donor-cell transformation is unknown. In more than a dozen cases a lymphoblastic lymphoma associated with Epstein-Barr virus genomes has occurred in donor cells. These highly fatal lymphomas have usually occurred in patients undergoing intensive treatment for GVHD.

Graft-versus-leukemia In recipients of allogeneic marrow grafts, evidence supporting the existence of a graft-versus-leukemia effect has been difficult to obtain because of the large number of deaths from other causes among patients with severe GVHD. Statistical methods have shown that the relative relapse rate for patients transplanted in relapse or for ALL in second remission was 2.5 times greater in recipients without GVHD than in those with GVHD. Recipients of allogeneic marrow who did not develop GVHD had approximately the same relapse rate as recipients of syngeneic marrow, indicating that subclinical GVHD did not reduce the relapse rate.

GENERALIZATIONS ABOUT MARROW TRANSPLANTATION Because of the complexity of the marrow grafting regimens, transplantation should be undertaken only by teams with all of the resources needed to ensure an optimal result. The number of such teams has increased rapidly over the past few years.

Marrow transplantation is obviously an expensive undertaking, primarily because of hospital costs, but cost has been reduced appreciably by transplantation earlier in the course of the disease when the patient is in relatively good condition. Cost analysis studies comparing marrow transplantation with combination therapy have found marrow transplantation to be more cost-effective.

The ethical problems of exposing a patient and donor to the marrow transplant regimen and the risk of death in the first 1 to 3 months after grafting have limited the use of marrow transplantation. However, the demonstration of better long-term survival rates with marrow transplantation compared to conventional therapy for several diseases and the cure of some diseases not cured by conventional therapy should alleviate the ethical concern. Extension of this form of therapy to other malignant diseases and to a variety of genetic disorders is being reported, and the current rapid rate of progress and the availability of unrelated volunteer donors may soon make a much broader application of marrow grafting a reality.

REFERENCES

APPELBAUM FR et al: Chemotherapy v. marrow transplantation for adults with acute nonlymphocytic leukemia: A five-year follow-up. Blood 72:179, 1988

BEATTY PG et al: Marrow transplantation from related donors other than HLA identical siblings. N Engl J Med 313:765, 1985

CLIFT RA et al: The treatment of acute non-lymphoblastic leukemia by allogeneic marrow transplantation. Bone Marrow Transplant 2:243, 1987

FEFER A et al: Treatment of chronic granulocytic leukemia with chemoradiotherapy and transplantation of marrow from identical twins. N Engl J Med 306:63, 1982

GOLDMAN JM et al: Bone marrow transplantation for chronic myelogenous leukemia in chronic phase. Ann Intern Med 108:806, 1988

MARTIN P et al: Effects of in vitro depletion of T cells in HLA-identical allogeneic marrow grafts. Blood 66:664, 1985

MEYERS JD, THOMAS ED: Infection complicating bone marrow transplantation, in *Clinical Approach to Infection in the Immunocompromised Host*, RH Rubin, LS Young (eds). New York, Plenum Press, 1981, p 507

O'REILLY RJ: Allogeneic bone marrow transplantation: Current status and future directions. Blood 62:941, 1983

PHILIP T et al: High-dose therapy and autologous bone marrow transplantation after failure of conventional chemotherapy in adults with intermediate-grade or high-grade non-Hodgkin's lymphoma. N Engl J Med 316:1493, 1987

RAPPEPORT JM et al: Application of bone marrow transplantation in genetic diseases. Clin Haematol 12:755, 1983

STORB R et al: Marrow transplantation for aplastic anemia. Semin Hematol 21:27, 1984

——— et al: Methotrexate and cyclosporine compared with cyclosporine alone for prophylaxis of acute graft versus host disease after marrow transplantation for leukemia. N Engl J Med 314:729, 1986

SULLIVAN KM et al: Chronic graft-versus-host disease in 52 patients: Adverse natural course and successful treatment with combination immunosuppression. Blood 57:267, 1981

THOMAS ED et al: Bone-marrow transplantation. N Engl J Med 292:832, 895, 1975

——— et al: Marrow transplantation for thalassemia. Lancet 2:227, 1982

——— et al: Marrow transplantation for the treatment of chronic myelogenous leukemia. Ann Intern Med 104:155, 1986

WEIDEN PL et al: Antileukemic effect of graft-versus-host disease in human recipients of allogeneic-marrow grafts. N Engl J Med 300:1068, 1979

YEAGER AM et al: Autologous bone marrow transplantation in patients with acute nonlymphocytic leukemia, using ex vivo marrow treatment with 4-hydroperoxycyclophosphamide. N Engl J Med 315:141, 1986

ZUTTER MM et al: Epstein-Barr virus lymphoproliferation after bone marrow transplantation. Blood 72:520, 1988

section 3 Neoplastic diseases

300 PRINCIPLES OF NEOPLASIA

JOHN MENDELSOHN

INTRODUCTION The past few years have witnessed remarkable progress in understanding the biologic and biochemical bases for cancer. Gains in the treatment of nonresectable cancer in adults have been gradual and have focused upon those malignancies characterized by unusual sensitivity to radiation and chemotherapy. These include primarily acute leukemia, the lymphoproliferative malignancies, testicular cancer, and breast cancer. New treatment modalities involving immunotherapy and agents that promote normal cell maturation remain experimental and are under intensive investigation. Meanwhile, the search has begun for compounds which can interact with oncogene products, gene regulators, and growth factors and their receptors. Research employing modern technology in molecular genetics and immunology promises to provide a new array of anticancer agents which could move rapidly into clinical trials. This is possible because understanding cancer as a pathologic process is buttressed by new knowledge of cancer as an acquired genetic derangement.

This chapter provides an overview of the biology, etiology, and clinical sequelae of the neoplastic process, followed by a description of the general methods for diagnosing cancer and determining its stage, or extent of spread. Oncogenes and the molecular genetics of malignant transformation are discussed in Chap. 10. Cancer treatment is presented in the following chapter, and the details of managing patients with specific types of malignant disease will be found in the chapters devoted to disorders of various specific organs.

Definition The terms cancer, neoplasia, and malignancy are usually used interchangeably in both the technical and popular literature. The disease called cancer is best defined by four characteristics which describe how cancer cells act differently from their normal counterparts.

1 *Clonality:* In most cases, cancer originates from a single stem cell which proliferates to form a clone of malignant cells.
2 *Autonomy:* Growth is not properly regulated by the normal biochemical and physical influences in the environment.
3 *Anaplasia:* There is a lack of normal, coordinated cell differentiation.
4 *Metastasis:* Cancer cells develop the capacity for discontinuous growth and dissemination to other parts of the body.

Properties similar to each of these characteristics *can* be expressed by normal, nonmalignant cells at certain appropriate times—for example, during embryogenesis and wound repair—but in cancer cells the characteristic is inappropriate or excessive. The process by which a normal cell is converted into one which exhibits these characteristic traits is termed *malignant transformation*.

THE CLINICAL PROBLEM One-third of all individuals in the United States will develop cancer. The 5-year relative survival rate for these patients (the probability of escaping death from cancer for 5 years following diagnosis) has risen to nearly 50 percent as a result of progress in the early diagnosis and the therapy of this disease. However, cancer remains second only to cardiac disease as a cause of death in this country. Twenty percent of Americans die from cancer; this amounted to 494,000 deaths in 1988. Half of the deaths were due to the three most common types of cancer: lung, breast, and colon-rectum. Lung cancer is more prevalent in males, while breast cancer is the commonest form of malignancy in females. Cancer of the colon and rectum is equally common in males and females.

Information is provided yearly by the American Cancer Society, summarizing the incidence and mortality rates for the common types of cancer. Table 300-1 and Fig. 300-1 present just a small portion of the extensive data available. Of particular importance is the clear documentation in Fig. 300-1 that deaths from lung cancer are increasing in the face of stable or falling rates for a number of other types of malignant disease.

Cancer typically presents to the physician as an abnormal growth, or tumor, which causes illness by production of biochemically active molecules, by local expansion, or by invasion into adjacent or distant tissue sites. The symptoms of the illness depend upon the specific molecular products and the location(s) of the tumor. Each type of cancer has a relatively distinctive natural history that describes the likely clinical course of the particular neoplastic process. Designing a proper treatment plan for an individual patient with malignant disease depends upon determining the extent of disease spread, together with a knowledge of the natural history and the available therapeutic alternatives for the particular type of cancer.

TUMOR CELL BIOLOGY AND BIOCHEMISTRY Since all cells in an organism originate from a single fertilized egg (zygote), all carry the identical genetic information. The proliferation and differentiation of this cell into an embryo, and eventually into a mature organism, involve selective and coordinated expression of the genomic repertoire. Control of gene expression is accomplished through incompletely understood molecular interactions which can be modulated, in part, by chemical influences in the environment. The genomic repertoire includes information which permits cells to expand clonally, to function with varying degrees of autonomy, to differentiate and dedifferentiate, and to move from one part of the organism to another in a coordinated way. In the adult, the process of wound

TABLE 300-1 Estimated new cases and deaths for major sites of cancer—1988

Site or type	Number of cases	Deaths
Lung	152,000	139,000
Colon-rectum	147,000	62,000
Breast	136,000	42,000
Prostate	99,000	28,000
Urinary tract	69,000	20,000
Uterus	47,000*	10,000
Lymphoma	39,000	18,000
Oral	30,000	9,000
Pancreas	27,000	25,000
Leukemia	27,000	18,000
Melanoma	27,000†	6,000
Stomach	25,000	14,000
Ovary	19,000	12,000
All sites‡	985,000	494.000

* Includes cervix. If carcinoma in situ is included, cases total over 97,000.
† Estimated new cases of skin cancer (nonmelanoma) = about 500,000.
‡ Includes additional sites.
NOTE: Estimates are based on rates from the N.C.I. SEER program 1982–1984.

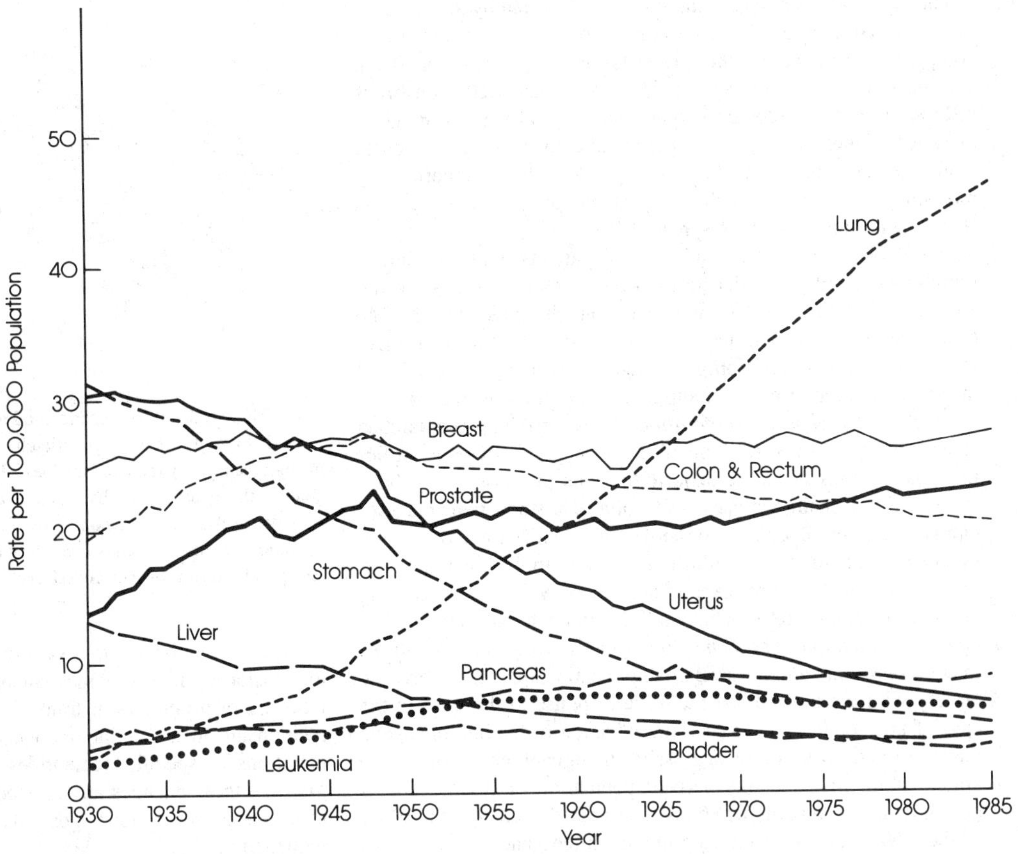

FIGURE 300-1 Cancer death rates by site in the United States, 1930 to 1985. *(Prepared by the American Cancer Society from data provided by the National Center for Health Statistics and the Bureau of the Census.)*

healing activates expression of these cellular characteristics in a more "embryo-like" fashion, but under well-coordinated control. In the case of malignancy, the normal control process is subverted or bypassed due to the anomalous activities of a select group of genes (oncogenes) which have central importance to the regulation of cellular activities. A detailed discussion of oncogenes is provided in Chap. 10.

Clonality Careful cytogenetic analysis of metaphase chromosome preparations from cancer cells has yielded a wealth of information about the neoplastic process. It has become clear that virtually all solid tumors and a majority of hematopoietic malignancies display abnormalities in the chromosomal karyotype which are inherited by the population of tumor cells. These may involve translocations of chromosomal fragments into new locations, as well as additions or deletions of parts of chromosomes or whole chromosomes. A particular karyotypic alteration often occurs in a substantial fraction of all patients with a form of cancer. The first and most well known example of this is the Philadelphia chromosome (Ph^1) observed in 85 percent of patients with chronic myelogenous leukemia (CML), in which the long arm of chromosome 22 is translocated onto the long arm of chromosome 9. This alteration is so characteristic of CML that when analysis of some cases of acute lymphocytic leukemia demonstrated the identical translocation, it was inferred that the disease represented an unusual conversion from CML (which usually progresses to acute myelocytic leukemia). Characteristic chromosomal rearrangements have been described in a number of other human cancers.

The observation of uniform karyotypic abnormalities in all cells within a tumor provides strong evidence for the clonal origin of the tumor. In turn, the chromosomal abnormalities serve as markers of the presence of a common malignant state in the individual cells.

A remarkable concordance between the chromosome locations of a number of human cellular oncogenes and the break points involved in chromosome translocations in human malignancies has been demonstrated. Furthermore, in many cases, these locations correlate with "fragile" sites in the chromosome. Treatment of cultured cells with agents that inhibit the DNA repair process induces chromosomal breaks far more frequently at many of these loci. A reasonable hypothesis, currently under investigation, links these phenomena and suggests that chromosome rearrangements may result in unregulated activation of cellular oncogenes. For example, in Burkitt's lymphoma, the typical translocation between chromosomes 8 and 14 places the cellular *myc* gene adjacent to the immunoglobulin heavy chain locus, a site of gene activation in the normal lymphocyte.

The new techniques of molecular genetics permit direct assessment of genetic alterations in DNA extracts from tissues suspected of harboring malignancy, using the method of *Southern blotting*. This involves restriction endonuclease digestion, agarose gel electrophoresis, and identification of specific DNA molecular species by hybridization with labeled specific probes. Changes in gene expression can be detected by a similar technique with RNA extracts known as *northern blotting*. The new technology of molecular genetics is more powerful than cytogenetics because (1) clonal genetic abnormalities can be identified in nondividing cells, (2) genetic rearrangements are detectable even when few tumor cells exist in a population of predominantly normal cells, and (3) the sensitivity of detection is greatly enhanced by obviating assays dependent on visual identification of altered staining patterns of chromosomes. The polymerase chain reaction takes advantage of the availability of appropriate primers for certain recombinant genes to amplify abnormal genetic material present in rare cells within a population, thereby enabling detection of genetic abnormalities in these cells by Southern blotting. These approaches to the diagnosis of genetic abnormalities are presented in detail in Chap. 6.

Clonal abnormalities in the genetic makeup of cells that can be detected with molecular techniques include gene mutation, rearrangement, translocation, deletion, and amplification. Some examples will serve to demonstrate the utility of these methods.

1 CML: The Ph^1 chromosome is formed by a translocation between chromosomes 9 and 22, with the break in chromosome 22 occurring in the break point cluster region (*bcr* region), which is the site of a gene. The translocation can therefore be identified by the presence of abnormal *bcr* bands on Southern blots. A fusion protein comprising portions of the products of *bcr* and c-*abl* (from chromosome 9) is expressed in CML cells, and detection of its mRNA by northern blotting is diagnostic. By taking advantage of these techniques, the presence of residual cells from the malignant clone can be detected in bone marrow that appears normal by morphologic criteria as well as by standard cytogenetic criteria (e.g., 30 normal metaphase spreads).

2 *Nodular lymphoma:* The majority of patients with low-grade lymphomas display translocations between chromosomes 14 and 18, involving the *bcl*-2 gene located on chromosome 18. The translocation can be detected by identification of either rearrangements in *bcl*-2 or the fusion gene product involving the *bcl*-2 and the immunoglobulin heavy chain gene from chromosome 14.

3 *Monoclonal lymphocyte proliferation:* Detection of kappa or lambda chain excess on the surface membranes of lymphocytes identifies malignant clones when the majority of cells in a population have identical light chain subtypes. Detection of a small percentage of clonally derived B cells is possible, by identifying clonal rearrangements of immunoglobulin genes. In a similar fashion, rearrangements of T-cell receptor genes are of value in diagnosing clonal proliferation of a malignant T-lymphocyte population.

4 *Gene amplification:* The N-*myc* oncogene is frequently amplified in neuroblastoma, and the level of amplification appears to correlate closely with the clinical stage and the response to therapy. In the case of breast adenocarcinoma, amplification of the *neu* oncogene may correlate with more aggressive malignant behavior. Gene amplification in a clonally derived population of tumor cells is detected directly on Southern blots as increased intensity of labeling of the DNA bands derived from the amplified gene.

Studies of the selective expression of the X-linked isoenzymes of glucose-6-phosphate dehydrogenase (G6PD) in heterozygotic patients have provided further evidence for the clonal origin of cancer from a single progenitor cell. Examination of both G6PD isoenzymes and chromosomal karyotypes in CML patients has demonstrated clonal abnormalities in erythroid, myeloid, and megakaryocytic cells, as well as B lymphocytes, suggesting that this malignancy originates in a precursor cell common to all of these cell lineages.

While there is convincing evidence for the origin of cancer from genetic alterations in a single cell, further heritable alterations commonly occur, resulting in the presence of a heterogeneous mixture of subclones in a mature tumor cell population which has proliferated enough to be clinically detectable. This heterogeneity can be demonstrated by assaying a variety of characteristics in the subpopulations within a tumor; for example, further abnormalities in the chromosomal karyotype, varied drug sensitivities and metastatic capacities, differences in growth rates, and the presence or absence of hormone receptors or particular cell surface glycoproteins. With time, therefore, the progressive accumulation of heritable abnormalities in tumor subpopulations typically results in highly significant phenotypic changes which have their clinical counterpart in development of resistance to previously effective therapy or in increased metastatic spread. The appearance of new chromosomal abnormalities in patients with Ph[1]-positive CML heralds the onset of a rapidly progressive, fatal phase of the disease. A schematic model of this process of clonal progression is shown in Fig. 300-2. It remains to be determined when in the life history of a typical malignancy the process of clonal progression occurs: the sequence of genetic alterations may occur early, with later expansion of selected subpopulations from a heterogeneous mixture of cells as circumstances change; alternatively the genetic alterations may occur close to the time when they are detected by changes in the behavior of the tumor cells.

Following the discovery of cellular oncogenes, evidence rapidly accumulated to show that unregulated activation of two or more of these genes may be the molecular genetic explanation for clonal progression in tumor cell subpopulations. Activation of cellular oncogenes may be due to a variety of genetic mechanisms in addition to translocation. These mechanisms include gene amplification, or insertion of promoters of transcription adjacent to (*cis*) or in a *trans* relationship to a cellular oncogene, with or without accompanying mutations of specific nucleotides in the oncogene DNA sequence. Many of these changes are undetectable in the karyotype, but can be identified by restriction digest analysis of cellular DNA or by DNA sequencing.

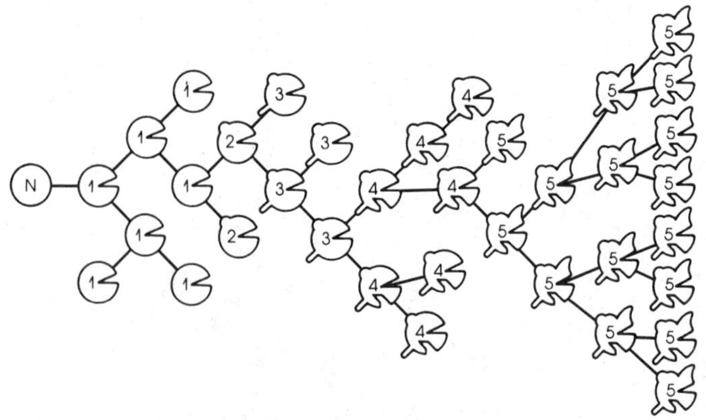

FIGURE 300-2 A schematic model of clonal progression. The N cell is normal. Five *hypothetical* genetic changes are noted. The first does not result in malignancy but the second does. The third adds invasiveness, the fourth confers the capacity to disseminate and produce metastases, and the fifth provides resistance to chemotherapy. Each may be accompanied by incremental alterations in the chromosomal karyotype, with an increasing tendency to aneuploidy during further clonal evolution.

Autonomy Environmental influences which regulate the proliferation of normal cells are circumvented when the process of malignant transformation occurs. This is demonstrable by a variety of experimental assays which document, in different ways, the capacity of the malignant cells to continue to proliferate under normally nonconducive conditions. These assays are listed in Table 300-2.

At least initially, the autonomy of human malignancies is relative rather than absolute. The well-known experiments of Huggins and associates in the 1950s led to a new form of cancer therapy which took advantage of the initial dependence of certain tumors upon the normal influences of sex hormones. The conversion of many prostatic and breast cancers from sensitivity to resistance to hormone therapy vividly demonstrates the further development of autonomy through clonal progression.

Many tumor cell lines can proliferate in culture medium without the usual requirement for serum, provided that a "cocktail" containing three to five essential growth factors and other growth-promoting agents is added. Examples of such factors are epidermal growth

TABLE 300-2 Experimental detection of malignant transformation

Assay	Normal cell	Transformed cell
Capacity of single cells to form colonies in agar suspension	Unsuccessful	Successful
Density-dependent inhibition of cell proliferation in liquid culture	Yes	No
Generations obtained by continuous division in liquid culture	Limited to about 50	Unlimited
Requirements for serum or growth factors	Invariable	Reduced or absent
Capacity to grow as xenografts	Absent	Present

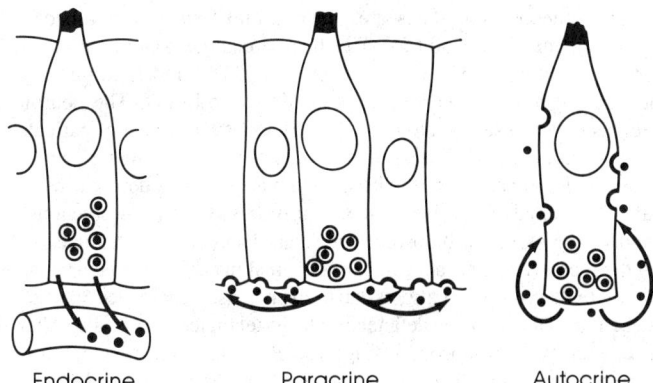

FIGURE 300-3 A diagrammatic representation of autocrine, paracrine, and endocrine secretion. Peptide growth factors are shown in latent form within the cell. The thickened, semicircular regions of the cell membrane represent receptor sites. *(From MB Sporn, GJ Todaro, N Engl J Med 303:878, 1980.)*

factor, platelet-derived growth factor, the carrier protein transferrin, and the hormone insulin. Malignant cells may obviate the requirements for even these essential factors. One mechanism, demonstrated experimentally and possibly of clinical significance, involves production of a growth factor (or its analogue) by the tumor cells themselves, a process called *autocrine secretion*. In this situation a polypeptide secreted by the tumor cells may have the capacity to bind to a receptor on the surface of the cells, resulting in autostimulation (Fig. 300-3). The first growth factor to be described with the potential for autocrine stimulation of tumor cells was transforming growth factor alpha, an analogue of epidermal growth factor (EGF), which also binds to the EGF receptor. Recent experiments have suggested that autocrine stimulation with platelet-derived growth factor (PDGF) may be accomplished by binding of ligand to the receptor intracellularly, prior to the expression of receptor on the cell surface. A second mechanism by which tumor cells can reduce dependence on growth factors involves expression of increased numbers of receptors on the cell surface. Increased expression of EGF receptors is a common event in epithelial tumors, occurring in all renal cell carcinomas and squamous lung carcinomas that have been examined, and in many other forms of malignancy. Tumor cells may develop a third mechanism for escaping regulation by a growth factor, by activating an internal biochemical process (e.g., a protein tyrosine kinase) ordinarily dependent upon binding of a specific growth factor to a cell surface receptor, thereby completely bypassing the need for exposure to the growth-promoting agent.

Anaplasia Lack of normal differentiation is a most useful characteristic in the pathologic diagnosis of malignancy. While cancer cells usually bear some of the morphologic characteristics of their normal mature counterparts, they display cellular and histologic abnormalities readily detectable with the light microscope. The cells tend to have large nuclei, with more apparent chromatin and prominent nucleoli. There are increased mitoses, as well as abnormal mitoses and giant cells containing multiple nuclei, reflecting aneuploidy and/or a failure of karyokinesis. The degree of morphologic derangement typically correlates with the extent of disease spread or the metastatic potential of the tumor. The histologic appearance of malignancy is one of disarray, with partial or complete loss of normal tissue architecture. Partial formation of structures such as glands or villi may be suggested, even in poorly differentiated malignancies.

Although the term is not used this way, the process of anaplasia may be expressed at a biochemical level as production of hormones or hormone-related peptides, which are either improperly regulated by normal feedback mechanisms (e.g., excessive corticosteroid production by an adrenal carcinoma), or are not appropriate for the particular cell type if it were normally differentiated (e.g., ACTH production by a carcinoma of the lung). In such cases, the genomic repertoire of the malignant cell is expressed inappropriately. Another example is the unregulated production of immunoglobulin (partial or complete chains) by neoplastic derivatives of B lymphocytes.

Histologic features which are abnormal but do not meet the criteria of anaplasia (loss of differentiation) are designated *dysplastic*. Such changes may be seen in "premalignant" situations, for example, in the epithelial lining of the bronchi of cigarette smokers. These abnormalities are often reversible. Cessation of smoking can lead to normalization of the lung epithelium over a period of 5 years.

Metastasis This term encompasses a number of phenotypic traits which together result in the clinical problem which most often leads to death from cancer. The cells lose their adherence and restrained position within an organized tissue, move into adjacent sites, develop the capacity both to invade and to egress from blood vessels, and become capable of proliferating in unnatural locations or environments. These changes in growth patterns are accompanied by biochemical alterations which have the capacity to promote the metastatic process. Invasive tumors may secrete, or may stimulate secretion of, a variety of tissue-degrading enzymes including collagenases and lysosomal hydrolases. Plasminogen activators which lead to promotion of fibrinolysis are also produced. Conversely, procoagulant compounds may be released into the environment of the tumor cells at stages when focal aggregation of cells might be of survival value. In experimental situations where tumor cells show a propensity to select a particular organ as a preferred site of metastasis, surface molecules on the metastatic cells appear to have a high affinity for endothelial cells in the vasculature of the specific target organ. The first step in tumor cell invasion probably involves attachment to the extracellular matrix, which is mediated by receptors on the cell plasma membrane that bind specifically to glycoproteins such as laminin and fibronectin. Additional biochemical steps are entailed in the progression of a tumor from a homogeneous proliferating clone to a group of heterogeneous subpopulations of cells, some of which have progressively accumulated the entire array of enzymes and surface molecules required for metastasis. It may be for this reason that the rate of metastasis is low during early tumor growth, in spite of the well-documented fact that malignant cells are often released from a tumor into the circulation continuously and in large numbers. Agents which could block critical steps in the metastatic process would be of great value in the armamentarium of antineoplastic agents.

It appears that clonal progression of a tumor generates biochemical or physiologic alterations which confer greater autonomy, greater degrees of anaplasia, and a greater capacity to metastasize. Because there is progressive selection for cells with increased tumorigenic capacity, the process has been called clonal evolution and has been compared to Darwinian evolution, in this case at a cellular level.

ETIOLOGY Patterns of cancer incidence vary with sex, race, and geographic location. In addition, the types of tumors observed vary with age. Hereditary traits and variations in the internal environments around cells explain some of the differences in cancer incidence. It is clear from epidemiologic investigations that variations in diet and exposure to chemical and physical agents in the external environment contribute to the development of neoplasia. The environmental agents which have been linked to the incidence of cancer fall into three broad categories: radiation, a variety of chemicals, and viruses.

Genetic factors Genetic alterations appear to play an essential role in oncogenesis. Several lines of evidence support this conclusion: (1) There are many examples of familial aggregation for specific histologic types of tumor (e.g., retinoblastoma). (2) Chromosomal abnormalities carried in the germ line confer increased risk of developing certain types of cancer (e.g., leukemia in trisomy 21). (3) Tumors often display specific somatic rearrangement of chromosomes or genes (e.g., CML). (4) Deficiency in the capacity to repair DNA damage by mutagens is accompanied by increased risk of malignancy (e.g., xeroderma pigmentosa). (5) The capacities for agents to mutate DNA and to elicit tumors are closely correlated, in studies of both bacteria and experimental animals (e.g., *Salmonella*/microsome test of Dr. Bruce Ames).

The molecular mechanisms explaining these genetic abnormalities are only beginning to be understood. They appear to fall into two categories: (1) genes which are deregulated and excessively expressed, displaying dominant genetic activity, such as the products of cellular proto-oncogenes; (2) genes which are suppressors of tumorigenic genetic activities and are recessive in that both alleles must be lacking for malignancy to occur, such as the retinoblastoma gene. The latter can appear to have a dominant inheritance pattern, because one of the alleles may be constitutionally deleted, so that a single genetic alteration (e.g., somatic mutation or loss) in the other allele results in neoplastic transformation. The retinoblastoma gene has been mapped to the q14 band of chromosome 13 and cloned. The cDNA has been used to demonstrate deletion of the retinoblastoma gene in some soft tissue sarcomas and other solid tumors.

There have been a number of reports of additional human malignancies which may be associated with chromosomal deletions and/or loss of restriction fragment length polymorphism (RFLP) alleles. These include Wilms's tumor (11p13), lung cancer (3p), renal cell carcinoma (3p), bladder cancer (11p), colorectal carcinoma (5q), and breast cancer (13). The nature of the information encoded by the genetic loci, in parentheses, is under intensive study. In the case of the retinoblastoma gene, the polypeptide product may bind to and inactivate a protein with enhancer-binding activity for DNA.

For many of the common malignancies, the incidence of cancer is higher among patients with positive family histories than among unselected patients, usually in the range of up to threefold. However, the risk can rise to as high as twenty-five- to thirtyfold in certain groups of patients with a familial history of breast cancer or bowel cancer. In addition, there are a number of uncommon inherited disorders involving either (1) a high risk for the occurrence of a particular neoplasm, or (2) the presence of multiple preneoplastic lesions that can progress to frank malignancy.

The hereditary neoplasms (Table 300-3) may occur as the only manifestation of a gene defect, or as part of a generalized syndrome involving multiple developmental abnormalities. The inheritance patterns in these disorders are generally autosomal dominant, with varying penetrance. Half of the children of patients with these disorders will inherit the gene defect.

TABLE 300-3 Hereditary cancer syndromes

I Hereditary neoplasms
- Retinoblastoma
- Nevoid basal cell carcinoma syndrome
- Multiple endocrine adenomatosis (Werner's syndrome)
- Pheochromocytoma and medullary thyroid carcinoma (Sipple's syndrome)
- Chemodectomas
- Polyposis coli
- Gardner's syndrome
- Tylosis with esophageal carcinoma

II Preneoplastic states
- *A* Hamartomatous syndromes
  - Neurofibromatosis
  - Tuberous sclerosis
  - von Hippel–Lindau syndrome
  - Multiple exostoses
  - Peutz-Jeghers syndrome
  - Cowden's multiple hamartoma syndrome
- *B* Genodermatoses
  - Xeroderma pigmentosum
  - Albinism
  - Werner's syndrome
  - Epidermodysplasia verruciformis
  - Polydysplastic epidermolysis bullosa
  - Dyskeratosis congenita
- *C* Chromosome breakage disorders
  - Bloom's syndrome
  - Fanconi's syndrome
- *D* Immune deficiency syndromes
  - Ataxia-telangiectasia
  - Wiskott-Aldrich syndrome
  - Late-onset immunologic deficiency
  - X-linked agammaglobulinemia

SOURCE: From JF Fraumeni, Jr, in JF Holland, E Frei.

The preneoplastic states are grouped into four major categories by Fraumeni (Table 300-3). The hamartomatous syndromes show autosomal dominant inheritance patterns. The most common is neurofibromatosis, occurring in 1 of 3000 live births. The neurofibromas undergo sarcomatous changes in about 10 percent of patients, with development of gliomas in the brain or optic nerve, meningiomas, acoustic neuromas, or pheochromocytomas. The genodermatoses are rare autosomal recessive genetic disorders which conspicuously involve the skin. Chromosome breakage disorders are characterized by the recessive inheritance of chromosomal instability and rearrangements of karyotypes; patients have an increased incidence of acute leukemia. The immune deficiency ataxic telangiectasia is also characterized by chromosomal fragility. Patients with hereditary or acquired immunodeficiency states have an increased incidence of neoplasia, most commonly the lymphoproliferative malignancies.

Race is a genetic factor in the incidence of cancer, but interpretation of epidemiologic data is made difficult by the concurrent effects of environmental and socioeconomic influences. Both the incidence and the death rate from cancer is higher in American blacks than in American whites, with all of the difference being accounted for by the higher cancer rate in black males. It is believed that later detection and less adequate treatment may account for part, but not all, of the difference in survival. The important effect of environmental factors is made clear by documented differences in cancer incidence for Asians living in Hawaii and in California.

Radiation It is estimated that less than 3 percent of cancers result from exposure to radiation. Radiation that can remove electrons from atoms is called ionizing radiation. It includes electromagnetic waves such as x-rays and gamma rays, as well as charged particles such as protons. The unit of radiation dose, the gray (Gy), measures the energy absorbed in matter as a result of exposure to radiation: 1 Gy = 100 rad.

Information on the capacity of radiation in relatively large doses to induce cancer in humans comes from studies on survivors of atomic bomb blasts, on individuals accidentally exposed to irradiation or radiative fallout, and on patients exposed to radiation for diagnostic purposes or for therapy. It has been learned that nearly all tissues are susceptible to tumor induction by radiation, but with variable sensitivity. The most sensitive tissues are the bone marrow, breast, and thyroid. The latent period is only 2 to 5 years for acute leukemia, and 5 to 10 years for most solid tumors. There is a higher incidence of leukemia in patients who have received radiation therapy for neoplastic diseases and for ankylosing spondylitis, and of thyroid cancer in children irradiated for thymic enlargement.

Solar radiation, resulting from exposure to electromagnetic radiation from the sun, is the primary risk factor in skin cancer. The evidence for this linkage comes from a variety of epidemiologic and experimental observations. Skin cancer is rare in blacks and the deeply pigmented racial groups, whereas it is especially common in fair-complexioned individuals. It occurs primarily on the parts of the body exposed to sunlight and has a higher incidence in outdoor workers. Patients with genetic diseases such as xeroderma pigmentosa and albinism, which are exacerbated by sunlight, have very high risks for the development of skin cancer.

The carcinogenic effect of solar irradiation is greatest in the spectral range of 290 to 320 nm (UV-B radiation), which produces delayed erythema in human skin (sunburn). This range of wavelengths correlates with the action spectrum for UV-induced damage to DNA.

Exposure to solar ultraviolet irradiation is also a risk factor in melanoma. As with skin cancer, there is a higher incidence of melanoma among populations living at a latitude nearer the equator, where exposure to UV irradiation is greatest.

Tobacco Numerous epidemiologic studies have demonstrated that the principal carcinogenic agent in our environment is inhaled tobacco smoke. The incidence of lung cancer is more than tenfold higher in male smokers than in nonsmokers. Furthermore, tobacco smoking is associated with increased rates of cancer of the oral cavity, esophagus, kidney, bladder, and pancreas. Particulate matter in

TABLE 300-4 Examples of occupational causes of cancer

Etiology	Site of malignancy
Arsenic (inorganic)	Lung, skin, liver
Asbestos	Mesothelium, lung
Benzene	Leukemia
Benzidine	Bladder
Chromium compounds	Lung
Radiation (mining, dial painting)	Numerous locations
Mustard gas	Lung
Polycyclic hydrocarbons (coal by-products)	Lung, skin
Vinyl chloride	Angiosarcoma of liver

tobacco smoke, known as "tar," contains a long list of chemicals, primarily polycyclic hydrocarbons, which have been shown experimentally to be contact carcinogens. In addition, the metabolic activation of tobacco components, for example, the cyclic *N*-nitrosamines, can produce carcinogens with the capacity to act upon the cells of internal organs. Tobacco-related malignancies account for one-third of all cancer deaths among men in the United States and for more than 10 percent of all female cancer deaths. Unfortunately, this figure is rising in females. As a result of increased use of tobacco by women in the period since World War II, the deaths from lung cancer in females exceeded deaths from breast cancer in 1988.

Clearly the single most effective action which could be taken against cancer at the present time involves not an application of molecular genetic research, but cessation of smoking. Fortunately, it appears that smoking cessation results in a gradual decrease in risk, so that after 10 to 15 years, exsmokers have nearly the same risk of lung cancer as nonsmokers. Because the habit of smoking is difficult to break, the physician's role in cessation of smoking is of critical importance. Doctors should deliver a *firm* antismoking message.

Occupational exposure The first report of cancer related to occupational hazards was Percival Pott's observation of an unusually high frequency of scrotal cancer among London chimney sweeps in 1775. It is now known that skin cancer (including scrotal) can be induced by a variety of coal tar products, such as the materials contacted in the London chimneys. Epidemiologic studies also have related lung cancer to exposure to coal by-products. Table 300-4 provides a partial listing of industrial agents which are known to cause cancer.

Air pollution It is clear that lung cancer incidence is increased by tobacco smoking and by certain industrial and occupational exposures (primarily related to coal tar and combustion by-products). Once the risks resulting from exposure to these factors are taken into account, the epidemiologic evidence that links ambient air pollution to lung cancer remains inconclusive. Studies correlating the incidence of lung cancer with increased levels of polycyclic hydrocarbons and benzo(a)pyrene in urban air are complicated by the difficulty of eliminating the contribution of exposure to these compounds through tobacco smoking as well as occupational exposure.

Medications Certain drugs and hormones have been shown to be carcinogenic. The synthetic nonsteroidal estrogen diethylstilbestrol (DES), which was used for a period of time to reduce fetal wastage in pregnant women, caused an increased incidence of vaginal and cervical cancer in daughters who were exposed in utero. Conjugated estrogens have been shown to increase the incidence of endometrial cancer in patients treated for menopausal symptoms. The use of progesterone concomitantly, together with decreased estrogen dose, may obviate this problem.

Alkylating agents have been shown to cause an increased incidence of acute myelocytic leukemia and probably other malignancies. They are used in therapeutic situations in which the poor prognosis of malignancy far outweighs the increased risk of an additional cancer in the future. However, because of this risk, new drug regimens which avoid the use of alkylating agents are being explored in situations where substantial long-term benefits from chemotherapy have been demonstrated, for example, in Hodgkin's disease.

The recipients of organ transplants who are treated with immunosuppressive agents, such as azathioprine and prednisone, have an increased incidence of histiocytic lymphoma as well as a variety of solid tumors. A similar increased incidence is observed in individuals with inherited and acquired immunodeficiency, for example, AIDS. This has been attributed to reduced immune surveillance, but a variety of other explanations are equally likely, such as activation of a latent oncogenic virus or chronic immunostimulation in conjunction with a compromised and malfunctioning immune system.

Diet The role of diet and nutrition in carcinogenesis has been the subject of intensive investigation and equally intensive controversy. There are numerous nutritional hypotheses of carcinogenesis. Some of these have led to unconventional forms of cancer therapy that are based upon no scientific evidence. Unfortunately, these putative dietary therapies are propagated upon a patient population for which proven treatment modalities are often unsuccessful in achieving cure, and at a time when there is a popular emphasis on healthful nutrition.

Epidemiologic analyses of international variations in cancer incidence and comparisons of the types and frequencies of cancer in populations with different dietary habits have yielded a great deal of evidence that cancers of most major sites are influenced by diet. These studies were reviewed in an authoritative publication, *Diet, Nutrition, and Cancer*. Interim dietary guidelines are suggested which are both consistent with good nutritional practices and likely to reduce the risk of cancer: (1) Reduce the intake of fat, saturated and unsaturated, from its present average level (40 percent) to 30 percent of total energy value in the diet. (2) Include fruits (especially citrus), vegetables (especially carotene-rich and cruciferous), and whole cereal grain (fiber) in the daily diet; these provide amounts of vitamins A and C as well as fiber adequate to obviate dietary supplements. (3) Minimize consumption of salt-cured or smoked food. (4) Use alcoholic beverages in moderation, since they increase the risk of certain cancers, especially when combined with cigarette smoking.

Experimental data lend support to the inferences from epidemiologic studies, but additional research is necessary to understand how dietary factors influence carcinogenesis. For example, epidemiologic evidence strongly correlates the intake of fat with the occurrence of cancer at several sites, especially the breast and colon. Possible explanations for this observation include increased adiposity, leading to greater conversion of androstenedione to estrone, which could influence carcinogenesis in the breast; and stimulation of increased bile salt excretion which could alter gut flora and thereby augment the production of carcinogenic substances by the bacteria in the colon. Vitamin C may act to prevent cancer by blocking endogenous formation of *N*-nitroso compounds in the gastrointestinal tract, but there are no data showing that taking vitamin C will prevent cancer in human beings. Dietary fiber enhances the rapid transit of potential carcinogens through the colon, which could explain the low incidence of bowel cancer and rectal cancer in tropical Africa.

It is important to stress that the accumulated scientific evidence does not support the anticarcinogenic value of particular vitamins, minerals, or nutritional supplements in amounts greater than provided by a prudent diet. Certainly their use in high doses in the therapy of established malignant disease is not indicated. The physician must be alert to the scientifically unproven dietary treatments which patients with cancer may be urged to undertake. Of course the greatest tragedy occurs when patients whose malignancy could be cured by proven therapeutic modalities are misled into depending upon such dietary manipulations.

Viruses Although there has been extensive research on viral oncogenesis with experimental murine tumors, viruses have been implicated as the direct cause of only one human cancer. Infection with human T-lymphotrophic virus I (HTLV-I) can lead to adult T-cell leukemia, an aggressive malignancy of T-lymphocytes, which has been reported in large series from Japan and the West Indies. The incidence of hepatocellular carcinoma in endemic regions of Asia and Africa is closely associated with previous infection with hepatitis B virus, followed by a carrier state, suggesting that a causal relationship is highly likely. Chronic hepatocyte infection by the virus might predispose to carcinogenesis in these cells. There may be a variety of contributing factors, including malaria, malnutrition, and exposure to aflatoxin. There also is a strong statistical correlation between herpes simplex 2 viral infection, which is sexually transmitted, and the incidence of cervical cancer. There are a number of situations in which viruses are linked to the occurrence of specific cancers with a high incidence in particular geographic locations, although a causative role has not been established. The Epstein-Barr virus is closely associated with African Burkitt's lymphoma as well as nasopharyngeal carcinoma in Asia. Cofactors in the development of these malignancies might be holoendemic malaria in African Burkitt's lymphoma, and a particular configuration of histocompatibility antigens in the case of nasopharyngeal carcinoma among Chinese. While the Epstein-Barr virus can infect human B lymphocytes (infectious mononucleosis) and transform them in cell culture, evidence is lacking that such a transformation is the cause of clinical malignancy.

Risk of cancer Knowledge of genetic and environmental factors that may contribute to cancer incidence can be utilized by the conscientious physician to identify patients who have an increased risk of malignancy. The presence of certain hereditary diseases in a patient's family may suggest procedures that can lead to early detection and prevention, for example, early surveillance by colonoscopy and prevention by prophylactic colectomy in persons who have familial polyposis of the colon. Environmental factors that increase cancer risks should be identified and avoided. It is evident, however, that changing an individual's life-style in order to avoid exposure to a carcinogen can require an extraordinary level of effort on the part of both the patient and the physician.

CLINICAL SEQUELAE The presence of a malignant lesion may not, in itself, cause symptoms in a patient with cancer. The primary lesion may, for a period of time, be unnoticed and unimportant for the normal maintenance of body functions, in which case its clinical significance is due to its potential for growth and spread. In addition, the presence of metastasis need not result in symptomatic illness. Patients with carcinoma of the bowel, whose disease may have spread beyond the limits of surgical curability, may live for many months or even years with easily detectable metastatic lesions in the lung or abdomen, yet remain free of symptoms until the function of a vital organ is compromised or obstructive problems appear.

Malignancies produce clinical symptoms in three general ways (Table 300-5): by direct effects resulting from invasion or compression of normal tissues; by release of cytokines, hormones, and other biologically active agents into the local and systemic environment; and by secondary psychological effects upon the patient. Each of these factors may contribute profoundly to the degree of illness experienced by the patient. Clinical symptoms resulting from released biologically active agents, as well as systemic problems caused by as yet undetermined mechanisms, are usually grouped under the category of "paraneoplastic syndromes."

TABLE 300-5 Symptoms caused by malignant diseases

I Mass effects
- *A* Ablation by crowding or by invasion
- *B* Obstruction of vessels, tubes, and ducts
- *C* Rupture of blood vessels

II Remote effects (paraneoplastic syndromes)
- *A* Ectopic hormone production
- *B* Neuropathies and CNS abnormalities
- *C* Dermatologic abnormalities
- *D* Metabolic disorders
  - *1* Anorexia, weight loss
  - *2* Fever
  - *3* Chronic inflammation
- *E* Hematologic disorders
- *F* Immunosuppression
- *G* Collagen vascular disorders

III Psychosocial effects
- *A* Loss of control
- *B* Acceptance of personal finitude
- *C* Fear of pain and mutilation
- *D* Separation and loneliness

Mass effects of malignancy In most cases tumors produce clinical problems as a result of local expansion, with obliteration of normal tissues, as the malignant cells proliferate within the confines of the involved organ: marrow replacement by leukemia results in reduced production of the normal cellular elements of the blood; lung cancer compromises oxygen exchange in involved alveoli; primary or metastatic cancer in bone causes weakened trabecular architecture, resulting in pathologic fractures; hepatomas replace normal hepatocytes and interfere with liver function. A second result of local expansion is compression of normal structures, with partial or complete obstruction of tubular organs, blood vessels, and lymphatics: colonic cancer may obstruct the gastrointestinal tract; lung cancer blocks airflow through bronchi and can obstruct pulmonary venous return; hepatic and biliary malignancies produce obstructive jaundice; a variety of intraabdominal neoplasms can encase the ureters, causing renal failure; in the extreme case, penetration of blood vessels can violate the integrity of the vasculature, resulting in hemorrhage. A third result of local expansion is pain, due to pressure on or stretching of nerve fibers. When neoplasia causes increased pressure on nervous tissue within the confines of the skull, the symptoms include headache and vomiting as well as seizure disorders and brain dysfunction.

Paraneoplastic syndromes The malignant process is felt to develop as a result of the unregulated and/or inappropriate expression of certain genes crucial to cell proliferation and differentiation. The aggressiveness of the malignant process is increased by the subsequent uncovering of additional genetic information. In this evolutionary process, abnormal genetic information may be expressed which results in severe physiologic effects upon the patient. As noted above, there may be excessive synthesis of a gene product which is normally found in the particular cell type, or the malignant cell may produce a molecule which does not ordinarily originate from its normal counterpart.

A common type of molecule produced by malignant tumors falls into the category of polypeptide hormones. The synthesis of vasopressin or ACTH by small cell carcinoma of the lung or parathormone by some squamous cancers are examples. These can produce clinical illness by mediating normal physiologic functions to an excessive degree. Other active molecules have been detected which are homologous with or identical to known growth factors. The potential for autonomous stimulation of proliferation mediated by production of essential growth-promoting agents has been discussed.

From this brief introduction, it can be seen that biologically active agents produced by malignant cells can be clinically important for a number of reasons:

1. They may serve as markers for the presence of a type of tumor. Detection of such markers early in the course of the disease might increase chances for cure. They also may be used to follow the clinical progress of the disease and anticipate recurrence.
2. They may produce symptoms as a result of their intrinsic biologic activity. In some cases these can become the major clinical problems determining survival (e.g., hypercalcemia).
3. They may serve to promote the growth of the tumor directly. In turn, growth-promoting agents of this type may become the focus of new approaches to anticancer treatment.

The paraneoplastic sequelae of cancer which involve ectopic hormone production are described in Chap. 309, and the neurologic manifestations of neoplasia in Chap. 310. Cutaneous manifestations of internal malignancy are discussed in Chap. 59. The association of malignancy with certain metabolic disorders, hematologic abnormalities, and immunosuppression will be further described here.

Metabolic disorders One of the major and most characteristic problems seen with cancer is weight loss, usually associated with anorexia. The extensive wasting which results is known as cachexia.

The cause for this commonly observed and often life-limiting disturbance remains to be determined in spite of the fact that many contributing factors have been identified. Abnormalities of taste and smell, physiologic malfunction of the gastrointestinal tract, excessive energy demands made by the tumor, and failure to adapt energy expenditure to the levels of nutrient intake have been implicated as causes of cachexia in patients with cancer. Biochemical abnormalities in energy metabolism have been well-characterized in these patients. Fatty acids are oxidized in preference to glucose, and anaerobic glucose metabolism is increased while oxidative phosphorylation is reduced. This results in an inefficient expenditure of ATP, which might lead to an energy deficit. However, none of these observations is felt to account for the magnitude of the problem.

Typically, the anorectic patient simply cannot ingest food, in spite of a clear understanding of the need for increased nourishment. The chief complaint is unpalatability. An aversion to meat has been clearly documented. While nausea may be a component of the syndrome, emesis occurs rarely. This may be because the patient feels so satiated that no food intake is tolerated.

Provision of alimentation through enteral tubes or by the intravenous route has the potential to provide total parenteral nutrition (TPN) to patients with cancer, and the techniques for performing these procedures have been well-described by investigators managing nonmalignant disease. At present there is no indication that the provision of nutritional support at this level can, by itself, affect the course of malignant disease. However, clinical trials have suggested a role for nutritional supplementation, including TPN, in preparing nutritionally deprived cancer patients for potentially beneficial surgical procedures or chemotherapy programs which otherwise might not have been tolerated due to the wasted state of the patient.

A polypeptide produced by macrophages has been isolated and named tumor necrosis factor (TNF), because of its capacity to cause lysis of certain types of tumor cells. Administration of TNF can mimic the syndrome of cachexia in experimental animals, and it is therefore also known as cachectin. Cytokines released by inflammatory cells and tumor cells are likely candidates as etiologic agents for the debilitation and wasting that accompany aggressive malignancy.

Fever is another sign associated with malignancy, and it is usually attributable to infection. Because of the debility which often accompanies cancer, and the depression in circulating granulocytes and mononuclear cells resulting from aggressive therapeutic measures, the types of infection seen may be unusual. Infection by endogenous bacteria, fungi, viruses, and protozoa must be considered when evaluating fever of unknown etiology in patients with malignancy (see Chap. 20). There remain unusual instances when fever cannot be explained by infection and must be attributed to a cause intrinsic to the neoplasm itself.

Hematologic abnormalities Anemia is found with increased incidence in advanced stages of malignant disease. The mechanisms accounting for anemia are, in nearly all cases, extrinsic to the tumor, and may be due to several mechanisms. Increased destruction of erythrocytes can result from hypersplenism, microangiopathic hemolysis, and autoantibodies, seen especially in the lymphoproliferative malignancies. Anemia due to occult bleeding is one of the cardinal signs of malignancy in the gastrointestinal tract. Decreased production of erythrocytes may result from iron deficiency related to bleeding, vitamin B_{12} or folate deficiency, erythron depletion due to tumor crowding in the marrow, toxicity secondary to chemotherapy or radiotherapy, and the anemia associated with chronic inflammatory disease.

Granulocytopenia is commonly associated with marrow infiltration by hematologic malignancies, and also results from chemotherapy. The etiologies of thrombocytopenia are comparable to those associated with anemia. Depression in one or all of the circulating hematopoietic elements may result from one of the various forms of marrow failure or aplastic anemia which are known to be preleukemic.

An increase in the formed elements of the blood may also occur. Erythrocytosis resulting from inappropriate production of erythropoietin is observed not only in polycythemia vera, but also in renal cell carcinoma, hepatoma, and cerebellar hemangioma. An elevated granulocyte count may result from marrow infiltration by tumor cells, or an inflammatory response to malignancy, and frank leukemoid reactions may be seen with nonhematopoietic tumors. Thrombocytosis unrelated to primary marrow disease is commonly associated with a systemic malignancy.

A hypercoagulable state is a rare clinical complication of malignancy, although it may be far more prevalent at a subclinical level. Mucin-producing tumors and adenocarcinomas, especially those of the pancreas and stomach, head the list of tumors reported to be associated with clinical disseminated coagulopathy (DIC). This may present as a migratory thrombophlebitis of unknown etiology, which can produce venous thrombosis as well as pulmonary embolism. Hypercoagulation also may be associated with marantic (nonbacterial) endocarditis and resultant thromboembolic episodes, which further complicate the clinical picture. The treatment of the primary malignancy is the only successful therapeutic attack on the problem. Anticoagulation, following the principles for treatment of DIC (Chaps. 62 and 289), may provide short-term benefits in acute situations, but with attendant risks.

Acute promyelocytic leukemia is often associated with abnormalities of hemostasis related to a hypercoagulable state. The malignant immature granulocytes can release procoagulant materials which initiate DIC. In this case, the addition of anticoagulation to the initial phase of antileukemia therapy results in an improved chance for a successful outcome.

Immunosuppression Advanced cancer is accompanied by abnormalities in immune function which can be demonstrated by skin testing against common antigens and by examination of lymphocyte responses to mitogenic stimulation in vitro. Moreover, in general, the extent of malignant disease correlates well with the degree of immune dysfunction. In spite of a vast experimental literature on this subject, the two significant questions concerning immunosuppression in cancer patients continue to be unanswered: (1) What is the mechanism(s) of inhibition? (2) Is the immunosuppression merely secondary to the malignant state, or could it play an etiologic role (failure of "immune surveillance")?

Experimental data have implicated defects in both T- and B-cell function, as well as abnormalities of macrophages, in the etiology of the reduced immune competence in cancer patients. Primary malignancies of lymphocytes are accompanied by abnormalities in the functioning of the particular cell type involved. Some of the lymphoproliferative malignancies are characterized by an increase in autoimmune reactions, most notably in 25 percent of patients with chronic lymphocytic leukemia. In addition, both chemotherapy and radiotherapy can produce long-standing suppression of immune function.

One approach to cancer treatment involves attempts to stimulate an effective immune response with the hope that immune antitumor activity can act alone or in concert with the standard therapeutic modalities to eliminate the malignant cell population. Monoclonal antibodies against antigens present in relatively increased quantities on tumor cells may provide ways to reconstitute or hyperconstitute immune responses to malignancy. Treatment with high concentrations of cytokines such as the interferons has produced responses in a number of types of malignancy, and this is especially effective in the therapy of hairy cell leukemia. Interleukin 2 (IL-2) is another cytokine which may produce antitumor responses in patients with melanoma and renal carcinoma, when administered in pharmacologic doses alone or in combination with lymphokine-activated killer (LAK) cells.

Psychosocial effects The diagnosis of cancer immediately raises in the mind of the patient and his or her family a host of questions and fears which require the undivided attention of an empathetic, considerate, and skilled physician. This is especially true when the particular form of cancer has a poor chance for cure, or when malignancy has recurred.

Of the variety of psychosocial problems experienced by patients, two which are particularly difficult to deal with are helplessness and loss of control. These involve both economic control and personal control of one's activity and one's future. Closely tied to these problems and adding to the feeling of helplessness is the difficulty of accepting personal finitude. A third major source of mental anguish is the fear of pain and mutilation. Finally, separation from loved ones, both anticipated and real, creates a void of loneliness and a fear of abandonment.

The reactions to the mental stresses which are produced by these problems can only be dealt with effectively by a professional who has become familiar with the patient's personality and his or her social and intellectual environment. Although one or another emotion may dominate at a particular time, the responses commonly observed include anger, denial, withdrawal, and depression. Added to these problems is the complexity resulting from the response of the patient's family to the illness and to the patient's own response to the illness. In spite of these stresses, some patients with incurable malignancies are able to adapt and reorient their lives in a creative and meaningful way. The intellectual and emotional challenge to the physician is obvious, and careful attention must be given to managing the patient's (and the family's) responses to malignancy in addition to providing specific treatment for the disease.

Does the patient's psychological attitude have a role in the cause or treatment of malignant disease? The question is a complex and controversial one. There is evidence, which is contested, that life stresses can predispose to systemic illness by producing anxiety or depression. One theory postulates that stress leads to a reduction in immunologic function, resulting in inadequate immune surveillance, but this explanation for the pathogenesis of cancer is not adequately supported by available clinical data. There are also claims that correction of emotional difficulties and development of positive attitudes can serve as effective anticancer therapy. In favor of psychological support and counseling is the clear benefit to the quality of life which can be achieved by helping patients with malignancy to develop positive attitudes and to gain some measure of control over *how* they are living. However, scientific evidence does not demonstrate that the patient's psyche can achieve regression or cure of the malignant process. Some of the strongest and most responsible advocates of counseling and attitudinal approaches to cancer patient management also stress the need for concurrent treatment with standard anticancer therapies.

DIAGNOSIS AND STAGING There are five general goals in evaluating a patient for the presence of malignancy. First, information must be gathered leading to biopsy of a candidate lesion, which alone can establish the pathologic diagnosis of neoplasia. The second goal is to determine as precisely as possible the extent of tumor spread, both at the site of origin and as metastases. The process of obtaining this information is known as *staging*. The third goal is to determine the growth rate and time course of the neoplasm in the particular patient undergoing diagnostic evaluation. The dictum that "every person is different" holds for cancers as well. Each malignancy is different, although there is a natural history which broadly characterizes each type of neoplasm. The rate of tumor growth can be determined by sequential assessment, using physical examinations or radiologic techniques, occasionally aided by the measurement of serum markers of tumor activity. The physician's ingenuity and persistence often come into play; an example is determining the existence of past radiologic studies, locating them, and obtaining them for review. The fourth goal in the evaluation is to determine the effects of the malignancy upon the health and performance of the patient. The importance of this in the design of a management plan is obvious, since control of symptoms and proper modification of acitivity levels will improve the well-being of the patient. In addition, it has become increasingly evident that the patient's performance status provides important data in predicting prognosis as well as response to anticancer therapy. The final goal in the diagnostic evaluation is the selection of appropriate anticancer therapy. The choice will depend on the information gathered as outlined, plus a knowledge of the treatment regimens which have the highest likelihood of producing cure, durable remission, or palliation. The principles of cancer therapy are presented in Chap. 301.

TABLE 300-6 Influence of pretreatment performance status on patients with inoperable lung cancer*

Performance status scale†				
ECOG	Karnofsky	Definitions	Median survival (weeks)	Patients in group (percent)
0	100	Asymptomatic, normal activity	34	2
1	80–90	Symptomatic, but ambulatory	24–27	32
2	60–70	Symptomatic, in bed less than 50% of day, needs minimal assistance	14–21	40
3	40–50	Symptomatic, in bed more than 50% of day, requires considerable assistance	7–9	22
4	20–30	100% bedridden, severely disabled	3–5	5

* N = 5022 males with inoperable lung cancer of all histologic types entered onto VA Lung Group protocols from 1968–1978.
† Eastern Cooperative Oncology Group (ECOG) performance status scale, and DA Karnofsky et al, Cancer 1:634, 1948.
SOURCE: Adapted from JD Minna et al, in VT DeVita, Jr et al.

There are two widely used clinical scales of performance status, the Karnofsky scale and a modification developed by the Eastern Cooperative Oncology Group. The influence of performance status upon prognosis is demonstrated by a report correlating performance and median survival in patients with inoperable lung cancer (Table 300-6).

Pathologic diagnosis The diagnosis of cancer is made by pathologic examination. While there are definite limitations to histologic and cytologic examination of tumor specimens, this procedure is essential in order to exclude inflammatory processes as well as hyperplasia or benign tumors. In addition, the tissue of origin of a malignancy must be known in order to select the appropriate therapy. Specimens for pathologic examination are usually obtained by biopsy of a suspicious lesion. The procedure may involve a surgical operation under general anesthesia, but in many cases tissue specimens can be obtained through local incision (e.g., breast cancer) or by removal of a piece of tissue under direct visualization (bronchoscopy, colonoscopy). When direct visualization is not possible because of the internal location of a suspected lesion, it is often possible to obtain tissue fragments or clumps of cells by fine-needle biopsy aspiration, guided by computed tomography or fluoroscopy. In addition, suitable cytologic preparations can be obtained by washing or scraping surface lesions, as is commonly done to evaluate lesions on the cervix or in bronchi. Finally, in the case of malignancy involving the hematopoietic system or growing in body cavities (e.g., ascites), needle aspiration of tumor cells in suspension can be performed.

To make the diagnosis of cancer the pathologist looks for histologic and cytologic features characteristic of the disease. These include pleomorphism of cellular and nuclear structure, a high rate of mitosis and the presence of large or multiple nuclei, disordered tissue architecture, destruction or invasion of normal tissue boundaries, and the presence of cells in inappropriate locations (metastases). Special stains are useful for identifying chemical components characteristic of particular cell types and tissues. Additional evidence can be brought to bear upon the pathologic diagnosis, using the results of immunohistochemical studies, flow cytometry data on cellular DNA content, chromosomal karyotype analysis, Southern blotting for detection of diagnostic abnormalities in rearranged or amplified genes, and electron microscopy. However, in the overwhelming majority of cases, the diagnosis is made with the light microscope, on the basis of morphologic evaluation of the cells individually and as organized into tissue structures.

After the pathologic diagnosis of malignancy is established, the description usually includes three characteristics which classify the neoplasia:

1 The tissue of origin (e.g., adenocarcinoma, epidermoid carcinoma, sarcoma, leukemia)
2 Anatomic origin (e.g., colon, lung, breast)
3 Degree of differentiation (e.g., well-differentiated or poorly differentiated)

Each of these characteristics gives the therapist information relevant to the selection of treatment and to the prognosis. Although this terminology for classification is followed in general, there are many examples of exceptions based upon customary nomenclature involving particular tissues of origin or on the use of eponyms (e.g., Hodgkin's disease, glioblastoma multiforme).

Staging of cancer The staging of a cancer patient involves the detection of the anatomic extent of the tumor, both in its primary location and in metastatic sites. This process is of critical importance in the clinical management for a number of reasons:

1 The optimal treatment plan for an individual patient is selected on the basis of the stage of disease.
2 By determining the presence of early metastatic disease, treatment can often be designed which can increase the chance for cure, or delay the development of symptoms even if cure is not achievable.
3 Staging provides information from which the physician can better evaluate the prognosis.
4 Because half of the cases of cancer cannot be cured by the therapies available today and because rapid advances in the development of anticancer treatment are occurring, management of an individual patient often involves new drugs or experimental procedures which are in the process of being evaluated for toxicity and efficacy. Staging to determine the extent of disease accurately is essential for evaluating factors influencing the results of such new treatments.

The anatomic extent of disease is best described and communicated to other professionals by a standardized nomenclature known as the TNM system. The three elements characterized in this system are the primary *t*umor, the regional lymph *n*odes, and *m*etastases (Table 300-7). The details of classification were decided upon by the International Union against Cancer (UICC) and the American Joint Committee for Cancer Staging (AJCCS). There is a scale of subcategories with designations ranging from 0 to 4 for each of the three tumor characteristics listed in the table. These scales were chosen because they can provide useful predictions of the clinical course. The primary tumor is classified by its size and the extent of local involvement. The involvement of lymph nodes is typically stratified by the spread to locations at a varying distance from the primary lesion and by the number of involved nodes. The most relevant information regarding metastases is their presence or absence. The details of stratification within the TNM system vary for each type of malignancy and are highly individualized. They depend on the characteristic growth patterns and lymphatic drainage patterns of neoplasms of the various organs. There is not always agreement about the definitions of the TNM characteristics, which can create confusion.

The stage of the tumor is typically divided into three or four categories (e.g., I to IV). For each type of malignancy, the various T, N, and M designations are assigned to one of four stages, in order to develop separation into groupings which correlate with data on prognosis and clinical responses to therapy. This is best described by mentioning a specific example. For the neoplasm with the highest mortality rate, non-small cell carcinoma of the lung, the therapy which has the best chance for curing the patient is surgery. The staging system for lung cancer (Table 300-8) is designed in a way which stratifies patients into groups, for which different treatment protocols are indicated. For the stages I and II patients, surgery is the treatment of choice. The extent of the surgical procedure depends on the extent of disease designated by the T and N classification within these two stages. Total excision of all tumor is the therapeutic goal, with 5-year postresection survival rates of 50 percent for stage I, 30 percent for stage II, and 15 percent for stage IIIa.

Clinical evaluation How does the clinician proceed to evaluate a patient for the presence of malignant disease? Early detection depends primarily on awareness of the hereditary and environmental factors contributing to the incidence of cancer, combined with thorough exploration for symptoms and signs which could lead to further diagnostic workup. The seven warning signals widely publicized by the American Cancer Society are useful to remember (Table 300-9) and are usually covered in a review of systems. A careful physical examination is especially useful in detecting early breast cancer, cancer of the colon, skin cancer, and head-and-neck cancers. Three diagnostic screening tests have proved of value in early detection: (1) the exfoliative cytology (''Pap smear'') screen for cervical cancer, (2) fecal occult blood testing, accompanied by periodic sigmoidoscopy, and (3) mammograms.

The prudent guidelines for early cancer detection provided by the American Cancer Society can be summarized as follows. A cancer-related checkup is recommended every 3 years for those 20 to 40 years of age. For breast cancer screening, an examination of patients in this age group by a physician is recommended every 3 years, a self-examination every month, and one baseline breast x-ray between the ages of 35 and 40. For detection of cervical and uterine cancer, an annual pelvic examination and Pap test are recommended, with a reduction in frequency after three normal examinations.

In the age group of 40 and over, a yearly cancer checkup is

TABLE 300-8 Stage Grouping of the New International Staging System for Lung Cancer*

Occult carcinoma	TX	N0	M0
Stage 0	TIS	Carcinoma in situ	
Stage I	T1	N0	M0
	T2	N0	M0
Stage II	T1	N1	M0
	T2	N1	M0
Stage IIIa	T3	N0	M0
	T3	N1	M0
	T1-3	N2	M0
Stage IIIb	Any T	N3	M0
	T4	Any N	M0
Stage IV	Any T	Any N	M1

* TX, positive cytology; TIS, carcinoma in situ; T1, less than or equal to 3 cm, no local invasion; T2, greater than 3 cm, more than 2 cm from carina; T3, direct extension to chest wall, diaphragm, pleura or pericardium; T4, invasion of mediastinum, intrathoracic organs, or vessels. N1, peribronchial or hilar nodes; N2, ipsilateral mediastinal nodes; N3, contralateral mediastinal nodes; M1, distant metastasis.

SOURCE: Mountain, CF: A new international staging system for lung cancer. Chest 89:225s–233s, 1986.

TABLE 300-7 TNM system of anatomic staging

T: Primary tumor
- T0 No evidence of primary tumor
- T1–4 Ascending degrees of increase in tumor size and involvement

N: Regional lymph nodes
- N0 No evidence of disease in lymph nodes
- N1–4 Ascending degrees of nodal involvement

M: Distant metastasis
- M0 No evidence of metastasis
- M1–4 Ascending degrees of metastatic involvement

TABLE 300-9 Cancer's seven warning signals

Change in bowel or bladder habits
A sore that does not heal
Unusual bleeding or discharge
Thickening or lump in breast or elsewhere
Indigestion or difficulty in swallowing
Obvious change in wart or mole
Nagging cough or hoarseness

SOURCE: American Cancer Society.

TABLE 300-10 Methods for diagnosis and staging

I History
II Physical examination, including examination of oropharynx, Pap test, and proctoscopy
III Radiologic studies
  A Roentgenogram
  B Ultrasound
  C Computerized axial tomography
  D Angiography and lymphangiography
  E Nuclear medicine
  F Magnetic resonance imaging
IV Laboratory studies
  A Hematologic evaluation
  B Chemical tests of internal organ function
  C Tumor markers
V Pathologic examination of tissue
VI Cytogenetics and molecular genetics

recommended by the American Cancer Society. Women over 40 are advised to have a professional breast examination every year, a self-examination every month, and a breast x-ray every 1 to 2 years for those 40 to 49 years of age, and every year for those 50 and over. For screening of cervical and uterine cancer in this age group, an annual pelvic examination and Pap test are recommended, with a reduction in frequency after three normal examinations. An endometrial tissue sample is recommended at menopause if the patient has high-risk factors. For colon and rectal cancer, a digital rectal examination is suggested every year after 40, and a stool occult blood test every year after 50 as well as a sigmoidoscopic examination every 3 to 5 years after two initial negative tests 1 year apart. It is estimated by the American Cancer Society that the 5-year survival rate for colorectal cancer could be increased from the current level of 55 percent to as high as 85 percent, if these early detection techniques were generally applied.

The three most common malignancies involve bowel, lung, and breast, and it is significant that screening tests are suggested for only two of these. Unfortunately, trials of mass screening for lung cancer with chest x-rays and sputum cytology have not resulted in reduced mortality, even when subjects believed to be at high risk were followed. However, the physician who is evaluating a patient in order to attempt to detect cancer early must learn whether or not the patient smokes cigarettes and should attempt to intervene.

The approach to a patient who presents to the physician with a history of symptoms or with abnormal physical findings which could be attributed to cancer involves selection of appropriate diagnostic procedures from a wide variety of available radiologic tests and laboratory studies (Table 300-10). The choice of diagnostic procedures used in the staging of cancer patients is guided by the natural history of the various types of malignancy. For example, knowledge that distant spread of breast cancer most frequently occurs to the lung, liver, bone, brain, and contralateral breast leads to consideration of studies of each of these organs as part of the staging workup. In addition, the diagnostician must know the probability of spread to these various metastatic sites in the presence or absence of abnormal findings in the history, physical examination, and standard blood studies. For the asymptomatic patient with breast cancer who has no abnormal physical findings outside of a small palpable breast lesion, and normal hematologic and blood chemistry values, a chest x-ray and a mammogram are the tests typically performed to stage the patient prior to a decision for definitive therapy. Similar considerations go into planning the diagnostic workup for patients with each of the various forms of malignancy. It is for this reason that a thorough familiarity with the natural history of malignancies of the various organs, as well as the efficacy of a wide variety of diagnostic procedures in detecting these cancers, is essential.

Tumor markers A tumor marker is an abnormality which is specific for a particular type of malignancy. For example, the Ph^1 chromosome abnormality in the karyotype is a marker for chronic myelogenous leukemia, and the exclusive presence of either κ or λ chains on the surface of a population of lymphocytes is a marker of the lymphoproliferative malignancies. Until recently there were no biochemical markers that were absolutely specific for and diagnostic of malignancy. However, utilization of molecular genetic technology has enabled detection of genetic alterations that are pathognomonic for particular malignancies (see discussion of "Clonality" above). In addition, recent reports demonstrate specific genetic abnormalities in a variety of types of cancer. Examples, some of which have been alluded to, include amplified *neu* or elevated *erb*B expression in breast cancer, elevated N-*myc* in neuroblastoma, overexpression of H-*ras* in bladder and prostate cancer, and amplified c-*myc* in small cell lung cancer. The term *marker* may also be used in a more restrictive sense, referring to molecules which are produced in abnormal amounts or under abnormal circumstances and are released into the circulation. The anaplasia and autonomy of the tumor cells permit production of molecules in greater than normal amounts or at inappropriate times in the life of the organism, and in this sense the abnormalities may become specific. Assays of such markers may be of great help to the clinician in a number of ways: (1) screening of high-risk individuals for the presence of malignancy, (2) diagnosis of malignancy, (3) monitoring of the effectiveness of therapy, (4) early detection of recurrence, and (5) immunodetection of metastatic sites, using radioactive-labeled antibodies against the markers.

The tumor marker of greatest use to the clinician is human chorionic gonadotropin (hCG), which has specificity because of its nearly exclusive production by the trophoblastic epithelium of the placenta under normal circumstances. The hCG levels rise during pregnancy. The hormone also may be secreted into the blood by trophoblastic tumors, as well as germ cell neoplasms of the testes and ovaries. Other neoplasms have been reported to be associated with elevated hCG levels, but the serum concentration rarely exceeds 10,000 ng/L (10 ng/mL) whereas trophoblastic tumors can produce concentrations over 100×10^6 ng/L (100,000 ng/mL). The usefulness of the assay for hCG is markedly enhanced by clinical data which show that changes in the serum hCG concentration in patients with secreting trophoblastic malignancies accurately reflect changes in the tumor burden. Therefore, decisions on the appropriate time to discontinue therapy can be based on the time course of serum levels, and decisions to reinstate therapy for recurrent disease are made on the basis of reappearance of hCG in the serum. The clinical test for hCG utilizes a radioimmunoassay for the beta subunit, to avoid cross reactivity with luteinizing hormone.

Two clinically useful tumor markers are products of genes which are expressed during the normal differentiation of fetal tissue but are partially or completely suppressed in the adult. These markers have been termed oncofetal antigens. Carcinoembryonic antigen (CEA) was originally thought to be specific for bowel cancer, but further studies have shown it to be a nonspecific tumor-associated antigen which also may be elevated in a variety of benign conditions. In the gastrointestinal tract, the molecule, a glycoprotein with a molecular weight of 180,000, is concentrated in the glycocalyx of epithelial cells, from which it is released into the lumen of the bowel. In the presence of malignancy, CEA concentrations may be elevated in the blood and other body fluids. Serum levels of CEA above the normal concentration of 2500 ng/L (2.5 ng/mL) are found in greater than 50 percent of neoplasms involving the colon, pancreas, stomach, lung, and breast. A variety of common nonmalignant conditions are associated with elevation of CEA, but typically not over 10,000 ng/L (10 ng/mL). These include cigarette smoking, chronic pulmonary disease, alcoholic cirrhosis, hepatitis, and inflammatory bowel disease. CEA is not selective for cancer, and measurements of its levels should not be used in screening for the presence of malignant disease. However, serial measurements of CEA levels in patients with secreting malignancies can provide valuable information on the efficacy of treatment and the recurrence of disease. The possibility that early elevation of serum CEA can predict recurrence of bowel cancer soon enough to allow further surgical resection for cure is under study.

The second clinically useful oncofetal antigen is alpha fetoprotein

(AFP), which is produced by the liver and gastrointestinal tract epithelium during gestation and which falls to levels less than 20,000 ng/L (20 ng/mL) after birth. Serum levels are elevated in 70 percent of patients with hepatocellular cancer, the majority of patients with nonseminomatous testicular cancer, and occasional patients with neoplasms of the gastrointestinal tract. As with CEA, the serum concentration of AFP may be elevated in benign conditions, especially in inflammatory disease of the liver. Its utility is in monitoring tumor activity, especially in the case of testicular tumors.

Elevation of either AFP or hCG is found in 80 to 90 percent of all nonseminomatous germ cell tumors of the testes. However, absence or normal levels of these biochemical markers of malignancy cannot be interpreted as proof that there is no tumor. Some tumors do not produce these marker molecules. Furthermore, because of tumor heterogeneity, it is possible for marker concentrations to fall in the presence of tumor, if a nonproducing subclone begins to grow preferentially. For this reason, recurrence of disease need not be accompanied by recurrence of elevated marker levels.

Other biochemical markers with clinical utility include calcitonin, with which familial medullary carcinoma of the thyroid can be detected in individuals who appear to be normal. Prostatic acid phosphatase levels are useful in determining the extent (stage) of prostatic cancer, and in monitoring the response to therapy.

There are many tumors which, because of increased cellular mass or loss of normal regulation, produce excessive quantities of polypeptides normally secreted into the circulation by the tissue of origin. Examples include the immunoglobulin molecules produced in multiple myeloma, and insulin or gastrin hypersecretion by islet cell tumors. In addition, tumors may secrete molecules which ordinarily are not produced in the tissue from which they are derived. This phenomenon has already been discussed in the description of the paraneoplastic syndromes, because in many cases these marker molecules have biologic activities which can produce clinical illness in the patient. In some cases of malignant disease, cultures of tumor cells have been found to secrete a variety of polypeptide hormones atypical of the tissue of origin. In addition, molecules related to normal hormones or to their precursor forms may be present in the patient's serum, in the absence of any demonstrable clinical effects. These observations provide evidence for the broad scope of genetic deregulation which may accompany the process of oncogene expression and carcinogenesis.

REFERENCES

CALABRESI P et al: *Medical Oncology: Basic Principles and Clinical Management of Cancer*. New York, Macmillan, 1985

CLINE MJ: Molecular diagnosis of human cancer. Lab Invest 61:368, 1989

DEVITA VT JR et al: *Cancer: Principles and Practices of Oncology*. Philadelphia, Lippincott, 1989

HOLLAND JF, FREI E: *Cancer Medicine*. Philadelphia, Lea & Febiger, 1982

MERKEL DE, MCGUIRE WL: Oncogenes and cancer prognosis, in *Important Advances in Oncology 1988*, VT DeVita Jr et al (eds). Philadelphia, Lippincott, 1988, chap 7

NORDENSKJOLD M, CAVENEE W: Genetics and the etiology of solid tumors, in *Important Advances in Oncology 1988*, VT DeVita Jr et al (eds). Philadelphia, Lippincott, 1988, chap 6

RUBIN P: *Clinical Oncology for Medical Students and Physicians*. New York, American Cancer Society, 1983

SCHOTTENFELD D, FRAUMENI JF JR: *Cancer Epidemiology and Prevention*. Philadelphia, Saunders, 1982

301 CANCER CHEMOTHERAPY

EDWIN C. CADMAN / HENRY J. DURIVAGE

In the United States cancer is the second leading cause of death and in 1988 resulted in an estimated 480,000 deaths. This translates to 167 deaths per 100,000 population per year, or an estimated 21 percent of all deaths in the United States in 1988. Thus, someone born in the United States in 1990 has a greater than 1 in 3 chance of developing cancer in his or her lifetime. However, while a decade ago only 10,000 patients per year with metastatic cancer were cured by chemotherapy, at present this rate has increased to 30,000 patients per year.

There has been a systematic approach to the development of cancer chemotherapy in the United States. Since the creation of the National Cancer Chemotherapy Program in 1955, over 700,000 compounds and extracts have been screened for antineoplastic properties. In 1945 there was only one drug known to be effective—namely, nitrogen mustard. Today, there are nearly 50 chemotherapeutic agents used, singly or combined, in the treatment of malignancy.

The introduction of cancer chemotherapy followed closely on the wave of excitement concerning the antibiotic treatment of infectious diseases. In 1943, after it had been observed that World War II soldiers exposed to nitrogen mustard gases had a reduction in the size of their lymph nodes, mechlorethamine hydrochloride (chlormethine) was first used to treat Hodgkin's disease. A rapid decrease in these patients' lymph nodes was documented, but the remissions were very transient. At about the same time, based on knowledge regarding certain antimetabolite antibiotics, the antifolate agent aminopterin (methotrexate) was first used in 1947 to treat acute lymphocytic leukemia. The use of methotrexate as a single agent in gestational choriocarcinoma in 1955 resulted in the first cancer cures.

The lack of cure in other cancers similarly treated prompted investigators to examine combinations of chemotherapeutic agents based on the concept of "therapeutic synergism" developed for the treatment of infections using a combination of antibiotics. The first empirical trials using combinations of antineoplastic drugs were reported in 1957 and 1960 in patients with bronchogenic carcinoma and testicular carcinoma. In the latter up to 22 percent complete responses were recorded. However, substantial toxicity and drug-related deaths were major deterrents. In 1958 the first randomized study in children with acute lymphocytic leukemia was reported, and remarkable responses were observed.

In 1964 Skipper and his colleagues began the first studies in which the scientific knowledge of drug combinations was specifically evaluated. They utilized the murine leukemia L1210 cell line to examine the growth characteristics of tumors in a mouse model and to characterize the response of cancer cells to chemotherapy. Their study also provided an experimental model for "cure." Because of their laboratory success, other researchers were prompted to scientifically study cancer growth and chemotherapy with the goal of improving our ability to destroy cancer cells.

This early research also included attempts at biochemical modulation. Drug combinations were tested in various cancer cell lines using the in vivo mouse model. Combinations of drugs were tested which were predicted to cause sequential blockade (of two different sequential enzymes in a pathway) or concurrent blockade (of two different enzymes not in sequence which would both contribute to a reduction in a needed common end product) and result in therapeutic synergy. The results were disappointing, in part because the predictions were incorrect, but also because individually the drugs did not have dramatic cytotoxic effects. But a precedent for further research was established, and from this work the basic principles of cancer chemotherapy have evolved. In many cancers, chemotherapy can result in (1) significantly improved survival, (2) reproducible palliation without significantly improved survival, or (3) occasional responses at the expense of substantial toxicity. There are a few cancers that remain totally unresponsive to chemotherapy—namely, malignant melanoma with visceral metastases, hypernephroma, pancreatic carcinoma, and metastatic adenocarcinomas of unknown primary. The capacity to cure disseminated cancer is dependent on combination chemotherapy alone, or together with biologic therapy, surgery and/or radiotherapy. Further progress in deriving more effective combinations is dependent on a rational and scientific approach to developing and screening chemotherapeutic drug combinations.

As shown in Fig. 301-1, many cancers can be cured by surgical resection. Chemotherapy for cancer is used primarily in the treatment of nonoperable or metastatic malignancy or as an adjunct to primary surgical therapy. The most widespread use of adjuvant chemotherapy is for breast cancer. Modest estimates are that an additional 5 percent of patients who otherwise would have relapsed and died of breast cancer are now cured because they were given adjuvant chemotherapy.

Although the primary goal for chemotherapy is to cure, most patients are, in fact, not cured. Nearly all patients have some tumor response to their therapy, but only a small number have their lives substantially prolonged. Therefore, to improve our ability to treat cancer, patients should be offered the choice of participating in clinical trials. The standard use of the terms "complete response" or "partial response" is an important clinical determinant for assessing the results of therapy.

CELL KINETICS Cancer is a clonal disease. A single cell becomes uninhibited in growth and continues to divide, leading to the formation of a tumor. The time for cellular division is generally quite long. The concept that all cancer cells multiply rapidly is incorrect. For example, breast cancer cells generally divide every 100 days. A simple series of mathematical evaluations yields compelling evidence that supports the contention that cancer has been present in any given individual for years prior to clinical detection. Given the average size of a cell of 1 μm, it will take 10^9 (1 billion) cells to form a 1-cm nodule, which is also equivalent to 1 g in weight. Assuming that all cells survived, it would take 30 cell doublings to achieve 1 billion cells from 1 cell; the first cancer cell divides to form two cancer cells; these two cells divide to form four cells, etc. This form of cell growth is exponential. If the time between doublings averages 100 days, then it will take almost 9 years for one cancer cell to result in a 1-cm nodule. A tumor which contains 10^{12} cells is equivalent to 1 kg. A cancer with this number of cells is a far-advanced malignancy which results in an extremely cachectic patient who is generally terminally ill. Only 10 more cell doublings are required to go from 10^9 cells to 10^{12} cells, which is approximately 3 years for a tumor whose cells divide every 100 days. Figure 301-2 describes tumor growth as a process that proceeds exponentially. Representative cancers and their doubling times, and the predicted time to form a 1-cm nodule, are presented in Table 301-1.

FIGURE 301-1 Estimation of cancer patient results for the 1990s.

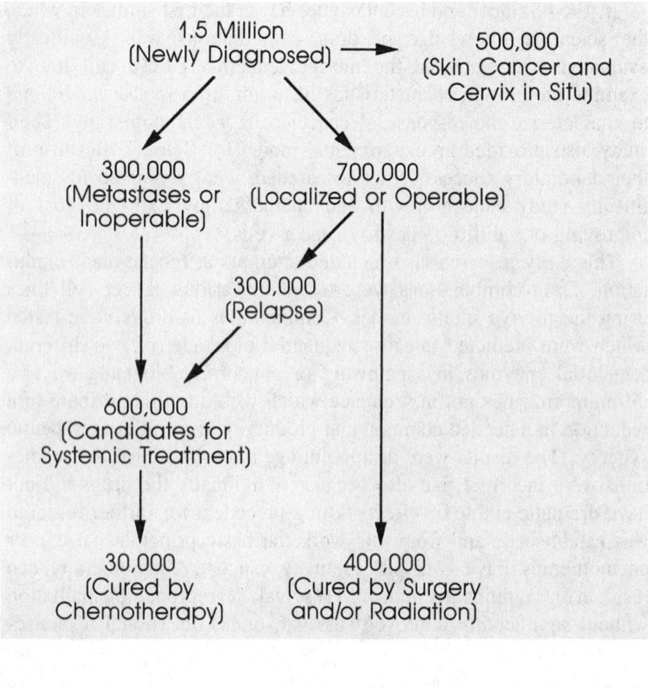

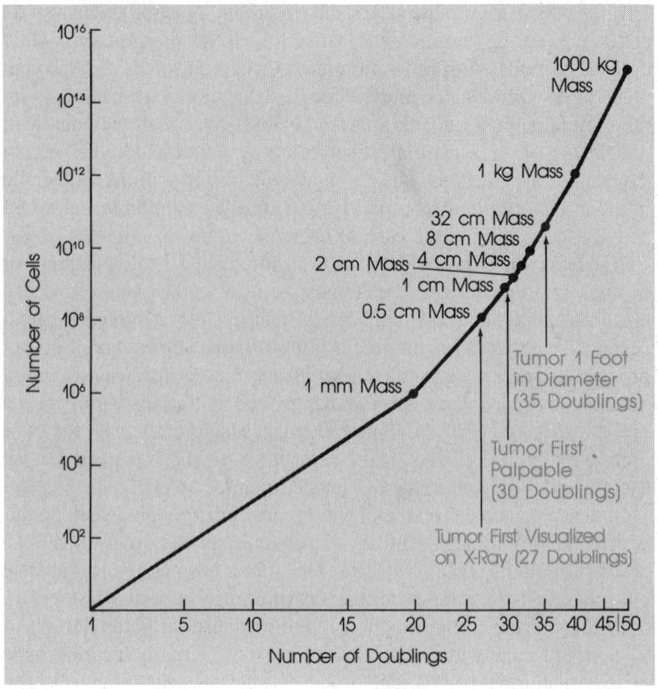

FIGURE 301-2 Schematic representation of the life cycle of a human tumor.

From this example, it is apparent that a small cancer is not a young tumor. Three-quarters of the cancer's "life" has been used to develop into a 1-cm lesion (30 doublings divided by 40 doublings). The actual growth kinetics of a cancer can vary considerably from this example, because this evaluation assumes linear growth and no natural cell loss. However, not all cells of a tumor divide simultaneously. The cell cycle (Fig. 301-3) consists of several phases, any of which contain various fractions of the cancer cell population.

Most chemotherapeutic agents affect cells during the synthesis of DNA. It is unclear if any of our current chemotherapeutic agents are effective in killing cells in G_0, or the resting phase. For example, methotrexate, which inhibits the formation of thymidylate (one of the four bases required for DNA synthesis), will not kill cells unless they are actively synthesizing this DNA precursor. Therefore, the success of chemotherapy is often highly dependent upon the cellular kinetics of the tumor at the time the drugs are administered.

The growth rate of malignant cells, which is exponential during the early phases of tumor growth, becomes less rapid in the later stages of tumor development. There are several reasons proposed for this reduction in the growth rate; these include (1) insufficient local nutrients (e.g., decreased blood supply) to support continued growth, (2) an increased rate of tumor cell death, and/or (3) fewer cells reentering the cell cycle. In general, the very small or undetected

TABLE 301-1 Tumor doubling times and duration of growth

Tumor	Doubling, days	Time to a 1-cm tumor
Burkitt's lymphoma	1–5	30–150 days
Testicular cancer	20	1.6 years
Diffuse (high-grade) lymphoma	12–25	1–2.1 years
Lung cancer	100	8.2 years
Colon cancer	100	8.2 years
Breast cancer	100–130	8.2–10.6 years

SOURCE: Adapted from G Gordon Steel, *Growth Kinetics of Tumors*, Oxford, Clarendon Press, 1977.

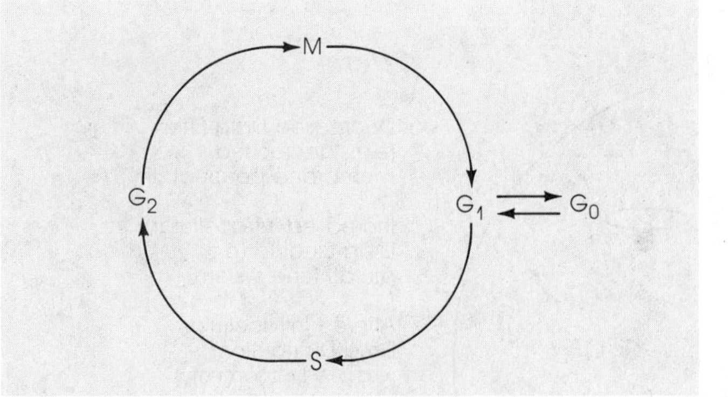

G_0 = resting phase (nonproliferation of cells)
G_1 = pre-DNA synthetic phase (12 h to a few days)
S = DNA synthesis (usually 2 to 4 h)
G_2 = post-DNA synthesis (2 to 4 h; cells are tetraploid in this stage)
M = mitosis (1 to 2 h)

FIGURE 301-3 The cell cycle.

cancers undergo a more rapid proliferation than the larger clinically apparent tumors.

Adjuvant chemotherapy refers to the administration of drugs following primary surgical therapy when residual tumor is small and clinically undetectable and the cells are more likely to be actively dividing. It is self-evident that it is easier to kill 10^3 than 10^9 cells; therefore, assuming that drugs kill the same percentage of cells each time they are given, it will also take less time to get rid of 10^3 than 10^9 cells. These assumptions apply only if the drugs are toxic to the cancer cells. *Neoadjuvant therapy* refers to the use of chemotherapy prior to or immediately after a curative resection of a malignancy.

PRINCIPLES OF CHEMOTHERAPY To achieve a cure of a malignancy, presumably all of the cancer cells must be destroyed. For this to occur with chemotherapeutic drugs (1) the cancer cells must be sensitive to the agent; (2) the drug must reach the malignant cell; (3) if the drug is effective only in a phase of the cell cycle, it must be given frequently enough that all the cancer cells enter this phase of the cell cycle while the drug is present; and (4) the malignant cells must be destroyed before drug resistance emerges. There are obvious exceptions to the validity of these concepts. Thus, an innocuous dose of a drug over a long period of time will never be effective. It is assumed that high drug dose over a short time period is effective because sufficient amounts of the drug remain within the cells or the tumor environment to be lethal, even though the drug may not be detectable in the serum.

Experimental and clinical studies have demonstrated the importance of dose intensity for effective cancer treatment. Dose intensity is the amount of drug given per unit time. In general, more drug given over a short time period is superior to the same amount over a longer time period. The clinical implications of this principle are quite important—namely, patients who are treated with chemotherapy should be given the maximum tolerated dose frequently. Low, nontoxic, and nontumoricidal doses favor the emergence of drug-resistant cancer cells.

Table 301-2 lists some of the general types of biologic and chemical agents used in the treatment of cancer. The first tumor to be cured by chemotherapy was choriocarcinoma. Methotrexate was effective and continues to be the treatment of choice for this malignancy except in far-advanced stages. This tumor divides rapidly; presumably very few cells are in the resting phase (G_0). However, it is not surprising that very few malignancies have been cured by the administration of a single dose. The use of drug combinations has enhanced the possibility of cure or remission. The theoretical advantage of combination therapy is that several drugs can be given

TABLE 301-2 Some types of biologic and chemical agents used in the treatment of cancer

Hormones
Cytokines
Interferons α, β, γ
Interleukins, especially IL-2
Tumor necrosis factor
Monoclonal antibodies coupled to tumoricidal agents
Cells
Lymphokine activated killer (LAK) cells
Tumor infiltrating lymphocytes (TIL)
Chemotherapeutic drugs

simultaneously or in close proximity to each other and thus lead to cell death by several mechanisms. This approach has been effective in the treatment of many cancers and reduces the emergence of drug-resistant cells. In general, if a cell is resistant to one drug, it is less likely also to be resistant to a second or third drug. However, certain caveats must be kept in mind. In selecting drug combinations, their site of action in the cell cycle is important. Thus, it makes little sense to use a drug that prevents DNA synthesis (viz., prevents cells from entering the S phase) together with an agent that is only effective on cells in the S phase. A negative aspect of combination therapy is that it is often associated with greater systemic toxicity.

Drug resistance The resistance of cancer cells to a cytotoxic drug is an inherent property of the cancer cell itself; it can be temporary or permanent. *Temporary resistance* can be due to environmental or local factors limiting cell killing as, for example, (1) by diminished blood supply to the tumor; (2) when cells are in "sanctuaries" such as the central nervous system and the drug does not cross the blood-brain barrier; or (3) when cells are in the wrong phase of the cell cycle.

The more significant problem, in general, is the development of genetic changes in the malignant cell leading to *permanent drug resistance*. Some of the major mechanisms include (1) increased intracellular inactivation of the drug; (2) increased efflux of the drug out of the cell by products of multidrug-resistant genes in the cell membrane (see below); (3) an increase in the number of target enzymes; (4) increased DNA repair, etc. (see Fig. 301-4).

Goldie and Coldman suggested in 1979 that just as bacteria mutate spontaneously to bacteriophage resistance, so cancer cells might develop resistance to drugs. They proposed that drug resistance was related to both *mutation rate* and *cell number* or size. Thus, if the intrinsic mutation rate is 10^{-6}, a tumor composed of 10^9 cells (approximately 1 cm in diameter) is very likely to develop a drug-resistant clone. Examples of this phenomenon probably occur in breast cancer, ovarian cancer, and acute leukemia with cancer cells responding initially but then becoming resistant with the emergence of resistant clones or cell lines.

A major clinical problem is that tumors of the visceral organs frequently are not responsive to chemotherapeutic agents. There may be several reasons for this. These tumors (e.g., colon, stomach, pancreas) may be inherently resistant due to the prior exposure of the normal tissue to the presence of these agents in the environment. Thus, they may have developed detoxification mechanisms to protect against the natural (? dietary) toxins from which many chemotherapeutic drugs have been developed. As shown in Fig. 301-2 the concept that a tumor 1 cm in size has gone through 30 doublings to reach 10^9 cells is based on exponential cell growth. This may not apply to all animal or human tumors. In fact, cell loss occurs in some tumors, and this may be as great as 90 percent. Thus, as many as 1200 doublings might be needed to reach 10^9 cells; this allows for an increased incidence of mutations to resistant cells, making it likely that the tumors are resistant to anticancer agents at the time of diagnosis.

A genetic mechanism leading to resistance of a wide range of drugs that have minimal, if any, relationship to each other involves pleiotropic or multidrug resistance (MDR). A single genetic step can

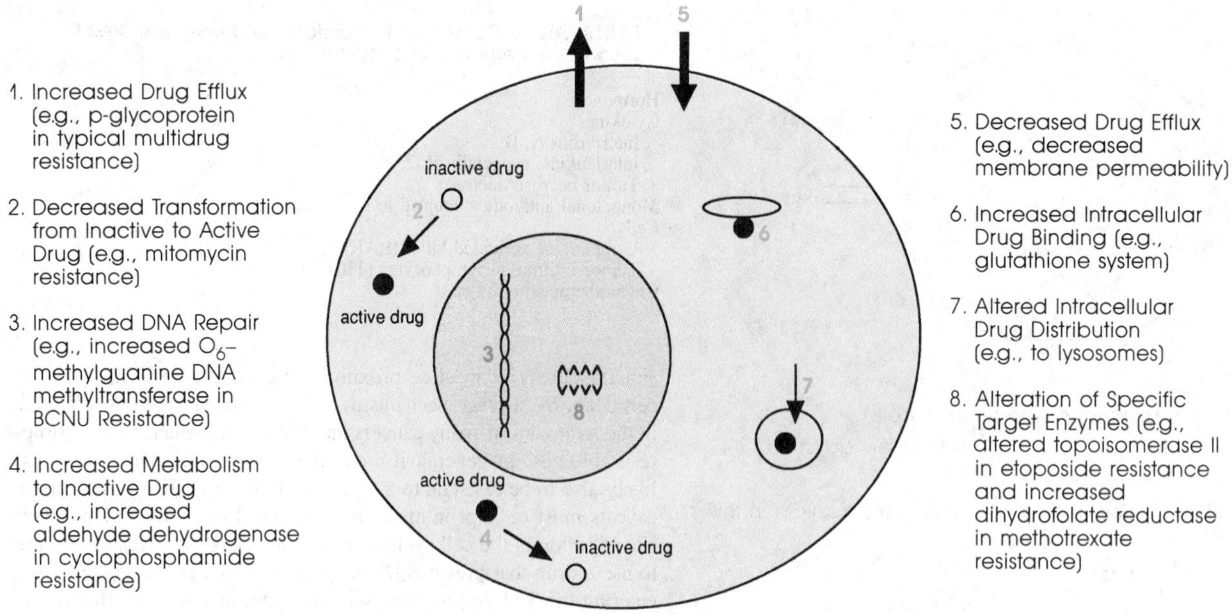

FIGURE 301-4 Potential sites for drug resistance at the cellular level.

make the cells resistant to the most effective and most used anticancer drugs. This genetic alteration leads to the expression on the cell surface of a 170-kDa glycoprotein (called P-glycoprotein, or P170). This protein leads to the increased drug efflux and, hence, reduced intracellular accumulation of the drug. However, a number of agents can reduce the actions of P170 and have been shown to potentiate the cytotoxic effects of certain drugs, at least in part by increasing their intracellular concentration. These agents include calcium channel antagonists, polyene antibiotics, and antiarrhythmic drugs (see Table 301-4).

Gene amplification can also be associated with drug resistance. This can occur as a result of gene reduplication if transcription is slowed down or stopped; it can also be induced by drugs that decrease DNA synthesis such as a low dose of alkylating agents or radiation. Therefore, giving a low dose or a weak antitumor agent or marginally effective x-radiation may induce resistance to drugs like methotrexate without any prior exposure to the drug. This reduplication or amplification of DNA may result in as many as 100 copies of a given region on a chromosome. This amplification may take either of two forms: (1) the duplicated DNA may be tandemly organized at a single site leading to a *homogeneously staining region* (HSR) by microscopy; or (2) it may exist as small, chromosome-like structures referred to as *double minutes* on stained chromosome preparations.

TABLE 301-3 Drugs that may modulate drug resistance

Drugs	Antineoplastic* drugs affected	Proposed mechanism of increased cytotoxicity
Calcium antagonists		
Verapamil	VCR, DNR,	Increased accumulation
Nifedipine	ADR	by blocking efflux
Nitrendipine		
Caroverine		
Calmodulin inhibitors		
Prenylamine	VCR, DNR	Same as above
Trifluoroperazine	ADR	
Clomipramine		
Amphotericin	ADR, ACT-D, BCNU	Alterations in lipid composition of plasma
Tween 80	ADR	membrane leading to
Perhexiline maleate	ADR	increased accumulation
Triparanol analogues		
Tamoxifen	ADR	Increased drug accumulation
Antiarrhythmic drugs		
Quinidine	ADR, VCR	Increased drug accumulation
Antihypertensive Reserpine	ADR	Increased drug accumulation
Thiol depleter		
Buthionine sulfoximine	L-PAM, PLAT, ADR	Drug inactivation, free radical metabolism, protection/repair of DNA

* ABBREVIATIONS: VCR, vincristine; DNR, daunorubicin; ADR, Adriamycin; L-PAM, melphalan; PLAT, cisplatin; BCNU, 1,3 bis(2 chloroethyl)1-nitrosourea; ACT-D, actinomycin D.

CLINICAL TRIALS The journey from basic research to clinically useful anticancer drugs takes many years. The time from a basic observation in the laboratory until sufficient information is obtained to support studies in human beings often ranges from 2 to 10 years. Once a drug has been proven safe and effective in rodents, it can enter clinical trials. The clinical trials program in this country is largely the result of coordinated efforts sponsored by the National Cancer Institute. There are three phases of clinical trials.

1 The purpose of phase 1 is primarily to determine the maximum tolerated dose and human pharmacology of the agent tested. Only patients with far-advanced cancer of any type for whom no further therapy is available or patients for whom no effective (''standard'') therapy exists may be eligible to receive phase 1 drugs.

2 The purpose of phase 2 is to determine for which cancers the new drug is effective. Only patients with measurable tumors for whom either no further therapy is available or for whom no initial therapy is known to be effective can elect to participate in this phase. The patient must not be terminally ill. In general between 15 and 30 patients with specific types of cancer are entered into these studies. Ideally each drug should be tested in 7 and 10 different types of tumors.

3 As a result of phase 2 studies, the drug may have been shown to be effective against a specific type of cancer. In phase 3 studies, the new drug is given to a more uniform group of patients with the type of cancer for which the drug was determined to be effective in the phase 2 study. These patients have usually not been treated, and randomization between the new treatment and the nonstandard treatment is done or the new agent is added to a standard effective therapy and compared to the standard therapy alone. If there is no standard effective treatment, then randomization is not performed; for example, there is no effective standard treatment for squamous cell cancer of the lung. Therefore, patients with this cancer type should be entered into a phase 3 study.

To determine if a drug is effective against a given cancer in a phase 2 study, we must rely on statistical analysis to assist in the decision-making process. If we assume that we wish to find only new drugs which have a minimum effectiveness of 20 percent, that is, that 20 percent of patients with cancer "X" will respond to the new drug, then projections to guide us can be made: Given this criterion, there is a 95 percent chance that in the first 14 patients with cancer "X" there will be at least 1 patient who responds to the new drug. If there is no response noted in the first 14 treated patients, then there is a 95 percent probability that the drug is not effective for the treatment of that type of cancer as defined by a minimum expected 20 percent response rate. The problem with this statistical reasoning is that it assumes that all 14 patients are similar. If a disparate group of patients (even if they have the same kind of cancer) is entered into the phase 2 study, the lack of response could be due to factors unrelated to the tumor type. Therefore, for a phase 2 study patients must be carefully selected.

Chemical and biologic agents in the treatment of cancer Many biologic and chemical agents can be given systemically to patients to produce destruction of cancer cells. These are shown in Table 301-4. As indicated above, in many instances these agents are used in combination rather than alone. Table 301-5 lists some drugs that are still investigational in the United States.

TABLE 301-4 Some commercially available anticancer drugs and hormones (dose-limiting effects are italicized)

Drug	Acute toxicity	Delayed toxicity*
Aminoglutethimide *Action:* Blocks steroidogenesis	Drowsiness; nausea; dizziness	Hypothyroidism (rare); bone marrow depression; fever; hypotension; masculinization
Asparaginase *Action:* Destroys essential amino acid (asparagine)	*Nausea and vomiting; fever;* chills; headache; hypersensitivity, anaphylaxis; abdominal pain; hyperglycemia leading to coma	CNS depression or hyperexcitability; acute hemorrhagic pancreatitis; coagulation defects; thrombosis; renal damage; hepatic damage
Bleomycin *Action:* Generates free radicals	*Nausea and vomiting; fever;* anaphylaxis and other allergic reactions	*Pneumonitis and pulmonary fibrosis; rash* and hyperpigmentation; stomatitis; alopecia; Raynaud's phenomenon; cavitating granulomas
Busulfan *Action:* Alkylates DNA	*Nausea and vomiting;* rare diarrhea	*Bone marrow depression;* pulmonary infiltrates and fibrosis; hyperpigmentation; alopecia; gynecomastia; ovarian failure; azoospermia; leukemia; chromosome aberrations; cataracts; hepatitis
Carboplatin *Action:* Cross-links DNA	*Nausea and vomiting*	*Bone marrow depression;* peripheral neuropathy (uncommon); hearing loss
Carmustine (BCNU) *Action:* Alkylates DNA	*Nausea and vomiting;* local phlebitis	*Delayed leukopenia and thrombocytopenia* (may be prolonged); pulmonary fibrosis (may be irreversible); delayed renal damage; gynecomastia; reversible liver damage; venoocclusive disease (hepatic or pulmonary) with high doses; leukemia
Chlorambucil *Action:* Alkylates DNA	Seizures; nausea and vomiting	*Bone marrow depression;* pulmonary infiltrates and fibrosis; leukemia; hepatic toxicity; sterility
Cisplatin (*cis*-DDP) *Action:* Cross-links DNA	*Nausea and vomiting;* anaphylactic reactions; fever; hemolytic-uremic syndrome	*Renal damage;* bone marrow depression; ototoxicity; hemolysis; hypomagnesemia; peripheral neuropathy; hypocalcemia; hypokalemia; Raynaud's disease; sterility; teratogenesis
Cyclophosphamide *Action:* Alkylates DNA	*Nausea and vomiting;* type 1 (anaphylactoid) hypersensitivity; facial burning with IV administration; visual blurring	*Bone marrow depression;* alopecia; hemorrhagic cystitis; sterility (may be temporary); pulmonary infiltrates and fibrosis; hyponatremia; leukemia; bladder cancer; teratogenesis; inappropriate ADH secretion
Cytarabine HCl *Action:* Inhibits DNA polymerase	*Nausea and vomiting;* diarrhea; anaphylaxis	*Bone marrow depression;* conjunctivitis; megaloblastosis; oral ulceration; hepatic damage; fever; pulmonary edema and central and peripheral neurotoxicity at high doses; rhabdomyolysis; pancreatitis when used with asparaginase
Dacarbazine *Action:* Alkylates DNA	*Nausea and vomiting;* diarrhea; anaphylaxis; pain on administration	*Bone marrow depression;* alopecia; flulike syndrome; renal impairment; hepatic necrosis; facial flushing; paresthesia; photosensitivity; urticarial rash
Dactinomycin *Action:* DNA intercalator	*Nausea and vomiting;* diarrhea; local reaction and phlebitis; anaphylactoid reaction	*Stomatitis; oral ulceration; bone marrow depression;* alopecia; folliculitis; dermatitis in previously irradiated areas
Daunorubicin HCl *Action:* DNA intercalator	*Nausea and vomiting;* diarrhea; red urine (not hematuria); severe local tissue damage and necrosis on extravasation; transient ECG changes; anaphylactoid reaction	*Bone marrow depression; cardiotoxicity;* alopecia; stomatitis; anorexia; diarrhea; fever and chills; dermatitis in previously irradiated arcas
Doxorubicin HCl *Action:* DNA intercalator; generates free radicals	*Nausea and vomiting;* red urine (not hematuria); severe local tissue damage and necrosis on extravasation; diarrhea; fever; transient ECG changes; ventricular arrhythmia; anaphylactoid reaction	*Bone marrow depression; cardiotoxicity;* alopecia; stomatitis; anorexia; conjunctivitis; acral pigmentation; dermatitis in previously irradiated areas
Estramustine phosphate sodium *Action:* Combination of estrogen and nitrogen mustard	Nausea and vomiting; diarrhea	Mild gynecomastia; increased frequency of vascular accidents; myelosuppression (uncommon); edema; dyspnea; pulmonary infiltrates and fibrosis; leukemia

(continued)

TABLE 301-4 Some commercially available anticancer drugs and hormones (dose-limiting effects are italicized) *(continued)*

Drug	Acute toxicity	Delayed toxicity*
Etoposide (VP16-213) *Action:* Inhibits topoisomerase II	*Nausea and vomiting;* diarrhea; fever; hypotension; allergic reactions	*Bone marrow depression;* alopecia; peripheral neuropathy; mucositis and hepatic damage with high doses
Floxuridine *Action:* Inhibits thymidylate synthesis	*Nausea and vomiting;* diarrhea	*Oral and gastrointestinal ulceration; bone marrow depression;* alopecia; dermatitis; hepatic dysfunction with hepatic infusion
Fluorouracil (5-FU) *Action:* Inhibits thymidylate synthesis	*Nausea and vomiting;* diarrhea; hypersensitivity reaction	*Oral and GI ulcers; bone marrow depression;* diarrhea (especially with fluorouracilleucovorin); neurologic defects, usually cerebellar; cardiac arrhythmias; angina pectoris; alopecia; hyperpigmentation; palmar-plantar erythrodysesthesia; conjunctivitis; heart failure
Flutamide *Action:* Antiandrogen	Nausea; diarrhea	Gynecomastia; hepatotoxicity
Hydroxyurea (hydroxycarbamide) *Action:* Inhibits ribonucleotide reductase	Nausea and vomiting; allergic reactions to tartrazine dye	*Bone marrow depression;* stomatitis; dysuria; alopecia; rare neurologic disturbances
Ifosfamide *Action:* Alkylates DNA	Nausea and vomiting; confusion; nephrotoxicity; metabolic acidosis	*Bone marrow depression; hemorrhagic cystitis* (prevented by concurrent mesna); alopecia; inappropriate ADH secretion; neurotoxicity (somnolence, hallucinations, blurring of vision, coma); teratogenesis
Interferon Alfa-2a, Alfa-2b *Action:* Multifaceted, increases HLA expression	Fever; chills; myalgias; fatigue; headache; arthralgias; hypotension	Bone marrow depression; anorexia; renal damage; hepatic damage
Leuprolide acetate (LHRH-releasing factor analogue) *Action:* LHRH analogue	Transient increase in bone pain and ureteral obstruction; hot flashes	Impotence; amenorrhea; testicular atrophy
Lomustine (CCNU) *Action:* Alkylates DNA	*Nausea and vomiting*	*Delayed (4 to 6 weeks) leukopenia and thrombocytopenia* (may be prolonged); transient elevation of transaminase activity; neurologic reactions; pulmonary fibrosis; renal damage; leukemia
Mechlorethamine HCl (nitrogen mustard) *Action:* Alkylates DNA	*Nausea and vomiting;* local reaction and phlebitis	*Bone marrow depression;* alopecia; diarrhea; oral ulcers; leukemia; amenorrhea; sterility
Melphalan *Action:* Alkylates DNA	Mild nausea; hypersensitivity reactions	*Bone marrow depression* (especially platelets); pulmonary infiltrates and fibrosis; amenorrhea; sterility; leukemia; inappropriate ADH secretion
Mercaptopurine *Action:* Hypoxanthine analogue	Nausea and vomiting; diarrhea	*Bone marrow depression; cholestasis and rarely hepatic necrosis; oral and intestinal ulcers; pancreatitis;* allopurinol and azathioprine increase overall toxicity
Mesna *Action:* Used in conjunction with ifosfamide; inhibits hemorrhagic cystitis	Nausea and vomiting; diarrhea	
Methotrexate (MTX) *Action:* Inhibits dihydrofolate reductase (DHFR)	*Nausea and vomiting;* diarrhea; fever; anaphylaxis; hepatic necrosis	*Oral and gestrointestinal ulceration,* perforation may occur; *bone marrow depression;* hepatic toxicity including cirrhosis; renal toxicity; *pulmonary infiltrates and fibrosis;* osteoporosis; conjunctivitis; alopecia; depigmentation; menstrual dysfunction; encephalopathy and anaphylactoid reactions with high doses
Mitomycin *Action:* Cross-links DNA	*Nausea and vomiting;* local reaction; fever	*Bone marrow depression* (cumulative); stomatitis; alopecia; acute pulmonary toxicity; pulmonary fibrosis; hepatotoxicity; renal toxicity; amenorrhea; sterility; hemolytic-uremic syndrome; bladder calcification
Mitotane (o, p′-DDD) *Action:* Inhibits steroidogenesis	*Nausea and vomiting;* diarrhea	*CNS depression;* rash; visual disturbances; adrenal insufficiency; brain damage with long-term high dosage; hematuria; hemorrhagic cystitis; albuminuria; hypertension; orthostatic hypotension; cataracts
Mitoxantrone HCl *Action:* DNA intercalator	Blue-green pigment in urine; blue-green sclera; nausea and vomiting; stomatitis	Bone marrow depression; cardiotoxicity; alopecia; white hair; skin lesions; hepatic damage; renal failure
Octreotide *Action:* Somatostatin analogue	Nausea; diarrhea; abdominal pain	Steatorrhea
Plicamycin *Action:* DNA intercalator	*Nausea and vomiting; diarrhea; fever*	*Hemorrhagic diathesis; bone marrow depression* (thrombocytopenia); coagulation abnormalities; hepatic damage; hypocalcemia and hypokalemia; stomatitis; renal damage

TABLE 301-4 Some commercially available anticancer drugs and hormones (dose-limiting effects are italicized) *(continued)*

Drug	Acute toxicity	Delayed toxicity*
Procarbazine HCl *Action:* Alkylates DNA	*Nausea and vomiting;* CNS depression; disulfiram-like effect with alcohol	*Bone marrow depression;* stomatitis; peripheral neuropathy; pneumonitis; leukemia; interacts with tyramine in food to cause hypertensive crisis
Streptozocin *Action:* Alkylates DNA	*Nausea and vomiting;* local pain; chills and fever	*Renal damage;* hypoglycemia; hyperglycemia; liver damage; diarrhea; bone marrow depression (uncommon); fever; eosinophilia; nephrogenic diabetes insipidus
Tamoxifen citrate *Action:* Antiestrogen	Nausea and vomiting; hot flashes; transient increased bone or tumor pain; hypercalcemia	Vaginal bleeding and discharge; rash; thrombocytopenia; peripheral edema; depression; dizziness; headache; decreased visual acuity; corneal changes; retinopathy
Thioguanine *Action:* Purine analogue	Occasional nausea and vomiting	*Bone marrow depression;* hepatic damage; stomatitis
Thiotepa *Action:* Alkylates DNA	*Nausea and vomiting;* local pain	*Bone marrow depression;* menstrual dysfunction; interference with spermatogenesis; leukemia
Vinblastine sulfate *Action:* Inhibits tubulin function	*Nausea and vomiting;* local reaction and phlebitis with extravasation	*Bone marrow depression;* alopecia; stomatitis; loss of deep tendon reflexes; jaw pain; muscle pain; paralytic ileus; inappropriate ADH secretion
Vincristine sulfate *Action:* Mitotic arrest; inhibits tubulin function	Local reaction with extravasation	*Peripheral neuropathy;* alopecia; mild bone marrow depression; constipation; paralytic ileus; jaw pain; inappropriate ADH secretion

* Cutaneous reactions (sometimes severe), hyperpigmentation, and ocular toxicity have been reported with virtually all nonhormonal anticancer drugs.
SOURCE: Adapted from *The Medical Letter,* June 2, 1989, with permission.

Hormonal therapy The growth of many tissues is influenced by hormones, and some tumors continue to possess receptors for them. Lymphoid tumors have receptors for glucocorticoids, estrogen, and progesterone; receptors are present on some breast cancers and endometrial cancers, and prostate cancers have abundant androgen receptors. Hormones bind to receptors in the cytoplasm and nucleus; this is associated with a conformational chance in the receptors that interact with the DNA in the nucleus leading to messenger RNA and protein synthesis.

Patients with breast cancer cells that have estrogen receptors have a greater than 50 percent chance of responding to hormonal agents such as tamoxifen, an antiestrogen (see Chap. 303). Endometrial

TABLE 301-5 Some investigational drugs (dose-limiting effects are in italics)

Drug	Acute toxicity	Delayed toxicity
Amsacrine (m-AMSA) *Action:* DNA intercalator	*Nausea and vomiting;* diarrhea; pain or phlebitis on infusion; anaphylaxis	*Bone marrow depression;* hepatic injury; convulsions; stomatitis; ventricular fibrillation; alopecia
Azacitidine *Action:* Inhibits DNA methylation	Nausea and vomiting; diarrhea; fever; drowsiness	Leukopenia (may be prolonged); thrombocytopenia; hepatic damage; muscle pain and weakness; bone marrow depression; possibly cardiotoxicity
Erythropoietin *Action:* Stimulates erythropoiesis	Fever; bone pain	Capillary leak; leukocytosis; local thrombosis
Hexamethylmelamine* (HMM) *Action:* Alkylates DNA	Nausea and vomiting	*Bone marrow depression;* visual disturbances (reversible); CNS depression; peripheral neuritis; visual hallucinations; ataxia
Interleukin 2 *Action:* Stimulates T-cell proliferation	*Fever; fluid retention;* rash; anemia; thrombocytopenia; nausea and vomiting; diarrhea; capillary leak syndrome; nephrotoxicity; myocardial toxicity; hepatotoxicity; erythema nodosum	Neuropsychiatric disorders; hypothyroidism
Mitoguazone (methyl-GAG; methyl glyoxal bis-guanylhydrazone; MGBG) *Action:* Alkylates DNA	*Nausea and vomiting;* fatigue	Myopathy; paresthesia; bone marrow depression; ventricular arrhythmias; stomatitis; gastrointestinal ulcerations
Pentostatin (2′-deoxycoformycin)	Nausea and vomiting; rash	Nephrotoxicity; CNS depression;
Semustine (methyl-CCNU) *Action:* Alkylates DNA	*Nausea and vomiting*	*Delayed leukopenia and thrombocytopenia* (may be prolonged); pulmonary fibrosis; renal failure; leukemia
Teniposide* (VM-26) *Action:* Multifactorial; mitotic arrest	Nausea and vomiting; diarrhea; phlebitis; anaphylactoid symptoms	Bone marrow depression; alopecia; peripheral neuropathy
Vindesine sulfate* *Action:* Inhibits tubulin function	Local reaction if extravasation; fever; nausea and vomiting; diarrhea	Bone marrow depression; alopecia; peripheral neuropathy; jaw pain

* Commercially available in Canada.
SOURCE: Adapted from *The Medical Letter,* June 2, 1989, with permission.

cancers may respond in one-third of patients to progestins; these hormones may also produce response in about 10 percent of patients with renal cancer, but the mechanism for this effect is not known.

Since prostate cancers grow under the influence of androgens, the hormonal treatment involves the use of agents with antiandrogen or estrogen properties. The development of nonsteroidal antiandrogens such as flutamide and antagonists of the hypothalamic releasing hormone LHRH such as leuprolide has produced promising clinical results in the treatment of prostatic cancer without the cardiovascular complications resulting from estrogen use.

Biologic agents Biologic approaches to the treatment of cancer are varied but in general can be divided into three categories: (1) agents augmenting the defenses of the host, (2) agents that are directly tumoricidal, and (3) agents that modify the behavior of the tumor.

CYTOKINES Agents that augment host defenses include the *cytokines* such as the interferons, interleukin 2, and tumor necrosis factor. *Interferons* (INF) are glycoproteins made by cells in response to viral infections. IFN-α is secreted by leukocytes, INF-β is secreted by fibroblasts, and IFN-γ is secreted by lymphocytes in response to mitogens. The mechanism by which IFNs are cytotoxic to cancer cells is not clear, but they inhibit cell proliferation and enhance T-cell cytotoxicity. IFN-α is the treatment of choice for hairy cell leukemia, producing a complete response in 50 percent of patients and a partial response in 90 percent. In addition, IFN-α has significant antitumor effects in renal cell carcinoma, ovarian cancer, melanoma, follicular lymphoma, and chronic myelogenous leukemia.

Interleukin 2 is a T-cell growth factor released by antigen-stimulated T cells. Purified IL-2 has been used to activate lymphocytes referred to as LAK cells (lymphokine activated killer cells) which differ from natural killer (NK) cells, to destroy tumor cells regardless of their immunogenicity. Clinical studies of so-called adoptive immunotherapy with concomitant administration of IL-2 and LAK cells have produced some complete and partial remissions in patients with advanced melanoma and renal cancers, with lesser responses in lung cancers. These studies suggest that tumor-infiltrating lymphocytes (TIL cells) plus IL-2 are somewhat more effective than LAK cells. However, there are significant systemic side effects associated with IL-2 administration, and this has limited its use.

Tumor necrosis factor (TNF) is produced and secreted by macrophages. It has been shown to have a direct cytotoxic effect against tumor cells, especially melanoma cells in culture. TNF has been cloned and produced in large quantities for clinical trials by recombinant techniques. However, in studies to date, TNF has not shown major cytotoxic activity in humans. Its toxicity is very similar to IL-2's.

Monoclonal antibodies Since the development of the hybridoma technique in 1975, many monoclonal antibodies have been produced against tumor-associated antigens. The theoretical advantage of these antibodies is their selectivity and specificity for given antigens and, in general, in their not binding to normal cells. They are being evaluated to assess their use alone (as complement-fixing antibodies) or conjugated with toxins (e.g., ricin, *Pseudomonas* toxin) or coupled with radioisotopes (e.g., ^{131}I). Most experience has been with murine antibodies. Clinical efficacy to date has been limited for a number of reasons including tumor cell heterogeneity, lack of cytotoxicity, and development of human antimouse antibodies.

Antineoplastic drugs One of the most important aspects of cancer chemotherapy trials in the 1960s and 1970s was the fact that drugs could *cure* some patients with cancer. Cancers can generally be grouped based on their response to antineoplastic drugs. Tables 301-6 to 301-8 list the tumors in which drugs have major, moderate, or minimal activity. In most cases maximum benefit is achieved by combination chemotherapy.

Antineoplastic drugs exert their cytotoxic effects by interfering with various cellular mechanisms involved in cell growth. The production of essential cellular components may be disrupted or damaged, or RNA and DNA synthesis and/or function may be altered. Figure 301-5 shows the major sites of action of most current antineoplastic drugs. The latter include alkylating agents, antineoplastic antibiotics, plant alkaloids, and antimetabolites.

Alkylating agents possess a characteristic alkyl moiety and exert their cytotoxic effects primarily by covalent bonding of the alkyl groups to cellular DNA or other molecules. Despite their apparent similarity, the alkylating agents exhibit a wide and varied spectrum of antitumor activity. Examples of alkylating agents are cyclophosphamide, the chlorethylnitrosoureas, and melphalan. *Antineoplastic antibiotics* have been isolated from microbial fermentation extracts. They also have a wide spectrum of antitumor activity and are largely responsible for the improved treatment of acute leukemias, lymphomas, and breast cancer. They include bleomycin, doxorubicin, mitomycin, and mitoxantrone. *Plant alkaloids* and other natural products have also yielded important antineoplastic drugs. The vinca alkaloids (e.g., vincristine, vinblastine) and podophyllotoxin derivatives (e.g., etoposide, teniposide) are examples of effective drugs derived from natural sources. *Antimetabolites* act by inhibiting crucial metabolic enzymes. Often prolonged exposure of these antimetabolites by continuous infusion is more effective than bolus administration. In general, antimetabolites such as 5-fluorouracil, methotrexate, and cytarabine are most effective on rapidly dividing cells.

SIDE EFFECTS OF CHEMOTHERAPEUTIC AGENTS AND THEIR MANAGEMENT Antitumor agents exert their actions by interfering with cellular structures and function, and there is often a narrow "window" between therapeutic and adverse effects. Most acute toxicities are expressed in rapidly dividing tissues or organs such as the bone marrow, intestinal mucosa, and hair follicles. The important side effects are described below along with approaches to anticipate, prevent, or ameliorate them.

MYELOSUPPRESSION Only a few anticancer agents directly suppress bone marrow stem cells. These include the alkylating drugs such as nitrogen mustard, cyclophosphamide, and the nitrosoureas. The reduction of the blood count for most other antineoplastic agents is the result of the inhibition of the proliferating committed cells in the marrow and not an effect on the nondividing stem cell. It is important to remember that a significant percentage of normal bone marrow cells are not actively dividing; this affords some selectivity in the choice of antitumor drugs.

In general, maximum bone marrow suppression occurs in the most actively dividing fractions such as platelets and granulocytes. Cell cycle–specific agents, such as the antimetabolites, seem to produce the most rapid granulocytopenic responses, but they are also associated with rapid recovery. For most anticancer drugs myelosuppression is the toxicity that determines the maximal dose that can be given. Only

TABLE 301-6 Diseases in which chemotherapy has major activity

Cancer	Drugs currently preferred	Alternative drugs
Acute lymphocytic leukemia (ALL)	Induction: vincristine + prednisone ± asparaginase ± doxorubicin or daunorubicin CNS prophylaxis: intrathecal methotrexate ± radiotherapy Maintenance: methotrexate + mercaptopurine Bone marrow transplant for chemotherapy failures	Etoposide + cytarabine, cyclophosphamide, cytarabine, thioguanine, teniposide,* mitoxantrone, etoposide, ifosfamide + mesna CNS prophylaxis: high-dose IV + intrathecal methotrexate, high-dose cytarabine, intrathecal cytarabine + methotrexate ± hydrocortisone Maintenance: doxorubicin and/or asparaginase in addition to methotrexate and mercaptopurine

TABLE 301-6 Diseases in which chemotherapy has major activity *(continued)*

Cancer	Drugs currently preferred	Alternative drugs
Acute myelogenous leukemia (AML)	Daunorubicin + cytarabine ± thioguanine Mitoxantrone + cytarabine ± daunorubicin Bone marrow transplant with cyclophosphamide plus either total-body irradiation or busulfan	High-dose cytarabine, mitoxantrone, amsacrine,* azacitidine,* etoposide, + eniposide,* ifosfamide + mesna
Breast cancer†,‡	Tamoxifen Cyclophosphamide + methotrexate + fluorouracil ± prednisone (CMF or CMFP) Cyclophosphamide + doxorubicin ± fluorouracil (AC or CAF)	Megestrol, leuprolide acetate, cisplatin ± vinblastine, ifosfamide + mesna, vincristine, mitomycin, mitoxantrone, etoposide, teniposide,* mitolactol,* estrogens, progestins, androgens, prednisone, aminoglutethimide
Choriocarcinoma	Methotrexate ± leucovorin ± dactinomycin	Vinblastine, chlorambucil, bleomycin, etoposide, cisplatin, methotrexate with leucovorin rescue
Embryonal rhabdomyosarcoma†	Vincristine + dactinomycin + cyclophosphamide (VAC) ± doxorubicin Vincristine + doxorubicin + cyclophosphamide	Methotrexate, cisplatin, ifosfamide + mesna
Ewing's sarcoma†	Cyclophosphamide + doxorubicin + vincristine (CAV)	Dactinomycin, etoposide ± ifosfamide with mesna
Hairy cell leukemia	Interferon or pentostatin*	Chlorambucil
Hodgkin's disease	Doxorubicin + bleomycin + vinblastine + dacarbazine (ABVD) ± cyclophosphamide ABVD alternated with MOPP Mechlorethamine + vincristine + procarbazine + prednisone (MOPP) Mechlorethamine + vincristine + procarbazine + doxorubicin + bleomycin + vinblastine (MOP/ABV) Chlorambucil + vinblastine + procarbazine + prednisone (CVPP) ± carmustine Marrow transplantation with lomustine, cyclophosphamide, etoposide	Lomustine, carmustine, etoposide, cisplatin + etoposide, teniposide,* streptozocin, methotrexate, ifosfamide + mesna, mitoguazone*
Lung, small cell (oat cell)	Cisplatin + etoposide (PE) Cyclophosphamide + doxorubicin + vincristine (CAV) PE alternated with CAV Cyclophosphamide + etoposide + cisplatin (CEP)	Methotrexate + doxorubicin + cyclophosphamide + lomustine (MACC) Ifosfamide + mesna, methotrexate,* cyclophosphamide, lomustine, carboplatin,* mechlorethamine
Non-Hodgkin's lymphoma, Burkitt's lymphoma	Cyclophosphamide Cyclophosphamide + vincristine + methotrexate Cyclophosphamide + high dose cytarabine ± methotrexate with leucovorin rescue	Carmustine, methotrexate, ifosfamide + mesna
Diffuse large cell lymphoma	Cyclophosphamide + doxorubicin + vincristine + prednisone (CHOP) Bleomycin + doxorubicin + cyclophosphamide + vincristine + prednisone (BACOP) Bleomycin + doxorubicin + cyclophosphamide + vincristine + prednisone + methotrexate with leucovorin rescue (M-BACOP) Prednisone + methotrexate-leucovorin + doxorubicin + cyclophosphamide + etoposide + mechlorethamine + vincristine + procarbazine + prednisone (ProMACE-MOPP) Bleomycin + doxorubicin + cyclophosphamide + vincristine + prednisone + procarbazine (COP-BLAM) Methotrexate with leucovorin + doxorubicin + cyclophosphamide + vincristine + prednisone + bleomycin (MACOP-B) Bone marrow transplantation with high-dose cyclophosphamide and total-body irradiation or with cyclophosphamide + carmustine + etoposide	Bleomycin, chlorambucil, lomustine, carmustine, cytarabine, etoposide, teniposide,* amsacrine,* methotrexate, high-dose cytarabine, ifosfamide + mesna, interferon (for follicular lymphomas), prednisone Cyclophosphamide + vincristine + methotrexate-leucovorin + cytarabine (COMLA) Dexamethasone sometimes substituted for prednisone
Osteogenic sarcoma†	Doxorubicin and high-dose methotrexate + leucovorin rescue ± cisplatin ± bleomycin ± cyclophosphamide ± dactinomycin	Ifosfamide + mesna, etoposide
Testicular	Cisplatin + etoposide ± bleomycin (PEB) Cisplatin + vinblastine + bleomycin (PVB) Vinblastine + dactinomycin + bleomycin + cyclophosphamide + cisplatin (VAB-6) Autologous marrow transplantation with carboplatin + etoposide	Cisplatin + ifosfamide with mesna + vinblastine or etoposide Doxorubicin, vincristine, ifosfamide + mesna, carboplatin,* etoposide, cyclophosphamide, methotrexate, plicamycin, dactinomycin
Wilms' tumor†	Dactinomycin + vincristine ± doxorubicin ± cyclophosphamide	Doxorubicin, cyclophosphamide, cisplatin, ifosfamide + mesna, etoposide

* Available in the USA only for investigational use.
† Drugs have major activity only when combined with surgical resection, radiotherapy or both.
‡ For adjuvant treatment of breast cancer, tamoxifen is generally preferred for postmenopausal patients and combinations of other drugs for premenopausal node-positive patients.
SOURCE: Adapted from *The Medical Letter*, June 2, 1989, with permission.

TABLE 301-7 Diseases in which chemotherapy has moderate activity

Cancer	Drugs currently preferred	Alternative drugs
Adrenocortical carcinoma	Mitotane or cisplatin	Doxorubicin, aminoglutethimide
Bladder	Cisplatin and/or doxorubicin ± methotrexate ± vinblastine* Instillation of BCG or thiotepa or doxorubicin or mitomycin	Fluorouracil, vinblastine, methotrexate, instillation of interferon
Brain		
Glioblastoma	Carmustine or lomustine	Semustine,* procarbazine, cisplatin, cyclophosphamide, etoposide
Medulloblastoma	Vincristine + carmustine ± mechlorethamine ± methotrexate Mechlorethamine + vincristine + procarbazine + prednisone (MOPP) Vincristine + cisplatin ± cyclophosphamide	
Cervix	Cisplatin + bleomycin ± methotrexate Bleomycin + mitomycin + vincristine ± cisplatin	Cyclophosphamide, vincristine, methotrexate, mitomycin, fluorouracil, doxorubicin, vinblastine; ifosfamide + mesna
Chronic lymphocytic leukemia	Chlorambucil ± prednisone	Cyclophosphamide, vincristine, pentostatin*
Chronic myelogenous leukemia (CML)		
Chronic phase	Busulfan Hydroxyurea, interferon Bone marrow transplantation with cyclophosphamide and total-body irradiation	Mitobronitol,* mercaptopurine, thioguanine, melphalan
Acute phase	Daunorubicin + cytarabine + vincristine + prednisone ± thioguanine High-dose cytarabine ± daunorubicin Vincristine + prednisone for lymphoid variant	Amsacrine,* azacitidine,* vincristine ± plicamycin
Endometrial	Megestrol acetate or hydroxyprogesterone caproate or medroxyprogesterone acetate Doxorubicin ± cyclophosphamide ± cisplatin	Fluorouracil, tamoxifen, carboplatin
Gastric	Fluorouracil + doxorubicin + cisplatin, ± semustine or mitomycin	Cisplatin ± etoposide, fluorouracil
Head and neck, squamous cell	Cisplatin + fluorouracil Belomycin + cisplatin ± methotrexate	Methotrexate, mitomycin, doxorubicin
Islet cell carcinoma	Streptozocin ± fluorouracil ± doxorubicin	Doxorubicin, dacarbazine, octreotide
Kaposi's sarcoma (AIDS-related)	Etoposide or interferon or vinblastine	Cyclophosphamide, vincristine
Mycosis fungoides	Combination chemotherapy as in Hodgkin's disease or non-Hodgkin's lymphoma Mechlorethamine (topical)	Carmustine (topical), photopheresis (psoralen + extracorporeal ultraviolet light) Vinblastine, methotrexate, interferon, pentostatin,* etretinate
Myeloma	Melphalan (or cyclophosphamide) + prednisone Melphalan + carmustine + cyclophosphamide + prednisone Dexamethasone + doxorubicin + vincristine (VAD)	Carmustine, vincristine, lomustine, doxorubicin, interferon
Neuroblastoma	Doxorubicin + cyclophosphamide + cisplatin + teniposide* Doxorubicin + cyclophosphamide Cisplatin + cyclophosphamide	Mechlorethamine, daunorubicin, dacarbazine, vinblastine, prednisone, cisplatin, teniposide,* etoposide Bone marrow transplantation
Non-Hodgkin's lymphoma		
Follicular lymphoma	Cyclophosphamide or chlorambucil, ± vincristine and prednisone, ± etoposide (combinations not demonstrably superior to single agents)	Cytarabine, asparaginase, methotrexate, interferon

* Available in the United States only for investigational use.
SOURCE: Adapted from *The Medical Letter*, June 2, 1989, with permission.

recently, with the availability of colony stimulating factors has there been the opportunity to give these drugs beyond their previously defined maximal doses. The use of colony stimulating factors following chemotherapy results in a resurgence of proliferation of the dormant stem cells causing a rapid repopulation of normal functional cells.

With most agents, when given as a single therapeutic dose, the nadir of granulocyte and platelet counts occurs 7 to 14 days later, with recovery occurring by day 21 to 28. However, with mitomycin and most of the nitrosoureas (e.g., lomustine and carmustine) maximum myelosuppression occurs 4 to 5 weeks after the initial dose, with recovery 2 to 3 weeks later. Other drugs, such as bleomycin and vincristine, are less myelotoxic and are generally safe to administer when blood counts are low.

Antineoplastic drugs often lead to levels of myelosuppression without clinical complications at granulocyte levels of about 1500 cells per microliter and platelet counts 50,000 per microliter. Significant myelosuppression, leading to infectious or bleeding complications, generally occurs as a result of intentional high-dose chemotherapy (e.g., leukemia induction regimen) or in patients with tumors that involve the bone marrow. It is of critical importance to make certain that recent blood counts are available and that drug dosages are calculated accurately before the drugs are given. Preferably drug dosages should be calculated by two individuals before administration.

NAUSEA AND VOMITING Most but not all anticancer drugs cause nausea and vomiting, and despite substantial advances in antiemetic therapy, prevention of chemotherapy-induced nausea and vomiting continues to be a therapeutic challenge. At present, the treatment of choice involves metoclopramide plus dexamethasone-containing regimens. However, their use does not always prevent or relieve nausea and vomiting induced by highly emetogenic chemotherapy. Factors which influence whether or not nausea and vomiting

TABLE 301-8 Diseases in which chemotherapy has minor activity

Cancer	Drugs currently preferred	Alternative drugs
Colorectal	Fluorouracil + levamisole Intraarterial floxuridine (hepatic metastases)	Semustine,* mitomycin, leucovorin, + fluorouracil
Liver	Doxorubicin or fluorouracil	Floxuridine, intraarterial floxuridine
Lung (non-small cell)	Cyclophosphamide + doxorubicin + cisplatin (CAP) Vindesine† or vinblastine + cisplatin ± mitomycin Cisplatin + etoposide	Methotrexate + doxorubicin + cyclophosphamide + lomustine (MACC) Fluorouracil + doxorubicin + mitomycin (FAM) Methotrexate, mitomycin, carboplatin*
Melanoma	Interleukin 2* ± lymphokine activated killer (LAK) cells*; dacarbazine; semustine*	Dactinomycin, carmustine, interferon
Pancreatic	Fluorouracil Fluorouracil + doxorubicin + mitomycin (FAM) Streptozocin + mitomycin + fluorouracil (SMF)	Mitomycin, leuprolide acetate
Renal	Interleukin 2* or interferon	Vinblastine, lomustine, progestins

* Available in the USA only for investigational use.
† Not available in United States.
SOURCE: Adapted from *The Medical Letter*, June 2, 1989, with permission.

will occur or will be serious include: (1) the nature of the drug, (2) drug dosage, (3) schedule of administration (i.e., daily vs. repeated single doses), (4) time of day the drug is given, (5) the rate of administration (when given intravenously), and (6) combination drug therapy.

FIGURE 301-5 Sites and mechanism of action of chemotherapeutic drugs.

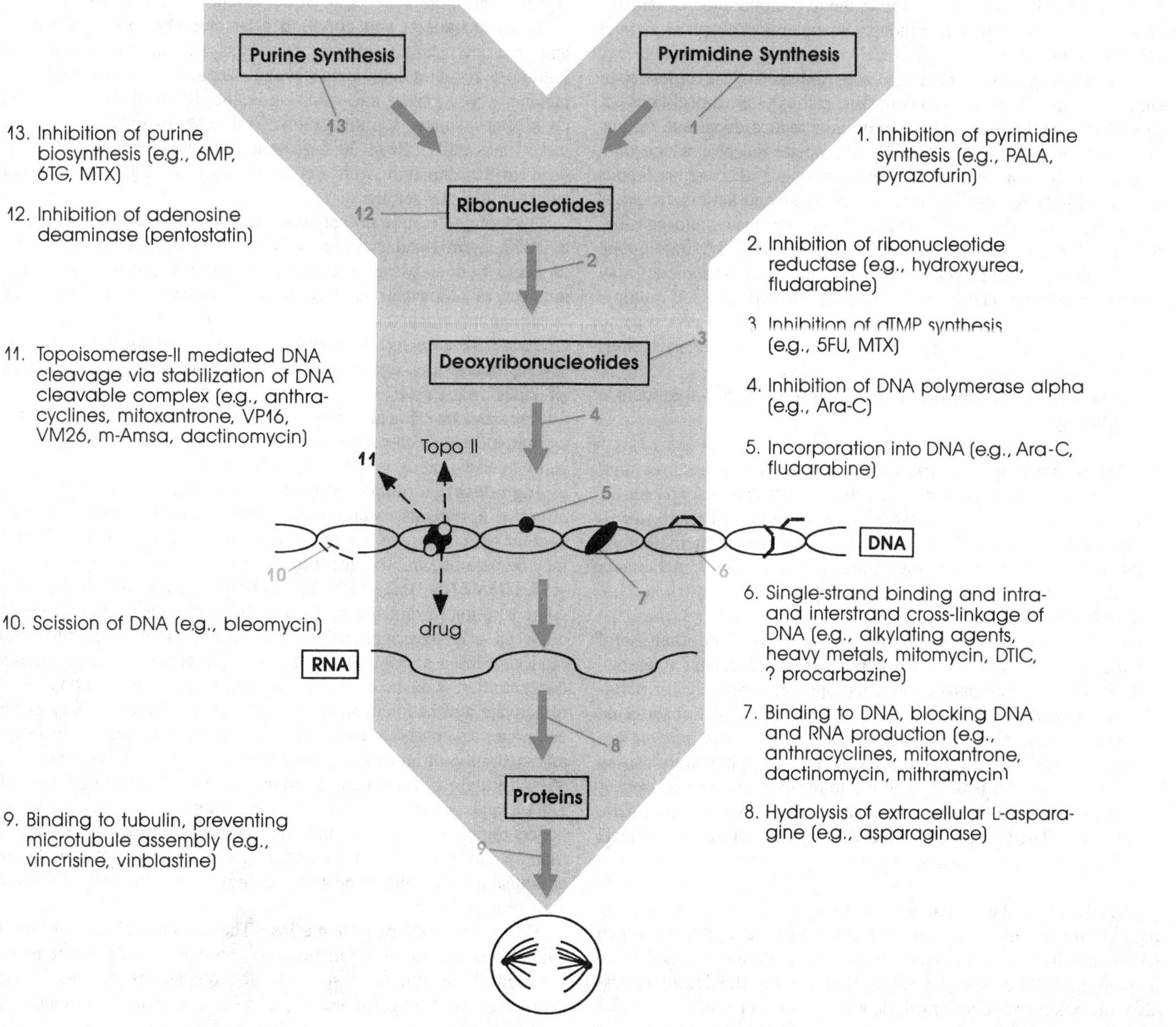

MECHANISMS OF NAUSEA AND VOMITING AND ANTIEMETIC PHARMACOLOGY The mechanisms by which antineoplastic drugs induce nausea and vomiting remain unclear, but the chemotrigger zone (CTZ) and emetic center of the brain appear to be involved. Emetogenic substances can reach the CTZ via the blood or cerebrospinal fluid. Dopamine release induced by these drugs and subsequent dopamine binding to specific receptors in the emetic center may initiate nausea and vomiting. Many antineoplastic drugs are thought to cause nausea and vomiting through stimulation of the CTZ. However, there are many other neurotransmitters in this region, and a combination of neurotransmitters may be responsible for initiating nausea and vomiting.

Stimuli from outside the central nervous system (e.g., gastrointestinal tract) can induce nausea and vomiting. Peripheral stimuli travel via vagal and sympathetic afferents directly to the vomiting center. In cats with a surgically ablated CTZ, mechlorethamine and cisplatin can induce vomiting, presumably by stimulation of peripheral gastrointestinal pathways which may involve an interaction with peripheral serotonin receptors. In animals and in human beings, some antiserotonergic compounds have been shown to delay and, in some cases, to prevent the emetic actions of cisplatin, cyclophosphamide, and doxorubicin.

The response to sight and smell of higher centers in the brain can lead to nausea and vomiting. When anticipatory nausea and vomiting is present, stimulation of these centers may be involved. Vestibular pathways influenced by motion or movement may also contribute to nausea and vomiting after chemotherapy. This may in part explain why inpatients often experience better emesis control than outpatients receiving identical treatment. Further evidence that vestibular pathways may play a role in the causation of nausea and vomiting is provided by the fact that the anticholinergic drug scopolamine has been shown to be a useful addition to the metoclopramide-dexamethasone antiemetic regimen, although scopolamine alone is not an effective antiemetic.

Enkephalin pathways have also been implicated, and it has been suggested that enkephalin and dopamine pathways are closely linked. Enkephalins and opiates such as morphine induce dopamine release through their interaction with a specific opiate receptor which may be involved in stimulating nausea and vomiting. Naloxone has a poor binding affinity for this receptor and possesses no antiemetic properties. However, the antiemetic actions of the opiates and possibly the cannabinoids may result from interaction with a separate opiate receptor that can be antagonized by naloxone. Thus, antiemetics may reduce or prevent nausea and vomiting by differing or multiple mechanisms; and combinations of antiemetics are often necessary to prevent nausea and vomiting caused by certain antineoplastic drugs or drug combinations.

The essential elements of antiemetic prescribing therefore include the following:

1 *Administration of antiemetics on a routine schedule.* Providing antiemetic therapy on a routine schedule because of expected or known onset of nausea and vomiting is essential. Single doses of antiemetics prior to the administration of emetogenic chemotherapy are seldom effective. The use of prn, or "as needed," antiemetic therapy for known emetogens is inappropriate and should be discouraged.

2 *Aggressive antiemetic therapy for new patients.* Too often useful antiemetics are not given in proper doses and dosing intervals. This conservative approach is inappropriate, especially for previously untreated patients who are to receive highly emetogenic chemotherapy, as it contributes to the loss of emesis prevention, which in turn contributes to the development of anticipatory nausea and vomiting. All patients who are to receive emetogenic chemotherapy for the first time should have an aggressive antiemetic approach. Their response or the development of adverse effects will influence future treatment strategies.

As discussed above, patients receiving a specific chemotherapy regimen for the first time should receive antiemetic therapy which has been shown to be effective against the antitumor regimen to be administered. When specific information is not available, an aggressive metoclopramide-dexamethasone regimen, or one of similar efficacy, should be described. The duration of antiemetic therapy will depend on the expected time course for the development of nausea and vomiting. Patients who previously experienced unsuccessful antiemetic therapy should have their previous regimen examined and optimized. If "optimal" antiemetic therapy was previously given and yet was unsuccessful, these patients should be considered for enrollment into clinical trials exploring new antiemetic treatments. Patients with refractory nausea and vomiting may benefit from heavy sedation and close inpatient monitoring during subsequent courses of chemotherapy.

ANTIEMETIC THERAPY FOR SPECIFIC ANTICANCER TREATMENTS **Cisplatin, first 24 h** Cisplatin is one of the most emetogenic antineoplastic drugs. Almost all patients receiving cisplatin will experience nausea and vomiting if no antiemetic protection is provided. However, metoclopramide plus dexamethasone regimens have been particularly effective. Major protection (fewer than two vomiting episodes) from cisplatin-induced nausea and vomiting occurs in 50 to 75 percent of the patients, but complete prevention rates are usually considerably lower.

Most commonly, metoclopramide, 2 mg/kg, is given intravenously every 2 h for four or five doses beginning 30 min prior to cisplatin administration. Dexamethasone, 10 to 20 mg intravenously, is also given 30 min before cisplatin and in many centers repeated with each metoclopramide dose. Alternatively, metoclopramide, 3 mg/kg, is given intravenously 30 min before and 1.5 h after cisplatin (with dexamethasone as above); this approach is as effective in a 2 mg/kg regimen and more suitable as an outpatient antiemetic regimen.

Delayed nausea and vomiting after cisplatin Delayed nausea and vomiting occurs frequently in patients who receive moderate- to high-dose cisplatin-containing chemotherapy; it is most common in patients whose nausea and vomiting is not prevented during the first 24 h after cisplatin administration. Oral doses of prochlorperazine, three times daily, 10 to 20 mg, or metoclopramide, 30 to 40 mg, used in combination with dexamethasone, 8 mg, have proved successful in this setting.

Cyclophosphamide and/or doxorubicin Cyclophosphamide (500 to 1000 mg/m^2) and doxorubicin (40 to 60 mg/m^2) chemotherapy regimens frequently cause nausea and vomiting that may not begin until several hours after the drugs have been administered. Aggressive metoclopramide plus glucocorticoid antiemetic regimens are often effective. Because the onset of nausea and vomiting is delayed for several hours after cyclophosphamide administration, an extended antiemetic regimen is desirable.

Dacarbazine Dacarbazine is a highly emetogenic agent. Metoclopramide alone or combined with a dexamethasone will prevent nausea and vomiting in approximately half of these patients.

High-dose cytarabine Metoclopramide antiemetic therapy is also effective in patients receiving high-dose cytarabine. Complete prevention of nausea and vomiting, after the first dose of cytarabine, may be obtained in 50 percent of patients.

ANTIEMETIC THERAPY BY INTRAVENOUS INFUSION The administration of antiemetics by a prolonged intravenous infusion is often an effective approach to the prevention of chemotherapy-induced nausea and vomiting. If a specific antiemetic drug plasma concentration is desired, continuous drug infusion is an optimal way to activate and maintain such concentrations. Moreover, because in any given patient the time at which nausea and vomiting occurs after administration of an antineoplastic drug may vary, intermittent bolus administration of antiemetic substances may not effectively control nausea and vomiting by failing to maintain the necessary plasma concentration of drug. In the case of metoclopramide prolonged therapy has been shown to be as effective as intermittent bolus administration, at the same time saving the nursing and pharmacy staff time and money.

Glucocorticoids as antiemetics The relative lack of short-term side effects caused by dexamethasone and methylprednisolone make them ideal antiemetics, especially for outpatients and for those receiving less emetogenic drugs, such as doxorubicin. Unfortunately, glucocorticoid antiemetic treatment alone is not optimal for patients receiving highly emetogenic drugs.

Benzodiazepines as adjuncts to antiemetic therapy The benzodiazepines have little, if any, antiemetic value by themselves. Their major effects are sedative, hypnotic, skeletal muscle relaxant, and amnesic; all of these may be desirable in some patients receiving emetogenic chemotherapy. Lorazepam is widely used as an adjunctive agent with metoclopramide-dexamethasone regimens; it lessens the anxiety associated with chemotherapy administration.

STOMATITIS AND MUCOSITIS Stomatitis is an inflammatory response of the oral mucosa and intraoral soft tissue structures that is not an uncommon response following the administration of cytotoxic drugs. Although there is much variability between individual patients, stomatitis is a complication of chemotherapy that is both drug- and dose-related. Almost all the anticancer drugs will cause stomatitis if a large enough dose is given. Patients undergoing induction chemotherapy for treatment of acute leukemia or as a preparative regimen before bone marrow transplantation are most likely to develop stomatitis. Some drugs, such as fluorouracil, cause stomatitis much more frequently than others. Stomatitis caused by methotrexate has been shown to be more a function of the duration of treatment rather than of peak drug plasma levels. The same is probably true for most, if not all, antitumor antimetabolites.

Early signs of stomatitis include mild erythema and edema of the buccal mucosa and/or tongue. This generalized inflammation may progress to painful ulcerations and secondary infections. Mouth sores usually occur 7 to 14 days after a dose of chemotherapy and take at least 7 days to heal after chemotherapy is discontinued. Stomatitis may lead to complications such as malnutrition (i.e., it may be too painful to eat), dehydration (i.e., pain on swallowing may prevent all oral intake), bleeding may be a sign of problems (such as thrombocytopenia), infection, and refusal of interruption of therapy.

The treatment of stomatitis includes good oral hygiene and providing pain relief. Topical anesthetics (e.g., viscous xylocaine) or mixtures containing a topical anesthetic may be needed, especially if the stomatitis interferes with eating. However, reducing subsequent doses of anticancer drugs may be necessary in patients with moderate to severe stomatitis.

ALOPECIA Antineoplastic drugs used singly or in combination often cause significant hair loss from the scalp. Although hair loss may seem relatively trivial compared to other side effects, it is often the most psychologically distressing complication of cancer chemotherapy. The hair loss produced by antineoplastic drugs is patchy and not similar to natural balding or thinning. It occurs over a few days, becoming maximal approximately 2 to 3 weeks after chemotherapy. The loss of hair is drug- and dose-dependent. The anthracyclines (doxorubicin and daunorubicin), cyclophosphamide, and vincristine commonly cause alopecia; but other drugs can also cause alopecia by themselves or in combination.

Scalp cooling undertaken for 30 to 60 min during and after treatment, can reduce hair loss. It is believed that when it works, it is due to decreased uptake of drugs by hair follicles.

REPRODUCTIVE EFFECTS Menstrual cycle changes (i.e., irregular periods, cessation of menses) in women and azoospermia in men, with elevation of serum follicle stimulating hormone (FSH), are relatively common side effects of chemotherapy. They occur more frequently with alkylating agents and patients receiving very intensive therapy. Men with Hodgkin's disease receiving 12 or more months of MOPP (mechlorethamine, oncovin, procarbazine, and prednisone) can all expect to become azoospermic. Sperm counts generally do not fully recover until 2 to 5 years after treatment has been discontinued. Ovarian dysfunction in women varies and appears to be related to age at the start of treatment, the specific drugs given, drug dose, and concomitant radiation therapy administered below the diaphragm. Almost all women with ovarian cancer receiving alkylating agents experience disruption of the menstrual cycle with a return to normal following completion of therapy.

In a retrospective study of over 2000 children who had received cancer chemotherapy during childhood or adolescence compared to a matched control group, fertility was not altered in the female group but was markedly decreased in males. Boys who received alkylating agents with or without radiation therapy below the diaphragm had a 60 percent decrease in fertility. This effect was greater if treatment was given after their fifteenth birthday than if given before.

Premenopausal women receiving adjuvant CMF (cyclophosphamide, methotrexate, fluorouracil) chemotherapy for breast cancer develop ovarian dysfunction that correlates with increasing age and duration of treatment. Nearly all women over 40 develop ovarian dysfunction after 4 to 6 months of treatment. Younger women may not have menstrual irregularities despite longer chemotherapy.

In men with testicular cancer, low sperm counts and/or abnormal sperm motility are often present before orchiectomy and may be accompanied by elevated levels of gonadotropins. Following aggressive cisplatin-etoposide (or vinblastine)-bleomycin chemotherapy, further impairment of spermatogenesis occurs, but is usually temporary. Full recovery of spermatogenesis is less likely in patients over age 30 receiving intensive chemotherapy and radiotherapy below the diaphragm.

REFERENCES

CUBEDDU LX et al: Efficacy of ondansetron (GR38032F) and the role of serotonin in cisplatin-induced nausea and vomiting. N Engl J Med 322:810, 1990

DEVITA VT JR: Principles of Chemotherapy, in *Cancer: Principles & Practice of Oncology*, 3d ed, VT DeVita Jr, S Hellman, SA Rosenberg (eds). Philadelphia, Lippincott, 1989, pp 276–300

DILLMAN RO: Monoclonal antibodies for treating cancer. Ann Intern Med 111:592, 1989

GOLDSTEIN LJ et al: Expression of a multidrug resistance gene in human cancers. J Natl Cancer Inst 81:116, 1989

GRECO FA, HAINSWORTH JD: The management of patients with adenocarcinoma and poorly differentiated carcinoma of unknown primary site. Semin Oncol 16:116, 1989

MUGGIA FM, NORRIS JR K: Future of cancer chemotherapy with cisplatin. Semin Oncol 16:123, 1989

302 THE MALIGNANT LYMPHOMAS

LEE M. NADLER

The malignant lymphomas, in contrast to leukemias, are neoplastic transformations of cells that reside predominantly in lymphoid tissues. The two major variants of malignant lymphoma are non-Hodgkin's lymphoma and Hodgkin's disease. Although both of these tumors infiltrate reticuloendothelial organs, their biologic and clinical behaviors suggest that they are probably not related. Table 302-1 compares non-Hodgkin's and Hodgkin's lymphomas with regard to cellular derivation, sites of disease, presence of systemic symptomatology, chromosomal translocations, and curability. This comparison supports the notion that they are fundamentally different diseases.

TABLE 302-1 The malignant lymphomas

	Non-Hodgkin's	Hodgkin's
Cellular derivation	90% B Cell 10% T Cell Rare monocytic	Unresolved
Sites of disease		
Localized	Uncommon	Common
Nodal spread	Discontiguous	Contiguous
Extranodal	Common	Uncommon
Mediastinal	Uncommon	Common
Abdominal	Common	Uncommon
Bone marrow	Common	Uncommon
B systemic symptoms*	Uncommon	Common
Chromosomal translocation	Common	Yet to be described
Curability	<25%	>75%

* Fever, night sweats, weight loss of greater than 10% of body weight.

CELLULAR AND DEVELOPMENTAL ASPECTS

To date, biologic studies have provided no clearcut explanations for the differences demonstrated in Table 302-1. It is important to examine the cellular origins of these tumors in an attempt to relate the neoplastic cell to its normal cellular counterpart. By understanding the lineage and corresponding normal stage of differentiation, it should be eventually possible to further group these tumors biologically according to cellular origin, ability to localize within specific microenvironments, propensity to further differentiate in vivo, production of cytokines, and response to therapy.

Non-Hodgkin's and Hodgkin's can be morphologically classified as shown in Tables 302-2 and 302-7. In order to understand the lineage derivation of these histologically defined subtypes, it is necessary to examine the normal populations of cells that reside in lymphoid tissues. To this end, B- and T-cell ontogeny will be reviewed and within this context the neoplastic lymphoma cell related to its normal cellular counterpart. Although histologic subtype is still the major basis for therapeutic decisions, the definition of immunologic phenotype is becoming more useful for classifying difficult cases.

Lymphocytes can be functionally subdivided into distinct populations by their expression of unique cell surface and molecular markers. In the past, human B cells were identified by their expression of cell surface or cytoplasmic immunoglobulin and their capacity to produce immunoglobulin. In contrast, human T lymphocytes were classically defined by the expression of sheep red blood cell receptors and their ability to regulate immune responses. During the past decade, the development of well-characterized monoclonal antibodies (MAbs) directed against T-cell surface molecules expressed on human lymphoid cells has led to very significant advances in both the phenotypic and functional characterization of these cells. MAbs have been useful in assigning cellular lineage and identifying normal stages of lymphoid differentiation. Similarly, molecular biologic techniques demonstrating gene rearrangements have been helpful in defining lineage, clonality, and, to a lesser extent, stage of differentiation.

NORMAL B-CELL ONTOGENY **Cell surface antigens** Normal B-cell ontogeny has been operationally divided into stages, namely pre-B cell, mature or resting B cell, activated/proliferating B cell, differentiating B cell, and plasma cell or secretory B cell (Fig. 302-1). These stages are delineated by the expression of unique cytoplasmic and cell surface antigens. Antigens can be clustered into pre-B, resting-B, activated-B, and plasma-cell subgroups. In addition, there are pan-B antigens. Several antigens have been useful in defining B-cell lineage since within the hematopoietic system they are uniquely expressed on B lymphocytes. Two of the most useful antigens are CD19 and CD20. Both are strongly expressed on the cell surface and, more importantly, their expression spans ontogeny from the early pre-B cells to the terminal stages of differentiation.

The most primitive pre-B cells have been defined by their coexpression of cell surface antigens, including Ia (of the major histocompatibility complex class II), CD19, and CD24. Stages of pre-B-cell ontogeny have been delineated by the sequential expression of CD10 (common acute lymphoblastic leukemia antigen, CALLA), CD20, and finally the appearance of cytoplasmic immunoglobulin mu (cμ) heavy chains without the expression of light chains. As pre-B cells mature, they are exported to the peripheral blood and lymphoid tissues where they reside until activated by antigen (mature B cell; Fig. 302-1).

Mature resting B cells continue to express cell surface Ia, CD antigens 19, 20, and 24, but no longer CD10. These cells also express cell surface immunoglobulins IgM and IgD (the B-cell antigen receptor); CD21, which is the receptor for the C3d cleavage fragment of complement and for Epstein-Barr virus (EBV); CD35, which is the C3b complement receptor; and CD22.

Following triggering by antigen or other signals of activation, mature resting B cells are activated and subsequently proliferate. In vitro, in vivo, and in situ studies show that the activation of resting B cells is accompanied by a sequence of cell surface antigenic changes. Resting B cells begin to lose cell surface IgD, CD21, and CD22. As these antigens are lost, a number of other antigens appear sequentially. These *activation antigens* are cell surface molecules involved in the regulation of cellular proliferation and/or differentiation or alternatively in the localization and binding of activated B cells. Activation antigens can be divided into those that are B-cell associated and those that are B-cell restricted. In the first group are CD71 (transferrin receptor), CD54 (ICAM-1, involved in homotypic aggregation), CD25 (low-affinity IL-2 receptor), CD5, and CD23 (low-affinity IgE receptor). Those that are B-cell restricted include B5, BB-1/B7, and Bac-1.

During differentiation there is a sequential loss of the B-cell activation antigens as well as pan-B-cell antigens, including Ia, CD19, -20, and -24. This stage is also characterized by the appearance of CD38 and PCA-1, which are expressed on plasma cells (secretory B cell).

Immunoglobulin gene rearrangements A vast variety and number of possible immunoglobulin molecules exist, each corresponding to a unique antigenic epitope. This diversity is thought to result from genetic recombination within the DNA of B lymphocytes. The germline DNA contains segments coding for different subunits of the immunoglobulin molecule. For the immunoglobulin heavy chain, these consist of a very large number of different variable (V) segments, a smaller number of different diversity (D) segments, a few joining (J) segments, and a constant region for each subclass of immunoglobulin.

The usual mechanism for achieving recombination of the immunoglobulin heavy chain genes involves joining together single V, D, and J segments with the appropriate constant region segment and excising the unused segments. Therefore, the numbers of potential recombinants of V, D, and J segments are enormous. Light chain

TABLE 302-2 Histologic classification of non-Hodgkin's lymphoma

Working formulation, malignant lymphoma	Rappaport terminology	Cellular origin, % B	Cellular origin, % T	Chromosomal abnormalities
Low-grade				
A Small lymphocytic cell	Diffuse well-differentiated lymphocytic (DWDL)	98	2	Trisomy 12 t(11;14) t(14;19)
B Follicular, predominantly small cleaved cell	Nodular poorly differentiated lymphocytic (NPDL)	100		t(14;18)
C Follicular mixed, small cleaved and large cell	Nodular mixed lymphocytic histiocytic (NM)	100		t(14;18) Trisomy 8
Intermediate-grade				
D Follicular, predominantly large cell	Nodular histiocytic (NH)	100		Trisomy 7
E Diffuse small cleaved cell	Diffuse poorly differentiated lymphocytic (DPDL)	80	20	
F Diffuse mixed, small and large cell	Diffuse mixed lymphocytic-histiocytic (DM)	90	10	Trisomy 3
G Diffuse large cell	Diffuse histiocytic (DH)	80	20	Trisomy 7,18 t(14;18)
High-grade				
H Large cell immunoblastic	Diffuse histiocytic (DH)	80	20	
I Lymphoblastic	Diffuse lymphoblastic (LL)	10	90	
J Small noncleaved cell; Burkitt's	Diffuse undifferentiated (DUL)	95	5	t(8;14)

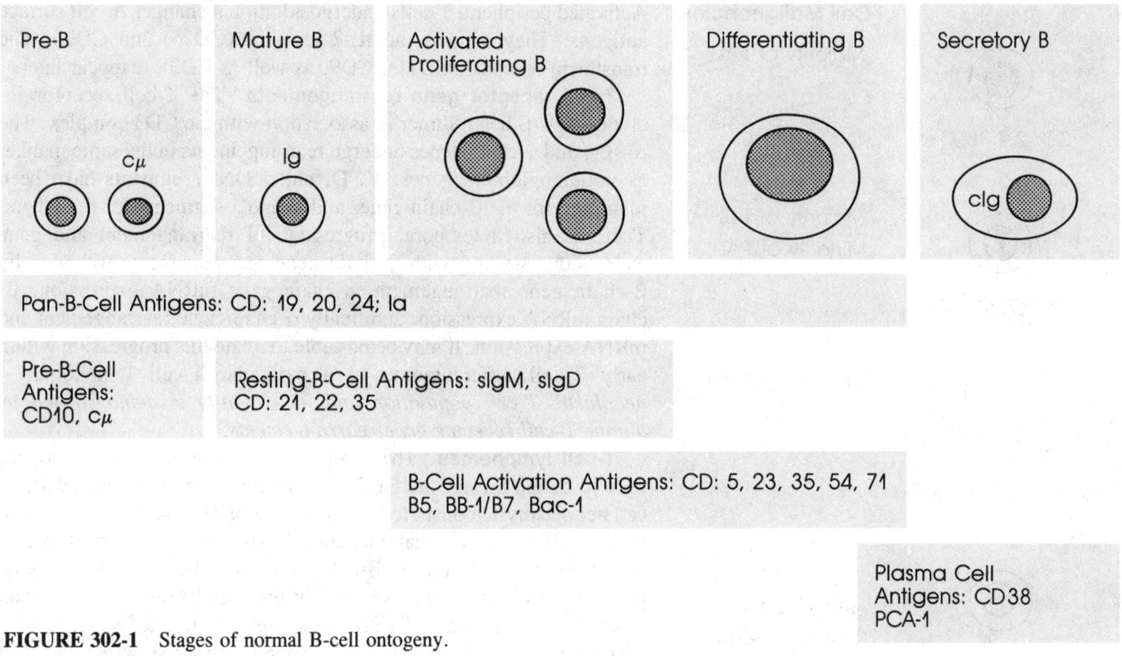

FIGURE 302-1 Stages of normal B-cell ontogeny.

genes lack D segments but have a similar mechanism of rearrangement. A functional rearrangement of a heavy or light chain gene prevents rearrangements of another gene of the same chain type (allelic exclusion); however, an abnormal heavy or light chain rearrangement that cannot be transcribed will allow the other heavy chain allele or one of the other light chain alleles, respectively, to attempt rearrangement. This functional allelic exclusion insures that only one immunoglobulin is allowed for any one B cell. The heavy chain gene undergoes rearrangement first, followed by the kappa and then the lambda light chain genes. Clonal rearrangement of immunoglobulin genes is consistent with a B-cell lineage derivation of a lymphoma.

MALIGNANT LYMPHOMAS OF B-CELL ORIGIN As seen in Table 302-2, more than 90 percent of all cases of non-Hodgkin's lymphomas are of B cell derivation. This observation is based upon the expression of B-lineage–restricted antigens as well as clonal rearrangements of immunoglobulin heavy and light chain genes. Non-T-cell acute lymphoblastic leukemias antigenically correspond to discrete stages of pre-B-cell development. It is noteworthy that no B-cell neoplasm phenotypically corresponds to the resting B lymphocyte (mature B). Myelomas correspond to secretory B cells. Although most investigators have attempted to relate B-cell lymphomas to major steps of B-lymphocyte development (Fig. 302-1), it is becoming increasingly clear that these tumors correspond to major and minor subpopulations of activated/proliferating or differentiating B cells. All B-cell non-Hodgkin's lymphomas express the pan-B-cell antigens including Ia, CD19, and CD20. Moreover, virtually all B-cell non-Hodgkin's lymphomas express one or more B-cell activation antigens. Although a common antigenic phenotype has been identified for each histologically defined subgroup, it should be stressed that significant antigenic heterogeneity exists within each subgroup. As indicated below, cell surface antigenic phenotype is considered within the context of the Working Formulation (Table 302-2). (MAbs commonly used in diagnosis of B-cell lymphomas are summarized in Table 302-3.)

TABLE 302-3 MAbs commonly used in diagnosis of B-cell lymphomas

CD	Common antibody terminology
5	Anti-T1, Leu 1, T101
10	J5, anti-CALLA, BA3
19	Anti-B4, anti-Leu 12
20	Anti-B1, anti-Leu 16, 1F5
21	Anti-B2
22	Anti-HD39 (anti-B3), SHCL-1
23	Anti-Blast-2 (anti-B5), MNM6
24	BA-1, J2
25	Anti-TAC, anti-IL-2R
38	Anti-T10
54	I-CAM-1
71	Anti-T9

Low-grade lymphoma The commonest low-grade lymphomas are the small lymphocytic and follicular small cleaved cell lymphomas. Small lymphocytic lymphomas, like B-cell chronic lymphocytic leukemias, appear to correspond to a unique population of activated B cells that express pan-B-cell antigens as well as CD21, B5, and CD5. In contrast, follicular small cleaved cell lymphomas are thought to correspond to subpopulations of germinal center B cells. These lymphomas express pan-B-cell antigens and CD21, B5, and CD10. When small lymphocytic lymphomas or follicular small cleaved cell lymphomas "transform" and morphologically resemble diffuse large cell lymphoma cells, they retain their CD5 and CD10 positivity, respectively.

Intermediate-grade lymphoma Within the intermediate-grade subgroup of B-cell lymphomas (Table 302-2), follicular large cell, diffuse large cell, and diffuse small cleaved cell lymphomas are immunologically distinct. Both subgroups of large cell lymphoma express pan-B-cell antigens and several B-cell activation antigens but less frequently express cell surface immunoglobulin or CD21. Follicular large cell, like follicular small cleaved cell lymphomas, express CD10, whereas B-cell diffuse large cell lymphomas are CD10 and CD5 negative. Diffuse small cleaved B-cell lymphomas morphologically and phenotypically resemble follicular small cleaved cell lymphomas. They both express pan-B-cell antigens and several of the B-cell activation antigens. Whereas follicular small cleaved cell lymphomas express CD10 and frequently demonstrate 14;18 translocations (see below), diffuse small cleaved cell lymphomas do not. A subgroup of diffuse small cleaved cell lymphomas, termed *mantle zone lymphomas,* are phenotypically identical to diffuse small cleaved cell lymphomas but also express CD5.

High-grade lymphoma Large cell immunoblastic lymphomas are phenotypically identical to B-cell diffuse large cell lymphomas. In contrast, Burkitt's lymphomas are related to follicular lymphomas in that they express pan-B-cell antigens, B-cell activation antigens, and CD10. African Burkitt's cells express CD21 whereas the American variation does not.

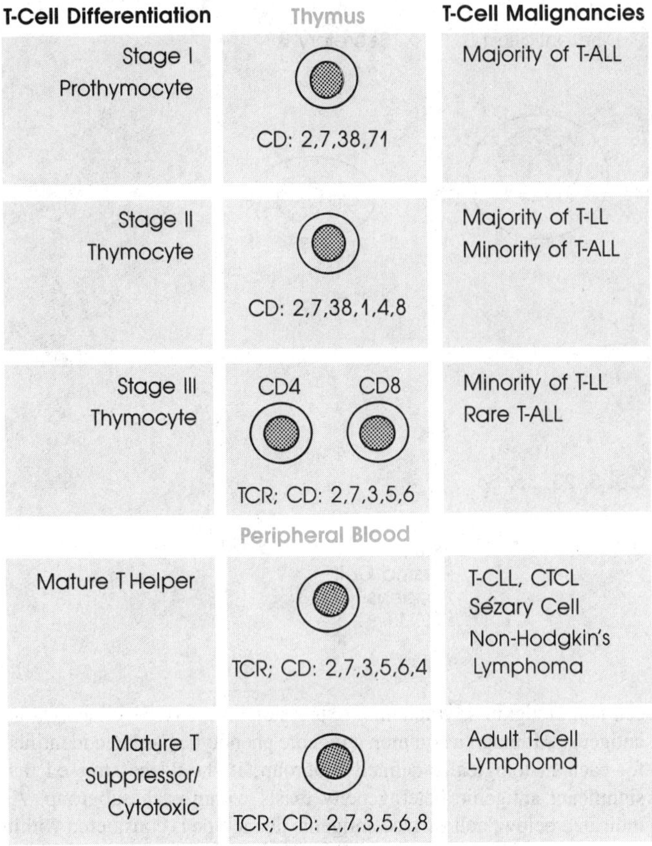

FIGURE 302-2 Correlation of T-cell differentiation and T-cell malignancies.

NORMAL T-CELL ONTOGENY **Cell surface antigens** A large number of MAbs have been developed that define cell surface antigens expressed on human T cells. These MAbs have been used to characterize the stages of T-cell ontogeny and differentiation, identify subsets of functionally distinct T cells, and elucidate the function of some of these cell surface antigens. Figure 302-2 summarizes the stages of normal T-cell ontogeny.

During embryonic and early postnatal development, bone marrow precursor cells migrate to the thymus. The thymic microenvironment provides a setting for the processing and eventual development of functionally competent T cells. These cells are subsequently exported into peripheral lymphoid tissues and the circulation. A sequence of changes in cell surface antigens identified by MAbs is observed to accompany intrathymic differentiation. The cells in the earliest stage (I) of intrathymic differentiation, which constitute 10 percent of the thymic lymphocytes, express CD2 (E-rosette receptor), CD71 (the transferrin receptor), CD38, and CD7.

Stage II thymocytes are characterized by the loss of CD71, the acquisition of CD1, and coexpression of CD4 and CD8. The population, coexpressing CD antigens 1, 2, 4, 7, 8, and 38, constitutes 70 percent of thymocytes.

With further maturation, cells lose CD1 and acquire mature T-cell antigens CD3, -5, and -6 (stage III). CD3 is a complex of chains that are noncovalently associated with the T-cell antigen receptor (TCR). In parallel with the expression of CD3, cells express TCR. It can exist as an α/β heterodimer and then recognizes antigen in the context of the major histocompatibility complex. A second T-cell receptor, also associated with CD3, is termed γ/δ. Cells that express the γ/δ TCR appear earlier in ontogeny than those expressing α/β. They are negative for CD4 and CD8 and are associated with natural killer cell (NK) activity.

When cells leave the thymus, they no longer express CD38 and are segregated into cells expressing either CD4 or CD8, constituting 60 to 70 percent and 30 to 40 percent of peripheral T cells, respectively. Activated peripheral T cells undergo additional changes in cell surface antigens. They express the IL-2 receptor (CD25) and CD26. The transferrin receptor (CD71), CD9, as well as CD38 reappear later.

T-cell receptor gene rearrangements The T-cell receptor includes an α/β heterodimer in association with the CD3 complex. The α-, β-, and γ-chain genes undergo rearrangements in the same manner as immunoglobulin genes. V, D, and J DNA segments have been identified for the β-chain gene, and V and J segments for the others. There is also a temporal progression of rearrangement and gene expression, starting with γ-chain gene rearrangement, followed by β-chain gene rearrangement, γ-chain gene mRNA expression, β-chain mRNA expression, and finally α-chain gene rearrangement and mRNA expression. It may be possible to relate this progression within early T-cell differentiation to a particular T-cell lymphoma. *A neoplastic T-cell population and its clonality is demonstrated by unique T-cell receptor gene rearrangements.*

T-cell lymphomas The most widely expressed T-cell antigens used to define lineage are CD2 and CD7. Moreover, as indicated, T-cell neoplasms demonstrate rearrangement of TCR genes. As depicted in Fig. 302-2, T-cell malignancies clearly reflect distinct stages of T-cell ontogeny. Similar to B-cell neoplasms, the common antigenic phenotype for T-cell neoplasms will be presented; however, significant heterogeneity is observed within histologically defined subgroups.

Lymphoblastic lymphomas correspond to stage II thymocytes and the majority express CD1, -2, -4, -7, and -8. The remainder of the T-cell lymphomas correspond to mature T-cell populations (mature helper cells or mature cytotoxic/suppressor T cells). Although these tumors express the phenotype of mature functional T cells, few neoplasms retain function in vivo. Diffuse small cleaved cell and diffuse large cell lymphomas variably express the mature T-cell antigens CD2, -3, -5, -6, and -7. Most express CD4; a small fraction express CD8. Cutaneous T-cell lymphomas also express a mature phenotype: CD2, -3, -4, -5, and -7. Sézary cells generally lack CD7 and Ia antigens, whereas cells infiltrating the skin are CD7 positive and invariably express CD25 and CD71. Adult T-cell lymphomas are similar to the cutaneous T-cell lymphomas in that they express CD2, -3, -4, -5, and -7.

CELLULAR ORIGIN OF THE REED-STERNBERG CELL Reed-Sternberg (RS) cells, in the appropriate cytoarchitectural milieu, are required for the diagnosis of Hodgkin's disease. The major obstacle to determining the cellular origin of Hodgkin's disease is the present inability to identify and isolate RS cells. Studies either have examined enriched populations of these cells or have examined them using immunologic staining techniques in tissue sections. As discussed below, evidence exists for both lymphoid and nonlymphoid origin. Unfortunately, these studies have been complicated by the contaminating effect of normal populations mixed with RS cells.

In Hodgkin's disease tissues the majority of cells are small lymphocytes with a "normal" T-cell phenotype (CD2, -3, -4 or -8, and -5) together with a variable number of presumably nonneoplastic B cells. Reed-Sternberg cells and their variants may be immunologically distinguished from the neoplastic cells of most non-Hodgkin's lymphomas by their lack of most T- and B-cell–associated antigens. Reed-Sternberg cells may contain intracellular immunoglobulin but this is polyclonal and is not thought to be produced by the RS cell. These cells express CD25 (low affinity IL-2 receptor) and the transferrin receptor (CD71), which are also expressed on activated B, activated T, and activated NK cells. They also express Ia antigens, certain antigens expressed on myeloid cells (e.g., CD13), receptors for peanut lectin, and the epithelial membrane antigen. Of great interest is the observation that RS cells of the lymphocyte-predominant form express the leukocyte common antigen (CD45R) whereas all other RS cells are negative.

Two unique antigens are expressed on the RS cell, and therefore MAbs directed against these antigens have proven to be diagnostically useful. The first is the Leu M1 antigen, which is expressed on RS cells in all subtypes of Hodgkin's disease except for the lymphocyte-predominant variant. The second antigen is the Ki-1 (CD30) antigen, which is expressed on virtually all RS cells. The Ki-1 antigen also is expressed on some activated B cells, activated T cells, EBV-transformed cell lines, and tumor cells isolated from some patients with immunoblastic lymphomas. Of great interest is the expression of CD30 on dendritic cells. Although these antigens are useful in the diagnosis of Hodgkin's disease, they have not been helpful in defining cellular lineage.

Recent molecular studies of RS-enriched populations have demonstrated immunoglobulin gene rearrangements in some specimens and T-cell β-chain rearrangements in others. Clonal rearrangements have not been seen in background lymphocytes. Although rearrangements of the T-cell γ-chain genes have been observed, they should not be misconstrued as evidence for a clonal T-cell origin since this gene may not provide evidence for clonality.

The lineage derivation of the RS cell is still unknown. Reed-Sternberg cells are not only observed in Hodgkin's disease but may be seen in small numbers in several variants of non-Hodgkin's lymphomas. Experts in the field believe that Hodgkin's disease is derived from subpopulations of activated B cells, activated T cells, or dendritic cells. The lack of expression of B- and T-lineage–restricted markers and lack of expression of the leukocyte common antigen suggest that they do not correspond to a known stage of B- or T-cell ontogeny. It is impossible to rigorously compare Hodgkin's to dendritic cells (either interdigitating or follicular) since these cells are also poorly characterized. Therefore, these studies support the notion that Hodgkin's and non-Hodgkin's lymphomas are derived from distinct cellular populations. Moreover, their distinct biologic and clinical behaviors (Table 302-1) are most probably a reflection of their divergent cellular origins.

NON-HODGKIN'S LYMPHOMA

EPIDEMIOLOGY About 30,000 new cases of non-Hodgkin's lymphoma occur each year in the United States and this number appears to be rising. Although the total number of patients is relatively small compared to some of the more common solid tumors, the malignant lymphomas are the commonest neoplasm of patients between the ages of 20 and 40. Moreover, they rank fourth in the total number of person-years of life lost each year from cancer. With the increasing incidence of acquired immunodeficiency syndrome (AIDS), the number of cases of non-Hodgkin's lymphoma has begun to increase sharply.

ETIOLOGY Animal studies suggest that lymphomas have a viral etiology. A herpesvirus has been isolated in avians, and C-type retroviruses have been identified in rodents, cows, and subhuman primates with lymphocytic lymphomas. In contrast, only endemic African Burkitt's lymphoma and adult T-cell lymphoma have been shown to have a viral etiology in humans. Thus, EBV has a strong association with the development of Burkitt's lymphoma, and the human T-cell leukemia virus appears to be the causative agent in adult T-cell lymphoma.

Although limited progress has been made in identifying agents that might be involved in inducing non-Hodgkin's lymphomas, exciting advances have been made in identifying those genes that appear to be involved in lymphomatous transformation. Cytogenetic abnormalities have been well documented in a number of non-Hodgkin's lymphomas (Table 302-2). DNA sequence analysis of several of these chromosomal translocations has demonstrated that genes that normally regulate heavy and light chain immunoglobulin synthesis have been juxtaposed to genes that regulate normal cellular activation and proliferation. It is postulated that these transforming genes or *oncogenes* have come under the control of those regulatory elements that normally control B-cell proliferation and differentiation. The best-studied example is the 14;8 translocation of Burkitt's lymphoma (see Chap. 7). In this disease, the c-*myc* oncogene on chromosome 8 is joined to the immunoglobulin heavy chain locus on chromosome 14. Another example is the 14;18 translocation commonly seen in follicular lymphomas where the oncogene termed *bcl*-2 (chromosome 18) is juxtaposed to the immunoglobulin heavy chain locus (chromosome 14). Table 302-2 summarizes the major chromosomal translocations associated with histologic subtypes of non-Hodgkin's lymphomas (see also Chap. 10).

TABLE 302-4 Diseases or exposures associated with increased risk of development of malignant lymphoma

Inherited immunodeficiency diseases
Klinefelter's syndrome
Chédiak-Higashi syndrome
Ataxia telangiectasia syndrome
Wiscott-Aldrich syndrome
Common variable immunodeficiency disease
Acquired immunodeficiency diseases
Iatrogenic immunosuppression
Acquired immunodeficiency syndrome
Acquired hypogammaglobulinemia
Autoimmune diseases
Sjögren's syndrome
Nontropical sprue
Rheumatoid arthritis and systemic lupus erythematosus
Chemical or drug exposures
Phenytoin
Radiation
Prior combination chemotherapy and radiation therapy
Viral association (other than HIV)
Epstein-Barr virus
Human T-cell leukemia virus

In a number of primary diseases, increasingly often there is subsequent development of non-Hodgkin's lymphoma and, to a lesser extent, Hodgkin's disease. As seen in Table 302-4, diseases of inherited and acquired immunodeficiency as well as autoimmune diseases are associated with an increased incidence of lymphoma. Non-Hodgkin's lymphomas that occur in the context of drug-induced immunosuppression, acquired or congenital immunodeficiency, and AIDS are frequently associated with EBV. The association between immunosuppression and induction of non-Hodgkin's lymphomas appears to be compelling since, if the immunosuppression can be reversed (e.g., discontinuing immunosuppressive agents following organ transplantation), a percentage of these lymphomas regress spontaneously. The incidence of lymphoma in iatrogenic immunosuppression, AIDS, and autoimmune disease argues strongly for immune dysregulation contributing to the development of lymphoma. Patients with certain environmental exposures have a higher incidence of lymphomas. Patients with Hodgkin's disease treated with radiation therapy and chemotherapy exhibit an increased risk of developing secondary large cell lymphomas. Lymphoma-like syndromes have also been found in patients treated with phenytoin. Although in most cases this disease regresses when the drug is stopped, a significant number of patients still develop true malignant lymphoma.

CLINICAL PRESENTATION AND DIFFERENTIAL DIAGNOSIS More than two-thirds of patients with non-Hodgkin's lymphoma present with persistent painless peripheral lymphadenopathy. At the time of presentation, differential diagnosis includes infections caused by bacteria, viruses (e.g., infectious mononucleosis, cytomegalovirus, and human immunodeficiency virus), and parasites (toxoplasmosis). In young patients, Hodgkin's lymphoma must be excluded. In older patients, other neoplasms must be considered. It is generally agreed that a firm spherical lymph node larger than 1 cm that is not associated with a documentable infection and that persists longer than 4 to 6 weeks should be biopsied. Certain clinical features suggest the diagnosis of non-Hodgkin's lymphoma. Involvement of Waldeyer's ring, epitrochlear, and mesenteric nodes are more suggestive of non-Hodgkin's lymphoma than Hodgkin's. Unlike patients with Hodgkin's disease, who can present with weight loss, fever, or night sweats (so-called B symptoms), it is less common for patients with non-Hodgkin's lymphoma to present with systemic complaints.

Non-Hodgkin's lymphoma patients also present with chest, abdominal, or extranodal symptomatology. Although much less commonly than with Hodgkin's disease, approximately 20 percent of patients with non-Hodgkin's lymphoma have mediastinal adenopathy. These patients most frequently present with persistent cough, chest discomfort, or without symptoms but having an abnormal chest x-ray. Occasionally a superior vena cava syndrome accompanies presentation, especially in patients with T-cell lymphomas and, to a lesser extent, in those with B-cell diffuse large cell lymphoma. Differential diagnosis includes infections (e.g., histoplasmosis, tuberculosis, or infectious mononucleosis), sarcoidosis, Hodgkin's disease, as well as other neoplasms. Involvement of retroperitoneal, mesenteric, and pelvic nodes is common in most histologic subtypes of non-Hodgkin's lymphoma. Unless massive or leading to obstruction, these nodes usually produce no symptoms. In contrast, patients who come to medical attention because of an abdominal mass, massive splenomegaly, or primary gastrointestinal lymphoma present with complaints similar to those caused by other abdominal space-occupying lesions. These complaints include chronic pain, abdominal fullness, early satiety, symptoms associated with visceral obstruction, or even acute perforation and gastrointestinal hemorrhage. Symptoms due to extralymphatic disease are common in some subtypes of diffuse non-Hodgkin's lymphoma but are uncommon in follicular lymphomas. Rarely, some patients present with symptoms of unexplained anemia. Those with diffuse non-Hodgkin's lymphomas can present with primary cutaneous lesions, testicular masses, acute spinal cord compression, solitary bone lesions, and rarely lymphomatous meningitis. Historically, primary non-Hodgkin's lymphoma of the central nervous system was a very rare form of diffuse non-Hodgkin's lymphoma. However with AIDS and the increasing use of high dose immunosuppressive therapy, lymphoma may soon be one of the most common types of primary brain tumors.

PATHOLOGIC CLASSIFICATION Rappaport and Working Formulation classification schemes The pathologic classification of non-Hodgkin's lymphomas has been difficult for both pathologists and clinicians. In 1966, Henry Rappaport presented the first clinically relevant classification scheme for non-Hodgkin's lymphomas. This classification was based on assessment of the overall pattern of lymph node architecture (low-power microscopy) as well as the cytology of the neoplastic cell (high-power microscopy). The Rappaport classification subdivides the non-Hodgkin's lymphomas into two major subtypes, namely *diffuse* and *nodular* (follicular). Nodular lymphomas retain some features of normal lymph nodes in that the neoplastic cells appear to form "germinal centers" (nodules). In contrast, in diffuse lymphomas, the normal cortical and paracortical lymph node architecture is largely effaced. Rappaport also divided non-Hodgkin's lymphomas into subgroups according to whether the malignant cell was (1) well differentiated, (2) poorly differentiated, or (3) histiocytic. This suggested that these tumors corresponded morphologically to distinct stages of lymphoid and monocytic differentiation. The importance of the Rappaport classification (Table 302-2) was that each histologically defined subtype of non-Hodgkin's lymphoma exhibited a unique natural history and response to therapy.

With the advent of modern immunology, the Rappaport classification proved to have several biologic defects. First, the term *histiocytic* was incorrect since virtually all of these tumors were of lymphoid origin. Second, certain clinical entities were not accounted for by the scheme. Therefore, in 1974 the Lukes and Collins and Kiel classification schemes were proposed. The strength of these two was that they were "immunologically correct." However, by the late 1970s, six independent pathologic schemes were in use throughout the world and therefore therapeutic trials could not be compared. Because of this confusion, a classification scheme termed the *Working Formulation* was proposed (Table 302-2). It incorporates the best features of the various classification systems and, more importantly, retains clinical relevance. The Working Formulation subdivides non-Hodgkin's lymphomas into *low-*, *intermediate-*, and *high-grade* subgroups, depending on their natural history. Low-grade lymphomas are characterized by an indolent clinical course; their natural history is not significantly altered by therapy. Intermediate- and high-grade lymphomas are associated with very short survivals. With the advent of aggressive combination chemotherapeutic regimens, some of these tumors demonstrate long-term disease-free survivals. Table 302-2 compares the Working Formulation and the Rappaport classifications. In clinical practice these classification schemes are frequently used interchangeably.

TABLE 302-5 Ann Arbor staging system

Stage I	Involvement in single lymph node region or single extralymphatic site.
Stage II	Involvement of two or more lymph node regions on the same side of the diaphragm. Can also include localized involvement of extralymphatic site (stage IIE).
Stage III	Involvement of lymph node regions or extralymphatic sites on both sides of the diaphragm.
Stage IV	Disseminated involvement of one or more extralymphatic organs with or without lymph node involvement.

NOTE: Substage A = asymptomatic patients; substage B = Patients with history of fever, sweats, or weight loss of greater than 10% bodyweight.

The histologic diagnosis of non-Hodgkin's lymphoma can only be reliably made on examination of lymph-node morphology. Since this is one of the most difficult areas of diagnosis, most cases should be reviewed by a hematopathologist. This is crucial, since therapeutic options are based on histologic subtype and only rarely by stage. The presence of follicular or diffuse patterns of the nodal architecture therefore predicts natural history and curability.

STAGING AND DISEASE DETECTION Conventional staging The Ann Arbor staging system developed for Hodgkin's disease has also been used in staging non-Hodgkin's lymphomas. This staging system focuses on the number of tumor sites (nodal and extranodal), location, and the presence or absence of systemic symptoms. Table 302-5 summarizes this staging system. In stages I and II sites of disease are on the same side of the diaphragm. Stage III disease involves both sides of the diaphragm, whereas stage IV is defined as extranodal lymphomatous involvement, most frequently of the bone marrow and liver. Systemic symptoms (fever, weight loss, and night sweats, i.e., B symptoms) are much less common in non-Hodgkin's lymphomas than in Hodgkins disease and therefore are not as useful in predicting prognosis. It must be emphasized that this classification scheme was specifically developed for Hodgkin's disease, which disseminates principally by contiguous lymphatic extension. Since non-Hodgkin's lymphomas most frequently disseminate hematogenously, for them this staging system has proven to be less useful.

The concept of staging is much less important in non-Hodgkin's lymphoma than in Hodgkin's disease. Since only 10 percent of patients with follicular lymphoma have localized disease, most advanced-stage patients are treated similarly. The majority of patients with diffuse lymphomas have advanced-stage disease and are therefore treated systemically. Thus, staging is undertaken in non-Hodgkin's lymphomas to identify the small number of patients who can be treated with local therapy and to stratify within histologic subtypes in order to prognosticate and to assess the impact of therapeutic regimens.

Staging procedures after biopsy diagnosis Staging must be undertaken in the context of the Working Formulation histologic grade. A suggested staging workup for patients with non-Hodgkin's lymphoma is summarized in Table 302-6. An organized approach to staging a patient with non-Hodgkin's lymphoma is mandatory. After the initial excisional biopsy and documentation of the pathologic and, when possible, immunologic subtype of disease, blood tests should be obtained, including complete blood count, routine chemistry, liver function test, and serum protein electrophoresis to document the presence of circulating monoclonal paraprotein. Indirect laryngoscopy is highly recommended. Waldeyer's ring involvement is often associated with intestinal involvement, and gastrointestinal contrast studies or endoscopy are indicated if the patient appears to have localized disease. Chest x-ray is used to exclude mediastinal and hilar adenopathy, pleural effusions, and pulmonary parenchymal infiltration. Chest

TABLE 302-6 Staging tests for malignant lymphomas

Test	Non-Hodgkin's	Hodgkin's
Essential		
1 Pathologic documentation by hematopathologist	X	X
2 Physical examination detailing nodal sites	X	X
3 Documentation of B symptoms	X	X
4 Laboratory evaluation of:		
a Complete blood counts	X	X
b Liver function tests	X	X
c Renal function tests	X	X
d Alkaline phosphatase	X	X
5 Chest roentgenogram	X	X
6 CT scan of abdomen and pelvis	X	X
7 Bone marrow biopsy—bilateral	X	—
Essential under certain circumstances		
1 Bilateral lymphogram of lower extremities	—	X
2 Bone marrow biopsy—bilateral	—	X
3 Whole chest CT scan (if chest roentgenogram is abnormal)	X	X
4 Exploratory laparotomy	—	X
5 Liver biopsy	X	X
Useful tests under certain circumstances		
1 Bilateral lymphogram of lower extremities	X	—
2 Exploratory laparotomy	X	—
3 Abdominal ultrasonogram	X	—
4 Radionuclide scans		
a Bone	X	X
b Liver-spleen	X	X
c Gallium	X	X
5 Head CT scan	X	—
6 Magnetic resonance imaging	X	X
7 Immunologic markers	X	X
8 Gene rearrangement studies	X	X
9 Chromosomal analysis	X	—

computed tomographic scan is used to assess more precisely the extent of disease and is not a required screening test. However, abdominopelvic CT scan is essential for accurate staging to assess lymphadenopathy in retroperitoneal, mesenteric, and retrocrural areas. Lymphangiography is less useful than in Hodgkin's disease, since common sites of disease in non-Hodgkin's lymphoma include nodes in the mesentery, hilum of liver, spleen, or kidneys, as well as nodes in the deep bony pelvis, none of which can be visualized by this procedure. The lymphogram may be an accurate predictor of intra-abdominal lymphoma since the majority of patients with a positive lymphogram also have disease in the liver and in abdominal nodes. The major advantage of lymphangiography over abdominopelvic CT scan is its ability to detect infiltrated but normal-sized retroperitoneal nodes. Bilateral percutaneous bone marrow biopsies must be performed, since the likelihood of lymphomatous involvement of the marrow is relatively high, especially in low-grade lymphoma, where marrow involvement occurs in 60 to 80 percent of cases. If there is any indication of hepatic abnormalities on blood tests or on liver scan, a liver biopsy is highly recommended.

More invasive tests are reserved for the uncommon presentation with stage I or II non-Hodgkin's lymphoma. While staging laparotomy may be performed in Hodgkin's disease, this is not so in the non-Hodgkin's lymphomas. In the diffuse non-Hodgkin's lymphomas, stages II, III, and IV can all be considered as reflecting disseminated disease and are therefore usually treated with chemotherapy. In contrast, only true stage I disease or, depending on the histologic subtype, stage II disease will be considered as localized and treated with radiation alone. Therefore, for most patients with non-Hodgkin's lymphoma it is less critical to ascertain the precise pathologic stage of disease. Moreover, it is common for these patients to exhibit disseminated disease after routine staging tests (e.g., bone marrow or liver biopsy), thus obviating laparotomy to prove dissemination. For example, within follicular lymphomas the poorly differentiated and mixed subgroups comprise more than 80 percent of patients. Following clinical staging and the minimally invasive techniques of bone marrow and liver biopsy, greater than 80 percent of these patients will have stage III or stage IV disease. Early in the staging process, only those diagnostic studies with low morbidity and a high probability of disclosing advanced disease should be employed. Bone marrow and liver biopsy, and, in selected patients, lymphangiography meet these requirements and usually obviate staging laparotomy. Thus, *surgical staging should never be considered a routine procedure in patients with non-Hodgkin's lymphoma.*

A number of other tests are becoming more important both in staging and in advancing our knowledge of the biology of non-Hodgkin's lymphoma. Radionuclide scans, especially with gallium, appear to have clinical utility. Gallium scans are commonly positive in intermediate- and high-grade lymphomas and in low-grade lymphomas that have converted to a higher histologic grade. Gallium, with high doses of isotope which permit delayed imaging, combined with single photon emission computed tomography (SPECT) are very sensitive in detecting tumor infiltration. These tests are also very useful in monitoring response to therapy and differentiating necrosis or fibrosis from active disease. The role of magnetic resonance (MR) imaging in detecting non-Hodgkin's lymphoma is under active investigation. Immunologic and molecular biologic studies are proving increasingly useful in confirming diagnosis. For example, in cases with difficult histopathologic patterns, cell surface markers can distinguish between non-Hodgkin's lymphoma and carcinoma (common leukocyte antigen, CD45-positive in lymphoma). Similarly, MAbs directed against lineage-restricted antigens and rearrangement of immunoglobulin or T-cell receptor genes are useful in identifying lymphoid tumors. Although therapeutic decisions are not currently made on the basis of lineage or state of differentiation of the neoplastic lymphocyte, these data may prove to be of prognostic importance. Moreover, delineation of the cell surface phenotype is becoming important because an increasing number of salvage treatment programs employ very high dose chemoradiotherapy and monoclonal-antibody–purged autologous bone marrow support (see below). Definition of a specific chromosomal abnormality may also have prognostic significance.

Sensitive techniques to detect minimal residual disease Monoclonal antibodies directed against cell surface antigens on lymphoid cells and molecular techniques to define immunoglobulin and T-cell-receptor gene rearrangements are very sensitive tools with which to assess tumor cell infiltration more accurately. Once the cell surface phenotype and genotype have been determined, one can examine other tissues for disease infiltration. The commonest and most accessible tissues to be tested include peripheral blood and bone marrow. Whereas conventional histologic analysis of the bone marrow can detect 1 lymphoma cell infiltrating 20 normal cells, immunologic flow cytometric and Southern blot analysis each improve this level of detection to approximately 1 lymphoma cell in approximately 100 normal cells. Similarly, flow cytometry has been used to detect "clonal excess" in the blood of patients with B-cell non-Hodgkin's lymphoma. More recently, newly developed molecular biologic techniques suggest that minimal disease detection can be markedly improved. For those non-Hodgkin's lymphomas with a known chromosomal translocation, it is now possible to identify a unique chromosomal "breakpoint." This has been most elegantly accomplished for the 14;18 translocation present in the majority of follicular lymphomas and in a smaller percentage of diffuse large cell lymphomas. This translocation, which occurs only in lymphoma cells, has been termed the *bcl*-2 breakpoint and its entire DNA sequence has been determined (see Chap. 10). Based on DNA sequence, it is possible to amplify this unique stretch of DNA using specific oligonucleotide primers and the polymerase chain reaction (PCR) (see Chap. 6). With this approach, 1 tumor cell in 100,000 cells can be detected. Thus, while other tests may be negative, PCR may demonstrate that the blood or bone marrow is contaminated by lymphoma cells. These biologic techniques are presently being compared to more conventional staging methods. Considering their sensitivity, they may be useful in more accurately assessing complete remission and, more importantly, determining whether treatment should be prolonged, altered, or intensified.

NATURAL HISTORY BY HISTOLOGIC SUBTYPE Considering the heterogeneity of non-Hodgkin's lymphoma and the unique clinical presentation and natural history within histologically defined subtypes, it is important to briefly review these subtypes.

Low grade SMALL LYMPHOCYTIC (DIFFUSE WELL-DIFFERENTIATED LYMPHOCYTIC) This disease is the lymphomatous presentation of chronic lymphocytic leukemia (CLL) and therefore occurs in middle- and older-aged patients. Patients usually present with generalized lymphadenopathy. Unlike CLL, the peripheral blood may be normal or reveal only a mild lymphocytosis (60 percent will have absolute lymphocytosis of >4000 per microliter at diagnosis). In contrast, the bone marrow is positive in 75 to 95 percent of cases. Serum paraprotein is found in about 20 percent of cases and hypogammaglobulinemia is common. Small lymphocytic lymphoma and CLL can convert to diffuse large cell lymphoma (Richter's syndrome, circulating large cell lymphoma). These patients usually present with abdominal masses and B symptoms and experience short survival.

FOLLICULAR, PREDOMINANTLY SMALL CLEAVED CELL (NODULAR POORLY DIFFERENTIATED LYMPHOCYTIC) Follicular lymphomas account for approximately 50 percent of the non-Hodgkin's lymphomas; the small cleaved cell variant is the most common subtype. Patients usually present with painless peripheral adenopathy in cervical, axillary, inguinal, and femoral regions. Patients frequently note that lymph node enlargement has been present for long periods of time and they have not sought medical attention because these nodes have "waxed and waned." Typically, there is enlargement of Waldeyer's ring, popliteal, and epitrochlear nodes. Some patients present with asymptomatic large abdominal masses with or without evidence of gastrointestinal and/or renal obstruction. Although patients may present with one or more sites of nodal disease, noninvasive workup usually demonstrates widely disseminated disease with involvement of spleen, liver, and bone marrow (80 to 90 percent with stage III or stage IV). Bone marrow involvement in follicular lymphoma reveals a unique pattern of paratrabecular infiltration. In contrast to diffuse lymphomas, very few patients present with extranodal disease and few present with B symptoms. The course of this disease is quite variable. Some patients can be observed with waxing and waning disease for 5 years without the need for therapy. Others demonstrate more disseminated and rapid growth and require treatment because massive nodal or organ enlargement leads to pain, lymphatic obstruction, organ obstruction, or, more rarely, neurologic symptoms. At the time of increasing generalized disease or rapid growth at a single site, involved nodes should be rebiopsied. At that time, a significant number of patients will demonstrate a "conversion" to a more aggressive histologic pattern, usually diffuse large cell. This conversion occurs in 60 percent of patients with follicular small cleaved cell lymphoma and is associated with infiltration of extranodal sites and, in some patients, with the development of systemic symptoms and a poorer prognosis, since the tumor is much less responsive to treatment. Late in the natural history of this disease, a number of patients circulate either small follicular cleaved cells or large cells as a leukemic phase. Historically, both disease-free and overall survivals of these patients have not changed in spite of many different therapeutic approaches. Few patients achieve complete remissions (noninvasively staged) with conventional single-agent or aggressive combination chemotherapy. However, these patients survive long periods of time with median survivals for patients with stages III and IV disease approaching 7 to 9 years.

FOLLICULAR, MIXED SMALL CLEAVED CELL AND LARGE CELL (NODULAR MIXED) This entity has similarities with both follicular small cleaved cell and follicular large cell lymphomas. Bone marrow infiltration at presentation is less common, but large abdominal masses are more commonly seen. It demonstrates a less favorable natural history with 35 percent disease-free survival at 2 years.

Intermediate grade FOLLICULAR, PREDOMINANTLY LARGE CELL (NODULAR HISTIOCYTIC) Although the follicular morphology is preserved, this disease behaves much more like diffuse large cell lymphoma. In contrast to other follicular lymphomas, this histologic variant has less infiltration of the marrow and liver and presents with larger masses. A finite cure rate has been reported. Most follicular large cell lymphomas that are not cured by treatment convert to diffuse large cell lymphomas.

DIFFUSE SMALL CLEAVED CELL (DIFFUSE POORLY DIFFERENTIATED LYMPHOCYTIC) This disease behaves like a follicular variant. Patients are middle-aged or older. At the time of presentation, most have stage IV disease with infiltration of the spleen, liver, and bone marrow. Marrow and hepatic infiltration occur in over 50 percent of patients. Later in the course of the disease, infiltration of other parenchymal organs (e.g., lung) is observed. Many patients present with massive splenomegaly and significant bone marrow infiltration. The overall survival is much shorter than observed in patients with low-grade lymphomas; however, like low-grade lymphoma, aggressive combination chemotherapy has not significantly changed the natural history of this disease.

DIFFUSE SMALL AND LARGE CELL (DIFFUSE MIXED) This tumor behaves most like diffuse large cell lymphoma. Some investigators consider these two tumors to be a spectrum of a single entity. Patients are usually older women with prominent extranodal disease, especially in the skin and gastrointestinal tract, and B symptoms are common. However, diffuse mixed lymphoma is a "wastebasket" of a number of pathologic entities and, therefore, it is difficult to compare clinical series with respect to disease presentation and response to treatment. In several clinical trials where patients with diffuse mixed and diffuse large cell lymphoma were treated identically, survival rates were comparable. However, in other series, a higher relapse rate was observed with diffuse mixed lymphoma.

DIFFUSE LARGE CELL (DIFFUSE HISTIOCYTIC) Patients present with either nodal enlargement (especially in the neck or abdomen) or extranodal disease (in the gastrointestinal tract, testes, bone, thyroid, salivary glands, skin, and brain). During the course of the disease, the liver, kidneys, and lung may be involved. Diffuse large cell lymphoma is highly invasive, with local compression of vessels or airways, involvement of peripheral nerves, and destruction of bone. Although bone marrow involvement initially is found in only 10 to 20 percent of patients, its detection is important because of its strong correlation with later spread to the central nervous system. Therefore, cytologic examination of spinal fluid is important in patients with bone marrow infiltration. Late in the disease, some patients demonstrate both extensive bone marrow infiltration and circulating large cell lymphoma cells. A number of clinical features reflect dissemination of disease and are considered to be associated with inability to achieve a complete remission and poor prognosis. These features include poor performance status, large tumor masses, bone marrow infiltration, multiple sites of extranodal disease, markedly elevated serum lactic dehydrogenase (LDH), and systemic B symptoms.

High grade LARGE CELL IMMUNOBLASTIC (DIFFUSE HISTIOCYTIC) This variant of diffuse large cell lymphoma demonstrates a unique pathologic appearance and the clinical course is usually fulminant. This disease usually occur in adults, commonly over age 50, and often in a setting of prior immune-mediated or lymphoproliferative disease (e.g., celiac disease, Hashimoto's thyroiditis, angioimmunoblastic lymphadenopathy, Sjögren's syndrome, Mediterranean lymphoma, cold aggulutinin disease, or Waldenström's macroglobulinemia). Anemia, lymphopenia, diffuse hypergammaglobulinemia, B symptoms, and advanced stage are common at presentation. Most patients present with extranodal disease and invasion of the bone marrow and central nervous system are common.

LYMPHOBLASTIC (DIFFUSE LYMPHOBLASTIC) Although lymphoblastic lymphomas represent a major subgroup of childhood non-Hodgkin's lymphomas, they are much less common in adults (less than 5 percent of adult non-Hodgkin's lymphomas). Patients are usually males in their twenties or thirties who present with lymphadenopathy in cervical, supraclavicular, and axillary regions (50 percent) or with a mediastinal mass (50 percent). In most patients the mediastinal mass is anterior, greater than 10 cm, and is associated with pleural effusions. Less commonly, patients present with extranodal disease (e.g., skin, testicular, or bony involvement). Greater than 90 percent of patients present with stage III or stage IV disease and half have B symptoms. Although the bone marrow is frequently normal at presentation, approximately 60 percent of patients develop bone marrow infiltration and a subsequent leukemic phase indistinguishable from T-cell acute lymphoblastic leukemia. Patients with bone marrow involvement have a very high incidence of CNS infiltration. Prior to current aggressive therapy, this disease was rapidly fatal.

SMALL NONCLEAVED CELL, BURKITT'S AND NON-BURKITT'S (DIFFUSE UNDIFFERENTIATED) Burkitt's lymphoma is a childhood tumor that has two major clinical presentations. The *African* endemic form presents as a jaw tumor that spreads to extranodal sites, especially to the bone marrow and meninges. The *American* form has an abdominal presentation with massive disease and ascites and, like the African form, also spreads to the bone marrow and central nervous system. Prior to aggressive therapeutic programs, all children died rapidly. These tumors are now treated with very aggressive chemotherapeutic programs with more gratifying results. True Burkitt's lymphoma is uncommon in adults but is occasionally seen in patients up to age 35. In contrast, small noncleaved cell, non-Burkitt's lymphomas are observed and are very aggressive and frequently present in extranodal sites. Like Burkitt's, these tumors have a very high propensity to invade the bone marrow and central nervous system.

Other subtypes AIDS-RELATED LYMPHOMAS Non-Hodgkin's lymphoma occurs in 5 to 10 percent of patients with AIDS. Most cases are grouped with high-grade tumors including small noncleaved cell and large cell immunoblastic. In these cases extranodal involvement is common with central nervous system, bone marrow, and gastrointestinal tract the most frequent sites. Most patients present with rapid nodal enlargement, appearance of an extranodal mass, or severe B symptoms. Primary CNS lymphoma is common in AIDS patients, and it is predicted that within 5 or more years this will be one of the commonest presenting CNS malignancies. These lymphomas have been associated with chromosomal translocations (8;14 and 8;22) and with EBV, although a causal relationship has not been definitively demonstrated. Although treated with the most aggressive combinations of chemotherapy, results have been poor.

CUTANEOUS T-CELL LYMPHOMAS Major variants include mycosis fungoides and Sézary syndrome. Both tumors are T-cell derived. Patients present with cutaneous manifestations, lymphadenopathy, and later with hepatic, splenic, and pulmonary infiltration. Infiltration of the bone marrow and circulating leukemia are also common late manifestations.

ADULT T-CELL LYMPHOMA This entity has been observed in Japan, the Caribbean, and in blacks in the southeastern United States and is associated with the human T-cell leukemia virus (HTLV-I) C type retrovirus. Patients present with generalized adenopathy, hepatosplenomegaly, cutaneous infiltration, hypercalcemia, lytic bone lesions, and a profound leukemia characterized by pleomorphic CD4-positive T-cells. This disease has a fulminant course and its natural history has been little altered by aggressive combination chemotherapy.

ANGIOIMMUNOBLASTIC LYMPHADENOPATHY (CLASSIFIED WITH LARGE CELL IMMUNOBLASTIC) This disease affects older adults who present with the acute onset of generalized lymphadenopathy, hepatosplenomegaly, and B symptoms. Immunologic abnormalities are common and include plasmacytosis, polyclonal hypergammaglobulinemia, and a positive Coombs test. Although this disease is progressive and frequently fatal, it is unresolved whether it is a hyperimmune disorder or a malignant lymphoma. Limited cytogenetic and clonal T-cell receptor β-chain rearrangements suggest a neoplasm akin to adult peripheral T-cell lymphoma.

TRUE HISTIOCYTIC LYMPHOMA This is a rare entity that is the neoplastic counterpart of the true histiocyte (macrophage) and exhibits the curious phenomenon of erythrophagocytosis. This disease has an abrupt onset with fever, progressive pancytopenia, splenomegaly, and mild lymphadenopathy.

THERAPY To decide the appropriate treatment regimen, the clinician must determine whether the histology is low-, intermediate-, or high-grade and whether the disease is localized or systemic. The next decision is whether or not to treat; if the treatment option is selected, whether the goal is to palliate symptoms or to cure. Although some general principles are agreed upon in the treatment of non-Hodgkin's lymphoma, therapeutic approaches for all histologic subtypes are actively being evaluated. Options to be chosen must consider age and the presence of comorbid diseases (cardiac, renal, pulmonary, etc.) that might significantly affect end-organ toxicity.

Radiotherapy Radiation has a very limited role in the primary treatment of non-Hodgkin's lymphoma. It should only be considered as a potential curative modality in patients whose disease has been exhaustively staged and found to be true stage I intermediate- or high-grade or true stage I or II low-grade non-Hodgkin's lymphoma. Most of the radiotherapeutic principles developed for the treatment of Hodgkin's disease (see below) also apply to non-Hodgkin's lymphoma. For patients with stage I disease, involved-field radiotherapy is employed with the dose dependent upon the histologic subtype. Doses of less than 3000 cGy are usually sufficient for low-grade disease whereas high-grade disease is frequently treated with 5000 cGy or greater. For patients with true stage I non-Hodgkin's lymphoma, the long-term disease-free survival ranges from 60 to 80 percent. In addition to its curative potential in stage I patients, radiotherapy is frequently used in conjunction with systemic therapy to treat sites of bulk disease. Moreover, in low-grade lymphomas it has been commonly used to palliate sites of symptomatic disease. The use of local radiotherapy for patients not being treated for cure must be carefully evaluated in view of its potential later use as total-body irradiation in salvage therapy (i.e., bone marrow transplantation).

Chemotherapy (See also Chap. 301 and Table 301-1 for abbreviations of standard regimens) This modality is used for most patients with stage II and all patients with stages III and IV non-Hodgkin's lymphoma. Chemotherapeutic options are dictated by grade and histologic subtype and therefore treatment regimens depend upon the Working Formulation.

LOW-GRADE LYMPHOMA For the most part, small lymphocytic (DWDL) and follicular small cleaved cell (NPDL) lymphomas are approached similarly. Traditionally, these tumors have not been treated until they produce symptoms. This was because single-agent chemotherapy or combinations of agents did not induce complete remissions and, more importantly, they did not change the overall survival of patients with these diseases. These regimens included the use of single alkylating agents like cyclophosphamide or chlorambucil or combinations like CVP (cyclophosphamide, vincristine, and prednisone) or CHOP (CVP plus adriamycin). More aggressive CHOP-like regimens (see intermediate-grade below) have produced more rapid and possibly higher percentages of complete remissions but unfortunately have not changed the overall survival rates for these diseases. In addition, attempts to treat patients for long periods of time with single-agent therapy or the addition of long-term "maintenance" treatment did not alter overall survival. If these diseases are to be cured, either more aggressive high-dose regimens must be evaluated or new therapeutic modalities must be employed. Recently, several institutions (e.g., National Cancer Institute, Dana Farber Cancer Institute, and St. Bartholomew's Hospital in London) have attempted to treat patients with advanced stage follicular lymphomas earlier in the course of their disease with aggressive chemotherapy combined with total nodal irradiation or with high-dose chemoradiotherapy and autologous bone marrow transplantation. These studies suggest that high complete-response rates in the range of 80 percent or greater are possible. However, the impact of these studies on long-term disease-free survival and possible cure is still uncertain.

INTERMEDIATE-GRADE LYMPHOMA The regimen used to treat diffuse large cell lymphoma is now also employed to treat follicular mixed, follicular large cell, and diffuse small cleaved cell lymphomas. *The treatment of diffuse large cell lymphoma is one of the major successes of modern chemotherapy.* These tumors were initially treated with single agents and then CVP. This regimen induced disease regression in most patients, but few complete responses or improvement in disease-free survival were observed. The first successful regimen was CHOP, which induced complete remissions in approximately 50 percent of patients and with long-term disease-free survival for more than half of the complete responders. Success with this and subsequent regimens required attention to administering full doses and adhering to schedules as strictly as possible. Over the past 15 years, attempts have been made to improve the percentage of complete remissions and overall cure rate. Additional agents have been added to CHOP, including bleomycin, methotrexate, procarbazine, nitrogen mustard, cytarabine hydrochloride (cytosine arabinoside), and etoposide (e.g., BACOD, m-BACOD, ProMACE-MOPP, COP-BLAM, COMLA, ProMACE/CytaBOM, MACOP-B). In addition to the complexity of the regimen, the duration of treatment has been prolonged for up to 12 months. With these approaches, the complete-remission rate now approaches 80 percent for the most aggressive regimens. However, not surprisingly, toxicities have also increased (e.g., infections as well as cardiac and pulmonary complications.) Patients who survive 2 years disease-free have an excellent chance of being cured. Prolonged ''maintenance'' therapy has not improved overall survival. With the various treatment options, and until randomized studies are completed, the selection of a treatment regimen for diffuse large cell lymphoma should be based on the therapist's experience with a particular regimen and its toxicities.

Both nodular mixed and nodular large cell lymphomas have been treated with CHOP-like regimens with high complete-remission rates and good evidence for long-term disease-free survival. In contrast, diffuse small cleaved cell lymphoma has been treated with most of the above aggressive regimens but while complete-response rates are high, relapse is rapid and cure is rare.

HIGH-GRADE LYMPHOMA These tumors have a very poor prognosis and need to be treated very aggressively. Lymphoblastic lymphoma and small noncleaved cell lymphomas have been treated with regimens even more aggressive than those used for diffuse large cell lymphoma. Although complete-remission rates are very high, the cure rate is still much less than is observed for diffuse large cell lymphoma. Groups with good prognostic features (bone marrow negative, low LDH) have better survival than those with poor prognostic characteristics. If there is CNS infiltration, intrathecal treatment or radiotherapy should be administered.

AIDS-RELATED LYMPHOMAS These tumors are among the most aggressive of the non-Hodgkin's lymphomas. Most are intermediate-grade diffuse large cell with some high-grade B-cell lymphomas also observed. These tumors are becoming increasingly more common and their response to therapy and prognosis is radically different compared to non-AIDS-related intermediate- and high-grade lymphoma despite their histologic resemblance. Aggressive regimens have had limited impact with fewer than 25 percent achieving complete remissions and few, if any, cures. Salvage regimens have also been very disappointing, with patients dying of lymphoma as well as complications of aplasia. Bone marrow transplantation has not been attempted.

Salvage chemotherapy Failure to achieve a complete remission or relapse following aggressive therapy is associated with short survival. Salvage chemotherapeutic regimens employing both higher doses and new drugs (e.g., ifosfamide, etoposide, and cisplatin) have therefore been used to induce remissions. Depending upon the histology and regimen, approximately one-third of patients attain a complete remission with partial remissions in another third. Unfortunately, these remissions tend to be short-lived with survival being less than 2 years.

Bone marrow transplantation (BMT) Patients whose disease is resistant to conventional or salvage therapeutic regimens can still be induced into a complete remission with very high dosages of chemotherapy or chemoradiotherapy. This treatment approach is complicated by very significant and prolonged myelosuppression. To overcome the latter, bone marrow can be infused from an identical twin, an HLA-matched relative, or from the patient following the completion of therapy. Bone marrow transplantation has become widespread in the treatment of patients with refractory or relapsed non-Hodgkin's lymphoma, and retrospective analysis demonstrates that a subgroup of patients clearly benefits from this approach. Patients whose disease has never responded to therapy or, following relapse, is resistant to all forms of salvage therapy, have less than 20 percent long-term disease-free survival. In contrast, those patients whose disease is still responsive to therapy achieve approximately 40 percent long-term disease-free survival with BMT. Studies with BMT have reported treatment-related deaths in the range of 20 to 30 percent; however, as patients are treated earlier in the course of their disease this mortality has significantly decreased (10 percent or less). This lower mortality has led some to use BMT as consolidation therapy in patients with incurable non-Hodgkin's lymphomas. Although this modality is clearly capable of curing some patients with relapsed non-Hodgkin's lymphomas, many issues still remain. These include optimal therapeutic regimen, optimal time of transplantation, source of bone marrow, the question of purging autologous bone marrow, as well as methods to minimize morbidity and mortality.

Newer modalities A variety of new therapeutic approaches have resulted from the advances in immunology and molecular biology. Over 10 years ago, MAbs directed against surface antigens expressed on non-Hodgkin's lymphoma cells were first used clinically in an attempt to specifically treat these tumors. The results of these studies suggest that MAbs by themselves do not induce significant tumor regressions. Although there was initial enthusiasm about using MAbs directed against unique idiotypes expressed on B-cell follicular lymphomas, many obstacles have been encountered. Some trials are evaluating MAbs coupled to radionuclides or toxins to specifically produce cytotoxic effects; other trials are using soluble factors (cytokines) that are potentially cytotoxic to tumor cells. The major cytokines being studied include the interferons, tumor necrosis factor, and interleukin 2 (IL-2). Recombinant hematopoietic growth factors that are responsible for growth of myeloid, lymphoid, and erythroid cells are also being tested. Conceptually, these growth factors will limit myelosuppression thereby permitting higher doses and more frequent administration of chemotherapeutic drugs. Early results are encouraging, and agents like granulocyte macrophage colony stimulating factor (GM-CSF) and G-CSF appear to hasten recovery of myeloid cells. The role of all of these agents in improving the treatment of lymphomas is being evaluated in many research centers.

HODGKIN'S DISEASE

EPIDEMIOLOGY AND ETIOLOGY Approximately 7500 new cases of Hodgkin's disease are diagnosed annually in the United States. The epidemiology of this disease has provided important information regarding the possible role of age, genetic, and environmental factors associated with its development. While the interpretation of epidemiologic factors remains controversial, these data still provide a context within which to examine the population at risk for Hodgkin's disease. In non-Hodgkin's lymphomas there is a linear increase in incidence with age. In contrast, in Hodgkin's disease in the United States and developed western nations, the age-specific incidence curve is characteristically bimodal with an initial peak in young adults (15 to 35 years) and a second peak after age 50. However, in Japan, there is an absence of the early peak, and in underdeveloped, tropical countries there is a shift of the first peak into childhood. Hodgkin's disease is more prevalent in males, and when the age-specific incidence curve is compared to the sex distribution of the patients, the increased male prevalence is most prominent in young adults. A disproportionate number of patients in the first modal peak exhibit nodular sclerosis histology. In childhood Hodgkin's disease, this male predominance is even more striking with over 80 percent of patients being male. This has led some investigators to hypothesize a sex-linked genetic or hormonally related increase in susceptibility.

Although controversial, clusters of patients with Hodgkin's have been reported. Increased risk has been associated with decreased number of siblings, single family dwellings, decreased number of playmates, early birth order, sibling with Hodgkin's, tonsillectomy, and certain HLA antigens. These findings have been used to suggest that Hodgkin's disease is caused by a virus possessing an oncogenic potential that is low but that increases with age at the time of infection. These observations suggest that genetic and environmental factors may be associated with the development of this disease. As in non-Hodgkin's lymphomas, there is an increased risk of Hodgkin's in patients with immunodeficiencies and autoimmune diseases (Table 302-4). The major obstacle to examining the etiology of Hodgkin's disease is the inability to isolate and study the "real" neoplastic cell. Unlike non-Hodgkin's lymphomas, no chromosomal abnormalities have been consistently demonstrated.

CLINICAL FEATURES AND DIFFERENTIAL DIAGNOSIS Patients with Hodgkin's disease usually present with localized disease that subsequently spreads to contiguous lymphoid structures; it ultimately disseminates to nonlymphoid tissues with a potentially fatal outcome. Patients commonly present with a newly detected mass or group of lymph nodes that are firm, freely moveable, and usually nontender. Approximately half present with adenopathy in the neck or supraclavicular area, and over 70 percent present with superficial lymph node enlargement. Because these are frequently not painful, detection by the patient may be delayed until the lymph nodes are quite large. Approximately 50 to 60 percent of patients present with mediastinal adenopathy. This is sometimes first detected on a routine chest x-ray. Hodgkin's nodes tend to be centripetal or axial in contrast to non-Hodgkin's lymphomas, which have a tendency to be centrifugal involving epitrochlear, Waldeyer's ring, and abdominal nodes. In 2 to 5 percent of patients, lymph nodes or other tissues involved with Hodgkin's disease can become painful after the ingestion of alcohol. The growth of lymph nodes may be quite variable; some lesions can remain stable for long periods of time, while spontaneous and temporary regression of some nodes may also occur.

The majority of patients presenting with Hodgkin's disease have few or no symptoms related to their disease. However, 25 to 40 percent of patients have some constitutional symptoms; the most common is low-grade fever which can be associated with recurrent night sweats. For some patients, night sweats may be the sole complaint. A small number of patients may have high fluctuating fevers accompanied by drenching night sweats (Pel-Ebstein fevers). These fevers can persist for several weeks followed by afebrile intervals. Fevers and night sweats are more commonly seen in older patients and in those with more advanced-stage disease. Some patients with extensive abdominal but limited peripheral adenopathy are first evaluated for fever and night sweats. They undergo a workup for fever of unknown origin and usually are found to have lymphocyte-depleted Hodgkin's disease. Another important presenting symptom is weight loss of greater than 10 percent. *Fever, night sweats, and weight loss are referred to as B symptoms.* Other frequent symptoms include fatigue, malaise, and weakness. Pruritus occurs in approximately 10 percent of patients at initial diagnosis; it is usually generalized and may be associated with a skin rash. Rarely, pruritus may be the only disease manifestation. Site-specific symptoms are also rare. However, mediastinal, pulmonary, pleural, or pericardial involvement may be associated with cough, chest pain, shortness of breath, or hypertrophic osteoarthropathy; bone involvement may be associated with bone pain. Occasionally a patient will present with obstruction of the superior vena cava as the first symptom. Sudden spinal cord compression can be a presenting complaint but is usually a complication of progressive disease. Headache or visual disturbances may be seen in the very rare patient with intracranial Hodgkin's disease, and abdominal involvement may result in abdominal pain, bowel disturbances, and even ascites.

Differential diagnosis is similar to that described for non-Hodgkin's lymphoma. Persistent lymph nodes larger than 1 cm present for 4 to 6 weeks should be biopsied. In patients with neck adenopathy, infections including bacterial or viral pharyngitis, infectious mononucleosis, and toxoplasmosis must be excluded. Other malignancies, such as non-Hodgkin's lymphomas, nasopharyngeal cancers, and thyroid cancers, can also present with localized neck adenopathy. Axillary adenopathy must be differentiated from non-Hodgkin's lymphoma and breast cancer. Since supraclavicular nodes drain both the thorax and the abdomen, regardless of infectious or neoplastic etiology, the left supraclavicular space is more commonly associated with lesions of the abdomen while the right side is more commonly associated with intrathoracic disease. Mediastinal adenopathy must be distinguished from infections, sarcoid, and other tumors. In older patients, the differential diagnosis includes tumors of the lung and mediastinum, specifically oat cell and epidermoid carcinomas. Reactive mediastinitis and hilar adenopathy from histoplasmosis can be confused with lymphoma since the former occurs in otherwise asymptomatic people. Primary abdominal disease with hepatomegaly, splenomegaly, and massive adenopathy is uncommon and may produce symptoms; other neoplastic diseases, especially non-Hodgkin's lymphoma, must be excluded under these circumstances.

DIAGNOSIS AND PATHOLOGIC CLASSIFICATION The diagnosis of Hodgkin's disease requires a biopsy that contains sufficient tissue to permit an accurate microscopic diagnosis. Biopsy specimens are usually from lymph nodes, but may occasionally be from other tissues. Needle aspirations or needle biopsies are not adequate for the histologic diagnosis of Hodgkin's disease.

The criteria for the diagnosis and classification of Hodgkin's disease have remained unchanged since 1966 when the Rye classification was adopted (Table 302-7). As indicated above, central to the diagnosis is the presence of the Reed-Sternberg cell, a large cell with a bilobed or multilobulated nucleus with prominent inclusion-like nucleoli. There are several morphologic variants of RS cells, and it is the frequency of these variants as well as the cellular and fibrous background of the proliferation that help to establish the histologic subtypes of Hodgkin's disease. It is important to note that RS cells may occasionally be found in other conditions such as infectious mononucleosis and non-Hodgkin's lymphoma. Thus, an accurate diagnosis of Hodgkin's disease depends on additional cellular and architectural features of the tissue and optimally also with supportive immunologic studies.

In the Rye classification, Hodgkin's disease is subdivided into four types: (1) lymphocyte-predominant, (2) nodular sclerosis, (3)

TABLE 302-7 Rye classification of Hodgkin's disease

Histologic subgroup	Incidence, %	Pathology: RS*	Pathology: Other	Prognosis
Lymphocyte-predominant	2–10	Rare	Predominance of normal-appearing lymphocytes	Excellent
Nodular sclerosis	40–80	Frequent "lacunae"	Lymphoid nodules, collagen bands	Very good
Mixed cellularity	20–40	Numerous	Pleomorphic infiltrate	Good
Lymphocyte-depleted	2–15	Numerous, often bizarre	Paucity of lymphocytes, pleomorphic, fibrosis	Poor

* RS = Reed-Sternberg cell.

mixed cellularity, and (4) lymphocyte-depleted. These variants define distinct entities with unique natural histories. Table 302-7 summarizes the major clinical characteristics of these types associated with the Rye classification. It is very important to stress that *treatment and prognosis in Hodgkin's disease are dependent on stage of disease* whereas *in non-Hodgkin's lymphoma, treatment and prognosis are largely based on histologic subtype.*

STAGING AND OTHER LABORATORY ABNORMALITIES **Ann Arbor classification** Following biopsy and histopathologic classification of Hodgkin's disease, one must define the extent of the disease (i.e., staging), which is essential for the selection of optimal therapy. In the Ann Arbor staging classification (Table 302-5), the patient receives both a clinical and a pathologic stage. The clinical stage is defined by the apparent extent of disease based on physical examination and other noninvasive studies. The pathologic stage is defined by data obtained from invasive tests including biopsy specimens obtained from different sites, usually during a staging laparotomy. The presence of localized extralymphatic disease is designated by the suffix E. Such extralymphatic involvement may include solitary involvement of lung, pericardium, or bone. Multifocal involvement in these organs usually is defined as disseminated disease. Bone involvement must be separated from bone marrow involvement, since bone marrow and liver involvement are always defined as stage IV disseminated disease.

The presence of systemic symptoms that are of prognostic importance is designated by the suffix B and their absence by the suffix A. B symptoms include loss of greater than 10 percent of body weight, fever, or night sweats. The presence of any of these symptoms results in a less favorable prognosis. As stated above, defining the pathologic stage is essential for determining optimal therapy. Patients with limited disease, such as pathologic stage IA or IIA, are effectively treated with radiotherapy alone, while patients with more disseminated disease, such as pathologic stage IIIB, IVA, or IVB, are most effectively treated with chemotherapy, alone or combined with radiotherapy.

Staging procedures after biopsy diagnosis The diagnostic studies recommended for complete staging are outlined in Table 302-6. There is general agreement on the studies that are considered to be essential. Detailed physical examination with attention to documentation of all sites of nodal involvement and splenomegaly is essential. The chest radiograph is usually sufficient to exclude mediastinal, hilar, pleural, and parenchymal involvement. However, in patients with demonstrable thoracic disease, chest CT scan more accurately defines extent of disease. A CT scan of the abdomen and pelvis has a definite place in the staging of Hodgkin's disease for the assessment of nodal, splenic, and hepatic disease. It can detect the exact location and extent of all enlarged nodes including parailiac, mesenteric, and retrocrural nodal areas as compared to a lymphogram, which evaluates only the paraaortic and common internal and external iliac nodes. However, the abdominopelvic CT scan has several limitations; it requires nodal enlargement for detection and is less sensitive in detecting splenic involvement (50 to 60 percent) or hepatic infiltration (25 percent).

A number of more invasive diagnostic tests are required if patients are clinically stage I, II, or IIIA. Lymphograms of the lower extremities are very useful to demonstrate paraaortic and iliac nodal enlargement; they are more sensitive than abdominopelvic CT scans since they can detect disease in normal-sized nodes. Moreover, lymphograms are useful prior to staging laparotomy to direct the surgeon to the nodes to be biopsied. However, the safety and accuracy of this procedure is highly dependent on the experience of the radiologist. If a staging laparotomy is considered, patients should undergo *bilateral bone marrow biopsies* and percutaneous *liver biopsy* to exclude stage IV disease. The role of staging laparotomy is still controversial. Historically, staging laparotomy with splenectomy has played an important role in understanding the biology of Hodgkin's disease. Staging laparotomy includes biopsy of selected lymph nodes in the retroperitoneum, splenectomy, and several needle and wedge biopsies of the liver. Traditionally, all patients without obvious stage IV disease underwent laparotomy, and nearly one-third had their initial clinical stage changed as a result of the procedure. For example, one-third of patients with normal-sized spleens had demonstrable tumor infiltration at laparotomy, whereas 25 percent of patients with clinical splenomegaly had no histologic evidence of disease. Similarly, hepatic infiltration by Hodgkin's disease is associated with splenomegaly. The liver is rarely involved when splenic involvement is not associated with splenomegaly. Liver involvement is present in as many as 28 percent of patients with positive lymphograms and enlarged spleens. Although very important, the routine use of staging laparotomy in all patients may not be appropriate. Laparotomies should be utilized in patients whose clinical stages make them a candidate for treatment with radiation therapy alone and in whom evidence of unsuspected abdominal disease will significantly change treatment. A staging laparotomy should not be performed in patients who are to receive chemotherapy based upon their clinical stage since it is rare for the clinical stage to be lowered after a laparotomy. A staging laparotomy with splenectomy should be performed by a surgeon who is skilled in this procedure, after careful review of clinical, laboratory, pathologic, and radiologic studies. In selected patients, laparoscopy performed by a skilled practitioner may substitute for a laparotomy. Finally, a number of ancillary studies may be very useful in selected patients and are listed in Table 302-6. Gallium scintigraphy is useful in following response to treatment and in differentiating residual or recurrent disease from bulky nodal fibrosis, particularly in the abdomen and mediastinum. A scan is necessary at the time of initial staging to determine whether the lymphoma is gallium-avid.

Laboratory abnormalities Routine blood counts, liver function tests, and renal function tests are all necessary parts of the medical workup, but do not provide information about the extent of Hodgkin's disease or of specific organ involvement. A moderate, normochromic, normocytic anemia associated with low serum iron and low iron-binding capacity, but with normal or increased iron stores in the bone marrow, may be present in patients with Hodgkin's disease as well as in those with other neoplastic and chronic diseases. A moderate to marked leukemoid reaction is common, particularly in symptomatic patients, and usually disappears with treatment. Mild peripheral absolute eosinophilia is not uncommon especially in patients with pruritus. Absolute monocytosis is also observed. Absolute lymphocytopenia (<1000 cells per cubic milliliter) usually occurs in patients with more advanced disease. Many tests have been evaluated as indicators of disease activity. To date, the erythrocyte sedimentation rate still is the best monitor but it suffers from its lack of specificity and can return to normal when residual disease is still demonstrable. Other abnormal tests include increased serum levels of copper, calcium, lactic acid, alkaline phosphatase, lysozyme, globulins, C-reactive protein, and other acute-phase reactants.

Immunologic abnormalities Hodgkin's disease is associated with a well-described but poorly understood immunologic defect. Untreated patients, including those with limited disease, have defective cellular immunity characterized by anergy to routine skin tests. They also have a reversal of the CD4:CD8 ratio, suggesting that this anergy may be due to increased numbers of suppressor cells as well as decreased numbers of CD4-positive cells. In several studies, decreased immune reactivity correlates both with advanced stages of disease and the presence of systemic symptoms. However, anergy to recall and neoantigen appear to have no prognostic significance. Following successful therapy, anergy reverses to recall antigens but is still present to neoantigens in some patients. In addition to anergy, other tests of T-cell function, including response to mitogens and suppressor-cell function, suggest a defect in immune function prior to and following treatment. Humoral immunity with antibody production to soluble antigens is normal in untreated patients. Thus, patients who undergo staging laparotomy and splenectomy will develop humoral immunity to pneumococcal antigens if immunized with the pneumococcal vaccine prior to therapy. The clinical impact of these immune defects is limited. Except for a higher than normal incidence of herpes zoster, these patients are not plagued by opportunistic infections.

NATURAL HISTORY ACCORDING TO HISTOLOGIC SUBTYPE Patients with lymphocyte-predominant Hodgkin's disease are usually asymptomatic at presentation and tend to have localized disease. These patients are usually young, rarely have systemic symptoms or mediastinal mass, and are predominantly males. Nodular sclerosis Hodgkin's disease is found most frequently in adolescents and young adults who usually have localized disease; a preponderance are young women who present with a large mediastinal mass. Lymphocyte-depleted Hodgkin's disease is usually disseminated at the time of diagnosis and occurs in older patients who frequently have systemic symptoms. The mixed cellularity type occurs in all age groups and stages and is only slightly more common in males. There is a tendency toward an older age peak than with nodular sclerosis (30 to 40 years) and approximately half of these patients have advanced disease. Patients with lymphocyte-predominant and nodular sclerosis Hodgkin's disease, if untreated, have a more indolent disease associated with a longer survival and are more likely to be cured with radiotherapy. However, all Hodgkin's patients receiving chemotherapy have comparable long-term survivals irrespective of their histologic subtype.

There are several variables that adversely affect the prognosis of Hodgkin's disease. The number of involved sites and presence of bulky disease are the most important variables since extensive disease is often associated with high frequency of drug-resistant tumor cells. Large masses in the chest (greater than one-third the chest diameter) do poorly with radiotherapy or chemotherapy alone, but respond better to combined treatment. The prognosis is generally poor if a patient's disease is resistant to primary therapy or if relapse occurs within 12 months. Increased age and systemic B symptoms are poor prognostic signs regardless of stage. Systemic B symptoms forbode very poor prognosis, especially when all three symptoms are present. Lymphocyte-depleted histology, although very uncommon, is associated with a poor prognosis. Finally, males appear to have poorer prognosis than women when corrected for age, stage, and histology.

TREATMENT OF HODGKIN'S DISEASE Essentially all patients can and should be treated with curative intent. Radiotherapy may cure over 80 percent of patients with localized Hodgkin's disease, and chemotherapy over 50 percent of those with disseminated disease. *The choice of treatment regimen is totally dependent on stage of disease*. Thus, it is critical that pretreatment evaluation be precise and thorough with the objective of defining optimal therapy. This requires an integrated multidisciplinary effort at major oncology centers. As with all neoplasms, the therapy of Hodgkin's disease is constantly being reevaluated to improve disease-free survival and decrease toxicity.

Radiotherapy Radiation therapy alone has been evaluated in patients with pathologic stages IA, IIA, IB, IIB, and in some patients with stage IIIA. While lower doses of therapy will cause tumor regression, it was the recognition that 4000 cGy delivered at the rate of 1000 cGy per week could eradicate local Hodgkin's disease that revolutionized the treatment of this disease and led to substantial cure rates in patients with localized disease. With the knowledge that Hodgkin's disease spreads by lymphatic contiguity, three types of radiation fields were devised—namely, the mantle field, paraaortic field, and pelvic irradiation. The mantle field includes the submandibular, cervical, supraclavicular, infraclavicular, axillary, mediastinal, and hilar lymph nodes. The paraaortic field covers the transverse processes of the abdominal vertebral bodies and the spleen, if the spleen has not been removed. Pelvic irradiation includes the common iliac, hypogastric, external iliac, and inguinal nodes. When there is gross pelvic nodal involvement, the femoral nodes are also treated. Sometimes the pelvic and paraaortic fields are treated as one unit and it is commonly called the *inverted Y* field. The use of pelvic irradiation has been recently reduced since stages I and II supradiaphragmatic Hodgkin's disease can be treated without pelvic irradiation, and for stage III disease, total nodal irradiation has only a limited role. Patients now receive mantle and paraaortic irradiation and only rarely total nodal irradiation. Patients receive doses of 3600 to 4000 cGy with an additional "cone down" dose for a total of 4000 to 4400 cGy to areas of bulk disease.

Patients with localized nodal Hodgkin's disease (pathologic stages IA and IIA) treated with mantle or paraaortic radiation therapy have a nearly 80 percent long-term disease-free survival. Patients with stages IB and IIB have reduced disease-free survival; however, most patients who relapse can be successfully treated with optimal combination chemotherapy. Early-stage patients with large mediastinal involvement appear to have a higher risk of relapse (disease-free survival of 40 to 55 percent) compared to patients with lesser or no mediastinal disease and should be managed with combined modality therapy.

Radiation therapy can lead to acute and late complications. Acute side effects of mantle irradiation include transient dry mouth, pharyngitis, fatigue, and weight loss; rarely, patients may develop transverse myelitis 9 months to several years later. Approximately 15 percent of patients within several months of mantle irradiation develop paresthesias in the lower extremities upon flexion of the neck or thighs (Lhermitte's syndrome). This syndrome usually resolves spontaneously; there is no correlation between this syndrome and irreversible spinal injury. With more recent techniques, including shielding and angling, this syndrome is rarely seen. Other long-term side effects include radiation pneumonitis (severe in less than 5 percent of patients) and subsequent pulmonary fibrosis. Late complications of mantle radiation include cardiac damage such as pericardial effusion with or without subsequent constrictive pericarditis and very rarely myocardial damage. Cardiac irradiation may also accelerate coronary artery disease and induce early myocardial infarctions. Chemical hypothyroidism may occur in up to 50 percent of patients with mantle irradiation. Paraaortic irradiation is rarely associated with significant side effects. Pelvic irradiation acutely induces transient diarrhea and bladder irradiation association with frequency. Chronic effects include potential long-term bone marrow suppression and sterility; therefore pelvic irradiation is less frequently employed. Moreover, increasing numbers of secondary tumors are being observed.

Chemotherapy By 1963 five agents had been identified as effective in the treatment of Hodgkin's disease, namely alkylating agents, vinca alkaloids, procarbazine, methotrexate, and prednisone. While disease regression occurred in 30 to 70 percent of patients, complete response occurred in only 10 percent. Based on the principles of dose, schedule, and combination chemotherapy, a four-drug combination regimen termed MOPP, meaning mechlorethamine (nitrogen mustard), Oncovin (vincristine), procarbazine, and prednisone, was introduced. In a "14 year median follow-up" of 188 patients, DeVita and his colleagues found that 84 percent had achieved a complete remission and 48 percent were alive. MOPP therapy has been associated with significant toxicity. Nearly all patients experience some degree of nausea and vomiting, which can be minimized by antiemetic therapy. Bone marrow suppression and associated leukopenia and occasional thrombocytopenia are frequently observed. Less commonly, absolute neutropenia occurs with increased susceptibility to infection. All males and nearly all older females become sterile following MOPP therapy, and all patients have a long-term risk of developing second malignancies.

Other multiple-drug regimens have been tested in the treatment of advanced Hodgkin's disease. However, none of the MOPP-derived combinations have been superior to the original MOPP administered at an optimal dose and schedule. Regimens have also been developed to treat MOPP-resistant patients. The best known of these is ABVD (adriamycin, bleomycin, vinblastine, and dacarbazine). A series of controlled clinical trials has demonstrated that ABVD is equivalent to MOPP in the successful treatment of primary advanced Hodgkin's disease. ABVD has also led to a significant number of prolonged complete remissions in MOPP treatment failures. Although most ABVD toxicities are identical to those from MOPP, the ABVD regimen produces only transient germ-cell toxicity in males, no drug-induced amenorrhea, and an apparent lower incidence of second tumors (although the data on this point are limited).

More recent studies have attempted to sequentially combine MOPP and ABVD to improve cure rate. The use of MOPP alternating with ABVD appears to produce higher complete remissions and disease-free survivals compared to MOPP alone, but longer periods of observations and more patients are necessary to confirm this observation.

Combined modality therapy In the past, combined modality therapy has been extensively employed in the treatment of intermediate- and advanced-stage Hodgkin's disease. Many patients received both MOPP and total nodal irradiation. Unfortunately, serious late consequences occurred. The most serious of these is the emergence of second malignancies, particularly acute nonlymphocytic leukemia and high-grade lymphomas. In patients treated with MOPP alone (or with one of its variants), the risk of leukemia within 10 years is 3 to 4 percent. The risk seems to be greater in patients over 40 years at the time of systemic treatment or when combined modality therapy is used (especially if salvage MOPP is administered after radiotherapy failure). The acute nonlymphocytic leukemia that occurs following MOPP differs from primary acute nonlymphocytic leukemia in that the former more commonly exhibits a preleukemia or myelodysplastic prodrome, a different cytogenetic profile with emphasis on partial or complete deletions of the 5th and 7th chromosomes, and a much lower response rate to antileukemia therapy. A recent study revealed an 18 percent cumulative actuarial risk of second tumors in 15-year survivors with Hodgkin's disease, and the risk of solid tumors appeared to continue to increase with time.

Salvage therapy After proper restaging, further radiotherapy can be delivered (if technically feasible) to patients who have shown relapse in areas outside a radiation port or following combination chemotherapy. In patients not achieving a complete remission or relapsing after MOPP, second line, non-cross-resistant regimens are available. If patients relapse more than 12 months after the completion of MOPP therapy, they should be retreated; if they relapse in less than 12 months, they should be treated with a salvage regimen. With ABVD as a salvage regimen, 50 percent of patients will achieve a complete remission and 20 percent will experience long-term disease-free survival. Selected chemotherapy patients who relapse after 12 months in limited nodal or pulmonary sites can be treated with salvage radiotherapy. Finally, as with non-Hodgkin's lymphoma, autologous or allogeneic bone marrow transplantation is an effective salvage treatment for some patients. Unlike in non-Hodgkin's lymphoma, total-body irradiation has minimal value and virtually all regimens include high-dose chemotherapy. Patients whose tumors are still sensitive to chemotherapeutic agents are more likely to experience long-term disease-free survival.

THERAPEUTIC RECOMMENDATION BY STAGE Stages IA and IIA, nonbulky disease Following staging laparotomy in patients with supradiaphragmatic disease, subtotal nodal irradiation is the treatment of choice. Rarely, in patients with subdiaphragmatic lymphoma, radiotherapy is delivered by an inverted Y field, including splenic pedicle in stage I disease and ranging through total nodal irradiation in stage II disease. Some suggest that treatment with involved-field radiotherapy combined with chemotherapy produces comparable results, but most do not consider this as an accepted treatment. For patients with subdiaphragmatic stage II disease of paraaortics, chemotherapy is recommended.

Stages IB and IIB, nonbulky disease The therapy is the same as for stages IA and IIA Hodgkin's disease; however, the relapse rate is higher. Relapse can usually be salvaged with chemotherapy. Previous studies have demonstrated that total nodal irradiation cures 80 percent and MOPP 60 percent of these patients. The combination of total nodal irradiation and MOPP is capable of producing a higher cure rate but also produces a significant incidence of second tumors and therefore is no longer recommended. If radiotherapy to the pelvis is considered, bone marrow harvesting prior to treatment should be undertaken.

Stage II, bulky disease Stage II disease with bulky mediastinal or hilar adenopathy should be managed with combined modality therapy. This should include chemotherapy and radiotherapy to sites of bulk disease.

Stage IIIA Patients who present with minimal splenic disease respond equally well to subtotal lymphoid irradiation, combination chemotherapy with irradiation, or chemotherapy alone, with equivalent results. For patients with extensive splenic disease or enlarged paraaortic and pelvic nodes, the recommended treatment is combination chemotherapy with or without irradiation to involved sites. Alternative therapy includes either total nodal irradiation or combination chemotherapy, although these approaches are more controversial.

Stage IIIB, stage IV Combination chemotherapy is recommended, with alternatives including combination chemotherapy with irradiation to involved sites or alternating combination chemotherapy and irradiation.

REFERENCES

ANDERSON KC et al: Monoclonal antibodies: Their use in bone marrow transplantation. Prog Hematol XV: 137, 1987

ARMITAGE JO: Bone marrow transplantation in the treatment of patients with lymphoma. Blood 73(7):1749, 1989

CANELLOS GP (ed): Advances in chemotherapy for Hodgkin's and non-Hodgkins lymphomas. Semin Hematol, 25(2):1, 1988

COSSMAN J: T-cell neoplasms and Hodgkin's disease, in *Malignant Lymphoma,* CW Berard, RF Dorfman, N Kaufman (eds). Baltimore, Williams & Wilkins, 1987, pp 104–123

DEVITA VT JR et al: Lymphocytic lymphomas, in *Cancer: Principles and Practice of Oncology,* 3d ed, VT DeVita Jr, S Hellman, SA Rosenberg (eds). Philadelphia, Lippincott, 1989, pp 1741–1798

FREEDMAN AS, NADLER LM: Cell surface markers in hematologic malignancies. Semin Oncol 14(2):193, 1987

——— et al: Expression of B cell activation antigens on normal and malignant B cells. Leukemia 1:9, 1987

GRIBBEN JG et al: Successful treatment of refractory Hodgkin's disease by high-dose combination chemotherapy and autologous bone marrow transplantation. Blood 73(1):340, 1989

HELLMAN S et al: Hodgkin's disease, in *Cancer: Principles and Practice of Oncology,* 3d ed, VT DeVita Jr, S Hellman, SA Rosenberg (eds). Philadelphia, Lippincott, 1989, pp 1696–1740

KAPLAN HS: *Hodgkin's Disease,* 2d ed. Cambridge, Harvard University, 1980

KORSMEYER S: Immunoglobulin and T-cell receptor genes reveal the clonality, lineage, and translocations of lymphoid neoplasms, in *Important Advances in Oncology 1987,* VT DeVita Jr, S Hellman, SA Rosenberg (eds). Philadelphia, Lippincott, 1987, pp 3–26

SELTZER, SE, JOCHELSON MS (eds): Lymphoma, part I. Semin Ultrasound, CT, MR. 6(4):347, 1985

———, ———: Lymphoma, part II. Semin Ultrasound, CT, MR. 7(1):1, 1986

SHOWE LC, CROCE CM: Chromosomal translocations in B and T cell neoplasias. Semin Hematol 23(4):237, 1986

SKLAR JL et al: Diagnostic molecular biology of non-Hodgkin's lymphoma, in *Malignant Lymphoma,* CW Berard, RF Dorfman, N Kaufman (eds). Baltimore, Williams & Wilkins, 1987, pp 204–221

303 BREAST CANCER

CRAIG HENDERSON

Breast cancer is both one of the most common and one of the most treatable of all human malignancies. The incidence of this disease provides a poor estimate of the frequency with which breast problems are brought to the attention of physicians of all specialties. For each patient diagnosed with breast cancer, another 5 to 10 women are biopsied for suspicious symptoms, and for each patient biopsied, dozens seek consultation because of symptoms or concern. Breast cancer is one of the few tumors for which there is conclusive evidence that screening will substantially decrease mortality. In the treatment of breast cancer radical surgical procedures have been almost entirely replaced by more limited forms of surgery, such as the modified radical mastectomy, and most breast cancer patients now have the option of combining breast-sparing procedures (e.g., partial mastectomy or lumpectomy) with radiation therapy as an alternative to mastectomy. However, medical therapies are now an important component of the treatment of almost all stages of invasive breast cancer.

ETIOLOGY AND RISK FACTORS

Epidemiologic data suggest that genetic, endocrine, and environmental factors may be involved in the initiation and/or the promotion of breast cancer growth. Although the principal value of these studies is the identification of etiologic factors that may prove useful in primary prevention programs, epidemiologic data are often used to identify high-risk groups of women to be targeted for intensive surveillance or even prophylactic mastectomy. It has not been established, however, that these strategies will decrease breast cancer mortality in these high-risk groups, and an inappropriate emphasis on risk factors may obscure the fact that 70 to 80 percent of all breast cancers occur in patients without identifiable risk factors.

In the United States the cumulative lifetime probability of developing breast cancer is 10.2 percent and of dying from breast cancer, 3.6 percent. Most of the risk of developing breast cancer is expressed after age 50, and the highest risk is after age 75 (Table 303-1). In counseling women regarding their risk of developing breast cancer, the use of 20- to 40-year interval probabilities may be more meaningful than the lifetime probability. For example, the probability of a woman without defined risk factors developing breast cancer between the ages of 50 and 70 is 4.67 percent; that of dying from breast cancer is 1.04 percent. A patient with a relative risk of 3 (e.g., a woman whose mother and sister have been diagnosed with breast cancer) would then have a 14 percent probability of developing breast cancer and a 3.1 percent probability of dying from breast cancer during this interval. This likely explains why no risk group with an observed cumulative incidence of breast cancer in excess of 30 to 40 percent or cumulative mortality in excess of 10 to 20 percent has been identified.

Genetic factors Although all relatives of breast cancer patients are at some increased risk of developing breast cancer, first-degree relatives (siblings, parents, children) have a two- to threefold increase in risk compared to the general population. Thus, the cumulative probability that a 30-year-old woman whose sister or mother had breast cancer will herself develop breast cancer by age 70 is somewhere between 8 and 18 percent. Some investigators have observed an even higher risk when two or more relatives are affected, when the affected patient is premenopausal, or when the patient has bilateral breast cancer, but these observations have not been consistent among epidemiologic studies.

Endocrine factors Early age of menarche, late onset of menopause, nulliparity, and late age at first pregnancy appear to be independently associated with an increased incidence of breast cancer. Since both diet and exercise may affect both age of menarche and the regularity of menses, it has been suggested that this effect of diet and exercise may explain, at least in part, variations in breast cancer incidence among women with different lifestyles. Age at first full-term pregnancy is a more important determinant of risk than the number of pregnancies. Compared to women with a first pregnancy before age 18, the relative risk of breast cancer is doubled if the first pregnancy is delayed until after age 24 and about quadrupled after age 30. Several investigators have observed that the risk of breast cancer is actually higher among women with their first pregnancies after age 30 than among nulliparous women, and it has been suggested that early pregnancy is protective while late pregnancy may promote development of the disease. These observations are consistent with the hypothesis that events between menarche and the first pregnancy are critical in determining the lifetime probability of developing breast cancer.

The effect of exogenously administered hormones has been extensively studied with conflicting results. Although most studies on the effects of oral contraceptives have failed to establish a firm association with incidence of breast cancer, prolonged administration (e.g., 4 years or more), administration prior to the first pregnancy, and observation after a long latency period have been associated with a significantly increased risk in some studies. The reasons for the contradictory results are not readily apparent, and this is an issue about which physicians must suspend judgment until there are more definitive data. The results of studies on the use of estrogen replacement are also contradictory, but a review of all of the evidence suggests that there is a cumulative dose effect. A recently published prospective study of 23,244 Swedish women demonstrated that the relative risk of developing breast cancer was significantly increased to 1.7 after a little more than 9 years of therapy. The use of estrogens and progestins in sequence did not lessen the increased risk from estrogen use alone and may actually have augmented the risk and shortened the average latent interval. The use of conjugated estrogens, such as those most commonly used in the United States, may be associated with less risk than that following the use of estradiol, the major estrogen replacement therapy in the Swedish study. Although the effects of postmenopausal estrogen replacement on breast cancer incidence are substantially less than its effects on the incidence of endometrial cancer, moderate doses of conjugated estrogen for 15 to 20 years might increase the cumulative relative risk of breast cancer to 1.5 to 2.0.

Environmental factors Studies of atomic bomb blast victims in Hiroshima and Nagasaki demonstrate a radiation dose effect in the induction of breast cancer after a latent period of about 20 years. The highest incidence was observed among women who were aged 10 to 14 at the time of the explosion, and there was almost no increase in breast cancer incidence among women who were aged 30 to 49 at the time.

Breast cancer incidence varies widely around the world, and the highest rates occur in affluent and westernized countries. The lowest incidence is among Asians, but both immigrant and second-generation Japanese women migrating to Hawaii and southern California have an increasing risk of developing breast cancer with their greater longevity in the west. The search for environmental factors that might explain this phenomenon have centered on diet, and especially dietary fat. There is an excellent correlation between international variation in dietary fat intake and breast cancer incidence, and rats fed high-fat diets have a greater tendency to develop mammary tumors. However, epidemiologic studies have thus far failed to reproducibly

TABLE 303-1 Probability of a white female developing and dying of breast cancer

Age interval, years	Risk of developing breast cancer, %	Risk of dying of breast cancer, %
Birth to 110	10.20	3.60
20–30	0.04	0.00
20–40	0.49	0.09
35–45	0.88	0.14
35–55	2.53	0.56
50–60	1.95	0.33
50–70	4.67	1.04
65–75	3.17	0.43
65–85	5.48	1.01

SOURCE: From Seidman et al, CA 35:36, 1985.

demonstrate an association between dietary fat and the development of breast cancer. Postmenopausal women who are obese have an increased risk of breast cancer. Moderate alcohol intake has been repeatedly shown to be associated with an increased risk of 40 to 60 percent, but the explanation for this is not readily apparent. While points of circumstantial evidence linking environmental factors and breast cancer risk are numerous, none is sufficiently well-established to warrant strongly urging women to change their lifestyle in any particular way. Of course, recommendations to reduce dietary fat content and to maintain ideal body weight may be prudent because of their beneficial effects on other organ systems even if the benefits in reducing risk of breast cancer are minimal.

BENIGN BREAST DISEASE In general, a woman's risk of subsequently developing breast cancer after a biopsy that demonstrates benign disease is increased relative to the total population of women. The most common histologic diagnosis assigned to these biopsy specimens is "fibrocystic disease," a poorly defined term that implies the presence of macroscopic, fluid-filled cysts and a nonspecific proliferation of epithelial and mesenchymal tissue. This has led many physicians to equate all lumps and irregularities detected on physical examination or mammography with "fibrocystic disease," suggesting that the women examined are at increased risk of developing breast cancer. It has not been demonstrated that women with lumpy breasts who have *not* had a biopsy have an increased risk of breast cancer, and it is estimated that most women (probably more than 80 percent) have at least some irregular tissue densities on examination and/or mammography. For these reasons the diagnosis of "fibrocystic disease" should not be based on nonhistologic findings, and the term should probably be abandoned by pathologists as well because of its lack of specificity.

The increased risk of breast cancer among women with benign breast disease seems to be confined entirely to that group of women who have histologic evidence of ductal or lobular cell proliferation on biopsy (about 30 percent of all patients biopsied for benign conditions), and especially those who have atypical hyperplasia (about 3 percent of biopsied patients). The relative risk for developing breast cancer in this group is 4.4 times that of an age-matched population of unselected women. In women with both atypical hyperplasia and a first-degree relative with a history of breast cancer, the risk of subsequent breast cancer is increased about ninefold. Such patients are rare (representing about 1 percent of all biopsies for benign disease), and the *observed* cumulative risk of a patient in this very high risk group developing breast cancer over a 25-year period is about 40 percent; the cumulative risk of a woman in this group dying of breast cancer is less than 10 percent.

IN SITU BREAST CANCER There are two histologically and clinically distinct variants of carcinoma in situ (CIS): ductal and lobular. Traditionally, both were considered the earliest detectable form of malignant transformation in the breast, but increasingly lobular CIS (or lobular neoplasia) is viewed as a risk factor akin to atypical hyperplasia. Lobular CIS does not form a palpable tumor and is usually found as an incidental finding in a premenopausal woman biopsied for some other condition. Additional biopsies will usually demonstrate additional foci of lobular CIS in the same or even the contralateral breast, and any attempt to totally excise lobular CIS by any method other than mastectomy is likely to be ineffective. Patients who have no further treatment after a diagnosis of lobular CIS have an increased lifetime risk of subsequently developing an invasive breast cancer with either a ductal or a lobular histology. Without treatment, the cumulative incidence of a subsequent breast cancer of any type (invasive or ductal in situ) is about 25 percent and the cumulative mortality somewhat less than 10 percent. Most of these cancers occur after a latent period of 5 to 20 years and occur as often in the contralateral as in the biopsied breast. For this reason, most physicians now routinely offer these patients one of two treatment options: careful observation or bilateral simple mastectomies and breast reconstruction. A patient's choice between these two disparate options is likely to depend on the anxiety generated by her perception of the risk associated with observation.

Ductal CIS (or intraductal carcinoma) may form palpable tumors. It occurs with almost equal frequency in premenopausal and postmenopausal women and is more often confined to one breast, even to one quadrant of the breast. Thus, it is possible to excise this type of cancer totally by more limited surgical procedures than mastectomy. Until recently, ductal CIS was uncommon, accounting for only about 1 percent of all cancers diagnosed in the United States. However, ductal CIS is often the cause of microcalcifications seen in mammograms, and it is estimated that ductal CIS constitutes almost 10 percent of all breast cancers now diagnosed in the United States due to the increased use of routine mammography. Because these changes in incidence and mode of diagnosis are recent, it is not certain that the natural history of the ductal CIS now being diagnosed is the same as that observed in earlier eras. The diagnosis of ductal CIS may be difficult. At one extreme, it may be mistaken for atypical hyperplasia, and at the other, microscopic foci of invasion may be overlooked. Electron microscopy will reveal additional areas of invasion, and this may account for the fact that axillary lymph node metastases are seen in 1 to 2 percent of patients with a diagnosis of ductal CIS.

The natural history of ductal CIS in patients treated with less than a mastectomy has been less extensively studied than that of lobular CIS. These patients, too, are at increased risk of developing a subsequent invasive cancer throughout life, but, unlike lobular CIS, this risk is more often expressed in the ipsilateral than in the contralateral breast. For this reason, a simple (or total) mastectomy *without node dissection* is still the standard treatment for this condition and is associated with a nearly 100 percent long-term survival. However, in recent years, wide excision alone, especially for very small tumors, or wide excision plus radiotherapy for larger tumors has been used in patients whose tumors can be totally excised. Although the initial results from these breast-conserving approaches are promising, more definite statements regarding the relative value of these treatments await longer follow-up and the completion of randomized trials in the United States and Europe.

Subsequent risk for invasive cancer in the contralateral breast after mastectomy The group of patients with the highest risk of developing breast cancer are those who have already had one breast cancer. The risk is lifelong and occurs at a rate of 0.5 to 1.0 percent per year of follow-up. Concurrent cancers in both breasts are diagnosed in about 4 percent of patients. However, the prognosis of a patient with two breast cancers, whether concurrent or sequential, is not measurably worse than that of a patient with only one breast cancer. Since the cancer with the worst clinical and pathologic stage determines the patient's overall prognosis, patients with a good prognosis after an initial diagnosis should be monitored carefully to detect a second cancer, should it occur, as early as possible.

SCREENING ASYMPTOMATIC PATIENTS

It has been firmly established by two randomized trials that periodic mammography performed in asymptomatic women will reduce breast cancer mortality by 20 to 30 percent. The only trial with follow-up in excess of 10 years was performed by the Health Insurance Plan (HIP) of New York. Patients in the study group of this trial were invited to undergo *both* mammography and physical examination at yearly intervals. Most of the benefits in the HIP trial derived from the physical examination, but this is likely due to the fact that the mammography equipment used was insensitive by modern standards. In the first reports from the HIP study, survival benefits were observed only for women in the study group over age 50. A more recent analysis has demonstrated a 24 percent reduction ($p < 0.05$) in mortality for all age groups at the end of 18 years of follow-up. The benefits of mammography in women 50 or over have been confirmed in almost all trials performed subsequent to the HIP study, and if the evidence from *all* of the available trials is considered together, there *may* be a much smaller but real benefit from screening women aged 40 to 49, as well. It is widely assumed that the benefits of screening are proportional to the patient's risk of developing breast cancer and that patients with a family history of breast cancer, benign breast disease, or those who are nulliparous should be screened at a younger age. These assumptions have not been prospectively or retrospectively evaluated in any study. Although yearly mammography and physical examination were used in the HIP trial, a Swedish trial demonstrated benefits of a similar magnitude in women over 50 years of age who received mammograms without physical examinations at 2- to 3-year intervals. No one has yet demonstrated that mortality is reduced by the use of a baseline mammography at age 35 or 40, even though many physicians employ this as a "halfway" measure.

Although there is an increasing tendency for professional societies in the United States to recommend yearly mammography for all women over the age of 40, some groups, such as the American College of Physicians and most European health services, have been more cautious in their interpretation of the available data. Large but still unpublished randomized trials from Great Britain and Canada may further alter the recommendations of these groups. However, based on the available evidence, the following guidelines appear reasonable:

1. Women age 50 and over should undergo an annual or biennial screening examination utilizing both mammography and physical examination.
2. Mammography should generally not be used in women under age 35.
3. Women between the ages of 40 and 49 may elect to undergo periodic screening examinations, but they should be informed about the controversies regarding the use of mammography in this age group.
4. Although not yet of proven value, it seems reasonable to recommend periodic screening mammography to high-risk patients over age 35. Mammography, with or without periodic physical examination, remains the only diagnostic tool of proven value in asymptomatic women. Although real, the risk of radiation-induced cancers is very small and is far outweighed by the benefits in women age 50 or over and probably in those age 40 to 49 as well. Ultrasound will not detect microcalcifications, often the only indication of tumor and especially of very small tumors. Thermography results in an unacceptably high false-positive and false-negative rate and has not even been shown to be helpful in identifying patients who should undergo mammography. Cancers appearing in patients who perform regular (e.g., monthly) breast self-examination (BSE) are, on average, smaller than those in patients who do not do BSE. The only known toxicity of BSE is the increased anxiety it causes some women. However, all published BSE studies have large length and lead-time biases. These biases occur because apparent survival advantages for patients whose cancers have been found by BSE may be due to a longer clinical observation period from diagnosis to death, or to the fact that slower growing tumors are more often detected by BSE, and not due to any improved efficacy of therapy, because the tumor was diagnosed before the onset of metastasis when it is theoretically more curable. It has not yet been shown in properly controlled trials that BSE will actually decrease breast cancer mortality.

DIAGNOSIS AND INITIAL EVALUATION

More than 80 percent of cancers are diagnosed because of a suspicious mass, usually a mass found by the patient. Pain without an immediately apparent mass is a less frequent presenting symptom, and increasingly breast cancer is being diagnosed on a routine mammogram in a totally asymptomatic patient. Nipple discharge is also an unusual presenting symptom. Most nipple discharges, whether serous or sanguineous, are caused by benign disorders, most commonly an intraductal papilloma. A nipple discharge with a negative test for hemoglobin is almost always benign, but breast cancer is the cause of a hemoglobin-positive discharge in less than 10 percent of such patients.

Physical examination should begin with a visual inspection of the breast while the patient is sitting. An underlying breast cancer may cause a protrusion, asymmetry in breast contour, or a subtle dimpling of the skin due to entrapment of Cooper's ligaments. Recent onset of nipple inversion may also be a sign of breast cancer, but both nipple inversion and asymmetry of breast size are common findings in the normal breast. Palpation of the breast is best performed when the patient is in a supine position. Breast cancers are most often described as irregularly shaped, firm or hard, painless nodules or masses, but in fact they may be of almost any shape or consistency. For this reason, any mass, lesion, or thickening that is distinctly different from the surrounding tissue (or "dominant") should be evaluated more carefully. The most common nonmalignant finding on breast examination is a diffuse, indistinct, and somewhat elastic amalgamation of lumps often mistakenly referred to as "fibrocystic disease" (see above). Well-defined cysts may be quite distinct but have a more elastic character than breast cancer. Benign fibroadenomas are often as firm as breast cancer but can be distinguished by their marblelike smoothness and slippery quality, their appearance in young women, and their recurrent nature. Fat necrosis and sclerosing adenosis, both benign conditions, can usually be distinguished from breast cancer only by biopsy. If there are signs of more locally advanced growth, mastectomy and/or radiotherapy are unlikely to substantially prolong a patient's life. These signs include fixation of the mass to the skin, the pectoralis muscle, or the chest wall, the presence of satellite skin nodules or ulcerations, the finding of matted axillary nodes, or the presence of any supraclavicular lymph nodes. Plugging of the dermal lymphatics will cause skin thickening and exaggeration of the usual skin markings, a process termed *peau d'orange*. When this is extensive and accompanied by inflammation, the patient usually has inflammatory breast cancer, a particularly virulent form of cancer best treated initially with chemotherapy and radiotherapy. Inflammatory breast cancer may be mistakenly diagnosed initially as mastitis, but infections or other inflammatory conditions of the breast are rare except in the first months postpartum or after trauma.

Further evaluation of a suspected cyst might include a repeat examination of the breast immediately following the next menstrual period in a premenopausal woman, the use of ultrasound to confirm the impression that the mass is fluid-filled, or removal of the cyst fluid with a fine-gauge needle *and reexamination of the breast to document that the cyst has disappeared.* The latter is the preferred approach in a symptomatic patient because it will usually relieve the pain and the patient will be reassured that this is not cancer, unless the cyst fluid is grossly bloody or reaccumulates rapidly.

Mammography If breast examination leads to any suspicion that a mass is malignant, biopsy should be performed. Biopsy should be *preceded* by a mammogram, which may better define the extent of the lesion, demonstrate other suspicious masses, and serve as a baseline obtained before distortion of normal breast architecture by biopsy. Abnormalities on mammogram that suggest a breast cancer include: (1) distinct, irregular, often crablike densities (Fig. 303-1), (2) *clusters* of five or more microcalcifications, each less than 1 mm in diameter and all in an area of less than 1 cm (Fig. 303-2), or (3) architectural distortion without a benign explanation such as a scar from a prior biopsy. Although more than 80 percent of suspicious microcalcifications are benign, cancers associated with such microcalcifications are usually the most curable of all breast cancers. Diagnosis can be made by radiologic placement of needles under local anesthesia and subsequent biopsy of tissue surrounding the needle ends. The excised tissue should be x-rayed to ensure that the calcifications or other suspicious lesions have been removed, and/or

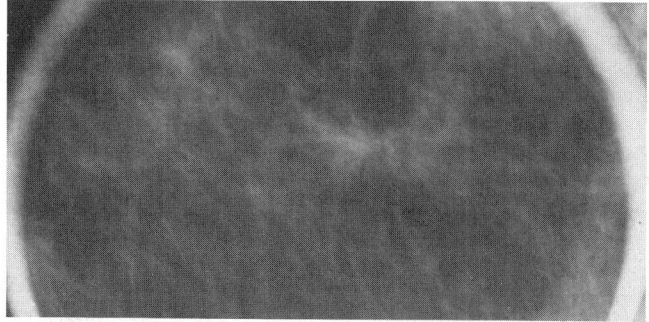

FIGURE 303-1 Focal compression mammogram shows a clinically occult 1-cm spiculated mass. Biopsy demonstrated infiltrating ductal breast cancer. *(Courtesy of Dr Paul Stomper.)*

the patient should have a repeat mammogram 4 to 6 weeks after biopsy when the breast is no longer tender.

In almost all instances, incisional or excisional biopsy of the breast may be performed under local anesthesia in a day surgery or an outpatient clinic, thus avoiding the additional risk of general anesthesia and permitting the patient to discuss and adjust to treatment options before undergoing definitive surgical treatment. Fine-needle aspiration and cytologic evaluation may also be diagnostic but is advisable *only* if an experienced cytologist is available and if all suspicious lesions read as negative are followed with a more definitive biopsy procedure. Tissue should be sent routinely for assay of estrogen and progesterone receptors. Additional staging procedures immediately following the diagnosis of breast cancer should include evaluation of those sites to which breast cancer most frequently metastasizes (see below).

NATURAL HISTORY AND PROGNOSTIC FACTORS

The natural history of breast cancer is characterized by long duration and marked heterogeneity. The median survival of patients who refuse all forms of treatment is between 2.5 and 3 years, but the survival of an untreated patient may exceed 20 years. Breast cancer is certainly among the more slowly growing tumors, and it has been estimated that the average tumor doubles about three times per year. If this applies to the preclinical (or prediagnostic) period of tumor growth, then the average breast cancer requires 10 years or more to grow from a single cell to 1 cm, the size at which it can be readily detected by most patients or physicians. Presumably metastases may occur during much of this preclinical period but likely with greatest frequency during the last 3 to 4 years of preclinical growth, when the tumor mass increases from 10^6 cells to more than 10^9 cells. Because microscopic or clinically undetectable micrometastases are well-established by the time of diagnosis, most breast cancer patients treated with local therapy only (i.e., surgery and/or radiotherapy) eventually die in spite of excellent local control of their disease. Because many patients' tumors metastasize late in the preclinical course, early detection with mammography will increase the patient's survival. Because the growth rate of the disease is so variable, comparisons of treatment effects in even well-defined patient cohorts are often erroneous unless the treatment groups have been defined by large, randomized controlled trials.

FIGURE 303-2 Mammogram shows a clinically occult 1-cm cluster of microcalcifications. Biopsy demonstrated infiltrating ductal breast cancer. *(Courtesy of Dr Paul Stomper.)*

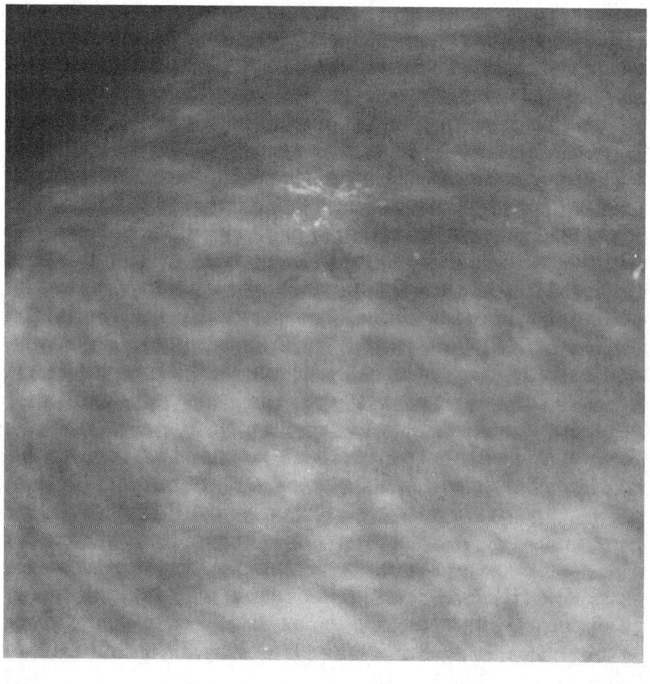

Clinical pathologic staging Clinical staging systems were developed by surgeons to identify *preoperatively* those patients unlikely to benefit from treatment with mastectomy. Although those with large tumor size and palpable axillary adenopathy were found to have a poorer long-term prognosis, the only patients categorically discouraged from undergoing mastectomy were those with signs of locally advanced disease (see above). About 25 to 35 percent of patients with axillary adenopathy will have no histologic evidence of tumor in lymph nodes, and the same percentage of patients without adenopathy *will* have histologic node involvement. Although information on histologic node involvement is of no value in deciding whether a patient should undergo mastectomy, this has proven to be the most accurate and reproducible prognostic factor worldwide. It is convenient to divide patients into three groups: those without node involvement, those with one to three positive nodes, or those with four or more positive nodes (Table 303-2). However, these divisions are arbitrary. A substantial number of node-negative patients will have recurrences and eventually die of breast cancer. Each additional positive node is associated with a worse prognosis, but some patients with more than 10 positive nodes will survive for 10 to 20 years or more. In general, the number of positive lymph nodes correlates with the time of recurrence as well as the probability of recurrence. For the data set shown in Table 303-2, the median time to recurrence was 2.1 years and the time to death 4 years for those patients with four or more positive nodes, compared to 4.1 years and >10 years, respectively, for those with one to three positive nodes. The hazard of recurrence decreased in all nodal subgroups after the first 3 years but remained fairly constant thereafter. This explains why the effects of therapy on recurrence rate, especially on recurrence in patients with many positive nodes, are apparent after a short follow-up, but the effects of therapy on survival may require much longer follow-up.

Patients with a larger breast mass or a higher clinical stage are more likely to have positive nodes, but within a single-node category the size of the breast cancer has independent prognostic value. This

TABLE 303-2 Ten-year survival and survival without recurrence relative to histologic node status at the time of radical mastectomy (no adjuvant systemic therapy given)

	Survival, %	
Node category	Overall	Without recurrence
All patients	60	47
Nodes negative	82	72
Nodes positive	40	25
1–3 nodes positive	54	34
4+ nodes positive	26	16

SOURCE: From Valagussa et al, CA 41:1170, 1978.

has led to the promulgation of staging systems that combine clinical and pathologic characteristics. However, these systems have changed so frequently and are used so differently by different specialists that the categorization of patients into one of four ''stages'' has lost all practical meaning. For example, a 3-cm tumor mass and no histologically involved lymph nodes is considered a stage II breast cancer, as is a 1-cm mass with eight positive nodes. Both the prognosis and the likely treatment of these two patients are substantially different. Therefore, a careful description of the patient's cancer, a precise measurement of tumor size, and a simple statement of the number of histologically positive lymph nodes will provide a more accurate description of ''stage'' than the use of stage numbers I to IV.

Histologic subtypes More than 80 percent of breast cancers are of the invasive ductal type. The next most common variety, infiltrating lobular, constitutes almost 10 percent of all cancers and has the same prognosis as infiltrating ductal carcinoma. Medullary carcinoma, representing about 5 percent of breast cancers, is less likely to metastasize to regional lymph nodes, but the prognosis of medullary cancers with nodal metastases is the same as that of the other major histologic groups with nodal metastases. The large number of histologic types that make up the remaining 5 percent of breast cancers are generally less malignant.

Tumor grade, defined by the degree of differentiation of cytoplasmic or nuclear features, has been shown repeatedly to correlate with the probability of recurrence or death from breast cancer. Other histologic characteristics that may be important include blood vessel or intramammary lymphatic vessel invasion, mitotic frequency, lymph node sinus histiocytosis, and tumor necrosis. However, the major limitation in the use of tumor histologic features is a lack of reproducibility from one pathologist to another, especially when the pathologist has not been specifically trained and is not very experienced in the use of these grading systems. For this reason, tumor grade is generally not used to make therapeutic decisions.

Estrogen receptors Tumors with an estrogen or progesterone receptor are more likely to respond to endocrine therapy used either as an adjuvant to mastectomy or radiotherapy soon after diagnosis or as a means of palliating metastatic disease symptoms later in a patient's course. In addition, most studies have demonstrated a significantly better disease-free survival and/or overall survival during the first 10 years of follow-up for patients who have one of these receptors. However, neither the estrogen nor the progesterone receptor identifies the 20 to 30 percent of node-negative patients likely to have recurrence, and at the end of 5 years, the difference in the recurrence rate among estrogen receptor–positive and –negative patients who are also node-negative is only about 5 percent.

Flow cytometry, ploidy, oncogenes The percentage of tumor cells undergoing mitosis has been shown in a number of experimental systems to be proportional to the growth fraction (i.e., the percentage of the tumor actually growing at any one point in time) and hence to the growth rate. This growth fraction can be estimated by thymidine labeling and autoradiography to obtain a thymidine labeling index (TLI) or by flow cytometry to estimate the fraction of cells in S phase (SPF). Clinical correlations have shown that a high TLI or high SPF is associated with early relapse and earlier breast cancer death, even after correction for other prognostic factors, such as lymph node and estrogen receptor status. However, as with other prognostic factors, these methods do not define distinct groups of patients, and, even though many clinical laboratories now routinely perform flow cytometry along with receptor determinations, there is still no standardization of methodology or established range of values associated with a particularly good or particularly poor prognosis. In general, patients with aneuploid tumors will have a worse prognosis than patients with predominantly diploid tumors, but early differences in relapse rate are not large, especially among node-negative patients.

Multiple genetic alterations have been described in breast cancers, including allelic deletions on chromosome 11 or 13 and amplification of the c-*myc* and *int*-2 genes. However, the most extensively studied is the amplification of the HER-2/*neu* (or c-*erb*B-2) gene. Some, but not all, studies have demonstrated a better survival among node-positive patients without amplification of this gene. The clinical importance of this relatively new area of study remains to be demonstrated, and the biologic importance of any of the known prognostic factors is still largely unexplored.

LOCAL THERAPY OF OPERABLE BREAST CANCER

Breast cancers are usually considered ''operable'' if it is technically possible to remove all cancerous tissue, if the tumor does not involve or has not become fixed to skin or structures deep to the breast, and if the tumor has not metastasized beyond the axillary or internal mammary lymph nodes. It has been demonstrated repeatedly in randomized clinical trials that more extensive surgical procedures will reduce the subsequent likelihood of tumor recurrence on the chest wall, in any remaining breast tissue, or in the nodal areas. However, these trials have failed to demonstrate that the type of surgery used will significantly affect patient survival. The evidence that local therapy has any effect on patient survival comes from the randomized trials of screening mammography (see above), in which it has demonstrated that early mastectomy results in a lower breast cancer mortality than late mastectomy.

The most extensive surgical procedure is the *radical mastectomy*, in which the breast is removed along with the pectoralis major and minor muscles and some overlying skin (at least 4 cm on each side of the tumor biopsy site), and there is an en bloc resection of all axillary contents, including lymph nodes beyond the subclavian vein. An *extended radical mastectomy* includes, as well, en bloc resection of the internal mammary nodes along with portions of the sternum and ribs. Because of the large cosmetic defect resulting from these procedures, neither is commonly used today, and it is doubtful whether their use is ever indicated, since the same or better local control of disease can be achieved with the use of radiotherapy added to less extensive surgical procedures. Most forms of the modified radical mastectomy leave the pectoralis major muscle intact, require the removal of less skin, and usually involve a less extensive node dissection. A *simple* or *total mastectomy* is the removal of the breast and a small amount of skin, but a simple mastectomy with node dissection approximates a modified radical mastectomy. Breast-conserving surgical procedures include wide excision, lumpectomy or tylectomy (Greek *tylos* = lump), segmental mastectomy, and quadrantectomy. These all require removal of the mass along with some normal surrounding tissue and differ only in the extent of the tissue excised. A separate excision for either a ''sampling'' of lymph nodes or a more complete lymph node dissection is possible with all of these procedures.

Radiotherapy When administered after a mastectomy, radiotherapy is usually referred to as ''adjuvant,'' while radiotherapy given after breast-conserving surgery is often called ''primary'' radiotherapy. Adjuvant radiotherapy is less commonly used now than it once was because it was not possible to demonstrate in multiple randomized trials that its use prolonged survival. In addition, a small but statistically significant increase in mortality from second tumors and/or cardiovascular disease has been reported in patients who survived more than 10 to 15 years after receiving adjuvant radiotherapy. However, this finding was observed primarily in patients treated with now-outdated radiotherapy techniques.

When breast-conserving therapy is used, the resection margins ideally should be microscopically free of tumor before radiotherapy is given. Usually 4500 to 5000 cGy is administered in divided fractions over about 5 weeks. The same doses of radiotherapy may be administered to the axillary, supraclavicular, and internal mammary nodes, and a boost of 1600 to 1800 cGy may be added to the tumor bed. The treatment of axillary nodal areas and the use of a boost is variable and depends on the tumor characteristics of an individual patient and the treatment philosophy of the radiotherapist. When all areas are treated, ''primary'' radiotherapy is as extensive as the radical mastectomy, and local tumor control is as good or better.

The choice between breast-conserving surgery plus radiotherapy and mastectomy will depend on the patient's assessment of the relative benefits and side effects associated with each procedure. The only real advantage of breast-conserving procedures is the greater sense of body integrity and improved cosmesis that may result. This advantage may be lost if the tumor mass is large relative to the size of the breast, thus necessitating almost total removal of the breast to obtain tumor-free margins. Under the best of circumstances the cosmetic results of limited surgery plus radiotherapy are excellent, and the treated breast may feel entirely normal and appear indistinguishable from the contralateral breast. More often the treated breast will be somewhat smaller with limited induration around the biopsy site; uncommonly (in less than 5 percent of patients) there will be marked induration, breast shrinkage, and distortion of normal breast architecture. Other complications from radiotherapy, including broken bones, brachial plexopathy, and pneumonitis, are uncommon and rarely either cause symptoms or are the source of more than transient symptomatology. There may be a subgroup of patients who have a relatively high recurrence rate (23 percent by the end of 5 years) if treated with breast-conserving surgery and radiotherapy. The histologic appearance of the tumors in these patients is characterized by extensive intraductal carcinoma in *both* the area of invasive carcinoma and adjacent tissues ostensibly free of invasive carcinoma. Although a small intraductal component in an invasive carcinoma is normal, the intraductal component comprises more than 25 percent of all tumor tissue in these patients and appears to be a marker of a tumor likely to be multifocal throughout the breast. Very limited data suggest that patients who have recurrences some years after initial surgery and radiotherapy with tumor confined entirely to the breast or breast and regional lymph nodes may be successfully treated with a secondary mastectomy and that this type of recurrence may not compromise survival.

Breast-conserving surgery *without* radiotherapy is generally not used because of the very high likelihood of local recurrence. In the only randomized trial addressing this issue, patients with tumor-free resection margins who were treated with segmental mastectomy alone had a local recurrence rate of 28 percent at the end of 5 years, compared to 8 percent for patients treated with segmental mastectomy plus radiotherapy. At the end of nearly a decade of follow-up, the survival of patients in these three groups is not significantly different.

Breast reconstruction Many patients will prefer mastectomy because it requires a shorter period of initial treatment and provides the patient with an added assurance that ''all the tumor has been removed.'' Psychological studies demonstrate that most mastectomy patients have fully recovered from the initial emotional trauma of mastectomy by the end of 1 year. Many patients feel that their lives are simplified and their sense of body integrity restored by surgical reconstruction of the breast. This may be performed at the time of mastectomy or many years later. The procedures used include simple placement of a submuscular (or less commonly, subcutaneous) silicon implant, the use of a tissue expander followed by silicon implant, the transposition of muscle and blood supply from either the back of abdomen using the latissimus dorsi or the lower rectus abdominis muscle (TRAM flap), or the creation of a free tissue flap using the gluteus maximus muscle anastomosed to the internal mammary vessels. The choice among these procedures will depend on the extent of the patient's prior surgery and radiotherapy, the patient's willingness to undergo additional surgical procedures, and the experience and philosophy of the plastic surgeon. Under the best of circumstances the reconstructed breast will appear to be exactly the same size and shape as the contralateral breast, but, in addition to reconstruction of a nipple, this may require mammoplasty on the contralateral breast and several surgical procedures.

Node dissection The main purpose of lymph node dissection is diagnostic, not therapeutic (see above). However, the morbidity associated with treatment of the lymph nodes is greater than with any other aspect of local therapy. Even with a limited node sampling or node dissection limited to levels I and II (i.e., the areas medial and inferior to the subclavian muscle), the patient often will complain of lifelong discomfort, hyperesthesia or hypalgesia, and/or a sense of pulling and contraction. When more extensive surgery is used, when the radiotherapy field includes the upper axilla, and especially when both modalities are used, these symptoms increase in frequency and severity. Patients may experience edema of the arm and hand, and on rare occasions the patient may totally lose use of the involved extremity. For this reason a full node dissection, as employed in the radical mastectomy, followed by radiotherapy, is usually contraindicated, and whenever possible surgical excision should be limited to lower nodes and radiotherapy to this area avoided altogether.

Summary recommendations for local therapy All patients with invasive operable breast cancer should receive some form of local therapy. In most cases this will be either a modified radical mastectomy (simple mastectomy plus node dissection) or breast-conserving surgery and limited node dissection followed by radiotherapy to the breast. Ideally, the patient will participate in the choice between these treatment alternatives and will see both a surgeon and a radiotherapist in the process of self-education regarding the benefits and limitations of these approaches.

ADJUVANT SYSTEMIC THERAPY

The use of systemic therapy, either chemotherapy or endocrine therapy, immediately after or as an ''adjuvant'' to local therapy will prolong the average time to recurrence of all patient groups. In addition, it has been reproducibly shown that the appropriate use of these therapies will significantly prolong the *survival* of some groups. Although theoretically possible, it has not yet been demonstrated that these therapies will ''cure'' any patient or group of patients not cured by local therapy alone.

An overview or meta-analysis of the large number of randomized adjuvant therapy trials has demonstrated that the use of adjuvant chemotherapy for some period in excess of 3 months will reduce a patient's odds of dying in the first 5 years after diagnosis by 14 ± 4 percent ($p = 0.003$). Although treatment prolongs the time to recurrence in women aged 50 and over as well as in those under age 50, adjuvant chemotherapy significantly improves survival only in those under 50 years of age. Among these younger women the odds of dying in the first 5 years may be reduced by 22 to 37 percent, and at the end of 5 years the survival of younger women given adjuvant chemotherapy was 7 to 9 percent higher than that of the control groups. The most commonly used and the most effective therapies in these studies were combinations that included cyclophosphamide, methotrexate, and 5-fluorouracil (CMF) (Table 303-3).

Adjuvant tamoxifen given for 1 year or more reduces the odds of death in the first 5 years after diagnosis by 16 ± 3 percent ($p <$

TABLE 303-3 Dose schedules of the drug regimens and endocrine therapies most frequently used to treat early and advanced breast cancer

Drug	Dose schedule
CMF(P) (28-day cycle)	
Cyclophosphamide	100 mg/m² PO days 1–14
Methotrexate	60 mg/m² IV days 1 and 8
5-Fluorouracil	600 mg/m² IV days 1 and 8
Prednisone (optional)	40 mg/m² PO days 1–14
CAF (21-day cycle)	
Cyclophosphamide	400–500 mg/m² IV day 1
Doxorubicin	40–50 mg/m² IV day 1
5-Fluorouracil	400–500 mg/m² IV days 1 and 8
Tamoxifen	10 mg PO bid
Megestrol acetate	40 mg PO qid
Aminoglutethimide	250 mg PO bid
+ hydrocortisone	10 mg PO qid

0.00001). However, when analyzed by age group, a significant survival benefit has been observed only in women aged 50 or more, where the reduction in the odds of death is 20 percent. At the end of 5 years the survival advantage for older, tamoxifen-treated women is about 6 percent. When tamoxifen was given from 2 to 5 years in these studies, it appeared to be more effective than when the duration of therapy was limited to 1 year.

Net benefit calculations There is no evidence that a patient who dies of breast cancer after mastectomy or radiotherapy has lived longer as a result of this local therapy. The patient is either cured or dies at about the same time she would have died without therapy. In contrast, systemic therapy may prolong life without curing the patient because systemic therapy causes a substantial but usually incomplete reduction in the size of tumor deposits at various metastatic sites. It is often erroneously assumed that a 10 percent survival advantage for the group of patients treated with adjuvant therapy means that *only* 10 percent of the patients have benefitted from therapy. In fact, the same survival difference between the treated and untreated patients can be obtained if *all* of the treated patients have a variable and transient prolongation of survival.

Calculation of the "average" size of this survival benefit requires long follow-up, and there is as yet no standard method for defining this average. However, it may be crudely estimated by subtracting the median survival of the patients randomized to the control group of a trial from the median survival of the treated group. When this is done for the premenopausal, node-positive patients randomized to receive 1 year of adjuvant CMF, the difference in median survivals exceeds 3 years, at least in one of the trials with the longest follow-up (the Milan trial). Of course, there is likely a wide range of effects around this average. Some patients may have had their lives shortened because of the toxicity of adjuvant chemotherapy. Some may have lived several decades longer as a result of treatment. The same calculations have been performed with data from a Scottish trial in which mostly postmenopausal, node-positive women were randomized to receive either 5 years of adjuvant tamoxifen or tamoxifen as first systemic therapy on relapse. The difference in median survival favored the treated patients and was just short of 2 years.

Most of these therapies, especially adjuvant chemotherapy, have well-known acute side effects and less well-defined delayed effects (see below). For this reason a real but small benefit may be outweighed by the toxicity of therapy. The expression of benefits as additional years of life eases this problem. For example, a premenopausal node-positive patient might subtract months during which CMF is administered (now usually about 6 months) and during which she experiences the toxicity of therapies from the 3 or more additional years of life gained from therapy to derive a "net" benefit of 2.5 or more years.

Node-negative patients Most of the early adjuvant trials included primarily or exclusively node-positive patients. However, since 20 to 30 percent of node-negative patients relapse and die of breast cancer in the first 10 years after diagnosis (Table 303-2), recent studies have included large numbers of node-negative patients, especially patients perceived as having the worst prognosis. Almost all of these trials demonstrate that adjuvant chemotherapy and adjuvant tamoxifen prolong the average time to recurrence of node-negative patients, but none of the large and more definitive trials has yet demonstrated a survival benefit. However, the interpretations of these trials are complicated by several additional considerations. Most node-positive patients eventually relapse and die of breast cancer, and therefore most node-positive patients will *potentially* benefit from adjuvant therapy. This is less true for node-negative patients, many of whom will be cured with local therapy and who will suffer the toxicities of therapy with no potential benefit. Further, the patients included in these trials had a higher relapse rate than that observed in previous studies of node-negative patients, suggesting that either previous studies have underestimated the virulence of breast cancer in node-negative patients or that the node-negative patients included in these adjuvant trials are not representative of all node-negative patients. The follow-up on these node-negative trials is still short, and it will be several years before the size of a survival benefit, if any, can be estimated or a cost-benefit analysis performed. Since the risk of death is smaller and peaks later after diagnosis among node-negative than among node-positive patients, the size of the survival benefit may be smaller and the importance of delayed side effects proportionally greater. Conversely, if node-negative patients have smaller micrometastatic tumor deposits, adjuvant therapy, and especially adjuvant chemotherapy, may cure some portion of these patients. The precise role of adjuvant therapy in node-negative patients will be uncertain for some years yet, and its use now requires mature clinical judgment and a well-informed patient.

Principles for the selection of an adjuvant chemotherapy regimen Combinations of drugs, such as CMF, are somewhat more effective than single agents, such as melphalan. Short durations of therapy in the range of 4 to 6 months have been shown to be as effective as more prolonged durations, such as 12 to 24 months. The optimal drug combination, dose, and schedule of the commonly used cytotoxic agents are not well defined, and it has not been reproducibly demonstrated that the use of tamoxifen or oophorectomy with chemotherapy will provide a substantial or significant survival benefit for premenopausal women or that the addition of chemotherapy to tamoxifen will be more effective than tamoxifen alone for postmenopausal women. Adjuvant systemic therapy is usually initiated as soon as possible after the completion of local therapy, and it has been argued, largely on theoretical grounds and from uncontrolled clinical observations, that adjuvant chemotherapy should be given before definitive surgery ("neoadjuvant," "protoadjuvant," or "primary chemotherapy"). However, in a large, randomized study, chemotherapy begun 1 month after surgery was as effective as chemotherapy begun within 36 h.

Principles for the use of adjuvant endocrine therapy Although there are theoretical reasons why longer durations of tamoxifen therapy might be more effective, there are no published data from randomized trials evaluating different durations of tamoxifen therapy. The survival benefits were most certain in two studies, one utilizing a 2-year and the other a 5-year course of therapy. Two British studies have suggested that estrogen receptor measurements do not define a group of patients who derive no benefit at all from adjuvant therapy, but no one outside of Great Britain has systematically looked for or observed a benefit from adjuvant tamoxifen in patients with receptor-negative tumors. Since the British observations are inconsistent with the well-documented role of these receptors in mediating tamoxifen effects, they should probably be viewed skeptically until further clinical trial data are available.

A series of randomized ovarian ablation trials conducted between 1948 and 1970 were interpreted *at that time* as providing insufficient survival benefit to justify the routine use of this form of endocrine therapy. However, these studies were conducted prior to the discovery of the estrogen receptor, and new trials evaluating ovarian ablation with luteinizing hormone–releasing hormone agonists have been initiated. The use of ovarian ablation in place of or in addition to chemotherapy for premenopausal women should await the completion of these studies.

Summary recommendations for adjuvant systemic therapy Premenopausal, node-positive patients should routinely receive some form of adjuvant therapy after completion of local therapy. If a formal trial is unacceptable to the patient, 6 months of therapy with CMF might be considered standard. Postmenopausal, node-positive, receptor-positive patients should routinely receive tamoxifen for 2 to 5 years, either as part of a formal protocol or independent of any ongoing trial. There is at present no established role for adjuvant systemic therapy in patients with in situ breast cancer or those with very small, node-negative tumors, especially those that are impalpable (e.g., found only on mammography or diagnosed with needle localization) or those that are minimally invasive. The treatment of other groups of patients should be undertaken only after full consideration of the limitations in our knowledge regarding survival benefits and delayed toxicities.

TREATMENT OF DISTANT METASTASES

Breast cancer can and frequently does metastasize to almost every organ in the body, but most commonly to skin, lymph nodes, lungs, liver, and bones. More than 10 percent of patients with any metastases will have CNS metastases at some point in the course of the disease, and new onset of frequent headache, personality change, otherwise unexplained vomiting, or localized neurologic dysfunction should lead to a prompt evaluation that includes a head CT scan (or MRI) and cytocentrifuge examination of cerebrospinal fluid. Isolated metastases to the leptomeninges are not uncommon, and visual disturbances may be due to breast cancer metastatic to the choroid. Choroid metastases can usually be seen on funduscopic examination. Breast cancer not infrequently metastasizes to the ovary and adrenal gland, and metastases to the abdomen may mimic ovarian cancer with diffuse peritoneal studding and the development of ascites. Metastases to the skin may occur anywhere and commonly appear on the scalp. A standard evaluation for metastases might include a complete blood count, platelet count, liver function studies, chest x-ray, bone scan, and marker study such as the carcinoembryonic antigen (CEA) and CA15-3 in addition to the investigation of specific signs and symptoms.

CHOOSING AMONG THERAPIES Breast cancer recurrences, even recurrences in the skin or the chest wall or along the mastectomy scar, represent bloodborne metastases and are *never* truly isolated recurrences. Other organs will eventually manifest disease, and the time interval from the first recurrence to the second will be roughly *proportional* to the interval from primary diagnosis to the appearance of the first metastasis, usually referred to as the disease-free interval (DFI). Although the treatment of metastases may prolong median survival by some months and have a profound effect on the survival of a few patients, the major value of treatment for metastatic disease is palliation of symptoms. Surgery and radiotherapy are more certain to shrink disease and palliate symptoms in a given area than systemic therapies. Systemic therapies are more likely to achieve long-term control of the disease throughout the body. Metastases to the brain and the choroid of the eye are almost always treated with radiotherapy. A local recurrence to the chest wall without evidence of distant disease might reasonably be treated with radiotherapy if the DFI is long. Malignant pleural effusions are best treated with complete chest tube drainage followed by sclerosis because the effusion may not clear even in a patient whose disease is otherwise responding to chemotherapy or endocrine therapy. The pain from bone metastases may be relieved by either systemic therapy or radiotherapy, but in a patient with multiple lesions or a short DFI an initial course of systemic therapy is preferred, since all lesions will be affected by the systemic therapy. If the bone cortex is severely eroded, a surgical approach with placement of stabilizing rods may be preferred since there is a long period of decreased tensile strength in a bone even after a response to radiotherapy or systemic therapy.

The median survival of all patients with metastatic breast cancer exceeds 2.5 years, and most patients will reach several, and some patients more than a dozen, decision points when treatment should or could be offered. Patients given extensive radiotherapy to bone metastases may not tolerate chemotherapy because of the effect of the radiotherapy on the bone marrow. Patients given chemotherapy may not benefit from endocrine therapy administered secondarily. There is no evidence that the treatment of asymptomatic metastases significantly prolongs survival, and a physician or patient may decide to hold therapy for some period of time both to avoid the toxicity of therapy and to better assess the pace of disease. An asymptomatic but anxious patient who wishes to "do something" might explore the use of new or more experimental therapies first and hold therapies with known efficacy in reserve.

Endocrine therapy versus chemotherapy The patient most likely to respond to endocrine therapy is one with an estrogen and/or progesterone receptor, a long DFI, disease limited to soft tissues (e.g., lymph nodes, breast, skin) or bone as opposed to viscera, and a prior documented response to endocrine therapy. The ideal patient for chemotherapy is anyone who is symptomatic and who is deemed a poor candidate for endocrine therapy. About two-thirds of all patients respond to chemotherapy. Although only one-third of unselected patients respond to endocrine therapy, two-thirds of patients with positive receptors and/or others of the characteristics listed above will respond to endocrine therapy. There is no evidence that a response to chemotherapy will occur more rapidly. The median duration of response to endocrine therapy, about 12 to 13 months, is somewhat longer than that to chemotherapy, about 9 to 12 months, but this likely reflects differences in the responding patient populations. Patients on either therapy may, on occasion, continue to respond for more than a decade. The choice between these two modalities will depend on the relative probability of benefit for an individual patient based on that patient's clinical characteristics.

ENDOCRINE THERAPY Patients who respond to one endocrine therapy frequently respond to a second, often to a third, and on occasion even to a fourth or fifth sequential endocrine manipulation. Patients who fail to respond at all are not likely to benefit from additional endocrine therapy. There is little difference in the efficacy of various forms of endocrine therapy, and for this reason, the least toxic therapy is usually used first. For postmenopausal women this is tamoxifen (Table 303-3); for premenopausal women it might be either tamoxifen or ovarian ablation by surgery or radiation. After response and progression of disease, a postmenopausal woman might be treated with either a progestin, such as megestrol acetate or medroxyprogesterone acetate, or aminoglutethimide plus hydrocortisone (Table 303-3).

Side effects of endocrine therapy More than 90 percent of patients treated with tamoxifen have no side effects at all. Others experience mild nausea that subsides after several weeks to a month, a flare reaction, menstrual disturbances if premenopausal, or hot flashes. The delayed side effects of tamoxifen, especially in patients receiving adjuvant tamoxifen, are still largely unknown. Preliminary evidence suggests that tamoxifen may decrease heart disease and osteoporosis while increasing the incidence of uterine cancer. Patients usually find weight gain due to increased appetite and fluid retention the most disturbing side effect of progestin therapies.

More than 10 percent of patients with metastatic breast cancer will experience hypercalcemia at some point in the course of their disease. Often this occurs soon after the initiation of endocrine therapy as part of a "flare." In addition to hypercalcemia, this syndrome is characterized by a sudden increase in bone pain, erythema around skin lesions, an increase in the number and intensity of lesions on bone scan, and an elevation of serum markers such as CEA and CA15-3. These signs and symptoms appear within hours to a few weeks after beginning endocrine therapy and subside by the end of a month. Unless hypercalcemia is life-threatening [calcium $\geq$ 3.5 mmol/L (14 mg/dL)], endocrine therapy should be continued and the underlying symptoms treated with pain medications, fluids, diuretics, and standard regimens for hypercalcemia (see Chap. 340).

CHEMOTHERAPY Although breast cancer responds to a long list of cytotoxic agents, three, and possibly four, appear to be especially effective and non-cross-resistant with each other: cyclophosphamide (C), doxorubicin (A, Adriamycin), mitomycin C, and vinblastine. Combinations of these drugs with each other and/or with methotrexate (M) and 5-fluorouracil (F) induce higher response rates and marginally improved survival compared to serial treatment with single agents. The most popular combinations are CMF, CMF plus prednisone, and CAF (Table 303-3). There is no evidence that survival is substantially improved by prolonged administration of these drugs, but the results of one randomized trial suggest that both response rate and quality of life are improved by some duration in excess of 3 months. A reduction of drug doses below those shown in Table 303-3 is likely to be associated with a lower response rate, but there is as yet no evidence of substantial benefit from exceeding these doses either. The use of very high dose therapy with autologous bone marrow support is an innovative therapy not yet proven to be beneficial in prolonging survival or improving quality of life.

Side effects of chemotherapy Although the acute side effects of chemotherapy often seem formidable, it has been repeatedly demonstrated in randomized trials that the efficacy of a regimen is a more important determinant of net quality of life than the side effects of treatment for patients with symptomatic, metastatic breast cancer. All of these drugs cause dose-related myelosuppression, thrombocytopenia, and, over some months, anemia. Gastrointestinal toxicity may include everything from mild nausea to protracted vomiting, severe mucositis, and diarrhea. Both myelosuppression and gastrointestinal toxicity are mitigated by the addition of prednisone to the regimen. Alopecia may be mild and gradual in onset with the use of CMF or abrupt and total with doxorubicin combinations. Doxorubicin cardiomyopathy occurs with increasing frequency after cumulative doses in excess of 450 mg/m^2 body weight have been given. All of these agents, and especially the alkylating agents, such as cyclophosphamide, are potential carcinogens, but it is still too early to fully assess the incidence of second tumors in patients given adjuvant chemotherapy.

SPECIAL PROBLEMS

Male breast cancer occurs with less than 1 percent of the frequency of female breast cancer. Predisposing risk factors include states of hyperestrogenism, such as Klinefelter's syndrome, schistosomiasis, a family history of breast cancer, and radiation exposure. Gynecomastia, in itself, is not an established risk factor (see Chap. 323). In other respects male breast cancer is nearly identical to female breast cancer with a similar prognosis, stage per stage. The primary lesion is usually treated with mastectomy since most men are not concerned with saving the breast. There are no data from controlled trials regarding the use of adjuvant systemic therapy for men, but the treatment of metastatic disease is nearly identical.

Cystosarcoma phylloides is a rare tumor more closely related to either benign fibroadenoma, from which it apparently arises in most cases, or sarcoma. It metastasizes in less than 5 percent of cases, but the local recurrence rate may exceed 20 percent, especially if it is treated inadequately. Treatment of the benign variety of cystosarcoma phylloides consists of wide excision, for the malignant variety, wide excision or simple mastectomy. Node dissection is rarely indicated.

Paget's disease of the nipple is often mistaken initially for a simple eczema and treated with glucocorticoids. However, a crusting, eroding, or scaling nipple lesion that does not respond promptly to conservative therapy should be biopsied. Histologically, Paget's disease is characterized by noninvasive or minimally invasive tumor cells growing on the undersurface of the nipple. In some cases there will be no other tumor in the breast, and some physicians now treat apparently localized disease with wide excision. However, in over half of the cases a mass will be found deep within the breast, in which case the prognosis and treatment of Paget's disease will depend on the size of the mass and the presence of involvement. The majority of the patients with Paget's disease will be treated like any other breast cancer patient.

Breast cancer is particularly difficult to diagnose and treat when it occurs *during pregnancy,* but stage per stage the prognosis approximates that of patients diagnosed in a nonpregnant state. There is no evidence that therapeutic abortion improves the prognosis. Mastectomy can be performed in the second and third trimesters, and chemotherapy has been given in the third trimester without observed damage to the fetus. *Pregnancy 2 years or more after diagnosis of breast cancer* is not associated with a higher recurrence rate or shortened survival, and counselling women regarding the advisability of pregnancy depends more on the patient's feelings regarding the possibility of not being able to see her child reach adulthood than about any potential risk to the patient from the pregnancy.

REFERENCES

General, natural history, prognostic factors

HARRIS JR, HENDERSON IC: Natural history and staging of breast cancer, in *Breast Diseases*, JR Harris et al (eds). Philadelphia, Lippincott, 1987, pp 233–258

HENDERSON IC et al: Breast Cancer, in *Cancer: Principles and Practice of Oncology*, VT DeVita Jr et al (eds). Philadelphia, Lippincott, 1989, pp 1197–1268

Familial incidence

ANDERSON DE, BADZIOCH MD: Risk of familial breast cancer. Cancer 56:383, 1985

Endocrine factors

BERGKVIST L et al: The risk of breast cancer after estrogen and estrogen-progestin replacement. N Engl J Med 321:293, 1989

HENDERSON BE et al: Estrogens as a cause of human cancer: The Richard and Hinda Rosenthal Foundation Award Lecture. Cancer Res 48:246, 1988

Dietary factors

WILLETT WC et al: Dietary fat and risk of breast cancer. N Engl J Med 316:22, 1987

Benign breast disease, in situ carcinoma

DUPONT WD, PAGE DL: Risk factors for breast cancer in women with proliferative breast disease. N Engl J Med 312:146, 1985

SCHNITT SJ et al: Ductal carcinoma in situ (intraductal carcinoma) of the breast. N Engl J Med 318:898, 1988

Screening

CHU KC et al: Analysis of breast cancer mortality and stage distribution by age for the Health Insurance Plan clinical trial. J Natl Cancer Inst 80:1125, 1988

EDDY DM et al: The value of mammography screening in women under age 50 years. JAMA 259:1512, 1988

Biology

LIPPMAN ME et al: Autocrine and paracrine growth regulation of human breast cancer. Breast Cancer Res Treat 7:59, 1986

Local therapy

HARRIS JR, HELLMAN S: Conservative surgery and radiotherapy, in *Breast Diseases*, JR Harris et al (eds). Philadelphia, Lippincott, 1987, pp 299–324

Adjuvant therapy

EARLY BREAST CANCER TRIALISTS' COLLABORATIVE GROUP: The effects of adjuvant tamoxifen and of cytotoxic therapy on mortality in early breast cancer: An overview of 61 randomized trials among 28,896 women. N Engl J Med 319:1681, 1988

HENDERSON IC: Adjuvant systemic therapy for early breast cancer. Curr Probl Cancer 11:125, 1987

PRITCHARD KI: Systemic adjuvant therapy for node-negative breast cancer: Proven or premature. Ann Intern Med 111:1, 1989

Systemic therapy

HENDERSON IC: Chemotherapy for advanced disease, in *Breast Diseases*, JR Harris et al (eds). Philadelphia, Lippincott, 1987, pp 428–479

———: Endocrine therapy of metastatic breast cancer, in *Breast Diseases*, JR Harris et al (eds). Philadelphia, Lippincott, 1987, pp 398–428

304 CARCINOMA OF THE OVARY

FRED J. HENDLER

The occurrence rate of ovarian cancer is relatively low, only 1.5 percent, and it is only the seventh most common cause of cancer in women. However, cancer of the ovary is the leading cause of death from gynecologic malignancies and the fourth most common cause of cancer-related death among women. Survival is excellent with early stage disease and poor when extensive disease is present. The apparent discrepancy between incidence and survival reflects the fact that most women at diagnosis have extensive disease. The high death rate associated with advanced disease has led to the development of aggressive multimodal therapy encompassing surgery, radiation, and/or chemotherapy. As a result, survival in patients with advanced

TABLE 304-1 Incidence and death rate of invasive gynecologic cancer

Tissue	Incidence, per year	Deaths, per year
Ovarian	20,000	12,000
Cervix, invasive	13,000	7,000
Uterine corpus and endometrium	34,000	3,000
Others	4,900	1,100

SOURCE: Modified from the *National Cancer Institute's Surveillance, Epidemiology, and End Results Program (1983–1985).*

disease has improved, and some advanced ovarian carcinomas may be cured.

INCIDENCE AND EPIDEMIOLOGY

Each year 20,000 new cases are diagnosed, and about 12,000 women die in the United States from ovarian cancer (Table 304-1). The disease is responsible for a fifth of all pathologically documented ovarian masses and is the most frequent ovarian mass detected in postmenopausal women. The peak incidence is in the sixth and seventh decades, with the disease eventually affecting 1 in 70 women. The incidence and death rate have remained fairly constant during the past 20 years, namely 14 and 9, respectively, per 100,000 women per year.

The epidemiology varies with histologic cell type. In the United States ovarian germ cell tumors are more frequent in young nonwhite women, and epithelial tumors are more common among postmenopausal white women. The epidemiology of epithelial tumors is similar to that of breast cancer. The highest incidence of ovarian cancer is in the western industrialized countries, and the lowest incidence is in Japan and the Mediterranean countries. The rate of ovarian cancer is increased in Japanese immigrants to the United States and in their descendants, suggesting that environmental factors are important epidemiologic variables. Hormones may also influence the incidence. Risk is higher in nulliparous women, women who have difficulty conceiving, and women with fewer pregnancies. However, no conclusive data link exogenous estrogen administration with an increased incidence. In fact, birth control pills may reduce the risk of developing ovarian cancer. Familial ovarian cancer is not as common as familial breast cancer. Women with either breast or ovarian cancer have a two- to fourfold greater risk of developing the other malignancy as well. Genetic disorders that affect the intestinal epithelium, such as Peutz-Jeghers syndrome, are associated with a five- to tenfold increased risk. Some chromosomal abnormalities (pure gonadal dysgenesis of the 46,XY type and mixed gonadal dysgenesis of the 46,XY/45,X type) are associated with an increased incidence of gonadoblastomas, while others (gonadal dysgenesis of the 46,XX and 45,X types) are not associated with ovarian malignancies (see Chap. 324). Chromosomal changes have been described in ovarian cancer tissue, but these appear to be acquired defects.

HISTOLOGIC CLASSIFICATION

Tumors can arise from all of the component cells of the ovary—epithelial, germinal, and stromal (Table 304-2). They may be benign, have a borderline malignancy (i.e., have some but not all the features of malignancy), or be truly neoplastic. Even in the neoplastic category, many gradations exist. The histologic grade of the tumor is based on the most aggressive cytologic and histologic pattern that is identified. Approximately 85 percent of ovarian carcinomas are of epithelial origin, derived from the coelomic epithelium or mesothelium from the embryonal gonadal ridge. The remaining 15 percent encompass a wide variety of cell types. In most, the tissue of origin can be identified, and, when more than one cell type is present, tumors are classified by the predominant cell type.

TABLE 304-2 Primary ovarian neoplasms

Cell type	Incidence, %
I Epithelial cell	85
A Serous	
B Mucinous	
C Endometrioid	
D Mesonephroid (clear cell)	
E Brenner	
F Undifferentiated	
G Carcinosarcoma	
II Stromal cell	<10
A Granulosa	
B Thecoma	
C Arrhenoblastoma	
D Sertoli	
E Gynandroblastoma	
F Lipoid	
III Germ cell	<5
A Teratoma	
1 Not otherwise specified	
2 Dermoid cyst	
3 Struma ovarii	
B Teratocarcinoma	
C Dysgerminoma	
D Embryonal carcinoma	
E Endodermal sinus	
F Choriocarcinoma	
G Gonadoblastoma	
H Mixed tumors	
IV Mesenchymal cell	2

EPITHELIAL TUMORS

CLINICAL FEATURES AND DIAGNOSIS Tumors derived from epithelial cells represent 85 percent of ovarian carcinomas. These malignancies most frequently occur in peri- or postmenopausal women. Frequently, the symptoms at presentation are nonspecific and usually include abdominal pain, increasing abdominal girth, and/or dysfunctional uterine bleeding. The symptoms have often been present for long periods and have been ignored. Thus, 75 percent of these tumors are widely disseminated at diagnosis. When the tumors are detected in premenopausal women, they may be more limited because menstrual abnormalities are associated with an earlier diagnosis.

Epithelial ovarian malignancies are rarely confined to one ovary and may be multifocal. Dissemination may occur early with small primary tumors. In limited disease, the tumors are confined to the ovaries and pelvic tissue. With extensive disease, the mode of spread is by diffuse peritoneal implantation of serosal surfaces and metastasis to regional lymphatics. The inferior surface of the right diaphragm is a frequent site for extrapelvic metastases. Hematogenous metastases are infrequent at the time of diagnosis. Careful examination of the entire abdominal cavity and retroperitoneal lymph nodes is required for accurate staging. Development of ascites with advanced disease is due to increased exudation and to blockage of diaphragmatic lymphatics.

PROGNOSTIC FACTORS Tumor stage A staging classification for all ovarian cancer was developed by the International Federation of Gynecology and Obstetrics (FIGO) in 1969 and revised in 1985. Tumor stage for epithelial carcinomas correlates the extent of disease with prognosis (Table 304-3). With a thorough and systematic diagnostic staging evaluation, many patients previously designated as stage I are now shown to have stage III disease. Similarly, malignant peritoneal washings in the presence of limited disease (stages Ic and IIc) probably indicate extensive disease outside the true pelvis, and such tumors should now be viewed as stage III. In short, many patients with apparent Ib, Ic, and IIc disease, when carefully staged, are at least stage III, and the prevalence of IIa and IIb disease has thereby been reduced. Apparently, only 20 to 30 percent of patients have limited ovarian cancer at presentation. By separating patients with previously unrecognized advanced disease, the prognosis in stages I and II has apparently improved to projected

TABLE 304-3 Pathologic staging of ovarian cancer

Stage	Extent of disease	Incidence, %	Projected 5-year survival, %
I	Involvement of ovaries only	15	80
a	Limited to one ovary, no ascites, external capsule intact		
b	Both ovaries involved, no ascites, external capsule intact		
c	Ia or Ib with tumor on surface of one or both ovaries or capsule ruptured or with malignant cells in peritoneal washings		
II	Ovarian involvement and extension into true pelvis	10	60
a	Extension or metastasis to uterus and/or tubes		
b	Extension to other pelvic tissues		
c	IIa or IIb with tumor on surface of one or both ovaries or capsule ruptured or with malignant ascites or with malignant cells in peritoneal washings		
III	Ovarian involvement with extension and/or metastasis into abdominal cavity including metastic implantation on the peritoneal surfaces of the liver and diaphragm and the serosal surface of the bowel	70	40
a	Tumor macroscopically limited to the true pelvis with negative nodes and with microscopic implantation on peritoneum		
b	Tumor limited to the true pelvis with negative nodes and with implantation on peritoneum none greater than 2 cm		
c	Retroperitoneal or inguinal node involvement or abdominal implants greater than 2 cm		
IV	Ovarian involvement with distant metastasis; pleural effusions must contain malignant cells; liver involvement must be parenchymal	5	0

cure rates of approximately 80 percent and 60 percent, respectively. In addition, the prognosis of patients with stage II disease has improved because patients with less bulky disease have been added to this stage. These stage shifts have no effect on true prognosis. Nevertheless, the staging system has documented the importance of the tumor burden to the prognosis. Furthermore, modern chemotherapy has altered the natural history of ovarian cancer, prolonging the time to relapse. As a result, 5-year survival may no longer be synonymous with cure.

Tumor burden Confined disease, although bulky, has a better prognosis than does disease of similar total burden that is diffusely distributed. Survival is better for stage Ia than for Ic, and survival for stage IIa is better than for IIb or IIc. When extensive disease is present (stages III or IV), survival correlates with the tumor burden at presentation and with the minimal residual tumor burden following surgical debulking (Table 304-4).

Histologic grade and cell type The histologic grade of the tumor is an important prognostic factor. Histologic grading systems are applied to tumors with proliferative activity (not borderline malignancies) and are based on the ability of tumors to form papillary structures and glands and on the degree of cellular atypia (Broder's classification). The histologic grade correlates with survival (Fig. 304-1). Tumors of borderline malignancy which are characterized by the presence of malignant cells and mitosis without evidence of tumor

TABLE 304-4 Five-year survival with respect to residual tumor size in stage III ovarian cancer

Tumor size, cm	Number of patients	Survival, % Two years	Five years
0	31	80	63
0–1	84	70	41
1–2	46	49	15
3–6	144	28	8
7	309	16	3

SOURCE: Smith and Day, 1979.

invasion have the best prognosis. Well-differentiated tumors (lower histologic grades) have a better prognosis than do poorly differentiated tumors (higher histologic grades). The tumors with higher histologic grade are usually stages III and IV at presentation and respond poorly to radiation and/or chemotherapy.

The histologic cell type similarly appears to be an important prognostic factor (Fig. 304-1). Mucinous and endometrial tumors with good prognosis can be distinguished from those with moderately poor prognosis, such as serous tumors, and from those more-undifferentiated carcinomas with poor prognosis.

Biologic markers Alpha fetoprotein and human chorionic gonadotropin (hCG) are useful tumor markers in germ cell tumors but not in epithelial carcinoma of the ovary. Carcinoembryonic antigen is often detectable in patients with epithelial cell tumors who have ascites and/or liver involvement, but it does not fluctuate consistently with tumor burden. Using a monoclonal antibody (OC125), a mucin-like glycoprotein (CA125) can be detected in normal coelomic epithelium, in normal müllerian duct cells, and in serum in about 80 percent of patients with epithelial ovarian malignancies. CA125 is

FIGURE 304-1 Prognosis factors in carcinomas of the ovary. *(From K Sigurdsson et al. Reprinted with permission.)*

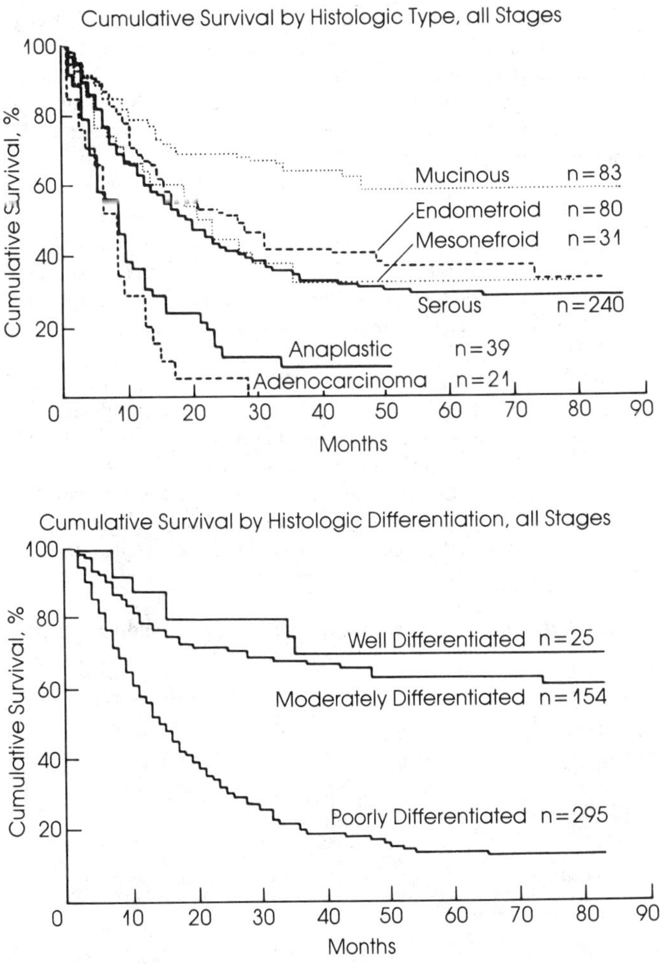

TABLE 304-5 Evaluation of epithelial ovarian carcinoma

I Staging evaluation
- *A* History and physical examination
- *B* Complete blood count, screening chemistries, CA125
- *C* Ultrasound, CT scan, or MRI of entire abdomen, including liver
- *D* Chest x-ray
- *E* Cystoscopy, intravenous pyelography, proctoscopy, and/or barium enema when indicated
- *F* Surgery
  - *1* Bilateral salpingo-oophorectomy
  - *2* Infracolic omentectomy, inspection of small bowel
  - *3* Periaortic node sampling
  - *4* Biopsy of liver, diaphragm, peritoneal gutters
  - *5* Peritoneal surface washing for cytologic examination

II Pathologic evaluation
- *A* Review of all tissue and peritoneal fluid blocks by at least two independent observers
- *B* Determination of histologic type
- *C* Determination of histologic grade
- *D* Review by ovarian cancer referral center

also present in serum from some patients with other adenocarcinomas, in some subjects with melanomas, and in some women who do not have carcinoma. The antigen level correlates with the extent of disease and fluctuates with therapy. However, the antigen level will often normalize while microscopic disease persists. In patients with known ovarian carcinoma an increase in the CA125 level in serum predicts recurrence.

STAGING EVALUATION A standard schema for evaluating suspected ovarian cancer is outlined in Table 304-5. Noninvasive diagnostic studies are of limited usefulness in detecting minimal abdominal involvement but are helpful in designing the surgical procedure.

The usual approach to staging an ovarian mass is to proceed directly to surgery once the diagnosis is suspected (Table 304-5). Paracentesis preoperatively is contraindicated in patients with ascites and a pelvic mass unless there is concern that the patient is infected. Once an epithelial cancer is diagnosed, the surgery should include (1) bilateral salpingo-oophorectomy, (2) hysterectomy, (3) omentectomy, (4) inspection and biopsy of the liver, diaphragmatic surfaces, and peritoneal gutters, and (5) cytologic examination of abdominal fluid and washings. Attempts should be made to remove all residual disease. When patients with bulk disease present following a diagnostic procedure, an aggressive surgical procedure should be undertaken. When patients present following an incomplete staging procedure with no clinical evidence of residual or bulk disease, peritoneoscopy should be performed; if disease is present, a second, more complete surgical procedure is indicated for complete staging and debulking.

THERAPEUTIC CONSIDERATIONS **Stage I** Stage I disease is adequately treated by a bilateral salpingo-oophorectomy and total abdominal hysterectomy done in the context of a staging procedure (Table 304-5). When the tumor is a borderline grade malignancy (approximately 25 percent of the stage I disease) and the patient is premenopausal and desires to have children, removal of the involved ovary and biopsy of the contralateral ovary may be adequate therapy. However, if the lesion is frankly malignant, if tumor involves both ovaries (Ib), or if ascites is present (Ic) a complete staging procedure should be performed. The prognosis for stage I disease treated with surgery alone may be as high as 90 percent for 5-year survival. Postoperative therapy has not been shown to be beneficial.

Stage II With a careful staging procedure less than 10 percent of epithelial tumors are stage II. Patients with a good prognosis (low histologic grade) tend to be treated similarly to stage I poor prognosis patients. Poor prognosis stage II (aggressive histologic grade) are treated as having advanced disease. Clinical trials evaluating the benefits of postoperative therapy in stage II disease are ongoing. Preliminary results suggest that postoperative therapy prolongs relapse-free survival. Survival at 5 years in patients treated with postnecrotic therapy may approach 80 percent.

Stages III and IV At least 70 percent of patients with ovarian carcinoma present with advanced disease. Multiagent chemotherapy results in improved survival if the total measurable tumor mass is reduced to less than 2 cm in diameter prior to chemotherapy. Reduction of the tumor mass to a diameter between 0.5 and 1.5 cm may be associated with additional survival benefits. When the tumor bulk is reduced to microscopic disease, some patients may be cured. If a complete remission is not achieved, cytoreductive surgery may prolong survival but not alter the cure rate.

Chemotherapy in advanced ovarian cancer has improved the 5-year survival to between 20 and 30 percent and altered the natural history of the disease. It can palliate most patients and probably can cure some patients with advanced disease. The chemotherapeutic regimens induce approximately a 60 percent complete clinical response rate, and 30 percent of patients attain a pathologic complete remission. About 20 percent of tumors of stages III and IV, typically histologic grade IV, do not respond. The most effective drugs are cisplatin, carboplatin, doxorubicin, alkylating agents (cyclophosphamide, melphalan, and chlorambucil), and hexamethylmelamine. Polychemotherapy which includes a platin derivative appears to be most effective, but an ideal drug regimen has not yet been developed (Table 304-6). Thus, patients with stages III and IV disease should be entered into cooperative group clinical trials.

To achieve complete remissions in patients with residual disease following cytoreductive surgery and chemotherapy, many modes of therapy have been evaluated. Radiation therapy can reduce mass disease in stages III and IV patients and has a role in the treatment of advanced disease. Furthermore, radiation therapy following cytoreductive surgery and multiagent chemotherapy may increase the remission rate in patients with bulk residual disease but has not improved survival or cure rates. Intraperitoneal administration of chemotherapeutic or radioactive agents requires further evaluation but may be useful in patients with only residual microscopic disease. Selection of appropriate chemotherapeutic agents in an assay utilizing cloned tumor cells has not been shown to be useful in most patients who fail conventional treatment. High-dose chemotherapy with either autologous bone marrow support or with supplemental hematologic growth factors is under investigation as an alternative approach in patients who have not achieved a complete response to conventional therapy.

TABLE 304-6 Responses to combination chemotherapy in advanced ovarian carcinoma

Regimen*	Investigators	No. of patients	Overall responses, %	Complete responses, %	Pathologic complete responses, %
Hexa-CAF	Young, 1978	40	75	—	33
H-CAP	Greco, 1981	46	96	76	30
CHAD	Vogl, 1983	26	92	42	22
PAC	Ehrlich, 1983	56	79	41	18
CHAP-5	Neijt, 1984	84	79	—	30
CHEX-UP	Louie, 1986	62	69	47	19

* Hexa-CAF: altretamine, cyclophosphamide, methotrexate, 5-fluorouracil; H-CAP: altretamine, cyclophosphamide, doxorubicin, cisplatin; CHAD: cyclophosphamide, altretamine, doxorubicin, cisplatin; PAC: cisplatin, doxorubicin, cyclophosphamide; CHAP-5: cyclophosphamide, doxorubicin, altretamine, cisplatin; CHEX-UP: cyclophosphamide, altretamine, 5-fluorouracil, cisplatin.

STROMAL TUMORS

Stromal tumors constitute only a tenth of ovarian malignancies but account for most of the hormone-secreting tumors. The majority have either masculinizing or feminizing effects, and the severity of the clinical syndrome is dependent in part on the patient's age (see Chaps. 54 and 322). Tumors that secrete hormones have a better prognosis because the tumors are relatively well-differentiated and because of the earlier clinical awareness that is associated with the hormonal effects. Feminizing tumors of the granulosa-theca cell variety are readily detected in prepubescent children because of the resultant precocious puberty, with breast development and uterine bleeding, and in postmenopausal women as a result of dysfunctional uterine bleeding. However, in the reproductive years these tumors are usually insidious since menstrual irregularities are often disregarded. Androgen-secreting tumors, which include arrhenoblastoma, lipoid and hilar cell tumors, adrenal-rest tumors, and gynandroblastomas, are more readily diagnosed because of the hirsutism and virilization (see Chap. 54). The endocrine syndromes may be caused by secretions of a steroid hormone that acts directly as an estrogen or an androgen (e.g., estradiol synthesis by granulosa cell tumors, testosterone synthesis by arrhenoblastomas), by secretion of a hormone that must be converted peripherally to active androgens or estrogens (e.g., androstenedione by thecomas), or by secretion of a peptide hormone that induces the synthesis of steroid hormones by uninvolved ovarian tissue (e.g., hCG by germ cell tumors).

As a result of the endocrine abnormalities, stromal tumors are detected at earlier stages than are epithelial tumors. Prospective clinical studies on the response to therapy are not available, but the prognosis for a given tumor stage appears to be no different than that of epithelial tumors (Table 304-3). When stromal tumors are confined to one ovary in reproductive or prepubescent women, a conservative approach is warranted. Removal of the involved ovary with a biopsy of the contralateral ovary may be adequate and will maintain ovarian and reproductive function without jeopardizing survival. Platin-based polychemotherapy may have some efficacy in granulosa cell tumors. All other stromal tumors appear to be basically unresponsive to either chemotherapy or radiation therapy. Thus, extensive disease and late recurrences are often managed by surgical debulking.

GERM CELL TUMORS

Germ cell tumors comprise less than 5 percent of ovarian malignancies, occur in young women, and have a higher incidence in blacks than in whites. They are usually unilateral with metastases to regional lymph nodes, hematogenous spread to the lungs, and direct extension to other pelvic organs. Peritoneal implantation and ascites are rare. Tumors that contain yolk sac epithelium produce alpha fetoprotein, and those with syncytiotrophoblasts produce hCG. These tumor markers make it possible to monitor the disease status and response to therapy. High levels of hCG are associated with feminizing syndromes and with hyperthyroidism because of structural similarities of the hCG alpha chain with alpha chains of follicle-stimulating hormone and thyroid-stimulating hormone (see Chap. 309). Hyperthyroidism also occurs in struma ovarii which are derived from specialized thyroid tissue within teratomas. Struma carcinoid tumors can arise from argentaffin tissue in teratomas. However, carcinoid syndrome is more frequently associated with metatasis to the ovary from a primary intestinal tumor than from strumal carcinoid (see Chap. 262). Pure choriocarcinoma of the ovary is rare and is due to a primary ovarian gestation, to metastasis from a choriocarcinoma of the uterus, or to direct germ cell derivation. Most commonly, elements of choriocarcinoma are observed as a component of a mixed germ cell tumor.

When germ cell tumors are clinically stage I, surgical removal of the involved ovary, biopsy of the contralateral ovary, and a limited node dissection should be performed. However, these tumors tend to be disseminated at presentation. They are responsive to multiagent chemotherapy and poorly controlled by surgery and radiation therapy. Historically, most patients with disseminated germ cell tumors have been treated primarily with vincristine, actinomycin D, and cyclophosphamide. However, cisplatin-containing chemotherapeutic regimens that are effective in testicular cancer appear to be similarly effective in ovarian germ cell tumors and are becoming the therapy of choice (see Chap. 305).

REFERENCES

BAST RC et al: A radioimmunoassay using a monoclonal antibody to monitor the course of epithelial ovarian cancer. N Engl J Med 309:883, 1983

BEREK JS et al: CA 125 serum levels correlated with second-look operations among ovarian cancer patients. Obstet Gynecol 67:685, 1986

DEMBO AJ: Abdominopelvic radiotherapy in ovarian cancer: A 10-year experience. Cancer 55:2285, 1985

FUKS Z et al: Chemotherapeutic and surgical induction of pathologic complete remission and whole abdominal irradiation for consolidation does not enhance the cure of stage III ovarian carcinoma. J Clin Oncol 6:509, 1988

HEINTZ APM et al: Epidemiology and etiology of ovarian cancer: A review. Obstet Gynecol 66:127, 1985

——— et al: Cytoreductive surgery in ovarian carcinoma: Feasibility and morbidity. Obstet Gynecol 67:783, 1986

HOWELL SB et al: Long-term survival of patients with small-volume disease treated with intraperitoneal chemotherapy. J Clin Oncol 5:1607, 1987

INTERNATIONAL FEDERATION OF GYNECOLOGY AND OBSTETRICS: Changes in definitions of clinical staging for carcinoma of the cervix and ovary. Am J Obstet Gynecol 156:236, 1987

O'CONNELL GJ et al: Predictive value of CA 125 for ovarian carcinoma in patients presenting with pelvic masses. Obstet Gynecol 70:930, 1987

OZOLS RF, YOUNG RC: Ovarian cancer. Curr Probl Cancer 11:59, 1987

——— et al: Advanced ovarian cancer: Correlation of histologic grade with response to therapy. Cancer 45:572, 1980

RUBIN SC, LEWIS JL JR: Second-look surgery in ovarian carcinoma. CRC Crit Rev Oncol Hematol 8:75, 1988

——— et al: Peritoneal cytology as an indicator of disease in patients with residual ovarian carcinoma. Obstet Gynecol 71:851, 1988

SIGURDSSON K et al: Prognostic factors in malignant epithelial tumors. Gynecol Oncol 15:370, 1983

SMITH JP, DAY TG: Review of ovarian cancer at the University of Texas System Cancer Center, MD Anderson Hospital, and Tumor Institute. Am J Obstet Gynecol 135:984, 1979

YOUNG RC: Initial therapy for early ovarian cancer. Cancer 60:2049, 1987

——— et al: Staging laparotomy in early ovarian cancer. JAMA 250:3072, 1983

——— et al: Cancer of the ovary, in *Cancer Principles and Pactice of Oncology*, VT DeVita Jr, et al (eds). Philadelphia, Lippincott, 1989, pp 1162–1196

305 TESTICULAR CANCER AND OTHER TROPHOBLASTIC DISEASES

MARC B. GARNICK

TESTICULAR CANCER

Carcinoma of the testis is a disease that serves as a model of a curable, solid neoplasm. Patients with localized forms of germinal cell cancer have a high cure rate when treated either with surgery or radiation therapy, and the advanced, metastatic forms, which in the past were almost universally fatal, are now also potentially curable. In 1977 testicular cancer was the third leading cause of cancer death in men between the ages of 15 and 34, but by 1981 the disease was no longer among the top five causes of cancer death in the same age group. The multidisciplinary principles and strategies that evolved for the management of patients with advanced testicular cancer are now being applied to other cancers.

Approximately 5700 new cases are diagnosed annually. The incidence in blacks is substantially lower than in whites. There is a peak frequency in early childhood and a larger peak incidence between 20 and 35 years. The disease is uncommon after age 40. A lesion suggestive of testicular neoplasm in a patient over the age of 50 should suggest a lymphoma rather than primary germinal cell carcinoma. This is especially true if there is bilateral involvement of the testes.

Several factors are known to predispose to development of testicular tumor. Men with a history of cryptorchid (undescended) testes have a several-fold increased risk, intraabdominal testes being more at risk than high inguinal testes. Both the cryptorchid testis itself and the contralateral normally descended testis are at risk, suggesting that some underlying testicular defect may predispose both to maldescent and to tumor development. Although the effectiveness of orchiopexy in reducing risk is not established, it is generally agreed that a high inguinal testis should be brought into the scrotum so that it can be followed carefully. Abdominal testes that cannot be treated in this manner should probably be removed. Other predisposing factors include a history of mumps orchitis, inguinal hernia in childhood, and testicular cancer in the contralateral testis. In the majority of cases no predisposing factor can be identified.

CLINICAL FEATURES AND DIAGNOSIS The manifestations of testicular cancer range from an asymptomatic nodule or swelling detected while performing testicular self-examination to dyspnea secondary to massive pulmonary metastases. Most testicular cancers are diagnosed because of symptoms related to the testes, but significant delay in making a diagnosis is common and is the result of oversight by physicians and by patients. Thus, high school health programs that teach testicular self-examination should be encouraged. Such programs have allowed early diagnosis, leading to more successful treatment outcomes. Most testicular cancers occur in men under age 40, and the public should be educated to the need to seek prompt medical advice for any change in previously normal testes, including the presence of a mass, a feeling of heaviness, pain, hardness, and swelling. Other causes of testicular masses include hydrocele, epididymitis, spermatocele, and orchitis, but to reduce delay in reaching a diagnosis, physicians should consider any testicular mass to be malignant until proven otherwise. Patients with testicular tumors may have pain because of associated nonneoplastic lesions, such as epididymitis.

Back or abdominal pain secondary to retroperitoneal adenopathy, weight loss, dyspnea secondary to pulmonary metastases, gynecomastia, supraclavicular lymphadenopathy, and urinary obstruction may also be present at diagnosis.

A testicular sonogram can aid in establishing the presence of a testicular parenchymal abnormality. Once the diagnosis of a testicular neoplasm is suspected, a blood sample should be set aside, prior to orchiectomy, for subsequent determination of the tumor marker glycoproteins, alpha fetoprotein (AFP) and human chorionic gonadotropin (hCG). The correct operative approach is a high radical inguinal orchiectomy. A transscrotal biopsy of the testis or a transscrotal orchiectomy should never be performed if the diagnosis of testicular cancer is likely. Because the lymphatic drainage of the testis (to the retroperitoneal lymphatics between L1 and L3) differs from that of the scrotum (to superficial and deep inguinal groin nodes), a scrotal incision in the presence of a testicular cancer may predispose to the development of local recurrences and metastases to the inguinal lymphatics. This rarely happens if a radical, high inguinal orchiectomy is performed.

CLASSIFICATION AND PATHOLOGY The most widely used classification of testicular tumors is that of Mostofi and is based on the cell type from which the tumor is derived, namely germinal or stromal (Leydig and Sertoli) cells (Table 305-1). Germinal cell tumors, the most common of these tumors and the focus of this chapter, can be subdivided into seminomas and nonseminomas. Seminomas are characterized by large cells with clear cytoplasm in a delicate fibrovascular stroma infiltrated with lymphocytes. Indeed, the granulomatous reaction around the tumor can be so intense as to suggest a graft-versus-host reaction. These tumors account for about half of all testicular neoplasms and can be divided into typical, spermatocytic, and anaplastic varieties. Germinal cell tumors of the nonseminoma type can be divided into embryonal cell tumors (yolk sac tumors), teratomas, and choriocarcinomas. Embryonal carcinomas are common in children and resemble embryonal carcinomas of the ovary. Choriocarcinomas contain syncytiotrophoblastic cells. Teratomas contain at least two types of germinal cell layers and in childhood are second in frequency to embryonal tumor. Mixed tumors that contain combinations of germinal cell types account for 40 percent of germinal cell tumors; the biology of such tumors is usually determined by the least differentiated (most malignant) elements. All four types of germinal cell tumors can also originate in extragonadal sites, most commonly the mediastinum or brain. Such extragonadal tumors are presumed to arise either from aberrant migration of germinal cells during embryogenesis or, alternatively, from some common precursor stem cell line that gives rise to the germinal cells, the thymus, and the pineal.

TABLE 305-1 Classification of testicular tumors

I Germinal cell tumors (95%)
- *A* Single cell tumors (60%)
  - *1* Seminomas
  - *2* Nonseminomas
    - *a* Embryonal cell tumors (yolk sac tumors)
    - *b* Teratomas
    - *c* Choriocarcinomas
- *B* Combination tumors (40%)

II Tumors of gonadal stroma (1–2%)
- *A* Leydig cell
- *B* Sertoli cell
- *C* Primitive gonadal structures

III Gonadoblastoma: germinal cell + stomal cell

SOURCE: After FK Mostofi, Cancer 45:1735, 1980.

From the clinical standpoint, the critical distinction is between *seminomas* and *nonseminomas*, based upon the histopathology of the orchiectomy specimen. The former must be in pure form; the latter may either be a mixed cancer with both seminomatous and nonseminomatous components or a pure form of a nonseminoma, such as embryonal cell carcinoma, teratoma, or choriocarcinoma. The term *teratocarcinoma* generally refers to a mixed nonseminomatous cancer consisting of teratoma and embryonal cell cancer.

The distinction between seminoma and nonseminoma is important because the staging evaluation and subsequent management in the two differ as a consequence of the relative radioresponsiveness of seminomas compared to the radioresistance of nonseminomas. Radiation therapy to the lymphatics of the abdomen and/or chest is the mainstay of therapy in patients with pure seminoma but is rarely utilized in patients with nonseminoma. In addition, seminomas usually spread via the regional lymphatics to the retroperitoneal nodes of the abdomen and/or to the mediastinal and supraclavicular lymph nodes before gaining access to other visceral structures. Pulmonary and other hematogenous metastases (e.g., hepatic, CNS, osseous) are more common in patients with nonseminomas than in patients with seminomas.

BIOLOGIC TUMOR MARKERS Germinal cell cancers of the testis often secrete biologic tumor markers that can be detected in the peripheral blood (see Chap. 309). Following orchiectomy, the presence of such markers in blood reflects the presence of metastatic disease. Such assays can also be valuable in monitoring therapy (marker levels fall with disease regression and increase with disease progression), and elevated levels in blood may predate the detection of new clinical or radiologic metastatic disease by weeks to months. The two most common markers are AFP and hCG. AFP is commonly secreted by embryonal cell cancer: its biologic half-life is approximately 6 days. AFP is not produced by pure seminoma, and its detection implies the presence of nonseminomatous elements, either in the primary lesion itself or in the metastatic site, even when the primary orchiectomy specimen is thought to be a pure seminoma. hCG is secreted by syncytiotrophoblastic giant cells, present most commonly in choriocarcinomas; such giant cells may be present in embryonal cell components and occasionally in so-called pure seminomas. The biologic half-life of hCG is approximately 24 h. hCG may be biologically active, and hCG-enhanced secretion of estrogen by the testis is the cause of gynecomastia in such patients (see Chap. 323).

STAGING EVALUATION The function of staging is to determine whether the cancer is localized to the testis or to regional lymphatics or is widely disseminated. Such information is necessary to determine if disease is amenable to local or regional therapy. If the disease is disseminated at presentation, the initial staging evaluation serves as a baseline in assessing subsequent response. Since the approach to staging and management is dictated by the pathologic diagnosis of the orchiectomy specimen, the appropriate evaluation will be outlined for each.

Pure seminoma The routine workup involves careful physical examination, an abdominal-pelvic computed tomographic (CT) scan to determine the presence of retroperitoneal adenopathy or visceral involvement, a chest x-ray with or without lung tomography, measurement of routine chemistries, and assessment of the biologic markers (AFP and hCG). In most cases, the biologic markers are undetectable. If AFP is elevated, the patient should be treated as having a nonseminoma, even though the pathologic interpretation is pure seminoma.

The portals for radiation therapy for pure seminomas were traditionally determined on the basis of bipedal lymphangiography. However, the necessity of lymphangiography for such purposes is less imperative today because CT scanning may provide similar information.

If plasma hCG is elevated in a patient with a diagnosis of pure seminoma, a search should be made for syncytiotrophoblastic giant cells. Otherwise, there may be some uncertainty of whether occult foci of nonseminomatous components are responsible for the hCG production. Also, if the physical or radiographic examinations fail to reveal any evidence of metastatic disease and the hCG is elevated before orchiectomy, it is necessary to follow the level of hCG sequentially. If the marker does not decline as predicted by its biologic half-life, the presence of occult metastatic cancer should be considered.

Nonseminoma The staging evaluation outlined for the seminoma is employed for the patient with a nonseminomatous germinal cell tumor of the testis. On the basis of these noninvasive staging studies, patients can be categorized as having stage I, early stage II, advanced stage II, or stage III disease. Patients with stage I disease have no clinical, radiographic, or marker evidence of tumor presence beyond the confines of the testis. Patients with early stage II have nonpalpable, small, retroperitoneal adenopathy on CT scans, usually measuring <4 to 5 cm. Advanced stage II is defined as retroperitoneal lymphadenopathy measuring >5 cm on CT scan or palpable retroperitoneal adenopathy with disease limited to lymphatics below the diaphragm. Stage III disease includes visceral involvement below the diaphragm (e.g., liver or bowel) or above the diaphragm (e.g., lung or supraclavicular lymphadenopathy). Furthermore, patients with stage III disease can be further subdivided according to anatomic location and extent of disease. Treatment decisions are often based on volume of disease in stage III patients.

Conceptually, patients with testicular cancer can be categorized pathologically as having either *seminoma* or *nonseminoma* and staged as having either "early" or "advanced" disease. Patients with *early* disease would be considered to have stage I and early stage II disease, while patients with *advanced* disease have advanced stage II or any form of stage III disease. This formulation allows rational decision making for nearly all categories of disease.

TREATMENT MODALITIES ACCORDING TO HISTOLOGY AND STAGE (Table 305-2) **Early seminoma** These patients have either a normal abdominal CT scan or retroperitoneal lymphadenopathy measuring less than 5 cm in greatest diameter. Most such patients

TABLE 305-2 Testicular cancer: General approach to management and cure rates*

	Seminoma	% Cure	Nonseminoma	% Cure
Stage I	XRT	95–97	RPLND or orchiectomy alone/observation	97
Early stage II	XRT	85–90	RPLND ± Chemo[a] or Chemo[a]	85–90
Advanced stage II Stage III	Chemo[a]	80–85	Chemo[a] ± TRS ± Chemo[b]	80–85

* XRT = radiation therapy, delivered to subdiaphragmatic lymphatics; RPLND = retroperitoneal lymph node dissection; chemo[a] = combination chemotherapy (see Table 305-3); TRS = tumor-reductive surgery; chemo[b] = additional chemotherapy given if surgical specimen reveals viable cancer.

are treated with abdominal radiotherapy, delivering 30 Gy (3000 rad) to the subdiaphragmatic lymph nodes and ipsilateral groin and a 6-Gy (600-rad) boost in areas of known disease. Although prophylactic mediastinal and supraclavicular radiation therapy was used in the past, this practice is generally not employed today. When treated with radiation following orchiectomy, patients with clinical stage I have a 95 to 97 percent cure rate, and patients with early stage II disease have an 85 to 90 percent survival rate.

Advanced seminoma In the past, patients with large retroperitoneal masses or mediastinal involvement were often treated with radiation therapy to fields including the subdiaphragmatic lymph nodes, whole abdomen, mediastinum, and supraclavicular nodes; however, survival rates were only 40 to 70 percent. If these patients subsequently suffered a relapse in an area outside the radiation therapy field, the ability to administer myelosuppressive combination chemotherapy was diminished and was associated with drug-related morbidity. Today, most patients with advanced forms of seminoma are treated initially with combination chemotherapy that includes cisplatin. Substantial tumor shrinkage occurs in the majority of patients. However, the proper management for partially regressed retroperitoneal masses following chemotherapy is controversial. Patients are restaged following chemotherapy, and depending upon the individual treatment protocol, further treatment with chemotherapy, surgery, or radiation therapy is addressed.

Stage I nonseminoma Patients with stage I nonseminoma are routinely treated with a retroperitoneal lymph node dissection (RPLND), using either a transabdominal or a thoracoabdominal approach. The rationale for this operation is based upon the inexact data generated from the noninvasive staging evaluation of the retroperitoneal lymphatics. The false-negative rate of abdominal CT scans in patients with clinical stage I is 35 to 40 percent. Thus, surgical removal of the retroperitoneal lymph nodes not only serves as therapy but also determines the need for possible additional therapy. If microscopic disease is detected and surgically removed, an 85 to 90 percent cure rate can be expected following RPLND.

More recently, a policy of orchiectomy followed by surveillance has been used for selected stage I nonseminoma patients. This strategy avoids a retroperitoneal lymph node dissection in a large percentage of patients. If relapse occurs, chemotherapy can then be instituted with achievement of greater than 90 percent cure rates.

Stage II nonseminoma The optimal management of patients with retroperitoneal lymphadenopathy measuring between 2 and 5 cm on the CT scan is controversial. While RPLND may be curative, a relapse rate of 30 to 45 percent can be expected. If relapse occurs after RPLND, combination chemotherapy can be administered, or chemotherapy may sometimes be given as an adjuvant to RPLND. Alternatively, combination chemotherapy can be given prior to RPLND. If complete resolution of disease is achieved following chemotherapy, RPLND would not be performed, obviating the need for the operation in this subset of patients.

Advanced stage (bulky stage II or stage III) nonseminoma Cisplatin-containing programs are in nearly universal use today, either with vinblastine and bleomycin (PVB), the combination of cisplatin

TABLE 305-3 Commonly used chemotherapy programs for advanced testicular cancer

PVB	VAB-6	BEP
Vinblastine Bleomycin Cisplatin	Vinblastine Bleomycin Cisplatin Cyclophosphamide Actinomycin D	Etoposide Bleomycin Cisplatin

with vinblastine, actinomycin D, bleomycin, and cyclophosphamide (VAB program) or with etoposide and bleomycin (BEP) (Table 305-3). The use of these agents is associated with complete remission in as many as 80 to 85 percent of patients when administered cyclically over a 9- to 12-week period.

Following such therapy, patients are then restaged (with physical, radiographic, and biochemical examinations) to assess the response of areas which previously contained disease and to determine the need for additional therapy. Large abdominal masses may undergo astonishing regression. Pulmonary nodules often resolve completely, and biologic markers frequently return to normal after chemotherapy. If a residual abdominal or pulmonary mass persists despite normal levels of plasma markers, surgical removal of the mass(es) should be undertaken. Table 305-4 outlines current recommendations. Preoperatively, it is difficult to determine the nature of such residual masses. Approximately 20 percent contain residual, viable cancer; 40 percent contain fibrosis, necrosis, or hemorrhage, and an additional 40 percent demonstrate the phenomenon of "teratomatous transformation." The latter is thought to result either from chemotherapy-induced differentiation of the primary mass into a teratoma or from the selective elimination of the more malignant elements of the mass but persistence of residual teratomatous components. If either fibrosis, hemorrhage, or teratoma is found following chemotherapy, additional postsurgical chemotherapy is usually not indicated. If, however, residual cancer is demonstrated, additional cisplatin combination chemotherapy is required.

If biologic markers are persistently positive following remission induction chemotherapy, additional chemotherapy is also indicated. "Tumor-reductive" surgery should not be attempted until biologic markers return to normal. Some patients experience complete resolution of physical, radiographic, and biochemical marker abnormalities after cisplatin-containing chemotherapy and may require no additional chemotherapy or surgery following their program of chemotherapy.

Testicular cancer which is refractory of PVB, VAB-6, or BEP programs may sometimes respond to the addition of ifosfamide. Ifosfamide has been approved by the FDA for third-line treatment with other antineoplastics for patients with refractory germ cell tumors. The combination of cisplatin, etoposide, and ifosfamide will result in a second or third remission, which may be durable, in approximately 25 percent of patients. On occasion, bone marrow transplantation may be considered.

FOLLOW-UP OF PATIENTS WITH TESTICULAR CANCER All patients with testicular cancer, regardless of pathology or stage, require meticulous follow-up with monthly physical exams, chest x-rays, and assessment of markers for 18 to 24 months. Patients with stage I nonseminoma who are treated with a surveillance policy following orchiectomy will need frequent abdominal-pelvic CT scanning in addition to the other follow-up evaluations. The frequency of these tests can be decreased in the third or fourth year following diagnosis. The goal is to detect relapse when the tumor burden is minimal. Most relapses from testicular cancer occur within the first 2 years following diagnosis, but late relapses do occur.

TABLE 305-4 Advanced testicular cancer, nonseminoma: Approach to management after initial chemotherapy

Biologic "markers"*	Radiographic abnormalities	Therapeutic choice
Positive	Present or absent	Additional chemotherapy†
Normal	Present	TRS‡ ± chemotherapy§
Normal	Absent	Observation

* Alpha fetoprotein and human chorionic gonadotropin.
† Chemotherapy with a "second-line" program, with attempts to "normalize" biologic markers.
‡ Tumor-reductive surgery.
§ Additional chemotherapy determined by presence of "viable" cancer in surgical specimen. Chemotherapy withheld if surgical specimen contains only fibrosis or teratoma.

SIDE EFFECTS OF THERAPY Radiation therapy and surgery Infertility can result both from radiation therapy and RPLND. Because these modalities are generally reserved for the management of early stage patients, a full discussion with patients about the potential loss of fertility is appropriate. Although of questionable benefit, the possibility of sperm banking should be considered prior to the initiation of either definitive radiation therapy for early stage seminomas or RPLND for early stage nonseminomas. Modifications in the surgical technique of RPLND (limited dissection) may decrease the incidence of fertility loss and ejaculatory disturbances.

Combination chemotherapy When standard cisplatin-vinblastine-bleomycin programs are employed, the major side effects are myelosuppression, potential for nephrotoxicity, nausea and vomiting, weight loss, anemia, ileus, pulmonary toxicity, ototoxicity, peripheral neuropathy, Raynaud's phenomenon, alopecia, hypomagnesemia, and stomatitis. Infertility is usual during therapy, although fertility may return years after completion of therapy. The use of the chemotherapy programs requires skill on the part of the treating physician and should not be attempted by the occasional user. With proper expertise these side effects can often be minimized. Hemorrhagic cystitis, which can occur with ifosfamide, can be minimized by concomitant use of the uroprotector mesna.

Bleomycin is known to cause pulmonary toxicity (see Chap. 205), and special precautions must be taken in patients who have received bleomycin and are scheduled for a surgical procedure. The acute respiratory distress syndrome has occurred in some and is thought to be related to excessive fluid overload and high inspired oxygen concentration ($F_{I_{O_2}}$) during the operative procedure. Current recommendations now call for the $F_{I_{O_2}}$ to be maintained at $\leq$24 percent and for patients to be kept in a hypovolemic or euvolemic state in the perioperative period. Such measures seem to minimize the postoperative pulmonary complications.

THE EXTRAGONADAL GERMINAL CELL SYNDROME Patients with extragonadal germinal cell tumors may present with a large anterior mediastinal mass, central nervous system abnormalities, or retroperitoneal disease. The response to therapy is generally lower when compared to primary testicular cancer, justifying the need for more intensive therapy. Many patients relapse years after the original diagnosis, leading to a lower cure rate compared to patients with primary testicular cancer. However, a proportion of these patients may be cured when treated with chemotherapy and tumor-reductive surgery. In addition, patients with "undifferentiated" cancer of the mediastinum or retroperitoneum may have an unrecognized form of extragonadal germinal cell cancer. Biologic markers and immunohistochemical staining of the biopsy material for AFP or hCG may provide useful clues. If positive, these patients should be treated as if they have potentially curable advanced testicular cancer.

OTHER TROPHOBLASTIC DISEASES

Trophoblastic tumors of females encompass all proliferative trophoblastic growths that develop from pregnancy and are, hence, entitled *gestational trophoblastic neoplasms*. Gestational trophoblastic tumors arise most commonly from antecedent molar pregnancies, but may also follow term and ectopic pregnancy and spontaneous abortions. The incidence of choriocarcinoma occurring during a term pregnancy is approximately 1 in 150,000 and approximately 75 percent of these patients demonstrate metastatic disease, the lungs being the most frequent site of metastases. The incidence of choriocarcinoma occurring with an ectopic pregnancy is approximately 1 in 5000; the incidence with spontaneous abortion is approximately 1 in 15,000.

Pathologically, the morphology of gestational trophoblastic neoplasms includes the complete and partial hydatidiform mole, invasive mole, and choriocarcinoma. The distinction between complete and partial is based upon gross and microscopic appearance and karyotype. Complete moles usually demonstrate the absence of fetal or embryonic tissue; such tissue is present in a partial mole. Most complete moles have a 46,XX chromosome pattern; partial moles generally have a triploid karyotype, with the extra set of chromosomes of paternal derivation.

Based upon data generated by the New England Trophoblastic Disease Center, presenting signs of patients with complete hydatidiform mole are abnormal vaginal bleeding (>90 percent), anemia (>50 percent), enlargement of the uterus (>50 percent), toxemia of pregnancy (25 percent), hyperemesis gravidarum (25 percent), and infrequently, hyperthyroidism and trophoblastic emboli to the lung. Patients with trophoblastic moles often present with the signs and symptoms of a spontaneous abortion, with vaginal bleeding being the most common feature.

Following evacuation of the molar pregnancy, approximately 15 percent of patients demonstrate localized uterine invasion, and 4 percent demonstrate metastatic disease, most often associated with choriocarcinoma.

Gestational trophoblastic neoplasms can be staged according to the FIGO staging system. Stage I is tumor localized to the uterus; stage II is tumor involving the pelvis and/or vagina; stage III is tumor involving the lung; stage IV is tumor involving other organs. The stage of the patient is generally determined after an extensive diagnostic evaluation, including a history and physical examination, measurement of hCG levels, and routine biochemical and hematologic evaluation. The metastatic workup generally includes a chest x-ray, abdominal-pelvic ultrasonography, evaluation of the liver for hepatic metastases, and, on occasion, angiography of abdominal or pelvic organs. In individuals with choriocarcinoma and documented metastases, hCG values are often measured in the cerebral spinal fluid to detect asymptomatic central nervous system involvement. Likewise, stool guaiac tests are often done to rule out lesions to the gastrointestinal tract.

The most important aspect of gestational trophoblastic neoplasms is the fact that there is a 100 percent cure rate in patients with stages I to III and approximately an 85 percent cure rate in patients with stage IV. Depending upon the extent of disease and the level of hCG in the bloodstream, individuals are treated with evacuation of their pregnancy or chemotherapy. For patients having a good prognosis, single-agent methotrexate or actinomycin D are generally employed, while high-risk patients are generally treated with combination chemotherapy, including methotrexate, actinomycin D, and cyclophosphamide. More recently, for patients with evidence of metastatic disease, more intensive programs, including vinblastine, bleomycin, and cisplatin, have been used with excellent success. Treatment is continued until baselines of hCG have returned to normal.

Many patients can expect normal reproductive function following treatment. There is, however, an increased incidence of repeat episodes of moles or gestational trophoblastic neoplasms in subsequent pregnancies. The sequential determination of hCG has been extremely valuable in the monitoring of such patients.

REFERENCES

BERKOWITZ RS, GOLDSTEIN DP: Management of molar pregnancy and gestational trophoblastic disease, in *Gynecologic Oncology*, RC Knapp, RS Berkowitz (eds). New York, MacMillan, 1986

BOSL GJ: Treatment of germ cell tumors at Memorial Sloan-Kettering Cancer Center: 1960 to present, in *Genitourinary Cancer: Contemporary Issues in Clinical Oncology*, vol 5, MB Garnick (ed). New York, Churchill Livingstone, 1985

EINHORN EH (ed): *Testicular Tumors: Management and Treatment*. New York, Masson, 1980

———, DONOHUE JP: Cis-diamminedichloroplatinum, vinblastine, and bleomycin combination chemotherapy in disseminated testicular cancer. Ann Intern Med 87:293, 1977

FUNG CY, GARNICK MB: Clinical stage I carcinoma of the testis: A review. J Clin Oncol 6:734, 1988

GARNICK MB: Advanced testicular cancer: Treatment choices in the "land of plenty" (editorial). J Clin Oncol 3:294, 1985

——— (ed): Contemporary Issues in urologic cancer. Semin Oncol vol 4, August, 1988

——— et al: The treatment and surgical staging of testicular and primary extragonadal germ cell cancer. JAMA 250:1733, 1983

HAINSWORTH JD, GRECO FA: Testicular germ cell neoplasms. Am J Med 75:817, 1983

POTTERN LM et al: Testicular cancer risk among young men: Role of cryptorchidism and inguinal hernia. J Natl Cancer Inst 74:377, 1985

STEPHENS RL, WILLIAMSON SK: Clinical stage I testicular cancer: Orchiectomy without node dissection [Editorial]. Ann Intern Med 109:179, 1988

WILLIAMS SD et al: Treatment of disseminated germ-cell tumors with cisplatin, bleomycin, and either vinblastine or etoposide. N Engl J Med 316:1435, 1987

——— et al: Immediate adjuvant chemotherapy versus observation with treatment at relapse in pathological stage II testicular cancer. N Engl J Med 317:1433, 1987

306 HYPERPLASIA AND CARCINOMA OF THE PROSTATE

ARTHUR I. SAGALOWSKY / JEAN D. WILSON

PROSTATIC HYPERPLASIA

Development of prostatic hyperplasia is an almost universal phenomenon in aging men. The prostate weighs only a few grams at birth; at puberty it undergoes androgen-mediated growth and reaches the adult size of about 20 g by age 20. It remains stable in size for about 25 years, and during the fifth decade a second growth spurt commences in the majority of men. Consequently, the disease affects men over the age of 45 and increases in frequency with age so that by the eighth decade more than 90 percent of men have prostatic hyperplasia at autopsy. Because of refinements in prostatic surgery, the disorder is not a major cause of death, but it is a leading cause of morbidity in elderly men. The prostate surrounds the urethra, and any enlargement is a potential cause of urinary tract obstruction; indeed, prostatic hyperplasia is the most common cause of obstruction to urinary outflow in men. Overall, about 10 percent of men at some time require prostatic surgery to relieve urinary tract obstructions. The disorder occurs in all populations but is less common in the orient. The mean age for development of symptomatic disease is about 65 years for whites and about 60 years for blacks. It is probable that prostatic hyperplasia does not predispose to the development of prostatic cancer.

PATHOGENESIS Unlike the pubertal growth spurt which involves the gland diffusely, prostatic hyperplasia begins in the periurethral region as a localized proliferation and progresses to compress the remaining normal gland. Histologically, the hyperplastic tissue is nodular and composed of varying amounts of glandular epithelium, stroma, and smooth-muscle elements. The hyperplastic process can compress and obstruct the urethra; rarely, the hyperplastic gland grows posteriorly to obstruct the rectum and cause constipation.

The pathogenesis is not well-understood, but two necessary features for the process are aging and the presence of testes; whether the testes play a direct or permissive role is not known, but the active androgen that mediates prostatic growth at all ages is dihydrotestosterone, which is formed within the prostate from plasma testosterone (see Chap. 321). In the castrated dog, hormonal therapy that increases dihydrotestosterone levels in the prostate causes prostatic enlargement comparable to that seen in spontaneous canine prostatic hyperplasia. Estradiol levels in men increase with age (absolutely or relative to testosterone levels), and in dogs estrogen acts synergistically with dihydrotestosterone to induce prostatic growth by enhancing the amount of androgen receptor protein in the tissue. Consequently, the role of aging in the development of prostatic hyperplasia in men would be explained if dihydrotestosterone is the mediator of the hyperplasia and if estradiol augments dihydrotestosterone action.

DIAGNOSIS Urethral obstruction results from the elongation, tortuosity, and compression of the posterior urethra, but there is no straightforward relationship between obstruction and prostatic size; indeed, severe obstruction can occur when the hyperplasia does not exceed the size of the normal gland. Early symptoms can be minimal because compensatory hypertrophy of the detrusor musculature of the bladder is capable of compensating for the increased resistance to urine flow. With increasing obstruction, diminution in the caliber and force of the urinary stream, hesitancy in initiating voiding, postvoiding dribbling, the sensation of incomplete emptying, and on occasion urinary retention supervene. These *obstructive* symptoms must be distinguished from *irritative* symptoms such as dysuria, frequency, and urgency that can result from inflammatory, infectious, or neoplastic causes. As the amount of residual urine increases, nocturia, overflow urinary incontinence, and a palpable bladder may be present. Eventually, the manifestations of chronic urinary retention and obstruction supervene, or acute urinary retention can be precipitated by infection, the ingestion of tranquilizing drugs, or alcohol. On occasion, profound obstruction can be compensated to the extent that symptoms are minimal or absent, and patients present with obstructive uropathy.

The prostate is palpated during digital rectal examination and should be characterized in regard to size, consistency, and shape. Hyperplasia commonly produces a smooth, firm, elastic enlargement, but it should be recognized that obstruction can occur in the absence of abnormalities on rectal examination. Ultrasonography with a rectal probe or magnetic resonance imaging allows a quantitative estimate of prostate size but ordinarily provides no information beyond that provided by rectal examination. An intravenous pyelogram with postvoiding film will document the degree of upper urinary tract obstruction and the extent of bladder emptying. To evaluate vesicle neck obstruction, cystourethroscopy is indicated. Measurement of urine flow rate and/or residual urine volume is recommended to document the degree of obstruction to outflow. More detailed urodynamic evaluation is occasionally required to rule out other causes of voiding dysfunction such as neurogenic bladder.

TREATMENT The treatment is surgical, and when surgery is indicated, transurethral prostatectomy is the usual procedure of choice. In the case of massive glands, open prostatectomy may be employed using either retropubic, suprapubic, or perineal approaches. Because the majority of men above age 60 have some degree of prostatic hyperplasia, the presence of the disorder is not an indication for treatment. Indications for surgery include decrease in urine flow of sufficient magnitude to cause men to seek relief, persistent residual urine, acute urinary retention due to obstruction with no reversible precipitating cause, and hydronephrosis. In men who lack definite indications for prostatectomy, it is advisable that they be examined periodically to determine the natural history of the process; many patients who receive no therapy experience no progression in symptoms over many years.

PROSTATIC CARCINOMA

Cancer of the prostate is the second most common malignancy in men and is the third most common cause of cancer death in men older than age 55 (after carcinomas of the lung and colon). In 1987 there were some 96,000 newly diagnosed cases and over 26,000 deaths from the disorder in the United States. Only about a third of cases identified at autopsy are manifest clinically. The disease is rare before age 50, and the incidence increases with advancing age.

The frequency varies in different parts of the world. In terms of age-adjusted mortality rates, the United States has 14 deaths per 100,000 men per year compared to 22 for Sweden and 2 for Japan. However, Japanese immigrants to the United States develop prostatic cancer at a frequency similar to other men in this country, suggesting that an environmental factor is the principal cause for population differences. The disease is more common among black men than white men in the United States; the reason for this difference is not known.

CLASSIFICATION Some carcinomas of the prostate are slow-growing and may persist for long periods without causing significant symptoms, whereas others behave aggressively. It is not known whether tumors can become more malignant with time. Insight into the natural history of a given tumor is provided by careful histopathologic grading of the lesion combined with surgical evaluation of the pelvic lymph nodes.

Histologic grading Over 95 percent of prostatic cancers are adenocarcinomas that arise in the prostatic acini. Adenocarcinoma may begin anywhere in the prostate but has a predilection for the periphery. The tumors are frequently multifocal. Variability in cellular size, nuclear and nucleolar shape, glandular differentiation, and the content of acid phosphatase and mucin may occur within a single specimen, but the most poorly differentiated area of tumor (i.e., the area with the highest histologic grade) appears to determine its biologic behavior. In the Gleason grading scheme the dominant and any other glandular histologic patterns are independently assigned numbers from 1 to 5 (best- to least-differentiated), and these numbers are summed to give a total score of 2 to 10 for each tumor. Such grading is reproducible and correlates with the course of the disease and with patient survival.

The remaining of prostatic cancers are divided among squamous-cell and transitional-cell carcinomas that arise in the prostatic ducts, carcinoma of the prostatic utricle (a müllerian duct remnant), carcinosarcomas that arise in the mesenchymal elements of the gland, and occasional metastatic tumors (usually carcinoma of the lung, melanoma, or lymphoma). These tumors will not be considered further.

Surgical staging Adenocarcinoma of the prostate may spread by three routes: direct extension, the lymphatics, and the bloodstream. The prostatic capsule is a natural boundary against growth of tumor into adjacent structures, but direct extension occurs upward into the seminal vesicles and bladder floor. Lymphatic spread can best be assessed by surgical exploration; the frequency with which it occurs correlates with the size and the histologic grade of the tumor. Only about one-tenth of tumors with a grade of less than 5 have lymph node involvement, while more than 70 percent of tumors with a Gleason grade of 9 or 10 have coexisting lymphatic invasion at the time of diagnosis. The route of lymphatic spread (in decreasing order) is to obturator, internal iliac, common iliac, presacral, and paraaortic nodes. Hematogenous metastases occur to bone (pelvis > lumbar vertebrae > thoracic vertebrae > ribs) more frequently than to viscera (lung > liver > adrenal gland). Diffuse pulmonary involvement is infrequent.

The standard staging scheme is that of Whitmore. Stage A represents cancer not detectable by rectal examination but found in a surgical specimen obtained during operation for prostatic hyperplasia or at autopsy. Stage A is subdivided into two groups: stage A_1, in which well-differentiated tumor is present in only a few transurethral chips from one lobe; and stage A_2, in which involvement is more diffuse. Stage B disease is palpable but confined to the prostate. Stage B_1 disease is a single nodule involving only one lobe and surrounded by tissue that is normal to palpation; stage B_2 involves the gland more diffusely. In stage C, palpable tumor extends beyond the prostate, but there are no distant metastases. In stage D, metastatic disease is present. Stage D_1 refers to involvement of pelvic nodes only with no other metastases, whereas in the D_2 category metastatic disease is more widespread. Any of the lower stages (A, B, or C) may progress directly to stage D. Failure to include pelvic lymphadenectomy in the staging process results in marked underestimation of the frequency of lymph node metastases; for example, about one-fifth of tumors tentatively classified as A_2 solely on the basis of prostate pathology actually constitute stage D disease when appropriate surgical staging is performed. The frequency with which early hematogenous metastases are missed with the current staging procedures is uncertain.

DIAGNOSIS **Symptoms and signs** Both early and advanced carcinoma of the prostate may be asymptomatic at the time of diagnosis, and more than 80 percent of patients have stage C or D disease at the time of diagnosis. In symptomatic subjects common presenting complaints (in descending order) include dysuria, difficulty in voiding, increased urinary frequency, complete urinary retention, back or hip pain, and hematuria. A high index of suspicion should be entertained in all men over age 40 with dysuria, frequency, or difficulty in voiding in the absence of mechanical urethral obstruction. Additional complications of advanced disease may include spinal cord compression for dual metastases, deep venous thrombosis and pulmonary emboli, and myelophthisis.

Palpation of the prostate is the most appropriate test for detection of all stages of disease other than stage A. Indeed, the importance of the rectal examination in the routine physical examination of men cannot be stressed too strongly. The posterior surfaces of the lateral lobes, where carcinoma begins most often, are easily palpable on digital rectal examination. Carcinoma characteristically is hard, nodular, and irregular, but induration may also be due to fibrous areas in benign prostatic hyperplasia, to focal infarcts, or to calculi as well as to tumor. The midline furrow between the lateral lobes may be obscured by either benign or malignant enlargement. Local extraprostatic extension of tumor into the seminal vesicles can also be detected by rectal exam. Scrotal and/or lower extremity lymphedema secondary to infiltration of pelvic lymph nodes are manifestations of extensive disease.

With the use of transrectal prostatic sonography, carcinoma is revealed as hypoechoic densities within the peripheral zone. The procedure is a sensitive means of identifying prostate cancer but is not specific enough for use as a screening test. Ultrasonography is useful for directing needle biopsy and for documenting the degree of extension of the tumor into bladder and seminal vesicles. Magnetic resonance imaging (MRI) and to a lesser degree computed tomography (CT) of the prostate may also be helpful in defining the extent of tumor and locating nodes for aspiration needle biopsy.

Biopsy Biopsy of the prostate is essential for establishing the diagnosis and is indicated when an abnormality is detected by palpation and/or by imaging or when lower urinary tract symptoms occur in men who have no known cause of obstruction. Core-needle biopsy may be performed transperineally or transrectally with less risk of bacterial contamination with the former and more precise sampling with the latter. Fine-needle aspiration cytology offers immediate diagnosis with minimal patient discomfort and morbidity. Open perineal biopsy is performed infrequently because it carries risk of at least temporary impotence and is a more extensive surgical procedure. Transurethral biopsy is also used infrequently because most early lesions are in the peripheral regions of the gland.

Biochemical markers Several biochemical markers provide ancillary information in diagnosing prostatic cancer. Elevation of serum prostate specific antigen (PSA) or acid phosphatase is present in some localized disease, more commonly with bony metastases. PSA is more sensitive than acid phosphatase in the identification of prostate cancer. However, no technique of assay for either the enzyme (including counterimmune electrophoresis and radioimmunoassay) or the antigen is sufficiently specific or sensitive for use in screening, and the major application of the assays is in following the progress of the disease. Likewise, none of the other biochemical markers studied—bone marrow acid phosphatase, hydroxyproline, cholesterol, isoleucine, glycine, aspartic acid, glutamic acid, methionine, or spermidine—has sufficiently high specificity or sensitivity for routine screening.

Assessment of metastic disease Bony metastases from prostatic carcinoma usually contain both osteoblastic and osteolytic components. The bony pelvis and lumbar vertebrae are involved most often, and metastases also occur in thoracic vertebrae, ribs, skull, and long bones. Skeletal survey has a low sensitivity of detection because a significant portion of bone must be involved to permit detection on a routine x-ray. Bone scans using radionuclides such as technetium 99 are more sensitive, but the specificity is not high because positive scans may occur in any metabolically hyperactive bone; this includes sites of inflammation, healing fractures, osteoarthritis, and Paget's disease. Therefore, when a positive radionuclide scan is obtained during an initial survey for bone metastases, the presence of other lesions must be excluded by conventional radiography of the affected site. Radionuclide bone scans are also useful for monitoring progression and response to therapy.

Surgical staging is the common modality for assessing lymph node involvement and determining therapy. The procedure usually includes removal of the external iliac, internal iliac, and obturator lymph node chains and is either performed by itself or in conjunction with prostatic surgery or implantation of radioactive beads. In some centers the initial procedure is either lymphangiography or pelvic CT scan of the pelvis, followed when positive by confirmatory thin-needle biopsy of the affected lymph nodes. When the CT scan or the lymphangiogram is negative, however, operative staging is mandatory.

TREATMENT **Surgery** Total prostatoseminovesiculectomy is the oldest treatment for carcinoma of the prostate. Radical perineal prostatectomy allows an easier vesicourethral anastomosis and less bleeding, while radical retropubic prostatectomy affords access to the pelvic lymph nodes. In experienced hands both procedures have a low risk of urinary incontinence (~ 1 percent for radical perineal and 1 to 4 percent for radical retropubic prostatectomy). Formerly both operations caused impotence in most patients. Improvements in surgical technique for the retropubic procedure allow preservation of the neurovascular supply to the corpora cavernosa and preservation of potency in the majority of patients without compromising the thoroughness of the operation.

Radical prostatectomy is not indicated for most stage A_1 cancer, since this disease usually is cured definitively by the simple prostatectomy at which the diagnosis is made. The role of radical prostatectomy in stage A_2 is unsettled. However, true stage A_2 disease in which pelvic nodes show no evidence of metastases may behave aggressively and be benefited by radical surgery, particularly when the neoplasm is anaplastic. Indeed, 5- and 10-year survivals equivalent to those of age-matched controls have been reported following such treatment for stage A_2 disease.

Radical prostatectomy has its clearest indication in stage B disease. Nearly all of the apparent surgical cures in this stage are in men who have 1- to 2-cm nodules involving only one lobe of the prostate (e.g., stage B_1), a group comprising only 5 percent of prostatic carcinoma patients. In addition, subjects with true stage B_2 disease may also be appropriate candidates for radical prostatectomy.

The effectiveness of radical prostatectomy for stage C disease is less certain. Morbidity rates from local pelvic symptoms, bladder outlet obstruction, hematuria, and ureteral obstruction may be decreased by radical prostatectomy in stage C disease, but controlled studies comparing morbidity rates after surgery with those following other therapies are lacking. Radical prostatectomy has little if any place in the treatment of stage D disease, and lymph node removal has no therapeutic benefit. Therefore, other means of therapy should be tried.

Radiation Radiation therapy was developed as a primary treatment in prostatic carcinoma because of a desire to avoid the impotence and occasional incontinence that followed radical prostatectomy. In most series, approximately 60 to 70 Gy (6000 to 7000 rad) are administered to the prostate over 6 weeks by a variety of delivery patterns. Radiation to the pelvic nodes may or may not be performed. Acute proctitis and urethritis are common side effects but are usually controllable by local measures and adjustments in radiation therapy. Chronic complications after full courses of external beam radiation include impotence in 30 to 60 percent; chronic proctitis in 10 to 15 percent; and occasional rectal stricture, rectal fistula, or rectal bleeding. It is not clear whether external beam radiation actually eradicates prostatic carcinoma, because many patients in whom progression of the tumor is slowed or halted have persistent tumor on rebiopsy, and the biologic potential of these persistent tumors is not clear.

The largest series on external beam radiation for prostatic cancer is that of Bagshaw; a variety of delivery techniques and doses were utilized in nearly 1300 patients, many of whom had received prior hormone manipulation. There was about 50 percent 10-year survival in stages A and B and a mean 10-year survival of 30 percent in stage C. The 5-year survival in stage D patients who received radiation to the pelvis as well was 58 percent. Several smaller studies have reported responses that in the aggregate are similar. The best results are obtained when the tumors are less than 2 cm in size at the time of therapy. There appears to be no consistent correlation between tumor grade and radiosensitivity.

Focal external beam radiation may be palliative for bone pain due to metastases. The duration of relief is variable. Radiation is less effective for alleviating ureteral obstruction secondary to metastatic tumor because the time lag for a successful response may be 6 to 8 weeks.

Interstitial radiation involves retropubic or perineal implantation of seeds of ^{125}I or ^{198}Au. This treatment avoids major extirpative surgery and provides a concentrated delivery of radiation to the target tissue. Successful seed implantation requires a well-defined primary tumor with a diameter less than 5 cm, a tumor volume less than 30 to 40 mL, and uniform distribution of seeds throughout the prostate. In the initial reports, 5-year survival following staging pelvic lymphadenectomy and retropubic implantation of ^{125}I or ^{198}Au seeds was comparable to survival rates after other forms of treatment, but the incidence of tumor progression is higher. Potency is preserved in more than 90 percent, and early complications are fewer and less severe than those after external beam radiation.

In summary, except for impotence following external beam radiation, serious morbidity is infrequent following either form of radiation therapy. Practical considerations make ^{125}I or ^{198}Au seed implantation most suited to stage B_1 disease. The long-term efficacy of either form of radiation as compared to radical prostatectomy for treatment of localized carcinoma (stages A_2, B_1, and B_2) is not clear, but current data suggest that radiotherapy may be less curative than radical prostatectomy.

Androgen deprivation Since growth of the normal prostate is dependent upon testicular androgens (see Chap. 321), it was logical to try androgen deprivation for treatment of prostatic cancer. Androgen deprivation can be achieved in four ways: (1) surgical extirpation of the glands that synthesize androgens (castration and adrenalectomy), (2) inhibition of pituitary gonadotropin (and/or adrenocorticotropic hormone, ACTH) production [estrogen therapy, hypophysectomy, or treatment with luteinizing hormone–releasing hormone (LHRH) analogues such as leuprolide or buserelin], (3) inhibition of androgen synthesis by the testes and adrenals (aminoglutethimide), and (4) inhibition of androgen binding to its receptor protein (cyproterone or flutamide).

The common means of achieving androgen deprivation at the clinical level are castration and estrogen therapy. Since testicular secretion accounts for more than 95 percent of testosterone production, bilateral orchiectomy results in a 90 percent decline of plasma levels. Estrogens such as diethylstilbestrol are potent inhibitors of the release from the pituitary gland of luteinizing hormone, the gonadotropin that regulates testosterone production, and consequently its administration also causes a fall in plasma testosterone to castration levels. Maximum depression of plasma testosterone is achieved with 3 mg of diethylstilbestrol per day. Other estrogens (conjugated estrogens, ethinyl estradiol, diethylstilbestrol diphosphate) are no more effective in lowering plasma testosterone than is diethylstilbestrol. Luteinizing hormone–releasing hormone analogues also inhibit leuteinizing hormone secretion and lower plasma testosterone levels.

Androgen depletion beyond that achieved by surgical castration, estrogen administration, or ACTH analogues can be accomplished by adrenalectomy. Since adrenal androgen production is under the control of ACTH, the adrenal sources of androgen can also be eliminated by hypophysectomy. The alternative to surgical ablation is the induction of a medical adrenalectomy and/or castration with drugs such as exogenous glucocorticoids that inhibit the synthesis of adrenal androgen or with agents such as flutamide that inhibit the binding of androgen to its cytoplasmic receptor protein. While these ancillary surgical and medical means have theoretical benefits for enhancing androgen deprivation, their usefulness in treating prostatic cancer is not established.

Androgen deprivation by means of bilateral orchiectomy, diethylstilbestrol therapy, or combined orchiectomy plus diethylstilbestrol was a standard form of treatment for carcinoma of the prostate for many years, based largely upon clinical reports comparing treatment groups with historical controls. Subsequently, in prospective control studies the effectiveness of high dose diethylstilbestrol or orchiectomy, alone or in combination, in enhancing survival in any stage of prostatic cancer was not clear cut. Furthermore, death from cardiovascular disease appeared to be more frequent in patients treated with large doses of diethylstilbestrol.

Even when there is no beneficial effect on survival, however, androgen deprivation decreases bone pain in two thirds of symptomatic stage D patients and hence constitutes a major therapy in the disease. Whether androgen deprivation therapy should be initiated early (asymptomatic phase) or late (symptomatic phase) in stage D disease is unsettled. Once the decision is made to institute such therapy, the choice must be made as to which form of androgen deprivation is appropriate. When acceptable to the patient, orchiectomy is safe and inexpensive and circumvents compliance problems. Diethylstilbestrol is also inexpensive and is usually safe in dosages of 3 mg per day or less in men who do not have preexisting cardiovascular disease. In men at risk for cardiovascular complications LHRH analogues appear to cause similar response rates and to have less cardiovascular complications than diethylstilbestrol. Hence, LHRH analogue treatment is an alternative to diethylstilbestrol and to orchiectomy.

Chemotherapy The age group at greatest risk for prostatic cancer has poor tolerance for chemotherapy. This feature, coupled with the variable course of the disease, makes it difficult to determine the effectiveness of such therapy. However, several comprehensive trials utilizing chemotherapy have been undertaken in stage D disease following relapse after hormonal treatment, a situation in which mean survival time is only 7 to 8 months. The agents studied most extensively are estramustine phosphate, prednimustine, and cisplatin; more limited trials have been conducted with 5-fluorouracil, melphalan, and hydroxyurea. Complete response is rare, and only one-tenth of stage D patients have an objective partial response. In other trials combinations of chemotherapeutic agents have been tested in stage D disease, most commonly estramustine phosphate plus prednimustine or cyclophosphamide plus another agent. Complete response is again rare, and only one-fourth of patients or fewer show any objective improvement. For progressive, symptomatic stage D prostatic cancer, endocrine ablation therapy should be undertaken first, but chemotherapeutic agents may provide some benefit when such patients relapse.

REFERENCES

Benign prostatic hyperplasia

WALSH PC: Benign prostatic hyperplasia, in *Campbell's Urology*, PC Walsh et al (eds). Philadelphia, Saunders, 1986, p 1248–1267

WILSON JD: The pathogenesis of prostatic hyperplasia. Am J Med 68:745, 1980

Carcinoma of the prostate

BAGSHAW MA: External radiation therapy of carcinoma of the prostate. Cancer 45:1912, 1980

BYAR DP, CORLE DK: VACURG randomized trial of radical prostatectomy for Stages I and II prostate cancer. Urology 17(4) (Suppl):7, 1981

Catalona WJ, Scott WW: Carcinoma of the prostate, in *Campbell's Urololgy*, PC Walsh et al (eds). Philadelphia, Saunders, 1986
Eisenberger M et al: A reevaluation of nonhormonal cytotoxic chemotherapy for the treatment of prostatic carcinoma. J Clin Oncol 3:827, 1985
Ercole CJ et al: Prostatic specific antigen and prostatic acid phosphatase in the monitoring and staging of patients with prostatic cancer. J Urol 138:1181, 1987
Guinan P et al: The accuracy of the rectal examination in the diagnosis of prostatic carcinoma. N Engl J Med 303:499, 1980
Hennricksson P, Johansson S-E: Prediction of cardiovascular complication in patients with prostatic cancer treated with estrogen. Am J Epidemiol 125:970, 1987
Herr HW: Iodine 125 implantation in the management of localized prostatic carcinoma. Urol Clin North Am 7:605, 1980
Jewett HJ: Radical perineal prostatectomy for palpable clinically localized, non-obstructive cancer. Experience at the Johns Hopkins Hospital, 1909–1963. J Urol 124: 492, 1980
Klein LA: Prostatic carcinoma. N Engl J Med 300:824, 1979
Leuprolide Study Group: Leuprolide versus diethylstilbestrol for metastatic prostate cancer. N Engl J Med 311:1281, 1984
Murphy GP et al: Current status of classification and staging of prostate cancer. Cancer 45:1889, 1980
National Institutes of Health Consensus Development Conference: The management of clinically localized prostate cancer. J Urol 138:1369, 1987
Schmidt JD: Chemotherapy of hormone-resistant stage D prostatic cancer. J Urol 123:797, 1980
Smith JA Jr: New methods of endocrine management of prostatic cancer. J Urol 137:1, 1987
Stamey TA: Cancer of the prostate. An analysis of some important contributions and dilemmas. 1982 Monographs in Urology 3:67, 1983
Walsh PC: Physiologic basis for hormonal therapy in carcinoma of the prostate. Urol Clin N Am 2:125, 1975
——— et al: Radical surgery for prostatic cancer. Cancer 45:1906, 1980

307 SKIN CANCER

NEIL A. SWANSON

Cancer of the skin is the most common neoplasm among adults in the United States; more than 500,000 new cases of nonmelanoma skin cancer occur annually. The majority of nonmelanoma skin cancers are basal cell carcinomas (BCC). The second most common are squamous cell carcinomas (SCC). This chapter will concentrate on BCC, describing its etiology, clinical and histologic presentation, and treatment modalities. Once these are understood, a logical choice of treatment can be offered providing a success rate of greater than 95 percent.

ETIOLOGY Exposure to sunlight, principally ultraviolet (UV-B spectrum), is a primary etiologic factor for nonmelanoma skin cancer. These cancers occur principally on sun-exposed skin, commonly on the head and neck. There is abundant evidence to support the combined effects of UV light, immune system function (as affected by UV exposure), and the protection afforded by melanin in skin cancer. Individuals with outdoor occupations, for instance, sailors and farmers, have a higher incidence of cancer than persons with indoor occupations. The incidence of solar keratosis, sun damage, and skin cancers on the hand and forearm of automobile drivers correlates with local driving practices and occupations: in the United States, the left side of the body; in Australia, the right side of the body. Skin type also plays a role. Fair-skinned Caucasian persons of Scottish, English, or Irish descent with red or light blond hair, blue eyes, and freckles are particularly susceptible.

Other predisposing factors include exposure to carcinogens, trauma or scarring, chronic radiation damage, viral infection, and immunosuppression. Arsenic is the most common chemical carcinogen; exposure is through medicine (Fowler's solution) or well water, which induces nonmelanoma skin cancers with a latent period of decades. Both BCC and SCC may arise in areas of chronic scarring as well as in areas of chronic x-ray damage. In most instances the radiation damage occurs following x-ray therapy administered several decades before for the treatment of acne or as a depilatory. Viral oncogenesis in nonmelanoma skin cancer probably contributes as a cocarcinogen. Many subtypes of human papilloma virus (HPV) have been found in verrucae, lesions of bowenoid papulosis, and genital neoplasms. HPV type 5 is most commonly found in benign lesions in patients with epidermal dysplasia verruciformis. HPV-5 has also been found in cancers developed from these lesions, and the papilloma virus, when combined with other oncogenic factors such as UV light and a decrease in cell-mediated immunity, can induce carcinomas. Defects in the immune system, seen most frequently with the use of immunosuppression in transplant patients, have produced a higher incidence of nonmelanoma skin cancers secondary to the immunosuppressive therapy. The behavior of these neoplasms is often aggressive. Lastly, genetic factors can play a role. The nevoid basal cell carcinoma syndrome is an autosomal dominant condition in which patients develop very large numbers of BCCs beginning in the second decade and eventually involving all parts of the skin. Xeroderma pigmentosum, an autosomal recessive disorder of defective DNA repair, is also associated with multiple cutaneous carcinomas.

CLINICAL PRESENTATION **Basal cell carcinoma** BCC usually occurs as a single lesion on hair-bearing and sun-exposed skin. There are five clinical types. The most common tumor is the *noduloulcerative* BCC. It usually presents as a raised, papular lesion that has translucent borders and exhibits telangiectasia and/or central ulceration. Histologic examination reveals circumscribed nests of tumor cells in the dermis with associated stromal retraction and palisading of the tumor cells at the periphery of the nests. Other clinical variants of BCC include *superficial* BCC, *pigmented* BCC, *morpheaform* BCC, and *keratotic* BCC. The superficial BCC can mimic chronic eczema in appearance, being red and scaly with a sharply marginated border. Pigmented BCC can have a smooth, somewhat translucent border with deep pigmentation, at times mimicking and being mistaken for malignant melanoma. More worrisome and difficult to treat, the morpheaform BCC often presents as a yellowish to white plaque-like lesion with telangiectasia, often mistaken clinically for morphea. It and the keratotic BCC (basosquamous carcinoma) are aggressive tumors with an infiltrative histology. BCC can recur within scar tissue, at the periphery of a scar or skin graft, or as a deep nodule. Care must be taken to examine any suspected recurrence and to biopsy and treat these lesions appropriately. BCC can recur up to 10 years after treatment, and there is a higher incidence of new primary nonmelanoma skin cancers in patients who have had a BCC than in individuals who have not. Therefore, long-term follow-up examination of the skin in these patients is important. The natural history of BCC is that of a slowly growing, locally invasive neoplasm. The degree of invasion depends on histologic subtype, with the morpheaform and keratotic BCCs as well as recurrent BCC being the most infiltrative and displaying more aggressive behavior. They also can be especially troublesome in immunosuppressed patients. Basal cell carcinoma rarely metastasizes; the incidence is less than 0.5 percent.

Squamous cell carcinoma SCC arises from epidermal keratinocytes. It commonly develops from sun-damaged skin or from a preexisting lesion such as chronic radiodermatitis, keratosis (solar or arsenical), chronic scar of any type (trauma), a lesion of lupus erythematosus, a chronic ulcer, a burn scar (Marjolin's ulcer), and other chronic inflammatory states. The red, scaly actinic keratosis can be premalignant, with SCC occasionally arising in a hypertrophic lesion.

SCC in situ occurs in the skin. It represents intraepidermal carcinoma consisting of atypical keratinocytes with pleomorphic nuclei confined to the epidermis. This clinically mimics chronic eczema but is more erythematous with a very sharply marginated border. Bowen's disease is the most common form of squamous cell carcinoma in situ. Erythroplasia of Queyrat is carcinoma in situ of the penis.

SCC can manifest as a noduloulcerative lesion with rolled margins. It can have satellite nodularity and can also be pigmented. Histologically the tumor has broad sheets and strands of atypical keratinocytes usually connected to the epidermis. These can infiltrate to the depths of the lower reticular dermis and subcutaneous tissue. Some pathologists grade SCC histologically as well, moderately, or poorly differentiated or as spindle cell tumor. This grading is not as critical as it is for other noncutaneous forms of SCC.

The natural history of SCC depends on its clinical nature, size, location, and depth of invasion. It has been stated that SCC arising in sun-exposed, actinically damaged skin has a lower metastatic rate than that arising on non-sun-exposed skin or in chronic scars and/or ulcers. This is probably true, but increasing evidence shows that this may be a result of the superficiality of actinically induced SCC. SCC that has infiltrated to the deep reticular dermis and fat, especially in the temple and periauricular areas, has a metastatic rate approaching that of de novo SCC, 10 to 30 percent. Mucocutaneous SCC, usually presenting on the lip, can metastasize in up to 12 percent of cases. Metastasis is usually angiolymphatic, presenting initially in local lymph nodes.

TREATMENT MODALITIES The treatment of BCC and SCC is similar, especially for small, histologically nonaggressive tumors. In order to determine the most appropriate type of treatment, a skin biopsy is necessary, not only to diagnose the tumor type, but also the histologic subtype. Incisional biopsies do not enhance metastasis, and a shave or punch biopsy can safely and adequately yield a diagnosis. In general, if the lesion is to be treated by a means other than excision, a shave biopsy is appropriate. A full-thickness biopsy, such as a punch, leaves a full-thickness scar that necessitates excision.

Treatment modalities used with basal cell carcinoma fall into the following groups: (1) excision, (2) electrodesiccation and curettage, (3) cryosurgery, (4) radiation therapy, and (5) Moh's surgery. A thorough discussion of these modalities is beyond the scope of this chapter. However, experience with all techniques, in conjunction with tumor type and clinical setting, is critical to ensure maximal therapeutic success while sparing as much normal tissue as possible. In most instances, SCCs are best treated with surgical excision or Moh's surgery. Actinic keratoses may be treated with topical liquid nitrogen.

REFERENCES

ALBRIGHT SD: Treatment of skin cancer using multiple modalities. J Am Acad Dermatol 7:143, 1982

FITZPATRICK TB et al (eds): Disorders of the dermis, in *Dermatology in General Medicine*, 3d ed. New York, McGraw-Hill, 1987, sect 16, pp 1033–1130

KOPF AW et al: Curettage-electrodesiccation treatment of basal cell carcinomas. Arch Dermatol 113:439, 1977

308 MELANOMA AND OTHER PIGMENTED SKIN LESIONS

ARTHUR J. SOBER / HOWARD K. KOH

Pigmented skin lesions are among the most common findings on physical examination. The challenge is to distinguish cutaneous melanoma, which may be lethal, from the remainder, which with rare exception are benign.

Melanoma originates from melanocytes, pigment cells present normally in epidermis and sometimes in dermis. This tumor affects approximately 28,000 individuals per year in the United States, resulting in 5800 deaths. The incidence has increased dramatically (700 percent increase in the past 40 years); it affects young individuals (onset from midteens); it has distinct clinical features which make it detectable at a time when cure by surgical excision is possible; and it is located on the skin surface, where it is visible. If the incidence continues to increase at the present rate, within a decade lifetime risk of melanoma will approximate 1 percent.

The reason for the increased incidence is uncertain, but may stem from increased recreational sun exposure especially early in life. Individuals of similar ethnic background who emigrate after childhood to areas of high sun exposure (Israel, Australia) have lower melanoma rates than individuals of similar age either born in these countries or who emigrated before age 10. Individuals most susceptible to development of melanoma are those with fair complexions, red or blond hair, blue or gray eyes, and freckles, and who are poor tanners and easy sunburners. In one literature survey 9 of 11 studies linked increased melanoma risk to history of sunburn. Other factors associated with increased risk include family history of melanoma (approximately 1 in 10 melanoma patients have a family member with melanoma), presence of a dysplastic nevus (atypical mole), a giant congenital melanocytic nevus, a small to medium-sized congenital melanocytic nevus (see below), and immunosuppression (Table 308-1). The presence of a large number of normal nevi may also be a risk factor for melanoma. A 64-fold increased risk for individuals with 50 or more nevi ≥ 2 mm in size has been reported. Melanoma is relatively infrequent in heavily pigmented peoples. Dark-skinned populations (natives of India, Puerto Rico), blacks, and Orientals have rates one-seventh to one-tenth that noted for lighter skinned Caucasians.

TABLE 308-1 Risk factors for cutaneous melanoma

High risk (>50-fold increased risk)
Persistently changing mole
Dysplastic nevi in patient with two family members with melanoma
Adulthood vs. childhood
>50 nevi ≥2 mm
Intermediate risk (~10-fold)
Family history of melanoma
Sporadic dysplastic nevi
Congenital nevi (?)
Caucasians vs. blacks or Orientals
Personal history of prior melanoma
Low risk (2- to 4-fold)
Immunosuppression
Sun sensitivity or excess exposure

SOURCE: Adapted from Rhodes et al.

CLINICAL CHARACTERISTICS There are four types of cutaneous melanoma (Table 308-2). Three of these—superficial spreading, lentigo maligna, and acral lentiginous melanoma have a period of superficial (radial) growth when the lesion increases in size but does not penetrate deeply. It is during the radial growth period that melanoma is most capable of cure by surgical excision. The fourth type, nodular melanoma, does not have a recognizable radial growth phase and usually presents as a deeply invasive lesion, fully capable of early metastasis. When tumors begin to penetrate deeply into the skin, they are in the vertical growth phase. Melanomas with radial growth phases are characterized by irregular and sometimes notched borders, variation in pigment pattern, and variation in color. Increase in size or change is noted by the patient in 70 percent of early lesions. Bleeding, ulceration, and pain are late signs and are of little help in early recognition. Nodular melanomas are dark brown–black to blue-black nodules. Melanoma may occasionally be amelanotic where the diagnosis of a new or changing skin nodule is established histologically as melanoma. Lentigo maligna melanoma confines itself to chronically sun-damaged, sun-exposed sites (face, neck, back of hands) in older individuals and appears to result from chronic solar damage similar to that seen with the nonmelanoma skin cancers (basal cell and squamous cell carcinomas). Acral lentiginous melanoma occurs on palms, soles, nail beds, and mucous membranes. While this type occurs in whites, it is most frequent (along with nodular melanoma) in blacks and Orientals. Superficial spreading melanoma (which in some cases may be deeply invasive) is most frequent in whites. Melanomas arising in dysplastic nevi (see below) are usually of this type. The back is the most common site for melanoma in men. In women the back and the lower leg from knee to ankle are frequent sites.

PROGNOSTIC FACTORS Prognostic factors are similar in white populations throughout the world (western Europe, United States,

TABLE 308-2 Clinical features of malignant melanoma

Type	Site	Average age at diagnosis, years	Duration of known existence, years	Color
Lentigo maligna melanoma	Sun-exposed surfaces, particularly malar region of cheek and temple	70	5–20* or longer	In flat portions, shades of brown and tan predominant, but whitish gray occasionally present; in nodules, shades of reddish brown, bluish gray, bluish black
Superficial spreading melanoma	Any site (more common on upper back and in women on lower legs)	40–50	1–7	Shades of brown mixed with bluish red (violaceous), bluish black, reddish brown, and often whitish pink, and the border of lesion is at least in part visibly and/or palpably elevated
Nodular melanoma	Any site	40–50	Months to less than 5 years	Reddish blue (purple) or bluish black; either uniform in color or mixed with brown or black
Acral lentiginous melanoma	Palm, sole, nail bed, mucous membrane	60	1–10	In flat portions, dark brown predominantly; in raised lesions (plaques) brown-black or blue-black predominantly

* During much of this time, the precursor stage, lentigo maligna, is actively confined to the epidermis.
SOURCE: Adapted from AJ Sober, in *Pathophysiology of Dermatologic Diseases*. NA Soter, HP Baden (eds), New York, McGraw-Hill, 1984.

Australia). The most important prognostic factor is stage at time of presentation. Five-year survival for clinical stage I (primary tumor; no clinical evidence of disease elsewhere) is about 85 percent. For clinical stage II (clinically palpable regional nodes that contain tumor), a 5-year survival of about 50 percent is noted when only one node is involved and about 15 to 20 percent when four or more nodes are involved. Five-year survival for clinical stage III (disseminated disease) is less than 5 percent. Fortunately, the majority of melanomas are diagnosed in clinical stage I. Within stage I, a gradient of prognosis can be delineated based on the thickness of the primary tumor (Table 308-3). This system is based on the rationale that the likelihood of metastasis should correlate with tumor volume. Thickness is the best single index of tumor volume. Melanomas less than 0.76 mm thick are usually cured by surgical removal (5-year survivals range from 96 to 99 percent). Approximately 40 percent of primary melanomas now fall into this low-risk category (thickness < 1 mm). When low-risk patients develop metastases, the primary tumors often exhibit either extensive microscopic features of regression or a small vertical growth phase. Approximately 60 percent of individuals with melanomas ≥ 3.65 mm thick will develop metastatic disease; most of these patients die from their melanoma. These thick tumors are almost always raised substantially above the plane of the skin. Two intermediate categories of thickness exist (Table 308-3). Certain anatomic sites appear to have more favorable prognoses, and some anatomic sites appear less favorable after adjusting for thickness. The favorable sites appear to be forearm and leg (excluding feet). Unfavorable sites include scalp, hands, feet, and mucous membranes. Survival for women in stage I is in general more favorable than for men, in part because of earlier diagnosis; women frequently have melanomas on the lower leg where self-recognition is more likely, and where prognosis is better. Older individuals, in general, have

TABLE 308-3 Prognosis of stage I melanoma by thickness (Breslow): 5-year survival rates for stage I

	Survival, %	
Thickness, mm	Overall	MCCG*
<0.76	96	99
0.76–1.49	87	95
1.50–2.49	75	84
2.50–3.99	66	70
≥4.00	47	44

* MCCG = Melanoma Clinical Cooperative Group.
SOURCE: From Balch.

poorer prognoses. This has been explained, in part, on delayed diagnosis (thicker tumors) and a higher proportion of acral melanomas (palmar-plantar), which have relatively less favorable prognoses. As in breast cancer, recurrence of melanoma may occur after many years. About 10 to 15 percent of first time recurrences develop after 5 years so that prolonged follow-up (at least 10 years) is warranted. The time to recurrence varies inversely with tumor thickness. Other prognostic factors for stage I melanoma include presence of an ulcer in the primary tumor, mitotic rate, and the presence of microscopic tumor satellites (foci of tumor ≥0.05 mm in diameter) in the reticular dermis or subcutaneous fat distinct from the main body of the tumor. The presence of microscopic satellites is also predictive of microscopic metastases to the regional lymph nodes. An alternate prognostic scheme for clinical stage I melanoma is based on determination of anatomic level of invasion within the skin. Level I is intraepidermal (in situ), level II penetrates the papillary dermis, level III fills the papillary dermis, level IV penetrates the reticular dermis, and level V penetrates into the subcutaneous fat. Survival at 5 years by level of invasion averages 100, 95, 82, 71, and 49 percent, respectively.

NATURAL HISTORY As noted above, stage I melanoma usually behaves in a predictable manner. Melanomas may spread by the lymphatic channels or the bloodstream. Earliest metastases are to regional lymph nodes. Drainage pathways can be predicted based on anatomic charts (which are frequently wrong) or on lymphoscintigraphy using technetium 99m injected around the primary tumor site. Surgical lymphadenectomy usually controls regional disease.

Liver, lung, bone, and brain are common sites of hematogenous spread, but unusual sites such as the anterior chamber of the eye may also occur. Most deaths result from brain metastases. Once metastatic disease is established, likelihood of cure is negligible.

MANAGEMENT The entire cutaneous surface including scalp and mucous membranes should be examined in each patient. Bright room illumination is important, and a 7- to 10× hand lens is helpful for evaluating variation in pigment pattern. A history of relevant risk factors should be elicited. Any suspicious lesions should either be biopsied, referred to a specialist, or recorded by chart and/or photography for follow-up. Examination of the lymph nodes and palpation of the abdominal viscera is part of the staging examination for suspected melanoma. The patient should be advised to have other family members screened if either melanoma or dysplastic nevi are present. The detection of early melanoma in relatives upon screening has been reported. Until other causes of melanoma are more clearly understood, protection from the sun should be practiced by the patient. Routine use of a sunblock of SPF ≥ 15, use of protective clothing, and avoiding intense midday ultraviolet exposure should be recommended. The patient should be educated in the clinical features of melanoma and advised to report any new growth or other change in a pigmented lesion. Patient education brochures are available from the American Cancer Society, the American Academy of Dermatology, and the Skin Cancer Foundation. Self-examination at 6- to 8-week intervals enhances the likelihood of detecting change between follow-up visits. The importance of routine follow-up visits for melanoma patients and patients with dysplastic nevi should be emphasized, since this facilitates early detection of new tumors.

PRECURSOR LESIONS A peculiar type of nevus termed the *dysplastic nevus* occurs in certain families affected by melanoma. In some families melanomas occur nearly exclusively in individuals with the dysplastic nevi. The nevi appear to be transmitted as an autosomal dominant trait. In other families the nevi may not be present in all individuals at risk of melanoma. The melanomas may arise within the dysplastic nevus (acting as a precursor) or in normal skin (the nevus acting as a marker of increased risk). An individual with dysplastic nevi and two family members with melanoma has a greater than 50 percent lifetime risk for developing melanoma. Table 308-4 lists the characteristic features of dysplastic nevi and their differentiation from benign acquired nevi. The number of dysplastic nevi may vary from one to several hundred. Dysplastic nevi usually look different one compared to another. The borders are often hazy and indistinct, and the pigment pattern is more highly variable than that in benign acquired nevi. Since the frequency of dysplastic nevi in melanoma-prone families is greater than 50 percent, some observers have suggested a polygenic inheritance rather than a single-gene pattern of inheritance. Of the 90 percent of melanoma patients regarded as sporadic (lacking a family history of melanoma), about 40 percent have dysplastic nevi, as compared to an estimated 5 percent of the population at large. Further studies to determine background frequency of dysplastic nevi are required once greater unanimity exists regarding the clinical and histopathologic features of dysplastic nevi. At present the diagnosis of dysplastic nevi is made microscopically. The fact that at least 20 percent of sporadic melanomas arise in association with a dysplastic nevus makes the dysplastic nevus the most important precursor for melanoma. Thus, recognition of the lesion is of paramount importance.

Less frequent precursors include the giant congenital melanocytic nevus and the small congenital melanocytic nevus. Congenital nevi are present at birth or appear in the neonatal period (tardive form). The giant melanocytic nevus, also called bathing trunk, cape, or garment nevus, is a rare malformation that affects perhaps 1 in 100,000 individuals. These nevi are usually greater than 20 cm in diameter and may cover more than half of the body surface. Giant nevi often occur in association with multiple small congenital nevi. The borders are sharp, and hair may be present. The lesions are usually dark brown and may have darker and lighter areas. Pigment is haphazardly displayed. The surface is smooth to rugose to cerebriform and may vary from one portion of the lesion to another. A lifetime risk of melanoma development of 6 percent has been estimated. The greatest risk is before age 5 and the next greatest period of risk is between ages 5 and 10. Early detection of melanoma is difficult in these lesions because of the deep dermal or subcutaneous origin of primary melanoma and because of the large and varied surface. Prophylactic excision early in life can be accomplished by staged removal with coverage by split-thickness skin grafts. The use of cultured keratinocytes for coverage appears promising.

The small to medium-sized congenital nevus, affecting approximately 1 percent of people, presents usually as a raised dark to medium brown lesion with a smooth or papillomatous surface. The border is sharp, and lesions may be oriented along lines of skin cleavage. Follicular hyper- and hypopigmentation may coexist in a salt-and-pepper configuration. The lesion may have an excess of thick coarse hairs. The risk of developing melanoma in these lesions is at present unknown; however, melanomas can arise in these lesions. From body surface area considerations, the coincidence of melanoma and small congenital nevi at the same site is probably higher than that calculated by chance. The remnants of a nevus with histopathologic features of a congenital nevus have been observed in 2 to 6 percent of melanomas. Management of small to medium-sized congenital nevi remains controversial, but at many medical centers consideration is given to prophylactic removal under local anesthesia in the early teen years. Melanomas in small congenital nevi appear to occur after this period of life.

DIFFERENTIAL DIAGNOSIS The aim of differential diagnosis is to separate benign pigmented lesions from melanoma and its precursors. If melanoma is a consideration, then biopsy or referral to a specialist is appropriate. It is appropriate to remove some benign look-alikes in order to decrease the chance of missing a melanoma. Table 308-5 summarizes the distinguishing features of benign lesions that may be confused with melanoma.

BIOPSY Any pigmented cutaneous lesion that has changed in size or shape or has other features suggestive of malignant melanoma should be biopsied. The recommended technique is a full-thickness excisional biopsy, as it facilitates pathologic assessment of the lesion, permits accurate measurement of thickness if the lesion is melanoma, and constitutes treatment if the lesion is benign. Shave biopsy or curettage of a suspected melanoma is contraindicated. For large lesions or lesions on anatomic sites where excisional biopsy may not be feasible (such as the face, hands, or feet), an incisional biopsy through the most nodular or darkest area of the lesion is acceptable; this should represent the vertical growth phase of the primary tumor. While there is a theoretical concern that an incisional biopsy might facilitate the spread of metastases, data from prospective studies do not support that concern.

STAGING Once the diagnosis of malignant melanoma has been confirmed, the tumor must be staged to determine prognosis and treatment. The history should probe for evidence of metastatic disease, such as malaise, weight loss, headaches, balance problem, visual difficulty, or bone pain. The physical examination should be especially directed to the skin, regional draining lymph nodes, central nervous system, liver, and spleen. In the absence of signs or symptoms of metastases, few laboratory or radiologic tests are indicated for staging purposes. Aside from a chest x-ray and, possibly, liver function tests, no other tests or scans are routinely indicated unless the history or physical examination suggests metastases to a specific organ. Specifically, liver-spleen scans and computed tomography have a low

TABLE 308-4 Clinical features distinguishing dysplastic nevi from benign acquired nevi

Clinical feature	Dysplastic nevi	Benign acquired nevi
Color	Variable mixtures of tan, brown, black, or red/pink within a single nevus; nevi may look very different from each other	Uniformly tan or brown.
Shape	Irregular borders; pigment may fade off into surrounding skin; macular portion at the edge of the nevus	Round; sharp, clear-cut borders between the nevus and the surrounding skin; may be flat or elevated.
Size	Usually more than 6 mm; may be more than 10 mm; occasionally smaller than 6 mm	Usually less than 6 mm in diameter.
Number	Often very many (more than 100), but occasionally may be only one	In a typical adult: 10 to 40 are scattered over the body; perhaps 15% of patients have no nevi.
Location	Sun-exposed areas; the back is the most common site, but dysplastic nevi may also be seen on the scalp, breasts, and buttocks	Generally on the sun-exposed surfaces of the skin above the waist; the scalp, breasts, and buttocks are rarely involved.

SOURCE: Modified from Friedman et al.

TABLE 308-5 Pigmented lesions that must be distinguished from cutaneous melanoma and its precursors

Lesion	Description
Blue nevus	Gun metal or cerulean blue, blue-gray. Stable over time. One-half occur on dorsa of hand and feet. Lesions are usually single, small, 3 mm to < 1 cm. Must be distinguished from nodular melanoma.
Compound nevus	Round or oval shape, well-demarcated, smooth-bordered. May be dome-shaped or papillomatous; colors range from flesh colored to very dark brown with individual nevi being relatively homogeneous in color.
Hemangioma	Dome-shaped reddish, purple, blue nodule. Compression with a glass microscope slide may result in blanching. Must be distinguished from nodular melanoma.
Junctional nevus	Flat to barely raised brown lesion. Sharp border. Fine pigmentary stippling noted especially upon magnification.
Lentigo Juvenile Solar	Flat uniformly medium or dark brown lesion with sharp border. Solar lentigenes are acquired lesions on sites of chronic solar exposure (backs of hands/face). Lesions are 2 mm to ≥1 cm. Solar lentigenes have reticulate pigmentation upon magnification.
Pigmented basal cell carcinoma	Papular border. May have central ulceration. Usually solar exposed surface in older patient. Patient usually has dark brown eyes and dark brown or black hair.
Pigmented dermatofibroma	Lesion is not well demarcated visually, is firm, and dimples downward when compressed laterally. Usually on extremities. Usually < 6 mm.
Seborrheic keratosis	Rough, stuck on, waxy feeling lesions with sharp borders ranging in color from flesh to tan, to dark brown. Presence of keratin plugs in surface of help in discriminating especially dark lesions from melanoma.
Subungual hematoma	Maroon (red-brown) coloration. As lesion grows out from nailfold, a curving clear area seen.
Tattoo (medical or traumatic)	In medical tattoo lesions are small pigmentary dots often blue or green which make a regular pattern (rectangle). Traumatic tattoos are irregular, and pigmentation may appear black.

yield and are not cost-effective. However, if signs of metastases exist, favored sites of spread, such as the liver, lungs, bone, and brain, should be scanned.

Staging categories are stage I (confined to the skin), stage II disease (spread to regional lymph nodes), and stage III (distant metastases). It is important to indicate whether staging was clinically or pathologically determined, or both—for example, the disease in a patient without palpable adenopathy but with microscopic disease found on biopsy would be classified as clinical stage I and pathologic stage II and has a different prognosis from one that is stage I by both clinical and pathologic criteria.

SURGICAL MANAGEMENT For a newly diagnosed stage I cutaneous melanoma, wide surgical excision of the lesion with a margin of normal skin is necessary to remove all malignant cells and minimize local recurrence. The "5-cm rule" states that the normal skin within 5 cm of the edge of the primary cutaneous melanoma should be excised. Such margins often require split-thickness skin grafts and are cosmetically disfiguring. Narrower margins have been regarded as more appropriate by some, as they allow for primary closure and may obviate the need for grafts or flaps. The appropriate width of the narrow margin is a source of controversy. Some literature suggests that while narrower surgical margins increase rates of local tumor recurrence, they have little to no effect on overall survival. A World Health Organization trial prospectively randomized between 1-cm and 3-cm margins in 612 patients with thin malignant melanomas (≤ 2 mm in thickness) reported that the thinner surgical margin resulted in higher rates of local recurrence but no difference in nodal metastases, distant metastases, disease-free survival, or overall survival after $4\frac{1}{2}$ years of follow-up. For thicker stage I lesions, definitive data are not available, but margins up to 3 cm appear to be reasonable. Once again, for lesions on the face, hands, and feet, strict adherence to margins must give way to individual considerations about the constraints of surgery and minimization of morbidity. In all instances, however, inclusion of subcutaneous fat in the surgical specimen allows for adequate thickness and assessment of surgical margins by the pathologist.

ELECTIVE REGIONAL NODE DISSECTION Elective regional node dissection in clinical stage I disease (without palpable adenopathy) has been advocated, based on the hypothesis that melanoma metastases disseminate in an orderly fashion from the skin to regional lymph nodes and finally to distant sites. Hence, surgical excision of nodal micrometastases could theoretically provide definitive treatment at a time of relatively low tumor burden and, hopefully, improve survival. The efficacy of this procedure remains unproven; while some retrospective series suggest a survival benefit, two randomized studies examining this question in patients with limb melanomas and clinical stage I disease showed no survival advantage between wide local excision followed by immediate elective regional node dissection and wide local excision followed by delayed dissection only if nodes became palpable. Furthermore, the procedure has associated morbidity and is complicated by the fact that many lesions, especially those on the trunk, have ambiguous nodal draining sites, making it difficult to decide which area to dissect. In situations of multiple draining sites, lymphoscintigraphy can be utilized to define the nodes that serve as the primary drainage area. Certainly, not all patients with clinical stage I disease require node dissections. Patients with lesions <0.75 mm thick have excellent prognoses and need no node dissection; at the other extreme, patients with lesions >3.50 mm have such a high risk for distant metastases that the possible benefit of an elective node dissection would be negated. A subset of patients with lesions of intermediate thickness may benefit the most from elective regional node dissection, but there is no consensus about which patients should undergo this procedure. Randomized studies may resolve this issue.

ADJUVANT THERAPY For patients free of disease but at high risk for metastases, adjuvant therapy that complements surgery is needed to destroy occult micrometastases, prolong disease-free survival, and improve cure rates. Many strategies have been tried, including chemotherapy, nonspecific immunotherapy such as immunization with bacillus Calmette-Guérin (BCG), chemoimmunotherapy, and radiation therapy. However, such studies have been hampered by improper stratification, lack of inclusion of those at high risk, lack of randomization, inadequate sample size, or inadequate length of follow-up. Hence, no consistent evidence documents adjuvant therapy as effective. Current trials are focused on specific active immunotherapy using viral antigens to induce tumor lysis. This is based on the hypothesis that the juxtaposition of strong viral antigens and putative weak tumor-associated or tumor-specific antigens can heighten a host immune response against micrometastases. Early studies are promising.

TREATMENT OF METASTATIC DISEASE Melanoma can metastasize to any organ, the brain being a particularly favored site. Metastatic melanoma is generally incurable, and survival is generally less than 1 year. Thus, the goal of treatment is usually palliative to improve the quality of life. Patients with soft-tissue and node metastases fare better than those with liver and brain metastases. If metastases are limited to regional nodes (stage II disease), a therapeutic lymph node dissection is indicated. Surgical excision of a single metastasis to the lung or surgically accessible brain site can also prolong survival. More often, however, patients have multiple brain metastases that require radiation and glucocorticoids. Radiation therapy is aimed at providing local palliation for recurrent tumors or metastatic sites. Chemotherapy has been generally disappointing, and the best single agent, imidazole carboximide (dacarbazine), has a response rate of only 20 to 25 percent and rarely induces complete remission. Combination chemotherapy does not result in consistent improvement in remission and survival rates compared to those of a single agent. Patients who have advanced regional disease isolated to a limb may benefit from hyperthermic limb perfusion with melphalan, which concentrates the chemotherapeutic agents and minimizes systemic leakage. In addition, in vitro and in vivo chemosensitivity tests may help select patients likely to benefit from chemotherapy. The lack of response to traditional treatments has spawned many trials using agents such as retinoids, high-dosage chemotherapy with autologous bone marrow transplantation, interferons, antipigmentary agents, and antibodies conjugated to isotopes, drugs, and toxins. Of all these investigational therapies, adoptive immunotherapy has the most promise; this treatment involves exposing lymphocytes from cancer patients to interleukin 2 (IL-2) to generate lymphokine-activated killer cells (LAK cells); the LAK cells are then reinfused in conjunction with IL-2 administration. This therapy may have particular relevance to melanoma because the immune system is suspected of having a critical role in the control of melanoma metastases. However, the early response rate appears to be only about 20 percent, most of these remissions are partial, are seen in patients with skin or lung metastases, and are of short duration. In addition, treatment with IL-2 has associated toxicities, especially related to increased capillary permeability. Research is now focusing on altering the administration of IL-2 to enhance the remission rate while minimizing the toxicity; trials include high-dose IL-2 either alone, with LAK cells, with even more potent tumor-infiltrating lymphocytes, or with other agents. The continued lack of curative treatment for metastatic disease underscores the importance of early detection and prevention of malignant melanoma to decrease avoidable mortality.

REFERENCES

Albert L et al: Dysplastic melanocytic nevi and cutaneous melanoma: Markers of increased melanoma risk for affected individuals and blood relatives. J Am Acad Dermatol (in press)

Armstrong BK: Epidemiology of malignant melanoma: Intermittent or total accumulated exposure to the sun. J Dermatol Surg Oncol 14:835, 1988

Balch CM et al (eds): *Cutaneous Melanoma: Clinical Management and Treatment Results Worldwide*. Philadelphia, Lippincott, 1985

Clark WH Jr et al: The histogenesis and biologic behavior of primary human malignant melanoma of the skin. Cancer Res 29:705, 1969

Friedman RJ et al: Early detection of malignant melanoma: The role of physical examination and self-examination of the skin. CA 35:130, 1985

Greene MH et al: Acquired precursors of cutaneous malignant melanoma: The familial dysplastic nevus syndrome. N Engl J Med 312:91, 1985

Illig L et al: Congenital nevi ≤ 10 cm as precursors to melanoma: 52 cases, a review, and a new conception. Arch Dermatol 121:1274, 1985

Koh HK et al: Adjuvant therapy of cutaneous malignant melanoma: A critical review. Med Ped Oncol 13:244, 1985

Kraemer KH et al: Risk of cutaneous melanoma in dysplastic nevus syndrome types A and B. N Engl J Med 315:1615, 1986

Rhodes AR: Neoplasms: Benign neoplasias, hyperplasias, and dysplasias of melanocytes, in *Dermatology in General Medicine*, TB Fitzpatrick et al (eds). New York, McGraw-Hill, 1987, pp 877–946

——— et al: Risk factors for cutaneous melanoma. JAMA 258:3146, 1987

Rigel DS et al: Dysplastic nevi. Markers for increased risk for melanoma. Cancer 63:386, 1989

Rosenberg SA et al: New approaches to the immunotherapy of cancer using interleukin-2. Ann Intern Med 108:853, 1988

Sober AJ et al: Early recognition of cutaneous melanoma. JAMA 242:2795, 1979

Swerdlow AJ et al: Benign melanocytic nevi as a risk factor for malignant melanoma. Br Med J 292:1555, 1986

Veronesi U et al: Delayed regional lymph node dissection in stage 1 melanoma of the skin of the lower extremities. Cancer 49:2420, 1982

——— et al: Thin stage 1 primary cutaneous malignant melanoma: Comparison of excision with 1 or 3 centimeters. N Engl J Med 318:1159, 1988

309 ENDOCRINE MANIFESTATIONS OF NEOPLASIA

LAWRENCE A. FROHMAN

Hormone secretion by tumors derived from nonendocrine tissue has been recognized for more than 50 years. Initially, the majority of reported cases were associated with hypoglycemia and hypercalcemia, but the term *ectopic hormone secretion* was first used in relation to Cushing's syndrome caused by adrenocorticotropic hormone (ACTH) secretion from a variety of tumors. The spectrum of ectopic hormone secretion has expanded as a result of increased clinical awareness and the availability of more sophisticated and sensitive assay techniques. However, the use of the term *ectopic* in this regard has been questioned with the recognition that hormones once believed to be tissue-specific may have widespread sites of production, i.e., gonadotropins are produced by the normal gonad and intestine, thyrotropin-releasing hormone (TRH) and ACTH by the pancreas, and somatostatin by the kidney and thyroid C cells. Nevertheless, the original term serves to distinguish tumor-associated hormone production from syndromes due to excess secretion of the major and characteristic hormone of a specific endocrine gland.

THEORIES OF ECTOPIC HORMONE SECRETION Several pathogenetic mechanisms have been proposed to explain ectopic hormone secretion. The "sponge" theory assumed a selective update of the circulating hormone by tumor tissue with subsequent release upon tumor cell death. This concept was abandoned, however, after the demonstration of arteriovenous differences of hormones across tumor vascular beds, of hormone mRNA in tumor tissue, and of hormone biosynthesis by tumors in vitro. The theory that random mutations resulted in altered DNA sequences and gene products was also discounted when it was established that the production of ectopic hormones by tumors is not random, i.e., that certain tumors commonly produce specific endocrinopathies. A third theory, that of gene derepression, proposed that regions of the genome not normally expressed become active and are transcribed in tumors, presumably as a result of loss of a normal suppressive mechanism during neoplastic transformation; in fact, however, there is no overall increase in gene transcription (derepression) in neoplastic cells. Two other explanations have also been proposed: *cellular dedifferentiation*, a theory that neoplastic cells revert to a more primitive level and again produce peptide hormones that were produced normally at an earlier developmental stage, and *arrested differentiation*, whereby hormone secretion is due to persistence of a function present during development because of a failure (arrest) of the developmental process. Arguments against these theories include an absence of evidence that cells can retrace their pathways of differentiation or that incompletely differentiated cells routinely secrete the hormone in question. Although the pathogenesis of ectopic hormone secretion is still unclear, the mechanism is likely the result of activation of selected gene expression by an oncogene.

CRITERIA FOR DIAGNOSIS Criteria for the diagnosis of ectopic hormone secretion have changed as more precise laboratory methodology made it possible to recognize clinically inapparent cases (Table 309-1). Although many of these criteria cannot be satisfied in individual cases, the majority have been fulfilled in the commonly recognized syndromes.

TUMOR TYPES ASSOCIATED WITH ECTOPIC HORMONE SECRETION Ectopic secretion of hormones is associated with a variety of tumors. Although original reports of these syndromes described primarily lung carcinomas, carcinoids, thymomas, and fibrosarcomas, virtually all tumors have the potential of hormone secretion. Nevertheless, the frequency of occurrence of ectopic hormone secretion among various tumor types is not random. The tumors most frequently associated with clinically recognized ectopic hormone production are small cell lung carcinomas, carcinoids, and pancreatic islet tumors.

TABLE 309-1 Criteria for establishing the diagnosis of ectopic hormone secretion

1 Association of a neoplasm with a syndrome attributable to excessive hormone secretion or with inappropriately elevated plasma and/or urine levels of a hormone not normally produced by the tissue from which the tumor is derived
2 Failure of plasma and/or urine hormone levels to respond to normal homeostatic suppression
3 Exclusion of other possible causal mechanisms for hormone hypersecretion
4 Reduction in hormone levels after tumor-specific therapy
5 Arteriovenous step-up gradients across tumor
6 Demonstration of hormone in tumor tissue
7 Biosynthesis and/or secretion of hormone by tumor tissue in vitro
8 Demonstration in the tumor of hormone-specific messenger RNA by cell-free translation or by hybridization with cDNA

Carcinoid tumors are generally found in the lung or the gastrointestinal tract. Gastrointestinal carcinoids may be present in either the foregut or the hindgut, though it is primarily foregut tumors that are hormonally active. In the lung these tumors are usually endobronchial and may remain undetected for long periods. There are many morphologic similarities between bronchial carcinoid tumors and small cell carcinoma of the lung. Indeed, the two types may have a common cell of origin, namely the Kulchitsky cell, a bronchial mucosal cell that has been called a neuroendocrine cell of the lung because of its peptide-containing granules observed on electron microscopy. A bombesin-like peptide (related to gastrin-releasing peptide) is present in Kulchitsky cells during fetal life and is the most frequent peptide produced by small cell carcinoma of the lung. Ectopic hormone secretion is also associated with other types of lung tumors, most commonly the squamous type of bronchogenic carcinomas.

In the 1960s Pearse proposed the theory that certain hormone-secreting cells are components of a "diffuse neuroendocrine system." Such cells were originally considered to be of neural crest or neuroectodermal origin and were designated APUD (amine precursor uptake and decarboxylation) cells on the basis of their ability to decarboxylate precursors of biogenic amines. Later it was discovered that many of these cells also produce the enzyme neuron-specific enolase and other neurosecretory cell markers. A corollary of the APUD theory was that tumors derived from APUD cells had the capability of hormone secretion. At present, there is doubt concerning the validity of the APUD theory on several grounds. First, all APUD cells are not of neuroectodermal origin. Second, the APUD function of these cells is not inherently linked with peptide hormone production, and third, some ectopic hormone-secreting tumors do not possess APUD characteristics. Nevertheless, the association of particular tumor types with the secretion of certain hormones is useful in evaluating these syndromes.

CHARACTERIZATION OF ECTOPIC HORMONES Type of hormone secreted Of the four classes of hormones—steroids, monoamines, substituted amino acids, and peptides/proteins—only the latter are secreted ectopically. Although the explanation is not known with certainty, the ectopic production of peptide/protein hormones may require less complicated derangements in cell metabolism. For example, an oncogene serving as an inducer or enhancer of gene transcription may be responsible for increasing the expression of a gene coding for a peptide hormone. In contrast, the synthesis of steroids, thyroid hormones, or monoamines requires multiple enzymatic steps and specifically targeted translocation of the precursor molecules through various cell compartments. The likelihood that this degree of cell specialization would occur as a consequence of neoplastic change is much less than the possibility that a process (protein synthesis) common to all cells might be initiated aberrantly.

Ectopic secretion of nearly all peptide hormones has been reported. These hormones may be grouped according to their usual site of origin (Table 309-2). The first group of hormones, common to the central nervous system and gastrointestinal tract, are most frequently secreted by carcinoids, small cell lung carcinomas, and pancreatic islet tumors. The second group, normally produced by the fetoplacental unit and/or the anterior pituitary, tends to be produced by gastrointestinal, hepatic, adrenal, and gonadal tumors. The third group, which includes insulin-like growth factors and parathyroid hormone–like factors, tends to be produced by mesenchymal, hepatic, genitourinary, and squamous cell lung tumors. In addition to the hormones listed, other humoral factors are believed responsible for tumor-associated syndromes such as hypertrophic osteoarthropathy, polyneuropathy, hypophosphatemic osteomalacia, and anorexia.

Relation to naturally secreted hormones The primary amino acid sequences of nearly all ectopically secreted hormones analyzed to date are identical to those of the native hormones. However, other differences in structure between ectopically secreted and native hormones can occur as a result of incomplete or abnormal processing of the precursor hormone. Several abnormal forms of ectopic hormones have been defined: (1) large-molecular-weight species due to incomplete enzymatic cleavage of the precursor (proopiomelanocortin); (2) small-molecular-weight fragments due to unregulated intracellular processing (fragments of growth hormone–releasing hormone); and (3) altered glycosylation species (microheterogeneity) due either to failed cleavage of carbohydrate residues during postribosomal hormone processing (glycosylated ACTH) or failure of normal glycosylation (the alpha subunit common to the gonadotropins and TSH). The usual consequence of such altered biosynthetic processing is a hormone variant with diminished biologic activity. If modification of hormone structure is sufficient to cause loss of all biologic activity, ectopic secretion is not accompanied by clinical manifestations. Even if a neoplastic cell can synthesize and store a biologically active hormone, a syndrome of hormone excess may not result if an intact secretory mechanism is absent. The frequency with which either an inactive hormone is synthesized or an active hormone is synthesized but not secreted is probably greater than that of classical ectopic hormone secretion since only a small percentage of tumors that contain ectopic hormones cause clinically recognizable syndromes attributable to hormone hypersecretion.

Other considerations Hormones may be secreted by both benign and malignant tumors. Although hormone secretion normally requires a high level of cellular differentiation, an incompletely differentiated tumor may still retain secretory capability. For example, the process of granule formation and hormone storage is not generally expressed by hormone-secreting tumors; consequently, the concentration of hormone in the tumor is usually low compared to that in endocrine glands. Overall hormone secretion per unit weight is also less and, as a result, considerable tumor mass is usually present before ectopic hormone secretion is clinically apparent. One notable exception is the relatively benign, highly differentiated neoplasm, usually a carcinoid or pancreatic islet tumor, that contains and secretes hormone at a level comparable to that of normal endocrine tissue and is sufficiently small to escape detection for long periods.

Many tumors produce multiple hormones. In some this is due to the existence of a common precursor for multiple hormones, e.g., ACTH, lipotropins, melanocyte-stimulating hormones (MSHs), and endorphins are all derived from a single precursor, proopiomelanocortin (POMC), and both vasoactive intestinal peptide (VIP) and peptide histidyl-methionine (PHM) are encoded in a single precursor. In other instances multiple hormones are produced in the absence of common precursors, e.g., production of ACTH, calcitonin, and somatostatin by medullary thyroid carcinoma and by small cell carcinoma of the lung. In some tumors separate cells secrete individual hormones, whereas in others multiple hormones are produced by the same cell. Furthermore, variation may occur in cell lines cloned from such tumors, suggesting that gene expression may be unstable in succeeding generations of tumor cells.

FREQUENCY The frequency of ectopic hormone secretion varies with the criteria used for its definition. The most frequently encountered syndromes are those of ACTH hypersecretion, hypercalcemia, and organic hypoglycemia. Ectopic ACTH secretion occurs in approximately 15 to 20 percent of patients with Cushing's syndrome. Thus, consideration of this diagnosis is of great importance. Similarly,

TABLE 309-2 Spectrum of ectopic hormone production

Group/hormone	Tumor type: Common	Tumor type: Infrequent
1 Neuroendocrine-gastrointestinal		
a ACTH, β-lipotropin, endorphins, MSHs, enkephalins	Lung carcinoma (small cell) Thymoma Pancreatic islet tumors Carcinoid Thyroid medullary carcinoma Pheochromocytoma Parotid tumor Prostatic carcinoma Renal carcinoma	Squamous cell, adenocarcinoma, and large cell carcinoma of the lung Breast carcinoma Colonic carcinoma Gallbladder tumors Testicular carcinoma Uterine carcinoma Laryngeal carcinoma Plasmacytoma Bladder small cell carcinoma
b Vasopressin, oxytocin, neurophysin	Lung carcinoma (small cell, anaplastic, adenocarcinoma) Carcinoid	Pancreatic carcinoma Duodenal carcinoma
c Corticotropin-releasing hormone	Lung carcinoma (small cell) Carcinoid	Pituitary gangliocytoma Medullary carcinoma of thyroid
d Growth hormone–releasing hormone	Carcinoid Pancreatic islet adenoma Lung carcinoma (small cell)	Adrenocortical adenoma Neurofibroma Endometrial carcinoma Pheochromocytoma Pituitary gangliocytoma
e Somatostatin	Lung carcinoma (small cell) Carcinoid Pheochromocytoma	
f Calcitonin	Lung carcinoma (small cell) Carcinoid	Breast carcinoma Pheochromocytoma
g Gastrin	Lung carcinoma (small cell)	Ovarian carcinoma
h Vasoactive intestinal peptide	Lung carcinoma (small cell) Pancreatic islet tumors	
i Insulin		Gastric carcinoma Lung carcinoma Carcinoid
j Glucagon		Lung carcinoma Carcinoid Renal carcinoma
k Gastrin-releasing peptide (bombesin-like)	Lung carcinoma Carcinoid	Medullary carcinoma of thyroid
2 Fetoplacental and/or anterior pituitary		
a Chorionic gonadotropin (and subunits)	Lung carcinoma Gastric carcinoma Ovarian carcinoma Adeno- and islet cell carcinoma of the pancreas Hepatoma Genitourinary tract tumors	Testicular carcinoma Ovarian carcinoma Adrenocortical carcinoma Breast carcinoma Melanoma Carcinoid
b Placental lactogen	Lung carcinoma (small cell)	Lymphoma Pheochromocytoma Hepatoma
c Growth hormone		Lung carcinoma (large cell) Carcinoid Pancreatic islet tumor
d Prolactin		Lung carcinoma Renal carcinoma Gonadoblastoma
3 Others		
a Tissue growth factors (somatomedins)	Mesenchymal tumors (i.e., fibrosarcoma) Hepatoma Adrenocortical carcinoma Pancreatic/bile duct carcinoma	Lung carcinoma Ovarian carcinoma Neuroblastoma Wilms's tumor
b Erythropoietin	Cerebellar hemangioblastoma Uterine fibroma Renal carcinoma	Adrenocortical carcinoma Hepatoma Pheochromocytoma
c Humoral hypercalcemic factor of malignancy, osteoclast-activating factor	Renal carcinoma Lung carcinoma (squamous) Hepatoma Pancreatic islet tumors	GI tract tumors Parotid tumors Genitourinary tract tumors Melanoma Breast carcinoma
d 1,25 Dihydroxy vitamin D	Lymphoma	

nearly half of patients with hypercalcemia unrelated to volume depletion, excess ingestion of vitamin D, or sarcoidosis have a malignancy rather than hyperparathyroidism, and of these about 70 percent secrete a hypercalcemic peptide that has parathyroid hormone–like biologic activity and is structurally similar, though not identical, to parathyroid hormone. In contrast, hypoglycemia due to ectopic production of an insulin-like growth factor is infrequent in patients suspected of having an insulinoma, and ectopic growth hormone–releasing hormone (GRH) secretion is a rare (<1 percent) cause of acromegaly.

CONSEQUENCES OF ECTOPIC HORMONE SECRETION The consequences of ectopic hormone secretion may be of greater significance than the tumor itself. This is particularly true for patients with benign or slowly growing malignant ACTH- or gastrin-producing tumors in whom fulminant Cushing's syndrome or bleeding peptic ulceration may be life-threatening. In others, the hormone may cause medical problems that shorten the life span beyond that attributable to the tumor itself, i.e., severe hypercalcemia, hyponatremia, or hypoglycemia.

The symptoms of ectopic hormone secretion may be the presenting manifestations of the neoplasm or occur late in the course of the disease. The rapidity of onset of the clinical features of hormone hypersecretion affects the frequency with which the syndrome is recognized. For example, excessive secretion of ACTH or vasopressin is clinically evident within weeks or months; thus, a fully developed syndrome can be associated with rapidly growing malignant as well as benign tumors. In contrast, acromegaly due to ectopic GRH secretion typically requires years to become apparent and therefore is observed only when caused by benign or slowly growing malignant neoplasms. Ectopic hormone secretion, once established, does not necessarily persist for as long as the tumor is present. Hormone secretion may cease or decline to clinically insignificant levels either spontaneously or in response to radiation or chemotherapy. Hormone secretion usually, but not invariably, recurs with tumor relapse.

In addition to effects on the host, ectopic hormone secretion has numerous important biologic implications. Since tumor-secreted factors that exhibit biologic effects are unlikely to be unique substances, their identification and characterization can assist in the search for the naturally occurring (eutopic) peptide. For example, tumor-secreted GRH was the source for the purification, isolation, and structural characterization of hypothalamic GRH. Relatively little attention has been given to possible effects of ectopically secreted hormones on the growth or survival of the tumor.

DIAGNOSIS Occasionally, the clinical manifestations of ectopic hormone secretion are so distinctive that they suggest the diagnosis before any hormone measurements have been performed. The development of gynecomastia in the absence of associated diseases such as cirrhosis or testicular failure may suggest the presence of ectopic gonadotropin secretion, while Cushing's syndrome and increased pigmentation or severe muscle weakness (due to hypokalemia) point to ectopic ACTH secretion.

More commonly, however, clinical manifestations of hormone excess are subtle or absent. In such instances basal serum levels of hormones, e.g., ACTH, may be elevated out of proportion to the biologic effects observed. This may be the result of ACTH precursor molecules that have little or no biologic activity. Identification of these hormonal forms can be accomplished by molecular sieve chromatography or by multiple, site-specific radioimmunoassays of serum. Similarly, disproportionate elevations of hCG may reflect the presence of the glycoprotein alpha subunit, which is biologically inactive but exhibits cross-reactivity in some radioimmunoassays. A specific alpha-subunit assay is used to confirm the diagnosis.

In other instances the diagnosis of ectopic hormone secretion may be suggested by finding suppressed levels of hormones that are subject to feedback inhibition. Low or undetectable levels of insulin or parathyroid hormone in the presence of hypoglycemia or hypercalcemia are suggestive of tumors that secrete an insulin-like growth factor or a humoral hypercalcemic factor of malignancy, respectively.

Alterations in normal feedback regulation may also provide clues that elevated circulating hormone levels are derived from ectopic sources. Patients with ectopic ACTH production do not respond to suppression by glucocorticoids or to stimulation by corticotropin-releasing hormone (presumably because of the absence of appropriate receptors in the tumor tissue), an observation that helps distinguish them from patients with pituitary-dependent Cushing's disease. Apparent suppression of ACTH, which has been noted in several case reports, could be explained by intermittent secretion of ACTH by the tumor (an uncommon and poorly understood phenomenon of ectopic hormone secretion) or by the coproduction of corticotropin-releasing hormone.

If the diagnosis is still in doubt, or if the source of ectopic secretion is unknown, selective venous catheterization may be an effective means of locating the tumor. As long as the tumor is actually secreting hormone at the time of study, a step-up gradient in the concentration of the hormone is of value in tumor localization and/or a search for metastases.

THERAPY Primary treatment of ectopic hormone–secreting tumors should be directed, if possible, toward removal of the tumor. Measurement of circulating hormone levels can serve as a marker for completeness of tumor excision or of the effect of radiation and chemotherapy for tumors considered inoperable, i.e., small cell carcinoma of the lung. In addition, recurrence of tumor may be heralded by reappearance of elevated hormone levels prior to clinical evidence of the tumor mass. However, occasional tumors may not secrete hormones at the time of recurrence, so that one cannot rely entirely on hormone measurements as a marker of tumor activity.

Frequently, the tumor cannot be removed or is already metastatic at the time of diagnosis. In such cases, two other approaches are available for eliminating the effects of ectopic hormone secretion. Pharmacologic agents may be used to inhibit hormone release. Octreotide, a long-acting somatostatin analogue, has been used effectively in inhibiting growth hormone–releasing hormone secretion, VIP secretion, and the clinical symptoms of the carcinoid syndrome.

The other approach involves blocking the action of the hormone when its secretion cannot be altered. Pharmacologic agents may interfere with hormone effects on target tissues. Examples include (1) demeclocycline to inhibit vasopressin action on the renal tubule in the syndrome of inappropriate antidiuretic hormone (SIADH) associated with malignancy, and (2) ketoconazole and/or mitotane to inhibit adrenal steroidogenesis in the ectopic ACTH syndrome. Alternatively, surgical removal of the target tissue may avoid life-threatening complications and permit relatively symptom-free long-term survival if the tumor itself is benign or is slowly growing. Examples include adrenalectomy for the ectopic ACTH syndrome and gastrectomy for recurrent gastrointestinal bleeding caused by gastrin-producing tumors. This form of therapy will be used with decreasing frequency as newer and more specific pharmacologic agents become available.

ECTOPIC HORMONES AS MARKERS FOR NEOPLASIA With the initial recognition of ectopic hormone secretion, it was hoped that by measuring these hormones a generally applicable means of screening for clinically silent tumors would become available. As knowledge of the spectrum of ectopic hormone secretion has increased, however, this hope has faded. The list of hormones that are secreted ectopically has lengthened to the point that cost considerations preclude the use of this form of screening. Even if the number of hormones were not as extensive, the limited correlation of tumor site and type with secretion of specific hormones necessitates an extensive workup to localize the tumor. Screening programs, when performed, have yielded relatively few positive results. Moreover evidence is lacking that earlier diagnosis, as a result of such procedures, reduces subsequent morbidity or mortality. Consequently, screening for ectopic hormone production is not justified as part of routine cancer detection programs.

REFERENCES

BOSTWICK DG et al: Expression of opioid peptides in tumors. N Engl J Med 17:1439, 1987

BROADUS AE et al: Humoral hypercalcemia of cancer.Identification of a novel parathyroid hormone-like peptide. N Engl J Med 319:556, 1988

FROHMAN LA, DOWNS TR: Ectopic GRH syndrome, in *Acromegaly*, R Robbins et al (eds). New York, Plenum, 1987

HEITZ PU et al: Ectopic hormone production by endocrine tumors: Localization of hormones at the cellular level by immunocytochemistry. Cancer 48:2029, 1981

HOWLETT TA, REES LH: Ectopic hormones. Spec Top Endocrinol Metab 7:1, 1985

INSOGNA KL, BROADUS AE: Hypercalcemia of malignancy. Annu Rev Med 38:241, 1987

KOHLER PC, TRUMP DL: Ectopic hormones syndromes. Cancer Invest 4:543, 1986

LOKICH JJ: The frequency and clinical biology of the ectopic hormone syndromes of small cell carcinoma. Cancer 50:2111, 1982

MELMED S et al: Acromegaly due to secretion of growth hormone by an ectopic pancreatic islet-cell tumor. N Engl J Med 312:9, 1985

———, RUSHAKOFF RJ: Ectopic pituitary and hypothalamic hormone syndromes. Endocrinol Metab Clin North Am 16:805, 1987

MUDDLE AH et al: Ectopic production of 1,25-dihydroxyvitamin D by B-cell lymphoma as a cause of hypercalcemia. Cancer 59:1543, 1987

ORTH D: Ectopic hormone production, in *Endocrinology and Metabolism*, 2d ed, P Felig et al (eds). New York, McGraw-Hill, 1987

SANO T et al: Growth hormone-releasing hormone-producing tumors: Clinical, biochemical, and morphological manifestations. Endocr Rev 9:357, 1988

SHAH VM et al: Ectopic beta human chorionic gonadotropin production by bladder urothelial neoplasia. Arch Pathol Lab Med 110:107, 1986

WYNICK D et al: Symptomatic secondary hormone syndromes in patients with established malignant pancreatic endocrine tumors. N Engl J Med 319:605, 1988

310 PARANEOPLASTIC NEUROLOGIC SYNDROMES

ROBERT H. BROWN, JR.

Neoplasms can derange neurologic function in a number of ways (Table 310-1, see also Chap. 353). Paraneoplastic neurologic syndromes, which occur in the setting of a remotely located neoplasm, can present in several forms (Table 310-2). These paraneoplastic syndromes share several characteristics. They are clinically dramatic, arising subacutely in weeks or even days to produce neurologic symptoms that may be profoundly disabling. These syndromes may precede detection of the neoplasm by months or even years; their recognition should prompt a timely search for carcinoma. Although more than one syndrome may arise with a given neoplasm, certain clinical manifestations are often associated with particular types of tumors (Table 310-2).

The diagnosis of a paraneoplastic neurologic disorder depends primarily on (1) the presence of a recognized clinical syndrome; (2)

TABLE 310-1 Effects of malignancy on the nervous system

I Direct invasion
II Metastatic invasion
 A Parenchymatous
 B Vascular (neoplastic angioendotheliosis)
 C Meningeal (meningeal carcinomatosis)
III Opportunistic infections
 A Bacterial (e.g., *Listeria*)
 B Nonbacterial
  1 Typical and atypical viral (e.g., progressive multifocal leukoencephalopathy)
  2 Fungal (e.g., cryptococcus)
IV Complications of antineoplastic therapy
 A Radiation (e.g., radiation necrosis)
 B Chemotherapy (e.g., vincristine neuropathy)
V Metabolic complications
 A Nutritional deficiency
 B Ectopic hormone production
VI Paraneoplastic syndromes

careful exclusion of other cancer-related disorders listed in Table 310-1; and (3) in some instances, confirmatory laboratory studies such as an electromyogram typical of myasthenia gravis or the presence in serum of antibodies with specific patterns of reactivity. Cerebrospinal fluid (CSF) may show protein elevation and a mild lymphocytic pleocytosis.

INCIDENCE Studies of the incidence of these syndromes are problematic because the syndromes are rare and classifications vary somewhat among studies. In one series, these syndromes were detected in about 7 percent of nearly 1500 patients with tumors, although recent studies suggest the incidence is somewhat lower. Among malignant tumors with paraneoplastic neurologic syndromes, the most common are lung (47 percent), stomach (12 percent), breast (12 percent), ovary (9 percent), and colon (6 percent). These syndromes are encountered in one-sixth of all ovarian tumors, one-seventh of lung tumors, and less frequently in stomach, prostate, and breast cancers.

PATHOLOGIC CHANGES Pathologic features of these syndromes have been well defined. One of the most common findings is encephalomyelitis characterized by perivascular lymphocytosis, microglial proliferation, and loss of neurons. To emphasize involvement of neurons in gray matter, the process is sometimes described as *polioencephalomyelitis*. While these changes may be diffuse throughout the neuraxis, they often predominate in a specific anatomic location that dictates the resulting clinical abnormalities. Thus, as outlined below, the manifestations of limbic encephalitis may differ from those of brainstem encephalitis. Inflammation may be evident in dorsal root ganglia or in gray and white matter of the spinal cord, producing, respectively, ganglioradiculitis or subacute poliomyelitis. A second striking pathologic finding is severe, focal degeneration or loss of neurons without inflammation. This is exemplified by the selective but widespread loss of Purkinje neurons in the cerebellum in subacute cortical cerebellar degeneration. This may occur in isolation or concurrently with findings of encephalomyelitis; thus, in cortical cerebellar degeneration there may be some accompanying cerebellar inflammation. As outlined below, some paraneoplastic syndromes are associated with pathologic changes in the peripheral nervous system such as multifocal demyelination, myonecrosis, or ultrastructural changes in the neuromuscular junction.

Autoimmune mechanisms have been implicated in several instances. Some paraneoplastic disorders are characterized by serum and spinal fluid antibodies that have highly specific patterns of reactivity with neural tissue or muscle. These are exemplified by the Lambert-Eaton myasthenic syndrome and myasthenia gravis, in which affected individuals have circulating antibodies that react with pre- and postsynaptic proteins (see Chap. 366). Both syndromes have been reproduced in animals by passive administration of fractionated immunoglobulins. As another example, in some cases of cortical cerebellar degeneration serum and spinal fluid antibodies react specifically with cerebellar cytoplasmic antigens. By contrast, immunoglobulins from patients with different paraneoplastic neurologic syndromes may show similar patterns of reactivity with neural tissue. Thus, antibodies recognizing neuronal nuclear antigens are common in patients with small cell carcinoma of the lung and several paraneoplastic syndromes such as subacute sensory neuropathy. In this instance, it appears that one or more pathogenic antibodies, possibly cross-reacting with antigens on the tumor, may provoke autoimmune neural injury in more than one region of the neuraxis. Detection of such antibodies may confirm that an evolving neurologic disorder is of paraneoplastic origin even though the antibodies are not diagnostic of a specific neurologic syndrome.

TREATMENT Treatment of the paraneoplastic disorders is not uniformly successful. The most consistently beneficial treatments are anti-immune therapy such as plasma exchange or immunosuppression in those disorders that are clearly autoimmune. In some instances, the paraneoplastic syndromes have regressed after resection of the carcinoma. Otherwise, therapy is largely symptomatic.

The following is an outline of the salient features of the major paracarcinomatous neurologic syndromes.

BRAIN, CEREBELLUM, AND SPINAL CORD

VISUAL PARANEOPLASTIC SYNDROMES Patients with carcinoma of the lung or cervix may develop progressive, painless loss of vision because of degeneration of the rods and cones. The electroretinogram is abnormal, and cells may be present in the spinal fluid. Lymphocytic inflammation of the retina accompanies loss of rods and cones. Paraneoplastic visual loss may also occur because of antibody-mediated loss of retinal ganglion cells. Sera of affected patients contain antibodies that react with antigens shared by the retinal ganglion cell and the tumor (e.g., small cell lung carcinoma).

LIMBIC ENCEPHALITIS Encephalitis of limbic structures such as the hippocampus and amygdala produces affective changes in personality including anxiety and agitated depression in association with selective, early memory loss suggestive of Korsakoff's psychosis, and occasionally confusion and hallucinations. In some cases the initial presentation is an amnesic syndrome. The affective disorder often prompts psychiatric evaluation. Abnormalities of the electroencephalogram or overt seizures may be present early in the syndrome. While cognition may initially be spared, dementia is common. As the disorder progresses, symptoms referrable to encephalitic involvement in other regions are often superimposed.

BRAINSTEM ENCEPHALITIS Symptoms of brainstem encephalitis relate directly to the distribution of the inflammation. Medullary involvement produces nausea, vomiting, nystagmus, possibly vertigo, and ataxia. A syndrome suggestive of progressive bulbar palsy with marked dysarthria and dysphagia is associated with pontine involvement. Mesencephalic inflammation and neuronal loss result in nuclear or internuclear eye movement abnormalities; diplopia and oscillopsia may be disabling. Rostral midbrain and nigral involvement may cause rigidity. Medullary symptoms typically predominate.

CEREBELLAR ENCEPHALITIS Inflammatory changes are rare in cerebellar cortex but may be severe in deep cerebellar nuclei such as the dentate nucleus. Inflammation within the dentate nucleus provokes myoclonus.

MYELITIS In paraneoplastic myelitis, the gray matter of the cord is diffusely inflamed with profound neuronal degeneration. This poliomyelitis may be widespread in the cord or restricted to a few segmental levels. Anterior horn cell destruction typically produces muscle weakness and neurogenic atrophy. Limb involvement is often asymmetric. There may be selective involvement of the neck and upper extremities or lower extremities alone. Corticospinal findings result from involvement of this tract in the cord or from brainstem disease. The corticospinal tract dysfunction and motor neuronopathy in these cases should not be confused with motor neuron disease; typical amyotrophic lateral sclerosis does not appear to arise on a paraneoplastic basis. The presence of sensory signs with cancer

TABLE 310-2 Paraneoplastic neurologic syndromes

Site	Evolution	Clinical features*	Cancer	Pathology
BRAIN AND CEREBELLUM				
Photoreceptor, retinal degeneration	Weeks to months	Painless visual loss progressing to blindness	Oat cell tumor; rarely cervical cancer	Loss of rods and cones; infiltration of retina with mononuclear cells
Limbic encephalitis	Weeks to months	Agitated, confusional state; memory loss followed by dementia[1]	Oat cell tumor of lung	Neuronal loss in medial temporal lobe and elsewhere in the limbic system; perivascular and meningeal lymphocytic infiltration
Brainstem encephalitis	Days to weeks	Nystagmus, diplopia, vertigo, ataxia, dysarthria, dysphagia[1]	Oat cell tumor	Neuronal loss in brainstem; inflammatory changes as above
Subacute cortical cerebellar degeneration	Weeks to months	Cerebellar ataxia, dysarthria[1,2]	Oat cell tumor; ovarian and breast cancer; Hodgkin's disease	Loss of Purkinje cells
Opsoclonus-myoclonus	Weeks	Dancing eyes and feet, cerebellar ataxia, and possibly encephalopathy	Neuroblastoma; bronchial carcinoma in adults	In adults, degeneration of dentate nuclei
SPINAL CORD				
Necrotizing myelopathy	Hours, days, or weeks	Para- or quadriplegia with areflexia; sensory loss and bladder dysfunction	Oat cell tumor, lymphoma	Severe necrosis of gray and white matter
Subacute motor neuronopathy	Weeks or months	Flaccid weakness and muscle atrophy; legs affected more than arms	Non-Hodgkin's lymphoma; loss of anterior horn cells	Inflammation of ventral horns
PERIPHERAL NERVE				
Acute demyelinating neuritis (Guillain-Barré, acute inflammatory demyelinating polyneuropathy, AIDP)	Hours to days	Ascending paralysis; areflexia; possibly ascending sensory loss; high CSF protein	Hodgkin's disease	Segmental demyelination; inflammation of peripheral nerves
Chronic inflammatory demyelinating polyneuropathy (CIDP)	Weeks to months	Chronic progressive or relapsing weakness with sensory loss; high CSF protein	Rarely lung, breast, and gastric cancer; lymphoma, myeloma	As in AIDP
Neuropathy with paraproteinemia	Weeks to months	Chronic; may be predominantly sensory[3] or motor[4]	Myeloma; osteosclerotic myeloma	As in CIDP
Subacute sensory neuronopathy	Weeks to months	Severe sensory loss with areflexia and ataxia; paresthesias, pain[1]	Oat cell and other lung tumors	Inflammation and neuronal degeneration in dorsal root ganglia; secondary axon loss
Sensorimotor neuropathy	Weeks to months	Distal motor and sensory loss[1]	Oat cell and other tumors	Axonopathy; some segmental loss of myelin
NEUROMUSCULAR JUNCTION				
Lambert-Eaton myasthenic syndrome	Weeks to months	Proximal weakness, fatigability; dry mouth; possibly ptosis[5]	Oat cell tumor, breast, prostate, stomach	Disruption of active zones on presynaptic terminals
Myasthenia gravis	Weeks to months	Weakness, fatigability, ptosis; diplopia[6]	Thymoma	Disruption of postsynaptic junctional membrane folds
MUSCLE				
Polymyositis	Months to years	Proximal weakness, myalgias, possibly cardiomyopathy; high creatine phosphokinase	Association with malignancy unclear; possibly breast, ovary, lung tumors; lymphoma	Lymphocytic inflammation of muscle interstitium; myofiber necrosis, phagocytosis
Necrotizing myopathy	Days to weeks	Rapidly progressive proximal weakness, possibly dysphagia, dyspnea	Bronchial carcinoma, Oat cell tumor	Severe myonecrosis with minimal inflammation or phagocytosis

* Superscript denotes possible immunoglobulin reactivity: (1) antineuronal nuclear antigen; (2) one or more cytoplasmic antigens expressed selectively in cerebellar Purkinje cells; (3) IgM M component reacting with myelin-associated glycoprotein; (4) IgG or IgA M component arising in association with osteosclerotic myeloma; (5) voltage-sensitive calcium channel at presynaptic terminal; (6) acetylcholine receptor on postsynaptic specialization.

denotes either dorsal root ganglioradiculitis or poliomyelitis involving the posterior horns.

NECROTIZING MYELOPATHY This syndrome, presenting clinically as a subacute transverse myelitis, often in a thoracic distribution, is distinguished from the less fulminant encephalomyelitis by the evolution of a densely necrotic, central thoracic cord lesion which tails off rostrally and caudally over several segmental levels. In some instances, there are multiple such lesions along the cord. Clinical findings include leg and possibly arm plegia, sensory loss, and loss of sphincter control. The lesion can initially be asymmetric, mimicking a Brown-Séquard syndrome. In severe cases, the spinal fluid protein and cell count are increased and myelography demonstrates focal cord swelling. Not all cases are associated with tumor; when present, the cancers are often lung, lymphoma, and leukemia.

OPSOCLONUS-MYOCLONUS This syndrome of opsoclonus, myoclonus, and ataxia, or "dancing eyes–dancing feet," occurs in children and adults. About one-half of affected children are found to have differentiated neuroblastomas, usually in the thorax. In adults, the syndrome may be associated with solid tumors such as bronchial carcinoma. The onset is subacute, and in some instances the syndrome lasts for months to be followed by permanent encephalopathy or retardation. Pathologic findings in adults include prominent neuronal degeneration in the dentate nucleus of the cerebellum suggesting a relationship to cortical cerebellar degeneration. Occasionally there is lymphocytic cuffing diffusely in the central nervous system and cerebrospinal fluid pleocytosis. Some adults and children respond to treatment of the cancer or to glucocorticoids.

SUBACUTE CORTICAL CEREBELLAR DEGENERATION (SCCD) This is a subacutely progressive cerebellar disorder characterized by profound truncal and appendicular ataxia arising within weeks in association with carcinoma, typically ovarian or oat cell of the lung. There often are superimposed symptoms potentially referable to the brainstem including vertigo, dysarthria, diplopia and nystagmus, or corticospinal signs. As a rule, any nonfamilial ataxia arising in patients over the age of 45 years should raise the suspicion of this entity. The predominant pathologic finding is widespread loss of cerebellar Purkinje cell neurons with some astrogliosis and secondary loss of Purkinje cell axons. Interestingly, in the purely degenerative disorder without inflammation elsewhere dentate neurons are largely spared, while they are often heavily damaged in encephalomyelitis. Many cases are associated with dementia for which an anatomic basis has not been established. The CSF commonly reveals a mild pleocytosis; cerebellar atrophy may be evident on neuroradiographic studies.

At least three types of anti-Purkinje cell antibodies have been detected in sera of patients with subacute cerebellar degeneration. Women with gynecologic cancer (breast, ovary) and SCCD have anti-Purkinje cell antibodies (APCA) recognizing cytoplasmic proteins of about 34 and 62 kDa. The former is a recently cloned, novel neuronal protein expressed selectively in cerebellar Purkinje cells. A different cytoplasmic antigen is recognized by immunoglobulins from patients with SCCD and adenocarcinoma of the lung; in this entity, the antibodies fail to recognize a specific protein on Western blots. In some patients with small cell carcinoma of the lung and SCCD, serum globulins ("anti-Hu" antibodies) stain nuclear antigens in many types of neurons. Anti-Hu antibodies are also detected in other paraneoplastic disorders (see below). APCA and anti-Hu antibody activities are of diagnostic significance as they help determine whether a neurologic syndrome is paraneoplastic. In addition, they underscore the likelihood that an antibody-mediated immunologic mechanism may underlie several of the paracarcinomatous syndromes.

PERIPHERAL NERVES

The diagnosis of peripheral neuropathy in association with cancer can be challenging. Paraneoplastic subacute sensory neuronopathy, arguably the most clinically distinctive, is a ganglioradiculitis which may arise with one or more other manifestations of encephalomyelitis. Other paraneoplastic neuropathies are difficult to distinguish from noncarcinomatous neuropathies. Their recognition is critical as they are relatively common and sometimes precede diagnosis of the underlying neoplasia. By electrodiagnostic criteria, neuropathy may be evident in as many as 50 percent of patients with lung cancer. In the evaluation of a possibly paracarcinomatous neuropathy, it is particularly helpful to ascertain whether the neuropathy (1) affects motor fibers, sensory fibers, or both; (2) predominantly involves axon or myelin; or (3) occurs with an abnormal serum paraprotein.

ACUTE INFLAMMATORY DEMYELINATING POLYNEURITIS (AIDP, GUILLAIN-BARRÉ) This syndrome, discussed in detail elsewhere (Chap. 363), is characterized by subacutely ascending paralysis, sensory loss which is often mild by comparison with the motor deficits, areflexia, and a characteristic elevation of CSF protein without pleocytosis. Histopathology reveals lymphocytic infiltration of nerves, segmental demyelination, and relative axonal sparing. AIDP may be associated with Hodgkin's disease.

CHRONIC INFLAMMATORY DEMYELINATING POLYNEUROPATHY (CIDP) This group of chronic progressive or relapsing, inflammatory demyelinative peripheral neuropathies is distinguished from acute polyneuritis by the time course, more prominent involvement of sensory nerves, lack of involvement of autonomic nerves, and responsiveness to immunotherapy. As in AIDP, the demyelinative nature of these neuropathies is defined physiologically by abnormalities such as slowed nerve conduction velocities or dispersion of compound muscle action potentials; as in AIDP, the pathologic hallmark is loss of myelin with relative preservation of axons or segmental demyelination. In some cases, physiologic studies may reveal only marginal slowing of conduction while the biopsy clearly demonstrates selective myelin loss. In other instances, a sural nerve biopsy may fail to reveal proximal demyelination detectable only with electrophysiologic methods. Elevation of the CSF protein helps confirm the diagnosis.

Rarely, CIDP occurs in association with solid tumors of lung, breast, and stomach. It also occurs with Waldenström's macroglobulinemia, gamma heavy chain disease, and lymphoma. In many instances, paraneoplastic CIDP is characterized by the presence of a serum paraprotein, typically a monoclonal immunoglobulin ("M component"). As many as 20 percent of patients with monoclonal gammopathies of undetermined significance develop significant hematologic disease, including malignancies.

Two chronic demyelinating neuropathies are particularly distinctive in this context. The first is associated with a monoclonal IgM that reacts with a myelin-associated glycoprotein (MAG) in peripheral nerve myelin. This pattern of reactivity occurs in about half of patients with an IgM gammopathy and neuropathy. This IgM anti-MAG neuropathy is more sensory than motor; it is only slowly progressive as compared to the subacute sensory neuronopathy (below). It remains to be established whether the anti-MAG antibody is a cause or consequence of the demyelination. The second distinctive subtype of CIDP occurs with osteosclerotic myeloma and monoclonal IgG or IgA antibodies that do not react with MAG. This polyneuropathy is predominantly motor and often quite indolent, although it may eventually produce severe limb wasting. Sensory and autonomic findings are unusual. A related group of CIDP patients develop polyneuropathy, organomegaly, endocrinopathy, the M protein, and skin changes (POEMS syndrome); one-half have osteosclerotic myeloma and IgG or IgA M proteins with lambda light chains. Some patients with demyelinative neuropathies and IgM M proteins respond well to immunosuppressive therapy. Those with osteosclerotic myeloma may improve after treatment of the underlying plasmacytoma, particularly if it is solitary.

SUBACUTE SENSORY NEURONOPATHY By contrast with AIDP and CIDP, many paraneoplastic neuropathies primarily affect the axon with relative sparing of myelin. The best example is the paraneoplastic subacute sensory neuronopathy which, as noted above, is a ganglioradiculitis. Inflammatory destruction of the sensory neuronal cell bodies (hence the term *neuronopathy*) in the dorsal root ganglia results in wallerian degeneration of axons both in peripheral nerve and ascending sensory long tracts (posterior columns of the spinal cord). Clinically, this is heralded by the subacute appearance of paresthesias and pain in the distal limbs and truncal sensory ataxia. Limb pain may be severe, and sensory ataxia may be profoundly disabling. Although initially restricted only to arms or legs, the symptoms eventually affect all four limbs. In many cases, the underlying malignancy is oat cell cancer of the lung; the paraneoplastic neuropathy often precedes the diagnosis of the tumor by more than a year. Some patients' sera possess antibodies (anti-Hu) reactive with a 35- to 40-kDa protein present both in nuclei of neurons and in small cell lung cancers.

SENSORIMOTOR NEUROPATHY This category of mixed sensory and motor axonopathies is perhaps the most common paraneoplastic neuropathy. Symptoms depend in part upon the severity, but may include muscle wasting and weakness or distal limb paresthesias and even pain. Pathologically, there is noninflammatory degeneration of axons and mild myelin loss, presumably secondary to the axonopathy. Paraneoplastic sensorimotor neuropathy has been reported with several types of tumors (lung oat cell, breast, stomach) and hematologic malignancies (Hodgkin's disease, lymphoma, multiple myeloma). In amyloidosis, itself often associated with myeloma, there may be an axonal neuropathy with intraneural deposition of amyloid fibrils derived from immunoglobulin light chains. Axonal neuropathy has been reported as a manifestation of occult insulinoma, possibly as a consequence of hypoglycemia. Infrequently, these neuropathies remit spontaneously; often they progress even with aggressive treatment of the underlying malignancy.

SUBACUTE MOTOR NEURONOPATHY A subacute motor neuronopathy causes slowly progressive weakness in patients with lymphoma. Many patients seem to improve following immunosuppressive therapy for the malignancy. In others, progression of the weakness may cease after several months independently of the status of the lymphoma. Some myelomas are associated with subacute motor neuronopathy. Pathologic lesions include loss of motoneurons in the anterolateral gray matter of spinal cord, gliosis, loss of myelin in ventral roots, and some Schwann cell proliferation. There is no clearly effective treatment for this condition.

NEUROMUSCULAR JUNCTION

LAMBERT-EATON MYASTHENIC SYNDROME (LEMS) This syndrome afflicts men more than women, occurs in association with either malignancy or autoimmune diseases, and is characterized by weakness, myalgias, and fatigability, typically more severe in the lower extremities and proximal muscles. Ptosis may be seen. Dysautonomic features are common, including dryness of the mouth and eyes, impotence, diminished sweating, and orthostatic symptoms. The incidence of associated malignancy is 70 percent in men and 25 percent in women. In most cases the tumor is a small cell carcinoma of the lung. There is striking reduction in strength at rest with transient improvement in power on repetitive maximal exertion. Tensilon may marginally improve strength. Electromyography demonstrates motor unit potentials whose amplitude is low at rest but increases with exercise or tetanic stimulation; this contrasts with the electromyographic findings in myasthenia gravis. Electron microscopy of the presynaptic motor nerve terminals at the neuromuscular junction reveals a decrease in numbers of active zones believed to correspond to voltage-sensitive calcium channels. LEMS is believed to be an autoimmune disorder associated with diminished quantal release of acetylcholine. It is associated with other autoimmune disorders and appears to be HLA-linked (B8 and DRw3 antigens). Passive transfer of LEMS immunoglobulin in mice reproduces the ultrastructural findings. Electrophysiologic studies of affected mouse diaphragms suggest there is down-regulation of the voltage-sensitive calcium channels. Moreover, LEMS immunoglobulin also diminishes potassium-induced (voltage-dependent) influx of calcium into tumor cells cultured from small cell lung cancer. Treatment is directed toward the underlying neoplasm or autoimmune disease, or toward augmentation of acetylcholine release with drugs that prolong presynaptic depolarization and thereby enhance calcium influx. Guanidine hydrochloride and aminopyridine may be beneficial either in autoimmune or paraneoplastic LEMS; plasma exchange and immunosuppression may also be effective.

MYASTHENIA GRAVIS This disorder, discussed elsewhere in detail (Chap. 366), is characterized by exercise-induced muscle weakness caused by an antibody-mediated reduction in the numbers of acetylcholine receptors at the postsynaptic junction. About 15 percent of cases are associated with thymoma; many arise concurrently with other autoimmune or thyroid disorders.

MUSCLE

POLYMYOSITIS-DERMATOMYOSITIS This subject is reviewed fully elsewhere (Chap. 364). While an increased incidence of malignancy in elderly patients with dermatomyositis has long been suggested, this concept has recently been challenged by a retrospective analysis of experience with polymyositis at the Mayo Clinic.

NECROTIZING MYOPATHY Carcinoma of the bronchus may rarely be associated with a subacute, widespread, necrotizing myopathy that involves all muscles including bulbar and diaphragmatic muscles, weakness of which is often fatal. Intrafusal muscle fibers are also involved. Deep tendon reflexes are preserved. Muscle undergoes degeneration without phagocytosis or significant inflammatory response. The cause of the necrotizing process is unknown.

OTHER

Several other neurologic syndromes have been reported to be paraneoplastic but are less well characterized. *Stiff-man syndrome*, or diffuse hypertonia due to loss of inhibitory spinal interneurons, may arise in association with carcinoma of the pharynx. In this context, it is of interest that in nonneoplastic stiff-man syndrome autoantibodies have been detected that react with glutamic acid decarboxylase. This enzyme is essential for the synthesis of γ-aminobutyric acid, a central nervous system inhibitory neurotransmitter. Nonfamilial, subacute *chorea and dystonia* occur with oat cell carcinoma of the lung, and *optic neuritis* may develop as a paraneoplastic disorder. In the latter disorder, it is difficult to exclude direct involvement of the optic nerve or chiasm by cancer cells, or indirect effects of the underlying malignancy, as in Table 310-1.

REFERENCES

ANDERSON NE et al: Paraneoplastic degeneration: Clinical-immunological correlations. Ann Neurol 24:559, 1988

——— et al: Autoantibodies in paraneoplastic syndromes associated with small-cell lung carcinoma. Neurology 38:1391, 1988

FURNEAUX HM et al: Characterization of a cDNA encoding a 34-kDa Purkinje neuron protein recognized by sera from patients with paraneoplastic cerebellar degeneration. Proc Natl Acad Sci USA 86:2873, 1989

GRAUS F et al: Sensory neuronopathy and small cell lung cancer. Am J Med 80:45, 1986

GRUNWALD GB et al: Autoimmune basis for visual paraneoplastic syndrome in patients with small cell lung carcinoma. Retinal immune deposits and ablation of retinal ganglion cells. Cancer 60:780, 1987

HENSON RA, URICH H: *Cancer and the Nervous System*. Oxford, Blackwell, 1982

KINSBOURNE M: Myoclonic encephalopathy of infants. J Neurol Neurosurg Psych 25:271, 1964

LAYZER RB: Stiff-man syndrome—an autoimmune disease? (editorial). N Engl J Med 318(16):1060, 1988

NAGEL A et al: Lambert-Eaton myasthenic syndrome IgG depletes presynaptic membrane active zone particles by antigenic modulation. Ann Neurol 24:552, 1988

POSNER JB: Paraneoplastic syndromes. Current Neurol 9:245, 1989

THIRKILL CE et al: Cancer-associated retinopathy (CAR syndrome) with antibodies reacting with retinal, optic-nerve, and cancer cells. N Engl J Med 321:1589, 1989

PART TWELVE ENDOCRINOLOGY AND METABOLISM

section 1 Endocrinology

311 HORMONES AND HORMONE ACTION

JEAN D. WILSON

Communication between cells is largely mediated by the endocrine and nervous systems. These two systems were originally considered distinct—information was thought to be carried either by neural impulses or by chemical mediators in the blood—but it is now clear that they constitute one coordinated network. Not only may neurotransmitters such as norepinephrine circulate in blood as hormones, but neural impulses have major effects on the release of chemical mediators such as testosterone and insulin. This interlocking relationship is most apparent in the hypothalamus, which serves as the highest integrative center for the two systems. Hence, one neuroendocrine system has evolved to integrate and coordinate the metabolic activities of the organism. Endocrinology deals largely with the chemical mediators in this system, but proper understanding of the role of hormones requires knowledge of the autonomic nervous system (Chap. 67) and of the metabolic capacities of cells.

The formulation of endocrinology has been blurred in additional ways. The term *hormone* originally referred to substances that are secreted into the circulation and act as chemical effectors in other tissues. However, the capacity to form such chemical mediators is not limited to so-called endocrine organs. Some hormones, such as angiotensins II and III, are formed in the bloodstream itself. Others, such as testosterone in women and dihydrotestosterone and estradiol in men, are in part secreted and in part formed in peripheral tissues from circulating precursors, so-called prohormones. Still other chemical mediators circulate only in restricted compartments such as the hypothalamic-pituitary portal system and do not reach the systemic circulation in appreciable quantities. Finally, certain hormones, such as insulin, dihydrotestosterone, and thyrotropin-releasing hormone (TRH), have paracrine actions in the same tissues in which they are formed and exert actions at distal sites, whereas other chemical mediators, such as müllerian-inhibiting substance, exert local actions exclusively.

BIOCHEMISTRY

SYNTHESIS The approximately 100 known mammalian hormones fall into three major categories—peptides or peptide derivatives, steroids, and amines. In the case of peptide hormones, genes code for messenger RNA, which is then translated into protein precursors. These proteins undergo posttranslational cleavage (preproparathyroid hormone → proparathyroid hormone → parathyroid hormone) and/or processing (thyroglobulin → thyroxine → triiodothyronine) to form the active hormone recognized by the target tissues. The distinct feature of peptide hormones is that one or a few structural genes code for the amino acid sequence of the peptide, and other genes are responsible for the alteration of the peptide to its final form. In the case of peptide hormones with subunits, the different subunits may be derived either from a single precursor (insulin) or from separate precursors [luteinizing hormone (LH)]. Furthermore, the same peptide hormone (somatostatin) can be formed from different prohormones encoded by distinct genes, individual prohormones such as proopiomelanocortin can be metabolized to different hormones in different cells, depending on the complement of processing enzymes in the cell in question, and the primary transcripts of genes such as that of the calcitonin gene can be alternatively spliced in different tissues to form messenger RNA for either calcitonin or calcitonin-related peptide. Peptide hormones may also be formed ectopically in malignancies of nonendocrine origin such as carcinoma of the lung and may be formed in small amounts in normal nonendocrine tissues (see Chap. 309).

In the case of steroid hormones the fundamental precursor—cholesterol (for most steroid hormones) or 7-dehydrocholesterol (for vitamin D metabolites)—undergoes a series of enzymatic transformations to form the final products. At least six enzymes and consequently a minimum of six genes are required to transform cholesterol to estradiol. Because of the number of enzymes required, the synthesis of steroids from cholesterol is unusual in malignancies of nonendocrine tissues. However, many tissues—malignant and nonmalignant—that cannot form steroid hormones de novo from cholesterol contain enzymes that convert circulating steroids to other hormones; examples are the conversion of androgens to estrogens by trophoblastic tumors and by normal adipocytes and the conversion of progesterone to deoxycorticosterone by the kidney.

Amine hormones are synthesized by a series of reactions similar to those involved in steroid hormone synthesis except that the precursors are amino acids. For example, tyrosine is the precursor for epinephrine and norepinephrine (see Chap. 67).

STORAGE Most tissues that synthesize hormones have a limited capacity to store the completed product. For example, the normal adult testes contain only about one-sixth of the quantity of testosterone needed for daily production, and consequently the testicular pool turns over several times to provide the normal daily output of hormone. Even when tissues have special storage organelles for hormone, the amount of hormone stored is usually limited: the insulin granules in the pancreatic beta cell ordinarily contain amounts of insulin sufficient only for short-term, reserve needs. (In contrast, nerve endings may contain a several-day supply of norepinephrine.) The limited capacity to store hormones in tissues is a chemical consequence of their unsuitability for incorporation into any of the three main storage compartments of the body (lipids, glycogen, or protein). For example, most steroid hormones are too polar to be stored in large quantities in lipid compartments, and peptide and amine hormones are unsuitable for incorporation into proteins. As a consequence of these factors the body pools of most hormones tend to be small. The major exceptions to this rule are those instances in which the precursor forms of hormone can be stored either as protein or in neutral lipid compartments; the normal thyroid gland contains the equivalent of a 2-week supply of thyroid hormones in the form of the protein thyroglobulin, and the precursor and intermediate forms of vitamin D can be stored in considerable quantity in hepatic lipid.

RELEASE The biochemical mechanisms involved in the release process are incompletely understood. In some instances they involve conversion of insoluble to soluble derivatives (proteolysis of thyroglobulin to thyroid hormones). In others, release is due to exocytosis of storage granules (insulin, glucagon, prolactin, growth hormone). Finally, release may involve passive diffusion of newly synthesized molecules such as steroid hormones down activity gradients into plasma; under this circumstance the rate of hormone release may be determined either by the rate of hormone synthesis or by the rate of blood flow to the tissue.

Because of the limited capacity for storage, most hormones are released into plasma at a pace reflecting the rates of formation. The pituitary trophic hormones [LH, adrenocorticotropin (ACTH), thyrotropin (TSH)] act in their target tissues to influence rates of both hormone synthesis and release. Even when peptide hormones are stored in granules, initial release of the stored material is followed by an enhanced rate of synthesis (as, for instance, the two-phase release of insulin induced by glucose infusion). For some hormones, major diurnal, sleep-related, developmental, and neural factors influence hormone release; again, it is assumed that in most of these instances synthesis and release are tightly linked.

The rate of hormone release in many instances is periodic or rhythmic, the cycle varying in frequency from minutes to hours (ultradian), to daily (circadian), to months or years (infradian). Hormones such as LH and follicle-stimulating hormone (FSH) are released in a pulsatile fashion with bursts of secretion occurring in a repetitive pattern: ACTH (and cortisol) release varies during a 24-h cycle, and thyroid hormone release can vary on longer cycles. Whether this intermittent release is a function of alterations in synthetic rates, changes in blood flow, or other mechanisms is uncertain, but most such cycles are under neurogenic control. In many instances the physiologic significance of pulsatile release is not fully understood, but in other instances changes in frequency or amplitude of the release pattern can have profound effects on hormone function; i.e., the pulsatile administration of luteinizing hormone–releasing hormone (LHRH) stimulates the release of LH by the pituitary, whereas the constant infusion of the same amount of hormone per unit time has the opposite effect. Furthermore, changes in frequency or amplitude of hormone release may characterize specific disease states; loss of the diurnal rhythm of cortisol release is characteristic of the early phase of Cushing's disease, and pulsatile release of LHRH is blunted in anorexia nervosa. Finally, understanding of the rhythms by which hormones are released is essential for interpreting plasma hormone levels.

TRANSPORT Hormones are transported via lymph, blood, and extracellular fluids from sites of synthesis to sites of cellular action and ultimately of metabolic inactivation and degradation. The plasma is probably a passive diluent for most peptide and amine hormones, and this feature explains the short half-lives (3 to 7 min) for most nonglycosylated peptide hormones. [Glycoprotein hormones such as human chorionic gonadotropin (hCG) have longer half-lives.] The more insoluble a hormone in water, the more important the role of transport proteins, and thyroid and steroid hormones are largely transported in protein-bound form. No transport protein yet characterized is exclusive; for example, testosterone can be transported both by a specific binding protein [testosterone-binding globulin (TeBG)] and by albumin; thyroxine can be transported both by prealbumin and by thyroxine-binding globulin (TBG). Protein-bound hormone (HP) cannot enter most cellular compartments and serves as a reservoir from which free hormone (H) is liberated for diffusion into intracellular compartments:

$$H + P \rightleftharpoons HP$$

Distribution of bound and free hormone in plasma is determined by the amount of hormone, the amount of binding protein, and the binding affinity of hormone for the protein. However, in the intact organism the effective level of free hormone is influenced by additional factors. When the rate of dissociation of a hormone from a binding protein is rapid (more rapid than the capillary transit time for a specific organ), the functional free fraction in vivo is also influenced by capillary transit time and membrane permeability.

Understanding the relation between free and bound hormone is essential for assessment of endocrine function. First, the free (dialyzable) fraction in vitro is generally less than the actual free fraction available in vivo because the portion of hormone bound to weak binding proteins such as albumin (in contrast to that protein bound to specific, high-affinity binding proteins) rapidly dissociates from the albumin as the free fraction diffuses from the capillary; consequently the albumin-bound hormone can function in vivo as a free fraction. Under some conditions, measurement of the dialyzable fraction does provide a useful index of the in vivo apparent free fraction. However, in hypoalbuminemic states, the in vitro free (dialyzable) fraction may increase when the in vivo free hormone level is actually diminished. In addition, in those tissue compartments such as liver in which proteins including hormone-transport protein complexes are cleared (in contrast to peripheral tissues in which only the free hormone enters the cell) free hormone levels have lesser effects on hormone uptake by the tissue.

Second, the distribution of hormones between plasma and tissue is a function of the balance between tissue binding proteins and plasma binding proteins. Therefore, levels of true or apparent free hormone may not reflect the amounts of hormone within cells.

Third, only the free hormone interacts with receptors in target cells and participates in the regulatory feedback mechanisms that control the rates of hormone synthesis. As a consequence, changes in the amount of transport protein alone cannot cause endocrine pathology in the steady state, provided the remainder of the endocrine feedback loop is intact. For example, profound elevations or decreases in TBG (either because of genetic or other factors) are both compatible with a euthyroid state. To illustrate, an increase in TBG would lower the level of free (dialyzable) hormone and lower the amount bound to albumin; as a consequence TSH secretion would increase, and the output of thyroxine by the thyroid would increase *until* TBG is again saturated so that the level of free hormone returns to the normal range, at which time TSH levels and thyroid hormone secretion also return to normal. Likewise, a decrease in TBG would temporarily increase the level of free hormone, and TSH secretion and thyroxine output would fall until the free level returns to normal.

To summarize, a change in the amount of a specific, high-affinity binding protein can cause profound alterations in hormone levels but by itself does not cause either a steady state hormone excess or deficiency, provided the regulatory feedback mechanisms that control hormone synthesis are intact. In contrast, alteration of the amount of a binding protein may cause endocrine pathology when hormone formation is not regulated by ordinary feedback control mechanisms or when feedback control mechanisms are deranged. For example, testosterone production in women is not regulated directly by testosterone levels, and alterations in TeBG levels in women may alter the steady state levels of free testosterone. Likewise, changes in TBG levels in a hypothyroid patient receiving a fixed dose of levothyroxine can cause alterations in free thyroxine levels.

DEGRADATION AND TURNOVER The plasma level (PL) of any hormone is dependent on two factors—the secretion rate (SR) of the hormone and the rates of metabolism and excretion, the so-called metabolic clearance rate (MCR):

$$PL = SR/MCR \quad \text{or} \quad SR = MCR \times PL$$

Metabolic clearance of hormones is accomplished by several mechanisms. Only small fractions of hormones are excreted intact in urine or bile. Degradation and inactivation of the hormone can take place in target tissues, in nontarget tissues such as liver and kidneys, or in both target and nontarget tissues. Peptide hormones are in general inactivated by proteases, largely in target tissues. Hormone metabolism frequently facilitates excretion of steroid and thyroid hormone by rendering them soluble in urine or bile. Thyroid hormones are deiodinated, deaminated, and deconjugated primarily by the liver. Steroid hormones are reduced, hydroxylated, and converted into glucuronide and sulfate conjugates. Biliary conjugates may be hydrolyzed in the gastrointestinal tract and reabsorbed into the circulation. The degradative mechanisms for different hormones have one common feature, namely, that alternative pathways exist for the catabolism of all hormones described to date.

Because of the nature of feedback control of hormone secretion, changes in rates of hormone degradation alone, like changes in plasma protein binding, do not cause endocrine pathology, provided the feedback loops that regulate synthesis are intact. For example, in severe liver disease and in myxedema, the degradation of glucocorticoids by the liver is impaired; as a consequence the turnover of cortisol slows, but the plasma level does not rise because secretion of ACTH is inhibited. Thus, a normal level of free hormone is maintained by decreasing the rate of cortisol secretion. The opposite is the case when glucocorticoid degradation is enhanced (as in thyrotoxicosis); in this situation cortisol secretion rises to keep the level of the hormone normal.

Although changes in rates of hormone degradation alone do not result in hormone deficit or excess, such changes may cause profound alterations in endocrine pharmacology. Thus, ordinary doses of glucocorticoids may cause the Cushing syndrome in patients with myxedema or liver disease, and consequently glucocorticoid dosage must be reduced in both conditions. Likewise, doses of glucocorticoids may have to be increased in the presence of hyperthyroidism. In addition, the development of hyperthyroidism in a patient with inadequate adrenal reserve can precipitate adrenal crisis by accelerating the rate of glucocorticoid catabolism. Thus, in circumstances in which the normal control mechanisms that regulate hormone synthesis are either circumvented or inoperative, changes in rates of hormone degradation may aggravate or cause pathology.

REGULATION OF HORMONE PRODUCTION

As stated above, fluctuations of hormone levels in the normal person are determined primarily by changes in rates of production. A unifying feature of all endocrine systems is the fact that the production of most hormones is regulated directly or indirectly by the metabolic activity of the hormone itself. This regulation is accomplished through a series of negative (and positive) feedback loops (Fig. 311-1). In some cases a fairly constant blood level of hormone is required, and some sensing device must exist to monitor either the hormone level itself or some related function such as plasma osmolality, blood glucose, plasma calcium, or body sodium content. For example, hormones produced in response to pituitary trophic hormones (cortisol, thyroxine, gonadal steroids) feed back on the hypothalamic-pituitary system to regulate their own rates of secretion. Similarly, parathyroid hormone and insulin are secreted in response to feedback signals from serum calcium and glucose levels, respectively. Feedback systems are generally more complex than this description indicates, sometimes operating indirectly by several steps; when the hormone itself acts as the direct regulator of feedback (testosterone on the hypothalamic-pituitary axis), the effect is mediated by the same

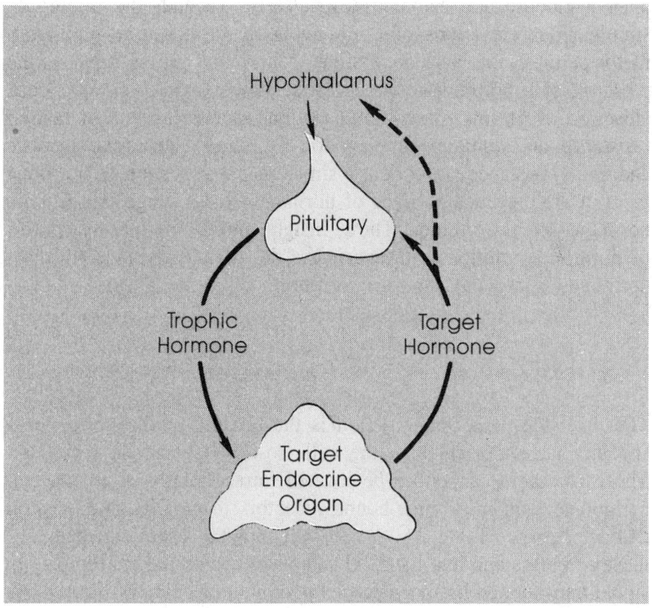

FIGURE 311-1 Feedback control of an endocrine organ such as the adrenal, thyroid, or gonads by the pituitary.

receptor-effector system by which the action of the hormone is accomplished in other target tissues. An example of positive feedback is the stimulation of LH release by estradiol prior to ovulation. Nonhormonal and environmental factors may alter both positive and negative feedback control mechanisms or the response to such control.

A usual feature of the feedback systems is rapidity of action; indeed, most respond within minutes or hours to varying metabolic demands to maintain homeostatic control within a narrow range. The main exceptions relate to gametogenesis in the ovary and testis (see Chaps. 321 and 322). In both instances, a complex differentiative process is involved. The steady state operation of these systems is such that sperm production tends to be relatively constant from day to day whereas ovulation is cyclic. However, spermatogenesis and export require approximately 2 months to complete so that changes in FSH levels may not result in altered levels of sperm in the ejaculate for long periods.

The fact that the secretion of hormones is under regulatory control has several important clinical implications. First, the significance of plasma levels of hormones may be interpretable only if the appropriate regulatory factors are taken into account (Fig. 311-2). The meaning of a borderline low plasma thyroxine may become clear only when thyroid-stimulating hormone (TSH) is measured simultaneously; likewise, plasma insulin and parathyroid hormone levels may be interpretable only in conjunction with simultaneous measurements of

FIGURE 311-2 Relation between target hormone level and trophic hormone level in normal and disease states (e.g., TSH and thyroid hormones, ACTH and cortisol, LH and testosterone).

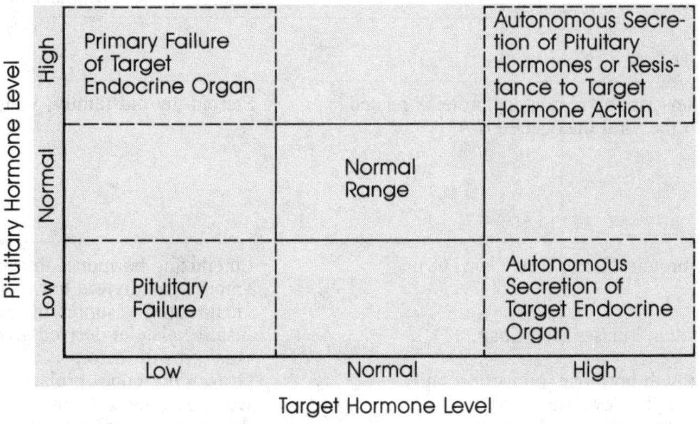

plasma glucose and calcium, respectively. Second, the finding of simultaneous elevations of hormone pairs (or hormone regulatory factor pairs) in the absence of signs of hormone excess suggests the presence of a hormone-resistance state. For example, simultaneous elevation of plasma glucose and insulin is characteristic of insulin resistance, and simultaneous elevation of LH and testosterone suggests androgen resistance. In contrast, simultaneous elevation of hormone pairs in the presence of signs of hormone excess suggests a trophic hormone–secreting tumor. Third, insight into the regulatory control of hormone secretion is the basis for the various dynamic tests of hormone reserve and hormone secretion.

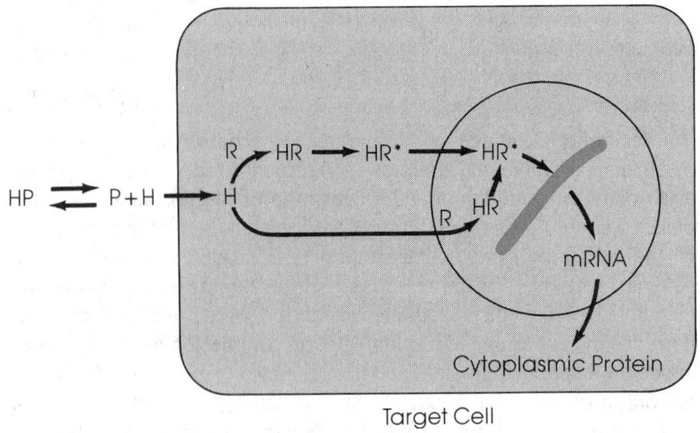

FIGURE 311-3 Mechanism of action of hormones with intracellular receptors. H = hormone; P = plasma transport protein; R = receptor; R* = activated receptor; mRNA = messenger RNA.

MECHANISMS OF HORMONE ACTION

The first step in hormone action is the binding of the hormone to specific macromolecules in the cell, so-called hormone receptors. These receptors can either be located intracellularly or in the cell membrane, and membrane-bound receptors in turn fall into several distinct classes (Table 311-1). Insight into the chemical nature of these receptors and into the mechanisms by which they participate in signal transduction has been accelerated by the cloning of the cDNAs and the genes that encode these proteins (see Chap. 6).

INTRACELLULAR RECEPTORS Most steroid and thyroid hormones are transported in plasma bound to carrier proteins (Fig. 311-3). The protein-bound hormones (HP) are in dynamic equilibrium with small amounts of free hormones (H) that diffuse by a passive mechanism into cells. In most instances the principal form of the hormone secreted into plasma (cortisol, progesterone, aldosterone, estradiol) undergoes no further metabolism within the cell and is responsible for hormone action within the target cell. Other hormones (thyroxine, testosterone) undergo chemical conversion to more active forms (triiodothyronine and dihydrotestosterone).

H binds to specific receptor proteins (R) in the cytoplasm or nucleus to form a hormone-receptor complex (HR). The hormone-receptor complex has the capacity to bind to specific regulatory sequences in DNA (so-called hormone regulatory elements) and thus acts as a regulator of transcription. As the result of this interaction with DNA new messenger RNAs (mRNAs) are formed, and the synthesis of cytoplasmic proteins is enhanced. The cytoplasmic proteins, in turn, mediate the effects of the hormone.

The cloning of the cDNAs for the various receptors revealed that receptors of this class bear a striking homology to the viral oncogene *erb*A and to each other. The fact that members of this family of hormone-dependent transcription factors are similar in structure suggests that these receptors have evolved from a common ancestral transcription factor. Each contains a hormone-binding domain, a DNA-binding domain, and an *N*-terminal variable or immunodominant domain (Fig. 311-4). An interesting feature of this class of receptors is that more than one receptor exists for certain hormones (thyroid hormones) and that candidate receptors have been identified for which no ligand is known. Elucidation of the structures of these receptors made it possible to analyze the mutations that impair hormone action and cause several hormone-resistance syndromes (see below).

MEMBRANE-BOUND RECEPTORS G protein family Receptors that bind GTP (G proteins) all work by similar mechanisms but are capable of mediating a complex range of actions. In every case, binding of ligand to the receptor produces a conformational change that causes GTP to bind to the protein at a special site. The active G protein then binds to a target protein and initiates a regulatory cascade involving one (or more) intracellular mediators including adenylate cyclase, phospholipase C, and arachidonic acid. The receptors of this class are monomeric proteins with an extracellular domain that binds ligand, an intracellular G protein–binding domain, and seven transmembrane-spanning regions. Elucidation of the molecular biology of the G protein has provided insight into the actions of drugs and signaling mechanisms in addition to hormones and into the pathophysiology of pseudohypoparathyroidism (see Chaps. 68 and 340 and below).

Protein kinases Receptors of this class are glycoproteins typically composed of two alpha subunits and two beta subunits which are linked by sulfhydryl bonds (Fig. 311-5). The alpha subunits are extracellular and contain the hormone binding site, and the beta subunits are transmembrane proteins. The beta subunit of the receptor is a hormone-regulated protein kinase capable of phosphorylating itself and other substrates on tyrosine residues using ATP as the phosphate source. In the case of insulin the tyrosine activity of the receptor is essential for hormone action. Point mutations in the coding sequence of receptor genes that prevent the protein kinase activity

TABLE 311-1 Classification of hormone receptors

Type	Characteristic hormones	Disease states due to mutant receptor components
INTRACELLULAR RECEPTORS		
Transcription regulatory proteins related to the viral oncogene *erb*A	Steroid-thyroid family, vitamin A	Testicular feminization and related syndromes; cortisol resistance; vitamin D–dependent rickets, type II; thyroid hormone resistance; pseudohypoaldosteronism
MEMBRANE RECEPTORS		
G-protein family (see Chap. 68)	Luteinizing hormone, thyroid-stimulating hormone, parathyroid hormone, epinephrine, somatostatin, vasopressin, glucagon	Pseudohypoparathyroidism, nephrogenic diabetes insipidus
Protein kinases (see Chap. 11)	Insulin, platelet-derived growth factor, epidermal growth factor	Diabetes mellitus with profound insulin resistance
Growth hormone–prolactin family	Growth hormone, prolactin	Laron dwarfism
Guanylate cyclase	Atrial natriuretic factor	
Ion channels (see Chap. 11)	Acetylcholine (nicotinic)	Myasthenia gravis

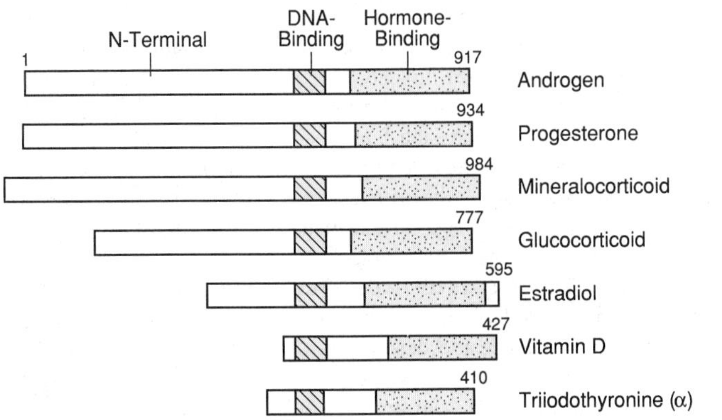

FIGURE 311-4 Intracellular receptors of the thyroid-steroid class. The areas of greatest homology (DNA-binding domain) are shown by the slanted bars, the areas of intermediate homology (hormone-binding domain) are shown by the stippled areas, and the areas with the least homology are shown by the open regions.

can cause profound resistance to insulin action (see below). Exactly how receptor kinase activity is transmitted into hormone action is not entirely clear. Several endogenous substrates of the enzyme have been identified, and physiologic effects of the hormone may either be indirect or direct consequences of the phosphorylation of the substrates or of the receptor itself.

Receptors of the growth hormone/prolactin class The growth hormone receptor is a protein of approximately 600 amino acids that contains a single, centrally located transmembrane domain. Interestingly, a high-affinity growth hormone–binding protein is present in the plasma; this protein corresponds to the extracellular hormone-binding domain of the growth hormone receptor and is believed to be cleaved from the receptor, but the role of the plasma protein in the regulation of growth is undefined. The growth hormone receptor shares approximately a 25 percent homology with the prolactin receptor (which may exist in more than one size) suggesting that the two receptors have evolved from a common ancestral gene. The mechanism(s) by which these receptors mediate hormone action is unclear. Mutations that impair the function of the growth hormone receptor are responsible for Laron dwarfism (see below).

FIGURE 311-5 Schematic representation of the insulin receptor. As the result of the binding of insulin to the alpha subunit the protein kinase function of the beta receptor is activated, and both exogenous protein substrates and the beta subunit itself are phosphorylated.

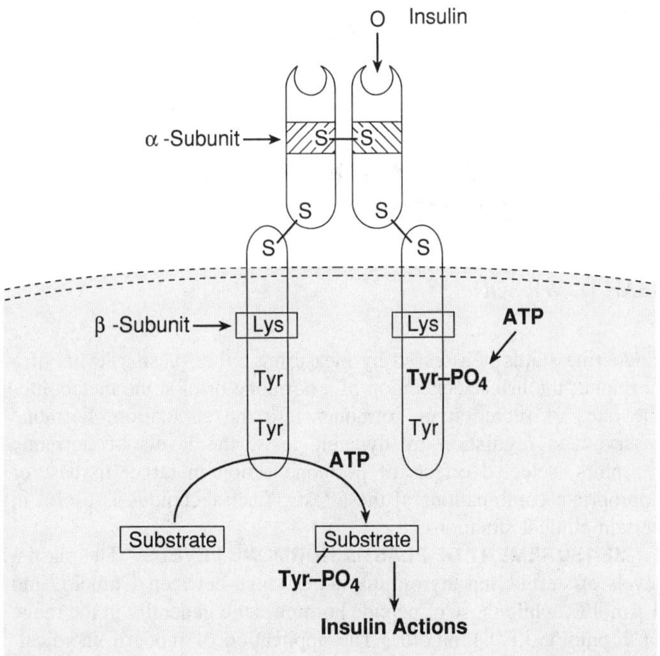

Other membrane-bound receptors The receptor for atrial natriuretic factor is a guanylate cyclase that spans the plasma membrane; the extracellular portion of the receptor binds the hormone, and the intracellular portion of the protein synthesizes guanosine-3′,5′-monophosphate (cyclic GMP) which serves as the second messenger for the hormone (see Chap. 68). The nicotinic acetylcholine receptor channel is a membrane-spanning complex of proteins that forms a true ion channel containing a central pore that can be opened and closed by ligand-binding-induced conformational change to allow sodium and potassium ions to cross the membrane and hence cause depolarization of cells that contain the receptors (see Chap. 11). Autoantibodies that block the function of this receptor cause myasthenia gravis (see Chap. 366).

ENDOCRINE DISORDERS

Endocrinopathy can result from hormone deficiency, hormone excess, or resistance to hormone action, and abnormalities in more than one endocrine system may coexist in the same individual.

DEFICIENCY STATES With few exceptions (calcitonin) hormone deficiency results in pathologic manifestations. The study of clinical disorders that result from hormone deficiency or absence played an important role in the evolution of endocrinology as a discipline. Such studies were followed by attempts to extract the responsible hormone from normal endocrine tissues, characterize the chemical nature (and ultimately synthesize the molecule), and administer the hormone to replace the deficit. The treatment of hypothyroidism by the administration of thyroid hormone is probably as successful as any therapeutic measure in medicine. Because clinical deficiency states can be induced in experimental animals by destruction or removal of the endocrine organ, an enormous amount is known about the pathophysiology of the deficiency states (diabetes mellitus, pituitary and adrenal insufficiency, hypothyroidism, and hypogonadism).

The nature of the destructive processes that cause failure of the endocrine organs is also understood in many instances; these include infections (adrenal insufficiency due to tuberculosis), infarction (postpartum pituitary failure) and tissue death of other causes (diabetes mellitus secondary to pancreatitis), tumors (chromophobe adenomas of the pituitary), autoimmune processes (Hashimoto's thyroiditis), dietary inadequacy (hypothyroidism due to iodine deficiency), and hereditary defects in hormone synthesis (pituitary dwarfism). In certain forms of diabetes mellitus, the cause may be a hereditary predisposition that renders the pancreas subject to destruction by several mechanisms (see Chap. 319). In other endocrine-deficiency diseases the etiology of the defect is unidentified (congenital anorchism).

HORMONE EXCESS With few exceptions (testosterone in men, progesterone in men and women) hormone excess causes pathologic effects. Four general types of hormone excess are recognized. In one, the hormone is overproduced by the gland that is the usual site of its production (hyperthyroidism, acromegaly, Cushing's disease); such excess production results from failure of circumvention of the feedback control mechanisms that regulate production of the hormone in the normal state, but the underlying mechanism is often obscure because animal models for the diseases are rare. The second type of hormone excess results when a hormone is produced by a tissue (usually malignant) that ordinarily is not a major endocrine organ (for example, ACTH production in oat cell carcinoma of the lung, thyroid hormone secretion by struma ovarii). Such hormone-excess states have been described for many hormones (see Chap. 309). A third type of hormone-excess state involves the overproduction of hormones in peripheral tissues from circulating precursors; for example, overproduction of estrogen in liver disease because of diversion of the precursor androstenedione from its usual sites of catabolism in the liver to sites of extraglandular estrogen formation. Finally, hormone excess all too commonly results from iatrogenic causes; for example, the complications resulting from glucocorticoid therapy (see Chap. 317).

Excess of a given hormone may result from more than one cause. Thyrotoxicosis can result from overproduction of hormone by the thyroid as a result of overproduction of TSH (rare); from stimulation by extrapituitary thyroid-stimulating factors; from autonomous thyroid hyperfunction; from leakage of preformed hormone from the thyroid due to an inflammatory injury; or from excess hormone from sources other than the thyroid itself, as in thyroid hormone overdosage, accidental ingestion of meats contaminated with thyroid tissue, or secretion by struma ovarii (see Chap. 316). The unraveling of the cause of specific hormone-excess states can be one of the most challenging problems of clinical endocrinology.

PRODUCTION OF ABNORMAL HORMONES In some instances abnormal hormones can cause endocrine disease. One form of diabetes mellitus is the result of a single-gene mutation that results in the production of an abnormal insulin molecule that is ineffective because of defective binding to the insulin receptor. In other cases, hormone precursors, hormone subunits, or incompletely processed peptide hormones may be released into the circulation, as is common in so-called ectopic hormone production of neoplasia (see Chap. 309). Alternatively, immunoglobulins may bind to hormone receptors and thus exert hormonal actions, for example, the thyroid-stimulating immunoglobulins that exert TSH-like actions in hyperthyroidism (see Chap. 316) or the antibodies to the insulin receptor that have insulin-like actions (see Chap. 319).

HORMONE RESISTANCE The concept that an endocrinopathy can result because the tissues cannot respond to normal (or increased) levels of a hormone evolved from the deduction that pseudohermaphroditism is due to peripheral resistance to the action of parathyroid hormone (see Chaps. 68 and 340). This concept has had far-reaching implications. First, the concept of hormone resistance served as a major stimulus for the study of how hormones act within cells. Second, more and more forms of hormone resistance have been identified, so that diseases are now recognized to result from resistance to most hormones. Such hormone resistance is frequently due to hereditary causes. Third, hormone resistance can be due to a variety of molecular abnormalities, including defects in receptors and in postreceptor effector mechanisms for hormones, development of antibodies to hormones or hormone receptors, and the absence of target cells. Fourth, abnormalities of receptors are now implicated in the pathogenesis of diseases outside the endocrine domain, such as familial hypercholesterolemia. Hormone resistance does not necessarily involve equally all target tissues for the hormone. For example, selective resistance to thyroid hormone can be restricted to the pituitary itself, and in one form of androgen resistance androgen action is more severely impaired in the testis than in other target tissues.

A common feature of hormone-resistance states is the coexistence of a normal or *elevated* level of the hormone in the circulation despite deficient hormone action. This feature is a consequence of the fact that most hormones are under regulatory feedback control and failure of hormone action usually leads to increased hormone production.

The elucidation of the structures of the various receptors and the cloning of the cDNAs for these proteins has made it possible to define the molecular defects in a number of hormone-resistance states (Table 311-1). Mutations of almost every class of receptor have now been identified, and several clinical implications are now apparent. First, in the past it was only possible to identify receptor defects that caused profound hormone resistance. Now that subtle defects in receptor function can be identified, hormone resistance may prove to be a common cause of human endocrinopathy. Second, when individual disorders are analyzed at the molecular level, it is apparent that the disorders are genetically heterogeneous. No two unrelated families with mutations of the insulin receptor, the growth hormone receptor, or the androgen receptor have proved to have identical disorders. Furthermore, in regard to individual receptors such as the androgen receptor, mutations may either be point mutations that cause single amino acid substitutions in the protein or premature termination codons that result in short molecules or gross deletions or rearrangements that cause complete disruption of the coding sequence. It is thus necessary to analyze each family separately. Third, the analysis of these mutations has provided major insight into hormone action—for example, establishing the critical importance of the tyrosine kinase function of the insulin receptor and making it possible to define the various domains of the intracellular receptors.

DISEASES AFFECTING MULTIPLE ENDOCRINE SYSTEMS The fact that disorders can affect more than one endocrine system has been known since the description of panhypopituitarism in the nineteenth century. Such disorders encompass diverse etiologies including autoimmunity (autoimmune polyglandular dysfunction, or Schmidt's syndrome), receptor abnormalities (gonadotropin and thyrotropin resistance in pseudohypoparathyroidism), tumors (multiple endocrine neoplasia, or MEN) and hereditary disorders of unknown etiology (lipodystrophies) (see Chap. 325). They may include both hypo- and hyperfunctioning states, and some clinical syndromes may occur in the context of more than one polyendocrine state (pheochromocytoma in MEN II, MEN III, and von Hippel–Lindau disease; diabetes mellitus in Schmidt's syndrome and lipodystrophy).

Because each endocrinopathy in such a constellation can also occur alone, all endocrine patients must be approached with a high index of suspicion for abnormalities of multiple systems. This is of particular importance because treatment of one condition may cause worsening of another (surgical procedures such as thyroidectomy can cause worsening of unrecognized pheochromocytoma) and because in certain of the familial syndromes it is mandatory to make systematic searches for the disease in potentially affected family members.

REFERENCES

EVANS RM: The steroid and thyroid hormone receptor superfamily. Science 240:889, 1988

GODOWSKI PG et al: Characterization of the human growth hormone receptor gene and demonstration of a partial gene deletion in two patients with Laron-type dwarfism. Proc Natl Acad Sci USA 86:8083, 1989

HABENER JF: Genetic control of hormone formation, in *Williams' Textbook of Endocrinology*, 7th ed, JD Wilson, DW Foster (eds). Philadelphia, Saunders, 1985, pp 9–32

KAHN CR, GOLDSTEIN BJ: Molecular defects in insulin action. Science 245:13, 1989

———, WHITE MF: The insulin receptor and the molecular mechanism of insulin action. J Clin Invest 82:1151, 1988

MARCELLI M et al: A single nucleotide substitution introduces a premature termination codon into the androgen receptor gene of a patient with receptor-negative androgen resistance. J Clin Invest Vol 85, 1990 In Press.

PARDRIDGE WM: Serum bioavailability of sex steroid hormones. Clin Endocrinol Metab 15:259, 1986

312 ASSESSMENT OF ENDOCRINE FUNCTION

JEAN D. WILSON

Endocrine status is assessed by measuring either plasma levels of a hormone, the urinary excretion of a hormone or of some metabolite, the rates of secretion of hormones into the circulation, hormone reserve and regulation by dynamic tests, the levels of hormone receptors, selected effects of hormone action in target tissues, or appropriate combinations of these tests. Each technique is useful in certain clinical situations.

MEASUREMENT OF PLASMA HORMONE LEVELS The plasma levels of steroid and thyroid hormones range between 1 nmol/L and 1 μmol/L, while those of peptide hormones are generally in the range of 1 pmol/L to 0.1 nmol/L. The application of modern chemical, chromatographic, radioreceptor, and radioimmunoassay techniques for the assessment of plasma constituents in low concentrations constitutes one of the significant advances of modern medicine and has made clinical endocrinology a more quantitative discipline. In the case of hormones whose plasma levels are relatively constant from moment to moment and day to day (thyroxine and triiodothyronine), the measurement of isolated plasma levels alone provides a reliable assessment of the hormone status in most clinical situations.

For several reasons, however, care must be exercised in assessing isolated plasma levels. First, for hormones with relatively simple structures (steroid and thyroid hormones) chemical and radioimmunoassay techniques are reliable so that measured values usually reflect the plasma levels as of a given moment. In the case of the more complex peptide hormones, however, considerable variability may exist in the structure of physiologically active hormone molecules in the circulation, some of which may be measured poorly in specific radioimmunoassay procedures; for example, standard radioimmunoassays for luteinizing hormone (LH) and for parathyroid hormone may on occasion either underestimate or overestimate the amount of biologically active hormone in plasma. In such situations, radioreceptor assays or in vitro bioassays may provide a better assessment of endocrine status.

Second, in the case of hormones that undergo pulsatile secretion (LH, testosterone) a single value is usually not representative of mean plasma levels. In these instances it is necessary either to measure levels in several samples drawn at random or to pool aliquots of three or more samples of plasma drawn at 20- to 30-min intervals for a single determination.

Third, when plasma levels exhibit a characteristic, predictable fluctuation such as the diurnal variation of plasma cortisol, the timing of plasma sampling can be designed to provide a useful index of the hormone status. Even here, however, it is important to recognize that plasma levels may exhibit diurnal variation only during certain phases of life (plasma LH levels in early puberty). In women appropriate interpretation of plasma gonadotropins, progesterone, and estradiol during the reproductive years requires reference to the corresponding phase of the ovulatory and menstrual cycles, and it may be necessary to obtain sequential studies over many days to provide interpretable data. Seasonal variations also occur in the levels of certain hormones (such as thyroxine and testosterone), but these changes are generally so small that they do not affect the interpretation of individual values. In some situations variation in hormone levels is not the result of any obvious rhythmicity but rather the consequence of waxing and waning of disease processes; repeated measurements of cortisol or of calcium and parathyroid hormone levels over many months may be necessary to establish a diagnosis of Cushing's syndrome or of hyperparathyroidism.

Fourth, in the case of steroids, thyroid hormones, and some peptide hormones such as growth hormone that are transported in plasma largely bound to proteins, measurement of total hormone concentration provides an index of endocrine status *only* to the extent that it allows a deduction of the level of the free or unbound hormone. Indeed, direct measurements of the free levels of these hormones (usually 1 percent or less of the total) can be done only in a few laboratories. Since the amount of free hormone is a function of the amount and the affinity of binding of transport proteins and the amount of hormone, the total hormone level reflects the amount of free hormone only as long as the amount of binding protein(s) remains constant or fluctuates only within narrow limits. In those instances in which the level of binding protein is increased [e.g., thyroid-binding globulin (TBG) and testosterone-binding globulin (TeBG, or sex steroid–binding globulin, SHBG) in pregnancy] or decreased [hereditary decreases in TBG and cortisol-binding globulin (CBG)] it is essential to utilize some other assessment of the amount of binding protein to allow estimation of the free hormone level (T_3 resin uptake for TBG or direct measurement of TBG, TeBG, or CBG).

Fifth, the range of plasma levels of most hormones within the normal population is broad. As a consequence, the level of a hormone in an individual may be halved or doubled (and thus be grossly abnormal for that person) but still be within the so-called normal range. For this reason it is frequently useful to assess appropriate hormone pairs simultaneously (LH and testosterone, thyroxine and thyroid-stimulating hormone); a borderline low testosterone level in the presence of elevated plasma LH is indicative of testicular failure, whereas the same level of testosterone in the presence of a normal LH implies that the endocrine status is normal (Fig. 311-2). Likewise, in women with increased testosterone production and secondary decrease in TeBG, plasma testosterone concentration may be normal despite increased production of the hormone.

URINARY EXCRETION The measurement of urinary excretion of a hormone or a hormone metabolite that reflects plasma levels or secretory rates offers certain advantages over the measurement of isolated plasma levels, e.g., the urinary excretion reflects average plasma levels over the time of collection. Thus, a 24-h urine free cortisol value may provide a better estimate of the function of the adrenal cortex than isolated measurements of plasma cortisol. Again, however, certain limitations of the use of urinary measurements must be kept in mind. (1) Urinary creatinine should be measured routinely to document the adequacy of the urine collection. Women excrete on average about 1 g, and men excrete about 1.8 g/d. Day-to-day variation should not exceed 20 percent. (2) The excretion of individual metabolites may not reflect changes in hormone secretion under all conditions. For example, the formation of the 18-oxo derivative of aldosterone may be influenced by drugs that do not alter secretion or plasma levels of the hormone. (3) Urine values are obviously meaningless for those hormones (thyroxine, triiodothyronine) excreted into bile. Of more importance is the fact that peptide hormones such as gonadotropins may be metabolized differently in different individuals prior to excretion into the urine so that establishment of the range of normal is difficult. (4) Hormones from more than one source may be excreted as common metabolites; urinary 17-ketosteroids are derived from both adrenal and gonadal androgens, and consequently the measurement is of little value in assessing testicular androgen production in men. (5) Changes in renal function may influence rates of hormone excretion into urine. Such changes can in part be corrected by measurement of urine creatinine, but in the case of metabolites or conjugates formed in the kidney itself excretion patterns may be distorted out of proportion to the decrease in creatinine clearance.

SECRETION AND PRODUCTION RATES The measurement of the actual secretion rate of a hormone circumvents most problems inherent in measurement of plasma levels and urinary excretion. Such measurements involve the administration of radioactive hormone and measuring the dilution that such a hormone undergoes as a consequence of mixture with endogenously secreted, nonradioactive hormone over a given period of time. In practice the plasma hormone itself or a unique metabolite of the hormone from urine is isolated, purified to radiochemical homogeneity, and used to calculate the amount of the hormone secreted during the time of study. In the case of hormones formed principally in peripheral tissues (estradiol and dihydrotestosterone in men, triiodothyronine in both sexes) radioactive precursors can be administered, and the rates of conversion to the metabolites in question can be measured for assessment of overall production rates. Alternatively, as described above, clearance rates of hormones can be measured and, together with mean plasma levels, used to estimate secretion rates. Unfortunately, these various techniques are complex and expensive to perform, require use of radioactive isotopes, and can be done in only a few centers.

DYNAMIC TESTS OF HORMONE RESERVE AND REGULATION When hypo- or hyperfunction is severe, measurement of the level of hormone in blood or urine may be satisfactory for making a diagnosis, particularly when the tests demonstrate appropriate feedback relationships; e.g., low plasma testosterone coupled with high plasma LH indicates primary testicular failure. In less clear-cut instances, however, stimulation tests are useful in establishing the significance of borderline low values. Likewise, suppression tests are used to document the presence of hyperfunction of endocrine systems. All such dynamic tests are designed to take advantage of the known feedback control mechanisms for various hormones (Fig. 311-1).

Two types of stimulation tests are in common use. In one, endogenous hormone production or action is blocked (cortisol production by metyrapone, estradiol action by clomiphene), and the capacity of the pituitary to respond by increasing endogenous production of the trophic hormone and/or the capacity of the target tissue to respond are then assessed; ideally such tests measure the integrity of an entire hypothalamic–pituitary–target tissue loop. In the other type of stimulation test, the trophic hormone itself is administered under some standardized regimen, and the capacity of the target tissue to respond is determined (cortisol levels before and after ACTH administration). Stimulation tests are particularly useful in four situations: (1) assessing hormone status when precise quantification of plasma levels is difficult or imperfect (ACTH), (2) assessing endocrine status when static tests are borderline low, (3) distinguishing primary from secondary (pituitary) causes of endocrine failure, and (4) assessing gonadal reserve in prepubertal patients in whom plasma gonadotropins and gonadal steroids are difficult to interpret.

Suppression tests are useful for the diagnosis of hyperfunction because the hyperfunctioning gland by definition does not operate under normal control mechanisms. Suppression can either be quantitatively or qualitatively abnormal. For example, the feedback control of the pituitary may be reset to respond to high levels of the suppressing hormone (pituitary ACTH secretion in Cushing's disease), or secretion can be autonomous (ACTH secretion by carcinoma of the lung). In principle, the feedback regulator is administered, and the degree of inhibition of hormone secretion is assessed for the endocrine system in question (change in ^{131}I uptake after administration of thyroid hormones, change in cortisol secretion after the administration of potent exogenous glucocorticoids, suppressibility of plasma growth hormone by glucose).

The clinical usefulness of dynamic tests of endocrine function is limited by the fact that they are altered by a multitude of secondary factors. Age, coexisting disease states, and concurrent drug regimens all interact to influence responsiveness and hence to limit the specificity of such tests. In particular, psychiatric disorders such as endogenous depression may impair endocrine dynamic tests in the absence of specific endocrine pathology.

HORMONE RECEPTORS AND ANTIBODIES The measurement of hormone receptors in biopsy material from target tissues or in fibroblasts propagated from biopsy material is useful—for example, in the diagnosis of partial hormone-resistance states such as rickets due to vitamin D resistance, hyperglycemia and hyperinsulinemia associated with insulin resistance, and male pseudohermaphroditism due to androgen resistance (see Chap. 311). In selected laboratories the cDNAs for some receptors can be sequenced to provide specific information about the structure of mutant proteins. Likewise, under selected conditions measurement of antibodies to hormones (such as antibodies to thyroid hormones that can cause hypothyroidism) or antibodies to target tissues (adrenal gland, gonads, thyroid) may be essential for the assessment of endocrine status. With certain exceptions (antibodies to thyroid tissue) these tests are not widely available.

TISSUE EFFECTS Perhaps the ideal hormone test is the measurement of the peripheral end result of hormone action in the target tissues for the hormone. For example, demonstration of the capacity to concentrate urine maximally following water restriction indicates that the hypothalamic control mechanisms are intact, that the posterior pituitary has a normal capacity to secrete vasopressin, that the vasopressin receptor is intact, and that the postreceptor effector mechanisms for the hormone are operative. Optimally such a test assesses the function of the entire pathway of hormone secretion and action. In practice, many such tests are imperfect. For example, even though vasopressin secretion is normal, intrinsic renal disease can result in a fixed low urine osmolality and thus distort the interpretation of the functional test of vasopressin action. In other instances the tests are difficult to perform and subject both to artifact and to influences from diverse parameters (for example, the metabolic rate is increased by fever even when thyroid function is normal). For these reasons, the identification of additional specific tissue markers for hormone action would be very useful.

IMAGING PROCEDURES Developments in imaging have had a profound impact in endocrinology and provide better means of identifying abnormalities in almost every endocrine system, from delineating small lesions of the pituitary and hypothalamus, to using bone densitometry for assessing metabolic bone disease, to the noninvasive localization of functioning parathyroid tissue in patients with persistent or recurrent hyperparathyroidism. Because the rate of technologic advance in the field is so rapid, the literature evaluating the effectiveness (and limitations) of up-to-date processes inevitably lags.

A major problem in the interpretation of imaging procedures stems from the fact that small nodules of no functional significance are known from autopsy studies to occur in the pituitary, the adrenal, and, less commonly, the testes. The natural history of these nonfunctioning adenomas is not well understood; the vast majority appear to remain limited in size and nonfunctional for life, but in rare instances they may evolve into autonomous and/or hyperfunctioning tumors. In addition, malignancies—both metastatic and primary—can occur in these tissues. Now such lesions can be recognized in life, and the incidental discovery of adrenal and pituitary masses is a common result of CT scans performed for other reasons. Several types of criteria have been proposed for deciding which of these masses are likely to be benign and which should be removed. For example, by one guideline solid, endocrinologically silent lesions of the adrenal smaller than 3.5 cm may be followed safely with serial CT scans whereas larger lesions deserve further workup such as sonographically guided percutaneous needle biopsy or exploratory surgery. Additional experience will be required to establish the validity of these and other criteria for the assessment of such masses.

Another unresolved issue stems from the fact that it is not always clear which imaging procedure is best in a given clinical situation. In some instances evidence will be accrued that will make clear the indications for one or another procedure. In other instances definite guidelines may be harder to develop, as in the choice of MRI versus CT scans for delineation of the anatomy of the hypothalamic-pituitary system. In some patients small lesions are best seen with MRI whereas in others lesions in the same areas—equally small and with similar histologic features—are better delineated with CT scans. As a consequence, there is a tendency in the workup of complicated cases to order both procedures routinely. Although this practice is justified in some cases, the costs of diagnostic workups are thereby inflated.

An unexpected dividend of the developments in imaging is that it is now possible to chart the natural history of endocrine disease in a different way, as in the occasional documentation of hemorrhage into a pituitary tumor that eventuates in development of the empty sella syndrome or the uncovering of a functioning adrenal adenoma in the absence of biochemical or clinical evidence of Cushing's disease.

REFERENCES

BELLDEGRUN A et al: Incidentally discovered mass of the adrenal gland. Surg Gynecol Obstet 163:203, 1986

GORDEN P, WEINTRAUB BD: Radioreceptor and other functional hormone assays, in *Williams Textbook of Endocrinology*, 7th ed, JD Wilson, DW Foster (eds). Philadelphia, Saunders, 1985, pp 133–146

GRIFFIN JE: Assessment of endocrine function, in *Textbook of Endocrine Physiology*, JE Griffin, SR Ojeda (eds). New York, Oxford University Press, 1988, p 56

HAMPER UM et al: Primary adrenocortical carcinoma: Sonographic evaluation with clinical and pathologic correlation in 26 patients. Am J Roentgenog 148:915, 1987

VAITUKAITIS JL: Hormone assays, in *Endocrinology and Metabolism*, P Felig et al (eds). New York, McGraw-Hill, 1987, p 165

YALOW RS: Radioimmunoassay of hormones, in *Williams Textbook of Endocrinology*, 7th ed, JD Wilson, DW Foster (eds). Philadelphia, Saunders, 1985, pp 123–132

313 NEUROENDOCRINE REGULATION AND DISEASES OF THE ANTERIOR PITUITARY AND HYPOTHALAMUS

GILBERT H. DANIELS / JOSEPH B. MARTIN

The pituitary, appropriately titled the master gland, produces six major hormones and stores an additional two hormones (Fig. 313-1). Growth hormone (GH) regulates growth and has important influences on intermediary metabolism (see Chap. 314). Prolactin (PRL) is necessary for lactation. Luteinizing hormone (LH) and follicle-stimulating hormone (FSH) control the gonads in men and women. Thyroid-stimulating hormone (TSH, thyrotropin) regulates thyroid function. Adrenocorticotropin (ACTH) controls glucocorticoid function of the adrenal cortex. These hormones are all synthesized in the anterior pituitary. Vasopressin (AVP; antidiuretic hormone, ADH) and oxytocin are produced in neurons of the hypothalamus and stored in the posterior lobe of the pituitary (see Chap. 315). Vasopressin (AVP) controls water conservation by the kidneys; oxytocin is necessary for milk let-down during lactation.

A feedback relationship exists between the anterior pituitary and its three target endocrine glands—the gonads, the adrenal cortex, and the thyroid. When the gonads fail or are removed, the concentrations of LH and FSH rise, a condition known as primary hypogonadism. When the adrenal cortex is removed or destroyed, primary adrenal insufficiency (or Addison's disease) results, and the serum ACTH concentration increases. Thyroid failure results in the characteristic rise in TSH of primary hypothyroidism.

When the pituitary gland is removed or destroyed, loss of the trophic hormones results in secondary hypogonadism, adrenal insufficiency, or hypothyroidism. Growth hormone and prolactin function are also lost. AVP and oxytocin function are not affected by destruction of the pituitary provided their site of origin in the hypothalamus is intact.

FIGURE 313-1 The relationship between the hypothalamus and pituitary. See text for details.

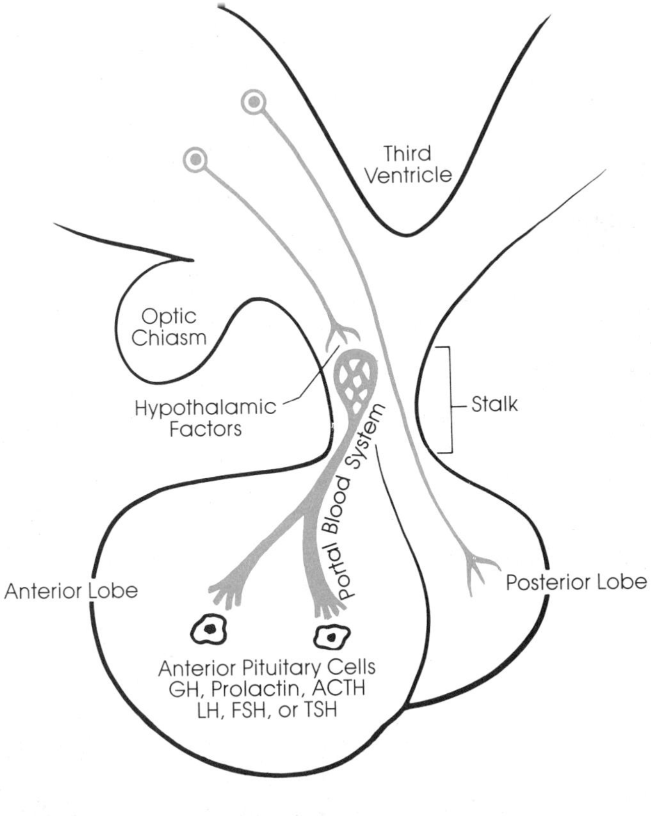

The pituitary is in turn under the control of the hypothalamus, which produces a number of chemical mediators. These hormones are synthesized in the hypothalamus and enter the portal vascular system which carries them through the pituitary stalk to the anterior lobe (Fig. 313-1). Interruption of the pituitary stalk is followed by reduction in the release of GH, LH, FSH, TSH, and ACTH from the anterior pituitary. This implies that stimulatory influences from the hypothalamus are necessary for release of these hormones. In contrast, the level of prolactin rises after interruption of the stalk, implying a normal tonic inhibitory hypothalamic influence on prolactin secretion. The rise in prolactin secretion indicates that stalk section does not lead to pituitary destruction. If the stalk section is not at too high a level, AVP and oxytocin release continue principally from axons that terminate in the median eminence of the hypothalamus. With hypothalamic ablation, the levels of GH, LH, FSH, TSH, ACTH, AVP, and oxytocin fall, whereas prolactin levels increase (Fig. 313-1).

Most hypothalamic factors that control secretion of the pituitary hormones are peptides (Table 313-1). Growth hormone–releasing hormone (GRH) is the dominant influence on GH release, and somatostatin acts as an inhibitory hormone for GH release. Although LH and FSH levels vary independently in physiologic states, one releasing hormone [luteinizing hormone–releasing hormone, LHRH, also called gonadotropin-releasing hormone (GnRH)] plays a major role in controlling their release. Thyrotropin-releasing hormone (TRH) controls TSH release and may also influence prolactin release. Corticotropin-releasing hormone (CRH) and other factors control ACTH release. In addition, dopamine acts as a prolactin inhibitory factor (PIF).

Pituitary tumors may lead to hormonal over- or underproduction or may cause mechanical problems by impinging on neighboring structures. The most common hormones produced by pituitary tumors are prolactin and GH. Prolactin excess leads to galactorrhea and/or hypogonadism; GH excess leads to gigantism and acromegaly. ACTH-secreting tumors produce Cushing's disease or Nelson's syndrome. TSH-secreting tumors are rare causes of hyperthyroidism. Gonadotropin-secreting tumors are paradoxically most often associated with hypogonadism. Large pituitary tumors may cause partial or complete hypopituitarism by compression of the adjacent normal gland or pituitary stalk and are associated with visual field disturbances due to compression of the optic chiasm with other neurologic disturbances caused by invasion of cavernous sinuses or cranial fossae.

TABLE 313-1 Anterior pituitary and hypophysiotropic hormones

	Hypophysiotropic hormones	
Pituitary hormone	Name	Structure
Thyrotropin (TSH)	Thyrotropin-releasing hormone (TRH)	Tripeptide
Adrenocorticotropin (ACTH)	Corticotropin-releasing hormone (CRH)	41 Amino acids
Luteinizing hormone (LH)	Luteinizing hormone–releasing hormone (LHRH)	Decapeptide
Follicle-stimulating hormone (FSH)	LHRH	Decapeptide
Growth hormone (GH)	Growth hormone–releasing hormone (GRH)	44 Amino acids
	Growth hormone release–inhibiting hormone* (somatostatin, GIH)	14 Amino acids
Prolactin	Prolactin release–inhibiting factor (PIF)	Dopamine
	Prolactin-releasing factor (PRF)†	Peptide ? Vasoactive intestinal polypeptide (VIP)

* Somatostatin also inhibits TRH-stimulated TSH release.
† TRH stimulates prolactin release.

Hypothalamic disease may cause hypopituitarism with the exception that secretion of prolactin may be increased. Diabetes insipidus due to AVP deficiency is virtually diagnostic of hypothalamic disease or of high interruption of the pituitary stalk. Disturbances of thirst, temperature regulation, appetite, and blood pressure may occur with hypothalamic disorders as well. Large hypothalamic masses may lead to visual field disturbances, obstruction of the third ventricle, and invasion of surrounding brain tissue.

ANATOMY AND EMBRYOLOGY

The pituitary gland (hypophysis) sits within the sella turcica (''Turkish saddle'') of the sphenoid bone at the base of the skull and is composed principally of the anterior (adenohypophysis) and posterior lobes (neurohypophysis). The intermediate lobe is rudimentary in humans. The normal pituitary gland weighs between 0.5 and 0.9 g.

The pituitary is separated from the brain by the diaphragma sella, an extension of the dura mater, and from the sphenoid sinus anteriorly and inferiorly by a thin layer of bone. The lateral walls of the sella abut on the cavernous sinuses, which contain the internal carotid arteries and cranial nerves III, IV, V, and VI. The optic chiasm is slightly anterior to the pituitary stalk, just above the diaphragma sella. Thus, tumors of the pituitary may lead to visual field defects, to cranial nerve palsies, or to invasion of the sphenoid sinus (Fig. 313-2).

The hypothalamus extends anteriorly to the margin of the optic chiasm and posteriorly to include the mammillary bodies. Superiorly, the hypothalamic sulcus of the third ventricle separates the thalamus from the hypothalamus. The rounded inferior base of the hypothalamus forms the tuber cinereum. The central portion of the base (termed the infundibulum or median eminence) is formed by the floor of the third ventricle and continues inferiorly to form the pituitary stalk. The releasing factors are synthesized in neurons that are along the margins of the third ventricle and that project fibers which terminate in the median eminence adjacent to the portal capillaries.

The cell bodies of the supraoptic and paraventricular nuclei of the hypothalamus produce vasopressin and oxytocin, which travel down nerve axons in the supraopticohypophysial and paraventriculohypophysial nerve tracts to reach the posterior lobe.

The communication between the hypothalamus and the anterior pituitary is chemical rather than physical. Releasing factors produced by hypothalamic neurons reach the anterior pituitary via the portal system to stimulate or inhibit hormone production. Some of the vasopressin-containing neurons also terminate in the median eminence, and vasopressin can stimulate release of ACTH and GH.

The anterior pituitary has the highest blood flow of any tissue in the body [0.8 (mL/g)/min]. The blood supply reaches the anterior pituitary by a circuitous route through the hypothalamus. Two derivatives of the internal carotid arteries, the superior hypophysial arteries (SHA), branch in the subarachnoid space around the pituitary stalk and terminate in the capillary network of the median eminence. These capillaries have a fenestrated endothelium which allows easy access to the hypothalamic releasing hormones. Transport of substances from the capillaries to the median eminence is also facilitated because the median eminence lies outside the blood-brain barrier. The capillaries then coalesce to form 6 to 10 straight veins known as the hypothalamic-pituitary portal circulation. These veins constitute the main blood supply to the anterior lobe and supply it with nutrients as well as information from the hypothalamus. A direct arterial blood supply to the anterior lobe is also present, but the magnitude and importance of that circulation are uncertain. The posterior pituitary is supplied entirely by blood from the inferior hypophysial arteries.

The anterior lobe is formed from the lateral proliferation of Rathke's pouch, an outpouching from the floor of the embryonic oral cavity. Rathke's pouch is met by a diverticulum from the floor of the third ventricle, which forms the posterior lobe.

Rathke's pouch is closed off by proliferation of the anterior and posterior lobe and forms a thin residual cleft in the gland (Rathke's cleft). This cleft may persist as a cyst lined with cuboidal or columnar epithelium. Since the pituitary rotates as it grows, these cysts usually lie in a position superior to the pituitary gland. The further growth and proliferation of these cysts can give rise to craniopharyngiomas, tumors that generally occupy a suprasellar position. Development of the sphenoid bone separates the pituitary from the oral cavity. Remnants of the pituitary, known as pharyngeal pituitaries, occa-

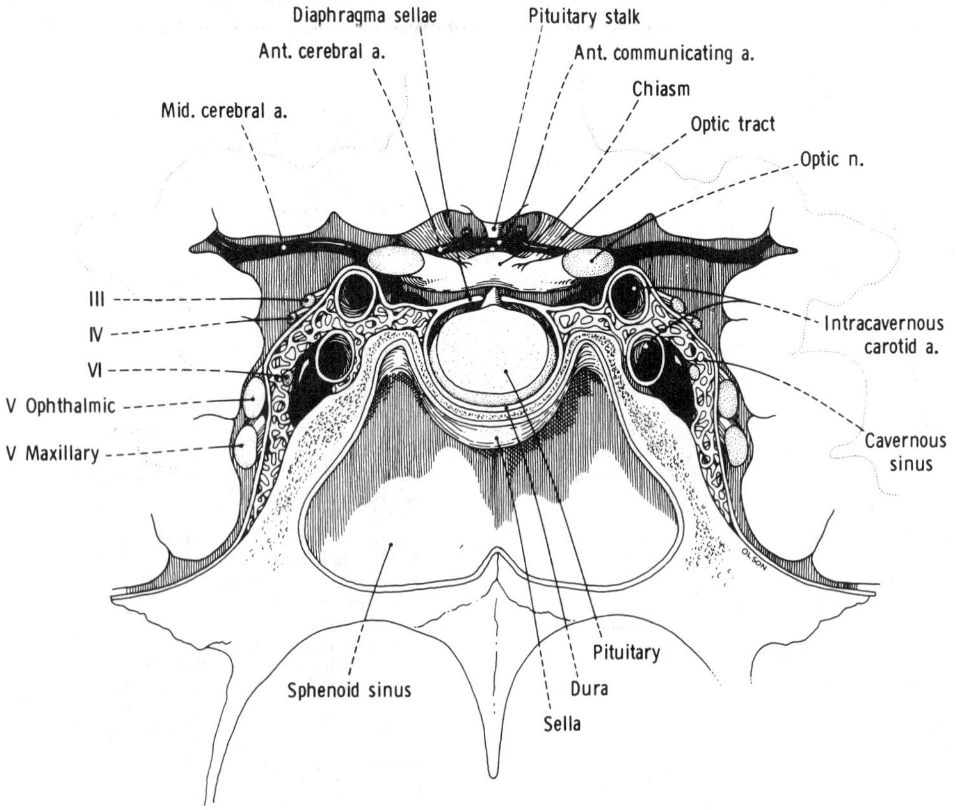

FIGURE 313-2 The relationship between the pituitary, cranial nerves, and the cavernous sinus as viewed in a coronal section through the sella. *(From JA Taren in RC Schneider et al (eds), Correlative Neurosurgery, 3d ed, Springfield, Ill., Charles C Thomas, 1982.)*

sionally persist within or below the sphenoid bone. These remnants may produce pituitary hormones and occasionally develop into pituitary tumors.

Five distinct cell types in the anterior pituitary secrete six different hormones: lactotrophs (prolactin), somatotrophs (GH), gonadotrophs (LH and FSH), thyrotrophs (TSH), and corticotrophs (ACTH).

PROLACTIN

PHYSIOLOGY The lactotrophs constitute 10 to 25 percent of the normal pituitary and increase to 70 percent during pregnancy. The prolactin gene on chromosome 6 codes for a precursor molecule that is larger than the circulating hormone. The predominant form of the processed hormone contains 198 amino acids (23,000 mol wt) in a single polypeptide chain containing three intrachain disulfide bonds. Higher-molecular-weight forms of prolactin, up to 100,000 mol wt (''big'' and ''big-big'' prolactin), may be present in small amounts in the circulation of normal persons and in larger amounts in patients with pituitary adenomas; these molecules react in prolactin radioimmunoassays but do not have normal biologic potency.

Prolactin is essential for lactation. Receptors for the hormone are present in human breast and gonads, whereas in other animals they are found in additional tissues. Prolactin promotes breast cancer in rodents; a similar connection has not been established in human breast cancer (see Chap. 303).

During pregnancy increasing estrogen production stimulates the growth and replication of the pituitary lactotrophs and causes increased prolactin secretion. The pituitary doubles in size during pregnancy and returns to normal after delivery. Prolactin during pregnancy prepares the breast for postpartum lactation. High estrogen levels inhibit prolactin action at the breast, so that lactation does not commence until estrogen levels decline post partum. Prolactin levels rise in the fetus beginning at about 25 weeks, probably owing to maternal estrogen transfer and stimulation of the fetal pituitary. The level falls rapidly after delivery, reaching a nadir by 2 to 4 weeks post partum. High concentrations of prolactin are present in amniotic fluid, although the origin and functional significance are unknown.

Under normal circumstances, prolactin secretion by the anterior pituitary is restrained by the hypothalamus. With hypothalamic destruction or pituitary stalk section, prolactin secretion increases, and serum concentrations rise. The hypothalamic inhibitory factor for prolactin appears to be dopamine, although peptide inhibitory factors have been described. The arcuate nucleus is the primary hypothalamic site of dopamine synthesis; dopamine travels down axons to nerve terminals in the median eminence where it is released (tuberoinfundibular dopamine system) into the portal circulation and reaches the anterior pituitary to inhibit prolactin release. The intravenous administration of dopamine (2 μg/min per kilogram of body weight) or the oral administration of dopamine precursors (e.g., levodopa) or dopamine agonists (e.g., bromocriptine) inhibits prolactin release. Increased blood prolactin appears to increase hypothalamic dopamine production, which in turn partially inhibits prolactin release via a ''short'' feedback loop.

The prolactin rise during suckling appears to require a prolactin-releasing factor, which has not yet been conclusively identified. Vasoactive intestinal peptide (VIP) may be responsible, as it is a potent stimulator of prolactin release. Suckling-induced prolactin rise is blocked by serotonin antagonists, such as methysergide, which suggests an influence of serotonin on prolactin release. TRH is also a potent stimulator of prolactin release; indeed, the lowest dose of TRH capable of stimulating TSH stimulates prolactin release as well. However, TSH and prolactin release are under independent control in most physiologic states; lactation does not lead to TSH elevation, and primary hypothyroidism is rarely associated with prolactin excess.

Prolactin concentrations rise during sleep, a phenomenon that requires the input of higher centers into the hypothalamus. Stress-related prolactin release can be blocked by opiate antagonists such as naloxone and is probably mediated by endogenous opioids. Morphine can stimulate prolactin release, which may contribute to the amenorrhea of narcotic addiction, but basal prolactin secretion is not influenced by opiate antagonists.

HYPERPROLACTINEMIA Clinical features Prolactin excess (hyperprolactinemia) has many causes, is associated with hypogonadism and/or galactorrhea, and may indicate the presence of a pituitary adenoma or hypothalamic disease. Of women with amenorrhea, 10 to 40 percent have hyperprolactinemia, and about 30 percent of women with amenorrhea and galactorrhea have prolactin-secreting pituitary tumors.

The hypogonadism associated with hyperprolactinemia appears to be due to inhibition of hypothalamic release of LHRH, resulting in a decrease in LH and FSH secretion. This functional hypogonadism can be regarded, in part, as a physiologic mechanism since breast feeding causes decreased fertility and delayed resumption of menses. In general, the higher the plasma prolactin, the greater the likelihood of amenorrhea. Milder degrees of hyperprolactinemia in women cause irregular menses or infertility due to a shortened luteal phase. Prolactin excess in men can cause impotence and infertility. In some series 8 percent of men with impotence and 5 percent of men with infertility have hyperprolactinemia. With prolactin elevation, FSH and LH levels in men decline, and serum testosterone is often low.

Galactorrhea, defined as milk production in a patient who is not post partum, is present in 30 to 90 percent of hyperprolactinemic women (see Chap. 323). The variation in incidence reflects, in part, variation in the intensity with which clinicians search for this finding. Galactorrhea may occur without hyperprolactinemia, particularly in parous women. However, galactorrhea is often a clue to prolactin excess; when galactorrhea is coupled with amenorrhea, hyperprolactinemia is present in 75 percent of patients. Hyperprolactinemia in men rarely causes gynecomastia or galactorrhea (see Chap. 323).

Differential diagnosis Prolactin excess has several mechanisms: (1) autonomous production (pituitary adenomas), (2) decreased dopamine or dopamine inhibitory action (e.g., due to hypothalamic disease or drugs that block dopamine synthesis, dopamine release, or dopamine action), (3) stimuli that overcome the normal dopaminergic inhibition (e.g., estrogens, possibly hypothyroidism), and (4) decreased clearance of prolactin (renal failure). No single suppression test can separate physiologic from pharmacologic or pathologic causes of hyperprolactinemia (Table 313-2).

Prolactin concentrations are slightly higher (<20 μg/L) in women than in men (<15 μg/L). During pregnancy, prolactin concentrations begin to increase during the second trimester and peak at term; maximal values are 100 to 300 μg/L, usually less than 200 μg/L. A pregnancy test is mandatory in all patients with hyperprolactinemic amenorrhea, as it is with amenorrhea alone. The mean prolactin level declines post partum but rises with each suckling episode. Over several months basal and suckling-stimulated prolactin concentrations diminish; by 4 to 6 months post partum, basal prolactin levels are normal, and the suckling-induced rise is absent despite continued nursing.

A careful drug history should be obtained in hyperprolactinemic patients. Dopamine-blocking drugs (e.g., phenothiazines, butyrophenones, metoclopramide) and dopamine-depleting drugs (e.g., methyldopa and reserpine) are important causes of hyperprolactinemia. Prolactin concentrations are rarely greater than 100 μg/L with these agents, provided renal failure is not present. Although high-dose estrogens cause hyperprolactinemia, oral contraceptives containing low doses of estrogen do not.

End-stage renal failure is associated with elevated serum prolactin in 70 to 90 percent of women and 25 to 60 percent of men. This contributes to hypogonadism in some patients with renal failure. Both decreased prolactin clearance and increased prolactin secretion may contribute to this elevation. The increased prolactin in cirrhosis of the liver has not been adequately explained.

Severe primary hypothyroidism may cause a mildly elevated serum prolactin, either due to elevated TRH or decreased dopaminergic

TABLE 313-2 Causes of hyperprolactinemia

I Physiologic states
  A Pregnancy
  B Nursing (early)
  C "Stress"
  D Sleep
  E Nipple stimulation
II Drugs
  A Dopamine receptor antagonists
    1 Phenothiazines
    2 Butyrophenones
    3 Thioxanthenes
    4 Metoclopramide
  B Dopamine-depleting agents
    1 Methyldopa
    2 Reserpine
  C Estrogens
  D Opiates
III Disease states
  A Pituitary tumors
    1 Prolactinomas
    2 Adenomas secreting GH and prolactin
    3 Adenomas secreting ACTH and prolactin (Nelson's syndrome and Cushing's disease)
    4 Nonfunctioning chromophobe adenomas with pituitary stalk compression
  B Hypothalamic and pituitary stalk disease
    1 Granulomatous diseases especially sarcoidosis
    2 Craniopharyngiomas and other tumors
    3 Cranial irradiation
    4 Stalk section
    5 Empty sella
    6 Vascular abnormalities including aneurysm
    7 Lymphocytic hypophysitis
  C Primary hypothyroidism
  D Chronic renal failure
  E Cirrhosis
  F Chest wall trauma (including surgery, *herpes zoster*)
  G Seizures

tone. Since primary hypothyroidism may also cause enlargement of the sella turcica, mimicking a pituitary adenoma, thyroid function tests are essential in all patients with elevated serum prolactin. Rarely, primary adrenal insufficiency causes reversible serum prolactin elevation.

If a hyperprolactinemic subject is not pregnant, post partum, cirrhotic, postictal, on medications, hypothyroid, or in renal failure, disease of the pituitary or hypothalamus is likely. Ectopic production of prolactin by nonpituitary tumors occurs rarely if at all. Diseases of the hypothalamus or pituitary stalk cause moderate prolactin elevation (usually less than 150 μg/L). Hyperprolactinemia occurs in 20 to 50 percent of patients with hypothalamic tumors.

Prolactin-secreting pituitary adenomas (prolactinomas) may either be small tumors in the parenchyma (so-called microadenomas) or cause enlargement of the pituitary (macroadenomas). Large, nonfunctioning pituitary adenomas may also cause modest prolactin elevation as a result of stalk compression and impedance of dopamine delivery to the gland. Acromegalics (25 to 45 percent) and patients with Nelson's syndrome (postadrenalectomy pituitary tumors in Cushing's disease) have elevated serum prolactin. Hyperprolactinemia is less common in untreated Cushing's disease.

Laboratory evaluation Serum prolactin levels should be measured in all patients with hypogonadism or galactorrhea. If basal prolactin concentration is elevated, further evaluation is warranted after establishing that minimal prolactin elevations (e.g., less than 30 μg/L) are not stress-related. Blood sampling from an indwelling catheter after a 90-min rest period will exclude "needle stick" hyperprolactinemia. Although there is no simple test to distinguish the various causes of hyperprolactinemia, a serum prolactin level of over 300 μg/L is diagnostic of a pituitary adenoma; a serum prolactin of over 100 μg/L in a nonpregnant patient is usually caused by a pituitary adenoma. Administration of dopamine agonists, such as bromocriptine, lowers prolactin regardless of the etiology and, therefore, is not useful as a differential test (Fig. 313-3). The majority of patients with prolactinomas have only a minimal or no rise in

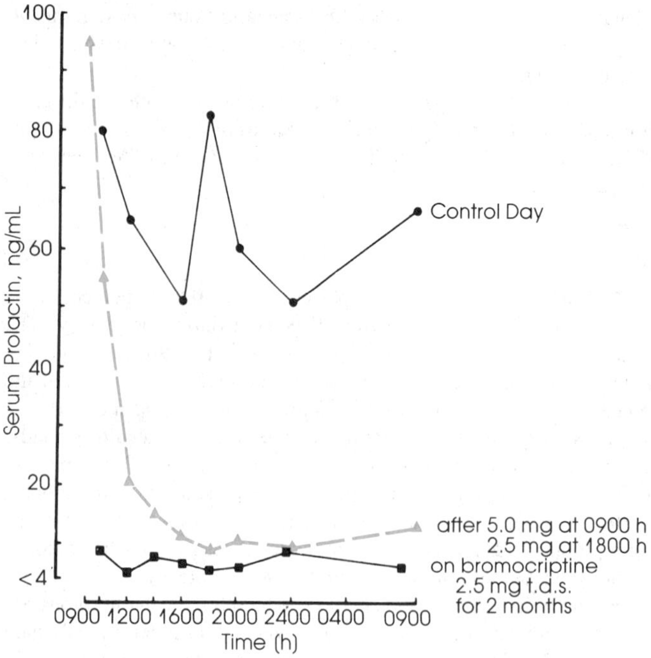

FIGURE 313-3 Changes in serum prolactin concentration in a woman with "idiopathic" hyperprolactinemia after an initial 5-mg dose of bromocriptine and when maintained on 7.5 mg daily. *(From GH Besser and MO Thorner, Postgrad Med J 52:66, 1976.)*

prolactin in response to TRH, as compared to the normal rise of 200 percent or more and the intermediate response (usually a doubling at serum prolactin) in patients with hypothalamic disease and those on dopamine-blocking agents. Unfortunately, the response to TRH is too variable to be of diagnostic value in individual patients.

In general, patients with unexplained hyperprolactinemia require contrast-enhanced computed tomography (CT) scanning of the hypothalamus and pituitary or magnetic resonance imaging (MRI) of this area. Pituitary macroadenomas are easily visualized on these scans, but microadenomas (<10 mm) may be more difficult to delineate. Patients with amenorrhea and minimal prolactin elevations may also have hypothalamic lesions (e.g., craniopharyngiomas) or large "nonfunctioning" pituitary adenomas. When no radiologic abnormalities are found the disorder is designated "idiopathic hyperprolactinemia," although a microadenoma may still be present. Sella tomography is not a useful screening test for small pituitary adenomas because of the high frequency of false-positive and false-negative results.

Microprolactinomas do not cause hypopituitarism (except for hypogonadism). If a small pituitary lesion is seen in a patient with hypopituitarism and hyperprolactinemia, sarcoidosis or other lesions involving the pituitary stalk should be suspected, rather than a microprolactinoma. In patients with macroprolactinomas or hypothalamic lesions, evaluation of pituitary function and formal visual field examinations are essential.

Prolactinomas PATHOLOGY Prolactinomas are the most common functional pituitary adenomas. Small unsuspected microadenomas are found in 5 to 20 percent of unselected autopsies; 40 percent of these small tumors contain prolactin by immunologic staining techniques, but the fraction that actually secrete prolactin is unknown. About 70 percent of macroadenomas previously thought to be nonfunctioning are, in fact, prolactinomas. Prolactin-secreting pituitary carcinomas are rare.

Prolactinoma size correlates with hormonal output; in general, the larger the tumor, the higher the prolactin levels. Large pituitary tumors with modest prolactin elevation (50 to 100 μg/L) are not true prolactinomas and differ in their biologic behavior. Microprolactinomas cause only hyperprolactinemia and hypogonadotropism, whereas macroprolactinomas may influence other pituitary hormones and cause headaches, visual field disturbances, and other structural problems.

CLINICAL PRESENTATION Microprolactinomas are more common than macroprolactinomas, and 90 percent of patients with microprolactinomas are women. In contrast, 60 percent of patients with macroprolactinomas are men. Irregular menses, amenorrhea, and galactorrhea are likely to result in early diagnosis, and this may explain the preponderance of microadenomas in women. Sexual dysfunction occurs in most men with prolactinomas, but this is the presenting complaint in 15 percent or less. Although delay in seeking medical help probably explains the larger tumors in men, more aggressive tumor behavior in men has not been excluded.

Estrogens promote the growth of lactotrophs, but an etiologic role has not been established for oral contraceptives in the pathogenesis of prolactinomas. Many women with prolactinomas first develop galactorrhea while on oral contraceptives or develop amenorrhea when the drug is discontinued. Some of these women may have been started on oral contraceptives for irregular menses that were the consequence of a prolactinoma. Although amenorrhea after discontinuing oral contraceptives is rare (about 2 percent), about a third of patients with postpill amenorrhea have prolactinomas. Development of galactorrhea in a woman on oral contraceptives mandates a prolactin determination. About 5 to 7 percent of prolactinoma patients have never menstruated (primary amenorrhea), making this an important treatable cause of primary amenorrhea. Prolactinomas may grow during pregnancy, and 15 percent of prolactinoma patients are first diagnosed in the postpartum period.

Women with prolactinomas who desire pregnancy need special consideration. Medical treatment of patients with microprolactinomas results in uneventful pregnancies 95 to 98 percent of the time; the remainder may develop headaches or visual field disturbances due to tumor enlargement that rarely requires therapy. Asymptomatic enlargement of microprolactinomas, as ascertained by radiologic studies, occurs in about 5 percent. With macroprolactinomas, the complications of tumor growth during pregnancy are more common. Symptomatic tumor enlargement occurs in about 15 percent of these patients, although individual series report complications in up to 35 percent. The majority of patients who develop symptoms do so during the first trimester.

In prolactinoma patients, the effect of pregnancy on prolactin secretion is variable. A further rise in prolactin during pregnancy may not occur even in patients in whom tumor growth occurs. Prolactin concentrations should be measured periodically throughout pregnancy in women with prolactinomas. If marked prolactin rise occurs (greater than 300 to 400 μg/L), then postpartum prolactin is usually greater than the prepartum level, and tumor growth is likely to have occurred. Patients with stable or declining prolactin concentrations during pregnancy may have lower prolactin concentrations after pregnancy than before. In such patients infarction or involution of the adenomas may have occurred during pregnancy. Rarely, macroprolactinomas in men grow as a consequence of replacement testosterone therapy, presumably as a result of extraglandular conversion of testosterone to estrogen.

THERAPY The therapy of prolactinomas is influenced by the natural history of the disorder. Although large pituitary adenomas must begin as small tumors, most microadenomas do not progress to macroadenomas. Knowledge of the natural history of untreated microprolactinomas is incomplete; 90 to 95 percent may remain stable or demonstrate decreased serum prolactin concentrations after 7 years of follow-up. Many patients with "idiopathic hyperprolactinemia" are presumed to harbor small microadenomas. Serum prolactin returns to normal in a third of patients with idiopathic hyperprolactinemia followed for 5 years without therapy; in two-thirds of such patients in whom the basal prolactin is less than 40 μg/L serum prolactin levels return to normal over this time span.

Not all patients with microprolactinomas need therapy. Women with microprolactinomas require therapy when they desire pregnancy, have decreased libido or troublesome galactorrhea, desire regular menses, or are at risk for osteoporosis. Men with microadenomas should be treated for decreased potency or libido or when infertility is a problem. Most patients with macroprolactinomas require therapy.

Dopamine agonist drugs lower prolactin concentrations in virtually all hyperprolactinemic patients (Fig. 313-3). Ovulatory menses and fertility are restored in 90 percent of premenopausal women, underscoring the direct relationship between hyperprolactinemia and amenorrhea. Bromocriptine, an ergot derivative with dopamine agonist actions, is the only effective prolactin-lowering agent licensed in the United States at this time. Bromocriptine should be given twice daily with food or a snack to prevent gastrointestinal irritation. Therapy should begin with 1.25 mg at bedtime to minimize the side effects of nausea, vomiting, fatigue, nasal stuffiness, and postural hypotension. The dosage is gradually increased to an average of 2.5 mg twice daily, although some patients can be treated with single daily doses. However, doses up to 15 mg/d may be required to return the prolactin concentration to normal in some patients with macroprolactinomas. Although the drug is expensive, it is effective in all forms of hyperprolactinemia and often abolishes nonhyperprolactinemic galactorrhea as well. Long-lasting (40-day) parenteral bromocriptine and long-lasting oral dopamine agonists are not licensed in the United States. Although these agents all have similar side effects, individuals may tolerate one but not the other.

Bromocriptine is the therapy of choice for patients with microprolactinomas who have one of the indications for treatment discussed above. Prolactin concentrations return to normal in almost all who tolerate the medication, usually within days of achieving full therapeutic dosages (Fig. 313-3). Menses usually resume within 2 months but may be delayed up to a year. Since pregnancy may occur without resumption of menses, a barrier contraceptive is recommended until menses become regular. In this way, bromocriptine can be stopped with the first missed period when pregnancy has occurred. Bromocriptine use during pregnancy is not, however, associated with an increased risk of congenital anomalies or fetal wastage. The effects of bromocriptine are usually not permanent, but a sixth of microprolactinoma patients maintain normal prolactin concentrations after stopping the drug.

In patients with macroprolactinomas, bromocriptine usually lowers the serum prolactin and may cause the tumor mass to shrink. In men testosterone concentrations usually begin to increase after 3 months of therapy and may reach normal levels by 6 to 8 months. Normal sperm counts are achieved in some.

One series of patients with large prolactinomas and suprasellar extension (mean prolactin of 1441 μg/L in women, 3451 μg/L in men) is of particular interest. Although prolactin levels fell to 10 percent of baseline in 96 percent of patients, most did not return to the normal range despite bromocriptine dosages of 7.5 to 20 mg/d. Visual field defects improved in 90 percent of those with field cuts. Tumor mass decreased by half or more in 60 percent of patients (see Fig. 313-4). When successful, bromocriptine alone is the therapy of choice in most patients with macroprolactinomas. With long-term (>2 years) therapy, the dosage of bromocriptine can often be reduced but rarely eliminated. In those patients in whom persistent hyperprolactinemia causes symptoms despite partial response to bromocriptine, radiation therapy and on occasion surgical debulking may be appropriate. In those women with large tumors who desire pregnancy, bromocriptine therapy during pregnancy should be considered, along with the alternatives of surgery or radiation therapy. Large nonfunctioning pituitary adenomas associated with hyperprolactinemia due to stalk compression usually do not shrink with bromocriptine therapy, although prolactin concentrations may on occasion return to normal. Patients with large prolactinomas, refractory to bromocriptine and other modalities of therapy, may partially respond to tamoxifen, an estrogen antagonist.

Following transsphenoidal resection of microprolactinomas, serum prolactin concentration returns to normal in up to 80 to 90 percent of patients, usually within 24 h. This procedure has low morbidity and mortality. Unfortunately, recurrence rates average 17 percent

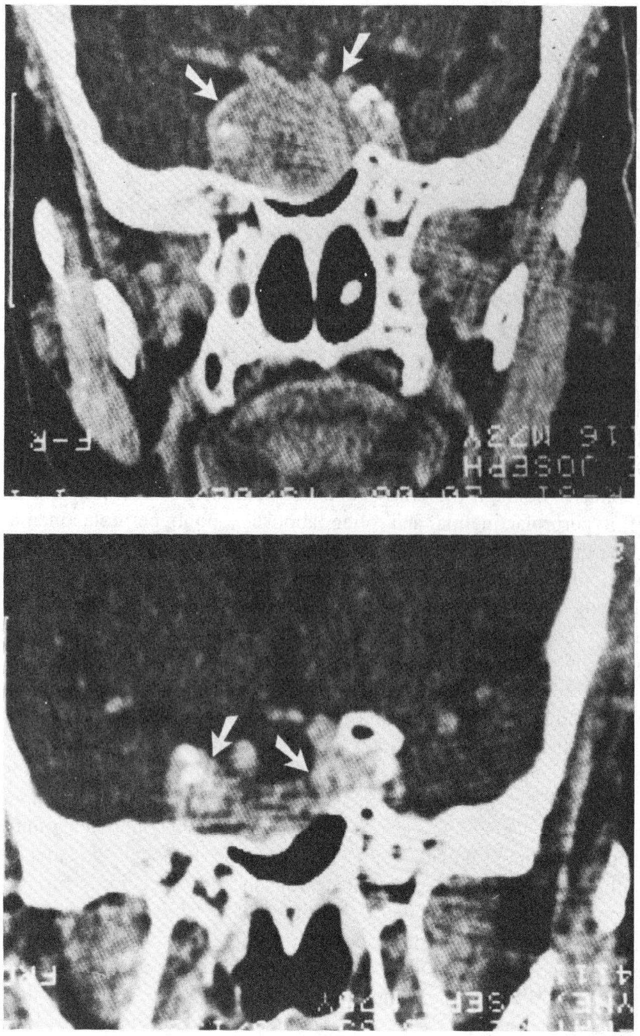

FIGURE 313-4 Frontal CT scan of a man with a large prolactin-secreting macroadenoma. *Top*, pretreatment scan. *Bottom*, scan after 1 year of treatment with bromocriptine. The upper border of the tumor is shown by arrows. (*From Molitch et al.*)

after "successful" surgery and may be as high as 40 percent after 6 years of follow-up. Surgery is appropriate for women with microprolactinomas who desire pregnancy and who cannot tolerate or do not wish to take dopamine agonist drugs.

Surgery, combined with bromocriptine and/or radiation therapy, is indicated for macroprolactinomas with suprasellar extension and persistent visual field defects and particularly in such patients desiring pregnancy. However, surgical resection, whether by transsphenoidal or transcranial approach, is rarely curative in patients with macroprolactinomas. Prolactin concentrations return to normal in about 30 percent, but even when they do, recurrence rates of up to 80 percent have been reported. In all patients in whom prolactin levels do not return to normal following surgery and in all with evidence of residual tumors after resection, long-term bromocriptine therapy and/or radiation should be given.

Conventional radiation therapy [4500 cGy (4500 rad) over 25 days] for prolactinomas causes a slow decline in serum prolactin concentration. Prolactin concentration returns to normal in about 30 percent of microprolactinoma patients 2 to 10 years after therapy. We do not favor this approach in patients with microprolactinomas because of the risk of their developing hypopituitarism. Radiation therapy is a useful adjunct to surgical or medical therapy in patients with macroprolactinomas; further growth is usually prevented, and shrinkage occurs in about half the patients. This therapy usually prevents tumor growth during subsequent pregnancies, but exceptions have been noted.

Heavy particle therapy with protons may be useful in treatment of macroprolactinomas without suprasellar extension or after surgical debulking of larger tumors. Occasional patients with microprolactinomas opt for this form of therapy. Long-term studies in prolactinoma patients are not available.

PROLACTIN DEFICIENCY Prolactin deficiency is manifested as an inability to lactate. Failure of lactation is often the earliest clue to panhypopituitarism resulting from pituitary infarction during the peripartum period. The lateral wings of the pituitary have a precarious blood supply; most lactotrophs reside in this area. During pregnancy, the hypertrophied and hyperplastic lactotrophs are at risk for necrosis. If systemic hypotension develops, as with postpartum hemorrhage, the hypertrophic and hyperplastic lactotrophs may infarct (Sheehan's syndrome). Patients with diabetes mellitus are susceptible to peripartum pituitary infarction even in the absence of significant hemorrhage. Autoimmune pituitary destruction (lymphocytic hypophysitis) may also occur during late pregnancy but often is associated with elevated prolactin levels.

Most prolactin radioimmunoassays cannot distinguish normal from low concentrations; hence, prolactin stimulation tests are needed to diagnose prolactin insufficiency. After administration of TRH or chlorpromazine, a rise in serum prolactin of less than 200 percent suggests prolactin deficiency. If prolactin deficiency is present, evaluation of other pituitary hormones is necessary as well to define other manifestations of hypopituitarism.

GROWTH HORMONE

PHYSIOLOGY Growth hormone (GH, somatotropin) is secreted by somatotrophs which make up about 50 percent of the anterior pituitary cells. The normal pituitary contains 3 to 5 mg of GH and secretes 500 to 875 μg of GH per day. The gene coding for GH is on chromosome 17; additional GH-related genes are of uncertain significance. Human growth hormone is a single polypeptide chain of 191 amino acids (22,000 mol wt) and contains two intrachain disulfide bonds. A larger (28,000 mol wt) precursor molecule is cleaved to yield GH. GH is stored in cytoplasmic granules in a high-molecular-weight polymeric form.

GH shares a 92 percent structural homology with human placental lactogen (hPL, chorionic somatomammotropin). GH and hPL genes are on the same chromosome and appear to have originated by gene duplication.

In the circulation, monomeric GH (22,000 mol wt) predominates. Larger molecular weight forms may represent dimers (i.e., "big" GH, 44,000 mol wt) that appear to be secreted by the pituitary gland into the circulation. Although "big" GH is measured by the GH radioimmunoassay, its biologic activity is reduced. Pulsatile release is characteristic. Circulating levels are immeasurably low for much of the day, punctuated by four to eight bursts after meals or exercise, during slow-wave sleep, or without obvious cause. The half-life of the hormone in plasma is 20 to 30 min.

GH is necessary for normal linear growth. Growth hormone deficiency causes short stature; growth hormone excess (prior to epiphyseal closure) leads to gigantism. GH does not appear to be the principal direct stimulator of growth but acts indirectly by stimulating the formation of other hormones. These factors, known as somatomedins (SM, somatotropin-mediating hormones) or insulin-like growth factors (IGF) are growth hormone–dependent and are responsible for growth stimulation (also see Chap. 314). Somatomedin C (insulin-like growth factor 1, IGF-1/SM-C), the most important somatomedin for postnatal growth, is produced in the liver and by other tissues as well. IGF-1/SM-C is a basic protein (7600 mol wt) that circulates bound to a large carrier molecule (140,000 mol wt). The complex has a half-life of 3 to 18 h, as compared to the half-life of 20 to 30 min for unbound hormone. As a consequence, the concentration of IGF-1/SM-C remains relatively constant throughout the 24 h period, in contrast to the fluctuating levels of GH itself. How the liver integrates GH pulses into somatomedin production is not known. Furthermore, local tissue generation of IGF-1/SM-C, particularly in bone, may play an important role in mediating growth through paracrine effects.

IGF-1 is structurally similar to proinsulin and exerts some insulin-like actions. Furthermore, GH is a trophic factor for insulin release, facilitating its release in response to various secretagogues, and GH-deficient individuals have impaired insulin release to glucose challenge. Technically, one might consider insulin a somatomedin.

During the prenatal and neonatal period growth is independent of GH, as shown by the normal birth length of GH-deficient children born to GH-deficient mothers. Nevertheless IGF-1/SM-C levels rise during pregnancy, and its concentration correlates with that of hPL, which may regulate somatomedin production. IGF-1/SM-C levels at birth are lower than those of adults and rise gradually during childhood to reach the adult range by age 8 to 10 years. IGF-1/SM-C levels are dependent upon nutritional status, declining in states of malnourishment. Elevated serum IGF-1/SM-C concentrations are present during the pubertal growth spurt, presumably accounting for the pubertal growth acceleration.

Although IGF-1/SM-C concentrations correlate with linear growth, the correlation is inexact, and therefore GH may have some direct influence on growth or cause somatomedin generation in target cells.

GH exerts additional metabolic effects, including stimulation of the incorporation of amino acids into protein. Although most of this action is somatomedin-mediated, GH can directly stimulate amino acid uptake in certain systems. Some amino acids, such as arginine, are potent stimuli for GH release.

GH may have a direct effect as an insulin antagonist. Patients with GH deficiency are prone to insulin-induced hypoglycemia; patients with GH excess develop insulin resistance. GH is one of the counterregulatory hormones that help restore a low blood sugar to normal (see Chap. 320). Hypoglycemia is a potent GH stimulus, and an acute rise in blood sugar inhibits GH release. GH increases free fatty acid release from adipocytes. The absence of this effect may be responsible for the pudgy appearance of children with GH deficiency. Increased serum free fatty acid concentrations tend to blunt GH release. GH opposes the action of insulin on sugar uptake and fatty acid release and complements the anabolic action of insulin on amino acid uptake.

GH is controlled by a dual hypothalamic regulation (Table 313-3). Secretion is stimulated by growth hormone–releasing hormone (GRH, somatocrinin) and inhibited by growth hormone release–inhibitory hormone (somatostatin, somatotropin release–inhibitory factor, SRIF). GRH appears to play the more important role, as stalk section leads to failure of GH release. In animals treated with anti-GRH antibodies the GH peaks disappear, and growth ceases; following treatment with antisomatostatin antibodies, the peaks remain, but the baseline values rise. After treatment with both anti-GRH and anti-somatostatin antibodies, the peaks disappear but the baseline rises. Although GRH- and somatostatin-containing neurons are separate, they have reciprocal interconnections.

Growth hormone–releasing hormone GRH has 44 amino acids, 29 of which are necessary for full potency. GRH belongs to a family of molecules that includes secretin, glucagon, vasoactive intestinal peptide (VIP), and gastric inhibitory peptide (GIP). The arcuate nucleus of the hypothalamus is the major site of GRH production, although a few such neurons are in the ventromedial nucleus as well. Axons containing the peptide project to the median eminence and terminate on the portal vessels. Whether GRH is also present in extracranial tissues is uncertain.

GRH stimulates GH release in vitro and in vivo, an effect that is calcium-dependent and appears to be mediated by cyclic adenosine monophosphate (cyclic AMP). Intravenous injection of GRH (0.1 to 3.3 μg/kg body weight) produces a peak GH response at 30 to 60 min with a return to baseline by 2 to 3 h postinjection (Fig. 313-5).

Somatostatin Somatostatin, a cyclic tetradecapeptide, is the most widely distributed of the hypothalamic releasing hormones.

TABLE 313-3 Growth hormone regulation

Class of agent	Stimulation	Inhibition
Hypothalamic factors	GRH	Somatostatin
Amines	Alpha-adrenergic stimuli (norepinephrine, clonidine)	Beta-adrenergic stimuli
	Beta-adrenergic blockers (propranolol)	Alpha-adrenergic blockers (phentolamine, dibenzyline)
	Dopaminergic stimuli (levodopa, bromocriptine, apomorphine)	Dopamine blockers (chlorpromazine)
	Serotonergic stimuli (L-tryptophan)	Serotonin blockers (methysergide, cyproheptadine)
Hormones	Decreased IGF-1/SM-C	Increased IGF-1/SM-C (obesity)
	Estrogen	Progestogens
	Vasopressin	Glucocorticoids
	Glucagon	
Fuels	Hypoglycemia*	Increased blood sugar
	Decreased free fatty acids	Increased free fatty acids
	Amino acids (arginine)*	
Others	Exercise*	
	Stress*	
	Sleep	

* Probably mediated through alpha-adrenergic stimulation.

The primary hypothalamic sources are the periventricular and medial preoptic areas of the anterior hypothalamus. Somatostatin is found in neurosecretory granules of axons that terminate in the median eminence. In addition to its function as a hormone, somatostatin is synthesized and distributed throughout the brain and serves as a neurotransmitter in many areas including the spinal cord, brainstem, and cerebral cortex. Somatostatin is also present in the gastrointestinal tract. Specific somatostatin-secreting cells (D cells) of the pancreatic islets participate in the regulation of insulin and glucagon secretion, an example of paracrine regulation by this hormone (see Chap. 319).

Somatostatin is produced by processing of a larger precursor molecule and exists in both 28– and 14–amino acid forms. The 28–amino acid somatostatin has a longer half-life and is a more potent inhibitor of GH and insulin secretion. Somatostatin 14 has a greater affinity for hypothalamic and cortical receptors and is more potent in inhibition of glucagon release. Somatostatin analogues are effective in the therapy of acromegaly, secretory pancreatic tumors, carcinoid syndrome, and other conditions.

Somatostatin inhibits GH secretion and decreases the GH response to secretagogues. Somatostatin also lowers serum TSH in normal and hypothyroid individuals and blunts TSH release in response to TRH. Somatostatin probably mediates the secondary hypothyroidism that may develop in GH-deficient children treated with GH. Somatostatin has no significant effect on the release of prolactin, gonadotropins, or ACTH in normal subjects but may lower ACTH concentrations in patients with Nelson's syndrome. Somatostatinomas are rare pancreatic islet cell or duodenal tumors that secrete somatostatin (see Chap. 262).

Growth hormone release is under complex physiologic control (Table 313-3). The various mediators appear to act through GRH and somatostatin. IGF-1/SM-C has an important feedback effect on GH secretion. An increased IGF-1/SM-C concentration inhibits GH release both through increased somatostatin production and by a direct action on the pituitary. A decrease in IGF-1/SM-C, as induced by starvation, leads to a compensatory increase in GH release.

A number of neurotransmitters influence GH release:

1 Hypothalamic dopamine, the important prolactin inhibitory factor, stimulates GH through an effect on GRH. Dopamine has a direct

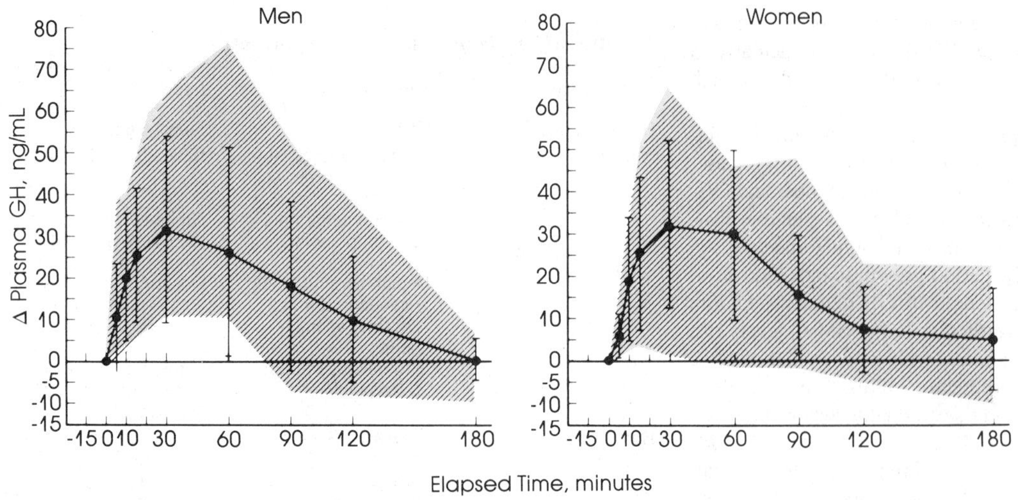

FIGURE 313-5 Response to GRH-44 (1 μg/kg) in eight men and eight women. The shaded area shows the full range of responses at each time point and the error bars indicate the mean ± 1 SD. *(From MC Gelato et al, J Clin Endocrinol Metab 59:200, 1984.)*

but weak inhibitory effect on GH release; this effect is overwhelmed by its hypothalamic stimulation of GRH secretion. Oral administration of dopamine precursors or agonists that cross the blood-brain barrier, such as levodopa, apomorphine, or bromocriptine, causes an increase in serum GH concentration. The effects of these stimuli can be utilized to test the adequacy of GH secretion (GH reserve).

2 Alpha-adrenergic agonists, such as clonidine, stimulate GRH and GH release whereas phentolamine, an alpha blocker, prevents the GH rise. A number of GH stimulators, including insulin hypoglycemia, arginine, and exercise, act through alpha-adrenergic mechanisms. Beta-adrenergic blockers potentiate the GH-stimulatory effect of clonidine (and of some other agents including levodopa), possibly by inhibiting somatostatin secretion.

3 Serotonin agonists stimulate GH release, and the nocturnal surge in GH secretion may be mediated by serotonin, as cyproheptadine (a serotonin antagonist) blocks the sleep-induced GH rise.

Obesity blunts GH release in response to many stimuli, including GRH itself. Weight reduction restores normal GH dynamics. In contrast, malnourished individuals, including women with anorexia nervosa, often have an increased GH concentration, probably as a result of decreased serum IGF-1/SM-C levels. Oral glucose administration decreases serum GH and the GH response to GRH.

A number of hormones influence GH release. Most factors that stimulate GH release are more potent in women than in men, an effect mediated by estrogen. In testing GH reserve in children, estrogen priming may be necessary before adequate GH release can be demonstrated. Although estrogen increases GH concentration, it decreases its biologic effect by blocking somatomedin production. This is similar to the estrogen effect on prolactin in which secretion is stimulated, but its action in promoting lactation is inhibited. Glucocorticoids inhibit GH release and may blunt somatomedin action as well, explaining the potent growth-inhibiting effects of these agents in children.

GROWTH HORMONE EXCESS: ACROMEGALY AND GIGANTISM **Clinical features** GH excess results in acromegaly, an insidious, chronic debilitating disease associated with bony and soft tissue overgrowth (Table 313-4). Acromegaly occurs most frequently in middle age. It is uncommon with a prevalence of 40 cases per million and an incidence of 3 cases per million per year. When GH excess develops prior to epiphyseal closure in children, increased linear growth and gigantism develop.

Most patients have soft tissue and bone enlargement which results in increased hand, foot, and hat size, prognathism, enlargement of the tongue, wide spacing of the teeth, and coarsening of facial features. Acromegalics are said to look more like each other than like their own family members (Fig. 313-6). Laryngeal hypertrophy and sinus enlargement lead to a hollow-sounding voice. A moist, doughy handshake, increased skin tags, acanthosis nigricans, and oily skin are common.

Acromegaly is more than a cosmetically disfiguring disease. Patients feel weak and tired. The basal metabolic rate increases, which in turn causes increased sweating. Obstructive sleep apnea may be an important cause of hypersomnolence. The majority have

TABLE 313-4 Acromegaly—manifestations

Location	Symptoms	Signs
General	Fatigue Increased sweating Heat intolerance Weight gain	
Skin and subcutaneous tissue	Enlarging hands, feet Coarsening facial features Oily skin Hypertrichosis	Moist, warm, fleshy, doughy handshake Skin tags Acanthosis nigricans Increased heel pad
Head	Headaches	Parotid enlargement, frontal bossing
Eyes	Decreased vision	Visual field defects
Ears		Otoscope speculum cannot be inserted
Nose-throat–paranasal sinuses	Sinus congestion	Enlarged furrowed tongue
	Increased tongue size	Tooth marks on tongue
	Malocclusion Voice change	Widely spaced teeth Prognathism
Neck		Goiter Obstructive sleep apnea Enlarged sinuses
Cardiorespiratory system	Congestive heart failure	Hypertension Cardiomegaly Left ventricular hypertrophy
Genitourinary system	Decreased libido Impotence Oligomenorrhea Infertility Kidney stones	
Neurologic system	Paresthesias Hypersomnolence	Carpal tunnel syndrome
Muscles	Weakness	Proximal myopathy
Skeletal system	Joint pains (shoulders, back, knees)	Osteoarthritis

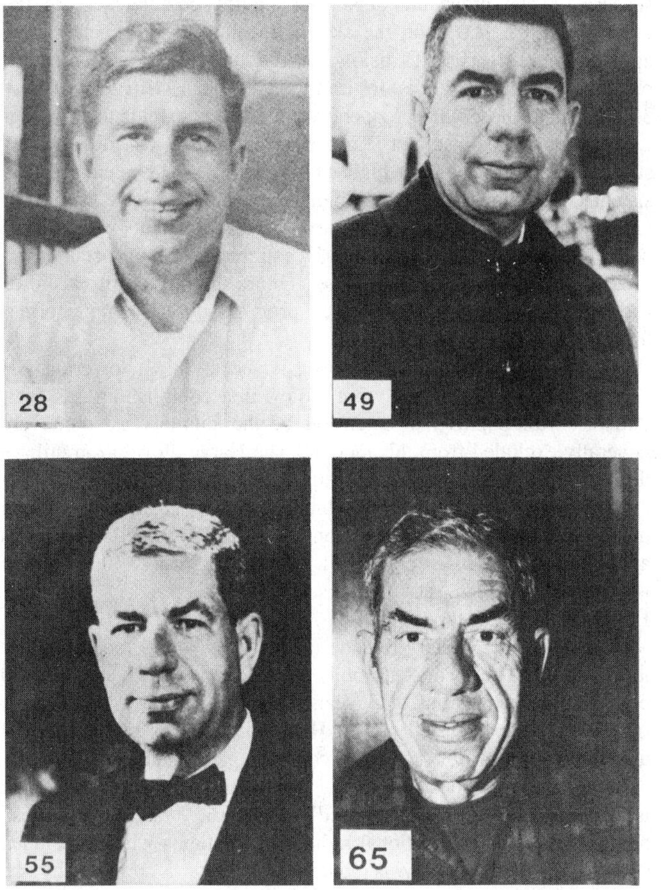

FIGURE 313-6 Serial photographs of a patient with acromegaly taken at ages 28, 49, 55, and 65 years, 6 months after removal of a GH-secreting adenoma. Note the gradual increase in the size of the nose, lips, and skin folds, particularly the nasolabial skin fold and forehead. *(From Reichlin, 1982.)*

neurologic and musculoskeletal symptoms including headaches, paresthesias (often due to carpal tunnel syndrome), muscle weakness, and arthralgias (particularly involving the shoulders, back, and knees). The cartilage hypertrophy and osseous overgrowth often lead to degenerative arthritis, and kyphoscoliosis may occur. Hypertension occurs in about one-third and is characterized by suppressed renin and aldosterone secretion associated with expansion of plasma volume and total body sodium. Almost all hypertensive acromegalics and about half of nonhypertensive acromegalics have increased left ventricular mass or left ventricular wall thickness. Although it is not established whether a specific cardiomyopathy occurs, acromegalics may develop congestive heart failure in the absence of other known underlying heart disease. Amenorrhea may occur with or without hyperprolactinemia, and hirsutism is often noted. Depression may persist after successful therapy for acromegaly. Many organs, including the liver and kidneys, increase in size with no evidence of functional impairment. Goiter is common, and 3 to 7 percent are hyperthyroid. Some series report abdominal pain and inguinal hernias each in about one-third of patients and nasal polyps in as many as 15 percent. Intracranial aneurysms coexist in 10 percent or less.

Patients with acromegaly probably have a shortened life expectancy with increased cardiovascular, cerebrovascular, and respiratory deaths. In studies in which modern therapy was available, effects on life expectancy are less striking. Patients with coexisting diabetes mellitus have increased mortality. Although increased prevalence of carcinoma has been reported in some series (including breast carcinoma in one series), the overall differences are not statistically significant. Skin tags appear to correlate with increased prevalence of colonic polyps and possibly with carcinoma of the colon.

Laboratory investigation Insulin resistance occurs in 80 percent, although abnormal glucose tolerance (20 to 40 percent) and clinical diabetes mellitus (13 to 20 percent) are less common. Hypercalciuria is frequent, apparently due to increased levels of circulating 1,25-dihydroxyvitamin D; renal stones occur in about one-fifth of patients. Hypercalcemia, when it occurs, is not due to acromegaly per se but suggests primary hyperparathyroidism as part of the multiple endocrine neoplasia I (MEN I) syndrome (see Chap. 325). GH causes increased renal tubular reabsorption of phosphate by an undefined mechanism. Elevation of serum phosphate occurs in about one-half. Hyperprolactinemia occurs in up to one-half of patients and is responsible for much of the associated galactorrhea, amenorrhea, and decreased libido.

Pathophysiology Well-defined pituitary adenomas are found in almost all patients with acromegaly and gigantism. The tumors tend to occur in the lateral wings of the sella where normal somatotrophs are found in abundance. Occasionally, tumors are found in ectopic locations along the lines of migration of Rathke's pouch, such as the sphenoid sinus or parapharyngeal regions.

GH levels correlate on average with tumor size. Tumors tend to be larger and may be more aggressive in younger patients. At the time of diagnosis 75 percent of somatotroph adenomas are macroadenomas, whereas two-thirds or more of prolactinomas are microadenomas at the time of diagnosis. Aggressive screening for acromegaly on the basis of subtle clinical clues might lead to early diagnosis while tumors are still small.

Immunohistochemical staining and electron microscopy of somatotroph tumors help to predict their behavior. Growth hormone–secreting carcinomas are rare and should be diagnosed only in the presence of distant metastases. Tumors that cause local invasion are called invasive adenomas.

Although hypothalamic GRH excess or somatostatin deficiency has been postulated to be the underlying abnormality leading to acromegaly, most acromegalics in fact have primary disease of the pituitary. Evidence for a pituitary etiology includes (1) low serum GRH in patients with acromegaly, (2) absence of somatotroph hyperplasia in the cells outside the adenomas, and (3) return of GH dynamics to normal upon successful removal of the somatotroph adenomas.

GRH-induced acromegaly is rare (less than 1 percent in a recent series). This diagnosis should be considered when pituitary somatotroph hyperplasia, rather than an adenoma, is diagnosed histologically. Bronchial carcinoids and pancreatic islet cell tumors are the most likely to secrete GRH, and certain of these tumors may cosecrete GH and/or IGF-1/SM-C as well. Hypothalamic gangliocytomas also produce GRH (as well as somatostatin) and may cause somatotroph hyperplasia and acromegaly. A number of other tumors (including small cell carcinoma of the lung, medullary carcinoma of the thyroid, and thymic carcinoid) contain GRH, but the amount of secretion from these tumors is unknown. These tumors also may be associated with ectopic ACTH production.

Isolated ectopic production of GH is rare but has been described in a patient with a pancreatic islet cell tumor; the tumor size in this instance (420 g) suggests inefficient GH production since GH-secreting pituitary tumors that cause acromegaly are usually much smaller.

Diagnosis Patients with acromegaly have symptoms for an average of 9 years and often see several doctors before the diagnosis is made. Newly consulted physicians are more likely to suspect the diagnosis than is a physician or family member who has watched the insidious progress of the disease. When suggestive facial features are noted, a comparison with old pictures may be helpful (Fig. 313-6).

Basal or random GH determinations may be elevated in normal persons, particularly in women, and should not be used to screen for acromegaly. A physiologic test of the capacity to inhibit GH release must be utilized. The standard screening test is the measurement of serum GH concentrations 60 to 120 min after the oral administration of 100 g glucose. A serum GH concentration of less than 5 μg/L is usually taken as a normal response, although a postsuppression value of less than 2 μg/L is a more rigorous criterion. Acromegalics usually have a GH concentration after glucose administration of greater than 10 μg/L; however, some suppress to values below 5 but rarely below 2 μg/L.

GH concentrations in acromegaly may vary during the day, although they are never undetectable as in normal persons. After glucose administration to acromegalics the GH concentrations usually are unchanged or increase, but some GH lowering may occur. GH levels increase in response to insulin-induced hypoglycemia and arginine infusion, and the response to GRH is enhanced in most acromegalics. Somatostatin infusion lowers GH concentration but usually not to normal values. In addition, GH-secreting pituitary tumors respond to stimuli that do not affect normal somatotrophs: TRH increases GH in the majority (80 percent), and LHRH increases GH in about 10 to 15 percent. Dopamine agonists stimulate GH release in normal persons but inhibit GH release in 75 percent of acromegalics. Somatotroph tumors that cosecrete prolactin are most likely to show GH stimulation with TRH and GH inhibition with dopamine agonists.

Measurements of serum IGF-1/SM-C concentrations correlate with disease activity even in patients with basal GH concentrations below 10 μg/L. IGF-1/SM-C values vary considerably between laboratories. The levels do not correlate well with basal GH concentrations but do correlate with mean 24-h GH levels.

All patients with large pituitary adenomas should be screened with GH measurements, preferably after glucose ingestion. In rare cases patients with elevated serum GH and IGF-1/SM-C concentrations may have large pituitary tumors, without clinical evidence of acromegaly. This syndrome is unexplained.

Radiologic investigation is necessary once the laboratory tests confirm the clinical suspicion of acromegaly. Conventional skull x-rays or coned-down views of the sella turcica are abnormal in 90 percent of patients with acromegaly. CT scanning or MRI provides better definition of tumor size and is necessary for appropriate therapeutic planning. Additional clues to the diagnosis of acromegaly can be found on conventional skull x-rays and include thickening of the skull with increased bone density, enlargement of the paranasal sinuses and proliferation of the mastoid air cells, and prognathism if the jaw is included. On bone x-rays one may see enlarged vertebral bodies with anterior lipping, tufting of the distal phalanges of the hands and feet, increased thickness and lengthening of the ribs and clavicles, and bowing of the femur, tibia, and fibula. Soft tissue x-rays demonstrate increased thickness of the heel pad (greater than 18 mm in women and 21 mm in men).

Testing of anterior pituitary function for hypopituitarism and for increased prolactin should be performed. Large somatotrope adenomas commonly cause neurologic abnormalities. In addition, acromegaly may be associated with hyperparathyroidism and pancreatic islet cell tumors in the MEN I syndrome and rarely with pheochromocytomas or hyperaldosteronism. The alpha subunit of the glycoprotein hormones may be oversecreted in acromegaly and may serve as an additional marker of tumor regrowth.

Therapy The objectives of therapy are (1) return of GH levels to normal, (2) stabilization or decrease in tumor size, and (3) preservation of normal pituitary function. The available modalities are variably successful in achieving these goals, and none is perfect. Although GH values of less than 5 μg/L are frequently interpreted as representing cures, a value of less than 2 μg/L is a better criterion; patients with GH values between 2 and 5 μg/L may have persistent symptoms and increased IGF-1/SM-C concentrations.

Transsphenoidal surgery has the advantage of producing a rapid therapeutic response; it is potentially curative and is the procedure of choice. Anesthesiologists should be alerted to the potential of a difficult intubation due to anatomic changes in the jaw, tongue, epiglottis, and larynx. GH concentrations may fall to normal within hours, and soft tissue (but not bony) enlargement may melt away, even before the patient has been discharged from the hospital. The success of this procedure depends upon the completeness of the resection and hence upon the size of the tumor. In expert hands, apparent cure rates (GH below 5 μg/L) average 75 percent in patients with preoperative GH levels of less than 40 μg/L but only 35 percent in those with preoperative GH levels greater than 40 μg/L. The occurrence of tumor regrowth and recurrent acromegaly after successful surgery may be higher than previously appreciated. Persistent GH response to TRH stimulation appears to have predictive value in assessing risk of relapse, even in those patients with normal postoperative GH concentrations. Hypopituitarism may occur in 10 to 20 percent of patients with larger tumors, but up to 10 percent of patients with pituitary insufficiency prior to surgery regain normal function.

Heavy particle pituitary radiation is successful in lowering GH concentrations in acromegaly but is slow in accomplishing this goal. Patients with suprasellar extension of the pituitary adenoma are generally excluded from this therapy. The Harvard cyclotron utilizes the Bragg peak with proton irradiation, achieving up to 12,000 cGy (12,000 rad) to the center of the pituitary adenoma. In patients with mean pretherapy GH concentration of 60 μg/L, GH concentrations are below 5 μg/L in 29 percent of patients at 2 years, 40 percent at 4 years, 75 percent at 10 years, and 92 percent by 20 years. Hypopituitarism occurs in about 20 percent.

Conventional pituitary radiation [4500 cGy (4500 rad)] also has its proponents. GH concentrations of less than 5 μg/L occur in 50 percent of acromegalics at 5 years and in 70 percent at 10 years (mean pretherapy GH 60 μg/L). Hypopituitarism is a sequela, and up to 50 percent of patients require replacement therapy. The hypopituitarism is most likely due to hypothalamic damage, which is less likely to occur with focused heavy particle radiation. We use heavy particle or conventional radiation in patients who have failed surgery or when surgery is contraindicated or is refused by the patient.

Bromocriptine is a useful adjunct to other modalities of therapy but rarely is successful alone. Clinical improvement is reported in up to 90 percent of patients with dosages of 20 to 60 mg/d. Objective decrease in hand and ring size as well as improvement in diabetes mellitus may occur in the absence of decreasing GH values. However, GH concentrations fall to less than 10 μg/L in only 35 percent, and values of less than 5 μg/L are achieved in only 15 percent. A decrease in tumor size occurs in a minority of patients.

A long-acting analogue of somatostatin (octreotide) lowers growth hormone to normal values in at least two-thirds of acromegalics and causes partial tumor regression (20 to 50 percent) in most. The drug must be administered subcutaneously (50 to 250 μg every 6 to 8 h). Side effects are minimal and include local pain, abdominal cramps, cholelithiasis, and temporary steatorrhea. This analogue is 40 to 50 times more potent in inhibiting GH secretion than in inhibiting insulin secretion, but abnormal glucose tolerance or worsening of diabetes mellitus occurs in some patients. Inhibition of TSH secretion does not appear to be a problem. It seems likely that this drug will be most useful as adjunctive therapy after external radiation or unsuccessful surgery. Indeed the success rate of surgery in acromegalic patients with invasive macroadenomas may be improved after octreotide pretreatment. The role of this agent as a primary treatment for acromegaly remains to be defined, but some patients have been treated successfully for as long as 2 years.

GH DEFICIENCY AND PITUITARY DWARFISM GH is often the first hormone to be lost in pituitary and hypothalamic disorders. In adults, GH deficiency is often cryptic and can only be diagnosed on the basis of stimulation tests for GH release. The consequences of GH deficiency in adults are still being explored. GH deficiency is probably responsible for the fine wrinkling of facial skin in patients with hypopituitarism. Diabetics with GH deficiency show a reduction in insulin requirements and may develop hypoglycemia. In children, GH deficiency leads to impaired growth and short stature and is often a consequence of hypothalamic GRH deficiency (see Chap. 314).

GONADOTROPINS

PHYSIOLOGY The gonadotropins, LH and FSH, are secreted by the gonadotrophs (also see Chaps. 321 and 322). These cells, which make up about 10 percent of the anterior pituitary, are dispersed throughout the anterior lobe, often situated close to the lactotrophs. Most gonadotrophs produce both LH and FSH, although a few cells produce only one hormone.

LH and FSH are glycoproteins of similar size (about 30,000 mol wt), which share a common alpha subunit [also present in TSH and human chorionic gonadotropin (hCG)] but have unique beta subunits. The alpha and beta chains are encoded in separate genes on separate chromosomes, and alpha chains are often produced in excess. The carbohydrate content of the molecules influences the biologic behavior and duration of action and may vary throughout the menstrual cycle. Although both FSH and LH are secreted in pulsatile fashion, the longer FSH half-life means that FSH concentrations fluctuate less throughout the day. FSH and LH regulate ovarian and testicular function.

FSH stimulates the growth of the granulosa cells of the ovarian follicle and controls the aromatase responsible for estradiol formation within these cells. LH stimulates the ovarian theca cells to produce androgens, which diffuse to the granulosa cells where they are converted to estrogens. Estradiol, the principal estrogen, peaks about 1 day prior to the LH surge, which in turn triggers ovulation. Postovulation, LH contributes to corpus luteum formation. Once conception has occurred, pituitary gonadotropin function is no longer necessary to sustain pregnancy.

In the testis LH is primarily responsible for controlling testosterone production in the Leydig cells. FSH, in conjunction with intratesticular testosterone, stimulates the seminiferous tubules to produce sperm. Thus LH and FSH are necessary for normal spermatogenesis, whereas testosterone production requires only LH.

Luteinizing hormone–releasing hormone [LHRH, also known as gonadotropin-releasing hormone (GnRH)], a decapeptide produced by the arcuate nuclei of the hypothalamus, is responsible for the release of both LH and FSH. Extrahypothalamic LHRH is present in other areas of the brain as well. Noradrenergic agonists appear to facilitate, whereas endogenous opioids inhibit, LHRH release.

LHRH stimulates and induces high-affinity pituitary receptors to stimulate LH and FSH production and release. The pituitary response to LHRH varies greatly throughout life. LHRH and the gonadotropins first appear in the fetus at about 10 weeks of gestation. During the first 3 months after birth, LHRH elicits a brisk gonadotropin rise. The sensitivity to LHRH then declines until the onset of puberty. Before puberty, the FSH response to LHRH is greater than that of LH. With the onset of puberty sensitivity to LHRH increases, and pulsatile LH secretion, first noted during sleep, ensues. Later in puberty and during the reproductive years, pulsations are present throughout the day, with LH responsiveness being greater than that of FSH. After the menopause FSH and LH concentrations rise, and postmenopausal FSH levels are higher than those of LH.

Pulsatile LHRH release results in pulsatile LH and FSH release. However, sustained infusion of LHRH and its analogues results in inhibition of LH and FSH release. This phenomenon has been utilized in the successful treatment of gonadotropin-mediated precocious puberty by the sustained administration of LHRH or its analogues. Conversely, in people with LHRH deficiency, the pulsatile administration of LHRH can restore a normal menstrual cycle or normal sperm and testosterone production.

The feedback relationship between the gonadal steroids and the hypothalamus and pituitary is detailed in Chaps. 321 and 322. Low doses of estrogens decrease the frequency of LHRH pulses and, more importantly, decrease the pituitary response to LHRH; this phenomenon is seen most clearly in postmenopausal women with elevated gonadotropins. However, sustained elevation of estrogens results in a positive feedback signal that stimulates LHRH and LH release; this phenomenon is responsible, in part, for the LH surge prior to ovulation. The sensitivity of LHRH to this positive feedback by estrogen increases during mid- to late puberty. Although progesterone decreases LHRH pulse frequency, the progesterone rise in the late follicular phase augments the pituitary LH response to LHRH and contributes to the LH surge. In castrated men, testosterone administration usually suppresses LH to undetectable levels and less often lowers FSH to normal (but not undetectable) concentrations. Inhibin, a peptide hormone produced by the testicular Sertoli cell and ovarian granulosa cell, is a potent inhibitor of FSH (but not LH) release. Its physiologic role is undefined. Testosterone decreases the frequency of LH pulsations, probably by a direct effect on LHRH release, and is converted in many tissues, including the brain, to estradiol, which inhibits the pituitary response to LHRH.

Gonadotropin measurements In postmenopausal women and men with primary hypogonadism, gonadal failure results in a marked increase in FSH and LH concentrations, providing an endogenous stimulation test. Such elevated gonadotropin concentrations ensure the adequacy of pituitary gonadotroph function. On the other hand, gonadotropin measurements are rarely indicated in a woman with ovulatory menses and in men with normal sperm counts. In evaluating gonadal failure associated with low testosterone concentrations in men or low estradiol levels in women, gonadotropin measurements help separate primary from central (secondary, hypogonadotropic) hypogonadism: high gonadotropin concentrations are indicative of primary gonadal failure; low or normal gonadotropin concentrations suggest hypothalamic or pituitary disease (see Chap. 312).

HYPOGONADOTROPIC (CENTRAL, SECONDARY) HYPOGONADISM Isolated gonadotropin deficiency may be present at birth as a congenital or hereditary disorder. Kallmann's syndrome is inherited as a single gene trait, afflicts men more severely than women, and is characterized by gonadotropin deficiency frequently associated with anosmia and midline anatomic defects. Kallmann's syndrome appears to be due to LHRH deficiency, as most patients secrete gonadotropins in response to LHRH administration after suitable priming. Acquired defects of LHRH production are common: hyperprolactinemia causes amenorrhea due to inhibition of LHRH release, possibly mediated by increased hypothalamic dopamine. Amenorrhea in anorexia nervosa, starvation, long-distance runners, and "stress" appears to be due to inhibition of LHRH release as well. Gonadotropin deficiency may be a relatively early defect in patients with large pituitary adenomas. Gonadotropin deficiency also occurs in patients with polyglandular endocrine deficiencies, presumably on an autoimmune basis (see Chap. 325) and in patients with hemochromatosis.

Patients with LHRH deficiency who desire fertility may respond to pulsatile therapy with LHRH or its agonists. When gonadotropin deficiency is due to pituitary disease, injections of FSH (menotropin) and chorionic gonadotropin (a hormone with LH-like activity) are necessary to achieve fertility.

ECTOPIC GONADOTROPIN SECRETION AND GONADOTROPIN-SECRETING TUMORS Ectopic gonadotropin production (usually hCG) can be associated with germinomas of the nonseminoma type (see Chap. 305), lung carcinomas, hepatomas, and other tumors. Children may develop precocious puberty, and men may develop gynecomastia. No distinct clinical syndrome occurs in women. Pituitary gonadotropin-secreting tumors are relatively common. Approximately 4 percent of all pituitary adenomas demonstrate gonadotropins or their subunits on immunologic staining; how often these tumors secrete gonadotropins is not clear.

FSH-secreting pituitary adenomas are large tumors, most commonly diagnosed in men with decreased libido, decreased serum testosterone, and normal prolactin levels. The finding of an increased FSH concentration may be misinterpreted as indicating primary hypogonadism if a pituitary adenoma is not suspected. The majority of these tumors overproduce intact FSH, but increased FSH beta and alpha subunits are common as well. About 40 percent demonstrate enhanced FSH secretion after TRH administration. Normal subjects and patients with primary hypogonadism do not have increased FSH secretion after TRH. Despite the normal or elevated LH concentrations in these patients, testosterone concentrations are low and respond normally to hCG administration. This suggests that the LH measured by radioimmunoassay is biologically inactive or that it represents immunologic cross-reactivity due to LH subunit overproduction.

LH-secreting pituitary adenomas are usually large tumors and are characterized by increased serum testosterone, elevated LH levels, and normal or low FSH concentrations, often with partial hypopituitarism. It is often difficult to diagnose gonadotropin-secreting pituitary adenomas in postmenopausal women because of the elevated gonadotropins associated with menopause. When faced with a large pituitary tumor and elevated plasma gonadotropin levels, with or without testosterone deficiency, the diagnosis is straightforward. However, differentiating primary hypogonadism (low testosterone with elevated FSH and LH) from the rare gonadotropin-secreting tumor of the pituitary with similar biochemistry presents a clinical dilemma. The preserved testicular response to exogenous hCG points toward a gonadotroph adenoma.

THYROTROPIN

PHYSIOLOGY TSH is a glycoprotein hormone (28,000 mol wt) composed of an alpha subunit which it shares with LH, FSH, and hCG and a unique beta subunit that confers specificity (also see Chap. 316). The genes coding for the alpha and beta subunits are on different chromosomes. TSH is produced by thyrotrophs which constitute about 10 percent of the cells of the anterior pituitary. TSH regulates the biosynthesis, storage, and release of thyroid hormones and determines thyroid gland size. TSH first appears in the fetal pituitary at about 10 weeks of gestation. TSH levels in normal subjects average 0.5 to 5.0 mU/L, with a slight increase in the nocturnal hours.

Thyrotropin-releasing hormone (TRH), the major hypothalamic mediator of TSH release, is a tripeptide found in highest concentrations in the medial division of the hypothalamic paraventricular nuclei and in the median eminence. Extrahypothalamic TRH is found in the posterior pituitary, in other parts of the brain and spinal cord, and in the gastrointestinal tract. TRH stimulates TSH secretion by increasing cytoplasmic free calcium; phosphatidylinositol and membrane phospholipids probably participate in TRH-stimulated TSH secretion. TRH stimulates the release of prolactin as well as that of TSH. The prolactin response is enhanced in hypothyroidism and diminished in hyperthyroidism. TRH-induced GH stimulation may occur in acromegaly, renal failure, depression, in many normal children, and in occasional normal adults.

The thyroid hormones thyroxine (T_4) and triiodothyronine (T_3) inhibit TSH production directly at the pituitary level. Both T_3 and T_4 bind to receptors on pituitary nuclei, but T_3 has a 40-fold greater affinity for these receptors than does T_4. Nevertheless, exogenous T_4 is more potent than T_3 in inhibiting TSH release because circulating T_4 is a more effective means of delivering T_3 to the pituitary than is T_3 itself. Half of intrapituitary T_3 is derived from T_4 conversion within the pituitary. The effects of T_4 and T_3 on hypothalamic TRH release in humans are unknown, but in animals they cause inhibition of TRH release. In hyperthyroidism TSH is suppressed, and the TSH response to TRH is absent; in primary hypothyroidism the basal TSH concentration is elevated, and the response to TRH is exaggerated.

Somatostatin decreases basal TSH release, the TSH response to TRH, and the nocturnal TSH peak. Dopamine and glucocorticoids decrease basal TSH concentration and the TSH response to TRH. Patients with untreated primary adrenal insufficiency may have slightly elevated TSH levels.

TSH concentrations can be interpreted only when serum thyroid hormone concentrations are known (see Chap. 312). In hyperthyroidism, thyroid hormone levels are elevated and TSH release is inhibited. Only sensitive TSH assays can differentiate between low and normal concentrations. A detectable serum TSH concentration by an ultrasensitive assay excludes conventional hyperthyroidism. Low thyroid hormone and elevated serum TSH concentrations are characteristic of primary hypothyroidism. Low thyroid hormone concentrations with a "normal" or "low" TSH concentration are found in central (secondary) hypothyroidism. The TRH stimulation test (no TSH response in hyperthyroidism, exaggerated TSH response in primary hypothyroidism) has largely been supplanted by sensitive TSH measurements. The TRH stimulation test is also not useful in the diagnosis of secondary hypothyroidism or in differentiating pituitary from hypothalamic disease.

PRIMARY HYPOTHYROIDISM Thyroid gland failure (primary hypothyroidism) leads to compensatory hypertrophy of the thyrotrophs. With thyroid failure of long duration, the pituitary gland and the sella turcica may enlarge. Although TSH-secreting tumors may develop in animals after thyroid gland removal, the increased TSH and pituitary size in human hypothyroidism is not autonomous and decreases with thyroid hormone replacement. Since hyperprolactinemia may also occur in patients with primary hypothyroidism, pituitary enlargement (hyperplasia) may be incorrectly diagnosed as a prolactinoma; however, the return to normal of prolactin concentrations with thyroid hormone therapy excludes that diagnosis. Severe primary hypothyroidism may occasionally cause impaired release of GH and ACTH after appropriate stimuli (so-called pituitary myxedema), and hypothyroid children may develop precocious puberty. These abnormalities are all corrected with thyroid hormone therapy.

SECONDARY HYPOTHYROIDISM Hypothyroidism due to pituitary or hypothalamic disease may be difficult to diagnose. With primary hypothyroidism serum TSH commonly rises before thyroid hormone concentrations decline below the normal range. No similar early laboratory clue exists in secondary hypothyroidism. Patients with central hypothyroidism usually do not have goiter, and many have deficiencies of other pituitary trophic hormones.

Some patients with hypothalamic hypothyroidism have mild TSH elevations, rather than normal or low concentrations as expected. Although the TSH elevations rarely exceed 10 mU/L, they are above the expected range for hypothyroidism due to TSH deficiency. Biologically inactive but immunologically active thyrotropin is present in such cases. After TRH injection, TSH concentration rises, and the biologic potency of the TSH is increased. This suggests an additional role for TRH in controlling the biologic activity of the TSH molecule by controlling its rate of glycosylation.

PITUITARY (TSH-INDUCED) HYPERTHYROIDISM Hyperthyroidism is not usually a disease of TSH overproduction. However, two types of TSH-mediated hyperthyroidism are recognized:

1 Pituitary tumors. These are usually macroadenomas with autonomous TSH secretion, unresponsive to thyroid hormone suppression or TRH stimulation. A hallmark of such tumors is overproduction of the glycoprotein hormone alpha subunit (TSH alpha), with a serum molar ratio of alpha to intact TSH of greater than 1:1. The free alpha subunit may be an important tumor marker and differs from the native alpha subunit in that one of its amino acids is carbohydrate-blocked and hence cannot combine with beta subunits. These tumors may produce other pituitary hormones in addition to TSH, most commonly GH. TSH and TSH alpha subunit secretion decrease with octreotide therapy.

2 Pituitary resistance to thyroid hormone. In this situation thyroid hormone fails to inhibit TSH secretion appropriately in the absence of a pituitary adenoma. Since TSH secretion is not inhibited, TSH rises and stimulates thyroid hormone overproduction. The peripheral tissues are not resistant to thyroid hormone, and clinical hyperthyroidism results. The pituitary resistance to thyroid hormone is incomplete since TSH can be suppressed with supraphysiologic levels of thyroid hormone and stimulated further with TRH; bromocriptine or octreotide may lower TSH as well. Pituitary resistance is usually diagnosed after thyroid gland ablation, when

TSH cannot be lowered to normal values with the usual therapeutic doses of thyroid hormone. However, once the hyperthyroidism has been treated, pituitary resistance is of no clinical consequence.

ADRENOCORTICOTROPIC HORMONE

PHYSIOLOGY ACTH is produced by corticotrophs which comprise about 15 percent of anterior pituitary cells, located principally in the central portion. ACTH is synthesized as part of a large precursor molecule termed pro-opiomelanocortin (POMC, 265 amino acids) (see Chap. 317). ACTH contains 39 amino acids, with near complete biologic activity residing in the *N*-terminal 26 amino acids. In the anterior pituitary POMC is cleaved to yield ACTH, β-lipotropin, and an *N*-terminal precursor.

ACTH controls the release of cortisol from the adrenal cortex. Although aldosterone is primarily controlled by the renin-angiotensin system, ACTH also stimulates aldosterone release acutely. Other derivatives of the POMC molecule, such as γ-melanocyte-stimulating hormone (γ-MSH), also influence aldosterone production and are found in increased concentrations in the plasma of patients with idiopathic hyperaldosteronism. Patients with ACTH deficiency have near-normal aldosterone production and do not require mineralocorticoid replacement therapy.

Corticotropin-releasing hormone (CRH) is the major but not exclusive regulator of ACTH release. CRH contains 41 amino acids on a single polypeptide chain. CRH is produced primarily by neurons of the paraventricular nuclei of the hypothalamus but is also present in other areas of the brain, including the limbic system and cortex, as well as in the pancreas, gut, and adrenal medulla. The placenta has the highest concentration outside the nervous system. CRH stimulates cyclic AMP production and regulates intracellular calcium and increases the concentration of POMC messenger RNA. Vasopressin potentiates the ACTH-releasing properties of CRH through a cyclic AMP–independent mechanism and may play a physiologic role in ACTH release. Beta-adrenergic stimuli and oxytocin cause ACTH release as well. Somatostatin blocks CRH-induced ACTH release.

ACTH is released in pulses with an overriding circadian rhythm. With a normal sleeping pattern, ACTH concentration is highest in the early morning (around 4 A.M.) and lowest in late evening. The characteristic diurnal rhythm of plasma cortisol occurs in response to these ACTH changes. In primary adrenal insufficiency (Addison's disease), cortisol concentrations fall and ACTH concentrations rise. This results in hyperpigmentation owing to the melanocyte-stimulating properties of ACTH. Cortisol administration inhibits ACTH release, a phenomenon dependent upon both the rate of rise of cortisol and its absolute concentration. Increased plasma cortisol inhibits CRH-induced ACTH release and may also inhibit CRH release. When supraphysiologic doses of glucocorticoids are given for prolonged periods, the hypothalamic-pituitary–adrenal cortex axis may remain suppressed for months after the drugs have been stopped, probably as the result of prolonged hypothalamic CRH suppression (see Chap. 317).

Stress, including hypoglycemia, surgery, and psychic distress, stimulates ACTH release, in part via increased CRH release. However, the magnitude of the ACTH release is greater than can be achieved during maximal stimulation with CRH. With severe illness, the requirements for cortisol may increase tenfold; failure to achieve these levels of cortisol during such periods may result in clinical adrenal insufficiency when adrenal reserve is impaired.

In normal persons ACTH circulates in low concentrations [2 to 18 pmol/L (10 to 80 pg/mL)]. It is difficult to measure ACTH in plasma and often not possible to separate low from normal values using commercial assays. Random ACTH measurements have little clinical significance. Tests for adrenal insufficiency and excess rely primarily on measurements of cortisol and its metabolites rather than on measurement of ACTH.

ACTH EXCESS (CUSHING'S DISEASE AND NELSON'S SYNDROME) Clinical features Cortisol excess is characterized by a central distribution of adipose tissue, muscle weakness, purplish striae, hypertension, amenorrhea, osteoporosis, fatigue, and psychiatric abnormalities. This syndrome may be caused by pituitary or ectopic ACTH overproduction, adrenal tumors, or exogenous glucocorticoid administration.

The presence of cortisol excess is established by the finding of increased excretion of urine free cortisol and/or 17-hydroxycorticosteroids that fails to decrease appropriately after either overnight (1 mg at midnight) or 2-day low-dose dexamethasone administration (0.5 mg every 6 h for eight doses). Additional suppression (and occasionally stimulation) tests are required to determine whether the Cushing's syndrome is due to a pituitary lesion. In patients with pituitary ACTH hypersecretion, either high-dose overnight (8 mg at midnight) or 2-day dexamethasone administration (2 mg every 6 h for 8 doses) results in suppression of urine 17-hydroxycorticosteroids and free cortisol and plasma cortisol, usually by greater than 50 percent. Urine 17-hydroxycorticosteroids increase after metyrapone administration in Cushing's disease. Plasma ACTH levels are normal or high-normal and show an exaggerated increase after CRH administration. Pituitary ACTH hypersecretion (Cushing's disease) is caused by a corticotroph microadenoma in 90 percent of patients and by a macroadenoma in most of the rest. Corticotroph hyperplasia has been documented in a few cases. The microadenomas are often small (3 mm or less) and may be difficult to find on CT or conventional MRI scanning. High-resolution MRI scanning with gadolinium may improve the localization of these tumors. Previously pituitary surgery was often recommended on the basis of dynamic testing alone. However, bilateral inferior petrosal sinus catheterization to localize the site of ACTH production can be used to confirm the pituitary source of ACTH production and to localize functioning adenomas when all imaging studies are negative.

Treatment Transsphenoidal microsurgery is successful in treating microadenomas in about 75 percent of patients. When surgery is successful, plasma cortisol concentrations fall almost to zero and often remain low for many months owing to delayed recovery of CRH and ACTH secretion by the hypothalamus and normal remaining pituitary. However, adrenal function eventually returns to normal in most patients. Cushing's syndrome may recur, however, even after apparently curative surgery. Previously, bilateral adrenalectomy was the therapy of choice for patients with pituitary Cushing's disease. Unfortunately, after this procedure enlarging pituitary adenomas with increased skin pigmentation (Nelson's syndrome) develop in 10 to 30 percent of patients.

Ectopic ACTH production is a relatively common disorder and can cause great difficulty in diagnosis (see Chaps. 309 and 317). When ACTH production is caused by rapidly growing tumors such as oat cell carcinoma of the lung, symptoms of Cushing's syndrome are blunted. Rather, patients have hypokalemia, muscle weakness, weight loss, and hyperpigmentation. ACTH concentrations often exceed 66 pmol/L (300 pg/mL) and do not change with dexamethasone administration. When slow-growing tumors such as thymic carcinoids, bronchial carcinoids, medullary carcinoma of the thyroid, and pancreatic islet cell tumors produce ACTH the typical features of Cushing's syndrome are common. In the latter group ACTH measurements and cortisol response to dexamethasone administration may mimic those found in patients with pituitary adenomas. However, with ectopic ACTH production ACTH concentrations generally do not change after CRH administration. When differentiation between pituitary and ectopic ACTH production is uncertain, bilateral inferior petrosal sinus catheterization is necessary. Cushing's syndrome can rarely be caused by ectopic production of CRH itself.

ACTH DEFICIENCY (SECONDARY ADRENAL INSUFFICIENCY) ACTH deficiency may be isolated or occur in association with other anterior pituitary hormone deficiencies. Reversible isolated ACTH deficiency is common after long-term glucocorticoid administration. If glucocorticoids are withdrawn suddenly in this situation or continued in physiologic doses when severe illness is present, adrenal insufficiency may occur (see Chap. 317). Symptoms include nausea, vomiting, fatigue, joint discomfort, and dizziness, and there may be fever, hypotension, hyponatremia, and hypoglycemia. Although cortisol is necessary for free water excretion, it is not needed for potassium excretion. Hence patients with ACTH deficiency are not hyperkalemic as are patients with primary adrenal insufficiency. Hyperpigmentation does not occur. These factors make diagnosis of secondary adrenal insufficiency more difficult than that of primary adrenal insufficiency. Isolated ACTH deficiency may occur without prior glucocorticoid therapy.

In general, patients undergoing pituitary surgery need to be treated with "stress" doses of glucocorticoids until normal adrenal function can be demonstrated postoperatively. All patients with pituitary macroadenomas or hypothalamic disease require testing of the pituitary-adrenal axis, but when pituitary surgery is planned testing can be limited in focus until after surgery is completed.

THE ENDOGENOUS OPIOID PEPTIDES

The endogenous opioid peptides, the enkephalins and endorphins, constitute approximately 10 to 15 substances that range in length from 5 to 31 amino acids (Fig. 313-7). Although these peptides are chemically unrelated to morphine, they bind to and act via the same opioid receptor. Although the opioid peptides have common chemical features, they arise via different biosynthetic pathways. In the pituitary β-endorphin, the most abundant endorphin, is synthesized as part of a larger precursor molecule (pro-opiomelanocortin, POMC) that also contains the full sequence of ACTH, α-melanocyte-stimulating hormone (α-MSH), β-MSH, and β-lipotropin (β-LPH) (Fig. 313-8). This precursor molecule also has the potential to generate other forms of endorphin, fragments termed α-endorphin and γ-endorphin. Cleavage sites within POMC allow the generation of each of the above-mentioned peptides in some anatomic sites. The biosynthetic pathway represents the only means by which the pituitary gland produces ACTH. Therefore, the biosyntheses of ACTH and β-endorphin are inextricably linked in the corticotroph cells of the pituitary by derivation from a single gene that encodes both hormones.

Different processing of POMC occurs within other tissues, depending on the enzymatic machinery within the tissues. For instance,

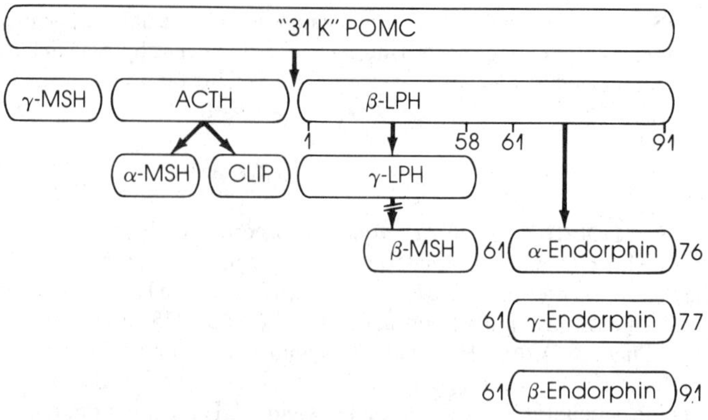

FIGURE 313-8 Biosynthetic pathway for β-endorphin in the pituitary gland. A single precursor protein, pro-opiomelanocortin (POMC) (molecular weight of approximately 31,000), is initially synthesized from translation of a gene that encodes the structure of adrenocorticotropin (ACTH), β-lipotropin (β-LPH), and β-endorphin. Prohormone-type cleavages can generate other hormones from the same precursor, although this occurs in tissues other than the pituitary. Abbreviations: MSH = melanocyte-stimulating hormone; LPH = lipotropin; CLIP = corticotropin-like intermediate peptide; ACTH = adrenocorticotropin.

although the pituitary does not metabolize ACTH to smaller fragments, the hypothalamus converts the precursor molecule to α-MSH. β-MSH is generated in the intermediate lobe of lower species. Humans lack an intermediate lobe and produce β-MSH in scattered cells within the pituitary. Although different cell types may synthesize the same primary gene product, the final profile of hormone secretion can differ completely.

The enkephalins are derived from different precursors. The adrenal glands synthesize enkephalins as part of a large protein, proenkephalin A, that contains six repeats of the Met-enkephalin sequence and one Leu-enkephalin structure. Dynorphins and enoendorphins are derived from a third distinct precursor molecule, proenkephalin B. Additional ("cryptic") peptides are encoded within the structures of these precursor proteins and have the potential to be released by "prohormone-type" cleavages. It is not known whether these peptides are secreted into the blood in vivo.

ACTH, β-endorphin, and β-LPH synthesis and secretion by the

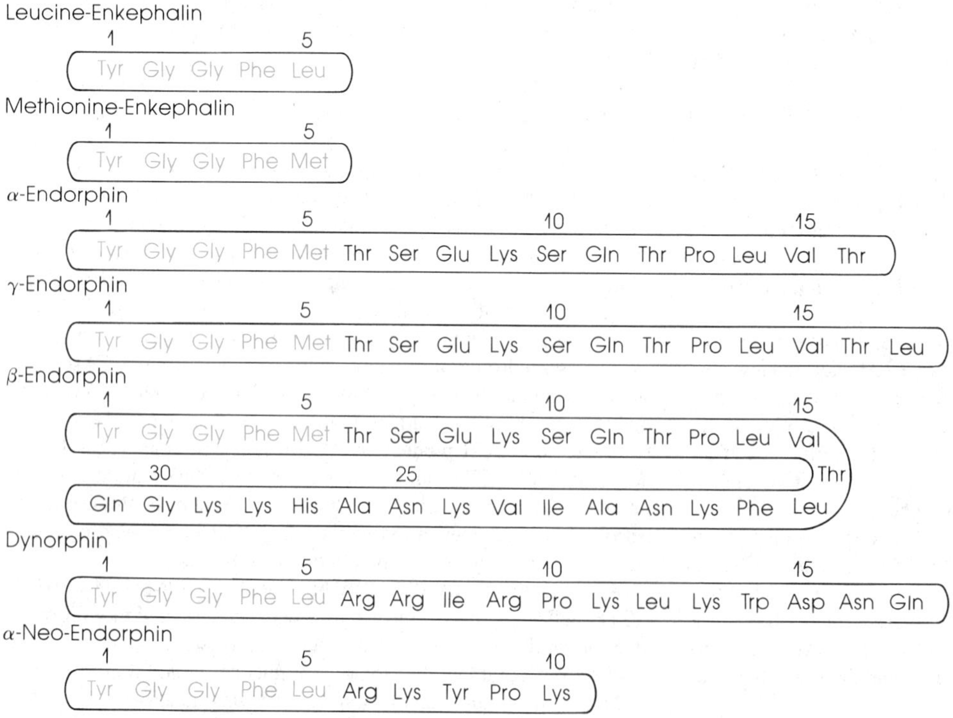

FIGURE 313-7 Structure of several endogenous opiate peptides. The amino-terminal (leftmost) four amino acids are identical in each peptide. At position 5, a methionine or leucine is found.

pituitary are linked both in normal and in abnormal states. Under normal conditions, β-LPH circulates in higher molar concentration than does β-endorphin, but the usual radioimmunoassays recognize both entities. Hence, levels of immunoreactive β-endorphin reflect the combined levels of β-endorphin and β-LPH. In adrenal insufficiency the plasma levels of both ACTH and β-endorphin are elevated; likewise, glucocorticoid replacement decreases the levels of both. Administration of corticotropin-releasing hormone (CRH) stimulates release of both ACTH and β-endorphin in a parallel manner, and in Nelson's syndrome the plasma levels of both ACTH and β-endorphin are elevated. Ectopic production of ACTH by tumors is also accompanied by β-endorphin excess. In the latter case, measurement of β-endorphin levels can be useful as a tumor marker and in some patients serves to monitor treatment. β-Endorphin and β-LPH have a longer half-life in blood than does ACTH, and measurement of plasma β-endorphin may be useful for the diagnosis of Cushing's disease.

The pituitary is the richest site of endorphin in the body. In the pituitary, ACTH and endorphin-containing cells are found in the anteromedial region of the anterior lobe, at the posterior boundary of the anterior lobe, and in nerve fibers of the posterior lobe. The hypothalamus also contains neurons that synthesize endorphin. These neurons have long projections to other regions of the brain. For example, regions of the brain associated with the limbic system contain substantial quantities of immunoreactive β-endorphin, suggesting a role in memory, learning, and emotions.

Neurons containing the enkephalins are even more widely distributed in the central nervous sytem. Levels are particularly high in the dorsal horn of the spinal cord, a region that contains opiate receptors and that is involved in the transmission of pain (see Chap. 15). Enkephalins are also present in the gastrointestinal tract. Concentrations in the myenteric plexus of the longitudinal muscles of the gut are higher than in the brain. Enkephalins are synthesized in the chromaffin cells of the adrenal medulla and packaged together with the catecholamines in the same secretory granules. Enkephalin is released as part of the sympathetic response to stress together with epinephrine and norepinephrine. Similarly, plasma enkephalin levels are high in pheochromocytoma.

Two general approaches have been employed to define the physiologic role of endorphins. One is to determine the effects of administration of endogenous opiate peptides to animals or humans. For example, the administration of β-endorphin produces an increase in the secretion of GH, prolactin, and vasopressin and a decrease in the secretion of ACTH, cortisol, LH, and FSH. The second approach is to assess the effects of antagonists of the opiates, such as naloxone. Such agents block the effects of endogenously secreted opiates, revealing the tonic or physiologic role of opiate peptides. Naloxone administration causes elevations in LH, FSH, and ACTH levels and prevents the stress-mediated rise in prolactin levels.

A variety of physiologic actions have been postulated for these hormones including: (1) morphine-like analgesic properties; (2) behavioral effects; and (3) neurotransmitter and neuromodulator functions. Indeed, these peptides may play a role in memory, learning, response to stress, reproduction, pain transmission, and regulation of appetite, temperature, and respiration. In addition, the placebo response, acupuncture-mediated analgesia, stress-induced amenorrhea, and the pathogenesis of shock may be mediated in part by enkephalins and the endorphins. Tranquilization, irritability, agitation, violent behavior, catalepsy, narcolepsy, catatonia, the smoking habit, alcoholism, and drug addiction may reflect biochemical abnormalities of the system.

DISEASES OF THE HYPOTHALAMUS AND PITUITARY

Diseases that affect the hypothalamus and pituitary can have both endocrine and nonendocrine manifestations.

HYPOTHALAMUS The human hypothalamus weighs about 4 g; hypothalamic dysfunction occurs only when disease is bilateral. Tumors in this region are often slow-growing and may achieve large size before symptoms appear. Signs of hydrocephalus or focal cerebral dysfunction may coexist with hypopituitarism and hypothalamic dysfunction. The hypothalamus exerts both endocrine and nonendocrine functions. Hypothalamic control of the pituitary gland has been discussed above. Nonendocrine functions are also influenced by the hypothalamus:

1 Food intake and feeding behavior. The basal hypothalamus controls maintenance of a stable weight. Several regions of the hypothalamus are implicated in hunger and satiety. The ventromedial nucleus is known to be involved in satiety, but it now appears that anterior hypothalamic regions are also concerned. Stimulation and termination of food ingestion appear to be affected by several neuropeptides, including the opioid peptides and neuropeptide Y. Hypothalamic obesity in humans is usually associated with lesions of the ventromedial nucleus; this obesity appears to involve a resetting of the weight set point. Marked hyperphagia, possibly related to rapid gastric emptying, occurs until the new weight set point is reached. Patients often demonstrate decreased activity and finicky eating once the new set point is reached. Other factors including thyroid and adrenal hormones also influence feeding behavior.

2 Temperature regulation. The anterior hypothalamus contains warm- and cold-sensitive neurons that respond to local and environmental thermal gradients. The posterior hypothalamus generates the signals necessary for heat dissipation. The temperature increase associated with infections is generated by the hypothalamus. Phagocytic cells throughout the body produce interleukin 1 (endogenous pyrogen) which stimulates the anterior hypothalamus to produce prostaglandin E_2. Prostaglandin E_2 raises the thermostat set point, leading to heat conservation (e.g., vasoconstriction) and increased heat production (e.g., muscle shivering) until blood and core temperatures match the new hypothalamic set point.

Abnormalities of temperature regulation may occur with hypothalamic disease. Hypothermia is a rare consequence of diffuse hypothalamic disease. Paroxysmal hypothermia with sweating, flushing, and a fall in body temperatures may occur, and sustained hyperthermia without tachycardia is reported with acute pathologic processes such as hemorrhage into the third ventricle. Poikilothermia (a change in body temperature of greater than 1°C with change in environmental temperature) is usually a consequence of posterior hypothalamic disease. Paroxysmal hyperthermia with episodic shaking chills, spiking fevers, and autonomic phenomena is a rare manifestation. It is important to remember that adrenal insufficiency can cause fever or hypothermia and that hypothyroidism may cause hypothermia.

3 Sleep-wake cycle. Lesions in the sleep center of the anterior hypothalamus result in insomnia. The posterior hypothalamus is important for arousal and maintenance of the waking state; posterior hypothalamic destruction due to ischemia, encephalitis, or trauma can result in a hypersomnolent state from which arousal is possible. Larger lesions extending to the reticular formation of the rostral midbrain cause coma (see Chap. 31).

4 Memory and behavior. Lesions of the ventromedial hypothalamus and premammillary region result in loss of short-term memory, often with Korsakoff's syndrome. Longer-term memory is often intact. Hypothalamic lesions may also cause a more typical picture of dementia. Rage reactions may result with ventromedial lesions, and lateral hypothalamic destruction may cause an apathetic state.

5 Thirst. The hypothalamus is the center for vasopressin production and for the control of thirst by serum osmolality, Impaired thirst may occur with hypothalamic lesions; rarely primary polydipsia without diabetes insipidus is a consequence of hypothalamic lesions.

6 Autonomic nervous system function. Parasympathetic pathways are stimulated by the anterior hypothalamus; sympathetic pathways are stimulated by the posterior hypothalamus. Diencephalic epilepsy is a rare syndrome associated with paroxysms of autonomic hyperactivity.

A diencephalic syndrome in children, characterized by emaciation, hyperkinesis and inappropriate affect, often with a cheerful disposition, can be caused by invasive tumors of the anterior and basal hypothalamus. Most of these children die by the age of 2 years, but in those who survive the clinical picture changes to one of increased appetite with obesity, irritability, and rage reactions.

In general, slow-growing tumors produce dementia, disturbances of food intake (obesity or emaciation), and endocrine dysfunction. Acute destructive processes are more likely to cause coma or disturbances of the autonomic nervous system.

Diseases of the anterior hypothalamus include craniopharyngiomas, gliomas of the optic nerve, sphenoid ridge meningiomas, granulomatous disease (including sarcoidosis), germinomas, and aneurysms of the internal carotid artery. Suprasellar pituitary adenomas and tuberculum sella meningiomas may grow into the hypothalamus as well. Lesions of the posterior hypothalamus include gliomas, hamartomas, ependymomas, germinomas, and teratomas.

Precocious puberty, particularly in males, can be associated with "pinealomas." However, these pinealomas actually are germinomas, and the precocious puberty appears to result from the ectopic production of chorionic gonadotropin by these tumors rather than from an effect on pituitary gonadotropins.

Craniopharyngiomas Craniopharyngiomas arise from remnants of Rathke's pouch. Most of these tumors are suprasellar, but about 15 percent are intrasellar. The tumors are usually cystic or partially cystic, often contain calcium, and are lined with stratified squamous epithelium. Although craniopharyngiomas are usually manifested in childhood, 45 percent of patients are over the age of 20, and 20 percent are over the age of 40 at the time of diagnosis.

Children usually present with signs of increased intracranial pressure due to hydrocephalus (80 percent) including headache, vomiting, and papilledema. Visual abnormalities such as loss of vision and field cuts are found in 60 percent. Short stature is sometimes found (7 to 40 percent), but retarded bone age is more common. Delayed sexual development occurs in about 20 percent, and diabetes insipidus may be present.

About 80 percent of adults present with visual complaints, and an additional 10 percent have visual abnormalities on careful testing. Papilledema is present in about 15 percent of adults. Headaches (40 percent), mental deterioration or personality change (26 percent), and hypogonadism (35 percent) are relatively common in adults. Hyperprolactinemia is present in one-third to one-half of patients, but prolactin levels rarely exceed 100 to 150 μg/L. Diabetes insipidus (15 percent), weight gain (15 percent), and panhypopituitarism (7 percent) may occur as well. Rarely, the cyst contents spill into the cerebrospinal fluid, causing a picture of aseptic meningitis.

Suprasellar calcification (see Fig. 313-13) in a flocculent, granular, or curvilinear pattern is present on skull x-rays in most children and in some adults with craniopharyngioma. Calcification is evident on CT scan in most of these adults, however. Hypothalamic germinomas may calcify as well. Skull x-ray abnormalities include calcification, sellar enlargement, and signs of increased intracranial pressure in 90 percent of children and 60 percent of adults.

Therapy of craniopharyngiomas is often unsatisfactory. Total removal often results in major functional deficits. We generally favor biopsy and partial resection followed by conventional radiation as a more conservative approach. Tumors less than 3 cm in diameter have a better prognosis.

Germ cell tumors Germinomas originate in the posterior third ventricle, anterior third ventricle (supra- or intrasellar), or in both locations (also see Chap. 305). Germinomas (also known as atypical teratomas) were previously confused with parenchymal tumors of the pineal (pinealomas); when located in the anterior third ventricle they were known as "ectopic pinealomas." Germinomas often infiltrate the hypothalamus and occasionally metastasize to the cerebrospinal fluid or distant sites.

The majority of patients have diabetes insipidus in association with variable anterior pituitary insufficiency. Precocious puberty may occur in boys, probably due to hCG production by these tumors. Diplopia, headache, vomiting, lethargy, weight loss, and hydrocephalus are common. The tumors usually begin in childhood but may be diagnosed in young adults. Because germinomas are radiosensitive, early recognition is important. When the tumor is located in the anterior third ventricle, biopsy by the transsphenoidal route is often possible. Tumors in the pineal region are more difficult to biopsy, leading some authors to recommend empirical radiation therapy or chemotherapy, whereas others prefer surgical biopsy or debulking followed by radiation and chemotherapy. Germinomas of the nonseminoma type may produce hCG and/or α-fetoprotein, whereas pure seminomas rarely produce tumor markers (see Chap. 305).

PITUITARY ADENOMAS Pituitary adenomas account for about 10 to 15 percent of intracranial neoplasms. They can cause anterior pituitary hormonal imbalance, structural problems related to invasion of surrounding structures, or syndromes of hormone excess. Occasionally, the diagnosis is the result of incidental findings during skull x-ray examinations. Small pituitary tumors are present in 6 to 20 percent of adults at autopsy.

Pathology Pituitary tumors were previously classified as basophilic, acidophilic, or chromophobic on the basis of hematoxylin and eosin staining. Corticotroph adenomas are generally basophilic; the more densely granulated prolactin-secreting tumors are acidophilic; the majority of prolactinomas, sparsely granulated GH-secreting tumors, TSH-secreting and gonadotropin-secreting tumors, and nonsecreting tumors are all chromophobic. Because this classification provides little insight into hormone production, it has been abandoned. Many nonfunctioning pituitary tumors are, however, still referred to as "chromophobes." Classification can also be based upon immunohistochemical staining or according to hormonal secretion, based upon hormone measurements in serum.

Furthermore, pituitary tumors have been classified by Hardy according to size and invasive characteristics. Stage I tumors are microadenomas (less than 10 mm in diameter) that may cause hormonal oversecretion but do not cause hypopituitarism and are not associated with structural problems. Stage II tumors are macroadenomas (greater than 10 mm) with or without suprasellar extension. Stage III tumors are macroadenomas that locally invade the floor of the sella and may cause sellar enlargement and suprasellar extension. Stage IV tumors are invasive macroadenomas with diffuse destruction of the sella, with or without suprasellar extension. The difficulty with this system of classification is that not all pituitary tumors fall neatly into one of these categories. For example, it may be difficult to separate thinning of the sellar floor (stage II) from erosion through the floor (stage III).

Endocrine manifestations Anterior pituitary hormone overproduction is suspected on clinical grounds and confirmed by appropriate laboratory evaluation (see Table 313-5). The most common secretory pituitary tumors are prolactinomas. They cause galactorrhea and hypogonadism, including amenorrhea, infertility, and impotence. GH-secreting tumors are the next most common secretory pituitary tumors and cause acromegaly or gigantism. Next in frequency are corticotroph (ACTH-secreting) adenomas which cause cortisol excess (Cushing's disease). Glycoprotein hormone–secreting pituitary adenomas (secreting TSH, LH, or FSH) are the least common. TSH-secreting adenomas are a rare cause of hyperthyroidism. Paradoxically, most patients with gonadotropin-secreting adenomas have hypogonadism.

About 15 percent of patients with tumors that come to surgery have adenomas that secrete more than one pituitary hormone. The most common combination is GH and prolactin, and other common patterns are GH-TSH, GH-prolactin-TSH, and ACTH-prolactin. Most of these tumors have one cell secreting two hormones (unimorphous), but some tumors have two or more cell types, each of which produces a single hormone (polymorphous).

Prolactinomas in women and corticotroph adenomas in both sexes are usually diagnosed while still microadenomas. In contrast, the

TABLE 313-5 Pituitary hormone evaluation

Hormone	Excess	Deficiency
Growth hormone	*1* Measurement of plasma growth hormone 1 h following glucose PO	*1* Measurement of plasma growth hormone 30, 60, and 120 min after one of the following: *a* Regular insulin 0.1 to 0.15 unit/kg IV *b* Levodopa 10 mg/kg PO *c* L-Arginine 0.5 mg/kg intravenously over 30 min
	2 Measurement of IGF-1/SM-C	*2* ?Measurement of IGF-1/SM-C
Prolactin	*1* Measurement of basal serum prolactin	*1* Measurement of serum prolactin 10 to 20 min after one of the following: *a* TRH 200 to 500 μg IV *b* Chlorpromazine 25 mg IM
TSH	*1* Measurement of T_4, free T_4 index, T_3, TSH	*1* Measurement of T_4, free T_4, free T_4 index, TSH
Gonadotropins	*1* Measurement of FSH, LH, testosterone, FSH beta, FSH response to TRH	*1* Measurement of basal LH, FSH in postmenopausal women; no measurements in menstruating, ovulating women *2* Testosterone, FSH, and LH in men
ACTH	*1* Measurement of urine free cortisol*	*1* Measurement of serum cortisol at 30 and 60 min following regular insulin 0.05 to 0.15 units per kilogram IV
	2 Dexamethasone suppression by one of the following: *a* Measurement of 8 A.M. plasma cortisol after administration of 1 mg dexamethasone at midnight *b* Measurement of 8 A.M. plasma cortisol or 24-h urine 17-hydroxysteroids or free cortisol after 0.5 mg dexamethasone PO q 6 h for 8 doses	*2* Metyrapone response by one of the following: *a* Measurement of plasma 11-deoxycortisol at 8 A.M. after 30 mg/kg body wt metyrapone at midnight (maximal dose 2 g) *b* Measurement of 24-h urinary 17-hydroxycorticoids or plasma 11-deoxycortisol day of and day after 750 mg metyrapone q 4 h for 6 doses *c* Measurement of 24-h urinary 17-hydroxycorticoids day of and day after 500 mg metyrapone q 2 h for 12 doses
	3 High-dose dexamethasone suppression by one of the following: *a* Measurement of plasma cortisol after 8 mg dexamethasone PO at midnight *b* Measurement of 8 A.M. plasma cortisol or 24 h urine 17-hydroxysteroids or free cortisol after 2 mg dexamethasone q 6 h for 8 doses *4* Metyrapone response (same protocol as for deficiency testing) *5* Response of plasma ACTH to ovine corticotropin releasing hormone (1 μg/kg body wt)	*3* ACTH stimulation test: Measurement of plasma cortisol and aldosterone at 0 and 60 min after IM or IV administration of 0.25 mg cosyntropin
Arginine vasopressin (AVP)	*1* Measurement of serum sodium and osmolality, urine osmolality in presence of normal renal, adrenal, thyroid function *2* Simultaneous measurement of serum osmolality and ADH levels	*1* Comparison of urine osmolality and serum osmolality under conditions of increased AVP secretion† *2* Simultaneous measurement of serum osmolality and AVP levels

* Tests 1 and 2 establish the diagnosis of Cushing's syndrome. Tests 3, 4, and 5 localize the Cushing's disease to the pituitary gland. Occasionally bilateral inferior petrosal sinus catheterization will be necessary.
† May be achieved by water deprivation or saline administration.

majority of patients with acromegaly and most men with prolactinomas have macroadenomas at the time of diagnosis. Glycoprotein hormone–secreting tumors are also usually quite large at the time of diagnosis.

About 25 percent of pituitary adenomas that come to surgery are apparently nonsecretory, although some stain immunologically for pituitary hormones. In some cases, particularly in the case of gonadotropin-secreting tumors, hormonal secretion is overlooked. Some of the ''nonfunctioning'' pituitary tumors, as well as some functional ones, secrete part of the glycoprotein hormone molecule, most commonly the alpha subunit. In general tumors without endocrine-related symptoms are large at the time of diagnosis and often cause structural problems. Alpha subunit excess is a frequent finding in patients with TSH-secreting adenomas, and FSH beta may be hypersecreted in patients with gonadotropin-secreting tumors.

Null cell tumors (no specific hormones identified by immunostaining) also are generally large when diagnosed, since no hormonal overproduction is present to provide early clues to diagnosis. Oncocytomas are nonsecretory pituitary adenomas with abundant mitochondria, commonly found in older men.

Pituitary adenomas are occasionally part of the multiple endocrine neoplasia (MEN I) syndrome (see Chap. 325). This dominantly inherited disease causes adenomas of the pituitary gland, secretory tumors of the endocrine pancreas, and hyperparathyroidism due to generalized parathyroid hyperplasia. Pituitary adenomas may secrete GH or prolactin or may be nonfunctioning. Insulinomas and gastrinomas are the most common tumors in MEN I. Pancreatic GRH-secreting tumors can cause acromegaly and pituitary hyperplasia.

Mass effects of pituitary tumors VISUAL FIELD DEFECTS The optic chiasm lies anterior and superior to the pituitary gland and in 80 percent of normal persons overlies the pituitary fossa; in about 15 percent the chiasm is anterior to the tuberculum sella (prefixed), and in 5 percent it overlaps the dorsum sella posteriorly (postfixed). The chiasm is found at a variable distance above the diaphragma sella, with up to 1 cm of separation in some patients. Since 90 percent of the chiasmal axons originate in the macula, loss of central vision is an early finding. Foggy or dim vision is also described by many patients.

The most common visual field defect in patients with pituitary adenomas is a bitemporal hemianopsia, and about 8 percent of patients develop complete loss of vision in one eye with a temporal defect in the opposite eye. Alternatively, patients may demonstrate bitemporal scotomas rather than hemianopsia, particularly with a rapidly growing lesion in association with a prefixed chiasm (see Chap. 23). For this reason visual field examinations must assess more than the lateral fields of vision. Of those patients with field defects about 9 percent have a single eye defect, most commonly a superior temporal defect. Occasionally, there is a monocular field loss such as a central scotoma that mimics nonpituitary lesions. When pituitary adenomas cause visual field defects, sellar enlargement is the rule.

OCULOMOTOR PALSIES Pituitary adenomas may extend laterally, invade the cavernous sinuses, and cause oculomotor palsies. When this occurs, visual field defects are usually not present. Involvement of the third cranial nerve is most common and may mimic diabetic third nerve neuropathy in that pupillary reactivity is usually preserved.

Additional findings associated with lateral extension of the adenoma may include involvement of the fourth and sixth cranial nerves, pain or numbness in the distribution of the fifth cranial nerve, and compression or obstruction of the carotid artery.

Headaches are common in patients with larger tumors and are also present in the majority of patients with acromegaly. Headaches may be exacerbated by coughing. Headaches are thought to be due to stretching of the diaphragma sella and may be referred to several locations, including the vertex of skull and to retroorbital, frontooccipital, frontotemporal, or occipital-cervical areas.

Very large pituitary tumors may invade the hypothalamus and cause hyperphagia, abnormal temperature regulation, loss of consciousness, and loss of hormonal input from the hypothalamus. Obstructive hydrocephalus involving the third ventricle is less common with pituitary adenomas than with craniopharyngiomas. Tumor invasion of the temporal lobe may cause complex partial seizures; invasion of the posterior fossa may be associated with brainstem dysfunction, and invasion into the frontal lobes causes alterations in mental state and frontal release signs.

PITUITARY APOPLEXY Acute hemorrhagic infarction of a pituitary adenoma may cause a dramatic syndrome including severe headache, nausea, vomiting, and depression of consciousness. Ophthalmoplegia, visual and pupillary disturbances, and meningismus may be present. Most of these symptoms are caused by direct pressure from the tumor, whereas meningismus results from blood in the CSF. The syndrome may either evolve slowly over a period of 24 to 48 h or may lead to sudden death.

Pituitary apoplexy is most commonly found in patients with somatotroph or corticotroph adenomas, but it may be the first clinical manifestation of a pituitary tumor. Both anticoagulation and radiotherapy predispose to hemorrhagic infarction. Rarely, pituitary apoplexy produces "autohypophysectomy" with "cure" of acromegaly, Cushing's disease, or hyperprolactinemia. Hypopituitarism is a common sequela; although hormonal measurements may be normal during the acute phase, cortisol and gonadal steroid concentrations decline over the ensuing days, and thyroxine concentrations decline over weeks. Diabetes insipidus is rare.

It is important to differentiate between pituitary apoplexy and a leaking aneurysm; angiography is often required in this situation. Acute pituitary apoplexy is generally considered a neurosurgical emergency and may require acute decompression of the pituitary, generally via the transsphenoidal route.

Therapy of pituitary adenomas Ideal therapy for pituitary adenomas would permanently correct hormonal hypersecretion without causing hypopituitarism and would shrink or remove the tumor mass without additional morbidity or mortality. Therapy for microadenomas may achieve both of these goals, whereas therapy for macroadenomas is usually less successful. In considering therapy it is critical to weigh the disability due to the tumor against any disability that may arise from the treatment. Regardless of tumor size the therapy should not be worse than the disease. Potentially serious diseases such as Cushing's disease or acromegaly may require more aggressive treatment than do prolactinomas.

MEDICAL THERAPY Bromocriptine, a dopamine agonist, is currently the therapy of choice for patients with microprolactinomas who require therapy. Bromocriptine corrects hyperprolactinemia in almost all patients with microprolactinomas; however, when the drug is stopped, prolactin levels often return to pretreatment levels.

Bromocriptine side effects of nausea, gastric irritation, and postural hypotension can be minimized by initially giving a low dose (1.25 mg) at bedtime with a snack. Other side effects include headache, fatigue, abdominal cramps, nasal congestion, and constipation. The dosage is gradually increased to a twice-daily schedule (most commonly 2.5 mg bid).

Bromocriptine is also effective in larger prolactin-secreting macroadenomas. Bromocriptine lowers prolactin levels by about 90 percent in most patients with large tumors but usually not to normal. Tumor shrinkage of 50 percent or greater occurs in about half the patients, and visual field defects may return to normal. Tumor shrinkage is occasionally accompanied by reversal of hypopituitarism. With giant adenomas, bromocriptine-induced tumor shrinkage may rarely cause a devastating intracranial hemorrhage. Unfortunately macroadenomas usually regrow when bromocriptine is stopped.

If visual field defects are not rapidly (within 1 month) returned to normal with bromocriptine, we usually recommend surgery. Symptomatic hyperprolactinemia with inadequate response to bromocriptine also requires surgery or radiation therapy. When pregnancy is desired, the decision whether to continue bromocriptine through pregnancy needs to be weighed against the consequences of additional therapy (radiation or surgery).

The somatostatin analogue octreotide (see p. 1664) is probably the adjunctive therapy of choice in acromegaly and may be appropriate for primary therapy in some patients. Bromocriptine is a useful therapeutic adjunct in some patients with acromegaly, particularly in those with coexistent hyperprolactinemia. GH concentrations rarely return to normal, but symptomatic improvement is common and tumor shrinkage may occur. Bromocriptine should be considered in acromegalic subjects whose GH levels remain elevated following surgery or who are waiting for radiation therapy to take effect. Nonfunctioning chromophobe adenomas usually do not shrink in response to bromocriptine, even when high doses are used.

Tamoxifen is occasionally useful as an adjunct in the therapy of large prolactinomas refractory to therapy with dopamine antagonists. Cyproheptadine, a serotonin antagonist, has been reported to induce remissions in occasional patients with corticotroph adenomas. Octreotide may also be useful adjunctive therapy in patients with TSH-secreting adenomas.

SURGERY Transsphenoidal surgery of pituitary microadenomas is safe and frequently corrects hormonal oversecretion. Hormonal overproduction is corrected within 24 h in 75 percent of patients with Cushing's disease due to corticotroph microadenomas, acromegaly with GH concentration less than 40 μg/L, and microprolactinomas associated with serum prolactin concentrations less than 200 μg/L. The initial success rate varies among institutions, with reported figures ranging from 50 to 95 percent. Unfortunately, after initially successful surgery hyperprolactinemia recurs in about 17 percent of patients followed for 3 to 5 years and possibly in 50 percent after 5 to 10 years. The recurrence rates after initially successful surgery in acromegaly and Cushing's disease are not established.

The mortality rate for transsphenoidal surgery of microadenomas is 0.27 percent with a morbidity rate of about 1.7 percent based on 2600 surgical procedures. Major complications include cerebrospinal fluid rhinorrhea, oculomotor palsy, and visual loss.

Pituitary surgery is less successful with larger secretory tumors. In patients with serum prolactin greater than 200 μg/L or GH greater than 40 μg/L, hormone concentrations return to normal in only 30 percent following surgery. Surgery is successful in about 60 percent of patients with Cushing's disease due to corticotroph macroadenomas. Recurrence rates with these secretory macroadenomas after a surgery-induced remission are uncertain; in the case of prolactin-secreting tumors, hyperprolactinemia recurs in 10 to 80 percent of patients. Pretreatment with octreotide in acromegalic patients with invasive macroadenomas may improve the surgical success rate.

Mass effects of large tumors are also rarely cured with surgery alone; in cases where surgery is the exclusive therapy, the 10-year recurrence of symptoms is 85 percent in patients not treated with radiation and/or bromocriptine. When radiation therapy is used in combination with surgery, the 10-year recurrence is 15 percent.

Surgery for macroadenomas has a mortality rate of around 0.86 percent and a morbidity rate of about 6.3 percent. Hypopituitarism occurs in an additional 10 percent of patients. Transient diabetes insipidus occurs in about 5 percent, and permanent diabetes insipidus occurs in 1 percent. Major complications of surgery for macroadenoma include cerebrospinal rhinorrhea (3.3 percent), permanent visual loss (1.5 percent), permanent oculomotor palsy (0.6 percent), and meningitis (0.5 percent).

RADIATION THERAPY Conventional radiation therapy is effective in preventing tumor growth (70 to 100 percent) but is unsatisfactory in the acute management of pituitary hyperfunction. Therapy consists of delivery of 4500 cGy (4500 rad) over 4.5 to 5 weeks, using rotational techniques. GH values of less than 5 μg/L can be achieved in half of acromegalics after 5 years and in 70 percent after 10 years. Conventional radiation alone is rarely successful in treating corticotroph adenomas in adults. Long-term efficacy of radiation in patients with prolactinoma is currently being studied. Complications of conventional radiation therapy include hypopituitarism in up to 50 percent of patients. This may be used as primary therapy for nonfunctioning tumors without structural problems or as an adjunct to surgery for functioning and nonfunctioning tumors.

Heavy particle therapy with proton beam or alpha particles is effective in treating secretory adenomas, but response is slow. Tumors with suprasellar extension or tissue invasion are generally excluded from such series. With proton beam therapy at the Harvard cyclotron, radiation doses of up to 14,000 cGy (14,000 rad) can be given safely without damage to surrounding structures. At 2 years, 28 percent of acromegalics achieve GH values of less than 5 μg/L; the cure rate increases to 56 percent at 5 years and 75 percent by 10 years. With Cushing's disease proton beam corrects the hypercortisolism in 55 percent at 2 years and in 80 percent by 5 years. Proton beam therapy effectively lowers ACTH and stops growth of most corticotroph adenomas in patients with Nelson's syndrome with the exception of adenomas that are invasive at the time of therapy. Long-term results for treatment of prolactinomas with proton beam therapy are not available.

Complications of heavy particle therapy include hypopituitarism in at least 10 percent of patients, although the exact long-term prevalence of this complication is uncertain. Visual field defects and oculomotor dysfunction, usually temporary, have been reported in about 1.5 percent of patients. The major draw-back of this form of therapy and of conventional radiotherapy is the length of time that must elapse before hormonal hypersecretion is corrected.

We generally treat microprolactinomas with bromocriptine. However, we recommend surgery for those patients with microprolactinoma who require therapy and are intolerant of dopamine agonists. Surgery generally does not result in hypopituitarism in this relatively benign disease. Surgery is usually our treatment of choice in patients with acromegaly or Cushing's disease because in most instances rapid reversal of hormonal hypersecretion is essential, and cure can often be achieved. Since Cushing's disease and acromegaly are serious diseases, more extensive surgery that results in hypopituitarism may be required.

Many patients with macroprolactinomas are treated with bromocriptine alone, and a trial of this agent should be given. We recommend transsphenoidal surgery and/or radiation therapy for patients with large prolactinomas who desire pregnancy, show persistent structural abnormalities or symptomatic hyperprolactinemia despite dopamine agonists, and who are intolerant of dopaminergic agents and as an alternative to continued bromocriptine in those who desire pregnancy. Patients with nonfunctioning pituitary adenomas with structural abnormalities require transsphenoidal surgery, generally followed by conventional radiation therapy. Heavy particle therapy is an effective alternative to surgery in patients with acromegaly or Cushing's disease who have contraindications to or refuse surgery. Heavy particle or conventional radiation therapy is effective in treating patients with persistent GH elevation after transsphenoidal surgery, as is octreotide. Heavy particle therapy is effective in persistent Cushing's disease as well. Proton beam therapy is effective in most patients with Nelson's syndrome and may be a desirable alternative to conventional radiation therapy in patients with macroprolactinomas and nonsecretory macroadenomas. Transfrontal surgery is occasionally required, particularly in patients with giant adenomas.

HYPOPITUITARISM *Hypopituitarism* refers to deficiency of one or more pituitary hormones and has many etiologies (see Table 313-6). Pituitary hormone deficiency may be congenital or acquired. Isolated GH or gonadotropin deficiency is common. Temporary ACTH deficiency as a consequence of long-term glucocorticoid therapy is also common, but permanent isolated deficiency of ACTH or TSH is rare. Deficiency of any of the anterior pituitary hormones may occur at the level of the pituitary gland or the hypothalamus. When diabetes insipidus is present, the primary defect is almost invariably in the hypothalamus or high pituitary stalk, often in conjunction with mild hyperprolactinemia and anterior pituitary hypofunction.

TABLE 313-6 Causes of hypopituitarism

A Isolated hormone deficiencies
- *1* Congenital or acquired deficiencies

B Tumors
- *1* Large pituitary adenomas
- *2* Pituitary apoplexy
- *3* Hypothalamic tumors, e.g., craniopharyngiomas, germinomas, chordomas, meningiomas, gliomas, and others

C Inflammatory diseases
- *1* Granulomatous disease, e.g., sarcoidosis, tuberculosis, syphilis, granulomatous hypophysitis
- *2* Eosinophilic granuloma
- *3* Lymphocytic hypophysitis (autoimmune)

D Vascular diseases
- *1* Sheehan's postpartum necrosis
- *2* ? Diabetic peripartum necrosis
- *3* Carotid aneurysm

E Destructive-traumatic events
- *1* Surgery
- *2* Stalk section
- *3* Radiation (conventional—hypothalamus; heavy-particle—pituitary)
- *4* Trauma

F Developmental anomalies
- *1* Pituitary aplasia
- *2* Basal encephalocoele

G Infiltration
- *1* Hemochromatosis
- *2* Amyloidosis

H "Idiopathic" causes
- *1* ?Autoimmune disease

Manifestations of hypopituitarism depend upon the specific pituitary hormones that are lacking. Growth failure due to GH deficiency is a common presenting complaint in children. GH deficiency in adults causes more subtle manifestations such as fine wrinkling around the eyes and mouth and in subjects with diabetes mellitus increased sensitivity to insulin. Complaints related to gonadotropin deficiency include amenorrhea and infertility in women and testosterone deficiency and decreased libido, decreased beard and body hair, and preservation of a youthful scalp hairline in men. TSH deficiency causes hypothyroidism with fatigue, cold intolerance, and puffy skin in the absence of goiter. ACTH deficiency results in cortisol deficiency, manifested by fatigue; decreased appetite; weight loss; decreased skin and nipple pigmentation; abnormal response to stress characterized by fever, hypotension, and hyponatremia; and a high mortality rate. Unlike primary adrenal insufficiency (Addison's disease) ACTH deficiency does not cause hyperpigmentation, hyperkalemia, or salt loss. With combined ACTH and gonadotropin deficiency, axillary and pubic hair may be lost. Children with combined GH and cortisol deficiency often develop hypoglycemia. AVP deficiency causes diabetes insipidus with polyuria and increased thirst. When pituitary adenomas impair anterior pituitary function, GH is often the first hormone to be compromised, followed by deficiencies of gonadotropins, TSH, and ACTH.

Etiology Damage to the anterior pituitary is commonly due to a pituitary adenoma (with or without infarction), pituitary surgery, heavy particle pituitary irradiation, closed head trauma, or infarction during the postpartum period (Sheehan's syndrome). Postpartum pituitary infarction occurs because the enlarged pituitary gland of pregnancy becomes vulnerable to ischemia; postpartum hemorrhage with systemic hypotension can destroy the pituitary gland. Inability to lactate is the most common initial clinical clue, and other symptoms of hypopituitarism may unfold over months or years. The condition is sometimes diagnosed years after the primary event. Although clinical diabetes insipidus is rare in this setting, a decreased vasopressin response to appropriate stimuli is common. Patients with diabetes mellitus are also prone to develop hypopituitarism late in pregnancy.

Another cause of hypopituitarism in women is lymphocytic hypophysitis, a syndrome that usually occurs during pregnancy or in the postpartum period. In this syndrome, a mass lesion is often seen on CT scanning which, when biopsied, consists of lymphocytic infiltration. Lymphocytic hypophysitis is due to autoimmune pituitary destruction and often occurs with other autoimmune diseases such as Hashimoto's (autoimmune) thyroiditis and gastric atrophy (see Chap. 325). Circulating antibodies to prolactin cells have been identified in some patients. Although only 30 cases of lymphocytic hypophysitis have been reported, about 7 percent of patients with other autoimmune diseases have prolactin antibodies in serum. It is not clear whether autoimmune hypophysitis is a common cause of ''idiopathic'' hypopituitarism in adults.

Hypothalamic or pituitary stalk damage has many causes (see Table 313-6). Certain lesions in this region, such as sarcoidosis, metastatic carcinoma, germinomas, histiocytosis, and craniopharyngiomas, commonly cause diabetes insipidus along with hypofunction of the anterior pituitary. Pituitary insufficiency, resulting from conventional radiation to the brain or the pituitary, is thought to be largely hypothalamic in origin, although diabetes insipidus generally does not occur.

Diagnosis (See Table 313-5) To diagnose GH deficiency, the most reliable GH stimulus is insulin-induced hypoglycemia in which the blood sugar declines to less than 2.2 pmol/L (40 mg/dL) (Fig. 313-9). A GH concentration of greater than 10 μg/L after hypoglycemia, levodopa, or arginine effectively excludes GH deficiency.

FIGURE 313-9 The insulin tolerance test. After an intravenous injection of regular insulin (0.1 unit/kg body weight) a fall in blood sugar and rise in plasma GH and cortisol is expected. This test permits evaluation of both GH and ACTH in patients with pituitary disease. *(After KJ Catt, Lancet 1:933, 1970.)*

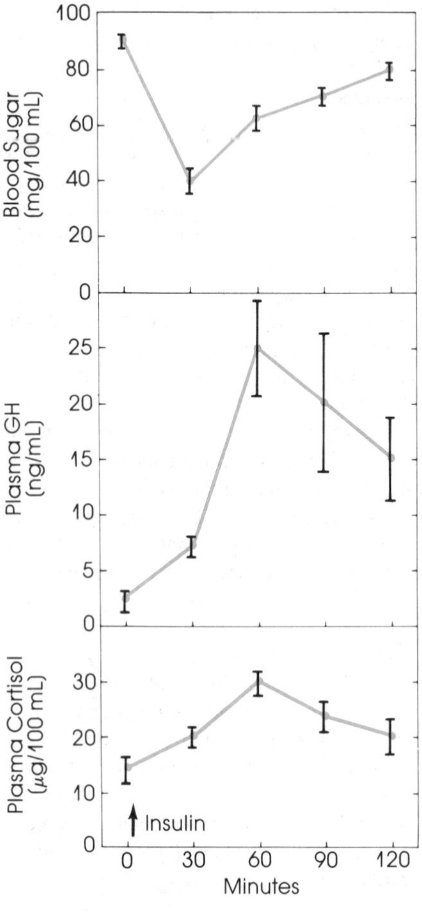

Measuring the basal GH or serum IGF-1/SM-C concentration is less reliable, because GH levels are undetectable in normal persons for much of the day and because IGF-1/SM-C concentrations in patients with GH deficiency may overlap the normal range.

Cortisol deficiency is potentially life-threatening. Basal cortisol function may be preserved in the face of extensive pituitary destruction; consequently, the ability of pituitary ACTH secretion to increase in response to ''stress'' must be assessed. Either the insulin tolerance test or the metyrapone test can be used to determine the adequacy of ACTH reserve; the ACTH stimulation test is a safer but less sensitive alternative.

The insulin tolerance test is safely performed on an outpatient basis in younger patients without heart disease or diseases predisposing to seizures (Fig. 313-9 and Table 313-5). Both cortisol and GH responses are measured. If hypopituitarism is strongly suspected, a lower dose of regular insulin (0.05 to 0.1 units per kilogram of body weight) should be employed. After adequate hypoglycemia, the peak plasma cortisol should be greater than 500 nmol/L (19 μg/dL), although other criteria have been suggested. Since the metyrapone test can precipitate acute adrenal insufficiency in patients with low basal cortisol secretory rates, it should always be performed in the hospital setting when the 8 A.M. basal plasma cortisol is less than 230 nmol/L (9 μg/dL). Furthermore, metyrapone administration in most patients should be preceded by a rapid ACTH stimulation test to ensure that the adrenals can respond to ACTH. A normal response to metyrapone administration (see Table 313-5) has been variably defined, but one criterion is an increase of plasma 11-deoxycortisol to greater than 200 nmol/L (7.5 μg/dL) and of the urinary 17-hydroxysteroids to at least twofold over baseline, usually to a value greater than 60 μmol/d (22 mg/d). The plasma cortisol must concomitantly fall to less than 110 nmol/L (4 μg/dL) to ensure that there has been an adequate stimulus for ACTH release if these criteria have not been met. Although ACTH responses to insulin-hypoglycemia and metyrapone have not been well-standardized, a peak ACTH concentration of greater than 40 pmol/L (200 pg/mL) is considered normal.

The rapid ACTH stimulation test (see Table 313-5) may be the safest and most convenient screening test for determining the adequacy of the pituitary-adrenal axis. Since the response of the adrenal gland to exogenous ACTH is dependent upon prior endogenous ACTH exposure, it follows that patients with profound ACTH deficiency will have a deficient adrenal response to exogenous ACTH stimulation. However, the rapid ACTH stimulation test may be normal in some patients with abnormal insulin tolerance tests and therefore may not detect all who are at risk for stress-induced adrenal insufficiency. Thus, whereas an abnormal ACTH stimulation test is indicative of an abnormal pituitary-adrenal axis, a normal response in the rapid ACTH stimulation test [cortisol greater than 500 nmol/L (19 μg/dL)] does not always establish that the pituitary-adrenal axis is normal.

Gonadotropin function is easier to evaluate. In women with regular menses gonadotropin secretion is normal, and gonadotropin measurements are superfluous. Likewise, a man with a normal serum testosterone and normal spermatogenesis need not have gonadotropins measured. In postmenopausal women gonadotropin levels are elevated (an endogenous stimulation test); ''normal'' levels suggest gonadotropin deficiency. Estrogen deficiency in women and testosterone deficiency in men in the absence of elevated gonadotropins imply gonadotropin deficiency.

To diagnose central hypothyroidism (thyrotropin deficiency), the serum T_4 and free T_4 (or T_3 resin uptake and free T_4 index) should first be measured. If these are in the midnormal range, TSH function is likely to be normal. If T_4 and free T_4 are low and the serum TSH is not elevated, central hypothyroidism is present. Minimal TSH elevation (with bioinactive TSH) can occur in hypothalamic hypothyroidism. Mild central hypothyroidism, a consideration in patients with known pituitary disease who have low-normal T_4 and free T_4 concentrations, remains a clinical diagnosis. Before considering the diagnosis of isolated TSH deficiency in patients with the biochemical features of central hypothyroidism without evidence of other pituitary hormone deficiency, it is important to exclude the thyroxine-binding globulin (TBG) deficiency syndrome (low T_4, increased T_3 resin uptake, low to low-normal free T_4 index, normal TSH) and the "sick euthyroid" syndrome (low T_4, low free T_4 or free T_4 index, normal TSH) (see Chap. 316).

Several diagnostic tests utilize hypothalamic-releasing hormones to assess pituitary reserve. While these tests are not helpful in assessing the adequacy of anterior pituitary function, they can be useful in certain situations. In patients with isolated gonadotropin deficiency, the gonadotropin response to gonadorelin (synthetic LHRH) may be useful in predicting which patients will respond to therapy with gonadorelin. CRH testing may be useful in the differential diagnosis of Cushing's syndrome but does not indicate whether the pituitary-adrenal axis will respond appropriately to stress. TRH stimulation testing is useful in some patients in supporting the diagnosis of hyperthyroidism or of acromegaly and in those cases in which documentation of prolactin deficiency is necessary to support a diagnosis of more generalized anterior pituitary hormone deficiency (e.g., mild central hypothyroidism). TRH testing is not necessary in the evaluation for central hypothyroidism and is not reliable in separating pituitary from hypothalamic hypothyroidism.

Therapy Multiple hormones must be replaced in patients with panhypopituitarism, but cortisol replacement is most important. We prefer prednisone for matters of convenience and cost, but many physicians use cortisone acetate. Prednisone (5 to 7.5 mg) or cortisone acetate (20 to 37.5 mg) can be given to some patients as a single morning dosage, whereas others require divided doses (two-thirds at 8 A.M., one-third at 3 A.M.). Hypopituitary patients may require lower daily glucocorticoid dosages than do patients with Addison's disease and do not require mineralocorticoid replacement. In stress situations or when preparing these patients for pituitary or other surgery, higher doses of glucocorticoids should be administered (e.g., for major surgery, hydrocortisone hemisuccinate 75 mg IM/IV every 6 h or methyl prednisolone sodium succinate 15 mg IM/IV every 6 h). Levothyroxine is the therapy of choice in central hypothyroidism (0.1 to 0.2 mg/d). Since thyroxine accelerates the degradation of cortisol and can precipitate adrenal crisis in patients with limited pituitary reserve, glucocorticoid replacement should always precede levothyroxine therapy in panhypopituitarism. Hypogonadism in women is treated with estrogen-progestogen combinations and in men with testosterone esters by injection. To achieve fertility gonadotropins must be administered by injection in patients with pituitary disease, whereas gonadorelin may be successful in those with hypothalamic disease. GH deficiency is not treated in adults; in children GH administration usually is required, but GRH injections may be effective in those with hypothalamic disease (see Chap. 314). Diabetes insipidus is treated with nasal desmopressin (usually 0.05 to 0.1 mL twice a day) (see Chap. 315).

RADIOLOGY OF THE PITUITARY Conventional posteroanterior and lateral skull x-rays define the contours of the sella turcica (Fig. 313-10). Abnormalities that may be identified on these films include enlargement, erosions, and calcifications in the region of the sella. CT scanning or magnetic resonance imaging (MRI) is necessary to define further intrapituitary and suprasellar lesions (Fig. 313-11). Angiography is routinely used when an aneurysm or vascular malformation is suspected as the cause of an enlarged sella and is occasionally necessary in patients with large pituitary or hypothalamic tumors. Intrasellar lesions can be visualized with direct coronal CT scanning, often with the aid of intravenous contrast material. High-resolution MRI scanning (sagittal and coronal views) using gadolinium (a paramagnetic MR contrast agent) provides comparable and in some cases superior information and avoids radiation exposure. The suprasellar region can be best visualized on axial CT views; however, the anatomic details of the optic chiasm obtained with MRI scanning make this the procedure of choice for imaging suprasellar pituitary tumors. Pneumoencephalography and metrizamide cisternography have been largely replaced by the newer modalities of CT and MR

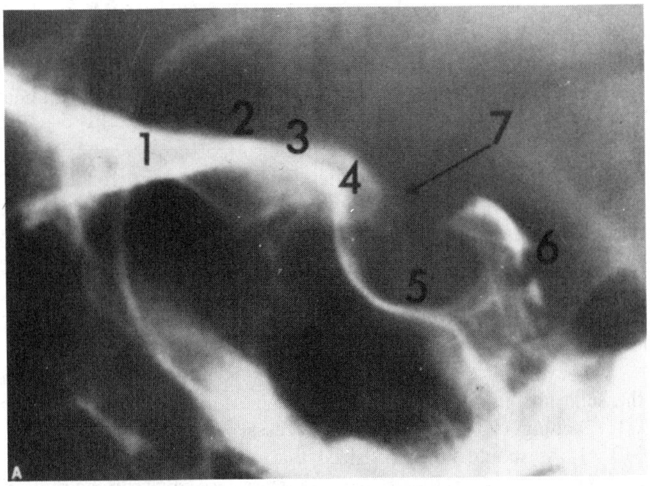

FIGURE 313-10 X-ray of the sella, lateral view. Note (1) planum sphenoidal, (2) limbus sphenoidal, (3) sulcus chiasmaticus, (4) tuberculum sellae, (5) sella floor with distinct lamina dura, (6) dorsum sellae, (7) anterior clinoid, and (8) sphenoid sinus. *(From SM Wolpert in Post et al.)*

FIGURE 313-11 Magnetic resonance imaging (MRI) in patient with a large pituitary adenoma. The arrow points to the adenoma which is seen on axial *(A)*, sagittal *(B)*, and coronal *(C)* views. *(From G Gerard et al, Hosp Pract 19:151, 1984.)*

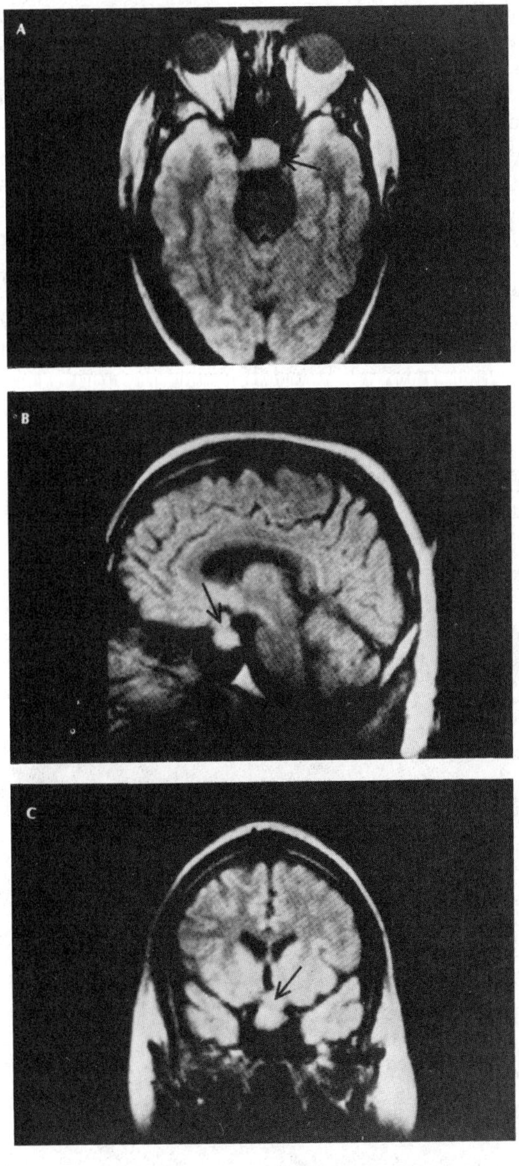

imaging. Sella tomography is not recommended, as it has a high frequency of false-positive and false-negative findings and exposes the lens of the eye to excessive radiation. Frontal tomography may be necessary for details of bony anatomy prior to transsphenoidal surgery.

The volume of the normal sella turcica (233 to 1092 mm^3, mean 594 mm^3) does not change in patients with pituitary microadenomas. With conventional radiography, pituitary microadenomas may be suspected on the basis of focal erosions or blistering of the floor of the sella, but these findings may also be present in normal individuals. Larger microadenomas may cause the floor of the sella to ''tilt'' when viewed in the frontal projection and may create the appearance of a double floor on lateral view (Fig. 313-12).

However, since most microadenomas neither affect the volume of the sella nor produce specific radiographic findings, high-resolution CT scanning or MR imaging is necessary for visualization (Fig. 313-13). It should be emphasized that localization of corticotroph adenomas in patients with Cushing's disease may be helpful in directing the surgical approach. In patients with modest prolactin elevations, however, the purpose of sella imaging is to exclude larger pathologic entities. Whether a microprolactinoma is actually visualized is less important, as this disorder is generally treated medically. On CT or MR images the normal pituitary gland has a height of 3 to 7 mm, although values up to 9 mm can be found in adolescents. The upper aspect is flat, concave, or, in younger patients, convex. The stalk is midline with a maximum diameter of 4 mm in axial sections. After intravenous contrast administration, the normal pituitary shows homogeneous enhancement on CT in 60 percent of patients and heterogeneous enhancement in 40 percent. Up to one-fifth of normal persons show discrete low-density areas on contrast-enhanced CT scanning. In random autopsies, one-fourth of individuals have small pituitary abnormalities (e.g., microadenomas, cysts, metastatic tumors, pituitary infarcts), but it is unclear whether such abnormalities correspond to the focal abnormal areas on CT scanning.

Microadenomas are best demonstrated on direct coronal CT scans taken in 1-mm sections after rapid infusion of contrast material or on sagittal or coronal MR images after intravenous gadolinium. On CT the normal pituitary enhances with contrast, as do the cavernous sinuses. Microadenomas, particularly microprolactinomas, usually appear hypodense with this technique (Fig. 313-13). T1-weighted coronal and sagittal views (MRI) and T2-weighted coronal views show the normal pituitary to be isointense with respect to cerebral white matter. A small, bright, high-intensity area is seen in the posterior sella on T1 images, corresponding to the posterior pituitary. Microadenomas appear as low-intensity focal areas on T1- and high-intensity focal areas on T2-weighted images. Small corticotroph adenomas are particularly difficult to visualize; however, even these can often be seen on MRI if a high-field-strength magnet (1.5 T) and gadolinium are used. The specificity of CT and MR diagnosis of microadenomas is enhanced when upward convexity of the diaphragma sellae, contralateral deviation of the pituitary stalk (Fig. 313-14), and/or bony erosion (CT scan) are also found.

Pituitary macroadenomas generally cause sella enlargement on conventional radiography, with or without bony erosion. However, an enlarged sella is not sufficient to diagnose a pituitary adenoma (see below). Additional findings in plain skull x-rays in patients with acromegaly may include prognathism, enlarged paranasal sinuses, hyperostosis of the external occipital protuberance, increased density of the central bone of the sella, and an enlarged square sella with tapered tuberculum. GH-secreting adenomas may calcify and regress to leave a pituitary calculus or stone. Larger corticotroph adenomas may cause depression of the central floor of the sella.

CT scanning of macroadenomas may reveal enlargement of the sella, a mass in the sella with contrast enhancement of the tumor or its capsule, and obliteration of the suprasellar cistern. An area of decreased density within an enhancing mass is present in about 20 percent of patients (CT) and suggests cystic degeneration of an adenoma. An additional one-fifth of patients with macroadenomas have a partially empty sella with CSF density within the sella (see below). Axial views are preferred if suprasellar extension is clinically

FIGURE 313-12 Lateral view of the sella turcica demonstrating a ''double floor'' due to downward displacement by a pituitary adenoma. Top arrow points to normal floor; bottom arrow points to floor displaced by tumor.

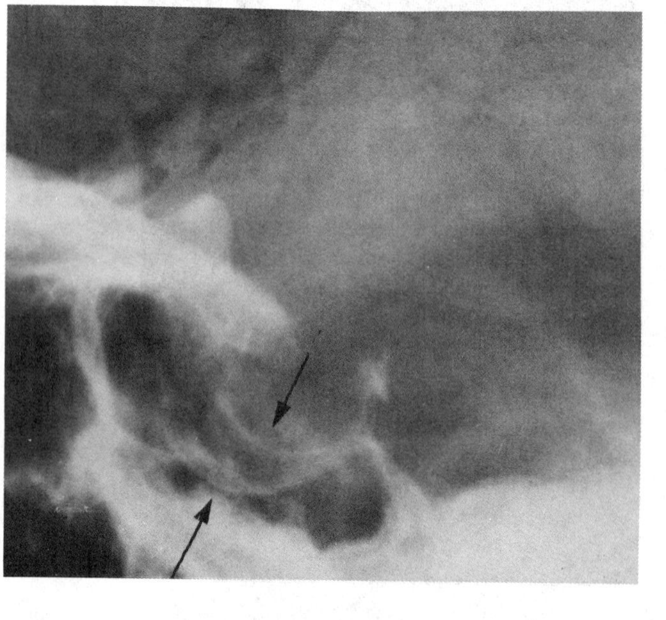

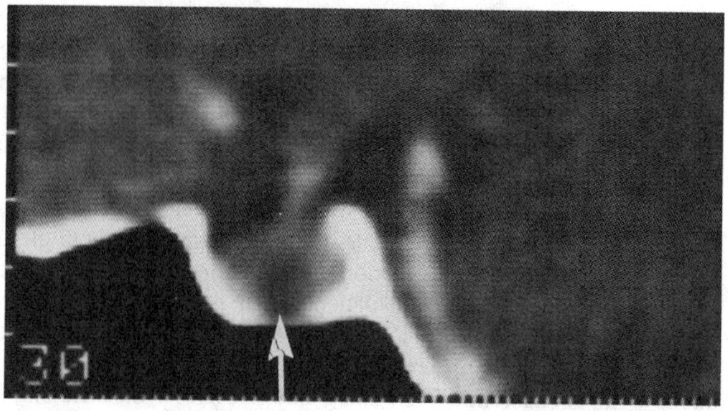

FIGURE 313-13 Sagittal CT scan of sella in patient with small microprolactinoma. The tumor has decreased density, and minimal erosion of the sella floor is demonstrated. Arrow points to tumor.

FIGURE 313-14 Coronal CT scan demonstrating 1.3-cm macroprolactinoma in a 30-year-old woman. Note decreased density of the tumor (arrow). The pituitary stalk is displaced to the left, and the floor of the sella slopes to the left as well.

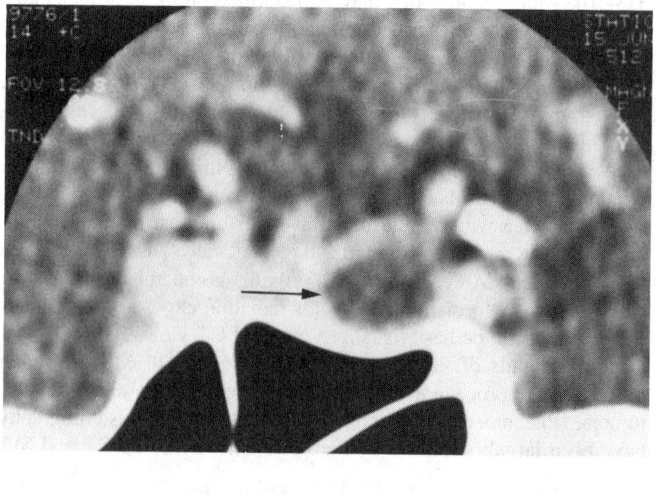

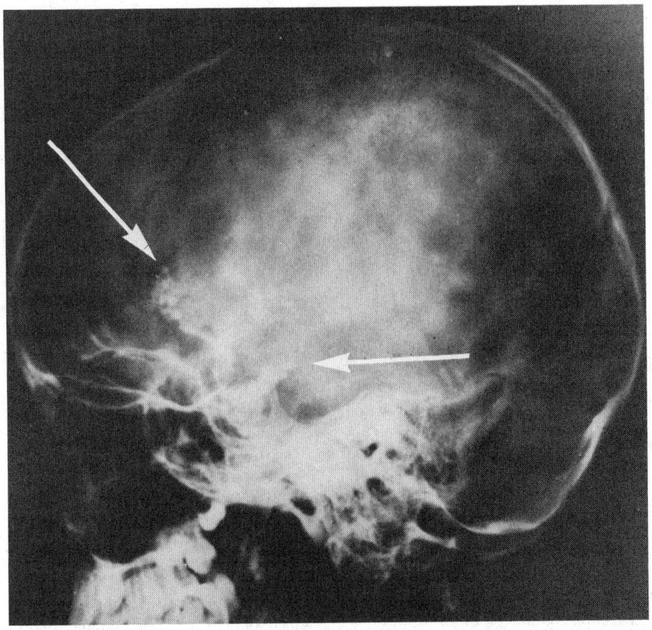

FIGURE 313-15 Lateral skull x-ray in a patient with a craniopharyngioma. Note dense calcification in suprasellar region (arrow).

suspected. On MRI, the adenomas are generally isointense on T1-weighted images and moderately hyperintense on T2-weighted images. Larger invasive tumors may extend into the cavernous sinus, sphenoid sinus, or any of the cranial fossae. Cavernous sinus invasion may be difficult to diagnose on CT and MRI; however, the flow void of the carotid artery on MRI does delineate tumors that surround the artery. Pituitary hyperplasia (e.g., thyrotroph hyperplasia in primary hypothyroidism or lactotroph hyperplasia during pregnancy) appears on CT as a full, enlarged sella that does not enhance after contrast administration.

Pituitary apoplexy is caused by a sudden increase in the size of a pituitary macroadenoma due to hemorrhage or infarction. Enlargement of the sella is almost always evident on plain films. In the case of hemorrhage, CT scanning reveals a high-density area within the adenoma during the acute phase and a decreased density, with or without marginal enhancement, as the hematoma is resorbed. With infarction, low-density areas are seen with or without enhancement. Two days after hemorrhage, MR scanning shows a high-intensity signal on T1 and T2 (due to methemoglobin) with some low-intensity signals intermixed (due to hemosiderin).

Craniopharyngiomas can often be suspected on plain skull x-rays on the basis of nodular or curvilinear calcification in the suprasellar region (Fig. 313-15). This calcification is visible in 80 to 90 percent of children but in less than one-half of adults. Although the sella may be enlarged and ballooned, the cortical bone is usually preserved. With intrasellar craniopharyngiomas, the dorsum sella is often displaced backwards. On CT scanning cystic components are present with ring or nodular calcification in most children and 80 percent of adults. The noncystic areas show variable enhancement in children. On MRI craniopharyngiomas may be either slightly hyper- or hypointense on T1 images and markedly hypointense on T2 images. Unfortunately calcification is usually not seen on MRI unless large amounts are present.

Most meningiomas of the sellar region cause abnormalities on routine skull films that include calcifications of the tumor and hyperostosis of the planum sphenoidale or of the chiasmatic sulcus. Meningiomas may also cause sella enlargement and thereby mimic pituitary adenomas. On CT scanning, meningiomas may give the appearance of an aneurysm because of their dense homogeneous enhancement. Angiography may be required to exclude an aneurysm and to delineate the feeding vessels. On MRI, meningiomas have the same intensity as brain on both T1- and T2-weighted images, but the mass effect usually allows the lesion to be seen. While this pattern may allow distinction between a meningioma and an aneurysm, angiography is diagnostic.

Aneurysms in the region of the sella contain concentric calcifications demonstrable on plain skull films in about 30 percent of patients. Aneurysms may cause sella enlargement, usually with lateral depression and erosion of the sella floor; a "double floor" is therefore seen on lateral films. On CT scanning the aneurysm is hyperdense with homogeneous contrast enhancement. Most patients with hyperdense lesions that enlarge the sella need to be studied with digital subtraction or conventional angiography. When aneurysms clot the CT appearance may change: new clots show no enhancement whereas old clots enhance like adenomas. Complete thrombosis of an aneurysm is sometimes indistinguishable by CT criteria from a pituitary adenoma. On MRI, a decreased signal due to flowing blood appears and can often demonstrate an aneurysm. Thrombus in the aneurysm has an MRI appearance similar to that of hemorrhage (see above).

On CT scans enhancing masses of the suprasellar region include optic chiasm or hypothalamic gliomas, metastases to the hypothalamus or pituitary stalk, germinomas, sarcoid granulomas, histiocytosis, aneurysms, and craniopharyngiomas. Nonenhancing suprasellar masses include dermoid tumors, epidermoid tumors, and arachnoid cysts.

THE ENLARGED SELLA–EMPTY SELLA SYNDROME Enlargement of the sella can be caused by pituitary adenomas, hypothalamic masses and cysts, aneurysms, primary hypothyroidism or hypogonadism, and increased intracranial pressure. It can also occur in patients with the primary empty sella syndrome (Fig. 313-16). In this situation the sella tends to be symmetrically ballooned without bony erosion. The suprasellar subarachnoid space herniates through an incomplete diaphragma sella (Fig. 313-16) so that the sella is filled

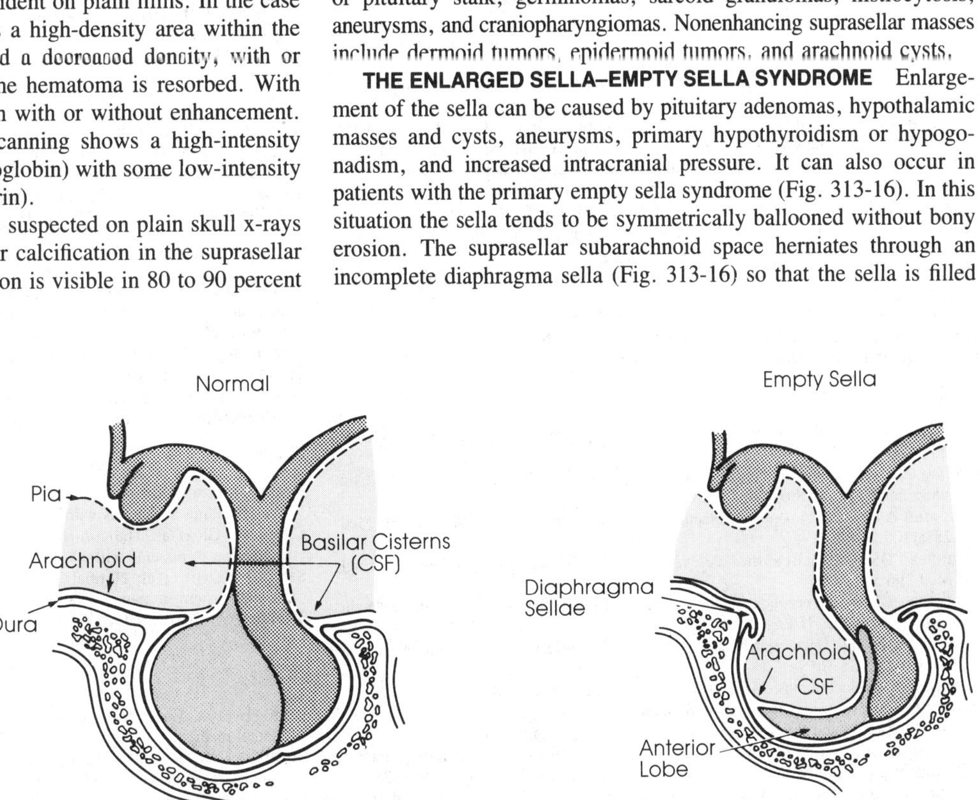

FIGURE 313-16 The findings in patients with the empty sella syndrome. *Left panel* shows the normal anatomic relationships. With the empty sella syndrome *(right panel)* ballooning of the sella results when an arachnoid diverticulum herniates through an incompetent diaphragma sellae. *(After Jordan et al.)*

with CSF within an arachnoid-lined sac. An incomplete diaphragma sella is thought to be a prerequisite. It is not clear whether transient or persistent increased CSF pressure is necessary to produce sella enlargement in these patients, but CSF pressure is generally normal when measured. The pituitary is flattened and pushed to one side but tends to function normally. The fact that the CSF fills the sella can be demonstrated with high-resolution CT scanning, MRI, or metrizamide cisternography.

It is important to differentiate the primary empty sella from the enlarged partially empty sella due to a degenerated pituitary adenoma. In the former the pituitary volume is usually normal, in the latter the pituitary volume is generally increased.

Most patients with the primary empty sella syndrome are obese, multiparous women with headaches; about 30 percent have hypertension. It is of interest that multiparity, obesity, and hypertension are associated with increases in CSF pressure. Selection bias cannot be excluded in case reports since skull x-rays may be obtained in patients with headaches, which in turn uncovers the enlarged sella. Endocrine symptoms are uncommon. Hyperprolactinemia occurs on occasion, possibly due to stalk stretching or coincidental microprolactinomas. GH secretory reserve is often abnormal in these patients, probably the result of obesity. Spontaneous CSF rhinorrhea and pseudotumor cerebri have each been reported in about 10 percent of the cases, but this may represent a bias of ascertainment. CSF rhinorrhea often requires surgical correction. Visual field defects have been reported and are thought to be caused by herniation of the optic chiasm into the sella turcica. Once the diagnosis of the empty sella syndrome has been established by CT scan, MRI, or metrizamide cisternography, further diagnostic studies are superfluous, and the therapy is reassurance.

REFERENCES

General

Abbound CF, Laws ER (Jr): Diagnosis of pituitary tumors. Endocrinol Metab Clin North Am 17:241, 1988

Besser GM: The hypothalamus and pituitary. Clin Endocrinol Metab 6:1, 1977

Black PMcL et al: *Secretory Tumors of the Pituitary Gland*. New York, Raven Press, 1984

Burrow GN et al: Microadenomas of the pituitary and abnormal sellar tomograms in an unselected autopsy series. N Engl J Med 304:156, 1981

Daniel PM, Prichard MML: The human hypothalamus and pituitary stalk after hypophysectomy or pituitary stalk section. Brain 59:813, 1972

Hollenhorst RW, Younge BR: Ocular manifestations produced by adenoma of the pituitary gland. Analysis of 1000 cases, in *Diagnosis and Treatment of Pituitary Tumors*, PO Kohler, GT Ross (eds). Amsterdam, Excerpta Medica, 1973, p 53

Imura H (ed): *The Pituitary Gland*. New York, Raven Press, 1985

Krieger DT, Martin JB: Brain peptides. N Engl J Med 304:876, 1981

Martin JB, Reichlin S: *Clinical Neuroendocrinology*, 2d ed. Philadelphia, Davis, 1987

Molitch ME (ed): Pituitary tumors: Diagnosis and management. Endocrinol Metab Clin North Am 16:3, 1987

Post KD et al (eds): *The Pituitary Adenoma*. New York, Plenum, 1980

Scanlon ME: Neuroendocrinology. Clin Endocrinol Metab 12:467, 1983

Vance ML et al: Bromocriptine. Ann Intern Med 100:78, 1984

Prolactin

Carter JN et al: Prolactin secreting tumors and hypogonadism in 22 men. N Engl J Med 299:847, 1978

Ferrari C et al: Functional characterization of hypothalamic hyperprolactinemia. J Clin Endocrinol Metab 55:897, 1982

Grossman A et al: Treatment of prolactinomas with megavoltage radiotherapy. Br Med J 288:1105, 1984

Kleinberg DS et al: Galactorrhea: 235 cases including 48 with pituitary tumor. N Engl J Med 296:589, 1977

Kleinberg DL et al: Pergolide for the treatment of pituitary tumors secreting prolactin or growth hormone. N Engl J Med 309:704, 1983

Klibanski A et al: Decreased bone density in hyperprolactinemic women. N Engl J Med 303:1511, 1980

Lawton NF: Prolactinomas: Medical or surgical treatment? Q J Med 243:577, 1987

Molitch ME: Hyperprolactinemia. Med Grand Rounds 1:307, 1982

———: Pregnancy and the hyperprolactinemic woman. N Engl J Med 321:1364, 1985

——— et al: Bromocriptine as primary therapy for prolactin-secreting macroadenomas: Results of a prospective multicenter study. J Clin Endocrinol Metab 60:698, 1985

Moriondo P et al: Bromocriptine treatment of microprolactinomas: Evidence of stable prolactin decrease after drug withdrawal. J Clin Endocrinol Metab 60:764, 1985

Schlecte J et al: Prolactin-secreting pituitary tumors in ammenorrheic women: A comprehensive study. Endocr Rev 1:294, 1980

Growth hormone

Asa SL et al: A case for hypothalamic acromegaly: A clinicopathological study of six patients with hypothalamic gangliocytomas producing growth hormone–releasing factor. J Clin Endocrinol Metab 58:796, 1984

Barkan AL et al: Treatment of acromegaly with the long-acting somatostatin analog SMS 201-995. J Clin Endocrinol Metab 66:16, 1988

——— et al: Preoperative treatment of acromegaly with long-acting somatostatin analog SMS 201-959: Shrinkage of invasive pituitary macroadenomas and improved surgical remission rate. J Clin Endocrinol Metab 67:1040, 1988

Clemmons DR et al: Evaluation of acromegaly by radioimmunoassay of somatomedin-C. N Engl J Med 301:1138, 1979

Eastman RC et al: Conventional supervoltage irradiation is an effective treatment for acromegaly. J Clin Endocrinol Metab 48:931, 1979

Eddy RL et al: Human growth hormone release: Comparison of provocative test procedures. Am J Med 56:179, 1974

Frohman LA, Jansson J-O: Growth hormone–releasing hormone. Endocrinol Rev 7:223, 1986

Gelato MC et al: Effects of a growth hormone releasing factor in man. J Clin Endocrinol Metab 57:674, 1983

——— et al: Effects of growth hormone-releasing factor on growth hormone secretion in acromegaly. J Clin Endocrinol Metab 60:251, 1985

Grossman A et al: Growth hormone releasing factor: Comparison of two analogues and demonstration of hypothalamic defect in growth hormone release after radiotherapy. Br Med J 288:1785, 1984

Lamberts SWJ: The role of somastostatin in the regulation of anterior pituitary hormone secretion and the use of its analogs in the treatment of human pituitary tumors. Endocr Rev 9:417, 1988

Lawrence JH et al: Successful treatment of acromegaly. Metabolic and clinical studies in 145 patients. J Clin Endocrinol Metab 31:180, 1970

Martin JB: Neural regulation of growth hormone secretion. N Engl J Med 288:1384, 1973

Melmed S et al: Pathophysiology of acromegaly. Endocr Rev 4:271, 1983

——— et al: Acromegaly due to secretion of growth hormone by an ectopic pancreatic islet-cell tumor. N Engl J. Med 312:9, 1985

Moses AC et al: Bromocriptine therapy in acromegaly. Use in patients resistant to conventional therapy and effect on serum levels of somatomedin C. J Clin Endocrinol Metab 53:752, 1981

Nabarro JDN: Acromegaly. Clin Endocrinol 26:481, 1987

Phillips LS, Vasilopoulou-Sellin R: Somatomedins. N Engl J Med 302:371, 1980

Reichlin S: Acromegaly. Med Grand Rounds 1:9, 1982

———: Somatostatin. N Engl J Med 309:1495, 1983

Sano T et al: Growth hormone–releasing hormone-producing tumors: Clinical, biochemical and morphological manifestations. Endocr Rev 9:357, 1988

Thorner MO et al: Somatotroph hyperplasia: Successful treatment of acromegaly by removal of a pancreatic islet tumor secreting a growth hormone releasing factor. J Clin Invest 70:965, 1982

——— et al: Extrahypothalamic growth-hormone-releasing factor (GRF) secretion is a rare cause of acromegaly: Plasma GRF levels in 177 acromegalic patients. J Clin Endocrinol Metab 59:846, 1984

Wright AD et al: Mortality in acromegaly. Q J Med 39:1, 1970

TSH

Beck-Peccoz P et al: Decreased receptor binding of biologically inactive thyrotropin in central hypothyroidism. Effect of treatment with thyrotropin-releasing hormone. N Engl J Med 312:1085, 1985

Bigos ST et al: Spectrum of pituitary alterations with mild and severe thyroid impairment. J Clin Endocrinol Metab 46:317, 1978

Gonadotropins

Cutler GB Jr: Therapeutic applications of luteinizing-hormone-releasing hormone and its analogs. Ann Intern Med 102:643, 1985

Marshall JC, Kelch RP: Gonadotropin-releasing hormone: Role of pulsatile secretion in the regulation of reproduction. N Engl J Med 313:1459, 1986

Snyder PJ: Gonadotroph cell adenomas of the pituitary. Endocr Rev 6:552, 1985

——— et al: Secretion of uncombined subunits of luteinizing hormone by gonadotroph cell adenomas. J Clin Endocrinol Metab 59:1169, 1984

ACTH

Borst GC et al: Discordant cortisol response to exogenous ACTH and insulin-induced hypoglycemia in patients with pituitary disease. N Engl J Med 306:1462, 1982

Chrousos GP et al: The corticotropin-releasing factor stimulation test: An aid in the evaluation of patients with Cushing's syndrome. N Engl J Med 310:622, 1984

Streeten DHP et al: Normal and abnormal function of the hypothalamic-pituitary-adrenal system in man. Endocr Rev 5:371, 1984

Taylor AL, Fishman LM: Corticotropin-releasing hormone. N Engl J Med 319:213, 1988

Endorphins

Imura H et al: Endogenous opioids and related peptides: From molecular biology to clinical medicine. J Endocrinol 107:147, 1985

Lundblad JR, Roberts JL: Regulation of proopiomelanocortin gene expression in pituitary. Endocr Rev 9:135, 1988

Marin WR: Pharmacology of opioids. Pharmacol Rev 35:283, 1984

Pfeiffer A, Herz A: Endocrine actions of opioids. Horm Metabol Res 16:386, 1984

Alpha Subunits

Klibanski A et al: Pure alpha subunit-secreting pituitary tumors. J Neurosurg 59:585, 1983

Hypothalamus

Bray GA, Gallagher TFJ: Manifestations of hypothalamic obesity in man: A comprehensive investigation of eight patients and a review of the literature. Medicine 54:301, 1974

Dinarello CA: Interleukin-1 and the pathogenesis of the acute phase response. N Engl J Med 54:301, 1984

———, Wolff SM: Molecular basis of fever in humans. Am J Med 72:799, 1982

Plum F, Van Uitert R: Nonendocrine diseases and disorders of the hypothalamus, in *The Hypothalamus*, S Reichlin et al (eds). New York, Raven Press, 1978, pp 415–473

Craniopharyngiomas

Banna M: Craniopharyngiomas in adults. Surg Neurol 1:202, 1973

———: Craniopharyngioma: Based on 160 cases. Br J Radiol 49:206, 1976

Hypopituitarism

Abboud CF: Laboratory diagnosis of hypopituitarism. Mayo Clin Proc 61:35, 1986

Arafah BM: Reversible hypopituitarism in patients with large nonfunctioning pituitary adenomas. J Clin Endocrinol Metab 62:1173, 1986

Asa SL et al: Lymphocytic hypophysitis of pregnancy resulting in hypopituitarism: A distinct clinicopathologic entity. Ann Intern Med 95:166, 1981

Edwards OM, Clark JDA: Post-traumatic hypopituitarism. Medicine 65:281, 1986

Veldhuis JD, Hammond JM: Endocrine function after spontaneous infarction of the human pituitary: Report, review, and reappraisal. Endocr Rev 1:100, 1980

Radiology

Bruneton JN et al: Normal variants of the sella turcica. Radiology 131:99, 1979

Heminghy S et al: Computed tomographic study of hormone-secreting microadenomas. Radiology 146:65, 1983

Jordan RM et al: The primary empty sella syndrome. Analysis of the clinical characteristics, radiographic features, pituitary function, and cerebrospinal fluid adenohypophysial hormone concentrations. Am J Med 62:569, 1977

Kucharczyk W et al: Pituitary adenomas: High-resolution MR imaging at 1.5 T. Radiology 161:761, 1986

Wolpert SM: The radiology of pituitary adenomas. Endocrinol Metab Clin North Am 16:553, 1987

314 DISORDERS OF GROWTH

RAYMOND L. HINTZ

NORMAL GROWTH Children may grow rapidly over relatively short periods of time, and the physician must be aware of normal standards for growth and development as a function of age. A record of these changes can be utilized as a sensitive indicator of general health. Minimal aberrations in health may initially be reflected in a deviation from the normal growth rate; conversely, an actively growing child seldom has a serious systemic disease. Thus, height and growth rate provide important information.

Both longitudinal and cross-sectional studies indicate that differences exist in growth among different ethnic groups. However, normal well-nourished children have remarkably similar growth patterns. For example, the average length of children, which at birth is about 50 cm, increases by about 25 cm in the first year of life, 12.5 cm in the second year, and 6.2 cm per year thereafter until puberty. This formula can be used to estimate average height up to about 10 years of age. Nomograms have been constructed to give a more accurate picture of average growth and the range of normal deviations from the mean (Figs. 314-1 and 314-2).

CONTROL OF GROWTH Growth involves both an increase in the total number of cells and the synthesis of macromolecules by individual cells. The relative importance of these processes varies from organ to organ and with age. The control and integration of growth also vary among tissues and with the stage of development.

Prenatal growth Prenatal development exemplifies the complexities of the integration and control of growth. During this time, a

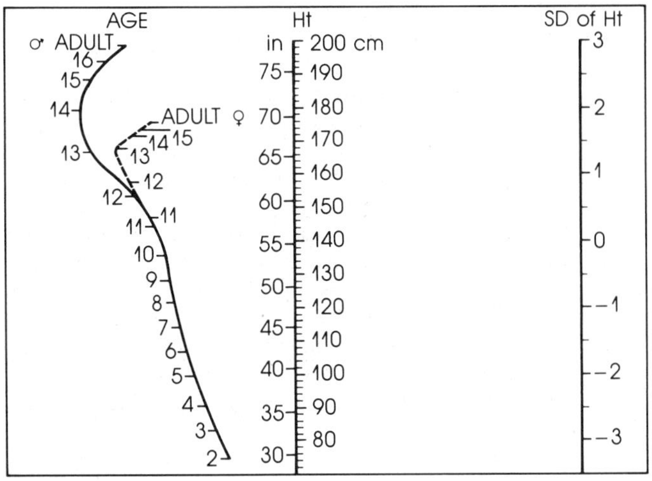

FIGURE 314-1 Nomogram for height of boys and girls.

single cell becomes a complex organism with billions of cells working in harmonious concert. The growth rate is astounding; the most rapid growth rate occurs during the second trimester. Prenatal growth may have different control mechanisms from those in the postnatal period. Growth hormone and thyroid hormone have relatively minor effects on growth during prenatal life. Prenatal growth rates are dependent on uterine blood flow and other maternal influences and are less dependent on the factors that determine ultimate stature. At birth the correlation between body length and adult height is weak ($r = 0.3$); by 2 years of age the correlation between body length and adult height is stronger ($r = 0.7$), indicating that the factors influencing adult stature begin operating early in postnatal life.

Genetic factors Stature is a polygenic trait (see Chap. 5), so that there is no simple method of predicting on the basis of genetic factors the adult height of any given child. However, on average there is a correlation between the mean height of parents and the mean height attained by their children.

Nutrition The next most important factor affecting growth is nutrition. Severe nutritional deprivation, as in marasmus or kwashiorkor (see Chap. 71), impairs growth. Selective deficiencies of vitamins and minerals, such as vitamin D, and subclinical deficiencies of nutrients may also retard growth. The trend toward increased adult stature in several countries over the last century may be due to improvement in diet, especially to an increase in protein intake during the growth period.

Hormones GROWTH HORMONE Growth hormone (GH, or somatotropin) plays the central role in the modulation of growth of children from birth until the completion of puberty. In the total

FIGURE 314-2 Nomogram for growth rate in boys and girls.

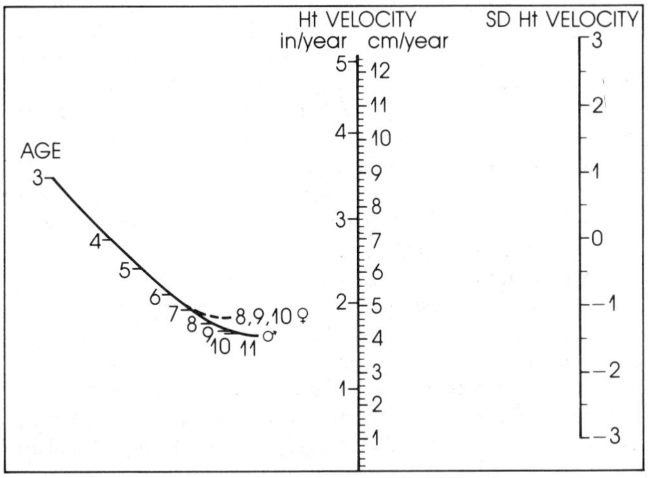

absence of GH, linear growth occurs at about half to a third the normal rate. GH may also play a role in the control of body anabolism throughout life.

GH is a member of a family of hormones that includes pituitary prolactin and human placental lactogen (hPL) (see Chap. 313). The most common form of GH in the pituitary and in the circulation is the 22,000-dalton ("22K") form. This is the hormone that was purified and sequenced from human pituitary glands. The second most common form is a 20,000-dalton ("20K") form. This variant is coded by the same gene sequence as the 22K growth hormone, but a segment of an exon (expressed part of the gene) in the growth hormone gene is not transcribed, thus resulting in a shorter hormone. Whether this variant fulfills some important metabolic function is not clear; the 20K form seems to have equivalent growth-promoting activity but may have a lesser effect on carbohydrate function than the 22K form.

GH secretion is under both positive and negative hypothalamic control (see Chap. 313). The somatotropin release–inhibiting factor (somatostatin, SRIF) is a 14-amino-acid peptide that is widely distributed in tissues outside the hypothalamus and is a potent inhibitor of the secretion of other hormones including insulin, glucagon, and gastrin.

The biologic action of GH-releasing hormone (GRH, somatocrinin) is contained in the first 29 amino acids of the 44-amino-acid peptide, and the aminoterminal amino acid is crucial for its biologic action. Patients with idiopathic GH deficiency may have a deficiency of GRH rather than an inability to make GH in the pituitary. Indeed, half or more of subjects with GH deficiency respond to prolonged pulsatile administration of GRH with an increase in plasma GH and with an accelerated growth rate.

The secretion of somatostatin and GRH, and hence the release of GH, is under the influence of several factors (Fig. 314-3). Higher centers in the central nervous system have synapses that terminate on hypothalamic cells that secrete somatostatin and GRH and exert both positive and negative influences. In addition, both GH and the GH-controlled somatomedin peptides influence the secretion or action of GRH and somatostatin. The secretion of GH is episodic with a relatively short (10- to 15-min) half-life in plasma. A significant proportion of GH in serum is bound to a binding protein that is structurally related to the GH receptor. Although small amounts of GH are secreted during waking periods, the major secretion of GH occurs during sleep, especially in association with third- and fourth-stage sleep.

THE SOMATOMEDINS Although GH may exert some direct effects on growth, the majority of its growth-promoting actions are mediated by the insulin-like growth factor or somatomedin peptides. Two IGF peptides from human plasma, IGF-I and IGF-II, have about 50 percent homology to the structure of human insulin and 70 percent homology to each other. Somatomedin C (SM-C) and IGF-I are structurally and functionally equivalent. The IGF peptides are bound tightly to specific plasma proteins and have half-lives of hours rather than minutes. IGF levels are dependent on GH secretion and are consequently high in acromegaly and low in hypopituitarism. In addition, the normal values are age-dependent, with low levels in early childhood, a peak during adolescence, and a decline in average values after the age of 50 years. The plasma levels of IGF-II are also dependent on the presence of a minimal amount of GH, but pathologic increases in GH do not result in a further increase in IGF-II. Thus, the values of IGF-II are low in hypopituitarism but are not elevated in acromegaly. The average levels of IGF-II are constant from 1 year of age to beyond the eighth decade of life.

THYROID HORMONE Unlike the pattern of growth seen with GH deficiency, the total absence of thyroid hormone leads to an almost complete cessation of linear growth. Thus, adequate thyroid hormone appears to be an absolute prerequisite for normal growth. There are several potential mechanisms for this phenomenon. Thyroid hormones exert direct effects on cell metabolism, and thyroid hormone deficiency results in diminished GH secretion in response to stimulation. Finally, the action of IGF-I on cartilage cells may be dependent on thyroid hormone.

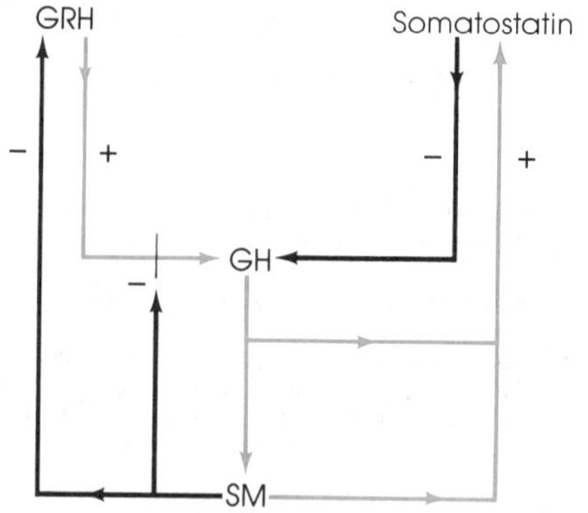

FIGURE 314-3 Feedback control of growth hormone secretion. GH = growth hormone; GRH = growth hormone–releasing hormone; SM = somatomedin. Stimulating influences are shown by arrows in color. Inhibitory influences are shown in black.

GONADAL STEROIDS Androgens and estrogens exert their major role in the stimulation of growth at the time of puberty. Much of the pubertal growth spurt is due to these hormones. Androgens have a direct stimulatory effect on the growth and maturation of bone, cartilage, and muscle. Estrogens appear to have a biphasic action, stimulating growth at low levels and inhibiting growth at high levels.

INSULIN Insulin has strong anabolic actions separate from its effects on carbohydrate metabolism. These actions include stimulation of protein synthesis and cell division. The excessive growth of some infants of diabetic mothers may be the consequence of high levels of plasma insulin in the fetus. The close structural relationship of insulin to the IGF group of growth factors and the ability of insulin to bind to the IGF-I receptor may explain some of these actions of insulin at high levels. However, insulin may also have growth-stimulating actions of its own at low levels in some cell types. The role of insulin in the control of normal growth is still unclear.

OTHER FACTORS Nerve growth factor which is structurally related to the insulin-IGF-I/SM-C family of peptides has actions on the development of sympathetic neurons and possibly on the maintenance and repair of other neurons. Epidermal growth factor has potent actions on the maturation of epidermal features but also acts on other cell types. Platelet-derived growth factor is released from platelets upon clotting and is also a potent mitogen in many cell culture systems. The plasma levels, control mechanisms, interactions with other growth-stimulating hormones, and physiologic roles of these growth factors remain to be elucidated.

DIAGNOSIS OF GROWTH DISORDERS Most individuals with short stature do not have a disease in the usual sense but exhibit some variation from the normal growth pattern (Table 314-1). Thus, the first step in dealing with growth disorders is to identify those individuals who have a normal variation in stature and who presumably do not require treatment.

Height and growth rate One of the most important factors in the differential diagnosis of short stature is the determination of the height percentile of the patient, derived by a comparison to others of

TABLE 314-1 Causes of short stature

Diagnosis	Usual practice, %	Referral center, %
Constitutional growth delay	98	80
GH deficiency	0.1	10
Hypothyroidism	0.2	4
Systemic disease	0.3	3
Chromosomal disorders	0.1	1
Bone-cartilage dysplasia	0.3	1
Psychosocial disorders	1	1

SOURCE: Modified from Horner et al, 1978.

his or her age (Fig. 314-1). A straightedge is placed on the patient's age and present height. The intercept on the right-hand scale estimates the number of standard deviations (SD) from the mean height for age. In general, the further away the patient is from the mean height for age, the more likely a disease is present. A height above the −2-SD level indicates that the patient is likely normal. The patient's growth rate also should be determined, if possible, either from existing growth data or by observation (Fig. 314-2).

Because of the large number of normal children with short stature, clinical judgment plays a large role in the approach to this problem. Individuals with severe short stature (> −3 SD for age) should undergo immediate evaluation, while those with less severe short stature may be serially observed so that the growth rate can be assessed. A consistently low growth rate should lead to further investigation. The diagnosis of constitutional delay is one of exclusion. In general, if the physician has excluded hypothyroidism, GH deficiency, and the more common systemic diseases, it is reasonable to observe the patient. However, the boundaries between "normal" and "disease" may be blurred, and the indications for treatment may change. Furthermore, continued failure to maintain a normal growth rate is an indication for reinvestigation.

History Important features in the history include the weight and gestational age at birth, growth and development in early infancy, and presence of systemic disease. It is also crucial to assess the stature of the parents and first- and second-degree relatives and to review the growth and pubertal development patterns of parents, siblings, and other relatives. A family history of late pubertal development may be helpful diagnostically.

Physical examination The body proportions must be evaluated. Relatively short limbs compared to the trunk suggest either long-standing hypothyroidism or one of the chondrodystrophies. Achondroplastic dwarfism is an extreme example of this, but more subtle forms of chondrodystrophy may elude the casual examination. It is also important to note the height-to-weight ratio. A short child who is underweight for height may have malnutrition or systemic disease. On the other hand, a child who is short but overweight is more likely to have endocrine disease. Patients with Cushing's syndrome, GH deficiency, or hypothyroidism are frequently relatively overweight for their height. Specific physical findings may suggest hypothyroidism, GH deficiency, or other specific syndromes (Table 314-2).

Laboratory evaluation Laboratory tests may either confirm the clinical impression or reveal unsuspected pathology. Assessment of bone age is useful to indicate possible pathology and to estimate final adult height. Because the manifestations of hypothyroidism may be minimal, a serum thyroxine should be obtained routinely. IGF-I measurements are also useful screening procedures, since most patients with GH deficiency have low values. There are also syndromes of GH resistance, such as Laron dwarfism, that are characterized by low IGF-I levels and high GH levels. Specific chemistries may be ordered to screen for other disease states. Any girl with unexplained short stature should have a chromosomal karyotype. Useful laboratory studies for the evaluation of short stature are summarized in Table 314-3. Abnormalities of these tests should lead to more specific investigations.

TABLE 314-2 Physical findings in syndromes of short stature

Syndrome	Specific physical findings
GH deficiency	Frontal bossing, central obesity, high-pitched voice
Hypothyroidism	Dry skin, coarse hair, immature facies
Cushing's syndrome	Central obesity, striae, hypertension
Gonadal dysgenesis	Webbed neck, multiple pigmented nevi, shield chest, delayed sexual development
Pseudohypoparathyroidism	Moon facies and obesity, short metacarpals, mental retardation
Bone-cartilage dysplasia	Abnormal proportions, macrocephaly
Russell-Silver dwarfism	Small at birth, "pointed" facies, asymmetry

TABLE 314-3 Screening laboratory investigations in short stature

Test or x-ray	Disorder
Serum thyroxine	Hypothyroidism
IGF-I	GH deficiency
Bone age	Constitutional delay, hypothyroidism, GH deficiency
Lateral skull film	Craniopharyngioma or other central nervous system lesion
Serum calcium	Pseudohypoparathyroidism
Serum phosphate	Vitamin D–resistant rickets
Serum bicarbonate	Renal tubular acidosis
Blood urea nitrogen	Renal failure
Complete blood count	Anemia, nutritional disorder
Sedimentation rate	Inflammatory disease of bowel
Chromosomal karyotype	Gonadal dysgenesis or other abnormality

TESTING OF GH SECRETION Because GH secretion is episodic and therefore variable, random measurements of plasma GH are not adequate tests of GH deficiency. Some GH stimulation tests for outpatient screening for GH deficiency are summarized in Table 314-4 (also see Chap. 313). Because of the long half-life of IGF-I, a random measurement of this hormone during the day is an accurate reflection of the mean plasma concentration. If care is taken to use age-related standards, measurement of IGF-I provides a reasonable screen for GH deficiency. Low levels of IGF-I should lead to more extensive evaluation. The other tests listed are indirect and largely nonphysiologic ways of provoking the release of GH. In our clinic, a GH level of 10 μg/L (10 ng/mL) after an exercise or clonidine test is interpreted as a normal response. If that level is not achieved, more definitive testing of GH reserve should be carried out as described in Chap. 313.

TREATMENT WITH GH GH deficiency The only established use of human GH is in the treatment of children who are GH-

TABLE 314-4 Screening tests for assessing GH secretion

1 IGF-I radioimmunoassay

Age-related normals (may vary with method):

Age, years	Range, units/mL
<1	0.17–0.62
1–5	0.14–1.44
6–11	0.50–2.06
12–17	0.78–3.73
18–25	0.92–2.06
26–40	0.70–2.04

2 Exercise test:

Vigorous exercise (running or stairsteps) for 20 min

20-min rest

Samples for measurement of GH by radioimmunoassay at 0, 20, and 40 min from beginning

Normal response: GH greater than or equal to 10 μg/L (10 ng/mL) on any sample

3 Clonidine test:

NPO after midnight

Administration of clonidine by mouth

Body weight, kg	Dose, mg
5 to 15	0.05
15 to 25	0.1
25 to 35	0.15
35 to 50	0.2
>50	0.25

Samples for measurement of GH by radioimmunoassay at 0, 60, and 90 min

Side effects: Postural hypotension and somnolence

Keep patient supine until after postural hypotension is gone

Normal response: Greater than or equal to 10 μg/L (10 ng/mL) on any sample deficient. Only between 1 in 4000 and 1 in 20,000 children have a GH deficiency. About half of these cases are due to idiopathic GH deficiency, and the other half are secondary to tumor and/or radiation therapy. In approximately one-third of the latter cases, only GH is deficient, and in the other two-thirds, there are multiple pituitary hormone deficiencies. If short stature is due to a systemic disease such as renal failure, treatment is directed toward the underlying disease state. Similarly, short stature due to hypothyroidism or cortisol excess is managed by treatment of the primary endocrine disorder. In general, the earlier the disorder is diagnosed and treated, the more successful the growth response will be; if treatment of the underlying disease is delayed until after puberty, little or no improvement in stature can be expected.

Unlike the broad species specificity of peptide hormones such as insulin, GH exhibits limited species specificity. Human GH stimulates linear growth in children with GH deficiency, whereas the bovine hormone is ineffective in humans. The collection of pituitary glands from autopsy material for the preparation of human GH did not supply adequate amounts of hormone for the treatment of all children who had GH deficiency, let alone provide sufficient material for the study of GH as a therapeutic agent for other conditions. Furthermore, the distribution of human pituitary GH in the United States and several other countries was discontinued in 1984 because of the development of Creutzfeldt-Jakob disease in four subjects who had been treated with human GH. The availability since 1985 of synthetic GH produced by recombinant DNA in bacteria has relieved the supply problem. Hormone is again available for patients with GH deficiency, and its relatively unlimited supply has allowed exploration of other therapeutic uses of GH, including the treatment of gonadal dysgenesis.

Most children with GH deficiency respond to GH treatment with an acceleration of growth rate to normal or even above normal rates. As with other peptide hormones, there is a dose-response curve to GH. The doses that have been tested range from 0.02 to 0.2 units (0.01 to 0.1 mg) per kilogram of body weight administered as an intramuscular injection three times a week. There is a wide variation in response, but the higher dosages in general result in higher average growth rates. It is possible that in selected clinical circumstances dosages of GH higher than those currently recommended should be administered. Treatment may be started at 0.06 or 0.1 units/kg body weight dosage. The majority of GH-deficient patients have a good growth response to this amount of GH. Daily subcutaneous injection of GH may be preferable; a starting dose of 0.025 or 0.05 units/kg body weight is used for daily therapy. If the patient fails to show an adequate growth rate, the dose can be increased until an adequate growth response is obtained or until the upper limit of 0.75 units/kg body weight per week is achieved. As doses of GH are increased above this level, the risk of glucose intolerance increases, particularly in children who are prediabetic.

An alternative method under study for the treatment of GH deficiency is the use of long-term, subcutaneous infusion of GH-releasing hormone (GRH). Since at least half of children with GH deficiency are able to secrete GH in response to GRH, this approach may ultimately be useful for those patients.

Short stature of other causes IDIOPATHIC SEVERE SHORT STATURE Growth hormone has been used for some patients with growth failure not due to GH deficiency. Many children with severe short stature (more than 2.5 SD below the mean for age) do not have GH deficiency. Some workers propose that a subgroup of children without GH deficiency but with low IGF-I levels are responsive to GH treatment. These patients are believed to have a relatively inactive GH or to have a partial defect in the control of GH secretion. For example, although they do not fulfill the usual criteria for GH deficiency, they may not have normal bursts of GH secretion during certain physiologic circumstances such as sleep. Whatever the etiology, some of these children have a short-term increase in growth rate in response to GH therapy; whether the final height of these children after GH treatment is greater than their predicted height is not established. Furthermore, it is not known whether there are serious side effects associated with the rise of GH levels to the supraphysiologic range.

GONADAL DYSGENESIS GH may also have a therapeutic role in the treatment of gonadal dysgenesis (see Chap. 7). The majority of women with gonadal dysgenesis have an average adult height between 135 and 142 cm. Androgens can cause a short-term increase in the rate of growth of girls with the disorder but do not result in an increase in final adult stature. The use of GH at modest doses is also associated with a small increase in the rate of growth. Results of a multicenter group study utilizing synthetic GH either alone or in combination with androgens are encouraging in terms of initial growth response. It is not known whether GH therapy results in an increase in adult stature, although predicted heights do increase.

SKELETAL DISORDERS Growth hormone has also been used to treat small numbers of subjects with a wide variety of other growth disorders including bone-cartilage dysplasias and other genetic syndromes associated with short stature. It is not clear whether GH is of use in any of these disorders.

REFERENCES

BROWN P: Potential epidemic of Creutzfeldt-Jacob disease from human growth hormone therapy. N Engl J Med 313:728, 1985

FRASIER SD: A review of growth hormone stimulation tests in children. Pediatrics 53:929, 1974

——— et al: A dose response curve for human growth hormone. J Clin Endocrinol Metab 53:1213, 1981

FURLANETTO R et al: Estimation of somatomedin-C levels in normals and patients with pituitary disease by radioimmunoassay. J Clin Invest 60:648, 1977

GERTNER J et al: Prospective clinical trial of human growth hormone in short children without growth hormone deficiency. J Pediatr 104:172, 1984

GRUMBACH M: Growth hormone therapy and the short end of the stick. N Engl J Med 319:238, 1988

HINDMARSH PC, BROOK CGD: Effect of growth hormone in normal short children. Br Med J 295:573, 1987

HINTZ RL: The somatomedins. Adv Pediatr 28:293, 1980

——— et al: Biosynthetic methionyl-human growth hormone is biologically active in adult man. Lancet 1:1276, 1982

HORNER JM et al: Growth deceleration patterns in children with constitutional short stature: An aid to diagnosis. Pediatrics 62:529, 1978

KASTRUP KW et al: Increased growth rate following transfer to daily sc administration from three weekly im injections of hGH. Acta Endocrinol (Copenh) 104:148, 1983

LANTOS J et al: Ethical issues on growth hormone therapy. JAMA 261:1020, 1989

LEWIS UJ et al: Human growth hormone: A complex of proteins. Recent Prog Horm Res 36: 477, 1980

RINDERKNECHT R, HUMBEL RE: Primary structure of human IGF-II. FEBS Lett 89:283, 1978

ROSENFELD RG et al: Three-year results of a randomized prospective trial of methionyl human growth hormone and oxandrolone in Turner's syndrome. J Pediatr 113:393, 1988

TANNER JM, ISREALSOHN WJ: Parent-child correlations for body measurements of children between the ages of one month and 7 years. Ann Hum Genet 26:245, 1963

——— et al: Effect of human growth hormone treatment for 1 to 7 years on growth of 100 children with growth hormone deficiency, inherited smallness, Turner's syndrome, and other complaints. Arch Dis Child 46:745, 1971

———, DAVIS PSW: Clinical longitudinal standards for height and height velocity for North American children. J Pediatr 107:317, 1985

THORNER MO et al: Acceleration of growth in two children treated with human growth hormone releasing factor. N Engl J Med 312:4, 1985

VIMPANI OV et al: Prevalence of severe growth hormone deficiency. Br Med J 2:427, 1977

WILSON DM et al: Subcutaneous versus intramuscular growth hormone therapy: Growth and acute somatomedin response. J Pediatr 76:361, 1985

315 DISORDERS OF THE NEUROHYPOPHYSIS

ARNOLD M. MOSES / DAVID H. P. STREETEN

There are two largely independent hypothalamic-neurohypophyseal systems composed of neurons in the supraoptic and paraventricular nuclei, from which axons extend through the pituitary stalk to the posterior pituitary. Hormones (vasopressin and oxytocin), formed within separate ganglion cells, migrate down the axons as part of precursor proteins. They are stored in secretory granules within the nerve terminals in the neurohypophysis and are released by exocytosis into the bloodstream in response to appropriate stimuli. Vasopressin or antidiuretic hormone (AVP or ADH) is predominantly concerned with the control of water conservation, and its release is coordinated with the activity of the thirst center that regulates fluid intake. Oxytocin stimulates uterine contractions and milk ejection.

VASOPRESSIN SYNTHESIS, RELEASE, AND ACTION

SYNTHESIS Vasopressin is synthesized in the magnocellular neurons of the anterior hypothalamus. It is translated as a preprohormone which is altered in the Golgi apparatus to form a prohormone. The prohormone is packaged into neurosecretory vesicles. While the prohormone is being transported to axonal terminals, enzymes generate the active nonapeptide (AVP), a 10,000 molecular weight protein called neurophysin, and a 39-amino acid glycopeptide. All three products are released into the peripheral circulation.

ACTIONS AVP conserves water by concentrating the urine. It binds to its V_2 receptor on the contraluminal surface of the distal tubular epithelium, mainly of the collecting ducts. At this site AVP enhances the hydrosmotic flow of water from the luminal fluid to the medullary interstitium and assists in maintaining constancy of the osmolality and volume of body fluids. High concentrations of AVP acting on V_1 receptors can cause vasoconstriction, as may occur in response to severe hypotension or to infusion of vasopressin for treatment of bleeding esophageal varices.

AVP, perhaps from axons that terminate in the cerebrum, may play a role in learning and memory, and AVP from fibers in the median eminence may influence corticotropin secretion.

NORMAL HORMONE LEVELS AVP concentrations in plasma and urine can be measured by radioimmunoassay. The results may be expressed either as units based on pressor activity in the rat or in terms of weight of purified vasopressin. Arginine vasopressin has a biologic activity of approximately 400 units per milligram (1 mU = 2.5 ng = 2.3 pmol). The neurohypophysis under conditions of random fluid intake contains approximately 8 units or 18 nmol (20 μg) of AVP. Under the same conditions peripheral plasma AVP concentration in ranges from 2.3 to 7.4 pmol/L (2.5 to 8 ng/L). At the latter level and above, urine osmolality is maximal. The AVP concentration of blood fluctuates, with a maximum late at night and in the early morning and a minimum in the early afternoon. Under conditions of normal hydration, healthy subjects release approximately 370 to 1400 pmol (400 to 1500 ng) from the pituitary and excrete 23 to 80 pmol (25 to 90 ng) AVP in urine in 24 h. During 24 to 28 h of dehydration the amount released increases three to five times with consequent increases in plasma and urinary levels.

METABOLISM Inactivation of AVP occurs largely in liver and kidneys, a major mechanism being the cleavage of the terminal glycinamide to produce a biologically inactive substance. Approximately 7 to 10 percent of secreted AVP is excreted in the urine as active hormone.

CONTROL OF AVP RELEASE The release of AVP is influenced by a number of stimuli.

Osmoregulation Under normal conditions AVP release is primarily regulated by osmoreceptors in the hypothalamus. Changes in the concentrations of plasma solutes to which the cellular membrane is impermeable cause alterations in the volume of the osmoreceptor cells, which in turn alter the electric activity of the neurons and control AVP release. Osmotic changes that stimulate release also enhance production of AVP. The servomechanism between effective plasma osmolality and AVP release normally maintains plasma osmolality within a very narrow range. The mean plasma osmolality of normal subjects following a water load of 20 mL per kilogram of body weight is 281.7 mosmol/kg, and the osmolality that initiates AVP release following infusion of hypertonic saline solution into water-loaded subjects is 287.3 mosmol/kg. Thus, the increase in plasma osmolality from full diuresis to the initiation of antidiuresis by hypertonic saline solution is only 5.6 mosmol/kg, or 2 percent.

The infusion of hypertonic saline solution at a constant rate into water-loaded subjects causes a linear rise in plasma osmolality with time. After an interval that depends on the infusion rate and the concentration of the saline solution, there is an abrupt, progressive fall in free water clearance without a significant change in solute or creatinine excretion. We have defined the osmotic threshold for AVP release as the plasma osmolality at the onset of antidiuresis under these conditions. In 73 normal subjects, this occurred at a mean plasma osmolality of 287 mosmol/kg. The osmotic threshold for AVP release may also be determined, with very similar results, by constructing a linear regression line between simultaneously obtained plasma osmolality and either plasma or urine AVP concentration during hypertonic saline infusion and extrapolating the regression line to the x-axis intercept (plasma osmolality).

Volume regulation Decreases in plasma volume, through effects on stretch receptors in the left atrium and perhaps in the pulmonary veins, stimulate the release of AVP by reducing the tonic inhibitory impulses from the left atrium to the hypothalamus. The neural impulses travel via the vagi to the reticular formation of the midbrain and diencephalon and thence to the supraoptic and paraventricular nuclei, where they are integrated with the other stimuli that affect AVP release. Positive pressure breathing, quiet standing, and vasodilatation due to a warm environment may activate this mechanism, which serves to restore plasma volume, even at times overriding osmotic inhibition of AVP release. Following volume contraction, circulating AVP concentrations may reach 10 times the levels induced by hypertonicity. Increased plasma volume inhibits AVP release by the reverse mechanisms, leading to a diuresis and correction of the hypervolemia. Negative pressure breathing, recumbency, lack of gravitational force (as occurs in space travel), submersion in water, and exposure to cold may activate this mechanism.

Baroreceptor regulation Activation of carotid and aortic baroreceptors in response to hypotension causes release of AVP. Hypotension due to blood loss is the most potent stimulus and may at times raise plasma levels of AVP to 2.3 nmol/L (2.5 μg/L). These concentrations of AVP may cause marked vasoconstriction, which probably plays a role in the restoration of blood pressure.

Neural regulation Many neurotransmitters and neuropeptides in the hypothalamus play a role in regulating and modulating the release of AVP. Acetylcholine stimulates AVP release by its nicotinic action on supraoptic neurons. Angiotensin II, histamine, bradykinin, and neuropeptide Y probably stimulate AVP release. Norepinephrine, prostaglandins, and dopamine stimulate or inhibit AVP release, depending on the experimental conditions. Gamma aminobutyric acid appears to act as an inhibitory neurotransmitter; serotonin and substance P are also present in the supraoptic nucleus, but their influence on magnocellular neuron activity is not clear. The regulatory action of opioid peptides on AVP release is unclear with reports indicating stimulation, inhibition, or no effect. Though the roles of these and other transmitters and peptides are still poorly defined, the antidiuretic actions of stress, emesis, and pain, and the diuretic actions of hypnosis, psychological conditioning, and inhalation of carbon dioxide certainly suggest an important influence of higher centers on the release of AVP.

Aging The aging process is associated with enhanced AVP release in response to a rising plasma osmolality and a progressive increase in plasma AVP concentration. These physiologic changes appear to place the older individual under greater risk of developing water retention and hyponatremia, despite a concomitant decline in maximal renal concentrating capacity in response to AVP, which is usually evident and progressive beyond 60 years of age.

Pharmacologic influences Pharmacologic agents that can stimulate AVP release include nicotine, morphine, vincristine, vinblastine, cyclophosphamide, clofibrate, chlorpropamide, and some of the tricyclic anticonvulsants and antidepressants. Ethanol has diuretic properties by inhibiting neurohypophyseal function under a variety of conditions. Some narcotic antagonists also inhibit AVP release. Experimentally chlorpromazine, reserpine, and phenytoin all diminish the loss of AVP from the pituitary and the rise in urinary excretion of AVP that result from water deprivation. In humans, phenytoin and chlorpromazine may inhibit AVP release and produce diuresis.

AVP RESPONSE TO WATER DEPRIVATION AND TO WATER LOAD Water deprivation provides both an osmotic and a volume stimulus to vasopressin release by increasing plasma osmolality and decreasing plasma volume. The maximum urinary osmolality after water deprivation varies, depending on renal medullary osmolality and other intrarenal factors. In response to fluid deprivation for 18 to 24 h, in normal individuals, plasma osmolality rarely rises above 292 mosmol/kg. The resultant stimulation of AVP release increases plasma AVP concentration to 14 to 23 pmol/L (15 to 25 ng/L).

The administration of water lowers plasma osmolality and expands blood volume, inhibiting the release of AVP via both the osmoreceptor and the atrial volume receptor mechanisms. An oral water load of 20 mL/kg in normal adults results in a fall in plasma osmolality to a mean of 281.7 mosmol/kg and causes a maximum diuresis in 1 to $1\frac{1}{2}$ h with free water clearance rising to approximately 12 mL/min and urine osmolality falling to 40 to 60 mosmol/kg. The delay in reaching maximal diuresis is accounted for by the time involved in absorption of water from the gut, in metabolizing previously secreted vasopressin, and in renal recovery from the action of vasopressin.

INTERACTION OF OSMOTIC AND VOLUME INFLUENCES Under conditions of water deprivation and of water loading, volume and osmotic influences act in parallel to influence AVP release. In other circumstances volume and osmotic influences may be competitive, and changes in plasma volume can modify the effects of hypertonic stimuli on AVP release. Osmotic factors ordinarily predominate to maintain plasma osmolality within a narrow range. Larger changes in blood volume, such as those induced by hemorrhage, may blunt and eventually overcome the osmotic influences, and hypotension can activate arterial baroreceptors and exert a powerful stimulus to the elaboration of AVP and override simultaneous inhibiting influences.

RELATION BETWEEN AVP RELEASE AND THIRST-INDUCED WATER INTAKE Under normal conditions there is close coordination between AVP release and thirst, both of which are regulated by small increases and decreases in plasma osmolality. The perception of thirst generally becomes apparent when plasma osmolality rises to values greater than 292 mosmol/kg. Thus, water intake is not stimulated until the urine is maximally concentrated. Angiotensin II increases thirst and AVP release under conditions of extracellular volume depletion. Normally, therefore, water losses lead to slight hypernatremia which increases thirst and fluid intake to an extent sufficient to restore and maintain normal plasma osmolality. In contrast, when there is loss of thirst perception (adipsia) fluid losses are uncorrected and hypernatremia occurs even though AVP release is adequate to concentrate the urine maximally.

EFFECTS OF GLUCOCORTICOIDS Hormones of the adrenal cortex and the posterior pituitary have antagonistic effects on water excretion. Cortisol elevates the osmotic threshold for AVP release elicited by hypertonic saline infusion in water-loaded normal subjects, and glucocorticoids protect against water intoxication and overcome the impaired response to water loading in adrenal insufficiency.

Although the subnormal ability to dilute the urine in adrenal insufficiency may in part be due to excessive circulating AVP, glucocorticoids can also act directly on the renal tubules to decrease water permeability and increase solute-free water in the absence of AVP.

CELLULAR MECHANISM OF AVP ACTIVITY The biochemical basis for the action of AVP on the renal tubule is shown in Fig. 315-1: (1) AVP binds to specific contraluminal V_2 receptor sites; (2) the receptor-hormone complex is coupled to and activates adenylate cyclase in the same contraluminal membrane via a guanine nucleotide binding stimulatory protein (see Chap. 68); (3) the production of cyclic AMP is increased; (4) the cyclic AMP is translocated to the luminal cell membrane where it causes the activation of membrane-bound protein kinase; (5) the activated protein kinase causes the phosphorylation of membrane proteins; and (6) permeability of the luminal membrane to water is increased. The AVP-generated cyclic AMP may be inactivated by a phosphodiesterase that converts cyclic AMP to 5′-AMP. AVP also stimulates prostaglandin E_2 production which, in turn, acts as a feedback inhibitor of adenylate cyclase activation.

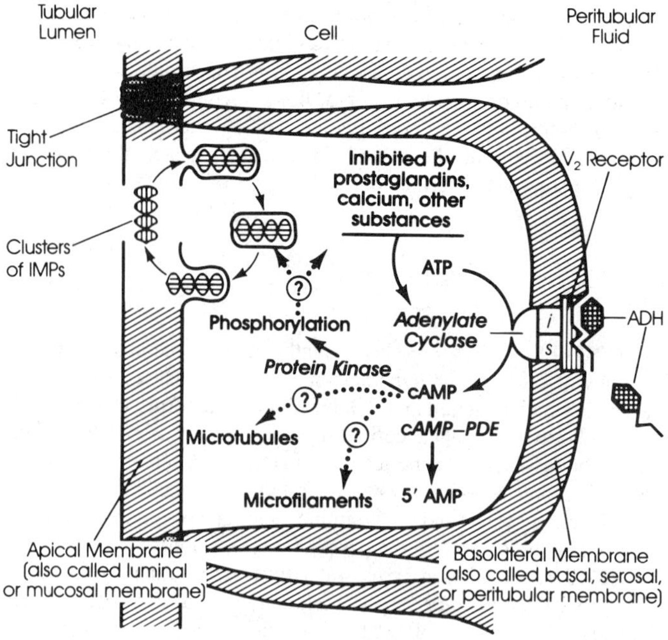

FIGURE 315-1 Schematic representation of the cellular action of vasopressin. The increased water permeability of responsive cells involves the V_2 receptor for vasopressin. Uninterrupted arrows denote steps that have been defined, interrupted arrows with question marks, postulated steps. ADH = antidiuretic hormone or vasopressin; i and s = inhibitory and stimulatory guanine nucleotide regulatory proteins; cAMP-PDE = phosphodiesterase; IMPs = intramembranous particles. *[From H Valtin, in Handbook of Physiology, Renal, Washington, DC, American Physiological Society (in press)]*

The final event in the transtubular movement of water is the appearance of particle aggregates in the luminal membrane of the cell (Fig. 315-2). These particles relieve the rate-limiting barrier to water flow. In the presence of the aggregates water molecules are able to move passively along an osmotic gradient. The transtubular movement of water depends also on the integrity of the microtubular system.

Various cations and drugs can influence the action of AVP. Calcium and lithium inhibit the adenylate cyclase response to vasopressin. Lithium also interferes with a subsequent biochemical action, as does potassium deficiency. Demeclocycline inhibits adenylate cyclase stimulation by AVP and also inhibits the cyclic AMP–dependent protein kinase. In contrast, chlorpropamide increases AVP-induced activation of adenylate cyclase.

DEFICIENCY OF VASOPRESSIN: DIABETES INSIPIDUS

Diabetes insipidus is a term which refers to the passage through the body of a large quantity of dilute fluid. This state of excessive water intake and hypotonic polyuria may be due to failure of AVP release in response to normal physiologic stimuli (central or neurogenic diabetes insipidus) or failure of the kidney to respond to AVP (nephrogenic diabetes insipidus).

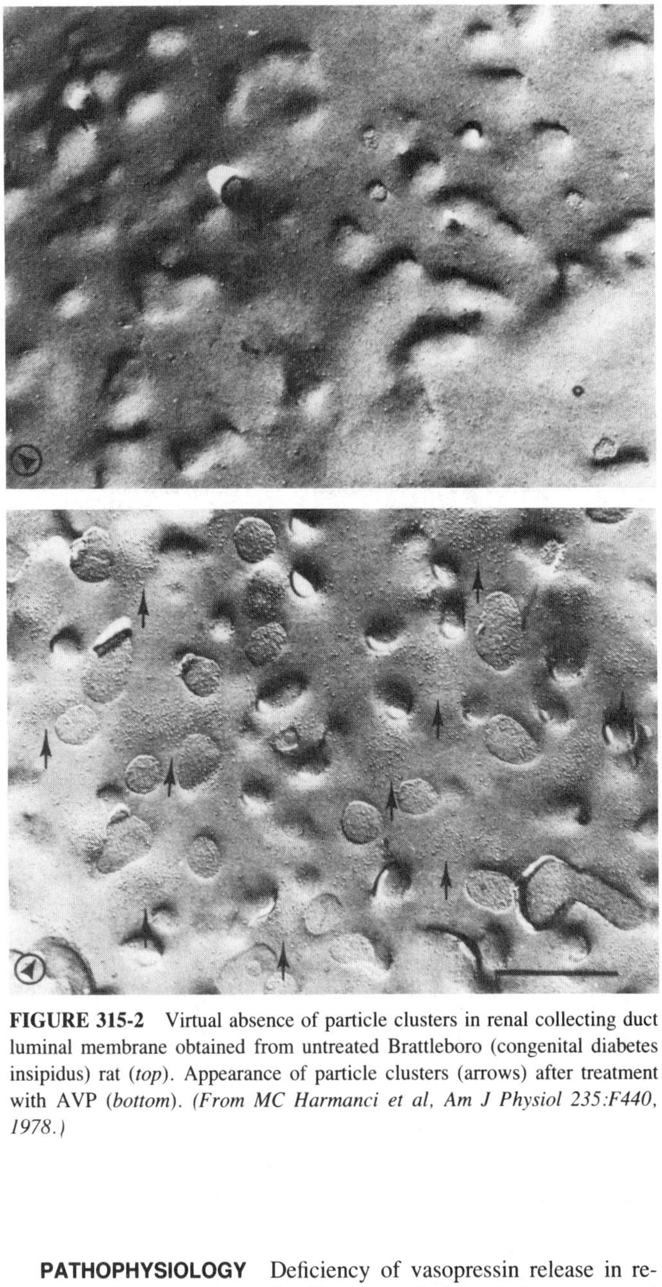

FIGURE 315-2 Virtual absence of particle clusters in renal collecting duct luminal membrane obtained from untreated Brattleboro (congenital diabetes insipidus) rat (*top*). Appearance of particle clusters (arrows) after treatment with AVP (*bottom*). *(From MC Harmanci et al, Am J Physiol 235:F440, 1978.)*

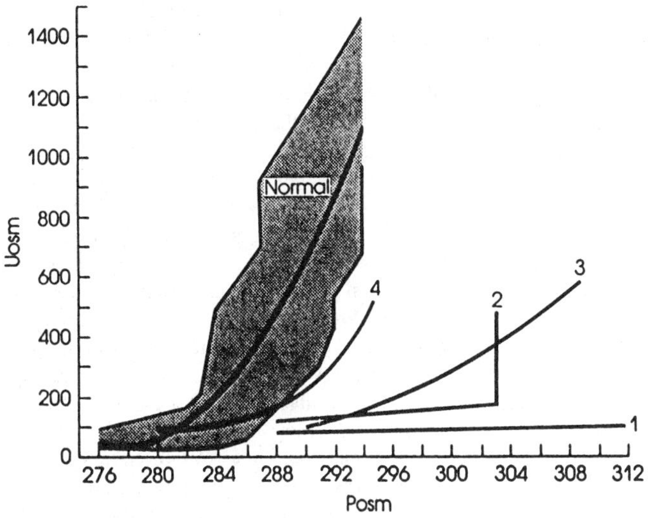

FIGURE 315-3 Relation of plasma and urinary osmolality during hydration and dehydration in normal adult subjects (shaded area) and in four types of patients with diabetes insipidus.

PATHOPHYSIOLOGY Deficiency of vasopressin release in response to the appropriate stimuli may result from lesions at several functional sites in the physiologic chain of events which regulates discharge of the hormone into the bloodstream. For conceptual purposes four types of central diabetes insipidus can be defined. Patients of the first type show very little rise in urine osmolality, even with a marked increase in plasma osmolality (1, Fig. 315-3) and no evidence of AVP release during hypertonic saline infusion. They are essentially devoid of releasable AVP. In the second type there is an abrupt increase in urine osmolality during dehydration (2, Fig. 315-3), but there is no evidence of an osmotic threshold during saline infusion. These patients have a defective osmoreceptor mechanism but are capable of releasing AVP in response to the hypovolemia of severe dehydration. The third type of patient has some rise in urine osmolality with increasing plasma osmolality (3, Fig. 315-3) and has an elevated osmotic threshold for AVP release. These patients have a sluggish release mechanism and may be said to have a high-set osmoreceptor. In the fourth type of patient, urine and plasma osmolality coordinates are shifted to the right of normal (4, Fig. 315-3). AVP release in these patients is initiated at a normal plasma osmolality but is subnormal in amount.

The second to fourth types of patients may develop a good antidiuresis in response to nausea, nicotine, methacholine, chlorpropamide, or clofibrate, indicating that the synthesis and storage of AVP are sufficient to allow for adequate urinary concentrating ability in the presence of an appropriate stimulus to release. In rare instances patients of the second to fourth types may present with asymptomatic hypernatremia associated with mild or absent evidence of diabetes insipidus.

ETIOLOGY The causes of central diabetes insipidus in 135 patients who satisfied the criteria described under "Diagnostic Tests" (below) and who had had diabetes insipidus for at least 6 months are shown in Table 315-1. Diabetes insipidus frequently starts in childhood or early adult life (median age of onset 21 years) and is more common in males than females. The major causes are as follows: (1) *Neoplastic or infiltrative lesions* of the hypothalamus or pituitary, including chromophobe adenomas, craniopharyngiomas, germinomas, pinealomas, metastatic tumors, leukemia, histiocytosis X, and sarcoidosis, caused diabetes insipidus in 37 patients. In approximately 60 percent of these patients evidence of partial or complete loss of anterior pituitary function was present. (2) *Pituitary or hypothalamic surgery or isotopic ablative therapy* caused diabetes insipidus in 32 patients and almost invariably was associated with anterior hypopituitarism.

TABLE 315-1 Characteristics of 135 cases of longstanding* central diabetes insipidus diagnosed by the authors at SUNY Health Science Center, Syracuse. Categories are arranged in order of increasing median age of onset.

Cause	Age of onset, years				Percent
	Median†	Range	Males	Females	of cases
Histiocytosis	2	1–30	3	2	4
Primary brain tumor —postoperative‡	15	6–50	9	11	15
Primary brain tumor —preoperative§	18	7–58	17	3	15
Idiopathic	20	<1–66	20	14	25
Head trauma	22	5–48	15	9	18
Nontraumatic encephalomalacia	43	15–73	3	4	5
Ruptured cerebral aneurysm	39	-	1	0	1
Post-hypophysectomy	42	24–68	4	8	9
Sarcoidosis	42		0	1	1
Metastatic cancer	56	32–72	6	5	8
			(58%)	(42%)	

* Longer than 6 months or until death.
† Median age of entire group = 24 years.
‡ 16 cases were of craniopharyngioma.
§ 5 cases were glioma, 7 germinoma, and 4 craniopharyngioma.

Surgically induced diabetes insipidus usually develops between 1 and 6 days after surgery and often disappears after a few days. It may remain absent or may recur and become chronic after an ''interphase'' of 1 to 5 days. Removal of the posterior lobe of the pituitary induces permanent diabetes insipidus only if the pituitary stalk is sectioned high enough to induce retrograde degeneration of most of the neurons of the supraoptic nucleus. (3) *Severe head injuries,* usually associated with fractures of the skull, caused diabetes insipidus in 24 patients and were associated with anterior hypopituitarism in only about one-sixth of patients. Spontaneous remissions of traumatic diabetes insipidus occasionally occur even after 6 months, presumably because of regeneration of disrupted axons within the pituitary stalk. (4) *Idiopathic diabetes insipidus* (in 34 patients) usually starts in childhood and is seldom (<20 percent) associated with anterior pituitary dysfunction. This diagnosis can be made only after a careful search has failed to reveal evidence of a tumor, infiltrative lesion, vascular lesion, or other presumptive cause of the AVP deficiency. The presence of anterior hypopituitarism or hyperprolactinemia or radiologic evidence of lesions within or above the sella should stimulate a continuing search for a causative lesion at 3- to 12-month intervals. The diagnosis of idiopathic diabetes insipidus is made with increasing confidence as the duration of negative findings on follow-up increases. A decrease in the number of neurons in the supraoptic and paraventricular nuclei has been reported in idiopathic diabetes insipidus, and circulating antibodies to hypothalamic nuclei may be present. In rare instances, dominant inheritance has been documented. (5) Seven patients had nontraumatic encephalomalacia from a variety of severe cerebral insults including shock, cardiopulmonary arrest, hypertensive encephalopathy, poisoning, and meningitis. All the patients were brain dead and had to be maintained on total life support systems.

CLINICAL MANIFESTATIONS *Polyuria, excessive thirst,* and *polydipsia* are almost invariably present in diabetes insipidus. Characteristically, these symptoms are sudden in onset, both when the disorder first presents itself and whenever the effects of administered vasopressin disappear during long-term therapy. In severe cases the urine is pale in color, and its volume may be immense (up to 16 to 24 L per day), requiring micturition every 30 to 60 min throughout the day and night. More frequently, however, the urine volume is only moderately increased (2.5 to 6 L per day), and occasionally it may be less than 2 liters per day, causing no complaints on the part of the patient. Urinary concentration (less than 290 mosmol/kg, specific gravity less than 1.010) is below that of the serum in severe cases but may be higher than that of serum (290 to 600 mosmol/kg) in patients with mild diabetes insipidus.

The slight rise in serum osmolality resulting from hypotonic polyuria stimulates thirst. Large volumes of fluid are imbibed, and cold drinks are preferred, patients often going to great trouble to secure cold fluids. Although thirst is probably secondary to loss of water, the administration of vasopressin often relieves or reduces thirst, even in the absence of fluid intake.

Normal function of the thirst center ensures that polydipsia closely matches polyuria, so that dehydration is seldom detectable except in the mild elevation of serum sodium concentration. However, when adequate replenishment of excreted water is interfered with, dehydration may become severe, causing weakness, fever, psychic disturbances, prostration, and death. These features are associated with a rising serum osmolality and serum sodium concentration, the latter sometimes exceeding 175 mmol/L. Adipsia is not found in idiopathic diabetes insipidus, but it may result from impaired function of the hypothalamic thirst center because of extension of the same abnormality that caused the diabetes insipidus. More frequently, dehydration occurs during unconsciousness produced by surgical anesthesia, head trauma, or other causes. It is particularly hazardous to administer large volumes of isotonic saline solution intravenously or of hyperosmolar protein by nasogastric tube unless adequate amounts of water are administered simultaneously in unconscious patients with untreated diabetes insipidus.

Hydronephrosis is a rare complication of the polyuria, especially in patients who fail to empty their bladders adequately because of bladder atony, uretheral strictures, or other causes.

DIAGNOSTIC TESTS The diagnostic procedures to establish the cause of hypotonic polyuria represent a pragmatic clinical approach in contrast to investigational studies on the pathophysiology of AVP release. Even though stimuli such as nausea, nicotine administration, hypoglycemia, and hypotension may release AVP, the results are clinically irrelevant. It is of little consequence to the patient with symptomatic diabetes insipidus that one or more of these nonosmotic stimuli retains its capacity to release AVP. The following procedures which utilize plasma and urine osmolality determinations are readily available, reliable, and safe and they allow the physician to establish the diagnosis rapidly and to initiate therapy. Measurement of plasma or urine AVP which are expensive and time-consuming are only occasionally needed, when osmolality measurements are inconclusive (Fig. 315-4). The tests should not be conducted in the presence of untreated thyroid or adrenocortical deficiency or in the presence of an osmotic diuresis (e.g., uncontrolled diabetes mellitus).

Assessment of the relation of plasma to urine osmolality The normal relationship between plasma osmolality (assuming no increase in blood urea or glucose) and urine osmolality is indicated in Fig. 315-3. If several simultaneously determined plasma and urine osmolalities in a patient with polyuria fall substantially to the right of the shaded area, the patient has central or nephrogenic diabetes insipidus. The latter diagnosis can be made if the response to injected vasopressin is subnormal (see ''Dehydration Test'' below) or if plasma or urinary AVP concentration is increased. The practice of relating plasma to urine osmolality is useful, particularly in postoperative neurosurgical cases or after head trauma, where its use can lead quickly to the differentiation of diabetes insipidus from parenteral fluid excess. In such patients, intravenous hydration can be slowed temporarily, and repeated plasma and urine osmolalities can be obtained and plotted as in Fig. 315-3, to determine whether the relationship is normal.

Dehydration test Comparison of the urinary osmolality after dehydration with that after vasopressin administration is a simple and reliable way of diagnosing diabetes insipidus and of differentiating vasopressin deficiency from other causes of polyuria. This test can and should be combined with the assessment of the relationship between plasma and urine osmolality.

FIGURE 315-4 Relationship between plasma osmolality (Posm) and urinary AVP excretion (U_{AVP}) in normal subjects (shaded area on left), patients with central diabetes insipidus (shaded area on right), and patients with nephrogenic diabetes insipidus (individual data points). Correlates in patients with SIADH fall to the left of the normal range. [*From AM Moses, in P Czernichow and AG Robinson (eds), Frontiers of Hormone Research, vol 13: Diabetes Insipidus in Man, Basel, Karger, 1985.*]

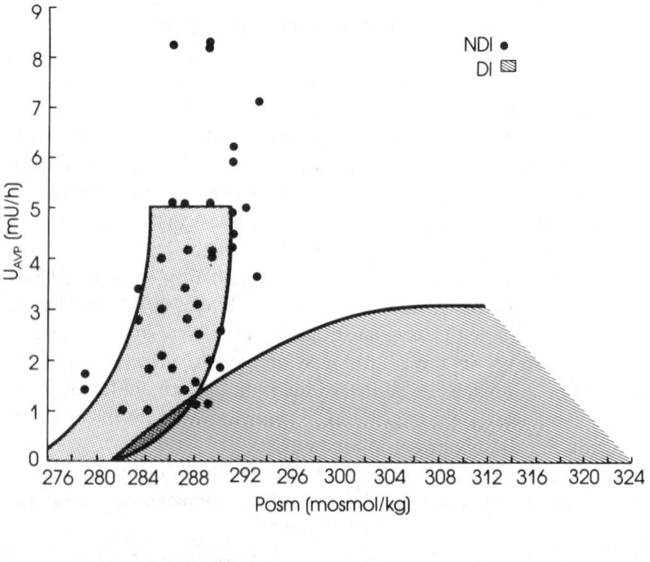

The maximal urinary concentrating capacity varies widely between individuals, and no absolute lower limits of "normal" can be defined in patients with nonspecific illnesses in whom AVP is produced in adequate amounts. It is impossible to distinguish between deficiency and sufficiency of AVP release solely by the level of the urinary osmolality attained after specified periods of water deprivation. On the other hand, if after prolonged dehydration vasopressin administration induces a further rise in urinary osmolality, there is a strong implication that vasopressin deficiency exists.

PROCEDURE

1 Fluids are withheld long enough to result in stable hourly urinary osmolalities (an hourly increase of <30 mosmol/kg for at least three successive hours). This is usually associated with a loss in body weight of at least 1 kg. In patients whose daily urinary volumes exceed 10 liters, the fluid deprivation should begin between 4 A.M. and 6 A.M. so that the patient can be carefully watched and the test terminated if weight loss exceeds 2 kg or the clinical condition deteriorates. In patients whose urinary volumes are only mildly increased or who are hyponatremic, water deprivation may be started about midnight.

2 Urine specimens are collected hourly for osmolality measurements from 6 A.M. at least until noon and preferably until the osmolality has been stable for three consecutive hours.

3 After the third hour of stable urinary osmolalities, the patient is given vasopressin as 5 units aqueous vasopressin or 1 μg desmopressin by subcutaneous injection or 10 μg desmopressin by nasal spray.

4 Plasma osmolality is determined immediately before the injection of vasopressin, and urinary osmolality is measured on the specimen collected between 30 and 60 min after the injection.

Vital signs should be monitored during the dehydration procedure, but when the test has been performed as described, adverse effects are rare.

INTERPRETATION In subjects with normal pituitary function, urinary osmolality does not rise by more than 9 percent after the injection of vasopressin, whatever the maximal urinary osmolality might be after dehydration alone. In central diabetes insipidus, the rise in urinary osmolality after vasopressin exceeds 9 percent. To ensure adequacy of dehydration, plasma osmolality before the vasopressin injection should be above 288 mosmol/kg. Patients who have polyuria from renal diseases, potassium depletion, or nephrogenic diabetes insipidus (see below) usually show little rise in urinary osmolality with dehydration and no further rise after vasopressin injection. Patients with compulsive water drinking (primary polydipsia) often require prolonged water deprivation before plasma osmolality reaches 288 mosmol/kg and before a plateau in urinary osmolality is reached; urinary osmolality rises by <9 percent after the administration of exogenous vasopressin.

Hypertonic saline infusions These tests are seldom necessary for the diagnosis of diabetes insipidus but are useful in the documentation of alterations in the osmotic threshold for AVP release; such changes may be of value in characterizing some cases of hypo- or hypernatremia. See references for details.

DIFFERENTIAL DIAGNOSIS Diabetes insipidus must be distinguished from other types of polyuria (Table 315-2). Several are recognizable by the history (e.g., recent lithium or mannitol administration, recent surgery under methoxyflurane anesthesia, or recent renal transplantation). In others the physical examination or simple laboratory procedures will indicate the diagnosis (evidence of glycosuria, renal disease, sickle cell anemia, hypercalcemia, or potassium depletion, including primary aldosteronism).

Congenital nephrogenic diabetes insipidus is a rare, usually familial, form of polyuria resulting from unresponsiveness to AVP. Females may have a less severe form of the disease than males, may concentrate urine reasonably well with water deprivation, and may be treatable with large amounts of desmopressin. One family with this disease has an abnormal gene located on the short arm of the X chromosome. Most patients studied appear to have a V_2-receptor abnormality, while some patients appear to have a postreceptor defect. All have normal V_1-receptor functions. Patients with congenital nephrogenic diabetes insipidus can be distinguished from those with vasopressin-deficient diabetes insipidus by the familial nature of the disorder (rare in central diabetes insipidus) and by lack of a dramatic reduction in daily urine volume when vasopressin or desmopressin is administered. When patients with nephrogenic and central diabetes insipidus cannot be differentiated with certainty by osmolality determinations alone, either elevated plasma, or urinary AVP concentration in relation to plasma osmolality (Fig. 315-4), or a high AVP concentration in relation to urine osmolality will allow the diagnosis of nephrogenic diabetes insipidus to be established.

TABLE 315-2 Major polyuric syndromes

I Primary disorders of water intake or output
- *A* Excessive water intake
  - *1* Psychogenic polydipsia
  - *2* Hypothalamic disease: histiocytosis X, sarcoidosis
  - *3* Drug-induced polydipsia
    - *a* Thioridazine
    - *b* Chlorpromazine
    - *c* Anticholinergic drugs (dry mouth)
- *B* Inadequate tubular reabsorption of filtered water
  - *1* Vasopressin deficiency
    - *a* Central diabetes insipidus
    - *b* Drug-induced inhibition of AVP release
      - *(1)* Narcotic antagonists
  - *2* Renal tubular unresponsiveness to AVP
    - *a* Nephrogenic diabetes insipidus (congenital and familial)
    - *b* Nephrogenic diabetes insipidus (acquired)
      - *(1)* Several chronic renal diseases, after obstructive uropathy, unilateral renal arterial stenosis, after renal transplantation, after acute tubular necrosis
      - *(2)* Potassium deficiencies, including primary aldosteronism
      - *(3)* Chronic hypercalcemias, including hyperparathyroidism
      - *(4)* Drug-induced: lithium, methoxyflurane anesthesia, demeclocycline
      - *(5)* Various systemic disorders: multiple myeloma, amyloidosis, sickle cell anemia, Sjögren's syndrome

II Primary disorders of renal absorption of solutes (osmotic diuresis)
- *A* Glucose: diabetes mellitus
- *B* Salts, especially sodium chloride
  - *1* Various chronic renal diseases, especially chronic pyelonephritis
  - *2* After various diuretics, including mannitol

Primary polydipsia Primary or psychogenic polydipsia is occasionally difficult to differentiate from diabetes insipidus and may occur in two forms. Chronic overingestion of water results in hypotonic polyuria and is often confused with diabetes insipidus. The intermittent ingestion of large quantities of fluid may also lead to water intoxication and dilutional hyponatremia even though there is normal urinary diluting capacity. This phenomenon is rare because normal adults can excrete between 10 and 14 mL/min of solute-free water, and it is an unusual circumstance which results in the ingestion of sufficiently more water than this to cause dilutional hyponatremia. The tendency to develop dilutional hyponatremia in these patients is increased because the chronic overingestion of fluids may limit their ability to excrete free water.

Polydipsia and polyuria are usually somewhat erratic, even in the chronic form of primary polydipsia. This is in contrast to the sustained polydipsia and polyuria of diabetes insipidus. These patients often have no nocturnal polyuria. Of 17 patients who were diagnosed as having sustained primary polydipsia, 10 were female and 7 were male with a median age of onset of 34 years (range 14 to 48). In three patients the onset of primary polydipsia followed head trauma, two had hypothalamic sarcoidosis, one was the sister of a patient with congenital nephrogenic diabetes insipidus, one was severely mentally retarded, and one had a hypothalamic lesion of unknown cause. The remaining nine patients had moderate to severe psychiatric disturbances and were frequently taking psychoactive drugs with anticholinergic properties. The syndrome has also been described in patients with anorexia nervosa who may drink huge quantities of

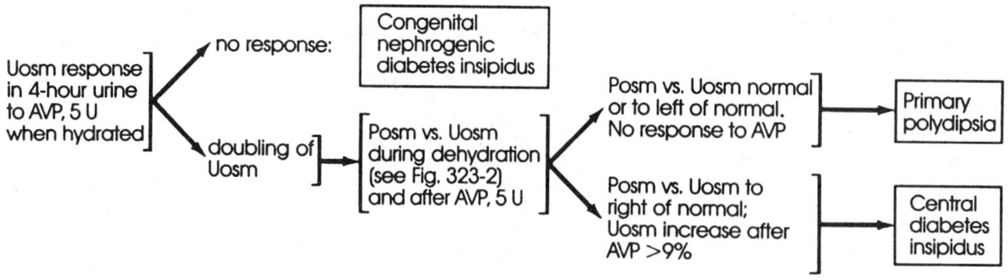

FIGURE 315-5 Approach to hypotonic polyurias

water; this consumption may markedly decrease when food intake increases. There is a predisposition toward dilutional hyponatremia in patients who ingest excessive fluids when urinary diluting capacity is impaired by therapeutic agents such as nonsteroidal anti-inflammatory drugs.

The diagnosis is usually evident from the combination of low plasma and urinary osmolalities. The relationship between urine and plasma osmolality during water deprivation is typically normal or supranormal (to left of normal in Fig. 315-3). There is an absent or minimal rise in urine osmolality after injection of vasopressin at the plateau of urine osmolality during the dehydration test. Because chronic overingestion of water may suppress release of AVP, and because chronic polyuria may cause a wash-out of the medullary osmotic gradient, urine osmolality may be subnormal in relation to plasma osmolality (to right of normal in Fig. 315-3). Therefore, it may be difficult, if not impossible, to differentiate patients with primary polydipsia from those with partial central diabetes insipidus. Indeed, there are probably patients with both problems. Attempts to treat these patients with vasopressin, even under close supervision, usually results in water intoxication.

A simple diagnostic approach to patients with hypotonic polyuria is shown in Fig. 315-5.

TREATMENT (See Table 315-3) Diabetes insipidus can be treated by hormone replacement. As is true of most peptides, oral administration of vasopressin is ineffective. Aqueous vasopressin may be administered subcutaneously in doses of 5 to 10 units and usually has a duration of action of 3 to 6 h. The main use of this preparation is in initial management of unconscious patients with acute onset of diabetes insipidus following head trauma or a neurosurgical procedure. Its short duration of action allows recognition of the recovery of neurohypophyseal function and prevents the development of water intoxication in patients receiving intravenous fluids.

Desmopressin has prolonged antidiuretic activity and is almost completely devoid of pressor effects. When used intranasally in amounts between 10 and 20 μg (0.1 to 0.2 mL) or by subcutaneous injection (1 to 4 μg), it has an antidiuretic action for 12 to 24 h in most patients. This analogue is the drug of choice in the treatment of most patients with diabetes insipidus. Lypressin is a nasal spray; a single application may result in an antidiuresis lasting approximately 4 to 6 h. Nasal absorption of both analogues may be decreased in the presence of an upper respiratory infection or allergic rhinitis with edema of the nasal mucosa. In such circumstances and in the unconscious patient with diabetes insipidus, desmopressin should be given by subcutaneous injection.

In the past, patients with an established diagnosis of diabetes insipidus were usually treated with intramuscular injections of vasopressin tannate in oil (2.5 or 5 units), which has an antidiuretic effect for 24 to 72 h. Since this material is a suspension of vasopressin tannate in peanut oil, it is essential that the ampul be warmed and then thoroughly shaken or inverted repeatedly until the brownish deposit of pituitary powder in the ampul is evenly distributed as a slightly cloudy suspension in the oil. A dry syringe should be used.

Patients with diabetes insipidus who have some residual releasable AVP (types 2 to 4) may respond to oral treatment with several nonhormonal agents. Chlorpropamide stimulates AVP release from the neurohypophysis and potentiates the action of submaximal amounts of AVP on the renal tubule, properties that make it of use in many patients with diabetes insipidus. Doses of 200 to 500 mg, usually taken once daily, are sufficient for an antidiuretic response. Its action starts within several hours of administration and usually lasts for 24 h. Chlorpropamide may also restore thirst perception and thus be useful in patients with thirst center defects. Hypoglycemia may occur but can usually be avoided by adherence to a regular schedule of meals. Clofibrate is capable of stimulating AVP release and has also been used in the treatment of diabetes insipidus. Doses of 500 mg four times a day often result in a prompt and sustained antidiuresis. In some patients, combined treatment with chlorpropamide and clofibrate results in complete restoration of water regulation to normal. Carbamazepine has also been observed to produce antidiuresis in patients with diabetes insipidus by stimulation of AVP release. Doses of 400 to 600 mg daily are effective, but the drug is not widely used owing to toxic side effects.

These therapeutic agents are effective only in central diabetes insipidus. In males with nephrogenic diabetes insipidus the only

TABLE 315-3 Agents used in treatment of diabetes insipidus

	Dose form	Usual dose	Duration of action, h
CENTRAL DIABETES INSIPIDUS			
Hormone replacement:			
Aqueous vasopressin	10 or 20 units/ampul	5–10 units subcutaneously	3–6
Desmopressin	2.5-mL intranasal preparation, 100 μg/mL; 1- or 10-mL ampul, for injection, 4 μg/mL	10–20 μg intranasally or 1–4 μg subcutaneously	12–24
Lypressin	5-mL bottle, 50 units/mL	2–4 units intranasally	4–6
Vasopressin tannate in oil	5 units/ampul	5 units intramuscularly	24–72
Nonhormonal agents:			
Chlorpropamide	100- and 250-mg tablets	200–500 mg daily	
Clofibrate	500-mg capsules	500 mg four times daily	
Carbamazepine	200-mg tablets	400–600 mg daily	
NEPHROGENIC DIABETES INSIPIDUS			
Hydrochlorothiazide	50-mg tablets	50–100 mg daily	
Chlorthalidone	50-mg tablets	50 mg daily	

agents of clinical value are thiazides and other diuretics. By producing sodium depletion, the diuretics cause a fall in glomerular filtration rate with enhanced reabsorption of fluid in the proximal portion of the nephron and decreased delivery of sodium to the ascending limb of the loop of Henle and consequently reduced capacity to dilute the urine. The therapeutic effect of diuretics in patients with nephrogenic diabetes insipidus is lost unless sodium intake is restricted. Some female patients with congenital nephrogenic diabetes insipidus and some patients with lithium-induced polyuria have been treated effectively with large doses of desmopressin.

PROGNOSIS The long-term prospects of a patient with diabetes insipidus are dependent primarily upon the underlying cause. In the absence of brain tumor or systemic disease, ready access to water and proper treatment of the polyuria usually lead to a normal life and life expectancy. Early recognition and treatment are important to prevent bladder distention, hydroureter, and hydronephrosis which may develop in patients with long-standing polyuria, particularly in patients with nephrogenic diabetes insipidus. The rare patient with adipsia or hypodipsia in association with diabetes insipidus is in danger of developing severe dehydration, which may lead to vascular collapse or central nervous system damage. Similarly severe complications may occur in patients with diabetes insipidus who develop impairment of consciousness. For this reason, all patients with diabetes insipidus should carry identification indicating the presence of the disorder and the necessity for treatment and fluid administration.

SYNDROMES ASSOCIATED WITH VASOPRESSIN EXCESS

Excessive blood levels or actions of vasopressin are associated with and probably cause water retention in several circumstances:

1 As a mechanism for *prevention of a rising plasma osmolality* which would otherwise result from sodium retention in edema, associated with congestive heart failure; cirrhosis with ascites; nephrosis; orthostatic edema; myxedema; and treatment with sodium-retaining drugs (fludrocortisone, nonsteroidal anti-inflammatory agents, and others)
2 As a mechanism of *defense against hypovolemia and/or hypotension* in adrenal insufficiency, excessive fluid losses (from vomiting, diarrhea, drug-induced diuresis, and excessive sweating), fluid deprivation, and probably positive pressure respiration
3 As a consequence of *drug- or disease-induced release of vasopressin from the neurohypophysis* caused by:
   a *Central nervous system disorders:* head trauma, subdural hematoma, subarachnoid hemorrhage, cerebral vascular thrombosis, brain tumor, cerebral atrophy, acute encephalitis, acute psychosis, tuberculous and other meningitides
   b *Drugs that release or potentiate the action of AVP:* chlorpropamide, vincristine, vinblastine, cyclophosphamide, carbamazepine, general anesthetics, tricyclic antidepressants
4 *In ectopic AVP production and release:*
   a *From neoplastic tissue:* oat cell carcinoma of lung, pancreatic carcinoma, lymphosarcoma, Hodgkin's disease, reticulum cell sarcoma, thymoma, carcinoma of duodenum or bladder
   b *From inflammatory lung diseases:* tuberculosis, lung abscess, pneumonias, empyema
5 *Other conditions:* Guillain-Barré syndrome, lupus erythematosus, acute intermittent porphyria, severe renovascular hypertension, and old age

SYNDROME OF INAPPROPRIATE AVP SECRETION OR SIADH SIADH is the term applied to vasopressin excess of types 3 to 5 above, associated with hyponatremia without edema (Table 315-4). In these patients the AVP excess is considered to be inappropriate since it occurs in the presence of plasma hypoosmolality. SIADH is analogous to abnormalities produced by administration of vasopressin and water to normal subjects. Although it might be conceptually valid to consider the AVP excess to be inappropriate in adrenal insufficiency and the edematous, hypovolemic, and hypotensive disorders listed in 1 and 2 above, their different pathogenic mechanisms and treatments make it clinically advisable not to consider these disorders as variants of the SIADH.

TABLE 315-4 Causes of SIADH

I Malignant neoplasms with autonomous AVP release
- *A* Oat cell carcinoma of lung
- *B* Carcinoma of pancreas
- *C* Lymphosarcoma, reticulum cell sarcoma, Hodgkin's disease
- *D* Carcinoma of duodenum
- *E* Thymoma

II Nonmalignant pulmonary diseases
- *A* Tuberculosis
- *B* Lung abscess
- *C* Pneumonia
- *D* Viral pneumonitis
- *E* Empyema
- *F* Chronic obstructive airways disease

III Central nervous system disorders
- *A* Skull fracture
- *B* Subdural hematoma
- *C* Subarachnoid hemorrhage
- *D* Cerebral vascular thrombosis
- *E* Cerebral atrophy
- *F* Acute encephalitis
- *G* Tuberculous meningitis
- *H* Purulent meningitis
- *I* Guillain-Barré syndrome
- *J* Lupus erythematosus
- *K* Acute intermittent porphyria

IV Drugs
- *A* Chlorpropamide
- *B* Vincristine
- *C* Vinblastine
- *D* Cyclophosphamide
- *E* Carbamazepine
- *F* Oxytocin
- *G* General anesthesia
- *H* Narcotics
- *I* Tricyclic antidepressants

V Miscellaneous causes
- *A* Hypothyroidism
- *B* Positive pressure respiration

Pathogenesis of SIADH The ectopic origin of authentic AVP from neoplasms and pulmonary tissue of the types listed above has been documented by tissue analysis. Neoplastic cells obtained from the lungs of patients with SIADH can synthesize, store, and release AVP, and in some patients AVP release is not entirely autonomous, being partially suppressible by water loading of the patient. Both AVP and its associated neurophysin are elevated in the plasma of over 60 percent of patients with small cell carcinoma of the lung. There is excellent correlation between the increases in plasma AVP and neurophysin concentrations on the one hand and the clinical responses to treatment or the recurrences of disease on the other. Vasopressin has also been demonstrated in tuberculous lung tissue. It seems likely, but has not been established, that intracranial lesions (meningitis, encephalitis, trauma, vascular accidents) may cause nonspecific irritative stimulation of AVP release from the neurohypophysis. Some drugs, such as vincristine, chlorpropamide, and carbamazepine, stimulate excessive release of AVP from the neurohypophyseal system and others (e.g., chlorpropamide and nonsteroidal anti-inflammatory agents) potentiate the antidiuretic action of secreted AVP on the renal tubular concentrating mechanism.

Excessive release or excessive renal tubular activity of vasopressin results in the excretion of a concentrated urine (with a urinary osmolality usually over 300 mosmol/kg) despite a subnormal plasma osmolality and serum sodium concentration. Sodium excretion in the urine is maintained (usually above 20 mmol/L) by hypervolemia, suppression of the renin-angiotensin-aldosterone system, and increased plasma concentration of atrial natriuretic peptide; and reduction in sodium concentration may be low if sodium intake is low, and urinary sodium concentration is higher if sodium intake is high.

Blood urea nitrogen and uric acid concentrations tend to fall because of plasma dilution and increased excretion of nitrogenous compounds. Because of the hypervolemia, blood pressure shows no orthostatic fall, but in spite of hypervolemia there is no recumbent hypertension (except when plasma angiotensin II is simultaneously elevated in angiotensinogenic hypertension) and no edema (for an unknown reason). The extracellular hypotonicity leads to intracellular edema, and severe symptoms may result from the consequent cerebral edema.

Clinical manifestations of SIADH In general, the rate of fall in serum sodium concentration is more important in producing the neurologic features of SIADH than the absolute magnitude of the fall. When SIADH is mild, with serum Na concentrations of 130 to 135 mmol/L, or developing gradually over several weeks, symptoms are often absent or may be limited to anorexia, nausea, and vomiting, such as occurs in other forms of hyponatremia. When hyponatremia is severe or acute in onset, body weight increases, and the symptoms of cerebral edema become predominant, including restlessness, irritability, confusion, coma, and convulsions associated with nonspecific EEG changes. Edema is almost always absent.

Diagnosis SIADH may be strongly suspected in patients who have hyponatremia and a concentrated urine (osmolality >300 mosmol/kg) associated with lethargy and in the absence of edema, orthostatic hypotension, and features of dehydration. The diagnosis of SIADH is made when other causes known to stimulate AVP release are excluded. The diagnosis is supported by the finding of blood urea nitrogen, serum uric acid, creatinine, and albumin concentrations in the low-normal or subnormal range. However, it is essential in making the diagnosis of SIADH to differentiate the condition from (a) the *dilutional hyponatremias* listed in 2 above, particularly adrenocortical insufficiency, in which orthostatic hypotension with tachycardia and an elevated or high-normal BUN are characteristic; (b) the *edematous states* listed in 1 above, particularly congestive heart failure with hyponatremia, and hypothyroidism; (c) *hypertensive states* associated with hyponatremia caused by renovascular stenosis or by diuretic therapy; (d) *primary polydipsia* which is always associated with a dilute urine (osmolality <150 mosmol/kg); (e) *pseudohyponatremia* associated with excessive plasma glucose, triglyceride, or protein concentrations [conditions (a) through (e) are easily recognizable by the associated plasma abnormalities]; and (f) the *"sick-cell" syndrome* in which hyponatremia is due to a subnormal setting of the hypothalamic osmoreceptors, associated usually with a chronic, debilitating disease and polyuria.

When the diagnosis of SIADH is not obvious after excluding other causes of hyponatremia, a positive diagnosis can usually be made with a *water-load test*. The water-load test is particularly useful in differentiating patients with a low-set osmoreceptor (who excrete the water normally) from all other hyponatremic states associated with a concentrated urine. This test should not be performed unless or until the serum sodium concentration has been elevated to a safe level (above 125 mmol/L) by restriction of water intake, and/or if necessary, saline administration. The patient is asked to drink the water load (20 mL per kilogram of body weight up to 1500 mL) in 10 to 20 min and urine is collected in hourly samples, with the patient recumbent between voidings, for 4 to 5 h in the morning. At least 65 percent of the water load should be excreted in 4 h or 80 percent in 5 h and the lowest urinary osmolality, usually reached in the second hour, should normally be below 100 mosmol/kg. It is essential, to prevent water intoxication in patients who have failed to excrete the water load normally, to allow no further water intake for the rest of that day. Failure to excrete the water load often occurs in adrenal insufficiency, or renal insufficiency, as well as in SIADH. It is important to appreciate, too, that SIADH cannot be diagnosed in the presence of severe pain, nausea, "stress," hypovolemia, hypotension, or other conditions that may stimulate AVP release even in the presence of plasma hypotonicity.

Measurements of plasma or urinary AVP (P_{AVP}, U_{AVP}) are useful adjuvants in establishing the diagnosis of SIADH. Plasma AVP is normally immeasurable in hyponatremic states but is detectable, even after a water load, in SIADH. The correlates of plasma osmolality (Posm) versus P_{AVP} or U_{AVP} concentration fall to the left of the normal values in SIADH (Fig. 315-4) and in any of the other hyponatremic states associated with a concentrated urine. Thus, in most patients with SIADH, P_{AVP} and U_{AVP} concentrations, which may fluctuate widely, are unrelated to concomitant changes in Posm. Occasionally, this lack of correlation between Posm and P_{AVP} or U_{AVP} may be inconsistent. Rarely, for instance, the baseline, unstimulated AVP level may be inappropriately elevated and may fail to change as Posm is raised until the Posm reaches the normal range. Further increases in Posm induced by hypertonic saline infusion or water deprivation may then result in normal or subnormal increases in P_{AVP} or U_{AVP}. This unusual phenomenon may reflect uncontrolled "leakage" of AVP from the neurohypophysis.

The diagnostic approach to SIADH is depicted in Fig. 315-6.

Treatment Restriction of fluid intake to 800 to 1000 mL daily is essential treatment. Since this intake will almost always be exceeded by urinary output plus insensible fluid loss, a negative water balance ensues that will result in gradual, daily reduction in weight, a progressive rise in serum Na concentration and osmolality, and symptomatic improvement. It is useful to verify the occurrence of these effects of fluid loss by documenting the changes in weight and serum Na concentration daily, until serum Na rises above 135 mmol/L.

Unless and until the underlying cause of the SIADH can be corrected, fluid intake should be appropriately restricted continuously, to maintain normonatremia. In addition to restriction of fluid intake, 5% sodium chloride solution, 200 to 300 mL, should be infused intravenously over 3 to 4 h in patients with severe confusion, convulsions, or coma. It is important to avoid the risk of inducing pontine myelinosis by not raising the serum Na concentration too rapidly. The possibility of causing congestive heart failure is remote

FIGURE 315-6 Approach to diagnosis of SIADH in patients with hyponatremia.

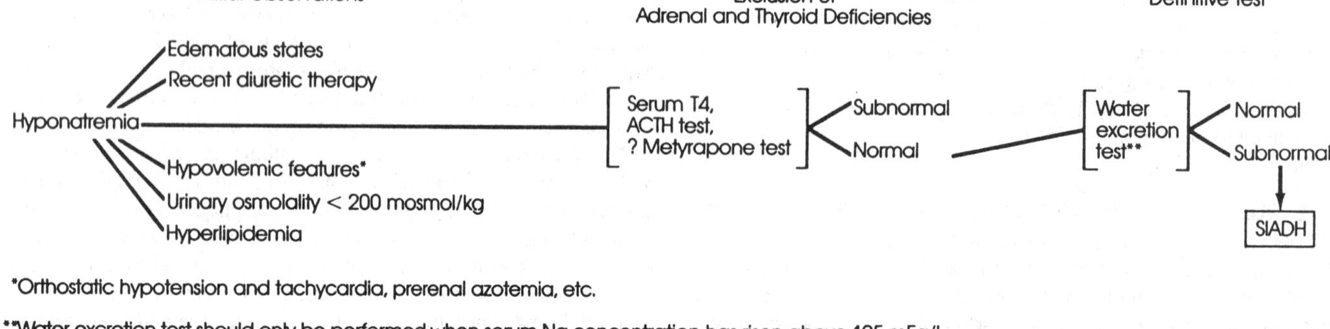

*Orthostatic hypotension and tachycardia, prerenal azotemia, etc.

**Water excretion test should only be performed when serum Na concentration has risen above 125 mEq/L, after water deprivation for as long as may be necessary.

as long as fluid is restricted, but this possibility may be further reduced by the simultaneous administration of furosemide, 40 mg intravenously.

Attempts should be made to identify and correct the cause of the SIADH as soon as possible. The administration of water-retaining drugs should be stopped. Treatment of hypothyroidism with thyroxine should be initiated. Pulmonary tuberculosis and other pulmonary infections should be appropriately treated, and meningitis or other CNS disorders should be sought and treated, if present. When a malignant tumor is the source of autonomous AVP release and SIADH, surgery, irradiation, and/or chemotherapy is often symptomatically beneficial even if the underlying neoplasm cannot be cured.

Antagonism of the release or actions of excessive AVP release is not often necessary and seldom successful. Although phenytoin inhibits AVP release, it is seldom effective in SIADH. Drugs that block the effect of AVP on the renal tubule may occasionally be useful in this syndrome. Demeclocycline is the most potent inhibitor of AVP action that is available for chronic administration, in doses of 900 to 1200 mg per day. Patients receiving demeclocycline should be carefully followed to detect any evidence of renal failure, bacterial superinfection, or excessive drug-induced water loss. Lithium salts interfere with AVP action on tubular water reabsorption and can cause polyuria by this mechanism. Unfortunately, lithium may have serious side effects in hyponatremic patients, and for this reason lithium salts are not recommended for treatment of SIADH.

Prognosis The prognosis of SIADH depends on the cause of the disorder. Drug-induced SIADH is rapidly and completely corrected by withdrawal of the causative agent. Similarly, the effective treatment of pulmonary or CNS infections results in improvement and eventual cure of SIADH caused by such lesions. Although SIADH resulting from oat cell carcinoma of the lung or other malignancies can often be controlled with vigorous restriction of fluid intake, the underlying malignancy determines the prognosis in these patients.

PARAVENTRICULAR-NEUROHYPOPHYSEAL SYSTEM AND OXYTOCIN

CHEMISTRY AND PHYSIOLOGY Oxytocin, a nonapeptide that differs by two amino acids from vasopressin, is produced predominantly in the cell bodies of the paraventricular nuclei and to a lesser extent in those of the supraoptic nuclei. It is synthesized and transported in neurosecretory granules by way of neuronal axons to the neurohypophysis, where it is stored or released, in conjunction with an oxytocin-specific neurophysin. Oxytocin release is stimulated by nerve impulses originating in the hypothalamus, which cause depolarization of the neurosecretory terminals of the posterior pituitary and subsequent release of oxytocin through a calcium-dependent process, similar to the mechanism for vasopressin. Estrogen stimulates release of oxytocin and its neurophysin. The secretion of oxytocin, as well as of vasopressin, is inhibited by ethanol. Some stimuli such as pain apparently release oxytocin and vasopressin simultaneously, but most stimuli release the two hormones independently. Oxytocin is primarily liberated during suckling, whereas vasopressin is released in much greater quantities than is oxytocin after an osmotic stimulus or hemorrhage. Manipulation or distention of the female genital tract, artificially or during parturition, is a more effective stimulus to oxytocin release than suckling.

Oxytocin acts on the membranes of myometrial and myoepithelial cells and results in an increased force of contraction. Sensitivity of the myometrium to oxytocin increases with the duration of pregnancy, but a role for oxytocin in the initiation and maintenance of labor is not established. Oxytocin may have survival value to the offspring since it may hasten the final stages of birth and lessen the chances of anoxia. Oxytocin also exerts a contractile action on the myometrium post partum and contracts the myoepithelial cells of the mammary alveoli, causing them to expel milk from the secretory tissue to the nipple. Oxytocin is 100 times more potent than vasopressin in its milk-ejecting activity in the human. In contrast, the antidiuretic potency of oxytocin relative to vasopressin is about 1:200. It is unlikely that oxytocin exerts any significant physiologic effect other than on the uterus and breast.

One milligram of purified preparation of oxytocin contains 450 IU of hormone, and the amount of oxytocin in the posterior pituitary ranges from 20 to 30 nmol (25 to 40 ng). In spite of the fact that there is no known role of oxytocin in the male, the male neural lobe stores oxytocin in amounts similar to those in the female. Plasma oxytocin concentration in both men and women exhibits episodic increases, with values ranging from a low of approximately 1 to 4 pmol/L (1.25 to 5 ng/L) but with no diurnal variation. In normal women there is a midcycle increase in plasma oxytocin concentration from a preovulatory value of approximately 2 pmol/L (2.5 ng/L) to a peak value of 4 to 8 pmol/L (5 to 10 ng/L) at the time of ovulation. During labor, plasma oxytocin concentrations may reach several hundred microunits per milliliter, with a rapid fall to prepartum levels after delivery. During suckling, plasma oxytocin levels of the mother vary but are usually about 10 to 20 pmol/L (12 to 25 ng/L). The half-life of oxytocin in plasma is about 3 to 5 min. Removal of oxytocin from the circulation is mainly by the kidneys and liver, although the uterus and mammary gland may remove some.

CLINICAL USE OF OXYTOCIN The clinical use of oxytocin is limited to the induction of labor, control of hemorrhage following incomplete abortion and curettage, and treatment of impaired milk ejection. For discussion of the obstetric uses of oxytocin, the reader is referred to textbooks on obstetrics. Care must be taken because oxytocin may cause uterine rupture and fetal death. The antidiuretic action of oxytocin can be elicited with single intravenous doses of as little as 100 mU. Maximal antidiuresis is reached with 40 to 50 mU/min. Since 10 to 40 units of oxytocin per liter of dextrose is often used in obstetric practice, water intoxication may result. The vasodilatory action of oxytocin may cause sudden death of obstetric patients with heart disease because of hypotension, tachycardia, and arrhythmias. Anesthetics may modify the cardiovascular responses to oxytocin. For instance, in patients under cyclopropane anesthesia, oxytocin produces more hypotension but less tachycardia than in unanesthetized subjects. The vasodilatory effect of oxytocin can be blocked by vasopressin.

REFERENCES

Bartter FC, Schwartz WB: The syndrome of inappropriate secretion of antidiuretic hormone. Am J Med 42:790, 1967

Cross BA, Leng G: *Progress in Brain Research*, vol 60: *The Neurohypophysis: Structure, Function and Control*. Amsterdam, Elsevier, 1983

Czernichow P, Robinson AG: *Frontiers of Hormone Research*, vol 13: *Diabetes Insipidus in Man*. Basel, Karger, 1985

Gash DM, Boer GJ (eds): *Vasopressin: Principles and Properties*. New York, Plenum, 1987

Knobil E, Sawyer WH (eds): *Handbook of Physiology*, sec 7: *Endocrinology*, vol IV: *The Pituitary Gland—Its Neuroendocrine Control*, part I. Washington, DC, American Physiological Society, 1974

Miller M et al: Recognition of partial defects in antidiuretic hormone secretion. Ann Intern Med 73:721, 1970

Moses AM: Osmotic thresholds for AVP release using plasma and urine AVP and free water clearance. Am J Physiol 256:R892, 1989

——— et al: Pathophysiologic and pharmacologic alterations in the release and action of ADH. Metabolism 25:697, 1976

——— et al: Marked hypotonic polyuria resulting from nephrogenic diabetes insipidus with partial sensitivity to vasopressin. J Clin Endocrinol Metab 59:1044, 1984

——— et al: Two distinct pathophysiological mechanisms in congenital nephrogenic diabetes insipidus. J Clin Endocrinol Metab 66:1259, 1988

Reichlin S: *The Neurohypophysis. Physiological and Clinical Aspects*. New York, Plenum, 1984

Robertson GL: The regulation of vasopressin function in health and disease. Rec Progr Hormone Res 33:333, 1977

316 DISEASES OF THE THYROID

LEONARD WARTOFSKY / SIDNEY H. INGBAR

Normal function of the thyroid gland is directed to the secretion of L-thyroxine (T_4) and 3,5,3′-triiodo-L-thyronine (T_3), iodinated amino acids that are the active thyroid hormones and that influence a diversity of metabolic processes (Fig. 316-1). Diseases of the thyroid are manifested by qualitative or quantitative alterations in hormone secretion, enlargement of the thyroid (goiter), or both. Insufficient hormone secretion results in *hypothyroidism* or *myxedema,* in which decreased caloric expenditure (hypometabolism) is a principal feature. Conversely, excessive secretion of hormone results in hypermetabolism and other features of a syndrome termed *hyperthyroidism* or *thyrotoxicosis*. Enlargement of the thyroid gland (normally 15 to 20 g in adults) may be generalized or focal. Generalized enlargements may not be symmetric, however, the right lobe tending to enlarge more than the left. They are associated with increased, normal, or decreased hormone secretion, depending upon the underlying disturbance. Focal enlargement usually reflects neoplastic disease, either benign or malignant, the former sometimes responsible for hypersecretion of hormone and hyperthyroidism, the latter rarely so. Any goiter may compress adjacent structures in the neck or mediastinum.

EMBRYOLOGY, ANATOMY, AND HISTOLOGY

The human thyroid originates embryologically from an evagination of the pharyngeal epithelium with some cellular contributions from the lateral pharyngeal pouches. Progressive descent of the midline thyroid anlage gives rise to the thyroglossal duct, which extends from the foramen cecum near the base of the tongue to the isthmus of the thyroid. Remnants of tissue may persist along the course of this tract as "lingual thyroid," as thyroglossal cysts or nodules, or as a structure contiguous with the thyroid isthmus called the *pyramidal lobe*. The latter is usually not discernible, except when the remainder of the gland is enlarged. Rarely, lingual thyroid may be the sole functioning thyroid tissue. In such cases, its secretion may or may not be sufficient to maintain a normal metabolic (euthyroid) state. Thyroid aplasia and functional failure of ectopic thyroid tissue are causes of sporadic neonatal hypothyroidism (1 in every 4000 or 5000 newborns), which responds to early treatment.

The fetal thyroid acquires the capacity to collect and organify iodine at about 10 weeks' gestation. Both T_4 and thyroid-stimulating hormone (thyrotropin, TSH) are detectable in the blood soon thereafter and increase in concentration during the second trimester. The increase in serum T_4 is due both to increasing thyroid secretion and to the appearance in plasma of thyroxine-binding globulin (TBG), and the increase in TSH is a reflection of the maturation of the fetal hypothalamus with resulting secretion of thyrotropin-releasing hormone (TRH). Maternal TRH readily crosses the placenta and could play a role in the development of the fetal pituitary-thyroid axis. Maternal TSH, by contrast, does not cross the placenta. T_3 is detectable in the blood later during the second trimester, but its concentration in blood and amniotic fluid remains low until shortly after parturition. By contrast, the concentration of its analogue, 3,3′,5′-triiodo-L-thyronine (reverse T_3, rT_3), is increased in fetal blood and amniotic fluid relative to that in maternal blood (Fig. 316-1). These differences are due to qualitative alterations in T_4 metabolism in the fetus. The low T_3 in fetal blood and amniotic fluid in the face of a high maternal concentration indicates that maternal-fetal transfer of T_3 is minimal, and the same is true of T_4. Hence, T_4 from the fetal thyroid is the major thyroid hormone available to the fetus. Except for the possible effect of maternal TRH, therefore, the fetal pituitary-thyroid axis is a functional unit distinct from that of the mother.

The normal adult thyroid contains two lobes joined by an isthmus and lies just anterior and caudad to the cartilages of the larynx. Fibrous septa divide the gland into pseudolobules which, in turn, are composed of vesicles, called *follicles* or *acini,* surrounded by a capillary network. Normally, the follicle walls are composed of cuboidal epithelium. The lumen is filled with a proteinaceous *colloid,* which contains a protein peculiar to the thyroid, *thyroglobulin,* within the peptide sequence of which T_4 and T_3 are synthesized and stored. The thyroid contains a smaller second population of cells, the C cells. They are the source of calcitonin and give rise to medullary thyroid carcinoma when they undergo malignant transformation.

THYROID HORMONE ECONOMY: NORMAL PHYSIOLOGY

The term *thyroid hormone economy* denotes the processes involved in the synthesis of hormones within the thyroid gland; their transport

FIGURE 316-1 Structural formulas of thyroxine, its precursors, and certain of its metabolites.

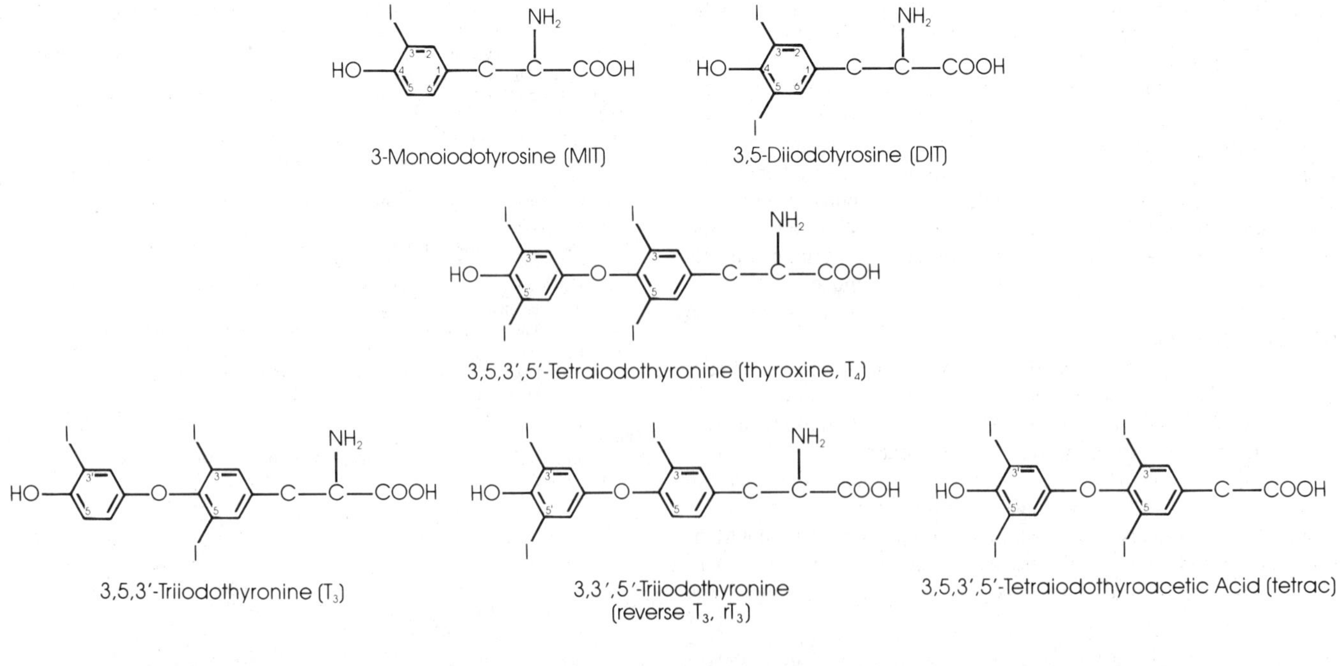

in the circulation; their action and metabolism within the peripheral tissues; and the regulatory mechanisms that maintain a normal supply of thyroid hormones. This section describes the normal physiology and biochemistry of the thyroid hormone economy. Abnormalities in transport, action, and metabolism are described in the sections dealing with laboratory tests or specific disorders.

HORMONE SYNTHESIS AND SECRETION Thyroid hormone synthesis depends on entry into the thyroid of adequate quantities of iodine, a constituent of T_4 and T_3; normality of iodine metabolism within the gland; and concurrent synthesis of a receptor protein for iodine, thyroglobulin. The structure of thyroglobulin favors iodinations and particularly formation of T_4 and T_3. Secretion of normal quantities of hormone, in turn, requires both a normal rate of hormone synthesis and the integrity of processes within the gland by which thyroglobulin is hydrolyzed and the active hormones liberated. Iodine enters the thyroid from the bloodstream in the form of inorganic or ionic iodide whose source is twofold: iodide derived either from the deiodination of thyroid hormones, from iodinated agents that the patient may have received, or from iodide ingested in food, water, or medication. Formerly, a dietary iodine intake of approximately 200 μg was considered normal in the United States, and this was sufficient to sustain a plasma iodide concentration of approximately 40 nmol/L (0.5 μg/dL). However, owing to iodine contamination of some foods, and to the widespread use of iodine in drugs, vitamin preparations, and antiseptic agents, the average iodine intake has increased to about 500 μg/d, and in some areas may be as high as 1000 μg daily, with corresponding increases in plasma iodide concentration. Iodide is removed from the plasma by the thyroid, kidneys, and salivary and gastrointestinal glands, but since iodide that enters gastrointestinal secretions is reabsorbed, net clearance is effected only by the thyroid and kidneys. In effect, the thyroid and kidneys compete for plasma iodide. Renal clearance is largely a function of glomerular filtration rate and is not influenced by humoral factors or plasma iodide concentration; the kidney is normally a passive participant in this competition. Hence, adjustments in the rate of entry of iodide into the thyroid relative to the rate of urinary excretion are mediated by changes in thyroid rather than renal avidity.

The synthesis and secretion of the active thyroid hormones can be divided into four sequential steps (Fig. 316-2). The first involves active transport of iodide from the plasma into the thyroid cell and follicular lumen. This occurs at a rate that exceeds passive diffusion of iodide out of the gland, with the result that the thyroid maintains concentration gradients for iodide (thyroid/plasma concentration ratios) of substantial magnitude (usually of 25 but up to 500 or more under certain conditions). Energy for iodide transport depends upon oxidative metabolism within the gland. The second step in hormone biosynthesis involves oxidation of iodide to a higher valence form that is capable of iodinating tyrosyl residues in thyroglobulin, a glycoprotein of approximately 660,000 mol wt that is synthesized within the follicular cell. Oxidation of iodide is effected by a peroxidase, which utilizes hydrogen peroxide generated during the course of oxidative metabolism within the gland. Organic iodinations occur at the cell-colloid interface, where they take place to a large extent in newly synthesized thyroglobulin undergoing exocytosis into the follicular lumen. The consequence is the formation of the peptide-bound, hormonally inactive precursors, monoiodotyrosine (MIT) and diiodotyrosine (DIT). Subsequently, these iodotyrosines undergo oxidative condensation, again through the mediation of peroxidase. This coupling reaction occurs within the thyroglobulin molecule and yields a variety of iodothyronines, including T_4 and T_3. Although minute quantities of thyroglobulin are detectable in the blood, most thyroglobulin is retained for a time within the gland, serving as a storage form of thyroid hormone, or "prohormone." Liberation of the active hormones into the blood involves pinocytosis of follicular colloid at the apical margin of the cells to form colloid droplets. The colloid droplets fuse with thyroid lysosomes to form "phagolysosomes," in which thyroglobulin is hydrolyzed by proteases and peptidases. The final step is release of the free iodothyronines, T_4

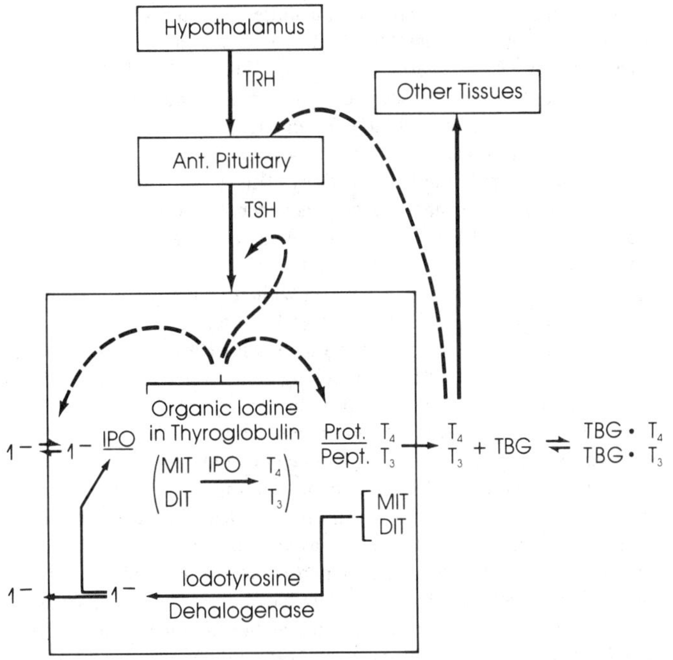

FIGURE 316-2 Schema depicting pathways in the synthesis and secretion of thyroid hormones and mechanisms for the suprathyroidal and intrathyroidal regulation of thyroid function. Small, solid arrows indicate pathways of iodine metabolism; open arrows indicate stimulation; cross-hatched arrows indicate inhibitory influences. TRH, thyrotropin-releasing hormone; TSH, thyroid-stimulating hormone; IPO, iodide peroxidase; prot., thyroid protease; peptid., thyroid peptidase; MIT, monoiodotyrosine; DIT, diiodotyrosine; T_4, thyroxine; T_3, 3,5,3′-triiodothyronine.

and T_3, into the blood. The thyroid gland is the only source of endogenous T_4; in contrast, thyroid secretion normally accounts for only about 20 percent of the T_3 produced, the remainder being generated in extraglandular tissues by the enzymatic removal of the 5′-iodine from the outer ring of T_4. Inactive iodotyrosines liberated by the hydrolysis of thyroglobulin are stripped of their iodine by an intrathyroid enzyme, iodotyrosine dehalogenase. Normally, iodide so liberated is reutilized in the synthesis of hormone, but a small proportion is lost into the blood (iodide leak); this proportion may become large under certain circumstances.

The thyroid is also capable of concentrating other monovalent anions such as pertechnetate, which is available as the radioactive isotope, sodium [^{99m}Tc]pertechnetate. Unlike iodide, little pertechnetate is organically bound; hence, its duration of stay within the thyroid is short. This property, together with its short physical half-life, makes pertechnetate a valuable radionuclide for imaging the thyroid by scintillation scanning.

The foregoing reactions are subject to inhibition by a variety of agents termed *goitrogens,* since, by virtue of their ability to inhibit hormone synthesis and indirectly stimulate TSH secretion, they induce goiter formation. Certain inorganic anions, notably perchlorate and thiocyanate, inhibit the iodide transport mechanism and thereby reduce substrate availability for hormone formation. The goiter and hypothyroidism that follow, however, can be prevented or relieved by doses of iodide sufficiently large to enable adequate quantities to enter the gland by passive diffusion. The commonly employed antithyroid agents, such as the derivatives of thiourea and mercaptoimidazole, exert more complex actions upon hormone biosynthesis. These agents, as well as certain aniline derivatives, inhibit the initial oxidation (organic binding) of iodide, decrease the proportion of DIT relative to MIT, and block coupling of iodotyrosines to form the hormonally active iodothyronines. The latter reaction is the most sensitive. Thus, it is possible for the synthesis of hormonally active iodothyronines to be decreased, although the total incorporation of iodine by the thyroid is inhibited but little. In contrast to the effect of the monovalent anions, the goitrogenic action of inhibitors of organic binding is not overcome by large quantities of iodine. Indeed, certain weak goitrogens, such as sulfonamides and antipyrine, are more potent when given with iodide, an effect not understood. Iodine itself, when given acutely in large doses, is capable of blocking the organic-binding and coupling reactions. This action (Wolff-Chaikoff effect) is normally transient, but in some otherwise normal individuals, prolonged administration of iodide is associated with continued inhibition of hormone synthesis and development of goiter, with hypothyroidism (iodide myxedema) or without hypothyroidism. Most patients with Graves' disease, especially after treatment with radioiodine or surgery, as well as patients with Hashimoto's disease, are inordinately sensitive to the blocking effect of iodide and develop hypothyroidism when given iodides chronically. The fetal thyroid is similarly sensitive, and pregnant women should not be given iodide in large amounts because of the danger of inducing goitrous hypothyroidism in the fetus. Iodide in large doses is capable of inhibiting proteolysis of thyroglobulin and hormone release, an effect readily demonstrable in hyperfunctioning thyroids and responsible for the ameliorative action of iodides in hyperthyroidism. Excess iodide may also induce thyrotoxicosis in susceptible individuals, as discussed below. Lithium, which is administered as the carbonate salt in some patients with depressive states, has several effects on intrathyroidal iodine metabolism, one of which is to inhibit hormone release. Dexamethasone in large doses also inhibits hormone release and, in conjunction with iodide, can effect a rapid reduction in the degree of thyrotoxicosis.

HORMONE TRANSPORT AND METABOLISM

HORMONE TRANSPORT In the blood, T_4 and T_3 are almost entirely bound to plasma proteins. T_4 is bound, in decreasing order of intensity, to a globulin, termed thyroxine-binding globulin (TBG), to a T_4-binding prealbumin (TBPA), and to albumin. By virtue of its intense affinity for T_4, TBG is the major determinant of normal binding. The interaction between T_4 and its binding proteins conforms to a reversible binding equilibrium in which the majority of the hormone is bound and a small proportion (normally about 0.03 percent) is free. T_3 is not significantly bound by TBPA and is bound less firmly than T_4 by TBG. As a consequence, the normal proportion of free T_3 (approximately 0.3 percent) is 8 to 10 times greater than that of T_4. Only the free or unbound hormone is available to tissues; therefore, the metabolic state correlates more closely with the concentration of free than with the concentration of total hormone in plasma, and homeostatic regulation of thyroid function is directed toward maintenance of a normal concentration of free rather than total hormone. Moreover, the relatively weak binding of T_3 accounts for its more rapid onset and offset of action. Disturbances of the thyroid hormone–plasma protein interaction are of two general types (see Table 316-1). In the first, the thyroid-pituitary axis is intrinsically normal, and the homeostatic control of thyroid hormone secretion is intact. Under these circumstances, disordered binding interactions result from alterations in thyroid hormone binding. For example, an increase in TBG initially lowers the concentration of free hormone and thus diminishes the quantity of hormone available to tissues. Total hormone concentration in serum then increases until the concentration of free hormone is restored to normal. At this time, the proportions of free T_4 and T_3 are decreased. The increase in total hormone concentration counterbalances the decrease in the free proportion; as a result, the absolute concentration of free hormone is normal, and the metabolic state of the patient is normal. Opposite changes occur when the concentration of TBG declines. Table 316-2 summarizes those states associated with primary alterations in the concentration of TBG. Primary disturbances in thyroid hormone binding also occur when other binding proteins in blood are increased, or when abnormal binding proteins appear. These are discussed below.

TABLE 316-1 Classification of the varieties of disordered thyroid hormone–plasma protein interactions

Type of abnormality	Serum T_4 and T_3	Percent FT_4 and FT_3 or RT_3U	FT_4 and FT_3 or FT_4I and FT_3I
I Primary abnormality in TBG			
A Increased concentration	↑	↓	N
B Decreased concentration	↓	↑	N
II Primary disorder of thyroid function			
A Hypothyroidism	↓		
B Hyperthyroidism	↑	↑	↑

NOTE: FT_4 = free T_4; FT_3 = free T_3; FT_4I = free T_4 index; FT_3I = free T_3 index; RT_3U = resin-T_3 uptake; TBG = thyroid-binding globulin.

The second type of disturbance of thyroid hormone–binding interactions results from a primary alteration in the concentration of thyroid hormones in the blood, as in hypothyroidism or thyrotoxicosis. Here, normal homeostatic control of thyroid hormone secretion is lost, either because of disease within the control mechanism itself or because an intact control mechanism is incapable of overcoming the effects of disease elsewhere. Under these circumstances, the concentration of TBG is changed little, if at all, and the concentration of free hormone varies directly with the total concentration of hormone. Since homeostatic mechanisms cannot restore the concentration of free hormone to normal, primary changes in thyroid function are associated with persistent changes in the concentration of total and free hormone, and, consequently, with alterations in the metabolic state. In these disorders, the proportion of free hormone changes in a direction similar to that of the change in hormone supply.

HORMONE METABOLISM Following penetration into the cell, T_4 and T_3 undergo a variety of reactions that lead ultimately to their excretion or inactivation. Thyroid hormones undergo metabolism mainly through the sequential removal of single iodine atoms (monodeiodinations) that ultimately yields the thyronine nucleus stripped of iodine. Deiodinative pathways account for approximately 70 percent of T_4 and T_3 disposal. In the case of T_4, the most important of these is the 5′-monodeiodination that leads to the generation of T_3. Since approximately 30 percent of T_4 is converted to T_3 and since T_3 has approximately three times the metabolic potency of T_4, virtually all of the metabolic action of T_4 can be ascribed to the action of the T_3 that it gives rise to. Normally, extraglandular formation accounts for about 80 percent of the T_3 in the blood and of overall T_3 production, the remainder coming from thyroid secretion. As a consequence, abnormal states and pharmacologic agents that impair T_3 formation lower the serum T_3 concentration (Table 316-3). When patients with thyroid hypofunction are treated with synthetic T_4 (levothyroxine) to sustain serum T_4 concentrations within or somewhat above the normal

TABLE 316-2 Circumstances associated with altered concentration of TBG

Increased TBG	Decreased TBG
Pregnancy	Androgens
Newborn state	Large doses of glucocorticoid
Oral contraceptives and other sources of estrogen	Chronic liver disease
Tamoxifen	Severe systemic illness
Infectious and chronic active hepatitis	Active acromegaly
Biliary cirrhosis	Nephrosis
Acute intermittent porphyria	Genetically determined
Perphenazine	Asparaginase
Genetically determined	

TABLE 316-3 States associated with decreased peripheral conversion of T_4 to T_3

I Physiologic
- *A* Fetal and early neonatal life
- *B* ? Old age

II Pathologic
- *A* Fasting
- *B* Malnutrition
- *C* Systemic illness
- *D* Physical trauma
- *E* Postoperative state
- *F* Drugs (propylthiouracil, dexamethasone, propranolol, amiodarone)
- *G* Radiographic contrast agents (ipodate; iopanoic acid)

range, normal or nearly normal serum T_3 concentrations are maintained. The generalization that the thyroid secretes relatively little T_3 does not apply to states in which the thyroid is hyperfunctioning or under increased stimulation by TSH or when thyroid iodine content is reduced. Under these conditions, the T_3/T_4 ratio of the secretory product and the serum concentration of T_3 relative to that of T_4 are increased. In addition, when T_4 production is decreased, as in early thyroid failure or iodine deficiency, the T_3/T_4 concentration ratio in blood is increased still further by an autoregulatory mechanism that leads to an increase in the efficiency of T_3 formation.

Approximately 40 percent of T_4 disposal is accounted for by monodeiodination at the 5 position of its inner ring to yield rT_3; this process accounts for nearly all rT_3 produced. rT_3 has little if any metabolic potency; therefore, the relative rates of outer- and inner-ring monodeiodination of T_4 determine the quantity of metabolically active hormone available. Factors that impair T_3 formation almost invariably increase serum rT_3 concentrations. This increase is not due to an increase in the production of rT_3 from T_4, but rather to a decrease in the 5′-monodeiodination of rT_3 to yield 3,3′-diiodothyronine (3,3′T_2), i.e., both the decreased conversion of T_4 to T_3 and the decreased degradation of rT_3 are due to a selective impairment of 5′-monodeiodination.

A second major pathway of metabolism of T_4 and T_3 and of their metabolites is conjugation in the liver, principally with glucuronate and sulfate. Conjugates either undergo deiodination locally or are secreted into the bile, but the magnitude of the enterohepatic circulation in humans is unknown. Reabsorption is incomplete at best, since the fecal excretion of T_4, T_3, and their iodine-containing metabolites accounts for approximately 20 percent of overall T_4 disposal. About 20 percent of T_4 and T_3 undergoes oxidative deamination and decarboxylation of the alanine side chain to yield tetraiodo- and triiodothyroacetic acid (tetrac and triac, respectively).

Under certain circumstances, changes in hormone accumulation and metabolism are the major determinant of changes in the rates of metabolic clearance of T_4 and T_3. Both phenobarbital and phenytoin increase the metabolic clearance of thyroid hormones without increasing the proportion of free hormone in the blood. Indeed, in the case of phenytoin, both total and free T_4 concentrations are diminished. Nevertheless, a normal metabolic state is maintained possibly because of an increase in T_3 formation.

HORMONE ACTION The thyroid hormones influence the growth and maturation of tissues, total energy expenditure, and the turnover of essentially all substrates, vitamins, and hormones, including the thyroid hormones themselves. The primary action of the hormone is exerted via binding to one or more intracellular receptor complexes which in turn bind to specific regulatory sites in the chromosomes to influence genomic expression (see Chap. 311). Other hormone actions may be mediated at the level of the mitochondrion to influence oxidative metabolism and at the level of the plasma membrane to influence the transcellular flux of substrates and cations.

REGULATION OF THYROID FUNCTION Regulation of thyroid function is effected by two general mechanisms, one suprathyroid and one intrathyroid in locus (Fig. 316-2). The proximate mediator of suprathyroid regulation is thyrotropin (thyroid-stimulating hormone, TSH), a glycoprotein secreted by basophilic (thyrotropic) cells in the anterior pituitary. TSH stimulates thyroid hypertrophy and hyperplasia; accelerates most aspects of intermediary metabolism in the thyroid; enhances synthesis of nucleic acid and protein, including thyroglobulin; and stimulates the synthesis and secretion of thyroid hormones. These actions of TSH result from binding of the hormone to specific receptors in the surface of the follicular cell and subsequent activation of the plasma membrane enzyme adenylate cyclase. The resulting increase in the cellular cyclic 3′,5′-adenosine monophosphate (cyclic AMP) concentration initiates most or all of the responses that characterize the action of TSH.

Regulation of TSH secretion, in turn, is effected by two opposing influences at the level of the thyrotropic cell. Thyrotropin-releasing hormone (TRH), a tripeptide of hypothalamic origin, stimulates the secretion and synthesis of TSH, whereas thyroid hormones both inhibit the TSH secretory mechanism directly and antagonize the action of TRH. Thus, homeostatic control of TSH secretion is exerted in a negative-feedback manner by thyroid hormones, and the threshold for feedback inhibition is apparently set by TRH. TRH is synthesized in the hypothalamus, reaches the pituitary via the hypophyseal portal blood system, and binds to specific receptors on the plasma membrane of the thyrotropic cell. Either activation of the adenylate cyclase system or a concomitant translocation of extracellular calcium into the cell initiates release of TSH. To what extent, if any, suprahypothalamic centers influence the secretion of TRH is uncertain. The negative-feedback effect of the thyroid hormones appears to take place entirely at the level of the thyrotropic cell. Thyroid hormones do not directly affect the hypothalamic secretion of TRH but reduce the number of TRH receptors on the thyrotropic cell, thus impairing its responsiveness to TRH. The negative-feedback action of the thyroid hormones is apparently mediated by a protein whose synthesis is induced by binding of the hormones to specific receptors in the nucleus of the thyrotropic cell. The principal arbiter of thyroid hormone action within the pituitary is T_3, both that generated locally from intrapituitary T_4 and that derived from the pool of free T_3 in the plasma. To what extent T_4 itself is effective within the pituitary is uncertain, but other factors modify the secretion of TSH and its response to TRH. Both somatostatin and dopamine appear to be physiologic inhibitors of TRH secretion. Estrogens enhance responsiveness to TRH, whereas glucocorticoids inhibit this function.

Intrathyroid regulation of thyroid function is also important. In some manner, changes in glandular organic iodine content cause reciprocal changes in thyroid iodide transport activity and regulate growth, amino acid uptake, glucose metabolism, and nucleic acid synthesis. These influences are evident in the absence of TSH stimulation and hence may be termed *autoregulatory*, but their most important role is to modify (iodine-enrichment inhibiting and iodine-depletion enhancing) the response to TSH, probably by modifying the generation of cyclic AMP consequent to TSH stimulation.

LABORATORY TESTS

Laboratory tests of thyroid hormone economy can be divided into five general categories: direct tests of thyroid function, tests related to the concentration and binding of thyroid hormones in blood, metabolic indexes, tests of the homeostatic control of thyroid function, and various tests that do not fit into other categories.

DIRECT TESTS OF THYROID FUNCTION Among all tests designed to assess thyroid status, only those that involve in vivo administration of radioactive iodine test glandular function per se, and measurement of the *thyroid radioactive iodine uptake* (RAIU) is the most common. ^{131}I has been used for this purpose, but ^{123}I is preferable because of the lower radiation dose that it delivers. The administered radioiodine mixes uniformly with the endogenous iodide in the extracellular fluid and, in the steady state, can be used to assess what percentage of the iodide entering and leaving the extracellular space per unit time is accumulated by the thyroid. The

RAIU is usually measured 24 h after administration of the isotope since it usually reaches a plateau value at this time, but in severe thyroid hyperfunction it may peak early. The RAIU varies inversely with the plasma iodide concentration and directly with the functional state of the thyroid. At usual levels of iodine intake in the United States (up to 1000 μg/d), the normal 24-h RAIU is approximately 5 to 30 percent of the administered dose. Consequently, this test discriminates poorly between normal and hypothyroid states. Values above the normal range, however, usually indicate thyroid hyperfunction and are useful in the diagnosis of hyperthyroidism. The RAIU is also a part of the thyroid suppression test (see below).

One valuable application of the RAIU is in the diagnosis of disorders in which thyrotoxicosis is associated with a low value of the RAIU. These include iodine-induced hyperthyroidism, thyrotoxicosis factitia, and the spontaneously resolving thyrotoxicosis that is associated with painless chronic thyroiditis or subacute thyroiditis.

TESTS RELATED TO HORMONE CONCENTRATION AND BINDING IN BLOOD Measurement of the concentration of T_4 and/or T_3 in serum, in conjunction with some assessment of hormone binding, is generally the means of confirming a diagnosis of hyperthyroidism or hypothyroidism. Highly specific and sensitive radioimmunoassays are used to measure *serum T_4* and *T_3* concentrations and when indicated for measuring *serum rT_3* concentration. The approximate normal ranges are 60 to 150 nmol/L (5 to 12 μg/dL) for T_4, 1 to 3 nmol/L (70 to 190 ng/dL) for T_3, and 0.2 to 0.6 nmol/L (10 to 40 ng/dL) for rT_3.

As mentioned above, alterations in the intensity of hormone binding by plasma proteins, as well as alterations in the rate of hormone secretion, influence the concentration of hormone in the blood. However, only alterations in hormone secretion lead to steady state alterations in the concentration of free hormone. Because they most consistently reflect the rate of hormone production, free hormone concentrations usually correlate better with the metabolic state than do total hormone concentrations. The free T_4 concentration (FT_4) can be measured by equilibrium dialysis of serum enriched with a tracer quantity of labeled T_4. The percent of T_4 that is dialyzable or free is thereby determined, and the product of this value and the total T_4 is the FT_4. However, since the dialysis technique is cumbersome, an indirect assessment of hormone binding, the *in vitro uptake test,* is simple to perform and usually provides the same information. Here, the serum is enriched with labeled T_4 or labeled T_3 and is then incubated with an insoluble, particulate matter, such as resin or charcoal, that binds free hormone. The percent of labeled hormone taken up by the particulate material varies inversely with both the concentration of unoccupied sites among the serum proteins and their affinity for the particular hormone being used. Labeled T_3 is usually used in preference to labeled T_4, since it is less strongly bound in the serum and hence yields higher, and therefore more nearly accurate, uptake values (resin T_3 uptake, RT_3U). In most clinical conditions, values of the RT_3U are proportionate to those of the percent of FT_4 and percent of FT_3. This proportionality reflects the fact that in normal serum T_4 and T_3 are mainly bound by a common binding site on TBG. Therefore, alterations in binding produced by an excess or deficiency of TBG or by an excessive or insufficient supply of T_4 do not seriously disturb the relationship between the intensity of T_4 binding and that of T_3. Under these conditions, therefore, one may calculate a *free T_4 index* (FT_4I) and a *free T_3 index* (FT_3I) as the product of the RT_3U and the total T_4 and T_3 concentrations, respectively, and these are proportional to the actual FT_4 and FT_3. (In practice, values of the FT_3 and FT_3I are rarely determined.)

Primary alterations in plasma TBG concentration (Table 316-2) produce changes in the RT_3U that are inverse and approximately proportionate to those in the serum T_4 and serum T_3; as a result, the FT_4I and FT_3I remain normal. By contrast, alterations in T_4 secretion cause changes in the percent FT_4 and RT_3U that are in the same direction as those in serum T_4. As a result, the FT_4 and FT_4I deviate from normal values more markedly than do the percent FT_4 and RT_3U alone. Immunoradiometric (IRMA) and chemiluminescent assay methods for the direct measurement of FT_4 have been developed; some provide reliable results in a wide range of disorders and may replace measurement of total T_4, RT_3U, and FT_4I in the diagnosis of thyrotoxicosis and hypothyroidism.

As noted earlier, several disorders are characterized by increased plasma binding of T_4 in which, because the protein involved is not TBG, the intensity of T_4 binding relative to that of T_3 is abnormal. Most commonly, binding of T_4 is enhanced, while that of T_3 is increased little, if at all. Included among these disorders is *familial dysalbuminemic hyperthyroxinemia (FDH)*, transmitted by autosomal dominant inheritance, in which the plasma concentration of an albumin variant with an unusually high affinity for T_4 is increased. As a result, the serum T_4 is markedly elevated, but, in keeping with the euthyroid state, FT_4 is normal. Because the RT_3U does not reflect the increase in the intensity of T_4 binding, calculated values of the FT_4I are greatly increased, often leading to a mistaken diagnosis of thyrotoxicosis. Similar findings occur when there is *increased T_4 binding by TBPA* or when the patient, usually one with autoimmune thyroid disease, develops *circulating antibodies* against T_4 itself.

In the foregoing disorders, in which the serum T_4 is increased owing to an increase in T_4 binding, the FT_4 and the metabolic state are normal. They are therefore classified among the disorders that lead to a state of *euthyroid hyperthyroxinemia,* a term that implies the presence of hyperthyroxinemia not caused by intrinsic thyroid disease (Table 316-4). The mechanism responsible for these findings is variable and in some cases uncertain. The increases in total T_4 do not appear to have any impact on the metabolic state, but the clinician should be aware of the causes of euthyroid hyperthyroxinemia lest hyperthyroidism be mistakenly diagnosed.

Some states are associated with an increased thyroid secretion of T_3, at least relative to the secretion of T_4. As a result, the serum T_3 concentration is disproportionately high relative to the prevailing serum T_4 concentration. This is apparently a consequence of hyperfunction of the follicular cell, since it is seen in all varieties of hyperthyroidism and in early thyroid failure, in which the gland is exposed to enhanced stimulation by TSH. Accordingly, the serum T_3 concentration and the derived FT_3I are generally superior to the corresponding values for T_4 in the diagnosis of hyperthyroidism. In *early* hypothyroidism, by contrast, the serum T_3 concentration and FT_3I may be normal despite subnormal values for the serum T_4 concentration and FT_4I. Consequently, the serum T_3 concentration is not reliable for the diagnosis of hypothyroidism.

Measurement of the serum rT_3 concentration is valuable in differentiating the "low T_3 syndrome" (see below) from intrinsic hypothyroidism; in the former the serum rT_3 concentration is increased, whereas in the latter it is usually subnormal.

METABOLIC INDEXES Tests in this category assess the metabolic impact of thyroid hormone in the peripheral tissues. Though tests of this type have value in the investigative setting, none of sufficient sensitivity, specificity, and ease of performance is available for routine use. Measurements of oxygen consumption in the basal state (basal metabolic rate, BMR) were once a mainstay in the diagnosis of thyroid disease but are now of historic interest. Several blood tests may be abnormal in patients with thyroid disease; their sensitivity may substantiate the diagnosis of thyroid dysfunction, but lack of specificity limits their utility. For example, serum concentrations of creatine phosphokinase and, less frequently, lactic dehydrogenase and aspartate aminotransferase are increased in hypothyroidism and may be slightly decreased in hyperthyroidism. The changes are nonspecific, and appreciation of them is important only in avoiding the inference that other diseases that produce similar changes are present. The concentrations in serum of testosterone-binding globulin (TeBG) and of angiotensin-converting enzyme are thyroid hormone–dependent and are, therefore, increased in thyrotoxicosis, but they are of no value in the diagnosis of thyroid disease. Increases in the *serum cholesterol concentration* are common in hypothyroidism of thyroid origin, and decreases in serum cholesterol are common in thyrotoxicosis. *Systolic time indexes,* such as the preejection period

TABLE 316-4 States associated with euthyroid hyperthyroxinemia

Disorder	FT_4	FT_4I	T_3	TSH	Comments
I Increased T_4 binding					
A Increased TBG	N	N	↑	N	See Tables 316-1 and 316-2
B FDH	N	↑	N,Sl ↑	N	Autosomal dominant inheritance
C Increased TBPA binding	N	↑	N	N	Increased concentration (islet-cell tumor) or affinity
D Anti-T_4 antibody	N	↑	N	N	Anti-T_3 antibody may be present
II Pituitary and peripheral thyroid hormone resistance	↑	↑	↑	↑	If only pituitary resistant, patient thyrotoxic
III Various disorders					
A Sick euthyroid syndrome	↑, N	↑	↓	N, ↓	Uncommon; poorly understood
B Acute psychiatric illness	↑, N	↑	N, ↑	N, ↑	Remits without treatment in several weeks
C Hyperemesis gravidarum	↑	↑	N	↓	Remits in several weeks
IV Drugs					
A Inhibitors of T_3-formation					
1 Radiographic contrast agents	↑	↑	↓	↑	Particularly ipodate and iopanoate
2 Propranolol	↑	↑	↓	N, ↑	Especially with large doses
3 Amiodarone	↑	↑	↓	↑	Increased TSH during first several months
B Heparin	↑	↑	N	—	Requires only small intravenous doses
C Levothyroxine therapy	↑	↑	N	↓	Hyperthyroxinemia in about 50% of cases

NOTE: FT_4 = free T_4 concentration; FT_4I = free T_4 index calculated from an in vitro T_3 uptake test; TSH = basal serum TSH concentration and response to TRH; N = normal; Sl = slightly.

and pulse-wave arrival time, are prolonged in hypothyroidism and shortened in hyperthyroidism. They are of value in monitoring thyroid replacement therapy in elderly patients or in patients with coexisting heart disease.

TESTS OF HOMEOSTATIC CONTROL Measurement of the basal *serum TSH concentration* is useful in the diagnosis of both advanced and subclinical hypothyroidism. The latter state represents a stage in the evolution of hypothyroidism, in which a structural or functional abnormality that impairs hormone synthesis is compensated for by hypersecretion of TSH. The normal TSH level is less than 5 mU/L. In thyrotoxic states, serum TSH concentration is almost always low or undetectable. While the conventional radioimmunoassays cannot distinguish between normal and subnormal values, immunoradiometric or chemiluminescent techniques employing monoclonal antibodies provide exquisite sensitivity. Thyrotoxic patients tend to have undetectable levels (<0.1 mU/L) while values in most normal subjects range between 0.3 and 3.0 mU/L in these assays (Fig. 316-3). Serum TSH concentrations are absolutely or inappropriately elevated, relative to serum FT_4 and FT_3 values, in patients with TSH-induced hyperthyroidism. This rare syndrome results either from a TSH-secreting pituitary adenoma or resistance of the TSH secretory mechanism to feedback inhibition by T_4 and T_3. Measurement of serum TSH is the best means of distinguishing between untreated hypothyroidism of thyroid origin, in which the values are invariably increased, and pituitary or hypothalamic hypothyroidism, in which the values are usually undetectable or within the normal range. Occasional patients with hypothyroidism of hypothalamic or pituitary origin secrete a form of TSH that is immunoactive but not bioactive. Here, serum TSH concentrations may be elevated rather than depressed.

The *thyrotropin-releasing hormone (TRH) stimulation test* assesses the functional state of the TSH-secretory mechanism, and has diagnostic value in diverse circumstances. Following the intravenous injection of TRH in normal subjects, the serum TSH begins to increase within minutes, reaches a maximum between 20 and 45 min, and then rapidly declines. The nature of the pituitary feedback mechanism is such that when hypothalamic-pituitary function is normal, one would expect an increased response to TRH when the thyrotropic cell senses a deficiency of thyroid hormone, particularly T_3, and a decreased or absent response when there is thyroid hormone excess. Thus, except in the rare instances of pituitary resistance to thyroid hormone, in which responses are usually normal, thyrotoxicosis is invariably accompanied by a blunted or absent TSH response to TRH. Owing to extreme sensitivity of the TSH-secretory mechanism to feedback inhibition, diminished responses to TRH commonly occur in apparently euthyroid patients with serum T_4 or T_3 levels within the normal range but with marginally increased T_4 or T_3 output from autonomously functioning toxic adenomas or toxic multinodular goiters. Blunted TRH responses may be also seen in some patients with euthyroid Graves' disease. In addition, responses to TRH are often decreased in elderly individuals, especially men. Despite these exceptions, a subnormal or absent response to TRH is an excellent confirmatory test for thyrotoxicosis. TRH tests are of less value in the diagnosis of hypothyroidism. Responses are increased in patients with primary hypothyroidism, but the magnitude of increase is generally proportional to the extent of increase in basal serum TSH. Some patients with pituitary hypothyroidism have subnormal responses, and some with TRH deficiency owing to hypothalamic disease have a near-normal response, but these expected responses are not seen consistently. Further, in as many as one-fourth of patients with hypothyroidism due to hypothalamic-pituitary disease, basal serum TSH concentrations are normal or slightly elevated, and the response to TRH is exaggerated, although some of this TSH may not be bioactive.

The *thyroid suppression test* is used to assess whether thyroid

FIGURE 316-3 Utility of sensitive TSH assay in evaluation of suspected thyroid dysfunction in ambulatory patients.

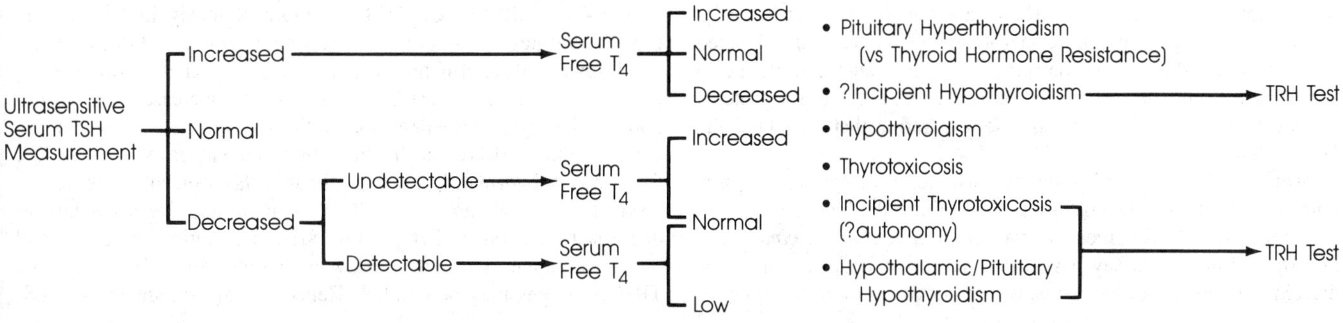

function is controlled by normal homeostatic mechanisms. Normally, exogenous thyroid hormone suppresses pituitary TSH secretion, resulting in a decrease in the RAIU. Since liothyronine is usually employed for the test (100 μg daily for 7 to 10 days), the resulting decline in serum T_4, as well as in the RAIU, can serve as an index of suppression. A normal suppressive response is a decrease of the RAIU to less than half of the control value and a decline of the serum T_4 to low normal or subnormal values. An abnormal suppression test is always present in hyperthyroidism, irrespective of the underlying cause; this indicates either autonomy of thyroid function, the presence of an abnormal (non-TSH) thyroid stimulator, or unremitting hypersecretion of TSH. A normal suppression test, on the other hand, is incompatible with and excludes a diagnosis of hyperthyroidism. An abnormal suppression test is not pathognomonic of hyperthyroidism, however, since it may persist after treatment of hyperthyroidism in Graves' disease and is seen in about half of the euthyroid patients with the ophthalmopathy of Graves' disease.

Because of the risk of adverse effects of exogenous thyroid hormone especially liothyronine in elderly patients and in those with cardiovascular disease, and since the TRH test is almost entirely devoid of undesirable side effects, the latter test has almost entirely supplanted the thyroid suppression test in the diagnosis of hyperthyroidism.

MISCELLANEOUS TESTS Various tests that do not assess thyroid function are of value in defining the nature of the thyroid disorder or in planning therapy. For example, high titers of *antimicrosomal antibodies* or *antithyroglobulin antibodies* are found in the serum of most adults with Hashimoto's disease and in many patients with primary thyroprivic hypothyroidism or Graves' disease. In the latter, the serum also contains antibodies against the TSH receptor on thyroid plasma membranes. In general, these are capable of inhibiting the receptor binding of TSH (TSH-binding inhibitory immunoglobulins, TBII) and of stimulating the production of cyclic AMP therein (thyroid-stimulating immunoglobulins, TSI). The clinical utility of tests for TBII and TSI stems from the fact that the disappearance of the factors from the serum during a course of antithyroid therapy implies the likelihood of a long-term remission of hyperthyroidism when therapy is withdrawn. In some patients, analogous antibodies have no intrinsic stimulatory effect but block the response to endogenous TSH and produce nongoitrous hypothyroidism. Both stimulatory and blocking anti-TSH receptor antibodies have the ability to cross the placenta and, as a consequence, to produce transient hyperthyroidism (neonatal Graves' disease) or hypothyroidism, respectively, in the newborn. Measurement of these antibodies during the last months of pregnancy makes it possible to assess the likelihood of the disorders developing in the neonate.

Some patients, most commonly those with autoimmune thyroid disease, develop *circulating antibodies against T_3 or T_4*, or both. In radioimmunoassays for these hormones, because the endogenous antibody competes with the exogenous antibody for binding of the added labeled ligand, spurious values for the concentration of the hormone are obtained. These may be grossly elevated or greatly depressed, depending on the technique of radioimmunoassay used. The true concentration of the hormone, as determined in extracts of the serum, is increased owing to the additional binding sites provided by the antibody, but antibody-bound hormone is unavailable for metabolic action. In the case of anti-T_3 antibodies, which are the more common, values of the RT_3U are low because endogenous antibody competes with the resin for binding of the added labeled T_3. Such antibodies can be detected by adding labeled hormone to serum, separating the immunoglobulins from other serum proteins by any of several techniques, and demonstrating that they bind the labeled hormone.

Along with several other thyroid disorders, differentiated carcinomas of the thyroid release thyroglobulin into the bloodstream. As a consequence, measurements of the *serum thyroglobulin concentration* by radioimmunoassay have value not in the initial diagnosis of thyroid carcinoma but in assessing the adequacy of initial therapy and in monitoring for recurrence or dissemination of the disease. In patients with thyrotoxicosis, subnormal serum thyroglobulin concentrations together with decreased values of the RAIU suggest the presence of thyrotoxicosis factitia.

Imaging by *scintiscanning* permits localization of sites of accumulation of radioiodine or sodium [^{99m}Tc]pertechnetate. This technique is useful for defining areas of increased or decreased function within the thyroid and for detecting retrosternal goiter, ectopic thyroid tissue, hemiagenesis of the thyroid, and functioning metastases of thyroid carcinoma. Ultrasonic examination of the thyroid is also a valuable technique for differentiating cystic nodules from those that are solid. Since ultrasonic scans provide an accurate indication of size, are noninvasive, and apparently have no injurious effects, sequential scans can be employed to assess changes in the size of the thyroid as a whole or of discrete nodules over time or in response to treatment.

SICK EUTHYROID SYNDROME

Severe illness, physical trauma, or physiologic stress can induce changes in one or more aspects of thyroid hormone economy, leading to findings referred to as the sick euthyroid syndrome (SES). Abnormalities in SES include alterations in the peripheral transport and metabolism of the thyroid hormones; the regulation of TSH secretion; and in some cases changes in thyroid function itself. Acting alone or together, these lead to changes in the concentrations of the circulating thyroid hormones, both total and free, that serve to define the several variants of the SES. Because of the frequency of illness in the general population and the nonspecificity of the disorders that cause it, SES is probably a more common cause of abnormalities in the concentration of thyroid hormones in the blood than intrinsic thyroid disease.

NORMAL-T_4 VARIANT OF SES Decreased production of T_3 owing to inhibition of the peripheral 5′-monodeiodination of T_4 is a consistent feature of the SES. This is reflected in a decrease in the serum total T_3 concentration that varies in severity with that of the illness. In moderately ill patients, serum total T_4 concentration is within the normal range. A decrease in the intensity of protein binding, greater for T_4 than T_3, is an additional accompaniment. As a result, values of the RT_3U are moderately increased, and the percent FT_4 is increased to a proportionately greater extent. As a consequence, values of the free T_4 index (FT_4I) and those of the free T_4 concentrations (FT_4) are often increased. Serum rT_3 concentrations are increased, owing to a decrease in the plasma clearance of rT_3 secondary to inhibition of its 5′-monodeiodination. The plasma clearance rate of T_4 is increased, probably as a result of decreased T_4 binding, and this, in the face of normal T_4 concentrations, indicates that the overall rate of T_4 degradation and production is increased. Production rates for T_3 are decreased, and those for rT_3 are normal. Serum TSH concentration and the response of serum TSH to TRH are generally normal, though they may increase to supranormal values and then return to normal as recovery from the illness takes place. Despite the reduction in the serum T_3 concentration, this variant of the SES can be separated from intrinsic thyroid disease because the serum T_4 and TSH are normal and because the serum T_3 is not useful for diagnosing hypothyroidism in any event.

LOW-T_4 VARIANT OF SES In more seriously ill patients, T_3 production rates and serum total and free T_3 concentrations decrease still further, and abnormalities in hormone binding increase in severity. As a consequence, serum T_4 concentrations decrease into the hypothyroid range, sometimes markedly so. This is partly but not entirely due to decreased T_4 binding since values of the FT_4 are frequently subnormal. These are probably the result of decreased T_4 production in the most severely ill patients and are secondary to decreased secretion of TSH. Serum TSH concentrations appear normal by conventional assay but are low with sensitive TSH assays, and TRH responses may be blunted. Hence, in this variant of the SES, there is an inappropriate hyposecretion of TSH, considering the low serum total and free T_4 and T_3 concentrations; its cause is unknown, but a diagnosis of pituitary hypothyroidism may be suggested. Production rates for rT_3 are diminished, owing to the decreased availability of its precursor T_4; nonetheless, serum rT_3 concentrations are increased, owing to retardation of its degradation, and this provides an important means of differentiating the SES from pituitary hypothyroidism, in which serum rT_3 concentrations are low. In patients with primary hypothyroidism who have associated illness, serum TSH concentrations remain elevated, though their concentrations are generally lower than they otherwise would be.

HIGH-T_4 VARIANT OF SES An unusual variant of the SES (approximately 1 percent of sick patients) is associated with increased serum total and free T_4 concentrations during acute illness and return to normal thereafter. This variant is most often seen in elderly women, many of whom have received medications that contain iodine. The principal source of diagnostic confusion is with the syndrome of "T_4 toxicosis," i.e., true thyrotoxicosis upon which illness has been superimposed, so that serum T_4 concentrations are increased and serum T_3 concentrations are normal. In the latter, however, serum rT_3 concentrations are higher, values of the serum total T_3 and FT_3I are higher, and TRH responses are blunted.

ABNORMALITIES IN HORMONE BINDING IN SES Multiple factors are responsible for the decreased binding of T_4 and, to a lesser extent, T_3 in the SES. Illness is associated with decreased synthesis of TBPA and a decrease in its serum concentration, but the extent to which this contributes to decreased T_4 binding is uncertain. In chronically ill patients, serum TBG concentration is subnormal. Most often, however, the extent of decreased T_4 binding cannot be explained by decreases in serum TBPA and TBG, and an inhibitor of hormone binding may be responsible. Its nature is uncertain, but it may be one or more fatty acids, which may also be responsible for diminished conversion of T_4 to T_3.

The importance of the SES is that the changes in circulating thyroid hormone concentrations that result should not be confused with those due to intrinsic thyroid or pituitary disease. Unresolved questions are whether the metabolic impact of thyroid hormone in peripheral tissues is decreased in the SES, whether the syndrome is a beneficial or adverse response to illness, and whether some patients would benefit from treatment with thyroid hormone.

SIMPLE (NONTOXIC) GOITER

Endemic goiter implies an etiologic factor or factors common to a particular geographic region. The term has been defined as the presence of generalized or localized thyroid enlargement in more than 10 percent of the population. *Sporadic* goiter arises in nonendemic areas as a result of factors that do not affect the population generally. Since these terms fail to define or distinguish the causes of such goiters and since thyroid enlargement of diverse etiology may exist in both endemic and nonendemic regions, it is prudent to employ a general term such as *simple* or *nontoxic goiter*. This all-inclusive category can be further subdivided into specific etiologic groups. Simple or nontoxic goiter can be defined as any enlargement of the thyroid gland that does not result from an inflammatory or neoplastic process and that is not initially associated with thyrotoxicosis or myxedema.

ETIOLOGY AND PATHOGENESIS Simple goiter is sometimes due to a definable cause of impaired thyroid hormone synthesis, such as iodine deficiency, ingestion of a goitrogen, or a demonstrable defect in a hormone biosynthetic pathway, but in most instances its cause is unknown. Whatever the cause, the clinical manifestations reflect the operation of a common pathophysiologic mechanism. Simple goiter occurs when one or more factors impair the capacity of the thyroid to secrete active hormones sufficient to meet the needs of the peripheral tissues. Although this has been presumed to lead to increased secretion of TSH, concentrations of TSH in the serum of patients with established simple goiter are usually normal. Hence, some other mechanism of goitrogenesis may be operative. A likely possibility is that depletion of glandular organic iodine accompanying impaired hormone synthesis increases the responsiveness of thyroid structure and function to levels of TSH that remain within the normal range. The resulting increases in both functioning thyroid mass and cellular activity overcome mild impairment of hormone synthesis; thus, the patient is metabolically normal, though goitrous. When the underlying disorder is severe, compensatory responses, now including hypersecretion of TSH, are inadequate to overcome the impairment, and the patient is both goitrous and hypothyroid. Thus, simple goiter cannot be clearly separated in the pathogenetic sense from goitrous hypothyroidism. Specific causes of simple goiter may exist with or without hypothyroidism (Table 316-5). Defective iodination of thyroglobulin may be an important cause in many patients. The possibility that goiter can be due to antibodies that stimulate thyroid growth but not function remains to be substantiated.

PATHOLOGY The histopathology of the thyroid in simple goiter varies with the severity of the etiologic factor and the stage at which the examination is made. In its initial stages, the gland exhibits a uniform hypertrophy, hyperplasia, and hypervascularity. As the disorder persists or undergoes repeated exacerbations and remissions, uniformity of thyroidal architecture is lost. Occasionally, the greater part of the gland may display a uniform involution or hyperinvolution with colloid accumulation. More often such areas are interspersed with patchy areas of focal hyperplasia. Fibrosis may demarcate hyperplastic or involuted nodules. These may resemble true neoplasms (adenomas). Areas of hemorrhage and irregular calcification may be present. The evolution of the multinodular stage is almost always accompanied by the development of functional autonomy. Indeed, heterogeneity of structure and function and a greater or lesser degree of functional autonomy are the hallmarks of the mature stage of this disorder.

CLINICAL MANIFESTATIONS In simple goiter the clinical manifestations arise solely from enlargement of the thyroid since the metabolic state is normal. In goitrous hypothyroidism, symptoms caused by thyromegaly are accompanied by signs and symptoms of hormonal insufficiency. Mechanical sequelae include compression and displacement of the trachea or esophagus, occasionally with obstructive symptoms if the goiter becomes sufficiently large. Superior mediastinal obstruction may occur with large retrosternal goiters. Signs of compression can be induced in the case of large retrosternal goiters when the patient's arms are raised above the head (Pemberton's sign); suffusion of the face, giddiness, or syncope may result from this maneuver. Hoarseness due to compression of the recurrent laryngeal nerve is rare in simple goiter and suggests neoplasm. Sudden hemorrhage into a nodule may lead to an acute, painful swelling in the neck and may produce or enhance compressive symptoms.

TABLE 316-5 Classification of the causes of hypothyroidism

I Thyroid
- *A* Thyroprivic
  - *1* Congenital development defect
  - *2* Primary idiopathic
  - *3* Postablative (radioiodine, surgery)
  - *4* Postradiation (lymphoma)
- *B* Goitrous
  - *1* Heritable biosynthetic defects
  - *2* Maternally transmitted (iodides, antithyroid agents)
  - *3* Iodine deficiency
  - *4* Drug-elicited (aminosalicylic acid, iodides, phenylbutazone, iodoantipyrine, lithium)
  - *5* Chronic thyroiditis (Hashimoto's disease)

II Suprathyroid (trophoprivic)
- *A* Pituitary
- *B* Hypothalamic

III Self-limited
- *A* Following withdrawal of suppressive thyroid therapy
- *B* Subacute thyroiditis and chronic thyroiditis with transient hypothyroidism (usually after a phase of thyrotoxicosis)

Hyperthyroidism may supervene in long-standing multinodular goiter (toxic multinodular goiter). In both endemic and sporadic multinodular goiter, the ingestion of excess iodide may result in the development of thyrotoxicosis (jod-Basedow phenomenon).

In regions where iodine deficiency is severe, goitrous enlargement may also be associated with varying degrees of hypothyroidism. Cretinism, both goitrous and nongoitrous, occurs with increased frequency in the children of goitrous parents in many countries where goiter is common. Although iodine deficiency is doubtless a factor in the etiology of endemic goiter, the frequency of goiter differs greatly among areas of equally severe iodine deficiency. In such instances, dietary or waterborne goitrogens appear to be important conditioning factors. In some areas, these goitrogens may be sufficient to cause goiter in the absence of iodine deficiency.

DIAGNOSIS The diagnosis of simple goiter requires, first, demonstration of a euthyroid state and, second, demonstration of normal serum T_4 and T_3 concentrations. The former may be difficult because manifestations of thyrotoxicosis may be subtle or atypical, especially among the elderly (see section on "Toxic Multinodular Goiter"). The latter may be problematic, since serum T_4 and especially T_3 concentrations may be near the upper limit of the normal range. In addition, the fact that serum T_3 concentrations decrease in the euthyroid elderly complicates interpretation of this test. The RAIU is usually normal but may be increased in the presence of iodine deficiency or a biosynthetic defect. Indeed, subclinical thyrotoxicosis may be present secondary to the significant functional autonomy of the goiter and consequently cause a decrease in both basal TSH and TSH response to TRH. Differentiation of nontoxic goiter from Hashimoto's disease is facilitated by the greater frequency of multinodularity in the former and by the presence of high titers of circulating antimicrosomal or antithyroglobulin antibodies in the latter. In some instances, emergence of a strongly dominant nodule may suggest the presence of a carcinoma. This is especially true if bleeding has caused it to increase in size rapidly and to lose the ability to accumulate iodine or pertechnetate.

TREATMENT The object of treatment is to reduce the size of the goiter, either by relieving external encumbrances to hormone formation or by providing sufficient quantities of exogenous hormone to inhibit TSH secretion and thereby put the thyroid gland almost completely at rest. In disorders characterized by decreased thyroid iodide stores, such as iodine deficiency or impairment of the thyroid iodide-concentrating mechanism, small doses of iodide may prove effective. Occasionally, a known extrinsic goitrogen can be withdrawn. Most commonly, however, no specific etiologic factor can be detected, and thyroid hormone therapy is required. For this purpose, levothyroxine (L-thyroxine) is the agent of choice. In the younger patient with the early diffuse stage of simple goiter, treatment can be instituted with 100 μg of levothyroxine daily, and the dose is increased over the next month or so to a maximum of 150 or 200 μg daily (average dose of 1.8 μg/kg body weight per day). Complete suppression would imply reduction of serum TSH to levels less than 0.1 mU/L by an ultrasensitive assay. Until uncertainties about the association of long-term excess thyroid hormone therapy and loss of bone mineral (osteopenia) are resolved, patients should be titrated to slightly less than a fully suppressive dose. Adequacy of suppression also may be assessed by measuring the RAIU, which should decrease to less than 5 percent of the administered dose at 24 h. Lesser decreases indicate only partial suppression, which may reflect the presence of autonomous foci demonstrable by scanning techniques. In the elderly or the patient with long-standing multinodular goiter, an ultrasensitive TSH measurement or a TRH stimulation test should be undertaken before initiating treatment with levothyroxine to determine whether significant functional autonomy is present. If such is indicated by an undetectable basal TSH or a diminished or absent TSH responsiveness to TRH, suppressive therapy with levothyroxine is contraindicated since such patients are or will eventually become thyrotoxic. Rather, consideration should be given to radioiodine ablation of the autonomous foci (see later section on "Toxic Multinodular Goiter"). On the other hand, if the TSH response to TRH is normal, excluding significant functional autonomy, treatment with levothyroxine can be initiated. In the elderly patient, the initial dose should not exceed 50 μg daily, and the dosage should be gradually increased, partial rather than complete suppression of the value for basal TSH and/or the RAIU being the end point. It is the practice to obtain a thyroid scan as part of the initial evaluation of all patients with multinodular goiter and to repeat the RAIU and scan (suppression scan), when practical, in patients receiving suppressive thyroid hormone therapy.

Results of therapy vary widely. The early diffuse, hyperplastic goiter responds well, with regression or disappearance in 3 to 6 months. In the authors' experience, the later, nodular stage responds less favorably, and significant reduction in gland size is achieved only in about one-third of the cases; however, in the remainder, suppressive treatment may forestall further glandular growth. Internodular tissue regresses more often than do nodules themselves. The latter may therefore appear to become more prominent during treatment. After maximum regression of the goiter, suppressive medication may be maintained for prolonged periods, reduced to minimal levels, or at times withdrawn. In an unpredictable manner, goiter may remain relieved or recur. In the latter instances, suppressive therapy should be reinstituted and continued indefinitely. In areas of endemic iodine deficiency, the size and prevalence of goiter and the frequency of cretinism can be reduced by the provision of iodized salt or water or the periodic injection of iodized oil.

Surgical therapy of simple goiter is physiologically unsound, but it may occasionally be necessary to relieve obstructive symptoms, especially those that persist after a trial of medical therapy. Surgical exploration of nodular goiter may be indicated in some individuals when evidence suggests carcinoma. However, the concept that subtotal resection of multinodular nontoxic goiter affords effective prophylaxis against the development of thyroid carcinoma is unsound. If for some reason subtotal thyroidectomy has been performed, levothyroxine in a usual dose of about 1.8 μg/kg body weight daily is recommended to inhibit regenerative hyperplasia and further goitrogenesis.

HYPOTHYROIDISM

Hypothyroidism can result from any of a variety of abnormalities that lead to insufficient synthesis of thyroid hormone. Hypothyroidism dating from birth and resulting in developmental abnormalities is termed *cretinism*. The term *myxedema* connotes severe hypothyroidism in which there is accumulation of hydrophilic mucopolysaccharides in the ground substance of the dermis and other tissues, leading to thickening of the facial features and doughy induration of the skin.

ETIOLOGY AND PATHOGENESIS A classification of hypothyroidism is presented in Table 316-5. Overall, the thyroid varieties account for approximately 95 percent of cases, only 5 percent or less being suprathyroid in origin. In thyroprivic hypothyroidism, loss of thyroid tissue leads to inadequate synthesis of thyroid hormone, despite maximum stimulation of any thyroid remnant by TSH. The most common cause of thyroprivic hypothyroidism is surgical or radioiodine ablation of the thyroid gland in the treatment of Graves' disease. Thyroprivic hypothyroidism may also occur as a primary idiopathic disorder. Primary hypothyroidism is frequently associated with circulating antithyroid antibodies and in some cases may result from the action of antibodies that block the TSH receptor. It may coexist with diabetes mellitus and other diseases in which circulating autoantibodies are found, such as pernicious anemia, systemic lupus erythematosus, rheumatoid arthritis, Sjögren's syndrome, and chronic hepatitis. In addition, hypothyroidism can be one manifestation of a polyglandular endocrine deficiency state in which autoantibodies cause variable insufficiency of thyroid, adrenal, parathyroid, and gonadal function (see Chap. 325). All these diseases, including isolated primary hypothyroidism, are associated with an increased frequency of specific HLA haplotypes and may be diverse reflections of disordered immune regulation. Finally, a developmental defect may result in failure of the gland to function adequately, leading to sporadic nongoitrous cretinism or juvenile hypothyroidism. A self-limited period of hypothyroidism is common in the course of subacute thyroiditis and in the syndrome of "painless thyroiditis," including the postpartum variant and usually after a temporary period of thyrotoxicosis. Owing to a persisting lack of TSH stimulation, intrinsically euthyroid subjects from whom chronic suppressive therapy is abruptly withdrawn experience a several-week period of thyroid hypofunction.

Impairment in the ability to synthesize adequate quantities of thyroid hormone leads to hypersecretion of TSH and hence goiter. If this compensatory response is inadequate, goitrous hypothyroidism ensues. The commonest cause of goitrous hypothyroidism in North America is Hashimoto's disease, in which defective organic binding of iodide and abnormal secretion of iodoproteins are frequent abnormalities. Iodide-induced goiter with or without hypothyroidism appears to arise from an intrinsic defect in the organic binding mechanism, which permits a persistent Wolff-Chaikoff effect. Euthyroid patients with Graves' disease, especially after surgery or radioiodine treatment, those with Hashimoto's disease, and the normal fetus are particularly susceptible to iodide-induced goiter. In view of the susceptibility of the fetal thyroid to iodide, with resulting goiter and hypothyroidism, iodine in large doses should not be given during pregnancy. Less common causes of goitrous hypothyroidism are hereditary defects in hormone biosynthesis and ingestion of drugs that induce defects in hormone biosynthesis, such as aminosalicylic acid and lithium. Finally, in areas of environmental iodine deficiency, goitrous cretinism and hypothyroidism can occur on an endemic basis. Diminished thyroid reserve occurs as a stage in the evolution of both thyroprivic and goitrous hypothyroidism.

In hypothyroidism of suprathyroid origin, the thyroid is intrinsically normal but is deprived of stimulation by TSH. Deprivation of TSH, most commonly the result of postpartum pituitary necrosis or a tumor of the pituitary or adjacent regions, results in pituitary hypothyroidism. Hypothalamic hypothyroidism is less common and results from inadequate secretion of TRH.

CLINICAL PICTURE The appearance of children with hypothyroidism depends on the age at which the deficiency began and the promptness with which replacement therapy was instituted. Cretinism may be manifested at birth but usually becomes evident within the first several months, depending upon the extent of thyroid failure. Hypothyroidism is present in approximately 1 of every 5000 neonates and manifests itself in persistence of physiologic jaundice, hoarse cry, constipation, somnolence, and feeding problems; since clinical diagnosis is difficult and early treatment is crucial for normal intellectual development, all neonates should be screened for hypothyroidism with measurements of the serum T_4 or TSH. In later months, delay in reaching the normal milestones of development becomes evident, and the physical characteristics of the cretin appear. These include short stature, coarse features with protruding tongue, broad flat nose, widely set eyes, sparse hair, dry skin, protuberant abdomen with an umbilical hernia, and impaired mental development. X-ray examination reveals retarded bone age, epiphyseal dysgenesis, and delayed dentition.

In the older child, the clinical manifestations of hypothyroidism are intermediate between those of infantile and adult hypothyroidism. Retardation of linear growth is manifested by shortness of stature, and retardation of sexual maturation results in delay in the onset of puberty. Poor performance at school may call attention to the diagnosis. The manifestations of adult hypothyroidism are present to a variable degree. X-ray examination reveals delayed union of the epiphyses.

In the adult, early symptoms of hypothyroidism are nonspecific and of insidious onset. They may include lethargy, constipation, cold intolerance, stiffness and cramping of the muscles, the carpal tunnel syndrome, and menorrhagia. Over the succeeding months, intellectual and motor activity slows, appetite declines, and weight increases. The hair becomes dry and tends to fall out, and the skin becomes dry. The voice becomes deeper and hoarse, and auditory acuity may deteriorate. Obstructive sleep apnea may occur. Ultimately, the clinical picture of florid myxedema appears, with dull expressionless face, sparse hair, periorbital puffiness, large tongue, and pale, cool skin that feels rough and doughy. Thyroid tissue is not readily palpable, except in the goitrous variety of hypothyroidism. The heart is enlarged owing to both dilation and pericardial effusion; if the heart is small, pituitary hypothyroidism (with adrenal insufficiency) should be considered. Adynamic ileus may result in megacolon or intestinal obstruction. Rarely, psychiatric symptoms or cerebellar ataxia may dominate the clinical picture. The relaxation phase of the deep tendon reflexes is characteristically prolonged, the so-called hung-up reflex. If left untreated, the patient with severe long-standing hypothyroidism may pass into a hypothermic, stuporous state (*myxedema coma*) that is frequently fatal. Respiratory depression is an important component of this state, and hence arterial P_{CO_2} may be increased. Factors that predispose to myxedema coma include cold exposure, trauma, infection, and administration of central nervous system depressants. Dilutional hyponatremia is common and results from impaired water excretion and from disordered regulation of vasopressin secretion.

LABORATORY TESTS The single most useful measurement is the serum TSH, which is invariably increased in the thyroprivic and goitrous varieties and is usually normal or undetectable in pituitary or hypothalamic hypothyroidism (Fig. 316-3). In the latter instances, hyposecretion of TSH is usually accompanied by hyposecretion of other pituitary hormones (see Chap. 313). A decrease in serum T_4 and in the FT_4I is common to all varieties of hypothyroidism. In the thyroid varieties, the serum T_3 may be decreased to a lesser extent than the serum T_4, the presumption being that the compensatory hypersecretion of TSH leads to a relative preponderance of T_3 secretion. In thyroprivic hypothyroidism the decreased RAIU is of limited diagnostic utility because of the low value for the lower limit of the normal range. In goitrous hypothyroidism, the RAIU may be increased or display an abnormal pattern of accumulation or retention.

Frequent manifestations of the hypothyroid state include an increased serum cholesterol in hypothyroidism of thyroid (but not pituitary) origin and increased concentrations in serum of creatine phosphokinase, aspartate transaminase, and lactic dehydrogenase. Systolic time intervals are altered in that the preejection period is prolonged, and the ratio of the preejection period to left ventricular ejection time is increased. Electrocardiographic changes include bradycardia, low-amplitude QRS complexes, and flattened or inverted T waves. In primary thyroprivic hypothyroidism, overt pernicious anemia occurs in about 12 percent of patients; histamine-fast achlorhydria and circulating antigastric parietal cell antibodies are more common.

Some patients who appear clinically euthyroid display laboratory evidence of early thyroid failure (subclinical hypothyroidism). In mild cases serum TSH and its response to TRH administration are increased while serum T_4 and T_3 concentrations are normal. When there is a greater degree of thyroid failure, serum T_4 concentration is decreased, but the serum T_3 concentration is normal or nearly so owing to TSH-induced hypersecretion of T_3 relative to T_4, and perhaps to more efficient conversion of T_4 to T_3. Subclinical hypothyroidism is most often seen in patients with Hashimoto's disease or those with Graves' disease who have been treated with ^{131}I or surgery and are usually stages in the evolution of frank hypothyroidism.

DIFFERENTIAL DIAGNOSIS Little difficulty will be experienced in diagnosing the classic picture of cretinism or juvenile and adult hypothyroidism. Occasionally, an infant with Down's syndrome may be confused with a cretin. However, the characteristic eye changes, Brushfield's spots in the iris, hyperextensibility of the joints, and normal skin and hair texture distinguish Down's syndrome from cretinism. Chronic nephritis and the nephrotic syndrome may simulate myxedema, particularly because of the facial puffiness and pallor. The nephrotic patient may have anemia, hypercholesterolemia, and anasarca, and the serum T_4 concentration may be decreased if there is significant loss of TBG into the urine. However, the FT_4I is normal or increased, the serum T_3 concentration is often subnormal, as in any severe systemic illness owing to impaired peripheral generation from T_4, and the serum TSH concentration is normal.

TREATMENT Two types of hormone are available for the treatment of hypothyroidism, synthetic hormone and thyroprotein derived from animal thyroids (Table 316-6). Synthetic hormones include levothyroxine (L-thyroxine), liothyronine (L-triiodothyronine), and liotrix (a combination of the two). The preparation of natural origin most commonly used is thyroid extract, USP. Because of their uniform potency, the authors prefer the synthetic preparations and specifically levothyroxine. Unlike liothyronine, liotrix, and even thyroid extract, ingestion of levothyroxine does not lead to abrupt increases in serum T_3 concentration, which can be dangerous in the older patient or in the patient with coexisting heart disease. Rather, a stable T_3 concentration is attained through continuous generation from administered levothyroxine.

In most instances, a normal metabolic state should be restored gradually, especially in the elderly or the patient with heart disease, since sudden increases in metabolic rate may tax cardiac or coronary reserve. In adults, an initial daily dose of 25 μg levothyroxine can be increased by 25- to 50-μg increments at 2- to 3-week intervals, until a normal metabolic state is attained. The dose necessary to sustain a normal metabolic state is usually about 1.8 μg/kg body weight per day, and this usually results in a serum T_4 at or somewhat above the upper limit of the normal range. The serum T_3 is superior to the serum T_4 as an indicator of the metabolic state in the patient receiving levothyroxine. Because of its long half-life, levothyroxine is administered as a single daily dose. The optimum dose for an individual should be based on clinical criteria and on measurements of serum TSH by an ultrasensitive assay or T_3. Elevations of the former indicate that treatment is insufficient and of the latter that it is excessive.

In neonatal, infantile, and juvenile hypothyroidism it is essential that full replacement therapy be begun as soon as possible; otherwise the chances of normal intellectual development and growth are poor. Infants and children require doses of levothyroxine that are disproportionately large in relation to body size. *In known or strongly suspected pituitary and hypothalamic hypothyroidism, thyroid replacement should not be instituted until treatment with hydrocortisone has been initiated,* since acute adrenocortical insufficiency may be precipitated by an increase in metabolic rate.

In some patients, hypothyroidism should be treated rapidly. This includes patients with myxedema coma and, because of the extreme sensitivity to central nervous system depressants, hypothyroid patients being prepared for emergency surgery. Here, intravenous administration of levothyroxine, in conjunction with the use of hydrocortisone, is indicated.

THYROTOXICOSIS

The term *thyrotoxicosis* denotes the clinical, physiologic, and biochemical findings that result when the tissues are exposed to, and respond to, an excess supply of thyroid hormone. Rather than a specific disease, thyrotoxicosis is a syndrome that can originate in a variety of ways (Table 316-7). The first, and most important, encompasses those diseases that lead to sustained overproduction of hormone by the thyroid gland itself. Here, hyperfunction of the gland variously results from excessive secretion of TSH, a rare cause associated with pituitary tumor or with resistance to thyroid hormone in the pituitary but not in peripheral tissues; the action of an abnormal, homeostatically unregulated thyroid stimulator of extrapituitary origin, as in Graves' disease, hyperthyroidism in association with Hashimoto's disease, or trophoblastic tumors; or the development of one or more areas of autonomous hyperfunction within the gland itself. The second category encompasses the thyrotoxic states associated with subacute thyroiditis and the syndrome termed *chronic thyroiditis with spontaneously resolving thyrotoxicosis;* an excess of preformed hormone leaks from the gland owing to the presence of inflammatory disease. New hormone formation is decreased, however, owing to the suppression of TSH secretion by the hormone excess, and in some cases to the inflammatory injury itself. Since the inflammatory disorders are transitory and since stores of preformed hormone are ultimately depleted, the thyrotoxicosis in these disorders is self-limited and is often followed by a transient period of thyroid hormone insufficiency. The third category of thyrotoxic state is one in which the source of excess hormone is outside of the thyroid gland itself, as in thyrotoxicosis factitia, the rare functioning metastatic thyroid carcinoma, or struma ovarii.

Although all of the foregoing disorders are associated with thyrotoxicosis, not all are associated with hyperthyroidism, a term which should be used to denote only those conditions in which sustained hyperfunction of the thyroid leads to thyrotoxicosis. Thus, thyrotoxic states can be classified according to whether or not they are associated with hyperthyroidism. This distinction has implications for diagnosis and for treatment. In hyperthyroidism, hyperfunction of the thyroid is reflected in an increased RAIU, whereas in the nonhyperthyroid thyrotoxic states, thyroid function (as reflected in the RAIU) is subnormal. Further, treatment of thyrotoxicosis by means intended to decrease hormone synthesis (antithyroid agents, surgery, or radioiodine) is appropriate in hyperthyroidism but is inappropriate and ineffective in other forms of thyrotoxicosis.

Though the specific diseases that cause thyrotoxicosis each make their own imprint on the clinical picture, the manifestations of the thyrotoxic state are largely the same. In the discussion that ensues, the major diseases that lead to a thyrotoxic state are individually described. Since the first considered and most important is Graves' disease, the common manifestations of thyrotoxicosis are described in relation to Graves' disease.

TABLE 316-6 Approximate therapeutic equivalence of various thyroid hormone preparations

Preparation	Average daily oral maintenance dose	Serum T_4
Thyroid extract, USP	120–180 mg	Normal
Levothyroxine	125 μg	Slightly increased
Liothyronine	50 μg	Decreased
Liotrix (T_4/ T_3 = 4:1)	2 units	Normal

TABLE 316-7 Varieties of thyrotoxicosis

I Disorders associated with thyroid hyperfunction*
- *A* Excess production of TSH (rare)
- *B* Abnormal thyroid stimulator
  - *1* Graves' disease
  - *2* Trophoblastic tumor
- *C* Intrinsic thyroid autonomy
  - *1* Hyperfunctioning adenoma
  - *2* Toxic multinodular goiter

II Disorders not associated with thyroid hyperfunction†
- *A* Disorders of hormone storage
  - *1* Subacute thyroiditis
  - *2* Chronic thyroiditis with transient thyrotoxicosis
- *B* Extrathyroid source of hormone
  - *1* Thyrotoxicosis factitia
  - *2* Ectopic thyroid tissue
    - *a* Struma ovarii
    - *b* Functioning follicular cacinoma

* Associated with increased RAIU unless body iodine burden is excessive.
† Associated with decreased RAIU.

GRAVES' DISEASE

Graves' disease, also known as Parry's or Basedow's disease, is a disorder with a triad of major manifestations: hyperthyroidism with diffuse goiter, ophthalmopathy, and dermopathy. Although part of the same disease complex, the three major manifestations need not appear together. Indeed, one or two need never appear, and, moreover, the three tend to run courses that are largely independent of one another.

PREVALENCE Graves' disease is a relatively common disorder that occurs at any age but is especially common in the third and fourth decades. The disease is more frequent in women than in men. In nongoitrous areas the ratio of predominance in women may be as high as 7:1. In areas of endemic goiter the ratio is lower. Genetic factors play an important role; there is an increased frequency of haplotypes HLA-B8 and -DRw3 in Caucasian, HLA-Bw36 in Japanese, and HLA-Bw46 in Chinese patients with the disease. Not surprisingly, there is a distinct familial predisposition to Graves' disease. In addition, among family members of patients with Graves' disease, a clinical and immunologic overlap exists with respect to Hashimoto's disease, primary thyroprivic hypothyroidism, and pernicious anemia and probably with respect to other diseases in which autoimmune features are prominent. In occasional patients, the disease picture may change from Graves' disease to Hashimoto's disease, or vice versa, and rarely patients with primary myxedema later become hyperthyroid. Thus, it is proper to consider Graves' disease, Hashimoto's disease, and primary myxedema as closely related autoimmune thyroid diseases.

ETIOLOGY AND PATHOGENESIS The cause is unknown. In view of the varied manifestations of Graves' disease and their differing courses, it is possible that no single factor is responsible for the entire syndrome. With respect to hyperthyroidism, the central disorder is a disruption of homeostatic mechanisms that normally adjust hormone secretion to meet the needs of peripheral tissues; if such were able to operate, hyperthyroidism could not be sustained. This homeostatic disruption results from the presence in plasma of an abnormal thyroid stimulator, first recognized when it was shown that the serum of patients with Graves' disease releases radioiodine from the prelabeled guinea pig or mouse thyroid. In view of its prolonged duration of action relative to that of TSH in this bioassay system, this material was designated the long-acting thyroid stimulator (LATS). LATS activity is present in one or more immunoglobulins of the IgG class elaborated by lymphocytes of patients with Graves' disease. LATS can be detected only in about half of patients with this disorder, and consequently its pathogenetic role was questioned. This failure to detect LATS in all patients with Graves' disease is due to the fact that the stimulator has variable actions in other species and is not uniformly detectable, therefore, in the conventional bioassay. When human thyroid tissue is used as the assay system, LATS-like responses can be demonstrated in the plasma of most patients. These responses and the corresponding names given to the responsible factors are as follows: prevention of the adsorption of LATS activity by human thyroid particulate fractions (LATS-protector, LATS-p), stimulation of colloid droplet or cyclic AMP generation in thyroid cells, slices, or membranes (thyroid-stimulating immunoglobulins, TSI), and inhibition of the binding of TSH to its receptors in human thyroid tissue (TSH-binding inhibitory immunoglobulins, TBII). These factors are probably antibodies against the thyroid TSH receptor. Activities of this type are also found in serum of some patients with euthyroid ophthalmic Graves' disease, an occasional patient with Hashimoto's disease, and some euthyroid relatives of patients with Graves' disease, though the reason for the absence of thyrotoxicosis in such instances is uncertain. Disappearance of these stimulatory factors from the serum during antithyroid treatment augurs well for long-term remission after treatment is withdrawn. Thus, while the basic cause of Graves' disease is not understood, an immunoglobulin or family of immunoglobulins directed against the TSH receptor mediates the thyroid stimulation of Graves' disease. A heritable abnormality in immune surveillance may permit particular lymphocytes to survive, proliferate, and secrete the stimulatory immunoglobulins in response to precipitating factors.

The pathogenesis of the ophthalmic component of Graves' disease is more enigmatic. One proposed mechanism is the development of antibodies against specific antigens in the extraocular muscles. Nothing is known of the pathogenesis of the dermopathy of Graves' disease.

PATHOLOGY In Graves' disease, the *thyroid gland* is diffusely enlarged, soft, and vascular. The essential pathology is that of parenchymatous hypertrophy and hyperplasia, characterized by increased height of the epithelium and redundancy of the follicular wall, giving the picture of papillary infoldings and cytologic evidence of increased activity. Such hyperplasia is usually accompanied by lymphocytic infiltration that reflects the immune aspect of the disease and that correlates in severity with levels of antithyroid antibodies in the blood. Following iodine medication, there is colloid storage, which sometimes causes enlargement and increased firmness of the gland. Graves' disease is associated with generalized lymphoid hyperplasia and infiltration and occasionally with enlargement of the spleen or thymus. Thyrotoxicosis may lead to degeneration of skeletal muscle fibers, enlargement of the heart, fatty infiltration or diffuse fibrosis of the liver, decalcification of the skeleton, and loss of body tissue (including fat deposits, osteoid, and muscle).

The *ophthalmopathy* is characterized by an inflammatory infiltrate of the orbital contents, exclusive of the globe, with lymphocytes, mast cells, and plasma cells. The orbital musculature is often enlarged, largely accounting for the increased volume of the orbital contents that causes the globe to protrude. Muscle fibers show degeneration and loss of striations, with ultimate fibrosis.

The *dermopathy* of Graves' disease is characterized by thickening of the dermis, which is infiltrated with lymphocytes and with hydrophilic, metachromatically staining mucopolysaccharides.

CLINICAL MANIFESTATIONS The manifestations comprise those that reflect the associated thyrotoxicosis and those specifically related to Graves' disease. The former vary in intensity with the severity of the thyrotoxicosis, the age of the patient, duration of the illness, and the presence of disease in other organs, such as the heart.

Manifestations of thyrotoxicosis Common manifestations include nervousness, emotional lability, inability to sleep, tremors, frequent bowel movements, excessive sweating, and heat intolerance. Weight loss is usual despite a well-maintained or increased appetite. Proximal muscle weakness is present with loss of strength often manifested by difficulty in climbing stairs. In premenopausal women, oligomenorrhea and amenorrhea tend to occur. Dyspnea, palpitations, and in older patients, enhancement of angina pectoris or cardiac failure may occur. In general, nervous symptoms dominate the clinical picture in younger individuals, whereas cardiovascular and myopathic symptoms predominate in older subjects.

Usually, the patient appears anxious, restless, and fidgety. The skin is warm and moist with a velvety texture, and palmar erythema is present. Separation of the fingernail from the nailbed (Plummer's nail) is common, especially on the ring finger. The hair is fine and silky. A fine tremor of the fingers and tongue, together with hyperreflexia, is characteristic. *Ocular signs* include a characteristic stare with widened palpebral fissures, infrequent blinking, lid lag, and failure to wrinkle the brow on upward gaze. These signs result from sympathetic overstimulation and usually subside when the thyrotoxicosis is corrected. They are to be distinguished from the *infiltrative ophthalmopathy* characteristic of Graves' disease, discussed below.

Cardiovascular findings include a wide pulse pressure, sinus tachycardia, atrial arrhythmias (especially atrial fibrillation), systolic murmurs, increased intensity of the apical first sound, cardiac enlargement, and, at times, overt heart failure. A to-and-fro, high-pitched sound may be audible in the pulmonic area and may simulate a pericardial friction rub (Means-Lerman scratch).

Manifestations of Graves' disease The distinctive manifestations of Graves' disease, diffuse hyperfunctioning goiter, ophthalmopathy, and dermopathy, appear in varying combinations and in varying frequency, goiter being the most common. Premature graying of the hair and patchy vitiligo are not specific to Graves' disease but are also common in other autoimmune disorders.

The *diffuse toxic goiter* may be asymmetric and lobular. The presence of a bruit over the gland usually signifies that the patient is thyrotoxic, but it may rarely be present in other disorders in which the thyroid is hyperplastic. Venous hums and carotid souffles should be distinguished from true thyroid bruits. An enlarged pyramidal lobe of the thyroid may be palpable.

The clinical signs associated with the *ophthalmopathy* of Graves' disease may be divided into two components: the spastic and the mechanical. The former includes the stare, lid lag, and lid retraction that accompany thyrotoxicosis and account for the "frightened" facies and classic eye signs previously described. These findings need not be associated with proptosis and usually return to normal after correction of thyrotoxicosis. The mechanical component includes proptosis of varying degrees with ophthalmoplegia and congestive oculopathy characterized by chemosis, conjunctivitis, periorbital swelling, and the potential complications of corneal ulceration, optic neuritis, and optic atrophy. When exophthalmos progresses rapidly and becomes the major concern in Graves' disease, it is termed *progressive* and, if severe, *malignant exophthalmos*. The term *exophthalmic ophthalmoplegia* refers to the ocular muscle weakness that commonly accompanies this disorder and results in impaired upward gaze and convergence and strabismus with varying degrees of diplopia. Exophthalmos may be unilateral early in the course of the disorder but usually progresses to bilateral involvement.

The *dermopathy* of Graves' disease usually occurs over the dorsum of the legs or feet and is termed *localized* or *pretibial myxedema*. It occurs in patients with past or present Graves' disease and is not a manifestation of hypothyroidism. About half of cases occur during the active stage of thyrotoxicosis. The affected area is usually well demarcated from normal skin by the fact that it is raised, thickened, has a *peau d'orange* appearance, and may be pruritic and hyperpigmented. The lesions are usually discrete, assuming a plaquelike or nodular configuration but in some instances becoming confluent. Clubbing of the fingers and toes with characteristic bony changes that differ from those of hypertrophic pulmonary osteoarthropathy may accompany the dermal changes (*thyroid acropachy*). This disorder is usually self-limited.

DIAGNOSIS When severe, Graves' disease presents little difficulty in diagnosis. Florid thyrotoxicosis is manifested by weakness, weight loss despite good appetite, nervous instability, tremor, intolerance to heat, sweating, palpitations, and hyperdefecation. When associated with diffuse thyroid enlargement, often accompanied by a bruit, and particularly when associated with ophthalmopathy, the clinical picture of Graves' disease is virtually unique. In such instances, laboratory tests documenting increased RAIU, serum T_4 and T_3, RT_3U, and FT_4I serve as baselines for evaluation of therapy, rather than necessary diagnostic aids. Occasionally, laboratory tests reveal a normal RAIU, normal serum T_4 and RT_3U, and elevated serum T_3 and FT_3I (T_3 toxicosis).

In less severe cases, particularly when ophthalmopathy is lacking, the diagnosis may be more difficult, since the symptoms of mild thyrotoxicosis are similar to those of other disorders (see "Differential Diagnosis" below). Presence of a goiter makes the diagnosis of hyperthyroidism likely, but careful palpation is necessary to determine whether toxic multinodular goiter, toxic adenoma, or subacute thyroiditis is present, since treatment of these disorders may differ from that of diffuse toxic goiter. Absence of thyroid enlargement makes the diagnosis of Graves' disease less likely but does not exclude it. In mild cases, confirmatory laboratory tests assume great importance. Unfortunately, mild thyrotoxicosis is often associated with marginal abnormalities in laboratory tests or values within the upper limit of the normal range. In such instances, an ultrasensitive TSH assay or the TRH stimulation test assumes crucial importance.

In a few (usually older) patients, the clinical picture may be one of apathy rather than hyperactivity, and evidence of hypermetabolism may be slight (*apathetic thyrotoxicosis*). In such patients, myopathic features may be pronounced. More often, cardiovascular manifestations predominate since mild hyperthyroidism may produce severe disability in patients with underlying heart disease. Hence, *all patients with unexplained cardiac failure or irregularities in rhythm, especially if atrial in origin, should be examined for thyrotoxicosis.* Clues to the diagnosis include a relatively rapid circulation time and resistance to the usual doses of digitalis, but laboratory confirmation is required.

DIFFERENTIAL DIAGNOSIS Signs and symptoms in a number of nonthyroid disorders may simulate certain aspects of the thyrotoxic syndrome. Anxiety is a prominent feature of thyrotoxicosis, and there is thus some overlap in the symptomatology of thyrotoxicosis with that of anxiety states of emotional origin. Tachycardia, tremulousness, irritability, weakness, and fatigue are common to both disorders. In anxiety of emotional origin, however, the peripheral manifestations of excessive thyroid hormones are absent; the skin is usually cold and clammy rather than warm and moist. Weight loss, when present in emotional anxiety, is characteristically accompanied by anorexia, whereas in thyrotoxicosis the appetite is generally increased. Thyrotoxicosis can occasionally be confused with such disorders as metastatic carcinoma, cirrhosis of the liver, hyperparathyroidism, sprue, myasthenia gravis, and muscular dystrophy. Hypokalemic periodic paralysis is more common in thyrotoxic patients, especially in Oriental and Latin American men. Signs and symptoms of thyrotoxicosis may overlap with those of pheochromocytoma, which can cause heat intolerance, excessive perspiration, tachycardia with palpitations, and a hypermetabolic state. In the above disorders and in other conditions considered in the differential diagnosis, the judicious application of laboratory tests usually makes it possible to differentiate them from thyrotoxicosis.

When bilateral ophthalmopathy is accompanied by goiter and thyrotoxicosis, the origin of the ophthalmopathy in Graves' disease is virtually certain. The presence of unilateral ophthalmopathy, even when associated with thyrotoxicosis, raises the possibility of some other intraorbital or intracranial disease. In the euthyroid patient with either unilateral or bilateral ophthalmopathy other causes must be excluded. These include cavernous sinus thrombosis, sphenoidal ridge meningioma, retrobulbar tumors, including leukemic deposits, and the rare granulomatous disorder pseudotumor oculi. Exophthalmos may also be seen in certain systemic disorders, such as uremia, accelerated hypertension, chronic alcoholism, chronic obstructive pulmonary disease, superior mediastinal obstruction, and Cushing's syndrome. Ophthalmoplegia in the absence of overt infiltrative manifestations can be confused with that which occurs in diabetes mellitus, myasthenia gravis, and myopathies. When doubt exists about the cause of ophthalmopathy, the demonstration of significant titers of TSI or TBII or of an abnormal TRH stimulation or thyroid suppression test suggests that the cause is Graves' disease, though not all patients with "euthyroid Graves' disease" demonstrate abnormal responses. In such cases, ultrasonography or computed tomography of the orbits is valuable in demonstrating characteristic thickening of the extraocular muscles.

When a thyrotoxic state occurs in a patient lacking the characteristic ophthalmopathy of Graves' disease, other causes of thyrotoxicosis must be considered. Careful palpation of the thyroid and studies with radioactive iodine are important in this regard. A symmetric, diffuse goiter of moderate or large size suggests the diagnosis of Graves' disease, especially if a bruit is present. However, the uncommon patient whose hyperthyroidism is secondary to an excess of TSH (associated with a *pituitary tumor* or resistance to feedback suppression of TSH secretion) or an abnormal stimulator of trophoblastic origin (*hydatidiform mole* or *choriocarcinoma of uterus* or *testis;* see Chap. 309) may present in this way. A single, prominent thyroid nodule or multiple nodules suggest *toxic adenoma* or *toxic multinodular goiter*, respectively. Tenderness of the thyroid associated with firm nodularity strongly suggests *subacute thyroiditis*, while a small, firm, nontender goiter is consistent with the syndrome of chronic thyroiditis with spontaneously resolving thyrotoxicosis. The foregoing disorders are discussed more fully in later sections. Absence of a palpable thyroid gland suggests an extrathyroid source of hormone, such as ectopic thyroid tissue *(struma ovarii)* or, more commonly, self-administration of hormone *(thyrotoxicosis factitia)*. Studies with radioactive iodine are also helpful. Except when hormone overproduction is secondary to increased iodine intake, values of the RAIU are increased in all disorders producing hyperthyroidism, and scintillation scanning may aid in differentiating among them. Conversely, thyrotoxicosis that is not the result of hyperthyroidism is characterized by subnormal values of the RAIU. Subacute thyroiditis and chronic thyroiditis with spontaneously resolving thyrotoxicosis are the most common. Ectopic thyroid tissue producing thyrotoxicosis is rare. Here, the RAIU, as measured over the thyroid, is low since TSH secretion is suppressed, but despite this, urinary excretion of the dose of ^{131}I is slowed, owing to accumulation of ^{131}I by the ectopic tissue. Functioning ectopic tissue can be located by direct counting or scintillation scanning. Thyrotoxicosis factitia most frequently occurs in medical or paramedical personnel or in those who have easy access to thyroid hormone preparations. The disorder resembles thyrotoxicosis caused by ectopic thyroid tissue in that the patient's thyroid gland is suppressed. Consequently, the RAIU is very low, and most of an administered dose of ^{131}I is excreted promptly in the urine. When the disorder is caused by ingestion of preparations containing T_4, such as levothyroxine or thyroid extract, the serum T_4 is increased. On the other hand, when caused by liothyronine, the serum T_4 is subnormal. Irrespective of the preparation, the serum T_3 is increased but more so when liothyronine is the offending agent. Measurement of serum thyroglobulin is useful to confirm thyrotoxicosis factitia. Levels are elevated in Graves' disease and thyroiditis but are subnormal with exogenous thyroid hormone suppression.

The demonstration of elevated titers of antithyroid antibodies or of TSI or TBII activity in the blood also provides strong evidence that Graves' disease is the cause of thyrotoxicosis.

TREATMENT Hyperthyroidism The hyperthyroidism in Graves' disease is often characterized by cyclic phases of exacerbation and remission, each of unpredictable onset and duration. Moreover, long-standing disease may be associated with progressive thyroid failure, probably consequent to chronic thyroiditis, with the result that hypothyroidism or decreased thyroid reserve supervenes. These characteristics of Graves' disease have important implications in the choice of and response to therapy.

The major approaches to the treatment are directed to limiting the quantity of thyroid hormones the gland can produce. The use of antithyroid agents interposes a chemical blockade to hormone synthesis, the effect of which is operative only as long as the drug is administered. Thus, the agents can control a given phase of active thyrotoxicity but probably do not prevent exacerbation at some subsequent period. The second major approach is ablation of thyroid tissue, thereby limiting hormone production. This may be achieved either by surgery or by means of radioactive iodine. Since these procedures induce permanent anatomic alterations of the thyroid, they can control the individual active phase and are more likely to prevent a later exacerbation or recurrence. On the other hand, surgery or radiation is more likely to lead to hypothyroidism, either shortly after treatment or with the passage of years.

Each therapy has advantages and disadvantages, indications and contraindications. The latter are more often relative than absolute. In general, a trial of long-term antithyroid therapy is desirable in children, adolescents, young adults, and pregnant women but may also be employed in older patients. Indications for ablative procedures include relapse or recurrence following drug therapy, a large goiter, drug toxicity, failure to follow a medical regimen, or failure to return for periodic examinations. Subtotal thyroidectomy may be elected for patients under the age of 40 in whom ablative therapy is required; however, opinions differ, and some authorities employ radioactive iodine in the treatment of patients in the second or third decades. Surgery is also preferable in patients with very large goiters or with a coincident nonfunctioning nodule, especially if there is a history of radiation to the head and neck. Radioactive iodine is the ablative procedure of choice in older patients, in patients who have had previous thyroid surgery, and in those in whom systemic disease contraindicates elective surgery.

In patients selected for *long-term antithyroid therapy*, satisfactory control can almost always be achieved if sufficient drug is administered. Most patients can be managed with propylthiouracil, 100 to 150 mg every 6 or 8 h. In occasional patients with severe disease, larger doses are required for initial control. Methimazole is at least as effective as propylthiouracil when administered in one-tenth the dosage. However, propylthiouracil has the advantage of inhibiting the peripheral conversion of T_4 to T_3, thereby bringing about more rapid symptomatic improvement. Once euthyroidism is achieved, the daily dosage may be reduced to the smallest doses that control the thyrotoxicosis. In some clinics the initial dose is continued and is supplemented with levothyroxine. By this latter regimen, hypothyroidism from overdosage of antithyroid drugs can be prevented. The undesirable consequences of hypothyroidism, such as enhancement of ophthalmopathy and enlargement of the goiter, may thereby be forestalled. The duration of therapy is difficult to predict in the individual patient and may be a function of the spontaneous course of the disease. The longer the course of therapy, the more likely it is that the patient will remain well when the drug is discontinued. In general a 12- to 24-month course is employed, following which one-third or one-half of patients remain well for a prolonged period or indefinitely. The likelihood of a prolonged remission is increased by a decrease in goiter size, reversion of the thyroid suppression test to normal, or disappearance of Graves' disease–related immunoglobulins (TSI and TBII) from the serum during treatment.

Leukopenia is the principal undesirable side effect of antithyroid drugs. A complete blood count should be obtained prior to initiating therapy to identify those patients with leukopenia related to Graves' disease. Mild transient leukopenia with antithyroid drugs may occur in approximately an additional 10 percent of patients and is not necessarily an indication for discontinuing therapy. When the absolute number of polymorphonuclear leukocytes reaches 1500 or less, antithyroid medication should be discontinued. Allergic rashes and drug sensitivity occur in a small percentage of patients. These may disappear with antihistamine therapy at the same or reduced dosage of antithyroid agent, but it is probably preferable when sensitivity reactions occur to change to another drug. On rare occasions (in less than 0.2 percent) agranulocytosis occurs. This may be sudden in onset. Hepatitis, drug fever, and arthralgias occur on occasion. In the authors' view, severe sensitivity reactions, including agranulocytosis, dictate the abandonment of antithyroid therapy, rather than recourse to an alternate drug.

Iodide inhibits the release of hormones from the hyperfunctioning thyroid gland, and its ameliorative effects occur more rapidly than those of agents that inhibit hormone synthesis. Hence, its main use is in patients with actual or impending thyrotoxic crisis and in patients with severe thyrocardiac disease. The response to iodide alone is often incomplete and transient. Furthermore, by expanding the thyroid store of hormone, iodide may prolong the latency of response to antithyroid therapy. Therefore, iodide is safely used only in conjunction with the antithyroid agents. If the clinical course is sufficiently severe to require iodide administration, antithyroid drugs are usually the primary therapeutic agents and should be given in large doses prior to iodide. Iodide is also useful in controlling thyrotoxicosis following ^{131}I administration, during the period in which the therapeutic effect of radioiodine has not yet taken place. Large doses of *glucocorticoids* (2 mg of dexamethasone every 6 h) reduce the serum

T_4 concentration and should be added to the regimen when relief of thyrotoxicosis is urgent. The iodinated x-ray contrast agent sodium ipodate has a similar effect. Iodine liberated from this agent inhibits thyroid secretion of T_4 and T_3, and serum T_3 is further reduced by the inhibition by ipodate of peripheral T_3 formation. Daily doses of 1 g orally are effective, but the same precautions concerning the use of iodine therapy are applicable to ipodate as well.

Owing to the pronounced adrenergic component in thyrotoxicosis, various *adrenergic antagonists* have been employed in its management. Of these, propranolol is the agent of choice because of its relative freedom from side effects. In doses of 40 to 120 mg daily, propranolol alleviates such adrenergic manifestations as sweating, tremor, and tachycardia and may reduce to some extent the conversion of T_4 to T_3. However, propranolol should be used only as adjunctive therapy rather than sole therapy, as some have suggested, since the underlying metabolic abnormalities are not affected. Moreover, although the diminution in heart rate and cardiac work may be beneficial, the blocking of adrenergic support of myocardial contractility requires caution in its use in the patient with coexisting heart failure, unless rate- or rhythm-related. As adjunctive therapy, the major usefulness of propranolol is during the period when the response to conventional antithyroid agents or to radioiodine therapy is being awaited and in the management of thyrotoxic crisis. It has been employed as the sole agent in preparation for thyroidectomy, but its use in this setting is not recommended since it does not render the patient euthyroid, with a likely greater risk of surgically induced crisis.

Radioactive iodine (*^{131}I*) affords a relatively simple, effective, and economical means of treating thyrotoxicosis. It can produce the ablative effects of surgery without the immediate operative and postoperative complications. The principal disadvantage of ^{131}I therapy, in the dosage usually employed, is its tendency to produce hypothyroidism with a frequency that increases with time. As many as 40 to 70 percent of patients may develop this complication within 10 years after treatment. Although hypothyroidism is treatable, once diagnosed, the insidious onset may obscure the diagnosis until serious complications have developed. Hence, some recommend that all patients be treated with large doses of ^{131}I to ensure relief of thyrotoxicosis and then placed on permanent physiologic replacement doses of thyroid hormone.

There is no evidence of carcinogenic or leukemogenic effects of radioiodine when it is given to adults in the doses commonly used in treating hyperthyroidism. However, the susceptibility to carcinogenesis may be increased in the thyroids of children. Mutagenic effects have not been reported and would be difficult to document. For these reasons, many physicians prefer to reserve radioiodine therapy for patients over 30 years of age or those unlikely to have children subsequently. Moreover, the longer the life expectancy after ^{131}I therapy, the greater the likelihood that hypothyroidism will develop. Among younger patients, therefore, only those with recurrent thyrotoxicosis following surgery, those who refuse surgery, and those with complicating illness that contraindicates surgery are candidates for radioiodine therapy. In elderly patients, treatment with large doses of radioiodine is the general method of choice, so that the undesirable effects of incomplete treatment or recurrence can be avoided.

The usual therapeutic dose of ^{131}I [approximately 5.9 MBq (160 μCi) per gram of estimated gland weight] has led to the disturbingly high frequency of hypothyroidism. As a result, though continuing to use this dose, some authorities regularly administer prophylactic replacement doses of thyroid hormone. On the other hand, others have administered smaller doses [approximately 3.0 MBq/g (80 μCi/g)]. However, this does not diminish the frequency of late hypothyroidism but merely delays its onset. Moreover, the smaller dose is less likely to relieve thyrotoxicosis within a relatively short period. Antithyroid agents can be employed, however, to speed the attainment of a eumetabolic state, and propranolol can be given to relieve symptoms, while the effect of the ^{131}I is taking hold. There is general agreement that patients with coexisting cardiac disease should receive ^{131}I in large doses in view of the hazard of recurrent thyrotoxicosis.

Radiation thyroiditis is an occasional immediate complication of ^{131}I therapy. When present, it commonly appears within 7 to 10 days and is associated with excessive release of hormone into the blood. Rarely, radiation thyroiditis may be so severe as to cause thyrotoxic crisis (see below); this complication is most likely in the elderly thyrotoxic patient with other systemic illness. For these reasons, patients with severe hyperthyroidism or underlying heart disease should be rendered eumetabolic with antithyroid agents before ^{131}I is administered. Interruption of antithyroid therapy for 3 to 4 days before and after ^{131}I treatment suffices to permit adequate accumulation and retention of administered ^{131}I. Propranolol may be used as an adjunct both before and after ^{131}I administration but should not be relied upon to provide adequate prophylaxis if given alone. The swelling that accompanies radiation thyroiditis may contraindicate the use of large doses of ^{131}I in patients with large retrosternal goiters.

Before radioactive iodine was introduced, *subtotal thyroidectomy* was the standard form of ablative therapy, and it is still employed in younger patients in whom antithyroid therapy is unsuccessful. Although precise preoperative programs differ, several general principles should be emphasized. Patients should first be rendered euthyroid by means of antithyroid agents. Only then should iodide (five drops of Lugol's solution a day for approximately 10 days) be administered concomitantly to effect an involutional response in the gland. Antithyroid drugs should not be discontinued merely because treatment with iodide is instituted. The response of the patient, and not the calendar, should dictate when surgery is performed.

Hazards of subtotal thyroidectomy include immediate complications, such as anesthetic accidents, hemorrhage sometimes leading to respiratory obstruction, and damage to the recurrent laryngeal nerve leading to vocal cord paralysis. Later complications include wound infection, hemorrhage, hypoparathyroidism, or hypothyroidism. Subtotal thyroidectomy should be performed by a surgeon experienced in this procedure; under this condition surgery is effective and relatively safe. Postoperative recurrences are uncommon. However, carefully conducted follow-up studies reveal that hypothyroidism follows surgery more frequently than previously suspected, although not as commonly as following treatment with conventional doses of ^{131}I.

The *treatment of hyperthyroidism during pregnancy* is a subject of some disagreement. Most physicians believe that antithyroid therapy is preferable to surgery, which should not be performed in any event during the first and third trimesters. Antithyroid agents carry less risk to the patient and the pregnancy. Further, since they traverse the placental barrier, they have the theoretical advantage of preventing fetal and neonatal hyperthyroidism when maternal titers of thyroid-stimulating IgG are high. As a clue to the risk of fetal hyperthyroidism, assays of such stimulators should be conducted in pregnant women with a history of Graves' disease, whether treated or not. On the other hand, the major disadvantage of antithyroid therapy is the possibility of inducing hypothyroidism in the fetus. T_4 and T_3 traverse the human placenta from mother to fetus only slowly, if at all, and simultaneous administration of thyroid hormone and antithyroid drugs to the mother will not protect the fetus from developing hypothyroidism. Hence, the cardinal rule in using the antithyroid agents in pregnancy is that the dosage should be the smallest necessary to control hyperthyroidism in the mother. From the laboratory standpoint, the physician should aim to keep the serum FT_4 concentration or the FT_4I within the normal limits, remembering that pregnancy is normally associated with some elevation of the serum total T_4, owing to an increase in serum TBG concentration. Since pregnancy appears to attenuate the severity of hyperthyroidism, control can often be achieved with maintenance doses of 200 mg propylthiouracil daily or less. At this dose level, fetal goiter or hypothyroidism has not been a problem. Patients who require doses of 300 mg daily or more during the first trimester should probably be treated by subtotal thyroidectomy during the middle trimester. The authors believe that patients carried through pregnancy on antithyroid agents should not be given propranolol as adjunctive treatment, in view of reports that the agent may cause fetal growth retardation and neonatal respiratory depression. Radioiodine should never be administered to a pregnant woman, and all women of childbearing age who are about to receive ^{131}I should have a pregnancy test performed first.

Ophthalmopathy, dermopathy When severe and progressive, ophthalmopathy is the most difficult component of Graves' disease to treat satisfactorily. Fortunately, in most patients the disorder runs a benign course that is largely independent of the course of the hyperthyroidism. In most instances, the activity of even moderately severe disease declines and disappears with time, although some exophthalmos and ophthalmoplegia may persist. In mild disease, considerable benefit may be obtained from simple measures, such as elevating the head at night, administering diuretics to reduce edema, and providing tinted glasses for protection from sun, wind, and foreign bodies. A 1% solution of methylcellulose or plastic shields may prevent corneal drying in patients unable to oppose the lids during sleep. In more severe cases, as evidenced by progressive exophthalmos, chemosis, ophthalmoplegia, or loss of vision, large doses of prednisone (120 to 140 mg daily) should be administered, since this is usually effective in reducing the edematous and infiltrative components. With improvement, the dosage is reduced to the lowest effective level, to minimize the effects of glucocorticoid excess. Orbital radiation may be helpful in some patients with acute, severe infiltrative manifestations. In cases that progress despite these measures, orbital decompression, i.e., removal of part of the bony orbit, is required to relieve intraorbital pressure. The management must always be conducted in concert with an ophthalmologist.

In general, treatment of associated hyperthyroidism should be carried out much as would be the case were ophthalmopathy not present, since the mode of treatment of the hyperthyroidism does not influence the course of the ocular disease. The suggestion that total thyroid ablation by surgery and large doses of ^{131}I is beneficial to the ophthalmic disease has not been borne out. It is agreed, however, that hypothyroidism be avoided.

Severe dermopathy can be alleviated by the topical application of glucocorticoids.

TOXIC MULTINODULAR GOITER

Toxic multinodular goiter is an occasional consequence of long-standing simple goiter, although the proportion of cases in which this complication arises is uncertain. In areas of nonendemicity, the etiology of nontoxic multinodular goiter is usually indeterminate. Hence, it is unclear whether a specific etiologic factor underlies those cases of nontoxic multinodular goiter that progress to thyrotoxic phase. Common to many nontoxic multinodular goiters, even in areas of iodine sufficiency, is a decrease in the iodine content of thyroglobulin, suggesting either a conditioned deficiency of iodine or an impairment of its normal incorporation into iodinated amino acids. There is no pathologic feature to distinguish the nontoxic from the toxic multinodular goiter. However, the transition from nontoxic to toxic nodular goiter involves the development of functional autonomy, i.e., independence from TSH stimulation in one or more areas of the gland. Scattered foci of functional autonomy are present, even early in the disease process. These increase in size and number as time passes so that even among seemingly euthyroid patients with nontoxic nodular goiter, approximately a fourth display, as evidence of functional autonomy, subnormal or absent responses to TRH administration. As judged from scintillation scanning, functional patterns may be of two types. In the first and more common, iodine accumulation occurs diffusely but in patchy foci throughout the gland. The second, less common, pattern is that of iodine accumulation in one or more discrete nodules within the gland, the remainder appearing to be essentially nonfunctional. Histologic and autoradiographic studies reveal marked heterogeneity of structure and function, the two being poorly correlated. In both endemic and sporadic nontoxic multinodular goiter, administration of iodides may lead to the development of thyrotoxicosis (jod-Basedow), a complication that is consonant with the functional autonomy that characterizes this disorder.

Because it arises in long-standing simple goiter, toxic multinodular goiter is a disease of the aging or elderly. For this reason and because of the nature of the underlying disease, the clinical presentation differs from that in Graves' disease. Ophthalmopathy is rare and would signal the emergence of Graves' disease superimposed on simple goiter. Some patients have typical thyrotoxicosis. Often, however, the degree of thyrotoxicosis is less severe than that in Graves' disease, although its physiologic impact upon specific organ systems may be great. Notable among these is the cardiovascular system, in which arrhythmias or congestive failure may be precipitated or accentuated by thyrotoxicosis that may be manifested only by subtle findings in other areas (apathetic hyperthyroidism). Weakness and wasting may predominate, frequently with loss of appetite rather than hyperphagia, suggesting the presence of a carcinoma.

In some patients, a definitive diagnosis of toxic nodular goiter is difficult to establish. On the one hand, enlargement or nodularity of the gland may escape detection because the patient has a short neck or is kyphotic or because the thyroid is substernal. When this is the case and when the clinical findings suggest thyrotoxicosis, RAIU and scintiscan may prove illuminating. On the other hand, even when a nodular goiter is palpable, the presence of mild but clinically significant thyrotoxicosis may be difficult to confirm, since values of the serum total T_4 and T_3, FT_4, and FT_4I, as well as the serum T_3, are often only near or slightly above the upper limit of the normal range. For example, a value for the serum T_3 that would be normal for a young adult may represent an increase in the elderly patient, since serum T_3 usually declines with age. Despite their value in situations such as this, thyroid suppression tests should not be undertaken in the elderly patient because of the hazard of adverse cardiovascular responses. Unfortunately, although a normal response to TRH would exclude a diagnosis of thyrotoxicosis in a patient with a nodular goiter, subnormal responses do not establish the diagnosis. Responses to TRH decline in the elderly, especially in men, and patients with nodular goiter who otherwise seem euthyroid may respond subnormally to TRH as a reflection of at least partial functional autonomy of the thyroid gland. An undetectable basal TSH and absent response to TRH by an ultrasensitive assay imply thyrotoxicosis (Fig. 316-3). When laboratory findings do not permit a clear diagnosis of thyrotoxicosis but suggestive clinical findings are present, a therapeutic trial of antithyroid drugs is indicated.

Radioactive iodine is the treatment of choice for toxic multinodular goiter. Large doses [740 to 1110 MBq (20 to 30 mCi)] are usually required, owing to the generally lower RAIU and to the variable degree of function throughout the gland. Moreover, the physiologic instability of the elderly patient makes definitive treatment desirable. For the same reason, it is usually wise to initiate therapy with antithyroid agents, withholding radioiodine until a euthyroid state is achieved, thereby forestalling an exacerbation of thyrotoxicosis should radiation thyroiditis occur. Unless contraindicated, propranolol is often useful in controlling manifestations of thyrotoxicosis both before and after radioiodine therapy, while its therapeutic effect is awaited. Hypothyroidism is an uncommon consequence of radioiodine treatment of toxic multinodular goiter, owing to the variable activity of differing portions of the gland, which permits previously quiescent areas to replace functionally those that have been destroyed by ^{131}I.

UNUSUAL VARIETIES OF THYROTOXICOSIS

In addition to Graves' disease and toxic multinodular goiter, thyrotoxicosis is seen in other disorders, including follicular adenoma of the thyroid and various forms of thyroiditis, which are discussed in later sections. This section will consider still other infrequent causes of thyrotoxicosis and unusual ways in which thyrotoxicosis may present from the laboratory standpoint.

UNUSUAL CAUSES OF THYROTOXICOSIS Rarely, hyperthyroidism and thyrotoxicosis are the result of sustained hypersecretion of TSH from either a *TSH-secreting pituitary adenoma* or a selective *resistance of the TSH-secretory mechanism* to feedback inhibition by thyroid hormones. The resistance syndrome may be a variant of a disorder in which both the pituitary and peripheral tissues are relatively resistant to thyroid hormones. TSH-secreting pituitary adenomas can be distinguished, in many cases, by radiologic evidence of pituitary tumor, by the fact that the concentration of free alpha subunits of TSH in serum is elevated, and by the fact that the response of the serum TSH to TRH is negligible. In the variant caused by pituitary resistance, subunit concentrations are not grossly elevated, and the TSH response to TRH is usually normal.

Patients with *trophoblastic tumor,* either choriocarcinoma or hydatidiform mole, frequently display elevations, sometimes marked, of serum total and free T_4 and T_3 concentrations. Clinical evidence of thyrotoxicosis may be lacking. Thyroid hyperfunction is caused by a circulating thyroid stimulator of trophoblastic origin, which is probably a variant of human chorionic gonadotropin (hCG), and abnormal thyroid function tests remit promptly after removal of the tumor.

Thyrotoxicosis factitia is a form of thyrotoxicosis without hyperthyroidism and results from purposeful or inadvertent ingestion of supraphysiologic quantities of thyroid hormone. The syndrome is usually a form of malingering and occurs most commonly in women with an underlying psychiatric disorder, usually paramedical personnel, or in patients who have taken thyroid hormones in the past or who have relatives that take thyroid hormones. In such patients, endogenous thyroid function is suppressed, as evidenced by subnormal values of the RAIU and serum thyroglobulin concentration. Both serum T_4 and T_3 concentrations are increased if the patient is taking a preparation that contains T_4, whereas the serum T_3 concentration is elevated and the serum T_4 depressed in patients taking T_3 alone. Factitious hyperthyroidism has also been described in people who ingest large quantities of ground meats contaminated with thyroid tissue.

Very rarely, thyrotoxicosis with a low RAIU is the result of excess hormone secretion by *ectopic thyroid tissue,* either widespread functioning metastases of thyroid carcinoma or struma ovarii.

The *jod-Basedow phenomenon* refers to the induction of thyrotoxicosis in a previously euthyroid patient as a result of exposure to increased quantities of iodine. It typically occurs in areas of endemic iodine deficiency when measures to increase iodine intake or body iodine stores are implemented. The presumption is that the supplemental iodine permits functionally autonomous thyroid tissue to produce and secrete excessive hormone. A similar phenomenon can occur in patients with nontoxic multinodular goiter who have received large doses of iodide. Since such patients tend to be elderly with the danger of serious cardiovascular manifestations should thyrotoxicosis ensue, large doses of iodine should not be given to those with multinodular goiter. Similarly, in such patients, pharmaceuticals containing iodine, most often x-ray contrast media, should be used only when indicated and with consideration of the possible hazard of inducing the jod-Basedow phenomenon. When a contrast study is indicated under these conditions, it may be judicious to administer large doses of propylthiouracil (450 to 600 mg/d) prior to and for a week after the procedure. Some patients may develop hyperthyroidism following exposure to large quantities of iodine despite the fact that after iodine is withdrawn, they recover, their thyroid function appears to be entirely normal, and evidence of functional autonomy is lacking.

UNUSUAL PRESENTATIONS OF THYROTOXICOSIS T_3 toxicosis Thyrotoxicosis in which serum T_4 is normal or low in the absence of a deficiency of TBG, while the serum T_3 is increased, is termed T_3 toxicosis. Although the production rate of T_3 is disproportionately increased relative to that of T_4 in patients with hyperthyroidism, in some this discrepancy is exaggerated. This may occur in association with Graves' disease, multinodular goiter, or hyperfunctioning adenoma. The diagnosis should be suspected in a patient with clinical manifestations of thyrotoxicosis in whom the serum T_4 and FT_4 are normal or low and the RAIU is normal or increased. This, together with the frequently palpable goiter, serves to differentiate this disorder from liothyronine-induced thyrotoxicosis factitia. In contrast to patients with nonthyroidal disorders that mimic thyrotoxicosis, patients with this disorder, as would be expected, demonstrate both nonsuppressibility of thyroid function in response to exogenous T_3 and blunted or absent responses to TRH. In many patients, thyrotoxicosis with increased serum T_3 and normal serum T_4 precedes emergence of typical increases in both, either during an initial episode of hyperthyroidism or more commonly during recurrence after previous treatment. In some patients in whom symptoms of thyrotoxicosis fail to regress completely during antithyroid therapy despite return of the serum T_4 concentration to normal, the serum T_3 concentration is persistently elevated. Such patients are prone to experience a recurrence of thyrotoxicosis when antithyroid therapy is withdrawn.

T_4 toxicosis In most patients with hyperthyroidism, the serum T_3 is increased to a relatively greater extent than is the serum T_4. This reflects the fact that in hyperthyroidism T_3 generated from T_4 peripherally is supplemented by release of substantial quantities of T_3 from the thyroid. However, thyrotoxicosis may sometimes be associated with a clear elevation of serum T_4 and a seemingly normal serum T_3 concentration. This syndrome of *T_4 toxicosis* occurs most commonly in patients who are elderly, ill, or both, and is, therefore, usually seen in a hospital setting. Presumably, the combination of high serum T_4 and normal serum T_3 concentration reflects inhibition of peripheral T_3 generation from T_4, with persistence of T_3 secretion along with T_4 from the thyroid.

MAJOR COMPLICATIONS OF THYROTOXICOSIS

CARDIAC DISEASE Thyrotoxicosis imposes a variety of burdens upon the heart. Hypermetabolism of the peripheral tissues increases both the metabolic and nonmetabolic (heat-loss) circulatory load, while direct effects of thyroid hormone on the myocardium increase the force, velocity, and rate of ventricular contraction. As a result, cardiac work and cardiac output are increased. Moreover, atrial irritability is enhanced, leading to arrhythmias, most importantly atrial fibrillation. In the patient with a normal heart, these burdens are usually tolerated. In the patient with underlying heart disease, however, cardiac insufficiency may be precipitated or aggravated. As would be expected, this complication is more common in the elderly patient and is common in the patient with toxic multinodular goiter, sometimes as the most prominent manifestation of the thyrotoxic state. In patients with cardiac insufficiency, clues to the presence of thyrotoxicosis include atrial fibrillation, relatively rapid circulation time, increased cardiac output (high-output failure), and resistance to the usual therapeutic doses of digitalis.

Treatment is directed at rapid alleviation of thyrotoxicosis and restoration of cardiac compensation. The former objective is best met by initiation of treatment with large doses of an antithyroid agent, followed by iodine if the clinical situation is urgent. In less severe cases, radioiodine treatment is preceded by antithyroid drug treatment alone. Management of the cardiac decompensation is carried out in the usual manner, employing larger than usual doses of digitalis but with care to avoid digitalis intoxication as thyrotoxicosis is alleviated. Adrenergic antagonists should not be employed in the presence of cardiac failure, unless failure is the consequence primarily of disturbance of cardiac rate or rhythm.

THYROTOXIC CRISIS Thyrotoxic crisis or storm causes a fulminating increase in the signs and symptoms of thyrotoxicosis. In the past, this disturbance was most often observed postoperatively in patients poorly prepared for surgery. However, with the preoperative use of antithyroid drugs and iodide and with appropriate measures directed to control of metabolic factors, weight, and nutritional status, postoperative thyrotoxic crisis should not occur. At present, so-called medical storm is more common and occurs in untreated or inadequately treated patients. It is precipitated by surgical emergency or complicating illness, usually sepsis. The syndrome is characterized by extreme irritability, delirium or coma, fever to 41°C or more, tachycardia, restlessness, hypotension, vomiting, and diarrhea. Rarely, the picture may be more subtle, with apathy, prostration, and coma, but with only slight elevation of temperature. Such postoperative complications as sepsis, septicemia, hemorrhage, and transfusion or drug reactions may mimic thyrotoxic crisis. The physiologic factor(s) that initiates thyrotoxic crisis is unknown. It does not appear to be an acute increase in the severity of thyroid hyperfunction. Rather, it may represent a shift from protein-bound to free hormone, secondary to circulating inhibitors to binding in systemic illness.

Treatment consists in providing general supportive therapy while undertaking measures for alleviating thyrotoxicosis as rapidly as possible. Supportive therapy includes treatment of dehydration and the intravenous administration of glucose and saline, vitamin B complex, and glucocorticoids. The latter are indicated because of the increased glucocorticoid requirements in thyrotoxicosis and because adrenal reserve may be reduced in this disorder. Patients should be placed in a cooled, humidified oxygen tent, and, if hyperpyrexia is present, a cooling blanket should be used. Digitalization is required to control ventricular rate in those with atrial fibrillation. If shock exists, intravenous pressor agents should be employed. Therapy of the hyperthyroidism consists of blockade of hormone synthesis by the immediate and continued administration of large doses of an antithyroid agent (e.g., 100 mg propylthiouracil every 2 h). If the patient is unable to swallow the medication, the tablets should be triturated and given by nasogastric tube, as parenteral preparations are unavailable. Following initiation of antithyroid therapy, inhibition of hormone release is sought through the administration of large doses of iodine intravenously or by mouth. The iodinated x-ray contrast agent sodium ipodate can be administered instead of iodine and has the added action of also inhibiting the peripheral conversion of T_4 to T_3. Doses of 1 g daily are effective. Adrenergic antagonists are an important, and perhaps critical, part of the therapeutic regimen, in the absence of cardiac failure. The beta-adrenergic blocking agent propranolol can be administered in doses of 40 to 80 mg every 6 h. If medications cannot be taken orally, 2 mg of propranolol may be given intravenously, with careful electrocardiographic monitoring. Large doses of dexamethasone (e.g., 2 mg every 6 h) should also be administered, since they inhibit hormone release, impair the peripheral generation of T_3 from T_4, and provide adrenal support. Indeed, with the combined use of propylthiouracil, iodine, and dexamethasone, the serum T_3 concentration generally returns to normal within 24 to 48 h. Antithyroid therapy, iodine, and dexamethasone must be continued until a normal metabolic state is approached, at which time iodine is progressively withdrawn and plans are made for definitive treatment.

NEOPLASMS

THYROID ADENOMAS True adenomas, as contrasted with localized adenomatous areas, are encapsulated and compress contiguous tissue. Adenomas vary in size and histologic characteristics and are classified into three major types: papillary, follicular, and Hürthle cell. The follicular adenomas can be subdivided according to the size of the follicles into colloid or macrofollicular, fetal or microfollicular, and embryonal varieties. There is variation in physiologic differentiation, as judged by the ability to concentrate radioiodine. The more highly differentiated adenomas (follicular) are the most common and are the most likely to mimic the function of normal thyroid tissue. Though their function may be responsive to TSH stimulation, usually it differs from that of normal thyroid tissue in being autonomous, i.e., the basal activity is independent of TSH stimulation. Adenomas of this type are usually unifocal, presenting as a single nodule. Often the patient reports that the nodule has grown slowly over many years. Initially, its function is insufficient to disturb hormonal equilibrium though its capacity to accumulate radioiodine is evident in scintiscans as an area of increased density within the still-functioning extranodular tissue (*"warm" nodule*). At this stage, demonstration of the inherent autonomy of the nodule's function requires scintiscanning while the patient is receiving suppressive doses of exogenous thyroid hormone (suppression scan). With time the nodule grows larger, its function increasing until it is sufficient to suppress TSH secretion. Consequently, the remainder of the gland undergoes atrophy and loss of function, and the scintiscan reveals radioiodine accumulation only in the region of the nodule (*"hot" nodule*). At this time, the patient may or may not be overtly thyrotoxic, but frank thyrotoxicosis usually supervenes eventually (*toxic adenoma*), particularly after iodine exposure. Relative to its overall rate of occurrence, hyperfunctioning adenoma is a frequent cause of T_3 toxicosis. Hyperfunctioning adenomas are amenable to ablation by surgery or ^{131}I. Large doses of the latter are usually required to bring about prompt cure. Before such treatment it is desirable to administer TSH and demonstrate by scintiscan the latent functional capacity of the extranodular tissue. Although it has been thought that radiation damage would be confined solely to the hyperfunctioning nodule being treated with ^{131}I, the remaining tissue being spared, this may not always be the case, since some patients with hyperfunctioning adenoma become euthyroid after treatment with ^{131}I only to become hypothyroid years later.

Hyperfunctioning nodules are rarely the seat of carcinoma. However, hyperfunctioning adenomas not infrequently undergo hemorrhagic necrosis. The resulting pain and nodularity may suggest subacute thyroiditis. Subsequently, there is loss of function and the appearance of a *"cold" nodule* on scintiscanning, since the remainder of the thyroid will have resumed function. When this happens, the nodule is likely to be mistaken for a carcinoma. Indeed, hypofunctioning, hemorrhagic adenomas and thyroid cysts account for the majority of cold nodules initially suspected of being carcinomas.

THYROID CARCINOMAS Thyroid carcinoma may be classified into two varieties, depending upon whether the lesion arises in thyroid follicular epithelium or from the parafollicular or C cells. The latter disorder, medullary thyroid carcinoma, has distinctive physiologic and clinical characteristics and is discussed separately (see Chap. 325). The thyroid may also be the site of lymphoproliferative disease or of carcinoma metastatic from a diagnosed or undiagnosed primary tumor elsewhere.

Carcinomas of follicular epithelium The three general histologic types differ in their clinical course. The least common, *anaplastic carcinoma,* is histologically undifferentiated, usually afflicts the elderly, and is highly malignant. The lesion is rapidly fatal, owing to extensive local invasion which is refractory to radiation. The second type of tumor, *follicular carcinoma,* histologically mimics normal thyroid tissue. This lesion usually undergoes early hematogenous spread, and the patient may present with a distant metastasis, usually in lung or bone. Follicular carcinoma or follicular elements in papillary carcinoma are responsible for those instances in which thyroid carcinoma, in situ or in metastases, accumulates significant quantities of ^{131}I. The third and most common type of tumor, *papillary carcinoma,* has a bimodal frequency, peaks occurring in the second or third decades and again in later life. This lesion is slowly growing and typically spreads to the regional lymph nodes, where it may remain indolent for many years. Acceleration of the disease may take place at any time. Follicular elements are usually present in both the primary lesion and its metastases.

DIAGNOSIS AND MANAGEMENT The diagnosis and management of thyroid carcinoma are interwoven with the management of the nodular goiter. In the past, this subject has evoked a wide disparity of views among authorities, stemming from seemingly contradictory data. On the one hand, surgically excised specimens of thyroid nodules, particularly solitary nodules, revealed a high frequency of carcinoma (as much as 20 percent in some series). On the other hand, despite the frequency of nodular goiter in the general population (approximately 4 percent), the frequency of thyroid carcinoma, either newly diagnosed or as a cause of death, is low. These respective data led either to vigorous or to conservative approaches to the management of nodular goiter. This discordance can be explained by the ability of the physician to select for surgery those patients who are at high risk of harboring thyroid carcinoma, with consequent weighting of statistics from surgical series. This capability has increased, the as yet unrealized aim being to operate on only those patients whose thyroids harbor carcinoma and to avoid surgery in patients whose thyroids do not.

Several features suggest the presence of carcinoma. Recent growth of a thyroid nodule or mass, especially if rapid and unaccompanied by tenderness and hoarseness, is a source of suspicion. Of particular importance is a history of x-ray to the head or neck or upper mediastinum in infancy or childhood, since this is associated with a high incidence of thyroid disease, including carcinoma, later in life. Nodular disease develops in approximately 20 percent of patients so exposed and may not be apparent until 30 years or more after the radiation exposure. Among patients in this group who have palpable nodules, approximately a third have thyroid carcinoma at surgery, often multicentric and sometimes metastatic.

Skillful palpation of the thyroid provides important information. A nodule in an otherwise normal gland (solitary nodule) creates more suspicion of thyroid tumor than does one nodule among many, since the latter is more likely to be part of a diffuse process, such as simple goiter. In addition, carcinomas are usually firm or hard in consistency and nontender. Fixation to surrounding structures and lymphadenopathy are late features. Since purely cystic lesions, especially those that are less than a few centimeters in diameter, are less likely to reflect malignancy than solid lesions, transillumination is sometimes helpful, and ultrasonograms (see below) are particularly so. Age and sex of the patient also influence the clinical decision. Benign nodular lesions are more common in women than in men, malignant nodular lesions less so. Hence, nodular lesions in men create more suspicion of carcinoma than in women.

Laboratory tests are of little assistance in differentiating between malignant and nonmalignant thyroid nodules. Overall thyroid function is usually normal. Except in patients with medullary thyroid carcinoma, in whom serum calcitonin concentrations may be elevated, tumor markers are of little value. Elevations of serum thyroglobulin are present in many patients with differentiated thyroid carcinoma but are not useful in the initial diagnosis, since they may be elevated in patients with benign adenoma, simple goiter, or Graves' disease. Soft-tissue x-rays of the neck may be of assistance, since finely stippled calcification within the thyroid suggests the presence of psammoma bodies within a papillary carcinoma and more dense calcifications may signify medullary carcinoma.

Fine-needle aspiration for cytology is the initial procedure of choice in the evaluation of most patients (Fig. 316-4). The technique is simple to learn, free of complications, and applicable to most nodules. Optimal application of that technique rests upon the availability of experienced histopathologic interpretation of the specimen obtained. When such is available, aspiration biopsy provides a reliable means of differentiating between benign and malignant nodules in all except highly cellular lesions or follicular lesions, where evidence of vascular invasion may be required to differentiate benign from malignant forms. Despite the occasional occurrence of false-positives and -negatives, the procedure can reduce the number of operations performed for nodules that prove to be benign. Further, a diagnosis of carcinoma permits planning of the surgery to be undertaken preoperatively and is often useful in providing an impetus to surgery when the patient or physician is uncertain if surgery should be performed.

While fine-needle aspiration for cytology is the keystone in the approach to the management of the patient with nodular goiter, scintillation scanning may be also useful. Although only approximately 20 percent of nonfunctioning thyroid nodules prove to be malignant, demonstration that a nodule is cold adds substantial weight to the other factors suggesting carcinoma. Nodules that are hyperfunctioning are rarely malignant. Ultrasonograms of the thyroid have value in demonstrating whether nodules are cystic, solid, or a mixture of the two. Cystic nodules can be aspirated, a procedure that is often curative, and their contents should be subjected to cytopathologic examination. Solid or mixed lesions are consistent with tumor but may be either benign or malignant.

When the cytologic results are equivocal, the physician must decide whether to continue to observe the patient; to administer suppressive doses of thyroid hormone in the hope that the suspect nodule will shrink or disappear—a hope that in the authors' experience is usually unrealized; or to proceed to excisional biopsy and thyroidectomy. There are some patients in whom the authors choose the latter course. In general, these include patients with a history of radiation to the thyroid and one or more clearly palpable nodules, as well as young men and women with solitary cold nodules, particularly if hard, nontender, and changing rapidly in size. In the remainder,

FIGURE 316-4

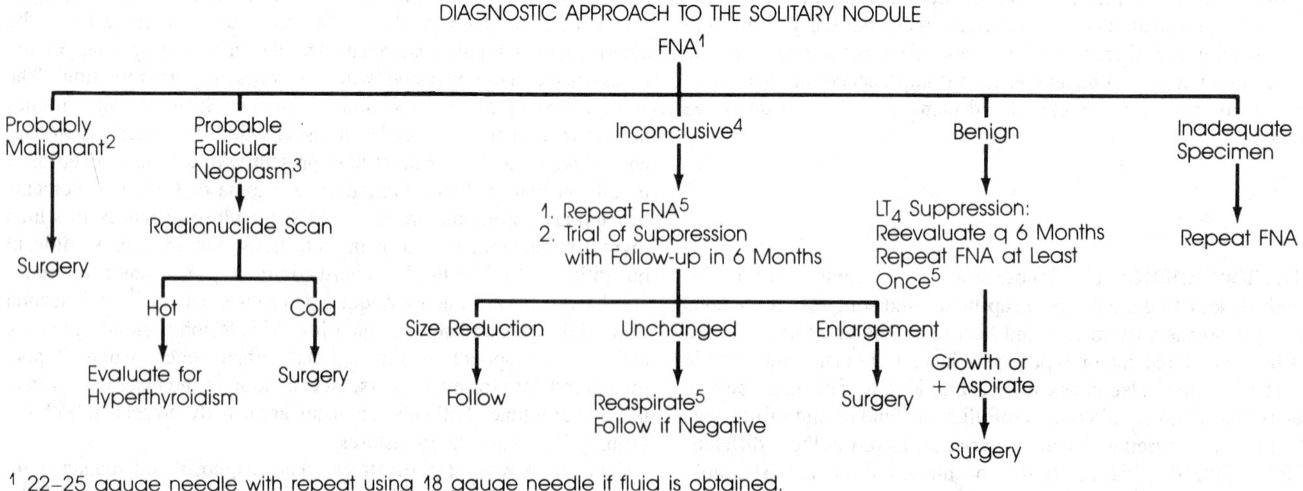

[1] 22–25 gauge needle with repeat using 18 gauge needle if fluid is obtained.
[2] Evidence of carcinoma (papillary, medullary, poorly differentiated, follicular) or lymphoma.
[3] e.g., sheets of follicular cells.
[4] e.g., small groups of uniform follicular cells with little colloid.
[5] Changes in cytologic findings redirect clinician to the appropriate arm of the algorithm.

the authors recommend thyroid hormone therapy with repeat aspiration cytology in 3 to 6 months.

Regardless of the operative procedure planned, surgery for thyroid carcinoma should be performed by a surgeon experienced in the procedure. Should surgery be delayed, suppressive therapy with levothyroxine is often recommended preoperatively to facilitate the operative procedure and perhaps to decrease the likelihood of tumor dissemination. In patients in whom a definitive preoperative diagnosis, such as by biopsy, has not been made, the suspected lesion is removed en bloc with a wide margin of surrounding tissue and is examined by frozen section. Opinions vary as to the type of procedure that is preferable when carcinoma is found. For lesions of 2 cm or less that are not multicentric and that have not metastasized, some recommend ipsilateral lobectomy, isthmectomy, and possibly contralateral partial lobectomy. Despite its higher rate of morbidity, the authors prefer that a near-total thyroidectomy be performed, especially for lesions >2 cm, in view of the frequency of seeding of tumor throughout the gland by transglandular lymphatic spread and of evidence that both recurrence rates and subsequent mortality are lower after the more extensive operation. Regional lymph nodes should be explored and removed if there is evidence of involvement, but radical neck dissection is not justified. If permanent sections reveal carcinoma when frozen sections had failed to do so and the initial procedure was limited, secondary surgery should be undertaken to remove residual thyroid tissue.

Approximately 3 weeks after surgery, liothyronine (50 to 75 μg daily) is substituted for levothyroxine, since it permits a more rapid return of TSH secretion when withdrawn some 3 weeks later. After an additional 2 or 3 weeks, when the serum TSH concentration has risen to the range of 50 mU/L, a large scanning dose of ^{131}I [185 to 370 MBq (5 to 10 mCi)] is administered and whole-body scans are obtained at 72 h. If residual thyroid tissue is found, as is usually the case, a thyroid ablating dose of 1850 MBq (50 mCi) of ^{131}I is administered, and if functioning metastases are present, the dose is doubled. Suppressive therapy with levothyroxine is reinstituted 24 to 48 h later. Approximately 1 week after administration of the second dose of ^{131}I, whole-body scans are repeated, as the larger dose of radioiodine may permit demonstration of functioning metastases not seen after the smaller initial dose. When this proves to be the case, some clinics withdraw suppressive therapy, administer an additional 3700 MBq (100 mCi) of ^{131}I, and then reinstitute suppressive therapy with levothyroxine.

Patients are reexamined approximately 6 months after the initial operation and at least every 6 months for several years thereafter. At these examinations, the neck is palpated for evidence of recurrence of metastases, which often can be treated with selective surgical removal. Blood is drawn for a serum thyroglobulin measurement, since elevated values in patients receiving suppressive therapy signal the presence of metastatic disease. At the initial 6-month examination, patients in whom metastases had previously been found are prepared for a whole-body scan as described above. Those in whom no metastases had been demonstrated by earlier scans are not rescanned unless the serum thyroglobulin is elevated but are rescanned approximately 1 year after the initial surgery. Patients in whom whole-body scans are positive are reentered into the therapeutic algorithm, as described above. Those in whom scans are negative continue to be reexamined and have measurements of serum thyroglobulin concentrations at regular intervals. If both serum thyroglobulin concentrations and scans are unrevealing, patients are scanned for the last time after approximately 3 years, unless serum thyroglobulin concentrations rise. In some patients, serum thyroglobulin may be elevated despite the absence of demonstrable functioning metastases. Such patients obviously cannot be treated with ^{131}I but should be studied with x-rays and bone scans to ascertain the site of the thyroglobulin-secreting metastases.

A program of this nature, involving near-total thyroidectomy, long-term suppressive therapy, and treatment of functioning metastases with radioiodine reduces the recurrence rate and prolongs survival in patients with papillary carcinoma of the thyroid. Follicular carcinoma should be treated with even greater vigor, since the results are generally less favorable. Because follicular carcinoma metastasizes to lung and bone, appropriate follow-up x-rays in addition to serum thyroglobulin are warranted. Treatment of anaplastic carcinoma is largely palliative; most patients die within 6 months of diagnosis.

THYROIDITIS

Thyroiditis embraces disorders of differing etiology. Two are exceedingly uncommon, *pyogenic thyroiditis* and *chronic fibrosing (Riedel's) thyroiditis.* Pyogenic thyroiditis is usually anteceded by a pyogenic infection elsewhere and is characterized by tenderness and swelling of the thyroid, redness and warmth of the overlying skin, and constitutional signs of infection. Treatment consists of antibiotic therapy and incisional drainage if a fluctuant area within the thyroid should occur. Riedel's thyroiditis is a disorder in which intense fibrosis of the thyroid and surrounding structures, leading to induration of the tissues of the neck, may be associated with mediastinal and retroperitoneal fibrosis. The principal importance of this disorder is that it requires differentiation from thyroid neoplasia. The other forms of thyroiditis, comprising subacute thyroiditis, chronic thyroiditis with transient thyrotoxicosis (CT/TT), and Hashimoto's thyroiditis, are more common. They are notable for their different clinical courses and for the fact that each can be associated, at one time or another, with a euthyroid, thyrotoxic, or hypothyroid state.

SUBACUTE THYROIDITIS This disorder, also termed *granulomatous, giant cell,* or *de Quervain's thyroiditis,* is viral in origin. Symptoms of thyroiditis usually follow those of an upper respiratory infection and include pronounced asthenia, malaise, and symptoms referable to stretching of the thyroid capsule, principally pain over the thyroid or pain referred to the lower jaw, ear, or occiput. Referred pain may predominate. These symptoms may smolder for weeks before the diagnosis is suspected. Less commonly, the onset is acute, with severe pain over the thyroid, accompanied by fever and occasionally symptoms of thyrotoxicosis. Physical findings include exquisite tenderness and nodularity over the thyroid, which may be unilateral but which usually involves other areas of the gland. Although local or referred pain is the commonest symptom, occasional patients have other features typical of the disease but have no pain.

Two laboratory findings are characteristic: a high erythrocyte sedimentation rate (ESR) and a depressed RAIU. Values for the remaining tests depend upon the stage of the disease in which they are obtained. Early, many patients are mildly thyrotoxic owing to leakage of hormone from the gland. The serum T_4 and T_3 are high. Later, as glandular hormone is depleted, the patient may pass through a hypothyroid phase, in which serum T_4 and T_3 are low and TSH increased. Diagnosis of the thyrotoxic phase is especially troublesome in the painless variant since the patient may be thought to have Graves' disease or toxic nodular goiter and therapy inappropriate for subacute thyroiditis may be instituted. Demonstration of a low RAIU usually serves to differentiate subacute thyroiditis from these other causes of hyperthyroidism. Differentiation of painless subacute thyroiditis from chronic thyroiditis with transient thyrotoxicosis is discussed below.

The disorder may smolder for months but eventually subsides with a return of normal thyroid function. In mild cases, aspirin suffices to control the symptoms. In more severe cases, glucocorticoid (prednisone, 20 to 40 mg daily) is generally effective. Propranolol can be used to control associated thyrotoxicosis. When the RAIU and serum T_4 return to normal, therapy can be withdrawn without recurrence of symptoms.

CHRONIC THYROIDITIS WITH TRANSIENT THYROTOXICOSIS This term denotes a disorder in which a self-limited episode of thyrotoxicosis is associated with a histologic picture of chronic lymphocytic thyroiditis that differs from that of Hashimoto's disease. This syndrome has been variously designated as painless thyroiditis, silent thyroiditis, hyperthyroiditis, chronic thyroiditis with spontaneously resolving hyperthyroidism, or, as the author prefers, chronic thyroiditis with transient thyrotoxicosis (CT/TT). Designations that imply the existence of hyperthyroidism are inappropriate, since ongoing production of thyroid hormone is negligible and the RAIU is decreased.

The syndrome occurs in patients of any age, and although it occurs mainly in women the female/male ratio is not as high as in Graves' disease. Manifestations of thyrotoxicosis are usually mild but may be severe. The thyroid is nontender, firm, symmetrical, and enlarged only slightly or moderately. Laboratory features include elevations of the serum T_4 and T_3 concentrations consonant with the thyrotoxicosis and a markedly depressed RAIU. The ESR is normal or only slightly elevated, rarely exceeding 50 mm/h, and antithyroid antibodies, when present, are present in low titer.

The etiology, pathogenesis, and pathophysiology of this disorder are unclear. Viral antibody titers show no characteristic patterns. It is presumed that thyrotoxicosis results from leakage of hormone from the gland, as in subacute thyroiditis. Low values for the RAIU, in turn, reflect suppression of TSH secretion, since urinary iodine excretion is not greatly elevated. Some degree of thyroid malfunction is indicated by failure of the RAIU to respond briskly to exogenous TSH stimulation.

Thyrotoxicosis in CT/TT usually abates within 2 to 5 months. Many patients have recurrent episodes of thyrotoxicosis of similar nature, sometimes following pregnancy (postpartum thyroiditis). The thyrotoxic phase may be followed in several months by a phase of self-limited hypothyroidism. The latter, which has been noted particularly in the postpartum period, may be the only component of the disease that is diagnosed because the thyrotoxic phase may be very brief. In Japan, as many as 5 percent of pregnant women may experience the syndrome post partum.

This disorder, in the thyrotoxic phase, needs differentiation, first, from Graves' disease; this can be accomplished by demonstration of a depressed RAIU and absence of increased urinary iodine excretion. The latter serves also to exclude the jod-Basedow syndrome. When these data are available, the disorder must be differentiated from other causes of thyrotoxicosis with a low RAIU, principally subacute thyroiditis. Lack of tenderness or nodularity of the thyroid and absence of marked elevation of the ESR tend to exclude the latter diagnosis. Patients with functioning ectopic thyroid tissue and thyrotoxicosis factitia characteristically respond to exogenous TSH stimulation with a brisk increase in RAIU. Definitive diagnosis of CT/TT can be made by thyroid biopsy.

Since the thyroid is not hyperfunctioning in this disorder, measures used in the treatment of hyperthyroidism are useless. Symptomatic treatment with propranolol or mild sedatives is administered until the thyrotoxicosis abates.

HASHIMOTO'S THYROIDITIS This disorder, also termed *lymphadenoid goiter,* is a common chronic inflammatory disease of the thyroid in which autoimmune factors play a prominent role. It occurs most frequently in women of middle age and is also the most common cause of sporadic goiter in children. Evidence of the participation of autoimmune factors includes the lymphocytic infiltration of the gland and the presence in the serum of increased concentrations of immunoglobulins and of antibodies against several components of thyroid tissue. Of these, the most important from the clinical standpoint are the antithyroglobulin antibody detected by the tanned red cell agglutination and the antimicrosomal antibody detected by immunofluorescence or complement fixation. This disorder also coexists with some frequency with other diseases of an autoimmune nature, including pernicious anemia, Sjögren's syndrome, chronic active hepatitis, systemic lupus erythematosus, rheumatoid arthritis, adrenal insufficiency, diabetes mellitus, and Graves' disease itself (see Chap. 325). These disorders, as well as Hashimoto's disease itself, also occur frequently in family members of patients with Hashimoto's disease.

Goiter is the outstanding feature. The enlargement involves the entire gland but not necessarily symmetrically. Typically, the consistency is rubbery, the margins are scalloped, and the general outline of the gland is preserved. The pyramidal lobe may be prominent. Early in the disease the patient is metabolically normal; however, even then decreased thyroid reserve is often manifest in an increase in serum TSH. The RAIU may be elevated early in the disease, reflecting the secretion of physiologically inactive iodoproteins, but the serum T_4 and T_3 are normal and the patient is euthyroid. As the disease progresses, thyroid failure, at first subclinical, may supervene owing to progressive replacement of thyroid parenchyma by lymphocytes or fibrous tissue. The thyroid failure is evident first in a rise in serum TSH concentration. With time, the serum T_4 concentration declines though the serum T_3 remains normal. Eventually, the serum T_3 concentration falls below normal, and frank hypothyroidism supervenes. High titers of antimicrosomal antibody are almost always present. High titers may also occur in other thyroid disorders, particularly primary thyroprivic hypothyroidism and Graves' disease but with lesser frequency. Although the foregoing findings usually suffice to permit a diagnosis, histologic confirmation by needle biopsy may be required. In view of the frequency with which hypothyroidism is either present or eventually develops, treatment with replacement doses of levothyroxine is indicated. In some patients, such therapy is associated with regression of goiter.

Occasional patients present with hyperthyroidism in association with a thyroid gland that is unusually firm and with high titers of circulating antithyroid antibodies, a combination which suggests, probably correctly, the concurrence of Graves' disease and Hashimoto's thyroiditis ("Hashitoxicosis"). In others, hyperthyroidism may supervene in a patient known to have Hashimoto's thyroiditis, presumably due to the emergence of clones of lymphocytes that produce stimulatory anti-TSH receptor antibodies. Hyperthyroidism in association with Hashimoto's thyroiditis is treated in a conventional manner, but ablative therapy is less commonly employed, since the associated chronic thyroiditis tends to limit the duration of thyroid hyperfunction and also predisposes the patient to the development of hypothyroidism after surgical or radioiodine treatment.

REFERENCES

Burman KD, Baker JR Jr: Immune mechanisms in Graves' disease. Endocr Rev 6:183, 1985

Burrow GN: The management of thyrotoxicosis in pregnancy. N Engl J Med 313:562, 1985

Fradkin JE, Wolff J: Iodide-induced thyrotoxicosis. Medicine 62:1, 1983

Hamburger JI: The autonomously functioning thyroid nodule: Goetsch's disease. Endocr Rev 8:439, 1987

Hay ID: Thyroiditis: A clinical update. Mayo Clin Proc 60:836, 1985

Hennessey JV et al: L-Thyroxine dosage: A re-evaluation of therapy with contemporary preparations. Ann Intern Med 105:11, 1986

Ingbar SH, Borges M: Peripheral metabolism of the thyroid hormones, in *Free Thyroid Hormones,* R Ekins et al (eds). Amsterdam, Excerpta Medica, 1979, p 17

Jacobson DH, Gorman CA: Endocrine ophthalmopathy: Current ideas concerning etiology, pathogenesis, and treatment. Endocr Rev 5:200, 1984

Oppenheimer JH et al: Advances in our understanding of thyroid hormone action at the cellular level. Endocr Rev 8:288, 1987

Rojeski MT, Gharib H: Nodular thyroid disease. N Engl J Med 313:428, 1985

Schneider AB et al: Sequential serum thyroglobulin determinations, ^{131}I scans, and ^{131}I uptakes after triiodothyronine withdrawal in patients with thyroid cancer. J Clin Endocrinol Metab 53:1199, 1981

——— et al: Radiation-induced thyroid carcinoma, clinical course, and results of therapy in 296 patients. Ann Intern Med 105:405, 1986

Smallridge RC: Thyrotropin-secreting pituitary tumors. Endocrin Metab Clin 16:765, 1987

Spencer CA: Clinical utility and cost effectiveness of sensitive thyrotropin assays in ambulatory and hospitalized patients. Mayo Clin Proc 63:1214, 1988

Stockigt JR, Barlow JW: The diagnostic challenge of euthyroid hyperthyroxinemia. Aust NZ J Med 15:277, 1985

Studer H, Ramelli F: Simple goiter and its variants: Euthyroid and hyperthyroid multinodular goiters. Endocr Rev 3:40, 1982

Wartofsky L, Oertel YC: Fine needle aspiration of thyroid nodules, in *Atlas of Nuclear Medicine,* D Van Nostrand, S Baum (eds). Philadelphia, Lippincott, 1988, p 193

———, Burman KD: Alterations in thyroid function in patients with systemic illness: The "euthyroid sick syndrome." Endocr Rev 3:164, 1982

317 DISEASES OF THE ADRENAL CORTEX

GORDON H. WILLIAMS / ROBERT G. DLUHY

BIOCHEMISTRY AND PHYSIOLOGY

STEROID NOMENCLATURE Steroids contain as their basic structure a cyclopentenoperhydrophenanthrane nucleus consisting of three 6-carbon hexane rings and a single 5-carbon pentane ring (Fig. 317-1). The carbon atoms are numbered in a sequence beginning with ring A. Adrenal steroids contain either 19 or 21 carbon atoms. The C_{19} steroids have methyl groups at positions C-18 and C-19. C_{19} steroids that have a ketone group at C-17 are termed *17-ketosteroids*. The C_{19} steroids have predominant androgenic activity. The C_{21} steroids have a 2-carbon side chain (C-20 and C-21) attached at position 17 and methyl groups at C-18 and C-19. C_{21} steroids that also possess a hydroxyl group at position 17 are termed *17-hydroxycorticosteroids*. The C_{21} steroids have either glucocorticoid or mineralocorticoid properties. *Glucocorticoid* signifies a C_{21} steroid with predominant action on intermediary metabolism; *mineralocorticoid* indicates a C_{21} steroid with predominant action on the metabolism of sodium and potassium.

BIOSYNTHESIS OF ADRENAL STEROIDS Cholesterol, derived from the diet and from endogenous synthesis, is the starting compound in steroidogenesis. The three major adrenal biosynthetic pathways lead to the production of glucocorticoids (cortisol), mineralocorticoids (aldosterone), and adrenal androgens (dehydroepiandrosterone). Separate zones of the adrenal cortex synthesize specific hormones; this reflects the enzymatic capacity of each zone to carry out certain transformations and hydroxylations (Fig. 317-2). The outer (glomerulosa) zone is mainly involved in aldosterone biosynthesis, and the inner (fasciculata-reticularis) zone is the site of cortisol and androgen biosynthesis.

STEROID TRANSPORT Some steroid hormones, e.g., testosterone and cortisol, circulate to a considerable extent bound to plasma proteins. Cortisol occurs in the plasma in three forms: free cortisol, protein-bound cortisol, and cortisol metabolites. *Free cortisol* refers to that quantity which is physiologically active but not protein-bound and, therefore, represents a form of cortisol acting directly on tissue sites. Normally, less than 5 percent of circulating cortisol is free. Only the unbound cortisol and its metabolites are filtrable at the glomerulus. Increased quantities of free steroid are excreted in the urine in states characterized by hypersecretion of cortisol, as the unbound fraction of plasma cortisol rises. *Protein-bound cortisol* is that reversibly bound to circulating plasma proteins. There are two cortisol-binding systems of plasma. One is a high-affinity, low-capacity alpha$_2$ globulin termed *transcortin* or *cortisol-binding globulin* (CBG), and the other is a low-affinity, high-capacity protein, *albumin*. The binding affinity of CBG for cortisol is reduced in areas of inflammation, thus increasing the local concentration of free cortisol. This phenomenon may be important in the glucocorticoid response to stress. Cortisol-binding globulin in normal humans can bind approximately 700 nmol of cortisol per liter of plasma (25 μg/dL). When the concentration of cortisol exceeds this level, the excess becomes bound in part to albumin, and a greater proportion circulates unbound. The CBG level is increased in high-estrogen states (e.g., pregnancy, oral contraceptive administration). The rise in CBG is accompanied by a parallel rise in protein-bound cortisol, with the result that the plasma cortisol concentration is elevated. However, the free cortisol levels probably remain normal, and signs and symptoms of glucocorticoid excess are absent. Most synthetic glucocorticoid analogues bind less efficiently to CBG (approximately 70 percent binding). This may explain the propensity of some synthetic analogues to produce cushingoid side effects at low dosage. *Cortisol metabolites* are biologically inactive and bind only weakly to circulating plasma proteins.

Aldosterone is bound to proteins to a smaller extent than either testosterone or cortisol, and an ultrafiltrate of plasma contains as much as 50 percent of the circulating aldosterone. The limited binding of aldosterone by plasma protein is significant in the metabolism of this hormone.

FIGURE 317-1 Basic steroid structure and nomenclature.

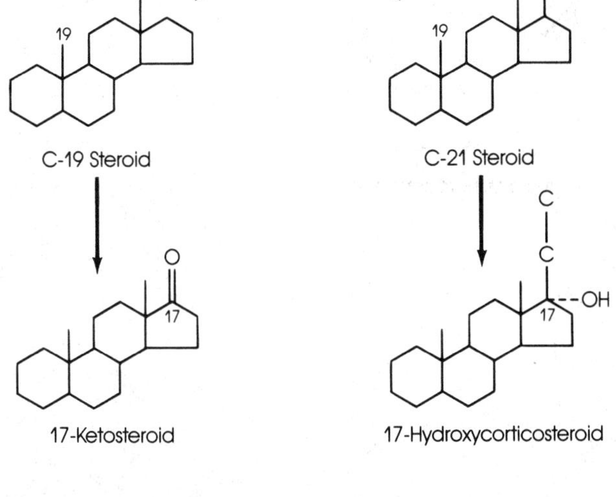

STEROID METABOLISM AND EXCRETION **Glucocorticoids** The daily secretion of cortisol ranges between 40 and 80 μmol (15 and 30 mg), with a pronounced diurnal cycle. Cortisol is distributed in a volume of body fluids approximating the total extracellular fluid space, with more than 90 percent in the protein-bound fraction. The plasma concentration of cortisol is determined by the rate of secretion, the rate of inactivation, and the rate of excretion of free cortisol. The liver is the major organ responsible for steroid inactivation, by reduction of ring A and conjugation of the reduced products with glucuronic acid at position C-3 to form water-soluble compounds. The 11-dehydrogenase system converts cortisol to the inactive cortisone and is influenced by the level of circulating thyroid hormone, the oxidative reaction being increased in hyperthyroidism.

Mineralocorticoids In normal subjects on a normal salt intake, the average daily secretion of aldosterone ranges between 0.1 and 0.7 μmol (50 and 250 μg). Since aldosterone is only weakly bound to proteins, its volume of distribution is larger than that of cortisol and approximates 35 liters. During a single passage through the liver, more than 75 percent of circulating aldosterone is normally inactivated by ring A reduction and conjugation with glucuronic acid. However, under certain conditions, such as congestive failure, this inactivation is reduced.

From 7 to 15 percent of aldosterone is excreted in the urine as a glucuronide conjugate, from which free aldosterone is released on standing at pH 1. This *acid-labile conjugate* is formed in the liver and in the kidney. For average salt intake, the 24-h urine excretion of the acid-labile conjugate ranges from 15 to 50 nmol (5 to 19 μg), that of the reduced derivative from 70 to 100 nmol (25 to 35 μg), and that of the nonconjugated, nonreduced free aldosterone from 0.5 to 2 nmol (0.2 to 0.6 μg).

Adrenal androgens The major androgen secreted by the adrenal is dehydroepiandrosterone (DHEA) and its C-3 sulfuric acid ester. From 15 to 30 mg of these compounds are secreted daily. Smaller amounts of Δ^4-androstenedione, 11β-hydroxyandrostenedione, and testosterone are secreted. DHEA is the major precursor of the urinary 17-ketosteroids. Two-thirds of the urine 17-ketosteroids in the male is derived from adrenal metabolites, and the remaining one-third comes from testicular androgens. In the female, almost all urine 17-ketosteroids are derived from the adrenal.

ACTH PHYSIOLOGY Corticotropin (ACTH) (see Chap. 313) is an unbranched polypeptide containing 39 amino acids. ACTH and a number of other peptides (lipotropins, endorphins, and melanocyte-stimulating hormones) are processed from a larger precursor molecule of 31,000 mol wt—pro-opiomelanocortin (POMC) (see Chap. 313 and Fig. 317-3). ACTH is synthesized and stored in basophilic cells of the anterior pituitary gland. The basophilic staining of the corticotrophs is the result of the glycosylation of ACTH and related peptides. Much of the potential for the corticotropic actions of ACTH is present in smaller polypeptide fragments; the *N*-terminal 18-amino-acid structure retains full biologic potency, and shorter *N*-terminal fragments exhibit partial biologic activity. Release of ACTH and

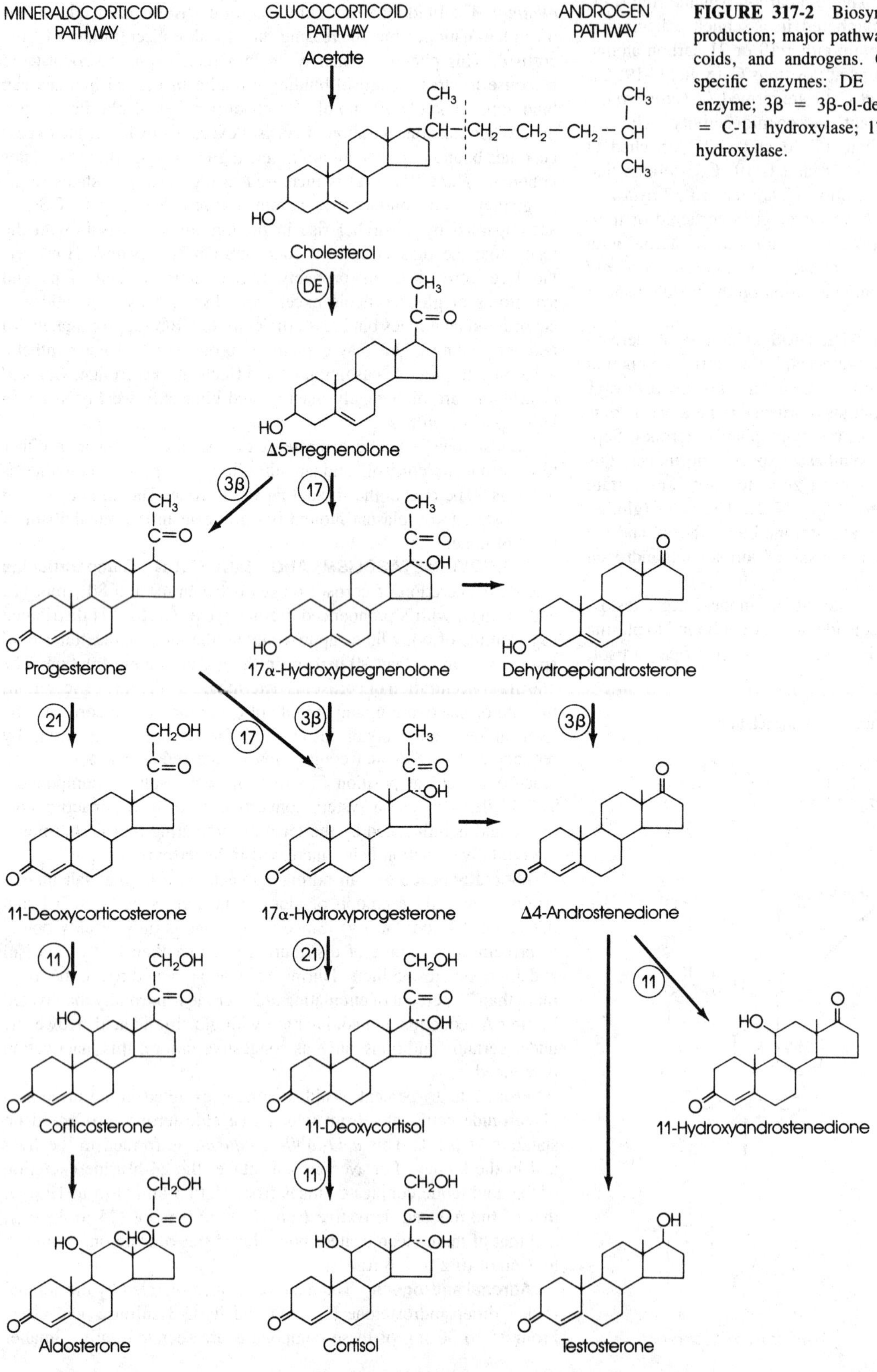

FIGURE 317-2 Biosynthetic pathways for adrenal steroid production; major pathways to mineralocorticoids, glucocorticoids, and androgens. Circled letters and numbers denote specific enzymes: DE = cholesterol side chain cleavage enzyme; 3β = 3β-ol-dehydrogenase with $\Delta^{4,5}$-isomerase; 11 = C-11 hydroxylase; 17 = C-17 hydroxylase; 21 = C-21 hydroxylase.

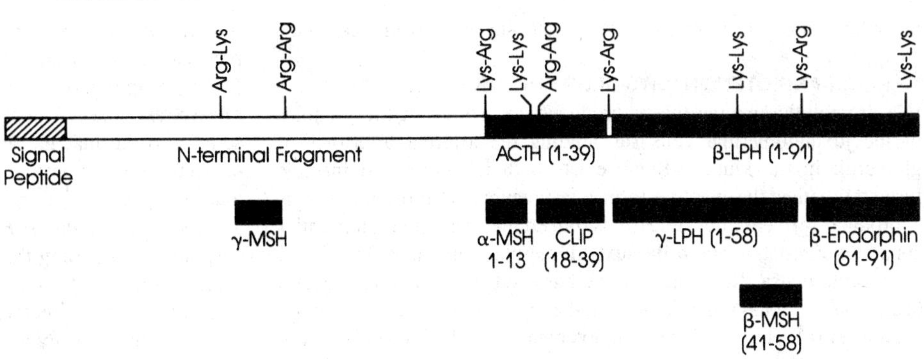

FIGURE 317-3 Schematic representation of the probable structure of the 31,000–mol wt pro-opiomelanocortin molecule. (*From DT Krieger, JB Martin, N Engl J Med 304:880, 1981. By permission of the New England Journal of Medicine.*)

related peptides from the anterior pituitary gland is governed by a "corticotropin-releasing center" in the median eminence of the hypothalamus, which upon stimulation releases a peptide with a chain of 41 amino acids (corticotropin-releasing hormone, CRH) that travels via the pituitary-stalk portal bloodstream to the anterior pituitary, where it effects the release of ACTH (Fig. 317-4). Some related peptides such as β-lipotropin (β-LPH) are released in equimolar concentrations with ACTH, suggesting enzymatic cleavage from the parent POMC prior to or concomitant with the secretory process. However, beta endorphin levels may vary disparately with circulating levels of ACTH depending on the nature of the stimulus. The functions and regulation of secretion of the related peptides derived from POMC are not understood.

The major factors controlling ACTH release include CRH, free cortisol concentration in plasma, stress, and the sleep-wake cycle (Fig. 317-4). The plasma level of ACTH varies during the day as a result of its pulsatile secretion but roughly follows a diurnal pattern, with a peak just prior to waking and a nadir before retiring. After several days on a new sleep-wake cycle, the pattern is altered to conform to the new cycle. ACTH and cortisol levels also increase in response to eating. Stress (e.g., pyrogens, surgery, hypoglycemia, exercise, and severe emotional trauma) can also enhance ACTH release. Stress-related secretion of ACTH abolishes circadian periodicity but is in turn suppressed by prior high-dose glucocorticoid administration. The secretion of ACTH following stress and the normal pulsatile, diurnal ACTH release are regulated by CRH; this is the so-called open feedback loop. CRH secretion, in turn, is influenced by hypothalamic neurotransmitters. For example, serotoninergic and cholinergic systems stimulate the secretion of CRH and ACTH; there is contradictory evidence regarding the inhibitory effects of α-adrenergic agonists and gamma-aminobutyric acid (GABA) on CRH release. In addition, there may be direct pituitary effects of these neurotransmitters. There is also evidence for peptidergic regulation of ACTH release. For example, beta endorphin and enkephalin inhibit and vasopressin and angiotensin II augment the secretion of ACTH. Finally, ACTH release is regulated by the free cortisol level in plasma. Cortisol decreases the responsiveness of adrenal corticotropic cells to CRH; i.e., in the presence of cortisol more CRH is required to produce a given increment of ACTH. The response of the POMC mRNA to CRH is also inhibited by glucocorticoids. In addition, glucocorticoids inhibit CRH release. This servomechanism establishes the primacy of blood cortisol concentration in the control of ACTH secretion. The inhibition of ACTH occurs in two phases: (1) an early fast feedback, possibly a membrane effect, lasting less than 10 min and dependent on the rate of increase of glucocorticoid levels; and (2) a time-dependent delayed feedback response, probably due to inhibition of synthesis of the precursor protein. The suppression of ACTH secretion that results in adrenal atrophy following *prolonged* glucocorticoid therapy may be primarily related to suppression of hypothalamic CRH release, since exogenous CRH administration in this circumstance produces a rise in plasma ACTH. Cortisol also exerts feedback on higher brain centers (hippocampus, reticular system, and septum) and perhaps on the adrenal cortex as well (Fig. 317-4).

The biologic half-life of ACTH in the circulation is less than 10 min. The action of ACTH is also rapid; within minutes of its release, the concentration of steroids in the adrenal venous blood increases. ACTH stimulates steroidogenesis via activation of the membrane-bound adenyl cyclase. Adenosine-3′,5′-monophosphate (cyclic AMP) in turn activates protein kinase enzymes, thereby resulting in the

FIGURE 317-4 The hypothalamic-pituitary-adrenal axis. The dominant feedback control of plasma cortisol is on the pituitary gland (1) and on the hypothalamic corticotropin-releasing center (2). Feedback of plasma cortisol may also act on higher nerve centers (3) and/or on the adrenal gland itself (4). There also may be a short feedback inhibition of CRH by ACTH (5). Hypothalamic neurotransmitters influence CRH release; serotoninergic and cholinergic systems stimulate the secretion of CRH and ACTH; alpha-adrenergic agonists and gamma-aminobutyric acid (GABA) probably inhibit CRH release. The opioid peptides, beta endorphin and enkephalin, inhibit and vasopressin and angiotensin II augment the secretion of CRH and ACTH. CRH = corticotropin-releasing hormone; β-LPH = beta lipotropin; POMC = pro-opiomelanocortin.

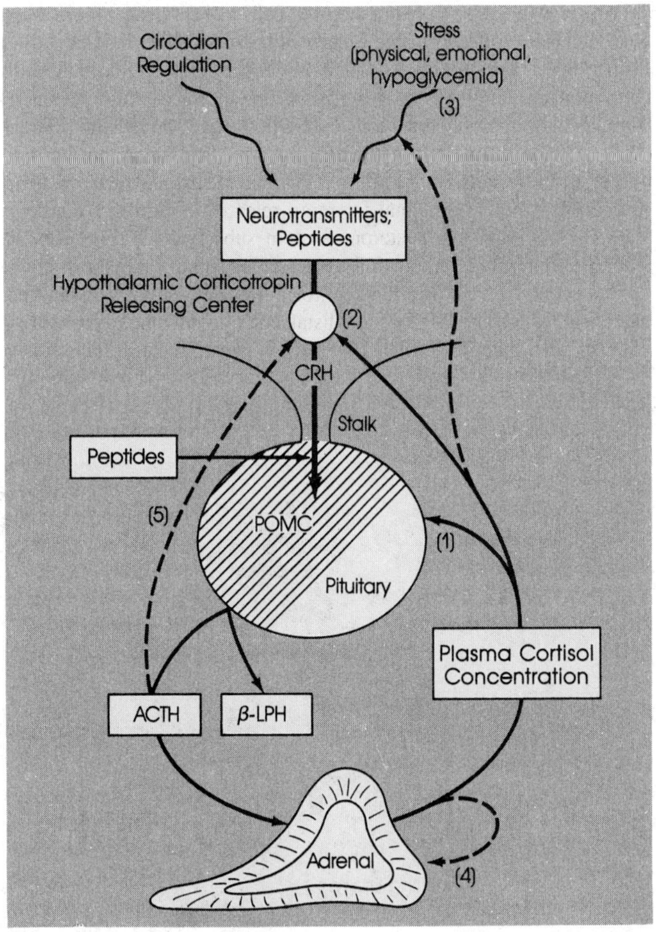

phosphorylation of proteins that activate steroid biosynthesis (see Chap. 68).

RENIN-ANGIOTENSIN PHYSIOLOGY (See also Chap. 196) Renin is a proteolytic enzyme that is produced and stored in the granules of the juxtaglomerular cells surrounding the afferent arterioles of glomeruli in the kidney. Renin exists both in active and inactive forms. Whether the inactive form is a precursor ("prorenin") or is a product formed after release is uncertain. The juxtaglomerular apparatus consists of both the juxtaglomerular cells and the cells of the macula densa. Renin acts on the basic substrate angiotensinogen (a circulating alpha$_2$ globulin made in the liver) to form the decapeptide angiotensin I (Fig. 317-5). Angiotensin I is then enzymatically transformed by converting enzyme, present in many tissues particularly in the pulmonary vascular endothelium, to the octapeptide angiotensin II by splitting off the two C-terminal amino acids. Angiotensin II is a potent pressor compound and exerts its pressor action by a direct effect on arteriolar smooth muscle. In addition, angiotensin II is a potent stimulus to the production of aldosterone by the zona glomerulosa of the adrenal cortex; the nonapeptide, angiotensin III, may also stimulate aldosterone production. Angiotensinases rapidly destroy angiotensin II (half-life approximately 1 min), while the half-life of renin is more prolonged (10 to 20 min). Other tissues, such as uterus, placenta, vascular tissue, brain, salivary glands, and adrenal cortex also produce renin-like substances, but the significance of these so-called tissue renins is not known.

Renal renin release is controlled by four interdependent factors, and the amount of renin released is a composite of the effects of all four. The *juxtaglomerular cells,* which are specialized myoepithelial cells cuffing the afferent arterioles, act as miniature pressure transducers, sensing renal perfusion pressure and corresponding changes in afferent arteriolar perfusion pressures. For example, under conditions of a reduction in circulating blood volume, there is a corresponding reduction in renal perfusion pressure and, therefore, in afferent arteriolar pressure (Fig. 317-5). This is perceived by the juxtaglomerular cells as a decreased stretch exerted on the afferent arteriolar walls. The juxtaglomerular cells then release increasing quantities of renin within the kidney circulation. This results in the formation of angiotensin I, which is converted in the kidney and peripherally to angiotensin II by converting enzyme. Angiotensin II stimulates the adrenal cortex to release aldosterone. Increasing plasma levels of aldosterone lead to increasing renal sodium retention and thus result in expansion of extracellular fluid volume, which, in turn, dampens the initiating signal for renin release. Within this context, the renin-angiotensin-aldosterone system subserves volume control by appropriate modifications of renal tubular sodium transport.

A second control mechanism for renin release centers in the *macula densa* cells, a group of distal convoluted tubular epithelial cells in direct apposition to the juxtaglomerular cells. They may function as chemoreceptors, monitoring the sodium (or chloride) load presented to the distal tubule, and such information may be conveyed to the juxtaglomerular cells, where appropriate modifications in renin release take place. Under conditions of increased delivery of filtered sodium to the macula densa, increasing release of renin is capable of decreasing glomerular filtration rate, thereby reducing the filtered load of sodium.

The *sympathetic nervous system* regulates release of renin in response to assuming the upright posture. The mechanism is either a direct effect on the juxtaglomerular cell to increase adenyl cyclase activity or an indirect effect on either the juxtaglomerular or the macula densa cells by way of a vasoconstrictive action on the afferent arteriole.

Finally, circulating factors may alter renin release. Increasing dietary *potassium* directly decreases renin release; decreasing potassium intake increases renin release. The significance of this potassium effect is unclear. *Angiotensin II* itself can exert a negative feedback control on renin release independent of alterations in renal blood flow, pressure, or aldosterone secretion. *Atrial natriuretic peptides* also may inhibit renin release. Thus, the control of renin release is complex, consisting of both *intrarenal* (pressor receptor and macula densa) and *extrarenal* (sympathetic nervous system, potassium, angiotensin, etc.) mechanisms. A given level of renin secretion probably reflects all these factors, with the intrarenal mechanism predominating.

GLUCOCORTICOID PHYSIOLOGY The division of adrenal steroids into glucocorticoids and mineralocorticoids is arbitrary in that most glucocorticoids have some mineralocorticoid-like properties, and vice versa (see Chap. 311). The descriptive term *glucocorticoid* is applied to those adrenal steroids with a predominant action on intermediary metabolism. The principal glucocorticoid is cortisol (hydrocortisone). Cortisol enters the target cell by diffusion, combines with high-affinity cytoplasmic receptor proteins, and is transferred to acceptor sites on the chromosomes, which then results in an increase in RNA synthesis and later in protein synthesis. One way of defining glucocorticoid effects is as those mediated by one class of high-affinity cytoplasmic receptors (so called type II or glucorticoid receptors) (see Chap. 311). The physiologic actions of the glucocorticoids on intermediary metabolism include the regulation of protein, carbohydrate, lipid, and nucleic acid metabolism. Glucocorticoids raise blood glucose by acting as an insulin antagonist and by suppressing the secretion of insulin, thereby inhibiting glucose uptake in peripheral tissues and promoting hepatic synthesis of glucose (gluconeogenesis). The actions on protein metabolism appear to be mainly catabolic in effect, with an increased protein breakdown and nitrogen excretion. Glucocorticoids increase hepatic glycogen content and promote the hepatic synthesis of gluconeogenesis. These actions are in large part explained by the mobilization of glycogenic amino

FIGURE 317-5 The interrelationship of the volume and potassium feedback loops on aldosterone secretion. Integration of signals from each loop determines the level of aldosterone secretion.

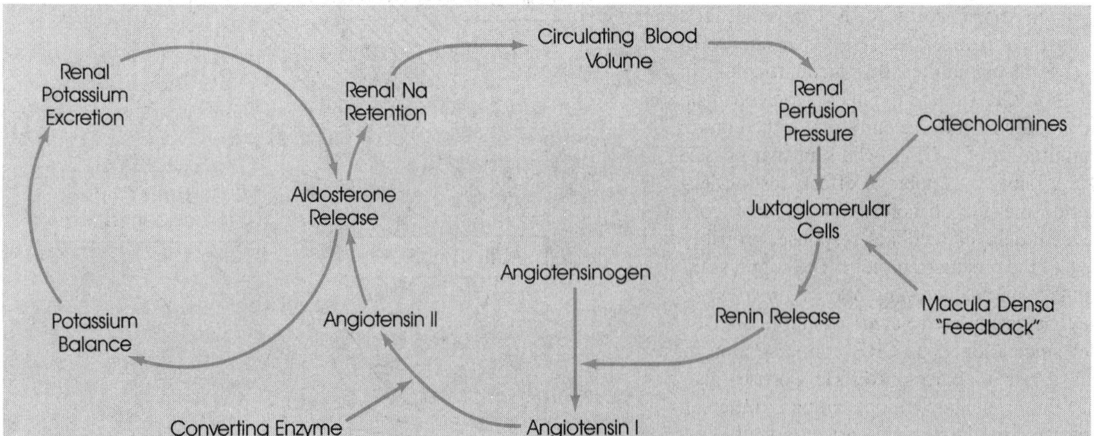

acid precursors from peripheral supporting structures, such as bone, skin, muscle, and connective tissue, due to protein breakdown and inhibition of protein synthesis and amino acid uptake. Glucocorticoid-induced hyperaminoacidemia also facilitates gluconeogenesis by stimulating glucagon secretion. Glucocorticoids act directly on the liver to stimulate the synthesis of certain enzymes, such as tyrosine amino transferase and tryptophan pyrrolase. Glucocorticoids inhibit the synthesis of nucleic acids in most body tissues, but in the liver RNA synthesis is stimulated. Glucocorticoids regulate fatty acid mobilization by enhancing activation of cellular lipase by lipid-mobilizing hormones (e.g., catecholamines and pituitary peptides).

The actions of cortisol on structural protein and on adipose tissue vary in different parts of the body. For example, pharmacologic doses of cortisol can deplete the protein matrix of the vertebral column (trabecular bone), but long bones (primarily compact bone) are affected only minimally; peripheral adipose tissue may diminish, whereas abdominal and interscapular fat may accumulate.

Glucocorticoids have anti-inflammatory properties, which are probably related to their actions on the microvasculature as well as to cellular effects. Cortisol maintains normal vascular responsiveness to circulating vasoconstrictor factors and opposes the increase in capillary permeability characteristic of acute inflammation. Glucocorticoids cause a polymorphonuclear leukocytosis; the circulating leukocyte mass is increased due to release from the bone marrow of mature cells as well as to inhibition of their egress through the capillary wall. Glucocorticoids produce a depletion of circulating eosinophils and of lymphoid tissue, specifically T cells (thymus-derived lymphocytes). The mechanism is by redistribution from the circulation into other compartments. Thus, cortisol impairs cellular-mediated immunity. Glucocorticoids also inhibit the production or action of the local mediators of inflammation such as the lymphokines and prostaglandins. These actions occur via the glucocorticoid receptors, and the effects are blocked by inhibitors of RNA and protein synthesis. Glucocorticoids inhibit actions and production of immune interferon by T lymphocytes, and the production of lymphocyte-activating factor (also known as interleukin 1) by macrophages. The action of glucocorticoids in suppressing fever may be explained by the latter effect since interleukin 1 appears to be identical to endogenous pyrogen, which can activate the hypothalamic fever center. Glucocorticoids also inhibit the production of T-cell growth factor (interleukin 2) by T lymphocytes. Glucocorticoids reverse macrophage activation and antagonize the action of migration-inhibiting factor (MIF), leading to reduced adherence of macrophages to vascular endothelium. Glucocorticoids inhibit prostaglandin and leukotriene production by inhibiting the activity of phospholipase A_2, thus blocking release of arachidonic acid from phospholipids. Finally, glucocorticoids inhibit the inflammatory actions induced by bradykinin and serotonin, such as increased vascular permeability. It is probably only at pharmacologic dosages that antibody production is reduced and lysosomal membranes stabilized, thereby suppressing the release of proteolytic acid hydrolases stored in these cytoplasmic organelles.

Cortisol levels are responsive within minutes to a variety of physical stresses (trauma, surgery, exercise) and psychological stresses (anxiety, depression). Hypoglycemia and fever are also potent stimuli of ACTH and cortisol secretion. The reasons why elevated glucocorticoid levels protect the organism under stress are not understood, but this action may be linked to the anti-inflammatory actions of cortisol in suppressing normal defense reactions, thus regulating the control of the inflammatory response in uninvolved tissues. In the absence of glucocorticoids, such stresses may cause hypotension, shock, and death. For these reasons, glucocorticoid administration should always be increased in individuals with hypofunction of the pituitary-adrenal axis during stress.

Cortisol has a major action on the distribution and excretion of body water. It subserves the extracellular fluid volume by retarding the migration of water into cells. It promotes renal water excretion by suppressing the secretion of vasopressin, increasing the rate of glomerular filtration, and acting directly on the renal tubule, the consequence being to guard against water intoxication by increasing solute-free water clearance. Glucocorticoids also have weak mineralocorticoid-like properties, and increasing doses produce renal tubular sodium reabsorption and increased urine potassium excretion. Glucocorticoids can also influence behavior; emotional disorders may occur with either excesses or deficits of cortisol. Lastly, cortisol suppresses the secretion of pituitary POMC and peptides derived from this precursor molecule (ACTH, beta-endorphin, and beta-lipotropin) as well as the secretion of hypothalamic CRH and vasopressin.

MINERALOCORTICOID PHYSIOLOGY The major mineralocorticoid, aldosterone, has two important activities: (1) It is a major regulator of extracellular fluid volume, and (2) it is a major determinant of potassium metabolism. These effects are mediated by binding of aldosterone to high-affinity type I or mineralocorticoid receptor proteins in target tissues (see Chap. 311). Volume is regulated through a direct effect on the renal tubular transport of sodium. Aldosterone acts predominantly at the distal convoluted tubule, where it causes a decrease in the excretion of sodium and an increase in excretion of potassium. The reabsorption of sodium ions causes a fall in the transmembrane potential, thus enhancing the flow of positive ions out of the cell into the lumen. The major intracellular singly charged positive ion is potassium. Since its concentration in the cell is forty- to eightyfold greater than in the lumen, potassium passively follows this relative electric gradient to restore the normal positive charge to the lumen. The reabsorbed sodium ions are then transported out of the tubular epithelial cells into the interstitial fluid of the kidney and from there into the renal capillary circulation. Water passively follows the transported sodium.

Hydrogen ion is also abundant in the tubular epithelial cell. Since its concentration is greater in the lumen than in the cell, it is actively secreted, but the reduced intraluminal positivity allows more hydrogen to be secreted with the same amount of energy. Aldosterone and other mineralocorticoids also act on the epithelium of the salivary ducts, sweat glands, and gastrointestinal tract to cause reabsorption of sodium in "exchange" for potassium ions.

When normal individuals are given aldosterone (or deoxycorticosterone), an initial period of sodium retention is followed by a natriuresis, and sodium balance is reestablished after 3 to 5 days. As a result, edema does not develop. This phenomenon is referred to as the "escape phenomenon," signifying an "escape" by the renal tubules from the sodium-retaining action of chronically administered aldosterone.

Three primary mechanisms control aldosterone release—the renin-angiotensin system, potassium, and ACTH (Table 317-1). The renin-angiotensin system is the major system for control of extracellular fluid volume, via regulation of aldosterone secretion (Fig. 317-5). In effect, the renin-angiotensin system maintains the circulating blood volume constant by causing aldosterone-induced sodium retention

TABLE 317-1 Factors regulating aldosterone biosynthesis

Factors	Effects
I Renin-angiotensin system	Stimulate
II Sodium ion	Inhibit (?physiologic)
III Potassium ion	Stimulate
IV Neurotransmitters	
A Dopamine	Inhibit
B Serotonin	Stimulate
V Pituitary hormones	
A ACTH	Stimulate
B Non-ACTH pituitary hormones (e.g., growth hormone)	Permissive (for optimal response to sodium restriction)
C Unidentified pituitary factors	Stimulate
D Beta endorphin	Stimulate
E γ-MSH	Permissive
VI Natriuretic factors	
A Atrial peptide	Inhibit
B Ouabain-like factors	Inhibit

during periods registered as volume deficiencies and by decreasing aldosterone-dependent sodium retention under conditions in which volume is registered as being ample.

Potassium ions directly regulate aldosterone secretion independently of the renin-angiotensin system (Fig. 317-5). In normal humans, oral potassium loading increases aldosterone secretion, excretion, and plasma levels. In addition, an increase in serum potassium of as little as 0.1 mmol/L increases plasma aldosterone levels under certain circumstances.

Physiologic amounts of ACTH acutely stimulate aldosterone secretion, but this action is not sustained if ACTH is infused for periods greater than 10 to 12 h. Most studies relegate ACTH to a minor role in the control of aldosterone. For example, subjects on high-dose steroid therapy for several years and with presumably complete suppression of ACTH have normal aldosterone-secretory responses to sodium restriction. Therefore, chronic ACTH deficiency per se does not alter glomerulosa cell responsiveness.

The prior dietary intake of both potassium and sodium can alter the magnitude of the aldosterone response to acute stimulation. Increasing potassium intake or decreasing sodium intake sensitizes the response of the glomerulosa cells to acute stimulation by ACTH, angiotensin II, and/or potassium.

Neurotransmitters (dopamine and serotonin) and some peptides, such as atrial natriuretic factor, γ-melanocyte-stimulating hormone (γ-MSH), beta endorphin, and an unidentified pituitary aldosterone-stimulating factor, also participate in the regulation of aldosterone secretion (Table 317-1). Thus, the control of aldosterone secretion involves both stimulatory and inhibitory factors.

ANDROGEN PHYSIOLOGY Androgens regulate male secondary sexual characteristics and can cause virilizing symptoms in women. They produce these actions by binding to high-affinity cytoplasmic receptors.

Steroids with predominant androgenic activity have 19 carbon atoms (Fig. 317-1). The principal adrenal androgens are dehydroepiandrosterone (DHEA), androstenedione, and 11-hydroxyandrostenedione. DHEA and its sulfate are *quantitatively* the major androgens secreted by the adrenal; DHEA and androstenedione are weak androgens, and they exert their effects via conversion in extraglandular tissues to the potent androgen, testosterone. The release of adrenal androgens is stimulated by ACTH, not by gonadotropins. With ACTH stimulation, 17-ketosteroids increase but to a lesser extent than do urine 17-hydroxycorticosteroids. It follows that adrenal androgens are suppressed by exogenous glucocorticoid administration.

LABORATORY EVALUATION OF ADRENOCORTICAL FUNCTION

The basic assumption in the measurement of plasma or urinary steroids is that they accurately reflect adrenal *secretory* rates of that steroid. A disadvantage of urine *excretion* values is that they may not truly reflect the secretion rate because of improper collection or altered metabolism. Measurement of the actual adrenal secretory rate of a given steroid would be preferable but is more difficult, involving isotope dilution techniques following administration of a radioactive steroid. Plasma levels reflect the level of secretion only at the time of measurement. The plasma level (PL) is dependent on two factors: the secretion rate (SR) of the hormone and the rate at which it is metabolized, i.e., its metabolic clearance rate (MCR). These three factors can be related mathematically as follows:

$$PL = \frac{SR}{MCR} \quad \text{or} \quad SR = MCR \times PL$$

BLOOD LEVELS (See Table 317-2) **Peptides** ACTH and angiotensin II can be measured by radioimmunoassay, but the measurements are technically difficult because of their low concentrations and their instability in human plasma. In addition, ACTH levels fluctuate from moment to moment, and a circadian rhythm is superimposed on basal ACTH secretion, with lower levels in the early evening than in the morning. Angiotensin II levels also vary diurnally but more importantly are influenced by dietary sodium intake and posture. Both upright posture and sodium restriction elevate angiotensin II levels.

TABLE 317-2 Range of normal values for tests of adrenal function

Test	Normal value, range
Plasma cortisol, nmol/L (μg/dL):	
8 A.M.	140–690 (5–24)
4 P.M.	80–330 (3–12)
Cortisol secretory rate, nmol/d (mg/d)	14–69 (5–25)
Urinary free cortisol, nmol/d (μg/d)	55–275 (20–100)
17-Hydroxycorticosteroids, μmol/d (mg/d)	5.5–28 (2–10)
Plasma testosterone, nmol/L (ng/mL):	
Men	10–35 (3–10)
Women	<3.5 (<1)
Plasma dehydroepiandrosterone (DHEA) nmol/L (μg/L)	7–31 (2–9)
Plasma DHEA sulfate, μmol/L (μg/L)	1.3–6.7 (500–2500)
Plasma 11-deoxycortisol (S), nmol/L (μg/dL)	<30 (<1)
Plasma 17OH progesterone, nmol/L (μg/L):	
Women	
Follicular phase	0.6–3 (0.2–1)
Luteal phase	1.5–10.6 (0.5–3.5)
Men	0.2–9 (0.06–3)
Plasma aldosterone, pmol/L (ng/dL) (100 mmol Na, 60–100 mmol K, supine, 8 A.M.)	<240 (<8)
Aldosterone secretion nmol/d (μg/d) (100 mmol Na, 600–100 mmol K)	140–690 (50–250)
Aldosterone excretion, nmol/d (μg/d) (100 mmol Na, 60–100 mmol K)	14–53 (5–19)
Plasma renin activity (μg/L)/h [(ng/mL)/h] (100 mmol Na, 60–100 mmol K, supine, 8 A.M.)	1–2.5 (1–2.5)
Plasma angiotensin II ng/L (pg/mL) (100 mmol Na, 60–100 mmol K, supine, 8 A.M.)	10–30 (10–30)
Plasma ACTH, pmol/L (pg/mL) (8 A.M.)	<18 (<80)

Most clinical determinations of the renin-angiotensin system, however, involve measurements of peripheral "plasma renin activity" (PRA) in which the renin activity is gauged by the generation of angiotensin I during a standardized incubation period. This method depends on the presence of sufficient angiotensinogen in the patient's plasma as substrate. The generated angiotensin I is then measured by radioimmunoassay. Plasma renin activity depends on dietary sodium intake and whether the patient is ambulatory. In normal humans a diurnal rhythm for PRA is characterized by peak values in the morning with decreases in activity in the afternoon.

Steroids Cortisol and aldosterone are both secreted episodically, and levels generally decline during the day with peak values in the morning and low levels in the evening. In addition, the plasma level of aldosterone, but not of cortisol, is increased by dietary potassium loading, sodium restriction, or assuming the upright posture. Measurement of the sulfate conjugate of DHEA is a useful index of adrenal androgen secretion since little is formed in the gonads and the half-life is 7 to 9 h.

URINE LEVELS The urine *17-hydroxycorticosteroid* assay measures steroids with a "dihydroxyacetone" C-17 side chain, i.e., with hydroxyl groups on C-17 and C-21 and a ketone group on C-20. Therefore, this determination includes cortisol, cortisone, tetrahydrocortisol, tetrahydrocortisone, and 11-deoxycortisol (Fig. 317-2). Normally, daytime (7 A.M. to 7 P.M.) excretion exceeds night values (7 P.M. to 7 A.M.).

The urine *17-ketosteroids* are those containing a ketone group at C-17 (Fig. 317-1). They originate either in the adrenal gland or the gonad. In normal women, 90 percent or more of total urinary 17-ketosteroids is derived from the adrenal gland, while in men only 60 to 70 percent is of adrenal origin. Urine 17-ketosteroid values are highest in young adults and decline with age.

The determination of urinary free cortisol is perhaps more useful than 17-hydroxysteroid measurements since elevated excretion values correlate with states of hypercortisolism, reflecting changes in the unbound, physiologically active, circulating levels of cortisol.

A carefully timed urine collection is a prerequisite for all excretory determinations. Urinary creatinine should be measured simultaneously to demonstrate the accuracy and adequacy of the collection procedure. Adjustments for body size can be made; e.g., normal subjects excrete 8 to 20 μmol (3 to 7 mg) of 17-hydroxycorticosteroids per gram of creatinine.

STIMULATION TESTS Stimulation tests are useful in documenting the existence of a hormonal deficiency state. A standardized and specific stimulus for the production and release of a given hormone is applied, and the quantity of the released hormone can then be measured.

Tests of glucocorticoid reserve Within minutes after initiation of an infusion of ACTH, cortisol levels increase in adrenal venous blood. This responsiveness of the adrenal gland to ACTH is utilized as an index of the "functional reserve" of the gland for production of cortisol. Under maximal ACTH stimulation the cortisol secretion increases tenfold to 800 μmol/d (300 mg/d). Such maximal stimulation can be obtained only with prolonged ACTH infusions. For clinical purposes, the functional adrenal reserve for cortisol production is standardized with a 24-h ACTH infusion. Synthetic α^{1-24}-ACTH (cosyntropin) is usually given in 500 to 1000 mL normal saline at a rate of 2 units per hour for 24 h. Normal subjects increase 17-hydroxysteroid excretion rates to at least 70 μmol/d (25 mg/d), and plasma cortisol levels exceed 1100 nmol/L (40 μg/dL). In patients with secondary adrenal insufficiency, the maximal 17-hydroxysteroid excretion rate is 8 to 55 μmol/d (3 to 20 mg/d), and the plasma cortisol value at 24 h ranges between 280 and 1100 nmol/L (10 and 40 μg/dL). Patients with primary adrenal insufficiency have smaller responses.

A screening test (the so-called rapid ACTH stimulation test) involves the administration of 25 units (0.25 mg) cosyntropin intravenously or intramuscularly and measurement of plasma cortisol levels before and 30 and 60 min later; the test can be performed at any time of the day. The most clearcut criterion for a normal response is a stimulated cortisol level >500 nmol/L (18 μg/dL), and the minimal stimulated normal increment of cortisol is >200 nmol/L (7 mg/dL) above baseline. However, ill patients with elevated basal cortisol levels may show no further increases following acute ACTH administration.

Tests of mineralocorticoid reserve and stimulation of the renin-angiotensin system Stimulation tests utilize protocols of programmed volume depletion, such as sodium restriction, diuretic administration, or upright posture. A simple potent test consists of severe sodium restriction and upright posture. After 3 to 5 days of a 10-mmol sodium intake, aldosterone secretion or excretion rates should increase two- to threefold over control. Supine morning plasma aldosterone levels usually increase three- to sixfold. In addition, plasma levels increase two- to fourfold in response to 2 to 3 h of upright posture.

Stimulation tests on normal dietary sodium intake may be carried out by the administration of a potent diuretic, such as 40 to 80 mg furosemide, followed by 2 to 3 h of upright posture. The normal response is a two- to fourfold rise in plasma aldosterone levels.

SUPPRESSION TESTS Suppression tests to document hypersecretion of adrenocortical hormones are based on the demonstration of a decrease in the target hormone following standardized suppression of its tropic hormone.

Tests of pituitary-adrenal suppressibility The ACTH release mechanism is sensitive to the circulating blood level of glucocorticoids. When such blood levels are increased in the normal individual, less ACTH is released from the anterior pituitary and less steroid is produced by the adrenal gland. The integrity of this feedback mechanism can be tested clinically by giving a potent glucocorticoid and judging suppression of ACTH secretion by analysis of urine steroid excretory values and/or plasma cortisol and ACTH levels. A potent glucocorticoid such as dexamethasone is utilized in order that the administered compound can be given in such small amounts that it does not contribute significantly to the steroids to be analyzed.

The best *screening* procedure is the overnight dexamethasone suppression test. This involves the measurement of plasma cortisol levels at 8 A.M. following the oral administration of 1 mg dexamethasone the previous midnight. The 8 A.M. value for plasma cortisol in normal subjects should be less than 140 nmol/L (5 μg/dL).

The definitive test of adrenal suppressibility is to administer 0.5 mg dexamethasone every 6 h for two successive days while collecting urine over a 24-h period for determination of creatinine, 17-hydroxysteroids, and/or free cortisol and/or measuring plasma cortisol levels. In a patient with a normal hypothalamic pituitary ACTH release mechanism, a fall in the urine 17-hydroxycorticosteroids to less than 8 μmol/d (3 mg/d) on the second day of dexamethasone administration, urinary free cortisol to less than 80 nmol/d (30 μg/d), or plasma cortisol to less than 140 nmol/L (5 μg/dL) is seen.

Normal responses to either of the suppression tests implies that the ACTH control of the adrenal glands is physiologically normal. However, an isolated abnormal result, particularly when the overnight suppression test is being used, does not in itself imply pituitary and/or adrenal disease.

Tests of mineralocorticoid suppressibility Mineralocorticoid suppression procedures have been devised using saline infusions, oral salt loading, or deoxycorticosterone administration for expansion of the extracellular fluid volume. With expansion of extracellular fluid volume, there is a decrease in renal renin release, a decrease in circulating plasma renin activity, and a decrease in aldosterone secretion and/or excretion. Various tests differ in the rate at which extracellular fluid volume is expanded. One convenient suppression test is the intravenous infusion of 500 mL normal saline solution per hour for 4 h, which normally suppresses plasma aldosterone levels to <220 pmol/L (<8 ng/dL) on a sodium-restricted diet or to 140 pmol/L (<5 ng/dL) on a normal sodium intake. This test should not be performed in potassium-depleted subjects.

TESTS OF PITUITARY-ADRENAL RESPONSIVENESS Stimuli such as insulin hypoglycemia, arginine vasopressin, and pyrogen, cause release of ACTH from the pituitary by an action on higher nerve centers, the hypothalamus, or the pituitary itself. By measuring plasma ACTH or plasma glucocorticoids the status of pituitary ACTH can be evaluated. Insulin-induced hypoglycemia is particularly useful, since the release of growth hormone and of ACTH is stimulated. In this test 0.05 to 0.1 unit of regular insulin per kilogram of body weight is administered intravenously as a bolus to reduce fasting glucose levels at least 50 percent below basal. The normal cortisol response is a rise to more than 500 nmol/L (18 μg/dL).

One of the best ways to test integrity of the pituitary-adrenal axis is the metyrapone test. Metyrapone is a drug that inhibits 11β-hydroxylase in the adrenal gland. As a result, the conversion of 11-deoxycortisol (compound S) to cortisol is interfered with, and increased amounts of 11-deoxycortisol accumulate while blood levels of cortisol decrease (Fig. 317-2). The hypothalamic-pituitary axis responds to the declining cortisol blood levels by releasing more ACTH. The metabolites of 11-deoxycortisol are excreted in increasing amounts in the urine, where they are measured as 17-hydroxycorticosteroids. Alternatively, changes in plasma 11-deoxycortisol levels can be measured. *Note that the adrenal glands must be capable of being stimulated by ACTH, since assessment of the response depends both on an intact hypothalamic-pituitary axis and on adrenal steroid production.*

While a number of modifications of the original metyrapone test have been described, we believe the best involves administering orally 750 mg of the drug every 4 h over a 24-h period and comparing the control and the post-metyrapone 17-hydroxysteroid excretion rates and/or plasma 11-deoxycortisol, cortisol, and ACTH levels. Normal individuals respond with at least a doubling of their basal 17-

hydroxysteroid excretion; 11-deoxycortisol levels in the blood should exceed 290 nmol/L (10 μg/dL) following metyrapone administration. The metyrapone test does not accurately reflect ACTH reserve if subjects are ingesting exogenous glucocorticoids or drugs that accelerate the metabolism of metyrapone (e.g., phenytoin).

A direct and selective test of the pituitary corticotrophs can be achieved with the investigational agent corticotropin-releasing hormone (CRH). The bolus injection of 1 μg per kilogram of body weight of ovine CRH stimulates ACTH and beta lipotropin secretion in normal human subjects within 60 to 180 min. However, the magnitude of the ACTH response is less than that produced by the insulin tolerance test, which implies that additional factors (such as vasopressin) augment stress-induced increases in ACTH secretion.

Although the rapid ACTH stimulation test reliably diagnoses primary adrenal insufficiency, normal cortisol responsiveness may be seen in a subset of patients with secondary adrenocortical insufficiency where there is a partial ACTH deficit and absence of adrenal atrophy. These patients have inadequate pituitary ACTH reserve and fail to increase ACTH secretion in response to stress such as surgery or hypoglycemia. Since a bolus of exogenous ACTH does not invariably exclude a diagnosis of secondary adrenocortical insufficiency, direct tests of pituitary ACTH reserve (metyrapone, insulin tolerance testing) should be used in the appropriate clinical setting. On the other hand, the rapid ACTH test can distinguish between primary and secondary adrenal insufficiency since aldosterone secretion is preserved in secondary adrenal failure by the renin-angiotensin system and potassium. Twenty-five units of cosyntropin is given intravenously or intramuscularly, and plasma cortisol and aldosterone levels are obtained before and 30 and 60 min later. Although the cortisol response is abnormal in both groups, patients with secondary insufficiency increase aldosterone levels above control by at least 140 pmol/L (5 ng/dL). No aldosterone response is seen in patients with primary adrenocortical insufficiency in whom the adrenal cortex is destroyed.

HYPERFUNCTION OF THE ADRENAL CORTEX

Distinct clinical syndromes are produced when excess adrenocortical hormones are secreted. Thus, excess production of cortisol is associated with Cushing's syndrome, excess production of aldosterone causes aldosteronism, and excess production of adrenal androgens causes adrenal virilism. These syndromes do not always occur in the "pure" form but may have overlapping features.

CUSHING'S SYNDROME Etiology Cushing described a syndrome characterized by truncal obesity, hypertension, fatigability and weakness, amenorrhea, hirsutism, purplish abdominal striae, edema, glucosuria, osteoporosis, and a basophilic tumor of the pituitary. As awareness of this syndrome increased, the diagnosis of Cushing's syndrome has been broadened into the classification shown in Table 317-3. Regardless of etiology, all cases of endogenous Cushing's syndrome are due to increased production of cortisol by the adrenal gland. Most are due to *bilateral adrenal hyperplasia*; the cause may be adrenocortical stimulation due to hypersecretion of pituitary ACTH or the production of ACTH by nonendocrine tumors. The incidence of pituitary-dependent adrenal hyperplasia in women is three times that in men, with the most frequent age of onset being the third or fourth decade. The cause of the hypersecretion of pituitary ACTH is still debated. Some speculate that the primary defect is the de novo development of a pituitary adenoma since in some reports tumors are found in over 90 percent of patients with pituitary-dependent adrenal hyperplasia. Alternatively, the defect may reside in the hypothalamus or in higher nerve centers, leading to release of CRH inappropriate to the level of circulating cortisol. The consequence would be that a higher level of cortisol is required to reduce ACTH secretion to normal. This primary defect would lead to hyperstimulation of the pituitary resulting in hyperplasia or tumor formation. As the pituitary tumor grows, it may become independent of the regulating influence of central nervous system factors and/or circulating cortisol levels. In surgical series most individuals with hypersecretion of pituitary ACTH have a microadenoma (<10 mm) (50 percent are 5 mm or less in diameter), but a macroadenoma (>10 mm) of the pituitary or diffuse hyperplasia of the corticotropic cells (hypothalamic-pituitary dysfunction) may also be found. The common finding of a microadenoma in pituitary-dependent adrenal hyperplasia does not rule out dysregulation of hypothalamic CRH as the defect in Cushing's disease. Long-term follow-up to determine the rate of recurrence following successful surgical resection is necessary to answer this issue. Traditionally, only an individual who has an ACTH-producing pituitary tumor has been defined as having *Cushing's disease*. However, in many centers, anyone who has hypersecretion of pituitary ACTH regardless of whether a tumor is identified by radiographic procedures is classified as having Cushing's disease. In this chapter we will use the traditional definition, although these definitions may become less distinct as small tumors are more easily diagnosed by high resolution scanning.

Nonendocrine tumors may secrete polypeptides that are biologically, chemically, and immunologically indistinguishable from either ACTH or CRH and that cause bilateral adrenal hyperplasia (see also Chap. 309). The ectopic production of CRH results in clinical, biochemical, and radiologic features indistinguishable from those caused by hypersecretion of pituitary ACTH. Often, but not invariably, the typical signs and symptoms of Cushing's syndrome are absent with ectopic ACTH production, and hypokalemic alkalosis and glucose intolerance are the prominent manifestations. The majority of these cases are associated with the primitive small-cell (oat cell) type of bronchogenic carcinoma or with tumors of the thymus, pancreas, or ovary, medullary carcinoma of the thyroid, or bronchial adenomas. The onset of Cushing's syndrome may be sudden, particularly in patients with oat cell carcinoma of the lung, and this feature accounts in part for the failure of these patients to exhibit the classic physical findings. On the other hand, patients with carcinoid tumors or pheochromocytomas have longer clinical courses and usually exhibit the typical cushingoid features. The secretion of ACTH by nonendocrine tumors is also accompanied by the accumulation of ACTH fragments in plasma and by elevated plasma levels of ACTH precursor molecules. Since such tumors may produce large amounts of ACTH, baseline steroid values are usually markedly elevated, and increased skin pigmentation is usually present. Indeed, hyperpigmentation in patients with Cushing's syndrome almost always points to an extraadrenal tumor, either in an extracranial location or within the cranium.

Approximately 20 to 25 percent of patients with Cushing's syndrome have primary overproduction of cortisol and other adrenal steroids due to an adrenal neoplasm. These tumors are usually unilateral, and about half are malignant. Occasionally, patients have biochemical features both of hypersecretion of pituitary ACTH and of an adrenal adenoma. These individuals usually have micro- or macro-nodularity of both adrenal glands resulting in *nodular hyperplasia*. In some this may be a familial autoimmune disorder often

TABLE 317-3 Causes of Cushing's syndrome

I Adrenal hyperplasia
- *A* Secondary to pituitary ACTH overproduction
  - *1* Pituitary-hypothalamic dysfunction
  - *2* Pituitary ACTH-producing micro- or macroadenomas
- *B* Secondary to ACTH or CRH-producing nonendocrine tumors (bronchogenic carcinoma, carcinoid of the thymus, pancreatic carcinoma, bronchial adenoma)

II Adrenal nodular hyperplasia

III Adrenal neoplasia
- *A* Adenoma
- *B* Carcinoma

IV Exogenous, iatrogenic causes
- *A* Prolonged use of glucocorticoids
- *B* Prolonged use of ACTH

seen in children and young adults (so-called pigmented multinodular cortical dysplasia).

The most common cause of Cushing's syndrome is *iatrogenic* administration of steroids for other reasons. While the clinical features bear some resemblance to those of individuals with an adrenal adenoma, these patients are usually readily distinguishable on the basis of history and initial laboratory studies.

Clinical signs, symptoms, and laboratory findings Many of the signs and symptoms of Cushing's syndrome logically follow from the known action of glucocorticoids (Table 317-4). As a result of mobilization of peripheral supportive tissue, muscle weakness and fatigability, osteoporosis, cutaneous striae, and easy bruisability result. The latter two signs are secondary to weakening and rupture of collagen fibers in the dermis. The osteoporosis may be so severe that collapse of vertebral bodies and pathologic fractures of other bones occur. Increased hepatic gluconeogenesis and insulin resistance can cause impaired glucose tolerance. Overt diabetes occurs in less than 20 percent of patients, probably in individuals with a familial predisposition to this disorder. Hypercortisolism promotes the deposition of adipose tissue in characteristic sites, notably in the upper part of the face, the typical "moon" facies; in the interscapular area, the "buffalo" hump; and in the mesenteric bed, where it produces the classic "truncal" obesity (Fig. 317-6). Rarely, there may be episternal fatty tumors and mediastinal widening secondary to fat accumulation. The reason for this peculiar distribution of adipose tissue is not known. The face appears plethoric, even in the absence of any increase in red blood cell concentration. Hypertension is common, and frequently there are profound emotional changes, ranging from irritability or emotional lability to severe depression, confusion, or even frank psychosis. In women, increased adrenal androgen secretion can cause acne, hirsutism, and oligomenorrhea or amenorrhea. The most common signs and symptoms in patients with hypercortisolism, i.e., obesity, hypertension, osteoporosis, and diabetes, are nonspecific and therefore less helpful in diagnosing this condition. On the other hand, easy bruising, typical striae, myopathy, and androgen effects (although less frequent) are, if present, more suggestive of Cushing's syndrome.

Except in iatrogenic Cushing's syndrome, plasma and urine cortisol and urinary 17-hydroxycorticosteroid levels are variably elevated. Occasionally, hypokalemia, hypochloremia, and metabolic alkalosis are present, particularly in individuals who have ectopic production of ACTH.

Diagnosis The diagnosis of Cushing's syndrome depends on the demonstration of increased cortisol production and the failure to suppress endogenous cortisol secretion normally when dexamethasone is administered. Once the diagnosis is established, further testing is designed to determine the etiology of the hypercortisolism (see Fig. 317-7 and Table 317-5).

For initial screening, the overnight dexamethasone suppression test is recommended (see above). In difficult cases (e.g., in obesity) measurement of a 24-h free cortisol excretion rate can also be used as a screening test. A level greater than 275 nmol/d (100 μg/d) is suggestive of Cushing's syndrome. The definitive diagnosis is then established by failure to suppress urinary cortisol to less than 80 nmol/d (30 μg/d), plasma cortisol to less than 140 nmol/L (5μg/dL), or 17-hydroxysteroid excretion to less than 8 μmol/d (3 mg/d) after a standard low-dose dexamethasone suppression test (0.5 mg every

TABLE 317-4 Incidence of signs and symptoms in Cushing's syndrome, percent

Typical habitus	97	Amenorrhea	77
Increased body weight	94	Cutaneous striae	67
Fatigability and weakness	87	Personality changes	66
		Ecchymoses	65
Hypertension (>150/90)	82	Edema	62
		Polyuria, polydipsia	23
Hirsutism	80	Hypertrophy of clitoris	19

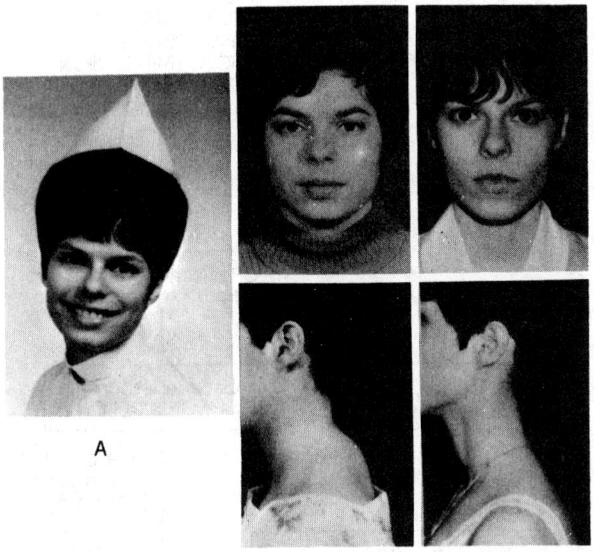

A B C

FIGURE 317-6 A 20-year-old woman with Cushing's syndrome due to a right adrenal cortical adenoma. *A*. Two years prior to surgery, age 18. *B*. One month prior to surgery, age 20. *C*. One year after surgery, age 21.

6 h for 48 h). Owing to diurnal variability, plasma cortisol and, to a certain extent, ACTH determinations are not meaningful when performed in isolation, but demonstration that the normal fall in P.M. levels of plasma corticoid does not occur may be useful.

Determining the etiology of Cushing's syndrome is complicated by the lack of specificity of all tests available and the spontaneous, sometimes clinical, changes in hormonal secretion, often dramatic, that may occur in the tumors producing this syndrome (periodic hormonogenesis). No test has a specificity greater than 95 percent, and it may be necessary to use a combination of tests to arrive at the correct diagnosis. A particularly useful first step is to determine the response of cortisol output to high-dose dexamethasone administration (2 mg every 6 h for 2 days). In most series, more than half of the patients so tested have a suppression of urine cortisol and/or 17-hydroxysteroid levels to less than 50 percent of basal values. These individuals usually have either an ACTH-secreting pituitary microadenoma or hypothalamic-pituitary dysfunction. Occasionally, in individuals with bilateral nodular hyperplasia and/or ectopic CRH production steroid output is also suppressed. Failure to suppress cortisol production after low- and high-dose dexamethasone administration (see Table 317-5) is usual in patients with adrenal hyperplasia secondary to an ACTH-secreting pituitary macroadenoma or ACTH-producing tumors of nonendocrine origin, and in adrenal neoplasms.

Theoretically, plasma ACTH levels should be useful in distinguishing the various causes of Cushing's syndrome, particularly in separating the ACTH-dependent from the ACTH-independent etiologies of the syndrome. In general, this is true for the ACTH-independent etiologies of the syndrome since most adrenal tumors have low or undetectable ACTH levels. Furthermore, ACTH-secreting pituitary macroadenomas and ACTH-producing nonendocrine tumors usually have elevated ACTH levels. In the ectopic ACTH syndrome, ACTH levels may be elevated above 110 pmol/L (500 pg/mL), with the majority above 40 pmol/L (200 pg/mL). In Cushing's syndrome, as the result of a microadenoma or pituitary hypothalamic dysfunction, ACTH levels range from 10 to 30 pmol/L (50 to 150 pg/mL) [normal $<$18 pmol/L ($<$80 pg/mL)], with half of values within the normal range. However, at least two problems hinder the utilization of ACTH levels in the differential diagnosis of Cushing's syndrome. First, reliable ACTH assays are still not widely available, and second, ACTH levels may be similar in individuals with hypothalamic-pituitary dysfunction, pituitary microadenomas, ectopic CRH pro-

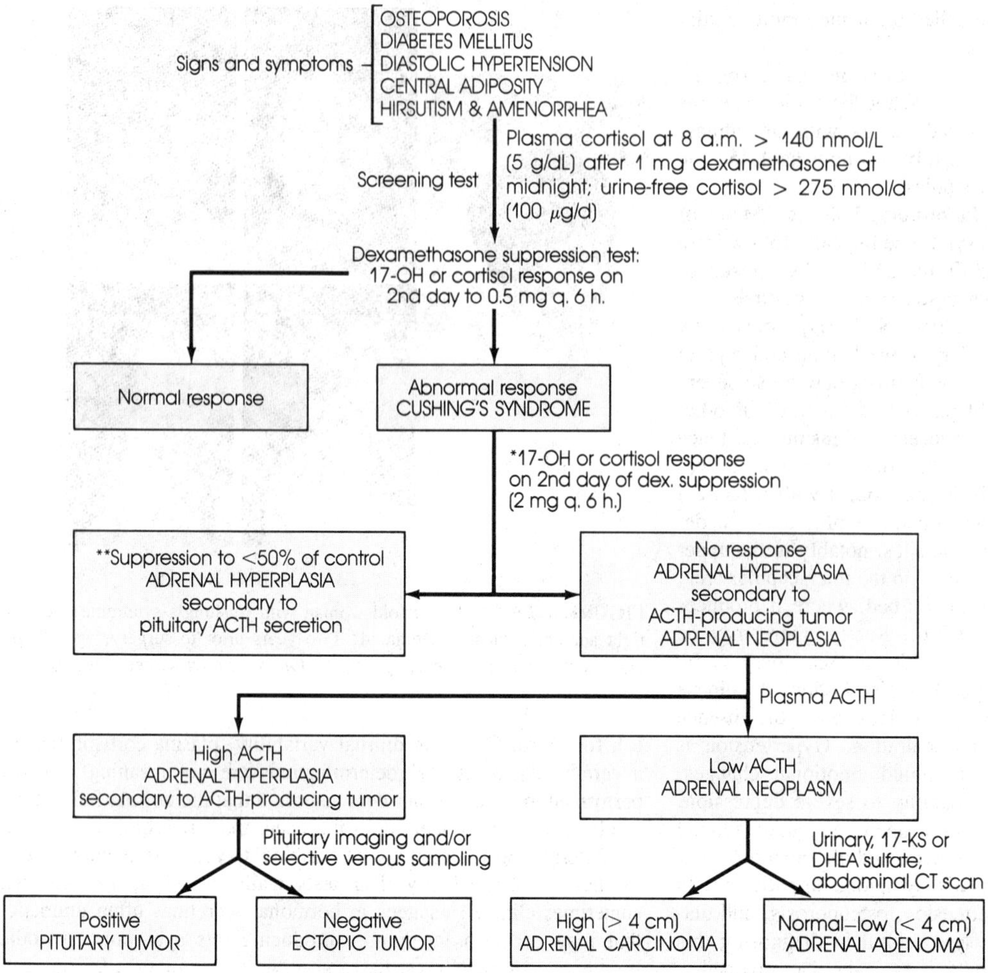

FIGURE 317-7 Diagnostic flowchart for evaluating patients suspected of having Cushing's syndrome.

*The 17-hydroxycorticosteroid response to metyrapone (750 mg given orally every 4 h for six doses) may be used as an alternative test to the high-dose dexamethasone test (2 mg given orally every 6 h). Increased urinary 17-hydroxycorticosteroid excretion following metyrapone occurs in the majority of patients with adrenal hyperplasia secondary to pituitary ACTH secretion; no response suggests an adrenal neoplasm or adrenal hyperplasia secondary to a nonendocrine ACTH-producing tumor.

**This group of patients probably contains subjects with both pituitary-hypothalamic dysfunction and pituitary microadenomas. In some instances, a pituitary microadenoma may be visualized by CT scanning of the sella turcica.

duction, and ACTH production from some nonendocrine tumors (especially carcinoid tumors) (Table 317-5).

Because of these difficulties, several additional tests have been advocated, e.g., the metyrapone and the CRH infusion tests. The rationales underlying these tests are similar: Steroid hypersecretion secondary to an adrenal tumor or the ectopic production of ACTH will suppress the hypothalamic-pituitary axis so that inhibition of pituitary ACTH release can be demonstrated by either test. Thus, most patients with pituitary-hypothalamic dysfunction and/or a microadenoma have an increase in steroid or ACTH secretion in response to metyrapone and CRH administration while most ectopic ACTH-producing tumors and adrenal tumors will not. Most pituitary macroadenomas also respond to CRH, while their response to metyrapone is variable. The utility of the CRH infusion test, however, is uncertain since only a limited number of studies have been performed and since CRH is not commonly available for testing. In addition, false-positive and -negative CRH tests in patients with nonendocrine and pituitary tumors have been reported.

TABLE 317-5 Diagnostic tests to determine the type of Cushing's syndrome

Test	Pituitary macroadenoma	Pituitary-hypothalamic dysfunction or microadenoma	Ectopic ACTH or CRH production	Adrenal tumor
Measurement of plasma ACTH	↑ to ↑↑	N to ↑	↑ to ↑↑↑	↓
Response to high-dose dexamethasone, %	<10	>80	<10	<10
Response to metyrapone, %	>80	>90	<10	<10
Response to CRH, %	>90	>90	<10	<10

NOTE: N, normal; ↑, elevated; ↓, decreased.

The major diagnostic dilemma in Cushing's syndrome is to distinguish between those individuals with microadenoma of the pituitary and/or pituitary hypothalamic dysfunction from some paraendocrine tumors (e.g., carcinoids or pheochromocytoma) that ectopically produced CRH and/or ACTH. Clinical manifestations are similar unless the ectopic tumor produces other symptoms, such as diarrhea and flushing from a carcinoid tumor or episodic hypertension from a pheochromocytoma. Sometimes one can distinguish between ectopic and pituitary ACTH production by using metyrapone or CRH tests as noted above. In these situations computed tomography (CT) scan of the pituitary gland is usually within normal limits. Magnetic resonance imaging (MRI) with the enhancing agent gadolinium may be superior to CT scanning in demonstrating a pituitary microadenoma in some patients with Cushing's disease. However, finding a structural feature consistent with an adenoma does not prove that the lesion is secreting ACTH. In fact, as the resolution of scanners becomes greater more variations of the normal pituitary anatomy will be imaged. For this reason selective venous sampling for ACTH is employed in some centers. Demonstration of a gradient between ACTH level in the petrosal sinus and in peripheral blood localizes the source of ACTH overproduction to the pituitary gland but does not distinguish pituitary dependent adrenal hyperplasia from pituitary hyperplasia secondary to a tumor producing CRH. No reliable test is available to make this distinction if the ectopic tumor is not seen or if it produces no other hormones.

The diagnosis of *cortisol-producing adrenal adenoma* is suggested by disproprtionate elevations in baseline urine 17-hydroxycorticosteroid or free-cortisol levels with only modest rises or suppression of urinary 17-ketosteroids or plasma DHEA sulfate. Adrenal androgen secretion is usually reduced in these patients owing to the cortisol-induced suppression of ACTH and subsequent involution of the androgen-producing zona reticularis.

The diagnosis of *adrenal carcinoma* is suggested by a palpable abdominal mass and by *markedly* elevated baseline values *both* of urine 17-hydroxysteroids and of plasma DHEA sulfate. Plasma and urine cortisol levels are variably elevated. Adrenal carcinoma is usually resistant to both ACTH stimulation and dexamethasone suppression. Markedly elevated adrenal androgen secretion often leads to virilization in the female. Feminizing estrogen-producing adrenocortical carcinoma in the male usually presents with gynecomastia. These adrenal tumors secrete increased amounts of androstenedione which is peripherally converted to the estrogens, estrone and estradiol (see Chap. 323). Functioning adrenal carcinomas that produce Cushing's syndrome are most often associated with elevated values for the intermediates of steroid biosynthesis (especially 11-deoxycortisol), suggesting inefficient conversion of the intermediates to the final product. Approximately 20 percent of adrenal carcinomas are not associated with endocrine syndromes and are presumed to be nonfunctioning or to produce biologically inactive steroid precursors. In addition, the excessive production of gonadal steroids is not detectable in certain situations (e.g., androgens in adult men).

Differential diagnosis PSEUDOCUSHING'S SYNDROME A variety of groups may present problems in diagnosis; these are patients with obesity, chronic alcoholism, depression, and acute illness of any type. Extreme *obesity* is uncommon in Cushing's syndrome; furthermore, with exogenous obesity, the adiposity is generalized, not truncal. On adrenocortical testing, abnormalities in patients with exogenous obesity are usually modest. Basal urine steroid excretion levels in obese patients are either normal or slightly elevated, a finding similar to their cortisol secretory values. Some patients have elevated conversion of secreted cortisol into excreted metabolites. *Urinary* and *blood cortisol* levels are normal, and the diurnal pattern in blood and urine levels is normal. Patients with *chronic alcoholism* and *depression* share similar abnormalities in steroid output: elevated urinary 17-hydroxysteroids, absent diurnal rhythm of cortisol levels, and resistance to suppression with dexamethasone (particularly overnight and low dose). In contrast to alcoholic subjects, depressed patients do not have clinical signs and symptoms of Cushing's syndrome. Following discontinuation of alcohol and/or improvement of the emotional status, steroid testing usually returns to normal. A normal cortisol response to insulin-induced hypoglycemia may distinguish these patients from subjects with Cushing's syndrome. *Acutely ill* subjects often have abnormal laboratory tests and fail to suppress with dexamethasone since major stress (such as pain or fever) interrupts the normal regulation of ACTH secretion. *Iatrogenic Cushing's syndrome,* induced by the administration of potent synthetic glucocorticoids, is indistinguishable by physical findings from endogenous adrenocortical hyperfunction. This situation can be distinguished by measuring blood or urine cortisol levels or urinary 17-hydroxysteroid excretion in a basal state where the levels are low secondary to suppression of the pituitary-adrenal axis. The severity of iatrogenic Cushing's syndrome is related to the total steroid dose, to the biologic half-life of the steroid preparation, and to the duration of therapy. Also, individuals on afternoon and evening doses of steroid develop Cushing's syndrome more readily and on smaller total daily steroid doses than do patients on a steroid program limited to morning doses only. The enzymatic disposition and binding of administered steroids also differ among patients.

Radiologic evaluation for Cushing's syndrome The preferred radiologic study to visualize the adrenals is CT scan of the abdomen (Fig. 317-8). This procedure has largely replaced previous invasive procedures (such as selective adrenal arteriography and venography) and 19-[^{131}I]iodocholesterol scanning; the CT scan is of value both in localizing adrenal tumors and in differentiating them from bilateral hyperplasia. All patients believed to have hypersecretion of pituitary ACTH should have a pituitary MRI scan with the contrast agent gadolinium (if available) to establish whether a pituitary tumor is present. Even with this technique small microadenomas may be undetectable; alternatively, false-positive masses due to nonsecretory, variations of the normal pituitary anatomy may be imaged.

Evaluation of asymptomatic adrenal masses With abdominal CT scanning, many incidental adrenal masses are discovered. This is not surprising, since 10 to 20 percent of subjects at autopsy have adrenal cortical adenomas. The first step in evaluating such patients is to determine if the tumor is functioning by appropriate screening tests. However, in 90 percent of the cases tumors detected incidentally at the time of abdominal CT scanning are nonfunctioning. Fortunately, they also are seldom malignant. Yet, nonfunctioning tumors raise difficult therapeutic questions. Since 20 percent of adrenal carcinomas are nonfunctioning, one could argue that all such lesions should be removed. However, the frequency of adrenal carcinomas is low compared with the frequency of benign cortical adenomas (less than 1 percent), and surgery is not indicated in most cases. The size of the tumor sometimes is of value: Adrenal carcinomas are rarely smaller than 3 cm in diameter, and adrenal adenomas are usually smaller than 6 cm (Fig. 317-8). If surgery is not performed, a repeat CT scan in 3 to 6 months is usually required for followup.

Therapy ADRENAL NEOPLASMS When an adenoma or carcinoma is diagnosed, adrenal exploration is performed with excision of the tumor. Because of the possible atrophy of the contralateral adrenal, the patient is treated pre- and postoperatively as if for total adrenalectomy even when a unilateral lesion is suspected, the routine being similar to that for an Addisonian patient undergoing elective surgery (Table 317-11).

Despite operative intervention, most patients with adrenal carcinoma die within 3 years of diagnosis. Metastases occur most often to liver and lung. The principal antitumor drug used to treat metastatic adrenocortical carcinoma is mitotane (*o,p'*-DDD), an isomer of the insecticide DDT. This drug suppresses cortisol production and decreases plasma and urine steroid levels. Although its cytotoxic action is relatively selective for the glucocorticoid-secreting zone of the adrenal cortex, the zona glomerulosa may also be inhibited. Because mitotane also alters the extraadrenal metabolism of cortisol, plasma and urinary cortisol levels must be assessed to titrate the effect. The drug is usually given in divided doses three to four times a day, with the dose increased gradually to 8 to 10 g daily. Almost all patients experience gastrointestinal side effects (anorexia, diarrhea, or vomiting) or neuromuscular side effects (lethargy, somnolence, or dizziness). All patients treated with mitotane should be placed on long-term maintenance glucocorticoid therapy, and in some mineralocorticoid replacement is appropriate. In approximately one-third of patients regression of both tumor and metastases occurs, but long-term survival is limited. In many patients, mitotane only inhibits steroidogenesis and does not cause regression of tumor metastases. Osseous metastases are usually refractory to the drug and should be treated with radiation therapy. Mitotane can also be given as adjunctive therapy after surgical resection of an adrenal carcinoma.

BILATERAL HYPERPLASIA Patients with hyperplasia have a relative or absolute increase in ACTH levels. Since therapy would logically be directed at reducing ACTH levels, the ideal primary treatment for ACTH- or CRH-producing tumors, whether in the pituitary or ectopic, is surgical removal. Occasionally, this is not possible because the disease, particularly with ectopic ACTH production, is often far advanced. In this situation "medical" or surgical adrenalectomy may be indicated to correct the hypercortisolism.

Controversy exists as to the proper treatment for bilateral adrenal hyperplasia when the source of the ACTH overproduction is not apparent. In some centers, these patients (especially patients with a positive high-dose dexamethasone suppression test) have surgical exploration of the pituitary via a transsphenoidal approach in anticipation of a microadenoma being found. These explorations prove fruitful in between 20 and 70 percent of the cases, depending on the skill of the surgeon and the ability of the radiologist to localize the

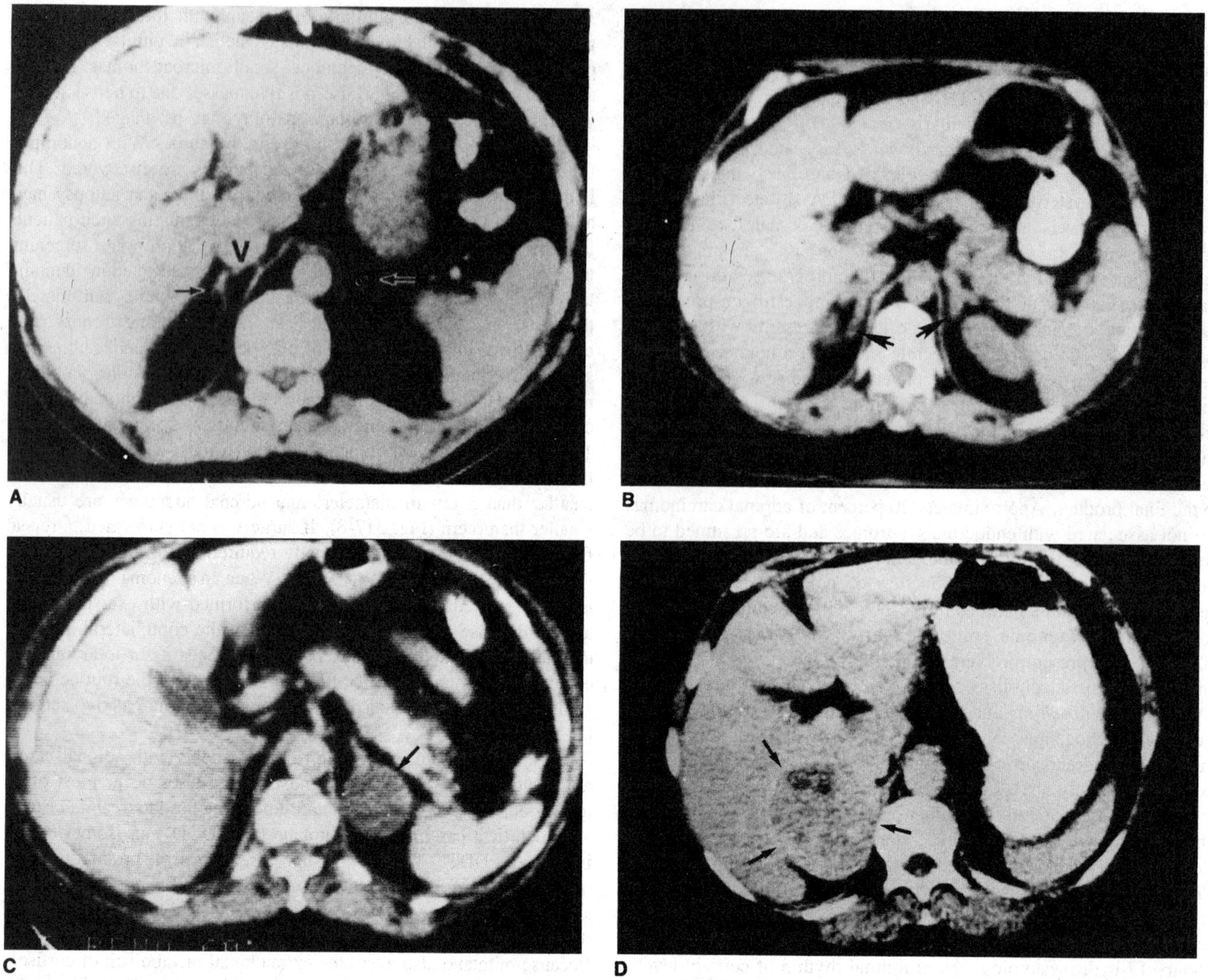

FIGURE 317-8 Computed tomography is the preferred method for visualizing the adrenal glands. The adrenal glands are indicated by arrows. *A*. The normal right adrenal gland is adjacent to the inferior vena cava (V) as it emerges from the liver. Approximately 90 percent of the right adrenal glands appear as linear structures extending posteriorly from the inferior vena cava into the space between the right lobe of the liver and the crus of the diaphragm. The normal left adrenal gland is lateral to the left crus of the diaphragm and below the stomach. The majority of left adrenal glands are shaped like an inverted "V" or "Y." *B*. Adrenal CT scan of a patient with ectopic ACTH production. Both adrenal glands (arrows) are enlarged (compare with A). In contrast, only 50 percent of patients with bilateral adrenal hyperplasia secondary to pituitary ACTH hypersecretion show enlargement of the adrenals when imaged by CT scan. *C*. CT scan of a patient with Cushing's syndrome with biochemical evidence only of cortisol overproduction. The left adrenal has been replaced by a racquet-shaped 2-cm tumor (arrow). Attenuation of the tumor is low because of its high lipid content. *D*. CT scan in a patient with Cushing's syndrome and biochemical evidence of an adrenal carcinoma. In contrast to *C*, the right-sided mass has a heterogeneous appearance and is larger in size—usual characteristics of an adrenal carcinoma.

microadenoma preoperatively. In equivocal circumstances selective venous sampling may be performed, or the patient may be referred to an appropriate center if the procedure is not locally available. In the event that a microadenoma is not found at the time of exploration, total hypophysectomy may be needed. Complications of transsphenoidal surgery include cerebrospinal fluid rhinorrhea, diabetes insipidus, panhypopituitarism, and optic or cranial nerve injuries. Furthermore, these pituitary neoplasms may recur if the primary abnormality actually resides in the hypothalamus.

In other centers, total adrenalectomy is the treatment of choice. Cure with this procedure is close to 100 percent. The adverse effects include the certain need for lifelong mineralocorticoid and glucocorticoid replacement therapy and a 10 to 20 percent probability of a pituitary tumor developing over the next 10 years, many requiring surgical therapy (Nelson's syndrome). It is uncertain whether in these individuals (see Chap. 313) the tumor develops de novo or is present prior to bilateral adrenalectomy but is so small that it is not detected by radiologic procedures. Periodic radiologic evaluation of the pituitary gland by CT scanning and serial ACTH levels should be obtained in any individual who has undergone bilateral adrenalectomy for Cushing's syndrome. Often, such pituitary tumors become locally invasive and impinge on the optic chiasm or extend into the cavernous or sphenoid sinuses. Thus, an aggressive surgical approach is often followed by postoperative irradiation.

In a few centers, pituitary irradiation is the primary treatment for pituitary ACTH overproduction, with the use of either conventional external or alpha (proton beam) radiation. The latter, while more effective, has a greater incidence of ocular motor palsy and hypopituitarism than does conventional radiation therapy. The long lag time between treatment and remission and the fact that the remission rate is less than 50 percent often contraindicate the use of external pituitary radiation in the presence of rapidly progressive or severe Cushing's syndrome.

Finally, in occasional patients in whom a surgical approach is not feasible, medical therapy directed at reducing hypothalamic CRH release either by administering the serotonin antagonist cyproheptadine or by administering an inhibitor of GABA transaminase, sodium valproate, has been successful in reducing cortisol secretion. Bromocriptine, a dopaminergic agonist, also suppresses ACTH output in occasional patients.

If ACTH levels cannot be successfully lowered by any of the above treatment modalities, then medical or surgical adrenalectomy may be indicated (Table 317-6). Inhibition of steroidogenesis may also be indicated in severely cushingoid subjects prior to surgical intervention. Chemical adrenalectomy may be accomplished by the administration of the inhibitor of steroidogenesis, ketoconazole (600 to 1200 mg/d). In addition, mitotane (2 or 3 g/d) and/or the blockers of steroid synthesis aminoglutethimide (1 g/d) and metyrapone (2 or 3 g/d) have been effective either singularly or in combination. Mitotane is slow in onset of action (over weeks). Hypoadrenalism is a risk with all these agents, and replacement steroids may be required.

ALDOSTERONISM Aldosteronism is a syndrome associated with hypersecretion of the major adrenal mineralocorticoid, aldosterone. *Primary* aldosteronism signifies that the stimulus for the excessive aldosterone production resides within the adrenal gland; in *secondary* aldosteronism the stimulus is extraadrenal.

Primary aldosteronism In the original case of excessive and inappropriate aldosterone production, the disease was the result of an *aldosterone-producing adrenal adenoma* (Conn's syndrome). The majority of cases involved a unilateral adenoma, usually small and occurring with equal frequency on either side. Rarely, primary aldosteronism occurs in association with adrenal carcinoma. It is twice as common in women as in men, occurs between the ages of 30 and 50, and is present in approximately 1 percent of unselected hypertensive patients. Many cases have clinical and biochemical features characteristic of primary aldosteronism, but a solitary adenoma is not found at surgery. Instead, these patients have *bilateral cortical nodular hyperplasia.* In the literature this disease has been alternatively termed "pseudo" primary aldosteronism, idiopathic hyperaldosteronism, or nodular hyperplasia. The cause is unknown.

SIGNS AND SYMPTOMS The continual hypersecretion of aldosterone increases the renal distal tubular exchange of intratubular sodium for secreted potassium and hydrogen ions, with progressive depletion of body potassium and development of hypokalemia. Most patients have diastolic hypertension, usually not of marked severity, and complain of headaches. The hypertension is probably due to the increased sodium reabsorption and extracellular volume expansion. Potassium depletion is responsible for the muscle weakness and fatigue and is related to the effect of potassium depletion on muscle membrane. The polyuria results from impairment of concentrating ability and is often associated with polydipsia. Electrocardiographic and roentgenographic signs of left ventricular enlargement are secondary to the hypertension. Electrocardiographic signs of potassium depletion, such as prominent U waves, cardiac arrhythmias, and premature contractions, are common. In the absence of associated congestive heart failure, renal disease, or preexisting abnormalities (such as thrombophlebitis), edema is characteristically absent. In cases of long duration, nephropathy with azotemia may be associated with congestive heart failure and edema.

LABORATORY FINDINGS Laboratory findings are dependent on both the duration and the severity of the potassium depletion. An overnight concentration test often reveals impaired ability to concentrate the urine, probably secondary to the hypokalemia. Urine pH is neutral to alkaline, because of excessive secretion of ammonium and bicarbonate ions to compensate for a metabolic alkalosis. Tests of glucocorticoid and androgen secretion are within the normal range.

Hypokalemia may be severe (less than 3 mmol/L) and reflects significant body potassium depletion, usually in excess of 300 mmol. *Hypernatremia* is due to both sodium retention and a concomitant water loss from polyuria. Metabolic alkalosis and elevation of serum bicarbonate are a result of hydrogen ion loss into the urine and migration into potassium-depleted cells. The alkalosis is perpetuated by potassium deficiency, which increases the capacity of the proximal convoluted tubule to reabsorb filtered bicarbonate. If hypokalemia is severe, serum magnesium levels are also reduced. In the absence of azotemia, serum uric acid is normal.

Total body sodium content and total exchangeable sodium are increased, while total exchangeable body potassium is usually reduced. The expanded extracellular fluid volume may be responsible for the reversed diurnal excretory pattern for salt and water, with predominant salt and water excretion occurring during the night.

DIAGNOSIS The diagnosis is suggested by persistent hypokalemia in a nonedematous patient on a normal sodium intake who is not receiving potassium-wasting diuretics (furosemide, ethacrynic acid, thiazides). If hypokalemia occurs in a hypertensive patient on a potassium-wasting diuretic, the diuretic should be discontinued and the patient should be given potassium supplements. After 1 to 2 weeks the potassium level should be remeasured, and if hypokalemia persists, the patient should be evaluated for a mineralocorticoid excess syndrome (Fig. 317-9).

The criteria for the diagnosis of primary aldosteronism are (1) diastolic hypertension without edema, (2) hyposecretion of renin (as judged by low plasma renin activity levels) that fails to increase appropriately during volume depletion (upright posture, sodium depletion), and (3) hypersecretion of aldosterone that fails to suppress appropriately during volume expansion (salt loading).

Patients with primary aldosteronism characteristically *do not have edema,* since they exhibit an "escape" phenomenon from the sodium-retaining aspects of mineralocorticoids. Rarely, pretibial edema may be present in patients with associated nephropathy and azotemia.

The estimation of plasma renin activity is of limited value in separating patients with primary aldosteronism from those with other causes of hypertension. While the failure of plasma renin activity to rise normally during volume-depletion maneuvers is a criterion for primary aldosteronism, suppressed renin activity also occurs in about 25 percent of patients with essential hypertension.

Since the determination of plasma renin responsiveness is not sufficient, the demonstration of lack of suppression of aldosterone secretion is necessary to diagnose primary aldosteronism (Fig. 317-9). The autonomy exhibited by aldosterone tumors in these patients refers only to the resistance to suppression of secretion during volume expansion; such tumors can and do respond in normal or above normal fashion to the stimuli of potassium loading or ACTH infusion.

Once hyposecretion of renin and failure to suppress aldosterone secretion are demonstrated, localization of aldosterone-producing adenomas should be determined preoperatively by abdominal CT scan or by percutaneous transfemoral bilateral adrenal vein catheterization with simultaneous adrenal venography. The latter technique permits radiologic localization, and, in addition, the adrenal vein sampling may demonstrate a two- to threefold increase in plasma aldosterone concentration on the involved side compared with the uninvolved side. In cases of hyperaldosteronism secondary to cortical nodular hyperplasia, no localization is found. It is important for samples to be obtained simultaneously if possible and for cortisol levels to be measured to ensure that false localization does not reflect an ACTH- or stress-induced rise in aldosterone levels.

DIFFERENTIAL DIAGNOSIS Patients with hypertension and hypokalemia may have primary or secondary hyperaldosteronism (see Fig. 317-10). A useful maneuver to distinguish between them is the

TABLE 317-6 Treatment modalities for patients with adrenal hyperplasia secondary to pituitary ACTH hypersecretion

I Reduce pituitary ACTH production
- *A* Transsphenoidal resection of microadenoma
- *B* Radiation
- *C* Treatment with hypothalamic serotonin antagonist (cyproheptadine) or GABA-transaminase inhibitor (sodium valproate)*

II Reduce or eliminate adrenocortical cortisol secretion
- *A* Bilateral adrenalectomy
- *B* Medical adrenalectomy (metyrapone, mitotane, aminoglutethimide, ketoconazole)*

* Not curative but effective as long as chronically administered in selected patients.

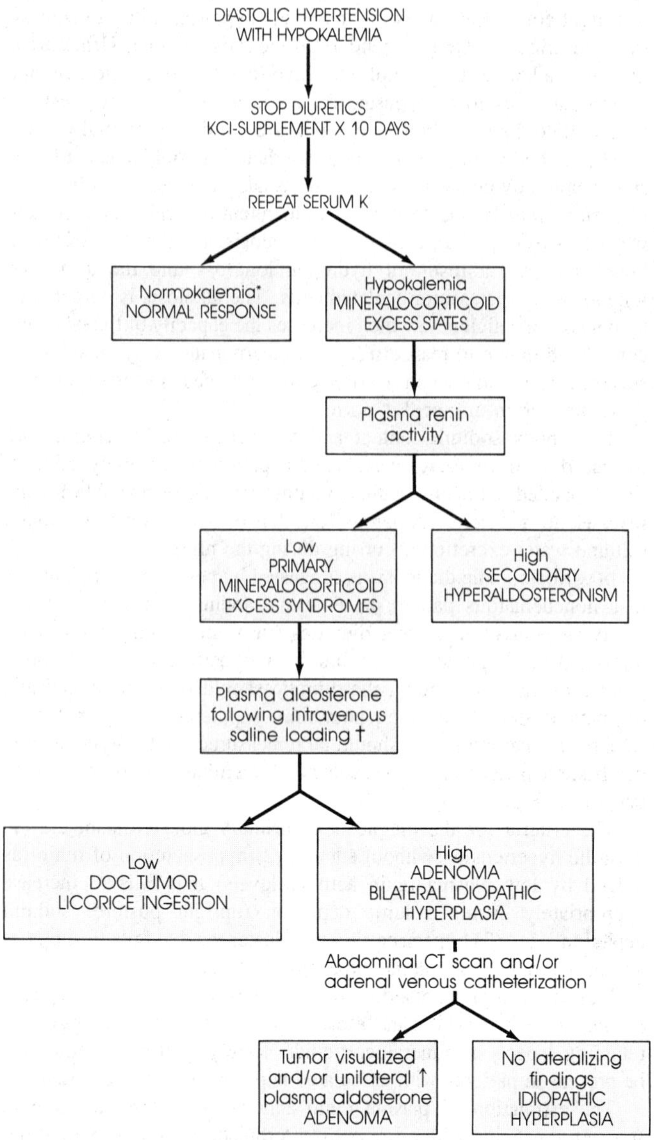

FIGURE 317-9 Diagnostic flowchart for evaluating patients with suspected primary aldosteronism.

*Serum K^+ may be normal in some patients with hyperaldosteronism who are taking potassium-sparing diuretics (spironolactone, triamterene) or ingesting low sodium–high potassium intakes.

†This step should not be taken if hypertension is severe (diastolic pressure >115 mmHg) or if cardiac failure is present. Also, serum potassium levels should be corrected before the infusion of saline solution. Alternative methods producing comparable suppression of aldosterone secretion include oral sodium loading (200 mmol/d for 3 days) or 10 mg deoxycorticosterone acetate (DOCA) intramuscularly every 12 h for 3 days.

measurement of plasma renin activity. Secondary hyperaldosteronism in patients with accelerated hypertension is due to elevated plasma renin levels; in contrast, patients with primary aldosteronism have suppressed plasma renin levels.

Primary aldosteronism must also be distinguished from other *hypermineralocorticoid states*. The common problem is to distinguish between hyperaldosteronism due to an adenoma and that due to idiopathic bilateral nodular hyperplasia. This is of importance, since hypertension associated with idiopathic hyperplasia is usually not benefited by bilateral adrenalectomy, whereas hypertension associated with aldosterone-producing tumors is usually improved or cured following removal of the adenoma. Although patients with idiopathic bilateral nodular hyperplasia tend to have less severe hypokalemia, lower aldosterone secretion, and higher plasma renin activity than do

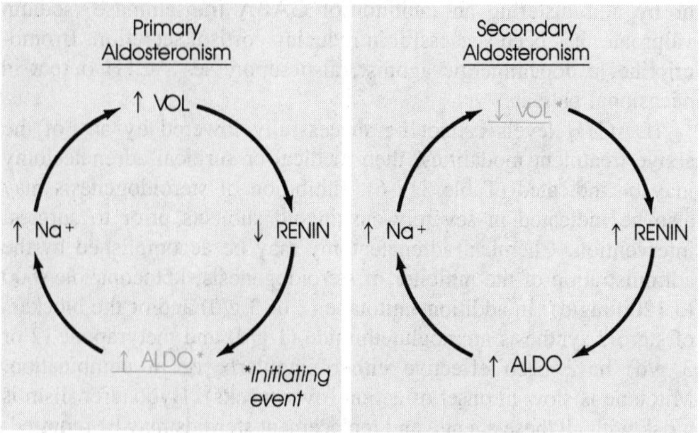

FIGURE 317-10 Responses of the renin-aldosterone volume control loop in primary versus secondary aldosteronism.

patients with primary aldosteronism, differentiation is impossible solely on clinical and/or biochemical grounds. An anomalous postural decrease in plasma aldosterone and elevated plasma 18-hydroxycorticosterone levels are present in the majority of patients with a unilateral lesion, but these tests are also of limited diagnostic value in the individual patient. A definitive diagnosis is best made by radiographic studies as noted above.

In a few instances, hypertensive patients with hypokalemic alkalosis have been found to have deoxycorticosterone (DOC)-secreting adenomas. Such patients have reduced plasma renin activity levels, but aldosterone measurements are either normal or reduced, suggesting the diagnosis of mineralocorticoid excess due to a hormone other than aldosterone. Rarely, hypermineralocorticoidism is due to a defect in cortisol biosynthesis, specifically 11- or 17-hydroxylation. ACTH levels are increased, with a resultant increase in the production of the mineralocorticoid 11-deoxycorticosterone. *Hypertension and hypokalemia can be corrected by glucocorticoid administration.* The definitive diagnosis is made by demonstrating an elevation of precursors of cortisol biosynthesis in the blood or urine. Occasionally, glucocorticoid administration produces normotension and normokalemia although a hydroxylase deficiency cannot be identified (Fig. 317-9). These patients have normal to slightly elevated aldosterone levels that do not fully suppress with saline but suppress after 2 to 8 weeks of dexamethasone (1 to 2 mg/d). The condition is familial and is termed *glucocorticoid suppressible hyperaldosteronism*.

Another rare cause of hyperkalemia and hypertension is 11 β-hydroxysteroid dehydrogenase deficiency in which cortisol cannot be converted to cortisone and hence binds to the mineralocorticoid type I receptor and acts as a mineralocorticoid (see Chap. 311). The ingestion of candies or chewing tobacco containing certain forms of licorice produces a syndrome mimicking primary aldosteronism. The sodium-retaining principle in such agent is glycyrrhizinic acid, which inhibits the 11 β-hydroxysteroid dehydrogenase and hence allows cortisol to act as a mineralocorticoid and causes sodium retention, expansion of the extracellular fluid volume, hypertension, depressed plasma renin levels, and suppressed aldosterone levels. The diagnosis is established or excluded by a careful history.

TREATMENT Primary aldosteronism due to an adenoma is usually treated by surgical excision. However, dietary sodium restriction and the administration of an aldosterone antagonist, spironolactone, are effective in many cases. Hypertension and hypokalemia are usually controlled by doses of 25 to 100 mg spironolactone every 8 h. Some patients have been successfully managed medically for years, but chronic therapy in men is usually limited by the development of gynecomastia, decreased libido, and impotence.

When bilateral hyperplasia is suspected, surgery is indicated only when significant, symptomatic hypokalemia cannot be controlled with medical therapy, e.g., by spironolactone, triamterene, or amiloride.

Dexamethasone, 1 mg every 12 h, may be tried for 4 to 6 weeks before surgery to rule out glucocorticoid-suppressible hyperaldosteronism. Hypertension associated with idiopathic hyperplasia is usually not benefited by bilateral adrenalectomy.

Secondary aldosteronism Secondary aldosteronism refers to an appropriately increased production of aldosterone in response to activation of the renin-angiotensin system (Fig. 317-10). The production rates of aldosterone are often higher in patients with secondary aldosteronism than in those with primary aldosteronism. Secondary aldosteronism usually occurs in association with the accelerated phase of hypertension or on the basis of an underlying edema disorder. Secondary aldosteronism in pregnancy is a normal physiologic response to estrogen-induced increases in circulating levels of renin substrate and plasma renin activity and to the antialdosterone actions of progestogens.

Secondary aldosteronism in hypertensive states either is secondary to a primary overproduction of renin (primary reninism) or is caused by an overproduction of renin which is secondary to a decrease in renal blood flow and/or perfusion pressure (Fig. 317-5). Secondary hypersecretion of renin can be due to a narrowing of one or both of the major renal arteries either by an atherosclerotic plaque or by fibromuscular hyperplasia. Overproduction of renin from both kidneys also occurs in association with severe arteriolar nephrosclerosis (malignant hypertension) or secondary to profound renal vasoconstriction (accelerated phase of hypertensive disease). The secondary aldosteronism is characterized by hypokalemic alkalosis, moderate to severe increases in plasma renin activity, and moderate to marked increases in aldosterone levels (see Chap. 196).

Secondary aldosteronism with hypertension can also be caused by a rare renin-producing tumor, in so-called primary reninism. These patients have the biochemical characteristics of renal vascular hypertension; however, the primary defect is renin secretion by a juxtaglomerular-cell tumor. The diagnosis can be made by the absence of changes in renal vasculature and/or demonstration of a space-occupying lesion in the kidney by radiographic techniques and documentation of unilateral increases in renal vein renin activity.

Secondary aldosteronism is present in many forms of *edema*. Increased aldosterone secretion rates are usual in patients with edema as a result of either cirrhosis or the nephrotic syndrome. In congestive heart failure, elevated aldosterone secretion varies depending on the severity of cardiac decompensation. The stimulus for aldosterone release in these conditions appears to be *arterial hypovolemia* and/or hypotension. Diuretic therapy often exaggerates the secondary aldosteronism via volume depletion; when this happens hypokalemia and on occasion alkalosis can become prominent features.

Secondary hyperaldosteronism rarely occurs without edema or hypertension (Bartter's syndrome). This syndrome is characterized by the signs of severe hyperaldosteronism (hypokalemic alkalosis) with moderate to marked increases in renin activity but normal blood pressure and absence of edema. Renal biopsy shows juxtaglomerular hyperplasia. The pathogenesis may be a defect in the renal conservation of sodium or chloride and/or an increased production of prostaglandins. The renal loss of sodium is thought to stimulate renin secretion and subsequent aldosterone production. Hyperaldosteronism produces potassium depletion, with the hypokalemia further elevating plasma renin activity. In some cases, the hypokalemia may be potentiated by a defect in renal conservation of potassium. Increased production of prostaglandins is present but is probably not a primary abnormality as administration of inhibitors of prostaglandin synthesis only temporarily reverses the features of this syndrome (see Chap. 231).

SYNDROMES OF ADRENAL ANDROGEN EXCESS The syndromes of adrenal androgen excess result from excess production of dehydroepiandrosterone and androstenedione, which are converted to testosterone in extraglandular tissues; the elevated testosterone levels account for most of the androgenic effects. Adrenal androgen excess may be associated with the secretion of greater or smaller amounts of other adrenal hormones and may, therefore, present as "pure" syndromes of virilization or as "mixed" syndromes associated with excessive production of glucocorticoids and some characteristics of Cushing's syndrome.

Clinical signs and symptoms The signs and symptoms of androgen excess can be divided into four areas: hirsutism, oligomenorrhea, acne, and virilization. Clinically, it is important to distinguish between simple hirsutism and hirsutism associated with virilization. In most cases of simple hirsutism, there is no known cause for the increased hair growth. On the other hand, if the patient is virilized as well as hirsute, increased levels of androgens are usually present (see Chap. 54). In general, the degree of virilization reflects both the duration and the degree of excess androgen secretion, although significant virilization can result from minimal changes in testosterone production, and a significant increase in testosterone production may be associated with minimal signs of virilization. The occurrence of oligomenorrhea in a hirsute patient increases the probability that an excess secretion of androgens will be found. Thus, the evaluation of the hirsute patient should include a careful history of the onset of menarche, past and present menstrual history, and reproductive capacity and a careful physical examination for signs and symptoms of androgen excess.

Etiology As in other states of adrenocortical hyperfunction, the syndromes associated with androgen excess may result from hyperplasia, adenoma, or carcinoma (the latter two having been discussed above). Adrenal androgen overproduction may also arise from *congenital adrenal hyperplasia*, owing to enzymatic defects. In these patients, increased adrenal androgen production is associated either with excess or decreased secretion of mineralocorticoids or decreased production of glucocorticoids. Since, in humans, cortisol is the principal adrenal steroid regulating ACTH elaboration, and since the ACTH stimulates both cortisol and adrenal androgen production, an enzymatic interference with cortisol synthesis may result in the enhanced secretion of adrenal androgens. In severe congenital virilizing hyperplasia, the adrenal output of cortisol may be so compromised as to cause glucocorticoid deficiency despite anatomic adrenal hyperplasia.

Congenital adrenal hyperplasia is the most common adrenal disorder of infancy and childhood. These children usually have severe enzyme deficiencies (see Chap. 324). The deficiency of enzymes is the result of autosomal recessive mutations. Partial adrenal enzyme deficiencies can be expressed after adolescence, predominantly in women with hirsutism and oligomenorrhea but minimal virilization. Late onset adrenal hyperplasia may account for 5 to 25 percent of women with hirsutism and oligomenorrhea, depending on the patient population.

Congenital adrenal hyperplasia is secondary to one of several defects in steroid synthesis. To date, defects have been described in the C-21, C-18, C-17, and C-11 hydroxylase enzymes, as well as in the 3β-ol-dehydrogenase enzyme (see Fig. 317-2). These enzyme deficits usually occur singly. C-21 hydroxylase deficiency is closely linked to the histocompatibility leukocyte antigen (HLA-B) locus of chromosome 6 so that HLA typing can be used to detect the heterozygous carriers in some affected families (see Chap. 14). The clinical expression in the different disorders is variable, ranging from virilization of the female (C-21 deficiency) to feminization of the male (3β-ol-dehydrogenase deficiency). (See also Chap. 324.)

Adrenal virilization in the female at birth is associated with ambiguous external genitalia (*female pseudohermaphroditism*). The onset of virilization is most probably after the fifth month of embryonic development. At birth there may be enlarged genitalia in the male infant and enlargement of the clitoris, partial or complete fusion of the labia, and sometimes a urogenital sinus in the female. If the labial fusion is nearly complete, the female infant has external genitalia resembling a penis with hypospadias. In the *postnatal* period, congenital adrenal hyperplasia is associated with virilization in the female and isosexual precocity in the male. The excessive androgens result in accelerated growth, with bone age exceeding chronologic age. Since epiphyseal closure is hastened by excessive androgens, growth stops, but truncal development continues, giving the characteristic appearance of a child of short stature with well-developed trunk.

The most common form of congenital adrenal hyperplasia (95 percent of cases) is a result of impairment of *C-21 hydroxylation*. In addition to cortisol deficiency, there is an associated reduction in aldosterone secretion in approximately one-third of the patients. Thus, with C-21 hydroxylase deficiency, adrenal virilization occurs with or without an associated salt-losing tendency due to aldosterone deficiency (see Fig. 317-2).

C-11 hydroxylase deficiency causes a "hypertensive" variant of congenital adrenal hyperplasia. Hypertension and hypokalemia occur because of the impaired conversion of 11-deoxycorticosterone to corticosterone, resulting in the accumulation of 11-deoxycorticosterone, a potent mineralocorticoid. Increased shunting again occurs into the androgen pathway.

The *C-17 hydroxylase* deficiency is characterized by hypogonadism, hypokalemia, and hypertension. This rare deficiency causes decreased production of cortisol and shunting of precursors into the mineralocorticoid pathway with hypokalemic alkalosis, hypertension, and suppressed plasma renin activity. Usually, 11-deoxycorticosterone production is elevated. Because C-17 hydroxylation is required for biosynthesis of adrenal androgens as well as for biosynthesis of gonadal testosterone and estrogen, this defect is associated with sexual immaturity, high urinary gonadotropin levels, and low urinary 17-ketosteroid excretion. Female patients have primary amenorrhea and lack of development of secondary sexual characteristics. Because of deficient androgen production, male patients either have ambiguous external genitalia or a female phenotype (male pseudohermaphroditism). Exogenous glucocorticoids can correct the hypertensive syndrome, and treatment with appropriate gonadal steroids results in sexual maturation.

With 3β-ol-dehydrogenase deficiency, conversion of pregnenolone to progesterone is impaired, with the result that pathways to both cortisol and aldosterone are "blocked," with shunting then occurring into the adrenal androgen pathway via 17α-hydroxypregnenolone to dehydroepiandrosterone. Since dehydroepiandrosterone is a weak androgen and because this enzyme deficiency is also present in the gonad, the genitalia of the male fetus may be incompletely virilized or feminized. Conversely, in the female, overproduction of dehydroepiandrosterone may produce partial virilization.

Diagnosis The diagnosis of *congenital adrenal hyperplasia* should be considered in all infants exhibiting "failure to thrive," particularly those having episodes of acute adrenal insufficiency or salt wasting or showing sustained hypertension. The diagnosis is further suggested by the finding of hypertrophy of the clitoris, fused labia, or urogenital sinus in the female and isosexual precocity in the male. In infants and children with a *C-21 hydroxylation block*, increased urine 17-ketosteroid excretion and increased plasma DHEA sulfate are typically associated with an increase in the blood levels of 17-hydroxyprogesterone and the urinary excretion of the metabolite of this steroid, pregnanetriol.

The diagnosis of a *salt-losing form of congenital adrenal hyperplasia* due to defects in C-21 hydroxylase enzyme is suggested by episodes of acute adrenal insufficiency with hyponatremia, hyperkalemia, dehydration, and vomiting. These infants and children often crave salt and exhibit laboratory signs of concomitant deficits in both cortisol and aldosterone secretion.

With the *hypertensive form of congenital adrenal hyperplasia* due to impaired C-11 hydroxylation, 11-deoxycorticosterone and 11-deoxycortisol accumulate. Both urine 17-ketosteroid and 17-hydroxycorticosteroid excretion may be elevated, since 11-deoxycortisol is included in the analysis. The diagnosis is secured by demonstrating increased levels of 11-deoxycortisol in the blood or increased amounts of tetrahydro-11-deoxycortisol in the urine.

The finding of very high levels of urine dehydroepiandrosterone with low levels of pregnanetriol and of cortisol metabolites in urine is characteristic of patients with 3β-ol-dehydrogenase deficiency. Marked salt wasting may also occur.

Patients with *late onset adrenal hyperplasia* (partial deficiency of C-21 hydroxylase) are characterized by normal or moderately elevated urinary 17-ketosteroids and plasma DHEA sulfate. A high basal level of a precursor of cortisol biosynthesis (such as 17-hydroxyprogesterone) or elevation of the precursor after ACTH stimulation confirms the diagnosis of a partial hydroxylase deficiency. It is uncertain how long the ACTH needs to be infused to unmask the enzyme deficiency, but it is likely that a 1-h infusion will pick up more than 75 percent and a 4-h infusion will detect more than 95 percent of those who have an enzyme deficiency documented with a 24-h ACTH infusion. Adrenal androgen output is easily suppressed by the standard low-dose (2 mg) dexamethasone test.

Differential diagnosis The causes of hirsutism can be divided into four broad categories: familial, idiopathic, androgen excess, and drugs. In general, the first two conditions are not associated with other signs of androgen excess, i.e., oligomenorrhea, significant acne, or virilization. Likewise, drug-induced hirsutism is usually not associated with other signs and symptoms of androgen excess, unless the drug is an androgen. The drugs that produce an increase in body hair include phenothiazines, minoxidil, and phenytoin. Each of these drugs, particularly minoxidil, produces a generalized increase in hair growth, not just an increase in hair growth in androgen target areas. The mechanism may be related to the ability of these drugs to convert vellus into terminal hair follicles.

If drugs are excluded, the only known causes of hirsutism amenable to treatment are those secondary to excess production of androgens by either the adrenal or the ovary.

In the female, the differential diagnosis of hirsutism and virilization is between adrenal and ovarian etiologies (Table 317-7). *Sudden onset of progressive hirsutism and virilization* suggests an adrenal or ovarian neoplasm. *Adrenal adenomas and carcinomas* may cause a pure or mixed virilizing syndrome. Since adrenal androgens are weak compared with gonadal androgens, adrenal virilization is characterized by *large increments in urine 17-ketosteroid excretion*. Virilizing adrenal adenomas are rare. *Virilizing adrenal carcinomas*, the most common adrenal tumors causing virilization, are associated with high plasma DHEA sulfate levels and high urinary 17-ketosteroid excretion rates; cortisol levels and 17 hydroxycorticosteroid excretion are normal or moderately elevated. Clinical differentiation between virilizing adrenal adenoma and carcinoma can usually be made preoperatively by CT scanning since carcinomas as a rule exceed 6 cm in size. Failure to reduce 17-ketosteroid levels and plasma DHEA sulfate levels to normal following dexamethasone suppression (0.5 mg given orally every 6 h for 2 days) further supports a diagnosis of virilizing adrenal tumor and excludes congenital adrenal hyperplasia. The most common virilizing *ovarian tumor* is the arrhenoblastoma, but other ovarian tumors, such as adrenal rest tumor, granulosa-cell tumor, hilar-cell tumor, and Brenner tumor, have been associated with virilization. Virilization due to ovarian tumors is usually characterized by normal levels of urinary 17-ketosteroids and DHEA sulfate, since the neoplasm usually secretes the potent androgen testosterone. Occasionally increases in 17-ketosteroid excretion occur

TABLE 317-7 Causes of hirsutism in women

I Familial
II Idiopathic
III Ovarian
- *A* Polycystic ovaries; hilus-cell hyperplasia
- *B* Tumor: arrhenoblastoma, hilus cell, adrenal rest

IV Adrenal
- *A* Congenital adrenal hyperplasia
- *B* Noncongenital adrenal hyperplasia (Cushing's)
- *C* Tumor: virilizing carcinoma or adenoma

in some patients with ovarian neoplasms, but baseline 17-ketosteroid excretion in excess of 100 μmol/d (30 mg/d) is rare with the exception of adrenal rest tumors. Like adrenal neoplasms, ovarian tumors are not suppressed by dexamethasone. With the exception of adrenal rest tumors, these tumors are largely independent of ACTH stimulation. Elevations of plasma testosterone or urinary testosterone excretion do not localize the neoplasm to the ovary, since testosterone can be elevated subsequent to peripheral conversion of adrenal precursors, such as DHEA (see Chap. 322).

The most common ovarian cause of excess androgen production is ovarian hyperthecosis or polycystic ovaries (see Chap. 322). As opposed to ovarian or adrenal tumors, virilization is less common with polycystic ovaries, whereas hirsutism is quite frequent. In most cases, the 17-ketosteroid excretion rate is greater than normal. Although the 17-ketosteroid excretion is partially reduced by dexamethasone, the residual level is often greater than in normal subjects. Plasma levels and production rates of androstenedione and to a lesser extent testosterone are usually increased. Follicle-stimulating hormone (FSH) levels tend to be lower than normal, and luteinizing hormone (LH) levels are tonically elevated, leading to the characteristic increased LH/FSH ratio. The laboratory findings in patients with hirsutism-virilizing syndromes are summarized in Table 317-8.

Treatment Treatment of adrenal virilism is dictated by the type of lesion. Patients with *congenital adrenal hyperplasia* have a fundamental defect of cortisol deficiency with resultant excessive ACTH stimulation, producing hyperplasia of the adrenal glands and causing additional "shunting" into the adrenal androgen pathway. Therapy in these patients consists of daily administration of glucocorticoids to suppress pituitary ACTH secretion. Because of its cost and intermediate half-life, prednisone is the drug of choice except in infants, when hydrocortisone is usually used. In adult patients with late-onset adrenal hyperplasia, a single bedtime dose of an intermediate-acting glucocorticoid, such as 2.5 or 5 mg of prednisone, suppresses pituitary ACTH secretion. The amount of steroid required by children with congenital adrenal hyperplasia is approximately 1 to 1.5 times the normal cortisol production rate of 33 to 35 μmol (12 to 13 mg) cortisol per square meter of body surface area per day and is given in divided doses two or three times per day. The dosage schedule is governed by repetitive analysis of the urinary 17-ketosteroids, plasma DHEA sulfate, and/or precursors of cortisol biosynthesis. Skeletal growth and maturation must also be closely monitored since overtreatment with glucocorticoid replacement therapy retards linear growth.

HYPOFUNCTION OF ADRENAL CORTEX

Adrenocortical hypofunction includes all conditions in which the secretion of adrenal steroid hormones falls below the requirements of the body. Adrenal insufficiency may be divided into two general

TABLE 317-9 Classification of adrenal insufficiency

I Primary adrenal insufficiency
- *A* Anatomic destruction of gland (chronic and acute)
  - *1* "Idiopathic" atrophy (autoimmune)
  - *2* Surgical removal
  - *3* Infection (tuberculous, fungus, viral–especially in AIDS patients)
  - *4* Hemorrhage
  - *5* Invasion: metastatic
- *B* Metabolic failure in hormone production
  - *1* Congenital adrenal hyperplasia
  - *2* Enzyme inhibitors (metyrapone, ketoconazole, aminogluteinimide)
  - *3* Cytotoxic agents (mitotane)

II Secondary adrenal insufficiency
- *A* Hypopituitarism due to hypothalamic-pituitary disease
- *B* Suppression of hypothalamic-pituitary axis
  - *1* Exogenous steroid
  - *2* Endogenous steroid from tumor

categories: (1) those associated with primary inability of the adrenal to elaborate sufficient quantities of hormone and (2) those associated with a secondary failure due to a primary failure in the elaboration of ACTH (Table 317-9).

PRIMARY ADRENOCORTICAL DEFICIENCY (ADDISON'S DISEASE) Addison's description of "general languor and debility, remarkable feebleness of the heart's action, irritability of the stomach, and a peculiar change of the color of the skin," summarizes the dominant clinical features of the disease. Advanced cases are usually easy to diagnose, but recognition of the disease in its earlier phases may present a real challenge.

Incidence Primary adrenocortical insufficiency is relatively rare. It may occur at any age and affects both sexes with equal frequency. Because of increasing therapeutic use of exogenous steroids, secondary adrenal insufficiency is relatively common.

Etiology and pathogenesis Addison's disease results from progressive adrenocortical destruction, which must involve more than 90 percent of the glands before signs of adrenal insufficiency appear. The adrenal is a frequent site for chronic granulomatous diseases, predominantly tuberculosis but also histoplasmosis, coccidioidomycosis, and cryptococcosis. In previous years, tuberculosis was found at postmortem examination in 70 to 90 percent of cases; however, the most frequent finding at present is *idiopathic* atrophy, and an autoimmune mechanism is probably responsible. Rarely, other lesions are encountered, such as bilateral hemorrhage, tumor metastases, amyloidosis, or sarcoidosis.

Half of patients have circulating adrenal antibodies. Some patients also have antibodies to thyroid, parathyroid, and/or gonadal tissue (see also Chap. 325). There is also an increased incidence of chronic lymphocytic thyroiditis (Hashimoto's disease) and an increased incidence of premature ovarian failure, type I diabetes mellitus, and Graves' disease in patients with idiopathic adrenal insufficiency. The occurrence of two or more of these autoimmune endocrine disorders in the same individual defines the polyglandular autoimmune syndrome

TABLE 317-8 Laboratory evaluation of hirsutism-virilizing syndromes

	Ovarian		Adrenal			
	PCO	Ovarian tumor	CAH	Adrenal neoplasm	Cushing's syndrome	Idiopathic
Urinary 17-ketosteroids, plasma DHEA sulfate	N↑	N	N↑	↑↑↑	N↑	N
Plasma testosterone	N↑	↑↑	N↑	N↑	N↑	N
LH/FSH ratio	N↑	N	N	N	N	N
Precursors of cortisol biosynthesis:						
Basal	N	N	N↑	N↑	N	N
Following ACTH infusion	N	N	↑↑	N↑	N	N
Cortisol following overnight dexamethasone suppresion test	N	N	N	↑	↑	N

NOTE: CAH, congenital adrenal hyperplasia; PCO, polycystic ovary syndrome; N, normal; ↑, elevated.

type II. Additional disorders in these patients include pernicious anemia, vitiligo, alopecia, nontropical sprue, and myasthenia gravis. Within families, multiple generations are affected by one or more of the above diseases. Type II polyglandular syndrome is the result of a mutant gene on the sixth chromosome and is associated with the HLA alleles B8 and DR3.

The combination of parathyroid and adrenal insufficiency and chronic mucocutaneous moniliasis constitutes a distinct familial syndrome (type I polyglandular autoimmune syndrome). Other autoimmune diseases also occur in higher frequency in these patients (e.g., pernicious anemia, chronic active hepatitis, alopecia, primary hypothyroidism, and premature gonadal failure). There is no HLA association; this syndrome is inherited in an autosomal recessive pattern, often with multiple affected siblings within a family. The type I syndrome usually presents during childhood, whereas the peak incidence of expression of the type II syndrome is in adulthood. The mechanisms by which genetic predisposition and/or autoimmunity interact in the pathogenesis of these disease states are unknown.

Clinical suspicion of adrenal insufficiency should be high in patients with acquired immunodeficiency syndrome (AIDS). Cytomegalovirus regularly involves the adrenal glands (so-called CMV necrotizing adrenalitis), and *mycobacterium avium-intracellulare*, *Cryptococcus*, and Kaposi's sarcoma involvement of the adrenals have also been reported. Clinical manifestations of adrenal insufficiency in AIDS patients may be uncommon, but tests of adrenal reserve are frequently abnormal. When interpreting tests of adrenocortical function, it is important to consider medications commonly used to treat AIDS patients that might potentiate or cause adrenal failure (rifampin, phenytoin, ketoconazole, and opiates).

Clinical signs and symptoms Adrenocortical insufficiency caused by gradual adrenal destruction is characterized by an insidious onset of slowly progressive fatigability, weakness, anorexia, nausea and vomiting, weight loss, cutaneous and mucosal pigmentation, hypotension, and occasionally hypoglycemia (Table 317-10). However, the spectrum may vary, depending on the duration and degree of adrenal hypofunction, from a complaint of mild chronic fatigue to the fulminating shock associated with acute massive destruction of the glands in the syndrome described by Waterhouse and Friderichsen.

Asthenia is the cardinal symptom. Early it may be sporadic, usually most evident at times of stress; as adrenal function becomes more impaired, weakness progresses until the patient is continuously fatigued, necessitating bed rest.

Hyperpigmentation may be a striking sign, but its absence does not exclude this diagnosis. It commonly appears as a diffuse brown, tan, or bronze darkening of both exposed and unexposed parts such as elbows or creases of the hand and of areas normally pigmented such as the areolas about the nipples. Bluish-black patches may appear on the mucous membranes. Some patients develop dark freckles, and occasionally irregular areas of vitiligo may appear paradoxically. As an early sign, patients may notice an unusually persistent tanning following exposure to the sun.

Arterial hypotension is frequent, and in severe cases blood pressures may be in the range of 80/50 or less. Postural accentuation of hypotension is common.

Abnormalities of gastrointestinal function often are the presenting complaint. Symptoms may vary from mild anorexia with weight loss to fulminating nausea, vomiting, diarrhea, and ill-defined abdominal pain, which at times may be so severe as to be confused with an acute abdomen. In addition, patients with adrenal insufficiency frequently have marked personality changes, usually in the form of excessive irritability and restlessness. Enhancement of the sensory modalities of taste, olfaction, and hearing is often present and is reversible with therapy. A decrease in axillary and pubic hair is common in women due to loss of adrenal androgen production.

TABLE 317-10 Incidence of symptoms and signs in Addison's disease, percent

Weakness	99	Hypotension (<110/70)	87
Pigmentation of skin	98	Abdominal pain	34
Pigmentation of mucous membranes	82	Salt craving	22
Weight loss	97	Diarrhea	20
Anorexia, nausea, and vomiting	90	Constipation	19
		Syncope	16
		Vitiligo	9

Laboratory findings In the early phase of gradual adrenal destruction, there may be no demonstrable abnormalities in the routine laboratory parameters, but adrenal reserve is decreased, that is, basal steroid output is normal but an increase does not occur in response to stress. Adrenal stimulation with ACTH uncovers abnormalities in this stage of the disease with a subnormal response and/or failure of cortisol levels to rise over basal. In more advanced stages of adrenal destruction, serum sodium, chloride, and bicarbonate are reduced while serum potassium is elevated. The hyponatremia is due to both loss of sodium into the urine (due to aldosterone deficiency) and movement into the intracellular compartment. This extravascular sodium loss depletes extracellular fluid volume and accentuates hypotension. Elevated plasma vasopressin and angiotensin II levels may be contributing factors to the hyponatremia through impairment of free water clearance. The hyperkalemia is due to a combination of aldosterone deficiency, impaired glomerular filtration, and acidosis. Basal levels of cortisol and aldosterone are subnormal and fail to increase following ACTH administration. Mild to moderate hypercalcemia occurs in 10 to 20 percent of patients; the reason for this is not understood. The electrocardiogram may show nonspecific changes, and the electroencephalogram exhibits a generalized reduction and slowing. There may be a normocytic anemia, a relative lymphocytosis, and usually a moderate eosinophilia.

Diagnosis The diagnosis of adrenal insufficiency should be made only with ACTH stimulation testing to assay the adrenal reserve capacity for steroid production (see above for ACTH test protocols). In *severe adrenal insufficiency* the cortisol secretory rate is markedly decreased, and this may be ascertained indirectly by the finding of low to absent 24-h urine cortisol, 17-hydroxycorticosteroids, and 17-ketosteroids. With *mild adrenal insufficiency* (decreased adrenal reserve), urine and blood steroid values overlap the normal range; thus, a diagnosis of adrenal insufficiency should never be excluded solely on the basis of normal basal urine steroid determinations. Plasma cortisol values vary from zero to the lower range of normal. Aldosterone secretion is usually low, resulting in salt wasting and secondary rises in plasma renin levels. In primary adrenal insufficiency, plasma ACTH and associated peptides (β-lipotropin) are elevated because of loss of the usual cortisol-hypothalamic-pituitary feedback relationship, whereas in secondary adrenal insufficiency, plasma ACTH values are low, or "inappropriately" normal (Fig. 317-11).

Differential diagnosis Since weakness and fatigue are common complaints, clinical diagnosis of early adrenocortical insufficiency is frequently difficult. However, mild gastrointestinal distress with weight loss, anorexia, and a suggestion of increased pigmentation make mandatory ACTH stimulation testing to rule out adrenal insufficiency, particularly before steroid treatment is begun. Weight loss is useful in evaluating the significance of weakness and malaise. Weight gain associated with lassitude is more characteristic of depressive syndromes. Racial pigmentation in many individuals may be a problem, but a *recent* and progressive *increase* is usually reported by the Addisonian patient with gradual adrenal destruction. However, hyperpigmentation is usually absent when adrenal destruction is rapid, as in bilateral adrenal hemorrhage. Hyperpigmentation in other diseases may also present a problem, but the appearance and distribution of pigment in Addison's disease are usually characteristic. When doubt exists, measurement of ACTH levels and testing of adrenal reserve with the infusion of ACTH provide clear-cut differentiation.

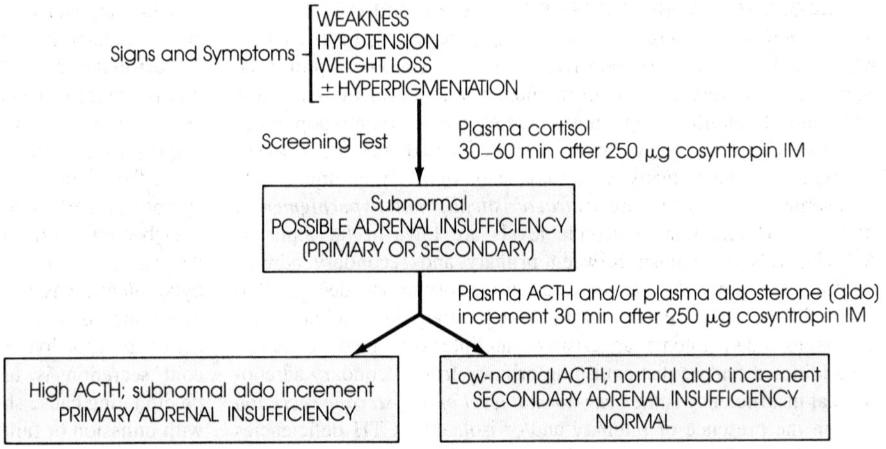

FIGURE 317-11 Diagnostic flowchart for evaluating patients with suspected adrenal insufficiency. Plasma ACTH levels are low in secondary adrenal insufficiency. In adrenal insufficiency secondary to pituitary tumors or idiopathic panhypopituitarism, other pituitary hormone deficiencies are present. On the other hand, ACTH deficiency may be isolated, as seen following prolonged use of exogenous glucocorticoids.

Since the isolated blood levels obtained in these screening tests may not be definitive, the diagnosis should always be confirmed by a continuous 24-h ACTH infusion. Normal subjects and patients with secondary adrenal insufficiency may be distinguished by insulin tolerance or metyrapone testing.

Treatment All patients with Addison's disease should receive specific hormone replacement. Like diabetics, these patients require careful and persistent education in regard to their disease. Since the adrenal gland elaborates three general classes of hormone, of which two, glucocorticoids and mineralocorticoids, are of primary clinical importance, replacement therapy should correct both deficiencies. Cortisone (or cortisol) is the mainstay of treatment. Cortisone dosage varies from 12.5 to 50 mg daily, with the majority of patients taking 25 to 37.5 mg in divided doses. Cortisol (30 mg daily) or prednisone (7.5 mg daily) in divided doses may also be given for substitution therapy. Patients are advised to take their glucocorticoid replacement medication with meals or, if this is impractical, with milk or an antacid because the drugs may increase gastric acidity. This is particularly important because if the steroid is biologically active, e.g., cortisol, prednisolone, and dexamethasone, it may exert local effects on the gastric mucosa. In addition, the larger proportion of the dose (e.g., 25 mg of cortisone) is taken in the morning, and the remainder (12.5 mg of cortisone) is taken in the late afternoon to simulate the normal diurnal adrenal rhythm. Some patients exhibit insomnia, irritability, and mental excitement after initiation of therapy; in these, the dosage should be reduced. Other indications for smaller amounts of glucocorticoids are hypertension, diabetes mellitus, or active tuberculosis.

Since this amount of cortisone or cortisol fails to replace the mineralocorticoid component of the adrenal gland, supplementary hormone is usually needed. This is accomplished by the daily oral administration of 0.05 to 0.1 mg fludrocortisone. Of course, patients should be instructed to ingest an ample intake of sodium (3 to 4 g/d). Adequacy of mineralocorticoid therapy can be assessed by measurement of blood pressure and serum electrolytes. Blood pressure should be normal and without postural change; serum sodium potassium, creatinine, and urea nitrogen should also be within the normal range.

Complications of glucocorticoid therapy, with the exception of gastritis, are *rare* in the dosage used in the treatment of Addison's disease. Complications of mineralocorticoid therapy occur more frequently and include hypokalemia, edema, hypertension, cardiac enlargement, or even congestive failure due to sodium retention. In the management of patients with Addison's disease, periodic measurements of body weight, serum potassium, and blood pressure are useful. All patients with adrenal insufficiency, including bilaterally adrenalectomized patients, should carry medical identification, should be instructed in the parenteral self-administration of steroids, and should be registered with a national medical alerting system.

Special therapeutic problems During periods of intercurrent illness, the dose of cortisone or cortisol should be increased to 75 to 150 mg/d. When oral administration is not possible, parenteral routes should be employed. Likewise, before surgery or dental extractions, supplemental glucocorticoids should be administered. Patients should also be advised to increase the dose of fludrocortisone and to add excess salt to their otherwise normal diet during periods of excessive exercise with sweating, during extremely hot weather, and with gastrointestinal upsets. For a representative program of steroid therapy for the patient with adrenal insufficiency who is undergoing a major operation, see Table 317-11. This schedule is designed to mimic on the day of surgery the output of cortisol in normal individuals undergoing prolonged major stress (10 mg/h, 250 to 300 mg/d). Thereafter, if the patient is progressing well and is afebrile, the dose of cortisol is tapered by 20 to 30 percent daily. Parenteral mineralocorticoid administration is unnecessary at cortisol doses greater than 100 mg/d because of the mineralocorticoid effects of cortisol at such dosages.

TABLE 317-11 Steroid therapy schedule for Addisonian patient undergoing a major operation*

	Cortisol phosphate (intramuscularly)		Cortisol infusion, continuous, mg/h	Cortisol (orally)		Fludrocortisone (orally),
	7 A.M.	7 P.M.		8 A.M.	4 P.M.	8 A.M.
Routine daily medication				20	10	0.1
Day before operation		50		20	10	0.1
Day of operation			10			
Postoperative:						
Day 1			5–7.5			
Day 2			2.5–5			
Day 3	50	50				
Day 4	50				20	0.1
Day 5				40	20	0.1
Day 6				20	20	0.1
Day 7				20	10	0.1

* All steroid doses are given in milligrams.

SECONDARY ADRENOCORTICAL INSUFFICIENCY Pituitary ACTH deficiency causes *secondary* adrenocortical insufficiency. ACTH deficiency may be selective, as is seen following prolonged administration of excess glucocorticoids, or may occur in association with multiple pituitary tropic hormone deficiencies (panhypopituitarism) (see Chap. 313). Patients with secondary adrenocortical hypofunction may have many symptoms and signs in common with Addisonian patients but are *characteristically not hyperpigmented* since ACTH and related peptide levels are low. In fact, plasma ACTH levels distinguish between primary and secondary adrenal insufficiency, since they are elevated in the former and decreased to absent in the latter. Patients with total pituitary insufficiency also have signs and symptoms suggestive of multiple hormone deficiencies. An additional feature distinguishing primary from secondary adrenocortical insufficiency is the *near-normal level of aldosterone secretion* seen in the presence of pituitary and/or isolated ACTH deficiencies (Fig. 317-11). Patients with pituitary insufficiency may present with hyponatremia, which may be dilutional or secondary to subnormal increments in aldosterone secretion in response to severe sodium restriction. However, the findings of severe *dehydration, hyponatremia,* and *hyperkalemia* are characteristic of severe mineralocorticoid insufficiency and favor a diagnosis of primary adrenocortical insufficiency.

Patients receiving long-term steroid therapy, despite physical findings of Cushing's syndrome, develop adrenal insufficiency because of prolonged pituitary-hypothalamic suppression and adrenal atrophy secondary to the loss of endogenous ACTH. Thus, these patients have two deficits, a loss of adrenal responsiveness to ACTH and a failure of pituitary ACTH release. These patients are characterized by low blood cortisol and ACTH levels, low baseline steroid excretion, and abnormal ACTH and metyrapone test results. Most patients with steroid-induced adrenal insufficiency eventually recover normal hypothalamic-pituitary-adrenal responsiveness, but individual response time varies from days to months. The rapid ACTH test can be used as a convenient assessment of recovery of hypothalamic-pituitary-adrenal function. Since the plasma cortisol concentrations after injection of cosyntropin and during insulin-induced hypoglycemia usually correlate closely, the rapid ACTH test assesses the integrated hypothalamic-pituitary-adrenal function (see "Tests of Pituitary-Adrenal Responsiveness," above). Additional testing to assess endogenous pituitary ACTH reserve includes the standard metyrapone and the insulin tolerance tests.

Substitution glucocorticoid therapy in patients with secondary adrenocortical insufficiency does not differ from that for Addisonian patients. Mineralocorticoid replacement therapy is usually not necessary, since aldosterone secretion is preserved. Otherwise, the same basic principles should be applied to patients with secondary adrenocortical insufficiency.

ACUTE ADRENOCORTICAL INSUFFICIENCY Acute adrenocortical insufficiency may result from several processes. One of these, termed *adrenal crisis,* is a rapid and overwhelming intensification of chronic adrenal insufficiency, usually precipitated by sepsis or surgical stress. Another involves an acute hemorrhagic destruction of both adrenal glands. In children this is usually associated with septicemia with *Pseudomonas* or meningococcemia (Waterhouse-Friderichsen syndrome). In adults, anticoagulant therapy or a coagulation disorder may result in bilateral adrenal hemorrhage in patients undergoing major stress where there is increased adrenocortical activity. Occasionally, bilateral adrenal hemorrhage in the newborn results from birth trauma. Hemorrhage also has been observed during pregnancy, following idiopathic adrenal vein thrombosis, and as a complication of venography (e.g., infarction of an adenoma). A third, and probably the most frequent, cause of acute insufficiency results from the rapid withdrawal of steroids from patients with adrenal atrophy secondary to chronic steroid administration. In the presence of severe stress, acute adrenocortical insufficiency may also occur in patients with congenital adrenal hyperplasia or those with decreased adrenocortical reserve when they are given pharmacologic agents that are capable of inhibiting steroid synthesis (mitotane, ketoconazole) or increasing steroid metabolism (phenytoin, rifampin).

Adrenal crisis The long-term survival of patients with Addison's disease largely depends upon prevention and treatment of adrenal crisis. Consequently, the occurrence of infection, trauma (including surgery), gastrointestinal upsets, or other forms of stress requires an immediate increase in hormone. In untreated patients, preexisting symptoms are intensified. Nausea, vomiting, and abdominal pain may become intractable. Fever may be severe or absent. Lethargy deepens into somnolence, and the blood pressure and pulse fail as hypovolemic vascular shock ensues. In contrast, patients previously maintained on chronic glucocorticoid therapy may not exhibit severe dehydration or hypotension until preterminally, since mineralocorticoid secretion is usually preserved. In all patients in crisis, a precipitating cause should be sought. Intercurrent infection associated with omission or failure to increase maintenance therapy is common.

Treatment is primarily directed toward the rapid elevation of circulating glucocorticoid and the replacement of the sodium and water deficits. Hence, an intravenous infusion of 5% glucose in normal saline solution should be immediately started with a bolus intravenous infusion of 100 mg cortisol followed by a continuous infusion of cortisol at a rate of 10 mg/h. Effective treatment of hypotension consists of aggressive repletion of sodium and water deficits. If the crisis was preceded by prolonged nausea, vomiting, and dehydration, several liters of saline solution may be required within the first few hours. Vasoconstrictive agents (such as dopamine) may be indicated in extreme conditions as adjuncts to volume replacement. With large doses of steroid, as for example 100 to 200 mg cortisol, the patient receives a maximal mineralocorticoid effect, and supplementary mineralocorticoid is superfluous. Following improvement, the patient can be offered oral fluids and the steroid dosage is tapered over the next few days to maintenance levels, with reinstitution of supplementary mineralocorticoid if needed (Table 317-11).

HYPOALDOSTERONISM

Isolated aldosterone deficiency accompanied by normal cortisol production occurs in association with hyporeninism, as an inherited biosynthetic defect, postoperatively following removal of aldosterone-secreting adenomas, during protracted heparin or heparinoid administration, in pretectal disease of the nervous system, and in severe postural hypotension.

The feature common to all patients with hypoaldosteronism is the inability to increase aldosterone secretion appropriately during salt restriction. Most patients present with unexplained hyperkalemia often exacerbated by restriction of dietary sodium intake. In severe cases urine sodium wastage occurs on a normal salt intake, whereas in milder forms excessive losses of urine sodium occur only during salt restriction.

Most cases of isolated hypoaldosteronism occur in patients with a deficiency in renin production (so-called hyporeninemic hypoaldosteronism). This syndrome is most commonly seen in adults with mild renal failure and diabetes mellitus in association with hyperkalemia and metabolic acidosis out of proportion to the state of renal impairment. Plasma renin levels fail to rise normally following sodium restriction and postural changes. The pathogenesis is uncertain. Possibilities include renal disease (most likely), autonomic neuropathy, extracellular fluid volume expansion, and a defect in conversion of presumed renin precursors into active renin. Aldosterone levels also fail to rise normally following salt restriction and volume contraction; this is probably related to the hyporeninism since biosynthetic defects in aldosterone secretion cannot usually be demonstrated. In these patients, aldosterone secretion increases promptly following ACTH stimulation, but it is uncertain whether the magnitude of the response is normal. On the other hand, the level of aldosterone appears to be subnormal in relationship to the hyperkalemia.

Hypoaldosteronism can also be associated with high renin levels. In many of these subjects, a biosynthetic defect has been noted where there is an inability to transform the C-18 methyl group of corticosterone to the C-18 aldehyde of aldosterone due to a deficiency of the enzyme 18-hydroxysteroid dehydrogenase. These patients manifest not only low to absent aldosterone secretion and elevated plasma renin levels but also elevated values for the intermediates of aldosterone biosynthesis (corticosterone and 18-hydroxycorticosterone). Severely ill patients may also exhibit the syndrome of hyperreninemic hypoaldosteronism. This selective hypoaldosteronism is seen in hypotensive critically ill patients. Patients with this syndrome have a high mortality rate (80 percent). Hyperkalemia is not part of this syndrome. Possible explanations for the hypoaldosteronism include adrenal necrosis (uncommon) or an adaptation to severe illness by a shift in steroidogenesis from mineralocorticoids to glucocorticoids, possibly related to prolonged ACTH stimulation.

Before considering the diagnosis of isolated hypoaldosteronism in a patient with hyperkalemia, "pseudohyperkalemia" (e.g., hemolysis, thrombocytosis) should be excluded by measuring plasma potassium. The next step is to demonstrate a normal cortisol response to ACTH stimulation. Then stimulated (upright posture, sodium restriction) renin and aldosterone levels are obtained. Low renin–low aldosterone levels establish a diagnosis of hyporeninemic hypoaldosteronism. High renin–low aldosterone levels are consistent with an aldosterone biosynthetic defect or a selective unresponsiveness of the glomerulosa to angiotensin II. Finally, elevated renin and aldosterone levels suggest primary renal unresponsiveness to aldosterone, so-called pseudohypoaldosteronism.

The aim of treatment of isolated hypoaldosteronism is to replace the mineralocorticoid deficiency. For practical purposes, the oral administration of fludrocortisone in a dose of 0.1 to 0.2 mg daily should restore electrolyte balance, if salt intake is adequate (e.g., 150 to 200 mmol/d). However, patients with hyporeninemic hypoaldosteronism usually require higher doses of mineralocorticoid to correct the hyperkalemia. This poses a risk in those patients who also may have hypertension and mild renal insufficiency and/or congestive heart failure. Therefore, an alternative approach is to administer furosemide, which can ameliorate the acidosis and the hyperkalemia, and reduce the salt intake. Occasionally a combination of these two approaches is efficacious.

NONSPECIFIC CLINICAL USE OF ADRENAL STEROIDS AND ACTH

The widespread utilization of glucocorticoids and ACTH emphasizes the need for a thorough understanding of the metabolic effects of these agents when used nonspecifically, if optimum effectiveness is to be obtained and if undesirable side reactions are to be minimized. Before instituting adrenal hormone therapy, the gains that can reasonably be expected should be weighed against the potentially undesirable metabolic actions of pharmacologic doses of hormone.

HOW SERIOUS IS THE DISORDER? In a patient whose life is threatened by unexplained shock or in whom other measures have failed, the physician need not hesitate to employ large-dosage steroid therapy. On the other hand, one should exercise restraint in administering steroids to a patient with early rheumatoid arthritis who as yet has not been exposed to the possible benefits of physiotherapy, analgesics, and a well-organized program of general medical care.

HOW LONG WILL GLUCOCORTICOID THERAPY BE REQUIRED? The use of intravenously administered steroids for a period of 24 to 48 h in the treatment of such life-threatening situations as status asthmaticus or pseudotumor cerebri has little or no contraindication, in contrast to the initiation of a program of chronic steroid therapy for asthma, arthritis, or psoriasis. In the latter instances, the almost certain complication of a Cushing's syndrome of some degree must be weighed against the potential benefit. These side effects should be minimized by a careful choice of steroid preparations, alternate-day or interrupted therapy programs, and the judicious use of supplementary adjuvants.

WHICH PREPARATION IS PREFERABLE? At least five considerations need to be taken into account in deciding which steroid preparation to use:

1 The biologic half-life of the compound. The rationale behind every-other-day therapy is to decrease the metabolic effects of the steroids for a significant amount of time over the 2-day period, yet at the same time to produce pharmacologic suppression of sufficient duration to maintain the disease in remission. Too long a half-life would defeat the first purpose, and too short a half-life would defeat the second. In general, the more potent the steroid, the longer its biologic half-life.

2 The importance of the mineralocorticoid effects of the steroid. Synthetic steroids have less mineralocorticoid effect relative to their glucocorticoid effect than do cortisol or cortisone (Table 317-12). This may be an important consideration in certain disease states.

3 The biologically active form of the steroid. Cortisone and prednisone, in contrast to the other glucocorticoids, have to be converted to biologically active equivalents before anti-inflammatory effects can occur. Because of this, in a condition in which steroids are known to be effective and when an adequate dose has been given without response, one should consider substituting cortisol or prednisolone for cortisone or prednisone.

4 The cost of the medication. This is a serious consideration if chronic administration is to be undertaken. Prednisone is the least expensive of available steroid preparations.

5 The variation in the manner in which preparations of glucosteroids are formulated. This factor may modify absorption. Thus, it is advisable for a patient whose steroid dosage has been standardized to continue to utilize the same pharmaceutical preparation to avoid relapse or overdosage.

ACTH VERSUS STEROIDS In general, adrenal steroid therapy is effective by mouth and can be regulated more accurately than ACTH therapy. The amount of steroid produced in response to ACTH varies from day to day, depending on the rate and extent of absorption of ACTH and on the state of the adrenal cortex. ACTH therapy stimulates the secretion of adrenal androgens as well as of hydroxysteroids. Sodium retention with ACTH is often more marked than with cortisone or prednisone therapy.

TABLE 317-12 Glucocorticoid preparations

	Estimated potency†	
Commonly used name*	Glucocorticoid	Mineralocorticoid
SHORT-ACTING		
Cortisol	1	1
Cortisone	0.8	0.8
INTERMEDIATE-ACTING		
Prednisone	4	0.25
Prednisolone	4	0.25
Methylprednisolone	5	<0.01
Triamcinolone	5	<0.01
LONG-ACTING		
Paramethasone	10	<0.01
Betamethasone	25	<0.01
Dexamethasone	30–40	<0.01

* The steroids are divided into three groups according to the duration of biologic activity. Short-acting preparations have a biologic half-life of less than 12 h; long-acting, greater than 48 h; and intermediate, between 12 and 36 h. Triamcinolone has the longest half-life of the intermediate-acting preparations.

† Relative milligram comparisons with cortisol, setting the glucocorticoid and mineralocorticoid properties of cortisol as 1. Sodium retention is insignificant in usual doses employed of methylprednisolone, triamcinolone, paramethasone, betamethasone, and dexamethasone.

TABLE 317-13 A "checklist" for use prior to the administration of glucocorticoids in pharmacologic dosages

1 Presence of tuberculosis or other chronic infection (chest x-ray, tuberculin test)
2 Evidence of glucose intolerance or history of gestational diabetes mellitus
3 Evidence of preexisting osteoporosis (spine x-ray or bone density assessment, if available, in postmenopausal patients)
4 History of peptic ulcer, gastritis, or esophagitis (stool guaiac test)
5 Evidence of hypertension or cardiovascular disease
6 History of psychological disorders

While some studies imply that ACTH may be superior to oral steroid therapy in the treatment of certain disorders such as dermatomyositis and multiple sclerosis, it is generally believed that the two agents are equally effective (or ineffective). Both ACTH and steroid therapy induce hypothalamopituitary suppression; however, in ACTH therapy adrenal gland size and activity are maintained, in contrast to the adrenal atrophy usually associated with steroid therapy.

EVALUATION OF PATIENT PRIOR TO INITIATING STEROID THERAPY (See Table 317-13) **Chronic infection** Three problems demand attention: (1) Any active infection, particularly tuberculosis, should be identified. If tuberculosis is present, steroid therapy can be employed, if indicated, in conjunction with antituberculous chemotherapy. (2) The chest film and tuberculin test provide baseline information for future comparison. Since high-dosage steroids minimize the tuberculin reaction, serial chest roentgenograms may be indicated. (3) Infection due to "opportunistic" low-virulence pathogens should be constantly considered in patients on high steroid dosage, especially when steroid therapy is combined with other immunosuppressive agents.

Diabetes mellitus Prolonged glucocorticoid therapy may unmask latent diabetes mellitus or aggravate preexisting disease. The presence of diabetes mellitus or the demonstration of impaired glucose tolerance may affect the decision to institute adrenal hormone therapy.

Osteoporosis All patients receiving long-continued steroid therapy are likely to develop some degree of osteoporosis. Indeed osteoporosis, with vertebral fractures or compression, is one of the most serious potential hazards of long-term steroid therapy. For patients at high risk (postmenopausal women, elderly men, and patients with restricted physical activity) initial films of the thoracolumbar segment of the spine are mandatory. Alternate-day or interrupted steroid therapy minimizes this complication (Table 317-14), and adjunctive therapies may be effective in the therapy of steroid osteoporosis (see Chap. 345).

Peptic ulcer, gastric hypersecretion, or esophagitis In conventional therapeutic doses (equivalent to 15 mg prednisone per day or less) glucocorticoids probably do not cause peptic ulceration; whether higher doses are associated with increased incidence of peptic ulcer disease is not established and probably depends on duration of treatment (as well as dose) and the presence of predisposing factors such as hypoalbuminemia or cirrhosis. However, even in conventional doses patients with a history of ulcer may experience aggravation of symptoms while receiving glucocorticoids. Consequently, all individuals with a positive history or with known risk factors should be given a vigorous "ulcer combating" program (antacids, cimetidine) along with glucocorticoids. *The development of anemia in a patient receiving glucocorticoids should suggest gastrointestinal bleeding as a cause, and patients should be cautioned to note black stools.*

TABLE 317-14 Supplementary measures to minimize undesirable metabolic effects of glucocorticoids

I Monitor caloric intake to prevent weight gain.
II Restrict sodium intake to prevent edema and minimize hypertension and potassium loss.
III Supplement potassium if necessary.
IV Give antacid therapy and/or histamine receptor antagonist therapy.
V Institute alternate-day steroid schedule if possible. Patients on steroid therapy over a prolonged period should be protected by an appropriate increase in hormone level during periods of acute stress. A rule of thumb is to *double* the maintenance dose.
VI Minimize osteopenia by (not proved effective):
  A Estrogen therapy for postmenopausal women; 0.625–1.25 mg conjugated estrogens, may be given "cyclically." Regular Papanicolaou smear and breast examination and mammography mandatory (see Chap. 322).
  B Consider supplementary vitamin D and calcium.

Hypertension or cardiovascular disease In general, the sodium-retaining propensity of many adrenal steroid preparations requires that caution be used when they are given to patients with preexisting hypertension or cardiovascular or renal disease. Use of preparations in which sodium-retaining activity is minimal, restriction of dietary sodium intake, and the use of diuretic agents and supplementary potassium salts will minimize the mineralocorticoid actions of steroid therapy. However, hypertension may still be exacerbated by several mechanisms, including steroid-induced increases in renin substrate and consequently in angiotensin II levels, and reduction in vasodilator prostaglandin production. Additionally, steroids accelerate atherogenesis by induction of hypertension, glucose intolerance, and unfavorable lipid profiles. Glucocorticoid-associated lipid abnormalities include hypertriglyceridemia and hypercholesterolemia, particularly increased LDL cholesterol levels.

Psychological difficulties Steroid therapy may be complicated by minor or severe psychological disturbances. In general, serious psychological disturbances are more closely related to the patient's personality structure than to the actual dose of hormone, although, as might be anticipated, larger doses of hormone are associated with more frequent serious reactions. At present there is no reliable method of determining beforehand a patient's psychological reaction to steroid therapy; moreover, previous tolerance of steroids does not necessarily ensure immunity to subsequent courses of therapy. Likewise, untoward psychological reactions on one occasion do not invariably mean that the patient will respond unfavorably to a second course of treatment; however, prophylactic treatment with lithium may be indicated.

Sleeplessness is a common complication and can be minimized by using the shorter-acting steroids and by prescribing the total dose as a single early-morning medication.

ALTERNATE-DAY STEROID THERAPY The single most effective measure in minimizing the cushingoid effects of glucocorticoid therapy is to administer the total 48-h dose as a *single* dose of *intermediate-acting steroid* in the morning, *every other day*. If symptoms of the underlying disorder can be controlled by this technique, the therapeutic program offers a distinct advantage. Three special considerations deserve mention: (1) The alternate-day schedule may be approached through a series of transition dose schedules that permit the patient an opportunity to adjust to the ultimate program. (2) The physician should provide the patient with supplementary nonsteroid medications, if required, on the "off day" to minimize symptoms of the underlying disorder. (3) The physician and the patient should recognize that many symptoms noted during the off day (e.g., fatigue, joint pain, muscle stiffness or tenderness, and fever) are those of relative adrenal insufficiency, rather than an exacerbation of the underlying disease. Knowing this is of vital importance, since the physician can reassure the patient and avoid giving up the program on the basis of a misconception.

The alternate-day concept capitalizes on the fact that cortisol secretion and plasma levels normally are highest in the early morning and lowest in the evening. The normal pattern is mimicked by administering an intermediate-acting steroid in the morning (7 to 8 A.M.) (Table 317-12).

Initially the steroid program often requires daily or more frequent doses of steroid to accomplish the desired anti-inflammatory or immunity-suppressing action. *Only after this desired effect has been achieved is an attempt made to switch over to an alternate-day program.* A number of programs may be employed for transferring a patient from a daily to an alternate-day program. The key points to be considered are flexibility in arranging a program and the use of supportive measures on the off day. One may attempt a transition by a series of gradations rather than by an abrupt complete changeover. One approach is to keep the steroid dose constant on one day and gradually reduce the level on the alternate day. Alternatively, the steroid dose can be increased on one day while being reduced on the alternate day. In any case it is important to anticipate that the patient will experience some increase in pain or discomfort between the 36 to 48 h following the last dose of steroid.

The general principles advocated in the long-term use of steroids and in implementing an alternate-day schedule are as follows:

1 Utilize intermediate-acting steroids such as prednisone or prednisolone.
2 Give the total daily steroid as a single morning dose.
3 Begin a transition program as soon as the manifestations of the diseases are under reasonable control.
4 If possible, eliminate steroid medication on the alternate day.

WITHDRAWAL OF GLUCOCORTICOIDS FOLLOWING THEIR LONG-TERM USE AS PHARMACOLOGIC AGENTS Complete withdrawal of steroids should be initiated by implementing an alternate-day schedule. Patients on an alternate-day program for a month or more experience less difficulty during a subsequent termination regimen as far as pituitary-adrenal function is concerned. The dosage is gradually reduced and finally discontinued after a normal replacement dosage has been reached (e.g., 5 to 7.5 mg prednisone). Complications rarely ensue unless undue stress is experienced, and patients should understand that for 1 year or longer after the complete withdrawal from long-term high-dosage steroid therapy, they should receive supplementary hormone in the presence of serious infection, operation, or injury.

In patients on high-dose daily steroid therapy, it is frequently advised to reduce total steroid dosage to approximately 20 mg prednisone daily before beginning the transition to every-other-day therapy. If a patient cannot tolerate an alternate-day program, it is debatable as to whether complete discontinuance should be considered. Under these circumstances a daily replacement dose of steroid should be continued, and at some future date another trial of gradual transition to the alternate-day schedule should be attempted. These patients will not require mineralocorticoid therapy, as aldosterone secretion is usually adequate.

REFERENCES

BECKER DM et al: Relationship between corticosteroid exposure and plasma lipid levels in heart transplant recipients. Am J Med 85:632, 1988

CHROUSOS GP et al: Late onset of 21-hydroxylase deficiency mimicking idiopathic hirsutism or polycystic ovary disease. Ann Intern Med 96:143, 1982

CROCK PA et al: Multiple pituitary hormone gradients from inferior petrosal sinus sampling in Cushing's disease. Acta Endocrinologica 119:75, 1988

HOLLENBERG SM et al: Primary structure and expression of a functional human glucocorticoid receptor cDNA. Nature 318:635, 1985

MAMPALAM TJ et al: Transsphenoidal microsurgery for Cushing disease: A report of 216 cases. Ann Intern Med 109:487, 1988

METZLER CH et al: Increased synthesis and release of atrial peptide during mineralocorticoid escape in conscious dogs. Am J Physiol 252:R188, 1987

MUJAIS SK et al: Modulation of renal sodium-potassium-adenosine triphosphatase by aldosterone. J Clin Invest 76:170, 1985

MUNCK et al: Physiological functions of glucocorticoids in stress and their relation to pharmacological actions. Endocr Rev 5:25, 1984

NEW MI, LEVINE LS: Recent advances in 21-hydroxylase deficiency. Ann Rev Med 35:649, 1984

NOLAN PM et al: Therapeutic problems with transsphenoidal pituitary surgery for Cushing's disease. Clev Clin Q 49:199, 1982

ORTH DN: The old and the new in Cushing's syndrome. N Engl J Med 310:649, 1984

OLDFIELD EH et al: Preoperative lateralization of ACTH-secreting pituitary microadenomas by bilateral and simultaneous inferior petrosal venous sinus sampling. N Engl J Med 312:100, 1985

PEDERSEN RC et al: Pro-adrenocorticotropin/endorphin-derived peptides: Coordinated action on adrenal steroidogenesis. Science 208:1044, 1980

PEMBERTON et al: Hormone binding globulins undergo serpin conformational change in inflammation. Nature 336:257, 1988

RABINOWE SL et al: la-Positive T lymphocytes in recently diagnosed idiopathic Addison's disease. Am J Med 77:597, 1984

ROSS EJ, LYNCH DC: Cushing's syndrome—killing disease: Discriminatory value of signs and symptoms aiding early diagnosis. Lancet 2:646, 1982

SCHAMBELAN M et al: Prevalence, pathogenesis and functional significance of aldosterone deficiency in hyperkalemic patients with chronic renal insufficiency. Kidney Int 17:89, 1980

SCHULTE HM et al: Continuous administration of synthetic ovine corticotropin-releasing factor in man: Physiological and pathophysiological implications. J Clin Invest 75:1781, 1985

STEWART PM et al: Mineralocorticoid activity of liquorice: 11-Beta-hydroxysteroid dehydrogenase deficiency comes of age. Lancet 2:821, 1987

STEWART PM et al: Syndrome of apparent mineralocorticoid excess. A defect in the cortisol-cortisone shuttle. J Clin Invest 82:340, 1988

SUDA T et al: Effects of corticotropin-releasing hormone and dexamethasone on proopiomelanocortin messenger RNA level in human corticotroph adenoma cells in vitro. J Clin Invest 82:110, 1988

TYRRELL JB et al: An overnight high-dose dexamethasone suppression test: Rapid differential diagnosis of Cushing's syndrome. Ann Intern Med 104:180, 1986

WEINBERGER MH: Primary aldosteronism: Diagnosis and differentiation of subtypes. Ann Intern Med 100:300, 1984

WILLIAMS GH, DLUHY RG: Control of aldosterone secretion, in *Hypertension*, 2d ed, J Genest et al (eds). New York, McGraw-Hill, 1983, p 320

WILLIAMS GH, DLUHY RG: Diagnostic imaging of the adrenal gland, in *Endocrinology*, 2d ed, LG DeGroot et al (eds). Orlando, FL, Grune and Stratton 1989, p 1633

WULFRATT NM et al: Immunoglobulins of patients with Cushing's syndrome due to pigmented adrenocortical micronodular dysplasia stimulate in vitro steroidogenesis. J Clin Endocrinol Metab 66:301, 1988

318 PHEOCHROMOCYTOMA

LEWIS LANDSBERG / JAMES B. YOUNG

Pheochromocytomas, also known as chromaffin tumors, produce, store, and secrete catecholamines. They are derived most often from the adrenal medulla but may develop from chromaffin cells in or about sympathetic ganglia (extraadrenal pheochromocytomas or paragangliomas). Related tumors that secrete catecholamines and produce similar clinical syndromes include chemodectomas derived from the carotid body and ganglioneuromas derived from the postganglionic sympathetic neurons.

The clinical features and morbidity of these tumors are due predominantly to the release of catecholamines. Hypertension is the most common manifestation, and hypertensive paroxysms or crises, often spectacular and alarming, occur in over half the cases.

Pheochromocytoma occurs only in approximately 0.1 percent of the hypertensive population, but it is, nevertheless, an important correctable cause of high blood pressure. Indeed, it is usually curable if properly diagnosed and treated, but may be fatal if undiagnosed or mistreated. Postmortem series indicate that the majority of pheochromocytomas are unsuspected clinically and that in many of these cases the tumor is related to the fatal outcome.

PATHOLOGY Location and morphology In adults approximately 80 percent occur as a unilateral solitary lesion, 10 percent are bilateral, and 10 percent are extraadrenal. In children a fourth of tumors are bilateral, and an additional fourth are extraadrenal. Solitary lesions inexplicably favor the right side. Although pheochromocytomas may grow to large size (over 3 kg), most weigh less than 100 g and are less than 10 cm in diameter. The tumors are highly vascular with an arterial supply derived from any of the three arteries that normally supply the adrenal.

The tumors are made up of large, polyhedral, pleomorphic chromaffin cells. Less than 10 percent are malignant. As with other endocrine tumors malignancy cannot be determined by the histologic appearance; local invasion of surrounding tissues or distant metastases indicate malignancy.

FAMILIAL PHEOCHROMOCYTOMA In approximately 5 percent of cases pheochromocytoma is inherited as an autosomal dominant trait either alone or in combination with other abnormalities such as multiple endocrine neoplasia (MEN) type IIa (Sipple's syndrome) or cosal neuroma syndrome) (see Chap. 325), von Reck- eurofibromatosis, or von Hippel–Lindau's retinal cer- angioblastomatosis. Bilateral adrenal pheochromocytomas mmon in the familial syndromes; within MEN kindreds over alf with pheochromocytomas have bilateral lesions. A familial syndrome should be suspected in any patient presenting with bilateral pheochromocytomas.

EXTRAADRENAL PHEOCHROMOCYTOMAS Extraadrenal pheochromocytomas have an average weight of 20 to 40 g and are usually less than 5 cm in diameter. Most are located within the abdomen in association with the celiac, superior mesenteric, and inferior mesenteric ganglia. Approximately 1 percent are in the thorax in relation to the paravertebral sympathetic ganglia, 1 percent are within the urinary bladder, and less than 1 percent are in the neck, usually in association with the sympathetic ganglia or the extracranial branches of the ninth or tenth cranial nerves.

Catecholamine synthesis, storage, and release Pheochromocytomas synthesize and store catecholamines by processes resembling those of the normal adrenal medulla (Chap. 67). Little is known about the mechanisms of catecholamine release from pheochromocytomas, but changes in blood flow and necrosis within the tumor may be the cause in some instances. These tumors are not innervated, and catecholamine release does not result from neural stimulation. Pheochromocytomas also store and secrete a variety of peptides including endogenous opioids, neuropeptide Y, and chromagranin A (see Chap. 67). The functional and clinical significance of these peptides is uncertain.

EPINEPHRINE, NOREPINEPHRINE, AND DOPAMINE Most pheochromocytomas contain and secrete both norepinephrine and epinephrine, and the percentage of norepinephrine is usually greater than in the normal adrenal. Most extraadrenal pheochromocytomas secrete norepinephrine exclusively. Rarely, pheochromocytomas produce epinephrine alone, particularly in association with MEN. Although epinephrine-producing tumors may be associated with a preponderance of metabolic and beta-receptor effects, in general the predominant catecholamine secreted cannot be predicted from the clinical presentation. Increased production of dopamine and homovanillic acid (HVA) is uncommon with benign lesions; the excretion of these precursors is, however, increased in some patients with malignant pheochromocytoma.

CLINICAL FEATURES Pheochromocytoma occurs at all ages but is most common in young to midadult life. Some series show a slight female preponderance. Although the presentation is characteristically unpredictable, most patients come to medical attention as a result of hypertensive crisis, paroxysmal symptoms suggestive of seizure disorder or anxiety attacks, or hypertension that responds poorly to conventional treatment. Less commonly, unexplained hypotension or shock in association with surgery or trauma will suggest the diagnosis.

Hypertension Hypertension is the most common manifestation. In approximately 60 percent of cases the hypertension is sustained, although significant blood pressure lability is usually present and half of patients with sustained hypertension have distinct crises or paroxysms. The other 40 percent have blood pressure elevations only during an attack. The hypertension is often severe, occasionally malignant, and usually resistant to treatment with standard drugs used for therapy of essential hypertension.

Paroxysms or crises The paroxysm or crisis is a typical manifestation, occurring in over half of patients. In an individual patient the symptoms are often similar with each attack. The paroxysms are commonly frequent but may be sporadic at intervals as long as weeks or months. With time the paroxysms usually increase in frequency, duration, and severity.

The attack usually has a sudden onset. It may last from a few minutes to several hours or longer. Headache, profuse sweating, palpitations, and apprehension, often with a sense of impending doom, are common. Pain in the chest or abdomen may be associated with nausea and vomiting. Either pallor or flushing may occur during the attack. The blood pressure is elevated, often to alarming levels, and is usually accompanied by tachycardia.

The paroxysm may be precipitated by any activity that displaces the abdominal contents. In some cases a particular stimulus may reproduce an attack in a characteristic fashion, but no clearly defined precipitating event may be found. Although anxiety may accompany the attacks, mental stress or psychological tension does not usually provoke a crisis.

Other distinctive clinical features Symptoms and signs of an increased metabolic rate, such as profuse sweating and mild to moderate weight loss, are common. Orthostatic hypotension is a consequence of diminished plasma volume and blunted sympathetic reflexes. Both of these factors predispose the patient with unsuspected pheochromocytoma to hypotension or shock during surgery or major trauma.

CARDIAC MANIFESTATIONS Sinus tachycardia, sinus bradycardia, supraventricular arrhythmias, and ventricular premature contractions have all been noted. Angina and acute myocardial infarction may occur even in the absence of coronary artery disease. Catecholamine-induced increase in myocardial oxygen consumption and, perhaps, coronary spasm may be involved in the pathogenesis of these ischemic events. Electrocardiographic changes, including nonspecific ST-T wave changes, prominent U waves, left ventricular strain patterns, and right and left bundle branch blocks may be present in the absence of demonstrable ischemia or infarction. Cardiomyopathy, either congestive with myocarditis and myocardial fibrosis or hypertrophic with concentric or asymmetric hypertrophy, may be associated with heart failure and cardiac arrhythmias. Noncardiogenic pulmonary edema may also occur in patients with pheochromocytoma, secondary to either shifts in extracellular fluid, altered pulmonary capillary permeability, or increased pulmonary venous tone.

CARBOHYDRATE INTOLERANCE Over half of patients have impaired carbohydrate tolerance due to suppression of insulin and stimulation of hepatic glucose output. The impaired glucose tolerance rarely requires specific treatment with insulin and disappears after removal of the tumor.

HEMATOCRIT Patients may have an elevated hematocrit secondary to diminished plasma volume. Rarely production of erythropoietin by the pheochromocytoma may cause a true erythrocytosis.

PHEOCHROMOCYTOMA OF THE URINARY BLADDER Pheochromocytoma within the wall of the urinary bladder may result in typical paroxysms in relation to micturition. The unique location of these tumors within the bladder wall is responsible for the production of symptoms while the tumors are quite small, and consequently, urinary catecholamine excretion may be normal or only minimally elevated. Hematuria is present in over half, and the tumor can often be visualized at cystoscopy.

Adverse drug interactions Severe and occasionally fatal paroxysms have been induced by opiates, histamine, ACTH, saralasin, and glucagon. These agents appear to release catecholamines directly from the tumor. Indirect-acting sympathomimetic amines, including methyldopa (when administered intravenously), may cause an increase in blood pressure by releasing catecholamines from the augmented stores within nerve endings. Drugs that block neuronal uptake of catecholamines, such as tricyclic antidepressants or guanethidine, may enhance the physiologic effects of circulating catecholamines. These drugs should be avoided in patients with known or suspected pheochromocytoma; indeed all medications should be carefully considered and cautiously administered in such patients.

Associated diseases Pheochromocytoma is associated with medullary carcinoma of the thyroid in the familial MEN syndrome types IIa and IIb and with hyperparathyroidism in MEN IIa (see Chap. 325). Hypercalcemia, resolving after tumor resection, has also been described in patients with pheochromocytoma in the absence of parathyroid disease, reflecting, in some cases, secretion of a non-PTH humoral factor by the tumor. Every member of MEN IIa and IIb kindreds should be screened periodically for pheochromocytoma by assay of a 24-h urine sample for catecholamines, including measurement of epinephrine. Pheochromocytoma should be excluded or removed before thyroid or parathyroid surgery.

The association of pheochromocytoma and neurofibromatosis is well recognized but not common. Nevertheless, since incomplete forms of neurofibromatosis may be associated with pheochromocytoma, minor manifestations such as five to six café au lait spots, vertebral abnormalities, or kyphoscoliosis should increase the suspicion of pheochromocytoma in a patient with hypertension. The incidence of pheochromocytoma in some kindreds with von Hippel–Lindau disease may be as high as 10 to 25 percent. Many of these are unsuspected clinically and diagnosed postmortem.

The incidence of cholelithiasis is about 15 to 20 percent in patients with pheochromocytoma. Cushing's syndrome is rarely associated with pheochromocytoma, usually a consequence of ectopic secretion of ACTH either by the pheochromocytoma or, less commonly, by a coexistent medullary carcinoma of the thyroid.

DIAGNOSIS The diagnosis is established by the demonstration of increased amounts of catecholamines or catecholamine metabolites in a 24-h urine collection. The diagnosis can usually be made by the analysis of a single 24-h urine sample, provided the patient is hypertensive or symptomatic at the time of collection.

Biochemical tests The determinations employed in the diagnosis include vanillylmandelic acid (VMA), the metanephrines, and unconjugated or "free" catecholamines (Chap. 67). Although much has been written about the relative specificity and sensitivity of the different measurements, they are probably equivalent provided the assays are properly performed. Accuracy of diagnosis is improved when two of the three determinations are employed, although this is not essential as a screening procedure. The following considerations apply to all the urinary tests: (1) Despite claims for the adequacy of determinations made on random urine samples and expressed per milligram of creatinine, analysis of a full 24-h urine sample is preferable. Creatinine should be determined as well to assess the adequacy of collection. (2) Where possible the collection should be obtained when the patient is at rest, on no medication, and without recent exposure to radiographic contrast media. Where it is not practical to discontinue all medications, those drugs known specifically to interfere in the assays (as noted above) should be avoided. (3) The urine collection should be properly acidified and kept cold during and after collection. (4) With specific high-quality assays dietary restrictions are minimal and should be specified by the laboratory performing the analyses. (5) Although most patients with pheochromocytoma excrete increased quantities of catecholamines and catecholamine metabolites, the yield is increased in patients with paroxysmal hypertension if a 24-h urine collection is initiated during a crisis.

FREE CATECHOLAMINES The upper limit of normal for total catecholamines is between 590 and 885 nmol (100 and 150 μg) per 24 h. In most patients with pheochromocytoma values in excess of 1480 nmol (250 μg) per day are obtained. Specific measurement of epinephrine is often of value since increased epinephrine excretion [over 275 nmol (50 μg) per 24 h] is usually due to an adrenal lesion and may be the only abnormality in cases associated with MEN. False-positive increases in catecholamine excretion result from exogenous catecholamines and related drugs such as methyldopa, levodopa, labetalol, and sympathomimetic amines, which may elevate catecholamine excretion for up to 2 weeks. Endogenous catecholamines from stimulation of the sympathoadrenal system may also increase urinary catecholamine excretion and result in a false-positive test. The relevant clinical situations include hypoglycemia, strenuous exertion, central nervous system disease with increased intracranial pressure, and clonidine withdrawal.

METANEPHRINES AND VMA In most laboratories the upper limit of normal is 7 μmol (1.3 mg) of total metanephrine and 35 μmol (7.0 mg) of VMA excretion per 24 h. In most patients with pheochromocytoma the increase in excretion of these metabolites is considerable, often more than three times the normal range. Metanephrine excretion is increased by exogenous and endogenous catecholamines and by treatment with monoamine oxidase inhibitors; propranolol may cause a spurious increase in metanephrine excretion, since a propranolol metabolite interferes in the commonly utilized spectrophotometric assay. VMA is less affected by endogenous and exogenous catecholamines but is spuriously increased by a variety of drugs, including carbidopa. VMA excretion is decreased by monoamine oxidase inhibitors.

PLASMA CATECHOLAMINES Measurement of plasma catecholamines has a limited application in the diagnosis. The care required in obtaining basal catecholamine levels (Chap. 67), the lack of readily available, reliable plasma catecholamine assays, and the satisfactory results obtained with urinary determinations make measurement of plasma catecholamines unnecessary in most cases. Plasma catecholamine levels are affected by the same drugs and physiologic perturbations that increase urinary catecholamine excretion. In addition, alpha- and beta-adrenergic receptor blocking agents may elevate plasma catecholamines by impairing catecholamine clearance.

In occasional patients, when the clinical features suggest pheochromocytoma and the urinary assays are borderline, measurement of plasma catecholamines may be worthwhile. Markedly elevated basal levels of total catecholamines support the diagnosis, although approximately one-third of patients with pheochromocytoma have normal or slightly elevated basal values. The usefulness of plasma catecholamine determinations may be increased by agents that suppress sympathetic nervous system activity. Clonidine and ganglionic blocking agents (Chap. 67) both markedly reduce plasma catecholamine levels in normal subjects and in patients with essential hypertension. These drugs have little effect on catecholamine levels in patients with pheochromocytoma. In patients with elevated or borderline basal catecholamine values, failure to suppress plasma or urinary levels with clonidine supports the diagnosis of pheochromocytoma.

Pharmacologic tests Reliable methods for the measurement of catecholamines and catecholamine metabolites in urine have rendered obsolete both the provocative and adrenolytic tests, which are nonspecific and entail considerable risk. A modified version of the adrenolytic test may be of some use, however, as a therapeutic trial in a patient in hypertensive crisis with features suggestive of pheochromocytoma. A positive response to phentolamine (5-mg bolus following a 0.5-mg test dose) is a reduction in blood pressure of at least 35/25 mmHg that becomes maximal after 2 min and persists for 10 to 15 min. The response to a pharmacologic agent is never diagnostic, and biochemical confirmation must always be obtained. Provocative tests in normotensive patients are potentially dangerous and rarely indicated. However, a glucagon provocative test may be of use in patients with paroxysmal hypertension and basal catecholamine levels below those usually found in patients with pheochromocytoma. Glucagon has a negligible effect on blood pressure or on plasma catecholamine levels in normal or hypertensive subjects. In patients with pheochromocytoma, on the other hand, glucagon may substantially increase both blood pressure and circulating catecholamine levels. The elevation in plasma catecholamine concentration, moreover, may occur in patients without a blood pressure response. It must be emphasized, however, that life-threatening pressor crises have occurred after administration of glucagon to patients with pheochromocytoma so that the test should never be performed casually. Careful continuous monitoring of the blood pressure is required, intravenous access must be adequate, and phentolamine must be at hand to terminate the test if a significant pressor reaction ensues.

Differential diagnosis Since the manifestations may be protean, the diagnosis must be considered and excluded in many patients with suggestive clinical features. In patients with essential hypertension and "hyperadrenergic" features such as tachycardia, sweating, and increased cardiac output, and in patients with anxiety attacks associated with blood pressure elevations, analysis of a 24-h urine collection is 've in excluding the diagnosis. Repeated determinations ted during attacks may be necessary, however, before sis can be excluded with certainty. The clonidine suppres- and glucagon stimulation tests may occasionally be helpful in excluding the diagnosis in difficult cases. Pressor crises associated with clonidine withdrawal or the use of monoamine oxidase inhibitors (Chap. 67) may mimic the paroxysms of pheochromocytoma. Factitious crises may be produced by self-administration of sympathomimetic amines in psychiatrically disturbed patients, particularly among those employed in the health care professions.

Intracranial lesions, particularly posterior fossa tumors or subarachnoid hemorrhage, may be associated with hypertension and increased excretion of catecholamines or catecholamine metabolites. While this is most common in patients who have suffered an obvious neurologic catastrophe, the possibility of subarachnoid or intracranial hemorrhage secondary to pheochromocytoma should be considered. Diencephalic or autonomic epilepsy may be associated with paroxysmal spells, hypertension, and increased plasma catecholamine levels. This rare entity may be difficult to distinguish from pheochromocytoma, but an aura, an abnormal electroencephalogram, and a beneficial response to anticonvulsant medications will often suggest the proper diagnosis.

MANAGEMENT **Preoperative management** The induction of stable alpha-adrenergic blockade is the basis of preoperative management and provides the foundation for successful surgical treatment. Once the diagnosis is established, the patient should be placed on phenoxybenzamine to induce a long-lived, noncompetitive alpha-receptor blockade. The usual initial dose is 10 mg every 12 h with increments of 10 to 20 mg added every few days until the blood pressure is controlled and the paroxysms disappear. Because of the long duration of action the therapeutic effects are cumulative, and the optimal dose must be achieved gradually with careful monitoring of supine and upright blood pressures. Most patients require between 40 and 80 mg of phenoxybenzamine per day although in some cases 200 mg or more may be necessary. Phenoxybenzamine should be administered for at least 10 to 14 days prior to surgery. Over this time the combination of alpha-receptor blockade and a liberal salt intake will restore the contracted plasma volume to normal. Before adequate alpha-adrenergic blockade with phenoxybenzamine is achieved, paroxysms may be treated with intravenous phentolamine. Prazosin, the selective $alpha_1$ antagonist, has been employed in the preoperative management of a small number of patients. Doses in the range of 1.5 to 2.5 mg every 6 h have effectively controlled blood pressure and paroxysms. The role of this agent in the management of pheochromocytoma has not been established; the relatively short duration of action may be a disadvantage compared with phenoxybenzamine. Prazosin may be useful as an antihypertensive agent in patients with suspected pheochromocytoma while workup is in progress, since it is usually better tolerated than phenoxybenzamine and prevents serious pressor crises if pheochromocytoma is present. Nitroprusside is the only other antihypertensive agent that reliably reduces blood pressure in patients with pheochromocytoma and may be useful on occasion.

Beta-adrenergic receptor-blocking agents should be given only after alpha blockade has been established, since administration of such agents by themselves may cause a paradoxic increase in blood pressure by antagonizing beta-mediated vasodilatation in skeletal muscle. Beta blockade is usually initiated when tachycardia develops during the induction of alpha-adrenergic blockade. Low doses often suffice, and a reasonable starting dose is 10 mg propranolol 3 to 4 times per day, increased as needed to control the pulse rate. Beta blockade is effective treatment for catecholamine-induced arrhythmias, particularly those potentiated by anesthetic agents.

Preoperative localization of the tumor Surgical removal of pheochromocytoma is facilitated if the location of the tumor, or tumors, can be established preoperatively. Once pheochromocytoma is diagnosed, localization should be undertaken while the patient is being prepared for surgery by the administration of alpha-receptor blocking agents. Computed tomography or magnetic resonance imaging of the adrenals is usually successful in identifying the intraadrenal lesions. Conventional chest roentgenograms and computed tomography of the chest usually suffice to identify intrathoracic lesions. If these studies are negative, abdominal aortography (once alpha-adrenergic blockade is complete) may be useful in identifying extraadrenal pheochromocytomas within the abdomen, since these lesions are often supplied by a large aberrant artery. If aortography and computed tomography fail to localize the lesion, venous sampling at different levels of the inferior and superior vena cava may reveal a step-up in catecholamine concentration in the region drained by the tumor; this area may then be restudied by selective angiography or directed scanning by computed tomography. An additional localization technique involves a radionuclide scintiscan after administration of an investigational radiopharmaceutical ^{131}I-metaiodobenzylguanidine (MIBG). This agent is concentrated by the amine uptake process and produces an external scintigraphic image at the site of the tumor. This type of scanning may be useful in characterizing lesions discovered by computed tomography when biochemical confirmation is indeterminate, as well as in localizing extraadrenal pheochromocytomas. Percutaneous fine-needle aspiration of chromaffin tumors is contraindicated; pheochromocytoma should be considered before adrenal lesions discovered by scanning techniques are aspirated.

Surgery Surgery is best performed in centers with experience in the preoperative, anesthetic, and intraoperative management of pheochromocytoma patients. In experienced hands surgical mortality is below 2 or 3 percent.

Adequate monitoring during the surgical procedure should include continuous recording of arterial pressure, central venous pressure, and electrocardiogram; in the presence of cardiac disease or if congestive failure has been present, pulmonary capillary wedge pressure should be monitored as well. Adequate fluid replacement is crucial. Intraoperative hypotension responds better to volume replacement than to the administration of vasoconstrictors. Hypertension and cardiac arrhythmias are most likely to occur during induction of anesthesia, intubation, and manipulation of the tumor. Intravenous phentolamine is usually sufficient to control the blood pressure, but nitroprusside may be required. Propranolol may be given in the treatment of tachycardia or ventricular ectopy.

PHEOCHROMOCYTOMA IN PREGNANCY Spontaneous labor and vaginal delivery in unprepared patients are usually disastrous for mother and fetus. In early pregnancy it seems reasonable to prepare the patient with phenoxybenzamine and remove the tumor as soon as the diagnosis is confirmed. The pregnancy need not be terminated, but the operative procedure itself may result in spontaneous abortion. In the third trimester, treatment with adrenergic blocking agents should be undertaken; when the fetus is of sufficient size cesarean section followed by extirpation of the tumor may be undertaken. Although the safety of adrenergic blocking drugs in pregnancy has not been established, these agents have been administered in several cases without obvious adverse effect.

UNRESECTABLE AND MALIGNANT TUMORS In cases of metastatic or locally invasive tumor or in patients with intercurrent illness that precludes surgery, long-term medical management is required. When the manifestations of pheochromocytoma cannot be adequately controlled by the chronic administration of adrenergic blocking agents, the concomitant administration of metyrosine may be required. This agent inhibits tyrosine hydroxylase, diminishes catecholamine production by the tumor, and often simplifies chronic management. Malignant pheochromocytoma frequently recurs in the retroperitoneum and metastasizes most commonly to bone and lung. Although these are resistant to radiotherapy, combination chemotherapy has had limited success in the treatment of the malignant tumors.

PROGNOSIS AND FOLLOW-UP The 5-year survival after surgery is usually over 95 percent, and the recurrence rate is less than 10 percent. After successful surgery catecholamine excretion returns to normal in about 1 week and should be measured to ensure complete tumor removal. Catecholamine excretion should be assessed at the reappearance of suggestive symptoms or yearly for several years, if the patient remains asymptomatic. In malignant pheochromocytoma the 5-year survival is less than 50 percent.

Complete removal of the pheochromocytoma cures the hypertension in approximately three-fourths. In the remainder hypertension recurs but is usually well controlled by standard antihypertensive agents. In this group either underlying essential hypertension or irreversible vascular damage induced by catecholamines may cause the persistence of the hypertension.

REFERENCES

AVERBUCH SD et al: Malignant pheochromocytoma: Effective treatment with a combination of cyclophosphamide, vincristine, and dacarbazine. Ann Intern Med 109:267, 1988
BRAVO EL, GIFFORD RW: Pheochromocytoma: Diagnosis, localization, and management. N Engl J Med 311:1298, 1984
BROWN MJ et al: Increased sensitivity and accuracy of phaeochromocytoma diagnosis achieved by use of plasma-adrenaline estimations and a pentolinium-suppression test. Lancet 1:174, 1981
DUNCAN MW et al: Measurement of norepinephrine and 3,4-dihydroxyphenylglycol in urine and plasma for the diagnosis of pheochromocytoma. N Engl J Med 319:136, 1988
ENGELMAN K: Phaeochromocytoma. Clin Endocrinol Metab 6:769, 1977
FUDGE TL et al: Current surgical management of pheochromocytoma during pregnancy. Arch Surg 115:1224, 1980
GLUSHIEN AS et al: Pheochromocytoma: Its relationship to the neurocutaneous syndromes. Am J Med 14:318, 1953
HAMILTON BP et al: Measurement of urinary epinephrine in screening for pheochromocytoma in multiple endocrine neoplasia type II. Am J Med 65:1027, 1978
HORTON WA et al: Von Hippel–Lindau disease: Clinical and pathological manifestations in nine families with 50 affected members. Arch Intern Med 136:769, 1976
JONES DH et al: The biochemical diagnosis, localization and followup of phaeochromocytoma: The role of plasma and urinary catecholamine measurements. Q J Med 49:431, 1980
KHAIRI MRA et al: Mucosal neuroma, pheochromocytoma and medullary thyroid carcinoma: Multiple endocrine neoplasia type 3. Medicine 54:89, 1975
LAURSEN K, DAMGAARD-PEDERSON K: CT for pheochromocytoma diagnosis. AJR 134:277, 1980
MACDOUGALL IC et al: Overnight clonidine suppression test in the diagnosis and exclusion of pheochromocytoma. Am J Med 84:993, 1988
MANGER WM, GIFFORD RW JR: *Pheochromocytoma*. New York, Springer-Verlag, 1977
MCCORKELL SJ, NILES NL: Fine-needle aspiration of catecholamine-producing adrenal masses: A possibly fatal mistake. Am J Roentgenol 145:113, 1985
PALUBINSKAS AJ et al: Localization of functioning pheochromocytomas by venous sampling and radioenzymatic analysis. Radiology 136:495, 1980
REINIG JW, DOPPMAN JL: Magnetic resonance imaging of the adrenal. Radiologe 26:186, 1986
REMINE WH et al: Current management of pheochromocytoma. Ann Surg 179:740, 1974
ROSS EJ et al: Preoperative and operative management of patients with pheochromocytoma. Br Med J 1:191, 1971
ST JOHN WM, GIFFORD RW JR: Prevalence of clinically unsuspected pheochromocytoma. Mayo Clin Proc 56:354, 1981
SISSON JC et al: Scintigraphic localization of pheochromocytoma. N Engl J Med 305:12, 1981
SJOERDSMA A et al: Pheochromocytoma: Current concepts of diagnosis and treatment. Ann Intern Med 65:1302, 1966
STEINER AL et al: Study of a kindred with pheochromocytoma, medullary thyroid carcinoma, hyperparathyroidism and Cushing's disease: Multiple endocrine neoplasia, type 2. Medicine 47:371, 1968
STEWART AF et al: Hypercalcemia in pheochromocytoma. Ann Intern Med 102:776, 1985

319 DIABETES MELLITUS

DANIEL W. FOSTER

Diabetes mellitus is the most common endocrine disease. The true frequency is difficult to ascertain because of differing standards of diagnosis but probably is between 1 and 2 percent. The disease is characterized by metabolic abnormalities; by long-term complications involving the eyes, kidneys, nerves, and blood vessels; and by a lesion of the basement membranes demonstrable by electron microscopy. Patients fulfilling these criteria are not homogeneous, and several distinct diabetic syndromes have been delineated.

TABLE 319-1 Classification of diabetes

A Primary
- *1* Insulin-dependent diabetes mellitus (IDDM, type 1)
- *2* Non-insulin-dependent diabetes mellitus (NIDDM, type 2)
  - *a* Nonobese NIDDM (type 1 IDDM in evolution?)
  - *b* Obese NIDDM
  - *c* Maturity-onset diabetes of the young (MODY)

B Secondary
- *1* Pancreatic disease
- *2* Hormonal abnormalities
- *3* Drug or chemical induced
- *4* Insulin receptor abnormalities
- *5* Genetic syndromes
- *6* Other

DIAGNOSIS The diagnosis of symptomatic diabetes is not difficult. When a patient presents with signs and symptoms attributable to an osmotic diuresis and is found to have hyperglycemia, essentially all physicians agree that diabetes is present. There is likewise little disagreement about an asymptomatic patient with persistently elevated fasting plasma glucose concentrations. The problem arises with the asymptomatic patient who for one reason or another is considered to be a potential diabetic but has a normal fasting glucose concentration in plasma. Such patients are often given an oral glucose tolerance test, and, if abnormal values are found, diagnosed as having "chemical" diabetes. There seems to be little question that normal glucose tolerance is strong evidence against the presence of diabetes; the predictive value of a positive test is less certain. Much evidence suggests that the standard oral glucose tolerance test overdiagnoses diabetes to a remarkable degree, probably because a variety of stresses can produce an abnormal response. The operative mechanism is thought to be epinephrine discharge. Epinephrine blocks insulin secretion, stimulates glucagon release, activates glycogen breakdown, and impairs insulin action in target tissues such that hepatic glucose production is increased and the capacity to dispose of an exogenous glucose load is impaired. Even anxiety over venipunctures may generate sufficient epinephrine to produce an abnormal test. Concomitant illness, inadequate diet, and lack of physical exercise also contribute to false-positive examinations.

In an attempt to deal with these problems, the National Diabetes Data Group of the National Institutes of Health in 1979 provided revised criteria for the diagnosis of diabetes following a challenge with oral glucose:

1 *Fasting (overnight)*: Venous plasma glucose concentration ≥7.8 mmol/L (140 mg/dL) on at least two separate occasions.[1]

2 *Following ingestion of 75 g of glucose:* Venous plasma glucose concentration ≥11.1 mmol/L (200 mg/dL) at 2 h and on at least one other occasion during the 2-h test; i.e., *two* values ≥11.1 mmol/L (≥200 mg/dL) must be obtained for diagnosis.

If the 2-h value is between 7.8 and 11.1 mmol/L (140 and 200 mg/dL) and one other value during the 2-h test period is equal to or greater than 11.1 mmol/L (200 mg/dL), a diagnosis of "impaired glucose tolerance" is suggested. The interpretation would be that persons in this category are at increased risk for the development of fasting hyperglycemia or symptomatic diabetes but that such progression is not predictable in an individual patient. Most patients (~75 percent) with impaired glucose tolerance never develop diabetes, and many subjects diagnosed as having diabetes by the second criterion may never manifest fasting hyperglycemia or symptomatic deterioration. Consequently, the oral glucose tolerance test is rarely indicated in clinical practice although it is useful as a research tool.

CLASSIFICATION A classification of diabetes is given in Table 319-1. The basic categories are those recommended by the National

[1] Venous whole blood concentrations are 15 percent lower than plasma values. Capillary whole blood, utilized in patient self-monitoring, is equivalent to venous plasma.

Group except for division into primary and secondary ary implies that no associated disease is present while in ndary category some other identifiable condition causes or ws a diabetic syndrome to develop. Insulin dependence in this classification is not equivalent to insulin therapy. Rather, the term means that the patient is at risk for ketoacidosis in the absence of insulin. Many patients classified as non-insulin-dependent require insulin for control of hyperglycemia although they do not become ketoacidotic if insulin is withdrawn.

The term *type 1* is often used as a synonym for insulin-dependent diabetes (IDDM), and *type 2* diabetes has been considered equivalent to non-insulin-dependent disease (NIDDM). This probably is not ideal since some patients with apparent non-insulin-dependent diabetes may in fact be destined to become fully insulin-dependent and prone to ketoacidosis. The subset of patients in this category are nonobese subjects who usually express HLA antigens associated with susceptibility to insulin-dependent diabetes and exhibit islet cell antibodies in the blood (see "Pathogenesis" below). For this reason it has been suggested that the classification shown in Table 319-1 be modified such that the terms *insulin-dependent* and *non-insulin-dependent* describe physiologic states (ketoacidosis-prone and ketoacidosis-resistant, respectively) while the terms *type 1* and *type 2* refer to pathogenetic mechanisms (immune-mediated and non-immune-mediated, respectively). Using such a classification three major forms of primary diabetes would be recognized: (1) type 1 insulin-dependent diabetes, (2) type 1 non-insulin-dependent diabetes, and (3) type 2 non-insulin-dependent diabetes. Category 2 can be considered as type 1 insulin-dependent diabetes in evolution; i.e., autoimmune beta-cell destruction occurs slowly rather than rapidly with the result that there is a delay in reaching the ketoacidotic threshold of insulin deficiency.

Secondary forms of diabetes encompass a host of conditions. *Pancreatic disease*, particularly chronic pancreatitis in alcoholics, is a common cause. Destruction of the beta-cell mass is the etiologic mechanism. *Hormonal causes* include pheochromocytoma, acromegaly, Cushing's syndrome, and therapeutic administration of steroid hormones. "Stress hyperglycemia," associated with severe burns, acute myocardial infarctions, and other life-threatening illnesses, is due to endogenous release of glucagon and catecholamines. Mechanisms of hormonal hyperglycemia include varying combinations of impairment of insulin release and induction of insulin resistance. A large number of *drugs* can lead to hyperglycemia, but most simply produce impaired glucose tolerance. Hyperglycemia and even ketoacidosis may occur as a result of abnormalities at the level of the *insulin receptor*. The dysfunction may be due to quantitative or qualitative defects in the receptor itself or to antibodies directed against it (see "Insulin Resistance," below). The mechanism is essentially pure insulin resistance. A number of *genetic syndromes* are associated with impaired glucose tolerance or hyperglycemia. The three most common are the lipodystrophies, myotonic dystrophy, and ataxia-telangiectasia. The final category, *other*, is poorly defined and is meant to include any condition which does not fit elsewhere in the etiologic scheme. The appearance of abnormal carbohydrate metabolism in association with any of the secondary causes does not necessarily indicate the presence of underlying diabetes although in some cases a mild, asymptomatic primary diabetes may be made overt by the secondary illness.

PREVALENCE Prevalence of diabetes is difficult to determine because various standards, many no longer acceptable, have been used in diagnosis. The National Diabetes Data Group, utilizing the 75-g oral glucose tolerance test as the diagnostic criterion, has estimated the prevalence of diabetes at 6.6 percent, with 11.2 percent of the population having impaired glucose tolerance. These figures are almost certainly too high. The estimate of 1 to 2 percent prevalence given at the beginning of this chapter is based on actual experience in long-term follow-up of patients who had a single abnormal glucose tolerance test suggestive of diabetes. Over a 5-year period less than a third of patients developed overt diabetes. Similar conclusions have been reached in Sweden where a prevalence of 1.5 percent has been estimated. Estimates for insulin-dependent diabetes are more reliable than for the non-insulin-dependent form since most patients are diagnosed after the abrupt appearance of symptoms. In England prevalence of the type 1 illness has been estimated to be 0.22 percent by age 16, and a study in the United States suggested a prevalence of 0.26 percent by age 20. If the prevalence of diabetes is about 1 percent, it follows that about one-fourth of cases have insulin-dependent disease while three-fourths are non-insulin-dependent. The relative frequency of insulin-dependent to non-insulin-dependent diabetes varies with age, being higher if a young population is studied and lower in the older age range. The cited prevalences are for the population as a whole. Certain subsets have different rates. For example, more than 40 percent of Pima Indians in the United States have type 2 NIDDM.

PATHOGENESIS OF TYPE 1 DIABETES MELLITUS By the time insulin-dependent diabetes mellitus appears, most of the beta cells in the pancreas have been destroyed. The destructive process is almost certainly autoimmune in nature, although details remain obscure. A tentative overview of the pathogenetic sequence is given in Table 319-2. *First,* genetic susceptibility to the disease must be present. *Second,* an environmental event ordinarily initiates the process in genetically susceptible individuals. Viral infection is believed to be a common triggering mechanism. The best evidence that an environmental insult is required comes from studies in monozygotic twins, in whom the concordance rate for diabetes is no more than 50 percent. If diabetes were a purely genetic illness, concordance rates would be approximately 100 percent. The *third* step in the sequence is an inflammatory response in the pancreas called "insulitis." The cells that infiltrate the islets are activated T lymphocytes. The *fourth* step is an alteration or transformation of the surface of the beta cell such that it is no longer recognized as "self" but is seen by the immune system as a foreign cell or "nonself." The *fifth* step is the development of an immune response. Because the islets are now considered "nonself," cytotoxic antibodies develop and act in concert with cell-mediated immune mechanisms. The end result is the destruction of the beta cell and the appearance of diabetes. Rarely, type 1 diabetes may develop from an exclusive environmental insult. An example is the ingestion of Vacor, a rat poison. It is also possible that in some cases autoimmune diabetes develops in the absence of an environmental trigger; i.e., it is purely genetic. Usually, however, the pathogenetic sequence is genetic predisposition → environmental insult → insulitis → conversion of beta cell from "self" to "nonself" → activation of the immune system → destruction of the beta cell → diabetes mellitus.

Genetics Although insulin-dependent diabetes aggregates in families, the mechanism of inheritance is unclear in mendelian terms. Transmission has been postulated to be autosomal dominant, recessive, and mixed, but none has been proven. The genetic predisposition is probably permissive and not causal.

Analysis of pedigrees shows a low prevalence of direct vertical

TABLE 319-2 The pathogenesis of type 1 diabetes mellitus

Step	Event	Agent or response
1	Genetic susceptibility ↓	HLAD region genes (T-cell receptor?)
2	Environmental event ↓	Virus (?)
3	Insulitis ↓	Infiltration of activated T lymphocytes
4	Activation of autoimmunity ↓	Self → nonself transition
5	Immune attack on beta cells ↓	Islet cell antibodies, cell-mediated immunity
6	Diabetes mellitus	>90 percent beta cells destroyed (alpha cells unopposed)

transmission. In one series of 35 families in which there was a child with classic insulin-dependent diabetes only four of the index cases had a parent with diabetes and two had a diabetic grandparent. Of the 99 siblings of these diabetic children only 6 had overt disease. Overall the chance of a child developing type 1 diabetes when another first-degree relative has the disease is only 5 to 10 percent. HLA identity of siblings (see below) increases the risk while nonidentity decreases it. Haploidentity (sharing of one HLA genotype) is an intermediate risk. The presence of non-insulin-dependent disease in a parent increases the risk for insulin-dependent diabetes in the offspring. It is not known whether the intermixing of IDDM and NIDDM in the same family represents a single genetic trait (i.e., the apparent NIDDM is really type 1 NIDDM) or whether two common genetic predispositions coexist in the same family by chance, each perhaps influencing the expression of the other. Low rates of transmission of IDDM make it difficult to discern mechanisms of inheritance through study of families but are reassuring to diabetic parents who may wish to have children.

One of the susceptibility genes in IDDM likely resides on the sixth chromosome in view of strong associations between diabetes and certain HLAs coded by the major histocompatibility region on this chromosome (see Chap. 14). Four loci designated by the letters A, B, C, and D (Fig. 319-1) are recognized with alleles at each site identified by numbers (e.g., DR3). A lower case w indicates that identification is provisional (e.g., DQw8). Gene products of the A, B, and C regions are called class I molecules while D-region products are called class II molecules. The D region is subdivided into DR, DP, and DQ and also contains several less well understood regions (DO, DX, DZ). HLA gene products are located in the plasma membranes of cells and are best considered as recognition and/or programming signals for initiation and amplification of immune responses in the body. Class I molecules are present on all nucleated cells and function primarily in defense against infections (especially viruses). They may also be involved in immune surveillance against malignancy. Class II molecules (also called Ia) are normally present on circulating and tissue macrophages, endothelial cells, B lymphocytes, and activated T lymphocytes. They function in the regulatory (helper-suppressor) T-cell system. They also are important in autoimmune diseases such as type 1 diabetes. Activation of the immune system is "MHC restricted." This means that antigens are recognized only if they reach the cell surface in association with a "self" HLA allele which "fits" the receptor on the responding T cell. Thus activation of cytotoxic T lymphocytes to fight a viral infection requires that a neoantigen be formed by the "self" class I molecule and the viral antigen. Similar restriction applies to antigen presentation by macrophages and B lymphocytes to helper T cells.

While definite associations exist between class I alleles and type 1 diabetes (B8, B15), the D locus is considered of primary importance with the class I loci involved through nonrandom associations with D (*linkage disequilibrium*). Because about 95 percent of white, type 1 IDDM patients express either DR3 or DR4 or the heterozygous DR3/DR4 configuration, it was initially thought that a susceptibility gene might be located nearby. Focus has now shifted to the DQ locus

FIGURE 319-1 A schematic representation of the major histocompatibility complex on chromosome 6. (*Courtesy of Dr. J. Harold Helderman.*)

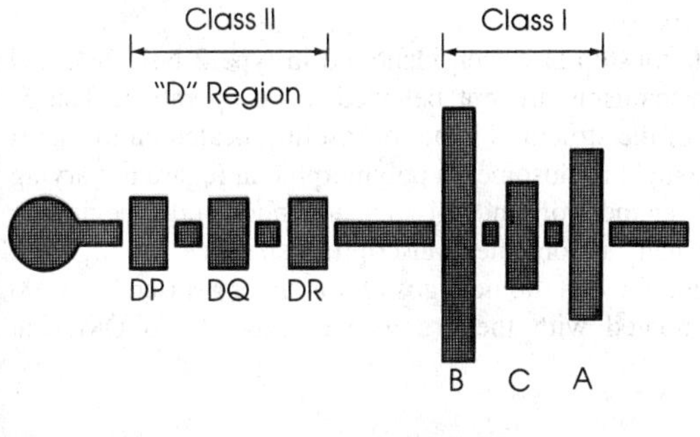

and to single amino acid changes in the gene product. Persons with alleles coding for aspartic acid in position 57 of the DQ_β chain have low susceptibility to type 1 diabetes, and persons who are homozygous $Asp_\beta57$-negative are at increased risk. A single $Asp_\beta57$ appears to exert intermediate protection in some populations but not in others. It is likely that other amino acids are also important because $Asp_\beta57$ does not appear to be protective in DR4/DR4 homozygotes. In these individuals the amino acid at position 45 appears crucial. At the time of this writing an extended allele designated DQw7 (previously DQw3.1) appears to confer protection while DQw8 (previously DQw3.2) confers maximum risk. DQw7 includes the code for $Asp_\beta57$. Interestingly, DR2/DR2 homozygotes also appear to be protected unless the DR2 clusters with a DQ_β susceptibility gene.

There seems to be little doubt that the HLA-D region is somehow involved in susceptibility to type 1 diabetes. The findings described above have narrowed the search, but other amino acid configurations may alter the function of class II molecules in such a way as to favor development of autoimmune diabetes. It is likely that allelic variation in the T-cell receptor is also involved in susceptibility to autoimmune disease, but understanding of these variations is less well developed than with the HLA side of the equation. How susceptibility or resistance is conferred remains unknown, although one theory proposes that induction of class II molecules on the surface of the beta cell (where they are normally not present) is important in initiating the destruction that leads to type 1 diabetes (see below).

Environmental event As noted earlier, the fact that a significant proportion of monozygotic twins remain discordant for diabetes (one twin with, the other without) has suggested that nongenetic factors are required for expression of diabetes in humans. Similar arguments derive from the fact that HLA identity or haploidentity does not ensure concordance.

The environmental factor in most cases is believed to be a virus capable of infecting the beta cell. A viral etiology was originally suggested by seasonal variations in the onset of the disease and what appeared to be more than a chance relationship between appearance of diabetes and preceding episodes of mumps, hepatitis, infectious mononucleosis, congenital rubella, and coxsackievirus infections. The viral hypothesis gained support from studies showing that certain strains of encephalomyocarditis virus cause diabetes in genetically susceptible mice. The isolation of a coxsackievirus B4 from the pancreas of a previously healthy boy who died following an episode of ketoacidosis and the induction of diabetes in experimental animals inoculated with the isolated virus also suggest that viruses can cause diabetes in humans. A rise in titer of neutralizing antibody to coxsackievirus over the weeks prior to death of the patient indicated that the virus was recently acquired. Further support for the viral theory comes from the observation that congenital rubella is associated with subsequent development of IDDM in about 20 percent of affected individuals in the United States. Cytomegalovirus genes have been found in the genome of a fifth of patients with type 1 diabetes. Presumably viral infections of the pancreas could induce diabetes by two mechanisms: direct inflammatory disruption of islets or induction of an immune response.

Despite its attractiveness, considerable caution should be reserved for the viral theory. Serologic studies seeking evidence of recent viral infection in patients with new-onset insulin-dependent diabetes are inconclusive at best.

Insulitis In animals activated T lymphocytes infiltrate the pancreatic islets prior to or simultaneous with development of diabetes. Lymphocytes are also found in the islets of young persons dying from new-onset diabetes, and radioactively labeled lymphocytes localize in the pancreas in humans with IDDM. These findings are in accord with the observation that immune endocrinopathies in general are associated with lymphocytic infiltration of the affected tissue. However, the insulitis might be an epiphenomenon not causally related to the pathogenetic sequence. This follows from the fact that in the low-dose streptozocin model of diabetes in rodents, which is immunologically mediated, loss of beta-cell mass occurs prior to t of insulitis. Moreover, experiments in mice with immune .dicate that T lymphocytes are not necessary for the beta- .ruction induced by low-dose streptozocin.

Conversion of the beta cell from "self" to "nonself" and activation of the immune system HLA-DR3 and -B15, known to be associated with immune endocrinopathy, are found with increased frequency in insulin-dependent diabetic subjects. There is a frequent coexistence of IDDM and other forms of autoimmune endocrinopathy such as adrenal insufficiency, Hashimoto's thyroiditis, hyperthyroidism, pernicious anemia, vitiligo, myasthenia gravis, and collagen-vascular disease (see Chap. 325). All of these conditions tend to run in families. In addition, islet cell antibodies are found in a high percentage of patients with insulin-dependent diabetes who are examined during the first year after diagnosis. These antibodies are also present in the blood of nonconcordant monozygotic twins or triplets destined to become concordant in the future. The same is true for siblings of patients with insulin-dependent diabetes mellitus. Killer T cells are present in 50 to 60 percent of recently diagnosed diabetic children, a value higher than in control populations. It is noteworthy that diabetes similar to human type 1 disease develops spontaneously in the BB rat. Affected animals exhibit insulitis, thyroiditis, and autoantibodies to pancreatic islets, smooth muscle, thyroid colloid, and gastric parietal cells. Diabetes in these animals can be prevented or reversed by immune modulation. The same is true for the NOD mouse.

What causes the autoimmune process? Early studies reported an increase in the ratio of helper to suppressor T cells in the circulation. The increase in this ratio was due to a deficiency of suppressor T cells. An unbalanced helper-T-cell population would predispose to exuberant antibody formation on exposure to antigen. Subsequent studies failed to confirm an increase in the ratio and noted lymphopenia with a greater diminution in CD4 (largely helper) than CD8 (largely suppressor) T lymphocytes. It is conceivable that early in the disease the CD4/CD8 ratio is high, changing as islet cell destruction proceeds, but this is not established.

The nature of the "self" to "nonself" transition that activates the autoimmune process remains a mystery. One theory is that the key event is an appearance of class II molecules on the surface of the insulin-producing beta cells. The idea is that these cells do not normally express D-region products but that in response to a virus (probably through production of γ-interferon) expression is induced. This would presumably allow the cell to function in antigen presentation utilizing either "self" or foreign antigens. Such antigen presentation would cause the cell to be recognized as "nonself." Whether this actually occurred would depend on the genetic makeup. Thus, if DQw7 were induced, autoimmunity and diabetes would not result, while a person bearing DQw8 would be vulnerable. Susceptibility is probably linked to the fit between newly appearing class II molecules, the requisite membrane antigen (foreign or autologous), and a particular form of the T-cell receptor on the helper T cell. This may account for the appearance of IDDM in the absence of high-risk HLA genes; i.e., in certain cases the class II molecule–T-cell receptor fit occurs even with an ordinarily low-risk allele. As attractive as the formulation is, it has been questioned because of discordant experiments that cannot be reviewed here. However, in the author's opinion it should not be dismissed, especially since alternative explanations have even more problems.

As is true in other immune-mediated endocrinopathies, evidence of an activated immune system may disappear with time. Thus, the islet cell antibodies present in newly diagnosed patients with type 1 IDDM disappear within a year or so. The presence of islet cell antibodies correlates with residual beta-cell mass as assessed in vivo by the capacity to release endogenous insulin in response to a fuel stimulus. As the capacity for endogenous insulin secretion disappears, so do islet cell antibodies. The implication is that as beta cells die, the stimulus to the immune response disappears.

Destruction of beta cells and development of IDDM Because persons developing insulin-dependent diabetes often have a rather abrupt onset of symptomatic hyperglycemia with polyuria and/or ketoacidosis, it was long assumed that beta-cell damage occurred rapidly. It is now believed that in most cases there is a slow loss of insulin reserve over a few to many years. This insight came from studies of discordant monozygotic diabetic twins and triplets where one twin or triplet developed diabetes long after the index case. In the slow course the earliest sign of abnormality is the development of islet cell antibodies at a time when there is no elevation of the blood sugar and glucose tolerance is normal. Insulin responses to a glucose load are intact. A phase then ensues in which the only metabolic abnormality is decreased glucose tolerance. Fasting blood sugar remains normal. In the third stage fasting hyperglycemia develops, but ketosis does not occur even when the diabetes is poorly controlled. The clinical appearance is that of non-insulin-dependent diabetes mellitus. With time, however, insulin dependence and ketoacidosis may develop, especially with stress. Many nonobese patients with non-insulin-dependent diabetes mellitus may have a slow autoimmune form of the disease as mentioned earlier.

The immune-directed destruction of beta cells probably involves both humoral and cell-mediated mechanisms, the latter being more important. Two types of antibodies have been identified: cytoplasmic and surface. Usually both are present simultaneously in a given patient, but either can occur alone. Islet cell surface antibodies have the capacity to fix complement and lyse beta cells. Surface antibodies appear to impair insulin release even before the beta cell is physically damaged. They interact with a membrane antigen that has not been precisely characterized. A 64,000-mol-wt peptide has received most attention, but other candidate antigens exist. One attractive target is the islet-specific glucose transport protein, since in all forms of diabetes loss of glucose-stimulated insulin secretion is the initial lesion. The fact that antibodies against insulin and proinsulin are often recognized early in the course has led some authors to feel that all such antibodies are secondary to leakage from damaged endocrine cells in the pancreas rather than a primary attack mechanism. At some point in the course cytotoxic T lymphocytes and antibody-dependent killer T cells participate in and complete the destructive process. Cytokines such as interleukin 1 (IL-1) and tumor necrosis factor (TNF-α) are likely also important. By the time overt diabetes appears, most insulin producing cells have disappeared. In one study pancreatic mass at autopsy averaged 40 g in type 1 diabetes versus 82 g in controls. Endocrine cell mass in subjects with IDDM decreased from 1395 to 413 mg, and beta cells, which averaged 850 mg in normals, were unmeasurable. Since alpha cells remained essentially intact, the ratio of glucagon- to insulin-producing cells approached infinity.

PATHOGENESIS OF TYPE 2 NON-INSULIN-DEPENDENT DIABETES Little progress has been made in understanding the pathogenesis of non-insulin-dependent diabetes mellitus. Although the disease runs in families, modes of inheritance are not known except for the variant known as *maturity-onset diabetes of the young* (MODY). This disease is manifested by mild hyperglycemia in young persons who are resistant to ketosis. Four lines of evidence suggest transmission as an autosomal dominant trait. First, three-generation direct transmission has been demonstrated in over 20 families. Second, a 1:1 ratio of diabetic to nondiabetic children is found when one parent has the disease. Third, about 90 percent of obligate carriers have diabetes. Fourth, direct male-to-male transmission excludes X-linked inheritance.

No HLA relationship has been identified in type 2 NIDDM, and autoimmune mechanisms are not believed to be operative. The 5′ flanking region of the structural gene for insulin, located on the short arm of the eleventh chromosome, is polymorphic in regard to varying number and arrangement of tandemly repeated nucleotides beginning some 363 base pairs before the transcription site (see Chap. 6). It was initially thought that homozygosity for a long insert (>1500 base pairs) correlated with the presence of type 2 NIDDM, but subsequent studies failed to confirm a unique relationship. Alcohol-induced flushing after priming with chlorpropamide has also been suggested as a genetic marker for certain forms of the type 2 illness. The fact that patients with IDDM given chlorpropamide also flush after alcohol ingestion has cast doubt on this assumption. Whatever its nature, the genetic influence is powerful, since the concordance rate for diabetes in monozygotic twins with type 2 disease approaches 100 percent. Risk to offspring and siblings of patients with NIDDM is higher than in type 1 diabetes. Nearly four-tenths of siblings and one-third of offspring eventually develop abnormal glucose tolerance or frank diabetes.

Patients with type 2 NIDDM have two physiologic defects: abnormal insulin secretion and resistance to insulin action in target tissues. The primacy of the secretory defect versus the insulin resistance is not established. Most patients with type 2 diabetes are obese, often massively so, and it has been speculated that obesity-induced insulin resistance leads to exhaustion of the beta cell; i.e., the secretory defect is secondary. On the other hand, many massively obese patients do not have diabetes or glucose intolerance, suggesting that obesity does not lead to diabetes in the presence of normal beta-cell responsiveness. The picture is further complicated by the observations that hyperglycemia per se may induce a beta-cell secretory defect and that relative insulin deficiency can cause insulin resistance. A period of aggressive dietary or insulin therapy leading to return of the blood sugar to normal may partially restore insulin secretory capacity as well as sensitivity to insulin action. Unfortunately this does not help in deciding primacy between a secretory defect and insulin resistance. The author favors the view that an islet cell abnormality is primary and necessary for development of diabetes but that acquired insulin resistance, usually obesity-related, is required for overt hyperglycemia to develop. Beta-cell mass is intact in type 2 NIDDM, in contrast to the situation with type 1 IDDM. The alpha-cell population is increased, resulting in an elevated alpha- to beta-cell ratio. This accounts for the excess of glucagon relative to insulin that characterizes NIDDM and that is a feature of all hyperglycemic states.

Although insulin resistance in type 2 NIDDM is associated with decreased numbers of insulin receptors, the bulk of the resistance is postreceptor in type (see below). Insulin resistance in NIDDM may exist independent of obesity. It has long been known that deposits of amyloid are found in the pancreas of patients with type 2 diabetes. This material is a 37-amino acid peptide termed *amylin*. Amylin is normally copackaged with insulin in secretory granules and is released simultaneously in response to insulin secretagogues. In animals amylin appears to induce insulin resistance. Its deposition in the islets may be the consequence of overproduction secondary to the insulin resistance to which it contributes. Alternatively, accumulation of amylin in the islets may contribute to the late failure of insulin production with longstanding NIDDM. The exact role of amylin is not defined.

A rare form of type 2 NIDDM, clinically mild, is due to production of an abnormal insulin that does not bind well to insulin receptors. Such persons respond normally to exogenous insulin.

CLINICAL FEATURES The manifestations of symptomatic diabetes mellitus vary from patient to patient. Most often medical help is sought because of symptoms related to hyperglycemia (polyuria, polydipsia, polyphagia), but the first event may be an acute metabolic decompensation resulting in diabetic coma. Occasionally, the initial expression is a degenerative complication such as neuropathy in the absence of symptomatic hyperglycemia. The metabolic derangements of diabetes are due to relative or absolute deficiency of insulin and relative or absolute excess of glucagon. Normally it is a rise in the molar ratio of glucagon to insulin that leads to metabolic decompensation. Changes in this ratio can be caused by a fall in insulin or a rise in glucagon concentration, separately or together. Conceptually alteration in biologic response to either hormone would have the same effect. Thus insulin resistance could cause metabolic effects expected of an elevated glucagon:insulin ratio even though the ratio assessed by immunoassay of the two hormones in plasma was not markedly abnormal or even decreased (the glucagon being biologically active, the insulin relatively inactive). The relationship between metabolic abnormalities and degenerative complications will be discussed subsequently. Typically, the clinical features of IDDM and NIDDM are distinctive.

TABLE 319-3 General characteristics of IDDM and NIDDM diabetes

	IDDM	NIDDM
Genetic locus	Chromosome 6	Chromosome 11 (?)
Age of onset	<40	>40
Body habitus	Normal to wasted	Obese
Plasma insulin	Low to absent	Normal to high
Plasma glucagon	High, suppressible	High, resistant
Acute complication	Ketoacidosis	Hyperosmolar coma
Insulin therapy	Responsive	Responsive to resistant
Sulfonylurea therapy	Unresponsive	Responsive

Insulin-dependent diabetes Insulin-dependent diabetes usually begins before the age of 40; in the United States peak incidence is around age 14. Some patients develop type 1 diabetes late in life, with the first episode of ketoacidosis occurring at age 50 or even later in rare instances. These patients, who on the basis of age should have type 2 NIDDM, are usually not obese. Onset of symptoms may be abrupt, with thirst, excessive urination, increased appetite, and weight loss developing over a several-day period. In some cases the disease is heralded by the appearance of ketoacidosis during an intercurrent illness or following surgery. As outlined in Table 319-3, type 1 patients vary from normal weight to wasted, depending on the length of time between onset of symptoms and start of treatment. Characteristically the plasma insulin is low or immeasurable. Glucagon levels are elevated but suppressible with insulin. Once symptoms have developed, insulin therapy is required. Occasionally an initial episode of ketoacidosis is followed by a symptom-free interval (the "honeymoon" period) during which no treatment is required. The likely explanation for this phenomenon is shown in Fig. 319-2.

FIGURE 319-2 Schematic representation of the "honeymoon" period. In this graph insulin secretory capacity is shown gradually decreasing in a patient destined to develop diabetes. At approximately 13½ years insulin would become insufficient to maintain plasma glucose in the normal range. An initial episode of ketoacidosis, for example, in association with acute appendicitis, is shown occurring in the twelfth year. Presumably stress-induced epinephrine release blocks insulin secretion and causes the syndrome. In normal subjects insulin reserve is such that hormone release is adequate, even in the face of stress. Following recovery from the stressful episode insulin secretory capacity returns to the previous level and remains sufficient for an additional year as indicated by the shaded area—the "honeymoon" period.

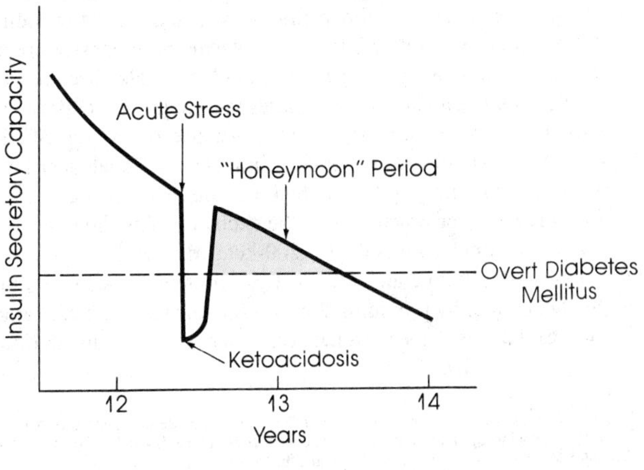

-dependent diabetes This disorder usually begins ‹eyond. The typical patient is overweight. Symptoms ...ually than in IDDM, and the diagnosis is frequently .. an asymptomatic person is found to have an elevated . glucose on routine laboratory examination. In contrast to ..sulin-dependent disease, plasma insulin levels are normal to high in absolute terms, although they are lower than predicted for the level of the plasma glucose; i.e., relative insulin deficiency is present. Stated in another way, if plasma glucose concentrations in nondiabetic subjects were raised to levels equivalent to those found in diabetic patients, insulin values would be higher in the normal group. This reflects the previously mentioned insulin secretory defect in NIDDM. Glucagon metabolism in non-insulin-dependent diabetes is complex. While the elevated fasting plasma concentrations can be lowered by large amounts of insulin, the exaggerated glucagon response to ingested nutrients cannot be suppressed; i.e., alpha-cell function remains abnormal. For unknown reasons non-insulin-dependent diabetics do not develop ketoacidosis. In the decompensated state they are susceptible to the syndrome of hyperosmolar, nonketotic coma. One hypothesis to explain the absence of ketoacidosis during stress is that the liver is resistant to glucagon so that malonyl-CoA levels remain high, inhibiting the fatty acid oxidation–ketogenic pathway (see below). If weight loss can be induced, patients may be managed by diet alone. The majority of patients failing dietary therapy respond to sulfonylureas, but improvement of hyperglycemia in many is not sufficient for control of diabetes. For this reason a high percentage of patients with NIDDM are treated with insulin.

TREATMENT Diet An estimate is made of the total energy intake needed per day based on ideal body weight (determined from life insurance tables). A decision is then made regarding carbohydrate, fat, and protein content, and an appropriate diet is constructed from the exchange system provided by the American Diabetes Association. Caloric recommendations from the Food and Nutrition Board for adults carrying out "average" activity decrease with age and range from 175 kJ per kilogram body weight (42 kcal/kg) in 18-year-old men to 140 kJ/kg (33 kcal/kg) for 75-year-old women. Intakes slightly less than official recommendations are usually preferable; 150 kJ/kg (36 kcal/kg) for men and 140 kJ/kg (34 kcal/kg) for women are reasonable initial values in most patients, but upward or downward adjustments may be necessary to achieve desired weight.

The minimal protein requirement for good nutrition is about 0.9 g per kilogram body weight per day. Recommended carbohydrate content is 40 to 60 percent of total energy intake, although fractional intakes as high as 85 percent have been prescribed. Protein and carbohydrate calories are supplemented with sufficient fat to bring energy intake to the desired level. Although sucrose is ordinarily not allowed in diabetic diets, a number of reports indicate that in moderation ordinary sugar does not exaggerate postprandial hyperglycemia. Currently most diabetic diets emphasize polyunsaturated fats as an antiatherogenic measure. Alternatively, monounsaturated fats can be used. A 50 percent fat diet containing 33 percent monounsaturated fatty acids and 35 percent carbohydrate reportedly lowers glucose levels, insulin requirements, and very low density lipoprotein concentrations while raising plasma high density lipoproteins. Fish oils containing omega 3 fatty acids have also been reported to be beneficial, but additional studies are required to draw firm conclusions. Increased amounts of fiber are also often prescribed.

Once the desirable caloric intake and the fractional distribution between fat, protein, and carbohydrate are decided, a diet has traditionally been constructed using the exchange lists shown in Table 319-4.[2] For example, a 9200-kJ (2200-kcal) diet with 50 percent of the calories as carbohydrate and 1 to 1.5 g protein per kilogram body weight can be met by providing 2 milk exchanges, 7 fruit exchanges, 12 bread exchanges, 8 meat exchanges, 4 fat exchanges, and unlimited type A vegetables (Table 319-5). In practice, precalculated diets of given caloric content prepared by the American Diabetes Association are usually used. Care must be taken to emphasize foods the patient likes and can obtain. As in any dietary regimen it is important to emphasize that it is the long-term, overall dietary pattern which counts. Deviation for one meal or two meals does not matter much. Thus a teenage diabetic may be allowed to eat a dessert, ordinarily forbidden, as a special treat with the understanding that resumption of the diet will be necessary the next day. Even in adults the "treat" technique often ensures better dietary cooperation than more rigid demands. Ideally patients should be trained by dieticians in a formal teaching program. Such classes are available in most large hospitals. If a patient is from a smaller community, it will probably be helpful to refer to a larger center for initial training.

In insulin-requiring diabetics the distribution of calories is also important if hypoglycemia is to be avoided. A typical pattern might include 20 percent of the total for breakfast, 35 percent for lunch, 30 percent for dinner, and 15 percent as a late-evening feeding. Occasionally a midafternoon snack is necessary. Different distributions may be required for different lifestyles; i.e., a person employed on a late-evening or night shift would not eat the major meal at noon. When regimens of meticulous control are attempted using multiple injections of insulin or insulin pumps, more frequent feedings are often prescribed. Thus one might recommend 20 percent of energy intake at both breakfast and lunch, 30 percent at dinner, and the remaining 30 percent as midmorning, midafternoon, and late-evening snacks depending on the pattern of plasma glucose during the day.

The traditional approach to dietary therapy has come under question as a result of experiments designed to measure actual blood sugar responses to ingested foods. It is now clear that the exchanges are not necessarily equivalent; i.e., foods of the same weight and similar fat, carbohydrate, or protein content may result in different postprandial increases in the plasma glucose. The term *glycemic index* has been coined to express these differences. In calculating a glycemic index the mean plasma glucose is measured over a 2- to 3-h period after ingestion of a test food and compared to the response with a reference standard of defined composition such as bread. Although

[2] Copies of *Exchange Lists for Meal Planning* may be ordered from the American Diabetes Association, National Service Center, 1660 Duke Street, P.O. Box 25757, Alexandria, VA 22313, or from any local affiliate of the association.

TABLE 319-4 Composition of food exchanges*

Exchange	kJ (kcal)	Carbohydrate, g	Fat, g	Protein, g
Milk	711 (170)	12	10	8
Vegetable†	146 (35)	7	—	2
Fruit	167 (40)	10	—	—
Bread	293 (70)‡	15	—	2
Meat	314 (75)‡	—	5	7
Fat	188 (45)	—	5	—

* Composition listed for one exchange.
† Type A vegetables contain little carbohydrate, fat, or protein and can be eaten in any amount. Exchange values are for type B vegetables.
‡ Calculated value for bread exchange is 285 kJ (68 kcal) and for meat exchange is 306 kJ (73 kcal) using 17 kJ/g (4 kcal/g) for carbohydrate and protein and 38 kJ/g (9 kcal/g) for fat.

TABLE 319-5 9400-KJ (2200 kcal) diabetic diet (50 percent carbohydrate)

Exchange	No.	kJ (kcal)	Carbohydrate, g	Fat, g	Protein, g
Milk	2	1420 (340)	24	20	16
Vegetable*					
Fruit	7	1170 (280)	70	—	—
Bread	12	3520 (840)	180	—	24
Meat	8	2510 (600)	—	40	56
Fat	4	750 (180)	—	20	—
Total		9370 (2240)	274 (50%)	80 (33%)	96 (17%)

* Type B vegetables include beets, carrots, onions, green peas, pumpkin, rutabagas, winter squash, and turnips. If these are desired, ½ to 1 cup can be substituted for one fruit exchange. All other common vegetables can be eaten as desired.

in principle the approach is attractive because it measures actual glycemic response to foods, its applicability to the general diabetic population is not established. One of the problems is that a glycemic index determined for a food ingested by itself may not apply in a normal mixed meal.

The importance of diet in the management of diabetes varies with type of disease. In insulin-dependent patients, particularly those on intensive insulin regimens, the composition of the diet is not of critical importance since adjustment of insulin can cover wide variations in food ingestion. In non-insulin-dependent patients not treated with exogenous insulin more rigorous adherence to a fixed diet is required since endogenous insulin reserve is limited. Such patients cannot respond to increased demand produced by excess calories or increased intake of rapidly absorbed carbohydrate.

Insulin Insulin is required for treatment of all patients with IDDM and many patients with non-insulin-dependent disease. If the physician does not use oral agents (see below), all diet-unresponsive NIDDM subjects must be given the hormone. It is fairly easy to control the symptoms of diabetes with insulin, but it is difficult to maintain a normal blood sugar throughout 24 h even if one utilizes multiple injections of regular insulin or infusion pumps. It is even more difficult to maintain normal blood sugars utilizing traditional insulin therapy given as one or two injections a day. Nondiabetic subjects maintain the plasma glucose concentration within a narrow range at all times despite episodic food intake. When a meal is eaten, a prompt rise in insulin release occurs such that absorbed carbohydrate is rapidly transported into the liver and other tissues. Even after meals, therefore, the plasma glucose in normal subjects does not rise into the hyperglycemic or glycosuric range. As the plasma glucose falls under the influence of insulin, release of the hormone is damped, and counterregulatory hormones enter the circulation to prevent hypoglycemia, ensuring smooth control of plasma glucose throughout the absorptive process. The diabetic treated with insulin by injection cannot reproduce these physiologic responses. If enough insulin is given to keep the postprandial glucose normal, inevitably too much insulin will be present during the postabsorptive phase and hypoglycemia will result. The same problem exists when insulin infusion pumps or multiple injections of insulin are utilized in an attempt to control diabetes tightly.

Because evidence suggests that some of the complications of diabetes may be prevented or partially reversed by maintenance of normal or near normal plasma glucose concentrations throughout the day, aggressive insulin therapy is frequently prescribed despite these difficulties. Three treatment regimens will be described: conventional, multiple subcutaneous injections (MSI), and continuous subcutaneous insulin infusion (CSII). *Conventional insulin therapy* involves the administration of one or two injections a day of intermediate acting insulin such as zinc insulin (lente insulin) or isophane insulin (NPH insulin) with or without the addition of small amounts of regular insulin. If the newly diagnosed diabetic is not in acute distress, therapy can be started as an outpatient, provided instruction in diet, insulin use, and monitoring are adequate and the physician can be reached by telephone for consultation. Adults of normal weight may be started on 15 to 20 units a day (the estimated daily insulin production rate in nondiabetic subjects of normal size is about 25 units a day). Obese patients, because of insulin resistance, may be started on 25 to 30 units a day. It is preferable to use the same quantity of insulin for several days before changing, the one exception being the hypoglycemic patient, for whom the dose should be immediately decreased unless a nonrecurrent cause of hypoglycemia (such as excessive exercise) is present. Generally changes should be no more than 5 or 10 units per step. It is probable that a single injection of insulin provides adequate control only in patients who have some residual capacity for insulin secretion. Poorly controlled patients should be placed on split therapy with about two-thirds of the total insulin given before breakfast and the remainder before supper. Two injections are almost always used when the total dose reaches 50 or 60 units a day but may be helpful at smaller doses as well since the peak action of intermediate insulins appears to be dose-related; i.e., a low dose may exhibit maximal activity earlier and disappear sooner than a large dose. Many physicians routinely add regular insulin to the intermediate dose even at initiation of therapy. Thus in a single-dose schedule one might begin with 20 units of intermediate and 5 units of regular insulin rather than 25 units of intermediate alone. This practice is based upon the concept that the regular insulin lowers the plasma glucose rapidly after which the more slowly absorbed insulin maintains the lowered level. Most patients on twice-daily insulin injections are also treated with a mixture of intermediate and regular insulin; e.g., 25 units NPH plus 10 units of regular before breakfast and 10 units of NPH plus 5 units of regular before supper. All patients should be taught to decrease insulin when significant extra activity or exercise is anticipated. The proper decrement must be determined by trial and error, although a reduction of 5 to 10 units is a reasonable first step. The blood glucose–lowering effect of exercise is primarily due to increased energy demands in previously non-contracting muscle; enhanced absorption of insulin from depot sites secondary to increased blood flow plays a minor role. Conversely a small amount of extra regular insulin can be taken before a meal that contains extra calories or food ordinarily not allowed (e.g., when the diabetic must eat out at a banquet or the teenager goes out on a date). For patients willing to self-monitor plasma glucose an algorithm for adjusting insulin can be provided. A typical protocol is shown in Table 319-6. Patients with complicated control problems may require hospitalization, where frequent plasma glucose determinations can guide therapy.

The *multiple subcutaneous insulin injection technique* most commonly involves administration of intermediate or long-acting insulin in the evening as a single dose together with regular insulin prior to each meal. Home glucose monitoring by the patient is necessary if the goal is the return of the plasma glucose to normal. One approach to initiation of therapy involves administration of 25 percent of the previous daily insulin dose in the patient's conventional regimen at bedtime as intermediate insulin [NPH or zinc (lente) insulin] with the other 75 percent given as regular insulin divided such that 40, 30, and 30 percent is given 30 min before breakfast, lunch, and supper, respectively. Alternatively, a three-injection schedule can be designated by omitting the night intermediate insulin and giving a long-acting insulin, such as insulin zinc extended (ultralente insulin) or protamine zinc insulin (PZI insulin), before the evening meal. Adjustments of dosage depend on response of the plasma glucose. A number of different protocols have been utilized, all of which represent sliding scales of insulin based on the plasma glucose. A typical schedule based on home monitoring of plasma glucose is shown in Table 319-7. Individual patients may require different dosages. For specific details the reader should consult one of the published papers utilizing the technique (e.g., Schriffrin and Belmonte). MSI can be effective in controlling the plasma glucose and in some studies appears to match goals achieved with CSII.

TABLE 319-6 Adjusting insulin dosage in conventional insulin therapy*

Blood glucose		Regular insulin, units	
mmol/L	mg/dL	Breakfast (to be mixed with intermediate dosage)	Supper
2.8–5.5	51–100	8	4
5.6–8.3	101–150	10	5
8.4–11.1	151–200	12	6
11.2–13.9	201–250	14	7
14.0–16.6	251–300	16	8
>16.6	>300	20	10

* Once the patient has most blood sugars in the reasonable range, a prescription can be written for varying the regular insulin dosage as illustrated. The prescription in this case was for a patient in reasonable control on 25 units of NPH plus 10 units of regular before breakfast and 10 units of NPH plus 5 units of regular before supper. Change in metabolic status may require adjustments in both intermediate insulin and the sliding scale of regular insulin.

Adjusting insulin dosage in a multiple-injection

..on of therapy
.6 to 0.7 units insulin per kilogram body weight
B 25% NPH at 9 P.M.; 75% regular in divided doses
(40% before breakfast, 30% before lunch, 30% before supper)
C Adjust NPH every 48 h based on fasting blood glucose
<3.3 mmol/L (<60 mg/dL) − 2 units
>5.0 mmol/L (>90 mg/dL) + 2 units
D Adjust regular insulin every 48 h based on 1-h postprandial glucose
<3.3 mmol/L (<60 mg/dL) − 2 units
>7.8 mmol/L (>140 mg/dL) + 2 units

II Daily therapy

Preprandial glucose		Regular insulin, units
mmol/L	mg/dL	
<33	<60	−2
3.4-5.0	61– 90	No change
5.1-6.7	91–120	+1
6.8-8.3	121–150	+2
8.4-11.0	151–200	+3
11.1-13.9	201–250	+4
>13.9	>250	+6

* With initiation of therapy insulin dosage is changed until target range is reached (see Table 319-8). After initial stabilization a variable insulin schedule is prescribed to maintain tight control. For example, if the patient after initiation is found to generally require 12 units of regular insulin before breakfast but has a prebreakfast blood sugar of 8.9 mmol/L (160 mg/dL), 15 units of regular insulin instead of the usual 12 would be taken.

SOURCE: Adapted from Schiffrin and Belmonte.

Continuous subcutaneous insulin infusion involves use of a small battery-driven pump that delivers insulin subcutaneously into the abdominal wall, usually through a 27-gauge butterfly needle. With CSII insulin is delivered at a basal rate continuously throughout the day with increased rates programmed prior to meals. Adjustments in dosage are made in response to measured capillary glucose values in a fashion similar to that used in MSI. Ordinarily about 40 percent of the total daily dose is given at the basal rate, the remainder being administered as preprandial boluses. There is little question that CSII can improve diabetic control relative to conventional therapy. Most patients report positive feelings of well-being as control improves. Nevertheless, although insulin infusion pumps have caught the attention of the public and many physicians, they should not be used indiscriminately. The danger of hypoglycemia is real, especially during the night in patients who maintain the plasma glucose consistently below 5.5 mmol/L (100 mg/dL). A fall in plasma glucose of 2.7 mmol/L (50 mg/dL) may not be important if the starting value is 8.3 mmol/L (150 mg/dL) but may be fatal if it occurs against a steady-state level of 3.3 mmol/L (60 mg/dL). Several deaths from hypoglycemia have occurred in pump users. Pumps should be prescribed only in disciplined and motivated patients who are followed by physicians with extensive experience in their use. Apart from problems of hypoglycemia, local insulin reactions and abscess formation may occur.

In some centers catheters for the insulin infusion pumps have been placed intravenously rather than subcutaneously. While few difficulties have been reported, this procedure appears unwise for routine use. Intraabdominal insulin pumps with reservoirs refillable from outside the body have been tried on experimental protocols. At present no advantage is apparent except that a pump does not have to be worn externally.

Alternative methods of insulin delivery are under study. One approach involves intranasal administration in a detergent carrier analogous to desmopressin for the treatment of diabetes insipidus. In animals insulin-secreting cells have been implanted in semipermeable membranes. The cells function for prolonged periods and respond in physiologic fashion to changing concentrations of plasma glucose. No similar human experiments have been reported.

Who should be recommended for meticulous control utilizing either MSI or CSII? There are only two absolute indications: pregnancy and renal transplantation. Maintenance of a normal plasma glucose during pregnancy prevents fetal macrosomy and respiratory distress and lowers perinatal mortality. Unfortunately, congenital malformations due to diabetes cannot be prevented by control of the blood sugar after conception occurs. This means that maximal safety for the fetus can only be provided by meticulous treatment of diabetes *prior* to impregnation. While a multicenter trial concluded that no relationship existed between degree of diabetic control and malformed fetuses, the author believes that routine treatment of diabetes in pregnancy is not an option; aggressive therapy should be initiated at the time pregnancy is planned. Inclusion of patients with renal transplants in the nonoptional category follows from the fact that diabetic nephropathy develops early in normal transplanted kidneys. The hope is that with improved metabolic control the acquired lesions can be slowed or prevented.

Meticulous control is an option for most other patients with insulin-dependent diabetes. Since the treatment schedules require much effort on the part of the patient, reliability and willingness to accept responsibility for self-care must be assessed ahead of time. Glucose monitoring is not inexpensive, and the financial status of the patient also has to be considered. Even if meticulous control does not achieve the goal of preventing late complications, in properly chosen patients it seems worthwhile in and of itself both because patients generally feel better when metabolically normal and because attention to clinical detail provides a sense of self-sufficiency and independence that is otherwise easily lost in diabetes. Meticulous control is rarely appropriate for patients whose life expectancy is shortened because of age, cardiovascular, cerebrovascular, or diabetic complications.

For surgical procedures in diabetic patients, intermediate insulin is omitted, and treatment is carried out with regular insulin alone. An effective method is to add 10 to 20 units of insulin to a liter of 5% glucose in water with infusion at a rate of 100 to 150 mL/h. Measurement of plasma glucose in capillary blood allows change of rate to avoid significant hypo- or hyperglycemia. It is also possible to administer 10 units of regular insulin subcutaneously and infuse 5 or 10% glucose at rates sufficient to avoid major changes in glucose concentration. Following surgery a sliding scale can be constructed for use in postoperative management.

Types of insulin A variety of insulins are available for use in the treatment of diabetes. Rapidly acting preparations are used in diabetic emergencies and in CSII and MSI programs. Intermediate preparations are used in conventional and MSI regimens. As noted, long-acting formulations are used in three-injection MSI schedules. Peak effects and duration vary from patient to patient and depend not only on route of administration but on dose. Hypoglycemic effects in insulin-treated diabetics appear to be delayed relative to normal subjects, probably because of the presence of anti-insulin antibodies in plasma. In one study in diabetics, regular insulin given subcutaneously had its onset of action at about 1 h, reached a peak at 6 h, and had measurable effects on average for 16 h, whereas in normal persons onset is within minutes, maximal action is around 2 h, and duration is only 6 to 8 h. With NPH insulin, diabetics exhibited an onset of action at 2.5 h, a peak at 11 h, and a total period of action of 25 h, more closely approximating values in normal subjects.

Commercial insulins are prepared in concentrations of 100 units per milliliter (U100) although higher concentrations can be obtained (e.g., U500). All commercial insulins are now "purified," meaning that they have a contamination with proinsulin <10 parts per million. Some preparations contain as little as 1 part per million. Animal insulins (beef, pork) are still in use, but insulin identical to the human molecule is now available. The advantages of purified animal insulins and "human" insulin are that insulin allergy, fat atrophy, and fat hypertrophy occur less frequently than with the previous preparations. It is possible that anti-insulin antibody (IgG) formation is slightly less with the "human" hormone. Given equivalent price structure it is appropriate to prescribe "human" insulin routinely. As stated above, the various insulins are available as rapid, intermediate, and long-acting preparations, although not all manufacturers offer all varieties. Lente and NPH insulin are used in most conventional therapy and are roughly equivalent in biologic effects, although lente appears to be slightly more immunogenic and to mix less well with regular insulin than does NPH.

Self-glucose monitoring For many years effectiveness of treatment for diabetes was followed by reviewing symptoms (such as frequency of nocturia) and measurement of glucose in the urine by semiquantitative techniques. Since the renal threshold for glucose in normal persons is in the range of 10 to 11 mmol/L (180 to 200 mg/dL) plasma glucose and may increase with the appearance of renal disease, assessment of glycosuria is of little value if the goal of therapy is to maintain the plasma glucose near normal. In consequence most insulin-requiring patients now monitor control and alter therapy based on self-measurement of the capillary blood sugar. In addition to the fact that such measurements are necessary in all treatment schedules utilizing variable insulin dosage the ability to assess the blood glucose as needed has other positive benefits. It bestows a sense of confidence and independence in the patient, has a reinforcing effect on therapeutic goals (for example, the effect of dietary indiscretion can be immediately seen), serves to give early warning of incipient hypoglycemia, and allows documentation of hypoglycemia when suggestive symptoms are present.

Although blood glucose can be estimated visually utilizing reagent strips, it is generally preferable to use an instrument for readings. This is because it is difficult for many patients to extrapolate accurately between the color changes and because subjective wishes may influence the extrapolation. It is harder to ignore a number appearing in a machine. A variety of glucose analyzers are available. The system chosen should be "dry" (i.e., not require washing of the reagent strip). In general, the cost of a machine, spring-driven lancet holder, and lancets is around $200, and many insurance carriers reimburse for the purchase. The patient needs to have supervised training in the technique, and simultaneous checks of the blood sugar in a laboratory should be done periodically to test accuracy of the self-analysis. Repeated studies show that patients can measure blood glucose accurately using these techniques.

Although urine testing for glucose is now rarely used to follow diabetes, the measurement of ketones in the urine remains important.

Goals of therapy Target levels for glucose control vary amongst diabetologists. The schedule shown in Table 319-8 lists the ranges considered acceptable and ideal by the author. The "acceptable" category would apply in conventional therapy utilizing a two-dose schedule of intermediate and regular insulin. The upper limit of 11.1 mmol/L (200 mg/dL) postprandially is arbitrary but is based on the finding in the Pima Indian population that complications of diabetes are rare if the 2-h value in the oral glucose tolerance test is less than 11.1 mmol/L. The "ideal" column represents values targeted in meticulous control regimens. Although some authors are more stringent and prefer the 1-h postprandial value to be no more than 7.8 mmol/L (140 mg/dL), the risk of hypoglycemia is greater under these circumstances. In general avoidance of serious hypoglycemia is more important than avoidance of hyperglycemia because the former has immediate consequences that may threaten the life of the patient or others (e.g., through an automobile accident) while the detrimental effects of hyperglycemia are long-term and less certain.

Hypoglycemia, the Somogyi effect, and the dawn phenomenon (See also Chap. 320) The problem of hypoglycemia is common in insulin-dependent diabetics, particularly when aggressive efforts are made to keep both the fasting plasma glucose and postprandial hyperglycemia within the normal range. Hypoglycemia may be caused by missing a meal or doing unexpected exercise but can occur in the absence of known precipitating events. Daytime episodes of hypoglycemia are usually recognized by autonomic symptoms, such as sweating, nervousness, tremor, and hunger. Hypoglycemia during sleep may produce no symptoms or cause night sweats, unpleasant dreams, and early-morning headache. In one study of insulin-dependent diabetic children monitored throughout 24 h, 18 percent had asymptomatic nocturnal hypoglycemia. If hypoglycemia is not aborted by the countercurrent regulatory mechanisms or by ingestion of carbohydrate, central nervous system symptoms ensue: confusion, abnormal behavior, loss of consciousness, or convulsions. As diabetes progresses, particularly with the development of neuropathy, epinephrine-induced symptoms may become blunted and lose their effectiveness as warning signals, with the consequence that central nervous system signs predominate. This syndrome has been dubbed *hypoglycemia unawareness*. Some authors have suggested that "human" insulin is more likely to cause unrecognized hypoglycemia than animal insulins, but this has not been observed in the United States. Up to 7 percent of deaths in insulin-dependent diabetic subjects are attributed to hypoglycemia.

TABLE 319-8 Goals for blood glucose in the control of diabetes*

Goal	Acceptable mmol/L	Acceptable mg/dL	Ideal mmol/L	Ideal mg/dL
Fasting	3.3–7.2	60–130	3.9–5.6	70–100
Preprandial	3.3–7.2	60–130	3.9–5.6	70–100
Postprandial (1 h)	<11.1	<200	<8.9	<160
3 A.M.	>3.6	>65	>3.6	>65

* Values for healthy patients below the age of 65. Goals my be shifted upward in older patients.

Protection against hypoglycemia is normally provided by two mechanisms as plasma glucose concentrations fall: cessation of insulin release and mobilization of counterregulatory hormones. The latter act to increase hepatic glucose production and decrease glucose utilization in nonhepatic tissues. Glucagon is the primary counterregulatory hormone, while epinephrine and norepinephrine released from the sympathetic nervous system serve as the major backup. Epinephrine is not required for maintenance of the plasma glucose provided glucagon is available but becomes critical in its absence. Cortisol and growth hormone do not function acutely but come into play with prolonged fasting or sustained hypoglycemia. Diabetic patients are vulnerable to hypoglycemia because of both insulin excess and counterregulatory failure. Since insulin is given by injection or infusion, the capacity to decrease plasma concentrations of the hormone as glucose levels fall is not available. Very early on the diabetic subject with type 1 insulin-dependent disease loses the capacity to increase glucagon release in response to hypoglycemia. Protection is thus dependent on epinephrine. Unfortunately, many patients subsequently also lose the capacity to release epinephrine and norepinephrine in response to hypoglycemia. In most circumstances catecholamine deficiency is probably due to diabetic autonomic neuropathy, but the defect may occur in the absence of clinically demonstrable nerve dysfunction. While failure of catecholamine release is usually a late event in diabetes, it can occur early. It is thought that beta-adrenergic blocking agents have the same effects as deficiencies of epinephrine, although a prospective clinical trial on the dangers of such agents in producing hypoglycemia under real life circumstances has not been carried out.

Counterregulatory hormone failure is especially dangerous when intensive insulin therapy is prescribed. The incidence of hypoglycemia is inversely related to the mean level of plasma glucose. Unfortunately there is no easy way to predict the occurrence of clinically significant counterregulatory failure. Experimentally an insulin infusion test can be used for this purpose but is probably not practical for routine use. In this test neuroglycopenic symptoms in the absence of autonomic signs or delay in return of plasma glucose from nadir after infusion of a standard amount of insulin are utilized to identify defects in the response system. Perhaps the best clinical clue to counterregulatory failure is the presence of frequent hypoglycemia not explicable by change in diet or exercise. Of additional concern are reports that intensive insulin therapy (meticulous control) may itself produce abnormal glucose counterregulation.

An important question is whether hypoglycemic symptoms can occur in the absence of low plasma glucose levels, for example, in response to a rapid fall in glucose concentrations. This question cannot be answered with certainty, but most evidence suggests that neither rate nor magnitude of the fall signals counterregulatory release, only a low plasma glucose. It has been traditionally believed that counterregulatory hormone release and autonomic symptoms are not triggered until the plasma glucose approaches 3 mmol/L (50 to 55 mg/dL). Careful studies in humans utilizing auditory or visual evoked potentials as a measure of cortical function in the brain have shown abnormalities at a level of 4 mmol/L glucose (70 to 72 mg/dL). A monitored drop of glucose of only 0.5 mmol/L (10 mg/dL) resulted in delay of the evoked potential and, with time, release of counterregulatory hormones. Whether the cumulative effect of mild, asymptomatic falls in plasma glucose could permanently damage the brain is unknown.

From time to time patients with diabetes report symptoms suggestive of catecholamine release in the presence of documented hyperglycemia. The cause of these episodes is unknown, but theories include simple anxiety, insulin-induced vascular permeability with hypotensive response, and sympathetic nervous system activation by insulin-enhanced carbohydrate utilization. Some authors have suggested that the threshold for CNS-stimulated autonomic activation is changed in subjects with chronic hyperglycemia, but no experimental support for this view is available.

Hypoglycemia can occur in diabetic patients consequent to other mechanisms. Diabetic renal disease is not infrequently accompanied by diminished insulin requirements and may lead to frank hypoglycemia if adjustments in dosage are not made. The mechanism is not known. Although half-times for insulin in plasma are increased in diabetic nephropathy, other factors doubtless play a role.

Hypoglycemia may be due to the development of autoimmune adrenal insufficiency as part of polyglandular autoimmune deficiency (see Chap. 325), which is more frequent in diabetics than in the population as a whole. Some patients develop hypoglycemia in association with high levels of circulating insulin antibodies. The exact mechanism has not been established. Occasionally an insulinoma may develop in a diabetic patient. Very rarely, permanent remission of apparently typical diabetes occurs. The reason is not known, but the initial sign may be frequent hypoglycemia in a previously well-controlled patient.

It must be emphasized that hypoglycemic attacks are dangerous and if frequent portend a serious or even fatal outcome. If the patient is conscious, sugar, candy, or a sugar-containing beverage can be given. If the patient is unarousable or unconscious, intravenous glucose is required. Patients should have a vial of glucagon available as well. If access to medical care is delayed, administration of 1 mg glucagon intramuscularly frequently aborts the attack.

The *Somogyi phenomenon* refers to rebound hyperglycemia following an episode of hypoglycemia due to counterregulatory hormone release. It should be suspected whenever wide swings in the plasma glucose occur over short time intervals even if symptoms are not reported. Such rapid changes contrast with the alterations seen following insulin withdrawal in previously well-controlled diabetic patients in whom hyperglycemia and ketosis develop gradually and smoothly over a 12- to 24-h period. Excessive hunger and weight gain occurring in the context of worsening hyperglycemia are clues that the insulin dosage may be too high, since poor control due to underinsulinization usually results in weight loss (because of osmotic diuresis and glucose wastage). If the Somogyi phenomenon is suspected, the insulin dose should be decreased as a trial, even when specific symptoms of overinsulinization are absent. The Somogyi phenomenon is probably rare in adults but may be more frequent in children.

The *dawn phenomenon* refers to an early morning rise in plasma glucose requiring increased amounts of insulin to maintain euglycemia. Although similar early morning hyperglycemia may result from hypoglycemia, as just described, the dawn phenomenon itself is thought to be independent of the Somogyi mechanism. The nocturnal surge of growth hormone release may be a factor. Increased clearance of insulin also occurs in the early morning hours, but the changes are probably not of major importance. Differentiation between the dawn phenomenon and posthypoglycemic hyperglycemia can usually be accomplished by measuring the blood glucose at 3 A.M. This is important since the Somogyi phenomenon is avoided by decreasing insulin dosages for the critical time period while the dawn phenomenon usually requires increased insulin to maintain glucose in the normal range.

Oral agents Non-insulin-dependent diabetes that cannot be controlled by dietary management often responds to sulfonylureas. The drugs are easy to use and appear to be safe. Fear that sulfonylureas might increase deaths from heart attacks, prompted by reports of the University Group Diabetes Program (UGDP), has largely dissipated because of questions about the design of that study and failure of other studies to confirm risks. On the other hand use of the oral drugs has decreased concomitant with the emphasis on better control as a possible means of slowing the development of late complications. While some patients with relatively mild disease have return of plasma glucose to normal on oral drugs, those with significant hyperglycemia tend to improve but do not approach the normal range. Thus a high percentage of non-insulin-dependent diabetics are now treated with insulin.

Sulfonylureas act primarily by stimulating release of insulin from the beta cell. They have the capacity to increase the number of insulin receptors in target tissues and also enhance insulin-mediated glucose disposal independent of an increase in insulin binding, but these effects are physiologically unimportant. Mean levels of plasma insulin do not increase following treatment with sulfonylureas despite significantly improved mean plasma glucose concentrations. The paradox of improved glucose metabolism in the absence of higher steady-state levels of insulin has been resolved by studies which show that elevation of plasma glucose to pretreatment values results in a rise of plasma insulin to levels higher than those seen pretreatment. Thus, the initial action of the drugs is to increase insulin release with lowering of the plasma glucose. As glucose concentrations fall, insulin levels also decrease since plasma glucose is the major stimulus to insulin release, thereby masking the initial stimulation of insulin secretion. The insulinogenic effect can then be unmasked by raising the plasma glucose to the previous elevated levels. The fact that sulfonylureas are ineffective in IDDM, where beta-cell mass is diminished, supports the pancreatic effect as primary, although as noted extrapancreatic mechanisms may play a minor role.

The characteristics of the sulfonylureas are summarized in Table 319-9. The newer drugs such as glipizide and glyburide are effective in smaller doses but otherwise differ little from agents in long use such as chlorpropamide and tolbutamide. In patients who have significant renal disease it is preferable to treat with tolbutamide or tolazamide since these agents are exclusively metabolized and inactivated by the liver. Chlorpropamide has the capacity to sensitize the renal tubule to antidiuretic hormone. It thus is helpful in some patients with partial diabetes insipidus but may cause water retention in patients with diabetes mellitus. Hypoglycemia is less common with oral agents than with insulin, but when it occurs it tends to be severe and prolonged. Some patients have required massive glucose infusions for days following the last dose of sulfonylurea. For this reason hospitalization is mandatory in patients with sulfonylurea-induced hypoglycemia.

The only other oral agents effective in the treatment of maturity-onset diabetes are the biguanides. They presumably lower plasma glucose by inhibiting gluconeogenesis in the liver although phenformin may increase the number of insulin receptors in some tissues. The drugs are ordinarily used only in combination with sulfonylureas under circumstances in which control is inadequate with sulfonylurea alone. Because of many reports linking phenformin to the appearance of lactic acidosis, the Food and Drug Administration removed the agent from routine clinical use in the United States. Phenformin and other biguanides are still used elsewhere in the world. Biguanides

TABLE 319-9 The sulfonylureas

Agent	Daily dose, mg	Doses per day	Duration of hyperglycemic action, h	Metabolism/excretion
Acetohexamide	250–1500	1–2	12–18	Liver/kidney
Chlorpropamide	100–500	1	60	Kidney
Tolazamide	100–1000	1–2	12–14	Liver
Tolbutamide	500–3000	2–3	6–12	Liver
Glyburide	1.25–20	1–2	Up to 24	Liver/kidney
Glipizide	2.5–40	1–2	Up to 24	Liver/kidney
Glibornuride	12.5–100	1–2	Up to 24	Liver/kidney

SOURCE: RH Unger, DW Foster.

should not be given to patients with renal disease and should be stopped if nausea, vomiting, diarrhea, or any intercurrent illness appears.

Two naturally occurring peptides are currently under investigation as adjuncts to treatment in NIDDM. Both insulin-like growth factor 1 (IGF-1, somatomedin C) and a product of the glucagon precursor gene called GLP-1 (glucagon-like peptide 1) or insulinotropin lower plasma glucose in normal subjects and in patients with type 2 diabetes. Their ultimate usefulness is not established.

Monitoring control of diabetes For those patients who measure blood glucose frequently for adjustment of insulin dosage an estimate of mean ambient glucose concentrations is readily available. For other patients, and as a check on accuracy of the self measurements, most diabetologists now measure hemoglobin A_{1c} to assess long-term control. Hemoglobin A_{1c}, a fast-moving minor hemoglobin component, is present in normal persons but increases in the presence of hyperglycemia. Its enhanced electrophoretic mobility is due to nonenzymatic glycation of the amino acids valine and lysine. The reaction is as follows:

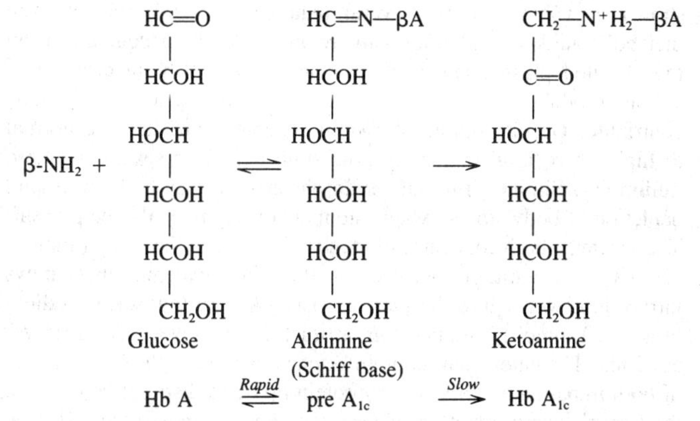

In this scheme β-NH_2 stands for the terminal valine of the β chain of hemoglobin. Aldimine formation is reversible so that pre-A_{1c} is labile while ketoamine formation is irreversible and thus stable. Pre-A_{1c} levels depend on the ambient glucose concentrations and do not reflect long-term control although they are measured in chromatographic methods for determining hemoglobin A_{1c}. Pre-A_{1c} must thus be removed to assess true Hb A_{1c} values accurately. Many laboratories employ high-performance liquid chromatography (HPLC) to make the measurement. A colorimetric method utilizing thiobarbituric acid also does not measure the labile pre-A_{1c} fraction. When properly assayed, the percent of glycated hemoglobin gives an estimate of diabetic control for the preceding 3-month period. Normal values must be obtained for each lab; on average nondiabetic subjects have Hb A_{1c} values of around 6 percent, and levels in poorly controlled diabetics may reach 10 to 12 percent. Measurement of glycated hemoglobin gives an objective assessment of metabolic control. Discrepancies between reported plasma glucose values and hemoglobin A_{1c} concentrations suggest either that measurement or reporting of the former is not accurate. Measurement of glycated albumin, because of its short half-life, can be used to monitor diabetic control over a 1- to 2-week period but clinically is rarely used.

ACUTE METABOLIC COMPLICATIONS In addition to hypoglycemia, diabetics are susceptible to two major acute metabolic complications: diabetic ketoacidosis and hyperosmolar, nonketotic coma. The former is a complication of insulin-dependent diabetes, while the latter usually occurs in the setting of non-insulin-dependent disease. Ketoacidosis rarely, if ever, develops in true type 2 diabetes.

Diabetic ketoacidosis Diabetic ketoacidosis appears to require insulin deficiency coupled with a relative or absolute increase in glucagon concentration. It is often caused by cessation of insulin intake but may result from physical (e.g., infection, surgery) or emotional stress despite continued insulin therapy. In the former case the concentration of glucagon rises secondary to insulin withdrawal, while in stress the operative stimulus is probably epinephrine and/or norepinephrine. In addition to stimulating glucagon secretion epinephrine presumably blocks release of the small amount of residual insulin found in some subjects with IDDM and inhibits insulin-induced glucose transport in peripheral tissues. These hormonal changes have multiple effects, but two are critical: (1) They induce maximal gluconeogenesis and impair peripheral utilization of glucose, causing severe hyperglycemia. Glucagon facilitates gluconeogenesis by inducing a fall in fructose-2,6-bisphosphate, an intermediate that stimulates glycolysis through activation of phosphofructokinase and blocks gluconeogenesis by inhibiting fructose bisphosphatase. When fructose-2,6-bisphosphate concentrations fall, glycolysis is inhibited, and gluconeogenesis is enhanced. The resultant hyperglycemia induces an osmotic diuresis that leads to the volume depletion and dehydration that characterize the ketoacidotic state. (2) They activate the ketogenic process and thus initiate development of metabolic acidosis. For ketosis to occur, changes must be produced in both adipose tissue and the liver. Free fatty acids from adipose stores represent the primary substrate for ketone body formation, and plasma levels of free fatty acids must rise if high rates of ketogenesis are to develop. However, fatty acids delivered to the liver are simply reesterified and stored as hepatic triglyceride or converted into very low density lipoproteins and transported back into the circulation unless the hepatic oxidative machinery for fatty acids is activated. While free fatty acid release is enhanced directly by insulin deficiency, accelerated fatty acid oxidation in the liver is primarily induced by glucagon, via action on the carnitine palmitoyltransferase system of enzymes responsible for the transport of fatty acids into the mitochondria following their esterification to coenzyme A. As shown in Fig. 319-3 carnitine palmitoyltransferase I transesterifies fatty acyl-CoA to fatty acylcarnitine, which then traverses the inner mitochondrial membrane via translocase. Reversal of the reaction occurs internally under the influence of carnitine palmitoyltransferase II. In the fed state carnitine palmitoyltransferase I is inactive, and, as a consequence, long-chain fatty acids cannot reach the β-oxidative enzymes for ketone body production. During starvation or uncontrolled diabetes the system is activated; under these circumstances the rate of ketogenesis is a first-order function of the concentration of fatty acids reaching transferase I.

Glucagon (or a change in the glucagon/insulin ratio) activates the

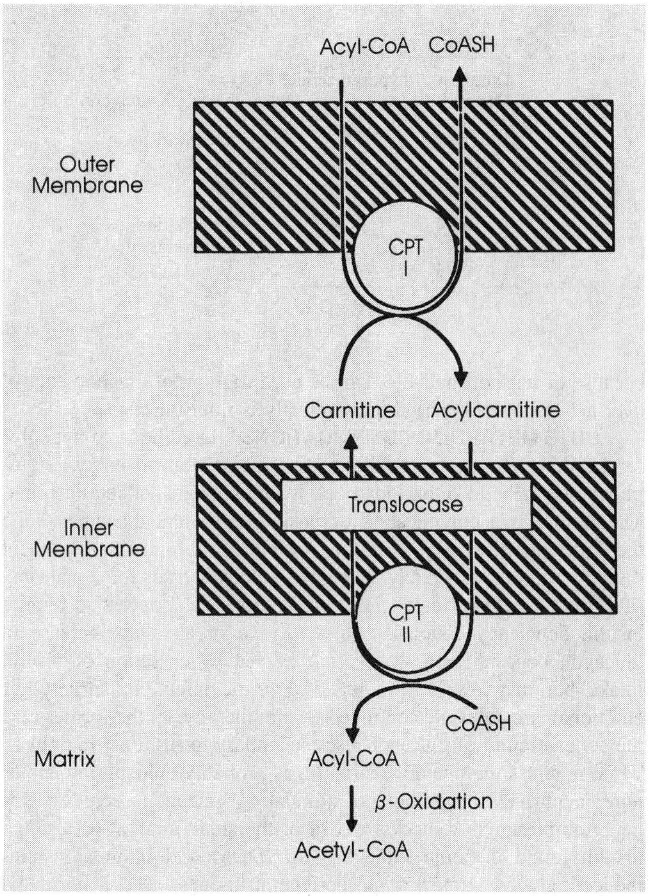

FIGURE 319-3 The carnitine palmitoyltransferase system. Long-chain fatty acyl-CoA molecules require transesterification to carnitine to traverse the inner mitochondrial membrane. Once across, the transesterification is reversed, and the fatty acyl-CoA is oxidized to either ketone bodies (liver) or CO_2 and water with the generation of ATP (nonhepatic tissues). CPT I is the rate limiting step, controlled by malonyl-CoA levels in tissue. CPT I, carnitine palmitoyltransferase I; CPT II, palmitoyltransferase II.

transport system in two ways. First, glucagon causes a rapid fall in hepatic malonyl-CoA content. It does so by interrupting the sequence glucose-6-phosphate → pyruvate → citrate → acetyl CoA → malonyl CoA via the previously mentioned decrease in fructose-2,6-bisphosphate. Malonyl-CoA, the first committed intermediate in the synthesis of fatty acids from glucose, is a competitive inhibitor of carnitine palmitoyltransferase I, and a fall in its concentration activates the enzyme. Second, glucagon causes a rise in hepatic carnitine concentration, which then drives the reaction toward fatty acylcarnitine formation by mass action. These events are summarized schematically in Fig. 319-4. At high plasma fatty acid concentrations hepatic uptake of fatty acids is sufficient to saturate both oxidative and esterifying pathways, resulting in fatty liver, hypertriglyceridemia, and ketoacidosis. Overproduction of ketones by the liver is the primary event in ketotic states, but limitation of peripheral utilization also plays a role at high concentrations of acetoacetate and β-hydroxybutyrate.

Clinically ketoacidosis begins with anorexia, nausea, and vomiting, coupled with an increased rate of urine formation. Abdominal pain may be present. If untreated, altered consciousness or frank coma may occur. Initial examination usually shows Kussmaul respiration, together with signs of volume depletion. Rarely the latter is sufficient to cause vascular collapse and renal shutdown. Body temperature is normal or below normal in uncomplicated ketoacidosis, and fever suggests the presence of infection. Leukocytosis, frequently very marked, is a feature of diabetic acidosis per se and may not indicate infection.

The characteristic metabolic abnormalities of diabetic coma are

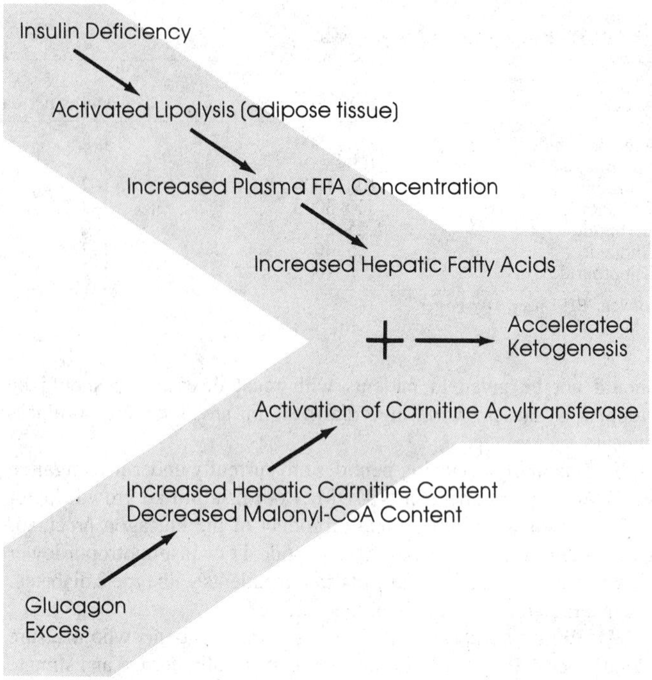

FIGURE 319-4 The regulation of ketogenesis. Significant production of acetoacetate and β-hydroxybutyrate by the liver requires provision of adequate free fatty acid substrate and activation of fatty acid oxidation. Lipolysis is primarily increased by insulin deficiency while the fatty acid oxidative sequence is activated primarily by glucagon. The immediate signal for oxidation is a fall in malonyl CoA content. *(After JD McGarry, DW Foster, Am J Med 61:9, 1976.)*

shown in Table 319-10. Several features deserve comment. The metabolic acidosis and anion gap are almost totally accounted for by the elevated plasma levels of acetoacetate and β-hydroxybutyrate, although other acids (e.g., lactate, free fatty acids, phosphates) contribute. Despite initial potassium concentrations that are normal to high, there is a total body potassium deficit of several hundred millimoles. Similarly, initial serum phosphorus may be high despite depletion of body stores. Magnesium deficiency may also be present. The serum sodium concentration tends to be low in the face of modest osmolar concentration because of the hyperglycemia that draws intracellular water into the plasma space. A very low serum sodium (e.g., 110 mmol/L) suggests an artifact due to severe hypertriglyceridemia. The latter is common in ketoacidosis and is the consequence of both impaired activity of lipoprotein lipase (a disposal defect) and the hepatic overproduction of very low density lipoproteins. If a fat meal has been ingested prior to the onset of ketoacidosis, chylomicrons

TABLE 319-10 Initial laboratory findings in diabetic ketoacidosis

Series	Dallas*	Los Angeles†	Washington‡
Age, y HL	38	36	43
Glucose, mmol/L (mg/dL)	26(475)	37(675)	41(733)
Sodium, mmol/L	132	131	132
Potassium, mmol/L	4.8	5.3	6.0
Bicarbonate, mmol/L	<10	6	10
BUN, mmol/L (mg/dL)	9(25)	11(32)	15(42)
Acetoacetate, mmol/L	4.8	—	—
β-Hydroxybutyrate, mmol/L	137	—	—
Free fatty acids, mmol/L	2.1	—	2.3
Lactate, mmol/L	4.6	—	—
Osmolarity, mosmol/liter	310	323	331

* Eighty-eight consecutive episodes of ketoacidosis at Parkland Memorial Hospital (DW Foster, unpublished observations).
† Mean data from 308 episodes of nonfatal ketoacidosis (PM Beigelman, Diabetes 20:490, 1971).
‡ Mean data from 10 episodes of ketoacidosis (JE Gerich et al, Diabetes 20:228, 1971).

may make up a major portion of the circulating fat. Lipemia is usually visible if triglyceride concentration is above 4.5 mmol/L (400 mg/dL). True hyponatremia may occur if the patient has vomited repeatedly and continued to drink water. Prerenal azotemia, reflecting volume depletion, is usually modest in degree and reversible with treatment. The serum amylase may be elevated, and frank pancreatitis can occur.

The diagnosis of ketoacidosis in a known diabetic is not difficult. Its appearance in a patient not previously known to have diabetes requires differentiation from the other common causes of metabolic acidosis with an anion gap: lactic acidosis, uremia, alcoholic ketoacidosis, and certain poisonings. The first step is to test the urine for glucose and ketones. If urine ketones are negative, another cause for the acidosis is likely. If positive, plasma examination is required to be certain that something more than starvation ketosis is present. Since quantitative determinations of acetoacetate and β-hydroxybutyrate are not routinely available, semiquantitative tests must be done using ketone reagent strips. Serial dilutions of plasma can be made and tested. A strong test may occur in undiluted plasma owing to starvation alone; a strong reaction beyond 1:1 dilution is presumptive evidence for ketoacidosis. Apart from diabetes the only other common ketoacidotic state is alcoholic ketoacidosis. This syndrome, which by definition occurs in chronic alcoholics, usually follows a debauch, but the patient may not have had alcohol for 24 h or longer. It never occurs in the absence of starvation and frequently is associated with severe vomiting and abdominal pain. Pancreatitis is present in up to 75 percent of patients. A plasma glucose of less than 8.3 mmol/L (150 mg/dL) was found in three-fourths of cases and in 15 percent was less than 2.8 mmol/L (50 mg/dL) on arrival at the hospital. Hyperglycemia may occur but is usually mild and rarely, if ever, above 17 mmol/L (300 mg/dL). Plasma free fatty acid concentrations are higher (mean 2.9 mmol/L) than in normal starvation (range 0.7 to 1.0 mmol/L), reaching levels seen in diabetic ketoacidosis. Presumably the liver is activated for ketogenesis by starvation in these patients and driven to maximal rates of ketone formation by the high fatty acid levels. Why some alcoholics mobilize fatty acids excessively is not known. In contrast to diabetic acidosis, the syndrome is rapidly reversible by the intravenous administration of glucose. As in all alcoholics given glucose, thiamine should be supplied to avoid precipitation of acute beriberi. (Other water-soluble vitamins, though not as critical, should also be infused.) Insulin is required only if hyperglycemia persists during therapy.

Diabetic ketoacidosis cannot be reversed without insulin. For decades 50 or more units of insulin were given per hour until ketosis was reversed, but now most patients are treated by "low-dose" insulin schedules in which 8 to 10 units of insulin are infused intravenously each hour. Most diabetic acidosis can be reversed adequately with low-dose treatment, but some patients do not respond. Presumably the insulin resistance that is characteristic of diabetic ketoacidosis is more pronounced in these patients than in responsive subjects. The problem is that resistant subjects cannot be identified prospectively. For this reason it is probably preferable to treat ketoacidosis with 25 to 50 units of regular insulin intravenously hourly until the acidosis is reversed. It can be given as a bolus or by constant infusion. There are no known toxic effects of larger insulin doses, since maximal physiologic response is obtained once insulin receptors are saturated regardless of how much insulin is given. The advantage of the higher dosage schedule is that it ensures saturation of the receptors in the face of competing antibodies or other resistance factors. High concentrations of insulin probably accelerate the reversal of ketoacidosis by acting via the IgF-1 receptor. Hormonal interaction with this receptor can lower plasma glucose by a mechanism independent of the insulin receptor. If physicians choose to use the low-dose insulin schedule, they should be alert to the possibility of resistance. Should acidosis persist unabated after several hours of treatment, larger amounts of insulin are clearly indicated. Ketoacidosis can also be adequately treated with intramuscular (but not subcutaneous) insulin.

Therapy of ketoacidosis also requires intravenous fluids. The usual fluid deficit is 3 to 5 liters, and both salt solutions and free water are needed. One to two liters of isotonic saline or Ringer's lactate should be given rapidly intravenously on arrival, with additional amounts determined by urine output and clinical assessment of the fluid state. When the plasma glucose falls to about 17 mmol/L (300 mg/dL), 5% glucose solutions should be given, both as a source of free water and as a prophylactic measure to prevent the late cerebral edema syndrome. The latter is a rare complication of ketoacidosis occurring most often in children. It is suspected when the patient remains comatose or lapses into coma following reversal of acidosis.

Potassium replacement is always necessary, but the time of administration will vary. The initial potassium is often high despite a total body deficit because of the severe acidosis. In this case the cation will ordinarily not be needed until 3 to 4 h after initiation of therapy, when reversal of acidosis and the action of insulin cause a shift of K^+ into intracellular water. On the other hand if the admission value is normal or low, potassium should be given early, since plasma concentrations fall rapidly during therapy, predisposing the patient to cardiac arrhythmias. In view of the phosphate depletion of ketoacidosis, potassium should be administered initially as the phosphate salt rather than as potassium chloride.

Bicarbonate therapy is indicated in severely acidotic patients (pH 7.0 or below), especially if hypotension is present (acidosis itself can cause vascular collapse). It is not used routinely in less acutely ill subjects since rapid alkalinization may have detrimental effects on oxygen delivery to tissues. The hemoglobin-oxygen dissociation curve is normal in diabetic ketoacidosis because of the opposing effects of acidosis and deficiency of red blood cell 2,3-diphosphoglycerate (2,3-DPG). If the acidosis is rapidly reversed, the deficiency of 2,3-DPG becomes manifest, increasing the avidity with which hemoglobin binds oxygen and impairing the release of oxygen in peripheral tissues. In a volume-depleted patient with poor tissue perfusion such a change theoretically could predispose to the development of lactic acidosis. It is also thought that bicarbonate may impair left ventricular function through paradoxical acidification due to more rapid entry of CO_2 than bicarbonate into intracellular water. If bicarbonate is given, the infusion should be stopped when the pH reaches 7.2 to minimize possible detrimental side effects and to prevent metabolic alkalosis as circulating ketones are metabolized to bicarbonate with reversal of ketoacidosis.

In following the response to treatment, two points should be emphasized. (1) Plasma glucose invariably falls more rapidly than plasma ketones. Insulin should not be stopped because glucose concentrations approach normal; rather, as mentioned, glucose should be infused and insulin continued until the ketosis has cleared. (2) Plasma ketone values are not very helpful. The testing materials measure acetoacetate and acetone but not β-hydroxybutyrate. Since β-hydroxybutyrate must be oxidized to acetoacetate prior to utilization, it is characteristic for the plasma ketones measured by reagent strip to remain stable or even rise early in therapy at a time when total ketone concentration (acetoacetate plus β-hydroxybutyrate) is steadily falling. Because β-hydroxybutyrate and acetoacetate represent a redox couple in equilibrium with mitochondrial NADH/NAD concentrations, vascular collapse or severe hypoxia may mask the presence of ketoacidosis as acetoacetate is reduced to β-hydroxybutyrate. Under these circumstances the β-hydroxybutyrate/acetoacetate ratio, normally about 3:1, may reach 7:1 or 8:1. Paradoxically, in such a situation, ketosis may seem to worsen as the patient gets better because of conversion of β-hydroxybutyrate to acetoacetate when the circulation is reestablished and tissue oxygenation is restored. The key parameters to follow are the pH and the calculated anion gap since these give a more accurate assessment of therapeutic progress. The usual picture is for the pH to rise and the anion gap to narrow even though the plasma bicarbonate remains low. The persistently low bicarbonate is the consequence of hyperchloremia that develops because of rapid infusion of sodium chloride, the loss of potential bicarbonate from the body in urine as ketones, and exchanges with intracellular buffers. Some patients demonstrate a persistent anion gap despite clinical improvement and a rising pH. Presumably, the unmeasured anion derives from tissue buffers. If the anion gap remains elevated and pH is persistently low, this indicates insulin resistance and requires aggressive increase in the amount of insulin administered. On the other hand, persistence of the anion gap does not indicate resistance when present in the face of clinical improvement and a rising pH.

All patients should be followed with a flow sheet outlining amounts and timing of insulin and fluids together with a record of vital signs, urine volume, and blood chemistries. Without such a record therapy tends to become chaotic.

Most patients with diabetic ketoacidosis recover when properly treated. While mortality in large series is reported to be around 10 percent, the majority of deaths result from late complications rather than from ketoacidosis itself. The major causes are myocardial infarction and infection, particularly pneumonia. Poor prognostic signs on admission include hypotension, azotemia, deep coma, and associated illness. In children, cerebral edema is a common cause of death (less frequent in adults). The cause of the brain swelling is not known. Theories include osmotic disequilibrium between brain and plasma as glucose is rapidly lowered, decreased plasma oncotic pressure due to infusion of large amounts of saline, and insulin-induced ion flux across the blood-brain barrier. Whatever the mechanism, mortality rates are high. Diagnosis is usually made by CT scan. Treatment involves the bolus infusion of 1 g mannitol per kilogram body weight in the form of a 20% solution. Although of questionable benefit, dexamethasone is also usually given: 12 mg initially then 4 mg every 6 h. If there is no response, hyperventilation to an arterial P_{CO_2} of about 28 mmHg should be carried out by an anesthesiologist or pulmonary specialist.

Other acute complications of ketoacidosis include vascular thrombosis and the adult respiratory distress syndrome. The former is induced by volume depletion, hyperosmolarity, increased viscosity of blood, and changes in clotting factors favoring thrombosis. The cause of the pulmonary lesion is not known; it is probably not related to the metabolic acidosis since respiratory distress syndrome occurs in hyperosmolar coma as well. Acute gastric dilatation is another rare complication. A rare infection associated with ketoacidosis is mucormycosis (see below). Table 319-11 summarizes the complications of diabetic ketoacidosis and its treatment.

Hyperosmolar coma Hyperosmolar nonketotic diabetic coma is usually a complication of non-insulin-dependent diabetes. It is a syndrome of profound dehydration resulting from a sustained hyperglycemic diuresis under circumstances in which the patient is unable to drink sufficient water to keep up with urinary fluid losses. Commonly an elderly diabetic—often living alone or in a nursing home—develops a stroke or infection, which worsens hyperglycemia and prevents adequate water intake. The full-blown syndrome probably does not occur until volume depletion has become severe enough to decrease urine output. Hyperosmolar coma has also been precipitated by therapeutic procedures such as peritoneal dialysis or hemodialysis, tube feeding of high-protein formulas, high-carbohydrate infusion loads, and the use of osmotic agents such as mannitol and urea. Phenytoin, steroids, immunosuppressive agents, and diuretics have also been reported to initiate the disorder.

The absence of ketoacidosis is important in the pathophysiology. When ketoacidosis occurs in an insulin-dependent diabetic, nausea, vomiting, and air hunger bring the patient to the physician before extreme dehydration can occur. Such a protective mechanism is not operative in the ketoacidosis-resistant, maturity-onset diabetic. Interestingly, hyperosmolar coma can occur in insulin-dependent diabetic patients given sufficient insulin to prevent ketosis but insufficient to control hyperglycemia. Although unusual, the same patient may present on one occasion with ketoacidosis and on the next with hyperosmolar coma.

The reason for the absence of ketoacidosis in maturity-onset diabetics is not known. The hepatic ketogenic machinery is not impaired since the patients frequently have ketone concentrations in the starvation range (2 to 4 mmol/L). Free fatty acid levels are lower in hyperosmolar coma than in ketoacidosis, and substrate deficiency may limit ketone formation. That this is the sole mechanism seems unlikely since some patients with hyperosmolar coma have high levels of free fatty acids in plasma. A more likely explanation is that insulin concentrations in the portal vein of type 2 diabetics are higher than those of insulin-dependent subjects and prevent full activation of the hepatic carnitine palmitoyltransferase system. Other possibilities include glucagon resistance, previously mentioned, and maintenance of high malonyl-CoA levels via increased Cori cycle activity. The Cori cycle refers to conversion of circulating glucose to lactate in peripheral tissues with return of lactate to the liver for gluconeogenesis. Lactate is also a precursor of malonyl-CoA.

Clinically patients present with extreme hyperglycemia, hyperosmolality, and volume depletion, coupled with central nervous system signs ranging from clouded sensorium to coma. Seizure activity—sometimes Jacksonian in type—is not unusual, and transient hemiplegia may be seen. Infections, particularly pneumonia and gram-negative sepsis, are common and indicate a grave prognosis. Pneumonia is often due to gram-negative organisms. A high index of suspicion for infection should be maintained, and routine culture of the blood and spinal fluid is indicated. Because of the extreme dehydration plasma viscosity is high, and widespread in situ thrombosis has been found at post mortem. Bleeding, probably the consequence of disseminated intravascular coagulation and acute pancreatitis, may accompany the illness.

The laboratory findings in two large series are shown in Table 319-12. Plasma glucose is generally around 55 mmol/L (1000 mg/dL), about twice the value seen in ketoacidosis. The serum osmolality is extremely high, but because of the hyperglycemia the absolute serum sodium concentration is often not elevated.[3] Prerenal azotemia with marked elevation of BUN and creatinine is characteristic. A mild metabolic acidosis is present, plasma bicarbonate on the average being about 20 mmol/L. The acidosis is due to a combination of

TABLE 319-11 Clues to complications in diabetic ketoacidosis

Complication	Clues
Acute gastric dilatation or erosive gastritis	Vomiting of blood or coffee-ground material
Cerebral edema	Obtundation or coma with or without neurologic signs, especially if occurring after initial improvement
Hyperkalemia	Cardiac arrest
Hypoglycemia	Adrenergic or neurologic signs; rebound ketosis
Hypokalemia	Cardiac arrhythmias
Infection	Fever
Insulin resistance	Unremitting acidosis after 4–6 h of adequate therapy
Myocardial infarction	Chest pain, appearance of heart failure; appearance of hypotension despite adequate fluids
Mucormycosis	Facial pain, bloody nasal discharge, blackened nasal turbinates, blurred vision, proptosis
Respiratory distress syndrome	Hypoxemia in the absence of pneumonia, chronic pulmonary disease, or heart failure
Vascular thrombosis	Strokelike picture or signs of ischemia in nonnervous tissue

SOURCE: Adapted from DW Foster, in *Current Therapy in Endocrinology and Metabolism 1985–1986*, DT Krieger, CW Bardin (eds). Toronto/Philadelphia, Decker, 1985.

[3] Serum osmolality can be estimated from the formula

$$\text{Serum osmolality (mosmol/L)} = 2\,([Na^+] + [K^+])(\text{mmol/L}) + \text{glucose(mmol/L)} + \text{BUN(mmol/L)}$$

In practice the contribution of the BUN is often ignored since it contributes to total osmolality but does not reflect the free water deficit. There are situations in which an increased osmolality is not equivalent to dehydration. Severe alcohol intoxication is one example, the ethanol itself providing the measured milliosmoles.

TABLE 319-12 Initial laboratory findings in hyperosmolar coma

Series	Brooklyn*	Washington†
Age, y HL	60	57
Glucose, mmol/L (mg/dL)	65(1166)	54(976)
Sodium, mmol/L	144	142
Potassium, mmol/L	5	5
Chloride, mmol/L	99	98
Bicarbonate, mmol/L	17	22
BUN, mmol/L (mg/dL)	31(87)	23(65)
Creatinine, mmol/L (mg/dL)	490(5.5)	—
Free fatty acids, mmol/L	0.73	0.96
Osmolarity, mosmol/L	384	374

* Mean data from 33 episodes of hyperosmolar coma (AA Arieff, HJ Carroll, Medicine 51:73, 1972).
† Mean data from 20 episodes of hyperosmolar coma (JE Gerich et al, Diabetes 20:228, 1971).

starvation ketosis, retention of inorganic acids secondary to the azotemia, and modest elevation of plasma lactate, the latter the consequence of volume depletion. If the bicarbonate is less than 10 mmol/L and plasma ketones are not elevated, it can be assumed that lactic acidosis is present.

The mortality rate in hyperosmolar coma is high (>50 percent). As a consequence immediate treatment is urgent. The most important measure is rapid administration of large amounts of intravenous fluids to reestablish the circulation and urine flow. The average fluid deficit is 10 liters. While free water will ultimately be needed, initial therapy should be with isotonic salt solutions, and 2 to 3 liters should be given over the first 1 to 2 h. Subsequently half-strength saline can be used. As the plasma glucose approaches normal levels, 5% dextrose can be given as a vehicle for free water. While hyperosmolar coma may be reversed by fluids alone, insulin should be given to control the hyperglycemia more rapidly. Many authors recommend small doses of insulin, but larger amounts may be necessary, particularly in the obese patient. Potassium salts are usually required earlier in the treatment of hyperosmolar coma than in ketoacidosis because the intracellular shift of plasma K^+ during therapy is accelerated in the absence of acidosis. If lactic acidosis is present, sodium bicarbonate should be given until tissue perfusion can be reestablished. Antibiotics are required if infection complicates the picture.

LATE COMPLICATIONS OF DIABETES The diabetic patient is susceptible to a series of complications that cause morbidity and premature mortality. While some patients may never develop these problems and others note their onset early, on average symptoms develop 15 to 20 years following the appearance of overt hyperglycemia. A given patient may experience several complications simultaneously, or a single problem may dominate the picture.

Circulatory abnormalities Arteriosclerosis of the type seen in nondiabetics occurs more extensively and earlier than in the general population. The cause for this accelerated atherosclerosis is not known, although, as discussed below, nonenzymatic glycation of lipoproteins may be important. Oxidized low density lipoproteins (LDL) are important in the generation of atherosclerosis. They bind not to the normal LDL receptor but to an alternative receptor (the acetyl LDL receptor). It is not known if diabetes enhances oxidation of LDL, although the ratio of high density lipoprotein (HDL) to LDL is altered (see below). Other factors of potential importance are increased platelet adhesiveness, possibly due to enhanced thromboxane A_2 synthesis, and decreased prostacyclin synthesis. Atherosclerotic lesions produce symptoms in a variety of sites. Peripheral deposits may cause intermittent claudication, gangrene, and, in men, organic impotence on a vascular basis. Surgical repair of large vessel lesions may be unsuccessful because of the simultaneous presence of widespread disease of the small vessels. Coronary artery disease and stroke are common. Silent myocardial infarction is thought to occur with increased frequency in diabetics and should be suspected whenever symptoms of left ventricular failure appear suddenly. Diabetes may also be associated with the clinical picture of cardiomyopathy, in which heart failure occurs in the face of angiographically normal coronary arteries and the absence of other identifiable causes of heart disease. As in nondiabetic subjects, smoking is a major risk factor for both coronary and peripheral vascular disease and should be avoided.

Retinopathy Diabetic retinopathy is a leading cause of blindness in the United States. On the other hand, most diabetics never become blind. Retinopathic lesions are divided into two large categories, *simple* (background) and *proliferative* (Table 319-13). The earliest sign of retinal change is an increased capillary permeability that is evidenced by leakage of dye into the vitreous humor after fluorescein injection. Occlusion of retinal capillaries follows, with subsequent formation of saccular and fusiform aneurysms. Arteriovenous shunts also occur. The vascular lesions are accompanied by proliferation of lining endothelial cells and a loss of the pericytes that surround and support the vessels. Hemorrhages into the inner retinal areas are dot-shaped, while bleeding into the more superficial nerve fiber layer causes flame-shaped, blot, or linear lesions. Preretinal hemorrhages characteristically have a boat-shaped appearance. Exudates are of two types. Cotton-wool spots can be shown by angiography to be microinfarcts—nonperfused areas surrounded by a ring of dilated capillaries. A sudden increase in the number of cotton-wool spots represents an ominous prognostic sign and may herald the appearance of rapidly advancing retinopathy. Hard exudates are more common than cotton-wool spots and probably represent leakage of protein and lipids from damaged capillaries.

The fundamental characteristics of proliferative retinopathy are new vessel formation and scarring. The stimulus for neovascularization may be hypoxia secondary to capillary or arteriolar occlusion. Two serious complications of proliferative retinopathy are vitreal hemorrhage and retinal detachment. Either may cause a sudden loss of vision in one eye.

The frequency of diabetic retinopathy appears to vary with the age of onset as well as the duration of the disease. Approximately 85 percent of patients eventually develop the complication, but some never develop lesions even after 30 years of disease. Retinopathy appears to develop earlier in older patients, but proliferative retinopathy is less common. Some 10 to 18 percent of patients with simple retinopathy progress to proliferative disease in a 10-year period. About half of patients with proliferative disease progress to blindness within 5 years.

Treatment for diabetic retinopathy is photocoagulation. Such treatment decreases the incidence of hemorrhage and scarring and is always indicated when new vessel formation occurs. Photocoagulation is also useful in treatment of microaneurysms, hemorrhages, and edema even if the proliferative stage has not begun. Panretinal photocoagulation is sometimes used to diminish retinal demands for oxygen in the hope that the stimulus for neovascularization will be decreased. In this technique several thousand lesions are produced

TABLE 319-13 Lesions of diabetic retinopathy

BACKGROUND
Increased capillary permeability
Capillary closure and dilatation
Microaneurysms
Arteriovenous shunts
Dilated veins
Hemorrhages (dot and blot)
Cotton-wool spots
Hard exudates
PROLIFERATIVE
New vessels
Scar (retinitis proliferans)
Vitreal hemorrhage
Retinal detachment

over a 2-week period. Complications of photocoagulation are within the acceptable range. Some loss of peripheral vision is inevitable with extensive burns. Another surgical technique, pars plana vitrectomy, is utilized for treatment of nonresolving vitreal hemorrhage and retinal detachment. Postoperative complications are more frequent than with photocoagulation and include retinal tears, retinal detachment, cataracts, recurrent vitreal hemorrhage, glaucoma, infection, and loss of the eye. Hypophysectomy, once widely performed for diabetic retinopathy, is no longer recommended. There is hope that inhibition of angiogenesis by drugs such as the experimental heparin analogue, beta-cyclodextrin tetradecasulfate, may prevent proliferative retinopathy. All patients with diabetic retinopathy should be followed by retinal specialists.

Diabetic nephropathy Renal disease is a leading cause of death and disability in diabetes. About half of end-stage renal disease in the United States is now due to diabetic nephropathy. Approximately 40 to 50 percent of patients with insulin-dependent diabetes develop this complication. Prevalence may be somewhat less with the non-insulin-dependent form of the disease, possibly because duration of illness tends to be shorter. However, two-thirds of diabetic Pima Indians (who have non-insulin-dependent diabetes) have diabetic glomerulosclerosis at autopsy. It is probable that nephropathy, like other complications, is influenced by the genetic background of the patient (it is rare in Japanese Americans with diabetes). Some families with multiple diabetic members rarely have renal disease while in others more than 80 percent of persons at risk have nephropathy.

Diabetic nephropathy involves two distinct pathologic patterns that may or may not coexist: diffuse and nodular. The former, which is more common, consists of widening of the glomerular basement membrane together with generalized mesangial thickening. In the nodular form large accumulations of PAS-positive material are deposited at the periphery of the glomerular tufts, the Kimmelstiel-Wilson lesion. In addition, there may be hyalinization of afferent and efferent arterioles, "drops" in Bowman's capsule, fibrin caps, and occlusion of glomeruli. Deposition of albumin and other proteins occurs in both glomeruli and tubules. The most specific lesions of diabetic glomerulosclerosis are hyalinization of afferent glomerular arterioles and the Kimmelstiel-Wilson nodules. Clinical renal dysfunction in diabetes does not correlate well with the histologic abnormalities.

Diabetic nephropathy may be functionally silent for long periods (~10 to 15 years). At onset of diabetes the kidneys are usually enlarged with "superfunction," i.e., glomerular filtration rates may be 40 percent above normal. The next stage is the appearance of *microproteinuria* (microalbuminuria), the excretion of albumin in the range of 30 to 550 mg/d. Normal persons excrete less than 30 mg/d. Microalbuminuria is not detected by reagent sticks for urinary protein, which generally become positive only when proteinuria is greater than 550 mg/d, a degree of leakage termed *macroproteinuria.* Since microalbuminuria is initially transient and can be induced by mechanisms other than diabetes, diagnosis requires an excretion rate of albumin greater than 15 μg/h (~30 mg/d) in two of three samples collected in a 6-month period. Persistent leakage of protein >50 mg/d is predictive of subsequent macroproteinuria. Once the macroproteinuric phase begins, there is a steady decline in renal function with glomerular filtration rate falling, on average, about 1 mL/min per month. A plot of the reciprocal of the serum creatinine against time usually results in a straight line and allows prediction of the rate of deterioration. Ordinarily azotemia begins about 12 years after diagnosis of diabetes. The nephrotic syndrome may occur prior to azotemia. Progression of renal disease is accelerated by hypertension.

There is no specific treatment for diabetic nephropathy. Meticulous control of diabetes can reverse microalbuminuria in some patients, but there is no evidence that diabetic nephropathy can be prevented by intensive insulin therapy. Hypertension must be treated aggressively whenever present. Low-protein diets may be useful, based on experimental studies in animals. A prospective study testing protein restriction in humans is underway. Once the azotemic phase is reached, treatment does not differ from other forms of renal failure. Chronic dialysis and renal transplantation are routine in patients with renal failure due to diabetes. Hyporeninemic hypoaldosteronism, which is associated with renal tubular acidosis, may require alkalinizing solutions (Shohl's solution) and avoidance of external potassium loads. Rarely, fludrocortisone may be required to control hyperkalemia.

Diabetic neuropathy Diabetic neuropathy may affect every part of the nervous system with the possible exception of the brain. While it is rarely a direct cause of death, it is a major cause of morbidity. Distinct syndromes can be recognized, and several different types of neuropathy may be present in the same patient. The most common picture is that of *peripheral polyneuropathy.* Usually bilateral, the symptoms include numbness, paresthesias, severe hyperesthesias, and pain. The pain, which may be deep-seated and severe, is often worse at night. It is occasionally lancinating or lightning in type, resembling tabes dorsalis (pseudotabes). Fortunately extreme pain syndromes are usually self-limited, lasting from a few months to a few years. Involvement of proprioceptive fibers leads to abnormalities of gait and development of typical Charcot joints, particularly in the feet. Loss of arch with multiple fractures of tarsal bones is a common finding by x-ray. On physical examination absent stretch reflexes and loss of vibratory sense are early signs. Diabetic neuropathy may also cause delay in return of the ankle reflex identical to that seen in hypothyroidism. *Mononeuropathy,* though less common than polyneuropathy, may also occur. Characteristically there is a sudden wrist drop, foot drop, or paralysis of the third, fourth, or sixth cranial nerves. Other single nerves, including the recurrent laryngeal, have been reported to be involved. Mononeuropathy is characterized by a high degree of spontaneous reversibility, usually over a several-week period. *Radiculopathy* is a sensory syndrome in which pain occurs over the distribution of one or more spinal nerves, usually in the chest wall or abdomen. The severe pain may mimic herpes zoster or an acute surgical abdomen. Like mononeuropathy, the lesion is usually self-limited. *Autonomic neuropathy* may present in a variety of ways. The gastrointestinal tract is a prime target, and there may be esophageal dysfunction with difficulty in swallowing, delayed gastric emptying, constipation, or diarrhea. The last is often nocturnal. Incompetence of the internal anal sphincter may mimic diabetic diarrhea. Orthostatic hypotension and frank syncope may occur. Cardiorespiratory arrest and sudden death, thought to be due solely to autonomic neuropathy, have been reported. Bladder dysfunction or paralysis is particularly distressing and often leads to the necessity of chronic catheter drainage. Impotence and retrograde ejaculation are additional manifestations in the male. Clues to autonomic neuropathy can be obtained by clinical tests such as measuring response of the heart rate to the Valsalva maneuver or standing. In both tests the subject has an electrocardiograph running for assessment of heart rate. In the former the subject blows against an anaeroid or mercury manometer to 40 mmHg pressure for 15 s. The test is performed three times with a rest period of 1 min in between. Normally the heart rate speeds during Valsalva such that the ratio of the longest interval between beats after release to the shortest interval during the test is >1.2. In autonomic neuropathy involving the parasympathetic system the ratio is <1:1. Similarly the ratio at the thirtieth beat after standing relative to that at the fifteenth beat should be >1.0. It is <1 in autonomic neuropathy. Diabetic *amyotrophy* is likely a form of neuropathy, although atrophy and weakness of the large muscles in the upper leg and pelvic girdle resemble primary muscle disease. Anorexia and depression may accompany amyotrophy. Because of the weight loss, such patients are often thought to have a paraneoplastic neuropathy.

Treatment of diabetic neuropathy is unsatisfactory in most respects. When pain is severe, it is easy for the patient to become habituated or addicted to narcotics or powerful nonnarcotic analgesics such as pentazocine. If the pain requires something stronger than aspirin, acetaminophen, or other nonsteroidal anti-inflammatory agents, codeine is the drug of choice. Phenytoin is used by some physicians, but others have not found it helpful. Combination therapy with amitriptyline and fluphenazine causes relief of pain in some patients and should always be tried. The recommended dosage is 75 mg amitriptyline at bedtime and 1 mg fluphenazine three times a day. Mononeuropathies and radiculopathies usually require no specific therapy since they are self-limited. Diabetic diarrhea often responds to treatment with diphenoxylate and atropine or loperamide. Orthostatic hypotension is best treated by having the patient sleep with the head of the bed elevated, avoidance of sudden assumption of the upright position, and the use of full-length elastic stockings. Occasionally volume expansion with fludrocortisone is required as in other forms of orthostatic hypotension.

Experimental therapy with aldose reductase inhibitors and myoinositol have failed to provide significant clinical benefit although enhanced regeneration of nerves has been reported in humans treated with an aldose reductase antagonist.

Diabetic foot ulcers A special problem in the diabetic patient is the development of ulcers of the feet and lower extremities. The ulcers appear to be primarily due to abnormal pressure distribution secondary to diabetic neuropathy. The problem is accentuated when there is bony distortion in the feet. Callus formation is usually the initial abnormality. Alternatively the ulcer may be initiated by ill-fitting shoes which cause blister formation in patients whose sensory deficits preclude recognition of pain. Cuts and punctures from foreign bodies such as needles, tacks, and glass are common, and a foreign body of which the patient is unaware may be found in the soft tissue. For this reason all patients with ulcers should have x-rays made of the feet. Vascular disease with diminished blood supply contributes to development of the lesion, and infection is common, often with multiple organisms. While no specific therapy is available for diabetic ulcers, aggressive supportive treatment can often lead to salvation of the leg without amputation. One approach is to simply put the patient to bed using hydrotherapy and debridement to remove nonviable tissue. Others recommend casting the leg with plaster to redistribute weight bearing and protect the lesion.

All diabetics should be instructed about proper foot care in an attempt to prevent ulcers. Feet should be kept clean and dry at all times. Patients with neuropathy should not be allowed to walk barefoot, even in the home. Properly fitted shoes are essential. This is a particular problem with women, since an adequate shoe for the diabetic is not often stylish. The feet should be carefully inspected daily for callus, infection, abrasions, or blisters and the physician consulted for any potentially troublesome lesion. Treatment with growth factors (e.g., fibroblast growth factor) may prove useful in the future.

What causes the complications of diabetes? The cause of diabetic complications is not known and may be multifactorial. Major emphasis has been placed on the polyol pathway wherein glucose is reduced to sorbitol by the enzyme aldol reductase. Sorbitol, which appears to function as a tissue toxin, has been implicated in the pathogenesis of retinopathy, neuropathy, cataracts, nephropathy, and aortic disease. The mechanism is perhaps best worked out in experimental diabetic neuropathy where sorbitol accumulation is associated with a decrease in myoinositol content, abnormal phosphoinositide metabolism, and a decrease in Na^+,K^+-ATPase activity. In experimental models primacy of the polyol pathway in initiating neuropathy was proven by showing that inhibition of aldol reductase prevented the fall in tissue myoinositol content and the decrease in ATPase activity. Myoinositol deficiency was not found in sural nerve biopsies from humans with diabetic neuropathy, in contrast to animals. Aldol reductase inhibition has also been shown to prevent experimental cataracts and retinopathy. It thus seems possible that neuropathy and retinopathy are primarily due to activation of the polyol pathway. It may also play a role in diabetic nephropathy.

A second mechanism of potential pathogenetic importance is glycation of proteins. (Current terminology uses *glycation* for nonenzymatic addition of hexoses to proteins and *glycosylation* for enzymatic addition.) The effect of such glycation on hemoglobin has been mentioned, but multiple proteins in the body are altered in the same way, often with disturbed functions. Examples include plasma albumin, lens protein, fibrin, collagen, lipoproteins, and the glycoprotein recognition system of hepatic endothelial cells. Particularly intriguing is the effect of glycation on lipoproteins. Glycated LDL is not recognized by the normal LDL receptor, and its plasma half-life is increased. Conversely, glycated HDL turns over more rapidly than native HDL. It has also been reported that glycated collagen traps LDL at rates two to three times greater than normal collagen. Conceivably the accelerated atherosclerosis of diabetes might be related to the combined effect of a glycated LDL that did not bind normally to LDL receptors but would be trapped to a greater than normal extent by macrophages and glycated collagen of blood vessels and other tissues. Dysfunctional HDL could contribute by diminishing cholesterol transport out of affected sites.

Glycated collagen is less soluble and more resistant to degradation by collagenase than native collagen. However, it is not clear that this is related either to the basement membrane thickening or the tight, waxy skin syndrome with limited joint mobility (scleroderma-like) seen in some patients with insulin-dependent diabetes (see "Miscellaneous Abnormalities," below). Although it is attractive to presume that nonenzymatic glycation of proteins plays a role in some degenerative complications, the evidence is less direct than with the polyol pathway. Linkage between the polyol pathway and the glycation sequence occurs as a result of the glycation of collagen and other proteins by fructose generated from sorbitol.

Increased blood flow has been postulated to play an initiating role in diabetic complications, possibly by increasing filtration of macromolecules that function as tissue toxins. There is supportive evidence for a role of hyperperfusion in diabetic nephropathy, but the hemodynamic hypothesis does not appear as attractive as the first two.

Can diabetic complications be prevented by meticulous control of diabetes? The critical question in diabetic therapy is whether hyperglycemia or some associated metabolic disorder causes or accelerates the development of the long-term complications just discussed. The alternative possibility is that complications are primarily determined by genetic factors independent of hyperglycemia. Perhaps the strongest evidence that the metabolic environment per se causes complications comes from the observation that kidneys from donors who have neither diabetes nor a family history of diabetes develop characteristic lesions of diabetic nephropathy within 3 to 5 years after transplantation into a diabetic recipient. Diabetic nephropathy did not develop when a kidney was transplanted into a diabetic subject whose disease had been reversed by pancreatic transplantation prior to renal transplantation. It has also been reported that kidneys with the lesions of diabetic nephropathy demonstrated reversal of the lesion when transplanted into normal recipients. All of these findings suggest that hyperglycemia or some other aspect of the abnormal metabolism of diabetes causes or influences the development of complications. On the other hand additional factors, probably genetic, must play a role. This follows from the fact that diabetic subjects with decades of poor control may escape the ravages of the late complications and from the fact that typical diabetic complications may be found in patients at the time of diagnosis of diabetes or even in the absence of hyperglycemia.

Meticulous control with insulin infusion pumps has been reported to decrease microalbuminuria, alter motor nerve conduction velocity, lower plasma lipoproteins, and decrease capillary leakage of fluorescein in the retina. Width of the capillary basement membrane in skeletal muscle has also been decreased. The changes are small in general, however, and of questionable biologic significance. Firm evidence does not exist to show that late complications can be either prevented or reversed by long-term near-normalization of the plasma glucose. Progression of retinopathy has been reported despite successful reversal of diabetes by pancreatic transplantation. Hopefully, definitive answers to this question may be forthcoming from a large multicenter trial now underway under the sponsorship of the National Institutes of Health.

Until the issue is clarified it is prudent to maintain the plasma glucose as near normal as possible in all diabetic patients. About this there appears to be no disagreement. The only question is whether insulin therapy should be routinely aggressive to the point where recurrent hypoglycemia occurs. A mild insulin reaction consisting of nervousness, tremor, hunger, and sweating that is rapidly interrupted by carbohydrate intake is probably not harmful except for the possibility of worsening diabetic control via the Somogyi reaction. Unfortunately, as stated earlier, many diabetics, particularly those with long-standing disease and autonomic neuropathy, do not have or do not recognize the usual warning signals and progress to altered central nervous system function with abnormal behavior, loss of consciousness, or even convulsions. The latter reactions are dangerous for both patient and society. Every effort should be made to control hyperglycemia, but the limit of therapy should be the appearance of hypoglycemic reactions. It does not seem wise to induce a condition that can cause immediate and irreversible damage to a patient in the unproven hope that late complications might be prevented.

Miscellaneous abnormalities of diabetes Diabetes affects almost every system in the body. Space limitations preclude discussion of all associated features, but several deserve comment. *Infections* in diabetics may not occur more frequently than in normal subjects, but they tend to be more severe. This may be due to impaired leukocyte function, a frequent accompaniment of poor control. In addition to common infections of the skin, urinary tract, lungs, and bloodstream, four unusual conditions appear to have specific relationship with diabetes. *Malignant external otitis,* usually due to *Pseudomonas aeruginosa,* tends to occur in older patients and is characterized by severe pain in the ear, drainage, fever, and leukocytosis. Soft tissues around the ear are swollen and tender. A mound of granulation tissue is characteristically present internally at the junction of the osseous and cartilaginous portions of the ear. The facial nerve becomes paralyzed in half the cases, and other cranial nerves may also be involved. Facial nerve paralysis is a poor prognostic sign, and mortality approximates 50 percent in this subset of patients. A 6-week course of ticarcillin or carbenicillin together with tobramycin is the treatment of choice. Surgical debridement is often necessary. *Rhinocerebral mucormycosis* is a rare fungal infection which usually develops in patients during or following an episode of diabetic ketoacidosis. Organisms are from the genera *Mucor, Rhizopus,* and *Absidia.* Onset is sudden with periorbital and perinasal swelling, pain, bloody nasal discharge, and increased lacrimation. The nasal mucosa and underlying tissues become black and necrotic. Cranial nerve palsies are not uncommon. There may be thrombosis of the internal jugular vein or sinuses of the brain. Proptosis, chemosis, and retinal vein engorgement indicate cavernous sinus thrombosis. Untreated, death usually occurs in a week to 10 days. Amphotericin B and aggressive debridement are the indicated therapies. *Emphysematous cholecystitis* tends to affect diabetic men (in contrast to ordinary cholecystitis, a disease predominantly present in women). Gangrene of the gallbladder is 30 times more frequent than in the usual forms, accounting for high rates of perforation and a mortality rate 3 to 10 times higher than in ordinary cholecystitis. Diagnosis is made when gas is seen in the gallbladder wall on plain films of the abdomen. Clostridial species are frequently cultured from bile, but other organisms may be present. Treatment is cholecystectomy coupled with broad-spectrum antibiotics. Clindamycin and an aminoglycoside are adequate coverage until cultures are returned. *Emphysematous pyelonephritis* is signalled by the presence of gas in the kidney or perirenal space. Antibiotic therapy is usually ineffective, and nephrectomy may be required. Mortality rates of 80 percent have been reported.

Hypertriglyceridemia is common in diabetes and is usually due to insulin deficiency. Both overproduction of very low density lipoproteins in the liver and a disposal defect in the periphery appear to be operative. The latter is a consequence of lipoprotein lipase deficiency, an insulin-dependent enzyme. Some diabetics exhibit hyperlipemia even when diabetic control is adequate, and these patients may have a primary familial hyperlipoproteinemia that is independent of diabetes. Patients who do not respond to dietary therapy should be treated for hypertriglyceridemia and hypercholesterolemia with drugs, as in nondiabetic subjects (see Chap. 326).

Some diabetics have *recurrent hyperkalemia* in association with hyperglycemia. Traditionally these patients have been considered to have hyporeninemic hypoaldosteronism although basal renin and aldosterone concentrations may be normal. Since the capacity to increase aldosterone production in response to stimulatory signals is impaired even when basal levels are normal, functional hypoaldosteronism probably plays a central role in the syndrome. With a deficiency of aldosterone, renal secretion of potassium is impaired and disposal of a potassium load is dependent on insulin-mediated transport of the cation into the intracellular space. Administration of potassium salts or triamterene to such patients may be dangerous. Whether potassium transport is directly regulated by insulin or is secondary to glucose movement is not clear. Affected subjects almost always have a hyperchloremic renal tubular acidosis.

A variety of skin lesions occur in diabetes. *Necrobiosis lipoidica diabeticorum* is a plaque-like lesion with a central yellowish area surrounded by a brownish border. It is usually found over the anterior surfaces of the legs. Ulceration may occur (see Fig. A1-28). *Diabetic dermopathy* (''shin spots'') is also usually located over the anterior tibial surface. The lesions are small rounded plaques with a raised border which may crust at the edges and ulcerate centrally. Several plaques may be arranged in linear fashion. Pigmentation is not prominent early, but as the lesion heals a depressed scar occurs with diffuse brown discoloration. A rarer abnormality is *bullosis diabeticorum.* The bullae may be superficial with clear serum or may be mildly hemorrhagic. The cause is unknown. *Infestations of the skin* with *Candida* and dermatophytes are common, and bacterial infections of a variety of types occur. In women *vaginal moniliasis* may be troublesome during hyperglycemic-glycosuric periods. While the symptoms respond to nystatin or gentian violet, recurrence is inevitable unless glycosuria is reversed. *Atrophy of adipose tissue* may occur at the site of insulin injections. The lipoatrophy is said to respond to injection of purified insulin into the atrophic area. Hypertrophy of fat may also occur, producing a lipoma-like lesion visible on physical examination.

Hyperviscosity occurs in diabetes, and *platelets aggregate abnormally.* The latter may be caused by increased prostaglandin synthesis. *Wound healing* is impaired in experimental diabetes but probably is not a major factor clinically. An interesting accompaniment of insulin-dependent diabetes is the presence of *joint contractures* (Dupuytren's contracture) coupled with *tight, waxy skin* over the dorsum of the hands. The hands resemble those in patients with scleroderma. The cause of the tendon contractures is unknown although alterations of cross-linking in collagen has been proposed. Patients with the joint contracture–waxy skin syndrome appear to have accelerated development of other diabetic complications. *Scleredema* is a common finding in diabetes. The lesion is a thickening of the skin over the shoulders and upper back that resembles scleroderma. The condition is benign.

NONROUTINE THERAPY Transplantation with whole pancreas or segments has cured diabetes in a number of patients but is usually performed only when kidney transplantation is required. Half the grafts have failed at 1 year. Islet cell transplantation has not been successful in humans. Prevention of type 1 diabetes by suppression of the immune system remains a hoped-for goal. Cyclosporine given within a 6-week period after the appearance of hyperglycemia may reverse the metabolic abnormalities and allow discontinuation of insulin therapy in a significant number of patients. However, its long-term use is too dangerous to be recommended. New immunosuppressive agents have considerable promise, however.

INSULIN RESISTANCE Insulin resistance in diabetic subjects is arbitrarily defined as the requirement of 200 or more units of insulin per day to control hyperglycemia and prevent ketosis. Relative insulin resistance is present in essentially all persons with diabetes when carefully looked for using the glucose clamp technique. It is the consequence of near complete insulin deficiency in IDDM, whereas in NIDDM the major problem is obesity.

Normal anabolic metabolism, mediated by insulin, requires the secretion of adequate amounts of normal hormone in response to meals. Insulin must then bind to a specific insulin receptor in target tissues (see Chap. 320). The insulin receptor is a tetrameric glycoprotein consisting of two alpha subunits and two beta subunits linked by disulfide bonds. The beta subunit is a tyrosine kinase that is activated when insulin binds to the alpha subunit. The tyrosine kinase autophosphorylates the insulin receptor and initiates subsequent intracellular phosphorylations that mediate the multiple actions of insulin. The only such action which is reasonably understood is glucose transport. Glucose enters the cell by facilitated diffusion utilizing "glucose transporter" molecules. While some of these are always present in the plasma membrane, insulin binding to the receptor initiates a rapid mobilization of intracellular stores of the transporter to the plasma membrane while simultaneously activating units already in place. In poorly controlled diabetes the number of stored transporters appears to be deficient.

Insulin resistance is characterized as *prereceptor* (abnormal insulin or insulin antibodies), *receptor* (decreased receptor number or diminished binding of insulin), or *postreceptor* (abnormal signal transduction, especially failure to activate the receptor tyrosine kinase). Combinations may exist. The nature of the molecular defect is known in some syndromes of insulin resistance but in many the defect has not been pinpointed.

In diabetic subjects with fullblown insulin resistance (>200 units of insulin per day) the problem is usually prereceptor resistance due to insulin antibodies. Insulin antibodies of IgG type are present in essentially all diabetics within 60 days of the initiation of insulin therapy. The titer of these antibodies fluctuates for reasons that are not clear. Although the correlation between antibody titer and functional resistance is not close, insulin binding by high levels of antibody is presumed to be the primary mechanism in most cases. Probably less than 0.1 percent of insulin-treated diabetics ever have significant resistance. The problem may appear within a few weeks of the start of therapy or many years later. The onset may be abrupt, resulting in ketoacidosis, but usually is gradual, with uncontrollable hyperglycemia being the major problem. About 20 to 30 percent of patients have concomitant insulin allergy. Therapy of the syndrome requires prednisone in large amounts—80 to 100 mg/d initially. Response often occurs in 48 to 72 h but may take longer. If no improvement has resulted after 3 to 4 weeks, it can be assumed that steroids will not be effective. Once insulin requirements begin to fall, prednisone dosage can be rapidly decreased by 10 to 20 mg every 3 to 7 days until a maintenance level of 5 to 10 mg/d is reached. These levels may be required for many months. Whether remission has occurred, allowing cessation of therapy, can only be determined by trial. Sulfated insulin may also be of benefit. On rare occasions insulin resistance in diabetics appears to be due to enhanced destruction of the hormone at the subcutaneous injection site. Such patients tend to respond normally to insulin given intravenously or intraperitoneally. In some patients addition of a protease inhibitor (aprotinin) to the insulin mixture has been helpful. When resistance is extreme, U500 regular insulin should be used in order to control the volume of the injection.

Insulin resistance occurs in diseases other than diabetes. In such disorders *acanthosis nigricans* is a physical sign of its presence. Acanthosis nigricans is a brown to black, velvety hyperpigmentation of the skin, most often present in the posterior and lateral folds of the neck. It is also found in the axilla, groin, umbilicus, and other areas. Acanthosis nigricans is common, occurring in 7 percent of 1412 children who made up the 6th and 8th grade populations of the public schools in one study. Higher prevalence was found in Hispanics and blacks than in whites. Although acanthosis nigricans may be a sign of occult malignancy, it is not associated with neoplasia in the insulin-resistant states. A list of the major syndromes of insulin resistance is given in Table 319-14.

Obesity is the most common cause of insulin resistance. It is associated with decreased receptor number, but the major problem is at the postreceptor level, where there is apparently a failure to activate the tyrosine kinase. *Werner's syndrome* is an autosomal recessive illness with a high incidence of hyperglycemia despite elevated concentrations of plasma insulin (see Chap. 325). There is little response to exogenous hormone. Other features include growth retardation, alopecia or premature graying of the hair, cataracts, hypogonadism, leg ulcers, atrophy of muscle, fat, and bone, soft-tissue calcification, and a high frequency of sarcomas and meningiomas.

Of the rare conditions associated with acanthosis nigricans, women with *insulin receptor abnormalities* have attracted the greatest interest. Type A patients are tall young women with a tendency to hirsutism and abnormalities of the reproductive tract who most probably have polycystic ovaries. However, other causes of androgen excess are associated with the syndrome. Most patients have an absolute decrease in the number of insulin receptors, but in some receptor function is qualitatively abnormal. At the molecular level defects range from a decrease in mRNA for the receptor to mutations that alter receptor processing or insertion into the membrane. Type B subjects are older women with evidence of immunologic disease. The clinical picture includes arthralgias, alopecia, enlarged salivary glands, proteinuria, leukopenia, and antinuclear and anti-DNA antibodies. Insulin resistance in these patients is due to blocking antibodies to the insulin receptor (not to insulin itself). Interestingly, antireceptor antibodies may also cause hypoglycemia. The determinant of agonist (hypoglycemia) or antagonist (insulin resistance) activity presumably depends on the site of binding to the insulin receptor. Both A and B patients have high plasma insulin concentrations.

Generalized and *partial lipodystrophies* are fat depletion syndromes differing primarily in the extent of fat atrophy (see Chap. 338). In the generalized form essentially all body fat is missing, while the more common partial type exhibits atrophy of fat in the face and trunk with normal or increased adiposity in the lower half of the body. The disease can be either congenital or acquired. Typically the patients develop hyperglycemia at puberty, but ketoacidosis never occurs. Marked hypertriglyceridemia with eruptive xanthoma is a frequent feature. Characteristic features are hepatomegaly, splenomegaly, cardiomegaly, hirsutism, lymphadenopathy, hypertrophy of the external genitalia, varicose veins, and (in the congenital forms) muscle hypertrophy. Mental retardation is common, and renal disease may develop. The term *lipoatrophic diabetes* is synonymous with total lipodystrophy. All patients have elevated plasma insulin levels. Resistance may be due to decreased number of receptors, diminished affinity of the receptor for insulin, or a postreceptor defect.

The *pineal hypertrophy syndrome* is characterized by insulin

TABLE 319-14 Insulin-resistant states

I Prereceptor resistance
  A Mutated insulins
  B Anti-insulin antibodies
II Receptor and postreceptor resistance
  A Obesity
  B Type A syndrome (absent or dysfunctional receptor)
  C Type B syndrome (antibody to insulin receptor)
  D Lipodystrophic states (partial or generalized)
  E Leprechaunism
  F Ataxia-telangiectasia
  G Rabson-Mendenhall syndrome
  H Werner syndrome
  I Alström syndrome
  J Pineal hyperplasia syndrome

resistance, early dentition with malformed teeth, dry skin, thick nails, hirsutism, and a peculiar sexual precocity with enlargement of the external genitalia. The latter may reach near adult size by age 3 or 4. The insulin resistance is severe, and ketoacidosis may occur despite high endogenous insulin levels. The *Alström syndrome* is a rare autosomal recessive disease characterized by childhood blindness due to retinal degeneration, nerve deafness, vasopressin-resistant diabetes insipidus, and, in males, hypogonadism with high plasma gonadotropin levels. The patients thus appear to have end organ resistance to multiple hormones. Other features include baldness, hyperuricemia, hypertriglyceridemia, and aminoaciduria. Superficially the patients may resemble subjects with the Lawrence-Moon-Biedl syndrome but can be differentiated on initial exam by the absence of polydactyly and mental deficiency. Insulin resistance in the Alström syndrome is mild. *Ataxia-telangiectasia* is characterized by cerebellar ataxia, telangiectasia, and a variety of abnormalities in the immune system in addition to insulin resistance. The *Rabson-Mendenhall syndrome* consists of dental dysplasia, dystrophic nails, premature puberty, and acanthosis nigricans. The insulin resistance is probably due to an insulin receptor abnormality. *Leprechaunism* is characterized by an elfin appearance of the face, hirsutism, absence of subcutaneous fat, thickened skin, and insulin resistance. The latter is probably due to abnormal receptor function. Not listed in Table 319-14 is insulin resistance due to hormone excess (acromegaly, Cushing's syndrome), myotonic dystrophy, and thalassemia major. The insulin resistance in these conditions is usually not clinically significant.

INSULIN ALLERGY Insulin allergy is due to IgE antibodies to insulin. Manifestations include immediate reactions with local stinging or itching, delayed local reactions with brawny swelling lasting up to 30 h, and generalized urticaria or frank anaphylaxis. Systemic reactions are usually seen in patients who have stopped insulin therapy for one reason or another and have then resumed treatment. The allergic reaction may occur as early as the second injection on resumption of therapy. Mild reactions can be treated with antihistamines. If the problem is severe, desensitization procedures are required. A 1-day insulin desensitization procedure is shown in Table 319-15. Once the patient is desensitized, insulin therapy should not be interrupted.

THE EMOTIONAL RESPONSE TO DIABETES Acceptance of the fact that a person has a chronic disease that requires a change in lifestyle is always difficult. This is particularly true in the case of diabetes since patients generally are aware that they are vulnerable to late complications and that life expectancy is shortened. It is not surprising that the emotional response to diabetes often hampers treatment. On the one hand, the primary reaction may be denial with an accompanying refusal to cooperate. At the other extreme is excessive preoccupation with the illness. The physician should make every effort to define a middle ground wherein the patient acknowledges his or her disease and responds prudently without becoming obsessed. The goal is to live with diabetes not for it. Diabetics are no different from other patients in that they may attempt to use their disease manipulatively with both family and physician. The problems are particularly acute with children and adolescents. While the psychiatric aspects of diabetes are not discussed here, most problems can be anticipated and handled if common sense is coupled with sympathy and firmness. It is also appropriate to offer cautious hope that the disease will be handled better in the future than is possible now.

TABLE 319-15 Insulin desensitization*

Time, h	Dose, units	Route
0	0.001	Intradermal
0.5	0.002	Intradermal
1	0.004	Subcutaneous
1.5	0.01	Subcutaneous
2	0.02	Subcutaneous
2.5	0.04	Subcutaneous
3	0.1	Subcutaneous
3.5	0.2	Subcutaneous
4	0.5	Subcutaneous
4.5	1	Subcutaneous
5	2	Subcutaneous
5.5	4	Subcutaneous
6	8	Subcutaneous

* Following desensitization, use 2 to 10 units of regular insulin every 4 to 6 h for 24 to 36 h after the 6-h injection before switching to intermediate-acting insulin.
SOURCE: *Schedule of JA Galloway*. For detailed information see JA Galloway, R Bressler, Med Clin North Am 62:663, 1978.

REFERENCES

General review

UNGER RH, FOSTER DW: Diabetes mellitus, in *Williams' Textbook of Endocrinology*, 8th ed, JD Wilson, DW Foster (eds). Philadelphia, Saunders, 1990, in press

Pathophysiology

BANERJI MA, LEBOVITZ HE: Insulin-sensitive and insulin-resistant variants in NIDDM. Diabetes 38:784, 1989

BOTTAZZO GF et al: In situ characterization of autoimmune phenomena and expression of HLA molecules in the pancreas in diabetic insulitis. N Engl J Med 313:353, 1985

EISENBARTH GS et al: The "natural" history of type 1 diabetes. Diabetes Metab Rev 3:873, 1987

HARRISON LC et al: MHC molecules and β-cell destructive immune and nonimmune mechanisms. Diabetes 38:815, 1989

KWOK WW et al: Mutational analysis of the HLA-DQ 3.2 insulin-dependent diabetes susceptibility gene. Proc Natl Acad Sci (USA) 86:1027, 1989

LEIGHTON B, COOPER GJS: Pancreatic amylin and calcitonin gene-related peptide cause resistance to insulin in skeletal muscle *in vitro*. Nature 335:632, 1988

REAVEN GM: Banting Lecture 1988. Role of insulin resistance in human disease. Diabetes 37:1595, 1988

SHEEHY MJ et al: Diabetes-susceptible HLA haplotype is best defined by a combination of HLA-DR and -DQ alleles. J Clin Invest 83:830, 1989

TODD JA et al: HLA-DQβ gene contributes to susceptibility and resistance to insulin-dependent diabetes mellitus. Nature 329:599, 1987

Acute complications

CARROLL P, MATZ R: Uncontrolled diabetes mellitus in adults: Experience in treating diabetic ketoacidosis and hyperosmolar nonketotic coma with low-dose insulin and a uniform treatment regimen. Diabetes Care 6:579, 1983

FOSTER DW, MCGARRY JD: The metabolic derangements and treatment of diabetic ketoacidosis. N Engl J Med 309:159, 1983

FRANKLIN B et al: Cerebral edema and ophthalmoplegia reversed by mannitol in a new case of insulin-dependent diabetes mellitus. Pediatrics 69:87, 1982

KITABCHI AE: Low-dose insulin therapy in diabetic ketoacidosis: Fact or fiction? Diabetes Metab Rev 5:337, 1989

Late complications

BROWNLEE M et al: Advanced products of nonenzymatic glycosylation and the pathogenesis of diabetic vascular disease. Diabetes Metab Rev 5:437, 1988

LOGERFO FW, COFFMAN JD: Vascular and microvascular disease of the foot in diabetes. N Engl J Med 311:1615, 1984

MOGENSEN CE, CHRISTENSEN CK: Predicting diabetic nephropathy in insulin-dependent patients. N Engl J Med 311:89, 1984

PARVING HH et al: Hemodynamic factors in the genesis of diabetic microangiopathy. Metabolism 32:943, 1983

RAMSAY RC et al: Progression of diabetic retinopathy after pancreas transplantation for insulin-dependent diabetes mellitus. N Engl J Med 318:208, 1988

ROSENSTOCK J, RASKIN P: Diabetes and its complications: Blood glucose control versus genetic susceptibility. Diabetes Metab Rev 4:417, 1988

SEQUIST ER et al: Familial clustering of diabetic renal disease. Evidence for genetic susceptibility and diabetic nephropathy. N Engl J Med 320:1161, 1989

WINEGRAD AI: Banting Lecture 1986. Does a common mechanism induce the diverse complications of diabetes? Diabetes 36:396, 1986

Treatment

COUSTAN DR: Pregnancy in diabetic women. N Engl J Med 319:1663, 1988

CRYER PE et al: Hypoglycemia in IDDM. Diabetes 38:1193, 1989

LEBOVITZ HE, FEINGLOS MN: The oral hypoglycemic agents, in *Diabetes Mellitus: Theory and Practice*, 3d ed, M Ellenberg, H Rifkin (eds). New Hyde Park, Medical Examination Publishing, 1983, pp 591–610

MECKENBURG RS et al: Long-term metabolic control with insulin pump therapy. N Engl J Med 313:464, 1985

SCHADE DS: Surgery and diabetes. Med Clin North Am 72:1531, 1988

SCHIFFRIN A, BELMONTE MM: Comparison between subcutaneous insulin infusion and multiple injections of insulin: A one year prospective study. Diabetes 31:255, 1982

SKYLER JS: Insulin pharmacology. Med Clin North Am 72:1337, 1988

SUTHERLAND DER: Who should get a pancreas transplant? Diabetes Care 11:681, 1988

ZINMAN B: The physiologic replacement of insulin. An elusive goal. N Engl J Med 321:363, 1989

Insulin resistance

FLIER JS et al: Acanthosis nigricans in obese women with hyperandrogenism. Characterization of an insulin-resistance state distinct from the type A and B syndromes. Diabetes 34:101, 1985

KAHN CR, WHITE MF: The insulin receptor and the molecular mechanisms of insulin action. J Clin Invest 82:1151, 1988

———, GOLDSTEIN BJ: Molecular defects in insulin action. Science 245:13, 1989

KURTZ AB, NABARRO JDN: Circulating insulin-binding antibodies. Diabetologia 19:329, 1980

STUART CA et al: Prevalence of acanthosis nigricans in an unselected population. Am J Med 87:269, 1989

320 HYPOGLYCEMIA

DANIEL W. FOSTER / ARTHUR H. RUBENSTEIN

Maintenance of the plasma glucose concentration within narrow bounds is essential for health. Hypoglycemia is dangerous (in the short run more serious than hyperglycemia) because glucose is the primary energy substrate of the brain. Its absence, like that of oxygen, produces deranged function, tissue damage, or even death if the deficit is prolonged. The vulnerability of the brain to hypoglycemia is due to the fact that it cannot utilize circulating free fatty acids as an energy source in contrast to other tissues of the body. Short-chain metabolites of the free fatty acids, acetoacetic and β-hydroxybutyric acids (''ketone bodies,'' ''ketoacids''), are efficiently oxidized by brain and can protect the central nervous system from damage by hypoglycemia when present at moderate concentrations in plasma. However, development of ketosis requires a number of hours in humans. Ketogenesis is not, therefore, an effective protective mechanism against acute hypoglycemia. Preservation of central nervous system function in the early phases of fasting or during hypoglycemia thus requires a prompt increase in the production of glucose by the liver. At the same time glucose utilization in other tissues is diminished by provision of free fatty acids as alternative substrate. These adaptive mechanisms are hormonally controlled and, under ordinary circumstances, are extremely effective. Occasionally, however, the system breaks down or is overwhelmed, resulting in the clinical syndrome hypoglycemia.

DEFENSE AGAINST HYPOGLYCEMIA The hypoglycemic states can best be understood as derangements of normal fuel metabolism. Under ordinary circumstances energy needs are met by exogenous substrate derived from food. Oxidation of the constituent molecules of food to carbon dioxide and water is accompanied by the generation of adenosine triphosphate (ATP), the principal high-energy compound of the body. In one sense, life can be defined as the continued ability to generate ATP (and related high-energy nucleotides) for the preservation of cellular integrity in all its manifestations. When caloric intake is greater than immediate oxidative needs, as after the usual meal, excess substrate is stored as fat, structural protein, and glycogen. Substrate flux in this phase of metabolism, called *anabolic,* proceeds from intestine to liver to utilization and storage sites. Insulin is the primary hormone mediating the anabolic phase, and counterregulatory hormone levels are suppressed.

The *catabolic* phase of metabolism begins about 5 to 6 h after a meal. Normally the only significant period of catabolism is during the overnight fast, but under some circumstances, particularly serious illness, it may be prolonged. During fasting/catabolism a series of metabolic adjustments maintain the plasma glucose in a safe range for central nervous system metabolism while at the same time providing energy for other tissues in the body. First, the liver is activated for glucose production, and second, a lipid economy is established for most other tissues of the body. Initially glucose from the liver is derived almost exclusively from hepatic glycogen. Because there is only about 70 g of glycogen available in the average human liver, glycogenolysis can only sustain the plasma glucose for a short time, ordinarily 8 to 10 h. Exercise may shorten the protective period, as may the stress of severe illness. To compensate for glycogen depletion gluconeogenesis begins early, with flux of substrate from muscle and adipose tissue stores to liver and then to utilization sites.

The precursors for hepatic glucose synthesis are lactate/pyruvate and amino acids (primarily alanine) derived from muscle and glycerol released from adipose tissue consequent to lipolysis. Amino acids constitute the primary substrate for gluconeogenesis. Most of the lactate is recycled from preformed glucose (*Cori cycle*), the only net contribution coming from the breakdown of muscle glycogen. Glycerol is initially a minor substrate but increases in importance with time. With prolonged fasting the kidney also becomes a gluconeogenic organ and contributes to total glucose production. The primary renal substrate is glutamine, not alanine. Proteolysis required to provide amino acids for gluconeogenesis accounts for the negative nitrogen balance of starvation. The same mechanism is operative in the stress of trauma, surgery, and severe infection. In quantitative terms the liver produces about 11 μmol/kg per min (2 mg/kg per min) of glucose in the initial phases of fasting. Higher glucose turnover indicates increased utilization of glucose, an important consideration in the differential diagnosis of hypoglycemia.

The switch to fat metabolism is accomplished by activation of the hormone-sensitive lipase in adipose tissue, which hydrolyzes stored triglycerides to long-chain fatty acids and glycerol. The long-chain fatty acids have two fates. The bulk (normally about 120 g/d) is utilized directly, and the remainder (about 40 g/d) is oxidized in the liver to acetoacetic and β-hydroxybutyric acids. Ketoacids can be utilized efficiently as an energy source by most tissues (liver only minimally), but their primary importance is as backup substrate for the brain, as noted above. The shift of most tissues to lipid metabolism is important since the preferential oxidation of free fatty acids and ketones in place of glucose spares the latter for utilization by the central nervous system.

Catabolic metabolism is initiated by a fall in insulin concentration in plasma coupled with secretion of the four counterregulatory hormones glucagon, epinephrine, cortisol, and growth hormone. In addition norepinephrine is released directly in tissues from sympathetic neurons. Glucagon is the primary hormone of glucose maintenance with epinephrine playing a backup or secondary role. The latter is particularly important in the defense against hypoglycemia in diabetes mellitus where the glucagon response is lost early (see Chap. 319). Cortisol and growth hormone function by antagonizing insulin action and act synergistically (''permissively'') with other hormones to promote mobilization of substrate and activation of gluconeogenesis.

The anabolic and catabolic phases of metabolism are summarized in Table 320-1. Breakdown in any of the adaptive mechanisms can lead to hypoglycemia.

SYMPTOMATOLOGY Symptoms of hypoglycemia fall into two main categories: those induced by an *excessive secretion of epinephrine* and those due to *dysfunction of the central nervous system.* Rapid epinephrine release causes sweating, tremor, tachycardia, anxiety, and hunger. Central nervous system symptoms include dizziness, headache, clouding of vision, blunted mental acuity, loss of fine motor skill, confusion, abnormal behavior, convulsions, and loss of consciousness. When the onset of hypoglycemia is gradual central nervous system symptoms predominate, and the epinephrine phase may not be recognizable. With more rapid drops in plasma glucose (as in insulin reactions), adrenergic symptoms are prominent. In the diabetic subject adrenergic symptoms may not be manifest if severe neuropathy is present.

The level of plasma glucose required to impair metabolism is not uniform. In nondiabetic persons acute lowering of the plasma glucose to around 2.8 mmol/L (50 mg/dL) produces autonomic nervous system symptoms and induces release of counterregulatory hormones.

TABLE 320-1 The feeding-fasting cycle

Phase	Primary hormone	Plasma substrates	Substrate flux	Active process
Anabolic*	Insulin	↑ Glucose ↑ Triglycerides ↑ Branched-chain amino acids ↓ Free fatty acids ↓ Ketones	Splanchnic bed → storage and utilization sites	Glycogen storage Protein synthesis Triglyceride formation
Catabolic†	Glucagon	↓ Glucose ↓ Triglycerides ↑ Alanine and glutamine‡ ↑ Free fatty acids ↑ Ketones	Storage sites → liver and utilization sites	Glycogenolysis Gluconeogenesis Proteolysis Lipolysis Ketogenesis

* Expected findings during the first several hours after ingestion of a mixed meal of fat, carbohydrate, and protein.
† The major catabolic phase occurs during the overnight fast, although partial catabolic cycles occur between meals.
‡ Arrows indicate plasma concentrations except for alanine and glutamine. While arterial concentrations of these amino acids are relatively constant, uptake by the liver and intestine is increased in the catabolic phase.

However, utilizing auditory evoked potentials as a sensitive indicator of central nervous system function, abnormalities can be seen in normal persons with a drop in glucose from 4.8 to 4.0 mmol/L (87 to 72 mg/dL). When blood glucose is sustained at 4.0 mmol/L (72 mg/dL) counterregulatory release eventually occurs (2 to 3 h) despite the fact that no symptoms are produced. Major symptoms of nervous system dysfunction may not occur until plasma glucose concentrations approximate 1 mmol/L (20 mg/dL). This is because normal persons have the capacity to increase cerebral blood flow sufficiently to deliver adequate glucose to the brain even with low concentrations. Cerebral atherosclerosis, with its nonelastic blood vessels, compromises this protective mechanism and allows symptomatic distress at higher glucose levels. Symptoms (adrenergic or CNS) due to hypoglycemia are unlikely with a plasma glucose above 3.0 mmol/L (60 mg/dL) in nondiabetic persons, recognizing that the physiologic sequence induced by hypoglycemia is subliminal CNS dysfunction, adrenergic symptoms, and then overt CNS dysfunction. Poorly controlled patients with diabetes mellitus appear to develop symptoms at higher glucose concentrations [4.3 mmol/L (80 mg/dL) in one report] while meticulously controlled diabetic patients have a lowering of the symptomatic threshold.

CLASSIFICATION It is traditional to classify hypoglycemia as either *postprandial* (reactive) or *fasting*. Pathologically low plasma glucose concentrations occur in the former only in response to meals, while in the latter only after fasting for a few to many hours. Patients with fasting hypoglycemia (particularly those with insulinomas) may exhibit a reactive component, but reactive patients do not have symptoms when food is withdrawn. Fasting hypoglycemia usually means that a disease process is associated with the lowered plasma glucose, but symptoms suggestive of postprandial hypoglycemia are often found in the absence of recognizable disease.

CAUSES OF HYPOGLYCEMIA Postprandial hypoglycemia The most common cause of postprandial hypoglycemia is alimentary hyperinsulinism (Table 320-2). Patients who have undergone gastrectomy, gastrojejunostomy, pyloroplasty, or vagotomy are subject to hypoglycemia following meals, presumably because of rapid gastric emptying with brisk absorption of glucose and excessive insulin release. Glucose concentrations fall more rapidly than insulin under these circumstances, and the resulting insulin-glucose imbalance leads to hypoglycemia. Ingestion of fructose or galactose induces hypoglycemia in children with fructose intolerance and galactosemia (Chap. 337), respectively. Leucine intake can rarely cause the syndrome in susceptible infants. Diabetes mellitus in its early phase is usually listed as a cause of reactive hypoglycemia, but in our experience symptomatic hypoglycemia as a premonitory symptom of diabetes is uncommon. Prediabetics, who by definition are normoglycemic, may have a late fall in plasma glucose after oral glucose tolerance testing, but this does not mean hypoglycemia. In fact, this pattern is similar to that frequently present in asymptomatic, healthy individuals (see below).

TABLE 320-2 Causes of postprandial (reactive) hypoglycemia

Alimentary hyperinsulinism
Hereditary fructose intolerance
Galactosemia
Leucine sensitivity
Idiopathic

Idiopathic alimentary hypoglycemia consists of two syndromes: *true hypoglycemia* and *pseudohypoglycemia*. In the former, adrenergic symptoms appear postprandially and are accompanied by a low plasma glucose at the time the symptoms appear spontaneously during everyday life. The symptoms are relieved by ingestion of carbohydrate, which raises the plasma glucose. Such patients are rare. The mechanism is unknown, although subtle (nonanatomic) dysfunction of the gastrointestinal tract might be operative. Some patients with true postprandial hypoglycemia turn out to have insulinomas (see below). *Pseudohypoglycemia* describes the condition of patients who reproducibly develop adrenergic symptoms suggestive of hypoglycemia 2 to 5 h after a meal but who do not have low plasma glucose concentrations when symptoms appear spontaneously in everyday life. The condition is often self-diagnosed with ''confirmation'' coming from a 5-h glucose tolerance test that reveals a lower than ''normal'' plasma glucose between 2 and 5 h.

Two questions have to be asked about pseudohypoglycemia. First, what are the symptoms (which may be incapacitating) due to? Second, can a valid diagnosis of hypoglycemia be made by a glucose tolerance test? The symptoms of nervousness, weakness, tremor, tachycardia, dizziness, and sweating reported by these patients are probably due to epinephrine release. Many otherwise normal persons experience similar symptoms at some time in their lives and may even have gained relief by eating. Patients with pseudohypoglycemia, on the other hand, develop the symptoms regularly and repetitively. In one study 80 consecutive subjects with reproducible postprandial symptoms by history were studied by 5-h glucose tolerance testing. Hypoglycemia was considered to be present if (1) the plasma glucose fell below 3.3 mmol/L (60 mg/dL) during the test, (2) symptoms or signs compatible with hypoglycemia were present, and (3) at least a doubling of plasma cortisol occurred 39 to 90 min after the nadir of plasma glucose (suggesting hypoglycemia sufficient to activate the hypothalamic-pituitary-adrenal axis). Only 18 of the 80 (23 percent) who by history were candidates for postprandial hypoglycemia fulfilled these criteria. Twenty-five percent of asymptomatic matched normal controls also met all three criteria. When the patients and controls were tested after a mixed meal, no subject in either group had a plasma glucose below 3.3 mmol/L (60 mg/dL), yet 14 of the 18 patients (78 percent) had symptoms typical of those occurring spontaneously and after glucose tolerance testing. The absence of hypoglycemia after mixed meals despite the presence of typical symptoms has been confirmed in other studies. *Pseudohypoglycemia* appears to be an accurate descriptive term for the syndrome and is preferable to "idiopathic postprandial syndrome" which has also been used. Many such patients are thought to have stress or anxiety as a predisposing factor. Presumably they have enhanced catecholamine release following a meal, although they might be abnormally sensitive to normal postprandial norepinephrine/epinephrine release.

Fasting hypoglycemia The causes of fasting hypoglycemia are many, but in all there is an imbalance between the production of glucose by the liver and its utilization in peripheral tissues. In some, hypoglycemia is due primarily to a defect in glucose production, while in others the problem is excess glucose utilization. Both defects may be present. For example, with insulin excess there is driven glucose utilization coupled with blunted hepatic glucose production. The latter is caused by insulin's capacity to block the glycogenolytic/gluconeogenic effects of the counterregulatory hormones. Dual defects are probably operative in disorders of fat oxidation and non-insulin-producing tumors as well.

Supply-side hypoglycemia (impaired production of glucose) characteristically requires much less glucose during therapy than does *demand-side hypoglycemia* (overutilization of glucose) (Table 320-3). As noted above, glucose production during a fast approximates 11 μmol/kg per min (2 mg/kg per min) in normal persons, but with insulin stimulation this increases to about 67 μmol/kg per min (12 mg/kg per min). Thus if more than 56 mmol (10 g) of glucose per hour is required to prevent or reverse hypoglycemia it can be assumed that overutilization is present.

UNDERPRODUCTION OF GLUCOSE As discussed earlier, the production of glucose by the liver initially involves the breakdown of stored glycogen and subsequently depends on gluconeogenesis, the synthesis of glucose from precursors delivered to the liver from peripheral tissues. The causes of inadequate production of glucose during fasting can be grouped into five categories: (1) hormone deficiencies, (2) defects in glycogenolytic or gluconeogenic enzymes, (3) inadequate substrate delivery, (4) liver disease, and (5) drugs. Hypopituitarism and adrenal insufficiency are the most common of the hormone deficiency states causing hypoglycemia. Defects in catecholamine or glucagon release are rare. Enzymic abnormalities causing hypoglycemia are generally seen in children and not adults. Glucose-6-phosphatase deficiency is the classic example of a defect in glycogen breakdown, but hypoglycemia may occur in young children with deficiencies of hepatic glycogen phosphorylase and in other forms of glycogen storage disease (Chap. 332). The inability to make glycogen because of inadequate glycogen synthetase activity also renders the infant susceptible to fasting hypoglycemia. In addition to glucose-6-phosphatase, three other enzymes are necessary for gluconeogenesis: pyruvate carboxylase, phosphoenolpyruvate carboxykinase, and fructose-1,6-bisphosphatase (fructose-1,6-diphosphatase) (Fig. 320-1). Hypoglycemia can occur with decreased activities of any of these enzymes, often in association with lactic acidosis. The cause of lactic acidosis in these disorders is not known, although impaired hepatic lactate uptake due to the gluconeogenic defect probably plays a role. Substrate deficiency appears to be one of the mechanisms operative in ketotic hypoglycemia of infancy, since alanine turnover in such patients is low. Inadequate substrate supply may also contribute to hypoglycemia in malnutrition, muscle-wasting states, chronic renal failure, and late pregnancy. Acquired liver disease can cause serious hypoglycemia. Hepatic congestion due to right-sided heart failure is particularly troublesome, but severe viral hepatitis or cirrhosis may also cause symptomatic hypoglycemia. Hypothermia, especially in association with alcohol, may cause very low levels of plasma glucose. Slowed enzymatic activity of the liver is the likely mechanism. The hypoglycemia of renal failure probably has multiple causes. In addition to impairing substrate delivery, uremic toxins may suppress hepatic gluconeogenesis. Decreased renal clearance of insulin and impairment of renal gluconeogenesis may contribute to the problem.

A number of drugs cause hypoglycemia. The most common, apart from insulin and sulfonylureas, is alcohol. Alcohol induces hypoglycemia only after a period of fasting sufficient to deplete liver glycogen stores. In this circumstance hepatic glucose production is dependent on gluconeogenesis. The oxidation of ethanol in the liver is accompanied by generation of high concentrations of NADH, the reduced form of nicotinamide adenine dinucleotide (NAD), in the cytosol of the cell. The increased NADH/NAD ratio diverts oxaloacetate into malate formation, diminishing its availability to the gluconeogenic sequence via the action of phosphoenolpyruvate carboxykinase (Fig. 320-1). The normal pathway of gluconeogenesis from pyruvate is thus blocked, leading to a drop in hepatic glucose output and hypoglycemia. Large amounts of ethanol are not required to produce this syndrome, and plasma alcohol concentrations may be as low as 5.4 mmol/L (25 mg/dL) at the time symptoms occur. Ethanol-induced hypoglycemia usually occurs in adults but can be seen in children who drink alcohol unknowingly. Salicylates (in children) and propranolol are the next most frequently involved drugs. Propranolol presumably causes difficulty in fasting patients or insulin-requiring diabetics by impairing the glycogenolytic response. In diabetes the drug may also prevent recognition of impending hypoglycemia by blunting the symptomatic response to epinephrine release. Other drugs have been reported to cause hypoglycemia in isolated cases, but the relationship is often unproved. Some drugs enhance glucose utilization. Pentamidine and disopyramide cause hyperinsulinism, the former by beta cell cytolysis ("insulin leak") and the latter by an unknown mechanism, perhaps as a direct insulin secretagogue. Quinine given in falciparum malaria has been reported to cause hyperinsulinemic hypoglycemia, but the issue is clouded because hypoglycemia occurs in untreated malaria as well, possibly secondary to malnutrition or liver involvement.

OVERUTILIZATION OF GLUCOSE Overutilization of glucose occurs in two settings. In the first, hyperinsulinism is present, and in the second, plasma insulin concentrations are low. There are basically

TABLE 320-3 Major causes of fasting hypoglycemia

I Conditions primarily due to underproduction of glucose
- *A* Hormone deficiencies
  - *1* Hypopituitarism
  - *2* Adrenal insufficiency
  - *3* Catecholamine deficiency
  - *4* Glucagon deficiency
- *B* Enzyme defects
  - *1* Glucose-6-phosphatase
  - *2* Liver phosphorylase
  - *3* Pyruvate carboxylase
  - *4* Phosphoenolpyruvate carboxykinase
  - *5* Fructose-1,6-diphosphatase
  - *6* Glycogen synthetase
- *C* Substrate deficiency
  - *1* Ketotic hypoglycemia of infancy
  - *2* Severe malnutrition, muscle wasting
  - *3* Late pregnancy
- *D* Acquired liver disease
  - *1* Hepatic congestion
  - *2* Severe hepatitis
  - *3* Cirrhosis
  - *4* Uremia (probably multiple mechanisms)
  - *5* Hypothermia
- *E* Drugs
  - *1* Alcohol
  - *2* Propranolol
  - *3* Salicylates

II Conditions primarily due to overutilization of glucose
- *A* Hyperinsulinism
  - *1* Insulinoma
  - *2* Exogenous insulin
  - *3* Sulfonylureas
  - *4* Immune disease with insulin or insulin receptor antibodies
  - *5* Drugs: quinine in falciparum malaria, disopyramide, pentamidine
  - *6* Endotoxic shock
- *B* Appropriate insulin levels
  - *1* Extrapancreatic tumors
  - *2* Systemic carnitine deficiency
  - *3* Deficiency in enzymes of fat oxidation
  - *4* 3-Hydroxy-3-methylglutaryl-CoA lyase deficiency
  - *5* Cachexia with fat depletion

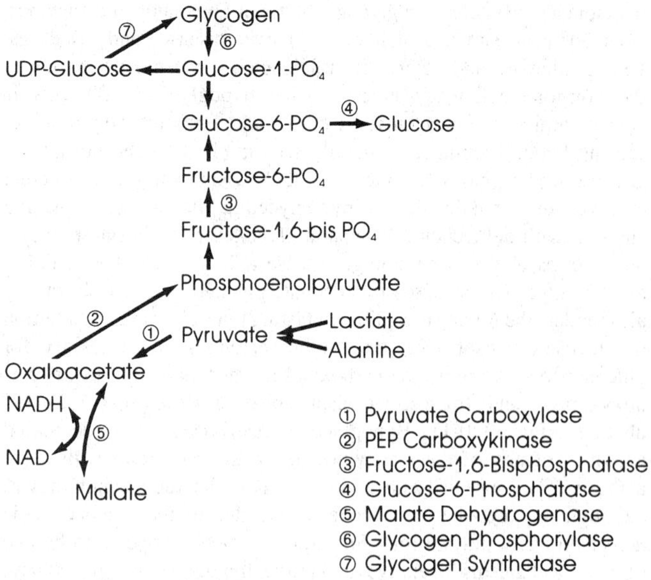

FIGURE 320-1 Scheme of hepatic carbohydrate metabolism. Only the sequence for gluconeogenesis, glycogen synthesis, and glycogenolysis is shown.

four causes of hyperinsulinemic hypoglycemia: insulinoma, exogenous insulin administration, sulfonylureas, and a peculiar form of insulin autoimmunity. Insulinoma is used generically here to include single solid tumors, microadenomatosis, and islet cell hyperplasia (nesidioblastosis), a rare syndrome in adults. Hypoglycemia in a diabetic taking prescribed insulin or oral agents is not a diagnostic problem. The difficulty comes when a nondiabetic subject induces hypoglycemia deliberately and surreptitiously because of psychiatric disturbance, raising the possibility of an insulin-producing tumor. The differential diagnosis between insulinoma and factitious hypoglycemia is considered below. Rarely hypoglycemia with hyperinsulinism occurs in autoimmune disease associated with antibodies to endogenous insulin. Mechanisms are not well understood, although dissociation of free insulin from hormone-antibody complexes at inappropriate times is probably most important. Idiotypic antibodies (antibodies against the anti-insulin antibodies) might also develop, functioning as insulin agonists with the insulin receptor. By binding insulin the antibodies may also induce excessive insulin release from the pancreas. Some patients have alternating insulin resistance/hyperglycemia and hypoglycemia. Insulin autoantibodies have been seen most frequently in subjects with hyperthyroidism treated with methimazole (thiamazole) but presumably they might arise in any autoimmune syndrome. Antibodies directed against the insulin receptor, usually a cause of insulin resistance, may also induce hypoglycemia with high plasma insulin levels. Under these circumstances conformational configuration of the antibody is thought to allow it to activate the insulin receptor, simultaneously blocking access of native insulin and impairing its clearance.

Sepsis with endotoxinemia causes hyperglycemia followed by hypoglycemia in experimental animals. Plasma insulin levels increase. Since hypoglycemia accompanying gram-negative sepsis has not been well studied in humans, its inclusion as a hyperinsulinemic state is tentative.

Hypoglycemia in the context of glucose overutilization and appropriately low plasma insulin concentrations occurs in two situations. The first is in association with solid extrapancreatic tumors, usually of large size. The most common are of mesothelial origin and include fibromas and sarcomas. The syndrome can also be seen with hepatomas, carcinomas of the gastrointestinal tract, and adrenal cancers. The mechanism of the hypoglycemia is not clear, although high levels of insulin-like growth factors may play a role. Indeed, in some studies insulin-like growth factors are present in essentially all such tumors. Presumably such factors, if present, act via the insulin receptor rather than by binding to their own receptors. One patient with tumor-associated hypoglycemia was reported to have an increased number of insulin receptors in liver, muscle, and circulating mononuclear cells, but the significance of the finding is not clear.

Symptomatic hypoglycemia due to overutilization may also occur in situations where free fatty acids and ketones are not available for oxidation in muscle and other tissues. Patients with *systemic carnitine deficiency* may have severe hypoglycemia. In this condition carnitine, which is necessary to transport fatty acids into mitochondria for oxidation, is low in plasma, muscle, liver, and other tissues. As a consequence, peripheral tissues cannot utilize fatty acids for energy production, and the liver cannot make ketone bodies as alternative substrate. The result is that all tissues become glucose-dependent, exceeding the capacity of the liver to meet the demand. Other features of systemic carnitine deficiency include nausea, vomiting, elevated blood ammonia levels, and hepatic encephalopathy. The illness thus constitutes one form of the Reye's syndrome. (In *myopathic carnitine deficiency* only muscle is involved, and a polymyositis-like syndrome without hypoglycemia is produced.) Nonketotic (or hypoketotic) hypoglycemia with secondary systemic carnitine deficiency and the Reye syndrome also accompany *deficiencies of medium- and long-chain acyl-CoA dehydrogenases and 3-hydroxy-3-methylglutaryl-CoA lyase (HMG-CoA lyase).* The first two enzymes operate in the fatty acid oxidative sequence while HMG-CoA lyase catalyzes the conversion HMG-CoA to acetoacetate and acetyl-CoA in the ketogenic cycle. Any time there is a block in fatty acid oxidation or ketone formation a secondary carnitine deficiency may develop. Accumulated acyl-CoA is transesterified to form acyl carnitine, which is then lost in the urine. Systemic carnitine deficiency in the absence of enzymic defect probably is due to a primary renal leak. It is not known whether the block in ketone production per se leads to hypoglycemia or whether secondary carnitine deficiency is required. If the former, ketones must become a primary (necessary) substrate during an extended fast. Hypoglycemia is less common with deficiency of *carnitine palmitoyltransferase,* the enzyme that transesterifies fatty acyl coenzyme A (CoA) to carnitine for oxidation. Presumably the defect is not complete in most patients, allowing some fatty acid oxidation to occur so that the tendency to hypoglycemia is minimized. The clinical picture is that of an exercise-induced myopathy with myoglobinuria. Hypoglycemia also occurs in patients with cachexia due to advanced cancer. At autopsy no recognizable triglyceride stores are present in adipose tissue, suggesting free fatty acid deficiency as the primary mechanism.

Causes of hypoglycemia in hospitalized patients Frequencies of diagnoses vary in unselected series. Drugs constitute the most common cause, the three most common agents being insulin, sulfonylureas, and alcohol. It has been estimated that 60 percent of the time one of these three agents is involved when hypoglycemia is diagnosed. Renal failure was present in nearly 30 percent of hypoglycemic episodes in hospitalized patients in one series but overall makes up about 15 percent of cases. Liver disease (about 15 percent), malnutrition (about 10 percent), and sepsis (about 5 percent) are the other common causes. A high index of suspicion for insulinoma, solid tumors, enzymatic defects, or hormonal deficiencies should be engendered by the finding of hypoglycemia in nondiabetic persons without uremia, liver disease, cachexia, or history of alcohol intake.

DIAGNOSIS **Fasting hypoglycemia** If a person with diabetes mellitus presents with symptoms of hypoglycemia, it is usually safe to conclude that no special diagnostic tests are needed since the hypoglycemia is almost always related to therapy. If a nondiabetic appears with similar symptoms—particularly if confusion, loss of consciousness, or convulsions are present—it is critical to draw blood for assay before intravenous glucose is administered. *The best time to obtain diagnostic laboratory tests with spontaneous hypoglycemia is at presentation.* The goal is to assess plasma insulin level and counterregulatory hormone response while the plasma glucose is low.

Assays should be carried out for glucose, insulin, insulin connecting peptide (C peptide), cortisol, drugs, and toxins, especially sulfonylureas and alcohol. It is often wise to freeze a separate sample of plasma for subsequent tests (e.g., proinsulin, carnitine, insulin antibodies, lactate) should the diagnosis not be clear from initial evaluation. Demonstration that hypoglycemia is accompanied by inappropriate insulin levels sharply narrows the clinical possibilities. Routine laboratory exams may also be helpful. For example, the absence of ketones or the presence of a metabolic acidosis may be clues to the primary problem.

Once the patient has become alert (assuming altered mental status is present on arrival), it is important to take a detailed history and carry out a physical examination. Special emphasis should be placed on food intake in the preceding 24 h and the possibility of drug ingestion. Signs of heart failure and hepatic congestion should be sought, and the presence and thickness of the adipose tissue mass should be noted. Pigmentation of the skin may suggest Addison's disease. Workup includes liver function studies and computed tomography (CT) scanning or abdominal sonography (to look for solid tumors in the retroperitoneal space or abdominal cavity). Patients with enzyme defects and rare hormonal deficiencies (epinephrine, glucagon) usually require evaluation in referral centers, since definitive assays for these hormones and enzymes are not routinely available. For reasons cited above it is important to quantitate the amount of glucose required to prevent recurrent hypoglycemia during acute phase therapy; i.e., if 8 to 10 g of glucose per hour is sufficient to prevent hypoglycemia, diminished glucose production is probably operative. A requirement for higher infusion rates suggests enhanced glucose utilization.

If the patient has a history compatible with hypoglycemia but does not have symptoms at the time of examination, hospitalization for fasting is generally required. The fast should be carried out for at least 72 h unless symptoms develop. Plasma glucose, insulin, C peptide, and cortisol should be measured every 6 h. Occasionally quantitation of plasma free fatty acids, glucagon, and total ketones is helpful. (For glucagon, a protease inhibitor such as aprotinin must be added.) Two points are at issue. First, does the patient have fasting hypoglycemia? Second, is the hypoglycemia associated with hyperinsulinism? Neither question is easy to answer. There is no definitive lower limit of plasma glucose that unequivocally defines pathologic hypoglycemia during a 72-h fast. Values of the nadir in one study are shown in Table 320-4. Women usually develop lower levels than men. Another series reported mean minimal levels of 3.4 mmol/L (62 mg/dL) in men and 2.9 mmol/L (52 mg/dL) in women during a 72-h fast. However, values as low as 1.2 mmol/L (22 mg/dL) may occur in normal women without symptoms. On balance, a presumptive diagnosis of hypoglycemia is probably justified if the plasma glucose falls below 2.8 mmol/L (50 mg/dL) in men and 2.5 mmol/L (45 mg/dL) in women at any time during the fast, provided typical symptoms are induced. The diagnosis of hypoglycemia is strengthened if symptoms are rapidly relieved by administration of carbohydrate. If symptoms are not produced, the diagnosis of hypoglycemia should be made with caution.

Absolute insulin values are not always helpful in diagnosing hyperinsulinism. In normal subjects when glucose concentrations rise insulin levels also increase, and when plasma glucose concentrations fall insulin release is inhibited. This means that plasma insulin concentrations must be interpreted in the light of the simultaneously determined glucose value. Thus, a "normal" absolute insulin level may be abnormal in the face of hypoglycemia, while high absolute levels may be appropriate if the glucose concentration is elevated. In an attempt to relate the two parameters the concept of the insulin/glucose ratio

$$\frac{\text{Plasma insulin } (\mu\text{U/mL})}{\text{Plasma glucose (mg/dL)}}$$

was developed utilizing conventional laboratory units. In normal persons the ratio is always less than 0.4, while most (but not all) patients with insulinoma have ratios greater than 0.4—often above 1.0. When the ratio is calculated in SI units [plasma insulin (pmol/L)/plasma glucose (mmol/L)] the normal value is less than 50. Patients with insulinoma may secrete insulin episodically; the ratio may, therefore, be normal on one occasion and abnormal on another. The insulin/glucose ratio tends to fall during fasting in normal individuals but increases in patients with insulinoma.

Plasma insulin concentration generally reaches background levels for the assay when the plasma glucose falls below about 4.4 mmol/L (80 mg/dL). While some studies have shown lower cutoff points, it is probable that any measurable insulin concentration should be considered suspicious if the plasma glucose is below 2.8 mmol/L (50 mg/dL) in men or 2.5 mmol/L (45 mg/dL) in women, regardless of the value of the insulin/glucose ratio. If hyperinsulinism is not demonstrated, one of the other causes of fasting hypoglycemia must be sought.

Should hypoglycemia not develop during fasting, insulinoma or other hypoglycemia-producing organic disease is unlikely, although insulinomas may rarely present solely as postprandial hypoglycemia with no depression of the plasma glucose even during a prolonged fast. Diagnosis usually is suspected in such cases because inappropriate insulin levels are shown during the postmeal episodes. Some authors recommend provocative tests with calcium, tolbutamide, glucagon, or leucine in suspected islet cell tumors, but overlap between normal subjects and patients with insulinoma is so great as to render the tests of little value in a given individual.

Postprandial hypoglycemia In patients presumed to have postprandial hypoglycemia the most widely used test has been a 5-h oral glucose tolerance examination. Since normal persons may have chemical hypoglycemia without symptoms in the glucose tolerance test while subjects with pseudohypoglycemia have symptoms in the absence of hypoglycemia following meal testing, the 5-h glucose tolerance test should be abandoned as a tool for diagnosis. The only unequivocal diagnostic test for true pseudohypoglycemia is the demonstration of a low plasma glucose concentration (less than 2.8 mmol/L or 50 mg/dL) during spontaneously developed symptoms. Some physicians utilize a home glucose analyzer in diagnosis. If no hypoglycemia is demonstrated during one week of testing (on arising,

TABLE 320-4 Mean plasma glucose and insulin during fasting

		Hours of fast				
Assay	Subjects	0*	24	36	48	72
Glucose mmol/L (mg/dL)	Men	4.7 (85)	4.6 (83)	4.3 (78)	4.3 (78)	3.9 (71)
	Women	4.6 (83)	3.5 (63)	2.8 (50)	2.6 (46)	2.7 (48)
Insulin pmol/L (μU/mL)	Men	100 (14)	64 (9)	57 (8)	57 (8)	43 (6)
	Women	86 (12)	43 (6)	29 (4)	21 (3)	29 (4)

* Zero values were obtained after overnight fast. Results are mean values for 20 normal men and 60 normal women.
SOURCE: TJ Merimee, JE Tyson, Diabetes 26:161, 1977.

TABLE 320-5 Differential diagnosis of insulinoma and factitious hyperinsulinism

Test	Insulinoma	Exogenous insulin	Sulfonylurea
Plasma insulin	High	Very high*	High
Insulin/glucose ratio	High	Very high	High
Proinsulin	Increased	Normal or low	Normal
C peptide	Increased	Normal or low†	Increased
Insulin antibodies	Absent	± Present‡	Absent
Plasma or urine sulfonylurea	Absent	Absent	Present

* Total plasma insulin in patients with insulinoma is rarely above 1435 pmol/L (200 μU/mL) in the basal state and often much lower. Values greater than 7175 pmol/L (1000 μU/mL) are highly suggestive of exogenous insulin injection.
† C peptide may be normal in absolute terms, but low in relation to the increased insulin value. See text for C-peptide suppression test.
‡ Insulin antibodies may not be present if only a few injections have been given, especially with purified insulins.

2 h after each meal, at bedtime, and during symptoms) the diagnosis of true postprandial hypoglycemia is rejected. Patients with pseudohypoglycemia usually have slightly elevated glucose concentrations during spontaneous attacks because of the hyperglycemic action of epinephrine, the stress hormone that induces the symptoms.

Insulinoma versus factitious hypoglycemia The self-induction of hypoglycemia by the injection of insulin or the ingestion of sulfonylureas is so common as to equal or exceed the incidence of insulinoma. The demonstration of hyperinsulinism during hypoglycemia cannot, therefore, be taken as definitive evidence of the presence of an islet cell tumor. Factitious disease should always be suspected when hypoglycemic symptoms appear in medical personnel or families of diabetic patients. Several tests are helpful in distinguishing insulinoma from factitious disease once hyperinsulinism has been established. Patients with insulinoma tend to have high concentrations of proinsulin in plasma (>20 percent of total insulin). Plasma proinsulin is not elevated by the administration of commercial insulin preparations or sulfonylureas. Measurement of the insulin connecting peptide (C peptide) will indicate whether the insulin circulating in plasma is of endogenous or exogenous origin. When insulin is cleaved from its precursor proinsulin molecule, C peptide is released into the portal vein in a 1:1 ratio with insulin. Thus, patients with insulinoma should have C-peptide concentrations that parallel the plasma insulin values. The characteristic pattern in factitious hypoglycemia due to insulin injection is a high circulating level of insulin with relatively suppressed C-peptide values because exogenous insulin suppresses endogenous insulin release in normal persons. Suppression does not usually occur in insulinoma. Some investigators recommend a C-peptide suppression test in equivocal situations. In this test 0.1 unit of insulin per kilogram of body weight is infused intravenously over 60 min. C-peptide concentration should be less than 1.2 ng/mL at the end of the test, provided the plasma glucose has dropped to 2.2 mmol/L (40 mg/dL) or less. Antibodies to insulin are helpful if present since they usually indicate chronic insulin injection. However, as noted earlier, autoantibodies directed against insulin may develop in hyperthyroidism and other autoimmune diseases. Anti-insulin antibodies cannot be taken as evidence of insulin injection under these circumstances. Sulfonylureas elevate both the C-peptide and insulin concentrations in plasma. Therefore, factitious hypoglycemia due to oral agents can only be diagnosed by a high index of suspicion coupled with assay of the drug in plasma or urine. The differential characteristics of insulinoma and the two types of factitious hypoglycemia are shown in Table 320-5.

TREATMENT The initial treatment of serious hypoglycemia (producing confusion or coma) is the intravenous administration of a bolus of 25 or 50 g glucose as a 50% solution followed by constant infusion of glucose until the patient is able to eat a meal. The importance of the meal resides in the fact that hepatic glycogen repletion is not effective with small quantities of intravenous glucose. Patients in the overutilization category may require large amounts of intravenous glucose to maintain consciousness. It is not enough to infuse 5% dextrose at a rate of 1 to 2 mL/min and assume the patient is protected (20 to 30% dextrose solutions may be required in some cases). Frequent measurement of capillary glucose concentrations should be carried out using glucose-sensitive reagent strips to assess effectiveness of glucose infusion rates. Intravenous glucose can usually be stopped once the patient has eaten, but this can only be determined by trial. Adrenergic reactions without central nervous system abnormalities can be treated with oral carbohydrate and do not require parenteral therapy.

Hypoglycemia from sulfonylureas may last for prolonged periods (days) (Fig. 320-2). It is common for patients to lapse back into coma if glucose infusions are stopped too soon. The reason for the prolonged effect is not always clear, though drug interactions, hepatic disease, and renal failure may play a role in some cases.

Surgery is the treatment of choice for insulinoma. Localization

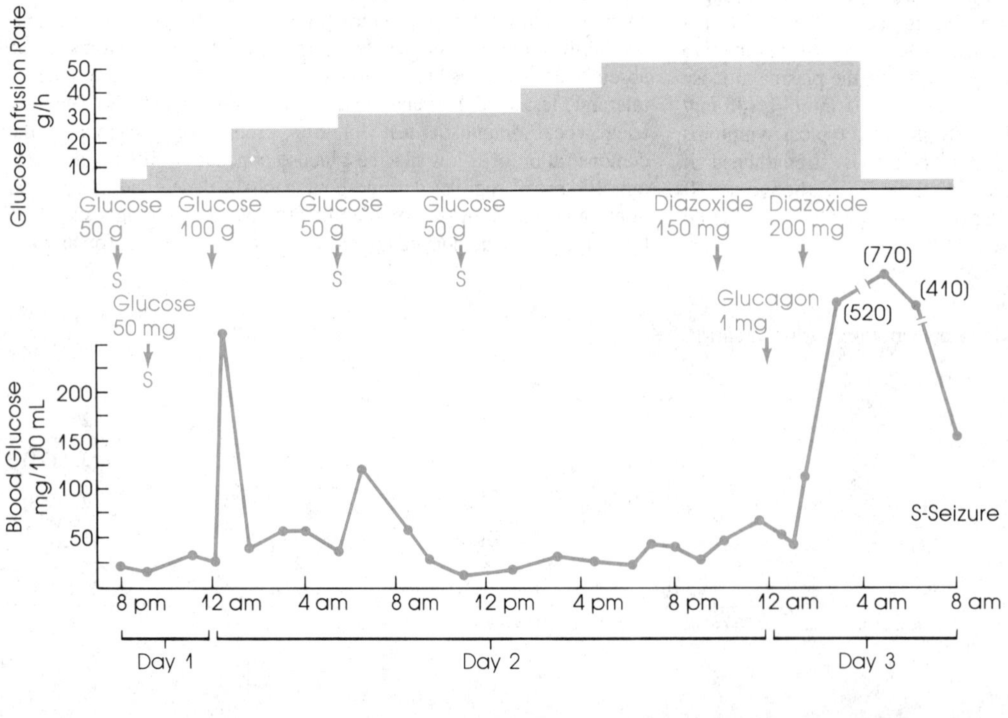

FIGURE 320-2 Prolonged and refractory hypoglycemia in factitious hypoglycemia due to chlorpropamide in an alcoholic. Note continued hypoglycemia despite the infusion of glucose at rates up to 50 g/h. *(From RM Jordan et al, Arch Intern Med 137:390, 1977. Copyright 1977, American Medical Association. Used by permission.)*

should be attempted with CT scan or sonography prior to exploration. Arteriography (celiac or superior mesenteric) is less effective. In some centers preoperative or operative sampling of insulin concentrations by selective pancreatic vein catheterization has been performed but appears to be of minimal benefit even if a rapid insulin assay is available. If the tumor cannot be palpated in the pancreas or located in an extrapancreatic site at the time of surgery, stepwise pancreatectomy (from tail to head) should be carried out with frozen sections made of sequential slices. Capillary glucose should be measured frequently (at each stage of the resection if the tumor is not obvious). A rise in plasma glucose may indicate removal of a small, nonpalpable lesion. In general, resection is stopped with an 85 percent pancreatectomy, even if the tumor is not found, to avoid malabsorptive complications. While a majority of patients are cured by surgery, as many as 15 percent have persistent hypoglycemia. Postoperative complications included acute pancreatitis, peritonitis, fistulas, pseudocyst formation, and chronic hyperglycemia (acquired diabetes).

Medical treatment is indicated in insulinoma only in preparation for surgery or after failure to find the tumor at operation. Two drugs are available, diazoxide and octreotide, a long-acting octapeptide analogue of somatostatin. Diazoxide can be given intravenously or orally in doses of 300 to 1200 mg/d and because of its salt-retaining properties must be accompanied by a diuretic. Octreotide is given subcutaneously in divided doses of 150 to 450 μg/d and may cause nausea and diarrhea and predispose to cholelithiasis. Treatment of metastatic insulin-producing carcinomas is unsatisfactory. Streptozocin, plicamycin, and doxorubicin have been tried in these malignancies, but the results are dismal. One multicenter trial reported improved results when streptozocin was combined with fluorouracil. Despite the generally poor prognosis, occasional patients with insulin-producing islet cell carcinomas survive for long periods.

Therapy of other forms of recurrent hypoglycemia, apart from hormone replacement in pituitary or adrenal insufficiency, is dietary. In most cases avoidance of fasting is all that is required. This is critical in diseases of fat oxidation or ketone synthesis. If intercurrent illness prevents eating, hospitalization for intravenous glucose is absolutely required. A high-protein, low-carbohydrate diet is frequently prescribed for patients with pseudohypoglycemia and often relieves symptoms. With true alimentary hypoglycemia it is probably important to keep the size of the individual meals small. The practice of giving massive amounts of vitamin E, crude adrenocortical extract, and trace metals to patients with pseudohypoglycemia is useless even if harmless (which has not been proved).

REFERENCES

AVRAM MM et al: Uremic hypoglycemia. A preventable life-threatening complication. NY State J Med 84:593, 1984

BERNSTEIN RK: Meaningful screening test for reactive hypoglycemia. Diabetes Care 10:792, 1987

BOYLE PJ et al: Plasma glucose concentrations at the onset of hypoglycemic symptoms in patients with poorly controlled diabetes and in nondiabetics. N Engl J Med 318:1487, 1988

CHARLES MA et al: Comparison of oral glucose tolerance tests and mixed meals in patients with apparent idiopathic postabsorptive hypoglycemia. Absence of hypoglycemia after meals. Diabetes 30:465, 1981

CLUTTER WE et al: Regulation of glucose metabolism by sympathochromaffin catecholamines. Diabetes/Metabolism Rev 4:1, 1988

COHEN RM et al: Proinsulin radioimmunoassay in the evaluation of insulinomas and familial hyperproinsulinemia. Metabolism 35:1137, 1986

DE FEO P et al: Modest decrements in plasma glucose concentration cause early impairment in cognitive function and later activation of glucose counterregulation in the absence of hypoglycemic symptoms in normal man. J Clin Invest 82:436, 1988

FERNER RE, NEIL HAW: Sulphonylureas and hypoglycaemia. Br Med J 296:949, 1988

FISCHER KF et al: Hypoglycemia in hospitalized patients. Causes and outcomes. N Engl J Med 315:1245, 1986

FOSTER DW, MCGARRY JD: Glucose, lipid and protein metabolism, in *Textbook of Endocrine Physiology*, JE Griffin, SR Ojeda (eds). New York, Oxford, 1988, pp 302–326

GERICH JE, CAMPBELL PJ: Overview of counterregulation and its abnormalities in diabetes mellitus and other conditions. Diabetes/Metabolism Rev 4:93, 1988

GIBSON KM et al: 3-Hydroxy-3-methylglutaryl-coenzyme A lyase deficiency: Report of five new patients. J Inher Metab Dis 11:76, 1988

GRUNBERGER G et al: Factitious hypoglycemia due to surreptitious administration of insulin. Diagnosis, treatment, and long-term follow-up. Ann Intern Med 108:252, 1988

HALE DE et al: Long-chain acyl coenzyme A dehydrogenase deficiency: An inherited cause of nonketotic hypoglycemia. Pediatr Res 19:666, 1985

MALOUF R, BRUST JCM: Hypoglycemia: Causes, neurological manifestations, and outcome. Ann Neurol 17:421, 1985

MERIMEE TJ: Insulin-like growth factors in patients with nonislet cell tumors and hypoglycemia. Metabolism 35:360, 1986

NAYLOR JM, KRONFELD DS: In vivo studies of hypoglycemia and lactic acidosis in endotoxic shock. Am J Physiol 248:E309, 1985

SERVICE FJ et al: Insulinoma. Clinical and diagnostic features of 60 consecutive cases. Mayo Clin Proc 51:417, 1976

TAYLOR TE et al: Blood glucose levels in Malawian children before and during the administration of intravenous quinine for severe falciparum malaria. N Engl J Med 319:1040, 1988

WASKIN H et al: Risk factors for hypoglycemia associated with pentamidine therapy for *Pneumocystis* pneumonia. JAMA 260:345, 1988

WEINSTOCK G et al: Islet cell hyperplasia: An unusual cause of hypoglycemia in an adult. Metabolism 35:110, 1986

321 DISORDERS OF THE TESTIS

JAMES E. GRIFFIN / JEAN D. WILSON

The testis produces sperm and the steroid hormones that regulate male sexual life. Both functions are under complex feedback control by the hypothalamic-pituitary system so that the testis has biosynthetic and regulatory features similar to those of the ovary and the adrenal. Testicular hormones are also responsible for the formation of the basic male phenotype during embryogenesis. The function of the embryonic testis and the disorders of sexual differentiation are described in Chap. 324.

PHYSIOLOGY AND REGULATION OF TESTICULAR FUNCTION

The testis consists of two components—a system of spermatogenic tubules for the production and transport of sperm and clusters of interstitial or Leydig cells that produce androgenic steroids.

THE LEYDIG CELL Testosterone synthesis The biochemical pathway by which the 27-carbon sterol cholesterol is converted to androgens and estrogens is depicted in Fig. 321-1. Cholesterol can either be synthesized de novo in the Leydig cell or derived from plasma lipoproteins. Five enzymatic transformations are required for the conversion of cholesterol to testosterone. In this process the side chain of cholesterol is cleaved in two steps to reduce the size from 27 to 19 carbons, and the A ring of the steroid is converted to the Δ^4-3-keto configuration. The five transformations are the 20,22-desmolase, the 3β-hydroxysteroid dehydrogenase-$\Delta^{4,5}$-isomerase-complex, 17α-hydroxylase, 17,20-desmolase, and 17β-hydroxysteroid dehydrogenase reactions. The first four reactions also take place in the adrenal.

The rate-limiting process in testosterone synthesis is the conversion of cholesterol to pregnenolone by the 20,22-desmolase reaction; luteinizing hormone (LH) from the pituitary regulates the activity of this enzyme and of other enzymes in the pathway. Other steroids including estradiol are synthesized in small amounts in the Leydig cell.

Testosterone secretion and transport Only about 70 nmol (20 μg) of testosterone is stored in the normal testes, so that the total hormone content turns over about 200 times each day to provide the average of 17 to 20 μmol (5 to 6 mg) that is secreted into plasma in normal young men (Fig. 321-2). Testosterone is transported in plasma bound to protein, largely to albumin and to a specific transport protein, testosterone-binding globulin (TeBG, also called sex hormone–binding globulin, SHBG). The bound and unbound fractions

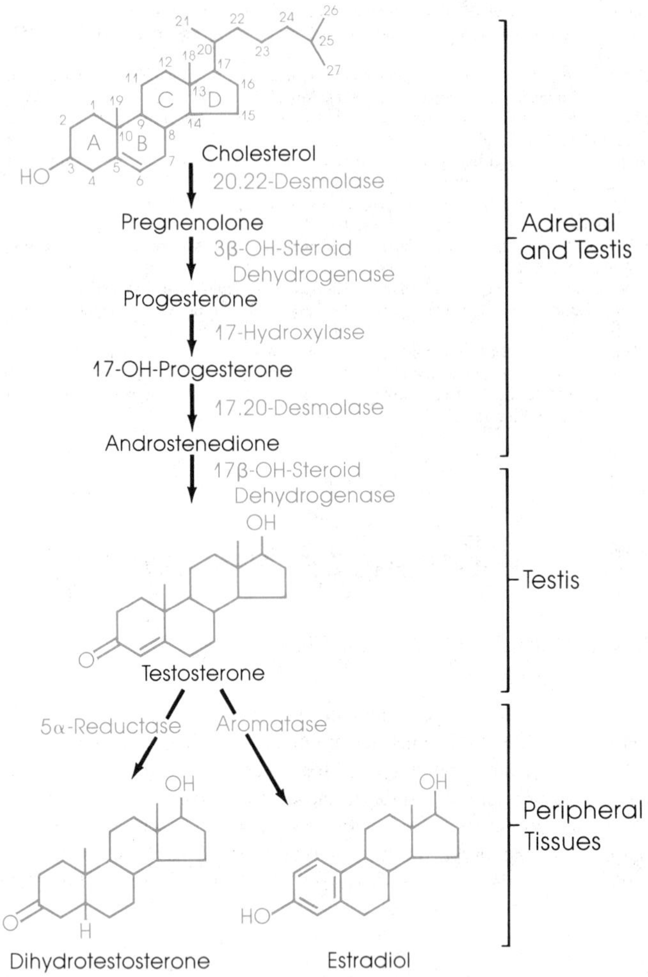

FIGURE 321-1 Pathways of androgen formation in the testis and the conversion of androgens to other active hormones in peripheral tissues.

in plasma are in dynamic equilibrium, only about 1 to 3 percent being present in the free fraction. The fraction of circulating testosterone available for entry into tissues approximates the sum of the free and albumin-bound fractions or about 40 to 50 percent of the total plasma testosterone.

Peripheral metabolism of androgens Testosterone serves as a circulating precursor (or prohormone) for the formation of two other types of active metabolites that mediate many of the physiologic processes involved in androgen action (Fig. 321-1). Testosterone can be 5α-reduced to dihydrotestosterone, which performs many of the differentiative, growth-promoting, and functional actions involved in male sexual differentiation and virilization. Circulating androgens in both sexes can also be converted to estrogens in extraglandular tissues. In men estrogens act in some instances in concert with androgens but can also have effects independent of or opposite to those of androgens. Thus, the physiologic effects of testosterone are the result of the combined effects of testosterone itself plus those of the active androgen and estrogen metabolites of the parent molecule. (In normal men small amounts of estradiol and dihydrotestosterone are also derived by direct secretion from the testis and indirectly from the weak adrenal androgen androstenedione.)

The quantitative relation between circulating androgens and the formation of estrogen in normal young men is illustrated diagrammatically in Fig. 321-2. The production rates of testosterone and androstenedione average about 20 and 10 μmol (6 and 3 mg), respectively, per day. All of estrone production [averaging about 240 nmol (66 μg) per day] can be accounted for by formation from circulating precursors. The mean estradiol production rate is about 170 nmol (45 μg) per day; about 35 percent of this amount is derived from circulating testosterone, 50 percent is derived from the weak estrogen estrone, and 15 percent is secreted directly into the circulation by the testes. When gonadotropin levels are elevated, the amount of estradiol secretion by the testis is increased.

The 5α-reduced and estrogenic metabolites can exert local (paracrine) actions in the tissues in which they are formed or enter the circulation and act as hormones at other sites. Circulating dihydrotestosterone is formed principally in the androgen target tissues, and estrogen formation takes place in many tissues, the most significant being adipose tissue. The overall rate of extraglandular estrogen formation increases with increasing amounts of adipose tissue and with age.

Plasma testosterone and its active metabolites are converted to inactive metabolites in the liver and excreted predominantly in the urine; approximately half of the daily turnover is excreted in the form of urinary 17-ketosteroids (primarily androsterone and etiocholanolone), and the remainder is excreted as a series of polar compounds (diols, triols, and conjugates).

Gonadotropin regulation and testosterone secretion Testosterone secretion is regulated by pituitary LH (Fig. 321-3). (For the details of pituitary function, see Chap. 313.) Follicle-stimulating hormone (FSH) may also augment testosterone secretion, possibly by inducing maturation of the Leydig cell. Testosterone also regulates the sensitivity of the pituitary to the hypothalamic-releasing factor luteinizing hormone–releasing hormone (LHRH, also called gonadotropin-releasing hormone, GnRH). Although the pituitary can convert testosterone to dihydrotestosterone and to estrogens, testosterone itself is the primary regulator of gonadotropin secretion. Testosterone also acts in the central nervous system to slow the rate of LHRH formation or secretion and consequently to decrease the frequency of pulsatile LH release. Under ordinary circumstances, LH secretion is exquisitely sensitive to the feedback effects of testosterone, with complete suppression following the administration of amounts of exogenous androgen that approximate the normal daily secretory rate of testosterone (about 20 μmol or 6 mg). However, prolonged elevation of plasma LH (as in testicular deficiency) renders the pituitary less sensitive to negative feedback control by exogenous androgen.

Neither the plasma concentration of testosterone nor that of LH is constant, each showing fluctuations of a pulsatile nature that reflect changes in secretory rates (Fig. 321-4). Major sleep-related surges in the pulsatile secretion of both LH and testosterone signal the initiation of male puberty. In the adult the diurnal variation in the magnitude of this episodic secretion of LH and testosterone is minor

FIGURE 321-2 Androgen and estrogen production in normal young men. Average production of androstenedione and testosterone are shown in the top boxes, and mean daily production of estrone and estradiol is shown in the lower boxes. Estrogen is formed by extraglandular aromatization (braces) or by direct secretion from the testes. Vertical arrows indicate the rates of extraglandular aromatization of androgens, and the horizontal arrows indicate the interconversion of androgen and estrogens by 17β-hydroxysteroid dehydrogenase. Thus estradiol arises from plasma testosterone, from estrone, and from direct secretion by the testes. *(Adapted from PC MacDonald et al.)*

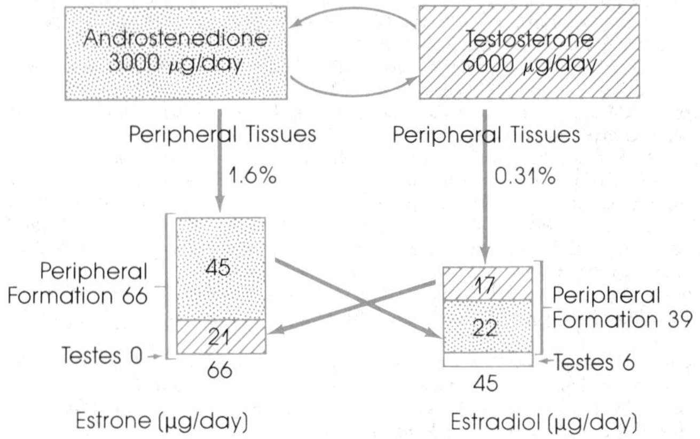

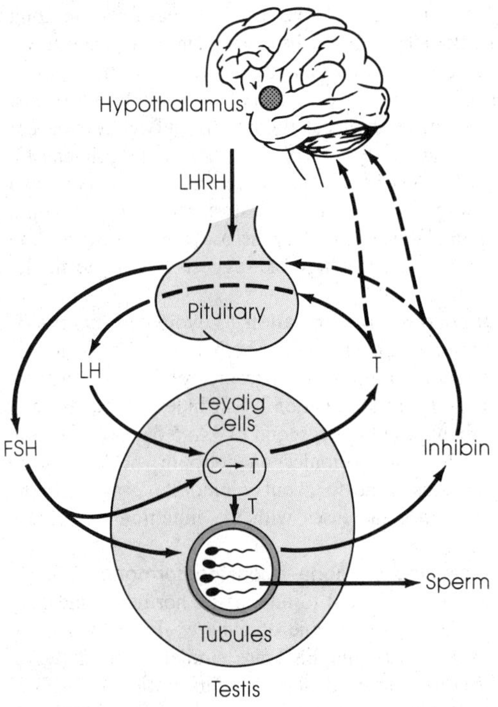

FIGURE 321-3 Regulation of testosterone and sperm production by LH and FSH. (C, cholesterol; T, testosterone.)

with peak morning levels only about 10 to 15 percent higher than during the rest of the day.

Androgen action The major functions of androgen are the regulation of gonadotropin secretion, the formation of the male phenotype during sexual differentiation, and the induction of sexual maturation and function following puberty. The cellular mechanisms by which androgens perform these functions are summarized schematically in Fig. 321-5. Testosterone (T) enters the cell by passive diffusion. Inside the cell T can be converted to dihydrotestosterone (D) by the 5α-reductase enzyme. T or D is then bound to the androgen-receptor protein in the cytosol (R). The hormone-receptor complex (TR or DR) is transformed to the DNA-binding state (TR* or DR*) and translocated to the nucleus, where it attaches to specific chromosomal sites; as a result, new messenger RNA is transcribed, and new protein appears within the cytoplasm of the cell. The androgen receptor protein is coded by a gene on the long arm of the X chromosome; it contains 917 amino acids and has a molecular mass of about 100 kDa. It is similar in structure to other steroid hormone receptors and has distinct hormone-binding, DNA-binding, and functional domains.

FIGURE 321-4 Twenty-four-hour pattern of plasma LH and testosterone in a normal man sampled every 20 min. *(Reprinted from Griffin and Wilson, 1985.)*

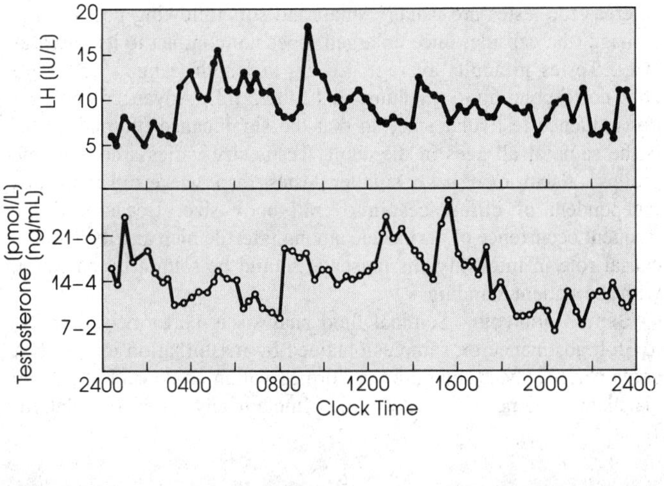

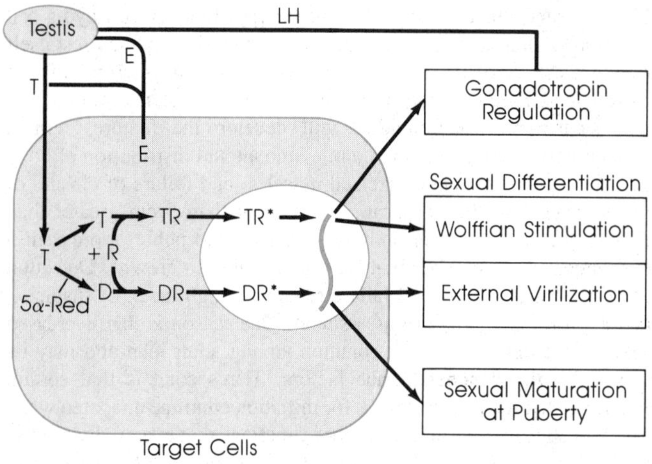

FIGURE 321-5 Current concepts of androgen action. (T, testosterone; D, dihydrostestosterone; E, estradiol; R, receptor protein; R*, transformed receptor protein; LH, luteinizing hormone; 5α-Red, 5α-reductase.)

Although testosterone and dihydrotestosterone bind to the same receptor, their physiologic roles differ. The testosterone-receptor complex regulates gonadotropin secretion and is responsible for the Wolffian stimulation phase of sexual differentiation (see Chap. 324), whereas the dihydrotestosterone-receptor complex is responsible for external virilization during embryogenesis and the major portion of androgen action during sexual maturation and adult sexual life, including the initiation and maintenance of spermatogenesis. The mechanism by which testosterone and dihydrotestosterone mediate these different functions is not known. The mechanisms by which estrogens act to augment or block androgen effects are also not known. It is presumed that estradiol acts by a mechanism similar to that of androgens but involving its own receptor protein (see Chap. 322).

THE SEMINIFEROUS TUBULE AND SPERMATOGENESIS Normal function of the seminiferous tubule is dependent on the pituitary and on the adjacent Leydig cells, both FSH and androgen being essential for initiating and maintaining normal spermatogenesis (Fig. 321-3). The major site of FSH action is the Sertoli cell in the seminiferous tubules. The seminiferous tubule also contains androgen receptors. Androgen appears to be essential for the initial phase of spermatogenesis, whereas FSH is required for the terminal phases of spermatid development. In the normal adult male this machinery produces more than 200 million sperm per day.

The Sertoli cell cannot synthesize steroid hormones de novo and is dependent on testosterone that diffuses in from adjacent Leydig cells. Sertoli cells can convert testosterone to estradiol and to dihydrotestosterone. The seminiferous tubules also produce the peptide hormone inhibin that regulates the secretion of FSH by the hypothalamic-pituitary axis (Fig. 321-3). Inhibin, a peptide hormone produced by Sertoli cells, is the primary physiologic regulator of FSH, but testosterone and estradiol also can inhibit FSH secretion.

The interlocking system in which two pituitary hormones regulate testicular function provides a precise dual-control mechanism by which Leydig cells and the spermatogenic tubules produce factors that feed back upon the hypothalamic-pituitary system to regulate their own function (Fig. 321-3).

ASSESSMENT OF TESTICULAR FUNCTION

LEYDIG CELL FUNCTION History and physical examination The assessment of Leydig cell function and androgen status should include inquiry about the presence at birth of developmental abnormalities of the urogenital tract, the timing and extent of sexual maturation at puberty, the rate of beard growth, and the current libido, sexual function, strength, and energy. Inadequate Leydig cell function or androgen action during embryogenesis may manifest itself by the presence of hypospadias, cryptorchidism, or microphallus. If Leydig cell failure occurs prior to puberty, sexual maturation will not occur, and the individual will develop the features termed eunuchoidism, including an infantile amount and distribution of body hair, poor development of skeletal muscles, and failure of closure of the epiphyses so that the arm span is more than 5 cm greater than the height, and the lower body segment (heel to pubic) more than 5 cm longer than the upper body segment (pubic to crown). Detection of postpubertal Leydig cell failure requires a high index of suspicion and appropriate laboratory assessment. One reason is that decreased sexual function is relatively common among adult men and may be caused by many nonendocrine factors. The second is that certain functions that require androgens for initiation continue unabated when Leydig cell failure occurs, and those functions that eventually regress may do so very slowly. For example, the frequency of shaving may not decrease for many months or even years because of the slow decline in rate of beard growth once established.

Plasma testosterone and dihydrotestosterone levels Plasma testosterone is measured by a specific radioimmunoassay. Testosterone is secreted into plasma in a pulsatile fashion every 60 to 90 min (Fig. 321-4); a single random sample provides a result within ±20 percent of the true mean value only two-thirds of the time while three equally spaced samples 15 to 20 min apart provide a more accurate assessment. The samples do not need to be assayed separately, and aliquots of the three samples can be pooled for a single determination. The range of plasma testosterone in normal adult men is 10 to 35 nmol/L (3 to 10 ng/mL). In adult men the plasma values vary slightly throughout the day and at different times of the year, but these variations are not as great as those for plasma cortisol and are not significant in routine clinical assessment. Plasma levels of testosterone correlate in general with testosterone secretory rates as measured by isotope infusion. Estimation of TeBG concentration is sometimes useful in the interpretation of total plasma testosterone levels. Such assays can be done either by measuring the binding capacity of radioactive androgen or with a specific radioimmunoassay. Estimates of bioavailable testosterone in plasma can be made by measuring the non-TeBG-bound fraction of testosterone.

The plasma testosterone value in prepubertal children is statistically higher in boys than girls, the range in both being 0.2 to 0.7 nmol/L (0.05 to 0.2 ng/mL). The rise in plasma testosterone at the start of puberty begins as a result of sleep-related nocturnal gonadotropin surges, so that during the initial phases plasma testosterone and LH are higher at night than during the day. The random daytime levels of plasma testosterone increase gradually as puberty progresses and reach adult levels at about age 17.

Dihydrotestosterone is also measured by radioimmunoassay. In normal young men the plasma dihydrotestosterone level is about one-tenth that of the testosterone value and averages around 2 nmol/L (0.5 ng/mL). In older men with benign prostatic hyperplasia, plasma dihydrotestosterone levels are higher and average about 3 nmol/L (0.9 ng/mL).

Urinary 17-ketosteroids The measurement of urinary 17-ketosteroids is not a valid way to assess testicular function. Urinary 17-ketosteroids are mainly weak adrenal androgens or their metabolites, and testosterone contributes only about 40 percent of daily 17-ketosteroid production in men.

Plasma LH Plasma LH is measured by specific radioimmunoassay. LH is also secreted in a pulsatile fashion and fluctuates more widely than does plasma testosterone so that in adult men an isolated random plasma LH is likely to be within ±20 percent of true mean value only a third of the time. Again, assay of a pool of plasma comprised of equal portions of three samples drawn 6 to 18 min apart as described above provides a value approaching the true mean. In early puberty plasma LH secretion increases only during sleep, but the pulsatile secretion in the adult is of similar magnitude during sleep and waking periods. The normal plasma LH values should be established for a given laboratory. The usual normal range in adult men is 5 to 20 IU/L. Bioactive LH can be assessed in some laboratories by the rat interstitial cell assay and may be detectable at times when the immunoreactive LH cannot be measured. A low plasma testosterone concentration can be interpreted correctly only if plasma LH is also measured simultaneously, and likewise the "appropriateness" of a given plasma LH must be interpreted in relation to the plasma testosterone. For example, a low plasma testosterone coupled with a low LH implies hypothalamic or pituitary disease, whereas the finding of a low plasma testosterone and a high LH suggests primary testicular insufficiency (see Chap. 312).

Response to gonadotropin stimulation Leydig cell function is difficult to assess prior to puberty when both LH and testosterone levels are low, and it is common to measure response of plasma testosterone to gonadotropin stimulation as an index of Leydig cell capacity. Normal prepubertal boys respond to 3 to 5 days of injection of 1000 to 2000 IU human chorionic gonadotropin (hCG) with an increase in plasma testosterone to about 7 nmol/L (2 ng/mL); the magnitude of the response increases with the initiation of puberty and peaks in early puberty.

Response to luteinizing hormone–releasing hormone The responsiveness of the pituitary gland to luteinizing hormone–releasing hormone (LHRH) changes at the time of puberty. Prior to puberty quantitative responses to LH and FSH are similar. With pubertal development the LH response to acute administration of LHRH increases while the FSH response remains the same. The amount of LH released following acute administration of LHRH probably reflects the amount of stored hormone in the pituitary. When 100 μg of LHRH is given subcutaneously or intravenously to normal men, there is, on average, a four- to fivefold increase in LH with the peak level at 30 min. However, the range of response is broad, with some normal men having less than a doubling of LH levels. In general, the peak LH following a single LHRH injection correlates with the basal levels. In patients with primary testicular failure measurement of basal LH is usually sufficient, and measurement of LHRH response adds little to aid the diagnosis. Men with either pituitary disease or hypothalamic disease may have a normal or an abnormal LH response to an acute dose of LHRH. Therefore, a normal response is of no diagnostic value, either in determining the presence or absence of disease or in distinguishing hypothalamic from pituitary disease. A subnormal response is of value in determining that an abnormality exists, even though the site is not determined. The LHRH test is most useful in the evaluation of men with secondary hypogonadism and subnormal LH response to an acute dose of LHRH. If daily infusions of LHRH for a week lead to the development of a normal LH response to an acute dose, a hypothalamic etiology is likely.

SEMINIFEROUS TUBULE FUNCTION **Examination of the testes** Evaluation of the testes is an essential portion of the physical examination. The seminiferous tubules account for about 60 percent of testicular volume. The prepubertal testis measures about 2 cm in length and 2 mL in volume and increases in size during puberty to reach the adult proportions by age 16. When damage to the seminiferous tubules occurs prior to puberty the testes are small and firm, whereas the testes are usually small and soft following postpubertal damage (the capsule, once enlarged, does not contract to its previous size). Testes in adults average 4.6 cm in length (range, 3.5 to 5.5 cm), corresponding to a volume of 12 to 25 mL. Advanced age does not influence testicular size, so that the significance of small testes is the same at all ages in the adult. Testis size varies among ethnic groups. Asian men have smaller testes than western Europeans, independent of differences in overall body size. Because of the frequent occurrence of varicocele among infertile men and its possible causal role in infertility, its presence should be sought by palpation with the patient standing.

Semen analysis Seminal fluid analysis is performed after 24- to 36-h abstinence on samples obtained by masturbation into a glass container. Analysis should be performed within an hour. The normal ejaculate volume is 2 to 6 mL. Immediately after ejaculation, coagulation of the seminal fluid occurs, followed within 15 to 30 min by liquefaction. Estimation of motility should be made on undiluted seminal fluid; more than 60 percent of the sperm should be motile and of normal morphology. The normal range for sperm density is generally considered to be greater than 20 million per milliliter with a total count per ejaculate of more than 60 million, but the definition of a minimally adequate ejaculate is not clear. Some men with low sperm counts are nevertheless fertile. This uncertainty as to the lower level of sperm density, percent motility, and percent normal forms in fertile semen stems from two issues. First, many factors produce temporary aberrations in sperm count, and in men who present with semen of equivocal quality it is necessary to examine three or more ejaculates to determine whether abnormal findings are permanent or temporary. Second, routine evaluation of the seminal fluid is dependent on tests that do not assess the functional capacity of the sperm. Although methods to measure sperm penetration of bovine cervical mucus and zona-free hamster ova have been developed, they are not sufficiently standardized to permit general use.

Plasma FSH Plasma FSH as measured by specific radioimmunoassay usually correlates inversely with spermatogenesis. In normal adult men, the range of plasma FSH is 5 to 20 IU/L. Men with intact hypothalamic-pituitary axes have elevations of FSH when damage to the germinal epithelium is severe.

Testicular biopsy Testicular biospy is useful in some patients with oligospermia and azoospermia both as an aid in diagnosis and as an indication of feasibility of treatment. For example, a normal testicular biopsy and a normal FSH in an azoospermic man suggest obstruction of the vas deferens, which may be surgically correctible. Tissue culture of the biopsy material with subsequent karyotypic analysis is necessary to identify those instances of Klinefelter syndrome secondary to chromosomal mosaicism in which the abnormality is limited to the testes. Testicular biopsy is often followed by a transient decrease in sperm counts, but there are no permanent adverse effects.

ESTROGENIC FUNCTION **Examination of the breasts** Breast enlargement (gynecomastia) is the most consistent feature of feminizing states in men (see Chap. 323). Gynecomastia is due to the proliferation of both glandular and adipose tissue. The presence of gynecomastia should be sought by examining the patient while he is in the sitting position using the fingers to grasp glandular tissue. Palpation with the flat of the hand while the patient is supine may result in failure to detect early or minimal breast enlargement. In obese men it is important to try to define the edge of the rim of glandular tissue that separates it from adipose tissue of the chest wall.

Plasma estrogen As discussed above, most of the estradiol and all of the estrone produced in normal men is formed by extraglandular aromatization of circulating androgens. Plasma estradiol is usually less than 180 pmol/L (50 pg/mL) in normal men; plasma estrone is somewhat higher but usually less than 300 pmol/L (80 pg/mL). Elevated estrogen production and elevated plasma levels can be due to elevations in plasma precursors (liver or adrenal disease), to increases in extraglandular aromatization (obesity), or to increased production by the testes (testicular tumors or androgen resistance).

PHASES OF NORMAL TESTICULAR FUNCTION

The phases of male sexual life can be defined in terms of the plasma testosterone value (Fig. 321-6). In the male embryo the production of testosterone by the testis commences at about 7 weeks of gestation. Shortly thereafter plasma testosterone attains a high value that is maintained until it falls late in gestation so that at the time of birth plasma testosterone is only slightly higher in males than in females. Shortly after birth, plasma testosterone in the male infant again begins to rise and remains elevated for approximately 3 months, falling to low levels by age 6 months to 1 year. The concentration then remains low (but slightly higher in boys than girls) until the onset of puberty,

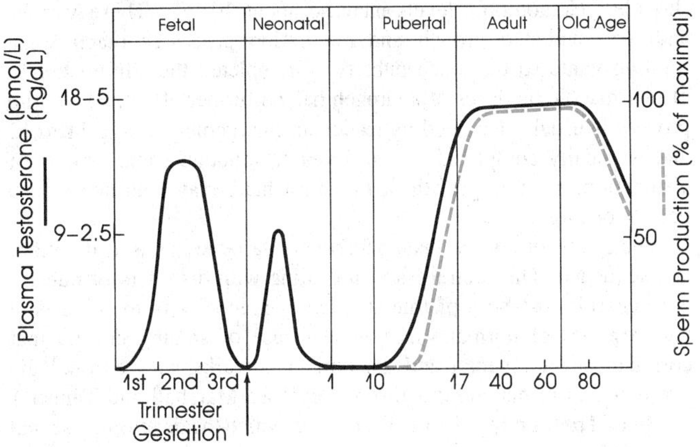

FIGURE 321-6 Phases of male sexual life. *(Reprinted from Griffin and Wilson, 1985.)*

when it begins to rise in boys, reaching adult levels by about age 17. The mean plasma level remains more or less constant in the adult until late middle age and then declines slowly during the later decades of life. During the third or adult phase of male sexual life sperm production becomes sufficient to allow reproduction to take place. The physiologic events that take place during these various phases differ, as do the pathologic consequences of derangements in testicular function at different stages of life. Male sexual differentiation during embryogenesis is considered in Chap. 324. The role of the surge of testosterone formation during the first year of life is unknown. The focus of this chapter is on testicular pathophysiology during puberty, mature sexual life, and old age.

ABNORMALITIES OF TESTICULAR FUNCTION

PUBERTY The factors that ultimately determine the onset of puberty are poorly understood and may reside in the hypothalamic-pituitary system, the testis, or the adrenal. Prior to the onset of puberty, gonadotropin secretion by the pituitary is low but appears to be under regulatory control by the testis, as prepubertal castration results in a rise in plasma gonadotropin levels. This suggests that prior to puberty the negative feedback control of gonadotropin secretion is exquisitely sensitive to the small amount of circulating testosterone. The onset of puberty is heralded by sleep-associated surges in gonadotropin secretion. Later in puberty the rises in LH and FSH persist throughout the day. Thus, with maturation the hypothalamic-pituitary system becomes less sensitive to negative feedback control, and the consequences are a higher mean plasma testosterone, maturation of the testes, and the onset of spermatogenesis. The rise in gonadotropin secretion is the consequence both of an increase in LHRH secretion and an increased sensitivity of the pituitary to LHRH. Plasma levels of bioactive LH increase even more than those of the immunoreactive hormone. The anatomic and developmental changes at the time of puberty are secondary to the rise in plasma testosterone. Maturation of the accessory organs of male reproduction (the penis, the prostate, the seminal vesicles, and the epididymides) accounts for about one-fourth of androgen-mediated nitrogen retention during puberty. The characteristic hair growth of male puberty involves development of mustache and beard, regression of the scalp line, appearance of body, extremity, and perianal hair, and extension of the pubic hair upward into a diamond-shaped pattern. Growth of axillary and pubic hair is initiated under the control of adrenal androgens and is promoted by testicular androgens. The larynx enlarges, and the vocal cords become thickened, resulting in a lowering of the pitch of the voice. Accelerated linear growth is accompanied by growth of muscle and connective tissue, accounting for the major portion of nitrogen retention at puberty. The principal androgen-sensitive muscles are those of the pectoral region and the shoulder. Hemoglobin levels increase about 10 g/L. These various androgen-mediated growth and maturation processes reach some limiting value so that once puberty is completed the administration of pharmacologic doses of androgen has no further effect. The entire process is usually heralded by testicular enlargement at age 11 to 12 and is usually completed within 5 years, although some aspects of virilization, such as growth of the chest hair, may continue over a decade or more.

The events of normal male puberty are variable in onset, duration, and sequence. The central issue in dealing with disorders of puberty is separating instances of true absence or precocity from subjects at the extremes of normal variation. The use of staging criteria that correlate developmental and anatomic landmarks with chronologic age is useful in making this distinction. (See Marshall and Tanner.)

Sexual precocity Those disorders in which the developing sexual characteristics are appropriate for the phenotype, i.e., virilization in boys, are termed *isosexual precocity*. *Heterosexual precocity* refers to feminizing syndromes in boys.

ISOSEXUAL PRECOCITY Sexual development prior to age 9 in boys is generally considered abnormal. *True precocious puberty* or *complete isosexual precocity* occurs when both premature virilization and spermatogenesis take place, and *precocious pseudopuberty* or *incomplete isosexual precocity* refers to virilization unaccompanied by spermatogenesis, indicating that androgen formation is not the result of premature activation of the hypothalamic-pituitary system. This distinction is blurred in practice because pure virilizing syndromes may cause activation of gonadotropin secretion secondarily and thus be followed by development of spermatogenesis. Furthermore, local androgen production in the testis, as in Leydig cell tumors, can cause local areas of spermatogenesis around the tumor and thus cause limited sperm production. We therefore prefer a simple two-part classification: virilizing syndromes (in which hypothalamic-pituitary activity is appropriate for age) and premature activation of the hypothalamic-pituitary system.

Virilizing syndromes can result from Leydig cell tumors, human chorionic gonadotropin (hCG)–secreting tumors, adrenal tumors, congenital adrenal hyperplasia (most commonly 21-hydroxylase deficiency), androgen administration, or Leydig cell hyperplasia. In all these situations plasma testosterone is inappropriately elevated for the age. Leydig cell tumors are rare in children but should be suspected when the testes are asymmetric in size (see Chap. 305). Virilizing adrenal tumors secrete large amounts of adrenal androgen (mainly androstenedione and dehydroepiandrosterone, some of which is converted to testosterone) and consequently cause elevated 17-ketosteroid secretion. Glucocorticoid administration does not suppress 17-ketosteroid excretion to normal in patients with testicular or adrenal tumors, in contrast to the prompt decrease that occurs following such treatment in congenital adrenal hyperplasia. Congenital adrenal hyperplasia leads to elevated 17-hydroxyprogesterone levels and as a consequence elevated androgen levels (see Chaps. 317 and 324). When this disorder is treated with glucocorticoids, true precocious puberty can then result if sufficient hypothalamic maturation has been produced by the increased androgen levels.

Gonadotropin-independent sexual precocity in boys may occur as a result of autonomous Leydig cell hyperplasia in the absence of Leydig cell tumor formation. The disorder is inherited as a male-limited autosomal disorder either from father to son or from mothers who are unaffected carriers. Virilization begins usually by age 2. Testosterone levels are elevated, often to the adult male range; however, immunoreactive and bioactive LH levels and the response to LHRH are prepubertal. Many of these boys were mistakenly thought to have true precocious puberty in the past because of the presence of spermatogenesis.

Premature activation of the hypothalamic-pituitary system may be "idiopathic" or due to central nervous system tumors, infections, or injuries. Such early hypothalamic-pituitary activation typically is associated with characteristics of normal puberty, i.e., sleep-related gonadotropin secretion, elevated plasma bioactive LH, and enhanced gonadotropin response to LHRH. Since the diagnosis of idiopathic true precocious puberty is one of exclusion, rare patients later prove to have been misclassified and to have an identifiable central nervous system abnormality. With improved means of diagnosis, such as computed tomographic scans and magnetic resonance imaging, delays in diagnosis will probably be less frequent.

Management of sexual precocity due to steroid- or gonadotropin-producing tumors, congenital adrenal hyperplasia, or an identified CNS abnormality is directed toward the primary disease. In boys with Leydig cell hyperplasia attempts have been made to lower plasma testosterone with medroxyprogesterone acetate or ketoconazole, but the long-term efficacy and safety of these agents is unknown. Idiopathic true precocious puberty and true precocious puberty due to inoperable CNS lesions are treated with LHRH analogue therapy, resulting in reversal of the pubertal maturation including decreased rate of skeletal development.

HETEROSEXUAL PRECOCITY Feminization in prepubertal boys can result from absolute or relative increases in estrogen due to a variety of causes (see Chap. 323).

Delayed or incomplete puberty The separation of failure of puberty from variants of normal is one of the most difficult problems in endocrinology. Some patients fail to show the normal spurt of growth and sexual development at the usual time but eventually commence puberty by age 16 or older. Adolescence may then either progress rapidly, or there may be a slow development and growth that continues until age 20 to 22. Many men with delayed onset of puberty attain heights within the normal adult range. At times the history reveals that a parent or sibling has shown a similar pattern of development. The major problem is to separate this group of patients with delayed puberty from patients with organic disorders that impair puberty. Panhypopituitarism and hypothyroidism can cause pubertal failure in males (see Chaps. 313 and 316). Absent puberty can also result from primary disease of the testis including defects in testicular development; this diagnosis is suspected on the basis of low plasma testosterone and elevated FSH and LH. Hereditary androgen resistance (in which plasma testosterone and LH are both high) usually results in hereditary male pseudohermaphroditism but in milder cases may be manifested by absent or incomplete puberty (see Chap. 324).

The most frequent finding in boys with absent puberty is both low plasma testosterone and low gonadotropin levels; in these patients it is necessary to distinguish those with delayed puberty from those with isolated gonadotropin deficiency or idiopathic *hypogonadotropic hypogonadism* (*the Kallman syndrome*). The manifestations of isolated gonadotropin deficiency vary from boys with eunuchoidal features and testes of prepubertal size to those with partial manifestations of LH and FSH deficiency and partial degrees of testicular enlargement and pubertal development. One less severe form of this disorder in which plasma FSH levels and spermatogenesis appear to be normal is termed the *fertile eunuch syndrome*.. Anosmia or hyposmia and cryptorchidism are common. Histologic examination of the testis reveals undifferentiated Leydig cells and immature germinal epithelium similar to a normal prepubertal testis. The disorder is inherited as an X-linked recessive trait or an autosomal dominant trait with variable expressivity. Serum FSH and LH levels are usually below the normal male range, and plasma testosterone levels are low for the age. The secretion of other pituitary hormones is usually normal. The defect appears to be in the synthesis or release of LHRH with the resultant gonadotropin pattern ranging from absence of pulsatile LH secretion to defects in amplitude and frequency of LH secretion; the administration of synthetic LHRH for a sufficient period corrects the endocrine abnormalities and initiates spermatogenesis. If untreated, these patients usually remain in the prepubertal state indefinitely. A prepubertal manifestation is microphallus, in which the size of the penis is below the fifth percentile for the age. Indeed, a fourth or more of isolated prepubertal microphallus is due to hypogonadotropic hypogonadism. Distinction between this disorder and delayed puberty is particularly difficult in patients of early or midpubertal age; the presence of microphallus, anosmia, or a family history of hypogonadotropic hypogonadism may help to establish the diagnosis. In the absence of such evidence, differentiation of the two states may become clear only after several years of observation. In some cases the response of plasma LH to LHRH stimulation may be helpful in suggesting that puberty is imminent.

ADULT ABNORMALITIES OF TESTICULAR FUNCTION At the completion of puberty, plasma testosterone levels reach the adult level of 10 to 35 nmol/L (3 to 10 ng/mL) throughout the day, plasma gonadotropins are 5 to 20 IU/L each for LH and FSH, and sperm production is sufficient to allow reproduction. The adult set of the complex regulatory system (Fig. 321-3) is sustained in the normal man for more than 40 years. However, the system is subject to a variety of influences, both at the level of the testis and of the hypothalamic-pituitary system. Spermatogenesis is exquisitely sensitive to alterations in temperature, and brief increases either in systemic or local temperature (as in a hot bath) can be followed by temporary decreases in sperm production. The system is likewise subject to influence by diet, drugs, alcohol, environmental agents, and psychological stress, all of which may cause temporary decreases in sperm count.

Persistent abnormalities of testicular function after the time of normal puberty can be due to hypothalamic-pituitary abnormalities (see Chap. 313), testicular defects, or to abnormalities of sperm transport. Certain of these conditions tend to affect Leydig cell function or spermatogenesis selectively, but most influence both aspects of testicular function and cause both underandrogenization and infertility (Table 321-1). The interlocking of defective Leydig cell function and infertility is a consequence of the dependence of spermatogenesis on androgen formation. Even partial decreases in testosterone production can cause infertility. Certain disorders (hyperprolactinemia, radiation, cyclophosphamide therapy, autoimmunity, paraplegia, androgen resistance) can cause either isolated infertility or a combined defect in testicular function in different subjects.

Hypothalamic-pituitary disorders Disorders of the hypothalamus and pituitary can impair secretion of gonadotropins (and cause as a consequence decreased androgen production and defective spermatogenesis) either as a portion of generalized disease of the anterior pituitary (see Chap. 313) or as an isolated defect, usually hypogonadotropic hypogonadism, in which secretion of both LH and FSH are impaired; hypogonadotropic hypogonadism can either be congenital or, rarely, an acquired idiopathic defect. Alternatively, gonadotropin secretion can be altered by factors other than hypothalamic pituitary pathology. For example, elevation of plasma cortisol in the *Cushing syndrome* can depress LH secretion independent of a space-occupying lesion of the pituitary. Some patients with *congenital adrenal hyperplasia* have suppressed gonadotropin secretion and consequent infertility. *Hyperprolactinemia* (either as the consequence of pituitary adenomas or of drugs such as phenothiazines) has been associated with combined Leydig cell and seminiferous tubule dysfunction, presumably the consequence of inhibition of LH and FSH secretion by prolactin. Occasionally, impaired fertility in hyperprolactinemia is associated with normal gonadotropin and androgen levels and is presumed to result from direct inhibition of sexual function or spermatogenesis by prolactin. *Hemochromatosis* impairs testicular function most commonly as the result of effects on the pituitary; less often it affects the testis directly (see Chap. 327). The use of *androgens* for purposes other than replacement therapy is often associated with impaired sperm production (see below). In several other conditions testosterone levels may be decreased in association with normal LH levels, and the mechanism is less clear. Men with massive obesity have decreased TeBG and decreased levels of total and bioavailable testosterone that return toward normal with weight loss. Obesity may be part of the mechanism for decreased testosterone levels in the subset of such men with Pickwickian syndrome (see Chap. 217). Some men with seizures of temporal lobe origin also have a hormonal pattern consistent with hypogonadotropic hypogonadism.

TABLE 321-1 Classification of abnormalities of testicular function in the adult

Site of defect	Presentation: Infertility with underandrogenization	Infertility with normal virilization
Hypothalamic-pituitary	Panhypopituitarism	
	Hypogonadotropic hypogonadism	Isolated FSH deficiency
	Cushing's syndrome	Congenital adrenal hyperplasia
	Hyperprolactinemia	Hyperprolactinemia
	Hemochromatosis	Androgen use
Testicular	Developmental and structural defects:	
	Klinefelter's syndrome*	Germinal cell aplasia
	XX male	Cryptorchidism
		Varicocele
		Immotile cilia syndrome
	Acquired defects:	
	Viral orchitis*	*Mycoplasma* infection
	Trauma	
	Radiation	Radiation
	Drugs (spironolactone, alcohol, ketoconazole, cyclophosphamide)	Drugs (cyclophosphamide)
		Environmental toxins
	Autoimmunity	Autoimmunity
	Granulomatous disease	
	Associated with systemic diseases:	
	Liver disease	Febrile illness
	Renal failure	Celiac disease
	Sickle cell disease	
	Neurologic diseases (myotonic dystrophy and paraplegia)	Neurologic disease (paraplegia)
	Androgen resistance	Androgen resistance
Sperm transport		Obstruction of the epididymis or vas deferens (cystic fibrosis, diethylstilbesterol exposure, congenital absence)

* The common testicular causes of underandrogenization and infertility in adults—Klinefelter's syndrome and viral orchitis—are associated with small testes.

Testicular defects Abnormalities of testicular function in the adult can be grouped into several categories: developmental and structural defects of the testes, acquired testicular defects, and disorders secondary to systemic and/or neurologic disease.

DEVELOPMENTAL ABNORMALITIES The *Klinefelter syndrome* (both the classic and mosaic forms) and the *XX male syndrome* are usually not recognized until after the time of expected puberty (see Chap. 324). Some developmental defects cause infertility in the presence of normal androgen production. These include varicocele, germinal cell aplasia, and cryptorchidism. *Varicocele* may be of etiologic importance in as much as one-third of all male infertility. It is caused by retrograde flow of blood into the internal spermatic vein that eventuates in progressive, often palpable dilatation of the peritesticular pampiniform plexus of veins. Varicocele occurs in about 10 to 15 percent in the general population and 20 to 40 percent in men with infertility and is thought to result from incompetence of the valve between the internal spermatic vein and the renal vein. It is more common on the left (85 percent). Unilateral varicocele increases the blood flow and the temperature of both testes as a result of the extensive anastomoses of the venous systems. The increased scrotal (and testicular) temperature is believed to be the cause of the poor-quality semen and infertility (the testes do not have the usual 2°C lower temperature than that of the abdominal cavity). The findings on semen analysis are usually nonspecific with all parameters showing some abnormality. In some studies, surgical resection results in improved fertility, with the best results (70 percent pregnancy rate) obtained in men whose preoperative sperm counts are over 10 million per milliliter.

Some patients with *germinal cell aplasia* (the Sertoli cell–only syndrome) have a positive family history and may constitute a specific entity in which the germinal epithelium is missing with resulting azoospermia; plasma testosterone and LH values are normal, and plasma FSH levels are elevated. Other patients with identical histologic and clinical findings have androgen resistance or a history of viral orchitis or cryptorchidism. Consequently a variety of conditions are commonly lumped under this term. The syndrome accounts for less than 10 percent of patients with azoospermia.

Unilateral *cryptorchidism,* even when corrected prior to puberty, is associated with abnormal semen in many individuals. This suggests that even in unilateral cryptorchidism the testicular abnormality is usually bilateral.

The *immotile cilia syndrome* is an autosomal recessive defect characterized by immotility or poor motility of the cilia of the airways and of the sperm. Kartagener's syndrome is a subgroup of the immotile cilia syndrome associated with situs inversus, chronic sinusitis, and bronchiectasis (see Chap. 208). The immotile sperm cannot fertilize. The structural abnormality leading to impaired motility of cilia can usually be defined by the electron-microscopic appearance. The specific defects that are known to cause the syndrome include defects in the dynein arms, spokes, or microtubule doublets. Cilia from epithelia and sperm tails from the same individual exhibit the same defects, but the pulmonary manifestations may be minor. *Other structural defects of sperm* that are less well understood can apparently lead to immotile sperm without involvement of cilia in the lung.

ACQUIRED TESTICULAR DEFECTS The most common cause of acquired testicular failure in the adult is *viral orchitis.* The responsible viruses include mumps virus, echovirus, lymphocytic choriomeningitis virus, and group B arboviruses. The orchitis is due to actual infection of the tissue by virus rather than indirect effects of the infection. Orchitis is the most common complication of mumps in adult men, occurring in as many as one-fourth of men who have the disease. In about two-thirds of the cases orchitis is unilateral, and in the remainder it is bilateral. It usually develops within a few days after the onset of parotitis but may precede it. The testis may return to normal size and function or undergo atrophy. Atrophy is believed to be due both to direct effects of the virus on the seminiferous tubules and to ischemia secondary to pressure and edema within the taut tunica albuginea. Semen analysis returns to normal in three-fourths of men with unilateral involvement and in only one-third of men with bilateral orchitis. Atrophy is usually perceptible within 1 to 6 months after the orchitis subsides, and the degree of atrophy is not necessarily proportional to the severity of the acute orchitis or the development of infertility. Unilateral atrophy occurs in approximately one-third of cases of mumps orchitis, and bilateral atrophy occurs in about one-tenth.

Trauma is the second most common cause of secondary atrophy of the testes. The exposed position of the testis in the scrotum renders it susceptible to both thermal and physical trauma—particularly in individuals with hazardous occupations.

Both the seminiferous tubules and the Leydig cells are sensitive to *radiation damage;* decreased secretion of testosterone appears to be a consequence of diminished testicular blood flow. Doses higher than 200 mGy (20 rad) cause increases in plasma FSH and LH levels and damage to the spermatogonia. After doses of about 800 mGy (80 rad) oligospermia or azoospermia develops. Higher doses may obliterate the germinal epithelium except for occasional stem and Sertoli cells. Fractionated radiation may have a more profound effect than single-dose radiation. Recovery of sperm density occurs in a dose-related fashion, and complete recovery of sperm density to preradiation levels may require as long as 5 years. Permanent infertility can occur after radiation therapy of malignant lymphoma in spite of shielding the testes. Permanent androgen deficiency in adult men is uncommon after doses of radiation in the therapeutic range; however, most boys receiving direct testicular radiation for acute lymphoblastic leukemia have permanently low plasma testosterone levels.

In general, *drugs* interfere with testicular function in one of four ways—inhibition of testosterone synthesis, blockade of the peripheral action of androgen, enhancement of estrogen levels, or direct inhibition of spermatogenesis. Certain drugs have multiple effects, and agents such as guanethidine that block the sympathetic nervous system can impair sexual function in men whose pituitary-testicular axis is normal.

Spironolactone and ketoconazole block the synthesis of androgen by interfering with the late reactions in androgen biosynthesis. Spironolactone and cimetidine compete with androgen for the cytoplasmic receptor protein and thus interfere with androgen action in the target cell. Testosterone levels may be low and estradiol levels may be elevated in patients taking large amounts of marijuana, heroin, or methadone, although the exact reasons are unclear. Alcohol, when consumed in excess for prolonged periods, causes decreased plasma testosterone, independent of liver disease or malnutrition. Elevated plasma estradiol and decreased plasma testosterone have been reported in men taking digitalis.

Antineoplastic and chemotherapeutic agents commonly interfere with spermatogenesis. Cyclophosphamide causes azoospermia or extreme oligospermia within a few weeks after the initiation of therapy. Cessation of therapy is followed by a return of spermatogenesis within 3 years in about half of patients. Combination chemotherapy for acute leukemia, Hodgkin's disease, and other malignancies may also impair Leydig cell function. In pubertal boys this is manifested by decreased serum testosterone and elevated LH levels while in adult men testosterone levels do not decline and the impaired Leydig cell function may only be detected as exaggeration of LH response to LHRH. The alkylating agents in the chemotherapeutic regimens seem to be responsible for the toxic effects on the Leydig cell.

Because of the potentially toxic effects of many physical and chemical agents on spermatogenesis, the occupational and recreational history should be carefully evaluated in all men with infertility. Known environmental hazards include chemicals, such as the nematocide dibromochloropropane, cadmium, and lead, microwaves, and ultrasound.

Testicular failure also occurs as a part of a generalized disorder of *autoimmunity* in which multiple primary endocrine deficiencies coexist (Schmidt's syndrome) and in which circulating antibodies to the basement membrane of the testes are present (see Chap. 325). Sperm antibodies are also a cause of isolated male infertility. In some instances such antibodies may be secondary phenomena resulting from duct obstruction or vasectomy. *Granulomatous diseases* can also destroy the testes, the most common such disorder being leprosy. Testicular atrophy occurs in 10 to 20 percent of men with lepromatous leprosy, the result of direct invasion of the tissue by the mycobacteria. The tubules are involved initially, followed by endarteritis and destruction of Leydig cells.

TESTICULAR ABNORMALITIES ASSOCIATED WITH SYSTEMIC DISEASE The common systemic diseases that cause underandrogenization and infertility are liver disease and renal failure. In *cirrhosis of the liver* a combined testicular and pituitary abnormality leads to decreased testosterone production independent of the direct toxic effects of ethanol. Although plasma LH is elevated, the level may be below the expected range given the degree of androgen deficiency. This is most likely the result of inhibition of LH secretion by the higher estrogen concentrations in patients with chronic liver disease. Increased estrogen production results from impaired hepatic extraction of adrenal androstenedione and subsequent increased peripheral conversion to estrone and estradiol. In effect there is shunting of estrogen precursors to sites of extraglandular aromatization. Testicular atrophy and gynecomastia are present in about half of men with cirrhosis, and many such men are impotent.

In chronic *renal failure* decreased androgen synthesis and diminution of sperm production develop in the setting of elevated plasma gonadotropins. The elevated LH is due to increased production as well as reduced clearance but is incapable of effecting normal testosterone production. In addition, about one-fourth of men with chronic renal failure have hyperprolactinemia. Low testosterone coupled with normal or increased plasma estrogen levels probably account for the presence of gynecomastia in about half of men on chronic hemodialysis. The role of the hyperprolactinemia in decreasing testosterone production is unclear. About half of men with renal failure on dialysis experience decreased libido and impotence. The etiology of the testicular abnormalities in renal failure is not well understood. Improvement in testosterone production with hemodialysis is incomplete, but successful transplantation may lead to return of testicular function to normal.

Men with *sickle cell anemia* usually have impaired secondary sexual development, and testicular atrophy is present in one-third. The defect may be either at the testicular or hypothalamic-pituitary level. Abnormalities in Leydig cell function, frequently accompanied by decreased sperm density, have been noted in a variety of chronic systemic diseases including protein-energy *malnutrition,* advanced *Hodgkin's disease* and *cancer* prior to chemotherapy, and *amyloidosis.* Most of these disorders cause a lowered plasma testosterone coupled with a normal to increased plasma LH, suggesting combined hypothalamic-pituitary and testicular defects. The low plasma testosterone is not the result of inhibitors that interfere with the binding to TeBG and hence is not analogous to the euthyroid sick syndrome. Similar hormone changes occur following *surgery, myocardial infarction,* and severe *burns,* and thus may be a nonspecific effect of illness.

The temporary decrease in sperm density after *acute febrile illness* usually occurs in the absence of any changes in testosterone production. Infertility in men with *celiac disease* is associated with a hormonal pattern typical of androgen resistance, namely elevated testosterone and LH levels. *Neurologic diseases* associated with altered testicular function include myotonic dystrophy and paraplegia. In myotonic dystrophy small testes may be associated with abnormalities of both spermatogenesis and Leydig cell function. Spinal cord lesions resulting in paraplegia lead to a temporary decrease in testosterone levels that tend to return to normal but persistent defects in spermatogenesis; some patients retain the capacity to obtain erection and to ejaculate.

ANDROGEN RESISTANCE Defects of the androgen receptor cause resistance to the action of androgen usually associated with defective male phenotypic development as well as infertility and underandrogenization (see Chap. 324). A less severe form of androgen resistance is associated with infertility due to oligo- or azoospermia in otherwise phenotypically normal men; this form of androgen resistance may cause a significant fraction of infertility previously classified as idiopathic azoospermia.

Impairment of sperm transport Disorders of sperm transport may lead to infertility in as many as 6 percent of infertile men with normal virilization. The obstruction may be unilateral or bilateral, congenital or acquired. In men with unilateral obstruction of sperm transport the infertility may result from antisperm antibodies. Obstructive azoospermia at the level of the epididymis also occurs in association with chronic infections of the paranasal sinuses and lungs. Tuberculosis, leprosy, and gonorrhea are rare causes of acquired obstruction of ejaculatory structures. Congenital defects of the vas deferens can occur as an isolated abnormality associated with absence of the seminal vesicles (and consequently absence of fructose in the ejaculate), in patients with *cystic fibrosis,* or in men whose mothers received *diethylstilbestrol* during pregnancy.

At least 40 percent of infertile men have infertility of unknown etiology; none of the above conditions is found on careful search. The therapy in all forms of male infertility except surgically correctable varicocele, vas deferens obstruction or treatable endocrinopathy, is unsatisfactory. Empirical therapy with androgens or gonadotropins has no significant effect on fertility. Although the semen quality may improve with such treatment, the pregnancy rate is usually no greater than in infertile men given no therapy (25 percent fertility in patients followed for a year). This latter fact should be kept in mind, namely that spontaneous resolution may occur in up to one-fourth of patients with idiopathic infertility followed with no treatment. Many forms of male infertility associated with some motile sperm in the semen can be treated by in vitro fertilization.

Fertility control in the male Although a variety of approaches to fertility control in men have been tried, including the condom as a safe barrier method that also prevents sexually transmitted disease, the most practical means is ligation of the vas deferens, a procedure that has been successful in large numbers of men and can be performed on an outpatient basis. The time required for azoospermia to occur following the operation depends upon the number of sperm in the terminal vas deferens and ejaculatory ducts at the time of surgery but is usually less than 40 days. Azoospermia should be documented in each case to prove effectiveness. No deleterious effects on either testosterone production or the hypothalamic-pituitary axis have been documented. Despite reports of immune-complex-associated accelerated atherosclerosis in vasectomized nonhuman primates, there does not appear to be any association between vasectomy and atherosclerosis in men. Vasectomy should only be recommended for men requesting permanent sterilization. Vasovasostomy for reanastomosis of the vas has a success rate of about 80 to 90 percent as judged by return of sperm to the ejaculate, but only about 30 to 40 percent subsequently achieve fertility. This discrepancy is possibly due to the development of antisperm antibodies as a consequence of the vasectomy.

OLD AGE Beginning at about age 60 mean plasma total and bioavailable testosterone concentrations decline. Nevertheless, though statistically lower than levels in young men, the concentrations of testosterone in elderly men usually remain within the normal range. The cause of the decreased testosterone level is likely decreased Leydig cell numbers in the testes. There is also a decline in seminiferous tubule function and decreased sperm production in older men. Plasma LH and FSH levels are usually increased in elderly men, and an increase in the rate of conversion of androgen to estrogen in peripheral tissues results in a decrease in the effective ratio of androgen to estrogen. These latter endocrine changes may play a role in the development of prostatic hyperplasia and possibly in development of gynecomastia in aging men (see Chap. 323). Male sexual function gradually declines after early adulthood, but there is no convincing evidence that hormonal changes have any direct bearing on changes in sexual function with age.

Prostatic hyperplasia See Chap. 306.

Cancer of the prostate See Chap. 306.

DISORDERS OF ALL AGES **Testicular tumors** (See Chap. 305) Chorionic gonadotropin is present in normal testes, and it is therefore not surprising that plasma gonadotropins are elevated in testicular tumors. Indeed, an elevated plasma level of the beta subunit of human chorionic gonadotropins (hCG-β) serves as a sensitive and specific marker of tumor activity in some men with germ cell tumors. Plasma levels of the beta subunit are elevated in all patients with choriocarcinoma, in one-third of embryonal carcinomas and teratocarcinomas, and rarely in seminomas. There is a good correlation between change in hCG-β levels and response to therapy.

Elevated estradiol and testosterone production in patients with testicular tumors can arise by at least two mechanisms. In trophoblastic tumors and in tumors of Leydig and Sertoli cells production of both hormones occurs autonomously in the tumor tissue itself; in these instances plasma gonadotropin levels and hormone production by the uninvolved portions of the testes are depressed, and azoospermia is common. However, when gonadotropins are secreted by the tumor, the gonadotropin acts to increase estradiol and testosterone production in the unaffected areas of the testes, and azoospermia is uncommon. When estrogens and androgens are formed (directly or indirectly) by the tumors, feminization, virilization, or no obvious change may result, depending on the pattern of hormones produced and the age of the patients. Other cellular markers of testicular tumor activity have been described in individual cases, including alpha fetoprotein.

Gynecomastia See Chap. 323.

HORMONAL THERAPY

ANDROGENS Pharmacologic preparations Effective androgen therapy requires the use of chemically modified analogues of testosterone. When testosterone itself is administered by mouth, it is absorbed into the portal blood and degraded promptly by the liver so that insignificant amounts reach the systemic circulation; when injected parenterally testosterone is rapidly absorbed from the injection vehicle so that it is difficult to sustain effective levels in the plasma. As a consequence, effective androgen therapy requires either the administration in a slowly absorbed form of testosterone (dermal patches or micronized oral preparation) or the administration of chemically modified analogues. Such chemical modifications either retard the rate of absorption or catabolism, so as to sustain effective blood levels, or enhance the androgenic potency of each molecule, so that full androgenic effects can be achieved at a lower blood level of the drug. Three types of modification of the molecule have received widespread clinical application (Fig. 321-7), namely esterification of the 17β-hydroxyl group, alkylation at the 17α position, and modification of the ring structure, particularly substitutions at the 2, 9, and 11 positions. Most agents actually contain combinations of ring structure alterations and either 17α-alkylation or esterification of the 17-hydroxyl. Esterification serves to decrease the polarity of the molecule. Consequently, the steroid is more soluble in the fat vehicles used for injection, and release of the steroid into the circulation is slowed. Most esters must be injected parenterally. The more carbon molecules in the acid esterified, the more prolonged the action. Currently available esters such as testosterone cypionate and testosterone enanthate can be injected every 1 to 3 weeks. Because the esters are hydrolyzed before the hormones act, the effectiveness of therapy can be monitored by assaying the plasma level of testosterone with time following administration.

FIGURE 321-7 Some of the androgen preparations available for pharmacologic use.

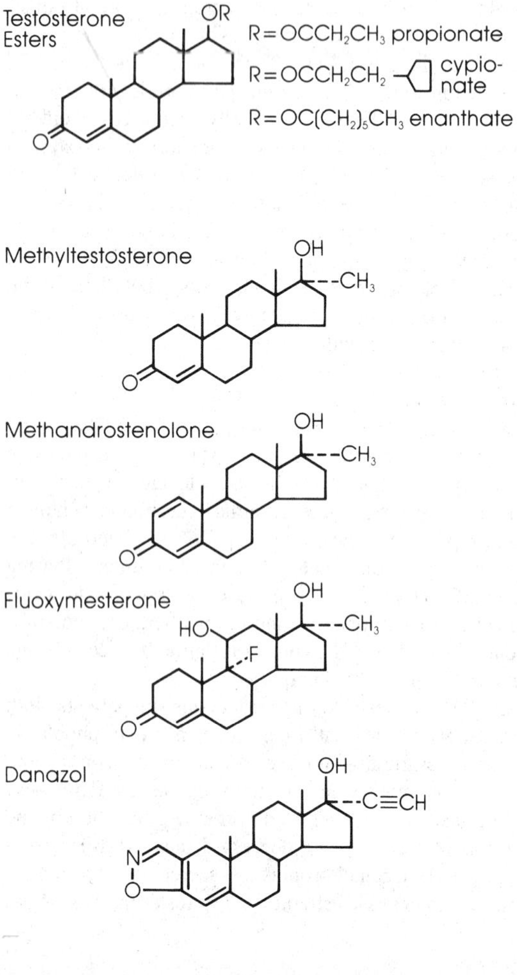

The effectiveness of 17α-alkylated androgens (such as methyltestosterone and methandrostenolone) when given by mouth is due to slower hepatic catabolism than occurs with testosterone itself so that the alkylated derivatives escape degradation by the liver and reach the systemic circulation. For this reason 17α-methyl or -ethyl substitution is a common feature of most orally active androgens. Unfortunately, all 17α-alkylated steroids may cause abnormalities of liver function, and for this reason they have a limited role in medicine.

Other alterations of the ring structure of the androgen molecule have been adopted empirically; in some instances the modification slows the rate of inactivation, in others it enhances the potency of a given molecule, and in still others it alters the conversion to other active metabolites. For example, the potency of fluoxymesterone may be due to the fact that, unlike most androgens, it is a poor precursor for conversion to estrogens in peripheral tissues. A transdermal therapeutic preparation of testosterone in which a testosterone-loaded film is applied each day to scrotal skin in the form of a patch makes it possible to sustain serum levels in the normal male range throughout the day. This therapy avoids the wide swings in serum testosterone values that occur between injections of testosterone esters.

Side effects of androgens All androgens carry the risk of inducing virilization in women. Among the early manifestations are acne, coarsening of the voice, and development of hirsutism. Menstrual irregularities are common. If treatment is discontinued as soon as these effects develop, the manifestations may slowly subside. With prolonged treatment, male-pattern baldness, worsening of the hirsutism and voice changes, and hypertrophy of the clitoris develop and are largely irreversible. There is considerable variation in the frequency and the degree to which these signs develop in women, probably because of individual differences in susceptibility, in steady-state blood levels among individuals, and in duration of therapy. In general, the younger the patient, the more striking the virilizing signs; nevertheless, florid virilization can also occur in adult women. At physiologic replacement doses testosterone esters have no known side effects in mature men. At supraphysiologic doses, however, gonadotropin secretion is inhibited, the testes decrease in volume, and the sperm count falls (indeed, low sperm counts may persist for as long as 9 months after such agents are discontinued). The so-called toxic side effects differ among the different agents and depending on the clinical setting in which they are used.

Retention of a limited amount of sodium is an inevitable consequence of androgen therapy, but in patients with underlying heart disease or renal failure or when androgens are administered in enormous amounts, as in some patients with carcinoma of the breast, the degree of sodium retention may lead to edema. Although androgens do not cause malignancy, they may promote growth of and intensify pain from carcinoma of the prostate and from breast carcinoma in men.

Feminizing side effects of androgen therapy in men are poorly understood. Testosterone itself can be converted (aromatized) in extraglandular tissues to estradiol. In contrast, 5α-reduction of the molecule precludes estrogen formation. The commonest manifestation of feminization is development of gynecomastia. Such breast enlargement is common in children given androgens and correlates with an increase in urinary estrogens, possibly because of a greater capacity to convert androgens to estrogens in childhood. The administration of testosterone esters to men results in an increase in plasma estrogen levels. In men with normal liver function, gynecomastia usually develops only after high doses of androgens.

All 17α-alkylated androgens can produce liver function abnormalities such as elevation of plasma alkaline phosphatase and conjugated bilirubin. The incidence of clinical liver disease probably depends upon the previous integrity of the liver, but jaundice may occur in the absence of preexisting liver disease. 17α-Alkylated drugs also cause an increase in a variety of plasma proteins that are synthesized in the liver. The most serious complications of oral androgen therapy are the development of peliosis hepatis (blood-filled cysts in the liver) and hepatoma. These disorders were initially described in patients with aplastic anemia, many of whom have Fanconi anemia, itself a predisposing factor for the development of malignancy. However, both lesions have also been reported in patients who received oral androgens for a variety of other causes, including use by athletes. There may be a similar increased incidence of hepatocellular neoplasms in women taking oral contraceptives. In some individuals these tumors regress and follow a benign course after discontinuation of the drugs, and in others the course is rapidly fatal.

One indication for the use of 17α-alkylated androgens is in hereditary angioedema; in this disorder the desired therapeutic benefit (increase in the level of the inhibitor of the first component of complement) may actually be a side effect of the 17-alkylated steroid rather than an effect of the parent androgen itself. As a consequence, weak androgens such as danazol are effective in this disorder (Fig. 321-7). Another indication for danazol is in the management of endometriosis (see Chap. 53).

Replacement therapy The aim of androgen therapy in hypogonadal men is to restore or bring to normal male secondary sexual characteristics (beard, body hair, external genitalia) and male sexual behavior and to mimic the hormonal effects on somatic development (hemoglobin, muscle mass, nitrogen balance, and epiphyseal closure). Since an assay for plasma testosterone is available for monitoring therapy, the treatment of androgen deficiency is almost universally successful. The parenteral administration of a long-acting testosterone ester such as 100 to 200 mg testosterone enanthate at 1- to 3-week intervals results in a sustained increase in plasma testosterone to the normal male range. Such esters act only through the release of testosterone itself into the circulation. If the hypogonadism is primary and of long duration (as in the Klinefelter syndrome) suppression of plasma LH to the normal range may not occur for many weeks, if at all. Considerable variability exists in the relation between plasma testosterone and male sexual behavior, but in postpubertal testicular failure (even of many years duration) resumption of normal sexual activity is usual following adequate replacement. Androgen does not restore spermatogenesis in hypogonadal states, but the volume of the ejaculate (derived largely from the prostate and seminal vesicles) and male secondary sex characteristics return to normal. The effects of endogenous androgen on hemoglobin, nitrogen retention, and skeletal development are also reproduced.

In patients of all ages in whom hypogonadism developed prior to expected puberty (such as patients with hypogonadotropic hypogonadism), it is appropriate to bring plasma testosterone slowly into the adult range. When therapy is commenced at the time of expected puberty in such patients, the normal events of puberty proceed in the usual fashion. If therapy is delayed until after the time of usual puberty, the degree to which normal virilization will occur is variable, but many patients undergo a relatively complete anatomic and functional maturation. Intermittent low-dose androgen therapy is indicated in prepubertal hypogonadal boys with microphallus to bring the external genitalia into the normal range. If such patients are monitored closely and given androgens only for short periods, such therapy usually has no adverse effects on somatic growth.

In boys of pubertal age with either isolated hypogonadotropic hypogonadism or primary testicular deficiency, the usual practice is to institute androgen therapy between the ages of 12 and 14 years, depending on the subjective need for sexual development. The initial administration of small doses of testosterone esters followed by a gradual increase to 100 to 150 mg/m^2 of body surface area every 1 to 3 weeks should result in a normal pubertal growth spurt. The time from the start of treatment to the appearance of secondary sex characteristics is variable. Penile development, deepening of the voice, and other secondary sexual characteristics usually commence during the first year of treatment. In normal boys puberty extends over several years, and treatment designed to replicate normal development does not shorten the process greatly.

Testosterone exerts its full action only in the presence of a balanced hormonal environment and, particularly, in the presence of adequate levels of growth hormone. Consequently, prepubertal boys who have coexisting growth hormone deficiency exhibit a diminished response to androgens both in regard to growth and to the development of secondary sex characteristics unless sufficient growth hormone is given simultaneously.

Pharmacologic uses Androgens have been used for a variety of disorders unassociated with hypogonadism, in the hope that potential benefits from the nonvirilizing actions of the agents (such as increase in nitrogen retention and muscle mass, increased hemoglobin, etc.) would outweigh any deleterious actions of the drugs. The most common nonreplacement uses of androgen have been attempts to improve nitrogen balance in catabolic states, self-administration by athletes in the belief that muscle mass and/or athletic performance will be improved, attempts to enhance erythropoiesis in refactory anemias including the anemia of renal failure, adjuvant therapy in carcinoma of the breast, treatment of hereditary angioedema and endometriosis, and management of growth retardation of various etiologies. Most expectations of beneficial effects in these disorders have been illusory for two reasons. First, pharmacologic doses of androgens do little if anything in men beyond the normal testicular androgen, and in women the virilizing side effects of androgens are formidable. Second, no androgen has been devised that exhibits only the nonvirilizing effects of the hormone. This is not surprising in view of the fact that all actions of androgens are mediated by a single high-affinity receptor protein in the cytoplasm (Fig. 321-5).

The most pervasive form of androgen abuse is by male athletes in the expectation that muscle development and athletic performance will be improved. In fact, however, in adequately controlled studies such therapy does not improve performance consistently, and in those rare instances in which it does, such improvement may be the consequence of sodium retention and expansion of the blood volume rather than of an effect on muscle development or strength. However, published trials of efficacy involve the administration of drugs at smaller doses than are usually taken by athletes; since the drugs at high dosage have multiple side effects, some of which preclude studies of efficacy in a double-blind fashion, it is not clear whether the question of efficacy can ever be resolved scientifically. Under no circumstances do putative benefits outweigh the risks associated with the use of oral androgens, a practice that cannot be condemned too harshly. At present, the only established indications for androgen therapy outside of male hypogonadism are in selected patients with anemia due to bone marrow failure, hereditary angioedema, or endometriosis.

Parenteral administration of testosterone esters to normal men results in little effects of any kind, except for the suppression of gonadotropin secretion by the hypothalamic-pituitary system and a consequent decrease in the production of sperm. There is no established contraindication to their administration to men with those disorders (such as short stature) where their use has been advocated, but the efficacy is not yet established. However, the virilizing side effects in women of androgens in usual dosages preclude their use in all except life-threatening situations. Even in potentially fatal diseases in women such as bone marrow failure and carcinoma of the breast great care must be exercised in androgen use.

GONADOTROPINS Treatment with gonadotropins is utilized to establish or restore fertility in patients with gonadotropin deficiency of all causes. Two gonadotropin preparations are available: human menopausal gonadotropins (hMG) (purified from the urine of post-menopausal women) and human chorionic gonadotropin (hCG) (purified from the urine of pregnant women). hMG contains 75 IU FSH and 75 IU LH per vial. hCG has little FSH activity and resembles LH in its ability to stimulate testosterone production by Leydig cells. Because of the expense of hMG, treatment is usually begun with hCG alone, and hMG is added later to stimulate the FSH-dependent stages of spermatid development. A high ratio of LH to FSH activity and a long duration of treatment (3 to 6 months) are necessary to bring about the maturation of the prepubertal testis. Once spermatogenesis is restored in hypophysectomized patients or initiated in hypogonadotropic hypogonadal men by combined therapy, it can usually be maintained with hCG alone.

Men with oligospermia of unknown etiology have also been treated with gonadotropins; the incidence of fertility in such patients is probably no greater than in similar groups of untreated controls.

The dosage of hCG required to maintain a normal testosterone level varies from 1000 to 5000 IU weekly. A variety of regimens have been utilized to induce maturation of spermatogenesis. Most involve starting with 2000 IU hCG three or more times a week until most of the clinical parameters, including plasma testosterone, indicate normal adult male development. hMG (usually one ampul) is then added three times a week to complete the development of spermatogenesis. After regression of spermatogenesis has occurred, the length of therapy required to restore spermatogenesis may be as long as 12 months.

LUTEINIZING HORMONE–RELEASING HORMONE LHRH (gonadorelin) is now available for endocrine testing. LHRH therapy is now used by some physicians for chronic therapy of the infertility of hypogonadotropic hypogonadism. It is necessary to administer LHRH in frequent boluses (25 to 200 ng/kg of body weight every 2 h), requiring the use of portable infusion pumps or periodic nasal application. In general, LHRH does not appear to be more efficacious than gonadotropin in returning sperm counts to normal.

REFERENCES

CARR BR, GRIFFIN JE: Fertility control and its complications, in *Williams' Textbook of Endocrinology*, 7th ed, JD Wilson, DW Foster (eds). Philadelphia, Saunders, 1985, pp 452–475

DAVIS JE: Male sterilization. Clin Obstet Gynaecol 6:97, 1979

DE KRETSER DM: The effects of systemic disease on the function of the testis. Clin Endocrinol Metabol 8:487, 1979

———, ROBERTSON DM: The isolation and physiology of inhibin and related proteins. Biol Reprod 40:33, 1989

GOLDZIEHER JW et al:Improving the diagnostic reliability of rapidly fluctuating plasma hormone levels by optimized multiple-sampling techniques. J Clin Endocrinol Metab 43:824, 1976

GRIFFIN JE, WILSON JD: Disorders of the testes and male reproductive tract, in *Williams' Textbook of Endocrinology*, 7th ed, JD Wilson, DW Foster (eds). Philadelphia, Saunders, 1985, pp 259–312

LAUE L et al: Treatment of familial male precocious puberty with spironolactone and testolactone. N Engl J Med 320:496, 1989

MACDONALD PC et al: Origin of estrogen in normal men and in women with testicular feminization. J Clin Endocrinol Metab 49:905, 1979

MARSHALL WA, TANNER JM: Variation in the pattern of pubertal changes in boys. Arch Dis Child 45:13, 1970

MASSEY FJ et al: Vasectomy and health: Results from a large cohort study. JAMA 252:1023, 1984

SANTORO N et al: Hypogonadotropic disorders in men and women: Diagnosis and therapy with pulsatile gonadotropin-releasing hormone. Endocr Rev 7:11, 1986

SHERINS RH et al: Male infertility, in *Campbell's Urology*, 5th ed, PC Walsh et al (eds). Philadelphia, Saunders, 1985, pp 640–699

SNYDER PF, LAWRENCE DA: Treatment of male hypogonadism with testosterone enanthate. J Clin Endocrinol Metab 51:1335, 1980

SPRATT DI, CROWLEY WF: Hypogonadotropic hypogonadism: GnRH therapy, in *Current Therapy in Endocrinology and Metabolism*, 3d ed, CW Bardin (ed). Toronto, Decker, 1988, pp 221–225

STYNE DM, GRUMBACH MM: Puberty in the male and female: Its physiology and disorders, in *Reproductive Endocrinology: Physiology, Pathophysiology and Clinical Management*, 2d ed, SSC Yen, RB Jaffe (eds). Philadelphia, Saunders, 1986, pp 313–384

WILSON JD: Androgen abuse by athletes. Endocr Rev 9:181, 1988

———, GRIFFIN JE: The use and misuse of androgens. Metabolism 29:1278, 1980

322 DISORDERS OF THE OVARY AND FEMALE REPRODUCTIVE TRACT

BRUCE R. CARR / JEAN D. WILSON

The ovary is the source of ova for reproduction and of the hormones that regulate female sexual life. The anatomic structure, response to hormonal stimuli, and secretory capacity of the ovary are different at different periods of life. This chapter will review normal ovarian physiology as a background for understanding the abnormalities of the ovary and other tissues of the female reproductive tract.

DEVELOPMENT, STRUCTURE, AND FUNCTION OF THE OVARY

EMBRYOLOGY During the third week of gestation the primordial germ cells arise from the endoderm lining the yolk sac at the caudal end of the embryo. The germ cells migrate to the genital ridge adjacent to the mesonephric kidney by the fifth week of gestation and undergo mitotic divisions. The gonads exist in an undifferentiated state until the seventh week of fetal life, at which time the primitive ovary can be differentiated from the testis (see Chap. 324). Estrogen formation in the ovary commences between weeks 8 and 10, and by 10 to 11 weeks of gestation some oogonia in the developing ovarian cortex begin developing into primary oocytes. The ovary contains a finite number of germ cells, the maximal number of about 7 million oogonia being reached by the fifth to sixth month of gestation. Afterward, the germ cells begin to decrease in number through a process of atresia such that only 1 million remain at birth, 400,000 are present at the time of menarche, and only a few remain at menopause. Two X chromosomes are required for normal development of the ovary; in individuals with a 45,X karyotype ovarian development occurs, but the rate of atresia is accelerated so that only a fibrous streak remains at the time of birth (see Chap. 324).

After the oogonia cease to proliferate, meiosis commences, proceeds until the diplotene stage of the first meiotic division is completed, and then remains stationary until the time of onset of ovulation at puberty. During the fifth month of fetal life, the primordial follicle consists of the primary oocyte arrested in meiosis, a single surrounding layer of granulosa cells, and a basement membrane that separates the primordial follicle from surrounding stromal (interstitial) tissues.

PUBERTAL MATURATION Final maturation of ovarian follicles commences during puberty. The two major hormones that regulate follicular development are the pituitary gonadotropins—follicle-stimulating hormone (FSH) and luteinizing hormone (LH) (Fig. 322-1). During the second trimester of fetal development the plasma gonadotropins rise to levels equivalent to those at menopause. This peak in gonadotropin levels may be causally related to the simultaneous peak in replication of oocytes. The hypothalamic-pituitary axis (the so-called gonadostat) undergoes maturation and becomes sensitive after the second trimester to negative feedback by circulating steroid hormones, particularly estrogen and progesterone produced in the placenta. The circulating gonadotropins decrease thereafter and are almost undetectable at the time of birth. In the neonate, concomitant with the decrease in estrogen and progesterone levels due to separation from the placenta at birth, there is a rebound increase in gonadotropin secretion that persists for the first few months of life. With continued maturation of the hypothalamic-pituitary system the gonadostat becomes sensitive to negative feedback control by the low levels of circulating steroid hormones, and plasma gonadotropins again decrease.

As the time of puberty nears, a decrease in the sensitivity of the gonadostat allows for increased secretion of FSH and LH, possibly

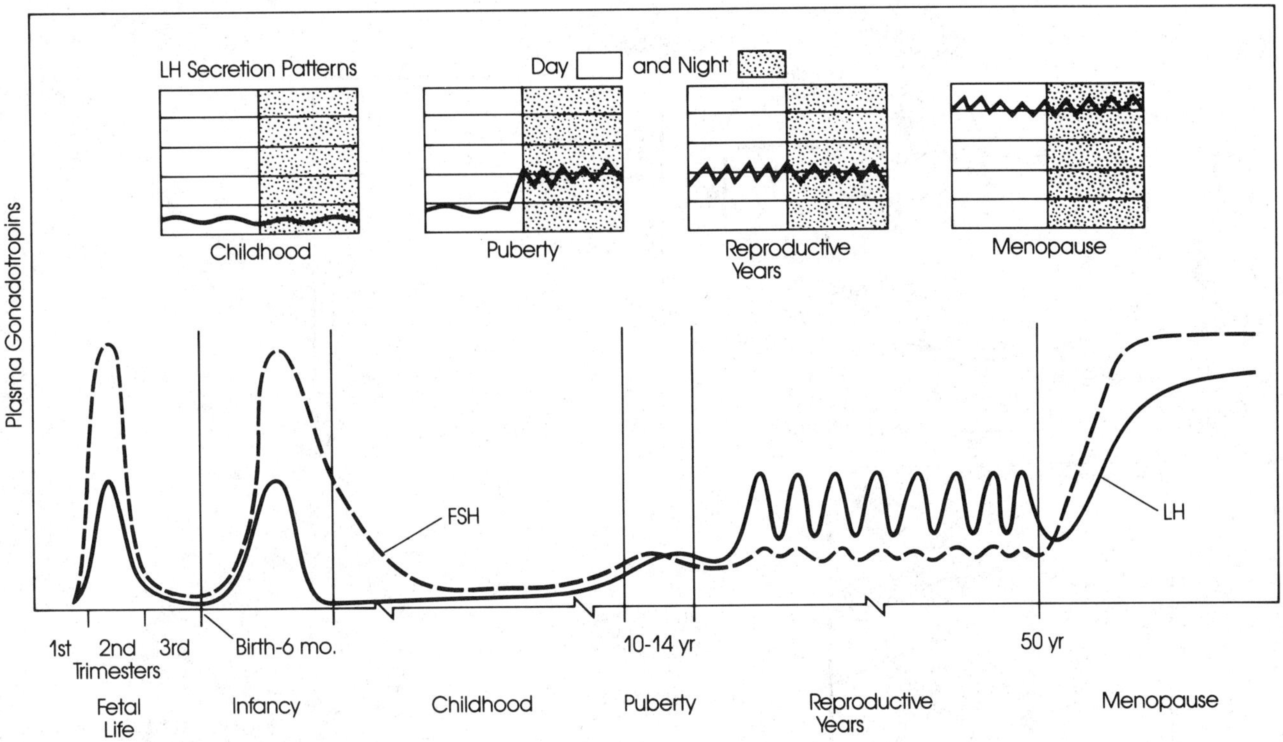

FIGURE 322-1 Pattern of gonadotropin secretion during different stages of life in women. FSH (follicle-stimulating hormone), LH (luteinizing hormone). The secretory patterns of LH during the waking hours (clear area) and night (stippled area) for each stage are indicated in the upper insets. (*After C Faiman et al.*)

secondary to increased episodic or pulsatile secretion of luteinizing hormone–releasing hormone (LHRH) by the hypothalamus (see Chap. 313). A sleep-induced, pulsatile pattern of LH secretion then ensues, the first step in the development of a cyclic pattern of gonadotropin secretion (Fig. 322-1). The increase in estrogen secretion subsequently exerts a positive feedback which leads to an exaggeration of the pulsatile release of LH and eventually to ovulation and the menarche, after which mean plasma gonadotropin concentrations reach adult values in which day and night levels are similar. After the menopause plasma gonadotropin levels rise, plateau 5 to 10 years later, and remain fairly constant until the eighth to ninth decade of life when the plasma levels may fall. Although ovarian function is regulated primarily by LH and FSH, the ovary is a source of several peptide and protein hormones and growth factors, raising the possibility that they play a role in ovarian pathophysiology.

With the development at puberty of decreased sensitivity of the hypothalamic-pituitary centers to circulating steroid hormones, LHRH release by the hypothalamus increases, gonadotropin secretion by the pituitary is enhanced, ovarian estrogen secretion increases, and the anatomic changes of puberty ensue. At age 10 to 11 the first secondary sexual characteristics begin to appear in girls, namely, development of the breast buds (thelarche), followed by the development of pubic hair (pubarche), and later by the development of axillary hair (adrenarche). The appearance of pubic and axillary hair is believed to be the result of an increase in adrenal androgens, commencing at approximately 6 to 8 years of age. A growth spurt ensues, and peak growth rate is attained at a mean age of 12 years.

The culmination of puberty is the onset of predictable, cyclic menses. The average time between the beginning of breast development and the onset of menses (menarche) is 2 years. During the first few years after menarche, menstrual cycles are often irregular and unpredictable due to anovulation. The age of menarche is variable and is determined in part by socioeconomic as well as by genetic factors and general health. In the United States the mean age of menarche is believed to have decreased at a rate of 3 to 4 months per decade over the last 100 years and is now around 13 years, a decrease believed to be due to an improvement in nutrition in the population at large. A critical body weight of around 48 kg or a critical combination of weight, body water, and body fat is associated with development of hypothalamic insensitivity to circulating steroids that leads to increased secretion of gonadotropins and finally to menarche. Obese girls with a body weight 20 to 30 percent above ideal have earlier menarche than do girls with normal weights. In contrast, participation in certain sports or ballet, malnutrition, and chronic debilitating disease commonly cause delayed menarche.

MATURE OVARY **Morphology** The anatomic components and function of the adult ovary are illustrated schematically in Fig. 322-2. Under the influence of gonadotropins, a group of primary follicles is recruited, and by day 6 to 8 of the menstrual cycle one follicle becomes mature or "dominant," a process characterized by accelerated growth of granulosa cells and enlargement of the fluid-filled antrum. The recruited follicles not destined to ovulate begin to undergo degeneration, similar to the atresia observed in other follicles during embryogenesis. Just prior to ovulation, meiosis resumes in the ova of the dominant follicle, and the first meiotic division is completed with formation of the first polar body. Rapid enlargement of the antrum (up to 10 to 25 mm in size) occurs with an associated increase in follicular fluid, followed by a thinning of the follicular surface and formation of a conical stigma. Ovulation from the dominant follicle occurs some 16 to 23 h after the LH peak or 24 to 38 h after the onset of the LH surge as the result of rupture of the follicular wall at the area of the stigma, followed by expulsion of the ovum together with a mass of surrounding granulosa cells called cumulus cells. The rupture is believed to result from the action of hydrolyzing enzymes on the surface of the follicle, possibly under the control of prostaglandins. The second meiotic division begins after the egg is fertilized by a sperm, and a second polar body is then extruded. Following ovulation, the formation of the corpus luteum begins in the retained remnant of the ovulated follicle; the remaining granulosa and theca cells increase in size and accumulate lipids and a yellow pigment, lutein, to become "luteinized." The basement membrane that separated the granulosa cells from the stroma

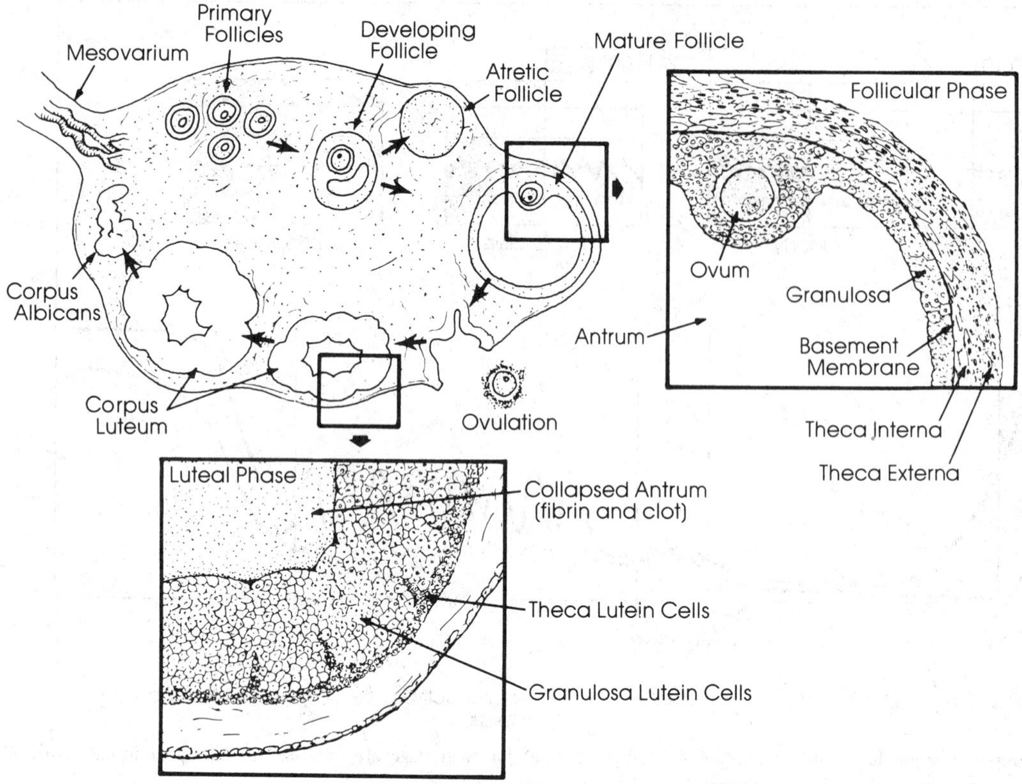

FIGURE 322-2 Developmental changes in the adult ovary during a complete 28-day cycle.

and blood vessels breaks, and capillaries, fibroblasts, and lymphatics from the theca invade the granulosa cells and reach the central cavity, thereby filling it with blood. After a period of 14 ± 2 days (the functional life of the corpus luteum) regression of vessels and atrophy of the corpus luteum commence and eventuate in replacement of the corpus luteum by a fibrous scar, the corpus albicans. The factors that limit the life span of the human corpus luteum are not known. However, if pregnancy occurs, the corpus luteum persists under the influence of placental or chorionic gonadotropins, and progesterone is produced by the corpus luteum for the support of early pregnancy.

Hormone formation STEROID HORMONES Like other steroid hormones, ovarian steroids are derived from cholesterol (Fig. 322-3). The ovary can synthesize cholesterol de novo from 2-carbon precursors and can also utilize cholesterol from circulating low-density lipoproteins (LDL) as substrate for steroid hormone formation (Fig. 322-4). Virtually all ovarian cells are believed to possess the complete enzymatic complement required for the conversion of cholesterol to estradiol (Fig. 322-3); however, different cell types within the ovary contain different amounts of these enzymes so that the predominant steroids produced differ in the various compartments. For example, the corpus luteum forms progesterone and 17-hydroxyprogesterone predominantly, whereas theca and stromal cells convert cholesterol to the androgens androstenedione and testosterone. Granulosa cells are particularly rich in the aromatase activity responsible for conversion of androgens to estrogen and utilize as substrates for this process androgens synthesized within the granulosa cells and in the adjacent theca cells.

The principal sites of action of LH and FSH are also illustrated in Figs. 322-3 and 322-4. LH acts primarily to regulate the first step in steroid hormone biosynthesis, namely the conversion of cholesterol to pregnenolone, and also induces subsequent enzymes in the pathway. FSH acts to regulate the final process by which androgens are aromatized to estrogens. As a consequence, in the absence of FSH, LH enhances substrate flow and the formation of androgens and/or progesterone, whereas FSH action is impeded in the absence of LH because of diminished substrate for aromatization.

Estrogens. Naturally occurring estrogens are 18-carbon steroids characterized by an aromatic A ring, a phenolic hydroxyl group at C-3, and either a hydroxyl group (estradiol) or a ketone (estrone) at C-17 (Fig. 322-3). (For the numbering of the steroid ring see Fig. 321-1.) The principal estrogen secreted by the ovary and the most potent naturally occurring estrogen is estradiol. Estrone is also secreted by the ovary, but the principal source of estrone is from extraglandular conversion of androstenedione in peripheral tissues. Estriol (16-hydroxyestradiol), the most abundant estrogen in urine, arises from the 16-hydroxylation of estrone and estradiol. Catechol estrogens are formed by hydroxylation of estrogens at the C-2 or C-4 position and may act as the intracellular mediators of some estrogen action. Estrogens promote development of the secondary sexual characteristics in women and cause uterine growth, thickening of the vaginal mucosa, thinning of the cervical mucus, and development of the ductular system of the breasts. The mechanism of estrogen action in target tissues is similar to that for other steroid hormones and involves the binding to a specific receptor protein, subsequent conformational change of the hormone-receptor complex, attachment of the complex to DNA, and initiation of the transcription of messenger RNA, which in turn causes increased protein synthesis in the cell cytoplasm (see Chap. 311).

Progesterone. Progesterone, a 21-carbon steroid (Fig. 322-3), is the principal hormone secreted by the corpus luteum and is responsible for progestational effects, namely induction of secretory activity in the endometrium of the estrogen-primed uterus in preparation for implantation of the fertilized egg. Progesterone also induces a decidual reaction in endometrium. Other effects include inhibition of uterine contractions, increased viscosity of cervical mucus, glandular development of the breasts, and increase in basal body temperature (thermogenic effect).

Androgens. The ovary synthesizes a variety of 19-carbon steroids including dehydroepiandrosterone, androstenedione, testosterone, and dihydrotestosterone, principally in stromal and thecal cells. The major ovarian 19-carbon steroid is androstenedione (Fig. 322-3), part of which is secreted into plasma and the remainder of which is converted to estrogen in granulosa cells or to testosterone in the interstitium.

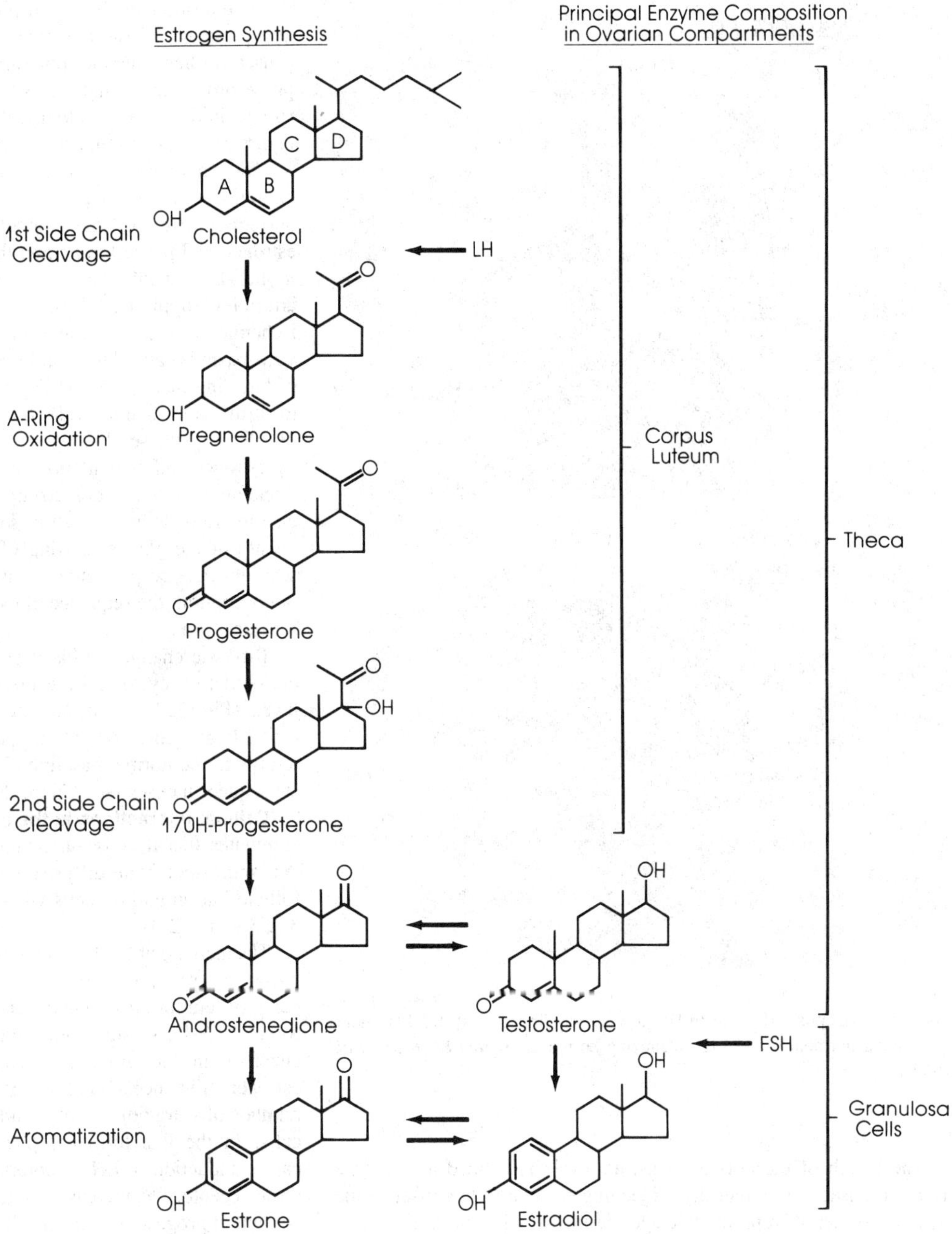

FIGURE 322-3 The principal pathway of steroid hormone biosynthesis in the ovary. Although every ovarian cell probably contains the complete enzyme complement required for the formation of estradiol from cholesterol, the amounts of the various enzymes and consequently the predominant hormones formed differ among the various cell types. The major enzyme complements for the corpus luteum, stroma, and granulosa cells are shown by the brackets; as a consequence these cells produce predominantly progesterone and 17-OH progesterone, androgen, and estrogen, respectively. The major sites of action of LH and FSH in mediating this pathway are shown in the horizontal arrows.

In peripheral tissues androstenedione can also be converted to testosterone and to estrogens. Only testosterone and dihydrotestosterone are true androgens with the capacity of interacting with the androgen receptor and thus inducing virilizing signs in women (see Chaps. 54 and 321).

OTHER HORMONES Other ovarian hormones play an uncertain role in human physiology. *Relaxin,* a polypeptide hormone produced by the human corpus luteum as well as by the decidua, causes softening of the cervix and loosening of the symphysis pubis in preparation for parturition in animals. *Oxytocin, vasopressin*, and other hypothalamic and pituitary hormones have also been found in granulosa and/or luteal cells, but their function in these cells is unknown. *Follicular inhibin* or *folliculostatin* (the equivalent of testicular inhibin) is secreted by the follicle and is believed to regulate the release of FSH by the hypothalamic-pituitary unit. *Follicle regulatory protein* (FRP) of human follicular fluid inhibits granulosa secretion and growth. *Gonadocrinins,* peptides purified from rat follicular fluid, stimulate the release of both FSH and LH from the pituitary in vitro and in vivo. Granulosa cells secrete *oocyte maturation inhibitor* (OMI), a factor that prevents premature ovulation. In addition, in the gonads of both sexes a *meiosis-inducing substance* (MIS) triggers the onset of meiosis, an event that occurs earlier in ovarian than in testicular development. A variety of growth factors produced locally (including IGF) have been shown to influence steroid secretion by the ovary.

The normal menstrual cycle The menstrual cycle is usually divided into a follicular or proliferative phase and a luteal or secretory phase (Fig. 322-5). The secretion of FSH and LH is fundamentally under negative feedback control by ovarian steroids (particularly estradiol) and probably by inhibin, but the response of gonadotropins to different levels of estradiol varies. FSH secretion is inhibited progressively as estrogen levels increase—typical negative feedback. In contrast, LH secretion is suppressed maximally by estrogen in low amounts and is enhanced in response to a rising and sustained elevation of estradiol—so-called positive feedback control. Negative feedback of estrogen involves both the hypothalamus and pituitary, whereas positive feedback operates primarily at the level of the pituitary.

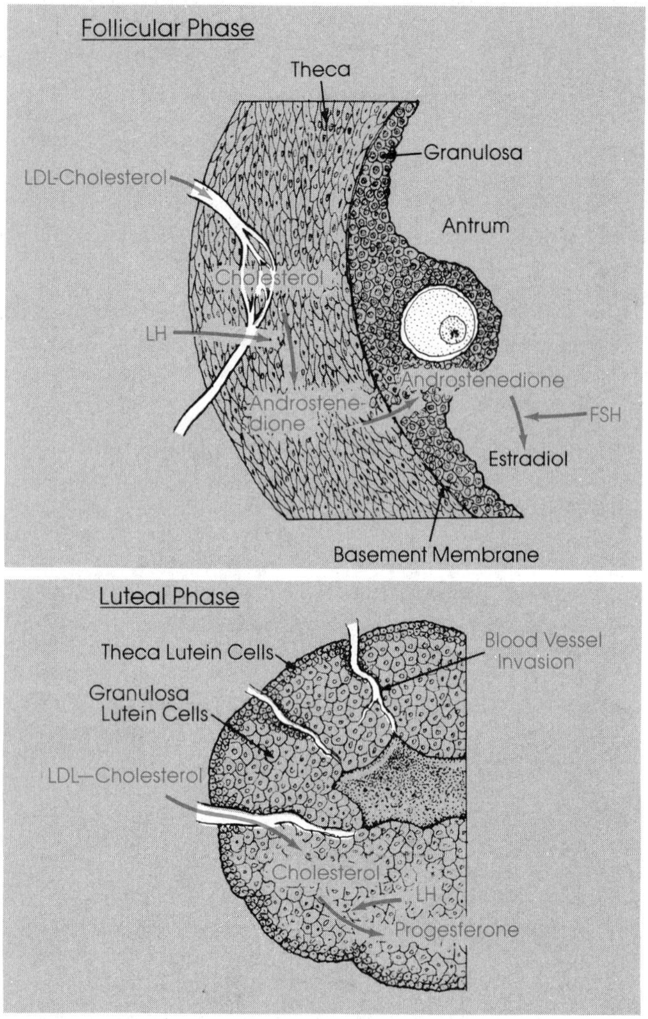

FIGURE 322-4 Cellular interactions in the ovary during the follicular phase (top) and luteal phase (bottom); LDL (low-density lipoprotein), FSH (follicle-stimulating hormone), and LH (luteinizing hormone). (*From BR Carr et al, 1982.*)

The length of the normal menstrual cycle is defined as the time from the onset of one menstrual bleeding episode to the onset of the next. In women of reproductive age the menstrual cycle averages 28 ± 3 days, and the mean duration of flow is 4 ± 2 days. Longer menstrual cycles (usually characterized by anovulation) occur at menarche and prior to menopause. At the end of one menstrual cycle and in the face of a waning corpus luteum, plasma levels of estrogen and progesterone fall, and circulating levels of FSH increase concomitantly. Under the influence of increasing levels of FSH, follicular recruitment is initiated to effect development of the follicle that will be dominant during the next cycle.

After the onset of menses, follicular development continues, but FSH levels decrease. Approximately 8 to 10 days prior to the midcycle LH surge, plasma estradiol levels begin to rise as the result of secretion of estradiol by the granulosa cells of the enlarging dominant follicle. During the second half of the follicular phase, LH levels also begin to rise (positive feedback). Just prior to ovulation, estradiol secretion reaches a peak and then falls. Immediately thereafter, a further rise in the plasma level of LH mediates the final maturation of the follicle, followed by follicular rupture and ovulation 16 to 23 h after the LH peak. Concomitant with the rise in LH is a smaller increase in the level of plasma FSH, the physiologic significance of which is unclear. Plasma progesterone also begins to rise just prior to midcycle and facilitates the positive feedback action of estradiol on LH secretion.

At the onset of the luteal phase plasma gonadotropins decrease, and plasma progesterone increases. A secondary rise in estrogens causes further gonadotropin suppression. Near the end of the luteal phase progesterone and estrogen levels fall, and FSH levels begin to rise to initiate the development of the next follicle (usually in the contralateral ovary) and the next menstrual cycle.

The endometrium lining the uterine cavity undergoes marked alterations in response to the changing plasma levels of ovarian hormones (Fig. 322-5). Concomitant with the decrease in plasma estrogen and progesterone and the decline of corpus luteum function in the late luteal phase, intense vasospasm occurs in the spiral arterioles supplying blood to the endometrium, followed by an ischemic necrosis, endometrial desquamation, and bleeding. This vasospasm is caused by locally synthesized prostaglandins. The onset of bleeding marks the first day of the menstrual cycle. By the fourth to fifth day of the cycle the endometrium is thin. During the proliferative phase glandular growth of the endometrium is mediated by estrogen. After ovulation increased progesterone leads to further thickening of the endometrium, but the rapid growth slows. The endometrium then enters the secretory phase characterized by tortuosity of the glands, curling of the spiral arterioles, and glandular secretion. As corpus luteum function begins to wane in the absence of conception, the sequence of events leading to menstruation is again set into action.

Biphasic changes in basal body temperature are characteristic of the ovulatory cycle and are mediated by alterations in progesterone levels (Fig. 322-5). An increase in basal body temperature of 0.3 to 0.5°C begins after ovulation, persists during the luteal phase, and returns to the normal baseline (36.2 to 36.4°C) after the onset of the subsequent menses (see Chap. 20).

Cellular interactions in the ovary during the normal cycle LH stimulates thecal cells surrounding the follicle to form androgens, and androstenedione diffuses across the basement membrane of the follicle into granulosa cells where it is aromatized to estrogen (Figs. 322-3 and 322-4).

The increase of FSH late in the preceding menstrual cycle stimulates growth and recruitment of the primary follicles by enhancing granulosa cell proliferation, resulting ultimately in the formation of the dominant follicle. FSH also stimulates activity and the amount of aromatizing enzymes in the granulosa cells that convert androstenedione to estrogen. Enhanced secretion of estradiol causes an increase in the number of estradiol receptors and further proliferation of granulosa cells. In the late follicular phase FSH, in concert with estradiol, causes induction of LH receptors on the granulosa cells. LH acts via these receptors to increase progesterone secretion at midcycle. The amount of progesterone formed by the follicle is believed to be limited by the availability of LDL-cholesterol to serve as substrate for steroidogenesis and by the fact that most of the progesterone formed is further metabolized to androstenedione by thecal cells. Prior to ovulation the granulosa cells of the follicle are bathed in follicular fluid but have limited access to circulating blood and consequently to plasma LDL. As depicted in Fig. 322-4, the granulosa cells become vascularized after ovulation, and plasma LDL-cholesterol becomes available to serve as the major substrate for progesterone synthesis by the corpus luteum. Thus, increased progesterone synthesis by the corpus luteum is the consequence of increased substrate availability. The peak in progesterone secretion by the corpus luteum is attained 8 days after ovulation at the time of maximal vascularization of the granulosa cells.

MENOPAUSE The menopause is defined as the final episode of menstrual bleeding in women. However, the term is used commonly to refer to the period of the female climacteric that encompasses the transitional period between the reproductive years up to and beyond the last episode of menstrual bleeding. During this period there is a gradual but progressive loss of ovarian function and a variety of endocrine, somatic, and psychological changes.

The median age of women at the time of cessation of menstrual bleeding is 50 to 51 years. Since the life expectancy in women is now close to 80 years, approximately one-third of life occurs after cessation of reproductive function. Preceding the menopause, the pattern of menstrual cycles is variable, but the interval between menses usually becomes longer. In addition, there is an increase in the mean levels of plasma FSH and LH, despite the continuation of ovulatory cycles. Thus, the ovary appears to become less responsive to gonadotropins prior to the menopause.

The menopause is the consequence of the exhaustion of ovarian follicles. The decrease in the number of ova begins in intrauterine life; by the time of the menopause few ova remain, and these appear to be nonfunctional. Only a small number of ova are lost as the result of ovulation during reproductive life, the majority of follicles and associated ova being lost by atresia. The cessation of follicular development results in a drop in the production of estradiol and other hormones, which in turn causes a loss of negative feedback on the hypothalamic-pituitary centers. In turn, the levels of plasma gonadotropins increase with FSH levels rising earlier and to a greater extent than those of LH (Figs. 322-1 and 322-6). The higher concentration of FSH than LH in postmenopausal women may result from the decrease in inhibin secretion by the ovary, from the fact that FSH is cleared from plasma less rapidly than LH due to its higher sialic acid content, and possibly from the loss of positive feedback on LH production by estradiol. Intravenous administration of LHRH to menopausal women results in a pronounced increase in the secretion of both FSH and LH, consistent with the enhanced hypothalamic-pituitary secretory activity in other forms of primary ovarian failure.

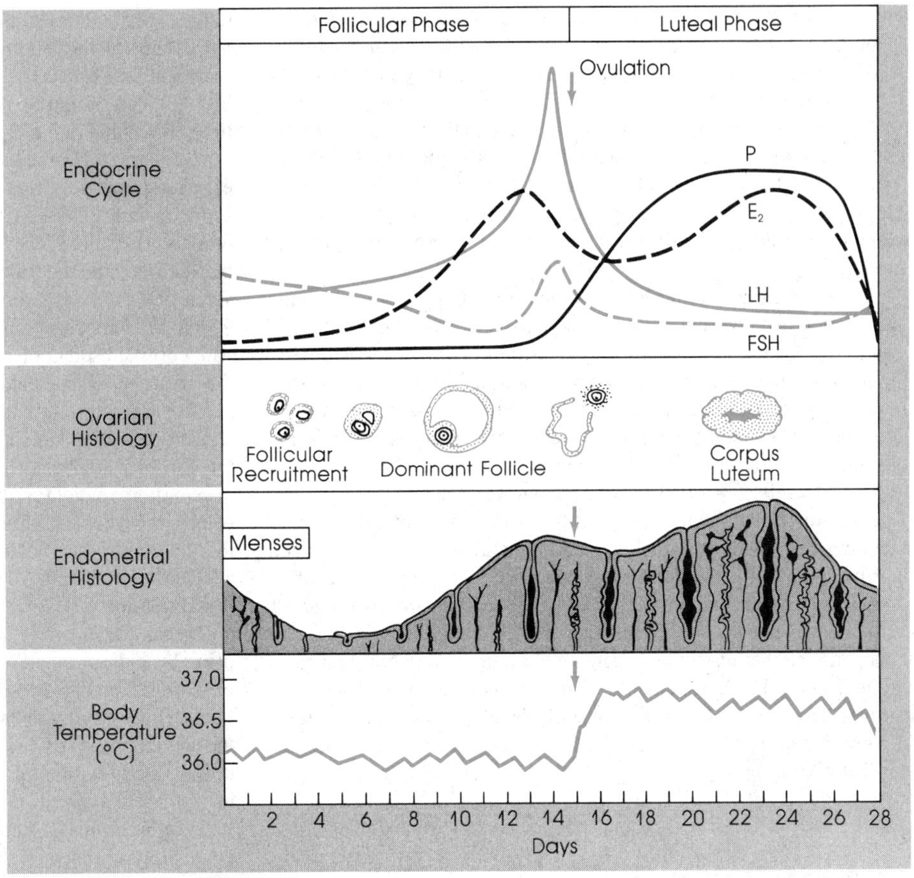

FIGURE 322-5 The hormonal, ovarian, endometrial, and basal body temperature changes and relationship throughout the normal menstrual cycle.

The ovaries of postmenopausal women are small, and the residual cells are predominantly stromal in type. Estrogen and androgen levels in plasma are reduced but not absent from the circulation (Fig. 322-6). Prior to the menopause, plasma androstenedione is derived almost equally from the adrenals and the ovaries; after menopause the ovarian contribution ceases so that the plasma levels of androstenedione fall by 50 percent (Fig. 322-6). However, the menopausal ovary continues to secrete testosterone, presumably formed in stromal cells.

Circulating estrogens in the ovulating woman are derived from two sources. Sixty percent of mean estrogen formation during the menstrual cycle is in the form of estradiol formed primarily by ovaries, and the remainder is estrone formed mainly in extraglandular tissues from androstenedione. After menopause, extraglandular estrogen formation becomes the major pathway for estrogen synthesis. Estrogen production by the menopausal ovary is minimal, and subsequent oophorectomy is not followed by any further decrease in estrogen levels. Plasma levels of estradiol, the principal estrogen secreted by the follicle, are lower in postmenopausal women than are the levels of estrone. The rate of peripheral formation of estrone increases somewhat in menopausal women so that estrone production is usually only slightly less than prior to the menopause, despite the fall in plasma androstenedione. Because a major site of extraglandular estrogen production is adipose tissue, peripheral estrogen formation may actually be enhanced in obese postmenopausal women, so that total estrogen production rates may be as great or greater than in premenopausal women. The predominant estrogen formed is estrone rather than estradiol.

The most common menopausal symptoms are those of vasomotor instability (hot flash), atrophy of the urogenital epithelium and skin, decreased size of the breasts, and osteoporosis. Approximately 40 percent of women in the postmenopausal period develop symptoms serious enough to seek medical assistance.

The pathogenesis of the hot flash is uncertain. There is a close temporal relationship between the onset of the hot flash and pulses of LH secretion; however, hot flashes occur in women with absence of pituitary function and following treatment with LHRH analogues where LH levels are absent or low. Alterations in catecholamine, prostaglandin, endorphin, or neurotensin metabolism in conjunction

FIGURE 322-6 Differences in hormone concentration in women during the reproductive years and in women during the menopause. FSH (follicle-stimulating hormone), LH (luteinizing hormone), E_2 (estradiol-17β), E_1 (estrone), Δ^4-A (androstenedione), T (testosterone). (*From SSC Yen and RB Jaffe, 1986, and from DR Mishell, Jr, and V Davajan.*)

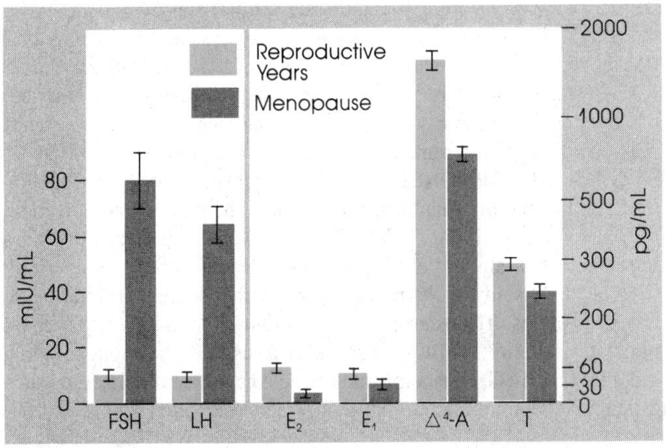

with low estrogen production may also play a role in this phenomenon. Other symptoms commonly associated with the hot flash, including nervousness, anxiety, irritability, and depression, may or may not be due to estrogen deficiency.

The decrease in size of the organs of the female reproductive tract and breasts during the menopause is the consequence of estrogen deficiency. The endometrium becomes thin and atrophic in most (although cystic hyperplasia may occur in one-fifth of postmenopausal women), and the vaginal mucosa and urethra also become thin and atrophic.

There is a close relationship between estrogen deprivation and the development of osteoporosis. Osteoporosis is one of the dread afflictions of aging. Approximately one-fourth of aging women and one-tenth of elderly men sustain a vertebral or hip fracture between the ages of 60 and 90, and the incidence appears to be greatest in elderly white women. Such fractures are a major cause of death and morbidity, and the fracture-related mortality increases from less than 10 percent in the 60- to 64-year age group to 30 percent or more in patients over 80. Many factors affect the development of osteoporosis including diet, activity, smoking, and general health, and estrogen deprivation is of particular importance in this regard. White postmenopausal women are more predisposed to osteoporosis and its consequences because bone density in such subjects is lower prior to menopause so that loss in bone density has more severe consequences in the group. Further evidence that osteoporosis is a disease of estrogen deprivation is suggested by early development of osteoporosis in women with premature menopause due either to natural causes or surgical castration.

LABORATORY AND CLINICAL ASSESSMENT OF HORMONAL STATUS

Assessment of the hormonal status of women can usually be made by obtaining a thorough history and physical examination. In general, presence of secondary sexual characteristics such as normal female breast development indicates adequate estrogen secretion in the past, and the presence of regular, predictable, cyclic menses implies that ovulation and the production of gonadotropins, estrogen, progesterone, and androgens are adequate and that the outflow tract is intact. Such a history may be more valuable than laboratory tests in evaluating ovarian hormone status. However, laboratory tests provide valuable ancillary information in the workup of women with endocrine dysfunction or infertility.

PITUITARY GONADOTROPINS Plasma gonadotropins are assessed by radioimmunoassay. Because both FSH and LH are secreted in pulsatile manner, the results obtained from a single serum sample may be difficult to interpret. Consequently, multiple samples at 20-min intervals for 2 h may be pooled to obtain a mean value. Serum gonadotropin measurements are of most use in evaluating women with suspected ovarian failure and in supporting the diagnosis of polycystic ovarian disease and hypogonadotropic hypogonadism. The normal ranges for serum LH and FSH in ovulating women are 5 to 25 IU/L and 5 to 30 IU/L, respectively. A persistent FSH above 40 IU/L is diagnostic of ovarian failure, and an LH value of less than 5 IU/L is suggestive of hypogonadotropic hypogonadism. In practice, however, gonadotropin values may be equivocal and must be interpreted in light of the remainder of the clinical findings.

OVARIAN HORMONES The mean plasma levels, production rates, and metabolic clearance rates of the principal ovarian hormones are presented in Table 322-1. The metabolic clearance rate of a hormone is that amount of plasma that is cleared of hormone per unit of time and is inversely proportional to the degree of binding to plasma proteins. Testosterone, which is tightly bound to testosterone-binding globulin (TeBG) (also known as sex hormone–binding globulin or SHBG), has a low metabolic clearance rate. Steroids such as androstenedione that are not tightly bound to carrier proteins have higher metabolic clearance rates. The production rate of a hormone is the sum of the amount of hormone produced by direct glandular secretion and by extraglandular conversion of prohormones and can be estimated by multiplying the concentration of hormone in plasma times the metabolic clearance rate of that hormone.

Estrogen Normal secondary sexual characteristics imply that estrogen production was adequate in the past. Indication of the current estrogen status can be obtained by pelvic examination. The presence of a moist, rugated vagina with copious, clear, thin cervical mucus that can be stretched and that exhibits arborization or ferning when spread on a slide is strong evidence of adequate estrogen production. Cytologic demonstration of mature vaginal epithelial cells and abundant cornified squamous epithelial cells with pyknotic nuclei confirms the presence of adequate estrogen levels.

The progesterone-withdrawal test provides a functional assessment of estrogen status. If menses appear within a week to 10 days after the end of a trial of medroxyprogesterone acetate (10 mg by mouth once or twice a day for 5 days) or after a single intramuscular injection of progesterone (100 mg), then prior estrogen priming was adequate to allow withdrawal bleeding.

Due to its variable level in plasma during the normal cycle and the difficulty of estimating the day of the cycle in women with abnormal cycles, the determination of estrogen levels in plasma or urine by radioimmunoassay is of little use in the routine assessment of estrogen status. Plasma estradiol is measured during attempts to induce ovulation with human menopausal gonadotropins to prevent the development of the ovarian hyperstimulation syndrome and is utilized along with ultrasound assessment to monitor follicular growth in women who are to undergo in vitro fertilization.

Progesterone Cyclic, predictable menses also imply that adequate progesterone is secreted during the luteal phase of the menstrual cycle. The indications for specific assay of progesterone are to document ovulation or evaluate the adequacy of the luteal phase in the evaluation of infertile women and to separate subjects with müllerian agenesis from those with the testicular feminization syndrome. Several functional assays of progesterone secretion can be utilized. The least expensive and most useful is the daily measurement of basal body temperature throughout a cycle. Due to the thermogenic properties of progesterone, documentation of the monthly biphasic curve with an elevated temperature for approximately 2 weeks after ovulation is a valid indication of progesterone secretion during the luteal phase (Fig. 322-5). Presence of viscous cervical mucus that does not stretch or fern and the presence of predominant intermediate cells on vaginal cytology or demonstration of a secretory epithelium in an endometrial biopsy during the luteal phase on day 20 to 22 of the cycle provide additional evidence of progesterone secretion. In

TABLE 322-1 Concentrations, metabolic clearance rates, and production rates of the major ovarian steroid hormones in blood of ovulatory women

Steroid	Binding	Phase of menstrual cycle	Plasma concentration nmol/L (ng/ml)	Production rate, μmol/d (mg/d)
Estradiol	TeBG and albumin	Follicular	0.07–2.6 (0.02–0.7)	0.3–3.6 (0.08–1.0)
		Luteal	0.7 (0.2)	0.9 (0.25)
Estrone	Albumin	Follicular	0.2–1.1 (0.05–0.3)	0.4–2.6 (0.1–0.7)
		Luteal	0.4 (0.1)	0.9 (0.24)
Progesterone	CBG and albumin	Follicular	3 (1)	6.4 (2)
		Luteal	16–80 (5–25)	80 (25)
Androstenedione	Albumin	—	5.6 (1.6)	10 (3)
Testosterone	TeBG and albumin	—	1.4 (0.4)	0.9 (0.25)

NOTE: TeBG, testosterone-binding globulin; CBG, cortisol-binding globulin; MCR, metabolic clearance rate.

SOURCE: Derived in part from MB Lipsett, in *Reproductive Endocrinology*, SSC Yen, RB Jaffe (eds). Philadelphia, Saunders, 1986.

addition measurement of serum progesterone by radioimmunoassay can be used to estimate progesterone secretion by the corpus luteum.

Androgen Under normal conditions the ovary secretes androstenedione, testosterone, and dehydroepiandrosterone. In conditions of androgen excess, hirsutism and/or virilization are common. The evaluation of androgen excess is discussed in Chap. 54.

DIAGNOSIS OF PREGNANCY Pregnancy is usually suspected and diagnosed on the basis of the history and findings on physical examination. Namely, a woman with previous cyclic, predictable menses develops amenorrhea accompanied by breast tenderness, malaise, lassitude, and nausea, and on physical examination a softening and enlargement of the uterus is found.

Laboratory assays of placental products excreted in urine facilitate the diagnosis of pregnancy. Human chorionic gonadotropin (hCG) is secreted by the trophoblastic cells of the placenta into the maternal plasma and excreted in the urine. Assays of urinary hCG make it feasible to detect the presence of functioning trophoblasts earlier than can be recognized by clinical assessments. Assays for measurement of hCG content of serum or urine utilize either antibody against hCG or receptor for hCG. With radioimmunoassays and simplified immunoassay kits it is possible to detect pregnancies 8 to 10 days after ovulation and before the first missed menstrual period. Radioimmunoassay of the β subunit of hCG in serum or urine makes it possible to differentiate between excess LH and hCG, an important distinction in evaluating women with trophoblastic disease such as hydatidiform mole or choriocarcinoma.

DISORDERS OF OVARIAN FUNCTION

PREPUBERTAL YEARS Puberty is said to be precocious if the onset of breast budding occurs before age 8 or if menarche commences before age 9. Those disorders in which the developing sexual characteristics are appropriate for the genetic and gonadal sex, i.e., feminization in girls or virilization in boys, are termed *isosexual precocity,* whereas *heterosexual precocity* occurs when sexual characteristics are not in accord with the genetic sex, namely virilization in girls or feminization in boys. Pubertal disorders of boys are described in Chap. 321.

Isosexual precocious puberty Isosexual precocious puberty in girls can be divided into three major categories (Table 322-2).

TRUE PRECOCIOUS PUBERTY True precocious puberty is characterized by an early but otherwise normal sequence of pubertal development, including increased secretion of gonadotropins and ovulatory menstrual cycles. Constitutional or idiopathic precocious puberty comprises 90 percent of cases. In these individuals no cause for the premature maturation of the central nervous system–hypothalamic-pituitary axis can be identified, and the diagnosis is one of exclusion. As many as half of these individuals have abnormal electroencephalograms. Premature appearance of secondary sexual characteristics and of ovulatory cycles with the accompanying risk of fertility may result in significant emotional disturbances. Therefore, prompt initiation of therapy is imperative. The usual treatment is medroxyprogesterone acetate in doses of 100 to 200 mg given intramuscularly every 2 to 4 weeks to suppress gonadotropin secretion. Such a regimen is usually effective in inhibiting ovarian estrogen production and ovulation but does not consistently control bone growth or prevent premature epiphyseal closure and the resultant short stature. LHRH analogues have been utilized to inhibit estrogen synthesis and thus inhibit precocious puberty, and there is evidence to suggest that they also prevent premature closure of the epiphyses.

About 10 percent of cases are due to organic brain diseases, including brain tumors (hypothalamic gliomas, astrocytomas, ependymomas, germinomas, and hamartomas), encephalitis, meningitis, hydrocephalus, head injury, tuberous sclerosis, and neurofibromatosis. It is essential to separate this group of patients from those with the idiopathic disorder, and patients designated as idiopathic occasionally

TABLE 322-2 Differential diagnosis of sexual precocity

I Isosexual precocity
- *A* True precocious puberty
  - *1* Constitutional
  - *2* Organic brain disease
  - *3* Congenital adrenal hyperplasia
- *B* Precocious pseudopuberty
  - *1* Ovarian tumors
  - *2* Adrenal tumors
  - *3* McCune-Albright syndrome
  - *4* Hypothyroidism
  - *5* Silver syndrome
  - *6* Estrogen-containing medications
- *C* Incomplete sexual precocity
  - *1* Premature thelarche
  - *2* Premature adrenarche
  - *3* Premature pubarche

II Heterosexual precocity
- *A* Ovarian tumors
- *B* Adrenal tumors
- *C* Congenital adrenal hyperplasia

prove to have such tumors. Fortunately, most patients with organic lesions serious enough to cause precocious puberty have obvious neurologic signs and symptoms. Evaluation of all patients with precocious puberty should include, at a minimum, skull films and computed tomography scans of the brain. The success of treatment depends upon the nature of the lesion, but surgical and radiation treatment of well-localized tumors is occasionally successful.

A rare cause of isosexual precocity is virilizing congenital adrenal hyperplasia due to 21-hydroxylase deficiency in girls in whom treatment is delayed until 4 to 8 years of age. After initiation of glucocorticoid replacement, such individuals may undergo true isosexual precocious puberty (see Chap. 317).

PRECOCIOUS PSEUDOPUBERTY Precocious pseudopuberty occurs when girls feminize as a consequence of enhanced estrogen formation but do not ovulate or develop cyclic menses. Ovarian cysts or tumors that secrete estrogen (granulosa-theca cell tumors) are the most frequent cause of precocious pseudopuberty. Granulosa-theca-cell tumors associated with intestinal polyps and pigmentation of the mucous membranes occur in the Peutz-Jeghers syndrome. Other ovarian tumors that secrete estrogens (or androgens that can be converted to estrogens at extraglandular sites) include dysgerminomas, teratomas, cystadenomas, and ovarian carcinomas (also see Chap. 304). Ovarian tumors can usually be detected by rectoabdominal examination, and sonography, computed tomography, and/or laparoscopy may also be of help. Ovarian teratomas and choriocarcinomas and other carcinomas that secrete hCG do not cause precocious puberty in girls unless there is concomitant secretion of estrogen by the tumor (hCG or LH in the absence of FSH does not induce ovarian estrogen production). Rarely, feminizing tumors of the adrenal cause isosexual precocious puberty, either by formation of estrogens directly or by secretion of weak androgens to serve as estrogenic precursors in extraglandular tissues.

Other causes of precocious pseudopuberty include the following: (1) The McCune-Albright syndrome (polyostotic fibrous dysplasia), characterized by café au lait spots, cystic fibrous dysplasia of bones, and sexual precocity. Some of these individuals have increased gonadotropin secretion, whereas others have functional ovarian cysts in the presence of low gonadotropins, which represents a form of gonadotropin-independent sexual precocity. Occasionally, this disorder leads to true precocious puberty (see Chap. 325). (2) Primary hypothyroidism in which secretion of thyrotropin-releasing hormone (TRH) as well as the secretion of other hypothalamic hormones is enhanced, leading to increased FSH levels and ovarian estrogen secretion, frequently with galactorrhea. (3) The Silver syndrome, or congenital asymmetry associated with short stature and precocious feminization. (4) Estrogen-containing medications including use of estrogen-containing creams for diaper rash or the ingestion of meat from estrogen-treated animals or poultry or any estrogen by mouth.

INCOMPLETE ISOSEXUAL PRECOCITY This term is used to describe the premature development of a single pubertal event and encompasses several entities. The appearance of breast budding prior to the age of 8 (premature thelarche) without other evidence of estrogen secretion and without premature bone maturation is believed to be due to a transient increase in estrogen secretion or a temporary increase in sensitivity to the small amounts of circulating estrogens formed prior to puberty. Usually the disorder is self-limited and resolves spontaneously. Occasionally axillary hair and/or pubic hair (so-called *premature adrenarche* and *pubarche*) appear without any other secondary sexual development. The phenomenon is associated with adrenal androgen secretion in the range of normal puberty and can be distinguished from syndromes of virilization by the absence of clitoromegaly. It requires no treatment, and patients enter puberty at about the average time.

Heterosexual precocity Virilization in a prepubertal female is usually due to congenital adrenal hyperplasia or to androgen secretion by an ovarian or adrenal tumor. The manifestations of virilization are described in Chap. 54. Virilization in girls with congenital adrenal hyperplasia usually takes place in a background of variable sexual ambiguity (see Chap. 324).

Evaluation of sexual precocity The evaluation of sexual precocity involves a careful history and physical examination including rectoabdominal examination, abdominal sonography, determination of bone age, and measurement of gonadotropins (and androgen or estrogen levels when appropriate). Skull films and further diagnostic tests are indicated if a neurologic disorder is suspected and no evidence of ovarian or adrenal tumor is found.

REPRODUCTIVE YEARS Disorders of the menstrual cycle ABNORMAL UTERINE BLEEDING Between menarche and the menopause, almost every woman experiences one or more episodes of abnormal uterine bleeding, here defined as any bleeding pattern that differs in frequency, duration, or amount from the pattern observed during a normal menstrual cycle. A variety of descriptive terms (such as *menorrhagia, metrorrhagia,* and *menometrorrhagia*) have been used to characterize patterns of abnormal uterine bleeding. A more logical approach is to divide abnormal uterine bleeding into those patterns associated with ovulatory cycles and those associated with anovulatory cycles.

OVULATORY CYCLES Normal menstrual bleeding with ovulatory cycles is spontaneous, regular, cyclic, and predictable and frequently associated with discomfort (dysmenorrhea). Deviations from this pattern associated with cycles that are still regular and predictable are most often due to organic disease of the outflow tract. For example, regular but prolonged and excessive bleeding episodes unassociated with bleeding dyscrasias (hypermenorrhea or menorrhagia) can result from abnormalities of the uterus such as submucous leiomyomas, adenomyosis, or endometrial polyps. Regular, cyclical, predictable menstruation characterized by spotting or light bleeding is termed *hypomenorrhea* and is due to obstruction of the outflow tract as from intrauterine synechiae or scarring of the cervix. Intermenstrual bleeding between episodes of regular, ovulatory menstruation is also often due to cervical or endometrial lesions. An exception to the association between organic disease of the uterus and abnormal uterine bleeding is the occurrence of episodes of regular bleeding more frequently than 21 days apart (polymenorrhea). These cycles may be a normal variant.

ANOVULATORY CYCLES Uterine bleeding that is unpredictable with respect to amount, onset, and duration and is usually painless is described as *dysfunctional uterine bleeding*. This disorder is not due to abnormalities of the uterus but rather to chronic anovulation and occurs when there is interruption of the normal progressive sequence of follicular and luteal phases under the influence of a dominant follicle and its resulting corpus luteum. As discussed above normal uterine bleeding in ovulatory cycles is due to progesterone withdrawal and requires that the endometrium first be primed with estrogen (when castrates or postmenopausal women are given progesterone withdrawal bleeding usually does not occur).

Dysfunctional uterine bleeding can occur in women who have a transient disruption of the synchronous hypothalamic-pituitary-ovarian patterns necessary for regular ovulatory cycles, most often at the extremes of the reproductive life, namely in the early menarche and in the perimenopausal period, but also as the secondary consequence of temporary stresses or intercurrent illnesses.

On the other hand, primary *dysfunctional uterine bleeding* can result from at least three pathophysiologic mechanisms.

1 *Estrogen withdrawal bleeding* occurs when estrogen is given to a castrate or postmenopausal woman and then withdrawn. As in other types of dysfunctional uterine bleeding, this form of menstrual bleeding is usually painless.
2 *Estrogen breakthrough bleeding* occurs when there is prolonged continuous estrogen stimulation of the endometrium not interrupted by cyclic progesterone secretion and withdrawal. This is the most common type of dysfunctional uterine bleeding and is usually due to anovulation associated with chronic acyclic estrogen production as in women with polycystic ovarian disease. Such women may have histories of irregular, unpredictable menses, oligomenorrhea, or amenorrhea (see below). Alternatively, estrogen breakthrough bleeding can occur in hypogonadal women given estrogens chronically rather than intermittently or in women with estrogen-secreting tumors of the ovary. Estrogen breakthrough bleeding may be profuse and is unpredictable with respect to duration, amount of flow, and time of occurrence. The endometrium is typically thin because its repair between episodes of bleeding is incomplete.
3 *Progesterone breakthrough bleeding* occurs in the presence of abnormally high ratios of progesterone to estrogen, for example, in women on continuous low-dose oral contraceptives.

The approach to a patient with dysfunctional uterine bleeding in the reproductive years begins with a careful history of menstrual patterns and prior hormonal therapy. Since not all bleeding from the urogenital tract is from the uterus, rectal, bladder, and vaginal or cervical sources must be excluded by physical examination. If the bleeding is from the uterus a pregnancy-related disorder such as abortion or ectopic pregnancy must also be excluded. Once the diagnosis of dysfunctional uterine bleeding is established a rational approach to management is as follows. During a first episode of dysfunctional bleeding the patient can simply be observed, provided the bleeding is not copious and no evidence of bleeding dyscrasia is present. If bleeding is moderately severe, control can be achieved with relatively high dose estrogen oral contraceptives for 3 weeks. Alternatively, a regimen of three or four low-dose oral contraceptive pills per day for 1 week followed by tapering to the usual dosage for up to 3 weeks is also effective. If uterine bleeding is more severe, hospitalization, bed rest, and intramuscular injections of estradiol valerate (10 mg) and 17α-hydroxyprogesterone caproate (500 mg) or intravenous or intramuscular conjugated estrogens (25 mg) usually control the bleeding. After initial treatment iron replacement should be instituted, and recurrence can be prevented by cyclic oral contraceptives for 2 to 3 months (or more if pregnancy is not desired). Alternatively, menses should be induced every 2 to 3 months with medroxyprogesterone acetate 10 mg by mouth once or twice a day for 10 days. If hormone therapy fails to control uterine bleeding, an endometrial biopsy or dilatation and curettage may be required for diagnosis and therapy. Indeed, uterine sampling may be indicated prior to hormone therapy in women at risk for endometrial cancer (i.e., in women approaching the age of menopause or in the massively obese); endometrial cancer is rare in ovulatory women of reproductive age.

AMENORRHEA An acceptable definition of amenorrhea is failure of menarche by age 16, irrespective of the presence or absence of secondary sexual characteristics, or the absence of menstruation for 6 months in a woman with previous periodic menses. However, women who do not fulfill these criteria should be evaluated if (1) the subject and/or her family are greatly concerned, (2) no breast development has occurred by age 14, or (3) any sexual ambiguity or virilization is present (Chap. 324). Amenorrhea is usually categorized as either primary (in a woman who has never menstruated) or secondary (in a woman in whom menstruation is present for a variable time and then ceases); some disorders can cause either primary or secondary amenorrhea. For example, most women with gonadal dysgenesis have primary amenorrhea, but occasional such patients have some follicles and ovulate for short periods so that pregnancies may rarely occur. Furthermore, patients with chronic anovulation (polycystic ovarian disease) most often have secondary amenorrhea but occasionally present with primary amenorrhea. For these reasons, categorization of amenorrhea into primary and secondary types is less helpful in the differential diagnosis than a classification based upon the major underlying physiologic derangements: (1) anatomic defects, (2) ovarian failure, and (3) chronic anovulation with or without estrogen present.

Anatomic defects. A variety of anatomic or structural defects of the female genital tract can preclude menstrual bleeding. Starting from the caudal end of the female genital tract, labial agglutination or fusion is often associated with disorders of sexual development, particularly female pseudohermaphroditism (congenital adrenal hyperplasia or exposure to maternal androgens in utero). (See Chap. 324.) Congenital defects of the vagina, imperforate hymen, and transverse vaginal septae can also cause amenorrhea. These women frequently have accumulation of menstrual blood behind the obstruction and may have cyclic, predictable episodes of abdominal pain.

More severe müllerian anomalies include müllerian agenesis (the Mayer-Rokitansky-Küster-Hauser syndrome) (see Chap. 324), second in frequency only to gonadal dysgenesis as a cause of primary amenorrhea. Women with this syndrome have a 46,XX karyotype, female secondary sex characteristics, and normal ovarian function, including cyclical ovulation, but have absence or severe hypoplasia of the vagina. The uterus usually consists of only rudimentary bicornuate cords, but if the uterus contains endometrium, cyclic abdominal pain and accumulation of blood may occur as in other forms of outlet obstruction. One-third of patients have abnormalities of the urogenital tract, and one-tenth have skeletal anomalies, usually involving the spine. The major diagnostic problem is separating müllerian agenesis from complete testicular feminization in which 46,XY genetic males with testes differentiate as phenotypic women with a blind vaginal pouch and an absent uterus. Women with testicular feminization have feminized breasts but a paucity of pubic and axillary hair. The disorder is due to a defect in the androgen-receptor protein that causes profound resistance to the action of testosterone (see Chap. 324). Testicular feminization can be diagnosed by demonstrating a male level of serum testosterone or a 46,XY karyotype, whereas the diagnosis of müllerian agenesis is established by demonstrating a 46,XX karyotype, biphasic basal body temperatures characteristic of ovulating women, and elevated levels of progesterone during the luteal phase.

A rare cause of absence of uterus in 46,XY phenotypic women who are sexually infantile is the so-called testicular regression syndrome or testicular agenesis (see Chap. 324).

Other abnormalities of the uterus that cause amenorrhea include obstruction due to scarring or stenosis of the cervix, often resulting from surgery, electrocautery, laser therapy, or cryosurgery. Destruction of the endometrium (Asherman's syndrome) may follow vigorous curettage, usually in association with postpartum hemorrhage or therapeutic abortion complicated by infection. This diagnosis is confirmed by hysterosalpingography or by direct vision of the endometrial scarring or synechiae using a hysteroscope.

Treatment of disorders of the outflow tract is surgical. Repair of vaginal agenesis results in normal menstruation and potential fertility only if an intact uterus is present.

Ovarian failure. Primary ovarian failure is associated with elevated plasma gonadotropins and can result from several causes. The most frequent cause is *gonadal dysgenesis*, in which the germ cells are lacking and the ovary is replaced by a fibrous streak. (Also see Chaps. 7 and 324.) Women with gonadal dysgenesis can be divided into two broad groups on the basis of chromosomal karyotype. The most common is due to deletion of genetic material in the X chromosomes and accounts for about two-thirds of gonadal dysgenesis. A 45,X karyotype is found in about half, and most have somatic defects including short stature, webbed neck, shield chest, and cardiovascular defects, collectively termed the Turner phenotype. The remainder of patients with identifiable abnormalities of the X chromosome have chromosomal mosaicism with or without associated structural abnormalities of the X chromosome. The most common form of mosaicism is 45,X/46,XX. Gonadal tumors are rare in 45,X patients, but gonadal malignancies have been reported in women with chromosomal mosaicism involving the Y chromosome. Therefore, a chromosomal analysis should be obtained in all cases of amenorrhea associated with ovarian failure, and the streak gonad should be removed if a Y chromosome is present. Approximately 90 percent of individuals with gonadal dysgenesis associated with deletion of genetic material in the X chromosome never have menstrual bleeding, and the remaining 10 percent have sufficient residual follicles to experience menses and, rarely, fertility; the menstrual and reproductive lives of such individuals are invariably brief.

A tenth of subjects with bilateral streak gonads have a normal 46,XX or 46,XY karyotype and are said to have *pure gonadal dysgenesis*. These individuals have either normal or above-average stature due to failure of estrogen-mediated epiphyseal closure in the presence of a normal chromosomal constitution. Pure gonadal dysgenesis does not constitute a phenotypic or chromosomally homogeneous disorder. Some are the result of X-linked or autosomal gene defects. Other possible causes include chromosomal mosaicism limited to gonadal tissue and destruction of germinal tissue in utero by environmental or infectious processes. Approximately one-tenth of such individuals with a 46,XY karyotype develop signs of virilization including clitoromegaly and have an increased incidence of tumors in the gonadal streaks; as a consequence gonadal streaks should be removed prophylactically as previously discussed when a Y chromosome is present. Approximately two-thirds of individuals with 46,XX karyotype experience no menses while the remainder have one or more menstrual episodes and are occasionally fertile.

Other causes of ovarian failure and amenorrhea include 17α-hydroxylase or 17,20-desmolase deficiency, premature ovarian failure, the resistant-ovary syndrome, and ovarian failure secondary to chemotherapy or radiation therapy for malignancy. *17α-Hydroxylase deficiency* is characterized by primary amenorrhea, sexual infantilism, and hypertension that is due to increased production of desoxycorticosterone (DOC), whereas women with 17,20-desmolase deficiency have primary amenorrhea and sexual infantilism with normal blood pressure (see Chaps. 317 and 324). The diagnosis of *premature ovarian failure* or *premature menopause* is applied to women who cease menstruating prior to the age of 40. The ovaries are similar to the ovaries of postmenopausal women, namely, paucity or absence of follicles as the result of accelerated follicular atresia. Premature ovarian failure due to ovarian antibodies may be one component of polyglandular failure together with adrenal insufficiency, hypothyroidism, and other autoimmune disorders (see Chap. 325). A rare form of ovarian failure is the *resistant-ovary syndrome* in which the ovaries contain many follicles arrested in development prior to the antral stage, possibly because of resistance to the action of FSH in the ovary. To differentiate this disorder from the 46,XX variety of pure gonadal dysgenesis, both of which are associated with sexual immaturity, it is necessary to perform ovarian biopsy. However, such a distinction is not clinically useful since the treatment of infertility in both conditions is usually unsuccessful.

CHRONIC ANOVULATION At least 80 percent or more of gynecologic endocrine problems result from chronic anovulation. Women with chronic anovulation fail to ovulate spontaneously but may ovulate with appropriate therapy. The ovaries of such women do not secrete estrogen in a normal cyclic pattern; it is clinically useful to differentiate those women who produce sufficient estrogen to have withdrawal bleeding after progesterone therapy from those who fail to produce enough estrogen to have progesterone withdrawal bleeding and who often have hypothalamic-pituitary dysfunction.

Chronic anovulation with estrogen present. Women with chronic anovulation who experience withdrawal bleeding after progesterone administration are said to be in a state of "estrus" due to the acyclic production of estrogen, largely estrone, by extraglandular aromatization of circulating androstenedione. The most common term for this disorder is *polycystic ovarian disease* (PCOD), a syndrome characterized by infertility, hirsutism, obesity, and amenorrhea or oligomenorrhea. When spontaneous uterine bleeding occurs in subjects with PCOD, it is unpredictable with respect to time of onset, duration, and amount, and on occasion the bleeding can be severe. The dysfunctional uterine bleeding is usually due to estrogen breakthrough (see above).

The disorder, which may be transmitted as an autosomal dominant or X-linked trait, was originally described by Stein and Leventhal as characterized by enlarged, polycystic ovaries, but the syndrome and its accompanying endocrine abnormalities are now known to be associated with a variety of pathologic findings in the ovaries, only some of which result in enlargement of the ovaries and none of which are pathognomonic. The most common finding is a white, smooth, sclerotic ovary with a thickened capsule, multiple follicular cysts in various stages of atresia, a hyperplastic theca and stroma, and rare or absent corpora albicans. Other ovaries have hyperthecosis in which the ovarian stroma is hyperplastic and may contain lipid-laden luteal cells. Thus, the diagnosis of PCOD is a clinical one, based upon the coexistence of chronic anovulation and varying degrees of androgen excess.

In most women with PCOD menarche occurs at the expected time, but uterine bleeding is unpredictable in onset, duration, and amount. Amenorrhea ensues after a variable time, although primary amenorrhea occurs in some women. Signs of androgen excess (hirsutism) usually become evident around the time of menarche. One formulation suggests that this disorder originates as an exaggerated adrenarche in obese girls (Fig. 322-7). The combination of elevated adrenal androgens and obesity would result in increased formation of extraglandular estrogen and lead to an acyclic positive feedback on LH secretion and negative feedback on FSH secretion so that the characteristic LH/FSH ratios in plasma would be greater than 2. The increased LH levels could then lead to hyperplasia of the ovarian stroma and theca cells and increased androgen production, which in turn would provide more substrate for peripheral aromatization and perpetuate the chronic anovulation. In the advanced state the ovary is the major site of androgen production, but the adrenal may continue to secrete excess androgen as well. The greater the obesity, the more this sequence would be perpetuated because adipose tissue stromal cells aromatize androgens to estrogens, which in turn exaggerates inappropriate LH release by positive feedback.

Thus, the fundamental defect in PCOD is viewed as one of inappropriate signals to the hypothalamus and pituitary. In fact, the hypothalamic-pituitary axis responds appropriately to high levels of estrogen, and ovulation can be induced with antiestrogens such as clomiphene citrate. Increased levels of plasma endorphins and inhibin may contribute to the perpetuation of the defect. The concept that the fundamental defect is one of inappropriate signals is supported by the findings in the ovary itself. Ovarian follicles from women with PCOD have low aromatase activity, but normal aromatase can be induced when the follicles are treated with FSH. In short, the anovulation is not due to an intrinsic abnormality in the ovary itself but rather the result of FSH deficiency and LH excess. An association exists between PCOD or hyperthecosis, acanthosis nigricans, and insulin resistance. The meaning of this association is not clear.

Treatment of PCOD is directed toward interrupting this self-perpetuating cycle and can be accomplished in several ways, including decreasing ovarian androgen secretion (wedge resection or oral contraceptive agents), decreasing peripheral estrogen formation (weight reduction), enhancing FSH secretion [administration of clomiphene, human menopausal gonadotropin (hMG), LHRH (gonadorelin) by portable infusion pump, or purified FSH (urofollitropin)]. The choice

FIGURE 322-7 Proposed mechanism for the initiation and perpetuation of chronic anovulation in polycystic ovarian disease (PCOD). This cycle may be entered or initiated via adrenal androgen excess or obesity, both of which result in enhanced extraglandular formation of estrogens. The therapy of PCOD involves interruption of the cycle at various sites. *(From SSC Yen and RB Jaffe, 1986, and from U Goebelsmann in DR Mishell, Jr, and V Davajan.)*

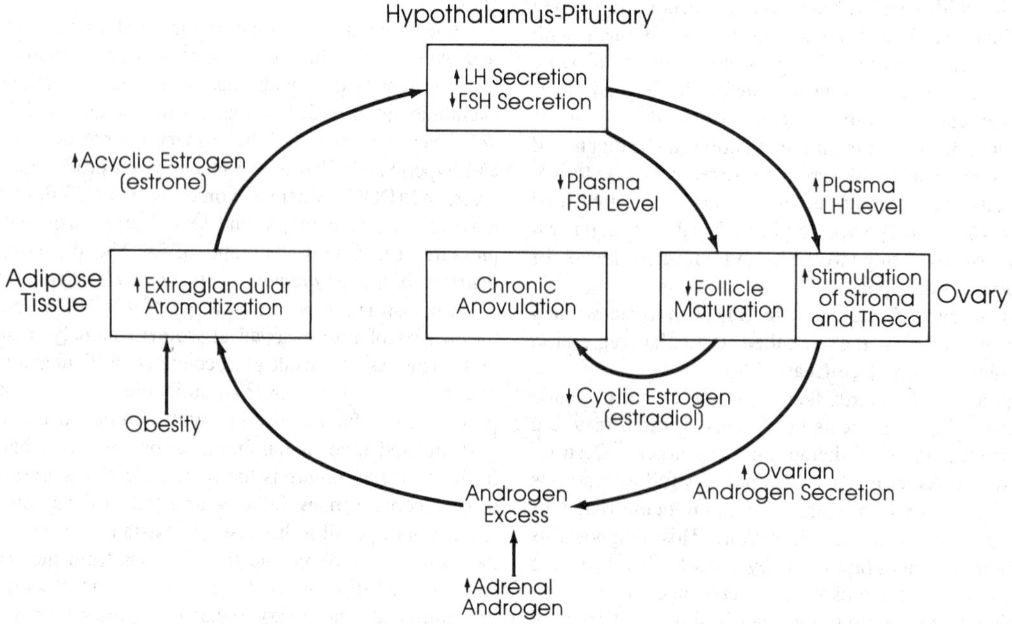

of therapy depends on the clinical findings and the needs of the patient. Attempt at weight reduction is appropriate in all who are obese. If the woman is not hirsute and does not desire pregnancy, periodic withdrawal menses can be induced with medroxyprogesterone acetate 10 days per month; such treatment prevents development of endometrial hyperplasia. If the woman is hirsute but does not desire pregnancy, the ovarian (and possibly the adrenal) component of androgen production can be suppressed with combined estrogen-progestogen oral contraceptive agents. Combined oral contraceptives are also indicated if prolonged or excessive menstrual bleeding is present. Once androgen excess is controlled, treatment of previously existing hair growth by shaving, depilatories, or electrolysis may be indicated (see Chap. 54). If the woman wants to become pregnant, induction of ovulation is necessary. The drug of choice for this purpose is clomiphene, which promotes ovulation in three-fourths of cases, or treatment with hMG, urofollitropin, or gonadorelin. Pretreatment with LHRH analogues prior to hMG, urofollitropin, or gonadorelin has been utilized to improve ovulation and pregnancy rates. Wedge resection of the ovaries is rarely indicated today because of the development of adhesions but may be successful on occasion.

Chronic anovulation with estrogen present may also occur with tumors of the ovary. These include granulosa-theca cell tumors, Brenner tumors, cystic teratomas, mucous cystadenomas, and Krukenberg tumors (also see Chap. 304). These tumors can either secrete excess estrogen themselves or produce androgens that can then be aromatized in extraglandular sites. As a result, chronic anovulation and the clinical features of PCOD are produced. Occasionally areas of the ovary not involved with tumors show the characteristic histologic changes of PCOD. Other causes of chronic anovulation with estrogen present include adrenal production of excess androgen (usually adult onset adrenal hyperplasia due to partial 21-hydroxylase deficiency) and various thyroid disorders.

Chronic anovulation with estrogen absent. Women with chronic anovulation who have low or absent estrogen production and do not experience withdrawal bleeding after progestogen treatment usually have hypogonadotropic hypogonadism due either to pituitary disease or to any of several organic or functional disorders of the central nervous system.

Isolated hypogonadotropic hypogonadism associated with defects of smell (olfactory bulb defects) is known as the Kallman syndrome (see Chaps. 313 and 321). Affected women are sexually infantile with a eunuchoid habitus and appear to have a defect in either the synthesis or release of LHRH. A variety of rare hypothalamic lesions can also impair LHRH production and cause hypogonadotropic hypogonadism; these include craniopharyngioma, germinoma (pinealoma), glioma, Hand-Schüller-Christian disease, teratomas, endodermal-sinus tumors, tuberculosis, sarcoidosis, and metastatic tumors that cause suppression or destruction of the hypothalamus. Central nervous system trauma and radiation can also cause hypothalamic amenorrhea and deficiencies in secretion of growth hormone, ACTH, vasopressin, and thyroid hormone.

More commonly, gonadotropin deficiency leading to chronic anovulation is believed to arise from functional disorders of the hypothalamus or higher centers. A history of a stressful event in a young woman is frequent. For example, chronic anovulation can begin suddenly in a woman who leaves home for the first time or experiences the death of a loved one. Gonadotropin and estrogen levels are in the low to low-normal range as compared to normal women in the early follicular phase of the cycle. In addition, rigorous exercise such as jogging or ballet and diets that result in excessive weight loss may lead to the development of chronic anovulation particularly in girls with a history of prior menstrual irregularity. The amenorrhea in these women does not appear to be due to weight loss alone but to a combination of a decrease in the percentage of body fat and chronic stress. An extreme form of weight loss with chronic anovulation is seen in anorexia nervosa. Anorexia nervosa is characterized by the development in a young woman of amenorrhea with associated severe weight loss, distorted attitudes toward eating and weight gain, self-induced vomiting, extreme emaciation, and distorted body image. Amenorrhea in anorexia nervosa can precede, follow, or appear coincidentally with the loss in body weight (see Chap. 73). During successful therapy gonadotropin changes recapitulate those observed during normal puberty (Fig. 322-1).

In addition, chronic debilitating diseases such as end-stage kidney disease, malignancy, or the malabsorption syndrome are believed to lead to development of hypogonadotropic hypogonadism via a hypothalamic mechanism.

Treatment of chronic anovulation due to hypothalamic disorders includes reversal of the stressful situation, reducing exercise, or correction of weight loss if appropriate. These women appear to be susceptible to the development of osteoporosis, and estrogen replacement therapy to induce and maintain normal secondary sexual characteristics and prevent bone loss is recommended in those who do not desire pregnancy, and gonadotropin or gonadorelin therapy is indicated when pregnancy is desired (see therapy section). When appropriate, therapy is directed at the primary disease of the hypothalamus.

Disorders of the pituitary can lead to the estrogen-deficient form of chronic anovulation by at least two mechanisms—direct interference with gonadotropin secretion by lesions that either obliterate or interfere with the gonadotropic cells (chromophobe adenomas, Sheehan's syndrome) or inhibition of gonadotropin secretion in association with excess prolactin (prolactinoma). *Pituitary tumors* make up approximately 10 percent of all intracranial tumors and may secrete no hormone, one hormone, or more than one hormone (see Chap. 313). In the past most pituitary tumors were assumed to be nonfunctional chromophobe adenomas, but prolactin levels are elevated in 50 to 70 percent of cases, either because of prolactin secretion by the tumor (prolactinomas) or interference by tumor mass with the normal inhibitory influence of the hypothalamus on prolactin secretion.

Prolactinomas can be divided into microadenomas (less than 10 mm in diameter) and macroadenomas (greater than 10 mm). Prolactin excess associated with low levels of LH and FSH constitutes a specific subgroup of hypogonadotropic hypogonadism. One-tenth or more of amenorrheic women have increased levels of serum prolactin, and more than half of women with both galactorrhea and amenorrhea have elevated prolactin levels. The amenorrhea in this disorder is most often associated with decreased or absent estrogen production, but prolactin-secreting tumors may on occasion be associated with normal ovulatory menses or chronic anovulation with estrogen present. Most prolactin-secreting adenomas grow slowly, and some cease growth after attainment of a certain size. The increased frequency of diagnosis of prolactin-secreting adenomas is probably due to several factors, including increased awareness, improved radiographic detection methods, and availability of radioimmunoassays for prolactin. However, since in older autopsy series a 9 to 23 percent prevalence of pituitary adenomas was observed in asymptomatic women, the clinical and prognostic significance of small microadenomas remains to be established. When tumors of any size are associated with symptoms of amenorrhea or galactorrhea, however, therapy should be considered, and when visual field defects or severe headaches are present bromocriptine therapy or neurosurgical evaluation is mandatory. The evaluation, differential diagnosis, and management of hyperprolactinemia is described in Chap. 313. In the latter half of pregnancy, prolactin-secreting pituitary tumors may expand, leading to headaches, compression of the optic chiasm, and blindness. Therefore, prior to induction of ovulation for the purposes of achieving pregnancy, it is mandatory to exclude the presence of a pituitary tumor.

Large pituitary tumors such as chromophobe adenomas—whether or not hyperprolactinemia is present—are likely to be associated with deficiency of hormones in addition to gonadotropins (Chap. 313).

Craniopharyngiomas, thought to arise from remnants of Rathke's pouch, account for 3 percent of intracranial neoplasms, occur most frequently in the second decade of life, and may extend into the suprasellar region. A large percentage of these tumors calcify and can be diagnosed by conventional skull films. Patients often present with sexual infantilism, delayed puberty, and amenorrhea due to gonadotropin deficiency. Craniopharyngioma may also result in impaired secretion of TSH, ACTH, growth hormone, and vasopressin.

Panhypopituitarism may occur spontaneously, result from surgical or radiation treatment of pituitary adenomas, or develop after postpartum hemorrhage (Sheehan's syndrome). The latter patients exhibit characteristic clinical manifestations including failure to lactate or ovulate, loss of genital and axillary hair, hypothyroidism, and adrenal insufficiency (see Chap. 313).

Evaluation of amenorrhea. A general schema for the evaluation of women with amenorrhea is given in Fig. 322-8. In the initial physical examination, special attention should be given to three features: (1) degree of maturation of the breasts, the pubic and axillary hair, and the external genitalia; (2) the current estrogen status; and (3) the presence or absence of a uterus. All women with amenorrhea should be assumed to be pregnant until proven otherwise. Even when history and physical examination are not suggestive, it is prudent to exclude pregnancy by a suitable screening test. Once this is done, the cause of amenorrhea can frequently be diagnosed by history and physical examination. For example, Asherman's syndrome is suggested by a history of curettage in a woman who previously menstruated; in women with primary amenorrhea and sexual infantilism the essential differential diagnosis is between gonadal dysgenesis and hypopituitarism, and, in addition, the diagnosis of gonadal dysgenesis (Turner's syndrome) or of anatomic defects of the outflow tract (müllerian agenesis, testicular feminization, and cervical stenosis) is frequently suggested on the basis of physical findings. When a specific cause is suspected, it is appropriate to proceed directly to confirm the diagnosis (such as obtaining a chromosomal karyotype or measurement of plasma gonadotropins). It is also useful to measure serum prolactin level during the initial evaluation.

Estrogen status is evaluated by determining if the vaginal mucosa is moist and rugated and if the cervical mucus can be stretched and shown to fern upon drying. If these criteria are indeterminate a progestational challenge is indicated, most often administration of 10 mg of medroxyprogesterone acetate by mouth once or twice daily for 5 days or 100 mg of progesterone in oil intramuscularly. (It should be emphasized that progestogen should never be administered until pregnancy is excluded.) If estrogen levels are adequate (and the outflow tract is intact) menstrual bleeding should occur within 1 week of ending the progestogen treatment. If withdrawal bleeding occurs, the diagnosis is chronic anovulation with estrogen present, usually polycystic ovarian disease.

If no withdrawal bleeding or only minimal vaginal spotting occurs, the nature of the subsequent workup is dependent on the results of the initial prolactin assay. If plasma prolactin is elevated or if galactorrhea is present, radiography of the pituitary should be undertaken. When the plasma prolactin is normal in the anovulatory woman with estrogen absent, plasma gonadotropins should be measured. If the gonadotropin levels are elevated, the diagnosis is ovarian failure. If the gonadotropins are in the low or normal range, the diagnosis is either hypothalamic-pituitary disorder or anatomic defect of the outflow tract. As indicated previously, the diagnosis of outflow tract disorder is usually suspected or established on the basis of the history and physical findings. When the physical findings are not clear-cut, it is useful to administer cyclic estrogen plus progestogen (1.25 mg of oral conjugated estrogens per day for 3 weeks with 10 mg of medroxyprogesterone acetate added for the last 7 to 10 days of estrogen treatment) followed by 10 days of observation. If no bleeding occurs, the diagnosis of Asherman's syndrome or other anatomic defect of the outflow tract is confirmed by hysterosalpingography or hysteroscopy. If withdrawal bleeding occurs following the estrogen-progestogen combination, the diagnosis of chronic anovulation with estrogen absent (functional hypothalamic amenorrhea) is suggested. Radiologic evaluations of the pituitary-hypothalamic areas may be indicated in the latter cases—irrespective of the prolactin level—because of the danger of overlooking a pituitary-hypothalamic tumor and because the diagnosis of functional hypothalamic amenorrhea is one of exclusion (see Chap. 313).

Infertility Infertility, the failure to become pregnant after 1 year of unprotected intercourse, affects approximately 10 to 15 percent of couples and is one of the common complaints for which women seek gynecologic assistance. Male factors account for 40 percent of infertility problems (see Chaps. 52 and 321). In women, failure of ovulation accounts for 30 percent, pelvic factors such as tubal disease and endometriosis account for half, and a cervical factor is implicated in about one-tenth of infertility evaluations. In 10 to 20 percent of infertile women no etiology is found. An immunologic cause may explain a portion of infertility in these couples. Finally, infertility in women may be due to *luteal phase dysfunction* in which ovulation is assumed to occur but progesterone formation is insufficient to allow preparation of the endometrium for implantation; the disorder

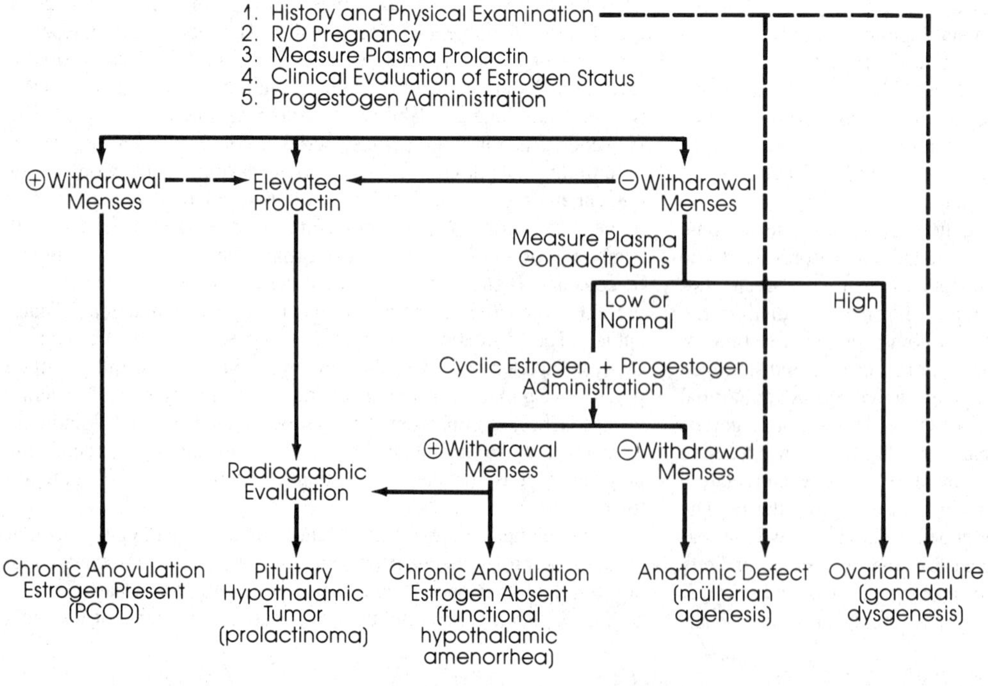

FIGURE 322-8 Flow diagram for the evaluation of women with amenorrhea. The most common diagnosis for each category is shown in parentheses. The dotted lines indicate that in some instances a correct diagnosis can be reached on the basis of history and physical exam alone.

is believed to be due to inadequate FSH secretion or action and consequent inadequate estrogen formation by the dominant follicle during the follicular phase.

The first diagnostic step in evaluation of the infertile couple is to determine whether the man or woman is the infertile partner, ordinarily by first obtaining a semen analysis in the man (see Chap. 321) and demonstration of presumed ovulation in the woman. Documentation of ovulatory cycles is obtained by daily measurement of basal body temperatures throughout the month. Occasionally, accurate basal body temperature records are not obtained, and demonstration of elevated serum progesterone levels during the luteal phase may be used as evidence of ovulation. Dating of endometrium by histologic examination of a biopsy sample is also useful for establishing ovulation or luteal phase dysfunction.

If the infertility is associated with amenorrhea, then the workup is that described in Fig. 322-8. If anovulation due to polycystic ovarian disease is the basis for infertility, ovulation can be induced utilizing clomiphene, gonadotropins, gonadorelin, or, on occasion, wedge resection of the ovaries. Bromocriptine is used to induce ovulation in cases of hyperprolactinemia. In the presence of prolactinomas the appropriate therapy prior to induction of ovulation remains controversial. Recommended therapies in this situation include observation, reinstitution of bromocriptine therapy, radiation therapy, or surgical resection of the tumor (see Chap. 313).

Hysterosalpingograms may be obtained to evaluate the fallopian tubes and uterine cavity. Further evaluation of tubal and ovarian disease is obtained by diagnostic laparoscopy and the demonstration of dye spillage from the fimbria after transcervical injection of dye during laparoscopy. Microsurgical repair of damaged or previously ligated fallopian tubes has resulted in an apparent increase in pregnancy rates. Removal of peritubular and fimbrial adhesions utilizing laser beam surgery is another treatment mode. Endometriosis can be diagnosed by laparoscopy, and treatment of endometriosis associated with infertility includes surgical resection of the endometrial implants or temporary gonadotropin suppression utilizing danazol (400 to 800 mg orally in divided doses for 4 to 6 months), LHRH analogues given by nasal spray or subcutaneous injection, or continuous low dose oral contraceptive agents to promote regression of the implants.

The cervical factor in infertility is evaluated by study of cervical mucus at an appropriate time after coitus. The test is preferably performed just prior to ovulation (day 12 to 13) when cervical mucus is thin and stretches and provides information as to the penetration and survival of the sperm in the female genital tract. Preferred treatment of infertility due to such abnormality is intrauterine insemination with washed sperm.

When other treatment modalities are unsuccessful, in vitro fertilization and embryo transfer (IVF-ET) may be tried. Indications for the use of IVF-ET in infertile couples include tubal obstructive disease, cervical factors, endometriosis, oligospermia, and unexplained infertility. Multiple follicles are induced with clomiphene and/or gonadotropins, and follicles are obtained by laparoscopy or transabdominal or transvaginal aspiration with ultrasound monitoring. After fertilization and cleavage, embryos are transferred to the uterine cavity. Although pregnancy rates vary, successful pregnancy has been reported in as high as 30 percent of cases after IVF-ET. Other techniques that have been successful include a modification of IVF-ET, known as gamete-intrafallopian transfer (GIFT) in which a mixture of sperm and ova are introduced into the end of the fallopian tube at laparoscopy, and intrauterine insemination after gonadotropin stimulation.

Medical aspects of pregnancy The possibility of pregnancy should be considered in all women of reproductive age who are evaluated for medical illness or considered for surgery. Procedures such as x-ray exposure, drugs, and anesthetics may be harmful to the developing fetus, and a variety of medical problems may worsen during pregnancy, including hypertension; diseases of the heart, lungs, kidney, and liver; and metabolic and endocrine disorders. Indeed, all women who present with abnormal vaginal bleeding or amenorrhea during the reproductive years should be assumed to have a complication of pregnancy, such as incomplete abortion, ectopic pregnancy, or trophoblastic disease (hydatidiform mole or choriocarcinoma). Women who present with these complications of pregnancy often have histories of abdominal pain and vaginal bleeding and may have evidence of intraabdominal hemorrhage.

Choriocarcinoma is a particular problem because of its protean manifestations. Half of these malignancies follow pregnancies complicated by hydatidiform mole, and the remainder occur after spontaneous abortion, ectopic pregnancy, or normal deliveries. Patients may present with intraabdominal bleeding due to rupture of the uterus, liver, or ovary, with pulmonary manifestations (cough, hemoptysis, pleuritic pain, dyspnea, and respiratory failure), or with gastrointestinal symptoms, usually chronic blood loss or melena. In addition, patients can present with cerebral metastases or renal involvement. The diagnosis can be established by demonstrating an elevated level of the β subunit of hCG in plasma. Treatment and cure are possible with chemotherapeutic agents (dactinomycin and/or methotrexate). (For manifestations of choriocarcinoma in men see Chap. 305.)

Ovarian tumors See Chap. 304.

TREATMENT

PROGESTOGENS The major use of progestogen is in conjunction with estrogen to ensure the full maturation of the endometrium, both in combination birth control pills and in the therapy of hypogonadal states. In certain circumstances, however, progestogen therapy is appropriate by itself—to induce a progestational effect on the estrogen-primed endometrium (diagnostic tests for the evaluation of amenorrhea), to inhibit pituitary gonadotropins (precocious puberty in girls, and the progestogen-only birth control pill), for prophylaxis to prevent hyperplasia in PCOD, and for palliation in endometrial and breast carcinoma or treatment of endometriosis. Even when a direct progestational effect is desired, the available oral drugs substitute a synthetic derivative for the naturally occurring hormone. Oral progestogens include medroxyprogesterone acetate, megestrol acetate, norethindrone, norgestrel, and micronized progesterone. Parenteral agents include progesterone in oil, medroxyprogesterone acetate suspension, and 17-hydroxyprogesterone caproate. Vaginal progesterone suppositories are used for treatment of luteal phase defects.

The most common undesirable side effect is breakthrough bleeding, which occurs when progestogens are used continuously. Other complications include nausea, vomiting, and hirsutism. Abnormal liver function is a side effect of those derivatives with alkyl substitution in the 17α position. Progestogens are contraindicated if pregnancy is known or suspected because of the risk of birth defects.

ESTROGENS Estrogenic drugs are used for three purposes—the treatment of gonadal failure, control of fertility, and in the management of dysfunctional uterine bleeding and carcinoma of the breast. (The use of estrogens in management of carcinoma of the breast is discussed in Chap. 303.) However, none of the presently available orally active or parenteral hormones replaces the pattern of concentration of estradiol characteristic of the normally cycling, premenopausal woman (Fig. 322-5). Estrogens that can be given by mouth are either nonsteroidal agents (such as diethylstilbestrol) that mimic the action of estradiol, estrogen conjugates that must be hydrolyzed before they become active (estrogen sulfates, predominantly estrone sulfate from pregnant mare's urine), or estrogen analogues that cannot be metabolized to estradiol (mestranol, quinestrol) (Fig. 322-9). Even when micronized estradiol is given orally, it is rapidly converted in the body to estrone. Because oral therapy neither replaces nor mimics the daily secretory pattern of the lost hormone, such therapy must be viewed as a pharmacologic substitution rather than a physiologic replacement. Likewise, the use of parenteral estrogens rarely mimics the physiologic situation. Parenteral preparations of conjugated es-

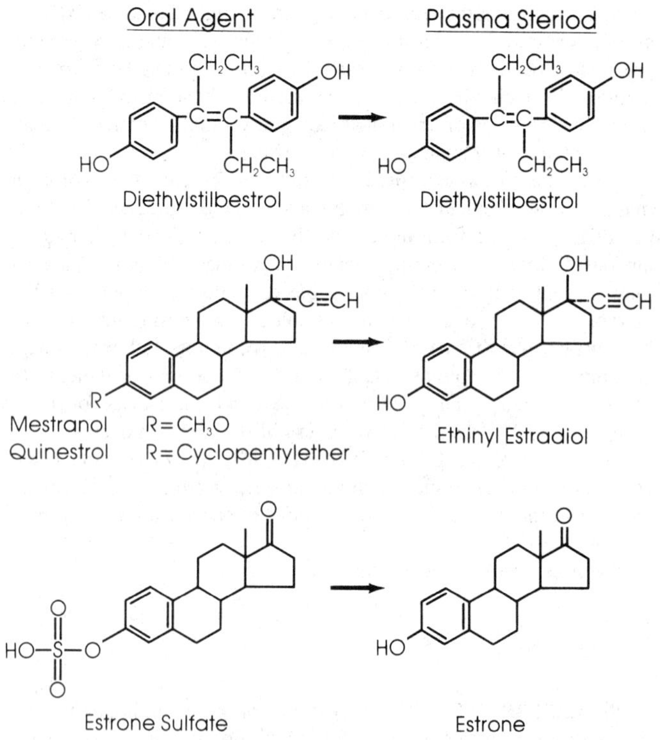

FIGURE 322-9 The circulating forms of administered estrogenic drugs.

trogens, like the oral derivatives, are poor precursors of estradiol, and estradiol esters (estradiol benzoate and valerate) rarely cause plasma estradiol levels that mimic the normal monthly secretory pattern of the hormone. Transdermal estrogen results in constant levels of blood estrogen and is effective in the treatment of menopausal symptoms. The side effects of estrogen substitution differ at various times of life.

Hypoestrogenism In women with decreased estrogen production, whether due to disease of the ovaries (gonadal dysgenesis) or to hypogonadotropic hypogonadism, treatment with cyclic estrogens should be instituted at the time of expected puberty for development and maintenance of female secondary sexual characteristics and prevention of osteoporosis. The most commonly used medications are conjugated estrogens (0.625 to 1.25 mg per day by mouth) or ethinyl estradiol or its precursors (0.02 to 0.05 mg by mouth). The addition of medroxyprogesterone acetate (5 to 10 mg daily) is recommended by most physicians during the last several days of monthly estrogen treatment to prevent development of endometrial hyperplasia during long-term estrogen treatment. Abnormal bleeding in women receiving estrogen replacement requires histologic evaluation of the endometrium. Such substitution therapy or the use of oral contraceptives (see below) may also be used for the purpose of suppressing pituitary gonadotropins, as in women with PCOD in whom the major therapeutic aim is suppression of ovarian androgen production prior to the time when fertility is desired.

Temporary administration of estrogens in larger quantities (up to two times the usual adult maintenance dose) may be necessary to induce full development of secondary sexual characteristics in girls and for the control of menopausal symptoms. Even larger doses of parenteral estrogens (10 mg of estradiol valerate or 25 mg of conjugated estrogen) in conjunction with progestogen may be required in some instances of dysfunctional uterine bleeding. Estrogen replacement (100 ng/kg) stimulates growth in women with gonadal dysgenesis, but at high doses (400 ng/kg) has no effect on growth. In addition to the potential long-term side effects of all estrogens (see below), these dosages may cause specific problems including nausea, vomiting, and edema.

Fertility control Since the use of all contraceptive methods is associated with diverse side effects, an understanding of the use, methods of actions, and consequences of these agents is important to all physicians. Furthermore, since pregnancy may aggravate a variety of chronic illnesses, fertility control should be recommended in many patients.

To be effective, fertility control requires patient acceptance and compliance. The most widely utilized methods include (1) rhythm and withdrawal techniques; (2) barrier methods including the condom, jellies, foam, suppositories, and diaphragms; (3) intrauterine devices (IUD); (4) hormonal contraceptives; (5) sterilization; and (6) abortion.

The rhythm and withdrawal technique and the barrier methods are effective if used correctly and consistently but in actual practice result in high failure rates because of imperfect compliance. Nevertheless, these methods carry the lowest incidence of side effects, and the side effects, when produced, are minor except for local allergic reactions. Their use should be recommended when there is a relative or absolute contraindication to other therapy.

The most widely utilized nonsurgical methods of contraception, the IUD and birth control pills, are effective but may be associated with significant side effects.

IUD The success rates of most IUDs are 95 to 98 percent. Only two devices are marketed in the United States. Both are T-shaped, cause minimal pain at insertion, and are associated with low expulsion rates. One of these IUDs contains copper, which enhances effectiveness, and is replaced at 4-year intervals. The other contains slow-release progesterone, which makes annual replacement necessary. The IUD is believed to prevent pregnancy by the induction of a chronic inflammatory reaction in the endometrium, resulting in an unfavorable environment for the implantation of the blastocyst.

Once the IUD is inserted, it is necessary to check periodically to be certain that the device is in place. Both minor and serious side effects can occur. Intermenstrual spotting and increased bleeding and pain or cramps at the time of menses are frequent causes of discontinuation of the IUD. In addition, the device may be expelled spontaneously during a menstrual period without the subject being aware of its loss. The most serious side effect is pelvic infection, occasionally leading to the development of tuboovarian abscess and subsequent infertility. The incidence of pelvic infection is more frequent than in users of oral or barrier contraceptives but no greater than in women using no contraception. Women with multiple sex partners are at greatest risk for pelvic infection. For this reason, use in nulligravida women is not advocated by many gynecologists. In addition, pregnancy with an IUD in place is more likely to be ectopic since intrauterine but not extrauterine pregnancies are inhibited. Because of the increased incidence of spontaneous and septic abortions when IUDs are in place, the device should be removed if pregnancy is detected. Any user who develops persistent, severe bleeding, lower abdominal pain, fever, or discharge should have the IUD removed.

ORAL CONTRACEPTIVES Oral contraceptive agents have been used by over 200 million women worldwide and by 1 out of 4 women in the United States under the age of 45. These agents are popular because of ease of administration, low pregnancy rate (less than 1 percent), and a relatively low incidence of side effects.

The most widely utilized oral contraceptive pills are either combination tablets or biphasic or triphasic formulations. A list of oral contraceptives marketed in the United States is given in Table 322-3. Combination oral contraceptive tablets contain one of two synthetic estrogens (mestranol or ethinyl estradiol) and one of five synthetic progestogens (norethindrone, norethindrone acetate, norethynodrel, norgestrel, or ethynodiol diacetate). The agents now available all contain no more than 50 μg ethinyl estradiol or its equivalent. The combination or biphasic or triphasic tablets are taken for 21 consecutive days followed by 7 days' rest. Progestogen-only tablets are taken continuously on a daily basis. Presumably, the ideal contraceptive contains the lowest amount of steroid to minimize side effects but an amount that is at the same time sufficient to prevent

TABLE 322-3 Composition of currently marketed oral contraceptives

Name	Estrogen	μg	Progestogen	mg
COMBINATION-TYPE				
Fixed type				
Estrogen content = 50 μg:				
Ortho-Novum 1/50	Mestranol	50	Norethindrone	1.0
Norinyl 1/50	Mestranol	50	Norethindrone	1.0
Ovcon 50	Ethinyl estradiol	50	Norethindrone	1.0
Ovral	Ethinyl estradiol	50	Norgestrel	0.5
Demulen	Ethinyl estradiol	50	Ethynodiol diacetate	1.0
Norlestrin 2.5/50	Ethinyl estradiol	50	Norethindrone acetate	2.5
Norlestrin 1/50	Ethinyl estradiol	50	Norethindrone acetate	1.0
Estrogen content <50 μg:				
Ortho-Novum 1/35	Ethinyl estradiol	35	Norethindrone	1.0
Norinyl 1+35	Ethinyl estradiol	35	Norethindrone	1.0
Modicon	Ethinyl estradiol	35	Norethindrone	0.5
Brevicon	Ethinyl estradiol	35	Norethindrone	0.5
Ovcon 35	Ethinyl estradiol	35	Norethindrone	0.4
Demulen 1/35	Ethinyl estradiol	35	Ethynodiol diacetate	1.0
Loestrin 1.5/30	Ethinyl estradiol	30	Norethindrone acetate	1.5
Loestrin 1/20	Ethinyl estradiol	20	Norethindrone acetate	1.0
Nordette	Ethinyl estradiol	30	Levonorgestrel	0.15
Lo-Ovral	Ethinyl estradiol	30	Norgestrel	0.3
Biphasic type				
Ortho-Novum 10/11				
First 10 days	Ethinyl estradiol	35	Norethindrone	0.5
Next 11 days	Ethinyl estradiol	35	Norethindrone	1.0
Triphasic type				
Ortho-Novum 7/7/7				
First 7 days	Ethinyl estradiol	35	Norethindrone	0.5
Second 7 days	Ethinyl estradiol	35	Norethindrone	0.75
Third 7 days	Ethinyl estradiol	35	Norethindrone	1.0
Tri-Norinyl				
First 7 days	Ethinyl estradiol	35	Norethindrone	0.5
Next 9 days	Ethinyl estradiol	35	Norethindrone	1.0
Next 5 days	Ethinyl estradiol	35	Norethindrone	0.5
Triphasil				
First 6 days	Ethinyl estradiol	30	Levonorgestrel	0.05
Second 5 days	Ethinyl estradiol	40	Levonorgestrel	0.075
Third 10 days	Ethinyl estradiol	30	Levonorgestrel	0.125
Tri-Levein				
First 6 days	Ethinyl estradiol	30	Levonorgestrel	0.05
Second 5 days	Ethinyl estradiol	40	Levonorgestrel	0.075
Third 10 days	Ethinyl estradiol	30	Levonorgestrel	0.125
PROGESTOGEN ONLY				
Micronor	None		Norethindrone	0.35
Nor Q.D.	None		Norethindrone	0.35
Ovrette	None		Norgestrel	0.075

pregnancy or breakthrough bleeding. The triphasic tablets containing 35 μg or less of estrogen and less than 1 mg of progestogen come closest to this goal.

Oral contraceptives inhibit ovulation by suppressing FSH and LH secretion. As a consequence, the secretion of all ovarian steroids is also suppressed, including estrogen, progesterone, and androgen (Fig. 322-10). These agents also exert minor direct inhibitory effects on the reproductive tract, altering the cervical mucus and thereby decreasing sperm penetration and decreasing the motility and secretions of the fallopian tubes and uterus.

The death rates associated with oral contraceptives and other forms of birth control are summarized in Table 322-4. Up to age 40 the mortality rates in women using oral contraceptives and IUDs are lower than in women using no form of contraception (this difference is because of the increased risk of death associated with pregnancy). The decrease in death rate below age 40 is even more striking in nonsmokers than in smokers using contraceptives. In fact, the death rates in nonsmoking women age 15 to 24 who use oral agents are lower than those with other forms of fertility control. The increased death rates in women using rhythm or barrier techniques probably results from the higher failure rate and the consequent risk of pregnancy in such women. Oral contraceptive agents are not recommended for smoking women after age 35, rarely in women after age 40, and women of all ages who are at increased risk for myocardial infarction.

Despite the overall safety of these agents, users are at risk for several serious side effects. In most retrospective and prospective studies an increased incidence has been found for *deep vein thrombosis* and *pulmonary embolism*. The relative increased risk varies from two- to twelvefold and is greater for women taking tablets containing more than 50 μg estrogen. The use of oral contraceptives is also associated with an increased risk of thromboembolism after surgery, and for this reason these agents should be discontinued at least 1 month prior to elective surgery. In retrospective studies there is a 3- to 9-times increased risk for *thromboembolic stroke* and a twofold greater risk for *hemorrhagic stroke* in users of oral contraceptives. However, three large prospective studies have demonstrated only a slight increase in hemorrhagic stroke in oral contraceptive users. Therefore, the drugs should be discontinued in women who experience visual complaints or severe headaches. Smoking and age increase the risk for stroke as well as the frequency of death from complications of deep venous thrombosis, pulmonary emboli, and myocardial infarction.

A small rise in blood pressure while taking oral contraceptives is common, and 5 percent of women develop significant *hypertension*

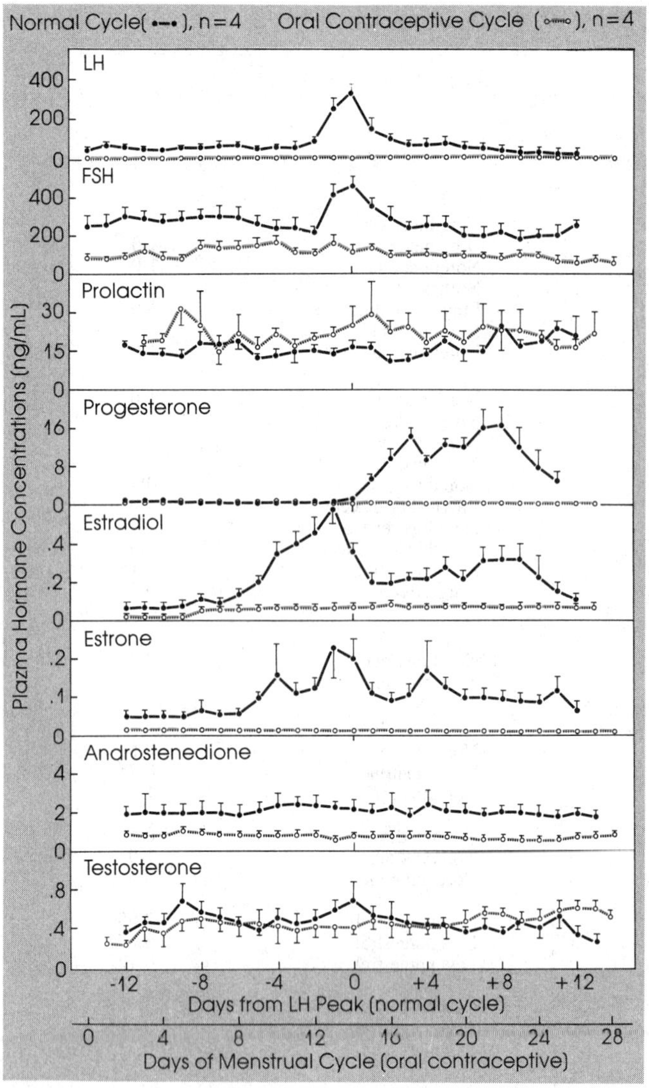

FIGURE 322-10 The mechanism of action of the birth control tablet. Mean daily plasma hormone concentrations during the ovarian cycle are shown for four ovulating women and four women treated with combination-type oral contraceptives. Data for the normal ovarian cycle are presented in relationship to the day of the LH peak; day 1 of the contraceptive cycle corresponds to the first day of uterine bleeding. The values are the mean ± SE obtained from four women. (*From BR Carr et al, 1979.*)

(blood pressure greater than 140/90) after 5 years of continuous use. Estrogens induce the synthesis of a variety of proteins by the liver including the renin substrate angiotensinogen. The resulting increased formation of angiotensin is believed to be involved in the development of hypertension. Alternatively, the progestogen component of oral contraceptives may be associated with increased risk of hypertension. In most cases, blood pressure returns to normal when oral contraceptives are discontinued.

Serum lipids and lipoproteins are altered in women on oral contraceptives, the nature of the change depending on the specific components of the oral contraceptives. In general, estrogens increase serum high-density (HDL) and very low density lipoproteins (VLDL). Progestogens depress the concentration of HDL.

A few women taking oral contraceptives develop *impairment of glucose tolerance* as manifested by abnormal glucose levels and elevated plasma insulin after an oral glucose load, both of which usually return to normal after discontinuing the agents. Because juvenile-onset and adult-onset diabetes may be associated with increased incidence of cardiovascular disease, it is also preferable to utilize other forms of contraception in these individuals.

Oral contraceptives should not be used by women with abnormal liver function tests or in women with acute or chronic liver disease. A rare complication linked to the long-term use of oral contraceptives is the development of peliosis hepatis, which can cause death due to sudden rupture and hemorrhage of the liver. Cholestatic jaundice may occur in those women predisposed to the development of the syndrome of recurrent jaundice of pregnancy.

Oral contraceptives cause an increased concentration of cholesterol in the bile, which is probably the cause for the twofold increase in *cholelithiasis* and cholecystitis in women on oral contraceptives.

Estrogens induce elevation of a variety of proteins secreted by the liver including cortisol-binding globulin (CBG), testosterone-binding globulin (TeBG), and thyroxine-binding globulin (TBG). Consequently, various laboratory tests of adrenal and thyroid function may be altered and must be interpreted with caution (see Chaps. 312 and 316). Oral contraceptives also slightly lower plasma ACTH levels, possibly due to an inhibitory effect on ACTH secretion or cortisol catabolism. Finally, serum prolactin levels are slightly elevated in women on oral contraceptives, but such treatment is not believed to play a role in the development of pituitary prolactinomas.

Other effects of oral contraceptive pills include minor dyspepsia, breast discomfort, weight gain, development of pigmentation of the face (chloasma), which is augmented by exposure to the sun, and a variety of psychological effects, such as depression and changes in libido. There is no convincing evidence that oral contraceptives are associated with an increased incidence of cancer of the uterus, cervix, or breast. In fact, oral contraceptives have many beneficial effects including control of dysmenorrhea and anovulatory bleeding, prevention of sexually transmitted diseases, and decreased incidence of endometrial and ovarian cancer.

The absolute contraindications to the use of oral contraceptives include previous thromboembolic disorders, cerebral vascular or coronary artery disease, known or suspected carcinoma of the breast or estrogen-dependent neoplasia, undiagnosed abnormal genital bleeding, or known or suspected pregnancy. Relative contraindications must be weighed against the risk-benefit ratio of the oral contraceptive pills and include hypertension, migraine headaches, diabetes mellitus, uterine leiomyomas, sickle cell anemia, hyperlipemia, and elective surgery.

OTHER STEROID CONTRACEPTIVES Types of steroid contraception

TABLE 322-4 Annual death rates associated with fertility control per 100,000 women

	Age group					
Contraceptive techniques	15–19	20–24	25–29	30–34	35–39	40–44
None (birth-related)	7.0	7.4	9.1	14.8	25.7	28.2
Oral contraceptives						
Smokers	2.4	3.6	6.8	13.7	51.4	117.6
Nonsmokers	0.5	0.7	1.1	2.1	14.1	32.0
IUD	1.3	1.1	1.3	1.3	1.9	2.1
Abortion	0.5	1.1	1.3	1.9	1.8	1.1
Barrier methods (birth-related)	1.5	1.4	1.0	0.8	1.3	7.6

SOURCE: Adapted from Ory.

other than the conventional oral contraceptives include (1) postcoital contraception and (2) injectable steroids. Use of high-dose estrogen for 5 days during the fertile part of the cycle (the morning-after pill) is an effective method of contraception, but is associated with significant side effects, particularly nausea. Administration of progestogens by injection, implants, or vaginal rings is used infrequently in the United States.

Estrogen treatment of the menopause The use of estrogens in postmenopausal women with osteoporosis is based on the belief that such therapy may relieve many of the disorders of the menopause and indeed of aging itself. In some parts of the United States by the mid-1970s as many as half of women in the menopausal age group used one or more forms of estrogen replacement for a median period of 5 years, accounting for more than 30 million prescriptions per year.

The menopause is not associated with a simple state of estrogen deprivation since some estrogens continue to be produced but is instead a state of altered estrogen metabolism; the predominant estrogen becomes estrone formed by extraglandular conversion of prehormone rather than estradiol secretion by the ovary. As is true for all estrogen therapy, the estrogen treatment of the menopause is actually a pharmacologic substitution of one or another estrogen analogue for the physiologic estradiol rather than a physiologic replacement of the missing steroid. Estrogens available for replacement therapy include conjugated estrogens, estrogen substitutes (diethylstilbestrol), synthetic estrogen (ethinyl estradiol or derivatives), micronized estradiol, estrogen-containing vaginal creams, and estrogen-containing dermal patches. Regimens associated with low risk of complications include (1) cyclic estrogen therapy in the lowest effective dose for 21 to 25 days per month, and (2) cyclic estrogens plus the addition of progestogen during the last 10 to 13 days of estrogen therapy.

The most clear-cut benefit of estrogen therapy in the menopause is the relief of vasomotor instability (hot flashes) and of atrophy of the urogenital epithelium and skin. Estrogen therapy ameliorates these symptoms in the majority of cases. When estrogen therapy is designed to treat hot flashes alone, such therapy should be continued for only a few years since hot flashes tend to diminish after 3 to 4 years in untreated women.

Several lines of evidence indicate that routine estrogen therapy is beneficial in preventing the complications of menopausal osteoporosis, especially in high-risk women (i.e., thin white women). First, in women undergoing premature menopause the incidence and complication rates of osteoporosis are increased, and long-term estrogen replacement appears to be beneficial. Second, estrogen therapy has short-term positive effects on calcium balance and long-term beneficial effects on bone density. Third, in women given estrogen therapy, the incidence of fractures is decreased.

Of the potential side effects, the possibility of an increased risk of endometrial carcinoma is perhaps most worrisome. The relative risk of developing endometrial adenocarcinoma in estrogen users is between 6 and 8. The risk is increased with duration and dosage of estrogen but is decreased in women given combination estrogen-progestogen therapy.

Despite the large body of evidence linking endometrial carcinoma and estrogen use, two types of doubt have been raised about the clinical significance of the association. First, some epidemiologists have argued that the increased risk associated with estrogens has been exaggerated because of problems inherent in obtaining adequate controls in retrospective analyses. Second, in spite of an increased incidence of endometrial carcinoma in the United States, there was no concomitant increased mortality from this disease. Indeed the increased incidence apparently involves low-grade malignancies which may be difficult to distinguish histologically from various forms of hyperplasia. These forms of malignancy have little effect on life expectancy.

Apprehension concerning worsening of hypertension and thromboembolic disease appears to be due to reports of the effects of estrogen-progesterone oral contraceptive pills during the reproductive years and not to estrogen use in menopausal women. There is no documented evidence that low-dose estrogen therapy in the menopause enhances the development or the severity of thromboembolic disease, breast cancer, or hypertension. Low-dose estrogen treatment in the menopause does not appear to influence the development of atherosclerosis, myocardial infarction, or stroke. Some evidence suggests that in fact estrogens may decrease the incidence of death from myocardial infarction. There is a slightly increased risk for the development of gallbladder disease with estrogen use in the menopause.

A reasonable approach to the use of estrogens in the menopause is as follows: (1) For long-term use, estrogens should be given in the minimal effective doses (0.625 mg conjugated estrogen or 0.01 to 0.02 mg ethinyl estradiol per day). Except when hot flashes preclude intermittent use, the agents are often prescribed for 25 days each month followed by a rest period. (For women with an intact uterus it is the practice in some clinics to give estrogens alone for 15 days, estrogen plus a daily progestogen for an additional 10 to 13 days, and nothing for a week.) (2) Such replacement therapy is indicated routinely in women undergoing premature menopause (surgically induced or spontaneous) at least until the age of normal menopause. (3) Estrogen therapy is also indicated routinely in women of all ages who have severe hot flashes or symptomatic atrophy of the urogenital epithelium. Hot flashes rarely persist for longer than 4 years, so that if given for this purpose the duration of therapy can be limited. (4) In women who have had prior hysterectomy potential benefits of treatment appear to outweigh the dangers. Whether estrogens should be given routinely to all women with intact uteri is unsettled, but the authors prescribe it routinely in the absence of contraindications in hopes of ameliorating osteoporosis (in combination with calcium). (5) Each woman receiving estrogens must be monitored indefinitely and frequently.

DRUGS TO INDUCE OVULATION The most common treatment for ovulation induction in women with PCOD is *clomiphene*. This antiestrogen is believed to act by binding to estrogen receptors in the hypothalamus and allowing FSH to rise to stimulate follicular development and ultimately result in ovulation. Clomiphene therapy is usually begun in a dose of 50 mg by mouth daily for 5 days commencing on the fifth day of progestin-induced uterine bleeding. If ovulation does not occur, the dose may be increased to 100 or 150 mg per day. Such treatment results in ovulatory cycles in 60 percent of women with PCOD. Additional regimens include clomiphene in combination with human menopausal gonadotropins (hMG), estrogen, glucocorticoids, or human chorionic gonadotropin (hCG).

The most commonly used gonadotropins for induction of ovulation are hMG, urofollitropin, and hCG. These agents are indicated in women who fail to ovulate on clomiphene. (For women with hypogonadotropic hypogonadism urofollitropin is not recommended.) The usual treatment regimen requires 1 to 3 ampuls of hMG or urofollitropin per day over an 8- to 12-day period to achieve adequate follicular stimulation and growth, followed by a single injection of 10,000 units of hCG 12 to 24 h after the last injection of hMG. For women with PCOD, pretreatment with LHRH analogues prior to hMG or urofollitropin appears to improve ovulation and pregnancy rates. Ovulation is successful in 90 percent of women, and pregnancy rates exceed 50 to 60 percent. Measurement of daily estrogen levels and frequent evaluation of ovarian size by ultrasound are indicated to prevent ovarian hyperstimulation. Ovarian hyperstimulation syndrome results from excessive stimulation of ovarian follicles with resultant enlargement of the ovaries and may progress to the development of ascites, hypotension, and shock. Therapy using hMG, urofollitropin, and hCG also carries a 20 percent risk of multiple pregnancies.

Bromocriptine is a dopamine agonist that is effective in inducing ovulation in women with elevated prolactin levels. Treatment is instituted at a usual dosage of 2.5 mg by mouth two or three times a day. Treatment should be discontinued as soon as pregnancy is diagnosed. The management of prolactin-secreting pituitary tumors is discussed in Chap. 313.

Luteinizing hormone–releasing hormone (LHRH, gonadorelin) and analogues Gonadorelin has been used successfully to induce ovulation in infertile women. The agent is infused subcutaneously or intravenously by a portable infusion pump which administers pulses at 90- to 120-min intervals for 10 to 20 days. After ovulation has occurred hCG is given to maintain corpus luteum function.

LHRH analogues that block ovulation have been used to treat a variety of gynecologic disorders; ovulation and ovarian steroidogenesis are inhibited due to down-regulation of LHRH receptors with a resultant decreased release of gonadotropins. Conditions in which these agents are under trial include fertility control, true precocious puberty, endometriosis, uterine leiomyomas, hirsutism, and, in combination with gonadotropins, ovulation induction and in vitro fertilization.

OTHER DISORDERS OF THE FEMALE REPRODUCTIVE TRACT

VULVA Most disorders of the vulva are due to venereal disease, most commonly syphilis (painless chancre), condyloma acuminata (venereal warts), and herpes vulvitis (painful ulcers) (see Chap. 93). All other lesions of the vulva, particularly in older women, must be biopsied. Early biopsy of cancer of the vulva is mandatory, because when it becomes symptomatic (pruritus and bleeding), it has often progressed to an advanced stage.

VAGINA Infections of the vagina usually present as vaginal discharge and pruritus. The most frequent organisms are *Trichomonas, Candida albicans,* and *Gardnerella vaginalis* (also see Chap. 93). The diagnosis is made by microscopic examination of the discharge, and appropriate therapy can be instituted utilizing vaginal or oral antibiotics.

Abnormalities of the vagina and cervix in female offsprings of women given diethylstilbestrol during pregnancy include adenosis of the vagina as well as structural abnormalities of the vagina, cervix, and uterus; the risk of developing a rare form of vaginal cancer (adenocarcinoma, clear cell type) is increased (2 per 10,000 exposed women). Periodic examination of women at risk should commence at age 12 to 14, and reevaluation should be undertaken after any episode of abnormal bleeding.

CERVIX Preinvasive lesions of the cervix (also known as cervical intraepithelial neoplasia) as well as invasive carcinoma of the cervix can be detected reliably by obtaining a Papanicolaou smear (Pap smear). Current recommendations by the American Cancer Society are that a Pap smear be obtained every 3 years after 2 negative Pap smears were obtained at yearly intervals. However, many gynecologists recommend yearly Pap smears especially in patients with more than one sexual partner.

UTERUS Only 40 percent of endometrial adenocarcinoma is detected by Pap smears. In women at high risk for endometrial carcinoma (obesity, history of chronic anovulatory cycles, diabetes, hypertension, estrogen treatment), yearly endometrial sampling should be performed. Low-dose oral estrogen therapy rarely causes breakthrough or withdrawal bleeding in menopausal women. Therefore, irrespective of whether the patient is on estrogen therapy, occurrence of postmenopausal bleeding makes it mandatory to obtain a tissue diagnosis to exclude endometrial cancer either by endometrial sampling or by curettage.

One of the most common disorders of the uterus and the most frequent tumor of women (1 of 4 women affected) is the uterine leiomyoma, or fibroid tumor. Three-fourths of women with leiomyoma are asymptomatic, and the diagnosis is made on routine pelvic examination. When associated with excessive menstrual blood loss, excessive size or rapid growth, or significant pelvic pain (see Chap. 53), the preferred treatment is surgical removal by hysterectomy if there is no desire for further childbearing. In young women myomectomy may on occasion be indicated when infertility or repeated fetal wastage is a manifestation or where future childbearing is desired.

FALLOPIAN TUBES AND OVARIES Infectious pelvic inflammatory disease is a common disorder of the fallopian tubes and usually becomes symptomatic after a menstrual period; the symptoms include fever, chills, abdominal pain, and vaginal discharge, and pelvic tenderness on physical examination is common. The initiating organism most often is *chlamydia trachomatis* or *Neisseria gonorrhoeae,* but tuboovarian abscess and sterility are probably caused by mixed aerobic and anaerobic superinfections and require wide-spectrum antibiotic treatment (see Chap. 94).

Endometriosis is a benign disorder characterized by the presence and proliferation of endometrial tissue (stroma and glands) outside the endometrial cavity. The clinical manifestations are variable. Endometriosis occurs most commonly between the ages of 30 to 40 and is found incidentally at the time of surgery in approximately one-fifth of all gynecologic operations. The fertility rate is significantly reduced in affected women. The disorder usually involves the posterior cul-de-sac or the ovaries and can give rise to ovarian enlargement (endometriomas), although it may also involve sites distant to the pelvis (lung, umbilicus). The most significant symptom is pelvic pain, characteristically dysmenorrhea (see Chap. 53). However, the frequency and degree of pelvic symptomatology correlate poorly with the extent of disease. Other symptoms include dyspareunia, pain with defecation, and infertility. The characteristic physical findings are multiple tender nodules palpable along the uterosacral ligament at the time of rectal-vaginal examination, a posteriorly fixed uterus, or enlarged cystic ovaries. The diagnosis can only be confirmed by direct visualization, usually at diagnostic laparoscopy. Treatment depends on the degree of involvement and the desires of the patient and includes observation for mild disease with no associated infertility or pain, hormonal suppressive therapy (see infertility), conservative surgery if fertility is desired, or removal of the uterus, tubes, and ovaries in severe disease. Endometriosis is rarely found after the menopause.

Any adnexal mass that persists for more than 6 weeks or is larger than 6 cm must be evaluated. Although ovarian cysts and neoplasms compose the largest group of pelvic adnexal masses (see above), tumors of the fallopian tubes, uterus, gastrointestinal tract, or urinary tract should also be considered. Sonography or radiographic evaluation is often helpful in identifying the nature of the adnexal mass prior to surgical exploration.

REFERENCES

Carr BR, Griffin JD: Fertility control and its complications, in *Williams' Textbook of Endocrinology*, 7th ed, JD Wilson, DW Foster (eds). Philadelphia, Saunders, 1985, pp 452–475

——— et al: Plasma levels of adrenocorticotropin and cortisol in women receiving oral contraceptive steroid treatment. J Clin Endocrinol Metab 49:346, 1979

——— et al: Plasma lipoprotein regulation or progesterone biosynthesis by human corpus luteum tissue in organ culture. J Clin Endocrinol Metab 52:875, 1981

——— et al: The role of lipoproteins in the regulation of progesterone secretion by human corpus luteum. Fertil Steril 38:303, 1982

Cunningham FG et al: *Williams' Obstetrics*, 18th ed. Norwalk, Appleton-Lange, 1989

D'Armiento M et al: McCune-Albright syndrome: Evidence for autonomous multiendocrine hyperfunction. J Pediatr 102:584, 1983

DiZerega GS, Hodgen GD: Folliculogenesis in the primate ovarian cycle. Endocrinol Rev 2:27, 1981

——— et al: The possible role for a follicular protein in the intraovarian regulation of steroidogenesis. Semin Reprod Endocrinol 1:309, 1983

Dmowski WP: Endocrine properties and clinical applications of danazol. Fertil Steril 31:237, 1979

Droegemuller W et al: *Comprehensive Gynecology*. St. Louis, Mosby, 1987

Erickson GF et al: Functional studies of aromatase activity in human granulosa cells from normal and polycystic ovaries. J Clin Endocrinol Metab 49:514, 1979

Faiman C et al: Patterns of gonadotropins and gonadal steroids throughout life. Clin Obstet Gynaecol 3:467, 1976

Frasier SD: *Pediatric Endocrinology*. New York, Grune & Stratton, 1980

Futterweit W: *Polycystic Ovarian Disease*. New York, Springer-Verlag, 1984

Gemzell C, Wang CF: Outcome of pregnancy in women with pituitary adenoma. Fertil Steril 31:363, 1979

GLUCKMAN PD et al: The human fetal hypothalamus and pituitary gland, in *Maternal-Fetal Endocrinology*, D Tulchinksy, KJ Ryan (eds). Philadelphia, Saunders, 1980

GOLDZIEHER JW: Polycystic ovarian disease. Fertil Steril 35:371, 1981

HATCHER RA et al: *Contraceptive Technology 1986–1987*. New York, Irvington, 1986

HSUEH AJW et al: Hormonal regulation of the differentiation of cultured ovarian granulosa cells. Endocr Rev 5:76, 1984

JONES HW JR et al (eds): *In Vitro Fertilization*. Baltimore, Williams & Wilkins, 1986

JUDD HL et al: Estrogen replacement therapy: Indications and complications. Ann Intern Med 98:195, 1983

KASE N, WEINGOLD A: *Principles and Practice of Clinical Gynecology*. New York, Wiley, 1983

KELCH RP: Management of precocious puberty. N Engl J Med 312:1057, 1985

KNOBIL E, NEILL JD (eds): *The Physiology of Reproduction*. New York, Raven , 1988

MATTINGLY RF, THOMPSON JD: *Operative Gynecology*. Philadelphia, Lippincott, 1985

MISHELL DR JR, DAVAJAN V (eds): *Reproductive Endocrinology, Infertility, and Contraception*, 2d ed. Philadelphia, Davis, 1986

PIEPER DR et al: Ovarian gonadatropin-releasing hormone (GnRH) receptors: Characterization, distribution, and induction by GnRH. Endocrinology 108:1148, 1981

RIGGS BL et al: Effect of the fluoride/calcium regimen on vertebral fracture occurrence in postmenopausal osteoporosis. N Engl J Med 306:446, 1982

ROSS GT: Disorders of the ovary and female reproductive tract, in *Williams' Textbook of Endocrinology*, 7th ed, JD Wilson, DW Foster (eds). Philadelphia, Saunders, 1985, pp 206–258

ROSS JL et al: A preliminary study of the effect of estrogen dose on growth in Turner's syndrome. N Engl J Med 309:1104, 1983

SCULLY RE: Ovarian tumors: A review. Am J Pathol 87:686, 1977

SEIBEL MM: A new era in reproductive technology. N Engl J Med 318:828, 1988

SHEARMAN RP (ed): *Clinical Reproductive Endocrinology*, Edinburgh, Churchill Livingston, 1985

SITTERI PK, MACDONALD PC: Role of extraglandular estrogen in human endocrinology, in *Handbook of Physiology*, sec 7, *Endocrinology*, SR Geiger et al (eds). Washington, DC, American Physiological Society, 1973, p 615

SPEROFF L: Menopause. Semin Reprod Endocrinol 1:1, 1983

——— et al: The ovary, in *Endocrinology and Metabolism*, P Felig et al (eds). New York, McGraw-Hill, 1981, p 669

——— et al: *Clinical Gynecologic Endocrinology and Infertility*, 4th ed. Baltimore, Williams & Wilkins, 1989

STEINGOLD KA et al: Treatment of hot flashes with transdermal estradiol administration. J Clin Endocrinol Metab 61:627, 1985

STUDD JWW, WHITEHEAD MI (eds): *The Menopause*. Oxford, Blackwell, 1988

STYNE DM, GRUMBACH MM: Puberty in the male and female: Its physiology and disorders, in *Reproductive Endocrinology*, SSC Yen, RB Jaffe (eds). Philadelphia, Saunders, 1986, pp 331–384

WALLACH EE, KEMPERS RD: *Modern Trends in Infertility and Contraception Control*, vol 3. Baltimore, Williams & Wilkins, 1985

WENTZ AC et al: *Gynecologic Endocrinology and Infertility*, Baltimore, Williams & Wilkins, 1988

YEN SSC: Neuroendocrine regulation of the menstrual cycle. Hosp Prac 14:84, 1979

———: Clinical application of gonadotropin-releasing hormone and gonadotropin releasing hormone analogs. Fertil Steril 39:257, 1983

———, JAFFE RB (eds): *Reproductive Endocrinology*, 2d ed. Philadelphia, Saunders, 1986

YING SY et al: Gonadocrinins: Peptides in ovarian follicular fluid stimulating the secretion of pituitary gonadotropins. Endocrinology 108:1206, 1981

323 ENDOCRINE DISORDERS OF THE BREAST

JEAN D. WILSON

Examination of the breasts is an important part of the physical examination. The breasts are the site of fatal and preventable disease in women and frequently provide clues to underlying systemic illness in both men and women. The internist frequently does not examine the male breast and is apt to refer the evaluation of the female breast to a gynecologist. It is the duty of every physician to distinguish the abnormal from the normal at the earliest possible stage and to call for assistance if there is any doubt. (For cancer of the breast see Chap. 303.)

ENDOCRINE CONTROL OF THE BREAST There is no histologic or functional difference in the breasts of boys and girls prior to the onset of puberty, but a profound sexual dimorphism in breast development ensues at the time of puberty. The endocrine control of female breast development is illustrated in Fig. 323-1. The pubertal growth of the female breast is dependent primarily upon the action

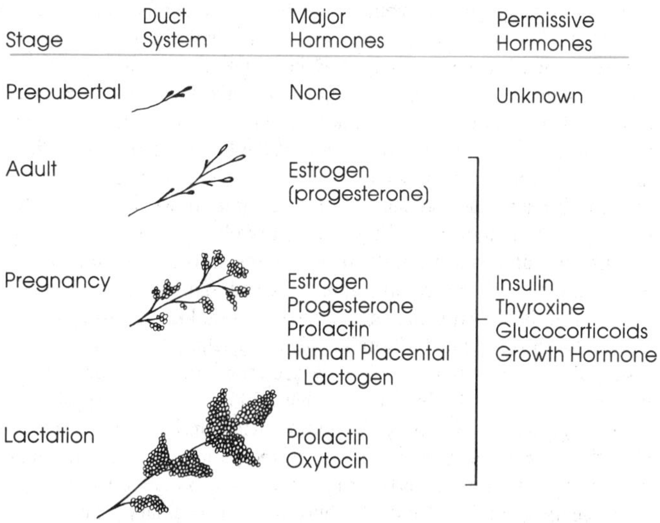

Stage
Duct System
Major Hormones
Permissive Hormones
Prepubertal
None
Unknown
Adult
Estrogen (progesterone)
Pregnancy
Estrogen
Progesterone
Prolactin
Human Placental Lactogen
Insulin
Thyroxine
Glucocorticoids
Growth Hormone
Lactation
Prolactin
Oxytocin

FIGURE 323-1 Endocrine control of female breast development and function at various stages of life.

of estradiol, which induces the growth, division, and elongation of the tubular duct system and maturation of the nipples. In men the administration of estrogen is equally effective in this regard. To produce true alveolar development at the ends of the ducts, however, the synergistic action of progesterone is required, a ratio of estrogen to progesterone of 1:20 to 1:100 being optimal. Once the anatomic development of the ducts and alveoli is complete, the continued action of estrogen and progesterone does not appear to be required for lactation itself.

The endocrine control of milk formation by the differentiated breast is complex, requiring, in addition to appropriate priming by estrogen and progesterone, specific lactogenic hormone and the permissive action of glucocorticoid, insulin, thyroxine, and in some species growth hormone. There are two lactogenic hormones. Human placental lactogen (hPL or chorionic somatomammotropin) is secreted in large amounts by the placenta during the latter phases of gestation and prepares the breast for milk production. It disappears from the fetal (and maternal) circulation shortly after termination of pregnancy. The pituitary hormone prolactin (see Chap. 313) plays the critical role in the initiation and maintenance of normal as well as inappropriate lactation. The plasma level of prolactin rises during pregnancy; during late pregnancy and lactation 60 to 80 percent of the anterior pituitary may consist of prolactin-secreting cells.

Unlike most pituitary hormones, the predominant regulation of prolactin secretion is negative, i.e., under ordinary basal conditions the hypothalamus secretes one or more inhibitory hormones, the most important being dopamine, which are delivered to the pituitary via the hypothalamic portal system and inhibit the release of prolactin into the blood (see Chap. 313). Most factors that influence prolactin secretion do so by affecting the synthesis or release of the inhibiting factors. Basal prolactin levels fall following delivery, but prolactin secretion is enhanced by stimulation of the breasts such as the act of nursing (the so-called sucking reflex), a phenomenon that is probably mediated by the reflex release of oxytocin. In the postgestational state the normal woman is capable of forming about a liter of milk per day containing 38 g fat, 70 g lactose, and 12 g protein. Normal lactation can be suppressed by the administration of estrogens or diethylstilbestrol, which inhibit milk production by direct effects on the breast, or bromocriptine, which inhibits prolactin secretion by the pituitary. Alternatively, if a woman does not nurse or empty her breasts post partum, lactation usually ceases of its own accord in 1 to 2 weeks.

GALACTORRHEA Exactly what constitutes nonpuerperal or inappropriate lactation is not always clearly defined in the literature. According to the studies of Friedman and Goldfein, it is not possible to demonstrate any breast secretion whatsoever in normal, regularly menstruating nulligravid women, but breast secretions can be demonstrated in a fourth of normal women who have been pregnant in the past; thus, breast secretions may be of no clinical significance in these instances. Spontaneous leakage of milk from the breasts is usually of more concern than milk that must be expressed. A second problem is related to the composition of the breast secretions. When the secretion is milky or white, it is safe to assume that it contains fat, casein, and lactose and is in fact milk; however, when the secretion is brown or greenish in color, it rarely contains normal milk constituents and consequently may not result from an underlying endocrinopathy. Furthermore, upon repeated sampling, the composition of milk constituents may increase from low, colostrum-like values to those typical of milk. Milky discharges must also be distinguished from blood or bloody secretions that may be present with neoplasms of the breast (see Chap. 303). With these problems in mind galactorrhea can be defined as inappropriate production of milk that is persistent or worrisome to the patient, recognizing that in some instances no underlying pathology will be demonstrated.

Since the action of a lactogenic hormone is a necessary requirement for the initiation of milk production, it is logical to consider galactorrhea as a manifestation of deranged prolactin physiology. However, as indicated above, a complex endocrinologic milieu is necessary for lactation, and in many instances in which prolactin is elevated, both in women who have not been appropriately primed and in men, no production of milk takes place. As a consequence, hyperprolactinemia is more common than galactorrhea. Furthermore, although enhanced prolactin secretion is necessary for the initiation of lactation, production can be maintained in the presence of minimally elevated or intermittently elevated prolactin levels so that basal plasma prolactin levels are not always elevated in patients with galactorrhea. For example, repeated stimulation of the nipples of women who have previously been pregnant can cause galactorrhea with minimal elevations of basal prolactin (the wet nurse phenomenon) similar to those in normal nursing mothers. Perhaps the strongest evidence that prolactin is always involved in galactorrhea is the fact that administration of bromocriptine, which suppresses plasma prolactin levels, causes a disappearance of galactorrhea even when the basal plasma prolactin levels are normal.

Differential diagnosis It is thus appropriate to consider galactorrhea as the result of a failure of the normal hypothalamic inhibition of prolactin release, of enhanced prolactin-releasing factor, or of autonomous prolactin secretion by tumors (Table 323-1). Pituitary stalk section in humans results in a striking increase in prolactin secretion, as the result of the inhibition of the delivery of prolactin inhibitory factors to the pituitary. Likewise, many drugs that influence the central nervous system (including virtually all psychotropic agents, methyldopa, reserpine, and antiemetics) cause enhanced prolactin release, presumably by inhibiting synthesis or release of dopamine or other prolactin inhibitory factors. Estrogens enhance prolactin levels by an uncertain mechanism. Extrapituitary central nervous system diseases can cause galactorrhea, presumably by interfering with delivery of the inhibitory factors to the pituitary (central nervous system sarcoidosis, craniopharyngioma, pinealoma, encephalitis, meningitis, hydrocephalus, hypothalamic tumors).

TABLE 323-1 A physiologic classification of galactorrhea

I Failure of normal hypothalamic inhibition of prolactin release
- *A* Pituitary stalk section
- *B* Drugs (phenothiazines, butyrophenones, methyldopa, tricyclic antidepressants, opiates, reserpine, verapamil)
- *C* Central nervous system disease, including extrapituitary tumors

II Enhanced prolactin-releasing factor
- Hypothyroidism
- Sucking reflex and breast trauma

III Autonomous prolactin release
- *A* Pituitary tumors
  - *1* Prolactin-secreting tumors
  - *2* Mixed growth hormone and prolactin-secreting tumors
  - *3* Chromophobe adenomas
- *B* Ectopic production of human placental lactogen and/or prolactin
  - *1* Hydatidiform moles and choriocarcinomas
  - *2* Bronchogenic carcinoma and hypernephroma

IV Idiopathic

In one pathologic state, primary hypothyroidism, galactorrhea results from enhanced prolactin-releasing activity. Thyrotropin-releasing hormone (TRH) stimulates prolactin release, and thyroid hormone replacement cures the galactorrhea. A similar mechanism, namely, enhanced secretion of oxytocin, may be involved in the galactorrhea of breast trauma.

Enhanced prolactin release can also occur from pituitary or nonpituitary tumors. Three types of pituitary tumors (see Chap. 313) may be associated with galactorrhea: pure prolactin-secreting tumors (micro- or macroadenomas), mixed tumors that secrete both growth hormone and prolactin and result in acromegaly with galactorrhea, and some chromophobe adenomas. The latter may either secrete prolactin or interfere with the delivery of inhibitory factors to the pituitary. Prolactin can also be secreted on occasion by other malignancies such as bronchogenic carcinoma, and hydatidiform moles and choriocarcinomas may secrete placental lactogen.

The known etiologies account for only a part of the cases of galactorrhea. In four published series totaling more than 500 carefully studied patients, a pituitary tumor was identified in about one-fourth of the patients, other known causes could be identified in another fourth or fifth, and the remaining half fall into the unknown category. Many patients may prove ultimately to have prolactin-secreting pituitary tumors, some probably have subtle disorders of hypothalamic function, and in others a drug-related cause may have been missed, but the fact remains that no satisfactory diagnosis is reached in many patients. When normal menses and galactorrhea coexist, the likelihood of establishing a diagnosis is poor.

Galactorrhea is unusual in men, even in the presence of profound elevations of plasma prolactin; when it does occur, it is usually upon the background of a feminizing state (see below).

Diagnostic evaluation If hyperprolactinemia is present, the workup is fundamentally that of a pituitary tumor once drug causes and hypothyroidism are excluded (see Chap. 313). Even when a specific cause cannot be identified and a diagnosis of idiopathic galactorrhea is made by exclusion, it is necessary to remember that pituitary tumors may subsequently become manifest. The higher the prolactin values and the more persistent the galactorrhea, the greater the likelihood of such a development.

Treatment The aim of treatment is to remove the source of the elevated prolactin, and resection of pituitary tumor, cessation of causative drugs, or correction of hypothyroidism is often followed by the disappearance of galactorrhea. Two other forms of therapy may have some usefulness. Breast binders can be effective in patients with mild galactorrhea of unknown etiology, presumably by preventing stimulation of the nipple and the consequent perpetuation of lactation. Bromocriptine, which suppresses plasma prolactin, has been used to treat patients with idiopathic hyperprolactinemia as well as patients with prolactin-secreting tumors of the pituitary. This drug not only suppresses lactation but may also cause resumption of normal menstrual cycles (and even fertility) in patients in whom amenorrhea accompanies galactorrhea.

GYNECOMASTIA A central issue in the evaluation of breast tissue in adult men is the separation of the normal from the abnormal. Whereas in autopsy data the incidence of active gynecomastia is between 5 and 9 percent, Nuttall and his colleagues have reported that approximately 40 percent of normal men and up to 70 percent of hospitalized men have palpable breast tissue. The reason for this discrepancy is not clear. On the one hand, it may be difficult to distinguish true breast tissue from masses of adipose tissue without true breast enlargement (lipomastia); in such cases true gynecomastia can be separated from lipomastia by mammography or by sonography. Alternatively, a true increase in the incidence of gynecomastia may have taken place, or the autopsy data may underestimate the frequency of palpable breast tissue. Regardless, we are left with major uncertainties; the finding of gynecomastia (distinct from lipomastia) could indicate underlying pathology or a normal variant. For the purposes of this discussion, we shall assume that any palpable breast tissue in men (except for the three so-called physiologic states) may reflect an underlying endocrinopathy and deserves a limited evaluation.

Early gynecomastia is characterized by proliferation in the breast of both the fibroblastic stroma and the duct system, which elongates, buds, and duplicates. As gynecomastia persists, progressive fibrosis and hyalinization are associated with regression of epithelial proliferation. Eventually the number of ducts decreases. Resolution occurs by reduction in size and epithelial content with gradual disappearance of the ducts, leaving hyaline bands that eventually disappear.

Growth of the breast in men, as in women, is mediated by estrogen and results from disturbances of the normal ratio of active androgen to estrogen in plasma or within the breast itself. As described in Chap. 321 estradiol formation in the normal man occurs principally by the conversion of circulating androgens to estrogens in peripheral tissues; the normal ratio of production of testosterone to estradiol in adult men is approximately 100:1 (6 mg versus 45 μg), and the normal ratio of the two hormones in plasma is about 300:1. Feminization results when there is a significant decrease in this effective ratio, as the result of diminished testosterone production or action, enhanced estrogen formation, or both processes occurring simultaneously. The predominant manifestation of feminization in men is enlargement of the breasts.

Enlargement of the male breast can occur as a normal physiologic phenomenon at certain stages of life or as the result of a variety of pathologic conditions (Table 323-2).

Physiologic gynecomastia In the *newborn* transient enlargement of the breast results from the action of maternal and/or placental estrogens. The enlargement ordinarily disappears in a few weeks but may persist longer. *Adolescent* gynecomastia occurs in many boys at some time during puberty. The median age of onset is 14; it is often asymmetric, occasionally unilateral for a portion of its course, and frequently tender, and it regresses so that by age 20 only a small number of men have palpable vestiges of gynecomastia in one or both breasts. Although the origin of the excess estrogen has not been identified, the onset of gynecomastia correlates with transient elevations of plasma estradiol prior to the completion of puberty so that the androgen/estrogen ratio is altered. *Gynecomastia of aging* also occurs in otherwise healthy men. Forty percent or more of aged men have gynecomastia. A likely explanation is the increase with age in the conversion of androgens to estrogens in extraglandular tissues. Abnormal liver function or drug therapy may be contributing causes to gynecomastia in such men.

Pathologic gynecomastia Pathologic gynecomastia can result from one of three basic mechanisms: deficiency in testosterone production or action (with or without a secondary increase in estrogen production), increase in estrogen production, or drugs (Table 323-2). Most of the individual disorders that cause primary and secondary testicular failure have been discussed in Chap. 321. The fact that a deficiency in testosterone production per se can cause gynecomastia is illustrated by the syndrome of congenital anorchia in which normal (or slightly low) estradiol production in the presence of profoundly decreased testosterone production results in florid gynecomastia. Such is the case in some patients with Klinefelter syndrome. In the inherited syndromes of androgen resistance, such as testicular feminization, deficient androgen action and increased testicular estrogen production are both present, although diminished androgen action is the more critical in inducing gynecomastia.

A primary increase in estrogen production can result from a variety of causes. Increased testicular estrogen secretion may result from elevations in plasma gonadotropins, for example, in cases of aberrant production of chorionic gonadotropin by testicular tumors or by bronchogenic carcinoma, from the ovarian elements in the gonads of men with true hermaphroditism, or as the result of direct secretion by testicular tumors (particularly Leydig cell and Sertoli cell tumors). Increased conversion of androgen to estrogens in peripheral tissues can either be due to increased availability of substrate for extraglandular estrogen formation or to increased amount of the enzymes of estrogen formation in peripheral tissues. Increased substrate availability for extraglandular conversion can result from increased production of androgens such as androstenedione (congenital adrenal hyperplasia, hyperthyroidism, and most feminizing adrenal tumors) or because of diminished catabolism of androstenedione by the usual pathways (liver disease). Increased amount of extraglandular aromatase can be caused by a rare hereditary abnormality or by tumors of the liver or adrenal gland.

Drugs can cause gynecomastia by several mechanisms. Many drugs either act directly as estrogens or cause an increase in plasma estrogen activity, for example, in men receiving diethylstilbestrol for prostatic carcinoma and in transsexuals in preparation for sex-change operations. Boys and young men are particularly sensitive to estrogen and can develop gynecomastia after the use of dermal ointments containing estrogen or after the ingestion of milk or meat from estrogen-treated animals. The gynecomastia of digitalis ingestion is usually attributed to an estrogen-like side effect of the drug, but in the experience of the author it is usually associated with abnormal liver function tests. A second mechanism by which drugs can induce gynecomastia is illustrated by gonadotropin, such as from human chorionic gonadotropin (hCG)–secreting tumors, which causes enhanced testicular secretion of estrogen. Other drugs cause gynecomastia by interfering with testosterone synthesis (ketoconazole and alkylating agents) and/or testosterone action, for instance by blocking the binding of androgen to its cytosol receptor protein in target tissues (spironolactone and cimetidine). Finally, drugs that cause gynecomastia by mechanisms which have not been defined include busulfan, ethionamide, isoniazid, methyldopa, tricyclic antidepressants, penicillamine, and diazepam, marijuana, and heroin. In some instances the feminization is due to effects of drugs on liver function.

Diagnostic evaluation The evaluation of patients with gyneco-

TABLE 323-2 Differential diagnosis of gynecomastia

PHYSIOLOGIC GYNECOMASTIA

- Newborn
- Adolescence
- Aging

PATHOLOGIC GYNECOMASTIA

- Deficient production or action of testosterone:
  - Congenital defects:
    - Congenital anorchia
    - Klinefelter syndrome
    - Androgen resistance (testicular feminization and Reifenstein syndrome)
    - Defects of testosterone synthesis
  - Secondary testicular failure:
    - Viral orchitis
    - Trauma
    - Castration
    - Neurologic and granulomatous diseases
    - Renal failure
- Increased estrogen production:
  - Estrogen secretion:
    - True hermaphroditism
    - Testicular tumors
    - Carcinoma of the lung and other tumors producing hCG
  - Increased substrate for extraglandular aromatase:
    - Adrenal disease
    - Liver disease
    - Starvation
    - Thyrotoxicosis
  - Increase in extraglandular aromatase
- Drugs:
  - Estrogens (diethylstilbestrol, birth control pills, digitalis, estrogen-containing cosmetics, estrogen-contaminated foods)
  - Drugs that enhance endogenous estrogen secretion (gonadotropins, clomiphene)
  - Inhibitors of testosterone synthesis and/or action (ketoconazole, metronidazole, alkylating agents, cisplatin, spironolactone, cimetidine)
  - Unknown mechanisms (busulfan, isoniazid, methyldopa, tricyclic antidepressants, penicillamine, diazepam, marijuana, heroin)
- Idiopathic

mastia should include the following procedures: (1) a careful drug history; (2) measurement and examination of the testes (if both are small, a chromosomal karyotype should be obtained; if they are asymmetric, an evaluation for testicular tumor should be instituted); (3) an evaluation of liver function; (4) an endocrine evaluation to include measurement of serum androstenedione or 24-h urinary 17-ketosteroids (usually elevated in feminizing adrenal states), measurement of plasma estradiol and hCG (helpful if elevated but usually normal), and measurement of plasma luteinizing hormone (LH) and testosterone. If LH is high and testosterone is low, the diagnosis is usually testicular failure; if LH and testosterone are both low, the diagnosis is most likely increased primary estrogen production (for example, a Sertoli cell tumor of the testis); and if both LH and testosterone are elevated, the diagnosis is either an androgen-resistance state or a gonadotropin-secreting tumor.

A satisfactory diagnosis can be made in only half or fewer of the patients referred for gynecomastia by using these various tests. This implies either that the diagnostic techniques are not sufficiently refined to recognize mild disturbances, that many causes of gynecomastia are as yet undefined, that the causes may be transient and difficult to diagnose, or, as suggested by Nuttall, that gynecomastia may in some instances be normal rather than due to a pathologic state. Because of the problem of separating the normal from the pathologic, gynecomastia should probably be routinely worked up only if the drug history is negative, if the breast is tender (indicating rapid growth), or if the breast mass is larger than 4 cm in diameter. In other instances a decision to perform an endocrine evaluation depends on the clinical context. For example, gynecomastia associated with signs of underandrogenization should be evaluated.

Treatment When the primary cause of the overestrogenization can be identified and corrected, the breast enlargement usually subsides promptly and eventually disappears. However, if the gynecomastia is of long duration (and fibrosis has replaced the original ductal hyperplasia), correction of the primary defect may not be followed by resolution. In such instances and when the primary cause cannot be corrected, surgery is the only effective therapy. Indications for surgery include several psychologic and/or cosmetic problems, continued growth, or a suspected malignancy. Although the relative risk of carcinoma of the breast is increased in men with gynecomastia, it is rare nevertheless. Prophylactic radiation of the breasts prior to the institution of diethylstilbestrol therapy is effective in preventing gynecomastia and has a low complication rate in elderly men. In rare patients who have painful gynecomastia and who are not candidates for other therapy, treatment with antiestrogens such as tamoxifen may be indicated.

REFERENCES

Galactorrhea

CHOTINER HC et al: Lactose and casein content of nonpuerperal breast secretion. J Reprod Med 22:267, 1979

DAVAJAN V: The significance of galactorrhea in patients with normal menses, oligomenorrhea, and secondary amenorrhea. Am J Obstet Gynecol 130:894, 1978

FRANTZ AG, WILSON JD: Endocrine disorders of the breast, in *Williams' Textbook of Endocrinology*, 8th ed, JD Wilson, DW Foster (eds). Philadelphia, Saunders, 1990, In press

FRIEDMAN S, GOLDFEIN A: Breast secretions in normal women. Am J Obstet Gynecol 104:846, 1969

JOHNSON DG et al: Prolactin secretion and biological activity in females with galactorrhoea and normal circulating prolactin concentrations at rest. Clin Endocrinol 22:661, 1985

KLEINBERG DL et al: Galactorrhea: A study of 235 cases, including 48 with pituitary tumors. N Engl J Med 296:589, 1977

KOPPELMAN MCS et al: Hyperprolactinemia, amenorrhea, and galactorrhea. A retrospective assessment of twenty-five cases. Ann Intern Med 100:115, 1984

KULSKI JK et al: Changes in the milk composition of nonpuerperal women. Am J Obstet Gynecol 139:597, 1981

RUIZ-VELASCO V: Hyperprolactinemia and mammary prostheses. A report of eight cases. J Reprod Med 31:267, 1986

SAUER HJ: Physiology of lactation and factors affecting lactation. Obstet Gynecol Clin North Am 14:615, 1987

TOLTS G: Prolactin: Physiology and pathology. Hosp Prac February 1980, p 85

TURKSOY RN et al: Diagnostic and therapeutic modalities in women with galactorrhea. Obstet Gynecol 56:323, 1980

Gynecomastia

ANDERSON JA, GROOM JB: Male breast at autopsy. Acta Pathol Microbiol Immunol Scand 90:191, 1982

CARLSON HE: Gynecomastia. N Engl J Med 303:795, 1980

CIMORA GA et al: Percutaneous oestrogen-induced gynecomastia: A case report. Br J Plast Surg 35:209, 1982

FASS D et al: Radiotherapeutic prophylaxis of estrogen-induced gynecomastia: A study of late sequela. Int J Radiation Oncology Bio Phys 12:407, 1986

FELDMAN D: Ketoconazole and other imidazole derivatives as inhibitors of steroidogenesis. Endocr Rev 7:409, 1986

FRANTZ AG, WILSON JD: Endocrine disorders of the breast, in *Williams' Textbook of Endocrinology*, 8th ed, JD Wilson, DW Foster (eds). Philadelphia, Saunders, 1990, In press

KORENMAN SG: The endocrinology of the abnormal male breast. Ann NY Acad Sci 464:400, 1986

MABUCHI K et al: Risk factors for male breast cancer. J Natl Cancer Inst 74:371, 1985

NIEWOEHNER CV, NUTTALL FQ: Gynecomastia in a hospitalized male population. Am J Med 77:633, 1984

NUTTALL FQ: Gynecomastia as a physical finding in normal men. J Clin Endocrinol Metab 48:338, 1979

PARKER LN et al: Treatment of gynecomastia with tamoxifen: A double-blind crossover study. Metabolism 8:705, 1986

324 DISORDERS OF SEXUAL DIFFERENTIATION

JEAN D. WILSON / JAMES E. GRIFFIN

Sexual differentiation is a sequential and ordered process. *Chromosomal sex,* established at the moment of fertilization, determines *gonadal sex,* and *gonadal sex* in turn causes the development of *phenotypic sex* in which the male or female urogenital tract is formed (Table 324-1). A disturbance of any step in this developmental process during embryogenesis may result in a disorder of sexual differentiation. Known causes of abnormalities in sexual development include environmental insults as in the ingestion of a virilizing drug during pregnancy, nonfamilial aberrations of the sex chromosomes as in 45,X gonadal dysgenesis, developmental birth defects of multifactorial etiology as in most cases of hypospadias, and hereditary disorders resulting from single gene mutations as in the testicular feminization syndrome.

Limitations of knowledge make it necessary to make empiric assignments as to the nature of the derangement in certain disorders. Nevertheless, a specific diagnosis can usually be made as the result of genetic, endocrine, phenotypic, and chromosomal assessment. As a consequence, appropriate gender assignment can be made, even in extreme instances of ambiguous genitalia, and tailoring of the phenotype can be undertaken when appropriate.

TABLE 324-1 Classification of disorders of sexual development

- Disorders of chromosomal sex:
  - Klinefelter syndrome
  - XX male
  - Gonadal dysgenesis
  - Mixed gonadal dysgenesis
  - True hermaphroditism
- Disorders of gonadal sex:
  - Pure gonadal dysgenesis
  - Absent testis syndrome
- Disorders of phenotypic sex:
  - Female pseudohermaphroditism:
    - Congenital adrenal hyperplasia
    - Nonadrenal female pseudohermaphroditism
    - Developmental disorders of müllerian ducts
  - Male pseudohermaphroditism:
    - Abnormalities in androgen synthesis
    - Abnormalities in androgen action
    - Persistent müllerian duct syndrome
    - Development defects of male genitalia

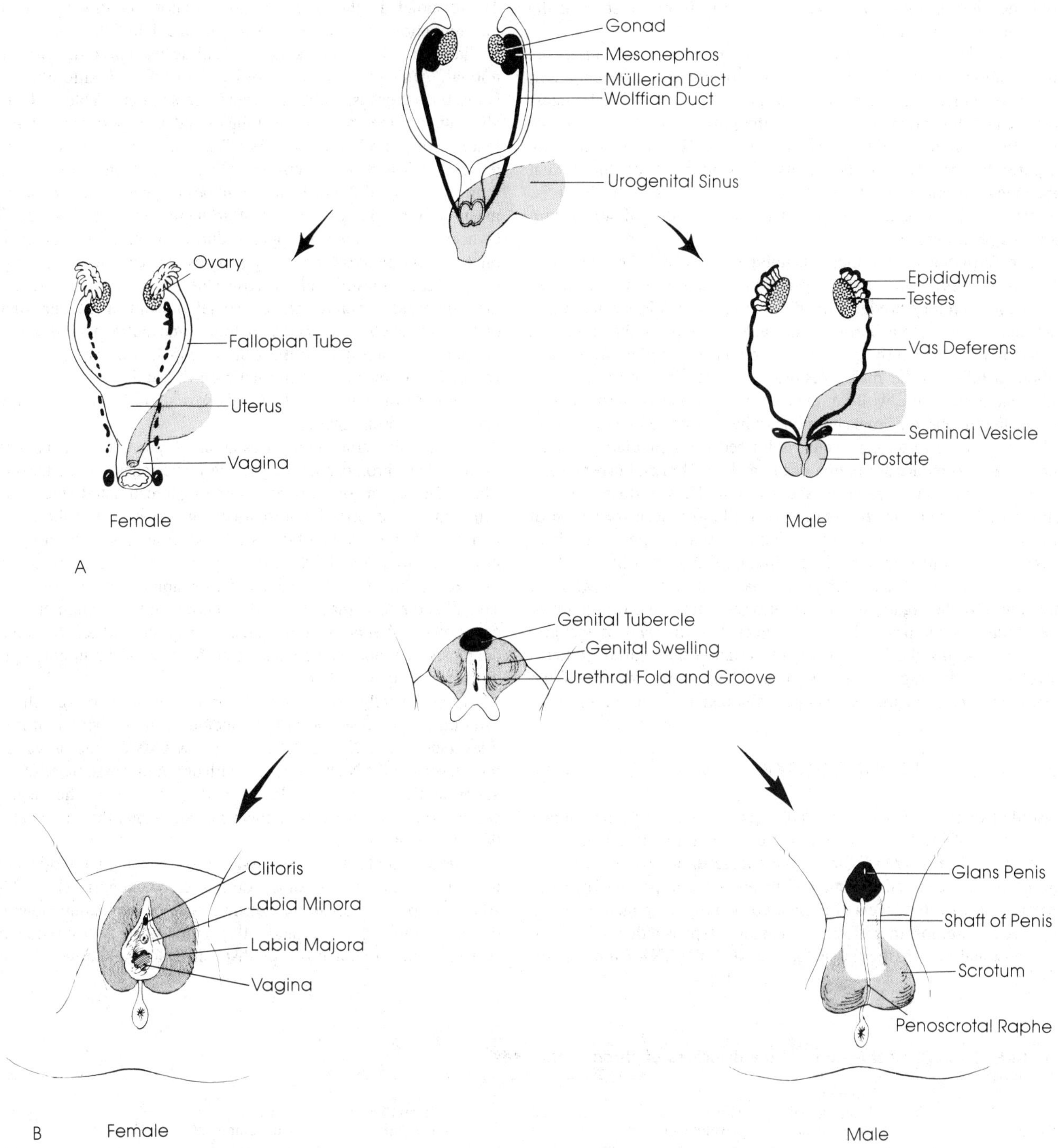

FIGURE 324-1 Normal sexual differentiation. *A*. Internal genitalia. *B*. External genitalia.

NORMAL SEXUAL DIFFERENTIATION

The first process in sexual differentiation is the establishment of chromosomal sex, the heterogametic sex (XY) being male and the homogametic sex (XX) female. The embryos of both sexes then develop in an identical fashion until approximately 40 days of gestation. The second phase of sexual differentiation is the conversion of the indifferent gonad into a testis or an ovary. The differentiation of the indifferent gonad into a testis is mediated by one or more testis determining factor (TDF) genes on the short arm of the Y chromosome; indeed, no matter how many X chromosomes are present (as in XXY, XXXY, etc.), a testis will develop as long as a Y chromosome is present. The final process, the translation of gonadal sex into phenotypic sex, is the direct consequence of the type of gonad formed and the endocrine secretions of the fetal gonads. The development of phenotypic sex results in the formation of the male and female urogenital tracts.

The internal genitalia are derived from the wolffian and müllerian ducts that exist side by side in early embryos of both sexes (Fig. 324-1*A*). In the male the wolffian ducts give rise to the epididymides, vasa deferentia, and seminal vesicles, and the müllerian ducts disappear. In the female the fallopian tubes, uterus, and upper vagina are derived from the müllerian ducts, and the wolffian ducts regress. The external genitalia and urethra in the two sexes develop from common anlage—the urogenital sinus and the genital tubercle, folds, and swellings (Fig. 324-1*B*). The urogenital sinus gives rise to the prostate and prostatic urethra in the male and to the urethra and lower portion of the vagina in the female. The genital tubercle is the origin of the glans penis in the male and clitoris in the female. The urogenital swellings become the scrotum or the labia majora, and the urethral folds develop into the labia minora or fuse to form the shaft of the penis and the male urethra.

In the absence of the testis, as in the normal female or in the male embryo castrated prior to the onset of gonadal differentiation, the development of phenotypic sex proceeds along female lines. Thus, masculinization of the fetus is the positive result of action of hormones from the fetal testis, whereas female development does not require the presence of the ovary. Development of the sexual phenotype normally conforms to the chromosomal sex. That is, chromosomal sex determines gonadal sex, and gonadal sex in turn controls phenotypic sex.

The formation of the male phenotype is vested in the action of three hormones. Two—müllerian-inhibiting substance and testosterone—are secretory products of the fetal testis. Müllerian-inhibiting substance is a protein hormone that acts to suppress the müllerian ducts and consequently prevents development of the uterus and fallopian tubes in the male. Testosterone acts directly to stimulate differentiation of the wolffian duct derivatives and is the precursor for the third embryonic male hormone, dihydrotestosterone (see Chap. 321). Dihydrotestosterone, which is formed from circulating testosterone, acts to induce formation of the male urethra and prostate and to cause formation of the penis and scrotum. Thus, testosterone and dihydrotestosterone function during fetal life to induce formation of the accessory organs of male reproduction by the same intracellular machinery by which they act in differentiated tissues (Chap. 321).

The secretion of testosterone by the fetal testis approaches a maximum by the eighth to tenth week of gestation, and formation of the sexual phenotypes is largely completed by the end of the first trimester. During the latter phases of gestation the ovarian follicles develop and the vagina matures in the female, and descent of the testes and growth of the external genitalia take place in the male.

DISORDERS OF CHROMOSOMAL SEX

Disorders of chromosomal sex (Table 324-2) occur when the number or structure of the X or Y chromosomes is abnormal (see Chap. 7).

KLINEFELTER SYNDROME **Clinical features** Klinefelter syndrome is characterized by small, firm testes, azoospermia, gynecomastia, and elevated levels of plasma gonadotropins in men with two or more X chromosomes. The common karyotype is either a 47,XXY chromosomal pattern (the classic form) or 46,XY/47,XXY mosaicism. The disorder is the most frequent major abnormality of sexual differentiation, the incidence being around 1 in 500 men.

Prepubertally, patients have small testes but otherwise appear normal. After puberty the disorder is manifest as infertility, gynecomastia, or occasionally underandrogenization (Table 324-3). Hyalinization of the seminiferous tubules and azoospermia are consistent features of the 47,XXY variety. The small, firm testes are characteristically less than 2.0 cm and always less than 3.5 cm in length (corresponding to 2 and 12 mL volume, respectively). The increased mean body height is the result of an increased lower body segment. Gynecomastia ordinarily appears during adolescence, is generally bilateral and painless, and may progress to become disfiguring (see Chap. 323). Obesity and varicose veins occur in one-third to one-half, and mild mental deficiency, social maladjustment, abnormalities of thyroid function, diabetes mellitus, and pulmonary disease may be more common than in the general population. The risk of breast cancer is 20 times that of normal men (but only about a fifth that in women). Most have a male psychosexual orientation and function sexually as normal men.

The mosaic variant comprises about 10 percent of the patients, as estimated by chromosomal karyotypes on peripheral blood leukocytes. The frequency of this variant may be underestimated since chromosomal mosaicism may be present only in the testes in subjects whose peripheral leukocyte karotype is normal. The mosaic form is usually not as severe as the 47,XXY variety, and the testes may be normal in size (Table 324-3). The endocrine abnormalities are also less severe, and gynecomastia and azoospermia are less common. Indeed, occasional patients with mosaicism may be fertile. In some the diagnosis may not even be suspected because of the minor degree of the physical abnormalities.

Approximately 30 additional karyotypic varieties of Klinefelter syndrome have been described, including those with uniform cell lines (such as XXYY, XXXY, and XXXXY) and a variety of mosaicisms of the X chromosome with or without associated structural abnormalities of the X. In general, the greater the degree of chromosomal abnormality (and in mosaic forms the more cell lines that are abnormal), the more severe the manifestations.

Pathophysiology The classic form is due to meiotic nondisjunction of the chromosomes during gametogenesis (Fig. 324-2). About 40 percent of the responsible meiotic nondisjunctions occur during spermatogenesis, and 60 percent occur during oogenesis. Advanced maternal age is a predisposing factor. The mosaic form is

TABLE 324-2 Clinical features of the disorders of chromosomal sex

Disorder	Common chromosomal complement	Gonadal development	External genitalia	Internal genitalia	Breast development	Comment
Klinefelter syndrome	47,XXY *or* 46,XY/47,XXY	Hyalinized testes	Normal male	Normal male	Gynecomastia	Most common disorder of sexual differentiation; tall stature.
XX male	46,XX	Hyalinized testes	Normal male	Normal male	Gynecomastia	Shorter than normal men; increased incidence of hypospadias. Similar to Klinefelter syndrome. May be familial.
Gonadal dysgenesis (Turner syndrome)	45,X *or* 46,XX/45,X	Streak gonads	Immature female	Hypoplastic female	Immature female	Short stature and multiple somatic abnormalities. May be 46,XX with structurally abnormal X chromosome.
Mixed gonadal dysgenesis	46,XY/45,X *or* 46,XY	Testis and streak gonad	Variable but almost always ambiguous; 60% reared as female	Uterus, vagina, and one fallopian tube	Usually male	Second most common cause of ambiguous genitalia in the newborn; tumors common.
True hermaphroditism	46,XX *or* 46,XY *or* mosaics	Testis and ovary or ovotestis	Variable but usually ambiguous; 60% reared as males	Usually a uterus and urogenital sinus; ducts correspond to gonad	Gynecomastia in 75%	May be familial.

TABLE 324-3 Characteristics of patients with classic versus mosaic Klinefelter syndrome*

	47,XXY, %	46,XY/47,XXY, %
Abnormal testicular histology	100	94†
Decreased length of testis	99	73†
Azoospermia	93	50†
Decreased testosterone	79	33
Decreased facial hair	77	64
Increased gonadotropins	75	33†
Decreased sexual function	68	56
Gynecomastia	55	33†
Decreased axillary hair	49	46
Decreased length of penis	41	21

* Table based on 519 XXY patients and 51 XY/XXY patients.
† Significantly different at $p < .05$ or better.
SOURCE: After Gordon et al.

thought to result from chromosomal mitotic nondisjunction after fertilization of the zygote and can take place either in a 46,XY zygote (Fig. 324-2) or a 47,XXY zygote. The latter defect or double nondisjunction (meiotic and mitotic) may be the usual cause and thus explain why the mosaic form is less frequent than the classic disorder.

Plasma follicle-stimulating hormone (FSH) and luteinizing hormone (LH) are usually high; FSH shows the best discrimination, and little overlap occurs with normals, a consequence of the consistent damage to the seminiferous tubules. The plasma testosterone averages half normal, but the range of values overlaps the normal range. Mean plasma estradiol levels are elevated, the cause of which is not entirely clear. Early in the course, the testes may secrete increased amounts of estradiol in response to the elevated plasma LH, but the testicular secretion of estradiol (and testosterone) eventually declines. Elevated plasma estradiol late in the course is probably due to a combination of a decreased metabolic clearance rate and an increased rate of conversion of testosterone to estradiol in extragonadal tissues. The net result both early and late is a variable degree of insufficient androgenization and enhanced feminization. The feminization, including gynecomastia, depends on the ratio of circulating estrogen to androgen (relative or absolute), and subjects with lower plasma testosterone and higher plasma estradiol levels are more likely to develop gynecomastia (see Chap. 323). The increase in plasma gonadotropins following the administration of luteinizing hormone–releasing hormone (LHRH) is exaggerated after the age of expected puberty, and the normal feedback inhibition of testosterone on pituitary LH secretion is diminished. Subjects with untreated Klinefelter syndrome may have "reactive pituitary abnormalities" in the form of enlarged or abnormal sella turcicas, presumably secondary to the persistent lack of gonadal feedback and hypertrophy of the gonadotrophs in response to stimulation by LHRH. It is not known whether actual adenoma formation occurs.

Management No method is available for reversing the infertility, and surgical removal is the only means for effective treatment of the gynecomastia. Some underandrogenized patients benefit from supplemental androgen, but such treatment may paradoxically worsen the gynecomastia, presumably by providing increased androgen substrate for the conversion to estrogens in the peripheral tissues. Androgen should be administered in the form of testosterone cypionate or testosterone enanthate. Following the administration of testosterone, plasma LH returns to normal only after several months, if at all.

XX MALE SYNDROME The incidence of a 46,XX karyotype in phenotypic males is approximately 1 in 20,000 to 24,000 male births. Affected individuals have absence of all female internal genitalia and male psychosexual identification. Indeed, the findings resemble those in the Klinefelter syndrome: the testes are small and firm (generally less than 2 cm), gynecomastia is frequent, the penis is normal to small in size, azoospermia and hyalinization of the seminiferous tubules are usual, mean plasma testosterone is low, plasma estradiol is elevated, and plasma gonadotropin levels are high. Affected individuals differ from typical Klinefelter patients only in that average height is less than in normal men, the incidence of mental deficiency is not increased, and the incidence of hypospadias is increased.

Four theories have been proposed to explain the pathogenesis of this disorder: (1) translocation of a portion of a Y chromosome to the X chromosome, (2) mosaicism for a Y chromosome in some cell lines or early loss of a Y chromosome, (3) mutation of an autosomal gene, or (4) deletion of genetic material on the X chromosome that normally has a negative regulatory effect on testis development. Mosaicism has not been documented, and no clearcut evidence has been adduced for an autosomal gene mutation. The majority of XX males whose DNA is probed with Y-chromosome DNA fragments containing the TDF gene are positive for Y-related DNA; thus, an X-Y interchange appears to be the common cause of the disorder. The management is similar to that of Klinefelter syndrome.

GONADAL DYSGENESIS (TURNER SYNDROME) Clinical features Gonadal dysgenesis is characterized by primary amenorrhea, sexual infantilism, short stature, multiple congenital anomalies, and bilateral streak gonads in phenotypic women with any of several defects of the X chromosome. This condition should be distinguished from (1) mixed gonadal dysgenesis in which a unilateral testis and a contralateral streak gonad are present; (2) pure gonadal dysgenesis in which bilateral streak gonads are associated with a normal 46,XX or 46,XY karyotype, normal stature, and primary amenorrhea; and (3) the Noonan syndrome, an autosomal dominant disorder of males and females characterized by webbed neck, short stature, congenital

FIGURE 324-2 Schema for normal spermatogenesis and fertilization showing effects of meiotic and mitotic nondisjunction leading to classic Klinefelter syndrome, Turner syndrome, and mosaic Klinefelter. The schema would be similar if the abnormal events took place during oogenesis.

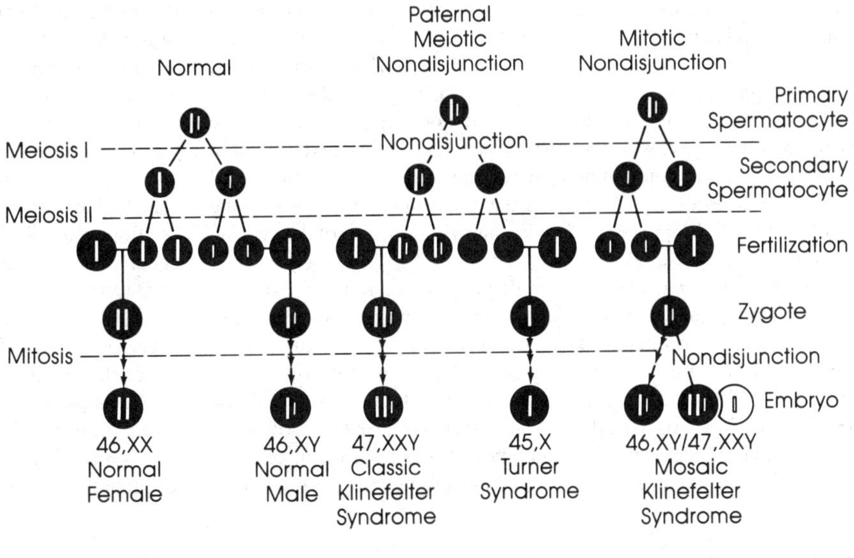

heart disease, cubitus valgus, and other congenital defects despite normal karyotypes and normal gonads.

The incidence is estimated at 1 in 2500 newborn females. The diagnosis is either made at birth because of the associated anomalies or more frequently at puberty when amenorrhea and failure of sexual development are noted in conjunction with the associated anomalies. Gonadal dysgenesis is the most common cause of primary amenorrhea, accounting for a third of such patients. The external genitalia are unambiguously female but remain immature, and there is no breast development unless the patient is treated with exogenous estrogen. The internal genitalia consist of infantile fallopian tubes and uterus and bilateral streak gonads located in the broad ligaments. Primordial germ cells are present transiently during embryogenesis but disappear as the result of an accelerated rate of atresia (see Chap. 322). After the age of expected puberty these streaks lack identifiable follicles and ova but contain fibrous tissue that is indistinguishable from normal ovarian stroma.

The associated somatic anomalies primarily involve the skeleton and connective tissue. Lymphedema of the hands and feet, webbing of the neck, low hair line, redundant skin folds on the back of the neck, a shield-like chest with widely spaced nipples, and a low birth weight are features that suggest the diagnosis in infancy. In addition, the facies may be characterized by micrognathia, epicanthal folds, prominent low-set or deformed ears, a fishlike mouth, and ptosis. Short fourth metacarpals are present in half, and 10 to 20 percent have coarctation of the aorta. In adults the average height rarely exceeds 150 cm. Associated conditions include renal malformations, pigmented nevi, hypoplastic nails, tendency to keloid formation, perceptive hearing loss, unexplained hypertension, and autoimmune disorders. Frank hypothyroidism is present in 20 percent.

Pathophysiology About half have a 45,X karyotype, approximately one-fourth have mosaicism with no structural abnormality (46,XX/45,X), and the remainder have a structurally abnormal X chromosome with or without mosaicism (see Chap. 7). The 45,X variety may result from chromosome loss during gametogenesis in either parent or a mitotic error during one of the early cleavage divisions of the fertilized zygote (Fig. 324-2). Short stature and other somatic features result from loss of genetic material on the short arm of the X chromosome. Streak gonads result when genetic material is missing from either the long or short arm of the X. In individuals with mosaicism or structural abnormalities of the X, phenotypes on average are intermediate in severity between that seen in the 45,X variety and the normal. In some patients with hypertrophy of the clitoris, there is an unidentified fragment of a chromosome present in addition to the X chromosome, assumed to be an abnormal Y; malignancy may develop in the streak gonads in this subset of patients. Rarely, familial transmission of gonadal dysgenesis can be the result of a balanced X-autosome translocation (see Chap. 7).

Assessment of sex chromatin was previously utilized as a means of screening for abnormalities of the X chromosome. Sex chromatin (the Barr body) in normal women is the result of inactivation of one of two X chromosomes, and women with a 45,X chromosome composition, like normal men, are said to be chromatin-negative. However, only about half of patients with gonadal dysgenesis (those with 45,X and those with the most extreme mosaicism and structural abnormalities) are chromatin-negative, and analysis of chromosomal karyotype is necessary to establish the diagnosis and to identify the fraction with Y chromosomal elements and a high chance of developing malignancy in the streak gonads.

Sparse pubic and axillary hair develop at the time of expected puberty, the breasts remain infantile, and no menses occur. Serum FSH is elevated in infancy, falls during midchildhood to the normal range, and increases to castrate levels at the age of 9 or 10. At this time, serum LH is also elevated, and plasma estradiol levels are low [<40 pmol/L (<10 pg/mL)]. Approximately 2 percent of 45,X subjects and 12 percent of mosaic subjects have sufficient residual follicles to allow some menstruation. Indeed, occasional pregnancy has been reported in minimally affected individuals; the reproductive life in such individuals is brief.

Management At the anticipated time of puberty replacement therapy with estrogen should be instituted to induce maturation of the breasts, labia, vagina, uterus, and fallopian tubes (see Chap. 322). Linear growth and bone maturation rates are approximately doubled during the first year of treatment with estradiol, but the eventual height of patients rarely approaches the predicted height. Treatment with growth hormone accelerates growth, but it is not established whether such therapy has an effect on final height (see Chap. 314).

Gonadal tumors are rare in 45,X patients but have occurred in several patients with mosaicism involving the Y chromosome; consequently, streak gonads should be removed in any patient with evidence of virilization or a Y-containing cell line.

MIXED GONADAL DYSGENESIS **Clinical features** Mixed gonadal dysgenesis is an entity in which phenotypic males or females have a testis on one side and streak gonad on the other. Most have 45,X/46,XY mosaicism, but the clinical entity is not confined to that chromosomal pattern. The incidence is unknown, but in most hospitals it is the second most common cause of ambiguous genitalia in the neonate after congenital adrenal hyperplasia.

About two-thirds are reared as females, and most phenotypic males are incompletely virilized at birth. The majority have ambiguous genitalia, including some degree of phallic enlargement, a urogenital sinus, and varying degrees of labioscrotal fusion. In most the testis is located intraabdominally; individuals with a testis in the inguinal or scrotal position are usually reared as males. A uterus, vagina, and at least one fallopian tube are almost invariably present.

The prepubertal testis appears relatively normal. The postpubertal testis contains abundant mature Leydig cells, but the seminiferous tubules lack germinal elements and contain only Sertoli cells. The streak gonad, a thin, pale, elongated structure located either in the broad ligament or along the pelvic wall, is composed of ovarian stroma. At puberty the testis secretes androgen, and virilization and phallic enlargement both occur. Feminization is rare; when it occurs, estrogen secretion from a gonadal tumor should be suspected.

Approximately a third exhibit the somatic features of 45,X gonadal dysgenesis, i.e., low posterior hairline, shield chest, multiple pigmented nevi, cubitus valgus, webbing of the neck, and short stature (height less than 150 cm).

Virtually all are chromatin-negative. In one series, two-thirds had the 45,X/46,XY karyotype, and in the remainder a 46,XY karyotype was present but mosaicism might have gone undetected or been limited to certain cell lines. The origin of 45,X/46,XY mosaicism is best explained by the loss of a Y chromosome during an early mitotic division of an XY zygote similar to the postulated loss of the X chromosome in the 46,XY/47,XXY mosaicism shown in Fig. 324-2.

Pathophysiology It has been assumed that the 46,XY cell line stimulates testicular differentiation whereas the 45,X stem leads to the development of the contralateral streak gonad, but actual comparisons between karyotype and phenotypic expression have failed to substantiate such a relationship. Furthermore, no clear correlation has been found between the percentage of cells cultured from blood or skin containing 45,X or 46,XY and the degree of gonadal development or of somatic anomalies.

Both masculinization and müllerian duct regression in utero are incomplete. Since Leydig cell function is normal at puberty, inadequate virilization in utero may be the result of delayed development of a testis that is ultimately capable of normal Leydig cell function. Alternatively, the fetal testis may simply be incapable of synthesizing adequate amounts of müllerian-inhibiting substance and androgen.

Management For the older child or adult in whom gender is fixed prior to diagnosis, the central issue in management is the possibility of tumor development in the gonads. The overall incidence of gonadal tumors is about 25 percent. Seminomas occur more frequently than gonadoblastomas, and the tumors may occur prior to puberty. The tumors occur most frequently in patients with a female phenotype who lack the somatic features typical of 45,X gonadal dysgenesis and are more common in intraabdominal testes than in the streak gonad. When the diagnosis is established in phenotypic females, early exploratory laparotomy and prophylactic gonadectomy should be undertaken both because gonadal tumors may occur in childhood and because the testis secretes androgen at puberty and thus causes virilization. Such subjects, like those with gonadal dysgenesis, are then given estrogen to induce and maintain feminization.

When the diagnosis is established in phenotypic males during late childhood or in adults the management is more complicated. Phenotypic males with mixed gonadal dysgenesis are infertile (no germinal elements are present in the testes) and have a high risk of developing gonadal tumors. Which testes can be safely conserved? In general the following observations apply: (1) tumors develop in scrotal streak gonads but not in scrotal testes, (2) tumors that develop in intraabdominal testes are always associated with ipsilateral müllerian duct structures, and (3) tumors in streak gonads are always associated with tumors in the contralateral abdominal testis. Based on these observations, it is recommended that (1) all streak gonads should be removed, (2) scrotal testes should be preserved, and (3) intraabdominal testes should be excised unless they can be relocated in the scrotum and are not associated with ipsilateral müllerian duct structures. Decisions as to reconstructive surgery of the phallus depend upon the nature of the defect.

When the diagnosis is established in early infancy and the genitalia are ambiguous, gender assignment is usually female. Resection of the enlarged phallus and gonadectomy can then be accomplished in infancy, sometimes in one procedure. If the decision is for male gender assignment, the same criteria apply as to which testes should be removed in infants as in older males.

TRUE HERMAPHRODITISM Clinical features True hermaphroditism is a condition in which both an ovary and a testis or a gonad with histologic features of both (ovotestis) is present. To justify the diagnosis there must be histologic documentation of both types of gonadal epithelium, the presence of ovarian stroma without oocytes not being sufficient. The incidence is unknown, but more than 400 cases have been reported. Three categories are recognized: (1) one-fifth are bilateral—testicular and ovarian tissue (ovotestes) on each side, (2) two-fifths are unilateral—an ovotestis on one side and an ovary or a testis on the other, and (3) the remainder are lateral—a testis on one side and an ovary on the other.

The external genitalia display all gradations of the male-to-female spectrum. Two-thirds are sufficiently masculinized to be reared as males. However, less than one-tenth have normal male external genitalia; most have hypospadias, and more than half have incomplete labioscrotal fusion. Two-thirds of phenotypic females have an enlarged clitoris, and most have a urogenital sinus. Differentiation of the internal ducts usually corresponds to the adjacent gonad. Although an epididymis usually develops adjacent to a testis, development of the vas deferens is complete in only one-third. Of the patients with an ovotestis, three-fourths have an epididymis, two-thirds have a fallopian tube, one-tenth have a vas deferens, and one-tenth have both a vas deferens and a fallopian tube. A uterus is usually present although it may be hypoplastic or unicornuate. The ovary usually occupies the normal position, but the testis or ovotestis may be found at any level along the route of embryonic testicular descent, frequently associated with an inguinal hernia. Testicular tissue is present in the scrotum or the labioscrotal fold in one-third, in the inguinal canal in one-third, and in the abdominal area in one-third.

Variable feminization and virilization ensue at puberty, three-fourths develop gynecomastia, and about half menstruate. In phenotypic men menstruation presents as cyclic hematuria. Ovulation occurs in approximately one-fourth and is more common than spermatogenesis. In men ovulation may present as testicular pain. Fertility has been reported in women following removal of an ovotestis and in a man who fathered two children. Congenital malformations of other systems are rare.

Pathophysiology About two-thirds of subjects have a 46,XX karyotype, a tenth have a 46,XY karyotype, and the remainder are chromosomal mosaics in which a Y cell line is present. The mechanism responsible for the gonadal development is unknown. Even though not demonstrable with conventional karyotyping methods, it was assumed that sufficient genetic material from the Y chromosome was present (as the result of translocation, nondisjunction, or mutation) to induce the development of testicular tissue. However, hybridization studies with Y chromosome–specific probes in the 46,XX disorder have failed to demonstrate the presence of DNA from the short arm of the Y. In rare instances multiple sibs with a 46,XX karyotype are affected, possibly the result of an autosomal or X-linked mutation.

Because corpora lutea are present in the ovaries of more than one-fourth of subjects, it can be deduced that a female neuroendocrine axis is present and functions normally in such individuals. Feminization (gynecomastia and menstruation) is the result of secretion of estradiol by the ovarian tissue present. In masculinized patients secretion of androgen predominates over secretion of estrogen, and some produce sperm.

Management When the diagnosis is made in a newborn or early infant, gender assignment depends upon the anatomic features. In older children and adults gonads and internal duct structures that are contradictory to the predominant phenotype (and the gender of rearing) should be removed, and when necessary the external genitalia should be modified appropriately. Although gonadal tumors are rare in true hermaphroditism, a gonadoblastoma has been reported in an individual with an XY cell line. Consequently, the possibility of future tumor development must be taken into account when the decision regarding conservation of gonadal tissue is made.

DISORDERS OF GONADAL SEX

Disorders of gonadal sex result when chromosomal sex is normal, but for one of several reasons differentiation of the gonads is abnormal. Thus, gonadal and phenotypic sex do not correspond to chromosomal sex.

PURE GONADAL DYSGENESIS Clinical features Pure gonadal dysgenesis is a disorder in which phenotypic females with gonads and genitalia identical to those with gonadal dysgenesis (bilateral streaks, infantile uterus and fallopian tubes, and sexual infantilism) have normal height, few if any congenital anomalies, and either a normal 46,XX or 46,XY karyotype. This disorder is only about one-tenth as common as gonadal dysgenesis. On genetic grounds this can be considered a separate disorder from gonadal dysgenesis, but it cannot be distinguished clinically from those instances of gonadal dysgenesis associated with minimal somatic abnormalities. The height is normal or greater than normal, some subjects being over 170 cm. Estrogen levels vary from profound deficiency typical of 45,X gonadal dysgenesis to some breast development and appearance of menses that terminate in an early menopause. About 40 percent have some feminization. Axillary and pubic hair are scanty, and the internal genitalia consist of müllerian derivatives only.

Tumors may develop in the streak gonads, particularly dysgerminoma or gonadoblastoma in the 46,XY disorder. Such tumors are frequently heralded by the development of virilizing signs or a pelvic mass.

Pathophysiology Although chromosomal mosaicisms have been described under this nosology, the designation here is restricted to subjects with uniform 46,XX or 46,XY karyotypes. (Those with mosaicism are variants of gonadal dysgenesis or mixed gonadal dysgenesis as described above.) The rationale for this restricted definition is based upon the fact that both the XX and XY varieties can result from single gene mutations. Several sibships have been reported in which more than one individual is affected with the 46,XX type of the disorder, frequently the result of consanguineous matings, suggesting an autosomal recessive pattern of inheritance. Familial occurrence of the 46,XY variety has also been described; in some the mutation appears to be inherited in an X-linked recessive pattern, while in other families the occurrence is compatible with a male-limited autosomal recessive inheritance. In some patients with the 46,XY form of the disorder, the TDF region of the Y chromosome is deleted. In both the 46,XX and the 46,XY forms the disorder prevents differentiation of ovary or testis, respectively; the development of the female phenotype is the consequence of the failure of gonadal development. As in all individuals with nonfunctional gonads, gonadotropin secretion is elevated, and estrogen secretion is low.

Management The management of the estrogen deficiency is identical to that in gonadal dysgenesis, namely, appropriate estrogen replacement therapy is initiated at the time of expected puberty and maintained in adult life (see Chap. 322). Because of the high frequency of gonadal tumors in the 46,XY variety, the streak gonads should be removed once the diagnosis is made. The development of virilizing signs is indication for immediate surgery. The natural history of the gonadal tumors in this disorder is uncertain, but the prognosis after surgical removal is usually good.

THE ABSENT TESTES SYNDROME (ANORCHIA, TESTICULAR REGRESSION, GONADAL AGENESIS, AGONADISM) Clinical features A spectrum of phenotypes has been described in 46,XY males with absent or rudimentary testes but in whom unequivocal evidence exists that endocrine function of the testis (e.g., invariable müllerian duct regression and variable testosterone synthesis) was present at some time during embryonic life. This rare disorder can be distinguished from pure gonadal dysgenesis in which no evidence can be inferred for gonadal function during embryonic development. The disorder varies in its manifestations from complete failure of virilization through varying degrees of incomplete virilization of the external genitalia to otherwise normal males with bilateral anorchia.

The purest form is represented by 46,XY phenotypic females with absent testes, sexual infantilism, and absence of both müllerian duct derivatives and accessory organs of male reproduction. Such individuals differ from 46,XY pure gonadal dysgenesis in that no gonadal remnant can be identified, including no streak gonad, and in the absence of müllerian derivatives. Testicular failure must have occurred between the onset of formation of müllerian-inhibiting substance and the secretion of testosterone, that is, after development of the seminiferous tubules but before the onset of Leydig cell function.

In others the testicular failure must have occurred later in gestation, and these individuals may constitute problems in gender assignment. In some, failure of müllerian regression is more pronounced than failure of testosterone secretion, but none exhibit normal müllerian development. In those with more extensive virilization the external genitalia are phenotypically male, but rudimentary oviducts and vasa deferentia may coexist internally.

At the final extreme is the syndrome of bilateral anorchia in which phenotypic men have absence of müllerian structures and gonads but male development of the wolffian system and external genitalia. Microphallus implies that failure of androgen-mediated growth occurred late in embryogenesis after anatomic development of the male urethra is complete. Persistent gynecomastia may or may not develop.

Pathophysiology The pathogenesis is not understood. The testicular regression could be the result of mutant genes, teratogen, or trauma. Multiple instances of agonadism in the same family have been reported, some of whom have unilateral and others bilateral defects.

The quantitative dynamics of gonadal steroid production have been studied in only a few patients. In two phenotypic women with primary amenorrhea, sexual infantilism, and no internal genital structures, androgen and estrogen kinetics were similar to those in gonadal dysgenesis; production rates of estrogen were low, and no glandular secretion of testosterone was found, confirming the functional as well as anatomic absence of the testes. In one phenotypic male with bilateral anorchia, testosterone and estrogen production was accounted for by peripheral conversion from plasma androstenedione. However, some subjects in whom no testes can be identified at laparotomy have blood testosterone values clearly above the castrate range, presumably derived from remnant testes.

Management The management of the two extremes is clearcut. Sexually infantile, phenotypic females should be treated like patients with gonadal dysgenesis, namely, given adequate estrogen to ensure appropriate breast and female somatic development, and any coexisting vaginal agenesis should be treated by surgical or medical means. Likewise, phenotypic males with anorchia should be given adequate androgen replacement to allow normal male secondary sexual development. The cases with incomplete virilization or ambiguous development of the external genitalia are more complex and require hormonal therapy at the time of expected puberty and individual assessment as to whether surgical therapy is appropriate.

DISORDERS OF PHENOTYPIC SEX

FEMALE PSEUDOHERMAPHRODITISM Congenital adrenal hyperplasia CLINICAL FEATURES The pathways by which glucocorticoids are synthesized in the adrenal gland and androgens are formed in the testis and adrenal are summarized in Fig. 324-3. Three reactions are common to the formation of glucocorticoids and androgens (20,22-desmolase, 3β-hydroxysteroid dehydrogenase, and 17α-hydroxylase); impairment of any of these reactions results in deficiency of glucocorticoid and androgen synthesis and consequently in both congenital adrenal hyperplasia (due to enhanced ACTH levels) and defective virilization of the male embryo (male pseudohermaphroditism). Two enzyme reactions are involved exclusively in androgen synthesis (17,20-desmolase and 17β-hydroxysteroid dehydrogenase); deficiency in either results in pure male pseudohermaphroditism with normal glucocorticoid synthesis. Deficiency of either of the terminal two enzymes of glucocorticoid synthesis (21-hydroxylase and 11β-hydroxylase) results in defective formation of hydrocortisone; the compensatory increase in ACTH secretion causes adrenal hyperplasia and a secondary increase in androgen formation that results in virilization in the female or precocious masculinization in the male.

The *adrenal insufficiency* in these disorders may produce equally severe and life-threatening problems in both sexes and is described in detail in Chap. 317. The major features of congenital adrenal hyperplasia are listed in Table 324-4. From the standpoint of *abnormal sexual development,* some defects in steroidogenesis result in female pseudohermaphroditism and some cause male pseudohermaphroditism. (One disorder, 3β-hydroxysteroid dehydrogenase deficiency, can cause either male or female pseudohermaphroditism, but since the more common genital defect is incomplete virilization of the male, it will be discussed as an abnormality of male phenotypic differentiation.)

Congenital adrenal hyperplasia due to 21-hydroxylase deficiency is the most common cause of ambiguous genitalia in the newborn, with an incidence of between 1:5000 and 1:15,000 in Europe and the United States. Virilization is usually apparent at birth in the female and within the first 2 to 3 years of life in the male. Manifestations in females include hypertrophy of the clitoris with ventral binding (chordee), partial fusion of the labioscrotal folds, and variable virilization of the urethra. The internal female structures and ovaries remain unaltered, and the wolffian ducts regress normally, probably because adrenal function begins relatively late in embryogenesis. The external appearance of affected females is similar to that of a male with bilateral cryptorchidism and hypospadias. The labioscrotal folds are bulbous and rugated and resemble a scrotum. Rarely the virilization is so severe that development of a complete male penile urethra and prostate results in errors in sex assignment at birth. Radiography following the injection of radiopaque dye into the external genital orifice is helpful in demonstrating the presence of a vagina, uterus,

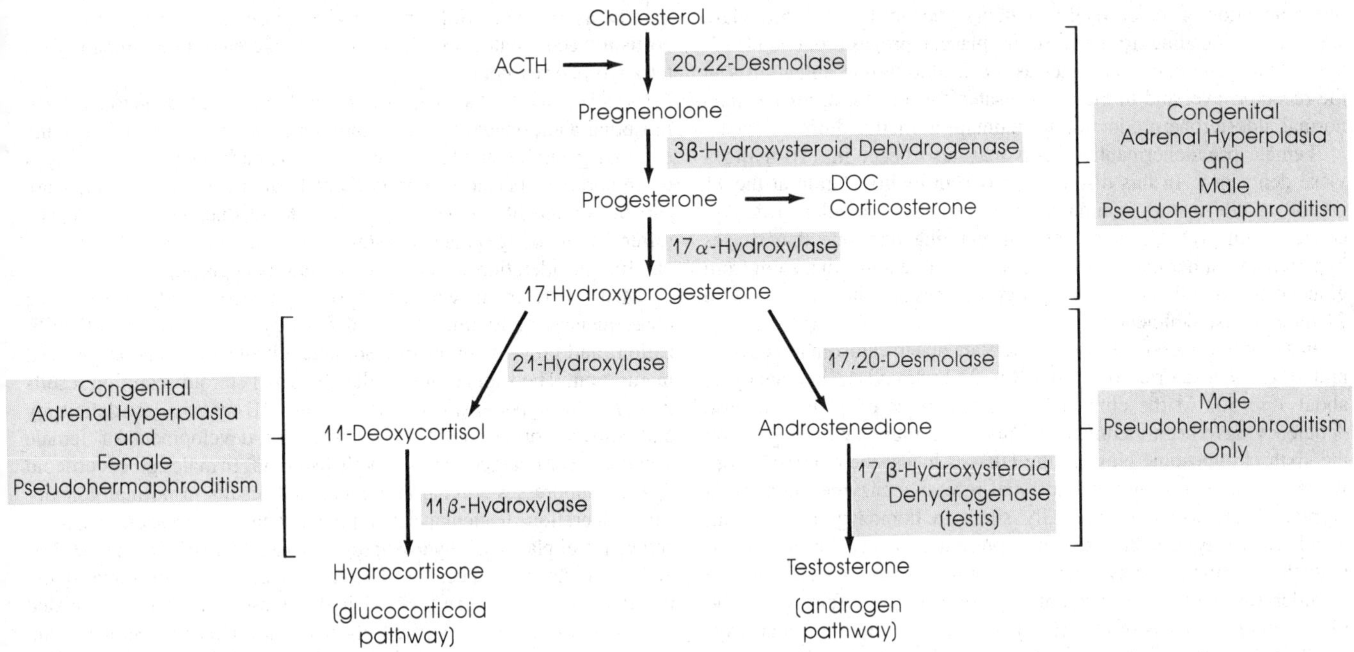

FIGURE 324-3 Pathways of glucocorticoid and androgen synthesis. Note abnormal conditions corresponding to impaired enzyme reactions.

and sometimes even fallopian tubes. In a few cases virilization of the female is slight or absent at birth and becomes evident in later infancy, adolescence, or adulthood, presumably as the result of allelic variation of the mutant genes (the so-called late-onset or adult form of the disorder). The untreated female with the congenital form of the disorder grows rapidly during the first year of life and has progressive virilization. At the time of expected puberty there is a failure of normal female sexual development and absence of menstruation. In both sexes rapid somatic maturation results in premature epiphyseal closure and a short adult height.

Since male phenotypic differentiation is normal, the condition is usually not recognized in the male at birth in the absence of overt adrenal insufficiency. However, early growth and maturation of the external genitalia, appearance of secondary sex characteristics, coarsening of the voice, frequent erections, and excessive muscular development are noticeable in the first few years of life. Virilization in the male can follow either of two patterns. Excessive adrenal androgens can inhibit gonadotropin production so that the testes remain infantile in size despite the acceleration of masculinization. Such untreated adult men are capable of erection and ejaculation but have no spermatogenesis. Alternatively, adrenal androgen secretion can activate a premature maturation of the hypothalamic-pituitary axis and initiate a true precocious puberty including early maturation of spermatogenesis (see Chap. 321). The untreated male is also subject to the development of ACTH-dependent "tumors" of the testis composed of adrenal rest cells.

In 21-hydroxylase deficiency, which accounts for about 95 percent of congenital adrenal hyperplasia, decreased production of hydrocortisone leads to increased release of ACTH, enlargement of the adrenal glands, and partial or complete compensation of the defect in the secretion of hydrocortisone. In about half the enzyme defect appears to be partial, and cortisol secretion is normal. This form is termed "simple virilizing" or "compensated." In the remainder there seems to be a more complete deficiency of the enzyme; the enlarged adrenal fails to produce adequate amounts of cortisol and aldosterone leading to severe salt wastage with anorexia, vomiting, volume depletion, and collapse within the first few weeks of life, the so-called salt-losing form of 21-hydroxylase deficiency. In all untreated patients

TABLE 324-4 Forms of congenital adrenal hyperplasia

Deficiency	Cortisol	Aldosterone	Degree of virilization of females	Failure of virilization in males	Dominant steroid secreted	Comment
21-Hydroxylase, partial (simple virilizing or compensated)	Normal	↑	+ + + +	0	17-Hydroxyprogesterone	Most common type (~95% of total); from one- to two-thirds salt losers
Severe (salt-losing)	↓	↓	+ + + +	0	17-Hydroxyprogesterone	
11β-Hydroxylase (hypertension)	↓	↓	+ + + +	0	11-Deoxycortisol and 11-deoxycorticosterone	Hypertension
3β-Hydroxysteroid dehydrogenase	0	0	+	+ + + +	Δ^5-3β-OH compounds (dehydroepiandrosterone)	Probably second most common, usually salt loss
17α-Hydroxylase	↓	↓	0	+ + + +	Corticosterone and 11-deoxycorticosterone	No feminization of female, hypertension
20,22-Desmolase (lipoid adrenal hyperplasia)	0	0	0	+ + + +	Cholesterol(?)	Rare, usually salt loss

overproduction of the cortisol precursors prior to the 21-hydroxylase step occurs, leading to increase in plasma progesterone and 17-hydroxyprogesterone. These act as weak aldosterone antagonists at the receptor level and in the compensated form result in greater than normal aldosterone production to maintain normal sodium balance.

Female pseudohermaphroditism may also occur in 11β-hydroxylase deficiency. In this disorder a block in hydroxylation at the 11 carbon results in the accumulation of 11-deoxycortisol and deoxycorticosterone (DOC), a potent salt-retaining hormone that causes hypertension rather than salt loss. The clinical features that stem from glucocorticoid deficiency and androgen excess are similar to those in 21-hydroxylase deficiency.

PATHOPHYSIOLOGY Both disorders are due to autosomal recessive mutations. The carrier frequency for 21-hydroxylase deficiency is about 1 in 50. At the clinical level three forms of 21-hydroxylase deficiency have been identified, all involving mutations of a gene on the sixth chromosome close to the HLA-B locus: the common type, which acts like an ordinary autosomal recessive enzyme mutation; a cryptic allele, which is clinically silent in homozygous form but which causes typical disease when present as a genetic compound with the common variety; and a late-onset variant. Carriers of the disorder (as well as homozygotes) within a given family can be identified on the basis of the HLA haplotype. At the molecular level the mutations that give rise to 21-hydroxylase deficiency are even more polymorphic; indeed, deletions of portions of the gene, conversion of the gene from a functional state to a form that is not transcribed normally, and point mutations have been characterized in different families with the disorder. 11β-Hydroxylase deficiency is due to mutation of the normal gene for the enzyme on chromosome 8.

For discussion of the endocrine pathology see Chap. 317. In brief, urinary excretion of ketosteroids is elevated, as is the excretion of the major metabolites that accumulate proximal to the enzymatic blocks. Plasma ACTH is elevated. In 21-hydroxylase deficiency, 17-hydroxyprogesterone accumulates in blood and is excreted predominantly as pregnanetriol. In 11-hydroxylase deficiency, 11-deoxycortisol accumulates in blood and is excreted predominantly as tetrahydrocortexolone.

MANAGEMENT Gender assignment should correspond to the chromosomal and gonadal sex, and appropriate surgical correction of the external genitalia should be undertaken as early as possible. This is of importance because appropriately treated men and women are capable of fertility. However, if the correct diagnosis is made late (after 3 years of age) gender assignment should be changed only after careful consideration of the psychosexual background.

Medical treatment with appropriate glucocorticoids prevents the consequences of hydrocortisone deficiency, arrests the rapid virilization, and prevents premature somatic advancement and epiphyseal maturation. The suppression of the abnormal steroid secretion results in cure of the hypertension in patients with 11β-hydroxylase deficiency and allows normal onset of menses and development of female secondary sex characteristics in both disorders. In males glucocorticoid therapy suppresses adrenal androgens and results in normal gonadotropin secretion, testicular development, and spermatogenesis. Measurements of plasma 17-hydroxyprogesterone, androstenedione, ACTH, and renin have all been used to assess adequacy of replacement therapy. In severe forms of 21-hydroxylase deficiency associated with salt loss or with elevated plasma renin activity treatment with mineralocorticoids is also indicated. In such patients the monitoring of plasma renin is useful for determining the adequacy of mineralocorticoid replacement.

Other causes of female pseudohermaphroditism Female pseudohermaphroditism may also occur in babies born to mothers who have virilizing tumors of the ovary (e.g., arrhenoblastomas or luteomas of pregnancy) and, rarely, to mothers with virilizing adrenal tumors. In the past, the administration to pregnant women of progestational agents with androgenic side effects (such as 17α-ethinyl-19-nor-testosterone) to prevent abortion resulted in masculinization of female fetuses.

TABLE 324-5 Anatomic, genetic, and endocrine profile of hereditary male pseudohermaphroditism

Disorder	Inheritance	Phenotype: Müllerian ducts	Wolffian ducts	Spermatogenesis	Urogenital sinus	External genitalia
DEFECTS IN TESTOSTERONE SYNTHESIS						
Five enzyme deficiencies	Autosomal or X-linked recessive	Absent	Variable development	Normal or decreased	Variable from male to female	Generally female
DEFECTS IN ANDROGEN ACTION						
5α-Reductase deficiency	Autosomal recessive	Absent	Male	Normal or decreased	Female	Clitoromegaly
Receptor disorders:						
Complete testicular feminization	X-linked recessive	Absent	Absent	Absent	Female	Female
Incomplete testicular feminization	X-linked recessive	Absent	Male	Absent	Female	Clitoromegaly and posterior fusion
Reifenstein syndrome	X-linked recessive	Absent	Variable development	Absent	Variable from male to female	Incomplete male development
Infertile male syndrome	X-linked recessive	Absent	Male	Absent or decreased	Male	Male
Undervirilized fertile male	X-linked recessive	Absent	Male	Normal or decreased	Male	Male
Receptor-positive resistance	Uncertain	Absent	Variable	Absent or decreased	Variable	Female to male
DEFECTS IN MÜLLERIAN REGRESSION						
Persistent müllerian duct syndrome	Autosomal or X-linked recessive	Rudimentary uterus and fallopian tubes	Male	Normal	Male	Male

Developmental disorders of müllerian ducts (congenital absence of the vagina, müllerian agenesis) CLINICAL FEATURES Congenital hypoplasia or absence of the vagina in combination with abnormal or absent uterus (the Mayer-Rokitansky-Kuster-Hauser syndrome) is second to gonadal dysgenesis as a cause of primary amenorrhea. Most patients are ascertained after the time of expected puberty because of failure to menstruate. The height and intelligence are normal, and the breasts, axillary and pubic hair, and habitus are feminine in character. The uterus can vary from almost normal, lacking only a conduit to the introitus, to the characteristic rudimentary bicornuate cords with or without a lumen. In some patients cyclical abdominal pain indicates that sufficient functional endometrium is present to result in retrograde menstruation and/or hematometra.

About one-third have abnormal kidneys, most commonly agenesis or ectopy. Fused kidneys of the horseshoe type and solitary ectopic kidneys located in the pelvis also occur. Skeletal abnormalities are present in one-tenth; two-thirds involve the spine, and limb and rib abnormalities account for the remainder. Specific bone abnormalities include wedge vertebrae, fused rudimentary or asymmetric vertebral bodies, and supernumerary vertebrae. The Klippel-Feil syndrome (congenital fusion of the cervical spine, short neck, low posterior hairline, and painless limitation of cervical movement) is a frequent association.

PATHOPHYSIOLOGY The karyotype is 46,XX. Most are believed to be sporadic in nature, but familial occurrence has been described. The pattern of inheritance in most familial cases is consistent with a sex-limited autosomal dominant mutation. Sporadic cases may represent new mutations of the type responsible for the familial disorder or be multifactorial in etiology. In the familial cases expressivity is variable; some affected family members have skeletal or renal abnormalities only, and some have other abnormalities of müllerian derivatives such as a double uterus. Bilateral renal aplasia in stillborn infants is commonly associated with absence of the uterus and vagina. Thus, the family history should be probed for isolated skeletal and renal abnormalities and for stillbirths that might result from congenital absence of both kidneys.

Documentation of ovulatory peaks of plasma LH and biphasic temperature curves during the cycle suggest that ovarian function is normal, and successful pregnancies have occurred after corrective vaginal surgery in patients with normal uteri.

MANAGEMENT Vaginal agenesis can be treated by surgical or nonsurgical means. Surgical repair generally utilizes a split-thickness skin graft around a solid rubber mold for the creation of an artificial vagina. Medical treatment consists of the repeated application of pressure against the vaginal dimple with a simple dilator to cause development of adequate vaginal depth. In view of complication rates of 5 to 10 percent in surgical series, medical treatment should be tried in most, and surgery should be reserved for patients in whom a well-formed uterus is present and the possibility of fertility exists. Frequent coitus or instrumental dilatation is essential for maintaining the neovagina formed by either technique.

MALE PSEUDOHERMAPHRODITISM Defective virilization of the male embryo (male pseudohermaphroditism) can result from defects in androgen synthesis, defects in androgen action, defects in müllerian duct regression, and uncertain causes. Four-fifths of male pseudohermaphrodites have normal androgen synthesis.

Abnormalities in androgen synthesis CLINICAL FEATURES- Enzymatic defects that result in defective testosterone synthesis (Fig. 324-3) can cause incomplete virilization of the male embryo during embryogenesis (Tables 324-4 and 324-5). Each of the defects blocks a step in the conversion of cholesterol to testosterone. Three (20,22-desmolase, 3β-hydroxysteroid dehydrogenase, and 17α-hydroxylase) are common to the synthesis of other adrenal hormones as well; consequently, their deficiency results in congenital adrenal hyperplasia (Table 324-4) as well as male pseudohermaphroditism. Two others (17,20-desmolase, and 17β-hydroxysteroid dehydrogenase) are unique to the pathway of androgen synthesis, and their deficiency results only in male pseudohermaphroditism. Since androgens are obligatory precursors of estrogens, synthesis of estrogen is also low in affected men and women in all but the terminal defect (17β-hydroxysteroid dehydrogenase deficiency)

The adrenal dysfunction is described in Chap. 317, and the present discussion concerns the abnormal sexual development. In 46,XY subjects there is usually no trace of uterus or fallopian tubes, indicating that the müllerian-inhibiting function of the testis during embryogenesis was normal. The masculinization of the wolffian ducts, urogenital sinus, and urogenital tubercle and the degree of virilization at puberty vary from almost normal to absent, and therefore, the clinical picture spans the range from phenotypic men with mild hypospadias to phenotypic women who prior to puberty resemble patients with complete testicular feminization. This variability is the consequence of varying severity of the enzymatic defects in different patients and of varying effects of the steroids that accumulate proximal to the metabolic blocks in the different disorders. In patients with partial defects and in whom plasma testosterone is normal the diagnosis can only be made by measuring the steroids that accumulate proximal to the metabolic block.

20,22-Desmolase deficiency (lipoid adrenal hyperplasia) is a form of congenital adrenal hyperplasia in which virtually no urinary steroids (either 17-ketosteroids or 17-hydroxycorticoids) can be detected. The defect is prior to the formation of pregnenolone and is assumed to involve the 20,22-desmolase (side-chain cleavage) enzyme responsible for the conversion of cholesterol to pregnenolone. The syndrome is associated with salt wasting and profound adrenal insufficiency, and most affected individuals die during infancy. At autopsy the adrenals and testes are enlarged and infiltrated with lipid. Affected males are incompletely masculinized whereas affected female infants have normal genital development. The gene for the human enzyme is located on chromosome 15.

3β-Hydroxysteroid dehydrogenase deficiency causes varying failure of masculinization and development of a vagina in male infants. Female infants may be modestly virilized at birth due to the weak

	Endocrine profile relative to normal male		
Breast	Testosterone production	Estrogen production	LH
Usually male	Normal to decreased	Variable	High
Male	Normal	Normal	Normal or increased
Female	High	High	High
Female	High	High	High
Female	High	High	High
Usually male	Normal or high	Normal or high	Normal or high
Female	Normal or high	Normal or high	Normal or high
Variable	Normal or high	Normal or high	Normal or high
Male	Normal	Normal	Normal

androgenic potency of dehydroepiandrosterone, the major steroid secreted. If the enzyme is absent in both the adrenal and testis, no urinary steroids contain a Δ^4-3-keto configuration, whereas in patients in whom the defect is partial or affects only the testis, the urine may contain normal or elevated levels of Δ^4-3-ketosteroids. Most patients have marked salt wasting and profound adrenal insufficiency, and long-term survival in untreated cases occurs only in states of partial deficiency. Affected males may experience an otherwise normal male puberty except for profound gynecomastia. In these individuals a low-normal blood testosterone level is accompanied by elevated Δ^5 precursors. The enzyme in different tissues must be under complex control since deficiency of the enzyme in the testis may be less severe than in the adrenal and since enzyme activity in the liver may be normal in the face of profound deficiency in the adrenal and testis. Individuals with normal liver enzymes can be mistakenly identified as having 21-hydroxylase deficiency if urinary Δ^5-pregnenetriol is not documented to be greater than urinary pregnanetriol.

17α-Hydroxylase–17,20-desmolase deficiency impairs the introduction of the 17 hydroxyl and the scission of the C-17,20 carbon bond that convert pregnenolone and progesterone to dehydroepiandrosterone and androstenedione, respectively. These reactions are mediated by a single cytochrome P_{450} enzyme encoded on chromosome 10, and it is unclear why both reactions occur in the ovary and testis whereas in the adrenal 17-hydroxy progesterone is largely converted to glucocorticoids and mineralocorticoids rather than the 19 carbon steroids. Likewise, it is unclear why some patients have selective impairment of either 17α-hydroxylase or 17,20-desmolase activity; the distinction between these activities must be functional and may involve the relative concentration of steroid substrates and competing enzymes. Whatever the explanation, the clinical consequences of 17α-hydroxylase and 17,20-desmolase deficiencies are different.

17α-Hydroxylase deficiency characteristically results in hypogonadism, absence of secondary sex characteristics, hypokalemic alkalosis, hypertension, and virtually undetectable hydrocortisone secretion in phenotypic women. The secretion of both corticosterone and desoxycorticosterone (DOC) by the adrenal is elevated, and urinary 17-ketosteroids are low. Aldosterone secretion is low due to high plasma DOC and depressed angiotensin levels and returns to normal after suppressive doses of hydrocortisone are administered. In 46,XX subjects amenorrhea, absent sexual hair, and hypertension are common, but, since gonadal steroids are not required for female development during embryogenesis, the phenotype is that of a normal prepubertal woman. In males the deficiency results in defective virilization that varies from complete male pseudohermaphroditism to ambiguous genitalia with perineoscrotal hypospadias and, in some, gynecomastia. Adrenal insufficiency does not develop, since the secretion of both corticosterone (a weak glucocorticoid) and DOC (a mineralocorticoid) is elevated. Hypertension and hypokalemia are prominent features of the disorder (even in the neonatal period) and remit after suppression of the DOC secretion by adequate glucocorticoid replacement.

17,20-Desmolase deficiency in males is associated with normal function of the adrenal cortex and a variable pattern of male pseudohermaphroditism. In the majority there is genital ambiguity at birth with some virilization at the time of expected puberty. Rare 46,XY patients have had a female phenotype and no virilization at the time of expected puberty. The disorder has been recognized in one 46,XX woman with sexual infantilism.

17β-Hydroxysteroid dehydrogenase deficiency involves the final step in testosterone biosynthesis, reduction of the 17-keto group of androstenedione. This is the most common of the enzymatic defects in testosterone synthesis. Affected 46,XY males usually have a female phenotype with a blind-ending vagina and absence of müllerian derivatives, but inguinal or abdominal testes and virilized wolffian duct structures are present. At the time of expected puberty, both virilization (with phallic enlargement and development of facial and body hair) and a variable degree of female breast development take place. In some untreated patients reversal of gender behavior from female to male occurs at puberty. Androgen and estrogen dynamics have not been elucidated in detail, but the 17-keto reduction of estrone to estradiol by the gonads is also low. 17β-Hydroxysteroid dehydrogenase is normally present in many tissues besides the gonads, and only the gonadal enzyme appears to be defective in this disorder. Plasma testosterone may be in the low-normal range, making it essential to document elevation in plasma androstenedione to make the diagnosis.

PATHOPHYSIOLOGY The available data for these various disorders are compatible with autosomal recessive inheritance. The pattern of steroid secretion and excretion depends on the site of the various metabolic blocks (Fig. 324-3). In general, gonadotropin secretion is high, and as a consequence many individuals with incomplete defects are able to compensate so that the steady-state levels of end products such as testosterone may be normal or almost normal.

In some cases of male pseudohermaphroditism testosterone formation is deficient for reasons other than a single enzyme defect in androgen synthesis. These include disorders in which Leydig cell agenesis (possibly due to absence of the LH receptor) or the secretion of a biologically inactive LH molecule is thought to be the primary defect. In addition, as described above, in several disorders including familial XY gonadal dysgenesis, sporadic dysgenetic testes, and the absent testis syndrome, deficient testosterone production is secondary to abnormal gonadal development.

MANAGEMENT Therapy with glucocorticoids and in some instances mineralocorticoids is indicated in those disorders causing adrenal hyperplasia. The decision as to the management of the genital abnormalities depends upon the individual case. Fertility has not been reported, and its consideration does not enter into sex assignment. In genetic females there is no problem (except in diagnosis) in that affected individuals are raised appropriately as females, and suitable estrogen replacement is administered at the time of expected puberty to promote development of normal secondary sex characteristics. The decision as to whether newborn males with ambiguous genitalia should be raised as males or females depends upon the anatomic defect; in general the more severely affected should be raised as females, and corrective surgery of the genitalia and removal of the testes should be undertaken as early as possible. In such subjects estrogen therapy is also indicated at the appropriate age to allow development of normal female secondary sex characteristics. In individuals raised as males, corrective surgery is indicated for any coexisting hypospadias, and monitoring of plasma androgens and estrogens should be undertaken at the time of expected puberty to determine whether supplemental testosterone therapy is appropriate.

Abnormalities in androgen action Several disorders of male phenotypic development result from abnormalities of androgen action. The spectrum of phenotypes is described in Tables 324-4 and -5. In these disorders testosterone formation and müllerian regression are normal, but male development is impaired to a variable degree as a result of resistance to androgen action in the target cells.

5α-REDUCTASE DEFICIENCY This autosomal recessive disorder is characterized by (1) severe perineoscrotal hypospadias; (2) a blind vaginal pouch of variable size opening either into the urogenital sinus or into the urethra; (3) testes with normal epididymides, vasa deferentia, and seminal vesicles, and termination of the ejaculatory ducts into the blind-ending vagina; (4) a female habitus without female breast development but with normal axillary and pubic hair; (5) the absence of female internal genitalia; (6) normal male plasma testosterone; and (7) masculinization to a variable degree at the time of puberty.

The fact that virilization during embryogenesis is defective only in the urogenital sinus and the external genitalia provided insight into the fundamental abnormality. Testosterone, the androgen secreted by the fetal testis, is responsible for differentiation of the wolffian duct into the epididymis, the vas deferens, and the seminal vesicle, whereas dihydrotestosterone mediates virilization of the urogenital sinus and the external genitalia. Consequently, a failure of dihydrotestosterone formation in a male embryo would be expected to cause the phenotype observed in this disorder, normal male wolffian duct derivatives with defective masculinization of the external genitalia and urogenital sinus. Since testosterone itself regulates LH secretion (see Chap. 321), plasma LH is usually normal or minimally elevated. As a result, testosterone and estrogen production rates are those of normal men, and gynecomastia does not develop.

The fact that the 5α-reductase enzyme is deficient in this disorder was established by assay of biopsied tissues and cultured fibroblasts from affected individuals. In most subjects the 5α-reductase is either profoundly deficient or functionally absent, and in others the enzyme protein is normal in amount but structurally abnormal.

RECEPTOR DISORDERS The androgen receptor is a typical member of the steroid/thyroid family of receptors with steroid-binding, DNA-binding, and functional domains and is encoded by a gene on the long arm of the X-chromosome. A variety of mutations of this gene impair receptor function and hence impair male phenotypic differentiation and/or virilization.

Clinical features. Complete testicular feminization is the most common form of male pseudohermaphroditism; estimates of frequency vary from 1 in 20,000 to 1 in 64,000 male births. It is the third most common cause of primary amenorrhea in phenotypic women after gonadal dysgenesis and congenital absence of the vagina. The features are characteristic. Namely, a woman is seen by the physician either because of inguinal hernia (prepubertal) or primary amenorrhea (postpubertal). The development of the breasts after puberty, the general habitus, and the distribution of body fat are female in character so that most patients have a truly feminine appearance. Axillary and pubic hair are absent or scanty, but some vulval hair is usually present. Scalp hair is that of a normal woman, and facial hair is absent. The external genitalia are unambiguously female, and the clitoris is normal. The vagina is short and blind-ending and may be absent or rudimentary. All internal genitalia are absent except for undescended testes that contain normal Leydig cells and seminiferous tubules without spermatogenesis.

The testes may be located in the abdomen, along the course of the inguinal canal, or in the labia majora. Occasionally, remnants of müllerian or wolffian duct origin are present in the paratesticular fascia or in fibrous bands extending from the testis. Patients tend to be rather tall and bone age is normal. Psychosexual development is unmistakably female in regard to behavior, outlook, and maternal instincts.

The major complication of undescended testes in this disorder as in all forms of cryptorchidism is the development of tumors (Chap. 305). Since affected individuals undergo a normal pubertal growth spurt and feminize successfully at the time of expected puberty and since testicular tumors rarely develop until after puberty, it is usual to delay castration until after the time of expected puberty. Prepubertal castration is indicated if the testes are present in the inguinal region or the labia majora and result in discomfort or hernia formation. (If hernia repair is indicated prepubertally, most physicians prefer to remove the testes at the same time to limit the number of operative procedures.) If the testes are removed prepubertally, estrogen therapy is required at the appropriate age to ensure normal growth and breast development. When castration is performed postpubertally, menopausal symptoms and other evidences of estrogen withdrawal supervene, and suitable estrogen replacement is indicated (see Chap. 322).

Incomplete testicular feminization is about one-tenth as frequent as the complete form. In the incomplete disorder there is a minor virilization of the external genitalia (partial fusion of the labioscrotal folds and some degree of clitoromegaly), normal pubic hair, and some virilization as well as feminization at the time of expected puberty. The vagina is short and blind-ending, but in contrast to the complete form, the wolffian duct derivatives are often partially developed. The management of patients with the complete and incomplete forms of testicular feminization differs. Since patients with the incomplete disorder virilize at the time of expected puberty, gonadectomy should be performed before the expected time of puberty in all prepubertal patients with clitoromegaly or posterior labial fusion.

Reifenstein syndrome is the term applied to forms of incomplete male pseudohermaphroditism initially described by a number of eponyms (Reifenstein syndrome, Gilbert-Dreyfus syndrome, Lubs syndrome). Each of these phenotypes was originally assumed to be a distinct entity, but these syndromes are now known to constitute variable manifestations of a single mutation. The most common phenotype is a man with perineoscrotal hypospadias and gynecomastia, but the spectrum of defective virilization in affected families ranges from men with azoospermia to phenotypic women with pseudovaginas. Axillary and pubic hair are normal, but chest and facial hair are minimal. Cryptorchidism is common, the testes are small, and azoospermia is present. Some have defects in wolffian duct derivatives such as absence or hypoplasia of the vas deferens. Since the psychological development in most is unequivocally male, the hypospadias and cryptorchidism should be corrected surgically. The only successful form of treatment of the gynecomastia is surgical removal.

The *infertile male syndrome* is probably the most common disorder of the androgen receptor and is not actually a form of male pseudohermaphroditism. Some such individuals are minimally affected subjects in families with Reifenstein syndrome with azoospermia as the only manifestation of the receptor abnormality. More commonly, the individuals present with male infertility and have negative family histories; indeed a disorder of the androgen receptor may be present in a fifth or more of men with idiopathic azoospermia. The *undervirilized fertile male* is an even less severe manifestation of an androgen receptor defect. In these families affected men have gynecomastia and undervirilization, and some are fertile.

Pathophysiology. The karyotype is 46,XY, and the mutant gene is X-linked. The frequency of a positive family history varies from about two-thirds of patients with testicular feminization and Reifenstein syndrome to only occasional patients with the infertile male syndrome. The patients with a negative family history are believed to be the result of new mutations.

Hormone dynamics are similar in all disorders of the androgen receptor. Plasma testosterone levels and rates of testosterone production by the testes are normal or higher than normal. The elevated testosterone production is caused by the high mean plasma level of LH, which in turn is due to defective feedback regulation caused by resistance to the action of androgen at the hypothalamic-pituitary level. Elevated LH concentration is responsible also for the increased estrogen production by the testes (see Chap. 321). (In normal men most estrogen is derived from peripheral formation from circulating androgens, but when plasma LH is elevated the testes secrete increased amounts of estrogen into the circulation.) Thus, resistance to the feedback regulation of LH secretion by circulating androgen results in elevated plasma LH levels, and this in turn results in the enhanced secretion of both testosterone and estradiol by the testes. Gonadotropin levels rise even higher (and menopausal symptoms may develop) when the testes are removed, indicating that gonadotropin secretion is under partial regulatory control. Presumably, in the steady state and in the absence of an androgen effect, estrogen alone regulates LH secretion, a control purchased at the expense of an elevated plasma estrogen concentration for a male. The hormonal changes in the infertile male syndrome are similar to those in the other receptor disorders but less marked. Some men with this syndrome do not have an elevation of plasma LH or plasma testosterone.

Feminization in these disorders is the result of two interlocking phenomena. First, androgens and estrogens have antagonistic effects, and virilization occurs in normal men when the ratio of androgen to estrogen is 100 to 1 or greater; in the absence of androgen action the cellular effect of estrogen is unopposed. Second, the testicular production of estradiol is greater than that of the normal male (although less than that of the normal female). Variable degrees of androgen resistance coupled with variably enhanced estradiol production result in different degrees of defective virilization and enhanced feminization in the four clinical syndromes.

Each of these syndromes is the result of an abnormality of the androgen receptor. Initially fibroblasts cultured from the skin of some subjects with complete testicular feminization were shown to have a near absence of high-affinity dihydrotestosterone binding. Subsequently, other individuals with complete testicular feminization as well as subjects with incomplete testicular feminization, Reifenstein syndrome, the infertile male syndrome, and undervirilization with fertility have been found to have either a decreased amount of an apparently normal receptor or a qualitatively abnormal androgen receptor. In some families, the fundamental defect is due to the deletion of a portion of the gene, in others the disorder is due to point mutations in the coding sequence, and in still others the defect appears to impair the transcription of the messenger RNA that encodes the receptor.

RECEPTOR-POSITIVE RESISTANCE A category of androgen resistance that does not appear to involve either the 5α-reductase or the androgen receptor was first identified in a family with the syndrome of testicular feminization. Subsequent patients have been described with phenotypes ranging from incomplete testicular feminization to the Reifenstein syndrome. The hormonal profile is similar to that in the receptor disorders. The site of the molecular abnormality in these patients is unclear. It could be due to receptor defects too subtle to be detected by the usual assay. If the defect is truly distal to the receptor, there could be failure of generation of specific messenger RNA or an abnormality of RNA processing. Indeed, the disorder may represent a heterogeneous group of molecular abnormalities.

Persistent müllerian duct syndrome Men with this disorder have testes and normal phenotypic development and in addition have bilateral fallopian tubes, a uterus, and an upper vagina, and variable development of the vas deferens. The subjects commonly present with inguinal hernias that contain the uterus, and cryptorchidism is common. Most have uninformative family histories, but in some families the condition is inherited either as an autosomal recessive or an X-linked recessive mutation. Because the external genitalia are well developed and the patients masculinize normally at puberty, it is assumed that during the critical stage of embryonic sexual differentiation the fetal testes produce a normal amount of androgen. However, müllerian regression does not occur for one of two reasons: some individuals fail to produce müllerian-inhibiting substance, and others produce normal amounts but do not respond to the hormone. To minimize the chance of tumor development and to maintain virilization, orchiopexy should be performed. Malignancy in the uterus or vagina has not been described, and because the vasa deferentia are closely associated with the broad ligaments, the uterus and vagina should be left in place to avoid disruption of the vasa deferentia during removal and consequently to preserve possible fertility.

Developmental defects of the male genitalia HYPOSPADIAS Hypospadias is a congenital anomaly in which the urethra terminates in an abnormal position along the midline of the ventral surface of the penis at some site between the normal urethral meatus and the perineum. This malformation is often associated with ventral contraction and bowing of the penis (chordee) and occurs in 0.5 to 0.8 percent of male births in the United States. It is common to categorize hypospadias as glandular (involving the glans penis), penile, or perineoscrotal. Since penile development is mediated by androgens, it is assumed that hypospadias results from some defect in androgen formation or androgen action during embryogenesis. Indeed hypospadias occurs in most disorders of male sexual differentiation. A rare cause of hypospadias is maternal ingestion of progestational agents early in pregnancy. However, the known causes (single gene defects, chromosomal abnormalities, and maternal drug ingestion) at best can account for only about one-fourth of cases, and the etiology of most remains unknown. The management is surgical.

CRYPTORCHIDISM The normal descent of the testis is perhaps the most poorly understood portion of male sexual differentiation, both in regard to the nature of the forces that result in the movement and to the hormonal factors that regulate the process. In anatomic terms testicular descent can be divided into three phases: (1) transabdominal movement of the testis from its site of origin above the kidney to the inguinal ring, (2) formation of the opening in the inguinal canal (processus vaginalis) through which the testis exits the abdominal cavity, and (3) actual movement of the testis through the inguinal canal to its permanent site in the scrotum. This entire process occurs over a 6- to 7-month period during gestation, beginning at about the sixth week and not completed in some normal individuals until after birth. Whatever its involvement, androgen is probably not the sole hormone responsible for normal descent. Failure of any of the above anatomic events can be responsible for the failure of descent of one or both testes. About 3 percent of full-term and 30 percent of premature male infants have at least one cryptorchid testis at birth but completion of descent can occur within the first few weeks of life so that the incidence of failure of descent by 6 to 9 months of age is only 0.6 to 0.7 percent. It is this latter category of maldescent that requires intervention.

Permanent cryptorchidism can be classified as intraabdominal (10 percent), canalicular (in the inguinal canal) (20 percent), high scrotal (40 percent), or obstructed (30 percent) in which maldescent is due to a physical barrier between the inguinal pouch and the inlet of the scrotum. These disorders must be distinguished from the temporarily retracted normal testis.

The cryptorchid testis functions poorly after puberty, but the extent to which maldescent is the result of an abnormality of the testis or the cause of abnormal function is unknown. Two general theories have been advanced as to the etiology—inadequate intraabdominal pressure and deficient endocrine function of the testis either because of deficient testosterone synthesis or inadequate formation of müllerian-inhibiting substance. Indeed, hereditary defects that result in inadequate development of intraabdominal pressure or inadequate development of the testes themselves can cause cryptorchidism. As is true for hypospadias, however, the known causes of cryptorchidism constitute only a small fraction of the cases, and the etiology in most remains to be identified. Two complications of cryptorchidism are important; spermatogenesis cannot occur at the temperature of the abdominal cavity, and it is therefore necessary to correct the process as early as possible to allow possible fertility. However, the fact that infertility is common in men who have been treated for unilateral as well as bilateral cryptorchidism suggests that maldescent is usually the consequence rather than the cause of the testicular malfunction. There is also a greater frequency of malignancy in undescended testis, and all should be surgically corrected for this reason (see Chap. 305).

REFERENCES

BROWN TR et al: Deletion of the steroid-binding domain of the human androgen receptor gene in one family with complete androgen insensitivity syndrome: Evidence for further genetic heterogeneity in this syndrome. Proc Natl Acad Sci USA 85:8151, 1988

DE LA CHAPELLE A: The etiology of maleness in XX men. Hum Genet 58:105, 1981

DONAHOE PK et al: Mixed gonadal dysgenesis, pathogenesis and management. J Pediatr Surg 14:287, 1979

EDMAN CD et al: Embryonic testicular regression: A clinical spectrum of XY agonadal individuals. Obstet Gynecol 49:208, 1977

GEORGE FW, WILSON JD: Sex determination and differentiation, in *The Physiology of Reproduction*, E Knobil, JD Neill (eds). New York, Raven, 1988, vol 1, pp 3–26

GORDON DL et al: Pathologic testicular findings in Klinefelter's syndrome. 47,XXY vs 46,XY/47,XXY. Arch Intern Med 130:726, 1972

GRIFFIN JE et al: Congenital absence of the vagina. The Mayer-Rokitansky-Kuster-Hauser syndrome. Ann Intern Med 85:224, 1976

———, WILSON JD: Disorder of sexual differentiation, in *Campbell's Textbook of Urology*, 5th ed, PC Walsh et al (eds). Philadelphia, Saunders, 1986, pp 1819–1855

———, The androgen resistance syndromes: 5α-Reductase deficiency, and related disorders, in *The Metabolic Basis of Inherited Disease*, 6th ed, CR Scriver et al (eds). New York, McGraw-Hill, 1989, pp 1919–1944

GRINO PB et al: A mutation of the androgen receptor associated with partial androgen resistance, familial gynecomastia, and fertility. J Clin Endocrinol Metab 66:754, 1988
GRUMBACH MM, CONTE FA: Disorders of sexual differentiation, in *Williams' Textbook of Endocrinology*, 7th ed, JD Wilson, DW Foster (eds). Philadelphia, Saunders, 1985, pp 312–401
GUERRIER D et al: The persistent müllerian duct syndrome: A molecular approach. J Clin Endocrinol Metab 68:46, 1989
LEONARD JM et al: The classification of Klinefelter's syndrome, in *Genetic Mechanism of Sexual Development*, HL Vallet, IH Porter (eds). New York, Academic, 1979
MILLER WL: Molecular biology of steroid hormone synthesis. Endocrinol Rev 9:295, 1988
NEW M et al: Congenital adrenal hyperplasia and related conditions, in *The Metabolic Basis of Inherited Disease*, 6th ed, CR Scriver et al (eds). New York, McGraw-Hill, 1989, pp 1881–1917
PAGE DC et al: The sex-determining region of the human Y chromosome encodes a finger protein. Cell 51:1091, 1987
RAMSAY M et al: XX True hermaphroditism in Southern African blacks: An enigma of primary sexual differentiation. Am J Hum Genet Vol 43:4, 1988
SIMPSON JL: Gonadal dysgenesis and sex chromosome abnormalities: Phenotypic-karyotypic correlations, in *Genetic Mechanisms of Sexual Development*, HL Vallet, IH Porter (eds). New York, Academic, 1979
——— et al: XY gonadal dysgenesis: Genetic heterogeneity based upon clinical observations, H-Y antigen status and segregation analysis. Hum Genet 58:91, 1981
ZAH W et al: Mixed gonadal dysgenesis. A case report and review of the world literature. Acta Endocrinol Suppl 197:3, 1975

325 DISORDERS AFFECTING MULTIPLE ENDOCRINE SYSTEMS

R. NEIL SCHIMKE

Multiple endocrine gland hyper- or hypofunction can result from mechanisms other than a primary abnormality in the hypothalamic-pituitary axis. While not common, certain of the conditions that affect multiple endocrine systems are inherited and thus have significance out of proportion to their frequency.

SYNDROMES WITH MULTISYSTEM HYPERFUNCTION

MULTIPLE ENDOCRINE NEOPLASIA, TYPE I (MEN I) This disorder, also termed the *Wermer syndrome*, comprises tumors or hyperplasia of the parathyroids, pancreatic islet cells, and pituitary. The clinical presentation is variable, depending on which of the potentially affected glands is hyperfunctioning at the time of diagnosis. About two-thirds of patients have adenomas of two or more endocrine systems, and one-fifth develop tumors of three or more systems.

The majority of affected subjects present with one of the following problems: (1) peptic ulcer and its complications, (2) hypoglycemia, (3) hypercalcemia and/or nephrocalcinosis, (4) complaints referable to pituitary dysfunction such as headaches, visual field defects, and secondary amenorrhea, and (5) multiple lipomas of the skin. A minority (probably <10 percent) come to medical attention with acromegaly, Cushing's syndrome, nonfunctional thyroid adenomas, hyperthyroidism, hepatomegaly (due to metastatic liver disease), or flushing (associated with the carcinoid syndrome).

Parathyroid involvement in MEN I may be asymptomatic for prolonged periods, although most patients eventually show signs of hyperparathyroidism. Tumors of the islet cells may elaborate excessive insulin or gastrin. Insulinomas cause hypoglycemia (Chap. 320), whereas excess gastrin secretion causes the Zollinger-Ellison syndrome with its multifocal or atypically located ulcers and massive hypersecretion of gastric acid. Symptoms may be identical with those of ordinary peptic ulcer, but there is a higher incidence of complications, including perforation, bleeding, and obstruction. Diarrhea is frequent, often with steatorrhea. Radiographic findings include giant gastric rugae, duodenal nodularity, ectopic ulcers in the esophagus, lower duodenum, and jejunum, and intestinal hyperperistalsis. Associated endocrine abnormalities consistent with the MEN syndrome are present in over one-quarter of patients with the Zollinger-Ellison syndrome and in half of the first-degree relatives of such patients. MEN I should be considered in a patient with the Zollinger-Ellison syndrome even when no other endocrine abnormalities are apparent.

Islet-cell tumors may also produce glucagon, vasoactive intestinal polypeptide (VIP), prostaglandins, adrenocorticotropic hormone (ACTH), parathyroid hormone, antidiuretic hormone (ADH), serotonin, somatostatin, calcitonin, and pancreatic polypeptide (also see Chap. 262). Glucagonomas cause hyperglycemia, weight loss, stomatitis, and a peculiar skin rash called *necrotizing migratory erythema*. VIP and prostaglandins have been implicated in the watery diarrhea (pancreatic cholera) syndrome sometimes seen in MEN I. Adrenal adenomas are common in MEN I but are rarely functional. Cushing's syndrome in patients with MEN I is usually of pituitary origin or due to ectopic ACTH or CRH secretion of an islet-cell or carcinoid tumor. Only a single aldosteronoma has been described in MEN I. Similarly, thyroid involvement is so variable and inconsistent that thyroid disease should not be considered intrinsic to MEN I. Other reported features of MEN I include small-intestinal and bronchial carcinoid tumors, schwannomas, thymomas, multiple lipomas, inclusion cysts, and cutaneous leiomyomas.

Patients with MEN I may develop symptoms at any age, but the condition presents rarely in childhood or after the age of 60. Affected individuals may demonstrate multiple endocrine system involvement simultaneously, or years may elapse between the discovery of one adenoma and the appearance of the next. Once the diagnosis is established, the patient must be surveyed periodically for appearance of new facets of the syndrome. By the same token, all first-degree relatives should be studied. A reasonable approach for screening relatives at risk is as follows: (1) review history for symptoms of peptic ulcer disease, hypoglycemia, renal calculi, lipomas, or hypopituitarism; (2) examine for multiple lipomas; (3) assay serum calcium, phosphorus, prolactin, and gastrin. Upper gastrointestinal series and sella turcica x-rays are of no proven value as screening tests. Serum pancreatic polypeptide determinations may be useful in centers where the assay is available.

The fundamental lesion in MEN I is unknown. Many classify MEN I as a neurocrestopathy thereby implicating faulty differentiation or regulation of the embryonic neural crest, which is the anlage of at least part of the endocrine system. The endocrine components of the neural crest have been classified into a subsystem of APUD cells, so named because of their capacity for amine precursor uptake and decarboxylation. The evidence supporting the contention that all APUD cells are derived from neural crest is not strong; instead, cells of diverse origin probably develop similar characteristics; i.e., they represent a structural-functional convergence. A circulating factor that has mitogenic factor for the parathyroid glands has been found in MEN I patients, suggesting a humoral cause for involvement of the parathyroids in the disorder. The MEN I gene has been tentatively mapped to chromosome 11.

The pituitary and parathyroid tumors in MEN I are usually benign, but pancreatic tumors are frequently malignant. Surgical removal of the affected gland is the usual therapy, although standard radiation techniques may be employed for the pituitary tumors, and bromocryptine is useful in prolactinomas. Hyperparathyroidism may be due to a single adenoma, but diffuse hyperplasia of more than one gland is more common. Since new adenomas may arise later, some have advocated removal of all the parathyroid glands with transplantation of extirpated fragments into the thigh or forearm, where they can be easily removed should hyperparathyroidism recur. Successful transplantation obviates the need for long-term therapy of hypoparathyroidism. In hypergastrinemia due to islet-cell lesions, total gastrectomy has been used to prevent recurrent peptic ulcers, and in rare cases distant metastases have regressed after this procedure. Histamine-2-receptor antagonists are efficacious in controlling the hyperacidity and diarrhea seen with hypergastrinemia.

MULTIPLE ENDOCRINE NEOPLASIA, TYPE IIa (MEN IIa OR MEN II) MEN IIa, also known as the *Sipple syndrome,* consists of pheochromocytoma (frequently bilateral and occasionally extraadrenal), medullary thyroid carcinoma (MTC), and, in about half of cases, parathyroid hyperplasia. MEN IIa can be related more directly to abnormal neural crest development than can MEN I, since both the adrenal medulla and the parafollicular or C cells of the thyroid originate in neural crest. However, there is no evidence that the parenchymal component of the parathyroid glands are so derived. The parafollicular cell elaborates calcitonin, the primary marker of medullary carcinoma of the thyroid. MTC is not common, comprising less than 10 percent of thyroid malignancies. At least 10 percent of MTC cases are familial, usually appearing as a component of MEN IIa or MEN IIb (see below). Medullary carcinoma may also occur in families without other associated endocrine dysfunction; this form is also transmitted as an autosomal dominant trait. MTC may present as a thyroidal mass or be clinically silent and undetectable by palpation or radioiodine scanning. The diagnosis is usually established by immunoassay of serum calcitonin, provided ectopic sites of calcitonin production can be excluded, e.g., breast, lung, and pancreatic islet-cell tumors. Occasionally, basal serum calcitonin levels are borderline in at-risk individuals, and measurement of plasma levels after calcium-pentagastrin infusion can be used to establish the diagnosis. MTC may on occasion secrete substances other than calcitonin, including ACTH, prolactin, serotonin, VIP, histamine, and various prostaglandins, resulting in a confusing array of symptoms.

The pheochromocytoma of MEN IIa may produce the classic signs of catecholamine excess as described in Chap. 318 or be asymptomatic. Approximately 5 percent of patients who present with pheochromocytomas also have MTC. Symptoms of hyperparathyroidism rarely bring the patient with MEN IIa to initial clinical attention.

Examination of cells from both the MTC and the pheochromocytoma components of MEN IIa using X-linked gene markers has led to the conclusion that the inherited defect produces multiple clones of abnormal cells; tumors then develop from a second mutation in the abnormal clone, accounting for the appearance of varying clinical patterns. The MEN IIa gene has been mapped to chromosome 10. Other tumors in MEN IIa include gliomas, glioblastomas, and meningiomas, all of which may be derived from the neural crest.

The age of the patient at the time of diagnosis varies from 2 to 67 years. C-cell hyperplasia of the thyroid may precede development of malignancy by many years, making early screening studies for calcitonin elevation mandatory in all family members at risk. The only effective therapy for MTC is surgical removal of the entire thyroid, as the tumors are multifocal in origin. Limited node dissection is often indicated since the cancer may progress slowly despite an aggressive histologic appearance, and prolonged survival is seen in patients with known metastatic disease. Serum calcitonin levels can be used to assess completeness of surgical removal of the tumor and in concert with selective venous catheterization may be utilized to locate metastases that are surgically accessible. Neither standard radioiodine nor x-ray therapy is helpful in disseminated medullary thyroid cancer, and chemotherapy has been of limited value (see Chap. 316). The pheochromocytomas are usually benign and are also treated surgically. Unresectable malignant pheochromocytoma requires long-term sympathetic blockade. A new radiopharmaceutical, *meta*-iodobenzyl guanidine, shows promise as both a diagnostic and a therapeutic agent.

MULTIPLE ENDOCRINE NEOPLASIA, TYPE IIb (MEN IIb OR MEN III) MEN IIb also consists of medullary thyroid carcinoma and pheochromocytoma, but affected individuals have striking dysmorphic features such as neuromas of the conjunctival, labial, and buccal mucosa, the tongue, the larynx, and the gastrointestinal tract; hence the alternate designation of the condition as the *mucosal neuroma syndrome*. Other physical findings include enlarged corneal nerves, "blubbery" lips, soft-tissue prognathism, and a habitus resembling that seen in the Marfan syndrome with hypotonia, lax joints, kyphoscoliosis, genu valgus, and pes cavus. The patients may have café au lait spots or a diffuse lentiginous type of skin pigmentation along with cutaneous neuromas or neurofibromas. Megacolon may occur.

MEN IIb and MEN IIa appear to be distinct syndromes. For example, both parathyroid hyperplasia and production of hormones other than calcitonin by MTC are rare in MEN IIb. The mean survival of patients with MEN IIb is around 30 years compared with 60 years for those with MEN IIa, suggesting a more malignant course in the former disorder, although histologically the thyroid tumors appear to be identical. As with MEN IIa treatment of the medullary carcinoma is surgical. The unusual physical features of MEN IIb should immediately suggest the diagnosis of underlying thyroid malignancy. MTC has been documented in asymptomatic children with MEN IIb, and C-cell hyperplasia has been found at operation as early as 15 months of age. Clinically, the associated pheochromocytomas behave as expected (Chap. 318). The MEN IIb gene has not been mapped.

McCUNE-ALBRIGHT SYNDROME This condition is characterized by the triad of polyostotic fibrous dysplasia, café au lait spots, and isosexual precocity, the latter occurring predominantly but not exclusively in females. The isosexual precocity may be hypothalamic in origin, but gonadotropin-independent ovarian function has been implicated in some cases (see Chap. 322). Cushing's syndrome, gigantism or acromegaly, and hyperprolactinemia may also occur in affected patients. The Cushing's syndrome may result from abnormal ACTH production or adrenal adenomas. Nodular toxic goiter and pheochromocytoma have also been reported. The bone lesion resembles that seen in hyperparathyroidism, and parathyroid hyperplasia has been described histologically but not clinically. The condition is usually sporadic, but pedigrees compatible with autosomal dominant inheritance have been seen. The cause of the condition is unknown (see Chap. 345).

SYNDROMES WITH MULTISYSTEM HYPOFUNCTION

POLYGLANDULAR AUTOIMMUNE SYNDROME TYPE I (CANDIDIASIS-ENDOCRINOPATHY SYNDROME) Features that differentiate this autoimmune condition from polyglandular autoimmune syndrome type II (see below) include childhood onset and extensive mucocutaneous monilial infection that becomes evident shortly after birth. Hypoparathyroidism is common, and adrenal insufficiency may develop acutely. Diabetes is rare. Organ-specific antibodies against a variety of endocrine glands may be detected early, and pernicious anemia, sprue, chronic active hepatitis, and membranoproliferative glomerulonephritis have been seen. Defective cellular immunity to *Candida albicans* is present; some have more generalized anergy. A cause-and-effect relationship between the monilial infection and the endocrinopathy has not been established. The disorder has occurred in sibs, occasionally from consanguineous unions, and the disease may be inherited as an autosomal recessive trait. No association with the HLA system has been demonstrated, but affected individuals may have a deficiency of immunoglobulin A and hypergammaglobulinemia. Suppressor T-cell function may be defective, but the immune profile can be variable even in sibs. The fungal infection is usually refractory to conventional chemotherapeutic drugs, although partial remission has been reported with a combination of ketoconazole and transfer factor. Amelioration of the candidiasis in no way affects the endocrinopathy, and conventional replacement therapy is required.

POLYGLANDULAR AUTOIMMUNE SYNDROME TYPE II (SCHMIDT SYNDROME) (See also Chaps. 316 and 317) This polyglandular deficiency state was first described by Schmidt in patients with both Addison's disease and lymphocytic thyroiditis. This syndrome has subsequently been expanded to include any combination of adrenal insufficiency, lymphocytic thyroiditis, hypoparathyroidism, and gonadal failure. Diabetes mellitus is frequent. The manifestations may be so extensive as to simulate panhypopituitarism; rarely, true pituitary deficiency has been described. The first evidence of endocrinopathy generally appears in adult life. The most significant laboratory feature, in addition to the low levels of circulating hormones, is the presence of antibodies to one or more endocrine glands. The antibodies may be directed against a clinically normal gland, but with time hypofunction usually supervenes. Additional evidence for an immune pathogenesis is provided by the increased frequency of antibodies to parietal cells of the stomach, with or without overt achlorhydria or pernicious anemia, and the presence of other disorders felt to have an autoimmune basis such as sprue, vitiligo, myasthenia gravis, pure red cell aplasia, and antibody-mediated immunoglobulin A deficiency. Hyperthyroidism may complicate the clinical picture.

The majority of affected individuals are female, and most cases are sporadic. A few reports have noted multiple affected family members, suggesting a genetic basis. Members of these families who show no endocrine disability frequently have serologic abnormalities indicative of a disturbance in immune function. Many of the component endocrine disorders in this syndrome are associated with the presence of certain HLA antigens, notably HLA-B8 and -Dw3 (in white populations). Other racial groups show different associations, e.g., hyperthyroidism with HLA-Bw35 in the Japanese. Because of this association it has been postulated that the basic lesion may reside in a mutation of an inherited immunologic mechanism. For example, a selective immunodeficient state might render an individual unduly susceptible to certain environmental antigens (e.g., viruses) that have a predilection for the endocrine system. Cell lysis or damage could result in release of intracellular contents and lead to development of autoantibodies. Such autoantibodies would not necessarily be pathogenic but could represent secondary phenomena, important as markers of potential clinical disease. Alternatively, the defect could reside in a genetically determined defect in suppressor T cells with consequent inadequate suppression of antibody synthesis. The syndrome is probably etiologically heterogeneous, and several pathogenetic mechanisms may be operative. At present, treatment is confined to providing hormone replacement.

LIPODYSTROPHIC SYNDROMES The lipodystrophic syndromes are described in Chap. 338. Insulin-resistant diabetes mellitus is common and may be associated with hyperlipoproteinemia, elevated growth hormone levels, and an increased incidence of polycystic ovarian disease.

DIABETES MELLITUS, DIABETES INSIPIDUS, AND OPTIC ATROPHY (WOLFRAM SYNDROME) This clinical triad has been noted in sibs and likely constitutes a rare autosomal recessive defect. Nerve deafness, usually mild, may also occur. The diabetes mellitus is of the early-onset insulin-dependent type. The diabetes insipidus usually appears prior to age 20. The varying manifestations are difficult to reconcile, and treatment requires replacement of the missing hormones.

OBESITY-HYPOGONADISM SYNDROMES A number of seemingly discrete entities share obesity, generally with frank diabetes mellitus, and hypogonadism that may be either primary or secondary. The *Laurence-Moon-Biedl syndrome* features retinitis pigmentosa, polydactyly, mental retardation, and renal anomalies along with obesity, hypogonadotropic hypogonadism, and in some patients, diabetes mellitus. There is sufficient resemblance between this syndrome and the *Alström syndrome* (retinitis pigmentosa, nerve deafness, diabetes mellitus, and primary gonadal failure) to cause

TABLE 325-1 Disorders with common polyglandular manifestations

		Type of endocrine involvement						
Condition	Clinical features	Hypothalamic-pituitary	Thyroid	Parathyroid	Pancreas	Adrenal	Gonads	Inheritance
Ataxia-telangiectasia	Early ataxia Oculocutaneous telangiectasia Immunologic deficiency	?Variably decreased pituitary reserve			Diabetes mellitus	Cortical hypoplasia	Dysgenetic gonads; gonadoblastomas later in females	Autosomal recessive
Pseudohypoparathyroidism	Short stature Short metacarpals and metatarsals Round facies Ectopic calcification	Variable deficiency of all pituitary hormones, including prolactin	Hypo- or hyperthyroidism	Elevated parathyroid hormone levels with either normo- or hypocalcemia	Diabetes mellitus		Ovarian failure	Probable X-linked dominant; heterogeneous
Myotonic dystrophy	Muscular dystrophy Premature baldness Mental retardation	Gonadotropin, growth hormone abnormalities, related to central integrative defect (?)	Hypothyroidism		Diabetes mellitus		Primary failure	Autosomal dominant
Noonan syndrome	Short stature Ptosis Webbed neck Pulmonary stenosis	Gonadotropin deficiency	Thyroiditis				Primary failure	Autosomal dominant
Fanconi syndrome	Short stature Bone marrow hypoplasia Abnormal skin pigmentation Radius malformations	Panhypopituitarism			Diabetes mellitus	Adrenal atrophy	Gonadal atrophy	Autosomal recessive
Werner syndrome	Premature aging of all organ systems Atrophic skin Cataracts Early osteoporosis		Papillary carcinoma		Diabetes mellitus		Gonadal atrophy	Autosomal recessive

frequent diagnostic confusion. Both are autosomal recessive disorders. However, polydactyly and mental retardation do not occur in the Alström syndrome. A similar condition is the *Biemond syndrome* in which obesity, diabetes mellitus, secondary hypogonadism, and postaxial polydactyly are combined with iris colobomata rather than pigmentary retinopathy. Patients with the *Prader-Willi syndrome* (obesity, hypogonadism, hypotonia, mental retardation) also have diabetes mellitus of the maturity-onset type. A genetic basis has not been established for the Biemond or the Prader-Willi syndromes. A small deletion of chromosome 15 is present in some patients with the latter disorder.

CHROMOSOMAL DISORDERS WITH ENDOCRINE DEFICIENCY (See also Chaps. 7 and 324) Patients with gonadal dysgenesis have hypogonadism and an increased incidence of diabetes mellitus and thyroiditis, thought to be on an autoimmune basis. In the Klinefelter syndrome an increased frequency of diabetes mellitus may occur along with gonadal failure. In the Down syndrome hypogonadism is probably universal in males, and menstrual irregularities and early menopause are common in women; in addition, increased prevalences of lymphocytic thyroiditis and diabetes mellitus have been reported.

OTHER CONDITIONS WITH MULTISYSTEM MANIFESTATIONS There are a number of other rare conditions in which involvement of more than one endocrine gland has been recorded often enough to constitute a significant facet of the syndrome. Some, like neurofibromatosis (von Recklinghausen's disease) and tuberous sclerosis, may show either hypo- or hyperfunction of endocrine glands because of interference with central regulatory mechanisms caused by the brain tumors characteristic of the diseases. By the same token, pheochromocytomas and carcinoid tumors may occur in neurofibromatosis because these tissues are ultimately derived from the same embryonic source.

Table 325-1 lists some additional conditions in which disorders of multiple endocrine systems have been seen. It is noteworthy that both primary and secondary failures have been reported within the diagnostic confines of the same syndrome. For example, both gonadotropin deficiency and primary testicular atrophy have been documented in patients with the Noonan syndrome and in unaffected members of the same families. Whenever a clinical condition like diabetes mellitus occurs in such distinct entities as myotonic dystrophy and ataxia-telangiectasia, the molecular mechanisms underlying the disease are probably heterogeneous. A better understanding of the genetic defect would provide insight into the function of the endocrine system.

REFERENCES

BRANDI ML et al: Parathyroid mitogenic activity in plasma from patients with familial multiple endocrine neoplasia type 1. N Engl J Med 314:1287, 1986

FARID NR (ed): *Immunogenetics of Endocrine Disorders*. New York, Liss, 1988

LEE PA et al: McCune-Albright syndrome. Long-term follow-up. JAMA 256:2980, 1986

LIPS CJM et al: Multiple endocrine neoplasia syndromes. CRC Crit Rev Oncol/Hematol 2:117, 1984

NEUFELD M et al: Two types of autoimmune Addison's disease associated with different polyglandular autoimmune syndromes. Medicine 60:355, 1981

RIMOIN DL, ROTTER JI: Genetic syndromes associated with diabetes mellitus and glucose intolerance, in *The Genetics of Diabetes Mellitus*, J Köbberling, R Tattersall (eds). New York, Academic, 1982, pp 149–181

section 2 Disorders of intermediary metabolism

326 THE HYPERLIPOPROTEINEMIAS AND OTHER DISORDERS OF LIPID METABOLISM

MICHAEL S. BROWN / JOSEPH L. GOLDSTEIN

The *hyperlipoproteinemias* are disturbances of lipid transport that result from accelerated synthesis or retarded degradation of lipoproteins that transport cholesterol and triglycerides through plasma. Elevated plasma lipoprotein levels are important clinically because they can cause two life-threatening diseases: atherosclerosis and pancreatitis. A reduction in cholesterol-carrying lipoproteins, achieved by diet and drugs, reduces the risk of myocardial infarction in subjects with hyperlipoproteinemia. Some hyperlipoproteinemias are the direct result of *primary* defects in the synthesis or degradation of lipoprotein particles. Other hyperlipoproteinemias are *secondary*, that is, the elevated plasma lipoprotein level occurs as part of a constellation of abnormalities caused by an underlying disorder in a related metabolic system, such as thyroid hormone deficiency or insulin deficiency. The primary hyperlipoproteinemias can be divided into two broad categories: (1) *single-gene disorders* that are transmitted by simple dominant or recessive mechanisms and (2) *multifactorial disorders* with complex inheritance patterns in which multiple variant genes, each having a subtle effect, interact with environmental factors to produce varying degrees of hyperlipoproteinemia in members of a family.

ROLE OF LIPOPROTEINS IN LIPID TRANSPORT The lipoproteins are globular particles of high molecular weight that transport nonpolar lipids (primarily *triglycerides* and *cholesteryl esters*) through the plasma. A general model for the structure of a lipoprotein particle is shown in Fig. 326-1. Each lipoprotein particle contains a nonpolar *core*, in which many molecules of hydrophobic lipid are packed to form an oil droplet. This hydrophobic core, which accounts for most of the mass of the particle, consists of triglycerides and cholesteryl esters in varying proportions. Surrounding the core is a polar *surface coat* of phospholipids that stabilize the lipoprotein particle so that it can remain in solution in the plasma. In addition to phospholipids, the polar coat contains small amounts of unesterified cholesterol. Each lipoprotein particle also contains specific proteins (termed *apoproteins*) that are exposed at the surface. The apoproteins bind to specific enzymes or transport proteins on cell membranes, thus directing the lipoprotein to its sites of metabolism.

Table 326-1 describes the characteristics of the five major classes of lipoproteins that normally circulate in human plasma. These lipoprotein classes differ in the composition of the nonpolar lipids in the core; in the composition of the apoproteins; and in density, size, and electrophoretic mobility.

Lipid transport: The exogenous pathway Figure 326-2 shows the pathways by which lipoproteins transport lipids in plasma. The largest amounts of lipoproteins are involved in the transport of dietary fat, which amounts to more than 100 g triglyceride and about 1 g

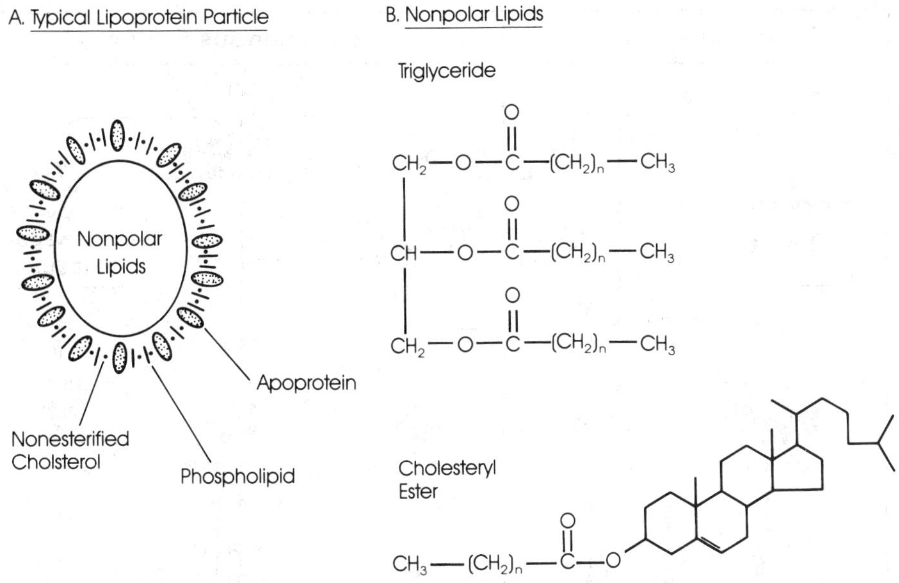

FIGURE 326-1 *A*. Diagrammatic representation of the structure of a typical plasma lipoprotein particle. The *core* of the spherical lipoprotein particle is composed of two nonpolar lipids, triglyceride and cholesteryl ester, which are present in different lipoproteins in varying amounts. The nonpolar core is surrounded by a *surface coat* composed primarily of phospholipids. Apoproteins are exposed at the surface and extend into the core. Variable amounts of unesterified cholesterol are interdigitated with the phospholipids of the surface coat. The qualitative composition of each of the five major classes of lipoprotein particles in human plasma is summarized in Table 326-1. *B*. Structures of the two nonpolar lipids, triglyceride and cholesteryl ester. In order for these nonpolar lipids to be assimilated into tissues, the ester bonds between the fatty acids and either glycerol (triglycerides) or cholesterol (cholesteryl esters) must be broken by lipoprotein lipase and the lysosomal cholesterol esterase, respectively.

cholesterol per day. Within intestinal epithelial cells, dietary triglycerides and cholesterol are incorporated into large lipoprotein particles called *chylomicrons*. The chylomicrons are secreted into the intestinal lymph and pass into the general circulation for transport to the capillaries of adipose tissue and skeletal muscle, where they adhere to binding sites on the capillary walls. While bound to these endothelial surfaces, the chylomicrons are exposed to the enzyme *lipoprotein lipase*. The chylomicrons contain an apoprotein, apoprotein CII, that activates the lipase, liberating free fatty acids and monoglycerides (Fig. 326-3). The fatty acids pass through the endothelial cells and enter the underlying adipocytes or muscle cells, where they are either reesterified to triglycerides or oxidized.

After the core triglycerides have been removed, the remainder of the chylomicron dissociates from the capillary endothelium and reenters the circulation. It has now been transformed into a particle that is relatively poor in triglyceride and enriched in cholesteryl esters. It has also undergone an exchange of apoproteins with other plasma lipoproteins. The net result is the conversion of the chylomicron to a *chylomicron remnant particle,* enriched in cholesteryl esters and apoproteins B48 and E. This remnant travels to the liver, where it is taken up with great efficiency. This uptake is mediated by the binding of apoprotein E to specific receptors, called *chylomicron remnant receptors,* on the surface of the hepatocytes. The surface-bound remnants are taken into the cell and degraded within lysosomes by a process called receptor-mediated endocytosis (Fig. 326-3). The overall result of the chylomicron transport process is to deliver dietary triglyceride to adipose tissue and cholesterol to the liver.

Some of the cholesterol that reaches the liver is converted to bile acids, which are excreted into the intestine to act as detergents and facilitate the absorption of dietary fat. In addition, some cholesterol is excreted into the bile without metabolism to bile acids. The liver also distributes cholesterol to other tissues by the endogenous pathway, which is discussed below.

Lipid transport: The endogenous pathway Triglyceride synthesis in the liver is enhanced when the diet contains excess carbohydrates. The liver converts the carbohydrate to fatty acids, esterifies the fatty acids with glycerol to form triglycerides, and secretes the triglyceride into the bloodstream in the core of *very low density lipoprotein (VLDL)*. The VLDL particles are relatively large, carry 5 to 10 times more triglycerides than cholesteryl esters, and contain a form of apoprotein B, designated B100, that differs from the apoprotein B48 of chylomicrons (Table 326-1).

The VLDL particles are transported to tissue capillaries, where they interact with the same lipoprotein lipase enzyme that catabolizes chylomicrons. The core triglycerides of the VLDL are hydrolyzed, and the fatty acids are used for triglyceride synthesis within adipose tissue. The remnants generated from the action of lipoprotein-lipase on VLDL are designated *intermediate-density lipoprotein (IDL)*. A portion of the IDL particles are catabolized by the liver through binding to receptors called *low-density lipoprotein (LDL) receptors,* which are distinct from the chylomicron remnant receptors. The remaining IDL remain in plasma, where they undergo a further transformation in which nearly all the residual triglycerides are removed. During this conversion, all the apoproteins are removed from the particle with the exception of apoprotein B100. The result is the transformation of the IDL particle into cholesterol-rich LDL. The core of LDL is composed almost entirely of cholesteryl esters, and the surface coat contains only one apoprotein, apoprotein B100. In humans a relatively high fraction of IDL escapes hepatic uptake, and consequently humans have relatively high circulating levels of LDL. Indeed, about three-fourths of the total cholesterol in normal human plasma is contained within LDL particles.

One function of LDL is to supply cholesterol to a variety of extrahepatic parenchymal cells, such as adrenal cortical cells, lymphocytes, and renal cells. These cells have *LDL receptors* localized on the cell surface. LDL that binds to this receptor is taken up by

TABLE 326-1 Characteristics of the major classes of lipoproteins in human plasma

Lipoprotein class	Major lipids	Apoproteins	Density, g/mL	Diameter, nm	Electrophoretic mobility
Chylomicrons and remnants	Dietary triglycerides	AI, AII, B48, CI, CII, CIII, E	<1.006	800–5000	Remains at origin
VLDL	Endogenous triglycerides	B48, CI, CII, CIII, E	<1.006	300–800	Pre-β
IDL	Cholesteryl esters, triglycerides	B100, CIII, E	<1.019	250–350	Slow pre-β
LDL	Cholesteryl esters	B100	1.019–1.063	180–280	β
HDL	Cholesteryl esters	AI, AII	1.063–1.210	50–120	α

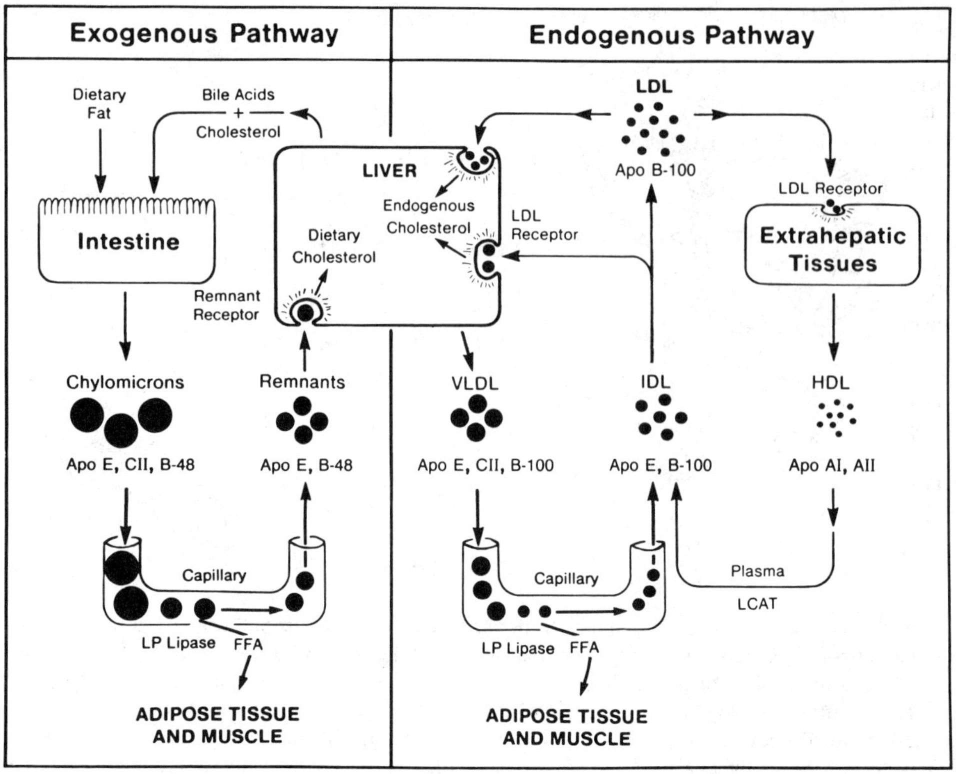

FIGURE 326-2 Model for plasma triglyceride and cholesterol transport in humans. The details of this model are described in the text. VLDL, very low density lipoprotein; IDL, intermediate-density lipoprotein; LDL, low-density lipoprotein; HDL, high-density lipoprotein; LCAT, lecithin:cholesterol acyltransferase; LP lipase, lipoprotein lipase; FFA, free fatty acids. The major apoprotein for each class of lipoproteins is shown. Other apoproteins are also present, and these are listed in Table 326-1.

receptor-mediated endocytosis and digested by lysosomes within the cells (Fig. 326-3). The cholesteryl esters of LDL are hydrolyzed by a lysosomal cholesteryl esterase (acid lipase), and the liberated cholesterol is used for membrane synthesis, as a precursor for steroid hormone synthesis, and as a regulatory molecule that suppresses the synthesis of new LDL receptors. Like extrahepatic tissues, the liver also has abundant LDL receptors; it uses the LDL-cholesterol for synthesis of bile acids and for generation of free cholesterol, which is secreted into the bile. In humans 70 to 80 percent of LDL is removed from the plasma each day by the LDL receptor pathway. Much of the remainder is degraded by a scavenger cell system in phagocytic cells in the reticuloendothelial system. In contrast to the receptor-mediated pathway for LDL degradation, the scavenger cell pathway is thought to function solely to degrade LDL when the lipoprotein reaches high concentrations in plasma rather than to supply cholesterol to cells.

As the membranes of parenchymal and scavenger cells undergo turnover and as cells die and are renewed, unesterified cholesterol is released into plasma, where it binds initially to *high-density lipoprotein* (*HDL*). This unesterified cholesterol is then coupled to a fatty acid in an esterification reaction catalyzed by the plasma enzyme *lecithin:cholesterol acyltransferase* (*LCAT*). The cholesteryl esters that are formed on the surface of HDL are transferred to VLDL and eventually appear in LDL. This establishes a cycle by which LDL delivers cholesterol to extrahepatic cells and by which cholesterol is returned to LDL from extrahepatic cells via HDL. Most of the cholesterol released from extrahepatic tissues is transported to the liver for excretion in the bile.

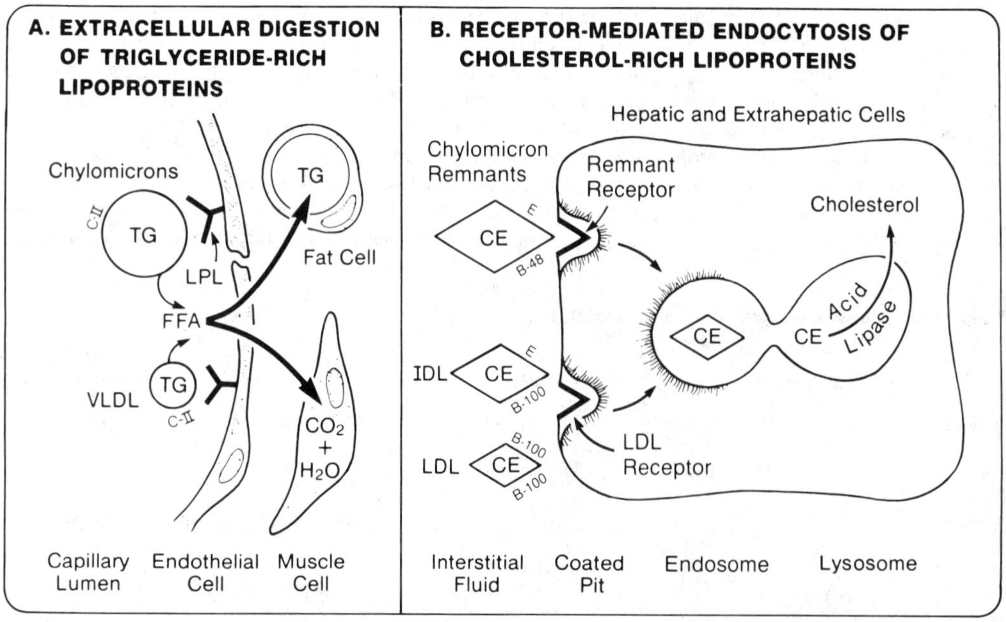

FIGURE 326-3 Comparison of the mechanisms by which triglyceride-rich lipoproteins and cholesterol-rich lipoproteins deliver their core lipids to target tissues. Triglycerides are hydrolyzed by an extracellular enzyme (LPL) that is attached to endothelial cells and operates at the endothelial surface. Cholesteryl esters are hydrolyzed by an intracellular enzyme, acid lipase, that is located in lysosomes and cleaves the esters that enter cells via receptor-mediated endocytosis. TG, triglycerides; LPL, lipoprotein lipase; VLDL, very low density lipoproteins; CE, cholesteryl esters; IDL, intermediate-density lipoproteins; LDL, low-density lipoproteins; FFA, free fatty acid. The apoproteins responsible for the interactions (CII, B, and E) are indicated.

TABLE 326-2 Patterns of lipoprotein elevation in plasma (lipoprotein types)

Lipoprotein pattern	Major elevation in plasma: Lipoprotein	Lipid
Type 1	Chylomicrons	Triglycerides
Type 2a	LDL	Cholesterol
Type 2b	LDL and VLDL	Cholesterol and triglycerides
Type 3	Chylomicron remnants and IDL	Triglycerides and cholesterol
Type 4	VLDL	Triglycerides
Type 5	VLDL and chylomicrons	Triglycerides and cholesterol

DIAGNOSIS OF HYPERLIPOPROTEINEMIA A variety of diseases cause elevations in the concentrations of one or more lipoprotein classes in plasma. In general, these abnormalities are detected by the finding of an elevated concentration of triglycerides or cholesterol in fasting plasma, a condition called *hyperlipidemia*. The value for plasma cholesterol represents the total cholesterol, which includes both cholesteryl esters and unesterified cholesterol. The plasma cholesterol and triglyceride levels provide information regarding the nature of the lipoprotein particle that is increased. An isolated elevation in plasma triglycerides indicates that the concentrations of chylomicrons or VLDL are increased. On the other hand, an isolated elevation of plasma cholesterol nearly always indicates that the concentration of LDL is increased. Frequently, both triglycerides and cholesterol are elevated. Such a combined abnormality may be produced by a marked elevation in chylomicrons or VLDL, in which case the ratio of triglyceride to cholesterol in plasma will be greater than 5:1. Alternatively, there may be an elevation of both VLDL and LDL, in which case the triglyceride/cholesterol ratio in plasma is usually less than 5:1.

The definition of hyperlipoproteinemia is arbitrary because plasma lipid and lipoprotein levels exhibit a bell-shaped distribution in the population, without clear separation between normal and abnormal values. Since lipoprotein concentrations are influenced by diet and other environmental factors, standards must be established for the population under consideration. Usually, arbitrary statistical limits of normal concentrations are selected, based on the examination of a large number of healthy-appearing subjects of different ages. The usual cut-off limit is the upper 5 to 10 percent of values (i.e., the 90th to 95th percentile values). However, analysis of blood lipid levels in individuals from industrialized and more agrarian cultures indicates that lipid and lipoprotein concentrations that are "normal" in a statistical sense are not necessarily healthy. As a working rule, hyperlipoproteinemia is considered to be present whenever the plasma cholesterol level exceeds 5.2 mmol/L (200 mg/dL) or the triglyceride level exceeds 2.2 mmol/L (200 mg/dL).

The various combinations of elevated lipoproteins that occur in disease states have been divided into six lipoprotein types or patterns (Table 326-2). Most of the lipoprotein types can be caused by several different genetic diseases (Table 326-3); conversely, some genetic diseases can produce more than one lipoprotein type. In addition, each of the abnormal lipoprotein types can occur as a secondary consequence of another metabolic disease (Table 326-4). Hence, the lipoprotein type must be considered a shorthand notation to describe an abnormal lipoprotein pattern in plasma and not a designation of a specific disease.

Ordinarily, the simple measurement of plasma lipid levels, coupled with a clinical assessment, is sufficient to classify the type of lipoprotein abnormality present (Table 326-2). Occasionally, electrophoresis of the plasma on agarose gels is useful either when an elevation in remnant particles is suspected (type 3 lipoprotein pattern giving a "broad beta" band on electrophoresis) or when chylomicronemia is a possibility (type 1 pattern). When the total cholesterol level exceeds 6.2 mmol/L (240 mg/dL), HDL levels should be measured, since low levels of this lipoprotein class are statistically associated with an increased risk of myocardial infarction (see Chap. 195). The level of HDL can be estimated in clinical laboratories using standardized lipoprotein separation techniques.

THERAPEUTIC APPROACHES The first approach for treatment of all hyperlipoproteinemias is dietary. Individuals who are overweight should be placed on a weight-reducing regimen. Virtually all patients with hyperlipoproteinemia, either primary or secondary, can be treated with a single diet that is low in cholesterol and saturated animal fats and relatively (but not absolutely) high in polyunsaturated vegetable oils, which reduce concentrations of plasma LDL.

The second therapeutic aim is to eliminate aggravating factors, such as diabetes mellitus, alcoholism, or hypothyroidism. Patients with hyperlipoproteinemia should also be encouraged to reduce all other risk factors that predispose to atherosclerosis. These include cessation of smoking, treatment of hypertension, maintenance of a good exercise and physical fitness program, and control of blood glucose in subjects with diabetes mellitus (see Chap. 195).

The final aspect of therapy involves the use of drugs that lower plasma concentrations of lipoproteins, either by decreasing their production or by increasing their removal from plasma. The drugs available for this purpose are discussed below.

TABLE 326-3 Characteristics of the primary hyperlipoproteinemias resulting from single-gene mutations

Genetic disorder	Primary biochemical defect	Plasma lipoprotein elevation (pattern)	Typical clinical findings	Lipoprotein pattern in affected relatives	Drug therapy: First choice	Drug therapy: Other
Familial lipoprotein lipase deficiency	Deficiency of lipoprotein lipase	Chylomicrons (1)	Eruptive xanthomas, pancreatitis	1	None	None
Familial apoprotein CII deficiency	Deficiency of apoprotein CII	Chylomicrons and VLDL (1 or 5)	Pancreatitis	1 or 5	None	None
Familial type 3 hyperlipoproteinemia	Abnormal apoprotein E of VLDL	Chylomicron remnants and IDL (3)		3, 2a, 2b, or 4	Gemfibrozil; clofibrate	Nicotinic acid
Familial hypercholesterolemia	Deficiency of LDL receptor	LDL (2a, rarely 2b)	Palmar and tuberous xanthomas; premature atherosclerosis	2a (rarely 2b)	Bile acid–binding resin plus lovastatin	Nicotinic acid; probucol
Familial hypertriglyceridemia	Unknown	VLDL (rarely chylomicrons) (4, rarely 5)	Tendon xanthomas; premature atherosclerosis	4 (rarely 5)	Gemfibrozil; nicotinic acid	Clofibrate
Multiple lipoprotein-type hyperlipidemia (familial combined hyperlipidemia)	Unknown	LDL and VLDL (2a, 2b, or 4, rarely 5)	(Eruptive xanthomas; premature atherosclerosis)	2a, 2b, or 4 (rarely 5)	Gemfibrozil; nicotinic acid	Lovastatin

TABLE 326-4 Clinical disorders associated with secondary hyperlipoproteinemia

Underlying disorder	Plasma lipoprotein elevation: Chylomicrons	IDL	VLDL	LDL	Lipoprotein type	Proposed mechanism for hyperlipoproteinemia	Associated abnormality of carbohydrate metabolism
ENDOCRINE AND METABOLIC							
Diabetes mellitus	+		+++		4 (rarely 5)	Increased secretion of VLDL; Decreased catabolism of VLDL and chylomicrons due to reduced lipoprotein lipase activity	Insulin deficiency or resistance
von Gierke's disease (glycogen storage disease, type I)	+		+++		4 (rarely 5)	Increased secretion of VLDL; Decreased catabolism of VLDL and chylomicrons due to reduced lipoprotein lipase activity	Hypoglycemia with decreased insulin secretion
Lipodystrophies (congenital and acquired forms)			++		4	Increased secretion of VLDL	Insulin resistance
Cushing's syndrome			+	++	2a or 2b	Increased secretion of VLDL with conversion to LDL	Insulin resistance
Sexual ateliotic dwarfism (isolated growth hormone deficiency)			++	++	2b	Increased secretion of VLDL with conversion to LDL	Insulin deficiency or resistance
Acromegaly			+		4	Increased secretion of VLDL	Insulin resistance
Hypothyroidism		+		+++	2a (rarely 3)	Decreased catabolism of VLDL and IDL	
Anorexia nervosa				++	2a	Reduced biliary excretion of cholesterol and bile acids	
Werner's syndrome				++	2a	Unknown	Insulin resistance
Acute intermittent porphyria				++	2a	Unknown	
DRUG-INDUCED							
Alcohol	+		+++		4 (rarely 5)	Increased secretion of VLDL in individuals genetically predisposed to hypertriglyceridemia	
Oral contraceptives	+		+++		4 (rarely 5)	Increased secretion of VLDL in individuals genetically predisposed to hypertriglyceridemia	Insulin resistance
Glucocorticoids			+	++	2a or 2b	Increased secretion of VLDL with conversion to LDL	Insulin resistance
RENAL							
Uremia			+++		4	Decreased catabolism of VLDL due to reduced lipoprotein lipase activity	Insulin resistance
Nephrotic syndrome			++	+++	2a or 2b	Increased secretion of VLDL; Direct secretion of LDL from liver; Decreased catabolism of VLDL and LDL	
HEPATIC							
Primary biliary cirrhosis and extrahepatic biliary obstruction					↑ Cholesterol; ↑ Phospholipids; ↑ Lipoprotein X	Diversion of biliary cholesterol and phospholipids into bloodstream	
Acute hepatitis (nonfulminant)			+++		4	Decreased hepatic secretion of lecithin: cholesterol acyltransferase (LCAT)	

TABLE 326-4 Clinical disorders associated with secondary hyperlipoproteinemia *(continued)*

Underlying disorder	Plasma lipoprotein elevation: Chylomicrons	IDL	VLDL	LDL	Lipoprotein type	Proposed mechanism for hyperlipoproteinemia	Associated abnormality of carbohydrate metabolism
HEPATIC *(continued)*							
Hepatoma				++	2a	Lack of feedback inhibition of hepatic cholesterol synthesis by dietary cholesterol	
IMMUNOLOGIC							
Systemic lupus erythematosus	++				1	Presence of IgG or IgM that binds heparin, thereby decreasing activity of lipoprotein lipase	
Monoclonal gammopathies (myeloma, macroglobulinemia, lymphoma)	++	++	++		3 or 4	Presence of IgG or IgM that forms immune complex with chylomicron remnants and/or VLDL, thereby decreasing their catabolism	
STRESS-INDUCED							
Emotional stress, acute myocardial infarction, extensive burns, acute gram-negative sepsis			++		4	Increased secretion and decreased catabolism of VLDL	

PRIMARY HYPERLIPOPROTEINEMIAS RESULTING FROM SINGLE-GENE MUTATIONS

FAMILIAL LIPOPROTEIN LIPASE DEFICIENCY This rare autosomal recessive disorder is attributable to the absence or marked reduction in the activity of the enzyme lipoprotein lipase. This deficiency leads to a metabolic block in the metabolism of chylomicrons, causing these lipoproteins to accumulate to massive levels in plasma.

Clinical features The disease usually presents in infancy or childhood with recurrent attacks of abdominal pain. The pain is caused by pancreatitis occurring as a consequence of the massive elevation of chylomicrons in plasma. Affected individuals intermittently develop eruptive xanthomas, small yellowish papules, frequently surrounded by an erythematous base, that appear predominantly on the buttocks and other pressure-sensitive surfaces. The xanthomas are caused by the deposition of large amounts of chylomicron triglycerides in cutaneous histiocytes. Triglycerides are also deposited in phagocytes of the reticuloendothelial system, producing hepatomegaly, splenomegaly, and foam cell infiltration of the bone marrow. When the level of chylomicrons in the blood is massively elevated [(i.e., plasma triglyceride level greater than 22 mmol/L (2000 mg/dL)], the blood appears pale and creamy and is said to be *lipemic*. When viewed with the ophthalmoscope, the retina is pale, and the retinal vessels are white, producing the appearance of lipemia retinalis. Despite the massive elevation of plasma triglycerides, accelerated atherosclerosis does not occur.

Pathogenesis Affected individuals are homozygous for a mutation that prevents normal expression of lipoprotein lipase activity. The primary genetic defect appears to involve the structure of the enzyme itself; the activator of lipoprotein lipase, apoprotein CII, is present in normal amounts. The parents are obligate heterozygotes for the lipoprotein lipase defect, but they are clinically normal. As a result of the deficiency of lipoprotein lipase in homozygotes, chylomicrons cannot be metabolized normally, and the level of chylomicrons in the blood rises to high levels after a fat meal. In normal individuals chylomicrons disappear from the blood after a 12-h fast. However, in affected patients high levels of chylomicrons are found in the plasma even after several days of fasting or ingestion of a fat-free diet.

The circulating chylomicrons inflame the pancreas when they pass through its capillaries. Within the capillary lumen in the pancreas, chylomicrons are exposed to small amounts of pancreatic lipase that leaks from the tissue. Partial hydrolysis of the triglycerides and phospholipids of the chylomicron produces toxic products, including fatty acids and lysolecithin, that break down tissue membranes, produce further leakage of lipase from the pancreatic acinar cells, and eventually cause fulminant pancreatitis.

Diagnosis The diagnosis of familial lipoprotein lipase deficiency is suggested by the finding of lipemic plasma in a young individual who has been fasting for at least 12 h. This lipemic plasma, when collected in the presence of EDTA, has a characteristic appearance after it has incubated overnight in a refrigerator at 4°C. A white layer of cream (which consists of chylomicrons) appears at the top of the tube. The layer beneath the cream is clear. The diagnosis of familial lipoprotein lipase deficiency is supported by the finding of a type 1 pattern on lipoprotein electrophoresis. It is confirmed by the demonstration that lipoprotein lipase levels in plasma fail to increase following the infusion of heparin. In normal individuals, intravenous heparin releases lipoprotein lipase from its binding sites within the capillary endothelium, and increased amounts of enzyme can then be assayed in the plasma. Gel electrophoresis of VLDL apoproteins in patients with lipoprotein lipase deficiency shows a normal amount of activator apoprotein CII, thus distinguishing these patients from those with the related disorder, familial apoprotein CII deficiency (see below).

Treatment The symptoms and signs of the disease recede when the patient is placed on a fat-free diet. Every attempt should be made to maintain the fasting plasma triglyceride level below 11 mmol/L (1000 mg/dL) to prevent pancreatitis. It has been found empirically that the chronic fat intake in affected adults must be less than 20 g/d to prevent symptomatic hyperlipemia. Since medium-chain triglycerides are not incorporated into chylomicrons, they have been employed to help achieve normal caloric intake. The diet should be supplemented with fat-soluble vitamins.

FAMILIAL APOPROTEIN CII DEFICIENCY This rare autosomal recessive disorder is due to the absence of apoprotein CII, an essential cofactor for lipoprotein lipase. Deficiency of this peptide creates a functional lipoprotein lipase deficiency, thus producing a syndrome that is similar but not identical to familial lipoprotein lipase deficiency (see above). Because of the apoprotein CII deficiency, lipoprotein lipase is not activated, and its two substrate lipoproteins, chylomicrons and VLDL, accumulate in the blood, thus causing hypertriglyceridemia (type 1 or type 5 lipoprotein pattern). The disorder is diagnosed in children or adults on the basis of recurrent attacks of pancreatitis or by milky plasma detected by chance. The diagnosis is made by showing an absence of apoprotein CII on gel electrophoresis of VLDL apoproteins. Transfusion of normal plasma (which contains abundant apoprotein CII) into the patient is followed by a dramatic fall in plasma triglyceride levels. Heterozygotes, who have 50 percent reduction in apoprotein CII levels, may exhibit slightly elevated triglyceride concentrations but do not have pancreatitis. Treatment involves use of a fat-restricted diet throughout life. In case of severe pancreatitis, transfusion of one or two units of normal plasma is helpful. As compared with patients with familial lipoprotein lipase deficiency, subjects with homozygous apoprotein CII deficiency are generally detected at a later age, accumulate more VLDL in their plasma, and rarely show cutaneous eruptive xanthomas. The reason for these clinical differences is not known.

FAMILIAL TYPE 3 HYPERLIPOPROTEINEMIA This is an inherited disorder in which the plasma concentrations of both cholesterol and triglycerides are elevated owing to the accumulation in plasma of remnant-like particles derived from the partial catabolism of VLDL. Also called familial dysbetalipoproteinemia, the disorder is transmitted by a single-gene mechanism, but its expression appears to require the presence of contributory environmental and/or genetic factors (discussed below).

Clinical features Affected individuals characteristically do not manifest hyperlipidemia or any clinical feature of the disease until after age 20. A unique clinical feature is the occurrence of two types of cutaneous xanthomas: xanthoma striata palmaris, which appear as orange or yellow discolorations of the palmar and digital creases, and tuberous or tuberoeruptive xanthomas, which are bulbous cutaneous xanthomas that may vary from pea to lemon size. The tuberous xanthomas are characteristically located over the elbows and knees. Xanthelasmas of the eyelids also occur but are not unique to this disorder (see "Familial Hypercholesterolemia" below).

Severe and fulminant atherosclerosis involves the coronary arteries, the internal carotids, and the abdominal aorta and its branches. The sequelae include premature myocardial infarctions, strokes, intermittent claudication, and gangrene of the lower extremities. Patients who develop clinical manifestations of this disorder often have hypothyroidism, obesity, or diabetes mellitus as aggravating factors.

Pathogenesis The hyperlipidemia is caused by the accumulation of large lipoprotein particles that contain both triglycerides and cholesteryl esters. These particles consist of chylomicron remnants produced from the catabolism of chylomicrons and IDL produced from the catabolism of VLDL through the action of lipoprotein lipase. In normal subjects, chylomicron remnant particles are rapidly taken up by the liver, and hence they are barely detectable in plasma. A portion of the IDL is also taken up by the liver while the rest is converted to LDL. In patients with type 3 hyperlipoproteinemia the uptake of IDL and chylomicron remnants by the liver is blocked, and these lipoproteins accumulate to high levels in plasma and tissues, producing xanthomas and atherosclerosis.

The mutation responsible for this disease involves the gene that encodes the structure of apoprotein E, a protein normally found in IDL and chylomicron remnants. This protein binds with very high affinity to both the chylomicron remnant receptor and the LDL receptor. Apoprotein E thus mediates the rapid uptake of chylomicron remnants and IDL by the liver. The gene for apoprotein E is polymorphic in the population. There are three common alleles, designated E^2, E^3, and E^4, with approximate frequencies of 0.12, 0.75, and 0.13 in the population. Each allele specifies a distinctive form of apoprotein E that differs from the others by a single amino acid substitution. This structural alteration allows each protein to be detected by isoelectric focusing. The three alleles create six genotypes: E^2/E^2, E^3/E^3, E^4/E^4, E^2/E^3, E^2/E^4, and E^3/E^4. Type 3 hyperlipoproteinemia occurs only in individuals who are homozygous for the E^2 allele (genotype, E^2/E^2). The protein produced by the E^2 allele is defective in its ability to bind to the liver receptors that mediate uptake of chylomicron remnants and IDL, as a result of which these particles accumulate in plasma.

The frequency of the E^2/E^2 genotype in the population is about 1 in 100. Yet the frequency of type 3 hyperlipoproteinemia is only about 1 in 10,000. Thus, only 1 percent of the individuals having genotype E^2/E^2 have symptomatic disease. It seems that most homozygotes for the E^2 allele are somehow able to compensate for the abnormal apoprotein E, because other apoproteins such as apoproteins B48 and B100 can also mediate binding to liver receptors, albeit less efficiently than apoprotein E. Familial type 3 hyperlipoproteinemia occurs only in those individuals who are homozygous for the E^2 allele and who are also unable to compensate for the abnormal function of the E protein. The inability to compensate may be caused by the independent inheritance of another defect in lipoprotein metabolism, such as familial hypercholesterolemia or multiple lipoprotein–type hyperlipoproteinemia (see below). When an individual is a heterozygote for one of these dominant diseases and is also homozygous for the E^2 allele, he or she expresses the syndrome of type 3 hyperlipoproteinemia. The expression of hyperlipoproteinemia is also brought out when an individual of genotype E^2/E^2 develops hypothyroidism, diabetes mellitus, or obesity. It should be emphasized that heterozygotes for the E^2 allele never show the clinical syndrome of familial type 3 hyperlipoproteinemia.

Diagnosis The diagnosis is suggested by the finding of palmar or tuberous xanthomas in a patient with elevated plasma levels of both cholesterol and triglyceride. Approximately 80 percent of symptomatic patients exhibit these xanthomas. The diagnosis is also suggested when a moderate elevation in the plasma concentration of both cholesterol and triglyceride occurs in such a way that the absolute concentrations of cholesterol and triglyceride are similar (e.g., the plasma cholesterol is about 7.8 mmol/L (300 mg/dL) and the triglyceride level is about 3.4 mmol/L (300 mg/dL). However, this finding does not always hold true and becomes especially unreliable when the disease is in severe exacerbation, in which case the plasma triglyceride tends to rise higher than the cholesterol.

The diagnosis is supported by the finding of a so-called broad beta band on lipoprotein electrophoresis (type 3 pattern). This appearance results from the presence of chylomicron remnants and IDL. The diagnosis can be established in specialized laboratories by two procedures. First, the plasma can be subjected to ultracentrifugation, and the chemical composition of the VLDL fraction can be measured. In affected patients, the VLDL fraction contains IDL and chylomicron remnants that have a relatively high ratio of cholesterol to triglyceride. Second, the diagnosis can be confirmed by the finding of homozygosity for the E^2 allele on isoelectric focusing of the proteins extracted from the remnant particles.

Treatment A vigorous search for occult hypothyroidism should be made, including measurement of plasma thyroid stimulating hormone (TSH) levels. If hypothyroidism exists, levothyroxine should be instituted. Patients who have hypothyroidism show a dramatic lowering of lipid levels with treatment. In addition, attempts should be made to control obesity and diabetes mellitus through diet and insulin treatment. If these measures are not successful, patients with type 3 hyperlipoproteinemia should be treated with a fibric acid, such as gemfibrozil or clofibrate. Affected patients usually show a dramatic and sustained reduction in plasma lipid levels when treated with these drugs. Nicotinic acid may be effective in the severely hyperlipidemic patient who does not respond to gemfibrozil or clofibrate.

FAMILIAL HYPERCHOLESTEROLEMIA This common autosomal dominant disorder affects approximately 1 in every 500 persons.

It is caused by a mutation in the gene for the LDL receptor. Heterozygotes manifest a two- to threefold elevation in the concentration of total plasma cholesterol which is attributable to an elevation in the level of LDL. Patients with two mutant LDL receptor genes (called familial hypercholesterolemia homozygotes) have six- to eightfold elevations in plasma LDL-cholesterol levels.

Clinical features Heterozygotes with familial hypercholesterolemia can be diagnosed at birth because their umbilical cord blood contains a two- to threefold increase in the concentration of LDL and hence a similar increase in total cholesterol. The elevated levels of plasma LDL persist throughout life, but symptoms typically do not develop until the third or fourth decade. The most important feature is the occurrence of premature and accelerated coronary atherosclerosis. Myocardial infarctions begin to occur in affected men in the third decade and peak in the fourth and fifth decades. By age 60, approximately 85 percent have experienced a myocardial infarction. In women the incidence of myocardial infarction is also increased, but the mean age of onset is delayed 10 years as compared with men. Heterozygotes for this disorder constitute about 5 percent of all patients who have a myocardial infarction.

Xanthomas of the tendons constitute the second major clinical manifestation of the heterozygous state. These xanthomas are nodular swellings that typically involve the Achilles and other tendons about the knee, elbow, and dorsum of the hand. They are formed by the deposition of LDL-derived cholesteryl esters in tissue macrophages. The macrophages are swollen with lipid droplets and form foam cells. Cholesterol is also deposited in the soft tissue of the eyelid, producing xanthelasma, and within the cornea, producing arcus corneae. Whereas tendon xanthomas are essentially diagnostic of familial hypercholesterolemia, xanthelasma and arcus corneae also occur in many adults with normal plasma lipid levels. The incidence of tendon xanthomas in familial hypercholesterolemia increases with age, and up to 75 percent of heterozygotes display this sign. The absence of tendon xanthomas does not rule out familial hypercholesterolemia.

Approximately 1 in 1 million persons in the general population inherits two copies of the familial hypercholesterolemia gene and is a homozygote for the disorder. These individuals have marked elevations in the plasma level of LDL from birth. A unique type of planar cutaneous xanthoma is often present at birth and always develops within the first 6 years of life. These xanthomas are raised, yellow, plaque-like lesions at points of cutaneous trauma, such as the knees, elbows, and buttocks. Xanthomas are almost always present in the interdigital webs of the hands, particularly between the thumb and index finger. Tendon xanthomas, arcus corneae, and xanthelasma are also characteristic. Coronary artery atherosclerosis frequently has its clinical onset before age 10, and myocardial infarction has been reported as early as 18 months of age. In addition, cholesterol deposition in the aortic valve may produce symptomatic aortic stenosis. Homozygotes usually succumb to the complications of myocardial infarction before age 20.

Obesity and diabetes mellitus do not occur with increased frequency in familial hypercholesterolemia. A slender body habitus is the rule.

Pathogenesis The primary defect resides in the gene for the LDL receptor. Studies of DNA from affected individuals suggest that at least 100 mutant alleles occur at this locus. These mutant alleles can be grouped into three classes. The most common, designated receptor-negative, specifies a gene product that is nonfunctional. The second most frequent mutant, designated receptor-defective, produces a receptor that has 1 to 10 percent of normal LDL binding activity. The third type, designated internalization-defective, produces a receptor that binds LDL normally but is unable to transport the receptor-bound lipoprotein into the cell. This rare allele produces the so-called internalization defect.

Phenotypic homozygotes possess two mutant alleles at the LDL receptor locus, and hence their cells show a total or near-total inability to bind or take up LDL. Heterozygotes have one normal allele and one mutant allele at the LDL receptor locus, and hence their cells are able to bind and take up LDL at approximately half the normal rate.

Because of the reduction in LDL receptor activity, LDL catabolism is blocked, and the level of LDL in plasma rises in a manner that is inversely proportional to the reduction in LDL receptors. In addition to the impaired catabolism of LDL, LDL production is increased. Enhanced production of LDL has been attributed to the lack of an LDL receptor on liver cells. The liver fails to remove IDL from the plasma normally, with the result that an increased amount of IDL is converted to LDL. This overproduction of LDL, together with its inefficient catabolism, accounts for the high concentrations in affected patients. The elevated LDL levels cause an increase in the uptake of LDL by scavenger cells, which accumulate at various sites in the body, producing xanthomas.

The accelerated coronary atherosclerosis in familial hypercholesterolemia results from the high LDL levels, which lead to an enhanced infiltration of LDL into the artery wall following episodes of endothelial damage. The large amounts of LDL that penetrate the artery wall cannot be cleared from the interstitial space by the scavenger cells, and atherosclerosis ultimately results. Some of the lipids in LDL may undergo oxidation when the lipoprotein enters the artery wall, and the resultant products may be toxic to endothelial cells, thereby accelerating the damage. High LDL levels may also act to accelerate platelet aggregation at sites of endothelial injury, thereby enhancing the growth of the atherosclerotic plaque (see Chap. 195).

Diagnosis The diagnosis of heterozygous familial hypercholesterolemia is suggested by the finding of an isolated elevation of plasma cholesterol, with a normal concentration of plasma triglycerides. Such an isolated elevation in plasma cholesterol is usually due to an elevation in the plasma concentration of LDL alone (type 2a pattern). However, most individuals in the general population with type 2a hyperlipoproteinemia do not have familial hypercholesterolemia. Rather, they have a form of polygenic hypercholesterolemia that puts them on the upper end of the bell-shaped curve for the general population (see "Polygenic Hypercholesterolemia" below). Type 2a hyperlipoproteinemia is also caused by multiple lipoprotein-type hyperlipidemia (discussed below). In addition, a variety of metabolic disorders, including hypothyroidism and nephrotic syndrome, can cause type 2a hyperlipoproteinemia (Table 326-4).

Among individuals who have a type 2a lipoprotein pattern, those with heterozygous familial hypercholesterolemia can be distinguished from those with polygenic hypercholesterolemia and multiple lipoprotein-type hyperlipidemia on several grounds. (1) In familial hypercholesterolemia the plasma cholesterol level tends to be higher. A plasma cholesterol level in the range of 9 to 10 mmol/L (350 to 400 mg/dL) is highly suggestive of heterozygous familial hypercholesterolemia. However, many patients with heterozygous familial hypercholesterolemia have cholesterol levels of 7 to 9 mmol/L (285 to 350 mg/dL), a range in which the other disorders cannot be excluded. (2) The occurrence of tendon xanthomas virtually establishes the diagnosis of familial hypercholesterolemia, since such xanthomas usually do not occur in patients with other forms of hyperlipidemia. (3) In cases in which the diagnosis is in doubt, other family members should be surveyed. In familial hypercholesterolemia half of the first-degree relatives show an elevated plasma cholesterol level. Hypercholesterolemia in relatives is particularly informative when it occurs in children, since elevated levels of cholesterol in childhood are characteristic of familial hypercholesterolemia but not of the other disorders.

Approximately 10 percent of heterozygotes with familial hypercholesterolemia have a concomitant elevation in plasma triglyceride levels (type 2b pattern). In these cases, the disease is difficult to differentiate from multiple lipoprotein-type hyperlipidemia. The finding of a tendon xanthoma or a hypercholesterolemic child in the family establishes the diagnosis of familial hypercholesterolemia.

The diagnosis of homozygous familial hypercholesterolemia ordinarily affords no problem, providing the physician is familiar with the clinical picture. Most patients are first seen by dermatologists in childhood because of the cutaneous xanthomas. Occasionally, the presentation is delayed until the onset of angina pectoris or until the child suffers a syncopal episode owing to the xanthomatous aortic stenosis. The finding of a cholesterol level greater than 16 mmol/L (600 mg/dL) with normal triglyceride values in a nonjaundiced child is highly suggestive of the diagnosis. Both parents should have elevated cholesterol levels and other features of heterozygous familial hypercholesterolemia.

In specialized laboratories the diagnosis of both heterozygous and homozygous familial hypercholesterolemia can be made by direct measurement of the number of LDL receptors on cultured skin fibroblasts or freshly isolated blood lymphocytes. Homozygous familial hypercholesterolemia has been diagnosed in utero by the absence of LDL receptors on cultured amniotic fluid cells. The mutant genes for the LDL receptor can also be visualized directly in genomic DNA from affected individuals by using restriction enzyme digests and Southern blots (see Chap. 6).

Treatment Inasmuch as the atherosclerosis in this disorder is a consequence of the long-standing elevation in plasma LDL levels, every effort should be made to lower the plasma LDL level into the normal range. Patients should be placed on a diet that is low in cholesterol, low in saturated fats, and high in polyunsaturated fats. This generally means the avoidance of milk, butter, cheese, chocolate, shellfish, and fatty meats and the addition of polyunsaturated cooking oils such as corn oil and safflower oil. With such a diet heterozygotes usually show a 10 to 15 percent drop in plasma cholesterol level.

Bile acid–binding resins, such as cholestyramine, should be added to the regimen when dietary therapy fails to lower the cholesterol levels to the normal range. These resins trap the bile acids excreted by the liver into the intestine and prevent their reabsorption. The liver responds to bile acid depletion by converting additional cholesterol into bile acids. This leads to an enhanced production of LDL receptors by the liver, which in turn lowers the plasma level of LDL. Unfortunately, affected subjects also respond to bile acid depletion by enhancing cholesterol synthesis in the liver, and this compensatory response ultimately limits the long-term success of bile acid sequestrant therapy. With the combination of diet and bile acid–binding resins, the extent of reduction in plasma cholesterol level usually is in the range of 15 to 20 percent in heterozygotes. The addition of nicotinic acid may help to block the compensatory increase in hepatic cholesterol synthesis, thus allowing a further lowering of the cholesterol. Major side effects of bile acid–binding resins include gastrointestinal bloating, cramps, and constipation. The major side effect of nicotinic acid is hepatotoxicity; it also produces flushing and headaches in most patients. Probucol has also been used for the treatment of familial hypercholesterolemia. Its mechanism of action is unknown.

A new class of drugs shows great promise for treatment of hypercholesterolemia. These drugs inhibit 3-hydroxy-3-methylglutaryl coenzyme A (HMG CoA) reductase, an enzyme in the cholesterol biosynthetic pathway. When cholesterol synthesis is inhibited, the production of LDL is diminished and the clearance of LDL by the liver is enhanced as a result of an increased production of LDL receptors. These two effects combine to lower plasma LDL levels by 30 to 50 percent. The HMG CoA reductase inhibitors are even more effective when given together with a bile acid–binding resin such as cholestyramine. One of the inhibitors, lovastatin, is available in the United States, and another inhibitor, simvastatin, is available in other countries. The major side effects of these drugs are myopathy (0.5 percent) and asymptomatic but persistent increases in plasma transaminases (1.9 percent). Both side effects are reversible on discontinuation of therapy. Myopathy is seen primarily in patients who are treated concomitantly with immunosuppressive drugs, gemfibrozil, or nicotinic acid.

Heterozygotes often show a moderate to marked lowering of plasma cholesterol level in response to the creation of an intestinal anastomosis that bypasses the ileum. This operation has the same functional effect as bile acid–binding resins, i.e., it accelerates the loss of bile acids in the stool. In certain patients in whom drug therapy is not tolerated, the creation of an ileal bypass may be indicated.

Homozygotes tend to be more resistant to treatment, probably because they are unable to increase production of LDL receptors. In general, combination therapy consisting of diet, a bile acid–binding resin, and nicotinic acid has little effect. Ileal bypass is uniformly ineffective. Several homozygous children have responded to surgical creation of a portacaval anastomosis. However, this procedure is still experimental. The use of a continuous-flow blood cell centrifuge to perform plasma exchanges at monthly intervals lowers the cholesterol in all homozygotes. After each plasma exchange, the plasma cholesterol level drops to about 8 mmol/L (300 mg/dL) and then gradually rises over the ensuing 4 weeks to the pretreatment level. If facilities are available, plasma exchange is the treatment of choice for homozygotes. One homozygous child has been treated with liver transplantation, which provided LDL receptors and lowered LDL levels by 80 percent.

FAMILIAL HYPERTRIGLYCERIDEMIA This is a common autosomal dominant disorder in which the concentration of VLDL is elevated in the plasma, causing hypertriglyceridemia.

Clinical features Affected individuals do not usually express hypertriglyceridemia until puberty or early adulthood. Thereafter, the fasting plasma triglyceride level tends to be moderately elevated in the range of 2 to 6 mmol/L (200 to 500 mg/dL) (type 4 lipoprotein pattern). The typical patient exhibits the clinical triad of obesity, hyperglycemia, and hyperinsulinemia. Hypertension and hyperuricemia are also frequent.

The incidence of atherosclerosis is increased. In one study affected patients constituted 6 percent of all individuals with myocardial infarction. However, it has not been established that the hypertriglyceridemia per se causes the increased atherosclerosis. As discussed above, many patients with this disease have diabetes, obesity, and hypertension. Each of these disorders by itself may predispose to atherosclerosis. Xanthomas are not a characteristic feature of familial hypertriglyceridemia.

Affected patients ordinarily have mild to moderate hypertriglyceridemia but may develop a severe exacerbation when exposed to a variety of precipitating factors. These include poorly controlled diabetes mellitus, excessive consumption of alcohol, ingestion of birth control pills containing estrogen, and the development of hypothyroidism. In response to any of these stimuli, the plasma triglyceride level can rise to more than 11 mmol/L (1000 mg/dL). During exacerbations such patients develop *mixed hyperlipidemia;* that is, they show an elevation in the concentration of both VLDL and chylomicrons (type 5 lipoprotein pattern). Whenever the concentration of chylomicrons rises to high levels, patients are predisposed to the formation of eruptive xanthomas and the development of pancreatitis. With treatment of the exacerbating condition, the chylomicron-like particles disappear from plasma, and the concentration of triglycerides returns to the moderately elevated basal condition.

In certain families some patients exhibit a severe mixed hyperlipidemia, even in the absence of known exacerbating factors. This is the so-called familial type 5 hyperlipidemia. Other individuals in the same family may have only the mild form of the disease with moderate hypertriglyceridemia and no hyperchylomicronemia (type 4 pattern).

Pathogenesis Familial hypertriglyceridemia is transmitted as an autosomal dominant trait, implying a mutation in a single gene. However, the nature of the mutant gene and the mechanism by which it produces hypertriglyceridemia have not been identified. It is likely that the disorder is genetically heterogeneous; that is, the hypertriglyceridemia phenotype in different families may result from different mutations.

Some patients with familial hypertriglyceridemia seem to have an underlying defect in the ability to catabolize the triglycerides of VLDL. When VLDL production rates become elevated due to obesity or diabetes, they are unable to increase the catabolism of VLDL proportionately, and hypertriglyceridemia results. The reason for this defect in catabolism is not apparent. Lipoprotein lipase activity increases normally in plasma after the administration of heparin, and no abnormalities of lipoprotein structure have been identified.

The increased prevalence of diabetes and obesity in this syndrome is believed to be fortuitous, owing to the fact that both conditions tend to increase VLDL production and hence to exacerbate hypertriglyceridemia. In family studies, one can find relatives who have diabetes without hypertriglyceridemia and relatives who have hypertriglyceridemia without diabetes, indicating that the two are inherited by independent mechanisms. When an individual inherits the gene(s) for diabetes as well as the gene for hypertriglyceridemia, the hypertriglyceridemia is more severe, and such a person is more apt to come to medical attention. Similarly, an individual with familial hypertriglyceridemia who has a normal weight usually has mild hypertriglyceridemia and is less likely to come to medical attention. However, if obesity develops, the hypertriglyceridemia worsens, and a diagnosis is more likely to be made.

Diagnosis A moderate elevation in the plasma triglyceride level, together with a normal cholesterol level, raises the possibility of familial hypertriglyceridemia. In most patients, the plasma is clear to somewhat cloudy on inspection. Chylomicrons typically are not found at the top of the plasma after overnight refrigeration. Electrophoresis of the plasma reveals an increase in the pre-β fraction (type 4 lipoprotein pattern). As mentioned above, an occasional patient exhibits severe hypertriglyceridemia with an elevation in both chylomicrons and VLDL. In this case, a cream layer develops on top (chylomicrons) and a cloudy infranatant (VLDL) is present after overnight storage of plasma in the refrigerator (type 5 lipoprotein pattern).

Given an individual who has an elevation in VLDL levels with or without an elevation in chylomicrons, there is no simple test to determine whether this subject has familial hypertriglyceridemia or hypertriglyceridemia due to some other genetic or acquired cause, such as multiple lipoprotein-type hyperlipidemia or sporadic hypertriglyceridemia. In a typical case of familial hypertriglyceridemia, half of the first-degree relatives have hypertriglyceridemia and no relatives have isolated hypercholesterolemia. Measurement of plasma lipid levels in children is not helpful inasmuch as the disease is typically not manifest until the time of puberty.

Treatment Attempts should be made to control all the exacerbating conditions. Caloric restriction is required in the obese subject. The dietary content of saturated fat should also be limited. Alcohol and oral contraceptives should be avoided. Diabetes mellitus, if present, should be treated vigorously. Thyroid function should be checked, and hypothyroidism treated if found. If the above measures fail, some patients respond to the administration of gemfibrozil or nicotinic acid. Clofibrate may also be useful in certain patients. The mechanism of action of neither drug is well defined. Patients with severe hypertriglyceridemia frequently show a dramatic response to a fish oil diet.

MULTIPLE LIPOPROTEIN-TYPE HYPERLIPIDEMIA This common disorder, which is also called familial combined hyperlipidemia, is inherited as an autosomal dominant trait. Affected individuals in a single family characteristically show one of three different lipoprotein patterns: hypercholesterolemia (type 2a), hypertriglyceridemia (type 4), or both hypercholesterolemia and hypertriglyceridemia (type 2b).

Clinical features Hyperlipidemia is not present in childhood. Elevations in the plasma cholesterol and/or triglyceride level appear at puberty and continue throughout life. The lipid elevations tend to be mild and vary from time to time so that affected individuals may have a mildly elevated cholesterol level at one examination and/or a mildly elevated triglyceride level at another time. Xanthomas are not a feature. However, premature atherosclerosis occurs, and the incidence of myocardial infarction in middle age is elevated in affected women as well as men.

Patients usually have a strong family history of premature coronary artery disease. This disorder is found in about 10 percent of all patients who have a myocardial infarction. The frequency of obesity, hyperuricemia, and glucose intolerance is increased in affected individuals, especially those with hypertriglyceridemia. However, this association is not as striking as in familial hypertriglyceridemia.

Pathogenesis The disease is transmitted within families as an autosomal dominant trait, implying a mutation in a single gene. Family studies show that about half of the first-degree relatives of an affected individual have hyperlipidemia. However, blood lipid levels are variable among affected individuals in the same family as well as in the same individual at different times. About one-third of hyperlipidemic relatives have hypercholesterolemia (type 2a lipoprotein pattern), one-third hypertriglyceridemia (type 4), and one-third both hypercholesterolemia and hypertriglyceridemia (type 2b). In most affected relatives the plasma lipid levels tend to be just above the 95th percentile for the population and to dip into the normal range intermittently.

While the extent (if any) of the genetic heterogeneity and the nature of the underlying biochemical mechanisms are not known, affected individuals may have an elevated rate of secretion of VLDL by the liver. Depending on the interplay of factors governing the efficiency of conversion of VLDL to LDL and the efficiency of catabolism of LDL, this overproduction of VLDL may manifest itself alternatively as an elevation in plasma VLDL levels (hypertriglyceridemia), an elevation in LDL levels (hypercholesterolemia), or both. The hyperlipidemia is worsened by diabetes, alcoholism, and hypothyroidism.

Diagnosis No clinical or laboratory methods exist by which to determine whether an individual with hyperlipidemia has the multiple lipoprotein-type disorder. The 2a, 2b, and 4 lipoprotein patterns can each occur in patients with several other diseases (see Tables 326-3 and 326-4). However, this disorder should be suspected in any individual whose hyperlipoproteinemia is mild and whose lipoprotein type changes with time. The diagnosis is supported by the finding of multiple abnormal lipoprotein types in relatives. The diagnosis can be ruled out by the finding of tendon xanthomas in the patient or the patient's relatives or by the finding of hypercholesterolemia in a relative under the age of 10 years.

Treatment Therapy should be directed at the predominant lipid elevated at the time of examination. General measures such as weight reduction, restriction of dietary saturated fat and cholesterol, and avoidance of alcohol and oral contraceptives are useful. Triglyceride elevations may respond to nicotinic acid or gemfibrozil. When only the cholesterol level is elevated, a bile acid–binding resin or lovastatin should be given. However, in some individuals the lowering of cholesterol levels with such a drug is accompanied by an increase in triglyceride levels.

PRIMARY HYPERLIPOPROTEINEMIAS OF UNKNOWN ETIOLOGY

POLYGENIC HYPERCHOLESTEROLEMIA By definition, 5 percent of individuals in the general population have LDL-cholesterol levels that exceed the 95th percentile and therefore have hypercholesterolemia (type 2a or type 2b lipoprotein patterns). On the average, among every 20 such hypercholesterolemic persons, 1 person has the heterozygous form of familial hypercholesterolemia, and 2 have multiple lipoprotein-type hyperlipidemia. The remaining 17 have a form of hypercholesterolemia, designated polygenic hypercholesterolemia, that owes its origin not to a single mutant gene but rather to a complex interaction of multiple genetic and environmental factors.

Most of the factors that place an individual in the upper part of the bell-shaped curve for cholesterol levels are not known. It is likely that subtle genetic differences exist among people with regard to many processes governing cholesterol metabolism. For example, among normal people there may be genetic polymorphisms in the proteins that govern the rates of intestinal cholesterol absorption, bile acid synthesis, cholesterol synthesis, and LDL synthesis or catabolism. Certain unfavorable combinations of these mildly altered proteins, coupled with an environmental challenge, such as a diet high in cholesterol or saturated fat, may raise the plasma cholesterol level.

Clinically, polygenic hypercholesterolemia can be distinguished from familial hypercholesterolemia and multiple lipoprotein-type hyperlipidemia in two ways: (1) family studies (hyperlipidemia is present in no more than 10 percent of first-degree relatives in polygenic hypercholesterolemia in contrast to 50 percent in the other two disorders) and (2) examination for tendon xanthomas (absent in both polygenic hypercholesterolemia and multiple lipoprotein-type hyperlipidemia but present in about 75 percent of adult heterozygotes with familial hypercholesterolemia).

Certain patients with polygenic hypercholesterolemia respond to dietary restriction of saturated fat and cholesterol. Other patients require drug therapy. A bile acid–binding resin with or without lovastatin or nicotinic acid may also be used.

SPORADIC HYPERTRIGLYCERIDEMIA In addition to the forms of primary hypertriglyceridemia that show familial aggregation, endogenous hypertriglyceridemia with or without hyperchylomicronemia is sometimes seen in individuals whose relatives do not manifest hyperlipidemia. For purposes of classification, this disorder is called sporadic hypertriglyceridemia. Affected patients comprise a heterogeneous group. Some would undoubtedly be classified under one of the genetic disorders described above if a larger number of relatives were available for lipid measurements. Other than an absence of hyperlipidemic relatives, patients with sporadic hypertriglyceridemia cannot be distinguished clinically from patients with the single-gene forms of primary hypertriglyceridemia. Inasmuch as patients with sporadic hypertriglyceridemia may develop hyperchylomicronemia and pancreatitis, they should be treated with diet and drugs as in the familial disease.

FAMILIAL HYPERALPHALIPOPROTEINEMIA This entity is characterized by elevated plasma levels of HDL, also called alpha lipoprotein. The plasma levels of LDL, VLDL, and triglycerides are normal. The elevated HDL causes a slight elevation in the total plasma cholesterol level. Although a selective elevation in plasma HDL cholesterol can be observed in individuals after exposure to chlorinated hydrocarbon pesticides, in alcoholism and after administration of estrogen, most cases of hyperalphalipoproteinemia have a genetic basis. In some families, hyperalphalipoproteinemia is inherited as an autosomal dominant trait, while in others a multifactorial or polygenic basis is suspected. Individual subjects with familial hyperalphalipoproteinemia show no distinctive clinical features.

Hyperalphalipoproteinemia is associated with a slightly increased longevity and an apparent protection against myocardial infarction. The mechanism for the increase in plasma HDL levels in this disorder has not been determined.

SECONDARY HYPERLIPOPROTEINEMIAS

A variety of clinical disorders produce secondary hyperlipoproteinemias. These are summarized in Table 326-4. The most frequently encountered forms of secondary hyperlipoproteinemia occur in association with diabetes mellitus, consumption of alcohol, and ingestion of oral contraceptives.

DIABETES MELLITUS Three distinct patterns of hypertriglyceridemia occur in patients with diabetes mellitus. Classic "diabetic hyperlipemia" consists of a massive elevation in the plasma triglyceride level that occurs in patients who have suffered from insulin deficiency or insulin resistance for many weeks or months. Such insulin-deprived patients develop a progressive increase in concentration of plasma VLDL and eventually of chylomicrons as well. Triglyceride levels as high as 280 mmol/L (25,000 mg/dL) are seen. Eruptive xanthomas, lipemia retinalis, and hepatomegaly can occur. Ketosis is frequently present, but severe acidosis is not characteristic. This form of massive hyperlipoproteinemia is seen only in partial insulin deficiency. Patients with this form of diabetic hyperlipidemia usually respond to a fat-free diet and to the administration of insulin, although triglyceride levels may not return entirely to normal.

The second type of hypertriglyceridemia in diabetics is associated with acute ketoacidosis. Such patients usually exhibit a mild hyperlipidemia with elevations of VLDL but not chylomicrons. On occasion, however, marked elevations of triglyceride are seen with lipemia retinalis. In this case both VLDL and chylomicrons are present.

The third type of hypertriglyceridemia is a mild to moderate elevation in plasma VLDL that persists even when patients appear to be adequately treated for their diabetes. This chronic triglyceride elevation generally occurs in patients who are obese. Inasmuch as most patients with well-controlled diabetes have normal plasma triglyceride levels, the occasional patient with persistent hypertriglyceridemia is likely to have an underlying familial hyperlipoproteinemic disorder. Indeed, family studies indicate that many of these patients have inherited the trait for familial hypertriglyceridemia in a pattern independent of the inheritance of diabetes mellitus.

The insulin deficiency or insulin resistance of diabetes produces a high VLDL level by two mechanisms. With acute insulin deprivation there is an increase in VLDL secretion from the liver as a secondary response to the increased mobilization of free fatty acids from adipose tissue. As the state of insulin deprivation becomes prolonged, the rate of removal of VLDL and chylomicrons from the circulation declines because lipoprotein lipase activity becomes diminished.

ALCOHOL CONSUMPTION In any individual the daily consumption of large amounts of ethanol can produce a mild, asymptomatic elevation in the plasma triglyceride level due to an elevation of VLDL. However, in a subgroup ethanol ingestion regularly produces massive and clinically significant hyperlipidemia with elevations in both VLDL and chylomicrons (type 5 lipoprotein pattern). In most of this group, the VLDL level remains mildly elevated (type 4 lipoprotein pattern), even in the basal state after recovery from the severe alcoholic hyperlipidemia. This suggests that these individuals have a form of familial hypertriglyceridemia or multiple lipoprotein-type hyperlipidemia that is exacerbated and converted to a type 5 pattern by the ethanol ingestion.

Ethanol elevates the plasma triglyceride level primarily because it inhibits fatty acid oxidation and enhances fatty acid synthesis in the liver. The excess fatty acids are esterified to triglyceride. Some of this excess triglyceride accumulates in the liver, producing the characteristic enlarged fatty liver of alcoholics. The remainder of the newly formed triglyceride is secreted into plasma, resulting in an increased secretion of VLDL. In those who develop massive alcoholic hyperlipidemia, there appears to be a partial defect in the catabolism of these VLDL particles. As the concentration of VLDL increases, the lipoprotein begins to compete with chylomicrons for hydrolysis by lipoprotein lipase, and the plasma concentration of chylomicrons also rises.

In severe alcoholic hyperlipidemia, eruptive xanthomas and lipemia retinalis are frequent. The most serious complication, pancreatitis, may be difficult to diagnose, since elevated triglyceride levels can interfere with the estimation of serum amylase. There is no evidence to indicate that pancreatitis can cause hyperlipidemia; rather the hyperlipidemia is the cause of the pancreatitis.

Plasma from patients with alcoholic hyperlipidemia is creamy in appearance. If a blood sample is drawn in calcium edetate and the plasma placed in the refrigerator at 4°C overnight, the chylomicrons float to the top, and the infranatant layer is turbid, owing to the combined elevation of VLDL and chylomicrons (type 5 pattern).

ORAL CONTRACEPTIVES The ingestion of estrogen-containing birth control pills causes an increase in the VLDL secretion rate from the liver. In most women the catabolism of VLDL also increases, so that the overall increase in plasma triglyceride level is modest. However, in women who have an underlying genetic disorder (such as familial hypertriglyceridemia or multiple lipoprotein-type hyperlipidemia) the plasma VLDL-triglyceride level can increase markedly, and hyperchylomicronemia can develop when estrogen-containing

TABLE 326-5 Rare autosomal recessive disorders of lipid metabolism

Disorder	Typical age of onset	Plasma lipid abnormality	Major clinical manifestations	Pathogenesis	Treatment
Abetalipoproteinemia	Early childhood	Very low cholesterol and triglyceride levels	Malabsorption of fat, ataxia, neuropathy, retinitis pigmentosa, acanthocytosis	Defective synthesis of apoprotein B leads to absence of chylomicrons, VLDL, and LDL in plasma	Vitamin E
Tangier disease	Childhood	Low cholesterol; triglycerides, normal to slightly elevated	Large orange tonsils, corneal opacities, relapsing polyneuropathy No premature atherosclerosis	Absence of HDL from plasma leads to generation of abnormal chylomicron remnants, which are taken up and stored as cholesteryl esters in phagocytic cells	None
Lecithin:cholesterol acyltransferase (LCAT) deficiency	Young adult	Total plasma cholesterol level variable with marked decrease in esterified cholesterol and increase in unesterified cholesterol; elevated VLDL level; structure of all lipoproteins is abnormal	Corneal opacities, hemolytic anemia, renal insufficiency, premature atherosclerosis	Decreased LCAT activity in plasma leads to accumulation of excess unesterified cholesterol in plasma and body tissues	Fat-restricted diet, kidney transplantation
Cerebrotendinous xanthomatosis	Young adult	None	Progressive cerebellar ataxia, dementia and spinal cord paresis, subnormal intelligence, tendon xanthomas, cataracts	Defective synthesis of primary bile acids in liver leads to increased hepatic synthesis of cholesterol and cholestanol, which accumulate in brain, tendons, and other tissues	None
Sitosterolemia	Childhood	Elevated levels of plant sterols in plasma, elevated or normal levels of cholesterol, normal triglyceride levels	Tendon xanthomas	Increased intestinal absorption of dietary cholesterol, sitosterol, and other plant sterols with accumulation in plasma and tendons	Diet low in plant sterols and cholesterol

medications are taken. These women generally have mild hypertriglyceridemia prior to the institution of oral contraceptive therapy, and they presumably are unable to increase VLDL catabolism in response to the stimulation of VLDL production. The elevated VLDL prevents the normal catabolism of chylomicrons by lipoprotein lipase, and secondary hyperchylomicronemia ensues. When the latter develops, severe pancreatitis can occur.

Ingestion of oral contraceptives may be a risk factor in promoting thromboembolic disease in young women, especially those with preexisting hypercholesterolemia. Thus, it is important to measure the plasma cholesterol and triglyceride levels prior to the institution of birth control therapy. The finding of hyperlipidemia is a contraindication to the use of these drugs.

RARE DISORDERS OF LIPID METABOLISM

Table 326-5 summarizes the clinical and pathophysiologic features of five rare autosomal recessive disorders of lipid metabolism. In two—abetalipoproteinemia and Tangier disease—the major effect of the abnormality is to cause a decrease in lipid levels in plasma. In two—cerebrotendinous xanthomatosis and sitosterolemia—the major effect of the inborn error is to cause an accumulation of unusual sterols in tissues. In LCAT deficiency, the underlying mutation produces both an abnormal pattern of lipoproteins in plasma and an accumulation of unesterified cholesterol in tissues.

REFERENCES

Brown MS, Goldstein JL: A receptor-mediated pathway for cholesterol homeostasis. Science 232:34, 1986

———, ———: Drugs used in the treatment of hyperlipoproteinemias, in *The Pharmacological Basis of Therapeutics*, 7th ed, AG Gilman et al (eds). New York, Macmillan, 1986, chap 34

Brunzell JD: Familial lipoprotein lipase deficiency and other causes of the chylomicronemia syndrome, in *The Metabolic Basis of Inherited Disease*, 6th ed, CR Scriver et al (eds). New York, McGraw-Hill, 1989, chap 45

Connor WE et al: Reduction of plasma lipids, lipoproteins and apoproteins by dietary fish oils in patients with hypertriglyceridemia. N Engl J Med 312:1210, 1985

Goldstein JL, Brown MS: Familial hypercholesterolemia, in *The Metabolic Basis of Inherited Disease*, 6th ed, CR Scriver et al (eds). New York, McGraw-Hill, 1989, chap 48

Havel RJ: Lowering cholesterol, 1988: Rationale, mechanisms and means. J Clin Invest 81:1653, 1988

Mahley RW, Rall SC: Type III hyperlipoproteinemia (dysbetalipoproteinemia): The role of apolipoprotein E in normal and abnormal lipoprotein metabolism, in *The Metabolic Basis of Inherited Disease*, 6th ed, CR Scriver et al (eds). New York, McGraw-Hill, 1989, chap 47

Scriver CR et al: *The Metabolic Basis of Inherited Disease*, 6th ed. New York, McGraw-Hill, 1989, chaps 44, 46, 49, 50, and 51

327 HEMOCHROMATOSIS

LAWRIE W. POWELL / KURT J. ISSELBACHER

DEFINITION Hemochromatosis is an iron-storage disorder in which an inappropriate increase in intestinal iron absorption results in deposition of iron with eventual tissue damage and functional impairment of the organs involved, especially the liver, pancreas, heart, and pituitary. In 1889, von Recklinghausen named the disease *hemochromatosis* and the iron-storage pigment *hemosiderin* because he believed that the pigment was derived from the blood. The terms *hemosiderosis* and *siderosis* are often used to describe the presence of stainable iron in tissues, but quantitative measurement of tissue iron is necessary for accurate assessment of body iron status (see below and Chap. 291). *Hemochromatosis* implies progressive iron overload leading to fibrosis and organ failure. Although there is debate about definitions, it seems logical to use the following terminology: (1) *genetic hemochromatosis*—the inherited disease now known to be associated with an abnormal gene tightly linked to the A locus of the HLA complex on chromosome 6, (2) *acquired hemochromatosis*—iron overload with tissue injury arising secondarily to other disease, usually an iron-loading anemia such as thalassemia or sideroblastic anemia, in which increased erythropoiesis is present. It should be emphasized, however, that in these acquired iron-loading disorders massive iron deposits in parenchymal tissues can lead to the same clinical and pathologic features that are seen in genetic hemochromatosis.

The metabolic defect leading to increased iron absorption in hemochromatosis is unknown. The genetic disease can now be recognized during its early stages when the iron overload is of lesser degree and organ damage is minimal. At this stage the disease is best referred to as *early* or *precirrhotic hemochromatosis* (see Fig. 327-1).

PREVALENCE Genetic hemochromatosis is now known to be one of the most common genetic diseases inherited as an autosomal recessive trait. In European Anglo-Saxon populations the gene frequency is approximately 5 percent, giving a disease (homozygote) frequency of approximately 0.3 percent, and a carrier (heterozygote) frequency of approximately 10 percent. However, expression of the disease is modified by several factors, especially blood loss associated with menstruation and pregnancies in women. The clinical expression of disease is 5 to 10 times more frequent in males than in females. Nearly 70 percent of patients develop their first symptoms between ages 40 and 60. The disease is rarely clinically evident below age 20, although with family screening (see below) asymptomatic subjects with iron overload can be identified, including young menstruating women.

FIGURE 327-1 Sequence of events in genetic hemochromatosis and their correlation with the serum ferritin concentration. Increased iron absorption is present throughout life. Overt, symptomatic disease usually develops between ages 40 and 60, but latent precirrhotic disease can be detected long before this.

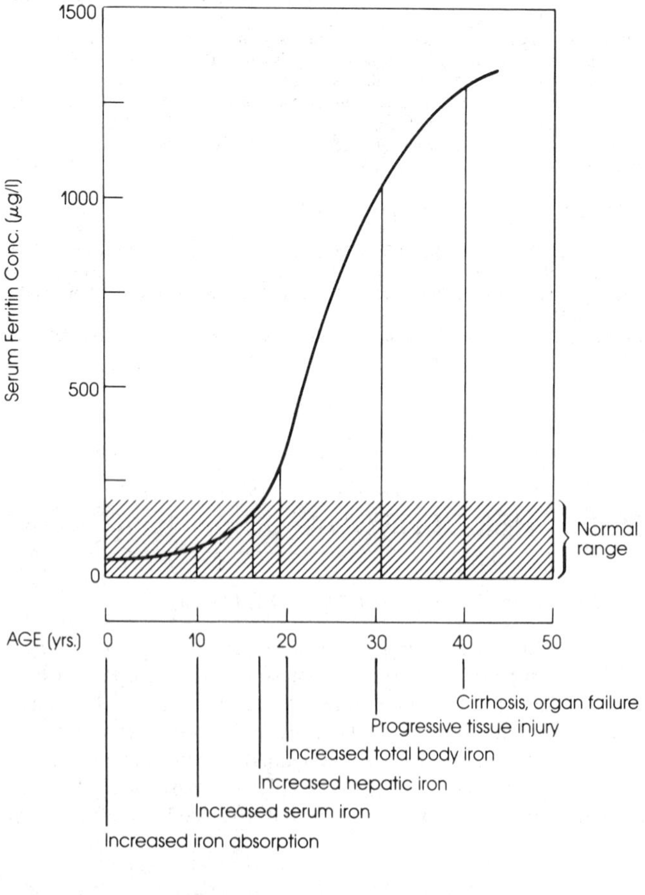

PATHOGENESIS Normally the body iron content of 3 to 4 g is maintained such that intestinal mucosal absorption of iron is equal to loss. This amount is approximately 1 mg per day in men and 1.5 mg per day in menstruating women. In hemochromatosis mucosal absorption is inappropriate to body needs, amounting to 4 mg per day or more. The resulting progressive accumulation of iron is reflected in an early elevation in the plasma iron and an increased saturation of transferrin. In advanced disease, the body may contain over 20 g iron. This excess iron is deposited mainly in parenchymal cells of the liver, pancreas, and heart. Iron in the liver and pancreas may increase 50 to 100 times; in the heart, 5 to 25 times; in the spleen, kidney, and skin, about 5 times. Tissue injury may result from disruption of iron-laden lysosomes and lipid peroxidation of subcellular organelles by excess iron. The demonstration of an association between hemochromatosis and the histocompatibility antigens HLA-A3, HLA-B14, and HLA-B7 has confirmed the genetic basis for the disease. The mode of inheritance is autosomal recessive, with homozygotes usually developing severe iron overload and symptomatic disease. In contrast, heterozygotes show no abnormalities or develop only minor derangements in iron metabolism without progressive iron overload or clinical evidence of the disease. In the absence of a genetic marker heterozygotes in the population cannot at this time be differentiated with certainty from normal subjects.

Gross parenchymal iron overload leading to *acquired* hemochromatosis occurs in association with chronic disorders of erythropoiesis, particularly in those with a defect in hemoglobin synthesis and ineffective erythropoiesis such as sideroblastic anemia and thalassemia. In this group of disorders the absorption of iron is increased, and these patients are also frequently treated with iron and blood transfusions. Porphyria cutanea tarda, a disorder characterized by a defect in porphyrin biosynthesis (Chap. 328), is also sometimes associated with excessive parenchymal iron deposits; however, the magnitude of the iron load is usually insufficient to produce tissue damage.

Alcoholic subjects with chronic liver disease may have increased tissue iron stores. They can be divided into two groups. The first group comprises patients who have a mild to moderate increase in stainable hepatic iron but relatively normal body iron stores. These patients have alcoholic liver disease (usually cirrhosis) but not hemochromatosis. The reason for the increased iron may be related in part to cell necrosis and uptake of iron released from adjacent Kupffer and parenchymal cells. The second (less common) group of alcoholic subjects with increased hepatic iron have gross iron deposition and increased body iron stores and are usually found to have genetic hemochromatosis with or without superimposed alcoholic liver disease. Hemochromatosis in a heavy drinker may be distinguished from alcoholic liver disease by two means: (1) measurement of hepatic iron concentration (see below and Table 327-1) and (2) studying relatives for evidence of the disease, including HLA typing of family members.

Excessive iron ingestion over many years has been reported to result in the clinical and pathologic features of hemochromatosis. This used to be common in certain South African blacks (Bantu) in whom the intake of excessive iron in an alcoholic beverage resulted from the practice of brewing fermented beverages in vessels made of iron. In other populations there are a few isolated reports of hemochromatosis developing in apparently normal subjects who have taken medicinal iron over many years, but it is probable that such individuals have the genetic trait. Family studies may be helpful.

The basic defect in hemochromatosis is not known but may involve the reciprocal relation between ferritin mRNA and transferrin receptor mRNA expression in the intestinal mucosa cell. Diagnosis is dependent

TABLE 327-1 Representative iron values in normal subjects, patients with hemochromatosis, and patients with alcoholic liver disease

Determination	Normal	Symptomatic hemochromatosis	Homozygotes with early, asymptomatic hemochromatosis	Alcoholic liver disease
Plasma iron, μmol/L (μg/dL)	9–27 (50–150)	32–54 (180–300)	Usually elevated	Often elevated
Total iron-binding capacity, μmol/L (μg/dL)	45–66 (250–370)	36–54 (200–300)	36–54 (200–300)	45–66 (250–370)
Transferrin saturation, percent	22–46	50–100	50–100	27–60
Serum ferritin, μg/L	10–200	900–6000	200–500	10–500
Urinary iron,* mg/24 h	0–2	9–23	2.5	Usually <5
Liver iron, μg/100 ng dry wt	30–140	600–1800	200–400	30–200

* After intramuscular administration of 0.5 g deferoxamine.

on the phenotypic expression of the disease (i.e., increased body iron stores), and the rate of iron accumulation may be modified by other factors such as blood loss and oral iron ingestion. The common denominator in all patients with hemochromatosis is the presence of *excessive amounts of iron in parenchymal tissues*. Parenteral administration of iron in the form of transfusions or iron preparations results in predominantly *reticuloendothelial cell* iron overload. This appears to lead to less tissue damage than iron loading of parenchymal cells.

PATHOLOGY At autopsy the enlarged, nodular liver and pancreas present a striking ochre color. Histologically iron is found in increased amounts in many organs, particularly in the liver and pancreas and to a lesser extent in the endocrine glands and the heart. A notable exception is the testis, the iron content of which is relatively low despite the fact that gonadal failure is a characteristic and early feature of the disease. In contrast, the pituitary gland is almost always involved. The epidermis of the skin is thin, and increased *melanin* is found in the cells of the basal layer. Deposits of iron are present around the synovial lining cells of the joints, and calcium pyrophosphate crystals may be seen to lie within deposits of calcium embedded in the synovial tissue.

The parenchymal deposits of iron in the liver of patients with genetic hemochromatosis are in the form of ferritin and hemosiderin. In the early stages, these deposits are found in the periportal parenchymal cells, especially within lysosomes in the pericanalicular cytoplasm of the hepatocytes. This stage progresses to perilobular fibrosis and deposition of iron in bile duct epithelium, Kupffer cells, and fibrous septa. Inflammatory cells are few in contrast to prominent proliferation of bile ductules. Wedge biopsy specimens show a characteristic pattern of fibrosis with dense fibrous septa surrounding groups of lobules somewhat analogous to the pattern in chronic biliary disease. In the advanced stage, a macronodular or mixed macro- and micronodular cirrhosis develops.

CLINICAL MANIFESTATIONS The symptoms and signs include skin pigmentation, diabetes mellitus, liver and cardiac impairment, arthropathy, and hypogonadism. The most frequently encountered initial symptoms are weakness, lassitude, weight loss, change in skin color, abdominal pain, loss of libido, and symptoms related to the onset of diabetes mellitus. Hepatomegaly, pigmentation, spider angiomas, splenomegaly, arthropathy, ascites, cardiac arrhythmias, congestive heart failure, loss of body hair, testicular atrophy, and jaundice are prominent physical signs in fully established disease.

The *liver* is usually the first organ to be affected, and hepatomegaly is present in more than 95 percent of symptomatic patients. Hepatic enlargement may exist in the absence of symptoms or in the presence of normal liver function tests. Indeed, over half the patients with symptomatic hemochromatosis have little or no laboratory evidence of functional impairment of the liver, in spite of hepatomegaly and fibrosis. Loss of body hair, palmar erythema, testicular atrophy, and gynecomastia are common. Manifestations of portal hypertension and esophageal varices occur less commonly than in Laennec's cirrhosis. Splenomegaly is present in approximately half the symptomatic cases. Hepatocellular carcinoma develops in about 30 percent of patients with cirrhosis. The incidence of this complication increases with age and is now the most common cause of death in treated patients. However, it appears to occur only in cirrhotic patients; hence the importance of early diagnosis and therapy.

Excessive *skin pigmentation* is present in about 90 percent of symptomatic patients at the time of diagnosis. Melanin deposition in the skin usually gives rise to bronzing. The characteristic metallic gray hue is believed to result from the presence of increased melanin or both melanin and iron in the dermis. Pigmentation usually is diffuse and generalized, but frequently it is deeper on the face, neck, extensor aspects of the lower forearms, dorsa of the hands, lower legs, genital regions, and in scars. In only 10 to 15 percent of cases is there demonstrable pigmentation of the oral mucosa. Pigmentation of the hard palate and retina has been described.

Diabetes mellitus occurs in about 65 percent of patients and is more likely to develop in patients with a family history of diabetes mellitus. The presence of a genetic predisposition and direct damage to the pancreas by iron deposition both contribute to the development of diabetes mellitus. The management of the diabetes mellitus is similar to that of other forms of diabetes mellitus except for a higher incidence of insulin resistance. Late degenerative sequelae are the same as in diabetes mellitus.

Arthropathy develops in 25 to 50 percent of patients. It most commonly occurs after the age of 50 but may occur at any time in the course of the disease, even as a first manifestation or long after therapy. The small joints of the hands, especially the second and third metacarpophalangeal joints, are commonly the first joints to be involved. A progressive polyarthritis involving wrists, hips, ankles, and knees may ensue. Acute brief attacks of synovitis may occur, associated with deposition of calcium pyrophosphate (chondrocalcinosis or pseudogout), chiefly in the knees. Roentgenologic manifestations consist of cystic changes of sclerosis of the subchondral bones, loss of articular cartilage with narrowing of the joint space, diffuse demineralization, hypertrophic bone proliferation, and calcification of the synovium. The mechanism of these abnormalities and their relationship to iron metabolism are not known.

Cardiac involvement is the presenting manifestation in about 15 percent of patients. The most common cardiac manifestation, congestive heart failure, occurs in about 10 percent of young adults with the disease. Symptoms of congestive failure may develop suddenly, with rapid progression to death if untreated. The heart is diffusely enlarged, and such cases may be misdiagnosed as idiopathic cardiomyopathy if other overt manifestations are absent. A variety of cardiac arrhythmias may be present, particularly supraventricular beats and paroxysmal tachyarrhythmias. Atrial flutter, atrial fibrillation, and varying degrees of atrioventricular block have also been described.

Loss of libido and *testicular atrophy* are common. The former may antedate other clinical manifestations of the disease. Testicular atrophy is usually due to the decreased production of gonadotropins associated with impaired hypothalamic-pituitary function due to iron deposition. Adrenal insufficiency, hypothyroidism, and hypoparathyroidism have been described but are rare.

DIAGNOSIS The association of (1) hepatomegaly, (2) skin pigmentation, (3) diabetes mellitus, (4) heart disease, (5) arthritis, and (6) evidence of hypogonadism should suggest the diagnosis of hemochromatosis. However, a parenchymal iron overload of comparatively short duration or modest degree may exist without any of these clinical manifestations, or with only some of them [e.g., in young subjects (see Fig. 327-1)]. Therefore, the diagnosis should be considered in any patient with unexplained hepatomegaly, idiopathic cardiomyopathy, abnormal skin pigmentation, loss of libido, diabetes mellitus, or arthritis.

The history should be particularly detailed in regard to disease in other family members, alcohol ingestion, iron intake, and the ingestion of large doses of ascorbic acid, which promotes iron absorption. The blood should be examined for evidence of anemia and abnormal erythropoiesis to rule out iron loading secondary to a hematologic disorder. Confirmation of the presence of liver, pancreatic, cardiac, and joint disease should be obtained by physical examination, roentgenography, and routine function tests of these organs. It then remains to be demonstrated that there is an increase in total-body iron stores and, in particular, an increased parenchymal iron concentration associated with tissue damage.

The methods available for the demonstration of excessive parenchymal iron stores include (1) measurement of serum iron and determination of percent saturation of transferrin, (2) estimation of chelatable iron stores using the agent deferoxamine, (3) measurement of serum ferritin concentration, (4) liver biopsy (Table 327-1), and (5) computed tomography and/or magnetic resonance imaging of the liver. Each has its inherent advantages and limitations. The serum iron level and percent saturation of transferrin are elevated early in the course of the disease, but their specificity is reduced by relatively high false-positive and false-negative rates. In particular, an increased serum iron concentration may be present in patients with alcoholic liver disease without iron overload; in this situation, however, the iron-binding capacity is usually not decreased as in hemochromatosis (Table 327-1). Population studies suggest that in otherwise healthy persons a fasting serum transferrin saturation greater than 62 percent strongly suggests homozygosity for hemochromatosis.

The serum ferritin concentration is usually a good index of body iron stores, whether they are decreased or increased. In most untreated patients with hemochromatosis, the serum ferritin level is greatly increased (Fig. 327-1 and Table 327-1). This test is also useful as a noninvasive screening test for the diagnosis of early disease, since it is usually abnormal before there is any morphologic evidence of liver damage and the ferritin concentration correlates with the magnitude of body iron stores.

These tests have, therefore, generally replaced the more cumbersome screening tests involving measurement of urinary iron excretion. However, in patients with inflammation and hepatocellular necrosis serum ferritin levels may be elevated out of proportion to body iron stores due to increased rate of release from tissues. A repeat determination of serum ferritin should therefore be carried out when any concurrent acute hepatocellular damage has subsided, e.g., in alcoholic liver disease. In some families serum ferritin levels in symptomatic relatives are normal despite increased iron stores; the reason for this finding is unclear, but it would appear to be unusual. In clinical practice, the *combined measurements* of the (1) percent transferrin saturation and (2) serum ferritin level provide the simplest and most reliable screening test for hemochromatosis, including the precirrhotic phase of the disease. If either of these tests is abnormal, liver biopsy should be performed since it is the *definitive* test for the diagnosis of hemochromatosis. It permits histochemical estimation of tissue iron, measurement of hepatic iron concentration, and assessment of the extent of tissue damage. Computed tomography shows increased density of the liver due to iron deposition. However, dual-energy scanning and experienced personnel are required, and the lower limits for accurate detection of increased tissue iron are still unclear. Magnetic resonance imaging may also detect increased tissue iron, but the sensitivity requires further evaluation.

When the diagnosis of hemochromatosis is established, it is of particular importance to examine family members at risk. Asymptomatic as well as symptomatic family members with the disease usually have an increased saturation of transferrin and an increased or increasing serum ferritin concentration. These changes occur even before the iron stores are greatly increased (see Fig. 327-1). A liver biopsy should then be performed, since it is imperative to establish the diagnosis and begin therapy before tissue damage occurs. Since the hemochromatosis allele lies close to the HLA-A locus on chromosome 6, HLA typing is helpful in evaluating families with the disease. Affected siblings (putative homozygotes) usually have both HLA haplotypes identical with those of the proband, and where children of a proband are affected, a homozygous-heterozygous mating probably occurred. Siblings sharing only one HLA haplotype with a patient (putative heterozygotes) will probably not develop progressive iron overload. Thus, HLA typing helps greatly in determining the probability of a sibling later developing the disease and therefore the desirable frequency of screening.

The distinction between hemochromatosis and alcoholic cirrhosis associated with increased tissue iron is usually not difficult if measurement is made of liver iron concentration and hepatic iron index (concentration divided by age) (Table 327-1). Where biopsy is not possible the deferoxamine excretion test can provide diagnostic information.

TREATMENT The therapy of genetic hemochromatosis involves the removal of the excess body iron and supportive treatment of damaged organs.

Iron is best removed from the body by weekly or twice weekly phlebotomy of 500 mL. Although there is an initial modest decline in the volume of packed red blood cells to about 35 mL/dL, the level stabilizes after several weeks. The plasma transferrin saturation remains increased until the available iron stores are depleted. In contrast, the plasma ferritin concentration falls progressively, reflecting the gradual decrease in body iron stores. Since one 500-mL unit of blood contains from 200 to 250 mg iron and about 25 g iron must be removed, weekly phlebotomy is usually required for 2 or 3 years. When the transferrin saturation and ferritin level become normal, phlebotomies are performed at such time intervals as are required to maintain these levels within the normal range. The measurements promptly become abnormal with iron reaccumulation. Usually one phlebotomy every 3 months will suffice.

Chelating agents such as deferoxamine, when given parenterally, remove 10 to 20 mg iron per day, less than half that mobilized by once weekly phlebotomy. Phlebotomy is also generally less expensive, more convenient, and safer for patients with genetic hemochromatosis, but chelating agents are indicated when anemia or hypoproteinemia is severe enough to preclude phlebotomy. Subcutaneous infusions of deferoxamine using a portable slow pump are the most effective means of administration.

The management of the hepatic failure, cardiac failure, and diabetes mellitus differs little from conventional management of these conditions. Loss of libido and change in secondary sex characteristics are partially relieved by parenteral testosterone or gonadotropin therapy (see Chap. 321).

PROGNOSIS The principal causes of death in *untreated* patients are cardiac failure (30 percent), hepatocellular failure or portal hypertension (25 percent), and hepatocellular carcinoma (30 percent).

Life expectancy of symptomatic patients is extended considerably by removal of the excessive stores of iron and maintenance of these stores at near-normal levels. The 5-year survival rate with therapy increases from 33 to 89 percent. With removal of iron by repeated phlebotomy, the liver and spleen decrease in size, liver function studies return to normal, pigmentation of skin decreases, and cardiac failure is reversed. Carbohydrate tolerance improves in about 40 percent. Removal of excess iron has little or no effect on hypogonadism or arthropathy. The fibrosis in the liver may decrease, but cirrhosis is irreversible. Hepatocellular carcinoma occurs as a late sequela in about one-third of patients who are cirrhotic at presentation despite adequate iron removal. The apparent increase in its incidence in treated patients is probably related in part to their increased life span. This complication does not appear to develop if the disease is treated in the precirrhotic stage, and the life expectancy of homozygotes diagnosed and treated before the development of cirrhosis does not differ significantly from that of the normal population. Hence, the importance of family screening and early therapy cannot be emphasized too strongly. Asymptomatic subjects who are detected by family studies should have phlebotomy therapy if iron stores are moderately to severely increased. Screening for increasing iron stores at appropriate intervals is also important. With this approach most manifestations of the disease can be prevented.

REFERENCES

BASSETT ML et al: HLA typing in idiopathic hemochromatosis: Distinction between homozygotes and heterozygotes with biochemical expression. Hepatology 1:120, 1981

——— et al: Value of hepatic iron measurements in early hemochromatosis and determination of the critical iron levels associated with fibrosis. Hepatology 318:24, 1986

EDWARDS CQ et al: Prevalence of hemochromatosis among 11,065 presumably healthy blood donors. N Engl J Med 318:1355, 1988

KLAUSNER RD, HARFORD JB: Cis-trans models for post-transcriptional gene regulation. Science 246:870, 1989

NEIDERAU C et al: Survival and causes of death in cirrhotic and in noncirrhotic patients with primary hemochromatosis. N Engl J Med 313:1256, 1985

POWELL LW, KERR JFR: The pathology of liver in hemochromatosis, in *Pathobiology Annual*, H Joacim (ed). New York, Appleton-Century-Crofts, 1975

——— et al: Expression of hemochromatosis in homozygous subjects: Implications for early diagnosis and prevention. Gastroenterology (in press) 1990

STEVENS RG et al: Body iron stores and the risk of cancer. N Engl J Med 319:1047, 1988

328 PORPHYRIAS

URS A. MEYER

The porphyrias are inherited or acquired disturbances in heme biosynthesis. Porphyrins are tetrapyrrole intermediates in this pathway and are formed from the precursors δ-aminolevulinic acid (ALA) and porphobilinogen. Heme, the ferrous iron complex of protoporphyrin IX, functions as a prosthetic group for hemoproteins such as hemoglobin, cytochromes, catalase, and tryptophan oxygenase. Heme biosynthesis is essential to life and is operative in all aerobic cells.

Each of the porphyrias is characterized by a unique pattern of overproduction, accumulation, and excretion of intermediates of heme biosynthesis. These patterns are the metabolic expression of deficiencies of specific enzymes of the heme biosynthetic pathway (Table 328-1, Fig. 328-1).

The main clinical manifestations are intermittent attacks of nervous system dysfunction and/or sensitivity of the skin to sunlight. The *neurologic syndrome* is characteristically precipitated by drugs such as barbiturates and results in abdominal pain, peripheral neuropathy, and mental disturbance. The neuropsychiatric symptoms occur only in those porphyrias in which there is great overproduction of the porphyrin precursors ALA and porphobilinogen. The pathogenesis of the neurologic lesion is unclear. The *skin photosensitivity* is related to increased porphyrin accumulation, although the lesions differ among the different disorders. When radiated with ultraviolet light of wavelength ≈400 nm, the conjugated double-bond structure of the tetrapyrrole nucleus causes porphyrins to become unstable, highly reactive oxidizing agents that react with molecules in the upper dermis and lower epidermis. The dominantly inherited human porphyrias exhibit variable expressivity. Only the biochemical or enzymatic abnormalities may be apparent. Such latent disease may occur as a phase or persist throughout life, or manifestations can be precipitated by factors such as drugs, hormones, or liver disease.

CLASSIFICATION The porphyrias are usually divided into two main groups, erythropoietic and hepatic, according to the two major sites of heme synthesis where the error of metabolism is predominantly expressed (Table 328-1). Erythropoietic forms of porphyria are the rare *congenital erythropoietic porphyria* (CEP) and *protoporphyria* (PP). But in some patients with PP, porphyrins accumulate both in erythropoietic and hepatic tissue. In *intermittent acute porphyria* (IAP), *hereditary coproporphyria* (HCP), and *variegate porphyria* (VP), heme biosynthesis is impaired predominantly in the liver, without affecting hemoglobin formation. *Porphyria cutanea tarda* (PCT) occurs both as a familial and as a sporadic disease. All patients with PCT have a deficiency of uroporphyrinogen decarboxylase in the liver. Acquired PCT occurs in individuals exposed to polyhalogenated hydrocarbons and in association with hepatic tumors. Poisoning with lead and hereditary tyrosinemia also produce abnormalities in porphyrin and heme synthesis (see Chap. 375). Small increases in urinary excretion of porphyrins or precursors and accumulation of porphyrins in erythrocytes may accompany numerous clinical conditions; these secondary phenomena do not produce symptoms or signs of porphyria.

BIOCHEMICAL CONSIDERATIONS The reactions that lead from the substrates glycine and succinyl coenzyme A to ALA, porphobilinogen (PBG), and finally heme are mediated by four mitochondrial and four cytosolic enzymes (Fig. 328-2). Differences exist in the regulation of heme biosynthesis among tissues.

In the liver ALA synthase catalyzes the rate-limiting reaction for heme formation under physiologic conditions. The enzymes subsequent to ALA synthase are present in excess. The principal regulation of ALA synthase is feedback repression by heme, the end product of the pathway. Increased demands for heme are met by the synthesis of ALA synthase. Hepatic ALA synthase can be induced by a large number of lipid-soluble drugs, steroids, and chemicals that are substrates and inducers of cytochrome P_{450} hemoproteins, the terminal oxidases in microsomal drug metabolism. This induction is modulated by genetic, metabolic, and environmental factors. The interdependence of heme synthesis and microsomal drug oxidation is important in several hepatic porphyrias where symptoms are precipitated by these drugs.

In the bone marrow ALA synthase is also rate-limiting in cells with fully expressed heme synthesis, but little is known of the role of the enzyme during division, differentiation, and maturation of erythroid cells. With maturation of erythroid cells the nuclei and mitochondria are extruded, and the mitochondrial enzymes of heme synthesis disappear, while the cytosolic enzymes catalyzing the reactions between ALA and coproporphyrinogen persist. Therefore, erythrocytes can be used for the diagnosis of porphyrias that are due to a defect in a cytosolic enzyme.

Control of heme synthesis differs in bone marrow and liver. The level of ALA synthase is the major determinant of heme formation in the liver, while heme synthesis in the bone marrow is triggered by the complex process of erythroid differentiation. These considerations probably explain the different manifestations of enzyme defects of heme synthesis in erythroid cells and liver.

The colorless and nonfluorescent porphyrinogens serve as intermediates between porphobilinogen and protoporphyrin. With the exception of protoporphyrin, porphyrins are by-products that have escaped from the biosynthetic path by irreversible oxidation of the corresponding porphyrinogen. Porphyrins do not possess physiologic function but are responsible, through their red-purple color and fluorescent properties, for the spectacular appearance of urine and erythrocytes in some patients.

The arrangement of two substituent side chains on the pyrrole ring of porphyrins determines the structural isomer types, numbered

TABLE 328-1 Characteristics of the porphyrias

	Erythropoietic porphyrias		Hepatic porphyrias				
	Congenital erythropoietic porphyria (CEP)	Protoporphyria (PP)	Intermittent acute porphyria (IAP)	Hereditary coproporphyria (HCP)	Variegate porphyria (VP)	Porphobilinogen synthase deficiency	Porphyria cutanea tarda (PCT)
Enzyme deficiency	Uroporphyrinogen III cosynthase (?)	Ferrochelatase	Porphobilinogen deaminase	Coproporphyrinogen oxidase	Protoporphyrinogen oxidase	Porphobilinogen synthase	Uroporphyrinogen decarboxylase
Inheritance	Autosomal recessive	Autosomal dominant	Autosomal dominant	Autosomal dominant	Autosomal dominant	Autosomal recessive	Autosomal dominant (familial form)
Metabolic expression	Erythroid cells	Erythroid cells and liver	Liver	Liver	Liver	Liver	Liver
Signs and symptoms:							
Photosensitive cutaneous lesions	Yes	Yes	No	Infrequent	Yes	No	Yes
Attacks of abdominal pain, neuropsychiatric syndrome	No	No	Yes	Yes	Yes	Yes	No
Laboratory abnormalities:							
Red blood cells:							
Uroporphyrin	+ + +	N	N	N	N		N
Coproporphyrin	+ +	+	N	N	N		N
Protoporphyrin	(+)	+ + +	N	N	N	+	N
Urine:							
δ-Aminolevulinic acid	N	N	(+ + +)	(+ + +)	(+ + +)	+ + +	N
Porphobilinogen	N	N	(+ + +)	(+ + +)	(+ + +)	+	N
Uroporphyrin	+ + +	N	+ +	+	+	+	+ + +
Coproporphyrin	+ +	(+)	N	+ +	+ +	+ + +	+
Feces:							
Coproporphyrin	+	(+)	N	+ + +	+	N	(+)
Protoporphyrin	+	+ +	N	+	+ + +	N	N

NOTE: N, normal; +, increased levels or excretion; + +, moderately increased; + + +, markedly increased; (+), increased in some patients only; (+ + +), frequently increased only during acute attacks.

I to IV. In nature only types I and III have been identified, and only type III is a substrate for the terminal steps of the pathway leading to protoporphyrin IX and heme. The catabolism of heme does not lead to porphyrins but to noncyclic tetrapyrroles referred to as *bile pigments*.

CONGENITAL ERYTHROPOIETIC PORPHYRIA

DEFINITION Congenital erythropoietic porphyria (CEP; Günther's disease, congenital photosensitive porphyria, erythropoietic uroporphyria) is a rare, recessively inherited defect that causes chronic photosensitivity with severe, mutilating skin lesions and hemolytic anemia.

GENETICS, INCIDENCE, AND PATHOGENESIS CEP is the rarest of the inherited porphyrias, less than 100 cases having been reported. Affected individuals are homozygous for an autosomal recessive gene; heterozygotes rarely have demonstrable abnormalities in porphyrin metabolism and appear normal. The underlying enzyme abnormality is a primary genetic deficiency of uroporphyrinogen III cosynthase with compensatory increases in the activities of ALA synthase and PBG deaminase in erythroid tissue. The defect is expressed solely in maturing erythroid cells and results in massive overproduction of uroporphyrinogen I while the production of uroporphyrinogen III is normal or slightly increased. Uroporphyrinogen I cannot be used for heme synthesis but is converted to coproporphyrinogen I. Uroporphyrin I, coproporphyrinogen I, and coproporphyrin I accumulate in tissues and are excreted in excess amounts in urine and feces.

CLINICAL PRESENTATION AND DIAGNOSIS Porphyrins accumulate in affected individuals during fetal development. Excretion of pink or red urine usually begins at or shortly after birth, whereas cutaneous photosensitivity, intermittent hemolysis, and splenomegaly may be manifested later. Hypertrichosis and red discoloration of the teeth (erythrodontia) and bones are common. Death may occur in childhood. With longer survival, severe scarring and mutilation occur, mostly affecting fingers, nose, and ears. The urine contains high concentrations of uroporphyrin I, coproporphyrin, and porphyrins with seven, six, five, and three carboxyl groups, whereas the excretion of ALA and PBG is normal. Large amounts of coproporphyrin I are found in the feces. Normoblasts, reticulocytes, and erythrocytes contain large quantities of uroporphyrin I and lower concentrations

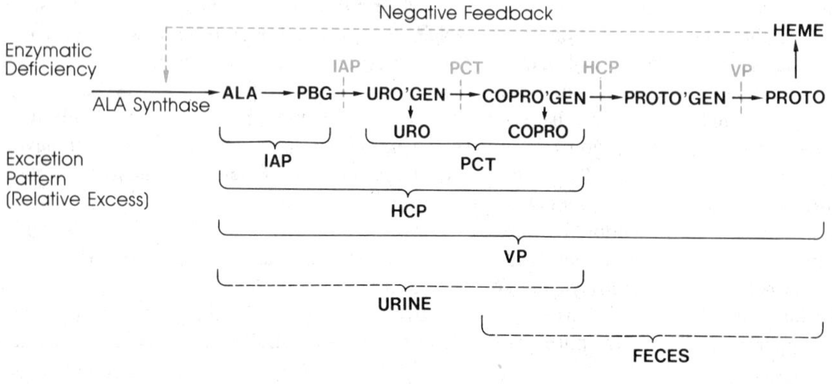

FIGURE 328-1 Patterns of urinary porphyrin and porphyrin precursor excretion in the hepatic porphyrias in relation to the enzymatic deficiency in the pathway of heme biosynthesis. Intermediates of the pathway excreted excessively during the acute phase of each of the hepatic porphyrias are within the respective brackets. (ALA, δ-aminolevulinic acid; PBG, porphobilinogen; URO'GEN, uroporphyrinogen; COPRO'GEN, coproporphyrinogen; PROTO'GEN, protoporphyrinogen; PROTO, protoporphyrin; IAP, intermittent acute porphyria; PCT, porphyria cutanea tarda; HCP, hereditary coproporphyria; VP, variegate porphyria.)

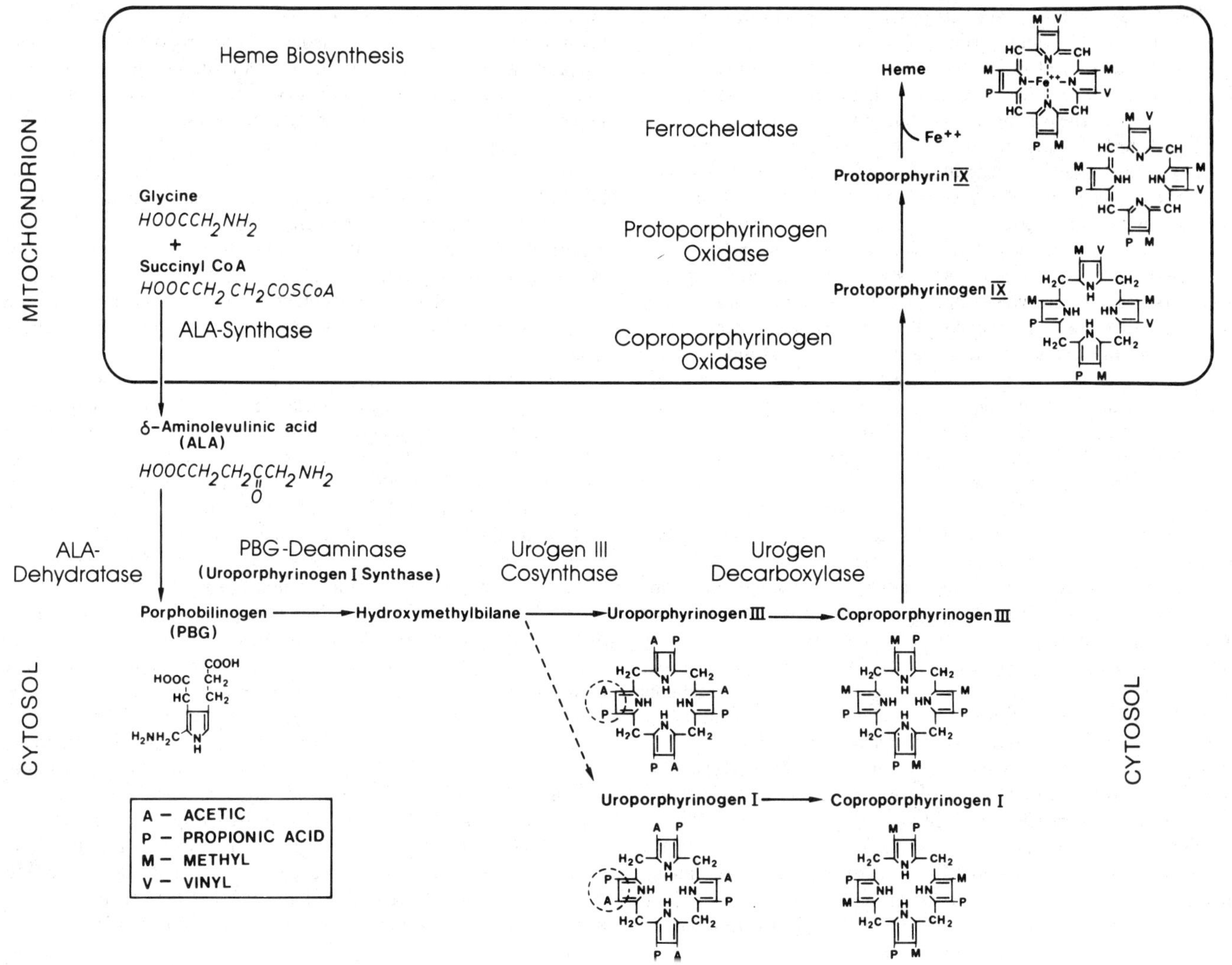

FIGURE 328-2 Outline of heme biosynthesis. (ALA, δ-aminolevulinic acid; PBG, porphobilinogen; URO'GEN, uroporphyrinogen.)

of coproporphyrinogen I. Normoblasts and reticulocytes exhibit intense red fluorescence. In accord with the normal excretion of ALA and PBG, neurologic disturbance does not occur.

TREATMENT Exposure to sunlight and trauma to the skin should be minimized. Oral carotenoids often decrease the photosensitivity (for details, see section on protoporphyria). In some cases, splenectomy has temporarily ameliorated hemolytic anemia, porphyrin excretion, and photosensitivity. The use of hematin infusions and packed erythrocyte transfusions to reduce hemolysis are other possibilities.

HEPATIC PORPHYRIAS

Three hepatic porphyrias, intermittent acute porphyria (IAP), hereditary coproporphyria (HCP), and variegate porphyria (VP), have many features in common. All are transmitted as autosomal dominants. Acute attacks of a life-threatening neurologic syndrome are precipitated by a variety of drugs, hormones, and other agents. During acute attacks increased urinary excretion of ALA and PBG occurs in all, but the patterns of porphyrins in urine and feces differ (Fig. 378-1). A recessively inherited deficiency of PBG synthase with extremely high urinary levels of ALA (but only slightly increased PBG) and a neurological syndrome identical to that of IAP, HCP, and VP has been described in a few homozygous patients (Table 328-1).

INTERMITTENT ACUTE PORPHYRIA Definition Intermittent acute porphyria [IAP, acute intermittent porphyria (AIP), pyrroloporphyria] is characterized by recurrent attacks of neurologic and psychiatric dysfunction. Photosensitivity does not occur. The primary defect is in porphobilinogen deaminase.

Genetics, incidence, and pathogenesis IAP is an autosomal dominant trait with variable expressivity. The frequency of the abnormal gene is estimated to be between 1 in 10,000 and 1 in 100,000, but in certain regions the incidence may be higher. Homozygous cases have not been observed. The defect consists of a partial (50 percent) deficiency of porphobilinogen deaminase, the enzyme that converts PBG to uroporphyrinogen I. Studies with antisera against human porphobilinogen deaminase suggest that at least four different classes of mutations can cause IAP. The most common mutation results in a decreased amount or absence of immunoreactive enzyme protein. The molecular defect at the gene level has not been defined. In the liver a partial deficiency of the enzyme leads to increased activity and/or inducibility of ALA synthase by drugs and other factors and, consequently, to increased formation and urinary excretion of ALA and PBG. Preformed porphyrins do not accumulate, and, therefore, cutaneous photosensitivity does not occur. Decreased porphobilinogen deaminase activity is observed in liver, erythrocytes, cultured skin fibroblasts, lymphocytes, and amniotic cells of patients with IAP. Thus, the enzymatic defect is present, albeit metabolically unexpressed, in tissues other than liver in most IAP patients examined. Deficiency of the enzyme does not necessarily result in clinical manifestations of acute porphyria without additional acquired factors, and only a third or less of individuals with the genetic defect ever experience an attack of porphyria. The relation between the genetic defect and the neurologic lesions is unknown.

Clinical presentation and diagnosis Symptoms rarely occur before puberty. Abdominal pain is frequently the initial and most prominent symptom of the porphyric attack. It may be moderate or severe, colicky, localized or generalized; radiation to the back or loins may occur. The pain probably results from autonomic neuropathy causing disturbed gastrointestinal motility with alternate areas of spasm and dilatation. The abdomen is usually soft, and tenderness is not marked. Because it is often accompanied by fever and leukocytosis, the acute porphyric attack can mimic any inflammatory abdominal disease. Severe vomiting and persistent constipation are common. Characteristically, the urine of patients with acute hepatic porphyria has a dark-red or "port-wine" appearance. Neurologic manifestations and mental disturbance are variable. Peripheral nerves, the autonomic nervous system, brainstem, cranial nerves, or cerebral function may be involved. Sinus tachycardia and labile hypertension with postural hypotension, urinary retention, and excessive sweating are frequent. Hypertension and tachycardia correlate with increased excretion of catecholamines. Peripheral neuropathy is predominantly motor, but sensory components may be present. Deep tendon reflexes are diminished or absent. Neuritic pain in the extremities, areas of hypesthesia and paresthesia, and foot and wrist drop are typical. Paraplegia or complete flaccid quadriplegia may ensue. Cranial nerve involvement may lead to optic nerve atrophy, ophthalmoplegia, and dysphagia. With more severe CNS involvement, delirium, coma, and seizures occur. Although the neuropathy is reversible to a surprising degree, residual paresis may last for years following an acute attack. Many patients have a long history of vague nervousness, emotional instability, and functional disturbances. Signs of mental disturbance occur in one-third, and an organic brain syndrome with restlessness, disorientation, and visual hallucinations may supervene. Hyponatremia can be severe. Multiple mechanisms (including gastrointestinal loss of sodium, imprudent fluid therapy, inappropriate secretion of antidiuretic hormone (vasopressin), and a sodium-losing nephropathy related to a toxic effect of ALA) have been implicated. Hypomagnesemia may cause tetany.

Acute attacks may last from days to months and vary in frequency and severity. In periods of remission symptoms may be slight or completely absent. Clinical (and biochemical) manifestations may be precipitated by usual therapeutic doses of barbiturates, anticonvulsants, estrogens, contraceptives, or alcohol. All these drugs are oxidized by hemoproteins of the cytochrome P_{450} system. Impaired hepatic metabolism of some of these drugs can occur during acute attacks. In some women, exacerbations correlate with the menstrual cycle, and latent porphyria may become manifest late in pregnancy or shortly after delivery. Prolonged periods of decreased caloric intake (fasting) and infections may also provoke attacks.

Laboratory findings Excessive excretion of ALA and PBG in the urine is characteristic during acute attacks and does not differentiate IAP from HCP and VP. The levels in urine do not correlate with the severity of the symptoms. The qualitative determination of porphobilinogen in the urine by the Watson-Schwartz or the Hoesch test is a simple and valuable screening aid for the diagnosis of an acute attack in IAP, HCP, and VP. These tests are almost always positive during episodes of neuropsychiatric dysfunction but are positive only when the concentration of PBG in the urine is three to five times the upper limit of normal; as a consequence, both assays may be negative in latent cases and in patients in whom urinary excretion of PBG becomes normal following recovery from an acute attack. In these instances urinary ALA and PBG excretion should be quantified by chromatographic methods. In latent IAP with normal excretion of ALA and PBG, diagnosis is possible by measuring the activity of porphobilinogen deaminase in erythrocytes, lymphocytes, or cultured skin fibroblasts. However, there is an overlap between the activities of the enzyme in erythrocytes from normals and patients with IAP, and definite diagnosis is not always possible.

In IAP the porphyrin precursors ALA and PBG are excreted in increased amounts, consistent with the enzymatic defect. Freshly passed urine is, therefore, usually colorless and contains little preformed uro- or coproporphyrin. The urine may darken on standing because PBG polymerizes spontaneously to uroporphyrin and porphobilin, a dark-brown pigment of unknown structure. However, some patients have enough nonenzymatically formed pigments to impart a dark-red appearance to freshly voided urine. The fecal porphyrin concentration is usually normal.

Conventional liver function tests are normal. A moderate reduction in red blood cell mass and blood volume and a transient normochromic, normocytic anemia are the only hematologic disturbances. Metabolic abnormalities during acute attacks include hypercholesterolemia with increased low-density lipoprotein levels, increased serum thyroxine, impaired glucose tolerance, and defective 5α-reduction of testosterone in liver. The relationship of these abnormalities to the genetic defect is unknown.

Treatment The treatment of the acute attack is identical in IAP, HCP, and VP. Some acute attacks seemingly can be aborted by administration of large quantities (500 g/d) of carbohydrates (glucose effect), although no objective study of the efficacy of this therapy has been performed. Intravenous administration of glucose at a rate of 20 g/h is recommended. If the patient does not improve within 48 h of continued glucose infusion or if neuropsychiatric symptoms progress, intravenous infusion of hematin (4 mg per kilogram of body weight infused over 10 to 15 min every 12 h for 3 to 6 days) should be tried. Hematin is commercially available in the United States as lyophilized powder (Panhematin); solutions are prepared immediately before infusion. Complications of hematin treatment seem to be rare. Thrombophlebitis at the site of infusion, a coagulopathy (manifested by thrombocytopenia, prolonged prothrombin time, abnormal partial thromboplastin time, and hypofibrinogenemia), and hemolysis have been reported. These complications apparently are caused by degradation products of unstable heme solutions. They occur less frequently or not at all with freshly prepared hematin or with stable solutions of heme-arginate, available in Europe (Normosang). Both hematin and glucose prevent the induction of hepatic ALA-synthase in animals, and both may reverse the biochemical abnormalities and cause improvement within 48 h. Supportive treatment with careful monitoring of fluid and electrolytes is important to prevent and/or correct hyponatremia, hypomagnesemia, and azotemia. Tachycardia and hypertension should be treated with beta-adrenergic blocking drugs. A list of agents considered to be "safe" or "probably safe" in patients with latent and acute IAP, HCP, and VP is given in Table 328-2. Acute attacks carry a substantial risk of fatality if

TABLE 328-2 Drugs considered to be safe (or probably safe) in patients with intermittent acute porphyria, hereditary coproporphyria, and variegate porphyria

Analgesics:
- Acetominophen, aspirin, ibuprofen
- Morphine and related opiates (meperidine, codeine)

Antibiotics:
- Penicillins, cephalosporins
- Methenamide, aminoglycosides

Psychoactive drugs:
- Phenothiazines (chlorpromazine), lithium, nortriptyline

Antihistamines:
- Diphenhydramine

Antihypertensives:
- Atenolol
- Propranolol
- Reserpine, thiazides

Miscellaneous:
- Atropine
- Cyclopropane, diethylether
- Neostigmine
- Propanidid
- Procaine
- Succinylcholine
- Nitrous oxide
- Glucocorticoids
- Oxazepam
- Chlordiazepoxide
- Insulin
- Heparin

the diagnosis is delayed and neurologic lesions progress, e.g., to respiratory paralysis. Complete recovery occurs in the majority, but neurologic deficits may require months or years to resolve. The most important measure in the management is prevention of acute attacks by instructing the patient to avoid provocative factors, such as drugs, steroids, alcohol excess, and deliberate fasting.

Some women with acute hepatic porphyria (IAP, HCP, or VP) have disabling premenstrual attacks with every cycle. These attacks can be prevented by daily intranasal or subcutaneous administration of a long-acting agonist of luteinizing hormone–releasing hormone (LHRH) such as leuprolide (leuproelin). The long-term effects of this treatment have not been evaluated.

HEREDITARY COPROPORPHYRIA Definition and genetics Hereditary coproporphyria (HCP) is a hepatic porphyria characterized by attacks of neuropsychiatric dysfunction identical with those of IAP and VP. Photosensitivity occurs in some. The primary genetic defect is a partial deficiency of coproporphyrinogen oxidase. The disease is inherited as an autosomal dominant trait. The incidence of HCP is uncertain since the majority of affected individuals remain asymptomatic.

Pathogenesis and clinical picture HCP is characterized by the excretion of large amounts of coproporphyrin III, mainly in feces but also in urine. Excretion of ALA and PBG is increased during acute attacks (positive Watson-Schwartz or Hoesch test) but usually returns to normal during remission. Acute attacks are indistinguishable from those of IAP and VP and are precipitated by the same factors. Skin photosensitivity occurs in approximately one-third of patients with overt disease. Its onset is frequently associated with intercurrent hepatic disease. A partial deficiency of coproporphyrinogen oxidase can be demonstrated in liver and other tissues.

Treatment Treatment is identical with that described for IAP.

VARIEGATE PORPHYRIA Definition Variegate porphyria (VP; South African genetic porphyria) is characterized both by acute attacks of neuropsychiatric dysfunction and by skin sensitivity to sunlight and to mechanical trauma. The primary enzymatic lesion in heme biosynthesis is a partial deficiency of protoporphyrinogen oxidase.

Genetics, incidence, and pathogenesis VP is inherited as an autosomal dominant trait. The disease is particularly common among the white population of South Africa, where its incidence is estimated at 1 in 400, and many cases have been identified as descendants of a woman who emigrated to Cape Town from the Netherlands in 1688. Elsewhere the disease is much less frequent, but VP has been recognized in many countries. The defect leads to the excretion of large amounts of protoporphyrin in bile and feces (with lesser increases in the fecal excretion of coproporphyrin) and to increased urinary excretion of ALA, PBG, and coproporphyrin during acute attacks.

Clinical presentation and diagnosis Overt cases with VP usually present in the second or third decade. The features include acute attacks of abdominal pain and neuropsychiatric symptoms, coupled with photocutaneous lesions. Neurologic and cutaneous manifestations may occur simultaneously or at different times. Most South African patients have cutaneous involvement, consisting of dermal abrasions, superficial erosions, and blister formation after trivial mechanical trauma. The mechanical fragility usually is limited to light-exposed parts of the skin. The lesions often leave depigmented or pigmented scars. Hyperpigmentation of the face and hands is common, and women often have hirsutism. The skin lesions are indistinguishable from those of porphyria cutanea tarda (PCT). Acute attacks of neuropsychiatric dysfunction are indistinguishable from those of IAP and HCP and are precipitated by the same factors. The characteristic chemical finding in VP is the continuous excretion of large amounts of proto- and coproporphyrin, even when clinical manifestations are minimal or absent. Urinary excretion of ALA, PBG, and porphyrins is either normal or moderately increased in asymptomatic patients or those who have only skin symptoms. During acute attacks the urinary excretion of ALA and PBG is increased (positive Watson-Schwartz or Hoesch test), and there also is increased urinary coproporphyrin and uroporphyrin. Erythrocyte porphyrins are normal, allowing distinction from protoporphyria.

Treatment Prophylactic measures and treatment of the acute attack with glucose and possibly hematin infusions are the same as for IAP and HCP, although the experience with hematin in VP is limited. Avoidance of exposure to direct sunlight and use of protective clothing (gloves, hats) are advocated. The prognosis is similar to or better than that of patients with IAP.

PORPHYRIA CUTANEA TARDA Definition Porphyria cutanea tarda (PCT; symptomatic cutaneous hepatic porphyria, symptomatic porphyria) is characterized by chronic lesions on light-exposed areas of the skin and a distinct pattern of urinary excretion of porphyrins. The disorder is caused by an inherited or acquired deficiency of hepatic uroporphyrinogen decarboxylase. Neurologic manifestations are absent.

Genetics, incidence, and pathogenesis There are at least four distinct types of PCT: (1) *familial PCT,* inherited as an autosomal dominant trait, in which uroporphyrinogen decarboxylase is decreased ≈50 percent in liver, erythrocytes, and other tissues; (2) *sporadic PCT,* associated with the use of alcohol or contraceptive steroids, in which a partial deficiency of uroporphyrinogen decarboxylase is restricted to the liver; (3) *hepatoerythropoietic porphyria (HEP),* which may represent a rare homozygous form of PCT, with a marked generalized decrease in uroporphyrinogen decarboxylase to <10 percent of normal and severe clinical manifestations beginning in infancy; (4) *toxic PCT,* occurring in individuals exposed to polyhalogenated hydrocarbons, notably hexachlorobenzene, and presumably also due to decreased hepatic uroporphyrinogen decarboxylase.

The incidence of the disease is not established, but sporadic PCT is the most commonly recognized type of human porphyria. It is unknown if decreased hepatic uroporphyrinogen decarboxylase in sporadic PCT is a consequence of a genetic or acquired (toxic) mechanism. Deficiency (of whatever etiology) in uroporphyrinogen decarboxylase, which catalyzes the conversion of uroporphyrinogen to coproporphyrinogen, may lead to a disturbance of hepatic heme synthesis and consequent skin photosensitivity only in the presence of additional factors such as iron overload, usually in association with alcoholic liver disease or the prolonged administration of estrogens. The mechanism by which iron overload and hormones cause clinical expression of latent PCT is unknown. In contrast to IAP, HCP, and VP, the enzymatic defect in PCT does not result in altered regulation of hepatic heme synthesis, and ALA synthase activity is normal or minimally increased even in overt cases. This probably accounts for the absence of acute neuropsychiatric attacks, the usually normal urinary ALA and PBG, and the lack of sensitivity to drugs such as barbiturates.

Clinical presentation and diagnosis Photosensitivity is the only major manifestation. The skin lesions are indistinguishable from those in VP. Skin symptoms usually begin insidiously, most often in men aged 40 to 60, and consist of enhanced facial pigmentation, increased fragility to trauma, erythema, and vesicular and ulcerative lesions. Sclerodermatous changes and increased hair on the forehead, malar region, or forearms are common.

Liver disease, frequently related to alcohol, is common, and hepatic siderosis is an almost constant finding, particularly in sporadic PCT, although the degree of iron deposition is variable and rarely severe. Spontaneous remission may occur. Estrogens (including contraceptive pills) or known hepatotoxic drugs may precipitate the clinical disease. The incidence of diabetes mellitus is increased in PCT, and association with systemic lupus erythematosus and other autoimmune syndromes has been noted.

The excretion in urine of uroporphyrin and, to a lesser extent, coproporphyrin is increased. The urine may be pink or brown. The excretion of ALA and PBG in urine is usually normal (negative Watson-Schwartz or Hoesch test). Although uroporphyrin is the major porphyrin in the urine, intermediary porphyrins (particularly hepta-carboxylic porphyrin) are also found. Increases in fecal porphyrins are less marked and usually restricted to the coproporphyrin fraction.

The diagnosis is established by the combined presence of skin photosensitivity, increased urinary uroporphyrin excretion, the lack of an increase in porphyrin precursors (ALA, PBG), and absence of a history of neuropsychiatric attacks.

Toxic acquired porphyria resembling PCT can occur in individuals accidentally exposed to polyhalogenated hydrocarbons, best documented for hexachlorobenzene. Moreover, PCT may occur in association with benign or malignant primary tumors of the liver. A syndrome apparently analogous to PCT but with no abnormalities of porphyrin excretion (pseudoporphyria) has been described in patients with chronic renal failure on hemodialysis.

Treatment Once the diagnosis of PCT is established, avoidance of alcohol, estrogens, and exposure to halogenated hydrocarbons often results in clinical and biochemical remission. Removal of hepatic iron by repeated phlebotomy may lead to long-lasting remissions within 6 to 9 months: 400 mL of blood (or the equivalent amount of erythrocytes) is removed weekly or less frequently with careful monitoring of the hemoglobin and plasma protein levels. For patients unable to tolerate phlebotomy, the administration of small doses of chloroquine (125 to 250 mg twice weekly) apparently removes uroporphyrins from the liver and has produced remissions. However, chloroquine carries the risk of hepatotoxicity. Chelation therapy with desferoxamine is another alternative to remove iron. Topical sunscreens and oral carotenoids are not effective in protecting against the skin lesions of PCT.

PROTOPORPHYRIA

DEFINITION Protoporphyria (PP; erythropoietic protoporphyria, erythrohepatic protoporphyria), a disorder in which mild skin photosensitivity is associated with high concentrations of protoporphyrin in erythrocytes, is due to a deficiency of ferrochelatase. Protoporphyrin may also accumulate in the liver.

GENETICS, INCIDENCE, AND PATHOGENESIS PP is inherited as an autosomal dominant trait with variable expressivity. The prevalence of PP is not established but seems to be similar to that of PCT. Activity of ferrochelatase, the mitochondrial enzyme that catalyzes the incorporation of ferrous iron into protoporphyrin, is deficient in bone marrow, peripheral blood, liver, and cultured skin fibroblasts. This deficiency results in the excessive accumulation of protoporphyrin in late normoblasts, reticulocytes, and young erythrocytes; protoporphyrin leaks into the plasma from erythrocytes as they age. Photosensitivity is mediated by protoporphyrin in plasma and skin and is evoked by visible light (380 to 560 nm). Skin photosensitivity shows seasonal variability. The liver participates in excess porphyrin production in some patients or, alternatively, may take up protoporphyrin from plasma. Many carriers of the defect remain clinically (and chemically) asymptomatic, and diagnosis may be possible only through enzymatic studies.

CLINICAL PRESENTATION AND DIAGNOSIS Mild photosensitivity usually begins in childhood. Exposure to sunlight for minutes or hours is followed by painful burning or stinging sensations, pruritus, erythema, and occasional edema (solar urticaria). The lesions subside over hours or days without scarring; alternatively, the initial skin lesions may progress to a chronic eczematous phase (solar eczema). There is no abnormal mechanical fragility or blister formation in skin as is characteristic for VP and PCT. Erythrodontia, hypertrichosis, and hyperpigmentation are absent. Attacks of neuropsychiatric dysfunction do not occur.

PP is generally benign, but may be associated with abnormalities of liver, biliary tract, or blood. The incidence of cholelithiasis is increased, and the gallstones contain protoporphyrin. Liver disease due to massive deposition of protoporphyrin may rarely progress to fatal cirrhosis. All patients therefore should have routine evaluation of liver function. Mild anemia is common.

PP is diagnosed by the detection of high concentrations of protoporphyrin in erythrocytes. Large numbers of red-fluorescing erythrocytes are seen by fluorescent microscopy. Protoporphyrin may also be elevated in plasma and feces, while urinary porphyrins, ALA, and PBG are usually normal.

TREATMENT Topical sunscreens usually are ineffective. Orally administered β-carotene (usually as a mixture of β-carotene and canthaxanthine) substantially improves the tolerance to sunlight. Serum β-carotene levels should be maintained between 10 and 15 μmol/L (600 and 800 μg/dL). The efficacy of carotenoid treatment is considered to be related to its ability to quench singlet oxygen and to act as free radical scavenger.

REFERENCES

BLOOMER JR: Protoporphyria, Semin Liver Dis: 2, 143, 1982

BONKOVSKY HL: Porphyria: Practical advice for the clinical gastroenterologist and hepatologist. Dig Dis 5, 179, 1987

KAPPAS A et al: The porphyrias, in *The Metabolic Basis of Inherited Disease*, 5th ed, JB Stanbury et al (eds). New York, McGraw-Hill, 1983

MASCARO JM (ed): The porphyrias. Semin Dermatol 5:69, 1986

MUSTAJOKI P, TENHUNEN R: Haem arginate in the treatment of hepatic porphyrias. Br Med J 293:538, 1986

PIERACH CA: Hematin therapy for the porphyric attack. Semin Liver Dis 2:125, 1982

PIMSTONE NR: Porphyria cutanea tarda. Semin Liver Dis 2:132, 1982

YEUNG LAIWAH AC, MCCOLL KEL: Management of attacks of acute porphyria. Drugs 34:604, 1987

329 GOUT AND OTHER DISORDERS OF PURINE METABOLISM

WILLIAM N. KELLEY / THOMAS D. PALELLA

GOUT

Gout is a term representing a heterogeneous group of diseases, which in their full development are manifested by (1) an increase in the serum urate concentration; (2) recurrent attacks of a characteristic acute arthritis, in which crystals of monosodium urate monohydrate are demonstrable in leukocytes of synovial fluid; (3) aggregated deposits of monosodium urate monohydrate (tophi) chiefly in and around the joints of the extremities and sometimes leading to severe crippling and deformity; (4) renal disease involving interstitial tissues and blood vessels; and (5) uric acid nephrolithiasis. These may occur singly or in combination.

PREVALENCE AND EPIDEMIOLOGY The serum urate value is elevated in an absolute sense when it exceeds the limit of solubility of monosodium urate in serum. At 37°C the saturation value of urate in plasma is about 415 μmol/L (7.0 mg/dL); a value above this represents supersaturation in a physicochemical sense. The serum urate concentration is relatively elevated when it exceeds the upper limit of an arbitrary normal range, usually defined as the mean serum urate value plus 2 standard deviations in a healthy population matched for age and sex. In most studies the upper limit is about 415 μmol/L (7.0 mg/dL) in men and 360 μmol/L (6.0 mg/dL) in women. In epidemiologic terms a serum urate value in excess of 415 μmol/L (7.0 mg/dL) carries an increased risk of gouty arthritis or renal stones.

Sex and age influence urate levels. In both boys and girls the serum urate concentration before puberty averages approximately 200 μmol/L (3.6 mg/dL). After puberty, levels increase in boys more than in girls. Values in men reach a plateau in the early twenties and are essentially stable thereafter. Values in women are constant from age 20 through 40, but with menopause the values rise and approach or equal those in men. These age and sex differences are thought to be related to differences in the renal clearance of urate, perhaps influenced by the levels of estrogens and androgens. Certain physiologic variables such as height, body weight, creatinine, blood urea nitrogen, serum creatinine, and blood pressure correlate with serum urate concentration. Other factors, including warm ambient temperature, alcohol intake, high social status, and achievement or intelligence also appear to correlate with a higher serum urate concentration.

Hyperuricemia by one or more of the above definitions is present in 2 to 18 percent of the population. In one hospitalized group, 13 percent of adult men exhibited a serum urate concentration in excess of 415 μmol/L (7.0 mg/dL).

The incidence and prevalence of gout are less than those of hyperuricemia. In most of the western world the overall prevalence is 0.13 to 0.37 percent of the population. The prevalence relates both to the degree of elevation of the serum urate and to the duration over which this elevation is sustained. Gout is therefore primarily a disease of adult men, and only about 5 percent of cases occur in women; it occurs rarely in the prepubertal child of either sex. The usual form is uncommon before the third decade, and the peak incidence is in the fifth decade.

INHERITANCE A family history of gout is obtained in 6 to 18 percent of gouty subjects, and figures as high as 75 percent are noted after persistent questioning. A precise definition of the inheritance of gout is complicated by the environmental factors that alter the serum urate concentration. In addition, the identification of several specific causes of gout indicates that the disorder is the common clinical manifestation of a heterogeneous group of diseases. Accordingly, analysis of the inheritance of hyperuricemia and gout in the population or even within families is difficult. Two specific enzymatic causes of gout, hypoxanthine-guanine phosphoribosyltransferase deficiency and 5-phosphoribosyl-1-pyrophosphate (PRPP) synthetase overactivity, are X-linked. In other families the inheritance is consistent with an autosomal dominant mode. More commonly, genetic studies suggest multifactorial inheritance.

CLINICAL FEATURES The full natural history of gout comprises four stages: asymptomatic hyperuricemia, acute gouty arthritis, intercritical gout, and chronic tophaceous gout. Nephrolithiasis may occur in any stage but the first.

Asymptomatic hyperuricemia Asymptomatic hyperuricemia is that stage in which the serum urate level is raised but arthritic symptoms, tophi, or uric acid stones have not yet appeared. In men vulnerable to classic gout, hyperuricemia begins at puberty, whereas in women at risk hyperuricemia is usually delayed until menopause. In contrast, patients with certain of the enzyme defects to be described later may be hyperuricemic from birth. While asymptomatic hyperuricemia may last throughout the lifetime with no recognizable consequences, the tendency toward acute gouty arthritis increases as a function of the level and the duration of hyperuricemia. The risk of nephrolithiasis also increases as serum urate values increase and correlates with the magnitude of uric acid excretion. While virtually all gouty subjects are hyperuricemic, only about 5 percent of hyperuricemics ever develop gout.

The phase of asymptomatic hyperuricemia ends with the first attack of gouty arthritis or nephrolithiasis. In most, gout comes before stone, usually after at least 20 to 30 years of sustained hyperuricemia. However, between 10 and 40 percent of gouty subjects have renal colic prior to the first episode of arthritis.

Acute gouty arthritis The primary manifestation of acute gout is exquisitely painful arthritis, at first usually monoarticular and associated with few constitutional symptoms but later often polyarticular and accompanied by fever. Estimates vary as to the percentage of patients in whom the initial gouty episode is polyarticular. Some authors' estimates are as high as 40 percent, and the majority of reports range from 3 to 14 percent. Attacks last a variable but limited period of time and are separated by asymptomatic intervals. In at least half the initial attack occurs in the first metatarsal phalangeal joint. Ultimately, 90 percent of patients experience an acute attack in the great toe (podagra).

Acute gouty arthritis is predominantly a disease of the lower extremities. The more distal the site of involvement the more typical are the attacks. Following the toe in order of frequency as sites of initial involvement are the insteps, ankles, heels, knees, wrists, fingers, and elbows. Acute attacks in the shoulder, hips, spine, sacroiliac, sternoclavicular, and mandibular joints are rare except in patients with established, severe disease. Gouty bursitis also occurs, the prepatellar and olecranon bursae being the most commonly involved sites. The patient may report trivial episodes of pain, often described as "twinges," preceding the first dramatic gouty attack. More commonly, the initial attack is unheralded and explosive. Often, the major attack begins at night, is exquisitely painful with inflamed joints, and may be triggered by a specific event such as trauma, alcohol ingestion, certain drugs, dietary excess, or surgery. The pain reaches peak intensity within several hours, and the associated signs of inflammation progress. The inflammatory response is typically so intense as to suggest pyogenic arthritis. Systemic signs may include fever, leukocytosis, and an elevated sedimentation rate. It is difficult to improve upon Sydenham's classic description:

The victim goes to bed and sleeps in good health. About two o'clock in the morning he is awakened by a severe pain in the great toe; more rarely in the heel, ankle, or instep. This pain is like that of a dislocation, and yet the parts feel as if cold water were poured over them. Then follow chills and shivers, and a little fever. The pain, which was at first moderate, becomes more intense. With its intensity the chills and shivers increase. After a time this comes to its height, accommodating itself to the bones and ligaments of the tarsus and metatarsus. Now it is a violent stretching and tearing of the ligaments—now it is a gnawing pain and now a pressure and tightening. So exquisite and lively meanwhile is the feeling of the part affected, that it cannot bear the weight of bedclothes nor the jar of a person walking in the room. The night is passed in torture, sleeplessness, turning of the part affected, and perpetual change of posture; the tossing about of the body being as incessant as the pain of the tortured joint, and being worse as the fit comes on. Hence the vain effort by change of posture, both in the body and the limb affected, to obtain an abatement of the pain.

The initial gouty episode indicates the serum urate concentration has been sufficiently elevated for a long enough period of time to result in tissue deposition of substantial amounts of urate.

Intercritical period The attack of gout may last only a day or two or up to several weeks but characteristically subsides spontaneously. No sequelae ensue, and resolution is complete. An asymptomatic phase termed the *intercritical period* then commences. The patient is totally free of symptoms during this stage, a feature that is diagnostically important. While approximately 7 percent never have a second attack, approximately 60 percent experience a recurrence within 1 year. However, the intercritical period may last up to 10 years and is terminated by successive attacks each of which may last longer and resolve less completely than its predecessors. Later attacks tend to be polyarticular, more severe, more prolonged, and associated with fever. In this stage gout may be difficult to differentiate from other types of polyarticular arthritis such as rheumatoid arthritis. Rare patients progress directly from the initial acute attack to chronic polyarticular disease with no remissions.

Tophi and chronic gouty arthritis In the untreated patient the rate of urate production exceeds the rate of urate disposition. As a result, the urate pool expands, and crystal deposits of monosodium urate eventually appear in cartilage, synovial membranes, tendons, and soft tissues. The rate of formation of these tophaceous deposits is a function of the degree and duration of hyperuricemia and of the severity of renal disease. The classic, but by no means the most common, location of a tophus is the helix or antihelix of the ear (Fig. 329-1). Tophi also commonly occur along the ulnar surface of the forearm, as saccular distensions of the olecranon bursae (Fig. 329-2), as enlargements of the Achilles tendon, or at other pressure points. Patients with the most severe tophi, interestingly, often have sparing of the helix and antihelix of the ear.

Tophi are difficult to differentiate from rheumatoid nodules and other types of subcutaneous nodules. They may ulcerate and exude chalky or pasty material rich in monosodium urate crystals. In contrast

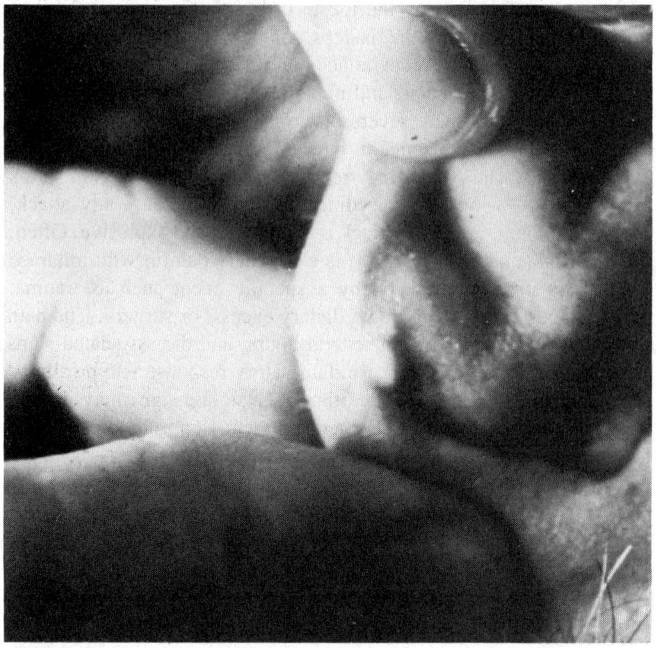

FIGURE 329-1 Tophus of the helix of the ear adjacent to the auricular tubercle.

to other subcutaneous nodules, tophi are rarely transient although they may resolve slowly in response to treatment of hyperuricemia. Documentation of monosodium urate crystals by polarizing microscopy of an aspirate establishes the nodule in question as a tophus. It is rare for a tophus to become infected. Patients with severe tophaceous disease appear to have milder and less frequent attacks of acute gouty arthritis than do nontophaceous subjects. Chronic tophaceous gout rarely occurs prior to the onset of gouty arthritis.

Effective therapy alters the natural history of the disease. Since the advent of effective antihyperuricemic therapy, only a minority of patients develop visible tophi, permanent joint changes, or chronic symptoms.

Nephropathy Some renal dysfunction occurs in up to 90 percent of subjects with gouty arthritis. Prior to the advent of chronic hemodialysis, renal failure accounted for 17 to 25 percent of deaths in the gouty population. The initial manifestation of renal involvement may be albuminuria or isosthenuria. If the patient presents in an advanced stage of renal failure it may be difficult to determine whether renal failure is a consequence of hyperuricemia or hyperuricemia is the result of renal disease.

FIGURE 329-2 Effusions of olecranon bursae of patient with gout. Note also the cutaneous deposits of urate and the minimal inflammatory response.

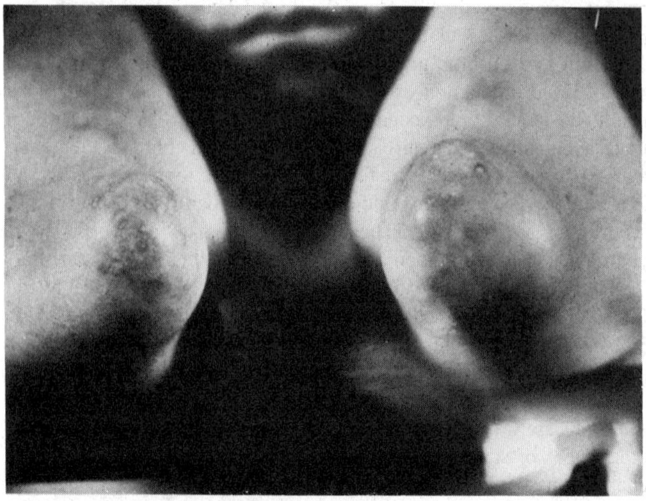

Two types of parenchymal renal damage have been described. The first, urate nephropathy, has been attributed to the deposition of monosodium urate crystals in the renal interstitial tissue. The second, obstructive uropathy, is due to the formation of uric acid crystals in the collecting tubules, renal pelvis, or ureter, with resulting blockage of urine flow.

There is considerable controversy over the pathogenesis of urate nephropathy. While crystals of monosodium urate have been demonstrated in the interstitium of kidneys from some gouty subjects, such crystals are not present in the kidneys of most people with gout. Conversely, renal interstitial urate deposition may occur in the absence of gout, although the clinical significance of such deposition is unclear. Unidentified factors may participate in the formation of urate deposits in the kidney. Further, there is a close correlation between the development of renal disease and the presence of hypertension in patients with gout. It is frequently not clear whether the hypertension causes the renal disease or the gouty renal disease is the cause of the hypertension.

Acute obstructive uropathy is a severe form of acute renal failure due to the precipitation of uric acid crystals in collecting ducts and ureters. Renal failure in this setting correlates more strongly with hyperuricaciduria than with hyperuricemia. This condition occurs most commonly in (1) patients with profound overproduction of uric acid, particularly subjects with leukemia or lymphoma who are subjected to aggressive chemotherapy, (2) patients with gout and marked hyperuricaciduria, and (3) (possibly) patients following severe exercise, rhabdomyolysis, or convulsions. Aciduria favors the formation of the relatively insoluble nonionized uric acid and, hence, may contribute to crystal precipitation in any of these conditions. Postmortem studies reveal intraluminal precipitates of uric acid with dilatation of proximal tubules. Therapy designed to decrease the formation of uric acid, accelerate urine flow, and increase the fraction of uric acid present as the more soluble ionized form, monosodium urate, is effective in the reversal of this process.

Nephrolithiasis While the prevalence of subjects with uric acid stones in the United States is about 0.01 percent, the prevalence in gouty subjects ranges from 10 to 25 percent. The major factor favoring formation of uric acid stones is the increased urinary excretion of uric acid. Hyperuricaciduria may be due to primary gout, inborn errors of metabolism resulting in the overproduction of uric acid, myeloproliferative disease, and other neoplastic disorders. When the urinary uric acid exceeds 6.5 mmol/d (1100 mg/d), the incidence reaches 50 percent. There is also correlation with increasing serum urate concentrations, the prevalence reaching approximately 50 percent at a serum urate value of 770 μmol/L (13 mg/dL) or above. Other factors contributing to the formation of uric acid stones include (1) undue acidity of the urine, (2) increased urine concentration, and (3) (perhaps) abnormalities of urinary constituents that affect the solubility of uric acid itself.

Gouty subjects also have an increased frequency of calcium-containing stones; the occurrence in gout is 1 to 3 percent, while that in the general population is about 0.1 percent. While the mechanisms for this association are unclear, there is a high frequency of hyperuricemia and hyperuricaciduria in patients seen because of calcium stones. Uric acid crystals may serve as a nidus for calcium stone formation.

Associated conditions Obesity, hypertriglyceridemia, and hypertension are common. The hypertriglyceridemia of primary gout is more closely associated with obesity or alcohol ingestion than with hyperuricemia itself. The incidence of hypertension in the nongouty population is correlated with age, sex, and obesity; when these factors are appropriately scored, there appears to be little or no direct relationship between hyperuricemia and hypertension. The increased frequency of diabetes is also probably related to factors such as age and obesity and not to hyperuricemia itself. In addition, the increased incidence of atherosclerosis has been attributed to the concomitant obesity, hypertension, diabetes, and hypertriglyceridemia.

Independent analysis of these variables suggests that obesity is

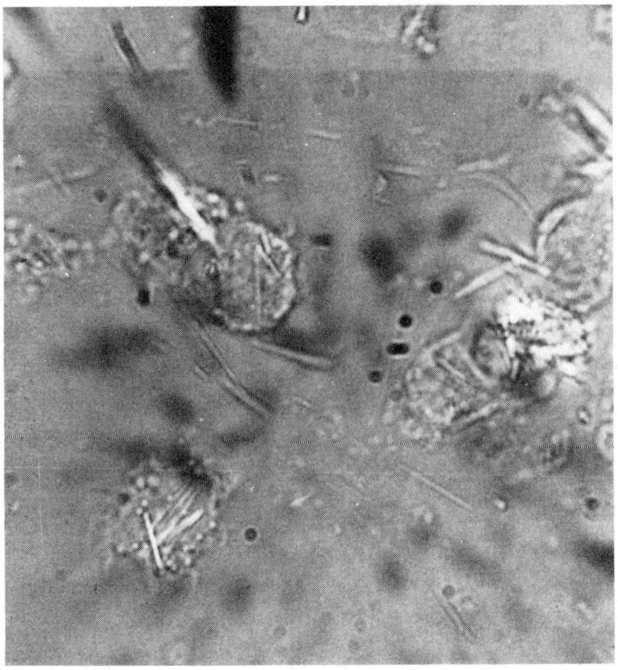

FIGURE 329-3 Crystals of monosodium urate monohydrate in joint aspirate.

most important. Hyperuricemia in the obese subject appears to be related to both increased production and reduced excretion of uric acid. Chronic alcohol ingestion also results in both overproduction and underexcretion of uric acid.

Rheumatoid arthritis, systemic lupus erythematosus, and amyloidosis rarely coexist with gout. The reasons for these negative associations are not known.

Acute gout should be suspected in any patient presenting with the sudden onset of monoarthritis, particularly in a distal joint of the lower extremity. Synovial aspiration should be performed in all such patients. The diagnosis of gout is established with certainty upon demonstration of monosodium urate crystals in leukocytes of synovial fluid from the involved joint by compensated polarized light microscopy (Fig. 329-3). The crystals are typically needle-shaped and negatively birefringent. Such crystals can be identified in synovial fluid of over 95 percent of patients with acute gouty arthritis. Failure to demonstrate urate crystals in synovial fluid after careful search under appropriate conditions makes the diagnosis unlikely. The presence of intracellular urate crystals establishes the diagnosis but does not exclude the possibility that another type of arthropathy is present concurrently.

Infection or pseudogout (calcium pyrophosphate dihydrate deposition) may coexist with gout. A Gram stain of the synovial fluid should be examined, and cultures should be obtained to exclude coexistent infection. Calcium pyrophosphate dihydrate is weakly positively birefringent and is more rectangular than monosodium urate. With polarized light microscopy, the crystals are easily differentiated. Synovial aspiration need not be repeated with subsequent episodes unless an alternative diagnosis is being considered.

During asymptomatic intercritical periods, synovial aspiration may still be helpful. Extracellular urate crystals can be found in more than two-thirds of aspirates from the first metatarsophalangeal joints of asymptomatic gouty patients Less than 5 percent of hyperuricemic patients without gout have such crystals.

Synovial fluid analysis may also be helpful in other ways. The total leukocyte count may be low or high. The predominant cell type is the polymorphonuclear leukocyte. As with other inflammatory fluids, the mucin clot is fair to poor. The concentrations of glucose and uric acid are the same as in serum.

In the patient in whom synovial fluid cannot be obtained or in whom intracellular crystals cannot be demonstrated, a presumptive diagnosis of gout can be seriously entertained if the patient has (1) hyperuricemia, (2) the classic clinical features described above, and (3) a dramatic response to colchicine. In the absence of crystals or this highly suggestive triad, the diagnosis of gout should be considered tentative. A dramatic therapeutic response to colchicine is strongly suggestive of the diagnosis of gouty arthritis but is not pathognomonic by itself.

Acute gouty arthritis must be differentiated from other causes of monarticular and polyarticular arthritis. A common initial presentation in the gouty patient is podagra, but many conditions mimic the painful, swollen big toe characteristic of the disease. These include soft tissue infection, pyogenic arthritis, inflamed bunions, local trauma, rheumatoid arthritis, degenerative arthritis with acute inflammation, acute sarcoidosis, psoriatic arthritis, pseudogout, acute calcific tendonitis, palindromic rheumatism, Reiter's disease, and sporotrichosis. Rarely, confusion may be caused by cellulitis, gonorrhea, fibrosis of the sole and heel, hematoma, and subacute bacterial endocarditis with embolization or suppurative arthritis. Gouty involvement of other joints such as the knee must also be differentiated from acute rheumatic fever, serum sickness, hemarthrosis, and the peripheral joint involvement of ankylosing spondylitis or inflammatory bowel disease.

Chronic gouty arthritis must be differentiated from rheumatoid arthritis, inflammatory osteoarthritis, psoriatic arthritis, enteropathic arthritis, and the peripheral arthritis associated with the spondyloarthropathies. A history of antecedent, self-limited monarticular arthritis, the presence of tophi, typical radiographic changes, and the demonstration of hyperuricemia add support to the diagnosis of chronic gout. Chronic gout can be similar to other inflammatory arthropathies. The existence of effective therapy for gout justifies a vigorous workup to establish or exclude this diagnosis.

PATHOPHYSIOLOGY OF HYPERURICEMIA **Classification** The biochemical hallmark and prerequisite of gout is hyperuricemia. The concentration of uric acid in body fluids is determined by the balance between rates of production and elimination. Uric acid is formed by oxidation of purine bases, which may be exogenous or endogenous in origin. About two-thirds of uric acid is excreted into the urine [1.8 to 3.6 mmol/d (300 to 600 mg/d)], and approximately one third is excreted into the gastrointestinal tract, where it is ultimately destroyed by bacteria. Hyperuricemia may be due to an excessive rate of uric acid production, a decrease in the renal excretion of uric acid, or a combination of both events.

Hyperuricemia and gout may be classified as metabolic or renal (Table 329-1). In those patients with hyperuricemia of metabolic origin, there is an increased production of uric acid, whereas in those with hyperuricemia of renal origin, decreased renal excretion of uric acid causes hyperuricemia. The distinction between metabolic and renal origins of hyperuricemia is not always clear-cut. A large number of gouty subjects have evidence of both mechanisms when thoroughly investigated. In such cases, the dominant component—renal or metabolic—directs classification. In the classification used here *primary* refers to those cases in which gout or hyperuricemia is the central manifestation of the disease, namely, gout that is neither secondary to another acquired disorder nor a subordinate manifestation of an inborn error that leads initially to a major disease unlike gout. While some cases of primary gout have a defined genetic basis, others do not. *Secondary* hyperuricemia or gout refers to those cases which develop in the course of another disease or as a consequence of drugs.

Overproduction of uric acid Overproducers of uric acid by definition excrete in excess of 3.6 mmol/d (600 mg/d) after a 5-day period of dietary purine restriction; such patients probably represent less than 10 percent of the gouty population. In these patients there is an acceleration in the rate of purine biosynthesis de novo or an increased turnover of purines. Understanding the basic mechanisms responsible for these abnormalities requires an understanding of purine metabolism (Fig. 329-4).

The purine nucleotides, adenylic acid (AMP), inosinic acid (IMP),

TABLE 329-1 Classification of hyperuricemia and gout

Type	Metabolic disturbance	Inheritance
Metabolic (10%):		
Primary		
Molecular defects undefined	Not established	Polygenic
Associated with specific enzyme defects		
PRPP synthetase variants, increased activity	Overproduction of PRPP and of uric acid	X-linked
Hypoxanthine-guanine phosphoribosyltransferase deficiency, partial	Overproduction of uric acid, increased purine biosynthesis de novo driven by surplus PRPP	X-linked
Secondary		
Associated with increased purine biosynthesis de novo		
Glucose-6-phosphatase deficiency or absence	Overproduction plus underexcretion of uric acid; glycogen storage disease, type I (von Gierke)	Autosomal recessive
Hypoxanthine-guanine phosphoribosyltransferase deficiency, "virtually complete"	Overproduction of uric acid; Lesch-Nyhan syndrome	X-linked
Associated with increased nucleic acid turnover	Overproduction of uric acid	
Renal (90%):		
Primary		
Secondary		

and guanylic acid (GMP), are the end products of purine biosynthesis. They can be synthesized in one of two ways: either directly from the purine bases, e.g., guanine to GMP, hypoxanthine to IMP, and adenine to AMP; or they may be synthesized de novo, beginning with nonpurine precursors and progressing through a series of steps to the formation of IMP, which is the common intermediate purine nucleotide. IMP can be converted either to AMP or to GMP. Once the purine nucleotides are formed, they are utilized for the synthesis of nucleic acids, adenosine triphosphate (ATP), cyclic AMP, cyclic GMP, and certain cofactors.

The various purine components are degraded to the purine nucleotide monophosphates. GMP is degraded via guanosine, guanine, and xanthine to uric acid. IMP is degraded through inosine, hypoxanthine, and xanthine to uric acid. AMP can be deaminated to IMP and further catabolized through inosine to uric acid, or it may be degraded to inosine by an alternate pathway with the intermediate formation of adenosine.

While the purine pathway is regulated in a complex manner, the intracellular concentration of 5-phosphoribosyl-1-pyrophosphate (PRPP) appears to be a major determinant of the rate of synthesis of uric acid in humans. Generally, when the concentration of PRPP in the cell is high, uric acid synthesis is elevated; when the concentration of PRPP is reduced, the synthesis of uric acid is also reduced.

Overproduction of uric acid in a small minority of adult gouty subjects occurs as either a primary or a secondary manifestation of an inborn error in metabolism. Hyperuricemia and gout occur as a primary manifestation of partial hypoxanthine-guanine phosphoribosyltransferase deficiency (reaction 2, Fig. 329-4) and of PRPP synthetase superactivity (reaction 3, Fig. 329-4). In the Lesch-Nyhan syndrome, the virtually complete deficiency of hypoxanthine-guanine phosphoribosyltransferase results in secondary hyperuricemia. These important inborn errors are discussed more fully below.

These two inborn errors of purine metabolism, hypoxanthine-guanine phosphoribosyltransferase deficiency and PRPP synthetase overactivity, account for less than 15 percent of all patients with primary hyperuricemia associated with an overproduction of uric acid. The cause of the overproduction in the majority of patients has not been defined.

There are numerous causes of secondary hyperuricemia associated with an increased production of uric acid. In some, the increased excretion of uric acid is related, as it is in primary gout, to an accelerated rate of purine biosynthesis de novo. Patients with glucose-

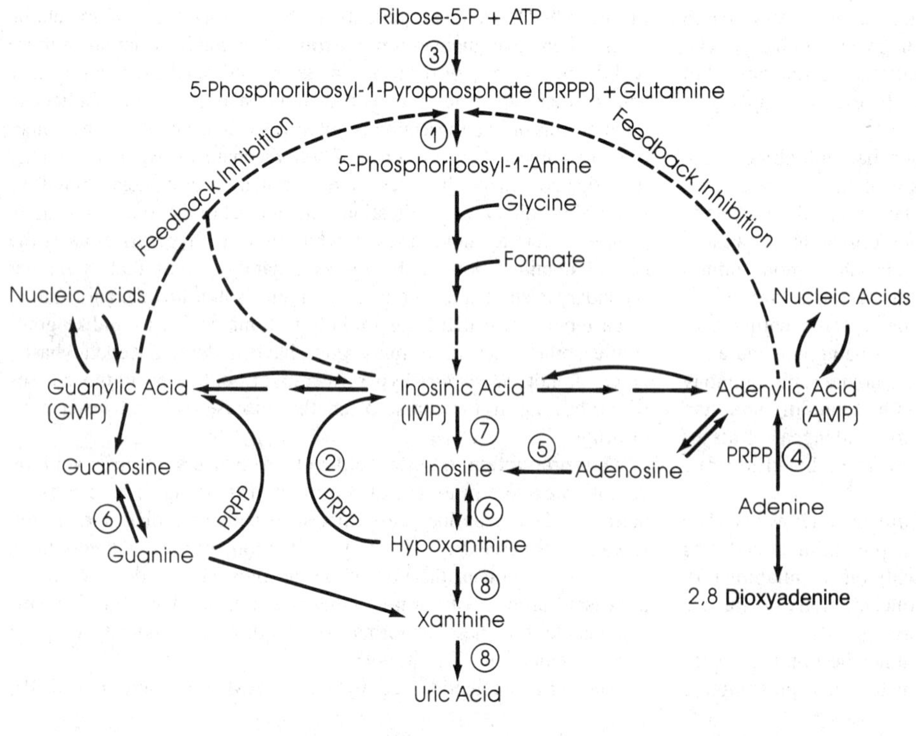

FIGURE 329-4 Outline of purine metabolism: (1) amidophosphoribosyltransferase; (2) hypoxanthine-guanine phosphoribosyltransferase; (3) PRPP synthetase; (4) adenine phosphoribosyltransferase; (5) adenosine deaminase; (6) purine nucleoside phosphorylase; (7) 5′-nucleotidase; (8) xanthine oxidase.

6-phosphatase deficiency (type I glycogen storage disease) uniformly exhibit an increased production of uric acid as well as an accelerated rate of purine biosynthesis de novo (see Chap. 332). Overproduction of uric acid in patients with this enzyme defect is multifactorial. An accelerated rate of de novo purine synthesis may be due in part to accelerated synthesis of PRPP. Additionally, accelerated degradation of purine nucleotides contributes to an increased rate of uric acid excretion. Both of these mechanisms are due to the deficiency of glucose as an energy source, and the production of uric acid can be decreased by the sustained correction of hypoglycemia in this disorder.

In the majority of patients with secondary hyperuricemia due to an overproduction of uric acid, the predominant abnormality appears to be an increased turnover of nucleic acids. A number of diseases, including the myeloproliferative and lymphoproliferative disorders, multiple myeloma, secondary polycythemia, pernicious anemia, certain hemoglobinopathies, thalassemia, other hemolytic anemias, infectious mononucleosis, and some carcinomas, may be associated with increased marrow activity or increased cell turnover in the marrow or at other sites and an associated increased turnover of nucleic acids. The increased turnover in nucleic acids leads in turn to hyperuricemia, hyperuricaciduria, and a compensatory increase in the rate of purine biosynthesis de novo.

Reduced excretion A large proportion of gouty subjects require a plasma urate value 60 to 120 μmol/L (1 to 2 mg/dL) higher than normal subjects to achieve a given rate of uric acid excretion (Fig. 329-5). This abnormality is most prominent in the gouty subject with a normal production of uric acid and is not present in most subjects with overproduction of uric acid.

The excretion of urate is dependent on glomerular filtration, tubular reabsorption, and tubular secretion. Uric acid appears to be completely filtered at the glomerulus and reabsorbed in the proximal tubule (i.e., presecretory reabsorption). Uric acid secretion then occurs in a subsequent segment of the proximal tubule, and partial reabsorption takes place at a second reabsorptive site in the distal portion of the proximal tubule (i.e., postsecretory reabsorption). While some uric acid reabsorption may also occur in the ascending limb of the loop of Henle and in the collecting duct, these latter two sites are thought to be quantitatively less important. The nature of these latter sites and the magnitude of their contribution to uric acid transport is not known.

FIGURE 329-5 Rate of uric acid excretion at various plasma urate levels in nongouty (solid symbols) and gouty (open symbols) subjects. Large symbols represent mean values; small symbols represent individual data of a few mean values selected to illustrate the degree of scatter within groups. Studies were conducted under basal conditions, after RNA feeding, and after infusions of lithium urate. *(From Wyngaarden. Reproduced by permission of Academic Press.)*

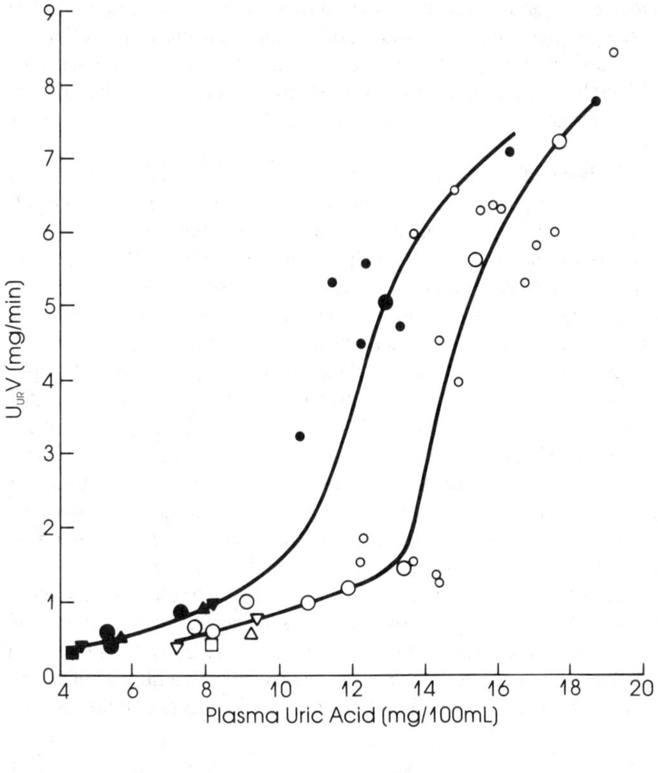

Theoretically, the altered renal excretion of uric acid exhibited by most patients with gout could be due to (1) reduced filtration of uric acid, (2) enhanced reabsorption, or (3) decreased secretion. No unequivocal data establish any one of these mechanisms as the basic defect, and it is likely that all three are operative within the gouty population.

Numerous secondary causes of hyperuricemia and gout can also be attributed to a decrease in the renal excretion of uric acid. A reduction in the glomerular filtration rate leads to a decrease in the filtered load of uric acid and thus to hyperuricemia; patients with renal disease are hyperuricemic on this basis. Other factors, such as decreased secretion of uric acid, have been postulated in patients with some types of renal disease (e.g., polycystic kidney disease and lead nephropathy). Gout is a rare complication of the secondary hyperuricemia due to renal disease.

Diuretic therapy is one of the most important causes of secondary hyperuricemia. Diuretic-induced volume depletion leads to enhanced tubular reabsorption of uric acid as well as decreased uric acid filtration. Decreased secretion of uric acid may also be a mechanism in diuretic-induced hyperuricemia. Other drugs lead to hyperuricemia by undefined renal mechanisms; these agents include low-dose aspirin, pyrazinamide, nicotinic acid, ethambutol, and ethanol.

Impaired renal excretion of uric acid is thought to be an important mechanism for the hyperuricemia associated with several disease states. Volume depletion may be important in patients with hyperuricemia associated with adrenal insufficiency and nephrogenic diabetes insipidus. In some situations hyperuricemia has been attributed to competitive inhibition of uric acid secretion by excess organic acids thought to be secreted by the same renal tubular mechanism responsible for uric acid secretion. Examples include starvation (ketosis and free fatty acids), alcoholic ketosis, diabetic ketoacidosis, maple syrup urine disease, and lactic acidosis of any cause. Hyperuricemia in conditions such as hyperparathyroidism, hypoparathyroidism, pseudohypoparathyroidism, and hypothyroidism may also have a renal basis, but the mechanism is unclear.

PATHOGENESIS OF ACUTE GOUTY ARTHRITIS The events leading to the initial crystallization of monosodium urate in a joint after an average of 30 years of asymptomatic hyperuricemia are not completely understood. Sustained hyperuricemia leads eventually to the development of microtophi in the synovial lining cells and perhaps to an accumulation in cartilage of monosodium urate on proteoglycans that have a high affinity for urate. By one of several mechanisms, probably including trauma with disruption of the microtophi and increased turnover of the cartilage proteoglycans, there is an episodic release of urate crystals into the synovial fluid. Other factors, such as a lower temperature in the joint space or an unequal reabsorption of water and urate from the synovial fluid, may accelerate urate precipitation.

A sufficient amount of crystals in the joint space triggers the acute attack by a process that appears to include (1) phagocytosis of the crystals by leukocytes with the rapid release of a chemotactic protein from the leukocytes, (2) activation of the kallikrein system, (3) activation of complement with the consequent formation of the chemotactic complement components, and (4) the ultimate urate-mediated disruption of lysosomes within the leukocytes, leading to destruction of white blood cells and release of lysosomal products into the synovial fluid. While progress in the understanding of acute gouty arthritis has occurred, questions about factors responsible for spontaneous resolution of the acute attack and the effect of colchicine remain to be answered.

TREATMENT The therapeutic aims in gout are (1) to terminate the acute attack as promptly and gently as possible; (2) to prevent recurrences of acute gouty arthritis; (3) to prevent or reverse complications of the disease resulting from deposition of monosodium urate crystals in joints, kidneys, and other sites; (4) to prevent or reverse associated features such as obesity, hypertriglyceridemia, or hypertension; and (5) to prevent formation of uric acid kidney stones.

Treatment of the acute gouty attack Acute gouty arthritis is treated with an anti-inflammatory agent. Colchicine is the drug most frequently employed. Standard therapy involves administration of 0.5 mg each hour or 1.0 mg every 2 h by mouth until one of three things occurs: (1) the patient improves, (2) gastrointestinal side effects develop, or (3) a maximum of 6 mg is taken without relief. Colchicine is most effective if therapy is begun shortly after the onset of symptoms. Over 75 percent of patients with gout show major improvement in symptoms within the first 12 h of treatment. However, as many as 80 percent of patients are unable to tolerate an optimal dose because of gastrointestinal side effects, which may precede or coincide with clinical improvement. Orally administered colchicine results in peak plasma levels in approximately 2 h. Consequently, it has been suggested that 1.0 mg every 2 h is less likely to lead to the accumulation of toxic levels before the onset of therapeutic effect. However, since therapeutic benefit relates to colchicine levels within leukocytes rather than plasma levels, the efficacy of this regimen requires further evaluation.

Intravenous administration of colchicine eliminates gastrointestinal side effects and provides a more rapid response. Colchicine levels become high in leukocytes, remain constant for 24 h, and are detectable for over 10 days after a single intravenous infusion. As an initial dose 2 mg should be given intravenously, followed by two additional doses of 1 mg at 6-h intervals if needed. Special care must be taken in the intravenous administration of colchicine. The drug is irritative and can lead to severe pain and necrosis if allowed to extravasate to surrounding tissues. It is important to make certain that the intravenous route is secure and that the drug is diluted with 5 to 10 volumes of normal saline solution and infused over a period of no less than 5 min. Colchicine by either oral or parenteral route may cause bone marrow depression, alopecia, hepatocellular failure, mental depression, seizures, ascending paralysis, respiratory depression, and death. Toxic effects are more likely in patients with hepatic, bone marrow, or renal disease and in those subjects on maintenance colchicine. The dosage should be reduced for these individuals, and the drug should not be used in neutropenic patients.

Other anti-inflammatory agents, including indomethacin, phenylbutazone, naproxen, and fenoprofen, are also effective in the treatment of acute gouty arthritis. Indomethacin may be given at a dose of 75 mg orally, followed by 50 mg every 6 h and continued at that dose for 24 h after relief is obtained. The drug is then tapered to 50 mg every 8 h for three doses and then to 25 mg every 8 h for three doses. Side effects of indomethacin include gastrointestinal toxicity, sodium retention, and complaints referable to the central nervous system. While the incidence of side effects may be as high as 60 percent in patients taking the doses described above, the drug is generally better tolerated than colchicine and probably is the treatment of choice in the patient with a well-established diagnosis of acute gouty arthritis. To improve the therapeutic response and thus diminish morbidity of the disease, the patient may be instructed to begin therapy with an anti-inflammatory agent at the first twinge of an acute attack. Uricosuric drugs and allopurinol have no role in the treatment of the acute gouty attack.

Systemic or locally administered (i.e., intraarticular) glucocorticoids are useful in treating acute gout particularly when colchicine and nonsteroidal anti-inflammatory drugs are contraindicated or ineffective. When given systemically, moderate doses should be administered either by the oral or intravenous route for several days at most before the drug is rapidly tapered and discontinued. An isolated monarthritis or bursitis can be terminated within 24 or 36 h by the intraarticular instillation of a long-acting steroid preparation (e.g., triamcinolone hexacetonide, 15 to 30 mg). This is particularly useful when standard drug regimens are not practical.

Prophylaxis Once the acute episode has resolved, a number of measures can reduce the likelihood of recurrence: (1) the institution of prophylactic daily colchicine or indomethacin, (2) controlled weight reduction for the obese patient, (3) avoidance of known precipitating factors such as heavy alcohol consumption or a diet rich in purines, and (4) the institution of antihyperuricemic therapy.

The administration of small daily doses of colchicine is effective prophylaxis against further acute attacks. A program of 1 to 2 mg colchicine a day is successful in about three-fourths of patients with gout and fails completely in only about 5 percent. In addition, this program is safe and essentially free of side effects. However, unless serum urate is maintained at normal levels, the patient is spared only acute arthritis and may develop other manifestations of gout. Maintenance colchicine therapy is particularly helpful during the first year or two after institution of antihyperuricemic drugs.

Prevention or reversal of the deposition of monosodium urate in tissues Antihyperuricemic agents are effective in reducing serum urate concentration and should be used in patients with (1) one or more attacks of acute gouty arthritis, (2) one or more tophi, and (3) uric acid nephrolithiasis. The aim of antihyperuricemic therapy is to maintain the serum urate below 415 μmol/L (7.0 mg/dL), the minimal concentration at which urate saturates the extracellular fluid. Reduction to these levels may be achieved by use of drugs that increase the renal excretion of uric acid or decrease uric acid production. Antihyperuricemic drugs generally do not have anti-inflammatory properties. Uricosuric agents reduce serum urate by enhancing the renal excretion. While a large number of drugs exhibit this property, the most effective agents available in the United States are probenecid and sulfinpyrazone. Probenecid is usually started in doses of 250 mg twice a day; it is increased over a period of several weeks to the dose necessary to achieve effective reversal of the hyperuricemia. A total dose of 1 g/d is appropriate for half of patients; the maximum dose should not exceed 3.0 g/d. Because the half-life is 6 to 12 h, it should be given in two to four evenly spaced doses per day. Hypersensitivity, skin rash, and gastrointestinal complaints are the major side effects. Although serious toxicity is rare, side effects may cause up to a third of the patients to discontinue probenecid.

Sulfinpyrazone is a metabolite of phenylbutazone with no anti-inflammatory activity. The drug is usually started at a dose of 50 mg twice a day and gradually increased to a maintenance level of 300 to 400 mg/d given in three or four divided doses. The maximum effective daily dose is 800 mg. Side effects are similar to those with probenecid, although the incidence of bone marrow toxicity may be higher. Approximately a fourth of patients stop the drug for one reason or another.

Probenecid and sulfinpyrazone are effective in most patients with hyperuricemia and gout. In addition to intolerance, failures can result from poor patient compliance, concomitant salicylate ingestion, or impaired renal function. Aspirin at any dose blocks the uricosuric effect of probenecid and sulfinpyrazone. These agents begin to lose effectiveness as the creatinine clearance falls below 80 mL/min and are ineffective when clearance reaches 30 mL/min.

During the negative urate balance induced by uricosuric therapy, the serum urate value drops and urinary uric acid excretion is elevated above pretreatment levels. With continuation of therapy excess urate is mobilized and eliminated, the serum urate falls, and uric acid excretion returns essentially to pretreatment levels. The transient increase in uric acid excretion, which usually lasts for only a few days, may lead to the development of renal calculi in a tenth of patients so treated. To avoid this complication uricosuric agents should be started at low doses and gradually increased as described. Maintaining an ample urine flow with adequate hydration and alkalinizing the urine with oral sodium bicarbonate alone or in combination with acetazolamide reduce the likelihood of stone formation. The ideal candidate for uricosuric agents is under 60 and has normal renal function, uric acid excretion of less than 700 mg/d on a general diet, and no history of renal stones.

Hyperuricemia may also be controlled by allopurinol, a drug that decreases uric acid synthesis. Allopurinol inhibits xanthine oxidase (reaction 8, Fig. 329-4), the enzyme that catalyzes the oxidation of hypoxanthine to xanthine and xanthine to uric acid. While allopurinol has a half-life in vivo of only 2 to 3 h, it is metabolized largely to oxipurinol, which also is an effective inhibitor of xanthine oxidase and has a half-life ranging from 18 to 30 h. In most patients 300 mg/d is an effective antihyperuricemic dose. Because of the long half-life of the major metabolite the drug may be administered once a day. Since oxipurinol is largely excreted in the urine, its half-life is prolonged in patients with renal insufficiency. The dose of allopurinol should, therefore, be reduced by half in patients with significant renal dysfunction.

Significant side effects of allopurinol include gastrointestinal distress, skin rashes, fever, toxic epidermal necrolysis, alopecia, bone marrow suppression, hepatitis, jaundice, and vasculitis. The overall incidence of side effects is about 20 percent; they are more common in the presence of renal insufficiency. In only 5 percent of patients the side effects are sufficient to force discontinuation of the drug. Important drug-drug interactions involving allopurinol include prolongation of the half-lives of mercaptopurine and azathioprine and enhancement of the toxicity of cyclophosphamide.

Specific indications for choosing allopurinol over a uricosuric drug include (1) an increased urinary uric acid excretion (greater than 700 mg/d on a general diet), (2) impairment of renal function with a creatinine clearance less than 80 mL/min, (3) tophaceous gout regardless of renal function, (4) uric acid nephrolithiasis, and (5) gout not controlled by uricosuric agents because of ineffectiveness or intolerance. Allopurinol and a uricosuric drug may be used simultaneously in the rare patient who cannot be controlled by a single medication. Such combination therapy requires no modification in the dosage of either agent and usually results in further lowering of the serum urate concentration.

Acute gouty arthritis may occur whenever there is a rapid and substantial change in the serum urate concentration. Thus, the initiation of antihyperuricemic therapy with any agent may precipitate acute gouty arthritis. In addition, recurrent attacks may occur for a year or longer when large tophaceous deposits are present, even if hyperuricemia is controlled. For these reasons, it is prudent to begin prophylactic therapy with colchicine prior to initiation of antihyperuricemic drugs and to continue it until the serum urate is controlled for at least a year or until all tophi have resolved. Patients should be warned of the possibility of flare-up during the early phase of therapy. While it is not necessary in most gouty patients, strict dietary purine restriction should be instituted in patients with severe tophaceous gout and/or renal failure.

Prevention and treatment of acute uric acid nephropathy Immediate and vigorous therapy is essential for acute uric acid nephropathy. The first step is to increase urine flow by vigorous hydration coupled with administration of a potent diuretic such as furosemide. The urine should be alkalinized to achieve conversion of uric acid to the more soluble monosodium urate. Alkalinization can be accomplished by the administration of sodium bicarbonate alone or in combination with acetazolamide. Allopurinol should also be administered to reduce uric acid formation. The initial dose in this setting should be 8 mg/kg body weight per day given as a single daily dose. The dose should be decreased after 3 or 4 days to 100 to 200 mg/d if renal insufficiency persists. Treatment for uric acid kidney stones is similar to that for acute uric acid nephropathy. In most cases allopurinol combined only with high fluid intake is effective.

WORKUP OF THE HYPERURICEMIC PATIENT Evaluation of the patient with hyperuricemia is directed toward (1) defining the cause of the hyperuricemia (which may disclose an important disease other than gout), (2) assessing the presence and extent of damage to tissues and organs, and (3) identifying associated abnormalities. From a practical standpoint these inquiries are pursued simultaneously, since decisions about the significance of hyperuricemia and about therapy depend on the answers to all of these.

The most important single test in the hyperuricemic patient is analysis of the urine for uric acid. If a history of stone disease is present, a flat plate of the abdomen and intravenous pyelogram may be indicated. If a renal stone is recovered, analysis for uric acid and other constituents is useful. If joint disease is present, synovial fluid analysis and x-rays of the involved joints are helpful. If there is a history of exposure to lead, measurement of urinary lead excretion after an infusion of calcium edetate may be useful in documenting the presence of gout due to lead exposure. In cases where the patient appears to be an overproducer, measurement of erythrocyte hypoxanthine-guanine phosphoribosyltransferase and PRPP synthetase levels may be indicated.

Management of asymptomatic hyperuricemia There is considerable controversy about the indications for therapy of the patient with asymptomatic hyperuricemia. Generally, treatment should be withheld unless the patient (1) becomes symptomatic; (2) has a strong family history for gout, nephrolithiasis, or renal failure; or (3) excretes large quantities of uric acid (greater than 6.5 mmol/d (1100 mg/d).

OTHER DISORDERS OF PURINE METABOLISM ASSOCIATED WITH HYPERURICEMIA AND GOUT

HYPOXANTHINE-GUANINE PHOSPHORIBOSYLTRANSFERASE DEFICIENCY STATES Hypoxanthine-guanine phosphoribosyltransferase catalyzes the conversion of hypoxanthine to inosinic acid and guanine to guanosinic acid (reaction 2, Fig. 329-4). PRPP serves as the phosphoribosyl donor. The deficiency of hypoxanthine-guanine phosphoribosyltransferase leads to decreased consumption of PRPP, which accumulates to higher than normal levels. The excess PRPP accelerates de novo purine biosynthesis and consequently increases uric acid production.

The Lesch-Nyhan syndrome is an X-linked disorder. The characteristic biochemical abnormality is a profound deficiency of the enzyme hypoxanthine-guanine phosphoribosyltransferase (reaction 2, Fig. 329-4). Affected patients have hyperuricemia and a profound overproduction of uric acid. In addition, they have a bizarre neurologic disorder characterized by self-mutilation, choreoathetosis, spasticity, and retardation of growth and mental function. The incidence is estimated at 1:100,000 births.

From 0.5 to 1.0 percent of adult gouty subjects with overproduction of uric acid have a partial deficiency of hypoxanthine-guanine phosphoribosyltransferase. These patients typically have the onset of gouty arthritis at a young age (15 to 30 years), a high incidence of uric acid stones (75 percent), and the occasional occurrence of mild neurologic dysfunction characterized by dysarthria, hyperreflexia, incoordination, and/or mental retardation. This disease is inherited as an X-linked trait so that men are affected through carrier females.

The enzyme whose deficiency results in these disorders, hypoxanthine-guanine phosphoribosyltransferase, is of considerable interest in genetics. With the possible exception of the globin gene family, the hypoxanthine-guanine phosphoribosyltransferase locus is the single most studied human gene.

Human hypoxanthine-guanine phosphoribosyltransferase has been purified to homogeneity, and its amino acid sequence has been determined. The normal enzyme has a native subunit molecular weight of 24,470 and consists of 217 amino acid residues. The normal enzyme is a tetramer with four identical subunits. The DNA sequence complementary to messenger RNA encoding hypoxanthine-guanine phosphoribosyltransferase has been cloned and sequenced as well. As a molecular probe, this cDNA sequence has been used to identify carrier status in a female at risk for whom conventional carrier detection techniques were not successful. The mutations that cause hypoxanthine-guanine phosphoribosyltransferase deficiency are heterogeneous. Protein sequencing techniques have been used to identify the amino acid substitutions in four variant forms of hypoxanthine-

TABLE 329-2 Structural and functional abnormalities in mutant forms of hypoxanthine-guanine phosphoribosyltransferase (HPRT)

		Mutation		Functional abnormalities			
						Michaelis constants	
Mutant enzyme	Clinical presentation	Nucleotide substitution	Amino acid substitution	Intracellular concentration, % normal	Maximal velocity	Hypoxanthine	PRPP
$HPRT_{Detroit}$	Lesch-Nyhan syndrome	T_{122}→C	Leu_{41}→Pro	ND	NM	NM	NM
$HPRT_{Toronto}$	Gout	ND	Arg_{51}→Gly	52	Normal	Normal	Normal
$HPRT_{New\ Haven}$	Lesch-Nyhan syndrome	G_{209}→A	Gly_{70}→Glu	50	NM	NM	NM
$HPRT_{Yale}$	Lesch-Nyhan syndrome	G_{211}→C	Gly_{71}→Arg	92	NM	NM	NM
$HPRT_{Flint}$	Lesch-Nyhan syndrome	C_{222}→A	Phe_{74}→Leu	<0.3	NM	NM	NM
$HPRT_{Arlington}$	Gout	A_{239}→T	Asp_{80}→Val	ND	NM	NM	NM
$HPRT_{Munich}$	Gout	C_{397}→A	Ser_{104}→Arg	79	↓	↑	Normal
$HPRT_{London}$	Gout	C_{329}→T	Ser_{110}→Leu	35–52	Normal	↑	Normal
$HPRT_{Midland}$	Lesch-Nyhan syndrome	T_{389}→A	Val_{130}→Asp	<0.3	NM	NM	NM
$HPRT_{Ann\ Arbor}$	Nephrolithiasis	T_{396}→G	Ile_{132}→Met	11	Normal	Normal	Normal
$HPRT_{Milwaukee}$	Gout	A_{481}→T	Ala_{161}→Ser	3	NM	NM	NM
$HPRT_{Kinston}$	Lesch-Nyhan syndrome	ND	Asp_{194}→Asn	72	Normal	↑	↑
$HPRT_{New\ Britain}$	Lesch-Nyhan syndrome	T_{595}→G	Phe_{199}→Val	<0.3	NM	NM	NM
$HPRT_{Ashville}$	Gout	A_{602}→G	Asp_{201}→Gly	4	NM	NM	NM

NOTES: PRPP denotes 5-phosphoribosyl-1-pyrophosphate; Ala, alanine; Arg, arginine; Asp, aspartic acid; Asn, asparagine; Glu, glutamic acid; Gly, glycine; Ile, isoleucine; Leu, leucine; Met, methionine; Phe, phenylalanine; Pro, proline; Ser, serine; Val, valine; ND, not determined; NM, not measured because of diminished catalytic activity; →, is replaced by; ↑, increased; ↓, decreased.

SOURCE: Wilson et al. and Davidson et al.

guanine phosphoribosyltransferase derived from deficient subjects: $HPRT_{Toronto}$, $HPRT_{Munich}$, $HPRT_{London}$, and $HPRT_{Kinston}$ (Table 329-2). More recently, recombinant techniques have been used to identify the actual mutation responsible for enzymic deficiency in more subjects. In each of the 14 examples in Table 329-2 a single amino acid substitution leads to either a catalytically incompetent protein or decreased steady-state concentration of hypoxanthine-guanine phosphoribosyltransferase as a result of diminished synthesis or accelerated degradation of the mutant protein. Although point mutations are the most common mechanism leading to hypoxanthine-guanine phosphoribosyltransferase deficiency, gene rearrangement, partial deletions, and insertions have also been described.

Human hypoxanthine-guanine phosphoribosyltransferase gene sequences have been transferred to mice via retroviral vector–infected bone marrow transplantation and by direct infection of brain tissue by recombinant herpes simplex virus type 1 vectors. A transgenic strain of mice that expresses the human enzyme has also been established. More recently, two strains of hypoxanthine-guanine phosphoribosyltransferase–deficient mice have been described. Neither strain displays the altered phenotype, and, therefore, these animals do not constitute an authentic model for the Lesch-Nyhan syndrome.

The associated biochemical abnormalities leading to the devastating neurologic consequences of the Lesch-Nyhan syndrome are incompletely understood. Evidence obtained from postmortem examination of brains from subjects with the Lesch-Nyhan syndrome indicates a specific defect in the central dopaminergic pathways, particularly those found in the basal ganglia and nucleus accumbens. Corroborating in vivo evidence is emerging from positron emission tomography studies of subjects deficient in hypoxanthine-guanine phosphoribosyltransferase. A defect in the metabolism of 2′-fluorodeoxyglucose in the caudate nuclei is present in the majority of subjects studied with this technique. The relationships between dopaminergic nervous system abnormalities and the aberrant metabolism of purines remain unknown.

The hyperuricemia resulting from partial or complete deficiency of hypoxanthine-guanine phosphoribosyltransferase can be successfully controlled with allopurinol, an inhibitor of xanthine oxidase. A few patients have developed xanthine stones with such therapy, but in the majority the renal stones and gout are effectively treated. No specific therapy exists for the neurologic abnormalities in the Lesch-Nyhan syndrome.

PRPP SYNTHETASE VARIANTS Several families are described in which there is increased activity of the enzyme PRPP synthetase (reaction 3, Fig. 329-4). The mutant enzymes, of which three different types are recognized, all exhibit increased activity, resulting in increased intracellular concentrations of PRPP, accelerated purine biosynthesis, and elevated excretion of uric acid. The inheritance pattern in this disease is also X-linked. These patients, like those with partial hypoxanthine-guanine phosphoribosyltransferase deficiency, generally develop gout in the second or third decade and have a high incidence of uric acid stones. Several kindred have been described in which nerve deafness is associated with PRPP synthetase overactivity groups.

OTHER DISORDERS OF PURINE METABOLISM **Adenine phosphoribosyltransferase deficiency** Adenine phosphoribosyltransferase catalyzes the conversion of adenine to AMP (reaction 4, Fig. 329-4). The first subjects described with a deficiency of this enzyme were heterozygous for deficiency of the enzyme and had no associated disease. It subsequently became apparent that heterozygosity for this deficiency is common, perhaps as frequent as 1:100. A homozygous deficiency of this enzyme has now been described in 11 patients with a history of renal stones composed of 2,8-dioxyadenine. Because of chemical similarity, 2,8-dioxyadenine may be confused with uric acid, and in each of these patients an incorrect diagnosis of uric acid nephrolithiasis was made initially.

Adenosine deaminase deficiency and purine nucleoside phosphorylase deficiency See Chap. 263.

Xanthine oxidase deficiency Xanthine oxidase catalyzes the oxidation of hypoxanthine to xanthine, xanthine to uric acid, and adenine to 2,8-dioxyadenine (reaction 8, Fig. 329-4). Xanthinuria, the first inborn error of purine metabolism to be defined at the enzyme level, is due to a deficiency of xanthine oxidase. As a result, affected patients with xanthinuria have hypouricemia and hypouricaciduria as well as an increased urinary excretion of the oxypurines, hypoxanthine, and xanthine. Half are asymptomatic, and a third have urinary xanthine stones. Several patients have been noted to have a myopathy. Three patients have been reported with polyarthritis, which may represent a crystal-induced synovitis. Precipitation of xanthine is thought to be the important factor in the development of each of these clinical manifestations.

Four patients have been described with combined congenital deficiencies of xanthine oxidase and sulfate oxidase. The clinical presentation is dominated by the serious neurologic abnormalities in the neonatal period seen in isolated sulfate oxidase deficiency. Although deficiency of a molybdate cofactor required by both enzymes has been postulated as the primary abnormality, therapy with ammonium molybdate has little effect on the neurologic manifestation. An acquired disorder mimicking combined xanthine oxidase and sulfate oxidase deficiency has been described in a patient on chronic total parenteral nutrition. Therapy with oral ammonium molybdate successfully restored enzymatic function and resulted in clinical resolution.

Myoadenylate deaminase deficiency Myoadenylate deaminase is an isozyme of adenylate deaminase found only in skeletal muscle. This enzyme catalyzes the conversion of adenylate (AMP) to inosinic acid (IMP). This reaction is a component of the purine nucleotide cycle and is probably important in the maintenance of energy production and utilization in skeletal muscle.

Deficiency of this enzyme is limited to skeletal muscle. The majority of deficient patients demonstrate exercise-induced myalgias, muscle cramps, and fatigue. Approximately one-third report weakness even in the absence of exercise. A few patients are apparently asymptomatic.

The disorder typically presents in childhood or adolescence. The clinical manifestations are those of a metabolic myopathy. Creatine kinase is elevated in less than half of subjects. Electromyograms and routine histology of muscle biopsies show nonspecific abnormalities. Presumptive evidence of adenylate deaminase deficiency can be obtained from performance of an ischemic forearm exercise test. Ammonia production is reduced in deficient patients since AMP deamination is blocked. The diagnosis must be confirmed by actual assay of AMP deaminase activity in a skeletal muscle biopsy since reduced ammonia production with exercise occurs in other myopathies. The disorder is slowly progressive, leading to mild disability in most cases. No specific therapy has been shown to be effective.

Adenylosuccinase deficiency Subjects deficient in adenylosuccinase are mentally retarded and often autistic. Additional neurologic abnormalities include seizures, psychomotor retardation, and other movement disorders. Urinary excretion of succinylamino-imidazole carboxamide riboside and succinyladenosine is elevated. Diagnosis depends upon demonstration of partial or complete absence of enzyme activity in liver, kidney, or skeletal muscle. Lymphocytes and fibroblasts show a partial deficiency. The prognosis is not known, and no specific therapy exists.

REFERENCES

Davidson BL et al: The molecular basis of HPRT deficiency in ten subjects determined by direct sequencing of amplified transcripts. J Clin Invest, 84:342, 1989

Kelley WN: Crystal-induced arthropathies, in *The Clinics in Rheumatic Diseases*. Philadelphia, Saunders, 1977, vol 3, pp 1–171

———, Fox IH: Antihyperuricemic drugs, in *Textbook of Rheumatology*, 3d ed, WN Kelley et al (eds). Philadelphia, Saunders, 1989, pp 884–899

——— et al: Gout and related disorders of purine metabolism, in *Textbook of Rheumatology*, 3d ed, WN Kelley et al (eds). Philadelphia, Saunders, 1989, pp 1395–1435

——— et al: Hypoxanthine-guanine phosphoribosyltransferase deficiency in gout. Ann Intern Med, 70:155, 1969

Palella TD, Fox IH: Hyperuricemia and gout, in *The Metabolic Basis of Inherited Disease*, 6th ed, CR Scriver et al (eds). New York, McGraw-Hill, 1989, chap 37

Talbott JH, Yu TF: *Gout and Uric Acid Metabolism*. New York, Grune & Stratton, 1976

Wilson JM et al: Hypoxanthine-guanine phosphoribosyltransferase deficiency: The molecular basis of the clinical syndromes. N Engl J Med 309:900, 1983

——— et al: A molecular survey of hypoxanthine-guanine phosphoribosyltransferase deficiency in man. J Clin Invest 77:188, 1986

Wyngaarden JB: Gout, in *Advances in Metabolic Disorders*, R Levine and R Luft (eds). New York, Academic, 1965, vol 2, pp 2–78

———, Kelley WN: *Gout and Hyperuricemia*. New York, Grune & Stratton, 1976

330 WILSON'S DISEASE

I. HERBERT SCHEINBERG

Wilson's disease is an autosomal recessive abnormality in the hepatic excretion of copper that results in toxic accumulations of the metal in liver, brain, and other organs. The disease occurs in populations of every ethnic and geographic origin and has a worldwide prevalence of about 1 in 30,000. Deficiency of the plasma copper protein ceruloplasmin is a characteristic feature.

NATURAL HISTORY Normal babies have low levels of plasma ceruloplasmin and high concentrations of hepatic copper. During the first year of life ceruloplasmin values rise and hepatic copper concentrations fall to normal adult levels. In contrast, serum ceruloplasmin changes very little in homozygotes for the Wilson's disease gene, and the concentration of hepatic copper remains elevated. However, clinical manifestations of copper excess are extremely rare before age 6, and about half of untreated patients remain asymptomatic through adolescence.

Wilson's disease presents with hepatic involvement in about half of patients. The toxic effects of copper in the liver may be manifest in four ways: as acute hepatitis, fulminant hepatitis, chronic active hepatitis, or cirrhosis. Acute hepatitis is often mistaken for viral hepatitis or infectious mononucleosis and is usually self-limited. Fulminant hepatitis, generally lethal, is characterized by progressive jaundice, malaise, ascites, hypoalbuminemia, and elevated plasma levels of liver enzymes. Sufficient copper may be released from necrosing hepatocytes to cause a hemolytic anemia. Parenchymal liver disease may persist following acute hepatitis or develop insidiously without prior acute disease into a clinical and histologic picture indistinguishable from chronic active hepatitis and always accompanied by cirrhosis. Finally, decades may elapse with no sign or symptom of liver disease but with the insidious development of cirrhosis. In all patients the past history of an episode of hepatitis can be overlooked unless they are questioned carefully.

In other patients the initial manifestations are extrahepatic. Neurologic or psychiatric disturbances are generally the first clinical signs in most of this group and are always accompanied by Kayser-Fleischer rings (Fig. A4-16). These green or golden deposits of copper in Descemet's membrane of the cornea do not interfere with vision but indicate that hepatic copper has been released and has caused brain damage. Rarely Kayser-Fleischer rings may be accompanied by sunflower cataracts. If a patient with frank neurologic or psychiatric disease does not have Kayser-Fleischer rings when examined by a trained observer using a slit lamp, the diagnosis of Wilson's disease can be excluded.

The primary neurologic manifestations are those of a movement disorder, particularly resting and intention tremors. Spasticity, rigidity, chorea, drooling, dysphagia, and dysarthria are common. Babinski responses and absent abdominal reflexes are occasionally noted; sensory changes, save for headache, never occur. Psychiatric disturbances, primarily due to the toxic effects of copper on the brain, but in some degree reactions to a life-threatening disease, are present in most patients with symptomatic disease. Syndromes indistinguishable from schizophrenia, manic-depressive psychoses, and classic neuroses may occur, and some bizarre behavioral disturbances defy classification. Improvement in the psychiatric state can occur with pharmacologic reduction of the copper excess, but psychotherapy is often also required.

In occasional patients the clinical onset reflects neither a hepatic nor a central nervous system disturbance. For example, primary or secondary amenorrhea may be the first evidence of disease in some young women; in others, repeated spontaneous abortions may be due to excess free copper in intrauterine secretions. Routine ophthalmo-

TABLE 330-1 Summary of analytic data in patients with Wilson's disease, heterozygous carriers, and control subjects

	Serum ceruloplasmin		Hepatic copper concentration	
Group	No. of patients	Mean ± SD, mg/L	No. of patients	Mean ± SD, μg/g dry weight
Wilson's disease:				
Asymptomatic	31	36±53	36	983.5±368
Symptomatic	84	59±71	33	588.3±304
Heterozygous carriers	95*	284±85	14	117.0±51
Normal subjects	180	307±35	16	31.5±6.8

* 71 parents of patients with Wilson's disease and 24 children, each of whom had one parent with Wilson's disease.
SOURCE: Sternlieb and Scheinberg, 1968.

logic examination in asymptomatic patients occasionally reveals Kayser-Fleischer rings, leading to the diagnosis.

PATHOGENESIS The metabolic defect in Wilson's disease is an inability to maintain a near-zero balance of copper. Excess copper, small amounts of which are essential to life, accumulates possibly because hepatic lysosomes lack the normal mechanism to excrete into bile the copper that has been catabolically cleaved from ceruloplasmin. This may cause deficiency of ceruloplasmin since a stoichiometric excess of copper in vitro inhibits the formation of ceruloplasmin from apoceruloplasmin and copper. The capacity of hepatocytes to store copper is eventually exceeded, and release into blood and uptake in extrahepatic sites occurs accompanied by a decrease in the hepatic copper concentration (Table 330-1).

Under normal circumstances essentially all tissue copper is present as the prosthetic element of copper proteins including cytochrome oxidase, tyrosinase, superoxide dismutase, and ceruloplasmin. There is normally little or no free (non-protein-bound) copper. In Wilson's disease more copper is present than can be bound by specific copper proteins; such copper is as toxic as excess iron, zinc, mercury, or lead. Toxicity of these cations is probably effected in large degree by pathologic combinations with proteins that ordinarily do not contain metal.

The pathologic consequences of the accumulated copper occur first in the liver. Abnormal fat and glycogen deposits are the earliest findings by light microscopy (Fig. 330-1). With electron microscopy mitochondrial abnormalities are observed early and appear to be specific for Wilson's disease (Fig. 330-2). Later, necrosis, inflammation, fibrosis, bile duct proliferation, and cirrhosis occur. Abnormalities in liver chemistries may be seen in any of these stages.

Death can occur from the effects of copper toxicosis in the central nervous system. In the brain the excess copper is distributed ubiquitously. Necrosis of neurons with cavitation may be preceded by the appearance of Opalski and Alzheimer type II cells; however, neither is specific for Wilson's disease.

Increased copper in the kidney produces little if any structural change and commonly does not alter renal function. Hematuria, proteinuria, the Fanconi syndrome, and renal tubular acidosis, though commonly seen in untreated patients, almost never lead to clinical renal disease. Pathologic effects in other organs and tissues are minor.

DIAGNOSIS The diagnosis is easy—*provided it is suspected.* Wilson's disease should be considered in any patient under the age of 40 with an unexplained disorder of the central nervous system, signs or symptoms of chronic active hepatitis, unexplained persistent elevations of serum transaminase, hemolytic anemia in the presence of hepatitis, unexplained cirrhosis, or in any patient who has a blood relative with Wilson's disease.

The diagnosis is confirmed in suspected cases by the demonstration either of (1) a serum concentration of ceruloplasmin less than 200 mg/L (20 mg/dL) and Kayser-Fleischer rings; or (2) a serum ceruloplasmin less than 200 mg/L (20 mg/dL) and a concentration of copper in a liver biopsy sample greater than 250 μg per gram of dry weight. Most symptomatic patients also excrete more than 100 μg copper per day in urine and exhibit histologic abnormalities on liver biopsy.

About 5 percent of patients have a serum concentration of ceruloplasmin greater than 200 mg/L (20 mg/dL), and some patients with other hepatic disorders, chiefly primary biliary cirrhosis, have elevated hepatic copper levels and, rarely, Kayser-Fleischer rings. In either circumstance measurement of the ability to incorporate radioactive copper into ceruloplasmin is useful as a discriminating test. Even in the presence of a normal concentration of ceruloplasmin, patients with Wilson's disease incorporate little or no isotope into the protein, while patients with other liver disorders and elevated hepatic copper incorporate the isotope normally.

TREATMENT Treatment consists of removing and detoxifying the deposits of copper as rapidly as possible and should be instituted once the diagnosis is secure whether the patient is ill or asymptomatic. The drug of choice is penicillamine. It is administered orally in an initial dose of 1 g daily, usually in divided doses 30 min before meals and at bedtime. Since penicillamine has an antipyridoxine effect in animals, 25 mg/d of vitamin B_6 is also given. Effectiveness of therapy should be assayed chemically and clinically. Initially, the

FIGURE 330-1 Fatty changes, glycogen deposits, and cellular infiltrates in a hematoxylin and eosin–stained section of liver from an asymptomatic boy with Wilson's disease.

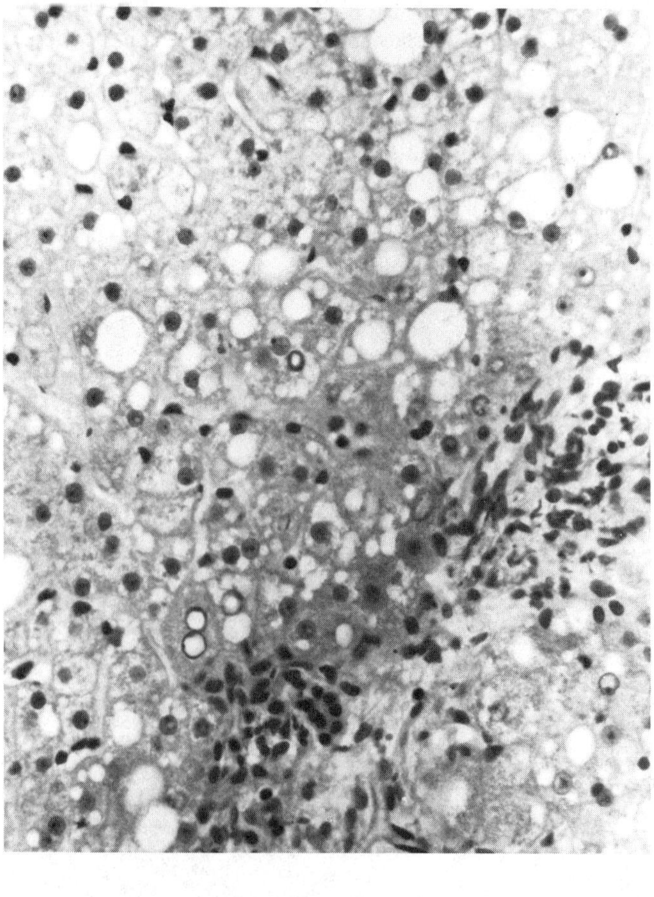

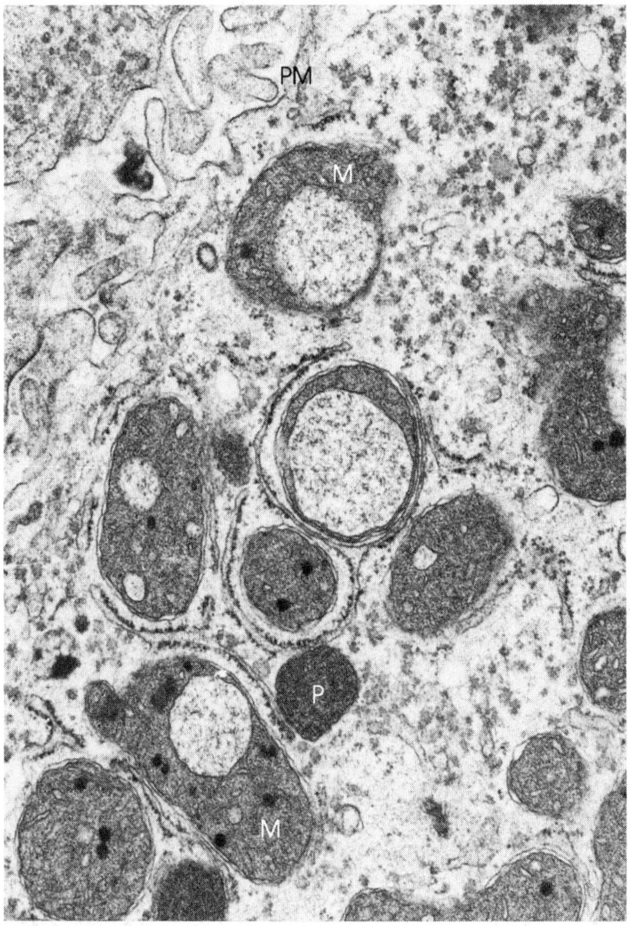

FIGURE 330-2 Electron micrograph of a liver biopsy sample from a 6-year-old asymptomatic boy. There are prominent vacuoles, containing granular material, in mitochondria (M). P, peroxisome; PM, plasma membrane.

24-h urinary excretion of copper should increase fivefold or more over the pretreatment level, and 1 to 3 mg copper per day may be excreted during the first months of therapy.

White blood cell and platelet counts, urinalysis, and body temperature should be monitored several times weekly for the first month of therapy and at intervals thereafter. Sensitivity to penicillamine usually appears within the first 14 days of treatment and may cause rash, fever, leukopenia, thrombocytopenia, lymphadenopathy, or proteinuria. Discontinuation of treatment is required if sensitivity develops. Therapy can often be resumed if the drug is reinstituted in small and gradually increasing dosage, although reactions are less likely to recur if 20 mg of prednisone is given daily for the first 2 weeks of penicillamine treatment and subsequently gradually discontinued. Reactions requiring a desensitizing regimen may recur several times before penicillamine can be administered without a steroid.

Lifelong and continual treatment is required. Inadequate treatment or interruption of therapy causes relapse that may be irreversible. Thus, of 11 patients who voluntarily discontinued penicillamine, after years of successful treatment, 8 died after an average survival of 2.6 years of noncompliance. Reinstitution of penicillamine after temporary interruption of therapy may be accompanied by the appearance or reappearance of sensitivity reactions. At any time—even after years of uneventful administration—granulocytopenia (or agranulocytosis), thrombocytopenia, the nephrotic syndrome, Goodpasture's syndrome, systemic lupus erythematosus, severe arthralgias, or myasthenia gravis may supervene. Toxicity is sometimes dose-related, and reduction of the dose to a level that is therapeutically effective but nontoxic may be possible. Continued low dosage of glucocorticoids may control penicillamine-associated lupus or arthralgias. After temporary interruption of the drug in patients with the nephrotic syndrome, it is sometimes possible to reinstitute therapy without recurrence of proteinuria. However, although irreversible intolerance to penicillamine is rare, the toxicity may be such that the drug must be withdrawn permanently and replaced by trientine, an orphan drug approved by the Food and Drug Administration in 1985.

After therapy with penicillamine has been successfully instituted, the patient should be seen indefinitely at 1- to 3-month intervals to detect drug toxicity and to manage the disease. Physical examination, including relevant neurologic assessment and inspection of the corneas with a slit lamp, and the patient's own evaluation provide the best indicators of the efficacy of treatment. Serial determinations of serum transaminase levels, albumin, and bilirubin are useful in following the course of liver function. Lack of clinical improvement or worsening of the disease may be due to irreversible damage present before therapy was begun, poor compliance, or inadequate dosage of penicillamine. Quantitative determinations of urinary copper excretion and of free copper in serum (total serum copper minus ceruloplasmin-bound copper) can help determine which is the case. After treatment for long periods, the level of urinary copper should be lower than at the onset of therapy, and rarely exceeds 1.5 mg/d. Even more helpful, the concentration of free serum copper is generally less than 2 μmol/L (10 μg/dL) in the adequately treated patient. After a patient has remained asymptomatic with no laboratory evidence of liver dysfunction for a year and in patients with minimal residual disease that has not changed, the dose of penicillamine may be reduced to 0.75 g/d.

Treatment of more than 100 asymptomatic patients with a confirmed diagnosis has established that continued administration of penicillamine can prevent virtually every manifestation of this disease.

REFERENCES

SCHEINBERG IH, STERNLIEB I: Wilson's disease, in *Major Problems in Internal Medicine*. Philadelphia, Saunders, 1984

——— et al: The use of trientine in preventing the effects of interrupting penicillamine therapy in Wilson's disease. N Engl J Med 317:209, 1987

——— et al: Penicillamine may detoxify copper in Wilson's disease. Lancet 2:95, 1987

STERNLIEB I: Evolution of the hepatic lesion in Wilson's disease (hepatolenticular degeneration), in *Progress in Liver Diseases*, H Popper et al (eds). New York, Grune & Stratton, 1972, vol IV, pp 511–526

———, SCHEINBERG IH: Prevention of Wilson's disease in asymptomatic patients. N Engl J Med 278:352, 1968

———, ———: Chronic hepatitis as a first manifestation of Wilson's disease. Ann Intern Med 76:59, 1972

WALSHE JM: Wilson's disease (hepatolenticular degeneration), in *Handbook of Clinical Neurology*, PJ Vinken et al (eds). New York, American Elsevier, 1976, vol 27

331 LYSOSOMAL STORAGE DISEASES

ARTHUR L. BEAUDET

GENERAL FEATURES

DEFINITION Lysosomes are cytoplasmic organelles that enclose an acidic environment and contain numerous enzymes capable of hydrolyzing most biologic macromolecules (Fig. 331-1). Primary lysosomes, the original bodies derived from the Golgi apparatus, may fuse with other membrane-bound vesicles to form secondary lysosomes. Secondary lysosomes contain material derived from outside the cell through endocytosis or material from within the cell through autophagy. A major function of the lysosome is degradation of used macromolecules related to normal turnover and tissue remodeling. Studies of the metabolism of vitamin B_{12}, lipoproteins, peptide hormones, and growth factors indicate that the lysosome is also important in the uptake of molecules through the process of adsorptive endocytosis. The initial cellular vacuole resulting from

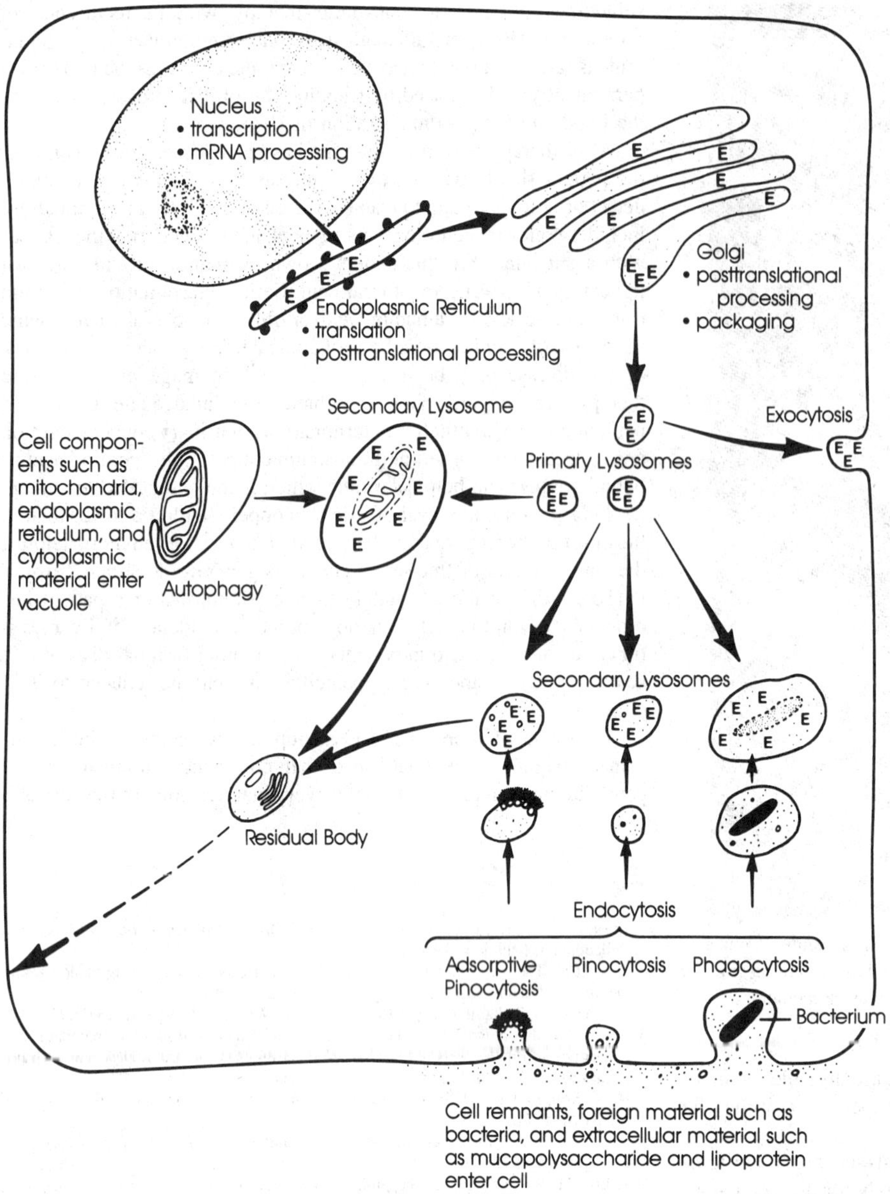

FIGURE 331-1 Biology of lysosomes. E represents lysosomal enzymes, including precursor forms. Lysosomal enzymes are synthesized in the endoplasmic reticulum and then undergo posttranslational processing that allows packaging into the primary lysosomes. The primary lysosomes can then undergo any of the several fates outlined.

adsorptive endocytosis is the receptosome, or endosome, and this vacuole fuses with lysosomes. The lysosomal enzymes are glycoproteins which are synthesized within the endoplasmic reticulum. The initial products of protein synthesis undergo extensive modification including proteolytic cleavage, addition of complex oligosaccharides, synthesis of recognition markers (mannose-6-phosphate in some instances), and compartmentalization into primary lysosomes. These processes occur in the endoplasmic reticulum, in the Golgi apparatus, and probably in the primary, if not secondary, lysosomes as well. (See Chap. 3 in Scriver et al. for more details of lysosomal biology and biogenesis.)

The concept of lysosomal storage diseases arose from the studies of type II (Pompe) glycogen storage disease. The demonstration of lysosomal accumulation of glycogen as the result of α-glucosidase deficiency and data from other disorders led Hers to define an inborn lysosomal disease as one in which (1) a single lysosomal enzyme is deficient and (2) abnormal deposits (of substrate) are present within vacuoles related to lysosomes. This definition can be modified to include single-gene defects affecting one or more lysosomal enzymes and thus encompass disorders such as the mucolipidoses and multiple sulfatase deficiency. The concept also can be expanded to include the deficiency of other proteins necessary for lysosomal function, such as sphingolipid activator proteins. Biochemical and genetic evidence indicates that these activator proteins are essential for hydrolysis of some substrates.

The lysosomal storage diseases include most of the lipid storage disorders, the mucopolysaccharidoses, the mucolipidoses, glycoprotein storage diseases, and others, as indicated in Table 331-1. The enzyme deficiencies have an autosomal recessive basis with the exception of Hunter's mucopolysaccharidosis II (MPS II), which is X-linked recessive, and Fabry's disease, which is X-linked with frequent manifestations in females. The target organs are determined by the usual sites of degradation for a macromolecule. For example, cerebral white matter is affected in patients with defects in degradation of myelin, hepatosplenomegaly develops in those with defects in degradation of glycolipids from red cell stroma, and generalized tissue involvement may occur in patients with defects in the degradation of ubiquitous mucopolysaccharides. The accumulated material often causes visceromegaly or macrocephaly, but secondary atrophy also can occur, particularly in brain or muscle. In simple terms, the symptoms appear to be due to damage from stored material, but exactly how this causes cell death or dysfunction often is unclear. All the disorders are progressive, and many are fatal in childhood or adolescence. Definitive diagnosis is accomplished best by specific enzyme assays on serum, leukocytes, or cultured skin fibroblasts, selecting the appropriate tests on clinical grounds. There is extensive phenotypic variation within disorders with infantile, juvenile, and adult forms of many entities. In addition, varying combinations of visceral, skeletal, and neurologic involvement can occur within a single enzyme disorder.

DIAGNOSIS A lysosomal storage disease is usually suspected on the basis of progressive neurologic dysfunction, visceromegaly, skeletal dysostosis, or some more specific finding, as outlined in Table 331-1. Progressive or degenerative disease is the hallmark of these disorders. The superimposition of degeneration upon normal childhood development results in a slowing of progress prior to loss of previously acquired abilities. The history should focus on the course of childhood development, neurologic symptoms, including seizures and visual or auditory impairment, the course of physical growth, and more specific findings such as coarsening facies, corneal clouding, exaggerated startle response, abdominal distention, joint pain, joint stiffness, hernias, and recurrent infection. The family history may reveal similarly affected siblings or consanguinity in autosomal recessive disease or other affected male family members in X-linked disorders. Ethnic background may be helpful because several lipid storage diseases are more frequent in Ashkenazi Jews, and mannosidosis and aspartylglucosaminuria may occur with increased frequency in Scandinavian populations. The juvenile form of sialidosis is frequent in the Japanese.

On physical examination the head circumference may be enlarged. Gigantism occurs early in the course of some mucopolysaccharidoses and glycoprotein storage diseases, while short stature is a later finding in many disorders. Ophthalmologic examination should include slit-lamp and careful funduscopic examination. Enlargement of the tongue, coarsening of the facies, and hepatosplenomegaly may occur. Skeletal findings may include gibbus deformity, broadening of the long bones, and joint stiffness. Cutaneous findings are rare except in fucosidosis, sialidosis, Fabry's disease, and Hunter's disease. Careful neurologic examination should attempt to distinguish the extent of involvement of gray matter, white matter, and peripheral nerves. Preliminary diagnostic studies should include examination of the peripheral blood smear for vacuolated or granulated leukocytes, urinary spot test for mucopolysaccharide, and radiologic bone survey. The preferred method of diagnosis is to use the above information to select specific enzyme assays in serum, leukocytes, or cultured skin fibroblasts. If a mucopolysaccharide screening test is positive or if clinical findings are suggestive, quantitative mucopolysaccharide analysis can be carried out. If a specific diagnosis is not readily established, biopsy of skin, bone marrow, rectal mucosa, liver, peripheral nerve, conjunctiva, or other tissue for light and electron microscopy can be helpful. Electron-microscopic findings can direct one toward or away from the general category of lysosomal storage diseases based on the presence or absence of engorged lysosomes. Again, enzyme assay is the proper method for diagnosis of the standard disorders. When significant evidence favors a lysosomal storage disease but no enzyme deficiency is demonstrable, chemical analysis of biopsy tissue from liver or brain may be an appropriate research starting point.

The diagnosis of lysosomal storage diseases in adults is often difficult, although studies such as bone marrow aspiration in Gaucher's disease and renal biopsy in Fabry's disease may be pathognomonic. The diagnosis is difficult in the face of insidious, slowly progressive neurologic and psychiatric symptoms as described below for deficiencies of aryl sulfatase A, hexosaminidase A, or β-galactosidase. Erroneous diagnoses are common in these disorders, and a high index of suspicion is required. Lysosomal α-glucosidase deficiency mimics muscular dystrophy (see Chap. 365).

HETEROGENEITY There is extensive clinical and biochemical heterogeneity within the lysosomal storage diseases. The biochemical genetic principles underlying this heterogeneity are reviewed in Chaps. 5 and 6. In general, a structural gene for lysosomal enzyme produces products that undergo posttranslational modification to become glycoproteins, often resulting in a series of electrophoretic variants, or isozymes. These isozymes may hydrolyze one or a variety of substrates, and the substrate specificity of particular isozymes may vary. Differences in substrate specificity also arise from the occurrence of similar but genetically distinct enzymes, for example, the β-galactosidases. Mutations within a gene may totally eliminate or reduce enzyme activity, alter posttranslational modification, or alter the activity of the enzyme for specific substrates.

In most instances different mutations within the structural genes for lysosomal enzymes account for varying degrees of severity from individual to individual as well as for the diverse combinations of visceral, skeletal, neurologic, ocular, and other manifestations. The heterogeneity is increased further by the recessive nature of most of the conditions in that each affected individual must have two mutant genes at the same locus. The exact mutation may vary in the two copies of the gene, making the patient a genetic compound heterozygote. In this instance either one or both genes may encode some form of residual enzyme activity for one or more substrates. Patients with intermediate clinical phenotypes with mucopolysaccharidosis type I (MPS I) have been cited as likely examples of compound heterozygotes. At a molecular level the majority of lysosomal storage disease patients might prove to be compound heterozygotes. Although it is useful to characterize clinical phenotypes as infantile, juvenile, adult, neuropathic, or nonneuropathic, the existence of different mutant alleles and of genetic compounds provides an explanation for those occasional patients who appear aberrant or intermediate as compared with the usual phenotype. Another type of heterogeneity is illustrated by MPS III A, B, C, and D, which are very similar disorders caused by different gene defects. Thus, biochemical heterogeneity can underlie apparent clinical homogeneity.

Further complexity results from the fact that certain enzyme activities are derived from complexes of nonidentical subunits. As a consequence, different mutations can cause deficiency of the same enzyme, for example, hexosaminidase A deficiency in Tay-Sachs and Sandhoff's diseases, and can explain multiple enzyme deficiencies due to a single-gene defect as in Sandhoff's disease. Genetic disorders that affect the posttranslational modification of lysosomal enzymes and defects in the lysosome itself may also cause lysosomal storage diseases. The mucolipidoses II and III are situations in which a single-gene defect alters the ability of a number of lysosomal enzymes to enter the lysosome. Thus, mutations outside the structural genes for the enzymes can account for further heterogeneity. Better understanding of the identity, subunit structure, posttranslational processing, and substrate specificities of lysosomal enzymes should provide further insight into phenotypic and genotypic heterogeneity.

Clinical diagnosis is facilitated but also somewhat complicated by the widespread use of synthetic substrates for measuring lysosomal enzyme activities. These substrates often measure a group of related activities attributable to different enzymes. Thus, the activity of β-galactosidase using an artificial substrate may represent the sum of various β-galactosidases encoded by different structural genes and having different substrate specificities. Clinical reliability generally is achieved by manipulating in vitro conditions to reflect that enzyme activity whose deficiency is characteristic of a clinical disorder. Genetic heterogeneity has, however, resulted in individuals with a mutant enzyme that either hydrolyzes the natural substrate and not the artificial substrate, or vice versa. This is exemplified by the normal individuals who have hexosaminidase A deficiency using artificial substrate and by patients with Tay-Sachs disease who have substantial levels of hexosaminidase A activity with artificial substrates. The presence or absence of disease correlates with ability to hydrolyze the natural G_{M2} ganglioside substrate. These phenomena have considerable significance for identification of affected patients, for heterozygote screening, and for prenatal diagnosis. They indicate the need to go beyond artificial substrate enzyme assays if normal results occur in the face of overwhelming clinical, electron-microscopic, or chemical evidence of a storage disease.

MANAGEMENT AND PREVENTION Specific therapy is not effective in lysosomal storage diseases at present, and care is largely symptomatic. The relentless, progressive course in many instances represents a tragic burden. Transplantation is effective in reversing

TABLE 331-1 Summary of lysosomal storage diseases

Disorder*	Heterogeneity (onset)	Enzyme deficiency	Stored material	Neurologic
G_{M1} gangliosidosis (71)	Infantile (birth) Juvenile (6–20 mo) Adult	β-Galactosidase	G_{M1} ganglioside Glycoproteins Keratan sulfate	Mental retardation, seizures, blindness; later in juvenile form, variable in adults
Tay-Sachs and variants, G_{M2} gangliosidosis (72)	Infantile (3–6 mo) Juvenile Adult forms	Hexosaminidase A	G_{M2} ganglioside	Mental retardation, seizures, blindness; later in juvenile form
Sandhoff, G_{M2} gangliosidosis (72)	Infantile (3–6 mo)	Hexosaminidase A and B	G_{M2} ganglioside Globoside	Mental retardation, seizures, blindness
G_{M2} gangliosidosis, AB variant (72)	Findings similar to Tay-Sachs except primary defect is a ganglioside activator protein.			
Krabbe, galactosylceramide lipidosis (68)	Infantile (2–6 mo) Late onset	Galactosylceramide β-Galactosidase	↑ Galactoscerebroside/sulfatide ratio	Mental retardation, leukodystrophy; variable in late onset
Metachromatic leukodystrophy, sulfatide lipidosis (69)	Late infantile (1–4 yr) Juvenile (4–20 yr) Adult	Arylsulfatase A (cerebroside sulfatase)	Galactosyl sulfatides	Mental retardation, leukodystrophy, psychosis and dementia in adults
Sphingolipid activator protein 1 deficiency (69)	Findings similar to metachromatic leukodystrophy except primary defect is activator protein.			
Niemann-Pick, sphingomyelin lipidosis (66)	Infantile neuropathic (1–4 mo) Late onset neuropathic Visceral	Sphingomyelinase in types A and B but not type C	Sphingomyelin Cholesterol	Mental retardation, ataxia, and seizures in neuropathic forms
Gaucher, glucosylceramide lipidosis (67)	Infantile (1–12 mo) Juvenile (2–6 yr) Adult	β-Glucocerebrosidase	Glucosylceramide	Mental retardation; spastic, later flaccid, ataxia in juvenile; no neurologic symptoms in adult form
Fabry, trihexosyl ceramidosis (70)	Hemizygous males Heterozygous females	α-Galactosidase A	Trihexosylceramide	Painful neuropathy
Acid lipase deficiency (64)	Infantile Wolman's disease (0–3 mo) Late onset cholesteryl ester storage disease (CESD)	Acid lipase	Cholesteryl ester Triglyceride	Mental retardation but mild related to growth failure in Wolman; none in CESD
Farber, ceramide deficiency (65)	Infantile (0–4 mo) Rare juvenile	Ceramidase	Ceramide	Occasional mental retardation, but may be secondary to somatic features
Pompe, glycogen storage type II (12)	Infantile (0–6 mo) Juvenile Adult	Acid maltase (α-1,4- and 1,6-glucosidase)	Glycogen	Probably normal mentally
Fucosidosis (63)	Infantile (3–12 mo) Juvenile	α-Fucosidase	Glycopeptides Glycolipids Oligosaccharides	Mental retardation
Mannosidosis (63)	Infantile (6–18 mo) Milder form	α-Mannosidase	Oligosaccharides	Mental retardation
Aspartylglucosaminuria (63)	Young adult onset	Aspartylglucosamine amidase	Aspartylglucosamine Glycopeptides	Mental retardation
Mucopolysaccharidosis IH and IS (61)	Infantile Hurler (6–12 mo) Intermediate Adult Scheie	α-Iduronidase	Dermatan sulfate Heparan sulfate	Mental retardation, absent in Scheie
Hunter, mucopolysaccharidosis II (61)	Severe infantile (6–12 mo) Mild juvenile	Iduronosulfate sulfatase	Dermatan sulfate Heparan sulfate	Mental retardation, less in mild form

* Numbers in parentheses refer to the chapters in Scriver et al. in which the disorder is discussed in detail.

TABLE 331-1 Summary of lysosomal storage diseases *(continued)*

Liver and/or spleen enlargement	Skeletal dysplasia	Ophthalmic	Hematologic	Genetics	Unique manifestations
+ + + + Less in juvenile, variable in adult	+ + + + Variable in juvenile and adult forms	Cherry-red spot in 50% of infantile; corneal clouding variable but more in adults	Foam cells Vacuolated lymphocytes	AR†	Coarse facies, edema, macroglossia, mucopolysacchariduria; early blindness in infantile, milder in juvenile; in adults often spondyloepiphyseal dysplasia +/− mucopolysacchariduria
0	0	Cherry-red spot in infantile form, rare in juvenile	0	AR	Macrocephaly, hyperacusis in infantile; increased in Ashkenazi Jews
0	0	Cherry-red spot	0	AR	Macrocephaly, hyperacusis, visceral histiocytosis
0	0	Optic atrophy	0	AR	Extreme irritability, ↑ CSF protein, fever, globoid cell neuropathology
0	0	Optic atrophy, less in juvenile and adult forms	0	AR	↑ CSF protein and early gait abnormalities in late infantile; peripheral neuropathy
+ + + + Less prominent in late onset forms	0	Macular degeneration and cherry-red spot in neuropathic forms	Distinctive foam cell Vacuolated lymphocytes	AR	Pulmonary infiltrates, brownish skin, infantile neuronopathic form increased in Ashkenazi Jews, sea-blue histiocytes
+ + + + Hypersplenism common	+ +	Usually normal	Distinctive foam cell	AR	Adult form includes ↑ acid phosphatase, pathologic fractures; Ashkenazi Jewish predilection
0	0	Corneal dystrophy, vascular lesions, cataracts	0	X-linked dominant	Cutaneous angiokeratoma, vascular thromboses, hypohidrosis
+ + +	0	0	Foam cells Vacuolated lymphocytes	AR	Adrenal calcification, anemia, vomiting and poor growth in Wolman; hepatic fibrosis and ↑ blood cholesterol in CESD
+/−	?	Mild macular degeneration	0	AR	Arthropathy—subcutaneous, periarticular and visceral nodules (lipogranulomatosis); ↑ CSF protein
Mild hepatomegaly	0	0	0	AR	Lethal skeletal and cardiac myopathy in infantile; primarily skeletal myopathy in adults
+ +	+ +	0	Vacuolated lymphocytes Foam cells	AR	Coarse facies, increased sweat electrolytes, angiokeratoma in juvenile
+ + +	+ +	Cataracts, corneal clouding	Vacuolated lymphocytes Granulated neutrophils	AR	Coarse facies, enlarged tongue
0	+ +	Lens opacities	Vacuolated lymphocytes	AR	Coarse facies, detectable by urine amino acid analysis
+ + +	+ + + +	Corneal clouding	Granulated lymphocytes	AR	Coarse facies, cardiovascular involvement, joint stiffness
+ + +	+ + + +	Retinal degeneration, no significant corneal clouding	Granulated lymphocytes	X-linked	Coarse facies, cardiovascular involvement, joint stiffness

† AR = autosomal recessive.

(Table continues next page)

TABLE 331-1 Summary of lysosomal storage diseases *(continued)*

Disorder*	Heterogeneity (onset)	Enzyme deficiency	Stored material	Neurologic
Sanfilippo A, mucopolysaccharidosis III A (61)	Late infantile (1–4 yr)	Heparan *N*-sulfatase (sulfamidase)	Heparan sulfate	Severe mental retardation
Sanfilippo B, mucopolysaccharidosis III B (61)	Late infantile (1–4 yr)	*N*-Acetyl-α-glucosaminidase	Heparan sulfate	Severe mental retardation
Sanfilippo C, mucopolysaccharidosis III C (61)	Late infantile (1–4 yr)	Acetyl-CoA:α-glucosaminide *N*-acetyltransferase	Heparan sulfate	Severe mental retardation
Sanfilippo D, mucopolysaccharidosis III D (61)	Late infantile (1–4 yr)	*N*-Acetylglucosamine-6-sulfate sulfatase	Heparan sulfate	Severe mental retardation
Morquio, mucopolysaccharidosis IV (61)	Some variation	*N*-Acetylgalactosamine-6-sulfate sulfatase	Keratan sulfate	0
Maroteaux-Lamy, mucopolysaccharidosis VI (61)	Variation in severity and cardiovascular involvement	*N*-Acetylhexosamine-4-sulfate sulfatase (arylsulfatase B)	Dermatan sulfate	0
β-Glucuronidase deficiency, mucopolysaccharidosis VII (61)	Few patients; infantile to adult forms	β-Glucuronidase	Dermatan sulfate ? Heparan sulfate	Mental retardation ? absent in some adults
Multiple sulfatase deficiency (69)	Late infantile (1–4 yr)	Arylsulfatases A, B, and C Other sulfatases	Sulfatides Mucopolysaccharides	Mental retardation
Sialidosis (63)	Congenital, infantile, juvenile, cherry-red spot myoclonus	Glycoprotein neuraminidase (sialidase)	Sialyloligosaccharides	Mental retardation, myoclonus
Galactosialidosis (71)	Infantile Juvenile	Protective glycoprotein	Sialyloligosaccharides	Mental retardation
Mucolipidosis II, I cell disease (62)	Infantile (0–3 mo)	UDP-*N*-acetylglucosamine (GlcNAc):glycoprotein GlcNAc-1-phosphotransferase	Glycoproteins Glycolipids	Mental retardation
Mucolipidosis III, pseudo-Hurler polydystrophy (62)	Late infantile (>2 yr)	UDP-*N*-acetylglucosamine (GlcNAc):glycoprotein GlcNAc-1-phosphotransferase	Glycoproteins Glycolipids	Mild mental retardation
Mucolipidosis IV (71)	Infantile	? Ganglioside neuraminidase	? Multiple	Mental retardation
Neuronal ceroid lipofuscinoses	Late infantile Juvenile Adult	Unknown	"Ceroid" "Lipofuscin"	Mental retardation, dementia variable in adults, seizures

* Numbers in parentheses refer to the chapters in Scriver et al. in which the disorder is discussed in detail.

the renal failure in Fabry's disease, and splenectomy may be helpful in adult Gaucher's disease. Considerable attention has been focused on enzyme replacement for lysosomal storage diseases using organ or fibroblast transplantation or the infusion of plasma, leukocytes, purified enzyme itself, or enzyme trapped in erythrocytes or liposomes. Although these approaches offer promise for treatment of manifestations outside the central nervous system, they are not of proven efficacy. The most distressing manifestations of lysosomal storage diseases involve the central nervous system, where the blood-brain barrier presents an additional obstacle to effective enzyme replacement therapy.

Genetic counseling is important in the management of these disorders. All the lysosomal storage diseases in which the specific enzyme deficiency is known either have been or presumably could be diagnosed in utero, since lysosomal enzyme activities are expressed in cultured amniotic fluid cells as well as in cultured skin fibroblasts. Prenatal diagnosis can also be made using chorionic villus biopsy. Although the incidence of miscarriage after this procedure may be slightly higher, the possibility of earlier diagnosis is attractive to families at risk. Heterozygote detection in close relatives is sometimes possible, although it can be difficult to achieve adequate statistical confidence for such determinations. Heterozygote detection is further complicated by random inactivation of X chromosomes in 46,XX carriers of X-linked diseases, but women at risk in such families should be counseled. More effective approaches to prevention require identification of heterozygous couples prior to the birth of an affected offspring. The feasibility of this approach has been demonstrated by heterozygote testing programs for Tay-Sachs disease. Such programs could result in a decreased frequency of these disorders through extensive testing and appropriate reproductive decisions by the rare couples at risk for affected offspring; the high frequency of the heterozygous state in Ashkenazi Jews and reliable methods for carrier detection for Tay-Sachs disease have facilitated this program. Efficient, accurate heterozygote detection methods would be needed to apply this approach to other diseases and to populations with lower heterozygote frequencies. Even under optimal conditions genetic variants may cause false-positive or false-negative results in any screening process.

TABLE 331-1 Summary of lysosomal storage diseases *(continued)*

Liver and/or spleen enlargement	Skeletal dysplasia	Ophthalmic	Hematologic	Genetics	Unique manifestations
+	+	0	Granulated lymphocytes	AR	Mild coarsening of facies
+	Severe, distinctive	Corneal clouding	Granulated neutrophils	AR	Severe deformity, odontoid hypoplasia, aortic regurgitation
+ +	+ + + +	Corneal clouding	Granulated neutrophils and lymphocytes	AR	Mild coarsening of facies, joint stiffness, valvular heart disease
+ + +	+ + +	Corneal clouding	Granulated neutrophils	AR	Coarse facies, ↑ vascular involvement
+	MPS features	Retinal degeneration	Vacuolated and granulated cells	AR	Icthyosis, combined MPS and metachromatic leukodystrophy phenotype
+ + Less in late form	+ + Less or absent in late form	Cherry-red spot	Vacuolated lymphocytes	AR	MPS phenotype in all but cherry-red spot myoclonus
+ + Less in juvenile	+ +	Cherry-red spot, corneal clouding	Vacuolated lymphocytes	AR	Angiokeratoma in juvenile; dysotosis multiplex
0/ +	+ + + +	Corneal clouding	Vacuolated and granulated neutrophils	AR	Coarse facies, inclusions in cultured fibroblasts, normal mucopolysacchariduria
0	+ + +	Corneal clouding	Vacuolated plasma cells	AR	Coarse facies, inclusions in cultured fibroblasts, joint contractures, valvular heart disease, normal mucopolysacchariduria
0	0	Corneal clouding, retinal degeneration	0	AR	Diagnosis based on electron microscopy; ? Ashkenazi Jewish predilection
0	0	Optic atrophy, macular degeneration, retinitis pigmentosa	Vacuolated lymphocytes Granulated neutrophils	AR	Electron microscopy helpful, degree of genetic heterogeneity unknown

MOLECULAR ANALYSIS Many of the lysosomal genes have been cloned. Specific mutations are being identified, and it may become possible to correlate severity of the phenotype with specific homozygous or compound heterozygous molecular genotypes. Molecular diagnosis is likely to supplement but not replace enzymatic diagnosis in most circumstances. It is also possible that availability of the cloned genes might allow for gene or enzyme replacement therapy.

SPECIFIC DISORDERS

SPHINGOLIPIDOSES G_{M1} gangliosidosis G_{M1} gangliosidosis is due to deficiency of β-galactosidase. The features of the infantile form are summarized in Table 331-1. The juvenile form is characterized by a later onset, survival to the latter half of the first decade of life, neurologic impairment and seizures, and milder skeletal and ocular findings. In adults, one phenotype (sometimes called Morquio B) includes corneal clouding, normal intelligence, and spondyloepiphyseal dysplasia similar to that seen in MPS IV. Other adults have minimal bony abnormalities but exhibit spasticity, ataxia, or myoclonus. Patients with slowly progressive extrapyramidal signs with prominent dystonia, cerebral and caudate atrophy, and absence of visceral findings have been misdiagnosed as juvenile parkinsonism. A high index of suspicion is necessary to recognize the diverse phenotypes caused by β-galactosidase deficiency in juvenile and adult patients, since a wide range of skeletal, ocular, neurologic, and visceral findings can occur. Isozymes of β-galactosidase occur, but the diversity of phenotypes is believed to be due to different mutations in the same structural gene. All forms of G_{M1} gangliosidosis have an autosomal recessive inheritance. The frequency of the disease is low, with fewer than 50 patients reported for any given phenotype. Patients with isolated β-galactosidase deficiency must be distinguished from those with combined deficiency of neuraminidase and β-galactosidase.

G_{M2} gangliosidosis Tay-Sachs disease is a relatively common inborn error of metabolism with thousands of documented cases. Although it is clinically very similar to Sandhoff's disease, the two are genetically distinct with deficiency of hexosaminidase A in the former and hexosaminidase A and B in the latter. An additional disorder, called the AB variant of G_{M2} gangliosidosis, occurs with normal hexosaminidase A and B activity. This variant is due to a deficiency of a protein factor (activator) necessary for activity of the enzyme against natural substrate. The presenting features are similar in all of the infantile disorders and include a developmental delay beginning in the third to sixth month with subsequent, rapidly progressive neurologic deterioration. Macrocephaly, seizures, retinal cherry-red spot, and an augmented startle response to sound suggest the diagnosis. The diagnosis is confirmed by enzyme assay. Most juvenile-onset patients with hexosaminidase deficiency present with dementia, seizures, and ocular findings, and some have an atypical spinocerebellar degeneration.

The neurologic manifestations of hexosaminidase A deficiency in adults are variable. Ataxia, dysarthria, lower motor neuron disease, pyramidal signs, and recurrent psychosis are common. Misdiagnoses have included Kugelberg-Welander spinal muscular atrophy, amyotropic lateral sclerosis, cerebellar or spinocerebellar ataxia, atypical Friedreich's ataxia, muscular dystrophy, dementia, schizophrenia, and others. The manifestations are slowly progressive, and, if considered, the diagnosis is easily established by serum enzyme assay.

Sandhoff's disease is nonallelic with Tay-Sachs disease, whereas the juvenile forms of hexosaminidase deficiency are usually allelic with Tay-Sachs disease. Tay-Sachs disease is the most frequent form of hexosaminidase deficiency, the risk being about 100 times higher in Ashkenazi Jews than in other ethnic groups. All forms of G_{M2} gangliosidosis are autosomal recessive. Hexosaminidase B is composed of β subunits whose structural locus is on chromosome 5, while hexosaminidase A is composed of α and β subunits with the structural locus for the α subunit on chromosome 15. Thus there is a defect in the α subunit in Tay-Sachs disease and in the β subunit in Sandhoff's disease.

Although no specific therapy is available, extensive programs for heterozygote detection to prevent Tay-Sachs disease have been carried out throughout the world. As of 1985, more than 530,000 people had been tested, and more than 21,000 heterozygotes and 527 couples at risk for Tay-Sachs in their offspring had been identified. Over 800 pregnancies had been monitored by prenatal diagnosis because of a previous affected child, and 602 pregnancies had been monitored based on results of carrier screening by 1985. The incidence of the disease has been reduced by 80 to 90 percent in the Jewish population in the United States and Canada.

LEUKODYSTROPHIES Krabbe's galactosylceramide lipidosis or globoid cell leukodystrophy is an infantile disease due to deficiency of galactosylceramide β-galactosidase. The clinical features are summarized in Table 331-1. Rapid neurologic deterioration and death occur within 1 to 2 years of onset. Premortem diagnosis is accomplished by enzyme assay. The presence of globoid cells in the brain is a characteristic postmortem finding. Galactosylceramide β-galactosidase is different from the β-galactosidase that is deficient in G_{M1} gangliosidosis. Krabbe's disease is an autosomal recessive disorder, and diagnosis can be made prenatally. Juvenile or adult forms are rare.

Deficiency of arylsulfatase A (cerebroside sulfatase) is the basis of metachromatic leukodystrophy, a lipid storage disease with a frequency of 1 in 40,000. The age of onset is later than that in Tay-Sachs disease or Krabbe's disease. Patients usually attain the ability to walk and frequently present with gait abnormalities in the second to fourth year of life. Initially the patients may be hypotonic with decreased deep tendon reflexes, the latter reflecting peripheral nerve involvement. The disease progresses over the first decade to include ataxia, increased muscle tone, decorticate or decerebrate posturing, and eventual loss of all contact with surroundings. Rare patients with a juvenile form of metachromatic leukodystrophy have the clinical onset between 4 and 20 years of age and progress more slowly.

The adult form deserves special mention as an example of the difficulties presented by subtle, slowly progressive forms of lysosomal storage diseases. The onset is in the second to fifth decade with a slowly progressive dementia. Emotional difficulties, motor dysfunction, and indistinct speech are often present. Even though conduction velocity in peripheral nerves is usually diminished, the deep tendon reflexes are often increased. Typical misdiagnoses include organic dementia, multiple sclerosis, and schizophrenia; psychiatric hospitalization is common. Premortem diagnosis was rare in the past, but the presence of periventricular hypodensities of white matter on computed tomography (CT) scan or abnormalities of periventricular white matter on magnetic resonance imaging (MRI) of the brain may suggest the diagnosis which should be confirmed by enzyme assay.

Although some diagnostic studies have been performed on urine, leukocytes or fibroblasts are preferable for diagnostic enzyme assay. Changes demonstrable on metachromatic staining of nerve tissue are nonspecific and not an adequate substitute for enzyme assay.

Arylsulfatase A is routinely measured using artificial substrate, and complexities involving low levels of activity in normal individuals and moderate levels of residual activity in symptomatic patients have been described. Heterogeneity involving mutations in multiple components of the cerebroside sulfatase activity may exist, but the majority of patients probably have simple allelic disorders on an autosomal recessive basis. A few patients with a phenotype similar to metachromatic leukodystrophy have been shown to have deficiency of a sphingolipid activator protein. Arylsulfatase A deficiency also occurs in multiple sulfatase deficiency.

NIEMANN-PICK DISEASE Niemann-Pick disease is a sphingomyelin lipidosis. In type A and B disease, there is a clear deficiency of sphingomyelinase, an enzyme that hydrolyzes sphingomyelin to yield ceramide and phosphorylcholine. The most common disorder, Niemann-Pick A, begins shortly after birth with hepatosplenomegaly, failure to thrive, and neurologic impairment. Retinal cherry-red spots occur, but seizures and hypersplenism are rare. The diagnosis can be made by recognition of the distinctive Niemann-Pick cell in the bone marrow but should be confirmed by enzyme assay. Niemann-Pick B disease is a relatively benign disorder with hepatosplenomegaly, sphingomyelinase deficiency, and sometimes pulmonary infiltrates; but there is no neurologic involvement. Niemann-Pick C disease is characterized by sphingomyelin lipidosis and progressive neurologic deterioration in childhood. Niemann-Pick C disease is not due to sphingomyelinase deficiency but is associated with a massive lysosomal accumulation of cholesterol due to an incompletely characterized defect in intracellular utilization of cholesterol.

GAUCHER'S DISEASE Gaucher's disease is a glucosylceramide lipidosis caused by deficiency of glucosylceramidase. An infantile form is characterized by early onset, marked hepatosplenomegaly, and severe neurologic progression to early death. A juvenile form with milder neurologic involvement exists. The type 1 or nonneuronopathic form (commonly called adult Gaucher's) is the most common lysosomal storage disease. The diagnosis of Gaucher's disease should be established by enzyme analysis. All forms of Gaucher's disease have an autosomal recessive genetic basis and are allelic disorders. Type 1 is about 30 times more frequent in Ashkenazi Jews, with an incidence in this group of about 1 in 2500 births. Absence of neurologic involvement is the criterion for inclusion in the type 1 or adult category.

Clinical manifestations include incidental discovery of painless splenomegaly; thrombocytopenia, anemia, or leukopenia secondary to hypersplenism; and bone pain. The course is variable, ranging from confinement to a wheelchair early in life to asymptomatic diagnosis in the ninth decade. Most patients have a mild course with relatively normal life expectancy. Partial or total splenectomy may be required. Pneumococcal vaccine should be administered prior to splenectomy. Careful management of postsplenectomy infection risks are important, and prophylactic antibiotics are recommended. The extent of bone disease is variable and includes bone pain, pathologic fractures, vertebral collapse, and aseptic necrosis of the femoral head. Bone pain with fever is termed pseudoosteomyelitis. MRI is particularly effective in demonstrating and differentiating bony abnormalities in Gaucher's disease. Moderate hepatic dysfunction is common, and, rarely, severe hepatic failure, portal hypertension, pulmonary infiltrates, and pulmonary hypertension may develop. Serum acid phosphatase is characteristically elevated. A distinctive storage cell is present in the bone marrow in all forms of Gaucher's disease, but enzyme assay should be performed because the Gaucher cell may also be found in patients with granulocytic leukemia and myeloma. Bone marrow transplantation may be considered in the rare case of life-threatening complications from the disease.

FABRY'S DISEASE Fabry's disease involves the accumulation of a trihexoside, galactosylgalactosylglucosylceramide, due to deficiency of α-galactosidase A. The disorder is X-linked. The most severe symptoms occur in hemizygous males with an incidence of about 1 in 40,000; milder symptoms occur in heterozygous females. Painful neuropathy is the most prominent symptom in younger men. The pain may be constant or cause intermittent crises of burning pain particularly in the palms and soles. Painful crises may mimic appendicitis or renal colic, and associated low grade fever may lead to misdiagnoses of inflammatory processes.

The diagnosis can be suggested by the astute dermatologist or ophthalmologist. Cutaneous manifestations include angiokeratoma and decreased sweating. The angiokeratoma occur as clusters of red angiectases in the superficial skin. They do not blanch with pressure and are located on the trunk, perineal area, penis, and scrotum. The anhidrosis or hypohidrosis can predispose to heat stroke with vigorous exercise, as in military training. A characteristic corneal opacity occurs in males and in most heterozygous females. Lenticular opacities and tortuosity of the conjunctival and retinal vessels also occur.

Cardiovascular manifestations include direct involvement of the myocardium with lipid deposition, arrhythmias, valvular dysfunction, and myocardial infarction. Cerebral vascular manifestations secondary to involvement of small vessels are not rare, and frank cerebral hemorrhage can occur. Deposition of lipid in the kidney results in progressive renal impairment with renal failure in middle age (see also Chap. 228). The mean age at death of males not treated for renal failure was 41 years in one study. The diagnosis is often recognized at renal biopsy on the basis of lipid vacuoles in glomerular and tubular epithelial cells.

Heterozygous females are affected more mildly, but corneal dystrophy and cutaneous manifestations may be seen on careful examination. Life expectancy is near normal in women, although the more serious complications occur rarely.

Therapeutic intervention of several types may be helpful. Counseling regarding the risks of hypohidrosis is important. Painful neuropathy frequently responds to administration of phenytoin. Renal failure can be treated by chronic dialysis, and the patients are acceptable candidates for transplantation since the donor kidney will not be impaired by the disease. The disease in the future might be amenable to enzyme replacement therapy, since the central nervous system is spared.

ACID LIPASE DEFICIENCY The infantile form of acid lipase deficiency, Wolman's disease, is listed in Table 331-1. Cholesteryl ester storage disease in adulthood and adolescence is a rare disorder with mild phenotypic features by comparison. The usual features are hepatosplenomegaly, lipid deposition in the liver, and increased plasma cholesterol. Hepatic fibrosis, esophageal varices, and poor growth may occur.

GLYCOPROTEIN STORAGE DISORDERS Fucosidosis, mannosidosis, and aspartylglucosaminuria are rare, autosomal recessive disorders involving hydrolases that degrade polysaccharide linkages. Glycolipids as well as glycoproteins are accumulated in fucosidosis. All are characterized by neurologic impairment and varying somatic involvements, as outlined in Table 331-1. Fucosidosis and mannosidosis are most often lethal disorders in childhood, while aspartylglucosaminuria presents as a late-onset lysosomal storage disease with prominent mental retardation and a prolonged course. Abnormal sweat electrolytes and cutaneous angiokeratomas are distinctive in fucosidosis, and an unusual cartwheel-type cataract occurs in mannosidosis. Aspartylglucosaminuria is remarkable in that urinary amino acid analysis is diagnostic with an increase of aspartylglucosamine; it is more frequent in the Finnish population. Sialidosis encompasses a group of phenotypes associated with glycoprotein neuraminidase (sialidase) deficiency. The phenotypes include an adult cherry-red spot myoclonus syndrome, infantile and juvenile presentations with mucopolysaccharidosis-like phenotypes, and a congenital presentation with hydrops fetalis. Many patients previously classified as having mucolipidosis I have been proven to have mannosidosis or sialidosis. Some patients with sialidosis have β-galactosidase deficiency as well as neuraminidase deficiency. The combined β-galactosidase and neuraminidase deficiency is due to a defect in a "protective protein." Each of the glycoprotein storage diseases can be diagnosed by appropriate enzyme assay.

MUCOPOLYSACCHARIDOSIS (MPS) The mucopolysaccharidoses represent a broad spectrum of disorders due to deficiencies of one of a group of enzymes which degrade three classes of mucopolysaccharides: heparan sulfate, dermatan sulfate, and keratan sulfate. The general MPS phenotype includes coarse facies, corneal clouding, hepatosplenomegaly, joint stiffness, hernias, dysostosis multiplex, mucopolysaccharide excretion in the urine, and metachromatic staining in peripheral leukocytes and bone marrow. Various components of the MPS phenotype are also found in the mucolipidoses, glycoprotein storage disorders, and other lysosomal storage diseases. Detailed clinical and radiologic evaluation and identification of the type of MPS excreted in the urine help to narrow the diagnostic possibilities. Definitive diagnosis requires assay of specific enzymes in various tissues such as cultured skin fibroblasts.

Hurler's or MPS IH disorder is the prototype MPS. Virtually all the components of the phenotype mentioned above are present and expressed in a severe degree. Nasal congestion and grossly visible corneal clouding are early features. Excessive growth during the first year of life is followed by poor growth late in the course. Radiologic features include enlargement of the sella turcica with a distinctive "shoe-shaped" fossa, broadening and shortening of the long bones, and hypoplasia and beaking of the vertebrae in the lumbar area. The vertebral beaking gives rise to an accentuated kyphosis or gibbus deformity. Death occurs within the first decade; postmortem findings include hydrocephalus and cardiovascular disease with occlusion of the coronary arteries. The biochemical defect is α-iduronidase deficiency with accumulation of heparan sulfate and dermatan sulfate.

MPS IS, or Scheie's syndrome, a clinically distinct disorder with childhood onset but adult survival, is characterized by joint stiffness, corneal clouding, aortic regurgitation, and usually normal intelligence. Surprisingly, this much milder disorder is also the result of α-iduronidase deficiency; it is allelic with Hurler's syndrome, as shown by lack of cross-correction of enzyme activity in cocultures of skin fibroblasts. Phenotypes occur that are clearly intermediate between Hurler's and Scheie's syndromes. It is believed that patients with an intermediate phenotype represent genetic compounds with one Hurler's allele and one Scheie's allele. Although genetic compounds must occur, in any one case their existence is difficult to distinguish from still other mutations of intermediate severity.

Hunter's, or MPS II, syndrome is distinguishable from Hurler's phenotype by the absence of gross corneal clouding and the X-linked recessive inheritance. The infantile form resembles the Hurler's disease phenotype, and a milder form allows survival into adulthood. The severe and mild forms may be allelic, since both are X-linked and share the same enzyme deficiency (iduronosulfate sulfatase).

Sanfilippo's mucopolysaccharidoses (MPS IIIA, IIIB, IIIC, and IIID) are distinguished by the accumulation of heparan sulfate without dermatan or keratan sulfate and by the marked central nervous system involvement with milder somatic involvement. Sanfilippo's mucopolysaccharidosis usually is diagnosed in the evaluation of mental retardation in childhood. Because the somatic features of this MPS are mild, the condition can be overlooked in the evaluation of an apparently isolated central nervous system problem. Death usually occurs during the second or third decade. The MPS III disorders are approximate genocopies. That is, four different enzyme deficiencies give rise to relatively indistinguishable clinical phenotypes with the same storage product. The four MPS III disorders can be diagnosed and distinguished by enzyme assay (Table 331-1).

Morquio's or MPS IV syndrome is distinguished by the absence of mental retardation and the presence of a distinctive bony dystrophy which can be classified as a spondyloepiphyseal dysplasia. Marked hypoplasia of the odontoid process can cause cervical dislocation and usually leads to some degree of spinal cord compression. Aortic regurgitation is frequent. The deficiency of *N*-acetylgalactosamine-6-sulfate sulfatase is the basis for this condition. Bone changes somewhat suggestive of Morquio's syndrome may also occur in β-galactosidase deficiency and in other forms of spondyloepiphyseal dysplasia. Maroteaux-Lamy's or MPS VI disorder is characterized by prominent osseous involvement, corneal clouding, and normal intellect. Allelic forms with variable severity but the same deficiency of arylsulfatase B (*N*-acetylhexosamine-4-sulfate sulfatase) have been described. MPS VII, or β-glucuronidase deficiency, has been described in only a few patients with a rather complete MPS phenotype. Extreme variability from a lethal infantile form to a mild adult disease occurs.

MUCOLIPIDOSES Mucolipidosis is a general term for lysosomal storage diseases involving some combination of MPS, glycoprotein, oligosaccharide, and glycolipids. The category of mucolipidosis I probably can be abandoned since most or all of these patients actually have a specific glycoprotein storage disease.

Mucolipidosis II, or I-cell disease, is an early onset disorder with mental retardation and an MPS phenotype. The distinctive features are striking inclusions in cultured skin fibroblasts and markedly elevated serum levels of lysosomal enzymes. The disorder has an autosomal recessive basis and is now known to represent a defect in the posttranslational processing of lysosomal enzymes. Mucolipidosis III, or pseudo-Hurler's polydystrophy, is a milder disorder with many aspects of the MPS phenotype, particularly dysostosis multiplex. The disorder presents in the first decade with joint stiffness, the diagnosis of rheumatoid arthritis often being considered. The major handicaps are progressive physical disabilities, particularly claw hand deformity and hip dysplasia. Mild mental retardation is common. Aortic and/or mitral valvular disease is routinely present, although often not functionally significant. Survival into adult life with possible stabilization of the condition is characteristic, with greater disability in males than in females. Inclusions in cultured skin fibroblasts and elevation of serum lysosomal enzymes are essentially identical with the findings in mucolipidosis II, suggesting that these are allelic disorders. The primary defect in mucolipidosis II and III is deficiency of UDP-*N*-acetylglucosamine (GLcNAc):glycoprotein GLcNAc-1-phosphotransferase, an enzyme involved in posttranslational synthesis of the oligosaccharide portion of the lysosomal enzymes.

NEURONAL CEROID LIPOFUSCINOSES The neuronal ceroid lipofuscinosis disorders include a wide clinical spectrum with onset in childhood, juvenile, or adult periods. It is uncertain if these disorders are true lysosomal storage diseases, indeed whether single or multiple biochemical genetic disorders are present. The clinical features include central nervous system deterioration with cerebral atrophy, usually commensurate with degree of impairment. Seizures, particularly myoclonic jerks, are prominent. Ocular involvement with optic atrophy, retinitis pigmentosa, and macular degeneration is present in the infantile and juvenile disorders but often absent in adult forms. Autosomal recessive inheritance is likely in most instances. The neuropathologic findings form the basis of the descriptive term for the disease. Electron microscopy demonstrates abnormal inclusions within lysosomes throughout a wide variety of tissues, despite the rather isolated neurologic clinical involvement. The presence of curvilinear bodies, electron-dense material, and fingerprint profiles on electron microscopy of white blood cells, liver biopsy, or muscle biopsy can be helpful diagnostically.

OTHER LYSOSOMAL STORAGE DISEASES Glycogen storage disease type II (Pompe's disease) is the prototype lysosomal storage disease. The predominant clinical features of skeletal and cardiac myopathy are described in Chap. 332. Some rarer disorders are included in Table 331-1. Multiple sulfatase deficiency is an autosomal recessive disorder characterized by a deficiency of five or more cellular sulfatases: aryl sulfatase A, aryl sulfatase B, other mucopolysaccharide sulfatases, and a nonlysosomal steroid sulfatase. The clinical picture combines features of metachromatic leukodystrophy, an MPS phenotype, and ichthyosis. Other neurodegenerative diseases may eventually be classifiable as lysosomal storage diseases. Disorders such as juvenile dystonic lipidosis, neuroaxonal dystrophy, Hallervorden-Spatz disease, Pelizaeus-Merzbacher disease, and other candidates exist. In addition, it is not unusual to identify patients with distinctive clinical features suggestive of lipidosis, mucolipidosis, or mucopolysaccharidosis, in which none of the present biochemically identifiable disorders can be identified. For these reasons, the number of distinct lysosomal storage diseases is likely to continue to increase.

REFERENCES

ARGOV Z, NAVON R: Clinical and genetic variations in the syndrome of adult GM_2 gangliosidosis resulting from hexosaminidase A deficiency. Ann Neurol 16:14, 1984

BEUTLER E: Gaucher disease. Blood Rev 2:59, 1988

DURAND P, O'BRIEN JS (eds): *Genetic Errors of Glycoprotein Metabolism*, Berlin, Springer-Verlag, 1982

LANIR A et al: Gaucher disease: Assessment with MR imaging. Radiology 161:239, 1986

SCRIVER CR et al (eds): *The Metabolic Basis of Inherited Disease*, 6th ed. New York, McGraw-Hill, 1989, chaps 12 and 61–72

TSUJI S et al: Genetic heterogeneity in type 1 Gaucher disease: Multiple genotypes in Ashkenazic and non-Ashkenazic individuals. Proc Natl Acad Sci USA 85:2349, 1988

WALTZ G et al: Adult metachromatic leukodystrophy. Arch Neurol 44:225, 1987

332 THE GLYCOGEN STORAGE DISEASES

ARTHUR L. BEAUDET

The glycogen storage diseases are a group of genetic disorders involving the pathways for storage of carbohydrate as glycogen and for its utilization to maintain blood sugar and to provide energy. Some forms are not associated with actual increases in glycogen content in tissues.

Glycogen is a highly branched polymer of glucose with the majority of residues in 1,4 linkage and with 7 to 10 percent of residues in 1,6 linkage. The treelike structure undergoes addition and removal of residues at its periphery. Glycogen molecules have molecular weights of many millions, and molecules may aggregate to form structures recognizable by electron microscopy. Liver generally contains less than 70 mg glycogen per gram of tissue, and muscle usually contains less than 15 mg/g, but these levels fluctuate as a consequence of feeding and hormonal stimuli. Abnormalities of glycogen structure can result either from decreased or increased branching.

The metabolic pathways involved in glycogen synthesis and breakdown are outlined in Fig. 332-1. These pathways differ among tissues; for example, certain reactions are active in liver but trivial or absent in muscle, and some enzyme functions are encoded by different genes in muscle and liver. Plasma glucose enters the cell and is phosphorylated by glucokinase or hexokinase. The former enzyme is found in liver where it accomplishes the majority of phosphorylation of glucose, while multiple hexokinases are distributed more widely in tissues. Glucose-6-phosphate (G6P) is converted to glucose-1-phosphate (G1P) in a reversible reaction catalyzed by phosphoglucomutase. Uridine diphosphate glucose (UDPG) is synthesized from G1P and UTP by UDPG pyrophosphorylase. Genetic

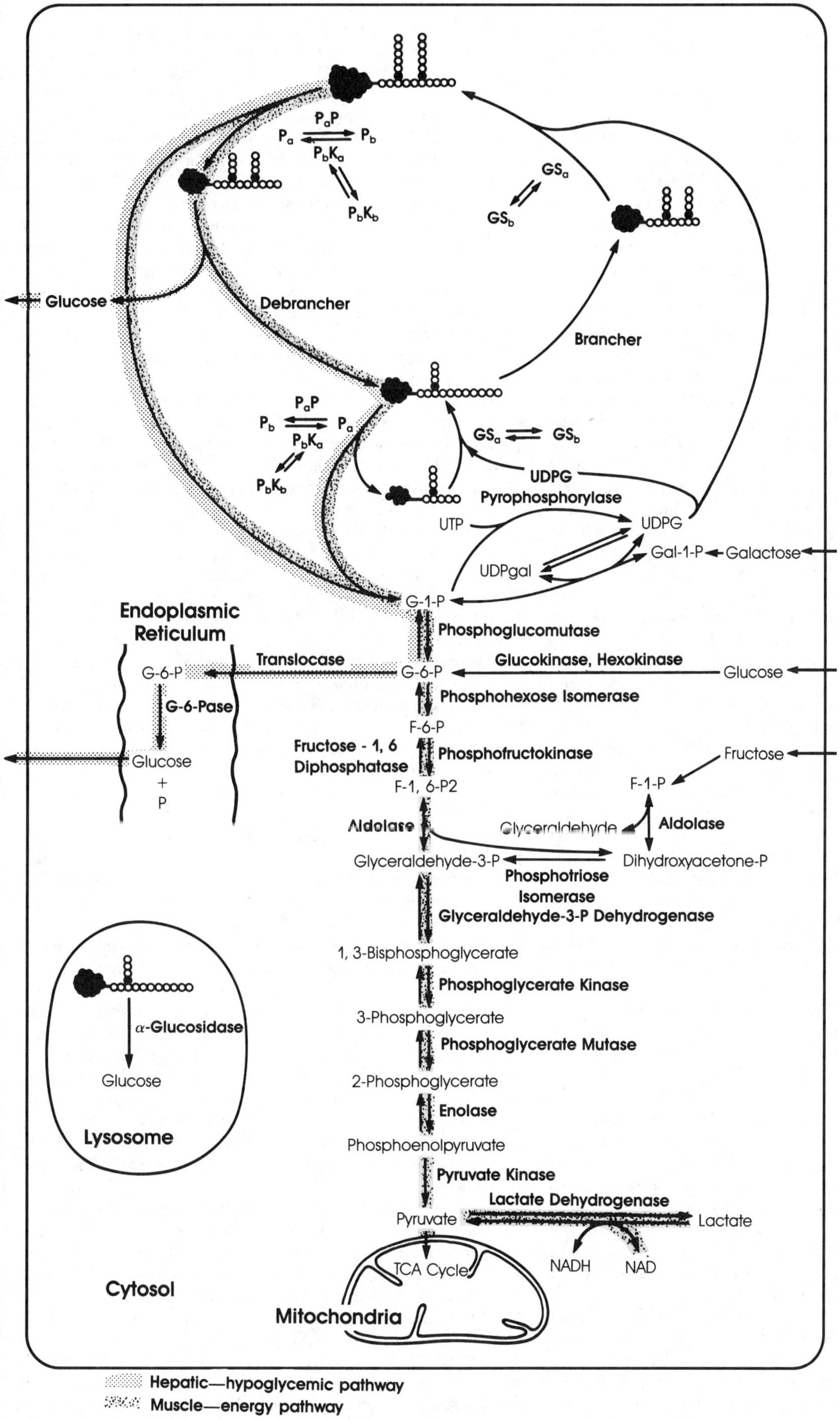

FIGURE 332-1 Metabolic pathways related to glycogen storage disease. A hypothetical composite cell is shown depicting both hepatic and muscle pathways. The shaded areas depict pathways that are blocked in the hepatic-hypoglycemic diseases or in the muscle-energy diseases. Nonstandard abbreviations are as follows: GS_a, active glycogen synthase; GS_b, inactive glycogen synthase; P_a, active phosphorylase; P_b, inactive phosphorylase; P_aP, phosphorylase *a* phosphatase; P_bK_a, active phosphorylase *b* kinase; P_bK_b, inactive phosphorylase *b* kinase.

deficiency has not been documented for any of these hepatic enzymes. Glycogen is then elongated by the addition from UDPG of individual glucose residues to an existing polymer. This reaction is catalyzed by glycogen synthase, which exists in an active dephosphorylated form and in an inactive phosphorylated form. Synthesis of a normally branched glycogen structure also requires the action of a branching enzyme (1,4-α-glucan:1,4-α-glucan-6-glucosyltransferase) which transfers a 1,4-linked oligosaccharide to a 1,6-linkage position.

Glucose is mobilized from glycogen by a complex group of enzyme reactions. Glycogen is acted upon directly by the active form of phosphorylase, phosphorylase *a,* to remove individual glucose units and yield G1P. Phosphorylase is encoded by different gene products in muscle and in liver. In both tissues, the enzyme can exist in an active phosphorylated form and in an inactive dephosphorylated form. Phosphorylase is a dimer of identical subunits, and both forms of the enzyme are subject to complex allosteric regulation. The inactive phosphorylase *b* is converted to the active form by phosphorylase *b* kinase. Phosphorylase *b* kinase also exists in an active phosphorylated form and in an inactive dephosphorylated form. Phosphorylase *b* kinase is composed of four nonidentical subunits $(\alpha,\beta,\gamma,\delta)_4$, and the δ chain is identical with the calcium-binding protein calmodulin. The rate of glucose mobilization by this system is regulated by a cascade of kinase reactions, including cyclic AMP–dependent protein kinase. Epinephrine and glucagon act to increase blood sugar via this cascade system by activation of phosphorylase and simultaneous inactivation of glycogen synthase. Glycogen also is acted upon directly by a debranching enzyme which carries out the debranching process by first transferring an oligosaccharide from a branch point to leave a single 1,6-linked glucose residue and then hydrolyzing the 1,6 linkage. Thus, the debrancher enzyme has both glucan transferase activity (oligo-1,4 → 1,4-transferase) and a glucosidase (amylo-1,6-glucosidase) activity and yields a single residue of glucose for each branch point removed. The G1P generated by phosphorylase, as mentioned above, must be further metabolized to G6P by phosphoglucomutase. In the liver G6P is transported by a specific translocase to the inner surface of the endoplasmic reticulum for hydrolysis by glucose-6-phosphatase. Glucose is then free to exit the hepatic cell to maintain blood levels. Many genetic deficiencies occur in the enzymes required for the conversion of glycogen to free glucose in the liver, and these cause the hepatic-hypoglycemic forms of glycogen storage disease.

If glycogen is used as a direct energy source, as in muscle, G6P and G1P must enter the pathways for glycolysis. Again, numerous enzymes are required in muscle for proper breakdown of glycogen and entry into the glycolytic pathway and tricarboxylic acid cycle. The enzymatic steps known to be associated with genetic deficiency states in muscle include muscle phosphorylase, debranching enzyme, muscle phosphofructokinase (PFK), and probably muscle phosphoglycerate mutase (PGAM) and lactate dehydrogenase (LDH) M subunit.

The lysosomal enzyme α-glucosidase, which is structurally and metabolically separate from the above-described pathways, is capable of degrading both 1,4 and 1,6 linkages in glycogen to give free glucose. This enzyme has widespread distribution in tissues, but its deficiency affects primarily skeletal and cardiac muscle.

CLASSIFICATION The clinical manifestations, diagnostic criteria, and therapy for glycogen storage diseases can be formulated in terms of the metabolic pathway outlined above (Table 332-1). According to this schema, two broad categories of disease can be delineated—those with a *hepatic-hypoglycemic* pathophysiology and those with a *muscle-energy* pathophysiology. Diseases with individualized pathophysiology also occur. It is suggested that disorders be designated by the specific protein deficiency, i.e., glucose-6-phosphatase deficiency. Although the roman numeral designations for types I through VII are in widespread use, numbering for higher types is confused and is to be avoided. Eponyms are of historical interest.

The hepatic-hypoglycemic disorders include glucose-6-phosphatase deficiency (type Ia), G6P microsomal translocase deficiency (type Ib), debrancher enzyme deficiency (type III), hepatic phosphorylase deficiency (type VI), and phosphorylase *b* kinase deficiency. Within this group, a distinction can be made between those disorders in which G6P and its metabolites are likely to be elevated (types Ia and Ib) and those disorders where G6P and related metabolites are likely to be decreased. This explains why increased glycolysis and lactic acidosis occur in types Ia and Ib disease but not in other forms of hepatic-hypoglycemic disease. Likewise, types Ia and Ib disease are distinct because gluconeogenesis, galactose, and fructose cannot contribute effectively to maintenance of blood sugar, in contrast to the other forms of hepatic-hypoglycemic disease. The glycemic response to epinephrine or glucagon tends to be blunted in the hepatic-hypoglycemic disorders. Dietary therapy with frequent feeding is a rational approach to the hepatic-hypoglycemic disorders and is tailored to reduce protein and to eliminate sources of galactose and fructose in types Ia and Ib disease.

The muscle-energy disorders include muscle phosphorylase deficiency (type V), phosphofructokinase deficiency (type VII), phosphoglycerate mutase deficiency, and LDH M-subunit deficiency. The clinical picture is one of muscle pain, myoglobinuria, and elevation of muscle enzymes in serum following vigorous exercise. The interruption of the pathway from glycogen to lactate with the accompanying failure to oxidize NADH is the unifying theme in these disorders. The failure of blood lactate to increase in response to exercise is a useful diagnostic test for the muscle-energy deficiency disorders. Debrancher enzyme deficiency constitutes an overlap syndrome; it presents primarily as a hepatic-hypoglycemic disorder in childhood, but serious muscle weakness occurs in some adults.

Two other disorders are best considered individually. Deficiency of lysosomal α-glucosidase is a lysosomal storage disease without major impact on either carbohydrate metabolism or maintenance of blood sugar (see Chap. 331). The major pathologic process in branching enzyme deficiency is a severe hepatic cirrhosis, possibly due to the harmful effects of the abnormal glycogen that accumulates. Glycogen content is generally normal, and the ability to maintain a normal blood sugar is not impaired.

HEPATIC-HYPOGLYCEMIC DISEASES Glucose-6-phosphatase deficiency, type Ia CLINICAL FEATURES Glucose-6-phosphatase deficiency, or von Gierke disease, is an autosomal recessive genetic disorder with an incidence of 1 in 100,000 to 400,000. The disorder is usually manifested during the first 12 months of life by symptomatic hypoglycemia or by the recognition of hepatomegaly. Occasional patients experience hypoglycemia in the immediate neonatal period, and rare patients never have hypoglycemia. Characteristic findings include a full-cheeked, rounded facial appearance; a protuberant abdomen due to marked hepatomegaly; and thin extremities. Hyperlipidemia may cause eruptive xanthomas and lipemia retinalis. Splenomegaly is usually mild or absent, although massive enlargement of the left lobe of the liver may be mistaken for enlargement of the spleen. Growth is usually normal for the first few months of life; growth retardation then supervenes, and adolescence is delayed. Mental development is usually normal except for injury from hypoglycemia.

The characteristic profound symptomatic hypoglycemia may be associated with blood glucose levels below 0.8 mmol/L (15 mg/dL). Liver enzymes are mildly elevated if at all. The presence of lactic acidosis is helpful in diagnosing this disorder, although blood lactate may be normal in the fed state in young infants. However, these patients are relatively resistant to development of ketosis. Hyperlipidemia is frequent and involves elevation of both cholesterol and triglycerides. Hypertriglyceridemia can be extreme with levels as high as 60 mmol/L (5000 mg/dL) or higher. Hyperuricemia due both to decreased renal excretion and increased production is frequent and often becomes more severe after adolescence. The rise in plasma glucose following administration of epinephrine or glucagon is impaired, as is the rise in blood glucose following administration of galactose by mouth. The pathogenesis of most of the metabolic

TABLE 332-1 Glycogen storage diseases

Type	Basic defect*	Clinical findings	Laboratory	Diagnosis	Treatment	Comments
DISORDERS WITH HEPATIC-HYPOGLYCEMIC PATHOPHYSIOLOGY						
Ia von Gierke	Glucose-6-phosphatase deficiency	Hypoglycemia, hepatomegaly, bleeding diathesis, short stature, delayed adolescence, hepatic adenomas, enlarged kidneys	Increased lactate, cholesterol, triglyceride, and uric acid	Enzyme assay on liver or intestine, increased glycogen with normal structure in liver	Frequent feeding, nighttime tube feeding, 60–70% carbohydrate, restrict sucrose and lactose, bicarbonate and allopurinol as needed	Common, severe, autosomal recessive
Ib	G6P microsomal translocase deficiency	As for Ia with addition of neutropenia and recurrent infection	As for Ia	Enzyme assay on liver with and without detergent	As for Ia	Rare, severe, autosomal recessive
III Cori	Debrancher enzyme deficiency	Hypoglycemia, hepatomegaly, some short stature and delayed adolescence, mild myopathy worsening in some adults	Normal lactate and uric acid; increased cholesterol, triglyceride, and SGOT	Enzyme assay on liver, muscle, or fibroblasts; leukocytes variable; increased glycogen with abnormal structure in liver and muscle	Frequent feeding, nighttime tube feeding, 50% carbohydrate and 15–20% protein	Common, intermediate severity, some hepatic fibrosis
VI Hers	Hepatic phosphorylase deficiency	Hepatomegaly, variable hypoglycemia	Minimal changes, ? hyperlipidemia	Enzyme assay on liver, increased hepatic glycogen with normal structure	Dietary therapy as for type III, often little treatment required	Rare and poorly characterized; ? autosomal recessive
Formerly VIb, VIII, or IX	Hepatic phosphorylase *b* kinase deficiency	Hepatomegaly, variable hypoglycemia, occasional findings in heterozygous females	Minimal changes	Enzyme assay on leukocytes, fibroblasts, or liver; increased hepatic glycogen with normal structure	Dietary therapy as for type III, often little treatment required	Very mild but may be fairly common, X-linked
DISORDERS WITH MUSCLE-ENERGY PATHOPHYSIOLOGY						
V McArdle	Muscle phosphorylase deficiency	Pain, cramps, and myoglobinuria on strenuous exercise	Increased CPK with episodes, deficient lactate production with ischemic exercise test	Muscle enzyme assay, increased muscle glycogen with normal structure	Avoid exercise, glucose or fructose before exercise	Some clearly autosomal recessive, male preponderance
VII	Muscle phosphofructokinase deficiency	As for type V, mild hemolytic anemia	As for type V	Muscle enzyme assay, increased muscle glycogen with normal structure	As for type V	Rare, autosomal recessive
	Muscle phosphoglycerate mutase deficiency	As for type V	As for Type V	Muscle enzyme assay, normal glycogen content	? As for type V	Based on one affected male
	LDH M-subunit deficiency	As for type V	Increased CPK with episodes; pyruvate but not lactate rises with ischemic exercise test	LDH isozymes on serum, erythrocytes or leukocytes; enzyme assay on muscle; ? glycogen content normal	? As for type V	Based on sibship of 3 males and 1 female affected
DISORDERS WITH INDIVIDUAL PATHOPHYSIOLOGY						
II Pompe	Lysosomal α-glucosidase deficiency	*Infantile:* hypotonia, muscle weakness, cardiac enlargement and failure, enlarged tongue, fatal early; *juvenile:* progressive skeletal muscle weakness; *adult:* progressive skeletal muscle weakness, pulmonary insufficiency presentation	Increased CPK, no hypoglycemia	Enzymes assay on muscle or fibroblasts, enzyme assay on leukocytes possible but pitfalls are serious	No effective treatment	Common, autosomal recessive, prenatal diagnosis available and widely utilized in infantile
IV Andersen	Brancher enzyme deficiency	Infantile failure to thrive, cirrhosis and liver failure, extreme hypotonia and weakness in some, fatal early	No hypoglycemia, changes of liver disease	Enzyme assay on liver, muscle, leukocytes or fibroblasts; glycogen content not remarkable but structure abnormal	No effective treatment	Very rare, autosomal recessive

* These defects provide the preferred nomenclature for the diseases.

abnormalities is not well understood; lactic acidosis may be due to increased glycolysis, and other abnormalities including poor growth may be the result of chronically altered levels of insulin and glucagon. Renal enlargement can be demonstrated by radiologic or sonographic techniques. Mild renal tubular dysfunction or the Fanconi syndrome may occur. Moderate anemia is usually due to recurrent nosebleeds and chronic acidosis but may become severe after prolonged acidosis. A bleeding diathesis is due to a platelet dysfunction.

Once type Ia disease is suspected clinically, the diagnosis is established by liver biopsy. Type Ia disease is suggested by lactic acidosis, an abnormal galactose tolerance test, or renal enlargement. Proper handling of biopsy material should be arranged to distinguish types Ia and Ib. Sufficient material for enzyme assay may be obtained by needle biopsy provided the bleeding time is normal, or alternatively, open liver biopsy provides more tissue for analysis. Microscopic examination of liver reveals increased glycogen in cytoplasm and nuclei; lipid vacuoles in hepatocytes are prominent, and fibrosis is usually absent.

The hypoglycemia and lactic acid acidosis may be life-threatening. Other troublesome features include short stature, delayed adolescence, and hyperuricemia. During adult years uric acid nephropathy and glomerulosclerosis may lead to renal failure. Hepatic adenomata are common after adolescence. There is a significant risk of hepatic malignant degeneration, often during the third decade, and subjects who live long enough are probably at increased risk for atherosclerosis.

TREATMENT The mainstay of management is frequent feeding. The most widely used approach in children has been the combination of frequent daytime feeding by mouth and continuous nighttime feeding by nasogastric tube (see Chap. 74). The regimen should include approximately 60 percent carbohydrate, and no significant portion of carbohydrate should come from sources containing galactose or fructose, which cannot be utilized effectively to maintain blood sugar. Raw cornstarch feeding provides a convenient, economical, and palatable source of slowly digested glucose polymer, and cornstarch therapy may become the primary dietary treatment for this disease. The ability of a family to carry out such a program is a significant variable, but in some instances the metabolic abnormalities and the rate of growth have improved substantially. Optimal management requires a team attentive to the dietary and psychosocial needs of patient and family. Control of elevated plasma urate may require the addition of allopurinol. This regimen provides a reasonably optimistic short-term prognosis, but it is not known whether the long-term risks of hepatic malignancy and atherosclerosis are ameliorated. Portacaval anastomosis is no longer used in the management of glycogen storage disease. Prenatal diagnosis is not possible at present.

G6P microsomal translocase deficiency, type Ib G6P microsomal translocase deficiency, historically referred to as *pseudo type I,* has an incidence of one-fifth to one-tenth that of type Ia. The term *microsomal translocase* describes the capacity to transport G6P into the endoplasmic reticulum. The clinical features are similar to those in type Ia, but unique features include neutropenia, impaired neutrophil migration, and recurrent pyogenic infections; in general, type Ib is more severe than Ia. Laboratory findings, responses to tolerance tests, and management are similar in the two disorders.

Type Ib disease was initially distinguished from type Ia by the presence of normal glucose-6-phosphatase activity on assay of biopsy tissue in the presence of detergent. However, glucose-6-phosphatase activity is low in type Ib disease when fresh tissue is homogenized and assayed in the absence of detergent. These results have been interpreted to imply a genetic deficiency of a microsomal G6P transport system as a primary defect in type Ib glycogen storage disease. The cause for the neutropenia and abnormal neutrophil migration is unknown, although the disease suggests a role for G6P transport in these cells.

Debrancher deficiency, type III CLINICAL FEATURES Debrancher enzyme deficiency, also known historically as Cori disease, is an autosomal recessive disorder and is one of the more frequent forms of glycogen storage diseases, occurring with a particularly high frequency in North African Jews. Symptomatic disease in the newborn period is unusual, and patients usually present with hypoglycemia or hepatomegaly during the first year of life. The physical findings are similar to those in type Ia, except that splenomegaly is more prominent, but the clinical course tends to be less severe. The skeletal or cardiac myopathy is usually mild or insignificant in childhood but may be disabling and progressive in adults. Some patients with myopathy are first diagnosed as adults because the features in childhood were mild and overlooked.

Fasting hypoglycemia occurs in about 80 percent of patients. The glucose response after glucagon or epinephrine is abnormal in the fasting state but may be normal shortly after eating since the terminal glucose residues in glycogen can be mobilized. The galactose tolerance test is usually normal. Ketosis is prominent, and blood lactate is normal. Serum transaminase is elevated, and further increases may occur with minor illnesses. Blood cholesterol and triglyceride are elevated in about two-thirds. Hyperuricemia is rare.

Two diagnostic modalities are used to establish the diagnosis—analysis of glycogen and measurement of debranching enzyme in tissue samples. The glycogen content of red blood cells and liver is increased in almost all, whereas glycogen content of muscle is increased only in some. Documentation of abnormal structure of glycogen with the use of spectrophotometric techniques is a more consistent finding than the increase in glycogen content. The establishment of the diagnosis by enzymatic assay is complicated both by methodologic problems and what is believed to be genetic heterogeneity. Both debrancher functions—the glucan transferase activity and glucosidase activity—are believed to reside in a single polypeptide, but as many as six subtypes of the disease may occur. While the diagnosis can be made in some patients using red cells, leukocytes, or fibroblasts, it is generally preferable to document the abnormal glycogen structure and the enzyme deficiency directly in biopsy material from liver or muscle. The pathologic findings in liver are similar to those in type Ia except for less lipid deposition and more prominent fibrous septae.

In regard to growth retardation and abdominal protuberance, the course is one of progressive improvement following adolescence, so that the adult appearance may be normal and hypoglycemia is less frequent. Liver tumors are not reported, and there is no information regarding the long-term risks of hyperlipidemia. The fraction of adult patients who develop a debilitating myopathy is probably low. Affected patients have had children.

TREATMENT Frequent feeding is also the mainstay of therapy for type III in childhood. Gluconeogenesis is normal and, as described above, patients can ingest galactose, fructose, or protein to help maintain blood glucose. Thus, dietary therapy can include a larger percentage of calories as protein, but carbohydrate intake should be 40 to 50 percent of the total. An evening feeding is often sufficient to avoid hypoglycemia, but nighttime nasogastric tube feeding or cornstarch therapy may be required in severely affected children. Attempts to lower blood lipids using dietary means are desirable. Prenatal diagnosis is possible.

Hepatic phosphorylase deficiency, type VI The diagnosis of hepatic phosphorylase deficiency, or Hers disease, was previously applied to a diverse group of patients with reduced hepatic phosphorylase levels due to a variety of causes but is now limited to patients in whom deficiency of hepatic phosphorylase is the primary defect. This nosologic difficulty is a consequence of the fact that phosphorylase exists in both active and inactive forms, and many factors may inhibit the activation of the enzyme secondarily. Consequently, diagnosis requires documentation that phosphorylase is absent and that the phosphorylase *b* kinase responsible for its activation is normal. The disorder is probably due to an autosomal recessive mutation.

Most patients have features similar to those in type III but in a milder form. The diagnosis is suspected because of hepatomegaly or hypoglycemia, and patients generally respond to dietary management similar to that employed in type III disease.

Phosphorylase *b* kinase deficiency Phosphorylase *b* kinase deficiency, now known to be a separate entity, was previously included in the type VI category. Various authors have designated this disorder as type VIa, type VIII, or type IX, but it is best termed *phosphorylase b kinase deficiency*. The best characterized form of the disorder is the X-linked variety, but there is potential for genetic heterogeneity, since the enzyme is composed of four nonidentical subunits. This disorder is relatively benign and is manifested in affected males by hepatomegaly, occasional fasting hypoglycemia, and some growth retardation, all of which tend to resolve spontaneously at the time of adolescence. Mild hepatomegaly may occur in female heterozygotes. The diagnosis can be established by specific enzyme assay of leukocytes or liver. Muscle phosphorylase *b* kinase is believed to be normal in this condition. Dietary management similar to that employed in type III can be employed for hypoglycemia or growth retardation. It is possible that this condition is relatively common and passes undiagnosed. Healthy adults with a history of abdominal protuberance in childhood are often identified during family studies of patients with this condition.

MUSCLE-ENERGY DISEASES (See also Chap. 365) In recognizing the various glycogen storage diseases that affect muscle, the *ischemic exercise test* is of particular use in the initial evaluation. A blood pressure cuff is inflated above arterial pressure, and the ischemic hand is exercised to maximum effort. The pressure cuff is released, and blood is drawn from the other arm at 2, 5, 10, 20, and 30 min for assay of lactate and pyruvate, muscle enzymes, and myoglobin.

Myophosphorylase deficiency, type V Myophosphorylase deficiency, or McArdle disease, is uncommon. Symptoms of pain and cramps after exercise usually develop during the second or third decade. A history of myoglobinuria is present in most, and on occasion myoglobinuria can cause renal failure. Affected individuals are otherwise healthy, without evidence of hepatic, cardiac, or metabolic disturbance. Performance of an ischemic exercise test usually causes painful cramping, which is helpful diagnostically. In addition, blood lactate does not rise whereas serum creatine phosphokinase is elevated after strenuous exercise.

The diagnosis is established by documentation of elevated glycogen content and reduced phosphorylase activity in biopsied muscle tissue. The glycogen is usually deposited in subsarcolemmal regions of the muscle. The gene for human myophosphorylase has been cloned and is located on chromosome 11, in keeping with the autosomal recessive nature of the disease. There is an excess of male patients, which may be due to better ascertainment in males, genetic heterogeneity, or other factors. A fatal infantile form of hypotonia in association with myophosphorylase deficiency also has been described.

Management of myophosphorylase deficiency requires the avoidance of strenuous exercise. Glucose or fructose ingestion prior to exercise can reduce symptoms.

Muscle phosphofructokinase deficiency, type VII There are two genetically distinct forms of phosphofructokinase. Activity in muscle is due to a distinct muscle isoenzyme, whereas activity in red cells is due both to a red cell isoenzyme and to the muscle form of the enzyme. A small number of families have been identified with deficiency of the muscle isoenzyme. Symptoms similar to those in myophosphorylase deficiency were present with pain and cramps, myoglobinuria, and elevated muscle enzymes in serum after strenuous exercise. Lactate production was impaired, and a mild nonspherocytic hemolytic anemia was present. Other patients have the anemia but no muscle symptoms; the latter phenomenon might be due to a qualitatively abnormal, unstable enzyme that rapidly disappears from the anucleate red cell but is replaced effectively in muscle cells and consequently prevents muscle symptoms.

Other muscle-energy diseases A group of even rarer familial metabolic disorders must be considered in the differential diagnosis of patients with myoglobinuria and elevated muscle enzymes in serum after exercise. These include phosphoglycerate mutase deficiency, LDH M-subunit deficiency, and carnitine palmityl transferase deficiency. (Older reports of phosphoglucomutase deficiency and phosphohexoseisomerase deficiency seem inconclusive by current standards.) When myophosphorylase, phosphofructokinase, or phosphoglycerate mutase are deficient, neither lactate nor pyruvate rises following exercise, whereas in deficiency of LDH M subunit there is a rise in pyruvate in the face of a failure of lactate production. Carnitine palmityl transferase deficiency is a disorder of lipid metabolism and is discussed in Chap. 320. Definitive diagnosis of these disorders must be established by enzyme assay of muscle tissue. Some patients with this clinical presentation have none of the above-mentioned enzyme deficiencies, and identification of other defects in muscle metabolism is likely in the future.

DISORDERS WITH INDIVIDUAL PATHOPHYSIOLOGY α-Glucosidase deficiency, type II Alpha-glucosidase deficiency, or Pompe disease, is a lysosomal storage disease, and the pathophysiology is discussed in Chap. 331. The incidence is not known but may exceed 1 in 100,000. The disorder is not associated with hypoglycemia, ketosis, or other abnormalities of intermediary metabolism.

The infantile form presents within the first 6 months of life and may be manifested at birth. Clinical features include skeletal muscle hypotonia and weakness, massive cardiac enlargement, enlargement of the tongue, and varying degrees of hepatomegaly. Muscle enzymes such as creatine phosphokinase and aldolase are usually elevated, and the ECG may show large QRS complexes and a shortened PR interval. Motor weakness and developmental delay may be present. Death occurs in the first 2 to 3 years in most cases due to the cardiac involvement.

The juvenile form has features suggestive of a progressive form of muscular dystrophy. These patients have gait abnormalities but no cardiac symptoms. Plasma creatine phosphokinase and aldolase are elevated, and the length of survival is variable. An even milder adult form presents as skeletal muscle weakness in the third to the fifth decade. Again, cardiac symptoms are absent, and serum muscle enzymes are elevated. Some patients have respiratory failure due to involvement of the muscles of respiration and are often misdiagnosed as having some form of muscular dystrophy.

Vacuolization of muscle and increased glycogen content are demonstrable on muscle biopsy. Electron-microscopic studies demonstrate membrane-bound vacuoles containing glycogen, a finding strongly suggestive of the disorder. Excessive glycogen is also found in other tissues including liver and central nervous system, particularly in the anterior horn cells of the spinal cord. Specific diagnosis is made by enzyme assay in biopsy material from muscle or liver or in cultured skin fibroblasts. In general, some residual enzyme activity is present in patients with the adult form of disease, but the exact level is not of prognostic significance. Prenatal diagnosis is reliable and has been used extensively for the infantile form. Various forms of enzyme infusion therapy have been tried but are ineffective.

Brancher deficiency, type IV Brancher enzyme deficiency, or Andersen disease, is a rare, autosomal recessive disorder. Features in infants include hepatomegaly, failure to thrive, and hypotonia in the first few months of life with subsequent development of progressive cirrhosis. In other patients the predominant feature is cardiac involvement and/or extreme hypotonia similar to that observed in spinal muscular atrophy and anterior horn cell degeneration. Death usually occurs within the first 2 or 3 years, although a more benign course is possible.

The symptoms are thought to be related primarily to the abnormal glycogen structure that results from a generalized deficiency of brancher enzyme. The presence of long outer chains on the glycogen molecules has led to the designation of the disease as amylopectinosis. The laboratory findings are generally those associated with severe liver disease except that hypoglycemia usually does not occur. The absence of hypoglycemia and the presence of normal glycogen content in the liver make the diagnosis difficult to establish. The diagnosis is suggested by finding abnormally structured glycogen in biopsy material and is established by direct assay of the enzyme in liver, leukocytes, or cultured skin fibroblasts. No effective treatment is known, but prenatal diagnosis is possible using cultured amniotic cells.

Other possible disorders of glycogen metabolism Deficiency of glycogen synthase has been reported in a small number of families. Affected patients usually have fasting hypoglycemia, seizures, and some degree of mental impairment. The presence of some hepatic glycogen, the increase in plasma glucose in response to glucagon or galactose, and the known lability of the activation system for glycogen synthase have all led to skepticism as to whether such a disorder actually exists. This syndrome may be confused with ketotic hypoglycemia of childhood (see Chap. 320).

There are also reports of more than one enzyme defect in the same patient and of different enzyme defects among siblings. Many of these reports may be related to difficulties inherent in measuring enzymes of glycogen metabolism in human pathologic tissue. At present no specific syndrome of multiple primary enzyme deficiency is documented.

REFERENCES

CHEN Y-T et al: Renal disease in type I glycogen storage disease. N Engl J Med 318:7, 1988

FERNANDEZ J et al: Glycogen storage disease. Recommendations for treatment. Eur J Pediatr 147:226, 1988

HERS H-G et al: Glycogen storage diseases, in *The Metabolic Basis of Inherited Disease*, 6th ed, CR Scriver et al (eds). New York, McGraw-Hill, 1989, p 425

MOSES SW et al: Neuromuscular involvement in glycogen storage disease type III. Acta Paediatr Scand 75:289, 1986

333 HERITABLE DISORDERS OF CONNECTIVE TISSUE

DARWIN J. PROCKOP

Heritable disorders that involve the major connective tissues of the body such as bone, ligaments, blood vessels, and skin are among the most common genetic diseases in humans. The three major categories of the diseases are osteogenesis imperfecta (OI), Ehlers-Danlos syndrome (EDS), and the Marfan syndrome (MS). This system of classification is in part historical and is in part based on the clusters of signs and symptoms in patients and in affected members of their families. Some patients are readily classified as OI because their bones are so brittle they suffer multiple fractures from minor trauma, and they have characteristic features such as blue sclerae and opalescent teeth. Some patients are easily recognized as EDS because their skin is grossly hyperelastic and ligaments are so loose that permanent dislocations develop in major joints. Similarly, many patients can be unequivocally classified as MS because of the characteristic triad of long and thin extremities, dislocations of the lenses, and life-threatening aortic aneurysms. However, many patients are difficult to classify because they have one or two cardinal features of one of the diseases but lack the others, and some patients have signs and symptoms of more than one of these diseases, e.g., blue sclerae suggestive of OI and joint dislocations suggestive of EDS. Attempts have been made to overcome these problems of nosology by defining a series of subtypes of the three major disease categories. However, the value of the more elaborate classification schemes has not been fully established. Many patients still cannot be precisely categorized. Moreover, many of the clinically defined types and subtypes do not reflect the mutations that cause the diseases. For example, most patients with OI have mutations that change the primary structure of type I procollagen. However, similar mutations changing the structure of type I procollagen occur in some patients with type VII EDS who have permanent joint dislocations but not fractures. At the same time, data on the molecular defects are not complete enough or readily enough available on individual patients to develop a new scheme of classification. Therefore, the current classification of OI, EDS, and MS based primarily on clinical criteria remains the best available system for diagnosis even though it will eventually be replaced by classifications based on the molecular defects that cause the diseases. Also, it is likely that additional information about the molecular defects will blur the distinction now made between OI, MS, and EDS and more common diseases of connective tissue such as familial forms of osteoporosis and aortic aneurysms.

DEFINITION AND CHEMICAL COMPOSITION OF CONNECTIVE TISSUES Connective tissues are loosely defined as the extracellular compartments and components that provide the structural support of the body and bind together its cells, organs, and tissues. The major connective tissues are bone, skin, tendons, ligaments, and cartilage. The term is also applied to blood vessels and to synovial spaces and fluids. Indeed, all organs and tissues contain some connective tissue in the form of membranes and septa.

Connective tissues contain large amounts of water, salt, albumin, and other components of plasma. The distinguishing feature of connective tissues, however, is that they contain a series of specific macromolecules that are assembled into a large and insoluble extracellular matrix (Table 333-1). The macromolecules include at least 13 different types of collagens, the related fibrous protein known as elastin, a series of proteoglycans, and additional components whose structure and function have been only partially defined.

Connective tissues such as bone, skin, and cartilage obviously differ both in appearance and function. The differences are in part explained by differences in their content of specific macromolecules. For example, tendons and ligaments consist primarily of type I collagen fibrils associated with other types of collagen that bind to and probably help organize the fibrils of type I collagen into larger fibers. Cartilage consists primarily of fibrils of type II collagen in the form of arcade-like structures that are distended by the presence of highly charged proteoglycans. Large blood vessels such as the aorta contain several different kinds of collagens and large amounts of elastin. The differences between the different connective tissues, however, also depend on variations in the size, orientation, and packing of collagen fibrils. The type I collagen fibrils in tendon are packed into thick, parallel bundles of fibers. In skin, type I collagen fibrils are randomly oriented in the plane of the skin. In cortical bone, type I collagen fibrils are deposited in intricate helical arrays around haversian canals. Therefore, the morphology and function of connective tissues are in part based on their content of specific macromolecules and in part on the three-dimensional organization of the macromolecules.

BIOSYNTHESIS OF CONNECTIVE TISSUE Assembly of the massive structures found in connective tissues is largely governed by the principle of *self-assembly*, whereby a molecular subunit of the correct size, shape, and surface properties binds to other molecules with the same structure, or with similar structures, in a spontaneous and highly ordered manner. Therefore, the molecular mechanisms and driving forces are similar to those involved in the formation of large inorganic crystals and organic polymers.

The principle of self-assembly of macromolecules in connective tissues is best illustrated by the assembly of collagen into fibrils. The collagen molecule is a long, thin rod consisting of three α-polypeptide chains wrapped into a rigid, ropelike triple helix not found in most other proteins (Fig. 333-1). Collagen has a triple-helical conformation, because each of the three α chains has a simple, repetitive amino acid sequence. Glycine (Gly) appears as every third amino acid. Therefore, the central sequence of 1,014 amino acids in each α chain can be designed as $(\text{-Gly-X-Y-})_{338}$, where X and Y represent amino acids other than glycine. It is essential that every third amino acid be glycine, the smallest amino acid, since this residue must fit in a sterically restricted space where the three chains of the triple helix

TABLE 333-1 Constituents of connective tissue in various tissues

Connective tissue	Known constituents	Approximate amounts (% dry wt)	Characteristics
Skin (dermis), ligaments, tendons	Type I collagen	80	Bundles of fibers of high tensile strength
	Type III collagen	5 to 15	Thin fibrils
	Type IV collagen, laminin, entactin, nidogen	<5	In basal laminae under epithelium and in blood vessels
	Types V to VII	<5	Distributions and functions unclear
	Fibronectin	<5	Associated with collagen fibers and cell surfaces
	Proteoglycans*	0.5	Provides resiliency
	Hyaluronate	0.5	Provides resiliency
Bone (demineralized)	Type I collagen	90	Complex organization of fibrils
	Type V collagen	1 to 2	Function unclear
	Proteoglycans	1	Function unclear
	Sialoproteins	1	Function unclear
	Osteonectin	2 to 3	Role in ossification
	Osteocalcin	1	Probable role in ossification
	α_2-Glycoprotein	1	Possible role in ossification
Aorta	Type I collagen	20 to 40	
	Type III collagen	20 to 40	Thin fibrils
	Elastin, microfibrillar protein	20 to 40	Amorphous, elastic fibrils
	Type IV collagen, laminin, entactin, nidogen	<5	In basal lamina
	Types V and VI collagens	<2	Functions unclear
	Proteoglycans	<3	Mucopolysaccharides, mainly chondroitin sulfate and dermatan sulfate; heparan sulfate in basal lamina
Cartilage	Type II collagen	40 to 50	Thin fibrils
	Types IX and X collagen	5 to 25	Possible role in maturation
	Proteoglycans	15 to 50	Provides resiliency
	Hyaluronate	0.5 to 2	Provides resiliency

* Proteoglycan structures are incompletely defined. About five different protein cores have been identified, and each has one or more kind of mucopolysaccharides attached. Major mucopolysaccharides of skin and tendon are dermatan sulfate and chondroitin-4-sulfate; of aorta, chondroitin-4-sulfate and dermatan sulfate; of cartilage, chondroitin-4-sulfate, chondroitin-6-sulfate, and keratan sulfate. Basal lamina contains heparan sulfate.

come together. The X- and Y-position amino acids are frequently the ring amino acids proline and hydroxyproline, which give rigidity to the triple-helical structure. The remaining X- and Y-position amino acids form clusters of hydrophobic and charged regions on the surface of the molecule that direct how one molecule spontaneously binds to other collagen molecules and thereby self-assembles into the large collagen fibrils found in tissues (Fig. 333-1).

About half of the 13 or so collagens in the body are called fibrillar because they form similar fibrils. Each contains three α chains that are folded into a triple helix. Type I collagen contains two identical

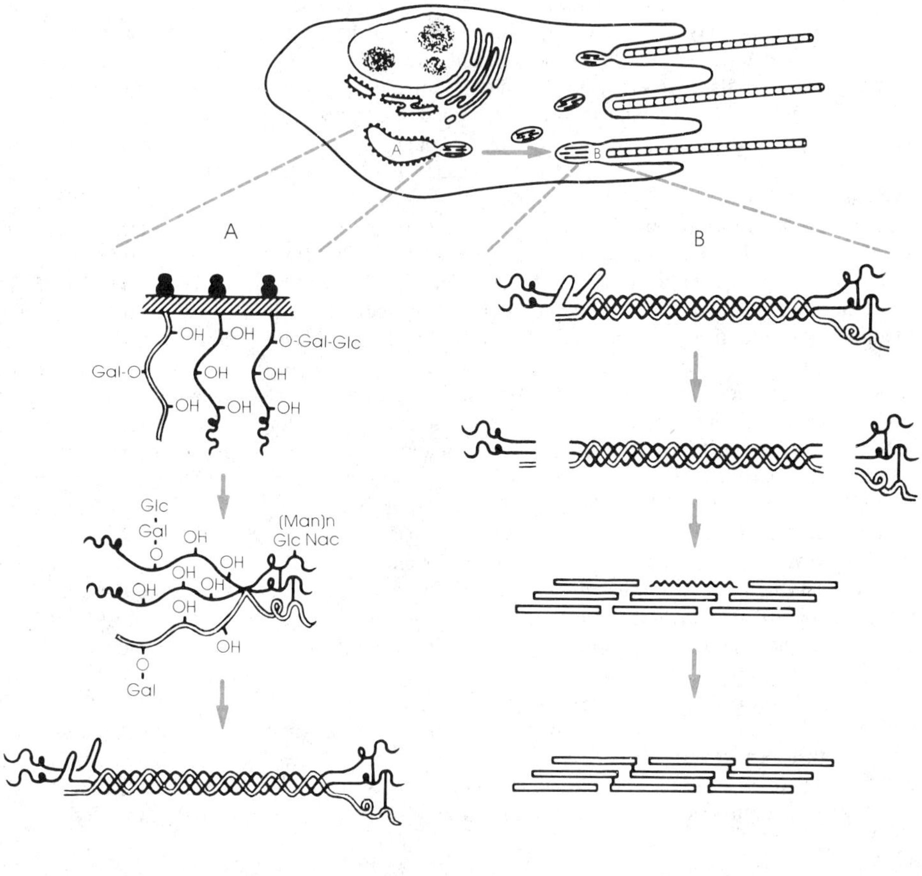

FIGURE 333-1 Schematic representation of synthesis of a type I collagen fibril by a fibroblast. *A*. Intracellular steps in the assembly of the procollagen molecule. Hydroxylations and glycosylations of the proα chains begin soon after the *N* termini pass into the cisternae of the rough endoplasmic reticulum and continue after the three chains associate through their *C*-propeptides and become disulfide-linked. *B*. Cleavage of procollagen to collagen, self-assembly of the collagen molecule into quarter-staggered fibrils, and cross-linking of the molecules in the fibrils. Cleavage of the propeptides may occur within crypts of the fibroblast, as shown here, or some distance from the cell. (*Reproduced with permission from Prockop and Kivirikko.*)

α chains called α1(I) and one slightly different chain called α2(I). Type II collagen and the type III collagen contain three identical chains called α1(II) and α1(III), respectively. About half of the known collagens are nonfibrillar. They are similar to the fibrillar collagens in that they contain -Gly-X-Y- sequences of amino acids that form triple-helical domains, but they also contain large globular domains. Self-assembly of most of the nonfibrillar collagens involves binding together of the globular domains to form networklike structures. For example, the type IV collagen found in basement membranes self-assembles into an amorphous network that provides a diffusion barrier and support for epithelial and endothelial cells in the renal glomerulus, skin, and most blood vessels.

Because fibrillar collagens spontaneously self-assemble into fibrils, they are first synthesized as larger and more soluble precursors called procollagens. The procollagen forms of type I, II, and III collagens are 1.5 times the mass of the corresponding collagens. The additional mass is in the form of amino acid sequences located at both the *N*-terminus and *C*-terminus of the molecule and called propeptides. To generate collagen fibrils, the *N*-terminal propeptides of procollagen must be cleaved by a specific procollagen *N*-proteinase, and the *C*-terminal propeptides must be cleaved by a specific procollagen *C*-proteinase. The cleavage of procollagens to collagens occurs after the molecules are secreted. The rates and order in which the propeptides are cleaved in different tissues probably influence the number of collagen fibrils formed and their morphology.

Assembly of the procollagens from the constitutive polypeptide chains, called proα chains, requires a large number of intracellular processing steps (Fig. 333-1). It also involves an unusual self-assembly step whereby the three chains fold into a triple-helical conformation. As the proα chains of procollagen are translated from mRNA on ribosomes, they pass into the cisternae of the rough endoplasmic reticulum. Hydrophobic "signal peptides" at the *N*-terminus are cleaved, and a series of additional posttranslational reactions begins. Proline residues in the Y position are converted to hydroxyproline by a specific prolylhydroxylase requiring ascorbic acid. Lysine residues in the Y position are similarly hydroxylated to hydroxylysine by a specific lysylhydroxylase also requiring ascorbic acid. The requirement for ascorbic acid by the two hydroxylases probably explains why wounds fail to heal in scurvy (see Chap. 76). Many of the hydroxylysine residues are further modified by glycosylation with galactose or with galactose and glucose. A large mannose-rich oligosaccharide is added to the *C*-terminal propeptide of each chain. As the last amino acids are incorporated into the proα chains, they are released into the cisternae of the rough endoplasmic reticulum. At this stage two proα1(I) and one proα2(I) chains associate through their *C*-propeptides. The association of the proα chains is directed by the structure and the surface properties of the globular *C*-propeptides. After the *C*-propeptides assemble correctly, the structure is locked in place by the formation of interchain disulfide bonds. Posttranslational modifications of the proα chains continue until each chain acquires a critical level of about 100 hydroxyproline residues. Then a few of the -Gly-X-Y- sequences at the *C*-terminus of the protein that are very rich in hydroxyproline fold into a triple-helical conformation. The short region of triple helix becomes a nucleus for self-assembly of the triple helix of the whole protein, much like a nucleus for crystallization, in that the triple-helical conformation in one -Gly-X-Y- sequence induces the next -Gly-X-Y- sequence to fold into the same conformation. As a result, the conformation is propagated from the nucleus until the entire α-chain domain becomes a continuous triple helix. Once the protein is folded, it passes from the rough endoplasmic reticulum to other membranous compartments, and it is secreted for processing to collagen and self-assembly of the collagen into fibrils.

The fibrils formed by the self-assembly of collagen have considerable tensile strength, and the strength is increased by cross-linking reactions that form covalent bonds between α chains in one molecule and α chains in adjacent molecules. The first step in cross-linking is oxidation by the enzyme lysyl oxidase of amino groups on lysine or hydroxylysine residues to form aldehydes. The aldehydes then interact to form stable covalent bonds.

The collagen fibrils and fibers in skin and tendon undergo repeated synthesis, degradation, and resynthesis during growth and development. They remain stable throughout most of adult life and turn over only with marked starvation or tissue destruction. The degradation of collagen fibers is initiated by specific collagenases found in fibroblasts, synovial cells, and other cell types. The collagenases cleave the collagen molecule at a point about three-quarters of the distance from its *N*-terminus. The cleavage triggers further degradation by other proteinases. In contrast to other connective tissue, collagen fibrils in bone undergo repeated degradation and synthesis throughout life as part of the continual remodeling of bone.

Essentially the same biosynthetic steps and the same posttranslational enzymes are involved in the biosynthesis of all collagens. Assembly of nonfibrillar collagens such as the type IV of basement membranes does not, however, involve cleavage of the globular domains at the ends of the protein since these are required for the self-assembly of the proteins into networklike structures. Elastin fibers are also assembled by a similar pathway. The elastin monomer, however, is a single polypeptide chain without a defined three-dimensional structure. It spontaneously self-assembles into amorphous elastic fibers, and the fibers then become tightly cross-linked through oxidation of lysine residues to aldehydes and complex interactions of the aldehydes.

Proteoglycan synthesis resembles collagen synthesis in that it involves a large number of posttranslational modifications. The synthesis begins with assembly of a core protein in the cisternae of the rough endoplasmic reticulum. The core protein then undergoes modifications by a series of sugar and sulfate transferases that generate large side chains of glycosaminoglycans. After secretion into the extracellular space, the core protein with its side chains binds to a smaller protein called a link protein. The complex of core protein and link protein then spontaneously binds to a long chain of hyaluronic acid to form a huge copolymer called a proteoglycan aggregate. Some of the four or more different kinds of proteoglycans in connective tissues bind to collagen fibrils and may thereby regulate the diameters of the fibrils. Others are closely associated with cell membranes and probably have an important role in the binding of cells to the extracellular matrix or in signal transduction from the matrix to the cell.

The assembly of bone follows much the same principles as the assembly of other connective tissues (see also Chap. 339). The first step is deposition of osteoid tissue that consists largely of type I collagen fibrils (Fig. 333-1). Mineralization of osteoid occurs by steps that are still incompletely defined; specific proteins probably bind to the collagen fibrils and then chelate calcium to initiate mineralization.

THE MUTATIONS THAT IMPAIR CONNECTIVE TISSUES Because of the large number of tissue-specific macromolecules in connective tissues, a large number of gene-protein systems are candidates for mutations that might cause disease. However, the situation may be simpler than originally assumed in that most forms of the disease appear to be caused by mutations in the structural genes for either type I or type III procollagens.

The most complete data are available on OI. About 90 percent of OI patients have mutations in either the gene for the proα1(I) chain or the gene for the proα2(I) chain of type I procollagen. A few of the mutations decrease expression of protein from one allele of the genes, but these are present in patients with the mildest form of the disease. Most of the mutations cause synthesis of a structurally abnormal but partially functional proα chain. Synthesis of abnormal proα chains from one mutant allele causes devastating effects because the abnormal proα chains interfere with assembly of normal proα chains into procollagen, the processing of procollagen to collagen, or the self-assembly of normal collagen into fibrils (Fig. 333-2). The mutations that underlie structurally abnormal proα chains include partial gene deletions, RNA splicing mutations, and a series of single

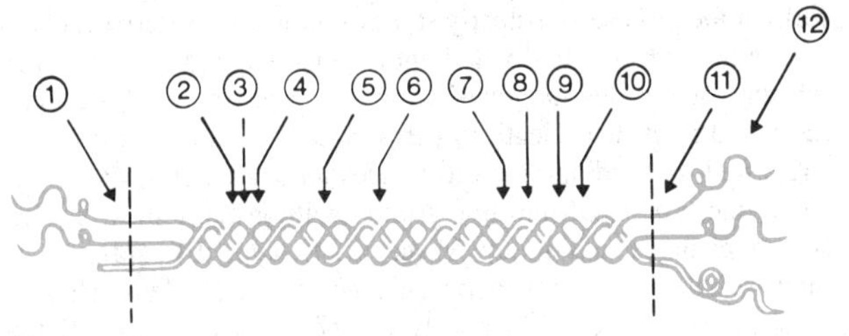

Pro α1

(1)	Splice Exon 6 (−24 aas)	EDS VII
(2)	Gly^{175} → Cys	OI
(3)	Insertion 50–70 aas	Lethal OI
(4)	Gly^{256} → Val	Lethal OI
(5)	Gly^{391} → Arg	Lethal OI
(6)	Deletion Exons 24–26 (−84 aas)	Lethal OI
(7)	Gly^{664} → Arg	Lethal OI
(8)	Gly^{748} → Cys	Lethal OI
(9)	Gly^{904} → Cys	Lethal OI
(10)	Gly^{988} → Cys	Lethal OI
(11)	Gly^{CT3} → Cys	OI
(12)	Frameshift Deletion of 5 bp	OI

FIGURE 333-2 Partial list of the mutations in the gene for the proα1(I) chain of type I procollagen that cause either OI or the type VII form of Ehlers-Danlos syndrome. Similar mutations have been found in the gene for the proα2(I) chains. *(Reproduced with permission from Prockop et al.)*

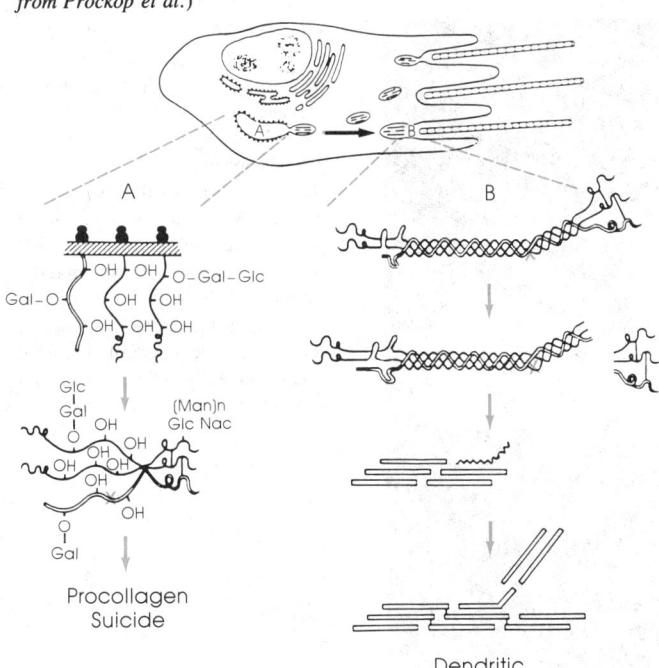

base mutations that substitute amino acids with bulkier side chains for glycines. The structurally abnormal proα chains exert their clinical effects through at least three molecular mechanisms (Fig. 333-3). First, the presence of an abnormal proα chain in a procollagen molecule containing two normal proα chains can prevent folding of the protein into a triple-helical conformation and lead to degradation of the whole molecule in a process called "procollagen suicide." Second, the presence of one abnormal proα chain in a procollagen molecule can interfere with cleavage of the *N*-propeptide from the protein by procollagen *N*-proteinase. The enzyme is unusual among proteinases in that it will not cleave procollagen substrate if the conformation of the cleavage site is disturbed. Therefore, mutations that change the amino acid sequence of a proα chain far from the cleavage site itself can markedly decrease or prevent cleavage of the *N*-peptide from all three chains. The persistence of the *N*-propeptide on a fraction of the molecules produced by fibroblasts interferes with the self-assembly of normal collagen produced by the same cell so that abnormally thin and irregular collagen fibrils are formed. Third, the substitution of a bulkier amino acid for glycine can produce a kink in the triple-helical structure. A small amount of collagen containing such a kink can cause assembly of abnormally branched or dendritic collagen fibrils.

FIGURE 333-3 Schematic summary of three mechanisms (see text) whereby mutations that cause biosynthesis of structurally abnormal proα1(I) or proα2(I) chains of type I procollagen interfere with either the assembly of the protein (*A*) or its processing to normal collagen fibrils (*B*). *(Reproduced with permission from Prockop et al.)*

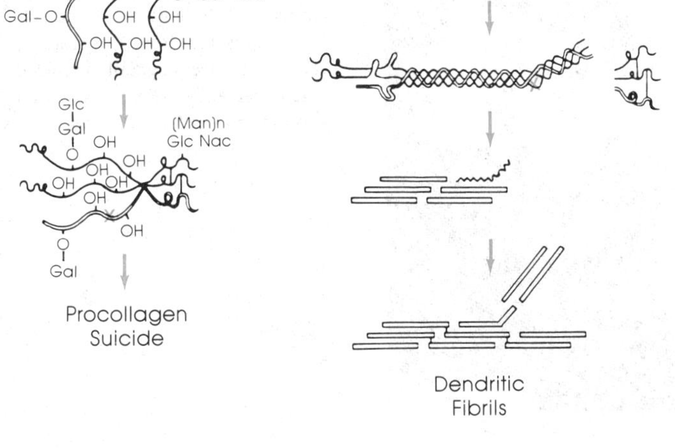

Type I procollagen genes harbor most of the mutations that cause OI for several reasons. One is that the collagen fibrils are a principal source of the structural strength of bone. Therefore, the whole structure is weakened by any mutation that drastically reduces the amount of collagen or distorts the normal geometry of collagen fibrils. A second reason derives from the extensive use of the principle of self-assembly in the synthesis of collagen fibrils. The advantage of the self-assembly principle is that highly ordered, large structures can be generated efficiently from small subunits with the correct properties. The disadvantage is that the presence of a few slightly flawed subunits can disrupt the process. In the assembly of procollagen, a flaw in one of 338 -Gly-X-Y- subunits in one proα chain can disrupt the triple-helix formed by all three proα chains and produce procollagen suicide. In the assembly of collagen into fibrils, the presence of a few incompletely processed or flawed collagen monomers can extensively distort the morphology of the fibrils formed. Hence, the two large genes for type I procollagen are highly vulnerable to disease-producing mutations in the sense that a mutation at any one of a large number of different sites can alter the assembly of collagen fibrils and produce an inherent weakness of bone and other connective tissues.

Over 30 mutations that cause synthesis of structurally abnormal type I procollagen and that produce OI have now been defined (Fig. 333-2). Similar mutations in the gene for type III procollagen are found in patients with the type IV variant of EDS, the most severe form of the disease that causes early death because of rupture of the aorta or other hollow organs. Data on one family indicate that some variants of the MS can also be produced by mutations in the type III procollagen gene that cause synthesis of structurally abnormal proα(III) chains. To date, the same mutation in a type I or type III procollagen gene has not been found in two unrelated people with OI, EDS, or MS. Similar mutations in the same genes and proteins can produce different disease syndromes, apparently because some features of the proteins are more important for the normal function of some connective tissues than others. There may, however, be more complex explanations for the marked differences among patients. Affected members of the same family tend to have the same manifestations and clinical course, but heterogeneity can be seen even within the same family. Because of the large size of the genes (20 to 40 kb), defining the mutation in a new patient or proband is a time-consuming process that can only be carried out in a research laboratory. Once the mutation in a family is found, however, it is relatively simple to use the polymerase chain reaction and appropriate primers together with allele-specific oligonucleotides to test other members of the same family.

Two forms of EDS are caused by mutations that are not in the structural genes for procollagen but instead are in the genes for two of the procollagen processing enzymes. Some variants of the ocular form of EDS (type VI) are caused by a deficiency of lysylhydroxylase, the enzyme that synthesizes the hydroxylysine in collagen. Some variants of type VII EDS are caused by deficiencies of procollagen *N*-proteinase. Such enzyme deficiencies appear to be rare causes of connective tissue diseases because, as with most enzyme deficiencies, a homozygous state in which the patient inherited two defective genes is necessary to reduce enzymic activity sufficiently to cause symptoms. To date, no mutations in genes for structural proteins other than collagens have been found to cause OI, EDS, or MS. This may in part be because detecting mutations in the genes is still technically difficult and in part because mutations in these genes may be so deleterious that they cause death at early stages of intrauterine development. Alternatively, mutations in the genes may be of less consequence than mutations in procollagen genes because less of the structure of the macromolecules they code for is essential for normal biologic function.

OSTEOGENESIS IMPERFECTA

General features The term osteogenesis imperfecta (OI) is used for heritable defects that make bones brittle. The increased fragility of bone is frequently associated with blue sclerae, characteristic dental abnormalities (dentinogenesis imperfecta), progressive hearing loss, and a family history of the disease. The most severe forms of OI produce death in utero, at birth, or shortly thereafter. The clinical course of more moderate forms is variable. Some patients have fractures at birth and then improve so that they have little incapacity in childhood or adulthood. Some appear normal at birth (see Fig. 333-4) and then become progressively worse. Some patients suffer from multiple fractures in childhood, improve after puberty, and begin to fracture more frequently later in life with a marked increase in women during pregnancy and after menopause. Some individuals from families with OI do not develop fracture until after menopause and their disease is difficult to distinguish from postmenopausal osteoporosis. Also, some individuals with osteoporosis are heterozygous carriers for gene defects that produce OI in homozygotes. Therefore, some forms of postmenopausal osteoporosis are in the same spectrum of diseases as OI.

Classification into types OI was initially classified as being either OI congenita or OI tarda, depending on whether fractures were present at birth or developed later. Currently, the most commonly used classification scheme for OI is the one developed by Sillence (Table 333-2). In the Sillence classification, type I is the mildest form of the disease and clearly shows a dominant pattern of inheritance in families. It is subdivided into types IA and IB depending on whether or not dentinogenesis imperfecta is also present. Type II is the lethal form with death in utero or shortly after birth. It has been suggested that radiograpic differences among patients can be used to subdivide type II OI into five groups, with group I showing the most severe changes and group V the least. Type III and type IV are intermediate in severity between types I and II. Type III is distinguished from type IV primarily on the basis that type III tends to become progressively severe with age. Also, type III is recessively inherited whereas type IV is dominantly inherited. The mode of inheritance, however, is frequently difficult to establish because many patients have sporadic mutations and, therefore, are the first affected member of the family. Also, many couples with one OI child elect not to have additional children, and most patients with type III or type IV OI do not have children.

Incidence Type I OI has both a birth incidence of 1:30,000 and a population frequency of 1:30,000. Type II OI has a birth incidence of about 1:60,000. Type III and type IV OI are less common.

Skeletal changes In type I OI the fragility of bones may be severe enough to limit physical activity or so mild that individuals are unaware of any debility. Radiographs of the skull of some patients with relatively mild syndromes show a mottled or wormian appearance, apparently because of small islands of irregular ossification. In type II OI, bones and other connective tissues are extremely fragile so that massive injuries can occur in utero or during delivery. Ossification of many bones is frequently incomplete. Continuously beaded ribs and crumpled long bones (accordian femora) are frequently seen radiographically. For reasons that are not apparent, the long bones may be either unusually thick or thin. In types III and IV, multiple fractures from minor physical stress can cause stunting of growth and skeletal abnormalities. Severe kyphoscoliosis may cause respiratory impairment and predispose to pulmonary infections. The appearance on radiographs of "popcorn-like" deposits of mineral on the ends of long bones is usually an ominous sign.

In all forms of OI, bone mineral density in unfractured bone is decreased compared to age-matched controls. However, the degree of intrinsic osteopenia is frequently difficult to evaluate, because recurrent fractures limit exercise and thereby exacerbate the decrease in bone mass. The healing of fractures appears to be as normal.

Ocular changes The sclerae can vary in color from normal to a slightly bluish or slate color to a bright blue. The blueness is probably

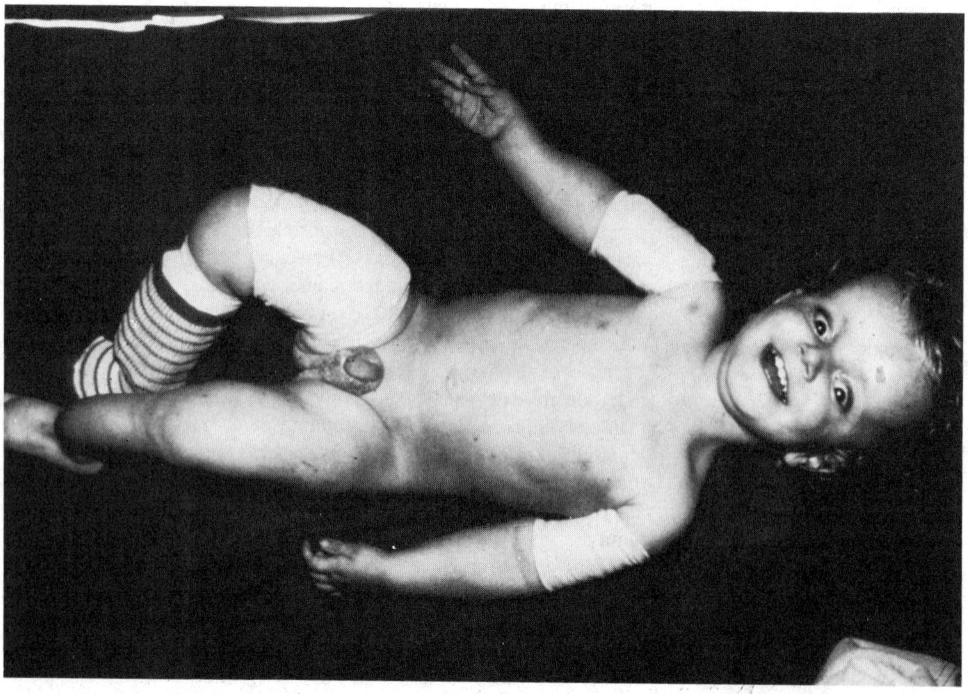

FIGURE 333-4 A 21-month-old boy with type III OI. Child was essentially normal at birth but then developed multiple fractures of arms and legs. He is homozygous for a four-base-pair deletion in the genes for proα2(I) chains that changes the sequence of the last 33 amino acids in these proteins. Therefore, the proα2(I) chains do not associate with proα1(I) chains, and the only type I procollagens formed are trimers of proα1(I) chains that have a partially unfolded *C*-terminal region. (*Reproduced with permission from Nicholls et al.*)

TABLE 333-2 Classification of osteogenesis imperfecta (OI) based on clinical manifestations and mode of inheritance as proposed by Sillence

Type	Bone fragility	Blue sclerae	Abnormal dentition	Hearing loss	Inheritance*
I	Mild	Present	Absent in IA, present in IB	Present in most	AD
II	Extreme	Present	Present in some	Unknown	AR or S
III	Severe	Bluish at birth	Present in some	High incidence	AR
IV	Variable	Absent	Absent in IVA, present in IVB	High incidence	AD

* AD, autosomal dominant; AR, autosomal recessive; S, sporadic.

caused by a thinness of the collagen layers of the sclerae that allows the choroid layers to be seen. Blue sclerae is an inherited trait in some families without evidence of increased bone fragility.

Dentinogenesis imperfecta The enamel of teeth is relatively normal, but the teeth frequently have a characteristic amber, yellowish-brown or translucent bluish-gray color because of improper deposition or deficiency of dentin. The deciduous teeth are usually smaller than normal, whereas permanent teeth are frequently bell-shaped and restricted at the base. The defect in dentin is directly attributable to the fact that the tissue is normally rich in type I collagen fibers. Some families show indistinguishable inherited teeth defects without any evidence of OI.

Hearing loss Deafness usually begins during the second decade of life, and hearing loss can be detected in 90 percent of patients over 30 years of age. The loss is primarily sensorineural, but the middle ear may also be involved. The histologic features include deficient ossification, persistence of cartilage in areas that are normally ossified, and abnormal calcium deposits.

Associated features Many patients and families show involvement of other connective tissues. Some patients have very thin skin and scar easily. Others have joint changes indistinguishable from those of EDS (see below). A few patients have cardiovascular manifestations such as aortic regurgitation, floppy mitral valves, mitral incompetence, and fragility of large blood vessels. For unknown reasons, some patients develop a hypermetabolic state with elevated serum thyroxine levels, hyperthermia, and excessive sweating.

Molecular defects Most patients with OI have mutations in one of the two genes for type I procollagen. In more severe forms of OI (types II, III, and IV), most of the mutations are dominant and cause synthesis of structurally abnormal proα chains whose effects are amplified by the three molecular mechanisms discussed above. The mutations that change the structure of the protein near the *N*-proteinase cleavage site tend to produce the extremely lax joints characteristic of type VII EDS rather than OI. Mutations that change the structure near the middle of the molecule or near the *C*-terminus tend to produce severe or lethal variants of OI. It has been difficult, however, to establish more extensive correlations between the site and nature of the mutation and the clinical phenotype. Also, a few patients with the mildest form of the disease (type I) have unidentified defects that decrease the rate of synthesis of proα1(I) chains. One patient was shown homozygous for a mutated allele for proα2(I) chains, and another patient was a compound heterozygote with independent mutations in two alleles for proα2(I) chains (Fig. 333-3). Such homozygous or compound heterozygous defects, however, tend to be rare. Data from one family suggest that heterozygous carriers for homozygous defects may be prone to osteopenia and perhaps osteoporosis.

Mosaicism in germline cells and in somatic cells The lethal variants of OI are, by definition, sporadic or new mutations. The frequency of a second child with lethal OI in the same family, however, is higher than the expected incidence of new mutations. Therefore, some parents of a child with type II OI apparently have mosaicism in their germline cells. Hence, they should be counseled that the chance of a recurrence is not negligible.

One asymptomatic woman was found to have mosaicism in her somatic cells for a mutation in a type I procollagen gene that produced lethal OI in one of her children. The woman subsequently had two normal children and had no evidence of any bone abnormalities at the age of 35. However, she was short compared to other members of her family, and she had temporal bossing and the triangular facies characteristic of many patients with OI. Such findings are frequently present in parents of children with OI and, therefore, somatic cell mosaicism may be more frequent than previously supposed.

Diagnosis The diagnosis is usually made on the basis of clinical criteria alone. The presence of fractures together with either blue sclerae, dentinogenesis imperfecta, or family history of the disease is usually sufficient to make the diagnosis. However, it is important to rule out other possible causes of fractures such as battered child syndrome, nutritional deficiencies, malignancies, and other heritable disorders including skeletal dysplasias and hypophosphatasia (Table 333-3). There is no consensus as to whether or not characteristic morphologic changes can be detected by electron microscopy of bone specimens. Procedures currently available in research laboratories can identify abnormal proα chains of type I procollagen by polyacrylamide gel electrophoresis of the protein synthesized by cultured fibroblasts in one-third or more of patients. Also, research procedures are available to identify mutations by analysis of mRNA or genomic DNA for type I procollagen; improvements in DNA technologies may make them generally available in the future. After a mutation in a type I procollagen gene has been definitively identified in a patient, a simple test based on polymerase chain reaction can be used to screen members of the same family and for prenatal diagnosis.

Treatment No convincing data have been presented that OI can be effectively treated. Many patients appear to be unusually intelligent and have successful careers in spite of severe deformities. Patients with mild forms may need little treatment after fractures decrease at the age of 15 to 20 years, but women may need special attention during pregnancy or after menopause when fractures again increase. More severely affected children require a comprehensive program of physical therapy, surgical management of fractures and skeletal deformities, and vocational education; emotional support for patients and parents is also necessary. Many of the fractures are only slightly displaced and have little soft tissue swelling. Therefore, they can be

TABLE 333-3 Partial differential diagnosis of OI

Age	Diagnosis	Distinguishing features
At birth	Hypophosphatasia	Unmineralized skull
	Achondrogenesis	Unmineralized vertebrae
	Thanatophoric dwarfism	H-shaped vertebrae
	Asphyxiating thoracic dystrophy	Cylindrical thorax
	Achondroplasia	Large head, short, tubular bones
Infancy	Battered child syndrome	Skull and rib fractures more common
	Immobilization osteogenesis	
	Scurvy	
	Congenital syphilis	
Childhood	Homocystinuria	Marfanoid appearance and mental deficiency
	Celiac disease	Steatorrhea, anemia
	Adrenal cortical tumor	
	Glucocorticoid therapy	

SOURCE: Modified from Smith et al., p. 126

treated with minimal support or traction for a week or two followed by a light cast. If fractures are relatively painless, physical therapy can be initiated early. A judicious amount of exercise is obviously important to prevent loss of bone mass secondary to physical inactivity. Some physicians advocate insertion of steel rods into long bones to correct limb deformities. The major rationale for the procedure is that correcting the deformities during childhood may make it possible to keep patients ambulatory. However, the risk-benefits and cost-benefits of the procedures are difficult to evaluate. A program for careful orthotic management developed by Bleck is a useful guide for the management of many patients.

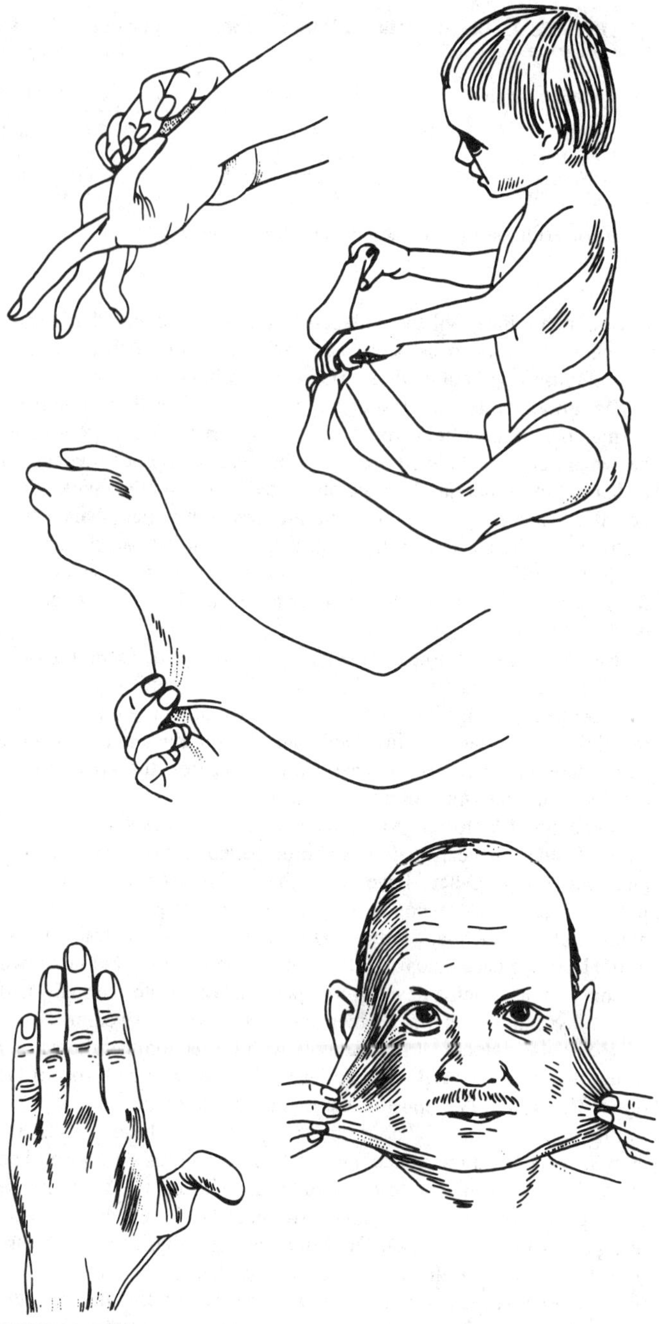

FIGURE 333-5 Schematic of the skin and joint changes in EDS. Girl in upper right has type VIIB EDS with dislocations of both hips that were not corrected by surgery. (*Reproduced with permission from Prockop and Guzman, Hosp Prac, 12(12):61, 1977.*)

EHLERS-DANLOS SYNDROME

General features The Ehlers-Danlos syndrome (EDS) describes a group of heritable disorders characterized by hypermobile joints and abnormalities of skin (Fig. 333-5). Beighton initially identified five types of EDS (Table 333-4). Type I is the classical, severe form of the disease with both joint hypermobility and characteristically velvety and hyperextensible skin. Type II is similar to type I but milder. In type III joint hypermobility is more prominent than the skin changes. Type IV is characterized by a striking thinness of skin and a predisposition to sudden death from rupture of large blood vessels or the large bowel. Type V is similar to type II but characterized by X-linked inheritance.

Types VI, VII, and IX were defined because of the presence of biochemical defects and phenotypes that did not fit into the types defined by Beighton. However, not all patients with these phenotypes have the molecular defect initially used to establish the classification. Type VIII was identified by the presence of generalized periodontitis together with moderate joint and skin changes. Because of overlapping signs and symptoms many patients and families cannot be assigned to any of the nine defined types of EDS.

Ligaments and joint changes Laxity and hypermobility of joints can vary from mild changes to changes severe enough to produce unreducible dislocations of hips and other joints. In milder forms, patients learn to reduce dislocations themselves or to avoid them by limiting physical activity. In more severe forms, surgical repair is required. Some patients have progressive difficulty with increasing age, but severe joint laxity can be compatible with a normal life span.

Skin The skin changes vary from a slight thinness and soft or velvety appearance to marked hyperextensibility or skin that is easily torn. Patients with several types of EDS also have easy bruisability. In patients with type IV EDS marked thinness of skin makes the subcutaneous blood vessels unusually prominent. Patients with type I EDS may have characteristic "cigarette-paper" scars of the skin from minor trauma. Similar but milder evidence of abnormal repair occurs in other forms, particularly type V. In type VIII, the skin is more fragile than hyperextensible, and it heals with atrophic, pigmented scars.

Associated changes Changes in connective tissues other than joints and skin include mitral valve prolapse, particularly in type I EDS. Pes planus and mild to moderate scoliosis are common. Extreme joint laxity and repeated dislocations may lead to early osteoarthritis. Hernias are frequent in those with types I and IX. Patients with type IV may have spontaneous rupture of the aorta or intestine. In type VI rupture of the eye with minimal trauma frequently occurs, and kyphoscoliosis can produce respiratory impairment. Also, sclerae are frequently blue in type VI. In type IX changes in joints and skin are minimal. This type is primarily defined by the presence of abnormalities in copper metabolism and includes diseases previously classified as X-linked cutis laxa, X-linked EDS, and Menkes's syndrome. Patients frequently have bladder diverticuli that can rupture, hernias, skeletal abnormalities that include characteristic occipital horns, and laxity of skin. In the variants formerly defined as cutis laxa, skin laxity is the most prominent finding and results in an appearance of premature senescence. These patients frequently develop pulmonary emphysema and pulmonary stenosis.

Molecular defects The molecular defects in the type I, type II, and type III variants of EDS are unknown. Electron microscopy of the skin from some patients has shown an unusual morphology of collagen fibers, but similar types of collagen fibrils are occasionally seen in normal skin.

Most patients with the type IV variant have a defect either in the synthesis or structure of type III procollagen. A defect in type III procollagen is consistent with the fact that these patients are prone to spontaneous rupture of the aorta and intestines, tissues that are rich in type III collagen. The mutations identified in the type III procollagen gene include partial gene deletions, RNA splicing mutations, and single-base mutations that convert codons for glycine to codons for amino acids with bulkier side chains. Therefore, most of

TABLE 333-4 Classification of EDS based on clinical manifestations and mode of inheritance

Type*	Joint hypermobility	Skin extensibility	Fragility	Bruisability	Other manifestations	Inheritance†
I	Marked	Marked	Marked	Marked	Skin characteristically soft, velvety; cigarette-paper scars; hernias; varicose veins; premature birth because rupture of fetal membranes	AD
II	Moderate	Moderate	Absent	Moderate	Milder than type I	AD
III	Marked	Minimal	Minimal	Minimal	Joint dislocations with minimal changes in skin	AD
IV	Small joints only	Minimal	Marked	Marked	Rupture of large arteries and bowel; thin skin with prominent venous network; characteristic facies in some	AD or AR
V	Moderate	Moderate	Absent	Moderate	Similar to type II	XL
VI	Minimal	Moderate	Moderate	Moderate	Similar to type II; intramuscular hemorrhage or keratoconus in some	XL
VII	Marked	Moderate	Moderate	Moderate	Multiple dislocations	AR or AD
VIII	Moderate	Moderate	Marked	Moderate	Advanced periodontitis; atrophic pigmented scars of skin	AD
IX	Mild	Mild	Absent	Absent	Bladder diverticuli with spontaneous rupture; hernias; skeletal abnormalities; skin laxity	XL

* Alternative designations; type I, gravis; type II, mitis; type III, benign familial hypermobility; type IV, ecchymotic or aortic; type V, X-linked; type VI, ocular; type VII, arthrochalosis multiplex congenita; type VIII, periodontal form; type IX, EDS with abnormal copper metabolism, Menkes's steely-hair syndrome (some variants) and cutis laxa (some variants).

† AD, autosomal dominant; AR, autosomal recessive; XL, X-linked.

the mutations lead to synthesis of abnormal but partially functional proα1(III) chains that produce "procollagen suicide," interfere with the processing of the *N*-propeptide, or alter fibril formation by the same mechanisms that amplify the effects of mutations in the genes for type I procollagen.

Type VI EDS was first characterized in two sisters by the fact that their collagen contained a decreased amount of hydroxylysine secondary to a deficiency of lysyl hydroxylase; a similar enzyme deficiency has been detected in other patients. Some patients with the clinical features of type VI EDS, however, do not have deficiency of lysyl hydroxylase.

Type VII EDS was first identified as a defect in the conversion of procollagen to collagen in patients with joint hypermobility and joint dislocations. At the molecular level, two kinds of genetic changes produce this disease. One, defined as type VIIA, is a deficiency of procollagen *N*-proteinase, the enzyme that removes the *N*-terminal peptide from type I procollagen. This form is inherited as an autosomal recessive trait. The second form, defined as type VIIB, involves a series of different mutations that make the type I procollagen resistant to cleavage by *N*-proteinase. The change in amino acid sequences of the proα chains of type I procollagen can be located as much as 90 amino acids away from the site at which the enzyme cleaves the protein. In both type VIIA and type VIIB variants, the persistence of the *N*-propeptide on the molecule causes the formation of fibrils that are unusually thin. Apparently, such thin fibrils can provide a scaffolding for bone but do not provide the necessary tensile strength for ligaments and joint capsules.

A defect in copper metabolism is present in most patients studied with type IX EDS (see Chap. 77). Low levels of serum copper and serum ceruloplasmin are accompanied by marked elevation of copper within cells. The molecular defects in some patients appear to be linked to synthesis of a diffusable factor involved either in regulation of the metallothionein gene or in some other aspect of copper metabolism.

Diagnosis Diagnosis is still based primarily on clinical evaluation of patients. Biochemical assays for known defects in EDS are still difficult and time-consuming. In type IV variants, incubation of cultured skin fibroblasts with radioactive proline or glycine followed by gel electrophoresis of the newly synthesized proteins will usually demonstrate a defect in the synthesis or secretion of type III procollagen. A protocol for observing both the secretion and the rate of processing of type I procollagen in cultures of skin fibroblasts provides a simple method of identifying deficiencies of procollagen *N*-proteinase and structural mutations that prevent cleavage of the *N*-propeptide. It should therefore be useful in the diagnosis of both type VIIA and type VIIB EDS. However, some patients with OI are also positive by this assay. In patients suspected of having type IX EDS, the assignment to this general category can be confirmed by assays of copper and ceruloplasmin in serum and in fibroblast cultures. Specific DNA tests should be available in the future for families in which the exact mutations in type I and type III genes have been defined.

Treatment There are no specific treatments for the disease. Surgical repair and tightening of the joint ligament require careful evaluation of individual patients since the ligaments frequently will not hold sutures. The cardiovascular status should be evaluated in all patients, particularly those suspected of having type IV. Patients with bruisability should be evaluated for specific bleeding disorders, but such tests are usually negative.

THE MARFAN SYNDROME

Diagnosis The Marfan syndrome is defined on the basis of characteristic changes in three connective tissue systems: the skeleton, the eyes, and the cardiovascular system. The disease is inherited as an autosomal dominant trait, and 15 to 30 percent of cases may be due to new mutations. "Skipped generations" due to variable expressivity is relatively common. Also, the typical marfanoid habitus, lens dislocations, and cardiovascular abnormalities can each be inherited independently in some families. Therefore, the diagnosis is usually not made unless at least one member of a family has characteristic changes in at least two of the three connective tissue systems.

Skeletal changes Patients are unusually tall compared to other members of the same family and have unusually long limbs. The ratio of the upper segment (top of head to top of pubic ramus) to the lower segment (top of pubic ramus to floor) is usually 2 standard deviations below mean for age, race, and sex. The patients usually have long and slender fingers and toes (called arachnodactyly or dolichostenomelia), but these are difficult to evaluate objectively. Because of longitudinal overgrowth of the ribs, many patients have chest deformities, including depression (pectus excavatum), protrusion (pectus carinatum), or marked asymmetry. Scoliosis is usually present, often accompanied by kyphosis.

Patients fall into three categories in terms of joint mobility. Most have moderate hypermobility of most joints. Some have marked hypermobility similar to that in EDS, but a few have exceptionally tight joints with contractures of hands and fingers. The group with the latter disorder, which is known as contractural arachnodactyly, appears to be less prone to cardiovascular problems.

Cardiovascular changes Mitral valve prolapse and aortic dilatation are common. Dilatation of the aorta begins in the root and is usually progressive so that dissection and rupture are common. Echocardiography is particularly helpful in evaluation.

Ocular changes The characteristic finding is subluxation of the lens (ectopia lentis), usually in an upward direction. The lens dislocation, however, may be detectable only by slit lamp examination. Displacement of the lens into the anterior chamber may cause glaucoma, but glaucoma is more frequent after surgical removal of the lens. The axial length of the globe is greater than normal, predisposing to myopia and retinal detachment.

Associated changes Striae may occur over the shoulders and buttocks. Otherwise the skin is normal. A number of patients develop spontaneous pneumothorax. High-arched palate and high pedal arches are frequent.

Molecular defects In spite of intensive efforts by many investigators, the molecular defects in most variants of MS are still unknown. Family studies with restriction fragment length polymorphisms have tended to rule out mutations in the genes for type I and type III procollagen. However, a mutation in the gene for proα2(I) chain of type I procollagen was found in one patient with an atypical form of the disease. A single-base mutation that converted a codon for glycine to a codon for arginine in the type III procollagen gene was found in one family with a history of early deaths from ruptured aortic aneurysms, arachnodactyly, easy bruisability, and bleeding tendencies.

Diagnosis The diagnosis is easiest to establish if the patient or members of the family have objective evidence of subluxed lenses, aortic dilatation, and severe kyphoscoliosis or chest deformities. The diagnosis is frequently made if ectopia lentis and an aneurysm of the ascending aorta are present without evidence of a Marfan habitus or a positive family history. All patients in whom the diagnosis is suspected should have a slit lamp examination and an echocardiogram. Also, homocystinuria (Table 333-3) should be ruled out by a negative cyanide-nitroprusside test for disulfides in the urine. Patients with types I, II, and III EDS may have ectopia lentis but lack the Marfan habitus and have characteristic skin changes not present in the Marfan syndrome.

Treatment There is no established treatment. Several investigators have recommended use of propranolol to delay or prevent the severe aortic complications, but the therapy is unproven. Surgical replacement of the aorta, aortic valve, and mitral valve has been undertaken in a number of patients.

The scoliosis tends to be progressive and should be treated by mechanical bracing and physical therapy if greater than 20° or by surgery if it continues to progress and becomes greater than 45°. Estrogen to induce menarche has been tried in girls with progressive scoliosis, but the results are inconclusive. The subluxated lens rarely requires surgical removal, but patients should be followed closely for signs of retinal detachment.

Counseling is based on a 50 percent probability of passing on the defective gene. Because of the heterogeneity of the disease, offspring may be more or less severely affected than the parents. Women should be advised that the cardiovascular risk of pregnancy is high.

REFERENCES

BLECK EE: Non-operative treatment of osteogenesis imperfecta: Orthotic and mobility management. Clin Orthop 159:115, 1981

BYERS PH et al: Ehlers-Danlos syndrome, in *Principles and Practice of Medical Genetics*, vol 2, AEH Emery, DL Rimoin (eds). New York, Churchill Livingston, 1983, p 36

McKUSICK VA: *Heritable Disorders of Connective Tissue*, 4th ed. St. Louis, Mosby, 1972

NICHOLLS AC et al: The clinical features of homozygous α-2(I) collagen deficient osteogenesis imperfecta. J Med Genet 21:257, 1984

PROCKOP DJ, KIVIRIKKO KI: Heritable diseases of collagen. N Engl J Med 311:376, 1984

——— et al: Type I procollagen: The gene-protein system that harbors most of the mutations causing osteogenesis imperfecta and probably more common disorders of connective tissue. Am J Med Genet 34:60, 1989

PYERITZ RE: Marfan syndrome, in *Principles and Practice of Medical Genetics*, vol 2, AEH Emery, DL Rimoin (eds). New York, Churchill Livingston, 1983, p 57

SILLENCE DO: Osteogenesis imperfecta: An expanding panorama of variance. Clin Orthop 191:11, 1981

———: Disorders of bone density, volume and mineralization, in *Principles and Practice of Medical Genetics*, vol 2, AEH Emery, DL Rimoin (eds). New York, Churchill Livingston, 1983, p 736

SMITH R et al: *The Brittle Bone Syndrome: Osteogenesis Imperfecta*. London, Butterworths, 1983

UITTO J, BAUER AE: Diseases associated with collagen abnormalities, in *Collagen in Health and Disease*, JB Weiss, MID Jayson (eds). New York, Churchill Livingston, 1982, p 289

334 INHERITED DISORDERS OF AMINO ACID METABOLISM

LEON E. ROSENBERG

All polypeptides and proteins are polymers of 20 different amino acids. Eight of these, referred to as *essential*, cannot be synthesized by humans and must be obtained from dietary sources. The others are formed endogenously. Although most of the body's amino acids are "tied up" in proteins, small intracellular pools of *free* amino acids are in equilibrium with extracellular reservoirs in plasma, cerebrospinal fluid, and the lumina of the gut and kidney. Physiologically, amino acids are more than mere "building blocks." Some (glycine, γ-aminobutyric acid) are neurotransmitters. Others (phenylalanine, tyrosine, tryptophan, glycine) are precursors of hormones, coenzymes, pigments, purines, or pyrimidines. Each has a unique degradative pathway by which its nitrogen and carbon components are used for the synthesis of other amino acids, carbohydrates, and lipids.

Current concepts of inherited metabolic diseases are based to a considerable degree on investigations of amino acid disorders. More than 70 such disorders are now known, the catabolic defects (approximately 60) discussed in this and the following chapter far outnumbering the transport abnormalities (approximately 10) considered in Chap. 336. Each of these disorders is rare—the incidences range from 1 in 10,000 for cystinuria or phenylketonuria to 1 in 200,000 for homocystinuria or alkaptonuria. Collectively, however, they occur in perhaps 1 in 500 to 1 in 1000 live births.

The salient features of inherited disorders of amino acid catabolism are summarized in Table 334-1. In general, these disorders are named for the compound which accumulates to highest concentration in blood (*-emias*) or urine (*-urias*). For many conditions (often called aminoacidopathie), the parent amino acid is found in excess; for others, generally referred to as organic acidemias, products in the catabolic pathway accumulate. Which compound(s) accumulates depends, of course, on the site of the enzymatic block, the reversibility of the reactions proximal to the lesion, and the existence of alternate pathways of metabolic "run-off." For some amino acids, such as the sulfur-containing or branched-chain molecules, defects at nearly each step in the catabolic pathway have been described. For others numerous gaps in our knowledge of defective reactions remain. Biochemical and genetic heterogeneity are common among the aminoacidopathies and the organic acidemias. Five distinct forms of hyperphenylalaninemia, seven forms of homocystinuria, and seven types of methylmalonic acidemia are recognized. Such heterogeneity reflects the presence of many different molecular defects and is of clinical importance as well as scientific interest.

The manifestations of these conditions differ widely (Table 334-1). Some, such as sarcosinemia or hyperprolinemia, appear to produce no clinical consequences. At the other extreme, complete deficiency of ornithine transcarbamylase or of branched-chain keto acid dehydrogenase causes neonatal death in the untreated patient. Central nervous system dysfunction, in the form of developmental retardation, seizures, alterations in sensorium, or behavioral disturbances, occurs in more than half of the disorders. Protein-induced vomiting, neurologic dysfunction, and hyperammonemia occur in many disorders of urea cycle intermediates. Metabolic ketoacidosis often accompanied by hyperammonemia is a frequent presenting finding in the disorders of branched-chain amino acid metabolism. Occasional disorders produce focal tissue or organ involvement such as liver disease, renal failure, cutaneous abnormalities, or ocular lesions.

The clinical manifestations in many of these conditions can be prevented or mitigated if diagnosis is achieved early and appropriate treatment (i.e., dietary protein or amino acid restriction or vitamin supplementation) is instituted promptly. For this reason, a growing number of aminoacidopathies and organic acidemias are screened for in mass newborn surveys which analyze blood or urine with an array of chemical and microbiologic techniques. Once a presumptive diagnosis is made, confirmation can be provided by direct enzyme assay on extracts of leukocytes, erythrocytes, or cultured fibroblasts. DNA-based diagnostic capability is possible for several disorders. For example, substitutions, deletions, and insertions have been used to diagnose and characterize phenylketonuria, ornithine transcarbamylase deficiency, citrullinemia, gyrate atrophy of the retina, propionic acidemia, and methylmalonic acidemia (see also Chap. 6). As additional genes are cloned, DNA-based analysis will become more common.

Several of these disorders (including branched chain ketoaciduria, isovaleric acidemia, propionic acidemia, methylmalonic acidemia, homocystinuria, cystinosis, phenylketonuria, ornithine transcarbamylase deficiency, citrullinemia, argininosuccinic aciduria) can be diagnosed prenatally by chemical analysis of amniotic fluid or by chemical, enzymatic, or DNA-based studies of fresh or cultured amniotic fluid cells. In addition to permitting selective termination of at-risk pregnancies, such diagnosis has led to improved postnatal treatment.

The remainder of this and the subsequent chapter focus on selected disorders that illustrate the principles, properties, and problems presented by the disorders of amino acid metabolism.

THE HYPERPHENYLALANINEMIAS

DEFINITION The hyperphenylalaninemias (Table 334-1), result from impaired conversion of phenylalanine to tyrosine. The most common and clinically important is phenylketonuria, which is characterized by an increased concentration of phenylalanine in blood, increased concentrations of phenylalanine and its by-products (notably phenylpyruvate, phenylacetate, phenyllactate, and phenylacetylglutamine) in urine, and severe mental retardation.

ETIOLOGY AND PATHOGENESIS Each of the hyperphenylalaninemias results from reduced activity of the enzyme complex called *phenylalanine hydroxylase*. In humans this complete enzyme system is expressed only in liver. Phenylalanine and molecular oxygen are substrates for the enzyme which requires a reduced pteridine, tetrahydrobiopterin, as a cofactor (Fig. 334-1). Tyrosine and dihydrobiopterin are the products of this catalytic system, the latter being reconverted to tetrahydrobiopterin by a second enzyme, dihydropteridine reductase. In classic phenylketonuria, activity of the hydroxylase apoenzyme, whose gene locus has been mapped to the q22–q24.1 region of chromosome 12, is almost totally deficient. Six different mutations leading to such complete deficiency are recognized. These include missense changes, splicing defects, and partial deletions. Benign hyperphenylalaninemia results from a less complete deficiency, whereas transient hyperphenylalaninemia (sometimes called transient phenylketonuria) is caused by a delayed maturation of the hydroxylase apoenzyme. In "malignant" hyperphenylalaninemia, however, persistently impaired hydroxylating activity results not from abnormality in the apohydroxylase but from a lack of tetrahydrobiopterin. The tetrahydrobiopterin deficiency has three metabolic causes: two distinct blocks in the pathway by which tetrahydrobiopterin is synthesized from GTP, or deficiency of dihydropteridine reductase, the enzyme that regenerates tetrahydrobiopterin from dihydrobiopterin (see Fig. 334-1). This reductase system is also needed by tyrosine hydroxylase and tryptophan hydroxylase.

As a group the hyperphenylalaninemias occur in about 1 in 10,000 births. Classic phenylketonuria, which accounts for nearly two-thirds of these, is an autosomal recessive trait and is widely distributed among whites and Orientals. It is rare in blacks. Phenylalanine hydroxylase activity in obligate heterozygotes is less than normal but distinctly higher than in affected homozygotes. Heterozygous carriers are clinically well but may have slightly increased phenylalanine concentrations in plasma. The other hyperphenylalaninemias are also inherited as autosomal recessive traits.

Phenylalanine accumulation in blood and urine and reduced tyrosine formation are direct consequences of the impaired hydroxylation. In untreated phenylketonuria and in its tetrahydrobiopterin-deficient variants, plasma concentrations of phenylalanine become sufficiently high [greater than 1200 μmol/L (20 mg/dL)] to activate alternate pathways of metabolism and lead to formation of phenylpyruvate, phenylacetate, phenyllactate, and other derivatives that are rapidly cleared by the kidney and excreted in urine. Plasma concentrations of several other amino acids are moderately reduced, probably secondary to inhibition of gastrointestinal absorption or impairment of renal tubular reabsorption by the excess phenylalanine in body fluids. The severe brain damage appears to be related to several consequences of phenylalanine accumulation: competitive inhibition of transport of other amino acids required for protein synthesis, impaired polyribosome formation or stabilization, reduced myelin synthesis, and inadequate formation of norepinephrine and serotonin. Phenylalanine is a competitive inhibitor of tyrosinase, a key enzyme in the pathway of melanin synthesis. This block plus reduced availability of the melanin precursor, tyrosine, accounts for the hypopigmentation of hair and skin.

CLINICAL MANIFESTATIONS No abnormalities are apparent at birth. Untreated children with classic phenylketonuria fail to attain early developmental milestones and demonstrate progressive impairment of cerebral function. Most require chronic institutionalization within a few years of birth because of the hyperactivity and seizures that accompany the severe mental retardation. Electroencephalographic abnormalities, "mousy" odor of skin, hair, and urine (due to phenylacetate accumulation), and a tendency to hypopigmentation and eczema complete the devastating clinical picture. In contrast, affected children who are detected at birth and treated promptly show none of these abnormalities. Children with transient hyperphenylalaninemia or with the benign variant are not at risk for any of the clinical consequences seen in untreated classic phenylketonuria. Those children with tetrahydrobiopterin deficiency, however, are the most unfortunate. Seizures appear early, followed by progressive cerebral

TABLE 334-1 Inherited disorders of amino acid catabolism

Amino acid(s) affected	Disorder or condition	Enzyme defect	Clinical manifestations*: Mental retardation	Neuropsychiatric dysfunction	Protein intolerance	Metabolic ketoacidosis
AROMATIC—HETEROCYCLIC						
Phenylalanine	Classic phenylketonuria	Phenylalanine hydroxylase	+	+	–	–
	Benign hyperphenylalaninemia	Phenylalanine hydroxylase	–	–	–	–
	Transient hyperphenylalaninemia	Phenylalanine hydroxylase	–	–	–	–
	Malignant hyperphenylalaninemia	Dihydropteridine reductase	+	+	–	–
	Malignant hyperphenylalaninemia	GTP cyclohydrolase	+	+	–	–
	Malignant hyperphenylalaninemia	6-Pyruvoyltetrahydrobiopterin synthase	+	+	–	–
Tyrosine	Hypertyrosinemia	Tyrosine aminotransferase (cytosol)	+	–	–	–
	Tyrosinosis	Tyrosine aminotransferase (?)	–	–	–	–
	Hereditary tyrosinemia	Fumarylacetoacetate hydrolase	–	–		–
	Alkaptonuria	Homogentisic acid oxidase	–	–	–	–
	Albinism (oculocutaneous)	Tyrosinase	–	–	–	–
	Albinism (ocular)	Unknown	–	–	–	–
Tryptophan	Tryptophanuria	Unknown	+	+	–	–
	Xanthurenic aciduria	Kynureninase	?	–	–	–
Histidine	Histidinemia	Histidine-ammonia lyase	±	±	–	–
	Urocanic aciduria	Urocanase	+	+	–	–
	Formiminoglutamic aciduria	Formiminotransferase	?	+	–	–
GLYCINE-IMINO ACIDS						
Glycine	Hyperglycinemia	Glycine cleavage	+	+	–	–
	Sarcosinemia	Sarcosine dehydrogenase	–	–	–	–
	Hyperoxaluria (type I)	Alanine: glyoxylate aminotransferase	–	–	–	–
	Hyperoxaluria (type II)	D-Glyceric acid dehydrogenase	–	–	–	–
Imino acids	Hyperprolinemia (type I)	Proline oxidase	–	–	–	–
	Hyperprolinemia (type II)	Δ'-Pyrroline dehydrogenase	–	–	–	–
	Hyperhydroxyprolinemia	Hydroxyproline reductase	–	–	–	–
	Iminopeptiduria	Prolidase	+	–	–	–
SULFUR-CONTAINING						
Methionine	Hypermethioninemia	Methionine adenosyltransferase	–	–	–	–
Homocystine	Homocystinuria	Cystathionine β-synthase	±	±	–	–
	Homocystinuria	5,10-Methylenetetrahydrofolate reductase	±	±	–	–
	Homocystinuria and methylmalonic acidemia (cbl C, D)‡	Cobalamin (vitamin B_{12}) reductase (cytosol) (?)	±	±	–	–
	Homocystinuria and methylmalonic acidemia (cblF)	Lysosomal efflux	+	+	–	–
	Homocystinuria (cblE, G)	Methyltransferase-associated cobalamin reductase (?)	+	+	–	–
Cystathionine	Cystathioninuria	Cystathionase	±	–	–	–
Cystine	Cystinosis	Lysosomal efflux	–	–	–	–
S-Sulfo-L-cysteine	S-Sulfo-L-cysteine, sulfite, and thiosulfaturia	Sulfite oxidase	+	+	–	–
CATIONIC						
Lysine	Hyperlysinemia (type I)	Lysine dehydrogenase	–	+	+	–
	Hyperlysinemia (type II)	Lysine: α-ketoglutarate reductase	±	±	–	–
	Saccharopinuria	Saccharopine dehydrogenase	–	–	–	–
	Hydroxylysinemia	Unknown	+	–	–	–
	Pipecolic acidemia	Unknown	+	+	–	–
	α-Ketoadipic aciduria	α-Ketoadipic acid decarboxylase	±	±	–	–
	Glutaric aciduria (type I)	Glutaryl CoA dehydrogenase	–	+	–	–
	Glutaric aciduria (type II)	Medium-chain acyl CoA dehydrogenase (?)	–	+	–	–

* +, Regularly present; ±, sometimes present; –, absent; ?, uncertain; all designations refer to manifestations in untreated disorder.
† AR, autosomal recessive; XL, X-linked; (AR), probably autosomal recessive.
‡ Designations in parentheses refer to complementation groups assigned by genetic analysis with cultured cells.

Ammonia intoxication	Other	Inheritance pattern†
–	Hypopigmented skin and hair, eczema	AR
–		AR
–		(AR)
–		(AR)
–		(AR)
–		AR
–	Palmar keratosis, corneal dystrophy	(AR)
–	Myasthenia gravis	?
–	Cirrhosis, hepatic failure, renal tubular dysfunction	AR
–	Ochronosis, arthritis	AR
–	Hypopigmentation of hair, skin, and optic fundus	AR
–	Hypopigmentation of optic fundus	XL
–	Photosensitive skin rash	AR
–		?
–	Hearing and speech deficit	AR
–		?
–		(AR)
–		AR
–		AR
–	Renal failure	AR
–	Calcium oxalate nephrolithiasis, renal failure	AR
–		AR
–		AR
–		AR
–	Crusting erythematous, ecchymotic dermatitis	AR
–		?
–	Dislocated lenses, osteoporosis, thrombotic vascular disease	AR
–		(AR)
–	Megaloblastic anemia	(AR)
–		(?)
–	Megaloblastic anemia	AR
–		AR
–	Fanconi syndrome, renal failure, photophobia	AR
–	Dislocated lenses	AR
+		?
–		AR
–		?
–		(AR)
–	Hepatomegaly, dysplastic optic disks	?
–		?
–		AR
–	Hypoglycemia	?

(Table continues next page)

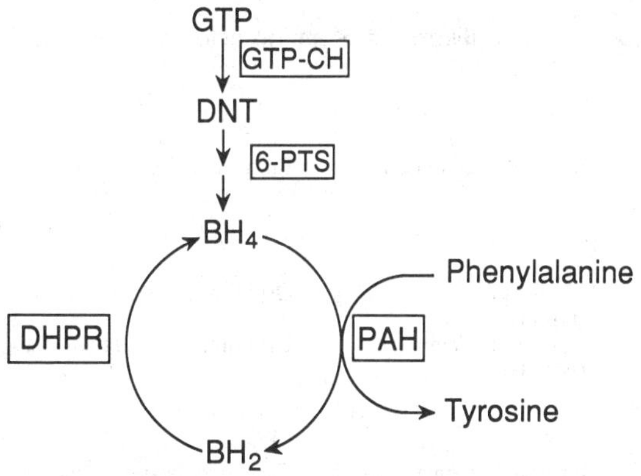

FIGURE 334-1 Pathways, enzymes, and coenzymes involved in the hyperphenylalaninemias. Blocked-in symbols highlight points of etiologic or therapeutic significance to the various genetic defects underlying these disorders. Abbreviations: GTP, guanosine triphosphate; GTP-CH, guanosine triphosphate cyclohydrolase; DNT, dihydroneopterin triphosphate; 6-PTS, 6-pyruvoyltetrahydropterin synthase; BH_4, tetrahydrobiopterin; BH_2, dihydrobiopterin; DHPR, dihydropteridine reductase; PAH, phenylalanine hydroxylase.

and basal ganglia dysfunction (rigidity, chorea, spasms, hypotonia). Most have succumbed to secondary infection within a few years despite early diagnosis and vigorous treatment.

A number of women with phenylketonuria who have been treated since infancy are now reaching adulthood and becoming pregnant. More than 90 percent of their offspring are markedly retarded, and many exhibit other congenital anomalies such as microcephaly, growth retardation, and congenital heart defects. Since these children are heterozygous, not homozygous for a phenylketonuria mutation, the clinical manifestations must be attributed to damage produced by the elevated maternal concentrations of phenylalanine to which they have been exposed in utero. This alarming syndrome is called maternal phenylketonuria.

DIAGNOSIS Plasma phenylalanine concentrations may be normal at birth in all the hyperphenylalaninemias but rise rapidly after institution of protein feedings and are usually abnormal by day 4. Since diagnosis and initiation of dietary treatment of classic phenylketonuria must be completed before the child is 30 days of age if developmental retardation is to be prevented, most newborns in North America and Europe are screened by determinations of blood phenylalanine concentration using the Guthrie bacterial inhibition assay. Infants with abnormal values are followed up with more quantitative fluorometric or chromatographic assays. In classic phenylketonuria and in tetrahydrobiopterin deficiency, values greater than 1200 μmol/L (20 mg/dL) are regularly observed. In transient or benign hyperphenylalaninemia concentrations are usually lower but above control values of less than 60 μmol/L (1 mg/dL). Distinction of classic phenylketonuria from its benign variants depends on following serial plasma phenylalanine concentrations as a function of age and dietary restriction. In transient hyperphenylalaninemia plasma values return to normal within 3 to 4 months. In benign hyperphenylalaninemia dietary restriction produces a more profound fall in plasma phenylalanine than that observed in classic phenylketonuria. Deficiency of tetrahydrobiopterin must be considered in any child with hyperphenylalaninemia who develops progressive neurologic impairment despite prompt diagnosis and dietary treatment. Diagnostic confirmation of these variants, which account for 1 to 5 percent of phenylketonuric children, can be achieved by enzyme assay on cultured fibroblasts. Of potentially greater therapeutic value, however, is the observation that administration of oral tetrahydrobiopterin loads can distinguish children with classic phenylketonuria (who show no chemical response) from those with tetrahydrobiopterin deficiency (who exhibit a sharp fall in plasma phenylalanine). Prenatal diagnosis of classic phenylketonuria is now feasible using DNA-based tests capable of detecting specific mutations or linked restriction fragment length

TABLE 334-1 Inherited disorders of amino acid catabolism *(continued)*

			Clinical manifestations*			
Amino acid(s) affected	Disorder or condition	Enzyme defect	Mental retardation	Neuropsychiatric dysfunction	Protein intolerance	Metabolic ketoacidosis
CATIONIC *()*						
Ornithine	Hyperornithinemia (type I)	Ornithine decarboxylase	+	+	+	−
	Hyperornithinemia (type II)	Ornithine aminotransferase	−	−	−	−
UREA CYCLE						
Carbamyl-phosphate	Hyperammonemia (type I)	Carbamylphosphate synthetase I	+	+	+	−
N-acetylglutamate	Hyperammonemia (type IA)	*N*-acetylglutamate synthetase	?	+	+	−
Ornithine	Hyperammonemia (type II)	Ornithine transcarbamylase	±	+	+	−
Citrulline	Citrullinemia	Argininosuccinate synthetase	+	+	+	−
Argininosuccinic acid	Argininosuccinic aciduria	Argininosuccinase	+	+	+	−
Arginine	Argininemia	Arginase	+	+	+	−
BRANCHED-CHAIN						
Valine	Hypervalinemia	Valine aminotransferase	+	+	+	−
Leucine, isoleucine	Hyperleucine-isoleucinemia	Leucine-isoleucine aminotransferase	+	+	+	−
Valine, leucine, isoleucine	Classic branched-chain ketoaciduria	Branched-chain ketoacid dehydrogenase	+	+	+	
	Intermittent branched-chain ketoaciduria	Branched-chain ketoacid dehydrogenase	±	−	+	+
Leucine	Isovaleric acidemia	Isovaleryl CoA dehydrogenase	±	±	+	+
	β-Methylcrotonyl glycinuria	β-Methylcrotonyl CoA carboxylase	+	+	−	+
	β-Hydroxy-β-methylglutaric aciduria	β-Hydroxy-β-methylglutaryl CoA lyase	−	+	+	+
Isoleucine, valine	α-Methylacetoacetic aciduria	β-Ketothiolase	±	±	+	+
	Propionic acidemia (pcc A, B, C)‡	Propionyl CoA carboxylase	±	±	+	+
	Propionic acidemia (bio)†	Holocarboxylase synthetase, biotinidase	+	±	+	+
	Methylmalonic acidemia (mut)‡	Methylmalonyl CoA mutase	±	±	+	+
	Methylmalonic acidemia (cbl A)‡	Cobalamin (vitamin B_{12}) reductase (mitochondrial) (?)	±	±	+	+
	Methylmalonic acidemia (cbl B)‡	Cobalamin (vitamin B_{12}): ATP adenosyltransferase	±	±	+	+
DICARBOXYLIC						
Glutamic acid	Glutathionemia	γ-Glutamyl-transpeptidase	+	−	−	−
5-Oxoprolinuria	Glutathione synthetase	±	±	±		

* +, Regularly present; ±, sometimes present; −, absent; ?, uncertain; all designations refer to manifestations in untreated disorder.
† AR, autosomal recessive; XL, X-linked; (AR), probably autosomal recessive.
‡ Designations in parentheses refer to complementation groups.

polymorphisms (RFLPs). Dihydropteridine reductase deficiency and the blocks in tetrahydrobiopterin synthesis can also be detected in utero using assays on cultured amniocytes.

TREATMENT Classic phenylketonuria is the first inherited metabolic disease in which it was demonstrated that mitigating the accumulation of the offending metabolite prevented the dire clinical consequences. This is accomplished by a special diet in which the bulk of protein is replaced by an artificial amino acid mixture low in phenylalanine. By supplementing this formula with a small amount of natural foods, an amount of dietary phenylalanine is provided that is sufficient for normal growth but is insufficient to produce markedly increased quantities of phenylalanine in blood. Ordinarily, plasma phenylalanine concentrations are maintained between 180 and 700 μmol/L (3 and 12 mg/dL).

To be maximally effective, such diet therapy must be instituted during the first month of life. Even then, modest nervous system dysfunction is often seen. Because uncontrolled hyperphenylalaninemia results in brain damage throughout childhood (and perhaps in adults), dietary restriction in classic phenylketonuria should be continued indefinitely. The transient and benign forms of hyperphenylalaninemia do not require long-term dietary restriction. As mentioned earlier, children with tetrahydrobiopterin deficiency deteriorate despite dietary phenylalanine restriction; efficacy of pteridine cofactor replacement is under study. Such patients may be helped, however, by a regimen in which dietary phenylalanine restriction is combined with supplements of levodopa and 5-hydroxytryptophan. Finally, the deleterious consequences of maternal phenylketonuria can be minimized by instituting dietary phenylalanine restriction prior to con-

Ammonia intoxication	Other	Inheritance pattern†
+		(AR)
−	Gyrate atrophy of choroid and retina	AR
+		AR
+		XL
+		AR
+		AR
+		AR
+		
−		?
−		?
−	"Maple syrup" odor	AR
−		AR
±	"Sweaty feet" odor	AR
−	"Cat's urine" odor	AR
−		?
+		AR
+		AR
−		?
+		AR
+		AR
+		AR
−		?
−		AR

ception and continuing such treatment throughout gestation. This means that women with phenylketonuria should stay on a phenylalanine-restricted diet from birth through the child-bearing years.

THE HOMOCYSTINURIAS

The homocystinurias are seven biochemically and clinically distinct disorders (Table 334-1), each characterized by increased concentration of the sulfur-containing amino acid, homocystine, in blood and urine. The most common form results from reduced activity of cystathionine β-synthase, an enzyme in the transsulfuration pathway by which methionine is converted to cysteine. All the other forms are the result of impaired conversion of homocysteine to methionine, a reaction catalyzed by homocysteine:methyltetrahydrofolate methyltransferase and two essential cofactors methyltetrahydrofolate and methylcobalamine (methyl–vitamin B_{12}). Depending on the underlying disorder, some patients with each of the homocystinurias show chemical and, in some instances, clinical improvement following administration of specific vitamin supplements (pyridoxine, folate, or cobalamin).

CYSTATHIONINE β-SYNTHASE DEFICIENCY **Definition** Deficiency of this enzyme leads to increased concentrations of methionine and homocystine in body fluids and to decreased concentrations of cysteine and cystine. The clinical hallmark is dislocated optic lenses. Mental retardation, osteoporosis, and thrombotic vascular disease are frequent.

Etiology and pathogenesis The sulfur atom of the essential amino acid methionine is transferred ultimately to cysteine by a series of reactions designated as the transsulfuration pathway (Fig. 334-2). In one of these steps, homocysteine condenses with serine to form cystathionine. This reaction is catalyzed by the pyridoxal phosphate–dependent enzyme, cystathionine β-synthase. The locus for this homodimeric enzyme has been mapped to the q21 region of chromosome 21. More than 600 patients have been described with deficiency of this enzyme. The condition is common in Ireland (1 in 40,000 births) but rare elsewhere (less than 1 in 200,000 births).

Homocysteine and methionine accumulate in cells and body fluids; cysteine synthesis is impaired, resulting in reduced concentrations of this amino acid and its disulfide form, cystine. In approximately half of patients synthase activity in liver, brain, leukocytes, and cultured fibroblasts is undetectable. In the remaining patients, tissues retain 1 to 5 percent of normal activity, and this residual activity can often be stimulated by pyridoxine supplementation. Heterozygous carriers of this autosomal recessive trait show no reproducible chemical abnormalities in body fluids but have reduced tissue synthase activity.

Homocysteine interferes with the normal cross-linking of collagen, an effect that likely plays an important role in the ocular, skeletal, and vascular complications. Altered collagen in the suspensory ligament of the optic lens and in bone matrix may account for the dislocated lenses and osteoporosis. Similarly, interference with normal ground substance metabolism in vascular walls may predispose to the arterial and venous thrombotic diathesis. Increased platelet adhesiveness may result from homocysteine accumulation, thereby contributing to the thrombotic occlusive disease so often observed. Recurrent cerebrovascular accidents secondary to thrombotic disease may account for the mental retardation, but direct chemical effects on cerebral cell metabolism have not been excluded.

Clinical manifestations More than 80 percent of homozygotes for complete synthase deficiency have dislocated optic lenses. This abnormality usually appears by 3 to 4 years of age and often results in acute glaucoma as well as impaired visual acuity. Mental retardation occurs in about half of such patients, often accompanied by ill-defined behavioral disturbances. Osteoporosis is a common radiologic finding (seen in two-thirds of patients by age 15) but rarely causes clinical disease. Life-threatening vascular complications, probably initiated by damage to vascular endothelium, are the major cause of morbidity and mortality. Occlusion of coronary, renal, and cerebral arteries with attendant tissue infarction can occur during the first decade of life. Nearly one-quarter of patients die of vascular disease before age 30. These vascular complications seem to be exacerbated by angiographic procedures. Importantly, pyridoxine-responsive patients have milder clinical manifestations in all regards. Heterozygous carriers for synthase deficiency (about 1 in 70 in the population) may be at increased risk for premature peripheral and cerebral occlusive vascular disease.

Diagnosis The cyanide-nitroprusside test is a simple way of demonstrating increased excretion of sulfhydryl-containing compounds in urine. Since cystine and *S*-sulfocysteine also give a positive test, other disorders of sulfur metabolism must be excluded, but this is usually possible on clinical grounds. Distinction of cystathionine β-synthase deficiency from other causes of homocystinuria can usually be accomplished by measurements of plasma methionine, which tend

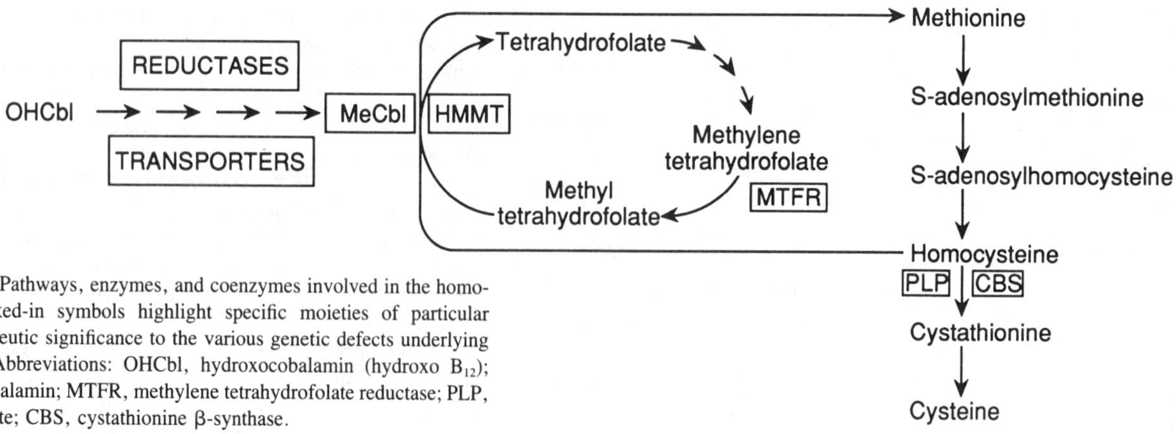

FIGURE 334-2 Pathways, enzymes, and coenzymes involved in the homocystinurias. Blocked-in symbols highlight specific moieties of particular etiologic or therapeutic significance to the various genetic defects underlying these disorders. Abbreviations: OHCbl, hydroxocobalamin (hydroxo B_{12}); MeCbl, methylcobalamin; MTFR, methylene tetrahydrofolate reductase; PLP, pyridoxal phosphate; CBS, cystathionine β-synthase.

to be increased in synthase-deficient patients and normal or low in those with impaired methionine formation (see below). Diagnostic confirmation depends on measurements of synthase activity in tissue extracts. Heterozygotes can be identified by measurement of peak serum homocystine after an oral methionine load and by measurement of tissue synthase activity.

Treatment As with classic phenylketonuria, effective treatment depends on early diagnosis. A number of infants diagnosed in the newborn period have been treated successfully with methionine-restricted, cystine-supplemented diets. Their clinical course has, thus far, been benign compared with that of untreated affected siblings. In approximately half of patients, oral supplements of pyridoxine (25 to 500 mg per day) produce a fall in plasma and urinary methionine and homocystine and an increase in cystine concentration in body fluids. This effect probably reflects a modest increase in synthase activity in cells of patients in whom the enzymatic defect is characterized by either reduced affinity for cofactor or accelerated degradation of mutant enzyme. Since such vitamin supplementation is simple and apparently harmless, it should be tried in all patients. There are no reports of the effect of pyridoxine supplementation therapy initiated soon after birth. Similarly, there are no data regarding pyridoxine supplements in heterozygous carriers.

5,10-METHYLENETETRAHYDROFOLATE REDUCTASE DEFICIENCY Definition In this form of homocystinuria, methionine concentrations in body fluids are normal or decreased because deficiency of 5,10-methylenetetrahydrofolate reductase leads to impaired synthesis of 5-methyltetrahydrofolate, a cofactor in the enzymatic formation of methionine from homocysteine (see Fig. 334-2). Central nervous system dysfunction occurs in most patients.

Etiology and pathogenesis 5-Methyltetrahydrofolate:homocysteine methyltransferase catalyzes the conversion of homocysteine to methionine. The methyl group transferred in this reaction comes from 5-methyltetrahydrofolate, which is converted to tetrahydrofolate in the process. 5-Methyltetrahydrofolate, in turn, is synthesized enzymatically from 5,10-methylenetetrahydrofolate by another enzyme, 5,10-methylenetetrahydrofolate reductase. Thus, reductase activity controls both methionine synthesis and tetrahydrofolate generation. This series of reactions is critical to normal DNA and RNA synthesis. A primary defect in the reductase activity results, secondarily, in deficient methyltransferase activity and impaired conversion of homocysteine to methionine. Methionine deficiency and impaired nucleic acid synthesis may contribute to the central nervous system dysfunction. The disorder appears to be inherited as an autosomal recessive trait.

Clinical manifestations More than 25 children with homocystinuria due to reductase deficiency have been reported. The most severely affected have presented with profound developmental retardation and cerebral atrophy early in life. Others manifested behavioral disturbances (catatonia) during the second decade or mild retardation. Presumably the severity of the clinical manifestations reflects the severity of the reductase deficiency.

Diagnosis and treatment The combination of increased concentrations of homocystine in body fluids with normal or decreased concentrations of methionine should suggest this entity. Serum folate concentrations are low in some patients. Confirmation requires direct reductase assays in tissue extracts (brain, liver, cultured fibroblasts). Although therapeutic experience is limited, one teenage girl with a catatonic psychosis responded dramatically, both chemically and clinically, to folate supplements (5 to 10 mg per day). When the folate was withdrawn, behavior worsened. This observation suggests that early diagnosis followed by folate supplementation may forestall neurologic or psychiatric disturbances.

DEFICIENCY OF COBALAMIN (VITAMIN B_{12}) COENZYME SYNTHESIS Definition Five other forms of homocystinuria also reflect impaired conversion of homocysteine to methionine. The primary defects in these entities, however, are in the synthesis of methylcobalamin, a cobalamin (vitamin B_{12}) coenzyme required by methyltetrahydrofolate:homocysteine methyltransferase (see Fig. 334-2). In some of these disorders methylmalonic acid accumulates in body fluids as well because synthesis of a second coenzyme, adenosylcobalamin, required for isomerization of methylmalonyl coenzyme A (CoA) to succinyl CoA is also impaired. These disorders are designated cblC, D, E, F, and G.

Etiology and pathogenesis As with 5,10-methylenetetrahydrofolate reductase deficiency, each disorder impairs remethylation of homocysteine. Since methylcobalamin is required for methyl-group transfer from methyltetrahydrofolate to homocysteine, impaired cobalamin metabolism leads to deficient methyltransferase activity. The defects responsible for impaired synthesis of methylcobalamin involve one of several steps in lysosomal or cytosolic activation of the vitamin precursor (see Fig. 334-2). In the cblF disorder, the transport of cobalamins out of lysosomes is impaired. In cblC and D, a reductase needed for formation of both methylcobalamin and adenosylcobalamin is deficient. In cblE and G, some component required to maintain a reduced form of cobalamin on the methyltransferase apoenzyme is impaired. Somatic cell genetic studies indicate that each of these abnormalities is distinct and imply that all are inherited as autosomal recessive traits.

Clinical manifestations The first reported patient with the cblC defect had profoundly arrested development and died of infection at age 6 weeks. More than 25 patients—mostly children—with these defects in cobalamin metabolism have been described subsequently. Although clinical manifestations vary considerably, neurologic and hematologic abnormalities include developmental delay, dementia, spasticity, megalobastic anemia, and pancytopenia. It is not possible to define a specific clinical syndrome for each of the five defects in cobalamin metabolism.

Diagnosis and treatment Homocystinuria, homocysteinemia, and hypomethioninemia are the chemical hallmarks. Methylmalonic acidemia, too, has been noted in those defects resulting from defective synthesis of both cobalamin coenzymes. These findings may also be present in juvenile- or adult-onset pernicious anemia in which intestinal cobalamin absorption is impaired. Measurement of serum cobalamin concentrations, low in pernicious anemia and normal in patients with defective conversion of cobalamin vitamin to coenzymes, helps in the differential diagnosis. Definitive diagnosis depends on demonstrating impaired coenzyme synthesis in cultured cells. Treatment of affected children with cobalamin supplements (1 to 2 mg per day) shows promise: homocystine and methylmalonate excretion fall to near normal values; the hematologic and neurologic deficits have also lessened to a variable degree in several patients. Intervention early in life seems to offer the best long-term prognosis.

REFERENCES

Boers GHJ et al: Heterozygosity for homocystinuria in premature peripheral and cerebral occlusive arterial disease. N Engl J Med 313:709, 1985

Fenton WA, Rosenberg LE: Inherited disorders of cobalamin transport and metabolism, in *The Metabolic Basis of Inherited Disease*, 6th ed, CR Scriver et al (eds). New York, McGraw-Hill, 1989, pp 2065–2082

Mudd SH et al: Natural history of homocystinuria due to cystathionine β-synthase deficiency. Am J Hum Genet 37:709, 1985

——— et al: Disorders of transsulfuration, in *The Metabolic Basis of Inherited Disease*, 6th ed, CR Scriver et al (eds). New York, McGraw-Hill, 1989 pp 693–734

Rosenberg LE, Scriver CR: Disorders of amino acid metabolism, in *Metabolic Control and Disease*, 8th ed, PK Bondy, LE Rosenberg (eds). Philadelphia, Saunders 1980, pp 583–776

Scriver CR et al: The hyperphenylalaninemias, in *The Metabolic Basis of Inherited Disease*, 6th ed, CR Scriver et al (eds). New York, McGraw-Hill, 1989, pp 495–546

335 STORAGE DISEASES OF AMINO ACID METABOLISM

LEON E. ROSENBERG

A number of inherited metabolic disorders are characterized by deposition or storage of particular metabolites in tissues. In most, storage reflects impaired degradation of the substance in question; in others, the mechanism is unknown. Many storage diseases involve large molecules such as glycogen, sphingolipids, mucolipids, cholesterol esters, and mucopolysaccharides (see Chaps. 332, 326, and 331); in others, metals such as iron and copper are deposited (see Chaps. 327 and 330). Finally, there is a group of storage diseases in which relatively small organic molecules are deposited. These include gout (see Chap. 329) and disorders of amino acid metabolism.

ALKAPTONURIA

DEFINITION Alkaptonuria is a rare disorder of tyrosine catabolism. Deficiency of the enzyme homogentisic acid oxidase leads to excretion of large amounts of homogentisic acid in urine and to accumulation of oxidized homogentisic acid pigment in connective tissues (ochronosis). After many years ochronosis produces a distinctive form of degenerative arthritis.

ETIOLOGY AND PATHOGENESIS Homogentisic acid is an intermediate in the catabolism of tyrosine to fumarate and acetoacetate. Activity of homogentisic acid oxidase, the enzyme that catalyzes the opening of the phenolic ring yielding maleylacetoacetic acid, is deficient in liver and kidney of patients with alkaptonuria, and homogentisic acid accumulates in cells and body fluids. Patients have minimally increased concentrations of homogentisic acid in blood because it is rapidly cleared by the kidney. As much as 3 to 7 g homogentisic acid may be excreted in the urine per day, but this is of little pathophysiologic significance. However, homogentisic acid and its oxidized polymers bind to collagen, leading to the progressive deposition of a gray to bluish-black pigment. The mechanism(s) by which degenerative changes develop in cartilage, intervertebral disk, and other connective tissues is unknown but may involve direct chemical irritation, impaired collagen cross-linking, disturbed articular chondrocyte metabolism, or some combination of factors.

Alkaptonuria was the first human disease shown to be inherited as an autosomal recessive trait. Affected homozygotes occur with a frequency around 1 in 200,000. Heterozygous carriers are clinically well and excrete no homogentisic acid in urine, even after loading doses of tyrosine.

CLINICAL MANIFESTATIONS Alkaptonuria may go unrecognized until middle life when degenerative joint disease develops in the majority. Prior to this time the tendency of the patient's urine to darken on standing may go unnoticed, as may slight discoloration of the sclerae and ears. The latter manifestations are generally the earliest external evidence of the disorder and develop after age 20 to 30. Foci of gray-brown scleral pigment and generalized darkening of the concha, antihelix, and, finally, helix of the ear are typical. Ear cartilages may be irregular and thickened. *Ochronotic arthritis* is heralded by pain, stiffness, and some limitation of motion of the hips, knees, and shoulders. Intermittent periods of acute arthritis, which may resemble rheumatoid arthritis, occur, but small joints are usually spared. Limitation of motion and ankylosis of the lumbosacral spine are common late manifestations. Pigmentation of heart valves, larynx, tympanic membranes, and skin occurs, and occasional patients develop pigmented renal or prostatic calculi. An increased incidence of degenerative cardiovascular disease may occur in older patients.

DIAGNOSIS A patient whose urine darkens to blackness on standing must be suspected of having alkaptonuria, but because of modern plumbing conditions this finding is not often observed. The diagnosis is usually made from the triad of degenerative arthritis, ochronotic pigmentation, and urine which turns black upon alkalinization. Homogentisic acid in urine may be identified presumptively by other tests: upon addition of ferric chloride, a purple-black color is observed; treatment with Benedict's reagent yields a brown color; addition of a saturated silver nitrate solution produces an immediate black color. These screening tests can be confirmed by chromatographic, enzymatic, or spectrophotometric determinations of homogentisic acid. X-rays of the lumbar spine are virtually pathognomonic. They show degeneration and dense calcification of the intervertebral disks and narrowing of the intervertebral spaces.

TREATMENT There is no specific treatment for ochronotic arthritis. Joint manifestations might be mitigated if homogentisic acid accumulation and deposition could be curbed by dietary restriction of phenylalanine and tyrosine, but the long course of the disease has discouraged such therapeutic attempts. Since ascorbic acid impedes oxidation and polymerization of homogentisic acid in vitro, its use has been suggested as a possible means of decreasing pigment formation and deposition. The efficacy of this form of treatment has not been established. Symptomatic treatment is similar to that for osteoarthritis (Chap. 281).

CYSTINOSIS

DEFINITION Cystinosis is a rare disorder characterized by the intralysosomal accumulation of free cystine in body tissues. This results in the appearance of cystine crystals in the cornea, conjunctiva, bone marrow, lymph nodes, leukocytes, and internal organs. Three variants have been identified: an infantile (nephropathic) form leading to the Fanconi syndrome and renal insufficiency in the first decade; a juvenile (intermediate) form in which renal disease becomes manifest during the second decade; and an adult (benign) form characterized by deposition of cystine in the cornea but not in the kidney.

ETIOLOGY AND PATHOGENESIS The basic defect in cystinosis involves impaired efflux of cystine from lysosomes rather than an abnormality in cystine catabolism. Lysosomal cystine efflux is an active, ATP-dependent process. The cystine content of tissues may be more than 100 times normal in the infantile form, more than 30 times normal in the adult form. Intracellular cystine appears to be located in lysosomes and does not exchange with other intracellular or extracellular pools of this amino acid. Neither plasma nor urinary concentrations of cystine are particularly elevated.

The extent of cystine crystal deposition varies from patient to patient, depending on the form of the disease and on the methods used to prepare pathologic specimens. Cystine accumulation in the kidney causes renal insufficiency in the infantile and juvenile forms. The kidneys are pale and shrunken, the capsule is adherent, and the corticomedullary junction is obscured. Microscopically, nephron organization is interrupted, glomeruli are hyalinized, connective tissue is increased, and the normal epithelium of the tubules is replaced by cuboidal cells. Narrowing and shortening of the proximal tubule produces the swan neck deformity that is characteristic of but not specific for cystinosis. Patchy depigmentation and degeneration of the peripheral retina occurs in the infantile and juvenile forms. Cystine crystals may also be deposited in the cornea, ocular conjunctiva, or uvea.

Each form of cystinosis appears to be inherited as an autosomal recessive trait. Obligate heterozygotes have intracellular cystine contents intermediate between those of normal persons and affected patients but are free of clinical abnormalities.

CLINICAL MANIFESTATIONS In the infantile form abnormalities are usually apparent by 4 to 6 months of age. Growth retardation, vomiting, fever, vitamin D–resistant rickets, polyuria, dehydration, and metabolic acidosis are prominent. Generalized proximal tubular dysfunction (the Fanconi syndrome) leads to hyperphosphaturia and hypophosphatemia, renal glycosuria, generalized aminoaciduria, hypouricemia, and often hypokalemia. Pyelonephritis may contribute, along with interstitial fibrosis, to progressive glomerular insufficiency. Death due to uremia or intercurrent infection usually occurs before age 10. Ocular manifestations are prominent. Photophobia is usually demonstrable within the first few years of life due to cystine deposits in the cornea, and retinal degeneration may appear even earlier.

In contrast, patients with the adult form manifest only ocular abnormalities. Photophobia, headache, and burning or itching of the eyes are major complaints. Glomerular and tubular function and the integrity of the retina are preserved. The findings in the juvenile variant fall between these extremes. These patients have both ocular and renal manifestations, but the latter do not become significant until the second decade. The renal lesion, albeit milder than that seen in the infantile form, eventually leads to renal insufficiency.

DIAGNOSIS Cystinosis must be considered in any child with vitamin D–resistant rickets, the Fanconi syndrome, or glomerular insufficiency. Hexagonal or rectangular cystine crystals can be detected in the cornea (by slit-lamp examination), in leukocytes from peripheral blood or bone marrow, or in biopsies of rectal mucosa. Diagnosis can be confirmed by quantification of cystine in peripheral blood leukocytes or cultured fibroblasts. The infantile form has been diagnosed prenatally by the demonstration of increased cystine content in cultured amniotic fluid cells.

TREATMENT The adult form is benign and requires no treatment. Symptomatic treatment of renal disease in the infantile or juvenile form of cystinosis does not differ from that of other forms of chronic renal insufficiency: maintenance of adequate fluid intake to prevent dehydration; correction of the metabolic acidosis; and ingestion of supplementary calcium, phosphate, and vitamin D to heal the rickets. Such measures are effective in maintaining growth, development, and well-being in affected children for a time. Two types of more specific therapy have been attempted. Cystine-restricted diets have not prevented progression of renal disease. This is not surprising given the nature of the primary defect and the large amount of cystine produced endogenously by cellular protein turnover. Whereas the early use of thiol reagents such as penicillamine and dimercaprol yielded no long-term benefits, administration of the free thiol, cysteamine, is helpful in slowing the progression of renal dysfunction, in improving growth, and in dissolving corneal cystine crystals. This compound acts in lysosomes by forming a mixed disulfide with cysteine that can be transported out of the organelle efficiently by a different transporter from that deficient in the disease.

The most successful form of therapy for nephropathic cystinosis is renal transplantation. Hundreds of affected children with end-stage renal disease have been so treated. Those patients who tolerated the procedure and did not develop immunologic problems have shown return of kidney function toward normal. The transplanted kidneys have not developed the functional abnormalities typical of cystinosis (i.e., the Fanconi syndrome or glomerular insufficiency). They may, however, continue to accumulate cystine in the cornea and other ocular tissues. Because the usual life span of a transplanted kidney is generally 15 to 20 years, some patients with the infantile form of cystinosis have received two or more transplanted kidneys.

PRIMARY HYPEROXALURIA

DEFINITION Primary hyperoxaluria is the designation for two rare disorders characterized by chronic excessive urinary excretion of oxalic acid and by calcium oxalate nephrolithiasis and nephrocalcinosis. Typically, patients with both forms develop renal insufficiency early in life and die of uremia. At postmortem examination, calcium oxalate deposits are widespread in renal and extrarenal tissues, a condition referred to as *oxalosis*.

ETIOLOGY AND PATHOGENESIS The metabolic basis for the primary hyperoxalurias involves pathways of glyoxylate metabolism. In type I hyperoxaluria, urinary excretion of oxalate and of the oxidized and reduced forms of glyoxylate is increased. The excessive synthesis of these substances results from a block in glyoxylate metabolism. The primary defect is deficiency of the hepatic peroxisomal enzyme, alanine:glyoxylate amino transferase. The resulting expansion of the glyoxylate pool leads to enhanced oxidation of glyoxylate to oxalate and to enhanced reduction of glyoxylate to glycolate. Each of these 2-carbon acids is then excreted in excess in the urine. In type II hyperoxaluria, L-glyceric acid is excreted in excess along with oxalate. In this condition, activity of D-glyceric acid dehydrogenase, which catalyzes the reduction of hydroxypyruvate to D-glyceric acid in the catabolic pathway of serine metabolism, is absent in leukocytes (and presumably other tissues). The accumulated hydroxypyruvate is instead reduced by lactic dehydrogenase to the L-isomer of glycerate, which is excreted in the urine. The reduction of hydroxypyruvate is coupled in some way to the oxidation of glyoxylate to oxalate, thus causing the formation of increased oxalate. Both disorders appear to be inherited as autosomal recessive traits. Heterozygotes are asymptomatic.

The pathogenesis of stone formation, nephrocalcinosis, and oxalosis relates directly to the insolubility of calcium oxalate. Extrarenal deposits of oxalate are prominent in the heart, walls of arteries and veins, male urogenital tract, and bone.

CLINICAL MANIFESTATIONS Nephrolithiasis and oxalosis may be manifest during the first year of life. Most patients experience renal colic or hematuria between ages 2 and 10 and succumb to uremia before age 20. With the onset of uremia, patients may develop severe peripheral arterial spasm and necrosis with resulting vascular insufficiency. Oxalate excretion falls as renal failure worsens. In patients with delayed onset of symptoms, survival to age 50 or 60 has been reported, despite recurrent nephrolithiasis.

DIAGNOSIS Oxalate excretion in normal children or adults is less than 0.5 mmol (60 mg) per 1.73 m^2 surface area per day. Patients with type I or type II hyperoxaluria generally excrete two to four times this amount. Distinction between the two types of primary hyperoxaluria depends on measurements of the other organic acids that identify them: glycolic acid in type I and L-glyceric acid in type II. Since patients with pyridoxine deficiency or chronic ileal disease may excrete excessive amounts of oxalate, these conditions must be excluded.

TREATMENT There is no satisfactory treatment. Urinary oxalate concentration can be transiently reduced by increasing the urinary flow rate. Large doses of pyridoxine (100 mg per day) may reduce urinary oxalate, but long-term effects are not dramatic. A diet high in phosphate content seems to reduce the frequency of attacks of renal colic, but oxalate excretion is unaffected. Finally, after renal transplantation renal function is lost because of calcium oxalate deposition in the transplanted kidney. The beneficial effects of combined liver-kidney transplantation observed in a single patient warrant additional study.

REFERENCES

GAHL WA et al: Lysosomal transport disorders, in *The Metabolic Basis of Inherited Disease,* 6th ed, CR Scriver et al (eds). New York, McGraw-Hill, 1989, pp 2619–2648

HILLMAN RE: Primary hyperoxalurias, in *The Metabolic Basis of Inherited Disease,* 6th ed, CR Scriver et al (eds). New York, McGraw-Hill, 1989, pp 933–944

LADU BN: Alcaptonuria, in *The Metabolic Basis of Inherited Disease,* 6th ed, CR Scriver et al (eds). New York, McGraw-Hill, 1989, pp 775–790

336 INHERITED DEFECTS OF MEMBRANE TRANSPORT

LEON E. ROSENBERG / ELIZABETH M. SHORT

The passage of certain molecules across plasma cell membranes depends on specific transport systems that owe their specificity to membrane receptor and "carrier" proteins. These membrane constituents recognize individual molecules or structurally related substances and catalyze their transmembrane movement by mechanisms poorly understood. The disorders considered in this chapter have three features in common: each is characterized by a specific defect in the transport of one or more compounds; each is inherited as a dominant or recessive trait, implying that a single genetic locus is involved; and each is presumed to reflect a primary alteration in a specific membrane protein. Many of these defects have been well characterized physiologically, but in none has the putative mutant transport protein been isolated. However, the cloning of the gene for the intestinal glucose transporter, whose deficiency underlies the glucose-galactose malabsorption syndrome, makes it possible to begin to characterize the molecular pathology in these syndromes.

More than 20 inherited disorders of membrane transport have been described in humans (Table 336-1). Most affect the gut and/or kidney only. Numerous classes of substrates are represented, including amino acids, sugars, cations, anions, vitamins, and water. Some are discussed elsewhere in this text. Those impairing the transport of amino acids, hexoses, urate, and chloride are discussed here as examples of the abnormalities encountered.

DISORDERS OF AMINO ACID TRANSPORT

As noted in Table 336-1, 10 disorders of amino acid transport have been described. Five of these (cystinuria, dibasicaminoaciduria, Hartnup disease, iminoglycinuria, and dicarboxylicaminoaciduria) show transport abnormalities for structurally related amino acids, thereby implying the existence of group-specific membrane receptors or carriers. With the exception of iminoglycinuria and dicarboxylicaminoaciduria, these defects have important clinical consequences. The remaining five disorders affect the transport of only one amino acid, implying the existence of substrate-specific transport systems. Each of these conditions affects transport in the kidney, gut, or both; none has been shown to alter transport in other tissues.

CYSTINURIA Definition Cystinuria, the most common inborn error of amino acid transport, is characterized by excessive urinary excretion of the dibasic amino acids: lysine, arginine, ornithine, and cystine. This aminoaciduria results from impaired tubular reabsorption of these amino acids. A similar transport defect exists in the intestinal mucosa. Because cystine is the least soluble of the naturally occurring amino acids, its overexcretion predisposes to the formation of renal, ureteral, and bladder calculi. Such calculi are responsible for the signs and symptoms of the disorder.

Etiology and pathogenesis Massive excretion of cystine and the other dibasic amino acids occurs only in classic cystinuria. The disorder, inherited as an autosomal recessive trait, is believed to result from alterations in a membrane carrier protein essential for transport of this group of amino acids in the apical brush border of proximal renal tubule and small intestinal cells. The putative protein has a greater affinity for ornithine and arginine than for lysine and cystine. Although the renal clearance of all four amino acids is increased in homozygotes, the presence of some residual transport capacity for these compounds plus the existence of three other disorders marked by selective excretion of members of this group (dibasicaminoaciduria, hypercystinuria, lysinuria) argues for the existence of at least three discrete renal transport systems for these amino acids: one for each amino acid alone; one shared by lysine, arginine, and ornithine; and one for all four amino acids.

Whereas urinary excretion patterns and renal clearance abnormalities in all homozygotes are similar, evidence for three allelic variants has come from studies of intestinal transport in homozygotes and of urinary excretion in obligate heterozygotes. Type I homozygotes lack mediated intestinal transport of cystine, lysine, arginine, and ornithine; heterozygotes have normal urinary amino acid excretion patterns. Type II homozygotes lack mediated lysine transport in the gut but retain some capacity for cystine transport; heterozygotes have moderately increased urinary excretion of each of the four amino acids. Type III homozygotes retain some capacity for mediated intestinal transport of the four involved substrates; heterozygotes have modestly increased urinary lysine and cystine.

Clinical manifestations Cystinuria is among the most common inborn errors, homozygotes occurring with a frequency of 1 in 10,000 to 1 in 15,000 in many ethnic groups. Two-thirds of adults with cystinuria are type I homozygotes. Cystine stones account for 1 to 2 percent of all urinary tract calculi. The maximum solubility of cystine in the physiologic urinary pH range of 4.5 to 7.0 is about 1200 μmol/L (300 mg/L). Since affected homozygotes regularly excrete 2400 to 7200 μmol (600 to 1800 mg) per day, crystalluria and calculus formation are a constant threat. Cystine stone formation usually becomes manifest in the second or third decade but may occur in the first year of life. Symptoms and signs are those typical of urolithiasis: hematuria, flank pain, renal colic, obstructive uropathy, and infection. Recurrent urolithiasis may lead to progressive renal insufficiency.

Diagnosis The presence of cystine in a urinary tract stone is pathognomonic of cystinuria. However, since 50 percent of the stones excreted by cystinuric subjects are of mixed composition and since as many as 10 percent may contain *no* detectable cystine, a urinary nitroprusside test should be done on all patients with urolithiasis to exclude this diagnosis. The nitroprusside test is also positive (appearance of a cherry red color) in some heterozygotes for cystinuria, in patients with hypercystinuria, homocystinuria, and cysteine β-mercaptolactate disulfiduria, and in the presence of acetone in the urine. When cystine content exceeds 1000 μmol/L (250 mg/L), cystine crystals may be seen in the sediment of acidified, concentrated, chilled urine. These hexagonal crystals are pathognomonic of cystine overexcretion in patients not taking sulfonamides.

Diagnostic confirmation of cystinuria depends upon the demonstration of the characteristic amino acid excretion pattern in the urine. Selective excretion of cystine, lysine, arginine, and ornithine can be demonstrated by paper chromatography or electrophoresis, and quantitative determinations can be made by column chromatography.

TABLE 336-1 Genetic disorders of membrane transport

Class of substance and disorder	Individual substrates	Tissues manifesting transport defect	Proposed molecular basis of defect	Major clinical manifestations	Mode of inheritance	Location of discussion
AMINO ACIDS						
Classic cystinuria	Cystine, lysine, arginine, ornithine	Proximal renal tubule, jejunal mucosa	Mutation of shared dibasic-cystine transport protein	Cystine nephrolithiasis	Autosomal recessive	Chap. 336
Dibasicaminoaciduria	Lysine, arginine, ornithine	Proximal renal tubule, jejunal mucosa	Mutation of dibasic transport protein	Type I: Benign Type II: Protein intolerance, hyperammonemia, retardation	Autosomal recessive	Chap. 336
Hypercystinuria	Cystine	Proximal renal tubule	Mutation of cystine transport protein	Some risk of cystine nephrolithiasis	Autosomal recessive	Chap. 336
Lysinuria	Lysine	Proximal renal tubule, jejunal mucosa	Mutation of lysine transport protein	Seizures, physical and mental retardation	Possible autosomal recessive	Chap. 336
Hartnup disease	Neutral amino acids	Proximal renal tubule, jejunal mucosa	Mutation of shared neutral amino acid transport protein	Constant neutral aminoaciduria, intermittent symptoms of pellagra	Autosomal recessive	Chap. 336
Tryptophan malabsorption	Tryptophan	Jejunal mucosa	Mutation of tryptophan transport protein	Indoluria, ?hypercalcemia, ?nephrocalcinosis	Probable autosomal recessive	Chap. 336
Methionine malabsorption	Methionine	Jejunal mucosa	Mutation of methionine transport protein	α-Hydroxybutyricaciduria, white hair, mental retardation, convulsions, hyperpneic attacks, edema	Probable autosomal recessive	Chap. 336
Histidinuria	Histidine	Proximal renal tubule, jejunal mucosa	Mutation of histidine transport protein	Mental retardation	Autosomal recessive	Chap. 336
Iminoglycinuria	Glycine, proline, hydroxyproline	Proximal renal tubule, jejunal mucosa	Mutation of shared glycine–imino acid transport protein	None	Autosomal recessive	Chap. 336
Dicarboxylicaminoaciduria	Glutamic acid, aspartic acid	Proximal renal tubule, jejunal mucosa	Mutation of shared dicarboxylic amino acid transport protein	None	Probable autosomal recessive	Chap. 336
HEXOSES						
Renal glycosuria	D-Glucose	Proximal renal tubule	Mutation of D-glucose transport protein	Glycosuria with normal blood glucose	Autosomal recessive	Chap. 336
Glucose-galactose malabsorption	D-Glucose D-Galactose	Jejunal mucosa, proximal renal tubule	Mutation of shared Na^+-dependent glucose-galactose transport protein	Watery diarrhea on feeding glucose, lactose, sucrose, or galactose	Autosomal recessive	Chaps. 240, 336
LIPIDS						
Familial hypercholesterolemia	Cholesterol	Fibroblasts, lymphoid lines, leukocytes	Mutation of membrane LDL–cholesterol receptor protein	Hypercholesterolemia, tendon xanthomas, arcus corneae, coronary artery atherosclerosis	Autosomal dominant	Chap. 326
URATE						
Hypouricemia	Uric acid	Proximal renal tubule	Mutation of urate transport protein	Hypouricemia, hyperuricosuria, ?hypercalcinuria	Autosomal recessive	Chap. 336
ANIONS						
Familial hypophosphatemic rickets	Inorganic phosphate	Proximal renal tubule, jejunal mucosa	Mutation of inorganic phosphate transport protein	Hypophosphatemia, phosphaturia, phosphatopenic rickets/osteomalacia	X-linked dominant	Chap. 341

TABLE 336-1 Genetic disorders of membrane transport *(continued)*

Class of substance and disorder	Individual substrates	Tissues manifesting transport defect	Proposed molecular basis of defect	Major clinical manifestations	Mode of inheritance	Location of discussion
ANIONS *(continued)*						
Congenital chloridorrhea	Chloride	Ileal and colonic mucosa	Mutation of Cl^-/HCO_3^- exchange pump carrier protein	Hydramnios, watery diarrhea, elevated fecal chloride, achloriduria, metabolic alkalosis with volume depletion, hyperaldosteronism	Autosomal recessive	Chaps. 240, 336
Familial goiter	Inorganic iodide	Thyroid gland, salivary gland, gastric mucosa	Mutation of iodide transport protein	Congenital hypothyroidism (cretinism), goiter	Probable autosomal recessive	Chap. 316
CATIONS						
Distal renal tubular acidosis (type I—gradient)	Hydrogen ion	Distal renal tubule	Mutation of distal tubule H^+ pump carrier protein	Hyperchloremic acidosis, hypokalemia, acquired nephrocalcinosis, and hypercalcinuria	Autosomal dominant	Chap. 231
Proximal renal tubular acidosis (type II—HCO_3^- wasting)	Hydrogen ion	Proximal renal tubule	Mutation of proximal tubule H^+ pump carrier protein	Hyperchloremic acidosis, bicarbonate wasting	Probable autosomal recessive	Chap. 231
Menkes' disease	Copper	Duodenal and jejunal intestinal cells	Possible serosal transport protein or intracellular transport defect	Severe mental retardation, pili torti (kinky hair), typical facies, arterial tortuosity, excess Wormian bones, thermal instability	X-linked recessive	Chaps. 77
Hereditary Spherocytosis Elliptocytosis Ovalocytosis Stomatocytosis	Sodium	Red blood cell (RBC) membranes	Mutation of membrane structure (? lipid or protein) resulting in increased sodium permeability	Increased RBC fragility resulting in variable degrees of hemolytic anemia, splenomegaly, and jaundice; RBC shape respectively spherocytic, elliptocytic, ovalocytic, or stomatocytic (target-shaped)	Each of these diseases of RBC morphology is a separately inherited autosomal dominant	Chap. 294
WATER						
Nephrogenic diabetes insipidus (AVP-resistant)	Water	Distal renal tubule	Lack of activation of AVP-responsive luminal membrane adenylate cyclase, possible defect in receptor or enzyme protein	Polyuria, polydipsia, hyposthenuria	X-linked recessive	Chap. 231
VITAMINS						
Juvenile pernicious anemia	Cobalamin (vitamin B_{12})	Ileal mucosa	Mutation of receptor for intrinsic factor–cobalamin complex	Megaloblastic anemia	Autosomal recessive	Chap. 292
Folate malabsorption	Folic acid	Small bowel	Mutation of folate transport protein	Megaloblastic anemia	Autosomal recessive	Chap. 292

Quantitation is important for differentiating some heterozygotes from homozygotes and documenting the reduction of free cystine excretion during therapy.

Treatment Medical management is aimed at reducing the concentration of cystine in urine. The most important treatment is maintenance of a large urine volume. Fluid ingestion in excess of 4 L/d is essential, and 5 to 7 L/d is optimal. Urinary cystine excretion should measure less than 1000 to 1200 μmol/L (250 to 300 mg/L). The daily fluid ingestion necessary to maintain this dilution of excreted cystine should be spaced over the waking hours, with one-quarter to one-third of the total volume ingested at bedtime. Stones can be prevented and even dissolved by such hydration. It must be made clear to the cystinuric subject that water is a drug. Solubility of cystine rises sharply in urine above pH 7.5, and urinary alkalinization can be therapeutic in some situations. Vigorous administration of sodium bicarbonate, acetazolamide, and polycitrates is required to maintain a persistently alkaline pH, but this measure introduces the danger of inducing formation of other "alkaline" stones (calcium oxalate, calcium phosphate, magnesium ammonium phosphate) and even of producing nephrocalcinosis.

Another treatment involves administration of penicillamine which undergoes sulfhydryl-disulfide exchange with cystine to form the mixed disulfide of penicillamine and cysteine. Since this disulfide is more than 50 times as soluble as cystine, penicillamine (in doses of 1 to 3 g per day) has the capacity to reduce free cystine excretion markedly, thereby preventing new stone formation and promoting dissolution of existing calculi. Unfortunately, allergic manifestations include acute serum sickness, agranulocytosis, pancytopenia, immune glomerulitis, and the Goodpasture syndrome. Thus, its use should be reserved for patients who fail to respond to hydration alone or who are in a high-risk category (one remaining kidney, renal insufficiency). Those patients unable to tolerate penicillamine may benefit from α-mercaptopropionylglycine, an experimental drug whose mechanism of action is similar to that of penicillamine but whose structure, and hence toxicity, is different. As many as two-thirds of patients unable to tolerate penicillamine may take α-mercaptopropionylglycine without ill effects. When medical management fails, urologic surgery is required. An occasional patient may require renal transplantation because of renal failure.

DIBASICAMINOACIDURIA Families have been described in which affected members have a defect in renal tubular reabsorption of lysine, arginine, and ornithine but *not* of cystine. The disorder almost surely reflects mutations in the genes coding for widely distributed transport protein used by the three dibasic amino acids only. Two variants have been observed, each apparently inherited as an autosomal recessive trait. Manifestations are related to the losses of ornithine, arginine, and perhaps lysine.

In the common form of dibasicaminoaciduria (type II), also known as lysinuric protein intolerance and much more common in Finland (1 in 60,000) than elsewhere in the world, homozygotes show defective intestinal transport of dibasic amino acids as well as exaggerated renal losses. The transport defect affects basolateral rather than luminal membrane transport. A defect in uptake of these substances by cultured fibroblasts and hepatocytes has also been reported. Affected patients present in childhood with hepatosplenomegaly, protein intolerance, and episodic ammonia intoxication. Plasma concentrations of lysine, arginine, and ornithine are reduced. The clinical findings have been attributed to hyperammonemia resulting from insufficient amounts of arginine and ornithine to maintain proper function of the urea cycle. Treatment includes dietary protein restriction and supplementation with citrulline, a neutral amino acid whose intestinal and hepatic transport are unimpaired, and which, when metabolized to arginine and ornithine, fuels the urea cycle. With 2.0 to 3.0 g of oral citrulline daily, dietary protein intake can be increased and growth improved in pediatric patients. Obligate heterozygotes are healthy and show no excess urinary loss of dibasic amino acids.

Type I dibasicaminoaciduria has been described in a large French-Canadian kindred. The female proband was moderately mentally retarded but had no clear history of protein intolerance or hyperammonemia. Her urinary losses of dibasic amino acids were not as great as those seen in type II homozygotes. The condition was distinguished from type II by the presence of modest excesses of dibasic amino acids in urine of both asymptomatic parents. A large number of chemically affected members of the family were also symptom-free. Other pedigrees containing asymptomatic heterozygotes have been identified by urinary screening programs. Type I disease may involve the same transport system as that impaired in the more common and severe type II disorder.

HARTNUP DISEASE Pellagra-like skin lesions, variable neurologic manifestations, and aminoaciduria for the monoaminomonocarboxylic amino acids with neutral or aromatic side chains characterize symptomatic Hartnup disease. Alanine, serine, threonine, valine, leucine, isoleucine, phenylalanine, tyrosine, tryptophan, glutamine, asparagine, and histidine are excreted in urine in quantities 5 to 10 times normal, and intestinal transport for these same amino acids is defective. The clinical manifestations result from nutritional deficiency of the essential amino acid tryptophan, caused by the combination of intestinal malabsorption and renal loss. Disease manifestations are episodic, related, at least in part, to metabolic demands for tryptophan. Only a small fraction of patients with the chemical findings typical of this disorder develop a pellagra-like syndrome, implying that onset of the clinical picture depends on factors over and above the transport defect.

The major pathway of tryptophan metabolism leads to the synthesis of niacin and nicotinamide-adenine dinucleotide (NAD). This pathway supplies about 50 percent of daily niacin needs. In patients with Hartnup disease, the renal and intestinal transport defect for tryptophan leads to niacin deficiency. The transport defect likely reflects abnormalities of a group-specific system for neutral amino acids. Some residual reabsorptive capacity persists for each involved amino acid. This suggests that they are transported by other carrier systems as well, a conclusion supported by the identification of patients with substrate-specific transport errors for tryptophan, methionine, and histidine.

Hartnup disease is inherited as an autosomal recessive trait. Homozygotes occur with a frequency of about 1 in 24,000 births. Heterozygotes exhibit no clinical or chemical abnormalities.

Pellagra is the clinical syndrome produced by dietary niacin deficiency, and its clinical features are those that characterize Hartnup disease (see Chap. 76). The diagnosis should be suspected in any patient with pellagra without a history of dietary niacin deficiency. The neurologic and psychiatric manifestations range from attacks of cerebellar ataxia to mild emotional lability to frank delirium and usually accompany exacerbations of the erythematous, eczematoid skin rash. Fever, sunlight, stress, and sulfonamide therapy provoke clinical relapses. Diagnosis is made by detection of the neutral aminoaciduria that does not occur in dietary niacin deficiency. Treatment is directed at niacin repletion and includes a high-protein diet and daily nicotinamide supplementation (50 to 250 mg).

IMINOGLYCINURIA This trait is characterized by excessive urinary excretion of glycine and the imino acids proline and hydroxyproline. Homozygotes for this autosomal recessive disorder occur with a frequency of about 1 in 16,000. The exaggerated renal clearance of glycine, proline, and hydroxyproline reflects a defect in the tubular transport system shared by these three compounds. An intestinal transport defect may also be present. This suggests that more than one mutation may lead to persistent iminoglycinuria, a thesis corroborated by the demonstration that obligate heterozygotes from some but not all families manifest glycinuria. No consistent clinical abnormalities have been reported in homozygotes, who are usually detected by urinary amino acid screening programs. Individuals with iminoglycinuria should be reassured as to the benign nature of the disturbance.

DICARBOXYLICAMINOACIDURIA Selective urinary loss and exaggerated endogenous renal clearance of glutamic and aspartic acids have been described in two unrelated children. Intestinal absorption of these dicarboxylic amino acids was impaired in one. This patient suffered from recurrent hypoglycemia; the other was asymptomatic.

SUBSTRATE-SPECIFIC DEFECTS IN AMINO ACID TRANSPORT Rare pedigrees exist in which individuals have defective renal tubular reabsorption and/or impaired intestinal absorption of a single free amino acid. These disorders, each apparently inherited as an autosomal recessive trait, suggest that transport of amino acids is catalyzed by substrate-specific as well as group-specific transport mechanisms.

Hypercystinuria Two siblings exhibited modest cystinuria without excessive urinary excretion of lysine, arginine, or ornithine. Fractional tubular reabsorption of cystine was reduced to about 80 percent of the filtered load, and up to 250 mg per day was excreted in the urine. Neither sibling showed any abnormality in intestinal absorption of cystine. Both were clinically well, although the cystine excretion places them at risk for cystine urolithiasis. Urinary cystine excretion by the parents was normal.

Lysinuria A child with selective impairment of renal tubular reabsorption of lysine has been described. Endogenous lysine clearance was increased; intestinal transport was impaired; plasma lysine was reduced. Mental and growth retardation and seizures were present. A lysine-supplemented diet stimulated growth. Urinary lysine excretion was normal in the parents.

Histidinuria Two siblings, each with mental retardation, exhibited a renal transport defect for histidine only. Urinary loss of histidine approached 40 to 50 percent of the filtered load, and an intestinal transport defect for histidine was also present. The clinically normal parents had normal urinary excretion but a modest defect in intestinal absorption of histidine. In two additional cases of isolated histidinuria myoclonic seizures occurred.

Methionine malabsorption Single children from two pedigrees have shown an intestinal transport defect for methionine. One may have had a renal transport defect as well. This disorder was detected because of urinary excretion of α-hydroxybutyric acid, a by-product of the intestinal bacterial breakdown of the unabsorbed methionine. This compound, which gives an odor resembling malt or dried celery to the urine, appears to be responsible for the white hair, attacks of hyperpnea, convulsions, edema, and mental retardation. Treatment of one of these children with a methionine-restricted diet caused improvement in all clinical manifestations.

Tryptophan malabsorption An isolated defect in intestinal absorption of tryptophan has been described in two siblings. The renal tubular reabsorption of tryptophan was normal. A variety of indoles were excreted in stool and urine. These compounds result from chemical degradation of unabsorbed tryptophan by intestinal bacteria and may be present in patients with Hartnup disease as well. Because of concomitant renal disease, hydrolytic enzymes were released into the urine, acted upon the indoles found there, and led to the formation of a blue pigment, indigotin. This sequence of events earned this condition the sobriquet ''blue-diaper syndrome.'' No pellagra-like symptoms were described. The mother also excreted indole compounds, suggesting that she is a carrier of this trait.

DISORDERS OF HEXOSE TRANSPORT

Nondiabetic melituria occurs in a number of conditions. Pentoses, hexoses, heptoses, and disaccharides have been identified in the urine; all except sucrose yield a positive test for reducing substances. Some melituria result from diffuse renal injury, others from ingestion of nonmetabolizable sugars. In still others the sugars accumulate in blood owing to deficient activity of catabolizing enzyme systems and ''spill'' into the urine. Only among the hexoses have specific inherited disorders of sugar transport been identified. The existence of renal glycosuria and intestinal glucose-galactose malabsorption as heritable, autosomal recessive disorders points to the existence of at least two specific carrier proteins for hexoses in human jejunal and renal brush border membranes: one for glucose and one shared by glucose and galactose.

RENAL GLYCOSURIA To avoid confusion with diabetes mellitus, Marble's criteria for the diagnosis of renal glycosuria should be followed: (1) glycosuria in the absence of hyperglycemia, (2) constant glycosuria with little fluctuation related to diet, (3) normal (or slightly flat) oral glucose tolerance test, (4) identification of urinary reducing substance as glucose, and (5) normal storage and utilization of carbohydrates. The Fanconi syndrome, in which renal glycosuria occurs as part of generalized proximal tubular dysfunction, should also be excluded. The condition is benign, but occasionally glycosuria may be great enough to cause polyuria and polydipsia. Even more rarely, dehydration or ketosis may develop under conditions of stress such as pregnancy or starvation.

In normal persons glucose is present in the glomerular filtrate at a concentration equal to that in plasma water and is reabsorbed throughout the proximal renal tubule by a sodium-dependent, phlorizin-inhibitable transport process. Reabsorptive capacity exceeds normal plasma glucose concentration. Thus, glucose does not appear in the urine until the threshold for reabsorption is reached. The plasma concentration at which filtered glucose begins to escape proximal tubular reabsorption is usually around 10 mmol/L (200 mg/dL). Maximal renal reabsorptive capacity is exceeded at a filtered load of around 2 mmol (325 mg)/min per 1.73 m^2 body surface area, and this value is defined as the tubular maximum for glucose (TmG).

Two patterns of glycosuria are recognized: type A characterized by a reduced tubular maximum reabsorptive capacity and type B showing a reduced threshold for glycosuria, an increased ''splay'' in the titration curve, and a normal TmG. Marked renal glycosuria occurs in individuals homozygous for either of these recessively inherited mutations and in genetic compounds for these presumably allelic mutations. Modest reduction in renal threshold or TmG is present in obligate heterozygotes in some pedigrees; modest glycosuria occurs in such family members when plasma glucose is elevated. The gene responsible for renal glycosuria segregates with the human histocompatibility leukocyte antigen (HLA) haplotype suggesting its location on chromosome 6. No linkage disequilibrium was observed, and no specific HLA antigens have been associated with renal glycosuria.

GLUCOSE-GALACTOSE MALABSORPTION In this condition, infants develop a profuse, watery diarrhea when fed milk or foods containing lactose, sucrose, glucose, or galactose. Fructose or carbohydrate-free formulas are well tolerated. A specific defect in intestinal absorption of glucose and galactose can be demonstrated by oral tolerance tests that produce little or no increase in plasma glucose or galactose. The primary defect involves the sodium/hexose cotransporter found in the intestinal and renal brush border. Active D-glucose and D-galactose transport are absent in affected children, and intermediate transport capacity is present in their parents. These findings confirm the specificity and the autosomal recessive inheritance of the disorder. Treatment with a glucose- and galactose-free diet leads to resolution of symptoms in childhood. Although the basic transport defect is present throughout life, most patients show an improved tolerance for glucose and galactose with age.

A number of these patients have renal glycosuria at normal plasma glucose concentrations. Renal titration studies generally demonstrate a reduced threshold for glucose reabsorption (type B renal glycosuria) with a normal TmG. Urinary glucose loss is not as severe as in isolated renal glycosuria. This finding suggests the presence of multiple glucose transport proteins in the kidney. One, responsible for the bulk of glucose reabsorption and specific for glucose only, is affected in renal glycosuria; another, shared by glucose and galactose and responsible for transporting less of the filtered load of glucose, is affected in glucose-galactose malabsorption. Either the former is not present in intestinal mucosa, or the shared system is more important in that tissue. In both disorders transport of sugars in all other tested tissues is normal, reflecting the multiplicity and tissue specificity of membrane transport proteins.

DEFECTIVE URATE TRANSPORT: HYPOURICEMIA

Individuals with a selective defect in renal tubular reabsorption of sodium urate have marked hypouricemia. Since little serum urate is bound to plasma proteins, failure to reabsorb filtered urate results in a serum urate ranging from 12 to 110 μmol/L (0.2 to 1.8 mg/dL). Moderate uricosuria is present, and half of patients have renal calculi.

Renal urate clearance normally averages 15 percent of glomerular filtration rate, and the excreted urate is composed both of filtered urate that has escaped reabsorption and secreted urate. Subjects with isolated hypouricemia have urate clearances averaging from 33 to 85 percent of the filtration rate; in some, urate clearance exceeds the glomerular filtration rate. Studies with probenecid, which blocks tubular reabsorption of urate, and pyrazinamide, which blocks tubular secretion, reveal that six of the eight families described have a presecretory urate reabsorptive defect, and two have defective transport affecting the entire tubule. In four families hypercalciuria due to enhanced intestinal calcium absorption is also present, but in others only uricosuria has been demonstrated. The defect is inherited as an autosomal recessive trait. Urate transport has not been studied in nonrenal tissue or in obligate heterozygotes. The defect is presumed to reflect mutation of one or both of the proximal renal tubular membrane proteins that transport sodium urate. The findings in these families support the hypothesis that renal urate reabsorption is controlled by more than one transport protein.

DEFECTIVE ANION TRANSPORT: CHLORIDORRHEA

This rare, autosomal recessive disease results from impairment of active transport of chloride in the ileum and colon. Absence of the chloride-bicarbonate ion exchange "pump" causes profound symptoms even before birth (polyhydramnios and absence of meconium). Massive watery diarrhea is apparent from the first days of life. This fluid loss, with its attendant impairment of electrolyte homeostasis, is life-threatening. A hypokalemic, hypochloremic, hyponatremic metabolic alkalosis develops with dehydration and secondary hyperaldosteronism. Fecal fluid contains an excess of chloride ion over the sum of the accompanying cations, sodium and potassium. Fecal chloride concentration always exceeds 90 mmol/L when volume and serum electrolyte disturbances are corrected, and this chloridorrhea is diagnostic. Renal chloride transport is normal. Decreased urine chloride results from the kidney's attempts to conserve salt and water.

Treatment requires adequate, life-long repletion of electrolyte and fluid losses, since no way has yet been found to mitigate the transport disorder. Exact replacement of water, sodium chloride, and potassium chloride can prevent the growth and psychomotor retardation and the development of progressive renal damage. The renal lesion, with hyalinized glomeruli, juxtaglomerular hyperplasia, calcifications, and arteriolar changes, is probably a result of chronic volume depletion. Treatment of hyperreninemia and hypokalemia with prostaglandin inhibitors may reduce renal damage but does not alter intestinal symptoms or the need for chronic sodium chloride repletion.

REFERENCES

DESJEUX JF: Congenital selective Na^+ D-glucose cotransport defects leading to renal glycosuria and congenital selective intestinal malabsorption of glucose and galactose, in *The Metabolic Basis of Inherited Disease,* 6th ed, CR Scriver et al (eds). New York, McGraw-Hill, 1989, pp 2463–2478

ELSAS LJ, ROSENBERG LE: Renal glycosuria, in *Strauss and Welt's Diseases of the Kidney,* 3d ed, LE Earley, CW Gottschalk (eds). Boston, Little, Brown, 1979, pp 1021–1028

HOLMBERG C, PERHEENTUPA J: Congenital chloride diarrhoea (CCD), in *Population Structure and Genetic Disorders,* AW Erikson et al (eds). New York, Academic, 1980, pp 596–599

KAMOUN PP et al: Renal histidinuria. J Inherited Metab Dis 4:217, 1981

LEVY HL: Hartnup disorder, in *The Metabolic Basis of Inherited Disease,* 6th ed, CR Scriver et al (eds). New York, McGraw-Hill, 1989, pp 2515–2528

ROSENBERG LE: Intestinal hexose transport in familial glucose-galactose malabsorption, in *Membranes and Disease,* L Bolis et al (eds). New York, Raven Press, 1976, pp 253–262

———, SCRIVER CR: Disorders of amino acid metabolism, in *Metabolic Control and Disease,* 8th ed, PK Bondy, LE Rosenberg (eds). Philadelphia, Saunders, 1980, pp 616–645

SEGAL S, THIER SO: Cystinurias, in *The Metabolic Basis of Inherited Disease,* 6th ed, CR Scriver et al (eds). New York, McGraw-Hill, 1989, pp 2479–2496

SHORT EM, ROSENBERG LE: Renal aminoaciduria, in *Strauss and Welt's Diseases of the Kidney,* 3d ed, LE Earley, CW Gottschalk (eds). Boston, Little, Brown, 1979, pp 975–1020

SIMELL O: Lysinuric protein intolerance and other cationic aminoacidurias, in *The Metabolic Basis of Inherited Disease,* 6th ed, CR Scriver et al (eds). New York, McGraw-Hill, 1989, pp 2497–2514

WEITZ R, SPERLING O: Hereditary renal hypouricemia: Isolated tubular defect of urate reabsorption. J Pediatr 96:850, 1980

337 GALACTOSEMIA, GALACTOKINASE DEFICIENCY, AND OTHER RARE DISORDERS OF CARBOHYDRATE METABOLISM

KURT J. ISSELBACHER

DEFINITION Galactosemia refers to any of three inborn errors of galactose metabolism. "*Classic*" *galactosemia* is due to the deficiency of galactose-1-phosphate uridyl transferase (GALT) and is typically associated with cataract formation, mental retardation, and cirrhosis. The second disorder, *galactokinase deficiency,* leads primarily to cataract formation. The third, *UDP-galactose-4-epimerase deficiency,* is the rarest of the group; few cases have been described, and the eventual outcome is uncertain.

PATHOGENESIS Lactose, the main carbohydrate in milk, is a disaccharide containing galactose and glucose; when ingested it is hydrolyzed by intestinal lactase. Normally the absorbed galactose is converted to glucose in the liver. The first reaction in this pathway is the phosphorylation of galactose to galactose-1-phosphate by galactokinase (specified by a gene on chromosome 17):

$$\text{Galactose} + \text{ATP} \xrightarrow{\text{galactokinase}} \text{galactose-1-phosphate}$$

The next step involves the conversion of galactose-1-phosphate to glucose-1-phosphate by GALT, the gene for which is on chromosome 9:

$$\text{Galactose-1-phosphate} + \text{UDP-glucose} \xrightarrow{\text{GALT}} \text{UDP-galactose} + \text{glucose-1-phosphate}$$

The uridine diphosphate (UDP) sugars can be reversibly interconverted by an epimerase reaction (UDP-galactose-4-epimerase):

$$\text{UDP-galactose} \longleftrightarrow \text{UDP-glucose}$$

Galactose can also be metabolized by alternative pathways. It can be converted (reduced) in the presence of NADPH (or NADH) to galactitol (dulcitol) by aldose reductase. It can also be oxidized to a limited extent by galactose dehydrogenase, leading to the formation of galactonic acid, xylulose, and CO_2. These pathways account for limited galactose metabolism in patients with galactosemia.

In galactokinase deficiency, galactose accumulates in the blood and tissues. In the lens galactose is converted by aldose reductase to galactitol, a sugar to which the lens is impermeable. As a consequence, excessive hydration occurs which, together with a decrease in glutathione in the lens, leads to cataract formation.

In classic galactosemia, GALT deficiency results in tissue accumulation of galactose-1-phosphate and galactose. As in galactokinase deficiency, cataracts develop secondary to galactitol accumulation in the lens. It is assumed that the cirrhosis and mental retardation of classic galactosemia are related to increased amounts of galactose-1-phosphate in these tissues. Elevated blood galactose levels may lead to a decreased hepatic output of glucose and hence to hypoglycemia. In the kidney and intestine accumulation of galactose and galactose-1-phosphate appears to lead to an inhibition of amino acid transport. In female homozygotes there is an increased incidence of hypergonadotrophic hypogonadism in which ovarian failure develops at an early age.

Both galactokinase and GALT deficiencies are transmitted as autosomal recessive traits. Heterozygotes for these disorders have half-normal enzyme levels but are asymptomatic. Maternal deficiency of galactokinase, together with lactose intake during pregnancy, may contribute to cataract formation during fetal development. However, not all persons with half-normal GALT enzymes in their cells are carriers of classic galactosemia. Some individuals homozygous for another gene, called the *Duarte variant,* normally have half-normal GALT levels and are asymptomatic. This group can be differentiated from classic galactosemia heterozygotes on the basis of the electrophoretic properties of the mutant enzyme. In both galactokinase deficiency and classic galactosemia there is a functional deficiency or absence of the involved enzyme. Classic galactosemia is due to a structural gene mutation, and the altered enzyme (GALT) protein does not function normally. Other clinical variants with altered enzyme electrophoretic mobility have been described.

The incidence of classic galactosemia is about 1 per 80,000 births in the white population. Approximately 0.8 to 1.3 percent of the population are heterozygotes for the galactosemia (GALT) gene, and about 10 percent carry the Duarte variant. During screening of newborns for galactosemia the most frequent cause of an abnormal result is compound heterozygosity for the Duarte variant and for classic galactosemia in which GALT levels are about 17 percent of normal. Such individuals are clinically asymptomatic.

CLINICAL FEATURES Symptoms of classic galactosemia usually begin within days to weeks after birth. The infant usually is reluctant to ingest breast milk or milk formulas, develops vomiting, shows poor nutrition, and fails to thrive. Jaundice, hepatomegaly, and evidence of liver disease may develop. Cataracts are usually not present at birth but develop gradually over weeks to months. Mental retardation becomes evident after 6 to 12 months and is usually not reversible. Infants with classic galactosemia are subject to bacterial sepsis (especially with *Escherichia coli*), and this may be the leading cause of death in the neonatal period. The only consistent feature of galactokinase deficiency is cataract formation.

DIAGNOSIS Galactokinase deficiency should be suspected in infants or children with cataract formation who have non-glucose-reducing substances in the urine. The diagnosis is made by demonstrating the deficiency of galactokinase in red blood cells.

Classic galactosemia must be considered when one or more of the clinical features described above are found. If the patient is ingesting milk, reducing sugar is present in the urine but gives a negative glucose oxidase reaction (i.e., is not glucose) and is identified as galactose by other techniques, such as chromatography. If the child is vomiting, has a poor food intake, or is on intravenous glucose feedings, galactose may not be present in the urine. The definitive diagnosis is made by demonstrating a lack or deficiency of red cell GALT by one of several techniques. The disease can also be diagnosed prenatally by enzyme studies on culture amniocentesis cells or by demonstrating increased galactitol in amniotic fluid. A nonenzymatic glycosylation of hemoglobin, analogous to that in diabetes mellitus, can be detected in patients with galactosemia as manifested by increased concentrations in the blood of Hb A_{Iab} rather than Hb A_{Ic}.

In the neonatal period galactosemia needs to be differentiated from primary liver disease. With liver damage, galactose removal from the blood is impaired, and elevated blood galactose levels and galactosuria may be present. However, GALT levels are normal in patients with liver damage.

TABLE 337-1 Some other disorders of carbohydrate metabolism

Disorder	Metabolic defect	Manifestations
Hereditary fructose intolerance	Deficiency of fructose-l-phosphate aldolase leads to accumulation of fructose-1-PO_4 in tissues.	Liver disease, renal tubular damage, and hypoglycemia.
Fructose-1,6-diphosphatase deficiency	Deficiency of the enzyme prevents gluconeogenesis from its normal precursors, lactate, glycerol, and alanine. Thus, maintenance of blood sugar is dependent upon exogenous glucose.	Lactic acidosis leads to hyperventilation, somnolence, and coma, usually with hypoglycemia and ketosis.

TREATMENT The treatment of galactosemia consists of the removal of galactose-containing foods from the diet, especially milk. Milk substitutes such as Nutramigen are often used. Although soybean preparations contain polysaccharide-bound galactose, they appear to be well tolerated because the bound galactose is not readily liberated. In general, the red cell levels of galactose-1-phosphate are not increased in affected infants fed soybean formulas.

The institution of a galactose-free diet usually leads to a dramatic improvement in all clinical features except for mental retardation. Patients should be kept on galactose-free diets indefinitely or at least until they have attained adequate physical and neurologic development.

OTHER DISORDERS OF CARBOHYDRATE METABOLISM Features of hereditary fructose intolerance and fructose-1,6-diphosphatase deficiency, two autosomal recessive disorders of fructose metabolism that lead to hypoglycemia, are summarized in Table 337-1 (also see Chaps. 332 and 320).

REFERENCES

ALLEN TJ et al: Evidence of galactosemia in utero. Lancet 1:603, 1980

BURMAN D et al (eds): *Inborn Errors of Carbohydrate Metabolism*. Lancaster, MTP Press, 1979

GITZELMANN R et al: Essential fructosuria, heredity fructose intolerance, and fructose 1,6-diphosphatase deficiency, in *The Metabolic Basis of Inherited Disease*, 5th ed, JB Stanbury et al (eds). New York, McGraw-Hill, 1983, p 118

KAUFMAN FR et al: Correlation of ovarian function with galactose-1-phosphate uridyl transferase levels in galactosemia. J Pediatr 112:754, 1988

NG WG et al: Transferase-deficiency galactosemia and the Duarte variant. JAMA 257:187, 1987

SARDHARWALLA IB, WRAITH JE: Galactosemia. Nutr Health 5:175, 1987

SEGAL S: Disorders of galactose metabolism, in *The Metabolic Basis of Inherited Disease*, 5th ed, JB Stanbury et al (eds). New York, McGraw-Hill, 1983, p 167

338 THE LIPODYSTROPHIES AND OTHER RARE DISORDERS OF ADIPOSE TISSUE

DANIEL W. FOSTER

This chapter is concerned with abnormalities in adipose tissue. The disorders are rare, the pathophysiology is frequently not clear, and only clinical descriptions can be given.

THE LIPODYSTROPHIES

The lipodystrophies are characterized by generalized or partial loss of body fat and metabolic abnormalities, including insulin resistance, hyperglycemia, and hypertriglyceridemia. A classification is shown in Table 338-1. In *generalized lipodystrophy* essentially all body fat is lost, while in *partial lipodystrophy* fat atrophy is limited. The

TABLE 338-1 The lipodystrophies

1 Generalized lipodystrophy
- *a* Congenital (familial or sporadic)
- *b* Acquired (sporadic)

2 Partial lipodystrophy
- *a* Common (sporadic)
- *b* Dominant (familial)
  - (*1*) Limb and trunk
  - (*2*) With Rieger anomaly

3 Localized lipodystrophy
- *a* Inflammatory
- *b* Noninflammatory

common acquired form of partial lipodystrophy ordinarily involves half the body, usually the upper segment. Dominantly transmitted partial lipodystrophy tends to spare the face. One variant is associated with eye and tooth malformations, the Rieger anomaly. *Localized lipodystrophy* may be either inflammatory or noninflammatory. The best-studied syndrome is *centrifugal lipodystrophy* in which fat atrophy begins in the groins or axillae of children under the age of 3 and spreads centrally to involve the entire abdomen. The edge of the lesion is red and scaly with an inflammatory infiltrate demonstrable on histologic examination. Fat atrophy usually disappears spontaneously when the patient is around 13 years of age.

GENERALIZED LIPODYSTROPHY Generalized lipodystrophy (also called lipoatrophic diabetes) may be either congenital or acquired. The congenital form is transmitted as an autosomal recessive trait. Males and females are equally affected. Rates of parental consanguinity are high. Loss of fat is usually obvious at birth, but the rest of the clinical picture may not appear until later (up to 30 years). The acquired disease often develops after some other illness. Measles, chicken pox, whooping cough, or infectious mononucleosis are common precipitating events, but hypothyroidism, hyperthyroidism, and pregnancy have been implicated. Some cases begin with the appearance of painful nodular swellings of adipose tissue resembling acute panniculitis (see below). The congenital and acquired forms are similar in clinical manifestations (Table 338-2).

Fat atrophy Loss of body fat is the characteristic feature. In congenital cases the skin of the face is tightly drawn over the bony structures, and the entire body is devoid of adipose tissue. Rarely, a small amount of breast fat remains. In the acquired form the face may be spared, but all other fat disappears. Adipose tissue cells can be identified microscopically, but they contain no triglyceride stores. Paradoxically the liver is engorged with fat, and the reticuloendothelial system contains lipid-laden macrophages (foam cells). The cause of the fat atrophy is not known. Fat-mobilizing polypeptides have been reported in the urine of patients with generalized lipodystrophy, but their role in the disease is uncertain.

A candidate molecule for the induction of lipodystrophy is a compound similar to cachectin (tumor necrosis factor), which is a potent inhibitor of lipoprotein lipase and causes fat depletion and hypertriglyceridemia when injected into animals. Lipoprotein lipase activity is low in generalized lipodystrophy, as would be predicted if a cachectin-like inducer were the cause. However, plasma levels of tumor necrosis factor were normal in two of the author's patients. Hepatic lipase is not impaired. Since triglyceride content of the adipocyte is the result of a balance between fat synthesis and fat breakdown, an alternative mechanism might involve activation of the hormone-sensitive lipase that catalyzes hydrolysis of triglycerides in the fat cell. For example, a defect in a natural inhibitor of the lipase, such as adenosine, could result in enhanced response to physiologic (nonelevated) concentrations of lipolytic hormones. Release of free fatty acids into plasma following norepinephrine infusion is impaired, but this may simply reflect the depleted triglyceride stores.

Although an inducing molecule could act as a circulating hormone in generalized lipodystrophy, such an etiology is unlikely in partial lipodystrophy where autotransplantation of adipocytes from an affected area to a nonaffected site resulted in reaccumulation of fat, and reverse transplantation from normal to affected site resulted in fat atrophy. An autocrine or paracrine function may be involved. In the former a cellular product would act on the cell of origin while in the latter a cellular product would act on adjacent cells, but in neither case would the putative inducer of lipodystrophy enter the circulation to act as a typical hormone.

Growth and maturation Linear growth is accelerated in the first few years of life in the congenital disorder and in acquired disease that begins early in childhood. Epiphyses close early, however, so that the final height is usually normal. True muscular hypertrophy is present, and patients may have an acromegalic appearance with coarse facial features and large hands and feet. The ears tend to be prominent in the congenital form. Many viscera are enlarged, and generalized lymphadenopathy may be present. The cause of the growth disorder is not known. Levels of growth hormone and insulin-like growth factor I (IGF-I, somatomedin C) are normal or low. Insulin-like growth factor II has not been systematically assessed. One possibility is that abnormal growth and pseudoacromegaly are due to high concentrations of insulin in plasma secondary to insulin resistance (see below). The elevated insulin might cross-react with the IGF-I receptor in muscle and cartilage and promote growth via this mechanism.

Liver Enlargement of the liver causes protuberance of the abdomen. Fatty liver may progress to cirrhosis, especially in the acquired disorder. Several patients have died from bleeding esophageal varices. Splenomegaly does not occur in the absence of portal hypertension.

Kidneys The kidneys are usually enlarged. Subjects with the acquired disorder may have proteinuria and the nephrotic syndrome, although not as frequently as in partial lipodystrophy. Moderate hypertension is common.

Genitalia The external genitalia (penis and testes in males, clitoris and labia majora in females) are usually hypertrophied in congenital disease. In women polycystic ovaries are common, resulting in the clinical picture of Stein-Leventhal syndrome. The cause of the genital abnormalities is not known. Systematic investigation of gonadotropin, estrogen, and androgen metabolism has not been carried out.

Skin Acanthosis nigricans is present in most. Hypertrichosis of face, neck, trunk, and limbs is frequent. Scalp hair is usually thick and curly, particularly early in life.

Central nervous system Mental retardation is present in about half the congenital cases. Dilatation of the third ventricle and basal cisterns has been demonstrated by pneumoencephalography. Central nervous system involvement appears to be less marked in the acquired disease, although two patients had astrocytomas arising in the floor of the third ventricle. Few patients have been examined with computed tomography or magnetic resonance imaging so that firm conclusions regarding CNS abnormalities cannot be drawn.

TABLE 338-2 Characteristics of the lipodystrophies

Finding	Congenital general	Acquired general	Acquired partial	Dominant partial
Inheritance	Autosomal recessive	Sporadic	Usually sporadic	Autosomal dominant
Age of onset	Infancy	Childhood to adult	Childhood to adult	Puberty
Sex incidence	Males and females equal	Female preponderance	Female preponderance	Female preponderance
Lipoatrophy	Face, trunk, limbs	Face, trunk, limbs	Face, upper trunk, upper limbs	Trunk and limbs
Liver involvement	+	+ +	Rare	0
Renal disease	+	+	+ +	0
Insulin resistance	+	+	+	+
Hyperglycemia	+	+	+	+
Hypertriglyceridemia	+	+	+	+
Acanthosis nigricans	+	+	Rare	+
Genital hypertrophy	+	+	Rare	+
Bone age	Accelerated	Normal to accelerated	Normal	Normal

Other abnormalities Bones tend to be sclerotic in generalized lipodystrophy, and cystic angiomatosis may be present. Cardiomegaly is common, but heart failure appears to be rare. Goiter is frequent. The associated abnormalities in generalized lipodystrophy are summarized in Table 338-3.

Metabolic and endocrine abnormalities Three major metabolic disturbances are characteristic.

1 *Insulin resistance.* Insulin resistance may be mild or severe. When severe the hyperglycemia may be difficult to control. Insulin and C-peptide concentrations are relatively or absolutely elevated, and response to exogenous insulin is impaired. Resistance is due to several causes, and affected siblings may exhibit different mechanisms. Increased insulin clearance, decreased number of insulin receptors, diminished affinity of the receptor for insulin, and postreceptor defects have all been reported. Insulin in the plasma of affected subjects is biologically active. Although glucagon levels are high (indicating insulin resistance in the alpha cell of the islets of Langerhans) and free fatty acid concentrations are elevated, ketoacidosis is unusual. One patient had recurrent epidoses of metabolic acidosis considered to be ketoacidosis, but concentrations of acetoacetate and β-hydroxybutyrate were characteristic of fasting ketosis, not ketoacidosis; presumably lactate or other organic acids were involved.

   Ketoacidosis may be infrequent because insulin resistance spares liver and skeletal muscle (or is less severe); glycogen levels in the liver are high (insulin stimulates glycogen synthesis), and branched-chain amino acids fall normally in response to injected insulin. Elevated insulin levels in portal vein plasma would counteract the actions of glucagon in the insulin-responsive hepatocyte. This would prevent activation of the ketone body synthesis in liver and assure utilization of incoming fatty acids for triglyceride synthesis and production of very low density lipoproteins. The elevated long-chain fatty acids in the plasma are of dietary origin and fall toward normal with restriction of dietary fat. The diabetes mellitus accompanying lipodystrophy appears to be typical apart from insulin resistance, including the propensity to develop late degenerative complications. High levels of insulin in plasma and resistance to ketoacidosis distinguish this condition from type I (autoimmune) insulin-dependent diabetes mellitus, although both conditions begin in childhood or early adult life. Some subjects with insulin resistance and lipodystrophy have point mutations of the insulin receptor (see Chap. 311).

2 *Hypertriglyceridemia with accumulation of both chylomicrons and very low density lipoproteins in the blood.* Eruptive xanthomas, lipemia retinalis, and recurrent pancreatitis may be seen. Although lipoprotein lipase is low, as noted, and there is a defect in disposal of triglycerides in the atrophied fat tissue, the major cause for the hypertriglyceridemia is overproduction of very low density lipoproteins (VLDL) in the liver. This overproduction is probably driven by the elevated free fatty acids in blood since dietary fat restriction results in a fall of VLDL production rates toward normal. Hyperinsulinemia may contribute by enhancing hepatic fat synthesis.

3 *A hypermetabolic state with normal thyroid function.* Basal metabolic rates are usually elevated although thyroid hormone values (thyroxine, triiodothyronine, reverse triiodothyronine) are normal. Patients do not gain weight with excessive caloric intake, indicating a facile capacity to waste calories as heat. Food intakes as high as 21,000 kJ (5000 kcal)/d are not unusual. One 16-month-old child ate 10,000 kJ (2400 kcal)/d. Following thyroidectomy in one patient, the basal metabolic rate decreased but did not return to normal; symptoms and signs of hypothyroidism supervened requiring treatment with thyroid hormone despite continued high metabolic rates. It thus seems clear that hypermetabolism is not due to hyperthyroidism. There is also no evidence of mitochondrial disease. Abnormal dietary thermogenesis, mediated by the sympathetic nervous system, is the likely cause of the increased metabolic rate. There is no evidence for adrenal medullary dysfunction.

TABLE 338-3 Accompanying abnormalities of lipodystrophy

Bone	Sclerosis, cystic angiomatosis
Brain	Mental retardation, third ventricle dilatation
Genitalia	Clitoromegaly, polycystic ovaries, penile hypertrophy
Heart	Cardiomegaly
Kidneys	Hypertrophy without renal failure
Liver	Hepatomegaly, fatty liver, cirrhosis, hepatic failure
Lymph nodes	Generalized lymphadenopathy
Skin	Acanthosis nigricans, hypertrichosis
Thyroid	Goiter, euthyroid state

Course and treatment Patients with generalized lipodystrophy may die at an early age. Hepatic failure, hemorrhage from esophageal varices, and renal failure are common causes of death. Despite the almost constant hypertriglyceridemia, symptomatic coronary artery disease is rare. There is no specific treatment for lipodystrophy, although dietary fat restriction is generally recommended. Medium-chain triglyceride supplementation has been reported to be of benefit. Pimozide therapy, hypophysectomy, and plasmapheresis are ineffective.

ACQUIRED PARTIAL LIPODYSTROPHY This is the most common of the lipodystrophies and usually affects women. Fat atrophy occurs in the upper half of the body, including the face, but spares the lower extremities. Rarely the lower half of the body is affected, leaving the upper torso intact. Occasionally the lesion affects only one side. The other anatomic features of generalized lipodystrophy are usually absent, and liver disease is unusual. Proteinuria, with or without the nephrotic syndrome, occurs more frequently than in other forms. The complement system is abnormal, and C3 levels tend to be low. C3 nephritic factor, a polyclonal IgG immunoglobulin that interacts with alternative pathway convertase to augment C3 activation, is present in serum. C3 levels may be low in unaffected first-degree relatives, but C3 nephritic factor is absent. Complement abnormalities disappeared after renal transplantation in one subject. Dermatomyositis and Sjögren's syndrome may occur. Rarely partial lipodystrophy progresses to the generalized form of the disease.

LIPODYSTROPHY WITH DOMINANT TRANSMISSION This variant is characterized by fat atrophy of the limbs and trunk with sparing of the face, which may actually be rounded. The neck may also be exempt. The disease usually begins at puberty but may not appear until middle age. Males are rarely affected. In families with the Rieger anomaly onset tends to be in infancy. Insulin resistance and hyperglycemia are usual, and severe hypertriglyceridemia with eruptive xanthoma may occur. The labia majora are hypertrophied, and polycystic ovaries may be seen. Acanthosis nigricans is usually present. Liver and renal disease do not occur.

LOCALIZED LIPODYSTROPHY Localized lipodystrophy takes several patterns. Centrifugal lipodystrophy (*lipodystrophia centrifugalis abdominalis infantilis*) has already been mentioned. Annular lipoatrophy is a bandlike ring of fat atrophy encircling a limb or the ankles. Occasionally only half the limb is involved, in which case the term often used is *lipoatrophia semicircularis.* On biopsy inflammatory infiltrates are usually present in the areas of fat atrophy. Localized lipodystrophy may also occur secondary to injection of insulin, iron dextrans, triamcinolone, and diphtheria/pertussis/tetanus vaccine.

MULTIPLE SYMMETRIC LIPOMATOSIS

Multiple symmetric lipomatosis, a disease found predominantly in men, is characterized by formation of multiple nonencapsulated lipomas in various areas. Two patterns of distribution are noted. In the *type I* variant, lipomas are primarily in the nape of the neck and in the supraclavicular and deltoid regions, resulting in an extraordinary bull-necked appearance (*Madelung collar*). Extension into the mediastinum may produce obstruction of the trachea or vena cava. Fat over the remainder of the body appears normal. In the *type II* pattern, lipomas are not localized to the neck but extend down over the body giving the appearance of simple obesity. Correct diagnosis requires recognition that the fat masses are symmetric and that the distal arms and legs are spared. Deep lipomatosis is absent in type II disease, and vena caval and tracheal compression do not occur.

Multiple symmetric lipomatosis may occur sporadically or in families. Autosomal dominant transmission has been postulated in the latter. Alcoholism is common. Coexisting folate deficiency, macrocytic anemia, and abnormal liver function may be due to alcohol and not lipomatosis. Neuropathy, which may be sensory, motor, or autonomic, is prominent, and neuropathic foot ulcers may be present. Histologic evidence from sural nerve biopsies suggests that the neuropathy is integral to the disease and not due to alcohol. The lesion is a chronic distal atrophy without the axonal degeneration and demyelination characteristic of alcohol injury.

Metabolic abnormalities include hyperuricemia, hypertriglyceridemia (VLDL, chylomicrons) and, paradoxically, an elevation of high-density lipoproteins (HDL) as well. Diabetes mellitus has not been reported, although hyperinsulinism may be present. A few patients have had renal tubular acidosis.

The cause of multiple symmetric lipomatosis is not known. The fat cells are slightly smaller than normal, suggesting hyperplasia. Isolated adipocytes appear to have a marked increase in lipoprotein lipase activity and a defect in adrenergic lipolysis. Lipolytic response to cyclic AMP is intact, suggesting an abnormality at the hormone receptor/adenylate cyclase unit. The biochemical abnormalities are not present in all cases.

There is no treatment except for surgical removal of lipomas that cause compression. They may also be removed for cosmetic reasons.

MEDIASTINO-ABDOMINAL LIPOMATOSIS

This syndrome may be a variant of multiple symmetric lipomatosis. The features include (1) exertional dyspnea due to compression of airways by lipomas of the mediastinum, (2) massive enlargement of the abdomen (pseudoascites) due to intraperitoneal and retroperitoneal fat, and (3) abnormal glucose tolerance or diabetes mellitus. The metabolic abnormalities and enzymic changes in adipocytes are identical with those in multiple symmetric lipomatosis except that HDL levels are not elevated.

ACUTE PANNICULITIS (NODULAR FAT NECROSIS)

The appearance of single or multiple crops of tender nodules in subcutaneous fat with a histologic picture of fat-cell necrosis, infiltration of inflammatory cells, and development of fat-filled macrophages (foam cells) is the hallmark of acute panniculitis. The nodules range in size from 0.5 to 10 cm and may be firm or fluctuant. They are usually, but not always, tender. On occasion they drain an oily solution, and suppuration may occur. Individual lesions last from 1 to 8 weeks before disappearing, and a pigmented depressed area may be left at the involved site. While some patients have only nodular panniculitis, which may or may not be relapsing, others develop fever, abnormal liver function, involvement of the bone marrow with leukemoid response, bleeding tendencies, nodular pulmonary lesions, and evidence of pancreatic disease with elevated plasma amylase and lipase levels. In the past this constellation of findings was called *Weber-Christian disease*. However, since painful or nonpainful panniculitis may result from a variety of conditions, Weber-Christian disease is not a specific entity, and the term should probably be abandoned.

It is not possible to develop a firm classification of acute panniculitis since the lesions may appear in sporadic fashion with many conditions. One classification system is given in Table 338-4.

TABLE 338-4 Causes of panniculitis

1 Panniculitis without systemic disease
  a Trauma
  b Cold
  c Subcutaneous fat necrosis of the newborn
2 Panniculitis with systemic disease
  a Connective tissue disorders (lupus erythematosus, scleroderma)
  b Lymphoproliferative disease (lymphoma, histiocytosis)
  c α_1-Antitrypsin deficiency
  d Pancreatic disease (cancer, pancreatitis)
  e Generalized lipodystrophy
  f Paraproteinemia with C_1 inhibition deficiency

Panniculitis without systemic disease is usually due to trauma (sometimes factitiously induced) or cold. For example, in equestrian cold panniculitis the lesions appear in the outer thighs of persons riding horseback for several hours in icy weather. One variant, subcutaneous fat necrosis of the newborn, may be due to a combination of obstetric trauma and hypothermia.

Panniculitis with systemic disease can be divided into several large categories. Collagen vascular disease is a frequent cause, although few patients with connective tissue disorders develop this complication. Lupus is probably most common, and scleroderma is second. About 2 to 3 percent of patients with lupus have nodular fat necrosis; it is more common in discoid lupus than in the systemic variant. Lymphomas and histiocytosis represent a second category. Histiocytic cytophagic panniculitis is a disease characterized by fever, serositis (pleural effusions), hepatosplenomegaly, panniculitis, anemia, leukopenia, thrombocytopenia, and coagulation defects. The characteristic lesion is the "beanbag" histiocyte containing ingested lymphocytes, red cells, and platelets. While some patients have a benign course, the majority have a fatal outcome due to hemorrhagic complications. Deficiencies of α_1-antitrypsin have been found in a number of patients with acute panniculitis and should be looked for in every suspected case. It is postulated that the α_1-antitrypsin deficiency predisposes to panniculitis secondary to trauma and induces a hyperactive immune response. Panniculitis with systemic symptoms, including fever and hepatitis, has also been seen with light-chain paraproteinemia and acquired deficiency of C_1 inhibitor in the classical complement-generating sequence. Severe pancreatic disease may also cause acute panniculitis. One distinct syndrome has been called *disseminated fat necrosis* and is described below. Finally, panniculitis may be associated with generalized lipodystrophy, especially the acquired type.

Acute panniculitis can be diagnosed only histologically. Once the lesion is identified a search for the cause must be made. If systemic symptoms are present and the course is rapidly downhill, the primary differential diagnosis is between collagen vascular disease, lymphoproliferative disorder, and pancreatitis or pancreatic cancer. Milder cases raise the possibility of α_1-antitrypsin deficiency.

Treatment is often unsatisfactory. Some patients with histiocytic cytophagic panniculitis respond to combined chemotherapy with cyclophosphamide, bleomycin, and prednisone. Patients with α_1-antitrypsin deficiency may respond to dapsone but should be given α_1-antiprotease concentrate (60 mg/kg body weight weekly) if this fails.

DISSEMINATED FAT NECROSIS

Disseminated fat necrosis (also called metastatic fat necrosis) is a syndrome in which patients with pancreatitis (two-thirds) or carcinoma of the pancreas (one-third) develop lesions that appear to be similar to or identical with nodular panniculitis. The fat necrosis has a predilection for periarticular sites. Fever is almost invariably present. Arthritis occurs in about 60 percent of cases and may be severe, resulting in destruction of the joint. Often there are sinus tracts running from the site of subcutaneous fat necrosis into the joint space, leading to deposition of necrotic material. Lytic bone lesions may underlie the site of fat necrosis. Polyserositis and vasculitis may be present. Since complement levels are low and immunofluorescent staining shows deposition of complement and IgG, the syndrome resembles, in some respects, lupus-associated panniculitis. Serologic studies for lupus have not been systematically carried out. Antinuclear antibody (ANA) and rheumatoid factor were negative in one patient.

Disseminated fat necrosis may be due to release of pancreatic enzymes into blood or lymph, and these enzymes may initiate fat necrosis at distal sites. Presumably free fatty acids released by pancreatic lipase and phospholipase A, both of which may be elevated in serum, induce tissue necrosis, with trypsin playing an ancillary role. Experimentally, necrosis can be induced in pericardial, subpleural, and subcutaneous fat by ligation of pancreatic ducts. Amylase and lipase levels may be elevated in pleural, pericardial, and ascitic fluid. These enzymes have also been found in fluid aspirated from subcutaneous nodules. A fistula developed between a pancreatic pseudocyst and the portal vein in one patient; shortly thereafter nodular fat necrosis appeared over most of the body. On the other hand an immune mechanism may be causal, given that polyserositis is common and that low complement levels and vasculitis may be present. The meaning of the eosinophilia that frequently accompanies disseminated fat necrosis is not known.

Mortality rates are high (even in the absence of pancreatic carcinoma), and death may occur in weeks to months. No treatment is known. Infusion of the protease inhibitor aprotinin appeared to have beneficial effects in one patient.

ADIPOSIS DOLOROSA

Adiposis dolorosa (Dercum's disease) is characterized by painful circumscribed adipose tissue deposits in subcutaneous tissues of the extremities and of other parts of the body. Juxtaarticular areas, particularly the knees, are the most common sites. Lesions vary from 0.5 to 5.0 cm. Pain and paresthesias may occur spontaneously or result from pressure. Affected subjects are frequently women (30:1). They are usually obese. The syndrome is associated with weakness, fatigue, emotional instability, and occasional dementia. The condition rarely begins until after menopause. Most cases are sporadic, but familial occurrence has been noted with a presumed dominant inheritance. Multiple associations have been reported, but they are probably chance phenomena. Autopsy reports from early in the century suggested abnormalities of the pituitary and other endocrine glands, but modern endocrinologic evaluations have not been undertaken.

Biopsy of affected sites may show no abnormalities, but granulomas with giant cell formations are usually seen. Fat necrosis is rare, thus separating the condition from acute panniculitis.

Treatment is unsatisfactory, although intravenous lidocaine has apparently provided relief in two cases.

REFERENCES

Lipodystrophy

BILLINGS JK et al: Lipoatrophic panniculitis: A possible autoimmune inflammatory disease of fat. Report of three cases. Arch Dermatol 123:1662, 1987

DUNNIGAN MG et al: Familial lipoatrophic diabetes with dominant transmission: A new syndrome. Q J Med 43:33, 1974

FRANKLIN B et al: Very low-density lipoprotein metabolism in an unusual case of lipoatrophic diabetes. Metabolism 33:814, 1984

LILLYSTONE D, WEST RJ: Lipodystrophy of limbs associated with insulin resistance Arch Dis Child 50:737, 1975

SEIP M: Generalized lipodystrophy, in *Ergebnisse der Inneren Medizin und Kinderheilkunde,* P Frick et al (eds). Berlin, Springer Verlag, 1971, pp 59–95

SOLER NG et al: Lipoatrophic diabetes: Endocrine dysfunction and the response to control of hypertriglyceridemia. Metabolism 31:19, 1982

WACHSLICHT-RODBARD H et al: Heterogeneity of the insulin-receptor interaction in lipoatrophic diabetes. J Clin Endocrinol Metab 52:416, 1981

WILSON DE et al: Eucaloric substitution of medium chain triglycerides for dietary long chain fatty acids in acquired total lipodystrophy: Effects on hyperlipoproteinemia and endogenous insulin resistance. J Clin Endocrinol Metab 57:517, 1983

Multiple symmetric lipomatosis

ENZI G: Multiple symmetric lipomatosis: An updated clinical report. Medicine 63:56, 1984

LEUNG NWY et al: Multiple symmetric lipomatosis (Launois-Bensaude syndrome): Effect of oral salbutamol. Clin Endocrinol 7:601, 1987

POLLOCK M et al: Neuropathy in multiple symmetric lipomatosis. Madelung's disease. Brain 111:1157, 1988

RUZICKA T et al: Benign symmetric lipomatosis Launois-Bensaude. Report of ten cases and review of the literature. J Am Acad Dermatol 17:663, 1987

Mediastino-abdominal lipomatosis

ENZI G et al: Mediastino-abdominal lipomatosis: Deep accumulation of fat mimicking a respiratory disease and ascites. Clinical aspects and metabolic studies *in vitro.* Q J Med 53:453, 1984

Acute panniculitis

ALEGRE VA, WINKELMANN RK: Histiocytic cytophagic panniculitis. J Am Acad Dematol 20:177, 1989

ARONSON IK et al: Panniculitis associated with cutaneous T-cell lymphoma and cytophagocytic histiocytosis. Br J Dermatol 112:87, 1985

PASCUAL M et al: Recurrent febrile panniculitis and hepatitis in two patients with acquired complement deficiency and paraproteinemia. Am J Med 83:959, 1987

PATTERSON JW: Panniculitis. New findings in the "third compartment," editorial. Arch Dermatol 123:1615, 1987

SMITH KC et al: Panniculitis associated with severe α_1 antitrypsin deficiency. Treatment and review of the literature. Arch Dermatol 123:1655, 1987

WINKELMANN RK: Panniculitis in connective tissue disease. Arch Dermatol 119:336, 1983

Disseminated fat necrosis

PHILLIPS MR JR et al: Inflammatory arthritis and subcutaneous fat necrosis associated with acute and chronic pancreatitis. Arthritis Rheum 23:355, 1980

WILSON HA et al: Pancreatitis with arthropathy and subcutaneous fat necrosis. Evidence for the pathogenicity of lipolytic enzymes. Arthritis Rheum 26:121, 1983

Adiposis dolorosa

ATKINSON RL: Intravenous lidocaine for the treatment of intractable pain of adiposis dolorosa. Int J Obes 6:351, 1982

section 3 Disorders of bone and mineral metabolism

339 CALCIUM, PHOSPHORUS, AND BONE METABOLISM: CALCIUM-REGULATING HORMONES

MICHAEL F. HOLICK / STEPHEN M. KRANE / JOHN T. POTTS, JR.

BONE STRUCTURE AND METABOLISM (See also Chap. 341) Bone is a dynamic tissue that is constantly remodeled throughout life. The arrangement of compact and cancellous bone provides a combination of strength and density suitable for mobility. In addition, bone provides calcium, magnesium, phosphorus, sodium, and other ions necessary for the support of homeostatic functions. The skeleton is highly vascular and receives about 10 percent of the cardiac output.

The properties of bone are a function of its extracellular components. The structure consists of a solid mineral phase in close association with an organic matrix of which 90 to 95 percent is type I collagen (see Chap. 333). The noncollagenous portion of the organic matrix contains proteins derived from serum (albumin and α_2-HS glycoproteins), α-carboxyglutamic acid (GLA)–containing proteins (*bone GLA protein,* or *BGP,* or *osteocalcin* and a matrix GLA protein), a glycoprotein called *osteonectin,* a phosphoprotein called *osteopontin,* sialoproteins, *thrombospondin,* and other less well characterized proteins. Some of these proteins may function in initiating mineralization and in binding of the mineral phase to the matrix. The mineral phase is made up of calcium and phosphate, best characterized as a poorly crystalline hydroxyapatite, although the calcium/phosphate molar ratio is less than the 1.67 of hydroxyapatite [empiric formula, $Ca_{10}(PO_4)_6(OH)_2$]. In addition, other ions are present, predominantly in the surface layers. The mineral phase of bone is deposited in intimate relation to the collagen fibrils and is found largely in specific locations within the ''holes'' of the collagen fibrils that result from the manner in which the collagen molecules are packed. This architectural organization of mineral and matrix results in a two-phase material uniquely suited to withstand mechanical stresses. The formation and the localization of the inorganic phase are probably determined in part by the organic matrix.

Bone is formed by cells of mesenchymal origin, *osteoblasts,* that synthesize and secrete the organic matrix. Mineralization of the matrix, particularly in *osteons* (haversian systems), begins soon after the matrix is secreted (primary mineralization) but is not completed until after several weeks (secondary mineralization). Osteoblasts are derived from mesenchymal stem cells and are characterized by their location and morphology, the presence of a specific skeletal form of alkaline phosphatase, receptors for parathyroid hormone (PTH) and 1,25-dihydroxyvitamin D [$1,25(OH)_2D$], and the ability to synthesize specific matrix proteins such as type I collagen, osteocalcin, and osteopontin. As an *osteoblast* secretes matrix which is then mineralized, the cell becomes surrounded by matrix and becomes an *osteocyte,* still connected with its blood supply through a series of canaliculi. Resorption of bone is carried out mainly by *osteoclasts.* Osteoclasts are multinucleated cells formed by fusion of precursor cells derived from a hematopoietic stem cell related to the mononuclear phagocyte series. Resorption of bone takes place in scalloped spaces (Howship's lacunae) where the osteoclasts are attached to the bone matrix through a ring of contractile proteins (clear zone) and form a specialized ruffled border. Mineral and matrix are removed in this space where the ruffled border is folded and is in contact with the bone. Proteins including a proton pump ATPase are found in the ruffled border membrane, which contributes to the production of a unique acid environment in the enclosed extracellular compartment and results in solubilization of the mineral phase. In addition to the proton pump, carbonic anhydrase (type II isoenzyme) is required to maintain the acid pH. Other features of osteoclasts include the presence of tartrate-resistant acid phosphatase, cell surface receptors for calcitonin, an integrin (vitronectin) receptor, and an ability to resorb mineralized bone. The bone matrix is resorbed in the acid environment adjacent to the ruffled border by acid hydrolyases following solubilization of the mineral phase. Several soluble ligands modulate the differentiation of osteoblasts or osteoclasts from precursor cells and modulate the function of the differentiated cells. Bone is a storehouse for growth regulatory factors. Some that affect osteoblast function include transforming growth factors (TGF-β I and II), acidic and basic fibroblast growth factors (FGF), platelet-derived growth factors (PDGF), and insulin-like growth factors (IGF-1 and -2). In addition, several proteins have the capacity to induce ectopic bone formation and may have a role in bone remodeling, e.g., osteoinductive factor, osteogenin, and bone morphogenic proteins. Other cytokines modulate resorption through effects on osteoclasts, e.g., interleukin 1 (IL-1), tumor necrosis factor (TNF), γ-interferon, and colony stimulating factors. Some of these effects on osteoclasts are mediated by osteoblasts and adjacent stromal fibroblasts in the marrow. For example, PTH receptors are not found on osteoclasts, and PTH increases osteoclastic bone resorption by first acting on osteoblasts or stromal fibroblasts. $1,25(OH)_2D$ receptors are found in precursor cells, which can differentiate into monocytes as well as osteoclasts, and $1,25(OH)_2D$ can induce differentiation along the osteoclast pathway. The effects of some cytokines such as IL-1 and TGF-α may be mediated by local production of prostaglandins. What had initially been termed *osteoclast-activity factor* is currently thought to reflect the presence of cytokines such as IL-1, TNF-α, TNF-β (lymphotoxin), and probably others as well.

In the embryo and in the growing child, bone develops either by remodeling and replacing previously calcified cartilage (endochondral bone formation), or it is formed without a cartilage matrix (intramembranous bone formation). New bone, whether in embryos or infants or that formed in adults during repair, has a relatively high ratio of cells to matrix and is characterized by coarse fiber bundles of collagen that are interlaced and randomly dispersed (woven bone). In adults, the more mature bone is organized with fiber bundles regularly arranged in parallel or concentric sheets (lamellar bone). In long bones, the lamellar bone is deposited in a concentric arrangement around blood vessels and forms the haversian systems. Growth in length of bones is dependent upon proliferation of cartilage cells and on the endochondral sequence at the growth plate. Growth in width and thickness is accomplished by formation of bone at the periosteal surface and by resorption at the endosteal surface with the rate of formation exceeding that of resorption. In adults, after the epiphyses close, growth in length and endochondral bone formation cease, except for some activity in the cartilage cells beneath the articular

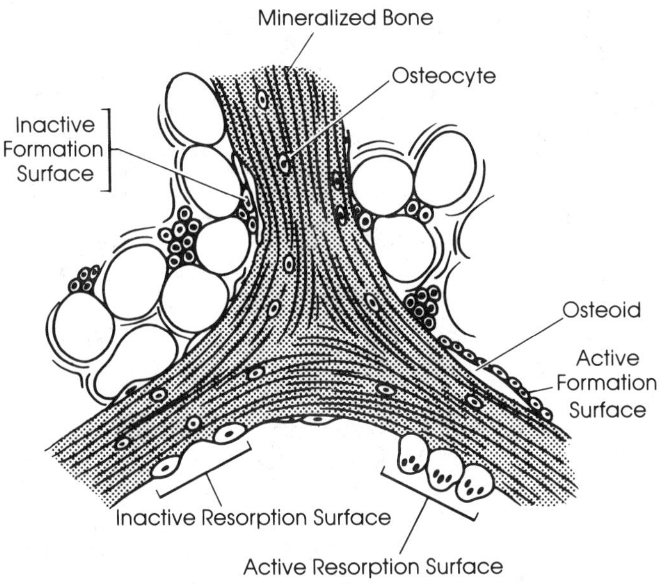

FIGURE 339-1 Schematic representation of bone remodeling surfaces in trabecular bone. Most bone surfaces in adults are involved in neither formation nor resorption. Such surfaces are usually smooth, have no osteoid seam, and are covered either by no visible cells or by flattened cells. Active formation surfaces are smooth and covered by osteoblasts which have an osteoid seam (clear), normally no thicker than 12 μm. The calcification front is located at the junction of the osteoid seam and mineralized bone (stippled). Inactive forming surfaces are not covered by osteoblasts but by only a few flattened cells. Active resorbing surfaces are irregular or scalloped and contain multinucleated osteoclasts. The latter are not seen on inactive resorbing surfaces.

surface. Even in adults, however, remodeling of bone (remodeling of haversian systems as well as trabecular bone) continues through life, as can be shown by microradiographic studies utilizing radioisotopes or fluorescence of tetracyclines fixed in bone in regions of new mineralization. Quantitative histomorphometric studies demonstrate that newly forming surfaces are characterized by smooth character, by uptake of tetracycline, and by relatively low mineral density. Actively forming surfaces are covered by active osteoblasts. The osteoid seam that results from the relative lag in mineralization of the newly formed organic matrix is normally no greater than about 12 μm. An index of the rate of bone formation can be obtained by examination of undemineralized sections of bone biopsies obtained from individuals who have received tetracycline for two periods separated by a drug-free interval. The distance between the fluorescent bands on the sections reflects the new bone formed. Resorption areas are characterized by their irregular configurations and the presence of osteoclasts (Fig. 339-1). Resorption precedes formation and is more intense, but it does not persist as long as formation. In adults, approximately 4 percent of the surface of trabecular bone (such as iliac crest) is involved in active resorption, whereas 10 to 15 percent of trabecular surfaces is covered with osteoid. Kinetic studies using isotopes such as radioactive calcium (^{47}Ca) provide estimates that as much as 18 percent of the total skeletal calcium may be deposited and removed each year. Thus, bone is an active metabolizing tissue that is dependent upon an intact blood supply. The remodeling of bone occurs in a manner somehow related to the continuous mechanical stresses to which it is subjected. Bone also serves as an important reservoir of mineral ions, particularly calcium, which are critical for a variety of processes.

The response of bone to injuries, such as fractures, infection, and interruption of blood supply, and to expanding lesions is relatively limited. Dead bone must be resorbed, and new bone must be formed, a process carried out in association with new blood vessels growing into the involved area. In injuries that disrupt the organization of the tissue, such as a fracture in which apposition of fragments is poor and motion exists at the fracture site, the osteoprogenitor stromal cells differentiate into cells with functional capacities other than those of osteoblasts, and repair is accompanied by formation of varying amounts of fibrous tissue and cartilage. When there is good apposition with fixation and little motion at the fracture site, repair occurs predominantly by formation of new bone without other scar tissue. Remodeling of this bone occurs along lines of force determined by mechanical stresses that are somehow translated into biologic response.

Expanding lesions in bone, such as tumors, induce resorption at the surface in contact with the tumor. A bowing deformity causes increased new bone formation at the concave surface and resorption at the convex surface, all seemingly designed to produce the strongest mechanical structure. Even in a disorder as architecturally disruptive as Paget's disease, remodeling is dictated by mechanical forces. Thus, the plasticity of bone is due to the response of cells interacting with each other and with the environment.

Mechanisms of bone formation and resorption Bone formation is an orderly process in which inorganic mineral is deposited in relation to an organic matrix. The mineral phase is composed of calcium and phosphorus, and the concentration of these ions in the plasma and extracellular fluid influences the rate at which the mineral phase is formed. In vitro, mineralization can proceed, and crystals of hydroxyapatite can grow at concentrations of calcium and phosphorus similar to those in an ultrafiltrate of plasma. However, the concentration of these ions at the sites of mineralization is unknown, and the cells involved (osteoblasts, osteocytes) may somehow regulate the local concentration of calcium, phosphorus, and other ions. Collagens from a variety of sources can catalyze the nucleation of a mineral phase of calcium and phosphorus from solutions of these ions, and the initial mineral phase is deposited in specific locations in the holes produced by the particular packing arrangement of the collagen molecules. The organization of collagen probably influences the amount and type of mineral phase formed in bone. There is one gene for each of the two $\alpha 1$ chains and the single $\alpha 2$ chain that make up type I collagen. The primary structures of type I collagen in skin and bone tissues are similar. There are differences, however, in posttranslational modifications of type I collagen such as hydroxylation, glycosylation, and the type, number, and distribution of intermolecular cross-links. In addition, the "holes" in the packing structure of the collagen are larger in normally mineralized collagen of bone and dentin than in unmineralized collagens such as tendon. The fact that single amino acid substitutions in the helical portion of either the $\alpha 1$ or $\alpha 2$ chains of type I collagen that result from mutations in the col1A1 or col1A2 genes in osteogenesis imperfecta markedly disrupt the organization of bone indicates the importance of the fibrillar matrix in the structure of bone (see also Chap. 333). The noncollagenous organic components such as osteocalcin, osteonectin, or osteopontin may also play a role in the formation of the mineral phase of bone. Alkaline phosphatase is a marker for osteoblasts, and cellular levels of this enzyme correlate with mineralization potential of osteoblasts. Although mineralization defects occur in individuals with decreased levels of alkaline phosphatase (hypophosphatasia), the function of alkaline phosphatase in the mineralization process is not completely understood. To explain how collagens from tissues that are normally not mineralized can catalyze nucleation of an inorganic phase from solutions similar to normal extracellular fluid, regulation of mineralization by inhibitory substances has been suggested. Inorganic pyrophosphate is a potent inhibitor of mineralization at concentrations below those necessary to bind calcium ions. Since alkaline phosphatase, present in osteoblasts and other cells, can catalyze the hydrolysis of inorganic pyrophosphate at neutral pH, this enzyme could regulate mineralization by controlling the concentrations of pyrophosphate. In addition, macromolecular inhibitors such as the proteoglycan aggregates may also influence the rate and extent of mineralization. In cartilage undergoing calcification, membrane-bound vesicles containing mineral are present outside the cells, and it has been suggested that this is the initial mineral phase.

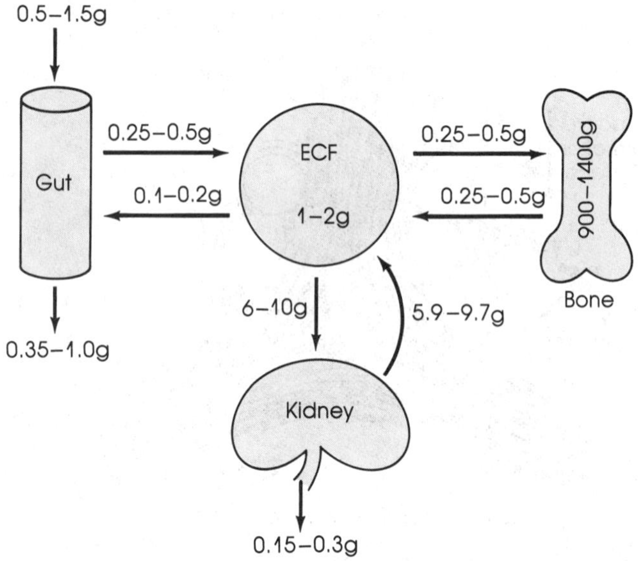

FIGURE 339-2 Calcium homeostasis. Schematic illustration of calcium content of extracellular fluid (ECF) and bone as well as of diet and feces; magnitude of calcium flux per day as calculated by various methods is shown at sites of transport in intestine, kidney, and bone. Ranges of values shown are approximate and chosen to illustrate certain points discussed in text. In intestine, absorption efficiency varies inversely with dietary calcium (chronic adaptation). This is reflected in typical quantities absorbed and excreted in feces; with 0.5-g intake, 50 percent absorption is depicted to occur (0.25 g), but at 1.5 g only 30 percent (0.5 g). Endogenous fecal calcium, the 0.1 to 0.2 g secreted into the intestinal lumen daily, is constant and does not vary with calcium intake or absorption. Quantities of calcium depicted as filtered, reabsorbed, and excreted at the kidney are chosen arbitrarily to indicate that at lower rates of filtration of calcium (expected at lower glomerular filtration rates), most is reabsorbed (e.g., 5.85 of 6 g), leading to urinary excretion of 150 mg; at higher rates of filtration (at high dietary calcium intake), slightly less is reabsorbed (e.g., 9.7 of 10 g), leading to a higher urinary excretion, 300 mg. In all situations, renal calcium reabsorption exceeds 95 percent of filtered load. Urinary calcium excretion is seen, therefore, to increase by only 150 mg despite a 1-g increase in dietary intake. In conditions of calcium balance, rates of calcium release from and uptake into bone are equal.

In bone, the calcium phosphate solid phase at the inception of mineralization is brushite ($CaHPO_4 \cdot 2H_2O$). As mineralization progresses, the solid phase is a poorly crystalline hydroxyapatite with a relatively low (~ 1.2) calcium/phosphate molar ratio. With age and maturation, the degree of crystal perfection increases as does the calcium/phosphate ratio. Fluoride ions, when incorporated into the mineral phase, decrease the proportion of amorphous calcium phosphate and increase crystallinity.

There is a limit for the concentration of calcium and phosphorus ions in the extracellular fluid below which mineralization will not occur. A "solubility product" for bone mineral is difficult to calculate since the mineral phase itself is of variable composition and the true nature of species in solution governing this solubility product is not known. Nevertheless, when the concentrations of calcium and phosphorus in extracellular fluid are excessive, a mineral phase may be formed in areas that are not normally mineralized.

When bone is resorbed, calcium and phosphorus ions from the solid phase are released into the extracellular space adjacent to the ruffled border of the osteoclast, and the organic matrix is then resorbed. The fact that bone resorption takes place in the region of the osteoclast adjacent to the bone surface, where the extracellular pH is low, lends support to the concept that this unique acid environment is required for solubilization of the bone mineral. The alkaline phosphatase of bone cells is an ectoenzyme that is released into the extracellular fluid. Increased circulating levels of the bone-derived enzyme are correlated with rates of bone formation. Other circulating markers of bone formation include osteocalcin and type I procollagen peptides. Markers for bone resorption are urinary excretion of hydroxyproline, hydroxylysine and its glycosides, and the bone-specific hydroxypyridinium collagen cross-links.

CALCIUM METABOLISM There is about 1 to 2 kg calcium in the average adult human body, of which over 98 percent is in the skeleton. The calcium of the mineral phase at the surface of the crystals is in equilibrium with ions of the extracellular fluid, but only a minor proportion of the total calcium (about 0.5 percent) is exchangeable. The calcium in the extracellular fluid is critical for a variety of functions, and it is remarkably constant. In normal adults, the range of plasma concentration is 2.2 to 2.6 mmol/L (8.8 to 10.4 mg/dL). The calcium in plasma is in three forms: as free ions, bound to plasma proteins, and, to a small extent, as diffusible complexes. The concentration of free calcium ions, mean 1.2 mmol/L (4.8 mg/dL), influences neuromuscular irritability and other cellular functions and is subjected to tight hormonal control, especially through parathyroid hormone, as described below. The concentration of serum proteins is an important factor in determining the concentration of calcium ions; most of the protein binding is to albumin. One formula that approximates the amount of calcium bound to proteins is

$$\% \text{ protein-bound Ca} = 0.8 \times \text{albumin (g/L)} + 0.2 \times \text{globulin (g/L)} + 3$$

Another correction is to subtract 0.25 mmol/L from the serum calcium concentration for every 10 g/L serum albumin lower than 40 g/L. Thus the concentration of ultrafiltrable calcium is usually about half the total calcium. In most laboratories only total calcium is determined, and knowledge of the concentration of proteins is essential to estimate concentration of calcium ions. Free ions can be measured directly with the use of calcium-specific electrodes.

Calcium ions inside the cell mediate a variety of cellular functions (see also Chap. 68). Most of the cellular calcium is in the form of insoluble complexes. The concentration of free calcium within the cell, which is critical for functional regulation, is low, approximately 0.1 μmol/L; thus, the gradient between plasma and intracellular free calcium is about 10,000 to 1. This gradient is tightly regulated. The concentration of calcium ions in the extracellular fluid is kept constant by the interaction of processes that constantly feed calcium into and withdraw calcium from the extracellular fluid. Calcium enters the plasma via absorption from the intestinal tract and by resorption of ions from the bone mineral. Calcium leaves the extracellular fluid via secretion into the gastrointestinal tract, urinary excretion, deposition in bone mineral, and, to a minor extent, via losses in sweat. Resorption and formation are usually tightly coupled, approximately 12 mmol (500 mg) calcium entering and leaving the skeleton daily (Fig. 339-2).

The average dietary calcium intake for adults in the United States when surveyed has been found lower than expected [15 to 20 mmol/d (0.6 to 0.8 g/d)]. However, with the heightened awareness of the role of adequate calcium intake for the prevention of osteoporosis, those on some type of supplement have an average intake of 20 to 37 mmol/d (0.8 to 1.5 g/d). In adults less than half of the calcium in the diet is absorbed. Calcium absorption increases during periods of rapid growth in children, in pregnancy, and in lactation and decreases with advancing age. If adequate vitamin D is available and vitamin D metabolism is normal, more dietary calcium is absorbed (adaptation). Most of the calcium is absorbed in the proximal small intestine, and the efficiency of absorption decreases in the more distal intestinal segments. Both active transport and diffusion-limited absorption are involved; the former is more important in the upper, and the latter is more important in the lower, intestine. Both are influenced by vitamin D through the action of its metabolites. All forms of calcium in the diet may not be equally absorbed; even with defined salts, calcium as the chloride is probably absorbed more efficiently than that in other preparations.

Calcium is also secreted into the lumen of the gastrointestinal tract. When isotopes of radioactive calcium are administered intravenously, radioactivity appears in the feces, making possible calculations of *endogenous fecal calcium* (Fig. 339-2). Higher estimates of calcium losses in intestinal juices have been made by other approaches. Secretion of calcium into the intestinal lumen is constant and independent of absorption. If calcium availability in the diet is low [less than 12 mmol/d (500 mg/d)], positive calcium balance requires an efficiency of absorption greater than 30 to 40 percent if intestinal uptake is sufficient to exceed losses via intestinal secretion and to match calcium losses through renal calcium excretion.

The urinary calcium excretion of normal adults on average calcium intakes ranges between 2.5 and 10 mmol/d (100 and 400 mg/d). When the dietary calcium is below 5 mmol (200 mg) daily, urinary calcium excretion is usually less than 5 mmol/d (200 mg/d). However, in most normal individuals the level of dietary intake over a wide range has relatively little effect on the urinary excretion of calcium. Hence, in individuals on diets low in calcium, this relative inefficiency of renal calcium conservation leads to negative calcium balance unless calcium absorption is maximally efficient (Fig. 339-2).

The amount of calcium in the urine is minute compared with that filtered through the glomerulus [about 150 to 250 mmol/d (6 to 10 g/d)]. The rates of reabsorption of the filtered calcium are high compared to rates of excretion. Reabsorption takes place predominantly in the proximal tubule (~60 percent) and in Henle's loop (~25 percent). Relatively small amounts of filtered calcium are reabsorbed in the distal tubule. It is not certain whether non-protein-bound, nonionic forms of calcium (e.g., calcium citrate) are cleared at different rates. The excretion of other electrolytes affects the urinary excretion of calcium. For example, urinary calcium is usually proportional to urinary sodium; sulfate also increases calcium excretion.

Maintenance of calcium balance (Fig. 339-2) is dependent upon the efficiency of intestinal absorption. Deficiency of parathyroid hormone or vitamin D, intestinal disease, or severe dietary calcium deprivation may provide challenges to calcium homeostasis that cannot be compensated adequately by renal calcium conservation, resulting in negative calcium balance. Increased bone resorption may protect against extracellular fluid calcium depletion even in states of chronic negative calcium balance but only at the expense of progressive osteopenia.

Pathophysiology Decrease in the concentration of free calcium ions in plasma results in increased neuromuscular irritability and the syndrome of tetany. This syndrome is characterized, when fully expressed, by peripheral and perioral paresthesias, carpal spasm, pedal spasm, anxiety, seizures, bronchospasm, laryngospasm, Chvostek's, Trousseau's, and Erb's signs, and lengthening of the QT interval of the electrocardiogram. In infants tetany may be manifested only by irritability and lethargy. The level of calcium ions that determines which features of tetany will be manifested varies among individuals. Tetany is also influenced by the concentration of other components of the extracellular fluid. For example, hypomagnesemia and alkalosis lower the threshold for tetany, whereas hypokalemia and acidosis raise the threshold.

Increases in total serum calcium are usually accompanied by increases in calcium ions and may be associated with anorexia, nausea, vomiting, constipation, hypotonia, depression, and occasionally lethargy and coma. Persistent hypercalcemia, especially when accompanied by normal or elevated levels of serum phosphate, may result in ectopic deposition of a solid phase of calcium and phosphate in walls of blood vessels, connective tissue about the joints, gastric mucosa, cornea, and renal parenchyma. Hypercalcemia per se alters renal function in addition to the pathologic effects of calcium-phosphate deposits in the lumen of renal tubules and in the interstitial areas of the kidney.

PHOSPHORUS METABOLISM Phosphorus is a major component of bone and of all other tissues and in some form is involved in almost all metabolic processes. The total amount of phosphorus in the normal adult is about 32 mol (1 kg), of which about 85 percent is in the skeleton.

In fasting plasma most of the phosphorus is present as inorganic orthophosphate in concentrations of approximately 0.9 to 1.3 mmol/L (2.8 to 4 mg/dL). In contrast to calcium, where about 50 percent is bound, only about 12 percent of the phosphorus in plasma is bound to proteins. Free HPO_4^{2-} and $NaHPO_4^-$ normally are about 75 percent of the total plasma phosphorus, and free $H_2PO_4^-$ is 10 percent. Since so many species are present, depending upon pH and other factors, it has been the convention to express concentrations in terms of mass of elemental phosphorus, i.e., milligrams phosphorus per deciliter, or molarity. Total phosphorus levels are higher in children and tend to rise in women after the menopause. There is a circadian variation of phosphorus concentration even during a 24-h fast, mediated in part by the adrenal cortex. The nadir occurs at about 9 A.M., and the maximum is at about 2 P.M. The magnitudes of the peaks and troughs vary with phosphorus intake but occur regardless of whether the intake is high or low. Despite changes in serum phosphorus levels of nearly twofold, serum ionized calcium levels do not change significantly.

During phosphate depletion, phosphaturia decreases before phosphatemia. This adaptive response of increasing tubular transport when luminal concentrations are decreasing can be observed in the coupled sodium/phosphorus transport of isolated renal tubular cells and is thus an intrinsic property of these cells. There is also heterogeneity of phosphorus transport among different segments of proximal renal tubules. Tubular fluxes of phosphorus rather than hypophosphatemia per se may be critical in modulating effects of hypophosphatemia such as the stimulation of 25(OH)D-1α-hydroxylase. Conversely, increased phosphorus loads and increased renal tubular phosphorus fluxes result in decreased renal tubular reabsorption of phosphorus and increased clearance and suppress the activity of 25(OH)D-1α-hydroxylase (see below). Ingestion of carbohydrate depresses serum phosphorus acutely by 0.3 to 0.5 mmol/L (1 to 1.5 mg/dL), presumably as the result of cellular uptake and formation of phosphate esters. Ingestion of phosphorus per se increases serum levels. Therefore, it is essential for the interpretation of serum levels and urinary clearances that samples be obtained in the fasting state. Decreases in plasma phosphorus also occur during induction of alkalosis.

Whereas only a small proportion of dietary calcium is absorbed from the intestine, phosphorus absorption is remarkably efficient. At low levels of dietary intake (less than 2 mg/kg body weight per day) 80 to 90 percent of ingested phosphorus is absorbed. Even with the higher levels of intake (greater than 10 mg/kg body weight per day) in the form of dairy products, cereals, eggs, and meat, absorption is about 70 percent. Hypophosphatemia due to deficient intestinal absorption is unusual except when excessive quantities of nonabsorbable antacids are consumed; the antacids bind phosphorus and prevent absorption from the intestinal lumen.

The major control of phosphorus economy is exerted at the level of the kidney. Phosphorus filtered through the glomerulus is largely reabsorbed in the proximal tubule (there is homeostatically important distal reabsorption as well) so that normally only about 10 to 15 percent of the filtered load is excreted. When filtered loads of phosphorus decrease, proximal tubular reabsorption increases. Conversely, when phosphorus loads are increased, tubular reabsorption decreases, and clearance rises. Thus, the urinary excretion of phosphorus normally reflects dietary intake, and conservation or elimination of excessive amounts of the ion depends upon adequate renal handling (Fig. 339-3). There is no good evidence for renal tubular phosphate secretion. Proximal reabsorption of phosphorus is dependent upon parallel sodium reabsorption, but whereas the sodium rejected by the proximal tubule may be reabsorbed distally, the rejected phosphorus is not. Therefore, the effects of volume expansion and decreased sodium reabsorption are to increase phosphorus clearance; similarly, diuretics such as acetazolamide, which act proximally, are phosphaturic parallel to the degree to which they are natriuretic.

Pathophysiology No direct symptoms result from hyperphosphatemia. However, when high levels are maintained for long periods, the driving force for mineralization is increased, and calcium phosphate may be deposited in abnormal sites. Ectopic calcification of

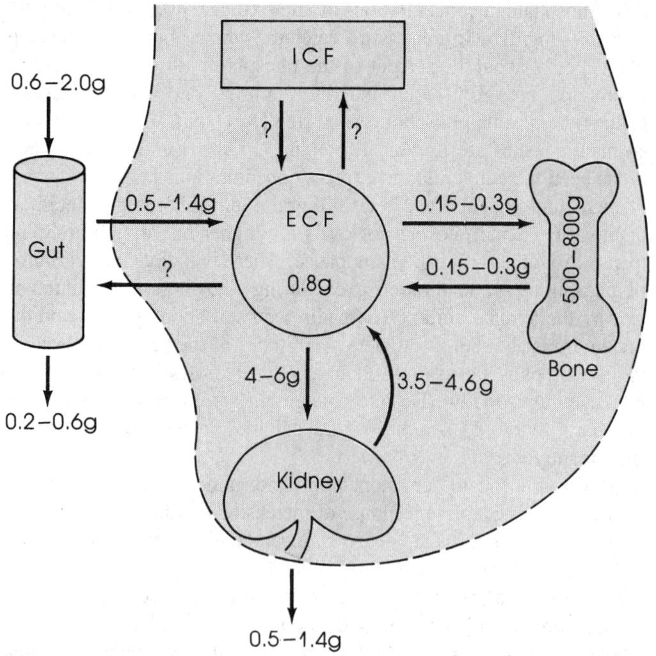

FIGURE 339-3 Phosphate homeostasis. Schematic illustration of inorganic phosphorus content (termed here phosphate) in extracellular fluid (ECF) and bone as well as diet and feces; magnitude of phosphorus flux per day as estimated by various methods is shown at transport sites in intestine, kidney, and bone. Range of values shown illustrates special features of phosphorus metabolism discussed in text. Intestinal phosphorus absorption is highly efficient, 85 percent at a lower intake (0.5 g of a 0.6-g intake) and 70 percent at a higher intake (1.4 g of a 2.0-g intake). Estimates of magnitude of endogenous fecal phosphate are less well established than for calcium. Contribution of at least 0.15 g is estimated to be added to the nonabsorbed phosphorus to provide a total of 0.2 g fecal phosphorus at the low intake level. At high phosphorus dietary intakes, no correction for endogenous fecal phosphate is calculated. Higher quantities of phosphorus are excreted in urine at all levels of dietary intake than for corresponding intakes of calcium; quantities excreted match closely the quantities absorbed, thereby maintaining phosphorus balance (no correction in this illustration is made for endogenous fecal phosphorus). Note that renal phosphorus reabsorption, in contrast to high and relatively invariant renal calcium reabsorption, varies from a low of 75 percent of filtered load to greater than 85 percent. The compartment labeled ICF refers to intracellular phosphorus, both organic and inorganic; rapid shifts of phosphorus into cells (and corresponding, possibly slower, efflux of phosphorus from cells) contribute to changes in ECF phosphorus. These shifts between ECF and ICF and phosphorus release from and uptake by bone are equal in conditions of phosphorus balance.

this type is thus encountered in untreated chronic renal failure with severe hypercalcemia and in vitamin D intoxication. *Tumoral calcinosis* is a rare heritable disorder in which ectopic calcification is associated with hyperphosphatemia and normal glomerular filtration rates (GFR). The disorder is characterized by high ratio of phosphorus tubule maximum (TmP) to GFR and increased serum levels of $1,25(OH)_2D$. The latter is a paradoxical finding and presumably is related to the abnormal renal tubular phosphate fluxes. Severe, acute hypophosphatemia may or may not be accompanied by symptoms such as anorexia, dizziness, bone pain, proximal muscular weakness, and waddling gait. Significant hypophosphatemia is encountered in severe alcoholics and is aggravated after repletion of nutrients, in the course of therapy of diabetic ketoacidosis, and for various reasons in severely ill, hospitalized elderly patients (see also Chap. 342). Myopathy may be present when hypophosphatemia is severe and may be accompanied by elevations in levels of serum creatinine kinase and rhabdomyolysis. Severe congestive cardiomyopathy has also been noted with chronic hypophosphatemia; restoration of phosphorus deficits leads to prompt reversal of the abnormalities. Respiratory muscle weakness is also common in the setting of severe hypophosphatemia and may improve with phosphate repletion. The bone pain and waddling gait are attributed to the osteomalacia which develops as a result of phosphate depletion. The muscular weakness may be due either to direct effects of hypophosphatemia on nerves and muscle or, in some instances, to the effects of hyperparathyroidism (either primary or secondary) which may have a role in the etiology of the hypophosphatemia. Defective growth in children may also be due to phosphate depletion. Hypophosphatemia results in decreased levels of 2,3-diphosphoglyceric acid and adenosine triphosphate (ATP) in erythrocytes which in turn alter the dissociation of oxyhemoglobin so that less oxygen is delivered in the periphery. Hemolytic anemia may be produced as the result of impairment of the ability of erythrocytes to deform in small vessels.

Negative phosphorus balance (Fig. 339-3) is rarely caused by inadequate phosphorus absorption in the intestine, and maintenance of normal phosphorus balance is dependent upon efficiency of renal excretion or conservation. In severe renal failure, hyperphosphatemia results from inadequate renal phosphorus clearance; heritable or acquired renal tubular defects may lead to hypophosphatemia due to inadequate renal conservation of phosphorus.

VITAMIN D

Vitamin D is a hormone, not a vitamin. With adequate exposure to sunlight, no dietary supplements are needed. The active principle of vitamin D is synthesized under metabolic control via successive hydroxylations in the liver and kidney and is transported through the blood to its target tissues (the small intestine and bone) to help maintain calcium homeostasis. Calcium and phosphate ions, parathyroid hormone, and possibly other peptide and steroid hormones play major roles directly or indirectly in the regulation of the renal metabolism of vitamin D. Analysis of hereditary and acquired defects in these metabolic processes have provided new insights into the pathophysiology of several disorders involving calcium, phosphorus, and bone metabolism. These discoveries have been the impetus for several advances, including the chemical synthesis of active vitamin D metabolites and analogues, the clinical use of 1α,25-dihydroxyvitamin D_3 [$1,25(OH)_2D_3$] (calcitriol) in many vitamin D–resistant disorders, the development and application of assays for measuring vitamin D metabolites in blood to define suspected abnormalities in vitamin D metabolism, and a growing interest in developing more potent vitamin D analogues for clinical use.

PHOTOBIOGENESIS OF VITAMIN D Vitamin D_3 is a derivative of 7-dehydrocholesterol (provitamin D_3), the immediate precursor of cholesterol. When skin is exposed to sunlight or certain artifical light sources, the ultraviolet radiation enters the epidermis and causes a variety of photobiochemical events. Among them is the transformation of 7-dehydrocholesterol to vitamin D_3. Wavelengths between 290 and 315 nm are absorbed by the conjugated double bonds at C_5 and C_7 of 7-dehydrocholesterol that result in the fragmentation of the B ring between C_9 and C_{10} to yield a 9,10-secosterol (*seco* means "split"), previtamin D_3 (Fig. 339-4). Previtamin D_3 is biologically inert but is thermally labile and spontaneously undergoes a temperature-dependent molecular rearrangement of its conjugated triene system (three double bonds) to form the thermally stable 9,10-secosterol, vitamin D_3 (Fig. 339-4). At body temperature it takes approximately 3 days for previtamin D_3 to convert completely into vitamin D_3. Large changes in the temperature of the surface of the skin do not affect the rate of this conversion because the process occurs in the actively growing layers of the epidermis where the temperature is relatively constant; changes in the core body temperature also have little effect on this reaction. Once vitamin D_3 is synthesized, it is translocated from the epidermis into the circulation by the vitamin D–binding protein. Thus, vitamin D_3 is made in the skin from previtamin for days after a single sun exposure (Fig. 339-4). Although melanin in the skin competes with 7-dehydrocho-

FIGURE 339-4 Photobiogenesis and metabolic pathways for vitamin D production and metabolism. Circled letters and numbers denote specific enzymes: *7* = 7-dehydrocholesterol reductase; *25* = vitamin D-25-hydroxylase; *1α* = 25(OH)D-1α-hydroxylase; *24R* = 25(OH)D-24R-hydroxylase; *26* = 25(OH)D-26-hydroxylase. The insert denotes the basic $\Delta^{5,7}$-diene steroid structures for the precursors of vitamin D_2 (ergosterol) and vitamin D_3 (7-dehydrocholesterol) and the 9,10-secosteroid structures of vitamin D_2 (ergocalciferol) and vitamin D_3 (cholecalciferol). Historically, the subscripts for vitamin D are related to the order in which the compounds were isolated and characterized. What was originally called vitamin D_1 is a mixture of compounds, and the term is no longer used. The next two vitamin D compounds, vitamin D_2 and vitamin D_3, were isolated, respectively, from the irradiation products of ergosterol (a $\Delta^{5,7}$-diene steroid found primarily in plants) and 7-dehydrocholesterol (a $\Delta^{5,7}$-diene steroid precursor of cholesterol present in animal tissues, including humans). Vitamin D_2 and D_3 differ in their side chains; the side chain for vitamin D_2 contains a Δ^{22} and a C_{24}-methyl group. Even though vitamin D_3 is the only endogenous form of vitamin D in skin, both vitamins D_2 and D_3 are metabolized identically and have equivalent biologic potencies in most mammals; in the absence of subscript the term vitamin D may refer to either compound.

In steroid nomenclature, substituents on the steroid ring skeleton that are spatially oriented below the plane of the molecule (drawn as a broken line) are called α *substituents*, and those substituents spatially oriented above the plane of the molecule (drawn as a solid line) are called β *substituents*. Because vitamin D is a structural derivative of a $\Delta^{5,7}$-diene steroid, by convention the numbering of the carbon atoms and the stereochemical designation of the functional groups remain the same as for the parent steroid. During the transformation $\Delta^{5,7}$-diene→previtamin D→vitamin D, the geometric position of ring A is altered, thereby changing the stereochemical orientation of its substituents; nonetheless, the original designation(s) of the hydroxyl function(s) on ring A of the steroid precursor are retained. The R,S notation, as in 24R,25-dihydroxy-vitamin D_3, specifies the spatial configuration of a substituent at an asymmetric carbon center.

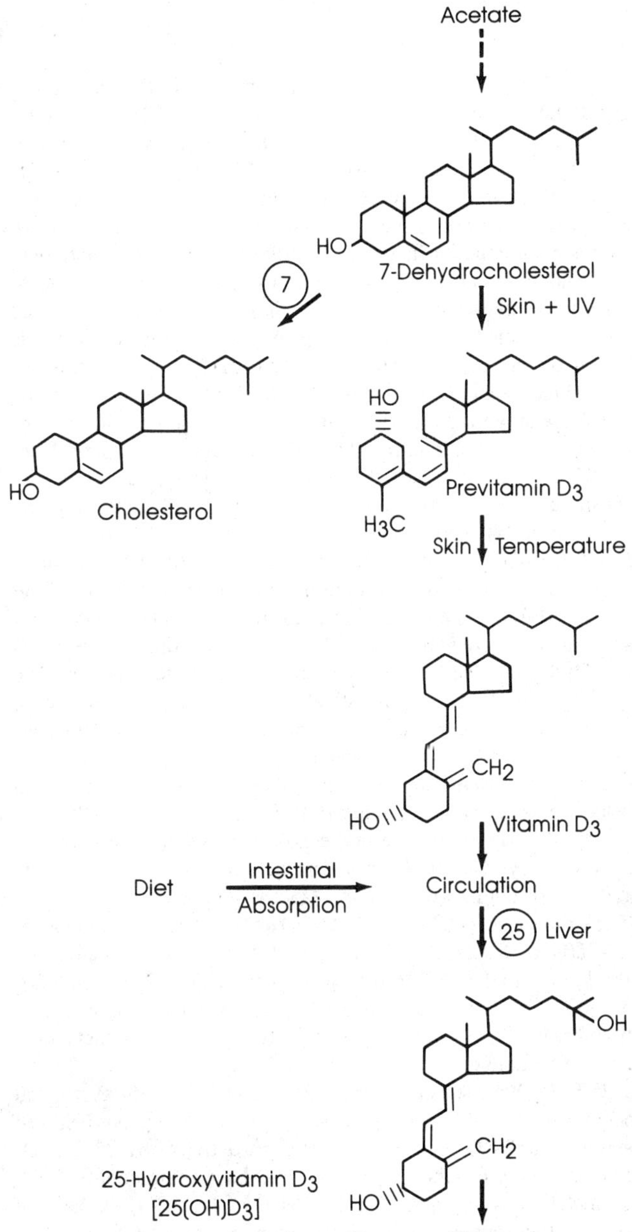

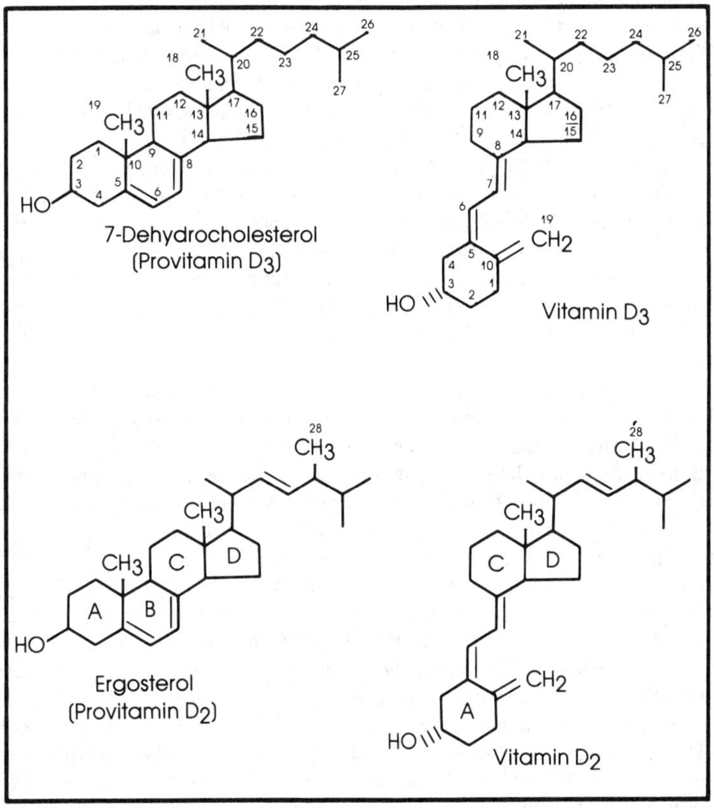

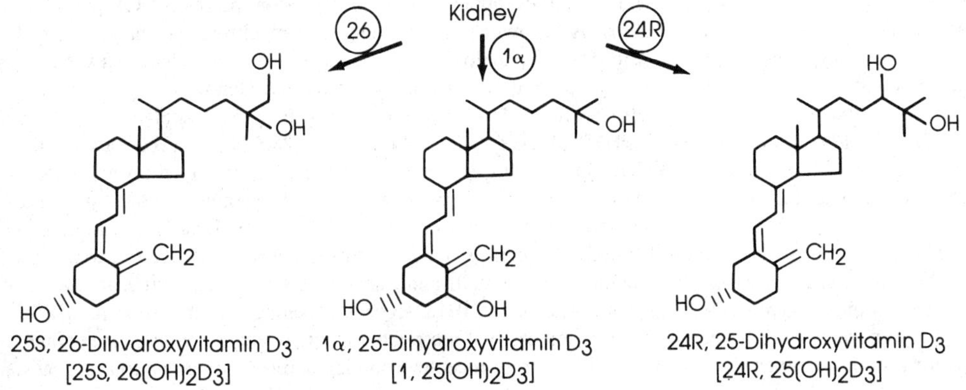

lesterol for ultraviolet photons and thus can limit the synthesis of previtamin D_3, the photochemical isomerization of previtamin D_3 to two biologically inert products (lumisterol$_3$ and tachysterol$_3$) appears to be more important in preventing excessive production of previtamin D_3 during prolonged exposure to the sun.

Aging decreases the capacity of the skin to produce vitamin D_3; greater than twofold reduction occurs after the age of 70 years. Topical sunscreens reduce cutaneous vitamin D_3 production by absorbing the solar radiation that is responsible for vitamin D_3 synthesis in the skin. Other factors that affect the cutaneous synthesis of vitamin D_3 include altitude, geographical location, time of day, and area of exposure. Latitude has profound effects on the cutaneous synthesis of vitamin D_3. As the zenith angle of the sun increases with approaching winter more of the high-energy ultraviolet photons responsible for previtamin D_3 synthesis are absorbed by the ozone layer. In Boston (42°N) and in Edmonton (52°N) the absorption of these photons is so complete that no vitamin D_3 is made in the skin between the months of November through February and October through March respectively. When the entire body is exposed to sufficient sunlight to cause mild erythema, the increase in the blood vitamin D is equivalent to consuming an oral dose of 10,000 international units (1 IU = 0.025 μg) of vitamin D_3. Only when skin radiation is insufficient to produce the required quantities of vitamin D_3 is there a need for dietary supplementation to prevent skeletal mineralization defects. Fish liver oils, a natural source of vitamin D, were used widely for the treatment of rickets early in this century. Crystalline vitamin D_2 (Fig. 339-4) or vitamin D_3 is now added to milk and cereals. Such supplementations prevent rickets and osteomalacia. The National Research Council of the United States recommends an intake of 200 IU per day for adults.

METABOLISM OF VITAMIN D Once vitamin D enters the circulation, either by its absorption from the diet or through the skin, it is transported to the liver bound to a specific alpha$_1$ globulin (vitamin D–binding protein). In the liver, vitamin D is metabolized to 25-hydroxyvitamin D [25(OH)D] by hepatic mitochondrial and/or microsomal enzyme(s) (Fig. 339-4). 25(OH)D is one of the major circulating metabolites of vitamin D, and its half-life is estimated to be about 21 days. The concentration of 25(OH)D and some of its metabolites in the serum is measured using competitive binding assays. The normal circulating concentration of 25(OH)D varies among different laboratories from 12 to 200 nmol/L (5 to 80 ng/mL). Individuals exposed to excessive sunlight may have concentrations of 25(OH)D up to 370 nmol/L (150 ng/mL) without adverse effects on calcium metabolism. Assays that employ chromatographic separation prior to binding analysis often have a lower normal range, possibly because other vitamin D metabolites simulate 25(OH)D in this assay. The normal range, apparently independent of method, is lower in Great Britain than in the United States; in Great Britain dietary supplements of vitamin D are not routine, and exposure to sunlight is less than in most regions of the United States. The serum 25(OH)D levels routinely measured reflect both 25-hydroxyvitamin D_2 [25(OH)D_2] and 25-hydroxyvitamin D_3 [25(OH)D_3]. The ratio of these two 25-hydroxylated derivatives depends on the relative amounts of vitamins D_2 or D_3 present in the diet and the amount of previtamin D_3 produced by exposure to sunlight.

The hepatic 25-hydroxylation of vitamin D is regulated by a product feedback mechanism. This regulation, however, is not tight; an increase in dietary intake or endogenous production of vitamin D_3 is reflected by elevations in 25(OH)D concentration levels in the serum. The levels can rise to greater than 1200 nmol/L (500 ng/mL) when the intake of vitamin D is increased. Serum 25(OH)D concentration levels are reduced in severe chronic parenchymal and cholestatic liver disease (Table 339-1).

25(OH)D is not biologically active at physiologic levels in vivo but is active in vitro at high concentrations. Normally, after formation in the liver, 25(OH)D is bound by the high-affinity vitamin D–binding protein that is synthesized in the liver and transported to the kidney for an additional stereospecific hydroxylation on either C_1 or C_{24} (Fig. 339-4). The kidney plays a pivotal role in the metabolism of 25(OH)D to the biologically active metabolite. The renal mitochondrial 25(OH)D-1α-hydroxylase activity is enhanced by hypocalcemia so that the rate of conversion of 25(OH)D to 1,25(OH)$_2$D increases. However, hypocalcemia may not control this hydroxylation directly. Any decrease in the serum concentration of calcium below normal is a stimulus for increased secretion of parathyroid hormone. Parathyroid hormone acts physiologically as a tropic hormone to increase the synthesis of 1,25(OH)$_2$D in the renal proximal convoluted tubule. The mechanism by which parathyroid hormone exerts its influence on the renal metabolism of 25(OH)D is not established; however, the renal production of 1,25(OH)$_2$D correlates with the effects of parathyroid hormone in lowering circulating concentrations (and presumably renal intracellular concentrations) of phosphate. 1,25(OH)$_2$D also influences the renal metabolism of 25(OH)D by diminishing 25(OH)D-1α-hydroxylase activity and enhancing the metabolism of 24R,25-dihydroxyvitamin D [24,25(OH)$_2$D].

TABLE 339-1 Serum concentrations of 25(OH)D in disorders of calcium, phosphorus, and bone metabolism

Disease states	Serum 25(OH)D
Vitamin D deficiency	↓
Intestinal malabsorption syndromes	↓
Liver disorders (chronic and severe)	↓
Nephrotic syndrome	↓
Osteopenia in the aged	N or ↓
Vitamin D intoxication	↑

NOTE: ↓ = decreased; N = normal; ↑ = increased.

24,25(OH)$_2$D is a circulating metabolite of 25(OH)D normally present in serum at a concentration of 1 to 10 nmol (0.5 to 5.0 ng/mL). 24,25(OH)$_2$D is also a substrate for renal 25(OH)D-1α-hydroxylase and is converted to 1α,24R,25-trihydroxyvitamin D [1,24,25(OH)$_3$D]. This trihydroxy metabolite is less potent than 1,25(OH)$_2$D in stimulating intestinal calcium transport; whether it has a physiologic role in maintaining calcium homeostasis is unclear. Cultured cells that possess nuclear receptors for 1,25(OH)$_2$D, such as chondrocytes, skin keratinocytes and fibroblasts, intestinal, and melanoma cells, also metabolize 25(OH)D to 24,25(OH)$_2$D. Although 24,25(OH)$_2$D may play a role in the expression of vitamin D action, it is more likely, that the C-24 hydroxylation is the first step in the degradation of both 25(OH)D and 1,25(OH)$_2$D.

The kidney also metabolizes 25(OH)D to 25S,26-dihydroxyvitamin D [25,26(OH)$_2$D]. 25,26(OH)$_2$D, like 24,25(OH)$_2$D, is metabolized by the kidney to 1α,25S,26-trihydroxyvitamin D [1,25,26(OH)$_3$D]. 1,25,26(OH)$_3$D is less active than 1,25(OH)$_2$D in inducing intestinal calcium transport, and the physiologic function of this metabolite remains to be defined.

1,25(OH)$_2$D is a substrate for the 25(OH)D–24R-hydroxylase and is metabolized to 1,24,25(OH)$_3$D, but this conversion is not believed to be important for the expression of biologic activity of 1,25(OH)$_2$D. More than twenty metabolites of vitamin D have been identified. All of the metabolites originate from 25(OH)D or 1,25(OH)$_2$D. Most of the metabolites appear to be degradation products. Of particular interest is the metabolic sequence that results in the inactivation of 1,25(OH)$_2$D by the oxidative cleavage of the side chain between C_{23} and C_{24} to yield a biologically inert and water-soluble product, 1α-hydroxyvitamin D–23-carboxylic acid (calcitroic acid).

PHYSIOLOGY OF VITAMIN D 1,25(OH)$_2$D, produced by the kidney and during pregnancy by the placenta, is the only known important metabolite of vitamin D; the potential roles of other metabolites have not been clarified. 1,25(OH)$_2$D bound to a vitamin D–binding protein is delivered to the intestine, where the free form is taken up by the cells and transported to a specific nuclear receptor protein. The 1,25(OH)$_2$D receptor belongs to the superfamily of steroid receptors that are related to the oncogene v-*erb*A (see Chap. 311). The vitamin-receptor complex activates transcription of genes;

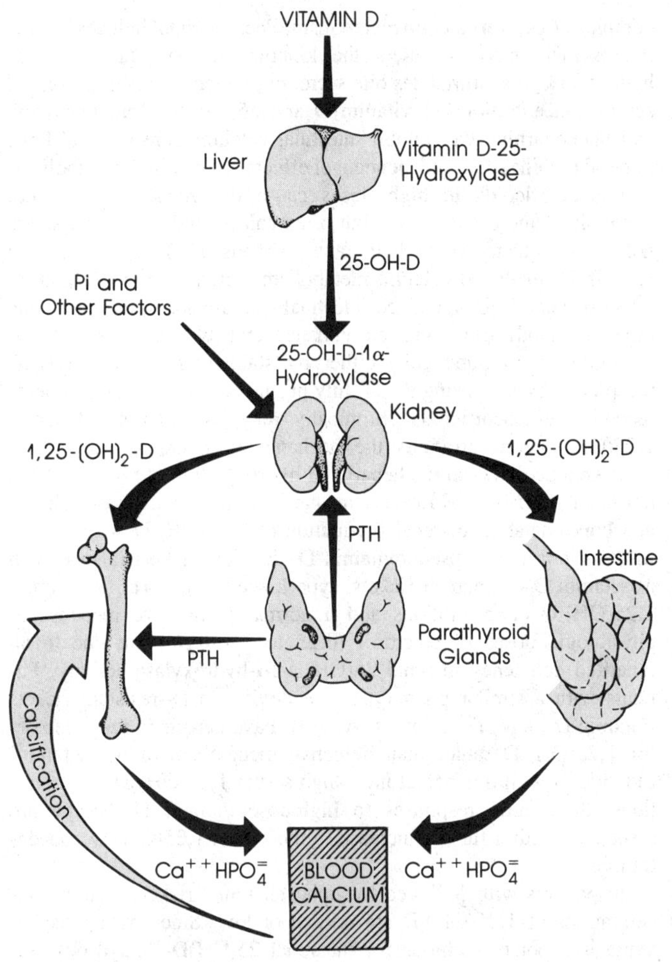

FIGURE 339-5 Schematic representation of the hormonal control loop for vitamin D metabolism and function. A reduction in the serum calcium below approximately 2.2 mmol/L (8.8 mg/dL) prompts a proportional secretion of parathyroid hormone that acts to mobilize calcium stores from the bone. Parathyroid hormone also promotes the synthesis of 1,25(OH)$_2$D in the kidney, which, in turn, stimulates the mobilization of calcium from bone and intestine. (*From MF Holick, Kidney Int 32:912, 1987.*)

in the intestine calcium-binding protein is synthesized, and in bone osteocalcin is produced. Some evidence suggests that 1,25(OH)$_2$D may also have nonnuclear effects on its target tissues; 1,25(OH)$_2$D increases the transport of calcium from the extracellular to intracellular space, and it can mobilize intracellular calcium concentrations from intracellular calcium pools. In the intestine the net effect of 1,25(OH)$_2$D is to stimulate calcium and phosphate transport from the small intestinal lumen into the circulation (Fig. 339-5). The effect of 1,25(OH)$_2$D on the enhancement of bone resorption is believed to be synergistic with parathyroid hormone. Mature osteoclasts do not possess receptors either for parathyroid hormone or 1,25(OH)$_2$D. Some evidence suggests that parathyroid hormone and 1,25(OH)$_2$D increase bone resorption activity by stimulating immature osteoclastic precursors that possess receptors for both parathyroid hormone and 1,25(OH)$_2$D to become mature osteoclasts and/or by interacting with osteoblasts to produce cytokines that enhance the activity of mature osteoclasts. The role of 1,25(OH)$_2$D on the renal handling of calcium and phosphorus remains uncertain.

Receptors for 1,25(OH)$_2$D are present in intestine, bone, and kidney and in tissues and cells that have not classically been recognized as target organs for this hormone, including skin, breast, pituitary gland, parathyroid glands, beta cells of the pancreatic islets, gonads, brain, skeletal muscle, circulating monocytes, and activated B and T lymphocytes. Although the physiologic role of 1,25(OH)$_2$D in these cells remains to be determined, 1,25(OH)$_2$D in vitro inhibits proliferation of human keratinocytes and fibroblasts, stimulates terminal differentiation of human keratinocytes, induces monocytes to produce interleukin 1 and to mature into macrophages and osteoclast-like cells, and inhibits interleukin 2 and immunoglobulin production by activated T and B lymphocytes, respectively. In addition, a variety of tumor cell lines including breast carcinomas, melanomas, and promyeloblasts possess receptors for 1,25(OH)$_2$D.

Cultured tumor cell lines that possess receptors for this hormone respond to the hormone by decreasing the rate of proliferation and by enhancing differentiation. For example, when malignant, receptor-positive human promyelocytic cells (HL-60) are exposed to 1,25(OH)$_2$D, the cells mature into functioning macrophages within 1 week. Although the mechanism of 1,25(OH)$_2$D induction of maturation is unknown, 1,25(OH)$_2$D decreases the expression of c-*myc* oncogene coincident with decreasing replication. This effect, however, is not a lasting one; when the metabolite is removed from maturing HL-60 promyelocytes, the cells revert to their original malignant state, and expression of c-*myc* oncogene is no longer suppressed.

The importance of 1,25(OH)$_2$D in the regulation of differentiation and immunoregulation is unknown. Patients with vitamin D–dependent rickets type II who are unable to respond to physiologic concentrations of 1,25(OH)$_2$D (because of insufficient or defective receptors for this hormone) appear to have no demonstrable in vivo defects in the cellular immune response and in the growth of skin (with the exception of the associated alopecia) and other tissues. It is also interesting that when these patients receive infusions of calcium the metabolic bone disease is reversed. Although the use of 1,25(OH)$_2$D (calcitriol) for the treatment of leukemia is not efficacious, the antiproliferative activity of calcitriol has been used for the treatment of psoriasis.

Most measurements of circulating 1,25(OH)$_2$D in humans in various physiologic or pathologic states utilize a receptor/competitive binding assay (Table 339-2). Serum concentrations of vitamin D and 25(OH)D vary with the season and with vitamin D intake. Serum concentrations of 1,25(OH)$_2$D, however, appear to be unaltered by seasonal variation, by increases in dietary vitamin D, or by exposure to sunlight; as long as vitamin D supplies and circulating concentrations of 25(OH)D are sufficient, metabolic influences operate on the renal

TABLE 339-2 Serum concentrations of 1,25(OH)$_2$D in disorders of calcium, phosphorus, and bone metabolism

Disease states	Serum 1,25(OH)$_2$D
Vitamin D deficiency	$\downarrow$ *
Renal failure:	
GFR > (30 mL/min)/1.7 m^2	$\downarrow$ or N
GFR < (30 mL/min)/1.7 m^2	$\downarrow$
Hypoparathyroidism	$\downarrow$ or N
Pseudohypoparathyroidism	$\downarrow$ or N
Vitamin D–dependent rickets:	
Type I	$\downarrow$ or N
Type II	$\uparrow$ or N
X-linked vitamin D–resistant rickets	$\downarrow$ or N
Tumor-induced osteomalacia	$\downarrow$
Oncogenic hypercalcemia	$\downarrow$
Some lymphomas	$\uparrow$
Hyperparathyroidism	$\uparrow$
Sarcoidosis, tuberculosis, silicosis	$\uparrow$
Idiopathic hypercalciuria	N or $\uparrow$
Williams' syndrome	$\uparrow$
Vitamin D intoxication	$\downarrow$ or N

* Serum 1,25(OH)$_2$D concentrations are normal or elevated in occasional patients with biopsy-proven osteomalacia and undetectable or low circulating concentrations of 25(OH)D. These patients also have secondary hyperparathyroidism, and they may represent a partially treated state; if a small amount of vitamin D is obtained from the diet or generated in the skin in these patients, the vitamin is efficiently converted to 1,25(OH)$_2$D. The net effect is low or undetectable circulating concentrations of 25(OH)D along with normal or elevated concentrations of 1,25(OH)$_2$D. However, in extreme vitamin D deficiency, circulating concentrations of 1,25(OH)$_2$D are low or undetectable.

NOTE: $\downarrow$ = decreased; N = normal; $\uparrow$ = increased; GFR = glomerular filtration rate.

25(OH)D-1α-hydroxylase to ensure a closely regulated circulating concentration of $1,25(OH)_2D$. The serum concentration of $1,25(OH)_2D$ ranges from 40 to 160 pmol/L (16 to 65 pg/mL). The serum half-life of $1,25(OH)_2D$ is from 3 to 6 h.

When the serum calcium falls below normal, secretion of parathyroid hormone is enhanced, resulting in increased production of $1,25(OH)_2D$. The principal physiologic regulation of the production of $1,25(OH)_2D$ appears to involve changes in serum calcium concentrations that result in reciprocal changes in secretion of parathyroid hormone, the latter controlling, possibly through actions on serum or tissue phosphorus concentrations, the rate of $1,25(OH)_2D$ production. Other factors that enhance $1,25(OH)_2D$ production in animals include estrogen, prolactin, and growth hormone. Humans adapt to increased calcium requirements during growth, pregnancy, and lactation by increasing the efficiency of intestinal calcium absorption, possibly by enhancing 25(OH)D-1α-hydroxylase activity. During the first two trimesters of pregnancy the concentrations of $1,25(OH)_2D$ increase proportional to increases in the concentrations of the vitamin D–binding protein; concentrations of free $1,25(OH)_2D$ do not change. During the last trimester when maximal mineralization of the fetal skeleton takes place, the increased demand for calcium is met by an increase in the free concentrations of $1,25(OH)_2D$, which in turn enhance maternal intestinal calcium absorption.

PATHOPHYSIOLOGY OF DISORDERS OF VITAMIN D NUTRITION AND METABOLISM *Hypovitaminosis D* results from inadequate endogenous production of vitamin D_3 in the skin, insufficient dietary supplementation, and/or the inability of the small intestine to absorb adequate amounts of vitamin D from the diet. Disease states equivalent to hypovitaminosis D result from (1) effects of drugs that antagonize vitamin D action, (2) alterations in the metabolism of vitamin D, or (3) deficient or defective receptors for $1,25(OH)_2D$. Hypovitaminosis D results in (1) disturbances of mineral ion metabolism and secretion of parathyroid hormone and (2) mineralization defects in the skeleton (e.g., rickets in children, osteomalacia in adults). The changes in the skeleton are described in Chap. 341. With regard to calcium metabolism, lack of vitamin D action leads to insufficient intestinal calcium absorption and to hypocalcemia. The latter stimulates the secretion of parathyroid hormone (secondary hyperparathyroidism), which enhances calcium release from bone and decreases calcium clearance by the kidney, and tends to blunt the hypocalcemia. (Late in the course of untreated hypovitaminosis D, severe hypocalcemia develops.) Hypophosphatemia is more marked than hypocalcemia, especially in early stages of vitamin D deficiency. The efficiency of intestinal phosphate absorption, similar to that of calcium absorption, is decreased. The increased secretion of parathyroid hormone, although partially effective in minimizing hypocalcemia, leads to urinary phosphate wasting through decreases in renal tubular reabsorption. This latter effect may be the most significant factor in causing hypophosphatemia. With an adequate glomerular filtration rate, the predominant changes in blood are severe hypophosphatemia, moderate or slightly low levels of calcium, and increased levels of parathyroid hormone. Blood levels of 25(OH)D are low (Table 339-1). As discussed in Chap. 341 defects in skeletal mineralization may accompany these disturbances in mineral ion metabolism.

Although the conversion of vitamin D to 25(OH)D is impaired in liver disease, there is no strong correlation between low serum 25(OH)D levels and osteopenia; multiple effects of the primary disease state seem to affect skeletal metabolism as well. Patients with nephrotic syndrome who excrete more than 4 g/d of protein in urine often have low 25(OH)D levels due to the loss in the urine of the vitamin D–binding protein with its associated tightly bound 25(OH)D. Circulating concentrations of 25(OH)D can also be decreased when 25(OH)D metabolism is increased, as in sarcoidosis and hyperparathyroidism. There is a relation between chronic anticonvulsant therapy and the development of osteomalacia or rickets; mineralization defects are worse in patients on multiple drug therapy and when vitamin D intake or exposure to sunlight is inadequate. Drugs have multiple and complex effects on calcium metabolism. Phenobarbital induces hepatic microsomal enzymes, alters the kinetics of the vitamin D–25-hydroxylase, and stimulates bile secretion, which results in decreased serum concentrations of vitamin D and 25(OH)D. Both phenytoin and phenobarbital can inhibit intestinal calcium transport and bone mineral mobilization, independent of effects of vitamin D metabolism.

Glucocorticoids in high doses cause disturbances in calcium metabolism and osteoporosis, but osteomalacia and rickets per se are not a consequence of such therapy. Actions of glucocorticoids on vitamin D–mediated calcium metabolism include a direct inhibitory effect of vitamin D–mediated intestinal calcium absorption and bone mineral mobilization and an enhancement of the sensitivity of $1,25(OH)_2D$ on bone cells either by stabilizing the $1,25(OH)_2D$ receptor or by increasing the affinity or number of receptors. Patients receiving glucocorticoids chronically may have depressed serum $1,25(OH)_2D$ concentrations; the mechanism(s) is unknown.

A genetic defect in the hepatic 25-hydroxylation of vitamin D has not been described. However, in one inherited disorder of calcium and bone metabolism renal production of $1,25(OH)_2D$ is defective. In the syndrome of pseudovitamin D–deficient rickets (also known as vitamin D–dependent rickets, type I; see Chap. 341), low serum $1,25(OH)_2D$ concentrations and a normal therapeutic response to physiologic doses of calcitriol (0.25 to 1.0 μg/d) are due to an inherited deficiency in renal 25(OH)D-1α-hydroxylase activity. Patients with a similar phenotype, pseudovitamin D–resistant rickets (vitamin D–dependent rickets, type II), have defects in the receptors for $1,25(OH)_2D$ rather than defective metabolism of the vitamin. Individuals with this defect have high serum $1,25(OH)_2D$ concentrations; therapeutic responses to high-dose vitamin D therapy are associated with a further increase in the serum $1,25(OH)_2D$ concentrations.

In patients with X-linked hypophosphatemic rickets, serum concentrations of $1,25(OH)_2D$ are normal or low. Since hypophosphatemia is a potent stimulus for the renal 25(OH)D-1α-hydroxylase, the serum $1,25(OH)_2D$ concentrations should be high. Thus, even a normal serum $1,25(OH)_2D$ concentration suggests a functional defect in the 25(OH)D-1α-hydroxylase system. In some cases, the combination of calcitriol and phosphate supplements offers a therapeutic advantage to phosphate therapy by itself (Chap. 341). In patients with mild to moderate chronic renal failure [glomerular filtration rate >0.5 mL/s (>30 mL/min)] and decreased phosphate clearance, hyperphosphatemia and acidosis play important roles in suppressing the renal production of $1,25(OH)_2D$ despite high circulating concentrations of parathyroid hormone. As the destruction of the renal cortex progresses, the reserves of the 25(OH)D-1α-hydroxylase are depleted to a point at which the kidney is unable to produce sufficient quantities of $1,25(OH)_2D$ to maintain calcium homeostasis, even when serum phosphorus concentrations are normal. Under these circumstances replacement therapy with calcitriol is most beneficial (Chap. 341). Aging decreases the responsiveness of the renal 25(OH)D-1α-hydroxylase to parathyroid hormone; this causes a slight lowering of $1,25(OH)_2D$ levels in the blood and may contribute to decreased calcium absorption in the elderly.

Patients with hypocalcemia due to hypoparathyroidism or pseudohypoparathyroidism have lower than normal mean serum concentrations of $1,25(OH)_2D$ although individual values may overlap with the normal range. In these patients favorable response to small replacement doses of calcitriol (0.25 to 1.0 μg/d; see Chap. 340) occurs even when the serum 25(OH)D concentrations are higher than normal. These observations are consistent with the concept that patients with absent or ineffective action of parathyroid hormone have defective function of renal 25(OH)D-1α-hydroxylase. It is not known to what extent serum $1,25(OH)_2D$ concentrations would be restored toward normal if the hyperphosphatemia were adequately controlled.

Patients with tumor-induced (oncogenic) osteomalacia have low serum phosphorus and $1,25(OH)_2D$ levels. These tumors presumably secrete a substance(s) that causes renal phosphorus wasting and inhibits the formation of 1,25$(OH)_2$D; after removal of the tumor the serum phosphorus and 1,25$(OH)_2$D levels return to normal.

In disease states equivalent to hypervitaminosis D such as sarcoidosis (and other chronic granulomatous disorders), lymphomas, idiopathic hypercalciuria, and Williams' syndrome there is an abnormality in the metabolism of 25(OH)D to 1,25$(OH)_2$D (Table 339-2). Hypercalcemia and hypercalciuria in sarcoidosis are associated with elevated circulating concentrations of 1,25$(OH)_2$D; sarcoid granulomas metabolize 25(OH)D to 1,25$(OH)_2$D in an unregulated manner, and pulmonary alveolar macrophages from patients with sarcoidosis synthesize 1,25$(OH)_2$D. In addition, normal pulmonary macrophages can be induced to metabolize 25(OH)D to 1,25$(OH)_2$D in vitro when exposed either to lipopolysaccharides from the cell wall of gram-negative bacteria or to γ-interferon. Most patients with tumor-induced hypercalcemia have low circulating concentrations of 1,25$(OH)_2$D (Table 339-2). The exceptions are patients with several types of lymphoma (including T-cell, mixed histiocytic-lymphocytic, and B-cell immunoblastic lymphomas) whose hypercalcemia is associated with elevated concentrations of 1,25$(OH)_2$D. In one report, surgical excision of a solitary splenic lymphoma resulted in rapid return of elevated serum 1,25$(OH)_2$D and calcium levels to normal suggesting that the lymphoma metabolized 25(OH)D to 1,25$(OH)_2$D in an unregulated manner. Hypercalcemic patients with elevated blood levels of 1,25$(OH)_2$D due to unregulated production of the hormone at an extrarenal site respond to glucocorticoid therapy with a decrease in the blood concentration of 1,25$(OH)_2$D and a return of the serum calcium level to normal. There is an association between elevated circulating concentrations of 1,25$(OH)_2$D in patients with primary hyperparathyrodisim, hypercalciuria, and renal stones. Similarly, in some instances of idiopathic hypercalciuria, intestinal calcium absorption is inappropriately increased. Approximately one-third of these patients have elevated circulating 1,25$(OH)_2$D. These findings are consistent with the hypothesis that excessive 1,25$(OH)_2$D production is responsible for the hyperabsorption of calcium by the small intestine. Infants with hypercalcemia associated with supravalvular aortic stenosis, mental retardation, and elfin facies (*Williams' syndrome*) also have elevated serum 1,25$(OH)_2$D concentrations. It is not clear whether the increased levels result from abnormal synthesis or degradation of 1,25$(OH)_2$D.

PHARMACOLOGY OF VITAMIN D AND ITS METABOLITES A variety of over-the-counter vitamin preparations contain 400 IU of either vitamin D_2 or vitamin D_3. More potent forms of vitamin D (calciferol) are available in capsule and tablet form (50,000 IU) as well as in oil (500,000 IU/mL) and in oral solution (8000 IU/mL). A single oral dose of 50,000 IU of vitamin D_2 increases the circulating concentrations of vitamin D from less than 25 nmol/L (10 ng/mL) to 130 to 260 nmol/L (50 to 100 ng/mL) within 12 to 24 h; the plasma half-life is about 2 days. Serum concentrations of 25(OH)D and 1,25$(OH)_2$D are not changed. For treatment of vitamin D deficiency, 50,000 IU of vitamin D twice a week for several weeks raises the circulating concentration of 25(OH)D into the normal range; in the presence of secondary hyperparathyroidism the circulating concentrations of 1,25$(OH)_2$D can increase to supranormal levels [(up to 600 pmol/L (250 pg/mL)]. 25$(OH)D_3$ (calcifediol) is available in capsules containing either 20 or 50 μg. This drug may be useful in treating vitamin D deficiency [low 25(OH)D concentrations] in patients with severe liver dysfunction. Pharmacologic doses are used to treat disorders of 25(OH)D metabolism; in pharmacologic doses 25$(OH)D_3$ is believed to be effective through its interaction with the receptor for 1,25$(OH)_2$D. 1,25$(OH)_2$D (calcitriol) is available in capsules containing 0.25 or 0.5 μg and as a solution for intravenous use (1.0 and 2.0 μg/mL). Calcitriol is efficacious in a variety of calcium metabolic disorders (see Chap. 340). 1α-Hydroxyvitamin D_3 [1$(OH)D_3$] is also a potent 1,25$(OH)_2D_3$ agonist. The structure of this analogue is identical to that of the natural renal hormone with the exception that it lacks a C_{25}-OH (Fig. 339-6). In humans, this analogue is rapidly metabolized by the liver to 1,25$(OH)_2D_3$. This analogue is used in Europe and Japan.

When vitamin D is chemically manipulated to rotate the A ring through 180 degrees, the C_3-β-OH assumes a geometric position that mimics the C_1-α-OH (Fig. 339-6). These compounds, called pseudo-1α-hydroxyvitamin D analogues, include dihydrotachysterol and 5,6-*trans*-vitamin D. These analogues are less effective in stimulating intestinal calcium transport on a weight basis than either vitamin D or 1,25$(OH)_2$D. However, because the pseudo-1α-hydroxyvitamin D analogues do not require a renal 1α-hydroxylation to be active on intestinal calcium transport, they are 3 to 10 times more potent than vitamin D in disease states that adversely affect the renal 25(OH)D-1α-hydroxylase, such as hypoparathyroidism and chronic renal failure. These analogues are efficiently metabolized in the liver to the corresponding 25-hydroxy derivatives, which are the biologically active forms.

PARATHYROID HORMONE Physiology The function of parathyroid hormone is to maintain extracellular fluid calcium concentration. The hormone acts directly on bone and kidney and indirectly on intestine through its effects on synthesis of 1,25$(OH)_2$D to increase serum calcium; in turn, parathyroid hormone production is closely regulated by the concentration of serum ionized calcium. This feedback system is one of the most important homeostatic mechanisms. Any tendency toward hypocalcemia, as might be induced by calcium-deficient diets, is counteracted by an increased rate of secretion of parathyroid hormone. This in turn (1) acts to increase the rate of dissolution of bone mineral, thereby increasing the flow of calcium from bone into blood, (2) reduces the renal clearance of calcium, returning more of the calcium filtered at the glomerulus into extracellular fluid, and (3) increases the efficiency of calcium absorption in the intestine. The relative physiologic importance in minute-to-minute calcium homeostasis of these three actions of parathyroid hormone, stimulation of calcium transport in bone, kidney, and intestine, is not clear, but most evidence suggests that immediate control of blood calcium is due to effects of the hormone on bone and, to a lesser extent, on renal calcium clearance. Maintenance of calcium balance, on the other hand, is probably due to the effects of the hormone on 1,25$(OH)_2$D levels and hence on the efficiency of intestinal calcium absorption. As much as 12 mmol (500 mg) calcium is transferred between extracellular fluid and bone each day (a large amount in relation to the total extracellular fluid calcium pool), and parathyroid hormone has a major effect on this transfer. The action of the hormone tends to preserve calcium concentration in blood acutely at the cost of bone destruction and bone mineral release. The action of parathyroid hormone on kidney to increase the reabsorption of filtered calcium may also contribute to rapid regulation of blood calcium concentration.

Parathyroid hormone has a dual action on bone, the *calcium replacement* and the *bone remodeling* effects. There is an increased rate of release of calcium from bone into blood after administration of parathyroid hormone, the time period needed to observe the change varying with the dose of hormone and the overall metabolic status (influenced by age, diet, etc.). Usually 30 min to 1 h is required to detect a significant increase in blood calcium, but with the use of radioisotopes changes in bone calcium release can be seen within minutes. When studied carefully in animals a rapid efflux of calcium out of blood into bone, presumably into bone cells, precedes the release of calcium. On the other hand, the more chronic effects of parathyroid hormone, mainly increase in the number of osteoclasts and a general increase in the remodeling of bone, are apparent only hours after the hormone is given. These latter actions, which involve increased protein synthesis, persist for hours after parathyroid hormone has been given. It is not clear whether the two effects of parathyroid action on bone represent a continuous spectrum with a common initiating biochemical event or whether they are separate actions.

Osteoblastic cells but not osteoclasts have receptors for parathyroid hormone. The action of PTH on osteoclasts is indirect, through cytokines released from osteoblasts to activate osteoclasts, e.g., osteoblasts must be present along with osteoclasts for PTH to activate osteoclasts to resorb bone.

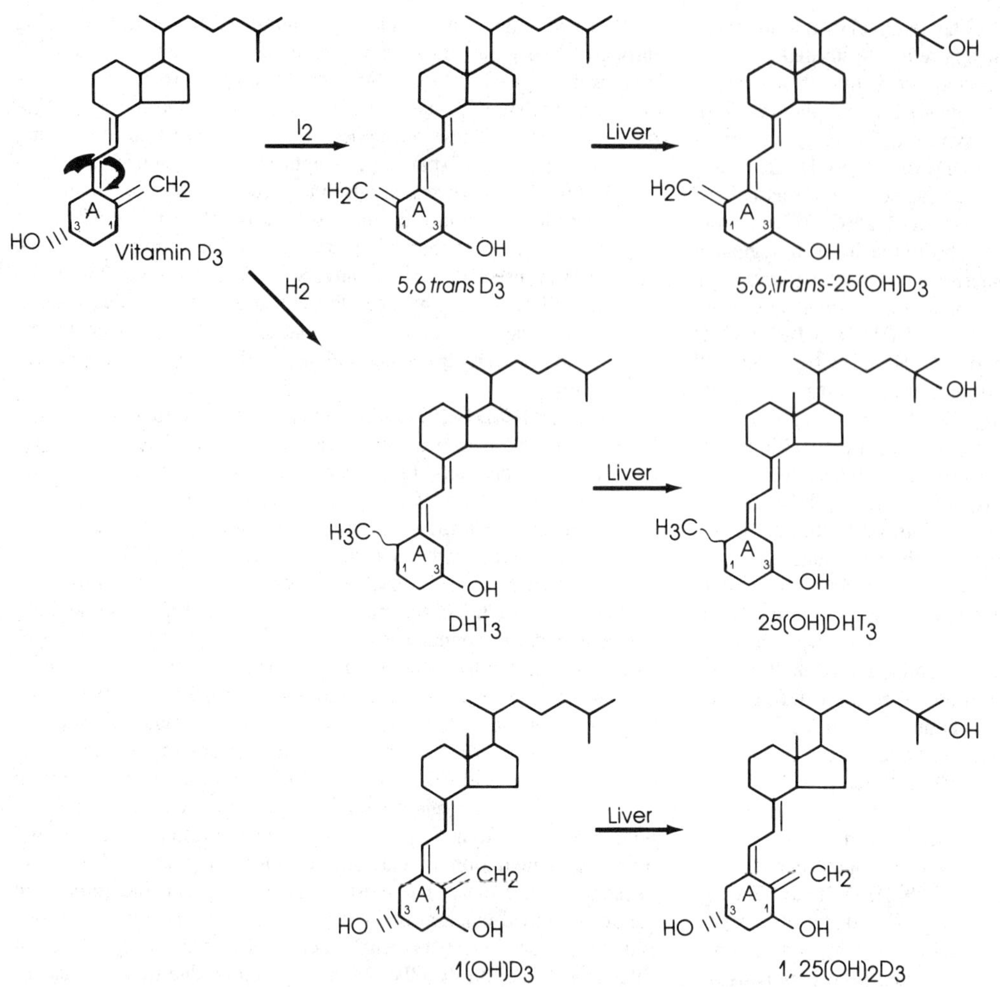

FIGURE 339-6 When vitamin D is treated with I_2 or reduced with H_2, ring A of the vitamin D molecule rotates 180° to reorient spatially the 3β-OH in a pseudo-1α-OH position. These analogues, 5,6-*trans*-vitamin D_3 and dihydrotachysterol, (DHT_3), are called pseudo-1α-hydroxy analogues. $1(OH)D_3$ is a synthetic analogue of $1,25(OH)_2D_3$ that lacks a C_{25}-OH. $1(OH)D_3$, 5,6-*trans*-vitamin D_3, and DHT_3 all undergo a hepatic C_{25}-hydroxylation before they are biologically active.

The nature of the cytokines that stimulate osteoclasts is a subject of major interest. IGF 1 and possibly other agents are candidates, but the definitive messenger(s) has not been determined.

Chemistry The complete amino acid sequences of the major forms of parathyroid hormone from cow, pig, rat, and human have been defined. The peptides consist of a single-chain structure composed of 84 amino acids. The molecules lack cysteine or cystine; the sequences of the four forms of the hormone are similar, as is illustrated in Fig. 339-7. The sequence of chicken parathyroid hormone has been deduced from the nucleotide sequence of the cloned cDNA. This molecule differs substantially from the mammalian hormones. One large sequence deletion in the middle of the molecule and a larger addition near the carboxy terminus result in a molecule of 88 rather than 84 amino acids. There is conservation in the amino-terminal portion needed for biologic actions of the molecule.

The structural requirements for the binding of the hormone to receptors and hence for its biologic activity have been defined. Synthetic fragments containing the amino-terminal sequence residues 1-34 or even shorter sequences, 2-26 being minimally active, exert the known biologic actions of the hormone on mineral ion transport in kidney and bone and by stimulating the renal 25-hydroxyvitamin D-1α-hydroxylase also exert the capacity of the hormone to stimulate intestinal calcium absorption. Since osteoblasts but not osteoclasts have receptors for parathyroid hormone, the effects of parathyroid hormone on stimulating osteoclastic bone resorption are indirect.

Fragments shortened at the amino terminus lose binding affinity more slowly than capacity to stimulate biologic response. The peptide 7-34 is a competitive inhibitor of the binding of active hormone to receptors in vitro and serves as a competitive inhibitor of the renal responses to the hormone, including the increased excretion of cyclic AMP and the enhanced clearance of phosphate. Rapid mobilization of calcium from bone is also blocked in certain test systems in vivo.

Biosynthesis, secretion, metabolism, and mode of action Several larger molecular forms have been identified in the biosynthetic sequence leading from gene transcription and translation to final packaging of the 84-amino acid peptide in secretory granules prior to secretion. The earliest detected precursor form, termed *prepro-parathyroid hormone,* consists of 115 amino acids; this molecular form is converted to an intermediate form of 90 amino acids termed *proparathyroid hormone,* then to the secreted product of 84 amino acids, parathyroid hormone. Parathyroid hormone shares, with other polypeptides and proteins destined for secretion from cells, this complex pattern of initial synthesis as a larger molecule which is then reduced in size by several cleavages prior to secretion. The regulation of these sequential steps in parathyroid hormone biosynthesis is unknown except by analogy with regulatory steps in biosynthesis, transport, and packaging of other proteins destined for secretion. The hydrophobic regions of the preproparathyroid hormone are similar to preprotein-specific regions of other cell-secreted proteins and serve a role in guiding transport of the polypeptide from sites of synthesis on polyribosomes through the endoplasmic reticulum to secretory granules. The genes for bovine, rat, and human parathyroid hormone have been cloned, and their structures have been determined. There are considerable homologies in the gene structures from these three species. Studies with cloned and expressed parathyroid hormone genes in vitro have demonstrated regions for control of gene expression at the transcriptional level, including sites for interaction and regulation by $1,25(OH)_2D$ and its receptor and "upstream" silencer elements as well as sites in which ambient calcium concentration regulates transcription. These in vitro observations are not well understood in terms of physiologic regulation of parathyroid hormone biosynthesis and secretion; the processing of hormone precursors (a posttranslational step of regulation of hormone production) may be more central to hormone availability than changes in transcription. It does not

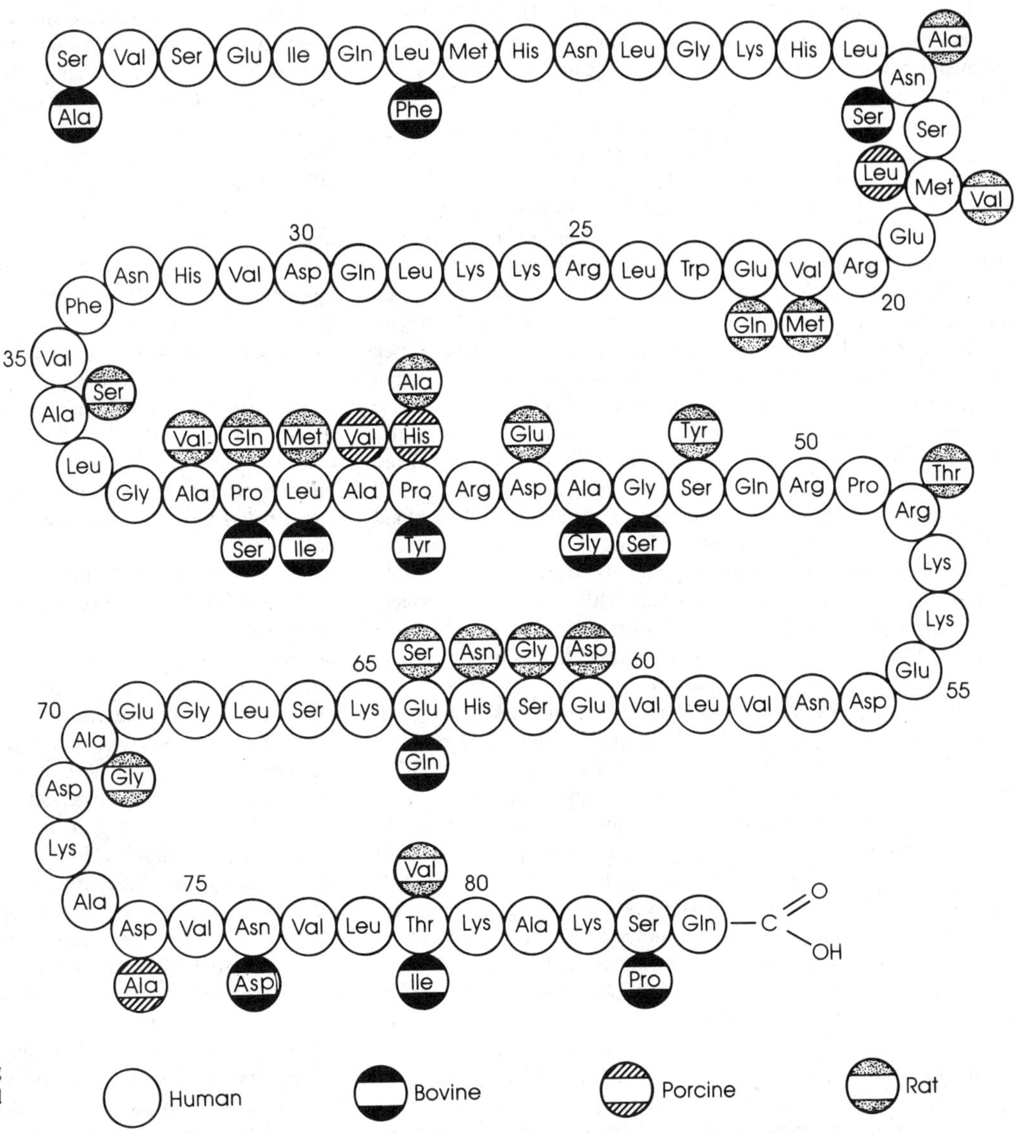

FIGURE 339-7 Model illustrating the sequence of human, cow, rat, and pig parathyroid hormone.

appear that changes in transcriptional activity of the parathyroid gene in the normal physiologic range of levels of blood calcium and $1,25(OH)_2D$ nor in short-term environmental stresses (e.g., fasting for 24 h) are important in control of blood levels of the hormone. Control is exerted by precise and rapid variation of rates of hormone secretion under the control of extracellular fluid calcium.

Blood calcium concentration over wide ranges controls the secretion of parathyroid hormone; the ionized fraction of blood calcium is the important determinant of hormone secretion. Hormone secretion increases steeply to a maximum value of fivefold above basal rates of secretion as calcium concentration falls from normal to the range of 1.9 to 2.0 mmol/L (7.5 to 8.0 mg/dL) (measured as total calcium). Beta-adrenergic agonists such as epinephrine and histamine-2 agonists may also increase hormone secretion, but the physiologic significance of these secretagogues is not established. Furthermore, drugs such as propranolol or cimetidine do not reproducibly decrease circulating parathyroid hormone levels.

Magnesium may influence hormone secretion in the same direction as calcium, but is a less potent secretagogue. It is unlikely that physiologic variations in magnesium concentration affect parathyroid secretion, but severe intracellular magnesium deficiency is associated with defective hormone secretion.

The hormone secreted in vivo from normal bovine and human parathyroid glands and from parathyroid adenomas is indistinguishable by immunologic criteria and by molecular size from the 84-amino acid peptide (molecular weight 9500) extracted from glands. However, much of the immunoreactive material found in the peripheral circulation of humans and animals (cow, dog) is smaller than the extracted or secreted hormone. The principal circulating fragments of immunoreactive hormone (approximate molecular weight 7000) lack a portion of the critical amino-terminal sequence required for biologic activity and, hence, are biologically inactive hormonal fragments. The nature of the cleavage process suggests that an endopeptidase cuts the molecule into two pieces.

Cleavage of the native peptide by an endopeptidase would be expected to result in formation of a second fragment, molecular weight 2000 to 3000, representing the amino-terminal, biologically active, portion of the hormone. There has been uncertainty concerning the presence or absence of such a circulating amino-terminal fragment. It has been also unclear (1) as to what extent peripheral metabolism accounts for the circulating fragment(s) of hormone as contrasted with intraglandular cleavage and subsequent secretion of hormone fragments and (2) whether peripheral metabolism is a purely catabolic process concerned only with hormone destruction or whether the peripheral cleavage results in formation of a metabolically active amino-terminal fragment of parathyroid hormone. Present evidence suggests that the liver and kidney are the principal sites at which peripheral metabolism of hormone occurs. Cleavages in these organs could regulate the concentration of hormonally active polypeptides in the circulation. Peripheral metabolism, in turn, may be affected by pathologic processes, such as renal failure or severe hepatic dysfunction. Certain conclusions can be made. There is no convincing evidence that circulating biologically active fragments are produced by peripheral metabolism; the latter process does not seem regulated by physiologic states (high vs. low calcium, etc.). Hence, peripheral metabolism of hormone, although responsible for rapid clearance of secreted hormone, appears to be a high capacity, metabolically invariant, catabolic process.

The rate of clearance of the secreted 84-amino acid peptide from blood is more rapid than the rate of clearance of the smaller, biologically inactive fragment(s) that results from peripheral metabolism. Hence, measurements of parathyroid hormone in blood by most immunoassays provide only an overall index of parathyroid gland activity rather than a direct measure of biologically active hormone, since biologically inert fragments rather than intact hormone are the principal circulating form of immunoreactive hormone. Changes in rate of production or clearance of fragments can change the concentration of immunoreactive hormone without involving corresponding changes in rate of hormone secretion. Such discordance between concentrations of immunoreactive hormone and biologically active peptide occurs, for example, in renal failure, since the kidney seems to be the principal route of excretion of hormone fragments. The problems inherent in accurate measurements of PTH in blood due to the heterogeneity of circulating forms of the molecule are now largely eliminated by use of double-antibody assays that detect only the intact molecule (as discussed in Chap. 340). Among other issues, the improved assays make it possible to make distinctions between excessive PTH production and excessive production of tumor-derived products that also elevate blood calcium.

One factor involved in humoral hypercalcemia associated with tumors has now been identified. The chemical features and biologic properties of the tumor factor (PTHrP, PTH-related peptide; HHM factor, humoral hypercalcemia of malignancy factor) have been deduced by use of recombinant DNA techniques and chemical peptide synthesis. PTHrP is a product of normal squamous epithelial cells in skin and may be involved in milk production in mammary tissue and in placental calcium metabolism in sheep. PTHrP is a larger molecule, 144 amino acids, and shares little homology with PTH except in the amino-terminal region; the genes for the two molecules are located on different chromosomes. The two peptides both interact with the PTH receptor. The tumor factor does affect certain biologic responses, however, that are different from those of PTH. For example, PTHrP stimulates bone resorption but has little effect on bone formation, unlike PTH which stimulates both processes.

The action of parathyroid hormone at the biochemical level involves effects on receptor(s) and second messengers in target cells. Stimulation of enzyme activity (adenyl cyclase, phospholipase C) during specific hormone–target cell membrane interaction leads to an increase in second messengers, intracellular cyclic AMP, and products of polyphosphoinositol metabolism (see also Chap. 68). Parathyroid hormone interacts with a specific receptor/adenylate cyclase complex on plasma membranes of target cells consisting of hormone receptor, enzyme catalytic unit (adenylate cyclase), and a guanyl nucleotide (GTP or GDP)–binding regulatory protein (G unit or N protein). The latter protein consists of α subunits that bind GTP or GDP and β subunits that dissociate when the α subunits bind GTP and reassociate when the α subunits bind GDP. The α subunit with bound GTP complexes with adenylate cyclase, thereby activating the enzyme to increase the rate of cyclic AMP production from ATP. Hydrolysis of the GTP to GDP on the α subunit leads to reassociation of the G units and reduction in adenylate cyclase activity. In short, hormone binding to its receptor initiates a cycle of α subunit/GTP binding and enzyme activation.

Following the administration of parathyroid hormone a rise in urinary cyclic AMP precedes any observable increase in phosphate excretion. Likewise, the effects on bone adenylate cyclase activity can be detected within 1 min of the addition of parathyroid hormone to a suspension of bone cells. In addition, administration of dibutyryl cyclic AMP simulates many of the actions of parathyroid hormone in parathyroidectomized animals. Dibutyryl cyclic AMP leads to a rise in serum calcium, a lowering of serum phosphate, and an increased excretion of calcium, phosphate, and hydroxyproline in urine. It is likely that PTH action involves more than one receptor, one guanyl nucleotide binding protein, and one messenger (cyclic AMP). In analogy with certain other peptide, adrenergic, and acetylcholine receptors, there is probably more than one chemically distinct PTH receptor. Differential responses with certain synthetic PTH analogues and antagonists and some distinctions between the biologic responses of PTH and PTHrP are best explained by the existence of more than one PTH receptor. The cDNA for the PTH receptor(s) has not been cloned, however; only successful cloning will make it possible to determine whether the suspected receptor heterogeneity is truly present.

Direct evidence exists for participation of the alternate second messenger system involving phospholipase C/polyphosphoinositol/inosine triphosphate (IP_3) and diacyl glycerol (DAG) in PTH action. There is also evidence for a PTH-mediated calcium channel response that is cyclic AMP independent. Presumably, a distinctive guanyl binding protein is involved in PTH-mediated responses in certain target cells, but this hypothesis also awaits testing (see also Chap. 68).

The mechanisms by which an increased intracellular concentration of cyclic AMP, IP_3, or DAG lead to changes in calcium and phosphate ion translocation is unknown. There is evidence for stimulation of protein kinases (protein kinase A, cyclic AMP; protein kinase C, DAG) that in turn cause phosphorylation of proteins that are believed to initiate the hormonal effect.

Pathophysiology In hyperparathyroidism there is an overproduction of parathyroid hormone by tumors of the parathyroid or hyperplasia involving all glands. The excess hormone results in hypercalcemia secondary to increased intestinal calcium absorption [increased synthesis of $1,25(OH)_2D$], reduced renal calcium clearance, and increased bone calcium release. Bone turnover increases in all patients, with resorption exceeding formation in many. Individual patients respond to the excess hormone variably at intestinal, renal, and bone target sites; the factors influencing the variable response from patient to patient are not known.

Hypophosphatemia results from the actions of the excessive parathyroid hormone on renal tubular phosphate reabsorption. Hypophosphatemia in turn aggravates the hypercalcemia in part by increasing the synthesis of $1,25(OH)_2D$ and by increasing the sensitivity of the bone to PTH action. The hypophosphatemia may also interfere with the normal mineralization of bone leading to a mixed picture of both increased resorption and deficient mineralization in adjacent skeletal sites.

Hypoparathyroidism causes hypocalcemia and hyperphosphatemia, a reversal of the response seen with hormone excess.

CALCITONIN (See also Chap. 325) Calcitonin is the potent hypocalcemic peptide hormone that, in many ways, acts as the physiologic antagonist to parathyroid hormone. Calcitonin reduces bone resorption and has opposing effects to parathyroid hormone on the kidney in that it increases renal calcium clearance. Calcitonin exerts at least some effects through stimulation of membrane-bound adenylate cyclase in receptor cells in kidney and bone. There is a variable hormonal responsiveness of renal tubular cells to calcitonin, parathyroid hormone, and vasopressin. In some portions of the nephron, there are cells that respond to all three hormones, whereas in other areas of the tubules the response is restricted to one or two of the hormones. In bone, osteoclasts possess calcitonin receptors, in contrast to the absence of receptors for PTH on osteoclasts. Indeed, direct effects of calcitonin on osteoclast morphology can be shown in vitro.

The thyroid gland is the major source of the hormone in mammalian species, and the cells involved in calcitonin synthesis arise from neural crest tissue. During embryogenesis these cells migrate into the ultimobranchial body. The latter body or gland arises from the last branchial pouch, hence the name *ultimobranchial body*. In submammalian vertebrates the ultimobranchial body remains as a discrete organ, anatomically separate from the thyroid gland. In mammals the ultimobranchial gland fuses with and is incorporated into the thyroid gland. Calcitonin is found in all vertebrate classes.

The naturally occurring calcitonins consist of a peptide chain of 32 amino acids. There is a considerable amount of variability in sequence among species. The entire chain of 32 amino acids appears to be required for biologic activity in the whole animal, although fragments function in in vitro systems. Calcitonin from salmon is 25 to 100 times more potent by weight in lowering serum calcium in animals than are mammalian forms of calcitonin; eel calcitonin is also highly potent. For example, the salmon hormone is at least 10 times more potent in humans than human calcitonin. Slow turnover may explain in part the greater biologic potency of salmon calcitonin, but the hormone binds more strongly to receptor sites as well. Calcitonin is synthesized as a precursor molecule, the parent molecule being four times larger than calcitonin itself. Analysis of the sequence of the coding portions of the gene for rat calcitonin indicates that at least two peptides flank calcitonin from which they are separated by basic residues. It is likely (in analogy with the common precursor for ACTH and endorphin) that these peptides are released along with calcitonin. Despite suggestions that one of the derivative peptides might have hypocalcemic action, there is, at present, no known biologic role for these noncalcitonin peptides.

There are two calcitonin genes, α and β, located on chromosome 11 in the general region of the beta globin and parathyroid hormone genes. The transcription of the calcitonin gene is complex. Two different messenger RNA molecules are transcribed from the α gene; one is translated into the precursor for calcitonin, and the other message is transcribed into an alternate product, calcitonin-gene-related peptide (CGRP). The two genes are sometimes called calcitonin/CGRP-1 and /CGRP-2 genes. CGRP is synthesized wherever the calcitonin message is expressed, for example, in medullary carcinoma of the thyroid. The β, or CGRP-2, gene is transcribed into the messenger RNA for CGRP in the central nervous system in animals; this gene is silent for calcitonin production. CGRP has cardiovascular actions and may serve a neurotransmitter or developmental role in CNS.

The secretion of calcitonin is under the direct control of blood calcium: an increase in calcium causes an increase and a decrease in calcium causes a decrease in calcitonin levels. Once secreted, calcitonin disappears rapidly from the circulation with a half-life of 2 to 15 min.

The concentration of calcitonin in the peripheral blood of normal humans is lower than in many other species. Basal and stimulated immunoreactive calcitonin levels are lower in women than in men and tend to decrease with age to a greater extent in women.

The physiologic role of calcitonin is incompletely understood. In animals calcitonin acts to lower both blood calcium and blood phosphate; the principal action is inhibition of bone resorption. The importance of calcitonin in increasing urinary calcium and phosphate clearance is synergistic with its effects on bone resorption. The actions of calcitonin on kidney and bone are in turn modulated by the regulation of calcitonin production by serum calcium. The view that calcitonin serves to protect against hypercalcemia is thus explained by the hypocalcemic effects of calcitonin triggered in response to hypercalcemia.

The role of calcitonin, if any, however, in normal adult humans is unknown. Changes in calcium and phosphate metabolism are not seen in humans despite extremes of variation in hormone production; there are no definite effects attributable to calcitonin deficiency (totally thyroidectomized patients receiving only replacement thyroxine) or excess (patients with the calcitonin-secreting tumor, medullary carcinoma of the thyroid). Patients with the latter disorder suffer multiple deleterious consequences of their malignancy (see Chap. 325), but no abnormalities in calcium or bone metabolism are recognized, perhaps because they become refractory to the skeletal effects of calcitonin.

Medical interest in calcitonin, therefore, at present is centered principally upon its use as a therapeutic agent and its usefulness, when deployed in radioimmunoassays, for detection of medullary carcinoma (Chap. 325). The use of calcitonin in the treatment of Paget's disease of bone is established (Chap. 344).

REFERENCES

Calcium, phosphorous, and bone metabolism

AVIOLI LV, KRANE SM (eds): *Metabolic Bone Disease and Clinically Related Disorders*. Philadelphia, Saunders, 1990

AZRIA M: The value of biomarkers in detecting alterations in bone metabolism. Calcif Tissue Int 45:7, 1989

BRINGHURST FR: Calcium and phosphate distribution, turnover, and metabolic actions, in *Endocrinology*, 2d ed, LJ DeGroot et al (eds). Philadelphia, Saunders, 1989, p 805

CANALIS E et al: Growth factors and the skeletal system. J Endocrinol Invest 12:577, 1989

COHN DV et al (eds): *Calcium Regulation and Bone Metabolism. Basic and Clinical Aspects*. Amsterdam, Excerpta-Medica, 1987

EPSTEIN S: Serum and urinary markers of bone remodeling: Assessment of bone turnover. Endocrine Rev 9:437, 1988

ERICKSEN EF: Normal and pathological remodeling of human trabecular bone: Three dimensional reconstruction of the remodeling sequence in normals and in metabolic bone disease. Endocrine Rev 7:379, 1986

EVERED D, HARNETT S (eds): *Cell and Molecular Biology of Vertebrate Hard Tissues*. Chichester, Wiley, 1988

GRAVELYN TR et al: Hypophosphatemia-associated respiratory muscle weakness in a general inpatient population. Am J Med 84:870, 1988

KANDERS B et al: Interaction of calcium nutrition and physical activity on bone mass in young women. J Bone Min Res 3:145, 1988

KLEEREKOPER M, KRANE SM (eds): *Clinical Disorders of Bone and Mineral Metabolism*. New York, Mary Ann Liebert, 1989

KRANE SM, SCHILLER AL: Metabolic bone disease. Introduction and Classification, in *Endocrinology*, 2d ed, LJ DeGroot et al (eds). Philadelphia, Saunders, 1989, vol 2, p 1151

LYLES KW et al: Correlations of serum concentrations of 1,25-dihydroxyvitamin D, phosphorus, and parathyroid hormone in tumoral calcinosis. J Clin Endocrinol Metab 67:88, 1988

MUNDY GR: Identifying mechanisms for increasing bone mass. J Natl Inst Health Res 1:65, 1989

O'GARA A: Peptide regulatory factors. Interleukins and the immune system 1. Lancet 1:943, 1989

PARFITT AM: The coupling of bone formation: A critical analysis of the concept and of its relevance to the pathogenesis of osteoporosis. Metab Bone Dis Relat Res 4:1, 1982

———: The cellular basis of bone remodelling. The quantum concept reexamined in light of recent advances in the cell biology of bone. Calcif Tissue Int 36:S37, 1984

PORTALE AA et al: Physiologic regulation of the serum concentration of 1,25-dihydroxyvitamin D by phosphorus in normal men. J Clin Invest 83:1494, 1989

POUILLES JM et al: Sensitivity of dual-photon absorptiometry in spinal osteoporosis. Calcif Tissue Int 43:329, 1988

RAISZ LG, KREAM BE: Regulation of bone formation. N Engl J Med 309:29, 1983

RECKER RR et al: Static and tetracycline-based bone histomorphometric data from 34 normal postmenopausal females. J Bone Min Res 3:133, 1988

RISTELI L et al: Radioimmunoassays for monitoring connective tissue metabolism. Rheumatology 10:216, 1986

TRACEY KJ et al: Peptide regulatory factors. Cachectin/tumour necrosis factor. Lancet 1:1122, 1989

URIST MR et al: Bone cell differentiation and growth factors. Science 220:680, 1983

Vitamin D

HOLICK MF: Vitamin D: Biosynthesis, metabolism, and mode of action, in *Endocrinology*, 2d ed, LJ DeGroot et al (eds). Philadelphia, Saunders, 1989, vol 2, chap 56

———: 1,25-Dihydroxyvitamin D_3 and the skin: A unique application for the treatment of psoriasis. Proc Soc Exper Biol Med 191:246, 1989

——— et al: Age, vitamin D, and solar ultraviolet. Lancet 2:1104, 1989

REICHEL H et al: The role of the vitamin D endocrine system in health and disease. N Engl J Med 320:981, 1989

WEBB AR et al: Influence of season and latitude on the cutaneous synthesis of vitamin D_3: Exposure to winter sunlight in Boston and Edmonton will not promote vitamin D_3 synthesis in human skin. J Clin Endocrinol Metab 67:373, 1988

Parathyroid hormone and calcitonin

ARNOLD A et al: Molecular cloning and chromosomal mapping of DNA rearranged with the parathyroid hormone gene in a parathyroid adenoma. J Clin Inv 83:2034, 1989

FRIEDMAN E et al: Clonality of parathyroid tumors in familial multiple endocrine neoplasia type 1. N Engl J Med 321:213, 1989

HOCK JM et al: Comparison of the anabolic effects of synthetic parathyroid hormone-related protein (PTHrP) 1-34 and PTH 1-34 on bone in rats. Endocrinology 25:2022, 1989

JUPPNER H et al: The parathyroid hormone-like peptide associated with humoral hypercalcemia of malignancy and parathyroid hormone bind to the same receptor on the plasma membrane of ROS 17/2.8 cells. J Biol Chem 263:8557, 1988

KHOSLA S et al: Nucleotide-sequence of cloned cDNAs encoding chicken preproparathyroid hormone. J Bone Min Res 3:689, 1988
MACINTYRE I: Calcitonin: Physiology, biosynthesis, secretion, metabolism, and mode of action, in *Endocrinology*, 2d ed, LJ DeGroot et al (eds). Philadelphia, Saunders, 1989, vol 2, chap 55
MANGIN M et al: Identification of a cDNA encoding a parathyroid hormone-like peptide from a human tumor associated with humoral hypercalcemia of malignancy. Proc Natl Acad Sci USA 85:597, 1988
NISHI M et al: Human islet amyloid polypeptide gene: Complete nucleotide sequence, chromosomal localization, and evolutionary history. Mol Endocrinol 3:11, 1775, 1989
NISSENSEN RA et al: Parathyroid hormone-like protein from human renal carcinoma cells: Structural and functional homology with parathyroid hormone. J Clin Invest 80:1803, 1987
RODDA CP et al: Regulation of fetal calcium metabolism: Evidence for a novel parathyroid hormone-related protein promoting placental calcium transport. J Bone Min Res 3 (Suppl):S213, 1988
ROSENBLATT M et al: Parathyroid hormone: Physiology, chemistry, biosynthesis, secretion, metabolism, and mode of action, in *Endocrinology*, 2d ed, LJ DeGroot et al (eds). Philadelphia, Saunders, 1989, vol 2, chap 54
RUSSELL J, SHERWOOD LM: Nucleotide sequence of the DNA complementary to avian (chicken) preproparathyroid hormone mRNA and the deduced sequence of the precursor. Mol Endocrinol 3:325, 1989
SUVA LJ et al: A parathyroid hormone-related protein implicated in malignancy hypercalcemia: Cloning and expression. Science 237:893, 1987
THAKKER RV et al: Association of parathyroid tumors in multiple endocrine neoplasia type 1 with loss of alleles on chromosome 11. N Engl J Med 321:218, 1989
THIEDE MA, RODAN GA: Expression of a calcium mobilizing parathyroid hormone-like peptide in lactating mammary tissue. Science 242:278, 1988
TRIMBLE ER et al: Secretin stimulates cyclic AMP and inositol trisphosphate production in rat pancreatic acinar tissue by two fully independent mechanisms. Proc Natl Acad Sci USA 84:3146, 1987
WAKELAM MJO et al: Activation of two signal-transduction systems in hepatocytes by glucagon. Nature 323:68, 1986
YAMADA H et al: Effects of human PTH-related peptide and human PTH on cyclic AMP production and cytosolic free calcium in an osteoblastic cell clone. Bone Min, 6:45, 1989

340 DISEASES OF THE PARATHYROID GLAND AND OTHER HYPER- AND HYPOCALCEMIC DISORDERS

JOHN T. POTTS, JR.

HYPERCALCEMIA

Hypercalcemia can be a manifestation of a serious illness such as malignancy or can be detected coincidentally by laboratory testing in a patient with no obvious illness. Management is a particular problem when the patient is asymptomatic. The number of patients recognized with asymptomatic hypercalcemia has increased severalfold in the last two decades. Does the hypercalcemia always require further evaluation? What are the most probable causes of hypercalcemia, and how can they be diagnosed? Can asymptomatic patients be followed, or is definitive therapy to eliminate the hypercalcemia the optimal medical management?

Whenever hypercalcemia is confirmed, a definitive diagnosis must be established. Although hyperparathyroidism, a frequent cause of asymptomatic hypercalcemia, is a chronic disorder in which manifestations, if any, may be expressed only over months or years, hypercalcemia can also be the earliest clue to the presence of malignancy, the second most common cause of hypercalcemia in the adult. The causes of hypercalcemia are numerous (Table 340-1), but hyperparathyroidism and cancer account for 90 percent of cases. Diagnosis can usually be established, but management of asymptomatic patients is still unsettled.

Before undertaking an evaluation of hypercalcemia, it is essential to be sure that true hypercalcemia, not a false-positive laboratory test, is present. Hypercalcemia is a chronic problem, and it is cost-effective to obtain several serum calcium measurements; these tests need not be in the fasting state. False-positive calcium tests are usually the result of inadvertent hemoconcentration during blood collection or elevation in serum proteins, particularly albumin. Measurement of ionized calcium is technically feasible, but there is no advantage, except in research applications, to measurement of ionized rather than total calcium.

TABLE 340-1 Classification of causes of hypercalcemia

Parathyroid-related:
1 Primary hyperparathyroidism
  a Solitary adenomas
  b Multiple endocrine neoplasia
2 Lithium therapy
3 Familial hypocalciuric hypercalcemia
	Vitamin D–related:
	1 Vitamin D intoxication
	2 ↑ $1,25(OH)_2D$; sarcoidosis and other granulomatous diseases
	3 Idiopathic hypercalcemia of infancy

Malignancy-related: *1* Solid tumor with metastases (breast) *2* Solid tumor with humoral mediation of hypercalcemia (lung, kidney) *3* Hematologic malignancies (multiple myeloma, lymphoma, leukemia)	Associated with high bone turnover: *1* Hyperthyroidism *2* Immobilization *3* Thiazides *4* Vitamin A intoxication Associated with renal failure: *1* Severe secondary hyperparathyrodism *2* Aluminum intoxication *3* Milk-alkali syndrome

Clinical features alone are helpful in differential diagnosis. Hypercalcemia in an adult who is asymptomatic is usually due to primary hyperparathyroidism. In most cases of malignancy-associated hypercalcemia the disease is not occult; rather, symptoms of the underlying malignancy bring the patient to the physician, and hypercalcemia is discovered during the workup. In patients with malignancy the interval between detection of hypercalcemia and death is often less than 6 months. Accordingly, if an asymptomatic individual has had hypercalcemia or some manifestation of hypercalcemia, such as kidney stones, for more than 1 or 2 years, it is unlikely that malignancy is the cause. As discussed below, however, differentiating primary hyperparathyroidism from *occult* malignancy can occasionally be a problem, and careful evaluation of patients is required, particularly when the duration of the hypercalcemia is unknown.

Hypercalcemia not due to hyperparathyroidism or malignancy can result from excessive vitamin D action, high bone turnover from any of several causes, or from renal failure (Table 340-1). The sensitivity and specificity of various diagnostic tests for the differential diagnosis were previously not optimal, but newer parathyroid hormone (PTH) immunoassays based on double-antibody methods are more reliable. Dietary history and a history of ingestion of vitamins and drugs are often helpful in recognizing some of the less frequent causes. Except in malignancy-associated hypercalcemia, acute management of the hypercalcemia is usually successful prior to the institution of definitive therapy. The type of treatment is based on the severity of the hypercalcemia and the nature of associated symptoms.

Hypercalcemia from any cause can result in fatigue, depression, mental confusion, anorexia, nausea, vomiting, constipation, reversible renal tubular defects, increased urination, alteration in the electrocardiogram (a short QT interval), and, in some patients, cardiac arrhythmias. There is a variable relation between the severity of hypercalcemia and the presence or absence of symptoms from one patient to the next. Generally, symptoms are more common at calcium levels above 2.9 to 3 mmol/L (11.5 to 12.0 mg/dL), but some patients, even at this level, are asymptomatic. When calcium exceeds 3.2 mmol/L (13 mg/dL), renal insufficiency and calcification in kidneys, skin, vessels, lungs, heart, and stomach may occur, particularly if blood phosphate levels are normal or elevated due to impaired renal function. Severe hypercalcemia, usually defined as 3.7 mmol/L (15 mg/dL) or above, is a medical emergency. When serum calcium is 3.7 to 4.5 mmol/L (15 to 18 mg/dL) or higher, coma and cardiac arrest can occur.

PARATHYROID-RELATED HYPERCALCEMIA Primary hyperparathyroidism NATURAL HISTORY AND INCIDENCE Primary hyperparathyroidism is a generalized disorder of calcium, phosphate, and bone metabolism that results from an increased secretion of parathyroid hormone. The excessive concentration of circulating hormone usually leads to hypercalcemia and hypophosphatemia. There is great variation in the clinical presentation. Patients may present with multiple signs and symptoms, including recurrent nephrolithiasis, peptic ulcers, mental changes, and, less frequently, extensive bone resorption. However, with greater awareness of the disease and wider use of multiphasic screening tests, including blood calcium determinations, the diagnosis is frequently made in patients who have no symptoms and minimal, if any, signs of the disease other than hypercalcemia and elevated levels of parathyroid hormone. If the frequency of diagnosis in referral centers reflects the incidence of the disease, hyperparathyroidism is more common than previously appreciated. In fact, the incidence of primary hyperparathyroidism may approximate *1 case per 1000 per year* in men over the age of 60 and *2 per 1000* in women 60 years of age or older. This incidence is greater than earlier estimates of *1 case per 10,000 persons per year* which were based on evaluation of patients with symptoms such as calcium-containing kidney stones. The clinical manifestations may be subtle, and the disease may have a benign course for many years or a full lifetime. Rarely, the disease seems to appear abruptly, and patients may exhibit severe complications, such as marked dehydration and coma, so-called hypercalcemic parathyroid crisis. The disease is most common in adults, with peak incidence between the third and fifth decades, but it occurs in young children and in the elderly.

ETIOLOGY AND PATHOLOGY <u>*Solitary adenomas*</u> The cause of hyperparathyroidism is one or more hyperfunctioning glands. The traditional view has been that a single abnormal gland is the cause in approximately 80 percent of patients; the abnormal gland is usually a benign neoplasm or adenoma and rarely a malignant tumor or parathyroid carcinoma. In a second group, approximately 15 percent, all glands are hyperfunctioning; this is termed *chief cell parathyroid hyperplasia*. The remaining few percent seem to have more than one abnormal gland but not necessarily all glands involved as in hyperplasia; this disorder is labeled *double or multiple adenoma*. There is considerable disagreement about this etiologic classification, particularly about the frequency of disorders involving single, several, and all-abnormal glands. This uncertainty has led to an associated disagreement about surgical management, in particular about how much tissue to remove to cure the disease and restore the euparathyroid state (discussed below).

Benign neoplasms are thought to be monoclonal, that is, one originally abnormal cell, losing growth control but not function, multiplies into an abnormal gland mass, or adenoma. In women, studies using X-linked markers that undergo random inactivation permit direct tests of monoclonality versus polyclonality of excised parathyroid tumors and indicate that adenomas are monoclonal; in turn a single abnormal gland is predicted in such patients. The tests have only been utilized in a few patients, however. In some series there are abnormalities in more than one but not all glands (*double adenoma*) in as many as 40 percent of patients or more. The functional significance of the enlarged glands is unknown—perhaps only one gland is truly hyperfunctioning. Tests of monoclonality versus polyclonality of the abnormal glands in this disorder have not been performed. The majority of evidence still favors a single, benign, monoclonal parathyroid adenoma as the cause of hyperparathyroidism in most patients because removal of a single gland usually restores the eucalcemic state.

Adenomas are most often located in the inferior parathyroid gland but are found in unusual locations in 6 to 10 percent of patients; such parathyroid adenomas may be located in the thymus, the thyroid, the pericardium, or behind the esophagus. Adenomas are usually 0.5 to 5 g in size but may be as large as 10 to 20 g (normal glands are 25 mg in weight on average). Chief cells are predominant in both hyperplasia and adenoma. The adenoma is sometimes encapsulated by a rim of normal tissue. Chief cell hyperplasia is especially common in familial cases of hyperparathyroidism and those that are part of the multiple endocrine neoplasia syndromes (see Chap. 325). With hyperplasia the enlargement may be so asymmetric that some involved glands appear grossly normal. In this case, histologic examination reveals a uniform pattern of chief cells and disappearance of fat even in the absence of an increase in gland weight. Thus, microscopic examination of biopsy specimens of several glands is essential to interpret findings at surgery. When an adenoma is present, the other glands are normal and contain a normal distribution of all cell types (rather than only chief cells) and normal amounts of fat.

Parathyroid carcinoma is usually not aggressive in character. Long-term survival without recurrence is common if at initial operation the entire gland is removed without rupture of the capsule. Even recurrent parathyroid carcinoma is usually slow-growing with local spread in the neck, and surgical correction of recurrent disease may be feasible. Occasionally, parathyroid carcinoma is more aggressive in character, with distant metastases (lung, liver, and bone) found at the time of initial operation. It may be difficult to appreciate initially that a primary tumor is carcinoma; increased numbers of mitotic figures and increased fibrosis of the gland stroma may precede invasive features. The diagnosis of carcinoma is often made in retrospect. Hyperparathyroidism from a parathyroid carcinoma may be clinically indistinguishable from other forms of primary hyperparathyroidism; a potential clue to the diagnosis, however, is provided by the degree of calcium elevation. Calcium values of 3.5 to 3.7 mmol/L (14 to 15 mg/dL) are frequent with carcinoma; this finding may alert the surgeon to remove the abnormal gland with care to avoid capsular rupture.

<u>*Multiple endocrine neoplasia*</u> Hyperparathyroidism may occur in a familial pattern without other endocrinologic abnormality. More often, however, hereditary hyperparathyroidism is part of a multiglandular endocrinopathy (see Chap. 325). There are several distinct syndromes of multiple endocrine neoplasia (MEN). The type I disorder (MEN I, Wermer's syndrome) consists of hyperparathyroidism and tumors of the pituitary and pancreatic islet cells, often associated with peptic ulcer and gastric hypersecretion (the Zollinger-Ellison syndrome). A mitogenic factor for parathyroid tissue is present in the sera of patients with MEN I. Another distinct constellation of endocrinologic abnormalities consists of hyperparathyroidism associated with pheochromocytoma and medullary carcinoma of the thyroid (MEN IIa). The pattern of inheritance is autosomal dominant. Tumors of the thyroid and adrenal medulla are not found in patients with MEN I, and pancreatic and pituitary tumors do not occur in patients with MEN IIa. Since the different endocrine tumors can develop at widely separated intervals, hyperparathyroidism and the related endocrine disorders should be carefully and repeatedly searched for in kindreds afflicted with the MEN syndromes.

SIGNS AND SYMPTOMS Half or more of patients with hyperparathyroidism are asymptomatic. These patients are either followed without therapy or are operated upon, eliminating the disease state. Manifestations of hyperparathyroidism involve primarily the kidneys and the skeletal system. Kidney involvement, due either to deposition of calcium in the renal parenchyma or to recurrent nephrolithiasis, was present in 60 to 70 percent of patients prior to 1970. With the increased frequency of detection of asymptomatic individuals, renal complications are less common.

Renal stones are usually composed of either calcium oxalate or calcium phosphate. Repeated episodes of nephrolithiasis or the formation of large calculi may lead to urinary tract obstruction and infection and may result in loss of renal function. Nephrocalcinosis may also cause decreased renal function and phosphate retention.

The unique bone involvement in hyperparathyroidism is osteitis fibrosa cystica. In the past osteitis fibrosa cystica occurred in 10 to 25 percent of patients with hyperparathyroidism. Histologically the pathognomonic features are a reduction in the number of trabeculae, an increase in the giant multinucleated osteoclasts in scalloped areas on the surface of the bone (Howship's lacunae), and a replacement of the normal cellular and marrow elements by fibrous tissues. Other bone changes include resorption of the phalangeal tufts and a replacement of the usually sharp cortical outline of the bone in the digits by an irregular outline (subperiosteal resorption). Loss of the lamina dura of the teeth is less specific. Tiny, ''punched-out'' lesions may be present in the skull, producing the so-called salt-and-pepper appearance.

Osteitis fibrosa cystica is now uncommon, even though the disease may be of long standing. The reduced frequency has not been explained. Other manifestations of bone disease, however, are frequent. Histomorphometric analyses of biopsied bone reveal an abnormality in bone turnover in most patients, even in those who do not evidence progressive loss of net bone mass; in such patients, rates of bone formation and bone restoration may be increased but balanced. In some patients, however, who do not have symptomatic bone disease or osteitis fibrosa cystica, rates of formation and resorption are not balanced so that a progressive loss of bone mineral mass causes osteopenia, indicating the need for surgery. There are no pathognomonic criteria to separate unequivocally parathyroid-dependent osteopenia from ''high-turnover'' osteoporosis as occurs in patients who are not hyperparathyroid.

Improved techniques are now available for monitoring bone mineral density. Computed tomography of the spine provides reproducible quantitative estimates (within a few percent) of spinal bone density. Similar, highly reproducible quantitation is also possible by photon densitometry for measurement of cortical bone density in the extremities, and dual-beam photometry can be used to estimate bone density in the spine or to measure total-body calcium. Serial measurements with these techniques can provide an early indication of whether or not progressive osteopenia is present. In some patients surgery is recommended because of progressive loss of bone, with the presumption that the progressive osteopenia is parathyroid hormone–dependent and hence treatable by correction of the hyperparathyroidism. Some patients have been followed for years, on the other hand, without evidence of loss of bone mass. Hence, bone disease with primary hyperparathyroidism can be quite variable.

Dysfunctions of the central nervous system, peripheral nerve and muscle, the gastrointestinal tract, and the joints also occur. An awareness of the signs and symptoms that may be seen in hyperparathyroidism may give the initial clue in the diagnosis. In some instances severe neuropsychiatric manifestations reverse after parathyroidectomy; in these patients there appears to be a cause and effect relationship. Generally, however, the fact that hyperparathyroidism is common in elderly patients, in whom there are often other problems, makes cause and effect of such problems as hypertension, renal deterioration, and depression uncertain and suggests caution in recommending surgery as a cure for hyperparathyroid patients. It is not apparent why some patients with hyperparathyroidism have no symptoms, while others with an equal degree of biochemical abnormality develop symptomatic disease.

Neuromuscular manifestations include proximal muscle weakness, easy fatigability, and atrophy of muscles. The clinical signs in these patients may be so striking as to suggest a primary neuromuscular disorder. The distinguishing feature is the complete regression of neuromuscular disease after surgical correction of the hyperparathyroidism.

Gastrointestinal manifestations of hyperparathyroidism are sometimes subtle and include vague abdominal complaints and disorders of the stomach and pancreas. Again, cause and effect are unclear, except in certain situations such as the multiple endocrine syndromes. In MEN I patients with hyperparathyroidism, duodenal ulcer is a result of the associated pancreatic tumors that secrete excessive quantities of gastrin (the Zollinger-Ellison syndrome). Pancreatitis has been reported in association with hyperparathyroidism, but the incidence and the mechanism are not established.

Chondrocalcinosis and pseudogout are said to be sufficiently frequent in hyperparathyroidism that screening of such patients is warranted. Occasionally, pseudogout is the initial manifestation.

DIAGNOSIS The diagnosis is made primarily on clinical grounds. The immunoassay for PTH is of particular value as a diagnostic test. Since hypercalcemia can be the presenting evidence for malignancy or other serious disease, a thorough evaluation of possible etiologies, including hyperparathyroidism, is indicated even in asymptomatic subjects. If the diagnosis of hyperparathyroidism is suspected after such an evaluation, a decision may be made to follow the patient for a time rather than to recommend surgery.

Hypercalcemia is the most common manifestation—either sustained or intermittent hypercalcemia. Careful consideration must be given to the justification for surgical exploration in the absence of hypercalcemia. So-called normocalcemic hyperparathyroidism, that is, surgically proven hyperparathyroidism accompanied by a normal calcium level but elevated values of immunoreactive PTH (iPTH), is rare in the absence of renal failure or gastrointestinal disease. If such patients have coexisting conditions that interfere with the calcium-elevating actions of PTH, such as chronic renal failure, severe malabsorption, or vitamin D deficiency, then the lack of calcium elevation need not argue against the presence of true hyperparathyroidism. Confusing situations can arise, however, in patients with recurrent kidney stones who are suspected of having hyperparathyroidism because of elevated iPTH levels but who have normal serum calcium. These patients may have true normocalcemic hyperparathyroidism. In situations in which the symptoms call for an early definitive diagnosis, it may be useful to search for postabsorptive hypercalcemia (detectable in certain patients when fasting hypercalcemia is absent) or to use a provocative test with benzothiadiazides (see below).

Hypercalciuria is common in hyperparathyroidism. However, PTH actually reduces calcium clearance, and the daily excretion of calcium in urine is lower than in patients with equivalent degrees of hypercalcemia from nonparathyroid causes.

Serum phosphate is usually low but may be normal, especially if renal failure has developed. Hypophosphatemia is a less useful diagnostic finding than hypercalcemia for two reasons. One, phosphate levels are influenced by dietary intake, diurnal variations, and other factors; to be useful, samples must be obtained in the morning under fasting conditions. Two, patients with severe hypercalcemia of all causes may have a low serum phosphate.

Many tests based on renal responses to excess parathyroid hormone (renal calcium and phosphate clearance; blood phosphate, chloride, magnesium; urinary or nephrogenous cyclic AMP) have been proposed and used in the past. These tests have low specificity for hyperparathyroidism and are not cost-effective; the improvement in the PTH immunoassay, long awaited, provide the more promising approach (as discussed below under differential diagnosis) in specificity and economy.

TREATMENT *Medical treatment* The medical treatment of hyperparathyroidism involves two separate issues. If hypercalcemia is severe and symptomatic, then the calcium must be lowered (the measures are described below. Hypercalcemia is not symptomatic in most patients with hyperparathyroidism, and it is usually not difficult to control the hypercalcemia. Simple hydration will often suffice to lower the calcium concentration to values below 2.9 mmol/L (11.5 mg/dL). There have been discussions in the past about whether chronic management of the hypercalcemia of hyperparathyroidism should be undertaken with oral phosphate therapy. Although the calcium concentration is lowered by phosphate in most patients, this is accompanied by an increase in iPTH levels in blood; it is unclear whether the increased PTH levels would cause more or less organ deterioration. There have been no systemic trials to evaluate effects of specific medical therapy for hypercalcemia.

Rather, the usual issue is to decide whether surgical intervention is required in a particular patient. If not, medical management consists of following the patient without specific therapy but monitoring bone and renal function periodically to ensure that silent osseous and renal deterioration does not occur. In postmenopausal women with hyperparathyroidism who are either unwilling or unable to undergo parathyroid surgery, estrogen therapy may retard demineralization of the skeleton and, in some, reduce blood and urinary calcium levels. If undesirable signs or symptoms occur, surgical intervention can then be recommended.

The natural history of the disease has been studied in several centers. Several hundred patients have been followed in attempts to afford a rational explanation for the benefits of surgery or the risks of medical observation. Large-scale randomized prospective clinical trials have not been undertaken, however. Rather, the long-term effects of hyperparathyroidism have been assessed in patients who do not have kidney stones, osteitis fibrosa cystica, or other clear-cut symptoms. Of principle concern is the possibility of progressive loss of bone density, a worrying problem in women who face the problem of age-dependent and estrogen-deficient bone loss in the absence of hyperparathyroidism. The concern is that such patients, even though asymptomatic, will suffer a degree of bone loss due to PTH excess that will leave them more vulnerable later in life to developing symptomatic osteoporosis. No generalization can be made in this regard other than that some patients, followed by noninvasive techniques for measuring bone density, show no evidence of substantial bone loss, while others show progressive bone loss. The reproducibility of the available noninvasive techniques for assessing bone density is 1 to 2 percent, and if progressive bone loss becomes significant, for example, in premenopausal women, surgery should be recommended to prevent further bone loss. Such decisions are more arbitrary in the elderly, in whom loss of bone may not be due to the hyperparathyroidism and bone loss may not cease once the patient is rendered euparathyroid. It is not that one can guarantee that parathyroidectomy will arrest progressive bone loss but rather that one cannot afford, except in a very elderly patient, to run the risk that persistent hyperparathyroidism may accelerate skeletal disease.

There are no indexes that help in predicting whether bone loss will be progressive or skeletal mass will remain stable. Hence, if patients wish to avoid surgery, bone mass must be monitored at intervals of 6 months to 1 year, then less frequently if bone mass is stable. Loss of renal function, on the other hand, occurs only rarely in the absence of kidney stones or infection.

No uniform recommendation can be made regarding medical (nonsurgical) management of patients with hyperparathyroidism. Decisions must be made in the light of the age of the patient and social and psychological factors. Most physicians believe it is appropriate to operate on young persons to avoid lifelong monitoring by time-consuming and expensive studies, particularly since surgical treatment is usually successful and does not carry a significant risk of mortality or morbidity. In patients over the age of 50, conservative evaluation without surgery is reasonable if the patient prefers and if progressive bone loss is not seen. The operation can be recommended for any patient in whom progressive bone loss is documented or in whom other symptoms of the disease appear, or for whom the stress of long-term follow-up is greater than the desire for surgical "cure." Estrogen therapy is appropriate for the management of postmenopausal women with hyperparathyroidism who are poor candidates for surgery; such therapy may not only protect the skeleton but also may reduce blood and urinary calcium levels.

Surgical treatment Parathyroid exploration is best undertaken by an experienced surgeon with the help of an experienced pathologist. Certain clinical features help in predicting the pathology; for example, in familial cases, multiple abnormal glands are likely. However, some critical decisions regarding management can be made only during the operation. The examination by frozen section of tissue removed at surgery helps direct the subsequent course of the operation.

As discussed under etiology there are many unresolved issues to consider in surgery for hyperparathyroidism. At the extreme of conservatism, the surgical approach is based on the view that typically only one gland (the adenoma) is abnormal. If an enlarged gland is found, a normal gland should be sought. If a biopsy of a normal-sized second gland confirms its histologic and therefore presumed functional normality, no further exploration, biopsy, or excision is needed. At the other extreme is the minority viewpoint that not only should all four glands be sought but also most of the total parathyroid tissue mass should be removed.

The concern with the former approach is that the rate of recurrence of hyperparathyroidism will be unnecessarily high because a second abnormal gland will sometimes be missed; the latter approach could involve unnecessary surgery and an unacceptable rate of hypoparathyroidism.

The majority viewpoint, judged by surgical reviews, is that conservative surgery, i.e., removal of what is usually only one enlarged gland after four-gland exploration, leads to cure in most cases.

Known hyperplasia, as predicted in familial cases, poses more difficult questions of surgical management. Once a diagnosis of hyperplasia is established, it is necessary to identify all the glands. It is usually recommended that three glands be totally removed and the fourth gland be partially excised; care should be taken to leave a good blood supply for the remaining gland. Some surgeons advocate transplantation of a portion of the removed, minced parathyroid tissue into the muscles of the forearm. Cryopreservation is also being explored. When parathyroid carcinoma is encountered, the tissue should be widely excised; care must be taken to avoid rupture of the capsule to prevent local seeding of the tumor.

If no glandular abnormalities are found in the neck, the issue of further exploration must be decided. There are documented cases of five or six parathyroid glands and, therefore, of unusual locations for adenomas. A variety of techniques have been developed to aid in the preoperative localization of the abnormal parathyroid tissue; usually these techniques are used in patients with unsuccessful neck explorations before further surgery is undertaken. The early techniques featured either selective intraarterial angiography or selective venous catheterization of the thyroid venous plexus and adjacent areas coupled with radioimmunoassay for PTH. The techniques were often successful, but the frequency of detection was less than or at least not higher than the rate of success of an experienced parathyroid surgeon in finding the abnormal tissue at the first operation, so the morbidity and expense of the procedures are not warranted. Noninvasive techniques have also been utilized for preoperative localization, including ultrasound, computed tomography of the neck and mediastinum, differential scanning after simultaneous radiothallium and technetium administration, and intraarterial digital angiography.

Ultrasound is reported to detect abnormal parathyroid tissue in 60 to 70 percent of cases and is most useful for lesions in the vicinity of the thyroid and less successful for lesions in the anterior mediastinum. The technique may assist the surgeon even in the initial operation by directing the surgery to the side of the neck where the abnormal gland is located. Computed tomography has a similar success rate and is more helpful with mediastinal glands, although false-positives are noted. The subtraction of the technetium image, which targets the thyroid, from the radiothallium image, which targets both thyroid and parathyroid, has led to successful preoperative localization in approximately half of patients undergoing a second exploration.

Several generalizations seem warranted. Localization and removal of a single abnormal parathyroid gland at the first operation is usually successful, depending upon the experience of the surgeon (greater than 90 percent success for experienced surgeons). Preoperative localization techniques, therefore, which are less than 90 percent successful, should be reserved for patients in whom initial exploration is unsuccessful. When a second parathyroid exploration is indicated, ultrasound, computed tomography, and thallium-technetium scanning should probably be combined with selective digital arteriography in one of the centers specializing in these techniques. At one center, there has been experience with angiographic ablation of mediastinal adenomas with reports of long-term cure using selective embolization or deliberate excessive injection of contrast material into the end-arterial circulation feeding the parathyroid tumor.

A decline in serum calcium occurs within 24 h after successful surgery; usually blood calcium falls to low normal values for 3 to 5 days until the remaining parathyroid tissue resumes hormone secretion. It may develop that intraoperative monitoring of parathyroid hormone levels by rapid PTH immunoassays will prove useful in guiding the surgery, as suggested by some studies (see below). Severe postoperative hypocalcemia is likely only if osteitis cystica is present or if injury to all the normal parathyroid glands occurs during surgery.

In general, patients with good renal and gastrointestinal function, who do not have symptomatic bone disease and a large deficit in bone mineral, have few problems with postoperative hypocalcemia. The extent of postoperative hypocalcemia varies with the surgical approach. If all glands are biopsied, hypocalcemia may be more prolonged and may be transiently symptomatic. Symptomatic hypocalcemia is more likely to occur after second parathyroid explorations, when normal parathyroid tissue may have been removed at the unsuccessful initial operation and when the manipulation and/or biopsy of the remaining normal gland has been more extensive in the search for the missing adenoma. Patients with hyperparathyroidism have efficient intestinal calcium absorption due to the increased levels of $1,25(OH)_2D$ stimulated by parathyroid excess. Once hypocalcemia signifies successful surgery, patients can be put on a high calcium intake or be given oral calcium supplements. Despite manifestations of mild hypocalcemia, most patients do not require parenteral therapy and do not experience severe symptoms. If the serum calcium falls below 2 mmol/L (8 mg/dL), *in particular if the phosphate level simultaneously rises,* the possibility of hypoparathyroidism must be considered. Coexistent hypomagnesemia should be checked for, as it interferes with PTH secretion and causes a relative hypoparathyroidism. Parenteral calcium replacement at a low level should be instituted if symptomatic hypocalcemia supervenes. Such symptoms include a general sense of anxiety and positive Chvostek and Trousseau signs coupled with serum calcium consistently below 2 mmol/L (8 mg/dL). For parenteral therapy, calcium (gluconate or chloride) solutions are prepared at a concentration of 1 mg/mL in 5% dextrose in water. The rate and duration of intravenous therapy are determined by the severity of the symptoms and the response of the serum calcium. A rate of infusion of 0.5 to 2 (mg/kg)/h or 30 to 100 mL/h of a 1 mg/mL solution usually suffices to relieve symptoms. Generally, parenteral therapy is required for only a few days. If symptoms become severe or if the need for parenteral calcium continues for more than 2 to 3 days, replacement therapy with vitamin D and/or oral calcium (2 to 4 g/d) should be started (see below). It is cost-effective to use calcitriol (doses of 0.5 to 1.0 μg per 24 h) because of the rapidity of onset and rapidity of cessation of action, in contrast to vitamin D per se (see below). A sudden rise in blood calcium after several months of vitamin D replacement may indicate restoration of parathyroid function to normal. This problem is minimized by use of calcitriol rather than vitamin D. It is also appropriate to monitor serum PTH serially to estimate gland function in such patients.

Magnesium deficiency may also complicate the postoperative course. Magnesium deficiency impairs the secretion of PTH, and, therefore, hypomagnesemia should be corrected whenever detected. Magnesium chloride is effective by mouth, but this compound is not widely available. Accordingly, repletion is usually parenteral. Only a fraction of body magnesium is present in extracellular fluid, but total-body magnesium deficiency is reflected by hypomagnesemia. Since the depressant effect of magnesium on central and peripheral nerve functions does not occur below 2 mmol/L (normal range, 0.8 to 1.2 mmol/L), parenteral replacement can be given rapidly. A cumulative dose as great as 0.5 to 1 mmol/kg body weight can be administered if severe hypomagnesemia is present; often, however, total doses of 12 to 15 mmol are sufficient. The magnesium is given either as an intravenous infusion over 8 to 12 h or in divided doses intramuscularly (magnesium sulfate, USP).

Lithium therapy Lithium, used in the management of bipolar depression and other psychiatric disorders, causes hypercalcemia in approximately 10 percent of patients. The parathyroids are involved in mediation of the hypercalcemia, and PTH levels may be elevated. The hypercalcemia is dependent on continued lithium treatment, remitting and recurring when lithium is stopped and restarted. In a few patients who were explored parathyroid adenomas were found. Histologic findings in the remaining parathyroid glands in these patients have not been described, but the implication is that there is a single abnormal gland.

The presence of hypercalcemia does not correlate with plasma lithium level, but the frequency with which hypercalcemia occurs is sufficiently high to support a causal relationship between lithium and the hypercalcemia, particularly the dependence of the hypercalcemia on the continuation of the lithium. It is presumed that in most cases an adenoma is not present, merely hyperfunctioning glands. Lithium, at the levels achieved in blood in treated patients, can be shown in vitro to shift the curve describing PTH secretion as a function of calcium level to the right, i.e., higher calcium levels are required to lower PTH secretion. It is logical to assume this effect can cause elevated PTH and consequent hypercalcemia in otherwise normal individuals. If careful studies were done, elevated PTH levels might be found in more patients treated with lithium than the 10 percent in whom frank hypercalcemia is detected. The adenomas reported in a few hypercalcemia patients with lithium therapy may reflect the presence of an independently occurring parathyroid tumor; an effect of lithium on parathyroid gland growth need not be implicated (although it is not excluded), since the majority of patients have complete reversal of hypercalcemia when lithium is stopped. Long-term follow-ups have not been reported; many patients are continued on lithium to treat psychiatric problems. These patients are presumably best managed according to the principles used in asymptomatic hypercalcemia independent of lithium administration. If troubling symptoms or unfavorable signs, such as rising blood calcium levels, progressive bone demineralization, or kidney stones, develop, it may be necessary to try alternate psychotropic medication. Since it is unclear how often parathyroid adenomas will be found, it does not seem wise to recommend parathyroid surgery unless the hypercalcemia and elevated PTH persist after lithium is discontinued.

Familial hypocalciuric hypercalcemia Familial hypocalciuric hypercalcemia (familial benign hypercalcemia; FHH) is transmitted as an autosomal dominant trait. Affected individuals are frequently discovered because of asymptomatic hypercalcemia; surgical exploration of the parathyroids is not indicated because parathyroidectomy does not cure the disorder. It is, therefore, important to separate such patients from those with primary hyperparathyroidism.

The pathophysiology is not understood, and there is no single biochemical marker to distinguish these patients from patients with primary hyperparathyroidism. Nonetheless, the aggregate evidence serves to separate FHH clearly from primary hyperparathyroidism. The majority of patients with primary hyperparathyroidism have less than 99 percent renal calcium reabsorption, and most patients with FHH exceed 99 percent reabsorption. The hypercalcemia may be detectable in affected members of the kindreds in the first decade of life, whereas hypercalcemia rarely occurs in primary hyperparathyroidism and the MEN syndromes under the age of 10 years. The iPTH values may be elevated in FHH, but the values are usually normal or lower than in patients with primary hyperparathyroidism. In patients who are inadvertently operated upon, hypercalcemia and hypocalciuria persist without elevated PTH; the hypercalcemia and hypocalciuria, therefore, do not seem PTH-dependent. Serum magnesium levels are, on average, higher in FHH than in primary hyperparathyroidism. The overall evidence favors some as yet uncharacterized non-parathyroid-dependent defect in calcium transport into or out of extracellular fluid.

Few clinical signs of symptoms are present in patients with FHH. Unlike the MEN syndromes, other endocrine abnormalities are not present. Most patients are detected as a result of family screening after the diagnosis has been made in one member of the kindred. All too commonly, the initial patient is operated upon without reversal of the hypercalcemia. At operation, the glands appear normal, or a moderate degree of hyperplasia of all parathyroid glands is seen. No patient has had reversal of hypercalcemia by surgery unless all of the parathyroid tissue has been inadvertantly removed, rendering the patient hypoparathyroid, a most undesirable result. The high renal calcium reabsorption and the prompt recurrence of hypercalcemia as long as any parathyroid tissue remains establish that there is some abnormality in the regulation of the ratio of extracellular-to-intracellular calcium concentration or some abnormal mechanisms of calcium sensing in cell membranes in the kidney and/or elsewhere independent of parathyroid hormone excess. The exact nature of this disorder and its natural history are not clear yet, but since the parathyroid glands are permissive rather than responsible for the syndrome, parathyroid surgery is not to be advocated, nor, in view of the lack of symptoms, is medical treatment needed to lower the calcium.

Malignancy-related hypercalcemia CLINICAL SYNDROMES AND MECHANISMS OF HYPERCALCEMIA Hypercalcemia due to malignancy is common (occurring with 10 to 15 percent of certain types of tumor, such as lung carcinoma), often severe and difficult to manage, confusing as to etiology, and sometimes difficult to distinguish from primary hyperparathyroidism. Traditionally, hypercalcemia in malignancy was thought to be due to a local invasion and destruction of bone by tumor cells and, only in a minority of cases, to the elaboration by the malignant cells of humoral mediators of hypercalcemia.

Although the presence of malignancy is often clinically obvious, hypercalcemia can occasionally be due to an occult tumor. With occult malignancy, diagnosis and definitive treatment must be accomplished quickly if the patient is to be protected from the complications of the underlying malignancy.

Humoral hypercalcemia of malignancy occurs in patients with cancers of the lung and kidney in which bone metastases are absent, minimal, or not detectable clinically. The clinical picture resembles primary hyperparathyroidism (hypophosphatemia accompanies hypercalcemia), and elimination or regression of the primary tumor leads to disappearance of the hypercalcemia. Ectopic production of PTH by the tumor was initially felt to be the mechanism of the hypercalcemia, but the disease mechanisms are now appreciated to be due to humoral mechanisms unrelated to ectopic PTH production.

Many patients with the humoral hypercalcemia of malignancy have elevated urinary nephrogenous cyclic AMP excretion, hypophosphatemia, and increased urinary phosphate clearance, findings compatible with the actions of a humoral agent that emulates PTH action. On the other hand, these patients not only have lower iPTH levels generally than patients with hyperparathyroidism but also high, rather than low, renal calcium clearance (relative to serum calcium when compared to true hyperparathyroidism), and low to normal levels of 1,25-dihydroxyvitamin D [$1,25(OH)_2D$], all consistent with mediation by humoral factors distinct from PTH.

The histologic character of the tumor is more important than the extent of skeletal metastases in predicting hypercalcemia. Small cell carcinoma (oat cell) and adenocarcinoma of lung, although the most common lung tumors associated with skeletal metastases, rarely cause hypercalcemia. By contrast, as many as 10 percent of patients with squamous cell carcinoma of the lung develop hypercalcemia. Histologic studies of bone in patients with squamous cell or epidermoid carcinoma of the lung, in sites invaded by tumor as well as areas remote from tumor invasion, reveal bone remodeling, including osteoclastic and osteoblastic activity. In contrast, minimal evidence of skeletal metabolic activation is seen despite extensive skeletal metastases of small cell (oat cell) carcinoma.

The cumulative findings suggest that agents other than PTH must be responsible for hypercalcemia and that only certain tumor types produce these factors. At least two general mechanisms of hypercalcemia are suspected. Most solid tumors associated with hypercalcemia, particularly squamous cell and renal tumors, produce and secrete cellular factors that are believed to cause increased bone resorption and to mediate the hypercalcemia through systemic actions on the skeleton as a whole by stimulation of bone resorption. Substances produced by cells involved in the marrow response to hematologic malignancies or breast carcinoma resorb bone through local destruction and may be identical or analogous to some of the known lymphokines and cytokines.

Classification of the hypercalcemia of malignancy is arbitrary (Table 340-2). Multiple myeloma and other hematologic malignancies involving the bone marrow have been typically classified as one group; bone destruction and hypercalcemia are believed to be caused through local mechanisms of malignant cells spread widely throughout the marrow spaces. Breast carcinoma is typical of solid tumors that cause hypercalcemia through *localized osteolytic destruction*, probably mediated by locally secreted tumor products different from those involved in multiple myeloma or lymphoma. Finally, solid tumors can cause hypercalcemia from secretion of one or more distinctive mediators (Table 340-2).

In addition to the bone-resorbing factors elaborated by malignant cells in patients with hypercalcemia of malignancy, there may be variable synergism and antagonism between various bone-active agents secreted by the tumors. In the humoral hypercalcemia of malignancy, osteoclastic resorption is generalized, and there is an absence of an osteoblastic or bone-forming response to the surge of bone resorption, implying some inhibition of the normal coupling of formation and resorption. Cooperativity and antagonism in the skeletal actions of locally released cytokines may include blockade of cytokine-induced bone resorption by interferon or related cytokines, both the bone-resorbing and bone-resorbing-blocking cytokines being secreted in response to interactions among tumor cells and host inflammatory cells. Thus, the interaction of more than one substance may determine whether hypercalcemia develops with a particular tumor.

Several hormones, hormone analogues, specific cytokines, and/or growth factors have been implicated as the result of clinical assays, in vitro tests, or chemical isolation. In some lymphomas, typically B-cell lymphomas, there is an increased blood level of $1,25(OH)_2D$. It is not clear whether the increased $1,25(OH)_2D$ is produced by stimulation of the renal 1α-hydroxylase or whether the metabolite is produced ectopically by lymphocytes; the latter seems likely, based on studies with the malignant cells. The principal interest in etiologic mechanisms in hematologic malignancies has focused on the production of distinctive bone-resorbing factors by activated normal lymphocytes and by myeloma and lymphoma cells. This factor(s), termed *osteoclast activation factor* (OAF), now appears to represent the biologic action of several different cytokines, probably interleukin 1 and lymphotoxin or tumor necrosis factor, two closely related cytokines.

In most instances, breast carcinoma is believed to cause hypercalcemia by local stimulation of osteoclasts directly by products secreted by the metastatic breast carcinoma cells and associated inflammatory cells. Breast carcinoma cells produce and secrete prostaglandins of the E series, which are potent local stimulators of bone-resorbing cells.

More than one factor may be responsible for humorally mediated hypercalcemia in patients with solid tumors, but, as discussed in the

TABLE 340-2 Classification of tumor hypercalcemia

1 Hematologic malignancies
- *a* Local bone destruction (OAF, interleukin 1, tumor necrosis factor, lymphotoxin)
  - Multiple myeloma
  - Lymphomas
- *b* Humoral mediation [$1,25(OH)_2D$, ?PTH-rP]
  - Lymphomas

2 Solid tumors
- *a* Local bone destruction (prostaglandin, E series)
  - Breast carcinoma
- *b* Humoral mediation (PTH-rP, ?other agents)
  - Lung (squamous cell)
  - Kidney
  - Urogenital tract
  - Other squamous tumors

preceding chapter, work by several laboratories has resulted in identification of a hitherto unrecognized factor that resembles but is distinct from PTH and fulfills criteria of a humoral agent for the hypercalcemia syndrome. The factor, termed PTH-rP (parathyroid hormone–related protein), competes with PTH for PTH receptor occupancy in binding and receptor labeling assays, stimulates cyclic AMP production in in vitro assays, causes bone resorption in vitro, and induces hypercalcemia in test animals. These data indicate that PTH-rP acts through activation of the PTH receptor(s).

Other lines of investigation point to the possible role of other factors in the genesis of tumor hypercalcemia. Levels of urinary cyclic AMP rise in test animals treated with synthetic PTH-rP, but $1,25(OH)_2D$ levels also rise, which is at variance with the fact that patients with the humoral syndrome have normal or depressed levels of $1,25(OH)_2D$. Tumor-derived growth factors, believed to act as autocrine regulators to maintain the transformation and growth of tumor cells, and cellular growth factors produced by nonmalignant cells are also potent bone-resorbing agents in vitro. Still other factors potentially involved in tumor hypercalcemia are known only by their bone-resorbing properties and lack of stimulation of renal or bone cell cyclic AMP production. Several of these factors stimulate production of prostaglandins of the E_2 type.

Thus, although identification of PTH-rP represents a singular advance, it is not established to what extent the substance constitutes the sole pathophysiologic mechanism in the humoral hypercalcemia of malignancy. Immunoassays or bioassays of sufficient sensitivity and specificity to detect the presence of the PTH-rP in the circulation of hypercalcemic cancer patients or any human subject are needed.

Diagnostic issues and treatment Ordinarily, the diagnosis of hypercalcemia secondary to tumor is not difficult to make because the tumor symptoms are prominent at the time the hypercalcemia is detected. Indeed, the hypercalcemia may be noted incidentally during the workup of a patient with known or suspected malignancy. Patients with malignancy and hypercalcemia may have a coexistent parathyroid adenoma, some reports suggesting an incidence as high as 10 percent. Laboratory testing becomes critical when occult carcinoma is suspected. Levels of iPTH by the newer double-antibody technique are undetectable or extremely low in tumor hypercalcemia, as would be expected with the mediation of the hypercalcemia by a nonparathyroid agent (the hypercalcemia suppressing the normal parathyroid glands). This improvement in the usefulness of the PTH assay is a significant advance in laboratory diagnosis. (Earlier assays gave equivocal results.) An assay that could detect PTH-rP should be helpful; low or undetectable PTH and elevated PTH-rP would serve to focus attention on the presence of an occult malignancy [although reports that PTH-rP is produced in parathyroid adenomas and that there are multiple forms of the protein produced through alternate gene splicing and tissue metabolism (Chap. 339) may mean that the utility of the PTH-rP assay would be limited].

Hypercalcemia in association with truly occult malignancy, however, is rare. Clinical suspicion that malignancy is the cause of the hypercalcemia is heightened when symptoms associated with the paraneoplastic syndromes, such as weight loss, fatigue, muscle weakness, and unexplained skin rash, or symptoms specific for a particular tumor are present. Squamous cell tumors are most frequently associated with hypercalcemia, and the tumors most frequently arise in the lung, kidney, and urogenital tract. X-ray examinations can focus on these areas when clinical evidence is unclear. Bone scans with technetium-labeled diphosphonate are useful for detection of osteolytic metastases; the sensitivity is high, but specificity is low; results must be confirmed by conventional x-rays to be certain that areas of increased uptake are due to osteolytic metastases per se. Bone marrow biopsies are helpful in patients with anemia or abnormal peripheral blood smears.

Treatment of the hypercalcemia of malignancy must be considered in the perspective of the history and presumed course of the individual patient. Control of the tumor is the principal objective, and reduction of tumor mass is usually also the key to satisfactory control of hypercalcemia. If a patient has severe hypercalcemia yet has an excellent chance for effective tumor therapy, treatment of the hypercalcemia should be vigorous. If hypercalcemia, on the other hand, is an accompaniment of the late stages of a tumor that is resistant to therapy, the treatment of the hypercalcemia should not be vigorous, as hypercalcemia can have a mild sedating effect. Standard therapies for hypercalcemia (discussed below) are applicable to patients with malignancy.

VITAMIN D–RELATED HYPERCALCEMIA Hypercalcemia related to abnormal vitamin D action can be due to *excessive ingestion* of vitamin D or *abnormal metabolism* of the vitamin. Abnormal metabolism of the vitamin is usually acquired in association with some widespread granulomatous disorder, but there is one, rare hereditary form of vitamin D sensitivity in infants associated with other developmental anomalies. As discussed in Chap. 339, vitamin D metabolism is carefully regulated, particularly the activity of the renal 1α-hydroxylase responsible for the production of $1,25(OH)_2D$. Many details of the regulation of 1α-hydroxylase remain unclarified, but the normal feedback suppression by $1,25(OH)_2D$ on the enzyme seems to work less well in infants than in adults and operates poorly, if at all, in ectopic sites, as distinct from the renal tubule; these facts explain the occurrence of hypercalcemia secondary to excessive $1,25(OH)_2D_3$ production in certain infants (Williams' syndrome) and in adults with granulomatous disease (sarcoidosis) or certain lymphomas.

Vitamin D intoxication The chronic ingestion of large doses of vitamin D, usually at least 50 to 100 times the normal physiologic requirement (doses in excess of 50,000 to 100,000 units per day), is required to produce hypercalcemia in normal individuals. In animals, vitamin D intoxication causes increased bone resorption as well as increased intestinal calcium absorption. In humans, excessive vitamin D action leads to an increase in intestinal calcium absorption, but it is not known whether increased bone resorption contributes to the hypercalcemia.

The immediate mechanism for the hypercalcemia is presumed to be an excessive production of $1,25(OH)_2D$ as a consequence of an increase in the substrate for the renal 1α-hydroxylase, namely, 25(OH)D production is less tightly regulated than is the production of $1,25(OH)_2D$. Hence, concentrations of 25(OH)D average 5 to 10 times above normal in patients on high-dose vitamin D, whether therapeutically, as in hypoparathyroidism, or accidentally, as in vitamin D intoxication. 25(OH)D has a definite, if low, biologic activity in intestine and bone. Hence, part of vitamin D intoxication may be attributable to the high levels of 25(OH)D itself, as well as supernormal levels of $1,25(OH)_2D$. Because of the infrequency of vitamin D intoxication, there have been few reports of the actual level of $1,25(OH)_2D$ in patients with vitamin D intoxication. Presumably, the presence of normal renal function and parathyroid reserve would lead to higher rates of formation of $1,25(OH)_2D$ than would occur in patients, for example, with impaired renal function or absence of PTH secretion in whom high doses of vitamins may be given to counter calcium deficiency.

The diagnosis is substantiated by documenting concentrations of 25(OH)D in excess of the upper limit of normal. Hypercalcemia is usually controlled by restriction of dietary calcium intake and appropriate attention to hydration. These measures, plus discontinuation of vitamin D, usually lead to satisfactory management, but vitamin D stores in fat may be substantial, and vitamin D intoxication may persist for weeks after vitamin D ingestion is terminated. Such patients are sensitive to glucocorticoids, which in doses of 100 mg of hydrocortisone per day, or its equivalent, return calcium levels to normal over several days.

Sarcoidosis and other granulomatous diseases Normal relations between 25(OH)D and the product, the active metabolite $1,25(OH)_2D$, are not maintained in patients with sarcoidosis and other granulomatous diseases. There is a positive correlation between 25(OH)D levels (reflecting vitamin D intake) and the circulating concentrations of $1,25(OH)_2D$; normally there is no increase in the active metabolite with increasing 25(OH)D levels. In patients with sarcoidosis, the site of synthesis of $1,25(OH)_2D$ is believed to be in macrophages or other cells associated with granulomatous deposits. Hypercalcemia has been reported in an anephric sarcoidosis patient in association with increased $1,25(OH)_2D$ levels. Macrophages obtained from granulomatous tissue form $1,25(OH)_2D$ at an increased rate when 25(OH)D is provided as substrate. Thus, the usual regulation of active metabolite production by calcium or PTH is circumvented in these patients, and hypercalcemia does not lead to a reduction in the blood levels of $1,25(OH)_2D$ in patients with sarcoidosis. PTH-independent production of $1,25(OH)_2D$ is suggested by normal $1,25(OH)_2D$ production in a patient with sarcoidosis and hypoparathyroidism. Clearance of $1,25(OH)_2D$ from blood may be decreased in sarcoidosis as well.

Even normocalcemic patients with sarcoidosis have unregulated production of $1,25(OH)_2D$ in response to vitamin D loading. Exposure to sunlight or administration of as little as 9000 units of vitamin D daily is followed by increased levels of the active metabolite. Treatment with moderate doses of steroids leads to a reversal of the hypercalcemia, as in other cases of excessive vitamin D action such as vitamin D intoxication, and reversal of the abnormal reponsiveness of $1,25(OH)_2D$ levels to vitamin D challenge. Presumably, steroid administration causes multiple effects in the disease, and both excessive production of the metabolite and the responsiveness to it in target organs are blocked.

Variation in reported frequency of hypercalcemia in sarcoidosis (10 percent or less in recent reports, 60 percent or more in older reports) is probably explained in part by the moderating influence of steroids used to control pulmonary complications and other manifestations of the granulomatous disease. Lytic lesions also occur in bone so that increased bone resorption could play a role in some cases. In most, however, hypercalcemia is directly related to an increased intestinal calcium absorption. Clinically, hypercalcemia is usually a manifestation of disseminated disease. Hence, pulmonary involvement is usual; chest x-ray may reveal a diffuse fibronodular infiltrate and/or prominent hilar adenopathy. Blood gamma globulin may also be elevated. The most useful diagnostic procedure is demonstration of noncaseating granulomas in liver or lymph node biopsy. The hypercalcemia of sarcoidosis can present a difficult problem in differential diagnosis, especially when many of the typical features of the disease are lacking (see Chap. 277).

Management of the hypercalcemia in these patients can be accomplished by avoiding excessive sunlight exposure and by limiting vitamin D and calcium intake; glucocorticoids in the equivalent of 100 mg hydrocortisone per day or less are sufficient to control hypercalcemia when it occurs. Presumably, however, the abnormal sensitivity to vitamin D and abnormal regulation of $1,25(OH)_2D$ synthesis will persist as long as the disease is active. PTH levels are usually suppressed and $1,25(OH)_2D$ levels are elevated, but primary hyperparathyroidism and sarcoidosis may occur in some patients.

Idiopathic hypercalcemia of infancy This unusual disorder, sometimes referred to as Williams' syndrome, consists of multiple congenital development defects, including supravalvular aortic stenosis, mental retardation, and an elfin facies, in association with hypercalcemia due to abnormal sensitivity to vitamin D. The syndrome was first recognized in England after the introduction of vitamin D fortification of milk. Hypercalcemia develops with vitamin D intakes as small as 2000 to 4000 units per day. Levels of $1,25(OH)_2D$ are elevated, ranging from 46 to 120 nmol/L (150 to 500 pg/mL). The mechanism of the abnormal sensitivity to vitamin D and of the increased circulating levels of $1,25(OH)_2D$ is unclear. The children become hypercalcemic because of excessive intestinal calcium absorption. The abnormality in vitamin D metabolism and the increased sensitivity to vitamin D intake are not seen after the first year of life. Treatment is restriction of calcium intake. Occasionally, the hypercalcemia can be severe, and calcium values above 4 mmol/L (16 mg/dL) are recorded. Treatment with glucocorticoids in the doses used for vitamin D intoxication or sarcoidosis, adjusted for body weight, rapidly reverses the hypercalcemia.

HYPERCALCEMIA ASSOCIATED WITH HIGH BONE TURNOVER

Hyperthyroidism Mild elevation of serum calcium is common in patients with hyperthyroidism, and hypercalciuria is even more common. As many as 20 percent of patients show high normal or mildly elevated serum calcium concentrations. The hypercalcemia seems due to increased bone turnover with bone resorption exceeding bone formation; direct effects of thyroid hormone on the skeleton seems to be responsible. Severe calcium elevations are not typical, however, and the presence of such suggests a concomitant disease such as hyperparathyroidism. Indeed, patients with thyrotoxicosis are more sensitive to the hypercalcemic effects of PTH. Usually, the hyperthyroidism is obvious, and the hypercalcemia is managed by specific therapy of the hyperthyroidism. Signs of hyperthyroidism may occasionally be occult, particularly in the elderly.

Immobilization Immobilization in adults is rarely associated with hypercalcemia in the absence of an associated disease, but may cause hypercalcemia in children and adolescents, particularly after spinal cord injury and paraplegia or quadriplegia. With resumption of some ambulation, the hypercalcemia in children usually returns to normal spontaneously.

The mechanism appears to involve a disproportion between rates of bone formation and bone resorption that results from the sudden loss of weight bearing. Hypercalciuria and increased mobilization of skeletal calcium can be seen in normal volunteers subjected to extensive bed rest, although hypercalcemia does not usually occur. An underlying disease associated with high bone turnover, such as Paget's disease, may cause hypercalcemia with immobilization even in older adults.

Thiazides Administration of benzothiadiazines (thiazides) can cause hypercalcemia in patients with high rates of bone turnover, such as patients with hypoparathyroidism treated with high doses of vitamin D. Traditionally, thiazides are associated with aggravation of hypercalcemia in primary hyperparathyroidism and have been used as a provocative test to bring out hypercalcemia that is borderline in patients suspected of having hyperparathyroidism. However, this effect can be seen in other high-bone-turnover states as well. The mechanism of action of the drugs is complex, but the overall result seems to be to impose a challenge to calcium homeostasis by actions on renal calcium excretion, on bone-calcium turnover, and on the efficiency of parathyroid action per se. Thiazide administration in normal individuals causes a transient increase in blood calcium (but usually within the high normal range) which reverts to preexisting levels after a week or more of continued administration. If normal hormonal function and calcium and bone metabolism are present, homeostatic controls are reset to counteract the calcium-elevating effect of the thiazides. In the presence of hyperparathyroidism or increased bone turnover from another cause, homeostatic mechanisms cannot be reset. The abnormal effects of the thiazide on calcium metabolism disappear within days of cessation of the drug.

Many aspects of the action of the thiazides in normal subjects and in patients with hyperparathyroidism remain unclear. The drug clearly augments PTH responsiveness on target cells of bone and renal tubule. Chronic thiazide administration leads to reduction in urinary calcium excretion; the hypocalciuric effect of the drug appears to reflect the enhancement of proximal tubular resorption of sodium and calcium in response to sodium depletion. Some of this renal action reflects augmentation of PTH actions and is clearly more pronounced in subjects with intact parathyroid secretion than, for example, in a group of hypoparathyroid patients whose renal calcium clearance initially was reported to be unresponsive. However, a substantial hypocalciuric effect can be achieved in hypoparathyroid patients on high-dose vitamin D and oral calcium replacement if sodium intake is restricted. This finding is the rationale for the use of thiazides as an adjunct to therapy in hypoparathyroid patients as discussed below.

Vitamin A intoxication Vitamin A intoxication is a rare cause of hypercalcemia. Most vitamin A intoxication results inadvertently

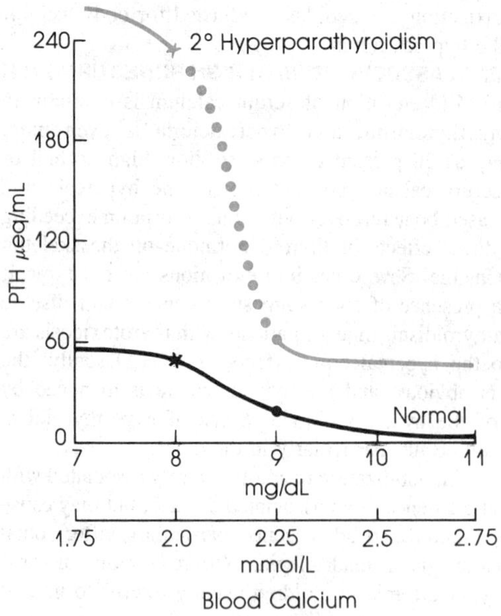

FIGURE 340-1 The relation between blood calcium and iPTH in normal subjects and subjects with secondary (2°) hyperparathyroidism. This model of secondary hyperparathyroidism assumes that there is an increased mass of parathyroid tissue. The lower line represents normal secretory patterns, and the upper line describes the exaggerated secretion (steeper slope) typical of secondary hyperparathyroidism. When calcium level in blood is raised by calcium infusion and multiple measurements of PTH and calcium are made, some portion of hormone secretion in normals is constant despite high calcium levels in blood (nonsuppressible secretion), and this secretion is higher in hyperparathyroidism. An elevation of blood calcium from low normal levels [(2 mmol/L (8 mg/dL)] to high normal levels [(2.2 mmol/L (9 mg/dL)] results in a reduction in PTH in both normal and hyperparathyroid individuals, but true involution of secondary hyperparathyroidism with treatment can be confirmed only by showing a return of the exaggerated response curve to normal.

from experiments with nutritional supplements. Calcium levels can be elevated into the 3 to 3.5 mmol/L (12 to 14 mg/dL) range after the ingestion of 50,000 to 100,000 units of vitamin A daily (10 to 20 times the minimum daily requirement). The patients have typical features of severe hypercalcemia that include fatigue and anorexia. They also have severe muscle pain and sometimes diffuse bone pain. The excess vitamin A intake is presumed to increase bone resorption.

Diagnosis can be established by history and by confirmatory measurements of vitamin A levels in serum, which may be increased severalfold above normal. Occasionally, skeletal x-rays reveal periosteal calcifications, particularly, in the hands. Withdrawal of the vitamin is usually associated with the prompt disappearance of the hypercalcemia and reversal of the skeletal changes. As in vitamin D intoxication, administration of 100 mg hydrocortisone or its equivalent per day leads to a rapid return of the serum calcium to normal.

HYPERCALCEMIA ASSOCIATED WITH RENAL FAILURE **Severe secondary hyperparathyroidism** Secondary hyperparathyroidism is the state in which excessive production of PTH is due to partial resistance to the metabolic actions of the hormone. Parathyroid gland hyperplasia with resultant increased secretion of PTH occurs because resistance to the normal level of the hormone leads to hypocalcemia which, in turn, is a stimulus to enlargement of the parathyroid glands by mechanisms direct or indirect, still not defined. This concept is based on animal and human studies, the former involving experimental renal failure with phosphatase retention and the latter involving treatment of patients with diphosphonates that block skeletal resorptive response. Figure 340-1 ilustrates the pathophysiology of hormone production in secondary hyperparathyroidism. When the parathyroid secretory reserve is tested by deliberately lowering blood calcium, the extent of rise in PTH for each milligram of decrement of plasma calcium is greater with parathyroid hyperplasia than with normal glands. There is, therefore, a higher concentration of hormone at any given level of calcium concentration. Since a portion of PTH secretion by each individual parathyroid cell is not suppressible by any degree of elevation of blood calcium concentration, larger glands (more cells) have a higher concentration of hormone output at the hypercalcemic end of the dose-response curve.

Secondary hyperparathyroidism occurs in patients with renal failure, osteomalacia (vitamin D deficiency), and pseudohypoparathyroidism (deficient response to PTH at the level of the receptor). The clinical manifestations of secondary hyperparathyroidism vary in these states. Hypocalcemia seems to be the common denominator in secondary hyperparathyroidism. Primary and secondary hyperparathyroidism can be distinguished by the autonomous nature of the growth of the parathyroid glands in primary hyperparathyroidism (presumably irreversible) and the adaptive increase in parathyroid gland size in secondary hyperparathyroidism (presumably reversible). In fact, reversal from an abnormal pattern of secretion, presumably accompanied by an involution of parathyroid gland mass to a normal pattern of function, may occur in patients treated with diphosphonate after the drug is withdrawn (Fig. 340-1).

In progressive kidney disease, the initial tendency to hypocalcemia seems attributable to two causes: phosphate retention that develops because of the reduced excretion of phosphate and reduced concentrations of $1,25(OH)_2D$ associated with progressive renal damage. The two disturbances reduce skeletal responsiveness to PTH. The deficient $1,25(OH)_2D$ also interferes with the absorption of calcium from the intestine, already impaired in uremia. The ultimate pathophysiologic consequences in any given patient with chronic renal failure represent the outcome of competing physiologic adaptations, stimuli that cause parathyroid gland hyperplasia (tendency toward hypercalcemia and excessive bone resorption) versus those that modify the hormonal responsiveness of the end organs—bone, gut, and residual renal tubules (tendency toward hypocalcemia, hyperphosphatemia, and reduced bone resorption). Typically patients with renal failure exhibit hyperphosphatemia (renal retention and increased bone breakdown) and a low normal or moderately low blood calcium (calcium-lowering action of the phosphate elevation and reduced availability of calcium from bone and gut). In patients with severe secondary hyperparathyroidism, hypercalcemia and hyperphosphatemia both develop due to an increase in bone resorption; parathyroid hypersecretion ''overshoots'' the degree of resistance to hormone action.

In addition to hypercalcemia and hyperphosphatemia, patients with symptomatic or severe secondary hyperparathyroidism may develop bone pain, ectopic calcification, and pruritus. The bone disease in patients with secondary hyperparathyroidism and renal failure is usually termed *renal osteodystrophy*. Concomitant osteomalacia (vitamin D and calcium deficiency) and osteitis fibrosa cystica (excessive PTH action on bone) may be seen. In fact, osteitis fibrosa cystica is now more common in untreated renal failure than in primary hyperparathyroidism.

Judicious medical therapy, which includes reduction of excessive blood phosphate by dietary phosphate restriction plus the use of nonabsorbable antacids and careful, selective addition of calcitriol (0.25 to 2.0 μg/d), may reverse severe secondary hyperparathyroidism. As illustrated in Fig. 340-1, involution of the parathyroids then occurs; reduction of increased cellular mass causes the exaggerated secretory response to return to normal. The level of PTH at any given level of blood calcium is now more appropriate, and excessive parathyroid action is reversed. Somewhat paradoxically, during successful medical reversal of secondary hyperparathyroidism, elevated serum calcium and phosphate levels return to normal despite the administration of increased amounts of calcium and vitamin D metabolites.

Aluminum intoxication Aluminum intoxication occurs in patients on chronic dialysis; manifestations include acute dementia and unresponsive, severe osteomalacia. Bone pain, multiple nonhealing fractures, particularly of the ribs and pelvis, and a proximal myopathy may occur. Hypercalcemia develops when attempts are made to treat these patients as one treats those with renal osteodystrophy due to renal failure, namely, by administration of vitamin D or calcitriol. Acute hypercalcemia occurs after administration of vitamin D because of impaired skeletal responsiveness. Aluminum is present at the site of osteoid mineralization, and osteoblastic activity is minimal. Presumably, these patients are unable to incorporate the increased blood calcium into the skeleton. Prevention is accomplished by avoidance of aluminum excess in the dialysis regimen; treatment involves mobilizing aluminum through the use of the chelating agent deferoxamine. Aluminum is mobilized from bone and, being tightly bound to the chelating agent, can be removed via dialysis. After aluminum toxicity is reversed, patients may show typical features of renal osteodystrophy and secondary hyperparathyroidism. They can then be managed like other patients with secondary hyperparathyroidism with renal disease. A failure to recognize the syndrome is associated with persistence of the disabling bone disease and a fatal course due to progressive features or to hypercalcemia inadvertently induced by treatment with vitamin D.

Milk-alkali syndrome The milk-alkali syndrome can cause several clinical presentations—acute, subacute, and chronic—all of which feature hypercalcemia, alkalosis, and renal failure. The syndrome is due to an excessive ingestion of calcium and absorbable antacids such as milk or calcium carbonate. The disorder is less frequent since nonabsorbable antacids and H-2 receptor antagonists such as cimetidine and ranitidine became available for the treatment of peptic ulcer disease.

Individual susceptibility must be important in pathogenesis, since many patients are treated with calcium carbonate without developing the syndrome. One variable is the fractional calcium absorption as a function of calcium intake. Some individuals absorb a high fraction of calcium, even with intakes as high as 2 g and more of elemental calcium per day, instead of reducing calcium absorption with high intake, as occurs in most normal subjects. Resultant, mild hypercalcemia after meals in such patients is postulated to be the critical factor in the generation of alkalosis. With the development of hypercalcemia, increased sodium excretion and some depletion of total-body water occurs. This phenomenon and perhaps, additionally, some suppression of endogenous PTH secretion due to mild hypercalcemia would lead to increased bicarbonate resorption. This bicarbonate retention then would lead to alkalosis in the face of continued calcium carbonate ingestion. Alkalosis per se causes selective enhancement of calcium resorption in the distal nephron, thus aggravating the hypercalcemia. The cycle of mild hypercalcemia → bicarbonate retention → alkalosis → renal calcium retention → severe hypercalcemia perpetuates and aggravates hypercalcemia and alkalosis as long as calcium and absorbable alkali are ingested.

Acute hypercalcemia and alkalosis occurring within days of beginning calcium and alkali ingestion, *acute milk-alkali syndrome,* is manifested by weakness, myalgia, irritability, and apathy. The impairment of renal function, including reduced renal concentrating ability and tubular dysfunction as well as hypercalcemia and alkalosis, reverse rapidly upon stopping the intake of calcium and alkali.

The far-advanced milk-alkali syndrome, sometimes referred to as *Burnett's syndrome,* is due to long-standing calcium and alkali ingestion. Severe hypercalcemia, irreversible renal failure, and phosphate retention may be accompanied by ectopic calcification. Some improvement may result when calcium and alkali ingestion is reduced, but prior to the availability of renal dialysis, renal failure led to death. There is an intermediate or subacute form in which the renal failure is reversible over a period of weeks after withdrawal of excessive calcium and alkali intake.

DIFFERENTIAL DIAGNOSIS: SPECIAL TESTS Differential diagnosis of hypercalcemia is best achieved by using clinical criteria, but the radioimmunoassay for PTH, as now modified, is useful in distinguishing among major causes. The clinical points that deserve major emphasis in arriving at a correct diagnosis are the presence or absence of symptoms or signs of disease and evidence of chronicity. If one discounts fatigue or depression, patients with *asymptomatic hypercalcemia* have primary hyperparathyroidism in well over 90 percent of instances; symptoms of malignancy are usually present when hypercalcemia is due to cancer. Disorders other than hyperparathyroidism and malignancy cause no more than 10 percent of hypercalcemia, and some of the nonparathyroid causes are associated with manifestations such as renal failure.

TABLE 340-3 Differential diagnosis of hypercalcemia: Laboratory criteria

	Blood*			
	Ca	P_i	$1,25(OH)_2D$	iPTH
Primary hyperparathyroidism	↑	↓	↑,↔	↑(↔)
Malignancy-associated hypercalcemia:				
Humorally mediated (HHM)	↑↑	↓	↓,↔	↓↔
Local destruction (osteolytic metastases)	↑	↔	↓,↔	↓↔

* Symbols in parentheses refer to values rarely seen in the particular disease.
NOTE: P_i = inorganic phosphate; iPTH = immunoreactive parathyroid hormone.

Chronicity is the second most important clinical criterion. If hypercalcemia has been manifest for more than 1 year, malignancy can usually (not always) be excluded as the cause of hypercalcemia. A striking feature of malignancy-associated hypercalcemia is the rapidity of the course, whereby signs and symptoms relatable to the underlying malignancy are evident within months of the first detection of hypercalcemia. Hyperparathyroidism is the likely diagnosis in patients with *chronic hypercalcemia.* Diseases such as sarcoidosis are rare, alternative causes of chronic hypercalcemia. A careful *history* of dietary supplements and drug use will often readily reveal intoxication with vitamin D or A or the use of thiazides.

Although clinical considerations are helpful in arriving at the correct diagnosis of the cause of hypercalcemia, appropriate laboratory testing is essential for definitive diagnosis (Table 340-3). Theoretically, the radioimmunoassay for PTH should separate hyperparathyroidism from all other causes of hypercalcemia, those with hyperparathyroidism having elevated levels of iPTH despite hypercalcemia and patients with malignancy and the other causes of hypercalcemia (except for other disorders mediated by parathyroid hormone such as lithium-induced hypercalcemia) having levels of hormone below normal or undetectable. Assays in use over the last two decades sometimes gave equivocal results, but assays based on the double-antibody method separate hypercalcemic patients with malignancy from those with primary hyperparathyroidism (Fig. 340-2), thus establishing the method as possessing the relevant specificity and sensitivity in the two disorders that account for more than 90 percent of all cases of hypercalcemia. $1,25(OH)_2D$ levels are elevated in many patients (but not all) with primary hyperparathyroidism and are also increased in states of vitamin D intoxication, particularly sarcoidosis. In other disorders associated with hypercalcemia, concentrations of $1,25(OH)_2D$ are low or, at the most, normal. Since not all patients with hyperparathyroidism, however, have elevated $1,25(OH)_2D$ levels and since not all nonparathyroid hypercalcemic patients have suppressed $1,25(OH)_2D$, the test is of low specificity and not cost-effective in differential diagnosis per se.

PTH levels are elevated in chronic renal failure; the elevation in older assays reflects, in part, accumulation of fragments secondary to renal failure rather than true parathyroid oversecretion. In general with the older type, single-antibody assays, those based on middle or carboxyl-region epitopes, give higher values than those based on amino-terminal recognition sites. The latter assays seemed to correlate better with other evidence of parathyroid overactivity such as osteitis fibrosa. Results with the double-antibody assay are similar to those seen with amino-terminal assays. Patients with sarcoidosis have low or undetectable levels of iPTH. No systematic surveys have been reported concerning double-antibody PTH radioimmunoassay results

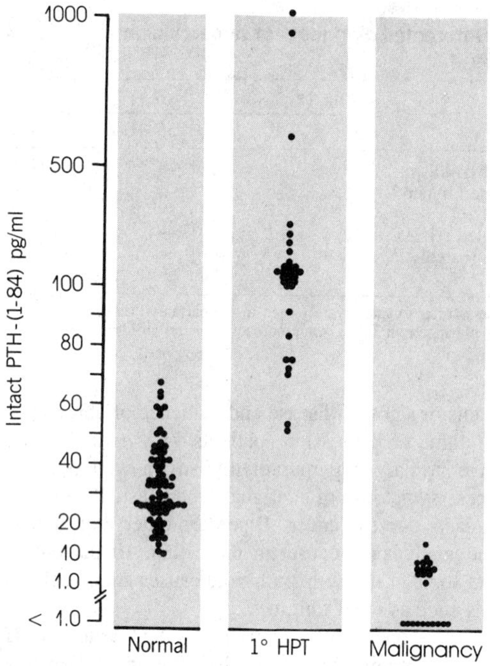

FIGURE 340-2 Levels of iPTH detected in normals, patients with primary hyperparathyroidism (1° HPT), and patients with hypercalcemia of malignancy by the double antibody assay. *(From SR Nussbaum et al: Highly sensitive two-site immunooradiometric assay of parathyrin and its clinical utility in evaluating patients with hypercalcemia. Clin Chem 33:1364, 1987.)*

in many of the other non-parathyroid-related causes of hypercalcemia shown in Table 340-1, largely because of the infrequency with which the disorders are encountered, but it is predicted they will be low or undetectable.

In summary, iPTH values are elevated in greater than 90 percent of parathyroid-related causes of hypercalcemia, undetectable or low in malignancy-related hypercalcemia, and undetectable or normal in vitamin D–related and high-bone-turnover-related causes of hypercalcemia (although there is a paucity of data for these latter categories); the same separation of groups is seen with measurements of $1,25(OH)_2D$ (Table 340-3).

Measurements of nephrogenous cyclic AMP are of limited value in distinguishing the two major causes of hypercalcemia: primary hyperparathyroidism and malignancy. Elevation of nephrogenous cyclic AMP occurs in some patients with malignancy and in essentially all patients with primary hyperparathyroidism. Specific laboratory tests are of utility in confirming the diagnosis of particular disorders (such as thyrotoxicosis); tests specific for tumor factors should be helpful when developed.

Some general recommendations can be made as to the differential diagnosis of hypercalcemia. Two independent causes of hypercalcemia in the same person, although reported, are rare. If a specific disease traditionally associated with hypercalcemia (Table 340-1) is clinically evident, it is reasonable to assume that the disease is responsible for the hypercalcemia. It is cost-effective in view of the specificity and speed of the PTH radioimmunoassay and the high frequency of hyperparathyroidism in hypercalcemic patients to measure the iPTH level in all hypercalcemic patients unless malignancy is clinically evident or a specific diagnosis of a nonparathyroid disease is obvious. If hypercalcemia disappears in response to control of hyperthyroidism, for example, or after reduction of excessive intake of fat-soluble vitamins or alkali and calcium, in the cases of vitamin D intoxication and milk-alkali syndrome, respectively, there is no need to search for a second cause of hypercalcemia. If specific treatment does not lead to a reversal of the hypercalcemia, a search for an additional cause, by detailed laboratory testing, must be undertaken. It also follows that if signs suggestive of malignancy are evident, the management of the patient focuses on management of the malignancy.

When no clues are evident as to the diagnosis, either because the patient is asymptomatic or because chronic illness obscures manifestations that might indicate the presence of malignancy, the following general approach can be used: If the patient is *asymptomatic* and if there is evidence by history of *chronicity* to the hypercalcemia, hyperparathyroidism is almost certainly the cause of the hypercalcemia. If iPTH levels (usually measured at least twice) are elevated, little additional evaluation is necessary. Hyperparathyroidism is never confirmed until abnormal parathyroid tissue is surgically removed and hypercalcemia is corrected, but patients with asymptomatic hypercalcemia who have the presumptive diagnosis on the basis of elevated concentration of iPTH can be followed without intervention but with careful monitoring or can be recommended for surgery with reasonable confidence of cure. If in such patients there is a family history suggestive of other endocrine abnormality, screening for multiple endocrine neoplasia should be undertaken in the patient and family.

If the patient does not have clear-cut symptoms and there is only a short history or no clue as to the duration of the hypercalcemia, *occult malignancy* must be considered with more care than if the hypercalcemia is known to be chronic. If the iPTH levels with the double-antibody technique are increased, the diagnosis of asymptomatic hyperparathyroidism is established.

If patients with a short history of hypercalcemia have clear-cut systemic symptoms and/or the iPTH levels are not elevated, then a thorough workup must be undertaken for malignancy, including chest x-ray, computed tomography of chest and abdomen, and bone scan. Attention should also be paid to clues for underlying hematologic disorders such as anemia, increased plasma globulin, and abnormal serum immunoelectrophoresis; bone scans can be negative in patients with multiple myeloma.

Finally, if a patient with *chronic hypercalcemia* is *asymptomatic* but iPTH values are not elevated and if malignancy seems unlikely on clinical grounds (*chronicity*), it is useful to search for other chronic illnesses that cause hypercalcemia, such as occult sarcoidosis.

MEDICAL TREATMENT OF HYPERCALCEMIA The acute treatment of hypercalcemia is usually successful. The serum calcium concentration can be decreased by 0.7 to 2.2 mmol/L (3 to 9 mg/dL) within 24 to 48 h in most patients, enough to relieve acute symptoms, prevent death from hypercalcemic crisis, and permit diagnostic evaluation. However, the chronic medical management of hypercalcemia is less satisfactory unless the underlying cause can be corrected because available therapies are inconvenient and may be toxic in chronic use.

Hypercalcemia develops because skeletal calcium release is excessive, intestinal calcium absorption is increased, or renal calcium excretion is inadequate. Understanding the particular pathogenesis helps guide therapy. For example, hypercalcemia in patients with osteolytic metastastes or acute immobilization is primarily due to excessive skeletal calcium release and is, therefore, minimally affected by restriction of dietary calcium. On the other hand, patients with vitamin D hypersensitivity or vitamin D intoxication have excessive intestinal calcium absorption, and restriction of dietary calcium is beneficial. Decreased renal function or extracellular fluid depletion decreases urinary calcium excretion. If additional abnormalities, such as increased bone breakdown, are present, hypercalcemia will develop. This may happen, for example, when patients with resorptive bone disease become dehydrated. In such situations, rehydration may rapidly reduce or reverse the hypercalcemia, even though excessive bone resorption and increased urinary calcium excretion continue.

Hydration, increased salt intake, mild and forced diuresis The first principle of treatment is to restore *normal hydration*. Many hypercalcemic patients are dehydrated because of vomiting, inanition, and/or hypercalcemia-induced defects in urinary concentrating ability. The resultant drop in glomerular filtration rate is accompanied by an additional decrease in renal tubular sodium and calcium clearance. Restoring a normal extracellular fluid volume corrects these abnormalities and increases urine calcium excretion by 2.5 to 7.5 mmol/d

(100 to 300 mg/d). Increased urinary sodium excretion to 400 to 500 mmol/d increases urinary calcium excretion even further than simple rehydration. Finally, after full benefits of simple rehydration have been achieved, saline can be administered or conventional doses of furosemide or ethacrynic acid can be given twice daily to depress the tubular reabsorptive mechanism for calcium (care must be taken to prevent the diuretic from provoking dehydration). The combined use of these therapies can increase urinary calcium excretion to 12.5 mmol/d (500 mg/d) or higher in most hypercalcemic patients. Since this is a substantial percentage of the exchangeable calcium pool, the serum calcium concentration usually falls 0.25 to 0.75 mmol/L (1 to 3 mg/dL) within 24 h. Precautions should be taken to prevent potassium and magnesium depletion during chronic therapy; calcium-containing renal calculi are a potential complication.

Under life-threatening circumstances, the above therapy can be pursued more aggressively, giving as much as 6 L isotonic saline (900 mmol sodium) daily plus furosemide or equivalent in doses up to 100 mg every 1 to 2 h or ethacrynic acid in doses to 40 mg every 1 to 2 h. Urinary calcium excretion may exceed 25 mmol/d (1000 mg/d), and the serum calcium may decrease by 1 mmol/L (4 mg/dL) or more within 24 h. Depletion of potassium and magnesium is inevitable unless replacements are given; pulmonary edema can be precipitated. The potential complications can be reduced by careful monitoring of central venous pressure and plasma or urine electrolytes; a bladder catheter may be necessary. The treatment approach should be immediately supplemented with agents to block bone resorption that become effective within a few days, since the forced diuresis therapy is difficult to sustain even in patients with good cardiopulmonary and renal function.

Plicamycin For the acute management of hypercalcemia, plicamycin (mithramycin), which inhibits bone resorption, is a useful therapeutic agent. Plicamycin must be given intravenously, either as a bolus injection or by slow infusion. The usual dose is 25 μg/kg body weight. In some patients, 10 μg/kg body weight can be given twice a week for chronic therapy. Treatment should not be repeated until hypercalcemia recurs, because the toxicity of the drug is dependent on the frequency of treatment and the total dosage. Careful monitoring is needed if repeated doses are used. The major side effects are thrombocytopenia, hepatocellular necrosis with increased lactic acid dehydrogenase (LDH) and aspartate aminotransferase (AST) levels, and decreased levels of clotting factors with resultant epistaxis, bruising, hemorrhage, and bleeding gums. Azotemia, proteinuria, and hypocalcemia may occur. Hypophosphatemia and hypokalemia may also develop, as may nausea, vomiting, stomatitis, and facial swelling. Toxicity is rare when only one or two doses are used and can be minimized by repeating single doses only when hypercalcemia recurs. Toxic effects other than hemorrhage can usually be reversed by stopping the drug.

Diphosphonates After an initial period of uncertainty relating to the divergent pharmacologic actions of this class of drugs (variable effects on bone formation vs. resorption and undesirable cellular effects—pyrexia, leukopenia), certain diphosphonates (bisphosphonates) are emerging as valuable, effective therapies with a favorable therapeutic/toxic ratio. Aminohydroxypropylidene diphosphonate (APD) is undergoing clinical trial. This drug acts primarily by blocking bone resorption without affecting bone formation. Diphosphonates, analogues of pyrophosphate, are "bone seeking" and have a long chemical half-life. The hypocalcemic action of APD lasts for weeks following intravenous administration to patients with hypercalcemia due to increased bone resorption such as in malignancy. If therapeutic actions are confirmed and toxicity remains minor, this drug class may be useful in the management of hypercalcemia; many new bisphosphonates are being evaluted.

Other therapies Glucocorticoids increase urinary calcium excretion and decrease intestinal calcium absorption when given in pharmacologic doses (e.g., 40 to 200 mg prednisone daily in divided doses), but they also cause negative skeletal calcium balance. In normal subjects and in patients with primary hyperparathyroidism, glucocorticoids neither increase nor decrease the serum calcium concentration. In patients with hypercalcemia due to certain osteolytic malignancies, however, glucocorticoids may be effective as a result of antitumor effects. The malignancies in which hypercalcemia responds to glucocorticoids are usually hematologic malignancies such as multiple myeloma, leukemia, Hodgkin's disease, and other lymphomas; carcinoma of the breast may also respond, at least early in the course. Glucocorticoids are effective in treating hypercalcemia due to vitamin D intoxication and in the vitamin D hypersensitivity of sarcoidosis. In all the above situations, the hypocalcemic effect develops over several days, and the usual glucocorticoid dosage is 40 to 100 mg prednisone (or its equivalent) daily in four divided doses. The side effects of chronic glucocorticoid therapy may be acceptable in some circumstances.

Prostaglandins of the E series may play a role in the hypercalcemia of certain malignancies, especially those metastatic or primary in bone marrow. Prostaglandin synthesis can be blocked by indomethacin or aspirin; these drugs may correct the hypercalcemia in a subset of patients with osteolytic lesions or even humoral hypercalcemia of malignancy. The analytical methods necessary to define prostaglandin excess are not widely available, and correlations between prostaglandin levels and hypercalcemia are usually not available. In those cases when a therapeutic trial has been reported to be successful, indomethacin, 25 mg every 6 h, or aspirin in sufficient doses to produce a serum salicylate level of 1.4 to 1.8 mmol/L (20 to 25 mg/dL) have been used to lower the serum calcium concentrations over several days.

Hypercalcemia complicated by severe failure is difficult to manage; dialysis is often the treatment of choice. Peritoneal dialysis can remove 5 to 12.5 mmol (200 to 500 mg) of calcium in 24 to 48 h and lower the serum calcium concentration by 0.7 to 3 mmol/L (3 to 12 mg/dL) if calcium-free dialysis fluid is used. Large quantities of phosphate are lost during dialysis, and serum inorganic phosphate concentrations usually fall, thus aggravating hypercalcemia. Therefore, the serum inorganic phosphate concentration should be measured after dialysis, and phosphate supplements should be added to the diet or to dialysis fluids if necessary. APD may be helpful in such situations.

Calcitonin decreases the skeletal release of calcium, phosphorus, and hydroxyproline within minutes of its intravenous injection. The subsequent changes in serum calcium and phosphorus depend upon the initial magnitude of skeletal resorption; subjects with the most rapid bone turnover show the greatest reduction in serum calcium concentration. Calcitonin also increases the renal clearance of calcium and phosphorus (and sodium). Unfortunately, escape from drug action occurs in patients and animals invariably after 12 to 24 h of high-dose continuous therapy or after several days of repeated therapy with calcitonin. The mechanism of escape is unknown; coadministration of glucocorticoids and calcitonin may prevent escape. This promising lead deserves further clinical evaluation, since calcitonin causes minimal toxicity. Calcitonin is effective by intravenous, intramuscular, or subcutaneous injection; doses used are 25 to 50 units every 6 to 8 h, usually in the form of salmon calcitonin.

Phosphate Patients with primary hyperparathyroidism are frequently hypophosphatemic, and hypercalcemia of other causes may also be complicated by hypophosphatemia. Hypophosphatemia decreases the rate of calcium uptake into bone, increases intestinal calcium absorption, and directly and indirectly stimulates bone breakdown. These effects aggravate hypercalcemia, and correcting hypophosphatemia lowers the serum calcium concentration. The usual treatment is 1 to 1.5 g phosphorus per day for several days, given in four divided doses to minimize the chances of developing hyperphosphatemia. Such therapy has been administered for prolonged periods in selected patients. It is generally believed but not established that toxicity will not occur if the phosphate therapy is limited to restoring serum inorganic phosphate concentrations to normal rather than making them supranormal.

Raising the serum inorganic phosphate concentration above normal

TABLE 340-4 Commercially available phosphate preparations

	1000 mg P	mmol Na	mmol K
Oral phosphate preparations:			
Neutraphos (1250-mg capsule)	4 caps	28.5	28.5
Neutraphos-K (1450-mg capsule)	4 caps	—	57
Phos-Tabs (860-mg tablet)	6 tabs	—	51
Fleets Phospho-Soda (liquid)	6.7 mL	40	—
Intravenous phosphate preparations:			
In-Phos	40 mL	65	8
Hyper-Phos-K	15 mL	—	50

SOURCE: After Neer and Potts (with permission).

does decrease serum calcium levels, sometimes strikingly. Intravenous phosphate is one of the most dramatically effective treatments available for severe hypercalcemia but is toxic and even dangerous so that it is used rarely and *only* in severely hypercalcemic patients with cardiac or renal failure. A dose of 1500 mg phosphate phosphorus or more intravenously over 6 to 8 h leads to a prompt decrease in serum calcium of as much as 1.2 to 2.5 mmol/L (5 to 10 mg/dL) in patients with initially normal serum inorganic phosphate concentrations. This therapy should be employed only in extreme emergencies for two reasons. First, fatal hypocalcemia can be produced by excessive dosage; frequent serum calcium determinations are necessary if intravenous phosphate is administered. Second, unlike sodium chloride, sodium phosphate does not remove calcium from the body. In fact, urine calcium generally declines and fecal calcium declines or remains the same. The decline in serum calcium reflects a redistribution of calcium within the body. There is a rapid efflux of calcium with no change in calcium influx to the circulation, findings indicative of precipitation of calcium phosphate salt. The calcium precipitates in bone, and metastatic calcification has also been reported in patients receiving oral or intravenous phosphate therapy for hypercalcemia. Indeed, hyperphosphatemia can cause metastatic calcification in normocalcemic animals. Thus, administration of intravenous phosphate in patients with compromised renal function who cannot have diuretic therapy is justifiable only as an emergency treatment.

Inorganic phosphate is commercially available for oral use in liquid, powder, and capsule form, and as a liquid for intravenous use. It is important to calculate doses in terms of phosphate phosphorus (see Table 340-4).

Anticancer drugs Several anticancer drugs have hypocalcemic effects independent of antitumor activity. Ethiofos (WR-2721), an organic thiophosphate, causes hypocalcemia in normocalcemic cancer patients; the action is attributed to inhibition of parathyroid hormone release. Extensive trials in vivo have not been reported.

Cisplatin has been tested in patients. The drug lowers serum calcium within days in the majority of treated patients with hypercalcemia and cancer; the beneficial effect lasts for weeks in most patients. The factors controlling responsiveness are unknown; the mode of action resembles that of mithramycin and diphosphonates: blockage of bone resorption. Similar effects and postulated mode of action have been reported with gallium nitrate, another experimental anticancer agent.

The ultimate utility of these agents is unclear, but their hypocalcemic effects represent a potentially useful therapy, especially in patients with malignancy.

Summary The various therapies for hypercalcemia are listed in Table 340-5. The choice depends upon the underlying disease, the

TABLE 340-5 Summary of treatments for hypercalcemia

Therapy	Therapeutic details	Indications	Complications	Precautions
MOST GENERALLY USEFUL THERAPIES				
Hydration	2 L or more	Universal	—	—
High salt intake	Achieve urine Na of 300 mmol/d or more	Universal	Edema	—
Furosemide or ethacrynic acid	40–160 mg/d 50–200 mg/d	Universal	↓K and ↓Mg	Measure serum K and Mg
Forced diuresis	4–6 L fluid IV/day containing 600–900 mmol Na plus furosemide every 1–2 h, plus at least 60 mmol K/day, plus at least 60 mmol Mg/day	Universal	Pulmonary edema; ↓K and ↓Mg	Intensive monitoring, including venous pressure and serum Mg and K
Oral phosphate	250 mg P every 6 h PO	Universal if serum P < 3 mg/dL	Ectopic calcification	Keep serum P below 5–6 mg/dL
Plicamycin	10–25 g/kg body weight IV, repeat PRN	Increased bone resorption	Liver; kidney; marrow toxicity	Monitor platelets, CBC, BUN, SCOT
Diphosphonate (aminohydroxypropylidene biphosphonate, APD)	15–30 mg IV every 2–6 h for 3–6 days or 1200 mg/d PO for 6 days	Increased bone resorption		
Prednisone or equivalent	5–15 mg every 6 h	Breast cancer, lymphomas, leukemias, multiple myeloma, vitamin D poisoning, sarcoidosis	Cushing's syndrome if chronic Rx	Alternate-day Rx for chronic use
SPECIAL THERAPIES FOR PARTICULAR USES				
IV phosphate	1500 mg P every 12 h until P is 2 mmol/L (6 mg/dL) or less	Severe hypercalcemia: diuresis or mithramycin contraindicated	Ectopic calcification: severe hypocalcemia	Monitor serum Ca and P closely
Calcitonin	2 units kg every 4 h subcutaneously	Adjunct in presence of bone reabsorption; paralysis; immobilization	—	—
Indomethacin	25 mg every 6 h PO	Certain types of pseudohyperparathyroidism	Na retention: GI bleeding; headache	Careful clinical monitoring
Dialysis	Lo-Ca bath	Acute renal failure	Multiple	Monitor serum P after dialysis

severity of the hypercalcemia, the serum inorganic phosphate level, and the renal, hepatic, and bone marrow function. Mild hypercalcemia [3 mmol/L (12 mg/dL) or less] can usually be managed by the sequence of hydration followed by intravenous sodium chloride and, if needed, small doses of furosemide or ethacrynic acid. Severe hypercalcemia [3.7 mmol/L (15 mg/dL)] requires rapid correction. Aggressive sodium-calcium diuresis with intravenous saline and large doses of furosemide and ethacrynic acid works but should be undertaken only if appropriate monitoring is available and cardiac function is adequate. Plicamycin has often been the drug of choice, but because of its potential toxicity plicamyin will probably be replaced by the diphosphonates, which also act by blocking bone resorption and, at present, seem safer and longer-acting.

There is a role for oral phosphate therapy in chronic management of hypercalcemia, unless its utility is superceded by the diphosphonates. Phosphate supplements should not be administered if hyperphosphatemia is present.

Severe dietary calcium restriction should be employed if intestinal absorption is enhanced (in sarcoidosis, vitamin D intoxication). Glucocorticoids and prostaglandin-synthesis inhibitors, even when effective in a particular disease, work slowly over several days and should not be relied upon as principal treatment for life-threatening hypercalcemia. Dialysis should be reserved for hypercalcemia complicating acute or chronic renal failure. There may be a role for calcitonin combined with glucocorticoids, but more experience is needed.

Chronic therapy of hypercalcemia poses greater problems of toxicity. One satisfactory regimen for chronic use is a combination of dietary calcium restriction, administration of sodium chloride with or without furosemide and ethacrynic acid, and moderate-dose oral phosphate (the patient is kept normophosphatemic). Some of the effective remedies (plicamycin, glucocorticoids, high-dose oral phosphate) may have significant toxicity when used chronically. Diphosphonates, if proven nontoxic, may become the chronic treatment of choice in cases of hypercalcemia where increased bone resorption is responsible for the disturbance in calcium metabolism.

HYPOCALCEMIA

PATHOPHYSIOLOGY OF HYPOCALCEMIA: CLASSIFICATION BASED ON MECHANISM *Chronic hypocalcemia* is less common than hypercalcemia; principal causes include chronic renal failure, hereditary and acquired hypoparathyroidism or vitamin D deficiency, and hypomagnesemia.

Critically ill patients may have *transient hypocalcemia* in association with severe sepsis, burns, acute renal failure, and extensive transfusions with citrated blood. In many instances, however, the hypocalcemia is more apparent than real. Although as many as half of patients in intensive care settings are reported to have calcium concentrations below 2.1 mmol/L (8.5 mg/dL), less than 10 percent have a reduction in ionized calcium. Patients with severe sepsis may have a decrease in ionized calcium (true hypocalcemia), but in other severely ill subjects hypoalbuminemia is the cause of the reduced total calcium concentration. Alkalosis, however, increases calcium binding to proteins, and in this setting direct measurements of ionized calcium should be made.

Medications such as protamine, heparin, and glucagon may cause transient hypocalcemia. These forms of hypocalcemia, apparent or real, are usually not associated with tetany and resolve with improvement in the overall medical condition. The transient hypocalcemia after repeated transfusions of citrated blood also usually resolves quickly.

Patients with acute *pancreatitis* have hypocalcemia that persists during the acute inflammation and varies in degree with the severity of the pancreatitis. The cause of hypocalcemia in pancreatitis remains unclear. Parathyroid hormone (PTH) values are variously reported to be low, normal, or elevated, and both resistance to PTH and impaired PTH secretion have been postulated, leaving no clear view as to the principal mechanism. Occasionally a chronic low total-blood calcium is detected in an elderly patient, with documented reduction in ionized calcium concentration but without obvious cause and with a paucity of symptoms of hypocalcemia; the pathogenesis is unclear.

TABLE 340-6 Functionally based classification of hypocalcemia (excluding neonatal conditions)

I PTH absent
- *A* Hereditary hypoparathyroidism
- *B* Acquired hypoparathyroidism
- *C* Hypomagnesemia

II PTH ineffective
- *A* Chronic renal failure
- *B* Active vitamin D lacking
  - *1* ↓ dietary intake or sunlight
  - *2* Defective metabolism:
    - Anticonvulsant therapy
    - Vitamin D–dependent rickets type I
- *C* Active vitamin D ineffective
  - *1* Intestinal malabsorption
  - *2* Vitamin D–dependent rickets type II
- *D* Pseudohypoparathyroidism

III PTH overwhelmed
- *A* Severe, acute hyperphosphatemia
  - *1* Tumor lysis
  - *2* Acute renal failure
  - *3* Rhabdomyolysis
- *B* Osteitis fibrosa after parathyroidectomy

Neuromuscular and neurologic symptoms are the most common manifestations of chronic hypocalcemia and include muscle spasms, carpopedal spasm, facial grimacing, and, in extreme cases, laryngeal spasm and convulsions. Respiratory arrest may occur. Increased intracranial pressure occurs in some patients with long-standing hypocalcemia, often in association with papilledema. Chronic mental changes include irritability, depression, and psychosis. The QT interval on the electrocardiogram is prolonged, in contrast to its shortening with hypercalcemia. Arrhythmias are reported, and digitalis effectiveness may be reduced. Intestinal cramps and chronic malabsorption may occur. Chvostek's or Trousseau's signs can be used to confirm latent tetany.

The classification of hypocalcemia shown in Table 340-6 is based on the premise that PTH is responsible for minute-to-minute regulation of plasma calcium concentration within narrow limits and, therefore, that the occurrence of hypocalcemia must mean a failure of the homeostatic action of PTH. The classification is offered for simplicity of approach to diagnosis. Failure of the PTH response can occur if PTH is absent due to hereditary or acquired gland failure, if the hormone is rendered ineffective by mechanisms that interfere with its action at target organs, or if the action of the hormone to raise blood calcium is overwhelmed by the loss of calcium from the extracellular fluid at a rate faster than it can be replaced.

PTH ABSENT Hypoparathyroidism, whether hereditary or acquired, has a number of common components. Acute and chronic symptoms that result from untreated hypocalcemia are shared by both types of hypoparathyroidism, although typically the onset of hereditary hypoparathyroidism is more gradual and acquired hypoparathyroidism lacks associated developmental defects seen in hereditary hypoparathyroidism. In earlier decades, acquired hypoparathyroidism secondary to surgery in the neck was more common than hereditary hypoparathyroidism, but the frequency of surgically induced parathyroid failure has diminished with the recognition of the importance of parathyroid gland preservation and the use of nonsurgical approaches in treatment of hyperthyroidism. Basal ganglia calcification and extrapyramidal syndromes occur in both hereditary and acquired hypoparathyroidism but are more common and earlier in onset in hereditary hypoparathyroidism. Pseudohypoparathyroidism, an example of ineffective PTH action rather than a failure of parathyroid gland production, shares several features with hypoparathyroidism, including extraosseous calcification and extrapyramidal syndromes such as choreoathetotic movements and dystonia. Papilledema and raised intracranial pressure occur in both states, as do chronic changes in fingernails and hair and lenticular cataracts, the latter usually reversible with treatment of hypocalcemia. Certain skin manifestations, including alopecia and candidiasis, occur exclusively in hereditary hypoparathyroidism.

Hypocalcemia associated with hypomagnesemia is associated both with deficient PTH release and impaired responsiveness to the hormone (also see Chap. 343). Patients with hypocalcemia secondary to hypomagnesemia have absent or low levels of circulating iPTH, indicative of diminished hormone release despite maximum physiologic stimulus by hypocalcemia. Plasma PTH levels return to normal with correction of the hypomagnesemia. Thus, hypoparathyroidism associated with low levels of PTH in blood can be due to hereditary gland failure, acquired gland failure, or acute but reversible gland dysfunction (hypomagnesemia). Patients with acquired or hereditary hypoparathyroidism also have hyperphosphatemia and absent or low levels of $1,25(OH)_2D$.

Hereditary hypoparathyroidism Hypoparathyroidism can occur as an isolated entity without other endocrine or dermatologic manifestations or, more typically, in association with other abnormalities such as defective development of the thymus or failure of other endocrine organs such as the thyroid or ovary (see Chap. 325). Hereditary hypoparathyroidism is often manifest within the first decade but may appear later.

One rare form of hypoparathyroidism due to congenital aplasia of the parathyroid glands is manifested shortly after birth. A linkage between defective development of the thymus and the parathyroid glands is recognized in the *DiGeorge syndrome,* which is also associated with congenital cardiovascular and other developmental defects. Most patients die in early childhood.

Hypoparathyroidism can occur in association with other diverse developmental defects or as part of a complex autoimmune syndrome involving failure of the adrenals, the ovaries, and the parathyroids in association with recurrent mucocutaneous candidiasis, alopecia, vitiligo, and pernicious anemia (see Chap. 325). In many cases, antibodies to endocrine organs are present; there is, in addition, a failure of cell-mediated immunity. The inheritance of the autoimmune syndrome appears to be autosomal recessive, and some unaffected family members show antibodies to endocrine tissue without evidence of endocrine failure. The disorder is usually referred to as autoimmune polyglandular deficiency.

Hereditary hypoparathyroidism occurs also as an isolated entity without any other defects. The mechanism of inheritance varies from one kindred to another. Autosomal dominant, autosomal recessive, and X-linked inheritance patterns have all been identified. In one pedigree, a structural abnormality in the parathyroid hormone gene is suspected, but for most families the defect appears to involve some other gene(s) in control of parathyroid gland function.

Treatment of hereditary hypoparathyroidism is similar to that for acquired hypoparathyroidism and pseudohypoparathyroidism, although specific features of each disease lead to additional treatments. Replacement therapy with vitamin D or calcitriol combined with a high oral calcium intake usually suffices to regulate blood calcium and phosphate levels satisfactorily. Oral calcium and vitamin D restore the overall calcium-phosphate balance but do not reverse the lowered urinary calcium reabsorption typical of hypoparathyroidism. Therefore, care must be taken to avoid excessive urinary calcium excretion due to excessive vitamin D and calcium replacement therapy; otherwise kidney stones could develop. Thiazide diuretics lower urine calcium by as much as 100 mg/d in hypoparathyroid patients on vitamin D, provided patients are maintained on a low-sodium diet. Use of thiazides seems to be of benefit in preventing severe hypercalciuria and in improving the management of certain patients (see above).

Acquired hypoparathyroidism *Acquired chronic hypoparathyroidism* is usually the result of inadvertent surgical removal of all the parathyroid glands; in some instances, not all of the tissue is removed, but the gland undergoes compromise of vascular supply secondary to fibrotic changes in the neck after surgery. In the past the most frequent cause of acquired hypoparathyroidism was surgery for hyperthyroidism. Chronic hypoparathyroidism now usually occurs after surgery for chief cell hyperplasia of the parathyroids where the surgeon, facing the dilemma of removing too little tissue and thus not curing the hyperparathyroidism, removes too much.

Parathyroid function is not totally absent in all patients with postsurgical hypoparathyroidism. Presumably, the persistence of some residual parathyroid activity reduces the amount of replacement therapy that is necessary, but suitable therapy varies greatly from patient to patient irrespective of the type of hypoparathyroidism or the question of residual parathyroid activity.

Other rare causes of acquired chronic hypoparathyroidism include radiation-induced damage subsequent to radioiodine therapy of hyperthyroidism or glandular damage in patients with hemochromatosis or with hemosiderosis after repeated blood transfusions. Although chronic infections may involve one or more of the parathyroids, they usually do not cause permanent hypoparathyroidism because all four glands are not usually involved.

Transient hypoparathyroidism is frequent following surgical exploration for hyperparathyroidism, particularly in patients in whom more than one exploration is required and in patients with multiple gland disease in which all glands must be identified and biopsied. Often, after a variable period of hypoparathyroidism, normal parathyroid function returns due to hyperplasia of remaining tissue. Occasionally, recovery occurs months after surgery. The management of transient, postoperative hypoparathyroidism is discussed under the surgical treatment of hyperparathyroidism. The treatment of chronic acquired hypoparathyroidism is similar to that used with idiopathic hypoparathyroidism: replacement with vitamin D and oral calcium.

Hypomagnesemia Hypomagnesemia of a severe degree is associated with severe hypocalcemia (also see Chap. 343). Restoration of the total-body magnesium deficits leads to rapid reversal of the hypocalcemia. There are at least two separate causes of the hypocalcemia—impaired secretion of PTH and reduced peripheral responsiveness to hormone action.

Hypomagnesemia is generally classified as primary or secondary; primary hypomagnesemia is due to hereditary defects in intestinal absorption or renal reabsorption of magnesium. Secondary hypomagnesemia, a more common condition, occurs on a nutritional basis or as a result of acquired intestinal or renal disorders. The most common causes of the secondary disorder are intestinal malabsorption syndromes, chronic alcoholism with poor nutritional intake, and parenteral nutrition in which magnesium replacement is omitted.

In experimental animals magnesium in extracellular fluid has effects similar to those of calcium on secretion of PTH; hypermagnesemia suppresses, and hypomagnesemia stimulates, PTH secretion. Effects of magnesium on hormone secretion are normally of little physiologic significance, however, because the effects of calcium dominate. Greater change in magnesium than in calcium is needed to influence hormone secretion. Nonetheless, hypomagnesemia, if it influences hormone secretion at all, might be expected to increase hormone secretion. It is, therefore, surprising to find that severe hypomagnesemia is associated with blunted secretion of PTH. The explanation for the paradox is that severe, chronic hypomagnesemia reflects intracellular magnesium deficiency; severe intracellular magnesium deficiency interferes with normal secretory mechanisms and normal peripheral responses to PTH. It is suspected that both effects involve function of adenyl cyclase in glandular and target tissues. Reduced intracellular stores of magnesium obscure any effects that might be brought about by acute changes in extracellular fluid magnesium in a magnesium-replete individual.

Severe hypocalcemia is often seen when serum magnesium is substantially below normal. Normal serum magnesium is 0.8 to 1.2 mmol/L (2 to 3 mg/dL). In most cases in which hypomagnesemia is associated with hypocalcemia, serum magnesium is below 0.4 mmol/L (1.0 mg/dL).

PTH levels are usually undetectable or inappropriately low despite the extreme stimulus of severe hypocalcemia. Even when iPTH levels are moderately elevated, acute repletion of magnesium leads to a further increase in iPTH concentration. The overall data indicate that PTH secretion is blunted in virtually all patients with severe hypomagnesemia; thus, absolute or relative hypoparathyroidism seems to be the rule in patients with hypocalcemia secondary to hypomagnesemia.

Diminished peripheral responsiveness to administered PTH can be shown in some patients with severe hypomagnesemia in addition. Some clinical reports document subnormal response in urinary phosphorus and urinary cyclic AMP excretion after administration of exogenous PTH to patients who are hypocalcemic and who have diminished PTH secretion. Both blunted PTH secretion and lack of renal response to administered PTH can occur in the same patient. Blunted skeletal responses have been claimed in many, but by no means all, patients studied with the hypomagnesemia-hypocalcemia syndrome. When acute magnesium repletion is undertaken, the restoration of PTH concentrations to normal or supranormal levels may precede by several days the restoration of normal serum calcium.

Overall, blunted PTH secretory response in hypomagnesemia seems the more important and invariant cause of hypocalcemia. The fact that impaired peripheral responsiveness, particularly renal response, is more variable from patient to patient may indicate that an even greater degree of magnesium deficiency is required to induce end organ resistance than to impair hormone secretion.

Several other features have been noted. The brisk response in hormone secretion following magnesium repletion, sometimes demonstrable within minutes of giving a large parenteral dose of magnesium, indicates that hormone biosynthesis is not impaired, only secretion. Serum phosphate levels are not elevated as they often are in patients with hypoparathyroidism, probably because phosphate deficiency is a frequent accompaniment of the nutritional deficiencies that cause hypomagnesemia. There have been a few reports of magnesium-wasting chronic renal disease; although magnesium is usually elevated in acute renal failure, increases in magnesium concentration are rare in chronic renal failure.

Repletion of magnesium is the cure of the condition, and attention must be given to restoring the intracellular deficiency, which may be considerable. After intravenous magnesium, serum magnesium may return to the normal range, but unless replacement therapy is continued, it will rapidly fall to subnormal levels again. If renal function is normal, a useful indicator of restoration of magnesium deficiency is the urinary magnesium excretion; magnesium is retained by the kidney until magnesium deficiencies are repleted. Intracellular deficits can be as great as 50 mmol or more, but in many cases parenteral administration of approximately 12 mmol magnesium reverses the signs of magnesium deficiency. Depending on the cause of the hypomagnesemia, treatment may have to be administered chronically to prevent recurrence.

PTH INEFFECTIVE PTH can be considered ineffective when the hormone's action to promote calcium absorption from the diet is interfered with because of a primary deficiency of vitamin D, because of conditions in which vitamin D is ineffective, or in chronic renal failure in which the calcium-elevating action of PTH is opposed by several different processes. Despite diverse pathophysiologic mechanisms, these conditions usually involve, but are not limited to, the unavailability of vitamin D as a cofactor for PTH. Hypocalcemia is usually mild rather than severe and is accompanied by hypophosphatemia. Typically, hypophosphatemia is more severe than hypocalcemia due to the increased secretion of PTH. Increased PTH is only partly effective in elevating blood calcium, yet it promotes renal phosphate excretion in a nearly unimpaired manner in vitamin D deficiency. Varying degrees of bone disease with impaired mineralization and/or frank osteomalacia are the more frequent and harmful consequences of chronic renal failure or inadequate or ineffective vitamin D action due to the hypophosphatemia.

Pseudohypoparathyroidism, on the other hand, is distinct in pathophysiology from the other disorders classified under ineffective PTH action. Pseudohypoparathyroidism resembles conditions in which there is an absence of PTH synthesis and secretion and is manifested, in the untreated state, by severe hypocalcemia and hyperphosphatemia. The cause of the disease, however, is inadequate peripheral response to PTH involving defective hormone binding to the receptor, deficient activation of guanyl nucleotide–binding proteins, and/or stimulation of adenyl cyclase to increase intracellular cyclic AMP (see Chap. 68).

Chronic renal failure Severe abnormalities in mineral ion and bone metabolism occur in chronic renal failure. Even prior to the initiation of extensive programs of dialysis, however, improved medical management of chronic renal failure and/or a more indolent course of the renal disease allowed many patients to survive for a sufficiently long period that renal osteodystrophy, the mixed bone disease associated with renal failure, became an important feature.

After the initiation of chronic dialysis programs, many of the impairments in mineral and bone metabolism became even more apparent. Now the roles of phosphate retention and impaired production of $1,24(OH)_2D$ are recognized as the principal factors responsible for inducing calcium deficiency, secondary hyperparathyroidism, and frequently a picture of severe bone disease. Less clearly, the uremic state appears to be associated with impairment of intestinal absorption by factors other than defects in vitamin D metabolism. Nonetheless, replacement of physiologic levels of $1,25(OH)_2$ usually leads to satisfactory calcium absorption, suggesting it is the lack of the vitamin D rather than intrinsic defects in intestinal cellular function that is the more important cause of the impaired mineral metabolism in chronic renal failure.

Hyperphosphatemia per se tends to lower blood calcium concentration by several actions; these include extraosseous deposition of calcium and phosphate, impaired sensitivity of the skeleton to the bone-resorbing action of PTH, reduced $1,25(OH)_2D$ production by surviving renal tissue, and reduction in calcium absorption due to trapping of calcium in insoluble form as calcium phosphate complexes. In animals, prevention of hyperphosphatemia by dietary means can block the development of secondary hyperparathyroidism, emphasizing the importance of phosphate retention in the pathogenesis of secondary hyperparathyroidism and the associated disorders of mineral and bone metabolism. Low levels of $1,25(OH)_2D$ are also critical in the hypocalcemia; the low levels of vitamin D metabolites are due to hyperphosphatemia and to destruction of renal tissue.

Therapy of chronic renal failure (see Chaps. 224 and 225) involves careful management of patients prior to dialysis as well as adjustment of dialysis regimens once this becomes necessary. Attention should be paid to restriction of phosphate in the diet, use of phosphate-binding antacids such as those based on aluminum hydroxide, provision of an adequate calcium intake by mouth, usually 1 to 2 g/d, and supplementation with calcitriol in doses of 0.25 to 1.0 μg/d. Each patient must be monitored closely. The aims of therapy are to restore normal calcium balance to prevent osteomalacia and secondary hyperparathyroidism. Renal osteodystrophy, as discussed above, is the principal disabling feature of chronic renal failure related to calcium metabolism. Reduction of hyperphosphatemia and restoration of normal intestinal calcium absorption by calcitriol can improve blood calcium concentration and reduce the manifestations of secondary hyperparathyroidism.

Vitamin D deficiency due to inadequate diet and/or sunlight Vitamin D deficiency is more common in the United States than previously recognized. Biopsies of bone in elderly patients with hip fracture (documenting osteomalacia) and abnormal concentrations of vitamin D metabolites, PTH, calcium, and phosphate have established that vitamin D deficiency may occur in as many as 25 percent of elderly patients, particularly in areas where there is little ambient sunlight. Concentrations of 25(OH)D are at the lower limits of normal or below normal in these patients. Quantitative histomorphometry of bone biopsy specimens reveals widened osteoid seams consistent with osteomalacia. PTH hypersecretion compensates for a tendency of the blood calcium level to fall, but with the consequence of inducing renal phosphate wasting and a combined mineral ion abnormality that results in osteomalacia.

The genesis of vitamin D deficiency is impaired intake of dairy products that are enriched with vitamin D, lack of vitamin supplementation, and reduced sunlight exposure in the elderly, particularly in winter in northern latitudes.

Treatment involves the administration of vitamin D and provision of 1 to 1.5 g calcium in the diet. Vitamin D supplementation should aim to provide several times the recommended daily requirement in younger people, which is probably a safe recommendation; a dosage of 1000 to 2000 units of vitamin D per day is satisfactory. Vitamin D is usually not available in multiple-dose forms. Hence, the administration of a capsule containing 50,000 units of vitamin D once-monthly is safe in elderly patients who have osteomalacia. The increased awareness of the importance of calcium supplementation, particularly in women, even without supplementation of vitamin D, may lessen the frequency of this problem. Severe hypocalcemia is rarely seen in the moderately severe vitamin D deficiency of the elderly, but vitamin D deficiency needs to be considered in the differential diagnosis of mild hypocalcemia.

Defective vitamin D metabolism ANTICONVULSANT THERAPY Anticonvulsant therapy with any of several agents induces a state of acquired vitamin D deficiency by increasing the turnover of vitamin D into inactive compounds. The more marginal the degree of vitamin D intake in the diet, the more likely that anticonvulsant therapy will lead to abnormalities in mineral and bone metabolism. The syndrome at its extreme involves several rickets with bone fractures, hypocalcemia, and hypophosphatemia. Occasionally, a severe proximal myopathy is reported. More often, frank hypocalcemia is not detected, and mild osteomalacia is the only clinical symptom. In other patients on long-term anticonvulsant therapy, no symptoms or signs are present, but bone density is lower than normal and responds favorably to vitamin D supplementation.

Anticonvulsants stimulate the hepatic microsomal mixed-oxidase enzymes and hence increase the rate of clearance of vitamin D and its metabolites. Phenytoin also impairs intestinal calcium absorption independent of effects on vitamin D; the drug also has deleterious effects on bone cell function in vitro including inhibition of collagen synthesis. All manifestations of the syndrome can nevertheless be reversed with adequate vitamin D supplementation.

Although $1,25(OH)_2D$ levels are lower for the degree of vitamin D intake in patients treated with chronic anticonvulsants than in the normal population, there is a great deal of variation. The greater prevalence of the disorder in some European populations and in children in homes for the mentally retarded probably reflects the lower vitamin D intake of those groups. Restoration of bone mineral mass and reversal of hypocalcemia, when seen, can be accomplished with vitamin D replacement plus added oral calcium. Adjustments in dose are indicated depending on the age and body size of the patient, but approximately 50,000 units of vitamin D weekly plus 1 g elemental calcium per day for several months are usually sufficient. Alternatively, administration of one 50,000-unit capsule of vitamin D monthly may be preventative if the anticonvulsant therapy must be given chronically.

VITAMIN D-DEPENDENT RICKETS TYPE I Rickets can be due to *resistance* to the *action* of vitamin D as well as to vitamin D deficiency. Vitamin D-dependent rickets type I, previously termed pseudo-vitamin D-dependent rickets, differs from vitamin D-resistant rickets in that it is less severe and in that the biochemical and radiographic abnormalities can be reversed with large doses of the vitamin.

Clinical features include hypocalcemia, often with tetany or convulsions, hypophosphatemia, secondary hyperparathyroidism, and osteomalacia, often associated with skeletal deformities and increased alkaline phosphatase. Doses of vitamin D or calcifediol, 100 to 1000 times above the usual amounts, are required to heal the bone disease, whereas physiologic amounts of calcitriol cure the disease. The disorder, an autosomal recessive trait, is due to a defect in conversion of 25(OH)D to $1,25(OH)_2D$. Plasma levels of $1,25(OH)_2D$ are low or undetectable even after administration of large doses of vitamin D or calcifediol. Response to high doses of vitamin D or calcifediol is probably due to direct actions of high levels of 25(OH)D. Treatment requires careful adjustment of calcitriol dose, particularly during growth periods.

Active vitamin D ineffective INTESTINAL MALABSORPTION Mild hypocalcemia, secondary hyperparathyroidism, severe hypophosphatemia, and a variety of nutritional deficiencies occur with gastrointestinal diseases. Hepatocellular dysfunction can lead to reduction in 25(OH)D levels, as in portal or biliary cirrhosis of the liver. Malabsorption of vitamin D and its metabolites, including calcitriol, may occur in a variety of intestinal diseases, hereditary or acquired. Hypocalcemia itself can lead to steatorrhea, due to deficient production of pancreatic enzymes and bile salts. Depending on the disorder, vitamin D or its metabolites can be administered parenterally, thereby guaranteeing adequate blood levels of active metabolites.

VITAMIN D-DEPENDENT RICKETS TYPE II Pseudo-vitamin D-dependent rickets can be due to defective response as well as to defective production of $1,25(OH)_2D$. This disorder, vitamin D-dependent rickets type II, results from any of several types of end organ resistance to the active metabolite, including absence or qualitative defects of the intracellular receptor protein for the hormone and postreceptor blocks in hormone action (see Chap. 311). The clinical features are similar to those with the type I disorder and include hypocalcemia, hypophosphatemia, secondary hyperparathyroidism, and rickets. Plasma levels of $1,25(OH)_2D$ are elevated at least three times above normal, in keeping with the refractoriness of the end organs. Severe alopecia totalis may commence early in life. Patients with this disorder usually require higher dose of vitamin D or vitamin D metabolites than with the type I disorder.

Pseudohypoparathyroidism Pseudohypoparathyroidism (PHP) is a hereditary disorder characterized by symptoms and signs of hypoparathyroidism, typically in association with distinctive skeletal and developmental defects. The hypoparathyroidism is due to a deficient end organ response to PTH. Excessive secretion of PTH is the consequence of hyperplasia of the parathyroids, a response to the resistance to hormone action. The entity is actually a syndrome in which various individuals and kindreds exhibit different aberrancies in hormone receptor complex response.

A working classification of the various forms of pseudohypoparathyroidism is given in Table 340-7. The classification scheme is based on the signs of ineffective parathyroid hormone action (low calcium and high phosphate), urinary cyclic AMP response to exogenous PTH, the presence or absence of Albright's hereditary osteodystrophy (AHO), and assays of the concentration of the G_s subunits of the adenylate cyclase enzyme (see Chap. 68). Using these criteria there are four types: pseudohypoparathyroidism (PHP) type I, subdivided into a and b categories; PHP-II; and pseudopseudohypoparathyroidism (PPHP). Individuals with PHP-I, the most common of the disorders, show a deficient response in urinary cyclic AMP following administration of exogenous parathyroid hormone. Pseudohypoparathyroidism type II refers to patients with hypocalcemia and hyperphosphatemia who have a normal urinary cyclic AMP response to PTH. These patients are assumed to have a defect in the response to PTH at a locus beyond that of cyclic AMP production, although at least some patients reported to have PHP-II may instead have occult vitamin D deficiency. Patients with the PHP-I syndrome are divided into type a, with reduced activity of the stimulatory G protein subunit (G_s) in in vitro assays, and type b, with normal amounts of G_s in erythrocytes. Subjects with PHP-Ia also have shortened metacarpals and metatarsals and the other features of Albright's hereditary osteodystrophy syndrome and commonly show resistance to hormones in addition to PTH. Patients with PHP-Ib have a normal phenotype without the AHO syndrome and do not show resistance to any hormones other than parathyroid hormone. Fibroblasts cultured from the skin of some patients with PHP-Ib show

TABLE 340-7 Classification of pseudohypoparathyroidism (PHP) and pseudopseudohypoparathyroidism (PPHP)

Type	Hypocalcemia, hyperphosphatemia	Response of Urinary cAMP to PTH	Serum PTH	G_s subunit deficiency	AHO	Resistance to hormones in addition to PTH
PHP-Ia	Yes	↓	↑	Yes	Yes	Yes
PHP-Ib	Yes	↓	↑	No	No	No
PHP-II	Yes	Normal	↑	No	No	No
PPHP	No	Normal	Normal	Yes	Yes	±

NOTE: ↓ = decreased; ↑ = increased; AHO = Albright's hereditary osteodystrophy.

a much reduced response of cyclic AMP accumulation to PTH but not to other agents that stimulate adenylate cyclase such as prostaglandins and forskolin, consistent with the presence of a defective receptor. A subset of these patients, however, have a normal response to cyclic AMP production in fibroblasts in vitro.

Patients with PPHP have typical features of the hereditary osteodystrophy syndrome despite normal serum calciums and normal response of urinary cyclic AMP to exogenous PTH. These individuals are usually first-degree relatives of patients with PHP-Ia, and patients initially classified as having PPHP have subsequently developed mild hypocalcemia. Patients with PPHP on average have levels of G_s subunits that are half normal. These various features suggest that PPHP is a mild variant of PHP-Ia and illustrate the heterogeneity of the defect in PTH responsiveness. Further studies will be necessary to clarify the pathogenesis of these disorders.

Little is known about the pathophysiology of the skeletal defects. The AHO syndrome includes round facies, short stature, obesity, brachydactyly, and heterotopic calcification. Mental deficiency is frequent.

The mode of inheritance in these various disorders is uncertain and may itself be heterogeneous. In some families the disorder may be an X-linked dominant defect, whereas in others the disorder appears to result from an autosomal dominant mutation with variable expressivity.

The mineral deposits in ectopic sites may include true bone, whereas bone formation in ectopic sites never occurs in idiopathic hypoparathyroidism. Amorphous deposits of calcium and phosphate are found in the basal ganglia in about half of patients. The defects in metacarpal and metatarsal bones are sometimes accompanied by abnormal phalanges as well, possibly reflecting premature closing of the epiphyses. The typical findings are abnormally short fourth and fifth metacarpals and metatarsals. The defects are usually bilateral. Exostoses and radius curvus are frequent. Impairments in olfaction and taste and unusual dermatoglyphic abnormalities have been reported. There is little improvement in mental status even after adequate therapy with calcium and vitamin D.

The diagnosis can usually be made without difficulty. Positive family history for developmental defects and/or the presence of developmental defects characteristic of PHP-Ia, including brachydactyly, in association with the signs of hypoparathyroidism, low calcium, and high phosphate, essentially make the diagnosis on clinical grounds. On the other hand, patients with PHP-Ib or PHP-II do not have phenotypic abnormalities. In PHP-Ib, administration of exogenous parathyroid hormone can lead to detection of the blunted cyclic AMP response; such tests are usually used to confirm the diagnosis even in PHP-Ia. Low levels of G_s subunits in erythrocyte membranes can also distinguish patients with PHP-Ia from those with PHP-Ib. Patients in both categories have elevated serum PTH, particularly if they are hypocalcemic. The diagnosis of PHP-II is more complex, in that cyclic AMP responses in urine are, by definition, normal. Since vitamin D deficiency itself can result in dissociation between phosphaturic and urinary cyclic AMP responses to exogenous PTH, vitamin D deficiency must be excluded before diagnosis of PHP-II can be made. PHP-II is separated from hypoparathyroidism by finding of elevated PTH levels; this finding per se, however, does not distinguish between secretion of abnormal PTH and a post-cyclic AMP receptor defect. Some patients with the PHP-II phenotype may actually have hypoparathyroidism secondary to secretion of an abnormal, biologically inactive PTH.

Treatment of PHP and PPHP is similar to that of hypoparathyroidism, except that the dose of vitamin D and calcium is usually lower than that required in true hypoparathyroidism. Variations in individual responses make it necessary to establish the optimal therapeutic program for each patient, based on maintaining the appropriate blood calcium concentration and urinary calcium excretion.

PTH Overwhelmed Occasionally, loss of calcium from the extracellular fluid is so severe that PTH cannot compensate. Such situations include severe, acute hyperphosphatemia, often in association with renal failure, or acute pancreatitis, conditions in which there is rapid efflux of calcium from extracellular fluid. Severe hypocalcemia can occur quickly; PTH rises in response to hypocalcemia but does not return blood calcium to normal. The chance of hypocalcemia is enhanced when renal failure is present.

Severe, acute hyperphosphatemia Severe hyperphosphatemia occurs in situations associated with extensive tissue damage or cell destruction (also see Chap. 342). The combination of an increased release of phosphate from muscle and an impaired ability to excrete phosphorus secondary to the renal failure causes moderate to severe hyperphosphatemia, the latter causing calcium loss from the blood and hypocalcemia of mild to moderate severity. Hypocalcemia is usually reversed with tissue repair and restoration of renal function as phosphorus and creatinine values return to normal. There may even be a mild hypercalcemic period in the oliguric phase of recovery of renal function. This sequence, severe hypocalcemia followed by mild hypercalcemia, reflects widespread deposition of calcium in muscle with subsequent redistribution of some of the calcium to the extracellular fluid after restoration of phosphate levels to normal.

Other causes of hyperphosphatemia that lead to hypocalcemia include hypothermia, massive hepatic failure, and hematologic malignancies, either because of high cell turnover as part of the malignancy or because of cell destruction when chemotherapy is instituted.

Treatment is directed toward lowering of blood phosphate by the administration of phosphate-binding antacids or dialysis, often needed for the management of renal failure. Although calcium replacement may be necessary if hypocalcemia is severe and symptomatic, calcium administration during the hyperphosphatemic period may increase extraosseous cellular calcium deposition, thereby aggravating ultimate tissue damage. Although the levels of $1,25(OH)_2D$ may be low during the hyperphosphatemic phase and may return to normal during the oliguric phase of recovery, mineral ion imbalance per se seems to be the principal pathophysiologic mechanism.

Osteitis fibrosa after parathyroidectomy Severe hypocalcemia after parathyroid surgery is less common now that osteitis fibrosa cystica is an infrequent manifestation of hyperparathyroidism. When osteitis fibrosa cystica is severe, however, bone mineral deficits can be large, and after parathyroidectomy, blood calcium levels can fall to the hypocalcemic range and remain depressed for days if calcium replacement is inadequate. The mechanism of the hypocalcemia is complex. Increased cellularity of bone in severe osteitis fibrosa cystica involves both osteoblastic and osteoclastic cells. High levels of PTH enhance bone-blood exchange, with resorption favored over formation; an abrupt decrease in PTH levels with surgery leaves bone formation favored over resorption. Calcium loss from blood is increased, and temporary hyporesponsiveness of bone to the bone-resorbing actions of PTH (lowered hormone levels after parathyroid surgery in the presence of receptor down-regulation) may add to the imbalance between bone resorption and bone formation. Treatment may require parenteral administration of calcium; addition of calcitriol and oral calcium supplementation may hasten the ability to withdraw parenteral calcium supplementation and/or reduce the amount needed.

DIFFERENTIAL DIAGNOSIS Care must be taken to ensure that true hypocalcemia is present; in addition, acute transient hypocalcemia can be a manifestation of a variety of severe, acute illnesses as discussed above. *Chronic hypocalcemia,* however, can usually be ascribed to a few disorders associated with an absence of PTH or its ineffectiveness. Important clinical criteria include the duration of the illness, signs or symptoms of associated disorders, and the detection of features that suggest a hereditary abnormality in calcium and bone metabolism. A nutritional history can be helpful in detecting a low intake of vitamin D and calcium in the elderly, and a history of excessive alcohol intake can be the clue to magnesium deficiency.

Hypoparathyroidism and pseudohypoparathyroidism are typically lifelong illnesses; hence, a recent onset of hypocalcemia in an adult is usually due to nutritional deficiencies, renal failure, or intestinal disorders that result in vitamin D deficiency or ineffective vitamin D action. A history of seizure disorder raises the issue of anticonvulsive medication. Neck surgery, even long past, can be associated with a delayed onset of postsurgical hypoparathyroidism. Developmental defects, particularly in childhood and adolescence, may point to the diagnosis of pseudohypoparathyroidism. Rickets and a variety of neuromuscular syndromes and deformities may indicate ineffective vitamin D action, either due to hereditary defects in vitamin D metabolism or rarely to vitamin D deficiency.

A pattern of *low calcium* with *high phosphorus* in the absence of renal failure or massive tissue destruction almost invariably means hypoparathyroidism or pseudohypoparathyroidism. A *low calcium* with a *low phosphorus* points to absent or ineffective vitamin D, thereby rendering the action of PHT on calcium metabolism ineffective. The relative ineffectiveness of PTH in vitamin D deficiency, anticonvulsant therapy, gastrointestinal disorders, and hereditary defects in vitamin D metabolism leads to secondary hyperparathyroidism as a compensation. The relatively unopposed action of the excess PTH on renal tubule phosphate transport, less dependent on vitamin D sufficiency than calcium transport, accounts for renal phosphate wasting and hypophosphatemia.

Exceptions to these patterns may occur. Most forms of hypomagnesemia are due to long-standing nutritional deficiency, and, despite the fact that the hypocalcemia is due principally to an acute absence of PTH, phosphate levels are usually low rather than elevated as in hypoparathyroidism. Chronic renal failure is often associated with hypocalcemia and hyperphosphatemia, despite secondary hyperparathyroidism.

Diagnosis is usually established by application of the PTH radioimmunoassay, tests for vitamin D metabolites, and measurements of the urinary cyclic AMP response to exogenous PTH. In hereditary and acquired hypoparathyroidism and severe hypomagnesemia, PTH is either undetectable or in the normal range, especially with double-antibody assays; this result in a hypocalcemic patient is supportive of hypoparathyroidism, as distinct from ineffective PTH action, in which even mild hypocalcemia is associated with elevated PTH levels. Hence, a failure to detect elevated PTH levels establishes the diagnosis of hypoparathyroidism; elevated levels suggest the presence of secondary hyperparathyroidism as found in many of the situations in which the hormone is ineffective due to associated abnormalities in vitamin D action. Assays for 25(OH)D and $1,25(OH)_2D$ can be quite helpful. Low or low normal 25(OH)D indicates vitamin D deficiency due to lack of sunlight, inadequate vitamin D intake, or intestinal malabsorption. A low level of $1,25(OH)_2D$ in the presence of elevated concentrations of PTH suggests ineffective PTH action, including chronic renal failure, severe vitamin D deficiency, vitamin D-dependent rickets type I, and pseudohypoparathyroidism. Recognition that mild hypocalcemia, rickets, and hypophosphatemia are due to chronic anticonvulsant therapy is made by history.

TREATMENT OF HYPOCALCEMIA The chronic management of hypoparathyroidism or pseudohypoparathyroidism, chronic renal failure, and hereditary defects in vitamin D metabolism all feature the use of vitamin D or vitamin D metabolites and calcium supplementation. Vitamin D itself is the least expensive form of vitamin D replacement and is frequently used in the management of uncomplicated hypoparathyroidism and disorders associated with ineffective vitamin D action. When vitamin D is used prophylactically, as in the elderly or in those with chronic anticonvulsant therapy, there is a wider margin of safety than with the more potent metabolites. On the other hand, most of the conditions in which vitamin D is used for chronic management of hypocalcemia require the use of 50 to 100 times the daily replacement doses, because the formation of $1,25(OH)_2D$ is deficient. In such situations, vitamin D is no safer than the active metabolite because intoxication does occur with high-dose vitamin D therapy. Calcitriol is more rapid in onset of action and also has a short biologic half-life; in high doses vitamin D is stored in body tissues and is cleared slowly.

One to five micrograms per day of vitamin D or calcifediol and slightly lower doses of calcitriol (0.25 to 1.0 μg/d) are required to prevent rickets. In contrast, 500 to 3000 μg of vitamin D_2 or D_3 is typically required in hypoparathyroidism; doses of calcifediol are also high (several hundred micrograms per day) compared with doses required in euparathyroid individuals. The dose of calcitriol is unchanged in hypoparathyroidism since the defect is in hydroxylation by the 1α-hydroxylase.

The slightly greater therapeutic efficacy of calcifediol than vitamin D_3 in conditions in which the metabolism of the vitamin is impaired may be due to superior metabolic availability for the renal 1α-hydroxylase or to direct action directly by 25(OH)D at receptors in target tissues. Vitamin D is metabolized to a variety of compounds other than the principal product, 25(OH)D. Calcifediol bypasses these alternate pathways and is directly available for metabolism to $1,25(OH)_2D$. In hypoparathyroidism and in hereditary defects in renal hydroxylase, the efficiency of formation of $1,25(OH)_2D$ from 25(OH)D is low, but some formation does occur with high substrate levels. Calcifediol has about 1 percent of the potency of calcitriol in in vivo and in vitro tests of vitamin D responsiveness.

Unless a loading dose is given, 2 to 4 weeks or even longer are required to achieve the maximum calcium replacement action of vitamin D or calcifediol; again, the onset of action of calcifediol is slightly more rapid. Calcitriol can be given for hypoparathyroidism at the same dose required for the prevention of rickets in euparathyroid individuals, 0.2 to 1.0 μg/d. Its onset of action is days rather than weeks. When vitamin D or calcifediol is withdrawn, weeks are required for the disappearance of the biologic effects, compared with a few days for calcitriol.

Patients with hypoparathyroidism should be given 2 to 3 g elemental calcium by mouth each day. The two agents, vitamin D (or vitamin D metabolites) and oral calcium, can be varied independently. Higher doses of vitamin D or its metabolites increase the efficiency of intestinal calcium absorption; higher intakes of oral calcium permit adequate calcium assimilation despite a lower efficiency of intestinal calcium absorption. In the event of hypercalcemia during the treatment of chronic hypocalcemia, the withdrawal of the supplemental oral calcium is effective in lowering calcium within 24 h, even more rapidly than withdrawal of calcitriol. Most patients with hypoparathyroidism can be managed with high-dose vitamin D therapy combined with 2 to 3 g oral calcium per day. If hypocalcemia alternates with episodes of hypercalcemia, then substitution of calcitriol will often make management easier.

The administration of thiazide diuretics in the usual antihypertensive doses and sodium restriction in patients with hypoparathyroidism lowers urinary calcium excretion. This hypocalciuric effect allows the calcium and vitamin D supplementation to be reduced. Patients will have a lower urinary calcium excretion at any given level of blood calcium on thiazides. The treatment also may protect against the development of kidney stones, a potential complication of the long-term management of hypoparathyroidism. If on dialysis, patients with chronic renal failure and hypocalcemia can have adjustments in dialysate calcium concentrations as an alternative to vitamin D and calcium supplementation. The doses of vitamin D and calcium required for the management of pseudohypoparathyroidism are usually lower than those required for hypoparathyroidism, reflecting incomplete resistance to the action of PTH in pseudohypoparathyroidism. The acute treatment of hypomagnesemia is discussed above; the use of magnesium chloride by mouth may be sufficient to restore blood magnesium.

REFERENCES

ADERKA D et al: Bacteremic hypocalcemia, a comparison between the calcium levels of bacteremic and nonbacteremic patients with infection. Arch Intern Med 147:232, 1987

AHN TG et al: Familial isolated hypoparathyroidism: A molecular genetic analysis of 8 families with 23 affected persons. Medicine 6502:73, 1986

AHONEN P : Autoimmune polyendocrinopathy–candidiasis–ectodermal dystrophy (APECED): Autosomal recessive inheritance. Clin Genet 27:535, 1985

BENSON L et al: Hyperparathyroidism presenting as the first lesion in multiple endocrine neoplasia type 1. Am J Med 82:731, 1987

BROADUS AE et al: Humoral hypercalcemia of cancer: Identification of a novel parathyroid hormone-like peptide. N Engl J Med 319:536, 1988

GARABEDIAN M et al: Elevated plasma 1,25-$(OH)_2D$ concentrations in infants with hypercalcemia and elfin facies. N Engl J Med 312:948, 1985

KIYOKAWA T et al: Hypercalcemia and osteoclast proliferation in adult T-cell leukemia. Cancer 59:1187, 1987

LAD TE et al: Treatment of cancer-associated hypercalcemia with cisplatin. Arch Intern Med 147:329, 1987

LEVINE MA et al: Activity of the stimulatory guanine nucleotide–binding protein is reduced in erythrocytes from patients with pseudohypoparathyroidism and pseudo-pseudohypoparathyroidism: Biochemical, endocrine, and genetic analysis of Albright's hereditary osteodystrophy in six kindreds. J Clin Endocrinol Metab 62:497, 1986

———, AURBACH GD : Pseudohypoparathyroidism, in *Endocrinology*, LJ DeGroot et al (eds). Philadelphia, Saunders, 1989, vol 2, chap 65

LIBERMAN UA et al: Resistance to 1,25-$(OH)_2$. Association with heterogenous defects in cultured skin fibroblasts. J Clin Invest 7:192, 1983

MALLETTE LE, EICHORN E : Effects of lithium carbonate on human calcium metabolism. Arch Intern Med 146:770, 1986

MARTIN P et al: Partially reversible osteopenia after surgery for primary hyperparathyroidism. Arch Intern Med 146:689, 1986

MAYNARD FM : Immobilization hypercalcemia following spinal cord injury. Arch Phys Med Rehabil 67:41, 1986

MUDDE AH et al: Ectopic production of 1,25-dihydroxyvitamin D by B-cell lymphoma as a cause of hypercalcemia. Cancer 59:1543, 1987

MUNDY GR et al: Tumor products and the hypercalcemia of malignancy. J Clin Invest 76:391, 1985

NEER RM, POTTS JT JR : Medical management of hyperparathyroidism and hypercalcemia, in *Endocrinology*, 2d ed, LJ DeGroot et al (eds). Philadelphia, Saunders, 1989, vol 2, chap 61

NORTON JA et al: Effect of parathyroidectomy in patients with hyperparathyroidism, Zollinger-Ellison syndrome, and multiple endocrine neoplasia type I: A prospective study. Surgery 1026:958, 1987

NUSSBAUM SR et al: Highly sensitive two-site immunoradiometric assay of parathyrin and its clinical utility in evaluating patients with hypercalcemia. Clin Chem 33:1364, 1987

ORWOLL ES : The milk-alkali syndrome: Current concepts. Ann Intern Med 97:242, 1982

SALUSKY IB, COBURN JW: The renal osteodystrophies, in *Endocrinology*, 2d ed, LJ DeGroot et al (eds). Philadelphia, Saunders, 1989, vol 2, chap 63

STUCKEY BGA et al: Fasting calcium excretion and parathyroid hormone together distinguish familial hypocalciuric hypercalcaemia from primary hyperparathyroidism. Clin Endocrinol 27:525, 1987

THEIBAUD D et al: Oral versus intravenous AHP,BP (APD) in the treatment of hypercalcemia of malignancy. Bone 7:247, 1986

WARRELL RP JR et al: Metabolic effects of gallium nitrate administered by prolonged infusion. Cancer Treat Rep 69:653, 1985

341 METABOLIC BONE DISEASE

STEPHEN M. KRANE / MICHAEL F. HOLICK

OSTEOPOROSIS

GENERAL CONSIDERATIONS *Osteoporosis* is the term used for diseases of diverse etiology that cause a reduction in the mass of bone per unit volume. The reduction in mass is not accompanied by a significant reduction in the ratio of the mineral to the organic phase, nor by any known abnormality in bone mineral or organic matrix. Histologically, the disorder is characterized by a decrease in cortical thickness and in the number and size of the trabeculae of cancellous bone with normal width of the osteoid seams. Osteoporosis is the most common of the metabolic bone diseases (disorders in which all the skeleton is involved) and is an important cause of morbidity in the elderly.

The remodeling of bone (its formation and resorption) is a continuous process. Any changes in the rates of formation and resorption that result in bone resorption exceeding bone formation can cause a decrease in bone mass. In osteoporosis the bone mass *is* decreased, indicating that the rate of bone resorption must exceed that of bone formation. Bone formation is higher in cortical than in cancellous bone. This difference is exaggerated by the normal menopause and exaggerated even further in patients with osteoporosis because rates of formation of cancellous bone tend to be lower in patients with osteoporosis, particularly in women after the menopause. The fact that about a third of postmenopausal women have high skeletal turnover, assessed by whole-body retention of ^{99m}Tc-methylene diphosphonate and by other biochemical markers, could reflect the greater relative contribution of cortical remodeling in this group. After closure of epiphyses and cessation of longitudinal growth, there is a period of consolidation with a decrease in cortical porosity. When peak adult bone mass is reached at about age 30 to 35 for cortical bone and probably earlier for trabecular bone, rates of bone formation and resorption are relatively low (compared to the period of growth spurt) and approximately equal. The normal balance between bone formation and resorption results in maintenance of skeletal mass. The rates of remodeling are different, however, not only in cortical compared to trabecular bone but also in individual bones or portions of bones. Most of the bone surfaces are "inactive" and not involved at any given time either in formation or resorption. Active surfaces may be randomly distributed, but formation and resorption are locally coupled as units. Resorption areas are covered by osteoclasts if active; bone formation surfaces are characterized by the presence of osteoid seams and are covered by active osteoblasts. Resorption precedes formation and is probably more intense, but it does not last as long as formation. As a consequence, there are normally more sites of active formation than of resorption. Bone turnover is high when there are many units active and low when there are few. Unless formation compensates for resorption, bone mass decreases. In both sexes after age 40 to 50 there is a slow rate of loss of cortical bone, of about 0.3 to 0.5 percent per year. In women around the menopause an accelerated loss of cortical bone is superimposed upon the age-related loss. Loss of trabecular bone begins at an earlier age in both sexes but is probably greater in degree in women. The rate of bone loss in women may also be accelerated around the time of menopause. These losses of bone mass range from 20 to 30 percent in men and 40 to 50 percent for some women. In general, the pattern of bone loss involves predominantly trabecular bone in the spine and distal radius in women and the spine and hip in both women and men. The loss in selected regions has been documented using techniques such as single- and dual-photon absorptiometry, quantitative computed tomography, x-ray-based dual-energy densitometry, and neutron activation analysis of total-body calcium. For example, the rate of loss is greater in the metacarpals, the femoral neck, and the vertebral bodies than in the midshaft of the femur, the tibia, and the skull.

Although, as noted, skeletal turnover may be increased, turnover is usually normal or low. Bone formation is low in the majority, but the degree of reduction varies with the different bone surfaces. The major remodeling abnormalities in patients with vertebral crush fractures are a reduced frequency of activation of remodeling units and a decrease in the function of osteoblasts. Even in those individuals with increased bone resorption, however, bone formation does not compensate. At some critical point if the difference between rates of formation and resorption is maintained, loss of bone substance may become so marked that the bone can no longer resist the normal mechanical forces to which it is subjected, and fracture results. Osteoporosis then becomes a clinical problem. The level of reduction in bone mass sufficient to result in fractures after minimal trauma is variable. The strength of bones such as the vertebrae may depend upon additional factors such as adequacy of ligamentous support and the age-related changes in the intervertebral disks. The normal trabecular architecture is also disturbed. For example, the horizontal trabeculae of the vertebral bodies are preferentially lost in osteoporosis. Microfractures are also frequent. In elderly individuals with osteoporosis, age-related impairment of vision, hearing, and other neurologic and intellectual functions are additional contributions to the occurrence of fractures.

In the process of remodeling of lamellar bone in adults, most of the net resorption occurs at the corticoendosteal surface. The abnormal remodeling in osteoporosis follows the same pattern; the bone loss includes cancellous bone, cortical bone at the endosteal surface, and intracortical bone, resulting in enlargement of the medullary cavity and thinning of the cortex. Since bone formation at the periosteum continues at a slow rate, the diameter of the bone does not decrease, and the periosteal surface retains its smooth configuration. In addition, the cancellous bone also undergoes progressive resorption, with some trabeculae being resorbed at rates faster than others, particularly those vertebral trabeculae with horizontal orientation.

The loss of bone that accompanies advancing age begins earlier and proceeds more rapidly in women than in men, and there is a trend toward acceleration of bone loss in women before the menopause. All of the reasons for this age-associated bone loss are not known, although several risk factors have been identified. In general, white women have a greater risk than black women, and white men have a greater risk than black men. One explanation for these population differences is that the bone mass at skeletal maturity is one determinant of the bone mass at subsequent ages. The lower incidence of osteoporosis and hip fracture in black men and women has been attributed to a higher bone mineral content in blacks than in whites. Of interest is that bone formation is lower in blacks. Since formation and resorption are usually closely coupled and since bone mass is increased, bone resorption (and turnover) must also be reduced. Osteoporotic subjects are frequently less muscular and have lower average body weight. Exercise may have a beneficial effect in maintaining bone mass. The facts that accelerated bone loss accompanies the menopause in some women and that premature osteoporosis occurs when bilateral oophorectomy is performed prior to the age of normal menopause suggest that estrogens play a major role in preventing bone loss. Furthermore, osteoporotic women as a group may have an earlier menopause than age-matched nonosteoporotic women. Osteoporotic women also have a higher incidence of smoking; cigarette smoking might directly affect bone remodeling or have secondary effects on ovarian function. Excessive alcohol consumption, which can result in decreased bone formation, also is a risk factor for osteoporosis. Dietary calcium intake and the efficiency of intestinal calcium absorption may also influence bone mass. Inability to synthesize adequate amounts of 1α,25-dihydroxyvitamin D [1,25$(OH)_2$D] may play a role in the decreased calcium absorption, possibly because of decreased parathyroid hormone levels, impaired activity of the renal 25(OH)D-1α-hydroxylase, or altered responsiveness of the enzyme to parathyroid hormone.

Although increased production of interleukin 1 by blood mononuclear cells in patients with osteoporosis may be a consequence of estrogen deficiency, the contributing role of interleukin 1 and other cytokines that may modulate bone resorption or bone formation in the genesis of osteoporosis has yet to be established. Although osteoporosis occurs with Cushing's syndrome, there is no established role of adrenal steroids in the osteoporosis associated with the menopause or advancing age.

It is also possible that excessive acid intake, particularly in the form of high-protein diets, results in "dissolution" of bone in an attempt to buffer the extra acid. Acidosis may also directly increase osteoclast function. Prolonged use of heparin as an anticoagulant is also associated with osteoporosis, and heparin potentiates bone resorption in vitro. Patients with osteoporosis have increased numbers of mast cells, presumably capable of producing heparin and other substances that modulate bone cell function, in the bone marrow. Circumscribed and diffuse areas of osteoporosis occur in patients with systemic mastocytosis.

As mentioned earlier, the remodeling of bone is responsive to mechanical forces of many types. The early response to immobilization in the normal skeleton is an increase in bone resorption while bone formation remains normal or is decreased; later there is a compensatory increase in bone formation. In osteoporosis, immobilization tends to aggravate the defect by increasing the gap between formation and resorption. A sedentary life in an individual with poor musculature may reduce mechanical forces exerted on the skeleton and increase the tendency to bone loss.

CLASSIFICATION (See Table 341-1) In some instances osteoporosis is a feature of another disease such as Cushing's syndrome. Osteoporosis (decreased bone mass with normal mineralization) is characteristic of certain heritable diseases of connective tissue such as osteogenesis imperfecta (see Chap. 333). In most osteoporosis, however, no other disease is apparent. This category of osteoporosis can be conveniently considered to comprise several forms. One form occurs in children or young adults of both sexes and with normal gonadal function. This form is frequently termed *idiopathic osteoporosis,* although most of the other forms are in fact also of unknown pathogenesis. So-called *type I osteoporosis* occurs in a subset of postmenopausal women who are between 51 and 75 years of age and is characterized by an accelerated and disproportionate loss of trabecular bone as contrasted with cortical bone. Fractures of vertebral

TABLE 341-1 Classification of osteoporosis

I Common forms of osteoporosis unassociated with other disease
- *A* Idiopathic osteoporosis (juvenile and adult)
- *B* Type I osteoporosis
- *C* Type II osteoporosis

II Disorders or conditions in which osteoporosis is a common feature
- *A* Hypogonadism
- *B* Hyperadrenocorticism
- *C* Thyrotoxicosis
- *D* Malabsorption
- *E* Scurvy
- *F* Calcium deficiency
- *G* Immobilization
- *H* Chronic heparin administration
- *I* Systemic mastocytosis
- *J* Adult hypophosphatasia
- *K* Associated with other metabolic bone diseases

III Osteoporosis as a feature of heritable disorders of connective tissue
- *A* Osteogenesis imperfecta
- *B* Homocystinuria due to cystathionine synthase deficiency
- *C* Ehlers-Danlos syndrome
- *D* Marfan's syndrome

IV Disorders in which osteoporosis is associated but pathogenesis not understood
- *A* Rheumatoid arthritis
- *B* Malnutrition
- *C* Alcoholism
- *D* Epilepsy
- *E* Diabetes mellitus
- *F* Chronic obstructive pulmonary disease
- *G* Menkes' syndrome

bodies and the distal forearm are the most common complications. Decreased parathyroid gland function may be compensatory to increased bone resorption. So-called *type II osteoporosis* is found in a large proportion of women and men over the age of 70. Fractures of the femoral neck, proximal humerus, proximal tibia, and pelvis are most common in this group. These skeletal sites contain both cortical and trabecular bone. Circulating levels of parathyroid hormone tend to be higher than normal. Both groups have decreased mean circulating levels of 1,25$(OH)_2$D.

GENERAL CLINICAL FEATURES Although osteoporosis is a generalized disorder of the skeleton, its major clinical sequelae result from fractures of the vertebrae, wrist, hip, humerus, and tibia, depending upon the pattern of the disease (type I or II osteoporosis). The most frequent symptoms from vertebral body fractures are pain in the back and deformity of the spine. Pain usually results from collapse of the vertebrae especially in the lower dorsal and upper lumbar regions, is typically acute in onset, and often radiates anteriorly around the flank into the abdomen. Such episodes may occur after sudden bending, lifting, or jumping movements that may seem to have been trivial; on some occasions they cannot be related to trauma. The pain may be increased even with slight movements such as turning in bed or by the Valsalva maneuver. Bed rest may relieve the pain temporarily, only for it to recur in spasms of variable duration. Radiation of pain down one leg is uncommon, and symptoms or signs of spinal cord compression are rare. The acute episodes of pain may also be accompanied by abdominal distention and ileus, thought to be due to retroperitoneal hemorrhage, but the use of narcotics at this stage also contributes to the ileus. Loss of appetite and apparent muscular weakness may also be present. Episodes of pain usually subside after several days to a week, and by 4 to 6 weeks patients may be fully ambulatory and able to resume normal activities. Although acute pain may be minimal, nagging, deep, dull, uncomfortable sensations may be localized to the area of fracture and brought about by straining or sudden changes in position. Patients may be unable to sit up in bed and have to arise by rolling over on the side and then propping themselves up. Most patients have disappearance or diminution of pain between episodes of vertebral body collapse. Others do not have acute episodes but complain of backache made worse by standing or moving suddenly. Tenderness is common over involved areas of the spinous processes or rib cage. The collapse fractures of the vertebral bodies are usually anterior, producing a wedge-shaped deformity and contributing to loss in height. This is particularly common in the middorsal region where collapse may be unassociated with pain but result in a dorsal kyphosis and exaggerated cervical lordosis described as a "dowager's" or "widow's" hump. Postural slumping with increase in existing curves also contributes to the loss of height. Scoliosis is also common in women with osteoporosis. Generalized skeletal pain is uncommon, and between fractures most patients are free of pain but may have other uncomfortable sensations in the back. Although recurrent episodes of collapse fractures of vertebral bodies, increasing spine deformity, and loss of height are common, the course in any one subject is not predictable, and there may be intervals of several years between fractures.

RADIOLOGIC FEATURES Prior to fracture and collapse the osteoporotic vertebral body shows a decrease in mineral density, increase in prominence of vertical striations due to a relatively greater loss of the horizontally oriented trabeculae, and prominence of the end plates. The bodies may become increasingly biconcave because of weakening of the subchondral plates and expansion of the intervertebral disks, resulting in the so-called codfish vertebrae. When collapse occurs it usually produces a decrease in the anterior height of the vertebral body and irregularity in the anterior cortex (Fig. 341-1). Older compression fractures may show reactive changes and osteophytes about the anterior margins. Most osteoporotic fractures occur in the middle and lower thoracic and upper lumbar vertebral bodies. Fractures of isolated vertebral bodies of T4 or higher should suggest malignancy. Although the cortices of long bones may be thin

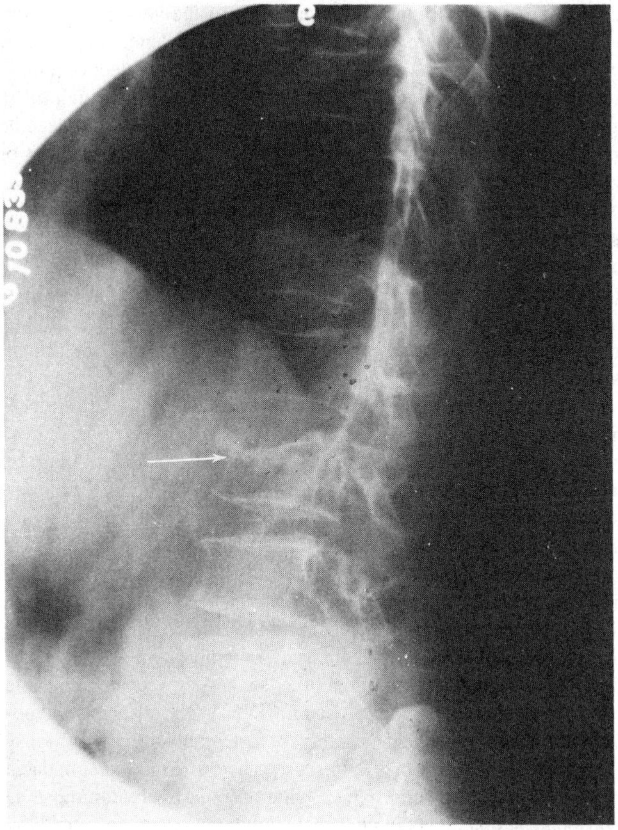

FIGURE 341-1 Lateral views of the lumbar spine of a 54-year-old man with idiopathic osteoporosis. A typical anterior compression fracture is indicated by the arrow.

because of excessive endosteal resorption, the outer margins are sharp in contrast to the typical effects of the subperiosteal resorption of hyperparathyroidism. Pseudofractures or Looser's zones are not present in osteoporosis in the absence of osteomalacia, but it may be impossible to distinguish osteoporosis from osteomalacia on radiologic grounds alone. In the absence of fractures standard roentgenograms are insensitive indicators of bone loss since as much as 30 percent decrease in bone mass may not be appreciated. Other procedures are required to establish whether a given individual has a sufficient decrease in bone mass to be at risk for fracture. These include single- and dual-photon absorptiometry, quantitative computed tomography, or neutron activation analysis of total-body calcium.

LABORATORY FINDINGS The concentrations of calcium and inorganic phosphorus in the blood are usually normal. Slight hyperphosphatemia is present in women who are past the menopause. The alkaline phosphatase in uncomplicated instances is normal, although slight increases may be seen after fractures. About 20 percent of postmenopausal women with osteoporosis have significant hypercalciuria. Urinary excretion of peptides containing hydroxyproline, an index of bone resorption, is usually normal or slightly increased in those with high-turnover osteoporosis. Serum levels of osteocalcin (bone GLA protein) and uptake of ^{99m}Tc-methylene diphosphonate also correlate with the rate of bone turnover.

DIFFERENTIAL DIAGNOSIS Since decrease in skeletal mass is a universal feature of aging, it is difficult to evaluate asymptomatic decreased bone density, determined radiographically, in older women, especially when unaccompanied by marked increase in biconcavity of vertebral bodies or fractures. Quantitative measurement of bone mass is, however, a predictor of future fractures. In the presence of bone pain with or without fracture or deformity, it is important to establish the presence or absence of known causes of osteoporosis as listed in Table 341-1 and to be certain that osteoporosis is the correct diagnosis. Malignancies of various types, particularly *multiple myeloma, lymphoma, leukemia,* and *carcinomatosis,* may result in diffuse loss of bone, especially the trabecular bone of the vertebral column, even in the absence of hypercalcemia. The absence of anemia, elevated erythrocyte sedimentation rate, abnormal electrophoretic patterns of serum proteins, and Bence Jones proteinuria is helpful in eliminating the possibility of multiple myeloma. However, needle bone biopsy or marrow aspiration may be appropriate in instances of severe osteoporosis with fractures. Quantitative histomorphometry on standard biopsy samples from the iliac crest is a research tool but is available in some referral laboratories. Bone biopsy samples must be properly fixed, not demineralized, and embedded in plastic to rule out osteomalacia, however.

Radiologic evidence of osteoporosis is common in patients with primary *hyperparathyroidism,* who may not have osteitis fibrosa (discrete lytic lesions of varying size and subperiosteal resorption) or elevation of serum alkaline phosphatase. Mild asymptomatic hyperparathyroidism is not a major risk factor for vertebral crush fractures, however. An element of secondary hyperparathyroidism may be present in some elderly patients with type II osteoporosis and in others with impairment of renal function, inadequate oral calcium intake, or decrease of intestinal calcium absorption. Increased numbers of osteoclasts may be present in bone biopsy specimens from such patients.

Osteomalacia may mimic osteoporosis or coexist with it, yet specific radiologic signs of osteomalacia may not always be present. Although the presence of abnormalities such as low or undetectable circulating levels of 25-hydroxyvitamin D [25(OH)D] and/or hypophosphatemia suggest the possibility of osteomalacia, bone biopsy may be essential for diagnosis, as discussed below. Since osteomalacia is more responsive to therapy (e.g., vitamin D in hypovitaminosis D or phosphate supplements in phosphate depletion) than the usual case of osteoporosis, such diagnostic procedures are often warranted.

In an occasional patient with *Paget's disease* the radiologic features may be almost purely lytic and be confused with osteoporosis. However, high alkaline phosphatase levels and moderately or markedly increased urinary excretion of hydroxyproline-containing peptides are clues to the presence of Paget's disease. Scanning procedures with bone-seeking isotopes are not helpful in differential diagnosis if fractures are present, because in any disease fractures demonstrate preferential uptake of isotope. However, in the absence of fracture, "hot spots" suggest tumor or early Paget's disease, particularly if present in the appendicular skeleton.

IDIOPATHIC OSTEOPOROSIS *Idiopathic osteoporosis* occurs in younger men and in premenopausal women in whom no other etiologic factor is detected. These patients probably have a number of different disorders with superficial resemblances. In some women the onset of the disease appears to be related to pregnancy and may represent a transient failure in homeostatic mechanisms such as failure to increase circulating levels of $1,25(OH)_2D$ and hence to protect the maternal skeleton from the stresses of childbirth (see Chap. 339). Some patients have low levels of serum alkaline phosphatase, though not low enough to fulfill diagnostic criteria for *hypophosphatasia.* Estrogens are ineffective in therapy. Losses of calcium and phosphorus are probably excessive, and it is unwise to permit women with osteoporosis to breast-feed since calcium losses via lactation are appreciable. Some patients have a disorder similar to mild forms of osteogenesis imperfecta, although such features as family history, blue scleras, and deafness are lacking. The course is variable; although recurrent episodes of fractures are characteristic, progressive deterioration does not occur in all patients, and in some the clinical problem is benign. Juvenile osteoporosis is a rare disorder with onset usually between the ages of 8 and 14 years and is characterized by the abrupt appearance of bone pain and fractures after minimal trauma. In many cases the disorder is self-limited, and recovery takes place spontaneously within 4 or 5 years.

GLUCOCORTICOID EXCESS Glucocorticoid excess does not appear to be involved in osteoporosis of the idiopathic variety or in the type I or II disorder. However, osteoporosis commonly accompanies Cushing's syndrome, both endogenous and exogenous, and in some instances is rapidly progressive, especially in children and in women over the age of 50. Bone loss of glucocorticoid excess is accounted for by a combination of low rates of bone formation (depressed osteoblastic oppositional rate) and high rates of bone resorption that accompany increased activation frequency of bone remodeling units. A part of the latter may be the result of glucocorticoid-induced secondary hyperparathyroidism, although increases in circulating parathyroid hormone have not been found consistently. Glucocorticoids, however, potentiate the effects of parathyroid hormone and $1,25(OH)_2D$ on bone cells in vitro. Glucocorticoids depress collagen synthesis in many tissues, as evidenced by delayed wound healing, thinning of the dermis, striae, and tendency to blue scleras. In some disorders in which glucocorticoids are administered in pharmacologic doses such as rheumatoid arthritis, a tendency to thin skin and osteoporosis is initially present, and the skeletal effects of the glucocorticoids may become particularly apparent. Even low dosages of glucocorticoids may accelerate bone loss in postmenopausal women as well as men with rheumatoid arthritis. Blood levels of 25(OH)D are normal or slightly decreased, and blood levels of $1,25(OH)_2D$ are usually normal. Glucocorticoids inhibit intestinal calcium absorption by a direct, vitamin D–independent action on the intestine. Osteomalacia is not observed histologically. Once osteoporosis develops in adults with Cushing's syndrome, the abnormality may persist indefinitely following alleviation of the glucocorticoid excess. In children, however, cure of the Cushing's syndrome may result in striking improvement in the appearance of the spine due to new endochondral bone formation around the less dense, older osteoporotic bone. Likewise, a striking increase in bone mass, increase in serum osteocalcin levels (indicative of increased osteoblastic function), and decrease in urinary hydroxyproline excretion may occur in young adults following therapy of Cushing's syndrome. Withdrawal of glucocorticoids or decrease of the dose by alternate-day schedule may thus be the only way to halt progression of the osteoporosis. Anabolic steroids are not effective in this regard. The defect in intestinal calcium absorption may be overcome by administering vitamin D in doses of 50,000 IU two times weekly plus supplemental oral calcium of 1 to 1.5 g per day. Vitamin D metabolites such as calcifediol [25(OH)D] may be more effective. When large doses of vitamin D are used, it is important to monitor serum and urinary calcium and serum 25(OH)D levels at intervals of 2 to 4 months, especially if glucocorticoid dosages are lowered. In Cushing's syndrome, spontaneous, symptomless fractures may occur in ribs and pubic and ischial rami even in the absence of marked osteoporosis of the spine. These fractures often heal partially with an exuberant calcified callus surrounding a radiolucent zone of nonunion, superficially resembling the pseudofractures of osteomalacia. If they appear in the thorax superimposed upon the lungs, they may be confused with nodules suggesting primary or metastatic tumor.

GONADAL DEFICIENCY Receptors for estrogens are in osteoblasts, and estrogens may function in these cells by stimulating production of substances that are anabolic for bone such as somatomedin C (insulin-like growth factor-1). Estrogen is deficient in the postmenopausal woman, and the administration of estrogen to such an individual reduces the negative calcium balance and decreases urinary hydroxyproline excretion. Estrogens are particularly useful in retarding the bone loss in women who have oophorectomy at an early age. Bone mass is also decreased in women athletes who are amenorrheic, such as marathon runners. Such women are particularly prone to tibial stress fractures. In patients of either sex castrated at an early age, the adult skeleton is smaller to begin with, and therefore age-related losses are more significant. Bone density is also decreased in women with hyperprolactinemia and in men with hypogonadism of all types.

THYROTOXICOSIS In many patients with hyperthyroidism, excessive bone resorption, occasionally marked in degree and far exceeding that in the usual patient with osteoporosis, can be associated with increased excretion of calcium and phosphorus in urine and feces. The excessive bone resorption is usually accompanied by a compensatory increase in bone formation. Parathyroid hormone secretion is decreased, and levels of $1,25(OH)_2D$ are normal or low. If the hyperthyroidism is of short duration, skeletal losses are inconsequential. However, in patients with chronic hyperthyroidism, especially in women after the menopause, this accelerated bone loss becomes clinically significant, and it is important to eliminate hyperthyroidism as a contributing cause of osteoporosis. Hypothyroid patients who are treated with excessive doses of levothyroxine may also have accelerated loss of bone mass. Although typical osteitis fibrosa (resorption lacunae containing osteoclasts and a fibrous stroma) may be seen on biopsy, the skeletal lesions have the radiologic appearance of osteoporosis.

ACROMEGALY Hypercalciuria and overall net negative calcium balance occur in acromegaly, and occasionally osteoporosis is an associated finding. The secondary panhypopituitarism and the associated gonadal insufficiency may be factors in production of the osteoporosis. In adult animals growth hormone decreases endosteal resorption and stimulates bone formation, and it is therefore unlikely that excessive secretion of growth hormone in itself produces osteoporosis.

DIABETES MELLITUS Individuals with juvenile or adult-onset diabetes mellitus have a decreased bone mass. In some series the incidence of hip fractures is increased, but studies of large groups of diabetic subjects have not revealed abnormal calcium metabolism or significant bone disease specifically attributable to the diabetes.

CALCIUM DEFICIENCY AND MALABSORPTION Although calcium deficiency may be a factor, it cannot be the sole or major cause in idiopathic, senile, or postmenopausal osteoporosis. Osteoporosis is an associated finding in a significant number of cases of steatorrhea, prolonged obstructive jaundice, and lactose intolerance and in patients following gastrectomy. Other patients may have a specific defect in calcium absorption or a failure to adapt adequately to a low-calcium diet either by increasing the percentage of dietary calcium absorbed or by decreasing urinary calcium excretion. Presumably, vitamin D is adequate in these instances to prevent osteomalacia.

HERITABLE DISORDERS OF CONNECTIVE TISSUE In the strict sense, the bone disease of osteogenesis imperfecta is osteoporosis (see Chap. 333). *Osteogenesis imperfecta* is clinically, genetically, and biochemically heterogeneous. Type I osteogenesis imperfecta is the autosomal dominant form characterized by mild to moderate bone fragility, blue sclerae, and premature deafness. The frequency of fractures tends to decrease around puberty, and another period of increased incidence occurs in women after the menopause. Type II is the lethal perinatal disorder. Type III is characterized by severe bone fragility, progressive bone deformity, and white sclerae. In type IV, sclerae are white, but other features are similar to those of type I disease. Many instances of osteogenesis imperfecta of all types have been linked to mutations in the *COL*1A1 and *COL*1A2 genes that encode type I collagen. Such linkage has been shown either by analysis of restriction fragment length polymorphisms (RFLPs) or by direct demonstration of mutations that produce amino acid substitutions or deletions. It is thought that the majority of patients with osteogenesis imperfecta will ultimately prove to have mutations in the type I collagen genes. In other individuals, defects in these genes may predispose to what is now diagnosed as idiopathic or postmenopausal osteoporosis, in the absence of other features of osteogenesis imperfecta. Osteoporosis also occurs in patients with *homocystinuria* due to cystathionine synthase deficiency, an autosomal recessive trait, associated with ectopia lentis, various deformities of the extremities, mental retardation, decreased pigmentation of hair and skin, and thromboembolism. The diagnosis is established by the finding of homocystine in urine. The osteoporosis may be due to the effect of homocysteine or other metabolites in interfering with the cross-linking of collagen.

THERAPY In considering treatment of osteoporosis, it should be emphasized that one is dealing with a group of disorders rather than a single entity. Even in patients within the same category, e.g., those with idiopathic osteoporosis, the etiologies may be different. It is also difficult to predict the course, especially in patients seen because of pain and collapse-fracture. Many patients in the idiopathic, postmenopausal (type I), and senile (type II) groups have a few episodes of vertebral body collapse but then go for many years without symptoms or further loss in height. Furthermore, the acute pain associated with vertebral body fracture tends to subside in weeks, and *any* treatment administered at that time might be considered efficacious. Although accurate estimation of bone mass can help determine efficacy of therapy, clinical benefit (diminution of bone pain, decrease in incidence of fractures) is more difficult to assess in view of variability in disease progression. It is generally agreed, however, that estrogen replacement in women is effective in preventing bone loss after oophorectomy or early in the menopause.

General measures Patients with acute pain secondary to fracture of vertebral bodies frequently require rest in bed in a position of maximum comfort, local heat, adequate analgesics, and avoidance of constipation. Use of traction or plaster jacket splints is not indicated. As soon as pain permits, the patient should attempt to move out of bed, slowly at first, perhaps with support of a walker or crutches. Braces are commonly employed, but their efficacy in preventing progression of spinal deformity has not been established. A well-made corset may provide support and comfort. Exercises to correct postural deformity and increase muscle tone are useful. Patients should be taught to avoid sudden painful movements such as jumping and how to lift and carry objects with minimal back strain. After the fractures have healed, a supervised exercise program that includes daily walking may be helpful in preventing further skeletal losses.

Estrogens and androgens The use of estrogens in postmenopausal women causes a decrease in urinary calcium and hydroxyproline excretion, especially during the first few months of treatment (see Chap. 322). Estrogens may have direct effects on osteoblasts and also decrease the rate of bone resorption, but bone formation usually does not increase and eventually decreases. Nevertheless, estrogens produce significant calcium retention, decrease the difference between bone formation and resorption, and retard bone loss. Although any restoration of skeletal mass is minimal, the use of estrogens effectively prevents bone loss following castration and in the menopause and decreases the incidence of osteoporotic fracture in postmenopausal women. The major role of estrogens is in preventing osteoporosis in menopausal women rather than treating clinical disease already developed, although they may also be effective in the woman with mild or moderate disease during the first 10 years following cessation of ovarian function. The common dosage is 0.625 mg/d as conjugated estrogens, usually in a cyclic fashion for the first 25 days of each month. (Lower doses of estrogens are usually ineffective.) Estradiol can also be administered in a percutaneous patch or gel for transdermal absorption (see Chap. 322). In women after hysterectomy progestogens are not necessary, but in women with a uterus, a progestogen (e.g., medroxyprogesterone 5 or 10 mg/d) may be added for the last 10 days of estrogen administration (see Chap. 322). Testosterone preparations are useful in treatment of osteoporotic men with gonadal deficiency, but there are no convincing reports of their efficacy in men with normal gonadal function. There is also no proven advantage to combinations of estrogens and androgens.

Calcium supplements, vitamin D metabolites, and thiazide diuretics Women who are estrogen-deprived require an average oral intake of 1500 mg/d of elemental calcium to remain in calcium equilibrium. The recommendation of the National Institutes of Health of 1000 mg elemental calcium per day for women on estrogen replacement and for men is reasonable. In postmenopausal women unable to take estrogens, the use of 1500 mg/d of oral calcium may have minor benefit in preserving cortical bone mass but has no effects on trabecular bone mass. Adequate calcium intake before age 30 to 35 may have beneficial effects on the attainment of peak bone mass, however. The content of elemental calcium of available preparations varies, depending upon the accompanying anion and the composition (Table 341-2). Vitamin D preparations have been used in osteoporosis because calcium absorption is impaired and levels of the active

TABLE 341-2 Elemental calcium content of various oral calcium preparations

Calcium preparation	Elemental calcium content
Calcium citrate	40 mg/300 mg
Calcium carbonate	400 mg/g
Calcium lactate	80 mg/600 mg
Calcium gluconate	40 mg/500 mg
Calcium carbonate + 5 μg vitamin D_2 (Os – Cal 250)	250 mg/tablet

metabolite, $1,25(OH)_2D$, are marginally low in serum. The efficacy of vitamin D itself has never been established, although reports have appeared indicating that oral administration of calcitriol [$1,25(OH)_2D$] can improve intestinal calcium absorption, suppress bone resorption, and prevent bone loss in patients with postmenopausal osteoporosis. Bone formation is not increased, however, and at the dose used in one study (mean, 0.8 μg/d) hypercalcemia and hypercalciuria were complications. To establish whether beneficial effects would be achieved with lower doses of calcitriol would require additional study. Thiazide diuretics are useful in patients with high-turnover osteoporosis associated with hypercalciuria and secondary hyperparathyroidism. In the absence of secondary hyperparathyroidism the thiazide diuretics lower urinary calcium excretion, suppress parathyroid gland function, inhibit synthesis of $1,25(OH)_2D$, and reduce intestinal calcium absorption.

Calcitonin Calcitonin decreases bone resorption, and the use of salmon calcitonin in established osteoporosis has been recommended in doses of 50 units subcutaneously every other day. Only patients with high-turnover osteoporosis (elevated levels of serum osteocalcin, increased urinary hydroxyproline excretion, and increased total body retention of ^{99m}Tc-methylene diphosphonate) appear to respond with improvement in bone mass. Another approach involves the use of salmon calcitonin administered by nasal spray (200 units per day) to avoid injections.

Fluoride Fluoride ions are deposited in the skeleton where they become incorporated into the crystal lattice of hydroxyapatite, substituting for hydroxyl ions. This process results in a mineral phase of greater crystallinity. Sodium fluoride is also the only therapeutic agent that can stimulate osteoblastic proliferation and function and increase bone formation. Indeed, chronic ingestion of high amounts of fluoride ions, usually in endemic areas where fluoride content of drinking water is very high, produces a form of hyperostosis, with dense bones, exostoses, neurologic complications due to bony overgrowth, and ligament ossification. Increased amount of bone with excessive osteoid is evidence of stimulation of bone formation, and a decrease in the rate of new vertebral fractures suggests that the new bone is of reasonable structure. Not all patients respond and some develop side effects including knee, foot, and ankle pain attributed to microfractures; other patients cannot tolerate sodium fluoride because of nausea. An oral slow-release form is better tolerated with fewer gastrointestinal and rheumatologic complications. Sodium fluoride has been recommended only for treatment of established vertebral osteoporosis with symptomatic crush fracture syndrome that would not likely respond to other therapies. Caution about fluoride has been raised in view of increased incidence of hip fractures in some series.

RICKETS AND OSTEOMALACIA

Rickets and *osteomalacia* are disorders in which mineralization of the organic matrix of the skeleton is defective (Table 341-3). In *rickets* the growing skeleton is involved; defective mineralization occurs not only in bone but also in the cartilaginous matrix of the growth plate. The term *osteomalacia* is usually reserved for the disorder in the adult in whom the epiphyseal growth plates are closed. A number of conditions result in rickets and/or osteomalacia such as inadequate dietary intake of vitamin D, inadequate exposure to solar ultraviolet radiation to form endogenous vitamin D, intestinal malabsorption of vitamin D, acquired and inherited disorders of vitamin D metabolism, inherited defects in the receptors for $1,25(OH)_2D$ in target tissues, chronic acidosis, renal tubular defects which produce hypophosphatemia or acidosis, aluminum intoxication, and chronic administration of anticonvulsants. In the renal tubular disorders rickets and osteomalacia develop in the presence of normal intestinal function and are not cured by treatment with doses of vitamin D adequate to cure deficiency rickets. Thus the term *vitamin D–resistant* (or

TABLE 341-3 Classification of rickets and osteomalacia

I Vitamin D deficiency
- *A* Dietary deficiency
- *B* Deficient endogenous synthesis

II Gastrointestinal
- *A* Small-intestinal diseases with malabsorption
- *B* Partial or total gastrectomy
- *C* Hepatobiliary disease
- *D* Chronic pancreatic insufficiency

III Disorders of vitamin D metabolism
- *A* Hereditary: pseudovitamin D deficiency or vitamin D dependency, types I and II
- *B* Acquired
  - *1* Anticonvulsants
  - *2* Chronic renal failure

IV Acidosis
- *A* Distal renal tubular acidosis (classic or type I)
- *B* Secondary forms of renal acidosis
- *C* Ureterosigmoidostomy
- *D* Drug-induced disease
  - *1* Chronic acetazolamide ingestion
  - *2* Chronic ammonium chloride ingestion

V Chronic renal failure

VI Phosphate depletion
- *A* Dietary: low phosphate intake plus ingestion of nonabsorbable antacids
- *B* Impaired renal tubular phosphate reabsorption
  - *1* Hereditary
    - *a* X-linked hypophosphatemic rickets (vitamin D–resistant rickets)
    - *b* Adult-onset vitamin D–resistant hypophosphatemic osteomalacia
  - *2* Acquired
    - *a* Sporadic hypophosphatemic osteomalacia (phosphate diabetes)
    - *b* Tumor-associated (oncogenous) rickets and osteomalacia
    - *c* Neurofibromatosis
    - *d* Fibrous dysplasia

VII Generalized renal tubular disorders (Fanconi's syndrome)
- *A* Primary renal
- *B* Associated with systemic metabolic abnormality
  - *1* Cystinosis
  - *2* Glycogenosis
  - *3* Lowe's syndrome
- *C* Systemic disorder with associated renal disease
  - *1* Hereditary
    - *a* Inborn errors
      - (*1*) Wilson's disease
      - (2) Tyrosinemia
    - *b* Neurofibromatosis
  - *2* Acquired
    - *a* Multiple myeloma
    - *b* Nephrotic syndrome
    - *c* Transplanted kidney
  - *3* Intoxications
    - *a* Cadmium
    - *b* Lead
    - *c* Outdated tetracycline

VIII Primary mineralization defects
- *A* Hereditary: hypophosphatasia
- *B* Acquired
  - *1* Diphosphonate (disodium etidronate) treatment
  - *2* Fluoride treatment

IX States of rapid bone formation with or without a relative defect in bone resorption
- *A* Postoperative hyperparathyroidism with osteitis fibrosa cystica
- *B* Osteopetrosis

X Defective matrix synthesis: fibrogenesis imperfecta ossium

XI Miscellaneous
- *A* Magnesium-dependent conditions
- *B* Axial osteomalacia
- *C* Parenteral alimentation
- *D* Aluminum intoxication

–refractory) rickets has been applied in these instances. Renal insufficiency, especially in children, and chronic hemodialysis per se are also associated with rickets or osteomalacia.

PATHOGENESIS AND HISTOPATHOLOGY For skeletal mineralization, sufficient calcium and phosphate must be present at the mineralization sites. Other conditions required for normal mineralization include intact metabolic and transport functions of osteoblasts and chondrocytes, adequate collagen matrix, possibly phosphorylation or other modifications of matrix components, and low concentrations of inhibitory substances such as proteoglycan aggregates or inorganic pyrophosphate. A specific function in the mineralization process for the γ-carboxyglutamic acid–containing proteins (e.g., osteocalcin, osteonectin, and phospho-sialoproteins) synthesized by bone cells has not been demonstrated, although they bind calcium ions. In cartilage the initial mineral phase is in membrane-bound extracellular vesicles. If the osteoblast continues to produce matrix components that cannot be adequately mineralized, rickets and osteomalacia result. If calcification continues to be inadequate, the production of organic matrix (osteoid) also gradually decreases. In bone there will be an increase in the fraction of the forming surface covered by incompletely mineralized osteoid, an increase in osteoid volume and thickness (the latter normally less than 12 to 14 μm), and a decrease in the calcification or mineralization front. The latter is detected in undemineralized sections by the fluorescence of previously ingested tetracycline or by special stains. There is a marked decrease in the rate of apposition of mineralized bone. A variety of methods are available to measure the thickness of the osteoid seams and the calcification front. In histologic sections stained with hematoxylin and eosin, the more heavily mineralized areas tend to appear violet or blue, whereas the osteoid seams appear pink. Subtle degrees of osteomalacia may not be appreciated with routine preparations, and undecalcified, thin sections (3 to 5 μm) stained, for example, with Goldner's trichrome method are necessary to establish its presence (Fig. 341-2). Rickets is also characterized by inadequate mineralization of the matrix of cartilage in the growing epiphyseal plate. Calcification in the interstitial regions of the hypertrophic zone is defective, the growth plate increases in thickness, the columns of cartilage cells (usually highly ordered) are disorganized, and there is a variable cupping of the epiphyses. The rachitic bones are often incapable of withstanding usual mechanical stresses and tend to undergo bowing deformities. If rickets is untreated, growth at the epiphyseal plates is slowed, and the eventual length of the long bones is diminished.

FIGURE 341-2 Photomicrograph of an undemineralized section stained with Goldner method of an iliac crest bone biopsy from a 45-year-old man with chronic renal failure maintained on hemodialysis. Almost the entire surface is covered by osteoid (O) readily distinguished from mineralized bone (MB). The thickness of the osteoid seams exceeds 100 μm in several areas.

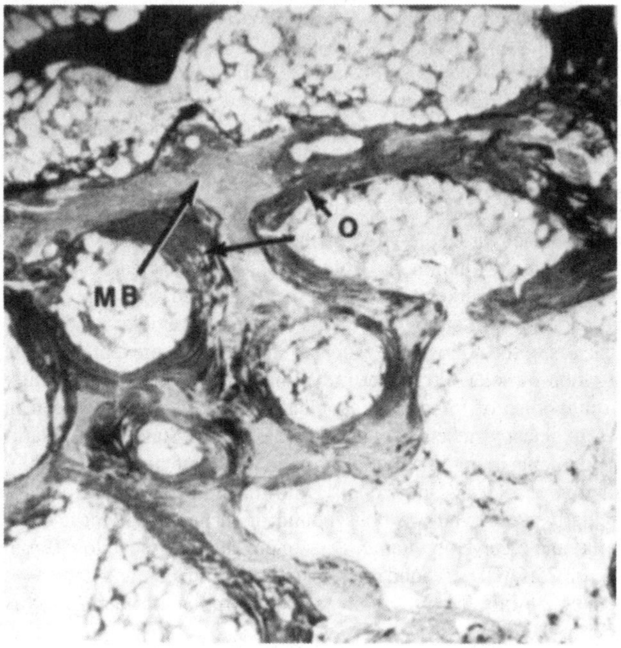

It has not been established whether vitamin D, through one of its metabolites, has a major direct effect on mineralization. Its primary roles after metabolic conversion to 25(OH)D and $1,25(OH)_2D$ are to regulate and enhance absorption of calcium ions from the intestinal lumen and, possibly, to enhance differentiation of stem cells to form osteoclasts. Insufficiency of the active metabolites of vitamin D leads to decreased intestinal absorption of calcium and decreased mobilization of calcium from bone, resulting in hypocalcemia. This stimulates increased synthesis and secretion of parathyroid hormone (PTH) and hyperplasia of the parathyroid glands. The increased circulating concentration of PTH tends to increase plasma calcium and enhances renal phosphate clearance, which, in turn, produces hypophosphatemia. When the concentration of phosphorus in the extracellular fluid falls below a critical level, mineralization cannot proceed normally. In severe vitamin D deficiency, normal levels of serum calcium cannot be maintained, and the driving force for mineralization is further decreased. The absence of some critical metabolite of vitamin D that acts directly on the skeleton may also play a role in the defective mineralization of rickets and osteomalacia.

Phosphate depletion alone can produce osteomalacia as in patients consuming large amounts of nonabsorbable antacids and in patients with excessive renal loss of phosphate due to decreased tubular reabsorption. Secondary hyperparathyroidism is usually not present in these patients. Hypophosphatemia per se produces mineralization defects despite its effect on increasing the activity of the renal 25(OH)D-1α-hydroxylase, but it cannot account for the osteomalacia in all the disorders listed in Table 341-3. In chronic renal failure, for example, plasma phosphate levels are not decreased and usually are increased. Similarly, plasma phosphorus levels are not depressed in infants and children with osteomalacia secondary to hypophosphatasia, a hereditary deficiency in alkaline phosphatase. Osteomalacia in some patients with chronic renal failure is associated with accumulation of aluminum in bone, and the aluminum probably plays a role in production of the mineralization defect.

CLINICAL FINDINGS The clinical manifestations of rickets are the result of skeletal deformities, susceptibility to fractures, weakness and hypotonia, and disturbances in growth. In extreme instances of vitamin D–deficiency rickets, hypocalcemia may be sufficient to produce tetany which, when severe, may be accompanied by laryngeal spasm and convulsive seizures.

In infants and young children features include listlessness, irritability, and often profound hypotonia and muscular weakness. As the disorder progresses, children become unable to walk without support. Abnormal parietal flattening and frontal bossing develop in the skull. The calvaria are softened (craniotabes), and sutures may be widened. Prominence of the costochondral junctions is called the "rachitic rosary," and the indentation of the lower ribs at the site of attachment of the diaphragm is known as *Harrison's groove*. If untreated, progressive deformities of the pelvis and extremities result, with bowing particularly common in the tibia, femur, radius, and ulna. Fractures are frequent, dental eruption is often delayed, and enamel defects are common.

The presentation of osteomalacia in adults usually is not as dramatic as in infants and children. The skeletal deformities may be overlooked, and the features of the underlying disorder may dominate, as, for example, in the vitamin D deficiency of adult celiac disease. Symptoms, when they occur, include diffuse skeletal pain and bony tenderness. Pain may be prominent about the hips and result in an antalgic gait. Muscular weakness may be difficult to distinguish from hesitancy to move because of skeletal pain. Proximal weakness may mimic that of primary muscle disorders and contribute to the waddling gait. Pain and weakness may be sufficient to cause patients to be confined to bed and chair. Many factors, including the secondary hyperparathyroidism, contribute to the myopathy. Clinical improvement in the myopathy usually results from specific therapy such as vitamin D repletion in nutritional osteomalacia, phosphate replacement in renal hypophosphatemia, or correction of acidosis. Fractures of involved bones may occur with minimal trauma. When the ribs are involved, severe deformities may develop in the thoracic cage, and the collapse of vertebral bodies may produce loss of height.

RADIOLOGIC FEATURES Radiologic changes reflect the pathologic changes. In rickets the alterations are most evident at the epiphyseal growth plate, which is increased in thickness, cupped, and hazy at the metaphyseal border due to decreased calcification of the hypertrophic zone and inadequate mineralization of the primary spongiosa. The trabecular pattern of the metaphyses is abnormal, the cortices of the diaphyses may be thinned, and the shafts may be bowed.

In osteomalacia decrease in bone density is usually associated with loss of trabeculae and variable thinning of the cortices. The radiologic changes may be indistinguishable from those in osteoporosis. Trabecular patterns may be blurred, producing a homogeneous ground glass appearance. The specific finding that suggests osteomalacia is the presence of radiolucent bands ranging from a few millimeters to several centimeters in length, usually perpendicular to the surface of the bones. They are particularly common at the inner aspects of the femur, especially near the femoral neck, in the pelvis, in the outer edge of the scapula, in the upper fibula, and in the metatarsals (Figs. 341-3 and 341-4). These radiolucent bands, called *pseudofractures* or *Looser's zones,* occur most often at sites where major arteries cross the bones and are thought to be due to the mechanical stress of the pulsation of these vessels. Subperiosteal erosions along the diaphyseal cortices are sometimes seen in secondary hyperparathyroidism.

FIGURE 341-3 Radiographs of the scapula of a 58-year-old woman with phosphate diabetes. The presence of a pseudofracture or Looser's zone is indicated by the arrow.

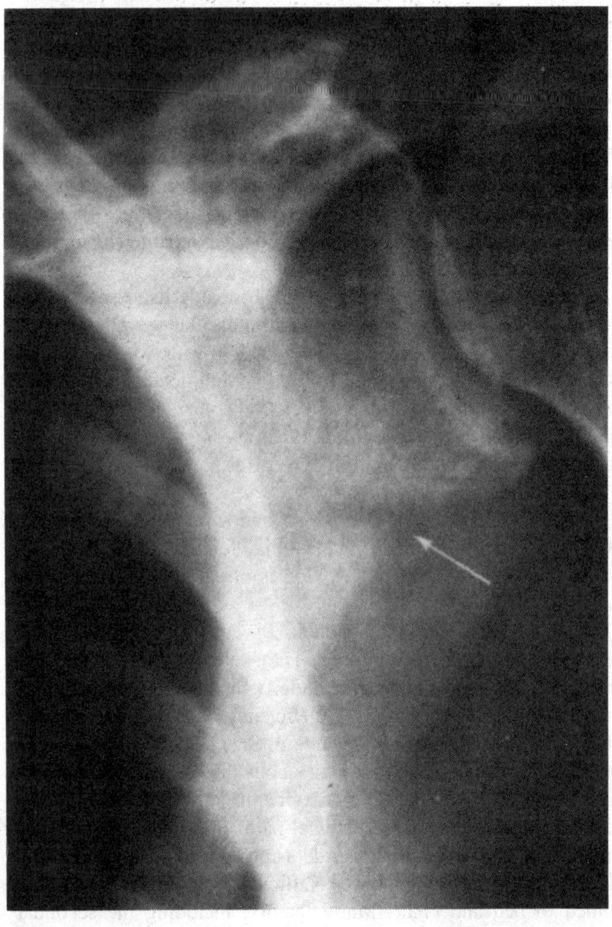

Increased rather than decreased density of bones may be observed in patients with renal tubular disorders rather than with vitamin D deficiency and may produce a striking thickening of the cortices and trabeculae of spongy bone. Despite the increase in mass of bone per unit volume, the trabeculae are covered with thickened osteoid seams typical of osteomalacia. Similar findings may occur in patients with chronic renal failure. The reason for the hyperostosis is unknown; the bone is architecturally abnormal and subject to fracture with minimal trauma.

LABORATORY FINDINGS Changes in serum concentrations of calcium, inorganic phosphorus, 25(OH)D, and $1,25(OH)_2D$ vary with the different disorders (see Chap. 339). In vitamin D deficiency, whether due to dietary lack, inadequate sunlight exposure, or intestinal malabsorption, serum calcium levels are normal or low, whereas phosphorus and 25(OH)D levels are characteristically low, the latter usually <12 nmol/L (<5 ng/mL) depending upon the assay. In contrast, levels of $1,25(OH)_2D$ may be normal or even elevated due to secondary hyperparathyroidism. Eventually, when levels of 25(OH)D become so low that there is inadequate substrate for the renal 25(OH)D-1α-hydroxylase, then the serum level of $1,25(OH)_2D$ will also decline. In adults the lower limit of serum phosphorus concentration is around 0.9 mmol/L (2.8 mg/dL); in children the lower limit of normal is closer to 1.3 to 1.5 mmol/L (4.0 to 4.5 mg/dL). In *severe* vitamin D depletion, hypocalcemia may be sufficient to produce tetany. Mild acidosis and generalized aminoaciduria also result from secondary hyperparathyroidism. As a rule, patients with renal tubular disorders maintain normal serum calcium levels, while hypophosphatemia is characteristic. Other laboratory findings such as glucosuria, aminoaciduria, acidosis, and hypouricemia reflect variable degrees of disturbance of proximal tubular function or features of the underlying disease (e.g., low plasma ceruloplasmin in Wilson's disease or abnormalities of immunoglobulins in multiple myeloma). In chronic renal failure hyperphosphatemia and some degree of hypocalcemia are usually accompanied by normal 25(OH)D and low $1,25(OH)_2D$ levels. In nephrotic syndrome serum 25(OH)D levels can be low due primarily to urinary losses of protein-bound 25(OH)D. Serum phosphorus levels are also normal or elevated in hypophosphatasia. Increased excretion of hydroxyproline-containing peptides occurs in those conditions in which secondary hyperparathyroidism and excessive bone resorption are associated with the defect in mineralization. Alkaline phosphatase levels in plasma are usually elevated in rickets or osteomalacia, but typical and even severe osteomalacia, especially that due to renal tubular disorders, may be accompanied by normal or only borderline elevations. Levels may increase during the early phases of therapy.

DIETARY VITAMIN D DEFICIENCY AND INADEQUATE ENDOGENOUS SYNTHESIS Most foods unfortified with vitamin D contain insufficient amounts of the vitamin to prevent rickets in growing children or osteomalacia in adults living in temperate-zone cities. As discussed in Chap. 339, in the absence of supplements, vitamin D must be formed endogenously through the ultraviolet irradiation of precursor 7-dehydrocholesterol in the skin. Many factors decrease the formation of vitamin D_3 from its precursor: increased melanin pigmentation, hyperkeratosis, sunscreens, limited exposure of the body, short days of sunlight, oblique angle of ultraviolet irradiation, and factors in the atmosphere, such as smog, which prevent adequate penetration of solar ultraviolet radiation. Since fortification of milk and routine use of vitamin D supplements for infants have been in effect, deficiency rickets is unusual in the United States. Poor, dark-skinned infants living in crowded northern cities are most susceptible. Furthermore, elderly individuals with insufficient sun exposure, particularly those who are housebound or in nursing homes, drink no milk, and receive no vitamin D supplements, may have low serum levels of 25(OH)D, secondary hyperparathyroidism, and increased frequency of hip fractures. Intestinal absorption of vitamin D is normal in the elderly.

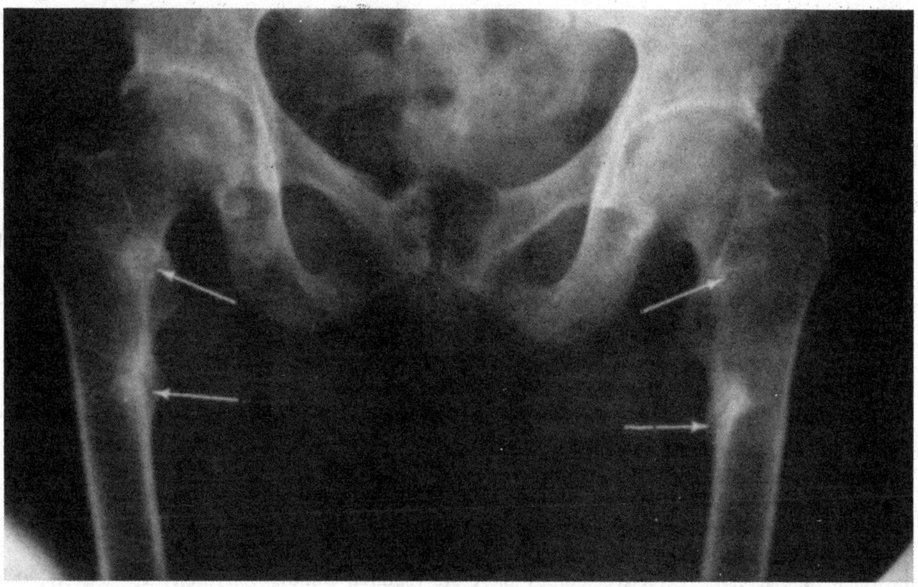

FIGURE 341-4 Radiograph of the femurs of a 47-year-old woman with Fanconi's syndrome of adult onset. The presence of multiple pseudofractures is indicated by the arrows.

VITAMIN D LOSS AND INTESTINAL MALABSORPTION Osteomalacia may be seen in patients with intestinal malabsorption such as in adult celiac disease and regional enteritis. Prior to the discovery of gluten sensitivity in some of these cases, celiac disease was among the more common disorders underlying osteomalacia. Vitamin D absorption, which normally occurs via chylomicrons, is impaired in diseases causing steatorrhea where emulsification of fat is disturbed, such as chronic biliary obstruction. Patients with cholestatic liver disease or extrahepatic biliary obstruction may have low serum levels of 25(OH)D and osteomalacia, due not only to poor vitamin D absorption but also to decreased hepatic production of 25(OH)D. Osteomalacia is less frequent in chronic pancreatic insufficiency. Patients who have had gastric surgery for peptic ulcer disease or gastric bypass for obesity may also develop osteomalacia, possibly due to malfunction of the proximal small bowel. Factors other than failure to absorb vitamin D may contribute to the osteomalacia in patients with small-bowel disease, such as inadequate absorbing surface and failure of intestinal cells to respond to the active metabolites of vitamin D. Secondary hyperparathyroidism is usually present in intestinal malabsorption, as it is in dietary lack of vitamin D, and may be particularly severe in patients who develop osteomalacia following intestinal bypass surgery. Some patients who lack vitamin D, usually associated with intestinal malabsorption, have normal circulating levels of $1,25(OH)_2D$, despite low or undetectable 25(OH)D. In these individuals the normal levels of $1,25(OH)_2D$ may be accounted for by ingestion of sufficient vitamin D in hospital diets to produce substrate 25(OH)D for 1α-hydroxylation by the renal enzyme that is increased in activity due to secondary hyperparathyroidism. In other patients, circulating $1,25(OH)_2D$ levels may not reflect levels at critical target cells.

ABNORMAL METABOLISM OF VITAMIN D Serum 25(OH)D levels are reduced in some instances of parenchymal and obstructive liver disease, but these findings have not yet been correlated with quantitative histologic studies of bone. Patients consuming anticonvulsant drugs such as phenobarbital, phenytoin, or carbamazepine may develop rickets or osteomalacia. For a given intake of vitamin D, patients receiving chronic anticonvulsant drugs have lower serum levels of calcium and 25(OH)D. Consumption of anticonvulsants may be especially important in individuals whose intake of vitamin D is marginal, who are nonambulatory and confined indoors, who have chronic recurrent infections, or in whom mild intestinal malfunction exists as in the postgastrectomy state. As discussed in Chap. 339 the anticonvulsant drugs have multiple actions on calcium homeostasis.

Two autosomal recessive syndromes associated with rickets have been termed *vitamin D–dependent rickets* (also see Chap. 311). Features of *type I vitamin D–dependent rickets* include hypocalcemia, hypophosphatemia, short stature, skeletal deformities of rickets, dental enamel hypoplasia, frequently marked elevations of serum alkaline phosphatase activity, generalized aminoaciduria, and secondary hyperparathyroidism. Treatment with massive doses of vitamin D or small doses of calcitriol reverses the abnormal biochemical findings, induces healing of the rickets, and restores the rate of skeletal growth. The abnormalities are due to mutations that impair the renal 25(OH)D-1α-hydroxylase. *Type II vitamin D–dependent rickets,* also termed *hereditary resistance to $1,25(OH)_2D$,* has many clinical features of the type I syndrome. Rickets is usually of early onset but varies in severity in different kindreds. Distinguishing features include alopecia, which may develop during the first few months of age, and multiple milia and epidermal cysts. The type II disorder is due to mutations that impair the $1,25(OH)_2D$ receptor. Different molecular abnormalities have been demonstrated in different kindreds including mutations that impair binding of the receptor to DNA and mutations that cause the formation of incomplete receptor molecules.

Abnormalities in vitamin D metabolism, not on a genetic basis, as well as osteomalacia may be found in patients on long-term total parenteral nutrition. Some of these individuals have hypoparathyroidism but this cannot account for the osteomalacia. Serum levels of 25(OH)D are normal although levels of $1,25(OH)_2D$ may be low. Aluminum has been detected in increased amounts in plasma, urine, and bone and may play a role in genesis of the osteomalacia similar to that postulated in patients with renal failure on chronic hemodialysis.

RENAL TUBULAR DISORDERS Rickets and osteomalacia occur in association with a variety of disorders of proximal renal tubular function. These disorders have in common increased renal clearance of inorganic phosphorus and hypophosphatemia with normal or near normal glomerular filtration rate. Increased phosphate clearance with resultant hypophosphatemia is usually an isolated defect with no other abnormalities except for increase in urinary glycine excretion (hyperglycinuria). X-linked hypophosphatemia (*phosphate diabetes* and *vitamin D–resistant rickets* are terms applied to these cases especially when the disorder presents in early childhood) is characterized by rickets that develops in an otherwise well-nourished, healthy-appearing child. When the child begins to walk and bear weight, lower limb deformities appear and become progressively worse. The rate of linear growth is at first normal and then slowed. The inheritance pattern is X-linked dominant. Many of these individuals develop a unique disorder of tendons, ligaments, and joint capsules characterized by calcification or, more probably, ossification of insertions of tendons and ligaments and joint capsules (enthesopathy). In some patients spontaneous remissions may be followed by recurrences in adult life associated, for example, with pregnancy and lactation. Hypophosphatemia is due to defective renal conservation of phosphate, which in turn is due to defective phosphate transport across the luminal membrane of proximal renal tubular cells. [A model of the human disease has been found in a strain of hypophosphatemic (Hyp) mice.] On the basis of analysis of RFLP studies in several kindreds of X-linked hypophosphatemia, the gene has been mapped to the short arm of the X chromosome (Xp22.31-p21.3). The sequence of the normal gene and the nature of the defect that leads to altered phosphate transport have not been elucidated. In affected individuals, the serum levels of 25(OH)D are normal, and the levels of $1,25(OH)_2D$ are in the low-normal range. Since the induction of hypophosphatemia in normal individuals results in stimulation of the 25(OH)D-1α-hydroxylase and an increase in the levels of $1,25(OH)_2D$, it has been proposed that altered renal tubular cellular phosphate fluxes that result from the mutation in X-linked hypophosphatemia fail to stimulate the hydroxylase. Thus, levels of $1,25(OH)_2D$, although in the normal range, are inappropriately low relative to the phosphate depletion. The skeletal mineralization defect is ascribable not only to the low ambient phosphate levels but also to an intrinsic defect in osteoblast function possibly related to that in the renal tubular cells. Effective therapy therefore requires combination of phosphate repletion with large amounts of oral phosphate, combined with supplements of calcitriol (see below). Combined therapy with calcitriol and inorganic phosphorus reverses the osteomalacia of trabecular bone surfaces, corrects the microscopic periosteocytic mineralization defects, and results in improvement in longitudinal growth. After the rickets is healed, however, defects in phosphate clearance and hypophosphatemia persist and medical therapy is still required. The effects of excessive calcitriol administration, such as nephrocalcinosis and nephrolithiasis, must be avoided. Adults with X-linked hypophosphatemia frequently have pseudofractures; osteoarthritis in the sacroiliac joints, wrists, knees, hips, and feet; and marked enthesopathy. Another variant of hereditary rickets has been termed *hereditary hypophosphatemic rickets with hypercalciuria*. Muscular weakness, not a feature of X-linked hypophosphatemia, may be present. These individuals, whose disorder is probably inherited as an autosomal recessive trait, have normocalcemia, hypophosphatemia, and striking absorptive hypercalciuria; the latter disappears after fasting and returns after oral calcium loading. Levels of $1,25(OH)_2D$ in serum are elevated in contrast to low-normal levels in X-linked hypophosphatemia. These elevations of serum $1,25(OH)_2D$ are an appropriate response of the 25(OH)D-1α-hydroxylase to phosphate depletion. Phosphate replacement induces healing of the rachitic lesions.

Sporadic cases of hypophosphatemia have also been described in adults in whom family histories are negative and where proximal muscle weakness is a prominent feature (also see Chap. 342). These patients also are best treated with a combination of calcitriol and inorganic phosphorus. As mentioned above, in most untreated patients with renal tubular disorders associated with rickets and osteomalacia, secondary hyperparathyroidism is not present.

In other patients the disorder in tubular function may be more widespread, involving (besides phosphorus) glucose, potassium, amino acids, and uric acid; the various combinations are termed the de Toni-Debré-Fanconi syndrome. The more complete renal tubular defects may occur sporadically or in families. In some instances the lesion is part of a more widespread disorder as in Wilson's disease and cystinosis. The acidosis of proximal tubular defects also plays a role in development of osteomalacia, possibly by altering metabolism of vitamin D or the renal handling of calcium and phosphorus. In this regard osteomalacia has accompanied the hyperchloremic acidosis of ureterocolic anastomosis.

TUMOR-ASSOCIATED (ONCOGENOUS) OSTEOMALACIA Osteomalacia and hypophosphatemia with high renal phosphate clearance occur with a variety of mesenchymal tumors. The latter have included giant cell tumors (benign or malignant), reparative granulomas, hemangiomas, fibromas, and other mesenchymal neoplasms. A similar syndrome occurs in patients with prostatic carcinoma. In some instances, removal of the tumor resulted in return of renal phosphorus clearance to normal, rise in serum phosphorus levels, and healing of the osteomalacia (or rickets in children). Serum $1,25(OH)_2D$ levels are low or undetectable, although chronic administration of sufficient calcitriol to raise circulating levels of this metabolite to normal does not alter renal phosphorus clearance or serum phosphorus concentrations. Humoral factors released by these tumors may impair proximal tubular functions such as 1α-hydroxylation of 25(OH)D *and* phosphate transport; removal of the tumor results in a return of serum $1,25(OH)_2D$ and phosphorus levels to normal.

CHRONIC RENAL FAILURE Osteomalacia is common in patients with chronic renal failure; it often tends to be the predominant type of renal osteodystrophy in younger patients and is more frequent in those with the lower plasma levels of calcium and phosphorus. A component of secondary hyperparathyroidism and osteitis fibrosa almost always accompanies the defect in mineralization. The defect itself probably involves a decreased conversion of 25(OH)D to $1,25(OH)_2D$ either because of insufficient viable renal cortical tissue or the inhibitory effect of hyperphosphatemia on renal 25(OH)D-1α-hydroxylase activity. In addition, there may be a primary defect in intestinal calcium absorption. Part of the secondary hyperparathyroidism may also be due to decreased phosphate clearance and subsequent hyperphosphatemia. Under circumstances of hyperphosphatemia and near-normal plasma concentration of calcium, the presence of inhibitors probably accounts for the defective mineralization. In some patients the osteomalacia responds to large doses of vitamin D or dihydrotachysterol or to small doses of calcitriol or calcifediol. However, some patients with renal osteodystrophy do not respond to pharmacologic doses of vitamin D or improve when given calcitriol. In some of these subjects accumulation of aluminum in the bone accounts for the vitamin D–refractory osteomalacia. Aluminum deposits can be identified at the mineralization fronts, and bone apposition rates are low. These individuals have high levels of aluminum accumulation and uncoupling of matrix deposition and mineralization. Individuals with lower amounts of aluminum develop a form of "aplastic" bone disease where matrix deposition and mineralization are more closely coupled. Deferoxamine can mobilize aluminum from bone and other tissues and is effective therapy of the aluminum osteodystrophy. In some patients with renal osteodystrophy the total bone mass may be increased (osteosclerosis), resulting in increased density of bone. This is particularly evident in the spine, where a characteristic appearance is that of dense bone at the superior and inferior margins of the vertebral bodies with more radiolucent central portions ("rugger jersey sign"). Histologically, although there is more bone per unit area, each trabecula is covered by an abnormally wide osteoid seam.

HYPOPHOSPHATASIA Rickets is a feature of a deficiency of alkaline phosphatase in infants and children, termed *hypophosphatasia*. There are four forms of hypophosphatasia, i.e., lethal perinatal, infantile, childhood, and adult. Rickets occurs in the infantile and childhood forms. In adults, the disorder may not be recognized until middle age, but there is frequently a history of early loss of deciduous or permanent teeth. Osteomalacia and calcium pyrophosphate deposition disease occur in the adult form. The severe perinatal and infantile forms are inherited as autosomal recessive traits; the pattern of inheritance in the other forms is uncertain. The low levels of circulating alkaline phosphatase activity are explained by a deficiency of the liver-bone enzyme due to defects in the alkaline phosphatase gene.

Although alkaline phosphatase is abundant in osteoclasts, its function in mineralization is not established. In hypophosphatasia there is increased urinary excretion of phosphoethanolamine and increased circulating levels of pyridoxal-5′-phosphate. The metabolic origin of the phosphoethanolanine is not established. Concentrations of pyridoxal-5′-phosphate are not elevated intracellularly, and the extracellular increases are consistent with the function of alkaline phosphatase as an ectoenzyme; whether alterations of pyridoxal-5′-phosphate metabolism contribute to the clinical abnormalities in hypophosphatasia is not known. Inorganic pyrophosphate (PPi) is a substrate for alkaline phosphatase, which accounts for increased levels of PPi in urine and plasma and for the increased incidence of calcium pyrophosphate deposition disease in hypophosphatasia. Since PPi can also function to inhibit growth of the calcium-phosphate mineral phase, excessive concentrations of PPi may cause the rickets and osteomalacia. There is no effective therapy.

OTHER DISORDERS ASSOCIATED WITH DEFECTIVE MINERALIZATION Disturbances in mineralization may be seen in patients consuming high doses of fluoride ion and in patients with Paget's disease treated with diphosphonates such as etidronate. Some decrease in mineralization of newly forming matrix, increase in surface covered by osteoid, and increase in the width of the osteoid seams occur in conditions that are not usually considered as osteomalacia except by these criteria. Biopsies in some of these conditions show a normal calcification front. Examples include patients with the osteitis fibrosa of hyperparathyroidism following surgical cure. In these circumstances there is a temporary imbalance between the rate at which mineral is supplied to bone and the rate at which bone matrix is formed. Wide osteoid seams and hypophosphatemia are also seen in children with osteopetrosis in whom there is inadequate resorption of bone and calcified cartilage but active bone formation.

A condition that resembles osteomalacia and is associated with a coarsened, mottled bony trabecular pattern, pseudofractures, and bone pain but normal plasma levels of calcium and phosphorus is *fibrogenesis imperfecta ossium.* The bone has a distinctive histologic appearance, with wide osteoid seams, distortion of the birefringent pattern of normal bone, and abnormal collagen fibers by electron microscopy. The nature of the abnormality is not known.

TREATMENT OF RICKETS AND OSTEOMALACIA In rickets and osteomalacia due to dietary absence of vitamin D or inadequate exposure to sunlight, vitamin D_2 (cholecalciferol) or vitamin D_3 (ergocalciferol) is given orally in doses of 2000 to 4000 IU (0.05 to 0.1 mg) daily for 6 to 12 weeks, followed by daily supplements of 200 to 400 IU, which are adequate to prevent the development of the disorder in otherwise normal subjects. In infants and children such treatment causes improvement in muscle tone and strength, increase in serum calcium and phosphorus, and decrease in alkaline phosphatase levels after several weeks. Radiologic evidence of healing is first noted within weeks and may be complete by a few months. Calcium supplements and larger initial doses of vitamin D may be necessary in infants and children with tetany. In adults with nutritional osteomalacia healing of pseudofractures may be evident within 3 to 4 weeks after therapy with as little as 2000 IU (0.05 mg) vitamin D daily. Healing is complete usually by 6 months.

Patients with osteomalacia due to intestinal malabsorption do not respond to the relatively small doses of vitamin D that can cure osteomalacia due to dietary absence or inadequate sunlight. In the presence of active steatorrhea, daily oral doses of vitamin D of 50,000 to 100,000 IU (1.25 to 2.5 mg) and large doses of calcium (e.g., 15 g calcium lactate or 4 g calcium carbonate orally per day) may be required. In some instances oral vitamin D is ineffective, and the parenteral route is required (e.g., 10,000 IU intramuscularly per day). Another approach is the use of artificial ultraviolet B irradiation or exposure to sunlight in addition to supplemental calcium. Small doses of calcitriol (0.5 to 1.0 μg daily) are usually effective in this form of osteomalacia. Inorganic phosphate therapy is not indicated either in deficiency or in intestinal malabsorption of the vitamin, since hypocalcemia will develop and intestinal calcium absorption will remain inadequate. In all patients in whom large doses of vitamin D are used, periodic monitoring of serum calcium and 25(OH)D levels is essential. Semiquantitative urinary calcium measurements alone are inadequate.

In patients on anticonvulsants, it is usually necessary to continue the drugs while adding supplemental vitamin D and to monitor levels of serum calcium and serum 25(OH)D until a therapeutic response (evidence of radiologic healing, improvement in symptoms) is obtained. Doses varying from 4000 to 40,000 IU daily have been recommended.

Treatment of rickets and osteomalacia in the presence of renal tubular disorders is more difficult. In the past, the X-linked form of hypophosphatemic osteomalacia was treated with large doses of vitamin D (from 50,000 to several hundred thousand IU or more daily), but skeletal responses were rarely complete. The use of dihydrotachysterol, a pseudo-1α(OH)D analogue, 0.2 to 0.6 mg orally per day, in place of vitamin D had the advantage of shorter onset and duration of action and more consistent skeletal healing. With vitamin D therapy alone radiologic evidence of healing in many patients is incomplete; some hypophosphatemia persists, linear skeletal growth remains abnormally slow, and bony deformities continue to develop. In addition, hypercalcemia and its consequences are potential hazards. Currently oral supplements of inorganic phosphate in divided doses of phosphorus, 1.0 to 3.6 g/d, and calcitriol, 0.5 to 2.0 μg/d, constitute the best regimen. Restoration of skeletal growth and healing of the bone disease result. In some adults, therapy with inorganic phosphate alone abolishes muscle weakness and bone pain and produces radiologic and histologic healing. The addition of calcitriol improves calcium balance and helps decrease secondary hyperparathyroidism and maintain a sufficient level of serum phosphorus to permit complete healing. In some patients there may be temporary increase in bone pain and rise in serum alkaline phosphatase during the early phases of treatment. In the osteomalacia associated with the chronic acidosis of renal tubular disorders, the use of alkali may be of value in supplementing therapy with phosphate and calcitriol. In patients with ureterosigmoidostomy, oral sodium bicarbonate can reverse acidosis, improve serum phosphate level, and heal the bone disease; with maintenance doses of alkali, recurrence of symptoms can be prevented.

Patients with nephrotic syndrome and low serum 25(OH)D levels benefit from modest vitamin D supplementation. In chronic renal failure high doses of vitamin D, similar to those needed to treat osteomalacia of renal tubular disorders, are used. Dihydrotachysterol at doses of 0.2 to 1.0 mg daily is effective in treating hypocalcemia and osteodystrophy resulting from chronic renal failure. Calcitriol in small doses is equally effective in most cases of renal osteodystrophy. The recommended initial dose is 0.25 μg/d. If after 2 to 4 weeks on this dose the biochemical parameters are unaltered, the dose is increased by 0.25 μg/d every 2 to 4 weeks until a satisfactory clinical biochemical response (including elevation of serum calcium levels and decrease in PTH levels) is obtained. The usual dose is 0.5 to 1.0 μg/d. Calcitriol may also be administered intravenously (1.0 to 2.5 μg three times weekly) in patients on dialysis, particularly to treat refractory osteitis fibrosa. Because there are no regulatory mechanisms to control the biological responses to calcitriol, there is a high incidence of transient hypercalciuria and hypercalcemia, especially initially. Thus, serum calcium should be monitored frequently during the first 1 to 2 months of therapy and less frequently once a stable dose has been established. Since calcitriol has a short duration of action and is not stored in fat depots, hypercalcemia usually resolves in 2 to 7 days after the dose is discontinued or decreased. Phosphate supplements are, of course, contraindicated in the usual patient with chronic renal failure. Occasionally, however, hypophosphatemia may result from the excessive use of nonabsorbable antacids or from excessive removal of phosphate through hemodialysis.

In patients who have had rickets in childhood, the abnormal mechanical stress of severe deformities may contribute to the development of degenerative joint disease, particularly in hips and knees. Osteotomies at the proper time after healing may prevent this complication and more extensive arthroplasties later in life.

REFERENCES

Osteoporosis

Aloia JF et al: Risk factors for postmenopausal osteoporosis. Am J Med 78:95, 1985

——— et al: Calcitriol in the treatment of postmenopausal osteoporosis. Am J Med 84:401, 1988

Avioli LV, Krane SM (eds): *Metabolic Bone Disease and Clinically Related Disorders*. Philadelphia, Saunders, 1990

Barzel US: Estrogens in the prevention and treatment of postmenopausal osteoporosis: A review. Am J Med 85:847, 1988

Bergkvist L et al: The risk of breast cancer after estrogen and estrogen-progestin replacement. N Engl J Med 321:293, 1989

Biller BMK et al: Mechanisms of osteoporosis in adult and adolescent women with anorexia nervosa. J Clin Endocrinol Metab 68:548, 1989

Boivin G et al: Fluoride content in human iliac bone: Results in controls, patients with fluorosis, and osteoporotic patients treated with fluoride. J Bone Min Res 3:497, 1988

Buchanan JR et al: Effect of excess endogenous androgens on bone density in young women. J Clin Endocrinol Metab 67:937, 1988

Cheema C et al: Effects of estrogen on circulating "free" and total 1,25-dihydroxyvitamin D and on the parathyroid-vitamin D axis in postmenopausal women. J Clin Invest 83:537, 1989

Civitelli R et al: Effects of one-year treatment with estrogens on bone mass, intestinal calcium absorption, and 25-hydroxyvitamin D-1α-hydroxylase reserve in postmenopausal osteoporosis. Calcif Tissue Int 42:77, 1988

——— et al: Bone turnover in postmenopausal osteoporosis. Effect of calcitonin treatment. J Clin Invest 82:1268, 1988

Cole WG et al: New insights into the molecular pathology of osteogenesis imperfecta. Q J Med 70:1, 1989

Dempster DW: Bone histomorphometry in glucocorticoid-induced osteoporosis. J Bone Min Res 4:137, 1989

Diamond T et al: Ethanol reduces bone formation and may cause osteoporosis. Am J Med 86:282, 1989

Drinkwater BL et al: Bone mineral content of amenorrheic and eumenorrheic athletes. N Engl J Med 311:277, 1984

Eastell R et al: Colles' fracture and bone density of the ultradistal radius. J Bone Min Res 4:607, 1989

Editorial: Risk factors in postmenopausal osteoporosis. Lancet 1:1370, 1985

Ettinger B et al: Postmenopausal bone loss is prevented by treatment with low-dosage estrogen with calcium. Ann Intern Med 106:40, 1987

Evans RA et al: Bone mass is low in relatives of osteoporotic patients. Ann Intern Med 109:870, 1988

Finkelstein JS et al: Osteoporosis in men with idiopathic hypogonadotropic hypogonadism. Ann Intern Med 106:354, 1987

Gallagher JC et al: Epidemiology of fractures of the proximal femur in Rochester, Minnesota. Clin Orthopaed Rel Res 150:163, 1980

Hedlund LR, Gallagher JC: Increased incidence of hip fracture in osteoporotic women treated with sodium fluoride. J Bone Min Res 4:223, 1989

Hodsman AB, Drost DJ: The response of vertebral bone mineral density during the treatment of osteoporosis with sodium fluoride. J Clin Endocrinol Metab 69:932, 1989

Holbrook TL et al: Dietary calcium and risk of hip fracture: 14-year prospective population study. Lancet 2:1046, 1988

Huppert LC: Hormonal replacement therapy. Benefits, risks, doses. Med Clin North Am 71:23, 1987

Jensen J et al: Cigarette smoking, serum estrogens, and bone loss during hormone-replacement therapy early after menopause. N Engl J Med 313:973, 1985

Kanis JA: Treatment of osteoporotic fracture. Lancet 1:27, 1984

Kelly TL et al: Quantitative digital radiography versus dual photon absorptiometry of the lumbar spine. J Clin Endocrinol Metab 67:839, 1988

Krane SM, Schiller AL: Metabolic bone disease, in *Endocrinology*, 2d ed, LJ DeGroot et al (eds). Philadelphia, Saunders, 1989, vol 2, p 1151

Krølner B et al: Physical exercise as prophylaxis against involutional vertebral bone loss: A controlled trial. Clin Sci Mol Med 64:541, 1983

Lindsay R et al: Prevention of spinal osteoporosis in oophorectomised women. Lancet 2:1151, 1980

Mamelle N et al: Risk-benefit ratio of sodium fluoride treatment in primary vertebral osteoporosis. Lancet 2:361, 1988

Marie PJ et al: Osteocalcin and deoxyribonucleic acid synthesis *in vitro* and histomorphometric indices of bone formation in postmenopausal osteoporosis. J Clin Endocrinol Metab 69:272, 1989

McDermott MT, Kidd GS: The role of calcitonin in the development and treatment of osteoporosis. Endocrine Rev 8:377, 1987

Mundy GR: Identifying mechanisms for increasing bone mass. J NIH Res 1:65, 1989

Nagant de Deuxchaisnes C: Therapy for skeletal disorders. Curr Opin Rheumatol 1:98, 1989

Pak CYC et al: Safe and effective treatment of osteoporosis with intermittent slow release sodium fluoride: Augmentation of vertebral bone mass and inhibition of fractures. J Clin Endocrinol Metab 68:150, 1989

Parfitt AM: Dietary risk factors for age-related bone loss and fractures. Lancet 2:1181, 1983

——— et al: Relationships between surface, volume, and thickness of iliac trabecular bone in aging and in osteoporosis: Implications for the microanatomic and cellular mechanisms of bone loss. J Clin Invest 72:783, 1985

Pocock NA et al: Recovery from steroid-induced osteoporosis. Ann Intern Med 107:319, 1987

Prockop DJ: Mutations in collagen genes: Consequences for rare and common diseases. J Clin Invest 75:783, 1985

Reeve J et al: The assessment of bone formation and bone resorption in osteoporosis: A comparison between tetracycline-based iliac histomorphometry and whole body ^{85}Sr kinetics. J Bone Min Res 2:479, 1987

Reginster JY et al: Relationship between whole plasma calcitonin levels, calcitonin secretory capacity, and plasma levels of estrone in healthy women and postmenopausal osteoporotics. J Clin Invest 83:1073, 1989

Riggs BL: Osteoporosis, in *Endocrinology*, 2d ed, LJ DeGroot et al (eds). Philadelphia, Saunders, 1989, vol 2, p 1188

———, Melton LJ III: Evidence for two distinct syndromes of involutional osteoporosis. Am J Med 75:899, 1983

———, ———: Involutional osteoporosis. N Engl J Med 314:1676, 1986

——— et al: Effect of the fluoride/calcium regimen on vertebral fracture occurrence in postmenopausal osteoporosis: Comparison with conventional therapy. N Engl J Med 306:446, 1982

——— et al: Changes in bone mineral density of the proximal femur and spine with aging: Differences between the postmenopausal and senile osteoporosis syndromes. J Clin Invest 70:716, 1982

——— et al: Incidence of hip fractures in osteoporotic women treated with sodium fluoride. J Bone Min Res 2:123, 1987

Riis B et al: Does calcium supplementation prevent postmenopausal bone loss? N Engl J Med 316:173, 1987

Sakhaee K et al: Postmenopausal osteoporosis as a manifestation of renal hypercalciuria with secondary hyperparathyroidism. J Clin Endocrinol Metab 61:368, 1985

Seeman E et al: Risk factors for spinal osteoporosis in men. Am J Med 75:977, 1983

——— et al: Effect of early menopause on bone mass in normal women and patients with osteoporosis. Am J Med 85:213, 1988

Silverberg SJ et al: Abnormalities in parathyroid hormone secretion and 1,25-dihydroxyvitamin D_3 formation in women with osteoporosis. N Engl J Med 320:277, 1989

Smith R et al: Osteoporosis of pregnancy. Lancet 1:1178, 1985

Spencer H et al: Chronic alcoholism: Frequently overlooked cause of osteoporosis in men. Am J Med 80:393, 1986

Steinberg KK et al: Sex steroids and bone density in premenopausal and perimenopausal women. J Clin Endocrinol Metab 69:533, 1989

Stepan JJ et al: Castrated men exhibit bone loss: Effect of calcitonin treatment on biochemical indices of bone remodeling. J Clin Endocrinol Metab 69:523, 1989

Stewart AF et al: Calcium homeostasis in immobilization: An example of resorptive hypercalciuria. N Engl J Med 306:1136, 1982

Weinstein RS, Bell NH: Diminished rates of bone formation in normal black adults. N Engl J Med 319:1698, 1988

Whitehead MI, Fraser D: Controversies concerning the safety of estrogen replacement therapy. Am J Obstet Gynecol 156:1313, 1987

Wilson RJ et al: Mild asymptomatic primary hyperparathyroidism is not a risk factor for vertebral fractures. Ann Intern Med 109:959, 1988

Osteomalacia

Andress DL et al: Osteomalacia and aplastic bone disease in aluminum-related osteodystrophy. J Clin Endocrinol Metab 65:11, 1987

——— et al: Intravenous calcitriol in the treatment of refractory osteitis fibrosa of chronic renal failure. N Engl J Med 321:274, 1989

Charhon SA et al: Effects of parathyroidectomy on bone formation and mineralization in hemodialyzed patients. Kidney Int 27:426, 1984

Delvin EE et al: Vitamin D nutritional status and related biochemical indices in an autonomous elderly population. Am J Clin Nutr 48:373, 1988

Fraser D, Scriver CR: Hereditary rickets and osteomalacia associated with abnormalities in vitamin D metabolism (calcipenic rickets) or phosphate homeostasis (phosphopenic rickets), in *Endocrinology*, 2d ed, LJ DeGroot et al (eds). Philadelphia, Saunders, 1989, vol 2, p 1080

Glorieux FH: Disturbances of phosphate metabolism—effects on bone, in *Metabolic Bone Disease: Cellular and Tissue Mechanism*, CS Tam et al (eds). Boca Raton, Fla, CRC Press, 1988, p 215

Godsall JW et al: Vitamin D metabolism and bone histomorphometry in patients with antacid-induced osteomalacia. Am J Med 77:747, 1984

Goldring SR, Krane SM: Disorders of calcification: Osteomalacia and rickets, in *Endocrinology*, 2d ed, LJ DeGroot et al (eds). Philadelphia, Saunders, 1989, vol 2, p 1165

Hardy DC et al: X-linked hypophosphatemia in adults: Prevalence of skeletal radiographic and scintigraphic features. Radiology 171:403, 1989

Harrell RM et al: Healing of bone disease in X-linked hypophosphatemic rickets/osteomalacia: Induction and maintenance with phosphorus and calcitriol. J Clin Invest 75:1858, 1985

Harvey JA et al: Lack of effect of 24,25-dihydroxyvitamin D_3 administration on parameters of calcium metabolism. J Clin Endocrinol Metab 69:467, 1989

Hochberg Z et al: 1,25-dihydroxyvitamin D resistance, rickets, and alopecia. Am J Med 77:805, 1984

rickets, and alopecia. Am J Med 77:805, 1984

Hodsman AB et al: Vitamin D–resistant osteomalacia in hemodialysis patients lacking secondary hyperparathyroidism. Ann Intern Med 94:629, 1981

——— et al: Bone aluminum and histomorphometric features of renal osteodystrophy. J Clin Endocrinol Metab 54:439, 1982

Kleerekoper M, Krane SM (eds): *Clinical Disorders of Bone and Mineral Metabolism*. New York, Mary Ann Liebert, 1989

Klein GL, Coburn JW: Metabolic bone disease associated with total parenteral nutrition. Adv Nutr Res 6:67, 1984

Kumar R: Hepatic and intestinal osteodystrophy and the hepatobiliary metabolism of vitamin D. Ann Intern Med 98:662, 1983

Lips P et al: The effect of vitamin D supplementation on vitamin status and parathyroid function in elderly subjects. J Clin Endocrinol Metab 67:644, 1988

Malloy PJ et al: Abnormal binding of vitamin D receptors to deoxyribonucleic acid in a kindred with vitamin D–dependent rickets, type II. J Clin Endocrinol Metab 68:263, 1989

Marie PJ, Glorieux FH: Relation between hypomineralized periosteocytic lesions and bone mineralization in vitamin D–resistant rickets. Calcif Tissue Int 35:433, 1983

McElduff A, Posen S: Parathyroid hormone sensitivity in familial X-linked hypophosphatemic rickets. J Clin Endocrinol Metab 69:386, 1989

Miyauchi A et al: Hemangiopericytoma-induced osteomalacia: Tumor transplantation in nude mice causes hypophosphatemia and tumor extracts inhibit renal 25-hydroxyvitamin-1-hydroxylase activity. J Clin Endocrinol Metab 67:46, 1988

Nordal KP, Dahl E: Low dose calcitriol versus placebo in patients with predialysis chronic renal failure. J Clin Endocrinol Metab 67:929, 1988

Parfitt AM et al: Metabolic bone disease with and without osteomalacia after intestinal bypass surgery: A bone histomorphometric study. Bone 6:211, 1985

Polisson RP et al: Calcification of entheses associated with X-linked hypophosphatemic osteomalacia. N Engl J Med 313:1, 1985

Portale AA et al: Physiologic regulation of the serum concentration of 1,25-dihydroxyvitamin D by phosphorus in normal men. J Clin Invest 83:1494, 1989

Ralphs JR et al: Ultrastructural features of the osteoid of patients with fibrogenesis imperfecta ossium. Bone 10:243, 1989

Reichel H et al: The role of the vitamin D endocrine system in health and disease. N Engl J Med 320:980, 1989

Ryan EA, Reiss E: Oncogeneous osteomalacia: Review of the world literature of 42 cases and report of two new cases. Am J Med 77:501, 1984

Whyte MP: Hypophosphatasia, in *The Metabolic Basis of Inherited Disease*, 6th ed, CR Scriver et al (eds). New York, McGraw-Hill, 1989, p 2843

342 DISORDERS OF PHOSPHORUS METABOLISM

JAMES P. KNOCHEL

Phosphorus is the most abundant intracellular anion and is critical for membrane structure, transport, and energy storage. The role of phosphate ions in tissues explains the systemic nature of cellular injury consequent to phosphorus deficiency.

At a plasma pH of 7.4, inorganic phosphate in plasma is a 4:1 mixture of HPO_4^{2-} and $H_2PO_4^-$. The sum of the products of the valences of these ions ($4 \times 2^- + 1 \times 1^-$) divided by the sum of the ions ($4 + 1$) is equal to 9/5 or an average valence of 1.8. Of the average 700 g of phosphorus in the body, 85 percent is in the skeleton, about 15 percent is in soft tissues, and 0.1 percent is in extracellular fluid. The phosphorus that is in extracellular fluid is in a freely diffusible form that (1) permits excretion of hydrogen ions as phosphate buffer into the urine and (2) is in diffusion equilibrium with cytosolic inorganic phosphate in cells.

A normal adult consumes approximately 1 g of phosphorus each day. Soluble phosphates in dairy products and meat are almost completely absorbed, predominantly in the midjejunum. Insoluble phosphates, in vegetables and seeds, are absorbable provided the phosphate can be digested from its ligand. For example, phosphorus in corn and oats is contained partly as phytic acid; these foods contain little phytase, which splits phytic acid into phosphate and inositol, and hence phosphorus from this source may be poorly absorbed. Thus, corn and oats may be rachitogenic in man if they comprise the major components of the diet.

Phosphorus absorption is under the influence of vitamin D, and phosphorus excretion is under the control of parathyroid hormone. Parathyroid hormone decreases tubular phosphate reabsorption and increases excretion into the urine. The effect of vitamin D on phosphate reabsorption by the kidney is relatively minor. The quantity of soluble phosphorus available for absorption from the diet varies, and excretion of phosphorus in the urine on a given day depends directly upon absorption. Accordingly, the range for phosphorus excretion in health is very broad.

HYPOPHOSPHATEMIA

CAUSES Hypophosphatemia has many causes (Table 342-1). The finding of hypophosphatemia is not always a reliable indicator of deficiency since a total-body deficiency of phosphorus may exist in the face of hyperphosphatemia as, for example, in diabetic ketoacidosis.

Hypophosphatemia can be moderate or severe. Decreased dietary intake is an unusual cause of hypophosphatemia because of the ubiquitous and abundant distribution of the mineral in foods. Decreased absorption of phosphorus from the small intestine occurs in a variety of malabsorptive states, but simple diarrhea is usually not a cause. One of the most common causes of hypophosphatemia is respiratory alkalosis. Indeed, discovery of hypophosphatemia should lead to a search for potentially serious causes of hyperventilation such as sepsis or otherwise unsuspected alcohol withdrawal. Reduction of intracellular P_{CO_2} and elevation of pH increase the activity of phosphofructokinase, the rate-limiting enzyme of glycolysis. Phosphorylation of glucose intermediates causes cellular uptake of phosphorus and hypophosphatemia. Administration of insulin or nutrients

TABLE 342-1 Causes of hypophosphatemia

I Decreased dietary intake
II Decreased intestinal absorption
- *A* Vitamin D deficiency
- *B* Malabsorption
- *C* Steatorrhea
- *D* Secretory diarrhea
- *E* Vomiting
- *F* PO_4-binding antacids

III Shifts from serum into cells
- *A* Respiratory alkalosis
  - *1* Sepsis
  - *2* Alcohol withdrawal
  - *3* Heat stroke
  - *4* Neuroleptic malignant syndrome
  - *5* Hepatic coma
  - *6* Salicylate poisoning
  - *7* Gout
  - *8* Panic attacks
  - *9* Psychiatric depression
- *B* Hormonal effects
  - *1* Insulin
  - *2* Glucagon
  - *3* Epinephrine
  - *4* Androgens
  - *5* Cortisol
  - *6* Anovulatory hormones
- *C* Nutrient effects
  - *1* Glucose
  - *2* Fructose
  - *3* Glycerol
  - *4* Lactate
  - *5* Amino acids
  - *6* Xylitol
- *D* Cellular uptake syndromes
  - *1* Recovery from hypothermia
  - *2* Burkitt's lymphoma
  - *3* Histiocytic lymphoma
  - *4* Acute myelomonocytic leukemia
  - *5* Acute myelogenous leukemia
  - *6* Treatment of pernicious anemia
  - *7* Hungry bone syndrome
    - *a* Following parathyroidectomy
    - *b* Acute leukemia

IV Increased excretion into the urine
- *A* Hyperparathyroidism
- *B* Renal tubular defects
  - *1* Renal rickets
  - *2* Polyostotic fibrous dysplasia
  - *3* Postrenal transplantation
  - *4* Oncogenic osteomalacia
- *C* Aldosteronism
- *D* Licorice ingestion
- *E* Volume expansion
- *F* Inappropriate secretion of vasopressin
- *G* Mineralocorticoid administration
- *H* Glucocorticoid therapy
- *I* Diuretics

TABLE 342-2 Causes of severe hypophosphatemia

Chronic alcoholism and alcohol withdrawal
Dietary deficiency and phosphate-binding antacids
Severe thermal burns
Recovery from diabetic ketoacidosis
Hyperalimentation
Nutritional recovery syndrome
Respiratory alkalosis
Therapeutic hyperthermia
Neuroleptic malignant syndrome
Recovery from exhaustive exercise
Renal transplantation
Acute renal failure

TABLE 342-3 Hypophosphatemic syndromes

Phosphate trapping
Rhabdomyolysis
Cardiomyopathy
Respiratory insufficiency
Erythrocyte dysfunction
Leukocyte dysfunction
Skeletal demineralization
Metabolic acidosis
Nervous system dysfunction

that stimulate insulin release is also a common cause of hypophosphatemia. Insulin stimulates phosphorus uptake by cells. Cellular phosphorus uptake also occurs in patients recovering from hypothermia as a result of reactivation of metabolism. Certain rapidly growing malignancies may take up enough phosphate to cause hypophosphatemia. Deposition of bone mineral following parathyroidectomy may also be a cause. Parathyroid hormone and volume expansion may independently reduce tubular reabsorption of phosphorus. A number of other conditions typified by chronic volume expansion may cause hypophosphatemia.

Severe hypophosphatemia is defined as phosphorus levels in serum below 0.3 mmol/L (1.0 mg/dL). Many of the conditions that result in such low levels are associated with prolonged hyperventilation with respiratory alkalosis or reflect rapid cellular uptake (see Table 342-2). Respiratory alkalosis does not cause phosphorus deficiency, but may reduce serum phosphorus values to 0.1 mmol/L (0.3 mg/dL) and urinary phosphorus excretion to virtually undetectable levels. Severe hypophosphatemia and severe total body deficiency of phosphorus occur in patients with poor dietary intake who consume phosphate-binding antacids. Similarly, treatment of diabetic ketoacidosis results in hypophosphatemia. Reduction of serum phosphorus below 0.3 mmol/L (1.0 mg/dL) suggests but does not prove the existence of serious phosphorus depletion. In chronic alcoholics, reduction of phosphorus content of skeletal muscle may be associated with reduction of muscle magnesium and potassium and accumulations of calcium, sodium, chloride, and water. These findings are not necessarily associated with elevations of creatine phosphokinase activity that would reflect acute muscle damage. However, during withdrawal from alcohol, phosphorus is often taken up rapidly into skeletal muscle or liver, resulting in severe hypophosphatemia, and in this instance hypophosphatemia may precipitate acute rhabdomyolysis.

Most patients with diabetic ketoacidosis are not severely depleted of phosphorus. Although, on the one hand, metabolic acidosis and insulin deficiency mobilize intracellular phosphate stores and lead to their excretion into the urine, most patients have not been sick long enough for severe phosphorus deficiency to occur. On the other hand, the existence of hypophosphatemia and hypokalemia, despite severe diabetic ketoacidosis, reflects severe body depletion of phosphorus and potassium that demands treatment. The history usually shows that this type of patient with diabetic ketoacidosis has been sick for many days, has not had significant vomiting, has been able to maintain a good intake of fluids, and has excreted phosphorus briskly for a period of many days, thus establishing severe deficiency. Such patients probably represent no more than 5 percent of all cases of diabetic ketoacidosis.

MANIFESTATIONS The major manifestations of phosphorus deficiency are listed in Table 342-3; it should be appreciated that many of these can occur simultaneously.

Phosphate trapping is an acute disorder resulting from reduction of intracellular inorganic phosphate concentration. The most common cause is administration of intravenous fructose. Fructose is metabolized by only three tissues in the body—the liver, the small bowel epithelium, and the proximal tubule of the kidney. When glucose is taken up into liver cells and phosphorylated by hexokinase, the resulting glucose-6-phosphate inhibits hexokinase, producing a smoothly regulated uptake of glucose that does not deplete or trap stores of inorganic phosphate. When fructose is administered intravenously, it is taken up into liver cells where it is converted to fructose-1-phosphate by the enzyme fructokinase. Fructose-1-phosphate does not inhibit fructokinase, thus permitting rapid uptake of fructose into liver cells and trapping of available stores of inorganic phosphate. Reduced intracellular phosphate concentration activates AMP deaminase and nucleotidase. The consequent reduction of adenylate compounds is reflected by increased uric acid production and hyperuricemia. Acute liver cell damage may occur. Disturbances of renal function may also occur after intravenous fructose. Hepatic and renal metabolic disturbances that follow fructose administration are preventable by infusing inorganic phosphate. Whether large concentrations of oral fructose affect intestinal epithelium in a similar manner has not been examined.

Rhabdomyolysis predictably occurs in chronic alcoholics who become acutely hypophosphatemic during the course of alcohol withdrawal. Hypophosphatemic rhabdomyolysis occurs rarely during treatment for diabetic ketoacidosis, during the course of hyperalimentation, or while refeeding patients with malnutrition. In alcoholics, evidence of muscle cell injury has preceded the occurrence of hypophosphatemia. Presumably, severe hypophosphatemia triggers induction of acute rhabdomyolysis. This syndrome can be reproduced experimentally. It does not occur if hypophosphatemia is prevented during hyperalimentation.

Cardiomyopathy occurs in severe phosphorus depletion. The usual manifestations include reduction in cardiac output, hypotension, impaired pressor responsiveness to catecholamines, and a reduced threshold to ventricular arrhythmias.

Respiratory insufficiency is a hypophosphatemic syndrome in malnourished patients receiving intravenous nutrients with inadequate phosphorus who become progressively hypophosphatemic over 8 or 10 days. Profound weakness causes failure of diaphragm function, hypoxia, and respiratory acidosis. Despite severe hypophosphatemia, these patients rarely develop rhabdomyolysis, presumably because they had no preexistent muscle damage. The initial clue to this complication may be inability to extubate a patient from a ventilator at the anticipated time. This syndrome is seldom seen in chronic alcoholics because rhabdomyolysis in such patients may correct hypophosphatemia spontaneously. Rapid correction of chronic respiratory acidosis may also cause hypophosphatemia and diaphragm weakness. In these patients, administration of phosphorus rapidly corrects muscle weakness and respiratory insufficiency.

Erythrocyte dysfunction is due to a decrease in 2,3-diphosphoglycerate (2,3-DPG) content. The red cell is the only tissue in the body that produces this substance. Both 2,3-DPG and ATP facilitate dissociation of oxyhemoglobin and promote oxygen delivery to tissue. Reduced 2,3-DPG and ATP both enhance affinity of oxygen for hemoglobin and reduce tissue oxygenation. This mechanism may explain central nervous system dysfunction in hypophosphatemia. Hemolysis due to phosphorus deficiency probably does not occur.

Leukocyte dysfunction due to phosphorus deficiency results in impaired phagocytosis and opsonization. As a result, chronic hypophosphatemia increases susceptibility to bacterial fungal infections.

Skeletal demineralization is an important effect of phosphorus deficiency, especially in patients with a poor dietary intake who simultaneously ingest phosphate-binding antacids. Under conditions of increased bone turnover, in normal children or in adults with Paget's disease, hyperparathyroidism, or bony metastases, demineralization may occur at such a rate as to cause hypercalcemia. Osteopenia, bone pain, and a syndrome resembling osteomalacia occur in chronic phosphorus deficiency.

Metabolic acidosis may occur in children or adults with phosphorus deficiency due to vitamin D deficiency. Reduced phosphorus intake results in mobilization of hydroxyapatite from bone that serves to maintain normal levels of serum phosphorus. Hypercalciuria occurs normally as a result of phosphorus deprivation. Severe hypophosphatemia has two important metabolic effects on the kidney. First, inorganic phosphate excretion into the urine falls so that hydrogen excretion as NaH_2PO_4 into the urine is eliminated. Second, phosphorus deficiency also elevates renal intracellular pH, which results in a profound decrease in ammonia production. The reduction in ammonia production eliminates hydrogen excretion as ammonium ions (NH^{4+}). Since excretion of hydrogen as phosphate buffer or ammonium accounts for nearly all of the kidney's capacity to secrete acid, it is surprising that phosphorus deficiency is only rarely associated with metabolic acidosis. The explanation lies in the fact that mobilization of hydroxyapatite from bone provides carbonate ions; they in turn buffer the retained hydrogen ions that otherwise would be excreted in the urine. Under conditions in which hydroxyapatite cannot be mobilized during phosphorus deprivation (e.g., vitamin D deficiency, severe magnesium deficiency, and perhaps aluminum poisoning), buffer cannot be mobilized adequately, and metabolic acidosis ensues.

Nervous system dysfunction is one of the most distinctive and predictable abnormalities in severe hypophosphatemia and phosphorus deficiency. This syndrome usually occurs in the setting of refeeding or hyperalimentation-induced hypophosphatemia that develops over the course of 8 to 10 days. Such patients become irritable and apprehensive and hyperventilate sufficiently to cause paresthesias and numbness. Profound muscular weakness is followed by dysarthria, confusion, obtundation, convulsive seizures, coma, and death. Alternatively, ascending motor paralysis with or without sensory disturbances may resemble the Guillain-Barré syndrome. In such cases, the cerebrospinal fluid is normal. Ophthalmoplegia, diplopia, and dysphagia suggest botulism, and poorly defined defects in color perception (metachromatopsia) suggests cerebral cortical dysfunction. In these patients, as in those with respiratory failure, spontaneous rhabdomyolysis does not occur despite severe hypophosphatemia.

TREATMENT Before initiating treatment for hypophosphatemia, the cause should be ascertained. Measurement of arterial pH and blood gases and of phosphorus concentration in the urine are helpful.

Milk is an excellent source of phosphorus, containing 33 mmol/L (100 mg/dL). Phosphate salts are also available for oral use. They are less likely to cause diarrhea in a phosphorus-deficient patient than in a normal person. Phosphorus salts cannot be given by intramuscular or subcutaneous injection, but sodium phosphate and potassium phosphate are available for intravenous use. The potassium salt should be given when hypokalemia and hypophosphatemia coexist. A safe dosage regimen for treatment of alcoholics who are hypophosphatemic, hypokalemic, and hypomagnesemic is the infusion each 8 to 12 h of 1 L of 0.5 normal NaCl in 5% glucose containing 9 mmol of potassium phosphate and 4.2 mmol $MgSO_4$ (2.0 mL of 50% $MgSO_4$ solution). Serum concentrations of potassium, magnesium, and phosphate should be closely monitored. Such infusions should be stopped when oral intake becomes possible.

Hyperphosphatemia should be avoided since it can cause severe hypocalcemia and crystal deposition in important structures including blood vessels, the eye, lung, heart, and kidney. Fatal alveolar diffusion block has occurred, especially if the patient is alkalotic.

HYPERPHOSPHATEMIA

Causes of hyperphosphatemia include renal insufficiency, hypoparathyroidism, pseudohypoparathyroidism, active untreated acromegaly, overmedication with phosphate salts, and acute tissue destruction. The latter instance occurs in rhabdomyolysis and during treatment for malignancy. Hyperphosphatemia in untreated diabetic ketoacidosis is best explained by cellular release of phosphorus because of acidosis and volume depletion.

Hyperphosphatemia is treated by dietary restriction, employment of phosphate-binding antacids, promotion of excretion by fluid administration, correction of acidosis, and administration of insulin.

REFERENCES

BLACHLEY JD et al: The harmful effects of ethanol on ion transport and cellular respiration. Am J Med Sci 289:22, 1985

BODE JC et al: Depletion of liver adenosine phosphates and metabolic effects of intravenous infusion of fructose or sorbitol in man and in the rat. Eur J Clin Invest 3:436, 1973

FULLER TJ et al: Reversible depression in myocardial performance in dogs with experimental phosphorus deficiency. J Clin Invest 62:1194, 1978

KNOCHEL JP : Hypophosphatemia in the alcoholic. Arch Intern Med 140:613, 1980

——— : The clinical status of hypophosphatemia. N Engl J Med 313:447, 1985

——— : Hypophosphatemia and phosphorus deficiency, in *The Kidney,* 4th ed, B Brenner, F Rector (eds). Philadelphia, Saunders, 1990

KONO N et al: Alteration of glycolytic intermediary metabolism in erythrocytes during diabetic ketoacidosis and its recovery phase. Diabetes 30:346, 1981

LOTZ M et al: Evidence for a phosphorus depletion syndrome in man. N Engl J Med 278:409, 1968

NEWMAN JH et al: Acute respiratory failure associated with hypophosphatemia. N Engl J Med 296:1101, 1977

VEECH RL et al: Cytosolic phosphorylation potential. J Biol Chem 254:6538, 1979

WEINSIER RL, KRUMDIECK CL : Death resulting from overzealous total parenteral nutrition: The refeeding syndrome revisited. Am J Clin Nutr 34:393, 1980

343 DISORDERS OF MAGNESIUM METABOLISM

JAMES P. KNOCHEL

Magnesium (Mg) is the most abundant intracellular divalent cation. The total magnesium content of a normal man is about 12.4 mmol (25 meq) per kilogram body weight. Of this, 1 percent is extracellular, 31 percent is in cells, and 67 percent is in bone. Serum magnesium ranges between 0.62 and 1 mmol/L (1.2 to 2.0 meq/L). Of this, the unbound diffusible concentration is about 0.6 mmol/L (1.2 meq/L). It exists in two forms in cells, one in solution which is in equilibrium with the diffusible form in plasma and a larger quantity bound to organic components. Since most magnesium inside cells is bound to ATP, in accordance with the principle of mass action, MgATP is in equilibrium with free magnesium ions. Thus, shifts in free magnesium concentration may help regulate stores of ATP. Since ATP is critical to nearly all metabolic transformations, a normal concentration of serum magnesium is essential for normal function. Magnesium ions may also act as cofactors that modify the activity of enzymes themselves.

The ideal intake of magnesium for an adult is 15 to 20 mmol (30 to 40 meq) per day. Foods rich in magnesium include seed grains, nuts, peas, and beans. Fresh meat, fish, and most fresh fruits contain relatively small amounts of magnesium. Magnesium is absorbed primarily in the jejunum and ileum, and healthy persons absorb about 30 to 40 percent of ingested magnesium. This may increase to 70 percent when intake is low or magnesium deficiency exists. The percentage of magnesium absorption is reduced by a high magnesium intake or, independently, by vitamin D deficiency. When magnesium intake is restricted, fecal excretion becomes neglible, and urinary excretion decreases to 0.5 to 1 mmol (1 to 2 meq) per day. Thus, magnesium retention by the kidney is very efficient. Magnesium excretion depends upon glomerular filtration of the unbound fraction, of which 25 percent is reabsorbed in the proximal tubule and 50 to 60 percent is reabsorbed in the loop of Henle. Loop diuretics, such as ethacrynic acid or furosemide, cause greater excretion of magnesium than do diuretics such as the thiazides that act on the distal tubule. Magnesium excretion is increased by expanding extracellular fluid volume by ingestion of water and salt, and aldosterone decreases reabsorption of magnesium by the renal tubule. Magnesium excretion increases sharply when the concentration in serum exceeds 0.85 mmol/L.

In health, slight hypomagnesemia occurs in highly trained individuals, hypermetabolic states such as cold acclimatization, or after experimental administration of thyroid hormone.

MAGNESIUM DEFICIENCY When any of the three major intracellular elements—magnesium, potassium, and phosphorus—has been deprived or lost, losses of the others usually follow. For this reason, deficiency of a single intracellular component almost never occurs. A diet devoid of magnesium causes depletion of phosphorus and potassium in skeletal muscle. Selective potassium deficiency may cause reductions in magnesium and phosphorus. Phosphorus deficiency may cause reductions in potassium and magnesium contents of tissue. The usual somatic responses to selective deprivation of one major intracellular element are anorexia, cellular atrophy, a negative nitrogen balance, and net loss of the other two major intracellular elements. Shrinkage of the cell and expulsion of the elements not deprived help to maintain a normal intracellular composition.

During hyperalimentation a different situation prevails. Provision of a diet that is otherwise replete but deficient in one major intracellular element promotes an anabolic state, and protoplasm is synthesized that has a major deficit of the ion being withheld. In these situations, serious derangements of cellular composition include accumulations of sodium, chloride, calcium, and water, suggesting a major interference with cellular ion transport. Indeed, elevation of cellular calcium, by activating proteases and phospholipases, may be an important cause of cellular injury under these conditions.

As in deficiencies of other major intracellular elements, deficiency of body magnesium can exist even when serum values are normal. In addition, magnesium deficiency may be organ-selective, since certain tissues become deficient before others. The definition of a true deficit of an intracellular element is reduction of its ratio with nitrogen in tissue. In muscle, this ratio is about 0.3 mmol (0.6 meq) magnesium per gram nitrogen. Red cell magnesium content appears to decrease in all species during magnesium deficiency. In contrast, muscle magnesium content remains perfectly normal in some species. Because of the inconsistency of tissue levels and because measurement of tissue magnesium is difficult, the clinician must rely upon serum or plasma magnesium levels to detect magnesium deficiency or excess.

The clinical physiology of magnesium deficiency Volunteers fed a diet deficient in magnesium eventually develop characteristic symptoms and findings. Within 3 to 7 days after reducing dietary magnesium intake to less than 0.5 mmol (1 meq) per day, renal excretion of magnesium declines to below 0.5 mmol (1 meq) per day. Anorexia, nausea, vomiting, lethargy, and weakness develop within weeks. Characteristic symptoms of magnesium deficiency consist of paresthesias, muscular cramps, irritability, decreased attention span, and mental confusion. These complaints may require months to appear.

The physical findings are manifestations of the associated hypocalcemia. These are a positive Trousseau test and a Chvostek's sign, peculiar movements of the fingers best described as athetoid tetany, and on occasion convulsive seizures. Muscle fasciculations may be precipitated by a sharp blow with a neurologic hammer to muscle. About half of patients with selective magnesium depletion become hypokalemic. In animals rhabdomyolysis may occur. Cardiac arrhythmias, disturbances of conduction, and even ventricular fibrillation and cardiac arrest can occur in patients with both hypokalemia and hypomagnesemia. In such instances, hypokalemia may be the cause of the associated ECG abnormalities. Digitalis potentiates the severity and potential danger of arrhythmias. In the presence of QT prolongation, polymorphic ventricular tachycardia (torsade de pointes) may occur that responds to magnesium salts. The causes of magnesium deficiency are shown in Table 343-1.

TABLE 343-1 Causes of hypomagnesemia

I Primary nutritional disturbances
- *A* Inadequate intake
- *B* Total parenteral nutrition
- *C* Refeeding syndrome

II Gastrointestinal disorders
- *A* Specific absorptive defects
- *B* Malabsorption syndromes
  - *1* Enteric fistulas
  - *2* Nontropical sprue
  - *3* Whipples disease
  - *4* Intestinal lymphoma
  - *5* Chronic pancreatic insufficiency
  - *6* Biliary diversion
  - *7* Giardiasis
  - *8* Short bowel syndrome
- *C* Prolonged diarrhea
- *D* Prolonged nasogastric suction
- *E* Pancreatitis

III Endocrine disorders
- *A* Hyperparathyroidism
- *B* Hypoparathyroidism
- *C* Hyperthyroidism
- *D* Primary hyperaldosteronism
- *E* Bartter's syndrome
- *F* Diabetic ketoacidosis
- *G* Alcoholic ketoacidosis
- *H* Administration of epinephrine
- *I* Syndrome of inappropriate secretion of antidiuretic hormone
- *J* "Hungry bones" syndrome after parathyroidectomy

IV Chronic alcoholism; alcoholic withdrawal

V Increased renal excretion
- *A* Idiopathic
- *B* Following renal transplantation
- *C* Cisplatin therapy
- *D* Aminoglycoside therapy
- *E* Amphotericin B therapy
- *F* Diuretics
  - *1* Furosemide
  - *2* Ethacrynic acid
  - *3* Acetazolamide
  - *4* Thiazides
  - *5* Chlorthalidone
  - *6* Osmotic agents
- *G* Recovery phase of acute tubular necrosis

Hypocalcemia usually does not develop until serum magnesium falls below 0.5 mmol/L (1.0 meq/L). Although mild magnesium deficiency may increase release of parathyroid hormone, severe hypomagnesemia [levels below 0.4 mmol/L (0.8 meq/L)] consistently blocks release of parathyroid hormone. The resulting hypocalcemia may be severe. In addition, magnesium deficiency impairs the normal calcemic response to parathyroid hormone at the level of the skeleton. Hypocalcemia can become sufficiently severe to cause tetany. Although tetany has been reported in patients with hypomagnesemia independently of hypocalcemia, both conditions usually exist in patients with this finding. The tetany does not respond to infusions of calcium but only to correction of magnesium levels. The hypocalcemia responds only to magnesium replacement therapy, usually requiring 2 to 7 days for correction. However, administration of magnesium salts intravenously to such a patient can cause prompt and sometimes explosive release of parathyroid hormone. In rare instances, acute hypercalcemia can occur.

Hypokalemia in patients with magnesium deficiency is less well understood. Aldosterone production may be enhanced, thus permitting loss of potassium into the urine. It is extremely difficult to correct the potassium deficiency with supplemental potassium salts. However, administration of magnesium salts sufficient to correct the hypomagnesemia promptly reduces potassium excretion and corrects the hypokalemia. For this reason, it should be kept in mind that hypokalemia refractory to KCl supplements may be due to magnesium deficiency. The causes of magnesium deficiency are shown in Table 343-1.

Gastrointestinal causes of magnesium deficiency Familial hypomagnesemia is manifested during childhood and is caused by reduced absorption of dietary magnesium. The most important cause of magnesium deficiency in adults is intestinal malabsorption and steatorrhea, as in nontropical sprue, the short bowel syndrome, chronic pancreatic insufficiency, or biliary diversion. Because of unabsorbed fat, complexes of nonabsorbable magnesium–fatty acid soaps are formed in the intestinal lumen. When long-standing, hypomagnesemia in such cases is often associated with hypocalcemia, hypokalemia, and hypophosphatemia. Because of steatorrhea, disorders related to malabsorption of fat-soluble vitamins, especially vitamins K, A, and D, may coexist. It is important to recognize that vitamin D deficiency associated with hypomagnesemia can cause severe weakness due to chronic proximal myopathy in association with pain in the lower back and hips reflecting osteomalacia. Such patients display multiple and complex nutritional deficiency.

Magnesium deficiency also occurs in patients undergoing prolonged nasogastric suction who have not received adequate supplies of magnesium salts. Acute hypomagnesemia, along with acute hypocalcemia, occurs in acute hemorrhagic pancreatitis because magnesium- and calcium-fatty acid soaps are formed in situ as a result of tissue necrosis.

Endocrine causes of hypomagnesemia Mild hypomagnesemia occurs in poorly controlled diabetes mellitus. Moderate hypomagnesemia may occur in hyperparathyroidism, hypoparathyroidism, hyperthyroidism, primary hyperaldosteronism, and during recovery from diabetic ketoacidosis. In primary hyperaldosteronism, aldosterone enhances magnesium excretion directly and acts via volume expansion to cause net losses of magnesium. These effects can be reversed by spironolactone. Hypomagnesemia may occur in hypokalemic and hyponatremic patients with the syndrome of inappropriate secretion of antidiuretic hormone (vasopressin). Presumably, this is the result of increased aldosterone production and overexpansion of the circulatory volume. Epinephrine and other potent beta agonists may cause transient hypomagnesemia. Experimentally, epinephrine administration causes uptake of magnesium ions into adipose tissue as fatty acids are released. Of interest, as catecholamines cause release of fatty acids into the blood, insoluble magnesium- and calcium-fatty acid complexes form. If serum is centrifuged, the precipitates settle to the bottom of the tube. As a result, spurious hypomagnesemia and hypocalcemia can be diagnosed. The latter event may explain the allegation that mild hypomagnesemia and hypocalcemia are common in seriously ill patients who have no predisposing cause for magnesium deficiency. Seriously ill patients often have elevated catecholamine levels in blood.

Hypomagnesemia associated with alcoholism Ethanol causes a transient loss of magnesium into the urine. Alcoholics with a reasonably normal nutrient intake and normal intestinal function usually have normal or only slightly depressed magnesium levels in blood. However, during alcoholic withdrawal, serum magnesium can decline in association with acute hypophosphatemia and acute hypokalemia. In animals, sustained ethanol administration in intoxicating doses causes severe depletion of phosphorus, moderate depletion of magnesium and potassium, and increases in intracellular sodium, chloride, water, and calcium. Selective depletion of phosphorus also causes magnesium wasting and muscle magnesium deficiency. Identical findings occur in muscles of severe alcoholic patients. In acute alcohol withdrawal, respiratory alkalosis and insulin release provoked by administration of nutrients act in concert to incorporate phosphate into cells. Increased ATP synthesis as a result of phosphate movement into cells may cause increased magnesium binding and coincident hypomagnesemia.

In alcoholics with intestinal malabsorption and steatorrhea, hypomagnesemia can be severe and is commonly associated with hypocalcemia, hypophosphatemia, and hypokalemia. Although a relationship has been claimed between hypomagnesemia and alcoholic withdrawal seizures, essentially all alcoholics in a withdrawal state display prominent respiratory alkalosis. Alkalosis lowers the threshold for seizure activity. Thus, the relationship of hypomagnesemia to seizures in this setting is far from clear. Furthermore, correction of hypomagnesemia in a withdrawing alcoholic appears to have no favorable effect on the withdrawal syndrome.

Magnesium deficiency may play a role in the temporary hypertension during alcohol withdrawal. Magnesium deficiency is associated with accumulation of calcium in smooth muscle. Accumulation of calcium potentiates the pressor response to circulating catecholamines. Withdrawing alcoholics nearly always have elevations of circulating catecholamines. The combined effects of magnesium depletion, calcium accumulation in cells, and hyperresponsiveness to catecholamines may explain the common occurrence of hypertension in this setting.

Magnesium deficiency due to increased renal excretion Hypomagnesemia can also result from impaired renal tubular reabsorption. Most of these states are associated with renal potassium wasting and hypokalemia, and some patients are hypercalciuric. Transient hypomagnesemia due to reduced renal tubular reabsorption may follow renal transplantation.

Aminoglycoside antibiotics, cisplatin, diuretics, and cyclosporine can cause magnesium wasting in the urine. Gentamicin causes hypomagnesemia and hypokalemia as a result of impaired tubular reabsorption. Hypomagnesemia develops after prolonged treatment and usually in patients who have received more than 8.0 g. Total recovery is the rule after the drug has been stopped. The majority of patients treated with cisplatin develop hypomagnesemia that can be severe; hypokalemia is less common. Even after cisplatin is withdrawn, the absorptive defect in the nephron may persist for months or years. About one-fourth of patients treated with cyclosporine and prednisone after renal transplantation develop serum magnesium levels below 0.5 mmol/L (1 meq/L). As mentioned above, loop diuretics are potent magnesuric agents, but significant hypomagnesemia in patients medicated with diuretics is infrequent. Patients receiving large doses of these drugs or patients receiving two diuretics acting at different sites in the nephron are more likely to develop hypomagnesemia.

Treatment of hypomagnesemia and magnesium deficiency Treatment of hypomagnesemia and its associated disorders should be aimed at correcting the cause. Patients with inadequate dietary intake or with diseases that either reduce intestinal absorption or cause excessive losses into the urine can often be corrected by oral administration of magnesium salts. Patients with potentially serious cardiac arrhythmias or with nausea and vomiting should be given intravenous magnesium sulfate. Magnesium sulfate heptahydrate ($MgSO_4 \cdot 7\ H_2O$) has a molecular weight of 234; thus, 1 mL of 50% solution contains 2.1 mmol (4.2 meq) magnesium. The usual adult dose of 50% magnesium sulfate is 2 mL every 6 h on the first day and half this quantity on each of the following 3 to 4 days. Magnesium sulfate may be given intramuscularly, but this is painful and may cause elevation of creatine phosphokinase levels reflecting muscle damage and thus blunting the value of measurements of the enzyme to detect rhabdomyolysis. It is preferable to infuse magnesium sulfate in a dose of 4.1 mmol (8.2 meq) each 6 h. Patients sufficiently ill to require intravenous magnesium sulfate are often hypokalemic and hypophosphatemic. Potassium phosphate and potassium chloride may be included with 50% magnesium sulfate in 0.5% saline containing 5% glucose. The total potassium content in each infusion bottle should represent one-fourth of the amount determined to be necessary each day. In patients who have an adequate urine flow, such solutions can be given in a quantity of 750 mL each 6 h until nausea and vomiting disappear and oral intake becomes possible. In patients with tetany due to magnesium deficiency, although hypocalcemia coexists, calcium is generally ineffective and infusions of magnesium salts usually require 2 h or more to relieve the tetany. Up to a full day may be required for all signs of latent tetany, such as Chvostek's or Trousseau's signs, to disappear completely. Several oral preparations of magnesium salts are available. Doses of 5 mL magnesium hydroxide containing antacids (Maalox, Gelusil, Mylanta) each contain 3.5 mmol (6.9 meq) magnesium. However, there are two theoretical objections to the use of these preparations. First, these compounds also contain aluminum salts that may be hazardous if the patient has renal impairment. Second, they bind phosphate in the gut, and it is known that phosphate deprivation by this method can itself promote loss of magnesium. Other preparations include magnesium chloride tablets, magnesium gluconate tablets, and commercially available magnesium oxide powder. Since both spironolactone and triamterene cause retention of magnesium and potassium, these drugs may be useful adjuncts to maintain normal serum magnesium levels in patients taking diuretics.

HYPERMAGNESEMIA Patients with end-stage renal disease frequently have modest hypermagnesemia and are at risk of developing significant hypermagnesemia in the event of the ingestion of magnesium-containing compounds such as antacids. Adrenal insufficiency may also cause modest hypermagnesemia. Symptomatic hypermagnesemia is uncommon and is usually precipitated by inadvertent overdose with magnesium salts or is deliberately induced to treat patients with eclampsia. Magnesium can reduce neuromuscular transmission and can act as a central nervous system depressant. Symptoms of hypermagnesemia usually correspond to serum levels. Nausea usually appears between 2 and 2.5 mmol/L (4 to 5 meq/L). Sedation, decreased deep tendon reflexes, and muscle weakness appear at levels of 2 to 3.5 mmol/L (4 to 7 meq/L). Hypotension, bradycardia, and diffuse vasodilatation appear between 2.5 to 5 mmol/L (5 to 10 meq/L). Areflexia, coma, and respiratory paralysis occur at levels between 5 and 7.5 mmol/L (10 and 15 meq/L). Patients treated for eclampsia must be observed very carefully for sequential signs of magnesium intoxication. If this occurs, symptoms and findings can be reversed very quickly by infusion of calcium salts since these ions electrically oppose one another at their sites of action.

REFERENCES

ALFREY AC et al: Evaluation of body magnesium stores. J Lab Clin Med 84:153, 1974

ANDERSON R et al: Skeletal muscle phosphorus and magnesium deficiency in alcoholic myopathy. Mineral Electrolyte Metab 4:106, 1980

CRONIN RE et al: Skeletal muscle injury after magnesium depletion in the dog. Am J Physiol 243:F113, 1982

———, KNOCHEL JP: Magnesium deficiency, in *Advances in Internal Medicine*, GH Stollerman (ed). Chicago, Yearbook Medical Publishers, 28:509, 1983

KNOCHEL JP: Hypophosphatemia in the alcoholic. Arch Intern Med 140:613, 1980

——— et al: The muscle cell in chronic alcoholism. The possible role of phosphate depletion in alcoholic myopathy. Ann N Y Acad Sci 252:274, 1975

KROENKE K et al: The value of serum magnesium determination in hypertensive patients receiving diuretics. Arch Intern Med 147:1553, 1987

QUAMME GA, DIRKS JH: Magnesium metabolism, in *Clinical Disorders of Fluid and Electrolyte Metabolism*, 4th ed, MH Maxwell, CR Kleeman, RG Narins (eds). New York, McGraw-Hill, 1987, chap 13, pp 297–316

RASMUSSEN HS et al: Magnesium and acute myocardial infarction. Arch Intern Med 146:872, 1986

SHILS ME: Experimental human magnesium depletion. Medicine 48:61, 1969

SHINE KI: Myocardial effects of magnesium. Am J Physiol 237:H413, 1979

TZIVONI D et al: Treatment of torsade de pointes with magnesium sulfate. Circulation 77:392, 1988

VELOSO D et al: The concentrations of free and bound magnesium in rat tissues. J Biol Chem 248:4811, 1973

VICTOR M: The role of hypomagnesemia and respiratory alkalosis in the genesis of alcohol withdrawal symptoms. Ann N Y Acad Sci 215:235, 1973

WHANG R et al: Frequency of hypomagnesemia in hospitalized patients receiving digitalis. Arch Intern Med 145:655, 1985

344 PAGET'S DISEASE OF BONE

STEPHEN M. KRANE

Paget's disease of bone (osteitis deformans) is usually focal but may be widespread. The initial event is excessive resorption of bone by cells such as osteoclasts, followed by the replacement of normal marrow by vascular, fibrous connective tissue. At some stage and to a variable degree, the resorbed bone is replaced by coarse-fibered, dense trabecular bone organized in haphazard fashion. The irregular and often rapid deposition of this new bone, to a great extent still lamellar, causes an increase in the number of prominent, irregular cement lines that give the bone its characteristic "mosaic" pattern. Most lesions show both excessive resorption and chaotic new bone formation.

INCIDENCE The prevalence is difficult to determine since it is often asymptomatic and is frequently detected when roentgenograms are obtained for other reasons or because of a high level of alkaline phosphatase on routine blood screening. On the basis of autopsy examination, the incidence is estimated to be about 3 percent in individuals over the age of 40; there is increased likelihood of occurrence with increasing age. The incidence varies in different parts of the world. Figures based on radiologic surveys indicate less than a 1 percent frequency in the adult populations in the United States, Great Britain, and Australia. In India, Japan, the Middle East, and Scandinavia, the disease is rare.

ETIOLOGY The etiology is unknown. No convincing evidence of endocrine abnormality has been produced. Likewise, although pagetic bone can be exceedingly vascular, it has not been established that the vascular abnormality is primary. Some of the manifestations can be suppressed with glucocorticoids, salicylates, and cytotoxic drugs, but there is no convincing evidence that the fundamental lesion is inflammatory. Intranuclear inclusions have been found by electron microscopy in osteoclasts in pagetic bone but not in osteoclasts or other bone cells in normal persons or patients with other bone diseases with the exception of pyknodysostosis. Some of the inclusions resemble nucleocapsids of viruses belonging to the measles group. Indirect immunofluorescence and immunoperoxidase studies using antibodies to measles virus support the suggestion that the inclusions are indeed measles virus nucleocapsids. Measles virus nucleocapsid mRNA has also been detected by in situ hybridization in bone cells from patients with Paget's disease. Other evidence suggests that the inclusions are due to respiratory syncytial virus. In one area of England ownership of dogs is more common in pagetic subjects than in controls, suggesting that a canine virus (for example, canine distemper) might be the infective agent. Thus, different viral agents might be responsible for Paget's disease in different patients.

PATHOPHYSIOLOGY The characteristic feature is increased resorption of bone accompanied by an increase in bone formation, which is usually adequate to compensate. In the early phase bone resorption predominates (for example, in the variant, *osteoporosis circumscripta*), and the bones are exceedingly vascular. This has been termed the *osteoporotic, osteolytic,* or *destructive phase* of disease in which the external calcium balance may be negative. Commonly the excessive resorption is followed closely by formation of new pagetic bone. In this so-called mixed phase of the disease, the rate of bone formation is so geared to that of bone resorption that the magnitude of the increase in bone turnover is not reflected in the overall calcium balance.

As the activity decreases, a progressive decrease in resorptive rate may occur, eventually leading to the occurrence of hard, dense, less vascular bone (the so-called *osteoplastic* or *sclerotic* phase) and a positive external calcium balance. The rates of bone turnover may be increased enormously in patients with active Paget's disease, occasionally more than 20 times normal. Quantitative histomorphometry of bone biopsies confirms the extent of remodeling with marked increase in resorption surfaces and deep scalloped lacunae containing giant osteoclasts with numerous nuclei and increased numbers of osteoblasts lining the edges. The calcification rate is also increased. The normal hematopoietic marrow is replaced by a loose stroma which may be highly vascular. The magnitude of the increase in turnover varies with the extent as well as the activity of the disease. The increase correlates with the increased plasma levels of bone alkaline phosphatase, which are higher in Paget's disease than in any other condition with the exception of hereditary hyperphosphatasia. Although increased bone resorption enhances release of calcium and phosphate ions from bone, utilization of these ions for new bone formation and, presumably, feedback control of parathyroid hormone secretion usually maintain the concentration of calcium ions in the plasma at normal levels. The concentration of phosphate in the plasma is normal or slightly elevated. When marked imbalance between bone formation and resorption occurs in favor of resorption, as after prolonged immobilization or fractures, urinary calcium excretion may be increased, and rarely hypercalcemia may occur. If, on the other hand, bone formation exceeds resorption (relatively uncommon), circulating levels of parathyroid hormone may be increased. Significant increases in trabecular bone resorption and osteoid surfaces in normal bone from patients with Paget's disease may be due to compensatory, secondary hyperparathyroidism. Resorption involves the organic phase of bone as well as the mineral phase. While the inorganic ions of the mineral phase are reutilized for bone formation, amino acids such as hydroxyproline and hydroxylysine are released during resorption of the collagen matrix of bone and are not reutilized for collagen biosynthesis. The urinary excretion of small peptides containing hydroxyproline is increased, reflecting the increased bone resorption. Peptides of about 1500 to 5000 mol wt containing hydroxyproline and other amino acids in proportions characteristic of collagen are also excreted in increased amounts in the urine and are correlated with increased bone formation. Other markers for increased matrix synthesis include elevated levels of osteocalcin (bone-GLA protein) (see Chap. 339) and procollagen extension fragments in plasma.

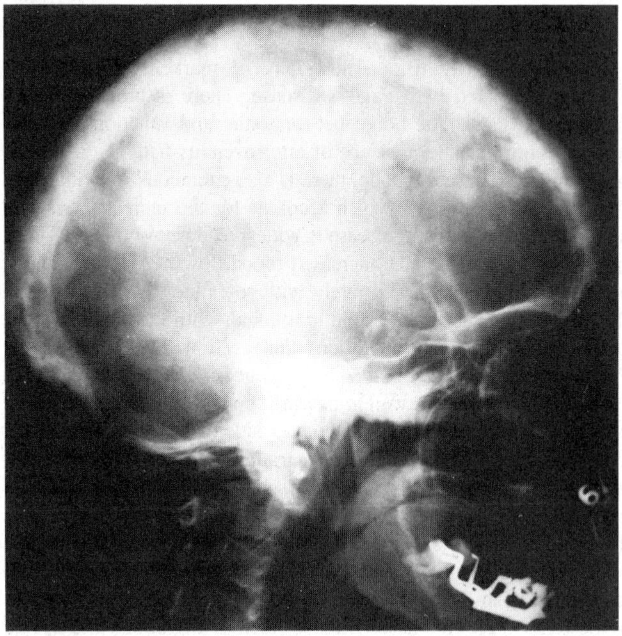

FIGURE 344-1 Lateral roentgenogram of the skull from a 58-year-old woman with Paget's disease of bone.

RADIOLOGIC CHANGES The radiologic findings reflect the underlying pathology and the phase of the disease that predominates at the time of the examination. The pelvic bones are most commonly involved, followed by the femur, skull, tibia, lumbosacral spine, dorsal spine, clavicles, and ribs; small bones are not as frequently diseased. The lytic phase of the disease may be overlooked except when it occurs in the skull as *osteoporosis circumscripta,* with areas of sharply demarcated radiolucency in the frontal, parietal, and occipital bones. In the long bones the lytic areas are usually first seen at one end, from which they progress toward the other end with a V-shaped advancing edge. The lesion may produce expansion of the cortex and exhibit features suggesting malignancy. Usually the lytic area is followed by a zone of increased density, representing the new bone formation of the mixed phase of the disease. In general, the bone shows enlargement with irregularly widened cortex in a coarse, striated pattern and increased density, occasionally focal in distribution. Perpendicular lines of radiolucency (cortical infractions) are frequent and occur on the convex side of bowed long bones, particularly the femur and tibia. Transverse fractures may also occur, some initiated at the sites of these cortical infractions. The remodeling of the pagetic bone usually follows the lines of stress produced by muscle pull or gravity, accounting for the characteristic lateral bowing of the femur or anterior bowing of the tibia and the tendency for most of the dense bone to be deposited on the concave side of the bowed bone. In the skull, in the mixed stage, there is enlargement and thickening, especially of the outer table, with irregular areas of increased density, often spotty (Fig. 344-1). Basilar invagination is common with involvement of the base of the skull. The changes in the pelvis also consist of bone resorption and new bone formation and are frequently accompanied by a characteristic thickening of the pelvic brim. In the sclerotic phase of the disease, the bone may show uniform increase in density, often in the absence of striations. This is common in the facial bones but is occasionally seen as well in the vertebrae where a homogeneous, dense pattern gives an "ivory" appearance similar to that typical of Hodgkin's disease, although the involved vertebrae are not enlarged in Hodgkin's disease. Computed tomography is useful in defining atypical lesions, particularly where neoplastic involvement is suspected. Technetium 99m diphosphonate bone scans are indicated to document the extent of disease when therapy is contemplated or to confirm the diagnosis when radiologic findings are inconclusive. Gallium 67 scans have also been used to define the extent of bone involvement.

CLINICAL PICTURE The clinical presentation is a function of the extent of the disease, the particular bones involved, and the presence of complications. Many patients are asymptomatic. In these individuals the disorder is discovered during radiologic examination of the pelvis or spine for an unrelated disease or complaint or because of the finding of an elevated level of plasma alkaline phosphatase. Other individuals may gradually become aware of a swelling or deformity of a long bone or develop a disturbance in gait due to unequal length of and change in the distribution of mechanical forces in the lower extremities. Enlargement of the skull is often not noticed by the patients, or they may be aware of increasing hat size. Pain in the face and headache are initial complaints in some; backache and pain in the lower extremities are common. The pain is usually dull but may be shooting or knifelike. Back pain is most common in the lumbar region and may radiate into the buttocks or lower extremities. This pain is probably due to the pagetic process itself, to distortion of articular facets, and to secondary osteoarthritis. Pain in the lower extremities may be associated with the transverse cortical infractions along the convex lateral surface of the femur or the anterior surface of the tibia. Often the new lytic lesions detected on bone scan are the most painful. Pain may also be due to involvement of the hip joint resembling degenerative joint disease and characterized by narrowing of the joint space, bony lipping at the margin of the acetabulum, and deepening of the acetabulum. Angioid streaks may be present in the retina. Hearing loss is due to direct involvement of the ossicles of the inner ear or of bone in the region of the cochlea or to impingement by bone on the eighth cranial nerve in the auditory foramen. More serious neurologic complications can result from overgrowth of bone at the base of the skull (platybasia) and compression of the brainstem. Compression of the spinal cord with paraplegia has been observed, particularly with involvement of the middorsal spine. Pathologic fractures of vertebrae may also produce spinal cord lesions.

COMPLICATIONS Blood flow may be markedly increased in extremities involved with Paget's disease. There is proliferation of blood vessels in pagetic bone, but anatomic and functional studies have not confirmed the presence of arteriovenous fistulas. Although blood flow is increased in bone, there is also cutaneous vasodilatation in the pagetic extremities, which accounts for the increased warmth noted clinically. When the disease is widespread, involving one-third or more of the skeleton, the increased blood flow may be associated with *high cardiac output* and rarely with so-called high-output heart failure. However, heart disease in individuals with Paget's disease is usually due to the same conditions that occur in other patients of similar age. *Pathologic fracture* may occur in the destructive phase of the disease. In the weight-bearing bones fractures are often incomplete, multiple, and on the convex side of the bone. They may occur spontaneously or follow slight trauma; the lesions are painful but heal spontaneously with no major disability. More serious fractures may also occur. Complete fractures are often transverse as if the bone were snapped like a piece of chalk. Under these circumstances the fracture may upset the delicate balance between bone formation and resorption in favor of resorption. At this stage the imbalance may be reflected by increased urinary calcium excretion, and in rare instances the serum calcium level may rise to dangerous levels.

There is no characteristic level of urinary calcium excretion, although calcium excretion tends to be higher when the resorptive phase predominates. This may be a factor which accounts for the somewhat higher incidence of *urinary stone* in these patients. Secondary changes in the cartilage of the hip joints and knees may result in articular symptoms. Hyperuricemia and gout commonly occur in men with Paget's disease, and calcific periarthritis may occur.

Sarcoma is the dread complication. The incidence is probably no greater than 1 percent, although higher incidence has been noted in some series that include many patients with polyostotic involvement. The sarcomas most frequently arise in the femur, humerus, skull, facial bones, and pelvis, and rarely in the vertebrae. In about 20 percent the tumors are multicentric. Histologically, they are usually osteosarcomas, although fibrosarcomas and chondrosarcomas have also been found. Increase in pain and swelling are the common complaints that lead to recognition of the sarcomas. The extent and character of the neoplastic involvement are established by computed tomography and/or magnetic resonance imaging. The level of alkaline phosphatase in the serum of patients with sarcomas usually reflects the activity and extent of the Paget's disease. In occasional patients an "explosive rise" of the phosphatase level may accompany the growth of the sarcoma, whereas in patients with limited Paget's disease, phosphatase levels may be only slightly elevated and give no clue to the development of the malignant lesion. The prognosis is poor following the development of sarcomas, and ablative surgery is rarely successful. Although chemotherapy is successful for treatment of some osteosarcomas in children, such regimens have little effect on survival of patients in whom osteosarcomas develop on the background of Paget's disease. Reparative granulomas resembling giant cell tumors may be locally destructive, but they do not metastasize.

THERAPY Most patients require no treatment, since the disease is localized and does not cause symptoms. Indications for therapy include persistent pain in involved bones, neural compression, rapidly progressive deformity resulting in disabling disturbance of posture and/or gait, high-output congestive heart failure, hypercalcemia, severe hypercalciuria with or without formation of renal stones, repeated fractures or nonunion, and preparation for major orthopedic surgery. *Aspirin* is an effective analgesic, and if it can be tolerated in large enough doses (3.6 to 4 g/d) for months or years, disease activity may be suppressed, as shown by decreases in the level of plasma alkaline phosphatase and urinary hydroxyproline excretion. Nonsteroidal anti-inflammatory drugs such as *indomethacin*, 25 mg three or four times daily, may also relieve pain, especially in the presence of hip involvement. *Glucocorticoids* suppress the disease but only in large doses (greater than 60 mg prednisone per day) which are usually not tolerated and, therefore, are not recommended. It is of interest that the high cardiac output of some patients may be reduced significantly after only a few days of glucocorticoid treatment. Orthopedic procedures also have a role in the management of selected cases. Total hip replacement may be indicated, and osteotomy may correct marked bowing deformities, particularly of the tibia. In patients with fractures or orthopedic procedures or in patients immobilized for any reason, urinary and serum calcium levels should be measured at intervals to anticipate the development of hypercalciuria and hypercalcemia. Early ambulation and adequate fluid intake are essential. Preparations of inorganic phosphate may reduce hypercalciuria under these circumstances (5 to 6 g/d neutral sodium phosphate in divided doses for 1 to 2 weeks).

Several agents reduce the excessive bone resorption of Paget's disease and are of possible therapeutic value. The administration of porcine, salmon, and human *calcitonins* for prolonged periods to pagetic patients may cause a decrease in plasma alkaline phosphatase and in urinary hydroxyproline excretion. Treatment with calcitonin causes variable decrease in bone pain, improvement in neurologic symptoms, and decrease in elevated cardiac output. Some patients have not continued to respond to porcine and salmon calcitonins, possibly because of the development of neutralizing antibodies. These individuals usually continue to exhibit a satisfactory response to human calcitonin. In others the development of secondary hyperparathyroidism has been postulated as the cause for a diminished response, although this cannot account for resistance in all cases. The calcitonins are probably most useful in patients with pain in areas of pagetic involvement, not due to associated joint disease. The dose of salmon calcitonin (the form available in the United States) is 50 to 100 MRC units daily given subcutaneously. In some cases it may be possible to reduce the dose to three times weekly. In severe cases alkaline phosphatase levels decrease, but not to the normal range. The disorder relapses after weeks or months when the calcitonin is discontinued. Some patients develop a sensation of warmth and/or nausea 30 min to several hours after injection. This may occur after initiating treatment or after months or years of therapy. The etiology is unknown, but the symptoms may be severe enough to discontinue the medication. Nasal spray and suppository formulations of calcitonin are efficacious and in the future may replace subcutaneous injection.

Cytotoxic drugs such as plicamycin and dactinomycin are potent agents in the disorder. Parenteral administration of plicamycin, 10 to 25 μg/kg body weight per day for 10 to 14 days, has produced striking decrease in urinary hydroxyproline excretion with subsequent decreases in plasma alkaline phosphatase level and clinical improvement. The indexes of active disease again become abnormal within weeks to months following completion of plicamycin therapy. Maintenance therapy may be administered as a weekly intravenous bolus. With doses of less than 15 μg/kg per week toxicity is low despite potential risks. Although the risks of plicamycin therapy appear to be low, it is seldom used in Paget's disease because of the availability of other effective, and even safer, agents.

Etidronate, a diphosphonate compound, given orally in doses up to 20 mg/kg body weight per day is effective in reducing bone resorption in almost all and in producing clinical improvement in some. Biochemical indices may be brought to normal, but in most the responses are incomplete. Serum alkaline phosphatase and urinary hydroxyproline excretion remain decreased for several months after withdrawal of the drug and only gradually return to pretreatment levels. In doses of 20 mg/kg body weight per day for periods of 6 months or longer and even with lower doses, mineralization of new bone may be inhibited and predispose to fracture. Some patients develop disabling pain over pagetic lesions within weeks or months of starting treatment that may be severe enough to warrant discontinuing the drug. Radiographs in some instances show an increase in bone lysis that heals when the drug is stopped. It is therefore recommended that doses of 5 mg or occasionally 10 mg/kg body weight per day be used for 6-month periods. Treatment could be reinstituted within 3 to 12 months if biochemical relapse occurs.

Other diphosphonate compounds such as the dichloromethylidene, 3-amino-1-hydroxypropylidine, aminohexane, or aminobutane derivatives have been introduced for therapy in Europe. The daily administration of these agents intravenously for 1 to 2 weeks or orally for several months produces rapid decrease in urinary hydroxyproline excretion and the characteristic delayed fall in serum alkaline phosphatase levels which, in contrast to experience with calcitonin or etidronate, usually reach the normal range. There is no inhibition of mineralization, and remission usually persists for 1 to 2 years or longer. Several of these highly effective agents are under trial in the United States. Although the diphosphonates and calcitonins act primarily to decrease bone resorption, the rate of new bone formation subsequently falls. As a result, the state of high bone turnover is shifted to a state of lower turnover, where rates of formation and resorption are still apparently geared to each other. In this lower turnover state, collagen fibers of the bone matrix are deposited in a more orderly fashion similar to normal bone.

REFERENCES

ALTMAN R, SINGER FR (eds): Proceedings of the Kroc Foundation Conference on Paget's Disease of Bone. Arthritis Rheum 23:1073, 1980

BASLÉ MF et al: Measles virus RNA detected in Paget's disease bone tissue by *in situ* hybridization. J Gen Virol 67:907, 1986

BIJVOET OLM et al: Paget's disease of bones: Assessment, therapy, and secondary prevention, in *Clinical Disorders of Bone and Mineral Metabolism,* M Kleerekoper, SM Krane (eds). New York, Mary Ann Liebert, Inc., 1989

HARINCK HIJ et al: Relation between signs and symptoms in Paget's disease of bone. Q J Med 226:133, 1986

HUVOS AG: Osteogenic sarcoma of bones and soft tissues in older persons. Cancer 57:1442, 1986

——— et al: Osteogenic sarcoma associated with Paget's disease of bone. A clinicopathologic study of 65 patients. Cancer 52:1489, 1983

KRANE SM: Etidronate disodium in the treatment of Paget's disease of bone. Ann Intern Med 96:619, 1982

MCDONALD DJ, SIM FH: Total hip arthroplasty in Paget's disease. J Bone Joint Surg 69A:766, 1987

MILLS BG et al: Gallium-67 citrate localization in osteoclast nuclei of Paget's disease of bone. J Nucl Med 29:1083, 1988

NAGANT DE DEUXCHAISNES C, KRANE SM: Paget's disease of bone: Clinical and metabolic observations. Medicine 43:233, 1964

REBEL A (ed): Symposium on Paget's disease. Clin Orthop Rel Res 217:1, 1987

SERET P et al: Sarcomatous degeneration in Paget's bone disease. J Cancer Res Clin Oncol 113:392, 1987

SINGER FR, KRANE SM: Paget's disease of bone, in *Metabolic Bone Disease,* LV Avioli, SM Krane (eds). Philadelphia, Saunders, 1990

STRICKBERGER SA et al: Association of Paget's disease of bone with calcific aortic valve disease. Am J Med 82:953, 1987

UPCHURCH K et al: Giant cell reparative granuloma of Paget's disease of bone. A unique clinical entity. Ann Intern Med 98:35, 1983

345 HYPEROSTOSIS, NEOPLASMS, AND OTHER DISORDERS OF BONE AND CARTILAGE

STEPHEN M. KRANE / ALAN L. SCHILLER

HYPEROSTOSIS

A number of disease states have in common an increase in the mass of bone per unit volume (hyperostosis) (Table 345-1). Such increase in bone mass is detected radiologically as increased density of the bone, often associated with a variable disturbance in the architecture of the tissue. In the absence of quantitative histomorphometric data, it is usually not possible to distinguish between an increase in bone mass due to excessive formation of new bone or to decreased resorption of bone already formed. When bone deposition is rapid, the new bone may be of the woven type, but if the process is more chronic, true lamellar bone is formed. The additional bone may be located at the periosteum, within the compact bone of the cortex, or in the trabeculae of the cancellous regions. In the medullary area, the new bone is deposited on and between the trabeculae and encroaches upon the medullary spaces. Typical examples of such responses are seen in areas adjacent to tumors or in association with infection. In some diseases, the increase in bone mass may be spotty, as in osteopoikilosis, whereas in others most of the skeleton may be involved, as in the malignant form of osteopetrosis in children. The increase in mass is usually not due to an excessive amount of mineral relative to matrix, except in disorders such as osteopetrosis where islands of calcified cartilage may persist. (The mineral density of calcified cartilage is greater than that of bone.) In some diseases, such as the osteosclerosis of renal insufficiency, the bone mass and radiodensity may be increased, even though the new bone formed is poorly mineralized and contains widened osteoid seams. Hyperostosis could be due to dysfunction of osteoblasts or osteoclasts. It is of interest, therefore, that infection of newborn mice produces an osteopetrosis-like phenotype in which osteoblast progenitors appear to induce increased bone formation. However, in human osteopetrosis of the relatively benign and sporadic type, viral nucleocapsid particles have been found in osteoclasts, and it is possible that viral infection causes disordered function in these cells to account for the excessive bone mass.

TABLE 345-1 Causes of hyperostosis

1 Endocrine disorders
- *a* Primary hyperparathyroidism
- *b* Hypothyroidism
- *c* Acromegaly

2 Radiation osteitis

3 Chemical poisoning
- *a* Fluoride
- *b* Elemental phosphorus
- *c* Beryllium
- *d* Arsenic
- *e* Vitamin A intoxication
- *f* Lead
- *g* Bismuth

4 Osteomalacic disorders
- *a* Renal tubular osteomalacia (vitamin D resistance or phosphate diabetes)
- *b* Chronic renal glomerular failure

5 Osteosclerosis (localized) associated with chronic infection

6 Osteosclerotic phase of Paget's disease

7 Osteosclerosis associated with carcinomatous metastases, malignant lymphoma, and hematologic disorders (myeloproliferative disorders, sickle cell disease, leukemia, multiple myeloma, systemic mastocytosis)

8 Osteosclerosis of erythroblastosis fetalis

9 Osteopetrosis
- *a* Infantile (malignant, autosomal recessive form)
- *b* Adult (benign, dominant form)
- *c* Intermediate form with carbonic anhydrase II deficiency and renal tubular acidosis

10 Unclassified diseases
- *a* Pyknodysostosis
- *b* Osteomyelosclerosis
- *c* Hyperostosis corticalis generalisata
- *d* Hyperostosis generalisata with pachydermia
- *e* Hereditary hyperphosphatasia
- *f* Progressive diaphyseal dysplasia (osteopathia hyperostotica multiplex infantilis; Camurati-Engelmann disease)
- *g* Melorheostosis
- *h* Osteopoikilosis
- *i* Hyperostosis frontalis interna

Several of these conditions are discussed in more detail in other chapters, although some generalizations are pertinent. Bone that is denser than normal may be seen occasionally in the osteitis fibrosa associated with hyperparathyroidism. When the hyperparathyroidism is successfully treated, the rate of bone resorption decreases abruptly out of proportion to the rate of bone formation; this imbalance may lead to the production of areas of bone density greater than in the surrounding skeleton, especially in the healing of brown tumors. In hypothyroidism, the rates of both bone formation and resorption may be decreased, but when the balance is in favor of formation bones are of increased density but normal architecture. Increased bone density also occurs in some instances of osteomalacia associated with disturbances in renal tubular function. The increased mass of bone occurs together with widened osteoid seams, as in chronic renal glomerular insufficiency. In the vertebral bodies the bone appears denser in transverse bands at the upper and lower margins, with a relatively radiolucent center. This "sandwich" appearance is similar to that seen in some patients with osteopetrosis and has been termed by the British the *rugger jersey sign*. Skeletal hyperostosis, including cortical hyperostoses, periostitis, and tendon and ligament ossification, is also a complication of long-term therapy with synthetic retinoids such as isotretinoin.

OSTEOPETROSIS Osteopetrosis (Albers-Schönberg or marble bone disease) is clinically, biochemically, and genetically heterogeneous. Although osteopetrosis has multiple causes, a defect in bone resorption is always the underlying mechanism. The most severe form in infants is due to defects in differentiation and/or function of osteoclasts. Several types of hereditary osteopetrosis which resemble the infantile human disease have been described in rodents, and in some the disorder can be cured by engraftment of hematopoietic cells from a normal donor. In humans infantile osteopetrosis is manifested in utero and progresses after birth with anemia, hepatosplenomegaly, hydrocephalus, cranial nerve involvement and death, often due to infections. In most of these instances the disorder is inherited as an autosomal recessive trait. Several attempts to transplant bone marrow from normal donors to provide normal osteoclast precursor cells have been successful, and osteopetrotic bone has been repopulated with functioning osteoclasts of donor origin that produce radiologic and/or bone biopsy evidence of bone resorption. One infant received a bone marrow transplant from a brother with successful response lasting more than 4 years, although vision was not restored. In other individuals with osteopetrosis, peripheral blood monocyte function is defective. In other cases of osteopetrosis, clinical improvement has been obtained using high doses of calcitriol.

Less fulminant forms of osteopetrosis are seen in older children and adults. In some of the latter the disorder is sporadic. In others the osteopetrosis is progressive with increasing age and is inherited as an autosomal dominant trait; anemia is not as severe, neurologic abnormalities are not as frequent, and recurrent pathologic fractures are the main feature. Although most cases are in infants and children, many are discovered first in adult life when roentgenograms are obtained because of fractures or unrelated diseases. There is no predilection for either sex. Even the inherited adult disorder is heterogeneous. Type I is characterized by increased thickness of the cranial vault, whereas rugger jersey sign and "endo bones" in the pelvis are features of type II. A defect in modeling of endosteal bone is present in both types, and there is an additional defect in the remodeling of trabecular bone in type II osteopetrosis.

In kindreds where it is associated with renal tubular acidosis and cerebral calcification, osteopetrosis is inherited as an autosomal recessive defect, is compatible with long survival, and is associated with a deficiency of one of the isoenzymes of carbonic anhydrase (carbonic anhydrase II). Carbonic anhydrase II is a major component of the enzyme system required for generation of the unique acid environment adjacent to the ruffled border of the osteoclast, and deficiency of carbonic anhydrase results in disordered bone resorption. Bone resorption is depressed. In some instances, islands of unresorbed calcified cartilage are encased in bone. The defect in remodeling results in disorganization of bone structure with thickened cortices and lack of funnelization of metaphyses. Despite increased density, the bone is abnormal mechanically and fractures readily. Osteomalacia or rickets is sometimes a component of the osteopetrosis in children (Fig. 345-1).

The histologic changes are reflected in the roentgenograms (Fig. 345-2), which reveal uniformly dense, sclerotic bone often without distinction between the cortical and cancellous regions. There is persistence of the primary spongiosa with central calcified cartilage cores surrounded by woven bone. Osteoclasts are often increased in number but apparently do not function properly. Osteoclasts may be morphologically normal or have loss of their ruffled borders suggesting that a spectrum of changes may occur. The variability may reflect heterogeneity in this syndrome, as in the osteopetrosis that occurs spontaneously in rodents. The long bones are usually involved, with increased density along the entire shaft. Foci of increased density

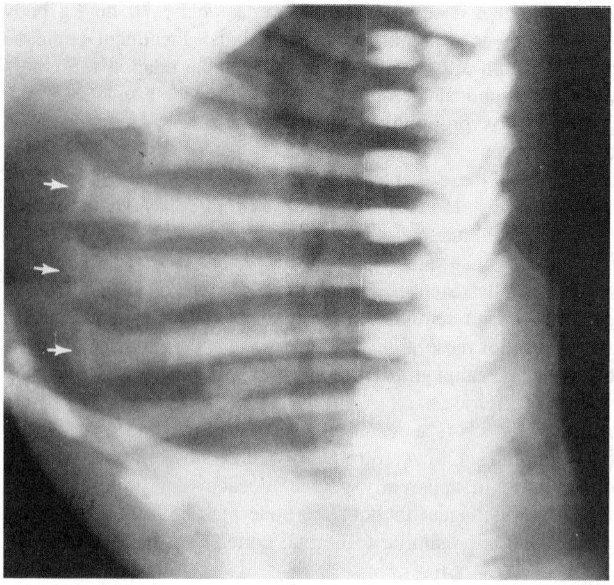

FIGURE 345-1 Lateral roentgenogram of the thorax of a 9-month-old boy with the "malignant" form of osteopetrosis. Note the uniform increase in mineral density of the vertebral bodies and the marked flaring of the ends of the ribs (arrows), indicative of rickets.

FIGURE 345-2 Roentgenogram of the spine and pelvis of a 55-year-old man with the more benign, dominant form of osteopetrosis.

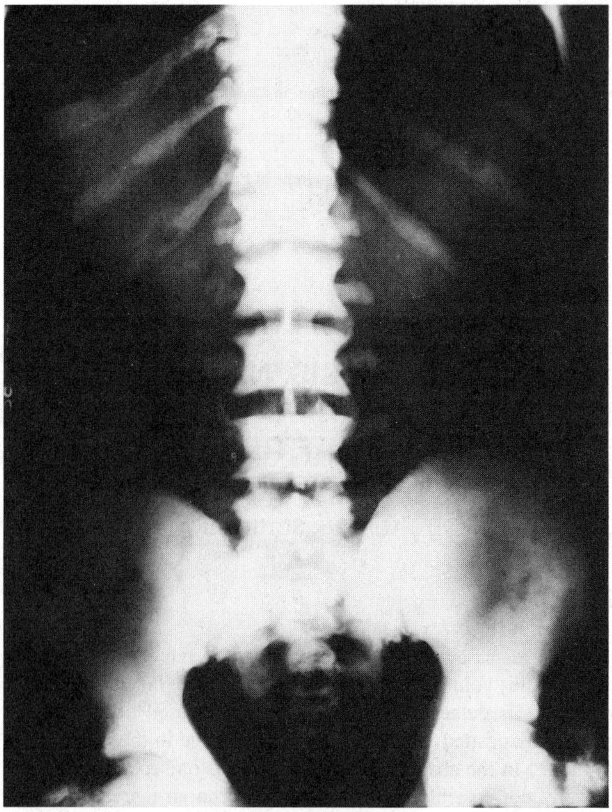

may be seen in the epiphyses corresponding to regions of unresorbed calcified cartilage. The metaphyses have a characteristic clubbed or splayed appearance. Horizontal bandings of increased density alternating with zones of decreased density in the long bones and vertebrae suggest that the defect is intermittent during periods of growth. The skull, pelvis, ribs, and other bones may be involved. The phalanges and the distal humerus may appear normal.

Encroachment of bone upon the marrow cavity, particularly in the malignant infantile disorder, is associated with anemia of the myelophthisic type with foci of extramedullary hematopoiesis in liver, spleen, and lymph nodes and enlargement of these organs. Neurologic abnormalities are associated with encroachment on cranial nerves and include optic atrophy, nystagmus, papilledema, exophthalmos, and impairment of extraocular motility. Facial paralysis and deafness are frequent; trigeminal lesions and anosmia are less common. In infants macrocephaly, hydrocephalus, and convulsions may occur, and infections such as osteomyelitis are frequent. Renal tubular acidosis is a feature of the form of osteopetrosis associated with a deficiency in carbonic anhydrase II.

In the milder dominant osteopetrosis, about half of the patients have no symptoms, and the disorder is discovered incidentally on roentgenograms. Other patients present because of fractures, bone pain, osteomyelitis, and cranial nerve palsies.

Fractures are a complication even with trivial trauma. Healing of such fractures is usually satisfactory, although delayed union may occur. When the disease is manifested first in adult life, fractures may be the only clinical problem. Levels of calcium and alkaline phosphatase in the plasma are usually normal in adults, although in children hypophosphatemia and, occasionally, moderate hypocalcemia have been noted. Serum acid phosphatase levels are usually increased.

The skeletal defect is not the same in all forms of osteopetrosis, and within a clinical subtype genetic and biochemical heterogeneity is common. As mentioned, several children with severe osteopetrosis have received bone marrow transplants from HLA-identical siblings which resulted in histologic and radiologic increases in bone resorption, accompanied by variable improvement in anemia, vision, hearing, and growth and development.

Unfortunately, it is not always possible to find appropriate donors for bone marrow transplantation, or patients may not be good candidates to receive transplants. Patients with the lethal forms have been treated with calcitriol. This therapy is associated with appearance of osteoclasts with normal ruffled borders and other evidence for increased bone resorption.

PYKNODYSOSTOSIS *Pyknodysostosis* resembles osteopetrosis but is a more benign condition not usually associated with hepatosplenomegaly, anemia, or cranial nerve involvement. In addition to a generalized increase in bone density, features include short stature, separated cranial sutures, hypoplasia of the mandible, kyphoscoliosis and deformities of the trunk, persistence of deciduous teeth, and progressive acroosteolysis of the terminal phalanges. Life span is usually unaffected, and the patient usually presents because of frequent fractures. Pyknodysostosis is inherited as an autosomal recessive trait. In one case levels of plasma calcitonin were intermittently elevated, and the response of the plasma calcitonin to infusions of calcium and glucagon was exaggerated. The gene that causes this disorder may be located on the short arm of a small acrocentric chromosome.

OSTEOMYELOSCLEROSIS *Osteomyelosclerosis* is a disorder in which the marrow cells are replaced by diffuse fibroplasia, occasionally accompanied by osseous metaplasia. When the latter is prominent, increased skeletal density is seen on roentgenograms. In early stages woven bone may be found in intratrabecular locations whereas in more advanced stages woven bone is observed in the medulla. The disorder is probably a phase in the course of the myeloproliferative disorders and is characteristically accompanied by extramedullary hematopoiesis.

Hyperostosis corticalis generalisata (van Buchem's disease) is characterized by osteosclerosis of the skull (base and calvaria), lower jaw, clavicles, and ribs, and thickening of the diaphyseal cortices of the long and short bones. Alkaline phosphatase levels in the serum are elevated, and the disorder may be due to increased formation of bone of normal structure. The major manifestations are due to neural compression and consist of optic atrophy, facial paralysis, and perception deafness. In *hyperostosis generalisata with pachydermia* (Uehlinger), the sclerosis is due to increased formation of subperiosteal spongy bone and involves the epiphyses, metaphyses, and diaphyses. Pain, swelling of joints, and thickening of the skin of the lower arms are common.

HEREDITARY HYPERPHOSPHATASIA This disorder is characterized by severe structural deformities of the skeleton with increase in thickness of the calvaria, large homogeneous areas of increased density at the base of the skull, and widening and loss of normal architecture of the shafts and the epiphyses of the long and short bones. There is a failure to deposit normal bone, with haphazard orientation of lamellae suggesting active remodeling that resembles Paget's disease of bone. Osteoclasts with multiple nuclei characteristic of Paget's disease and the typical "mosaic" pattern of faceted units of lamellar bone are not found, however. Levels of plasma alkaline phosphatase and urinary excretion of hydroxyproline peptides and other collagen degradation products are markedly increased. The disorder is apparently inherited as an autosomal recessive trait. Calcitonin therapy may be of value in some of these patients.

PROGRESSIVE DIAPHYSEAL DYSPLASIA A disorder in which a symmetric thickening and increased diameter of the diaphyses of long bones occurs, particularly in femurs, tibias, fibulas, radii, and ulnas, has been termed *progressive diaphyseal dysplasia* (Camurati-Engelmann disease). Pain over affected areas, fatigue, abnormal gait, and muscle wasting are the major manifestations. Serum alkaline phosphatase levels may be elevated and, on occasion, hypocalcemia and hyperphosphatemia may be found. Other abnormalities include anemia, leukopenia, and elevated erythrocyte sedimentation rate. Clinical and biochemical improvement may result from the use of glucocorticoids.

MELORHEOSTOSIS This rare condition usually begins in childhood and is characterized by a slowly progressive linear hyperostosis in one or more bones of one limb, usually in a lower extremity. All segments of the bone may be involved, with sclerotic areas that have a "flowing" distribution. The involved limb is often extremely painful.

OSTEOPOIKILOSIS This benign disorder is usually discovered by chance and is not associated with symptoms. It is characterized by dense spots of trabecular bone less than a centimeter in diameter, usually of uniform density, that are located in the epiphyses and adjacent parts of the metaphyses. All bones may be involved except the skull, ribs, and vertebrae.

HYPEROSTOSIS FRONTALIS INTERNA *Hyperostosis frontalis interna* is an abnormality of the inner table of the frontal bones of the skull consisting of smooth, rounded enostoses covered by dura and projecting into the cranial cavity. These enostoses are usually less than 1 cm at their greatest diameter and usually do not extend posteriorly beyond the coronal suture. The abnormality is found almost exclusively in women, who are frequently obese, hirsute, and who have a variety of neuropsychiatric complaints (Morgagni-Stewart-Morel syndrome). However, hyperostosis frontalis interna also occurs in women with no obvious illness or particular associated disease. The finding in the skull may be a manifestation of a generalized metabolic disorder.

NEOPLASMS OF BONE

Primary neoplasms of the skeletal system reflect in their histology the cellular and extracellular components of the skeleton. However, it is not always possible to prove that a tumor arises from the same type of tissue that it produces. The precursor cells of bone tissue are probably derived from distinct cell lines in which the osteoclasts arise from hematopoietic cells and the osteoblasts arise from the stromal cell system. The primitive stromal cell could differentiate into chondroblasts and fibroblasts as well as osteoblasts. Neoplasms can arise from all these cell types. Each of these cells can produce its characteristic extracellular matrix, and neoplasms arising from them may thus be recognized. Primary neoplasms of bone can arise also from other hematopoietic, vascular, and neural elements.

PATHOPHYSIOLOGY Neoplasms in bone induce resorption of skeletal tissue. This bone resorption results from production by the tumor cells of factors that stimulate osteoclast function and/or recruitment and differentiation of the osteoclast hematopoietic precursor cells. One of the factors produced by the tumor cells is the parathyroid hormone–related peptide (PTHrP) that interacts with the PTH receptor (see also Chap. 340). Other factors that induce bone resorption by modulating recruitment, differentiation, and/or activation of osteoclasts include cytokines such as transforming growth factor alpha, interleukins 1 and 6, tumor necrosis factor, and lymphotoxin derived from the tumor, resident bone cells, or infiltrating mononuclear inflammatory cells. What was initially termed ''osteoclast activating factor'' is now known to include cytokines such as interleukin 1 and lymphotoxin produced by monocytes and lymphocytes. Prostaglandin production by some tumors may also mediate bone resorption. T lymphocytes infected with some viruses can metabolize circulating 25(OH)D to $1,25(OH)_2D$, which may also stimulate bone resorption. Tumors may also alter blood supply to bone by obstructing vessels or inducing angiogenesis. Tumors may also produce reaction in surrounding bone and alter the normal contour. The epiphyseal plate, articular cartilage, cortex, and periosteum of bone often offer a barrier to the spread of neoplastic tissue. Alteration of the contour of the cortex is not due to ''expansion'' but to remodeling of the bone in the area and formation of new bone with the new contour. Some tumors induce primarily an osteoblastic or sclerotic reaction in surrounding bone, which results in increased radiodensity. Primary neoplasms may be less radiopaque than surrounding bone or more radiopaque, depending upon the degree of calcification or ossification of the matrix and the density of the tissue. Bone tumors may be recognized because of (1) the presence of a mass in the soft tissues, (2) deformity of a bone, (3) pain and tenderness, or (4) pathologic fractures. Tumors of bone may also be detected incidentally on roentgenograms obtained for other reasons. Although it is usually possible to classify bone tumors as benign or malignant, prediction of the clinical outcome on histologic and radiologic criteria is not always possible.

The extent of the lesions should be defined by standard and computed tomographic techniques and magnetic resonance imaging, if available. Lesions can also be assessed by bone scans utilizing ^{99m}Tc polyphosphonate. There are numerous pitfalls in the clinical diagnosis and interpretation of histologic features of tumors of bone. However, proper evaluation and selection of therapy require evaluation of both radiographic and histologic features. Management, therefore, requires cooperation of the orthopedist, oncologist, radiologist, radiotherapist, and pathologist.

BENIGN TUMORS The most common benign tumors are *osteochondromas* (exostoses) and *endochondromas* (which may be multiple in Ollier's disease), *benign giant cell tumors, unicameral bone cysts, osteoid osteomas,* and *nonossifying fibromas* (fibrous cortical defects). As a rule benign tumors are not painful except for osteoid osteomas, benign chondroblastomas, and benign chondromyxoidfibroma. The usual clinical problem is that of slowly progressing mass, pathologic fracture, or deformity. Treatment is usually accomplished by resection or curettage and bone grafting. When wide resection of tissue is necessary, insertion of metal and plastic prostheses or allograft transplantation may preserve limb function.

MALIGNANT TUMORS The most common malignant tumor of bone is multiple myeloma (see Chap. 265). Primary lymphoma may also arise locally in bone. Malignant tumors of nonhematopoietic origin include osteosarcomas, chondrosarcomas, fibrosarcomas, and Ewing's tumor. Giant cell tumors may be included here since they may metastasize and are locally destructive. *Osteogenic sarcomas* are presumed to arise from osteoprogenitor cells and have a wide variation in histopathology, with at least six histologic types. These tumors always contain woven bone at least in small foci, and may contain in addition cartilaginous and fibrous elements. They are most common in the second and third decades and are less common under the age of 10 and over the age of 40. Genetic factors are important in the genesis of osteosarcomas particularly in children. Between 30 and 40 percent of patients with retinoblastoma have a hereditary predisposition to the tumor as well as to other cancers, particularly osteosarcomas. This predisposition is determined by a genetic locus within the q14 band of chromosome 13 that can be detected by analysis of restriction fragment length polymorphisms. Homozygosity for the mutant allele at the retinoblastoma locus in the osteoblast precursor could lead to osteosarcoma in the same way that homozygosity for the allele in a retinoblast could lead to retinoblastoma. In contrast, when osteosarcomas occur in older individuals, some predisposing cause is usually present such as Paget's disease, prior exposure to ionizing radiation, or a bone infarct. In primary osteogenic sarcomas the lesions usually arise in the metaphyseal region of long bones, especially in the distal femur, proximal tibia, and proximal humerus. The most common symptoms are pain and swelling which may be present for weeks or months. The roentgenographic features of osteosarcomas depend upon the degree of bone destruction, the extent to which mineralized bone is formed by and within the tumor, and the type of reaction in the surrounding bone. Thus, the lesions may vary from purely lytic lesions to dense areas containing radiopaque lumps, clouds, or spicules of tumor bone in varying patterns of organization. Discontinuities may occur in the cortex surrounding the lesion. In other cases, hyperostotic periosteal reactions may involve grossly layered bone. If the tumor grows rapidly, it may destroy the cortex and penetrate the soft tissue surrounding the bone; it leaves only a cuff of periosteal new bone at the peripheral margin of the tumor, just at the point of penetration (Codman's triangle). High plasma alkaline phosphatase levels in those sarcomas that are predominantly osteogenic parallel the course of the tumor. In general, high levels of serum alkaline phosphatase activity correlate with a poor prognosis. When lesions are adequately treated by amputation, chemotherapy, or radiation, the level of alkaline phosphatase falls, and when metastases appear, the level rises again, often reaching values higher than those present initially. When values are initially high, the course is often rapidly fatal. Metastases occur primarily by the hematogenous route especially to the lung.

The prognosis of osteosarcoma was very poor prior to development of effective chemotherapy, with radiologic evidence of pulmonary metastases usually occurring within a year following surgical amputation that was potentially curative. The course varies with the type of tumor; for example, a ''telangiectatic'' variant has a very poor prognosis, unless treated with aggressive chemotherapy, whereas the less common low-grade intramedullary type has a better prognosis. In the typical intramedullary type of osteosarcoma, death occurs within 6 months from the onset of detectable pulmonary metastases, suggesting that the lesions in the lungs were present at the time of amputation or that cells were shed from the tumor during the operation.

Several chemotherapeutic programs are efficacious. The disease-free and overall survival rates after 4 to 5 years in patients with no demonstrable metastases have increased from about 20 percent with ablative surgery alone to 80 percent or higher with current treatment programs. Since microscopic metastatic foci must be present when the bone tumors are first recognized, aggressive adjuvant chemotherapy is now routine. Chemotherapeutic programs include high-dose methotrexate with leucovorin rescue and various combinations of doxorubicin, cisplatin, bleomycin, cyclophosphamide, and dactinomycin. Amputation or surgical resection of the sarcoma leaving a wide margin of normal tissue is generally carried out. More frequently, a limb-sparing procedure is attempted, particularly in distal femoral osteosarcomas, with allograft bone and cartilage transplants and/or prosthetic devices used to preserve the joint. Resection of isolated pulmonary metastases combined with chemotherapy may also improve survival in younger individuals with primary osteosarcomas. The prognosis of osteosarcoma occurring on the background of Paget's disease in adults is still poor despite chemotherapy.

Chondrosarcomas are distinguishable from osteogenic sarcomas. In contrast to the latter, chondrosarcomas usually arise in adulthood and old age, with the peak incidence in the fourth, fifth, and sixth decades. Most are located in the pelvic girdle, ribs, and diaphyseal portions of the femur and humerus; distal portions of the extremities are involved rarely. Chondrosarcomas probably arise by malignant transformation in enchondromas and more rarely in the cartilaginous cap of osteochondromas. As a rule, chondrosarcomas are slow growing and slow to recur. Radiographically the lesions appear destructive, with mottled increases in radiodensity which reflect the variable degree of calcification of cartilaginous matrix and ossification. Radical excision is the treatment of choice. Histologic grading of the tumor can be valuable for predicting prognosis and determining appropriate surgical therapy.

Ewing's tumor This is a malignant sarcoma composed of small, round cells that occurs most frequently in the first three decades of life. Most are located in the long bones, although any bone may be involved. Ewing's sarcoma is highly malignant with a low incidence of cure by ablative surgery with or without radiation. However, radiation therapy to the primary site and site(s) of metastases combined with chemotherapy with doxorubicin, cyclophosphamide, vincristine, and dactinomycin improves survival of patients with Ewing's sarcoma, including some with metastatic disease.

TUMORS METASTATIC TO BONE The skeleton is a common site for metastases from carcinomas and occasionally even from sarcomas. Skeletal metastases may be silent or produce symptoms by the same mechanisms as primary tumors, i.e., pain, swelling, deformity, encroachment on hematopoietic tissue in the marrow, compression of spinal cord or nerve roots, and pathologic fractures. In addition, rapidly lytic skeletal metastases can result in hypercalcemia. The bones involved most commonly are the vertebrae, proximal femur, pelvis, ribs, sternum, and proximal humerus, in that order of frequency. The carcinomas that most frequently metastasize to bone arise in prostate, breast, lung, thyroid, kidney, and bladder. Malignant cells reach the skeleton via the bloodstream. Those that survive may proliferate and distort the normal architecture, probably by production of substances that cause dissolution of both mineral phase and organic matrix.

Osteolysis most often results from modulation of osteoprogenitor cells to osteoclasts in the surrounding bone. Some mediators involved in induction of osteoclasts were described earlier in this section. Some carcinoma cells may also act directly to resorb bone. Carcinomatous metastases (which are usually predominantly osteolytic) arise from thyroid, kidney, and lower bowel. Other tumors induce an *osteoblastic* response in which the new bone does not arise from the tumor itself, but is induced from normal skeletal cells by some product(s) of the tumor cells. The resulting lesion may be more dense than the surrounding tissue. Occasionally the increase in radiodensity is uniform, simulating osteosclerosis. Carcinoma of the prostate characteristically produces osteoblastic metastases. Carcinoma of the breast can cause both osteolytic and osteoblastic metastases. Malignant carcinoid tumors arising from the embryonic foregut and hindgut metastasize to bone with high frequency, producing an osteoblastic reaction. Hodgkin's disease in bone also produces an osteoblastic response both focal and diffuse. More malignant lymphomas in bone produce predominantly destructive lesions. As a rule, osteolytic metastases are the ones associated with hypercalcemia, hypercalciuria, and increased excretion of hydroxyproline-containing peptides (reflecting matrix destruction); they are usually associated with normal or only slightly increased levels of serum alkaline phosphatase. Osteoblastic metastases, on the other hand, may cause more marked elevations of serum alkaline phosphatase and may be associated with hypocalcemia. With some metastases (as in carcinoma of the breast) there may be phases in which osteolysis predominates (with hypercalciuria, hypercalcemia, and normal alkaline phosphatase levels) alternating with phases in which alkaline phosphatase levels rise and the skeletal lesions become more sclerotic.

Treatment of skeletal metastases is usually palliative. In slowly growing localized lesions (as in some instances of carcinoma of the thyroid or occasionally in carcinoma of the kidney), local radiation is useful to relieve pain or reduce compression of surrounding structures. Many patients with carcinomas of breast or prostate survive for years even after extensive skeletal metastases are recognized. Castration and estrogen therapy or receptor antagonists may slow the progress of the lesions in patients with metastatic prostatic carcinoma (see Chap. 306). When patients with mammary cancer are treated with estrogens or androgens, the character of the reaction to the metastases may temporarily shift from a predominantly osteoblastic to a lytic phase with resultant hypercalcemia (see Chap. 303). Plicamycin, which inhibits osteoclast function and is effective in treating hypercalcemia associated with malignant disease, may also be useful in palliation of osteolytic metastases. The diphosphonates, which decrease bone resorption in Paget's disease, are useful in reducing bone metastases and the accompanying morbidity, such as bone pain, pathologic fractures, and hypercalcemia. The newer derivatives, such as the dichloromethylene and the aminohydroxypropylidene analogues, as well as etidronate are effective, presumably by decreasing the ability of the tumor to establish itself in bone by blocking bone resorption. The bone pain in patients with metastatic carcinoma may also be relieved by the use of levodopa. Hypercalcemia in patients with malignant tumors is not due solely to skeletal metastases, although this is the most common cause. Production of circulating stimulators of osteoclast differentiation, such as PTHrP, is another cause of the humoral hypercalcemia of malignancy. Hypercalcemia per se, whether spontaneous or induced by therapy, may produce anorexia, polyuria, polydipsia, depression, and eventually coma. In addition, nephrocalcinosis can result from hypercalcemia, and death may result from renal insufficiency.

OTHER DISORDERS OF BONE AND CARTILAGE

FIBROUS DYSPLASIA (McCUNE-ALBRIGHT SYNDROME) This syndrome is characterized by osteitis fibrosa disseminata, areas of pigmentation, and endocrine dysfunction, with precocious puberty in females. The bony lesions, called *fibrous dysplasia,* may occur in the absence of the other features. The fundamental nature of the disorder is unknown; the disease does not appear to be heritable, although it has been reported to affect monozygotic twins. The disease occurs with equal frequency in both sexes.

Incidence The disease may be divided into three main categories: (1) monostotic, (2) polyostotic, and (3) McCune-Albright syndrome and its variants. The monostotic form is the most common. The lesions can be asymptomatic, associated with local pain, or predispose to pathologic fracture. The majority of the lesions are in the ribs or in the craniofacial bones, especially the maxillas. Many other bones may be affected, however, such as metaphyseal or diaphyseal portions of the proximal femurs or tibias. Monostotic fibrous dysplasia is most often diagnosed between 20 and 30 years of age. There are usually no associated skin lesions. Approximately a quarter of the individuals with the polyostotic form have more than half the skeleton involved by disease. One side of the body may be affected, and the lesions may be distributed segmentally in a limb, particularly in the lower extremities. Craniofacial lesions are present in approximately half of patients with the polyostotic form. Whereas the monostotic form is usually detected in young adults, fractures and skeletal deformities occur in childhood in the polyostotic form; the disease is generally more severe and deforming with early clinical onset. Lesions, especially monostotic lesions, may become quiescent around the time of puberty and may worsen during pregnancy. McCune-Albright syndrome is more common in females. Short stature is ascribed to premature closure of the epiphyses. The most frequent extraskeletal manifestations are the skin lesions.

Pathology All forms of fibrous dysplasia have an identical histologic appearance, although cartilage is more commonly involved in the polyostotic form. The marrow cavity is filled by gritty, gray-pink, rubbery tissue that replaces the normal cancellous bone. Often, the endosteal cortical surface is scalloped. Histologically, the lesions contain benign-appearing fibroblastic tissue arranged in a loose whorled pattern (Fig. 345-3). The grittiness is due to irregularly arranged woven bone spicules, most of which lack osteoblastic palisading or rimming, which are embedded in the fibrous tissue. These bone spicules may also have prominent cement lines. In approximately 10 percent of cases, islands of hyaline cartilage are present, and more rarely, myxoid tissue may predominate in young patients. Examination by polarized light and with the use of special stains indicates a contiguity of collagen fibers of the osseous and marrow tissue. In the polyostotic form cystic degeneration may be characterized by the presence of hemorrhage with hemosiderin-containing macrophages and osteoclast-type giant cells in the periphery of the cyst. Malignant transformation of either monostotic or polyostotic fibrous dysplasia occurs but with a frequency of less than 1 percent. The malignant change is usually detected in the third or fourth decades in individuals who have had lesions first identified in childhood. In about a third of the cases the neoplasms arise in previously radiated lesions. Ossifying fibroma of long bones is a peculiar fibroosseous cortical lesion which may be a variant of fibrous dysplasia. It is most common in the tibial shaft of teenagers. Although benign, the lesion has a tendency to recur if not adequately excised.

Radiologic changes The roentgenographic appearance of the lesions is that of a radiolucent area with a well-delineated, smooth or scalloped border, typically associated with focal thinning of the cortex of the bone (Fig. 345-4). Fibrous dysplasia and Paget's disease of bone are two disorders that can cause a bone to become larger than normal. The lesions of fibrous dysplasia are not usually cysts in the strict sense, since they are not fluid-filled cavities. They occasionally appear multiloculate. The so-called ground glass appearance reflects the content of the thin spicules of calcified, woven bone. Frequently, deformities are present such as coxa vara, shepherd's-crook deformity of the femur, bowing of the tibia, Harrison's grooves, and protrusio acetabuli. Involvement of facial bones, usually with lesions of increased radiodensity, may create a leonine appearance (leontiasis ossea) superficially resembling leprosy. Fibrous dysplasia of the temporal bones can cause progressive loss of hearing and obliteration of the external ear canal. Advanced skeletal age in females is correlated with sexual precocity but may also be seen in males without sexual precocity. The lesions tend to spare the epiphyseal regions before puberty, but in older individuals fibrous dysplasia may develop in the epiphyses. Occasionally, a focus of fibrous dysplasia may undergo cystic degeneration with an enormous distortion of the shape of the bone, and mimic the so-called aneurysmal bone cyst.

FIGURE 345-3 Photomicrograph of the lesion of fibrous dysplasia. Note spicules of dark-staining woven bone (WB) surrounded by loose fibroblastic tissue.

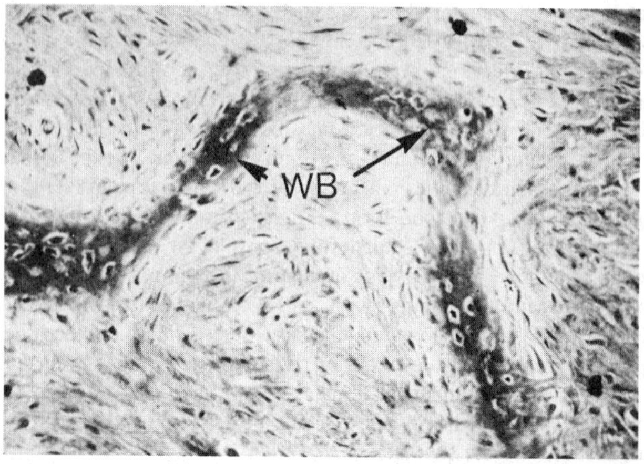

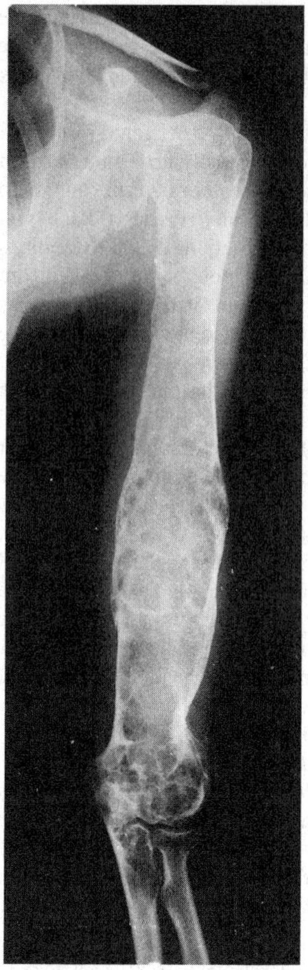

FIGURE 345-4 Roentgenogram of the upper extremity from a 33-year-old woman with fibrous dysplasia of bone. Typical lesions involve the entire humerus as well as the scapula and proximal ulna.

Clinical picture The clinical course is variable. Skeletal lesions are usually detected because of localized pain, deformities, or fractures. Other symptoms ascribable to bone involvement are headache, seizures, cranial nerve abnormalities, hearing loss, narrowing of the external ear canal, or even spontaneous scalp hemorrhages if there is craniofacial bone disease. In some females and even less commonly in males, sexual precocity is the presenting complaint, occasionally before the appearance of skeletal symptoms. Serum calcium and phosphorus values are usually normal. In approximately one-third of patients, levels of serum alkaline phosphatase may be elevated to high values, and urinary hydroxyproline excretion is often increased. In some subjects, high cardiac output similar to that in extensive Paget's disease may be found. In general, patients with extensive involvement have widespread disease when symptoms first appear, whereas when disease is mild at the onset extensive disease does not usually develop.

The cutaneous pigmentation in most patients with McCune-Albright syndrome consists of isolated dark-brown to light-brown macules which tend to remain on one side of the midline (Fig. 345-5). The border is usually, although not always, irregular or jagged (''coast of Maine'') in contrast to the smooth borders of the pigmented macules of neurofibromatosis (''coast of California''). As a rule there are fewer than six of the lesions, which range in size from 1 cm to those covering very large areas, particularly the back, buttocks, or sacral regions. When the lesions are present in the scalp, the overlying hair may be more deeply pigmented than that over the remainder of the scalp. Localized alopecia is associated with osteomas of the skin, and such lesions tend to have concordance with the skeletal lesions. The pigmentation tends to be on the same side as the skeletal lesions and actually overlie them.

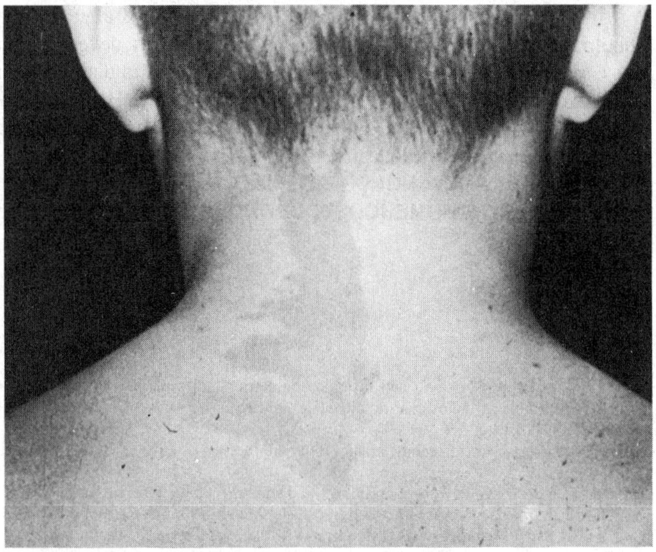

FIGURE 345-5 Typical pigmented café au lait lesion of the skin in an 11-year-old boy with polyostotic fibrous dysplasia. The border has the jagged "coast of Maine" appearance that is characteristic of McCune-Albright's syndrome. Note that the lesion is limited to one side (left) of the body.

The sexual precocity of unknown cause is found in females and rarely in males (see also Chaps. 321 and 322). Premature vaginal bleeding and development of axillary and pubic hair and of breasts are the main features. In the few ovaries that have been examined, no corpora lutea have been seen. The cause of the precocious sexuality is still not clear. In the few cases where measurements have been reported, the girls have high estrogen levels and low or undetectable gonadotropins. Autonomous hyperfunction of ovarian cysts may account for the high estrogen levels and sexual precocity. Estrogen receptors have been measured in the bone lesions. It is therefore not surprising that precocious sexuality is not limited to patients with cranial involvement. The characteristic pigmented macules are usual but not invariable. Another endocrine abnormality with increased frequency is hyperthyroidism. Rarer associations include Cushing's syndrome, acromegaly, possibly hypogonadotropic hypogonadism, and soft tissue myxomas. Hypophosphatemic osteomalacia may also accompany fibrous dysplasia and resembles the disorder associated with other skeletal and nonskeletal tumors. As mentioned, sarcomatous degeneration may rarely occur in fibrous dysplasia.

Although the lytic lesions of fibrous dysplasia resemble the brown tumors of hyperparathyroidism, the age of the patient, normal calcium levels, increased density of bone in the skull, and areas of cutaneous pigmentation identify the former condition. However, fibrous dysplasia and hyperparathyroidism may coexist. Neurofibromas may involve bone and produce cutaneous pigmentation as well as nodules in the skin. The pigmented macules of neurofibromatosis are more numerous and more widely distributed than in fibrous dysplasia, usually have smooth borders, and tend to involve areas such as the axillary folds. Other lesions that have roentgenographic features similar to those of isolated fibrous dysplasia are unicameral bone cysts, aneurysmal bone cysts, and nonossifying fibromas. Leontiasis ossea is most often due to fibrous dysplasia, although other disorders may also produce this appearance such as craniometaphyseal dysplasia, hyperphosphatasia, and, in adults, Paget's disease.

Treatment Fibrous dysplasia is not curable. The symptoms, however, can be managed using a variety of orthopedic procedures such as casting, osteotomy with internal fixation, curettage, and bone grafting depending upon the lesion and the age of the patient. Indications for such procedures include progressive deformity, nonunion of fractures, and pain unresponsive to conservative treatment. Calcitonin may be effective in treatment of widespread disease associated with bone pain and high serum alkaline phosphatase levels (see Chap. 344).

DYSPLASIAS AND CHONDRODYSTROPHIES A variety of diseases of bone and cartilage have been called *dystrophies* or *dysplasias*. The *osteochondrodysplasias* are heritable disorders of connective tissue that are characterized by primary abnormalities of cartilage that lead to disturbances in cartilage and bone growth and development. They comprise more than 100 distinct entities, which can be distinguished based on clinical, genetic, and radiologic features. The biochemical (and genetic) defects have been identified in few of these conditions. The greatest success has been in delineation of errors in metabolism of glycosaminoglycans (acid mucopolysaccharides) to explain the pathogenesis, for example, of Hunter's and Hurler's syndromes (see Chap. 331). Some reports suggest the presence of abnormalities in type II collagen in disorders such as Stickler's syndrome, Kniest dysplasia, and forms of achondrogenesis. In a related syndrome, spondyloepiphyseal dysplasia, a fragment of 36 amino acids in the helical region of type II collagen is deleted. A biochemical explanation for many of these conditions will permit more than a descriptive classification. At present, however, a useful scheme is that proposed by Rubin based on the consideration of errors in modeling of bone and cartilage (Table 345-2). Other clinical and genetic features form the basis of a classification by Rimoin. Pathologic processes in the skeletal dysplasias may be expressed as a deficiency (hypoplasia) or excess (hyperplasia) in relation to normal development.

Spondyloepiphyseal dysplasia The spondyloepiphyseal dysplasias are disorders in which abnormalities of growth occur in various bones including the vertebrae, pelvis, carpal and tarsal bones, and the epiphyses of tubular bones. On the basis of roentgenographic findings, this group can be divided into (1) those with generalized platyspondyly, (2) those with multiple epiphyseal dysplasias, and (3) those with epiphysometaphyseal dysplasias. *Morquio's syndrome,* in which there is a defect in degradation of glycosaminoglycans (therefore a "mucopolysaccharidosis") is inherited as an autosomal recessive trait and is associated with corneal opacities, dental defects, variable disturbances in intellect, and increased urinary excretion of keratosulfate, belongs in the first group. Other forms of spondyloepiphyseal dysplasia, some of which are accounted for by defects in type II collagen, may not be recognized until late in childhood or young

TABLE 345-2 Working classification of bone dysplasias

- *I* Epiphyseal dysplasias
  - *A* Epiphyseal hypoplasias
    - *1* Failure of articular cartilage: spondyloepiphyseal dysplasia, congenita and tarda
    - *2* Failure of ossification of center: multiple epiphyseal dysplasia, congenita and tarda
  - *B* Epiphyseal hyperplasia
    - *1* Excess of articular cartilage: dysplasia epiphysialis hemimelica
- *II* Physeal (growth plate) dysplasias
  - *A* Cartilage hypoplasias
    - *1* Failure of proliferating cartilage: achondroplasia, congenita and tarda
    - *2* Failure of hypertrophic cartilage: metaphyseal dysostosis, congenita and tarda
  - *B* Cartilage hyperplasias
    - *1* Excess of proliferating cartilage: hyperchondroplasia
    - *2* Excess of hypertrophic cartilage: enchondromatosis
- *III* Metaphyseal dysplasias
  - *A* Metaphyseal hypoplasias
    - *1* Failure to form primary spongiosa: hypophosphatasia, congenita and tarda
    - *2* Failure to absorb primary spongiosa: osteopetrosis, congenita and tarda
    - *3* Failure to absorb secondary spongiosa: craniometaphyseal dysplasia, congenita and tarda
  - *B* Metaphyseal hyperplasia
    - *1* Excessive spongiosa: familial exostosis
- *IV* Diaphyseal dysplasias
  - *A* Diaphyseal hypoplasias
    - *1* Failure of periosteal bone formation: osteogenesis imperfecta, congenita and tarda
    - *2* Failure of endosteal bone formation: idiopathic osteoporosis
  - *B* Diaphyseal hyperplasias
    - *1* Excessive periosteal bone formation: Engelmann's disease
    - *2* Excessive periosteal bone formation: hyperphosphatasia

adult life. Flat vertebral bodies are associated with other abnormalities in shape and alignment. The disordered development of the capital femoral epiphyses leads to irregularities in shape and flattening of the femoral heads and early onset of osteoarthritis of the hips.

Achondroplasia *Achondroplasia* is a physeal dysplasia in which dwarfism results from decrease in the proliferation of cartilage in the growth plate. This disorder is among the more common types of dwarfism and is inherited as an autosomal dominant trait. Histologic sections through the growth plate show a thin zone of cartilage cells with absence or abbreviation of the normal columnar arrangement and zone of provisional calcification, although endochondral ossification may not be completely disorganized. Formation of the primary spongiosa is reduced since there is often a transverse bar of bone sealing off the plate from further endochondral ossification. However, formation and maturation of the secondary ossification centers and articular cartilage are not disturbed. Appositional growth at the metaphysis continues, with resulting flare in this region of the bone; intramembranous bone formation at the periosteum is normal. The abnormal proliferation at the growth plate, leaving other areas relatively unaffected in the tubular bones, causes production of short bones that are proportionately thick. However, the length of the spine is almost always normal. The appearance of short limbs with a normal trunk is characteristically accompanied by a large head, saddlenose, and an exaggerated lumbar lordosis. The disease is usually recognized at birth. Those who survive the period of infancy usually have normal mental and sexual development, and life span may be normal. However, spinal deformity may lead to cord compression and nerve root encroachment, especially in those with kyphoscoliosis. Homozygous achondroplasia is a more serious disorder and a cause of neonatal death. In view of the observations in spondyloepiphyseal dysplasia, several of the achondroplasias may also eventually be explained on the basis of defects in genes encoding extracellular matrix components of cartilage such as proteoglycan core protein, types II or IX collagens, or link protein.

Enchondromatosis (dyschondroplasia, Ollier's disease) This is also a disorder affecting the growth plate in which the hypertrophic cartilage is not resorbed and ossified in a normal fashion. It results in masses of cartilage with disorderly arrangement of the chondrocytes showing variable proliferative and hypertrophic changes. These masses are located in the metaphyses in close association with the growth plate in very young patients but often are diaphyseal in teenagers and young adults. The disorder is usually recognized in childhood by the appearance of deformities or retardation in growth. The most common sites of involvement are the ends of long bones, usually in the region where rate of growth is most marked. The pelvis is often involved, but ribs, sternum, and skull are seldom affected. There is also a tendency toward unilateral involvement. Chondrosarcoma develops occasionally in the enchondromata. The association of enchondromatosis and cavernous hemangiomata in the soft tissues including the skin is known as Maffucci's syndrome.

Multiple exostoses (diaphyseal aclasis or osteochondromatosis) This is a disorder of the metaphysis, inherited as an autosomal dominant character, in which areas of the growth plate become displaced, presumably by growing through a defect in the perichondrium or so-called ring of Ranvier. The spongiosa forms within the mass as vessels invade the cartilage. Therefore, the diagnostic radiographic finding is the direct continuity of the mass to the marrow cavity of the parent bone with absence of underlying cortex. Usually the growth of these exostoses ceases when growth of the adjacent plate ceases. The lesions may be solitary or multiple and are usually located in the metaphyseal areas of long bones with the apex of the exostosis directed toward the diaphysis. Often the lesions produce no symptoms, but occasionally interference with the function of a joint or tendon or compression of nerves may result. Dwarfism may occur. The metacarpals may be shortened, resembling those seen in McCune-Albright's hereditary osteodystrophy. Multiple exostoses are sometimes seen in patients with pseudohypoparathyroidism.

An exostosis may suddenly begin to enlarge long after growth should have ceased, and rarely chondrosarcomas may develop from the cartilage cap of an exostosis. Pregnancy may stimulate growth of an exostosis that clinically may mimic malignancy. However, the lesion merely undergoes exuberant endochondral ossification and cartilage hyperplasia without malignant changes.

RELAPSING POLYCHONDRITIS See Chap. 284.

TIETZE'S SYNDROME (COSTOCHONDRAL SYNDROME) See Chap. 284.

REFERENCES

Hyperostosis

Bollerslev J et al: Structural and histomorphometric studies of iliac crest trabecular and cortical bone in autosomal dominant osteopetrosis: A study of two radiological types. Bone 10:19, 1989

Bostman OM et al: Osteosarcoma arising in a melorheostotic femur. J Bone Joint Surg 69A:1232, 1987

Canalis E et al: Dynamic bone morphology and studies on the effects of serum on bone metabolism in vitro in a case of pycnodysostosis. Metab Bone Dis Rel Res 2:99, 1981

Caudle RJ et al: Melorheostosis of the hand. A case report with long-term follow-up. J Bone Joint Surg 69A:1229, 1987

Chan Y-L et al: Dialysis osteodystrophy: A study involving 94 patients. Medicine 64:296, 1985

Coccia PF et al: Successful bone-marrow transplantation for infantile malignant osteopetrosis. N Engl J Med 302:701, 1980

——— et al: Cells that resorb bone. N Engl J Med 310:456, 1984

Coindre JM et al: Histomorphometric analysis of sclerotic bone from idiopathic myeloid metaplasia (nine cases). J Pathol 144:163, 1984

Crisp AJ, Brenton DP: Engelmann's disease of bone—a systemic disorder? Ann Rheum Dis 41:183, 1982

DiGiovanna JJ et al: Extraspinal tendon and ligament calcification associated with long-term therapy with etretinate. N Engl J Med 315:1177, 1986

Einhorn TA et al: Hyperphosphatasemia in an adult. Clinical, roentgenographic, and histomorphometric findings and comparison to classical Paget's disease. Clin Orthop 204:253, 1986

Gennant HK et al: Osteosclerosis in primary hyperparathyroidism. Am J Med 59:104, 1975

Jacobson HG: Dense bone—too much bone: Radiological considerations and differential diagnosis. Part II. Skeletal Radiol 13:97, 1985

Johnson CC et al: Osteopetrosis: A clinical, genetic, metabolic and morphologic study of the dominantly inherited benign form. Medicine 47:149, 1968

Kaplan FS et al: Successful treatment of infantile malignant osteopetrosis by bone-marrow transplantation. J Bone Joint Surg 70A:617, 1988

Key L et al: Treatment of congenital osteopetrosis with high-dose calcitriol. N Engl J Med 310:409, 1984

Kraemer KH et al: Prevention of skin cancer in xeroderma pigmentosum with the use of oral isotretinoin. N Engl J Med 318:1633, 1988

Kumar R et al: An unusual case of pycnodysostosis. Arch Dis Child 63:558, 1988

Manzke E et al: Skeletal remodeling and bone-related hormones in two adults with increased bone mass. Metabolism 31:25, 1982

Mills BG et al: Osteoclasts in human osteopetrosis contain viral-nucleocapsid-like nuclear inclusions. J Bone Min Res 3:101, 1988

Schmidt J et al: Retrovirus-induced osteopetrosis in mice. Effects of viral infection on osteogenic differentiation in skeletoblast cell cultures. Am J Pathol 129:503, 1987

Shapiro F et al: Variable osteoclast appearance in human infantile osteopetrosis. Calcif Tissue Int 43:67, 1988

Sheldon J et al: Engelmann's disease (progressive diaphyseal dysplasia): A review and presentation of two cases with abnormal phosphate retention. Metab Bone Dis Rel Res 2:307, 1981

Sly WS et al: Carbonic anhydrase II deficiency in 12 families with the autosomal recessive syndrome of osteopetrosis with renal tubular acidosis and cerebral calcification. N Engl J Med 313:139, 1985

Thompson RC Jr et al: Hereditary hyperphosphatasia. Am J Med 47:209, 1969

Van Buchem FSP et al: Hyperostosis corticalis generalisata. Am J Med 33:387, 1962

Neoplasms of bone

Bacci G et al: Therapy for primary non-Hodgkin's lymphoma of bone and comparison of results with Ewing's sarcoma. Ten years' experience at the Istituto Ortopedico Rizzoli. Cancer 57:1468, 1986

——— et al: Neoadjuvant chemotherapy for osteosarcoma of the extremity. Clin Orthop 224:268, 1987

Charhon SA et al: Parathyroid function and vitamin D status in patients with bone metastases of prostatic origin. Mineral Electrolyte Metab 11:117, 1985

Dryja TP et al: Chromosome 13 homozygosity in osteosarcoma without retinoblastoma. Am J Hum Genet 38:59, 1986

Ettinger LJ et al: Adjuvant adriamycin and cisplatin in newly diagnosed, nonmetastatic osteosarcoma of the extremity. J Clin Oncol 4:353, 1986

Fechner RE et al: A symposium on the pathology of bone tumors. Pathol Ann 19(Part 1):125, 1984

Goorin AM et al: Osteosarcoma: Fifteen years later. N Engl J Med 313:165, 1985

Han M-T et al: Aggressive thoracotomy for pulmonary metastatic osteogenic sarcoma in children and young adolescents. J Pediatr Surg 16:928, 1981

HAYES FA et al: Metastatic Ewing's sarcoma: Remission induction and survival. J Clin Oncol 5:1199, 1987

VAN HOLTEN-VERZANTVOORT AT et al: Reduced morbidity from skeletal metastases in breast cancer patients during long-term bisphosphonate (APD) treatment. Lancet 2:983, 1987

HUVOS AG: Osteogenic sarcoma of bones and soft tissues in older persons. A clinicopathologic analysis of 117 patients older than 60 years. Cancer 57:1442, 1986

——— et al: Osteogenic sarcoma associated with Paget's disease of bone. A clinicopathologic study of 65 patients. Cancer 52:1489, 1983

KANIS JA (ed): Clodronate—a new perspective in the treatment of neoplastic bone disease. Bone 8(Suppl 1):S1, 1987

KLEEREKOPER M, KRANE SM (eds): *Clinical Disorders of Bone and Mineral Metabolism*. New York, Mary Ann Liebert, pp 1–649, 1989

MANKIN HJ, GEBHARDT MC: Advances in the management of bone tumors. Clin Orthop Rel Res 200:73, 1985

——— et al: The use of frozen cadaveric allografts in the management of patients with bone tumors of the extremities. Orthop Clin North Am 18:275, 1987

MISER JS et al: Preliminary results of treatment of Ewing's sarcoma of bone in children and young adults: Six months of intensive combined modality therapy without maintenance. J Clin Oncol 6:484, 1988

SCHILLER AL: Diagnosis of borderline cartilage lesions of bone. Semin Diag Pathol 2:42, 1985

SIMON MA, NACHMAN J: The clinical utility of preoperative therapy for sarcomas. J Bone Joint Surg 68A:1458, 1986

——— et al: Limb-salvage treatment versus amputation for osteosarcoma of the distal end of the femur. J Bone Joint Surg 68A:1331, 1986

SUIT HD et al: Treatment of the patient with stage M_0 soft tissue sarcoma. J Clin Oncol 6:854, 1988

SUTOW WW et al: Survival after metastasis in osteosarcoma. Natl Cancer Inst Monogr 56:227, 1981

UNNI KK et al: Conditions that simulate primary neoplasms of bone. Pathol Ann 15(Part 1):91, 1980

WIGGS J et al: Prediction of the risk of hereditary retinoblastoma, using DNA polymorphisms within the retinoblastoma gene. N Engl J Med 318:151, 1988

WINKLER K et al: Neoadjuvant chemotherapy of osteosarcoma: Results of a randomized cooperative trial (COSS-82) with salvage chemotherapy based on histological tumor response. J Clin Oncol 6:329, 1988

YUNIS EJ, BARNES L: The histologic diversity of osteosarcoma. Pathol Ann 21(Part 1):121, 1986

Other disorders of bone and cartilage

AKESON WH et al: *Symposium on Heritable Disorders of Connective Tissue*. St. Louis, Mosby, 1982

ALBRIGHT FA et al: Syndrome characterized by osteitis fibrosa disseminata, areas of pigmentation and endocrine dysfunction, with precocious puberty in females. Report of five cases. N Engl J Med 216:727, 1937

BENEDICT PH: Endocrine features in Albright's syndrome (fibrous dysplasia of bone). Metabolism 11:30, 1962

——— et al: Melanotic macules in Albright's syndrome and in neurofibromatosis. JAMA 205:618, 1968

GEFFNER ME et al: Treatment of acromegaly with a somatostatin analog in a patient with McCune-Albright syndrome. J Pediatr 111:740, 1987

GRABIAS SL, CAMPBELL CJ: Fibrous dysplasia. Orthop Clin North Am 8:771, 1977

HARRIS RI: Polyostotic fibrous dysplasia with acromegaly. Am J Med 78:539, 1985

HARRIS WH et al: The natural history of fibrous dysplasia: An orthopaedic, pathological and roentgenographic study. J Bone Joint Surg (Br) 44A:207, 1962

KAPLAN FS et al: Estrogen receptors in bone in a patient with polyostotic fibrous dysplasia (McCune-Albright syndrome). N Engl J Med 319:421, 1988

LEE B et al: Identification of the molecular defect in a family with spondyloepiphyseal dysplasia. Science 244:978, 1989

NAGER GT et al: Fibrous dysplasia: A review of the disease and its manifestations in the temporal bone. Ann Otol Rhinol Laryngol 91(suppl 92):1, 1982

PALOTIE A et al: Predisposition to familial osteoarthrosis linked to type II collagen gene. Lancet 1:924, 1989

RIMOIN DL: The chondrodystrophies. Adv Hum Genet 5:1, 1975

RUBIN P: *Dynamic Classification of Bone Dysplasias*. Chicago, Year Book, 1964

SAMBROOK PN et al: Synovial complications of spondylepiphyseal dysplasia of late onset. Arthritis Rheum 31:282, 1988

SILLENCE DO et al: Neonatal dwarfism. Pediatr Clin North Am 25:431, 1978

STEPHENSON RB et al: Fibrous dysplasia. An analysis of options for treatment. J Bone Joint Surg 69A:409, 1987

YABUL SM et al: Malignant transformation of fibrous dysplasia. A case report and review of the literature. Clin Orthop 281, 1988

PART THIRTEEN NEUROLOGIC DISORDERS

346 IMPACT OF NEUROBIOLOGY ON NEUROLOGY AND PSYCHIATRY

JOSEPH B. MARTIN

Advances in molecular genetics, neurobiology, and brain imaging are having a major impact on neurology and psychiatry. These advances are changing our understanding of how the brain is constructed and of the way it functions. They are also expanding the repertoire of experimental approaches, some of which may be successful in solving both basic and clinical problems. The discoveries imply the possibility of defining a rational taxonomy for many of the inherited diseases affecting the nervous system, enable new approaches for understanding the molecular basis of development (and degeneration) of the nervous system, and permit analysis of cognitive brain function in ways not previously possible.

The advances have occurred on several fronts, which are now beginning to coalesce into a general move forward. The identification of genes responsible for several of the inherited neuropsychiatric diseases has provided insight into their pathogenesis. Research in molecular structure has disclosed several proteins that subserve receptor and membrane channel functions (see Chap. 11). Elucidation of neurotransmitter signal transduction has modified our perception of intercellular and intracellular communication. These discoveries have major implications for drug development by permitting identification of more selective receptor agonists and antagonists. There is also new insight into the mechanisms of cellular injury and neuronal death. The ability to analyze neuronal structure and function extends also to the intact brain. Positron emission tomography (PET) and in vivo magnetic resonance spectroscopy now provide means for analysis of the functional organization of the brain.

The impacts of some of these efforts are reviewed in this chapter.

MOLECULAR GENETICS Applications of molecular biology have already had a major effect on the clinical neurosciences. In the case of inherited neurologic diseases, there is the use of DNA probes that demonstrate restriction fragment length polymorphisms (RFLPs), which can be combined with linkage analysis in affected pedigrees (see Chap. 6). These tools have made possible the chromosomal localization of the mutant gene in Huntington's disease (see Chap. 359), some cases of familial Alzheimer's disease (see Chap. 359), neurofibromatosis (see Chap. 358), Friedreich's ataxia (see Chap. 359), spinal muscular atrophy, torsion dystonia, Wilson's disease, and several types of familial CNS tumors including retinoblastoma and von Hippel–Lindau disease (see Table 346-1). The use of linkage analysis with chromosome-specific RFLPs is the first step toward characterization of the abnormal gene product, a process referred to as "reverse genetics," i.e., analysis of gene structure makes possible studies of the abnormal cellular protein (see Chap. 285).

In two conditions this approach has already affected clinical practice. In Duchenne's dystrophy, an X-linked disorder, the muscle abnormality results from failure to encode for a membrane protein, *dystrophin,* which is absent from skeletal muscle in virtually all patients with the disorder (see Chap. 365). This discovery has proved of theoretical importance in a less severe allied condition, Becker's dystrophy, where dystrophin is present but in abnormal amounts or of abnormal size. Dystrophin is also present in smooth muscle, cardiac muscle, and brain. Its presence in the brain presumably accounts in some way yet to be defined for the frequent occurrence of mental retardation in individuals with Duchenne's dystrophy. The precise function of dystrophin remains to be elucidated, but it is now known to be a membrane-associated structural protein that appears to function as a strut to maintain membrane integrity during muscular contraction. The discovery of dystrophin demonstrates elegantly the power of reverse genetics. Decades of effort attempting to define the protein abnormality in Duchenne's dystrophy had been unsuccessful. The quantities of dystrophin present in muscle are so minute that it could not have been characterized by current biochemical approaches.

In retinoblastoma, identification of the protein encoded by the normal allele of the gene (a growth suppressor gene) that is absent from the tumor has provided insight into cellular growth. It is postulated that an inherited mutation affects one allele of the normal gene. If this is followed by a "second hit" mutation that eliminates the function of the second allele in one of the cells in the developing retina, the cell growth suppressor cannot be synthesized. The consequence is the abnormal division of cells in the retina and tumor formation (see also Chap. 10). Another tumor associated with hereditary retinoblastoma is osteosarcoma. A similar mechanism for tumor formation may be involved in Wilms' tumor (on chromosome 11) and in the von Hippel–Lindau syndrome, which leads to hemangioblastoma, pheochromocytoma, and renal cell carcinoma (shown by RFLPs to be located on chromosome 3) (see Table 346-1).

The application of RFLPs has provided new approaches to presymptomatic and prenatal diagnosis of Huntington's disease (Fig. 346-1), Duchenne's dystrophy, retinoblastoma, and von Hippel–Lindau disease (see also Chap. 353).

CHARACTERIZATION OF NEW NEUROTRANSMITTER CANDIDATES More than 60 neurotransmitter candidates have been identified in brain based upon localization within synaptic vesicles, release with depolarization, and interactions with postsynaptic receptors. The functions of these agents, many of which are small-molecular-weight peptides (neuropeptides), remain obscure in many cases. But some are known to modulate functions such as pain transmission (opioid peptides), satiety (cholecystokinin), and thirst (angiotensin).

The discovery of these molecules has made possible new approaches to defining neuronal populations in the human brain by immunohistochemical staining, autoradiography, and in situ messenger RNA hybridization. This information has made it possible to delineate the subclasses of cells affected in neurodegenerative diseases, such as Alzheimer's, Parkinson's, and Huntington's disease. Realization that dopamine cells are affected in Parkinson's disease led to the idea of therapy with levodopa. In Huntington's disease, it has been possible to define the subsets of neurons affected by the degenerative process in the striatum and to show selective sparing of other cell types (see Chap. 359). Although this has not led yet to specific theories about the mechanisms of cell death, it has resulted in speculations about potentially beneficial therapeutic strategies.

Many of these newly discovered neuropeptides appear to share

TABLE 346-1 Chromosomal localization and gene abnormalities in selected neurologic diseases

Genetic classification and disease	Chromosome	Gene defect	Comments on genetic heterogeneity
AUTOSOMAL DOMINANT			
Charcot-Marie-Tooth disease (type 1)	1p22–1q23	Unknown	Unknown
von Hippel–Lindau disease	3p	Unknown (possible deficiency in growth suppressor gene)	None demonstrated in over 10 pedigrees
Huntington's disease	4p16.3	Unknown	None demonstrated in over 100 pedigrees
Spinocerebellar ataxia (one form)	6p21.2–q12	Unknown	Unknown
Torsion dystonia	9q32–q34	Unknown	None demonstrated
Retinoblastoma	13q14	Absence of Rb protein	Allelic heterogeneity
von Recklinghausen's neurofibromatosis (NFI)	17q11.2	Unknown	None demonstrated in over 25 pedigrees
Familial amyloidotic polyneuropathy	18q11.2–q12.1	Single-base pair substitution in mRNA for transthyretin	Allelic heterogeneity
Myotonic dystrophy	19–centromere	Unknown	None demonstrated
Benign familial convulsions	20q13.2	Unknown	Unknown
Familial Alzheimer's disease	21q21	Unknown (not amyloid protein)	Probable heterogeneity
Bilateral acoustic neurofibromatosis (NF2)	22q11–q13	Unknown	Unknown
AUTOSOMAL RECESSIVE			
Gaucher's disease	1q21	Amino acid substitution in glucocerebrosidase	Allelic heterogeneity
Spinal muscular atrophy	5q11.2–q13.3		None demonstrated
Friedreich's ataxia	9p22–centromere	Unknown	None found in 23 pedigrees
Ataxia-telangiectasia	11q22–23	Unknown	None found in 31 families
Wilson's disease	13q14.11	Unknown (not ceruloplasmin)	Unknown
G_{M2} gangliosidosis			
Tay-Sachs disease (type 1)	15q22–q25	Mutation in gene encoding α chain of hexosaminidase	Allelic heterogeneity
Sandhoff's disease (type 2)	5q13	Mutation in gene encoding β chain of hexosaminidase	Allelic heterogeneity
X-LINKED RECESSIVE			
Duchenne's dystrophy	Xp21.21	Absence of dystrophin	Multiallelic heterogeneity
Becker's dystrophy	Xp21.21	Defect in dystrophin	Multiallelic heterogeneity
Pelizaeus-Merzbacher disease	Xq21–q22	Defect in myelin proteolipid protein	Unknown
Adrenoleukodystrophy	Xq27–q28	Unknown	Unknown
Lesch-Nyhan syndrome	Xq27	Hypoxanthine-guanine phosphoribosyltransferase deficiency	Multiallelic heterogeneity
Emery-Dreifuss dystrophy	Xq28	Unknown	Unknown
MITOCHONDRIAL DISEASES WITH MATERNAL TRANSMISSION			
Mitochondrial myopathy		Deletion in mitochondrial DNA	
Leber's hereditary optic atrophy		Amino acid substitution in NADH dehydrogenase, subunit 4	

SOURCE: Modified from JB Martin, 1989. Reproduced with permission.

nerve terminals and often even secretory vesicles with conventional neurotransmitters. It appears likely that neuropeptides exert profound modulatory effects on the actions of the primary neurotransmitter. In other cases the peptide may influence neuronal plasticity, growth, or differentiation.

BIOCHEMICAL CLASSIFICATION OF RECEPTOR SUBTYPES Some of the most important insights from the new biology have resulted from the cloning of the genes of several neurotransmitter and hormone receptors that were identified originally by pharmacologic means. Based on pharmacologic analysis alone it was difficult to account for the diverse effects mediated by molecules of low molecular weight. For example, acetylcholine has many diverse effects that on pharmacologic analysis were divided into muscarinic and nicotinic effects. With the biochemical elucidation of acetylcholine receptor subtypes and through the use of molecular cloning techniques and molecular probes, it is now established that multiple forms of muscarinic (M1, M2, M3, M4, and M5) and nicotinic (N1 and N2) receptors exist in the brain and that their distribution varies from region to region. Thus, differences in receptor subtypes expressed in different regions of the brain can account for the complex multiple effects of the medications acting on cholinergic receptors. The molecular specificities of the various receptor subtypes provide sensitive systems with which to search for selective agonists and antagonists. For example, M1 agonists may facilitate memory. Regional differences in the distribution of the subtypes of the nicotinic cholinergic receptor in the central nervous system make it possible to explore the neurologic basis of nicotine addiction.

Identification of the subclasses of the alpha- and beta-adrenergic receptors, of serotonin receptors, and of gamma-aminobutyric acid (GABA) receptors makes it possible to correlate structure and function and provide a rational basis for molecular classification of drug actions. In the case of the GABA receptor, structural features that account for the interaction of barbiturates and benzodiazepines can now be elucidated (see Snyder).

Subclasses of glutamate receptors that mediate excitatory amino acid neurotransmitter effects have also been defined. Glutamate, one of the most abundant of all neurotransmitters in the brain, functions to promote rapid neurotransmitter depolarization by opening membrane channels that permit diffusion of sodium and potassium ions. These rapid effects are mediated by two receptor subtypes, identified by ligand binding with kainate and quisqualate. The identification of an additional subtype of glutamate receptor which binds *N*-methyl-D-aspartate (the *NMDA receptor*) made possible identification of additional glutamate functions. The NMDA receptor appears to mediate other functions that heretofore were classed in the category of plasticity, a process considered important, for example, in memory and learning. The NMDA subtype of glutamate receptor is linked to a voltage-sensitive channel that responds to repetitive activation by the opening of an ion channel (Fig. 346-2; see also Chap. 11). The actions of calcium permit transduction of electrical events into

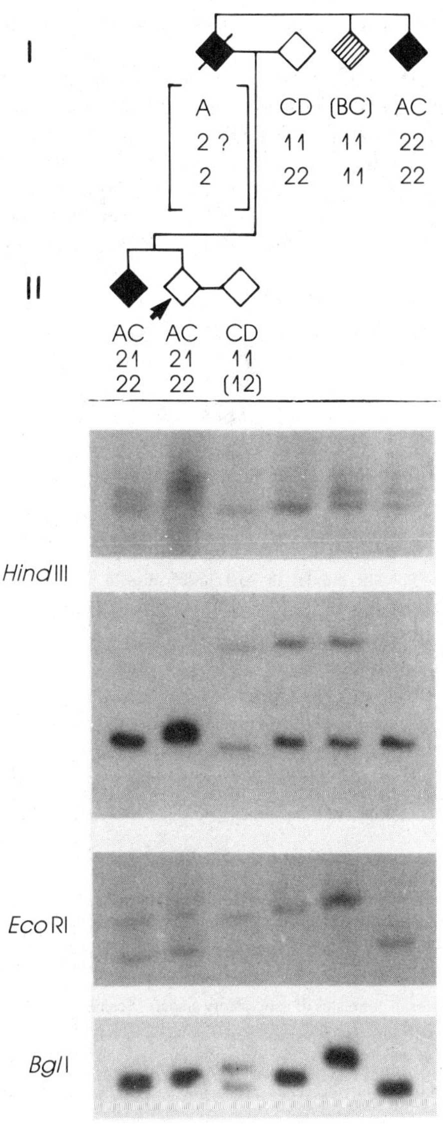

FIGURE 346-1 Sample family pedigree and Southern blot for a positive predictive test for Huntington's disease. Solid symbols denote a person with Huntington's disease; a diagonal line, a dead person; and crosshatched symbols, a person suspected to have Huntington's disease; the arrow indicates the family member who requested the predictive test. *Hind*III, *Eco*RI, and *Bgl*I were employed to detect alternate forms of RFLPs. *Hind*III recognized two different RFLPs, producing A, B, C, and D patterns, whereas *Eco*RI and *Bgl*I recognized only one RFLP (1 or 2). In cases in which the combination of alleles grouped together on a specific chromosome or phase could not be specified, alleles with alternative possible phases are depicted in parentheses (i.e., C11/D12 could be C12/D11 for subject II-3). Markers reconstructed for a deceased subject are enclosed in brackets. The affected sibling (I-4) of the affected parent (I-1) and the affected sibling (II-1) of the participant (II-2) had only the A22 haplotype (set of alleles located on same chromosome) in common; therefore, the Huntington's disease gene appeared to segregate with A22. A sibling (I-3) of the affected parent with neurologic symptoms that were suspected of indicating the presence of Huntington's disease did not have the A22 form of the marker. The participant inherited from the affected parent the A22 form of the marker allele apparently linked to the Huntington's disease gene, since the C12 was inherited from the unaffected parent. *(From GJ Meissen et al, with permission.)*

molecular changes that can alter neuronal function permanently, i.e., change cellular function to subserve a memory or learning response.

It now appears, on the basis of quite definitive experimentation, that activation of the NMDA receptor can also have deleterious effects on the cell, whereby calcium entry induces *neurotoxicity* that, if sufficiently severe, can lead to neuronal cell death. This mechanism may explain some of the extensive neuronal cell damage that occurs in ischemia, hypoxia, epilepsy, and, perhaps, neurodegenerative diseases (see Choi).

These findings have resulted in great interest in the development of new drugs that might selectively block the NMDA receptor, thereby minimizing the effects of ischemia or hypoxia that occur in stroke or after cardiorespiratory arrest. The profound potential of this work is illustrated by the demonstration that NMDA receptor blockade induced even several hours after the neuronal insult may be "neuroprotective."

Cloning of cellular membrane channels (sodium, potassium, calcium) has also had a profound effect on defining mechanisms of neuronal excitability. It can be expected that these findings will also be translated into discovery of more effective neuroactive drugs.

BRAIN IMAGING The development of computed tomography and proton imaging by magnetic resonance has revolutionized our ability to define lesions in the brain and spinal cord (see Chap. 348). Other techniques have been developed to make it possible to study brain function as well as structure by the application of positron emission tomography (PET), single photon emission computed tomography (SPECT), and nuclear magnetic resonance spectroscopy (NMRS).

PET scanning involves the use of positron-emitting radionuclides with short half-lives in which particle disintegration is captured in a three-dimensional array by multiple sensors positioned about the head. With the use of radioisotopes for carbon (^{11}C), oxygen (^{15}O), and fluorine (^{18}F), it is possible to measure cerebral blood flow, cerebral oxygen metabolism, and cerebral glucose uptake (with ^{18}F-labeled deoxyglucose). The last technique uses the principles devel-

FIGURE 346-2 Model of proposed mechanisms of activation and deactivation of glutamate (GLU) *N*-methyl-D-aspartate (NMDA) receptor-channel complex. *A* and *B*. Glutamate attaches to receptor to cause opening of channel, first to Na^+ and K^+ and, after membrane depolarization, to Ca^{++}. Glycine (GLY) modulates effects of GLU. *C*. Competitive receptor antagonists, such as AP5 can prevent GLU activation. *D*. Other drugs and ions can block an opened channel by noncompetitive antagonism. These drugs include phencyclidine (PCP) and an experimental neuroprotective drug, MK801. Mg^{++} can also block the channel.

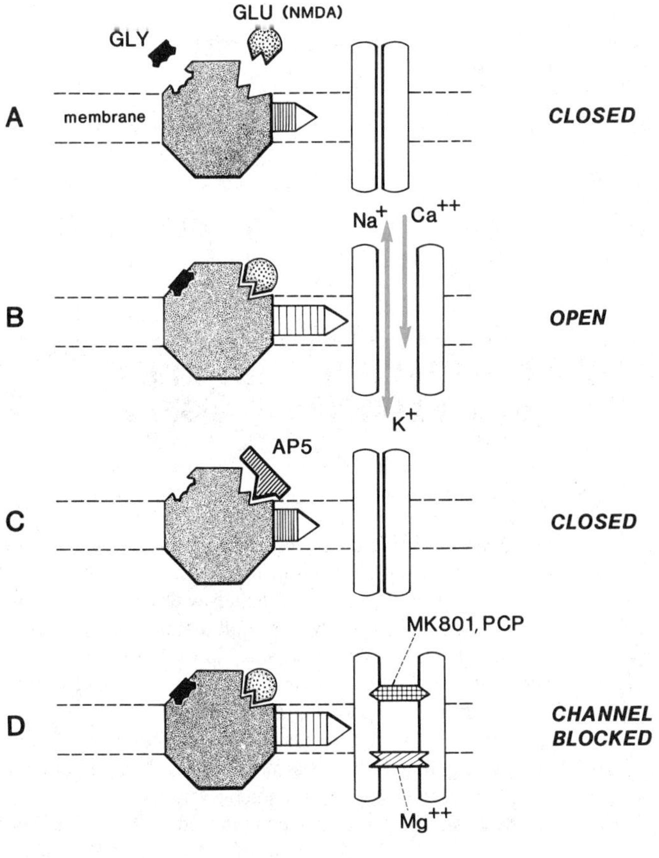

oped by Sokoloff and colleagues, who first used the technique of labeled deoxyglucose combined with tissue section autoradiography. PET scanning is also used to define regional changes in cerebral function associated with stroke, Alzheimer's disease, Huntington's disease, and schizophrenia, and it identifies foci of hyperactivity associated with seizures.

Perhaps the most creative use of PET techniques has been analysis of language function. Two theories of language had emerged from studies in neurology and linguistics. The first proposed that language function occurs serially, i.e., an object is first seen in the occipital lobes, its name is recalled by the temporal lobes, and the information is then sent to the frontal lobes, which direct formation of speech. PET studies have now confirmed the second of these hypotheses, which suggested from linguistic analysis that language occurs in a parallel array. Posner and colleagues, using subtraction techniques to isolate activity associated with a particular language task, have shown clearly that brain processing occurs simultaneously in several of the regions underlying a set of neurologic functions. These kinds of analyses now permit regionalized functional study of the brain in a manner not hitherto expected by the physical limits set by three-dimensional imaging using positron emitters. Regional studies of this kind have also shown that brain blood flow changes that occur in panic disorder and anticipatory anxiety correlate with anatomic loci in the temporal lobes.

There have also been important advances in the use of radioligands for neurotransmitter receptors. The imaging of dopamine and of dopamine receptors in the basal ganglia has been achieved in both normals and in patients with Parkinson's disease and with 1-methyl-4-phenyl-1,2,3,6-tetrahydropyridine (MPTP) poisoning. In the latter case deficits in basal ganglion function in asymptomatic subjects exposed to MPTP raise the possibility of identifying subclinical deficits and of following subjects over time to determine eventual outcome and prognosis.

SPECT imaging has been made possible by refinements in detection systems for single photon emitters. The resolution of SPECT does not yet reach the capacity of PET, but the longer half-lives of the isotopes and the simplicity of the detection systems make it less expensive and potentially more widely available. Its potential includes measurement of radioligand binding to receptors and determination of cerebral blood flow. Thus far, studies with SPECT have delineated regional changes in brain metabolism and blood flow in the neurodegenerative diseases.

NMR spectroscopy offers an opportunity to assess brain function at the subcellular molecular level. The technique uses natural emissions from atomic nuclei activated by magnetic fields to measure endogenous molecules. Potential nuclei include ^{31}P, ^{13}C, ^{23}Na, ^{7}Li, in addition to ^{1}H. The promise of analysis of ^{31}P is the closest to realization. It is possible to quantitate several phosphate-containing compounds (phosphocreatine, ATP, ADP, and inorganic phosphorus). The combination of spectral analysis with topical NMR permits localization within superficial regions of brain. It can be anticipated that further refinements of this technique will make possible measurement of brain metabolism with spatial resolution that may exceed that of PET.

REFERENCES

BREAKEFIELD XO, CAMBI F: Molecular genetic insights into neurologic diseases, in *Annual Review of Neuroscience*, vol 10, WM Cowan et al (eds). Palo Alto, Annual Reviews, 1987, pp 535–594

BROWN GG et al: In vivo ^{31}P NMR profiles of Alzheimer's disease and multiple subcortical infarct dementia. Neurology 39:1423, 1989

BUCKLEY NJ et al: Antagonist binding properties of five cloned muscarinic receptors expressed in CHO-K1 cells. Molec Pharmacol 35(4):469, 1989

CHOI D: Glutamate neurotoxicity and diseases of the nervous system. Neuron 1:623, 1989

COOPER JR et al: *The Biochemical Basis of Neuropharmacology*. New York, Oxford University Press, 1986

GUSELLA JF et al: DNA markers for nervous system diseases. Science 225:1320, 1984

MARTIN JB: Molecular genetics: Applications to the clinical neurosciences. Science 238:765, 1987

———: Molecular genetic studies in the neuropsychiatric disorders. Trends Neurosci 12:130, 1989

MEISSEN GJ et al: Predictive testing for Huntington's disease with use of a linked DNA marker. N Engl J Med 318:535, 1988

PETTEGREW JW et al: ^{31}P nuclear magnetic resonance studies of phosphoglyceride metabolism in developing and degenerating brain: Preliminary observations. J Neuropathol Exp Neurol 46:419, 1987

POSNER MI et al: Localization of cognitive operations in the human brain. Science 240:1627, 1988

REIMAN EM et al: Neuroanatomical correlates of anticipatory anxiety. Science 243:1071, 1989

ROWE CC et al: Localization of epileptic foci with postictal single photon emission computed tomography. Ann Neurol 26:660, 1989

SNYDER SH: Drug and neurotransmitter receptors: New perspectives with clinical relevance. JAMA 261:3126, 1989

section 1 The central nervous system

347 APPROACH TO THE PATIENT WITH NEUROLOGIC DISEASE

JOSEPH B. MARTIN

Symptoms and signs of disordered nervous system function are among the most frequent and complex in clinical medicine. Because neurologic disorders may affect cognitive function with disturbances in language, perception, and memory, as well as produce specific symptoms referable to subcortical structures, spinal cord, peripheral nerve, or muscle, the array of symptoms and signs presented to the physician are numerous and diverse. A careful assessment of the character and pattern of the symptoms, their temporal profile, and associated complaints, together with a focused neurologic examination, permit a conclusion to be reached among various alternatives.

These considerations are made more complicated by the difficulties that often arise in distinguishing so-called neurologic from psychiatric diseases. In general, the neurologist has defined disease of the nervous system as any condition that produces a visible anatomic or definable biochemical lesion. However, it is now recognized that many primary neurologic disorders, which present with severe clinical manifestations, fail to show any demonstrable neuropathologic or neurochemical abnormality, even when scrutinized by the most modern techniques of neurobiology. The conditions of dystonia musculorum deformans, spasmodic torticollis, tardive dyskinesia, and Gilles de la Tourette's syndrome, for example, are considered to be neurologic disorders, yet no defined structural abnormality has been reported. The possibility that such disorders are caused by abnormalities of neurotransmitter release or of receptor function is currently viewed as likely because of their partial response to various neuropharmacologic drugs. In other disorders traditionally treated by the psychiatrist, in particular the major psychoses of schizophrenia and of manic-depressive disease, accumulated evidence based on genetic analysis, responses to neuroactive agents, and documented neuroendocrine-biochemical abnormalities suggest that these, too, are primary disorders of nervous system function. This conclusion is supported further by observations that similar psychotic symptoms can be observed in patients with readily identifiable lesions of the nervous system (chronic temporal lobe seizures, brain tumor) or after the administration of certain drugs, such as lysergic acid or amphetamines.

Despite the importance of these areas of overlap between neurology and psychiatry, most neurologic conditions for which a patient seeks general medical care are due to readily demonstrated disease processes. It is the task of the clinician to develop a neurologic method of analysis that will result in accurate diagnosis of the site of the disorder and of its likely cause. Only then can effective approaches to management and treatment be developed.

In this and the subsequent sections, neurology and psychiatry are considered separately because many of the approaches to diagnosis and treatment remain distinct even today. In the chapters that follow, neurologic disorders and diseases are described as they present to the neurologist or general internist. Currently accepted explanations in terms of anatomy, physiology, pharmacology, and chemistry are offered. The section on psychiatric disorders is found in Chaps. 368 and 369. Dependency syndromes are described in Chaps. 370 to 373.

THE NEUROLOGIC METHOD OF CLINICAL EVALUATION The strategy used in evaluating a patient with neurologic illness is to begin with the question, Where is the lesion that is causing the neurologic symptoms? The first clues to answering this question appear in the history, and the examination is then "tailor-made" to clarify uncertainties or to make distinctions suggested by the history. Thus, optokinetic nystagmus might be an important part of the examination in a patient with a left hemiparesis and dressing apraxia, but irrelevant to the examination of a patient complaining of burning feet. In a patient who presents with the history of ascending paresthesia and weakness, the examination must be *directed* to deciding, among other things, if the location of the lesion is the spinal cord or peripheral nerves. Notations regarding muscle stamina or endurance might be crucial to the examination of a patient with myasthenia gravis, as opposed to the usual tests of peak muscle power. What one does with the neurologic examination depends on what the questions are; the questions are formulated by a properly taken history.

Deciding "where the lesion is" accomplishes the task of delimiting the number of possible etiologies to a manageable, finite size. In addition, this strategy safeguards against making really tragic errors. Symptoms of recurrent vertigo, diplopia, and nystagmus should not trigger "multiple sclerosis" as an answer (etiology), but "brainstem" or "pons" (location); then a diagnosis of brainstem arteriovenous malformation will not be missed because it is not considered. The combination of optic neuritis and spastic, ataxic paraparesis should not be memorized as "multiple sclerosis"; then central nervous system syphilis and vitamin B_{12} deficiency (both treatable) will not be overlooked.

Only after the clinician decides "where the lesion is," should the question "what the lesion is" be asked.

The neurologic history A bewildering array of clinical abnormalities require documentation and interpretation during the neurologic evaluation of a patient. The analysis becomes difficult because similar symptoms and signs may present in a patient with any of several disorders. A number of general principles relevant to obtaining a complete neurologic history are important for the physician, whether a generalist or a specialist. Careful attention to the description of the symptoms as experienced by the patient and substantiated by family members or friends permits, in many instances, an accurate localization and determination of the probable cause of the complaints even before an examination of the patient has been undertaken. Two principles should be followed. First, each complaint ought to be chased down as far as possible in an effort to delineate (before the examination) where the lesion might be or, more importantly, *to formulate a set of questions to be answered by the examination.* A patient complains of weakness of the right upper limb. What are the associated features? Is this weakness for brushing the hair or opening a twist-top can? Second, in neurology—where many of the diseases are due to *anatomically restricted* lesions—*negative* associations may be crucial. A patient with a right hemiparesis without a language deficit likely has a different lesion (and likely etiology) than a patient with a right hemiparesis and aphasia. Several of the important factors that aid greatly in defining the nature of the neurologic disorder include:

1 *Temporal course of the illness.* It is particularly important to ascertain the precise rate of appearance and progression of the symptoms experienced by the patient. A paroxysmal onset of a neurologic complaint, occurring within seconds or minutes, usually indicates a cerebrovascular lesion or a seizure. Attention to the temporal march of symptoms may help define a focal seizure, a transient cerebral ischemic attack (TIA), or the onset of a migraine. For example, the onset of sensory symptoms located in one extremity that spreads over a few seconds to adjacent portions of that extremity and then to the other limb or to the face suggests a seizure. A more gradual onset involving less discrete regions of the extremities points to the possibility of a TIA. A similar, but slower progression of sensory change occurring in a young person together with other symptoms of headache, nausea, or visual disturbance suggest migraine. In general, the march of a migraine is slower than that of seizure, and a TIA tends to be more generalized in location on the side of the body or extremities. The presence of positive sensory symptoms or motor movements suggests a seizure; in contrast, transient loss of a function (negative symptom) suggests a TIA. A stuttering onset where symptoms appear, stabilize, regress, and then progress over hours or days also suggests the presence of impending vascular ischemia. In some cases, a demyelinating process may produce new symptoms over the course of a few hours. Progressing symptoms associated with the systemic manifestation of fever, stiff neck, and altered level of consciousness or awareness suggest the possibility of an infectious process. The course of the illness over years in terms of remissions and exacerbations offers additional clues to the nature of the process. Recurrent neurologic symptoms involving any level of the neuraxis with partial or complete recovery suggest the possibility of multiple sclerosis. Slowly progressive disorders without remissions tend to be characteristic of the neurodegenerative processes that affect the nervous system.

2 *Subjective descriptions of the complaint.* It is wise for the physician to recall that patient vocabularies are often limited and that symptoms are interpreted within the experience of the patient. Descriptions are highly introspective and subject to the patient's degree of intelligence and general familiarity with medical terminology. The same words often mean very different things to individual patients. For example, dizziness may be a description applied by the patient to impending syncope, to a sense of giddiness, or to true vertigo. Numbness may mean a complete loss of feeling, a positive sensation of tingling, or paralysis. Blurring of vision may be used to describe unilateral visual loss, as in amaurosis fugax, or diplopia. It is important to determine the level of understanding that the patient exhibits with respect to the complaint in order to assess accurately the precise significance of the symptom.

3 *Corroboration of the history by other close associates.* It is often useful to obtain additional information from family, friends, or observers to corroborate or expand the patient's description. Memory loss, personality change, drug abuse, excess alcohol intake, and other factors may severely impair the ability of patients to describe accurately their subjective experiences or prevent them from being completely open and forthright about the factors that have contributed to the illness. Complaints of loss of consciousness that may be due to syncope or seizures necessitate seeking details from patients and family to ascertain the exact circumstances. It is often important to recognize the major manifestations of depression and anxiety that may mask or color the presentation given by the patient. Failure to note these underlying factors which

interfere with the patient's performance may result in the incorrect interpretation that a variety of complaints are actually due to structural disease of the brain.

4 *Family history.* Many neurologic disorders, particularly those presenting in childhood or early adulthood, are familial or inherited conditions. It is important to ascertain the familial frequency of occurrence of systemic diseases such as hypertension, heart disease, or stroke, which may affect the nervous system. It is essential to inquire about the possibility of consanguinity of the parents or of the existence of similar symptoms in other members of the family. These may provide clues to a propensity toward a hereditary neurologic condition. It is critical to distinguish between a *negative* family history and an *incomplete* family history. It is insufficient to simply ask, Is there any similar illness in any member of your family? A negative response to such an inquiry may mean that there is, in fact, no such illness in the patient's family, but it may also mean that the patient is unfamiliar with relatives or their medical histories. It is wise to elicit specific positive or negative data about relatives as follows: Are your parents living? If so, are they well? If not, what illness did they have and how did they die? It should always be remembered that maternity is a fact, but paternity is only an assumption.

It is also important to elicit family history data regarding all illnesses rather than just neurologic and psychiatric disorders. Many familial neurologic illnesses are associated with signs and symptoms in other systems (e.g., the phakomatoses, hepatocerebral disorders, neuroophthalmic syndromes, etc.).

5 *Medical illnesses.* Many neurologic illnesses occur in the context of systemic disorders. A history of allergy and asthma may suggest the onset of polyarteritis, with mononeuritis multiplex. Previous or current medical illnesses such as diabetes mellitus, hypertension, and abnormalities of blood lipids may be relevant to evolving symptoms that affect the nervous system. Similarly, the presence of systemic diseases that have an increased association with peripheral neuropathy should be explored. Most patients with coma in a hospital setting can be shown to have a metabolic, toxic, or infectious process.

6 *The patient's perception of the disease.* It is frequently helpful to ask patients what they perceive to be wrong. Do they have a particular fear about a disease like Alzheimer's disease, a brain tumor, or multiple sclerosis? Increasingly, patients who complain of failing memory are concerned about early symptoms of Alzheimer's disease. Patients with headaches may fear that a tumor or an impending stroke is a possibility. Patients with sensory symptoms frequently are concerned about the possibility of multiple sclerosis. Or the patient may seek attention because a relative or friend has been diagnosed with a serious neurologic illness.

7 *Drug use and abuse and toxin exposure.* It is essential to inquire about the history of drug use, both prescribed and illicit. Complaints of yellow vision may occur with digitalis administration. Excessive vitamin administration may lead to peripheral neuropathy, as has been demonstrated in the case of pyridoxine. Aminoglycoside antibiotics may exacerbate symptoms of weakness in patients with disorders of neuromuscular transmission, such as myasthenia gravis. Dizziness may be secondary to ototoxicity caused by the aminoglycosides. In eliciting a history of drug use it is often necessary to be quite specific and to use lay terminology. Most patients are, for example, unaware that over-the-counter sleeping pills, cold preparations, and diet pills are actually drugs. Alcohol, the most prevalent neurotoxin, is often not recognized as such by patients. History of environmental or industrial exposure to neurotoxins may provide the essential clue; consultation with the patient's family or employer may be required.

8 *History of malignancy.* Because malignant tumors may present with nervous system metastases or occasionally with any of several paraneoplastic syndromes, it is important to determine whether any history of malignancy exists and whether chemotherapy or radiotherapy was given. Patients with prior malignancy can present with unexpected and unusual neurologic complications.

9 *Formulating an impression of the patient.* Use the opportunity while taking the history to form an impression of the patient. Is there evidence of anxiety, depression, hypochondriasis? Are there any clues to defects of language, memory, inappropriate behavior, or secondary gain? The neurologic assessment begins as soon as the patient walks into the room and the first introduction is made.

The neurologic examination After obtaining a complete medical and neurologic history, the physician should have reliable clues to the portions of the nervous system to be examined. By the elicitation of specific signs it is then determined whether the nervous system is affected, and, if so, to what degree and which part. The anatomic localization of the lesion assumes special significance in neurology, as certain diseases are known to affect certain regions of the nervous system and not to involve others. Recognition of a constellation of symptoms and signs (a syndrome) points to the possible existence of certain diseases and to the exclusion of others.

A systematic neurologic examination should encompass a survey of all functions from the cerebrum to peripheral nerve and muscle, i.e., from the mental status examination to the simplest reflexes. Such a detailed examination requires the performance of a series of physical tests aimed at eliciting the functional capacities of each part of the nervous system. The examiner must acquire skills that come only from the repeated use of the same techniques and instruments on a large number of normal and abnormal individuals. Errors and serious omissions are avoided if the examination procedure is orderly and systemic, beginning with mental (cerebral) functions and continuing with cranial nerves, then with motor, reflex, and sensory functions of the arms, trunk, and legs, and finishing with an analysis of posture and gait.

The mental status is already appreciated while the history is being taken. But rather profound disorders of recent memory or of spatial organization may be missed unless specifically tested for. Faults of memory, incoherence of thought, dominating ideas, peculiarities of mood and outlook, aphasic errors, problems of articulation, and loss of insight and judgment should be sought. If abnormalities are noted, a more formal analysis of these functions is undertaken along the lines suggested in Chaps. 29, 30, 32, and 33. The function of each cranial nerve is then examined in order, beginning with olfaction (see Chaps. 22, 23, 24, and 360). Examination of the motor system should include estimates of power of each of the major muscle groups, evidence of atrophy or fasciculation, and assessment of the tone of the musculature during passive manipulations, looking for signs of spasticity, rigidity, or hypotonia (as outlined in Chaps. 25 and 362). Speed and coordination of the limbs are assessed. Next, prevailing postures and the stance and gait are evaluated (Chap. 26). The tendon reflexes are examined for evidence of increased or decreased (or absent) response or of asymmetry between right and left sides or between arms and legs. The superficial cutaneous reflexes, abdominal and plantar, are then evaluated. Touch, pain, vibration, and joint-position sense are tested as the final part of the examination (see Chap. 28).

This detailed neurologic examination is undertaken only if there are symptoms of disturbed nervous system functioning. If none are present, it suffices to do an abbreviated examination which includes evaluation only of pupils, ocular movements, optic fundi, facial movements, speech, strength of arm and leg muscles, tendon and plantar reflexes, pain and vibratory sensation in hands and feet, and gait. All of this can be completed in 3 to 5 min. The findings, even in the short examination, should be recorded in the patient's record for future reference.

Two additional points about the examination are worth noting. First, in recording observations it is important for the physician to describe what is found, rather than to apply a poorly defined medical term (i.e., "patient groans to sternal rub" rather than "obtunded").

Second, if the patient's complaint is brought out by some activity, reproduce the activity in the office. If the complaint is of dizziness when raising the right arm and turning the head to the left, have the patient do it. If pain occurs after walking two blocks, have the patient demonstrate it and repeat the examination.

Experience teaches that the neurologic examination may be normal even in patients with a serious neurologic disease, such as one which causes seizures or syncope. Or the patient may arrive in a coma with no available history, and the examination proceeds along the lines described in Chap. 31. An inadequate history may to some extent be replaced by a succession of examinations from which the course of the illness may be plotted.

The formulation of the problem and establishment of an etiologic diagnosis The clinical data obtained from the history and the examination are assembled into one of the known syndromes and are interpreted and translated in terms of neuroanatomy and neurophysiology. From the syndrome the physician should be able to determine the anatomic localization(s) that best explains the clinical findings. The anatomic localization, mode of onset and course of illness, other medical data, and laboratory findings are then integrated. Finally, the etiologic diagnosis is reached, and therapy appropriate for the disorder is proposed.

The proper selection of laboratory tests which will assist in arriving at an anatomic, but more particularly at an etiologic, diagnosis poses another set of problems for the clinician. In Chaps. 348 and 362 are described the principal tests and when they should be used. Radiologic imaging techniques, utilizing computed tomography (CT) scanning, and magnetic resonance imaging (MRI) have had a major impact on the neurologic assessment. It cannot be overemphasized, however, that the anatomic method of physical diagnosis should proceed together with imaging studies for localization of the site of the disorder. There are commonly great discrepancies between the findings on examination and on brain imaging which are resolved only after continued careful assessment of the patient, together with further radiologic study. Assiduous attention to the clinical method in neurology remains as important today as it ever was.

REFERENCES

Adams RD, Victor M: *Principles of Neurology*, 4th ed. New York, McGraw-Hill, 1989

DeJong RN: *The Neurologic Examination*. New York, Harper and Row, 1979

Swanson PD: *Symptoms and Signs in Neurology*. Philadelphia, Lippincott, 1984

348 IMAGING OF THE NERVOUS SYSTEM

KENNETH R. DAVIS / JOSEPH B. MARTIN

Imaging of the brain and spinal cord has revolutionized the ability to visualize lesions that cause neurologic dysfunction. These developments have occurred as a result of the application to clinical problems of computed tomography (CT) scanning in the 1970s, magnetic resonance imaging (MRI) in the 1980s, and positron emission tomography (PET) and single-photon emission computed tomography (SPECT) in the past 5 years. Nuclear magnetic resonance spectroscopy (NMRS) has promise for the study of function in the central nervous system (CNS) to complement those currently available with PET and SPECT.

COMPUTED TOMOGRAPHY CT scanning provides a sensitive and reproducible method for evaluating suspected lesions in the CNS. It is often the procedure of choice whether or not MRI is available and may also be complementary in circumstances where MRI is available. Its principal utility is when rapid information about the state of the CNS is desired, and it is particularly important for decisions related to emergent surgical versus medical management of patients with the sudden onset of a neurologic deficit. Such conditions include acute head or spinal trauma, stroke where a differentiation between hemorrhage and infarction is important, and other circumstances where a decision as to immediate operative intervention is important. CT continues to have an advantage over MRI in emergency settings in patients with acute neurologic deterioration. It has high specificity, particularly for the demonstration of acute hemorrhage, where its imaging capacity exceeds that of MRI.

The CT scan is also widely used for the evaluation of lesions that involve bone, such as metastatic disease at the base of the skull. However, the radionuclide bone scan provides a more sensitive and generalized evaluation for bone metastases than CT or MRI. Calcification within lesions of the brain is demonstrated best by CT rather than MRI. CT is also the better imaging method for fractures of the face, temporal bone, and base of the skull. It is also an important imaging technique for evaluating fractures of the spine, although soft tissue encroachment upon the spinal cord is better visualized by MRI.

MAGNETIC RESONANCE IMAGING MRI is useful in the following circumstances:

1 Screening for metastatic disease. With the administration of intravenous contrast material, such as gadolinium-DTPA, metastatic tumors can be visualized within the brain parenchyma, as well as primary tumors that cause a breakdown of the blood-brain barrier (Fig. 348-1). Imaging with gadolinium-DTPA may be more sensitive for these conditions than noncontrast MR or CT scanning with contrast. It is also the preferred method for visualization of pituitary tumors, acoustic neurinomas (Fig. 348-2), and other posterior fossa tumors, where CT artifacts from dental fillings on coronal scans of the sellar region and from nearby bony structures in the posterior fossa may prevent clear delineation of the lesion.

2 Imaging of demyelinating diseases such as multiple sclerosis (MS) and other white matter disorders of the brain and spinal cord (Fig. 348-3). It is possible to visualize small (2 to 5 mm) white matter lesions and to watch their progress over time. Contrast enhancement may make it possible to determine the acute perivascular involvement of new active lesions in MS. It is also the method of choice for evaluation of the leukodystrophies and for other white matter diseases such as Binswanger's disease (see Chap. 351).

3 Screening for the presence of arteriovenous malformation (AVM) and aneurysms, particularly when family members at risk require evaluation (Fig. 348-4). MRI is followed by angiography if more detailed visualization is necessary in preparation for surgical intervention, or if the findings are equivocal. Development of MRI methods for evaluation of blood flow (MRI angiography) promises to improve the ability to delineate blood flow and vascular lesions, including encroachment upon the lumen by atheromatous plaques in the carotid and vertebral basilar systems (Fig. 348-5).

4 Evaluation of congenital and developmental abnormalities of the CNS. These include the Chiari malformation, porencephalic cysts, as well as a variety of inherited abnormalities affecting the CNS (e.g., tuberous sclerosis).

5 Detection of posterior fossa vascular lesions. Small lacunes can be visualized within the brainstem that are not visible on CT scan (see Chap. 351). It is also the procedure of choice for the demonstration of small hemorrhages more than several days old in the posterior fossa. MRI angiography is capable of visualizing basilar and vertebral artery flow (Fig. 348-5).

6 Lesions intrinsic to the spinal cord. Particularly advantageous is the ability to examine the entire spinal cord and canal, a technique that has led to improved management, particularly of thoracic disc syndromes. Myelopathy should be evaluated first with an MRI to differentiate intramedullary from extramedullary lesions. Metastatic

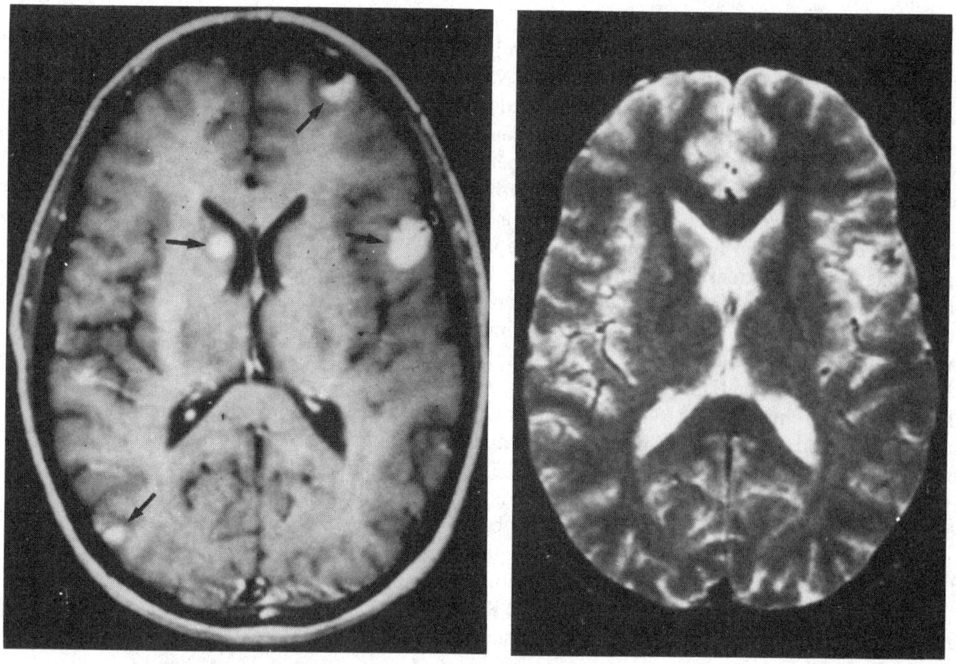

A B

FIGURE 348-1 Cerebral metastases. Magnetic resonance scan of the brain showing many more obvious enhancing lung metastases on the T1-weighted image (*arrows*) with intravenous contrast material (*A*) than on the T2-weighted image prior to contrast injection (*B*).

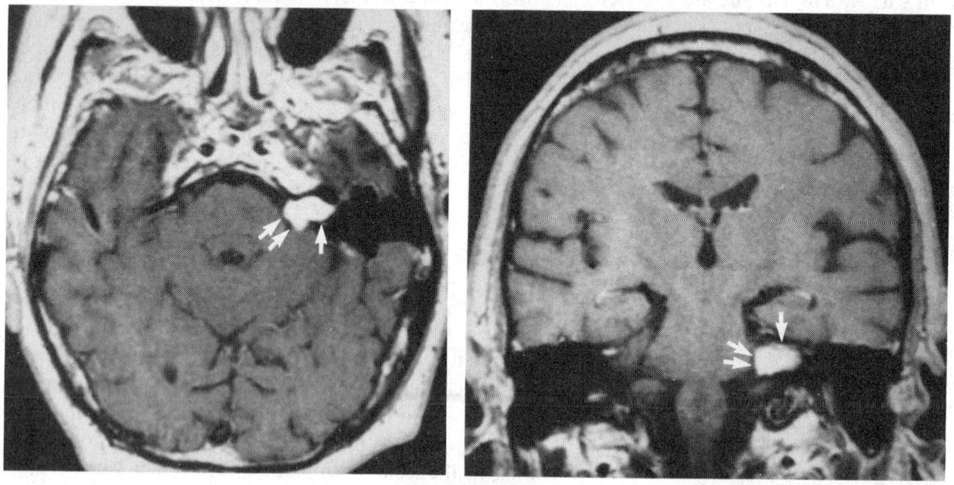

A B

FIGURE 348-2 Acoustic neurinoma. MRI with intravenous contrast material clearly depicts the intracanalicular (*arrow*) and cerebellopontine angle cistern (*double arrows*) components of an acoustic neurinoma on axial (*A*) and coronal (*B*) views. (*Courtesy of R.G. Gonzalez, M.D.*)

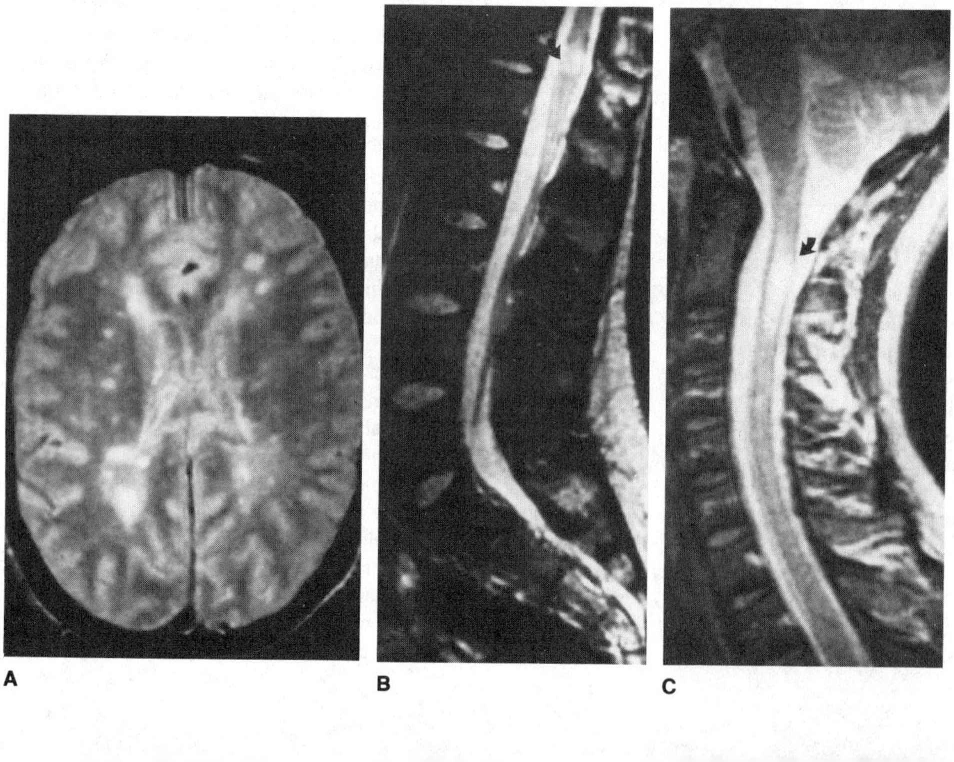

A B C

FIGURE 348-3 Multiple sclerosis. *A.* A proton-density MRI reveals multiple periventricular hyperintense multiple sclerosis plaques. The T2-weighted MRI of the spine shows a hyperintense plaque within the conus medullaris (*B*) and the upper cervical cord (*C*), respectively (*arrows*), in different patients. (*Courtesy of S. Sweriduk, M.D.*)

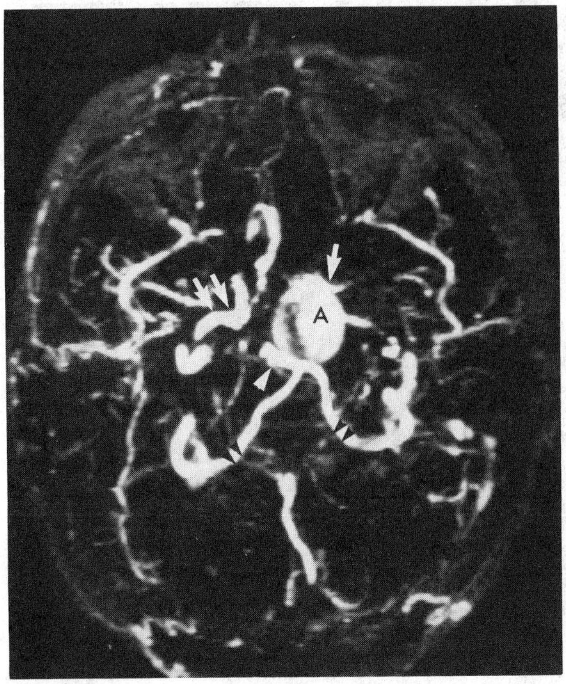

FIGURE 348-4 Cerebral aneurysm. MR angiography indicates the presence of a large aneurysm originating from the left internal carotid artery. A, aneurysm. Single arrow: left carotid artery. Double arrows: right carotid artery. Angle arrowhead: basilar artery. Double arrowheads: vertebral arteries. (*Courtesy of D. Mikulis, M.D.*)

disease affecting the spinal cord from an epidural location is easily visualized by MRI. It is also the best method for the demonstration of intrinsic spinal cord lesions including tumors (Fig. 348-6), syringomyelia, and areas of demyelination (Fig. 348-3). Use of intravenous contrast material may provide increased sensitivity or improved characterization of a lesion (Fig. 348-7). As compared to the myelogram, MRI allows visualization within and around the entire cord. The postmyelography CT scan is limited in the full evaluation of the spine because a large number of slices, and hence excessive time, are required. MRI is the choice for acute spinal cord syndromes caused by extramedullary lesions, including epidural abscess and metastases. Osteomyelitis of the spine and secondary abscess are readily visualized by MRI (Fig. 348-8).

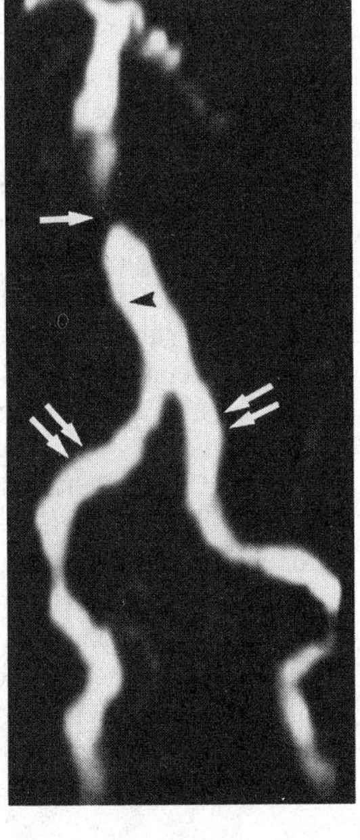

FIGURE 348-5 Basilar artery stenosis. MR angiogram of the vertebral basilar circulation showing stenosis of the mid-basilar artery (*arrow*) with turbulent flow artifact above the stenosis. Double arrows: vertebral arteries. Arrowhead: normal lower basilar artery. (*Courtesy of Gilbert Vezina, M.D.*)

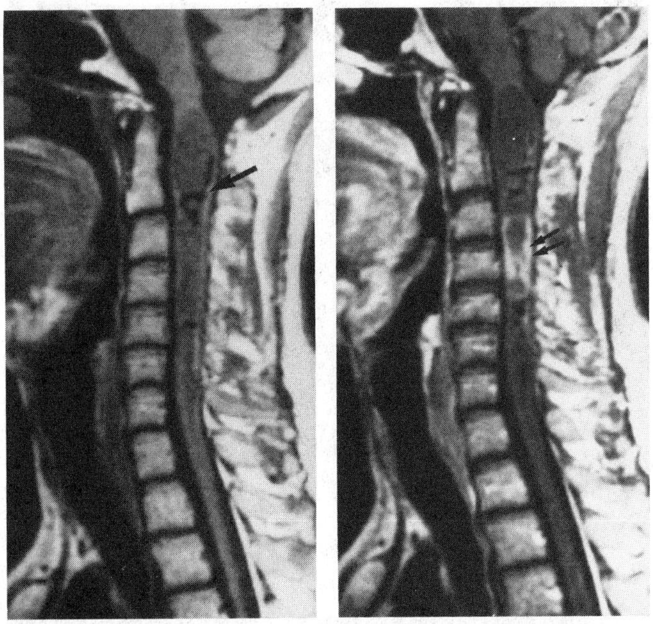

A B

FIGURE 348-6 Ependymoma. *A*. A T1-weighted sagittal MRI of the cervical spine made without intravenous contrast shows expansion of the cervical cord by an ependymoma (*arrow*) with mixed hypointense signal intensities. *B*. Following intravenous injection of gadolinium DTPA contrast, the T1 image shows enhancement of a portion of the tumor (*double arrows*) that would be most likely to yield a positive biopsy.

7 Although MRI is useful in the evaluation of all vertebral disc and spondylosis problems, it is particularly valuable for patients who have had previous back surgery. Following the administration of intravenous contrast material, it is possible to visualize extradural granulation tissue and to determine whether fibrosis (scarring) or recurrent disc protrusion is contributing to root symptoms. Fibrous granulation tissue usually shows early enhancement following intravenous contrast material, whereas a disc fragment may show delayed slight enhancement 15 to 20 min after injection.

8 Developmental lesions of the spinal cord such as syringomyelia, tethered cord, lipomas, and cavernous hemangiomas. MRI can demonstrate vascular lesions that subsequently may require angiography for definition, but may also demonstrate small intramedullary lesions that are not visible on the angiogram.

However, the problems of taking care of patients in the MRI scanner, particularly those who are unconscious on life support systems, who have gunshot wounds, or who are in MRI-incompatible tongs or halos for spinal traction or immobilization, limits the use of MRI. In these circumstances, it may be necessary to obtain a myelogram performed with a water-soluble, nonionic contrast material that permits a subsequent CT-myelogram.

MYELOGRAPHY If the MRI is insufficient to account for the clinical presentation, it may be necessary to perform a myelogram or CT-myelogram in which a water-soluble, nonionic contrast material is instilled into the subarachnoid space. Films are usually taken at the time of contrast injection and followed by a CT scan of the appropriate regions. The procedure is particularly useful in cervical spondylosis where an MRI may not demonstrate detail of a herniated disc or osteophyte. The safety of new nonionic, water-soluble contrast materials has made myelography a more feasible procedure associated with less risk. Iophendylate myelography, now rarely performed, does not permit subsequent CT evaluation. Furthermore, residual iophendylate after myelography may produce artifacts on subsequent MR scans. A CT-myelogram may be particularly useful in cervical disc disease and spondylosis to demonstrate narrowing of the neural foramen and to differentiate an osteophyte (hard disc) from soft disc

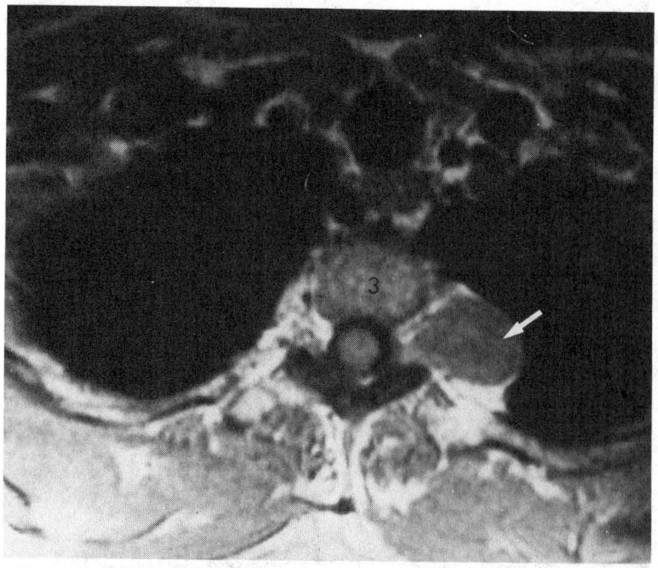

A

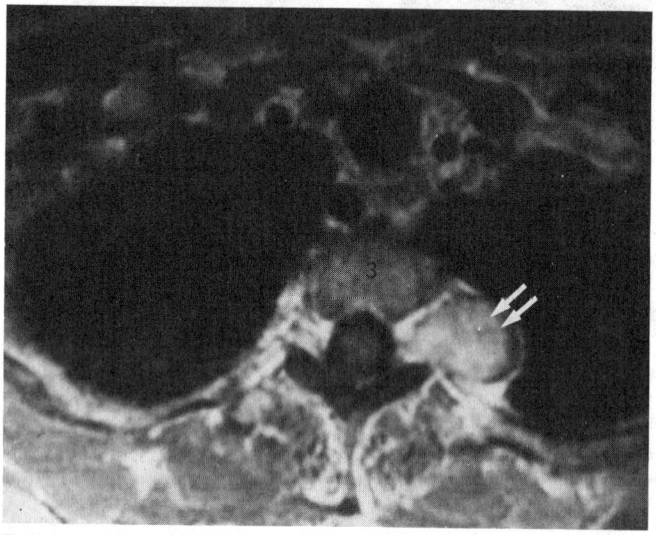

B

FIGURE 348-7 Neurofibroma. T1-weighted axial MRI of the spine through the D2-3 neural foramen reveals a hypointense foraminal and extraforaminal neurofibroma (*arrow*) extending into the left paraspinal region (*A*) that enhances (*double arrows*) with intravenous contrast (*B*).

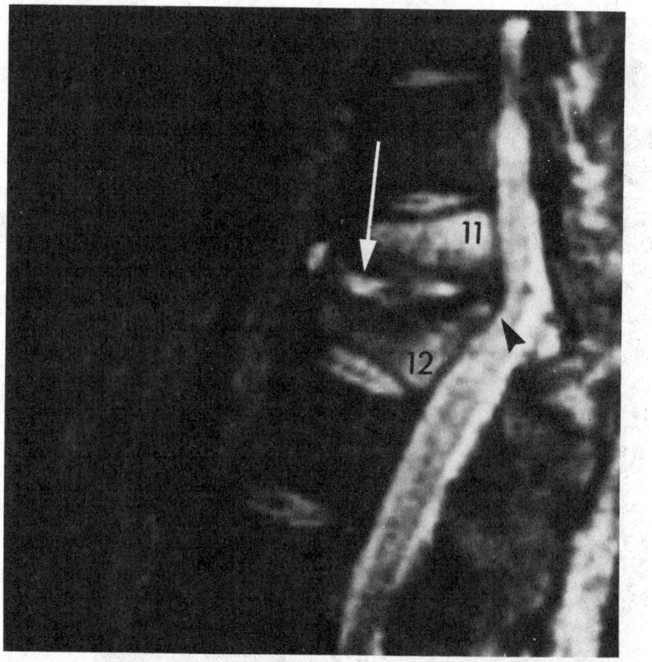

FIGURE 348-8 Osteomyelitis of the spine. A T2-weighted sagittal MRI indicates hyperintense signal of the remaining D11-12 disc space (*arrow*) between the collapsed, slightly hyperintense surrounding vertebral bodies. These findings are caused by disc space infection and surrounding osteomyelitis. Posterior extension of the epidural mass represents epidural abscess (*arrowhead*).

material. This may not always be optimally visualized on MRI. For tumors of the vertebral foramen, such as neurofibromas, a myelogram and CT-myelogram are not often necessary, given the availability of MRI and use of intravenous contrast material (see Fig. 348-9). Seeding of tumors along roots in the cauda equina is often visualized on MRI, but these may be too small to be identified or not enhance with intravenous contrast material. In this circumstance, a myelogram followed by a CT-myelogram may be the best choice. Herniated lumbar disc is usually detected by MRI (Fig. 348-9), but some physicians still prefer to have the anatomic details confirmed by CT and myelography prior to surgery. If the MRI is normal or equivocal, a myelogram may demonstrate enlarged veins in cases of suspected AVM of the cord, prior to deciding on spinal angiography. MRI may detect flow voids of the AVM and an abnormal signal within the cord. In such cases where AVM is suspected, a spinal angiogram rather than a myelogram will be the next step after an unremarkable MRI. Finally, a CT myelogram may be the examination of choice in spinal cord injury where ferromagnetic metal stabilization has been used and MRI-incompatible life-support systems are required. In these circumstances, it is difficult to perform an adequate MRI.

INTERVENTIONAL RADIOLOGY It is now possible to navigate into small vessels using maneuverable microcatheters and to visualize the vasculature and microcatheter by high-resolution, digital fluoroscopic equipment with real-time roadmapping capabilities. The decrease in the time required for microcatheter entry and visualization of target vessels results in faster studies at lower risk. The studies are usually performed by transfemoral retrograde catheterization using specialized coaxial microcatheters that can enter small vessels in the distribution of the anterior, middle, and posterior cerebral, vertebral, basilar, external carotid, or spinal circulations. This technique, along with availability of polymerizing glues such as *n*-butyl-cyanoacrylate, microcoils, and various particulate agents, make endovascular embolization treatment of AVMs possible. Treatment may be partial, to facilitate surgical resection, or primary and definitive. The development of detachable balloons that are attached to microcatheters has made possible the endovascular treatment of fistulas, such as carotid-cavernous or vertebral-venous fistulas. Detachable balloons can also be used to occlude aneurysms or the parent feeding vessel. Nondetachable balloons are used to predict deficiencies of neurologic function that may follow permanent surgical or balloon occlusion of vessels. For example, selective microcatheterization of a vessel supplying an AVM followed by injection of amobarbital can be used to test for adverse neurologic effect prior to embolization. Nondetachable balloons may be used to dilate and treat certain cases of vasospasm secondary to subarachnoid hemorrhage from an aneurysm. Finally, preoperative embolization is often used to reduce vascularity in tumors such as meningiomas, glomus jugulare, and angiofibromas prior to surgical removal.

POSITRON EMISSION TOMOGRAPHY PET is based upon three-dimensional reconstruction of brain sections using positron-emitting radionuclides. By utilization of a number of individual radionuclides and radiolabeled moieties, it provides an opportunity to measure quantitatively: regional cerebral blood flow, blood volume, oxygen metabolism, glucose transport and metabolism, and neurotransmitter metabolism; and it permits neurotransmitter receptor localization (see Table 348-1.) PET can provide spatial resolution, approaching 3 to 5 mm definition in sequential slices.

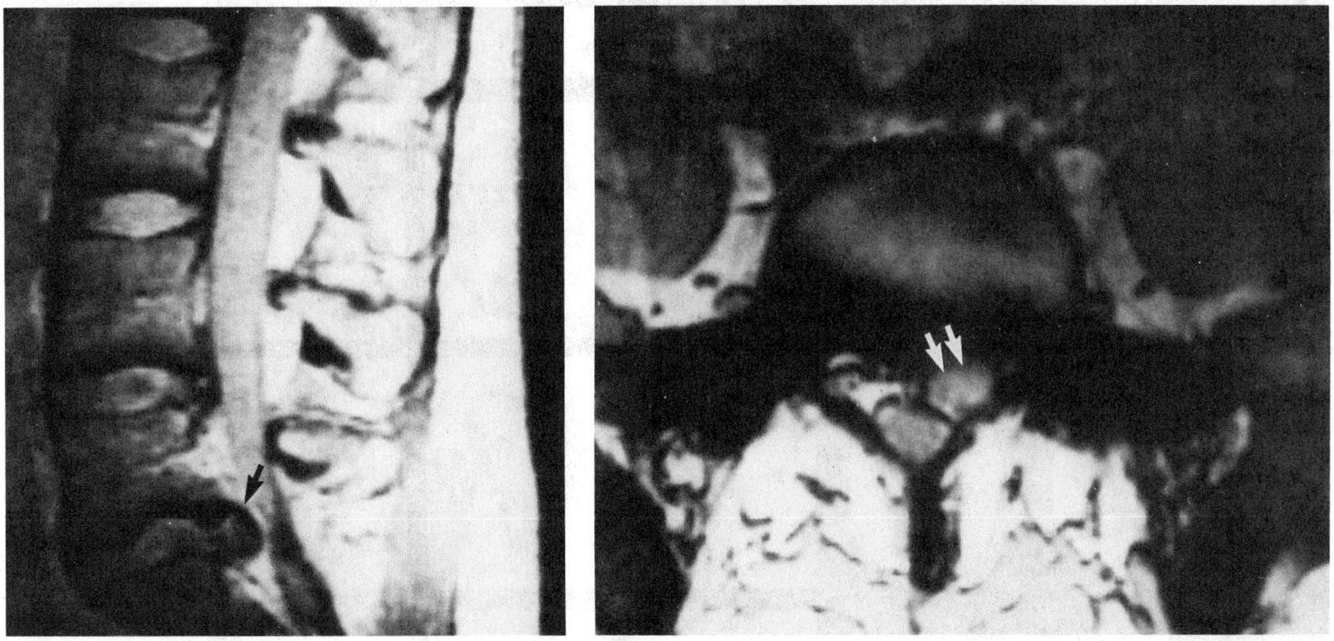

A B

FIGURE 348-9 Herniated and extruded disc at L5-S1. *A*. The sagittal proton density MRI shows the abnormal hypointense disk (*arrow*) producing a large extradural defect. *B*. Using a 110-degree flip angle, the axial multiplanar gradient echo image shows the disc lateralized to the left (*double arrows*) compressing the S1 root sleeve and thecal sac as well as extruding caudally into the lateral recess of S1.

Cerebrovascular disease In acute ischemic injury to the brain, PET studies demonstrate functional alterations in blood flow and oxygen metabolism when the CT scan may be normal; however, the difficulty in obtaining emergency PET studies limits its usefulness in this setting. MRI scans do show acute changes in stroke more readily than CT and are now widely used. In the assessment of long-term neurologic dysfunction after a stroke, PET scanning with deoxyglucose may show focal abnormalities that extend well beyond the lesions seen on CT or MRI. Analysis in such circumstances may provide insight into neural connections important for cognition (Chap. 346).

TABLE 348-1 Examples of tracers used in positron emission tomography of brain

Process	Tracer
Blood flow	$H_2{}^{15}O$, $C^{15}O_2$, ^{11}C-alcohols
Blood volume	$C^{15}O$-RBC, ^{11}CO-RBC, ^{68}Ga-labeled EDTA
Tissue pH	^{11}C-DMO, $^{11}CO_2$
Transport and metabolism	
Oxygen	^{15}O-O_2
Glucose, glucose analogues, carbohydrates	2-deoxy-2-^{18}F-fluoro-D-glucose, 2-^{11}C-deoxy-D-glucose, ^{11}C-D-glucose, ^{11}C-lactate, -pyruvate, -acetate, -succinate, -oxaloacetate
Amino acids: ^{13}N	L-^{13}N-glutamate, -glutamine, -alanine, -aspartate, -leucine, -valine, -isoleucine, -methionine
Amino acids: ^{11}C	L-^{11}C-aspartate, -glutamate, -valine, -leucine, -phenylalanine, -methionine
Molecular diffusion	^{68}Ga-EDTA
Protein synthesis	L-1-^{11}C-leucine, -methionine, -phenylalanine, L-^{11}C-methylmethionine
Receptor systems	
Dopaminergic	^{18}F-spiperone, ^{11}C-spiperone, ^{11}C-raclopride, ^{75}Br- and ^{76}Br-*p*-bromospiperone, ^{18}F-haloperidol, ^{11}C-pimozide, ^{11}C-methyl, -ethylspiperone, L-^{11}C-dopa, 6-^{18}F-fluoro-L-dopa, ^{18}F-ethylspiperone
Cholinergic	^{11}C-imipramine, ^{11}C-QNB
Benzodiazepine	^{11}C-flunitrazepam, -diazepam, -RO15-1788, ^{18}F-fluorovalium
Opiate	^{11}C-etorphine, N-methyl-^{11}C-morphine, ^{11}C-heroin, -carfentanil
Adrenergic	^{11}C-norepinephrine, -propranolol
Anticonvulsants	^{11}C-valproate, -phenytoin

SOURCE: Adapted from Phelps and Mazziotta, with permission.

Epilepsy The PET application most useful in epilepsy is assessment of glucose metabolism by measurement of brain uptake and phosphorylation of [^{18}F]fluorodeoxyglucose (FDG). The methods are based on those developed by Sokoloff and colleagues for 2-deoxyglucose autoradiography in tissue sections. The PET scan summates approximately 40 min of local cerebral glucose metabolism and allows assessment of regional variations. PET studies have been most useful in patients with focal seizures. About 70 percent of patients with partial (focal) seizures that are refractory to medical treatment show zones of decreased glucose metabolism in the interictal state. The site of hypometabolism correlates with the epileptic focus in many patients. The same region often shows enhanced glucose metabolism if it is measured during a seizure discharge. In patients with temporal lobe seizures, it is common to find hypometabolism in one lobe.

The application of FDG-PET to evaluation of epilepsy patients undergoing consideration for surgical treatment is useful for confirming the unilaterality of sites producing electrical discharges and, in some cases, rendering intracerebral recordings unnecessary (Fig. 348-10).

Neurodegenerative diseases Parkinson's disease, caused by degeneration of the dopaminergic nigra-striatal pathway, can be demonstrated by [^{18}F]6-fluoro-L-dopa (^{18}F-FD) and PET. Decreased accumulation of ^{18}F-FD occurs in the striatum in Parkinson's disease and during normal aging. 6-Fluoro-L-dopa is decarboxylated to 6-fluoro-L-dopamine by the enzyme aromatic L-amino acid decarboxylase, and the product then enters nerve terminals. PET allows visualization of the entrapped labeled dopamine. Decreased dopamine levels have been demonstrated in patients with Parkinson's disease induced by 1-methyl-4-phenyl-1,2,3,6-tetrahydropyridine and in asymptomatic drug addicts exposed to the drug, who presumably have subclinical degeneration of the nigra-striatal pathway.

Abnormalities can also be detected by FDG-PET in the basal ganglia in Huntington's disease (decreased metabolism) and in the brainstem and cerebellum in degenerative diseases such as olivopontocerebellar degeneration and Friedreich's ataxia (decreased metabolism). Decreased oxygen extraction and metabolism in the cerebral

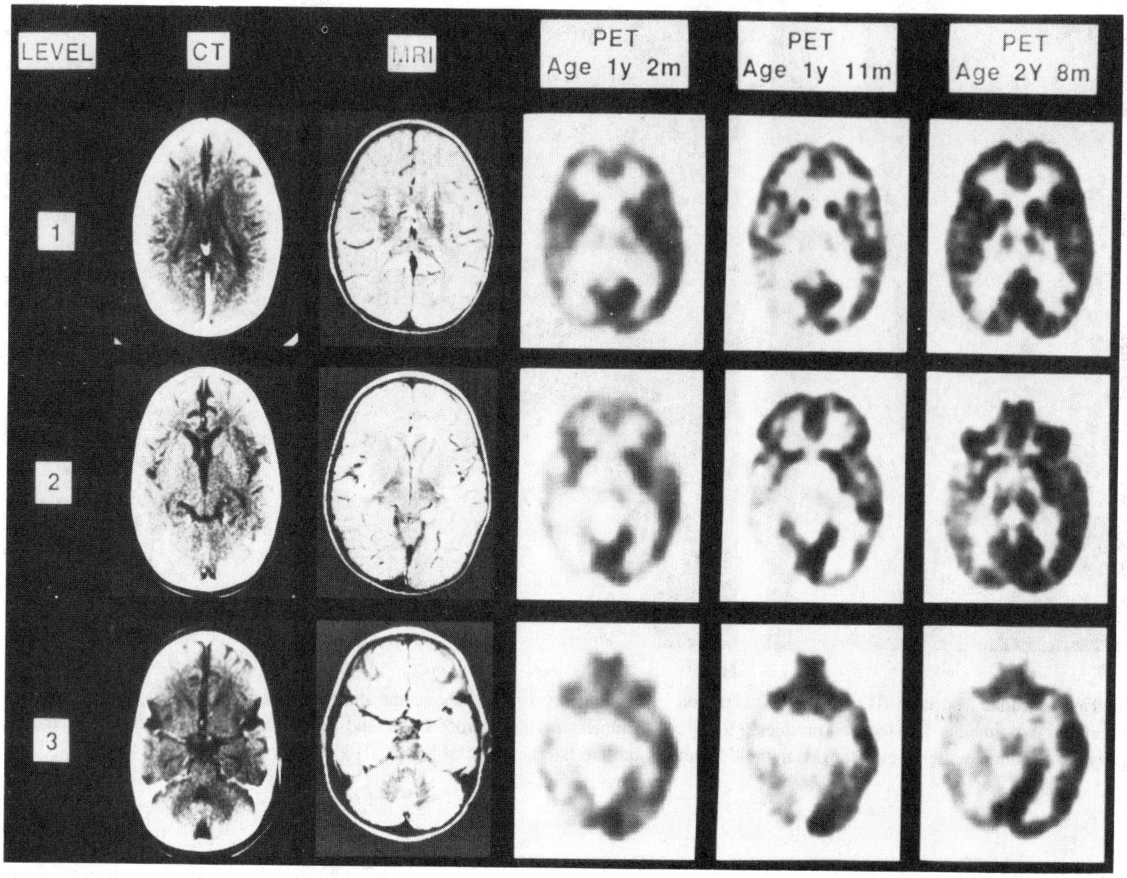

FIGURE 348-10 Preoperative CT, MRI, and FDG-PET images of a patient with infantile spasms (epilepsy). The right side of the brain is to the viewer's left. Both CT and MRI failed to show abnormalities. Interictal PET studies performed at ages 1 year 2 months, 1 year 11 months, and 2 years 8 months revealed right occipitotemporal hypometabolism, corresponding to the surface EEG localization of interictal discharges. (*Used with permission of Harry Chugani and Annals of Neurology.*)

cortex may be demonstrated in Alzheimer's disease and in schizophrenia. Abnormalities in dopamine receptors have also been documented in schizophrenia. PET studies are also valuable in neuropsychological studies (see Chap. 346).

Although PET is at present primarily a research tool, its increasing availability in medical centers for cardiac imaging (see Chap. 178) makes likely more widespread application to other neurologic and psychiatric diseases.

SINGLE-PHOTON EMISSION COMPUTED TOMOGRAPHY SPECT depends on gamma-emitting radionuclides attached to molecules that can readily cross the blood-brain barrier. SPECT allows for concurrent blood flow determination and visualization of neurotransmitter receptors (see also Chap. 346). For example, [^{123}I]isopropyl amphetamine (IMP) and [^{99}Tc]m-d, 1-hexamethyl-propylene-amine-oxime–labeled iodoamphetamine have been used to demonstrate abnormalities in epilepsy, Alzheimer's disease, and Parkinson's disease. However, present SPECT technology is relatively nonquantitative and insensitive in demonstrating changes, and its spatial resolution is considerably less than that of PET. On the other hand, SPECT is less expensive and more widely available. It is now widely acknowledged as a potentially important diagnostic tool for differentiation of dementia caused by Alzheimer's disease from that caused by vascular disease (multi-infarct dementia) (see Chap. 30).

NUCLEAR MAGNETIC RESONANCE SPECTROSCOPY NMRS offers the potential of assessing brain function at metabolic and molecular levels. NMRS uses naturally occurring nonradioactive measurements of ^{31}P, ^{13}C, ^{23}Na, ^{7}Li, and ^{1}H. The ^{31}P NMR spectrum can detect tissue concentrations of the phosphomonoesters phosphocholine and inorganic orthophosphate, the phosphodiesters glycerol-3-phospho-ethanolamine and glycerol-3-phosphocholine, the triphosphate ATP, and other phosphorus-containing molecules including phosphocreatinine. The ^{31}P NMR spectrum gives quantitative analysis of these compounds in vivo with the potential of three-dimensional resolution within the brain. At present, much of the work in this area is experimental (see also Chap. 346).

REFERENCES

Brant-Zawadski M, Norman D (eds): *Magnetic Resonance Imaging of the Central Nervous System*. New York, Raven, 1987

Chugani HT et al: Infantile spasms: I. PET identifies focal cortical dysgenesis in cryptogenic cases for surgical treatment. Ann Neurol (1990)

Duara R et al: Positron emission tomography in Alzheimer's disease. Neurology 36:879, 1986

Felix R et al: Brain tumors: MR imaging with gadolinium-DTPA. Radiology 156:681, 1985

Johnson KA et al: Single photon emission computed tomography in Alzheimer's disease: Abnormal iofetamine I 123 uptake reflects dementia severity. Arch Neurol 45:392, 1988

Junck L et al: PET imaging of human gliomas with ligands for the peripheral benzodiazepine binding site. Ann Neurol 26:752, 1989

Latchaw RE (ed): *Computed Tomography of the Head, Neck and Spine*. Chicago. Year Book, 1985

Lee SH, Rao KCVG (eds): *Cranial Computed Tomography and MRI*, 2d ed. New York, McGraw-Hill, 1987

McGeer PL et al: Positron emission tomography in patients with clinically diagnosed Alzheimer's disease. Can Med Assoc J 134:597, 1986

Modic MT, Masaryk TJ, Ross JS (eds): *Magnetic Resonance Imaging of the Spine*. Chicago, Year Book, 1989

Pettegrew JW et al: ^{31}P nuclear magnetic resonance study of the brain in Alzheimer's disease. J Neuropath Exp Neurol 47:235, 1988

Phelps ME, Mazziotta JC: Positron emission tomography: Human brain function and biochemistry. Science 228:799, 1985

Ross JS et al: Magnetic resonance angiography of the extracranial carotid arteries and intracranial vessels: A review. Neurology 39:1369, 1989

Williams AL, Haughton VM (eds): *Cranial Computed Tomography. A Comprehensive Text*. St. Louis, Mosby, 1985

Wong DF et al: Positron emission tomography reveals elevated D_2 dopamine receptors in drug-naive schizophrenics. Science 234:1558, 1986

Zawadzki MB, Norman D: *Magnetic Resonance Imaging of the Central Nervous System*. New York, Raven, 1987

349 CLINICAL ELECTROPHYSIOLOGY AND OTHER DIAGNOSTIC METHODS

KEITH CHIAPPA / BHAGWAN SHAHANI / JOSEPH B. MARTIN

Clinical neurophysiologic techniques provide an objective, quantitative measure of function of the central and peripheral nervous systems (CNS and PNS), including the autonomic nervous system. These studies have proved useful in the investigation and understanding of a variety of neurologic disorders. Because many of the procedures are time-consuming and costly, they should be undertaken only when they can shed new light on the clinical problem by providing data that are otherwise unavailable. Clinical neurophysiologic studies are also useful for monitoring and following the progression or recovery of patients with certain neurologic disorders.

NEUROPHYSIOLOGIC STUDIES OF MUSCLE AND NERVE

ELECTROMYOGRAPHY Electromyography refers to several diagnostic procedures in which electrical activity of nerve and muscle is studied. Strictly speaking, the term *electromyography* (EMG) is used when a needle electrode is inserted into a skeletal muscle to study changes in electric potential (voltage) during a state of complete relaxation and with graded voluntary activity. There are no EMG wave forms that are diagnostic for a particular disease entity, and it is not possible to sample every muscle in the body. Electromyography is an extension of the clinical neurologic examination and, by itself, cannot be used to arrive at a specific clinical entity. Clinical applications of EMG and conventional nerve conduction studies for the diagnosis of disorders affecting skeletal muscles, peripheral nerves, and neuromuscular junctions are described in Chap. 362.

Newer EMG techniques for evaluation of nerve conduction Methods for study of electrical conduction in proximal nerve segments include measurements of latencies for F responses, H reflexes, and blink reflexes. These techniques determine conduction times in nerves from the periphery (of a limb or the face) to the central nervous system (spinal cord or brainstem) and back again.

The *F response* measures the time required for a stimulus applied to the axon of an alpha motor neuron to propagate antidromically to the anterior horn of the spinal cord and then to return orthodromically down the same axon. The *H reflex* measures the time required for orthodromic conduction up the nerve via group IA sensory fibers, through the spinal monosynaptic connection with the alpha motor neuron, and then orthodromically down the motor axon. Conduction along proximal sensory and motor nerves and spinal roots can be measured. The application of these techniques to the measurement of proximal nerve conduction has increased recognition of abnormal conduction velocity in patients with peripheral neuropathy to between 80 and 90 percent. These studies are also useful in documenting a *conduction block* in proximal segments of peripheral nerves and roots in patients with inflammatory and demyelinating neuropathies (e.g., Guillain-Barré syndrome).

The *blink reflexes* measure conduction in branches of the trigeminal and facial nerves. The blink reflex is evoked by electric stimulation of the supraorbital branches of the trigeminal nerve and measures latency to blink response. It permits localization of lesions in the distribution of the facial or trigeminal nerve.

Nerve conduction studies, both conventional (see Chap. 362) as well as the late-response studies described here, only give information regarding large-diameter fast-conducting axons and do not provide information regarding conduction in intermediate and small-diameter nerve fibers. By applying physiologic principles of collision of nerve impulses evoked by stimulation at two different sites (proximal and distal) in the same nerve, it is possible to measure conduction in motor axons with small diameters. Abnormal conduction velocities of intermediate size fibers can be demonstrated in some patients with metabolic and nutritional neuropathies in whom conventional methods and late-response studies are normal.

Single-fiber EMG and macro EMG In addition to conventional EMG with concentric needle electrodes, specialized techniques permit the recording of the EMG of single fibers or of the entire motor unit (macro EMG). Single-fiber techniques, by recording *jitter* (variations in potentials) in individual fibers, can measure accurately, within microseconds, the performance of individual neuromuscular junctions. Characteristic quantitative abnormalities are found in patients with myasthenia gravis, Lambert-Eaton syndrome, and other disorders of neuromuscular transmission. Single-fiber EMG studies are also used to calculate *fiber density*, the number of single muscle fiber action potentials belonging to one motor unit within the recording area of the single-fiber EMG electrode (approximately 200 μm). Fiber density values are increased after disorders that cause denervation followed by reinnervation.

Macro EMG techniques presumably measure summated electrical activity of all fibers belonging to a motor unit and allow estimation of true motor unit size. The amplitude and area of macro EMG motor unit potentials is increased in reinnervation and decreased in primary muscle diseases that cause reduction in the number of muscle fibers per motor unit.

EMG in disorders of the CNS The application of EMG and nerve conduction studies to evaluation of CNS function is termed *central EMG*. Since the motor unit is the final common path for all nerve impulses controlling skeletal muscles, disorders of motor control produced by lesions of the CNS may result in abnormal discharge patterns of motor neurons that can be documented by electrophysiologic techniques. For example, surface EMG recordings from pairs of agonist and antagonist muscles, analysis of single motor unit recruitment patterns, and microneurographic studies are useful in evaluating different types of tremor, including rest tremor of Parkinson's disease, familial essential tremor, and physiologic tremor (see Chap. 25). Cerebellar ataxia can usually be differentiated from other tremors and from sensory ataxia. Asterixis can be distinguished from tremor, and different types of myoclonus can be documented. Studies of proprioceptive and exteroceptive reflexes are helpful in the differential diagnosis of movement disorders and in differentiating spasticity from other types of disorders of tone, such as rigidity. Studies of the H reflex and F responses provide information regarding the excitability of the motor neuron pool. The effect of vibration on the H reflex has been used to evaluate *presynaptic inhibition* in different neurologic disorders. *Silent-period studies* have been used to evaluate function of proprioceptive input from muscle spindles. Mismatching of information from muscle spindles and joint receptors can result in an apparent "cerebellar" ataxia in patients with acute inflammatory polyneuropathy (Fisher syndrome) due to a lesion in the peripheral nervous system. EMG recordings and blink reflexes are useful in documenting clinically inapparent lesions of the brainstem in multiple sclerosis and in localizing early compressive lesions of trigeminal and facial nerves produced by small posterior fossa tumors.

QUANTITATIVE SENSORY TESTING Light touch and vibratory sensation are mediated by large-diameter myelinated nerve fibers (see Chaps. 28 and 363). Small myelinated nerve fibers convey messages encoded by cold receptors and some nociceptors, and unmyelinated sensory pathways transmit impulses generated by warmth receptors and polymodal nociceptors. A reproducible quantitative examination of several sensory modalities can be performed in approximately 1 h.

Vibratory perception can be determined by a hand-held vibrator equipped with an indicator for monitoring the pressure applied to the skin. The stimulus strength is measured by peak-to-peak displacement of the vibratory rod and the perception and disappearance thresholds for vibratory sensation are recorded at least three times. The technique of vibrametry is now used widely to assess and follow patients with peripheral neuropathies, including those in whom sensory nerve action potentials are absent.

Thermal threshold determination is performed with a special probe in which temperature varies at a constant rate. The probe is either warmed or cooled. The thermal stimulator is applied to the skin at different sites, and the temperature of the probe measured by a thermocouple is recorded. Thresholds for cold and warmth perception and for cold and heat pain are obtained by asking the subject to press a button when a given perception is felt. Using quantitative thermal testing in patients with Guillain-Barré syndrome, for example, it is possible to document impairment of cold perception thresholds (small myelinated fibers) and preservation of warmth perception thresholds (unmyelinated sensory fibers). Sensory pathways, which are inaccessible to conventional electrophysiologic testing, can be studied by this technique.

AUTONOMIC TESTING Two simple electrophysiologic techniques are often used to evaluate function of the autonomic nervous system. The *sympathetic skin response* (SSR), which is a voltage change recorded from the skin, is evoked by a variety of stimuli, including an electrical stimulus, a loud noise, or deep inspiration. The SSR can be easily recorded from hands and feet of all normal subjects. Using a commercially available EMG machine provided with bandpass filters to include low frequencies (low-frequency cutoff of 0.16 Hz), SSR evaluates function of a subset of sympathetic nerve fibers that mediate sudomotor (sweating) function. SSR abnormalities are more commonly associated with axonal neuropathies than with demyelinating neuropathies. Quantitative in vitro studies of a group of patients with sural nerve biopsy has shown that absent SSR is due to loss of unmyelinated nerve fibers.

Using standard EMG equipment the QRS complex can be recorded through surface electrodes placed over the dorsum of each hand. By superimposing pairs of QRS complexes, it is possible to measure *RR-interval variation* at rest and during deep breathing. RR-interval variation is abnormal in many patients with Guillain-Barré syndrome who have involvement of small myelinated nerve fibers in the vagus nerve.

In most patients with clinical symptoms and signs of dysautonomia, one of these two electrophysiologic tests is abnormal. Both the SSR and RR-interval tests are simple and reproducible and they are useful to rule out involvement of the autonomic nervous system in patients referred to the laboratory for evaluation of peripheral neuropathy.

ELECTROENCEPHALOGRAPHY

The electroencephalographic (EEG) examination is part of the clinical study of many patients suspected of having disease of the CNS, either primary or secondary to a systemic medical illness. The conventional EEG recording should include the resting record and a number of *activating procedures* as follows: (1) The patient is requested to breathe deeply 20 times a minute for 3 min. The resulting alkalosis and cerebral vasoconstriction may activate characteristic seizure patterns or other abnormalities. (2) A powerful light (a stroboscope) is placed over the patient's face and flashed at frequencies from 1 to 20 per s with the patient's eyes open and closed. The EEG may then show abnormal discharges in photosensitive patients. (3) The EEG is recorded after the patient is allowed to fall asleep naturally or following sedative drugs given by mouth or by vein. Procedures 1 and 2 are routinely employed, but sleep may be extremely helpful in bringing out certain abnormalities, especially where temporal lobe epilepsy and other seizures are suspected. Sleep deprivation the night prior to the EEG study is useful when a sleeping record is desirable.

Certain preparations are necessary if EEG is to be most useful. The patient should not be sedated and should not have been for a long time without food, for both sedative drugs and relative hypoglycemia modify the normal EEG pattern. The same may be said of mental concentration, extreme nervousness, or drowsiness, all of which tend to suppress the normal alpha rhythm and increase muscle artifacts. When dealing with patients suspected of having epilepsy who are already being treated for it, most physicians prefer to record the first EEG while the patient continues to receive drugs.

TYPES OF NORMAL RECORDINGS The normal EEG in adults shows somewhat asymmetric 8- to 12-Hz, 50-μV sinusoidal *alpha waves* in both occipital and parietal regions. These waves wax and wane spontaneously and usually disappear promptly when patients open their eyes or fix their attention on something. Waves faster than 13 Hz and of lower amplitude (10 to 20 μV), called *beta waves,* are also seen symmetrically in the frontal regions. Very slow waves *(delta waves),* sharp waves, or other unusual patterns are absent in a normal record. When normal subjects fall asleep, the rhythm slows symmetrically, and characteristic waveforms (*vertex sharp waves* and *sleep spindles*) appear (see Chap. 34 for a more detailed description of polysomnography and the EEG in sleep); if the sleep is induced by barbiturates or benzodiazepines, an increase in the fast frequencies is seen and is considered to be normal. Excessive fast activity should raise the possibility that a patient is receiving one of these classes of compounds. In addition, there are many common and uncommon normal variants that should not be mistaken for abnormalities (e.g., drowsy hypersynchrony, 14 + 6 positive spikes, 6 per s spike-wave, rhythmic midtemporal discharge, and benign epileptiform transients of sleep).

The most pathologic finding of all is "electrocerebral inactivity," which means that the electrical activity of the cortical mantle, measured at the scalp, is below 2 μV and probably absent. Acute intoxication with anesthetic levels of drugs, such as barbiturates, and extreme hypothermia [<21°C(<70°F)] can also produce this sort of isoelectric EEG. However, in the absence of CNS depressants or extreme hypothermia, a record that is "flat" at highest recording sensitivity all over the head (except for artifacts such as EKG whose presence is a biologic calibration that indicates that the recording system is functioning properly) is the result of cerebral hypoxia, ischemia, or widespread cortical destruction. Such a patient, without EEG activity, reflexes (other than spinal), spontaneous respiration, or muscular activity of any kind for 6 h or more, is said to be in "irreversible coma." The brain of such patients is largely necrotic. There is no chance for neurologic recovery, and the patient may be considered dead, despite the preservation of vegetative (cardiovascular) functions supported by mechanical means, such as respirators (see also the discussion of brain death in Chap. 31). There has been no exception to this statement in over 1000 patients examined at the Massachusetts General Hospital in the past 20 years. Although the demonstration of electrocerebral silence by EEG should not be a legal requirement for the determination of brain death, it can be a very useful confirmation of the clinical conclusion.

Localized regions with absence of EEG activity may rarely be seen when there is a large area of infarction or an extensive surface tumor clot lying between the cerebral cortex and the electrodes. The localization of this abnormality is precise, but of course the nature of the lesion cannot be ascertained by EEG. Most such lesions, however, are too small, relative to the recording arrangement, to be visible, and the EEG may then record abnormal waves arising from functional, though [illegible]-anged, brain at the borders of the lesion. These abnormal waves are slower and of higher amplitude (50 to 350 μV) than normal. Those which are less than 4 Hz are called *delta waves;* those from 4 to 7 Hz are called *theta waves;* and the higher-voltage, faster waves are known as spikes or sharp waves. These fast and slow waves may be combined, and when a series of them suddenly interrupts relatively normal EEG patterns in a paroxysmal fashion, they are highly suggestive of epilepsy.

NEUROLOGIC CONDITIONS WITH ABNORMAL EEG In the following groups of neurologic disorders, the EEG may be of considerable help in reaching the correct diagnosis.

Epilepsy EEG correlates of the epilepsies are discussed in Chap. 350, and the review of this topic by Engel is highly recommended.

Brain tumor, abscess, and subdural hematoma Clinically significant intracranial space-occupying lesions are characteristically associated with abnormalities in the EEG, depending on their type and location, in some 90 percent of patients. In addition to diffuse changes, the classic abnormalities are focal or localized slow waves (usually delta), or, occasionally, seizure activity and decreased amplitude and synchronization of normal rhythms. As a rule, those lesions which expand more rapidly (abscess, some metastases, glioblastoma), especially when situated supratentorially, have the greatest frequency of EEG abnormalities (90 to 95 percent of the latter two and virtually 100 percent of abscesses). Slower growing tumors (astrocytomas) and particularly those outside the cerebral hemispheres (meningiomas, pituitary tumors) may produce no change in the EEG, though they may be very evident clinically or on imaging. The EEG abnormality has the correct lateralization in as many as 75 to 90 percent of patients with supratentorial tumors or abscesses. The EEG may be focally abnormal at a time when a cerebral metastasis is not yet visible on a computed tomography scan. A normal EEG and CT scan together almost exclude the presence of a supratentorial brain tumor or abscess. The EEG may be normal, however, in 20 to 25 percent of patients with infratentorial tumors.

Cerebrovascular disease Both the diffuse and localized EEG changes produced by vascular lesions such as cerebral infarcts and intracranial hemorrhages depend on their location and size rather than their type. The EEG has been shown to be useful in the differential diagnosis of vascular hemiplegia. If the lesion responsible is in the internal carotid or a major cerebral artery, an area of decreased normal activity and excessive slowing is practically always seen acutely in the appropriate region. If the hemiplegia is due to small vessel disease, i.e., a lacunar infarction deep in the cerebrum or brainstem (see Chap. 351), the EEG is usually normal. Large hemispheral lesions associated with acutely depressed levels of consciousness also produce widespread, diffuse, slow-wave activity of a nonspecific type as is seen with stupor or a coma from any cause. Resolution begins after a few days, cerebral edema subsides, and focal activity may then be seen (slow-wave activity or suppression of normal background rhythms). Smaller infarctions are associated with acute focal abnormalities that lateralize the lesion well but do not localize it precisely. In contrast with tumors, further resolution continues, and after 3 to 6 months roughly 50 percent of patients with cerebrovascular accidents have a normal EEG despite the persistence of clinical abnormalities. Under these circumstances the prognosis for further recovery is poor. Persistence of moderate- to high-voltage EEG abnormalities after this time period, particularly if spikes or sharp waves are present, suggests the presence of abnormally functioning tissue, which might be epileptogenic. The EEG may be of lateralizing value in acute subarachnoid hemorrhage, depending upon the extent to which the adjacent cerebrum is affected.

Brain injury Cerebral contusion or laceration produces EEG changes similar to those described for cerebrovascular disease. Diffuse changes often give way to focal ones, especially if the lesions are on the lateral or superior surface of the brain, and these in turn usually disappear over a period of weeks or months unless seizures supervene. Sharp waves or spikes sometimes emerge as the focal slow-wave abnormality resolves. These or failure of the EEG to "normalize" usually precede the occurrence of posttraumatic epilepsy. Following head injury, therefore, serial EEGs may be of prognostic value as regards the prospect of epilepsy.

Diseases that cause coma and states of impaired consciousness The EEG is abnormal in almost all conditions in which there is some impairment of consciousness. With hypothyroidism the rhythms are normal in configuration but are usually slow. In general, the more profound the change in consciousness, the more abnormal the EEG recording. In these latter situations slow waves (delta) are bilateral, are of high amplitude, and tend to predominate over the frontal regions. This pertains to such differing conditions as acute meningitis or encephalitis, severe disorders of blood gases, glucose, electrolyte and water balance, uremia, diabetic coma, liver coma, or impairment of consciousness accompanying the large cerebral lesions discussed above. In hepatic coma, the degree of abnormality in the EEG corresponds to the degree of confusion, stupor, or coma. Moreover, paroxysms of bilaterally synchronous large, sharp "triphasic waves" are characteristic, though they may also be seen with other metabolic encephalopathies associated with renal or pulmonary failure. Diffuse diseases (e.g., Alzheimer's disease) affecting the cerebral cortex are accompanied by a relatively slight degree of diffuse, slow-wave abnormality in the theta (4- to 7-Hz) range. Certain more rapidly progressive ones, such as subacute sclerosing panencephalitis (SSPE), Creutzfeldt-Jakob disease, and to a lesser extent the cerebral lipidoses, have, in addition, very characteristic, almost pathognomonic EEG changes consisting of recurring complex bursts of sharp and slow activity. A focal, temporal EEG abnormality in a patient suspected of having herpes simplex encephalitis may indicate the side for cerebral biopsy or may be sufficient confirmation to allow initiation of antiviral therapy. A normal EEG in a patient who is apathetic, slow, depressed, or forgetful is a point in favor of the diagnosis of an affective disorder or schizophrenia.

An EEG may also assist the physician in caring for a comatose patient when the pertinent history is unavailable. It may point to such otherwise unexpected causes as hepatic encephalopathy (bilaterally synchronous triphasic waves), intoxication with barbiturates or benzodiazepines [(excess fast activity), clinically inapparent continuous epileptic discharges (status epilepticus), a large space-occupying lesion, or diffuse anoxia-ischemia ("burst-suppression") pattern with repetitive generalized complexes separated by periods with very little EEG].

Other diseases of the cerebrum There are many disorders of nervous function that cause little or no alteration in the EEG. Multiple sclerosis and other demyelinating diseases are examples, though as many as 50 percent of advanced cases will have an abnormal record. Delirium tremens, Wernicke-Korsakoff disease, transient global amnesia, and withdrawal seizures, despite the dramatic nature of the clinical picture, cause little or no changes in the EEG. Some degree of slowing often accompanies confusional states. Interestingly, anxiety states and psychoses, such as manic-depressive disorders or schizophrenia, abnormal states due to hallucinogenic drugs such as LSD, and the majority of cases of mental retardation are associated with no important modification of the normal record or with nonspecific abnormalities.

SPECIAL APPLICATIONS OF THE EEG Because the EEG provides information about the status and function of the brain, it is useful as a monitor in the operating room to ensure the presence of a viable brain during the increasingly extensive procedures of modern cardiovascular surgery. The presence of EEG patterns appropriate to the depth of anesthesia and the agents in use is the final common denominator and confirms the adequacy of cerebral blood flow and oxygenation. It is routine practice now for the EEG to be monitored continuously during carotid endarterectomies in patients with stenotic or ulcerative carotid artery disease. Characteristic EEG changes (particularly marked voltage attenuation) signal the need for a temporary bypass shunt to maintain sufficient cerebral blood flow to preclude ischemic cerebral damage during surgery. Observing EEG changes may eventually be shown to be useful in monitoring the cerebral status of all patients during surgical anesthesia.

In the neurosurgical operating room the EEG can be recorded from exposed brain (electrocorticogram), and seizure patterns can be localized more precisely than from the scalp so that resection of such physiologically abnormal tissue may be undertaken (see Chap. 350).

The routine EEG can be of value in the diagnosis of hysterical blindness. Similarly, a response evoked by noise during light sleep can be helpful in confirming the presence of hearing in a patient who feigns total deafness. These responses may also be useful in evaluating hearing and vision in infants. Ambulatory EEG monitoring over a 24-h period, in which a miniature EEG recorder allows the patient to engage in normal daily activities at home or work, may assist in the evaluation of unexplained episodes of disturbed consciousness.

EVOKED RESPONSES

An evoked response (sometimes termed an evoked potential) is the record of electrical activity produced by groups of neurons within the cord, brainstem, thalamus, or cerebral hemispheres following stimulation of one or another sensory system by means of visual, auditory, or tactile input. The amplitude of these potentials, as recorded from the scalp using ordinary EEG electrodes, ranges from less than 0.5 to 20 μV. Because of their extremely small size, they can rarely be recognized on the ink-written EEG record with the background of ongoing EEG activity, which itself is usually 50 μV or more in amplitude. Therefore, special techniques, requiring simple computers, must be used to extract the evoked response waveform that one is interested in, from the continuous background EEG activity. These techniques are called "averaging" because the process involves repeating 100 to 1000 precisely timed stimuli and recording the electrical activity during a certain brief interval following each stimulus. The random ongoing EEG activity which, at any given point in time following the stimulus, is sometimes negative and at other times positive in polarity, tends to cancel out with sufficient repetition. The evoked response, however, is time-locked to the stimulus, and at a given time following the stimulus always has the same electrical sign as well as shape. The evoked response thus grows larger with repetition while the background averages out and becomes smaller. It is important to have special amplifiers, to apply the electrodes to the surface of the scalp with great care, and to time stimuli precisely with a minimum of accompanying electrical artifact. These evoked responses provide sensitive, objective extensions of the clinical neurologic examination of the related sensory system, but they are no more specific etiologically and must be carefully integrated into the clinical situation by a physician familiar with the clinical use of the test. The physician must decide if other procedures are indicated to differentiate the possible causes of the conduction abnormality.

VISUAL EVOKED RESPONSES Visual evoked responses produced by a pattern shift (PSVER) have the longest history of clinical usefulness. During this test, patients are asked to watch an alternating black and white checkerboard pattern which is projected on a screen. When patients watch this pattern shift, it produces a characteristic waveform which can be recorded from the scalp over the posterior portion of the head. Under normal circumstances, this triphasic wave has a distinctive positive peak at 95 to 115 ms latency (usually called P100) from the time of pattern reversal. This latency, the duration of the response, and the amplitude of the peak are measured; the latency is the most important parameter clinically. Each eye is tested independently. A purely monocular abnormality indicates that the conduction defect is anterior to the chiasm.

Many diseases processes affecting the optic nerve fibers in their intraocular, orbital, or cranial portions produce abnormalities of this potential. Glaucoma, compression of the optic nerve, chiasm, or tract by various space-occupying lesions, and degenerative disease of this system often produce a reduction in amplitude and/or prolonged latency of the PSVER. If the visual system is sufficiently affected, no response may be recorded by stimulation of one or both eyes. In a general hospital setting, however, the most common cause of abnormality in this response is optic neuritis, frequently associated with multiple sclerosis. Demyelination of the optic nerve fibers, as a primary demyelinating disease or due to one of the lesions listed above, slows conduction in the nerve fibers so that the latency of the positive peak of the PSVER is prolonged (115 to 200 ms). In fact, almost all patients with optic neuritis, even after the visual acuity has returned to normal, continue to show distinct abnormalities in this PSVER at a time when detailed ophthalmologic evaluations reveal no abnormality. In multiple sclerosis, if the PSVER is normal, the neuroophthalmologic examination is almost always normal (we have had no exceptions to this rule in more than 225 patients). Even when the PSVER is abnormal, the visual fields, visual acuity, pupillary reactions, and optic fundus examination are normal in a considerable number of patients.

Approximately one-half of the patients with multiple sclerosis who have never had visual symptoms also show abnormalities, and this accounts for one of the most useful aspects of the test. If a patient presents with what appears to be the first episode of a neurologic illness in which the lesion is in the brainstem or spinal cord, a demonstration by means of an abnormal PSVER of another clinically unsuspected lesion in a different part of the central nervous system (the optic nerves) makes the diagnosis of multiple sclerosis more likely and may spare the patient certain neuroradiologic procedures.

Abnormalities in visual acuity have no effect on the PSVER unless the acuity is so poor that the patient cannot see the checkerboard pattern—patients with acuity of 20/200 or better are suitable for testing. The only other requirement is that the patient be cooperative enough to sit still for 20 min and watch the pattern. Infants and children can also be tested by using special techniques.

BRAINSTEM AUDITORY EVOKED RESPONSES Brainstem auditory evoked responses (BAERs) are more difficult to obtain than PSVERs because BAERs are much smaller, of the order of 0.5 μV. These are produced by clicks transmitted to one of a patient's ears through earphones. The patient may be alert or comatose and need not be particularly cooperative except that excess movement or muscle artifact makes the response even more difficult to obtain. BAERs of essentially normal appearance can be recorded from infants and children. BAERs consist of a series of seven waves which appear within the first 10 ms after the click. These (named I to VII) are considered to represent successive activation of the auditory nerve (I) and the brainstem auditory pathways (cochlear nucleus, II; superior olivary complex, III; lateral lemniscus, IV; inferior colliculus, V; and higher auditory centers, VI, VII). A lesion at or between any of these levels either obliterates or delays the appearance of waves from successively higher levels. The same is true of other lesions affecting the brainstem, such as small vascular lesions, central pontine myelinolysis or hypoxic damage. The waves that arise from structures caudal to the lesion are perfectly normal in latency, whereas those arising from structures cranial to the lesion are either obliterated or delayed. This allows one to pinpoint quite accurately the level of the lesion within the brainstem auditory pathways and provides a very neat opportunity for correlation of clinical observations with neurophysiologic and occasionally pathologic data. This test is useful as a screening test for patients with acoustic neuromas (who almost always show an abnormality), for patients suspected of having multiple sclerosis, for comatose patients in whom the level of lesion within the central nervous system is not clear, and for other patients in whom documentation of brainstem lesions is important. Hearing loss can often be recognized in this test, since changes in the latency of the first (and, therefore, subsequent) waves are produced, and these must be taken into consideration in the evaluation of the results obtained. Interwave latencies, which are the parameters used to measure central conduction, are not affected by hearing loss or stimulus intensity. The test is also useful in screening high-risk infants for hearing defects.

SOMATOSENSORY EVOKED RESPONSES Somatosensory evoked responses (SERs) are produced by small painless electrical stimuli administered to large sensory fibers in mixed nerves of the hand or leg. The afferent volley is recorded at many levels as it ascends the somatosensory pathways, and a series of waves can be recorded which reflect activity in peripheral nerve trunks, tracts in the spinal cord, gracile and cuneate nuclei, pontine and/or cerebellar structures, thalamus, thalamocortical radiations, and primary sensory fields of the cortex. Lesions of the pathways at any level affect the subsequent waves, thus providing localizing and confirmatory data in a similar fashion to the BAER.

Evoked responses can be used for a single evaluation of patients (looking for lesions in the various pathways discussed) or as a quantitative method for following a patient's course to document functional improvement or deterioration as time passes, following therapy, and so on. They also prove useful for on-line monitoring of function in optic nerve, brainstem, or spinal cord during neurosurgical procedures that involve manipulation of those structures. Since BAERs and SERs are unaffected by general anesthesia and high-dose barbiturates, they also can be used to follow CNS function in comatose patients. Longer latency auditory and somatosensory evoked responses have been studied for a number of years. These are largely cortically produced responses, dramatically affected by drowsiness, inattention, and other poorly controllable variables, and have not proven to be clinically useful. Neither have most visual evoked responses produced by stroboscopic flashes. They are very useful in evaluation of visual pathways in infants and young children who are not cooperative enough to watch the checkerboard pattern and in adults during surgery or when comatose. Under other circumstances, pattern-shift PSVERs afford a much more reliable and reproducible response.

MOTOR EVOKED RESPONSES In conventional motor nerve conduction studies, recordings are made from peripheral muscles and the nerve is stimulated at various sites between the muscle and the spinal cord. The rostral limit of such studies has been determined by the accessibility of the proximal parts of the peripheral nervous system to stimulation. Magnetic stimulators developed over the last few years induce sufficient current flow in conductive tissues to allow the motor cortex itself to be stimulated painlessly through the intact skull in humans. The resultant compound motor action potential, measured over peripheral muscles, has a very high amplitude (compared to SEP waveforms) and does not require signal averaging. Stimulation of the motor pathways at multiple sites allows the conduction properties of the intervening motor tracts, including central ones, to be studied in health and disease. This provides objective, numerical data relating to the functioning of central motor pathways, previously amenable only to peripheral tests usually dependent on patient cooperation (e.g., grip strength).

Clinical applications of these motor evoked responses have been reported and they show very good correlations with motor disabilities in multiple sclerosis and motor neuron diseases. In the latter disease, the motor cortex may be unexcitable by the transcranial magnetic stimulator, despite moderate preservation of voluntary strength.

LUMBAR PUNCTURE AND CEREBROSPINAL FLUID EXAMINATION

The information yielded by the examination of the cerebrospinal fluid (CSF) is often of crucial importance in diagnosis and treatment.

INDICATIONS FOR LUMBAR PUNCTURE Lumbar puncture is performed for the following reasons:

1 To obtain pressure measurements and to secure a sample of CSF for cellular, chemical, and bacteriologic examination.

2 To aid in therapy by the administration of spinal anesthetics and occasionally antibiotics or antitumor agents.

3 To inject air for air contrast myelography or, very rarely, for pneumoencephalography; a radiopaque substance or a water-soluble contrast medium for myelography; or a radioactive substance [e.g., indium or radioactive iodinated serum albumin (RISA)] for the study of CSF dynamics and to aid in the diagnosis of hydrocephalus or CSF leak.

Lumbar puncture carries a risk if the CSF pressure is high (evidenced by headache and papilledema), for it increases the possibility of fatal cerebellar or tentorial herniation. In doubtful cases, it is wise first to obtain a CT or magnetic resonance image (MRI) to exclude a mass lesion before proceeding to perform a lumbar puncture. However, if it seems important in a given case of suspected increased intracranial pressure to have the information yielded by CSF examination, the lumbar puncture may be performed with a fine-bore (no. 22 or 24 gauge) needle as the last part of the clinical study. (Note that if the pressure is over 400 mmHg, one should obtain the necessary sample of fluid, remove the needle, and then, according to the suspected clinical disease and patient's condition, administer mannitol in a dose of 0.75 to 1.0 mg/kg.) Dexamethasone should be started in a dose of 4 to 6 mg every 6 h in cases of tumor, cerebral trauma, hemorrhage, and certain types of encephalitis (acute hemorrhagic leukoencephalitis, herpes simplex encephalitis).

Cisternal puncture and lateral cervical puncture (C1–C2), although safe in the hands of the expert, are too hazardous to entrust to those without experience. The lumbar puncture is to be preferred except in obvious instances of spinal block requiring a sample of cisternal fluid or myelography above the lesions, or in rare instances where infection of the skin or subcutaneous tissue render needle penetration dangerous.

Experience teaches the importance of meticulous technique. Lumbar puncture should always be done under sterile conditions. If procaine is injected in and beneath the skin, the procedure should be painless. Failure to enter the lumbar subarachnoid space after two or three trials can usually be corrected by doing the puncture with patients in the sitting position and then assisting them to lie on their side for pressure measurements and fluid removal. The "dry tap" is more often due to an improperly placed needle than to a pathologic obliteration of subarachnoid space by compressive lesion of the spinal cord or chronic adhesive arachnoiditis. A bloody tap due to transfixation of a meningeal vessel may result in hopeless confusion of the diagnosis if it is falsely interpreted as indicating hemorrhage in the subarachnoid spaces and ventricles. Lumbar puncture should be undertaken with particular care in patients with thrombocytopenia or disorders of blood coagulation because serious hemorrhage into the extradural or intradural space may occur.

EXAMINATION PROCEDURES Once the lumbar puncture is successful, some or all of the following aspects of the CSF should be studied: (1) pressure and "dynamics"; (2) gross appearance of CSF including centrifugation, if blood is present, to examine the supernatant for xanthochromia; (3) number and type of cells and presence of microorganisms; (4) protein, sugar, and, in special instances, analysis of pigments; (5) exfoliative cytology using Millipore filters; (6) Wassermann reaction and appropriate serologic precipitation reactions (including cryptococcal antigen in patients with immunologic suppression, e.g., AIDS); (7) protein immunoelectrophoresis for determination of gamma globulin levels, and other special biochemical tests (for NH_3, pH, CO_2, enzymes, etc.); and (8) bacteriologic cultures and virus isolation. See the appendix for normal values of CSF constituents.

REFERENCES

Chiappa KH (ed.): *Evoked Potentials in Clinical Neurology*, 2nd ed. New York, Raven Press, 1989

Ebersole JS, Bridgers SL: Ambulatory EEG monitoring, in *Recent Advances in Epilepsy*, TA Pedley, BS Meldrum (eds). New York, Churchill Livingstone, 1986, pp 111–135

Engel J, Jr: *Seizures and Epilepsy*. Philadelphia, F.A. Davis, 1989

Engel J Jr: A practical guide for routine EEG studies in epilepsy. J Clin Neurophysiol 1(2):109, 1984

Hess CW et al: Magnetic brain stimulation: Central motor conduction studies in multiple sclerosis. Ann Neurol 22:744, 1987

Kimura J: *Electrodiagnosis in Diseases of Nerve and Muscle*, 2d ed. Philadelphia, F.A. Davis, 1989

Niedermeyer E, Lopes da Silva F (eds): *Electroencephalography*, 2d ed. Baltimore, Urban & Schwarzenberg, 1987

Oh SJ: *Electromyography, Neuromuscular Transmission Studies*. Baltimore, Williams & Wilkins, 1988

Shahani BT (ed): *Electromyography in CNS Disorders: Central EMG*. Boston, Butterworth, 1984

Spehlmann R: *EEG Primer*. New York, Elsevier Biomedical Press, 1981

Stalberg E, Young RR (eds): *Clinical Neurophysiology*. London, Butterworth, 1981

350 THE EPILEPSIES AND CONVULSIVE DISORDERS

MARC A. DICHTER

The *epilepsies* are a group of disorders characterized by chronic, recurrent, paroxysmal changes in neurologic function caused by abnormalities in the electrical activity of the brain. They are estimated to affect between 0.5 and 2 percent of the population, and can occur at any age. Each episode of neurologic dysfunction is called a *seizure*. Seizures may be *convulsive* when they are accompanied by motor manifestations, or may be manifest by other changes in neurologic function (i.e., by sensory, cognitive, emotional events). Epilepsy can be acquired as a result of neurologic injury or a structural brain lesion and can also occur as a part of many systemic medical diseases. Epilepsy also occurs in an *idiopathic* form in an individual with neither a history of neurologic insult nor other apparent neurologic dysfunction. Isolated, nonrecurrent seizures may occur in otherwise healthy individuals for a variety of reasons, and under these circumstances, the individual is not said to have epilepsy.

CLASSIFICATION OF SEIZURES

The neurologic manifestations of epileptic seizures are varied, ranging from a brief lapse of attention to a prolonged loss of consciousness with abnormal motor activity. The proper classification of the kinds of seizures which an individual is experiencing is important for an appropriate diagnostic workup, prognostic evaluation, and selection of therapy. The classification of epileptic seizures provided in this chapter is based on the International Classification of Epileptic Seizures. It emphasizes the clinical seizure type and ictal (seizure-associated) and interictal (between seizure) electroencephalographic pattern (Table 350-1), whereas etiology, anatomic substrate, and pathways of spread are not major considerations. The older terminology of grand mal, petit mal, and psychomotor or temporal lobe epilepsy has been integrated into the current scheme. In addition to identifying the seizure types which an individual is experiencing, it is also useful to categorize the clinical context within which the seizures occur. Epilepsy syndromes that take into account the age of the patient, types of seizures, presence of underlying neurologic lesion, etc., help define groups of patients with relatively predictable prognoses and for whom specific therapies are indicated.

The major underlying premise of the seizure classification is that some seizures (partial or focal seizures) start in one area of the brain (cortex) and either remain localized or generalize (that is, spread throughout the brain), whereas other seizures appear to be general from their earliest manifestation.

PARTIAL OR FOCAL SEIZURES Partial or focal seizures begin with the activation of neurons in one area of the cortex. The specific clinical symptoms depend on the area of cortex involved and imply dysfunction in a limited area of the cortex. The lesion may be due to birth injury, postnatal trauma, tumor, abscess, infarction, vascular malformation, or some other structural abnormality. The abnormal area of the cortex underlying the seizure activity can be identified by the specific neurologic phenomena observed during the focal seizure. Partial seizures are classified as "simple" if there is no alteration of consciousness or awareness of the environment and "complex" if there is such a change.

Simple partial seizures Simple partial seizures can occur with motor, sensory, autonomic, or psychic symptoms. A simple partial seizure with motor signs consists of recurrent contractions of the muscles of one part of the body (finger, hand, arm, face, etc.) without loss of consciousness. Each muscular contraction is caused by the discharge of neurons in the corresponding area of the contralateral motor cortex.

TABLE 350-1 Classification of epileptic seizures

I Partial or focal seizures
- *A* Simple partial seizures (with motor, sensory, autonomic, or psychic signs)
- *B* Complex partial seizures (psychomotor or temporal lobe seizures)
- *C* Secondary generalized partial seizures

II Primary generalized seizures
- *A* Tonic-clonic (grand mal)
- *B* Tonic
- *C* Absence (petit mal)
- *D* Atypical absence
- *E* Myoclonic
- *F* Atonic
- *G* Infantile spasms

III Status epilepticus
- *A* Tonic-clonic status
- *B* Absence status
- *C* Epilepsia partialis continua

IV Recurrence patterns
- *A* Sporadic
- *B* Cyclic
- *C* Reflex (photomyoclonic, somatosensory, musicogenic, reading epilepsy)

The muscle activity of a partial seizure ("ictus") may remain confined to one area or may spread from the affected area to involve contiguous ipsilateral body parts (i.e., right thumb to right hand to right arm to right side of face). This "Jacksonian march," first described by Hughlings Jackson, is caused by a demonstrable progression of epileptiform discharges in the contralateral motor cortex and may occur over seconds or minutes. The EEG manifestations of this form of seizure are often very striking and consist of regularly occurring spike discharges in the appropriate area of the motor cortex. Between seizures (interictal period) this region may give rise to irregular spike discharges in the EEG.

Simple partial seizures may have other behavioral manifestations if the seizure discharges occur in other cortical regions. Thus, sensory symptoms (paresthesias, vertiginous feelings, simple auditory or visual hallucinations) occur with epileptiform discharges in the contralateral sensory cortex, and autonomic and psychic symptoms [i.e., the sensation of having experienced something before (déjà vu), unwarranted sense of fear or anger, illusions, and even complex hallucinations] occur with discharges in temporal and frontal lobes.

Complex partial seizures (temporal lobe or psychomotor seizures) Complex partial seizures are episodic changes in behavior in which an individual loses conscious contact with the environment. The onset of these seizures may consist of any of a variety of auras: an unusual smell (as of burning rubber), a feeling that the current experience has happened before (déjà vu), a sudden intense emotional feeling, a sensory illusion such as that of objects growing smaller (micropsia) or larger (macropsia), or a specific formed sensory hallucination. Patients may come to recognize these as heralding their seizures, or the memory of the aura may be lost in the postictal amnesia, which often occurs if the seizure becomes generalized. During complex partial seizures there may be a cessation of activity with some minor motor activity, such as lip smacking, swallowing, walking aimlessly, or picking at one's clothes (automatisms). Complex partial seizures may also be accompanied by the unconscious performance of highly skilled activities such as driving a car or playing complicated musical pieces. When the seizure ends, the individual is amnesic for events which took place during the seizure and may take minutes or hours to recover full consciousness.

Patients with complex partial seizures have EEGs that exhibit unilateral or bilateral spikes, sharp waves, or slow wave discharges over temporal or frontotemporal regions both interictally and during seizures. Most of these seizures originate from epileptiform activity in the temporal lobes—especially the hippocampus or amygdala—or other parts of the limbic system, but others have been shown to originate from mesial parasagittal or orbital frontal regions. Epilepsy manifest by these kinds of seizures is also referred to as "temporal lobe epilepsy'' and ''psychomotor epilepsy'' in older classification schemes.

Although often showing spike discharges or focal slowing during complex partial seizures, exceptionally the surface EEG may be normal. Sphenoidal electrodes may record the abnormal discharges, but in some cases only depth electrodes in the hippocampus or amygdala or other limbic structures will show seizure discharges. The occasional discrepancy between surface and depth electrophysiologic events is a particularly difficult problem when trying to use the surface EEG to determine the nature of an abnormal behavior in an individual susupected of having complex partial seizures. (See ''Differential Diagnosis of Seizures,'' below.)

Secondary generalization of partial seizures Simple or complex partial seizures can progress to generalized seizures with loss of consciousness and often with convulsive motor activity. This may occur immediately or after many seconds or a minute or two. In addition, many patients with focal seizures have generalized seizures without an obvious initial focal component which are difficult to distinguish from primary generalized seizures. The presence of an aura or the observation of any focal feature (twitching of one extremity, aphasia, tonic eye deviation) at the onset of the generalized seizure or the presence of a postictal focal neurologic deficit (Todd's paralysis) are important clues to a focal origin to the seizure.

PRIMARY GENERALIZED SEIZURES Tonic-clonic (grand mal) One of the most common kinds of epileptic paroxysms is the generalized tonic-clonic seizure. Some of these appear to be primary generalized seizures and others are the result of secondary generalization from partial seizures. In either case, the seizures follow a common pattern. The primary generalized seizures usually start without warning, although some individuals sense a vague, nonspecific sense of the impending event. The onset is heralded by a sudden loss of consciousness, a *tonic* contraction of the muscles, a loss of postural control, and a cry produced by a forced expiration caused by contraction of the respiratory muscles. The individual falls to the floor in an opisthotonic posture, often sustaining injury, and remains rigid for many seconds. There may be cyanosis as respiration is inhibited. Soon a series of rhythmic contractions of all four limbs occurs. This *clonic* phase can last for a variable period of time and ends when the muscles relax. The individual remains unconscious and unarousable for a period of minutes or longer. There is usually a gradual return to consciousness, and often a period of disorientation during recovery. The patient may even be combative if restrained. During the seizure, urinary or fecal incontinence and tongue biting may occur. Postictally there is amnesia for the seizure, and sometimes a retrograde amnesia as well. Headache and drowsiness are common sequelae, and the individual may not return to baseline functioning for days.

The EEG in patients with tonic-clonic seizures shows low-voltage fast (10-Hz or more) activity during the tonic phase, which converts gradually to slower, larger sharp waves throughout both hemispheres. During the clonic phase there are bursts of sharp waves associated with the rhythmic muscular contractions and slow waves coincident with the pauses. Often the excessive muscular activity of the seizure causes artifacts which interfere with ictal EEG recordings. Interictally, the EEG is often abnormal, with polyspike (or spike) and wave or occasionally sharp and slow wave discharges; interictal EEGs may also be normal.

Tonic seizures Tonic seizures are a less common form of primary generalized seizure which consist of the sudden occurrence of a rigid posturing of the limbs or torso, often with deviation of the head and eyes toward one side. They are not followed by a clonic phase, and are often of shorter duration than tonic-clonic seizures.

Absence seizures (petit mal) Pure absence seizures consist of the sudden cessation of ongoing conscious activity without convulsive muscular activity or loss of postural control. Such seizures may be so brief as to be inapparent. Usually they last for seconds and, occasionally, for as long as several minutes. The brief lapses of consciousness or awareness may be accompanied by minor motor manifestations such as eyelid fluttering, small chewing movements of the mouth, or mild shaking of the hands. During longer absences, automatisms may occur which may be difficult to distinguish from complex partial seizures. At the end of the absence seizure, the patient regains awareness of the environment very quickly, and there is usually no period of postictal confusion.

Absence seizures almost always begin in younger children (6 to 14 years of age) and rarely appear for the first time in adults. These brief seizures may occur hundreds or more times per day and go on for weeks or months before it is recognized that the child is having seizures. Absence seizures may first be recognized when the child begins having learning difficulties in school.

The EEG is pathognomonic in this form of seizure disorder. Brief 3-Hz spike and wave discharges, which appear synchronously throughout all the leads, occur interictally, but become clinically significant as absence seizures when they last more than several seconds. Interictal EEG background activity is otherwise normal. Often the EEG demonstrates that the child is having more seizures than was thought from clinical observation alone.

Absence seizures usually occur in otherwise neurologically normal children. These seizures are usually sensitive to antiepileptic drugs (see below). Children with this condition often do quite well once it is treated. Approximately one-third outgrow the seizure disorder, one-third continue to have only absence seizures, and one-third have concomitant generalized tonic-clonic seizures.

Absence seizures can be differentiated from absence-like attacks which occasionally occur in complex partial seizures by the lack of aura, immediate recovery from the absence, and typical 3-Hz spike and wave EEG pattern.

Atypical absence Atypical absence seizures are similar to absence seizures but coexist with other forms of generalized seizures, such as tonic seizures, myoclonic seizures, or atonic seizures (see below). The EEG is more heterogeneous, containing spike and wave discharges at 2 or 4 Hz during the absence attacks and poorly developed background with spike or polyspike activity during interictal periods.

Atypical absence seizures commonly occur in children with some other form of underlying neurologic dysfunction and tend to be resistant to medication. In the most severe form of this disorder, the Lennox-Gastaut syndrome, children have several kinds of generalized seizures and often have intellectual impairment.

Myoclonic seizures Myoclonic seizures are sudden, brief, single or repetitive muscle contractions involving one body part or the entire body. In the latter case, the seizure is accompanied by a violent fall, without a loss of consciousness. Myoclonic seizures often coexist with other seizure types but may occur alone. The EEG shows polyspike and wave discharges or sharp and slow waves, both ictally and interictally. Although often idiopathic, myoclonic seizures occur as a major neurologic symptom in a variety of medical conditions including uremia, hepatic failure, Creutzfeldt-Jakob disease, subacute leukoencephalopathies, and a hereditary degenerative condition, Lafora body disease.

Juvenile myoclonic epilepsy (of Janz) has been identified as a distinct syndrome which begins in adolescence and which has a genetic component. It often begins with postawakening myoclonic seizures, and later in its course, these may be followed by generalized tonic-clonic seizures.

Atonic seizures Atonic seizures are brief losses of consciousness and postural tone not associated with tonic muscular contractions. The individual may simply drop to the floor without apparent cause. Atonic seizures usually occur in children and are often accompanied by other forms of seizures. The EEG contains polyspikes and slow waves. The ''drop attacks'' of atonic seizures need to be distinguished from cataplexy seen in narcolepsy (where the patient remains conscious), transient brainstem ischemia, or sudden rises in intracranial pressure.

Infantile spasms or hypsarrhythmia These primary generalized seizures occur in infants between birth and approximately 12 months of age and consist of several types of brief synchronous contractions of the neck, torso, and both arms (usually in flexion). Infantile spasms often occur in children with underlying neurologic diseases, such as anoxic encephalopathy or tuberous sclerosis, but can rarely occur in an otherwise apparently normal infant. The prognosis for children with this form of seizure disorder is grave, and approximately 90 percent develop mental retardation in addition to their seizures. The EEG is characterized by a very disorganized background, random high-voltage slow waves, spikes, and burst suppression (hypsarrhythmia). The spasms and hypsarrhythmia tend to disappear over the first 3 to 5 years of life only to be replaced by other forms of generalized seizures. Infantile spasms sometimes respond to treatment with ACTH or valproic acid.

STATUS EPILEPTICUS Prolonged or repetitive seizures without a period of recovery between attacks can occur with all forms of seizures and is defined as "status epilepticus." When tonic-clonic seizures are involved, this state can be life-threatening (see "Treatment of Seizures"). Absence status, on the other hand, may proceed for some time before it is recognized, because the patient does not lose consciousness or have convulsive movements. Status epilepticus of partial seizures is called *epilepsia partialis continua* and may occur with partial motor, sensory, or visceral seizures. Complex partial seizures may also present as status epilepticus.

RECURRENCE PATTERNS All classes of recurrent seizures can occur sporadically or randomly, with no apparent triggering event, or can occur cyclically, i.e., in concert with the sleep-wake cycle or the menstrual cycle (catamenial epilepsy). Epileptic seizures can also occur as evoked reactions to a specific stimulus (reflex epilepsy), although this is relatively infrequent. Examples are seizures triggered by photic stimulation (photomyoclonic or photoconvulsive epilepsy), specific musical compositions (musicogenic epilepsy), tactile stimulation (somatosensory-induced epilepsy), or reading (reading or language epilepsy). The latter usually consists of brief myoclonic jerks of the jaw, cheek, and tongue which occur during silent or oral reading and may progress to generalized tonic-clonic seizures.

PATHOPHYSIOLOGY OF EPILEPSY

Epileptic seizures can be induced in any normal human (or vertebrate) brain with a variety of different electrical or chemical stimuli. The ease and rapidity with which these seizures can occur and the stereotyped nature of the seizures produced suggest that the normal brain, particularly the cerebral cortex, contains within its fine anatomic and physiologic structure a mechanism which is inherently unstable and which can be influenced in many different ways to produce a seizure. Thus, many different kinds of metabolic abnormalities and anatomic lesions of brain can produce seizures, and conversely, there is no pathognomonic lesion of the epileptic brain.

The hallmark of the altered physiologic state of epilepsy is a rhythmical and repetitive hypersynchronous discharge of many neurons in a localized area of the brain. A reflection of this hypersynchronous discharge can be observed in the electroencephalogram. The EEG records the integrated electrical activity generated by synaptic potentials in neurons in the superficial layers of a localized area of cortex. Normally, the EEG records unsynchronized activity during periods when the mind is actively working, or mildly synchronized activity when the mind is in a restful state (i.e., alpha waves during relaxation with closed eyes) or during various stages of sleep. In the epileptic focus, neurons in a small area of the cortex are activated for a brief period (50 to 100 ms) in an unusually synchronized manner, and this produces a larger, sharper waveform in the EEG—the spike discharge. If the synchronous neuronal discharge occurs over several seconds, a focal seizure follows; if it spreads through the brain and lasts for many seconds or minutes, a complex partial or generalized seizure (the ictus) will occur and the EEG can have a variety of appearances, depending on which areas of brain are involved and how the primary discharging areas project to the superficial cortex. During the seizure the EEG may display low-voltage fast activity or high-voltage spikes or spike and wave discharges throughout both hemispheres.

During the interictal spike discharge, the neurons in the epileptic focus undergo a large membrane depolarization (the depolarizing shift, or DS) accompanied by action potential generation. After the DS, the neurons hyperpolarize and stop firing for several seconds. In areas around the discharging focus, the neurons are also inhibited. Thus, it appears as if the epileptic discharge is limited to a localized area of cortex by a ring of inhibition around the focus and slightly delayed inhibition within the focus. When the epileptic focus undergoes a transition from the isolated discharges to a seizure, the post-DS inhibition disappears and is replaced by a depolarizing potential. Neurons in contiguous areas and in synaptically connected distant areas are then recruited into the seizure and become activated. Local cortical circuits, long association pathways (including callosal), and subcortical pathways are all utilized for the spread of the discharges. Thus, a focal seizure can spread locally or generalize throughout the brain. Widely ramifying thalamocortical pathways are likely to be responsible for the rapid generalization of some forms of epilepsy, including absence seizures.

A number of metabolic events occur within the brain during the epileptic discharges which may contribute to the development of the focus, to the transition to seizures, or to postictal dysfunction. During the discharges, extracellular potassium concentration increases and extracellular calcium concentration decreases. Both of these changes have profound effects on neuronal excitability and neurotransmitter release and on neuronal metabolism. Neurotransmitters and neuropeptides are also released in unusually large amounts during seizure discharges. Some of these substances can have prolonged actions on central neurons and may be responsible for prolonged postictal phenomona such as Todd's paralysis. In addition to the ionic effects, seizures produce increases in cerebral blood flow to the primary involved areas, increases in glucose utilization, and alterations in oxidative metabolism and local pH. It is possible that these events are not just consequences of the seizures but actually contribute to the development of the seizure activity and that manipulation of such factors could become an effective means for controlling seizures.

There are many mechanisms by which seizures can develop in either normal or pathologic brains. Three common mechanisms include (1) diminution of inhibitory mechanisms, especially synaptic inhibition due to gamma-aminobutyric acid (GABA), (2) enhancement of excitatory synaptic mechanisms, especially those mediated by the *N*-methyl-D-aspartate (NMDA) component of glutamate responses, and (3) enhancement of endogenous neuronal burst firing (usually by enhancing voltage-dependent calcium currents). Different forms of human epilepsy may be caused by any one or combination of these mechanisms. For example, in some forms of chronic focal epilepsy, inhibitory interneurons appear to be preferentially lost; in other models, and possibly in cases of human hippocampal sclerosis, aberrant recurrent excitatory connections may form among surviving neurons. In primary generalized absence epilepsy, thalamic neurons with large, low-threshold, transient, voltage-dependent calcium currents may be responsible for generating the diffusely synchronous cortical spike and wave activity.

Currently available antiepileptic drugs appear to operate on several of these mechanisms. Phenytoin, carbamazepine, barbiturates, and valproic acid all appear able to block voltage-dependent sodium channels in a use-dependent manner, such that individual action potentials are relatively unaffected but high-frequency repetitive firing is reduced. The barbiturates and benzodiazepines can enhance GABA-mediated inhibition. Ethosuximide appears to block a low-threshold, transient calcium current in neurons. At present, no drugs are available for clinical use which specifically block excitatory synaptic systems, but much effort is being expended in this direction.

Electrical stimulation is another mechanism by which seizures can easily be produced in a normal brain. At certain current strengths and stimulus frequencies, seizure discharges are produced and become self-sustaining beyond the original stimulus. Generalized tonic-clonic seizures result. At lower stimulus parameters, seizure afterdischarges may not occur. However, if a stereotyped subthreshold stimulus is repeated at regular intervals (which may even be as infrequent as one stimulation per day), there is a gradual buildup of response until generalized seizures occur to the same stimulus which was originally subthreshold. Eventually spontaneous seizures may occur without any further electrical stimulation. This phenomenon has been called "kindling." Its relationship to the pathophysiology of posttraumatic epilepsy or to the issue of whether the occurrence of seizures themselves tends to foster the continued development of a seizure focus in human beings has not been resolved.

THE CAUSES OF EPILEPSY

The likely etiology of a given seizure depends on the age of the patient and the type of seizure (Table 350-2). In young infants, anoxia or ischemia before or during birth, intracranial birth injury, metabolic disturbances such as hypoglycemia, hypocalcemia, and hypomagnesemia, congenital malformations of the brain, and infections are the most common causes of seizures. In the young child, trauma and infections are common causes of epilepsy, although idiopathic seizures account for the majority of patients.

Genetic factors can influence the development of epilepsy and have also been shown to affect EEG patterns in general. Patients with primary generalized seizures, especially absence and myoclonic seizures, have a higher familial incidence of epilepsy than is found in the normal population, and relatives of such patients have higher incidences of dysrhythmic EEGs, even when they do not have seizures. The mode of inheritance of epilepsy susceptibility appears complicated and probably represents multiple genes with variable penetrance. Even in the highest risk group, however, the chance of a sibling or a child of an individual with generalized seizures also having epilepsy is below 10 percent.

Young children also frequently (approximately 2 to 5 percent of the population) develop seizures with febrile illnesses. These febrile convulsions are short generalized tonic-clonic convulsions which occur during the early phases of a febrile illness in children between the ages of 3 months and 5 years. Febrile seizures must be distinguished from seizures which are triggered by central nervous system infections which coincidentally produce fever (meningitis or encephalitis). There is minimal likelihood that the child will develop epilepsy or any neurologic impairment from the febrile convulsion if the seizure lasts less than 5 min, is generalized rather than focal, and is not associated with any interictal EEG abnormalities or abnormalities on neurologic examination. There may be a family history of this kind of febrile seizure. Febrile seizures of this kind are probably best treated with quick and relatively vigorous attempts to keep children from developing excessive fevers during various childhood illnesses but without specific antiepileptic medication. Some pediatricians prefer to maintain children susceptible to febrile convulsions on phenobarbital medication; others advocate administration of benzodiazepines at the first signs of illness. On the other hand, if the febrile convulsion is prolonged or focal or is associated with an abnormal EEG, or if the child has a neurologic abnormality, there is a significant risk of subsequent epilepsy. These children should be treated with chronic antiepileptic therapy.

TABLE 350-2 The causes of seizures

Infant (0–2)	Paranatal hypoxia and ischemia Intracranial birth injury Acute infection Metabolic disturbances (hypoglycemia, hypocalcemia, hypomagnesemia, pyridoxine deficiency) Congenital malformation Genetic disorders
Child (2–12)	Idiopathic Acute infection Trauma Febrile convulsion
Adolescent (12–18)	Idiopathic Trauma Drug, alcohol withdrawal Arteriovenous malformations
Young adult (18–35)	Trauma Alcoholism Brain tumor
Older adult (>35)	Brain tumor Cerebrovascular disease Metabolic disorders (uremia, hepatic failure, electrolyte abnormality, hypoglycemia) Alcoholism

In adolescents and young adults, head trauma is a major cause of focal epilepsy. Epilepsy can be caused by any kind of serious head injury, with the likelihood of developing recurrent seizures being proportional to the extent of the damage. Injuries which either cause dural penetration or produce posttraumatic amnesia of more than 24-h duration may result in a 40 to 50 percent incidence of later epilepsy, while the incidence with closed head injuries with cerebral contusion varies from 5 to 25 percent. Brief concussions or nonpenetrating head injuries without loss of consciousness are not usually epileptogenic. Seizures which occur immediately or within the first 24 h of injury are not associated with a poor prognosis, whereas seizures occurring after the first day and within the first 2 weeks indicate a high likelihood of posttraumatic epilepsy. Most recurring seizures develop by 2 years after the injury. Approximately 50 percent of patients with posttraumatic seizures spontaneously recover, 25 percent have medically controllable seizures, and 25 percent have seizures that are much more intractable to antiepileptic medication. The effectiveness of prophylactic anticonvulsant medication after head trauma still requires adequate documentation, although many physicians treat such patients (and other postoperative neurosurgical patients) with phenytoin or phenobarbital to attempt to prevent the development of posttraumatic seizures.

In the adolescent or young adult age group, generalized tonic-clonic seizures tend to be idiopathic or are associated with drug (especially barbiturate) or alcohol use or withdrawal. Arteriovenous malformations may present as focal seizures in this age group. Between ages 30 and 50, brain tumors become more common causes of seizures and may be present in 30 percent of patients with new focal seizures. In general, the incidence of seizures is higher with slowly growing brain tumors involving the cerebrum, such as meningiomas or low-grade gliomas, than with the more malignant types. However, seizures can occur in individuals with any kind of central nervous system mass lesion, including highly malignant metastatic tumors or completely benign vascular malformations.

Above age 50, cerebrovascular disease is the most common cause of focal or generalized seizures. Seizures can occur acutely in patients with an embolus, hemorrhage or, more rarely, a thrombosis but occur more often as a late sequel to these lesions. Seizures can also result from "silent" cerebral infarctions in patients with no known cerebrovascular disease. Brain tumors, either primary or metastatic, also present with seizures in the older age group.

At any age, a variety of medical diseases can produce metabolic disturbances which may present as seizures. Uremia, hepatic failure, hypo- or hypercalcemia, hypo- and hyperglycemia, or hypo- and hypernatremia may be associated with myoclonic seizures or generalized tonic-clonic seizures.

EVALUATION OF THE PATIENT WITH A SEIZURE

Individuals with seizures present to physicians either in an emergency room setting during the acute attack or in an office setting days after the epileptic event. In the former case, the seizure may be the presenting symptom of a serious central nervous system disorder which requires immediate diagnosis and therapy. In the latter case, the seizure may be a symptom of a more chronic neurologic dysfunction and a different approach is warranted.

Initial emergency evaluation is directed toward ensuring adequate ventilation and perfusion and stopping the seizure (see "Treatment"). Once the patient is medically stable, the investigation is directed at determining the cause of the seizure. Often a careful history (either from the patient, if recovered, or from a friend or relative), a physical examination, and a few blood studies can provide the diagnosis.

A history suggesting a recent febrile illness accompanied by headaches, change in mental status, or confusion suggests an acute CNS infection (either meningitis or encephalitis) and indicates the need for urgent examination of the CSF. In this context, a complex partial seizure may be the presenting symptom of herpes simplex encephalitis. A history of headache and/or change in mental functioning preceding the seizure, coupled with either signs of increased intracranial pressure or a focal neurologic deficit, suggests an underlying mass lesion (tumor, abscess, arteriovenous malformation) or a chronic subdural hematoma. Seizures with a clear focal onset or aura are especially worrisome in this regard. An MRI or CT scan should be performed for a more definitive diagnosis.

The general physical examination may provide important etiologic information. Gum hyperplasia is usually the result of chronic phenytoin therapy. Exacerbation of a chronic seizure disorder due to intercurrent infection, alcohol, or cessation of therapy is a common cause of patients presenting to an emergency room. Skin examination may reveal the port wine facial stain of Sturge-Weber disease (with accompanying cerebral calcifications), the stigmata of tuberous sclerosis (adenoma sebaceum and shagreen patches), or neurofibromatosis (subcutaneous nodules, café au lait spots). Body or limb asymmetries may indicate hypotrophic somatic development contralateral to a congenital or infantile cerebral lesion.

The history or physical examination may also reveal evidence of chronic alcoholism. Heavy alcohol users commonly have seizures for any of several reasons—old cerebral contusion (from falls or fights), chronic subdural hematoma, metabolic derangements of undernutrition and liver disease, CNS infection, or alcohol withdrawal ("rum fits"). Seizures occurring during alcohol use or withdrawal, in the absence of other causes, are usually brief generalized tonic-clonic seizures which occur singly or in a flurry of two or three. Once the flurry is over, chronic antiepileptic treatment is unnecessary, since they are usually self-limiting. Seizures in alcoholics which occur at other times should be treated, but this group of patients presents a particular challenge because of lack of compliance and metabolic problems which complicate drug therapy.

Routine blood studies will indicate if the seizure was caused by hypoglycemia, hypo- or hypernatremia, or hypo- or hypercalcemia. These biochemical abnormalities should be corrected and the cause determined. In addition, other less common causes of seizures can be sought with appropriate tests: thyrotoxicosis, acute intermittent porphyria, and lead or arsenic intoxication.

In the older patient, a seizure may indicate an acute cerebrovascular accident or may be a delayed effect of an old cerebral infarct (even a silent one). The manner in which further evaluation proceeds is dictated by the patient's age, cardiovascular status, and accompanying symptoms.

Generalized tonic-clonic seizures can occur in neurologically normal individuals after moderate sleep deprivation. Such seizures can be seen in individuals working double shifts, in college students around examination time, and in soldiers returning from short leaves of absence. After the first seizure, if all investigations are normal, such individuals do not require further treatment.

If the patient's history, physical examination, and blood chemistries are all normal after a seizure, it is likely that the seizure was "idiopathic" and was not caused by a serious underlying CNS lesion. However, tumors or other mass lesions may be entirely asymptomatic, and every adult with an unexplained seizure should have an EEG and an MRI or CT scan (both without and with contrast) and should be reexamined at regular intervals (3 to 6 months).

The EEG is important in relation to the differential diagnosis of the seizure, the determination of the cause of the seizure, and the proper classification of the seizure. When the diagnosis of a seizure is in doubt, as, for example, when trying to distinguish seizures from syncope, the presence of a paroxysmal EEG abnormality supports the diagnosis of epilepsy. For this purpose, special activation procedures (sleep recording, photic stimulation, or hyperventilation), special EEG leads (sphenoidal, nasopharyngeal, or nasoethmoidal) for recording from deep structures, or prolonged monitoring, even on an ambulatory basis, can be employed. The EEG can also reveal focal abnormalities (spikes, sharp waves, or focal slow waves) which would indicate the possibility of a focal neurologic lesion even if the seizure symptomatology appeared generalized from the outset.

The EEG is also used to help classify seizures. It can distinguish focal seizures with secondary generalization from primary generalized seizures and is especially useful in the differential diagnosis of brief lapses of consciousness. Absence seizures are always accompanied by bilateral spike and wave discharges, whereas complex partial seizures are accompanied by either focal paroxysmal spikes or slow waves or by a normal surface EEG. In cases of absence seizures, the EEG may reveal that the patient is having many more small seizures than was clinically apparent and may help in monitoring antiepileptic drug therapy.

In the past, lumbar puncture, skull x-rays, arteriography, and pneumoencephalography were important adjuncts to the evaluation of the seizure patient. Lumbar puncture is still employed in those situations where acute or chronic CNS infections or subarachnoid hemorrhage are suspected. MRI and CT scans can now provide more definitive information about anatomic lesions than the older, invasive techniques.

DIFFERENTIAL DIAGNOSIS OF SEIZURES

SYNCOPE VERSUS SEIZURE Sudden loss of consciousness, usually without convulsive movements, presents a common diagnostic problem in both children and adults (see Chap. 21). Faints are often preceded by a feeling of light-headedness, of the room spinning, or of a flush, and are often, but not always, precipitated by an environmental stimulus such as prolonged standing in a hot, crowded area, the sight of blood, a fright, etc. In older people, pure syncope is most often secondary to cardiovascular problems, such as Stokes-Adams attacks, tachyarrhythmias, or orthostatic hypotension, and these may occur with or without a warning. A clear focal onset of the event (i.e., abnormal smell, head turning, staring, etc.) favors seizure as the cause. In addition, convulsive muscular contractions, tongue biting, or incontinence commonly accompany seizures but are much less common with fainting spells. Occasionally vasovagal or other types of fainting episodes can be accompanied by either clonic movements or brief generalized tonic-clonic seizures. If the original loss of consciousness can be ascribed to a clear nonepileptic cause (e.g., the patient was having blood drawn or a dental procedure at the time), it is not necessary to regard the episode as a manifestation of epilepsy, and antiepileptic drug therapy is not indicated.

When the origin of a syncopal episode is in doubt, the patient should undergo a complete cardiovascular evaluation, an EEG with sleep recording, and, if available, a prolonged ambulatory EEG monitoring. If the EEG shows paroxysmal activity (which is often brought out by drowsiness and sleep onset), and the patient has no signs of cardiac arrhythmia with ECG monitoring or of valvular disease on echocardiogram, it is likely that the syncopal episode represented a seizure and the patient should be evaluated and treated accordingly.

TRANSIENT ISCHEMIC ATTACKS AND MIGRAINE Transient ischemic attacks (TIAs) and migraine episodes can present as a transient alteration in neurologic function (usually without loss of consciousness) which may be confused diagnostically with focal seizures. Neurologic dysfunction due to ischemia (TIA or migraine) is often a negative symptom (i.e., loss of feeling, numbness, visual field deficit, paralysis), whereas deficits due to focal seizure activity are often positive (twitching, paresthesias, visual distortion, or hallucination), although this distinction is not absolute. Brief stereotyped episodes which conform to dysfunction in a single vascular territory in an individual with either known vascular disease, heart disease, or with risk factors for vascular disease (diabetes, hypertension) are more likely TIAs. However, since cerebral infarcts are a common cause of subsequent seizures in older patients, a paroxysmal EEG focus should be sought.

Classic migraine headaches with a visual aura, unilateral headache, and gastrointestinal upset are usually easy to distinguish from seizures. However, some migraine patients have only "migraine equivalents" such as a hemiparesis, numbness, or aphasia and may not have subsequent headache. These episodes, especially when they occur in older individuals, are hard to distinguish from TIAs, but may also represent focal seizures. The presence of loss of consciousness after some forms of vertebrobasilar migraine and the common occurrence of headaches after seizures makes this differential diagnosis more difficult. The slower development of neurologic dysfunction in migraine (often occurring over minutes) is the most helpful point. Nevertheless, occasionally such patients need to be investigated for all three problems with an MRI or CT scan, carotid studies, and specialized EEG procedures before a diagnosis can be made. In some cases, a therapeutic trial with antiepileptic drugs (which, interestingly, can prevent migraines as well as seizures in some patients) will be necessary for the final diagnosis.

PSYCHOMOTOR VARIANTS AND "HYSTERICAL" SEIZURES As remarked above, patients with complex partial seizures often have bizarre behavioral manifestations of their seizures. These may consist of abrupt changes in personality, feelings of impending doom or of undirected fear, abnormal bodily sensations, episodic forgetfulness, or brief repetitive motor activities such as picking at one's clothes or stamping a foot. Many of these patients also have personality disorders and a significant proportion have had psychiatric intervention. It is common, especially if these patients do not have tonic-clonic seizures or loss of consciousness and when these patients appear emotionally disturbed, for these episodes of psychomotor seizures to be called "psychopathic fugues" or "hysterical seizures." This incorrect diagnosis is often reinforced by a "normal EEG" interictally, or even during one of these episodes. It must be emphasized that seizures can arise from foci deep in temporal lobe structures with *no* surface EEG manifestations. This has been repeatedly demonstrated with depth electrode recordings. Moreover, deep temporal seizures can be manifest only by the kinds of phenomena described above and may be free of the usual seizure phenomena of motor convulsions and loss of consciousness.

In a small number of cases, individuals present with seizure-like events which upon investigation turn out to be hysterical "pseudoseizures" or frank malingering. Often these individuals have had true seizures in the past or are acquainted with an individual with epilepsy. Such pseudoseizures can be quite difficult to distinguish from true seizures. Hysterical seizures are characterized by nonphysiologic events such as a progression of twitching from one hand to the other without spread to subjacent ipsilateral face or leg areas, twitching of all four extremities without loss of consciousness (or with surreptitious loss of consciousness), or careful attention to avoiding injury by moving away from a wall or bed edge while having motor convulsions. In addition, hysterical seizures, especially in adolescent girls, may have frankly sexual overtones, with pelvic thrusting or genital manipulation. While many forms of temporal lobe seizures can occur with normal surface EEGs, generalized tonic-clonic seizures always produce abnormal EEGs both during and after the seizure. Most generalized tonic-clonic seizures and many complex partial seizures of moderate duration are accompanied by rises in serum prolactin (during the immediate 30-min postictal period), whereas "hysterical" seizures are not. Although not an absolute distinguishing point, such measurements, especially if positive, can be very helpful in characterizing the origin of a given "spell." After careful observation, especially with video-EEG monitoring, and after establishing a relationship with the patient, pseudoseizures can sometimes be elicited by suggestion. Frequently, when patients are appropriately confronted with this diagnosis, they respond well, and the pseudoseizures are eliminated or greatly reduced in frequency.

TREATMENT OF SEIZURES

Treatment of the patient with a seizure disorder is directed at eliminating the cause of the seizures, suppressing the expression of the seizures, and dealing with the psychosocial consequences which may occur as a result of the neurologic dysfunction underlying the seizure disorder or from the presence of a chronic disability.

If the seizure disorder is a result of a metabolic disturbance, such as hypoglycemia or hypocalcemia, restoration of normal metabolic function is usually accompanied by cessation of the seizures. If the seizures are caused by a structural brain lesion, such as a brain tumor, arteriovenous malformation, or cerebral cyst, removal of the offending lesion may eliminate the seizures. However, long-standing lesions, even nonprogressive ones, can result in gliosis and chronic denervation. These changes may lead to chronic epileptic foci which will not be eliminated by the subsequent removal of the original lesion. In such cases, surgical extirpation of the epileptic brain regions may be necessary for control of the epilepsy (see "Neurosurgical Approaches to Epilepsy," below).

There is complex interrelationship between the limbic system and neuroendocrine function which may have significant implications for patients with epilepsy. Normal hormonal fluctuations may influence the frequency of seizures, and epilepsy can cause changes in neuroendocrine function. For example, some women will have a marked change in the pattern of their seizures during particular parts of the menstrual cycle (catamenial epilepsy), while others may have changes in seizure frequency in response to oral contraceptives or pregnancy. In general, estrogens tend to exacerbate seizures, while progesterones tend to be more protective. On the other hand, some patients with epilepsy, especially complex partial seizures, may also have an associated reproductive endocrine dysfunction. Disorders in sexual interest, especially hyposexuality, are frequently observed. In addition, women may have polycystic ovary disease, and men may have disturbances in potency. Some patients with these endocrine disorders have not had clinical seizures but have significantly abnormal EEGs (often with temporal discharges). Whether the epilepsy causes the endocrine and/or behavioral dysfunction or whether the two conditions are separate manifestations of a common underlying neuropathologic process is not known. However, endocrine manipulation can sometimes be useful in controlling some forms of seizures, and antiepileptic medication may be a useful adjunct for treating some forms of endocrine dysfunction.

PHARMACOLOGIC CONTROL OF EPILEPSY The fundamental modality for the treatment of epilepsy is pharmacologic therapy. The goal is to protect the patient from having seizures without interfering with normal cognitive function (or, in the child, with development of normal intellectual function) and without producing harmful systemic side effects. If possible, the individual should be treated with the lowest possible dose of a single antiepileptic medication. Precise knowledge of the kind of seizure the patient is having, the spectrum of action of the available antiepileptic medications, and a few basic pharmacokinetic principles can result in the complete control of approximately 60 to 75 percent of patients with epilepsy. Many patients appear to be resistant to medications or develop unnecessary side effects because the medications chosen are not appropriate for the kind(s) of seizure or are not administered in the optimum doses.

The availability of serum levels of antiepileptic drugs makes it possible to optimize dosage regimens for individual patients and to monitor drug compliance. Thus, patients can be placed on a medication and after a suitable equilibration period (usually several weeks, but at least five "half-lives"), the amount of medication in the serum can be determined and compared to standard therapeutic ranges established for each drug. Utilizing blood levels to adjust doses can compensate for individual patient variability in absorption or metabolism of drugs.

Many antiepileptic drugs are bound by serum proteins, and it is the unbound, or "free," drug which is in equilibrium with extracellular spaces within the brain; this level correlates best with seizure control. However, "total" drug is measured in the serum by conventional assays. Under most circumstances, this is adequate for determining if the antiepileptic drug is in the therapeutic range. Occasionally, serum antiepileptic drug levels will be high, yet the patient continues to have seizures without any physiologic side effects of the drug. In these cases, it is possible that serum protein binding is higher than expected and that the patient is undermedicated in relation to the free drug available. Increase in dose may produce control without any untoward side effects (despite a blood level above the therapeutic range). Similarly, individuals with impaired liver or renal function may have low serum proteins or circulating "toxins," which reduces drug binding. In this case, toxicity may appear at unusually low serum levels because of a relatively higher free level of drug.

Intensive long-term EEG and video monitoring have demonstrated that careful characterization of seizures and selection of antiepileptic drugs can significantly increase seizure control in many patients whose seizures had previously been considered intractable to conventional antiepileptic drugs. In fact, often these patients can have one or more of their multiple drugs removed while still achieving better control.

INDICATIONS FOR USE OF SPECIFIC DRUGS Generalized tonic-clonic seizures (grand mal) There are four medications which are of proven value in this very common form of seizure—phenytoin (or diphenylhydantoin), carbamazepine, phenobarbital (and other long-acting barbiturates), and valproic acid (Table 350-3). Most patients will be controlled by adequate doses of any one of these, although individual patients may respond better to one or another. The choice among them often relates to minimizing undesirable side effects.

Phenytoin can often produce effective control with no sedation and very little, if any, intellectual impairment. However, phenytoin produces gum hyperplasia in some individuals, coarsening of facial features, and mild hirsutism, all of which can lead to long-term changes in appearance, which is especially unpleasant for young women. Phenytoin may produce lymphadenopathy and, in very high doses, may be toxic to the cerebellum.

Carbamazepine is equally effective and does not have many of the side effects seen with phenytoin. Cognitive function appears as well or even better preserved than with phenytoin. However, carbamazepine can cause gastrointestinal upset and may cause bone marrow depression with mild to moderate falls in peripheral white count (3.5 to 4 $\times$ 10^3 per microliter) which can occasionally become severe and which must be watched carefully. In addition, carbamazepine can produce hepatotoxicity. For these reasons, a complete blood count (CBC) and liver function tests should be performed before starting carbamazepine, and at 2-week intervals for a period after initiating therapy.

Phenobarbital is also effective against tonic-clonic seizures and has none of the side effects mentioned above. It commonly causes sedation and a dulling of intellect, however, especially early in its use, and this may lead to poor compliance. The sedation is dose-dependent and may limit the amount of drug which can be given to achieve complete control. However, if control can be achieved with nonsedative doses of phenobarbital, it may be the safest chronic regimen. Primidone is a barbiturate which is metabolized to phenobarbital and phenylethylmalonamide (PEMA). In children, the barbiturates can produce a state of hyperactivity and hyperirritability which will limit their usefulness. Barbiturates may also exacerbate depression.

Valproic acid (sodium valproate) has also been shown to be effective for tonic-clonic seizures. It can cause gastrointestinal irritation, bone marrow suppression (especially thrombocytopenia), hyperammonemia, and hepatic dysfunction (including rare instances of fatal progressive hepatic failure which appear to be idiosyncratic rather than dose-related and are more common in children under 2 years of age). A CBC with platelet count and liver function tests should be performed before beginning therapy and at biweekly intervals after initiating therapy for a suitable period until the safety of the drug is established in the individual patient.

In addition to their systemic side effects, all four of these drugs have neurologic toxicities at higher doses. Nystagmus is common at therapeutic blood levels but ataxia, dizziness, tremor, intellectual dulling, forgetfulness, confusion, and even stupor may occur with increasing blood concentrations. These are reversible when blood levels fall back to therapeutic levels.

Partial seizures, including complex partial seizures (temporal lobe epilepsy) Three of the four groups of drugs which are useful for tonic-clonic seizures are also effective for partial seizures. Carbamazepine and phenytoin are the drugs of choice while the barbiturates may also be effective. In general, complex partial seizures are difficult to control, and patients with these seizures may require more than one medication (i.e., carbamazepine and a barbiturate, or phenytoin and a barbiturate, or any one of the primary drugs and high doses of methsuximide) and may become candidates for neurosurgical intervention. These are the kinds of seizures for which many epilepsy centers are conducting trials of new antiepileptic drugs.

Other primary generalized seizures [absence (petit mal), atypical absence, myoclonic] These seizures respond to different classes of medications than either tonic-clonic or focal seizures. For simple absence, ethosuximide and valproic acid are the drugs of choice. Side effects of ethosuximide include gastrointestinal upset, behavior changes, dizziness, and lethargy but are not often troublesome. For more difficult to control atypical absence seizures and for myoclonic seizures, valproic acid is the drug of choice. Clonazepam (a benzodiazepine) can also be used for atypical absence and myoclonic seizures. It can cause drowsiness and irritability, but usually does not cause other systemic side effects. Trimethadione was one of the first antiabsence drugs but is now rarely used because of its potential toxicity.

Approximately one-third of children who present with "pure" absence seizures also have tonic-clonic seizures at some later time. The question of whether these children should be treated prophylactically with an anti-tonic-clonic seizure medication has not been resolved. Since valproic acid has actions against both classes of seizures, its use has been increasing in children with absence. The concurrent use of phenobarbital with antiabsence drugs for this purpose should be avoided, as it may interfere with therapy for the absence.

Status epilepticus Generalized tonic-clonic status epilepticus is a life-threatening medical emergency, but overzealous and incautious treatment can produce more harm than good. Patients are in danger from hyperpyrexia and acidosis (from prolonged muscle activity) and less commonly, hypoxia or compromise of respiratory function. Immediate treatment for status is protection of the airway, protection of the tongue (with a soft object, large enough not to be swallowed, between the clenched teeth), protection of the head, and then establishment of a secure parenteral (intravenous) access. A bolus of 50% glucose in water (after blood is drawn for analysis), even if hypoglycemia is not expected, may stop the seizures. All further intravenous medication should be given after preparation for respiratory and circulatory support is available.

Phenytoin, 1000 to 1500 mg (18 to 20 mg/kg) in a slow intravenous

TABLE 350-3 Commonly used antiepileptic drugs

Generic name	Trade name	Principal uses	Dosage	Half-life	Therapeutic range	% Protein bound	Toxic effects: Neurologic	Toxic effects: Systemic	Drug interactions
Phenytoin (diphenylhydantoin)	Dilantin	Tonic-clonic (grand mal) Focal Complex partial	300–400 mg/d (3–5 mg/kg, adult) (4–7 mg/kg, child)	24 h (wide variation)	10–20 μg/mL	90	Ataxia Incoordination Confusion Cerebellar Skin rash	Gum hyperplasia Lymphadenopathy Hirsutism Osteomalacia Facial coarsening	Level increased by isoniazid, dicumarol, sulfonamides Level decreased by carbamazepine, phenobarbital Altered folate metabolism Folate interferes with effects
Carbamazepine	Tegretol	Tonic-clonic Focal Complex partial	600–1200 mg/d (20–30 mg/kg, child)	13–17 h	4–12 μg/mL	80	Ataxia Dizziness Diploplia Vertigo	Bone marrow suppression Gastrointestinal irritation Hepatotoxicity	Level decreased by phenobarbital, phenytoin
Phenobarbital	Luminol	Tonic-clonic Focal	60–120 mg/d (1–5 mg/kg, adult) (3–6 mg/kg, child)	90 h (shorter in children)	10–50 μg/mL	40–60	Sedation Ataxia Confusion Dizziness Decreased libido Depression	Skin rash	Level increased by valproic acid, phenytoin Enhances metabolism of other drugs via liver enzyme induction
Primidone	Mysoline	Tonic-clonic Focal	750–1000 mg/d (10–25 mg/kg)	Primidone, 8 h Phenylethylmalonomide, 24–48 h Phenobarbital, 90 h	Primidone, 2–10 μg/mL Phenobarbital, 10–50 μg/mL	Small for primidone or phenylethylmalonomide	Same as phenobarbital		
Sodium valproate (valproic acid)	Depakane Depakote	Absence Atypical absence Myoclonic Tonic-clonic	750–1250 mg/d (30–60 mg/kg)	15 h	50–100 μg/mL	80–94	Ataxia Sedation Tremor	Hepatotoxicity Bone marrow suppression Gastrointestinal irritation Weight gain Transient alopecia Hyperammonemia	May precipitate absence status if given with clonazepam Increases free phenytoin Decreases phenobarbital Increases active carbamazepine metabolites
Ethosuximide	Zarontin	Absence (petit mal)	750–1250 mg/d (20–40 mg/kg)	60 h, adult 30 h, child	40–100 μg/mL	Small	Ataxia Lethargy	Gastrointestinal irritation Skin rash Bone marrow suppression	
Methsuximide	Celontin	Absence (complex partial)	600–1200 mg/d	38–50 h	10–30 μg/mL (*N*-desmethyl methsuximide)	Small	Ataxia Lethargy	Same as ethosuximide	Increases phenytoin level Increases phenobarbital from primidone
Clonazepam	Clonopin	Absence Atypical absence Myoclonic	1–12 mg/d (0.1–0.2 mg/kg)	24–48 h	5–70 ng/mL	50	Ataxia Sedation Lethargy	Anorexia	May precipitate absence status if given with valproic acid
Trimethadione	Tridione	Absence Atypical absence (intractable seizures only)	900–2100 mg/d (20–60 mg/kg)	6–13 days (for dimethadione)	700 μg/mL (for dimethadione)	Small	Sedation Blurred vision	Skin rash Bone marrow suppression Nephrosis Hepatitis	

''push'' (not in 5% dextrose in water—phenytoin precipitates in this low pH solution) no faster than 50 mg/min, is one of the drugs of choice. It does not depress respiration but may produce mild atrioventricular block and, if given too rapidly, can cause a serious fall in blood pressure. Blood pressure and EEG should be monitored.

The benzodiazepines, diazepam, 10 mg, or lorazepam, 4 mg (followed by another 4 mg if necessary), are also effective in stopping status epilepticus when administered intravenously. However, these drugs may depress respiratory function (or even cause respiratory arrest), and measures for respiratory support should be available before they are administered. The use of a benzodiazepine after phenobarbital administration carries a particular risk. The benzodiazepines are short-acting drugs in these circumstances, and after they are administered, a second, longer-acting antiepileptic such as phenytoin is usually required to prevent recurrence of seizures.

Phenobarbital, in a dose of 10 to 20 mg/kg (up to 1 g), divided into two to four doses at 30- to 60-minute intervals, can also be administered for status epilepticus. Phenobarbital also causes respiratory depression and should not be used immediately after treatment with intravenous diazepam.

If tonic-clonic seizures cannot be controlled within 30 to 60 min with the above sequence, the likelihood of serious neurologic sequelae or death becomes very high. Serious consideration needs to be given to anesthetizing the patient with barbiturates or inhalation anesthetics, with EEG monitoring to ensure that cessation of electrical seizure activity accompanies cessation of motor convulsions.

After stopping the seizures, it is imperative to determine the cause of the status epilepticus in order to prevent its recurrence. In most adults the cause can be determined and is usually tumor, vascular disease, infection, cerebral damage, or precipitous withdrawal from alcohol or antiepileptic medication. In children, the incidence of idiopathic status is higher (approximately 50 percent), and the remaining cases are divided between acute brain illnesses such as purulent meningitis, encephalitis and dehydration with electrolyte disturbances, and chronic encephalopathies. Tonic-clonic status epilepticus is a dangerous condition; the mortality may be over 10 percent with another 10 to 30 percent of patients being left with permanent neurologic sequelae.

NEUROSURGICAL TREATMENT OF EPILEPSY If a structural lesion (i.e., tumor, cyst, abscess, etc.) is causing recurrent seizures, the removal of that lesion and nearby diseased brain will often eliminate the seizures or make them easier to control. Some patients, however, have uncontrollable seizures without a demonstrable structural lesion. These are often complex partial seizures with ictal and interictal EEG abnormalities emanating from one or both temporal lobes. Many surgical series have shown that if the epileptogenic lesion can be clearly localized to one temporal lobe, neurosurgical removal of that temporal lobe can result in significant improvement in 60 to 95 percent of the patients. Localization often depends on intensive EEG monitoring and may require intracranial recordings from the temporal or frontal lobes. In a high percentage of cases the removed temporal lobe can be shown to have microscopic pathology, such as hippocampal (or "Ammon's horn") sclerosis (loss of pyramidal cells in the hippocampus), a hamartoma, or cortical ectopia.

Some individuals with complex partial seizures also develop a psychiatric illness characterized most often as a borderline personality with certain specific behavioral manifestations including hypergraphia, hyperreligiosity, lack of sense of humor, and disordered sexuality. The psychiatric aspects of this illness may result from the epilepsy or may be independently produced by the same underlying brain lesion which produces the epilepsy. The personality disorder may not significantly change after epilepsy surgery, even if the seizures are controlled.

TREATMENT OF A SINGLE SEIZURE Some individuals present with a single, brief, generalized tonic-clonic seizure and, after complete evaluation, are found to have a normal EEG and no underlying cause for the seizure. Some of these individuals (between 40 and 70 percent, depending on the series) go on to have recurrent seizures. The decision to treat such a patient with several years (at least) of antiepileptic medication must be made on an individual basis, considering the patient's lifestyle, risks from a sudden loss of consciousness, and feelings about medications.

CESSATION OF ANTIEPILEPTIC DRUG THERAPY Many patients with epilepsy require antiepileptic drug therapy for life. However, a large proportion of epileptic patients become seizure-free on appropriate medication, and approximately half of such patients can eventually stop their medications and remain seizure-free. The patient who has had no seizures for 4 years, who had had relatively few seizures before control was attained, who only required a single medication, who has a normal neurologic exam and no structural lesion causing the seizures, and who has a normal EEG at the end of the therapeutic period has the best chance of remaining seizure-free if medication is slowly tapered (over 3 to 6 months). An abnormal EEG is not a contraindication to discontinuing medication. When considering the discontinuance of antiepileptic therapy, the consequences of the recurrence of seizures must be carefully considered. One inopportune seizure in a previously well-controlled patient who is not used to taking precautions may be a life-threatening event or lead to loss of a driver's license or loss of employment. Nevertheless, since all medications carry some risk of toxicity and since medication compliance in a healthy individual is often variable, it is worth a careful trial of medication tapering in individuals who meet the above criteria and are willing to accept the risk.

EPILEPSY AND PREGNANCY Most women with epilepsy can undergo uneventful pregnancies and deliver healthy babies—even those taking antiepileptic medications. During the pregnant state, however, body metabolism changes, and close attention must be given to antiepileptic drug levels. Sometimes relatively high doses have to be given to ensure therapeutic levels. Most women who are well controlled before pregnancy will remain so during pregnancy and delivery. Women whose seizures are not under good control before becoming pregnant are at higher risk for having increased difficulties during the pregnancy.

One of the most serious complications of pregnancy, toxemia, often presents as a generalized tonic-clonic convulsion in the third trimester. This seizure is a symptom of a severe neurologic disturbance and is not a manifestation of epilepsy, nor is it more common in epileptic women. The toxemic state must be treated in order to control the seizures.

There is a two- to threefold higher incidence of significant fetal malformations in offspring of epileptic women, and this is likely due to a combination of a low incidence of medication-induced malformation and of genetic predisposition in this population. Among those malformations which do occur, a fetal-hydantoin (which is not unique to babies exposed to phenytoin) syndrome consisting of cleft lip and palate, heart defects, digital hypoplasia, and nail dysplasia has been identified.

Although it would be ideal for women contemplating pregnancy to have their antiepileptic drugs discontinued, it is likely that for a large number of women this would result in recurrence of seizures which would, in the long run, be more harmful for both mother and baby. If patients meet the criteria for discontinuance of medication, this should be done with a suitable interval before pregnancy is to occur. Other patients should be tapered to a minimal effective dosage and, if possible, maintained on only one medication. There are no clear data indicating differences in safety for phenobarbital, phenytoin, or carbamazepine when used alone. Less experience is available for valproate. Phenobarbital, primidone, or phenytoin can cause transient and reversible deficiency in vitamin K–dependent clotting factors in the neonate, and these should be promptly treated. Babies exposed to chronic barbiturates in utero are often transiently sluggish, hypotonic, jittery, and often show signs of barbiturate withdrawal. These babies should be considered at risk for neonatal problems and should be slowly withdrawn from barbiturates and closely observed in the nursery during the neonatal period.

DRIVING AND EPILEPSY Each state has its own regulations for determining when an individual with epilepsy can obtain a driver's license, and several states have laws about the physician's obligations in either reporting epileptic patients to the registry or informing the patients of their responsibilities to do so. In general, patients can drive after a seizure-free interval (on or off medications) which ranges from 6 months to 2 years. In some states there is no fixed interval, but the individual is required to have a physician's letter attesting to seizure control. It is the physician's responsibility to warn the epileptic patient of the risks of driving when seizures are not under control.

SOCIAL AND EDUCATIONAL REHABILITATION Most people with epilepsy attain adequate control of their seizures and are able to attend school and obtain employment and live a relatively normal life. Children with epilepsy tend to have more problems in school than their peers, but every effort should be made to keep these children integrated into the mainstream of the educational process while supplying additional help in the form of academic tutoring or psychological counseling.

REFERENCES

AIRD R et al: *The Epilepsies: A Critical Review*. New York, Raven, 1984

CALLAGHAN N et al: Withdrawal of anticonvulsant drugs in patients free of seizures for two years. N Engl J Med 318:942, 1988

COMMISSION ON CLASSIFICATION AND TERMINOLOGY OF THE ILAE: Proposal for revised clinical classification of epileptic seizures. Epilepsia 22:489, 1981

DICHTER M, AYALA GF: Cellular mechanisms of epilepsy: A status report. Science 237:157, 1987

EMERSON R et al: Stopping medication in children with epilepsy. N Engl J Med 304:1125, 1981

ENGEL J JR: *Seizures and Epilepsy*. Philadelphia, Davis, 1989

——— (ed): *Surgical Treatment of the Epilepsies*. New York, Raven, 1987

LAIDLAW J, RICHENS A (eds): *A Textbook of Epilepsy*, 3d ed. London, Churchill Livingstone, 1988

LEVY R et al (eds): *Antiepileptic Drugs*. 3d ed. New York, Raven, 1989

MATTSON R et al: Comparison of carbamazepine, phenobarbital, phenytoin, and primidone in partial and secondarily generalized tonic-clonic seizures. N Engl J Med 313:145, 1985

351 CEREBROVASCULAR DISEASES

J. PHILIP KISTLER / ALLAN A. ROPPER / JOSEPH B. MARTIN

Cerebrovascular disease, the third leading cause of death after heart disease and cancer in developed countries, has an overall prevalence of 794 per 100,000. Five percent of the population over 65 are affected by a stroke, and, in the United States, it is estimated that more than 400,000 patients are discharged each year from hospitals after a stroke. The loss of these patients from the work force and the extended hospitalization they require during recovery make the economic impact of the disease one of the most devastating in medicine.

PATHOGENESIS AND PATHOLOGY OF STROKE Cerebrovascular disease is caused by one of several pathologic processes involving the blood vessels of the brain. The process may (1) be intrinsic to the vessel, as in atherosclerosis, lipohyalinosis, inflammation, amyloid deposition, arterial dissection, developmental malformation, aneurysmal dilation, or venous thrombosis; (2) originate remotely, as occurs when an embolus from the heart or extracranial circulation lodges in an intracranial vessel; (3) result from decreased perfusion pressure or increased blood viscosity with inadequate cerebral blood flow; or (4) result from rupture of a vessel in the subarachnoid space or intracerebral tissue.

A *stroke* is the acute neurologic injury occurring as a result of one of these pathologic processes. Other secondary symptoms may accompany stroke and vascular disease including pressure on cranial nerves from an aneurysm; vascular headache; or increased intracranial pressure with a venous thrombosis.

Normal brain function requires continuous supply of oxygenated blood. Cardiac arrest results in unconsciousness within 10 s; in animal experiments, total cessation of blood flow produces irreversible cerebral infarction within 3 min. Reduced blood flow may interfere with brain function, but the brain can remain viable for more prolonged periods. For example, patients who suffer cerebral embolism or cerebral vasospasm following subarachnoid hemorrhage often recover partially or completely, suggesting that focal areas of brain can remain functionless and ischemic for hours, even days, yet recover. This has led to the notion of an ischemic zone (penumbra or halo) that surrounds an infarct. There are also several secondary phenomena that may contribute to ongoing neuronal death. These include excitotoxins released by damaged neurons, cerebral edema, and alterations in local blood flow.

An infarcted brain is pale initially. Within hours to days, the gray matter becomes congested with engorged, dilated blood vessels and minute petechial hemorrhages. When an embolus blocking a major vessel migrates, lyses, or disperses within hours, recirculation into the ischemic area causes hemorrhagic infarction and may aggravate subsequent edema formation after the blood-brain barrier has been disrupted. A primary intracerebral hemorrhage, on the other hand, damages the brain by directly injuring tissue at the site of the hemorrhage and by compressing the surrounding tissue.

After an ischemic stroke, intracerebral hemorrhage, or transient episode of cerebral ischemia has occurred, the prelude to therapy is a precise diagnosis. The evaluation of a stroke must include clear definitions of the character and location of the lesion, the vascular pathologic process producing the symptoms, and the anatomy of spared collateral circulation to the ischemic area. The brain repairs itself only by forming fibrogliotic scar tissue at the site of an infarction or hemorrhage; therefore, therapeutic efforts after a stroke can only hope to minimize secondary loss. Such efforts should attempt to protect both the normal and ischemic brain from either initial or recurrent pathologic processes, as well as from the secondary effects of the stroke itself, e.g., brain compression from intracranial hemorrhage or edema. Such preventive therapy has three broad goals: (1) to reduce risk factors, thus attenuating the pathologic process; (2) to prevent recurrent stroke by removing the underlying pathologic process; and (3) to minimize secondary brain damage by maintaining adequate perfusion to marginally ischemic areas, and by reducing edema formation. Except for the elimination of risk factors, all aspects of therapy remain controversial. Because proof of efficacy is lacking for many therapies, current therapy is largely empirical and based on the physician's knowledge of the risks associated with various diagnostic procedures and therapeutic initiatives.

Strokes can be classified according to their pathophysiologic mechanism. The most important factor is an accurate assessment of the initial clinical presentation and temporal profile, which are determined by the pathologic process and the size and location of the diseased vessel and by the availability of collateral circulation (Figs. 351-1*A*–*C* and 351-2). The most important source of collateral flow for the internal carotid and vertebrobasilar arteries is the circle of Willis. When arteries distal to the circle of Willis, the middle, anterior, or posterior cerebral arteries are involved, collateral flow is limited to anastomoses over the cortical surface of the brain, the brainstem, or cerebellum. In these circumstances, or when the circle of Willis collateral is inadequate (Fig. 351-2, I–IV), factors that affect blood viscosity and clotting become increasingly important determinants of the extent of the stroke.

TIA syndrome The term *transient ischemic attack (TIA)* has usually been applied to any sudden focal neurologic deficit that clears completely in less than 24 h. This definition is probably too broad, because it includes other disease entities that are not necessarily caused by ischemia per se, e.g., a focal epileptic manifestation or a migraine attack with neurologic symptoms. Furthermore, ischemic symptoms that persist longer than an hour are usually accompanied by tissue injury, even though clinical recovery frequently occurs. Therefore, it is advisable to consider focal but totally reversible episodes lasting minutes to an hour as TIAs.

The specific symptoms of a TIA point to the particular arterial territory involved (carotid, middle cerebral, vertebrobasilar, or small penetrating artery). The duration, stereotypic nature, and frequency of repetitive spells suggest the underlying pathophysiologic mechanism. For example, repetitive (up to 5 to 10 per day), short-lived (15 min or less), stereotypic spells of hand and arm weakness suggest

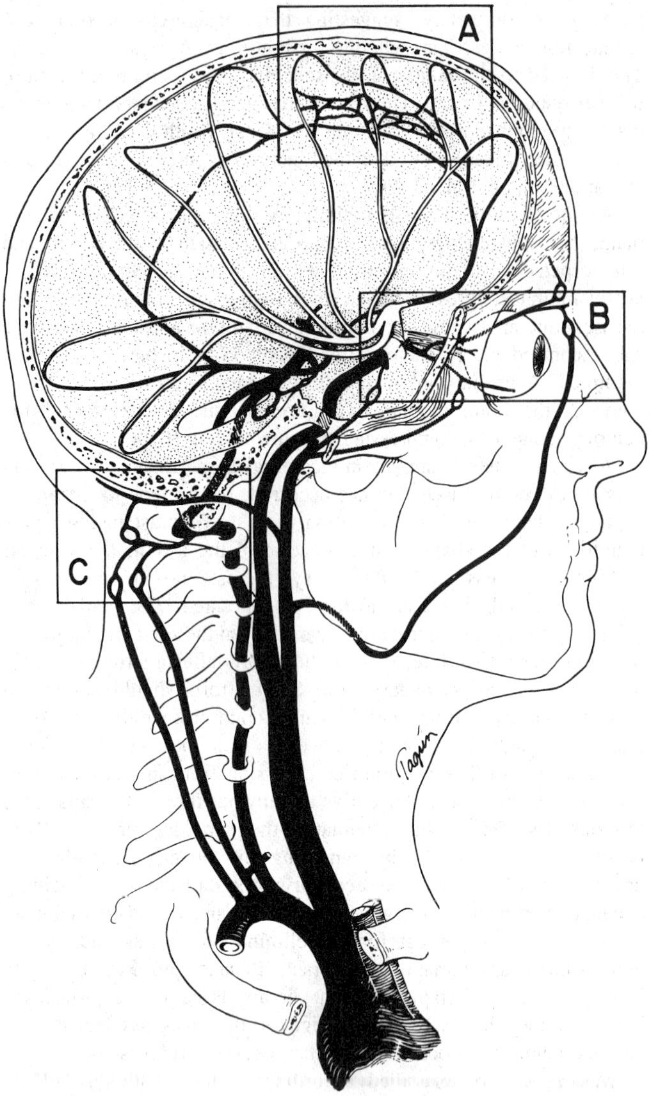

FIGURE 351-1 Arrangement of the major arteries of the right side carrying blood from the heart to the brain. Also shown are vessels of collateral circulation that may modify the effects of cerebral ischemia *(A,B,C)*. Not shown is the circle of Willis which also provides a source for collateral circulation. *A*. The anastomotic channels between the distal branches of the anterior and middle cerebral artery, termed borderzone or watershed anastomotic channels. Note that they also occur between the posterior and middle cerebral arteries and the anterior and posterior cerebral arteries. *B*. Anastomotic channels occurring through the orbit between branches of the external carotid artery and ophthalmic branch of the internal carotid artery. *C*. Wholly extracranial anastomotic channels between the muscular branches of the ascending cervical arteries and muscular branches of the occipital artery that anastomose with the distal vertebral artery. Note that the occipital artery arises from the external carotid artery, thereby allowing reconstitution of flow in the vertebral from the carotid circulation. *(Courtesy of C.M. Fisher, M.D.)*

that proximal arterial narrowing or occlusion have produced transient focal ischemia (''low flow'') in the contralateral motor cortex. In contrast, a single episode of speech difficulty with or without hand, arm, or face weakness lasting 12 h suggests an embolic TIA in the contralateral frontal lobe. A transient short-lived episode (12 to 24 h) of pure motor hemiparesis—face, arm, leg, and foot—occurring *without* dysphasia or hemineglect suggests transient ischemia in the internal capsule or in the corticospinal tract of the ventral pons, territories supplied by penetrating arteries arising from larger parent vessels (a ''lacunar TIA''). TIA in the vertebrobasilar system often presents with short-lived, repetitive episodes of dizziness, diplopia, and dysarthria. The repetitive, short-lived nature of these spells suggests transiently reduced blood flow rather than embolism.

The mechanism of embolic TIA is obvious, and only the source needs to be considered in deciding therapy. The mechanism of focal ''low-flow'' TIAs or lacunar TIAs, however, remains less certain. A critically stenotic or occluded artery can probably reduce flow to a focal region of brain. Poor collateral circulation contributes to the ischemia, but factors such as blood viscosity, vessel wall compliance, and other unknown factors may explain the transient reduction. Although TIAs resolve completely, they warn that a stroke may follow. Therefore, it becomes important to consider the pathophysiologic mechanisms of stroke and TIA together.

The terms *stroke in evolution* (also called *progressive stroke*) and *completed stroke* need special mention. Stroke in evolution refers to a neurologic deficit that progresses or fluctuates while the patient is under observation, whereas completed stroke implies that no further deterioration will occur. Several mechanisms have been proposed to explain stroke in evolution, among them progressive narrowing of an artery by thrombus, development of cerebral edema, thrombus propagation obliterating collateral branches to the ischemic brain, and systemic factors, e.g., arterial hypotension. Although these may have a role in some cases, it is more likely that fluctuating neurologic deficits are the result of emboli propagating, migrating, lysing, and dispersing, or are caused by recurrent artery-to-artery embolization, fluctuating collateral flow through the circle of Willis, through border zone anastomotic channels, or through orbital or cervicovertebral collaterals (Figs. 351-1*A–C* and 351-2). Fortunately, refinement in clinical diagnosis and new diagnostic techniques usually allow prediction of the type and location of strokes and their underlying vascular lesions, making a more focused approach to therapy both possible and mandatory.

Risk factors in stroke Cerebral vascular disease is associated with several risk factors. An atherothrombotic stroke often indicates that the patient has cardiovascular or peripheral vascular disease. Atrial fibrillation, valvular heart disease, myocardial infarction, and bacterial endocarditis are sources of emboli, and their presence suggests embolism as the diagnosis. Severe hypertension is linked to small-vessel lipohyalinotic disease, lacunar strokes, and the formation of atherothrombotic lesions at the carotid bifurcation, in the middle cerebral artery stem, and in the vertebrobasilar system. Hypertension also predisposes to deep intracerebral hemorrhages. The advent of antihypertensive therapy is the principal factor accounting for the declining incidence of stroke. Smoking and familial hyperlipidemia, although less important than hypertension, are also associated with an increased risk of atherothrombotic disease and stroke. Racial differences predispose to specific types of stroke and may affect stroke incidence independently of other factors. Ischemic strokes occur more often in the early morning hours, whereas hemorrhages tend to occur during waking hours.

ISCHEMIC CEREBROVASCULAR DISEASE: GENERAL REMARKS

Ischemic cerebrovascular disease results from arterial narrowing or thrombosis or from arterial occlusion by embolism. Cerebral arterial thrombosis secondary to atherosclerosis and cerebral embolism cause similar symptoms and signs, but with different temporal profiles. Differences in symptomatology are discussed in the section on cerebral embolism.

Of the many causes of ischemic stroke listed in Table 351-1 and discussed elsewhere, thrombosis complicating atherosclerosis of intra- and extracranial vessels ultimately accounts for most cases. Atherosclerosis affects each artery at specific locations. In general, atheromatous plaques tend to form at branchings and curves of large vessels, and thrombosis is likely to occur at the site of maximal luminal narrowing.

The details of the process that superimposes thrombosis on artherosclerosis are discussed in Chap. 195. The damage that atherosclerotic thrombosis causes to the brain is determined by the

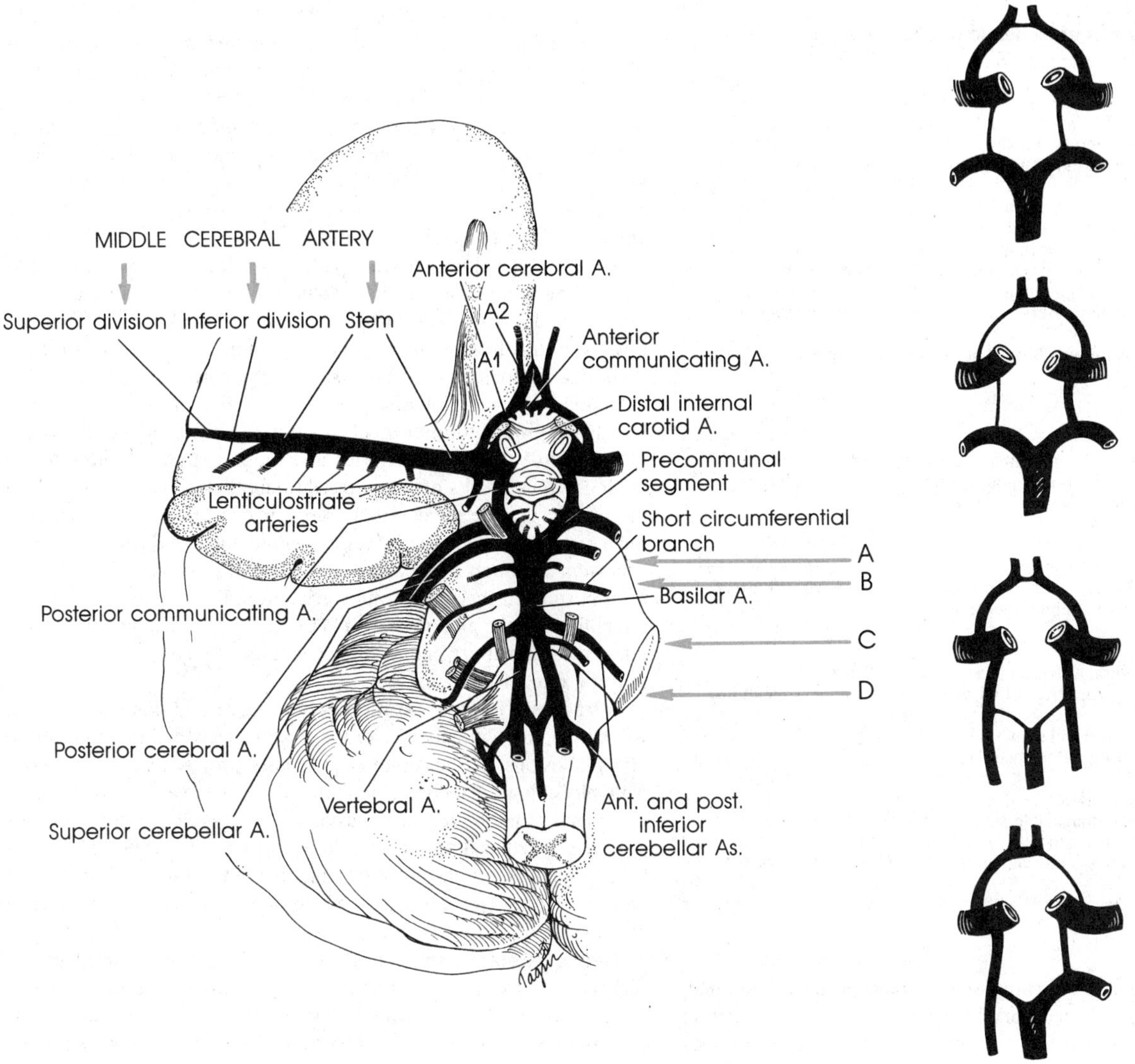

FIGURE 351-2 Diagram of the brainstem, cerebellum, inferior right frontal lobe, and temporal lobe transected. Principal branches of the vertebral basilar arterial system are pictured. Small branches of the vertebral and basilar artery that penetrate the medulla and pons are not pictured. The stem of the middle cerebral artery with its small, deep penetrating lenticulostriate arteries and the circle of Willis with its small, deep penetrating branches are shown. Roman numerals I, II, III, and IV represent some of the possible variations of the Circle of Willis due to atresia of one or more of its arterial components. *A, B, C,* and *D* arrows point to the four cross-sections of the brainstem diagrammed below (*D* = Fig. 351-7, *A* = Fig. 351-8, *B* = Fig. 351-9, *C* = Fig. 351-10). Although typical vascular syndromes of the pons and medulla have been designated by the shaded areas in Figs. 351-7 to 10, the shading is arbitrary. Great variability in infarct size and location occurs when the basilar or vertebral arteries, or one of their penetrating branches, becomes occluded. This variability is because of variation in arterial anatomic location and available collateral circulation. Thus the stroke syndromes produced are often atypical, incomplete, or merge with one another. *(Courtesy of C.M. Fisher, M.D.)*

available collateral flow, the speed of thrombotic occlusion, and by embolism distal to the thrombosis (''artery-to-artery'' embolus). The clinical symptoms and signs resulting from occlusion of a particular artery differ from one patient to another, and many syndromes are partial representations of an idealized complete stroke in an arterial distribution. The following descriptions apply to infarction and ischemia in specific arteries due to thrombosis, recognizing that similar clinical pictures may occur after embolism. Occasionally, hemorrhage within these vascular territories also causes similar symptoms and signs.

ATHEROTHROMBOTIC DISEASE OF THE INTERNAL CAROTID ARTERY AND ITS BRANCHES

The origin of the carotid artery is the most common site of artherosclerosis and superimposed atherothrombosis that lead to TIA or stroke. Less often, disease at the siphon (S-shaped portion of the internal carotid artery in the cavernous sinus) or in the proximal segment (stem) of the middle or anterior cerebral arteries may be responsible for the symptom (rarely, the origin of the common carotid artery may be the site). The natural history of asymptomatic atherosclerotic stenosis or of ulcerated lesions at these locations is unknown. Presumably, in most instances the disease is progressive.

Internal carotid artery Atherosclerosis in the proximal internal carotid artery is usually most severe in the first 2 cm and arises from the posterior wall, often extending downward into the common carotid artery. Disease in this area is usually heralded by a minor stoke or TIA caused by embolism from the carotid artery to its intracranial branches or to a ''low-flow'' hemodynamic crisis. Emboli rather than low flow, however, probably cause most strokes or TIAs from carotid disease.

When *emboli* arise from a stenotic or ulcerated atherosclerotic lesion at the origin of the internal carotid artery, symptoms may result from occlusion of the ophthalmic artery, the middle cerebral artery stem or one or more of its branches, or, less often, the anterior cerebral artery. Small platelet emboli may occlude either only the ophthalmic artery or the very distal vessels of the middle cerebral artery, causing transient monocular blindness (*amaurosis fugax*) or small asymptomatic infarctions in the cerebral arterial watershed,

TABLE 351-1 Causes of ischemic stroke

THROMBOSIS

A Atherosclerosis
*B** Arteritis: Temporal arteritis, granulomatous arteritis, polyarteritis, Wegener's granulomatosis, granulomatous arteritis of the great vessels (Takayasu's arteritis, syphilis)
*C** Dissections: Carotid, vertebral, or intracranial arteries at the base of the brain (spontaneous or traumatic)
*D** Hematologic disorders: Polycythemia first-degree or second-degree, sickle cell disease, thrombotic thrombocytopenic purpura, etc.
*E** Cerebral mass effect compressing intracranial arteries: Tentorial herniation—post-cerebral artery; giant aneurysm—middle cerebral artery compression
F Miscellaneous: Moyamoya disease, fibromuscular dysplasia, Binswanger's disease

VASOCONSTRICTION

*A** Cerebral vasospasm following subarachnoid hemorrhage
*B** Reversible cerebral vasoconstriction: Etiology unknown, following migraine, trauma, eclampsia of pregnancy

EMBOLISM

A Atherothrombotic arterial source: Bifurcation common carotid artery, carotid siphon, distal vertebral artery, aortic arch
*B** Cardiac source
- *1* Structural heart disease
  - *a Congenital:* Mitral valve prolapse, patent foramen ovale, etc.
  - *b Acquired:* following myocardial infarction, marantic vegetation, etc.
- *2* Dysrhythmia, atrial fibrillation, sick sinus syndrome, etc.
- *3* Infection: acute bacterial endocarditis

*C** Unknown source
- *1* Healthy child or adult
- *2* Associations: hypercoagulable state secondary to systemic disease, carcinoma (especially pancreatic), eclampsia of pregnancy, oral contraceptives, lupus, anticoagulants, factor C deficiency, factor S deficiency, etc.

* May occur in patients under 30.

respectively. Larger emboli composed of platelet-fibrin clot may occlude the primary and secondary branches of the middle cerebral artery leading to discrete and easily recognizable neurologic syndromes that suggest the area involved. Some emboli are large enough to occlude the proximal "stem" of the middle cerebral artery, leading to devastating ischemia of the entire middle cerebral territory (deep white matter, lenticular nuclei, and cortical surface). Other emboli large enough to occlude the middle cerebral stem may cause only deep infarction because collateral flow through the cortical surface is sufficient (Fig. 351-1*A*). Large emboli may not entirely occlude a major vessel or may migrate or lyse and disperse, causing a neurologic deficit that fluctuates (stroke in evolution) or resolves.

In a few symptomatic patients, an ulcerated plaque may be the only lesion in the carotid bifurcation, but far more often there is a stenotic lesion with a residual lumen diameter of less than 2 mm. The incidence of large embolic strokes resulting from an ulcerated lesion alone is undetermined, but it is probably low and mostly associated with large ulcers (4 mm or greater). *A nonstenotic or slightly stenotic carotid lesion in conjunction with a stroke or a single prolonged TIA suggests the heart as the source of the embolus.* Atheromatous lesions at the origin of the great vessels in the aortic arch can also produce cerebral emboli that cause transient ischemia or infarction, but the incidence of this mechanism, thought to be low, is also undetermined.

Internal carotid artery occlusion or severe stenosis ($\leq$ 1 mm) may be entirely asymptomatic if collateral circulation through the circle of Willis is adequate. Inadequate collateral circulation may lead to a stroke or TIA. When *low arterial flow* results in cerebral infarction or transient ischemia, it does so in the border zone or "watershed" areas, approximately between the cortical surface branches of the middle cerebral and the anterior or posterior cerebral arteries (Fig. 351-1*A*). Two anatomic conditions contribute to this complication. First, the residual lumen diameter of carotid artery stenosis is typically less than 1.5 mm (80 to 90 percent occluded). Second, collateral flow to the ipsilateral middle cerebral artery is impaired, usually because of an incomplete circle of Willis (Fig. 351-2), occlusion of the contralateral internal carotid artery, or, infrequently, because of concomitant vertebrobasilar circulation insufficiency. Occasionally, the external carotid ophthalmic channels (Fig. 351-1*B*) or cortical surface vessels (Fig. 351-1*A*) can supply enough collateral flow to minimize the ischemic area, even if the circle of Willis is inadequate.

Other explanations of the pathophysiology of low-flow TIAs include intermittent spasm that occludes a severely stenotic lesion in the carotid artery or intermittent decompensation of cortical collateral flow resulting from transient spasm, hypotension with cardiac arrhythmia, or increased blood viscosity (in polycythemia, thrombocythemia, or macroglobulinemia). In arterial occlusion, a clot may propagate upward from the occlusion through the siphon to the origin of the middle or anterior arteries and cause a stroke. More often, a fresh embolus breaks off from the thrombotic material and lodges in the middle or anterior cerebral artery or one of its distal branches. Such distal embolism usually occurs within hours or days after carotid occlusion although it may develop 6 months or more later. It has been postulated that emboli may arise from the proximal stump and travel through the external carotid circulation to reach the intracranial internal carotid artery and its branches (Fig. 351-1*B*), but this process must be rare, if it occurs at all.

Intracranial internal carotid artery The carotid siphon is involved less commonly with atherosclerosis than the proximal internal carotid artery. Lesions in the siphon can cause strokes and TIAs whose pathophysiologic and clinical features duplicate those discussed above. In general, siphon stenosis is asymptomatic until the atheromatous process has reduced the residual lumen to 1.5 mm or less. Collateral flow around the circle of Willis undoubtedly influences the natural history of these lesions and their response to medical or surgical therapy.

Middle cerebral artery In contrast to the internal carotid artery, occlusion of the middle cerebral artery stem or one of its major branches is usually due to embolus (artery-to-artery, cardiac, or of unknown source) rather than atherothrombosis. Atheromatous lesions in the middle cerebral stem may cause ischemic symptoms either by narrowing the artery or by occluding the origin of one or more of the lenticulostriate arteries supplying the deep white matter and basal ganglia. Symptomatic atheroma rarely occurs distal to the first bifurcation of the middle cerebral artery. Because the circle of Willis is proximal to the origin of the middle cerebral artery, collateral blood flow to the middle cerebral artery territory must arise from small cortical-surface border zones and anastomotic vessels of the anterior and posterior cerebral arteries. Clinical evidence indicates that TIAs in the middle cerebral artery territory usually warn of vessel narrowing prior to thrombotic occlusion.

Anterior cerebral artery Atheromatous deposits in the proximal segment of the anterior cerebral artery rarely cause symptoms because the occlusion is circumvented by collateral circulation through the anterior communicating artery. However, if the anterior communicating artery is congenitally atretic or if the atheromatous lesion occurs distal in the anterior cerebral artery, TIAs and stroke may occur.

CLINICAL SYNDROMES Middle cerebral artery The cortical branches of the middle cerebral artery supply the lateral surface of the hemisphere except for (1) the frontal pole and a strip along the superomedial border of the frontal lobe supplied by the anterior cerebral artery, and (2) the lower temporal and occipital pole convolutions, which are in the territory of the posterior cerebral artery (Fig. 351-3).

The proximal middle cerebral artery gives rise to penetrating branches that supply the putamen, outer globus pallidus, posterior limb of the internal capsule above the plane of the upper border of the globus pallidus, the adjacent corona radiata, and the body, upper, and lateral head of the caudate nucleus. In the sylvian cistern, the

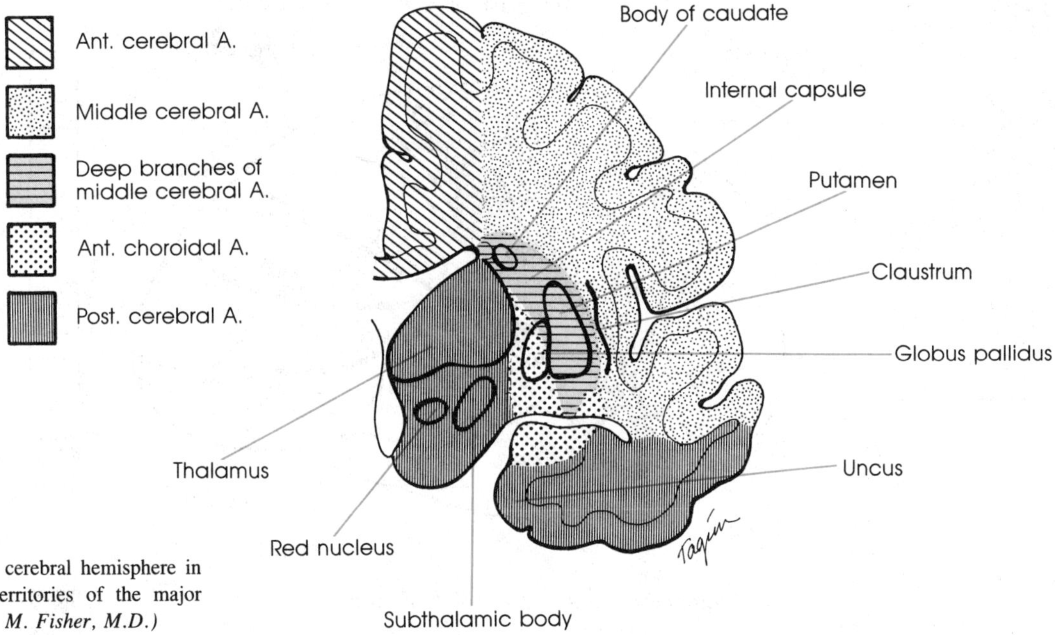

FIGURE 351-3 Diagram of a cerebral hemisphere in coronal section, showing the territories of the major cerebral vessels. *(Courtesy of C. M. Fisher, M.D.)*

middle cerebral artery stem in most patients divides into *superior* and *inferior divisions*. Branches of the inferior division supply the inferior parietal and temporal cortex, and those from the superior division supply the frontal and superior parietal cortex (Fig. 351-4). There is considerable variability in the parietal lobe supply between the two divisions, with about two-thirds of individuals having an inferior division that supplies regions above the angular gyrus.

If the entire middle cerebral artery is occluded at its stem, blocking both the penetrating and cortical branches, the clinical findings are contralateral hemiplegia and hemianesthesia. If the dominant hemisphere is involved, global aphasia is also present. If the nondominant hemisphere is affected, apractagnosia and anosognosia are found (Fig. 351-4). Dysarthria may also occur.

Complete middle cerebral territory syndromes occur most often when an embolus occludes the stem of the artery. Cortical collateral blood flow and differing arterial configurations are probably responsible for the development of partial middle cerebral artery syndromes. Partial middle cerebral territory syndromes may also be due to an embolus that enters the middle cerebral artery stem without complete occlusion or that lyses and moves distally. Symptoms and signs may fluctuate in such patients (stroke in evolution).

Partial syndromes resulting from embolic occlusion of a single branch include hand, or arm and hand, weakness alone (brachial syndrome), or facial weakness with motor aphasia, with or without arm weakness (frontal opercular syndrome). A combination of sensory disturbance, motor weakness, and motor aphasia suggests that an embolus has occluded the proximal superior division branch and infarcted large portions of the frontal and parietal cortices (Fig. 351-4). If Wernicke's aphasia occurs without weakness, the inferior division of the middle cerebral artery supplying the posterior part (temporal cortex) of the dominant hemisphere is probably involved (Fig. 351-4). Jargon speech and an inability to comprehend written and oral language are prominent features, often accompanied by a contralateral superior quadrantanopsia. Hemineglect or spatial agnosia without weakness indicates that the inferior division of the middle cerebral artery in the nondominant hemisphere is involved.

Anterior cerebral artery The anterior cerebral artery is divided into two segments: the precommunal (A1) circle of Willis, or stem, which connects the internal carotid artery to the anterior communicating artery, and the postcommunal (A2) segment distal to the anterior communicating artery (Fig. 351-2). The A1 segment of the anterior cerebral artery gives rise to several deep penetrating branches that supply the anterior limb of the internal capsule, the anterior perforate substance, amygdala, anterior hypothalamus, and the inferior part of the head of the caudate nucleus (Fig. 351-3).

Infarction in the territory of the anterior cerebral artery is uncommon and most often due to embolism rather than artherothrombosis. Occlusion of the A1 segment of the anterior cerebral artery is usually well tolerated, because of collateral flow. If both A2 segments arise from a single anterior cerebral stem (contralateral A1 segment atresia), then the occlusion affects both hemispheres. Profound abulia (a delay in verbal and motor response) and bilateral pyramidal signs with paraplegia result. Occlusion of a single A2 segment of the anterior cerebral artery results in the contralateral symptoms noted in the legend of Fig. 351-5.

Anterior choroidal artery This artery arises from the internal carotid artery and supplies the posterior limb of the internal capsule and the white matter posterolateral to it, through which pass some of the geniculocalcarine fibers (Figs. 351-3 and 351-6). The complete clinical syndrome of anterior choroidal artery occlusion consists of contralateral hemiplegia, hemianesthesia (hypesthesia), and homonymous hemianopsia. However, because this territory is also supplied by penetrating vessels of the middle cerebral stem, the posterior communicating, and posterior choroidal arteries, syndromes with minimal deficits may occur and patients frequently recover partially or completely.

Internal carotid artery The clinical picture of internal carotid occlusion varies depending upon whether the cause of ischemia is propagated thrombus, embolism, or low flow. The cortex supplied by the middle cerebral territory is most often affected. With a competent circle of Willis, however, occlusion can be entirely asymptomatic. Less often, there is massive infarction of the deep white matter and cortical surface from propagation of a thrombus up the internal carotid artery, into the middle cerebral stem, or from embolization to the stem of the middle cerebral artery. Symptoms are identical to middle cerebral stem occlusion (see above). When the origins of both the anterior and middle cerebral arteries are occluded by embolus to the top of the carotid artery, abulia and/or stupor occurs with hemiplegia, hemianesthesia, and aphasia or anosognosia. When the posterior cerebral artery arises from the internal carotid artery (an unusual configuration called a fetal posterior cerebral artery), it also may become occluded and give rise to symptoms referable to its peripheral territory (Figs. 351-5 and 351-6).

Carotid occlusion may cause low-flow infarction if the circle of Willis is incomplete. The territory of the distal cortical branches of

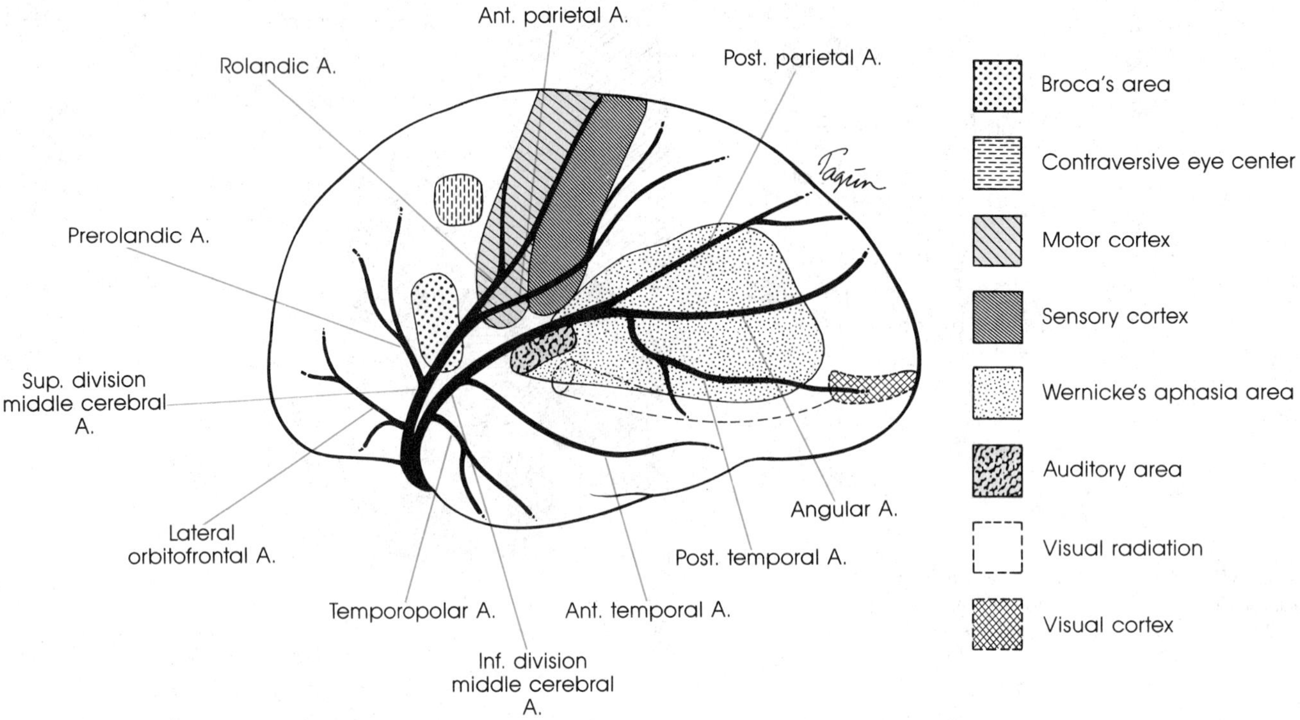

FIGURE 351-4 Diagram of a cerebral hemisphere, lateral aspect, showing the branches and distribution of the middle cerebral artery and the principal regions of cerebral localization. Note the bifurcation of the middle cerebral artery into a superior and inferior division (*Courtesy of C. M. Fisher, M.D.*)

Signs and symptoms	*Structures involved*
Paralysis of the contralateral face, arm, and leg; sensory impairment over the same area (pinprick, cotton touch, vibration, position, two-point discrimination, stereognosis, tactile localization, barognosis, cutaneographia)	Somatic motor area for face and arm and the fibers descending from the leg area to enter the corona radiata and corresponding somatic sensory system
Motor aphasia	Motor speech area of the dominant hemisphere
Central aphasia, word deafness, anomia, jargon speech, sensory agraphia, acalculia, alexia, finger agnosia, right-left confusion (the last four comprise the Gerstmann syndrome)	Central, suprasylvian speech area and parietooccipital cortex of the dominant hemisphere
Conduction aphasia	Central speech area (parietal operculum)
Apractognosia of the minor hemisphere (amorphosynthesis), anosognosia, hemiasomatognosia, unilateral neglect, agnosia for the left half of external space, dressing "apraxia," constructional "apraxia," distortion of visual coordinates, inaccurate localization in the half field, impaired ability to judge distance, upside-down reading, visual illusions (e.g., it may appear that another person walks through a table)	Nondominant parietal lobe (area corresponding to speech area in dominant hemisphere); loss of topographic memory is usually due to a nondominant lesion, occasionally to a dominant one
Homonymous hemianopsia (often homonymous inferior quadrantonopsia)	Optic radiation deep to second temporal convolution
Paralysis of conjugate gaze to the opposite side	Frontal contraversive field or fibers projecting therefrom

the middle cerebral artery tends to be involved, giving rise to transient or stepwise, progressive hip, shoulder, or arm weakness. Other TIAs suggestive of carotid insufficiency include recurrent unilateral tongue, lip, cheek, or hand numbness, with or without motor weakness.

In addition to supplying the ipsilateral brain, the internal carotid artery perfuses the optic nerve and retina via the ophthalmic artery (Fig. 351-1). In about 25 percent of symptomatic internal carotid disease, transient recurrent monocular blindness (TMB or amaurosis fugax) warns of the lesion. Patients may describe a shade that seems to sweep up, down, or across the field of vision or may say that the periphery of vision fades away. They may also complain that their vision was blurred in that eye or that the upper or lower half of vision disappeared. In most cases, these symptoms last only a few minutes. Rarely, ophthalmic or central retinal artery occlusion develops at the time of stroke.

Common carotid artery All the neurologic symptoms and signs of internal carotid occlusion may also be present with occlusion of the common carotid artery. Bilateral common carotid arterial occlusion at their origin may occur in "pulseless disease," or the aortic arch syndrome (see Chap. 197). Clues to this condition are absence of pulsation in carotid and radial arteries, faintness on arising from the horizontal position, recurrent loss of consciousness, headache, neck pain, transient blindness (unilateral or bilateral), dim vision with exercise, premature cataracts, retinal atrophy and pigmentation, atrophy of the iris, leukomas, peripapillary arteriovenous anastomoses, optic atrophy, and/or claudication of the jaw muscles. An incomplete aortic arch syndrome has been reported consisting of various combinations of carotid, subclavian, or innominate stenosis or occlusion (see below).

LABORATORY INVESTIGATION Several diagnostic techniques are available for evaluating patients with a carotid bruit, carotid-territory stroke, or TIA.

Noninvasive carotid tests Noninvasive carotid tests reliably determine the severity and location of carotid atherothrombotic disease in over 90 percent of patients. Indirect assessment of pressure in the internal carotid artery is made by ophthalmodynamometry, oculoplethysmography, and directional supraorbital Doppler examination. Ultrasound techniques define directly the bifurcation of the common carotid artery by real-time B-mode imaging and analysis of the Doppler-shift signal of the returning echo of flowing blood. Ultrasound

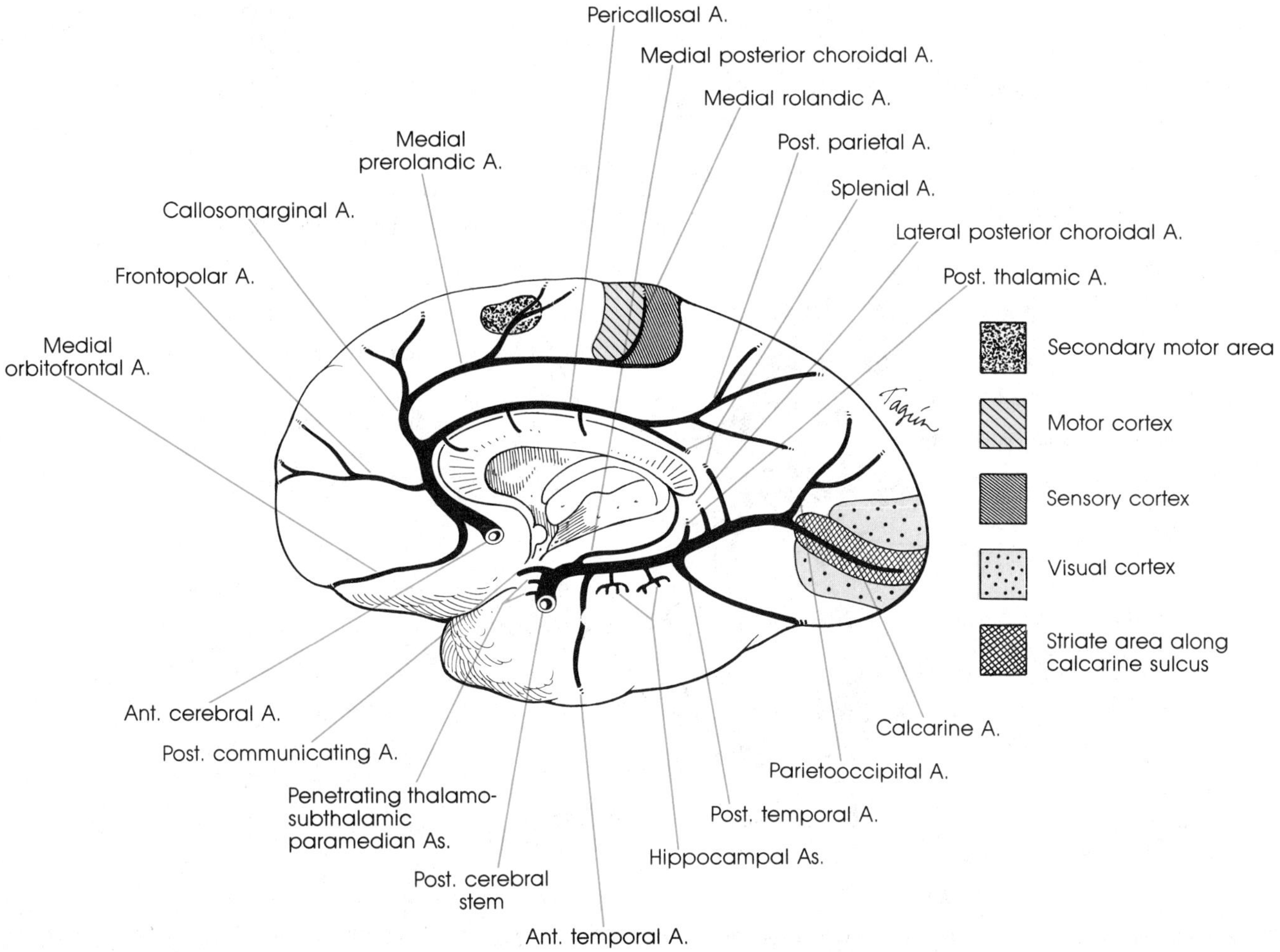

FIGURE 351-5 Diagram of a cerebral hemisphere, medial aspect, showing the branches and distribution of the anterior cerebral artery and the principal regions of cerebral localization. (*Courtesy of C. M. Fisher, M.D.*)

Signs and symptoms	*Structures involved*
Paralysis of opposite foot and leg	Motor leg area
A lesser degree of paresis of opposite arm	Involvement of arm area of cortex or fibers descending to corona radiata therefrom
Cortical sensory loss over toes, foot, and leg	Sensory area for foot and leg
Urinary incontinence	Sensorimotor area in paracentral lobule
Contralateral grasp reflex, sucking reflex, gegenhalten (paratonic rigidity)	Medial surface of the posterior frontal lobe (?) supplemental motor area
Abulia (akinetic mutism), slowness, delay, intermittent interruption, lack of spontaneity, whispering, reflex distraction to sights and sounds	Uncertain localization—probably cingulate gyrus and medial inferior portion of frontal, parietal, and temporal lobes
Impairment of gait and stance (gait apraxia)	Frontal cortex near leg motor area
Dyspraxia of left limbs, tactile aphasia in left limbs	Corpus callosum

imaging can reliably identify most atheromatous lesions at the common carotid bifurcation. Atherosclerotic stenotic lesions alter normal laminar flow to rapid disturbed flow with a broad range of velocities immediately distal to the stenosis. These changes can be detected by continuous-wave or range-gated pulsed-Doppler techniques. Errors arise when calcification in a plaque prevents penetration of the ultrasound beam, and when a soft thrombus has the same density as flowing blood. Duplex ultrasound scanning combines B-mode images of the artery with range-gated pulsed-Doppler analysis of flowing blood at each point in the image. Recently, Doppler technology has been developed to allow analysis of intracranial blood flow in the middle and anterior cerebral artery stems, the distal internal carotid and ophthalmic arteries, and in the basilar and vertebral arteries (*transcranial Doppler*). Such studies of intracranial arterial flow are particularly helpful in assessing collateral flow in the circle of Willis, identifying middle cerebral artery stem stenosis or vasospasm, and in documenting the direction and velocity of blood flow in the vertebral or basilar arteries.

Experience suggests that an optimal set of noninvasive tests includes (1) direct assessment of the bifurcation of the common carotid artery by B-mode ultrasound imaging and spectral analysis of the Doppler shift signal to give a semiquantitative assessment of the severity of the stenotic lesion (best expressed as residual lumen diameter) and (2) oculoplethysmography and transcranial Doppler analysis to provide an assessment of the hemodynamic significance of internal carotid origin or carotid siphon stenosis. Positive tests are more diagnostic than apparently normal patterns. However, none of these tests distinguishes reliably between a completely occluded internal carotid origin and one that is nearly completely occluded. Noninvasive testing is most helpful in assessing the carotid artery in patients with middle or anterior cerebral artery stroke or TIA of uncertain cause, in following the progress of a carotid stenosis

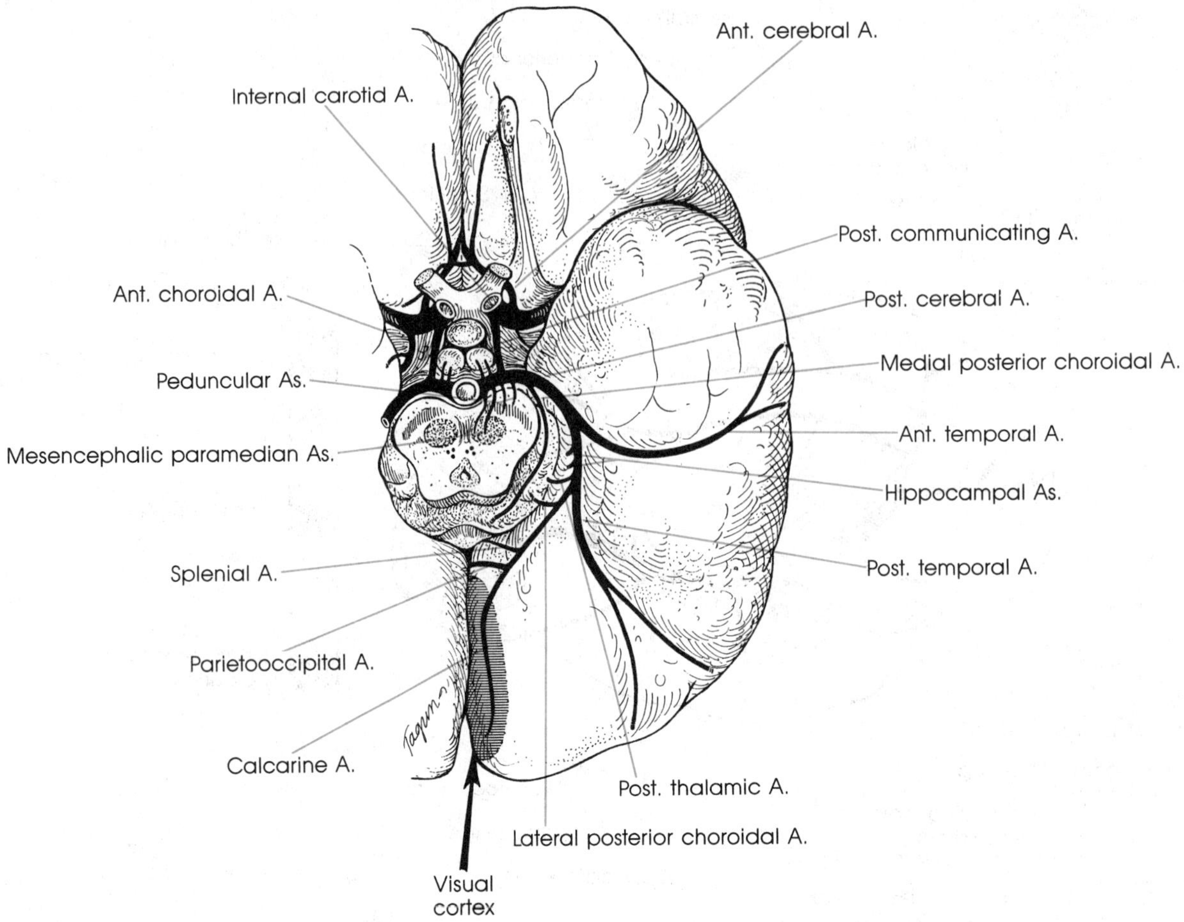

FIGURE 351-6 Inferior aspect of the brain with the branches and distribution of the posterior cerebral artery and the principal anatomic structures shown. (*Courtesy of C. M. Fisher, M.D.*)

Signs and symptoms	*Structures involved*
Peripheral territory (see also Fig. 351-5)	
Homonymous hemianopsia (often upper quadrantic)	Calcarine cortex or optic radiation nearby
Bilateral homonymous hemianopsia, cortical blindness, awareness or denial of blindness; tactile naming, achromatopsia (color blindness), failure to see to-and-fro movements, inability to perceive objects not centrally located, apraxia of ocular movements, inability to count or enumerate objects, tendency to run into things which the patient sees and tries to avoid	Bilateral occipital lobe with possibly the parietal lobe involved.
Verbal dyslexia without agraphia, color anomia	Dominant calcarine lesion and posterior part of corpus callosum
Memory defect	Hippocampal lesion bilaterally or on the dominant side only
Topographic disorientation and prosopagnosia	Usually with lesions of nondominant, calcarine, and lingual gyrus
Simultagnosia, hemivisual neglect	Dominant visual cortex, contralateral hemisphere
Unformed visual hallucinations, peduncular hallucinosis, metamorphopsia, teleopsia, illusory visual spread, irreminiscence, paliopsia, distortion of outlines, central photophobia	Calcarine cortex
Complex hallucinations	Usually nondominant hemisphere
Central territory	
Thalamic syndrome: sensory loss (all modalities), spontaneous pain and dysesthesias, choreoathetosis, intention tremor, spasms of hand, mild hemiparesis	Posteroventral nucleus of thalamus; involvement of the adjacent subthalamus body or its afferent tracts
Thalamoperforate syndrome: crossed cerebellar ataxia with ipsilateral third nerve palsy (Claude's syndrome)	Dentatothalamic tract and issuing third nerve
Weber's syndrome: third nerve palsy and contralateral hemiplegia	Third nerve and cerebral peduncle
Contralateral hemiplegia	Cerebral peduncle
Paralysis or paresis of vertical eye movement, skew deviation, sluggish pupillary responses to light, slight miosis and ptosis (retraction nystagmus and "tucking" of the eyelids may be associated)	Supranuclear fibers to third nerve, interstitial nucleus of Cajal, nucleus of Darkschewitsch, and posterior commissure
Contralateral rhythmic, ataxic action tremor; rhythmic postural or "holding" tremor (rubral tremor)	Dentatothalamic tract (?)

detected by other means such as an asymptomatic bruit, or in assessing the patency of the middle cerebral stem or vertebrobasilar system in patients with appropriate symptoms.

Cerebral angiography Cerebral angiography performed by selective extracranial injection after transfemoral catheterization remains the most reliable method of assessing the cerebrovascular system. It can (1) detect ulcerative lesions, severe stenosis, and formation of a mural thrombus at the carotid bifurcation, (2) directly visualize atherothrombotic disease or dissection in the siphon and intracranial vessels, (3) demonstrate collateral circulation around the circle of Willis and on the cortical surface, and (4) show embolic occlusion of cerebral branch vessels. Although angiography cannot measure blood flow directly, it reflects relative pressures in major vessels and can suggest compromised flow in the internal carotid system. Computerized enhancement techniques have improved the resolution of angiography and reduced the amount of dye injections necessary.

However, the advantages of selective cerebral angiography must be assessed in the context of its risks. Complications range from 2 to 12 percent in various studies. The principal risks are aortic or carotid artery dissection and embolic stroke. Although rare, cholesterol microemboli from aortic arch atheroma can cause watershed cerebral infarction and renal failure. A skilled angiographer and careful attention to hydration can reduce these risks. Patients with recurrent headaches or a history of migrainous phenomena have been given glucocorticoids before angiography, but their value in preventing ischemic complications has not been established. In some patients the less risky technique of brachial artery injection offers as much relevant information as selective intracranial angiography from transfemoral catheterization.

Intravenous digital subtraction angiography is a computer-reconstruction method developed to circumvent problems inherent in arterial catheterization. However, its poor resolution and the need for large amounts of contrast material have made it virtually obsolete. Magnetic resonance techniques that image intracranial vessels are being developed (see below).

Cerebral imaging Brain imaging remains the most important acute test once a stroke has occurred. The extent and location of infarcted brain tissue can be assessed by CT scanning, which provides an estimate of extent and location of supratentorial cerebral infarction, including small 0.5- to 1.0-cm lacunar infarctions. In addition, CT scans immediately exclude hemorrhage as the cause of focal stroke and can detect surrounding edema, and less consistently, hemorrhagic infarction. *CT, however, cannot detect most cerebral infarctions for at least 48 h.* It does not reliably identify infarction of the cortical surface gray matter at any age. Furthermore, when infarction occurs in the brainstem—i.e., in the vertebral or basilar territories—CT is even less reliable because of bone and motion artifacts and the small size of many infarcts (see also Chap. 348).

Magnetic resonance imaging reveals more than CT scanning in patients with stroke. Within hours of onset, with MRI the extent and location of infarction on the cortical surface and small lacunar infarctions in the posterior fossa can be easily identified. The hemorrhagic components of infarction can be detected using high-field-strength magnets (1.5 to 4 tesla) and different pulse sequencing. Blood flow in many intracranial arteries can be detected by varying the image plane and using variable pulsing techniques. Future applications are likely to expand the angiographic capability. Tomographic assessment of cerebral blood flow and metabolism using nuclear magnetic spectroscopy may soon be possible (Chap. 348).

Xenon blood flow and positron emission tomography can assess cerebral blood flow and metabolism qualitatively and quantitatively. These methods remain time-consuming and expensive and are used largely to conduct research rather than to guide therapy (see Chap. 348).

THERAPY FOR CAROTID TERRITORY TIA Anticoagulant therapy Heparin has been used when impending carotid or middle cerebral occlusion is suspected as the cause of TIA, but in the absence of established clinical proof of efficacy its use must be considered empirical. Heparin may be useful in the short term in stemming additional TIAs and in preventing complete occlusion of a tightly stenotic lesion while the patient is awaiting angiography, surgery, or oral anticoagulation. Heparin prevents clot formation and propagation by inhibiting the activation of prothrombin and by accelerating the rate of neutralization of several clotting factors and thrombin. However, in a few cases it has been thought to promote thrombosis, presumably by platelet activation and consumption in the clotting process. Thrombocytopenia may occur as a side effect.

The use of chronic anticoagulant therapy with sodium warfarin (coumadin) is even more controversial and problematic. Most studies of efficacy of chronic anticoagulant therapy to prevent stroke or to decrease TIAs are difficult to appraise for a number of reasons, e.g., lack of randomization, small number of patients, and lack of uniformity in the diagnosis of the cause of the TIA. In some studies, the inclusion of patients with other transient neurologic symptoms unrelated to ischemia have further complicated assessment of the results. Many believe that chronic anticoagulation therapy benefits patients with carotid-territory TIAs who are not candidates for surgery either because of medical conditions or because the lesion is surgically inaccessible (carotid siphon or middle cerebral stem). Because of the often devasting effect of middle cerebral artery occlusions, anticoagulation is similarly recommended when patients present with TIAs or minor strokes from a tightly stenotic lesion in the stem of the middle cerebral artery.

To minimize the bleeding complications of warfarin, it has been suggested that the prothrombin time should be maintained between 1.3 and 1.5 times control value (see "Embolism," below). Contraindications to anticoagulant therapy include an actively bleeding ulcer, malignant hypertension, uremia, hepatic failure, or poor patient compliance. Relative contraindications are old age, systolic blood pressure above 180 mmHg, or a history of bleeding ulcer, or bleeding diathesis.

Antiplatelet therapy Studies of the effect of antiplatelet agents on the natural history of TIAs and minor strokes can be criticized for the same reasons as the anticoagulation studies. Aspirin has been the agent most widely investigated in the prevention of stroke. Eight randomized trials have considered either aspirin alone or aspirin in combination with another antiplatelet agent. The two largest have suggested that aspirin alone may be beneficial in preventing further TIAs and strokes in symptomatic patients. Another study, in which angiography was performed routinely, suggested that aspirin benefitted patients who had TIAs associated with a lesion in the internal carotid artery, but not those who had a single TIA and no carotid lesion, i.e., those thought to have emboli from the heart. In these studies, aspirin has reduced the stroke risk over 3 years from approximately 19 to 12 percent. But endarterectomy, not aspirin, is the treatment of choice for most TIAs resulting from severe atherothrombotic disease of the internal carotid artery. Most physicians agree that aspirin may be used when TIAs are caused by inoperable carotid artery lesions or, perhaps, by ulcerative plaques.

There are theoretical reasons to avoid the excessive use of aspirin. Paradoxically, aspirin inhibits platelet formation of thromboxane A_2, a platelet-aggregating, vasoconstricting prostaglandin, but also inhibits the formation of prostacyclin, an antiaggregating vasodilating prostaglandin derived from endothelial cells. Aspirin in low doses predominantly inhibits the production of thromboxane A_2; therefore, many physicians recommend aspirin in doses of 300 mg or less per day.

Dipyridamole acts by inhibiting platelet phosphodiesterase, which is responsible for breakdown of cyclic adenosine monophosphate. The resulting elevation in platelet cyclic AMP level inhibits aggregation of platelets. Sulfinpyrazone inhibits the platelet-release reaction and interferes with platelet adhesion to subendothelial tissues. However, there is no compelling clinical evidence to suggest that dipyridamole, sulfinpyrazone, or other antiplatelet agents such as clofibrate or ibuprofen are better than aspirin in preventing recurrent TIAs or stroke in patients with symptomatic atherothrombotic cerebral vascular disease. Ticlopidine is thought to inhibit platelet binding to fibrinogen, and recent studies have compared its efficacy to aspirin's in preventing stroke in patients with TIAs or stroke. Unfortunately, these studies, like the aspirin studies, suffer from their failure to define precisely the cause of the cerebral symptoms. Ticlopidine has the disadvantage of producing a small risk of leukopenia, diarrhea, and rash.

Carotid endarterectomy Carotid endarterectomy remains the main therapy for TIAs caused by severe internal carotid stenosis, though its indications are being carefully scrutinized in several current studies. First introduced in 1954, the procedure has been associated with a morbidity ranging from 1 to 20 percent, depending on the patient population and the experience of surgeons and physicians. Although many studies suggest that this procedure is effective in preventing additional TIAs or strokes, its value has yet to be confirmed by a well-designed, controlled, randomized clinical trial. To make these surgical trials valid, the more threatening ($\leq$ 1.0-mm) lesions must be accurately identified. *Unless the acute combined complication rate of angiography and surgery is less than approximately 3 to 5 percent, carotid surgery is unlikely to be more effective than no treatment.*

Patients with a tightly stenotic lesion in one carotid artery and either an occlusion of the contralateral carotid artery or an inadequate circle of Willis are at somewhat higher risk of intraoperative stroke during endarterectomy. Intraoperative electroencephalographic or evoked potential monitoring can detect cerebral ischemia during the procedure and warn the surgeon to take steps to improve circulation.

Most patients who undergo endarterectomy have hypertensive arteriosclerotic cardiovascular disease and peripheral vascular disease. Active coronary diseases such as unstable angina, recent myocardial infarction (within 6 months), or congestive heart failure are contraindications to surgery. Severe hypertension is often corrected before surgery, but excessive lowering of the blood pressure should be avoided with tight carotid artery stenosis, because it can lead to vessel occlusion and stroke.

Stenosis can recur after surgery, although it seldom does. Poor surgical technique, excessive scar formation, and active arteriosclerotic disease have been implicated. Within the first year, the underlying pathologic process appears to be largely the proliferation of fibrous tissue; after the first year, of fibrous tissue and atherosclerosis. When stenosis recurs and gives rise to symptoms, surgery, although feasible, becomes more difficult technically.

Tandem stenotic lesions of the internal carotid artery—one at the carotid bifurcation and one at the carotid siphon—require special consideration. If the siphon stenosis has a residual lumen diameter of more than 2 mm and the lower carotid a diameter of less than 2 mm, then endarterectomy can generally be recommended. If the siphon narrowing is more severe, the value of endarterectomy is less certain. Anticoagulant or antiplatelet therapy may be preferable. But there is no consensus about the efficacy of either therapy in this setting.

Anastomosis of a superficial temporal branch of the external carotid artery to a cortical surface branch of the middle cerebral artery (EC/IC bypass) can provide collateral flow to the middle cerebral territory. Such surgery has been considered in patients with an occluded carotid artery or a tightly stenotic lesion of the carotid siphon or middle cerebral stem who present with recurrent TIAs or minor strokes. However, the results of a worldwide randomized study failed to prove greater benefit of surgical compared to anticoagulation or antiplatelet therapy in these conditions.

THERAPY FOR CAROTID TERRITORY STROKE The severity of a recent stroke in the territory of the internal carotid artery is an important factor in the decision about therapy. If there is a complete hemiplegia, severe aphasia, or anosognosia, indicating involvement of the major portions of the middle cerebral territory, the prevention of additional strokes in that arterial distribution becomes moot. Instead, careful attention to maintenance of adequate blood pressure and prevention of delayed cerebral edema becomes important. There is little evidence to support the use of anticoagulant therapy once a "completed" or static major stroke deficit exists. However, if marked clinical improvement occurs during the first hours after onset or if the deficit is small, some anecdotal evidence suggests that short-term anticoagulation (heparin) prevents further damage, i.e., benefits "stroke in evolution." Given the pathophysiologic mechanisms of carotid stroke, many physicians use short-term anticoagulation in a patient with a slight stroke from a recently occluded or tightly stenotic internal carotid artery, hoping to prevent a second, possibly more devastating, event. In such patients, small ischemic infarcts may become hemorrhagic, but they rarely develop frank hemorrhages that act as a mass. Nonetheless, this possibility and the theoretical risk of thrombosis promotion make the timing and benefit of early heparinization controversial.

Even though no controlled studies exist, endarterectomy can tentatively be recommended for patients with tightly stenotic internal carotid lesions who present with a minor stroke in the territory distal to the lesion. The risk of surgery in experienced hands may be as low as 2 percent if the patient has no medical contraindications. When the contralateral carotid artery is tightly stenotic or occluded, endarterectomy of the ipsilateral carotid artery has a higher morbidity. Comparison of the natural history of cases of symptomatic tight carotid stenosis with surgical results has not been made, but some experience suggests that additional strokes develop in more than 3 percent of patients who are not treated surgically. Surgical trials will hopefully assess the degree of stenosis accurately enough to analyze separately the tightly stenotic ($\leq$ 1.0-mm) lesions.

Hemorrhage into a cerebral infarct is rare following internal carotid endarterectomy and probably occurs no more frequently than it would without surgery if postoperative hypertension is avoided. Nevertheless, most surgeons advise that carotid endarterectomy be delayed 2 to 6 weeks after a stroke. Earlier surgery, although controversial, may be preferable when the neurologic deficit is small or transient.

Surgery has also been performed in some cases of acute carotid artery occlusion, usually less than 8 h old, but the results are generally unsatisfactory once a major neurologic deficit is present. For most patients with a mild to moderate stroke and demonstrated occlusion of the internal carotid artery, alternative therapies include anticoagulants or antiplatelet agents, or neither. Some physicians prescribe warfarin for 6 months in hopes of preventing embolization of the propagated thrombus. In exceptional circumstances, endarterectomy of the external carotid artery or the contralateral stenotic internal carotid artery may be considered, depending on the findings at angiography and the nature of the recurrent clinical symptoms. An embolism from an occluded carotid artery suggests that the use of anticoagulation therapy may be helpful in preventing a second stroke, whereas recurrent symptoms suggestive of diminished blood flow in a hemisphere that is isolated from collateral sources of blood supply warrant consideration of surgery.

Therapy for stenosis of the carotid siphon or the middle cerebral stem associated with stroke or recurrent TIAs remains controversial. Because of the failure of external carotid–internal carotid (EC/IC) bypass surgery to reduce risks of ischemic stroke, antiplatelet therapy (aspirin) or anticoagulant therapy (warfarin) is recommended in most cases. In the absence of randomized studies to indicate which is more efficacious, antiplatelet therapy is usually recommended first for carotid siphon stenosis followed by anticoagulation if recurrent symptoms occur. Because of the potentially devastating effects of middle cerebral artery occlusion, anticoagulation with warfarin is recommended for symptomatic middle cerebral stem stenosis. In cases where recurrent symptoms occur in spite of this therapy, lowering of the blood viscosity may be helpful. Fortunately, with time, recurrent symptoms often diminish despite the treatment choice.

The unusual case of atherothrombotic stenosis or occlusion of the proximal anterior cerebral artery may cause intermittent symptoms involving the contralateral leg. Antiplatelet or anticoagulation therapy has been recommended, but no studies have documented the natural history of atherothrombotic disease at this location, and no surgical procedure protects the distal territory of the anterior cerebral artery from ischemia caused by proximal stenosis.

Experimental therapies Although much attention has been directed toward the investigation of the opioid-like substance naloxone in the treatment of acute ischemic infarction, it has yet to be shown to be efficacious. Several earlier studies suggested a beneficial effect on outcome with hemodilution, but randomized trials have given conflicting results. Reducing blood viscosity is a more promising innovative therapy for ischemic stroke. If the blood pressure remains constant, reduction of whole-blood viscosity (mainly by reduction in hematocrit and serum fibrinogen) results in increased flow through a stenotic lesion. In theory, this form of therapy increases flow to the ischemic zone (penumbra) that lies between infarcted and normal brain. This therapy has little risk. Preliminary work with drugs that block calcium influx into ischemic cells, either conventional calcium channel blockers or glutamate receptor blockers, has also had variable success in patients with stroke and in animal models.

ASYMPTOMATIC CAROTID BIFURCATION STENOSIS WITH BRUIT The natural history of an atherosclerotic lesion of the carotid bifurcation that causes a bruit but has not caused either a TIA or stroke is unknown. The available studies have examined small populations, and most failed to localize and quantitate the severity of the stenotic lesion. The studies of asymptomatic patients with cervical bruits who are about to undergo major surgical procedures have the same deficiencies. Although in some studies patients with cervical bruits were found to be at increased risk of heart disease, stroke, and death, the strokes did not necessarily occur in the vascular territory of the carotid giving rise to the bruit. At the present time, given these facts, there is little justification for operating on the carotid artery in such patients.

However, patients with tightly stenotic lesions at the origin of the internal carotid artery (1.5 mm or less) that reduces flow in the distal internal carotid artery may be at higher risk of thrombotic occlusion. Although such patients have reduced flow in the distal internal carotid artery, they may remain asymptomatic because of adequate collateral flow across the anterior circle of Willis. When stroke occurs, it is usually the result of ipsilateral artery to artery embolism. A high pitched prolonged bruit fading into diastole is often associated with a tightly stenotic lesion at the origin of the internal carotid artery. It may become fainter as the stenosis progresses and flow is reduced and may disappear altogether when occlusion is imminent. Noninvasive carotid testing can often identify tightly stenotic lesions (see above). Two randomized trials are in progress to assess efficacy of surgery in patients with asymptomatic carotid stenosis. Surgery is considered only when hemodynamically significant stenotic lesions can be demonstrated. Antiplatelet therapy or observation is therefore recommended in most patients.

ATHEROTHROMBOTIC DISEASE OF THE VERTEBROBASILAR–POSTERIOR CEREBRAL ARTERY SYSTEM

The two vertebral arteries join to form the basilar artery at the pontomedullary junction. The basilar artery divides into two posterior cerebral arteries in the interpeduncular fossa (Fig. 351-2). Each of these major arteries gives rise to long and short circumferential branches and to smaller deep penetrating branches that supply the cerebellum, medulla, pons, midbrain, subthalamus, thalamus, hippocampus, and medial temporal and occipital lobes. Atherosclerosis has a predilection for the origin and the distal segments of the vertebral arteries, the proximal basilar artery, and the origin of the major and minor branches of the vertebral, basilar, and posterior cerebral arteries. Predictably, atheromatous disease at each site carries its own unique natural history, produces its own clinical syndromes, and has its own specific therapeutic implications.

POSTERIOR CEREBRAL ARTERY Pathophysiology In 70 percent of cases, both posterior cerebral arteries arise from the bifurcation of the basilar artery; in 22 percent, one or the other comes from the ipsilateral internal carotid artery; in 8 percent, both come from the ipsilateral internal carotid artery (Fig. 351-2) via the posterior communicating arteries. The precommunal segment (mesencephalic portion) of the true posterior cerebral artery is atretic in such cases (Fig. 351-2).

Atheroma formation at the top of the basilar artery or along the precommunal segment of the posterior cerebral artery may cause symptoms by narrowing one or more of the small brainstem-penetrating branches (Figs. 351-2 and 351-6) that supply the middle cerebral peduncles, the substantia nigra, red nucleus, oculomotor nuclei, midbrain reticular formation, subthalamic nucleus of Luys, decussation of superior cerebellar peduncles, the medial longitudinal fasciculus, and the medial lemniscus. The artery of Percheron (the posterior thalamosubthalamoparamedian artery), is a single artery that arises from either the right or the left precommunal segment of the posterior cerebral artery. It divides in the subthalamus to supply the inferior medial and the anterior portions of the thalamus and subthalamus bilaterally. The thalamogeniculate branches, which also originate from the precommunal portion of the posterior cerebral artery, supply the dorsal, dorsomedial, anterior, and inferior thalamus and the medial geniculate body. The medial posterior choroidal artery supplies the superior dorsomedial and dorsoanterior thalamus and the medial geniculate body in addition to the tela choroidea of the third ventricle. The lateral posterior choroidal artery supplies the choroid plexus of the lateral ventricle.

Atheroma in the posterior cerebral artery distal to the junction with the posterior communicating artery (Fig. 351-6) may occlude small circumferential branches that course around the midbrain to supply the lateral part of the cerebral peduncles, medial lemniscus, tegmentum of the midbrain, superior colliculi, lateral geniculate body, and posterior lateral nucleus of the thalamus, choroid plexus, and hippocampus. On the rare occasions when atheroma occur more distally in the posterior cerebral artery (Fig. 351-6), occlusion may produce ischemia and infarction in the medial inferior temporal lobe, parahippocampal and hippocampal gyri, and occipital lobe—including the calcarine cortex and the visual association areas 18 and 19.

Clinical manifestations The site of atheromas and the degree of narrowing determine the clinical syndrome. Although factors of collateral circulation or serum viscosity may play a role in some cases, embolic occlusion is the usual cause of stroke in this vascular territory. Two syndromes are commonly observed: (1) midbrain, subthalamic, and thalamic signs, which are due to disease of the precommunal segment of the posterior cerebral artery or of its penetrating branches; and (2) cortical temporal and occipital lobe syndromes, due to occlusion of the postcommunal segment.

PROXIMAL PRECOMMUNAL SYNDROMES (CENTRAL TERRITORY) If the proximal posterior cerebral artery is occluded, infarction usually occurs in the ipsilateral or bilateral subthalamus and medial thalamus and in the ipsilateral cerebral peduncle and midbrain, producing concomitant signs (Fig. 351-6). If the posterior communicating artery is atretic, the peripheral territory supplied by posterior cerebral artery is also affected (Fig. 351-6). If the posterior cerebral artery is completely occluded at its origin, hemiplegia secondary to infarction of the cerebral peduncle occurs. Involvement of the red nucleus and/or dentatorubrothalamic tract can produce contralateral ataxia. A third nerve palsy with contralateral ataxia (Claude's syndrome) or with contralateral hemiplegia (Weber's syndrome) may result. If the subthalamic nucleus of Luys is involved, contralateral hemiballismus may occur. Occlusion of the artery of Percheron produces paresis of upward gaze and drowsiness and is often associated with abulia. Extensive infarction in the midbrain of the subthalamus occurring with bilateral posterior cerebral stem occlusion is usually secondary to embolism. Coma, bilateral pyramidal signs, and "decerebrate rigidity" occur in this setting.

Atheromatous occlusion of the penetrating branches of the thalamic and thalamogeniculate arteries produces less extensive thalamic and thalamocapsular lacunar syndromes. The *thalamic syndrome of Dejerine and Roussy* is the best known. Its main feature is contralateral hemisensory loss of both superficial sensation (pain and temperature) and deep sensation (touch and proprioception). Occasionally, it may affect only pain and temperature or vibration and joint position sense. After a few weeks or months, an agonizing, searing pain may develop in the affected areas. Patients describe the pain as tight, drawing, icy, and knifelike. It is devastatingly persistent and responds poorly to analgesics. Occasionally, anticonvulsants are beneficial. If the posterior limb of the internal capsule is involved, hemiparesis or hemiplegia may accompany the hemisensory syndrome. Other associated motor signs include hemiballismus, choreoathetosis, intention tremor, incoordination, and posturing of the hand and arm, particularly while walking.

POSTCOMMUNAL SYNDROMES (PERIPHERAL OR CORTICAL TERRITORY) (Fig. 351-6) Occlusion of the posterior cerebral artery causes infarction of the cortical surface of the medial temporal and occipital lobes. Contralateral homonymous hemianopsia is the usual manifestation. Occasionally, only the upper quadrant of the visual field is involved. If the visual association areas are spared and only the calcarine cortex is involved, the patient is aware of visual defects. Central vision may be spared if middle cerebral artery branches supply the macular region of the occipital pole. Medial temporal lobe and hippocampal involvement may cause an acute disturbance in memory, particularly if it occurs in the dominant hemisphere, but the defect usually clears because memory has bilateral representation. If the dominant hemisphere is affected and the infarct extends to involve the splenium of the corpus callosum, the patient may demonstrate alexia without agraphia. Visual agnosia for faces, objects, mathematical symbols, and colors and anomia with paraphasic errors (amnestic aphasia) may also occur in this setting even without callosal involvement. Occlusion of the posterior cerebral artery can produce peduncular hallucinosis (visual hallucinations of brightly colored scenes and objects).

Bilateral infarction in the distal posterior cerebral arteries produces cortical blindness. The patient is often unaware of the blindness. The clinical clue to the site is a finding of normal pupillary reaction to light. Tiny islands of vision may persist; and the patient then reports that vision fluctuates as images are captured in the preserved portions. Rarely, only peripheral vision is lost and central vision is spared; resulting in "gun-barrel" vision. A constellation of symptoms termed *Balint's syndrome* can occur with unilateral or bilateral visual association area lesions. It includes optic ataxia (inability to visually guide limb movements), ocular ataxia (inability to direct eyes to a precise point in the visual field), inability to enumerate objects in a picture or extract meaning from a picture, and inability to avoid objects seen in one's path. Balint's syndrome is most often seen with bilateral infarctions, secondary to low flow in the distal posterior and or middle cerebral "watershed" territories as occurs after arrest. Embolic occlusion of the top of the basilar artery can produce a clinical picture that includes any or all of the central or peripheral territory symptoms. Its hallmark is suddenness of onset and bilaterality of symptoms including ptosis and somnolence (see above in the discussion of the artery of Percheron).

Laboratory evaluation Infarction in the peripheral territory of the posterior cerebral artery can be easily documented by CT or MRI. Infarction in the central territory of the posterior cerebral artery, particularly in territories supplied by the penetrating branches of the posterior cerebral artery, is not reliably detected by CT scanning. MRI can detect infarctions greater than 0.5 cm in this area.

Therapy Because infarction in the territory of the posterior cerebral artery is usually secondary to embolism from the vertebrobasilar system or from the heart, treatment with anticoagulants to prevent further embolic events is appropriate. Transient ischemic symptoms in the territory of the posterior cerebral artery may result from atherothrombotic stenosis of its proximal portion or one of its penetrating branches (lacunar TIA). The natural history of such atheromatous disease is unknown. Thus, the efficacy of anticoagulants vs. antiplatelet therapy vs. no medication is still uncertain. In general, antiplatelet therapy seems safest in this setting.

VERTEBRAL AND POSTERIOR INFERIOR CEREBELLAR ARTERIES The *vertebral artery,* which arises from the innominate artery on the right and the subclavian artery on the left, divides into four anatomic segments. The first segment extends from its origin to its entrance into the sixth or fifth transverse vertebral foramen. The second segment traverses the vertebral foramina from C6 to C2. The third segment passes through the transverse foramen and circles around the arch of the atlas to pierce the dura at the foramen magnum. The fourth segment courses upward to join the other vertebral artery to form the basilar artery; only the fourth segment gives rise to branches that supply the brainstem and cerebellum. The *posterior inferior cerebellar artery* in its proximal segments supplies the lateral medulla and, in its distal branches, the inferior surface of the cerebellum. Anastomotic channels exist among the ascending cervical arteries, the thyrocervical arteries, the occipital artery (branch of the external carotid artery), and the second segment of the vertebral artery (Fig. 351-1). In 10 percent of patients, one vertebral artery is too small to contribute significant blood to the brainstem.

Atherothrombotic lesions have a predilection for the first and fourth segments of the vertebral artery. Although the atheromatous narrowing in the first segment (the origin) may be significant, it seldom produces brainstem ischemic strokes. Collateral flow from the contralateral vertebral artery or the ascending cervical and ascending thyrocervical or occipital arteries is usually sufficient to prevent ischemia (Fig. 351-1*D*). When one vertebral artery is atretic and an atherothrombotic lesion threatens the origin of the other, the only avenues for collateral circulation are through the ascending cervical artery, the thyrocervical artery, and the occipital artery, or by retrograde flow down the basilar artery via the posterior communicating artery (Fig. 351-2 and 351-6). In this setting, low flow in the vertebrobasilar system exists and TIAs may occur. In addition, incipient thrombosis in the proximal basilar or distal vertebral system may occur. If the subclavian is blocked proximal to the origin of the vertebral artery, exercise of the left arm may draw blood from the vertebrobasilar insufficiency (*subclavian steal*). It rarely leads to significant vertebrobasilar ischemia.

Atheroma in the fourth segment of the vertebral artery can occur proximal to or distal to the origin of the posterior inferior cerebral artery, as well as at the junction with the other vertebral artery to form the basilar artery. When it is proximal to the origin of the posterior inferior cerebral artery, a critical narrowing can threaten the lateral medulla and posterior inferior surface of the cerebellum.

Although atheromatous disease rarely narrows the second and third segments of the vertebral artery, this region is subject to dissection, fibromuscular dysplasia, and rarely to encroachment by osteophytic spurs within the vertebral foramina.

Clinical manifestations *Transient cerebral ischemic attacks* resulting from vertebral artery insufficiency cause dizziness or vertigo, numbness of the ipsilateral face and contralateral limbs, diplopia, hoarseness, dysarthria, and dysphagia. Hemiparesis is rare. Such TIAs are usually short (up to 10 to 15 min) and repetitive.

When *infarction* ensues, it most often affects the lateral medulla with or without the posterior inferior cerebellum (Wallenberg's syndrome). Its features are listed in Fig. 351-7. In 70 to 80 percent of the cases, the syndrome occurs after ipsilateral vertebral artery occlusion; in the remainder it results from posterior inferior cerebellar artery occlusion. Atherothrombotic occlusion of the medullary penetrating branches of the vertebral or posterior inferior cerebellar artery results in partial syndromes of the ipsilateral, lateral, or medial medulla.

Rarely, a medial medullary syndrome occurs in which the pyramid becomes infarcted, causing a contralateral hemiparesis of the arm and leg, sparing the face. If the medial lemniscus and emerging hypoglossal nerve fibers are involved, contralateral loss of joint position sense and ipsilateral tongue weakness occur.

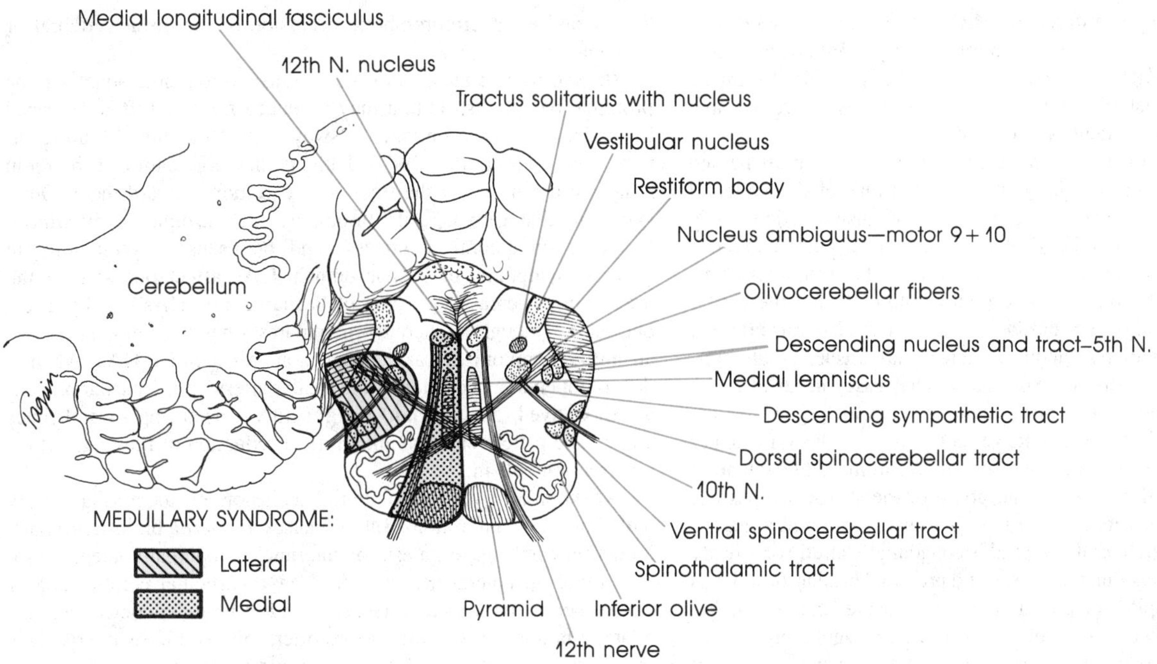

FIGURE 351-7 *(Courtesy of C. M. Fisher, M.D.)*

Signs and symptoms	*Structures involved*
1 Medial medullary syndrome (occlusion of vertebral artery or of branch of vertebral or lower basilar artery)	
On side of lesion:	
Paralysis with atrophy of half the tongue	Ipsilateral twelfth nerve
On side opposite lesion:	
Paralysis of arm and leg sparing face; impaired tactile and proprioceptive sense over half the body	Contralateral pyramidal tract and medial lemniscus
2 Lateral medullary syndrome (occlusion of any of five vessels may be responsible—vertebral, posterior inferior cerebellar, superior, middle, or inferior lateral medullary arteries)	
On side of lesion:	
Pain, numbness, impaired sensation over half the face	Descending tract and nucleus fifth nerve
Ataxia of limbs, falling to side of lesion	Uncertain—restiform body, cerebellar hemisphere, cerebellar fibers, spinocerebellar tract (?)
Nystagmus, diplopia, oscillopsia, vertigo, nausea, vomiting	Vestibular nucleus
Horner's syndrome (miosis, ptosis, decreased sweating)	Descending sympathetic tract
Dysphagia, hoarseness, paralysis of palate, paralysis of vocal cord, diminished gag reflex	Issuing fibers ninth and tenth nerves
Loss of taste	Nucleus and tractus solitarius
Numbness of ipsilateral arm, trunk, or leg	Cuneate and gracile nuclei
On side opposite lesion:	
Impaired pain and thermal sense over half the body, sometimes face	Spinothalamic tract
3 Total unilateral medullary syndrome (occlusion of vertebral artery): Combination of medial and lateral syndromes	
4 Lateral pontomedullary syndrome (occlusion of vertebral artery): Combination of lateral medullary and lateral inferior pontine syndromes	
5 Basilar artery syndrome (the syndrome of the lone vertebral artery is equivalent): A combination of the various brainstem syndromes plus those arising in the posterior cerebral artery distribution	
Bilateral long tract signs (sensory and motor; cerebellar and peripheral cranial nerve abnormalities)	Bilateral long tract; cerebellar and peripheral cranial nerves
Paralysis or weakness of all extremities, plus all bulbar musculature	Corticobulbar and corticospinal tracts bilaterally

Cerebellar infarction with edema formation can lead to *sudden respiratory arrest* due to raised intracranial pressure in the posterior fossa. Drowsiness, Babinski signs, dysarthria, and bifacial weakness may be absent or present only briefly before respiratory arrest ensues. Gait unsteadiness, dizziness, nausea, and vomiting may be the only early symptoms and signs and should arouse suspicion of this impending complication.

Laboratory evaluation When TIAs occur in the territory of the lateral medulla, it becomes important to determine the adequacy of blood flow in the distal vertebral artery and the posterior inferior cerebellar artery. Angiography is therefore considered if the diagnosis is unclear. CT scanning may detect a large cerebellar infarction in the territory of the posterior inferior cerebellar artery. MRI can detect cerebellar infarction earlier and, with high-resolution scanning, can detect lateral medullary infarction. MRI can also image blood flow in the fourth segment of the vertebral artery. With the further development of MRI technology, it may be possible to image atherothrombotic material in the vertebral and basilar arteries and determine if they are patent or occluded.

Therapy Four important therapeutic issues arise in managing patients with ischemia or infarction in the territory of the vertebral or posterior inferior cerebellar artery. First, the ensuing edema may be life-threatening. It should be treated with osmotic agents (mannitol); surgical decompression may be necessary. Second, thrombosis of the fourth segment of the vertebral artery may send clots into the basilar artery or emboli into the basilar or posterior cerebral arteries. Symptoms or signs of basilar insufficiency may ensue. Acute anticoagulation with heparin is advocated in such cases in an effort to prevent clot propagation. Third, some physicians argue for the prophylactic use of heparin in acute vertebral artery occlusion whether or not basilar artery symptoms have occurred. Chronic anticoagulation is not recommended after the acute phase of the stroke has passed. Fourth, when one vertebral artery is symptomatic with atheromatous disease and the contralateral vertebral is congenitally atretic or already occluded, basilar ischemia may ensue and proximal basilar thrombosis may develop. Despite its potential hazards, acute anticoagulation with heparin, followed by chronic warfarin anticoagulation, is recommended in such patients. When the same circumstance occurs but the symptomatic vertebral atherothrombotic lesion lies immediately proximal to the posterior inferior cerebellar artery, occipital-to–posterior inferior bypass grafting has been recommended. The efficacy of this surgery is unproven, and it should be considered only after anticoagulation therapy has failed.

BASILAR ARTERY Pathophysiology Branches of the basilar artery supply the base of the pontis and superior cerebellum and fall into three groups: (1) paramedian, seven to 10 in number, which supply a wedge of pons on either side of the midline; (2) short circumferential branches, five to seven in number, which supply the lateral two-thirds of the pons and middle and superior cerebellar peduncles; and (3) two bilateral long circumferential arteries (superior cerebellar and anterior inferior cerebellar arteries) which course around the pons to supply the cerebellar hemispheres.

Atheromatous lesions can occur anywhere along the basilar trunk, but are most often in the proximal basilar and distal vertebral segments. Typically, lesions occlude either the proximal basilar and one or both vertebral arteries. The clinical picture varies depending on the availability of retrograde collateral flow from the posterior communicating arteries.

Although atherothrombosis occasionally occludes the top of the basilar artery, emboli from the heart or proximal vertebral or basilar segments are more common.

Clinical manifestations Because the brainstem contains many structures in close approximation, a diversity of clinical syndromes may emerge with ischemia. Involvement of the corticospinal tracts, corticobulbar tracts, medial and superior cerebellar peduncles, spinothalamic tracts, and cranial nerve nuclei cause the common symptoms and signs (see Figs. 351-8 to 351-10).

Unfortunately, the symptoms of transient ischemia or infarction in the territory of the basilar artery often do not indicate whether the basilar artery itself or one of its branches is diseased, yet the distinction has important implications for therapy. The picture of complete basilar insufficiency, however, is easy to recognize. A combination of bilateral long tract signs (sensory and motor) with signs of cranial nerve and cerebellar dysfunction suggest this diagnosis. A "locked-in" state of quadriplegia occurs with bilateral basis pontis infarction. Coma due to dysfunction of the reticular activating system and quadriplegia with cranial nerve signs suggest complete and devastating pontine and upper midbrain infarction. The therapeutic goal, however, is to recognize impending basilar occlusion before such a devastating infarction occurs. A series of TIAs or a slowly progressive, fluctuating stroke become extremely significant when they herald an atherothrombotic occlusion of the distal vertebral or proximal basilar artery.

TRANSIENT ISCHEMIC ATTACKS Transient ischemic attacks in the proximal basilar distribution may produce dizziness (often described by patients as "swimming," "swaying," "moving," "unsteadiness," or "lightheadedness"). Patients may complain that the room is upside down or that the floor seems to move toward them. Other symptoms that warn of basilar thrombosis include diplopia, dysarthria, facial or circumoral numbness, and hemisensory symptoms. In general, symptoms of basilar branch TIAs affect one side of the brainstem, whereas symptoms of basilar artery TIAs usually affect both sides, though a "herald" hemiparesis has been emphasized as an initial symptom of basilar occlusion. Most often TIAs, whether due to impending occlusion of the basilar artery or of a basilar branch, are short-lived (5 to 30 min) and repetitive, occurring several times a day. The pattern suggests intermittent reduction of flow rather than recurrent embolism.

INFARCTION Atherothrombotic occlusion of the basilar artery with brainstem infarction usually causes *bilateral* brainstem signs. Sometimes only gaze paresis or internuclear ophthalmoplegia associated with ipsilateral hemiparesis, i.e., a particular combination of cranial nerve and long tract (sensory and/or motor) deficits, signifies bilateral brainstem ischemia. More often, bilateral basis pontis signs coexist with unilateral or bilateral pontine tegmental signs.

Symptomatic atherothrombotic occlusion of a branch of the basilar artery usually causes *unilateral* symptoms and signs involving motor, sensory, and cranial nerves. Occlusions of the two long circumferential branches of the basilar artery produce specific clinical syndromes depending on the artery involved.

SUPERIOR CEREBELLAR ARTERY Occlusion of the superior cerebellar artery results in severe ipsilateral cerebellar ataxia (middle and/or superior cerebellar peduncles), nausea and vomiting, dysarthria, and contralateral loss of pain and temperature sensation over the extremities, body, and face (spino- and trigeminothalamic tract). Partial deafness, ataxic tremor of the ipsilateral upper extremity, Horner's syndrome, and palatal myoclonus may rarely occur. Partial syndromes occur frequently (see Fig. 351-8).

ANTERIOR INFERIOR CEREBELLAR ARTERY Occlusion of the anterior inferior cerebellar artery produces variable degrees of infarction because the size of this artery and the territory it supplies vary inversely with those of the posterior inferior cerebellar artery. The principal symptoms include ipsilateral deafness, facial weakness, true vertigo (whirling dizziness), nausea and vomiting, nystagmus, tinnitus and cerebellar ataxia, Horner's syndrome, and paresis of conjugate lateral gaze. The opposite side of the body loses pain and temperature sensation. An occlusion close to the origin of the artery may cause corticospinal tract signs (see Fig. 351-10).

Occlusion of one of the five to seven short circumferential branches of the basilar artery affects the lateral two-thirds of the pons and/or middle or superior cerebellar peduncle, whereas occlusion of one of the seven to ten paramedian branches of the basilar artery affects a wedge-shaped area on either side of the medial pons (Figs. 351-8 to 351-10). Many syndromes of brainstem syndromes with cranial nerve abnormalities and crossed hemiplegia have been given eponyms, e.g., Weber, Claude, Benedict, Foville, Raymong-Cestan, Millard-Gubler.

Laboratory evaluation MRI scanning can detect brainstem infarction due to either basilar artery or basilar branch occlusion. Application of defined pulse sequences can detect blood flow in the basilar artery. MRI scanning combined with transcranial Doppler analysis may eventually replace conventional angiography in documenting basilar artery potency. CT scanning is not reliable in detecting brainstem infarcts but can show hemorrhages and assess mass effect after large cerebellar infarctions.

Selective cerebral arteriography remains the best method to define atherothrombotic disease of the basilar artery. Since arteriography entails potential morbidity and may precipitate the very stroke one is seeking to prevent, it is recommended only when the information

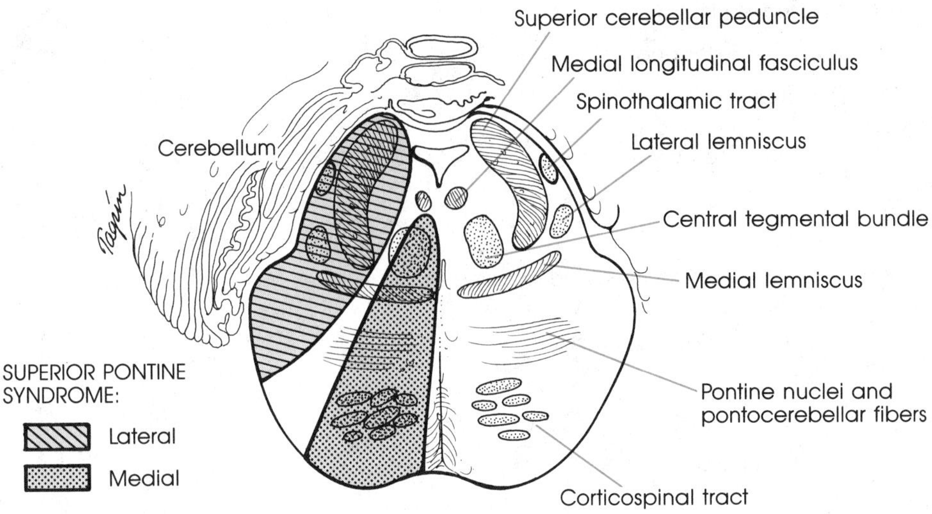

FIGURE 351-8 (*Courtesy of C. M. Fisher, M.D.*)

Signs and symptoms	*Structures involved*
1 Medial superior pontine syndrome (paramedian branches of upper basilar artery)	
On side of lesion:	
Cerebellar ataxia (probably)	Superior and/or middle cerebellar peduncle
Internuclear ophthalmoplegia	Medial longitudinal fasciculus
Myoclonic syndrome, palate, pharnyx, vocal cords, respiratory apparatus, face, oculomotor apparatus, etc.	Localization uncertain—central tegmental bundle (?), dentate projection (?), inferior olivary nucleus (?)
On side opposite lesion:	
Paralysis of face, arm, and leg	Corticobulbar and corticospinal tract
Rarely touch, vibration, and position are affected	Medial lemniscus
2 Lateral superior pontine syndrome (syndrome of superior cerebellar artery)	
On side of lesion:	
Ataxia of limbs and gait, falling to side of lesion	Middle and superior cerebellar peduncles, superior surface of cerebellum, dentate nucleus
Dizziness, nausea, vomiting; horizontal nystagmus	Vestibular nucleus
Paresis of conjugate gaze (ipsilateral)	Pontine contralateral gaze
Skew deviation	Uncertain
Miosis, ptosis, decreased sweating over face (Horner's syndrome)	Descending sympathetic fibers
Static tremor reported in one case	Dentate nucleus (?), superior cerebellar peduncle (?)
On side opposite lesion:	
Impaired pain and thermal sense on face, limbs, and trunk	Spinothalamic tract
Impaired touch, vibration, and position sense, more in leg than arm (there is a tendency to incongruity of pain and touch deficits)	Medial lemniscus (lateral portion)

provided will assist in the management of the patient. Occasionally, injection of angiographic dye in the posterior circulation precipitates a delirious state sometimes associated with cortical blindness. This reversible state can last for 24 to 38 h or, rarely, several days.

Therapy Impending basilar occlusion causing transient or fluctuating symptoms should be treated with short-term anticoagulation with intravenous heparin, after MRI or CT scanning has excluded hemorrhage. When basilar artery stenosis or occlusion is associated with minor or improving stroke, long-term anticoagulation with warfarin is recommended. If, on the other hand, basilar branch disease is the cause, then the rationale for using warfarin is uncertain. While embolism from the heart or from atheroma in the distal vertebral system may occlude a penetrating basilar branch, this is unlikely. Therefore, long-term control of blood pressure and antiplatelet therapy are recommended as preventive measures in the management of small-vessel basilar branch disease. Because of the long-term accumulative risk of anticoagulation therapy, it is generally reserved for symptomatic large-vessel atherothrombotic disease.

LACUNAR DISEASE

The term *lacunar disease* refers to atherothrombotic and lipohyalinotic occlusive disease of the penetrating branches of the circle of Willis, middle cerebral artery stem, and vertebral and basilar arteries.

PATHOPHYSIOLOGY The middle cerebral artery stem, the arteries comprising the circle of Willis (A1 segment of the anterior cerebral artery, anterior and posterior communicating arteries, and precommunal segment of the posterior cerebral arteries), the basilar, and the vertebral arteries all give rise to 100- to 300-μm-diameter branches that penetrate the deep gray and white matter of the cerebrum or brainstem (Fig. 351-2). Each of these small branches can be thrombosed either by atherothrombotic disease at its origin or by the development of lipohyalinotic thickening. Thrombosis of these vessels causes small infarcts that are referred to as *lacunes*. They range in size from as small as 3 to 4 mm to 1 to 2 cm. Hypertension is the principal risk factor for such small-vessel disease. Lacunar infarcts represent approximately 10 percent of all strokes.

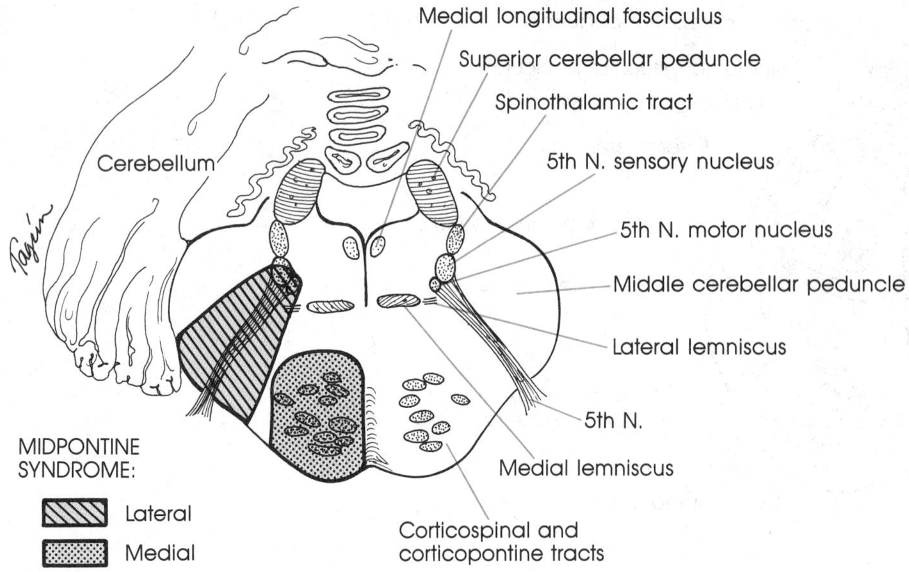

FIGURE 351-9 *(Courtesy of C. M. Fisher, M.D.)*

Signs and symptoms	*Structures involved*
1 Medial midpontine syndrome (paramedian branch of midbasilar artery)	
On side of lesion:	
Ataxia of limbs and gait (more prominent in bilateral involvement)	Pontine nuclei
On side opposite lesion:	
Paralysis of face, arm, and leg	Corticobulbar and corticospinal tract
Variable impaired touch and proprioception when lesion extends posteriorly	Medial lemniscus
2 Lateral midpontine syndrome (short circumferential artery)	
On side of lesion:	
Ataxia of limbs	Middle cerebellar peduncle
Paralysis of muscles of mastication	Motor fibers or nucleus of fifth nerve
Impaired sensation over side of face	Sensory fibers or nucleus of fifth nerve
On side opposite lesion:	
Impaired pain and thermal sense on limbs and trunk	Spinothalamic tract

CLINICAL MANIFESTATIONS Lacunar infarcts cause recognizable stroke syndromes that usually evolve over hours or longer. Transient symptoms (lacunar TIAs) may herald a lacunar infarct; they may occur several times a day, and last only a few minutes. When infarction occurs, it usually causes a sudden deficit, but may evolve in a progressive fashion over a few days. Recovery often begins within hours or days after the infarct, and over weeks or months may be complete or result in minimal residual deficit. In some cases significant disability persists.

The most common lacunar syndromes are the following:

1 Pure motor hemiparesis from an infarct in the posterior limb of the internal capsule or basis pontis. Here, the face, arm, leg, foot, and toes are almost always involved. The weakness may be intermittent (TIA), progress in a stepwise manner, or appear abruptly, and may progress to complete paralysis, but improvement occurs in many cases.

2 Pure sensory stroke from an infarct in the ventrolateral thalamus.

3 Ataxic hemiparesis from an infarct in the base of the pons or *dysarthria and a clumsy hand or arm* due to infarction in the base of the pons or in the genu of the internal capsule.

4 Pure motor hemiparesis with "motor aphasia" due to thrombotic occlusion of a lenticulostriate branch supplying the genu and anterior limb of the internal capsule and adjacent white matter of the corona radiata.

Before the advent of hypertensive therapy, multiple lacunes often caused *pseudobulbar palsy* with emotional instability, a slowed abulic state, and bilateral pyramidal signs. This syndrome is now uncommon.

Other lacunar syndromes have been described, some not correlated with arterial occlusion. An anarthric pseudobulbar syndrome due to bilateral infarctions in the internal capsule can occur from disease in the lenticulostriate arteries. Syndromes resulting from occlusion of the penetrating arteries of the proximal posterior cerebral artery were discussed above. Syndromes resulting from occlusion of the penetrating arteries of the basilar artery (Figs. 351-8 to 351-10) include ipsilateral ataxia and crural (leg) paresis, pure motor hemiparesis with horizontal gaze palsy, and hemiparesis with a crossed sixth nerve palsy. Lower basilar branch syndromes include sudden internuclear ophthalmoplegia, horizontal gaze palsy, and appendicular cerebellar ataxia.

Syndromes resulting from vertebral branch occlusions include pure motor hemiparesis sparing the face by involving the medullary pyramid, and syndromes that involve the lateral pontomedullary area, which may include vertigo, vomiting, facial weakness, Horner's syndrome, ipsilateral trigeminal numbness, and contralateral spinothalamic sensory loss.

LABORATORY EVALUATION The CT scan documents most supratentorial lacunar infarctions, and MRI successfully documents both supratentorial and infratentorial infarctions when the lacunes are 5 mm or greater. Lacunar infarction is diagnosed when the infarct size is less than 2 cm, and its location is attributable to occlusion of a small penetrating arterial branch of a major parent vessel. Larger

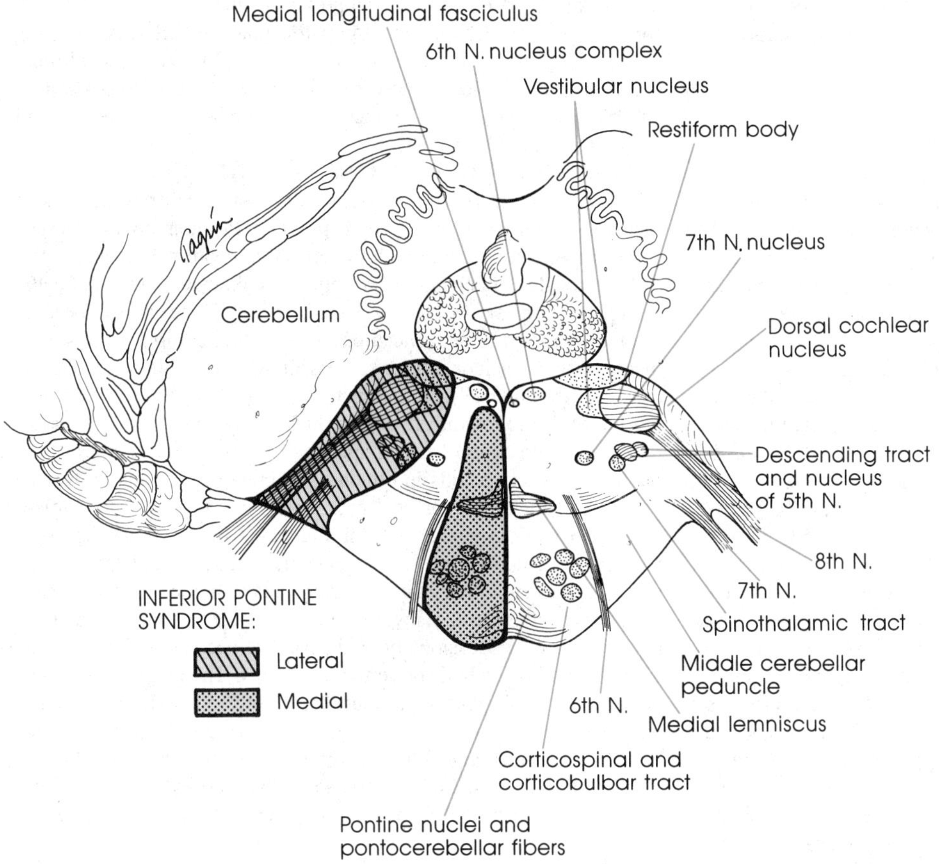

FIGURE 351-10 *(Courtesy of C. M. Fisher, M.D.)*

Signs and symptoms	*Structures involved*
1 Medial inferior pontine syndrome (occlusion of paramedian branch of basilar artery)	
On side of lesion:	
Paralysis of conjugate gaze to side of lesion (preservation of convergence)	"Center" for conjugate lateral gaze
Nystagmus	Vestibular nucleus
Ataxia of limbs and gait	Middle cerebellar peduncle (?)
Diplopia on lateral gaze	Abducens nerve
On side opposite lesion:	
Paralysis of face, arm, and leg	Corticobulbar and corticospinal tract in lower pons
Impaired tactile and proprioceptive sense over half of the body	Medial lemniscus
2 Lateral inferior pontine syndrome (occlusion of anterior inferior cerebellar artery)	
On side of lesion:	
Horizontal and vertical nystagmus, vertigo, nausea, vomiting, oscillopsia	Vestibular nerve on nucleus
Facial paralysis	Seventh nerve
Paralysis of conjugate gaze to side of lesion	"Center" for conjugate lateral gaze
Deafness, tinnitus	Auditory nerve or cochlear nucleus
Ataxia	Middle cerebellar peduncle and cerebellar hemisphere
Impaired sensation over face	Descending tract and nucleus fifth nerve
On side opposite lesion:	
Impaired pain and thermal sense over half the body (may include face)	Spinothalamic tract

deep white matter infarcts in the territory of the middle cerebral artery (so-called giant lacunes) are probably due to embolism or large atherosclerotic plaques that occlude the mouths of several adjacent penetrating vessels. The electroencephalogram (EEG) is usually normal, or nearly so, in lacunar infarction but abnormal in cortical surface infarction.

THERAPY Lacunar strokes may present with a fluctuating progressive course, and acute reduction in blood pressure may worsen symptoms. Antihypertensive therapy is begun after the patient's symptoms become stable. Whether anticoagulant or antiplatelet agents benefit patients with lacunar TIAs and fluctuating stroke is unknown. Some studies suggest that thalamic lacunes may be associated with minor hemorrhage, since hemosiderin-laden macrophages are sometimes seen at autopsy. This circumstance increases the risk of using heparin. On the other hand, some patients with fluctuating hemiparesis from atherothrombotic disease of a basilar branch or of the middle cerebral stem lenticulostriate arteries may improve coincident with heparin administration. Most physicians, however, do not use anticoagulation in patients with typical lacunar strokes. Long-term therapy after lacunar stroke requires careful control of hypertension to prevent progression of vascular disease.

OTHER CAUSES OF CEREBRAL INFARCTION

VENOUS THROMBOSIS (Table 351-1) Lateral or sagittal sinus thrombosis or thrombosis of small cortical veins occurs as a complication of sepsis, intracranial infections (meningitis), conditions associated with hypercoagulable states such as polycythemia and sickle cell anemia, or during pregnancy or administration of oral contraceptives. Venous thromboses may cause an increase in intracranial pressure, headaches, focal seizures, and focal neurologic signs affecting the legs more than the arms. Massive venous infarction with secondary edema may be fatal. The CT scan shows hemorrhagic infarction underlying the occluded veins, and may show clot in the posterior sagittal sinus, but the definitive diagnosis is made with angiography.

DISSECTION OF THE CERVICOCEREBRAL ARTERIES Dissection of the large extracranial arteries may cause cerebral infarction, and is a frequent cause of stroke in children and young adults. The dissection divides the media of the vessel or separates the intima from the media. TIAs and infarction occur when the vessel is critically narrowed or occluded or when dissection causes emboli. Trauma, either severe or trivial, accounts for a substantial proportion of cases. Spontaneous dissection also occurs in atheromatous lesions and can occur in association with fibromuscular dysplasia, homocystinuria, or arteritis. The internal carotid artery is the most common site. An oculosympathetic palsy (Horner's syndrome) occurs in over half the cases. A self-audible bruit may appear, and tenderness over the carotid bulb may be present. In carotid dissection, transient monocular blindness or TIAs often precede embolic or "low-flow" watershed infarction, leaving time for therapeutic intervention. When the patient has only oculosympathetic palsy, TIAs, or a minor stroke, anticoagulation with heparin is recommended. Surgical exploration is only considered for patients with increasingly severe TIAs or a mild stroke that is worsening. After the patient's symptoms have stabilized, anticoagulation with warfarin is recommended for 6 months. Repeat angiography often demonstrates a reestablished lumen in the formerly occluded vessel.

Patients with symptomatic vertebral, middle cerebral, or posterior cerebral artery dissection may also be managed in the acute phase with heparin and later with warfarin.

FIBROMUSCULAR DYSPLASIA OF THE CERVICAL VESSELS Fibromuscular dysplasia of the cervical vessels occurs mainly in young women. The carotid or vertebral arteries show multiple rings of segmental narrowing alternating with dilatation. Occlusion is usually incomplete. The process is often asymptomatic, but occasionally is associated with an audible bruit, TIAs, or stroke. Hypertension, if present, may be the result of renal artery stenosis. The cause and natural history of fibromuscular dysplasia is unknown (see Chap. 230). Transient ischemic symptoms or embolic stroke generally occur only when the residual lumen diameter of the narrowed portion of the artery is less than 2 mm. Surgical dilatation of the cervical internal carotid artery is possible in symptomatic cases but is associated with considerable morbidity. Anticoagulation may be more successful than surgery in patients with TIAs of increasing severity.

ARTERITIS Arteritis due to bacterial or syphilitic infection is no longer a common cause of cerebral thrombosis. Other arteritides are rare but can cause cerebral thrombosis (see below and Chaps. 269 and 276). Necrotizing or granulomatous arteritis, occurring alone or in association with generalized polyarteritis nodosa or Wegener's granulomatosis, involves the distal small branches (less than 2-mm-diameter) of the main intracranial arteries and produces small ischemic infarcts in the brain, optic nerve, or spinal cord. The disease, although rare, is relentlessly progressive. The CSF often has cells. In some cases, glucocorticoid therapy (prednisone, 40 to 60 mg/d) has been helpful, and recently, immunosuppressive drugs have been used with some success (see Chap. 276). Idiopathic giant cell arteritis involving the great vessels arising from the aortic arch (Takayasu's syndrome) may, on rare occasions, cause carotid or vertebral thrombosis. It is an infrequent cause of the aortic arch syndrome in the western hemisphere (see Chap. 197).

TEMPORAL ARTERITIS (CRANIAL ARTERITIS) (See Chap. 276) This is a relatively common affliction of elderly persons in which the external carotid system, particularly the temporal arteries, is the site of a subacute granulomatous inflammation with an exudate of lymphocytes, monocytes, neutrophilic leukocytes, and giant cells. Usually the most severely affected parts of the artery become thrombosed. Headache or head pain is the chief complaint. Systemic manifestations include anorexia, loss of weight, malaise, and polymyalgia rheumatica. The inflammatory nature of the illness is indicated by one of the following: fever, slight leukocytosis, increased erythrocyte sedimentation rate, and anemia. Occlusion of branches of the ophthalmic artery results in blindness in one or both eyes in over 25 percent of patients. Occasionally, an ophthalmoplegia due to involvement of ocular nerves occurs. An arteritis of the aorta and its major branches, including carotid, subclavian, coronary, and femoral arteries, has been found at postmortem examination in some cases. Significant inflammatory involvement of intracranial arteries is rare, but strokes occur occasionally on the basis of occlusion of the internal carotid, middle cerebral, or vertebral arteries. The diagnosis depends on the finding of a tender thrombosed or thickened cranial artery and the demonstration of the lesion in a biopsy specimen. Glucocorticoids bring striking subjective relief and often prevent blindness. Prednisone is most often used, beginning with large daily doses of 80 to 120 mg and then tapering after 2 to 4 weeks using the erythrocyte sedimentation rate as a guide.

MOYAMOYA DISEASE Moyamoya disease is a poorly understood occlusive disease involving large intracranial arteries, especially the internal carotid artery and the stem of the middle and anterior cerebral artery. The lenticulostriate arteries develop a rich collateral flow circulation around the middle cerebral occlusive lesion that on cerebral angiography gives the impression of a puff of smoke (*moyamoya*). Other collaterals include transdural anastomoses between the cortical surface branches of the middle cerebral artery and the scalp arteries. The disease mainly occurs in the oriental population, but should be suspected when TIAs or stroke occur in children or young adults. Its etiology is unknown. Few pathologic studies have been made; they suggest that hyalinotic fibrous-type material is associated with the arterial narrowing. Because of the occurrence of subarachnoid hemorrhage from rupture of the transdural anastomotic channels, anticoagulation is not recommended in all symptomatic cases. Extracranial-intracranial (EC/IC) bypass grafting has been recommended in some cases, but its efficacy is not established.

ISCHEMIC DISEASES ASSOCIATED WITH HYPERCOAGULABLE STATE Certain diseases have been associated with ischemic infarction in special clinical circumstances through a mechanism of a hypercoagulable state (see Chaps. 287 and 288). They include polycythemia vera, thrombotic thrombocytopenic purpura, idiopathic thrombocytosis, hyperproteinemia, and sickle cell anemia. Furthermore, circulation of anticardiolipin antibodies ("lupus anticoagulant") has been associated with stroke in young adults, although its relative frequency is controversial. Some cases may be due to cerebral embolism (see below), but others seem to be caused by local arterial thrombosis.

REVERSIBLE CEREBRAL SEGMENTAL VASOCONSTRICTION Reversible, widespread cerebral segmental vasoconstriction has been noted in patients with severe headache and fluctuating neurologic symptoms and signs. Sometimes cerebral infarction has ensued. The cause is unknown. Eclampsia, the postpartum period, head injury, migraine, and sympathomimetic intoxication have all been associated with this entity. Angiography is the only means of establishing the diagnosis. The CSF is normal in most cases but an elevated protein and slight lymphocytic pleocytosis has been found in some cases.

No effective therapy is known. Maintenance of normal systemic arterial pressure or even increasing it modestly with adequate hydration seems important on empiric grounds. Glucocorticoids and vasodilators such as calcium channel blocking agents or intravenous nitroglycerin may be considered.

BINSWANGER'S DISEASE Binswanger's disease (chronic progressive subcortical encephalopathy) is a rare condition in which the subcortical white matter becomes subacutely infarcted. The CT or MRI scan detects periventricular areas of white matter disruption and gliosis. There is lipohyalinosis in the small arteries of the deep white matter, as in hypertension. There are usually associated lacunar or embolic strokes. Binswanger's disease may represent a type of border zone ischemic infarction in the deep white and gray matter between the penetrating arteries of the circle of Willis and of the cortex. Unfortunately, the pathophysiologic basis of the disease remains unknown, and the underlying microvascular pathology may be different in younger patients without hypertension and typical cases in older patients with severe long-standing hypertension. Binswanger's disease is one of the causes of gait disability and abulia in the elderly.

ORAL CONTRACEPTIVE AGENTS Oral contraceptive agents have been associated with an increased incidence of stroke in young women (13.2:100,000 among women who take oral contraceptives compared to 2.8:100,000 among those who do not). In most cases, there is no vascular occlusion on angiography; or if there is occlusion, it is found to have opened later, suggesting embolism as the cause of the stroke. The source of the embolus, however, is uncertain. Pathologic examination has shown that the affected arteries and the heart are normal. Migraine and cigarette smoking have been associated with increased frequency of strokes in young women on oral contraceptives and suggest that hypercoagulability may predispose to thrombosis formation and/or embolization.

CEREBRAL EMBOLISM

PATHOPHYSIOLOGY Cerebral embolism is the most common cause of ischemic stroke. The heart is the most common source of embolic material, with artery-to-artery embolism, usually arising from an atherothrombotic lesion in the carotid or vertebrobasilar system, a somewhat less frequent source (see above). Other causes, such as thrombus in the pulmonary vein, fat emboli, tumor emboli, marantic endocarditis, air emboli, paradoxical emboli, and complications of neck or thoracic surgery (Table 351-1), may occasionally be responsible. Frequently, however, embolic cerebral infarction occurs without an obvious source.

"Unknown source" cerebral embolism poses one of the most perplexing problems in cerebrovascular disease. Patients with hypercoagulability states due to oral contraceptive agents, anticardiolipin antibody, chronic illness, antithrombin 3 deficiency, or metastatic tumor may develop sudden cerebral embolism. In some patients, examination may fail to disclose potential sources of embolism such as the opening snap of mitral stenosis or intermittent atrial fibrillation. Many patients, especially those in the second to fifth decade, suffer sudden embolic strokes that leave no clue to their etiology.

The size, site, and to some extent the pathologic nature of the fragment determines the size, location, and character of the ensuing infarct. Emboli from the heart lodge in the middle cerebral artery or one of its branches 80 percent of the time, in the posterior cerebral artery or its branches 11 percent of the time, and in the vertebral or basilar arteries or the branches in the remainder. Cardiac emboli infrequently go to the anterior cerebral artery. Emboli large enough to occlude the stem of the middle cerebral artery (2 to 3 mm) lead to a large stroke, one that involves both deep gray and white matter as well as the cortical surface and its underlying white matter. A smaller embolus may occlude a small cortical or penetrating arterial branch. Characteristically embolic platelet fibrin clot has a tendency to migrate, lyse, and disperse, accounting for fluctuations in symptoms and, in some cases, complete recovery of the ischemic deficit. The location and size of an infarct also depends on the extent of spared collateral circulation.

Because emboli migrate and lyse, recirculation into the infarcted brain may cause petechial hemorrhages (*hemorrhagic infarction*). On rare occasions, petechial hemorrhages coalesce to form a significant hemorrhagic mass (*hemorrhage into infarction*). This is more likely to occur when the stem of the middle cerebral artery is occluded and large areas of infarction develop before recirculation occurs.

Many types of heart disease, including cardiac arrhythmias or diseases due to cardiac structural abnormalities, may produce cerebral emboli.

Cardiac arrhythmias of all types have been associated with cerebral and systemic embolism. Emboli associated with the sick sinus syndrome and atrial fibrillation are particularly common. There is a high incidence of cerebral embolism associated with atrial fibrillation in patients with rheumatic valvular disease. However, recent studies show that patients with atrial fibrillation from any cause are at risk of embolization. The incidence in patients with atrial fibrillation without valvular disease is estimated at 4 to 7 percent per year, and in most cases, the initial stroke causes severe disability.

Mural thrombus formation with embolism occurs relatively frequently in patients with arteriosclerotic cardiovascular disease and myocardial infarction.

Postsurgery embolization is a high risk in intracardiac surgery and prosthetic valve replacement (Starr-Edwards and Bjork-Shiley valves have been particularly implicated). Thoracic surgery (pulmonary vein embolism) and head-and-neck surgery (aortic or carotid artery-to-artery emboli) have an uncommon but definite association with cerebral embolism. Long bone fracture and thoracic surgery or angiography are associated with cerebral fat embolism and air embolism, both of which give rise to multiple areas of petechial hemorrhage. The principal complication of the use of artificial hearts is cerebral embolism. The overall risk of stroke after any type of general surgery is 0.2 to 1 percent.

Congenital septal defects may give rise to paradoxical embolism. Material (thrombus, tumor, infective or fibrous marantic vegetation) accumulating on a valve or the endocardial surface may become displaced. Vegetations on the aortic and mitral valves from rheumatic or marantic endocarditis are associated with systemic or cerebral emboli and can be diagnosed by a combination of history, physical examination, and laboratory tests. Typically flat vegetations under the mitral and, to a lesser extent, aortic valve leaflets have been noted in patients with systemic lupus erythematosus (Libman-Sacks vegetations). There may give rise to cerebral embolism but more often are a nidus for bacterial endocarditis.

The *vegetations of acute and subacute bacterial endocarditis* give rise to septic embolism (see Chap. 188) and can cause large areas of infarction similar to noninfective embolic infarction if they occlude a major intracranial artery. Alternatively, they may give rise to small septic infarcts with microscopic abscesses. Large brain abscesses, however, are not associated with embolization from subacute bacterial endocarditis. Mycotic aneurysms caused by septic embolism give rise to subarachnoid or intracerebral hemorrhage. Endocarditis should always be considered and ruled out when cerebral embolism is suspected.

Atrial myxoma results in tumor emboli arising from the endocardial surface. Physical signs of pulmonary hypertension or a high erythrocyte sedimentation rate together with signs of systemic illness (fever, malaise) may help in the differential diagnosis. *Mitral valve prolapse* with mural thrombus formation has been associated with cerebral embolism, but insufficient data exist based on the natural history of this abnormality to predict the incidence of recurrent embolism (presumably low). Echocardiography establishes this diagnosis.

CLINICAL MANIFESTATIONS The onset of the neurologic deficit from embolism is sudden and usually maximal. This temporal profile with a neurologic syndrome corresponding to the distribution of a major branch vessel points to cerebral embolism. Sometimes, however, the neurologic deficit may not be complete and after its sudden onset, may fluctuate. The neurologic signs may wax and wane, lasting only a few minutes or hours, then partially or completely disappear, suggesting an embolic TIA, or a mild deficit may progress to complete major infarction over hours. The neurologic deficit corresponds to the cerebral cortex supplied by the arterial territory affected. The resulting deficits resemble those caused by occlusive atheromatous lesions (see sections on atherothrombosis and lacunar stroke). Certain neurologic syndromes strongly suggest embolism as their cause. In the middle cerebral artery territory these include (1) the frontal opercular syndrome, in which there is facial weakness and severe aphasia or dysarthria; (2) the brachial or hand plegia syndrome, in which the arm and hand, or the hand is paralyzed with or without cortical sensory abnormalities; (3) the syndromes of Broca's or Wernicke's aphasia alone, when the dominant hemisphere is involved; or (4) the syndrome of left visual neglect, when the nondominant parietal lobe is involved; (5) a sudden hemianopic field defect, which suggests a posterior cerebral territory embolus; or (6) a sudden foot incoordination or weakness, suggesting an anterior cerebral territory embolus. Sudden gait unsteadiness may suggest a cerebellar embolus. Sudden sleepiness and an inability to look up associated with bilateral ptosis suggests an embolus to the top of the basilar artery, specifically to the artery of Percheron (the small vessel supplying both sides of the medial subthalamus and thalamus arising from the top of the basilar artery).

Seizures following cerebral infarction occur most often after embolic infarction and are not associated with deep white matter lacunar infarction. They are associated with supratentorial cortical surface infarction but are infrequent at the onset and are more often the result of gliotic scar that matures months or more after stroke. Seizures after infarction are rare before 6 months and peak in incidence at 12 to 18 months. Many cases of idiopathic epilepsy in the elderly are probably the result of silent cortical infarction.

LABORATORY EVALUATION Although early CT scanning is usually negative in embolic stroke, it serves to exclude hemorrhage. MRI scanning is better to document the extent and location of the embolic infarction, both supratentorially and infratentorially. Although endocarditis is rarely the cause of cerebral embolism, laboratory evaluation should include a sedimentation rate and blood cultures. Noninvasive carotid studies combined with transcranial Doppler analysis can exclude hemodynamically significant carotid stenosis as the source of emboli if there is any clinical or circumstantial reason to consider this source. Cerebral angiography is considered only when endarterectomy is considered and/or noninvasive tests for significant carotid stenosis have produced equivocal results. Twenty-four hours after cardiogenic cerebral embolism, angiography is often negative, indicating that the embolus has lysed and dispersed. An ECG may show an arrhythmia or myocardial infarction that may have contributed to the source of embolism. Echocardiography or more sophisticated techniques for imaging the ventricular chambers are often used to determine whether a cardiac thrombus was the source of embolism. These techniques are generally insensitive to small clots and are positive in less than 20 percent of patients who have had cerebral emboli. Even after extensive evaluation, including ECG, echocardiography, coagulation studies, etc., the majority of emboli have no evident source.

THERAPY Therapy of patients with embolic cerebral infarction consists of managing the stroke itself, in both the acute and chronic phases, and in preventing further embolic strokes. When cerebral embolism is suspected, the immediate goal is to keep cerebral perfusion in the ischemic area as adequate as possible. The blood pressure should not be lowered even if hypertension is found unless it is malignant hypertension (see Chap. 196). If the blood pressure is low, raising it is probably advisable in the hours after stroke. An excessive rise above normal may, however, aggravate edema formation. Approximately 5 percent or less of patients with middle cerebral artery strokes have enough *secondary cerebral edema* to cause clinical problems. These few patients who are at risk from edema have large regions of low density and slight mass effect on early CT scans, often involving both the middle and anterior cerebral artery territories. Once infarction becomes evident, edema seldom becomes problematic until the second or third day but can then cause mass effect for up to 10 days. Two observations governing the severity of the edema associated with cerebral embolism seem to apply. First, in instances of supratentorial embolic infarction, the larger the area of infarct, the more likely that edema formation will become a problem. Emboli that lodge in the middle cerebral artery stem are much more likely to cause symptomatic edema formation that leads, in a few patients, to coma and death than are emboli in a distal branch of the middle cerebral artery. Second, small amounts of edema formation in the cerebellum following embolic infarction, usually in the territory of the posterior inferior cerebellar artery (inferior cerebellum), can lead to an acute increase in intracranial pressure in the posterior fossa. The resulting compression of the brainstem may result in sudden coma and respiratory arrest requiring emergency surgical decompression. Water restriction and agents that raise the serum osmolarity should be considered early in both instances. Intravenous mannitol is most frequently used to raise the serum osmolality to approximately 300 mosmol/L; it is given as often as every 2 to 4 h. The acute management of artery-to-artery embolus, in either the carotid or vertebral territory, is discussed above (see "Ischemic Cerebrovascular Disease").

When the deficit is large enough to suggest that the embolus has lodged in the middle cerebral artery stem with corresponding infarction of the basal ganglion, deep white matter, and cortical surface, acute anticoagulation with heparin is generally avoided. On rare occasions symptomatic basal ganglion hemorrhage into infarcted tissue occurs. But when the stroke is smaller and involves the cortical surface or when the deficit fluctuates, suggesting partial arterial occlusion, then acute anticoagulation should be considered. For future stroke prevention, chronic anticoagulation with warfarin is general recommended beginning 2 to 5 days after the stroke. A second embolism is rare in the first 3 days. The usual duration of anticoagulation is 6 months or longer if chronic ventricular failure or ventricular aneurysms are present. Lifelong anticoagulation with warfarin may be legitimately instituted in patients who have evidence of recurrent embolism or embolism associated with chronic, intermittent, or sustained atrial fibrillation. Prophylactic anticoagulation for chronic atrial fibrillation without embolism remains controversial. It is the subject of several current randomized, controlled trials.

The appropriate dosage of warfarin has been debated. At the moment, the standard is "low-dose" warfarin (prothrombin time 1.3 to 1.5 times control), the exception being that prothrombin time in patients with prosthetic heart valves and high risk of embolism is often maintained at two times control. The minimal effective antithrombotic warfarin dose has yet to be determined. This determination may require newer, more sensitive methods for monitoring the hemostatic system or more sensitive, uniform thromboplastin reagents.

INTRACRANIAL HEMORRHAGE: GENERAL REMARKS

Of the many causes of nontraumatic intracranial hemorrhage, four are particularly common: deep hypertensive or spontaneous lobar intracerebral hemorrhage, ruptured saccular aneurysm, and bleeding from an arteriovenous malformation. Hemorrhage associated with a bleeding disorder and rupture of a mycotic aneurysm are less common. Rare causes include idiopathic brain purpura, brainstem (Duret) hemorrhages associated with brainstem compression during herniation, and small multifocal hemorrhages associated with hypertensive encephalopathy.

HYPERTENSIVE INTRACEREBRAL HEMORRHAGE

PATHOPHYSIOLOGY Hypertensive hemorrhages typically occur in one of four sites: (1) the putamen and adjacent internal capsule, (2) the thalamus, (3) the pons, and (4) the cerebellum. They rarely originate in the central white matter of the hemispheres. A penetrating artery arising from the middle cerebral artery stem, basilar artery, or circle of Willis is generally the source of hemorrhage, the same vessels that are known to be damaged by hypertension.

The hemorrhage begins as a small oval mass, then spreads by dissection, growing in volume, displacing and compressing adjacent brain tissue. Rupture or seepage into the ventricular system may occur. Primary intraventricular hemorrhage is rare.

Most hypertensive intracerebral hemorrhages develop over a few minutes, but some evolve over 30 to 60 min, and others, particularly those associated with anticoagulant therapy, may evolve for as long as 24 to 38 h. Once bleeding stops, it has generally been thought not to start again, but some larger clots have been shown by sequential CT scanning to have originated as smaller hemorrhages, and it is believed that the frequency of rebleeding or enlargement has been underestimated in the past. Edema in the compressed tissue around the hemorrhage often leads to increasing mass effect and, in some cases, worsening of the clinical state. Within 48 h, macrophages begin to phagocytize the hemorrhage at its outer surface. After 1 to 6 months, the hemorrhage mass is generally resolved to a slitlike orange cavity lined with glial scar tissue and hemosiderin-laden macrophages.

CLINICAL MANIFESTATIONS Hypertensive intracerebral hemorrhages are most common in patients with prolonged sustained hypertension. Although not particularly associated with exertion, intracerebral hemorrhages almost always occur while the patient is awake and sometimes when under stress. Unlike the sudden onset of embolism, these strokes usually evolve over a few minutes, with the neurologic signs and symptoms dependent on the site and size of the extravasation. Vomiting and headache are hallmarks of acute hemorrhages that distinguish them from other strokes. Seizures are uncommon but occur in a few instances.

Putamenal hemorrhage, the most common hypertensive hemorrhage, invariably disrupts the internal capsule adjacent to the basal ganglia. Contralateral hemiplegia is therefore the sentinel sign, but when these hemorrhages are large, the patient may become comatose within a few minutes. In milder cases, over 5 to 30 min, the face sags on one side, speech becomes slurred, the arm and leg gradually weaken, and *the eyes deviate away from the side of the hemiparesis.* The paralysis may worsen until the affected limbs become flaccid or extend rigidly with a Babinski sign on the same side. In the worst case, drowsiness gives way to stupor as signs of upper brainstem compression appear. Coma ensues, accompanied by deep, irregular, or intermittent respiration, a dilated and fixed ipsilateral pupil, bilateral Babinski signs, and decerebrate rigidity. Edema formation in the adjacent brain may cause progressive deterioration over 12 to 72 h.

Thalamic hemorrhages also produce a hemiplegia or hemiparesis from pressure on or dissection through the internal capsule adjacent to the thalamus. A prominent sensory deficit involving all modalities is usually present. Aphasia, often with preserved verbal repetition, may occur after hemorrhage into the dominant (left) thalamus, and apractagnosia or mutism occurs in some cases of nondominant hemorrhage. There also may be a transient homonymous visual field defect. Thalamic hemorrhages cause several typical ocular disturbances by virtue of extension medially into the upper midbrain. These include most characteristically: deviation of the eyes downward and inward, so they appear to be looking at the patient's nose; unequal pupils with absence of light reaction; skew deviation, with the eye opposite the hemorrhage displaced downward and medially; ipsilateral ptosis and miosis (Horner's syndrome); absence of convergence; paralysis of vertical gaze; an assortment of lateral gaze abnormalities (paresis or pseudoparesis of the sixth nerve), and retraction nystagmus.

In *pontine hemorrhages,* deep coma with quadriplegia usually occurs over a few minutes. There is often prominent decerebrate rigidity, and small (1-mm) pupils that react to light. There is impairment of reflex horizontal eye movements evoked by head turning (doll's-head or oculocephalic maneuver) or by irrigation of the ears with cold water (see Chap. 31). Hyperpnea, severe acute hypertension, and hyperhidrosis are common. Death usually occurs within a few hours, but there are exceptions where consciousness is retained because the hemorrhage is limited to the tegmentum.

Cerebellar hemorrhages usually develop over several hours with repeated vomiting and inability to walk or stand. In mild cases there may be no other neurologic signs; therefore it is imperative to test gait. Occipital headache and dizziness or vertigo may be prominent symptoms. There is often paresis of conjugate lateral gaze toward the side of the hemorrhage, forced deviation of the eyes to the opposite side, or an ipsilateral sixth nerve palsy. Other less frequent ocular signs include blepharospasm, involuntary closure of one eye, ocular bobbing, and skew deviation. There may be little or no evidence of the usual signs of cerebellar disease, and only a minority of cases show nystagmus or ataxia of the limbs. A mild ipsilateral facial weakness and a diminished corneal reflex are common. Dysarthria and dysphagia may occur. There are no Babinski signs until late in the evolution of the hemorrhage as it expands to brainstem. As the hours pass, and occasionally with unanticipated suddenness, the patient becomes stuporous, then comatose as a result of brainstem compression, at which point reversal of the syndrome by surgical removal of the clot is seldom successful.

In summary, ocular signs have been highlighted as a method of rapidly localizing hemorrhages. In putamenal hemorrhage, the eyes are deviated to the side opposite the paralysis; in thalamic hemorrhage, the eyes are deviated downward and the pupils may be 3 to 4 mm and unreactive; in pontine hemorrhage, the reflex lateral eye movements are impaired and the pupils are less than 1 mm yet reactive; and in cerebellar hemorrhage, the eyes may be deviated laterally (to the side opposite the lesion) in the absence of paralysis.

LABORATORY EVALUATION The CT scan reliably detects all acute hemorrhages of 1 cm or more in diameter in the cerebral or cerebellar hemispheres. After the first 2 weeks, x-ray attenuation values of clotted blood diminish until they become isodense with surrounding brain. Mass effect and edema may remain. In some cases, a surrounding rim of contrast enhancement appears after 2 to 4 weeks and may persist for months. Small pontine hemorrhages may not be identified because of motion and bone artifact that obscure structures in the posterior fossa. MRI, though more sensitive for delineating posterior fossa lesions, is not necessary in most instances. Proper pulse sequences on MRI can, however, differentiate a hematoma mass from edema. Images of flowing blood on MRI scan may identify arteriovenous malformations as the cause of the hemorrhage. Angiography is used when the etiology of intracranial hemorrhage is uncertain, particularly if the hematoma is not in one of the four usual sites for hypertensive hemorrhage. For example, hemorrhage into the temporal lobe suggests rupture of a middle cerebral artery berry aneurysm. Lumbar puncture carries considerable risk after intracerebral hemorrhage and should generally be avoided unless CT scanning is not available.

THERAPY The size and location of the hematoma determine the treatment and prognosis. Supratentorial hematomas greater than 5 cm in largest diameter generally have a poor prognosis, and infratentorial pontine hematomas greater than 3 cm in size are usually fatal. The occurrence of edema in the week after the intracerebral hemorrhage often worsens the prognosis. The tissue surrounding the hematoma is displaced and compressed but not necessarily infarcted. Hence, in survivors, improvement can result as the hematoma is reabsorbed and the tissue regains its function. Careful management of the patient during the critical acute phase of the cerebral hematoma can lead to considerable recovery.

Surgical removal of an acute supratentorial clot is controversial, but most surgeons have found it necessary on rare occasions. In stuporous patients who still have reflex eye movements and some pupillary reaction, surgery may prevent temporal lobe herniation and irreversible brainstem compression. One important randomized trial has shown a benefit of surgery, though marginal, only in patients in this state. Lifesaving surgery may nonetheless leave major neurologic residua. In contrast, surgical treatment of acute cerebellar hemorrhage is usually recommended because it prevents secondary brainstem compression that is the mechanism of death and it offers an excellent prognosis for recovery. If patients are alert without focal brainstem signs and if the cerebellar hematoma is small, acute surgical removal may not be necessary.

Mannitol and other osmotic agents reduce intracranial pressure that has been raised by the volume of the hematoma and edema (see Chap. 352). Steroids are of uncertain value in curtailing edema from intracerebral hematoma. Monitoring of the intracranial pressure may help to assess medical therapy. Both excessive hypo- and hypertension should be avoided. Toxemia of pregnancy and malignant hypertension associated with acute hemorrhage should be treated cautiously to avoid excessive or precipitous lowering of the blood pressure.

LOBAR INTRACEREBRAL HEMORRHAGE

As control of hypertension in the general population has improved, the relative proportion of hemorrhages outside the basal ganglia and thalamus has increased. These ''lobar hemorrhages'' appear on CT scan as oval or circular clots in the subcortical white matter. The role of chronic hypertension in their genesis is controversial, but many occur without a history of increased blood pressure. A number of other underlying conditions are found in almost half the cases, the most common being arteriovenous malformation. Others are due to bleeding diathesis, often associated with warfarin administration; hemorrhages into tumor, usually a melanoma or glioma; aneurysms of the circle of Willis that bleed into brain substance; and there are a large number whose causes remain undetermined even after extensive study including arteriography. Many of these are presumed to be from arteriovenous malformations that have become obliterated or are angiographically occult.

Amyloid angiopathy, a cause of both single and recurrent lobar hemorrhages in the elderly, can only be diagnosed by postmortem demonstration that cerebral vessels stain strongly with Congo red. Amyloid is deposited in the walls of the cerebral arteries, but not elsewhere in the body. Patients may have multiple hemorrhages, with months between occurrences.

CLINICAL MANIFESTATIONS The neurologic symptoms and signs of lobar hemorrhage appear suddenly, over one to several minutes. Most lobar hemorrhages are small enough to cause a restricted clinical syndrome that simulates an embolus to a vessel supplying one lobe. For example, the major neurologic deficit of occipital hemorrhage is hemianopsia; of left temporal hemorrhage, aphasia and delirium; of parietal hemorrhage, thalamic-like hemisensory loss; and of frontal hemorrhage, arm weakness. Large hemorrhages may be associated with stupor or coma if they secondarily compress the lower thalamus and midbrain, but the greater distance of lobar clots from these vital structures makes coma result less frequently than putamenal or thalamic hemorrhages.

Most patients with lobar hemorrhages have focal headaches that are attributable to the innervation of adjacent dural vessels: occipital hemorrhage causes pain over the ipsilateral eye; temporal hemorrhage, over the area around or anterior to the ipsilateral ear; frontal hemorrhage, over the forehead or diffusely in the frontal quadrant; and parietal hemorrhage, over the temple region. Stiff neck or seizures are uncommon, but more than half the patients vomit or are initially drowsy.

TREATMENT In awake or drowsy patients, surgical evacuation offers little benefit over medical management with fluid restriction, and osmotic agents. Stuporous or comatose patients who do not respond rapidly to medical therapy for raised intracranial pressure should generally have the clot evacuated.

SUBARACHNOID HEMORRHAGE—SACCULAR ANEURYSM

Rupture of an intracranial saccular aneurysm is the most common cause of subarachnoid hemorrhage, followed by arteriovenous malformation. Although autopsy studies have estimated that 5 percent of the population harbor aneurysms, the incidence of bleeding is about 4:100,000 per year. This devastating disease causes a greater than 10 percent mortality during the first day, and another 25 percent succumb in the first 3 months. Of those who survive, more than half are left with major neurologic deficits as a result of the initial hemorrhage or of a delayed complication, such as rehemorrhage, infarction from cerebral vasospasm, or hydrocephalus. Given these alarming figures, the major therapeutic emphasis should be on preventing the initial rupture and, if rupture occurs, preventing the predictable early complications.

PATHOPHYSIOLOGY Saccular aneurysms occur at the bifurcations of the large arteries at the base of the brain and rupture into the subarachnoid space of the basal cisterns. The common sites of saccular aneurysms include the junction of the anterior communicating artery with the anterior cerebral artery, the junction of the posterior communicating artery and the internal carotid artery, the bifurcation of the middle cerebral artery, the top of the basilar artery, the junction of the basilar artery and the superior cerebellar artery or the anterior inferior cerebellar artery, or the junction of the vertebral artery and the posterior inferior cerebellar artery. Approximately 85 percent of cases occur in the anterior circle of Willis; 10 to 30 percent of patients have multiple aneurysms; 10 to 20 percent occur in bilateral identical locations.

As an aneurysm develops, it often forms a neck with a dome. The length of the neck and the size of the dome, factors that are important in planning microsurgical obliteration, vary greatly. The arterial internal elastic lamina disappears at the base of the neck. The media thins, and connective tissue replaces smooth-muscle cells. At the site of rupture (most often the dome) the wall thins to less than 0.3 mm, and the tear that allows bleeding is often no more than 0.5 mm long.

It is not possible to determine which aneurysms are likely to rupture, but limited data suggest that those larger than 7 mm may warrant prophylactic surgical obliteration.

CLINICAL SYMPTOMS, EVOLUTION, AND MANAGEMENT
Prodromal symptoms Prodromal symptoms may suggest the location of an unruptured aneurysm and suggest that it is progressively enlarging. A third nerve palsy, particularly when associated with pupillary dilatation, loss of light reflex, and focal pain above and behind the eye, indicates an expanding aneurysm at the junction of the posterior communicating artery and the internal carotid artery. Prompt surgery is indicated. A sixth nerve palsy may indicate an aneurysm in the cavernous sinus, and visual field defects can occur with an expanding supraclinoid carotid aneurysm. Occipital and posterior cervical pain may signal a posterior inferior cerebellar artery (PICA) or anterior inferior cerebellar artery (AICA) aneurysm. Pain in or behind the eye and in the low temple can occur with an expanding middle cerebral aneurysm.

It is not known for certain if an aneurysm can cause small intermittent bleeding into the subarachnoid space—so-called warning leaks. However, the importance of recognizing the smallest aneurysmal rupture or leak is undeniable. Sudden unexplained headache at any location should raise suspicion of subarachnoid hemorrhage and be investigated by a CT scan to look for blood in the basal cisterns. Often a small subarachnoid hemorrhage will not be seen by CT scan, necessitating a lumbar puncture to detect subarachnoid blood.

Initial clinical presentation: Acute major subarachnoid hemorrhage At the moment of aneurysmal rupture, with major subarachnoid hemorrhage, the intracranial pressure approaches the mean aterial pressure and cerebral perfusion pressure falls. This may account for the sudden transient loss of consciousness that occurs in up to 45 percent of cases. Sudden loss of consciousness may be preceded by a brief moment of excruciating headache, but most patients first complain of headache upon regaining consciousness. In 10 percent of cases, aneurysmal bleeding may be severe enough to cause loss of consciousness for several days. In about 45 percent of cases, severe headache, usually associated with exertion, is the presenting complaint. The headache is often called by the patient "the worst headache of my life." Words like "explode" or "burst" may be used. It may be "all over" or "in the back of the head and neck." Vomiting is a prominent symptom and when coupled with sudden headache should always raise the question of acute subarachnoid hemorrhage.

Although sudden headache in the absence of focal neurologic symptoms is the hallmark of aneurysmal rupture, focal neurologic deficits may occur (in addition to direct cranial nerve compression by the enlarging aneurysm as noted above). Anterior communicating artery aneurysms or middle cerebral bifurcation aneurysms may rupture into the subdural space, into the basal cisterns of the subarachnoid space, or directly into the underlying brain and form a clot large enough to produce a localized mass effect. The common deficits that result include hemiparesis, aphasia, anosognosia (hemineglect), memory loss, and abulia. An unusual acute unilateral hemispheric swelling with associated focal neurologic signs and stupor occurs rarely, immediately following aneurysmal rupture. Transient interruption of the cerebral circulation, possibly from acute vascular spasm, may underlie this complication.

Initial evaluation Over 75 percent of cases have evidence of a subarachnoid clot on a noncontrast CT scan obtained within 72 h of aneurysmal rupture. The extent and location of subarachnoid blood may help locate the underlying aneurysm and identify the cause of the initial neurologic deficit. The clot in the subarachnoid space may also help predict the delayed neurologic deficits due to cerebral vasospasm. *A noncontrast CT scan should be done first because arterial enhancement in the basal cisterns may be mistaken for clotted blood.* A later contrast CT scan may improve the definition of an aneurysm or demonstrate an unsuspected arteriovenous malformation. If the CT scan neither establishes the diagnosis of subarachnoid hemorrhage nor demonstrates a mass lesion or obstructive hydrocephalus, a lumbar puncture should be performed to establish the presence of subarachnoid blood. Lumbar puncture prior to scanning is indicated only if the CT scan is not available at the time of the suspected subarachnoid hemorrhage. MRI scanning may complement (or soon supplement) CT in the initial evaluation, but it is contraindicated postoperatively if metallic surgical clips were used.

Once the diagnosis of subarachnoid hemorrhage from ruptured saccular aneurysm has been established, angiography is generally delayed until just prior to surgery (though the time of surgery is becoming increasingly earlier). Angiography is performed to localize and define the anatomic details of the aneurysm and to determine if there is focal cerebral vasospasm. If an arteriovenous malformation or mycotic aneurysm is suspected because of the location of blood on CT, angiography should be done earlier.

The ECG frequently shows ST-segment and T-wave changes similar to those associated with ischemic coronary heart disease. Prolonged QRS complex, increased QT interval, and prominent "peaked" or deeply inverted symmetric T waves, although suggesting primary cardiac disease, are usually secondary to the intracranial hemorrhage. The cause of these changes is debated, but there is evidence that structural myocardial lesions may occur after acute hemorrhage.

Serum electrolyes are obtained because hyponatremia may develop from urinary sodium loss, possibly due to natriuretic peptides released by the brain or heart.

Initial management Following subarachnoid hemorrhage, a stuporous or comatose patient may have increased intracranial pressure. Care is required to maintain adequate cerebral perfusion pressure while avoiding excessive elevation of mean arterial pressure. Frequent arterial blood-gas determinations are helpful to assess alveolar ventilation. If hypercapnia exists, mechanically assisted ventilation is necessary. If a subdural or intracerebral hematoma mass is causing neurologic deterioration, its surgical removal and, if feasible, obliteration of the aneurysm are undertaken.

Because rebleeding is possible all patients are put on bed rest in a quiet, preferably darkened room and are given adequate stool softeners to prevent constipation. If headache or neck pain is severe, mild sedation and analgesics are prescribed. Aspirin, an antiplatelet agent, is inappropriate, but acetaminophen, meperidine and phenobarbitol, or other sedatives may be used. Extreme sedation is generally avoided because it can obscure the assessment of initial or delayed neurologic deficits.

Seizures are uncommon at the onset of aneurysmal rupture. The quivering, jerking, and extensor posturing that usually accompany loss of consciousness are probably related to the sharp rise in intracranial pressure. However, phenytoin or phenobarbitol are sometimes given as prophylactic therapy, since a seizure may cause rebleeding.

Glucocorticoids may help reduce the head-and-neck ache caused by the irritative effect of blood in the subarachnoid space, but there is no evidence to suggest they help in treatment of the cerebral edema that is sometimes seen in patients immediately after a subarachnoid hemorrhage, and they are generally omitted.

DELAYED NEUROLOGIC DEFICITS There are three major causes of delayed neurologic deficits: *rerupture, hydrocephalus,* and *cerebral vasospasm.* Recognizing each of these depends upon knowing precisely the cause and character of the initial neurologic findings.

Rerupture The incidence of rerupture in the first 3 weeks following subarachnoid hemorrhage is 10 to 30 percent. Because rerupture is associated with death and poor outcome, numerous clinical investigations of the effects of antifibrinolytic agents have been undertaken. Most have demonstrated a reduced rebleeding rate but also an increased incidence of ischemic stroke, presumably from vasospasm.

In general, when a thick clot is seen in the basal cisterns on the CT scan 24 to 48 h after hemorrhage (see below), symptomatic vasospasm is likely to develop and the use of antifibrinolytic agents is probably inappropriate. On the other hand, minimal or no blood on the initial CT scan or on the 24- to 48-h scan suggests that the blood in the basal cisterns has washed out and that delayed vasospasm is unlikely. Antifibrinolytic therapy may then be considered in selected cases, particularly if surgery is delayed.

Hydrocephalus Acute hydrocephalus can cause stupor and coma and requires emergency ventricular drainage. More often, subacute hydrocephalus over a few days or a few weeks causes progressive drowsiness or abulia with incontinence. Differentiating hydrocephalus from symptomatic cerebral vasospasm in the anterior communicating arteries is often difficult. It may clear spontaneously or require temporary ventricular drainage. Permanent ventricular drainage, if necessary, is usually done at the time of aneurysmal surgery. A chronic hydrocephalus similar to normal-pressure hydrocephalus may appear a few weeks to months after subarachnoid hemorrhage. It may present with gait difficulty, incontinence, or slowed mentation (abulia). The clue to the diagnosis may be a lack of initiative in conversation or a failure to recover independence after the aneurysm has been surgically clipped. Ventricular shunting is the treatment of choice.

Cerebral vasospasm Narrowing of the arteries at the base of the brain following subarachnoid hemorrhage from ruptured saccular aneurysm (*cerebral vasospasm*) can lead to delayed cerebral ischemia and infarction. This *symptomatic cerebral vasospasm* after subarachnoid hemorrhage occurs in approximately 30 percent of patients and is the major cause of delayed morbidity or death. Signs of ischemia usually appear 4 to 14 days after the initial subarachnoid hemorrhage, most frequently at about 7 days. The new deficits may fluctuate and correspond to ischemia in specific arterial territories. The severity and distribution of vasospasm determines whether cerebral infarction will develop.

Clinical evidence suggests that the extent and location of clotted blood on CT scans can be used to predict the incidence, location, and severity of cerebral vasospasm in patients after subarachnoid hemorrhage. A high incidence of symptomatic cerebral vasospasm in the middle and anterior cerebral artery territories has been found in patients with early CT scans showing globular subarachnoid clots larger than 5 × 3 mm in the basal cisterns, or layers of blood 1 mm thick or greater in the cerebral fissures. CT scans less reliably predict vasospasm in the vertebral, basilar, or posterior cerebral arteries. The CT scan should be obtained between 24 and 96 h following subarachnoid hemorrhage since blood present initially can disappear or ''wash out'' on a scan obtained after 24 h. With the further passage of time, x-ray attenuation values of clotted blood diminish so that its full extent and location may not be reliably detected after 96 h.

Cerebral vasospasm is a local phenomenon related to the presence of blood in the cerebrospinal fluid, surrounding a basal vessel. Its cause is unknown. Laboratory studies have suggested that substances such as serotonin, prostaglandins, and catecholamines can produce arterial narrowing. However, all these compounds break down rapidly in vivo, and only large amounts produce spasm in vitro. More sustained arterial vasospasm has been produced by experiments with incubated whole blood and erythrocyte breakdown products. The best current hypothesis suggests that a clot encases the artery; then after a few days spasmogenic hemoglobin breakdown products induce spasm. Once the vessel is in spasm, high-energy phosphate metabolism becomes impaired, because the surrounding clot prevents cerebrospinal fluid from nourishing the vessels. Vasa vasorum are not present in the vessels at the base of the brain or over the cortical surface. The reduction in local ATP may prevent the artery from relaxing.

CLINICAL SYNDROMES Symptomatic severe cerebral vasospasm presents with symptoms referable to the specific arterial territories involved. For example, spasm of the middle cerebral stem or its main branches causes contralateral hemiparesis, dysphasia (dominant hemisphere), anosognosia, or apractagnosia (nondominant hemisphere). Even severe vasospasm may not produce ischemic symptoms if sufficient collateral blood flow develops through border zone anastomotic channels (Fig. 351-1*A*). Proximal anterior cerebral artery vasospasm is associated with abulia and incontinence while severe vasospasm of the posterior cerebral artery is associated with hemianopic visual field defects. Severe spasm of the basilar or vertebral arteries occasionally produces focal brainstem ischemia. All of these focal neurologic symptoms may develop over a few days, fluctuate, or present abruptly.

TREATMENT Therapeutic efforts to prevent or treat symptomatic cerebral vasospasm have been universally disappointing. The failure to find a satisfactory therapy for cerebral vasospasm has prompted a search for prophylactic measures to prevent or minimize its occurrence. Treatment with the calcium channel blocking agent nimodipine has been reported in several studies to have beneficial effects, but patients in both the treated and untreated groups developed symptomatic vasospasm.

The most commonly accepted form of therapy for symptomatic cerebral vasospasm is to increase the cerebral perfusion pressure by raising mean arterial pressure through plasma volume expansion and the judicious use of pressor agents, ordinarily phenylephrine or dopamine. Raised perfusion pressure has been associated with symptomatic improvement in some patients, but high arterial pressure may risk rebleeding. The therapies generally require monitoring the central venous pressure, arterial pressure, and, in severe cases, the intracranial and pulmonary artery wedge pressure. Angioplasty is currently under investigation.

Severe cerebral edema in patients with infarction from vasospasm may increase the intracranial pressure enough to reduce cerebral perfusion pressure. Treatment, as outlined in Chap. 352, is with mannitol and hyperventilation. Plasma osmolality is usually raised to approximately 300 mosmol/L. As a last resort, barbiturate-induced coma has been used to reduce intracranial pressure in some patients; it has not been proven to improve outcome.

Surgical treatment of saccular aneurysms The advent of the operating microscope has made microsurgical obliteration of a ruptured aneurysm a safe and effective means of preventing disastrous rerupture. Some neurosurgeons delay surgery for at least 10 to 14 days, although the trend has been toward earlier surgery. Operation is undertaken when the patient is clinically stable. Delayed surgery allows cerebral swelling from the initial rupture time to resolve and minimizes the risk of symptomatic vasospasm in the postoperative period.

The wisdom of delaying surgery has been questioned, especially if the patient is neurologically intact. Surgery within the first 48 h eliminates the problem of rebleeding, can remove potentially spasmogenic clots from the basal cisterns, theoretically preventing vasospasm, and allows volume expansion or hypertensive therapy for vasospasm to be conducted without the risk of rebleeding. While it is technically possible to remove local clots and obliterate aneurysms early, some subarachnoid clots are too extensive for safe, complete removal. The timing of aneurysm surgery, still controversial, should therefore be tailored to the individual patient. Intravascular catheter techniques to obliterate aneurysms are investigational but may have a role in management of aneurysms considered to have a high surgical risk.

Giant aneurysms Giant aneurysms larger than 2 cm in diameter occur at the same sites as small aneurysms. The three most common locations are the intracranial internal carotid, middle cerebral bifurcation, and top of the basilar arteries. Although they can bleed, they usually cause symptoms by compressing the adjacent brain or cranial nerves. Edema formation in the compressed brain can be relentless, compounding the mass effect. It is resistant to treatment and may be fatal. This progression is particularly likely if a giant aneurysm occurs at the bifurcation of the middle cerebral artery. Surgical decompression, until recently was the only adequate therapy. It is extremely difficult technically and carries a high morbidity in the presence of edema. Newer interventional neuroradiologic procedures may prove helpful (see Chap. 348).

Mycotic aneurysms Mycotic aneurysms are located distal to the first bifurcation of major arteries of the circle of Willis. Emboli from bacterial endocarditis should be suspected and appropriate blood cultures taken. Because of their distal location in the arterial tree they rarely leave significant amounts of clotted blood in the basal cisterns, and severe cerebral vasospasm is infrequent. Mycotic aneurysms, however, are subject to rerupture. Although antibiotic therapy may reduce this risk, surgical obliteration remains the definitive treatment.

OTHER CAUSES OF INTRACRANIAL HEMORRHAGE

ARTERIOVENOUS MALFORMATION An angioma, or hemangioma, consists of a tangle of abnormal vessels forming an abnormal communication between the arterial and venous systems. Most are developmental arteriovenous fistulas in which the constituent vessels enlarge and grow with the passage of time. Angiomas vary in size from a small blemish a few millimeters in diameter to a huge mass of tortuous channels composing an arteriovenous shunt of sufficient magnitude to raise the cardiac output. Hypertrophic dilated arterial ''feeders'' approach the main lesion, disappear below the cortex, and break up into a network of thin-walled blood vessels which connect directly with draining veins. These often form huge, dilated, pulsating channels, carrying away arterial blood. The blood vessels forming the tangle interposed between arteries and veins are usually abnormally thin and do not have a normal structure. Angiomas occur in all parts of the brain, brainstem, and spinal cord, but the larger ones are most frequently in the posterior half of the hemispheres, commonly forming a wedge-shaped lesion extending from the cortex to the ventricular lining.

Angiomas are more frequent in men and may occur in more than one member of a family in the same or successive generations. Although the lesion is present from birth, bleeding or other complaints are most common between the ages of 10 and 30, occasionally as late as the fifties.

The chief clinical symptoms and signs are headache, seizures, and those associated with rupture. When headache occurs (without bleeding), it may be hemicranial and throbbing, like migraine, or diffuse. There may be hemiplegia with headache, resembling hemiplegic migraines. Focal seizures that become generalized occur in about 30 percent of cases and are usually well managed with anticonvulsants. In half of cases, arteriovenous malformations become evident as intracerebral hemorrhages. In most of these cases, the hemorrhage is mainly intraparenchymal with a small amount of spillage into the subarachnoid space. Blood is usually not deposited in the basal cistern, and symptomatic cerebral vasospasm is therefore rare. The threat of rerupture in the first 3 weeks is low, so that there is no need to consider the use of antifibrinolytic agents. The hemorrhage may be massive, leading to death acutely, or may be as small as 1 cm in diameter, leading to minor focal symptoms or no deficit. In either case, the hemorrhagic mass may compress the arteriovenous malformation so completely that angiography cannot detect the malformation. Hence, when arteriovenous malformation (AVM) is suspected, angiography is best postponed until the hematoma has completely resolved, i.e., after 6 to 8 weeks. Rarely the angioma is large enough to steal blood away from adjacent normal brain tissue, rendering the surrounding brain ischemic. This deprivation is most often seen when large AVMs in the middle cerebral–posterior cerebral system or middle cerebral–anterior cerebral system extend from the cortical surface to the ventricular system. Hydrocephalus may result when the vein of Galen enlarges as a channel for drainage from the AVM.

Large AVMs of the carotid–middle cerebral system may be associated with a systolic and diastolic bruit (sometimes self-audible) over the eye, forehead, or neck where a bounding, forceful carotid pulse may be perceived. Headache at the onset of AVM rupture is not as prominent or as common as it is with a ruptured saccular aneurysm. Contrast CT scan can often detect the channels of an AVM prior to rupture; newer MRI techniques may prove more sensitive.

Although many AVMs eventually rupture, definitive surgical therapy is usually reserved until after the first episode of hemorrhage; the threat of rerupture is 3 percent per year thereafter. When surgery is not feasible because of the location and size of AVMs, other therapeutic options being evaluated include endovascular embolization and proton beam irradiation.

TRAUMA Head injury can result in intracerebral (especially temporal lobe and inferior frontal) hematoma and infratentorial hematomas, subarachnoid bleeding, acute and chronic subdural hematoma formation, and acute epidural hematoma formation. Trauma must be considered in any patient with an unexplained acute neurologic deficit (hemiparesis, stupor, or confusion), particularly if the deficit occurred in the context of a fall. These entities and their distinction from spontaneous hemorrhage are discussed more fully in Chap. 352.

HEMATOLOGIC DISORDERS Intracerebral hemorrhage associated with hematologic disorders (leukemia, aplastic anemia, thrombocytopenic purpura) can occur at any intracranial site and may present as multiple intracerebral hemorrhages. Skin and mucous membrane bleeding is usually evident and offers a diagnostic clue. Intracerebral hemorrhage associated with anticoagulant therapy can occur at any location, often lobar, and may evolve slowly over 24 to 48 h. Fresh frozen plasma and vitamin K are usually given immediately. When intracerebral hemorrhage is associated with aspirin, fresh platelet transfusions may be required.

BRAIN TUMORS Hemorrhage into a brain tumor may be the first manifestation of neoplasm. Choriocarcinoma, malignant melanoma, renal cell carcinoma, and bronchogenic carcinoma are among the most common metastatic tumors associated with intracerebral hemorrhage. Glioblastoma multiforme in adults and medulloblastoma in children may also have areas of intracerebral hemorrhage.

OTHER CAUSES Primary intraventricular hemorrhage is rare. It usually begins intraparenchymally and dissects into the ventricular system without leaving signs of intraparenchymal hemorrhage. Sepsis can cause small petechial hemorrhages through the cerebral white matter. There is no blood in the spinal fluid, and this condition should not be confused with a stroke. Inflammatory disease of the arteries and veins, especially polyarteritis nodosa and lupus erythematosus, can produce hemorrhage into the central nervous system. Most of the time it is associated with hypertension. An intensely inflammatory and hemorrhagic white matter process termed *Hurst's hemorrhagic leukoencephalitis* is probably a type of hyperacute multiple sclerosis. Moyamoya, mainly an obliterative disease that causes ischemic symptoms, may also have multiple small aneuysms that rupture in a small percentage of patients. Hemorrhages into the spinal cord are usually the result of an AVM or metastatic tumor. Epidural spinal hemorrhage usually compresses the cord rapidly and produces a transverse myelopathy (see Chap. 361).

HYPERTENSIVE ENCEPHALOPATHY (See Chap. 196)

In this acute syndrome, severe hypertension is associated with headache, nausea, vomiting, convulsions, confusion, stupor, and coma. Focal or lateralizing neurologic signs, either transitory or lasting, may occur but are infrequent and always suggest some other form of vascular disease (hemorrhage, embolism, or atherosclerotic thrombosis). By the time neurologic manifestations appear, the hypertension has usually reached the malignant state, with retinal hemorrhages, exudates, papilledema (hypertensive retinopathy grade IV), and evidence of renal and cardiac disease. In many, but not all, cases the cerebrospinal fluid pressure and the protein values are both elevated. The hypertension may be essential or due to chronic renal disease, acute glomerulonephritis, acute toxemia of pregnancy, pheochromocytoma, Cushing's syndrome, or ACTH toxicity. Lowering of the blood pressure with hypotensive drugs may reverse the process in several days if permanent damage is not severe. Neuropathologic examination may reveal a cerebral swelling or hemorrhages of various sizes from massive to petechial. A cerebellar pressure cone reflects increased pressure in the posterior fossa, and in some instances lumbar puncture has been fatal. Microscopically there are small hemorrhages, clusters of microglial cells, minute cerebral infarcts, and necrosis of arterioles.

The term *hypertensive encephalopathy* should be reserved for this syndrome and not for chronic recurrent headaches, dizziness, epileptic seizures, recurrent TIAs, or small strokes, which often occur in association with high blood pressure.

REFERENCES

AUSMAN JI et al: Vertebrobasilar insufficiency: A review. Arch Neurol 42:803, 1985

BAUER KA, ROSENBERG RD: The pathophysiology of the prethrombotic state in humans: Insights gained from studies using markers of hemostatic system activation. Blood 70:343, 1987

BOUGHNER DR, BARNETT HJM: The enigma of the risk of stroke in mitral valve prolapse. Stroke 16:175, 1985

BOUSSER MG et al: "AICLA" controlled trial of aspirin and dipyridamole in the secondary prevention of athero-thrombotic cerebral ischemia. Stroke 14:5, 1983

CALL G et al: Correlation of continuous-wave Doppler spectral flow analysis with gross pathology in carotid stenosis. Stroke 19:584, 1988

CANADIAN COOPERATIVE STUDY GROUP: A randomized trial of aspirin and sulfinpyrazone in threatened stroke. N Engl J Med 299:53, 1978

CAPLAN LR: "Top of the basilar" syndrome. Neurology 30:72, 1980

CEREBRAL EMBOLISM STUDY GROUP: Immediate anticoagulation of embolic stroke: Brain hemorrhage and management options. Stroke 15:779, 1984

CHAMBERS BR et al: Outcome in patients with asymptomatic neck bruits. N Engl J Med 315:860, 1986

EC/IC BYPASS STUDY GROUP: Failure of extracranial-intracranial arterial bypass to reduce the risk of ischemic stroke: Results of an international randomized trial. N Engl J Med 313:1191, 1985

Fisher CM: Occlusion of the internal carotid artery. Arch Neurol Psychiatry 65:346, 1951
——— et al: Lateral medullary infarction: The pattern of vascular occlusion. J Neuropathol Exp Neurol 20:323, 1961
——— et al: The arterial lesions underlying lacunes. Acta Neuropathol (Berl) 12:1, 1969
———: Clinical syndromes in cerebral thrombosis, hypertensive hemorrhage, and ruptured saccular aneurysm. Clin Neurosurg 22:117, 1975
——— et al: Atherosclerosis of the carotid and vertebral arteries—extracranial and intracranial. J Neuropathol Exp Neurol 24:455, 1965
——— et al: Cerebral vasospasm with ruptured saccular aneurysm: The clinical manifestations. Neurosurg 1:245, 1977
——— et al: Spontaneous dissection of cervico-cerebral arteries. Can J Neurol Sci 5:9, 1978
——— et al: The correlation of cerebral vasospasm and the amount of subarachnoid blood detected by computerized cranial tomography after ruptured aneurysm. Neurosurg 6:1, 1980
———: Late-life migraine accompaniments as a cause of unexplained transient ischemic attacks. Can J Neurol Sci 7:9, 1980
———: Lacunar strokes and infarcts: A review. Neurology 32:871, 1982
Hinton RC et al: Influence of etiology of atrial fibrillation on incidence of systemic embolism. Am J Cardiol 40:509, 1977
——— et al: Symptomatic middle artery stenosis. Ann Neurol 5:152, 1979
Hirsh J et al: Optimal therapeutic range for oral anticoagulants. Chest (Suppl) 95(2):5s, 1989
Kistler JP: Cardiac embolic cerebrovascular disease. Primary Care 6:745, 1979
——— et al: Vertebral basilar territory stroke. Delineation by proton nuclear magnetic resonance imaging. Stroke 15:417, 1984
——— et al: Therapy of ischemic cerebral vascular disease due to atherothrombosis. N Engl J Med 311:27, 100, 1984
Mohr JP: Valvular disease, cardiac arrest, systemic hypotension, and cardiac surgery, in *Handbook of Clinical Neurology*, GW Bruyn, PJ Vinken (eds). Amsterdam, North-Holland, 1978
——— et al: The Harvard Cooperative Stroke Registry: A prospective registry. Neurology 28:754, 1978
———: Lacunes. Stroke 13:3, 1982
Phillips SJ: An alternative view of heparin anticoagulation in acute focal brain ischemia. Stroke 20:295, 1989
Ropper AH, Davis KR: Lobar cerebral hemorrhages: Acute clinical syndromes in 26 patients. Ann Neurol 8:141, 1980
Welin L et al: Analysis of risk factors for stroke in a cohort of men born in 1913. N Engl J Med 317:521, 1987
Wilkins RH: Natural history of intracranial vascular malformation: A review. Neurosurg 16:421, 1985
Wolf PA et al: Atrial fibrillation, a major contributor to stroke in the elderly: The Framingham study. Arch Intern Med 147:1561, 1987

352 TRAUMA OF THE HEAD AND SPINAL CORD

ALLAN H. ROPPER

Head injuries are frequent in industrialized countries, affecting many patients in the prime of life. To appreciate the medical and social magnitude of this problem it needs only to be recognized that almost 10 million Americans have head injuries yearly, about 20 percent serious enough to cause brain damage. Among men under 35 years old, accidents, usually motor vehicle collisions, are the chief cause of death, and over 70 percent of these involve head injury. Minor head injuries are so common that almost all physicians encounter patients requiring immediate care or suffering from various sequelae. Traumatic spinal cord injuries often occur in conjunction with head injury. The two are best considered together in the context of trauma to the nervous system.

In the past two decades, declining mortality from head and spinal cord injuries can be attributed mainly to public health measures, such as use of seat belts and motorcycle helmets, and the development of ambulance systems with trained personnel. A systematic approach to the evaluation of patients with head and spine trauma, beginning at the scene of the accident, has improved outcome. An understanding of the pathologic lesions produced by trauma is essential for diagnosis and to provide a framework for management.

TYPES OF HEAD INJURIES

SKULL FRACTURES A blow to the skull causes fractures if the elastic tolerance of the bone is exceeded. Significant intracranial lesions accompany two-thirds of skull fractures, and the presence of a skull fracture increases manyfold the chances of an underlying subdural or epidural hematoma. Consequently, fractures assume importance primarily as markers of the site and severity of injury. They also cause cranial nerve injuries and produce entry pathways to the cerebrospinal fluid (CSF) for bacteria (meningitis) and air (pneumocephalus), or for leakage of CSF. Fractures are classified as linear, basilar, compound, or depressed; linear fractures account for 80 percent of all skull fractures and are most often associated with subdural or epidural hematomas. Linear fractures usually extend from the point of impact toward the base of the skull.

Basilar skull fractures are often extensions of adjacent fractures over the convexity of the skull but may occur independently due to stresses on the floor of the middle cranial fossa or occiput. They are usually located parallel to the petrous bone or along the sphenoid bone toward the sella turcica and ethmoidal groove. Most are uncomplicated, but they may cause CSF leak, pneumocephalus, or cavernous-carotid fistula. Fractures of the basal skull bones are often accompanied by signs of hemotympanum (blood behind the tympanic membrane), delayed ecchymosis over the mastoid process (Battle's sign), or periorbital ecchymosis (''racoon sign''). Because routine x-ray examination can fail to disclose basilar fractures, they should be suspected in the presence of these clinical signs. Cerebrospinal fluid may also leak through the cribriform plate or the adjacent sinus and present as a watery discharge from the nose (CSF rhinorrhea). Persistence of rhinorrhea or recurrent meningitis is an indication for a surgical repair of torn dura underlying the fracture. The site of the leak is often difficult to determine, but useful diagnostic tests include metrizamide instillation into thc CSF with subsequent computed tomography (CT) scans, or radionuclide or fluorescein injection into the CSF followed by assessment of uptake by absorptive nasal pledgets. The site of intermittent leaks is rarely delineated; most resolve spontaneously. Sellar fractures can also be radiologically occult, although they are sometimes associated with serious neuroendocrine dysfunction. Occasionally, fractures of the dorsum sella cause sixth or seventh nerve palsies or optic nerve damage. An air-fluid level in the sphenoid sinus suggests a fracture of the sellar floor.

About 20 percent of petrous bone fractures, usually along the long axis of the bone, are associated with facial palsy. Disruption of ear ossicles and CSF otorrhea are other complications. Transverse petrous fractures are less common, almost always damaging the cochlea or labyrinths and often the facial nerve. External bleeding from the ear can result from petrous bone fractures, though local laceration of the external canal from abrasions is more common. Frontal bone fractures are often depressed, involving the frontal and paranasal sinuses and the orbits; anosmia frequently follows if the olfactory filaments in the cribriform plate are disrupted.

Depressed skull fractures are often compound but are commonly asymptomatic, except for amnesia due to concussions, because the impact energy is dissipated in breaking the bone. Some cause brain contusions and focal neurologic signs appropriate to the underlying cortical area. Surgical repair and bone elevation with exploration of the dura is required in most cases. Delayed or incomplete debridement of the wound leads to a high incidence of infection. If the skin is lacerated over a skull fracture and the underlying meninges are torn, or if the fracture passes through the posterior wall of a nasal sinus, bacteria or air may enter the cranial cavity resulting in meningitis, abscess formation, or pneumocephalus.

CRANIAL NERVE INJURIES Cranial nerves liable to injury with basilar skull fractures are the olfactory, optic, oculomotor, trochlear, first and second branches of the trigeminal, facial, and auditory. Anosmia and an apparent loss of taste (actually a loss of perception of aromatic flavors, with elementary tastes retained) occurs in approximately 10 percent of serious head injuries, particularly with falls on the back of the head. This results from displacement of the brain and shearing of the olfactory nerve filaments. Recovery usually occurs with residual hyposmia, but if bilateral anosmia persists for several months, the prognosis is poor. Fractures of the sphenoid bone may bruise or transect the optic nerve, resulting in unilateral partial or complete blindness, and an unreactive pupil usually equal in size to the other side, with a preserved consensual light response. Partial optic nerve injuries from closed trauma result in blurring of vision, central or paracentral scotomas, or sector defects. Prognosis for recovery of vision varies widely. Direct orbital injury may cause short-lived blurred vision for close objects because of reversible iridoplegia. Oculomotor nerve injury causes the globe to turn outward with loss of adduction and vertical movement and a fixed dilated pupil; vision is preserved. Diplopia only on looking down, which suggests trochlear nerve damage from fracture of the lesser sphenoid wing, is not uncommon as an isolated problem from minor injury and may be delayed in appearance for several days. Patients report correction of the diplopia by tilting the head away from the affected eye. Direct facial nerve injury by a basal fracture is present immediately in 3 percent of severe injuries or may also be delayed 5 to 7 days. Petrous fractures, particularly the less common transverse type, are liable to produce this injury. Delayed facial palsy has a good prognosis; its mechanism is not known. Injury to the eighth cranial nerve with fractures of the petrous bone causes loss of hearing, vertigo, and nystagmus immediately after injury; the nystagmus is frequently positional. Deafness due to nerve injury must be distinguished from rupture of the eardrum, blood in the middle ear, or disruption of the ossicles from fracture through the middle ear. A high-tone hearing loss occurs with direct cochlear concussion.

CONCUSSION Concussion refers to an immediate but transient loss of consciousness often described as dazed or "star-struck" and associated with a short period of amnesia. It typically occurs after blunt impact or deceleration of the frontal or occipital areas that creates sudden movement of the brain within the skull. In severe cases, a brief convulsion, or autonomic symptoms and signs such as facial pallor, bradycardia, faintness with mild hypotension, or sluggish pupillary reaction may occur, but most patients are neurologically normal. Higher primates are particularly susceptible to concussion; in contrast, billy goats, rams, and woodpeckers can tolerate impact velocity and deceleration a hundred times greater than that experienced by humans. The mechanism of loss of consciousness in concussion is believed to be transient electrophysiologic dysfunction of the reticular activating system in the upper midbrain caused by rotation of the cerebral hemispheres on the relatively fixed brainstem. The mechanism of the associated amnesia is not known. Gross and light microscopic changes in the brain are usually absent after concussion, but biochemical and ultrastructural changes such as mitochondrial ATP depletion and local disruption of the blood-brain barrier suggest that complex abnormalities occur. The CT and MRI scans are normal, and there are usually no red blood cells in the CSF as occurs with more severe injuries. Approximately 3 percent of patients who have sustained concussions will have an intracranial hemorrhage (subdural, epidural, or parenchymal), but the presence of a skull fracture increases the risk manyfold.

Amnesia after concussion typically follows a few moments of unresponsiveness after impact. Rarely there is no loss of consciousness. The memory loss spans the time of, and moments before, mild impact injuries but may encompass previous weeks (rarely months) in more severe trauma. Any anterograde amnesia is usually brief and disappears rapidly in alert patients. The extent of retrograde amnesia has been suggested as a coarse measure of the severity of injury. Improvement usually occurs in an orderly progression from most distant to recent memories, with islands of amnesia occasionally remaining in severe cases. Hysterical posttraumatic amnesia is not uncommon. It should be suspected when abnormalities of behavior occur, such as a tendency to recount events that cannot be recalled on later testing, bizarre affect, a person forgetting his or her own name, disproportionate or selective memory loss, or exaggerated anterograde deficit in comparison to the degree of injury.

A single uncomplicated head injury has not been shown to produce permanent neurobehavioral changes in most patients who are free of preexisting psychiatric problems and substance abuse. In some patients, however, there has been increasing attention to minor problems in memory and concentration that may have an anatomical correlate in small shearing lesions (see below).

CONTUSION, BRAIN HEMORRHAGES, AND SHEARING LESIONS **Hemispheral lesions** Contusions on the surface of the brain and deeper hemorrhages result from mechanical forces that move the hemispheres relative to the skull. Deceleration of the brain against the inner skull causes contusions, either under a point of impact (coup lesion) or in the antipolar area (contrecoup lesion). Trauma sufficient to cause prolonged unconsciousness beyond concussion usually produces contusions varying from small superficial cortical petechiae to hemorrhagic and necrotic destruction of large portions of a hemisphere. Because the motion of the hemispheres brings them into contact with the prominences of the sphenoid and other frontal basal bones, blunt impact, as from an automobile dashboard, typically causes contusions on the orbital surfaces of the frontal lobes and the anterior and basal portions of the temporal lobes. The anterior corpus callosum may also be bruised from striking the falx. With lateral forces, as from the doorframe of a car, contusions occur on the convexity of the hemispheres.

Contusions are visible on CT scan, appearing early as smudged hyperlucencies from scattered cortical and subcortical blood and a mass that distorts adjacent structures, most prominently the lateral ventricles. After several hours the surrounding edematous tissue appears as a ring of lower density. Confluent, roughly spherical contusions can be distinguished from spontaneous cerebral hemorrhages because the former characteristically extend to the cortical surface. After a week some contusions have a surrounding ringlike contrast-enhancing density that may be mistaken for tumor or abscess. Glial and macrophage reactions begin within 2 days, years later resulting in scarred hemosiderin-stained depressions on the surface (*plaques jaune*) that are one source of posttraumatic epilepsy. Large single hemorrhages after minor trauma are found in patients with a bleeding diathesis or in the elderly, sometimes related to cerebrovascular amyloidosis.

The clinical signs produced by contusions vary with their location and size; most often a hemiparesis or gaze preference is seen, similar to a middle cerebral artery stroke. Bilateral large contusions produce coma with extensor posturing; when contusions are limited to the frontal lobes, an abulic-taciturn state or inappropriate jocularity and indifference occur. Contusions of the temporal lobes cause an aggressive combative syndrome, described below. With large contusions the secondary effect of progressive edema is the most threatening aspect of the injury. Coma and signs of secondary brainstem compression (pupillary enlargement) then dominate the examination. Seizures soon after trauma are rare with contusions, as indeed they are for several weeks after most acute head injuries.

Deep hemorrhages in the central white matter may result from confluent contusions in the depths of a sulcus. However, ganglionic, diencephalic, and other deep hematomas due to torsion or shearing forces in the brain often occur independently of surface damage. The areas around these hematomas may become edematous, resulting in enlargement of the affected region and progressively raised intracranial pressure.

Another type of white matter, or "shearing," lesion consists pathologically of widespread acute disruption of axons. Axonal shearing occurs at, or soon after, impact. The affected areas of white matter are replaced with glial proliferation over a period of several months. There are characteristically small areas of tissue disruption in the corpus callosum and dorsolateral pons. Widespread axonal shearing lesions in the deep white matter of both hemispheres may explain persistent coma or vegetative state, but small hemorrhages in the midbrain and diencephalon are as often the cause. Shearing lesions are not usually visualized by CT scanning, but in severe cases small hemorrhages of the corpus callosum and centrum semiovale are seen.

On occasion, head trauma causes diffuse brain swelling within a few hours after injury. Most instances are due to widespread contusion though CT scanning fails to reveal significant focal lesions or hemorrhage. The edema creates a mass effect with disastrous consequences. This problem is encountered in children and young adults who may develop a virtually instantaneous generalized edema probably due to microvascular disruption, hypertension, and greatly increased cerebral blood flow.

Deep cerebral hemorrhages may occur several days after severe injury. Sudden neurologic deterioration, often in already comatose patients, or a sustained and unexplained rise in intracranial pressure should prompt a CT scan to detect delayed hemorrhage.

Brainstem hemorrhages A syndrome with coma, midposition or larger pupils unreactive to light, and impaired or absent oculocephalic reflex eye movements results from small linear or oval-shaped hemorrhages in the high midbrain, visible on CT scan, though often delayed in appearance. Though extensor posturing occurs with stimulation, the limbs are otherwise flaccid. This clinical syndrome should be suspected even in the initial absence of a hemorrhage on CT scan. These acute midbrain hemorrhages may be the result of primary injury from rotational forces in the upper midbrain. They also occur from secondary compression of the brainstem by supratentorial hematomas and lateral tissue shifts or pressure from the adjacent temporal lobes. Magnetic resonance image (MRI) scanning shows many other small brainstem and hemispheric white matter lesions that are related to mechanical disruption of tissue, similar to shearing. In pathologic material from severe, acutely fatal injuries, small linear and oval hemorrhages are found in the low thalamic and subthalamic regions and throughout the midline of the brainstem (termed *Duret hemorrhages*).

Residual symptoms and signs of primary or secondary brainstem hemorrhages or ischemic lesions include tremor, pupillary enlargement, eye movement abnormalities, or the "locked-in" syndrome (see Chap. 31). Midbrain or diencephalic hemorrhages are the only well-defined traumatic brainstem lesions responsible for coma. Most other cases of coma without fixed pupils and unexplained by CT scan are probably due to diffuse axonal shearing injuries in the cerebral hemispheres.

SUBDURAL AND EPIDURAL HEMATOMAS In severe head injury, hemorrhages beneath the dura (subdural) or between the dura and skull (epidural) may be combined with contusions and other injuries, making it difficult to determine their relative contribution to the clinical state. However, subdural and epidural hematomas often occur as the primary lesion, each with a characteristic clinical and radiologic appearance. Because the mass effect of the hemorrhage and rise in intracranial pressure may be life-threatening, it is important to make an immediate diagnosis by CT scanning and carry out surgical evacuation.

Acute subdural hematoma Acute subdural hematomas become symptomatic in minutes to hours after injury. Up to one-third of patients have a lucid interval before coma supervenes, but the majority are drowsy or comatose from the moment of injury. Arousable patients complain of unilateral headache and frequently have a slightly enlarged pupil on that side. Stupor or coma with unilateral pupillary enlargement are the major signs in larger hematomas. Pupillary dilation is ipsilateral in most, but 5 to 10 percent are contralateral to the hematoma. Lateralizing signs such as a hemiparesis are helpful in only a few patients and may be ipsilateral to the clot. Acute seizures or isolated hemianopsias are uncommon. The CT scan shows the clot, allowing early evacuation. MRI scans may fail to demonstrate an acute collection of blood. Angiography with oblique projections can also outline subdural hematomas and has been used if CT scanning is unavailable. In an acutely deteriorating patient with rapidly diminishing alertness and pupillary enlargement, burr holes or an emergency craniotomy are sometimes appropriate without prior radiographic confirmation of subdural hematoma. A subacute syndrome is seen in alcoholics and in the elderly, with drowsiness, headache, confusion, or mild hemiparesis occurring days to 2 weeks after injury.

Direct trauma or surface contusions are not required for the formation of acute subdural hemorrhage; acceleration forces alone, as from whiplash, are adequate, especially in the elderly. Most subdural hematomas are small crescentic collections over the hemispheral convexity, adjacent to variable degrees of surface hemorrhagic contusions. Larger clots are thought to be primarily venous in origin, though additional arterial bleeding sites are often found, and some, when explored surgically, appear to be exclusively arterial. Most are located over the frontotemporal region, less often in the inferior middle fossa or over the occipital poles. Less common instances of interhemispheric, posterior fossa, or bilateral convexity clots are difficult to diagnose clinically, although drowsiness and the signs expected for each region can be detected. Small subdural hematomas may be asymptomatic and usually do not require therapy.

Acute epidural hematoma Epidural hematomas evolve more rapidly and therefore can be more treacherous. They occur in 1 to 3 percent of all head injuries and in up to 10 percent of severe ones. They are less often associated with underlying cortical damage than subdural hematomas. The majority of patients are unconscious when first seen, often with associated injuries of subdural clot and contusion. A "lucid interval" of several minutes to hours before coma supervenes is said to be most characteristic of epidural hemorrhage, though it is not common and by no means the only cause of this temporal profile. The findings of drowsiness progressing to coma, pupillary enlargement, and hemiplegia are similar in some respects to subdural hematoma, but occur more rapidly.

The location of epidural hematomas is explained by their origin from torn dural vessels, most commonly the middle meningeal artery. Epidural clots therefore overlie the lateral temporal convexity. The majority of patients have fractures of the squamous portion of the temporal bone, through the path of the torn vessel. Frontal, inferior temporal, or occipitoparietal epidural hematomas are less frequent, occurring when fractures disrupt branches of the middle meningeal artery. Dural laceration over the sagittal or lateral sinuses or rupture of small diploic veins can rarely cause venous epidural hemorrhages. Epidural hematomas strip the tightly attached dura from the inner table of the skull, producing a characteristic lenticular-shaped clot on CT scan. They may be relatively less frequent in the elderly because of the tighter attachment of dura to skull that occurs with aging. Posterior fossa epidural hematomas are rare and difficult to detect clinically (most result from surgery such as resection of an acoustic neuroma).

Chronic subdural hematoma In chronic subdural hematoma, a preceding traumatic cause is less often clear; 20 to 30 percent of patients fail to give a history of injury. Elderly patients or those with a bleeding diathesis seemingly form clots spontaneously. The causative injury may be trivial (striking the head against the branch of a tree, a sudden stop in a car with lurching forward, or striking the head during a fall or faint) and is often forgotten because it was remote in time. A period of weeks, or even months, follows when headaches (common but not invariable), slowed thinking, confusion, changes in personality, seizures, or a mild hemiparesis are the main findings. Fluctuation in the severity of the headache is typical, often with positional changes. Many chronic subdural hematomas are bilateral and give particularly misleading clinical syndromes. The initial clinical impression is often a stroke, brain tumor, drug intoxication, or a depressive, senile, or other type of dementia, the latter because disturbances of consciousness (drowsiness, inattentiveness, incoherence of thought) are more prominent than focal or lateralizing signs such as hemiparesis. Hemianesthesia or hemianopsia are seldom observed, probably because the anatomic structures subserving these functions are deep and not easily compressed. The diagnosis should be considered in dementias of apparently rapid onset, particularly if headache is present. The condition does not usually progress. When it does, the patient may become comatose with fluctuations of alertness and pupillary dilation as occurs in acute subdural hematoma. Acute bleeding is superimposed on the chronic hematoma in these cases. Occasionally patients present with "spells" of hemiparesis or aphasia typically lasting more than 10 min, sometimes indistinguishable from a transient ischemic attack. Patients with undetected small bilateral subdural hematomas seem to tolerate surgery, anesthesia, and nervous system depressive drugs poorly, often remaining drowsy or confused for long periods postoperatively.

Skull x-rays are usually normal except for a shift of a calcified pineal body to one side or an occasional unexpected fracture. The CT scan without contrast infusion typically shows a low-density mass over the convexity of the hemisphere, but may show only a shift of the midline structures and compression of the lateral ventricles because the clot becomes isodense to adjacent brain after 2 to 6 weeks. Bilateral chronic hematomas are often missed because of the absence of lateral tissue shifts. A "hypernormal" CT scan with absent cortical sulci and small ventricles in an older patient should suggest the diagnosis of bilateral isodense hematomas. Contrast infusion demonstrates the chronic fibrous capsule in some cases. MRI scans are very reliable in identifying a clot. The CSF may be clear, bloody, or xanthochromic, depending on the presence or absence of recent or old contusion and subarachnoid hemorrhage, and the pressure is usually elevated. However, lumbar puncture is not recommended for diagnosis because of risk of worsening tissue shifts. Chronic subdural hematomas can gradually expand, and then behave clinically like a tumor. Treatment with glucocorticoids alone is sufficient in some cases, but surgical evacuation is most often successful. Fibrous membranes (pseudomembranes) grow from the dura and encapsulate the region. Craniotomy and removal of the membranes is required if there is recurrent fluid accumulation. Small hematomas are largely resorbed, and only the organizing membranes remain, becoming calcified after many years.

PENETRATING INJURIES, COMPRESSIONS, AND LACERATIONS Tangential scalp wounds from bullets can produce neurologic signs or delayed seizures due to small hemorrhages or contusions, even in the absence of missile penetration. Bullets entering the brain cause considerable damage because of tremendous kinetic energy. A cylindrical area of necrosis surrounds the bullet track. Injuries differ with varying projectiles; soft civilian bullets typically shatter on impact and leave a track of metallic fragments with disproportionately less parenchymal damage. Military bullets, because of high velocity and energy, disrupt tissue at great distances from the track and produce massive brain destruction.

Penetrating bullet injuries cause a rapid increase in intracranial pressure for several minutes followed by a drop depending on the volume of secondary hemorrhage and the degree of developing edema. Infection is a risk mainly from shell fragments, shrapnel, grenades, and mines, because such small projectiles carry surface bacteria and dirt into the brain. Nevertheless, most neurosurgeons administer systemic antibiotics prophylactically and perform local debridement in all types of penetrating injuries. Traumatic aneurysms can form due to disruption of vessel walls from the shock wave of the projectile; facial-orbital entrance wounds have the highest incidence. The aneurysms have an unpredictable course; most that rupture do so in the first month. The prognosis for survival after missile injuries is good if consciousness is preserved and poor if coma is present from the outset.

Other intracranial foreign bodies from knives, picks, studguns, or high-speed tool bits may be missed unless skull x-rays are taken after minor penetrating injuries. Surgical removal, debridement, and extensive exploration for hemorrhage and necrotic tissue is required. Simply removing a protruding object is not sufficient.

TRAUMATIC VASCULAR OCCLUSION AND DISSECTION Minor, sometimes unnoticed, neck trauma can produce dissection (stripping of the intima or the media) of the internal carotid or vertebral arteries. Chiropractic neck manipulation accounts for some cases. Severe blunt trauma to the neck can initiate a dissection several centimeters above the origin of the internal carotid artery. In awake patients there is usually local neck pain over the internal carotid artery, a Horner's syndrome, and headache over the ipsilateral anterior cranium. Some patients with carotid dissection subsequently have large middle cerebral artery strokes with hemiplegia, visual field and sensory deficits, and if the dominant hemisphere is affected, aphasia. In drowsy or comatose patients evidence of dissection or subsequent stroke is difficult to discern but is suggested by unexplained hemiplegia, unilateral miosis, or the appearance of cerebral infarction on CT scan. Angiography demonstrates either the typical "string sign" characterized by an elongated narrowed lumen extending over 5 to 10 cm, or complete occlusion of the carotid artery beginning several centimeters distal to the bifurcation, sometimes accompanied by a distal embolus in the middle cerebral artery. On rare occasion, basilar skull fractures cause carotid dissection beginning at the point of entry of the artery into the skull. Traumatic "false" aneurysms of the cervical carotid artery result from deep penetrating, and occasionally from nonpenetrating, blunt trauma of the neck. A pulsatile mass and bruit over the artery establish the diagnosis and mandate surgical repair. Traumatic vertebral artery dissection can produce vertigo, vomiting, suboccipital or supraorbital headache, and other signs of lateral medullary ischemia. These symptoms are frequently attributed to vestibular concussion. In drowsy or comatose patients the only indication of vertebral artery occlusion may be inferior cerebellar infarction on CT scan.

Intracranial vascular damage is rare except in penetrating injuries. High-velocity projectiles, as discussed above, disrupt vessel walls, leading to aneurysms of large vessels in the vicinity of the wound, usually a surface branch of the middle cerebral artery. Preexisting saccular aneurysms may rupture after basilar skull fractures, and this diagnosis should be considered if subarachnoid hemorrhage is profuse and inadequately explained by accompanying subdural blood on CT scan. Vasospasm from traumatic subarachnoid blood may be involved in the development of infarction after head injury.

Cavernous sinus arteriovenous fistulas are serious complications in patients surviving severe head injury. They are first evident as a self-audible bruit (many are also audible to the examiner), proptosis, conjunctival injection, or visual impairment. Angiography shows early filling of the cavernous sinus and its draining tributaries. The fistula generally enlarges, causing increasingly severe local changes around the eye and orbit and decreased chances of visual recovery. About 10 percent, mostly small fistulas, resolve spontaneously. Many surgical approaches have been tried including ligation of the carotid artery, direct obliteration of the fistula or cavernous sinus, and angiographic-guided balloon embolization. A detachable balloon technique has proved successful in many cases (see Chap. 348).

INTRACRANIAL PRESSURE AND CEREBRAL BLOOD FLOW

The pathophysiology of intracranial pressure (ICP) regulation and its relationship to cerebral blood flow (CBF), which is applicable to many pathologic processes including cerebral hemorrhage, encephalitis, and brain edema after stroke, is best understood in the context of head trauma. The components of the intracranial compartment are brain, CSF, and blood. Because the skull limits total intracranial content, the volume of these compartments is compromised by expanding lesions within the cranial cavity. The brain is virtually incompressible; therefore CSF and blood serve as the main buffers of increasing intracranial volume. The relationship between increments in intracranial volume and the associated rises in ICP, termed *compliance,* approximates an exponential function after the volume buffering capacity of CSF and blood are exceeded. ICP is normally between 2 and 12 mmHg. Raised ICP in the range 15 to 40 mmHg, while not harmful by itself, can rapidly result in secondary damage, either by precipitously decreasing global cerebral perfusion when ICP exceeds blood pressure in the cranium, or by associated shifts of brain tissue that damage the thalamus and brainstem. The global damage from increased ICP is therefore ischemic in nature and related to the arithmetic difference between ICP and blood pressure in the major cerebral arteries. This difference is termed *cerebral perfusion pressure,* or CPP. Cerebral perfusion pressure below 40 to 60 mmHg is considered detrimental to nerve cells; therapy is therefore directed toward maintaining perfusion above this range. The rationale for keeping CPP even higher (i.e., bringing ICP below 15 to 20 mmHg) is to afford a margin of safety should transient increases in ICP occur. Physiologic changes or medications that increase blood pressure do not necessarily improve CPP because increased vascular pressures exacerbate brain edema in damaged areas and induce plateau waves (see below), resulting in further increases in ICP that ultimately lower perfusion.

The most important secondary complication of head injury is raised intracranial pressure arising from the added volume of contusions, hematomas, and the progressive edema surrounding them. A close relationship exists between clinical outcome and ICP in patients with closed head injury. At least 50 percent of patients who die as a result of head injury do so solely because of uncontrolled rises in ICP, and outcome is inversely related to the level of ICP after acute injury. Aggressive treatment of raised ICP in modern intensive care units is believed to improve survival after severe head injury. The role of direct monitoring of ICP to guide therapy is controversial.

Resting ICP, CPP, and compliance are spontaneously interrupted by rises in ICP termed *plateau waves.* They often are precipitated by iatrogenic maneuvers such as suctioning, physical therapy, excess fluid administration, or pain. Such plateau waves (lasting 1 to 10 min, and ranging from 25 to 60 mmHg) are most pronounced in patients with diminished intracranial compliance. They are best observed on continuous recordings of ICP. Plateau waves are probably due to a loss of cerebrovascular tone with a resultant increase in cerebral blood volume. Signs of apparent transtentorial herniation such as pupillary enlargement may occur after plateau waves (they more often do not), and occasionally brain death ensues. The proximate cause of deterioration is probably a reflex rise in blood pressure, part of the Cushing reflex (hypertension and bradycardia), greatly increasing intracranial blood volume and cerebral edema.

There is little consensus about the importance of alterations in cerebral blood flow caused by head injury. For several minutes to an hour after acute head injury, cerebral blood flow may increase in some patients although metabolic demands and oxygen consumption are diminished. Autoregulation, the ability of the cerebral vasculature to keep blood flow constant in response to decreased or increased perfusion pressure, is also impaired in damaged regions. Vascular factors have been found to account for approximately two-thirds of the rise in ICP after severe head injury. The blood-brain barrier also becomes more permeable after head injury in badly damaged regions, making edema formation more likely.

There is a complex relationship between raised ICP and clinical signs such as coma and pupillary enlargement that accompany supratentorial masses. ICP represents the accommodation of intracranial contents to additional mass; clinical signs are a parallel barometer of tissue shifts, particularly affecting structures around the tentorial opening. Raised ICP per se does not cause signs (including coma) until it reaches levels that preclude cerebral perfusion; it then causes global ischemia in a fashion similar to acute hypotension. Coma and other secondary signs resulting from tissue shifts in the region of the tentorial opening are described in Chap. 31. Horizontal midline shift at the level of the pineal body is closely related to the level of consciousness with acute unilateral mass lesions.

Other secondary phenomena after severe head injury cause brain damage and alter outcome. Hypoxia, for example, is common from a number of causes, and when severe, is associated with a poorer outcome.

CLINICAL SYNDROMES AND TREATMENT OF HEAD INJURY

MINOR INJURY A fully alert and attentive patient presenting after head injury with one or more symptoms of headache, faintness, nausea, a single episode of emesis, difficulty with concentration, or slight blurring of vision has a good prognosis with little risk of subsequent deterioration. Such patients have sustained a concussion or have been dazed, and have a brief amnestic epoch surrounding the moment of impact. Occasionally, vasovagal syncope occurs several minutes to an hour after the injury and causes concern. Constant generalized or frontal headache is common in the days following trauma; it is often throbbing or hemicranial in nature, like migraine. The majority of patients with a minor syndrome do not have a skull fracture on skull x-ray, or hemorrhage on CT scan. The decision to obtain these tests depends largely on the availability of CT or MRI scanning and clinical signs suggesting that the impact was severe (e.g., prolonged concussion, periorbital or mastoid hematoma, repeated vomiting, etc). Children and young adults are particularly prone to drowsiness, vomiting, and irritability, sometimes delayed for several hours after apparently minor injuries. After a period of observation for several hours, arrangements may be made for the patient to be accompanied home to be observed by family or friends.

Persistent severe headache and repeated vomiting in the context of normal alertness and no focal neurologic signs are usually benign, but CT or MRI scanning and/or skull x-rays should be obtained. Skull fractures increase the likelihood of a subdural or epidural hematoma. Patients with these exaggerated signs, even if they follow minor injury, deserve observation in the hospital for 24 h. Clinical judgment, the presence of associated noncranial injuries, the availability of others at home, and the examiner's certainty of a normal neurologic examination should guide the need for further surveillance.

INJURY OF INTERMEDIATE SEVERITY Patients who are not comatose but who have persistent confusion, behavioral changes, less than normal alertness, extreme dizziness, or focal neurologic signs such as hemiparesis should be admitted to the hospital and have a CT scan. The clinical syndromes most common in this group, in addition to postconcussive headache and dizziness, unsteadiness, photophobia, and vomiting of minor injury, include (1) delirium with a disinclination to be examined or moved, expletive speech, and resistance if disturbed, most often associated with anterior temporal lobe contusions; (2) a quiet, disinterested, slowed mental state (abulia) with dull facial appearance and slight irascibility if bothered, the patient lying quietly with eyes closed when undisturbed, seen with inferior and frontopolar frontal contusions (usually without grasp responses); (3) severe memory loss with poor retrograde and anterograde performance, headache, and photophobia, with medial temporal lobe contusions or diffuse injury; (4) a focal deficit such as aphasia or mild hemiparesis (hemianopsia is rare as an isolated posttraumatic finding), suggesting subdural hematoma or convexity contusion; (5) global confusion with inattention, poor performance on simple mental tasks, fluctuating or slightly erroneous orientation, associated with several types of injuries including the first two described above as well as medial frontal contusions and interhemispheric subdural hematoma; (6) repetitive vomiting, nystagmus, drowsiness, and unsteadiness, usually from a labyrinthine concussion, but occasionally due to a posterior fossa subdural hematoma or vertebral artery dissection; (7) drowsiness alone or with muteness, often unassociated with significant CT scan abnormalities; and (8) diabetes insipidus with or without a frontal-temporal lobe syndrome, from damage to median eminence or pituitary stalk and adjacent medial cortex.

The syndromes of intermediate severity are usually preceded by brief loss of consciousness and many are associated with skull fractures. A CT scan is required to exclude surgically remediable subdural or epidural hematomas and to define areas of contusion that later enlarge with edema, or coalesce to form intraparenchymal hemorrhages. Paroxysmal or rhythmic EEG abnormalities, in contrast to acute convulsions, are common over the region of a large contusion. Many intermediate injuries are complicated by drug or alcohol intoxication, making toxic screening important.

Close clinical observation in a well-staffed setting is advisable in order to detect increasing drowsiness, change in respiratory pattern or pupillary enlargement, and to ensure fluid restriction. Fully awake or slightly drowsy patients with small subdural hematomas may be treated with glucocorticoids and fluid restriction; larger clots, especially with fluctuating or worsening alertness, require surgery. Epidural hematomas causing compression of adjacent brain should be evacuated in patients who have a good chance of recovery from other injuries. Free water intake should be limited, allowing serum osmolarity to rise spontaneously toward 290 mosmol/L. Fever must be treated assiduously with antipyretics or a cooling blanket, and its source must be identified (usually aspiration). So-called central fever is rare. The routine, acute administration of phenytoin is controversial. About half of neurosurgeons advocate its use, particularly in children and young adults, in the belief that it may reduce the incidence of posttraumatic epilepsy. Glucocorticoids may be useful if there is a contusion, hemorrhage, or edema on the CT scan; otherwise they complicate management and should be omitted. The possibility of associated cervical spine injuries should be considered in all patients with syndromes of intermediate severity. The neck should be immobilized, and adequate x-rays of the spine should be obtained.

The majority of patients with intermediate injury improve over 1 to 6 weeks. During the first week alertness, irascibility, memory, and mental performance fluctuate. Behavioral changes such as agitation are most evident at night and sometimes seem to be worsened by large doses of glucocorticoids or CNS-depressant drugs. Haloperidol is useful when used sparingly. Subtle abnormalities of intellectual function particularly attention, spontaneity, and memory, tend to return to normal later, and frequently do so abruptly.

SEVERE HEAD INJURY AND COMA Patients who are stuporous or comatose from the outset require immediate neurologic attention and often, resuscitation. There is often pupillary enlargement or asymmetry. Persistent unresponsiveness is a grave sign. After the patient is intubated and the blood pressure is stabilized, attention is given to life-threatening noncranial injuries, followed by a survey neurologic examination.

The possibility of cervical injuries should not be overlooked, and the cervical spine must be immobilized during the initial assessment. The depth of coma and the size of the pupils are most important. Most severely injured patients hyperventilate. Extensor limb posturing and bilateral Babinski signs, combined with apparently purposeful movements, are common. Asymmetry in limb posture, limb movement, or gaze perference suggest a subdural or epidural hematoma or a large contusion.

As soon as vital functions permit and cervical spine x-rays and a CT scan have been obtained, the patient should be taken to a critical care unit. The finding of an epidural or subdural hematoma or large intracerebral hemorrhage are usually indications for surgery and intracranial decompression. In one large series the time between injury and evacuation of acute subdural hematomas was the major determinant of outcome. If such lesions are not present and the patient is still comatose and critically ill, attention is directed toward treating raised ICP. Patients with abnormal CT scans showing contusions, hemorrhages, or tissue shifts are the best candidates for ICP monitoring. The lumbar CSF pressure does not accurately reflect the intracranial pressure and may increase the risk of brain herniation, therefore the practice in most head injury treatment centers is to use one of several devices that is inserted intracranially to measure ICP. The pressure can be monitored continuously, disturbances in compliance and falling CPP can be identified, and appearance of plateau waves can be noted.

The treatment of raised ICP is best guided by direct measurement but may proceed on a presumptive basis using clinical status and CT scan as guides. All potentially exacerbating factors must be eliminated. Hypoxia, hyperthermia, hypercarbia, awkward head positions, and high mean airway pressures from mechanical ventilation all increase cerebral blood volume and ICP. Many, but not all, patients will have lower ICPs when the head and trunk are elevated. If raising the patient's head lowers blood pressure, then cerebral perfusion pressure may be optimal in the supine position. Active management of raised ICP includes induced hypocarbia to an initial level of 28 to 33 mmHg P_{CO_2} and hyperosmolar dehydration with 20% mannitol (0.25 to 1 g/kg every 3 to 6 h), preferably using directly measured ICP as a guide. Otherwise, a serum osmolality of 305 to 315 mosmol/L is desirable, as is ventricular or subarachnoid fluid drainage when it is possible.

Persistently raised ICP after inception of this conservative therapy generally indicates a poor outcome, but the addition of high-dose barbiturates may further lower ICP and salvage a small number of patients. In many instances barbiturates cause a parallel reduction in ICP and blood pressure without resulting in net improvement in cerebral perfusion. The beneficial effects of barbiturates, aside from their sedative and anticonvulsant activities, are not established, and they can cause disastrous hypotension so that their routine use in severe head injury remains controversial. Further details of treatment of raised ICP are given in Chap. 31. Systolic blood pressure should be maintained above 100 mmHg by vasopressor agents, if necessary, but when pressors are required to support barbiturate use, there is usually little improvement in CPP. Mean blood pressure levels above 110 to 120 mmHg may exaggerate brain edema and are associated with plateau waves; hypertension may be treated with diuretics and beta-adrenergic blocking agents, or intermittent doses of barbiturates. A number of other antihypertensive drugs, including some calcium-channel blockers, are relatively contraindicated because they may lower blood pressure while leaving ICP unchanged, or raising it. Fluid and electrolytes must be administered cautiously, and free water administration should be limited. Administration of phenytoin or phenobarbital to prevent seizures is recommended by many neurosurgeons. Hourly antacids by nasogastric tube to keep gastric pH above 3.5, and administration of sucralfate or cimetidine are used to prevent gastrointestinal bleeding. The use of large doses of glucocorticoids in severe head injury has not been shown to improve outcome. Several recent studies suggest that early nutritional support results in earlier neurologic recovery from head injury. If the patient remains comatose, it is worthwhile to repeat the CT scan to exclude a delayed surface or intracerebral hemorrhage. Intensive care salvages some critically ill head-injured patients by concentrating efforts on simple treatments that avoid medical complications, particularly pneumonia and sepsis, and preventable increases in ICP. Whether more assiduous control of ICP and CPP will produce better results remains to be proved.

ASSOCIATED DERANGEMENTS OCCURRING WITH SEVERE HEAD TRAUMA Injuries outside the cranium should be searched for at the outset, because they are likely to be forgotten if not initially noted. In particular, associated spinal, long bone, and abdominal injuries may cause delayed difficulties in management. However, secondary medical complications dominate the intermediate-term intensive care of head trauma patients.

Fluids and electrolytes Over half of patients who persist in coma for 24 h after head injury develop abnormalities of electrolytes or fluid balance. Frequently these are a consequence of therapy, but the metabolic responses to head trauma are similar to those produced by trauma elsewhere and are important in planning treatment. Daily input-output records and body weights, when possible, are important in management. Water restriction and osmotic agents render most patients hyperosmolar and hypovolemic, requiring monitoring of serum osmolality and sodium concentrations. Diabetes insipidus should be suspected if urine output increases and urine specific gravity is low. Replacement of water losses suffices for mild cases, but vasopressin may be required in persistent cases. Serum osmolality above approximately 325 mosmol/L should be avoided because of the associated decrease in cardiac output.

Aldosterone and antidiuretic hormone (ADH) secretion in response to stress favor sodium and free water retention, respectively. The latter usually predominates, leading to mild hypervolemic hyponatremia in untreated patients, but is obscured by concomitant administration of osmotic agents. Severe hyponatremia results from excessive ADH secretion, which may occur with raised ICP, basilar skull fractures, and after prolonged mechanical ventilation. Potassium is lost in head injury because of trauma-induced aldosterone hypersecretion, therapeutic osmotic diuresis, and glucocorticoids. Because potassium is predominantly an intracellular ion, hypokalemia is frequently manifested as a hypochloremic alkalosis with normal or minimally depressed serum potassium and requires adequate replacement therapy with KCl.

Respiratory complications Some patients with head injuries have hypoxia acutely after injury without obvious pulmonary infiltrates. Aspiration pneumonia presents a great risk; acid burn injury from aspirated gastric contents, infection, and atelectasis may combine to produce the adult respiratory distress syndrome (ARDS) and severe arteriovenous shunting. Some evidence suggests that agents that coat the gastric lining without reducing pH, such as sucralfate, are associated with less aspiration pneumonia than are conventional prophylactic agents for gastric bleeding. ARDS can also occur due to disseminated intravascular coagulopathy, fat embolism, or rarely "neurogenic" pulmonary edema. Treatment is similar to other cases of ARDS with positive end-expiratory pressure (PEEP) to allow lowered inspired oxygen concentrations and to prevent further atelectasis. The effect of PEEP on ICP is complex, but PEEP should not be withheld if necessary for oxygenation.

Atelectasis is common in all poorly responsive patients and is treated with chest physical therapy and adequate ventilator tidal volumes. Pulmonary embolism is also a major threat to bedridden patients, and intermittent pneumatic calf compression or modest doses of subcutaneous heparin may be useful prophylaxis. The latter has not predisposed to intracerebral or gastrointestinal bleeding. Early recognition of deep leg vein thrombosis and aggressive treatment by occlusion of the inferior vena cava may prevent later emboli.

Gastrointestinal hemorrhage The majority of patients with severe head injuries develop gastric erosions, but only a few have clinically significant hemorrhages. Gastrointestinal bleeding usually occurs in the first days to 1 week. Unlike most patients in shock or with stress ulceration, head-trauma patients often have elevated gastric acidity. The synergistic effect of glucocorticoids in causing upper tract hemorrhage has been questioned, but the incidence of viscus perforation, particularly of the cecum, is elevated. Prophylactic treatment with gastric coating agents, as discussed above, with cimetidine, or with frequent antacid administration to keep gastric pH high (above 3.5) reduces gastric hemorrhage in other stress states and is commonly used in head trauma.

Fat embolism Patients with severe long bone injuries are subject to widespread cerebral fat embolism. This complication is seen less often than previously, perhaps due to better fluid replacement. In the typical case, head injury is a minor part of the overall trauma; in a few, severe cranial injury masks the syndrome. Several days after the bone fractures, restlessness, delirium, or drowsiness progressing to coma in severe cases, seizures, generalized brain edema, and hypoxia develop. About half have retinal and conjunctival punctate hemorrhages or visible fat in retinal vessels. A petechial rash, prominent in the anterior axillary folds and supraclavicular fossae, diffuse interstitial infiltrates on the chest x-ray, fat in the urine, or renal failure occur in some patients. Severe reduction in arterial oxygen content is common from widespread lung injury (ARDS). Cerebral fat embolism causes cerebral purpura, mainly in the white matter, due to capillary occlusion by fat globules. There is evidence that cases recognized and treated early have a better prognosis. Massive doses of glucocorticoids, reduction of ICP, and administration of positive-pressure ventilation with high end-expiratory pressures have been claimed to be useful. Heparin or intravenous alcohol are no longer recommended.

Cardiovascular changes Acute head trauma may cause transient apnea and cardiac arrest. In the absence of overwhelming brain damage recovery from the arrest is the rule. Subsequently, raised ICP may cause systemic hypertension, either with the classically associated bradycardia (Cushing response) or, almost as frequently, with tachycardia. Cardiac arrhythmias are common, most notably sinus bradycardia, supraventricular tachycardias, nodal rhythm, and heart block. T-wave inversion and alterations in the ST segment may simulate subendocardial ischemia.

Neurogenic pulmonary edema is a form of ARDS in which the alveoli fill with fluid as they would in congestive heart failure but left ventricular end-diastolic pressure (measured by pulmonary capillary wedge pressure) is normal. A pulmonary vascular leak may be produced when a sudden shift of intravascular volume occurs from the systemic to pulmonary circulation, as occurs transiently with suddenly raised ICP. Once the pulmonary vasculature has been damaged, an alveolar capillary leak may continue despite return of blood pressure to normal. The result is pulmonary edema with normal central venous and wedge pressures after the initial injury.

Hematologic complications A large number of patients demonstrate a mild coagulopathy, and 5 to 10 percent have various degrees of disseminated intravascular coagulation. A correlation may exist between the severity of injury and the level of increased fibrin degradation products in blood. The cause of the coagulopathy is thought to be the release of highly thromboplastic material into the systemic circulation from the damaged brain.

PROGNOSIS Extensive work by Jennet's group in Glasgow and others has provided data on the outcome in severe head injury (Table 352-1). Verbal output, eye opening, and the best motor response are important predictors of ultimate outcome. Eighty-five percent of patients with aggregate Glasgow Coma Scale scores of 3 or 4 die 24 h after injury. Yet a number of patients with a poor initial prognosis, including absent pupillary light responses, survive, suggesting that aggressive management is justified in virtually all patients. Patients below approximately 20 years of age, particularly children, may make remarkable recoveries after grave early neurologic signs. In one large study of severe head injury, 55 percent of children had a good outcome at 1 year, compared to 21 percent of adults.

Evoked potentials have prognostic value in head injury, and their accuracy probably exceeds clinical observations and ICP measurements. Somatosensory evoked potentials are the most useful, with bilaterally absent cortical potentials (with more caudal potentials present) being predictive of death or a vegetative state in 85 to 95 percent of patients. Prediction of a good functional outcome in the presence of normal or mildly abnormal tests is less certain.

TABLE 352-1 Glasgow Coma Scale for head injury

Eye opening (E):	
Spontaneous	4
To loud voice	3
To pain	2
Nil	1
Best motor response (M):	
Obeys	6
Localizes	5
Withdraws (flexion)	4
Abnormal flexion posturing	3
Extension posturing	2
Nil	1
Verbal response (V):	
Oriented	5
Confused, disoriented	4
Inappropriate words	3
Incomprehensible sounds	2
Nil	1

NOTE: Coma score = E + M + V. Patients scoring 3 or 4 have an 85 percent chance of dying or remaining vegetative, while scores above 11 indicate 5 to 10 percent likelihood of death or vegetative state and 85 percent chance of moderate disability or good recovery. Intermediate scores correlate with proportional chances of patients recovering.

SPINAL CORD TRAUMA

Approximately 10,000 patients a year in the United States, mostly young and otherwise healthy, become paraplegic or quadriplegic because of spinal cord injuries. There are an estimated 200,000 quadriplegics in the country. The majority of cord injuries in civilian life result from damage to the surrounding vertebral column, from fracture, dislocation, or both. Vertical compression with flexion is the main mechanism of injury in the thoracic cord, and hyperextension or flexion is the main cause of injury in the cervical cord. Preexisting spondylosis, a congenitally narrowed spinal canal, hypertrophied ligamentum flavum (see Chap. 361), or instability of the apophyseal joints of adjacent vertebrae from diseases such as rheumatoid arthritis, predispose to severe spinal cord damage after minor degrees of injury.

PATHOPHYSIOLOGY AND PATHOLOGY OF CORD INJURY

Much damage to the spinal cord is due to secondary phenomena in the minutes and hours following injury. Even when a complete transverse myelopathy is evident immediately after impact, some secondary changes are avoidable, and the resultant damage may be reversible. The immediate injury causes pericapillary hemorrhages that coalesce and enlarge, particularly in the gray matter. Infarction of gray matter and early white matter edema are evident within 4 h of experimental blunt injury. Eight hours after injury there is global infarction at the injured level, and only at this point does necrosis of white matter and paralysis below the level of the lesion become irreversible. The necrosis and central hemorrhages enlarge to occupy one or two levels above, and below, the point of primary impact. Gliosis in these regions results in necrotic areas over several months and may cavitate causing a progressive syringomyelic syndrome.

The early phases of injury are associated with reduced regional blood flow from direct capillary damage and a more prolonged secondary ischemia. A number of interventions including opiate antagonists, thyrotropin-releasing hormone, local cord cooling, dextran infusion, adrenergic blockade, glucocorticoids, and hyperbaric oxygen are of uncertain clinical usefulness. More importantly, the critical factor for recoverable function is the time from injury to institution of therapy. Complete axonal disruption from the immediate trauma or secondary phenomena precludes recovery.

TYPES OF SPINAL CORD INJURY AND THEIR MANAGEMENT

Any patient with severe head injury potentially has an associated instability of the spinal column. The care of such patients begins at the scene of the accident. The neck should be immobilized to prevent cord damage, and care should be taken during transport and during the physical and radiologic examinations to avoid neck extension or rotation and to prevent torsion-rotation of the thoracic spine. Blood pressure, respiratory status, and systemic injuries are attended to rapidly. Most patients can be intubated, if necessary, by blind nasotracheal technique without neck extension. High thoracic or cervical cord trauma regularly cause mild hypotension and bradycardia because of functional sympathectomy (often corroborated by bilateral ptosis and miosis—Horner's syndrome) that responds to infusion of crystalloid or colloid.

The neurologic examination in the awake patient focuses on neck or back pain, diminished limb power, a sensory level on the trunk, and deep tendon reflexes, usually absent below the level of an acute cord injury. Injuries above C5 cause quadriplegia and respiratory failure. At C5 and C6 the biceps are also weak, and at C4 and C5 the deltoid and supra- and infraspinatus are weak. C7 injuries cause weakness of the triceps, wrist extensors, and forearm pronators. Injuries at T1 and below cause paraplegia; the precise level can be determined from the level of sensory loss. Compression in the low thoracic and lumbar region causes a conus medullaris or cauda equina syndrome (see Chap. 361). Cauda equina injuries are usually incomplete, involving peripheral nerves rather than spinal cord, and therefore are surgically remediable for longer periods after injury than spinal cord compression. In a comatose patient absent reflexes should be sought in the legs, or in all the extremities, associated in the latter case with small pupils or paradoxical breathing from high cervical cord injury.

The next priority is to exclude a surgically remediable and potentially reversible cord compression due to dislocation of a vertebral body. Many traumatic myelopathies have no clearly associated fracture or dislocation. If x-rays suggest any aberration in the position of vertebrae, then reduction should be quickly undertaken. The role of myelography is controversial, but many neurosurgeons instill a few drops of Pantopaque into the spinal subarachnoid space to demonstrate a block to the flow of CSF. At present, examination by CT and MRI are more useful. Decompression within 2 h of severe injury may lead to some recovery of cord function. With incomplete myelopathies, especially if the limbs are becoming progressively weaker, early decompression is strongly recommended, even many hours after injury. Surgical approaches to decompressing the spinal column depend upon the specific nature of the injury. In complete transverse myelopathies beyond 6 to 12 h in duration, decompressive laminectomies are usually unsuccessful in restoring function.

The concerns with spinal column fractures, with or without myelopathy, are threefold: (1) detection of vertebral dislocations causing cord compression, (2) instability caused by fractures that will lead to misalignment and cord compression in the future, and (3) the proper treatment of fractures through the pedicles, facets, or vertebral bodies. Some fractures heal with immobilizaton and time, usually 2 to 3 months; others require surgical fusion to ensure stability.

Atlantoaxial dislocations can cause immediate death from respiratory failure, an event that may occur with no neurologic signs. Rheumatoid arthritis predisposes to this injury. Atlantooccipital dislocations occur predominantly in children and are almost always fatal. "Jefferson's fractures" are burst fractures of the ring of the atlas resulting from a force descending on the vertex of the skull as in diving accidents; they are usually asymptomatic. "Hangman's fractures" are produced by hyperextension and longitudinal distraction of the upper cervical spine, as occurs with penal hanging or striking the chin on a steering wheel in head-on collisions. These are usually fractures through the pedicles of C2 with subluxation anteriorly of C2 on C3. Traction reduction and immobilization allow proper healing.

Hyperflexion dislocation of the cervical vertebrae commonly causes traumatic quadriplegia. Occasionally, a markedly displaced injury is unassociated with neurologic dysfunction, presenting only with neck pain. In most cases, however, minor subluxation is associated with a severe neurologic deficit. Ligamentous disruption presumably allows compression of the cord at the moment of impact, but the vertebral bodies return closer to their original stations afterward. Therefore, any degree of subluxation must be treated as potentially unstable.

Compression fractures of the cervical spine can cause neurologic damage if a bone fragment is driven backward (burst fracture) into the spinal cord. "Teardrop fractures" with crushing of a vertebral body, leaving a fragment of bone anteriorly, are usually associated with ligamentous disruption and spinal instability. Single compression fractures of the thoracic spine are usually stable because the thoracic cage provides support, but they may be associated with anterior cord compression and require decompression and stabilization with the insertion of metal rods.

Mild hyperextension injuries may cause only disruption of supporting ligamentous structures and be well tolerated. More severe injuries cause vertebral displacement and cord compression. The "central cord syndrome" is produced by brief compression of the cord and disruption of the central gray matter usually occurring in patients with an already narrow spinal canal, either congenitally or from cervical spondylosis. There is weakness of the arms, often with pinprick loss over the arms and shoulders, and relative sparing of leg power and sensation on the trunk and legs. Abnormality of bladder function is variable. The prognosis for recovery is good.

Thoracolumbar fractures are produced by impact in the high or midback, usually while the patient is bent over. Impingement on the spinal canal results in a complex combination of cauda equina and conus medullaris dysfunction. Pure lumbar fractures produce cauda equina compression. Myelography, MRI, or CT scan allows precise localization, and surgical decompression is usually recommended, even with complete deficits, because the potential for recovery of peripheral nerves is great.

The subsequent care of patients with spinal cord injury is best undertaken in specialized centers. General principles of medical and urologic management are discussed in Chap. 361.

REFERENCES

ADAMS JH et al: Diffuse brain damage of the immediate impact type. Brain 100:489, 1977

BAKAY L, GLASSAUER FE: *Head Injury*. Boston, Little, Brown, 1980

BECKER DP et al: Outcome from severe head injury with early diagnosis and intensive management. J Neurosurg 47:491, 1977

DACEY RG et al: Neurosurgical complications after apparently minor head injury. J Neurosurg 65:203, 1986

EISENBERG HM et al: High-dose barbiturate control of elevated intracranial pressure in patients with severe head injury. J Neurosurg 69:15, 1988

GOLDSTEIN M: Traumatic brain injury: A silent epidemic. Ann Neurol 27:327, 1990

JENNET B et al: Predicting outcome in individual patients after head injury. Lancet 1:1081, 1976

LANGFITT TW, GENARELLI TA: Can the outcome from head injury be improved? J Neurosurg 56:19, 1982

LEVIN HS et al: Neurobehavioral outcome following minor head injury: A three center study. J Neurosurg 66:234, 1987

MARSHALL LF et al: The outcome with aggressive treatment in severe head injury. I: The significance of intracranial pressure monitoring. II: Acute and chronic barbiturate administration in the management of head injury. J Neurosurg 50:20, 1979

ROPPER AH et al (eds): *Neurological and Neurosurgical Intensive Care*, 2d ed. Baltimore, Aspen, 1988

353 NEOPLASTIC DISEASES OF THE CENTRAL NERVOUS SYSTEM

FRED HOCHBERG / AMY PRUITT

Tumors of the brain, of its meningeal coverings, and of the spinal cord are estimated to cause the death of 90,000 patients in the United States each year. Of these tumors, more than three-quarters are *secondary* metastases arising in patients undergoing treatment for systemic cancer. *Primary* tumors arising within the meninges or the parenchyma of the brain or spinal cord are common at all ages of life. Brain neoplasms claim a disproportionate share of hospital beds, diagnostic tests, and other medical resources. One-fourth of the annual $4 billion cost for care of cancer patients in the United States is allocated to patients with neoplasms of the central nervous system.

Although the specialized care of such patients is usually delegated to the neurosurgeon, radiotherapist, or neurooncologist, with the advent of new imaging techniques the internist is increasingly involved in the initial diagnosis. Late in the course of the disease, such patients again may come under the care of a general physician. The proper care of patients with primary or metastatic tumors of the central nervous system requires a systematic approach that enables the physician to (1) distinguish tumor from other causes of neurologic dysfunction such as infection, metabolic derangement, pseudotumor cerebri, or subdural hematoma; (2) make proper use of sophisticated diagnostic techniques such as magnetic resonance imaging (MRI), computed tomography (CT), and of more invasive tests such as arteriography; (3) provide early therapy to control cerebral edema and avoid seizure activity; (4) exclude systemic malignancy prior to referring the patient for a biopsy; and (5) recognize the medical complications of the tumor and of its therapy.

APPROACH TO THE PATIENT WITH CENTRAL NERVOUS SYSTEM TUMORS

CLASSIFICATION OF TUMORS Tumors of the CNS may originate in the brain or spinal cord (primary tumors) or may spread from systemic sites of cancer (metastatic tumors). Both benign and malignant primary CNS tumors are capable of producing neurologic impairment. Primary tumors arise from glial cells (astrocytoma, oligodendroglioma, glioblastoma), ependymal cells (ependymoma), or supporting tissue (meningioma, schwannoma, papilloma of the choroid plexus). In childhood, tumors arise from more primitive cells (medulloblastoma, neuroblastoma, chordoma). Malignant astrocytoma or glioblastoma is the most common type of primary tumor in adults over age 20. A classification of intracranial tumors is given in Table 353-1.

CLINICAL MANIFESTATIONS OF INTRACRANIAL TUMOR Intracranial tumors may be located within the brain substance (intraaxial) or in close proximity to the brain (extraaxial). The latter produce symptoms by compression or infiltration of brain. Many of the symptoms caused by intracranial masses reflect tumor expansion within a fixed bony vault into space normally occupied by brain, blood, and cerebrospinal fluid (CSF). The nature and severity of these symptoms depend on the location of the tumor and the rate of its growth. Although brain tissue can accommodate the presence of slowly growing tumors, masses larger than 3 cm in diameter compress the brain, its blood supply, and CSF pathways. This compression is increased by peritumoral edema (vasogenic cerebral edema). Neurologic deterioration occurs as the tumor infiltrates or displaces normal brain structures; as the tumor develops areas of hemorrhage, necrosis, or cyst formation; or as the tumor obstructs the normal flow of CSF, producing hydrocephalus.

Papilledema, or choking of the optic nerve head, emerges in the setting of impaired retinal venous return or axoplasmic flow along the optic nerve. Increasing intracranial pressure caused by a mass in one hemisphere may displace the medial temporal lobe (uncus) through the tentorial notch. As the uncus is forced inferiorly (*uncal herniation*) the midbrain is displaced and the third cranial nerve is compressed. The clinical signs of a unilateral third-nerve palsy—fixed, dilated pupil followed shortly thereafter by depression of consciousness, dilation of the opposite pupil, and hemiparesis on the opposite side of the original pupillary abnormality—should alert the physician to uncal herniation. A mass located more centrally in the supratentorial region produces a less specific picture called *central herniation*. In this situation the patient develops depression of consciousness as supratentorial structures compress the diencephalon and upper midbrain. Cheyne-Stokes respiration develops, but there is preservation of pupillary activity until late in the course of the deterioration (see Chap. 31).

Cerebellar masses may cause the cerebellar tonsils to herniate into the foramen magnum. As the tonsils are pushed inferiorly, the medulla and portions of the cervical spinal cord are compressed or infarcted.

TABLE 353-1 Classification of intracranial tumors

Type of tumor	Percent of total	
Glioma:	40	
Glioblastoma		20
Astrocytoma grades I and II		10
Ependymoma		6
Medulloblastoma		2
Oligodendroglioma		1
Papilloma of choroid plexus		1
Metastases	23	
Meningioma	17	
Pituitary adenoma	5	
Schwannoma	5	
Lymphoma	3	
Miscellaneous (congenital tumors, PNETs*)	7	

* Primitive neuroectodermal tumors.

Abnormalities of cardiovascular regulation ensue. The resulting bradycardia and hypertension are followed by irregularity or cessation of respiration. Posterior fossa lesions of small size may produce early hydrocephalus by obstruction of CSF flow at the level of the fourth ventricle or aqueduct of Sylvius.

Symptoms of intracranial tumor may develop in patients with previously diagnosed systemic cancer or in those not known to harbor a malignancy. Patients with intracranial tumor usually present with one or more of the following groups of symptoms: (1) headache with or without evidence of increased intracranial pressure; (2) progressive generalized decline in cognitive abilities or impairment of specific neurologic functions affecting speech and language, gait, or memory; (3) adult-onset seizures or increased frequency or severity of previously documented seizure activity; or (4) focal neurologic symptoms reflecting the particular anatomic site of the tumor, such as those caused by acoustic schwannoma (neuroma) in the cerebellopontine angle or by meningioma of the olfactory groove, sella, or parasellar areas.

Headache is the initial symptom in half of patients with brain tumors. Traction on the dura, blood vessels, or cranial nerves results from local compression, elevation of intracranial pressure, edema, or hydrocephalus. In most patients with supratentorial tumor, pain radiates to the side of the tumor mass, whereas patients with posterior fossa masses describe retroorbital, retroauricular, or occipital pain. Emesis or hiccups, often without nausea, signals development of increased intracranial pressure and is especially common in patients with masses located beneath the tentorium.

Tumors of the frontal lobes may attain considerable size before symptoms develop, and then symptoms often are nonspecific. Subtle, progressive disturbances of mentation, slowness of comprehension, loss of acuity in business affairs, memory disorders, or apathy, lethargy, and drowsiness may be reported. Spontaneity of thought and activity is lost. Incontinence of urine and disordered gait may be seen by family members. The development of a true dysphasia and/or motor weakness signal progression of the tumor or its associated edema into motor cortex and speech areas of the frontoparietal region.

Masses in the temporal lobes are associated with personality changes that may resemble affective or psychotic thought disorders. Various combinations of auditory hallucinations, abrupt shifts in mood, and altered sleep, appetite, and sexual functions are soon interspersed with complex partial seizures possibly accompanied by visual field defects in the superior quadrants contralateral to the tumor.

Disorders of communication and vision characterize parietooccipital masses. Receptive aphasia with contralateral hemianopsia characterizes left parietal tumors, while a combination of spatial disorientation, constructional apraxia, and left homonymous hemianopsia bespeaks right parietal tumors.

Tumors of the diencephalon often present with a combination of failure of pupillary constriction to light, failure of upward gaze, and neuroendocrine abnormalities. Hydrocephalus due to obstruction to CSF flow at the level of the third ventricle leads to headache. Syndromes suggesting tumors of diencephalon or posterior fossa origin are more fully discussed in the section of this chapter devoted to neoplasms of these regions.

Cerebellar and brainstem lesions lead to a combination of cranial nerve palsies and incoordination of limbs or gait with or without accompanying signs of hydrocephalus. (See Chap. 360 for discussion of cranial nerve symptoms and signs.)

Seizures occur as the initial symptom in 20 percent of patients with brain tumors. Patients with new onset of epilepsy after the age of 35 must be evaluated for brain tumor. Similar high-risk groups of new seizure patients include those with previously diagnosed systemic cancer, longstanding neurologic diseases (including such neuroectodermal disorders as von Recklinghausen's disease and tuberous sclerosis), or acute or atypical psychiatric disorders. A carefully obtained history may uncover disordered time perceptions (déjà vu or déjà jamais), paroxysms of fear, and clinging "viscous" personality changes in addition to obvious features such as "complex partial" (temporal lobe) seizures or personality changes that antedate the diagnosis by years. Occasionally, the first symptom simulates a transient ischemic attack with no residual deficit or discernible seizure, but more commonly the pattern of clinical seizures provides localizing information. Thus, the "Jacksonian march" of tonic-clonic seizure points to frontal tumors and a sensory march characterizes tumors of the sensory parietal cortex. Metastatic tumors, occupying the junction of gray and white matter, are more likely than are primary tumors to produce acute symptoms evolving in days to weeks. Even more rapid onset of symptoms reflects hemorrhage in tumors of lung, melanoma, renal cell, choriocarcinoma, or thyroid origins. In contrast, with the exception of oligodendroglioma and malignant astrocytoma, primary brain tumors are unlikely to hemorrhage.

PHYSICAL EXAMINATION OF THE PATIENT WITH SUSPECTED CNS TUMORS When the physician examines a brain tumor suspect who is not previously known to have a systemic cancer, the general examination should include (1) a survey of the skin for stigmata of neurocutaneous syndromes or melanoma, (2) a search for enlarged lymph nodes, (3) an examination of the abdomen for hepatic or splenic enlargement, (4) a rectal examination with stool guaiac test, (5) a breast and pelvic examination in female patients, and (6) a cardiopulmonary examination.

The neurologic examination of the patient with suspected brain tumor should focus first on an evaluation of the mental status. The examiner should look for evidence of specific localizing cognitive deficits, such as dysphasia, dyspraxia, or memory loss, in addition to gleaning a sense of any personality change which has occurred. The patient is examined for increased intracranial pressure (papilledema or sixth cranial nerve paresis) and for other cranial nerve abnormalities. Asymmetries of strength, sensation, visual fields, and reflex activity should be sought. Attention should be paid to the constellation of signs suggestive of tumors in specific supratentorial, diencephalic or posterior fossa sites (see above). Combinations of cranial nerve abnormalities and corticospinal or lumbosacral radicular signs raise suspicion of leptomeningeal metastases (see below).

INVESTIGATION OF THE PATIENT WITH INTRACRANIAL TUMOR Advances in neuroradiology have contributed greatly to the diagnosis and management of patients with suspected neoplastic disease of the CNS. A plan for appropriate diagnostic studies based on the initial MRI or CT scan results is outlined in Table 353-2. The language of neurooncology differs from that of medical oncology, familiar terms such as "benign," "malignant," and "metastasizing" taking on different connotations when the tumor involves the CNS. Benign and malignant tumors are not differentiated in the scheme of Table 353-2 because the initial clinical approach is identical. Although many primary CNS tumors exhibit microscopic characteristics classifiable as "benign" because they are well-differentiated histologically and grow slowly, they are, nevertheless, incurable. Tumors of identical histology may have very different prognoses, depending upon their location and amenability to resection. Secondary CNS tumors are malignant in the conventional sense, since they represent metastases and invade normal tissue. Both benign and malignant tumors may produce profound, irreversible neurologic impairment. Primary brain tumors, with rare exceptions, do not metastasize outside the CNS; however, virtually all primary brain tumors are capable of diffuse seeding to the leptomeninges. Thus, the approach to *all* intracranial tumors, summarized in Table 353-2, relies on the clinical history and physical examination and on information provided by MRI scan and CT.

The laboratory evaluation of intracranial tumors MRI and contrast-enhanced CT scanning have now largely replaced the combination of skull x-ray, electroencephalogram, radionuclide brain scan, and arteriography as the principal tests for the evaluation of patients with suspected brain tumor.

MAGNETIC RESONANCE IMAGING (MRI) MRI is the procedure of choice for the evaluation of neurologic dysfunction in a patient suspected of having cancer. MRI delineates most metastatic and

TABLE 353-2 Evaluation following MRI or CT scan of the patient with suspected neoplastic disease of the brain and spinal cord

CT/MRI result	Possible diagnosis	Pretreatment evaluation	Primary treatment	Secondary treatment
KNOWN SYSTEMIC CANCER: BRAIN				
Normal				
No focal deficits on examination	Infection, metabolic abnormality	Lumbar puncture, exclude infection or metabolic problem	See text	———
Focal deficits on examination	Vascular disease, carcinomatous meningitis, seizure, paraneoplastic syndrome, complications of therapy	Lumbar puncture, follow-up MRI 4–6 weeks, gadolinium MRI	See text	Glucocorticoids as needed
Solitary mass	Radioresistant or radiosensitive tumor, unrelated tumor	MRI (Gd-DTPA)*, metastatic evaluation, surgical opinion	Glucocorticoids, radiation if radiosensitive tumor or active systemic disease found	Glucocorticoids as needed
Multiple masses	Metastases	None	Glucocorticoids, radiation	Glucocorticoids as needed, radiation, chemotherapy as indicated
NO KNOWN SYSTEMIC CANCER: BRAIN				
Normal	No disease	Repeat MRI (Gd-DTPA) in 8–12 weeks if symptoms persist		———
Solitary mass	Neoplastic disease, primary or secondary tumor, benign or malignant tumor	Metastatic evaluation, surgical opinion, MRI (Gd-DTPA)	Glucocorticoids, biopsy, radiation	Glucocorticoids as needed
Multiple masses	Neoplastic disease, primary or secondary tumor	Metastatic evaluation	Glucocorticoids and radiation if systemic tumor identified Glucocorticoids, biopsy, and radiation if no systemic tumor is found	See text
KNOWN SYSTEMIC CANCER: SPINAL CORD				
Normal	Nonneoplastic disease Carcinomatous meningitis Paraneoplastic	CSF analysis CSF cytology CT/myelogram	See text	See text
Abnormal	Metastases vs. tumor vs. nonneoplastic	CSF cytology, CT/myelogram, metastatic evaluation, surgical opinion	Glucocorticoids, chemotherapy (meningeal disease), Radiation	See text
NO KNOWN SYSTEMIC CANCER: SPINAL CORD				
Normal	No disease	Further evaluation in 8–12 weeks if symptoms persist (EMG)	See text	
Abnormal	Metastases vs. primary tumor vs. nonneoplastic	Metastatic evaluation, CSF analysis and cytology, angiography, CT/myelogram, MRI (Gd-DTPA)	See text	———

* Gd-DTPA = gadolinium diethylenetriamine pentaacetic acid.

primary tumors of the nervous system (see also Chap. 348). Lesions of the skull base and those in the brainstem, cerebellum, and spinal cord are visualized with greater detail with MRI than with CT, myelographic, or radionuclide images (Fig. 353-1). In addition to great sensitivity and delineation of anatomic detail, MRI offers the advantages of requiring no radiation exposure or administration of contrast material. The "flow-void" characteristic of MRI images provides a measure of tumor vascularity and may be reconstructed to create an MRI angiogram that often removes the need for preoperative arteriography. Hemorrhage, seen in metastatic melanoma and glioblastoma, is easily identified as hemoglobin products or as ferritin. Tumors which contain fat (epidermoid, lipoma, craniopharyngioma) are recognized by their "bright" T2 signals as are those growths with cysts containing high concentrations of protein. The interpretation of MRI abnormalities can be very vexing, however. Many patients harbor unexplained white matter abnormalities ("unidentified bright objects," or UBOs) in close proximity to the ventricular system. Extensive areas of T2 signal abnormality on MRI are not clearly correlated with the extent of tumor on CT nor with the histologic tumor margin. These areas, reflecting cerebral edema, infarction, tumor necrosis, and the effects of prior irradiation and surgery, hinder the physician's attempt to use MRI for treatment planning.

Paramagnetic contrast with intravenous gadolinium diethylenetriamine pentaacetic acid (gadolinium DTPA) produces contrast changes in MRI similar to those observed following the use of organic iodides in CT. The combination of paramagnetic agents and higher energy MRI units may provide better separation of tumor from nontumor tissue and better resolution of the spinal cord and brachial plexus. Gadolinium DTPA administration occasionally produces hypotension and nausea or emesis. The agent is cleared through the kidneys and must be used with caution in hepatic failure because of altered iron metabolism. As red cell morphology may be altered, gadolinium DTPA should be used with caution in hemolytic anemia.

CT SCAN Contrast-enhanced CT imaging delineates intracranial masses as small as 0.5 cm in diameter. Certain tumors whose density exceeds that of normal brain parenchyma, including meningioma, melanoma, and primary lymphoma, and tumors with spontaneous hemorrhage can be visualized without contrast enhancement. CT scanning may be better than MRI for definition of meningiomas and other calcium-containing tumors such as oligodendroglioma and pineal region tumors. Tumors commonly appear as homogeneous or ring-

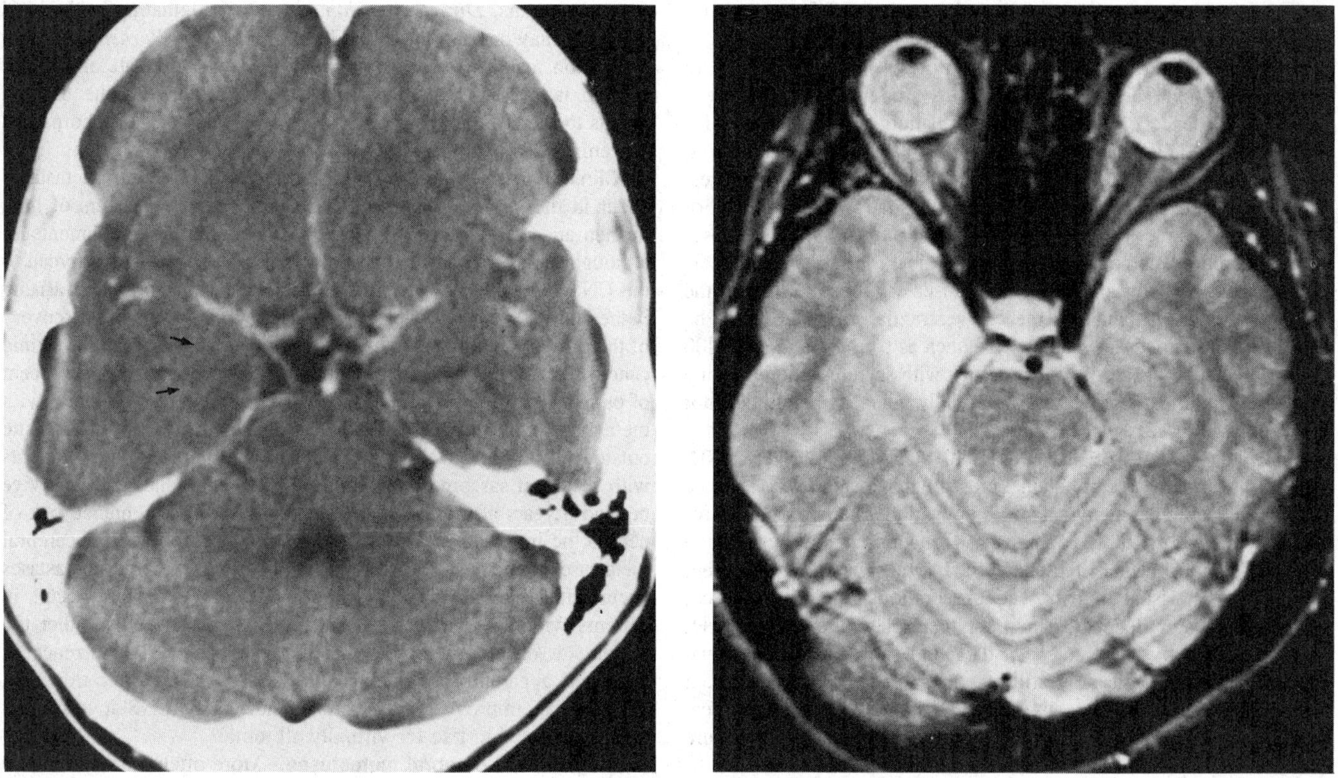

A B

FIGURE 353-1 CT and MRI scans in a 57-year-old woman with a long history of temporal lobe epilepsy. *A.* Contrast-enhanced CT scan showed decreased absorption in the medial left temporal lobe (arrows) with no sign of contrast enhancement. Lesion was present on a CT scan taken 5 years earlier. *B.* Recent T2-weighted image shows a hyperintense circumscribed mass in the same lobe. Biopsy revealed a low-grade astrocytoma.

enhancing masses surrounded by variable amounts of edema. Reconstructions in coronal and sagittal planes and magnification of focal regions allow detection of 95 percent of intracranial masses and definition within 1 cm of the histologic border of the tumor. Although not a substitute for biopsy diagnosis, the CT often correctly predicts the histology of the tumor. Despite MRI advances CT remains the technique of choice for irradiation treatment planning and for the evaluation of the response of brain tumors to therapy.

Initial CT studies may show no abnormality in meningeal carcinomatosis, small metastases, primary brain lymphoma, or some glial tumors that emerge in the setting of chronic seizure activity. Repeat CT scanning, using single or double doses of contrast, 4 to 5 weeks later, usually provides tumor detection. However, if the initial CT scan of a patient with suspected CNS cancer is negative, MRI should be performed. The clinician should be wary of attributing all CT or MRI scan masses to tumor, as ringlike abnormalities may occur in abscesses, in recent cerebral infarction, in the plaques of multiple sclerosis, as a consequence of encephalitis, and in certain vascular malformations with or without hemorrhage. Asymptomatic meningioma and aneurysm are sometimes detected incidentally during evaluation for brain tumors.

Before MRI, brainstem, cerebellar, and spinal cord masses could be further defined by a combination of CT and subarachnoid administration of water-soluble contrast agents. MRI has largely supplanted this procedure except for the delineation of intradural lesions of the spinal cord.

ANGIOGRAPHY Transfemoral arteriography provides selective visualization of internal carotid and vertebral arteries and their branches. Vessels of malignant tumors are characterized by an angiographic "blush" with enlarged early draining veins, features not seen in association with an intracerebral hemorrhage, infarction, or abscess. The identification on MRI of "flow-voids" has diminished the requirement for arteriograms. Preoperative neurosurgical planning is often aided by knowledge of the vascular anatomy or by embolization of excessively vascularized tumors such as meningioma (see Chap. 348).

MANAGEMENT OF INTRACRANIAL TUMORS Surgery: Biopsy and resection Surgical exploration allows tumor identification in patients with either solitary or multiple intracranial masses. Surgical exploration may be necessary to obtain a diagnosis in patients with multiple CT masses in whom a thorough systemic evaluation, including hemogram, liver function studies, carcinoembryonic antigen, chest x-ray, sputum cytology, radionuclide bone and liver scans, and perhaps intravenous pyelography is unrewarding. Of patients with multiple CNS metastatic lesions, 20 percent have no evidence of systemic cancer.

Tumor biopsy is performed through an open craniotomy or with CT-guided stereotaxic techniques. The establishment of a diagnosis is important to determine prognosis and treatment. *Resection* is undertaken and may be curative for some primary tumors such as meningioma, ependymoma, oligodendroglioma, and low-grade astrocytoma (see below) in nondominant, frontal, anterior temporal, or occipital locations or in the ventricular system. *Partial resection* improves patient symptoms, often including better seizure control; by diminishing cerebral edema, it reduces dependence on glucocorticoids. Although resection offers little to patients with multiple intracranial lesions, such as those with brain lymphoma, it may be of value for solitary metastases. Resection of a *solitary tumor* in patients with known systemic cancer may be considered if (1) there is a greater than 2-year interval without known residual systemic malignancy, (2) relief of specific symptoms such as hydrocephalus is required, (3) the tumor is known to be radioresistant as in the case of melanoma, sarcoma, and renal or colonic carcinomas, (4) symptomatic tumor recurs after radiation and (5) the patient's systemic disease is under good control and the cerebral tumor is the limiting factor in quality of survival. For selected patients, this approach offers survival free of neurologic disease of more than 1 year.

Acute treatment of intracranial tumors Clinical evidence of acute or subacute deterioration, such as stupor, focal neurologic signs, or evidence of transtentorial herniation, requires aggressive management. Treatment is directed to reducing cerebral edema, lowering intracranial pressure, and reducing the risk of seizures. Treatment with daily doses of dexamethasone 30 to 60 mg or methylprednisolone 120 to 200 mg in four to six divided doses reduces cerebral edema and associated surgical morbidity. Glucocorticoids may not control symptoms caused by obstruction of the ventricular system, and emergency ventricular drainage may be required. Anticonvulsant medications, such as phenytoin (300 to 400 mg/d), are usually prescribed for patients with seizures, though many physicians administer them prophylactically when intracranial tumor has been diagnosed.

PSEUDOTUMOR—BENIGN INTRACRANIAL HYPERTENSION Symptoms of increased intracranial pressure may occur in the absence of demonstrable parenchymal or leptomeningeal tumor or hydrocephalus. However, little distinguishes the symptomatic presentation of true tumor from that of pseudotumor, which includes headache, neck stiffness, visual blurring and obscurations, diplopia, nausea, and vomiting. Papilledoma, which may be unilateral or asymmetric, is accompanied by enlargement of the blind spot and altered visual acuity. Pseudotumor usually afflicts young, often obese women; it occurs most often in the absence of systemic cancer and focal neurologic difficulties. The marked increases in intracranial pressure may reflect impaired venous drainage within the brain or skull or may accompany the hormonal alterations of pregnancy, oral contraceptive use, or obesity. Less-common predisposing endocrinologic illnesses include both hypo- and hyperthyroidism, hypoparathyroidism, adrenal insufficiency, and both endogenous and exogenous excess of adrenocorticoids. Rare associations occur with sarcoidosis and lupus erythematosis. A variety of drugs have been implicated, including supplemental vitamin A, tetracycline, nalidixic acid, nitrofurantoin, sulfa preparations, lithium, indomethacin, phenytoin. The diagnosis is confirmed by the exclusion of an intracranial mass lesion or meningeal cancer. In the presence of a normal or small ventricular system on CT scan, lumbar puncture carries no risk for brain herniation. Cerebrospinal fluid is invariably under increased pressure but is otherwise unremarkable. Treatment is aimed at prevention of visual deficits and lasting symptoms by reducing the CSF volume by repetitive lumbar punctures. The removal of an offending drug or metabolic cause will reverse symptoms within 1 week's time. Patients refractory to this may benefit from acetazolamide, furosemide, or short-term glucocorticoid therapy. Lumboperitoneal shunting and surgical subtemporal decompression or optic nerve sheath fenestration are reserved for patients with progressive visual impairment who have failed medical therapy. The outlook for most patients is excellent—fully 80 percent respond to conservative therapy, but as many as 10 percent experience permanent or recurrent visual deficits.

SYSTEMIC CANCER AND THE CENTRAL NERVOUS SYSTEM

CEREBRAL METASTASES The most common CNS tumors are metastatic. The following section discusses the approach to patients who present with a CNS tumor where systemic cancer must be considered.

Pathogenesis and pathology Cerebral metastases occur in one-quarter of patients with systemic cancer. Spread to the calvarium, brain parenchyma, and subarachnoid space occurs through several mechanisms. *Hematogenous tumor embolism* from intermediate sites such as lung and liver is the most common mechanism in solid tumors of the breast and lung and in melanoma. Spread into the spinal canal via the *perivertebral venous system* occurs with uterine, colonic, and prostatic tumors. *Direct extension* of tumors originating in the head and neck may occur through the base of the skull. *Paraspinal direct* infiltration may occur with lymphoma and with prostate and breast carcinomas. *Tumor passage from the eye* or through the choroid plexus to the brain and subarachnoid space occurs in lymphoma and leukemia.

Clinical manifestations Sixty percent of cerebral metastases occur in the setting of diagnosed systemic cancer. Cancers of lung in men and of breast in women account for the largest percentage, although melanoma is the tumor with highest likelihood of spread to the CNS. Of patients with a cerebral metastasis (most often arising in the lung) 20 percent develop neurologic symptoms before discovery of the primary malignancy. At some point after diagnosis of systemic cancer, 25 percent of patients with lung carcinoma, 6 to 20 percent of patients with breast carcinoma, and about 50 percent of those with melanoma (when this last tumor has already metastasized to a site outside the CNS) develop tumors in brain or spinal cord. Patients with recurrent sarcoma or ovarian or colorectal cancer who survive beyond 3 years after the original diagnosis face a heightened risk of neurologic involvement. These tumors rarely accounted for cerebral metastases in the past. In the majority of patients, cerebral metastases occur with systemic relapse (Table 353-3). An exception occurs in patients with lung cancer, where the CNS is frequently either the initial site of presentation or of first demonstrated recurrence in otherwise apparently well-controlled disease. As systemic treatment continues to improve survival, the incidence of CNS involvement can be expected to rise for virtually all tumors.

Diagnosis of cerebral metastases More often than is the case with primary brain tumors, those of metastatic origin occur in a setting of seizure activity, increasingly severe head pain, and motor weakness. These difficulties often evolve in days to weeks. MRI or contrast-enhanced CT scan is the procedure of choice for evaluating patients with known systemic cancer and new neurologic symptoms (Table 353-2). Tumors appear with equal frequency as multiple ring-shaped lesions or solitary masses. Three categories of patients without neurologic symptoms or signs are initially evaluated by MRI or CT scanning. First, patients with lung carcinoma for whom attempted cure with pulmonary lobectomy is planned should have a scan preoperatively, since 5 percent of such patients will have clinically unsuspected cerebral metastases. Second, prophylactic brain radiation for small cell carcinoma of the lung should be preceded by a scan. Third, patients with widely disseminated cancer due to breast or testicular tumors, sarcoma, or melanoma who are about to receive systemic chemotherapy should have a scan to stage the disease.

Ten percent of patients with cancer develop neurologic difficulties in the absence of an intracranial mass on CT scan. Most of these will be found to have an abnormality on MRI scan. Focal motor or cranial nerve symptoms, headache, or impaired intellectual performance may reflect cerebrovascular lesions known to be associated with systemic cancer, unwitnessed seizures, meningeal carcinomatosis, paraneoplastic syndromes, or complications of tumor therapy (Table 353-4).

Patients with systemic neoplasms can develop several types of cerebrovascular disease. Multiple cerebral infarctions are the most frequent in patients with solid tumors. Patients with lymphoma or leukemia may develop diffuse encephalopathic difficulties from infarcts due to disseminated intravascular coagulation; or may develop focal findings from emboli of nonbacterial thrombotic endocarditis, hemorrhage in the setting of clotting abnormalities, or thrombocytopenia. In the absence of an etiology, laboratory studies should be done to exclude a circulating anticoagulant.

Focal deficits in patients with negative MRI or CT scans may result from seizures due to undetectable metastatic disease or may be manifestations of meningeal carcinomatosis or paraneoplastic syndromes (see Chap. 310). Gadolinium DTPA MRI or repeat CT scan in 4 to 6 weeks often discloses the tumor if present. A lumbar puncture with cytologic examination is mandatory in such patients both to exclude infection and to search for leptomeningeal tumor (see

TABLE 353-3 Interval between diagnosis of cancer and occurrence of brain metastases

Tumor	Patients with brain metastases, percent: At diagnosis of primary	Sometime during course of tumor growth	At autopsy	Interval from diagnosis of primary tumor to diagnosis of brain metastasis, percent
Lung tumor	10–15	22–30	15–30	90 after 3 months
Breast tumor	1	6–20	15–30	90 after 1 year
Melanoma	6	50	40–80	80 after 1 year
Renal tumor	4	11–13	8–20	90 after 1 year
Colorectal tumor	1	—	1	75 after 2 years
Sarcoma	1	36	—	90 after 1 year

SOURCE: L Weiss et al, *Brain Metastases*, Boston, Hall, 1980; M Deutsch et al, Cancer 34:1607, 1974.

below). CSF pleocytosis with mild elevation of protein may be found with paraneoplastic disorders.

Treatment The common assumption that brain metastases represent a uniform disease has been proved invalid. Therapeutic decisions must be based on the type, extent, and radiosensitivity of the primary tumor, the morbidity produced, and the number and location of metastases.

Patients with solitary lesions and little or no active systemic disease may require surgery, whereas for those with advanced, widespread systemic cancer, comfort is the prime consideration. Steroids may be used in such patients to maximize neurologic function and to reduce headache (see "Acute Treatment of Intracranial Tumors").

RADIATION THERAPY After acute symptoms are treated, most patients with multiple cerebral metastases or unresectable solitary lesions receive radiation therapy. A common approach is palliative whole-brain radiation totaling about 30 Gy (3000 rad) given in 10 to 15 equal fractions. Three-quarters of patients improve clinically and by CT; over one-half are able to discontinue their steroid medication for a time. However, only 30 percent of patients who complete radiation therapy survive 6 months and fewer than 20 percent are alive at 1 year. Two-thirds of the latter patients die from recurrent systemic tumor and not from cerebral disease. Treatment is less effective in the elderly, in those with advanced systemic cancer, and in patients with radiation-resistant tumors such as melanoma and gastrointestinal and lung tumors. Reinstitution of glucocorticoids may be useful when progressive neurologic deterioration recurs.

TABLE 353-4 Complications of chemotherapy

Neurologic problem	Drug(s)	Route
Encephalopathy	Glucocorticoids	PO/IM/IV
	L-Asparaginase	IV
	Procarbazine	PO/IV
	Nitrosoureas	PO/IV/IA/HDIV
	Cytosine arabinoside	HDIV
	Cisplatin*	IV
Leucoencephalopathy	Methotrexate	HDIV/IT
Cerebral edema	Cisplatin	IA
	Nitrosoureas	IA/HDIV
Optic nerve damage	Nitrosoureas	IA/HDIV
Cerebellar ataxia	5-Fluorouracil	IV
	Cytosine arabinoside	IT
Cranial neuropathy	Vincristine	IV
	Cisplatin*	IV/IA
Myelopathy/radiculopathy	Thio-TEPA	IT
	Methotrexate	HDIV/IT
	Cystosine arabinoside	HDIV/IT
Peripheral neuropathy	Vincristine†	IV
	Cisplatin	IV
Myopathy	Glucocorticoids	PO/IM/IV
	Vincristine	IV

* Ototoxicity and vestibular toxicity.
† Autonomic neuropathy may be seen as well.
NOTES: IA = intraarterial; IM = intramuscular; IV = intravenous; PO = per os; IT = intrathecal; HDIV = high dose intravenous.
SOURCE: Modified from Young.

CHEMOTHERAPY Systemic (intravenous or intraarterial) chemotherapy has been used with some success to treat cerebral metastases of lung (small cell), breast, and testicular origin. Anecdotal reports of brain metastases of breast origin responding to tamoxifen or other systemic chemotherapy have appeared.

LEPTOMENINGEAL METASTASES Pathogenesis and pathology Eight percent of patients with cancer develop diffuse infiltration of the meninges. The cranial and spinal nerve roots are usually affected. Tumors that commonly invade the meninges include non-Hodgkin's lymphoma, leukemia, melanoma, and adenocarcinoma of breast, lung, or gastrointestinal origin.

Clinical manifestations The common symptoms are headache, alteration in mentation, cranial nerve abnormalities, and lumbosacral radiculopathies. Patients may also present with seizures. The MRI or CT scan usually is normal, but may reveal enlarged ventricles. With contrast injections, scans may reveal diffuse enhancement of the meninges over the cerebral hemispheres and at the base of the brain.

A lumbar puncture is required for diagnosis. Three-quarters of patients show a modest CSF mononuclear pleocytosis of 5 to 100 cells. Elevation of protein and lowered glucose content may occur, but demonstration of malignant cells is required to confirm the diagnosis. Repeat lumbar or cervical subarachnoid punctures may be necessary to obtain positive cytology. In the past, myelography was often done in such patients because of back pain and radicular symptoms; it often disclosed multiple small nodules on the nerve roots. MRI studies using surface coils provide equal sensitivity providing that arachnoiditis is not present. Larger lesions can be detected and treated with radiation.

Treatment Treatment of meningeal carcinomatosis usually requires a combination of cranial radiation and intrathecal administration of chemotherapeutic agents. Chemotherapy is given either into the lumbar subarachnoid space or (more effectively) into a reservoir connected to the lateral ventricle. Agents commonly used include methotrexate, triethylenethiophosphoramide (thio-TEPA), cytosine arabinoside, and methylprednisolone either alone or in combination.

About one-half of patients with breast carcinoma respond initially to these treatments, but the median survival is only 7 months. The prognosis is particularly grave for meningeal carcinomatosis of melanoma or lung tumor origin; few responses are seen. A much better prognosis is expected in patients with lymphoma or leukemia with control for 2 or more years being common. Treatment failures reflect tumor drug resistance, poor circulation of drug within the subarachnoid space, and complications arising from chemotherapy and radiation (see Table 353-4).

TOXIC EFFECTS OF CANCER TREATMENT Chemotherapy Chronic glucocorticoid therapy may induce insulin-dependent diabetes mellitus, myopathy, and aseptic necrosis of the hip and may predispose to thrombophlebitis. In the early stages the muscle changes reverse with steroid taper and intensive physical therapy. Administration of anticonvulsants is associated with cutaneous allergies. Anticonvulsant doses may need to be adjusted in patients receiving glucocorticoids. Allergy to an anticonvulsant may be masked while the patient receives glucocorticoids and revealed later when the steroid medication is tapered. Table 353-4 summarizes the neurologic toxicities of currently used *chemotherapeutic agents*.

Radiation therapy Radiation therapy may cause toxic effects on the CNS. Acute changes include lethargy, loss of appetite, alterations in mental status, or exacerbation of previous symptoms and signs. These develop within 1 to 2 weeks of its initiation. These effects are usually attributable to worsening cerebral edema and are best treated with increased doses of glucocorticoids. Subacute changes that develop between 3 and 18 months after treatment are ascribed to radiation-induced demyelination and are unresponsive to steroids. Reappearance of previous neurologic impairment and the appearance of a mass which is indistinguishable from recurrent tumor on MRI or CT scan may occur. These areas of radiation necrosis may be visualized by hypometabolism following the injection of positron-emitting ^{18}F-deoxyglucose (PET scan). Patients who have received spinal radiation may develop Lhermitte's phenomenon with tingling in the back and legs following flexion of the neck.

Between 18 and 60 months after radiation, still other less reversible changes occur. These include retarded growth rate and impaired intellectual development in children who have received more than 30 Gy (3000 rad) of whole-brain radiation. At doses above 50 Gy (5000 rad), adults may exhibit cortical atrophy, communicating hydrocephalus, and hypothalamic dysfunction with elevated prolactin levels and amenorrhea or impotence. Dementia resulting from these changes is irreversible and in the case of hydrocephalus is usually unimproved by ventricular shunting.

The peripheral nervous system can also be affected by radiation therapy. Localized dysfunction of the brachial or lumbosacral plexus may follow radiation in excess of 40 Gy (4000 rad), usually appearing more than 1 year after treatment (see Chap. 363). Unlike peripheral nerve problems due to tumor invasion, radiation plexopathy is commonly painless. Additional tests, including CT scan, may be necessary to distinguish tumor invasion from radiation toxicity. Glucocorticoids may afford some benefit.

PRIMARY BRAIN TUMORS

In the following section, the most common primary brain tumors in adults are discussed by histologic type. Other tumors which occur in characteristic locations and whose presenting symptoms therefore reflect site rather than specific histology are then discussed by location. These include tumors located in the diencephalon-third ventricle, the posterior fossa, and the skull base.

MALIGNANT ASTROCYTOMA (GLIOBLASTOMA) Definition Malignant astrocytoma or glioblastoma (also known as malignant glioma or grade 3 or 4 astrocytoma) and the less malignant anaplastic astrocytoma account for about one-quarter of the 5000 intracranial gliomas diagnosed yearly in the United States; 75 percent of gliomas in adults are of this category. Because of its profound and uniform morbidity, it contributes more to the cost of cancer on a per capita basis than does any other tumor. The patient, commonly stricken in the fifth decade of life, enters a cycle of repetitive hospitalizations and operations while experiencing the progressive complications associated with relatively ineffective treatments of radiation and chemotherapy.

Pathogenesis and pathology Epidemiologic studies offer few clues to the etiology of malignant astrocytoma. Some tumors arise in patients with longstanding seizure disorders or personality disorders resulting from temporal lobe dysfunction and in scars incurred from head trauma, suggesting that in certain instances the malignant cells emerge from a more benign glial proliferation. There are rare instances of malignant tumors occurring in families, suggesting a genetic propensity. At least four human oncogenes (*sis, myc, src,* n-*myc*) have been identified in cell lines derived from primary brain tumors, and there is overexpression for the receptors of both platelet-derived (PDGF) and epidermal (EGF) growth factors. Small clusters of tumors have appeared in certain occupational settings, notably in the petroleum processing industry. The tumor has an appearance similar to that produced by a variety of viral agents inoculated into animals. On gross examination, the surrounding normal brain is distorted and infiltrated by yellow tumor tissue containing areas of necrosis, cysts, and hemorrhage. Microscopic examination reveals a highly cellular composite of heterogeneous glial cells with elongated or rounded astrocytes whose processes stain for glial fibrillary acidic protein. Giant cells may be seen along with mitotic figures and the proliferation of small capillaries.

Clinical manifestations Patients commonly present with a subacute progressive neurologic deficit exhibiting either focal signs or personality changes. Prior mental changes or seizures may antedate tumor diagnosis by months to years. Clinical symptoms may occur abruptly with seizures or with sudden deficits secondary to tumor hemorrhage. The CT scan reveals a heterogeneous pattern of tumor enhancement interspersed with hypodense foci presumably corresponding to tumor necrosis and edema. Multiple tumors can occur but are uncommon. MRI scans often define more extensive tumor involvement than is indicated on the CT scan.

Malignant astrocytoma can arise in the brainstem, cerebellum, or spinal cord in addition to the more common locations within the white matter of the cerebral hemispheres. The prognosis for any site, unfortunately, has not changed greatly in the last 20 years. Following treatment, less than 6 months of useful function can be expected for most patients before progression of symptoms signals recurrent tumor. Death results in 80 percent of patients from tumor recurrence within 6 to 12 months. Progressive neurologic deterioration is followed by stupor and coma. In patients who survive over 1 year, often young adults, CNS dissemination can occur to the meninges or the ventricular ependyma. Metastasis outside the CNS is extremely rare.

Treatment Confirmation of histology by biopsy should be performed in most patients; debulking of tumor is recommended if the tumor is located in an area that permits an extensive operation.

Therapeutic modalities are not highly effective. The average life expectancy of 17 weeks for untreated patients is improved by postoperative external beam radiation alone to 47 weeks and by radiation combined with chemotherapy to 62 weeks. A subgroup of young patients under age 50 obtains significant improvement in quality and duration of life. Such patients have a 20 percent 2-year survival after cranial radiation of 55 to 60 Gy (5500 to 6000 rad) combined with adjunctive chemotherapy with the nitrosoureas carmustine (BCNU) or lomustine (CCNU).

Efforts to improve prognosis for this malignancy include radiotherapy trials of implanted radiation sources of isotopic iodine (^{125}I brachytherapy). Current chemotherapeutic trials are based on the localized nature of the tumor and of its recurrence and involve local arterial infusions of cisplatin prior to radiation or at the time of tumor recurrence. Experimental approaches include the use of β-interferon, interleukin-stimulated lymphocyte killer cells (LAK) or monoclonal antibodies.

ASTROCYTOMA Definition Low-grade astrocytomas occur throughout the brain and spinal cord. The subcortical white matter is the most common site in adults. In children and young adults astrocytomas arise in the optic nerves, cerebellum (cystic, juvenile, pilocytic astrocytoma), and brainstem (pontine glioma). These tumors are also associated with neurofibromatosis and tuberous sclerosis and are found in 20 percent of patients undergoing temporal lobectomy for control of chronic seizure disorders.

Pathogenesis and pathology The tumors are avascular without necrosis and contain homogeneous populations of well-differentiated astrocytes. The astrocytomas are divided into those with good prognosis (80 percent survivorship at 5 years) (cystic cerebellar, "juvenile" pilocytic, giant cell subependymoma) and those with likely recurrence after surgery (infiltrating, gemistocytic, anaplastic).

Clinical manifestations The tumors evolve slowly over several years, producing symptoms by displacement of normal brain or by invasion of white matter tracts. Optic nerve gliomas cause progressive, monocular or bitemporal visual field defects leading eventually to

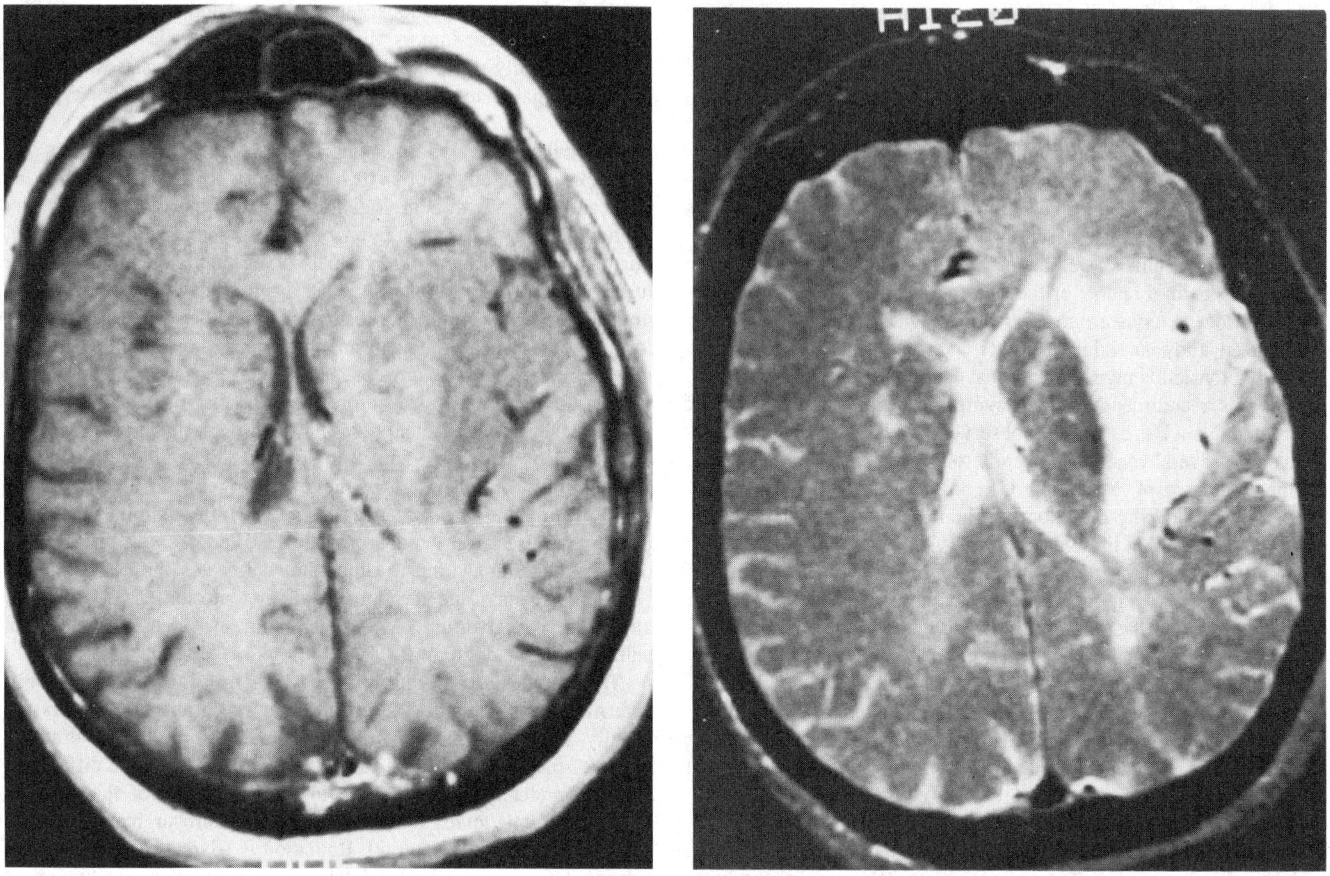

A

B

FIGURE 353-2 *A*. Gadolinium-DTPA-enhanced T1-weighted axial image demonstrating a decreased signal in the right temporoparietal region with no evidence of contrast enhancement. Mild effacement of the body of the left lateral ventricle without midline shift is present. Biopsy showed low-grade glioma. *B*. T2-weighted axial MRI of same tumor showed area of hyperintense signal corresponding to low signal area seen on T1 study.

blindness and sometimes proptosis. Hypothalamic compression may cause endocrine dysfunction. Hydrocephalus is rare. In the brainstem, such tumors typically involve several cranial nerves (often the abducens, facial, and trigeminal) and later impinge on corticospinal fibers and medial lemniscal and spinothalamic tracts. These symptoms must be distinguished from those caused by multiple sclerosis, arteriovenous malformations, cysts of cysticercosis and echinococcal origin, and extramedullary tumors such as schwannomas or meningiomas. Cerebellar astrocytomas cause progressive incoordination and gait ataxia combined with abnormalities of eye movements. In supratentorial locations, these tumors may produce seizures before any focal abnormality appears on clinical examination. In *gliomatosis cerebri,* slow infiltration of white matter occurs with atypical individual astrocytes without evidence of localized tumor.

Early use of MRI scanning may allow for earlier diagnosis and intervention (see Figs. 353-1, 353-2, and 353-3). MRI often demonstrates white matter abnormalities in patients with normal CT scans and is the preferred procedure for early diagnosis and follow-up. A stable clinical course is common with astrocytoma and repeat radiologic studies may show little change. The characteristic CT appearance is an indistinct mass that is hypodense with respect to surrounding brain and exhibits little or no contrast enhancement, calcification, or evidence of edema. Malignant degeneration of astrocytomas is heralded by rapid progression of symptoms and signs, evidence of expanded size or altered MRI T2 or CT signal, or the presence of new enhancement on MRI with gadolinium DTPA or CT with iodine contrast.

Treatment Because up to half of nonenhancing CT masses may be aggressive gliomas, many surgeons argue for early biopsy. This is especially true in the setting of seizure progression or increase in

FIGURE 353-3 Brainstem glioma in a 9-year-old boy. The medulla and cervical spinal cord are twice as wide as normal. Focal areas of cystic degeneration are seen as hypodense T1 signals. Biopsy revealed an astrocytoma.

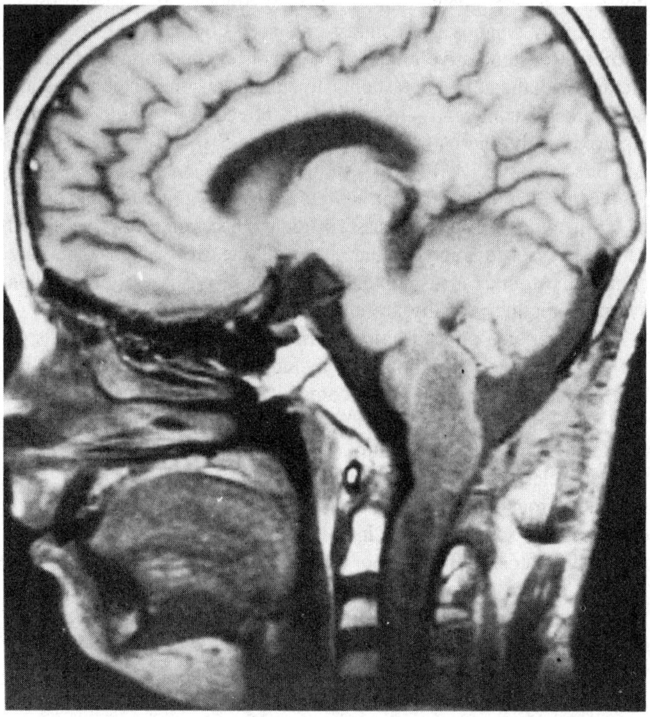

the size of the lesion. Surgical excision can be curative for some cerebellar, optic nerve, and lobar astrocytomas. Cyst drainage and partial resection are feasible for many. Biopsy should be obtained for supratentorial tumors but is less frequently considered for brainstem or spinal cord gliomas. Exceptions to the latter are tumors that have a cystic or extraaxial component. Postoperative radiation is recommended for incompletely resected tumors and for those involving the brainstem (for which multiple daily doses are often provided). Its role in the treatment of excised supratentorial tumors is less clear. The possible benefits of radiation therapy are weighed against the known long natural course of the astrocytoma and the complications of irradiation. A consortium of treatment groups has placed under randomized study the value of "early" versus "delayed" irradiation of newly biopsied benign astrocytoma. Until this study is completed, radiation is recommended when symptoms and signs progress or enlargement on CT or MRI is observed. Radiation may be safely delayed for several years in apparently totally resected tumors because of the accuracy of MRI and CT scans. The judicious use of glucocorticoids during radiation or when symptoms recur improves function. The median life expectancy is 67 months for supratentorial tumors and 89 months for cerebellar tumors. Average survivals of 15 months after radiation are reported for patients with brainstem tumors. However, the 5-year survival is only 30 percent. Chemotherapy, currently under investigation for brainstem tumors, may offer some improvement in survival.

OLIGODENDROGLIOMA Definition This tumor of oligodendroglial origin may develop in isolation or may be mixed with other glial cells. An uncommon tumor, it represents less then 10 percent of all gliomas.

Pathology Microscopic examination discloses rounded cells containing darkly staining nuclei with poorly staining cytoplasm, the "fried egg" appearance. The tumor is prone to spontaneous hemorrhage. Both "benign" and "malignant" forms are seen.

Clinical manifestations Presentation is most commonly in the third or fourth decade and tumors are most frequently in the frontal lobes or within the ventricles. CT reveals a well-defined, low-attenuation mass with fine speckled calcium deposits and small cysts.

Treatment Although the oligodendroglioma is histologically benign, resection is curative in only one-third of patients. The role of postoperative radiation is uncertain; it is recommended only for incompletely resected tumors or those with mixed glial features or with evidence of progression after operation. Some oligodendrogliomas have malignant features. Such malignant transformation is more readily diagnosed if contrast-enhanced CT is used. Prospective studies of postoperative radiation have not been performed. Chemotherapy with the nitrosoureas lomustine or carmustine (in combination with procarbazine and vincristine) is effective in some patients. Approximately one-half of patients survive 5 years after diagnosis, and one-third survive 10 years.

MENINGIOMA Definition Meningiomas account for 20 percent of brain tumors. They can arise in either the cranium or the spinal canal. They occur more frequently at all sites in women. They are commonly found as asymptomatic tumors at postmortem. When symptomatic they usually present in the fifth or sixth decades.

Pathogenesis and pathology Meningiomas arise from cells of the pia-arachnoid. Common sites include the midline along the falx cerebri and the lateral cerebral convexity, the olfactory groove and along the sphenoid ridge, the tuberculum sellae, foramen magnum, and tentorium of the cerebellum. They also arise on occasion within the ventricles, where on radiographic examination they are indistinguishable from a papilloma of the choroid plexus. Meningiomas may coexist with schwannomas in patients with the central form of neurofibromatosis. Both tumor types are related to the loss of a "tumor suppressor" gene on chromosome 22. They occur more frequently in women with breast cancer; some meningiomas contain estrogen and progesterone receptors.

On the basis of microscopic characteristics, meningiomas are divided into seven categories: syncytial, transitional, fibroblastic, microcystic, psammomatous, angioblastic, and malignant meningiomas. Malignant tumors display mitoses, invade normal brain, and occasionally develop CNS and extraneural metastases. Angioblastic and malignant forms are more likely than the other types to recur.

Clinical manifestations The clinical presentation reflects the slow expansion of tumor in the characteristic locations within the skull and spine, with neurologic deficits evolving over many years. Tumors of the parasellar region produce a combination of second, third, fourth, fifth, and sixth cranial nerve deficits. Cerebellopontine tumors may produce a syndrome similar to that of acoustic schwannomas (see "Tumors of the Posterior Fossa" below). Early hearing loss is not a typical finding in meningioma. Parasagittal and frontal tumors may produce seizures or may be entirely asymptomatic, often growing to enormous size before they are discovered. Parasagittal lesions that attain sufficient size may cause spastic paraparesis and incontinence. Falx meningioma should be considered in the differential diagnosis of gait disorders in the middle-aged and elderly. In all locations, meningiomas must be distinguished from similar-appearing dural metastases from breast, prostate, and lung. The CT scan often discloses calcium within a tumor and delineates the close relation between the mass and the dura, falx, or tentorium, as well as the altered bony calvarium. MRI often shows isodense masses that enhance with gadolinium-DTPA.

Treatment Tumor site, rather than histology, is the major determinant of outcome. Intraventricular or parasagittal tumors are usually resectable and recurrence is rare. Those in the olfactory groove, sphenoid ridge, and parasellar locations are more difficult to resect completely and are prone to recur. Tumors of the foramen magnum may be totally removed with microneurosurgical techniques (see "Spinal Tumors" below). Radiation is advocated for malignant meningiomas and for incompletely excised symptomatic tumors of other histologic subtypes. Chemotherapy is without apparent efficacy.

PAPILLOMA OF THE CHOROID PLEXUS Definition Neoplasms derived from choroid plexus epithelium are rare, representing only 0.5 percent of all intracranial tumors.

Pathogenesis and pathology In children most such tumors occur in the lateral ventricles, whereas in adults the fourth ventricle is the most common site. The histologic structure resembles normal choroid plexus, with a connective tissue core covered by a single layer of cuboidal epithelium.

Clinical manifestations Very rare examples of malignant transformation have been described. Metastases to the leptomeninges may occur. The tumor may secrete excessive CSF leading to communicating hydrocephalus.

Treatment Surgery is the treatment of choice and is usually highly successful.

LIPOMA Lipoma can develop anywhere within the brain or spinal cord, though the corpus callosum is the most common location. The association of lipomas with partial or complete agenesis of this structure and with other dysplastic or hamartomatous anomalies such as ectopias, colloid cysts, and epidermoids supports the theory that they are the result of disorders of development. Intraspinal lipomas are most common in the thoracic region and are associated with spina bifida in one-third of cases. All lipomas can be easily demonstrated by MRI. The treatment of symptomatic cranial and spinal lipomas is excision.

DERMOID AND EPIDERMOID TUMOR Definition The distinction between dermoid tumors and epidermoids (true cholesteatomas) is often difficult. Both result from inclusion of ectodermal tissue at the time of closure of the neural groove and soon thereafter.

Pathology and pathogenesis Cholesteatomas are slowly growing tumors that most often afflict young adults, occurring commonly in lateral or midline locations within the skull, i.e., the cerebellopontine angle, the suprasellar region, the fourth ventricle, the pineal region, and over the hemispheres. No clear relationship has been established between cholesteatoma of the cerebellopontine angle and middle ear infection. Dermoid tumors, which are frequently cystic, occur largely in the posterior fossa or in the lumbosacral region. Rarely they are found in suprasellar or pineal regions.

Clinical manifestations Symptoms vary according to the location of these tumors, the general pattern being slow evolution of defects attributable to the specific area with seizures interspersed when the tumor occupies cortical regions. MRI provides excellent delineation.

Treatment Treatment of the cholesteatoma is total surgical removal of the tumor together with its capsule. Dermoid tumors similarly are curable if total surgical excision is possible.

PRIMARY LYMPHOMA OF THE CENTRAL NERVOUS SYSTEM

Definition Primary lymphomas are now recognized to be relatively common in the CNS. Before 1972, fewer than 25 cases had been identified at the Massachusetts General Hospital over a 50-year period. Since 1977, 10 cases per year have been diagnosed. Primary lymphoma is distinguished from the more frequent secondary involvement of the meninges that occurs in patients with poorly differentiated non-Hodgkin's lymphomas.

Pathogenesis and pathology The tumor is uncommon in patients without immunologic compromise. It is usually seen in patients with mixed humoral and cellular immune deficits. Three such disorders are recognized: inherited disorders of immunity such as combined immunodeficiency disease, selective IgM deficiency, or selective IgA abnormalities seen with combined immunodeficiency and Wiskott-Aldrich syndrome; acquired immunodeficiency syndrome (AIDS); and therapeutic immunosuppression following organ transplantation or treatment of autoimmune disorders. The demonstration of Epstein-Barr virus (EBV) DNA within primary lymphoma in some affected patients raises the possibility that this agent may play a role in the pathogenesis of this disease.

The tumor may be focal or multicentric in the subcortical white matter, the walls of the ventricles, or the subarachnoid space. Tumor cells are always found in a perivascular distribution. At biopsy, tumor cells are often indistinguishable from normal lymphocytes, leading to an erroneous early diagnosis of "encephalitis" or "nonspecific perivascular inflammation." The B-cell populations may be characterized as malignant by monoclonal antibodies to immunoglobulin surface proteins. The tumors contain cells defined histologically as diffuse histiocytic or poorly differentiated lymphocytes by the Rappaport system and as follicular center cells and small cleaved cells by the Lukes-Collins system (see Chap. 302). Burkitt-type lymphomas are rarely reported.

Clinical manifestations A history of personality change, focal deficits, or seizures evolving over several weeks in an immunosuppressed patient should raise the suspicion of cerebral lymphoma. Obviously, in these circumstances infection must be excluded. Patients with HIV infection are often treated presumptively for toxoplasmosis and brain lymphoma. The CT scan typically reveals multiple periventricular masses which enhance with contrast. Similar lesions are seen on T2-weighted MRI sections. These may persist when CT abnormalities have disappeared. A characteristic feature, rarely observed with other types of intracranial tumor, is the marked reduction or disappearance of lesions after a few weeks of high-dose glucocorticoid therapy (dexamethasone 6 to 10 mg four times daily). When both symptoms and CT abnormalities resolve after glucocorticoid therapy, remissions lasting several months are common, and steroids can be tapered. Spontaneous remissions without glucocorticoid therapy have been described. The usual clinical course is recurrence after 4 to 6 months, with resistance to steroid administration. The tumor may seed the meninges in one-quarter of patients. Systemic lymphoma is found in less than 10 percent of patients and occurs late in the course of the disease. However, uveitis or vitreitis may occur at the time of presentation or early in the evolution of the disease; when present, it is helpful in the initial diagnosis.

Treatment After biopsy or diagnosis by CSF cytology, the recommended treatment is chemotherapy consisting of high-dose methotrexate and glucocorticoids, alone or in combination with cyclophosphamide, doxorubicin, and vincristine, followed by radiation. Chemotherapy provides therapeutic drug levels in brain parenchyma and most importantly, in the CSF. Partial or complete remission occurs in over three-quarters of patients. When methotrexate is administered prior to radiation, there is a reduced risk of radiation or drug-induced white matter damage. The median survival following irradiation is 17 months. Radiation treatment is recommended for patients with brain lymphoma.

TUMORS OF THE THIRD VENTRICLE AND PINEAL REGION

Several categories of tumors occur in close proximity to the diencephalon, hypothalamus, and third ventricle; these are pituitary adenoma, craniopharyngioma, germ-cell neoplasms, pineal tumors, and glial, meningeal, or metastatic tumors.

Uncommon tumors of the pineal region include astrocytomas, glioblastomas, meningiomas, and metastases. Nonneoplastic masses occurring in this region include colloid cysts of the third ventricle (see "Colloid Cysts" below) and parasitic cysts (cysticercosis).

Pituitary adenomas These tumors are described in Chap. 313.

Craniopharyngiomas These tumors arise from remnants of Rathke's pouch, derived from the primitive stomatodeum. They are usually suprasellar in location and cause symptoms related to neuroendocrine dysfunction or visual compromise (see also Chap. 313). They are easily identified by a "bright" T2 signal on MRI (Fig. 353-4).

Germ-cell tumors DEFINITION Germ-cell tumors, which account for half of all pineal region neoplasms, arise primarily during childhood or early adolescence and include germinoma, teratoma, embryonal carcinoma, endodermal sinus tumor, and choriocarcinoma.

CLINICAL MANIFESTATIONS The most common of these germ-cell tumors is the germinoma. It may occur in the pineal region or at the base of the hypothalamus. It occurs more frequently in males,

FIGURE 353-4 This 39-year-old woman presented with headaches and gait disturbance (caused by a craniopharyngioma). On a T1-weighted coronal MRI, a large, lobulated hyperdense mass is visualized in the suprasellar cistern compressing the inferior third ventricle. There is enlargement of the frontal and temporal ventricles.

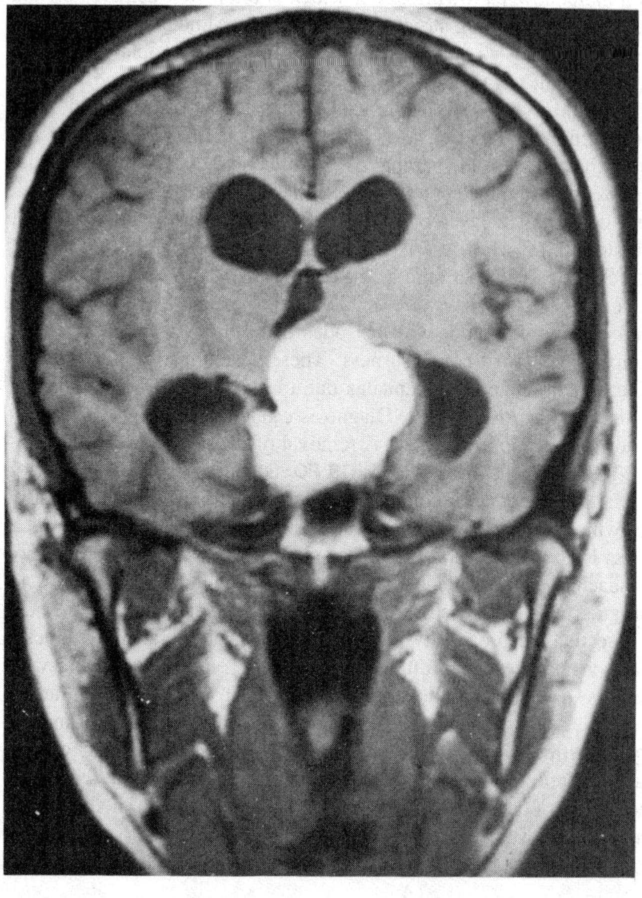

who present with findings of diabetes insipidus and other neuroendocrine deficiences, bitemporal visual field defects, paralysis of upward gaze (see Chap. 23), and sometimes hydrocephalus. The typical features of pineal masses occur more commonly with nongerminomatous germ-cell tumors. Findings include Parinaud's syndrome—a failure of upward gaze and pupillary dilatation with deficiencies in response to light. Rarely, other signs such as nystagmus retractorius or brainstem signs due to compression may occur. Diagnosis may be assisted by the finding of elevated serum and CSF levels of alphafetoprotein (AFP) and of human chorionic gonadotropin (hCG) in germinomas. MRI and CT scans identify tumors of the pineal region *but offer no histologic differentiation.*

TREATMENT Following biopsy by transcallosal or suboccipital route, radiation is given. Germinomas are radiosensitive; up to 80 percent are cured by well-tolerated doses of cranial radiation. Craniospinal irradiation is provided when tumor invades the ventricles or subarachnoid space, or is found outside the pineal region. Other histologic subtypes have poorer prognoses and recurrence is common, often with seeding of the cranial nerves and meninges. Recurrences sometimes respond to drug treatment with etoposide, cisplatin, and doxorubicin, which are beneficial in testicular tumors of similar histology.

Pineoblastoma and pineocytoma These tumors account for 20 percent of growths in the pineal region.

PATHOGENESIS AND PATHOLOGY Pineoblastoma and pineocytoma arise from pineal organ cells. The pineoblastoma is a primitive malignant tumor of childhood and early adult life and is indistinguishable both in appearance and natural history from primitive neuroectodermal tumors that arise elsewhere in the CNS. The tumor may contain astrocytic or neuronal elements. Recurrence is invariable and dissemination through the ventricular system and subarachnoid space is frequent.

TREATMENT Brain and neuraxis radiation are recommended, and chemotherapy as outlined above for germ-cell tumors has been successful in producing remissions in a few patients. Chemotherapy prior to irradiation is reserved for pineoblastoma. The pineocytoma is a more slowly growing tumor which is often well-demarcated and resembles the normal structure of the pineal. Although histologically benign, it tends to recur, probably because of incomplete removal. It is resistant to radiation.

Colloid cysts PATHOGENESIS AND PATHOLOGY Colloid cysts arise within the anterior third ventricle and are considered to develop from the anlage of the paraphysis, a component of the third ventricle, or possibly from the ependyma itself. The cysts are well-encapsulated and consist of a layer of connective tissue covered with columnar ciliated cells. The cyst is filled with glycoproteinaceous material which stains with periodic acid Schiff (PAS).

CLINICAL MANIFESTATIONS Symptoms occur usually in adults and may be dramatic, with episodes of headache, weakness of the limbs, and loss of consciousness. These symptoms are attributed to intermittent acute hydrocephalus due to blockage of the foramen of Monro by the mobile cyst. Diagnosis cannot be made with certainty prior to operation; treatment is removal of the cyst.

TUMORS OF THE POSTERIOR FOSSA Tumors of the posterior fossa pose special problems in diagnosis and treatment. Rapidly growing tumors may cause obstructive hydrocephalus, and even small mass lesions in the posterior fossa may result in vomiting, lethargy, headache, and papilledema. Slowly growing tumors give rise to progressive signs which are recognized by rather specific syndromes. These include progressive unilateral hearing loss, facial weakness, pain or numbness, and a unilateral sixth nerve deficit occurring with tumors in the cerebellopontine angle. Gait ataxia and unilateral cerebellar signs occur with hemangioblastoma, medulloblastoma, or cystic astrocytoma of the cerebellum. Progressive diplopia, cranial nerve abnormalities, and crossed corticospinal tract and reflex abnormalities occur in brainstem glioma. Nuchal and occipital pain are common with all tumors of the posterior fossa. Corticospinal signs develop with further tumor enlargement and encroachment on the brainstem.

Acoustic schwannoma DEFINITION The acoustic schwannoma (synonymous with acoustic neuroma) is composed of myelin-forming Schwann cells that cover the acoustic nerve fibers. Schwann cells normally replace oligodendroglia as the nerve leaves the brainstem to enter the internal auditory meatus.

PATHOGENESIS AND PATHOLOGY Schwannomas are slow-growing masses that compress rather than invade normal tissue. When bilateral, they represent an inherited form of schwannoma which is diagnostic of "central" neurofibromatosis. Other CNS tumors associated with neurofibromatosis or von Recklinghausen's disease are schwannomas of spinal and other cranial nerves, intracranial and spinal meningiomas, gliomas, and ependymomas (see Chap. 358).

CLINICAL MANIFESTATIONS AND TREATMENT Early detection of acoustic schwannomas at a time of minimal hearing deficit and minimal facial motor difficulty is essential, as hearing may be spared by microneurosurgical intervention while the tumor is still restricted to the canal. Brainstem auditory-evoked responses, CT and MRI studies, especially with contrast injection, have replaced metrizamide cisternography by enhancing the physician's ability to detect these tumors in their early stages.

Hemangioblastoma DEFINITION The cerebellar hemangioblastoma is an uncommon tumor that may be solitary but is frequently multiple. When the tumors are multiple, they are considered part of von Hippel-Lindau disease. This autosomal dominant disorder, linked to chromosome 3, typically consists of retinal, cerebellar, and spinal hemangioblastomas and visceral lesions, usually renal and/or pancreatic tumors or cysts. Polycythemia may be present.

PATHOGENESIS AND PATHOLOGY Hemangioblastomas are well-circumscribed and often cystic. The tumor may consist solely of a small nodule attached to the wall of a large cyst. The lesion is usually highly vascular and may be mistaken for an arteriovenous malformation. The microscopic appearance is one of numerous capillary vessels separated by sheets of clear cells with an abundance of intracytoplasmic vacuoles. The tumors are probably derived from capillary endothelial cells.

CLINICAL MANIFESTATIONS Dizziness, ataxia of gait or of the limbs, and symptoms of raised intracranial pressure are characteristic features of the cerebellar hemangioblastoma. The tumors may bleed spontaneously, resulting in a paroxysmal onset of headache and neurologic deficit. The MRI may show vascular "flow voids" or ferritin suggesting old hemorrhage.

TREATMENT Craniotomy with opening of the cerebellar cyst and excision of the mural tumor may be curative. Though the tumor is histologically benign, postoperative recurrences and the appearance of less operable spinal lesions worsen the prognosis. Patients with the von Hippel-Lindau syndrome should have periodic ophthalmologic evaluation for the appearance of retinal angiomas and general medical follow-up for early detection of renal tumors.

Ependymoma PATHOGENESIS AND PATHOLOGY These are glial tumors that occur chiefly in childhood and young adulthood, with a typical cranial location in the fourth ventricle. The tumor is composed of uniform ependymal cells surrounding a central lumen. Spinal ependymomas, which are more common, arise within the dura of the lumbar spine and represent more than half of spinal intramedullary gliomas. In this location, the prognosis is excellent. Supratentorial tumors are often more aggressive in rate of growth.

TREATMENT Resection and radiation to the tumor site results in 5-year survival in excess of 80 percent for spinal cord lesions and between 30 percent and 50 percent for posterior fossa tumors. The role of chemotherapy in the treatment of local recurrences and of seeding within the subarachnoid space is not established.

PRIMITIVE NEUROECTODERMAL TUMORS (PNET) Several histologic varieties of tumor arise from primitive neuroectodermal tumors (PNET) which contain cells with a capacity to differentiate into medulloblasts, astrocytes, oligodendrocytes, ependyma, ganglion cells, or skeletal muscle. Some tumors have several cell types, but all PNETs share a propensity for local invasion, subarachnoid dissemination, and extraneural metastases. The initial evaluation should include CT scan and myelography with CSF cytology.

Medulloblastoma DEFINITION The *medulloblastoma* is the most common variety of PNET. It accounts for 25 percent of childhood brain tumors. However, one-fourth of medulloblastomas occur in patients over age 20.

PATHOGENESIS AND PATHOLOGY In children the tumor is usually located in the midline, in the inferior portion of the vermis of the cerebellum. In adults the cerebellar hemisphere is most often the site of occurrence. It is composed of small, densely staining cells which elicit a brisk glial response. Invasion of the meninges, ventricles, and subarachnoid space is common.

CLINICAL MANIFESTATIONS The common presentation is occipital headache, vomiting, and trunkal ataxia. Hydrocephalus is frequent. With enlargement of the tumor other signs of brainstem compression emerge. As spinal axis dissemination occurs in one-third of patients CSF cytologic examination and myelography are advocated during initial evaluation.

TREATMENT Resection of the tumor is usually attempted, followed by radiation in doses of 45 to 50 Gy (4500 to 5000 rad) to the posterior fossa, together with 40 Gy (4000 rad) to the whole brain and 35 to 40 Gy (3500 to 4000 rad) to the spinal cord. Chemotherapy prior to irradiation has not been shown to be effective, although it is used with some success in recurrent tumors. Nitrosourea, procarbazine, and vincristine combined with prednisone and intrathecal methotrexate are advocated. Five-year survival is nearly 75 percent. The posterior fossa remains the major site for recurrence. A pessimistic outlook exists for children under 3 years, those with large tumors, and those with subarachnoid spread. Metastases to lung, liver, vertebrae, and pelvis are reported. Some medulloblastomas may take on features reminiscent of neuroblastoma.

Neuroblastoma DEFINITION The neuroblastoma, a relatively common adrenal tumor, can rarely occur as a primary CNS tumor. Eighty percent of cases present during the first decade of life.

PATHOGENESIS AND PATHOLOGY Microscopically, neuroblastoma resembles medulloblastoma because of its small dense cells. Variations in pathology occur. Some tumors show differentiation to ganglion cells but do not have a better prognosis. These tumors appear to form a spectrum of tumors of embryonal origin, ranging from the aggressive, poorly differentiated PNETs to the very well differentiated and quite slow growing neurocytomas. The intraparenchymal tumors found in children resemble in clinical behavior the PNETs, with neuroaxis spread and occasional extraneural metastases. CT reveals a hypodense mass with dense uniform enhancement after contrast administration as well as variable hemorrhage and calcification. These tumors may present as slowly growing intraventricular masses in adults and may grow to large size before discovery.

TREATMENT The rarity of these tumors has prevented any randomized therapeutic trials. Optimal treatment may consist of radical excision with postoperative radiation, though definitive evidence that radiation increases survival is lacking. Because of the frequency of local recurrence and CSF metastases, prophylactic spinal irradiation may be justified. A trial of chemotherapy, either pre- or postirradiation may be worthwhile, especially in younger patients with more aggressive-appearing tumors. Long-term follow-up is complete but appears to have a greater than 30 percent 5-year survival. The survival of adults with intraventricular tumors may be better than that of other primitive CNS tumors.

TUMORS OF THE SKULL BASE Tumors in this region produce characteristic clinical presentations that pose unique diagnostic difficulties even with advanced neuroradiologic procedures. Meningiomas, tumors of bone (including epidermoid and dermoid tumors and osteomas), chordomas, schwannomas (neurofibromas) of the cranial nerves, nasopharyngeal carcinoma, and metastases may all present with pain localized to the lower face, ear, or occiput and with involvement of one or more cranial nerves making exit from the skull. Metastases arise commonly from the lung, breast, nasopharynx, testicle, and prostate. Multiple myeloma and occasionally lymphoma may appear at this site. The mass may be palpable or may be visualized on polytomography, CT scan, or MRI; however, even a combination of all three studies may be negative. These studies usually differentiate successfully other erosive processes of the skull base, including fibrous dysplasia, Paget's disease, xanthomatosis, and osteitis fibrosa cystica. Enlargement of specific cranial nerve foramens may be the first evidence of schwannomas or of *glomus* tumors of the chromaffin cells in the jugular bulb. These last tumors invade temporal and occipital bone and produce hearing abnormalities and lower cranial nerve deficits.

Chordomas arise from remnants of the notochord. Of these, 60 percent are localized in the clivus, 30 percent in the sacral region, and the remaining 10 percent along the extent of the spine and skull base. The chordoma is not easily distinguished in appearance from radiation-sensitive chondrosarcomas and chondroid chordoma. They are highly invasive, expanding along the skull base and causing serial cranial nerve compression, sometimes with invasion of the nasopharynx. Up to one-third may metastasize via the subarachnoid space. A cauda equina syndrome (see ''Spinal Tumors'') results from sacral tumors. Clivus tumors may be difficult to visualize adequately on CT scan but are clearly delineated by MRI. Complete removal is rarely feasible and postoperative radiation therapy is recommended. Radiation with cyclotron-derived protons is followed by 80 percent survival at 5 years and 63 percent at 10 years with minimal complications.

Metastases to the skull base are treated with radiation therapy. In the presence of characteristic patterns of pain and cranial nerve deficit, radiation may be considered to treat presumptive metastases in patients with known systemic malignancy even when radiographic examinations are inconclusive.

SPINAL TUMORS **Pathogenesis and pathology** Tumors of the spinal canal and of the cord are only one-quarter as common as are intracranial tumors. Spinal neoplasms arise from the same types of cells as their counterparts in the cerebrum. They are classified according to location as intramedullary (within the substance of the spinal cord), extramedullary (or intradural), and extradural. Some tumors, such as schwannomas, may be both extradural and intradural. The most frequent location for all types of spinal neoplasms is in the thoracic cord, presumably reflecting its greater total length. These tumors arise from cells of the spinal cord, nerve roots, meninges, vascular structures, or the vertebral column. Tumors of the spinal cord parenchyma are relatively infrequent compared to lesions arising outside the substance of the cord. In one large series, nerve sheath tumors (schwannomas) accounted for 29 percent of all spinal tumors, meningiomas for 25.5 percent, gliomas for 22 percent, and sarcomas for 12 percent. Metastatic lesions represent about 13 percent of all spinal tumors, but as with intracranial tumors, these figures reflect neurosurgical service statistics and metastases are likely underrepresented.

Clinical manifestations Any lesion that narrows the spinal canal sufficiently to encroach on neural structures can give rise to neurologic symptoms. Dysfunction may arise from direct compression of the spinal cord and its nerve roots or from interference with blood supply. The rapid growth of metastatic lesions leads to motor and sensory symptoms over a period of days to weeks, whereas slowly growing astrocytomas and ependymomas produce symptoms over a period of months to years.

Extramedullary tumors (both intradural and epidural) cause symptoms by compressing the spinal cord or nerve roots. The initial symptoms are usually focal back pain and paresthesias followed by sensory loss below the level of the pain, weakness, and bladder and bowel dysfunction. Intramedullary lesions usually extend over several spinal cord segments, and their symptoms and signs are more varied than those of extramedullary tumors. A common pattern is dissociated sensory loss, with pain and temperature sensation impairment in the segments of tumor origin and with sparing of posterior column sensory function. Later, as the tumor grows peripherally, spinothalamic tracts may be involved. Since, in the thoracic and cervical regions, the sacral pain and temperature fibers lie superficial to those fibers representing more rostral regions, the sacral segments may be spared. Atrophy in the appropriate segments due to anterior horn cell involvement may combine with corticospinal tract signs.

These clinical presentations are not diagnostic of spinal cord neoplasm. Transverse myelitis from multiple sclerosis or other causes can lead to rapid onset of spinal cord dysfunction associated with pain, paresthesias, and weakness (see Chap. 361). A similar syndrome can occur as a paraneoplastic process, resulting from a necrotic myelopathy (see Chap. 310). Syringomyelia can produce a chronic syndrome indistinguishable from that produced by intramedullary neoplasms. Other diseases that can lead to a progressive spinal cord syndrome include combined system degeneration due to vitamin B_{12} deficiency, amyotrophic lateral sclerosis, cervical spondylosis, arachnoiditis, vascular anomalies, meningeal carcinomatosis, and spinal stenosis due to a combination of degenerative disk disease and hypertrophy of the ligamentum flavum (see Chap. 361).

Additional specific clinical syndromes occur in two other locations within the spinal canal. *Foramen magnum tumors* may extend into the cervical region or rostrally into the posterior fossa. A combination of signs and symptoms referrable to lower cranial nerves, sensory loss in the distribution of the second cervical segment, posterior headache, and asymmetric sensory and motor involvement of the limbs leads to the suspicion of such a tumor, most commonly a meningioma. *Tumors of the conus medullaris or cauda equina* produce pain in the back, rectum, and/or both legs and may mimic lumbosacral disk disease. With tumor growth, muscle atrophy in the legs associated with sphincter dysfunction and reflex changes usually point to the correct site of involvement.

Diagnosis of spinal cord tumors MRI has replaced all other modalities in the evaluation of the patient with cancer suspected to exist outside of or within the dura of the spinal canal (Fig. 353-5). In most centers MRI can be performed as an emergency procedure.

FIGURE 353-5 Sagittal T1-weighted MRI image of the conus medullaris (arrow) in a 26-year-old male with malignant primitive neuroectodermal tumor.

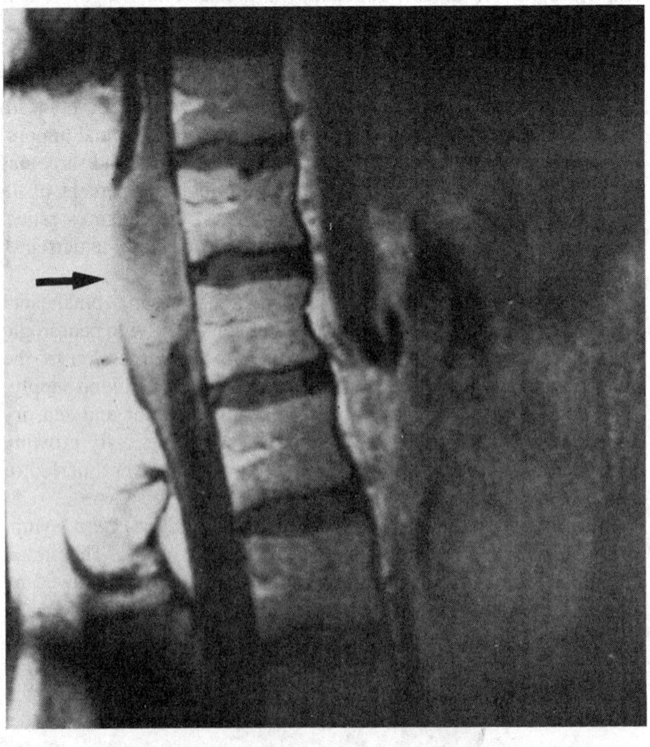

With or without gadolinium, these studies delineate the site, number, and extent of *extradural* deposits, while providing definitive information concerning the enlargement of neural foramens (which occur with schwannomas), distortion of paraspinal tissues with masses that have grown into the spinal canal from extraneural sites (as with lymphomatous spread), and the intricate anatomy of the cervicomedullary junction (as with meningioma or skull-base chordoma or nasopharyngeal metastases). MRI pictures have supplanted confusing arguments regarding ''complete'' or ''incomplete'' myelographic block. By identifying multiple extradural lesions needless surgery can be avoided and irradiation fields appropriately applied. Intradural, leptomeningeal metastases or tumors within the spinal cord or its roots are equally amenable to MRI visualization, especially when used following injection of gadolinium.

Myelography following the subarachnoid injection of nonionic contrast materials is often used to complement MRI studies or when they are unavailable. A small amount of contrast injected prior to CT evaluation of the spine is used to elucidate the coexistence of extradural tumor *and* calcified disk fragment, compression fracture of the bony vertebrae, osteomyelitis, or defects from prior surgery or irradiation. Similarly these CT studies identify intradural processes including arachnoiditis, lipomatous masses, and syrinx for which MRI experience remains scanty.

Cerebrospinal fluid removed at the time of myelography should be analyzed for cell count, protein content, and cytology. A specimen stained with Wright's stain should be analyzed and cells examined further after cytocentrifugation. The cell count is usually normal in spinal tumors unless there is meningeal tumor, but protein content is increased in virtually all cases of high-grade spinal cord block. The CSF glucose is usually normal unless there is meningeal tumor invasion.

Treatment Once the diagnosis of spinal cord tumor is established, rapid treatment is mandatory to maximize neurologic recovery. Extramedullary primary neoplasms are treated with microneurosurgery, and complete resection is usually possible. The most common intramedullary tumors, ependymomas and astrocytomas, usually can only be partially resected and are likely to recur. The role of radiation therapy for slowly growing tumors of this class is not well established; for high-grade astrocytomas a course of postoperative radiation is recommended. Glucocorticoids may improve function temporarily. There is no established role for chemotherapy of spinal neoplasms.

EPIDURAL CANCER: THE PATIENT WITH CANCER AND BACK PAIN Spinal epidural cancer should be suspected in patients with back pain and known systemic malignancy even in the absence of neurologic signs. Progressive paraparesis with bladder dysfunction and development of a sensory deficit may be avoided by early intervention. High doses of glucocorticoids (up to 100 mg dexamethasone per day) are administered immediately and radiation therapy is usually recommended. The results of treatment in the large series of patients with epidural cancer reported by Gilbert has led to the conclusion that radiation therapy is as effective as surgery in the relief of symptoms. The clinical condition of the patient at the time of diagnosis is the most important factor in prognosis; only 3 percent of patients paraplegic at the time of treatment, regardless of type of therapy, regain ambulation. Reconsideration is being given to surgical decompression as a primary mode of treatment in patients with radioresistant malignancies such as melanoma and lung, prostatic, and colonic cancers and in the setting of paraparesis of recent onset.

REFERENCES

Brant-Zawadzki M: MR imaging of the brain. Radiology 166:1, 1988

Bullard DE et al: Oligodendroglioma. An analysis of the value of radiation therapy. Cancer 60:2179, 1987

Byrne TN, Waxman SG: *Spinal Cord Compression; Diagnosis and Principles of Management.* Philadelphia, FA Davis 1990

Corbett JJ et al: Visual loss in pseudotumor cerebri. Arch Neurol 39:461, 1982

Gilbert RW et al: Epidural spinal cord compression from metastatic tumor: Diagnosis and treatment. Ann Neurol 3:40, 1978

GUTIN PH: Recurrent malignant gliomas: Survival following interstitial brachytherapy with high activity iodine 125 sources. J Neurosurg 67:864, 1987
HART R et al: Acoustic tumors: Atypical features and recent diagnostic tests. Neurology 33:211, 1983.
HESSELINK JR, PRESS GA: MR contrast enhancement of intracranial lesions with Gd-DTPA. Radiol Clin North Am 26:873, 1988
HOCHBERG FH, MILLER DC: Primary central nervous system lymphoma. J Neurosurg 68:835, 1988
HUGHES EN et al: Medulloblastoma at the Joint Center for Radiation Therapy between 1968 and 1984. The influence of radiation dose on the patterns of failure and survival. Cancer 61:1992, 1988
JENNINGS MT et al: Intracranial germ cell tumors: Natural history and pathogenesis. J Neurosurg 63:155, 1985
LAWS ER et al: Neurosurgical management of low grade astrocytomas of the cerebral hemispheres. J Neurosurg 61:665, 1984
LINSTADT D et al: Radiotherapy of primary intracranial germinomas: The case against routine craniospinal irradiation. Int J Radiat Oncol Biol Phys 15:291, 1988
MIRA JG et al: Outcome of prophylactic and therapeutic cranial irradiation in disseminated small cell lung carcinoma. Int J Radiat Oncol Biol Phys 14:861, 1988
RECHT L et al: Central nervous system metastases from non-Hodgkin's lymphoma: Treatment and prophylaxis. Am J Med 84:425, 1988
SMOKER WR et al: The role of MR imaging in evaluating metastatic spinal disease. Am J Radiol 149:1241, 1987
SUNDAESAN N, GALICICH JH: Surgical treatment of brain metastases. Cancer 55:1382, 1985
WALKER MD (ed): *Cancer Treatment and Research Series, Oncology of the Nervous System*, WL McGuire (series ed). Boston, Martinus Nijhoff, 1983
——— et al: Randomized comparison of radiation therapy and nitrosoureas for the treatment of malignant glioma of the brain. N Engl J Med 303:1323, 1980
WASSERSTROM WR: Diagnosis and treatment of leptomeningeal metastases from solid tumors. Cancer 49:759, 1982
YOUNG DP: Neurology complications of chemotherapy, in *Neurological Complications of Therapy*, A Silverstein (ed). Mount Kisco, NY, Futura Publishing, 1982, p 57

354 BACTERIAL MENINGITIS AND BRAIN ABSCESS

DONALD H. HARTER / ROBERT G. PETERSDORF

Pyogenic infections of the cranial contents originate in one of two ways, by hematogenous spread or by extension from surface structures, paranasal sinuses, osteomyelitic foci in the skull, penetrating cranial injuries, congenital sinus tracts, or following neurosurgical procedures.

ACUTE BACTERIAL MENINGITIS

DEFINITION Bacterial meningitis may be defined as an inflammation in response to bacterial infection of the pia-arachnoid and the fluid residing in the space which it encloses and also of the fluid in the ventricles of the brain. Since the subarachnoid space is continuous around the brain, spinal cord, and the optic nerves, an infective agent (or tumor cells or blood) gaining entry to any one part of it may extend immediately to all of it, even its most remote recesses; therefore, meningitis is always *cerebrospinal*. It also reaches the ventricles, either directly from the choroid plexus or by reflux through the basal foramens of Magendie and Luschka.

PATHOLOGY The effect of bacteria or other organisms in the subarachnoid space is to cause an inflammatory reaction in the pia and arachnoid and in the cerebrospinal fluid (CSF); in pyogenic meningitis, pus accumulates in this space. The infective agent or its toxin (gram-negative endotoxins, pneumococcal cell wall fragments), if allowed sufficient time to act, injures those structures which lie within the subarachnoid space (cranial and spinal roots) or ventricles (choroid plexuses) and adjacent to it (pial arteries and veins, underlying cerebral and cerebellar cortices, subpial white matter of the spinal cord, peripheral fibers of optic nerves, ependymal and subependymal tissues). In addition, purulent material may interfere with the flow of CSF from the ventricles or along the subarachnoid space over the brainstem, with resulting obstructive hydrocephalus. Although the outer arachnoidal membrane proves to be a remarkably effective barrier to the extension of infection, some reaction in the cranial subdural space and even in the inner surface of the dura and the spinal epidural space may occur. This happens more often in infants, approximately 15 percent of whom develop subdural effusions in response to meningitis, than in adults.

ETIOLOGY The causes of bacterial meningitis vary with age as follows:

1 *Streptococcus pneumoniae* (see Chap. 99) causes 30 to 50 percent of cases in adults, 10 to 20 percent in children, and up to 5 percent of cases in infants.
2 *Neisseria meningitidis* (see Chap. 109) causes from 10 to 35 percent of cases in adults and from 25 to 40 percent in children up to age 15. It is a rare cause in infants.
3 *Haemophilus influenzae,* type B (see Chap. 115) is responsible for 40 to 60 percent of cases in children, but for only 1 to 3 percent in adults and for virtually none in infants.

Also important in the etiology of meningitis are *Staphylococcus aureus* and *Staph. epidermidis* (see Chap. 100); the latter accounts for 75 percent of infections associated with shunting procedures for hydrocephalus. *S. aureus* meningitis occurs largely in postoperative neurosurgical patients, in patients with vertebral infection, and as a complication of *S. aureus* endocarditis. Other causative organisms include group B streptococci, particularly in infants; anaerobic or microaerophilic streptococci and gram-negative bacilli, usually in association with brain abscess, epidural abscess, head trauma, neurosurgical procedures, or cranial thrombophlebitis; *Escherichia coli* and other Enterobacteriaceae such as *Klebsiella-Enterobacter, Proteus, Citrobacter, Pseudomonas,* and *Acinetobacter calcoaceticus* (see Chap. 111), usually as a consequence of head trauma, neurosurgical procedures, spinal anesthesia, lumbar puncture, or shunting procedures to relieve hydrocephalus. Heretofore, gram-negative bacilli were associated most often with neonatal meningitis, but the spectrum has shifted to adults with debilitating diseases and other predisposing causes. Almost one-fifth of bacterial meningitis cases occurring in persons 50 years of age or older are due to gram-negative enteric bacteria. The outcome in this group has been notoriously poor. Rare meningeal pathogens include *Salmonella, Shigella, Clostridium perfringens,* and *Neisseria gonorrhoeae.*

The changing etiology of bacterial meningitis is reflected by the appearance of *Listeria monocytogenes* as a major pathogen, particularly in infants or elderly, debilitated patients or in those with immunosuppression secondary to transplantation, those who are receiving therapy for cancer, or those with connective tissue diseases. Alcoholism and high-dose steroids also appear to be predisposing factors. *Listeria* meningitis accounts for approximately 2 percent of all reported cases of bacterial meningitis in the United States. The mortality rate in the adult group with severe underlying disease is 70 percent (see Chap. 103).

EPIDEMIOLOGY AND CLINICAL SETTING The incidence of bacterial meningitis is between 4.6 and 10 cases per 100,000 persons per year. More than 2000 deaths due to bacterial meningitis are reported in the United States every year. *H. influenzae* is the most frequent cause, followed by *N. meningitidis* and *S. pneumoniae.* About 70 percent of all cases occur in children under the age of 5. Pneumococcal, *H. influenzae,* and meningococcal infections have a worldwide distribution, tending to occur more often in males and during the fall, winter, and spring. *H. influenzae* meningitis is the most frequent meningeal infection in children between 2 months and 3 years of age. Meningococcal infections occur most often in children and adolescents, but they are also encountered throughout most of adult life with a sharp decline after age 50. Meningococcal meningitis differs from other forms of meningitis because it may occur in epidemics. Pneumococcal meningitis predominates in adults over 40 years of age.

A variety of factors apart from age predispose to the development of certain types of acute bacterial meningitis. Acute otitis media and mastoiditis occur in about 25 percent of patients with pneumococcal meningitis, and pneumonia occurs in another 25 percent. Recent head injury is recorded in 10 to 20 percent of patients with pneumococcal meningitis and may give rise to recurrent meningitis because of persistent cerebrospinal fluid rhinorrhea. Pneumococcal meningitis also occurs in patients with sickle cell disease, Hodgkin's disease, or multiple myeloma; in urban general hospitals many adults who develop pneumococcal infections suffer from chronic alcoholism. Immunoglobulin deficiency (whether congenital or acquired), splenectomy, and renal or bone marrow transplantation also predispose patients to pneumococcal infection. Adults who develop *H. influenzae* meningitis should be suspected of harboring an anatomic defect (dermal sinus tract, old skull fracture) or have abnormal immune defenses. Meningitis caused by *Staph. aureus* usually follows neurosurgical procedures, a penetrating cranial wound, vertebral osteomyelitis, epidural abscess, and bacterial endocarditis. This organism and *Staph. epidermidis* account for the majority of cerebral ventricular shunt infections and occasionally neonatal omphalitis and meningitis. Gram-negative bacillary infections also complicate neurosurgical operations and other nosocomial diseases; they are assuming progressively greater importance in meningitis in adults.

PATHOGENESIS The three most common meningeal pathogens are invasive and depend upon antiphagocytic capsular or surface antigens for survival in the tissues of the infected host; all express their pathogenicity largely in the form of extracellular proliferation. All three are inhabitants of the nasopharynx in a significant part of the population. It is evident from the frequency with which the carrier state is detected that nasal colonization is not a sufficient explanation for infection of the meninges. The factors which predispose the colonized patient to bloodstream invasion, which is the usual route by which bacteria reach the meninges, are obscure. They include (1) antecedent viral infections of the upper respiratory passages; (2) in the case of the pneumococcus, infections in the lung and the absence of bactericidal antibodies; and (3) deficiencies in the terminal components of complement in *H. influenzae* and meningococcal infection (see Chaps. 109 and 115). Once bloodborne, the factors that lead to meningeal localization of bacteria are unknown, but it has been postulated that pneumococci, *H. influenzae,* and meningococci possess a unique predilection for the meninges. Other possibilities are that the entry of bacteria into the subarachnoid space is facilitated by disruption of the blood-CSF barrier by trauma, circulating endotoxin, inflammatory cytokines (see Chap. 20), or an initial viral infection of the meninges. Once CSF entry occurs, bacterial replication proceeds readily because levels of immunoglobulins and complement are too low to permit opsonization and/or bacteriolysis and phagocytosis by neutrophils is impaired.

Avenues other than the bloodstream by which bacteria can gain access to the meninges include congenital neuroectodermal defects, craniotomy sites, diseases of the middle ear and paranasal sinuses, and cranial trauma, notably skull fractures. Occasionally brain abscesses may rupture into the subarachnoid space or ventricles, infecting the meninges. The isolation of anaerobic streptococci, *Bacteroides* spp., or *Actinomyces* or of a mixture of microorganisms in the CSF should suggest the possibility of a brain abscess occurring as an antecedent to meningitis.

Once developed, characteristic features of bacterial meningitis include an increase in intracranial pressure, disruption of the blood-brain barrier, cerebral edema, and alterations in cerebral blood flow.

SYMPTOMATOLOGY Fever, headache, photophobia, seizures, vomiting, impairment of consciousness, and stiff neck and back are common to bacterial meningitis irrespective of its etiology. When the initial symptoms are only pain in the neck or abdomen, a confusional state, or delirium, the diagnosis is difficult. Three patterns of onset have been documented. In approximately 25 percent of patients, meningitis has a fulminant onset and patients become seriously ill within 24 h, usually without antecedent respiratory tract infections. In over 50 percent, meningitis develops over 1 to 7 days and is associated with respiratory symptoms. Slightly less than 20 percent have meningeal symptoms after 1 to 3 weeks of respiratory symptoms.

In children, the onset is often nonspecific. Fever and vomiting are more frequent than headache. There is a higher incidence of seizures, and the error of misinterpreting seizures as febrile convulsions is greater. The classic signs of meningitis may be minimal in elderly, debilitated patients in whom low-grade fever and changes in mental status may occur without headache or nuchal rigidity.

There are certain special clinical features that correlate with particular types of meningitis. Meningococcal meningitis should always be suspected in epidemics of meningitis; when the evolution is extremely rapid; when the onset is attended by a morbilliform, petechial, or purpuric skin eruption, larger ecchymoses, and lividity of skin in the lower parts of the body; and when circulatory collapse has occurred. Since a rash accompanies approximately 50 percent of meningococcal infections, its presence should dictate immediate institution of therapy for a neisserial infection, even though similar rashes may be observed with echovirus type 9 meningitis and rarely with staphylococcal, *H. influenzae,* and streptococcal meningitis. Recurrent systemic infections with meningococcus or *Haemophilus* should lead to the suspicion of complement deficiency. A family history of fulminant meningococcal disease in males in skipped generations suggests properdin deficiency. Pneumococcal meningitis is usually preceded by an infection in the lungs, ears, and sinuses, and, rarely, endocarditis. In addition a pneumococcal etiology should be suspected in patients suffering from alcoholism, sickle cell disease, basal skull fracture, following splenectomy or organ transplantation, or when there are multiple recurrences of bacterial meningitis following head trauma. *H. influenzae* meningitis may follow upper respiratory and ear infections in young children.

The signs of meningeal irritation—stiff neck or positive Kernig's and Brudzinski's signs—may be absent in the very young, the very old, or the severely obtunded. Signs of focal cerebral disease, although seldom prominent, are more frequent in pneumococcal and *H. influenzae* meningitis and are associated with a comparatively poor prognosis. Seizures are encountered most often in children with *H. influenzae* meningitis. In some instances they are caused by hypoglycemia, hyponatremia, or penicillin neurotoxicity. Some of the more transitory focal cerebral signs may represent postictal phenomena (Todd's paralysis); stable, local, cerebral lesions are probably the result of vasculitis and occlusion of cerebral veins with infarction of cerebral tissue, or they may connote localization of pus as occurs in brain abscess or subdural empyema. Abnormalities involving the third, fourth, and sixth as well as other cranial nerves are particularly frequent with pneumococcal meningitis.

LABORATORY FINDINGS The alterations of the cerebrospinal fluid are diagnostic. The *number of leukocytes* in the CSF ranges between 1000 and 100,000 per milliliter but averages between 5000 and 20,000. Cell counts above 50,000 per milliliter raise suspicion of the possibility of a brain abscess having ruptured into the ventricle (ventricular empyema). Neutrophilic leukocytes generally predominate, but an increasing proportion of mononuclear cells are found in the exudate as the infection continues, especially in partially treated meningitis. CSF lymphocytosis occurs in about one-third of bacterial meningitis patients with CSF cell counts of 1000 per milliliter or less. In the early stages careful cytologic examination may reveal some of the mononuclear cells to be myelocytes or young neutrophils. Later, as treatment takes effect, the proportions of lymphocytes, plasma cells, and histiocytes steadily increase. Early in meningococcal meningitis with fulminant meningococcemia, or more rarely with pneumococcal meningitis, the cellular response may be minimal or absent despite the presence of bacteria.

The CSF *pressure* is so consistently elevated (above 180 mmH_2O) that a normal or low pressure on the initial lumbar puncture in a case of suspected bacterial meningitis should raise the possibility that the needle was partially occluded or that the spinal arachnoid space was blocked.

The *protein levels* of CSF are higher than 45 mg/dL in 90 percent of cases, and most determinations fall in the range of 150 to 500 mg/dL.

The *sugar concentration* of CSF is depressed, usually to a level lower than 40 mg/dL or less than 40 percent of the blood sugar concentration (measured concomitantly), provided the latter is less than 250 mg/dL. However in atypical or "culture-negative cases," other conditions associated with a depressed CSF glucose should be considered. These include hypoglycemia from any cause, sarcoidosis of the central nervous system, meningeal carcinomatosis or gliomatosis, fungal or tuberculous meningitis, and subarachnoid hemorrhage. In acute cases of pyogenic meningitis, the CSF glucose concentration often approaches zero.

Gram stain of sedimented CSF permits identification of the causative agent in most cases of bacterial meningitis; it will be positive in about three-fourths of patients with untreated bacterial meningitis. Pneumococci and *H. influenzae* are identified more readily than are meningococci. Small numbers of gram-negative diplococci present within leukocytes may be indistinguishable from nuclear material which may also be gram-negative and of the same shape. In such cases a thin film of uncentrifuged CSF may lend itself more readily to morphologic interpretation than will a smear of sedimented CSF. The commonest errors in reading Gram-stained smears of CSF are misinterpretation of precipitated dye or debris as gram-positive cocci and confusion of pneumococci with *H. influenzae*. *Haemophilus* organisms may stain heavily at the poles so that they resemble gram-positive diplococci, and older pneumococci often lose their capacity to take a gram-positive stain. *Listeria monocytogenes* may be misidentified as a "diphtheroid" or hemolytic streptococcus in the microbiology laboratory. Staining with acridine orange and examination under a fluorescence microscope may demonstrate bacteria not observed with the Gram stain.

Cerebrospinal fluid cultures are positive in 70 to 80 percent of cases. When brain abscess is suspected, anaerobic cultures should be made, and meningococci should be cultured under 10% CO_2 (see Chap. 80). Partially treated meningitis poses a most difficult problem in diagnosis because cultures are often negative. The measurement of bacterial antigen in the CSF by latex agglutination, countercurrent immune electrophoresis (CIE), radioimmunoassay, or enzyme-linked immunosorbent assay (ELISA) to determine the presence of a specific capsular polysaccharide associated with *H. influenzae* type B, *S. pneumoniae*, and meningococcal serogroups A, B, C, and Y has been helpful. It has limited value in *E. coli* and streptococcal group B infections. Latex agglutination tests typically have a sensitivity of 90 to 100 percent, compared to 65 to 75 percent for CIE. Detection of antigen in the serum or urine of bacterial meningitis patients is not a sensitive diagnostic method. The concentration of bacterial antigen diminishes as treatment progresses. Failure to detect antigen does not rule out bacterial meningitis.

In addition to CSF cultures, *blood cultures* should always be obtained because they are positive in 40 to 60 percent of patients with *H. influenzae* and with meningococcal and pneumococcal meningitis and may provide the only definitive clue to the causative agent (if CSF cultures are negative). Routine cultures of the pharynx or external ear are as often misleading as helpful because pneumococci, *H. influenzae*, and meningococci are such common inhabitants of these locations. However, culture of pus from the middle ear or sinuses is often helpful.

The *blood leukocyte count* is generally elevated, and usually there is a shift to the left. Most patients with meningitis are sufficiently ill to require determination of blood urea nitrogen and serum electrolytes. These may be abnormal because of severe dehydration and may reveal inappropriate secretion of antidiuretic hormone (AVP) with resultant hyponatremia.

ROENTGENOGRAPHIC STUDIES Patients with bacterial meningitis should have x-rays of the chest, skull, and sinuses as soon as possible after admission. Chest x-rays are particularly important because they may reveal a silent area of pneumonitis or abscess. Sinus and skull films may provide clues to the presence of cranial osteomyelitis, paranasal sinusitis, or skull fracture. Computed tomography (CT scan) is usually not necessary in bacterial meningitis and is normal early in most infections. It is indicated when there is a suspicion of purulent sinusitis, mastoiditis, or epidural and brain abscess and always in the presence of focal neurologic deficits. In severe cases it may show cerebritis, vascular occlusions, and encephalomalacia. Later in the course, CT will detect hydrocephalus, brain abscess, and subdural effusions or subdural empyema. If bacterial meningitis is suspected and the patient does not have papilledema or focal neurologic findings, lumbar puncture should not be delayed while waiting for a CT scan to be done. When, in the presence of suspected meningitis, a CT scan is indicated to exclude lesions that might cause herniation, antibiotics may be instituted after blood cultures have been obtained. Most of the time this preliminary antibiotic treatment will not interfere with isolation and identification of the organism from the CSF.

COMPLICATIONS OF BACTERIAL MENINGITIS The longer the duration of meningitis and the less effective the treatment, the greater the chances that complications and neurologic residua will develop. The cranial nerve palsies, usually third, sixth, seventh, and eighth nerves, which occur in some 10 to 20 percent of cases usually disappear within a few weeks. Approximately 10 percent of infants and children who have bacterial meningitis will be left with persistent unilateral or bilateral sensory hearing loss. Deafness is especially frequent with pneumococcal, *H. influenzae*, and meningococcal meningitis. If focal and lateralizing neurologic signs last for some days or occur late in the course of meningitis, they are usually indicative of a vasculitis and cerebral infarction. Such lesions are most extensive in children with *H. influenzae* meningitis who are inadequately treated. If these lesions are extensive, they may leave the child retarded and epileptic. Persistent coma is more common in pneumococcal meningitis in adults. In infants or very young children with bacterial meningitis (particularly due to *H. influenzae*), prolonged alteration in state of consciousness or increased intracranial pressure (ICP) should raise the suspicion of obstructive hydrocephalus and subdural effusions. Approximately 30 percent of children who have had bacterial meningitis later will turn out to have subtle learning deficits.

DIFFERENTIAL DIAGNOSIS The diagnosis of bacterial meningitis is not difficult, providing a high index of suspicion is maintained. All febrile patients with lethargy, headache, or confusion of sudden onset, even if only low-grade fever is present, should be subjected to lumbar puncture. It is particularly important to consider meningitis in febrile, confused alcoholic patients. Too often the symptoms are mistakenly ascribed to inebriation, delirium tremens, or hepatic encephalopathy until the CSF reveals a meningitis.

Bacterial meningitis can be diagnosed definitively only by examination of the CSF. Viral meningoencephalitis and tuberculous, leptospiral, and fungal meningitides often enter into the differential diagnosis. Also to be considered are Behçet's syndrome, a disease characterized by recurrent oral and genital ulcers along with meningitis, and Mollaret's meningitis, which consists of recurrent episodes of fever, headache, and meningeal irritation accompanied by a leukocytosis in the CSF.

Tuberculous meningitis is discussed in Chap. 125. The diagnosis of other intracranial suppurative diseases is detailed below.

PROGNOSIS The case fatality rate for bacterial meningitis in the United States approximates 14 percent; it is highest for gram-negative and miscellaneous causes of meningitis. Of the three common forms of meningitis, pneumococcal meningitis is the most lethal. The triad of pneumococcal meningitis, pneumonia, and endocarditis has a particularly high fatality rate. The case fatality rate of *H. influenzae* or meningococcal meningitis has remained fixed at 5 to 15 percent for many years. Also in meningococcal infection, because of the fulminating nature of the disease and the often complicating adrenocortical necrosis (Waterhouse-Friderichsen syndrome), the mortality rate remains significant. Old age, infancy, abrupt onset, bacteremia, coma, seizures, and a variety of concomitant diseases including alcoholism, diabetes mellitus, multiple myeloma, and head trauma all worsen the prognosis.

It is often impossible to explain the death of the patient or at least to trace it to a single specific mechanism. Bacteremia with hypotension or brain swelling and bilateral temporal and/or cerebellar herniation are clearly implicated in the deaths of some patients during the initial 48 h. These events may occur in bacterial meningitis of any etiology; however, some observations suggest that they are more important in meningococcal infection. There is experimental evidence that acute centrally mediated respiratory failure (rather than circulatory collapse) is the major mechanism of early death. Deaths occurring later during the course of illness may be due to necrosis of brain tissue and respiratory failure, often consequent to aspiration pneumonia.

TREATMENT **Antimicrobials** Bacterial meningitis is a medical emergency; the rapid destruction of bacteria in the meninges and in the CSF is essential to survival. For this reason, drugs and dosages which achieve bactericidal activity in the CSF should be used where possible. The following therapeutic regimens are recommended: [NOTE: Dosage reductions of the penicillins, cephalosporins, and trimethoprim-sulfamethoxazole are needed in patients with renal failure (see Chap. 85).]

1 For adults with pneumococcal, meningococcal, or *Listeria monocytogenes* meningitis, penicillin G, 18 to 24 million units intravenously each day in four to six divided doses, is recommended; for children the dose of penicillin G should be 300,000 to 400,000 units per kilogram per day in divided doses every 4 h. Ampicillin (12 to 18 g daily intravenously in divided doses) or chloramphenicol (4 to 6 g given intravenously in divided doses) are alternative treatment regimens in adults. Ampicillin can also be used in children at a dosage of 300 to 400 mg/kg per day. The third-generation cephalosporins, cefotaxime (2 g IV every 4 h), or ceftriaxone (2 g IV once daily) are effective in pneumococcal and meningococcal but *not* in *Listeria* meningitis. Trimethoprim-sulfamethoxazole (160 mg TMP/800 mg SMX intravenously every 6 h) or chloramphenicol should be used to treat *Listeria* meningitis in penicillin-allergic patients.

2 For children over 2 months of age with *H. influenzae* or uncomplicated meningitis of unknown etiology, cefotaxime, 200 mg/kg per day in divided doses every 4 to 6 h, or ceftriaxone, 100 mg/kg per day up to a maximum of 2 g/d as a once-daily dose, should be administered. The use of these cephalosporins has largely replaced, in the United States, the combination of ampicillin and chloramphenicol, although the two regimens are of equivalent efficacy. For the older regimen, ampicillin, 300 to 400 mg/kg per day intravenously in divided doses, plus chloramphenicol, 75 to 100 mg/kg per day intravenously, should be given. The reason for the use of two drugs is that 15 to 25 percent of *H. influenzae* isolates are resistant to ampicillin, and chloramphenicol-resistant *H. influenzae* have also been reported. In order to avoid interference between the two drugs, ampicillin should be given 30 min before chloramphenicol. Once the causative microorganism has been recovered and its sensitivity to antimicrobials has been determined, chloramphenicol can be discontinued if the organism is sensitive to ampicillin. If the isolate is resistant to both ampicillin and chloramphenicol or if the child is intolerant to chloramphenicol, cefotaxime or ceftriaxone should be used. In adults with *H. influenzae* meningitis, the doses of ampicillin (12 to 18 g/d) and chloramphenicol (4 to 6 g/d) are administered intravenously either as a constant infusion or in divided doses. Alternatively, therapy with cefotaxime or ceftriaxone as outlined for pneumococcal infections can be employed.

3 Adult patients with pneumococcal, meningococcal, or *H. influenzae* meningitis who may be allergic to the penicillins can be treated with chloramphenicol in dosage of 4 to 6 g/d, or with a third-generation cephalosporin as outlined above. If the history of penicillin allergy is one of acute anaphylaxis, chloramphenicol is the preferred choice.

4 In meningitis due to gram-negative enteric bacilli, the organism is usually susceptible to treatment with a third-generation cephalosporin or a combination of antibiotics. Therapy can be started with cefotaxime, 2 g intravenously every 4 h, ceftazidime, 2 g intravenously every 6 h, or ceftriaxone 2 g/d, and an aminoglycoside (gentamicin or tobramycin, 3 to 5 mg/kg per day). Intrathecal therapy with gentamicin (8 to 10 mg/d) should be considered. When the bacterial species has been identified and its sensitivity to antimicrobials determined, the antibiotic regimen can be modified. If *Pseudomonas aeruginosa* or *Acinetobacter calcoaceticus* is identified, parenteral and intrathecal gentamicin or tobramycin should be given in conjunction with ceftazidime. Trimethoprim-sulfamethoxazole may provide a useful alternative for gram-negative meningitis (except that caused by *P. aeruginosa*) when the causative agent is resistant to third-generation cephalosporins.

5 Meningitis due to *Staphylococcus aureus* should be treated with a penicillinase-resistant penicillin rather than penicillin G because over 80 percent of isolates are penicillin-resistant. Nafcillin or oxacillin in daily doses of 12 to 18 g can be used in adults. Patients with staphylococcal meningitis who are allergic to penicillin can be given vancomycin intravenously (1 g every 8 to 12 h to adults) and intrathecally 10 to 20 mg/d.

6 When the etiology of meningitis is unknown, the drugs of choice are as follows: in adults, ampicillin, 12 to 18 g/d, or penicillin, 18 to 24 million units per day in divided doses, plus cefotaxime or ceftriaxone. In the penicillin-allergic patient chloramphenicol, 75 to 100 mg/kg per day in divided doses, may be substituted. In children, a third-generation cephalosporin administered as outlined for treatment of *H. influenzae* is recommended; in neonates, ampicillin, 200 mg/kg per day, and an aminoglycoside, usually gentamicin (2.5 to 5.0 mg/kg per day), are recommended.

7 Foci of infection in the paranasal sinuses or mastoids, in an infected shunt, or in cranial osteomyelitis should be identified so that appropriate drainage may be carried out when the acute episode of meningitis has subsided. Removal of shunts or reservoirs should be considered and is often necessary.

8 In most patients bacterial meningitis need not be treated for longer than 10 days except when there is a persistent parameningeal focus of infection. Antibiotics should be administered in full doses parenterally (preferably intravenously) throughout the period of treatment to avoid treatment failures due to inadequate concentrations of antibiotic in the plasma and CSF. Meningitis caused by *P. aeruginosa* or *Listeria monocytogenes* is usually treated for 3 weeks to prevent relapse.

9 Repeated lumbar punctures are not necessary to follow the course of therapy as long as the patient is doing well and the pathogen has been identified. The CSF sugar may remain low for a number of days after cultures become negative and should cause concern only if bacteria are present. Likewise, persistent but steadily diminishing mononuclear pleocytosis following pyogenic meningitis is the rule. CSF examination at the end of treatment for bacterial meningitis in patients who have recovered clinically from pneumococcal, meningococcal, or *H. influenzae* meningitis is not useful because it may lead to unnecessarily prolonged hospitalization; relapse after recommended therapy is extremely unusual. In meningitis caused by enteric gram-negative bacilli, in particular, *P. aeruginosa,* periodic repeat CSF examinations are indicated to follow the therapeutic response and confirm culture negativity. Similarly, repeat CSF examination is indicated in patients with meningitis complicating shunt or reservoir insertion and can determine the need for removal of the foreign body.

Adrenocortical steroids The few controlled studies available have demonstrated that steroids exert no beneficial effects in pyogenic meningitis, except in children with meningitis caused by *H. influenzae,* in whom the incidence of postmeningeal nerve deafness is reduced by the administration of dexamethasone. For adults these drugs should not be used except as an adjunct to intravenous mannitol in severe cerebral edema.

Other forms of therapy Intrathecal administration of enzymes to lyse excessive subarachnoid cellular exudate which may be associated with spinal block or hydrocephalus in the subacute stages of bacterial meningitis is of no value. There is also no evidence to support the therapeutic efficacy of repeated drainage of CSF. In fact, increased CSF pressure in the acute phases of bacterial meningitis is largely a consequence of CSF outflow blockage, increased intracranial blood volume, and later cerebral edema. In this situation lumbar puncture may predispose to temporal lobe or cerebellar herniation and death. Mannitol and urea have been employed apparently successfully in some cases of severe brain swelling with unusually high initial CSF pressures (>400 mmH_2O). Either should be accompanied by dexamethasone in relatively high doses (4 to 10 mg intravenously every 6 h). An adequate but not excessive amount of parenteral fluids should be given, and phenytoin should be given to control seizures. In children care should be taken to avoid hyponatremia and water intoxication—a cause of brain swelling. Subdural effusions usually resolve spontaneously but must be followed by serial CT scans. Drainage is rarely necessary.

RECURRENT MENINGITIS

Recurrent attacks of bacterial meningitis usually follow in the wake of trauma. The interval between the traumatic episode and the initial bout of posttraumatic meningitis may be as long as several years. *S. pneumoniae* is the usual bacterial pathogen. Often it proves to be one of the higher serologic types, reflecting the predominance of such strains in nasal carriers. *CSF rhinorrhea* is present in most of these patients but may be transient. The patient with recurrent meningitis of inapparent origin should always be suspected of having a fistulous connection between the nasal sinuses and the subarachnoid space. The fistula is usually traumatic (old basal skull fracture), and the site is the frontal or ethmoid sinuses or the cribriform plate. The rhinorrhea may be difficult to demonstrate except by injecting a radioactive tracer into the CSF and watching for its appearance in nasal secretions. Cerebrospinal fluid rhinorrhea may also be detected by measuring the glucose concentration of nasal secretions. The usual mucous secretions contain little glucose, but in CSF rhinorrhea the amount approximates that in the CSF. The prognosis in recurrent meningitis is remarkably benign, and the mortality is much lower than in ordinary pneumococcal meningitis. Nevertheless, vaccination of these patients with pneumococcal vaccine is indicated, and long-term prophylactic chemotherapy with penicillin V should be considered. Treatment of recurrent meningitis is similar to that for first bouts. Attempts to demonstrate CSF rhinorrhea should be made only after the acute infection has subsided; if evidence of a fistula is found, surgical repair should be considered.

Other causes of recurrent meningitis include congenital bony abnormalities of the inner ear, congenital dermal sinus tract, and tumors at the base of the skull.

SUBDURAL EMPYEMA

DEFINITION Subdural empyema is a suppurative process in the cranial subdural space between the inner surface of the dura and the outer of the arachnoid. The proper term for this condition is not *abscess* but *empyema,* indicating suppuration in a preformed space. Subdural empyema accounts for approximately one-fifth of all localized intracranial infections. About three-fourths of cases are unilateral, and the remainder bilateral.

ETIOLOGY The infection usually gains entry to the subdural space from the frontal or ethmoid sinuses or, less often, from the mastoid cells. These cases are termed *primary* subdural empyema. The subdural space may also become infected by extension of bacteria from a contiguous site of osteomyelitis or from a brain abscess. Septic thrombophlebitis and venous drainage of bacteria to the subdural space may be important in its development. Rarely has it been observed with bloodstream infections. Secondary subdural empyema usually follows neurosurgical drainage of a chronic subdural hematoma.

The bacterial flora in subdural empyema closely resembles that seen in chronic sinusitis and brain abscess; it may be polymicrobial. Isolates in order of decreasing frequency include aerobic streptococci, staphylococci, microaerophilic and anaerobic streptococci, aerobic gram-negative rods, and other anaerobes.

PATHOLOGY A collection of subdural pus in quantities of a few milliliters to 100 to 200 mL lies over the cerebral hemisphere. It is often mistaken for meningitis. The arachnoid, when cleared of exudate, is cloudy, and thrombosis of meningeal veins may be seen. The underlying cerebral hemisphere is depressed, and in fatal cases there is often an ipsilateral temporal lobe pressure cone. Microscopic studies demonstrate various degrees of organization of the exudate on the inner surface of the dura and infiltration of the underlying pia with small numbers of neutrophilic leukocytes, lymphocytes, and mononuclear cells. There is superficial thrombophlebitis; the thrombi in cerebral veins appear to begin on the outer side (toward the empyema). The thrombosis extends to other dural sinuses, and the superficial layers of the cerebral cortex undergo ischemic necrosis, which probably accounts for the unilateral seizures and signs of disordered cerebral function.

SYMPTOMATOLOGY AND LABORATORY FINDINGS The usual history includes chronic sinusitis or otitis with a recent flare-up and evidence of local pain and increase in purulent nasal or aural discharge. The illness is severe and progressive. Generalized headache, fever, vomiting, and a depressed sensorium are the first indications of intracranial spread. They are followed within a few days by localizing signs including focal motor seizures, hemiplegia, hemianesthesia, and aphasia. Papilledema is present in one-half of the patients at the time of diagnosis. Stupor or coma develops rapidly as the cerebral symptoms progress. Fever is usually present, but the neck is not always stiff. There is a leukocytosis and increased erythrocyte sedimentation rate. Lumbar puncture poses a distinct risk because it may precipitate transtentorial herniation. It is generally contraindicated if the diagnosis of subdural empyema is suspected and certainly should not be performed in advance of a CT scan of the head. The CSF shows increased pressure, a raised white blood cell count in the range of 50 to 1000 per milliliter including both neutrophils and lymphocytes, elevated protein (75 to 300 mg/dL), and normal sugar values. Unless subdural empyema is complicated by bacterial meningitis, no bacteria can be recovered from the CSF. In the type of subdural empyema that follows drainage of a chronic subdural hematoma, the onset is more indolent, fever is lower, and there is usually a local wound infection.

DIAGNOSIS Skull films may show involvement of the sinus or mastoid. CT scanning is the method of choice for establishing the diagnosis and location of a subdural empyema. The usual CT scan appearance is a crescentic or elliptical hypodense area lying directly below the cranial vault or adjacent to the falx cerebri. After administration of contrast, the CT scan may demonstrate an intense line of enhancement between the subdural collection and cerebral cortex. False-negative CT scans have been reported. When there is question about the diagnosis after CT scanning, magnetic resonance imaging may be required to define the lesion; cerebral angiography is rarely necessary or useful. In secondary empyemas, CT scan is invariably positive. Several conditions need to be distinguished clinically from subdural empyema: cerebral thrombophlebitis, brain abscess, viral encephalitis, acute hemorrhagic encephalitis (see Chap. 355), and bacterial meningitis with localizing neurologic findings or seizures.

TREATMENT Drainage of pus is the single most important part of treatment. In particular, it is important to institute drainage early because delaying it sharply increases the mortality rate. Specimens of pus obtained at surgery should be transported to the laboratory in oxygen-free containers and cultured both aerobically and anaerobically. Initial treatment should be guided by the Gram stain of the pus. In the absence of an identifiable organism, appropriate empiric antibiotic therapy consists of 20 million units of penicillin per day plus chloramphenicol, 4 g/d, administered intravenously. If a foul odor is present suggesting anaerobic infection, metronidazole, 500 mg intravenously every 6 h, may be substituted for chloramphenicol. If staphylococcal infection is suspected, nafcillin should be substituted for penicillin G (12 to 18 g/d in divided doses for adults). In postoperative neurosurgical patients the possibility of methicillin-resistant *S. aureus* or *S. epidermidis* should be considered and vancomycin administered as described for meningitis. Without such massive antimicrobial therapy and surgery, most patients will die, usually within 7 to 14 days, often while the unsuspecting physician and surgeon are waiting for better localization of an assumed cerebral abscess, the most commonly mistaken diagnosis. Antibiotic therapy can be altered when final culture and sensitivity results are available. It should be continued for 3 to 6 weeks. Drugs to reduce cerebral edema and to prevent seizures should be given. Mortality in subdural empyema is now between 10 and 20 percent. Long-term sequelae include seizures, hemiparesis, and dysphasia.

CRANIAL EXTRADURAL ABSCESS

This condition is almost invariably associated with osteomyelitis in a cranial bone which originates from an infection in the ear or paranasal sinuses. Pus and granulation tissue accumulate on the outer surface of the dura, separating it from the cranial bone. Symptomatically, the effects are those of a local inflammatory process: frontal or auricular pain, purulent discharge from the sinuses or ear, and fever and local tenderness. Unrelenting headache is a frequent complaint. Focal neurologic signs are uncommon. A cranial epidural abscess characteristically enlarges too slowly to cause sudden neurologic abnormalities. The CSF is usually clear and under normal pressure but may contain a few lymphocytes and neutrophils (20 to 100 per milliliter) and slightly raised protein concentration. CT scan is the diagnostic procedure of choice. False-negative scans have been reported; the diagnosis can then be made by contrast-enhanced CT scan or magnetic resonance imaging (MRI). Treatment consists of prompt surgical drainage of the epidural space, debridement of infected bone, and appropriate systemic antibiotics. The primary sinusitis or mastoiditis, from which the extradural infection has arisen, may also require surgical drainage.

SPINAL EPIDURAL ABSCESS

This type of abscess possesses unique clinical features and constitutes an important neurologic and neurosurgical emergency. It is discussed in Chap. 361.

INTRACRANIAL THROMBOPHLEBITIS

The lateral, cavernous, and superior longitudinal sinuses are relatively uncommon sites of infection. Usually there is evidence that the intracranial process has extended from the middle ear and mastoid cells, the paranasal sinuses, and skin around the upper lip, nose, and eyes.

LATERAL SINUS THROMBOPHLEBITIS In lateral sinus thrombophlebitis, which usually follows otitis media and mastoiditis, the earache and mastoid tenderness are succeeded, after a period of days to a few weeks, by fever, headache, nausea, and vomiting due to increased ICP. There may be swelling over the mastoid region, distention of veins, and tenderness of the jugular vein in the neck. With jugular vein involvement, there may be neck pain and restriction of movement. Drowsiness and coma are common. Papilledema (unilateral in some patients) is seen in about one-half of cases. Convulsions occur, but focal neurologic findings are infrequent. Abducens nerve paralysis and trigeminal nerve involvement (Gradenigo's syndrome) are found when there is spread to the inferior petrosal sinus.

CAVERNOUS SINUS THROMBOPHLEBITIS In this condition, which is usually secondary to oculonasal infections, the clinical syndrome is one of orbital edema, chemosis, venous congestion, and evidence of palsy of the third, fourth, ophthalmic fifth, and sixth cranial nerves. Later spread through the circular sinus to the opposite cavernous sinus results in bilateral symptoms and signs. The posterior part of the cavernous sinus may be infected via the superior and inferior petrosal veins without the occurrence of orbital edema or ophthalmoplegia. The patient appears acutely ill with high fever, headache, nausea, and vomiting. There is eye pain and the orbits are tender to pressure. Chemosis, edema, and cyanosis of the upper face are present; the bulbs are proptosed. Sensorium may remain clear until late in the infection. Ophthalmoplegia, pupillary changes, retinal hemorrhages, papilledema, and sensory changes in the ophthalmic division of the trigeminal nerve may be present. The CSF is usually normal unless there is associated meningitis or subdural empyema. The only effective therapy in the fulminant variety, associated with thrombosis of the anterior portion of the sinus, has been antimicrobial therapy usually aimed at coagulase-positive staphylococci (see Chap. 100), anaerobic or microaerophilic streptococci (see Chap. 108), and occasionally gram-negative pathogens. Anticoagulants have been used occasionally, but their value has not been proven. Cavernous sinus thrombosis must be differentiated from mucormycosis, which may cause a similar clinical picture in uncontrolled diabetics or in immunosuppressed patients (see Chap. 151).

SUPERIOR LONGITUDINAL SINUS THROMBOPHLEBITIS The superior sagittal sinus may become infected by spread from the lateral or cavernous sinuses or by extension from the nasal cavities, from a focus of osteomyelitis, or from epidural or subdural infection. General signs include fever, headache, and papilledema. Edema of the forehead and anterior part of the scalp occur. The typical neurologic picture is one of unilateral convulsions and hemiplegia, first on one side of the body, then on the other, because of extension into the superior cerebral veins. The paralysis may be predominantly monoplegic and involve mainly the legs.

Cerebral angiography with particular attention to the late filling of venous sinuses is the most specific diagnostic test. Digital subtraction angiography has been useful in the diagnosis of sagittal sinus thrombosis. CT scans show normal or small ventricles, hemorrhages, low-density lesions, and a high density lesion in the involved sinus. Postcontrast CT scan may demonstrate a filling defect in the involved sinus. Radionuclide dynamic and static scans may indicate termination of isotope activity in the midportion of the sinus. MRI may be the best and safest diagnostic approach.

All types of thrombophlebitis, especially those related to ear and paranasal sinus infection, may be complicated by other forms of intracranial suppuration including bacterial meningitis, subdural empyema, or brain abscess. The proper treatment of major sinus thrombosis due to infection is the systemic administration of antibiotics against organisms isolated from blood or pus or presumed to be present in the primary focus of infection. Antibiotics should be used in high dosage, and surgical drainage of infected bone and tissues should be carried out. The initiating focus should be brought under control by surgery if necessary. To operate on the primary focus before medical treatment is instituted is to court disaster. The better plan is to institute antibiotic therapy; surgery on the ears or sinuses should be decided upon only after the infection is controlled. In general, anticoagulants should be avoided because brain hemorrhage may result. Residual neurologic deficits are frequent, but the prognosis for recovery is good when optimal treatment is given early in the illness.

ASEPTIC THROMBOSIS OF INTRACRANIAL VENOUS SINUSES This may develop after sinus and ear infections and may lead to an obscure increase in intracranial pressure because of the occlusion of one lateral or superior sagittal sinus. The more common conditions which may be accompanied by aseptic thrombosis are postpartum and postoperative states, which are often characterized by thrombocytosis and hyperfibrinogenemia; use of oral contraceptive drugs;

congenital heart disease and marasmus in infants; systemic cancer; Behçet's disease; sickle cell disease; primary or secondary polycythemia; disseminated intravascular coagulation; and cryofibrinogenemia.

MALIGNANT EXTERNAL OTITIS

This paracranial infection is found in elderly patients with diabetes mellitus. Beginning in the external auditory canal, it spreads from the outer ear to the soft tissues below the temporal bone and invades the parotid gland, temporomandibular joint, masseter muscle, and temporal bone. *Pseudomonas aeruginosa* is responsible for the infection. The high mortality rate (initially reported at 40 percent) led to the term *malignant* for the condition; the adjective *necrotizing* or *invasive* may be preferable.

Symptoms and signs include pain in the ear with or without a purulent discharge, swelling of the parotid gland, trismus, and paralysis of the sixth to twelfth cranial nerves. Death is usually due to the development of meningitis. CT scan findings include obliteration of the normal fat planes in the subtemporal area and patchy destruction of the bony cortex of the mastoid. Radionuclide scans using Tc 99m or Ga 67 citrate are helpful in the initial identification of the disease and in following the course of the infection.

Prolonged intravenous administration of tobramycin, ticarcillin, ceftazidime, or imipenem is necessary to treat this condition. The choice of the β-lactam is determined by antimicrobial sensitivity testing. Antibiotics should be given for 6 weeks or for at least 2 weeks after all symptoms have resolved. Treatment for basal skull involvement may need to last at least 3 months, and, for prolonged treatment, oral ciprofloxacin may be a convenient and effective approach. Surgical debridement may be necessary.

BRAIN ABSCESS

PATHOGENESIS Most of the focal suppurative intracranial processes of this type are linked to chronic ear and sinus or pulmonary infections. About 25 percent of brain abscesses are due to disease of the middle ear, mastoids, or paranasal sinuses. Infection spreads to the brain directly across bone and dura mater or through vascular channels by septic thrombophlebitis or arteritis.

With frontal or ethmoid sinusitis, the abscess forms in the frontal lobe; with middle ear or mastoid infection, the abscess localizes to the temporal lobe or cerebellum. Of the remaining cases, about 25 percent are due to contaminated penetrating wounds or postoperative infections and about 25 percent are metastatic. Of these, about half are traceable to pleuropulmonary disease—usually bronchiectasis, empyema, lung abscess, or bronchopleural fistula. In the rest, the source of infection may be skin, bone, teeth, or heart. In about 20 percent of cases, the source cannot be ascertained. Brain abscess is seldom a consequence of bacterial meningitis. Brain abscess also occurs in patients whose immune systems are defective or suppressed. In these instances, *Nocardia* or nonbacterial causes such as fungi, protozoans, and helminths may be recovered from the abscess.

Brain abscess is particularly frequent in congenital heart disease with right-to-left shunts (e.g., tetralogy of Fallot) and may also complicate arteriovenous vascular abnormalities of the lung, as in cases of familial telangiectasia (Osler-Rendu-Weber syndrome). When brain abscess is associated with a right-to-left cardiac shunt, it is frequently single. With cranial trauma, the location of the abscess will depend on the site of the penetrating wound. In contrast to the otogenic and rhinogenic abscesses, abscesses of hematogenous origin are frequently multiple and may occur anywhere in the brain.

Bacterial endocarditis rarely gives rise to brain abscess. Instead, the picture is one of focal embolic encephalitis with or without signs of embolic vascular disease elsewhere (see Chap. 90). In subacute endocarditis the emboli are sterile and cause only infarction and mycotic aneurysms. The CSF may contain a small number of neutrophilic leukocytes, lymphocytes, and red blood cells; the protein level may be elevated, but cultures are sterile and sugar values remain normal. In acute bacterial endocarditis caused by *S. aureus*, miliary abscesses and purulent meningitis may develop. There may be infarcts and subarachnoid or intracerebral hemorrhages secondary to rupture of a mycotic aneurysm. Rarely do the miliary abscesses progress to large ones. Rapidly evolving cerebral signs in endocarditis are nearly always caused by embolic infarction or hemorrhage.

ETIOLOGY Streptococci, including *S. milleri* (a member of the viridans group), other viridans and nonhemolytic streptococci, enterococci, β-hemolytic streptococci, and peptostreptococci, are the most commonly isolated group of microorganisms (see Chap. 108). Next in order of frequency are members of the *Bacteroides* group, Enterobacteriaceae (*Proteus, Escherichia coli, Klebsiella*), and *S. aureus*. Pneumococci, meningococci, and *H. influenzae* rarely cause brain abscess. In addition to *Bacteroides* and anaerobic streptococci, anaerobic actinomyces, veillonellae, and fusobacteria have been isolated. Bacterial species vary with the site of the abscess—staphylococcal abscesses are usually a consequence of penetrating head trauma or bacteremia; enteric organisms are almost always associated with ear infections; anaerobic streptococci are commonly metastatic from the lung. Two or more species of bacteria are identified in a single abscess in approximately 25 percent of cases, and mixtures of aerobes and anaerobes may be found. *Nocardia* species can cause brain abscesses. They often occur in association with pulmonary involvement and complicate immunosuppressive disease or therapy (see Chap. 152).

PATHOLOGY The location of brain abscess in decreasing order of frequency is in frontal, parietal, temporal, and occipital lobes, followed by cerebellum and basal ganglia. Abscesses rarely occur in the pituitary gland or brainstem. Localized inflammatory necrosis and edema, septic thrombosis of vessels, and aggregates of degenerating leukocytes (suppurative encephalitis) represent the early reaction of bacterial invasion of the brain. This is followed by encapsulation of the liquefied brain and of accumulated pus. The lesion becomes encapsulated by fibroblasts and newly formed vessels, and the capsule thickens over a period of weeks. The meninges adjacent to the abscess, especially near the point of entry of infection, are infiltrated by neutrophils, lymphocytes, and plasma cells. Cerebral edema associated with the abscess and products of bacterial metabolism (such as anaerobically produced gas) result in increased ICP. The evolution of cerebral abscess can be divided into four stages: early cerebritis (1 to 3 days), late cerebritis (4 to 9 days), early capsule formation (10 to 13 days), and late capsule formation (14 days and later).

CLINICAL MANIFESTATIONS Most patients have symptoms for less than 2 weeks. Characteristically the clinical presentation is more like that of an expanding intracranial mass lesion than an infectious process. In patients with chronic ear, sinus, or pulmonary infections, a recent reactivation of the infection usually precedes the onset of cerebral symptoms. In a number of patients, evidence of CNS invasion is acute, and headache, vomiting, increasing obtundation, seizures, and a variety of localizing neurologic signs appear within a few days. In other patients, bacterial invasion of the brain substance may be asymptomatic or may be attended only by a slowly developing focal neurologic disorder. Sometimes stiff neck accompanies generalized headache, suggesting the diagnosis of meningitis. Early symptoms may subside or appear to respond to antimicrobials. Within a week or two, recurrent headache, slowness in mentation, focal or generalized convulsions, progressive neurologic defects, and obvious signs of increased intracranial pressure provide evidence of a mass in the brain. At this stage, the symptoms of infection are not conspicuous. Fever is present in less than half of the patients. Symptoms are usually progressive in their intensity. On presentation less than half of patients will have altered consciousness with lethargy, irritability, confusion, or coma. Hemiplegia is the most common focal finding. Seizures, either focal or generalized, occur in about one-third of patients; papilledema and neck stiffness are present in about one-quarter of patients.

Patients demonstrate focal neurologic signs related to location of the abscess as described below.

Frontal lobe abscess Headache, drowsiness, inattention, and general impairment of mental function are prominent. Hemiparesis with unilateral motor seizures and expressive aphasia are the most frequent neurologic signs.

Temporal lobe abscess Headache is usually on the side of the abscess and is localized to the frontotemporal region. If the abscess lies in the dominant hemisphere, there is aphasia and anomia (inability to name objects). A homonymous upper quadrantic field defect may also be demonstrable owing to interruption of the inferior portion of the optic radiation. This may be the only sign in abscess of the right temporal lobe. Contralateral motor or sensory defects in the limbs tend to be minimal, though weakness of the lower face is often observed.

Cerebellar abscess Headache in the postauricular or suboccipital region is usually the first symptom and may at first be ascribed to infection in the mastoid cells. Coarse nystagmus and gaze weakness to the side of the lesion and a cerebellar ataxia of the ipsilateral arm and leg are present in most patients. As a rule, the signs of increased ICP are more prominent than those of focal cerebral disease. Mild contralateral or bilateral pyramidal signs may provide evidence of ipsilateral brainstem compression.

DIAGNOSIS The diagnosis of a brain abscess depends on (1) a demonstrated source of infection in the ears, sinuses, or lungs or the presence of a right-to-left cardiac shunt, (2) evidence of increased ICP, and (3) focal cerebral or cerebellar signs. Clues to the origin of the abscess are often present on initial evaluation. They include chronic ear disease with discharge, sinus infection, orbital cellulitis, pharyngitis, infected skin wound, and chest infection.

Lumbar puncture in suspected brain abscess is potentially dangerous, particularly when the ICP is obviously elevated, and the information to be derived is not specific enough to justify the risk. Routine x-rays of the skull may demonstrate gas in an abscess cavity. The electroencephalogram (EEG) is usually abnormal with focal changes.

The CT scan is the most valuable procedure for visualizing brain abscess(es). It also demonstrates ventricular distortion, surrounding edema of white matter, and the thickness of the capsule; it enables close follow-up of therapy. Injection of iodine-containing contrast material will enhance the selectivity of the CT scan and will permit the visualization of an abscess from the early stage of focal cerebritis to a densely encapsulated mass demonstrated as a ''ring'' that is sharply demarcated both internally and externally with a homogeneous central area of decreased attenuation. Generally only a CT scan is required to make the diagnosis. Peripheral ring enhancement may also be found in tumor, cerebral infarction, resolving hematoma, radiation necrosis, and recent surgery; these conditions may enter into the differential diagnosis of the CT scan findings. Although MRI is more sensitive than CT in the detection of changes produced by early cerebritis, the improved sensitivity of MRI is rarely clinically significant. If CT scanning is not available, radionuclide brain scan is a reliable method for localizing brain abscess. If both CT and radionuclide scans are negative, there is little likelihood of cerebral abscess. Scanning procedures have supplanted arteriography in nearly all instances.

When the typical clinical picture is present and CT scan corroborates the presence of a mass lesion, the diagnosis is easy. If there is no source of infection and there are only signs and symptoms of a mass lesion, the diagnosis may be difficult. Sometimes only surgical exploration will settle the issue.

TREATMENT During the stage of acute suppurative cerebritis, intracranial operation accomplishes little and probably causes only additional trauma and swelling of brain tissue. If a predisposing factor is present and the presumed offending organism has been successfully cultured, there is good evidence that many brain abscesses visible by CT scanning can be cured at this stage by the administration of adequate doses of antimicrobials. Since the bacteriologic diagnosis must be presumptive, the most widely used regimen for adults consists of 20 to 30 million units of penicillin G and 2 to 4 g of metronidazole, both drugs given intravenously in divided doses. Cefotaxime or ceftriaxone may be added empirically in dosages similar to those for meningitis. Chloramphenicol, 4 to 6 g/d in divided doses, may be substituted for penicillin in allergic patients. This choice of antimicrobial agents is based on the preponderance of anaerobic streptococci and *Bacteroides* that are usually isolated from brain abscess. Treatment should be continued for 6 to 8 weeks, and if there is clinical improvement and recovery during antibiotic treatment, surgical intervention can be withheld.

For well-defined brain abscesses, selection of specific antimicrobials requires recovery of the responsible microorganism(s). Pus from the abscess cavity can be obtained by needle puncture at the time of craniotomy or by CT-guided percutaneous stereotactic operation, a procedure that is performed under local anesthesia with a 1 percent mortality rate. The specimen should be sent to the laboratory for Gram stain and for routine and anaerobic bacteriologic and fungal cultures. Specimens must be handled in a way that will not kill fastidious bacteria. Once the infecting bacteria have been identified and their sensitivities determined, the appropriate antibiotic regimen can be chosen.

Serial CT scanning and prompt, aggressive antibiotic treatment have avoided surgical intervention in cases of well-formed, small (<3 cm) abscesses, particularly when an organism has been isolated elsewhere. The indications for medical management include presence of multiple abscesses after one has been aspirated for diagnosis and culture, small abscesses located in deep brain structures, concomitant meningitis or ependymitis, the presence of a ventricular shunt, and an uncorrectable bleeding diathesis. In many instances, surgery should be performed to confirm the diagnosis, culture the organism, and treat the condition. Since the advent of CT-directed stereotactic surgery entails minimal risk, the only absolute contraindication to surgery is a bleeding diathesis.

ICP monitoring may be useful in the management of some brain abscesses, but is not usually employed. Initial elevation of ICP and threatening temporal lobe or cerebellar herniation should be managed by the prompt intravenous injection of mannitol or dexamethasone. Persistence or progression of high ICP manifested by deepening coma requires operation, regardless of the stage of the abscess. Likewise, clear-cut evidence of a mass lesion that is not improving with antimicrobial therapy is an indication for surgery. Gas-containing abscesses should be aspirated surgically or excised. The usual methods of treatment of an abscess are total excision or drainage by aspiration. If the abscess is superficial and encapsulated, total excision is sometimes attempted; if it is deep, aspiration of the abscess is the least traumatic treatment but might have to be repeated.

PROGNOSIS With the availability of CT scanning, more effective antimicrobials, and improved surgical techniques, abscesses have been treated earlier and more effectively. Mortality has fallen to approximately 10 percent. Neurologic abnormalities, particularly focal epilepsy, are rare, troublesome sequelae to brain abscess surgery. Following successful treatment of cerebral abscess in patients with congenital heart disease, correction of the cardiac anomaly is indicated to prevent recurrence.

REFERENCES

Anon JB, Miller GW: Malignant external otitis. South Med J 77:1541, 1984

Blaquiere RM: The computed tomographic appearances of intra- and extracerebral abscesses. Br J Radiol 56:171, 1983

Cherubin CE, Eng RHK: Experience with the use of cefotaxime in the treatment of bacterial meningitis. Am J Med 80:398, 1986

Dagbjartsson A, Ludvigsson P: Bacterial meningitis: Diagnosis and initial antibiotic therapy. Pediatr Clin North Am 34:219, 1987

Durack DT: Prevention of central nervous system infection in patients at risk. Am J Med 76(5A):231, 1984

GARVEY G: Current concepts of bacterial infections of the central nervous system: Bacterial meningitis and bacterial brain abscess. J Neurosurg 59:735, 1983
GORDON JJ et al: Meningitis due to *Staphylococcus aureus*. Am J Med 78:965, 1985
GORSE GJ et al: Bacterial meningitis in the elderly. Arch Intern Med 144:1603, 1984
HARRISON MJG: The clinical presentation of intracranial abscess. Q J Med 204:461, 1982
KAUFMAN DM et al: Subdural empyema: Analysis of 17 recent cases and review of the literature. Medicine 54:485, 1975
LEBEL MH et al: Dexamethasone therapy for bacterial meningitis. Results of two double-blind, placebo-controlled trials. N Engl J Med 319:964, 1988
LEFROCK JL et al: Gram-negative bacillary meningitis. Med Clin North Am 69:243, 1985
MANAPLANT TJ, ROSENBLUM MI: Trends in the management of bacterial brain abscesses: A review of 102 cases over 17 years. Neurosurgery 23:451, 1988
MARTON KI, GEAN AD: The spinal tap: A new look at an old test. Ann Intern Med 104:840, 1986
MAYHALL CG et al: Ventriculostomy-related infections: A prospective epidemiological study. N Engl J Med 310:553, 1984
POLLOCK SS et al: Infection of the central nervous system by *Listeria monocytogenes*: A review of 54 adult and juvenile cases. Q J Med 211:331, 1984
RAO KCVG et al: Computed tomographic findings in cerebral sinus and venous thrombosis. Radiology 140:391, 1981
ROSENBLUM ML et al: Controversies in the management of brain abscesses. Clin Neurosurg 33:603, 1986
SCHAAD UB et al: A comparison of ceftriaxone and cefuroxime for the treatment of bacterial meningitis in children. N Engl J Med 322:142, 1990
SZE G, ZIMMERMAN RD: The magnetic resonance imaging of infections and inflammatory diseases. Radiol Clin North Am 26:839, 1988

355 VIRAL DISEASES OF THE CENTRAL NERVOUS SYSTEM: ASEPTIC MENINGITIS AND ENCEPHALITIS

DONALD H. HARTER / ROBERT G. PETERSDORF

Viruses can affect the central nervous system in a variety of ways. Although much is known about the nature and replication of viruses, the correlation between viral properties and the type of the neurologic disease produced is inadequate or incomplete. Viruses that differ widely in their morphology, chemical composition, and replication can provoke identical clinical and pathologic changes in the CNS.

It is helpful to consider the time between the patient's first exposure to the viral agent and the appearance of disease, that is, to distinguish between CNS infections of a "fast" or "slow" nature. In fast or acute viral disease, neurologic changes occur very shortly after the patient first becomes infected by the virus. The illness follows a course of one to several weeks. In slow viral disease, the neurologic changes appear months to years after viral invasion, are insidious in development, and progress slowly.

ACUTE VIRAL CNS DISEASE

GENERAL CONSIDERATIONS Most viral CNS infections are the end result of preceding infection in other tissues and organs. There is usually a phase of extraneural viral replication before the nervous system becomes involved. Acute viral CNS infections are classified according to the clinical findings presented by the patient or, more indirectly, by the part of the nervous system involved by the disease process. In these terms, acute viral CNS disease is defined as meningitis, encephalitis, or myelitis, depending on the patient's symptoms and signs and the location of the infection. It is often difficult, however, to arrive at a single satisfactory localization on the basis of clinical findings alone. This leads to the use of compound terms such as meningoencephalitis or encephalomyelitis to describe the disease. This manner of classification is less than satisfactory because it gives no clear idea about the virus causing the condition.

Viruses vary in size, morphology, chemical composition, and effect on the host (see Chap. 133). Their common characteristics include a genome, which is either RNA or DNA surrounded by a protective protein shell; the fact that they multiply only inside the cell; and that the initial step in replication involves separation of the genome from its protective shell. They are divided into two broad categories on the basis of their nucleic acid content and then into major families and genera (Table 355-1). Certain common properties of viruses are important determinants of the disease they produce. Herpesviruses have a tendency to remain latent in cells. Togaviruses and bunyaviruses are transmitted by insect vectors. Enteroviruses replicate in the gastrointestinal tract and are transmitted by the oral-fecal route. Myxoviruses contain a segmented genome which is prone to genetic recombination. Selection of the most effective methods of virus isolation depends in great measure on the virus's properties. Knowledge of a virus's biochemical composition is of help in determining whether antiviral therapy can be used. Understanding the biologic features of viruses within the major families and genera permits associations which are impossible when the location of the disease process is considered alone (see Chap. 133).

ASEPTIC OR VIRAL MENINGITIS Etiology The term *aseptic meningitis* designates a disease characterized by an acute onset, meningeal symptoms, fever, cerebrospinal fluid (CSF) pleocytosis, and bacteriologically sterile cultures. The illness has a relatively benign clinical course of short duration, and recovery is the rule. With the introduction of more refined methods of viral isolation and the use of new culture techniques to define other microorganisms, it has become clear that aseptic meningitis is a syndrome of multiple etiologies. When viral infection produces the syndrome, the condition should be referred to as viral meningitis.

Epidemiology Aseptic meningitis affects between 9000 and 12,000 persons in the United States every year. Although all ages are involved, more than 90 percent of the patients are under age 30. The peak incidence of aseptic meningitis is in the late summer. The majority of cases seen in the summer are due to picornaviruses other than polioviruses, such as the coxsackie- and echoviruses. Mumps meningitis occurs more often in the winter and late spring. Both sexes are affected equally by enteroviruses, but there is a 2:1 or 3:1 male predominance in mumps meningitis. Acute aseptic meningitis may occur in the course of infection with Epstein-Barr virus (EBV) (see Chap. 137), cytomegalovirus (CMV) (see Chap. 138), herpes simplex virus type 2 (HSV-2) (see Chap. 135), varicella-zoster virus (VZV) (see Chap. 136), and human immunodeficiency virus (HIV) (see below and Chap. 264).

TABLE 355-1 Viruses of vertebrates

RNA-containing		DNA-containing

Picornavirus*
  Enterovirus*
  Cardiovirus
  Rhinovirus
  Aphthovirus
  Hepatitis A
	Paramyxovirus*
	  Paramyxovirus*
	  Morbillivirus*
	  Pneumovirus
		Hepadnavirus

		Parvovirus

		Papovavirus*
		  Papillomavirus
		  Polyomavirus*

	Orthomyxovirus
	  Influenzavirus
	  Influenza C virus	

Calicivirus		Adenovirus

Togavirus*
  Alphavirus*
  Rubivirus*
  Pestivirus
  Arterivirus
	Bunyavirus*
	  Bunyavirus*
	  Phlebovirus
	  Nairovirus
	  Uukuvirus
	  Hantavirus
		Herpesvirus*
		  Alphaherpesvirus*
		  Betaherpesvirus*
		  Gammaherpesvirus*

		Poxvirus
Flavivirus*		Iridovirus
Coronavirus	Arenavirus*	

Rhabdovirus*
  Vesiculovirus
  Lyssavirus*
	Reovirus	

	Birnavirus	

Filovirus	Retrovirus*
	  Oncovirus
	  Spumavirus
	  Lentivirus*	

* Virus genera and families associated with neurologic illnesses.

Clinical picture The symptoms and signs of viral meningitis are similar irrespective of the particular virus involved. The onset of illness is acute. There may be a prodromal "flulike" illness before the onset of meningitis, as in lymphocytic choriomeningitis. This biphasic pattern of illness also may be observed in young children with poliomyelitis or in illness due to other insect-borne viruses (see Chaps. 148 and 149). CNS involvement is manifested by an intense frontal or retroorbital headache. Malaise, nausea and vomiting, listlessness, and photophobia may be present. As a rule, there is little impairment of consciousness. The patient may be drowsy and slightly confused but is usually oriented and rational. Stupor and coma occur rarely. The temperature is usually elevated in the range of 38 to 40°C. There is neck stiffness on forward flexion. Kernig's and Brudzinski's signs are present in most cases but may be absent in patients with minimal meningeal irritation. Extension of the spine may be such that a child will sit with the head retracted and the arms extended posteriorly in the form of a tripod. Signs of focal damage to the central nervous system are rarely present. Occasionally, strabismus or diplopia, asymmetry of tendon reflexes, and an inconstant extensor plantar response may be found.

Clinical findings outside the nervous system may provide clues to the virus involved in the infection. Parotitis in association with viral meningitis suggests mumps. Skin rash has been a prominent feature of coxsackievirus or echovirus infections (see Chap. 144). Blotchy or punctate maculopapular rashes that involve the extremities and which occur chiefly in the summertime are commonly due to echovirus. Herpangina (large, painful vesicles in the posterior one-third of the oropharynx) are usually caused by coxsackieviruses. Sharp pains in the chest aggravated by deep respiration or coughing suggest the pleurodynia seen with Coxsackie B viruses. Infection with VZV, HSV, or EBV is usually dominated by nonneurologic manifestations.

Laboratory findings The lumbar CSF is usually under increased pressure and clear or slightly turbid in appearance. Slight turbidity can be demonstrated by holding a tube containing CSF to the light and agitating the fluid with a gentle finger tap. CSF usually contains 10 to 100 cells per microliter. At times, the cell count rises to levels of 3000 per microliter or greater. The cells are usually more than three-fourths lymphocytes or mononuclear cells. Polymorphonuclear cells may predominate in the early phases of aseptic meningitis. The CSF protein and sugar concentrations are usually normal. Isolated instances of depressed CSF sugar in patients with infections due to mumps or HSV have been reported but are rare. If the patient presents with CSF that contains less sugar than expected, meningitis due to bacteria, mycobacteria, or fungi should receive first attention. Oligoclonal IgG bands may be found in the CSF of patients with viral meningitis. Gram stain and india ink preparations fail to identify an organism; bacterial and fungal cultures are negative. Although certain viruses (such as mumps, HSV, VZV, and CMV) can be recovered from CSF with relative ease, in most cases of viral meningitis, it is usually impossible to recover the responsible viral agent from the patient's CSF. The white cell count in the blood is usually normal, but leukopenia is present in about one-third of patients.

The specific viral diagnosis can usually be made by performing serologic tests on acute and convalescent sera and by attempting to isolate viruses from feces, urine, and throat washings. With the exception of CMV and HIV, performance of a Monospot test or specific measurement of antibodies to EBV can lead to the diagnosis of aseptic meningitis complicating infectious mononucleosis (see Chap. 137). Other useful tests can include CSF cytologies, a nontreponemal antibody test for syphilis (see Chap. 128) and serologies for *Borellia burgdorferi* (see Chap. 132). Attempts to isolate the agent from blood are usually unsuccessful.

Differential diagnosis The syndrome of viral or aseptic meningitis can be caused by a number of different infectious and noninfectious agents. The majority of cases of viral origin are due to picornaviruses, togaviruses, herpesviruses, paramyxoviruses, and arenaviruses. The list of nonviral infectious causes of the aseptic meningitis syndrome is extensive. It includes intracranial infections located near the meninges (otitis, mastoiditis, vertebral osteomyelitis); brain abscess; partially treated bacterial meningitis; and mycobacterial, spirochetal, fungal, rickettsial, protozoan, or helminthic infections.

Noninfectious causes of the aseptic meningitis syndrome include the intrathecal introduction of drugs and agents for diagnostic tests and tumors in close proximity to the cerebral ventricles or that invade the subarachnoid space. Cytologic examination of cells in the CSF will distinguish neoplastic meningeal infiltration from viral meningitis. Systemic diseases such as sarcoidosis, disseminated lupus erythematosus, and infective endocarditis may be associated with aseptic meningitis.

Also, there are a number of infrequently encountered systemic diseases in which the CSF findings resemble viral meningitis. These include (1) Behçet's disease, characterized by uveitis, genital and oral ulcers, and focal neurologic abnormalities; (2) Vogt-Koyanagi and Harada's diseases, which combine uveitis, depigmentation of the hair and skin about the eyes, loss of eyelashes, and deafness; (3) Mollaret's meningitis; and (4) Lyme disease.

Treatment The treatment of viral meningitis is symptomatic. Antiviral agents are not indicated in uncomplicated cases. Fever and other symptoms resolve in 3 to 5 days, and patients are usually entirely well within 2 weeks. CSF abnormalities are most pronounced from the fourth to sixth day, but the CSF white blood cell count may remain elevated for several weeks in patients who are otherwise asymptomatic. Initial therapy with antimicrobial agents may be appropriate if the initial elevation is not completely typical for viral infection. In most instances, patients recover from viral meningitis without sequelae. A limited number of patients may develop muscular weakness and other forms of motor disability. A very small number of patients may have recurrent attacks of viral meningitis; the multiple episodes are often due to different viruses. Acyclovir treatment can shorten the course of infection with HSV and VZV (see Chaps. 135 and 136).

Prognosis It is important to recognize that viral meningitis is an acute and self-limited illness and to realize that it may mimic life-threatening CNS infections which are potentially treatable. Most important to appreciate is the similarity between viral meningitis and partially treated bacterial meningitis, tuberculous meningitis, or fungal meningitis. If the CSF changes are not completely characteristic of viral meningitis or if the patient's clinical response is atypical, it is important to perform repeated lumbar punctures and to reexamine the CSF within a relatively brief period of time, until the clinical picture becomes clear.

VIRAL ENCEPHALITIS **Definition** The term *encephalitis* is used when there is clinical and/or pathologic evidence of involvement of the cerebral hemispheres, brainstem, or cerebellum by the infectious process. It is customary to divide viral encephalitis into primary and postinfectious or parainfectious forms and to consider whether the disease is sporadic or epidemic. The *primary* form of the disease occurs when the encephalitis is the presenting form of the disease and is due to direct invasion and replication of virus within the CNS. The term *postinfectious* or *parainfectious* is used to describe an encephalitis that follows or occurs in combination with other viral illnesses or administration of certain vaccines (see Chap. 356). The cause of the encephalitis in such cases is believed to be a hypersensitivity reaction. The pathologic picture is typical of multifocal perivenous demyelination. The virus cannot be recovered from the CNS. If the inflammatory condition extends into the spinal cord, the term encephalomyelitis is used.

Clinical picture When encephalitis is the primary illness, such as with togaviruses and herpesviruses, there may be a minor illness consisting of such systemic symptoms as headache, myalgia, malaise, and upper respiratory symptoms. These nonspecific symptoms may occur several days before neurologic complaints and signs are recognized.

The onset of neurologic symptoms is abrupt. There is alteration in the patient's state of consciousness with lethargy, drowsiness, or stupor. The patient's behavior may be abnormal as a consequence of confusion, disorientation, and hallucinations. A convulsion or series of convulsions may occur at the start of the illness, and seizures may be the sole presenting symptom. The patient usually complains of headache, nausea, and vomiting. Fever is usually present, and there may be stiffening of the neck on forward bending. Focal neurologic abnormalities are found, depending on the portion of the nervous system involved by the inflammatory process. Involvement of the cerebral hemispheres may result in aphasia, signs of corticospinal and corticobulbar tract lesions, involuntary movements, ataxia, sensory defects, and loss of retentive memory.

Laboratory examinations General laboratory tests are usually of little help in the diagnosis of encephalitis. They may provide evidence of systemic disease, such as abnormal lymphocytes in infectious mononucleosis and elevated amylase and transaminase levels in mumps and certain picornavirus infections.

Lumbar puncture, followed by examination of the CSF, is the most important diagnostic test. The CSF is usually under normal or slightly elevated pressure, clear or slightly turbid, and contains an increased number of white cells (in the range of 50 to 500 per microliter), a slight-to-moderate elevation of protein content, and a normal glucose level. There may be a predominance of polymorphonuclear leukocytes in the early phase of the illness. The protein content will often rise as the total cell count diminishes. In encephalitis caused by HSV-1, the CSF may be slightly bloody or xanthochromic and contain a significant number of red blood cells. This reflects the sometimes hemorrhagic nature of HSV encephalitis. Occasionally a viral encephalitis may exist without CSF abnormalities, which makes the diagnosis even more difficult.

The electroencephalogram may be of diagnostic help in suspected encephalitis. Diffuse or bilateral abnormalities can be defined by the EEG in patients who present with focal or unilateral neurologic deficits. A number of EEG changes may be seen, but the most common pattern is a diffuse slow wave activity with disruption of normal rhythms, punctuated at times with periodic high-amplitude bursts and spike-and-wave complexes. Computed tomography (CT), magnetic resonance imaging (MRI), and radionuclide scans may be helpful in demonstrating intracranial mass lesions or localized foci of infection about or within the brain. The cerebral cortex may be enhanced diffusely. Because of its sensitivity to altered water content, MRI detects changes of viral encephalitis before CT.

Diagnosis When presented with a patient with suspected viral encephalitis, it is important to exclude nonviral infections for which potential treatment is available. A number of conditions can mimic viral encephalitis (Table 355-2). It is imperative to consider these alternative causes when the patient is first evaluated. Once the

TABLE 355-2 Nonviral conditions mistaken for acute viral encephalitis

Infection:	
Bacterial	Early or imperfectly treated meningitis Brain abscess Parameningeal infections Illness due to mycobacteria, spirochetes, *Mycoplasma*
Fungi	*Cryptococcus, Coccidioides immitis, Histoplasma, Candida, Nocardia, Blastomyces*
Rickettsia	Rocky Mountain spotted fever
Protozoa	"Fresh water" amebiasis, malaria, toxoplasmosis
Metazoa	Cysticercosis, trichinosis, and others
Intoxication	Salicylates, barbiturates, heavy metals, tick paralysis
Endocrine and metabolic disorders	Acute sodium, calcium, or carbohydrate imbalance; porphyria, pheochromocytoma
Systemic diseases	Sarcoidosis, hyperglobulinemia, collagen disease, neoplasms, endocarditis with embolization
Acute psychotic disorders	

SOURCE: After Brown.

diagnosis of primary viral encephalitis is secure, it is important to determine if the illness is occurring as part of an epidemic or as an isolated sporadic event. Knowledge of the seasonal, geographic, and age group occurrence of the disease can often furnish enough information to make an informed guess about the correct viral etiology. During the summer and early fall, togaviruses, bunyaviruses, and picornaviruses may prevail. Some of these viruses may produce milder disease than others; some, such as western equine and California encephalitis viruses, affect a predominantly young age group. In the winter, epidemic encephalitis is more often associated with paramyxovirus, VZV, EBV, or rubella virus infection. HSV is responsible for more cases of nonepidemic sporadic encephalitis cases than any other virus.

The course of viral encephalitis is variable. It may be a short-lived, benign illness or a devastatingly severe one which leaves the patient with pronounced impairment of cerebral functions. Severe sequelae may be associated with certain viruses (HSV-1, eastern equine encephalitis, Japanese encephalitis, and St. Louis encephalitis). Other viruses cause milder disease (California encephalitis, western equine encephalitis). The acute phase of the disease usually lasts a few days to a week. Resolution can be abrupt or gradual. The disease may be complicated by a salt-wasting syndrome resulting from hypothalamic involvement and/or alterations in temperature or respiratory control centers owing to brainstem involvement. These events may occur rapidly and require prompt recognition and correction. Neurologic defects may continue to improve over a period of weeks to months.

In most instances of epidemic encephalitis, the viral diagnosis is made by serologic tests of acute and convalescent phase sera. Three major serologic tests are employed: complement-fixation, hemagglutination-inhibition, and neutralization. Because the serologic test is crucial for viral diagnosis, it is imperative to obtain an acute-phase serum as soon as the diagnosis of viral encephalitis is suspected. In vector-transmitted encephalitis which does not result in fatality, the blood is the most likely tissue source of viral isolation. Isolation of virus from blood is difficult, however, because viremia is usually brief and occurs before the onset of neurologic symptoms. In fatal cases, the virus can often be isolated from brain and spinal cord by inoculation of susceptible animals and tissue culture.

When HSV encephalitis is suspected, greater urgency is required in arriving at a viral diagnosis because there is a definite advantage in initiating antiviral therapy as quickly as possible (see Chap. 135). Serologic tests are not helpful. A number of patients with HSV encephalitis present with fever and neurologic findings compatible with a bilateral space-occupying lesion of the medial parts of the temporal and the orbital parts of the frontal lobes. A severe retentive memory defect is a frequent sequelum. HSV can be best demonstrated in brain tissue obtained by biopsy. Examination of the tissue by light, electron, and immunofluorescence microscopy and inoculation of a brain homogenate into cell cultures and animals permit a specific diagnosis of HSV early in the course of the patient's illness. However, many neurologists object to biopsy as a diagnostic procedure because the risks and sequelae outweigh the dangers of treatment. Moreover, enhanced CT scans, MRI, and radionuclide brain imaging often reveal the temporal lobe lesions which, when added to the clinical picture and a CSF pleocytosis, make the diagnosis fairly certain and permit treatment without brain biopsy. MRI may improve the sensitivity by detecting hemorrhage in certain HSV encephalitis patients.

Encephalitis may present as an infrequently encountered manifestation of a systemic disease such as measles, varicella, or neoplasia. When this is the case, the encephalitis occurs after the more characteristic features of the disease have become evident. Rarely, the systemic disease may appear after the diagnosis of encephalitis has been established.

UNUSUAL FORMS OF VIRAL ENCEPHALITIS *Acute cerebellar ataxia* may be associated with a number of different viruses (picornaviruses, VZV, and EBV). The illness usually afflicts children between the ages of 1 and 5 years. The majority of patients have had a preceding mild infectious illness a week or so before the onset of neurologic signs. The onset of the illness is characteristically abrupt with prominent ataxia of the trunk and limbs. Complete recovery is the rule, but a permanent cerebellar deficit may ensue in patients when ataxia is profound in the early stages of the illness. In some instances of VZV infection, the cerebellar lesions are of the parainfectious, demyelinating type (see Chap. 356).

Acute hemorrhagic leukoencephalitis is an infrequently encountered hyperacute disease of cerebral white matter which is often preceded by some form of systemic viral illness, most often an upper respiratory tract infection. The disease is marked by an acute onset, progressively deepening disturbance of consciousness, fever, seizures, and focal cortical abnormalities. Cerebral involvement is frequently unilateral. The course is rapid and usually fatal. There is a peripheral leukocytosis, and the CSF frequently contains mononuclear and polymorphonuclear leukocytes. The presence of mass effect or increased absorption coefficient on CT scan within the first 3 days of encephalitis should suggest this diagnosis. The cause of the disease is unknown. It has not been linked to infection by a specific virus or group of viruses and may well be allergic in nature. A virus has not been recovered from brain tissue. Treatment includes vigorous control of intracranial pressure and seizures and aggressive use of glucocorticoids in high dosage (see Chap. 356).

Limbic encephalitis is a form of encephalitis localized to the temporal and frontal lobes—the limbic part of the brain. It is encountered as a remote effect of malignancy—most commonly carcinoma of the lung. A viral etiology has been suspected but never proved. Patients with limbic encephalitis have marked impairment of recent memory manifested by a confabulatory-amnestic state, and generalized seizures. The patient's CSF often contains a limited number of lymphocytes and mononuclear cells. The EEG is characterized by paroxysmal and/or slow waves over one or both temporal lobes. Pathologic changes are most pronounced in the hippocampal formation and amygdaloid nuclei. Encephalitis with predilection for the brainstem has also been reported as a remote effect of tumor (see Chap. 310).

Encephalitis lethargica (von Economo's disease) first occurred during and for about 10 years after World War I. A causative viral agent was never identified, but the clinical and pathologic features were those of a viral infection of the thalamus and midbrain. The disease was characterized by pronounced somnolence and ophthalmoplegia. A high proportion of survivors developed a parkinsonian syndrome months or years after the encephalitis (see Chap. 359). Sporadic case reports of patients with the clinical features of encephalitis lethargica appear even to the present time.

MYELITIS Viral infection of the central nervous system may localize in the parenchyma of the spinal cord producing myelitis. Poliovirus infection with damage to spinal motor neurons is the prototype of a viral infection localized chiefly to the spinal cord. Vaccination has markedly reduced but not eliminated poliomyelitis because patients who have not been vaccinated remain susceptible. Progressive muscular weakness, fasciculations, and atrophy occur in some patients many years after an acute episode of poliomyelitis. The cause of this ''postpolio'' syndrome is still uncertain; it may be a recrudescence of viral activity (see Chap. 144).

Spinal paralytic disease has also been described with other enteroviruses (coxsackieviruses and echoviruses). The illness is characterized by an asymmetric flaccid paralysis of the limbs; it is usually less severe and has a higher rate of recovery from muscular weakness than poliomyelitis.

Other viruses have also been reported to affect the spinal cord directly. Herpesvirus type 2 infection in the genital and perineal region has been associated with paralysis of sphincter function, probably indicative of direct viral involvement of the sacral spinal cord. Myelitis due to VZV (aside from the ganglionitis and unilateral poliomyelitis) is another very rare cause of a leukomyelitis resulting in bilateral weakness of the legs with occasional ankle clonus or extensor plantar responses. Sphincter disturbances are present in two-thirds of patients and a sensory level in about one-half of patients. The CSF contains from 25 to 125 cells per microliter; the protein content may be normal or elevated. Recovery of function is the rule.

There may also be delayed involvement of the white matter of the spinal cord following viral infection. This is a parainfectious demyelinative process that interrupts sensory and motor tracts at one level and is termed an acute transverse myelitis. It begins with the abrupt onset of bilateral weakness of the legs and concomitant involvement of ascending sensory pathways. Urinary bladder and bowel functions are usually disturbed early in the course of the illness. An exanthem or respiratory infection not uncommonly precedes neurologic symptoms. Acute myelitis in the absence of encephalitis has been described in association with measles, VZV, echovirus, HSV, and infectious mononucleosis. It has also been observed after rabies and smallpox vaccination. Virus isolation from CSF has been unsuccessful. A small proportion of patients with acute transverse myelitis will later develop multiple sclerosis. Acute spinal epidural abscess should be considered and excluded in patients who present with an acute nontraumatic transverse spinal cord syndrome. Rarely schistosomiasis may present with transverse myelitis (see Chap. 170).

TREATMENT Of the various viruses that cause acute encephalitis, HSV is the most responsive to antiviral chemotherapy. The drug of choice is acyclovir, given intravenously. Details of therapy are given in Chap. 86.

CNS DISEASES DUE TO SLOW VIRUS INFECTION

In slow virus infections, a protracted period, often months or years, passes between the introduction of the infectious agent and the appearance of clinical illness. Once neurologic disease is established, it may progress slowly over many months or years. The reasons why a certain virus will cause acute illness in one patient and slow infection in another are still largely unknown. Viruses causing slow infections do not appear to share any common features. No single virus property can be correlated with the slow virus disease process. The factors invoked to explain slow virus infections include (1) a defect in the composition of the virus; (2) a change in the virus's antigenicity, (3) an altered or defective host immune response; (4) a special property of the virus which permits it to remain latent or to become integrated in the host cell's genome; or (5) a yet incompletely understood and possibly unique method of replication.

Slow virus CNS diseases affect the parenchyma of the cerebral hemispheres and, in some instances, the cerebellum, brainstem, and spinal cord. These infections are not grouped by their topography, i.e., the part of the nervous system that they damage, or by their clinical presentation. Some slow viruses provoke a mild conventional inflammatory response during the time they are clinically silent; others are able to reside within cells for long periods without causing detectable cytopathic changes. The role of immunity in slow virus infection is largely unknown. Some slow virus infections occur in the presence of elevated levels of circulating antibodies; in others, there may be no detectable immune response.

Because infective agents causing some human slow CNS diseases have not been demonstrated to contain nucleic acid, the slow viral CNS infections are divided into those due to conventional viruses and those due to unconventional agents whose viral nature has not been fully established (Table 355-3). There are currently nine well-defined neurologic diseases caused by slow viruses. No consistently effective therapy is now available for any of them. Conventional viruses have been recovered from the CNS of patients with subacute sclerosing panencephalitis (SSPE), progressive multifocal leukoencephalopathy (PML), progressive rubella encephalitis, tropical spastic paraparesis (TSP), and persistent viral infection in immunodeficient patients. Each of these is based on an inflammatory reaction in the CNS. Kuru, Creutzfeldt-Jakob disease (CJD), and Gerstmann-Sträussler-Scheinker (GSS) disease share common neuropathologic features

TABLE 355-3 Slow virus diseases of the CNS

Conventional viruses	Subacute sclerosing panencephalitis (SSPE) Progressive multifocal leukoencephalopathy (PML) Progressive rubella encephalitis Tropical spastic parapheresis (TSP) Persistent infection in immunodeficiency: Congenital or primary Acquired or induced
Unconventional viruslike agents	Kuru Creutzfeldt-Jakob disease (CJD) Gerstmann-Sträussler-Scheinker disease (GSS)

which are noninflammatory. They produce fine vacuolation of nervous tissue and hence are referred to as the subacute spongiform virus encephalopathies. Although these diseases have been shown to be of infectious etiology by the transmission of neurologic illness to higher primates, their causative agents remain incompletely characterized. They are classified as the slow virus infections due to unconventional agents.

The best studied of the unconventional transmissible agents is scrapie, a neurologic disease of sheep. The true nature of the scrapie agent has not been defined. There is evidence that a surface membrane protease-resistant protein (PrP) is involved in the development of the disease. Concentrated and partially purified scrapie agent contains a sialoglycoprotein of approximately 27,000 to 30,000 mol wt, designated PrP 27-30, as a major component. PrP 27-30 is recovered from scrapie-infected brain; the protein is not found in normal brain. Because of this association, the term *prion* was introduced as an operational name for the putative infectious agent. Prion is defined as a small proteinaceous infectious particle that is resistant to inactivation by most procedures that modify nucleic acids.

PrP is a host-specified protein that is encoded by a single exon that can be expressed in both normal and diseased animals. Brains of scrapie-infected animals contain two isomorphs of PrP, a scrapie form (PrP^{Sc}) and cellular form (PrP^{C}). The two proteins have different physical differences that appear to be due to posttranslational modification. After proteolysis, PrP^{Sc} loses an amino-terminal peptide to become PrP 27-30. Homogenates of tissue culture cells expressing the cloned PrP gene fail to induce clinical signs of scrapie when inoculated into susceptible mice. PrPs have been recovered from the brains of patients with CJD and GSS disease and have been named PrP^{CJD} and PrP^{GSS}, respectively.

SUBACUTE SCLEROSING PANENCEPHALITIS (SSPE) This progressive and ultimately fatal disease of children and adolescents had been suspected to be of viral origin since its initial description as inclusion body encephalitis. Measles virus or a virus very closely related to measles virus has been recovered from the brains of patients with the disease. The disorder may be considered to be a slow form of measles encephalitis (see Chap. 141).

SSPE occurs in patients between the ages of 4 and 20; 80 percent are under 11. The disease affects boys 3 to 10 times as frequently as girls. Mean annual incidence rates have fallen rapidly in the last two decades; the drop in incidence roughly parallels the decline in the number of measles cases diagnosed since the introduction of live attenuated measles vaccine. Most patients are from rural areas or small towns. Characteristically, they are entirely well until the disease begins. The onset of usually insidious mental deterioration, often expressed by a decline in the patient's schoolwork, is the presenting symptom. Incoordination, ataxia, and myoclonic jerks develop within a few months along with abnormalities of the pyramidal and extrapyramidal motor systems. Cortical blindness, papilledema, and optic atrophy may be present; focal chorioretinitis has been described. A few cases have occurred in association with infectious mononucleosis.

The patient becomes bedridden within 6 to 9 months. Death results from superimposed pulmonary or urinary tract infections or from decubiti. Signs of meningeal irritation are absent. The differential diagnosis includes cerebral storage diseases, nonstorage poliodystrophies, leukodystrophies, and demyelinating diseases of childhood.

The CSF gamma-globulin level, as determined by electrophoresis, quantitative immunochemical assay, or colloidal gold curve, is elevated, but the fluid is otherwise normal. The EEG typically shows a "burst suppression" pattern characterized by synchronous and symmetrical spike and high-voltage slow wave activity followed by electrical inactivity. Elevated levels of measles antibody are found in the serum and CSF. CT scan abnormalities correlate with the stage and duration of the disease. They include lateral ventricular dilatation, cortical atrophy, low parenchymal attenuation, and brainstem and cerebellar atrophy.

Pathologic findings include lymphocyte and mononuclear infiltrations about small cerebral arteries and veins, intranuclear and intracytoplasmic inclusions in neurons and glial cells, and varying degrees of destruction of medullated nerve fibers. The lesions occur in the cerebral gray and white matter, brainstem, and cerebellum.

Measles virus is the etiologic agent. Electron-microscopic studies show that the intranuclear inclusions in brain cells are composed of hollow tubular filaments resembling the internal nucleocapsid component of a paramyxovirus. Staining of brain tissue from patients with the disease demonstrates measles virus antigen in the inclusions. An agent serologically identical with measles virus and having the properties of measles virus has been recovered from brain by cocultivating cell cultures originating from brain tissue with established laboratory cell lines.

Attempts to transmit the disease to animals have met with variable results. Ferrets inoculated with suspensions of brain from patients with the disease develop a nonfatal neurologic disorder with EEG changes.

There is evidence that SSPE patients have clinical measles at an unusually early age, but SSPE appears many years after the patient's initial rubeola infection. A few reported cases may have been related to measles vaccination. The risk of SSPE following measles vaccination is far less, however, than the risk of encephalitis or SSPE following natural measles.

SSPE patients lack antibody to one of the measles virus proteins (the M or matrix protein) despite high titers of antibodies to the other viral proteins. Extracts of SSPE-infected brain lack significant quantities of M antigen. The M protein is a nonglycosylated protein localized to the inner surface of the viral membrane; it is important in the assembly of the virus particle at the cell surface. SSPE brain cells do not appear capable of synthesizing the M protein even in normal amounts. The molecular reasons for the absence of M polypeptide in terminal SSPE may involve decreased transcription and translation of M messenger RNA.

Isoprinosine has been reported by some to affect the course of the disease favorably in an open therapeutic trial, but there is controversy about its effectiveness. The drug has not been approved by the Food and Drug Administration. Other forms of treatment (including interferon and plasmapheresis) have been ineffective.

PROGRESSIVE MULTIFOCAL LEUKOENCEPHALOPATHY (PML) This rare neurologic condition usually occurs in patients who have leukemia, malignant lymphoma, carcinomatosis, acquired immunodeficiency syndrome (AIDS), or a variety of other chronic disease processes, or who are involved with immunosuppressive therapy. The disease is consistently associated with disorders of cell-mediated immunity with which deficits in humoral antibody response may or may not coexist.

The disease affects adults of both sexes, and its duration from onset of symptoms to death is 1 to 6 or more months. The neurologic signs and symptoms reflect a diffuse, asymmetric involvement of the cerebral hemispheres. Hemiplegia, hemianopsia, aphasia or dysarthria, and organic mental changes are frequent; visual field abnormalities and complete or incomplete transverse myelitis may develop. Headache and convulsive seizures are rare, but EEG abnormalities consisting of diffuse or focal abnormalities are often present. Lesions in the white matter may be recognized on CT scans. MRI is helpful in demonstrating white matter destruction. CSF is normal. Specific diagnosis can be made by brain biopsy.

The pathologic changes consist of multiple areas of demyelination with little or no perivascular infiltration and abnormal mitotic figures in astrocytes. The presence of distinctive intranuclear inclusions in oligodendrocytes first suggested that the disease was of a viral etiology. Electron-microscopic observations show the intranuclear inclusion bodies to be composed of closely packed spheres, which have the physical dimensions and properties of the polyomavirus genus of the papovaviruses.

By employing tissue cultures derived from human fetal brain, it has been possible to recover a new human polyomavirus serotype (JC virus) from the brains of PML patients. Abundant virus particles are present in brain. Rapid identification of the virus in brain is possible using fluorescent antibody staining or electron-microscopic agglutination with monospecific hyperimmune rabbit serum. Serologic diagnosis using the patient's serum is unreliable. The virus has not been demonstrated in tissues other than brain; the disease has not been transmitted to animals. There are isolated reports of clinical remission with cytarabine hydrochloride, but no cures. Death usually occurs within 6 months of onset.

PML may result from the activation of a polyomavirus which has been latent in brain or other tissues since childhood infection. Alternatively, there may be certain individuals who fail to acquire immunity in childhood and have their first encounter with the virus when a disease that interferes with cell-mediated immunity develops.

PROGRESSIVE RUBELLA ENCEPHALITIS A chronic progressive encephalitis developing in boys with the typical stigmata of the congenital rubella syndrome (Chap. 142) and sharing some of the features of SSPE was first described in 1974. Fewer than 20 patients have been reported.

The illness begins in the second decade and is characterized by dementia, cerebellar ataxia, spasticity, and seizures. The CSF has an increased cell count, and the protein and IgG levels are elevated. High titers of antibody to rubella virus can be detected in both the serum and CSF. Rubella virus has been recovered from the brain by use of the cocultivation technique.

Unlike SSPE, patients with rubella panencephalitis have the stigmata of congenital rubella before the onset of progressive disease. Myoclonus is less constant, and the EEG does not show the burst suppression observed in SSPE. Histologic examination of the brain shows mineralization of old lesions and an inflammatory reaction, but not the inclusion bodies characteristically found in SSPE.

The clinical picture of progressive rubella encephalitis also resembles the rare case of juvenile paresis that may occur in patients with congenital syphilis. The immune status of patients with rubella encephalitis has not been fully defined, and the pathogenesis of the disease remains obscure.

TROPICAL SPASTIC PARAPARESIS (TSP) This slowly progressive disorder of the spinal cord has been described in patients living in circumscribed regions located in equatorial latitudes. It appears to be caused by infection with the human retrovirus, HTLV-I, an agent that is transmitted by sexual contact, from mother to fetus, by intravenous drug abuse, and by blood transfusion. HTLV-I virus is also the etiologic agent of adult T-cell leukemia. Foci of the disease have been encountered in the Caribbean, South India, South Africa, the Seychelles, and Colombia. A similar disease known as HTLV-I–associated myelopathy (HAM) has been reported in Japanese patients. The disease affects about 10 to 100 persons per 100,000 in a tropical HTLV-I endemic area. TSP afflicts both men and women in their middle age. The disease is slow in onset, chronically progressive, and characterized by a spastic weakness of both legs with pyramidal tract signs as well as bilateral symmetric loss of vibratory sensation distally in the feet. Achilles tendon reflexes are absent in about one-fourth of patients. There is no pleocytosis in the CSF, but the protein content is increased. Increased levels of CSF gamma globulin and oligoclonal bands are often detected.

Pathologic changes are observed in the lateral and anterior columns of the spinal cord where there is loss of myelin and axons. Perivascular and parenchymal infiltration with lymphocytes and macrophages, as well as astrocytosis, are found in the white and gray matter of the spinal cord. Lymphocytes also infiltrate the spinal cord's blood vessels and subarachnoid space.

Antibodies to HTLV-I have been demonstrated in sera and CSF from patients with TSP and HAM. Cultured peripheral blood lymphocytes from TSP patients form multinucleated giant cells and react with sera and monoclonal antibodies to HTLV-I. An HTLV-I-like virus has been isolated from T-cell lines derived from peripheral blood and CSF of TSP patients

PERSISTENT VIRAL DISEASE IN IMMUNODEFICIENT PATIENTS Persistent or chronic neurologic infections of the nervous system may occur in immunodeficient patients. The immunodeficiency state may be congenital (primary) or acquired. Enteroviruses may be recovered from the CSF of patients with primary agammaglobulinemia over a period of many years, during which time there is a persistent CSF pleocytosis. A chronic or subacute encephalitis has also been described in children with congenital hypogammaglobulinemia. A specific virus has not been associated with this disorder.

NEUROLOGIC CONDITIONS RELATED TO INFECTION WITH HUMAN IMMUNODEFICIENCY VIRUS (HIV-1) Involvement of the nervous system by HIV-1 produces complex clinical findings resulting from a primary neurotropic disorder as well as the immunologic compromise that permits other viruses to replicate in and damage nerve tissue.

The immunocompromised patient with AIDS is susceptible to a variety of infectious agents that can attack the CNS. The most common viral agents that assert themselves belong to the HSV and papovavirus groups, i.e., viruses that may remain latent until there is dysfunction of normal immunologic processes. The most commonly isolated viruses from these groups include HSV, CMV, and the PML agent (JC virus). Infection with these viruses in the patient with AIDS can produce a variety of neurologic conditions—most notably atypical aseptic meningitis, acute or subacute encephalitis, PML, and viral myelitis. In addition to viral encephalitis and PML, the patient with AIDS may also develop toxoplasma brain abscess and primary CNS lymphomas. Differentiation from PML is often difficult solely on the basis of CT, MRI, and other laboratory tests. Because treatment for these conditions varies, it may be necessary to perform a brain biopsy and obtain a specimen of the cerebral lesion to make the correct diagnosis.

Neurologic disease may be the only clinical manifestation of HIV infection. It can be expressed as subacute dementia, aseptic meningitis, peripheral neuropathy, or vacuolar myelopathy. Subacute encephalitis is the most frequent cause of neurologic abnormality in AIDS patients. Because of the terminal nature of overt CNS infection in patients with AIDS, brain biopsy is usually reserved for patients who have failed empiric treatment for toxoplasmosis and in whom the possibility of reversible disease exists.

There is evidence that HIV-1 replicates in brain, probably in macrophages. HIV-1 has been recovered from CSF, brain, spinal cord, and sural nerve, suggesting that the AIDS dementia, myelopathy, and peripheral neuropathy may be caused by infection with the retrovirus.

AIDS dementia is insidious in onset and progresses gradually. The early manifestations include an inability to recall, loss of capacity to concentrate, and difficulty in performing complex sequential tasks. There is slowing of verbal and motor responses; spontaneity and animation are reduced. The condition may be difficult to differentiate from depression. As the disease advances, there may be gait unsteadiness, leg weakness, impaired handwriting, and tremor. In the advanced stage, there is global cognitive impairment and pronounced psychomotor slowing. Initially, CT and MRI scans appear normal. As the disease progresses, cortical atrophy and enlargement of the ventricles may become prominent. The MRI scan may disclose only atrophy, but hyperintense abnormalities may be visualized in the central white matter of some patients with AIDS-associated dementia. The CSF may contain mononuclear cells and have mildly elevated protein content.

The brains of patients with AIDS demonstrate moderate to marked cerebral atrophy and histologic changes involving the white matter and subcortical structures; the cortical gray matter is largely spared. The microscopic findings include multifocal perivascular rarefaction and focal vacuolation of the white matter with perivascular and parenchymal collections of macrophages and multinucleated giant cells. Neuronal loss is present only in the most severe cases.

Clinical trials, some still in progress, suggest that zidovudine (formerly AZT) improves functional status in some patients with AIDS dementia.

KURU Kuru, or "trembling with fear," is a progressive and fatal neurologic disorder that occurs exclusively among natives of the New Guinea highland. The disease is rare and seems to be disappearing; its elucidation represented a major hallmark in microbiology.

Difficulty in walking is usually the first sign of kuru. This usually progresses from a minor disturbance in gait to marked ataxia with lurching and staggering. Eventually, ambulation becomes so incoordinated that patients are unable to walk independently or to use their limbs because of intention tremor. Patients display an inability to perform rapid alternating movements, hypotonia, and abnormal involuntary movements which take the form of myoclonus, athetosis, or chorea. Slurring of speech and convergent strabismus appear as the disease progresses. There are no abnormalities in the blood or CSF. Dementia develops in the later phases of the disease. The illness terminates fatally in 4 to 24 months, usually from decubitus ulcers or bronchopneumonia. Kuru was common in male and female children and in adult women, but rare in adult men. The incubation period may be longer than 20 years in older patients.

Pathologic changes are limited to the CNS and include widespread neuronal loss, intense astrocytosis and microglial proliferation, loss of myelinated fibers, and the presence of plaquelike bodies. Perivascular cuffing by lymphocytes and mononuclear cells is rarely present.

It was the close similarity between the neuropathologic and clinical findings found in kuru and in scrapie that suggested the possibility that kuru might be caused by a virus or some closely related infectious agent. The infectious origin of kuru was confirmed subsequently by the transfer of a kurulike syndrome in chimpanzees 10 to 82 months after intracerebral inoculation of suspensions of brain from human cases. Disease has also been produced in chimpanzees by inoculation of tissues other than brain. The clinical illness in chimpanzees appears 3 to 11 months after inoculation. The disease has also been successfully transmitted to a number of new world and old world monkeys as well as to other animals. The specific agent responsible for the disease has not been fully characterized.

Cannibalism is the probable mode of transmission of kuru. Native custom in New Guinea dictated that bone marrow, viscera, and brain be cooked and eaten. The agent may be introduced by conjunctival, nasal, or skin contamination during the practice of ritual cannibalism. The marked predilection of kuru for the adult female may be explained by the observation that cannibalism appears more prevalent among women and that males who practice cannibalism seldom eat the bodies of women. The recent influx of foreign settlers into the kuru area has led to increasing rejection of cannibalistic practices and this in turn may be responsible for the progressive decline in the number of cases of kuru since 1960.

CREUTZFELDT-JAKOB DISEASE (CJD) CJD is an invariably fatal degenerative disease of the CNS that usually afflicts persons between the ages of 50 to 75 years and presents as a rapidly evolving dementia with myoclonus. Unlike kuru, the disease is not geographically limited and has been reported from over 50 countries around the world. The annual incidence is about one case per million inhabitants in metropolitan areas. The majority of cases occur between the ages of 50 and 75, but patients as young as 16 and as old as 80 have been reported.

Although CJD may have diverse clinical presentations, it usually begins with gradually progressive mental deterioration in the form of memory loss, mood changes, and errors in judgment. Disturbances of stance, gait, motor control, visual disturbances, and dizziness and vertigo may be prominent in the early stages of the disease. Some patients complain of headache. The patient may experience distortions in the shape and appearance of objects. Higher cortical function deficits, such as aphasia or apraxia, may occur. Hallucinations, delusional ideas, and confusion may appear as the disease progresses. In certain patients, cerebellar signs and visual abnormalities may predominate and may be confused initially with cerebrovascular insufficiency. As the condition worsens, the patient becomes mute, stuporous, spastic, and rigid. Myoclonic jerks and other abnormal movements become more prominent as the disease progresses. Visual deterioration may advance to cortical blindness. Disturbances of oculomotor control and of the autonomic nervous system have been noted.

The disease progresses rapidly. The majority of patients die within 6 months, most often 2 to 3 months after the onset of their disease. About 5 to 10 percent of cases will have an illness lasting 2 years or more.

Only rarely has a second member of a family been affected. Fifteen percent of CJD patients have a family history of the disease consistent with an autosomal dominant transmission; the onset of the illness in familial cases is earlier than in sporadic cases. A family history of presenile dementia can be obtained in about 10 percent of CJD patients.

The EEG is often helpful in making the correct diagnosis. During the early stages, it may only show mild, excessive generalized slowing more marked over one hemisphere or even focal. As the disease progresses, distinctive repetitive sharp waves with a characteristic interval of 0.5 to 1.0 s are seen. The sharp waves may first be unilateral, resembling periodic lateralized epileptiform discharges (PLEDS), but eventually they become bilateral and synchronous. In the final stages of the disease, all background EEG activity becomes progressively slower and of lower amplitude, sometimes with the persistence of periodic complexes. Repetitive sharp waves are also occasionally seen in the EEGs of patients with dementia due to other illnesses such as Alzheimer's disease or Binswanger's subcortical encephalopathy, but not with the regular rate found in CJD patients. Serial EEG tracings are helpful in questionable cases.

A CT scan of the brain is usually normal, but sulcal widening, ventricular enlargement, and moderate cortical atrophy may be visualized. Rapid progressive atrophic changes on serial CT scans may suggest the diagnosis. MRI scanning may demonstrate bilateral cortical atrophy without apparent white matter changes. Positron emission tomography (PET) has demonstrated temporal lobe hypometabolism with hemispheric asymmetry. The CSF is usually normal except for a slight elevation in the protein content. No immunologic response, either humoral or cellular, to the CJD agent has been demonstrated in the blood.

The cerebrum and cerebellum are affected predominantly. The brain may show cerebral atrophy. Microscopic examination demonstrates widespread status spongiosus, nerve cell loss, and intensive gliosis. Vacuoles are located within the neuropil, i.e., within axons, dendrites, and glial fibers. There is no inflammatory reaction.

Electron-microscopic observations in CJD have disclosed membrane fragments in vacuoles. Abnormal fibrils similar in appearance to the scrapie-associated fibrils (SAF) have been observed in CJD brain fractions. The exact composition of these fibrils is unclear. CJD brains have been shown to contain protease-resistant proteins (PrP^{CJD}) with molecular weights ranging from 10,000 to 50,000. These CJD proteins reacted with antibodies raised against the scrapie PrP 27-30. Immunologic identification by western blots provides a diagnostic adjunct to neuropathologic examination and animal transmission experiments. Protein polymers in CJD brain aggregate to form plaques with the staining properties of amyloid; these amyloid collections can be stained by antiserum to hamster scrapie PrP 27-30. The SAF and PrPs present in CJD brain resemble those observed in other naturally occurring and experimentally induced spongiform encephalopathies of humans and other animals. It is uncertain if they represent a form of the infectious agent or modified pathologic products.

Sixty percent of patients with kuru and CJD demonstrate an autoimmune antibody directed against 10-nm neurofilaments. The antibody usually appears late in the disease. It can occasionally be found in normal subjects. The significance of this antibody is unclear.

CJD may be mistaken for Alzheimer's disease with myoclonus. In this situation, the presence of cerebellar signs provides strong evidence against the possibility of Alzheimer's disease. At times, CJD can be confused with multi-infarct dementia, alcoholic or nutritional deficiency syndromes, or primary brain tumors. The hallmarks of the disorder (mental deterioration, multisystem neurologic signs, myoclonus, and typical EEG changes) evolving over a period of months in a middle-aged patient usually secures the diagnosis.

The CJD agent has been found in lymph nodes, liver, kidney, spleen, lung, cornea, and CSF of patients with the disorder. The way the disease is acquired naturally is unknown. Incubation periods as long as 20 years may occur in natural transmission. The higher incidence of CJD among Israelis of Libyan origin who eat sheep's eyeballs has led to speculation that the disease may be naturally transmitted by the ingestion of scrapie-infected meat. There is an unexpectedly high incidence of previous brain or eye operations among CJD patients. Human-to-human transmission has occurred by corneal transplantation, by the implantation of contaminated stereotactic electroencephalographic electrodes, by cadaveric dura mater graft, and by the parenteral administration of growth hormone prepared from cadaveric human pituitary glands. Transmission of CJD has not been linked to blood transfusion.

There is no evidence of an increased risk among spouses, friends, and medical or nursing personnel caring for CJD patients. The patient's CSF and blood should be considered, however, as potential sources of infection. Precautions should be taken to avoid autoinoculation with needles, scalpels, or other instruments that have been contaminated by the patient's tissues. Maximum care should be taken to avoid accidental percutaneous exposure to blood, CSF, or tissue. Contaminated skin can be disinfected by a 5- to 10-min exposure to 1 *N* sodium hydroxide followed by extensive washing with water. Contaminated material should be steam-autoclaved for 1 h at a temperature of at least 132°C or immersed for 1 h in 1 *N* sodium hydroxide or a 10% sodium hypochlorite solution. More detailed guidelines for the handling of materials from patients with these disorders have been developed by the Centers for Disease Control. These should be applied to all patients who have evidence of rapid intellectual deterioration, particularly when it is associated with myoclonus.

There is no effective treatment for CJD. Claims that amantadine hydrochloride is effective have not been substantiated.

GERSTMANN-STRÄUSSLER-SCHEINKER (GSS) DISEASE GSS disease is an inherited autosomal dominant illness characterized by spinocerebellar ataxia with dementia and plaquelike deposits of amyloid in the brain. Inoculation of brain tissue from GSS disease produces spongiform encephalopathy in nonhuman primates. PrP and PrP-immunoreactive amyloid plaques accumulate in the brains of these patients. The putative gene for the syndrome is linked to the PrP gene, codon 102, on the short arm of chromosome 20. A substitution of leucine for proline at this codon may lead to the development of the GSS disease. The usual onset of the disease is in the fifth decade. GSS disease follows a lengthy course, usually on the order of 2 to 10 years. Ataxia is prominent in the early phase of the illness; dementia follows later. The patient's symptoms and signs are reminiscent of olivopontocerebellar atrophy. Pathologic changes include spinocerebellar and corticospinal tract degeneration, extensive amyloid deposits, and spongiform degeneration. Like other human spongiform encephalopathies, there is no effective treatment for GSS disease.

There have been isolated reports that brain tissues for a restricted number of patients with familial Alzheimer's disease induced neurologic disease and spongiform changes in chimpanzees. Numerous other transmission attempts from patients with both familial and nonfamilial Alzheimer's disease have been negative. At present, there is no direct evidence to indicate that Alzheimer's disease is caused by a slow virus.

REFERENCES

Berger JR et al: Progressive multifocal leukoencephalopathy associated with human immunodeficiency virus infection. A review of the literature with a report of sixteen cases. Ann Intern Med 107:78, 1987

Bockman JM et al: Creutzfeldt-Jakob disease prion proteins in human brains. N Engl J Med 312:73, 1985

Brown P: Acute viral encephalitis, in *Current Diagnosis* 7, RB Conn (ed). Philadelphia, Saunders, 1985, p 918

——— et al: The epidemiology of Creutzfeldt-Jakob disease: Conclusion of a 15-year investigation in France and review of the world literature. Neurology 37:895, 1987

Dyken PR: Subacute sclerosing panencephalitis. Current status. Neurol Clin 3:179, 1985

Gabuzda DH, Hirsch MS: Neurologic manifestations of infection with human immunodeficiency virus: Clinical features and pathogenesis. Ann Intern Med 107:383, 1987

Gajdusek DC: Unconventional viruses and the origin and disappearance of kuru. Science 197:943, 1977

Griffith JF, Ch'ien LT: Herpes simplex virus encephalitis. Diagnostic and treatment considerations. Med Clin North Am 67:991, 1983

Ho DD, Hirsch MS: Acute viral encephalitis. Med Clin North Am 69:415, 1985

Hudson AJ et al: Gerstmann-Sträussler-Scheinker disease with coincidental familiar onset. Ann Neurol 14:670, 1983

Johnson RT: The pathogenesis of acute viral encephalitis and postinfectious encephalomyelitis. J Infect Dis 155:359, 1987

Prusiner SB: Scrapie prions. Ann Rev Microbiol 43:345, 1989

Ratzan KR: Viral meningitis. Med Clin North Am 69:399, 1985

Roman GC, Roman LN: Tropical spastic paraparesis. A clinical study of 50 patients from Tumaco (Colombia) and review of the worldwide features of the syndrome. J Neurol Sci 87:121, 1988

Rosenberg RN et al: Precautions in handling tissues, fluids, and other contaminated materials from patients with documented or suspected Creutzfeldt-Jakob disease. Ann Neurol 19:75, 1986

Walker DL: Progressive multifocal leukoencephalopathy, in *Handbook of Clinical Neurology*, JC Koetsier (ed). Amsterdam, Elsevier Science Publishers 1985, vol 3(47), p 503

Weil ML et al: Chronic progressive panencephalitis due to rubella virus simulating subacute sclerosing panencephalitis. N Engl J Med 292:994, 1975

Whitley RJ et al: Vidarabine versus acyclovir therapy in herpes simplex encephalitis. N Engl J Med 314:144, 1986

356 DEMYELINATING DISEASES

JACK P. ANTEL / BARRY G. W. ARNASON

The demyelinating diseases comprise a group of neurologic disorders important both because of the frequency with which they occur and the disability that they cause. Demyelinating diseases have in common the pathologic feature of focal or patchy destruction of myelin sheaths in the central nervous system accompanied by an inflammatory response. Some degree of axonal damage may occur as well, but demyelination always predominates. Multiple sclerosis is the most common of the demyelinating diseases. Its cause is not known. Current opinion holds that autoimmunity, perhaps induced by viral infection, is likely to be implicated in its pathogenesis. Acute disseminated encephalomyelitis and its hyperacute variant, acute hemorrhagic leukoencephalitis, are acute and monophasic immune-mediated demyelinating diseases. HTLV-I–associated myelopathy provides an example of a virus-initiated chronic demyelinating disease.

Myelin loss occurs in other conditions as well, but in these others an inflammatory response is lacking. Included are genetically determined defects in myelin metabolism, exposure to toxins such as carbon monoxide, and opportunistic viral infection of oligodendrocytes (e.g., progressive multifocal leukoencephalopathy) against a background of immune incompetence. These entities, which are usually not classified as demyelinating diseases, are discussed in Chaps. 355 and 359.

MULTIPLE SCLEROSIS

This disease usually presents in the form of recurrent attacks of focal or multifocal neurologic dysfunction, reflecting lesions within the central nervous system (CNS). Attacks occur, remit, and recur, seemingly randomly over many years. The disease begins most commonly in early adult life. The frequency of flare-ups is greatest during the first 3 to 4 years of disease, but a first attack, which may have been so mild as to escape medical attention and can barely be recalled, may not be followed by another attack for 10 to 20 years. During typical episodes, symptoms worsen over a period of a few days to 2 to 3 weeks and then remit. Recovery is usually rapid over a period of weeks, although at times it may extend over several months. The extent of recovery varies markedly between patients and from one attack to the next in the same person. Remission may be complete, particularly after early attacks; often, however, remission is incomplete and as one attack follows another, a stepwise downward progression ensues with increasing permanent deficit.

In perhaps as many as one-third of cases the disease declares itself as a slowly but inexorably progressive illness. This is particularly likely to be the case if onset is after age 40. Although occasional patients die within the first few years of disease onset, most do not, and the average survival from multiple sclerosis (MS) is better than 30 years after onset of disease.

Multiple sclerosis is pleomorphic in its presentations. The clinical picture is determined by the location of foci of demyelination within the CNS. Classic features include impaired vision, nystagmus, dysarthria, decreased perception of vibration and position sense, ataxia and intention tremor, weakness or paralysis of one or more limbs, spasticity, and bladder problems.

Criteria which must be satisfied to establish a diagnosis of clinically definite MS include a reliable history of at least two episodes of neurologic deficit and objective clinical signs of lesions at more than one site within the CNS. Demonstration of additional lesions by laboratory tests [e.g., evoked potentials, urologic studies, computed tomography, or, most sensitively, magnetic resonance imaging (MRI)], in concert with one objective clinical lesion, also fulfills the criteria. A finding of increased cerebrospinal fluid immunoglobulin with oligoclonal bands supports the diagnosis but will not substitute for the above criteria. Clinically probable MS is defined as either two attacks with clinical evidence of one lesion or one attack with clinical evidence of two lesions (or one clinical and one paraclinical lesion). Follow-up studies of probable MS patients indicate considerable diagnostic imprecision in this category. When signs pointing to damage of white matter tracts in optic nerves, brainstem, and spinal cord are present together and more than one attack is known to have occurred, a diagnosis of multiple sclerosis can be made with greater than 95 percent certainty. In the early years of the disease, when few relapses have occurred and fixed deficits are mild, the diagnosis may prove difficult, and single or multiple focal lesions due to other causes must be excluded.

PATHOLOGY Many scattered, discrete areas of demyelination, termed *plaques,* are the pathologic hallmark of multiple sclerosis. Macroscopically, plaques appear as gray-pink sharply defined areas which stand out against the surrounding white matter of the central nervous system. Lesions may extend into gray matter, although nerve cell bodies are seen to be preserved on microscopic examination. Plaques vary in size from a few millimeters to several centimeters; larger ones form by coalescence of smaller ones and by expansion of their margins. Plaques may be found anywhere in the white matter but typically occur in the paraventricular areas of the cerebrum and subpially, and within the brainstem and spinal cord. Their topography conforms to that of the venous drainage of the brain and spinal cord, and no particular anatomic structures are respected. The peripheral nervous system is not affected. The number of plaques found at autopsy invariably exceeds the number expected on the basis of physical signs. Many plaques, therefore, are clinically silent; this establishes that substantial impulse conduction occurs across regions of demyelination. In fact, autopsy studies indicate that 20 percent of multiple sclerosis cases are clinically silent during life.

The microscopic features of multiple sclerosis lesions depend on their age. Typically lesions of different ages and evidence of new activity about the margins of old lesions are encountered. Active multiple sclerosis lesions feature T-lymphocyte and monocyte-macrophage accumulations about venules and at plaque margins where myelin is being destroyed. The inflammatory cells that invade the white matter and the soluble mediators that they release (lymphokines and monokines) are held responsible for the myelin breakdown. Macrophages also function as scavengers of myelin debris; fat-laden macrophages may persist for months, perhaps for years, after the acute inflammatory response has subsided. Plasma cells accumulate within plaques and are usually found at or near their centers.

An astroglial response at or just beyond the margins of acutely demyelinating lesions is characteristic. In established, inactive plaques, a thick mat of fibrillary gliosis throughout the demyelinated regions is usual, and only a few residual perivascular macrophages are found. Oligodendrocyte number has been said to be normal or increased at the plaque margin. Yet, oligodendrocyte number is reduced within plaques, indicating that ultimately, this cell type is lost in multiple sclerosis. Indeed, damage to oligodendrocytes may be the primary event.

Only limited regeneration of myelin occurs in multiple sclerosis (shadow plaques). Absent remyelination, mechanisms responsible for recovery from an MS attack along segmentally demyelinated axons are likely multiple. Resolution of edema, as documented by MRI or CT scan, may permit return of saltatory conduction along segmentally demyelinated axons. Restoration of conduction may also relate, in part, to insertion of K^+ channels along the length of denuded axonal segments rather than exclusively at the nodes of Ranvier as is the situation in myelinated nerve.

Axons within plaques tend to be spared, although in acute lesions frank necrosis with loss of axons sometimes occurs. At least 10 percent of multiple sclerosis plaques show marked axonal loss, and ultrastructural studies indicate that loss of axons may be more general than can be appreciated by routine histology. All gradations of pathologic change between the extremes described above are encountered.

The pathologic features of MS fail to account for the hour-to-hour and day-to-day waxings and wanings in function so characteristic of the disease. Conduction of impulses through demyelinated nerve is compromised and is further altered by transient changes in the internal milieu such as alterations in temperature and in electrolyte balance or by stress. Fever, or even minor increases in body temperature, such as may follow a hot bath or exercise, may cause a failure of conduction through demyelinated regions and lead to evanescent symptoms and signs. The mechanism of this axonal fatigability is unknown, but some type of conduction block is assumed to occur. It is important to distinguish transient fluctuations in symptomatology of the type just described from attacks of disease.

ETIOLOGY The cause or causes of MS remain unknown. A role for immune-mediated or infectious factors has been proposed, but data to support these postulates are fragmentary and indirect. Isolation of HTLV-I–related viral components from CNS tissue in patients with MS is reported, but the etiologic significance of these findings remains uncertain (see Waksman).

Epidemiology Epidemiologic studies have established several facts which will ultimately have to be incorporated into any coherent theory of the disease. Average age of onset of the first clinical episode of MS falls within the third and fourth decades. Females account for 60 percent of cases. For disease to begin in childhood or beyond the sixth decade is uncommon but not unknown.

In general, incidence in temperate climatic zones exceeds that in tropical zones; but variations within regions with similar climates do exist; hence the effect is not simply one of latitude or temperature. The incidence of MS in northern Europe, Canada, and the northern United States is approximately 10 new cases each year per 100,000 persons between the ages of 20 and 50. The incidence in Australia, New Zealand, and the southern United States is one-third to one-half of that; in Japan, elsewhere in the Orient, and in Africa MS is rare. Some epidemiologic evidence also suggests that persons migrating from high- to low-risk regions as children may be partially protected from MS. The data are consistent with the existence of an environmental factor, possibly a virus, and perhaps geographically restricted, that influences development of MS.

Genetic factors The incidence of MS among American Indians and blacks is lower than that among whites living in the same regions. This suggests that genetic factors also influence disease susceptibility. Blood relatives of MS patients (children, siblings) have an at least fifteenfold increased risk of developing MS. This could reflect an interplay of several genetic factors, shared exposure to an environmental factor, or a combination of the two. Concordance for MS between identical twins (25 percent) is markedly greater than for fraternal twins (2 to 3 percent). Family studies have failed to reveal any predictable genetic pattern but do argue persuasively for a genetically determined predisposition to disease.

Certain histocompatibility antigens (HLA) are overrepresented in patients with MS. Among whites with the disease the HLA-B7, -DR2, and -DQW1 alleles occur with increased frequency. Most illnesses with which an HLA association has been shown are autoimmune or infectious in nature, a finding in keeping with current thought about the etiology of MS. Many American blacks with MS express the DW2 allele; this allele is rare in blacks in Africa, among whom MS is virtually unknown. It follows that an HLA-linked genetic factor which predisposes to MS exists, but inasmuch as the vast majority of persons bearing DR2 or DQW1 do not develop the disease, additional genetic or environmental factors must play a role. Paradoxically, siblings concordant for MS have concordance rates for HLA haplotypes little above those expected by chance. The HLA-B12 allele is less frequent in MS than in the population at large. This finding suggests that genetically determined protective factors may operate in MS.

Autoimmune factors The lesions of MS are mimicked by those of experimental allergic encephalomyelitis (EAE), an autoimmune disease induced in animals by immunization with myelin. Lesions of EAE are demyelinating, perivenular, plaque-like, occur in chronic and recrudescent forms, and have an inflammatory infiltrate composed of lymphocytes, macrophages, and plasma cells. T lymphocytes sensitized to specific myelin antigens (myelin basic protein or proteolipid protein) can adoptively transfer the disease. In MS, sensitivity to these myelin antigens cannot be demonstrated. Chronic demyelination can be a consequence of viral infection in animals. Demyelination follows infection of mice with Theiler's murine encephalomyelitis virus; infected animals do not exhibit sensitivity to myelin antigens. Attempts to find any antigen to which only MS patients react have failed.

Attacks of MS are associated with changes in peripheral blood monocyte and lymphocyte properties. Reported changes include heightened prostaglandin secretion by macrophages (which may in turn influence lymphocyte properties), reduced suppressor cell function, an increased number of activated T cells as evidenced by their expression of certain surface antigens, heightened T-cell–dependent in vitro immunoglobulin secretion, deficient interferon secretion, and possibly reduced natural killer (NK) cell function. Whether these changes relate to the etiology of MS is not known.

Within the cerebrospinal fluid (CSF), T-cell activation is apparent during active disease. Excessive IgG production within the CNS is characteristic of MS at all stages of disease; whether this reflects the presence of some stimulator of B cells in the brain in MS or is the result of a defect in immune regulation is not known. Viral infection of brain remains a possible cause of MS, despite the fact that all attempts to isolate, rescue, or "passage" a virus from MS brains or to visualize a virus within them have failed.

Precipitating factors Most attacks of MS occur without any evident antecedent. There is a modestly increased risk for an attack following viral infections. Injury and even emotional upsets have been claimed to precipitate attacks of MS; evidence in support of these claims remains anecdotal and nonpersuasive. The probability that an attack of MS will occur during the first 6 months after pregnancy is greater than chance would predict, but this observation is counterbalanced by a decreased risk of an attack during the second and third trimesters of pregnancy. In established cases, trauma, including lumbar puncture, myelography, and surgery, has not been shown to relate to attacks or to progression of disability nor has emotional turmoil been shown to alter the tempo at which the disease evolves. Experience has also shown that vaccinations do not provoke attacks of MS.

CLINICAL MANIFESTATIONS The first attack of MS may declare itself as a single symptom or sign (45 percent) or as more than one (55 percent). Approximately 40 percent of MS patients will have an episode of optic neuritis, either as their first difficulty or at some point along the course of their disease. Optic neuritis presents as loss of vision, partial or total, usually in one eye, seldom in both, and is often associated with pain on movement of the eye. Macular vision tends to be most affected (central scotoma), but a wide range of field defects may occur. Disturbances of color perception sometimes provide an early indication of mild disease. Fewer than half of optic neuritis patients will show evidence of an inflamed optic nerve head (papillitis); most show no changes in the optic disc at the outset, indicating that the demyelinating lesion is developing some distance behind the nerve head (retrobulbar neuritis). Both forms of optic neuritis will be followed by optic nerve atrophy, detected as pallor of the optic disc.

It is important to recognize that cases of optic neuritis occur as an isolated event. Nonetheless, 35 percent of men and 75 percent of women with optic neuritis go on to develop MS in the ensuing 15 years. Unfortunately, it is difficult to predict who will and who will not develop the disease, although presence of oligoclonal bands in the CSF and of multifocal cerebral lesions on MRI scanning are seemingly unfavorable findings. Whether optic neuritis occurring alone and for unknown reasons constitutes a *forme fruste* of MS with but a single attack is not known. Approximately one-third of patients with optic neuritis recover completely, one-third partially, and one-third little or not at all. Visual evoked response testing reveals prolonged latencies of the evoked potentials in more than 80 percent of established cases of MS; less than half of these can describe an antecedent optic neuritis. Clearly subclinical involvement of the optic pathways is common.

Symptoms and signs of neurologic dysfunction arising from brainstem, cerebellar, and spinal cord lesions are frequent in MS. Diplopia may occur either because the third, fourth, or sixth cranial nerve pathways are damaged along their course within the CNS or because an internuclear ophthalmoplegia (INO) has developed (see Chap. 23). An INO reflects involvement of the medial longitudinal fasciculus. The sign consists of an inability to adduct one eye on attempted lateral gaze together with full abduction of the other eye, which shows horizontal nystagmus. Bilateral INO in a young adult is virtually diagnostic of MS, although a few instances of bilateral INO in systemic lupus erythematosus are on record. Another clinical feature of brainstem involvement is either facial hypesthesia or tic douloureux (fifth cranial nerve). When tic douloureux occurs in a young adult, the possibility of underlying MS should be seriously entertained. Bell's palsy or hemifacial spasm (seventh cranial nerve), vertigo, vomiting, and nystagmus (vestibular connections of the eighth cranial nerve) are also frequent; less commonly there is complaint of deafness. Involvement of cerebellar connections results in ataxia which can affect speech (scanning), head or trunk (titubation), limbs (intention tremor), and stance and gait. Cerebellar ataxia may be combined with sensory ataxia due to involvement of the spinal cord.

Spinal cord lesions produce a myriad of motor and sensory problems. Corticospinal tract interruption results in the classical features of upper motor neuron dysfunction (weakness, spasticity, hyperreflexia, clonus, Babinski response, loss of abdominal skin reflexes). Posterior column lesions cause loss, or diminution, of joint-position and vibration senses as well as the frequently encountered complaints of tingling or tightness of the extremities and of bandlike sensations about the trunk. Less often pain and temperature sensations are lost or diminished, reflecting spinothalamic tract involvement. Partial lesions of sensory tracts or of the root entry zones of sensory nerves can produce painful dysesthesias as well as interruption of reflex arcs. On occasion, spinal cord lesions will result in paroxysmal symptoms including tonic spasms which can be painful.

Symptoms of bladder dysfunction, including hesitancy, urgency, frequency, and incontinence, are common features of spinal cord involvement. Equally common is bowel dysfunction, particularly constipation. Males with MS, if questioned, often complain of sexual impotence; methods exist to distinguish physical from psychogenic causes. Patients with MS may experience an electric shock-like sensation on flexion of the neck, called Lhermitte's sign.

Severe spinal cord lesions can result in loss of function, sometimes total, below the level of the lesion; less complete lesions can result in the hemicord syndrome of Brown-Séquard (see Chap. 361). When either of these events occurs, it is referred to as a transverse myelitis. A single episode of transverse myelitis not followed by subsequent progression of disease may, as with an isolated episode of optic neuritis, represent a *forme fruste* of MS, although less than 10 percent of acute transverse myelitis cases develop MS. Again as with optic neuritis, approximately one-third of patients with transverse myelitis recover completely, one-third partially, and one-third not at all. Spinal cord involvement is the predominating feature in most advanced cases of MS.

Cerebral symptoms may occur in MS due to extensive involvement of subcortical and central white matter. With extensive lesions of brain, intellect may suffer, sometimes disastrously. By far the most frequent emotional feature of MS is depression. Euphoria, when it occurs, indicates widespread cerebral disease and is often associated with dementia and pseudobulbar palsy. Three to five percent of patients (twice the expected rate) will have one or more epileptic seizures, presumably because of extension of plaques into gray matter. Focal neurologic signs of cerebral origin, such as hemiparesis, homonymous hemianopsia, and dysphasia, while seen in MS, are rare.

Neuromyelitis optica and MS An ill-defined symptom complex known as Devic's syndrome, or neuromyelitis optica, is considered by some to be an entity distinguishable from MS. The complex is characterized by acute optic neuritis, usually bilateral, which is followed, or less frequently preceded, within hours to weeks by transverse myelitis. The cerebrospinal fluid (CSF) may show a pleocytosis with polymorphonuclear cells and a protein content that is higher than is usual for MS. Pathologic examination in fatal cases reveals more tissue destruction and cavitation than is expected in MS, although this may bespeak no more than the intensity of the process.

COURSE OF ILLNESS AND PROGNOSIS The clinical course of MS is unpredictable. In general, symptoms which appear acutely and those referable to sensory paths and the cranial nerves have a more favorable prognosis than those developing insidiously or involving motor and especially cerebellar function. According to McAlpine, 80 percent of patients who have a purely exacerbating and remitting disease have unrestricted function after 10 years. Of cases in which exacerbations and remissions are superimposed on a progressive tempo of evolution, 50 percent are disabled after 10 years. In cases that have a purely progressive course from the outset (in these the brunt of the disease usually falls on the spinal cord) long-term prognosis for ambulation is poor.

Rarely MS may be fulminant and fatal within weeks to months. Such cases, which are referred to as acute MS, show intense inflammatory responses within the plaques. Onset in such patients may be with headache, vomiting, delirium, convulsions, even coma, plus an array of signs indicating severe compromise of cortical, brainstem, optic nerve, and spinal cord function. Distinction from acute disseminated encephalomyelitis may be difficult in life; at autopsy the lesions are larger and more like those of MS.

DIFFERENTIAL DIAGNOSIS The diagnosis of MS becomes secure when signs referable to multiple lesions of CNS white matter have developed and remitted at different times. Particularly in the early phases of disease, the neurologic symptoms may suggest discrete dysfunction of the nervous system, and other causes of focal disease must be excluded. An excellent clinical rule is that MS should not be diagnosed when all the patient's symptoms and signs can be explained by a single lesion. A common aphorism is that MS presents with symptoms in one leg and signs in both.

Conditions to be excluded vary depending on the sites of the lesions. Abrupt monocular loss of vision may result from impaired vascular supply to the optic nerve, including embolic and thrombotic occlusion of the carotid, ophthalmic, or central retinal arteries, or as an accompaniment of migraine. When monocular visual loss is more gradual, compressive lesions affecting the optic nerve or an optic nerve glioma need to be considered.

In patients presenting with acute or progressive spinal cord disease, the presence of focal lesions affecting the cord and of degenerative-nutritional diseases which selectively affect spinal cord tracts should be considered (see Chaps. 357 and 361). Patients with progressive spastic paraplegia should be evaluated for the presence of intrathecal or extradural neoplasm, vascular malformations, and for cervical spondylosis. Such evaluation often requires a CT body scan, MRI, or myelography. Hereditary ataxias can present as degeneration of multiple CNS tracts, with or without involvement of the peripheral nervous system. Degeneration of posterior columns and corticospinal and spinocerebellar tracts is common in these disorders. Hereditary ataxias are slowly progressive and feature stereotyped symmetric involvement as well as a family history consistent with autosomal dominant, or recessive, inheritance. Amyotrophic lateral sclerosis (ALS) usually presents with prominent lower motor neuron signs (atrophy, weakness, and fasciculations) in addition to pyramidal signs (spasticity, hyperreflexia) and without sensory abnormalities. Subacute combined degeneration of the cord can be excluded by symmetry of spinal symptoms and by a normal serum vitamin B_{12} level, a normal bone marrow, and a normal Schilling test.

When progressive brainstem dysfunction occurs, posterior fossa tumor as well as brainstem encephalitis should be excluded. Single cranial nerve palsies, particularly Bell's palsy, trigeminal sensory neuropathy, or tic douloureux may occur as part of the MS picture, but evidence of multifocal disease must be present before they can be ascribed to MS. When vertigo is the complaint and nystagmus is detected, inner ear disease should be considered as well as the possibility that barbiturates or phenytoin have been taken.

There are several multifocal and recrudescent diseases of the central nervous system which may mimic MS. Systemic lupus erythematosus and other vasculitides may cause scattered and recurring lesions within brain, brainstem, and spinal cord, as can the mitochondrial encephalopathies (MELAS syndrome) (see Chap. 365). Behçet's disease is characterized by recurrent episodes of focal brain disease, CSF pleocytosis, oral and genital ulcers, and uveitis. Other disorders to be excluded include meningovascular syphilis, cryptococcosis, toxoplasmosis, other chronic nervous system infections, and sarcoidosis. Lyme disease can present with focal neurologic signs in the absence of antecedent skin lesions, arthralgias, or peripheral neuropathy (see Chap. 132). HTLV-I–induced disorders are described below. AIDS encephalopathy and myelopathy need also to be considered in progressive cases.

When complaints are vague and findings minimal, a diagnosis of conversion reaction (hysteria) may come to mind. This diagnosis should always be made on the basis of positive criteria for hysteria and never as a "diagnosis by exclusion." Early in its course, MS is mislabeled as hysteria with distressing frequency. Patients with MS may develop superimposed hysterical phenomena adding to the complexity of the clinical syndrome.

A few patients present with pain as their principal symptom. Awareness of its occurrence in MS and careful attention to a thorough examination will usually clarify the diagnosis.

A firm diagnosis of MS should only be made when the evidence is unequivocal. Aside from the distress that such a diagnosis causes, it will serve to explain almost any subsequent neurologic event and may divert attention away from other possibly treatable diseases.

LABORATORY TESTS Although the diagnosis of MS continues to depend on its clinical features, laboratory aids have become increasingly useful as supports for the diagnosis. In the vast majority of patients with MS, one or more tests will be abnormal, although normal results do not rule out the diagnosis.

The CSF in MS patients typically reveals only a slight or no increase in cell number. Ninety percent of patients show fewer than 10 cells per microliter in their CSF; cell counts greater than 50 are rare. The cells in the CSF are predominantly T lymphocytes, although rare plasma cells may be found. Some correlation exists between the extent of pleocytosis and disease activity. Higher cell counts also are more typical in early stages of disease. Evidence that the lymphocytes in the CSF are activated not only during exacerbations of disease but also during seeming remission has been presented; this indicates that disease activity smolders at all times, even though neither the physician nor the patient may be able to detect changes. T-cell lines specifically reactive with various viral and nonviral antigens can be derived from the CSF of MS patients, again suggesting that a heterogeneous immune response is ongoing (see discussion of oligoclonal bands below). The CSF of 90 percent of patients contains less than 60 mg/dL of total protein; protein of greater than 100 mg/dL should raise questions about whether the diagnosis is correct.

The most characteristic CSF finding in MS is an increase in immunoglobulin G (IgG) which contrasts with relatively normal total protein and albumin concentrations. IgG levels are increased in 80 percent of MS patients; the increase is greatest in long-standing cases with severe neurologic deficits. Early in the disease, when the diagnosis is most in doubt, IgG values can be normal. IgG levels do not change in any meaningful way with relapses and remissions. Most of the IgG in the CSF is synthesized within the central nervous system. The increased IgG fraction in the CSF explains the first-zone abnormality of the colloidal gold curve, a test of historical interest.

When the CSF IgG from MS patients is subjected to electrophoresis or isoelectric focusing, it fractionates into a restricted number of bands (termed oligoclonal bands). Oligoclonal banding of IgG has also been found in the CSF in a number of acute and chronic central nervous system infections; in subacute sclerosing panencephalitis cases, these bands have been shown to be antibodies to the infective agent. In MS, the IgG bands have not been shown to be directed against any single viral or intrinsic brain antigen; more likely they represent a heterogeneous group of antibodies directed against many antigens. The number of bands in the CSF is greater in those with longer disease duration. It has also been suggested that high levels of IgG and many oligoclonal bands are associated with a severe course. The overall IgG shows further restrictions in its heterogeneity, with the IgG1 being mainly of the $G1m_1$ allotype. Rare cases of MS without increased CSF IgG synthesis or oligoclonal bands have been documented at autopsy.

Within CSF, myelin debris as well as myelin basic protein fragments appear during attacks of disease. Myelin basic protein levels can be measured by radioimmunoassay; the level seems to reflect the extent of myelin breakdown since levels also increase in other disorders associated with white matter breakdown such as stroke.

Conduction of nerve impulses along axons denuded of their myelin is slowed. Evoked response testing provides a sensitive means to detect slowed conduction of visual, auditory, or somatosensory impulses. Such tests employ repetitive sensory stimuli and utilize computer averaging techniques to record the electric responses evoked during the conduction of these stimuli along visual, auditory, or somatosensory afferent pathways. In normal subjects, the pattern of the evoked responses and time for conduction are highly predictable. One or more of the evoked response tests will reveal slowing of conduction in 80 percent of MS patients; in 30 to 40 percent of patients, abnormal evoked responses are detected without any clinical symptoms or signs in the involved pathway being apparent. Evoked response testing may confirm the presence of additional sites of disease in suspected cases with only a single clinically detectable lesion (see Chap. 349).

Computed tomography (CT) of the brain may reveal low-density lesions within white matter, usually in a paraventricular or subcortical distribution. Enhancement of lesions following intravenous infusion of iodine with delayed scanning indicates the presence of acute lesions with disruption of the blood-brain barrier. Enhancement may disappear as the clinical symptoms resolve. Cortical atrophy with enlarged ventricles is also found in some patients. The incidence of such abnormalities discovered by CT scanning is approximately 25 percent.

MRI is the most sensitive means of detecting lesions of MS. More than 90 percent of patients with clinically definite MS show multifocal cerebral white matter lesions on MRI, better seen with spin-echo (T2-weighted) than with inversion recovery (T1-weighted) images. Serial MRI studies of MS patients with relapsing disease indicate that the frequency of lesion formation, either arising de novo or as an expansion of a preexisting lesion, far exceeds clinical relapse rate. New lesion formation is also observed in progressive MS patients. Lesions typically develop over several weeks and resolve over 2 to 3 months; such resolving lesions likely reflect inflammation and edema rather than demyelination and gliosis. IV administration of gadolinium DTPA can enhance detection of ''active'' lesions on T1-weighted images (see Chap. 348). MRI lesions suggest that the MS disease process rarely ''sleeps.'' Coalescence of MRI lesions appears to correlate with development of progressive disease. Multifocal cerebral white matter lesions are detected by MRI in 60 to 75 percent of cases of isolated optic neuritis and chronic progressive myelopathy. Technical advances now permit direct detection of inflammatory demyelinating lesions within the optic nerves and spinal cord.

Elevated CSF IgG, abnormal evoked responses, and lesions on CT scans and MRI provide useful adjuncts in evaluation of the patient with suspected MS; however, the clinical findings remain paramount in establishing the diagnosis.

TREATMENT OF MS No effective treatment for MS is known. Therapeutic efforts are directed toward (1) amelioration of the acute episode, (2) prevention of relapses or progression of disease, and (3) relief of symptoms.

In acute flare-ups of disease, glucocorticoid treatment may lessen the severity of symptoms and speed recovery; however, ultimate recovery is not improved by this drug nor is the extent of permanent disability altered. Glucocorticoids likely act chiefly via mechanisms other than modulation of the immune response. They may improve the ability of demyelinated nerve to conduct and reduce edema and inflammation within plaques. Usual regimens utilize either ACTH, to stimulate endogenous glucocorticoid synthesis, or prednisone. ACTH is preferred by many clinicians since the only controlled trials that demonstrated the efficacy of glucocorticoid therapy in flare-ups of MS and in acute optic neuritis were performed with this drug. ACTH is commonly given in a dose of 80 units daily intravenously for 3 to 7 days, followed by intramuscular injections in periodically decreasing doses over the next 2 to 3 weeks. Prednisone, 15 mg qid, is sometimes given rather than ACTH, again, over 3 to 7 days with gradually tapering doses over the next 2 to 3 weeks. Since prednisone is taken by mouth, the treatment is simpler than with ACTH, and an admission to the hospital may sometimes be avoided. Use of long-term daily or alternate-day steroids is not advised.

Immunosuppressive agents such as azathioprine and cyclophosphamide have been claimed to reduce the number of relapses in several series, but there is no consensus about the efficacy of these drugs. Plasma exchange in combination with immunosuppression, total-lymphoid irradiation, cyclosporine A, α-interferon, β-interferon, or copolymer I remains under active investigation. γ-Interferon provokes exacerbations.

Symptomatic treatment should address both the physical and psychological needs of patients. Patients should avoid excess fatigue and extremes of temperature and eat a balanced diet. Diets containing low levels of saturated fats have been advocated. The use of belladonna alkaloids and bethanechol chloride can help bladder dysfunction. Periodic checks for urinary tract infection should be performed. Bowel training can alleviate disorders of bowel function. Drugs available for the treatment of spasticity include diazepam, baclofen, and dantrolene sodium. Painful dysesthesias, facial twitching, tic douloureux, and tonic spasms may respond to carbamazepine or phenytoin. Occasionally trigeminal root injection is required to relieve tic douloureux (see Chap. 360).

ACUTE DISSEMINATED ENCEPHALOMYELITIS

Acute disseminated encephalomyelitis (ADEM) may be defined as a monophasic encephalitis or myelitis of abrupt onset characterized by symptoms and signs indicative of damage chiefly of the white matter of the brain or spinal cord. The process may be severe, and even fatal, or mild and evanescent. Pathologic features are those of innumerable minute foci of perivenular lymphocyte and mononuclear cell infiltration with demyelination. The topography of the demyelination corresponds to that of the inflammatory infiltrates. The condition most commonly follows vaccinations against rabies or smallpox or acute infectious illnesses, especially measles, but may occur without any obvious antecedent. The cause is uncertain but is believed by some to represent a hypersensitivity, perhaps to myelin basic protein, and to be the human counterpart of experimentally induced EAE.

ETIOLOGY The entity has been described after two types of vaccination: after rabies vaccination with the Semple vaccine, which contains brain tissue, now seldom used, and after vaccination against smallpox, now seldom performed.

Shortly after introduction of rabies vaccination by Pasteur, it became evident that neuroparalytic accidents could follow this procedure. After a course of injections a sudden encephalitic or myelitic catastrophe might occur coincident with hypersensitivity-type reactions at the sites of vaccine injection. The process clearly involved hypersensitivity to nervous system antigens. The incidence was variously reported as between 1 in 1000 and 1 in 5000 persons vaccinated. An identical syndrome has followed inoculation with noninfected brain material, indicating that killed rabies virus was not the cause; with the introduction of duck embryo killed rabies virus vaccine (which is free of myelinated nervous tissue), the condition has markedly decreased in incidence, although cases continue to be reported from countries where Semple-type vaccines remain in use. Neuroparalytic accidents were most frequent in young adults, the peak age of occurrence corresponding to that of onset of MS. In some cases cellular immune sensitivity to myelin basic protein has been demonstrated.

Smallpox vaccination was also followed by an incidence of ADEM averaging perhaps 1 case per 5000 persons vaccinated but with marked differences between vaccination programs. The complication almost always occurred in conjunction with a primary take rather than a booster-type response. The encephalitis usually followed the peak of the vaccination response by a few days to a week or more but on occasion preceded it. The complication was unknown in children less than 2 years of age; in infants, smallpox vaccination was sometimes associated with an encephalopathy with brain swelling, i.e., toxic encephalopathy.

One case of measles in 1000 is followed by neurologic complications, which are often severe. The mortality rate averages 20 percent, and half the survivors are left with residual damage. The syndrome usually follows the rash by a few days. It bears no relationship to the severity of measles itself. Systemic lymphocyte sensitivity to myelin basic protein has been demonstrated in some patients. All attempts to isolate a virus have failed. Abnormal CSF and changes in the electroencephalogram are observed in perhaps half the children who contract measles, suggesting that subclinical neurologic involvement may be much more widespread than is usually appreciated. A subtle decline in performance and changes in behavior following measles may reflect this inapparent nervous system involvement. Measles vaccination has drastically reduced the frequency of this complication.

An identical clinical picture was seen formerly as a complication of smallpox and is still encountered during or following chickenpox and extremely rarely as a complication of rubella. Demyelinating encephalomyelitis is very rare in mumps; instead there is often a true viral meningitis. A clinical picture identical to postinfectious encephalomyelitis has been described after mycoplasma infections. Despite its striking association with measles, the occurrence of the same clinical picture after several different infections fits better with the postulate that the basic process involves hypersensitivity rather than a direct viral infection of the brain and spinal cord.

CLINICAL MANIFESTATIONS The disease usually begins abruptly. Headache and delirium may give way to lethargy and coma. Coma has an ominous prognosis. Seizures at the onset or shortly thereafter are not infrequent. There may be stiffness of the neck, other signs of meningeal irritation, and fever. Focal signs may be engrafted on this picture, and spinal cord involvement with flaccid paralysis of all four limbs is particularly common. Monoparesis and hemiplegia are also seen. Tendon reflexes may be lost initially only to become hyperactive later; extensor plantar responses are the rule, and sphincter control is generally lost. Sensory loss is variable but may be extensive and severe. Brainstem involvement may be reflected by nystagmus, ocular palsies, and pupillary changes. Some cases may present as a purely spinal cord syndrome and in mild instances with minor signs such as a facial palsy. Chorea and athetosis are rare. Cerebellar signs may predominate, particularly in cases associated with chickenpox. Involvement of motor and sensory peripheral nerves can be documented clinically and electromyographically in some patients. The CSF almost always shows an increase in protein (50 to 100 mg/dL) and lymphocytes (10 to several hundred cells); rarely it is normal. The mortality is 20 percent, and perhaps half the survivors have residual deficits. Recurrences are almost unknown.

The diagnosis is not difficult if there is a history of rabies or smallpox vaccination or of measles. In cases without such a history, distinction from viral encephalitis may be difficult and at times not possible. Reye's syndrome may be difficult to distinguish from acute disseminated encephalomyelitis. Vomiting at onset, a normal CSF, hyperammonemia, and raised intracranial pressure should suggest Reye's syndrome; frequent convulsions and focal signs argue against it. A distinction from acute MS may not be possible.

PREVENTION AND TREATMENT Since smallpox has been eradicated, there is no longer reason to vaccinate against it. Use of duck embryo and human diploid vaccine in rabies prophylaxis has almost eliminated neuroparalytic accidents, and measles vaccination has drastically reduced what used to be the largest group of postinfectious encephalomyelitides.

Administration of high doses of glucocorticoids every 4 to 6 h is the treatment of choice though controlled trials have not been carried out.

ACUTE NECROTIZING HEMORRHAGIC ENCEPHALOMYELITIS

Acute necrotizing hemorrhagic encephalomyelitis is a rare tissue-destructive disease of the CNS which occurs with explosive suddenness within a few days of an upper respiratory infection. The pathologic findings are distinctive. On sectioning the brain, much of the white matter of one or both hemispheres is seen to be destroyed almost to the point of liquefaction. The involved tissue is pink or yellowish-gray and flecked with multiple small hemorrhages. Sometimes similar changes are localized to the brainstem or spinal cord. On histologic examination the core lesion resembles that of acute disseminated encephalomyelitis in showing perivenular foci of demyelination, all of like age. As in acute disseminated encephalomyelitis lymphocytes and macrophages are present in the regions of myelin loss, but superimposed on and dominating the picture is an intense polymorphonuclear infiltrate, in keeping with the necrotizing nature of the process. The vessels themselves are partially necrotic; they may contain platelet or fibrin thrombi within their lumens and fibrin deposits beyond their walls. Multiple small hemorrhages at sites of vessel damage are an invariable feature as is a violent inflammatory reaction in the meninges. Large necrotic foci form by coalescence of smaller lesions in the hemispheres, brainstem, or spinal cord.

The clinical course of the illness resembles that of acute disseminated encephalomyelitis save for its apoplectiform onset and rapidity of progress, sometimes leading to death within 48 h. Neurologic signs are frequently unilateral, reflecting disease in one cerebral hemisphere, but may be bilateral. It is probable that certain patients showing an explosive myelitic illness are suffering from a necrotizing myelitis of similar type, but pathologic evidence in support of this view has been difficult to obtain. The CSF examination discloses a more intense reaction than in other demyelinating diseases. Often a polymorphonuclear pleocytosis of up to 2000 cells and a considerable increase in amount of protein are detected. In cases of slower evolution the cell counts are lower and cells are mainly of the mononuclear type.

The etiology of this disease is not established; however, the entire clinical-pathologic entity bears a close resemblance to a hyperacute form of EAE that can be induced in animals by administration of endotoxin, pertussis vaccine, or the vaccine's histamine-sensitizing factor coincident with or shortly after injection of myelin in adjuvant. The lesions in this experimental disease can perhaps be considered as those of a Sanarelli-Shwartzman reaction within the brain superimposed on an acutely demyelinating process. Rarely a lesion like acute necrotizing hemorrhagic encephalomyelitis occurs in MS.

The differential diagnosis of this disorder includes acute encephalitis, particularly those types causing tissue necrosis (herpes simplex, arbovirus), acute bacterial cerebritis, septic embolic occlusion of an artery, thrombophlebitis, and suppurative brain abscess. The similarity of acute necrotizing hemorrhagic encephalomyelitis to acute disseminated encephaloymyelitis suggests that steroid therapy may be beneficial.

HTLV-I–ASSOCIATED MYELOPATHY (HAM)–TROPICAL SPASTIC PARAPARESIS (TSP)

HAM-TSP presents as a syndrome of progressive spasticity of the lower limbs associated with variable amounts of low back pain, bowel and bladder dysfunction, and disrupted superficial and proprioceptive sensations. The illness develops on a background of HTLV-I infection.

PATHOLOGY The characteristic features are a chronic inflammatory response within the gray and white matter and the meninges, demyelination with relative axonal sparing, proliferation of small blood vessels with perivascular cuffing, and reactive astrocytosis; the above are more marked in the lateral columns of the spinal cord than in the spinothalamic and spinocerebellar tracts. In severe cases, focal spongiosus of tissue is found. Pathologic changes can extend into the brainstem, cerebellum, and cerebrum.

ETIOLOGY Evidence that HTLV-I is the cause of this syndrome includes presence of serum and CSF anti-HTLV-I antibodies, isolation of HTLV-I from systemic and CSF white blood cells, and detection of viral particles within the CNS by electron microscopy. The fact that the immune response is activated coupled with the apparent response of HAM cases to glucocorticoid therapy argues for an immune component in the pathogenesis of tissue injury.

EPIDEMIOLOGY HAM describes the progressive myelopathy syndrome endemic to southern Japan, a temperate climate zone; TSP describes the same etiologic syndrome occurring in tropical regions of the Caribbean, South America, and Africa, affecting mainly, but not exclusively, individuals of black ethnic origin. Peak age of onset of clinical symptoms ranges from 30 to 60 years; childhood onset cases are rare but have been reported from Japan. Females are affected more frequently than males. In endemic areas, prevalence of serum HTLV-I antibodies in the population range from 5 to 20 percent, far exceeding the number of symptomatic individuals. Routes of disease transmission include sexual transmission from male to female, maternal-fetal passage, and blood transfusion. The latency period ranges from 2 years in transfusion cases to many years in maternal-fetal cases. Association of the neurologic syndrome with HTLV-I–induced adult T-cell leukemia is rare. HTLV-I–associated neurologic syndromes have begun to be reported in nonendemic areas.

GENETICS In Japan, specific HLA-region haplotypes are associated with development of the neurologic syndrome; other haplotypes are associated with leukemia.

CLINICAL FEATURES Initial symptoms are usually those of leg weakness with or without back pain. Less frequent complaints are leg paresthesias and bladder dysfunction. Clinical findings include spastic lower limbs with hyperreflexia and Babinski reflexes. In 10 to 60 percent of cases posterior column sensations (proprioception, vibration) are impaired, as are superficial sensations, sometimes with a sensory level that is less well defined than in spinal cord compression syndromes. Less frequent signs include upper limb weakness and spasticity, cerebellar dysfunction, and cranial nerve palsies.

CLINICAL COURSE The progressive myelopathy typically evolves over many years; cases with a more rapid evolution and cases with apparent arrest are also observed.

DIFFERENTIAL DIAGNOSIS Within endemic areas, other causes of myelopathy must be included. Epidemics of "TSP" are on record; such cases are often associated with optic neuropathy and deafness and may be attributable to toxin exposures, particularly with cyanide-containing cassava, malnutrition, or other infectious agents endemic to specific regions, such as treponema. The syndrome of tropical ataxic neuropathy (TAN), characterized by sensory ataxia and slowed peripheral nerve conduction velocities, is also induced by chronic cyanide intoxication (cassava) combined with dietary deficiency. Cases of MS within the endemic TSP-HAM regions do not demonstrate serologic evidence of HTLV-I infection. The severe HTLV-I cases associated with spongiosus of spinal cord need be distinguished from HIV-associated vacuolar myelopathy.

LABORATORY TESTS Within the peripheral blood, T-cell ratios are usually normal, although occasional patients show inverted CD4/CD8 ratios. An increased proportion of T cells express activation antigens compared to controls. Some patients, particularly Japanese, have mild cellular responses within the CSF (up to 50 to 100 cells); in such cases, occasional leukemia-like cells may be found. CSF protein is modestly increased in about 50 percent of cases. Increased CSF immunoglobulin with oligoclonal banding is characteristic. In more than 80 percent of suspected cases, HTLV-I antibodies are detectable in serum and CSF. Virus can be isolated from peripheral blood and CSF. Cerebral lesions are observed on MRI in a minority of cases.

THERAPY Beneficial response to glucocorticoid therapy is claimed in HAM cases; response is less in TSP cases. Viral-directed therapies are under study.

REFERENCES

GONZALEZ-SCARANO F et al: Multiple sclerosis disease activity correlates with gadolinium-enhanced magnetic resonance imaging. Ann Neurol 21:300, 1987

HEMACHUDHA T et al: Myelin basic protein as an encephalotigen in encephalomyelitis and polyneuritis following rabies vaccination. N Engl J Med 316:369, 1987

PATY DW et al: MRI in the diagnosis of MS: A prospective study with comparison of clinical evaluation, evoked potentials, oligoclonal banding, and CT. Neurology 38:180, 1988

POSER CM et al: New diagnostic criteria for multiple sclerosis: Guidelines for research protocols. Ann Neurol 13:227, 1983

RIZZO JF, LESSELL S: Risk of developing multiple sclerosis after uncomplicated optic neuritis: A long-term prospective study. Neurology 38:185, 1988

SEVER JL, GIBBS CJ (eds): *Retroviruses in the Nervous System, Proceedings of a Symposium Sponsored by the National Institutes of Health.* Ann Neurol (Suppl) 23, 1988

WAKSMAN BH: Multiple sclerosis—relationship to a retrovirus? Nature 337:599, 1989

WEINER HL, HAFLER DA: Immunotherapy of multiple sclerosis. Ann Neurol 23:211, 1988

357 NUTRITIONAL AND METABOLIC DISEASES OF THE NERVOUS SYSTEM

MAURICE VICTOR / JOSEPH B. MARTIN

Included under the title of this chapter is a large and diverse number of neurologic disorders that fall into two distinct types—acquired and inherited. In this chapter, emphasis will be on the *acquired* diseases, insofar as they are essentially disorders of adult life and a major source of concern to internist and neurologist alike. The *inherited* metabolic and nutritional diseases, on the other hand, are predominantly disorders of infancy and childhood and are more appropriately considered in a textbook of pediatrics (see also Chaps. 331 to 335). However, a small proportion of the inherited diseases permit survival to adolescence or early adult life or may even have their onset during these periods. These latter instances, which need to be differentiated from certain degenerative and acquired metabolic diseases, are discussed here briefly and in other chapters of this book to which the reader will be referred.

DISEASES DUE TO NUTRITIONAL DEFICIENCY

The general aspects of deficiency disease have been presented in Chap. 76, which should be reviewed as an introduction to the discussion of deficiency diseases of the nervous system. The term *deficiency* will be used here in its strictest sense, to designate those diseases or syndromes resulting from the *lack of an essential nutrient in the diet or from a conditioning factor that increases the need for that nutrient.* The neurologic diseases in this category are the following:

1 Wernicke's disease and Korsakoff's psychosis
2 "Alcoholic" cerebellar degeneration
3 Nutritional polyneuropathy
4 Pellagra
5 Deficiency amblyopia (nutritional optic neuropathy)
6 The syndrome of amblyopia, painful neuropathy, and orogenital dermatitis (Strachan's syndrome)
7 Subacute combined degeneration of the spinal cord (vitamin B_{12} deficiency)
8 Folic acid deficiency
9 Vitamin E deficiency

A number of general principles are applicable to all of the diseases under consideration. Of the known vitamin deficiencies, it is essentially the B deficiencies that are of importance in neurologic disease. Thiamine chloride, nicotinic acid, pyridoxine, pantothenic acid, and possibly folic acid and riboflavin each plays a role in carbohydrate metabolism, upon which the CNS depends for its principal source of energy. These vitamins function as coenzymes in the Krebs tricarboxylic acid cycle; in addition, thiamine is involved in the hexosemonophosphate shunt. Vitamin B_{12} is required for the conversion of methylmalonyl to succinyl coenzyme A and for the conversion of homocystine to methionine. Vitamin E deficiency is a rare cause of central nervous system disease.

Except for subacute combined degeneration of the spinal cord and other manifestations of vitamin B_{12} deficiency, it is not possible to relate the deficiency diseases in humans to the lack of one particular vitamin. For example, polyneuropathy may result from any one of several vitamin deficiencies [thiamine chloride (vitamin B_1), pyridoxine (vitamin B_6), pantothenic acid, and probably B_{12}]. Moreover, pellagra, beriberi, and Strachan's syndrome are probably related to a deficiency of several vitamins. These generalizations should not obscure the fact that certain manifestations of deficiency disease are related to the lack of a specific nutrient (e.g., the ocular signs of Wernicke's disease to a deficiency of thiamine).

In the western world, deficiency diseases of the nervous system occur most often in the alcoholic population of large urban centers. Alcohol acts mainly by displacing food in the diet, but it also increases the demand for B vitamins, which are necessary to metabolize the carbohydrate furnished by alcohol itself, and it may impair the gastrointestinal absorption of vitamins. Dietary faddism, impaired absorption of dietary nutrients (as occurs in sprue, after gastric plication for the treatment of obesity, or resection of stomach and small bowel), and the use of certain drugs (e.g., isoniazid and hydralazine, which interfere with the enzymatic function of pyridoxine) account for a small number of cases of deficiency disease.

Each of the deficiency diseases may occur in pure form and will be so described. More often they occur in various combinations. Stated in another way, deficiency diseases usually involve both the central and peripheral nervous systems, an attribute that they share with few other categories of disease. Also, the examination of patients with deficiency disease frequently discloses nonneurologic signs of malnutrition such as general wasting, lesions of the skin and mucous membranes, and circulatory abnormalities.

WERNICKE'S DISEASE OR ENCEPHALOPATHY Wernicke described an illness of acute onset characterized by mental disturbance, paralysis of eye movements, and ataxia of gait. Swelling of the optic discs and retinal hemorrhages were also present, and there was a progressive depression of the state of consciousness, leading to death, so that a fatal outcome was at one time considered a universal feature of this disease. Wernicke described focal vascular lesions in the gray matter around the third and fourth ventricles and aqueduct of Sylvius. He regarded the disease as inflammatory in nature and suggested the name *acute superior hemorrhagic polioencephalitis*. Since Wernicke's time, views regarding this disease have undergone considerable modification.

Symptoms and signs The most readily recognized abnormalities are the ocular motor signs, and it is difficult to make the clinical diagnosis without them. The usual ocular abnormality is a weakness or paralysis of abduction (sixth nerve palsy) which is invariably bilateral though rarely symmetric and is accompanied by horizontal diplopia, strabismus, and nystagmus. Three types of nystagmus may occur, conjugate horizontal or vertical gaze–evoked nystagmus being the most frequent. An asymmetric horizontal gaze–evoked nystagmus in the abducting eye is characteristic of internuclear ophthalmoplegia. Rarely, one sees a primary position upbeat or downbeat nystagmus with oscillopsia. Each of these abnormalities may be present alone, but far more often a constellation of signs of disordered motility is present, including supranuclear paralysis of gaze. Horizontal gaze palsy is more frequent than vertical gaze palsy. Rarely an isolated paralysis of downgaze or an isolated paralysis of convergence or divergence occurs. In advanced disease there may be complete loss of ocular movement, and the pupils, which ordinarily are spared, may become miotic and nonreacting. Ptosis is rare. The parenteral administration of thiamine in the early stages results in dramatic improvement of the eye movement disorders although horizontal nystagmus may persist.

The *ataxia* affects stance and gait predominantly. The patient may be unable to stand or walk without support. With specific treatment the disorder of equilibrium improves, and the patient is left with a wide-based, uncertain gait. The mildest degree of ataxia is brought out only by heel-to-toe walking. In contrast to the gross disorder of locomotion, an intention (cerebellar) tremor of the limbs is relatively infrequent. The latter abnormality, when present, affects the legs more than the arms. Scanning speech is present only in isolated cases.

A derangement of mental function is found in about 90 percent of patients and takes one of several forms: (1) The most common is a *global confusional-apathetic state,* characterized by profound listlessness, inattentiveness, indifference to the surroundings, and disorientation. Unconsciousness or deep stupor as the initial abnormality is distinctly rare, but drowsiness is common. Spontaneous speech is minimal. Many questions directed to the patient go unanswered, or the patient may fall asleep while being questioned, a state from which he or she can be readily aroused, however. Whatever questions the patient answers betray disorientation in time and place, misidentification of those nearby and an inability to grasp the meaning of the illness or immediate situation. Many of the patient's remarks are irrational and show no consistency from one moment to another. Under these circumstances a more extensive evaluation of intellectual function is seldom possible. (2) Some patients show a disproportionate disorder of retentive memory, i.e., the Korsakoff amnesic state (see Chap. 30 and later in this chapter). (3) A relatively small number of patients (less than 20 percent in our series) show the symptoms of alcohol withdrawal, either delirium tremens or a variant thereof.

The symptoms of Wernicke's disease may appear simultaneously and rather acutely, but more often ophthalmoplegia and/or ataxia precede the mental signs by days or weeks.

Wernicke's disease is usually associated with other nutritional disorders, both neurologic and nonneurologic. In more than 80 percent of patients, a *polyneuropathy* of varying degrees of severity is evident. Rarely, *amblyopia* or *spinal spastic ataxia* may be present. Many patients in the chronic stage demonstrate impaired olfactory discrimination, a defect that is most likely related to the diencephalic lesions (see below).

Full-blown beriberi heart disease occurs rarely in patients with Wernicke's disease, although indications of *disordered cardiovascular function* such as tachycardia, exertional dyspnea, postural hypotension, and minor ECG abnormalities are common. Occasionally patients die suddenly, the mode of death suggesting "cardiovascular collapse," and Wernicke's disease is characterized by a state of high cardiac output which is out of proportion to the oxygen consumption. This is probably due to an abnormal state of peripheral vasodilatation, which in turn may be related to thiamine deficiency. Postural hypotension and syncope are related to impaired function of the automatic nervous system, more specifically to a defect in sympathetic regulation.

Ancillary findings Vestibular function, as measured by the response to standard caloric testing, is always impaired bilaterally and more or less symmetrically in the acute stages of Wernicke's disease (*vestibular paresis*). The cerebrospinal fluid (CSF) is normal or shows only a modest elevation of protein content; protein values above 1.0 g/L (100 mg/dL) or a pleocytosis should always suggest the presence of a complicating illness. In untreated cases of Wernicke's disease, there is invariably an elevation of the *blood pyruvate,* and a marked reduction in the *blood transketolase* (a thiamine-dependent enzyme of the hexose monophosphate shunt). Diffuse slowing of the EEG, mild to moderate in degree, occurs in about one-half of the patients. On the other hand, total cerebral blood flow and cerebral oxygen and glucose consumption may be greatly reduced in the acute stages and persist for several weeks after the institution of treatment.

Course of the illness Death occurs in 15 to 20 percent of hospitalized patients and is usually due to a complicating infection (pneumonia, pulmonary tuberculosis, and septicemia being the most common) or to hepatic failure.

Patients who recover do so in a characteristic manner. Ocular palsies may *begin to improve* within hours after the administration of thiamine and practically always within several days. Failure to respond in this manner raises doubts about the diagnosis of Wernicke's disease. Sixth nerve palsies, ptosis, and vertical gaze palsies recover completely, within a week or two in most cases, but vertical gaze–evoked nystagmus may persist for months. Horizontal gaze palsies recover completely as a rule, but a fine horizontal gaze–evoked nystagmus usually remains as a permanent sequela of the disease.

Ataxia improves somewhat more slowly than the ocular motor abnormalities. Approximately half the patients recover incompletely and are left with a slow, shuffling, wide-based gait and inability to walk tandem. The residual gait disturbance and horizontal nystagmus provide a means of identifying obscure and chronic cases of dementia as alcoholic-nutritional in origin. Vestibular function, as measured by caloric testing, improves at about the same rate as the ataxia of stance and gait, i.e., over a period of weeks or months, and recovery is usually but not always complete.

The symptoms of apathy, drowsiness, and confusion recede gradually, and as they do, the *defect in retentive memory and learning (Korsakoff's psychosis;* see Chap. 30) stands out more clearly. It is important to emphasize that Wernicke's disease and Korsakoff's psychosis are not separate diseases, but that the changing ocular and ataxic signs and the transformation of the global confusion state into an amnesic syndrome are successive stages in the recovery of a single disease process. Stated in another way, Korsakoff's psychosis is the psychic component of Wernicke's disease. Hence the symptom complex should be called Wernicke's disease when the amnesic state is not evident and the Wernicke-Korsakoff syndrome when both the ocular-ataxic and amnesic symptoms can be recognized.

The outcome of Korsakoff's psychosis varies. Complete or almost complete recovery occurs in less than 20 percent of patients. In the remainder recovery is slow and incomplete. Depending on the severity of the residual symptoms, the patient may or may not be able to lead a supervised existence out of a hospital. The residual mental state is characterized by large gaps in memory, without confabulation, and an inability of the patient to sort out events in their proper temporal sequence. This late stage of the disease, when the ocular and ataxic signs have receded or are not recognized, is often loosely referred to as "alcoholic deteriorated state" or "alcoholic dementia."

Pathologic changes Patients who die in the acute stages of Wernicke-Korsakoff disease have symmetrically placed lesions in the paraventricular regions of the thalamus and hypothalamus, the mamillary bodies, periaqueductal region of the midbrain, floor of the fourth ventricle, and anterior-superior folia of the cerebellum, particularly of the vermis. Lesions are invariably found in the mamillary bodies and less consistently in the other areas. Microscopically, the principal change consists of varying degrees of necrosis of parenchymal structures. Many nerve cells and fibers are destroyed; others remain intact and are seen against a background of reactive glial elements, both astrocytes and microgliocytes. The blood vessels are prominent, owing to adventitial and endothelial proliferation. Hemorrhagic lesions are present in a small proportion of cases and are usually of recent origin. The oculomotor and vestibular nuclei are regularly involved, but to a lesser degree.

Clinical-pathologic correlations The ocular motor signs are attributable to lesions in the brainstem affecting the abducens nuclei and eye movement centers in the pons and rostral midbrain (see Chap. 23). The lesions of the vestibular nuclei are probably responsible for the loss of caloric responses and gross abnormality of equilibrium that characterize the initial stage of the disease. The lack of significant destruction of nerve cells in these lesions accounts for the rapid improvement in oculomotor and vestibular function.

The persistent ataxia of stance and gait is related to the loss of neurons in the superior vermis of the cerebellum; extension of the lesion into the anterior parts of the anterior lobes accounts for the ataxia of individual movements of the legs. These cerebellar lesions are indistinguishable from those of so-called *alcoholic cerebellar degeneration* (see below).

The amnesic defect is related to lesions in the diencephalon, more specifically to those in the medial dorsal nuclei of the thalami. Lesions in the mamillary bodies are probably not critical in respect to memory function since they are found in patients with Wernicke's disease who had shown no disorder of memory during life.

Etiology and pathogenesis Nutritional deficiency is the causal factor. Wernicke's disease has been encountered in prisoners-of-war and in patients with wasting diseases of varied origin, i.e., circumstances in which alcohol played no part. The specific factor responsible for most, if not all, of the symptoms of the Wernicke-Korsakoff syndrome is a deficiency of thiamine. The marked sensitivity of the ocular abnormalities to the administration of thiamine accounts for their rapid abatement after the ingestion of a meal or two. The quality of prompt reversibility indicates that the ocular signs are due to a biochemical abnormality and not to irreversible structural changes. On the other hand, the slow and incomplete recovery of the memory defect suggests that this symptom is due to irreversible structural changes, presumably in the medial dorsal nuclei.

The mechanism whereby thiamine deficiency causes brain lesions is not established. Thiamine is a cofactor for several enzymes including transketolase, pyruvate dehydrogenase, and α-ketoglutarate dehydrogenase. Thiamine deficiency produces a diffuse decrease in cerebral glucose utilization, and lesions in thiamine-deficient experimental animals are diminished by antagonists that block *N*-methyl-D-aspartate–preferring glutamic acid receptors. This latter finding suggests that the neurotoxicity of thiamine deficiency may be mediated by excitotoxicity evoked by glutamic acid release (see also Chaps. 346 and 359).

The selective vulnerability of certain periventricular regions to a deficiency of thiamine is not understood. McEntee and Mair have pointed out that the lesions lie in the monoamine-containing pathways and have presented evidence that 3-methoxy-4-hydroxyphenylglycol (MHPG), the primary brain metabolite of norepinephrine, is decreased in the CSF of alcoholic patients with Korsakoff's psychosis; moreover, the administration of clonidine, an $alpha_2$-adrenergic agonist, seemed to improve the memory disorder in these patients. These authors have theorized that damage to the ascending norepinephrine-containing neurons in the brainstem and diencephalon is the basis for the amnesia.

The topography of the lesions caused by thiamine deficiency has been studied in rhesus monkeys. Witt and Goldman-Rakic found that the severity and number of brain nuclei affected are related to the duration and number of bouts of thiamine deficiency.

Treatment of the Wernicke-Korsakoff syndrome Wernicke's disease represents a medical emergency, and its recognition demands the immediate administration of thiamine. A delay of a few hours may be crucial in determining whether the patient with ocular and ataxic signs will be prevented from developing Korsakoff's psychosis and whether the patient with early Korsakoff's changes will be restored to a state of mental competency. Although 2 to 3 mg of thiamine may modify the ocular signs, much larger doses are needed to replenish the thiamine stores—50 mg intravenously and 50 mg intramuscularly, the latter dose being repeated each day until the patient resumes a normal diet. The other B vitamins may be given by mouth in the dosages outlined in Chap. 76. If the patient cannot or will not eat, parenteral feeding and administration of B vitamins become necessary.

A particular danger attends the treatment of the severely depleted alcoholic patient with intravenous glucose solutions. Such infusions may exhaust the patient's reserve of B vitamins and either precipitate Wernicke's disease in a previously unaffected patient or cause a rapid worsening of an early form of the disease. For this reason, B vitamins must be administered to all alcoholic patients requiring parenteral glucose. The cardiovascular status of each patient should be monitored carefully. Since these patients are confused and forgetful, they must be supervised continually, preferably on a medical ward.

A special problem arises when the patient recovers from the acute phase of the illness and the amnesic psychosis becomes prominent. The disposition of the patient to family, nursing home, or mental institution should be made on the basis of the severity of the mental illness as well as the capacity of the family unit and social circumstances.

NUTRITIONAL POLYNEUROPATHY (See also Chaps. 76 and 363) Nutritional polyneuropathy is usually a disease of the alcoholic population. As mentioned above, it is present in most patients with the Wernicke-Korsakoff syndrome, but it may occur as the only manifestation of deficiency disease. The peripheral neuropathy of alcoholics ("alcoholic polyneuropathy") does not differ in any fundamental way from that of beriberi. The clinical features of nutritional polyneuropathy and its identity with beriberi are discussed in Chaps. 76 and 363. A deficiency of thiamine chloride, pyridoxine, pantothenic acid, vitamin B_{12}, and perhaps folic acid has been demonstrated in individual cases to cause nutritional polyneuropathy. In the alcoholic patient it is usually not possible to incriminate a particular vitamin.

"ALCOHOLIC" CEREBELLAR DEGENERATION This is the term applied to a common, stereotyped, nonfamilial form of cerebellar ataxia that occurs on a background of prolonged ingestion of alcohol. Usually the symptoms evolve in subacute fashion, i.e., over several weeks or months, sometimes more rapidly. In some patients the symptoms are present in mild but stable form and worsen after an attack of pneumonia or delirium tremens.

The signs are those of cerebellar dysfunction, affecting stance and gait predominantly. The legs are involved more severely than the arms, and nystagmus and speech disturbances occur relatively infrequently. Once established, the signs change very little, although some improvement of gait may follow the cessation of drinking, due probably to improvement in general nutrition and recovery from associated polyneuropathy.

The pathologic changes consist of degeneration of varying severity of all the neurocellular elements of the cerebellar cortex, particularly of the Purkinje cells, with a striking topographic restriction to the anterior and superior aspects of the vermis and adjacent parts of the anterior lobes of the cerebellum. The disorder of stance and gait is related to the lesion in the vermis, and the ataxia of the limbs is due to the involvement of the anterior lobes. A similar clinical-pathologic syndrome is observed occasionally in nutritionally depleted nonalcoholic patients.

Central nervous system disorders in alcoholism not associated with vitamin deficiency A number of alcohol-associated disorders are not attributable to nutritional deficiency or trauma. There appears to be an increased incidence of hypertension in alcoholics and probably of strokes, both ischemic infarction and spontaneous subarachnoid hemorrhage. Alcoholics as a group also show dilatation of the lateral ventricles and widening of sulci on CT or MRI scans. The nature of these changes is obscure. They do not correlate with any mental abnormality, nor do they represent cerebral atrophy insofar as partial and sometimes complete reversal occur with sustained abstinence. Some believe that alcohol can cause intellectual deterioration separate from effects due to nutritional deficiency, but an entity of "alcoholic dementia" has never been established on the basis of clinical and neuropathologic studies. A syndrome of progressive myelopathy occurring in alcoholics has also been described. Such patients are said to show no evidence of nutritional deficiency (B_{12} or folic acid) or of liver disease. The nature of the spinal cord disease is unknown, and a causal relationship to the toxic effects of alcohol remains to be established.

PELLAGRA This disease is described in Chap. 76. Neurologic manifestations are quite diverse. Pellagra is essentially an encephalopathy, although involvement of the spinal cord and peripheral nerves may occur. The early mental symptoms—insomnia, fatigue, anxiety, nervousness, irritability, and depression—may be mistaken for a psychiatric disorder. However, as the disease advances, slowing and inefficiency of mental processes and impairment of memory become clear-cut. Pellagra may not only cause psychiatric manifestations but occasionally may result from them because certain mental illnesses, including alcoholism, cause anorexia and dietary deficiency.

The spinal cord involvement in pellagra has not been clearly delineated, perhaps because the mental state of the patients has precluded accurate testing. In general, there is both posterior and lateral column involvement, predominantly the former. Neuropathic signs are difficult to distinguish from other types of nutritional polyneuropathy. Other manifestations such as tremor, extrapyramidal rigidity, suck and grasp reflexes, and coma (referred to in the past as "nicotinic acid–deficiency encephalopathy") have indiscriminately been included in the pellagra syndrome, as have various disorders of the special senses.

A *spastic paretic syndrome,* apart from the other symptoms and signs of pellagra, may be a rare manifestation of nutritional deficiency. The chief signs are spastic weakness of the legs with absent abdominal and increased tendon reflexes, clonus, and extensor plantar responses. These signs are usually accompanied by other manifestations of nutritional deficiency, such as Wernicke's disease, amblyopia, and peripheral neuropathy.

Pathologic features The distinctive neuropathologic changes in pellagra are most readily discerned in the large Betz cells of the motor cortex, although the same changes are seen to a lesser extent in the smaller pyramidal cells of the cerebral cortex and cells of the basal ganglia, cranial motor and dentate nuclei, and anterior horns of the spinal cord. The affected cells appear swollen and rounded with eccentric nuclei and loss of Nissl staining. This *central neuritis of pellagra,* as it is called, appears to represent a primary affection of the whole motor cell. The spinal cord lesions take the form of a symmetric degeneration of the dorsal columns, especially the fasciculus gracilis, and to a lesser extent of the corticospinal tracts. The posterior column degeneration is probably secondary to degeneration of specific dorsal root ganglion cells.

DEFICIENCY AMBLYOPIA (NUTRITIONAL OPTIC NEUROPATHY, TOBACCO-ALCOHOL AMBLYOPIA) These terms refer to a characteristic form of visual impairment that complicates nutritional disease and is due to a lesion in the optic nerve, more or less confined to the zone of the papillomacular bundle. The cornea and other parts of the refractive mechanism are uninvolved, hence the term *amblyopia.*

The main symptoms are dimness or blurring of vision for near and distant objects and impairment of color vision, which worsens progressively and insidiously for several days or weeks. In addition to a reduction in visual acuity, examination discloses the presence of bilateral and roughly symmetric central or centrocecal scotomas, which are larger for colored than for white test objects. Pallor of the temporal portion of the optic disc is observed in some cases. Untreated, this condition progresses to irreversible optic atrophy.

Deficiency amblyopia was common in prisoners of war. Although this form of amblyopia had previously been described in association with beriberi (due to thiamine deficiency) and pellagra (due to niacin deficiency), the peak incidence among prisoners coincided with neither of these syndromes but with the syndrome of orogenital dermatitis and "burning feet" ("Strachan syndrome," see below).

In the United States, most, if not all, of the cases of retrobulbar neuropathy attributed to the toxic effects of alcohol or tobacco—so-called tobacco-alcohol amblyopia—are of nutritional origin. Optic neuropathy may occur as the only manifestation of vitamin deficiency, but more often it is combined with other evidence of nutritional deficiency, such as peripheral neuropathy and the Wernicke-Korsakoff syndrome.

Although the nutritional origin of this type of amblyopia has been established, the specific vitamin deficiency can rarely be determined. Observations in both humans and experimental animals indicate that a deficiency of thiamine (vitamin B_1), vitamin B_{12}, or perhaps riboflavin may cause lesions in the optic nerves. Two causative mechanisms for the pathogenesis of tobacco amblyopia have been proposed: (1) chronic cyanide (generated in tobacco smoke) poisoning; and (2) alterations of fatty acid metabolism resulting from derangement of proprionate metabolism in the central nervous system. The notion that cyanide or other substances in tobacco smoke have a toxic effect upon the optic nerves is not supported by experimental data. And, since fatty acids take part in the formation and preservation of myelin, the biochemical consequences of vitamin B_{12} deficiency may be sufficient to account for both ophthalmologic and other neurologic involvement. However, in only a small proportion of patients with this type of amblyopia can a vitamin B_{12} deficiency state be established.

Treatment consists of the administration of a balanced diet, supplemented with B vitamins, and the interdiction of alcohol where this is the cause of nutritional deficiency.

SYNDROME OF AMBLYOPIA, PAINFUL NEUROPATHY, AND OROGENITAL DERMATITIS (STRACHAN'S SYNDROME) There have been many reports of a neurologic syndrome that is undoubtedly nutritional in origin but cannot be fitted into the boundaries of beriberi or pellagra. Strachan attributed the disorder to malaria. Originally known as "Jamaican neuritis," the syndrome occurs among the undernourished populations of many tropical countries. Large numbers of patients with this syndrome were observed also in the besieged population of Madrid during the Spanish Civil War and among prisoners of war during World War II in the Middle and Far East. In the United States, occasional alcoholic patients have this syndrome.

Strachan's syndrome is essentially a disorder of the peripheral and optic nerves. The peripheral nerve disorder is characterized mainly by sensory symptoms and signs (painful paresthesias of the feet, loss of superficial and deep sensation, and ataxia). On the other hand, foot drop and muscle weakness occur rarely. A frequently associated disorder is failing vision, which may go on to complete blindness and pallor of the optic discs. Deafness and vertigo are rare, but among some prisoners of war these symptoms were so prominent as to earn the epithet "camp dizziness." In these respects the syndrome differs from beriberi. Along with the neurologic signs there may be varying degrees of stomatoglossitis, corneal degeneration, and genital dermatitis. These mucocutaneous lesions are spoken of together as the *orogenital syndrome*. Because the genital dermatitis and stomatoglossitis are typical of pellagra and the ocular lesions, of vitamin A deficiency, it is possible Strachan's syndrome can be accounted for by multiple vitamin deficiencies.

There have been few pathologic studies of this syndrome. Aside from the damage to the papillomacular bundle in the optic nerve, the most consistent abnormality has been a loss of myelinated fibers in the posterior columns (fasciculus gracilis) of the spinal cord. This indicates a systematized degeneration of the central processes of the large bipolar sensory neurons of the lumbosacral spinal ganglia. Degeneration of the peripheral processes of these neurons probably accounts for the loss of pain and temperature sensation. There are no reliable data concerning the specific vitamin deficiencies that cause this disease.

SUBACUTE COMBINED DEGENERATION (SCD) OF THE SPINAL CORD (See also Chap. 76) This term designates the spinal cord disease that is due to vitamin B_{12} deficiency. The brain, optic nerves, and peripheral nerves may also be affected but far less often than the spinal cord. The neurologic and hematologic manifestations (pernicious anemia) are distinctive insofar as they are caused not by a lack of vitamin B_{12} in the food but by an inability to transfer this nutrient across the intestinal mucosa. Such a nutritional disorder is referred to as a *conditioned deficiency,* since it depends upon the lack of an intrinsic factor in the gastric secretions (see Chap. 292). Rarely neurologic symptoms due to vitamin B_{12} deficiency occur in patients with disease of the distal small intestine (Crohn's disease, lymphoma) or after surgical resection.

Clinical manifestations Neurologic symptoms are present in the majority of patients with vitamin B_{12} deficiency. The patient first notices general weakness and paresthesias, consisting of tingling, "pins-and-needles" feelings, or other vaguely described sensations in the distal parts of the limbs; the lower extremities may be involved before the upper ones or vice versa. The paresthesias tend to be constant, to progress steadily, and to be the source of much distress. As the illness progresses, the gait becomes unsteady, and movements of the limbs, especially the legs, become stiff and awkward.

Early in the course of the illness, when only paresthesias are present, there may be no objective signs. Later, the neurologic examination discloses a disorder of the posterior and lateral columns of the spinal cord, predominantly the former. Loss of vibration sense, the most consistent sign, is more pronounced in the legs than in the arms, and frequently it extends over the trunk. Position sense is involved to a somewhat lesser extent. The motor defects are usually limited to the legs and include loss of power, spasticity, changes in the tendon reflexes, clonus, and extensor plantar responses. At first the patellar and Achilles reflexes may be diminished, increased, or absent. With treatment, the reflexes may return to normal or become hyperactive. The gait at first is predominantly ataxic, later ataxic and spastic. If the disease remains untreated, an ataxic paraplegia with variable degrees of spasticity and contracture may develop.

A loss of superficial sensation below a segmental level on the trunk, implicating the spinothalamic tracts, occurs rarely, but such a finding should always suggest the possibility of some other disease of the spinal cord. More often the sensory defect takes the form of a blunting of tactile, painful, and thermal sensation over the distal segments of the lower limbs, implicating the peripheral nerves, but such findings are uncommon.

The nervous system involvement in vitamin B_{12} deficiency is characteristically, though not perfectly, symmetric. A definite asymmetry of motor or sensory findings, maintained over a period of weeks or months, should always cast doubt on the diagnosis.

Mental signs are frequent, ranging from irritability, apathy, somnolence, suspiciousness, and emotional instability to a marked confusional or depressive psychosis, or even to intellectual deterioration. Optic neuropathy with impaired acuity and cecocentral scotoma has been reported with virtually all forms of vitamin B_{12} deficiency. In all cases, variable improvement in acuity occurs once systemic vitamin B_{12} is administered. Although dementia and amblyopia are relatively uncommon manifestations of vitamin B_{12} deficiency, each may occasionally be the initial manifestation of the disease.

Pathology and pathogenesis The pathologic process takes the form of a diffuse, though uneven, degeneration of the white matter of the spinal cord and sometimes of the brain. At first there is swelling of myelin sheaths, characterized by separation of myelin lamellae and formation of intramyelinic vacuoles. This is followed by a coalescence of small foci of tissue destruction into larger ones, giving the tissue a vacuolated appearance. The myelin sheaths and the axis cylinders are both affected, the former perhaps earlier and to a greater extent than the latter. Astrocytic gliosis is minimal in the early lesions, but in the more chronic ones gliosis is pronounced. The changes begin in the posterior columns of the lower cervical and upper thoracic cord and spread from this region up and down the cord, as well as forward into the lateral columns. The lesions are not limited to specific systems of fibers within the posterior and lateral funiculi but are scattered irregularly through the white matter. The changes in the optic nerves are similar to those in other types of nutritional neuropathy, i.e., a degeneration of myelinated fibers in the territory of the papillomacular bundles.

The *pathogenesis* of the nervous system lesions in vitamin B_{12} deficiency is not well understood. Impairment of DNA synthesis probably accounts for the hematologic abnormalities and the production of megaloblasts; however, since neurons do not divide, this mechanism cannot be invoked to explain the central nervous system changes. One of the better-understood functions of vitamin B_{12} is its role as a coenzyme in the methylmalonyl CoA mutase reaction. Impairment of this metabolic step may lead to the production of abnormal fatty acids, which are important building blocks of cell membranes and of myelin. However, Carmel et al. have described a hereditary form of cobalamin deficiency, in which methylmalonyl CoA mutase activity was normal despite the presence of typical neurologic abnormalities. These authors attributed the neurologic abnormalities to an impairment of methionine synthase activity. These and other hypotheses have been reviewed by Beck.

Diagnosis and treatment The chief obstacle to early diagnosis is the lack of parallelism between the hematologic and neurologic signs. This is particularly true of patients who have received folic acid, which serves to maintain a hematologic remission for an indefinite period while the neurologic signs worsen, often to an irreversible stage. Under these circumstances the most reliable diagnostic procedures are the measurement of the serum B_{12} concentration and the two-stage Schilling test (see Chap. 292). In rare instances, even these tests may be inconclusive, in which case the finding of high serum concentrations of cobalamin metabolites—methylmalonic acid and homocysteine—may be diagnostically useful.

The treatment of the neurologic manifestations of vitamin B_{12} deficiency differs in no way from the treatment of the hematologic ones. Patients whose vitamin B_{12} stores have been depleted require large doses of cobalamin—1000 μg intramuscularly each day during hospitalization, then weekly for a month, and then monthly for the remainder of the patient's life.

The most important factor influencing the *response to treatment* is the duration of the neurologic disease. Recovery may be complete if therapy is instituted within a few weeks of the onset of symptoms. For this reason SCD and the other neurologic complications of vitamin B_{12} deficiency represent medical emergencies. If symptoms have been present for longer than a month or two, only partial recovery can be expected, and in long-standing cases the best that can be expected is the arrest of progression of the symptoms.

FOLIC ACID DEFICIENCY Despite the frequent occurrence of folic acid deficiency, a role in the pathogenesis of nervous system disease has not been established beyond doubt. The polyneuropathies that occasionally complicate sprue and other malabsorption syndromes and the chronic administration of phenytoin have been attributed, on uncertain grounds, to folate deficiency. With respect to folate deficiency and spinal cord disease, the data are equally limited. Cases have been described (see Pincus) in which the neurologic signs of subacute combined degeneration were attributed to folic acid deficiency. In these cases there was no evidence of vitamin B_{12} deficiency but there was a resolution of both the hematologic and neurologic abnormalities after the institution of folate therapy.

VITAMIN E DEFICIENCY A rare neurologic disorder of childhood, consisting essentially of a spinocerebellar degeneration in association with a polyneuropathy and pigmentary retinopathy, has been related to a deficiency of vitamin E that develops after prolonged intestinal malabsorption (Satya-Murti et al.). The same mechanism has been proposed to explain the neurologic disorders that sometimes complicate abetalipoproteinemia, fibrocystic disease, and extensive intestinal resections (Harding et al.). Vitamin E deficiency also occurs in young children with chronic cholestatic hepatobiliary disease. Ataxia, loss of tendon reflexes, ophthalmoparesis, proximal muscle weakness with elevated serum creatine phosphokinase, and decreased sensation are the usual manifestations. These symptoms are referable to parts of the nervous system and musculature known to be involved in animals deprived of vitamin E—degeneration of Clarke's columns, spinocerebellar tracts, posterior columns, nuclei of Goll and Burdach, and sensory roots (Nelson et al.). In affected children neurologic function improves after the long-term correction of vitamin E deficiency.

NEUROLOGIC SYNDROMES CAUSED BY HYPERVITAMINOSIS Acute toxicity with vitamin A causes symptoms of headache, dizziness, irritability, and drowsiness. Chronic hypervitaminosis A can give rise to chronic increased intracranial pressure (pseudotumor cerebri) (see Chap. 76).

The ingestion of pyridoxine in excessive amounts (2 g or more daily) can cause a sensory neuropathy characterized clinically by progressive ataxia, impairment of position and vibration sense, and loss of deep tendon reflexes. Motor strength is preserved. The syndrome is reversible with discontinuation of pyridoxine.

ACQUIRED (SECONDARY) METABOLIC DISEASES OF THE NERVOUS SYSTEM

In this important category of neurologic disease, disturbance of cerebral function is due to disease in some other organ system—heart (and circulation), lungs (and respiration), kidneys, liver, endocrine glands, and possibly pancreas. Each of these diseases affects the nervous system in somewhat different ways.

ANOXIC-ISCHEMIC ENCEPHALOPATHY This common and often disastrous condition is caused by a lack of oxygen to the brain, resulting from hypotension or respiratory failure. Sometimes both are responsible, and one cannot say which predominates—hence, the ambiguous designation in clinical records, as "cardiorespiratory failure." The conditions that most often lead to anoxic-ischemic encephalopathy are (1) myocardial infarction; (2) cardiac arrest; (3) hemorrhage, with shock and circulatory collapse; in these situations vascular supply to the brain is compromised before respiration; (4) shock; (5) suffocation (from drowning, strangulation, aspiration of vomitus or blood, compression of the trachea by hemorrhage or a surgical pack, or a foreign body in the trachea); (6) diseases that paralyze the muscles of respiration or compromise the central nervous system respiratory drive (trauma, vascular disease of the brain, epilepsy), causing respiratory failure followed by cardiac failure; and (7) carbon monoxide (CO) poisoning, in which respiration fails first and then cardiovascular functions. Hypoxia alone may induce different clinicopathologic consequences than a combination of hypoxia and hypoperfusion (ischemia).

Clinical manifestations Mild degrees of hypoxia cause inattentiveness, impaired judgment, and motor incoordination but have no lasting effects. With severe hypoxia or anoxia, as occurs with cardiac arrest, consciousness is lost within seconds, but recovery will be complete if breathing, oxygenation of blood, and cardiac action are restored within 3 to 5 min. If anoxia persists beyond this time, there is serious and permanent injury to the brain, particularly to those parts in which the efficiency of circulation is marginal (globus pallidus, cerebellum, hippocampus, and the "borderzone regions" of the parietooccipital lobes). Clinically, it is difficult to judge the precise degree of hypoxia-ischemia since slight heart action or an imperceptible blood pressure may serve to maintain the circulation to some extent. Hence some individuals have made an excellent recovery after cerebral anoxia that allegedly lasted 8 to 10 min or longer. *An important clinical rule is that degrees of hypoxia which at no time abolish consciousness rarely if ever cause permanent damage to the nervous system.* P_{O_2} as low as 2.7 kPa (20 mmHg) is well tolerated if it develops gradually and blood pressure is normal. Also, subjects who demonstrate intact brainstem function (as indicated by normal ciliospinal, oculovestibular, and pupillary light responses, and intact doll's-head eye movements) usually have a better outlook for recovery of consciousness and perhaps all of their faculties. Conversely, absence of these reflexes and the presence of pupils that are persistently fixed to light indicate a grave prognosis.

Extreme or sustained global ischemia causes brain death (see Chap. 31). Immediately after resuscitation from cardiorespiratory arrest, the physical findings may suggest brain death (dilated, unresponsive pupils, absent brainstem reflexes and respiration, and isoelectric EEG), yet full recovery may occur. However, persistence of the unresponsive state for more than an hour or two invariably carries a poor prognosis. The diagnosis of brain death must be made with caution because anesthesia, drug intoxication, and hypothermia may also cause deep coma, absent brainstem reflexes, and an isoelectric EEG but permit recovery. The problem of brain death has been brought increasingly to public attention because of ethical and moral issues that surround the question of discontinuing supportive medical therapy. Issues of management are most difficult in the patient who has suffered severe but lesser degrees of cerebral anoxia.

Patients who suffer a severe anoxic encephalopathy, but one that falls short of causing "brain death," often stabilize breathing and heart action. Neurologic evaluation shows the patient to be profoundly comatose, with eyes slightly divergent and motionless but with reactive pupils, flaccid or intensely rigid limbs, and diminished tendon reflexes. Within a few minutes after cardiac action and breathing have been restored, generalized convulsions and isolated or grouped twitches of muscles (myoclonus) may supervene. Decerebrate or decorticate postures may be present or occur upon pinching the limbs, and bilateral Babinski signs can be evoked. In the first 24 to 48 h death may occur in a setting of rising temperature, deepening coma, and circulatory collapse. Or, with somewhat lesser degrees of injury, where the cerebral and cerebellar cortices are partly or completely destroyed but brainstem-spinal structures remain intact, the individual may survive in a state referred to as "irreversible coma" or "persistent vegetative state" (see Chap. 31). The latter patients remain mute, unresponsive, and unaware of their environment for weeks, months, or years. Criteria to predict accurately the outcome of anoxic encephalopathy early in the comatose period have been developed (see Chap. 31). If intoxication can be excluded, the presence of fixed dilated pupils and paralysis of eye movement for 24 to 48 h, along with marked slowing of the EEG, usually signifies irreversible cerebral damage. Deep coma of this type, lasting more than a few days, is rarely attended by full recovery.

Patients with lesser degrees of injury improve after a period of coma. Consciousness is regained, and then various degrees of confusion, visual agnosia, extrapyramidal rigidity, or movement disorder (action or intention myoclonus, choreoathetosis, cerebellar ataxia) become manifest. Some of these patients quickly pass through this posthypoxic phase and proceed to make full recovery; others are left with permanent neurologic sequelae. The *posthypoxic syndromes* observed most frequently are (1) *persistent coma or stupor;* and, with lesser degrees of cerebral injury, (2) *dementia,* with or without extrapyramidal signs; (3) *visual agnosia;* (4) *parkinsonism;* (5) *choreoathetosis;* (6) *cerebellar ataxia;* (7) *intention or action myoclonus;* and (8) *Korsakoff's amnesic state. Seizures* may continue to be a problem but are uncommon.

A relatively uncommon and unexplained phenomenon is *delayed postanoxic encephalopathy.* Initial improvement, which appears to be complete, is followed after a variable period of time (several days to a week or longer) by a relapse, characterized by apathy, confusion, irritability, and occasionally agitation or mania. A few patients have recovered from this second episode, but in most the neurologic syndrome progresses, with shuffling gait, diffuse rigidity and spasticity, coma, and death after 1 to 2 weeks. Postmortem examination of these patients has shown the major abnormality to be widespread cerebral demyelination. Exceptionally, another delayed syndrome occurs, in which a period of hypoxia is followed by a slow, deteriorating state, affecting basal ganglia more than cerebral cortex and white matter and progressing for weeks to months until the patient is mute, rigid, and helpless.

The essential *mechanism* in hypoxic encephalopathy is a neuronal lack of oxygen and an arrest of all aerobic metabolic processes necessary to sustain the Krebs tricarboxylic cycle and the electron transport system. Lactic acid accumulates in the tissues. The pathophysiology of delayed progression is not understood. Experimental observations suggest that glutamate release from hypoxic-ischemic brain tissue can induce neurotoxicity by actions exerted through one subclass of glutamate receptor, the *N*-methyl-D-aspartate (NMDA) receptor.

Diagnosis This depends on (1) the history of a hypoxic-ischemic event and evidence of reduced oxygenation of arterial blood [P_{O_2}<5.3 kPa (40 mmHg)], CO intoxication (indicated by its spectroscopic band or cherry-red color of the skin for a few minutes to hours after the episode), blood pressures below 9.3 kPa (70 mmHg) systolic, or cardiac arrest; and (2) as outlined above, the typical clinical sequence of events after a possible hypoxic-ischemic episode has terminated. Renal damage (anuria) and myocardial infarction may also have occurred and provide corroborative evidence of hypoxia.

Treatment The treatment of anoxic encephalopathy is directed mainly at the prevention of a critical degree of hypoxic injury. After a clear airway is secured, artificial respiration, external thoracic cardiac massage, the use of a cardiac defibrillator or pacemaker, and open chest surgery all have their place, and every second counts in their prompt utilization. Once cardiac and pulmonary function are restored, there is no evidence that any pharmacologic measure enhances recovery. Barbiturates, glucocorticoids, dimethyl sulfoxide, and benzodiazepines have been given without proof of benefit. A small proportion of patients develop secondary complications of diffuse brain swelling after cardiac arrest; this condition is more common in children. This is detected by compression of the lateral ventricles and cisterns on CT scan, or by very high lumbar CSF pressure. Seizures should be controlled by anticonvulsants. Posthypoxic myoclonus may respond to oral administration of clonazepam 8–12 mg/d. Other details of treatment are considered in Chap. 31.

HYPERCAPNIC ENCEPHALOPATHY Chronic emphysema and fibrosing lung disease and, in rare instances, an inadequacy of central respiratory drive lead to chronic respiratory acidosis, with an elevation of P_{CO_2} and a reduction in arterial P_{O_2}. Secondary polycythemia and cor pulmonale often accompany these pulmonary diseases.

Clinical Manifestations The clinical syndrome consequent upon hypercapnia (and hypoxia) consists of generalized or bilateral frontal or occipital headache, often intense and persistent for hours; papilledema; mental dullness, drowsiness, confusion, stupor, and coma; a fast-frequency action tremor and coarse twitching of all muscles, which are in a state of sustained contraction; and inability to maintain a fixed posture or interruption of a voluntary movement because of brief lapses of sustained muscle contraction (asterixis). Intermittent drowsiness, indifference and inattention to the environment, reduction of psychomotor activity, imperception of the sequence of events, and forgetfulness constitute the more subtle manifestations of this syndrome.

In fully developed cases, the cerebrospinal fluid (CSF) is under increased pressure, P_{CO_2} may exceed 10 kPa (75 mmHg), and oxygen saturation of the arterial blood ranges from 85 to 40 percent. The EEG reveals slow activity in the delta and theta range, sometimes bilaterally synchronous. The mechanism of the cerebral disorder is said to be CO_2 narcosis, but the biochemical mechanism is not known. The danger of administering morphine or sedatives, which blunt the respiratory drive (already depressed by the CO_2 retention), or inhaled O_2, which removes the sole stimulus (low P_{O_2}) to the respiratory center, is now widely recognized.

Treatment Forced ventilation with an intermittent positive-pressure respirator, treatment of heart failure with digitalis and diuretics, venesection to reduce the viscosity of the blood, and antibiotics to combat pulmonary infection are the most effective therapeutic measures. If stupor or coma persists, the arterial O_2 level should be rechecked; it may be critically reduced, and needs to be raised by controlled O_2 administration to a point [6.7 to 7.3 kPa (50 to 55 mmHg)] where consciousness is improved but the stimulus to respiratory drive is not removed. Also, the pH of the CSF may be very low, in the range of 7.15 to 7.25. In CO_2 narcosis, correction of the acidosis of blood is easier than that of CSF, which tends to lag. The management of respiratory failure is discussed in detail in Chap. 210.

Differential diagnosis Unlike pure hypoxic encephalopathy, hypercapnia rarely causes prolonged coma and is not a cause of irreversible brain damage. Papilledema and asterixis are important diagnostic features. (Asterixis is also characteristic of liver failure and uremia, and occasionally it is observed in other metabolic disorders.) The syndrome of hypercapnia is apt to be mistaken for brain tumor, a confusional psychosis of nondescript type, or a chronic extrapyramidal syndrome causing myoclonus or chorea.

HYPOGLYCEMIC ENCEPHALOPATHY (See also Chaps. 319 and 320) This condition is a frequent and important cause of episodic confusion, convulsions, coma, and sometimes of hemiparesis and other focal neurologic signs. The essential biochemical abnormality is a critical lowering of the blood glucose concentration to less than 1.4 mmol/L (25 mg/dL) (lower in infants), which, if it lasts for many minutes, leads to exhaustion of cerebral glucose reserve. As cerebral oxidation proceeds without exogenous glucose, the lipid and protein components of neurons are metabolized, and irreversible damage occurs. The severely hypoglycemic patient becomes deeply comatose before permanent damage occurs. Consequently prompt treatment is important.

Etiology The most common causes of hypoglycemic encephalopathy are (1) accidental or deliberate overdose of insulin or an oral antidiabetic agent, (2) islet cell, insulin-secreting tumor of the pancreas or retroperitoneal sarcoma, (3) ethanol ingestion, (4) acute, nonicteric hepatic encephalopathy of childhood (Reye's syndrome), and (5) an idiopathic syndrome occurring in the neonatal period. In the past, hypoglycemic encephalopathy was a frequent complication of "insulin shock" therapy of schizophrenia.

Clinical manifestations As the concentration of blood glucose decreases to about 1.7 mmol/L (30 mg/dL), the initial symptoms appear—nervousness, hunger, flushed facies, headache, palpitation, anxiety, sweating, and trembling—and these gradually give way to confusion, drowsiness, focal neurologic signs, and occasionally excitement or overactivity. In the next stage, forced sucking, grasping, motor restlessness, muscular spasms, and finally decerebrate rigidity occur, in that sequence. Myoclonic twitching and convulsions may develop in some patients. Blood levels of approximately 0.6 mmol/L (10 mg/dL) are associated with deep coma, dilatation of the pupils, pallor, shallow respirations, bradycardia, and hypotonicity of limb musculature—the so-called medullary phase of hypoglycemia. If glucose is administered before the medullary phase is reached, the patient is restored to normal within a few minutes, retracing the aforementioned steps in reverse order. Once the medullary phase appears, and particularly if it persists for a time before the hypoglycemia is corrected, neurologic recovery is delayed for a period of days or weeks and may be incomplete.

A huge dose of insulin that produces severe hypoglycemia, even of relatively brief duration (30 to 60 min), is more dangerous than a series of less severe hypoglycemic episodes from smaller doses of insulin, possibly because in the former the counterregulation mechanisms are likely to be less effective. In this situation massive amounts of glucose may have to be infused in order to maintain plasma glucose levels in the normal range (see Chap. 320).

Pathology The major *neuropathologic effect* is on the cerebral cortex; nerve cells degenerate and are replaced by microgliocytes and astrocytes. The distribution of lesions is similar though not identical to that in hypoxic encephalopathy (the cerebellar cortex is relatively spared in hypoglycemic encephalopathy). The sequelae of the two disorders are also much alike.

Episodes of chronic hypoglycemia may give rise to two other syndromes, both relatively uncommon. One, termed *subacute hypoglycemia,* is characterized by drowsiness and lethargy, diminution in psychomotor activity, deterioration of social behavior, and confusion. Oral or intravenous glucose immediately alleviates the symptoms. In the other, *more chronic syndrome,* there is gradual deterioration of intellectual function, raising the question of a presenile dementia, and in some reported instances there have been tremor, chorea, rigidity, cerebellar ataxia, and rarely signs of lower motor neuron involvement ("hypoglycemic amyotrophy"). These subacute and chronic forms of hypoglycemia have been observed with islet cell hyperplasia or tumor, carcinoma of the stomach, fibrous mesothelioma, carcinoma of the cecum, and hepatoma.

Differential diagnosis The major clinical differences between hypoglycemia and hypoxia are in the clinical setting and mode of evolution of the neurologic disorder. Hypoglycemia usually disturbs cerebral function more slowly than hypoxia, over a period of 30 to 60 min rather than in a few seconds or minutes. The recovery phase and sequelae of the two conditions are much the same. *Recurrent hypoglycemia,* as occurs with an islet cell tumor, may masquerade for some time as an episodic confusional psychosis or convulsive illness, and diagnosis awaits a period of demonstrably low blood glucose or hyperinsulinism (see Chap. 320).

Correction of the hypoglycemia at the earliest moment is the obvious therapy. It is not known whether hypothermia or other measures will increase the safety period in hypoglycemia or alter the outcome.

HYPERGLYCEMIC COMA Two hyperglycemic syndromes occur, mainly in the diabetic: (1) hyperglycemia with ketoacidosis and

(2) hyperosmolar nonketotic hyperglycemia. These are described in Chap. 319.

ACUTE HEPATIC ENCEPHALOPATHY Chronic hepatic insufficiency with portacaval shunting of blood is often punctuated by episodes of stupor, coma, and other neurologic symptoms, a state referred to as hepatic coma or portal-systemic encephalopathy. Also, hereditary hyperammonemic syndromes of infancy may lead to episodic coma with or without seizures. A special type of nonicteric hepatic encephalopathy (Reye's syndrome) occurs in children, presenting as acute brain swelling, in conjunction with rapid enlargement of the liver, fine droplets of fat in hepatocytes, high serum aspartate aminotransferase (AST, SGOT) and other liver enzymes, and very high levels of serum ammonia (see Chap. 256).

Clinical features The central feature of acute hepatic encephalopathy in the adult is a derangement of consciousness, presenting first as mental confusion with increased or decreased psychomotor activity, followed by progressive drowsiness, stupor, and coma. The confusional state that occurs before coma intervenes is frequently combined with characteristic lapses of sustained muscle contraction (asterixis). The EEG becomes abnormal during the earliest stages of the confusional state. Paroxysms of bilaterally synchronous delta waves, characteristically triphasic and prominent in the frontal regions, are at first interspersed with alpha activity and later, as the coma deepens, displace all normal activity. A variable, fluctuating rigidity of the trunk and limbs, grimacing, suck and grasp reflexes, exaggeration or asymmetry of tendon reflexes, Babinski signs, and focal or generalized seizures round out the clinical picture.

The syndrome usually evolves over a period of days to weeks and often terminates fatally. At times it does not advance beyond the stage of drowsiness and confusion with asterixis and EEG changes. This relatively mild form needs to be differentiated from other forms of acute confusional psychosis and delirium. If the metabolic disorder persists for months and years, a mild dementia and a disorder of posture and movement may gradually appear (grimacing, tremor, dysarthria, ataxia of gait, choreoathetosis), and the condition must then be distinguished from other dementing and extrapyramidal syndromes (see further on in this chapter).

Pathology and pathogenesis The striking *neuropathologic finding* in patients who die in a state of hepatic coma is a diffuse increase in the number and size of the protoplasmic astrocytes (Alzheimer type II astrocytes) in the deep layers of the cerebral cortex and in the lenticular nuclei, with little or no alteration in the nerve cells or other parenchymal elements.

The *pathogenesis* of hepatic encephalopathy is not fully understood. The most plausible theory relates it to an abnormality of nitrogen metabolism, wherein ammonia and/or other amines, which are formed in the bowel by the action of urease-containing organisms on dietary protein and are carried to the liver in the portal circulation, fail to be converted into urea, either because of hepatocellular disease or portal-systemic shunting of blood, or both. As a result, these substances reach the systemic circulation, where they interfere with cerebral metabolism in some obscure way. Other theories of causation have been discussed in Chap. 254 and have recently been reviewed by Zieve and by Cooper and Plum.

Treatment Despite an incomplete understanding of the genesis of hepatic coma, the most effective means of treating this disorder consists of restriction of dietary protein; mechanical cleansing of the colon; oral administration of antibiotics that suppress or eliminate urease-producing organisms in the bowel; and the use of lactulose, an inert sugar that acidifies the colonic contents. Additional methods of treatment, the practicality of which remain to be established, are discussed in Chap. 254.

In acute hepatitis, delirious, confusional, and comatose states also occur, but their mechanisms are not understood. Blood ammonia levels are usually elevated but of unclear significance, because of other associated metabolic abnormalities.

CHRONIC HEPATIC ENCEPHALOPATHY (ACQUIRED HEPATOCEREBRAL DEGENERATION) Clinical manifestations Patients who survive an episode or several episodes of hepatic coma are occasionally left with residual neurologic abnormalities, such as tremor of the head or arms, asterixis, grimacing, choreatic twitching of the limbs, dysarthria, ataxia of gait, or impairment of intellectual function, and these symptoms may worsen with repeated attacks of stupor and coma. In other patients with hepatic failure, these neurologic abnormalities become manifest in the absence of discrete episodes of hepatic coma. In either event, patients thus afflicted deteriorate neurologically over a period of months or years. As the condition evolves, a chronic characteristic dysarthria, mild ataxia, wide-based, unsteady gait, and choreoathetosis, mainly of the face, neck, and shoulders, are joined in a common syndrome. Mental function is slowly altered—a simple dementia with lack of concern and indifference to the illness evolves. A coarse rhythmic tremor of the arms, appearing with certain sustained postures, mild corticospinal tract signs, and diffuse EEG abnormalities complete the clinical picture. Other less frequent signs are muscular rigidity, grasp reflexes, tremor in repose, nystagmus, asterixis, and action or intention myoclonus. Many of the neurologic abnormalities that occur as part of acute hepatic encephalopathy may also be observed in patients with chronic hepatocerebral degeneration, the only difference being that the abnormalities are evanescent in the former and irreversible in the latter.

The chronic cerebral symptoms, like the transient ones, may occur with all varieties of chronic liver disease. Portacaval shunts are always present; jaundice, ascites, and esophageal varices are manifest in most of the cases.

Pathology Chronic hepatocerebral degeneration, like acute and subacute hepatic encephalopathy, is characterized by a widespread hyperplasia of protoplasmic astrocytes in the deep layers of the cerebral and cerebellar cortices as well as in the thalamic and lenticular nuclei and many other nuclear structures of the brainstem. In addition, in the chronic disease, medullated fibers and nerve cells are destroyed in the affected areas, and polymicrocavitation is prominent at the corticomedullary junction, in the striatum (particularly in the superior pole of the putamen), and in the cerebellar white matter. Protoplasmic astrocytic nuclei contain periodic acid Schiff (PAS)–positive glycogen granules. Nerve cells may appear swollen and chromatolyzed, accounting for the so-called Opalski cells. The similarity of these lesions to those observed in the familial form of hepatocerebral disease (Wilson's disease) suggests a common hepatogenesis.

UREMIC ENCEPHALOPATHY Episodic confusion and stupor and other neurologic symptoms may accompany any form of severe renal disease. In addition, a number of neurologic syndromes complicate chronic hemodialysis and kidney transplantation. Chronic polyneuropathy, the most common neurologic complication of renal failure, is discussed in Chap. 363.

Acute uremic encephalopathy The initial cerebral symptoms attributable to uremia consist of apathy, fatigue, inattentiveness, and irritability; later, confusion, disturbances of sensory perception, hallucinations, and stupor supervene. The later symptoms are practically always associated with twitching of the muscles and myoclonic jerks, and the patient may convulse.

Uremic encephalopathy, if associated with irreversible and progressive renal disease, can only be managed with dialysis or renal transplantation (see Chap. 225). Convulsions, which occur in about one-third of cases, often preterminally, respond to relatively low plasma concentrations of phenytoin and phenobarbital.

The brains of patients with uremic encephalopathy and the twitch-convulsive syndrome show hyperplasia of protoplasmic astrocytes in some cases but never to the degree observed in hepatic encephalopathy. Cerebral edema is notably absent. Restoration of renal function corrects the neurologic syndrome, attesting to a biochemical rather than a structural abnormality. Whether this is caused by the retention of organic acids, elevation of phosphate in the CSF, or by the action of other toxins has never been settled.

"Disequilibrium syndrome" and dialysis encephalopathy These terms refer to syndromes that commonly complicate hemodialysis or peritoneal dialysis. The *disequilibrium syndrome* is characterized by headaches, nausea, muscular cramps, nervous irritability, agitation, drowsiness, and convulsions. The headache develops in approximately 70 percent of patients, while the other symptoms are observed in 5 to 10 percent, usually in those undergoing rapid dialysis or in the early stages of a dialysis program. The symptoms tend to occur in the third to fourth hour of dialysis and last for several hours. Sometimes the symptoms appear 8 to 48 h after completing dialysis (see Chap. 225).

Dialysis encephalopathy or *dialysis dementia* is an uncommon complication of chronic hemodialysis. It begins with stuttering and dysarthria, coupled with a predominantly motor aphasia, to which are added facial and generalized myoclonus, focal and generalized seizures, personality changes and psychotic episodes, intellectual decline, progressive aphasic disorder, and EEG abnormalities. The latter consist of bisynchronous, predominantly frontal or multifocal bursts of slow wave discharges, associated with spikes and sharp waves. The CSF is usually normal. At first these symptoms are intermittent, occurring during or immediately after dialysis and lasting for only a few hours, but gradually they become more persistent and eventually permanent. Once established, the syndrome is usually steadily progressive over a 1- to 15-month period (average survival of 6 months in 42 cases analyzed by Lederman and Henry). A few patients have a waxing and waning course and survive for several years. In some patients the myoclonus and seizures subside for several months under the influence of clonazepam or diazepam.

The neuropathologic changes are subtle and consist of a mild microcavitation of the upper layers of the cerebral cortex. Although the changes are diffuse, the left (dominant) hemisphere is affected more than the right, and the left frontotemporal operculum more than other parts of the cortex (Winkelman). The predominant affection of the operculum would explain the striking disturbance of speech and language. Alfrey and his associates found that the cerebral gray matter of patients who died with dialysis encephalopathy contained a much greater amount of aluminum than analogous tissue from dialysis patients without encephalopathy. The aluminum was derived from both the dialysate and orally administered aluminum gels. The concept that dialysis encephalopathy represented a form of aluminum intoxication was supported by the observations that (1) the frequency of dialysis dementia was related to the concentrations of aluminum in the dialysate and (2) deionization of the water used in the dialysate prevented the occurrence of new cases. The possibility that other trace elements contribute to the syndrome has not been excluded.

Kidney transplantation is associated with an increased risk of developing primary cerebral lymphoma, Wernicke's encephalopathy, and central pontine myelinolysis. Systemic fungal infections are common at autopsy in patients who have had renal transplants and long periods of immunosuppressive treatment, and in some of these patients there is involvement of the central nervous system. *Cryptococcus, Listeria, Aspergillus, Candida, Nocardia,* and *Histoplasma* are the usual organisms. Other central nervous system infections that complicate transplantation are toxoplasmosis and cytomegalic inclusion disease.

ENCEPHALOPATHIES DUE TO ELECTROLYTE AND ENDOCRINE DISTURBANCES Brief reference to these important groups of metabolic encephalopathies is given here. More detailed accounts are found in the cross-referenced chapters.

Metabolic acidosis [(arterial pH<7.30, P_{CO_2}<4.7 kPa (<35 mmHg), HCO_3 <10 mmol/L)] due to diabetes mellitus, renal failure, lactic acidosis, or poisoning with an acid substance produces a syndrome characterized by drowsiness, stupor, and coma with dry skin and Kussmaul breathing, described in Chap. 51. Extreme degrees of *hyperosmolality* of the blood may develop in the course of diabetes mellitus [blood glucose>22 mmol/L (>400 μg/dL)] and in extreme hypernatremia, resulting in either case in tremulousness, convulsions, and coma. In some instances the movement disorder resembles chorea or the myoclonic twitching of uremia. *Hypokalemia* is characterized by extreme muscular weakness associated with a stuporous-confusional state, and sometimes by striking changes in personality and behavior (see Chap. 51).

Hyponatremia, usually with water intoxication, is another cause of episodic coma, especially in infants. Among the many causes, the syndrome of inappropriate secretion of antidiuretic hormone (SIADH) is of special importance, since it commonly complicates neurologic diseases of many types—head trauma, bacterial meningitis and encephalitis, cerebral infarction and subarachnoid hemorrhage, neoplasm, and sometimes Guillain-Barré disease (see Chap. 315). The diagnosis of SIADH should be suspected in any critically ill neurologic or neurosurgical patient who excretes urine that is hypertonic relative to the plasma. As the hyponatremia develops, there is a decrease in alertness, which progresses through stages of confusion to coma, often with convulsions. Lack of recognition of this state may allow the serum Na^+ to fall to dangerously low levels, 100 mmol/L or lower. Treatment is described in Chap. 315. Replacement with intravenous NaCl in severe cases must be done cautiously because vigorous and rapid correction of severe hyponatremia has been incriminated in the pathogenesis of central pontine myelinolysis (CPM) and related brainstem, cerebellar, and cerebral lesions (Laureno). Ayus and colleagues emphasize the risks of persistent severe hyponatremia and suggest the following therapeutic guidelines: serum Na^+ above 120 mmol/L does not require immediate correction. If Na^+ is >105 mmol/L, it can be safely corrected to a level of 125 to 130 mmol/L at a rate of administration of Na^+ of 2 mmol/h. If serum Na^+ is less than 105 mmol/L, it is corrected by 20 mmol/L at a rate of 2 mmol/h and then permitted to return slowly to normal. More prospective studies are needed to determine the safest method of correcting severe hyponatremia.

In children more than adults, cholera being an exception, extremely *severe diarrhea* may be attended by an encephalopathy. Irritability, weakness, headache, seizures, stupor, and coma may develop over a period of 2 to 3 days and carry a grave prognosis unless promptly relieved. Presumably this is a metabolic encephalopathy due to loss of fluids and electrolytes and can be corrected by their replacement.

In the *endocrine encephalopathies* the clinical phenomena are even more abstruse. Confusional states may be combined with agitation, hallucinations, delusions, anxiety, and depression. And the duration of the illness may be measured in weeks and months, rather than days. Derangement of higher nervous function may follow the *administration of ACTH or glucocorticoids,* and the same symptoms have been reported in *Cushing's disease* (see Chap. 317). The neurologic manifestations of *thyrotoxicosis* are particularly elusive. Allusions to thyrotoxic psychosis are widely recorded in the medical literature; mental confusion, seizures, manic or depressive attacks, delusions, and chorea occur in various combinations with muscular weakness and atrophy, periodic paralysis, and myasthenia (see Chap. 316). Treatment of the hyperthyroidism gradually restores the patient to a normal mental state. *Myxedematous patients* may show slow mentation and depression, and in a small proportion there is a major change in cerebral function, taking the form of inattentiveness, apathy, and drowsiness or extreme somnolence. These symptoms can usually be reversed within weeks to months by thyroid medication. The association of myxedema and cerebellar ataxia is well documented, but the neuropathologic basis of this disorder remains unclear. In *hyperparathyroidism,* when the serum calcium levels reach 3.7 mmol/L (15 mg/dL) or higher, the patient sinks into a quiet state of inattentiveness, lethargy, and confusion. Stupor, coma, and death may be caused by extreme degrees of hypercalcemia such as occur occasionally in cases of hypervitaminosis D and metastatic tumors of the bones. Chronic *hypoparathyroidism,* either idiopathic or following thyroid or parathyroid resection may rarely give rise to intracranial calcifications and an extrapyramidal motor syndrome. Adrenal insufficiency may be attended by episodic confusion, stupor, or coma, without special identifying features (see Chap. 317).

The term *pancreatic encephalopathy* describes a syndrome of agitation and confusion, sometimes with hallucinations and clouding of consciousness, dysarthria, and changing rigidity of the limbs, in association with acute pancreatic disease. The status of this entity is uncertain. A uniform neuropathologic change has not been discerned. We agree with Pallis and Lewis who suggest that before such a diagnosis can be seriously entertained in a patient with acute pancreatitis, one should exclude delirium tremens, the cerebral effects of shock, renal or hepatic failure, hypoglycemia, diabetic acidosis, hyperosmolality, hypokalemia, hypo- or hypercalcemia, any one of which may complicate the underlying disease(s).

Lactic acidosis can cause encephalopathy in patients who undergo jejunoileostomy for treatment of morbid obesity. Such patients report episodes of confusion, ataxia, and slurred speech. D-Lactate, an isomer not normally found in the blood and a product of intestinal bacteria, is present in serum, urine, and stool in these patients. D-Lactate causes encephalopathy by interfering with pyruvate metabolism. Diagnosis is dependent upon recognition of metabolic acidosis associated with hyperchloremia and measurement of elevated D-lactate (see Dahlquist; Cross). A more common cause of encephalopathy in patients with jejunoileal shunting is hepatic (see Chap. 72).

HEREDITARY METABOLIC DISEASES OF LATE ONSET

Inherited metabolic disorders affecting amino acid metabolism (Chaps. 334 and 335), lysosomal enzyme functions (Chap. 331), and cerebral lipids (Chap. 331) are generally rare and first become manifest during infancy or childhood. In this chapter are described a small number of hereditary metabolic disorders that may have their onset in late adolescence and adulthood and may present diagnostic problems because of the similarity of clinical presentation to other more common acquired and degenerative diseases of the nervous system. Noteworthy attributes of these diseases are their chronicity and progressive nature.

METACHROMATIC LEUKODYSTROPHY (See Chap. 331) Probably the most common member of this category is *adult metachromatic leukodystrophy (MLD)*. While the majority of cases appear in early childhood, approximately 25 percent manifest their first symptoms after age 21. Cases among men outnumber those in women 2:1. The mode of inheritance is autosomal recessive in almost all instances. The onset is insidious, and the course is protracted, over 20 or more years.

Mental symptoms tend to dominate the clinical picture. Failing scholastic performance, forgetfulness, and irrationality occur early in the illness but may be obscured by peculiarities of personality, such as suspiciousness, delusional thinking, and bizarre actions. These latter qualities may raise the question of schizophrenia or immature (''borderline'') personality development. Sooner or later a mild cerebellar ataxia presenting as awkwardness and falling, mild pyramidal signs, masked facies, and bizarre postures stamp the illness as neurologic. Eventually mental processes deteriorate to the point where the patient is helpless, demented, mute, incontinent, and bedfast.

Specific diagnostic tests include (1) the demonstration of a diminished arylsulfatase A activity in white blood cells, serum, and urine, (2) increased excretion of sulfatides in the urine, (3) slowed conduction velocity in nerves, and (4) deposits of metachromatic material in nerve biopsies. No treatment is available.

ADRENOLEUKODYSTROPHY In this X-linked metabolic disorder, either adrenal insufficiency or cerebral symptoms may be the initial manifestation. The cerebral lesions may present as a homonymous hemianopsia, cortical blindness, hemiparesis, aphasia, or dementia. Usually the signs are asymmetric at first and progress intermittently. Relatively pure polyneuropathic and myelopathic forms have also been described. The diagnosis is usually made by the finding of a low blood cortisol level in a man with cerebrospinal demyelinating disease, although a purely spinal type, taking the form of a progressive spastic paraparesis, has been described in the heterozygote (female carrier). Increased urinary concentration of C22-C26 fatty acids is diagnostic. Glucocorticoid replacement therapy helps the symptoms of adrenal insufficiency but has no effect on the neurologic disorders. The latter progress intermittently over a few years, and usually the outcome is fatal.

ADULT LIPID STORAGE DISEASES G_{M2} *gangliosidosis* (hexosaminidase A deficiency) has been observed in young adults. Many are from non-Jewish families, and males and females in the same generation are equally affected. Generalized seizures may mark the beginning of a cerebral disorder that later is evidenced by alterations of behavior and intellectual decline. A progressive ataxia and mild signs of corticospinal disease, the combination of which interferes with independent locomotion, clarifies the diagnosis. The fundi and visual function are normal in most cases, but typical cherry-red macular spots are seen occasionally. The liver and spleen are normal or slightly enlarged. The CSF protein is normal. CT scans of the brain reveal a modest ventricular enlargement. A slowly developing dementia, cerebellar ataxia, polymyoclonus, and failing vision may characterize the clinical picture in some cases. In yet others, the presenting syndrome has consisted of prominent motor neuron involvement accompanied by muscle cramps, suggesting a diagnosis of spinal muscular atrophy or amyotrophic lateral sclerosis (see Chap. 359). G_{M2} ganglioside is increased in tissue obtained by cerebral biopsy. Membranous cytoplasmic bodies are visualized by electron microscopy of rectal, appendicular, and cortical neurons. *Gaucher's* and *Niemann-Pick* diseases are yet other storage diseases that may present in adult life. (See Chap. 331.)

Ceroid lipofuscinosis The Kufs type of *ceroid lipofuscinosis* is a lipid storage disease that only becomes evident in adolescence or early adult life. Usually the disease begins with mental deterioration, followed by seizures, ataxia, increasing rigidity, athetotic posturing, and corticospinal signs. Skin and conjunctival biopsies, examined by electron microscopy, show lipofuscin storage material in fibroblasts and endothelial cells.

SUBACUTE NECROTIZING ENCEPHALOMYELOPATHY (LEIGH'S DISEASE) Some cases of this disease begin in adolescence and take the form of a progressive polymyoclonus with seizures and cerebellar ataxia and relatively mild impairment of intellectual function.

SUMMARY These rare forms of hereditary metabolic diseases should be considered whenever an adolescent or young adult becomes demented, shows a psychiatric syndrome with decline in cognitive functions, has seizures (especially with polymyoclonus), failing vision, and cerebellar ataxia in combination with corticospinal signs or a progressive polyneuropathy.

REFERENCES

ADAMS RD, FOLEY JM: The neurological disorder associated with liver disease of the nervous system. Proc Assoc Res Nerv Ment Dis 32:198, 1953

———, VICTOR M: *Principles of Neurology*, 4th ed. New York, McGraw-Hill, 1989

ALFREY AC et al: The dialysis encephalopathy syndrome: Possible aluminum intoxication. N Engl J Med 294:184, 1976

AYUS JC et al: Treatment of symptomatic hyponatremia and its relation to brain damage: A prospective study. N Engl J Med 317:1190, 1987

BECK WS: Cobalamin and the nervous system. N Engl J Med 318:1752, 1988

BLASS JP, GIBSON GE: Abnormality of a thiamine-requiring enzyme in patients with Wernicke-Korsakoff syndrome. N Engl J Med 297:1367, 1977

BRAIN RESUSCITATION CLINICAL TRIAL I STUDY GROUP: Randomized clinical study of thiopental loading in comatose survivors of cardiac arrest. N Engl J Med 314:397, 1986

CARDINALE GJ et al: Effect of methylmalonyl coenzyme A: A metabolite which accumulates in vitamin B_{12} deficiency on fatty acid synthesis. J Biol Chem 245:3771, 1970

CARMEL R et al: Hereditary defect of cobalamin metabolism (*cblG* mutation) presenting as a neurologic disorder in adulthood. N Engl J Med 318:1738, 1988

CHARNESS ME et al: Ethanol and the nervous system: Medical Progress. N Engl J Med 321:442, 1989

COOPER AJL, PLUM F: Biochemistry and physiology of brain ammonia. Physiol Rev 67:440, 1987

CREMER GM et al: Myxedema and ataxia. Neurology 19:37, 1969

CROSS SA, CALLOWAY WC: D-Lactic acidosis and selected cerebellar ataxias. Mayo Clin Proc 59:202, 1984

DAHLQUIST NR et al: D-Lactic acidosis and encephalopathy after jejunoileostomy: Response to overfeeding and to fasting in humans. Mayo Clin Proc 59:141, 1984

——— et al: D-Lactic acidosis and encephalopathy after jejunoileostomy: Response to overfeeding and to fasting in humans. Mayo Clinic Proc 59:141, 1984
HARDING AE et al: Spinocerebellar degeneration associated with a selective defect of vitamin E absorption. N Engl J Med 313:32, 1985
KLATSKY AL et al: Alcohol consumption and blood pressure. N Engl J Med 296:1194, 1977
KOLODNY EH, BOUSTANY RM: Storage diseases of the reticuloendothelial system, in *Hematology of Infancy and Childhood,* 3d ed, D Nathan, F Oski (eds). Philadelphia, Saunders, 1986
LAURENO R: Central pontine myelinolysis following rapid correction of hyponatremia. Ann Neurol 13:232, 1983
LEDERMAN RS, HENRY CE: Progressive dialysis encephalopathy. Ann Neurol 4:199, 1978
LINDENBAUM J et al: Neuropsychiatric disorders caused by cobalamin deficiency in the absence of anemia or macrocytosis. N Engl J Med 318:1720, 1988
MCENTEE WJ, MAIR RG: Memory enhancement in Korsakoff's phychosis by clonidine: Further evidence for a nonadrenergic deficit. Ann Neurol 7:466, 1980
MARKS R, ROSE FC: *Hypoglycemia.* Oxford, Blackwell, 1965
MOSER HW et al: Adrenoleukodystrophy: Studies of the phenotype, genetics and biochemistry. Johns Hopkins Med J 147:217, 1980
NELSON JS et al: Progressive neuropathologic lesions in vitamin E–deficient rhesus monkeys. J Neuropathol Exp Neurol 40:166, 1981
PALLIS CA, LEWIS PD: *The Neurology of Gastrointestinal Disease.* Philadelphia, Saunders, 1974
PINCUS JH: Folic acid deficiency. A cause of subacute combined system degeneration, in *Folic Acid in Neurology, Psychiatry, and Internal Medicine,* MI Botez, EH Reynolds (eds). New York, Raven, 1979, pp 427–433
PLUM F, POSNER JB: *Diagnosis of Stupor and Coma,* 3d ed. Philadelphia, Davis, 1980
POTTS AM: Tobacco amblyopia. Surv Ophthalmol 17:313, 1973
RASKIN NH, FISHMAN RA: Neurologic disorders in renal failure. N Engl J Med 294:143, 204, 1976
SAGE JI et al: Alcoholic myelopathy without substantial liver disease. A syndrome of progressive dorsal and lateral column dysfunction. Arch Neurol 41:999, 1984
SATYA-MURTI S et al: The spectrum of neurologic disorders from vitamin E deficiency. Neurology 36:917, 1986
SCHAUMBURG HH et al: Sensory neuropathy from pyridoxine abuse. A new megavitamin syndrome. N Engl J Med 309:445, 1983
SERDARU M et al: The clinical spectrum of alcoholic pellagra encephalopathy. Brain 111:829, 1988
SHIMOJYO S et al: Cerebral blood flow and metabolism in the Wernicke-Korsakoff syndrome. J Clin Invest 46:849, 1967
VICTOR M: Polyneuropathy due to nutrional deficiency and alcoholism, in *Peripheral Neuropathy,* 2d ed, PJ Dyck et al (eds). Philadelphia, Saunders, 1984, pp 1899–1940
———, ADAMS RD: On the etiology of the alcoholic neurologic diseases: With special reference to the role of nutrition. Am J Clin Nutr 9:379, 1961
——— et al: A restricted form of cerebellar degeneration occurring in alcoholic patients. Arch Neurol 1:577, 1959
——— et al: Deficiency amblyopia in the alcoholic patient: A clinicopathologic study. Arch Ophthalmol 64:1, 1960
——— et al: The acquired (nonwilsonian) type of chronic hepatocerebral degeneration. Medicine 44:345, 1965
——— et al: *The Wernicke-Korsakoff Syndrome and Related Neurologic Disorders Due to Alcoholism and Malnutrition.* Philadelphia, Davis, 1989
WILKINSON DS, PROCKOP LD: Hypoglycemia: Effects on the nervous system, in *Handbook of Clinical Neurology,* PJ Vinken, BW Bruyn (eds). Amsterdam, North-Holland, 1976, vol 27, pp 53–78
WINKELMAN MD, RICANATI ES: Dialysis encephalopathy: Neuropathologic aspects. Hum Pathol 17:823, 1986
WITT ED, GOLDMAN-RAKIC PS: Intermittent thiamine deficiency in the rhesus monkey. I. Progression of neurological signs and neuranatomical lesions. Ann Neurol 13:376, 1983
ZIEVE L: Pathogenesis of hepatic encephalopathy. Metab Brain Dis 2:147, 1987

358 NEUROCUTANEOUS SYNDROMES AND OTHER DEVELOPMENTAL DISORDERS OF THE CENTRAL NERVOUS SYSTEM[1]

VERNE S. CAVINESS, JR.

Developmental disorders that involve the nervous system and are encountered in adult life are the emphasis of this chapter. The discussion is arranged according to broad phenotypic groupings, namely, *neurocutaneous syndromes* in which abnormalities of the nervous system are associated with abnormalities of osseous structures and the skin, *developmental disorders principally affecting the nervous system,* and *neuroskeletal disorders.*

[1]This is in part the revision of the chapter in the 11th edition by GR DeLong and RD Adams.

NEUROCUTANEOUS SYNDROMES

A large number of neurocutaneous disorders (also *phakomatoses* from Greek *phakos,* "lentil," "mole," or "freckle") are expressed in a patchy fashion in affected tissues. The most commonly encountered of these, reviewed below, are transmitted by autosomal dominant inheritance. The chromosomal linkage group has been (provisionally) identified for four of these dominantly transmitted forms (Table 358-1).

NEUROFIBROMATOSIS (VON RECKLINGHAUSEN'S DISEASE) The dominating feature of this disorder is the neurofibroma, a tumor that arises from the Schwann cells and fibroblasts of the neurilemmal sheath of the peripheral nerve. Two nonallelic heritable forms are now recognized. *Neurofibromatosis type 1,* carried on chromosome 17, is the classic autosomal dominant neurocutaneous disorder in which tumors involving the sheaths of peripheral nerves are associated with characteristic cream-brown cutaneous lesions (café-au-lait spots). The neurofibromas themselves are only occasionally symptomatic, as when they result in entrapment of a nerve root at the intervertebral foramina. The disorder may be associated with other tumors of the central nervous system including optic glioma, glioblastoma, and meningioma, and rarely with pheochromocytoma (see also Chap. 318). Other associated aberrations include hamartomas of the iris (Lisch nodules), freckling concentrated around the nipples and in the axillae, stenosis of the aqueduct of Sylvius, leading to obstructive hydrocephalus, and mild degrees of mental retardation, related presumably to developmental abnormalities of the cerebral cortex. *Neurofibromatosis type 2,* carried on chromosome 22, is also an autosomal dominant disorder in which neurofibromas involve the acoustic nerves exclusively and usually bilaterally. The acoustic neurinomas may produce deafness and other symptoms and signs of a cerebellopontine angle lesion (see Chap. 353). They may also be associated with meningiomas and astrocytomas.

TUBEROUS SCLEROSIS (BOURNEVILLE'S DISEASE) In this condition, cutaneous lesions of multiple types are associated with malformation and tumors of the central nervous system. Mental deficiency, though not invariable, may be profound and associated with a remarkably intractable seizure disorder. The earliest lesions to emerge are leaf-shaped hypopigmented spots ("white spots") scattered over the trunk and limbs. These are seen most clearly under ultraviolet light (Wood's lamp). The adenoma sebaceum, a hallmark of the disorder, is an angiofibroma, distributed in a butterfly pattern over the cheeks, chin, and forehead. The individual adenomas vary in size from 0.1 to 1.0 cm and are elevated and pinkish or pinkish-yellow in color. The skin over the lumbosacral region of the back

TABLE 358-1 Chromosomal locations of dominant mutant genes in the phakomatoses*

Disorder	Chromosome	Phenotypic signature	Mental retardation	Tumors
NF-1	17	Café-au-lait spots, neurofibromas	Occasionally	Multiple types: CNS, PNS, viscera
NF-2	22	Bilateral acoustic neuromas	No	Acoustic neuromas; other CNS
TS	9	White spots, adenoma sebacea	Frequent	CNS: tubers, gliomas; viscera
VH-L	3	Cerebral hemangioblastomas, retinal angiomas	No	Angiomas of viscera; renal cell carcinomas

* NF-1 and NF-2 are neurofibromatosis types 1 and 2; TS, tuberosclerosis; VH-L, von Hippel-Lindau; CNS and PNS, central and peripheral nervous systems.

may be marked by a rough thickening which is yellowish in color like sharkskin or pigskin (shagreen patch). The cutaneous lesions may provide the earliest clue to the causation of mental retardation or infantile epilepsy. Rhabdomyoma of the heart and tumorous malformations (angioleiomyomas) of the kidney, liver, adrenal glands, and pancreas are also characteristic of this disorder. The disorder can be inherited as an autosomal dominant trait: linkage studies with restriction fragment length polymorphisms (RFLPs) in some pedigrees have located the mutant gene to chromosome 9.

In the brain multiple nodular tumors, composed of abnormal neurons and glial cells, often lie in the plane of the cerebral cortex itself. These can be diagnosed accurately in T2-weighted magnetic resonance scans. If calcified, they may also be visualized by CT scans or skull x-rays. Calcified nodules occur in brain subependymal regions adjacent to the ventricles. If large, they may obstruct the foramen of Monro, causing a unilateral or bilateral hydrocephalus. Masses of subependymal glial tissue forming nodules are likened to "candle gutterings" on the walls of the ventricles. The electroencephalogram is usually abnormal but without specific pattern. The only treatment is symptomatic. When severe epilepsy and mental retardation are present, prognosis for life beyond the third decade is poor. Death is usually due to seizures, associated tumors, or intercurrent diseases.

CEREBELLORETINAL HEMANGIOBLASTOMATOSIS (VON HIPPEL–LINDAU SYNDROME) This syndrome of retinal and cerebellar hemangioblastoma is inherited as an autosomal dominant disorder (encoded on chromosome 3) (see Table 358-1). The retinal lesions are capillary angiomas, usually multiple, causing progressive loss of vision. The cerebellar hemangioblastomas, which may be multiple, are slowly growing cystic tumors. These may also occur in the medulla or in the spinal cord where they may be associated with a syrinx. Enlargement of cerebellar tumor may lead to obstructive hydrocephalus with headache, papilledema, and cerebellar ataxia. Only rarely do tumors become symptomatic before adolescence, but the diagnosis must be considered in all adults with a cerebellar tumor. Tumors of the central nervous system are a part of a constellation including agiomas and cysts of the liver, pancreas, and kidneys and tumors of the epididymis and kidney. The latter may be lethal. Pheochromocytomas may occur in this as in other kinds of phakomatoses (see Chap. 318). An association with renal cell carcinoma led to localization of the mutant gene on chromosome 3. Polycythemia, presumably the consequence of ectopic production of erythropoietin by the hemangioblastoma, may disappear after excision of the tumor.

ENCEPHALOTRIGEMINAL SYNDROME (STURGE-WEBER DISEASE) Capillary or cavernous hemangiomas, within but not always limited to the cutaneous distribution of the trigeminal nerve, co-occur with a predominantly venous hemangioma that can spread through subjacent leptomeninges. The adjacent cerebral cortex is progressively destroyed, perhaps as a consequence of interruption of local blood flow. The first neurologic symptom is usually a focal seizure on the side opposite the skin lesion. Sensorimotor paralysis or permanent visual field defect, the most common sequelae, may be either of sudden or of insidious onset with progression. In time calcium is deposited within the area of involved cortex and may be visualized as a characteristic "railroad track" in conventional x-rays or CT scans. If the skin lesion is within the area of supply of the ophthalmic division of the trigeminal nerve, the occipital lobes are more commonly involved. A facial nevus is more often associated with involvement of the parietal and frontal lobes. The intracranial and cutaneous lesions may also occur separately. The disease is usually sporadic; a familial occurrence consistent with autosomal dominant inheritance is exceptional. Deeply situated arteriovenous malformations rarely coexist. Blindness in the eye on the side of the nevus is nearly always due to glaucoma. Most patients with this malformation survive for many years, often with mental defects and hemiparesis.

Hemangioma of the trunk or upper or lower extremity may be associated with a spinal cord vascular malformation (Klippel-Trenaunay syndrome) and with hypertrophy of the involved extremity. The cord lesion may cause infarction in nervous tissue, producing a spinal sensorimotor paralysis. Surgical exploration and decompression are seldom beneficial.

DEVELOPMENTAL DISORDERS OF THE CENTRAL NERVOUS SYSTEM

Developmental disorders expressed largely or even exclusively as disturbance of neurologic functions afflict a substantial portion of the population. Certain of these, particularly when neurologic disability is severe, are complicated secondarily by restricted general somatic growth, articulatory contractures, and general medical disorders resulting from limited mobility and poor personal care. The discussion will be focused upon developmental disorders expressed predominantly as malfunction of the forebrain, particularly the cerebral hemispheres. Three general syndromes emerge: mental retardation, where the disability is predominantly in the domains of cognition, language, and memory; autism, where socialization is the prominently defective characteristic; and "cerebral palsy," where disability largely relates to motor function.

MENTAL RETARDATION Mental retardation specifies an IQ less than 70 resulting from a pathophysiologic process affecting the cerebrum during the developmental period. If IQ is normal, the diagnosis is not applied to more restricted learning disabilities including dyslexia, incompetence with mathematics, and a variety of developmental language disorders. Mental retardation, even if it is the predominant disability, is often conjoined with a complex of other disabilities which include disordered motor function, abnormalities of special senses, such as hearing and sight, and a variety of medical problems.

Etiology and pathogenesis The specific cause of abnormal cerebral development cannot be defined for as many as half of all mentally retarded persons. For many, the disorder is familial and may be due to either single-gene defects or polygenic inheritance. Among the remaining half in whom the cause can be identified, the recognized causes include the 21 trisomy and fragile X syndromes and intrauterine exposure to alcohol (see Chap. 7). Collectively these few disorders are responsible for a third of mental retardation in this country. Prevalence for each approximates 1:1000 live births. Other identifiable causes include encephaloclastic processes, such as infection, hypoxia-ischemia, trauma, and hydrocephalus, occurring either before or after birth. Intrauterine exposures to infectious and pharmacologic teratogenic agents are also common, including exposure to HIV infection or to cocaine and other "recreational" drugs. Malnutrition, hypothyroidism, and other metabolic disorders may also cause mental retardation if the conditions occur during intrauterine and postnatal life. Among the general medical conditions is a substantial list of heritable disorders of metabolism. The list is long and includes enzymopathies relating to amino acid, carbohydrate, organic acid, and lipid processing such as phenylketonuria (see Chap. 334), galactosemia (see Chap. 337), proprionic aciduria, and disorders of lysosomal enzyme function such as neuronal ceroid lipofuscinosis, the gangliosidoses, and the mucopolysaccharidoses (see also Chaps. 331 and 333).

Many chromosomal and single-gene disorders of metabolism may be diagnosed prenatally. Where diagnosis is made postnatally, it may be critical to do so expeditiously in the case of treatable CNS infections and correctable or manageable metabolic disorders, i.e., cretinism or phenylketonuria. During the first 2 years of life diagnosis and intervention are also critical for malnutrition, a state usually coupled to other socioeconomic deprivations. These deprivations may result in retarded brain growth and mental development that persist into adult life. If, however, such children are "rescued" by refeeding and placement in a stimulating and supportive environment, the effects of early malnutrition are largely reversible, and normal mental development can result.

Clinical manifestations The defining characteristic of this domain of cerebral disturbance, subnormal IQ, is an inexact but a meaningful predictor of behavioral capabilities. Severely retarded children, those with IQs of less than 20, are virtually unable to look after themselves. Often they never sit up, walk, or stand. Language is rudimentary; at most a few words are understood and uttered. They exhibit only primitive emotional reactions, and sphincteric control may never be achieved. Motor mannerisms such as rhythmic rocking, rolling, head banging, and bouncing movements are typical and often are accompanied by bleating sounds and squeals. Music may encourage rhythmic movements. The physical appearance may be unremarkable. However, if the insult to the brain occurs in utero or early in postnatal life, a variety of physical deformities, particularly microcephaly and variable degrees of joint contracture, are common in this group.

If the mental defect is less pronounced, that is, there is an IQ of 20 to 50, and if specific motor defects do not coexist, then sitting, walking, and speech are acquired, often after a delay. The existence of a cerebral defect may be noted for the first time when the child fails to speak normally during the second and third year of life and seems not to be able to learn the usual household tasks and play activities as well as other children. However, delay in speech development by itself is not a mark of mental retardation, for some children who are intelligent and show remarkable talent in communicating by gesture are slow in talking. Also the deaf child may be singled out by indifference to noise and reduced vocalization but otherwise normal development. Toilet training also may be difficult to accomplish in the retarded child, but again it may be delayed in an otherwise normal child.

The least severely retarded of these individuals (IQ of 50 to 70) grow and develop, in many ways not differently than the normal child during the early years of life. Their abilities and adaptations merge imperceptibly with those of the general population. Often there is neither somatic nor other specific neurologic abnormality. That such a child is handicapped may not be evident until it is apparent that scholastic pursuits are relatively unsuccessful. There may be manifest inability to learn with poor school progress, and the child with an IQ of 60 to 70 is generally unable to pass the sixth grade. Vocational training is of more value than other types of education. The mildly retarded child may be able to acquire useful occupational skills and to work under careful supervision.

Whereas IQ is a useful index of competence, the clinical and behavioral characteristics of individuals with retarded development cannot be adequately described by this single attribute. In particular, social competence, which may vary in ways that are not predicted by IQ, may largely determine the life expectations of retarded children. This aspect of behavior should be an organizing theme for education and training. Some mentally retarded persons are pleasant and amiable and achieve a satisfactory social adjustment. At the opposite extreme is the poorly understood syndrome of autism, associated with varying degrees of retardation, in which the child or older person fails to manifest any kind of interpersonal, social contact (see "Autism," below). Many retarded individuals are dull, apathetic, and underactive. Others display an incessant hyperactivity, characterized by a very short attention span, a restless inquisitive searching of the environment, and low frustration tolerance; they may be destructive or recklessly fearless and may seem strangely impervious to injury. As with the mentally normal but hyperactive, inattentive child, improvement in these children can often be achieved by using stimulants and desipramine.

Three specific disorders associated with mental retardation deserve separate description.

Fetal alcohol syndrome The fetal alcohol syndrome may be the most prevalent cause of defective cerebral development in industrialized nations. Its estimated frequency in the United States, 1:700 live births, is probably less than the actual occurrence and is even greater than the occurrences of trisomy 21 (Down's syndrome) and the fragile X syndrome. The fully developed disorder includes marked growth retardation, microcephaly, and cardiac valvular lesions. Characteristic facial features include hypotelorism, small palpebral fissures, small nasal bridge, and reduction of the vermillion border of the upper lip. Mental retardation may be profound. However, the less severely affected may have IQs in the normal range but be significantly disabled by attention deficit disorder with hyperactivity and learning disabilities. The severity of the disorder is related to alcohol dose, and the threshold for clinical expression appears to lie in the ingestion of 30 to 60 mL of absolute alcohol equivalent per day. Additional risk factors including exposure to multiple drugs or venereally transmitted infectious agents may interact with alcohol abuse. The potential risk to successive offspring is obvious.

Fragile X syndrome The fragile X chromosome anomaly is a phenotype that combines dysmorphic somatic characteristics with mental retardation. Cytogenetic analysis shows constriction of the terminal segment of the long arm of the affected X chromosome, and the fragile link is subject to breakage. Expression of the anomaly in standard tissue culture conditions is enhanced by folate deficiency and other modifications. The characteristic phenotype is expressed in approximately 80 percent of males and in 35 percent of females carrying a single affected X chromosome. It remains uncertain whether the chromosome anomaly is a determinant of, or simply marker for, the phenotypic anomalies. Stigmata include macroorchidism in males, possibly large ovaries in females, prognathism, and large everted ears. The skull is narrow and elongate. Mental retardation is usually mild to moderate and associated with dysphonic, sometimes echolalic speech. The association of the fragile X chromosome anomaly and autism in males (see below) has been estimated to be as high as 10 to 15 percent. A therapeutic response to treatment with folate has not been substantiated.

Down's syndrome (See Chap. 7) Down's syndrome accounts for about 1 percent of all mental retardation. Trisomy of chromosome 21 or translocation of parts of this chromosome is responsible for the disorder. Older mothers are more apt to have babies with Down's syndrome than are young mothers. The mean age of the mother is 37.

The degree of mental retardation in Down's syndrome varies from mild to severe and is associated with a characteristic facial appearance and small stature. Many stigmata can be recognized in the neonatal period. The head tends to be small and round, with sloping forehead. The ears are set low and are oval, with small lobules. The eyes slant slightly upward and outward owing to the presence of a medial epicanthal fold, which partly covers the angle of the palpebral fissure. The bridge of the nose is poorly developed. The mouth tends to hang open, and the tongue is usually enlarged, heavily fissured, and protruding. Gray-white specks of depigmentation are seen in the iris (Brushfield's spots). The little fingers are often short and curved inward (clinodactyly), owing to a hypoplastic middle phalanx. The hands are broad with a single transverse palmar crease. Lenticular opacities and congenital heart lesions (septal defects) are found in some cases. At birth these children are of average size, but at later periods of life they are characteristically small. The brain is of reduced weight with a relatively simple convolutional pattern. Of the patients who survive to puberty, many live to middle adult life and may develop a premature Alzheimer's type cerebral degeneration (onset in the majority by the age of 40) (see Chap. 359).

CRETINISM (See also Chap. 316) Cretinism and childhood hypothyroidism occur endemically in parts of the world where there is iodine deficiency and in infants everywhere with congenital disorders of thyroid function. The frequency is greater than that of phenylketonuria. For iodine deficiency to produce cretinism the mother must be lacking in iodine during the pregnancy, especially in the first trimester. Diagnosis rests with the clinical picture, for in the iodine-deficient state routine measures of thyroid function may be normal. Jaundice, umbilical hernia, noisy respirations, hypotonia, depression of reflexes, and lethargy are present at birth. Coarse facial features, large tongue, and constipation become manifest later. Among those with endemic cretinism, the neurologic abnormality consists of mental deficiency, deaf-mutism (or lesser degrees of hearing loss), and a combination of flexed posture with spasticity and rigidity of proximal limb musculature. These deficits persist throughout adult life.

AUTISM Autism is a mysterious and provocative condition. Long considered primarily psychiatric or a childhood form of schizophrenia, it is now generally thought to represent an organic defect in brain development characterized by failure to develop communicative language or other form of social communication. Some autistic persons often show motor and other skills far beyond that expected of a mentally retarded person. Often they are obsessively preoccupied with inanimate objects, such as lights, running water, or spinning objects. Most children with autism prove later to be retarded, and the ultimate level of disability depends largely on the IQ. Some gradually acquire language and may then exhibit certain exceptional talents, such as in mathematics (idiot savant). Upon reaching adult life they retain all the above characteristics. Not more than 1 in 20 improves significantly.

The etiology is unknown and there are likely to be multiple causes. A few detailed histopathologic studies identify abnormalities of forebrain limbic structures, and a reduction in volume of the midline region of the cerebellum is observed in CT and MR images. The abnormality of limbic structures is consistent with our understanding of the role of the medial temporal lobes in mediating language, affective, motivational, and social behavioral functions in human beings and also consistent with the finding that up to 30 percent of autistic children eventually manifest temporal lobe epilepsy. There is no specific therapy.

ABNORMALITIES OF MOTOR FUNCTION (CEREBRAL PALSY) *Cerebral palsy* refers to a developmental disorder of motor function that is present from infancy or early childhood and that is due to a nonprogressive cerebral disorder. The more commonly encountered conditions are spastic diplegia (affecting the legs), hemiplegia (affecting the arm and leg on the same side), and heterogeneous extrapyramidal syndromes. Cerebral infarction resulting from hypoxia and/or ischemia is one determinant of these disorders. For most the abnormal state has its origins before birth in events that go unrecognized. The insult may occur perinatally as a result of obstetrical mishap in 20 percent or less of cases. For some few an encephaloclastic event occurs in early childhood.

Spastic diplegia resulting from a prenatal or perinatal insult to the brain may not attract attention until several weeks or months after birth. There may be a delay in all normal developmental sequences, especially those that depend on the motor system. Once walking is attempted, usually much later than in the normal child, the characteristic stance and gait become manifest. The legs are advanced stiffly in short steps, each describing part of the arc of a circle: adduction is often so strong as to lead to actual crossing (scissors gait), with lower legs slightly splayed out and the feet flexed and turned in, the heels not touching the ground. Crural paraparesis is the rule, though in general it is associated with at least a mild affection of the arms as well. In the adolescent and adult, the legs tend to be short and small, but the muscles are not markedly atrophic, as in infantile muscular atrophy and dystrophy. Less commonly there may also be pseudobulbar dysarthria and athetosis.

Hemiplegia is a not uncommon condition of infancy and childhood, and a difference in function of the right and left extremities may be noticed soon after birth or during the first 6 to 12 months of life. The parents may be the first to notice that movements of prehension and exploration are carried out with only one arm. The affection of the leg is usually recognized later, i.e., during the first attempt to stand and walk. Mental defect is even less common than with cerebral diplegia and less common than in bilateral hemiplegia. Convulsions occur in 35 to 50 percent of children with congenital hemiplegia and may persist throughout life. If the hemiplegia is acquired during childhood, seizures often accompany the onset. They may be generalized but are frequently unilateral and limited to the hemiplegic side. Often, after a series of seizures, the affected side will be weak for several hours or longer (Todd's paralysis).

In *double hemiplegia,* a less frequent condition, the bilateral weakness of face, arms, and legs arises at any age under conditions of more severe acquired cerebral disease. The arms are severely affected, in contrast to their minimal involvement in cerebral diplegia. A quadriplegic state may occur without bulbar involvement. The condition is relatively rare and may result from a bilateral cerebral lesion or a high cervical cord lesion. Although this may occasionally result from cysts, tumors, and other malformations, it is usually produced in the infant by fracture-dislocation of the cervical spine, induced during a difficult breech delivery. Similarly, in paraplegia, with weakness or paralysis limited to the legs, the lesion may be either a cerebral form of diplegia or a spinal one. Sphincteric disturbances and a loss of sensation below a certain level on the trunk favor a spinal localization.

The spastic and rigid cerebral diplegias discussed above shade almost imperceptibly into the congenital extrapyramidal syndromes. Many such patients are found in every cerebral palsy clinic and ultimately reach adult medical clinics. Pyramidal tract signs may be absent. The nonprogressive extrapyramidal cases considered here are generally attributable to severe perinatal hypoxia; others represent separate diseases such as erythroblastosis fetalis with kernicterus. These are to be distinguished from the progressive acquired or hereditary postnatal syndromes such as familial athetosis, dystonia musculorum deformans, and cerebellar ataxia.

Congenital choreoathetosis (double athetosis) is probably the most frequent representative of this group. Like the spastic states, it may be recognized only after several months or a year have elapsed. Syndromes may be mixed, however. All combinations of chorea, athetosis, ballismus, myoclonus, and dystonia may be found in a single case, or one or another type of movement disorder may predominate. However, in all instances there is, in addition, a primary defect in voluntary movement. Choreoathetosis varies in severity. In some the disorder is so mild that the abnormal movements are misinterpreted as restlessness or "the fidgets"; in others, every voluntary act is marred by intense involuntary movements, leaving the patient nearly helpless. The severely handicapped patients, even with the help of rehabilitation clinics and corrective orthopedic operations, rarely achieve a degree of motor control that permits them to lead an independent life, and they need supportive treatment and help as adults. Intelligence may be preserved.

Kernicterus was a more common cause of abnormal cerebral development prior to the contemporary practice of restraining early postnatal serum bilirubin concentrations to levels below 250 μmol/L (15 mg/dL). The majority of infants with this disorder die within the first week of two of life, and those who survive are often mentally retarded, deaf, and totally unable to sit, stand, or walk. However, exceptional patients, obviously less damaged, are mentally normal or at most only slightly backward. Either athetosis or ataxia may be present. A few have rigid limbs and a picture not too different from that of cerebral spastic diplegia with involuntary movements. Kernicterus should always be suspected if an extrapyramidal syndrome is accompanied by bilateral deafness and palsy of upward gaze.

NEUROSKELETAL DISORDERS

The skull and vertebral column normally enlarge coordinately with growth of the central nervous system. Abnormalities in the size of the skull can occur secondary to underlying abnormalities of brain development. Abnormalities resulting primarily from derangements of osseous development may lead to aberrations in skull shape and to entrapment of the enclosed nervous system, as in the Chiari and related malformations.

SECONDARY MACROCRANIA AND MICROCRANIA Alterations in the circumference of the head greater than (macrocrania) or less than (microcrania) the 98th percentiles are considered abnormal. Macrocrania may result from potentially correctable hydrocephalus and is associated with headache, mental dullness, depression, visual blurring, difficulty walking, and urinary incontinence. Limited ability to elevate the eyes, ataxia of gait, hyperreflexia in the legs, and Babinski responses are common signs.

Developmental causes of *noncommunicating hydrocephalus* include aqueductal stenosis, the Dandy-Walker malformation in which the cerebrospinal fluid escape from the fourth ventricle is obstructed, and the Chiari malformations (see below). Neoplasms or cysts, particularly when located within the ventricular system or impinging upon structures of the posterior fossa, must be excluded. *Communicating hydrocephalus* may develop after recovery from disorders that cause scarring of the leptomeninges, such as intraventricular hemorrhage in the perinatal period, especially in premature infants, and meningitis. Localized head enlargement, associated with mental slowing and contralateral long tract signs, may complicate porencephalic cerebral defects resulting from a focal cerebral injury in the perinatal period or early childhood.

Macrocrania may also be the result of an abnormally large brain (macrocephaly). Benign, or asymptomatic, macrocephaly may be familial. Macrocephaly and a characteristic triangular face, moderate impairment of cognitive functions, and macrosomia constitute the syndrome of cerebral gigantism (Soto), which in some families appears to be transmitted by autosomal dominant inheritance. Symmetric or asymmetric macrocephaly, seizures, and cognitive impairment may occur with neurofibromatosis. Macrocephaly can also occur in certain lysosomal storage disorders that affect the brain, but such individuals rarely reach adulthood.

Microcrania is most commonly secondary to microcephaly. Typically this is a consequence of lack of brain growth and may result from virtually any heritable or acquired disorder that affects the developing brain. *Microcephaly vera* is a rare but distinctive disorder transmitted by autosomal recessive inheritance and associated mental retardation and brain weight less than 500 g. The face and facial features are distinctively prominent in relation to the small cranium.

PRIMARY DISORDERS OF SKELETAL DEVELOPMENT The Chiari malformations are among the most prevalent and complex neuroskeletal malformations. The characteristic feature is entrapment and compression of the rhombencephalon within an underdeveloped posterior cranial fossa (see Marin-Padilla). In the severest forms, typically apparent at birth, the cerebellar vermis, medulla, and fourth ventricle are herniated or extruded into the upper cervical canal (Chiari type II) or protrude exteriorly as an occipital encephalocele at the base of the skull (Chiari type III). Hydrocephalus and hydromyelia may be associated with meningomyelocele arising from the lumbosacral spinal cord. Milder degrees of herniation of the posteroinferior region of the cerebellum ("tonsils") into the cervical canal with little or no downward displacement of the fourth ventricle (Chiari type I) or milder degrees of the Chiari II deformity may become symptomatic only in adolescence or adult life. Symptoms typical of adult expression of the Chiari malformation include pain that is localized to the cranial-cervical junction, which is aggravated by head movement or Valsalva maneuver. There may be unsteadiness of gait, dysarthria, and dysphagia, corresponding to compromise of cerebellar-related connections and lower cranial nerve paresis. Downbeat nystagmus is characteristic.

Syringomyelia and *syringobulbia* occur in association with the Chiari malformations. Syringomyelia, a disorder of the cervical region of the spinal cord, can be viewed as a progressive destructive expansion of a central cavitation of the spinal cord. A variable number of segments of the upper cervical and thoracic cord, or of the medulla and pons in the case of syringobulbia, may be involved. Typically, the commissure and the posterior horns of the central gray and the axonal fascicles of the posterior and lateral columns of the cord are damaged. The neurologic manifestations include impairment of pain and temperature perception in a capelike distribution and impairment of perception of vibration and joint displacement and spasticity in the lower extremities. To the extent that anterior horn cells are destroyed at cervical segmental levels, muscle atrophy and weakness appear in the upper extremities (see Chap. 361). Extension of the cystic cavity upwards into the brainstem can cause facial pain, nystagmus, and lower cranial nerve deficits.

Other disorders of the axial skeleton and the lower spinal cord and cauda equina are also characteristically associated with the Chiari malformation but may occur independently. The osseous anomalies include aberrations of the primary pattern of formation (absence or fusion) or the size of vertebrae, hemivertebrae, or fusion of vertebra and scapula (Sprengel's deformity). The Klippel-Feil deformity is a complex of osseous and visceral anomalies that include low hairline, platybasia, fusion of cervical vertebra with short neck, and deafness. These malformations may entrap and damage the brain and spinal cord. The disorders of the lower vertebral region may become symptomatic with rapid growth in adolescence or in adult life. Diastematomyelia, the protrusion of a bony spur into the vertebral canal, is of particular importance in adults because it represents a treatable form of deficit. Intermittent, generally progressive disturbances of somatic and visceral motor function, typically associated with pain, may be subtle clues to the diagnosis.

A cauda equina syndrome, that is, impairment of both somatic and visceral sensory and motor functions referable to the lower lumbar and sacral roots, may result from lipomas or dermoid cysts within the lower vertebral canal. A dimple or tuft of hair near the midline in the lumbar region or within the gluteal crease may suggest the persistence of a sinus tract or a deeper-lying anomaly affecting vertebral canal and spinal roots. Tethering of the cord to the lower end of the vertebral canal by fibrous bands may result in traction that becomes symptomatic with growth in adolescence. Stenosis of the lumbar vertebral elements may be associated with claudication, that is, symptoms of a cauda equina syndrome that develop with walking.

CT and MRI, particularly when utilized in conjunction with myelography for syrinx and other spinal disorders, are sensitive and efficient diagnostic procedures. Images obtained in the midsagittal plane are particularly appropriate for diagnosis of the Chiari malformation and syrinx and for abnormalities of the lumbosacral region. In principle, treatment is surgical. Decompression is appropriate for entrapment and compression; shunting is required for hydrocephalic (or syringomyelic) states. Mass lesions and bony spurs are excised.

SYNOSTOSES AND CRANIOFACIAL DEFORMITIES Cranial synostosis and some other craniofacial anomalies affect principally the rostral region and the vault of the skull. Premature closure of the sagittal suture results in an elongate (scaphocephalic) skull, and premature closure of the coronal sutures causes a broad and foreshortened (brachycephalic) skull. If all major sutures close prematurely, a tower (turricephalic) skull results, manifest by shallow orbits with bulging eyes. Other combinations may affect one or more sutures. Synostosis, particularly when generalized, may result in cerebral compression and hydrocephalus. Less extensive disorders are cosmetically disfiguring. Early surgical correction of the disorders is appropriate.

REFERENCES

Adams RD: Neurocutaneous disease, in *Dermatology in General Medicine*, 3d ed, TB Fitzpatrick et al (eds). New York, McGraw-Hill, 1986

———, Lyon G: *Neurology of Hereditary Metabolic Diseases of Children*. New York, McGraw-Hill, 1982

Caviness VS Jr: The Chiari malformations of the posterior fossa and their relation to hydrocephalus. Dev Med Child Neurol 18:103, 1976

Chasnoff IJ et al: Cocaine use in pregnancy. N Engl J Med 313:666, 1985

Ho HZ et al: The fragile-X syndrome. Dev Med Child Neurol 30:257, 1988

Lamiell JM et al: Von Hippel-Lindau disease affecting 43 members of a single kindred. Medicine 68:1, 1989

Marin-Padilla M: Clinical and experimental rachischisis, in *Handbook of Clinical Neurology*, PJ Vinken, GW Bruyn (eds). Amsterdam, North Holland, 1978, pp 159–191

Martuza RL, Eldridge R: Neurofibromatosis 2 (bilateral acoustic neurofibromatosis). N Engl J Med 318:684, 1988

Riccardi VM: Von Recklinghausen neurofibromatosis. N Engl J Med 305:1617, 1981

Seizinger BR et al: Models for inherited susceptibility to cancer in the nervous system: A molecular-genetic approach to neurofibromatosis. Dev Neurosci 9:144, 1987

SMITH DW: *Recognizable Patterns of Human Malformation*, 3d ed. Philadelphia, Saunders, 1982
SWAIMAN KF: *Pediatric Neurology: Principles and Practice*. St. Louis, Mosby, 1989
VOLPE JJ: *Neurology of the Newborn*. Philadelphia, Saunders, 1987

359 DEGENERATIVE DISEASES OF THE NERVOUS SYSTEM

M. FLINT BEAL / EDWARD P. RICHARDSON, JR. / JOSEPH B. MARTIN

In classifying diseases of the nervous system, it is customary to designate a group of them as *degenerative*, indicating that they are characterized by gradually evolving, relentlessly progressive neuronal death occurring for reasons that are still largely unknown. The identification of these diseases depends upon exclusion of such possible causative factors as infections, metabolic derangements, and intoxications. A considerable proportion of the disorders classed as degenerative are genetic, with either dominant or recessive inheritance. Others, however, occur only sporadically—as isolated instances in a given family.

Classification of the degenerative diseases cannot be based upon any exact knowledge of cause or pathogenesis; their subdivision into individual syndromes rests on descriptive criteria based largely upon neuropathologic and clinical aspects. This group of diseases presents as several distinct clinical syndromes, the recognition of which can assist the clinician in arriving at a diagnosis.

GENERAL CONSIDERATIONS The degenerative disorders usually begin insidiously and run a gradually progressive course over many years. Their course is generally more protracted than that of the hereditary metabolic diseases of the nervous system (see Chap. 357). The earliest changes may be so subtle that it often is impossible to assign any precise time of onset. At times the history suggests an abrupt onset of disability—particularly when an injury or some other event in the patient's life has occurred to which illness might conceivably be related. By careful questioning, it is frequently evident that the patient or family has suddenly become aware of a condition that had, in fact, already been present but had passed unnoticed.

The family history is of great importance, and denial of familial occurrence cannot always be taken at face value. Some patients or their relatives are hesitant to disclose that a neurologic disease afflicts the family. In other cases, the extent of the disease affecting other family members may be so slight as to go unnoticed by the family—as may occur, for instance, in the group of the hereditary ataxias. Moreover, small sibships in a family may prevent well-established hereditary diseases from being recognized. Familial occurrence, of course, does not always mean that a disease is hereditary; it may indicate instead that there has been a common exposure to an infective or toxic agent.

Many of the degenerative nervous system diseases progress uninfluenced by therapeutic measures. Caring for such patients is often an anguishing experience for all concerned. In others, such as persons with Parkinson's disease, symptoms can often be alleviated by wise and skillful management. The physician's caring attention may be of great help even when curative measures cannot be offered.

The symptoms and signs of this group of diseases tend to have a bilaterally symmetric distribution. This aspect alone may help to distinguish the disorder from other varieties of neurologic disease. In some patients, in the early stages, one side of the body, or one limb, may become involved in the presence of normal findings elsewhere. Eventually, despite the asymmetric beginning, the inherently bilateral nature of the process generally asserts itself.

A striking characteristic of the degenerative disorders is that particular anatomic or physiologic systems of neurons may be selectively affected, leaving others entirely intact. This is exemplified in amyotrophic lateral sclerosis, in which the disease process is limited to cerebral and spinal motor neurons, and in some forms of progressive ataxia in which only the Purkinje cells of the cerebellum are affected. In Friedreich's ataxia and some other syndromes, the disease process affects multiple neuronal systems.

In this respect certain degenerative neuronal diseases resemble others of known cause, particularly intoxications, where similarly circumscribed effects occur. Diphtheria toxin, for example, produces selective breakdown of peripheral nerve myelin, triorthocresyl phosphate affects the corticospinal tracts in the spinal cord together with the peripheral nerves, and the neurotoxin 1-methyl-4-phenyl-1,2,3,6-tetrahydropyridine (MPTP) brings about death of dopamine-containing neurons in the substantia nigra. Selective involvement of particular neuronal systems is not, however, characteristic of all of the degenerative diseases; some are characterized by pathologic changes that are diffuse and unselective.

Typically, the pathologic process in the nervous system is one of slow involution of nerve cell bodies or their axonal extensions, unaccompanied by any intense tissue reaction or cellular response, although the loss of neurons and fibers is often accompanied by hyperplasia of fibrillary astrocytes (gliosis). The cerebrospinal fluid (CSF) shows little if any change—at most a slight elevation of protein, without abnormalities in specific proteins, cell count, or in other constituents. Moreover, since these diseases invariably result in tissue loss, rather than in new tissue formation, radiologic visualization of the brain, the ventricular system, or subarachnoid space shows either no change or an enlargement of the CSF compartments. These negative laboratory findings thus help to distinguish the degenerative disorders from the other large classes of progressive diseases of the nervous system—tumors and infections.

CLASSIFICATION Since etiologic classification is impossible, subdivision of the degenerative diseases into individual syndromes rests on descriptive criteria based largely on their clinical aspects and pathologic anatomy. Many of these syndromes are named after distinguished neurologists and neuropathologists. A useful classification is outlined in Table 359-1.

SYNDROMES IN WHICH PROGRESSIVE DEMENTIA PREDOMINATES

In the disease entities that follow, the clinical picture is dominated by gradual loss of intellectual capacities, i.e., by dementia. Other neurologic abnormalities, except in the terminal stages, are absent or relatively insignificant. (For further discussion of dementia, including its clinical evaluation, Chaps. 29, 30, and 32 should be consulted.)

ALZHEIMER'S DISEASE Alzheimer's disease is perhaps the most important of all the degenerative diseases because of its frequent occurrence and devastating nature. It is the commonest cause of dementia in the elderly, with all that this implies in the way of distress for patients and families, and economic loss in the form of the costs entailed in the long-term care of patients totally disabled by the disease. Historically, the term *Alzheimer's disease* was applied to progressive dementia coming on in late middle life but preceding the senile period, following the original description by Alois Alzheimer in 1907, in which the illness of a woman dying at the age of 55 was depicted clinically and pathologically. It became usual to classify cases of this kind under the heading of *presenile dementia*. Meanwhile, it became increasingly apparent that very old people dying with progressive mental deterioration, generally referred to as *senile dementia*, showed cerebral lesions that were identical to those found in cases of presenile dementia. Such cases are now designated as *senile dementia of the Alzheimer type*. Current evidence indicates that the disease process is the same, regardless of the age of onset. At the same time, Alzheimer's disease is clearly age-related. It is extremely uncommon in young people and rare in middle age; as age advances, however, it is increasingly frequent, such that its prevalence

TABLE 359-1 Clinical classification of the degenerative diseases of the nervous system

I Disorders characterized by progressive dementia in the absence of other prominent neurologic signs
- *A* Alzheimer's disease
- *B* Senile dementia of the Alzheimer type
- *C* Pick's disease (lobar atrophy)

II Syndromes combining progressive dementia with other prominent neurologic abnormalities
- *A* Mainly in adults
  - *1* Huntington's disease
  - *2* Multiple system atrophy combining dementia with ataxia and/or manifestations of Parkinson's disease
  - *3* Progressive supranuclear palsy (Steele-Richardson-Olszewski)
  - *4* Diffuse Lewy body disease
  - *5* Corticodentatonigral degeneration
- *B* Mainly in children or young adults
  - *1* Hallervorden-Spatz disease
  - *2* Progressive familial myoclonic epilepsy

III Syndromes of gradually developing abnormalities of posture and movement
- *A* Paralysis agitans (Parkinson's disease)
- *B* Striatonigral degeneration
- *C* Progressive supranuclear palsy (see *II, A, 3* above)
- *D* Torsion dystonia (torsion spasm; dystonia musculorum deformans)
- *E* Spasmodic torticollis and other restricted dyskinesias
- *F* Familial tremor
- *G* Gilles de la Tourette syndrome

IV Syndromes of progressive ataxia
- *A* Cerebellar degenerations
  - *1* Cerebellar cortical degeneration
  - *2* Olivopontocerebellar atrophy (OPCA)
- *B* Spinocerebellar degenerations (Friedreich's ataxia and related disorders)

V Syndrome of central autonomic nervous system failure (Shy-Drager syndrome)

VI Syndromes of muscular weakness and wasting without sensory changes (motor neuron disease)
- *A* Amyotrophic lateral sclerosis
- *B* Spinal muscular atrophy
  - *1* Infantile spinal muscular atrophy (Werdnig-Hoffmann)
  - *2* Juvenile spinal muscular atrophy (Wohlfart-Kugelberg-Welander)
  - *3* Other forms of familial spinal muscular atrophy
- *C* Primary lateral sclerosis
- *D* Hereditary spastic paraplegia

VII Syndromes combining muscular weakness and wasting with sensory changes (progressive neural muscular atrophy; chronic familial polyneuropathies)
- *A* Peroneal muscular atrophy (Charcot-Marie-Tooth)
- *B* Hypertrophic interstitial polyneuropathy (Dejerine-Sottas)
- *C* Miscellaneous forms of chronic progressive neuropathy

VIII Syndromes of progressive visual loss
- *A* Pigmentary degeneration of the retina (retinitis pigmentosa)
- *B* Hereditary optic atrophy (Leber's disease)

in persons over 80 years old is estimated at more than 20 percent. Advancing age is unmistakably a predisposing factor, but it is incorrect to consider Alzheimer's disease as the inevitable accompaniment of aging. Many elderly people remain mentally unimpaired into the ninth and tenth decades. Genetic predisposition to Alzheimer's disease emerges as a clear-cut pattern in some families, particularly in those with early age of onset. There are well-documented familial cases, some following an autosomal dominant pattern of inheritance. An exception to the statement that Alzheimer's disease is rare in young people occurs in the instance of Down's syndrome (trisomy 21), which leads to the development of the characteristic lesions of Alzheimer's disease in the majority of the patients after 40 years of age.

Pathology The outstanding pathologic feature is death and disappearance of nerve cells in the cerebral cortex. This leads ultimately to extensive convolutional atrophy, especially in the frontal, parietal, and medial temporal regions. There is a corresponding enlargement of the ventricular system, but this is usually not extreme.

Two kinds of microscopic lesions are distinctive for the disease. The first, originally described by Alzheimer, consists of intraneuronal accumulations of filamentous material in the form of loops, coils, or tangled masses—referred to as *Alzheimer neurofibrillary tangles*. Their nature is currently under active investigation. The neuropathologic evidence strongly suggests that these fibrillar masses are of major importance in bringing about the death of neurons. Electron microscopy reveals accumulations of paired helical filaments that differ from normal neurofilaments and microtubules. Recent studies have shown that a major component is an abnormally phosphorylated form of the microtubule protein tau. Alzheimer neurofibrillary tangles also contain ubiquitin, a protein that marks cells for proteolysis.

Neurofibrillary tangles tend to be most abundant, together with the most extreme degrees of neuronal loss, in the hippocampus and adjacent parts of the temporal lobe—structures that have been found to be of greatest importance in memory function.

The other histopathologic change that characterizes Alzheimer's disease is the presence of intracortical clusters of thickened neuronal processes, both axons and dendrites (collectively referred to as *neurites*), generally in the form of an irregular ring surrounding a spherical deposit of amyloid fibrils. These lesions, which had been recognized before Alzheimer's description of the neurofibrillary change, were termed *senile plaques*. Recent elucidation of their structure has led to their current designation as *neuritic plaques*. They have been shown to contain paired helical filaments identical to those found in the perinuclear cytoplasm of the diseased neurons. One form of plaque, the *diffuse plaque,* consists of amorphous amyloid without neurites. The nature and origin of the amyloid component are being intensively studied. It is now evident that amyloid, identified by its staining reactions and ultrastructural features, is not a uniform substance; instead, its tinctorial and morphologic character depends upon a particular molecular spatial configuration (beta-pleated sheet fibrils) that can be brought about with various proteins, some of immunologic origin, some not.

There is another aspect to the problem of cerebral amyloidosis in Alzheimer's disease. In many, but not all, cases identical amyloid deposits may be found in the walls of small meningeal and intracortical arteries, and the question has arisen as to whether this cerebrovascular amyloidosis (often called *cerebral amyloid angiopathy* or *congophilic angiopathy* because of the characteristic staining of amyloid with the dye Congo red) has a close relationship, perhaps even causative, to plaque amyloidosis. The amyloid in the blood vessels in Alzheimer's disease, as well as that in the core of neuritic plaques, has been isolated and sequenced. The amyloid peptide (β- or A_4-peptide) gene is on chromosome 21, on which the familial Alzheimer's disease gene also has been localized in some families. However, the two loci are not identical. Antibodies against the cerebrovascular amyloid cross react with the amyloid in neuritic plaques. It is as yet unclear where the amyloid in plaques originates—whether from neurons or blood vessels; most investigators favor the former.

Biochemical studies show that choline acetyltransferase, the key enzyme required for the synthesis of acetylcholine, is decreased in the cerebral cortex in Alzheimer's disease. The major source of neocortical cholinergic innervation is a group of neurons situated in the basal part of the forebrain just beneath the corpus striatum—the nucleus basalis of Meynert. Careful neuropathologic investigations have shown that in Alzheimer's disease, this nucleus is a site of major neuronal loss and of frequent Alzheimer neurofibrillary tangles. These studies suggest that impairment of cholinergic transmission may play a part in the clinical expression of the disease. However, attempted therapy with cholinomimetic agents has been largely unsuccessful. Less consistent reductions in cortical norepinephrine and serotonin appear to be caused by neuronal loss in the locus coeruleus and raphé nucleus, respectively. Loss of peptidergic neurons in the cerebral cortex is associated with reduced cortical concentrations of somatostatin and corticotropin releasing factor. Reduction in CSF concentrations of somatostatin is also reported.

It is anticipated that investigations of the biochemistry of the cerebral lesions in Alzheimer's disease will lead ultimately to an understanding of their pathogenesis. The remarkable discovery that one form of progressive dementia, Creutzfeldt-Jakob disease, is the result of infection with a transmissible virus-like agent has led to the question as to whether Alzheimer's disease and other neuronal degenerations might be due to a similar form of infectious agent. All attempts to transmit Alzheimer's disease have failed, however, so that currently an infective basis is thought unlikely.

Clinical manifestations The onset is insidious and subtle, with changes most noticeable first in memory for recent happenings and in other aspects of mental activity. Emotional disturbances such as depression, anxiety, or odd, unpredictable quirks of behavior, may be salient features in the early stages. Progression is usually slow and gradual, and unless other medical conditions supervene, it may smolder on for 10 or more years.

In the milder cases, including those of the senile period, the noteworthy features are those of simple dementia, as described in Chap. 32. More unusual disorders of thought and intellect, including aphasia, apraxic disturbances, and abnormalities of space perception, may be seen, especially in the presenile group. Exceptionally, and only in the advanced stages of the disease, extrapyramidal signs appear; the patient walks in a shuffling manner with short steps, and there is a generalized stiffness of the musculature with slowness and awkwardness of all movements. In some patients, sudden jerklike contractions of various muscles (myoclonus) may occur in the presence of otherwise typical Alzheimer's disease, but this is unusual and should immediately raise the suspicion of Creutzfeldt-Jakob disease (Chap. 355). Terminally the patient may become nearly decorticate, losing all ability to perceive, think, speak, or move.

Laboratory investigations, including blood and CSF determinations, do not yield any conclusive or pertinent data. There is a diffuse slowing in the electroencephalogram in the more advanced stages of the disease. Enlargement of the ventricular system and subarachnoid space resulting from brain atrophy can be demonstrated by computed tomography (CT) scan and by magnetic resonance imaging (MRI). These imaging procedures, however, are not decisive for making the diagnosis, especially in the earlier stages, because the degree of cerebral atrophy demonstrated may be no more than that seen in patients of a similar age group who are functioning normally. Recent studies with positron emission tomography have shown decreased glucose metabolism in the temporal and parietal lobes. During the course of the illness, occasional convulsive seizures may occur, but they are relatively rare and should raise suspicion of other diseases. Terminally, the patient dies from intercurrent disease, in a state of total helplessness. Institutional care is usually necessary long before the end.

Differential diagnosis The physician should recognize that treatable conditions may at first appear to be dementia of the Alzheimer type. Space-occupying lesions, such as chronic subdural hematoma or slowly growing frontal neoplasms (meningioma or glioma) should be excluded. CT and MRI scanning usually demonstrate mass lesions of these kinds, as well as an unsuspected hydrocephalus, which, when treated by a shunt procedure for ventricular decompression, may lead to dramatic improvement in the patient's state. Other treatable conditions producing a dementia-like state include metabolic derangements (liver disease), vitamin B_{12} deficiency, and hypothyroidism. Elderly people may be unusually susceptible to the sedative effects of medications, so that chronic drug intoxication may need to be considered. Cerebrovascular disease is not ordinarily a cause of uncomplicated dementia, but finding multiple small infarcts on CT or MRI scanning raises the possibility of multi-infarct dementia. Depression can mimic dementia, particularly in the elderly, in whom it may be all too easy to attribute deficits in thinking, motivation, and memory to cerebral disease (see Chaps. 29 and 30). Depression may show a most gratifying response to appropriate treatment (see Chap. 368).

The evidence that cholinergic innervation may be impaired in Alzheimer's disease has led to attempts to correct the deficiency pharmacologically, but so far none of these has proved to be effective.

Practical measures that may help in the management of cases of Alzheimer's disease are suggested in Chaps. 29 and 30.

PICK'S DISEASE (LOBAR ATROPHY) This remarkable form of cerebral disease, characterized by circumscribed cerebal atrophy (lobar sclerosis), enters in the differential diagnosis of dementia in the presenile period. It is, however, an extremely rare condition as compared with diffuse cerebral atrophy of the Alzheimer type. Hereditary transmission (as a dominant trait) is frequent in Pick's disease, and women are more frequently affected than men. The age distribution is similar in both of these varieties of progressive dementia.

Pathology So striking are the gross pathologic changes in the brain that in typical cases the diagnosis can be made at a glance. Severe atrophy of the anterior portions of the frontal and temporal lobes occurs, and there is a curiously sharp line of demarcation between the atrophied portions and the remainder of the brain, which appears normal or nearly so. In some cases, the frontal atrophy is more prominent; in others, the temporal lobes are more severely involved; in general, both regions are affected. Rarely, the disorder has a predominantly unilateral localization—as in cases described originally by Pick. Atrophic changes also occur in subcortical structures: caudate nucleus, putamen, thalamus, and substantia nigra, and in the descending frontopontine fiber system. There are striking changes in nerve cells in the affected regions in most cases. These consist of fibrillary deposits within the cytoplasm—masses of straight fibrils, differing from the paired helical filaments of Alzheimer's disease. In some neurons, densely packed spherical aggregates (Pick bodies) can be seen with silver-impregnation methods. In other affected neurons, the fibrils are more widely dispersed, and the neuronal cytoplasm takes on a rounded, distended appearance, forming ballooned cells. Recent evidence suggests that despite the morphologic differences, these neuronal changes are biochemically related to those in Alzheimer's disease, as indicated by common antigenic properties. In rare instances of Alzheimer's disease, disproportionate atrophy of the frontal and temporal lobes may suggest Pick's disease, but in such cases the distinguishing feature is the presence of the characteristic plaques and neurofibrillary tangles, which are not found in Pick's disease.

Clinical manifestations If Pick's disease has any distinctive clinical features, they consist of unusually severe signs of frontal lobe or temporal lobe dysfunction (see Chap. 32). Typical early manifestations are a general impoverishment of mental function, changes in behavior patterns, and a striking lack of insight. The later phases of the disease are characterized by loss of retentive memory (with temporal lobe involvement), loss of all language functions, and, when the frontal lobes are mainly affected, prominent grasp and sucking reflexes. In CT and MRI scans the shrinkage of the cortex and the low density of the white matter in the affected lobes may be diagnostic. Progression, as in Alzheimer's disease, is slow and relentless, the average duration being about 7 years. In the late stages, rigidity, dystonic postures, and perhaps tremor may be prominent features; these can be ascribed to extension of the disease process into the basal ganglia.

Differential diagnosis The considerations already noted with regard to Alzheimer's disease apply to Pick's disease as well.

SYNDROMES COMBINING DEMENTIA WITH OTHER NEUROLOGIC SIGNS

HUNTINGTON'S DISEASE This disorder, characterized by a combination of choreoathetotic movements and progressive dementia usually beginning in midadult life, is transmitted as an autosomal dominant disease. Recent genetic studies have shown that the determining gene is located on the terminal segment of the short arm of chromosome 4. The classic description is that of George Huntington, who, together with his father and grandfather, all physicians, made clinical observations on familial cases living near their home on Long Island, New York. Huntington, writing in 1872, entitled his paper "On Chorea"; subsequently the disorder described by him came to be known as *Huntington's chorea.* The more general term used in this chapter—Huntington's disease—is preferable, since the disease state comprises more than abnormal movements, and the motor abnormalities often are more complex than would be implied by the unqualified term *chorea*.

Because of its distressing and incapacitating nature, and its implications for members of any family in which it appears (50 percent risk in all children of an affected parent), the disease has attracted attention in recent years and has been found to be considerably more frequent and widely distributed than once was thought. It is estimated that there are approximately 25,000 cases in the United States alone. In virtually all cases that come to the notice of a physician, there is a family history of the disease, although occasionally patients present with typical symptoms and no documentable family history; no proven case of a new mutation has occurred. Some of these cases are classified as senile chorea, where family members have died of other causes before the disease became manifest.

Pathology Distinctive for Huntington's disease is atrophy of the caudate nucleus and, to a lesser extent, other structures of the basal ganglia (putamen and globus pallidus), out of proportion to any other changes in the brain. The degree of atrophy is directly related to the severity and duration of the disease. In the late stages, the caudate nucleus, which normally forms a convexly rounded eminence in the lateral wall of the lateral ventricle, takes on instead a flattened or concave appearance. As the result of the tissue loss, the ventricular system becomes correspondingly widened, especially the frontal horns. Along with these changes in the basal ganglia, there characteristically is diffuse gyral atrophy, most severe over the convex aspect of the brain.

The atrophy of the caudate nucleus and putamen is seen microscopically to be due to extensive loss of neurons, which stands out in contrast to the intactness of adjacent structures such as the nucleus accumbens septi, the nucleus basalis of Meynert (so strikingly involved in Alzheimer's disease), and the thalamus.

There are no morphologically distinctive or characteristic cytopathologic alterations in the neurons in Huntington's disease such as occur in Alzheimer's and some other diseases. Neurochemical studies have shown a striking decrease of γ-aminobutyric acid (GABA) and of its synthesizing enzyme, glutamic acid decarboxylase, in the caudate nucleus, putamen, globus pallidus, and pars reticulata of the substantia nigra, and some decrease also in choline acetyltransferase in the caudate nucleus. The loss of GABA can be attributed to depletion of the abundant medium-sized *spiny* neurons within the striatum. Spiny neurons are characterized in Golgi studies by a large number of dendritic spines and have been shown to constitute the projection neurons of the striatum. They provide efferents to both the globus pallidus and substantia nigra. In contrast *aspiny* neurons, with few dendritic spines, are striatal interneurons with locally arborizing axons. In addition to GABA, other neurotransmitters contained within striatal spiny neurons, including substance P, enkephalins, and dynorphin, are similarly depleted in the striatum and its sites of projection.

Recent observations indicate that the peptide neurotransmitters somatostatin and neuropeptide y are relatively increased in the caudate nucleus and putamen in Huntington's disease, and cells identifiable as somatostatin–neuropeptide y neurons (*aspiny* neurons) are selectively preserved—in striking contrast to the loss of other neurons in the same regions. The large aspiny neurons containing acetylcholine are also preserved. The pathophysiologic meaning of this sparing is not clear as yet; its occurrence emphasizes the fact that in Huntington's disease, as in other neuronal-system degenerations, selective vulnerability of neurons occurs in a particular region with preservation of others. The pattern of resistance of certain neuronal groups has provided clues to a possible underlying pathogenesis of the disease. The susceptible spiny neurons have dense glutamate inputs from the cerebral cortex. The pattern of cell death can be reproduced experimentally by glutamate receptor agonists that act on the *N*-methyl-D-aspartate subclass of glutamate receptors (see Chaps. 11 and 346). These observations have led to the hypothesis that striatal neurons die as a result of glutamate-induced neurotoxicity.

The progressive dementia of Huntington's disease is still not well characterized neuropathologically. Pathologic examination reveals shrinkage of cortical volume, but it has been difficult to document cell loss. Biochemical studies, however, are consistent with a mild neuronal loss, particularly in the frontal cortex. Further correlative biochemical and neuropathologic studies, using careful quantitative methods, will be needed to resolve this issue.

Clinical aspects The disorder has a prevalence in Europe and North America of 7 to 10 per 100,000 population. The movement disorder generally makes its appearance in early to middle adult years (average age of onset about 35 to 40 years). It is characteristic of the disease that younger patients, with onset of symptoms in the age group of 15 to 40 years, suffer a more severe form of the disorder than older patients, with onset in the 50s and 60s, and the neuropathologic changes in the brain are correspondingly more extensive and severe in the younger as compared with the older patients. Huntington's disease is occasionally manifest in childhood (even before the age of 4); in such cases transmission usually occurs through the father. Such cases are rare and tend to be characterized more by rigidity than by chorea and by other atypical features such as convulsive seizures and cerebellar ataxia (Westphal's variant).

The involuntary movements (bizarre grimacing, respiratory irregularity, faulty articulation of speech, and irregular, arrhythmic, unpatterned movements of the limbs, imparting to the gait a peculiar dancing quality) tend to be less quick and more athetoid than in Sydenham's chorea (see Chap. 25). Some reported cases that on genealogic and pathologic grounds must be classified with Huntington's chorea have shown progressive rigidity rather than choreiform movements, even in the adult. As a general rule, dementia runs parallel with the motor disorder. Occasionally it may appear before or after chorea; very rarely it may be slight or lacking altogether. Neuropsychiatric manifestations of depression, erratic behavior, and emotional outbursts often seriously handicap the patient before dementia or the movement disorder are severe. The advance of the disease is slow, with death on average occurring 15 to 20 years after onset of symptoms. Increasing disability from involuntary movements and mental changes result in death from intercurrent infection or, not rarely, by suicide.

Differential diagnosis There is no difficulty in the recognition of typical cases. The relatively late onset, the slowly progressive course, the prominent dementia, and lack of association with rheumatic fever help to exclude Sydenham's chorea. Patients with Parkinson's disease when overdosed with levodopa may develop a widespread chorea or choreoathetosis, and this, combined with the early dementia that occurs in some patients, can reproduce the picture of Huntington's disease. Phenothiazine drugs may induce generalized chorea, unassociated with dementia, and the movement disorder may persist for months or years after the medication is discontinued (tardive dyskinesia). Typically, tardive dyskinesia spares the forehead and does not impair gait in contrast to the findings in Huntington's disease. Finally, there is a form of self-limited chorea, which, like other localized dyskinesias, may appear in older persons without identifiable cause. Hepatolenticular degeneration (Wilson's disease) and nonfamilial forms of hepatocerebral degeneration may display clinical abnormalities resembling those of Huntington's disease, but the specific changes characteristic of these disorders, including liver disease, corneal Kayser-Fleischer rings (in Wilson's disease), and the typical biochemical abnormalities, are absent in Huntington's disease (see Chap. 330). Choreoathetosis appearing during the second postnatal year and lasting throughout life is due to hypoxic birth injury or kernicterus. Sporadic cases of choreiform movements beginning in middle or late life may present a difficult problem in exact diagnosis. The occasional cases of violent choreiform movements produced by vascular lesions, classically in the subthalamic region, are characterized by sudden onset, unilateral distribution (hemiballismus), and a tendency to improve after a period of initial severity. A few cases of acute choreoathetosis have accompanied hyperthyroidism. Virus encephalitis may occasionally be associated with choreiform movements; acute development, fever, and pleocytosis in the CSF help in recognition of such cases. Hereditary acanthocytosis is a rare condition which can mimic Huntington's disease.

Treatment No form of treatment has as yet been devised that halts the relentless progression of this disease, and therapeutic attempts to alleviate the abnormal movements have generally been unsatisfactory. Dopamine receptor antagonists (butyrophenones or phenothiazines) may partially ameliorate the chorea, but the side effects characteristic of this class of drugs limit their use. The depression, which is so common in many patients, usually responds to tricyclic antidepressants. The application of molecular genetic probes for presymptomatic and prenatal testing is available in several centers. However, until the gene itself is discovered, testing can only be performed in families by linkage analysis (see Chaps. 6 and 346).

MULTIPLE SYSTEM ATROPHY General experience has indicated that cases of multiple affection of neuronal systems may occur in which progressive dementia is combined with varying degrees of ataxia, dysarthria, and parkinsonian dyskinesia, depending upon the pattern of anatomic distribution of the pathologic changes. For cases of this kind, the general term *multiple system atrophy* or *degeneration* has been applied. In some, loss of neurons in the cerebellar cortex and in the pontine nuclei and inferior olivary nuclei results in the predominating picture of *olivopontocerebellar degeneration,* to be discussed below as one of the syndromes of progressive ataxia. These changes may be combined with similar neuronal loss in the substantia nigra (and in the striatum in striatonigral degeneration), resulting in parkinsonian features (discussed below under "Parkinson's Disease"). Pathologically, the disease process is characterized by death and disappearance of the affected cells and an accompanying reactive gliosis, without intracellular inclusions or other distinctive features. The cerebral cortex generally shows little discernible change, so that it may be difficult to ascribe a definite pathoanatomic basis for the dementia, which, for this reason, is sometimes designated as *subcortical.* Typically multiple system atrophy is a disorder of late adult life, occurring sporadically in some instances and genetically transmitted in others. Further details of individual syndromes are given in later sections.

PROGRESSIVE SUPRANUCLEAR PALSY (STEELE-RICHARDSON-OLSZEWSKI SYNDROME) This disorder is discussed below among the syndromes characterized by gradually developing abnormalities of posture and movement. It is mentioned here because progressive dementia may accompany the other neurologic abnormalities, although it appears late in the course and generally is not severe.

DIFFUSE LEWY BODY DISEASE Diffuse lewy body disease is a rare illness that presents with progressive dementia or psychosis. Parkinsonian signs, which may be absent or mild at the onset, eventually become common, and rigidity is usually severe. Tremor is often absent. Other features include involuntary movements, myoclonus, quadriparesis in flexion, orthostatic hypotension, and dysphagia in some cases. Lewy bodies are found profusely in the brainstem, basal forebrain, hypothalamic nuclei, and neocortex. The course of the illness is relentlessly progressive over several years.

CORTICODENTATONIGRAL DEGENERATION Corticodentatonigral degeneration with neuronal achromasia is a rare illness which has also been termed cortical-basal ganglionic degeneration. Watts and colleagues have studied seven cases. The illness begins at age 55–75 and the initial symptoms are loss of dexterity in one limb (usually an arm) combined with rigidity and often a tremor in the limb. The illness then progresses steadily over several months to involve the other limbs with rigidity, postural imbalance, and masked facies. Dyspraxia is a prominent clinical feature but dementia is usually mild or absent until late in the clinical course. The findings at autopsy are severe neuronal loss and gliosis in cerebral cortex which is greatest in the perirolandic regions and mild neuronal loss and gliosis in the substantia nigra. In cortical areas many of the pyramidal neurons are swollen with indistinct nuclei and poorly stained pale cytoplasm ("achromasia").

HALLERVORDEN-SPATZ DISEASE This unusual disorder, often affecting several siblings in a family in a manner suggesting an autosomal recessive trait, is associated with a rather variable clinical picture in which abnormalities of posture and muscle tone, involuntary movements, and progressive dementia predominate. Pathologically, there are characteristic abnormalities in the basal ganglia, suggesting a localized disorder of metabolism. The features of the condition were classically described in an affected family by Hallervorden and Spatz (1922).

Pathology Distinctive for this condition is the accumulation of large amounts of pigmented material in the globus pallidus and pars reticulata of the substantia nigra, resulting in grossly visible brownish discoloration of these regions. Microscopically, there are irregular pigmented, ferruginous concretions and granules of varying brownish or greenish hues, depending on the stains used. Although much of this pigment contains iron, serum iron and ferritin are normal, and there is no systemic disorder of iron metabolism. There also is loss of nerve cells. Another feature of the disease is the presence of focal swelling of axons, most probably in their terminal portions; this is especially pronounced in the regions affected by the pigmentary disorder, but typically can be found at all levels of the central nervous system, including the cerebral cortex. This neuroaxonal change may link the disease with childhood neuroaxonal dystrophy.

Clinical aspects The disorder typically makes its appearance in childhood or adolescence, with abnormalities in muscle tone and movements, such as rigidity and choreoathetosis. Abnormal postures of the trunk characteristic of torsion spasm (dystonia) may be seen, or the clinical picture may be reminiscent of parkinsonism. Cerebellar ataxia is also present in some instances. Speech becomes indistinct, and there is progressive intellectual impairment. Eventually, the involuntary movements give way to increasing generalized rigidity, and death comes as a rule about 10 years after onset. A few cases of late onset have shown a parkinsonian syndrome.

Differential diagnosis No feature of the clinical picture serves to distinguish this particular disorder from other conditions showing dementia with extrapyramidal motor abnormalities. Wilson's disease must be excluded by appropriate laboratory tests. The clearly progressive course sets this condition apart from clinically similar abnormalities resulting from accidents or illnesses at birth or in the neonatal period. It has lately been demonstrated that following intravenous injection of labeled ferrous citrate, there is a selective uptake of radioactive iron in the region of the basal ganglia; possibly a study of this kind would be helpful in diagnosis. In an advanced case, CT scanning may show extreme atrophy of the brain, especially including the structures of the basal ganglia, but the pigmented deposits do not show any increased radiographic density. In some cases there is lucency in the putamen and globus pallidus. MRI scans show a characteristic pattern of increased density in the globus pallidus surrounded by low density on T2-weighted images. This sign has been termed "eye of the tiger." At present no effective treatment is known. Treatment with a chelating agent, deferoxamine mesylate, has not shown definite benefit, and levodopa and other antiparkinsonian medications, tryptophan, and megavitamin therapy have been of only temporary and questionable help.

PROGRESSIVE FAMILIAL MYOCLONIC EPILEPSY There are several neurologic disorders that can result in a syndrome of convulsive seizures, myoclonic jerklike contractions of the musculature, and progressive dementia. Those most frequently encountered in practice are subacute sclerosing panencephalitis in children, adolescents, and young adults (Chap. 355), and subacute spongiform encephalopathy (Creutzfeldt-Jakob disease) in older adults (Chap. 355). The syndrome can also occur in some of the rare forms of metabolic familial disorders: neuraminidase deficiency associated with macular cherry-red spots (Chap. 331) and ceroid-lipofuscinosis (Chap. 338). When these and other disorders of known cause can be excluded from consideration, there remain some clinicopathologic entities which can appropriately be considered under the heading of the hereditary degenerative diseases. Several families presenting this syndrome have been carefully studied in northern Europe (Sweden and Finland), but there is no specific geographic distribution.

Lafora's disease This variety of recessively inherited progressive myoclonic epilepsy is characterized by distinctive intracytoplasmic inclusions in cerebral neurons, called Lafora bodies following their original description by Gonzalo Lafora (1911). These have been found to be composed of polymers of glucose (polyglucosans) and thus indicate a disorder of carbohydrate metabolism, but the biochemical defect that leads to their accumulation is unknown. The Lafora bodies are widely distributed, but most numerous in the thalamus, substantia nigra, and dentate nucleus of the cerebellum. Subsequent to Lafora's reports, similar polysaccharide deposits have been found in myocardial and skeletal muscle fibers, skin, and in the liver, and it is now possible to establish the diagnosis in the presymptomatic phase by skin or liver biopsy.

The disorder characteristically makes its appearance during childhood or adolescence in the form of recurrent seizures (generalized or restricted), or uncontrollable myoclonic jerks, or combinations of the two. With the passage of time, the myoclonic phenomena become increasingly severe, and there is deterioration of all intellectual functions. Death from intercurrent infection generally occurs before the age of 25. Anticonvulsive treatment may help in controlling the seizures, but there currently is no effective treatment for the underlying disease.

Unverricht-Lundborg disease This is a rare autosomal recessive illness with onset in adolescence of myoclonic and tonic-clonic seizures. Dementia is mild or absent at the outset, but eventually there is a gradual intellectual decline as well as dysarthria, ataxia, and intention tremor. Survival into adulthood is usual. Pathologic studies show widespread degenerative changes without evidence of storage material.

Other varieties of myoclonic epilepsy When Lafora's disease and the metabolic and infective disorders mentioned above have been excluded, there remains a rather heterogeneous group of progressive neurologic illnesses having in common autosomal recessive inheritance, myoclonic phenomena, convulsive seizures, and mild dementia. Ataxia of stance, gait, and limb movements is a prominent feature in most cases—so much so that the term introduced by Ramsay Hunt, *dyssynergia cerebellaris myoclonica,* is often applied. In a few cases, including some of those originally described by Hunt, there is an overlap with Friedreich's ataxia, or with chronic sensorimotor neuropathies (see Chaps. 361 and 363). The neuropathologic changes in the few cases that have come to postmortem examination have varied from case to case. In some, atrophy of the dentate nucleus and its fiber projections has been prominent; in others, there has been loss of neurons, especially Purkinje cells, in the cerebellar cortex; in still others, changes have been confined to long-tract degeneration (posterior columns and spinocerebellar tracts) in the spinal cord; a few patients have had cortical, basal-ganglionic, or retinal lesions. Variations also occur in the age of onset and the rate of progression. Until more is known about the biochemistry and genetics of this group of disorders, no satisfactory classification is possible. For further details of these syndromes, general reference works on neurology, such as that of Adams and Victor, should be consulted.

Treatment with appropriate anticonvulsant medications has been helpful in some mild cases, but phenytoin is contraindicated. L-Tryptophan and carbidopa or valproic acid have ameliorated myoclonus in a few cases.

SYNDROMES OF ABNORMAL POSTURE, TREMOR, AND INVOLUNTARY MOVEMENT

PARALYSIS AGITANS (PARKINSON'S DISEASE) This is a common condition first named and described by James Parkinson in 1817. His remarkably complete account gives this definition:

Involuntary tremulous motion, with lessened muscular power, in parts not in action and even when supported; with a propensity to bend the trunk forward, and to pass from a walking to a running pace, the senses and intellects being uninjured.

Typically, Parkinson's disease is a disorder of middle or late life, with very gradual progression and a prolonged course. Although it has been seen to occur in families (the estimated familial incidence is 1 to 2 percent), it usually is sporadic. It is well recognized, however, that the epidemic encephalitis of von Economo, which occurred in a worldwide distribution in the years following World War I, was followed by a syndrome clinically almost indistinguishable from paralysis agitans. It is usual in such instances to speak of postencephalitic parkinsonism, whereas the term *Parkinson's disease* should be reserved for true paralysis agitans of unknown cause. Parkinson's disease bears no consistent relation to any known disease process such as arteriosclerosis, trauma, or intoxication (except for MPTP, see below), although such conditions have often been invoked as etiologically significant and may at times produce somewhat similar clinical manifestations.

Pathology Despite the general medical familiarity with the condition and an extensive literature on the subject, it cannot be said that the pathologic changes of paralysis agitans are yet fully understood. The most regularly observed changes have been in the aggregates of melanin-containing nerve cells in the brainstem (substantia nigra, locus coeruleus), where there are varying degrees of nerve cell loss with reactive gliosis (most pronounced in the substantia nigra) along with distinctive eosinophilic intracytoplasmic inclusions (Lewy bodies). Similar changes are seen in the nucleus basalis of Meynert. Lesions in pigmented nuclei, but without Lewy bodies, characterize the pathologic findings in postencephalitic parkinsonism, in striatonigral degeneration, and in the Shy-Drager syndrome (discussed below).

Biochemical studies show a decrease of dopamine in the caudate nucleus and putamen, emphasizing the point that Parkinson's disease can be considered an example of neuronal system disease, involving mainly the nigrostriatal dopaminergic system. Confirmation of the importance of the nigrostriatal dopaminergic system arose from observations of the effects of accidental intoxication of drug users by self-injection with 1-methyl-4-phenyl-1,2,3,6-tetrahydropyridine (MPTP), which selectively destroys dopaminergic neurons of the substantia nigra. The typical clinical manifestations of this disease resemble closely those of Parkinson's disease. The pathologic features of MPTP-induced Parkinson's disease, however, differ from those of idiopathic cases in the absence of Lewy bodies and the lack of neuronal loss in the locus coeruleus, but the mechanism by which the drug kills substantia nigra neurons may provide new insights about the pathogenesis of the idiopathic illness.

Clinical apsects In its fully developed form, Parkinson's disease cannot be mistaken for any other. The stooped posture, the stiffness and slowness of movement, the fixity of facial expression, and the rhythmic tremor of the limbs, which subsides on active willed movement or complete relaxation, are familiar to every clinician. Although symmetric in the later stages, the disorder typically begins asymmetrically, e.g., as a slight tremor of the fingers of one hand or in one leg. Also typical are more or less general hypokinesia and stiffness of the musculature so that even where tremor is inapparent, the disease may betray itself by a somewhat staring and immobile facial expression, a monotonous voice, a general slowness and diminution of all motor activity, and a curious lack of the little spontaneous movements of postural adjustment that are so characteristic of the normal individual. When tremor is minimal, patients often are able to alleviate it by relaxation or by movement or to hide it by keeping their hands in their pockets. The tremor is generally most pronounced in the hands but may involve the legs (and thus secondarily the trunk), lips, tongue, and neck muscles, and is easily seen in the eyelids when they are lightly closed. Its frequency is 4 to 5 per second, but another faster (action) tremor (7 to 8 per second) predominates in some patients. There is never total paralysis, although this is implied by the name of the disease; nevertheless, general enfeeblement of voluntary movement is characteristic of the fully developed disorder. Generally accompanying the stooped attitude is the typical festinating gait, whereby the patient, prevented by the abnormality of postural tone from making the appropriate reflex adjustments required for effective walking, progresses with quick shuffling steps at an accelerating pace as if to catch up with the body's center of gravity. Clinical examination of the tendon and plantar reflexes discloses no abnormalities. There are no sensory changes, although deep aching in joints and muscles is common. Eventually, patients may become so incapacitated by rigidity and tremor as to be helpless in caring for themselves. It has often been observed, however, that even severely disabled patients may, when excited or under great emotional stress, perform complex motor acts quickly and efficiently. Although the temporary alleviation under extreme provocation can never be long maintained, it is nevertheless true that the severity of the symptoms is considerably influenced by emotional factors, being aggravated by anxiety, tension, and unhappiness, and minimal when the patient is in a contented frame of mind. Despite the inherently progressive nature of the condition, much can be achieved with good medical management, and patients may continue for years to live effective, happy lives.

Although intellectual deterioration is not a consistent feature of early Parkinson's disease, dementia has been increasingly recognized to be a feature of advanced Parkinson's disease. It eventually afflicts up to one-third of all cases. The dementia is typically insidious in onset and may be heralded by disorientation at night. In advanced cases patients may suffer from vivid auditory and visual hallucinations, often precipitated by levodopa therapy.

Differential diagnosis In typical cases, this is not difficult. The extrapyramidal syndromes associated with most diseases of known cause or established nature, such as cerebrovascular disease, cerebral hypoxia (including carbon monoxide asphyxia), or metallic poisoning, differ from paralysis agitans in a number of respects, such as atypical behavior or tremor, presence of signs of corticospinal tract deficit, or early onset of dementia. The differentiation from postencephalitic parkinsonism may be impossible; a clear history of an attack of epidemic encephalitis (prolonged somnolence, disturbance of consciousness, diplopia) and relatively early age of onset of the disorder and the presence of tics, localized spasms, and oculogyric crises may be the only clues to this diagnosis. A neurologic disorder similar to some degree to Parkinson's disease occurs with the prolonged administration of large amounts of reserpine and phenothiazine drugs, as the result of their blocking action on dopaminergic transmission. This drug-induced syndrome usually subsides on discontinuation or decrease in the dosage of the drug, but it may continue indefinitely in the syndrome of *tardive dyskinesia*. MPTP-induced parkinsonism persists because of the destructive effects of the drug on the nigral dopaminergic neurons. Parkinsonism very rarely is produced by cerebral neoplasms or other focal lesions, but then only when the nigrostriatal system has been largely destroyed, with relative sparing of the corticospinal projections.

Some Parkinson-like postural and motor abnormalities may be seen following the repeated blows to the head sustained by boxers—in the "punch drunk" syndrome, in which lesions of the substantia nigra are one of the neuropathologic components. In this condition, dementia, ataxia, dysarthria, and inappropriate behavior are prominent, and neuronal cell loss with neurofibrillary tangles is evident in the cerebral cortex.

Multiple bilateral infarcts in the corticospinal pathways and central structures of the brain may induce a syndrome that in some ways resembles paralysis agitans (so-called arteriosclerotic parkinsonism), but careful clinical assessment of the history and findings, particularly the reflex status, serves to distinguish this disorder from true Parkinson's disease. Striatonigral degeneration is a rare syndrome which can be clinically indistinguishable from Parkinson's disease but which does not respond to dopaminergic agents (see below). Progressive supranuclear palsy may also present as a parkinsonian syndrome; however, eventually the characteristic abnormalities of eye movement become manifest.

Treatment Although there is no treatment that is known to halt or reverse the neuronal degeneration that presumably underlies Parkinson's disease, methods are now available which can bring about a considerable degree of relief from symptoms in many patients. An important part of any therapeutic program is the maintenance of optimum general health and neuromuscular efficiency by planned programs of exercise, activity, and rest; expert physical therapy may be of great help in achieving these ends. In addition, the patient often needs much emotional support in meeting the stress of the illness, in comprehending its nature, and in carrying on courageously in spite of it. Along with these general supportive measures, which are applicable to many chronic illnesses, patients generally require a carefully thought-out program of treatment specifically aimed at counteracting the pathophysiologic disorder that produces their disabilities.

Drug therapy should be adapted to the patient's needs, which vary with the stage of the disease and the predominant manifestation(s). Usually anticholinergic drugs are most effective in suppressing tremor at rest, and propranolol or primidone is best for action tremor. Levodopa improves akinesia and postural imbalance; anticholinergic drugs have little effect on these two abnormalities.

The decision about whether to treat with a drug and the choice of drug(s) are influenced by the stage of the disease. The scale of Hoehn and Yahr is recommended:

Stage I: Unilateral involvement.
Stage II: Bilateral involvement but no postural abnormalities.
Stage III: Bilateral involvement with mild postural imbalance; the patient leads an independent life.
Stage IV: Bilateral involvement with postural instability; the patient requires substantial help.
Stage V: Severe, fully developed disease; the patient is restricted to bed and chair.

For patients with mild disease (stages I and II), no medication may be required, or only an anticholinergic drug, or amantadine (a dopamine agonist), or a combination of both. Levodopa is required for stages III, IV, and V. In each instance, one uses the lowest dose that gives satisfactory benefit; this decreases the chances of unwanted side effects such as dyskinesias, the on-off phenomenon, and mental confusion, as well as of loss of efficacy of the drug.

The anticholinergic drugs in use share the capacity to block muscarinic receptors and thereby to reduce cholinergic transmission. They are effective not only in relieving the rest tremor of mild Parkinson's disease but also may be combined with levodopa in the treatment of the severe forms of the disease. The anticholinergic drugs also reverse the dystonia and parkinsonian symptoms of neuroleptic drugs.

Currently available anticholinergic drugs are trihexyphenidyl, benztropine, biperiden, and procyclidine. The usual dose of trihexyphenidyl is 1 to 2 mg qid. Benztropine has both anticholinergic and antihistaminic properties; the usual dose is 0.5 to 1.0 mg tid. The optimal dose of all these medications varies for each patient and often needs adjusting. Low doses of these drugs cause dry mouth but few if any other side effects. Larger doses should be given with caution for in the elderly they may cause confusion, visual and tactile hallucinations, narrow-angle glaucoma, and urinary retention. Anticholinergic drugs may exacerbate dementia and should be withdrawn when dementia becomes clinically evident.

Propranolol, a beta-adrenergic antagonist, is helpful in suppressing the fast-frequency action tremor in Parkinson's disease and in the hereditary tremor syndrome. The usual dose is 40 to 80 mg tid. In large doses, it may slow the heart rate and lower blood pressure, which are disadvantages in patients with a tendency to orthostatic hypotension. Metoprolol, a specific beta-adrenergic antagonist, is also effective and is safer in patients with suspected asthma. Primidone in a dose of 50 mg at bedtime has also been shown to be effective. If the tremor is not improved after 1 week, the dose can be increased up to 250 mg daily. Many clinicians now initiate therapy with this regimen.

Amantadine was found by accident to be helpful in Parkinson's disease. Its effect is achieved by its capacity to release stored dopamine from presynaptic terminals; thus it is efficacious in the earlier stages of the disease, before the majority of the dopaminergic neurons in the midbrain have degenerated. It tends to be especially beneficial for tremor. The usual dosage is 100 mg bid; larger doses may produce side effects such as skin changes (livedo reticularis), ankle edema, and mental confusion. In some patients, the addition of amantadine to levodopa achieves better results than either medication alone.

Levodopa, which increases the dopamine levels in the striatum and restores neurotransmitter balance between dopamine and acetylcholine, improves akinesia and postural disorders (and sometimes rest tremor) in 75 percent of patients. Levodopa is now given in combination with a dopa-carboxylase inhibitor (carbidopa) which prevents destruction of levodopa in the bloodstream and peripheral tissues but does not pass the blood-brain barrier. This combination therefore makes it possible to achieve optimum effects with a smaller dosage of levodopa than would otherwise need to be used. In this way, some of the side effects of levodopa, particularly nausea and vomiting, can be greatly reduced. The combination (Sinemet) is available in ratios of 1:4 carbidopa to levodopa (25 mg/100 mg) or 1:10 (10/100, 25/250). A total dosage of levodopa from 300 to 2000 mg daily can be used; the relative amounts of carbidopa and levodopa, and the timing of the medications, should be adjusted according to the needs of the individual patient. Although levodopa now is the cornerstone of therapy, it can be combined with an anticholinergic drug, with amantadine, or with bromocriptine.

Bromocriptine is a dopamine agonist which acts directly upon dopamine receptors, unlike levodopa, which requires enzymatic transformation into dopamine within the brain. It has been found to be helpful in the treatment of Parkinson's disease, generally in combination with levodopa. When used alone, patients with mild early disease will often respond to doses of 15 to 30 mg daily. However, more advanced patients may need a dosage range of 50 to 100 mg daily. When given in combination with other drugs, smaller quantities should be used, beginning with 2.5 mg tid. Doses of bromocriptine ranging from 20 to 30 mg daily have been effective as an adjunct to levodopa therapy. Whether or not to use bromocriptine and the dosage are matters that must be decided on the basis of what seems best for an individual patient. The side effects are much the same as those with levodopa.

It must be said that although the modern treatment of Parkinson's disease is more successful than any that was available before the introduction of levodopa, including stereotactic surgery, there are still many problems. Underlying much of the difficulty undoubtedly is the fact that none of these therapeutic measures has an effect on the underlying disease process, which consists of neuronal degeneration. Ultimately a point seems to be reached where pharmacotherapy can no longer compensate for the loss. The major difficulties consist of fluctuations or sudden variations in the response to the drugs used (the on-off response), the development of weakness or immobility (akinesia), and dyskinesias, which increasingly become a problem as the years go by. The dyskinesias consist of choreiform or choreoathetotic movements, which in the late stages of the disease alternate with paralyzing akinesia depending upon a very narrow dosage variation (50 to 100 mg) of levodopa. Interference with absorption of levodopa may be partially responsible since continuous intravenous infusions of levodopa result in a stable clinical state. Loss of therapeutic efficacy also occurs: a single dose which at one time was effective for 5 to 6 h may last only an hour or so. Giving smaller amounts of medication more frequently is sometimes efficacious. In addition, agents acting directly on the postsynaptic receptor, such as bromocriptine, are sometimes more effective. It has recently been shown that temporary levodopa withdrawal, advocated as a method of dealing with the long-term complications of Parkinson's disease, carries some risk and does not result in improved efficacy of levodopa.

Progressive dementia, which eventually overtakes one-third to one-half of the patients in later years, may render them less tolerant to medication. Visual and tactile hallucinations are especially prominent in this group of patients.

As many as one-half of patients with Parkinson's disease have depressive symptoms. They should be treated along the lines suggested in Chap. 369.

The introduction of stereotaxic surgery, with the placement of precisely localized focal lesions in central structures in the brain—mainly the ventrolateral thalamus, or globus pallidus contralateral to the side of the major symptoms—was an important advance in the attempt to relieve the symptoms of Parkinson's disease. The success that has been achieved with levodopa has largely supplanted these procedures, which, although very beneficial in well-chosen cases, were not without risk and at times were followed by severe disability. Neurosurgical treatment of this kind can still be recommended for patients who are relatively young and who have a severe unilateral disabling or disfiguring tremor. Recent interest has focused on adrenal medullary transplants to the striatum. Although initial reports indicated favorable responses, subsequent experience in many centers has failed to confirm the earlier report. Fetal tissue transplants containing substantia nigra neurons may be more effective. Clinical trials indicate that deprenyl (a monoamine oxidase B inhibitor) can retard clinical progression of the disease.

STRIATONIGRAL DEGENERATION This rare syndrome closely resembles Parkinson's disease clinically, but clearly differs from it pathologically. The classic clinicopathologic description is that of Adams, van Bogaert, and Van der Eecken, who encountered the disorder in four middle-aged patients with no family history of similar disease. Three of the patients showed the typical clinical picture of Parkinson's disease; orthostatic hypotension was observed in one of them, and cerebellar ataxia in another.

The principal neuronal cell loss is in the striatum and substantia nigra. There is an association in some cases with a progressive ataxic disorder resembling olivopontocerebellar degeneration, and in others with degeneration of spinal cord neurons of the autonomic nervous system, similar to the Shy-Drager syndrome, in which postural hypotension is a major component (see below). The degree to which parkinsonian symptoms occur probably depends on the extent of the nigral lesions as balanced against those in the cerebellum and its connections. Cases of this kind represent examples of multiple system degeneration as described above.

The disorder characteristically occurs in late middle age. Treatment with anti-Parkinson's disease medications has usually not been successful. For measures which control hypotension see under "Shy-Drager Syndrome" (below and Chap. 21).

PROGRESSIVE SUPRANUCLEAR PALSY (STEELE-RICHARDSON-OLSZEWSKI SYNDROME) This disorder, first clearly described in 1963 by Richardson, Steele, and Olszewski, occurs in elderly individuals in approximately the same age period as paralysis agitans. Moreover, it is among the group of parkinsonian patients that most of the examples of this disease are to be found.

Pathology A loss of neurons and gliosis are found on postmortem examination in the tectum and tegmentum of the midbrain, the subthalamic nuclei of Luys, the vestibular nuclei, and to some extent the ocular nuclei. A characteristic finding is the presence of neurofibrillary tangles similar to those of Alzheimer's disease on light-microscopic examination, but differing from them on electron microscopy in that they are composed of straight rather than paired helical filaments. The cause of the disease is unknown. A slow virus has been suspected, but attempts to transfer it to monkeys by the intracerebral inoculation of brain tissue have failed.

Clinical manifestations The clinical features are quite distinctive: disturbances of balance and gait with unexpected falls; rigidity of the neck and other trunk muscles, resembling Parkinson's disease; "masking" of the face; reduction in the volume of the voice; extreme flexion or extension dystonia of the neck; and difficulty in looking down—all these are early symptoms and any one of them may first bring the patient to a physician. Ophthalmoplegia has been regarded as the cardinal clinical sign of the disease. Typically there is initial impairment of vertical saccadic movements and a loss of the fast component of optokinetic nystagmus usually affecting downward more than upward gaze. With progression of the disease horizontal eye movements are affected, with oculovestibular reflexes preserved. Symptoms progress over months and years, until the patient becomes virtually anarthric with total loss of voluntary control of eye movements, and severe cervical and truncal rigidity. Dementia is usually mild with forgetfulness, slowing of thought processes, apathy, and impaired ability to manipulate acquired knowledge. There are no impairments of vision, hearing, somatic sensation, or voluntary power, and signs of corticospinal involvement are minimal or absent. The diagnosis should be considered whenever an elderly patient begins to fall repeatedly and inexplicably and has extrapyramidal symptoms with a rigid neck and paralysis of conjugate or vertical gaze.

Treatment Treatment has been unsuccessful. Relatively little benefit comes from the administration of the antiparkinsonian group of drugs, although they should be tried. Occasionally levodopa, or a combination of levodopa with an anticholinergic drug, has helped to diminish some of the symptoms.

NORMAL-PRESSURE HYDROCEPHALUS Normal-pressure hydrocephalus (NPH) is a syndrome of communicating hydrocephalus in which intracranial hypertension is either absent or not recognized. It is discussed here because of the common association of the condition with dementia and abnormalities of gait.

Pathology and pathophysiology Although it is recognized that delayed hydrocephalus can occur after meningitis, head injury, or subarachnoid hemorrhage, the majority of patients presenting with NPH give no history of such an illness. Studies of isotope cisternography indicate that NPH is a communicating hydrocephalus presumed to be due to partial obliteration of the subarachnoid space with defective CSF reabsorption through the arachnoid villi. Whether episodes of increased intracranial pressure occur during the course of the illness is debated. Some patients monitored continuously show fluctuations in CSF pressure including so-called plateau waves.

Clinical manifestations Typically, the patient or family describe a subacute onset, over weeks, months, or sometimes years, of progressive intellectual deterioration accompanied by slowness and restriction of movements, particularly of gait. No single diagnostic gait disorder occurs (see description, Chap. 26). A broad-based stance with hesitant initiation of walking is common. In some patients ataxic features are present. Hyperreflexia in the legs and extensor plantar responses may be found. Urinary incontinence is noted in less than one-half of patients.

Differential diagnosis Parkinson's disease can be differentiated by its clinical features and the response to carbidopa-levodopa (Sinemet). Bifrontal disease due to tumor (butterfly glioma), metastases, or cerebral infarction can be identified by CT or MRI. Multi-infarct dementia with gait disórder can be recognized by focal, often asymmetric, neurologic signs and by CT changes. Aqueductal stenosis may present occasionally in late adulthood with hydrocephalus, headaches, dementia, and incontinence. The CT or MRI usually will demonstrate an enlarged third ventricle with normal fourth ventricle.

Treatment The diagnosis can be difficult because of the common association of ventricular enlargement and gait disorder in patients with degenerative brain conditions, particularly Alzheimer's disease. CSF pressure in NPH is usually in the normal range of 80 to 150 mmH_2O. Isotope cisternography demonstrating reflux into the ventricular system may be helpful in some cases. However, the finding of ventricular reflux has not proved to determine reliably which patients are likely to improve following a surgical shunt. Temporary benefit in the gait disorder after removal of 25 to 30 mL of CSF has been noted in some patients. When the history of dementia and gait disorder is subacute in onset and accompanied by considerable ventricular dilatation, surgical shunting is warranted. Ventricular-peritoneal shunting is the procedure most commonly performed. Between 40 and 70 percent of patients show benefit after surgery. The gait disorder tends to show a better response to shunting than the dementia (see Black et al. for review).

TORSION DYSTONIA (TORSION SPASM; DYSTONIA MUSCULORUM DEFORMANS) This is a syndrome of sustained muscular contraction frequently causing twisting and repetitive movements that result in abnormal, at times bizarre, postures of the limbs and trunk. Eventually these postures become more or less fixed. Underlying the clinical disorder may be any of several pathologic conditions, such as the lesions of neonatal hypoxia, Wilson's disease, the pigmented lesions of Hallervorden-Spatz disease (described above), GM_1 gangliosidosis, ataxia-telangiectasia, or kernicterus. There is, in addition, an important group of cases with a variable pattern of genetic transmission. Occasionally, a similar disorder occurs sporadically in late adult life. It is to these cases, both hereditary and sporadic, that the term *torsion dystonia* (torsion spasm, dystonia musculorum deformans) is correctly applied. In these conditions, the course tends to be progressive, and the cause and pathogenesis remain unknown. Genetic linkage studies have shown a positive correlation to markers on chromosome 9 and the mechanism is autosomal dominant inheritance.

Pathology Few cases of dystonia musculorum deformans not due to one of the definable disease processes indicated above have been adequately studied neuropathologically. Reported results from these cases has led to uncertainty as to what the pathologic-anatomic basis of the clinical state might be, although it was generally assumed that the basal ganglia were diseased. A careful study by Zeman and Dyken, which included comparison of the findings in patients with the disease with control material, failed to demonstrate any neuropathologic abnormality to which the clinical changes could reasonably be attributed. These negative findings, which are perhaps surprising, must not be interpreted as indicating that there is "no disease" in the brain, but rather that the pathologic state is not one that can be disclosed by the usual histopathologic techniques. It may well be that more careful quantitative assessments of certain populations of neurons and studies of the pathophysiology of neurotransmitters will result in further elucidation of this disease.

Clinical manifestations The motor abnormalities are described in Chap. 25. In the early stages, the involuntary muscular contractions are intermittent and variable in location and severity, but typically interfere with motor performance by superimposing an unwanted posture upon parts in use. One leg may briefly be pulled into a flexed or extended position or one shoulder elevated. Later the lingual, pharyngeal, neck, and thoracic muscles participate, and grimacing may occur. These latter may also be the first and only signs of disease for several years. Progression may be relatively rapid in cases with onset during early childhood, but is slow in those beginning in late childhood or adult life. The end result is extreme disability, with grossly distorted postures of the trunk and contractures of the limbs. Affection of face and tongue muscles results in faulty articulation of speech, which eventually becomes incomprehensible. The tendon and plantar reflexes are normal.

The most severe type, which occurs almost exclusively in Ashkenazi Jews, characteristically makes its appearance in childhood after a preceding period of normalcy. Typically it becomes first evident in the lower limbs and then evolves, sometimes relatively rapidly, into the generalized state of severe incapacity described above. The manner of genetic transmission—whether autosomal recessive or dominant with variable penetrance—is still not wholly settled. In the recognized autosomal dominant type, which occurs mainly in non-Jewish populations, the disorder comes on later (often in midadult life) and takes a milder form. It tends to appear first in the upper limbs and to remain more restricted in its extent than the early-onset variety, and progression is less relentless. The late-life sporadic cases are generally similar in character to those of the autosomal dominant form; here, the possibility of dominant transmission with incomplete penetrance cannot always be excluded.

FOCAL DYSTONIAS In addition to the generalized dystonias noted above, there is a group of focal or segmental dystonias which appear sporadically in adult life. Their clearly involuntary nature, and lack of susceptibility to willed control by the patient, distinguish them from the common tics, habit spasms, and mannerisms described in Chap. 25. They have often been erroneously interpreted as manifestations of hysteria. If the muscle contraction is frequent and prolonged, aching pain accompanies it—for which the spasm may mistakenly be blamed.

The most frequent and familiar type of focal dystonia is *spasmodic torticollis*. This is a disorder of adults that afflicts women somewhat more frequently than men. It consists of an involuntary turning of the head to one side—intermittent at first, then gradually worsening to the point of being more or less continuous. In some cases, torticollis is the first manifestation of a generalized dystonia, but more usually it remains focal and segmental.

Another frequent focal dystonia of adults is exemplified by *writer's cramp,* in which the dystonic postures and movements occur only during the performance of specific acts, to the extent that carrying out the act in the usual way, such as writing with a pen or pencil, becomes impossible, while other motor activities using the same musculature are unimpaired. An analogous disorder sometimes afflicts musicians.

The combination of blepharospasm and oromandibular dystonia—*cranial dystonia*—is sometimes referred to as Meige's syndrome. When the throat and respiratory muscles are involved, this interferes with speech production, resulting in spastic dysarthria. The muscles of the neck are variably affected. It should be recalled that similar dystonic states (facial-cervical and more extreme dyskinesias) can result from the use of phenothiazine and similar drugs. This sometimes persists after discontinuation of the medication as *tardive dyskinesia*—a troublesome condition that may resist all forms of treatment.

Differential diagnosis Hepatolenticular degeneration (Wilson's disease) should be seriously considered in any case presenting these motor symptoms and appropriate measures should be undertaken for its investigation (see Chap. 330). The progressive course, and possibly the family history, differentiate the degenerative group from the "symptomatic" dystonias resulting from infections or metabolic disorders occurring at birth or later. Hallervorden-Spatz disease, however, cannot be distinguished on clinical grounds alone. Rare instances of GM_1 gangliosidosis or other lipid storage diseases may begin in adult life with a dystonic syndrome, and drug-induced (tardive) dyskinesia must be considered in all cases of focal or generalized dystonia in adults, especially if they have or have had a psychiatric illness.

Treatment This is extremely difficult and often unsatisfactory. In the generalized dystonias, pharmacotherapy should certainly be attempted and, in most patients, needs to be individualized. Marsden and Fahn, whose experience with this disorder is extensive, suggest beginning with an anticholinergic agent such as trihexyphenidyl or ethopropazine and very gradually increasing the dosage until either benefit ensues or intolerable side effects appear. They found that the response in children (who may be able to take as much as 80 mg/d of trihexyphenidyl) was better than in adults, who tolerated the high doses less well, generally because of mental disturbances. In their experience, the next best group of drugs for ameliorating dystonic spasms are the benzodiazepines (such as diazepam) which likewise are used in high dosage after a very gradual introduction and increase (up to 80 mg of diazepam daily). Again, children are more tolerant of the side effects (mainly drowsiness). A combination of anticholinergics and benzodiazepines may work out best. Other drugs—both dopaminergic agonists and antagonists—have been used, occasionally with success.

Stereotaxic surgical operations have been used in the past to treat generalized dystonias, with insufficient benefit to counterbalance the risks. Cervical cord stimulation, a less hazardous procedure, has helped some patients; referral to a neurosurgeon with experience in the technique should be considered when medical treatment has failed.

The symptoms of the focal dystonias, if not severe, may be more acceptable to the patient than prolonged trials with various drugs or surgical intervention. Biofeedback techniques are sometimes helpful. Denervative surgical procedures may at times be beneficial if only a very restricted group of muscles is involved (as in torticollis). Blepharospasm has recently been successfully treated temporarily with local injection of botulinum toxin into the orbicularis oculi muscles. Beneficial effects last on average for 10 to 12 weeks. Neuroleptics (dopamine-antagonists) such as haloperidol or perphenazine may be useful in the treatment of focal dystonias. Here again, the program of management must be adapted to the individual patient's needs.

FAMILIAL TREMOR One of the commonest hereditary disorders of the human nervous system is that which gives rise to a fast-frequency (6 to 8 per second) action tremor. This may appear at any age but more often during adolescence and adult years; once started, it lasts throughout life. The heredity is dominant. Probably all cases are not the same, for some patients have tremors of slower frequency, looking more like those of Parkinson's disease, but lacking the slowness of movement, rigidity, and flexed postures of that disorder. In patients of advanced age it is called *senile tremor*. Consumption of alcohol suppresses the fast-frequency forms, as does a beta-adrenergic blocking agent (propranolol) in doses of 20 to 40 mg three times daily. The slightly slower rhythmic action tremors with frequencies of approximately 6 per second do not consistently respond to propranolol or alcohol. Primidone 50 mg at bedtime has recently been found to be effective and has been advocated for use as initial therapy. If there is no response after 1 week the dose should be increased gradually up to 250 mg at bedtime. Usually the tremor is the only abnormality, but in a few patients a cerebellar ataxia or an extrapyramidal syndrome may appear years later. The pathologic basis is unknown.

GILLES DE LA TOURETTE SYDROME This condition, of unknown cause and uncertain pathology, presents with multiple tics, associated with snorting, sniffing, and involuntary vocalizations. It begins in childhood, usually as isolated tics, which are at first difficult to distinguish from habit spasms. Progression occurs over years, and other behavioral findings appear; compulsive touching of others, repeating of words or phrases, and explosive utterance of obscenities (coprolalia). Careful attention to other members of the family has given evidence that the disease is hereditary, with an autosomal dominant pattern of transmission. Obsessive compulsive disorder appears to be an alternate phenotypic expression of the gene in these families.

The course of the illness is unpredictable. In some cases associated mild neurologic abnormalities are found with hyperactivity, disorders of attention, and abnormal psychologic tests. Dementia does not occur. In some patients the condition abates, in others it progresses, leading to serious disability. Treatment is only partially satisfactory. Haloperidol has received the most clinical attention, but should be used only in severe cases, and in the smallest effective dosage: 0.25 to 0.5 mg daily. Clonidine has proved effective in some cases.

SYNDROMES OF SLOWLY DEVELOPING ATAXIA

These conditions are distinguished clinically by progressive unsteadiness in standing and walking, along with impaired coordination of the limbs. Pathologically, they are characterized by degeneration of the cerebellum and/or its related fiber systems, and thus constitute classic examples of the system diseases. Although sporadic instances occur, hereditary transmission is an outstanding feature in most cases; as a result, this group of disorders is often referred to as the *hereditary ataxias*. Their subdivision into more or less separate entities is largely arbitrary, with pathologic changes of varying distribution underlying clinically indistinguishable symptom complexes. As yet, not enough is known about the underlying basis for the pathophysiologic alterations for a more satisfactory classification to be established.

Attempts to establish a classification on a genetic basis, on the presumption that a defective gene expressed as a progressive ataxia would produce a distinctive clinicopathologic picture, have not been successful. Instead, the phenotypic expression of the genetic abnormality commonly varies widely among affected members of an individual family. Because of these difficulties, the most that a clinician can do when confronted with a case is to exclude infective, toxic, metabolic, or neoplastic diseases for which there might be effective treatment, to search for evidence of genetic factors, and to assess the state of the patient as precisely as possible. There are now indications that some of the hereditary ataxic disorders may be associated with an identifiable biochemical abnormality though at present it is not possible to make use of this information in a way that would correct the abnormality and benefit the individual patient.

Nevertheless, if one takes a broad view of the whole group of hereditary ataxias, it turns out that there are certain clinicopathologic groupings that allow a very simplified descriptive classification. According to this principle, three main categories may be emphasized: (1) *cerebellar cortical degeneration*, (2) *olivopontocerebellar atrophy*, and (3) *spinocerebellar degenerations*, including *Friedreich's ataxia*.

CEREBELLAR CORTICAL DEGENERATION In this disorder, the principal neuropathologic feature is loss of neurons (mainly of Purkinje cells) in the cerebellar cortex. Cases of this kind characteristically occur in late adult life. Although the condition can occur sporadically, in the majority it is inherited as an autosomal dominant trait.

Pathology The loss of Purkinje cells tends to be most severe in the superior vermis and adjacent parts of the cerebellar cortex, but can be more extensive. The granule neurons are less affected. In long-standing cases, there is an associated atrophy of neurons in the olivary nuclei of the medulla, apparently representing a transsynaptic retrograde degeneration resulting from the loss of Purkinje cells, to which the olivocerebellar fibers project. In advanced cases atrophy of the cerebellar cortex can be readily demonstrated by CT scanning. In the purest forms of this disorder, as exemplified by the cases of late onset, slow progression, and dominant inheritance, other neuronal systems remain relatively intact.

Clinical manifestations Incoordination first appears in the legs, resulting in abnormal stance and an unsteadiness of gait of a wavering, lurching character typical of cerebellar ataxia (see Chap. 26). This gait disturbance is a consequence of degenerative changes in the superior vermis of the cerebellum and adjacent parts of the cerebellar cortex. With more extensive cerebellar involvement, a disturbance in articulation and rhythm of speech occurs and the arms become ataxic. There may be nystagmus. The illness progresses gradually, often extending over two or three decades, without appreciably curtailing the life span. Dementia tends to be mild or a late feature of this circumscribed cerebellar atrophy of late life. However, cerebellar cortical degeneration with very similar features may occur as a component in many of the ataxic disorders.

In addition to this slowly evolving, relatively circumscribed form of cerebellar cortical degeneration, there is a subacutely developing diffuse cerebellar cortical degeneration that affects all parts of the cerebellar cortex indiscriminately, often in association with some inflammatory changes. This disorder occurs in the presence of malignant neoplastic diseases of various kinds and is referred to as *carcinomatous cerebellar degeneration* (see Chap. 310). It is now apparent that this is one of a number of interrelated neurologic degenerative syndromes that occur on the background of malignant disease but do not result from any direct effect of the neoplasm on the nervous system such as invasion or metastasis. These so-called paraneoplastic disorders are etiologically unclarified; an immunologic or viral attack on neural structures has been postulated, but never proven. Paraneoplastic cerebellar degeneration produces a striking clinicopathologic syndrome that tends to stand out as a particular entity (see Chap. 310).

OLIVOPONTOCEREBELLAR ATROPHY (OPCA) Grouped under this category are a number of similar disorders characterized by a combination of cerebellar cortical degeneration, atrophy of the inferior olivary nuclei secondary to this, and degeneration and disappearance of the neurons of the pontine nuclei and their fiber projections in the basis pontis and middle cerebellar peduncles. Konigsmark and Weiner distinguished five varieties on the basis of differences in the form of hereditary transmission and in the extent of other abnormalities both within and outside of the nervous system. Most instances of OPCA can now be considered to represent various forms of multiple system degeneration in which admixtures of parkinsonism, dementia, spasticity, choreoathetosis, retinal degeneration, myelopathy, and peripheral neuropathy may be encountered, sometimes obscuring the ataxic component. For present-day views of the classification of OPCA and the features of the various forms of disease brought under this heading, the monograph edited by Duvoisin and Plaitakis may be usefully consulted. The introduction of the new techniques of imaging—CT and MRI—now make it possible to visualize clearly the pontocerebellar lesions and some of the other atrophic changes in the central nervous system.

Autosomal dominant inheritance is characteristic in many families—most notably the Schut family, on which information extending over five generations has been obtained. Genetic linkage has shown localization to chromosome 6 in this family. Families of Portuguese ancestry, mainly from the Azores, who manifest the various syndromes that have been brought together under the heading of Joseph's disease have also been extensively studied. These families illustrate with striking clarity the varied phenotypic expression of what may turn out to be a single genetic abnormality.

Recessively transmitted OPCA has on the whole been less distinctly established than the dominant (or sporadic) forms, but of particular interest is a group of families with an autosomal recessive disorder and late-adult onset of neurologic symptoms, in whom the disease is characterized by multiple system degeneration, including a prominent OPCA component, and in which deficiency of glutamic acid dehydrogenase has been demonstrated in leukocytes and cultured fibroblasts from affected family members. Glutamate, among its other functions, acts as an excitatory neurotransmitter and is involved in the excitatory input to the Purkinje cells from the granule cells of the cerebellar cortex. In excess, this transmitter has neurotoxic effects, which might be the basis of the Purkinje cell degeneration that is so prominent in OPCA. These observations, and other biochemical leads that have opened up in connection with some of the dominant forms of OPCA, suggest a promising field of research that may give new etiologic and pathophysiologic insights into a wide group of neuronal degenerative diseases and may ultimately suggest avenues for therapeutic approach.

Pathology OPCA and the disorders related to it exemplify clearly the phenomenon of selective premature neuronal death, and of affection of particular, vulnerable neuronal systems with sparing of others. The distribution of neuronal lesions that characterizes OPCA as distinct from other neuronal system degenerations has already been indicated. The neuronal changes are in no way distinctive or specific in OPCA. Rather, it is the particular location of the neuronal loss that determines the clinicopathologic picture. Still not fully clarified in this group of disorders is what determines the dementia that so often accompanies them. It has been generally assumed that abnormalities occur in the cerebral cortex, but examination of the cortex in typical cases discloses insufficient abnormality to account for the cognitive and behavioral alterations. On the other hand, the lesions of the cerebellum and related systems provide a reasonable explanation for the incoordination (ataxia) that is observed; the lesions in the basal ganglia and substantia nigra (equivalent to striatonigral degeneration) underlie the features of parkinsonism and of other postural and movement disorders that are so frequently seen as manifestations of OPCA; and involvement of the peripheral motor neurons, similar to what occurs in the motor neuron disease group to be discussed later, produces the severe muscular weakness and atrophy that may be encountered. The disturbances of ocular motility that typify some cases still are in need of further anatomic elucidation.

Clinical manifestations There is great clinical variation among cases of OPCA. Some present a picture of a relatively pure cerebellar ataxia indistinguishable from that seen in cases with atrophy of the cerebellar cortex (and secondarily of the inferior olivary nuclei) alone. Others are characterized by parkinsonian features. Superimposed is an evolving dementia. For accounts of these varied forms of clinical expression, general neurologic reference works and specialized monographs (such as that edited by Duvoisin and Plaitakis) should be consulted.

SPINOCEREBELLAR DEGENERATIONS (FRIEDREICH'S ATAXIA) This group of ataxic disorders is characterized by degeneration of long ascending and descending fiber systems in the spinal cord, including the spinocerebellar tracts, and concomitant degeneration of peripheral axons and myelin sheaths in the form of chronic peripheral neuronopathy.

The classic form of hereditary ataxia, first clearly depicted by Nikolaus Friedreich of Heidelberg in 1863, constitutes a relatively distinct symptom complex which generally runs true to form, although it overlaps other heredodegenerative syndromes, particularly other types of spinocerebellar atrophy. In some families, the disorder occurs with dominant inheritance; usually it is a recessive trait. Recent studies have linked the recessive form of the disease to chromosome 9.

Pathology The principal changes are cell loss in the dorsal root ganglia and secondary degeneration in the posterior columns and spinocerebellar tracts of the cord and in the peripheral nerves. Degeneration is also evident in the corticospinal tracts in most cases. The cerebellum is variably affected. In addition to these neuropathologic changes there is in some cases a peculiar form of myocardial degeneration resulting in fiber loss and fibrosis. There are no other associated visceral lesions.

Clinical manifestations As with other progressive ataxias, the disorder first appears in the legs, affecting the individual during late childhood. The patient, previously healthy, begins to stagger and lurch in walking and is unsteady on standing. Clumsiness and cerebellar tremor of the hands and arms appear later along with dysarthria and abnormal rhythm (scanning) of speech. These symptoms result from changes in the dorsal root ganglia, the spinocerebellar tracts, and cerebellum; it is not easy to ascertain the relative contribution of lesions in each structure to the ataxia. The limbs, in addition to being ataxic, generally show considerable weakness. Examination usually discloses nystagmus and skeletal deformities: kyphoscoliosis, the basis of which is not certain, and a peculiar foreshortening of the feet (pes cavus) with cocking of the toes, best ascribed to atrophy and contractures of the musculature of the feet at a time when the bones of the feet are malleable. Typically, there is the unusual combination of total absence of tendon reflexes with extensor plantar reflexes (Babinski sign). This results from the presence of degeneration of the corticospinal tracts together with the involvement of peripheral sensory neurons that relay afferent signals from muscle spindles. Impairment of position and vibration sense in the extremities is prominent and, in some patients, sensation of pain, temperature, and light touch is diminished in a distal and roughly symmetric distribution consistent with an axononeuropathy affecting small nerve fibers. Mentation is usually preserved, though a few of the patients have been of low intelligence or have become demented late in the course of the disease. Survival beyond early adult life is rare, with death frequently the result of associated cardiomyopathy.

Occasionally very mild or fragmentary forms of the disorder (such as pes cavus and absent or hyperactive tendon reflexes) may be encountered with little, if any, disability or progression. Such abnormalities are most likely to be seen in other members of the family of a patient afflicted with the fully developed form of the disease. A related syndrome, the Roussy-Lévy syndrome, shows similarities to Friedreich's ataxia and to peroneal muscular atrophy. Mild ataxia, pes cavus, absent ankle and knee tendon jerks, and atrophy of lower leg muscles occur. In some well-documented cases the peripheral nerves show hypertrophy due to proliferation of Schwann cells (see Chap. 363). Chronic familial polyneuropathies are particularly difficult to distinguish since they also give rise to sensory ataxia, but signs of pyramidal tract disease are absent (see Chap. 363). Hereditary forms of cerebellar ataxia with corticospinal signs (hyperactive tendon reflexes) and sensory disturbances are also known to occur in the adolescent or adult. Familial spastic paraplegia with or without optic atrophy (Behr's syndrome) is another closely related disease. In the absence of a family history, and with atypical clinical findings, further diagnostic studies to exclude congenital malformation, spinal cord compression, foramen magnum tumor, and multiple sclerosis will be necessary.

No treatment is of proven value. Earlier reports of disturbed pyruvate metabolism have not been confirmed.

DIFFERENTIAL DIAGNOSIS OF THE ATAXIAS The slow but relentless progression in the absence of abnormalities in other parts of the nervous system and in the CSF distinguishes the hereditary group from other diseases and other forms of cerebellar ataxia such as may occur with hereditary metabolic diseases, or with neoplastic, infectious, or demyelinative disease, or with drug intoxications (e.g., phenytoin) or with hyperpyrexia. The degenerative disorders under discussion tend to develop slowly over many years in a setting of otherwise good general health, and in the absence of other neurologic symptoms and signs; this, together with the other clinical differences, distinguishes them from such hereditary metabolic diseases as juvenile Gaucher's disease, juvenile Niemann-Pick disease, and juvenile hexosaminidase deficiency and from alcoholic cerebellar ataxia or nutritional deficiency disease, with or without Wernicke-Korsakoff syndrome. Alcoholic cerebellar degeneration usually develops over a few days to weeks, and then may remain more or less unchanged for the remainder of the patient's life (Chap. 357). A prolonged deficiency of vitamin E can result in progressive ataxia, incoordination of the limbs, areflexia, and distal loss of proprioception and vibratory sense, mimicking spinocerebellar degeneration. Most cases are associated with fat malabsorption

In the cases associated with carcinoma, the tempo of evolution of the process is relatively rapid, with severe disability coming on within a period of months. Vertigo, diplopia, and nausea may be prominent. In an occasional patient, the neurologic symptoms have appeared before there was any obvious evidence of carcinoma. Opsoclonus (rapid side-to-side jerking of the eyes) and oscillopsia (movement back and forth of objects seen) may be conjoined. In contrast to the consistently normal CSF findings in the forms of cerebellar degeneration noted above, the CSF in paraneoplastic degeneration may show increased lymphocytes and protein.

TREATMENT No specific treatment is available for any of the progressive ataxias, although encouragement to remain active is beneficial to health in general. Gait training is of relatively little value in enabling patients to compensate for their disability. In cases where parkinsonian features are prominent, antiparkinsonian medications should be tried (see above), but the response in the group of multiple system degenerations is generally unsatisfactory. Trauner has reported that baclofen in high dosage may help control involuntary movements in some cases of OPCA, but the ataxia is not benefited.

IDIOPATHIC AUTONOMIC FAILURE (IDIOPATHIC ORTHOSTATIC HYPOTENSION, SHY-DRAGER SYNDROME)

Abnormalities of central autonomic nervous system functions manifest principally by failure to maintain blood pressure and by urinary incontinence are now recognized to be caused in some cases by a progressive degenerative disorder of the CNS that affects several systems; in some patients the peripheral nervous system is also involved (postganglionic sympathetic neurons). Bradbury and Eggleston in 1925 called attention to the combination of postural hypotension, incontinence, impotence, and abnormality of sweating (anhidrosis). Symptoms of central neurologic origin develop later in many of these patients consisting predominantly of extrapyramidal or cerebellar dysfunction.

PATHOGENESIS AND PATHOLOGY The cause of the disorder is unknown. In 1960 Shy and Drager described neuropathologic changes in the brainstem and basal ganglia, and subsequently others showed a prominent loss of neurons in central regions of the autonomic nervous system, affecting in particular the cells of the intermediolateral column of the thoracic spinal cord. Abnormalities have also been found in peripheral autonomic ganglia (cell loss). In the brainstem and basal ganglia there is widespread symmetric neuronal degeneration affecting the caudate nucleus, substantia nigra, locus coeruleus, olivary nuclei, dorsal vagal nuclei, and in some cases affecting the cerebellum. Cell loss is accompanied by gliosis; Lewy bodies typical of Parkinson's disease are present in some cases. For these reasons many neurologists consider the Shy-Drager syndrome to be a unique form of multisystem degeneration resembling but distinct from either Parkinson's disease or OPCA.

Clinical manifestations The onset is insidious, usually in the sixth or seventh decade. Men are more frequently affected than women. Disturbances of urinary bladder function, including hesitancy and incontinence, postural dizziness and syncope, impotence, and decreased sweating are the presenting manifestations. Later symptoms of extrapyramidal dysfunction resembling parkinsonism or cerebellar findings may emerge. The condition becomes severely disabling over the course of 5 to 7 years in most patients. The hallmark of the condition is postural hypotension, defined as a fall in blood pressure greater than 30/20 mmHg on standing upright from a supine position (see Chap. 21). Despite this fall in blood pressure there is usually a total failure of compensatory tachycardia, the pulse rate remaining unchanged. Autonomic signs of pupillary asymmetry, partial Horner's syndrome, or partial parasympathetic denervation occur in some patients. Anhidrosis is common and can be demonstrated by placing the individual in a warm room after application of a starch-iodine mixture to the skin. The parkinsonian manifestations may be identical to those of idiopathic parkinsonism, although in many patients rigidity and bradykinesia are more prominent than tremor. Cerebellar gait ataxia and mild limb ataxia may be evident. Other findings include laryngeal paralysis and sleep apnea.

Treatment The treatment is symptomatic. The postural hypotension is usually the most disabling initial symptom. Antigravity stockings to minimize pooling of venous blood in the legs are recommended. A leotard that covers the lower abdomen may provide additional benefit. Pharmacologic agents are given to expand blood volume and to enhance vascular responsivity. Increased NaCl intake combined with fludrohydrocortisone 0.05 to 0.2 mg twice daily is usually beneficial (see Chap. 21). In severe cases, adrenergic drugs such as ephedrine, levodopa, or amphetamine may improve the disability. The parkinsonism symptoms often respond initially to Sinemet or bromocriptine, but later in the course most patients become refractory to these agents. Centrally acting alpha agonists (e.g., yohimbine or clonidine) may also be beneficial.

SYNDROMES OF MUSCULAR WEAKNESS AND WASTING WITHOUT SENSORY CHANGES: MOTOR NEURON DISEASE

AMYOTROPHIC LATERAL SCLEROSIS (ALS) ALS is the most frequently encountered form of progressive motor neuron disease, and it presents a clinical syndrome that is generally familiar to physicians who see patients with neurologic diseases. It is characteristically a disorder of late middle age. Most patients are older than 50 when symptoms begin. The disease rarely develops before the third decade, and patients whose symptoms begin in the late teenage years often seem to have an inherited variant of the disorder. Men are more frequently affected than women. Because of its restriction to motor neurons of the central nervous system, ALS represents another prime example of a neuronal system disease. It occurs sporadically in most instances. Familial occurrence, with transmission as an autosomal dominant trait, is observed in about 10 percent of cases and differs in some clinical and pathologic aspects (Table 359-2).

TABLE 359-2 Categories of degenerative motor neuron diseases

I Amyotrophic lateral sclerosis
- *A* Spinal muscular atrophy
- *B* Bulbar palsy
- *C* Primary lateral sclerosis
- *D* Pseudobulbar palsy

II Heritable motor neuron diseases
- *A* Autosomal recessive spinal muscular atrophy (SMA)
  - *1* Type I: Werdnig-Hoffmann, acute
  - *2* Type II: Werdnig-Hoffmann, chronic
  - *3* Type III: Kugelberg-Welander
  - *4* Type IV: Adult onset
- *B* Familial amyotrophic lateral sclerosis
- *C* Other
  - *1* Arthrogryposis multiplex congenita
  - *2* Progressive juvenile bulbar palsy (Fazio-Londe)
  - *3* Neuroaxonal dystrophy

III Associated with other degenerative disorders
- *1* Olivopontocerebellar atrophies
- *2* Peroneal muscular atrophy

Pathology The disease is characterized by progressive loss of motor neurons, both in the cerebral cortex and in the anterior horns of the spinal cord, together with their homologues in some motor nuclei of the brainstem. It typically affects both upper and lower motor neurons, although variants may predominantly involve only particular subsets of motor neurons, particularly early in the course of the illness. Thus, in bulbar palsy and spinal muscular atrophy (or progressive muscular atrophy) the lower motor neurons of brainstem and spinal cord, respectively, are most severely involved while pseudobulbar palsy and primary lateral sclerosis affect upper motor neurons innervating the brainstem and spinal cord. The loss of motor neurons is not accompanied by any distinctive or unique cytopathologic features. The affected cells undergo shrinkage, often with some excessive accumulation of the pigmented lipid (lipofuscin) that normally develops in these cells with advancing age, and they eventually disappear. Focal enlargement of proximal motor axons is frequently seen; ultrastructurally, these "spheroids" are composed of accumulations of neurofilaments. Beyond some astroglial proliferation, which is the inevitable accompaniment of all disintegrative processes in the central nervous system, the interstitial and supportive tissues and the macrophage system remain largely inactive, and there is no inflammation. The death of the peripheral motor neurons in the brainstem and spinal cord leads to denervation and consequent atrophy of the corresponding muscle fibers. Histochemical and electrophysiologic evidence indicate that in the early phases of the illness denervated muscle can be reinnervated by sprouting of nearby distal motor nerve terminals, although reinnervation in this disease is considerably less extensive than in most other disorders affecting motor neurons (e.g., poliomyelitis, peripheral neuropathy). As denervation progresses, there is shrinkage of the musculature and a fiber atrophy that is readily recognized in muscle biopsies. It is this muscular atrophy that is designated by the term *amyotrophy,* which appears in the common name for the disease. The loss of motor neurons in the cortex results in disappearance of the long axons and their myelin sheaths that make up the corticospinal tracts, which travel via the internal capsule and extend through the brainstem, including the pyramids of the medulla oblongata, to the lateral (and a portion of the anterior) white matter columns of the spinal cord. The loss of fibers in the lateral columns, together with the fibrillary gliosis which imparts a particular firmness (sclerosis) to the affected tissues, makes up the lateral sclerosis component of the disease. The fact that the nerve fiber loss is more extensive in the distal parts of the affected tracts in the lower spinal cord rather than the more proximal parts, such as the internal capsule, suggests that the affected neurons first undergo disintegration at their distal terminals and the disease process proceeds in a centripetal direction until ultimately the parent cell body dies, a phenomenon referred to as "dying back." The disease clearly affects the large pyramidal neurons (Betz cells) of the motor cortex in the precentral gyrus, but in some cases the extent of degeneration in the long projection pathways provides evidence that many other neurons involved in voluntary movement, both in the cortex and in subcortical nuclei, are also affected.

A remarkable feature of the disease is the selectivity of neuronal cell death. The entire sensory apparatus, the regulatory mechanisms for the control and coordination of movement, and the components of the brain that are needed for intellect and thinking, remain intact. There is also some consistent selectivity in motor system involvement. The motor neurons required for ocular motility remain unaffected as do the parasympathetic neurons in the sacral spinal cord (the nucleus of Onufrowicz, or Onuf) which innervate the sphincters of the bowel and bladder.

Clinical manifestations The first evidence of the disease is manifest as insidiously developing asymmetric weakness, usually first apparent in one of the limbs. Fatigue and easy cramping of affected muscles can be prominent. The weakness is accompanied by visible wasting and atrophy of the muscles involved; particularly in the early stages of the disease, affected muscles may display focal twitchings—fasciculations—when not concealed by overlying adipose tissue. Virtually any muscle group may be the first to show signs of the disease, but as time passes, more and more muscles become involved until ultimately the disorder takes on a symmetric distribution in all regions, including the muscles of chewing, swallowing, and movements of the face and tongue. Early involvement of the muscles of respiration may lead to death before the disease is far advanced elsewhere; otherwise the disorder generally is terminated by pulmonary infection secondary to the profound generalized weakness.

The corticospinal component of the disease becomes apparent in the form of hyperactivity of the muscle-stretch reflexes (tendon jerks) and, often, spastic resistance to passive movements of the affected limbs. With corticospinal involvement the plantar reflex will be upgoing (the Babinski sign) until—as often occurs—lower motor neuron dysfunction in the legs advances sufficiently that extensor movement of the great toes is impossible. The disease process in the corticobulbar projections innervating the brainstem results in dysarthria and exaggeration of the motor expressions of emotion leading to involuntary weeping or laughter (so-called pseudobulbar affect), or strange admixtures of both. Ocular motility is spared, even when other brainstem functions are greatly impaired. Throughout the evolution of the disease, awareness and intellectual abilities typically remain intact. Dementia is not usually a component of ALS; when it occurs, it is due to the superimposition of another disease process.

The course is relentlessly progressive and leads ultimately to death, but the total duration of the illness is variable. In recent studies approximately 50 percent of patients can be expected to die within 3 to 5 years from the onset of the disease; some may live considerably longer. Very rarely, what seems to be ALS may become stabilized, or even regress to the point of recovery.

Differential diagnosis Because the underlying process in ALS is currently untreatable, it is imperative that potentially remediable causes of motor neuron dysfunction be excluded (see Table 359-3), particularly in atypical cases. Compression of the cervical cord or cervicomedullary junction from tumors in the cervical region or at the foramen magnum, or from cervical spondylosis with osteophytes projecting into the vertebral canal, can at times give rise to weakness, wasting, and fasciculations in the upper limbs and spasticity in the legs, thus closely resembling ALS. The absence of cranial nerve involvement may be helpful in differentiation, although some compressive lesions in the foramen magnum may implicate the twelfth cranial (hypoglossal) nerve, with resulting affection of the tongue. Absence of pain or of sensory changes, normal function of bowels and bladder, normal roentgenographic studies of the spine, and absence of changes in the composition or dynamics of the cerebrospinal fluid are all points in favor of ALS against spinal cord compression. Where doubt exists, MRI scans and contrast myelography should be performed in order to visualize the cervical spinal cord.

TABLE 359-3 Etiology and investigation of secondary motor neuron disorders

Diagnostic categories	Investigations
I Structural lesions	
A Parasagittal or foramen magnum tumors	MRI/CT scan—head, spine including foramen magnum
B Cervical spondylosis	MRI/CT scan or myelogram
C Chiari malformation or syrinx	
D Spinal cord arteriovenous malformation	
II Infections	
A Bacterial—tetanus	CSF exam
B Viral—poliomyelitis, herpes zoster	Antibody titers
III Intoxications, physical agents	
A Toxins—lead, aluminum, other metals	24-h urine for lead, mercury arsenic, thallium, aluminum
B Drugs—strychnine, phenytoin, dapsone	
C Electric shock	
D X-irradiation	Serum lead and aluminum
IV Immunologic mechanisms	
A Plasma cell dyscrasias	Complete blood count, sedimentation rate
B Autoimmune polyradiculoneuropathy	Immunoprotein electrophoresis, antinuclear antibody (ANA), cryoglobulins (+/−) bone marrow biopsy
V Paraneoplastic	
A Paracarcinomatous	
B Paralymphomatous; Hodgkin's disease	
VI Metabolic	
A Hypoglycemia	Fasting blood sugar (FBS)
B Hyperparathyroidism	Routine chemistries including calcium, magnesium, phosphate
C Hyperthroidism	Thyroid functions
D Vitamin B_{12}, Vitamin E deficiency	Vitamin B_{12}, folate, vitamin E levels
E Malabsorption	Stool fat (72-h; spot), carotene, prothrombin time (PT)
VII Hereditary biochemical disorders	
A Hexosaminidase A deficiency	Lysosomal enzyme screen
B α-Glucosidase deficiency (Pompe's)	
C Hyperlipidemia	Lipid electrophoresis
D Hyperglycinuria	Urine and serum amino acids
E Methylcrotonylglycinuria	CSF amino acids

Other treatable disorders that occasionally can mimic ALS are chronic lead poisoning and thyrotoxicosis. These may be suggested by the patient's social or occupational history or by unusual clinical features. When the family history is positive, inherited enzyme disorders such as hexosaminidase A or α-glucosidase deficiency must be excluded (see Chap. 357). These can readily be identified by appropriate laboratory tests. Benign fasciculations are occasionally a source of concern because on inspection they resemble the fascicular twitchings that accompany motor neuron degeneration. The absence of weakness or atrophy, and of denervation phenomena on electrophysiologic examination, excludes ALS or other serious neurologic disease. Poliomyelitis is now recognized to result in a delayed progressive deterioration of motor neurons which presents clinically with progressive weakness, atrophy, and fasciculations. Its cause is unknown but is thought to reflect prior sublethal injury to motor neurons by the poliovirus.

Treatment There is no treatment that has influence on the underlying pathologic process in any form of motor neuron disease. Modern rehabilitative measures, including mechanical aids of various kinds, can do much in helping patients to overcome the effects of their disabilities and often, with respiratory support, to survive longer than would otherwise have been the case. Initial observations (reviewed by Tandan and Bradley) showed that intravenous (or intrathecal) infusions of thyrotropin releasing hormone (TRH) result in transitory improvement of motor functions in some patients with ALS. Unfortunately TRH has not shown any long-term benefits. A recent report showed beneficial effects of treatment with branched chain amino acids; this will require verification.

SPINAL MUSCULAR ATROPHY (SMA) In the varieties of motor neuron disease that are grouped under this heading, the peripheral motor neurons are affected without evidence of involvement of the corticospinal motor system (Table 359-2). In comparison with ALS, SMA in general occurs in a younger age group, runs a slower, more protracted course (except in the infantile form), and tends to be hereditary (usually autosomal recessive) rather than sporadic. The SMA group undoubtedly includes several distinct disease processes that differ from one another genetically and phenotypically.

Infantile SMA (Werdnig-Hoffmann disease) This rapidly fatal disorder is characterized by autosomal recessive transmission. Not infrequently, infantile SMA (sometimes also referred to as SMA type I) is apparent even before birth, as indicated by decreased fetal movements in comparison with what normally would be expected. The afflicted infants are weak and floppy (hypotonic), though alert, and muscle-stretch reflexes are absent. Weakness progresses relatively rapidly, and death ensues generally within the first year of life; rarely, the child survives to 3 years of age.

Neuropathologically, Werdnig-Hoffmann disease is characterized by extensive loss of the large motor neurons. Sections of the muscles show extreme degrees of denervation atrophy. During life, the diagnosis is made by electrophysiologic studies and by muscle biopsy, which shows the characteristic denervational pattern rather than an intrinsic myopathy or inflammatory disease of muscle. There is no effective treatment, but a family that has had an affected infant may be helped by genetic counseling.

There is another form of infantile muscular atrophy, also characterized by autosomal recessive inheritance, which appears to be distinct from Werdnig-Hoffmann disease in that the evolution is considerably slower, with survival into preadolescence or even into adult life. This disorder, which has been called *chronic childhood SMA*, or SMA type II, is considerably rarer than Werdnig-Hoffmann disease.

These motor neuron diseases can be distinguished from benign congenital hypotonia, which is a nonprogressive form of myopathy, by electrophysiologic assessment and by muscle biopsy.

Juvenile SMA (Wohlfart-Kugelberg-Welander disease) This disorder, also referred to as SMA type III, manifests itself during late childhood and runs a slow, indolent course. Typically the muscles of the trunk and the proximal parts of the limb are earliest and most severely involved—a picture that closely resembles that of progressive muscular dystrophy, even to the presence of pseudohypertrophy of the calf muscles in some cases. Electrophysiologic and biopsy evidence of denervation in the affected muscles serves to distinguish this disease from any of the myopathic syndromes.

Other genetically determined varieties of SMA In individual families, other syndromes characterized by SMA in varying patterns have been described. An infantile variety involving mainly the musculature innervated by the brainstem is referred to as the *Fazio-Londe syndrome*. In some juvenile cases, the distribution is distal, rather than proximal, as in the Wohlfart-Kugelberg-Welander variety. In addition, there is a slowly evolving adult form of SMA, sometimes called SMA type IV (Table 359-2). Depending upon the family, autosomal dominant, autosomal recessive, or X-linked recessive patterns of heredity may be discerned.

A component of SMA may also be found in some of the multiple system degenerations that have already been referred to, e.g., in Joseph's disease and in some of the syndromes characterized by olivopontocerebellar degeneration. Some of the recognized familial metabolic disorders also present a striking picture of progressive symmetric muscular weakness and atrophy, for instance, adult hexosaminidase A deficiency (the enzymopathy that results in Tay-Sachs disease in infancy) and adrenomyeloneuropathy. For details and more extensive discussions of these disorders, specialized monographs (such as that edited by Rowland), reviews (Tandan and Bradley), and general reference works on neurology (Adams and Victor) should be consulted.

Primary lateral sclerosis (PLS) It might be thought that this is a variant of ALS in which the amyotrophic component is lacking, but the few cases of this disorder that have been described have been encountered in remarkably pure form. It occurs as a sporadic disease of late life, affecting the same age group that is prone to develop ALS. The course may be similar to that of ALS with approximately 3 years from onset to death. Clinically, the illness is characterized by progressive spastic weakness of the limbs, preceded or followed by spastic dysarthria and dysphagia, indicative of corticobulbar tract involvement. Fasciculations, amyotrophy, and sensory changes are absent. On neuropathologic examination, there is selective loss of large pyramidal cells in the precentral gyrus and degeneration of the corticospinal and corticobulbar projections; the peripheral motor neurons and other neuronal systems are spared.

It may be necessary to consider PLS in the differential diagnosis of late-life progressive spastic paresis of the limbs, but obviously it is necessary, by appropriate studies of CSF and radiographic investigations, to exclude treatable disorders such as parasagittal intracranial tumors, neoplasms of the spinal cord, cervical spondylosis, or inflammatory diseases.

HEREDITARY SPASTIC PARAPLEGIA This is a very rare disorder which differs from PLS in several respects. Instead of occurring sporadically, it is characterized by genetic transmission—as an autosomal dominant trait in the majority of cases. Several families are on record in which it has appeared in many successive generations. It appears at a younger age, usually in the fourth decade, and the course is very slowly progressive, to the extent that patients often live out a full life span. The condition is probably genetically heterogeneous; the group with onset in childhood or adolescence can be distinguished from those in whom the disease does not appear until the age of 35 years or older; as might be expected, there is considerable overlap between these groups. In a few families, a clinically indistinguishable disorder shows a pattern of autosomal recessive inheritance.

Pathology Neuropathologically, there is degeneration of the corticospinal (pyramidal) tracts, which appear almost normal at brainstem levels but become increasingly atrophic as they descend through the spinal cord. In addition, the ascending tracts in the posterior columns and the spinocerebellar tracts show some loss of fibers so that the picture resembles to some degree the findings in Friedreich's ataxia. In fact, some individual cases of what seems to be a fairly pure spastic paraparesis may actually represent an incomplete form of Friedreich's ataxia. In such families spastic paraparesis is the outstanding phenotypic expression of Friedreich's ataxia.

Clinical manifestations As the name implies, the lower limbs are affected earliest and most severely. The major cause of disability is spasticity rather than weakness. There is concomitant exaggeration of the muscle stretch reflexes. Late in the course, urinary urgency and incontinence, and sometimes fecal incontinence, may occur; sexual potency tends to be preserved. In pure forms of the disorder, ataxia and amyotrophy are absent or minimal. In some patients, minor sensory changes (in the form of impaired vibration and position sense) may be observed in the late stages.

It is important in cases of otherwise unexplained progressive spastic paraparesis, despite a negative family history, to examine as many family members as possible. Members of a family with minimal degrees of the disease may be asymptomatic and unaware of its presence, even though they can be shown on examination to have spasticity and hyperreflexia.

SYNDROMES COMBINING MUSCULAR WEAKNESS AND WASTING WITH SENSORY CHANGES

PROGRESSIVE NEURAL MUSCULAR ATROPHY The degenerative disorders characterized by progressive weakness and wasting of skeletal muscles combined with sensory changes are usually chronic diseases of peripheral nerves, often occurring as hereditary conditions. Although clinical and pathologic subvarieties exist, there is no sharp dividing line between them, and they are best considered together under the designation given above, in which the term *neural* emphasizes the peripheral nerve affection. Chronic peripheral neuropathy is an associated disorder in some of the hereditary ataxias and is regularly encountered in the classic form of Friedreich's ataxia. It is also a component of adrenomyeloneuropathy and other leukodystrophies (see Chap. 331). In some cases of progressive neural muscular atrophy, other genetically determined CNS diseases may occur such as progressive optic atrophy or pigmentary degeneration of the retina. The peripheral neuropathy begins distally and progresses in a centripetal fashion with the feet and legs first affected, and involvement of the hands and more proximal parts only after a considerable interval, usually several years.

The two most frequent forms of hereditary polyneuropathy, *peroneal muscular atrophy* (Charcot-Marie-Tooth disease) and *hypertrophic interstitial polyneuropathy* (Dejerine-Sottas disease), are described in Chap. 363. Brief reference is also made there to a rare condition known as *Refsum's disease*.

Although no specific treatment is available (except in Refsum's disease, as indicated in Chap. 363), patients whose disease is of slow progression and in whom conditions are otherwise favorable may be greatly helped by measures to ensure a stable walking surface, such as corrective shoes, braces to prevent foot drop, and even orthopedic procedures to stabilize the joints.

SYNDROMES OF PROGRESSIVE VISUAL LOSS Although the preceding discussion of the various hereditary progressive nervous system disorders categorized as degenerative has emphasized the intellectual, motor, and peripheral sensory derangements that result from these, many of these syndromes are accompanied by concomitant loss of the neural structures subserving vision. The hereditary ataxias, including Friedreich's, and hereditary spastic paraplegia stand out as examples. The pathologic changes, viewed broadly, take on two forms: selective degeneration of retinal ganglion cells with secondary optic atrophy, and a more diffuse degenerative process involving all retinal components, with subsequent migration of the melanin-containing cells of the pigment epithelium into the superficial retinal layers, resulting in the picture of *pigmentary degeneration of the retina* (formerly, but erroneously—since there is no inflammation—called retinitis pigmentosa). Occasionally, the peripheral visual system is the major, or only, site of disease resulting in progressive blindness without other neurologic defects. The major entities of this kind, including Leber's *hereditary optic atrophy*, are described in Chap. 360. A more complete review, with references to the pertinent literature, is given by Adams and Victor.

REFERENCES

General

ADAMS RD, VICTOR M: *Principles of Neurology*, 4th ed. New York, McGraw-Hill, 1989

——— et al: Striatonigral degeneration. J Neuropathol Exp Neurol 23:584, 1964

ASBURY AK et al: *Diseases of the Nervous System*, vols I and II. Philadelphia, Ardmore Medical Books, Saunders, 1986

GILMAN S et al: *Disorders of the Cerebellum*. Philadelphia, Davis, 1981

Greenfield's Neuropathology, 4th ed, JH Adams et al (eds). New York, Wiley, 1984

MARSDEN CD, FAHN S (eds): *Movement Disorders*. London, Butterworth, 1982

ROSENBERG RN: *Neurogenetics: Principles and Practice*. New York, Raven, 1986

Alzheimer's disease

BALL MJ: Alzheimer's disease: A challenging enigma. Arch Pathol Lab Med 106:157, 1982

FRIEDLAND RP et al: Alzheimer's disease: Clinical and biochemical heterogeneity. Ann Intern Med 109:298, 1988

GLENNER GG: On causative theories in Alzheimer's disease. Human Pathol 16:433, 1985

HAXBY JV et al: Heterogeneous anterior-posterior metabolic patterns on dementia of the Alzheimer type. Neurology 38:1853, 1988

HYMAN BT et al: Alzheimer's disease: Cell-specific pathology isolates the hippocampal formation. Science 225:1168, 1984

JOACHIM CL et al: Clinically diagnosed Alzheimer's disease: Autopsy results in 150 cases. Ann Neurol 24:50, 1988

KATZMAN R: Alzheimer's disease. N Engl J Med 314:964, 1986

PERL DP, BRODY AR: Alzheimer's disease: X-ray spectrometric evidence of aluminum accumulation in neurofibrillary tangle-bearing neurons. Science 208:297, 1980

PETRY S et al: Personality alterations in dementia of the Alzheimer type. Arch Neurol 45:1187, 1988

SCHEINBERG P: Dementia due to vascular disease—A multifactorial disorder. Stroke 19:1291, 1988

SELKOE DJ: Biochemistry of altered brain proteins in Alzheimer's disease. Ann Rev Neurosci 12:493, 1989

ST. GEORGE-HYSLOP PH et al: The genetic defect causing familial Alzheimer's disease maps on chromosome 21. Science 238:664, 1987

WHITEHOUSE PJ et al: Alzheimer's disease and senile dementia: Loss of neurons in the basal forebrain. Science 215:1237, 1982

Huntington's disease

FERRANTE RJ et al: Selective sparing of a class of striatal neurons in Huntington's disease. Science 230:561, 1985

HAYDEN MR: *Huntington's Chorea*. Berlin, Springer-Verlag, 1981

MARTIN JB, GUSELLA JF: Huntington's disease: Pathogenesis and management. N Engl J Med 315:1267, 1986

MEISSEN GJ et al: Predictive testing for Huntington's disease with use of a linked DNA marker. N Engl J Med 318:535, 1988

VONSATTEL JP et al: Neuropathological classification of Huntington's disease. J Neuropathol Exp Neurol 44:559, 1985

Parkinson's disease

FABBRINI G et al: Motor fluctuations in Parkinson's disease: Central pathophysiological mechanisms, part I. Ann Neurol 24:366, 1988

FAHN S et al (eds): *Recent Advances in Parkinson's Disease*. New York, Raven, 1986

GROWDON JH: Medical treatment of extrapyramidal diseases, in *Update III: Harrison's Principles of Internal Medicine*, KJ Isselbacher et al (eds). New York, McGraw-Hill, 1982

HOEHN MM, YAHR MD: Parkinsonism: Onset, progression and mortality. Neurology 17:427, 1967

LANGSTON JW et al: Chronic parkinsonism in humans due to a product of meperidine-analog synthesis. Science 219:979, 1983

MARTTILA RJ et al: Parkinson's disease in a nationwide twin cohort. Neurology 38:1217, 1988

MAYEUX R et al: Reappraisal of temporary levodopa withdrawal ("drug holiday") in Parkinson's disease. N Engl J Med 313:724, 1985

MOURADIAN MM et al: Motor fluctuations in Parkinson's disease: Central pathophysiological mechanisms, part II. Ann Neurol 24:372, 1988

NUTT JG et al: The "on-off" phenomenon in Parkinson's disease: Relation to levodopa absorption and transport. N Engl J Med 310:438, 1984

PARKINSON STUDY GROUP: Effect of deprenyl on the progression of disability in early Parkinson's disease. N Engl J Med 321:1364, 1989

Cerebellar degeneration

DUVOISIN RC, PLAITAKIS A (eds): *Advances in Neurology*, vol 41, *The Olivopontocerebellar Atrophies*. New York, Raven, 1984

KONIGSMARK BW, WEINER LP: The olivopontocerebellar atrophies: A review. Medicine 49:227, 1970

TRAUNER DA: Olivopontocerebellar atrophy with dementia, blindness, and chorea. Arch Neurol 42:757, 1985

Motor neuron disease

MITSUMOTO H et al: Amyotrophic lateral sclerosis: Recent advances in pathogenesis and therapeutic trials. Arch Neurol 45:189, 1988

PLAITAKIS A et al: Pilot trial of branched-chain amino acids in amyotrophic lateral sclerosis. Lancet 1:1015, 1988

ROWLAND LP (ed): *Advances in Neurology*, vol 36, *Human Motor Neuron Diseases*. New York, Raven, 1982

TANDAN R, BRADLEY WG: Amyotrophic lateral sclerosis: Part 1, Clinical features, pathology, and ethical issues in management. Ann Neurol 18:271, 1985

———, ———: Amyotrophic lateral sclerosis: Part 2, Etiopathogenesis. Ann Neurol 18:419, 1985

Miscellaneous

BAUMANN RJ et al: Lafora disease: Liver histopathology in presymptomatic children. Ann Neurol 14:86, 1983

BERKOVIC SF et al: Progressive myoclonic epilepsies: Specific causes and diagnosis. N Engl J Med 315:296, 1986

BLACK PM et al: CSF shunts for dementia, incontinence and gait disturbance. Clin Neurosurg 32:632, 1985

BURKHARDT CR et al: Diffuse Lewy body disease and progressive dementia. Neurology 38:1520, 1988

HARDING AE: Hereditary "pure" spastic paraplegia: A clinical and genetic study of 22 families. J Neurol Neurosurg Psychiatry 44:871, 1981

——— et al: Spinocerebellar degeneration associated with a selective deficit of vitamin E absorption. N Engl J Med 313:32, 1985
HENSON RA, URICH H: *Cancer and the Nervous System*. Blackwell Scientific, 1982
IIVANAINEN M, HIMBERG J-J: Valproate and clonazepam in the treatment of severe progressive myoclonus epilepsy. Arch Neurol 39:236, 1982
JANKOVIC J, ONMAN J: Botulinum A toxin for cranial-cervical dystonia: A double-blind, placebo-controlled study. Neurology 37:616, 1987
KRAMER PL et al: Dystonia gene in Ashkenazi Jewish population is located on chromosome 9q32–34. Ann Neurol 27:114, 1990
LOGIGIAN EL et al: Myoclonus epilepsy in two brothers: Clinical features and neuropathology of a unique syndrome. Brain 109:411, 1986
MCGEER EG, MCGEER PL: The dystonias. Can J Neurol Sci 15:447, 1988
MCLEOD JG, TUCK RR: Disorders of the autonomic nervous system: Part 2. Investigation and treatment. Ann Neurol 21:519, 1987
MESULAM MM, PETERSEN RC: Treatment of Gilles de la Tourette syndrome: Eight-year, practice-based experience in a predominantly adult population. Neurology 37:1828, 1987
MUNOZ-GARCIA D, LUDWIN SK: Classic and generalized variants of Pick's disease: A clinicopathological, ultrastructural, and immunocytochemical study. Ann Neurol 16:467, 1984
PAULS OL, LECKMAN JF: The inheritance of Gilles de la Tourette syndrome and associated behaviors. N Engl J Med 315:993, 1986
SETHI KD et al: Hallervorden-Spatz syndrome: Clinical and magnetic resonance imaging correlations. Ann Neurol 24:692, 1988
STEELE JC: Progressive supranuclear palsy. Brain 95:693, 1972
TISSOT R et al: *La Maladie de Pick*. Paris, Masson et Cie, 1975
WATTS RL et al: Corticobasal ganglionic degeneration. Neurology 35:178, 1985
ZEMAN W, DYKEN P: Dystonia musculorum deformans: Clinical, genetic and pathoanatomical studies. Psychiatr Neurol Neurochir 70:77, 1967

360 DISORDERS OF THE CRANIAL NERVES

MAURICE VICTOR / JOSEPH B. MARTIN

The cranial nerves are susceptible to disorders that rarely affect the spinal peripheral nerves, and for this reason deserve to be considered separately. This chapter describes the principal syndromes of disordered function and the diseases that cause them. Cranial nerve disorders of taste and smell, vision and ocular movement, and vertigo and deafness are also discussed in Chaps. 22 to 24.

OLFACTORY NERVE (See Chap. 24)

OPTIC NERVE

TRANSIENT MONOCULAR BLINDNESS (AMAUROSIS FUGAX) (See also Chap. 351) **Definition** Amaurosis fugax is the name applied to an attack of transient painless loss of vision in one eye. Frequently it is recurrent. (The term *amaurosis* refers to blindness from any cause, in distinction to *amblyopia,* which refers to a loss of vision from disease of structures other than the eye itself.)

Clinical manifestations Amaurosis fugax is a common clinical symptom indicative of transient retinal ischemia, usually associated with ipsilateral internal carotid artery stenosis or to embolism of the retinal arteries. In some cases the basis for the symptom cannot be discerned.

Typically, the episode of blindness evolves swiftly, in a matter of 10 to 15 s, and is described as a shade that falls smoothly and painlessly over the field until the eye is completely blind. Or, a similar obliteration of the visual field may occur from below. The blindness lasts for a few seconds or minutes, sometimes longer, then clears slowly and uniformly, the patient's vision returning in the reverse direction from that in which it was lost. Sometimes there is only a generalized dimness of vision, rather than a complete loss, or only a segment of the visual field may be involved. Many patients who experience amaurosis fugax on the basis of carotid stenosis also have transient attacks of contralateral hemiparesis, but it is uncommon for the two types of attack to occur simultaneously.

Diagnosis The transient visual loss that accompanies classic migraine is of a different type. Often it begins with unformed flashes of light (photopsia) or dazzling zigzag lines (fortification spectra or teichopsia), which move across the visual field for several minutes, leaving scotomatous or hemianopic defects. The patient with migraine may complain of blindness in one eye, but examination usually shows the defects to be bilateral and homonymous, i.e., they occupy corresponding halves of both visual fields. The latter symptoms point to an origin in the visual cortex of one occipital lobe. In so-called basilar migraine, in which the neurologic symptoms are referable to the territory of the basilar artery, the transient visual disturbances may occupy the whole of both visual fields.

Investigation and treatment Amaurosis fugax is most commonly a manifestation of ipsilateral internal carotid artery disease. Attention should be directed to carotid bruits, and noninvasive tests for carotid blood flow and lumen diameter should be carried out in every case. The decision of when to proceed to angiography is discussed in Chap. 351. Definitive treatment is dependent upon the results of these investigations. In the absence of carotid disease other possible sources of emboli (cardiac or aortic) should be sought. Amaurosis fugax may sometimes herald occlusion of the central retinal artery or anterior ischemic optic neuropathy due to giant cell arteritis or to nonarteritic (arteriosclerotic) disease. The sedimentation rate is usually elevated in giant cell arteritis (Chap. 276).

RETROBULBAR OPTIC NEUROPATHY OR NEURITIS Definition This syndrome is characterized by the rapid development (hours or days) of impaired vision in one or both eyes. In the latter case the eyes may be affected either simultaneously or sequentially. The visual loss in such cases is usually the result of acute demyelinative disease of optic nerves, although a number of other causes of unilateral or bilateral optic nerve disease must be sought (see below).

Clinical manifestations The most frequent setting is one in which a child, adolescent, or young adult notes a rapid diminution of vision in one eye (as though a veil or haze covered every object seen). The condition may progress to severe loss of vision (<20/100) within a few days, but complete blindness is rare. The optic disc and retina may appear normal, but in some patients the optic disc is hyperemic and elevated with blurring of the disc margins (papillitis). Peripapillary hemorrhages are seen infrequently, and the veins are not engorged. *Papillitis* is distinguished from *papilledema* due to increased intracranial pressure by the acute and often marked reduction of visual acuity that accompanies the former. Also, in retrobulbar neuropathy, there is often pain on movement of the eye or on pressure on the globe. After a few days or weeks the other eye may become similarly involved, with loss, typically, of central vision but with some preservation of peripheral vision. The pupillary light reflex is impaired. In a high percentage of patients, no cause can be found, and after days or weeks there is spontaneous recovery of vision. In the majority of patients the visual acuity returns to normal or near normal within months of the attack. Sometimes a small central scotoma persists. The optic disc later becomes slightly pale due to demyelination, often most prominent in the temporal region. The CSF may be normal or may contain from 10 to 20 lymphocytes, and the protein content, particularly the gamma globulin portion, may be increased. Oligoclonal bands are found in some patients.

About 50 percent of such patients will develop other symptoms and signs consistent with multiple sclerosis within 10 to 15 years, and even more will do so if the patients are observed for longer periods (see Chap. 356). Less is known about children with retrobulbar neuropathy, but the prognosis for them is considerably better than that for adults. Multiple sclerosis is the most common cause of a *unilateral retrobulbar neuritis.* Bilateral optic neuritis may occur a few days or weeks in advance of an attack of transverse myelitis. This combination is called neuromyelitis optica or Devic disease (Chap. 356).

Diagnosis Other causes of unilateral optic neuropathy, all of them rare, include postinfectious or disseminated encephalomyelitis, posterior uveitis, and, more commonly, vascular lesions of the optic nerve. *Anterior ischemic optic neuropathy* (*AION*) is a condition caused by interruption of blood supply to the optic nerve secondary to atherosclerotic or inflammatory disease of the ophthalmic artery or its branches (see Chap. 23). It presents clinically as acute, painless, visual loss in one eye, usually accompanied by an altitudinal visual field defect. In severe cases visual loss is complete and permanent. The fundus shows a pale swollen optic disc surrounded by splinter-shaped peripapillary hemorrhages. Occasionally only a section of the disc is pale and swollen. The macula and the retina are normal. Investigations are directed toward excluding temporal arteritis (see Chap. 276). Rarely, microemboli can cause occlusion of the posterior ciliary arteries and AION; for example, following open heart or coronary artery bypass surgery.

Central retinal artery occlusion (*CRAO*) also presents with sudden blindness. In this entity the optic disc initially appears normal. The retina is infarcted and appears pale with accentuation of the macular cherry-red spot. In all cases of unilateral involvement of the optic nerve, tumor (glioma, von Recklinghausen neurofibromatosis, meningioma) needs to be ruled out.

Treatment Acute optic neuropathy due to demyelination usually resolves without specific treatment. Severe visual loss is commonly treated with prednisone 40 to 80 mg daily in divided doses for 7 to 10 days with gradual tapering over a few days. Some physicians recommend ACTH treatment. Both forms of treatment may hasten recovery from an individual attack, but do not prevent further attacks or modify their severity.

TOXIC-NUTRITIONAL OPTIC NEUROPATHY Simultaneous impairment of vision in the two eyes, with central or centrocecal scotomas, occurring over a period of days or weeks, is usually due to a toxic or nutritional disorder rather than to a demyelinative process (see Chap. 357). Impairment of vision due to *methyl alcohol intoxication* is abrupt in onset and is characterized by large symmetric central scotomas, as well as by symptoms of systemic disease and acidosis (see Chap. 374). The lesion is in the retinal ganglion cells and their axons, which project into the optic nerve. The most important treatment is intravenous administration of sodium bicarbonate. Hemodialysis is a useful adjunct because of the slow rate of oxidation of methyl alcohol. Other drugs with proven but less devastating toxic effects on the optic nerve include chloramphenicol, ethambutol, isoniazid, streptomycin, sulfonamides, digitalis, ergot, disulfiram, and heavy metals.

Degenerative diseases may affect the retina or the optic nerves, taking the form of optic atrophy. There are several types of hereditary optic atrophy, the most frequent being the Leber type, which is sex-linked, occurring in males (see Chap. 23). An autosomal dominant form of congenital or early infantile optic atrophy and optic atrophy with diabetes mellitus and deafness are described. Senile macular degeneration and various forms of retinitis pigmentosa are important causes of visual loss (see Chap. 23).

BITEMPORAL HEMIANOPSIA This type of visual disorder is usually related to suprasellar extension of a pituitary adenoma (often with an enlarged sella), but may also be due to a craniopharyngioma, saccular aneurysm of the circle of Willis, meningioma of the tuberculum sellae (normal sella or thickened tuberculum by radiography), and rarely sarcoidosis, metastatic carcinoma, and Hand-Schüller-Christian disease (see Chap. 313). The lesion involves the decussating nasal fibers from each retina.

OCULOMOTOR, TROCHLEAR, AND ABDUCENS NERVES (See Chap. 23)

TRIGEMINAL NERVE

The trigeminal nerve supplies sensation to the skin of the face and half of the vertex of the skull and motor innervation to the masseter and pterygoid masticatory muscles.

PAROXYSMAL FACIAL PAIN (TRIGEMINAL NEURALGIA, TIC DOULOUREUX) Definition The most striking disorder of trigeminal nerve function is tic douloureux, a condition characterized by excruciating paroxysms of pain in the lips, gums, cheek, or chin, and, very rarely, in the distribution of the ophthalmic division of the fifth nerve. The disorder occurs almost exclusively in middle-aged and elderly persons. The pain seldom lasts more than a few seconds or a minute or two but may be so intense that the patient winces, hence the term *tic*. The paroxysms recur frequently, both day and night, for several weeks at a time. Another characteristic feature is the initiation of pain by obvious stimuli applied to certain areas on the face, lips, or tongue (the so-called trigger zones) or by movement of these parts. Sensory loss cannot be demonstrated. In studying the relations between stimuli applied to the trigger zone and the paroxysm of pain, it is found that the adequate stimulus for precipitating an attack is a tactile one and possibly tickle, rather than a noxious or thermal stimulus. Usually a spatial and temporal summation of impulses is necessary to trigger an attack, which is followed by a refractory period of up to 2 or 3 min.

The diagnosis of this disorder rests upon these strict clinical criteria, and the condition must be distinguished from other forms of facial and cephalic neuralgia and pain arising from diseases of the jaw, teeth, or sinuses. Tic douloureux is usually without assignable cause; occasionally it is a manifestation of multiple sclerosis when it appears in younger adults and may be bilateral. Very rarely it may occur with herpes zoster or a tumor. To a degree that remains uncertain and controversial, pain of tic douloureux may be caused by a redundant or tortuous blood vessel in the posterior fossa, causing an irritative lesion of the nerve or its root. Usually, however, space-occupying lesions, such as aneurysms, neurofibromas, or meningiomas affecting the nerve, produce a loss of sensation (trigeminal neuropathy).

Treatment The initial treatment of tic douloureux is pharmacologic. Carbamazepine is the drug of choice and is effective initially in 75 percent of patients. Unfortunately, up to one-third cannot tolerate the drug in the doses required to alleviate pain. Carbamazepine should be started gradually, 100 mg with food, as a single dose, and increased to 200 mg qid. Doses greater than 1200 to 1600 mg provide no additional benefit.

If drug treatment fails, surgical therapy should be offered. The most widely applied procedure is percutaneous retrogasserian rhizotomy accomplished by radiofrequency lesions. Relief is obtained by one to three procedures in more than 95 percent of patients. Later recurrences affect 7 to 31 percent of patients. Complications and morbidity are infrequent in experienced hands. The procedure results in partial numbness of the face and carries a risk of corneal denervation with secondary keratitis when used for first division trigeminal neuralgia.

A second treatment, microvascular dissection, requires a suboccipital craniectomy, a major procedure requiring about 1 week of hospitalization. It has an 80 percent efficacy but is accompanied by a 5 percent major complication rate. Not all patients operated upon have a demonstrated vascular or other compressive lesion of the trigeminal nerve. The most troublesome complication of all surgical treatments is the development of anesthesia dolorosa or denervation hypersensitivity. This condition responds poorly to treatment. Tricyclic antidepressants or phenothiazines are usually given with only partial success in alleviating the discomfort.

TRIGEMINAL NEUROPATHY A variety of diseases may affect the trigeminal nerve in addition to those mentioned above. Most present with sensory loss on the face or with weakness of the jaw muscles. Deviation of the jaw on opening indicates weakness of the pterygoids of the side to which the jaw deviates. Tumors of the middle cranial fossa (meningiomas), of the trigeminal nerve (schwannomas), or of the base of the skull (metastatic) may cause a combination of motor and sensory signs. Lesions in the cavernous sinus can affect the first and second divisions of the trigeminal nerve, and lesions of the superior orbital fissure can affect the first (ophthalmic) division. The accompanying corneal anesthesia increases the risk of ulceration (neurokeratitis).

Anesthesia and analgesia of the face have been reported after treatment with stilbamidine (formerly used in the treatment of kala azar and multiple myeloma). Pain and itching may occur during recovery. Rarely, an idiopathic form of trigeminal neuropathy is observed. It is characterized by feelings of numbness and paresthesias, sometimes bilaterally, with loss of sensation in the territory of the trigeminal nerve but without weakness of the jaw. Recovery is the rule, but the symptoms may be troublesome for many months, or even years. Leprosy may involve the trigeminal nerves.

Tonic spasm of the masticatory muscles, known as *trismus,* is symptomatic of tetanus (see Chap. 105). It may also occur as an idiosyncratic reaction in patients treated with phenothiazine drugs; lesser degrees may be associated with disease of the pharynx, temporomaxillary joint, teeth, and gums.

FACIAL NERVE

FACIAL PALSY AND FACIAL SPASM The seventh cranial nerve supplies all the muscles concerned with facial expression. The sensory component is small (the nervus intermedius of Wrisberg); it conveys taste sensation from the anterior two-thirds of the tongue and probably cutaneous impulses from the anterior wall of the external auditory canal. The motor nucleus of the seventh nerve lies anterior and lateral to the abducens nucleus. After leaving the pons the seventh nerve enters the internal auditory meatus with the acoustic nerve. The nerve continues its course through the middle ear to exit from the skull via the stylomastoid foramen. It then passes through the parotid gland and subdivides to supply the facial muscles.

A complete interruption of the facial nerve at the stylomastoid foramen paralyzes all muscles of facial expression. The corner of the mouth droops, the creases and skin folds are effaced, the forehead is unfurrowed, and the eyelids will not close. Upon attempted closure of the lids, the eye on the paralyzed side is seen to roll upward (Bell's phenomenon). The lower lid sags also, and the punctum falls away from the conjunctiva, permitting tears to spill over the cheek. Food collects between the teeth and lips, and saliva may dribble from the corner of the mouth. The patient complains of a heaviness or numbness in the face, but no sensory loss is demonstrable and taste is intact.

If the lesion is in the middle ear portion, taste is lost over the anterior two-thirds of the tongue on the same side. If the nerve to the stapedius is interrupted, there is hyperacusis (painful sensitivity to loud sounds). Lesions in the internal auditory meatus may also affect the adjacent auditory and vestibular nerves, causing deafness, tinnitus, or dizziness. Intrapontine lesions that paralyze the face usually affect the abducens nucleus and often the corticospinal and sensory tracts.

If the peripheral facial paralysis has existed for some time and recovery of motor function has begun but is incomplete, a kind of contracture (actually a continuous diffuse contraction) of facial muscles may appear. The palpebral fissure becomes narrowed and the nasolabial fold deepens. With the passage of time, the face and even the tip of the nose become pulled to the unaffected side. Attempts to move one group of facial muscles result in contraction of all of them (associated movements, or *synkinesis*). Facial spasms may develop and persist indefinitely, being initiated by every facial movement (hemifacial spasm). This condition may represent a transient or permanent sequela to a Bell's palsy but may also be due to an irritative lesion of the facial nerve (e.g., an acoustic neuroma, an aberrant artery which compresses the nerve and is relieved by surgery, or a basilar artery aneurysm). However, in the most common form of hemifacial spasm, the cause and pathology are unknown. Anomalous regeneration of the seventh nerve fibers may result in other curious disorders. If fibers originally connected with the orbicularis oculi come to innervate the orbicularis oris, closure of the lids may cause a retraction of the mouth; or if fibers originally connected with muscles of the face later innervate the lacrimal gland, anomalous tearing (crocodile tears) may occur with any activity of the facial muscles, such as eating. Yet another unusual facial synkinesia is one in which jaw opening causes a closure of the eyelids on the side of the facial palsy (jaw-winking).

BELL'S PALSY Definition The most common form of facial paralysis is idiopathic, i.e., *Bell's palsy*. The incidence rate of this disorder is about 23 per 100,000 annually, or about 1 in 60 or 70 persons in a lifetime. The pathogenesis of the paralysis is unknown. The few autopsied cases of this disease have shown only nondescript changes in the facial nerve and not inflammatory changes, as is commonly presumed.

Clinical manifestations The onset of Bell's palsy is fairly abrupt, maximum weakness being attained by 48 h as a general rule. Pain behind the ear may precede the paralysis for a day or two. Taste sensation may be lost unilaterally, and hyperacusis may be present. In some cases there is mild CSF lymphocytosis. Fully 80 percent of patients recover within a few weeks or months. Electromyography may be of value in distinguishing a temporary conduction defect from a pathologic interruption in the continuity of nerve fibers. Evidence of denervation after 10 days indicates that there has been axonal degeneration and that there will be a long delay before regeneration occurs, and that it may be incomplete. The presence of incomplete paralysis in the first week is the most favorable prognostic sign.

Treatment Protection of the eye during sleep, massage of the weakened muscles, and a splint to prevent drooping of the lower part of the face are the measures generally employed in the management of such cases. A course of prednisone beginning with 60 to 80 mg daily during the first 5 days and then tapered over the next 5 days may be beneficial. Unroofing of the facial nerve in the facial canal has been practiced, but there is no evidence that this measure is helpful, and it may be harmful.

Differential diagnosis There are many other causes of facial palsy. Tumors that invade the temporal bone (carotid body, cholesteatoma, dermoid) may produce a facial palsy, but the onset is insidious and the course progressive. The *Ramsay Hunt syndrome,* presumably due to herpes zoster of the geniculate ganglion, consists of a severe facial palsy associated with a vesicular eruption in the pharynx, external auditory canal, and other parts of the cranial integument; often the eighth cranial nerve is affected as well. *Acoustic neuromas* frequently involve the facial nerve by local compression (see Chap. 353). Infarcts and tumors are the common pontine lesions which may interrupt the facial nerve fibers. Bilateral facial paralysis (facial diplegia) occurs in acute inflammatory polyradiculoneuritis (Guillain-Barré disease) and in a variety of sarcoidosis known as *uveoparotid fever* (*Heerfordt syndrome*). The *Melkersson-Rosenthal syndrome* consists of a rarely encountered triad of recurrent facial paralysis, recurrent—and eventually permanent—facial (particularly labial) edema, and less constantly, plication of the tongue; many causes of this rare syndrome have been suggested, but none has been established. Leprosy frequently involves the facial nerve.

A puzzling disorder is the *facial hemiatrophy of Romberg*. It occurs mainly in females and is characterized by a disappearance of fat in the dermal and subcutaneous tissues on one side of the face. It usually begins in adolescence or early adult years and is slowly progressive. In its advanced form the face is gaunt and the skin is thin, wrinkled, and rather brown. The facial hair may turn white and fall out, and the sebaceous glands become atrophic. The muscles and bones are not involved as a rule. Sometimes the atrophy becomes bilateral. The condition is a form of lipodystrophy, and the localization within a dermatome suggests a disorder of some neural trophic factor of unknown nature. The treatment is transplantation of skin and subcutaneous fat by a plastic surgeon.

Facial myokymia is a fine fibrillary activity of the facial muscles which may be caused by a plaque of multiple sclerosis. *Blepharospasm* is an involuntary recurrent spasm of both eyelids that occurs in elderly persons as an isolated phenomenon or with varying degrees of spasm of other facial muscles (see Chap. 25). Relaxant and sedative drugs are of little help, although in many patients this disorder subsides spontaneously. In severe persistent cases of blepharospasm or hemifacial spasm, an effective treatment has been differential facial nerve section of selected branches of the nerve or nerve decompression (from vessels) intracranially. Cases are now successfully treated by local injection of botulinus toxin into the orbicularis oculi; the spasms are relieved for 3 to 4 months, and the injections can be repeated without morbidity.

All these forms of nuclear or peripheral facial palsy must be distinguished from the supranuclear type. In the latter the frontalis and orbicularis oculi muscles are involved less than those of the lower part of the face, since the upper facial muscles are innervated by corticobulbar pathways from both motor cortices, whereas the lower facial muscles are innervated only by the opposite hemisphere. In supranuclear lesions there may be a dissociation of emotional and voluntary facial movements, and often some degree of paralysis of the arm and leg or an aphasia (in dominant hemisphere lesions) is conjoined.

VESTIBULAR NERVE

The eighth cranial nerve has two components, vestibular and auditory. Symptoms and signs of involvement of the vestibular portion are discussed in Chap. 22 and in this section. The auditory nerve and its disorders are discussed in Chap. 24.

MÉNIÈRE'S SYNDROME Definition and clinical manifestations Ménière's disease, or Ménière's syndrome, is the name applied to recurrent vertigo accompanied by tinnitus and deafness. The latter symptoms may be absent during the initial attack(s) of vertigo, but they invariably appear as the disease progresses and are increased in severity during an acute attack. With milder forms of the syndrome the patient may complain more of head discomfort, slight instability, and difficulty in concentration than of vertigo and may be considered to be anxious or depressed. Provided that deafness is not complete, the recruitment phenomenon can be demonstrated (see Chap. 24).

Ménière's disease has its onset most frequently in the fifth decade of life, though younger adults and the elderly are not spared. The pathologic changes are said to consist of a dilatation of the endolymphatic system which leads to a degeneration of the delicate vestibular and cochlear hair cells. The relation of these pathologic changes to the paroxysmal disorder of labyrinthine function is unknown.

Treatment During an acute attack, rest in bed is the most effective treatment, since the patient can usually find a position in which vertigo is minimal. Dimenhydrinate, cyclizine, or meclizine in doses of 25 to 50 mg tid is useful in the more protracted cases. A low-salt diet is still used in treatment, but its value is difficult to judge. Mild sedative drugs may help the anxious patient between attacks. Usually the deafness is unilateral and progressive, and when it is complete, the vertiginous attacks cease. However, the course is variable, and if the attacks persist in a severe manner, permanent relief can be obtained by surgical destruction of the labyrinth or section of the vestibular portion of the eighth nerve intracranially.

BENIGN POSITIONAL VERTIGO Another disorder of labyrinthine function is characterized by the occurrence of paroxysmal vertigo and nystagmus with the assumption of certain critical positions of the head. This is the positional vertigo of Bárány, of the so-called benign paroxysmal type (see Chap. 22). In refractory cases, in which attacks continue, vestibular exercises may be beneficial.

DIFFERENTIAL DIAGNOSIS OF VERTIGO There are many other causes of acute vertigo, such as purulent labyrinthitis complicating meningitis, serous labyrinthitis due to infection of the middle ear, "toxic labyrinthitis" due to drug intoxication (e.g., with alcohol, quinine, streptomycin, gentamicin, and other antibiotics), motion sickness, trauma, and hemorrhage into the internal ear. In these instances the attacks of vertigo tend to last longer than in the recurrent form, but in other respects the symptoms are similar. Streptomycin or gentamicin may damage the fine hair cells of the vestibular end organs and cause a permanent disorder of equilibrium (as well as hearing), especially in older patients.

There has been described a dramatic clinical syndrome, characterized by the abrupt onset of severe vertigo, nausea, and vomiting, without tinnitus or hearing loss. The vertigo persists for several days or weeks, and labyrinthine function is permanently ablated on one side. Occlusion of the labyrinthine division of the internal auditory artery would logically explain this syndrome, but pathologic or angiographic confirmation of this hypothesis has so far not been obtained.

Vertigo of vestibular nerve origin may occur with diseases that involve the nerve in the petrous bone or the cerebellopontine angle. Except that it is less severe and is less frequently paroxysmal, it has many of the characteristics of labyrinthine vertigo. The adjacent auditory division of the eighth cranial nerve may also be affected, which explains the frequent association of vertigo with tinnitus and deafness. The function of the eighth cranial nerve may be disturbed by tumors of the lateral recess (especially acoustic neuroma), less frequently by meningeal inflammation in this region and rarely, by an abnormal vessel that compresses the nerve.

Vestibular neuronitis and *benign recurrent vertigo* are the names that have been applied to a clinical syndrome that occurs mainly in middle-aged and young adults (sometimes in children) and is characterized by the abrupt onset of vertigo, nausea, and vomiting, without impairment of hearing. The attacks are brief and leave the patient for some days with a mild positional vertigo. They may occur only once or recur in varying degrees of severity. The cause is unknown. The medical treatment is the same as for Ménière's disease.

A particular variety of paroxysmal vertigo affects children. The attacks occur in a setting of good health and are of sudden onset and brief duration. Pallor, sweating, and immobility are prominent manifestations, and occasionally vomiting and nystagmus occur. No relation to posture or movement of the head has been observed. The attacks are recurrent but tend to cease spontaneously after a period of several months or years. The outstanding abnormal finding is demonstrated by caloric testing, which shows impairment or loss of vestibular function, bilateral or unilateral, frequently persisting after the attacks have ceased; cochlear function is unimpaired, however. The pathologic basis of this disorder has not been determined.

GLOSSOPHARYNGEAL NERVE

GLOSSOPHARYNGEAL NEURALGIA Glossopharyngeal neuralgia resembles trigeminal neuralgia in many respects but is much less common. The pain is intense and paroxysmal; it originates in the throat, approximately in the tonsillar fossa. In some cases the pain is localized in the ear or may radiate from the throat to the ear, because of implication of the tympanic branch of the glossopharyngeal nerve (Jacobson's nerve). Spasms of pain may be initiated by swallowing. There is no demonstrable sensory or motor deficit. Cardiac symptoms of bradycardia with hypotension and fainting have been reported. A trial of carbamazepine or phenytoin is the recommended therapy, but if this is unsuccessful, division of the glossopharyngeal nerve near the medulla is the definitive treatment. Percutaneous rhizotomy of glossopharyngeal and vagal fibers in the jugular foramen alleviates pain in some patients.

Very rarely, herpes zoster may involve the glossopharyngeal nerve. Glossopharyngeal neuropathy in conjunction with vagus and accessory nerve palsies may occur due to a tumor or aneurysm in the posterior fossa or in the jugular foramen. Hoarseness due to vocal cord paralysis, some difficulty in swallowing, deviation of the soft palate to the intact side, anesthesia of the posterior wall of the pharynx, and weakness of the upper part of the trapezius and sternocleidomastoid muscles make up the syndrome (see Table 360-1, jugular foramen syndrome).

TABLE 360-1 Cranial nerve syndromes

Site	Cranial nerves involved	Eponymic syndrome	Usual cause
Sphenoid fissure (superior orbital)	III, IV, first division V, VI	Foix	Invasive tumors of sphenoid bone; aneurysms
Lateral wall of cavernous sinus	III, IV, first division V, VI, often with proptosis	Foix Tolosa-Hunt	Aneurysms or thrombosis of cavernous sinus; invasive tumors from sinuses and sella turcica; benign granuloma responsive to steroids
Retrosphenoid space	II, III, IV, V, VI	Jacod	Large tumors of middle cranial fossa
Apex of petrous bone	V, VI	Gradenigo	Petrositis; tumors of petrous bone
Internal auditory meatus	VII, VIII		Tumors of petrous bone (dermoids, etc.); infectious processes; acoustic neuroma
Pontocerebellar angle	V, VII, VIII, and sometimes IX		Acoustic neuroma; meningioma
Jugular foramen	IX, X, XI	Vernet	Tumors and aneurysms
Posterior laterocondylar space	IX, X, XI, XII	Collet-Sicard	Tumors of parotid gland, carotid body, and metastatic tumor
Posterior retroparotid space	IX, X, XI, XII and Horner syndrome	Villaret Mackenzie Tapia	Tumors of parotid gland, carotid body, lymph nodes; metastatic tumor; tuberculous adenitis

SPINAL ACCESSORY NERVE

Isolated involvement of the eleventh cranial nerve can occur anywhere along its route, resulting in partial or complete paralysis of the sternocleidomastoid and trapezius muscles. More commonly, involvement occurs in combination with deficits in the ninth and tenth cranial nerves in the jugular foramen or after exit from the skull (see Table 360-1).

VAGUS NERVE

DYSPHAGIA AND DYSPHONIA Complete interruption of the intracranial portion of one vagus nerve results in a characteristic paralysis. The soft palate droops ipsilaterally and does not rise in phonation. There is loss of the gag reflex on the affected side, as well as the "curtain movement" of the lateral wall of the pharynx, whereby the faucial pillars move medially as the palate rises in saying "ah." The voice is hoarse, slightly nasal, and the vocal cord lies immobile in the cadaveric position, i.e., midway between abduction and adduction. There may also be a loss of sensibility at the external auditory meatus and back of the pinna. Usually no change in visceral function can be demonstrated.

Complete interruption of both vagi is said to be incompatible with life, and this is probably true if the nuclei are involved in the medulla by poliomyelitis or some other disease. However, in the cervical region, both vagi have been blocked with procaine (Novocain) for the treatment of intractable asthma, without mishap. The pharyngeal branches of both vagi may be affected in diphtheria; the voice has a nasal quality, and regurgitation of liquids through the nose occurs during the act of swallowing.

The vagus nerve may be implicated at the meningeal level by neoplastic and infectious processes and within the medulla by tumors and vascular lesions, e.g., the lateral medullary syndrome of Wallenberg, and by motor neuron disease. This nerve may be involved by the inflammatory lesion of herpes zoster. Polymyositis and dermatomyositis, which cause hoarseness and dysphagia by direct involvement of laryngeal and pharyngeal muscles, may be confused with diseases of the vagus nerves. Also dysphagia is a symptom in some patients with myotonic dystrophy (see Chap. 42 for discussion of nonneurologic forms of dysphagia).

The recurrent laryngeal nerves, especially the left, are most often damaged as a result of intrathoracic disease. Aneurysm of the aortic arch, an enlarged left atrium, and tumors of the mediastinum and bronchi are much more frequent causes of an isolated vocal cord palsy than are intracranial disorders.

When confronted with a case of laryngeal palsy, the physician must attempt to determine the site of the lesion. If it is intramedullary, there are usually other signs, such as ipsilateral cerebellar dysfunction, loss of pain and temperature sensation over the ipsilateral face and contralateral arm and leg, and an ipsilateral Horner syndrome. If the lesion is extramedullary, the glossopharyngeal and spinal accessory nerves are frequently involved (see discussion of the jugular foramen syndrome above). If it is extracranial in the posterior laterocondylar or retroparotid space, there may be a combination of ninth, tenth, eleventh, and twelfth cranial nerve palsies and a Horner syndrome. Combinations of these lower cranial nerve palsies have a variety of eponymic designations, listed in Table 360-1. If there is no sensory loss over the palate and pharynx and no palatal weakness or dysphagia, the lesion is below the origin of the pharyngeal branches, which leave the vagus nerve high in the cervical region; the usual site of disease is then the mediastinum.

HYPOGLOSSAL NERVE

The twelfth cranial nerve supplies the ipsilateral muscles of the tongue. The nucleus of the nerve or its fibers of exit may be involved by intramedullary lesions (tumor, poliomyelitis, or motor neuron disease). Lesions of the basal meninges and the occipital bones (platybasia, Paget's disease) may compress the nerve in its extramedullary course or in the hypoglossal canal. Isolated lesions of unknown cause can occur. Atrophy and fasciculation of the tongue develop weeks to months after interruption of the nerve.

MULTIPLE CRANIAL NERVE PALSIES

Several cranial nerves may be affected by the same disease process. In this situation, the main clinical problem is to determine whether the lesion lies within the brainstem or outside of it. Lesions that lie on the surface of the brainstem are featured by involvement of adjacent cranial nerves (often occurring in succession) and late and rather slight involvement of the long sensory and motor pathways and segmental structures lying within the brainstem. The opposite is true of intramedullary, intrapontine, and intramesencephalic lesions. The extramedullary lesion is more likely to cause bone erosion or enlargement of the foramens of exit of cranial nerves. The intramedullary lesion involving cranial nerves often produces a crossed sensory or motor paralysis (cranial nerve signs on one side of the body and tract signs on the opposite side).

Involvement of multiple cranial nerves outside the brainstem is frequently the result of trauma (sudden onset), localized infections such as herpes zoster (acute onset), granulomatous disease such as Wegener's granulomatosis (subacute onset), Behçet's disease, or tumors and enlarging saccular aneurysms (chronic development). Of the tumors, neurofibromas, meningiomas, chordomas, cholesteatomas, carcinomas, and sarcomas have all been observed to implicate a succession of lower cranial nerves. Owing to their anatomic relationships, the multiple cranial nerve palsies form a number of distinctive syndromes, listed in Table 360-1. Sarcoidosis has been found to be the cause of some cases of multiple cranial neuropathy, and chronic glandular tuberculosis (scrofula) the cause of a few others. Malignant granuloma of the nasopharynx may also affect multiple cranial nerves, as do nasopharyngeal tumors, platybasia, and basilar invagination of the skull, and the Chiari malformation that becomes evident in adult life. A purely motor disorder without atrophy always raises the question of myasthenia gravis (see Chap. 366). Guillain-Barré syndrome commonly affects the facial nerves bilaterally (facial diplegia). In the Fisher variant of the Guillain-Barré syndrome oculomotor paresis occurs with ataxia and areflexia in the limbs. Wernicke encephalopathy can cause a severe ophthalmoplegia combined with other brainstem signs (see Chap. 357).

A benign idiopathic form of multiple cranial nerve involvement on one or both sides of the face is occasionally seen. The disease may recur over a period of years with variable degrees of recovery between attacks. The condition is called *polyneuritis cranialis multiplex*.

REFERENCES

Adams RD, Victor M: *Principles of Neurology*, 4th ed. New York, McGraw-Hill, 1989

Baloh RW: Vertigo, in *Current Therapy in Neurologic Disease* 2d ed, RT Johnson (ed). Philadelphia, Decker, 1987, pp 7–10

Brodal A: The cranial nerves, in *Neurological Anatomy in Relation to Clinical Medicine*, 3d ed. New York, Oxford, 1980, chap 7, pp 448–577

Brownstone PK et al: Bilateral superior laryngeal neuralgia. Arch Neurol 37:525, 1980

Dalessio DJ: Trigeminal and glossopharyngeal neuralgia, in *Current Therapy in Neurologic Disease*, 2d ed, RT Johnson (ed). Philadelphia, Decker, 1987, pp 62–65

Durelli L et al: The Melkersson-Rosenthal syndrome: A case with increased CNS IgG synthesis. Ann Neurol 18:623, 1985

Eisen A, Bertrand G: Isolated accessory nerve palsy of spontaneous origin: A clinical and electromyographic study. Arch Neurol 27:496, 1972

Elston JS: Botulinum-toxin treatment of hemifacial spasm. J Neurol Neurosurg Psychiatr 49:824, 1986

Glaser JS: *Neuro-ophthalmology*. Hagerstown, Harper & Row, 1978

Groves J: Bell's (idiopathic) facial palsy, in *Scientific Foundations of Otolaryngology*, R Hinchcliffe, D Harrison (eds). London, Heinemann, 1976, pp 446–459

Hauser WA et al: Incidence and prognosis of Bell's palsy in the population of Rochester, Minnesota. Mayo Clin Proc 46:258, 1971

Karnes WE: Diseases of the seventh cranial nerve, in *Peripheral Neuropathy*, 2d ed, PJ Dyck et al (eds). Philadelphia, Saunders, 1984, chap 55, pp 1266–1299

Kaye AH, Adams CBT: Hemifacial spasm: A long-term follow-up of patients treated by posterior fossa surgery and nerve wrapping. J Neurol Neurosurg Psychiatry 44:1100, 1981

Lecky BRF et al: Trigeminal sensory neuropathy. Brain 110:1463, 1987

Liebold JE: Drugs having a toxic effect on the optic nerve. Intern Ophthalmol Clin 11:137, 1970

Selby G: Diseases of the fifth cranial nerve, in *Peripheral Neuropathy*, 2d ed, PJ Dyck et al (eds). Philadelphia, Saunders, 1984, chap 54, pp 1244–1265

Sweet WH: The treatment of trigeminal neuralgia (tic douloureux). N Engl J Med 315:174, 1986

———: Percutaneous methods for the treatment of trigeminal neuralgia and other faciocephalic pain; comparison with microvascular decompression. Semin Neurol 8:272, 1988

361 DISEASES OF THE SPINAL CORD

ALLAN H. ROPPER / JOSEPH B. MARTIN

Diseases of the spinal cord are frequently devastating, causing permanent and severe neurologic disability. Small lesions can produce quadriplegia, paraplegia, and sensory deficits far beyond the damage they would inflict elsewhere in the nervous system because the spinal cord contains, in a small cross-sectional area, almost the entire motor output and sensory input systems. Many spinal diseases are reversible, particularly extrinsic cord compression, making acute spinal cord lesions among the most critical of neurologic emergencies.

The stereotypic organization of the spinal cord, innervating the limbs and trunk segmentally through 31 pairs of spinal nerves, makes anatomic diagnosis relatively straightforward. A sensory level, paraplegia, or other typical syndromes usually permit recognition of a spinal cord process. Full assessment of cord disease requires a careful examination supplemented by laboratory tests, including magnetic resonance imaging (MRI), computed tomography (CT) scanning, myelography, analysis of cerebrospinal fluid (CSF), and somatosensory evoked responses. Most deficiencies in evaluating patients with signs of spinal cord disease result from cursory physical examination or inadequate x-rays. Computed tomography and MRI are replacing conventional myelography because of their ease of performance and better resolution; MRI gives particularly valuable information about intrinsic cord structure.

SPINAL COLUMN AND SPINAL CORD ANATOMY RELEVANT TO CLINICAL SIGNS The spinal cord is organized in a uniform somatotopic fashion throughout its length, giving rise to easily identifiable syndromes (see Chaps. 15, 25, and 28). The longitudinal location of lesions is established by the uppermost level of sensory and motor dysfunction. However, the relationship between the vertebral bodies of the spinal column (or their surface markers, the vertebral spines) and the cord segments that underlie them at times complicates the anatomic interpretation of signs of spinal cord diseases. Spinal cord syndromes are described according to the cord segment affected rather than by the surrounding vertebrae. During embryologic development the growth of the cord lags behind that of the spinal column, so that the cord ends behind the first lumbar vertebral body and the lower nerves must take an increasingly oblique downward course to exit near their targets in the limbs or viscera. The upper cervical cord segments lie behind the same numbered vertebral body, whereas the lower cervical segments are located one above each corresponding vertebral body, the upper thoracic cord two segments higher, and the lower thoracic cord, three segments higher. The lumbar and sacral cord segments, which form the conus medullaris, are located behind the ninth thoracic to first lumbar vertebrae. The cervical roots (except C8) exit from neural foramina above their respective vertebral bodies, while thoracic and lumbar roots exit below each body. In judging encroachment by various extrinsic masses, particularly spondylosis, careful radiographic measurement of the sagittal diameters of the spinal canal is often useful; they are normally 16 to 22 mm in the cervical and thoracic spine, 15 to 23 mm from L1 to L3, and 16 to 27 mm below.

CLINICAL SYNDROMES OF SPINAL CORD DISEASE The principal clinical signs of spinal cord damage are a "sensory level," i.e., loss of sensation below a circumferential horizontal line on the trunk, and weakness in the extremities innervated by the descending corticospinal fibers. Sensory symptoms, particularly paresthesias, may begin in the feet (or in one foot) and ascend, giving the impression early on of a polyneuropathy before a static sensory level is apparent. Lesions that disrupt descending corticospinal and bulbospinal tracts at a single cord level cause paraplegia or quadriplegia, with the characteristics of increased muscle tone, enhanced deep tendon reflexes, and Babinski signs. A careful examination often also elicits segmental signs that are approximate indicators of the location of a transverse lesion, such as a band of altered sensation at the rostral extent of the sensory level (hyperalgesia or hyperpathia), and isolated flaccidity, atrophy, or a single diminished deep tendon reflex. The sensory level to pinprick and temperature sensation is generally one or two segments below the level of an asymmetric lesion, but is at the level of the lesion in bilateral lesions. This is a result of the course of sensory fibers which ascend and cross to the opposite spinothalamic tract after synapsing in the dorsal horn. Midline back pain is also an accurate localizing sign, particularly in the thoracic region, where interscapular pain may be the first sign of cord compression. Radicular pain marks the primary site of a more laterally placed spinal lesion. Pain from lower cord (conus medullaris) lesions is often referred to the low back.

Early in the course of a severe and acute transverse lesion there may be flaccidity of the limbs rather than spasticity, due to so-called spinal shock. This state may last for several weeks and be mistaken for extensive segmental damage, but the reflexes later become increased. Brief clonic or myoclonic limb movements often precede paralysis in acute transverse lesions, particularly those due to infarction. Autonomic dysfunction, mainly urinary retention, is another prominent sign in transverse spinal lesions and should call attention to cord disease if it occurs in conjunction with spasticity or a sensory level.

Much is made of the clinical distinction between intramedullary (within the cord) and extramedullary compressive lesions, but most rules are approximations that do not distinguish one from the other dependably. Features that favor extramedullary lesions include radicular pain; a Brown-Séquard hemicord syndrome (see below); asymmetric lower motor neuron signs in one or two segments; early corticospinal signs; marked sacral sensory loss; and early, prominent CSF abnormalities. On the other hand, poorly localized burning pain, dissociated loss of pain sensation with sparing of joint position sensation, sparing of sensation in the perineal and sacral areas, late and less prominent corticospinal signs, and normal or minimally altered CSF generally favor an intramedullary lesion. ''Sacral sparing'' refers to the preservation of pinprick and temperature sensation in the sacral dermatomes, usually S3 to S5, with more rostral areas affected up to the sensory level. This is usually a dependable sign of intrinsic cord disease damaging the innermost fibers of the spinothalamic tracts while sparing those placed more laterally which subserve sacral sensation.

The *Brown-Séquard syndrome* is an eponym given to a hemicord syndrome consisting of ipsilateral mono- or hemiplegia, accompanied by ipsilateral loss of joint position and vibration sense, with contralateral loss of pain and temperature (spinothalamic) sensation. The segmental level for pain and temperature loss is sometimes one or two levels below the anatomic lesion. Segmental signs, such as radicular pain, muscle atrophy, or decreased tendon reflexes when they occur, are often unilateral.

Lesions limited to, or primarily within, the central portion of the cord preferentially damage gray matter neurons and segmental tracts crossing at that level. Traumatic contusion, developmental syringomyelia, tumors, and vascular lesions in the territory of the anterior spinal artery are the most common lesions localized to the central cord. Inflammatory diseases occur in this distribution less frequently. In the cervical cord, the central cord syndrome gives arm weakness out of proportion to leg weakness and a ''dissociated'' sensory loss signifying analgesia (loss of pin sensation), in a cape distribution over the shoulders, lower neck, and upper trunk without anesthesia (loss of touch sensation) or pallanesthesia (loss of vibration sense).

Lesions located in the region of the first lumbar vertebral body or below compress the spinal nerves of the cauda equina and cause a flaccid, areflexic, asymmetric paraparesis usually accompanied by bladder and bowel dysfunction. A sensory level is found in a saddle distribution up to L1, corresponding to the roots carried in the cauda equina. The Achilles and patellar reflexes are diminished or absent. Pain is common and projected to the perineum or thighs. With conus medullaris lesions pain is less prominent than in cauda equina lesions, and bladder and prominent bowel symptoms occur earlier. Compressive lesions may involve both the cauda and conus causing a combined syndrome of lower motor neuron signs and some hyperflexia or a Babinski sign.

The classic syndrome of the foramen magnum is weakness of the shoulder and arm followed by weakness of the ipsilateral leg, then contralateral leg, and finally, contralateral arm. Masses in this region sometimes produce suboccipital pain spreading to the neck and shoulders. A Horner's syndrome is another clue to a high cervical cord lesion; it does not occur with lesions below T2.

A few nontraumatic diseases are capable of producing sudden ''strokelike'' myelopathy without preceding symptoms. They include epidural hemorrhage, hematomyelia, cord infarction, nucleus pulposus embolism, and compression by spinal subluxation.

SPINAL CORD COMPRESSION **Tumors of the cord** Tumors in the spinal canal may be primary or metastatic, and are classified as extradural (''epidural'') or intradural, and the latter as intra- or extramedullary (see Chap. 353). The majority of neoplastic lesions are epidural arising from metastases to the adjacent spinal column. Neoplasms originating in the prostate, breast, and lung, and lymphoma and plasma cell dyscrasias are particularly common, though virtually every malignant tumor has been reported to cause metastatic epidural cord compression. The initial symptom in epidural compression is usually local back pain, often worse in the recumbent position, and causing the patient to awaken at night. Radiating radicular pain exacerbated by coughing, sneezing, or straining may accompany the back pain. Pain and local tenderness often precede other symptoms by many weeks. Neurologic signs commonly evolve over several days to a few weeks. The cord syndrome begins with progressive weakness, eventually acquiring all the hallmarks of a transverse myelopathy with paraparesis and a sensory level. A plain radiograph may show lytic or blastic changes, or a compression fracture at the level appropriate to the cord syndrome; radionuclide bone scans are more frequently positive. CT scan, myelography, and particularly MRI remain the optimal way of demonstrating cord compression. A horizontally widened and flattened cord from extrinsic compression is seen at the margins of the subarachnoid block, and the adjacent vertebral body is usually abnormal (Fig. 361-1).

In the past, emergency laminectomies were considered necessary to treat epidural cord compression by tumor, but treatment with high-dose glucocorticoids and rapid, fractionated radiation therapy has been as successful. Outcome is most closely related to the tumor type and its radiosensitivity. Paraparesis frequently improves within 48 h of the administration of glucocorticoids. Some incomplete or early transverse cord syndromes may still be better treated surgically, but each case must be analyzed individually taking into account the radiosensitivity of the tumor, distribution of other metastases, and the patient's general medical condition. Whichever therapy is chosen, it is wise to proceed quickly and use glucocorticoids as soon as the diagnosis of cord compression is suspected.

Intradural, extramedullary tumors are a less frequent cause of spinal cord compression and evolve more slowly than extradural

FIGURE 361-1 Sagittal section MRI showing compression deformity of the T12 vertebral body from metastatic adenocarcinoma (below arrows), and compression and displacement of the spinal cord. *(Courtesy of Greg Shoukimas, M.D., Department of Radiology, Massachusetts General Hospital.)*

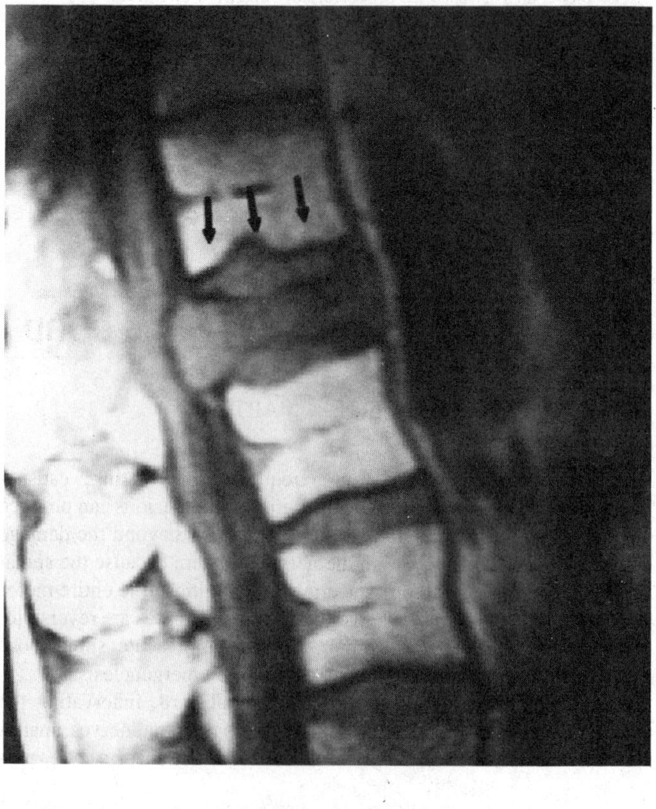

lesions. Meningiomas and neurofibromas are most common. Symptoms usually begin with radicular sensory changes and an asymmetric spinal cord syndrome. Radiologic studies show the typical appearance of dislocation of the cord to one side and an outline of the tumor within the subarachnoid space. Primary intramedullary tumors of the spinal cord are discussed in Chap. 353.

Neoplastic compressive myelopathies of all types initially cause minimal elevation of CSF protein, but with complete block of the subarachnoid space CSF protein concentration rises to the 1 to 10 g/L (100 to 1000 mg/dL) range due to impaired CSF circulation from the caudal sac to the intracranial subarachnoid space. There are usually few or no cells, cytology for malignant cells is often negative, and CSF glucose concentration remains normal unless there is accompanying widespread carcinomatous meningitis (see Chap. 353).

Epidural abscess This is a treacherous lesion, often misdiagnosed at first (see Chap. 354). The predisposing clinical settings are furunculosis of the back or scalp, bacteremia, or minor back injury. The condition can occur as a complication of local operation or very rarely after lumbar puncture. Spinal osteomyelitis acts as the nidus for the formation of an abscess that subsequently enlarges to compress the cord. The osteomyelitis is usually small and not often evident on plain radiographs. For several days to 2 weeks there may be only unexplained fever and mild spinal ache with local tenderness; later, radicular pain occurs. As the abscess expands, it rapidly causes cord compression with a transverse and usually complete transection syndrome. The proper treatment is rapid decompression by laminectomy and drainage, followed by appropriate antibiotics determined from culture of the purulent material. Incomplete drainage is not uncommon, resulting in a chronic granulomatous and fibrous reaction that may be sterilized with antibiotics but continues to act as a compressing mass. Tuberculous pyogenic abscess formation, more common in the past, is still a common cause of epidural abscess in developing countries.

Epidural hemorrhage and hematomyelia Hemorrhage into the spinal chord (hematomyelia) or epidural space produces an acute transverse myelopathy evolving over minutes or hours, accompanied by severe pain. Although these hemorrhages may originate from an arteriovenous malformation, or from hemorrhage into a tumor during anticoagulation with warfarin, they are more commonly spontaneous. Epidural hematoma may occur in the setting of minor trauma, lumbar puncture, warfarin anticoagulation, or secondary to coagulation disorders. Back and radicular pain can precede weakness by several minutes to hours, and be so severe that patients may be perceived to act in a peculiar, exaggerated fashion. Lumbar epidural hematoma results in loss of both knee and ankle reflexes, whereas retroperitoneal hematomas usually cause only absence of the knee reflexes. A myelogram or MRI defines the mass; CT scan is sometimes normal because the clot cannot be distinguished from adjacent bone. Subdural and subarachnoid clots are particularly painful and may occur spontaneously or under circumstances similar to those causing epidural hemorrhages. The CSF with epidural hemorrhage is usually clear or contains a few red blood cells; in subarachnoid or subdural hemorrhage the CSF is grossly bloody at first and later becomes discolored to a deep yellow-brown characteristic of blood pigments present in the CSF. There may be, in addition, a pleocytosis and lowered CSF glucose, giving the impression of bacterial meningitis.

Acute disk protrusion Lumbar disk herniation, a common disorder, is discussed in Chap. 19. Thoracic or cervical disk protrusion is less often a cause of spinal cord compression, usually occurring after direct trauma to the spinal column. Degeneration of cervical disk spaces with adjacent osteoarthritic hypertrophy causes a subacute spondylytic-compressive myelopathy in the cervical, and less often the thoracic region, discussed below. Embolism from nucleus pulposus material causing acute spinal cord infarction is also described below.

Other unusual compressive lesions Patients with iatrogenic or primary Cushing's syndrome have a tendency to form increased epidural fat tissue that rarely can reach a size large enough to compress the thoracic cord. Extramedullary hematopoiesis has caused cord compression in a number of hematologic diseases. Eroding aortic aneurysms, echinococcal or other parasitic cysts, gummas, lymphomatoid-granulomatosis, mucopolysaccharidoses, and other rare lesions can also compress the cord.

Arthritic diseases of the spine occur in two clinical forms: a lumbar or cauda equina compression from ankylosing spondylitis, or cervical cord compression from destruction of the cervical apophyseal or atlantoaxial joints in rheumatoid arthritis. Spinal complications arising as one component of severe generalized joint disease in rheumatoid arthritis are often overlooked. Forward subluxation of cervical vertebral bodies, or of the atlas on the axis, can cause a devastating, even fatal, acute cord compression after minor trauma such as whiplash, or it may present as a chronic compressive myelopathy similar to cervical spondylosis. Separation of the odontoid process from the axis may narrow the upper spinal canal compressing the cervicomedullary junction, particularly in flexion movements.

NONCOMPRESSIVE NEOPLASTIC MYELOPATHIES Intramedullary metastasis, paracarcinomatous myelopathy, and radiation myelopathy In the context of known cancer most myelopathies are compressive. However, when radiologic studies fail to show compression, there is often difficulty distinguishing between several less common entities: intramedullary metastasis, paracarcinomatous myelopathy, and radiation myelopathy. In a patient with known metastatic cancer and a progressive myelopathy shown to be noncompressive, intramedullary metastasis is the most likely diagnosis since paraneoplastic myelopathy is rarer (see Chap. 310). Back pain is the most common initial symptom with intramedullary metastasis, though it is not invariable, followed by progressive spastic paraparesis and, less often, paresthesias. Dissociated sensory loss or sacral sparing, though characteristic of intrinsic compression, is uncommon, and asymmetric paraparesis with incomplete sensory loss is typical. Myelography, CT scan, or MRI may show a swollen cord without extrinsic compression; in almost half of patients CT or myelography are normal; MRI is more successful in outlining a metastatic mass or primary intramedullary tumor (Fig. 361-2). Intramedullary metastases usually

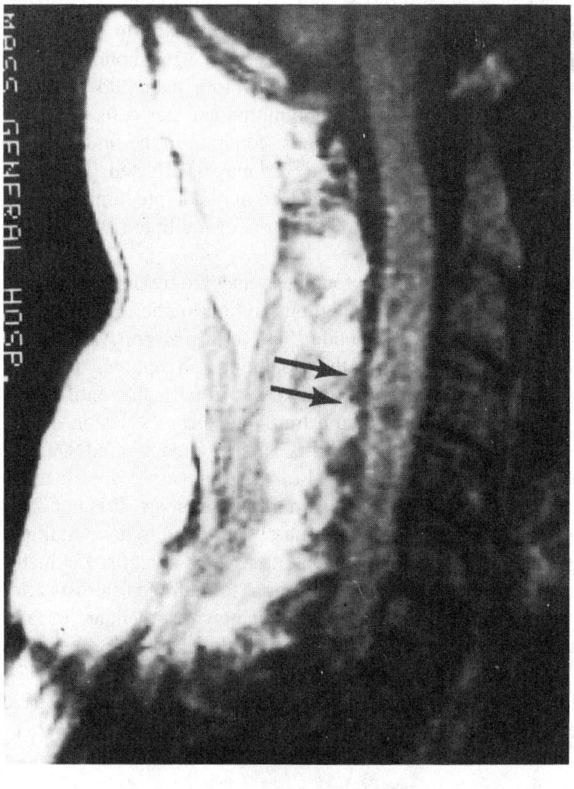

FIGURE 361-2 Sagittal MRI showing intrinsic fusiform enlargement of the cervical spinal cord from an intramedullary tumor. The tumor displays a low-density signal (arrows). *(Courtesy of Greg Shoukimas, M.D., Department of Radiology, Massachusetts General Hospital.)*

arise from bronchogenic carcinoma and less often from breast cancer and other solid tumors. Metastatic melanoma, an uncommon cause of extrinsic cord compression, more often presents as an intramedullary mass. The pathology of the metastasis is usually a single eccentrically placed nodule that presumably arrived hematogenously. Radiation therapy may be helpful in appropriate circumstances.

Carcinomatous meningitis, a common form of CNS invasion in malignancy, does not cause a myelopathy unless there is extensive subpial infiltration from adjacent roots causing nodules with secondary compression or infiltration of the cord. An incomplete, painless cauda equina syndrome can result from carcinomatous root infiltration (see Chap. 353). Headache is common, and repeated CSF examinations eventually reveal malignant cells, an elevated protein, and, in some cases, reduced CSF glucose concentration.

A progressive necrotic myelopathy associated with a paucity of inflammation can occur as a remote effect of cancer, usually with solid tumors. The radiologic studies and CSF are normal, or there may be slightly elevated protein. A subacute progressive spastic paraparesis evolves over days or weeks, usually asymmetrically, with distal paresthesias ascending to establish a sensory level, and late bladder dysfunction. Several adjacent segments of cord are involved.

Radiation may produce a delayed subacute progressive myelopathy due to microvascular hyalinization and vascular occlusion (see Chap. 353). It frequently presents a differential diagnostic problem when the cord lies within radiation portals used to treat other structures such as the mediastinal lymph nodes. Differentiation from paracarcinomatous myelopathy or intramedullary metastasis is difficult except by circumstantial history of prior radiation.

INFLAMMATORY MYELOPATHIES **Acute myelitis, transverse myelitis, and necrotic myelopathy** These are a group of related diseases marked by intrinsic inflammation of the cord and a clinical syndrome evolving over several days to 2 or 3 weeks. There may be a transverse or virtually complete spinal syndrome (transverse myelitis) or incomplete variants such as a posterior column myelopathy with ascending paresthesias and a sensory level for vibration; ascending, predominantly spinothalamic findings; or a Brown-Séquard syndrome with leg paresis and contralateral spinothalamic-type sensory changes. Many cases follow a viral illness. The most common presenting findings in transverse myelitis are back pain, progressive paraparesis, and asymmetric ascending paresthesias in the legs, later affecting the hands if the disease progresses, creating confusion with Guillain-Barré syndrome. Radiologic studies are necessary to exclude a compressive lesion. The CSF contains 5 to 50 lymphocytes per microliter in most patients; occasionally more than 200 cells per microliter are found, and rarely, polymorphonuclear cells predominate. The inflammatory process is most common in the mid and low thoracic regions, but any level of the cord may be affected. A chronic progressive cervical myelitis has been described, predominantly in older women, and is believed to be a form of multiple sclerosis (see Chap. 356).

In some cases necrosis is profound and may progress intermittently for several months to involve contiguous portions of the cord, reducing much of it to a thin gliotic ribbon. The term *progressive necrotic myelopathy* has been given to this condition. Exceptional cases of necrotic myelopathy progress to involve virtually the entire cord (necrotic panmyelopathy). When a transverse necrotic lesion occurs before or shortly after optic neuritis, it has been termed Devic's disease or neuromyelitis optica. All of these processes appear to be related to, and many are variants of, multiple sclerosis. It is not clear what proportion of patients will ultimately be found to have multiple sclerosis after a single episode of acute transverse myelitis. Estimates have been 15 to 80 percent, a range similar to multiple sclerosis after optic neuritis. The postinfectious demyelinating disorders are usually monophasic and only rarely recur, though fluctuation of symptoms related to a single level of the cord is common (see Chap. 355). Systemic lupus erythematosus and other autoimmune disorders have also been associated with myelitis.

Infectious myelopathy Direct viral infection of the cord produces specific types of myelitis. In the past, the most common form was poliomyelitis. Herpes zoster, preceded by radicular symptoms, is presently the most common cause of viral myelitis. The pathologic process is not restricted to the gray matter as is polio. Lymphocytes are always found in the CSF.

The human retroviruses HTLV-I and HIV may be associated with myelopathies (see Chap. 355). HTLV-I causes a chronic progressive, noninflammatory cord syndrome with symmetric spastic paraparesis and mild sensory and bladder disturbances. The disease is endemic in several areas where the virus is endemic, including areas of the Caribbean, South America, and southern Japan. It was identified as "tropical spastic paraparesis" before the virus was known. A myelopathy with vacuolar pathologic changes has been associated with HIV. There is generally no clear sensory level in the retroviral myelopathies.

Intramedullary cord abscesses caused by bacteria or mycobacteria arising in the context of systemic infection have been reported. Chronic meningitic lesions due to syphilis may produce a secondary subpial myelitis and radiculitis that evolve slowly (see below). An intense granulomatous, necrotic, and inflammatory myelitis is peculiar to infestation by *Schistosoma mansoni,* caused by a local response to tissue-digesting enzymes produced by ova from the parasite. Toxoplasmosis may also rarely cause a focal myelopathy.

Toxic myelopathy A toxic noninflammatory myelopathy, sometimes with optic atrophy, has been reported, mainly in Japan, and linked to ingestion of iodochlorhydroxyquinoline. Most patients have recovered, but many have persistent paresthesias.

Arachnoiditis This is a nonspecific term referring to inflammation, scarring, and fibrous thickening of the arachnoid membrane capable of compressing nerve roots or, rarely, the spinal cord. It is usually a postoperative complication or results from instillation of radiographic dye, antibiotics, or noxious chemicals into the subarachnoid space. The CSF contains many cells and an elevated protein concentration soon after the inciting event, but the inflammation then subsides. There may be slight fever in acute cases. Bilateral asymmetric radicular limb pain is the most prominent feature, with additional signs of root compression, such as reflex loss. Back pain and radicular symptoms are attributed to lumbar arachnoiditis, perhaps more often than justified. Arachnoiditis is not often responsible for cord compression (see Chap. 19). Treatment is controversial; laminectomy has led to improvement in some patients. Multiple meningeal cul-de-sacs, or arachnoid cysts, along nerve roots, occur as a congenital process that may produce severe radicular pain in midadulthood when the cysts enlarge and distort or exert traction on spinal nerve roots or ganglia. An unexplained delayed paraplegia has been reported after the use of chymopapain for the treatment of disk herniation.

SPINAL CORD INFARCTION Because the anterior or posterior spinal arteries are not usually involved by atherosclerosis, and only occasionally are affected by angiitis or emboli, most infarctions of the spinal cord are due to ischemia secondary to distant vascular occlusions. Aortic thrombosis or dissection causes cord infarction by interrupting the entire radicular and direct arterial supply to the anterior and posterior spinal arteries. The infarction typically occurs in a vascular watershed region of the thoracic cord between the large tributary to the spinal cord arising from the lower aorta, the artery of Adamkiewicz, and the anterior spinal artery arising from the vertebral arteries. The anterior spinal artery syndrome usually appears abruptly, like a stroke, or emerges postoperatively if the proximal aorta has been clamped. In some cases, however, symptoms progress over 24 to 72 h making diagnosis difficult. Spinal infarction has been reported rarely with systemic arteritis, immune reactions of serum sickness, and after intravascular contrast injection, heralded in the latter by severe back pain at the time of injection.

Cord infarction caused by microscopic fragments of herniated nucleus pulposus may occur after minor trauma, frequently during athletic activities. There is sharp local pain followed by a rapid paraplegia and a transverse cord syndrome evolving over several minutes to an hour. Pulposus tissue is found in small intramedullary vessels and often within the marrow of the adjacent vertebral body. The route from the disk space to marrow and thence to the cord is uncertain. This entity should be suspected in young adults with catastrophic transverse cord syndromes after back injury or exercise.

VASCULAR MALFORMATION OF THE SPINAL CORD Arteriovenous malformations (AVM) of the spinal cord are among the most difficult lesions to detect because of their great clinical variability. They may simulate multiple sclerosis, transverse myelitis, spinal cord stroke, or neoplastic compression. AVMs are most often found in the low thoracic or lumbar cord in middle-aged men. The majority begin with an incomplete progressive cord syndrome that may advance subacutely or episodically, like multiple sclerosis, producing bilateral corticospinal, spinothalamic, and posterior column symptoms and signs in any combination. Almost all patients are paraparetic and unable to walk within several years. About one-third have an abrupt syndrome with a single acute transverse myelopathy from bleeding, which simulates acute myelitis; others present with several acute exacerbations. About half have back or radicular pain, a few have a claudication syndrome similar to lumbar canal stenosis, and rare patients describe an acute onset with severe, localized back pain. Fluctuation of pain or neurologic signs with exercise, posture, or menses is helpful in suspecting the diagnosis. Bruits over the lesion are rare but should be sought at rest and after exercise. Most patients have mild elevation of CSF protein and a few show CSF pleocytosis. Bleeding into the cord or CSF may occur. Myelography, CT or MRI shows a lesion in 75 to 90 percent of cases. The anatomic details of most AVMs can be demonstrated with selective spinal angiography, a procedure requiring experience for safe and efficacious performance.

The pathogenesis of the myelopathy caused by AVMs (that have not bled) is incompletely understood, but appears to be a necrotic noninflammatory process consistent with ischemia. A dorsal AVM with a prominent progressive intramedullary syndrome (Foix-Alajouanine) has been reported with an adjacent necrotic myelopathy. The abnormal vessels have a characteristic thickened, hyalinized wall. Since any necrotic process within the cord may give rise to neovascularization and thick walled vessels, the pathologic basis of this vascular malformation remains controversial. Arteriovenous fistulas outside the spinal cord, including in visceral organs, have been associated with a vascular myelopathy due to large draining veins that traverse the spinal canal.

CHRONIC MYELOPATHIES **Spondylosis** This is a general term for several related degenerative changes of the spine giving rise to compression of the cervical cord and adjacent roots. Cervical spondylosis is primarily a disease of older patients, affecting men more often than women, and consisting of a combination of (1) narrowing of intervetebral disk spaces with nucleus pulposus herniation or annulus bulging, (2) osteophytic spur formation on the dorsal (posterior) aspect of the vertebral bodies, (3) partial subluxation of vertebrae, and (4) hypertrophy of the dorsal spinal ligament and dorsolateral facet articulations (see Chap. 19). The bony changes are reactive in nature, but there is no true arthritis. The most important feature causing spinal cord symptoms and signs is a "spondylitic bar" formed by osteophytes arising from the dorsal surfaces of adjacent vertebral bodies resulting in a horizontal compression of the ventral cord (Fig. 361-3*A* and *B*). Extension of the bar laterally, accompanied by articulatory hypertrophic changes or encroachment on the neural foramina, often causes additional radicular symptoms. The sagittal diameter of the spinal canal may be narrowed further by actual disk protrusion, or by hypertrophy or buckling of the dorsal spinal ligament, particularly during neck extension. Although the radiographic findings of spondylosis are common in the elderly, only a few patients develop myelopathy or radiculopathy, often dependent upon a congenitally narrow canal.

Neck and shoulder pain with stiffness are early symptoms; pressure on nerve roots is associated with radicular arm pain, most often in a C5 or C6 distribution. Compression of the cervical cord produces a slowly progressive spastic paraparesis, at times asymmetric, and often accompanied by paresthesias in the feet and hands. Vibratory sense is substantially diminished in the legs in most patients, and occasionally there is a sensory level for vibration on the upper thorax. Coughing or straining often produces leg weakness or radiating arm or shoulder pain. Dermatomal sensory loss in the arms, atrophy of intrinsic hand muscles, increased deep tendon reflexes in the legs, and asymmetric Babinski signs are common. Urinary urgency or incontinence do not occur unless the process is well-advanced. The reflexes in the arms are often diminished at some level, notably the biceps, corresponding to C5–C6 cord compression or root involvement. Either radicular, myelopathic, or combined signs may predominate. The diagnosis should be considered in cases of progressive cervical myelopathy, paresthesias of feet or hands, or wasting of the

FIGURE 361-3 *A*. Lateral x-ray of the cervical spine showing spondylitic "bar" formation from the junction of adjacent osteophytes at C6–C7 (arrow). *B*. Horizontal CT section at C6 from patient shown in *A*, after instillation of water-soluble dye into the subarachnoid space. A spur of the bony osteophyte compresses and distorts the spinal cord (arrows).

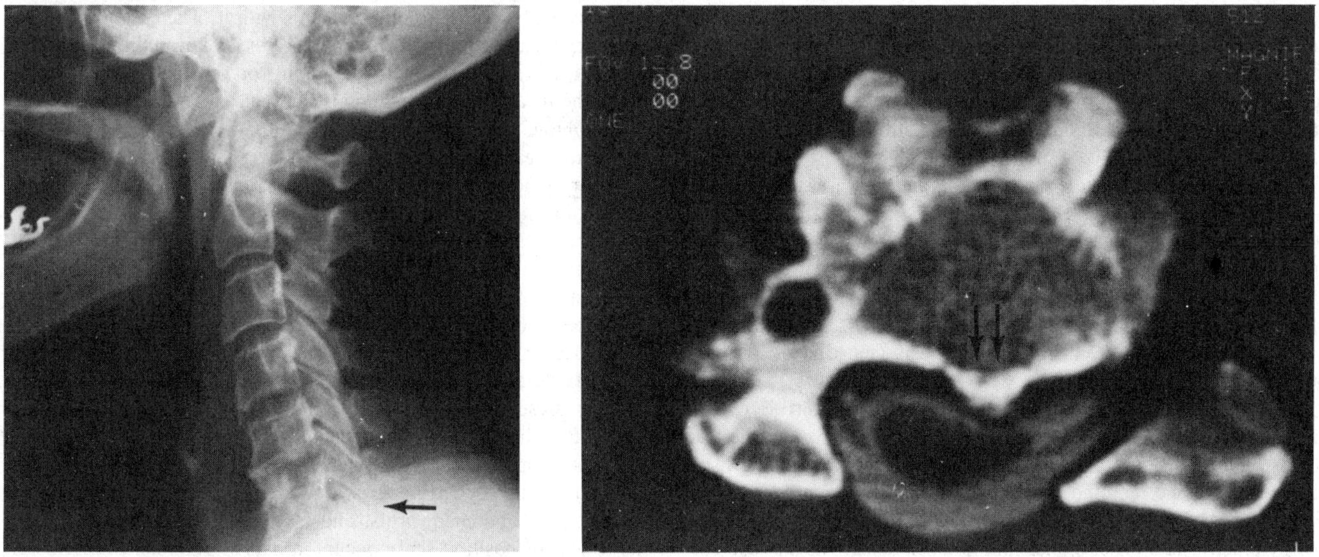

A **B**

hands. Spondylosis is also one of the most common causes of gait difficulty in the elderly, often causing an otherwise unexplained increase in leg reflexes or Babinski signs.

Plain radiographs demonstrate spondylitic bars, intervertebral narrowing and subluxations, reversal of the normal cervical spine curvature, and reduction of the sagittal diameter of the canal to less than 11 mm, or to 7 mm with neck extension (Fig. 361-3*A*). The CSF is usually normal or shows a slightly elevated protein concentration. Somatosensory evoked potentials can be very helpful by demonstrating normal conduction in peripheral large sensory fibers and a delay in central conduction in the mid or high cervical cord. Electromyography may also be useful in demonstrating radicular compression.

Cervical spondylosis is both an under- and overdiagnosed disease. Many patient with intrinsic cord processes, particularly amyotrophic lateral sclerosis, multiple sclerosis, and subacute combined degeneration, have had cervical laminectomies in the belief that spondylosis was responsible. There may be temporary improvement suggesting that there was an element of spondylolytic compression, but the underlying intrinsic myelopathy soon progresses. A mild progressive gait disorder with sensory symptoms in the feet and hands caused by cervical spondylosis may also be incorrectly attributed to peripheral neuropathy.

Rest and cervical immobilization with a soft collar are helpful in minor cases, traction may be helpful in others, but an operation is advisable if there are advanced symptoms of gait difficulty, severe hand weakness, or bladder difficulty, particularly if there is a virtually complete block of the subarachnoid space on myelography or CT scan.

Lumbar stenosis (also discussed in Chap. 19) is an intermittent and chronic compression of the cauda equina usually based on congenital narrowing of the lumbar spinal canal, which is further compromised by disk protrusion or spondylitic changes. Exercise brings about an aching pain in the buttocks, thighs, and calves, frequently sciatic in distribution, ceasing with rest and thereby simulating vascular-induced claudication. During the peak of pain, deep tendon reflexes and sensation may be reduced as compared to the resting state; peripheral vascular studies are normal. Lumbar stenosis and cervical spondylosis commonly occur together, the former probably explaining occasional lower extremity fasciculations in cervical spondylosis.

Degenerative and inherited myelopathies The prototype of the inherited disorders causing spinal cord syndromes is Friedreich's ataxia, a progressive, recessively inherited, leg and truncal ataxia of late childhood onset. Intention tremor, clumsiness of the arms, and, later, dysarthria occur. Kyphoscoliosis and pes cavus are common. Areflexia, Babinski signs, and severely impaired vibratory and joint position sense loss are found on examination. Fragmentary or milder forms of the illness occur and overlap with other syndromes including spastic paraparesis (Strümpell-Lorrain), cerebellar cortical degeneration with ataxia, and olivopontocerebellar atrophy (see also Chap. 359).

Amyotrophic lateral sclerosis (motor neuron disease) must be considered in patients with symmetric spastic paraparesis without sensory findings. It causes a pure motor syndrome with combined corticospinal, corticobulbar, and anterior horn cell involvement. Clinical or electromyographic evidence of widespread muscle fasciculations and denervation, in contrast to the limited segmental denervation of spondylosis, confirms the diagnosis (see Chaps. 359 and 362).

Subacute combined degeneration due to vitamin B_{12} deficiency This treatable myelopathy causes a progressive spastic and ataxic paraparesis and neuropathy, usually with prominent distal paresthesias of the feet and hands. It should be considered in cases simulating cervical spondylosis, late-onset degenerative myelopathies, and symmetric late-onset spinal multiple sclerosis. The disease can also involve the peripheral and optic nerves, and the brain. The diagnosis is confirmed by low B_{12} serum concentration and a positive Schilling test. This entity and related nutritional degenerations are discussed in Chap. 357. Whether folate or vitamin E deficiencies can produce a similar syndrome is controversial. Rarely, multiple sclerosis and B_{12} deficiency myelopathy are found in the same patient.

Syringomyelia Syringomyelia is a progressive myelopathy characterized pathologically by cavitation of the central spinal cord. It is often idiopathic or developmental (see Chap. 358) but may result from trauma, primary intramedullary tumors, extrinsic compression with central cord necrosis, arachnoiditis, hematomyelia, or necrotic myelitis. The developmental type usually begins in the midcervical cord and extends upward to the medulla or downward as low as the lumbar cord. It commonly takes an eccentric position often causing unilateral long tract signs or reflex asymmetries. Many cases occur in association with craniovertebral abnormalities, most commonly the Arnold-Chiari malformation, but also including myelomeningocele, basilar skull impression (platybasia), atresia of the foramen of Magendie, or Dandy-Walker cysts (see Chap. 358).

The cardinal clinical signs of syringomyelia correspond to a central high cervical cord syndrome and depend on the extent of the syrinx and associated abnormalities such as the Arnold-Chiari malformation. The classic presentation is (1) sensory loss, usually of a dissociated type (loss of pain and temperature and preservation of touch and vibration senses), which is ''suspended'' over the nape of the neck, shoulders, and upper arms (cape distribution), and eventually extends to the hands, (2) wasting of muscles in the lower neck, shoulders, arms, and hands, with asymmetric or absent reflexes, and (3) high thoracic kyphoscoliosis. The majority begin asymmetrically with unilateral sensory loss. A number of patients develop loss of pin sensation on the face attributed to damage to the descending tract of the trigeminal nerve in the upper cervical cord. Cough-induced headache and neck pain are common with associated Arnold-Chiari malformations.

Symptoms in idiopathic cases begin in adolescence or early adulthood, progress irregularly, and frequently arrest for several years. A few patients escape major disability, but over half become wheelchair-bound. Analgesia leads to injuries, burns, and trophic ulcers in the fingertips. Charcot joints in the shoulders, elbows, or knees are common in advanced cases. Prominent lower extremity weakness or hyperreflexia suggest an associated abnormality at the craniovertebral junction. Syringobulbia results from extension of the cavity into the medulla, or rarely the pons, usually occupying the lateral medullary tegmentum. Palatal and vocal cord paralysis, dysarthria, nystagmus, episodic dizziness, tongue weakness, and Horner's syndrome may occur.

Slow enlargement of the cavity may create a narrowing or complete block of the subarachnoid space. The cavity is separate from the central canal but usually communicates with it. The diagnosis can be made dependably from the clinical features, confirmed by finding an enlarged cervical cord on myelography or on delayed CT images several hours after subarachnoid instillation of metrizamide or another water-soluble contrast material (Fig. 361-4*A*). Syrinx cavities are shown to greatest advantage by MRI (Fig. 361-4*B*). The cervicomedullary junction should be examined for associated developmental abnormalities.

Therapy is directed at decompressing the cavity to prevent progression of damage and decompressing the spinal canal if the cord is distended. Laminectomies and suboccipital decompression are sometimes recommended when an Arnold-Chiari malformation accompanies an enlarged cervical cord.

Tabes dorsalis Tabes and meningovascular syphilis of the spinal cord are presently rare but at one time had to be considered in the differential diagnosis of most spinal cord syndromes. The most common symptoms of tabes are characteristic fleeting and repetitive, lancinating pains occurring mostly in the legs, less commonly in the back, thorax, abdomen, arms, and face. Severe gait and leg ataxia due to loss of position sense occurs in half of patients. Paresthesias, bladder disturbances, and acute abdominal pain with vomiting (visceral crisis) occur in 15 to 30 percent. The cardinal signs of tabes are loss

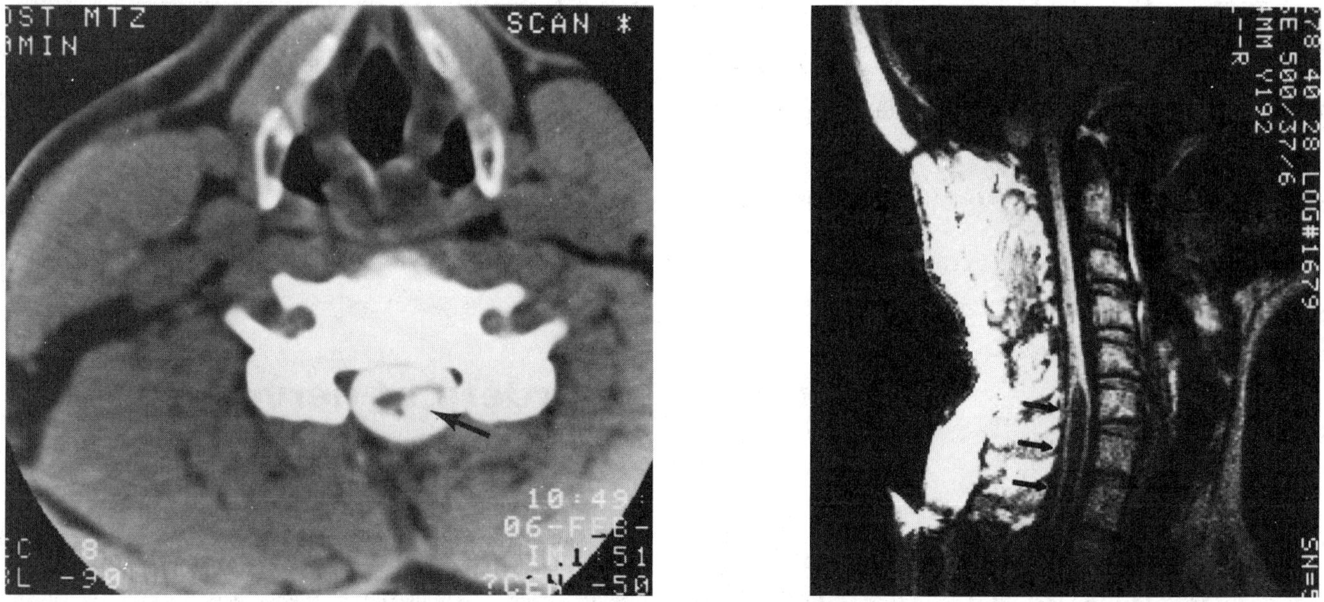

A

B

FIGURE 361-4 *A*. Horizontal CT section 1 h after subarachnoid instillation of water-soluble contrast medium showing the cervical spinal cord surrounded by contrast and dye in a large intramedullary syrinx cavity (arrow). *B*. Sagittal MRI of same patient shown in *A* showing the syrinx cavity and enlargement of the spinal cord (arrows). *(Courtesy of Greg Shoukimas, M.D., Department of Radiology, Massachusetts General Hospital.)*

of reflexes in the legs, impaired position and vibratory sense, Romberg's sign, and bilateral, Argyll Robertson pupils, which fail to constrict to light but react with accommodation.

Traumatic spinal cord lesions and compression of the cord secondary to orthopedic disorders are discussed in the chapter on cranial and spinal injury (Chap. 352).

GENERAL CARE OF THE PATIENT WITH ACUTE PARAPLEGIA OR QUADRIPLEGIA Protection from secondary damage to the urinary tract is a high priority in the acute stages of paraplegia. The bladder is areflexic, retains urine, and the patient is unaware of bladder distention, making damage to the detrusor muscle from overdistention possible. Urologic rehabilitation requires bladder drainage and avoidance of urinary infection. This is best accomplished by intermittent catheterization by trained personnel. Continuous closed system urinary drainage, which is associated with a higher infection rate than intermittent catheterization, or suprapubic drainage are less desirable alternatives. Patients with acute lesions, especially those causing spinal shock, frequently need special cardiovascular care because of paroxysmal hypertension or hypotension. Ileus and gastric stress ulcers are other potential acute medical problems in patients with complete transverse cord lesions. Cimetidine, ranitidine, or sucralfate may be useful in these circumstances. Pulmonary embolism due to immobilization is a grave early risk occurring in approximately one-third of patients after acute cord trauma. Subcutaneous heparin may reduce the risk of early embolic complications. Rarely spinal injury patients have become hypercalcemic from immobilization.

High cervical cord lesions cause varying degrees of mechanical respiratory failure requiring artificial ventilation. In cases of incomplete respiratory failure with forced vital capacities of 10 to 20 mL/kg, chest physical therapy is useful, and a negative pressure cuirass may be used to alleviate atelectasis and fatigue, particularly if the major lesion is below C4. With severe respiratory failure, tracheal intubation (performed over an endoscope if the spine is unstable), followed by tracheostomy, provides tracheal access for ventilation and suctioning. A promising new technique is phrenic nerve pacing in patients with lesions at C5 or above.

As clinical signs stabilize, attention should be directed to the psychological state of the patient and the development of a rehabilitation plan framed by realistic expectations. An aggressive program is often remarkably successful with younger and middle-aged patients allowing return to home and a productive lifestyle.

Chronic nursing care problems can be handled by patients with varying degrees of assistance. The major issues are related to immobilization: skin breakdown over pressure points, urinary sepsis, and autonomic instability, and the potential for pulmonary embolism. Early care includes frequent repositioning, application of skin emollients, and soft bed coverings. Specialized beds turn the patient or distribute body weight evenly rather than predominantly on bony prominences. If the sacral cord segments are undamaged, then a large degree of automatic voiding can be entrained. Patients initially void reflexly between catheterizations and later learn to induce voiding with various maneuvers. If residual urinary volumes lead to infection, surgical procedures or an indwelling catheter may be necessary. Bowel regimens and disimpaction are necessary in most patients to ensure at least biweekly evacuation and avoid colonic distention or obstruction.

Severe hypertension and bradycardia occur in response to noxious superficial stimuli, bladder or bowel distention, or surgery, particularly in patients with cervical and high thoracic cord lesions. Flushing and diaphoresis above the level of the lesion may accompany the hypertension. The mechanism of this dysautonomia is not well understood. A potent antihypertensive agent may be necessary, particularly during surgery, but beta-blocking drugs should probably be avoided. Some patients become severely bradycardic with tracheal suctioning; this can be prevented with small doses of atropine.

Detailed aspects of the physical therapy, rehabilitation, and orthotics related to severe spinal cord diseases may be found in specialized texts. The orthopedic stabilization of the spine in relation to cord trauma is discussed in Chap. 344.

REFERENCES

Adams CBT, Logue V: Studies in cervical spondylitic myelopathy. Brain 94:579, 1971
Aminoff MJ, Logue V: Clinical features of spinal vascular malformations. Brain 97:197, 1974
Auld AW et al: Metastatic spinal epidural tumors: An analysis of 50 cases. Arch Neurol 15:100, 1966
Baker AS et al: Spinal epidural abcess. N Engl J Med 293:463, 1975
Barnett HJM et al: *Syringomyelia.* Philadelphia, Saunders, 1973

BYRNE TN, WAXMAN SG: Spinal cord compression. Contemporary Neurology Series, vol 33. Philadelphia, Davis, 1990
EDELSON R et al: Intramedullary spinal cord metastasis. Neurology 22:1222, 1972
GILBERT RW et al: Epidural cord compression from metastatic tumor: Diagnosis and treatment. Ann Neurol 3:40, 1978
GREENBERG HS et al: Epidural spinal cord compression from metastatic tumor: Results with a new treatment protocol. Ann Neurol 8:361, 1980
HARDY AG, ROSSIER AB: *Spinal Cord Injuries: Orthopedic and Neurological Aspects.* Stuttgart, Thieme, 1975
JOHNSON RT, MCARTHUR JC: Myelopathies and retroviral infections. Ann Neurol 21:113, 1987
LOGUE V: Angiomas of the spinal cord: Review of the pathogenesis, clinical features, and results of surgery. J Neurol Neurosurg Psychiatr 42:1, 1979
———, EDWARDS MR: Syringomyelia and its surgical treatment. J Neurol Neurosurg Psychiatr 44:273, 1981
MCILROY WJ, RICHARDSON JC: Syringomyelia: A clinical review of 75 cases. J Can Med Assoc 93:731, 1965
ROPPER AH, POSKANZER DC: Prognosis of acute and subacute transverse myelopathy based on early signs and symptoms. Ann Neurol 4:51, 1978
ROSSIER AB et al: Posttraumatic cervical syringomyelia. Brain 108:439, 1985
SRIGLEY JR et al: Spinal cord infarction secondary to intervertebral disc embolism. Ann Neurol 9:296, 1981

section 2 Disorders of nerve and muscle

362 APPROACH TO THE PATIENT WITH NEUROMUSCULAR DISEASE

ROBERT C. GRIGGS / WALTER G. BRADLEY / BHAGWAN SHAHANI

The neuromuscular diseases are disorders of the *motor unit* and of the sensory and autonomic peripheral nerves. Each motor unit consists of: (1) the *motor neuron cell body,* located in either the spinal cord anterior horn (for muscles innervated by the spinal cord) or a cranial nerve nucleus (for ocular, facial, bulbar musculature); (2) the *axon* of the motor neuron in the peripheral (or cranial) nerve; (3) the *neuromuscular junction;* and, (4) the *muscle fibers* innervated by the motor neuron. The sensory peripheral nerves comprise (1) the *sensory neuron* cell body in the posterior root ganglion; (2) the *central axon* passing to the spinal cord in the posterior root; (3) the *distal axon* in the peripheral nerve; and (4) the *sensory nerve terminal* in skin, muscle, joint capsule, etc. The autonomic nerves are divided into *sympathetic* and *parasympathetic* fiber systems. The sympathetic preganglionic fibers arise from cell bodies in the intermediolateral column of the spinal cord and enter the sympathetic ganglia, where postganglionic fibers arise to innervate blood vessels or viscera. The parasympathetic preganglionic neurons lie in the brainstem and sacral spinal cord, and axons terminate in the viscera, special sensory organs, or skin, which contain the postganglionic neurons and their nerve terminals. Neuromuscular diseases are classified into four groups depending upon which portion of the motor unit is involved (see Table 362-1).

The major symptoms of diseases of the motor unit are muscle weakness, fatigue, cramps, pain, or stiffness. Symptoms of peripheral nerve disease include, in addition, decreased sensation (hypesthesia or hypalgesia), abnormal sensations (paresthesias), or painful sensations (dysesthesias) (see Chap. 28). Symptoms of autonomic nervous system disease include postural dizziness, and abnormal cardiac, visceral, and ocular function, and changes in sweating. The symptoms of neuromuscular disease, particularly those of weakness or sensory disturbance, do not necessarily distinguish disorders of the peripheral nervous system from those of the central nervous system. Most neuromuscular diseases are relatively symmetric in contrast to the asymmetry of many central nervous system diseases.

CLINICAL ASSESSMENT

History and physical examination will lead to a diagnosis in a majority of patients with neuromuscular disease. Failure to arrive at a diagnostic impression before routine and sophisticated laboratory studies often leads to diagnostic inaccuracy and confusion. Few of the biochemical, histologic, and electrodiagnostic studies used to evaluate patients with neuromuscular disease are pathognomonic since nerve and muscle can respond to disease processes in only a limited number of ways.

CLINICAL HISTORY Weakness and fatigue (See Chap. 25) The patient with weakness, particularly when of gradual onset, may not recognize it, emphasizing the useful axiom that "signs of muscle weakness precede symptoms of weakness." Words such as numbness, deadness, tiredness, or fatigue may be used by a patient unfamiliar with what is taking place. On the other hand, some complaints of "weakness" result from systemic rather than neuromuscular disease. In such patients, strength is often normal or only mildly reduced, since the complaint is usually loss of stamina and endurance. The patient with fatigue should be asked to distinguish between true weakness and the less specific symptoms of lassitude and asthenia. If the patient is unable to perform a normal activity, true weakness is suggested. Objective evidence of weakness is established if symptoms exceed the bounds of normal variation (e.g., double vision, drooping eye lids, difficulty in swallowing, aspiration of food or liquids into the airway) as opposed to the more subjective complaints of inability to lift, carry, or push an object.

The time-course and severity of weakness must be quantitated by questions concerning alterations in functional abilities: for the legs, difficulty in rising from a chair or commode, rising from a squatting position, or climbing up and down stairs, and a history of frequent tripping, stumbling, or falling; for the trunk, difficulty in sitting up from supine in bed; or for the arms, difficulty in washing the hair, opening jars, fastening buttons, or raising objects onto a shelf.

Abnormalities of sensation (See Chaps. 28 and 363) Sensory symptoms suggest peripheral nerve disease although, as with weakness, sensory abnormalities can occur with disease at any level of the nervous system. The characteristics and localization of sensory symptoms in the various peripheral nerve syndromes and diseases

TABLE 362-1 Classification of neuromuscular disease

Site of involvement	Typical example
Anterior horn cell	
Without upper motor neuron involvement	Spinal muscular atrophy
With upper motor neuron involvement	Amyotrophic lateral sclerosis
Peripheral nerve	
Unifocal	Carpal tunnel syndrome
Multifocal	Mononeuritis multiplex (e.g., polyarteritis nodosa)
Diffuse	Diabetic neuropathy
Neuromuscular junction	Myasthenia gravis
Muscle	Duchenne muscular dystrophy

are discussed in Chap. 28. In contradistinction to weakness, it is axiomatic that "sensory symptoms precede objective sensory signs."

Muscle pain (See Chap. 27) Muscle aches and pains may suggest inflammatory or metabolic muscle disease but are far commoner in bone, joint, and nerve disease. Persistent muscle pain in a patient with normal strength usually results from a cause other than myopathy. Intermittent muscle pain, however, particularly when precipitated by exercise, should raise a consideration of a substrate utilization defect such as a glycogen or lipid storage myopathy or the purine nucleotide cycle disorder, myoadenylate deaminase deficiency. It is important to determine if other factors, such as fasting, precipitate pain and then to inquire about associated findings such as dark urine which may be indicative of myoglobinuria.

Autonomic dysfunction The most common complaint is "dizziness," or "blackouts," which prove to be precipitated by the patient standing up from sitting or lying. Loss of potency in the male is frequent in autonomic neuropathies. Explosive diarrhea or cyclical diarrhea-constipation are sometimes present, as is partial urinary retention.

PHYSICAL EXAMINATION **Strength testing** Reliable testing of strength requires that the examiner have an adequate frame of reference for normal strength and that the patient be motivated and able to cooperate with testing. As with history taking, it is helpful to quantitate the ability to perform tasks required in daily living. The legs are particularly easy to test by observing: walking on heels and toes; rising from a chair, noting whether there is a need to use the arms; rising from a squat; and stepping up on to a chair. It is also important to examine the legs for a *knee extension lag,* the inability to fully extend the leg against gravity. The number of degrees of extension lag can be measured with a goniometer. Patients with even a minor extension lag almost invariably report frequent tripping and falling. The converse is also true: patients with muscle weakness who report frequent falls usually have quadriceps muscle weakness producing a knee extension lag. Trunk and neck muscles can be tested by having the patient sit up from supine; extending the head over the edge of an examining table is a sensitive method of detecting neck weakness. The arms are not as easily evaluated with function testing: inspection of shoulders for scapular winging as the arms are elevated and watching the patient lift the arms above the head test shoulder girdle function. Hand strength can be judged by determining the degree of difficulty in extracting two fingers from the grip of the patient and by noting the ability of the patient to blanch the knuckles when making a tight fist. When the lesion affects a specific region, e.g., the brachial plexus or the ulnar nerve, it is essential to test each individual muscle of the arm or hand.

Formal muscle testing, assigning a numerical grade to muscle strength, is usually based on the MRC (Medical Research Council of Great Britain) 0 to 5 scale:

5—normal
4—able to oppose gravity plus resistance
3—able to move fully against gravity but not resistance
2—able to move with gravity eliminated
1—trace movement
0—no movement

An important assessment is whether a muscle is indeed *weaker than one would expect,* after making allowances for age, male-female differences, inactivity, or generalized illness. If one has a limited time for the testing of muscle strength, the assessment of function is likely to be of more value than formal muscle testing.

Muscle bulk Muscle atrophy and hypertrophy are often difficult to recognize because of wide variation among normals. The problem is accentuated in young children and in obese patients because of overlying adipose tissue. Atrophy is easier to appreciate when asymmetric. Muscle enlargement or hypertrophy is a normal accompaniment of physical activity. It is occasionally a sign of disease in patients with long-standing spasticity or myotonic disorders. So-called pseudohypertrophy, in which the muscles become enlarged by replacement with connective tissue or fat, may be prominent in certain of the muscular dystrophies but is also seen with spinal muscular atrophy and other denervating conditions. Actual hypertrophy of muscle fibers may also be present in these patients. Muscle enlargement may also be caused by infiltration with substances such as amyloid or by parasitic infestation (e.g., cysticercosis).

Focal muscle swelling may be due to inflammatory infiltrates, calcium deposits, or tendon rupture. Preservation of some parts of a muscle, while other parts atrophy, may occur in spinal muscular atrophy and some forms of muscular dystrophy, giving an appearance of a focal swelling during muscle contraction ("belly hypertrophy"). Single or multiple muscle masses in a patient without weakness may indicate a neoplastic process. Other causes of muscle enlargement include focal myositis, sarcoidosis, ectopic ossification, and tendon rupture.

Pathologic fatigue Patients with disorders of neuromuscular transmission such as myasthenia gravis can usually be shown to fatigue on examination. Sustained upward gaze produces gradual ptosis of the eyelids (curtain sign); eye movements become disconjugate on sustained horizontal gaze; the voice may become hoarse, slurred, or nasal with prolonged speech; or a smile may rapidly become a sneer when the patient cannot maintain facial muscle activity. Inability to sustain limb activity is less easily quantitated since patients who are weak from any cause may have decreased endurance.

Sensory testing Patients with peripheral neuropathy usually have sensory loss. The distribution of sensory disturbance as well as the modalities affected are often of diagnostic importance (see Chaps. 28 and 363).

Autonomic testing A fall of systolic blood pressure of more than 20 mmHg from lying to standing indicates impaired autonomic control of peripheral blood vessels. A greater fall often occurs with exercise in the erect position. The pulse rate does not increase normally in response to this hypotension if there is an autonomic neuropathy. Similarly, there is no slowing of the heart rate following a sustained Valsalva maneuver.

Other findings Myotonia, fasciculations, myokymia, and other spontaneous activity (Chap. 27) should be sought. Certain disorders such as myotonic dystrophy and facioscapulohumeral dystrophy have distinctive and virtually pathognomonic facial features. Less diagnostic but significant facial weakness is found in other myopathies and in myasthenia gravis. Contractures, particularly of the Achilles tendons, limitation of hip joint movement, and scoliosis may indicate that weakness is of long duration.

DIFFERENTIAL DIAGNOSIS Weaknesses produced by diseases of the motor unit are distinguishable from each other by their distribution, by the time-course of the illness, and by accompanying clinical findings such as muscle bulk and tone, reflexes, and sensory findings. The portion of the motor unit involved by a disease process is usually evident from clinical findings (Table 362-2). Motor neuron diseases (Chap. 359) are suggested in the patient whose weakness is accompanied by prominent atrophy, fasciculations, and lack of sensory involvement. The reflexes may be disproportionately depressed if anterior horn cell disease alone is present or pathologically increased if there is coexistent upper motor neuron disease, such as amyotrophic lateral sclerosis. Peripheral neuropathy (Chap. 363) is suggested by the presence of distal weakness associated with sensory involvement. In general, patients with peripheral neuropathy have depressed reflexes; preservation of reflexes in the presence of significant weakness suggests a cause other than neuropathy. Neuromuscular junction disorders (Chap. 366) are suggested if ocular and bulbar weakness is prominent, particularly if there is *diurnal variation,* with the patient becoming weaker as the day progresses. Pathologic fatigue can usually be demonstrated. Reflexes are preserved in most neuromuscular junction disorders, particularly myasthenia gravis.

Myopathy versus other neuromuscular disease Clinical features which suggest myopathy in contrast to other motor unit diseases include a proximal distribution of weakness, relative preservation or

TABLE 362-2 Presenting clinical features of the neuromuscular diseases

	Anterior horn cell	Peripheral nerve	Neuromuscular junction	Muscle
Distribution of weakness	Asymmetric limb or bulbar	Symmetric distal	Extraocular, bulbar, proximal limb	Symmetrical limb (bulbar in some)
Atrophy	Marked and early	Moderate	None	Slight early; marked later
Sensory involvement	None	Paresthesias, hypesthesia	None	None
Characteristic features	Fasciculations, cramps, tremor	Combined sensory and motor abnormality	Diurnal fluctuation	
Reflexes	Variable (depending on degree of upper motor neuronal involvement)	Decreased out of proportion to weakness	Normal	Decreased in proportion to weakness

increase of muscle bulk, and the preservation of reflexes. Table 362-3 presents a classification of primary muscle diseases. Many patients with muscle symptoms, however, have disorders that do not fit into this table because evaluation discloses disease in another portion of the motor unit or in another system (see Chap. 25). For example, a patient with a denervation produced by nerve root damage from a lumbar disc protrusion may have muscle cramps, pain, and weakness in muscles innervated by those nerve roots. Furthermore, fatigue, weakness, and pain are common accompaniments of derangements of cardiac, hematologic, gastrointestinal, pulmonary, renal, or hepatic function. Despite complaints of weakness and fatigue and the finding of atrophy, it is relatively infrequent for patients with pulmonary or cardiac disease to be mistaken for those with primary muscle disease.

Proximal weakness is so characteristic of myopathies that, by a somewhat circular argument, proximal weakness is usually attributed to "myopathy." In fact, neuropathies such as acute or chronic inflammatory polyneuropathy, the neuromuscular junction disorders, and many anterior horn cell diseases have predominantly proximal weakness. Proximal weakness, occurring in disorders such as hyperthyroidism and hyperparathyroidism and as a result of glucocorticoid administration, is often termed "myopathic," despite the fact that the underlying pathophysiology of the muscle disorders in these conditions has not been defined.

Acute generalized weakness Weakness developing over the course of less than an hour is usually caused by a metabolic or toxic disorder affecting either the neuromuscular junction or muscle. A sudden alteration in circulating potassium, calcium, sodium, magnesium, or phosphate may result in partial or complete paralysis of muscle. Acute failure of neuromuscular junction transmission may occur with botulism and other toxins, hypermagnesemia, aminoglycoside antibiotics, and other medications. Weakness developing over the course of 24 h may occur in electrolyte, metabolic, and toxic disorders; in periodic paralysis (Chap. 367); and in acute inflammatory myopathies, particularly those related to viral and parasitic infection (Chap. 364) and certain acute polyneuropathies (Chap. 363). Occasionally, patients with more chronic disorders first realize that they are weak when the insidious progression of their weakness produces an abrupt change in function.

TABLE 362-3 Classification of primary muscle diseases

I Hereditary
- *A* Muscular dystrophy (Chap. 365): Duchenne, myotonic, facioscapulohumeral, limb-girdle, oculopharyngeal, scapuloperoneal, congenital, distal, and ocular
- *B* Congenital myopathies (Chap. 365): Central core, nemaline, centronuclear, fiber-type disproportion
- *C* Metabolic myopathies (Chap. 365):
  - *1* Glycogen: Deficiencies of phosphorylase, phosphofructokinase, phosphoglyceromutase, acid maltase, others
  - *2* Lipid: Defective synthesis or transport of carnitine; deficiency of carnitine palmityl transferase
  - *3* Purine nucleotide cycle: Deficiency of myoadenylate deaminase
- *D* Myotonia (Chap. 365): Congenita, paramyotonia
- *E* Periodic paralysis (Chap. 27 and 367): Hypokalemic, hyperkalemic

II Inflammatory (Chap. 364)
- *A* Collagen disease: Systemic lupus erythematosus, rheumatoid arthritis, scleroderma, mixed-connective tissue
- *B* Sarcoidosis, carcinoid, neoplastic
- *C* Infections: Numerous, especially viral (influenza B), protozoal (toxoplasmosis), parasitic (trichinosis)
- *D* Idiopathic: Polymyositis, dermatomyositis

III Endocrine and metabolic (Chap. 365)
- *A* Electrolyte abnormalities: Calcium, phosphate, magnesium, sodium, potassium
- *B* Endocrine: Hypo- and hyperfunction of thyroid, adrenal, parathyroid, pituitary

IV Toxic (Chap. 365): Alcohol, opiates, pentazocine, clofibrate, others

V Tumors and masses: Primary and metastatic neoplasms, infection, sarcoidosis, myositis ossificans, calcinosis, muscle rupture and hemorrhage

Subacute weakness Weakness developing over days is more common in peripheral nerve or neuromuscular junction diseases than in muscle or anterior horn cell disease. Acute inflammatory polyneuropathy (Guillain-Barré syndrome) and porphyric, diphtheritic, and toxic neuropathies are of subacute onset. Myasthenia gravis and other neuromuscular junction diseases must also be considered in the differential diagnosis. Subacute weakness can occur in severe polymyositis and dermatomyositis (see Chap. 364). Weakness from endocrine disorders and certain muscle toxins (Table 362-3) may also develop subacutely (Chap. 365). Of the anterior horn cell disorders only infections with poliomyelitis and other viruses commonly evolve subacutely. Amyotrophic lateral sclerosis occasionally pursues a subacute, severe course.

Slowly progressive weakness *Slowly progressive proximal weakness* evolving over weeks to months may be caused by polymyositis or dermatomyositis or an unsuspected endocrinopathy. When the course has extended for a year or more, however, one of the muscular dystrophies, spinal muscular atrophy, or a neuromuscular junction defect such as myasthenia gravis may be present. Neuropathies are seldom proximal, the major exceptions being acute and chronic inflammatory polyneuropathy, porphyric neuropathy, and diabetic proximal mononeuropathy. *Slowly progressive distal weakness* is more characteristic of peripheral nerve or anterior horn cell disorders than of disorders of muscle or the neuromuscular junction. The only commonly encountered distal myopathy is myotonic dystrophy. Less common disorders such as distal muscular dystrophy, nemaline and centronuclear myopathies, and a variant of polymyositis known as inclusion body myositis may present with distal weakness. Prominent distal lower limb weakness is also present in the facioscapulohumeral and scapuloperoneal muscular dystrophies, but proximal involvement is invariably also present in such patients. *Slowly progressive bulbar weakness* is more typical of anterior horn cell or neuromuscular junction disorders than of myopathies. Bulbar weakness (difficulty in speaking, coughing, and swallowing) occurs commonly in motor neuron disease (especially amyotrophic lateral sclerosis) and neuromuscular junction disorders. It is also seen in oculopharyngeal dystrophy, myotonic dystrophy, and polymyositis or dermatomyositis. *Ocular muscle weakness and ptosis* do not occur in motor neuron disease and are uncommon in peripheral neuropathy. Ophthalmoparesis is typical of myasthenia gravis and may occur in myotonic and oculopharyngeal dystrophies. Weakness limited to or predominantly ocular in location (*progressive external ophthalmoplegia*) occurs in disorders such as the Kearns-Sayre syndrome (Chap. 365).

LABORATORY ASSESSMENT

Patients with significantly impaired strength and sensation merit thorough diagnostic study. The sequence of investigations should be based on the test's diagnostic specificity and sensitivity, level of patient discomfort, and cost. Hematologic, renal, and hepatic function and serum electrolytes should be evaluated. In many instances, thyroid, adrenal, and other endocrine studies may be indicated. Other useful diagnostic tests are the serum creatine kinase (CK) level, nerve conduction studies, electromyography, and in many instances muscle biopsy. Nerve biopsy is a more specialized technique with a relatively small number of specific indications (see Chap. 363). Repetitive stimulation of nerve with recording from muscle should be obtained when a neuromuscular junction defect is suspected. Since many diagnostic tests are uncomfortable and expensive, it is important to consider what information is being sought in requesting each test. Confounding features in the investigations must also be understood. For instance, muscle necrosis and inflammation and an elevated serum CK may occur after minor muscle trauma such as is caused by electromyography and intramuscular injection. Electromyography and muscle biopsy obtained from a muscle affected by past nerve root disease (e.g., from a herniated disk) may show neuropathic abnormalities unrelated to a new disease process. A patient complaining of weakness and fatigue who is found on examination to have no weakness should be examined during exercise. Some of these patients have a metabolic myopathy. Others may have a neuromuscular junction, central nervous system, or psychological problem requiring appropriate investigations.

BIOCHEMICAL EVALUATION OF NEUROMUSCULAR DISEASE Certain enzymes, especially CK, occur in high concentrations in the sarcoplasm of muscle, and may leak into blood to serve as an indicator of muscle damage. The serum CK, aldolase, lactic dehydrogenase (LDH), aspartate aminotransferase (AST, SGOT), and alanine aminotransferase (ALT, SGPT) may be elevated in the serum of a patient with active muscle destruction. Since several of these enzymes are used for screening for abnormalities of organs other than muscle, it is not uncommon for a patient with muscle disease to be first identified by an unexpected elevation in one of these enzymes. The clue to the muscle origin of the increased enzyme levels is that the degree of abnormality decreases in the order CK > aldolase > LDH > SGOT > SGPT. The serum CK level is the most sensitive test and may be very high (raised more than tenfold) in diseases with muscle fiber necrosis, such as the muscular dystrophies, polymyositis, and rhabdomyolysis. It is frequently slightly elevated in spinal muscular atrophy, amyotrophic lateral sclerosis, and other motor neuron disorders and is usually normal in peripheral neuropathies and neuromuscular junction disorders. Strenuous exercise in normal individuals can elevate the level of serum CK for 6 h or more. Three isoenzymes of CK occur: MM, MB, and BB. MM predominates in skeletal muscle, MB occurs mainly in cardiac muscle, and BB is mainly in brain. Elevations of CK-MB levels are used to indicate the presence of myocardial damage. CK elevation caused by acute muscle injury is usually due to the MM isoenzyme. However, in many patients with long-standing necrotizing muscular diseases and in athletes, the proportion of MB in skeletal muscle rises and in consequence the proportion of CK-MB in blood is elevated.

MUSCLE COMPOSITION AND MASS Computed tomography and magnetic resonance imaging can differentiate between muscle fibers, fat, and connective tissue and may show distinctive differences between muscular dystrophy and the other forms of muscle disease. The high cost and the nonspecificity of the findings limit the role of these techniques. Estimations of total muscle mass are of some importance in metabolic studies. A simple decline in muscle mass without weakness is indicative of a process other than a neuromuscular disease, for example, aging, neoplasm, impaired nutrition, renal or hepatic disease. The 24-h urinary creatinine excretion is the most widely available technique used to estimate muscle mass; it is decreased in patients with wasting from any cause.

METABOLIC, ENDOCRINE, AND OTHER STUDIES Hypo- and hyperkalemia, hypernatremia, hypo- and hypercalcemia, hypophosphatemia, and hypermagnesemia can all cause severe, usually acute, weakness. Serum potassium levels are labile and subject to rapid shifts induced by acidosis or alkalosis. The intracellular concentration of potassium is high, so that hemolysis during blood collection may spuriously elevate the potassium level. The extensive muscle damage in rhabdomyolysis may produce a true hyperkalemia. Such elevations in serum potassium are generally not greater than 0.1 meq/L, however, unless the serum is stained with hemoglobin, as occurs with hemolysis, or the urine with myoglobin, as occurs with rhabdomyolysis.

Chronic endocrine disorders, either hypo- or hyperfunction of thyroid, adrenal, or parathyroid glands, may cause weakness in the absence of other clinical evidence of endocrinopathy. Rheumatoid arthritis, systemic lupus erythematosus, scleroderma, and the polymyalgia rheumatica syndrome may be complicated by muscle weakness. Tests for these diseases are usually indicated in the evaluation of unexplained muscle pain and weakness. The weakness in most of these disorders is related to disuse atrophy and joint pain; muscle inflammation and evidence of muscle destruction are uncommon. Disorders of muscle mitochondrial function may cause a high plasma lactate level. Other laboratory investigations that may be indicated in patients with peripheral neuropathy include tests for diabetes mellitus; levels of serum vitamin B_{12}, folate, and lipids; serum protein electrophoresis; urinary and serum immunoelectrophoresis; lipoprotein electrophoresis; and urinary porphyrins and heavy metal levels. Diagnostic enzyme determinations are available in white blood cells in certain neuromuscular disorders, such as aryl sulfatase and acid maltase deficiencies.

MYOGLOBINURIA Acute muscle destruction, *rhabdomyolysis* associated with myoglobinuria, occurs with acute toxic, metabolic, inflammatory, infectious, and traumatic muscle damage (see Chap. 364). The molecular weight of myoglobin is lower than that of hemoglobin, so that the urine rather than the serum changes color in extensive rhabdomyolysis. Myoglobinuria causes a positive urine test for blood in the absence of urinary erythrocytes. Confirmatory testing for myoglobin uses a specific immunoassay.

EXERCISE TESTING (See Chap. 365) Patients with substrate utilization defects characteristically have decreased exercise tolerance and muscle pain and weakness during or following exercise. Most defects in the enzymatic pathways of glycolysis result in the failure of muscle to generate adenosine triphosphate (ATP) from glycogen and a diminished or absent production of lactic acid. Patients with these disorders can be evaluated with a forearm exercise test to evaluate the level of venous lactic acid. Patients with disturbance of fatty acid metabolism (such as carnitine palmityl transferase deficiency, in which long-chain fatty acids cannot be transferred into mitochondria for beta oxidation) generate lactic acid normally. Patients with myoadenylate deaminase deficiency generate lactate in normal or increased amounts but fail to produce ammonia in the exercise test (Chap. 365). Measurement of specific muscle enzymes can define the cause of the disorder.

ELECTROPHYSIOLOGIC STUDIES OF NEUROMUSCULAR DISEASE

NORMAL MOTOR UNIT PHYSIOLOGY The motor unit is the final common pathway for motor activity of the nervous system, and muscle is the final effector of the motor unit. All movement, posture, and reflex activity result from integrated discharge of large numbers of motor units by spinal and supraspinal mechanisms. The strength of a muscle contraction depends upon the number of motor units recruited, the frequency of motor unit discharge, the speed of contraction of muscle fibers in the motor unit, and the nature of the motor unit (whether fatigue-resistant or fatigue-prone). The number of motor units varies greatly among muscles, ranging from as few as 10 in the extraocular muscles, to approximately 100 in the intrinsic muscles of the hands, to nearly 2000 in leg muscles such as the gastrocnemius. The number of muscle fibers per muscle varies up to a thousandfold, from 1000 in extraocular muscles to over 1 million in large leg muscles. The muscle fibers of the motor unit are dispersed randomly within a muscle, and fibers innervated by the same anterior horn cell are generally not contiguous. An understanding of the organization of motor units and their patterns of firing is important in the interpretation of clinical and laboratory findings in normal and diseased muscle.

The physiologic characterization of the muscle fibers relate importantly to the exercise capacity of muscle. Motor units that innervate type 1, slow-twitch muscle fibers are designed for continuous and prolonged activity, since their energy supply is derived from the oxidative metabolism of mitochondria. These motor units are smaller and are activated (*recruited*) by low-intensity efforts. High-intensity effort or rapid muscle contraction, such as lifting of a heavy weight or sprinting, recruits larger motor units that innervate rapid-twitch type 2 muscle fibers, which derive their energy supply from anaerobic glycolysis.

As muscles relax, the cessation of firing of individual motor units occurs in a groupwise fashion so that a patient exerting an inadequate effort owing to functional weakness (e.g., malingering), lack of motivation, or pain will frequently have a ratchet-like or "give-way" quality on muscle testing. This may permit the distinction between true and feigned weakness.

ELECTROMYOGRAPHY The normal electromyogram The measurement of electric activity arising from muscle fibers is usually performed by inserting a needle electrode percutaneously into a muscle. The electric activity from this electrode is then displayed on a cathode-ray oscilloscope and can be made audible through a loudspeaker. Such studies provide only an average picture of the local electric activity of muscle, and normal electric activity in one area does not exclude the possibility of pathologic phenomena close by.

In a single muscle fiber, as the action potential travels from the neuromuscular junction toward the ends of the muscle fiber, current flows outward through the normally polarized region of the muscle membrane (*sarcolemma*) toward the depolarized zone (Fig. 362-1). The recording electrode initially becomes slightly positive relative to the reference electrode. When the depolarized region moves under the recording electrode, a negative deflection occurs. As the active region moves away from the electrode, the membrane under the electrode become repolarized. The net result is a triphasic action potential (Fig. 362-1). The motor unit comprises many such fibers, and hence firing of many fibers of the motor unit produces a more complex wave form (*the motor unit action potential*) resulting from summation of individual action potentials. Normal muscle is electrically silent when at rest, once *insertional activity,* produced by the trauma of placing the needle, has died down. When a muscle is voluntarily contracted, motor unit action potentials appear. With increasing strength of contraction, the number and size of the motor unit action potentials increase, until with full contraction individual motor unit potentials can no longer be distinguished, and a *complete recruitment (interference) pattern* is produced.

The abnormal electromyogram SPONTANEOUS ACTIVITY DURING COMPLETION RELAXATION Persistent insertional activity occurs in myotonic disorders, in polymyositis, and in denervated muscles. Spontaneous activity of a single muscle fiber is called *fibrillation,* and of part of or an entire motor unit, *fasciculation.* Triphasic fibrillation potentials and biphasic positive sharp waves can be seen 7 to 25 days after denervation of muscle fibers (depending upon the distance of denervated muscle fibers from the site of the nerve lesion), and may persist for several years unless reinnervation occurs. Fibrillation appears with destruction of the motor neuron or its axon and in muscle diseases where a portion of a muscle fiber is separated from its innervated portions by segmental necrosis.

Fasciculations are seen with slowly progressive disease of the anterior horn cells such as amyotrophic lateral sclerosis and progressive spinal muscular atrophy, with compressive nerve root lesions, and in some motor neuropathies. In the syndrome of *benign fasciculations,* the same motor unit tends to fire at a regular rate that is usually faster than that of fasciculations indicative of disease.

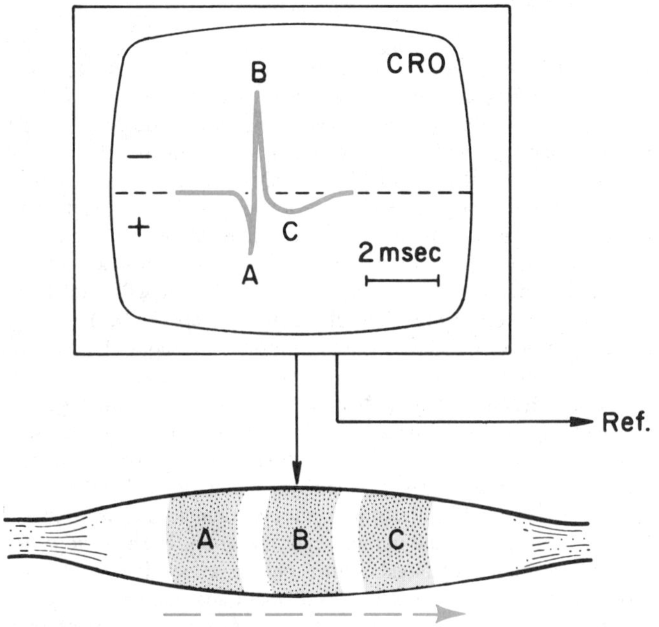

FIGURE 362-1 The triphasic muscle action potential. The shaded area represents the zone of the action potential, which is negative to all other points on the fiber surface. It is shown at three points in its course (from left to right) along the fiber. At each point, the correspondingly lettered portion of the triphasic muscle action potential displayed on the cathode ray oscilloscope (CRO) reflects the potential difference between the active (vertical arrow) and reference (Ref.) electrodes. Polarity in this and subsequent figures is negative upward as depicted. The time calibration is on the CRO screen. (For further details see text.)

In *myotonia,* the sarcolemma is irritable, and repeated muscle depolarization and contraction occur despite voluntary relaxation (see Chap. 365). Such patterns occur in myotonic congenita, myotonic dystrophy, and the periodic paralyses. On electromyography (EMG), myotonia causes high-frequency repetitive discharges that wax and wane in amplitude and frequency, producing a "dive bomber" or "motorcycle" sound on the loudspeaker. Bizarre, *repetitive high-frequency discharges* without waxing and waning are seen in many disorders affecting the motor neurons or muscle. *Coupling of action potentials* into doublets, triplets, or higher multiples of single units occurs in tetany, hemifacial spasm, and myokymia and indicates instability in repolarization of the nerve fiber. Electric silence characterizes *contracture,* as in McArdle's disease and malignant hyperthermia.

ABNORMALITIES IN MOTOR UNIT POTENTIALS Early in the course of denervation, the remaining motor units are normal, but with the development of reinnervation, the remaining motor units increase in amplitude and become longer in duration and polyphasic (see Fig. 362-2). Conversely, in diseases such as polymyositis, the muscular dystrophies, and other myopathies that destroy scattered fibers within a motor unit (Fig. 362-2), the motor unit action potentials are of lower amplitude and shorter duration and are polyphasic.

In diseases of the central or peripheral nervous system, a *reduced recruitment (interference) pattern* results from maximum voluntary effort because fewer motor units are activated. Conversely, in patients with primary muscle disease, maximum voluntary effort produces a *full recruitment pattern* despite marked weakness. Because fewer muscle fibers are active, however, the amplitude of the pattern is reduced from normal.

A number of advanced electromyographic techniques, such as single-fiber EMG and macro EMG (see Chap. 349), have been

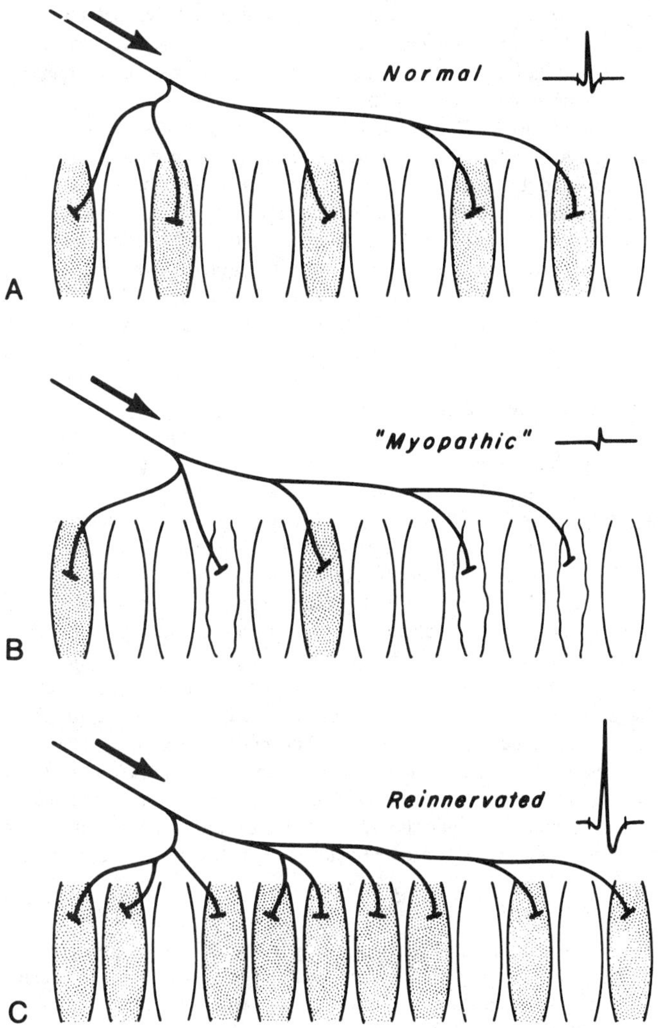

FIGURE 362-2 Motor unit potentials. The shaded muscle fibers are functional members of one motor unit; the axon, which enters from the upper left, branches terminally to innervate the appropriate muscle fibers. The motor unit action potential produced by each motor unit is seen in the upper right; its duration is measured between the two small vertical lines. The normal-appearing but unshaded fibers belong to other motor units. *A*. The normal situation, with five muscle fibers in the active unit. *B*. In this myopathic unit, only two fibers remain active; the other three (shrunken) have been affected by a muscle disease. *C*. Four fibers which belonged to other motor units and had been denervated have now been reinnervated by terminal axon sprouting from the healthy motor unit. Both the motor unit and its action potential are now larger than normal. Note that only under these abnormal circumstances do fibers in the same unit lie next to one another.

developed to investigate the stability of neuromuscular junction and motor unit reinnervation; their description is beyond the scope of this presentation.

Nerve conduction studies Stimulation of the larger peripheral motor and sensory nerves permits the recording of their action potentials and provides objective quantitative data of *latency* and *conduction velocity*. The technique is performed by stimulating the nerve with surface electrodes placed over the nerve. The resulting *compound action potential* is recorded by electrodes placed over the nerve proximally in the case of large sensory nerve fibers, or over the muscle distally in the case of motor nerve fibers in a mixed motor sensory nerve (see Fig. 362-3). The normal maximum motor and sensory nerve conduction velocities vary from 40 to 80 m/s in different peripheral nerves. Values are approximately half in newborn infants, and reach the adult range by 3 to 4 years of age. Normal values have been defined for *distal* or peripheral latencies that represent conduction time from the most distal stimulating electrodes, measured in milliseconds from the stimulus artifact to the onset of the response. It is important that the limb be kept warm during nerve conduction studies because subnormal temperatures cause slower conduction velocity. The *compound muscle action potential* obtained by stimulating a mixed motor nerve is of relatively high amplitude (5 to 10 mV) because of the amplification produced by the large number of muscle fibers in each motor unit. Sensory nerve action potentials, lacking this amplification, are of low amplitude (10 to 50 μV), and hence are more difficult to record. In abnormal nerves, sensory nerve action potentials may be small or absent, and sensory conduction measurements may be impossible to record. In contrast, reliable measurement of motor conduction velocities are usually possible even though only a few functional nerve fibers remain intact.

Maximum nerve conduction velocity measurements reflect the status of the best surviving of the largest myelinated nerve fibers and may be normal despite extensive loss of nerve fibers. Hence, nerve conduction velocity is normal or only slightly below normal in many neuropathies, though the amplitude of the evoked action potential is often reduced. In diseases of peripheral nerves causing severe segmental demyelination, such as chronic inflammatory polyneuropathy, diphtheria, metachromatic leukodystrophy, and the hypertrophic neuropathies, the maximum nerve conduction velocities may be reduced to below half of normal. Focal compressions of nerve, as in entrapment syndromes, produce localized slowing of conduction because of demyelination and narrowing of axons at the site of compression. The conduction of proximal segments of the nerves and nerve roots can be studied by F waves and H reflexes (see Chap.

FIGURE 362-3 Measurement of nerve conduction velocity. The median nerve is stimulated through the skin at the wrist (1) or in the antecubital fossa (2), and the resultant compound muscle action potential is recorded as the potential difference between a surface electrode over the thenar eminence (vertical arrow) and a reference electrode (Ref.) more distally. Sweep 1′ on the cathode ray oscilloscope (CRO) depicts the stimulus artifact (moment of stimulation at 1) followed by the muscle potential. The distal latency is the time A′ on the CRO sweep (3.0 ms, for example) which corresponds to conduction over distance A in the hand. The same is true for sweep 2′ where stimulation is at point 2, and the time from artifact to response is A′ + B′. The maximal motor conduction velocity from points 2 to 1 is obtained by dividing distance B by time B′.

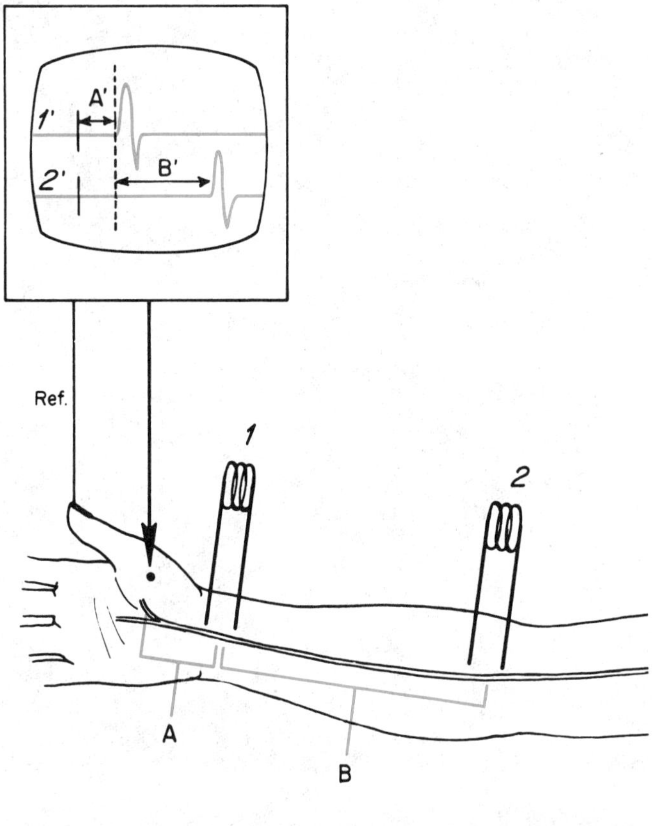

349), or by stimulation of nerve roots by a needle electrode or magnetic stimulator.

Repetitive stimulation tests In myasthenia gravis, a disorder of the neuromuscular junction, the size of the initial compound muscle action potential produced by a supramaximal electric stimulus to the nerve may be normal. However, after a few stimuli at rates of 2 to 3 Hz the amplitude of compound muscle action potential declines. It then increases again after the fourth or fifth stimulus. This pattern of decrement followed by increment is characteristic of myasthenia gravis. This defect resembles the partial blockade produced by curare and reflects a postjunctional disorder of synaptic function. The defect is reversed by administration of anticholinesterase medications such as intravenous edrophonium hydrochloride (5 to 10 mg). A progressive decline in the compound muscle action potential with repetitive stimulation may also occur in poliomyelitis, amyotrophic lateral sclerosis, myotonia, and other diseases of the motor unit; however, the typical pattern of decrement-increment seen in myasthenia gravis is not present in other disorders.

In the Lambert-Eaton (myasthenic) syndrome, repetitive stimulation causes a facilitation of transmission. Rapid stimulation of nerve (20 to 30 Hz) results in a progressive increase in the amplitude of the muscle action potential, which is small at the first stimulus, to a nearly normal amplitude. This facilitation response is not affected by anticholinesterase drugs.

HISTOPATHOLOGY OF MUSCLE AND NERVE

MUSCLE BIOPSY Biopsy is useful in (1) distinguishing between neurogenic and myopathic processes; (2) recognizing specific disorders of muscle such as muscular dystrophy or the congenital myopathies; (3) identifying specific metabolic defects of muscle by histochemical or biochemical techniques; and (4) diagnosing diseases of connective tissue and blood vessels, such as polyarteritis nodosa, and infections such as trichinosis or toxoplasmosis.

Muscle biopsy is performed under local anesthesia. In children and in adults with diffuse conditions, an adequate specimen can often be obtained by needle biopsy. Open biopsy may be necessary to obtain sufficient tissue to diagnose focal, patchy processes such as myositis or vasculitis. In all instances, the muscle chosen for sampling must be appropriate for the condition suspected, and the specimen must be handled by a laboratory skilled in the evaluation of muscle biopsies. If the biopsy is taken from a muscle that has recently been traumatized by an EMG needle or that has been affected by a preexisting disease (e.g., coincidental nerve root compression), misleading information will be obtained.

Muscle fibers are subdivided into two types which have different staining characteristics with the myosin ATPase reaction at pH 9.4. Type 1 fibers (fatigue-resistant and rich in oxidative enzymes) stain lightly with this reaction, and type 2 fibers (fast-contracting, fatigue-prone, and rich in glycolytic enzymes) stain darkly. Normal muscle has a random distribution of fibers of the two histochemical types.

Denervation, reinnervation A denervated muscle fiber undergoes atrophy, and in the initial stages myofibrils are lost to a greater degree than is sarcoplasm containing the mitochondria, so that muscle fibers appear "super dark" with stains for oxidative enzymes (Fig. 362-4). Such denervated fibers are squeezed by adjacent innervated fibers and therefore become angulated and atrophic. In the initial stages of denervation, because of motor unit overlap, denervated atrophic fibers are distributed randomly throughout the muscle. Remaining motor axons sprout to reinnervate such fibers, eventually producing fiber type grouping. With subsequent death of such enlarged motor units,

FIGURE 362-4 *A*. Normal skeletal muscle biopsy stained for myosin ATPase, pH 9.4. Type 1 fibers are light and type 2 dark. *B*. Chronic denervation-reinnervation showing fiber type grouping. Myosin ATPase, pH 9.4. *C*. Chronic denervation-reinnervation in amyotrophic lateral sclerosis, preparation stained for mitochondrial enzyme, NADH-TR. There are groups of reinnervated type 2 fibers (light), and of denervated angulated atrophic fibers, many of them "superdark" and showing target-fiber changes. *D*. Type 2 fiber atrophy. Myosin ATPase, pH 9.4.

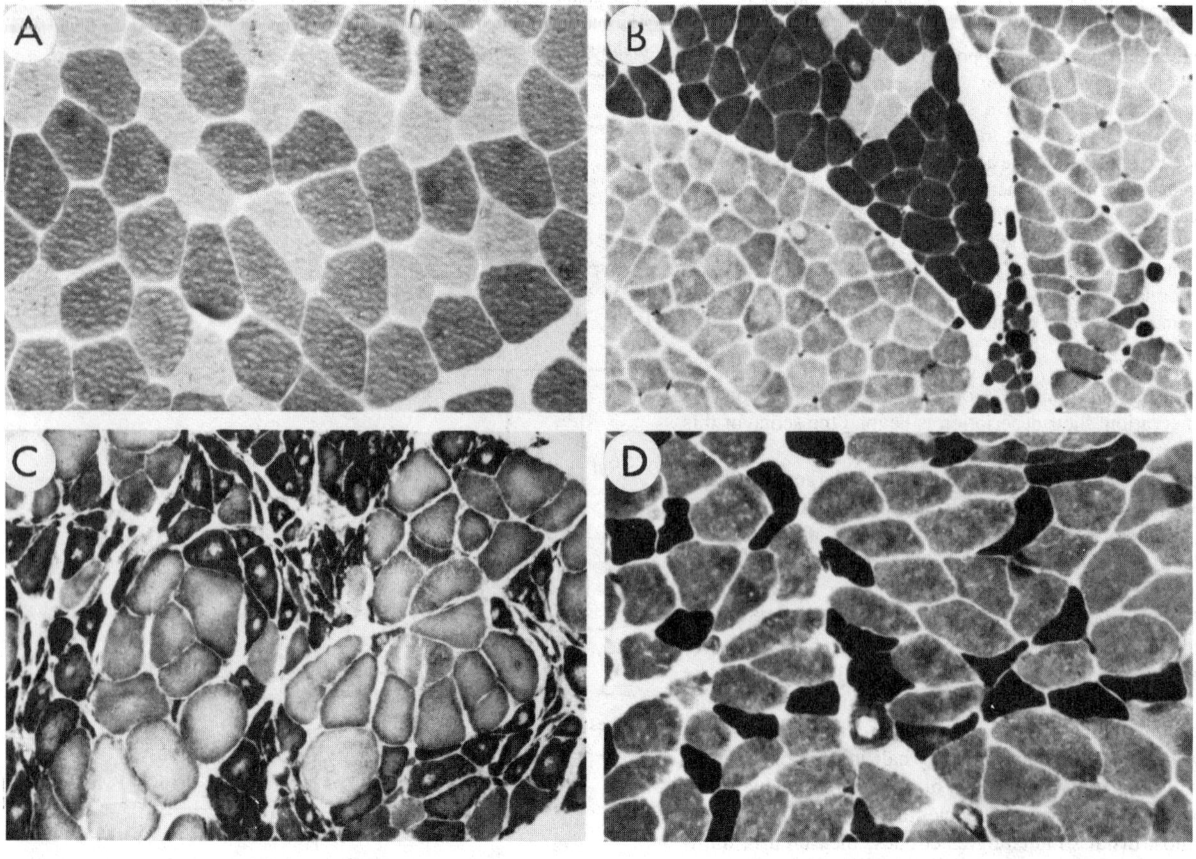

grouped fiber atrophy occurs. The typical appearance of a denervated and reinnervated muscle is shown in Fig. 362-4*B* and *C*. The fiber diameter distribution in chronically denervated and reinnervated muscle is bimodal, with the atrophic denervated fibers making up one population and the normal size (or hypertrophied) innervated fibers making up the other population.

Muscle fiber necrosis and regeneration Damage of the sarcolemma of the muscle fiber allows entry of calcium at high extracellular concentration into the low-calcium environment of the sarcoplasm. Calcium entry activates a neutral protease, initiating proteolysis. Calcium also deranges mitochondrial function and can cause cell death. Invading macrophages phagocytize the muscle fibers. Satellite cells, which provide the basis for regeneration of muscle fibers, are spared in most of the processes that damage muscle. They proliferate and fuse to produce multinuclear myotubes leading to regeneration of the muscle fiber. Characteristically, regenerating fibers are small, are basophilic owing to an increased concentration of RNA, and have large vesicular internal nuclei. The distribution of muscle fiber diameters in a typical chronic myopathy is broad and unimodal, very different from the bimodal diameter distribution of denervated and reinnervated muscle.

Muscle fiber necrosis and regeneration are common in trauma, Duchenne muscular dystrophy, polymyositis, and dermatomyositis. Eventually, if the necrosis is sufficiently chronic, regeneration may fail, causing progressive loss of muscle fibers and replacement with fat and fibrous tissue. A chronic myopathy, Duchenne muscular dystrophy, is illustrated in Fig. 362-5. Differences in the extent and tempo of these processes allow histologic distinction among the muscular dystrophies, inflammatory myopathies, and acute rhabdomyolysis.

Structural changes in muscle fibers Degeneration of muscle fibers without frank necrosis produces structural alteration of individual muscle fibers; disorganization of myofibrils and sarcoplasm produces target fibers (Fig. 362-4*C*), ringbinden (appearance of a portion of the myofibrils wrapped transversely around the remaining longitudinal myofibrils), central cores, cytoid bodies, and nemaline bodies. In one congenital myopathy the fibers resemble myotubes (centronuclear myopathy). In others, abnormal mitochondria suggest an abnormality of mitochondrial biochemistry, while the presence of vacuoles suggests a disturbance of glycogen or lipid metabolism. Rimmed vacuoles (accumulations of degenerating phospholipid material between myofibrils) occur particularly in oculopharyngeal muscular dystrophy and inclusion body myositis.

Inflammatory changes Perivascular and interstitial inflammatory cell infiltration with lymphocytes and macrophages is characteristic of polymyositis and dermatomyositis. Necrosis and regeneration of muscle fibers are also present. In some instances, atrophy of the fibers located on the periphery of muscle fasciculi (*perifascicular atrophy*) is prominent and can be an indicator of inflammatory myopathy, even though a focus of inflammation is not present in the muscle taken at biopsy. Muscle biopsy may show vasculitis in patients with collagen diseases or granulomas in patients with sarcoidosis.

Changes specific to fiber type Pathologic changes may be restricted to one fiber type in the muscle. The most common such condition is type 2 fiber atrophy (Fig. 362-4*D*), which occurs in a wide range of disorders that limit activity such as disuse, muscle pain, joint pain, and upper motor neuronal dysfunction. Atrophy of type 1 fibers is less frequent and occurs in myotonic dystrophy, rheumatoid arthritis, and some congenital myopathies.

NERVE BIOPSY Nerve biopsy is more difficult and more traumatic than muscle biopsy and is useful in a limited number of specific circumstances (see Chap. 363). The sural nerve in the leg or the superficial radial nerve at the wrist are the usual biopsy sites. Both are sensory nerves and may show no changes in pure motor neuropathies. The biopsy procedure is performed under local anesthesia, and specimens are obtained for light and electron microscopy and for teasing of individual nerve fibers. Nerve biopsy aids in (1) distinguishing between segmental demyelination and axonal degeneration; (2) identifying inflammatory neuropathies; and (3) establishing specific diagnoses such as amyloidosis, sarcoidosis, leprosy, vasculitis, and several metabolic neuropathies. Full evaluation of the nerve biopsy requires the facilities of a laboratory with special interest and experience in peripheral nerve pathology. Light microscopic examination of biopsied nerves is of limited value, showing only gross changes such as vasculitis, inflammation, infiltration by granuloma or amyloid, loss of axons, and axonal degeneration. More information is obtained by electron microscopy and studies of single teased nerve fibers. Some diseases affect specific fiber types. For instance, large myelinated fibers are affected in Friedreich's ataxia and unmyelinated fibers in familial amyloidosis. Quantitative morphometry (measurement of the number of fibers and the distribution of their diameters) can therefore be of additional help. Two basic pathologic processes may be seen in nerve biopsies.

Segmental demyelination Diseases may attack either myelin or the Schwann cell, causing the myelin sheath to undergo degeneration but leaving the axon essentially unchanged. Healing of this segmental demyelination proceeds through a phase of abnormally thin myelin sheaths, which may eventually return to normal thickness. However, even after apparent recovery of segmental demyelination, single teased nerve fiber studies demonstrate short and variable lengths of the internodes (distance between the nodes of Ranvier). If this process is progressive, *onion-bulb formation* occurs with thinly remyelinated fibers lying at the center of concentric lamellae of redundant Schwann cell cytoplasm.

Axonal degeneration Death of the nerve cell body or section of the axon at any level will lead to degeneration of the distal parts of the axon with secondary degeneration of the myelin sheath. If the nerve cell body remains intact proximally there is attempted axonal

FIGURE 362-5 *A*. Normal muscle. Hematoxylin-eosin. *B*. Duchenne muscular dystrophy, showing hyalin fibers, fiber degeneration, loss of fibers and fibrosis. Hematoxylin-eosin.

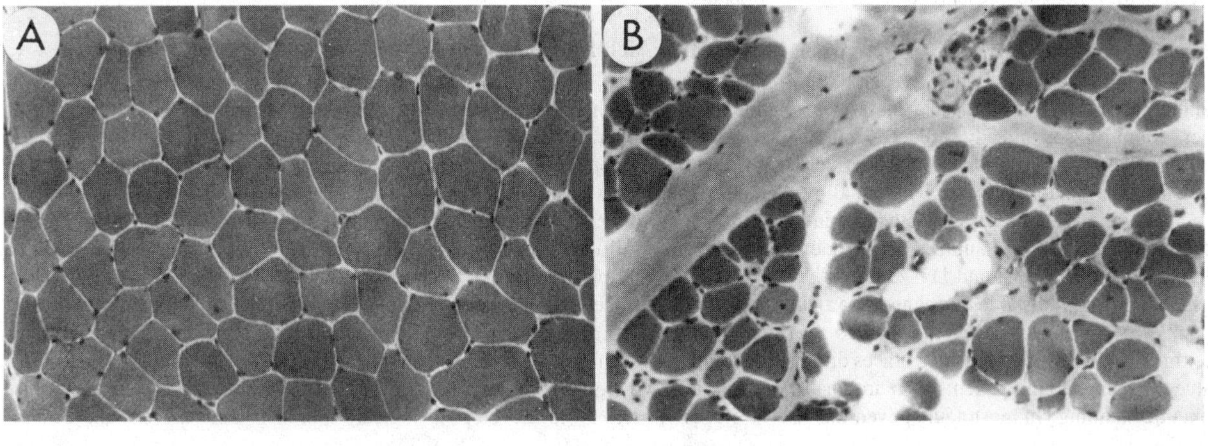

regeneration with sprouting. Such nerve sprouts (*clusters*) are characteristic of degenerating and regenerating axonal neuropathy.

Pathologic changes in neuropathies Axonal degeneration is most common in toxic, inherited, traumatic, and ischemic diseases. Segmental demyelination may occur in the inherited and autoimmune inflammatory disorders; in the latter condition inflammatory cell infiltration may be seen. A mixed picture of axonal degeneration and segmental demyelination, together with a vasculopathy, is characteristic of diabetes mellitus. Some specific pathologic changes may indicate the probable etiology of a neuropathy. The deposition of IgM on the myelin-associated glycoprotein of the myelin sheaths in IgM gammopathies can be detected by immunofluorescence techniques. The deposition leads to an increase in myelin periodicity. Amyloid fibrils are present in amyloid neuropathy. Specific inclusions may be seen in the Schwann cells in metachromatic leukodystrophy and adrenomyeloleukodystrophy.

GENERAL THERAPEUTIC CONSIDERATIONS

Cardiac Most disorders of skeletal muscle also involved cardiac muscle. Symptomatic cardiac dysfunction is relatively uncommon, however, perhaps because the limited exercise capacity of the patient with weakness decreases demands on cardiac performance. Relatively specific electrocardiographic abnormalities occur in Duchenne dystrophy and infantile acid maltase deficiency. Cardiac conduction disorders including complete heart block occur in patients with myotonic dystrophy. An electrocardiogram should be obtained in all patients with neuromuscular disease, particularly in patients with myopathies.

Respiratory Diminished pulmonary function in patients with acute or chronic neuromuscular disease may progress to ventilatory failure. The earliest manifestation of respiratory muscle weakness is a decrease in maximum expiratory and inspiratory pressures. Diaphragmatic weakness, in particular, may be substantial in patients with neuromuscular disease and should be evaluated by examining pulmonary function both while the patient is supine and sitting. Diaphragmatic weakness causes a decrease in pulmonary function when measured in the supine compared with the erect position. Paradoxical abdominal movements may be evident. Patients with chronic respiratory failure may be maintained with home respiratory support. The possible occurrence of cor pulmonale from insidious respiratory failure should be considered in any patient with neuromuscular disease who develops ankle edema or other signs of heart failure.

Physical therapy Physical therapy is of greatest value in patients with muscle weakness when joint contractures are developing and when enforced immobility, such as an injury, results in decreased activity. Exercises may increase strength in muscles weakened by disease as in normal persons, but there is little evidence that exercise improves functional abilities. However, therapeutic standing in patients with marginal leg and trunk function has considerable psychological benefit and may help to preserve bone mineralization and cardiovascular reflexes.

Dietary modification Dietary restriction is often necessary in patients with muscle weakness since caloric expenditure is decreased because of immobility and loss of muscle mass. Development of obesity further compromises already reduced mobility, worsens pulmonary function, and may depress ventilatory drive. Unless there is specific evidence for malabsorption of vitamin B_{12} or vitamin E neither these nor any other vitamin has a specific role in the treatment of neuromuscular disease. Certain vitamins are hazardous in excessive dosages, including vitamins B_6, A, and D (see Chaps. 76 and 340).

Bracing In patients with distal leg weakness, particularly of foot dorsiflexion, ankle-foot orthoses can restore gait to nearly normal. With more proximal weakness, however, leg braces diminish mobility and are of value only in enabling patients who are unable to walk to perform therapeutic standing. In most adults, even this use of braces is impractical because such standing in braces usually requires assistance.

Scoliosis Spinal deformity complicates many neuromuscular diseases, particularly those that occur before puberty. Duchenne dystrophy, spinal muscular atrophy, and congenital myopathies are particularly liable to this complication. Once full long-bone growth has been achieved, many of these patients should have surgical correction of the scoliosis. Severely impaired pulmonary function is a contraindication to such therapy; therefore, patients with progressive scoliosis need careful sequential follow-up to determine the appropriate timing for surgery.

GENETIC EVALUATION AND COUNSELLING (See also Chap. 365) Management of the patient with hereditary muscle disease should include careful family pedigree analysis and genetic counselling. The family history may initially be negative in many patients with autosomal dominant diseases such as Charcot-Marie-Tooth disease, myotonic dystrophy, and facioscapulohumeral dystrophy because of the variable expressivity of the disorders. The availability of chromosomal markers for linkage analysis has made carrier detection, antenatal diagnosis, and early diagnosis of disease feasible in several hereditary neuromuscular diseases (e.g., in Duchenne and myotonic dystrophy). The availability of therapy for disorders such as periodic paralysis, myotonia, and certain metabolic myopathies and of preventive measures in disorders such as malignant hyperthermia provides a strong impetus for early diagnosis. History alone is often inadequate for family evaluation. Physical examination or inspection of photographs of family members will often identify mildly afflicted individuals, providing clues to the characteristic facial or other features of the disorder. Molecular biologic techniques now permit specific diagnosis of certain neuromuscular diseases by identification of an abnormal or missing gene product. Thus, the protein dystrophin is lacking in muscle of patients with Duchenne dystrophy (see Chap. 365).

REFERENCES

Brooke MH: *A Clinician's View of Neuromuscular Disease*, 2d ed. Baltimore, Williams and Wilkins, 1986

Carpenter S, Karpati G: *Pathology of Skeletal Muscle*. New York, Churchill Livingstone, 1984

Engel AG, Banker BQ (eds): *Myology*, New York, McGraw-Hill, 1986

Kimura J: *Electrodiagnosis in Diseases of Nerve and Muscle*, 2d ed. Philadelphia, Davis, 1989

Oh SJ: *Electromyograph; Neuromuscular Transmission Studies*. Baltimore, Williams and Wilkins, 1988

Riggs JE et al: The periodic paralyses. Neurol Clin 6:485, 1988

Schaumburg HH et al: *Disorders of Peripheral Nerves*. Philadelphia, Davis, 1983

363 DISEASES OF THE PERIPHERAL NERVOUS SYSTEM

ARTHUR K. ASBURY

Peripheral neuropathy is a general term indicating disorder of peripheral nerve of any cause; therefore, knowing that a peripheral neuropathy is present in a particular patient should instigate a search for its basis.

The basic processes affecting nerve and muscle and the approach to diseases of nerve and muscle are fully set forth in Chap. 362. The first purpose here is to build upon that base by providing an overview of the wide array of peripheral neuropathies that afflict humans. Disorders of peripheral nerve exhibit such a bewildering and complex set of manifestations that it is difficult for the physician to know where to begin and how to proceed. Therefore the second purpose here is to develop a logical approach and assessment scheme (summarized in Fig. 363-1) which will guide the examiner to correct diagnoses and management decisions.

GENERAL DESCRIPTION OF NEUROPATHIC SYNDROMES The prototypical picture of polyneuropathy occurs with acquired toxic or metabolic neuropathic states. From a symptom standpoint, the first noticeable features tend to be sensory and consist of tingling, prickling, burning, or bandlike dysesthesias in the balls of the feet or tips of the toes, or in a general distribution over the soles. Symmetry of symptoms and findings in a distal graded fashion is the rule, but occasionally dysesthesias appear in one foot a brief time before the other or may be more pronounced in one foot. Some care and judgment is needed to avoid confusion with mononeuropathy multiplex. If the polyneuropathy remains mild, no objective motor or sensory signs may be detectable.

With progression, pansensory loss is usually found over both feet, ankle jerks are lost, and weakness of dorsiflexion of the toes, best demonstrated in the great toe, may be present. In some instances, the process begins with weakness in the feet, usually dorsiflexion of the toes and feet without subjective sensory symptoms. As worsening occurs, sensory loss moves centripetally in a graded "stocking" fashion, and the patient may complain that the feet have a numb or "wooden" feeling or may say "I feel as though I'm walking on stumps." Patients experience difficulty walking on their heels during examination and their feet may slap while walking. Later, the knee jerk reflex disappears and foot drop becomes more apparent. By the time sensory disturbance has reached the upper shin, dysesthesias are usually noticed in the tips of the fingers. The degree of spontaneous pain varies, but is often considerable. Light stimuli to hypesthetic areas, once perceived, may be experienced as extremely uncomfortable (hyperpathia). Unsteadiness of gait may be out of proportion to muscle weakness because of proprioceptive loss.

Worsening proceeds in a centripetal, symmetrically graded manner with muscle atrophy, pansensory loss, and areflexia and with motor weakness that is usually greater in the extensor muscles than in corresponding flexor groups. When the sensory disturbance reaches mid thigh, generally a tent-shaped area of hypesthesia on the lower abdomen may be demonstrated. This will grow broader, and the apex will extend rostrally toward the sternum as the neuropathy worsens. By this time, patients generally cannot stand or walk or hold objects in their hands.

In the most extreme cases, ventilatory capacity may be impaired along with sphincteric function. Hypesthesia at the crown of the scalp may be present and spread radially into both the trigeminal and C2 distribution. Considering the entire sequence, nerve fibers are affected according to length of axon without regard to root or nerve trunk distribution—hence, the aptness of the term "stocking-glove" to describe the pattern of sensory deficit. In general, the motor deficit is also graded, distal, and symmetric.

Variations on the general sequence outlined above are manifold and explain the diversity of clinical syndromes encountered. Variations include the rate of evolution; fluctuations in the course; the eventual degree of severity; the presence or absence of positive motor and sensory symptoms; the symmetry of features and their distribution in terms of proximal versus distal, arms versus legs, and motor versus sensory; the relative proportion of dysfunction attributable to large fiber deficit and to small fiber deficit; and the determination, mainly by electrodiagnostic examination, of axonal versus demyelinating processes.

ASSESSMENT AND DIAGNOSIS OF NEUROPATHY **Taking the first step** Clues to the diagnosis of specific peripheral neuropathies often lie in unnoted or readily forgotten events occurring weeks or months prior to the onset of symptoms. Inquiry should be made about recent viral illnesses; other systemic symptoms; institution of new medications; potentially toxic exposures to solvents, pesticides, or heavy metals; the occurrence of similar symptoms in family members or coworkers; habits concerning alcohol; and the presence of known

FIGURE 363-1 Flowchart approach to the evaluation of peripheral neuropathies. (*After Asbury, 1983.*)

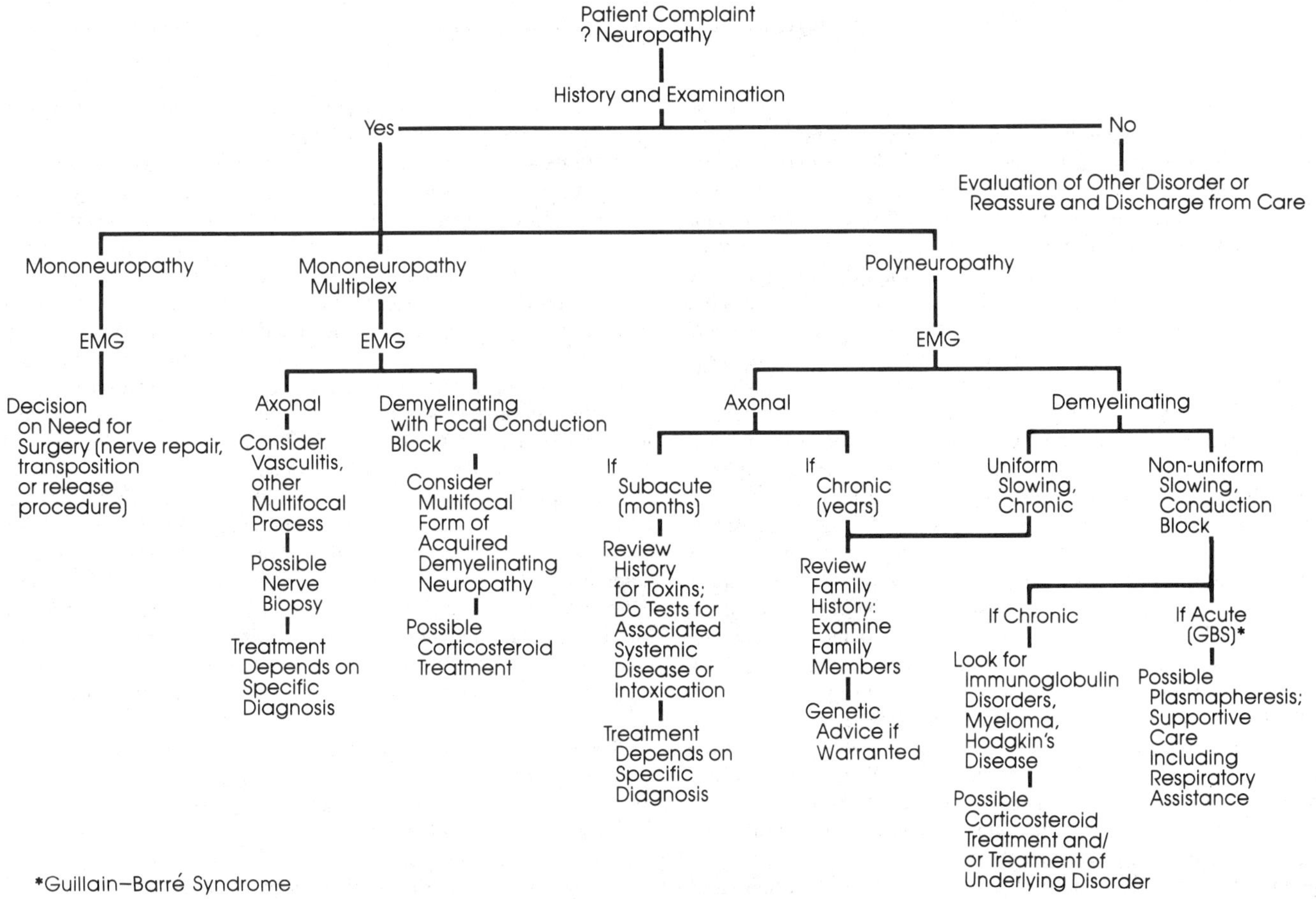

preexisting medical disorders. It is also useful to ask patients if they would otherwise feel well if free of their neuropathic symptoms, to obtain an idea of the presence or absence of an underlying systemic illness.

It is important to learn how symptoms first appeared. Even with distal polyneuropathies, symptoms may appear in the sole of one foot a few days or a week before the other, but usually the patient will describe a distal graded disturbance that moves evenly and symmetrically in centripetal fashion. Tingling dysesthesias will appear in the fingertips only when similar symptoms have reached the level of the knees. It is most important to determine whether symptoms first appeared in the distribution of individual digital nerves involving only one-half of a digit at a time and then gradually spread to become coalescent. This pattern of onset raises strong suspicions of a multifocal process (mononeuropathy multiplex) such as might be encountered with a systemic vasculitis or cryoglobulinemia.

The evolution of neuropathy ranges from rapid worsening over a few days to an indolent process extending many years. Polyneuropathies with a slowly progressive course lasting more than 5 years are most likely to be genetically determined, particularly if the major manifestations are distal atrophy and weakness with few or no positive sensory symptoms. Exceptions are diabetic polyneuropathy and paraproteinemic neuropathies in which the progression may be insidious over 5 to 10 years. Axonal degenerations of toxic or metabolic origin tend to evolve over several weeks to a year or more, and the rate of progression of demyelinating neuropathies is highly variable, ranging from a few days in Guillain-Barré syndrome to many years in others.

Major fluctuations in the course of neuropathy bring to mind two possibilities: (1) relapsing forms of neuropathy, or (2) repeated toxic exposures. A slow fluctuation in symptoms taking place over weeks or months (reflecting changes in the activity of neuropathy) should not be confused with day-to-day variation or diurnal undulation of symptoms. The latter are common to all neuropathic disorders. An example is carpal tunnel syndrome in which dysesthesias may be prominent at night but absent during the day.

In polyneuropathies, the findings can be expected to be quite symmetric on both sides of the body. If only one foot slaps when the patient walks, the process is not symmetric and the possibility of a multifocal process is raised. In addition, in acquired symmetric polyneuropathies, the muscles of extension and abduction tend to be weakened to a greater extent than the muscles of flexion and adduction. Hence, weakness in lower legs often affects the peronei and anterior tibial muscles, with attendant foot drop, more than the gastrocnemius group or foot inverters. In most polyneuropathies the legs are more severely affected than the arms and the distal muscles more than the proximal ones. There are exceptions to this rule, as in lead neuropathy, in which manifestations of bilateral wrist drop may predominate, and occasionally in porphyric neuropathy, in which arms may be more affected than legs and proximal muscles more than distal.

Palpation of the nerve trunk to detect enlargement is a frequently forgotten part of the neurologic examination. In mononeuropathies, the entire course of the nerve trunk in question should be explored manually for focal thickening; the presence of neurofibroma, point tenderness, or Tinel's phenomenon (generation of a tingling sensation in the sensory territory of the nerve by tapping along the course of the nerve trunk); and elicitation of pain by putting the nerve trunk on stretch. In leprous neuritis, fusiform thickening of nerve trunks is frequent, and beading of nerve trunks may be encountered in amyloid polyneuropathy. Certain genetically determined neuropathies of the hypertrophic variety may be attended by uniform thickening of all nerve trunks, often to the caliber of a clothesline or larger.

Most neuropathies involve nerve fibers of all sizes, but on occasion selective damage restricted to large or to small fibers predominates. In a polyneuropathy affecting mainly small fibers, diminished pinprick and temperature sensation, often with burning painful dysesthesias, may predominate along with autonomic dysfunction but with relative sparing of motor power, balance, and tendon jerks. Selected cases of amyloid and distal diabetic polyneuropathies fall into this category. In contrast, large-fiber polyneuropathy is characterized by areflexia, imbalance, relatively minor cutaneous sensory deficit, and variable but often severe motor dysfunction.

In addition to taking a history and doing a physical examination that bears in mind the points made above, certain other measures can be undertaken routinely in the evaluation of a patient with neuropathy. Electrodiagnostic examination is a key procedure in all patients. For patients with polyneuropathy or mononeuropathy multiplex, standard tests should include a complete blood count and erythrocyte sedimentation rate, urinalysis, chest x-ray, postprandial blood glucose, and serum protein electrophoresis. Further tests should be dictated by the formulation arrived at via the combined history and physical and electrodiagnostic examination (see Fig. 363-1).

Taking the next step The next step is electrodiagnostic examination. It is not generally possible to make the distinction between axonal versus demyelinating disorders on clinical examination alone; here electrodiagnostic analysis is particularly useful. Electrodiagnostic features of demyelination are slowing of nerve conduction velocity (NCV), dispersion of evoked compound action potentials (CAPs), conduction block (major decrease in amplitude of muscle CAP upon proximal stimulation of its nerve as compared to distal stimulation), and marked prolongation of distal latencies. In contrast, axonal neuropathies are characterized by a reduction in amplitude of evoked CAPs with relative preservation of NCV. The distinction between a primarily demyelinating neuropathy from one which is primarily axonal is crucial because of the differing approaches to diagnosis and management. If in a particular instance of progressive polyneuropathy or subacute or chronic evolution the electrodiagnostic findings are those of an axonopathy, a long list of metabolic states and exogenous toxins come into consideration (see Tables 363-1 and 363-2). If the course is protracted over several years, it raises the likelihood of the neuronal (axonal) form of peroneal muscular atrophy (HMSN-II); family members must be examined and additional attention given to the family history.

Alternatively, if the electrodiagnostic findings are more indicative of primary demyelination of nerve, the approach is entirely different. The possibilities then include acquired demyelinating neuropathy, thought to be immunologically mediated, and genetically determined neuropathies, some of which are marked by uniform and drastic slowing of nerve conduction velocities.

With these considerations in hand, a flowchart can be constructed (Fig. 363-1) which summarizes the clinical and electrodiagnostic approach to the evaluation and management of a neuropathic disorder. Using this scheme, the clinician determines for each patient the tempo, distribution, severity, and functional impairment, and other features previously discussed, making a clinical judgment as to whether the problem represents a mononeuropathy, a mononeuropathy multiplex, or a polyneuropathy. Often this distinction is obvious. With the sum of clinical and electrodiagnostic information in hand, the differential diagnostic possibilities and management options will have been narrowed to only a few. The remainder of this chapter deals with the details of this formulation.

Electrodiagnosis As seen in Fig. 363-1, electrodiagnosis is a key part of the evaluation of any neuropathy. See Chap. 362 for details of technique and interpretation. For example, electrodiagnosis helps one to be certain about the presence or absence of a sensory deficit when this is not clear by clinical examination alone. It provides information about the distribution of subclinical findings, thus sharpening the diagnostic focus. A listing of the general questions which may be posed by the clinician to the electrodiagnostician includes

1 The distinction between disorders primary to nerve or to muscle (neuropathy versus myopathy).
2 The distinction between root or plexus involvement and more distal nerve trunk involvement.
3 The distinction between generalized polyneuropathic processes and widespread multifocal nerve trunk affection.

TABLE 363-1 Polyneuropathy associated with systemic diseases

		Axonal†			Demyelinating†					
Systemic disease	Occurrence*	Acute	Subacute	Chronic	Acute	Subacute	Chronic	Sensory vs. motor‡	Autonomic†	Comment
Diabetes mellitus	C	—	±	+	—	±	+	S, SM, rarely M	± to +	Mixed axonal demyelination often seen; see Table 363-4
Uremia	S	±	+	+	—	—	—	SM	±	Controllable with proper dialysis; curable with successful renal transplant
Porphyria (3 types)	R	+	±	—	—	—	—	M	± to +	May be proximal > distal and may have atypical proximal sensory deficits
Hypoglycemia	R	±	+	±	—	—	—	M	—	Usually with insulinoma; arms often > legs; ? anterior horn cells affected
Vitamin deficiency, exclude B_{12}	S	—	+	+	—	—	—	SM	±	Involves at least thiamine, pyridoxine, folate, pantothenic acid; probably others
Vitamin B_{12} deficiency	S	—	±	+	—	—	—	S	—	Peripheral nerve involvement variable; often overshadowed by myelopathy
Chronic liver disease	S	—	—	—	—	—	+	S or SM	—	Usually mild or subclinical
Primary biliary cirrhosis	R	—	±	+	—	—	—	S	—	Epineurial and subperineurial xanthomatous deposits
Primary systemic amyloidosis	R	—	±	+	—	—	—	SM	+	Also seen with amyloidosis associated with myeloma or macroglobulinemia
Hypothyroidism	R	—	—	—	—	±	+	S	—	May respond to thyroid replacement
Chronic obstructive lung disease	R	—	±	+	—	—	—	S or SM	—	Few reports; a questionable entity
Acromegaly	R	—	—	+	—	—	—	S	—	Carpal tunnel syndrome also frequent
Malabsorption (sprue, celiac disease)	S	—	±	+	—	—	—	S or SM	±	Basis for neuropathy unclear; deficiency suspected
Carcinoma (sensory)	R	—	+	+	—	—	—	Pure S	—	Carcinomatous sensory neuropathy; due to gangliitic neuronopathy; mostly breast carcinoma; paraneoplastic; relatively rare
Carcinoma (sensorimotor)	S	—	+	+	—	—	—	SM	±	Sensorimotor axonal neuropathy; mostly with lung carcinoma; more common than pure sensory, but still infrequent
Carcinoma (late)	C	—	+	+	—	—	—	S>M	±	Mild, late axonal neuropathy, probably related to weight loss and wasting
Carcinoma (demyelinating)	S	—	—	—	+	+	±	SM	—	Acute or relapsing demyelinating neuropathy sometimes seen with carcinoma
Lymphoma including Hodgkin's	S	—	+	+	+	+	±	See above	±	Same as carcinomatous types, although pure sensory type is even rarer
Polycythemia vera	R	—	±	+	—	—	—	S	—	Also many CNS manifestations; often shooting pains in limbs
Multiple myeloma lytic type	S	—	±	+	—	—	—	S, M, or SM	±	Symptomatic neuropathy uncommon, subclinical neuropathy frequent
Multiple myeloma§: osteosclerotic or solitary plasmacytoma	S	—	—	±	—	±	+	SM	—	Although may show severe slowing of nerve conduction velocity recent work suggests this is secondary demyelination

See Footnote next page. *(continued)*

TABLE 363-1 Polyneuropathy associated with systemic diseases (*continued*)

Systemic disease	Occurrence*	Axonal† Acute	Axonal† Subacute	Axonal† Chronic	Demyelinating† Acute	Demyelinating† Subacute	Demyelinating† Chronic	Sensory vs. motor‡	Autonomic†	Comment
Benign monoclonal gammopathy:	S									
IgA		—	±	+	—	—	—	SM	—	IgM_{κ} (or occasionally IgM_{λ}) may bind to myelin-associated glycoprotein or glycolipids
IgG		—	±	+	—	—	—	SM	—	
IgM		—	—	—	—	±	+	SM	—	
Macroglobulinemia	R	—	—	±	—	—	+	SM	—	Usually but not always axonal
Cryoglobulinemia	R	—	±	+	—	—	—	SM	—	May be mononeuropathy multiplex in presentation

* R = rare; S = sometimes; C = common.
† ± = sometimes; + = usual.
‡ S = sensory; M = motor; SM = sensorimotor.
§ Some cases associated with POEMS syndrome (see text).

4 The distinction between upper and lower motor neuron weakness.
5 The distinction, in a given generalized polyneuropathic process, between primary demyelinating neuropathy and axonal degeneration.
6 The assessment, in both primary axonal and demyelinating neuropathies, of many factors bearing on the nature, activity, and likely prognosis of the neuropathy.
7 The assessment, in mononeuropathies, of the site of the lesion and its major effect on nerve fibers, especially the distinction between demyelinating conduction block and wallerian degeneration.
8 The characterization of disorders of the neuromuscular junction.
9 The identification, often in muscle of normal bulk and strength, of chronic partial denervation, fasciculations, and myotonia.
10 The analysis of cramp, and its distinction from physiologic contracture.

Nerve biopsy The sural nerve at the ankle is the preferred site for cutaneous nerve biopsy. There are few indications to employ this invasive technique. The main one is in asymmetric and multifocal neuropathic disorders producing a clinical picture of mononeuropathy multiplex, the basis of which is still unclear after other laboratory investigations are complete. Diagnostic considerations include vasculitis, amyloidosis, leprosy, and occasionally sarcoidosis. Nerve biopsy is also helpful when one or more cutaneous nerves are palpably enlarged. Another clinical application is in establishing the diagnosis in some genetically determined childhood disorders such as metachromatic leukodystrophy, Krabbe's disease, giant axonal neuropathy, and infantile neuroaxonal dystrophy. In all of these recessively inherited diseases, both the central nervous system (CNS) and the peripheral nervous system (PNS) are affected.

There is a tendency to carry out sural nerve biopsy in distal symmetric polyneuropathies of subacute or chronic evolution. This practice is discouraged because it is a low-yield measure. Nerve biopsy in this situation is only useful as part of an approved research protocol when the biopsy will provide crucial information not otherwise obtainable.

POLYNEUROPATHY Although this term connotes a widespread symmetric process, usually distal and graded, polyneuropathies

TABLE 363-2 Polyneuropathy associated with drugs or environmental toxins

	Axonal* Acute	Axonal* Subacute	Axonal* Chronic	Demyelinating* Acute	Demyelinating* Subacute	Demyelinating* Chronic	Sensory vs. motor†	Autonomic*	CNS*	Comment
DRUGS										
Amiodarone (antiarrhythmic)	—	—	+	—	—	+	SM	—	—	Dose-dependent neuropathy, reversible by decreasing dose; lysosomal dense body accumulation
Aurothioglucose (antirheumatic)	±	±	—	+	+	—	SM	—	—	Idiosyncratic reaction, ? immune-mediated
cis-Platinum (antineoplastic)	—	+	+	—	—	—	S	—	—	Severe sensory neuropathy, ? neuronopathy; also ototoxicity; dose-related
Dapsone (dermatologic including leprosy)	—	±	+	—	—	—	M	—	—	Dose-related pure motor neuropathy
Disulfiram (antialcohol)	±	+	+	—	—	—	SM	—	±	Usually occurs after months of treatment
Hydralazine (antihypertensive)	—	±	+	—	—	—	S>M	—	—	A pyridoxine antagonist; only rarely neurotoxic
Isoniazid	—	±	+	—	—	—	SM	±	—	A pyridoxine antagonist; neurotoxic in slow acetylators

* ± = sometimes, + = usual.
† S = sensory; M = motor; SM = sensorimotor.

TABLE 363-2 Polyneuropathy associated with drugs or environmental toxins *(continued)*

	Axonal*			Demyelinating*			Sensory vs. motor†	Autonomic*	CNS*	Comment
	Acute	Subacute	Chronic	Acute	Subacute	Chronic				
DRUGS *(continued)*										
Metronidazole (antiprotozoal	—	—	±	—	—	—	S	—	+	Dose-related central-peripheral distal axonopathy
Misonidazole (radiosensitizer)	—	±	+	—	—	—	S	—	+	Neurotoxicity is the limiting factor
Perhexilene (antiarrhythmic)	—	—	±	—	—	+	SM	±	—	Dose-related neuropathy; lysosomal dense body accumulation
Phenytoin (anticonvulsant)	—	—	+	—	—	—	S>M	—	—	Large-fiber neuropathy, mild, after 20–30 years of phenytoin use
Pyridoxine (vitamin)	—	±	+	—	—	—	S	—	—	Occurs with large intake; >500 mg per day
Thalidomide (antileprous)	—	—	+	—	—	—	S>M	±	+	Red skin and brittle nails; also teratogenic; recovery from neuropathy poor
Vincristine (antineoplastic)	—	+	+	—	—	—	S>M	—	—	Mild sensory neuropathy is nearly universal, hands>feet; motor signs should prompt cessation of treatment
Nitrofurantoin (urinary antiseptic)	—	±	+	—	—	—	SM	—	—	Generally total dose-related; presence of renal failure may enhance toxicity
TOXINS										
Acrylamide (flocculant; grouting agent)	—	±	+	—	—	—	S>M	±	+	Large-fiber neuropathy; sensory ataxia
Arsenic (herbicide; insecticide)	±	+	+	—	—	—	SM	±	±	Skin changes and Mees' lines in nails; if acute intoxication, many systemic effects
Buckthorn (toxic berry)	—	—	—	+	+	—	SM	—	—	Only occurs where berries grow; may mimic GBS
Carbon disulfide, CS_2 (industrial)	—	—	+	—	—	+	SM	—	+	Neurofilamentous accumulation in axons; demyelinating features are secondary
Diphtheria	—	—	—	+	+	—	SM	—	—	Clinically very rare now; can be confused with GBS
Dimethylamino propionitrile (industrial)	—	—	+	—	—	—	S>M	+	—	Small-fiber neuropathy with prominent bladder symptoms and impotence in males
γ-Diketone hexacarbons (solvents)	—	±	+	—	—	+	SM	±	+	Same features as CS_2; these solvents now in restricted use
Inorganic lead	—	—	+	—	—	—	M>S	—	±	Selective motor neuropathy with prominent wrist drop
Organophosphates	—	±	+	—	—	—	SM	—	+	Brain and spinal cord are also affected, the latter irreversibly
Thallium (rat poison)	—	+	+	—	—	—	SM	—	+	Also alopecia, Mees' lines in nails; ? selective damage to neural mitochondria

* ± = sometimes, + = usual.
† S = sensory; M = motor; SM = sensorimotor.

present a high degree of diversity because of the extreme variability of tempo, severity, mix of sensory and motor features, and presence or absence of positive symptoms. The patient with a fulminant, severely dysesthetic sensory neuropathy and alopecia who is in the early phases of thallium intoxication bears little similarity to the patient with a 40-year history of insidiously progressive clumsiness of gait whose findings are foot drop, lower leg atrophy, pes cavus, and minimal asymptomatic distal sensory deficit (i.e., peroneal muscular atrophy, either type I or II; see Table 363-3). These two patients fall near opposite ends of the spectrum of polyneuropathy.

The classification of peripheral neuropathies has become increasingly complex as the capacity to discriminate new subgroups and identify new associations with toxins and systemic disorders improves. Further, our grasp of the pathophysiologic basis for the clinical phenomena observed in neuropathy has increased rapidly (see Chap. 362). But these advances are primarily descriptive; little or no progress has been made in illuminating the fundamental pathogenetic events in nervous tissue which eventuate in any one of the polyneuropathies.

The important features of each major grouping of polyneuropathies are summarized below and key aspects of specific polyneuropathies may be found in Tables 363-1 to 363-4.

TABLE 363-3 Genetically determined neuropathies

Genetic disorder	Inheritance pattern	Age of onset	Basic process	Other features*	Other systems involved	Metabolic defect	Comment
Peroneal muscular atrophy (HMSN-I)†	Dominant	Decades 2–3	Demyelinating	Hypertrophic change with onion bulb formation; marked ↓ NCV	Some families—Duffy locus linkage	Unknown	Pes cavus, congenital hip problems, motor deficit predominates
Peroneal muscular atrophy (HMSN-II)†	Dominant	Decades 3–5	Axonal	Marked ↓ NAP; NCV sl. decreased	—	Unknown	Same as HSMN-I
Hereditary amyloid neuropathies	Dominant	Decades 3–4	Axonal	Small fiber involvement; endoneurial amyloid deposition	Some families—cornea	Amino acid mutation in transthyretin (prealbumin)	Dysautonomia may be prominent. Genetic defect on chromosome 18.
Hereditary sensory neuropathy (HSN-I)	Dominant	Decades 1–3	Neuronopathic	DRG neurons selectively involved	Sensorineural deafness, some families	Unknown	Frequent distal mutilation—hands and feet
Porphyric neuropathy	Dominant	Adult life	Axonal	Neuropathy part of attacks; may be recurrent	Widespread cellular abnormality	Enzyme defects in porphyrin pathway	Acute intermittent porphyria, variegate porphyria, and erythropoietic porphyria
Hereditary liability to pressure palsy	Dominant	Decades 2–3	? Demyelinating	Tomaculous changes in myelin	—	Unknown	Ulnar, peroneal, and brachial plexus involvement particularly
Fabry's disease	X-linked	Young males	Neuronopathic	Sensory neuronopathy, small DRG neurons	Kidney, skin, lung	Accumulation of ceramide-trihexoside	Neuropathy painful; often die of renal failure
Peroneal muscular atrophy (Phillips et al., 1985)	X-linked	Infancy to 2d decade	Axonal or demyelinating	Heterozygote females may have symptoms		Unknown	Localizes to long arm of X chromosome
Adrenomyeloneuropathy	X-linked	Young males	? Axonal	Mild neuropathy, spastic paraparesis, baldness, hypogonadism	Adrenal cortex, cerebral white matter, spinal cord	Accumulation of very long chain fatty acids	Phenotypic variant of adrenoleukodystrophy; dietary therapy possible
Hereditary sensory neuropathy (HSN-II)	Recessive	Decades 1–3	Neuronopathic	DRG neurons selectively involved	—	Unknown	May be less severe than HSN-I
Déjerine-Sottas neuropathy (HMSN-III)	Recessive	1st decade	Demyelinating	Hypertrophic change with onion bulb formation	May be mentally retarded	Unknown	Marked nerve trunk enlargement
Refsum's disease	Recessive	1st or 2d decade	Demyelinating	Hypertrophic change with onion bulb formation	Retinitis pigmentosa, ichthyosis, sensorineural deafness	Defect in α-oxidation of β-methylated fatty acids	Low phytanate diet, plasmapheresis therapy
Ataxia-telangiectasia	Recessive	Decade 1 or 2	Axonal	Neuropathy moderate	Cell nuclear aneuploidy, skin and scleral telangiectasia, cerebellar atrophy, immunopathy	Basic defect unknown	High incidence of early neoplasia

* DRG, dorsal root ganglia; NAP, nerve action potential; sl, slightly; HMSN, hereditary motor-sensory neuropathy; HSN, hereditary sensory neuropathy.
† Both forms are also collectively referred to as Charcot-Marie-Tooth neuropathy.

TABLE 363-3 Genetically determined neuropathies *(continued)*

Genetic disorder	Inheritance pattern	Age of onset	Basic process	Other features*	Other systems involved	Metabolic defect	Comment
Abetalipoproteinemia	Recessive	Decade 1 or 2	Neuronopathic	Large DRG neurons	Retinitis pigmentosa, acanthocytosis of red blood cells	Absence of all lipoprotein-containing apo B	Proprioceptive disturbance marked, minimal small fiber deficit
Giant axonal neuropathy	Recessive	1st decade	Axonal	Massive segmented accumulation of neurofilaments in axons	Slowly progressive encephalopathy with Rosenthal fibers	Generalized disorder of 10-nm filaments	Intermediate filament masses in other cell types
Metachromatic leukodystrophy	Recessive	1st decade	Demyelinating	Schwannopathy with cerebroside accumulation	Cerebral white matter disease predominates	Defect of arylsulfatase A	Infantile, juvenile, and adult onset forms
Globoid cell leukodystrophy	Recessive	1st decade	Demyelinating	Schwannopathy with galactocerebroside accumulation	Cerebral white matter disease predominates	Defect of β-galactosidase	Characteristic clefts in Schwann cell cytoplasm
Friedreich's ataxia	Recessive	1st decade	Axonal	Spinocerebellar and corticospinal tracts involved; also 1° sensory neuron	Cardiomyopathy; usual cause of death	Controversial	Ataxia is both sensory and cerebellar

* DRG, dorsal root ganglia; NAP, nerve action potential; sl, slightly; HMSN, hereditary motor-sensory neuropathy; HSN, hereditary sensory neuropathy.
† Both forms are also collectively referred to as Charcot-Marie-Tooth neuropathy.

Acute axonal polyneuropathy In this setting the term acute means evolution over days, making these neuropathies relatively uncommon. Included are porphyric neuropathy and massive intoxications, often suicidal or homicidal in intent. For example, an individual receiving a large dose of arsenic (e.g., 100 mg of arsenous oxide) will become violently ill in a few hours with vomiting, diarrhea, and circulatory collapse. In 1 to 3 days serious renal and liver failure will ensue, and between 14 and 21 days polyneuropathy will appear, often as the systemic disorder abates. Progression occurs for 2 or 3 weeks, but following a plateau, recovery requires months.

Subacute axonal polyneuropathy Subacute, meaning to evolve in weeks, characterizes many instances of toxic and metabolic polyneuropathy, but perhaps even more of these are chronic in evolution (months). Scanning the appropriate columns in Tables 363-1 and 363-2 provides many possibilities. Management in almost all instances involves removing from contact the offending agent or treating the associated systemic order.

Chronic axonal polyneuropathy This category includes many more types of polyneuropathy, in part because the term chronic subsumes neuropathies that have progressed over a period as short as 6 months to as long as 60 years. As a rough approximation, slow worsening for more than 5 years, absence of positive symptoms, mainly motor deficit, and absence of systemic disorder all favor a genetically determined neuropathy. Although these are mostly autosomal dominant in inheritance pattern, recessively inherited and X-linked varieties also occur, including a form phenotypically resembling dominantly inherited peroneal muscular atrophy (HMSN-II) and also adrenomyeloneuropathy (see Table 363-3). To complete the picture, an array of rare autosomal recessive neuropathies occur in childhood.

TABLE 363-4 Classification of diabetic neuropathies

A Symmetric
- *1* Distal, primarily sensory polyneuropathy
  - *a* Mainly large fibers affected
  - *b* Mixed*
  - *c* Mainly small fibers affected*
- *2* Autonomic neuropathy
- *3* Chronically evolving proximal motor neuropathy*†

B Asymmetric
- *1* Acute or subacute proximal motor neuropathy*†
- *2* Cranial mononeuropathy†
- *3* Truncal neuropathy*†
- *4* Entrapment neuropathy in the limbs

* Often painful.
† Recovery, partial or complete, is likely.

Acute demyelinating polyneuropathy For all practical purposes, this category is synonymous with Guillain-Barré syndrome (GBS). This acute, frequently severe and fulminant polyneuropathy occurs at a rate of one case per million population per month, or approximately 3500 cases per year in the United States and Canada. Incidence patterns are similar world-wide. In over two-thirds, a viral infection, either clinically overt or evidenced by serum titer rise, precedes the onset of neuropathy by 1 to 3 weeks. Herpes infections [cytomegalovirus, Epstein-Barr virus (EBV)] account for a large proportion of virus-triggered cases. Another 5 to 10 percent of cases occur within 1 to 4 weeks of a surgical procedure. GBS occurs on a background of lymphoma, including Hodgkin's disease, and in lupus erythematosus more frequently than can be attributed to chance alone. Although the weight of evidence suggests that GBS is immune-mediated, the immunopathogenesis remains obscure. In 1976 to 1977, a flurry of some 500 cases followed in the wake of the national swine flu vaccination program in the United States. This exceeded by severalfold the baseline incidence expected in this period among the vaccines. The epidemiologic features of this outbreak resembled a point-source epidemic with an "incubation" period of 1 to 6 weeks. The reason why swine flu vaccine appeared to trigger GBS in 1976 to 1977 has never been discovered. In subsequent annual flu vaccine programs in the United States, no excess cases of GBS have been identified.

The clinical features of GBS typically include areflexic motor paralysis with mild sensory disturbance coupled with an acellular rise of total protein in the cerebrospinal fluid by the end of the first week of symptoms. Most patients with GBS require hospitalization, and about one-fourth will need ventilatory assistance at some point during the illness. The prognosis is good; approximately 85 percent of patients make a complete or nearly complete recovery. The mortality rate is 3 to 4 percent. Management is generally supportive care, but plasmapheresis also has a role. Large, multicenter, controlled trials in North America and Europe have demonstrated a beneficial effect of plasmapheresis, especially when initiated in the first 2 weeks of illness. In contrast, the utility of glucocorticoid treatment is unproved, and it is generally considered not to be effective.

Other acute demyelinating polyneuropathies are rare and include buckthorn berry intoxication and diphtheritic polyneuritis (see Table 363-2).

Subacute demyelinating polyneuropathy Neuropathies in this category are heterogeneous in origin, although all are acquired. Most common is a relapsing and remitting neuropathy which has many clinical features in common with GBS, but differs from GBS in tempo, course, and absence of discernible triggering events. Previously mentioned toxins (buckthorn berry, diphtheria toxin, aurothioglucose) may also induce a picture of widespread subacute demyelination of peripheral nerves (see Table 363-2).

Chronic demyelinating polyneuropathy Although more common than the subacute neuropathies, chronic polyneuropathy with demyelinating features encompasses a wide diversity of disorders, including hereditary neuropathies, inflammatory neuropathies, and other acquired neuropathies associated with diabetes mellitus, dysproteinemias, other metabolic states, and some chronic intoxications. To complicate matters, many of these disorders present an electrodiagnostic picture of mixed axonal-demyelinative findings. Frequently it is difficult to determine which process, axonal degeneration or demyelination, is the primary event. Aspects of many of these neuropathies are included in Tables 363-1 to 363-3 and in the sections below.

SPECIAL CATEGORIES OF NEUROPATHY **Hereditary neuropathies** The major characteristics of this highly variegated group of disorders are summarized in Table 363-3. With the exception of the porphyric neuropathies, the onset of neuropathic dysfunction is insidious and progression is indolent over years or decades. Most of these diseases are quite rare with the striking exception of the dominantly inherited peroneal muscular atrophies (HMSN-I and HMSN-II; see Table 363-3). In peroneal muscular atrophy, phenotypic expression is often variable, so that affected family members of a propositus may have no symptoms and minimal neurologic findings but (in HMSN-I) may still show severe reduction of nerve conduction velocity.

Neuropathies with inflammation Acquired inflammatory demyelinating neuropathies fall into two major groups, the acute form called Guillain-Barré syndrome and more chronic forms, usually referred to as chronic inflammatory demyelinating polyradiculoneuropathy (CIDP). The entire group of acquired inflammatory demyelinating neuropathies constitutes a significant proportion of all cases of polyneuropathy and shares a distinctive clinical, electrophysiologic, and pathologic pattern. The diagnosis rests upon recognition of the clinical pattern and of other features, including elevated cerebrospinal fluid protein level, electrophysiologic changes (marked slowing of conduction velocities, delayed late responses, prolonged distal latencies, dispersion of evoked responses, and evidence of conduction block), and pathologic changes of low-grade inflammation and demyelination-remyelination of peripheral nerves. The course of GBS is acute and monophasic, whereas the more chronic forms pursue either a slowly progressive or a relapsing course. Cases with an intermediate course occur frequently enough to blur the diagnostic delimitation of GBS from the more chronic types of acquired inflammatory demyelinating neuropathy.

Pathogenetically, this group of inflammatory neuropathies is generally agreed to be immune-mediated, but the specific antigens involved and the crucial events of the immune response and why it is activated are uncertain.

Management of chronic, acquired CIPD involves a judicious mix of glucocorticoid therapy, other immunosuppressants, and plasmapheresis. These powerful agents are used only if the disorder is severe enough to threaten walking.

Diabetic neuropathies Classifications of the neuropathies of diabetes mellitus are found in Table 363-4. Although this provides a satisfactory frame of reference, the limitations inherent in classifying diabetic neuropathies should be understood. The most serious limitation is that most patients will not fit neatly into any single category, but rather will have overlapping clinical features of several. For instance, many diabetics with distal, primarily sensory polyneuropathy also can be shown to have autonomic dysfunction, usually in the form of vasomotor disturbance in the limbs and abnormalities of sweating. Similarly, patients who develop a proximal motor syndrome may have dysautonomic features (including sexual impotence in males) and some degree of distal sensory polyneuropathy. To compound matters, such patients appear at risk to develop a cranial mononeuropathy.

Classifying the diabetic neuropathies tells us nothing of the pathogenesis of the neuropathic lesion. Rather, attempts at classification represent an educated guess at identifying the apparent anatomic sites of disorder and the critical clinical features. Pain is a frequent feature of diabetic neuropathies (see Table 363-4) but is variable in incidence and degree and is subjective in nature. The term diabetic amyotrophy should be avoided because of its ambiguity.

Diabetic neuropathies tend to occur in the setting of long-standing hyperglycemia (decades) whether insulin-dependent or not. By far the most common neuropathies related to diabetes mellitus are the diffuse sensory and autonomic types (categories 1 and 2 under "Symmetric" in Table 363-4). Sensory and autonomic polyneuropathy, chronic and indolent in evolution, may first be noticed in the third or fourth decade in patients with juvenile-onset diabetes but tends to occur after age 50 in patients with adult-onset diabetes. Focal and multifocal types of neuropathy are less common but quite dramatic (categories 1, 2, and 3 under "Asymmetric" in Table 363-4). They rarely occur before the age of 45 and are usually subacute or acute in onset. Cranial mononeuropathies refer to isolated sixth or third nerve palsies. The latter spares the pupil in three-fourths of cases, and some local pain or headache occurs in one-half. Truncal, or thoracoabdominal, neuropathy is painful, involves one or more intercostal or lumbar nerves unilaterally, and frequently coexists with the asymmetric proximal motor neuropathy. Femoral and obturator nerve–innervated muscles (quadriceps femoris, iliopsoas, adductor magnus) and loss of knee jerk on that side are the most evident features of asymmetric proximal motor neuropathy. Sensory deficit is minor, but pain in the hip and anterior thigh may predominate. Common to all of these multifocal and focal neuropathies is the strong likelihood for subsidence of pain within weeks to a year and partial or complete recovery of function. The same is true of symmetric proximal motor neuropathy (category 3 under "Symmetric" in Table 363-4).

Focal and multifocal diabetic neuropathies are considered to be ischemic in origin, and the basis for symmetric polyneuropathies, thought by some to involve abnormality of nerve metabolism, includes the possibility of ischemia.

Management of diabetic neuropathies is directed toward optimal control of hyperglycemia and symptomatic pain suppression. The role of aldose reductase inhibitors in preventing or reversing diabetic complications, including neuropathy, remains unclear. Entrapment neuropathies are frequently amenable to surgical decompression procedures.

Neuropathies with dysproteinemia An association between polyneuropathy and both multiple myeloma and macroglobulinemia has been recognized for many years. With commonly encountered multiple myeloma (MM) having either lytic or diffuse osteoporotic bone lesions, clinically overt polyneuropathy is relatively infrequent, occurring in approximately 5 percent of patients. These neuropathies are sensorimotor, may be severe, and generally do not reverse with successful suppression of the myeloma. In most cases, electrodiagnostic and pathologic features are consistent with a process of axonal degeneration.

In contrast, myeloma with osteosclerotic features, although representing only 3 percent of all myelomas, is associated with polyneuropathy in almost one-half of cases. These neuropathies, which may also occur with solitary plasmacytoma, seem to be different from those linked to MM in that they (1) often respond to radiation or removal of the primary lesion, (2) are more frequently demyelinating in character, (3) are associated with different monoclonal proteins and light chains (almost all lambda as opposed to mostly kappa in MM), and (4) frequently occur in association with other systemic findings. These include skin thickening, hyperpigmentation, hypertrichosis, organomegaly, endocrinopathy, anasarca, papilledema, and clubbing of fingers. (POEMS syndrome: *p*olyneuropathy, *o*rganomegaly, *e*ndocrinopathy, *m* protein, and *s*kin changes.) A great deal of attention has been paid to this curious syndrome in Japan, where it is prevalent, but the underlying mechanism remains unknown.

Benign monoclonal gammopathy with an IgM serum spike, and usually with kappa light chains, is described in association with demyelinating polyneuropathy that often follows a protracted course and indolent progression. In about one-quarter of cases, the monoclonal serum protein binds to normal human peripheral myelin, specifically to myelin-associated glycoprotein. Immunocytochemical studies show binding of IgM to nerve obtained at biopsy or autopsy of these patients, but in a pattern different from that seen following incubation of sections of nerve with the IgM serum. Incubated nerves show uniform staining of the entire expanse of compact myelin sheath, but in vivo deposited IgM can be demonstrated to localize more selectively, probably at sites of myelin splitting, the latter a phenomenon characteristic of most dysglobulinemic neuropathies. Whether the IgM bound to nerve in vivo plays a role in damaging nerve is unresolved.

Autonomic neuropathy The autonomic nervous system regulates the visceral organs and vegetative functions. Many pharmacologic agents modify specific autonomic functions, but autonomic neuropathy (dysautonomia) with structural changes in pre- and postganglionic neurons can also occur. Usually autonomic neuropathy is a manifestation of a more generalized polyneuropathy also affecting somatic peripheral nervous function, as in diabetic neuropathy, GBS, and alcoholic polyneuropathy, but occasionally syndromes of pure pandysautonomia are encountered. Symptoms of dysautonomia are mainly negative (i.e., loss of function) and include postural hypotension with faintness or syncope, anhidrosis, hypothermia, bladder atony, obstipation, dry mouth and dry eyes from failure of salivary and lacrimal glands to secrete, blurring of vision from lack of pupillary and ciliary regulation, and sexual impotence in males. Positive phenomena (hyperfunction) may also occur and include episodic hypertension, diarrhea, hyperhidrosis, and either tachycardia or bradycardia.

Plexopathy This term refers to disorders of either the brachial or lumbosacral plexus. Lesions of the brachial plexus are characterized by motor and sensory signs different from those expected either in mononeuropathies of the upper limb or in polyneuropathies. The usual causes are direct trauma to the plexus, idiopathic brachial neuritis (also called neuralgic amyotrophy), cervical rib or band, infiltration by malignant tumor, or prior radiation therapy. When the upper parts of the brachial plexus, arising from cervical roots 5 through 7, are affected, weakness and atrophy of shoulder girdle and upper arm muscles occur. Injuries to the lower brachial plexus, arising from the eighth cervical and first thoracic roots, produce distal arm weakness, atrophy, and sensory deficit in the forearm and hand. In general, idiopathic brachial neuritis, radiation damage [greater than 60 Gy (6,000 rad)] and particular types of trauma (arm jerked downward) result in damage to the upper portions of the brachial plexus. In contrast, infiltration by malignant tumor, cervical rib or band, and certain other types of trauma (arm jerked upward) cause damage to the lower brachial plexus. Lumbosacral plexopathies are less common; they may be due to idiopathic lumbosacral plexitis, retroperitoneal hemorrhage, malignant tumor infiltration, or occur in association with long-standing diabetes mellitus.

Miscellaneous causes of neuropathy Ischemia of nerve severe enough to produce clinical symptoms has as its basis the widespread compromise of blood flow in the vasa nervorum. Typically, this is the result of small-vessel disease involving the vasa nervorum directly, as occurs with vasculitis, rather than large-vessel disease, such as atherosclerosis. Clinically, widespread disease of the vasa nervorum produces mononeuropathy multiplex, which electrodiagnostically has the features of a patchy axonal process.

Cold exerts deleterious effects on peripheral nerve directly without an intermediate step of ischemia being necessary. Cold injury to nerve occurs after prolonged exposure, usually of a limb, to moderately low temperatures, as with immersion of the feet in seawater; actual freezing of tissue is not required. Axonal degeneration of myelinated fibers is the pathologic expression of cold injury. Frequently limbs affected by cold injury to nerve show sensory deficit and dysesthesias, cutaneous vasomotor instability, pain, and marked sensitivity to minimal cold exposure, which persist for many years. The pathophysiology of these phenomena is uncertain.

TROPHIC CHANGES IN SEVERE NEUROPATHY The array of observable changes in completely denervated muscle, bone, and skin, including hair and nails, is well known, if incompletely understood. It is unclear what portion of the changes is due purely to denervation versus that caused by disuse, immobility, lack of weight bearing, and particularly recurrent, unnoticed, painless trauma. Considerable evidence favors the view that ulceration of skin, poor healing, tissue resorption, neurogenic arthropathy, and mutilation are the result of repeated heedless injury to insensitive parts. This sequence of events is avoidable with proper attention to and care of the insensitive parts by both patient and physician.

RECOVERY FROM NEUROPATHY In contrast to axons in the central nervous system, peripheral nerve fibers have an excellent capability to regenerate under proper circumstances. The process of regeneration following axonal degeneration may take from 2 months to more than a year, depending on the severity of the neuropathy and the length of regeneration required. Whether regeneration takes place depends upon the subsidence of the initial basis for neuropathy. This could be removal from contact with a neurotoxic substance or correction of an abnormal metabolic state. A deficit secondary to demyelination may recover rapidly since intact axons may remyelinate in just a few weeks. For example, a patient with GBS, in whom demyelination but no secondary axonal degeneration has occurred, may recover to normal strength from bedfastness and paralysis of arms and legs in as little as 3 to 4 weeks.

MONONEUROPATHY MULTIPLEX (MULTIFOCAL NEUROPATHY) This term means simultaneous or sequential involvement of individual noncontiguous nerve trunks, either partially or completely, evolving over days to years. Since the disease process underlying mononeuropathy multiplex involves peripheral nerves in a multifocal and random fashion, there is a tendency, as worsening occurs, for the neurologic deficit to become less patchy and multifocal and more confluent and symmetric. Some patients present initially with a distal symmetric neuropathy. Attention to the pattern of early symptoms is therefore important in making the judgment that a particular neuropathy is indeed a mononeuropathy multiplex.

Once that issue is settled, the next question is whether the process is primarily axonal or demyelinating. Almost one-third of all adults with the clinical syndrome of mononeuropathy multiplex have a clear-cut picture of a demyelinating disorder usually with multiple foci of persistent conduction block by electrodiagnostic examination. More intensive study of this subgroup suggests that the multifocal demyelinating neuropathy represents part of the spectrum of chronic acquired demyelinating neuropathy, that is, CIDP. Management of this multifocal subgroup is the same as for CIDP. (See ''Neuropathies with Inflammation'' above.)

The remaining two-thirds of patients with mononeuropathy multiplex have a picture by electrodiagnostic examination of axonal involvement that is heterogeneously distributed. Although ischemia would be suspected as the basis for neuropathy in these patients, only about one-half can be shown to have a process, usually vasculitis, affecting the vasa nervorum. The others remain undiagnosed even on follow-up, and the basis for their mononeuropathy multiplex is uncertain. Management in this group is conservative, but the management of those with proven vasculitis of vasa nervorum is the same as treatment for systemic vasculitis (see Chap. 276).

In individuals in whom vasculitic change in vasa nervorum can be demonstrated, any one of a large number of underlying disorders may be responsible. The primary vasculitides of the polyarteritis nodosa group constitute the most frequent basis, followed closely by the vasculitis syndrome occurring in the course of other connective tissue disorders. In descending order of frequency, the latter are rheumatoid arthritis, systemic lupus erythematosus, and mixed connective tissue disease. Other rarer causes of mononeuropathy multiplex due to nerve ischemia from occlusion of vasa nervorum include mixed cryoglobulinemia, Sjögren's syndrome, Wegener's granulomatosis, progressive systemic sclerosis, Churg-Strauss allergic granulomatosis, and hypersensitivity angiitides. Management of the neuropathy in each instance is predicated upon the appropriate treatment of the responsible disease.

Mononeuropathy multiplex syndrome may also be seen as a manifestation of leprosy, sarcoidosis, certain types of amyloidosis, hypereosinophilia syndrome, cryoglobulinemia, and multifocal types of diabetic neuropathy.

MONONEUROPATHY Mononeuropathy means focal involvement of a single nerve trunk and therefore implies a local causation.

TABLE 363-5 Some common mononeuropathies

Nerve	Origin (spinal segments)	Muscles innervated	Usual site of lesion	Clinical features	Comments
UPPER EXTREMITY					
Suprascapular	C5,C6	Supraspinatus Infraspinatus	Suprascapular notch of scapula	Weakness of lateral rotation of the humerus	No sensory deficit
Long thoracic	C5–C7	Serratus anterior	Variable	Winging of scapula	No sensory deficit
Axillary	C5,C6	Deltoid, teres minor	Near shoulder joint	Weakness of shoulder abduction; atrophy of shoulder	Sensory deficit similar to C5 dorsal root lesion (see Figs. 28-2 and 28-3)
Radial	C5–T1	Triceps, brachioradialis, wrist, finger, and thumb extensors	Spiral groove of humerus	Wrist drop most obvious, also finger and thumb extensors paralyzed	Saturday night palsy (acute compression) is frequent cause
Posterior interosseous branch	C7,C8	Finger and thumb extensors	Edge of supinator muscle below elbow	Finger drop; wrist relatively spared	No sensory deficit
Ulnar	C8,T1	Ulnar flexor of the wrist, long flexors of 4th and 5th digits, and most intrinsic hand muscles	Ulnar groove at the elbow	Weakness of finger adduction and abduction and thumb adduction (see text); interosseous atrophy, claw-hand	May be acute or insidious; sensory symptoms/signs are distinctive (Figs. 28-2 and 28-3); also see text
			Cubital tunnel	Same as above	Often pain over medial proximal forearm (cubital tunnel)
			Medial base of palm	Intrinsic hand muscles only, interosseous atrophy	No sensory deficit
Median	C6–T1	Abductor pollicis brevis; more proximal muscles include forearm pronator, long finger and thumb flexors	Carpal tunnel	Characteristic sensory symptoms and deficit and inability to make a circle with thumb and index finger	Sensory deficit as per Figs. 28-2 and 28-3 (see text); known as carpal tunnel syndrome
Anterior interosseous branch	C7–T1	Long flexors of thumb and index and middle fingers	Anterior interosseus branch below the elbow	Weakness of pinch; pain in volar forearm	No sensory deficit
LOWER EXTREMITY					
Femoral	L2–L4	Iliopsoas (hip flexor) and quadriceps femoris (knee extensor)	Proximal to inguinal ligament	Knee buckling; absent knee jerk; weak anterior thigh muscles with atrophy	Association with diabetes mellitus; sensory disturbance as per Fig. 28-2
Lateral femoral cutaneous branch	L2,L3	None	Inguinal ligament	Dysesthetic hyperpathia of lateral thigh	Known as meralgia paresthetica
Obturator	L3,L4	Thigh adductors	Intrapelvic or at pubis	Weakness of hip adduction	Sensory deficit on medial thigh
Sciatic	L4–S3	Hamstring muscles, hip abductor and all muscles below the knee	Near sciatic notch	Severe lower leg and hamstring weakness; flail foot; severe disability	Uncommon except from war wounds
Posterior tibial	L5–S2	Calf muscles (proximally), toe flexors and other intrinsic foot muscles	Tarsal tunnel, near medial malleolus	Pain and numbness of sole, weak toe flexors	Known as tarsal tunnel syndrome
Peroneal	L4–S1	Dorsiflexors of toes and foot, evertors of foot	At neck of fibula	Foot drop and weakness of foot eversion	Sensory deficit is similar in distribution to L5, S1 sensory roots

Direct trauma, compression, and entrapment are the usual causes. Ulnar neuropathies, due to lesions either at the ulnar groove or in the cubital tunnel, and median neuropathy due to compression in the carpal tunnel constitute the great majority of mononeuropathies encountered in clinical practice. These are described below, and other common mononeuropathies are listed in Table 363-5.

In the absence of a history of trauma to the nerve trunk, factors favoring conservative management include sudden onset, no motor deficit, few or no sensory findings even though pain and sensory symptoms might be present, and no evidence of axonal degeneration by electrodiagnostic criteria. Factors favoring surgical intervention include chronicity and worsening neurologic deficit on examination, particularly if motor, and electrodiagnostic evidence that the lesion has produced a degree of wallerian degeneration.

Ulnar nerve Complete ulnar paralysis results in a characteristic claw-hand deformity owing to wasting of the small hand muscles and hyperextension of the fingers at the metacarpophalangeal joints and flexion at the interphalangeal joints. The flexion deformity is most pronounced in the fourth and fifth fingers. Sensory loss occurs over the fifth finger, the ulnar aspect of the fourth finger, and the ulnar border of the palm. The superficial location of the nerve at the elbow makes it a common site of pressure palsy. The ulnar nerve may also become entrapped just distal to the elbow in the cubital tunnel formed by the aponeurotic arch linking the two heads of the flexor carpi ulnaris. Prolonged pressure on the base of the palm, as occurs with use of hand tools or bicycle riding, may result in damage to the deep palmar branch of the ulnar nerve, causing weakness of the small hand muscles but no sensory loss.

Median nerve The median nerve in the carpal tunnel lies in close quarters with nine tendons. Entrapment of the nerve at the wrist (carpal tunnel syndrome) may be secondary to excessive use of the wrist, tenosynovitis with arthritis, or local infiltration, for example, by a thickening of connective tissue and deposit of amyloid with multiple myeloma or one of the mucopolysaccharides. Other systemic diseases associated with an increased incidence of carpal tunnel syndrome are acromegaly, hypothyroidism, rheumatoid arthritis, and diabetes mellitus, but these account for only a small fraction of all cases. The main symptoms of carpal tunnel syndrome are nocturnal paresthesias of thumb, index, and middle fingers. With worsening, numbness demonstrable by pin examination occurs in that distribution, and eventually weakness and atrophy of the abductor pollicis brevis (thenar eminence) becomes evident. Treatment of carpal tunnel syndrome is surgical section of the carpal ligament. Incomplete lesions of the median nerve between the axilla and wrist may result in causalgia (a particularly severe type of burning pain; see Chap. 15).

OTHER FOCAL NEUROPATHIES Peripheral nerve tumors These are mostly benign and can arise on any nerve trunk or twig. Although peripheral nerve tumors occur anywhere in the body including the spinal roots and cauda equina, many are subcutaneous in location and present as a soft swelling, sometimes with a purplish discoloration of the skin. Two major categories of peripheral nerve tumors are recognized: neurilemmoma (schwannoma) and neurofibroma. Neurilemmomas are usually solitary and grow within the nerve sheath, rendering the tumor relatively easy to dissect free. In contrast, neurofibromas tend to be multiple, grow within the endoneurial substance, rendering them difficult to dissect, may undergo malignant changes, and are the hallmark of von Recklinghausen's neurofibromatosis. This disease is characterized by an autosomal dominant inheritance pattern, any number of neurofibromas from one to thousands, five or more café au lait–pigmented skin lesions greater than 1.5 cm (80 percent of patients), axillary freckles (93 percent of patients), and an increased incidence of seizure disorder and mental retardation (see Chap. 358).

Herpes zoster This is a sensory neuritis of viral cause characterized by acute inflammation of one or more dorsal root ganglia, due to varicella-zoster virus infection. Lancinating pain and hyperalgesia over the skin surface supplied by affected roots occur for 3 to 4 days, followed by the appearance of herpetic eruption in the same segment characterized by painful raised blisters on reddened bases. If the inflammatory process spreads to involve adjacent motor roots of anterior horns of the cord, segmental motor weakness and wasting appear. Paralysis of the oculomotor nerves may occur in conjunction with ophthalmic division involvement of the trigeminal ganglion (ophthalmoplegic zoster). Facial paralysis may occur with involvement of the geniculate ganglion and herpetic eruption on the ipsilateral tympanic membrane or external ear canal (Ramsay Hunt syndrome).

Leprous neuritis This is a major worldwide cause of neuropathy. *Mycobacterium leprae* organisms readily invade Schwann cells in cutaneous nerve twigs, particularly those associated with unmyelinated nerve fibers. Two major forms of leprous neuritis are recognized, tuberculoid and lepromatous, which actually represent the far ends of a spectrum of disease, the middle of which is called dimorphous leprosy (patchy and multifocal involvement of skin and nerve). Treatment depends upon where in the spectrum a given case is classified (see Chap. 126). Tuberculoid (high-resistance) leprosy is restricted to a single patch of hypesthetic or anesthetic skin in any location. The skin patch is frequently thickened, reddened, or hypopigmented. If a superficially placed nerve trunk, typically a cutaneous nerve, courses just beneath the area of affected skin, it may be engulfed in the inflammatory reaction, resulting in an associated mononeuropathy. Such a nerve may be palpably enlarged and beaded. Lepromatous (low-resistance) leprosy is marked by immunologic tolerance and widespread skin thickening, cutaneous anesthesia, and anhidrosis, sparing only the warmest parts of the body, notably the axilla, groin, and beneath the scalp hair. Motor signs (focal weakness and atrophy) result from damage to mixed nerves lying close to the skin, particularly the median, ulnar, peroneal, and facial nerves.

Bell's palsy This is due to inflammation of the facial nerve in the facial canal, the basis for which remains obscure. Edema may play a part leading to compression of nerve fibers, with resulting acute unilateral paralysis of facial muscles (see Chap. 360).

Sarcoidosis This may involve single or multiple peripheral nerves, producing asymmetric mononeuritis or polyneuritis. Unilateral or bilateral facial paralysis is described in association with parotitis and uveitis (Heerfordt's syndrome).

Polyneuritis cranialis This is a relapsing and remitting mononeuropathy multiplex restricted to cranial nerves. It is usually associated with indolent tuberculous cervical adenitis (scrofula) or sarcoidosis. Treatment of the underlying condition will halt the cranial nerve palsies.

Acknowledgment

By arrangement with the publishers, portions of this section also appear in substantially the same form in Asbury AK: Diseases of peripheral nerve, in *Diseases of the Nervous System*, AK Asbury, GM McKhann, WI McDonald (eds). Philadelphia, Saunders, 1986, and London, Heinemann, 1986.

REFERENCES

ASBURY AK: New aspects of disease of the peripheral nervous system, in *Harrison's Textbook of Internal Medicine, Update IV*. McGraw-Hill, New York, 1983, 211–229

———, GILLIATT RW: *Peripheral Nerve Disorders: A Practical Approach*. London, Butterworth, 1984

BENSON MD: Familial amyloidotic polyneuropathy. Trends Neurosci 12: 88, 1989

BROWN MJ (eds): Neuropathy. Semin Neurol 7:1, 1987

DAWSON DM et al: *Entrapment Neuropathies*. Boston, Little, Brown, 1983

DYCK PJ et al (eds): *Peripheral Neuropathy*, 2d ed. Philadelphia, Saunders, 1984

———: *Diabetic Neuropathy*. Philadelphia, Saunders, 1987

LAYZER RB: *Neuromuscular Manifestations of Systemic Disease*, vol 25: *Contemporary Neurology Series*. Philadelphia, Davis, 1984

SPENCER PS, SCHAUMBURG HH (eds): *Experimental and Clinical Neurotoxicology*. Baltimore, Williams & Wilkins, 1980

STEWART JD: *Focal Peripheral Neuropathics*. New York, Elsevier, 1987

364 DERMATOMYOSITIS AND POLYMYOSITIS

WALTER G. BRADLEY / RUP TANDAN

Dermatomyositis and polymyositis are conditions of unknown etiology in which the skeletal muscle is damaged by a nonsuppurative inflammatory process dominated by lymphocytic infiltration. The term *polymyositis* is applied when the condition spares the skin and the term *dermatomyositis* when polymyositis is associated with a characteristic skin rash. One-third of cases are associated with various connective tissue disorders, such as rheumatoid arthritis, lupus erythematosus, mixed connective tissue disorder, and scleroderma, and one-tenth with a malignancy.

ETIOLOGY The cause of these diseases is unknown. The two main theories are that the diseases are due to a viral infection of the skeletal muscle or to an autoimmune disorder (Chap. 276). Experimental viral myositis can be induced in animals by coxsackievirus. A mild inflammatory myopathy can occur with influenza. The numerous electron-microscope observations of virus-like particles in muscle fibers in dermatomyositis or polymyositis have not been confirmed by virus isolation, rising titers of antiviral antibodies have not been demonstrated, and the disease has not been passed into animals by injection of extracts of affected muscles. One-third of cases have elevated serum antibodies to toxoplasma, but the disease does not generally respond to therapy against toxoplasmosis. A lymphocyte-mediated disease resembling polymyositis has been reported in laboratory animals injected with sterile muscle extracts together with Freund's adjuvant (experimental allergic myositis). Immunohistochemical studies of muscle have shown that fiber necrosis probably results from the action of activated T cells and macrophages in polymyositis, and from T-helper-cell-dependent stimulation of B cells with resultant antibody-mediated cytotoxicity in dermatomyositis. A small proportion of patients have deposition of immunoglobulins on intramuscular blood vessels, suggesting that circulating antibodies may play some role in the disease. The close association of polymyositis and diseases of connective tissue favors the notion of a common autoimmune etiology or pathogenesis. In older patients dermatomyositis is frequently associated with a malignancy. Thus, dermatomyositis-polymyositis is a syndrome which probably has a number of different causes.

CLASSIFICATION The classification of the dermatomyositis-polymyositis group which is most widely used is given in Table 364-1. This classification is based partly on known differences in etiology and has a number of drawbacks, as noted below. Other uncommon associations of polymyositis are sarcoidosis, giant cell myositis with thymoma, and myositis in systemic infections due to viruses, toxoplasma, or parasites. A focal infective myositis due to streptococcal or staphylococcal infection is mostly seen in the tropics. Focal nodular myositis is a variant of polymyositis where focal areas of myositis cause hot, often painful, multifocal muscle masses. Inclusion body myositis is an inflammatory myopathy with characteristic clinical and pathologic features (see below).

INCIDENCE Current estimates that the annual incidence of the inflammatory myopathies is about five per million of the population are probably too low.

TABLE 364-1 Classification of polymyositis-dermatomyositis

Group I:	Primary idiopathic polymyositis
Group II:	Primary idiopathic dermatomyositis
Group III:	Dermatomyositis (or polymyositis) associated with neoplasia
Group IV:	Childhood dermatomyositis (or polymyositis) associated with vasculitis
Group V:	Polymyositis (or dermatomyositis) with associated collagen vascular disease

SOURCE: Classification suggested by Bohan et al.

CLINICAL MANIFESTATIONS Group I: Primary idiopathic polymyositis This group comprises about one-third of all cases of inflammatory myopathy. It is insidiously progressive over weeks, months, or even years. Rarely the disease is acute, producing severe muscle weakness in a matter of days. The disease may develop at any age and in either sex. Females outnumber males 2:1.

The patients first become aware of weakness of the proximal limb muscles, especially the hips and thighs, and find difficulty in arising from the squatting or kneeling position and in climbing or descending stairs. When shoulder girdle muscles are involved, placing an object on a high shelf or combing the hair becomes difficult. Occasionally the disease is more restricted, affecting only the neck, the shoulder, or the quadriceps muscles. Pain of an aching type in the buttocks, thighs, and calves is experienced in about 10 percent of the cases, and tenderness on palpation in another 20 percent. Early symptoms of dysphagia and weakness of flexor muscles of the neck in a patient with a chronic myopathy suggest the diagnosis of polymyositis.

When the patient is first seen, there may be weakness of the muscles of the trunk, the pectoral and pelvic girdles, the upper arms and thighs, the anterior neck, more so than the posterior, and the pharynx. Ocular muscles are almost never affected except in a rare association with myasthenia gravis. The distal muscles are spared in about 75 percent of cases. Muscle atrophy, contractures, and diminished tendon reflexes are rare in early myositis and never as pronounced as in muscular dystrophies and denervating conditions. When the reflexes are disproportionately reduced, carcinoma with polymyositis and polyneuropathy or the Lambert-Eaton syndrome should be considered. Occasionally, the reflexes may be paradoxically brisk in dermatomyositis-polymyositis, perhaps due to irritation of muscle spindle receptors by the inflammation.

At presentation about 25 percent of patients have dysphagia, about 5 percent have significant respiratory impairment, and 5 percent are unable to walk. Dysphagia is due to involvement of striated muscles of the pharynx and upper esophagus. At some time in the course of the disease cardiac abnormalities are observed in about 30 percent of cases; these include ECG changes, arrhythmias, and heart failure secondary to myocarditis. About half of the fatal cases have pathologic evidence of cardiac disease with necrosis of myocardial fibers, usually with only modest inflammatory reaction. The frequency of myocardial infarction may be increased in those treated for long periods with glucocorticoids. In a few cases there is dyspnea due to lymphocytic pneumonitis, pulmonary edema, or pulmonary fibrosis. Arthralgia, Raynaud's phenomenon, and, rarely, low-grade fever may also be present.

Group II: Primary idiopathic dermatomyositis This group comprises just over one-third of all cases of myositis. The skin changes may precede or follow the muscle syndrome and include a localized or diffuse erythema, maculopapular eruption, scaling eczematoid dermatitis, or, rarely, an exfoliative dermatitis. The classic lilac-colored (heliotrope) rash is on the eyelids, bridge of the nose, cheeks (butterfly distribution), forehead, chest, elbows, knees and knuckles, and around the nail beds. Itching may be troublesome in some cases. The skin lesions may be subtle and easily overlooked. Periorbital edema is frequent, particularly in acute cases. The skin lesions may occasionally ulcerate. Subcutaneous calcification may occur, especially in children.

The typical rash and myositis allow a diagnosis of dermatomyositis, and such cases may be placed in this category (group II, Table 364-1) if idiopathic and into groups III, IV, and V if there are other features, namely malignancy, vasculitis in children, and an established collagen vascular disease. There should be concern about an underlying malignancy in patients with dermatomyositis over the age of 60.

Group III: Polymyositis or dermatomyositis with neoplasia This syndrome, which comprises about 8 percent of all cases of myositis, is categorized separately, although muscle and skin changes are indistinguishable from those in the other groups. Malignancy, however, is uncommon in myositis seen in children and in association with a connective tissue disorder. The malignancy may antedate or postdate the onset of the myositis by up to 2 years. The incidence of this paraneoplastic syndrome is higher in patients with dermatomyositis over the age of 60; therefore, in such patients a thorough history and clinical examination (including breast and rectal) must be supplemented by hemogram, biochemical profile, urine analysis for blood and cytology, stool samples for occult blood, chest x-ray, and sputum for cytology seeking clues for an underlying malignancy. This relatively inexpensive search often uncovers most malignancies; undirected radiologic screening procedures are costly and unhelpful in improving the yield. The most common malignancies are lung, ovary, breast, gastrointestinal tract, and myeloproliferative disorders. The myositis is a paraneoplastic syndrome, the cause of which may lie in an altered immune status or an occult viral infection of the muscle.

Group IV: Childhood polymyositis and dermatomyositis associated with vasculitis This group comprises about 8 to 20 percent of all cases of myositis in various series. Inflammatory myopathy in childhood is frequently associated with skin involvement and clinical or pathologic evidence of vasculitis in skin, muscles, gastrointestinal tract, and other organs. There are degeneration and loss of capillaries in a perifascicular distribution in the skeletal muscles; often necrotizing lesions of the skin; and ischemic infarction of kidneys, gastrointestinal tract, and rarely brain. Consequently, some authors have reported mortality rates of up to one-third in childhood dermatomyositis, though most have found that the prognosis is better than in adult dermatomyositis-polymyositis. One limitation of the classification of Bohan et al. is that it is not clear whether or not all cases of childhood myositis should be included in group IV. Subcutaneous calcification is frequently present in childhood dermatomyositis.

Group V: Polymyositis or dermatomyositis with an associated connective tissue disorder This "overlap group" comprises about one-fifth of all cases of myositis. Scleroderma, rheumatoid arthritis, mixed connective tissue disease, and lupus erythematosus are the most common associated conditions; polyarteritis nodosa and rheumatic fever are more rarely associated. Criteria for placement in the overlap group combine the demonstration of the appropriate clinical and laboratory abnormalities required for the diagnosis of the connective tissue disorder together with clinical and laboratory evidence of myositis. The diagnosis of myositis is often difficult in patients with connective tissue disorders producing arthritis, since this may often produce muscle weakness with type II fiber atrophy. Moreover, perivascular inflammatory foci are common in muscle in connective tissue disorders. Demonstration of increased serum creatine kinase (CK), electromyography (EMG), and muscle biopsy are often required to make this diagnosis. Though patients in this overlap group usually respond to glucocorticoid therapy, the prognosis for recovery of function is poorer than in pure dermatomyositis-polymyositis. Dysphagia in group V patients with scleroderma is often due to involvement of the smooth muscle of the distal third of the esophagus.

Other disorders associated with myositis SARCOIDOSIS AND POLYMYOSITIS The skeletal muscle contains noncaseating granulomas with Langhans-type multinuclear giant cells in at least one-quarter of patients with sarcoidosis. Symptomatic polymyositis is, however, uncommon. Regenerating multinuclear myoblasts resemble Langhans' giant cells, which has led to misdiagnosis in many of the cases reported in the literature to have "sarcoid myositis." Giant cell or granulomatous polymyositis and myocarditis, sometimes associated with myasthenia gravis, have been recorded in patients with thymomas.

FOCAL NODULAR MYOSITIS A syndrome of acutely developing and painful focal inflammatory nodules, sometimes occurring sequentially in different muscles, has been termed *focal nodular myositis*. The pathologic appearance and response to therapy are similar to those in generalized polymyositis. The differential diagnosis includes, when single, a muscle tumor (sarcoma or rhabdomyosarcoma) and, when multiple, muscle infarcts such as can occur in polyarteritis nodosa.

INFECTIOUS POLYMYOSITIS Rare cases of polymyositis have clear-cut evidence of being due to known pathogens such as toxoplasma (Chap. 162), viruses (Chap. 144), and spirochetes (Lyme disease). Antibody screening will suggest the diagnosis in such cases. Polymyositis occurs in homosexual men infected with the human immunodeficiency virus (HIV), sometimes as the presenting feature and rarely due to therapy with zidovudine (AZT). Raised serum CK, EMG evidence of a myopathy, and muscle fiber necrosis with or without inflammatory infiltrates are seen. Trichinosis may be confused with iodiopathic polymyositis, particularly if the history of raw pork ingestion is not obtained. The symptoms of trichinosis are variable and depend upon the parasitic load. Low-grade fever, muscle pain of variable degree, conjunctival and periorbital edema, and fatigue are frequent. Weakness is generally mild. Heavy infestation is often associated with central nervous system symptoms of delirium, coma, or focal neurologic deficit. The frequent myocardial involvement is manifested by tachycardia and ECG changes. The diagnosis is made by the history of ingestion of undercooked pork, marked eosinophilia, sensitivity to intradermal *Trichina* antigen, and the appearance of serum antibodies to *Trichina* during the course of the disease. Occasionally the diagnosis is not recognized until a muscle is biopsied. Pyomyositis, a suppurative inflammation of muscle due to staphylococcus or streptococcus, is mainly seen in the tropics. The presentation is that of a diffuse abscess of the muscle.

INCLUSION BODY MYOSITIS The clinical features of this condition are similar to those of chronic idiopathic polymyositis, except that focal and distal muscle involvement are more frequent. Muscle biopsy shows interstitial and occasionally perivascular inflammatory infiltration, necrosis, and regeneration of muscle fibers, but in addition there are "rimmed vacuoles" in the fibers. Electron microscopy reveals paramyxovirus-like filaments in the nuclei and sarcoplasm. The nature of these filaments is still in dispute. This disorder responds poorly to immunosuppressive therapy, and the prognosis is for a chronically progressive disorder with loss of ambulation about 5 to 10 years after presentation.

EOSINOPHILIC MYOSITIS This rare disease probably represents one manifestation of the spectrum of hypereosinophilic syndrome. Subacute onset of muscle pain and proximal weakness, elevated serum CK, myopathic features on electromyogram, and histologic appearances of a myositis with an eosinophilic inflammatory infiltrate are characteristic. Some patients may respond to glucocorticoids, methotrexate, or leukapheresis.

EOSINOPHILIC FASCIITIS This disorder is characterized by painful swelling and thickening of the skin in the extremities, limitation of movement due to contractures, and mild muscle weakness. Raised sedimentation rate, peripheral eosinophilia, hypergammaglobulinemia, and mildly elevated CK are seen. The EMG may show myopathic features. Histologically there is marked thickening and infiltration of the deep fascia with mononuclear cells and eosinophils, some involvement of the epimysium and perimysium, and varying but not striking degeneration of muscle. Most patients respond to treatment with glucocorticoids.

RELAPSING EOSINOPHILIC PERIMYOSITIS In this disease there are recurrent painful and tender areas in the neck or lower extremities, but without muscle weakness. Raised sedimentation rate and peripheral eosinophilia are frequent, serum CK is sometimes raised, and pathologically there is eosinophilic infiltration of the perimysium. Response to glucocorticoids is usually good.

LABORATORY FINDINGS In all forms of polymyositis there may be elevated serum levels of the enzymes present in skeletal muscle, such as CK, aldolase, serum glutamic oxaloacetic transaminase (SGOT), lactic acid dehydrogenase (LDH), and serum glutamic pyruvate transaminase (SGPT). The degree of rise decreases from the first to the last in this series of enzymes, and the pattern is the reverse of that seen in liver disease. Tests for circulating rheumatoid factor and antinuclear antibodies are positive in less than one-half of the cases. Myoglobin can be found in the urine when muscle destruction is acute and extensive; rarely, acute polymyositis causes the full syndrome of rhabdomyolysis and myoglobinuria. The erythrocyte sedimentation rate is elevated in about two-thirds of cases. Most other hematologic indexes are normal. In about 40 percent of cases the electromyogram reveals a markedly increased insertional activity (muscle irritability), together with the typical myopathic triad of motor unit action potentials which are of low amplitude, are polyphasic, and have an abnormally early recruitment. In a further 40 percent of the patients only myopathic changes are present. The ECG is abnormal in about 5 to 10 percent of the cases at presentation. Since the pathologic process in myositis is patchy, greater diagnostic yield is obtained by taking the biopsy from two clinically affected muscles and by skip serial sectioning of all specimens. Muscles recently used for EMG or intramuscular injection must be avoided as these procedures can produce inflammatory changes and muscle fiber damage, leading to false-positive results. In about two-thirds of cases, the biopsies will demonstrate the typical pathologic changes of myositis, but despite following the above recommendations, about 10 percent of cases have normal muscle biopsy.

Skeletal muscle pathology The principal changes in muscle consist of infiltrates of inflammatory cells (lymphocytes, macrophages, plasma cells, and rare eosinophils and neutrophils) and destruction of muscle fibers with a phagocytic reaction. Perivascular (usually perivenular) inflammatory cell infiltration is the hallmark of polymyositis. Interstitial inflammatory cell infiltration is also a prominent feature of the disease, but lesser degrees of it may be seen in other conditions as a secondary reaction (e.g., in facioscapulohumeral and Becker's muscular dystrophy). The inflammatory infiltrates contain activated T cells of the helper-inducer and cytotoxic-suppressor types, with accompanying macrophages in polymyositis, and B cells in dermatomyositis. Evidence of muscle fiber degeneration and regeneration is almost invariably present. Many of the residual muscle fibers are small, with increased numbers of sarcolemmal nuclei. Either the degeneration of muscle fibers or the infiltration of inflammatory cells may predominate in any given biopsy specimen. Blood vessel changes and perifascicular atrophy are prominent in childhood dermatomyositis, but less so in adult dermatomyositis and polymyositis. Capillary loss due to endothelial cell necrosis occurs particularly in the periphery of fascicles and may explain the perifascular atrophy. Other features include reduplication of capillary basement membrane and the presence of tubular inclusions within endothelial cells. Type II muscle fiber atrophy and muscle infarcts may also be found. Vasculitis is also seen in polymyositis or dermatomyositis associated with connective tissue disorders.

DIAGNOSIS Patients with dermatomyositis with the characteristic skin rash, muscle weakness, and evidence of muscle damage by EMG and elevation of serum CK may not require a muscle biopsy to confirm the diagnosis. In the case of idiopathic polymyositis, however, a firm diagnosis must be based on the presence of a typical clinical picture, a typical EMG, elevation of serum CK, and a diagnostic muscle biopsy. All four criteria are required to be certain of the diagnosis, since inflammatory changes may occasionally occur in other myopathies (e.g., facioscapulohumeral muscular dystrophy) and in other connective tissue disorders without clear muscle weakness. However, in less than one-third of cases of polymyositis are *all* these criteria satisfied. It may be particularly difficult to obtain a diagnostic muscle biopsy because of the patchy nature of the disease. Thus, a therapeutic trial of glucocorticoids should be given when full investigation of a patient with significant disability leaves a diagnosis of "possible polymyositis," usually because of a nondiagnostic muscle biopsy.

DIFFERENTIAL DIAGNOSIS The clinical picture of skin rash and proximal or diffuse muscle weakness has few causes other than dermatomyositis. However, proximal muscle weakness without skin involvement can be due to many conditions other than polymyositis and necessitates detailed investigation to establish the correct diagnosis.

Subacute or chronic progressive muscle weakness This may be due to denervating conditions such as the spinal muscular atrophies or amyotrophic lateral sclerosis. Upper motor neuron signs in the latter in addition to the muscle weakness aid in the diagnosis. The muscular dystrophies, such as those of Duchenne and Becker and the limb-girdle and facioscapulohumeral types, may appear similar to polymyositis (Chap. 365). However, the muscular dystrophies usually develop more slowly, rarely present after the age of 30, usually involve the pharyngeal and posterior neck muscles only in their later course, and have a pattern of muscle involvement which is selective, involving some muscles such as the biceps and brachioradialis early in the course of the disease, and sparing others, such as the deltoid. Nevertheless, in rare patients it may be difficult, even with a muscle biopsy, to distinguish chronic polymyositis from a rapidly advancing muscular dystrophy. This is particularly true of facioscapulohumeral muscular dystrophy, where interstitial inflammatory cell infiltration is commonly found early in the disease. Such doubtful cases should always be given an adequate trial of glucocorticoid therapy. Dystrophia myotonica produces a characteristic facies with ptosis, facial myopathy, temporalis muscle wasting, and grip myotonia (Chap. 365). Some of the metabolic myopathies, including glycogen storage disease due to myophosphorylase deficiency and the lipid storage diseases due to carnitine and carnitine palmityltransferase deficiency, produce exertional cramps, rhabdomyolysis, and muscle weakness; diagnosis rests upon biochemical studies of the muscle biopsy (Chap. 365). Glycogen storage disease due to acid maltase deficiency also requires muscle biopsy for diagnosis. The endocrine myopathies such as those due to hypercorticosteroidism, hyper- and hypothyroidism, and hyper- and hypoparathyroidism require the appropriate laboratory investigations for diagnosis. Muscle wasting in patients with an underlying neoplasm may be true polymyositis, but it can be due to a protein-wasting state (cachexia), a paraneoplastic neuropathy, or type II fiber atrophy.

Muscle weakness with marked exercise-induced fatigue Fatigue without much muscle wasting may be due to the neuromuscular junction disorders, myasthenia gravis, or the Lambert-Eaton syndrome. Repetitive nerve stimulation studies aid in the diagnosis of these conditions (Chap. 366).

Acute muscle weakness This may be caused by an acute neuropathy such as that due to the Guillain-Barré syndrome or a neurotoxin. When combined with painful muscle cramps, rhabdomyolysis, and myoglobinuria, it may be due to known metabolic disorders including some of the glycogen storage diseases such as myophosphorylase deficiency (McArdle's disease), carnitine palmityltransferase deficiency, and myoadenylate deaminase deficiency. Acute viral infections may cause a similar syndrome. Chronic alcoholics may develop a painful myopathy with myoglobinuria after a bout of heavy drinking or may present with a painless acute hypokalemic myopathy which is completely reversible, or may show an asymptomatic elevation of serum CK and myoglobin. Acute muscle weakness with myoglobinuria may occur in prolonged severe hypokalemia due to potassium loss, or with hypophosphatemia and hypomagnesemia, often seen in chronic alcoholics and in patients on nasogastric suction receiving parental hyperalimentation. An acute necrotizing myopathy with myoglobinuria can rarely accompany hypernatremia and hyponatremia.

Drug-induced myopathies Rhabdomyolysis and myoglobinuria have been associated with intake of amphotericin B, ϵ-aminocaproic acid, fenfluramine, heroin, and phencyclidine. A predominantly hypokalemic myopathy may result from prolonged use of diuretics, carbenoxolone, and azathioprine. Penicillamine has been reported to produce a myositis. The use of clofibrate, cimetidine, chloroquine, emetine, and, recently, AZT has been associated with a myopathy. Toxic myopathies usually have a different pathology from polymyositis and require a careful drug history for diagnosis. In other cases investigation reveals no etiology, and these may be due to a true acute autoimmune polymyositis or to an as yet undiscovered metabolic defect.

Pain on movement and muscle tenderness Patients with muscle pain and little or no weakness may be thought to be neurotic or hysterical. A number of conditions including *polymyalgia rheumatica* (Chap. 276) and arthritic disorders of adjacent joints enter into the differential diagnosis of polymyositis. The muscle biopsy either is normal or discloses type II fiber atrophy, but in polymyalgia rheumatica the temporal artery biopsy may show giant cell arteritis (Chap. 276). *Fibrositis* and *fibromyalgia* are syndromes which frequently enter into the differential diagnosis of polymyositis. Patients complain of focal or diffuse muscle tenderness, aching, and weakness, which is sometimes poorly separated from joint pain. In other patients there may be minor signs of a collagen vascular disorder, such as an increased erythrocyte sedimentation rate, antinuclear antibody (ANA), or rheumatoid factor, and occasionally there is slight elevation of the serum CK. The muscle biopsy occasionally shows a few interstitial inflammatory cells. Where there is a focal "trigger point," biopsy may show inflammatory infiltration of the connective tissue. Rarely does this syndrome develop into frank polymyositis, and the prognosis is therefore more benign than that of polymyositis (see below). Many such patients show some response to nonsteroidal anti-inflammatory agents, though most continue to have indolent complaints.

TREATMENT Glucocorticoids in high dosage are the accepted treatment for severe dermatomyositis-polymyositis, though there is no controlled trial to prove their effectiveness. The best results are obtained from the use of prednisone, starting at a dose of 1 to 2 mg/kg body weight per day (60 to 100 mg/d for adults). Improvement may begin within 1 to 4 weeks, though in some patients treatment may need to be continued for 3 months before improvement occurs. When there is significant improvement in the weakness, the daily dose may be reduced by 5 mg every 4 weeks. Repeated manual muscle testing and serum CK determinations should be performed to ensure that the myositis does not relapse. At about 40 mg/d, the schedule is changed gradually to 80 mg every other day in order to reduce the incidence of glucocorticoid side effects. There is some evidence that the use of alternate-day glucocorticoids from the outset may be effective, particularly in patients with milder disease. Children and patients with acute to subacute dermatomyositis-polymyositis tend to improve more rapidly than those with chronic polymyositis. If the dose is reduced too rapidly, or to too low a level, relapse will occur, necessitating return to high dosage. Prednisone therapy may have to be continued for several years, but an attempt should be made every year to withdraw the therapy from patients who are clinically stable in order to determine if the disease is still active.

Cytotoxic drugs should be tried when the disease is severe, when the response to glucocorticoids is inadequate after 1 to 3 months, or when relapses are frequent. Azathioprine (2.5 to 3.5 mg/kg body weight per day in divided doses) is the most commonly used cytotoxic drug in this disease, and in combination with glucocorticoids in preliminary studies has shown a better response than glucocorticoids alone. Cyclophosphamide and methotrexate have also been used with benefit. The aim of cytotoxic therapy with azathioprine or cyclophosphamide is to lower the total lymphocyte count to about 750 per microliter, while maintaining the hemoglobin level above 12 g/dL, the total white cell count above 3000 per microliter, and the platelet count above 125,000 per microliter. Weekly blood counts are required to monitor the cytotoxic drug therapy. Methotrexate is effective at doses that do not produce lymphopenia. The combined use of prednisone and a cytotoxic drug usually allows a lower dose of prednisone to be used. In preliminary studies total-body irradiation has been successfully used in some patients with disease refractory to glucocorticoids and immunosuppressants, but long-term follow-up is lacking. Bed rest has been recommended in the acute phase of the disease but is harmful in the long term. Physiotherapy and rehabilitative devices are important in the long-term treatment of patients with dermatomyositis-polymyositis.

Elderly patients, particularly those with dermatomyositis, should be followed closely for the possibility of malignant disease, and any new symptoms or signs must be appropriately investigated by a directed approach. If a malignant lesion is found, it should be treated, since the muscle weakness may disappear if the neoplasm is eradicated. However, a response to glucocorticoids can usually be obtained even in patients with polymyositis associated with a malignancy.

The serum CK activity is useful for following patients during reduction of immunosuppressant therapy, since a rise in level generally indicates an incipient clinical relapse. However, it cannot be used to indicate initial response in patients being treated with prednisone for dermatomyositis-polymyositis, since this drug lowers the serum CK activity in a way which is not fully understood, but which is not related to the suppression of muscle inflammation.

Side effects of high-dose daily glucocorticoid therapy (see Chap. 317) are relatively common in patients treated for polymyositis, and these may limit therapy. However, these can be minimized by appropriate use of alternate-day therapy. When patients who have been stable on a static dose of prednisone develop increasing muscle weakness, this may be due to either a relapse of the myositis or to glucocorticoid myopathy. An EMG, serum CK measurement, and, rarely, muscle biopsy may help in differentiating these two conditions if the changes of myositis are present. However, often the only way to separate them is to reduce the dose of prednisone slowly; if glucocorticoid myopathy is the cause of the weakness, it will improve; if a relapse of the myositis is responsible, the weakness will increase.

Side effects of cytotoxic drugs include marrow suppression, alopecia, gastrointestinal tract disorders, damage to the testes and ovaries (including potential genetic damage), disorders of chronic immunosuppression, and potential for malignancy.

PROGNOSIS The overall mortality rate of individuals with dermatomyositis-polymyositis is about four times that of the general population; death is due usually to pulmonary, renal, and cardiac complications. Females, blacks, and those severely affected at presentation have a worse prognosis. Evidence from several series suggests that patients seen at tertiary referral centers may have less favorable outcome when compared with patients seen at smaller community hospitals, probably because they represent a population with more severe disease which shows poorer response to therapy. Nevertheless, the 5-year survival rate is about 75 percent overall, and is better than this in children. The majority of patients improve with therapy. Many patients make a full functional recovery, though some weakness of the shoulders and hips, usually not disabling, remains at the conclusion of treatment. Relapse may occur at any time. Glucocorticoids should not be discontinued too soon, for the relapse which may follow is often more difficult to treat than the original presentation. About one-half of the patients with this disease recover and can discontinue therapy within 5 years after the onset of the symptoms; about 20 percent still have active disease requiring continued therapy. The remaining 30 percent have inactive disease but residual muscle weakness.

REFERENCES

Arahata K, Engel AG: Monoclonal antibody analysis of mononuclear cells in myopathies. V. Identification and quantitation of T8^{+} cytotoxic and suppressor cells. Ann Neurol 23:493, 1988

Banker BQ, Engel AG: The polymyositis and dermatomyositis syndromes, in *Myology*, AG Engel, BQ Banker (eds). New York, McGraw-Hill, 1986, pp 1385–1422

Bohan A et al: A computer-assisted analysis of 153 patients with polymyositis and dermatomyositis. Medicine 56:255, 1977

Bradley WG, Tandan R: Inflammatory diseases of muscle, in *Textbook of Rheumatology*, 3d ed, WN Kelley et al (eds). Philadelphia, Saunders, 1988, chap 72

Carpenter S, Karpati G: *Pathology of Skeletal Muscle*. New York, Churchill Livingstone, 1984, pp 515–592

Curie S: Inflammatory myopathies. Part I: Polymyositis and related disorders, in *Disorders of Voluntary Muscle*, 4th ed, JN Walton (ed). London, Churchill Livingstone, 1981, chap 15

DeVere R, Bradley WG: Polymyositis: Its presentation, mortality, and morbidity. Brain 98:637, 1975

Mastaglia FL, Ojeda VJ: Inflammatory myopathies. Ann Neurol 17:215, 317, 1985

Plotz PH et al: Current concepts in the idiopathic inflammatory myopathies: polymyositis, dermatomyositis, and related disorders. Ann Int Med 111:143, 1989

Richardson JB, Callen JP: Dermatomyositis and malignancy. Med Clin North Am 73:1211, 1989

365 MUSCULAR DYSTROPHY

JERRY R. MENDELL / ROBERT C. GRIGGS

Most myopathies including the hereditary, inflammatory, endocrine, metabolic, and toxic disorders can result in chronic weakness. The approach to differential diagnosis of these disorders is summarized in Chap. 362.

HEREDITARY MYOPATHIES

Muscular dystrophy refers to a group of disorders that have little in common except for their name and the fact that they are inherited. Each type of muscular dystrophy has unique phenotypic and genetic features (Table 365-1).

DUCHENNE MUSCULAR DYSTROPHY This disorder was first described by Edward Meryon (1852) but the disease bears the name of the French neurologist Duchenne. Duchenne's dystrophy is an X-linked recessive disorder affecting males almost exclusively. Estimates of incidence range from 13 to 33 per 100,000 live-born males. In one-third or more of cases the family history is negative, suggesting that many are due to new mutations.

Molecular genetics The gene and gene product, called dystrophin, have recently been identified. The gene, an estimated 2000 kilobases in size, is the largest identified human gene. Dystrophin is a protein of about 400 kDa localized to the plasma membrane of the muscle fiber. Recognition of the gene and gene product was an outgrowth of a series of studies beginning with the recognition that rare females with the Duchenne phenotype had translocations on the short arm of the X chromosome at the Xp21 site. Independent studies accomplished through genetic linkage employing restriction fragment length polymorphisms (RFLPs) as genetic markers confirmed the Duchenne locus at Xp21. In 1985, Kunkle and colleagues isolated the DNA from a male patient with Duchenne's dystrophy who had a large deletion on the X chromosome. The patient also had retinitis pigmentosa, chronic granulomatous disease, and the McCleod red blood cell phenotype. The same year Worton and colleagues cloned the DNA spanning a translocation junction in a female with a Duchenne dystrophy phenotype who had an X;21 translocation. DNA from these patients served as the starting points for chromosomal walking which led to the identification of the Duchenne gene and gene product.

Clinical manifestations Clinical manifestations usually begin at 3 to 5 years of age. The boys fall frequently and have difficulty keeping up with their friends when playing. Running, jumping, and hopping are invariably abnormal. Motor milestones may be delayed even before age 2, but if there is no family history the diagnosis is often not suspected. By age 5 muscle weakness is obvious by muscle testing. On getting up from the floor the patient uses his hands to climb up himself (Gowers' maneuver). In younger children, the calf muscles are usually enlarged from true muscle hypertrophy; later, calf enlargement is appropriately called *pseudohypertrophy* since muscle is replaced by fat and connective tissue.

Contractures of heel cords and iliotibial bands become apparent by age 7 to 8, when toe walking is associated with lordotic posture.

TABLE 365-1 Progressive muscular dystrophies

Type	Usual inheritance	Clinical features	Other organ system involvement
Duchenne's (pseudohypertrophic)	X-linked recessive	Onset by age 5 Progressive weakness of girdle muscles Inability to walk after age 12 Kyphoscoliosis Respiratory failure in second to third decade	Cardiomyopathy Mental impairment
Becker's (benign pseudohypertrophic)	X-linked recessive	Onset in early to late childhood Slowly progressive weakness of girdle muscles Ability to walk after age 15 Respiratory failure after fourth decade	Cardiomyopathy
Myotonic	Autosomal dominant	Onset any decade Slowly progressive weakness of eyelids, face, neck, distal limb muscles Myotonia	Cardiac conduction defects Mental impairment Cataracts Frontal baldness Gonadal atrophy
Facioscapulohumeral	Autosomal dominant	Onset second to fourth decade Slowly progressive face, shoulder girdle, foot dorsiflexion weakness	Hypertension
Limb-girdle (may include several disorders)	Autosomal recessive	Onset early childhood to adult Slowly progressive weakness of shoulder and hip girdle muscles	Cardiomyopathy
Oculopharyngeal	Autosomal dominant (French-Canadian or Hispanic background)	Onset fifth to sixth decade Slowly progressive weakness of extraocular, eyelid, face, and pharyngeal muscles Cricopharyngeal achalasia	
Less well-characterized forms of muscular dystrophies:			
Congenital (may include several disorders)	Autosomal recessive	Onset at birth Hypotonia, contractures and delayed milestones Early respiratory failure in some; others have static course	Cerebral
Distal (may include several disorders)	Autosomal recessive	Onset second to third decade Slowly progressive weakness of legs beginning with foot drop	
Scapuloperoneal (may include several disorders)	Autosomal dominant	Onset third to fifth decade Progressive shoulder girdle and foot dorsiflexor weakness	Cardiomyopathy

Loss of muscle strength is progressive with predilection for proximal limb muscles and the neck flexors; leg involvement is more severe than arm involvement. Between ages 8 and 10 walking usually requires the use of braces; joint contractures and limitations of hip flexion and knee, elbow, and wrist extension are made worse by prolonged sitting. By age 12 most patients are confined to a wheelchair. Contractures become fixed and a progressive scoliosis often develops which may be associated with considerable discomfort. The chest deformity associated with scoliosis further impairs pulmonary function which is already diminished by the muscle weakness. By age 14 to 18 patients develop serious, sometimes fatal, pulmonary infections. Other causes of death include aspiration of food and acute gastric dilatation.

A cardiac cause of death is uncommon despite the existence of a cardiomyopathy in almost all patients. Congestive heart failure seldom occurs except with severe stress such as pneumonia. Cardiac arrhythmias are rare. The typical ECG shows an increased net RS in lead V_1; deep narrow Q waves in the precordial leads; and RSR′ or polyphasic R waves in V_1.

Intellectual impairment in Duchenne's dystrophy is common and in contrast to the muscle disease is nonprogressive. One-third of patients have intelligence quotients below 75 and the mean is estimated at 85. The intellectual impairment is not the result of physical limitations since verbal skills are impaired before weakness is severe. Its basis is not known but recent findings that dystrophin is found in the brain raise questions about the relationship of intellectual impairment to deficits in the gene product.

Laboratory investigation Laboratory confirmation includes assessment of serum CK level, which is invariably elevated between 20 and 100 times normal. The levels are abnormal at birth, making it possible to diagnose an affected boy early in life. Serum CK activity remains high until late in the disease, when levels decline because of inactivity and loss of muscle mass.

Myopathy can be demonstrated by electromyography (EMG). The muscle biopsy shows muscle fibers of varying size as well as small groups of necrotic and regenerating fibers (see Fig. 362-4). Connective tissue and fat replaces lost muscle fibers.

The understanding of the gene defect in Duchenne's dystrophy has greatly expanded the possibilities for carrier detection and prenatal diagnosis. Serum CK testing is nevertheless still an important initial step and will be elevated in about 50 percent of female carriers. In addition, since about 60 percent of Duchenne boys have a deletion or duplication of one or more exons within the gene, complementary DNA probes are now available for testing potential carriers and for use on amniotic fluid cells or chorionic villi in prenatal diagnosis. In families without deletions or duplications, linkage analysis using probes recognizing RFLPs is also available.

Treatment There is no definitive treatment for Duchenne's dystrophy. Some clinicians advocate administration of glucocorticoids.

BECKER'S MUSCULAR DYSTROPHY This less severe form of X-linked recessive muscular dystrophy was described by Becker and Keiner in 1955. It is often called the benign form of pseudohypertrophic muscular dystrophy. The presentation is similar to that of Duchenne's dystrophy except that the time course is slower. The incidence of Becker's dystrophy is approximately one-tenth that of the Duchenne type. The condition is not usually recognized before age 5 and walking continues well beyond age 15, sometimes into the fourth decade. Calf muscle enlargement is prominent. Death from complications similar to those of Duchenne's dystrophy may occur after age 40.

Until the isolation of the gene for dystrophin, it was not known whether Becker's and Duchenne's dystrophies represented genetically distinct disorders. Recent investigations indicate that these two conditions result from defects of the dystrophin gene and that differences in severity can be attributed to the amount and type of dystrophin deficiency in the muscle.

Carrier detection methods are identical for Duchenne's and Becker's dystrophies. Unlike Duchenne's dystrophy, Becker patients reach child-bearing age; while none of their sons will be affected, the daughters of the Becker patient will all be carriers.

Laboratory confirmation of Becker's dystrophy is the same as that for Duchenne's dystrophy in that high serum CK levels are present early in the course and then gradually decline. The EMG and muscle biopsy changes are similar to those of Duchenne's dystrophy.

FACIOSCAPULOHUMERAL MUSCULAR DYSTROPHY This slowly progressive disorder is usually inherited as an autosomal dominant disorder, affecting males and females equally. It is extremely variable in severity and may start at any age, commonly in the third or fourth decade. Cases starting earlier in life tend to have a worse prognosis. Some patients may remain asymptomatic throughout life. As the name implies, there is characteristic weakness of facial, shoulder girdle, and proximal arm muscles. Scapular winging and sloping shoulders reflect weakness of the serratus anterior, trapezius, and rhomboid muscles; later, the biceps and triceps muscles are affected; the deltoid muscles are usually relatively spared. Facial involvement often produces a lifelong inability to whistle, an expressionless face, and a sullen appearance. Foot drop may occur early in the disease from peroneal and anterior tibial muscle weakness. Leg weakness may eventually progress to loss of ambulation.

Other systems are usually unaffected in facioscapulohumeral dystrophy. Cardiac disease and respiratory compromise are rare, and their occurrence usually suggests a coincidental illness. Patients frequently appear to have exophthalmos but thyroid function is normal; a mild but labile hypertension is common. Intellectual function is intact and life span may be normal.

Diagnostic studies may be unnecessary in typical cases, particularly when a family history is present. CK level may be normal or slightly elevated; EMG and muscle biopsy tend to have mixed features of myopathy and neuropathy and may be misleading. No specific treatment is available; ankle-foot orthoses are occasionally helpful for foot drop. Scapular stabilization procedures improve scapular winging but may not improve function.

LIMB-GIRDLE DYSTROPHY This term encompasses more than one disorder. Inheritance is usually by autosomal recessive transmission. Proximal muscle weakness may begin in either the legs or the arms but usually progresses to all extremities. Weakness may begin before age 5 or as late as the third decade and may be associated with hypertrophy of calf and other muscles. Ambulation continues for over 20 years after the disease first appears. In some patients cardiac involvement results in congestive heart failure or arrhythmias; occasional patients may present with a cardiomyopathy. Respiratory failure ensues after 30 or more years of disease. Intellectual function remains normal. Diagnosis requires the exclusion of inflammatory and metabolic myopathies as well as the phenotypically similar spinal muscular atrophies. The serum CK is elevated in limb-girdle dystrophy although the values are usually lower than in Duchenne's and Becker's dystrophies; the EMG pattern is that of a myopathy. The muscle biopsy shows active myopathy but is not specific.

MYOTONIC DYSTROPHY **Clinical manifestations** This autosomal dominant disorder affects muscle and numerous other tissues. The incidence is estimated to be 1 per 10,000 and may be higher since many cases escape recognition. Associated features include intellectual impairment, hypersomnia, cardiac disease, posterior subcapsular cataracts, gonadal atrophy, respiratory failure, and gastrointestinal disease. Weakness initially involves eyelid, temporalis, facial, and neck flexor muscles, as well as the distal extremity muscles. Myotonia is demonstrable in hand grip or by percussion of the tongue, the wrist extensors, or the thenar eminence. Disease onset is usually in the second and third decade, but affected individuals may remain free of signs or symptoms throughout life. A severe form of the disease, *congenital myotonic dystrophy,* occurs in some infants of affected mothers and is characterized by severe facial and bulbar weakness; neonatal respiratory insufficiency may occur but is usually self-limited. Affected infants are frequently intellectually impaired.

Molecular genetics The disorder is transmitted by a mutant gene on the long arm of chromosome 19 which is linked to the genes for apolipoprotein C2, secretor substance, the Lutheran blood group, peptidase D, and the third component of complement. Several RFLPs have been identified that are closely linked to the myotonic dystrophy locus. Early disease detection and antenatal diagnosis are now possible in selected families using linkage techniques.

Diagnosis Diagnosis is often self-evident because of the distinctive facial appearance; the characteristic pattern of weakness and the abnormalities cause the typical narrow, "hatchet" face; premature frontal balding is frequent. The presence of distal weakness and myotonia confirm the diagnosis. Diagnosis can be made before the onset of symptoms in affected family members by clinical and EMG evaluation for myotonia and by slit-lamp examination for the characteristic cataracts. The CK activity is normal or slightly elevated. Muscle biopsy often shows distinctive type I fiber atrophy; severely involved muscles may have a characteristic appearance including ring fibers, sarcoplasmic masses, and numerous central nuclei.

Cardiac involvement most commonly affects the conduction system; first-degree heart block is present in a majority, and complete heart block may require pacemaker implantation. Since sudden death may occur, patients must be monitored carefully for conduction disturbances, though precise criteria for the timing of pacemaker implantation are lacking. Tachyarrhythmias and congestive failure are less frequent. Respiratory muscle weakness may be severe even in patients with minor limb weakness. Impaired ventilatory drive and hypersensitivity to the depressant effects of small doses of opiates and sedatives may result in sudden ventilatory failure, particularly in the pre- or postoperative setting. Sleep apnea may occur on both a central and peripheral basis (Chap. 217). Chronic hypoxia may lead to cor pulmonale and is the usual cause of heart failure for the patient.

Treatment Myotonia is seldom so disabling as to require treatment; phenytoin is the therapy of choice since the other antimyotonia agents, quinine and procainamide, may worsen cardiac conduction.

MYOTONIA CONGENITA This disorder occurs in autosomal dominant (Thomsen) and autosomal recessive forms (Chap. 27). Patients with the autosomal recessive form may develop slight weakness; patients with the dominant form do not develop weakness. Myotonia can be markedly alleviated by antimyotonia agents including quinine, procainamide, phenytoin, acetazolamide, or tocainide. These patients have no involvement of heart or other organs.

OCULOPHARYNGEAL DYSTROPHY The term *progressive external ophthalmoplegia* describes disorders characterized by slowly progressive ptosis and limitation of eye movements with the sparing of pupil and muscles of accommodation. Patients usually do not complain of diplopia, in contrast to conditions with a more acute onset of ocular muscle weakness. *Oculopharyngeal dystrophy* is an autosomal dominant disorder in which ophthalmoplegia appears in the fifth or sixth decade. Many patients are of French-Canadian or Hispanic ancestry. Pharyngeal weakness leads to cricopharyngeal achalasia, progressive difficulty in swallowing, and frequent, often asymptomatic, aspiration. Severe malnutrition may develop but can be alleviated by surgical correction of cricopharyngeal achalasia.

Additional types of *ocular myopathies* are associated with mitochondrial abnormalities in muscle (see discussion of metabolic myopathies below).

CONGENITAL MUSCULAR DYSTROPHY This rare disorder appears to represent more than one disease. In most cases inheritance is autosomal recessive but instances of autosomal dominant inheritance have been reported. The usual picture of infantile hypotonia and muscle weakness and wasting is associated with joint contractures. Facial and neck weakness is common with sparing of extraocular muscles. Serum CK is usually elevated and the muscle biopsy shows features typical of muscular dystrophy. The condition is relatively nonprogressive, but many patients are never able to walk. A more severe form of the condition may lead to death from respiratory failure.

In some patients with congenital muscular dystrophy there is also cerebral involvement with hypomyelination of the deep white matter of the brain detectable by computed tomography (CT). Many patients show no clinical manifestations of hypomyelination. A more severe form of congenital muscular dystrophy, associated with cerebral involvement, occurs in Japan, and is called the Fukuyama-type. It is often associated with generalized convulsions, global developmental delay, and death by 10 years of age.

DISTAL MUSCULAR DYSTROPHY This rare disorder has at least three separate variants. The most frequent is an autosomal recessive or sporadic disorder that presents with distal leg weakness in the second or third decade. Slow progression affecting more proximal muscles occurs. The CK level is markedly elevated. Other distinct forms of a distal myopathy include an autosomal dominant Scandinavian form (Welander) which begins in the hands, and a late-onset (fourth to fifth decade) autosomal dominant disorder that begins in the legs and in which cardiomyopathy is frequent.

SCAPULOPERONEAL DYSTROPHY Several forms of neuromuscular disease cause foot drop and winging of the scapulas. An autosomal dominant form presents in the third to fifth decade and is variable in its progression; respiratory failure is uncommon, but cardiomyopathy may occur. An X-linked recessive form (Emery-Dreifuss) begins in early childhood and is associated with prominent joint contractures and cardiac conduction disorders. Certain cases of facioscapulohumeral dystrophy may lack facial weakness and resemble scapuloperoneal dystrophy.

CONGENITAL MYOPATHIES

These rare disorders are distinguished from muscular dystrophies by the presence of specific histochemical and structural abnormalities in muscle. A nonprogressive course is common but not invariable. The typical infant has hypotonia and delayed motor milestones. Pectus excavatum, kyphoscoliosis, hip dislocation, and pes cavus are common. The diagnosis is important, since the long-term prognosis and management differ from that of the muscular dystrophies.

Four major forms of congenital myopathies have been described: central core disease, nemaline (rod) myopathy, myotubular (centronuclear) myopathy, and congenital fiber-type disproportion.

CENTRAL CORE DISEASE This disease, the first congenital myopathy described, was identified by Shy and Magee in 1956. The disorder is inherited as an autosomal dominant disorder but sporadic cases also occur. In infancy hypotonia and delayed motor milestones are typical, but the diagnosis may come to attention in an adult with muscle weakness or skeletal abnormalities.

Short, slender stature and skeletal abnormalities including congenital hip dislocation, scoliosis, pes cavus, and pectus excavatum are characteristic. Weakness of the muscles of the face and limbs, particularly the legs, is mild. The muscle biopsy is diagnostic; it shows fibers with single or multiple central or eccentric discrete zones (cores) devoid of oxidative enzymes. Other laboratory studies are less helpful since the serum CK and the EMG may be normal. Patients with this disorder may be predisposed to develop malignant hyperthermia (Chap. 20).

NEMALINE MYOPATHY This disorder, also called rod myopathy, was described by Shy and colleagues in 1963. Inheritance is usually as an autosomal dominant trait but it may be recessive or sporadic. Infantile hypotonia is frequent, and death may occur from respiratory failure. The skeletal abnormalities are striking; they include a long face, high arched palate, and slender musculature. Kyphoscoliosis, pectus excavatum, and pes cavus may be present. Muscle weakness affects the face, palate, and limb muscles. The prognosis is variable, with some patients progressing to wheelchair confinement or respiratory failure while in others the disease does not progress.

Muscle histology shows clusters of small rod or nemaline (thread-like) bodies for which the condition was named. Rods, derived from Z-band material, are usually found in type I fibers, and the muscle often shows type I predominance. The serum CK level may be normal or mildly elevated, and the EMG usually shows myopathy.

MYOTUBULAR MYOPATHY This disorder was described by Spiro, Shy, and Gonatas in 1966. The histologic abnormality in myotubular myopathy resembles the embryonic or developmental myotube stage of a muscle fiber. Others have preferred to call the disease *centronuclear myopathy,* arguing that the fibers are not embryonic. The condition is usually sporadic, but inheritance may be as an autosomal dominant, recessive, or X-linked recessive trait. Infantile hypotonia and weakness are common and may cause death. Presentations at an older age include features similar to nemaline myopathy with a long narrow face, pes cavus, and scoliosis. Muscle bulk is reduced, and proximal and distal weakness is of varying severity. The feature that separates these patients from those with other congenital myopathies is the presence of external ophthalmoplegia. The course may or may not be progressive.

Serum CK activity is normal or slightly elevated. The EMG is usually abnormal with excessively recruited small motor unit potentials associated with fibrillations and positive sharp potentials. Muscle biopsy shows muscle fibers with rows of central nuclei often surrounded by a perinuclear clear zone. Type I fibers may be preferentially affected and may be atrophic.

CONGENITAL FIBER-TYPE DISPROPORTION Clinical features of this disorder include hypotonia, weakness, delayed milestones, and skeletal deformities similar to those of other congenital myopathies. The diagnosis is established by the muscle biopsy which shows an increased number of small type I fibers and normal or hypertrophied type II fibers. The pathogenesis is poorly understood. The prognosis is generally good, with most patients showing improvement with age although some residual motor impairment commonly persists; occasional patients may have progressive weakness.

DISORDERS OF MUSCLE ENERGY METABOLISM

Skeletal muscle utilizes two principal sources of energy—fatty acids and glucose. Abnormalities in either glucose or lipid utilization can be associated with distinct clinical features. The more dramatic feature is an acute muscle pain syndrome which can evolve into severe rhabdomyolysis and myoglobinuria. The other is progressive muscle weakness simulating muscular dystrophy. The explanation for the different clinical syndromes is often unknown.

GLYCOGEN STORAGE AND GLYCOLYTIC DEFECTS There are four disorders of glycogen metabolism (types II, III, IV, and V) and four disorders of glycolysis (types VII, IX, X and XI) associated with significant skeletal muscle manifestations (see also Chap. 332).

Acid maltase deficiency (type II glycogenosis) Acid maltase is a lysosomal enzyme, an acid hydrolase, having α-1,4- and α-1,6-glucosidase activity which breaks down glycogen to glucose; however, the enzyme has no well-defined role in carbohydrate metabolism. Three clinical forms of acid maltase deficiency are each inherited as autosomal recessive traits. The biochemical basis for the different clinical presentations is not understood.

In infancy, acid maltase deficiency has features of a generalized glycogenosis. No abnormalities are noted at birth, but shortly thereafter severe muscle weakness, cardiomegaly, hepatomegaly, and tongue enlargement develop. Glycogen accumulation in motor neurons of the spinal cord and brainstem contribute to the muscle weakness. Death usually occurs by 1 year of age.

In children and adults, the picture resembles muscular dystrophy. The childhood form is associated with delayed developmental milestones, proximal limb muscle weakness, and calf enlargement and may progress to respiratory failure and death before the end of the second decade. Cardiac involvement may be present, but hepatomegaly and macroglossia are infrequent.

The adult form begins in the third or fourth decade and may be misdiagnosed as limb-girdle dystrophy or polymyositis. Respiratory failure from diaphragmatic weakness may be the initial manifestation of the disease. The heart, liver, and tongue are not involved. The diagnosis is suggested by muscle biopsy which shows vacuoles containing glycogen and the lysosomal enzyme, acid phosphatase. By electron microscopy, membrane-bound and free tissue glycogen are found. Definitive diagnosis is established by muscle biochemistry. Acid maltase activity is also reduced in the urine. Serum CK level may be as high as ten times normal. EMG distinguishes acid maltase deficiency from muscular dystrophy by the occurrence of bizarre high-frequency and myotonic discharges accompanying short-duration motor unit potentials, fibrillations, and positive sharp potentials.

Debrancher enzyme deficiency (type III glycogenosis) Muscle weakness is uncommon in debrancher enzyme deficiency. This mild disease of childhood is dominated by hepatomegaly, growth retardation, and hypoglycemia. These findings usually diminish or disappear after puberty, and muscle weakness and wasting associated with decreased exercise tolerance may develop. Diagnosis is suggested by a failure of lactic acid level to rise following exercise of the forearm. The serum CK level is elevated. EMG shows myopathy which may be accompanied by membrane irritability with myotonic discharges. Muscle biopsy shows a vacuolar myopathy with increased glycogen. Definitive diagnosis requires muscle biochemistry.

Brancher enzyme deficiency (type IV glycogenosis) Brancher enzyme deficiency is a severe fatal disorder of infancy in which skeletal muscle manifestations are relatively minor in the face of the chronic liver failure. The muscle hypotonia and wasting may, however, suggest the possibility of a primary muscle disease or spinal muscular atrophy.

Muscle phosphorylase deficiency (type V glycogenosis) Exercise intolerance is the dominant feature of muscle phosphorylase deficiency, first described in 1951 by McArdle. The disorder, usually inherited as an autosomal recessive trait, has an unexplained predilection for males. Painful muscle cramps and fatigue after intense exercise such as running or lifting heavy objects usually develops after adolescence. Early infantile and late onset variants have been described. Many patients report a "second wind" phenomenon if they rest briefly or slow down during exercise, which allows them to continue an activity for a longer period of time. Overexertion may lead to rhabdomyolysis and myoglobinuria, and renal failure can result. Persistent weakness and wasting of muscle is rare, and examination of the patient between attacks is usually normal. Other organs are not affected.

Serum CK levels fluctuate widely and may be elevated even during symptom-free periods. The forearm exercise test shows no rise in lactic acid. The EMG is often normal except when taken following an episode of rhabdomyolysis. Muscle biopsy often shows subsarcolemmal blebs containing glycogen. Muscle phosphorylase deficiency can be recognized by a histochemical stain and confirmed by biochemistry. Patients can remain moderately active once they establish their limitations. Dietary supplementation with either glucose or fructose has not alleviated symptoms.

Phosphofructokinase deficiency (type VII glycogenosis) This disorder resembles muscle phosphorylase deficiency and is also an autosomal recessive trait with a male predominance. The precipitating events and the laboratory features also resemble phosphorylase deficiency. A histochemical stain for phosphofructokinase (PFK) can demonstrate the deficiency. Definitive diagnosis requires biochemical analysis of muscle enzymes. Some patients with PFK deficiency have mild hemolysis, increased reticulocyte count, and elevated bilirubin because of a deficiency of a PFK subunit shared by muscle and red blood cells.

New glycolytic enzyme deficiency syndromes Since 1981 deficiencies of three additional glycolytic enzymes have been identified: phosphoglycerate kinase (PGK) deficiency (type IX), phosphoglycerate mutase (PGAM) deficiency (type X), and lactate dehydrogenase deficiency (LDH) (XI). The clinical pictures of the three are similar. In each, episodic myoglobinuria and myalgias precipitated by intense exercise begin in childhood or adolescence. Autosomal recessive inheritance is probable in each disorder. Serum CK level may be elevated during and between episodes. In PGAM and LDH deficiencies, the rise in lactic acid following forearm exercise is lower than normal. PGK deficiency shows no rise in lactate and closely resembles muscle phosphorylase and PFK deficiencies. The muscle histology is unremarkable in these disorders with little evidence of glycogen storage. Diagnosis requires muscle biochemistry.

DISORDERS OF LIPID METABOLISM

Lipid is an important muscle energy source during rest and prolonged, moderately intense exercise (Fig. 365-1).

CARNITINE DEFICIENCY Carnitine deficiency occurs in myopathic and systemic forms.

Myopathic carnitine deficiency is associated with generalized muscle weakness, usually beginning in childhood. The clinical features overlap with muscular dystrophy and polymyositis. Most cases are sporadic, but the inheritance pattern is thought to be autosomal recessive. Cardiomyopathy may be present. Serum CK level is slightly elevated, and the EMG shows myopathy. The muscle biopsy shows striking lipid accumulation. Serum carnitine is normal. The cause for decreased muscle carnitine is not understood. A defect of transport into muscle has been postulated. Some patients respond to oral carnitine supplements; this should be tried in all cases. Other patients have responded to prednisone for unknown reasons. A diet substituting medium-chain for long-chain triglycerides has been helpful in some cases. Rare patients have also responded to riboflavin.

Systemic carnitine deficiency, an autosomal recessive disease of infancy and early childhood, is characterized by progressive weakness and episodes of hepatic encephalopathy with nausea, vomiting, confusion, coma, and early death. The low *serum* carnitine level distinguishes this condition from the myopathic form. No single cause has been identified to explain the low serum carnitine level. Decreased synthesis explains some cases while increased urinary excretion is seen in others. Serum CK level may be slightly elevated. The muscle biopsy shows lipid storage. In some cases the liver, heart, and kidney also show increased lipid. Treatment with oral carnitine supplements or glucocorticoids has helped some but not all patients.

FIGURE 365-1 Free fatty acids for muscle energy are derived from triglycerides stored in muscle and from circulating very low density lipoproteins (VLDL) which are broken down by endothelial lipoprotein lipase (1) in the capillary. Carnitine, an essential substrate for lipid metabolism, is made in the liver and transported to muscle. In muscle, free fatty acids combine with coenzyme A (CoA-SH) through the action of fatty acylsynthetase (2) found in the outer mitochondrial membrane forming fatty acylcoenzyme A (F-acyl-CoA). Transport through inner mitochondrial membrane requires transfer to carnitine by carnitine palmityltransferase 1 (CPT I) bound to the outer surface of the inner mitochondrial membrane (3). Inside the mitochondrion, fatty acylcarnitine (F-acylcarnitine) is regenerated by CPT II (4) bound to the inner surface of the inner mitochondrial membrane. The fatty acylcoenzyme A then proceeds to beta oxidation.

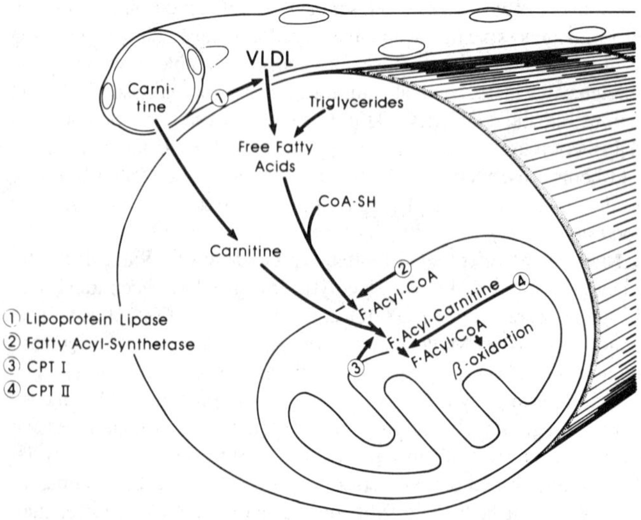

CARNITINE PALMITYLTRANSFERASE DEFICIENCY Deficiency of carnitine palmityltransferase (CPT) presents with recurrent myoglobinuria. It is not known if CPT I or CPT II activities are selectively deficient; the deficiency apparently results from disordered regulatory properties of an abnormal enzyme. Rhabdomyolysis may follow prolonged exercise such as soccer, football, or a long hike, but at times no precipitating cause can be found. Initial symptoms often commence in childhood. In contrast to defects in glycolysis where muscle cramps follow short intense bursts of exercise, the muscle pain in CPT deficiency does not occur until the limits of energy utilization have been exceeded and muscle breakdown has begun. Episodes of rhabdomyolysis may produce severe weakness, and some patients require ventilatory assistance. In contrast to carnitine deficiency, strength is normal between attacks and the muscle biopsy does not show lipid accumulation. The diagnosis requires direct measurement of muscle CPT. Treatment consists of increased carbohydrate intake before exercise or of substituting medium-chain triglycerides in the diet. Neither has been entirely satisfactory.

MYOADENYLATE DEAMINASE DEFICIENCY The enzyme adenylate deaminase converts 5′-adenosine monophosphate (5′AMP) to inosine monophosphate (IMP) with liberation of ammonia and may play a role in regulating adenosine triphosphate (ATP) levels in muscle. In 1978 a group of patients with myalgias and exercise intolerance were found to be deficient in the muscle isoenzyme, adenylate deaminase. The deficiency, however, occurs in as many as 1 percent of the population and can be detected by histochemical staining of muscle tissue as well as by biochemical analysis. Muscle ammonia production is decreased following forearm exercise. Since the original description, a less consistent clinical picture has emerged. Patients with other neuromuscular disorders including anterior horn cell disease, muscular dystrophy, and myasthenia gravis occasionally have the same enzyme deficiency. The full clinical significance of adenylate deaminase deficiency is not established.

MITOCHONDRIAL MYOPATHIES A heterogeneous group of disorders is characterized by abnormal mitochondria in "ragged-red fibers," named for their appearance in the trichrome stain of biopsied muscle. The most common disorder is characterized by progressive ptosis, external ophthalmoplegia, and proximal weakness and was initially called oculocraniosomatic neuromuscular disease with ragged-red fibers when described by Olson et al. in 1972. Many of these cases show autosomal dominant inheritance. In other cases of sporadic onset, beginning in childhood and referred to as the *Kearns-Sayre syndrome,* there are accompanying cardiac conduction defects which may cause complete heart block, retinal pigmentary degeneration, short stature, and gonadal defects. Another disorder recently assigned the acronym *MERRF syndrome,* because of its myoclonic epilepsy and ragged-red fibers, presents between the first and fifth decades with generalized seizures, myoclonus, dementia, hearing loss, and ataxia. A third disorder, the *MELAS syndrome,* is a slowly progressive disease characterized by mitochondrial myopathy, encephalopathy, lactic acidosis, stroke-like episodes including alternating hemiparesis, hemianopsia or cortical blindness, and focal or generalized seizures.

There is evidence that some of the mitochondrial myopathies are related to abnormalities in mitochondrial, as opposed to nuclear, DNA which appears to be derived solely from the mother through the ovum. In MERRF syndrome which is associated with a defect in cytochrome oxidase, an enzyme of the respiratory chain critical for oxidative phosphorylation, there is unequivocal evidence for maternal inheritance. Affected males do not transmit the condition. In Kearns-Sayre syndrome isolated muscle mitochondria show deletions in mitochondrial DNA, although no examples of transmission of disease to offspring have been reported.

INFLAMMATORY MYOPATHIES

Polymyositis and dermatomyositis (Chap. 364) develop slowly over the course of months. The presence of a characteristic skin rash usually makes the diagnosis of dermatomyositis straightforward. Chronic polymyositis, with slowly progressive proximal weakness, may be impossible to separate on clinical grounds from sporadic cases of limb-girdle dystrophy. Even with detailed EMG and biopsy studies it may prove difficult to establish the diagnosis of polymyositis with confidence. A subgroup of subacute or chronic inflammatory myopathy is termed *inclusion body myositis* because of distinctive cytoplasmic and nuclear inclusions consisting of abnormal filaments. Inclusion body myositis does not respond to glucocorticoid therapy. Chronic myositis may also occur with any of the collagen-vascular diseases and with sarcoidosis.

ENDOCRINE AND METABOLIC MYOPATHIES

Many endocrine disorders cause weakness. Muscle fatigue is more common than true weakness. The cause of weakness in these disorders is not well-defined. It is not even clear that weakness results from disease of muscle as opposed to another part of the motor unit since the CK level is often normal and the muscle histology is characterized by atrophy rather than by destruction of muscle fibers. Nearly all respond to appropriate endocrine management.

THYROID DISORDERS (See Chap. 316) *Hyperthyroidism* may occasionally present as muscle weakness, and the majority of patients are weak. *Hypothyroidism* commonly presents with muscle weakness and pain. The serum CK is often elevated and levels as high as 100 times normal may occur even with minimal clinical evidence of muscle disease. Adult patients may have muscle hypertrophy with cramps (Hoffmann's syndrome) and in children with cretinism a distinctive myopathy with muscle hypertrophy may occur (Kocher-Debré-Sémélaigne syndrome).

PARATHYROID DISORDERS (See Chap. 340) *Hyperparathyroidism* is often associated with muscle weakness and atrophy and may be accompanied by "muscle" pain which is probably from associated bone disease. Hyperreflexia is characteristic. *Hypoparathyroidism* frequently presents with neurologic involvement. The neuromuscular manifestations are usually those of tetany, but since the serum CK level is often elevated such patients are occasionally considered to have polymyositis. Hyporeflexia or areflexia is usually present despite the presence of Chvostek's and Trousseau's signs.

ADRENAL DISORDERS (See Chap. 317) Endogenous elevations of glucocorticoids may produce severe muscle weakness and wasting. Adrenal insufficiency is frequently associated with lassitude and weakness although there is usually little objective reduction in strength.

PITUITARY DISORDERS (See Chap. 313) Acromegaly is occasionally associated with muscle enlargement. Myopathic weakness may occur, but weakness usually results from associated endocrine abnormalities or from neuropathy. The weakness of panhypopituitarism is probably due to coexisting adrenal or thyroid insufficiency.

DIABETES (See Chap. 319) Proximal weakness in the patient with diabetes is usually the result of neuropathy. The finding of evidence on EMG or biopsy for myopathy or of a markedly elevated serum CK level usually suggests coincidental illness.

VITAMIN DEFICIENCY Severe malabsorption, particularly when it occurs in early childhood, may lead to a vitamin E deficiency myopathy. Vitamin E otherwise has no role in the treatment of muscle weakness (Chap. 76). Vitamin D deficiency (Chap. 341), from either decreased intake or decreased absorption, as well as impaired vitamin D metabolism, such as occurs in renal disease, may lead to chronic muscle weakness; pain probably reflects underlying bone disease. Deficiency of other vitamins does not cause myopathy.

OTHER METABOLIC DISORDERS Systemic illnesses such as malignancy and chronic respiratory, cardiac, hepatic, and renal failure are frequently associated with severe muscle wasting and complaints of weakness. Strength testing often demonstrates only mild weakness in such patients, and the problem is often a lack of endurance. Evidence for active muscle degeneration is usually lacking. Electrolyte disturbances such as chronic hypokalemia, hypercalcemia, and hypocalcemia from various causes may produce chronic muscle weakness.

TABLE 365-2 Toxic myopathies

I Focal myopathies: Pentazocine, meperidine
II Generalized myopathies
- *A* Inflammatory: Cimetidine, D-penicillamine, procainamide
- *B* Muscle weakness and myalgias: Chloroquine, clofibrate, colchicine, glucocorticoids, emetine, ϵ-aminocaproic acid, labetalol, perhexilene, propranolol, vincristine
- *C* Rhabdomyolysis and myoglobinuria: Alcohol, azathioprine, heroin, amphetamine, clofibrate, ϵ-aminocaproic acid, phencyclidine, barbiturates, cocaine
- *D* Malignant hyperthermia: Halothane, ethylene, diethyl ether, methoxylflurane, ethyl chloride, trichloroethylene, gallamine, succinylcholine, lidocaine, mepivacaine

TOXIC MYOPATHIES

A classification of toxic myopathies is shown in Table 365-2. Drugs and chemicals may produce focal or generalized damage of skeletal muscle.

The most common cause of focal damage is the injection of narcotic analgesics. Two agents in particular, pentazocine and meperidine, may cause a severe fibrotic reaction in muscle. Common injection sites include deltoid, triceps, gluteus maximus, and quadriceps muscles. The muscles become indurated and hard and may have local abscess formation. Cutaneous ulcerations and depressions may occur. Severe joint contractures may develop.

Other drugs may induce generalized muscle weakness, particularly affecting the proximal muscles. In most cases the exact mechanism of drug toxicity is poorly understood. D-Penicillamine induces a condition simulating the clinical and pathologic picture of dermatomyositis and polymyositis. A similar condition has been reported with cimetidine. Procainamide may cause myositis as part of a systemic lupus-like reaction. After many months of treatment, chloroquine produces a distinctive vacuolar myopathy that may involve the heart. Clofibrate is associated with muscle pain and weakness either shortly after the start or following several months of treatment. Serum CK elevation may be the only clofibrate-induced abnormality. Emetine hydrochloride (used for treatment of amebiasis), ϵ-aminocaproic acid (an antifibrolytic agent), and perhexilene (used for angina pectoris) have all been observed to cause weakness and muscle fiber necrosis following several weeks of therapy.

Drug-induced myopathy accompanied by proximal weakness occurs with glucocorticoid therapy. Those fluorinated in the 9α-position, such as triamcinolone, dexamethasone, and betamethasone, are most likely to cause weakness, but chronic administration of all glucocorticoids including prednisone cause weakness. Divided-dose as opposed to single-morning-dose therapy produces more severe weakness. A single-dose, alternate-day regimen has the greatest muscle-sparing effect (Chap. 317). The clinical diagnosis of steroid-induced muscle weakness can be difficult if the medication is being used to treat an underlying inflammatory myopathy. The presence of a normal serum CK level, minimal or no changes of myopathy on EMG, and type II muscle fiber atrophy on biopsy are helpful in suggesting steroid-induced weakness.

In some instances toxic myopathy may be more catastrophic, causing rhabdomyolysis and myoglobinuria. A very serious drug-induced condition, *malignant hyperthermia* (Chap. 20), occurs in susceptible individuals following exposure to certain general anesthetics and depolarizing muscle relaxants (Table 365-2). In local anesthesia, amides including lidocaine and mepivacaine have been implicated as precipitating agents.

REFERENCES

Banker BQ: The congenital myopathies, in *Myology*, AG Engel, BQ Banker (eds). New York, McGraw-Hill, 1986, vol 2

BROOKE MH: *A Clinician's View of Neuromuscular Disease*, 2d ed. Baltimore, Williams & Wilkins, 1985
DIMAURO S et al: Disorders of lipid metabolism in muscle. Muscle Nerve 3: 369, 1980
ENGEL AG: Acid maltase deficiency, in *Myology*, AG Engel, BQ Banker (eds). New York, McGraw-Hill, 1986, vol 2
GRIGGS RC, MOXLEY RT (eds): Metabolic myopathies. Semin Neurol, 3: 225, 1983
KOENIG M et al: Complete cloning of the Duchenne muscular dystrophy (DMD) cDNA and preliminary genominic organization of the DMD gene in normal and affected individuals. Cell 50: 509, 1987
RIGGS JE (ed): *Neurologic Clinics*, vol 6: *Muscle Disease*. Philadelphia, Saunders, 1988
WALLACE DC et al: Familial mitochondrial encephalomyopathy (MERRF): Genetic, pathophysiological, and biochemical characterization of a mitochondrial DNA disease. Cell 55: 601, 1988

366 MYASTHENIA GRAVIS

DANIEL B. DRACHMAN

Myasthenia gravis (MG) is a neuromuscular disorder characterized by weakness and fatigability of skeletal muscles. The underlying defect is a decrease in the number of available acetylcholine receptors (AChRs) at neuromuscular junctions, due to an antibody-mediated autoimmune attack. Treatment now available for MG is highly effective, although a specific cure has remained elusive.

PATHOPHYSIOLOGY To diagnose and manage patients with MG, it is essential to understand the basic function of the neuromuscular junction and the changes that occur as a result of the disease process (see Fig. 366-1). Acetylcholine (ACh) is synthesized in the motor nerve terminal and stored in vesicles (quanta) containing approximately 10,000 molecules each. Quanta of ACh are released spontaneously, giving rise to miniature end-plate potentials. When an action potential reaches the nerve terminal, ACh from 150 to 200 vesicles is released and combines with AChRs that are densely packed at the peaks of postsynaptic folds. Channels in the AChRs are opened, permitting the rapid entry of cations, chiefly sodium, which produces depolarization at the end-plate region of the muscle fiber. If the depolarization is sufficiently large, it initiates an action potential that is propagated along the muscle fiber, triggering muscle contraction. This process is rapidly terminated by diffusion of ACh away from the receptor, and hydrolysis of ACh by acetylcholinesterase (AChE).

In MG, the fundamental defect is a decrease in the number of available AChRs at the postsynaptic muscle membrane. In addition, the postsynaptic folds are flattened, or ''simplified'' (Fig. 366-1*B*). These changes result in decreased efficiency of neuromuscular transmission. Therefore, although ACh is released normally, it produces small end-plate potentials which may fail to trigger muscle action potentials. Failure of transmission at many neuromuscular junctions results in weakness of muscle contraction.

FIGURE 366-1 Diagrams of (*A*) normal and (*B*) myasthenic neuromuscular junctions. V = vesicles; M = mitochondria. See text for description of normal neuromuscular transmission. The MG junction shows reduced number of AChRs (stippling); flattened, simplified postsynaptic folds; a widened synaptic space; and a normal nerve terminal.

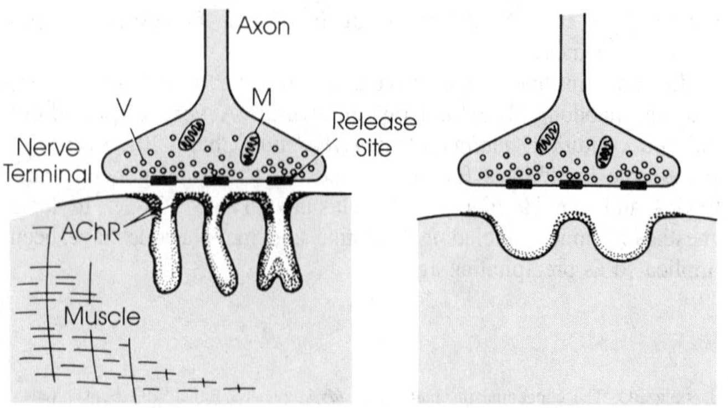

The amount of ACh released per impulse *normally* declines on repeated activity (termed *presynaptic rundown*). In the myasthenic patient, decreased efficiency of neuromuscular transmission combined with the normal rundown results in the activation of fewer and fewer muscle fibers by successive nerve impulses and, hence, increasing weakness, or *myasthenic fatigue*. This mechanism also accounts for the decremental response to repetitive nerve stimulation seen on electrodiagnostic testing.

The neuromuscular abnormalities in MG are brought about by an autoimmune response mediated by specific anti-AChR antibodies. The anti-AChR antibodies reduce the number of available AChRs at neuromuscular junctions by three distinct mechanisms: (1) AChRs may be degraded at an accelerated rate by a mechanism involving cross-linking of the receptors; (2) the active site of the AChR, i.e., the site that normally binds ACh, may be blocked by the antibodies; (3) the postsynaptic muscle membrane may be damaged by the antibody in collaboration with complement.

How the autoimmune response is initiated and maintained in MG is not completely understood. However, the thymus appears to play a role in this process. The thymus is abnormal in approximately 75 percent of patients with MG: in about 65 percent of patients the thymus is ''hyperplastic,'' with the presence of active germinal centers, while 10 percent of patients have thymic tumors (thymomas). Musclelike cells within the thymus (myoid cells), which bear AChRs on their surface, may serve as a source of autoantigen and trigger the autoimmune reaction within the thymus gland.

CLINICAL FEATURES Myasthenia gravis is not rare, with a prevalence rate of at least 1 in 10,000. It may affect individuals in any age group, but there are peaks of incidence in women in their twenties and thirties and in men in their fifties and sixties. Overall, women are affected more frequently than men, with a ratio of approximately 3:2. The cardinal features are *weakness* and *fatigability* of muscles. The weakness increases during repeated use (fatigue) and may improve following rest or sleep. The course of MG is often variable. Exacerbations and remissions may occur, particularly during the first few years after the onset of the disease. Remissions are rarely complete or permanent. Unrelated infections or systemic disorders often lead to increased myasthenic weakness, and may precipitate so-called crisis (see below).

The distribution of muscle weakness has a characteristic pattern. The cranial muscles, particularly the lids and extraocular muscles, are often involved early, and diplopia and ptosis are common initial complaints. Facial weakness produces a ''snarling'' expression when the patient attempts to smile. Weakness in chewing is most noticeable after prolonged effort, as in chewing meat. Speech may have a nasal timbre caused by weakness of the palate or a dysarthric ''mushy'' quality due to tongue weakness. Difficulty in swallowing may occur as a result of weakness of the palate, tongue, or pharynx, giving rise to nasal regurgitation or aspiration of liquids or food. In approximately 85 percent of patients, the weakness becomes generalized, affecting the limb muscles as well. The limb weakness in MG is often proximal and may be asymmetric. Despite the muscle weakness, deep tendon reflexes are preserved. If weakness of respiration or swallowing becomes so severe as to require respiratory assistance or intubation, the patient is said to be in *crisis*.

DIAGNOSIS AND EVALUATION The diagnosis is suspected on the basis of weakness and fatigability in the typical distribution described above, without loss of reflexes or impairment of sensation or other neurologic function. The suspected diagnosis should always be confirmed definitively before treatment is undertaken; this is essential because (1) other treatable conditions may closely resemble MG, and (2) the treatment of MG may involve surgery and the prolonged use of drugs with adverse side effects.

Anticholinesterase test Drugs that inhibit the enzyme AChE allow ACh to interact repeatedly with the limited number of ACh receptors, producing improvement in the strength of myasthenic muscles. Edrophonium is used most commonly, because of the rapid onset (30 s) and short duration (about 5 min) of its effect. It is essential that an objective endpoint be used to evaluate the effect of edrophonium. The examiner should focus on one or more unequivocally weak muscle groups and evaluate their strength objectively. For example, weakness of extraocular muscles, impairment of speech, or the length of time that the patient can maintain the arms in forward abduction may be useful measures. An initial dose of 2 mg edrophonium is given intravenously. If definite improvement occurs, the test is considered positive and terminated. If there is no change, the patient is given an additional 8 mg intravenously. The dose is administered in two parts because some patients react to edrophonium with unpleasant side effects such as nausea, diarrhea, salivation, fasciculations, and rarely syncope. Atropine (0.6 mg) should be at hand for intravenous administration if these symptoms become troublesome.

False-positive tests occur in occasional patients with other neurologic disorders, such as amyotrophic lateral sclerosis, and in placebo-reactors. False-negative or equivocal tests may also occur. In some cases it is helpful to use a longer-acting drug such as neostigmine, given orally, since this permits more time for detailed evaluation of strength. In virtually all instances, it is desirable to carry out further testing to establish the diagnosis of MG definitively.

Electrodiagnostic testing *Repetitive nerve stimulation* often provides helpful diagnostic evidence of MG. Anticholinesterase medication should be stopped at least 6 h prior to testing. It is best to test weak muscles or proximal muscle groups. Electric shocks are delivered at a rate of 3 or 5 per second to the appropriate nerves, and action potentials are recorded from the muscles. In normal individuals, the amplitude of the evoked muscle action potentials does not change at these rates of stimulation. However, in myasthenic patients there is a rapid reduction in the amplitude of the evoked responses of more than 10 to 15 percent. As a further test, a single dose of edrophonium may be given to prevent or diminish this decremental reaction.

Antiacetylcholine receptor antibody As noted above, anti-AChR antibodies are detectable in the serum of approximately 80 percent of all myasthenic patients, but in only about 50 percent of patients with weakness confined to the ocular muscles. The presence of anti-AChR antibodies is virtually diagnostic of MG, but a negative test does not exclude the disease. The measured level of anti-AChR antibody does not correspond well with the severity of MG in different patients. However, in an individual patient, a treatment-induced fall in the antibody level often correlates with clinical improvement.

Differential diagnosis Several other conditions that cause weakness of the cranial and/or somatic musculature must be considered in the differential diagnosis of MG; these include drug-induced myasthenia, Lambert-Eaton myasthenic syndrome, neurasthenia, hyperthyroidism, botulism, intracranial mass lesions, and progressive external ophthalmoplegia. Treatment with *penicillamine* may result in true MG, but the weakness is mild, and recovery occurs within weeks or months after discontinuing its use. Other drugs such as *aminoglycoside antibiotics* in very large doses and *procainamide* can cause neuromuscular weakness in normal individuals or exacerbation of weakness in myasthenic patients.

The *Lambert-Eaton myasthenic syndrome* is a presynaptic disorder of the neuromuscular junction that can cause weakness similar to that of MG. The proximal muscles of the lower limbs are most commonly affected, but other muscles may be involved as well. Cranial nerve findings, including ptosis of the eyelids and diplopia, occur in up to 70 percent of patients and resemble features of MG. However, the two conditions are readily distinguished as patients with Lambert-Eaton syndrome have depressed or absent reflexes, autonomic changes such as dry mouth and impotence, and show incremental responses on repetitive nerve stimulation. It is now known that Lambert-Eaton syndrome is caused by an autoantibody directed against calcium channels on the motor nerve terminals, resulting in impaired release of ACh. A majority of patients with this syndrome have an associated malignancy, most commonly small cell carcinoma of the lung, which is thought to trigger the autoimmune response. The diagnosis of Lambert-Eaton syndrome may signal the presence of the tumor long before it would otherwise be detected, permitting early removal. Treatment of the neuromuscular disorder involves plasmapheresis and immunosuppression, as for MG.

Neurasthenia may present with weakness and fatigue, but muscle testing usually reveals the "jerky release" characteristic of nonorganic disorders, and the complaint of fatigue in these patients means tiredness or apathy rather than decreasing muscle power on repeated effort. *Hyperthyroidism* is readily diagnosed or excluded by tests of thyroid function, which should be routinely carried out in patients with suspected MG. It is worth noting that abnormalities of thyroid function (hyper- or hypothyroidism) may increase myasthenic weakness. *Botulism* can cause myasthenic-like weakness, but the pupils are often affected and repetitive nerve stimulation gives an *incremental,* rather than decremental, response. Diplopia that mimics the symptoms of MG may occasionally be due to *intracranial mass lesions* that compress nerves to the extraocular muscles (e.g., sphenoid ridge meningioma), but computed tomography (CT) or magnetic resonance imaging (MRI) scanning of the head and orbits usually reveals the lesion.

Progressive external ophthalmoplegia is a rare condition resulting in weakness of the extraocular muscles, which may be accompanied by weakness of the proximal muscles of the limbs, and a variety of other systemic features that are beyond the scope of this chapter. Most patients with this condition have mitochondrial disorders that can be detected on muscle biopsy (see Chap. 365).

Search for associated conditions Myasthenic patients have an increased incidence of several associated disorders. *Thymic abnormalities* occur in approximately 75 percent of patients, as noted above. Neoplastic change (thymoma) may produce enlargement of the thymus, which is best detected by CT or MRI scanning of the anterior mediastinum. Enlargement of the thymus in a patient over 40 years of age is highly suspicious of thymoma. *Hyperthyroidism* may occur in 3 to 8 percent of patients and may aggravate the myasthenic weakness. Tests of thyroid function should be obtained. Because of the *association with other autoimmune disorders,* blood tests for rheumatoid factor and antinuclear antibodies should be carried out in all patients. Chronic infection of any kind can exacerbate MG and should be carefully sought. Finally, measurements of *ventilatory function* are valuable because of the frequency and seriousness of respiratory impairment in myasthenic patients.

Because of the side effects of glucocorticoids and other immunosuppressive agents used in the treatment of MG, a thorough medical investigation should be made, searching specifically for evidence of chronic or latent infection (such as tuberculosis or hepatitis), hypertension, diabetes, renal impairment, and glaucoma.

MEDICAL AND SURGICAL THERAPY The prognosis has improved strikingly as a result of advances in treatment; virtually all myasthenic patients can be returned to full productive lives with proper therapy. The most important methods used in the treatment of myasthenia gravis include anticholinesterase medications, immunosuppressive agents, thymectomy, and plasmapheresis.

Anticholinesterase medications Most myasthenic patients can be improved, but few can be brought completely to normal by anticholinesterase medication. There is no substantial difference in efficacy among the various anticholinesterase drugs; oral pyridostigmine is most widely used in the United States. As a rule, the beneficial action of oral pyridostigmine begins within 15 to 30 min and lasts for 3 to 4 h, but the individual response may vary. Treatment is begun with a moderate dose, e.g., 60 mg 3 to 5 times daily. Adjustment of the dosage, i.e., frequency and amount, should be tailored to the patient's individual requirements throughout the day. For example, patients with weakness in chewing and swallowing may benefit by taking the medication before meals so that optimal strength coincides with mealtime. Long-acting pyridostigmine tablets may be helpful to get the patient through the night, but should never be used for daytime medication because of their variable absorption. The maximum useful dose of pyridostigmine rarely exceeds 120 mg every 3 h during daytime. Overdosage with anticholinesterase medication may cause increased weakness and other side effects. In some patients, muscarinic side effects of the anticholinesterase medication (diarrhea, abdominal cramps, salivation, nausea) may limit the dosage tolerated. In these cases, atropine may be used to block the autonomic side effects without altering the beneficial effects on skeletal muscle.

Thymectomy Two separate issues should be distinguished: surgical removal of thymoma and thymectomy as a treatment for myasthenia gravis. In the case of thymoma, surgical removal is necessary because of the possibility of local tumor spread, although most thymomas are benign. In the absence of a tumor, the available evidence suggests that up to 85 percent of patients improve after thymectomy, and 35 percent may achieve drug-free remission. However, the improvement may begin as long as 1 to 10 years after surgery. The advantage of thymectomy is that it offers the possibility of long-term benefit, in some cases diminishing or eliminating the need for continuing medical treatment. In view of these potential benefits and of the negligible risk in skilled hands, thymectomy has gained widespread acceptance in the treatment of MG. It is the consensus that thymectomy should be carried out in all patients with generalized MG between the ages of puberty and at least 55. Whether thymectomy should be recommended as a rule in children, in adults over 55 years of age, and in patients with weakness limited to the ocular muscles is still a matter of debate. Thymectomy must be carried out in a hospital where this procedure is performed regularly, and where the staff is experienced in the pre- and postoperative management, anesthesia, and surgical techniques of total thymectomy.

Immunosuppression Immunosuppression using glucocorticoids, azathioprine, and other drugs is effective in nearly all patients with MG. The choice of which drugs to use should be guided by their relative benefits and risks for the individual patient. In general, clinical improvement begins somewhat more rapidly with steroid treatment than with the other immunosuppressive agents. The side effects of each drug may preclude its use in some patients, as indicated below.

STEROID THERAPY Glucocorticoids, when used properly, produce improvement in myasthenic weakness in the great majority of patients. The initial dose of prednisone should be relatively low (15 to 25 mg/d) to avoid the early weakening that occurs in about one-third of patients treated initially with a high-dose regimen. The dose is increased stepwise, as tolerated by the patient (usually 5 mg/d at 2- to 3-day intervals), until there is marked clinical improvement or the dose of 50 mg/d is reached. This dose is maintained for 1 to 3 months and then is gradually modified to an alternate-day regimen over the course of an additional 1 to 2 months, until the dosage of 100 mg on alternate days is reached. Generally, patients begin to improve within a few months after reaching the maximum dose, and improvement continues to progress for months or years. The prednisone dosage may gradually be reduced, but usually months or years may be needed to determine the minimum effective dose and close monitoring is required by patient and doctor. *Few patients are able to do without prednisone entirely.* Patients on long-term glucocorticoid therapy must be carefully followed to prevent or treat adverse side effects. The commonest errors in the steroid treatment of myasthenic patients include:

1 Insufficient persistence; improvement may be delayed and gradual

2 Too early, too rapid, or excessive tapering of steroid dosage

3 Lack of attention to prevention and treatment of side effects

The management of patients treated with glucocorticoids is discussed in Chap. 317.

OTHER IMMUNOSUPPRESSIVE DRUGS Azathioprine, cyclosporine (ciclosporin), or occasionally cyclophosphamide is effective in many patients, either alone or in combination with glucocorticoid therapy. Azathioprine is the most widely used because of its relative safety in most patients. Its therapeutic effect may add to that of glucocorticoids and/or allow the steroid dose to be reduced. However, up to 10 percent of patients are unable to tolerate azathioprine because of idiosyncratic reactions consisting of flulike symptoms of fever and malaise, bone marrow depression, or abnormalities of liver function. An initial dose of 50 mg/d should be used to test for adverse side effects. If this is tolerated, the dose is gradually increased until the white blood count falls to approximately 3000 (except in patients concomitantly receiving steroids), or the lymphocyte count falls below 1000 per microliter. The typical dosage range is 2 to 3 mg/kg body weight. The beneficial effect of azathioprine takes at least 3 to 6 months to begin and even longer to reach a maximum level.

Cyclosporine is approximately as effective as azathioprine. It is usually reserved for patients who cannot tolerate azathioprine, as its use is more complicated, requiring measurement of blood levels, and the side effects (particularly nephrotoxicity) are more problematic. Cyclophosphamide is reserved for patients refractory to the other drugs because of the relatively high risk of adverse side effects, including late development of malignancies.

Plasmapheresis In view of the antibody-mediated pathogenesis of MG, plasmapheresis has been used therapeutically. The plasma, which contains the pathogenic antibodies, is mechanically separated from the blood cells, which are returned to the patient in a suitable fluid medium. Plasmapheresis produces a short-term reduction in anti-AChR antibodies, with clinical improvement in many patients. Thus, it is useful as a temporary expedient in seriously affected patients, or to improve the patient's condition prior to surgery (e.g., thymectomy). The long-term treatment of myasthenic patients requires other methods of therapy outlined in this chapter.

Management of myasthenic crisis Myasthenic crisis is defined as an exacerbation of weakness sufficient to endanger life. The usual serious threats to life are respiratory failure, caused by diaphragmatic and intercostal weakness, and aspiration, secondary to pharyngeal weakness. Treatment should be carried out in an intensive care unit staffed with physicians experienced in the management of myasthenia gravis, respiratory insufficiency, infectious disease, and fluid and electrolyte therapy. The possibility that the deterioration could be due to excessive anti-ChE medication (''cholinergic crisis'') is best excluded by temporarily stopping anti-ChE drugs. The most common cause of crisis is intercurrent infection. This should be treated immediately, because the mechanical and immunologic defenses of the patient can be assumed to be compromised. The myasthenic patient with fever and early infection should be treated like other immunocompromised patients. Early and effective antibiotic therapy, respiratory assistance, and pulmonary physiotherapy are essentials of the treatment program. As discussed above, plasmapheresis is frequently helpful in hastening recovery.

REFERENCES

DRACHMAN DB: Biology of myasthenia gravis. Ann Rev Neurosci 4:195, 1981

——— (ed): Myasthenia gravis: Biology and treatment. Ann NY Acad Sci 505:1, 1987

ENGEL AG et al: The motor endplate in myasthenia gravis and in experimental autoimmune myasthenia gravis: A quantitative ultrastructural study. Ann NY Acad Sci 274:60, 1976

FAMBROUGH DM et al: Neuromuscular junction in myasthenia gravis: Decreased acetylcholine receptors. Science 182:293, 1973

LINDSTROM J et al: Myasthenia gravis. Advances in Immunol 42:233, 1988

TANDAN R et al: Metastasizing thymoma and myasthenia gravis. Favorable response to glucocorticoids after failed chemotherapy and radiation treatment. Cancer 65:1286, 1990

TOYKA KV et al: Myasthenia gravis: Study of humoral immune mechanisms by passive transfer to mice. N Engl J Med 296:125, 1977

367 PERIODIC PARALYSIS

ROBERT C. GRIGGS

Disorders that cause patients of normal strength to become weak intermittently are not common. In contrast, the complaint of intermittent weakness is frequently encountered. The evaluation of such symptoms is challenging because the examination is often normal between attacks and because reliance on history is crucial for diagnosis. This chapter considers the primary periodic paralyses. Other disorders that cause episodic weakness are considered elsewhere (see Chap 27).

All primary periodic paralyses have some features in common. In most patients the disorders are inherited as autosomal dominant traits. Symptoms usually begin early in life and rarely commence after age 25. Attacks typically follow rest or sleep and almost never occur in the midst of vigorous activity, although antecedent exercise frequently provokes weakness. Patients remain alert during the attacks. Early in the course of these disorders interattack strength is normal but after years of attacks progressive weakness may develop. All forms of periodic paralysis are amenable to treatment and progressive weakness can be prevented and even reversed.

Diagnosis is based upon patient history and confirmed by appropriate evaluation of serum electrolytes during attacks and by evaluating the response of strength to provocative testing with glucose, insulin, potassium, and cold.

HYPOKALEMIC PERIODIC PARALYSIS This disorder occurs as an autosomal dominant condition in two-thirds of cases and as sporadic cases in one-third. Males are more frequently and more severely affected. Attacks of weakness characteristically begin in adolescence but may commence in the first decade. Onset after age 25 is rare; the new onset of episodic paralysis in older individuals is almost never due to periodic paralysis.

Attack frequency varies from daily to yearly. Attacks last from 3 to 4 h to as long as a day or more. Meals high in carbohydrate or high in sodium may provoke attacks. Paralysis involves limb muscles, usually proximal more than distal; rarely ocular, bulbar, or respiratory muscles are weakened, and bulbar and respiratory involvement may prove fatal. Reflexes become hypoactive, and cardiac arrythmias may occur during attacks. Patients may develop persistent proximal weakness after years of attacks. Examination during attack-free intervals is otherwise normal except for the frequent presence of eyelid myotonia.

Diagnosis is established by demonstrating a low serum potassium during a paralytic attack and by excluding secondary causes of hypokalemia (Chap 27). Electrocardiograms during attacks show characteristic features of hypokalemia. Electromyography is not helpful in diagnosis, but muscle biopsy often shows the presence of single or multiple centrally placed vacuoles. Patients whose attacks are so infrequent as to preclude the study of a spontaneous attack require provocative testing with glucose and insulin administration. Such tests are potentially hazardous, and patients must be carefully monitored during their performance. Since these disorders are rare such testing is most appropriately carried out in referral centers.

Pathogenesis The pathogenesis of paralytic attacks is incompletely understood. There is evidence for an abnormality of muscle membrane, possibly in sodium transport in hypokalemic and other forms of periodic paralysis. The contractile apparatus is normal. Distinctive abnormalities in potassium regulation occur in hypokalemic periodic paralysis. Patients with hypokalemic periodic paralysis often have a decrease in total body potassium but this may reflect muscle wasting. There is no increased excretion of potassium in the urine before or during attacks, but there is excessive flux of potassium from blood into muscle, possibly owing to an abnormality of muscle membrane that causes muscle to become electrically inexcitable. Muscle from these patients is abnormally sensitive to the effect of insulin on potassium uptake; the significance of this increased sensitivity is not known since weakness is often severe at levels of serum potassium that do not affect normal individuals. Moreover, attacks may occur when insulin levels are low. Therefore, factors other than hypokalemia per se are important in the induction of weakness.

Treatment ACUTE ATTACKS The acute paralysis improves following the administration of potassium salts. Oral KCl (0.2 to 0.4 mmol/kg) should be given to patients with severe weakness and repeated at 15 to 30 min intervals depending on the response of the ECG, serum potassium, and muscle strength. Milder attacks usually resolve spontaneously; resolution of weakness is hastened by exercising affected muscles. When patients are unable to swallow or are vomiting, intravenous therapy may be necessary. Small, repeated bolus therapy with KCl (0.1 mmol/kg) may be administered over 5 to 10 min with careful monitoring of the ECG and serum potassium. If potassium is administered as a dilute solution (20 to 40 mmol/L) in 5% glucose or in physiologic saline solution, serum potassium may decline, and weakness may worsen. Mannitol is the preferred vehicle for administering intravenous potassium in such situations since it facilitates rapid return of serum potassium to normal and avoids the hazard of lowering of serum potassium as may occur when glucose or saline solution are given.

PREVENTION OF ATTACKS The goal of therapy is the elimination of attacks, which also prevents interattack weakness and may improve interattack weakness after it has developed. Prior to availability of effective means of attack prevention, chronic progressive interattack weakness frequently caused serious disability. Prophylactic administration of potassium salts, even in large dosage, does not prevent attacks but acetazolamide (125 to 1000 mg/d in divided dosage) abolishes attacks in the majority of cases. The mechanism of action of acetazolamide is not fully understood, but it may block the flux of potassium from serum into muscle. The metabolic acidosis that it produces may underlie its beneficial effect. Paradoxically, acetazolamide lowers serum potassium; to achieve an adequate response in some patients it may be necessary to give supplementary potassium along with acetazolamide and to avoid high-carbohydrate meals. Chronic acetazolamide treatment may be associated with renal calculi, and patients should be monitored for this complication. In occasional patients attacks may not respond to or may even be worsened by acetazolamide. In such patients triamterene (25 to 100 mg/d or spironolactone 25 to 100 mg/d) may prevent attacks.

THYROTOXIC PERIODIC PARALYSIS Attacks of hypokalemic periodic paralysis can occur in subjects with thyrotoxicosis, most commonly in young Latin American or oriental men where up to 10 percent of thyrotoxic patients may have periodic paralysis. In many patients thyrotoxicosis has also been overlooked for many months; periodic paralysis has also occurred with T_3-toxicosis and with exogenous thyroid hormone administration. The usual age of onset of the disorder is that of thyrotoxicosis; otherwise the clinical features resemble familial hypokalemic periodic paralysis. Acute attacks respond to potassium administration. Treatment of underlying thyrotoxicosis abolishes attacks and β-adrenergic blocking agents reduce the frequency and severity of attacks while measures to control thyrotoxicosis are being instituted. Acetazolamide is not helpful in preventing attacks. The pathogenesis of thyrotoxic periodic paralysis is uncertain but there is evidence for a decrease in the activity of the calcium pump. The pathogenesis of thyrotoxic periodic paralysis is likely to be different from that of nonthyrotoxic periodic paralysis since thyroid hormone does not worsen the latter.

HYPERKALEMIC PERIODIC PARALYSIS This disorder differs from hypokalemic periodic paralysis in that attacks are usually brief (1 to 2 h or less) and more frequent; clinical or electromyographic myotonia is often demonstrable. Attacks are usually precipitated by fasting or by rest following exercise. The disease onset is usually at an earlier age than for hypokalemic periodic paralysis, and attacks or myotonia may be evident in the first year of life. The disorder is usually transmitted as an autosomal dominant defect; rare sporadic cases occur.

The name "hyperkalemic" is misleading since patients are often normokalemic during attacks. It is the fact that attacks are *precipitated by potassium administration* that best defines the disorder. "Potassium-sensitive" periodic paralysis is probably preferable terminology. Moreover, the serum potassium is often slightly elevated when patients are not having attacks of weakness. Attacks are characterized by limb weakness predominantly, though cranial and respiratory muscle involvement may occur. Cardiac arrythmias occur occasionally. Paresthesias and muscle pain are present during many attacks, and Chvostek's sign is often present during attacks.

Diagnosis is suggested by a modest elevation of serum potassium during attacks in nearly half of patients; at times, however, the serum potassium is normal or even low. Intravenous glucose-insulin loading does not precipitate weakness but potassium-loading tests (0.05 to 0.15 g/kg) will provoke weakness in such patients. Myotonia may be increased. Potassium-loading tests are potentially hazardous and are contraindicated in patients with renal disease and diabetes. Random serum potassium measurements may suggest the diagnosis since potassium elevations are frequent during attack-free intervals. Electromyographic evidence of myotonia and the finding of vacuoles on muscle biopsy provide supporting data.

Pathogenesis Hyperkalemia during attacks of hyperkalemic periodic paralysis seldom reaches levels that would be expected to produce paralysis. Furthermore, serum potassium may remain within the normal range. Factors other than hyperkalemia are clearly important in the pathogenesis of attacks. An abnormality of the sarcolemma may cause spontaneous depolarization of the muscle cell and lead both to myotonia and to paralysis. Increased permeability of the muscle membrane to sodium has been noted; a decreased activity of the sodium-potassium pump may be involved in the spontaneous depolarization.

Treatment Attacks of weakness are seldom severe enough to require emergency treatment and are never fatal. Oral glucose or other carbohydrate hastens recovery. Since interattack weakness may develop after repeated attacks, prophylactic treatment is usually indicated. Remarkably, acetazolamide (125 to 1000 mg/d), the treatment of choice for hypokalemic periodic paralysis, was first found to be beneficial for hyperkalemic periodic paralysis, possibly because of its kaliopenic effect. Thiazide diuretics (e.g., chlorothiazide 250 to 1000 mg/d) are usually more effective and have fewer side effects.

NORMOKALEMIC PERIODIC PARALYSIS Most subjects with periodic paralysis in whom potassium is normal during attacks, behave like those with typical "hyperkalemic" periodic paralysis, since they are similarly sensitive to potassium administration. In fact, the so-called hyperkalemic and normokalemic forms of this disorder may be a single entity. Treatment is the same as for hyperkalemic periodic paralysis.

Rarely, patients with episodic normokalemic paralysis are not potassium sensitive, but they usually show evidence of muscle destruction or other features suggesting that they should not be classified as having a primary periodic paralysis.

PARAMYOTONIA WITH PERIODIC PARALYSIS Attacks of paralysis may occur in the paramyotonias, either provoked by cold or spontaneously. Paramyotonia congenita is characterized by paradoxical (i.e., worsening with activity) myotonia, cold provocation, spontaneous attacks, and family history compatible with an autosomal dominant defect. The cold provocation of weakness and muscle stiffness distinguishes this disease from other periodic paralyses. A therapeutically useful subclassification of the paramyotonias has been proposed: (1) paramyotonia congenita, in which spontaneous attacks of weakness are associated with a lowering of serum potassium and in which measures that decrease serum potassium provoke weakness; and (2) paralysis periodica paramyotonia in which spontaneous attacks may be associated with hyperkalemia and may be provoked by oral potassium administration. This potassium sensitivity has led in the past to the classification of this disorder as a variant of hyperkalemic or normokalemic periodic paralysis.

Diagnosis depends upon the provocation of weakness and stiffness with cold. Glucose and insulin loading and potassium challenges aid in the subclassification of the disorder and provide assistance in the choice of medication for treatment.

Pathogenesis The two types of paramyotonia probably have different etiologies. In paramyotonia congenita cooling of muscle results in an abnormal depolarization, leading first to myotonia and then to inexcitability. Both forms of paramyotonia are characterized by an abnormal uptake of potassium by muscle. Sodium and potassium conductance become abnormal with cooling of muscle. An abnormality of sodium channels with a resulting increase in sodium permeability may account for this alteration.

Treatment Spontaneous attacks of periodic paralysis in paramyotonia congenita are relatively infrequent. Many patients do not require prophylactic treatment for prevention. In the case of paramyotonia congenita, patients with severe and frequent attacks of weakness may respond to spironolactone, and subjects with paralysis periodica paramyotonica may respond to acetazolamide or thiazides. Acetazolamide may provoke weakness in paramyotonia congenita. Myotonia in both types of paramyotonia improves with 400 to 1200 mg/d of tocainide or with mexiletine hydrochloride (150 to 900 mg/d). These antiarrhythmic agents may work in myotonia by blocking abnormal sodium channels; tocainide also improves weakness and decreases the abnormal uptake of potassium by muscle.

REFERENCES

GRIGGS RC et al: Intravenous treatment of hypokalemic periodic paralysis. Arch Neurol 40:539, 1983

MOXLEY RT et al: Potassium uptake in muscle during paramyotonic weakness. Neurology 39:952, 1989.

RESNICK JS et al: Acetazolamide prophylaxis in hypokalemic periodic paralysis. N Engl J Med 278:582, 1968

RIGGS JE: The periodic paralyses. Neurologic Clinics 6:485, 1988

STREIB EW: Paramyotonia congenita: Successful treatment with tocainide. Clinical and electrophysiological findings in seven patients. Muscle Nerve 10:155, 1987

PART FOURTEEN PSYCHIATRY

section 1 Psychiatric disorders

368 PSYCHIATRY AND MEDICINE

This chapter's coverage is divided into major mood disorders (by Lewis L. Judd), schizophrenia (by David L. Braff), anxiety disorders (by Karen Thatcher Britton, S. Craig Risch, and J. Christian Gillin), and personality disorders (by Igor Grant).

MAJOR MOOD (AFFECTIVE) DISORDERS[1]

For centuries it was recognized that some individuals are subject to extremes in mood but, until recently, distinguishing mood alterations that are pathologic from those that are not was elusive. The realization that major mental disorders are psychobiologic phenomena resulting from abnormal brain mechanisms together with the development of an objective, empirically based diagnostic classification system has now made it possible for clinicians to distinguish consistently between abnormal mood states and the normal evanescent changes in emotions that are a part of everyday life.

Recent epidemiologic research has shown that at any instant about 5 percent of the adult population in this country is suffering from clinically significant mood (or affective) disorders. Traditionally, mental disorders in this category were designated as *affective* disorders; however, this has now been replaced by the term *mood* disorder, because the latter refers to a sustained rather than fluctuating emotional state. The mood disorders are a heterogeneous group of mental disorders characterized by extreme exaggerations and disturbances of mood and affect associated with physiologic (vegetative), cognitive, and psychomotor dysfunctions. There is a marked tendency to periodicity and recurrence throughout the patient's lifetime, in which diagnosable affective episodes appear and remit and are followed by symptom-free periods (euthymia) lasting weeks, months, or years. Indeed, recent studies have shown that the disability resulting from mood disorders, even those that are minimally symptomatic, exceeds that of most major chronic medical disorders such as diabetes, arthritis, and angina. The most prevalent and important diagnostic syndromes among the mood disorders are *major depression* (unipolar disorders) and *manic-depressive illness* (bipolar disorders).

The unipolar-bipolar division is a useful distinction in regard to clinical characteristics, life course, and treatment. Evidence continues to accumulate indicating that unipolar and bipolar depressions are, in all likelihood, psychobiologically different but very closely related disorders. For example, bipolar disorders tend to begin, on the average, a decade earlier, pursue a more recurrent course relative to unipolar depression, and respond better to lithium.

An additional distinction that has been helpful in reducing heterogeneity among these disorders is that of primary-secondary. The rationale behind this is that affective disorders occurring in a pure form are likely to be more homogeneous than affective disorders that coexist with other psychiatric or medical conditions. A major affective disorder is *primary* when the affective episode (manic or depressive) is the first-appearing psychiatric illness in a patient's lifetime and is not associated with other psychiatric or medical illnesses. Conversely, a mood disorder is classified as *secondary* when it appears in conjunction with other psychiatric or medical conditions. Depressive episodes can be observed in conjunction with virtually every mental disorder, including schizophrenia, anxiety disorders, alcoholism, substance abuse, dementia, and personality disorders.

Mood disorders can also be associated with such medical diseases as the following: endocrinopathies (Cushing's disease, hyper- or hypothyroidism, hyperparathyroidism), collagen diseases (systemic lupus erythematosus), cardiovascular disease (congestive heart failure, myocardial infarction), neurologic diseases (stroke, Parkinson's disease, Alzheimer's disease, brain tumors, or multiple sclerosis), infections (hepatitis, influenza), malignancies (pancreatic adenocarcinoma, disseminated carcinomatosis), metabolic disorders (porphyria), and vitamin deficiencies (vitamin B_1, nicotinic acid). In addition, the chronic administration of the following medications can also precipitate an affective episode: glucocorticoids, α-methyldopa, propranolol, benzodiazepines, reserpine derivatives, levodopa, neuroleptics, cimetidine, indomethacin, cycloserine, and anti-cancer drugs. Withdrawal from CNS stimulants such as amphetamines or drugs of abuse like cocaine may also be a precipitating factor. It should be noted, however, that even though an affective episode may be classified as being secondary, it can be the most important and compelling aspect of a patient's clinical picture requiring immediate and specific therapeutic intervention (see also Chap. 29).

DIAGNOSTIC CATEGORIES OF MOOD DISORDERS The diagnosis of a clinically significant affective episode is based upon the criteria contained in the revised third edition of the *Diagnostic and Statistical Manual* (DSM-IIIR). This method of diagnostic classification has been developed and approved by the American Psychiatric Association and is the official standard diagnostic system used in this country today. Two general types of affective episodes can be observed: major depressive episodes (sustained for at least 2 weeks) and manic episodes (sustained for at least 1 week). The diagnostic criteria for major depressive episodes and manic episodes are included in Tables 368-1 and 368-2.

Major depression The diagnosis of major depression is made when the patient presents with the necessary signs and symptoms of a major depressive episode (see Table 368-1). The diagnostic category of major depression represents the unipolar form of the mood disorders, in which patients manifest only the single pole of affect, that of depression. The diagnosis of recurrent major depression is made when major depressive episodes are repeated throughout a patient's lifetime and is synonymous with the term recurrent unipolar depres-

[1] By Lewis L. Judd. The author gratefully acknowledges the contributions of Robert M. A. Hirschfeld, M.D., Hagop Akiskel, M.D., Robert M. Post, M.D., and Nancy L. Ostrowski, Ph.D.

TABLE 368-1 Diagnostic criteria for major depressive episode*

A At least five of the following symptoms have been present during the same 2-week period and represent a change from previous functioning; at least one of the symptoms is either (1) depressed mood, or (2) loss of interest or pleasure. (Do not include symptoms that are clearly due to a physical condition, mood-incongruent delusions or hallucinations, incoherence, or marked loosening of associations.)
- *1* Depressed mood (or can be irritable mood in children and adolescents) most of the day, nearly every day, as indicated either by subjective account or observation by others
- *2* Markedly diminished interest or pleasure in all, or almost all, activities most of the day, nearly every day (as indicated either by subjective account or observation by others of apathy most of the time)
- *3* Significant weight loss or weight gain when not dieting (e.g., more than 5% of body weight in a month), or decrease or increase in appetite nearly every day (in children, consider failure to make expected weight gains)
- *4* Insomnia or hypersomnia nearly every day
- *5* Psychomotor agitation or retardation nearly every day (observable by others, not merely subjective feelings of restlessness or being slowed down)
- *6* Fatigue or loss of energy nearly every day
- *7* Feelings of worthlessness or excessive or inappropriate guilt (not merely self-reproach or guilt about being sick)
- *8* Diminished ability to think or concentrate, or indecisiveness, nearly every day (either by subjective account or as observed by others)
- *9* Recurrent thoughts of death (not just fear of dying), recurrent suicidal ideation without a specific plan, or a suicide attempt or a specific plan for committing suicide

B
- *1* It cannot be established that an organic factor initiated and maintained the disturbance
- *2* The disturbance is not a normal reaction to the death of a loved one (uncomplicated bereavement)†

C At no time during the disturbance have there been delusions or hallucinations for as long as 2 weeks in the absence of prominent mood symptoms (i.e., before the mood symptoms developed or after they have remitted).

D Not superimposed on schizophrenia or schizophreniform, delusional, or psychotic disorders.

*A major depressive syndrome is defined as criterion *A* above.
†Morbid preoccupation with worthlessness, suicidal ideation, marked functional impairment or psychomotor retardation, or prolonged duration suggest bereavement complicated by major depression.
SOURCE: Adapted from DSM-IIIR.

sion. Following the first episode, between 50 and 80 percent of patients will have at least one more major depressive episode. Approximately 20 percent will have a subsequent manic episode, at which point the patient is then reclassified as having a bipolar disorder (manic depressive illness). Major depression is approximately twice as common in women as men. The 1-month prevalence in the adult population (18 years and over) is 2.9 percent for women and 1.6 percent for men. Age at first onset is most often in the late twenties and the thirties, but major depression can occur at any age. Most natural-course studies indicate that unipolar patients average two to three major depressive episodes during their lifetimes, although some patients have only single episodes and others have many more. The average duration of an untreated depressive episode is 8 to 9 months with a range of 1 to 12 months. There is no clear-cut relationship between risk for major depression and socioeconomic class, race, education, or occupation.

There are two other important subtypes of unipolar depression that should be noted: dysthymia and atypical major depression. *Dysthymia* is a chronic, milder form of depression. The diagnosis of dysthymia requires that the range of symptoms has been present for at least 2 years, but often patients describe many years of suffering (see Table 368-3). In the adult population dysthymia is twice as frequent in women as in men, and its 1-month prevalence is 3.3 percent. Clinical studies during the past decade have found that dysthymia occurs in conjunction with a major depression in about 25 percent of patients, a condition labeled *double-depression*. Double-depression is associated with substantially increased risks of recurrence and chronicity for major depression.

The symptoms of *atypical depression* actually match those of "typical" major depression but are distinguished from the latter by the following: reverse vegetative symptoms (e.g., overeating and

TABLE 368-2 Diagnostic criteria for manic episode*

A A distinct period of abnormally and persistently elevated, expansive, or irritable mood.

B During the period of mood disturbance, at least three of the following symptoms have persisted (four if the mood is only irritable) and have been present to a significant degree:
- *1* Inflated self-esteem or grandiosity
- *2* Decreased need for sleep, e.g., feels rested after only 3 h of sleep
- *3* More talkative than usual or pressure to keep talking
- *4* Flight of ideas or subjective experience that thoughts are racing
- *5* Distractibility, i.e., attention too easily drawn to unimportant or irrelevant external stimuli
- *6* Increase in goal-directed activity (either socially, at work or school, or sexually) or psychomotor agitation
- *7* Excessive involvement in pleasurable activities that have a high potential for painful consequences, e.g., the person engages in unrestrained buying sprees, sexual indiscretions, or foolish business investments

C Mood disturbance sufficiently severe to cause marked impairment in occupational functioning or in usual social activities or relationships with others, or to necessitate hospitalization to prevent harm to self or others

D At no time during the disturbance have there been delusions or hallucinations for as long as 2 weeks in the absence of prominent mood symptoms (i.e., before the mood symptoms developed or after they have remitted).

E Not superimposed on schizophrenia or schizophreniform, delusional, or psychotic disorders.

F It cannot be established that an organic factor initiated and maintained the disturbance.†

* A manic syndrome is defined as including criteria *A*, *B*, and *C* above. A hypomanic syndrome is defined as including criteria *A* and *B*, but not *C*, i.e., no marked impairment.
† Somatic antidepressant treatment (e.g., drugs, electroconvulsive therapy) that apparently precipitates a mood disturbance should not be considered an etiologic organic factor.
SOURCE: Adapted from DSM-IIIR.

hypersomnia), interpersonal rejection sensitivity, a sense of "leaden paralysis," or the experience of a significant amount of concurrent anxiety, and/or excessive responsiveness to environmental changes. It is clinically important to identify atypical major depression as distinct from typical major depression, because the former is often very responsive to monoamine oxidase inhibitor (MAOI) antidepressants. Non-psychiatric physicians must be fully aware that the classic manifestations of major depression and the variations described above are primarily based on studies in psychiatric settings. Recent evidence suggests that in medical, especially primary care, setting, many depressed patients initially present with minimal or no psychologic symptoms (e.g., dysphoric mood, low self-esteem, intense guilt, etc.) and instead focus on somatic complaints (e.g., fatigue, bodily

TABLE 368-3 Diagnostic criteria for dysthymia

A Depressed mood (or can be irritable mood in children and adolescents) for most of the day, more days than not, as indicated either by subjective account or observation by others, for at least 2 years (1 year for children and adolescents).

B Presence, while depressed, of at least two of the following:
- *1* Poor appetite or overeating
- *2* Insomnia or hypersomnia
- *3* Low energy or fatigue
- *4* Low self-esteem
- *5* Poor concentration or difficulty making decisions
- *6* Feelings of hopelessness

C During a 2-year period (1-year for children and adolescents) of the disturbance, never without the symptoms in *A* for more than 2 months at a time.

D No evidence of an unequivocal major depressive episode during the first 2 years (1 year for children and adolescents) of the disturbance.*

E Has never had a manic episode or an unequivocal hypomanic episode (see Table 368-2).

F Not superimposed on a chronic psychotic disorder, such as schizophrenia or delusional disorder.

G It cannot be established that an organic factor initiated and maintained the disturbance, e.g., prolonged administration of an antihypertensive medication.

* There may have been a previous major depressive episode, provided there was a full remission (no significant signs or symptoms for 6 months) before development of the dysthymia. In addition, after these 2 years (1 year in children and adolescents) of dysthymia, there may be superimposed episodes of major depression, in which case both diagnoses are given.
SOURCE: DSM-IIIR.

aches and pains, sleep problems, impotence, etc.). Some uninformed clinicians may refer to these patients somewhat pejoratively as "cracks." Frequently, these patients may initially deny subjective feelings of depression and may even appear superficially cheerful. Diagnosing these individuals is difficult, especially if the clinician is not alert to the possibility of a depressive episode. However, a previous personal history or the presence of a family history of typical mood disorders is an important diagnostic clue that a current mood disorder may be present. The importance of these patients to the primary care physician should not be underestimated as recent studies have indicated that this patient population presents the fourth most common set of complaints in primary care settings. Further, early diagnosis and treatment are vital; these patients and their families experience a great deal of personal suffering with patients often experiencing occupational difficulties, becoming big users of medical services, and tending toward substance abuse (especially alcohol) in misguided attempts at self-medication. Finally, and more ominously, data from "psychological" autopsies of suicide victims indicate that a significant percentage have sought medical advice for the same type of ill-defined somatic complaints previously noted and were unfortunately not diagnosed and hence not treated appropriately.

Bipolar disorders Bipolar disorders are diagnosed using the criteria for both manic and major depressive episodes. In this category of mood disorder, both the affective poles of mania and depression are present. Bipolar disorders are diagnosed as bipolar disorder, manic, if the current episode meets criteria for a manic episode and as bipolar disorder, depressed, if the episode meets criteria for a major depressive episode. Bipolar patients who have depressive and manic features simultaneously (e.g., extreme fatigue with racing thoughts, hypersomnia with increased sexual drive, etc.) are classified as bipolar disorder, mixed. Bipolar depression is slightly more frequent in women than men. Men have significantly more manic than depressive episodes, whereas women have significantly more depressive than manic episodes. The age of risk for bipolar disorder extends from as early as 6 to 7 years to over 65, but the peak age of onset in both men and women for the first attack is in the late twenties and early thirties, with a mean age of onset of 32.5 years. The illness can begin with either a manic or depressive episode. About two-thirds of first episodes are manic and approximately 60 percent of these patients will have a predominantly manic course, while the remaining 25 to 30 percent manifest primarily depressive episodes. Most natural-course studies of untreated bipolar patients generally agree that they will average nine diagnosable affective episodes during their lifetimes (range 1 to more than 20). The pattern is that the cycle length, which is measured from the onset of one episode to the onset of the next, will decrease and the number of episodes will increase over time. For example, in untreated bipolar patients the time between the first and second episode averages from 3.5 to 4 years, between the second and third episodes about 2 years, and between episodes three and four somewhere between 12 and 18 months. Episode duration is from 4 to 13 months, and the average is about 8.5 months but may be shorter during manic phases. Attempts have been made to categorize affective episodes in the bipolar patient based on how often the episodes occur in juxtaposition to those of opposite polarity. The vast majority of episodes are uniphasic, i.e., a manic or depressive episode is preceded by a symptom-free period; however, approximately 10 or 15 percent are biphasic with a depressive episode more often preceding the manic.

There is a small but distinct group of bipolar patients who manifest very rapid cycling patterns (bipolar disorder, mixed). The rapid cycler is a patient who presents with more than four or five episodes in 1 year, but there are patients who have considerably more episodes and there are case reports of patients cycling every 24 h. The rapid-cycling bipolar patient has eight times the number of affective episodes in his or her lifetime in comparison to slow cyclers. Eighty percent of rapid cyclers are women, and the appearance of rapid cycling may be related to impaired thyroid function. Although it is still controversial, there is evidence in a special subgroup of bipolar patients that rapid cycling may be related to previous treatment with tricyclic antidepressants and can only be effectively controlled after the patient is removed from tricyclics and treated with thyroid supplement.

The life-long intensity of illness in bipolar disorder, even among the slow cyclers, is much more extreme than it is in unipolar disorder. Bipolar patients have significantly more episodes of illness, more hospitalizations, spend more total time in the hospital during their lifetimes, are more likely to divorce and, if left untreated, are at significantly higher risk to commit suicide.

ETIOLOGY AND PATHOPHYSIOLOGY OF THE MAJOR MOOD DISORDERS Considerable progress has been made in identifying and characterizing the etiologic factors in major mood disorders, but a comprehensive and detailed understanding of the etiology of these disorders has yet to be achieved. Tremendous advances in knowledge during the past 25 years have provided excellent leads for focused scientific inquiry into the causes of these disorders; these leads, in turn, have led to the development of very specific and effective treatments. Like many other human diseases, the mood disorders are the result of interactions between the patient's genetic makeup and the environment. Evidence continues to mount that significant genetic factors are involved in these disorders, but the genetic components do not appear to be so overwhelming that the disorder is manifested without any environmental challenges. In general, the cause of a major affective episode can be conceptualized by two intersecting continua both with progressive intensities. One involves the patient's inherited constitutional predisposition to develop affective episodes; this interacts with the second continuum of the environmental stresses and life events to which the patient is exposed. Thus, there are those individuals with very high genetic predispositions for mood disorders in whom the disorder will be manifested seemingly without precipitating events. In contrast, there are patients with lower genetic predisposition in whom the disorder is manifested only when the patient is exposed to more serious precipitating life events and cumulative life stresses.

Genetic factors Data derived from virtually every methodologic strategy in human genetics strongly suggest significant genetic influences in the major mood disorders, but as yet the mode of genetic transmission has not been established. The degree of genetic expression varies considerably from patient to patient, and in some patients marked predictable genetic factors are present; in other genetic expression appears to be significantly less influential. *Twin studies* have been used by psychiatric geneticists to attempt to quantify genetic loading in various psychiatric diseases. Studies of mood disorders in twins have reported concordance rates among monozygotic (MZ) twins ranging from 33.3 to 75 percent, with an average of approximately 65 percent. In contrast, the concordance rates for dizygotic (DZ) twins range from 9 to 23 percent, averaging 15 percent. The difference in concordance rates between MZ and DZ twins strongly suggests inherited genetic vulnerability. The concordance rate is highest for recurrent (>3 episodes) mood disorders, which also suggests that the less recurrent mood disorders have less genetic influence. Although no definitive studies are available using the *adoption study* strategy, there is a trend indicating that adoptees with mood disorders have a greater incidence of affective illness in their biologic parents than in their adopted parents.

A large number of *family studies* have been conducted in the mood disorders. The standard paradigm is to make independent and blind diagnoses in the first-degree relatives of mood disorder patients, anticipating that if genetic components are present, the consanguineous relatives will manifest an increased risk for affective illness. First-degree relatives of bipolar patients have a morbidity risk for bipolar disorder ranging from 2.8 to 17.7 percent and a risk of up to 22.4 percent for unipolar depression. The first-degree relatives of unipolar patients have a risk of 6.4 to 17.0 percent for unipolar depression and of 0.3 to 29.0 percent for bipolar disorder. Thus, bipolar patients have both unipolar disorders among their blood relatives, whereas unipolar patients have increased incidence of unipolar, but not bipolar, disorders in their relatives. There is growing evidence that bipolar disorders are an excellent model for molecular genetic investigations. There are a large number of ongoing studies combining careful diagnostic and family pedigree studies with molecular genetics in an attempt to identify the linkage between specific gene markers and the manifestation of major mood disorder in an afflicted or informative family. Several years ago a group reported a genetic linkage on the short arm of chromosome 11 with bipolar disorders in a pedigree of the Old Order Amish. However, a more recent study on an expanded number of subjects in the same pedigree has failed to confirm the original observation. More recently a linkage on the X chromosome has been reported for bipolar disorder in an Israeli pedigree; to date this has not been confirmed by replication studies. In addition, a small subgroup of bipolar patients has been found who have a linkage between protan-deutan (red-green) color blindness, glucose-6-phosphate dehydrogenase deficiency, and the presence of bipolar disorder. Unfortunately this latter pattern has not been present in other families similarly afflicted with bipolar disorders.

In summary, the genetic studies strongly indicate the inheritance of a vulnerability to mood disorders, especially bipolar illness, but the genetic expression is heterogeneous and the degree of vulnerability varies significantly. There is evidence that the genetic factors are stronger in bipolar disorder than in unipolar depression. There is enormous promise for continued molecular genetic studies in the bipolar disorders, but as yet a definitive replicated linkage has not been identified.

Neurotransmitter systems The earliest investigations of etiologic mechanisms in the mood disorders involved studies of the various neurotransmitter systems in the brain. The original biogenic amine hypothesis focused primarily on the central nervous system (CNS) neurotransmitters norepinephrine, serotonin, and dopamine, attributing depression and mania, respectively, to the deficiency or excess of these neurotransmitters at important synaptic sites in the brain. This hypothesis has stimulated and directed research in the field for many years, and data consistent with the hypothesis continue to emerge. Urinary and cerebrospinal fluid (CSF) studies of norepinephrine, its metabolite 3-methoxy-4-hydroxyphenethyleneglycol (MHPG), and the catalytic enzyme dopamine β-hydroxylase have been reported as being increased or decreased in the predictable direction during depressive and manic episodes. More recently, increases in norepinephrine have been described in both mania and depression. Recent studies identifying alterations in serotonin metabolism have focused attention on 5-hydroxyindole acetic acid (5-HIAA), a serotonin metabolite, that has been found to be reduced in the CSF of depressed patients who make frequent impulsive and aggressive suicide attempts. Deficits in other neurotransmitters such as dopamine and gamma-aminobutyric acid (GABA) have also been identified in some patients with major depression. Finally, another neurotransmitter hypothesis that has directed research in the affective disorders is the cholinergic hypothesis, which postulates increased central cholinergic tone in depression, decreased cholinergic tone in mania, and an imbalance between the cholinergic and adrenergic neurotransmitter systems as being a central pathophysiologic mechanism in affective disorders.

Within the past 10 years, there has been a shift of research focus from the neurotransmitter biosynthetic, storage, and release mechanisms in the presynaptic neuron to the study of receptors on postsynaptic neurons. There is growing evidence that postsynaptic receptor kinetics and activity are predictably and consistently altered during affective episodes and by the psychotropic medications known to ameliorate these disorders. Current research in the pathophysiology of the affective disorders is being concentrated on the role of postsynaptic receptor systems and especially the cascade of intraneuronal molecular and biochemical events that occur in the postsynaptic neuron following the binding of the neurotransmitter to the receptor.

In summary, there is general agreement in the large number of studies that have been conducted to date that the relative functional underactivity of neurotransmitter and/or the down-regulation of postsynaptic receptors have often been correlated with depressive episodes. However, the reciprocal changes that one would predict have not been consistently identified in manic episodes, in part because of the difficulties encountered in the study of these patients, who are extremely hyperactive and noncompliant. Nevertheless, the cumulative data present unequivocal evidence of dysfunctional brain mechanisms in the mood disorders, but a full and precise understanding of the pathophysiology is not yet available.

Environmental factors There is little systematic data available indicating what role environmental stresses and untoward life events play or what types of stressors might be etiologically significant in the development of major affective episodes. Attempts have been made, for example, to relate early childhood loss and parental separation as predisposing factors for the future development of an affective illness, but the data are inconsistent. In general, studies have shown an overall temporal relationship between stressful and negative life events and the subsequent appearance of affective episodes. Research attempting to characterize qualitative differences in the impact of life stress have been disappointing, although serious life events such as the death of a child or a spouse, job loss, marked changes in social status, and even severe assaults on self-esteem have been linked to affective episodes. While the relationship between environmental stresses and the appearance of affective episodes has not always been demonstrated, generally speaking most experts agree that a single severe or multiple severe adverse events in life can interact with the constitutional predisposition of a patient and result in the triggering of an affective episode.

In further support of the influence of environmental events are the studies that have been conducted in higher primates. In these studies, phenomena that resemble or are analogous to the depressive states in humans are seen in monkeys using both mother/infant and peer separation paradigms. Interestingly, the monkey's "despair" response to the separation can be predictably enhanced by drugs known to specifically alter central concentrations and metabolism of various relevant CNS neurotransmitters (e.g., norepinephrine, dopamine), suggesting that psychosocial and CNS biochemical factors interact in the genesis of affective episodes.

Brain-environmental interactions One of the brain's most important and central functions is to receive incoming stimuli from the environment for purposes of storage, integration, and interpretation, which in turn provides the basis for an organized and appropriate response. Thus, it should not be surprising to find that environmental events do exert consistent and powerful influences on brain function. However, there is a genuine paucity of testable hypotheses available that offer a plausible explanation of how environmental events could trigger the pathophysiologic brain processes that have been identified with recurrent mood disorders. One of the exceptions is the "kindling" hypothesis of Post and colleagues. From data based on animal models, including stimulant-induced behavioral sensitization (i.e., cocaine-induced seizures) and electrophysiologic kindling (increased sensitivity to electrically induced seizures), the suggestion has been made that a similar sensitization process may be involved in the recurrent episodes characteristic of the cyclic bipolar disorders. This hypothesis is consistent with the observations that spontaneous recurrences of affective episodes late in the progression of the illness seem, at times, to occur without precipitating factors; patients respond differently to pharmacotherapies at different stages of the disorder; there is frequently an increased sensitivity to anticonvulsant medications (i.e., carbamazepine combined with lithium) in some patients at late stages; and there is an increased rate of cycling as the disease progresses. One implication of this line of research is that prophylactic use of pharmacotherapy may be justifiable early in the treatment of unipolar and bipolar mood disorders.

Biologic rhythms The marked tendency of major mood disorders to periodic manifestation and possibly to seasonal variations has stimulated hypotheses that suggest that the dysregulation of biologic rhythms may be centrally involved in the pathophysiology of affective disorders. There are reports of desynchronization of circadian rhythms in some bipolar patients in which these patients manifested both rapid free-running circadian rhythms (e.g., 23- versus 24-h rhythms) and a phase delay in their rhythms. There is also a special subgroup of patients with major depression in which the depressive episodes are manifested at specific seasons of the year. The most consistently studied groups are those with so-called "winter" depression (also called *seasonal affective disorder*). These patients, while residing in more northern latitudes, experience major depressive episodes during the winter when days are significantly shorter and periods of darkness more prolonged; they do not experience depression of this type when residing in latitudes where the environmental light/dark cycle is not as extreme. Controlled treatment studies, using intense white light (>2000 lux) presented at a specified time during the day and for a precise period of time, have proven to be therapeutically effective in some patients with this syndrome.

BIOLOGIC CORRELATES AND LABORATORY STUDIES **Neurohormonal correlates** For a number of years probes into the pathophysiologic mechanisms of the affective disorders have used various neurohormones whose secretion is regulated by one or more of the CNS neurotransmitters. One consistent finding from these studies has been that a significant subpopulation of patients with major depression hypersecrete cortisol and have abnormal cortisol circadian secretion patterns. Recent investigations with corticotropin-releasing hormone (CRH) stimulation have yielded blunted adrenocorticotropic hormone (ACTH) responses, suggesting that the corticosteroid abnormality is of central origin. In addition, even though it is now controversial, the dexamethasone suppression test (DST) has been useful in both diagnosis and monitoring of treatment. The standard DST used in psychiatry involves the administration of 1 mg of dexamethasone at 2300 hours with subsequent cortisol determinations at 1600 and 2300 hours the following day. The nonsuppression of cortisol is an abnormal or positive response [>140 nmol/L (>5 μg/dL) cortisol concentration in the 1600 or 2300 sample]. Initial studies reported that up to 50 percent of patients with serious major depression were nonsuppressors on the DST. Further investigations indicate that DST nonsuppression is most likely a state marker, which is positive during the depressive episode but returns to normal after successful resolution of the episode. False positives on the DST occur in patients with alcoholism, malnutrition, obesity, pregnancy, major physical illnesses, anticonvulsant use, excessive caffeine intake, and in patients over 65 years and this has eroded the usefulness of the test. In addition, more recently a number of studies have appeared in the literature reporting a much smaller percentage of DST nonsuppressors associated with major depressive episodes and an increased percentage in many other psychiatric illnesses. DST nonsuppression among depressed patients has now been reported as low as 10 to 15 percent, especially among depressed outpatients, making this test of no value as a screening test for depression. While the status of this diagnostic marker is still controversial, it is useful in monitoring treatment efficacy in DST-positive depressives, since the DST response reverts to normal when the episode remits. Failure of DST to normalize despite apparent clinical recovery has, in some studies, been associated with suicide.

Other neuroendocrine markers have also been explored, but none as widely as the DST. In major depression, between 25 and 30 percent of patients respond to thyrotropin-releasing hormone (TRH) with blunted thyroid-stimulating hormone (TSH) responses. TSH blunting is not specific to depressive episodes, but an exaggerated TSH response to TRH suggests borderline hypothyroidism and might be useful in identifying those refractory or rapid-cycling bipolar patients who would benefit from thyroid supplementation (e.g., T_3 or T_4). Small subgroups of depressed patients have manifested blunted growth hormone responses to the following challenge agents: clonidine, amphetamine, levodopa, 5-hydroxytryptophan, and hypoglycemia (insulin tolerance test). Even though 15 to 25 percent of depressed patients have blunted growth hormone responses, it has not proved to be diagnostically useful. More recently, blunted prolactin responses to both TRH and opiate alkaloid challenges have also been reported in subpopulations of depressed patients; while these findings may be of interest in terms of pathophysiologic mechanisms, they are not useful diagnostically.

Sleep studies The disruption of sleep patterns is present in virtually every patient with major affective disorder, and polysomnographic studies of sleep in these patients have proved to be of interest. In approximately 60 percent of cases of major depression there is a significantly shortened time period between the onset of sleep and the appearance of the first rapid eye movement (REM) (i.e., decreased REM latency). In addition, the density of the REM epoch, measured by the number of eye movements, is increased; there is a tendency for the REM epoch to be increased in duration, and there is a shift of REM activity to an earlier part of the night. These findings from all-night EEG sleep recordings have remained among the most consistent biologic markers for major depression, although they lack specificity, since short REM latency has also been reported in anorexia nervosa, obsessive-compulsive disorders, sleep apnea, and narcolepsy.

Neurotransmitter metabolites and enzymes The neurotransmitter hypotheses of mood disorders have stimulated a number of studies correlating biogenic amine metabolites with manic and depressive episodes. The data are inconsistent and have not been consistently useful either diagnostically or therapeutically. The one possible exception is MHPG, a metabolite of norepinephrine. Some workers have reported low MHPG excretion as predicting a positive therapeutic response to the antidepressants imipramine, desipramine, etc., and high MHPG excretion as predicting a response to amitriptyline, nortriptyline, etc. While these data are of interest and with further study may result in the identification of biochemical subtypes in major depression, these findings have not been regularly replicated in other laboratories.

Investigators who have examined the levels of the enzyme monoamine oxidase (MAO) in platelets, report it to be low in bipolar disorders and high in subjects with anxiety. Further, ^{3}[H]imipramine-binding studies in platelets also have been found to be low in major depressives who were suicidal. Again, these findings, although of interest, lack specificity, since similar results have also been reported to be altered in other psychiatric conditions such as alcoholism, anorexia and bulimia, and impulse control disorders.

TREATMENT OF THE MAJOR MOOD DISORDERS Important advances have been made in the treatment of the major mood disorders, and the majority of these patients can now be treated with a high degree of specificity and success. The most important discoveries have been in the development of potent psychotropic medications for both major depression and the bipolar disorders. The central therapeutic tools in the treatment of the major affective disorders are the antidepressants and lithium. The use of these psychotropic medications is specifically covered in much greater detail in Chap. 369.

Because major affective disorders have strong tendencies for recurrence, an important aspect of the patient's treatment is the comprehensive education of patients and their families about the disorder. It should be emphasized to the patient that these are psychobiologic disorders that involve altered biochemical states in the brain, and that episodes can be triggered by adverse events and stresses in the environment but may occur spontaneously as well. Each patient should be urged to become an expert on his or her own disorder, concentrating on how it manifests and what early signs and symptoms may herald an impending manic or depressive episode. The patient and the family must be urged to take on the responsibility for the early recognition of the impending episode, since the earlier a patient presents for treatment, the easier it is to remediate the episode. The absolute necessity of medication compliance must be emphasized, and the patient must understand thoroughly the need to take the medications precisely as prescribed and to be aware of side effects and of the potential medical sequelae from the medications.

The counseling and therapeutic techniques the physician uses in dealing with patients who are suffering acute manic or depressive episodes are simple and relatively straightforward. During the acute phase of these episodes, patients respond better to short (10 to 20 min) visits one to three times per week. During these visits the general focus is on monitoring the medication and side effects, but it is also essential that the physician be very reassuring and supportive to the patient. Because patients are functioning essentially in an altered state secondary to the depressive or manic episode, the treatment must be sustained by the physician's optimism and knowledge that, with time, these episodes can be abated or successfully terminated if the right medication and dose are prescribed. Virtually all the mood-stabilizing and -ameliorating psychotropic medications have a significant delay between the time the patient begins the medication and the time of achieving full therapeutic benefits. It is during this time that supportive reassurance and encouragement from the physician is particularly important in sustaining the patient in treatment.

There are approximately 30,000 suicides a year in this country, and clinical surveys have indicated that approximately 70 percent of these patients have major affective disorders. Suicidal ideation is one of the important symptoms that accompany major depression, in both bipolar and unipolar disorders; considerations of suicidal lethality are significant components of the management of these patients. Although it is not possible to distinguish precisely between patients who will attempt suicide and those who will not, there are some factors which should be considered. Generally speaking, many experts agree that patients who have given detailed thought to the method of suicide, who have concomitant alcoholism or drug abuse, and who are socially isolated with few (if any) social supports, in addition to elderly males and patients with terminal medical illnesses, have a greater potential risk for suicide. On the other hand, all of the above characteristics lack true specificity in the assessment of suicidal risk. However, one of the most important risk factors, recently identified, is the presence of an undiagnosed and untreated mental disorder, especially a mood disorder.

Once the acute depressive or manic episode is under control, the switch from supportive to more insight-oriented psychotherapy is a useful adjunct to the pharmacotherapy. Recent studies have established that the combination of psychotherapy with pharmacotherapy is significantly better than either of these two modalities alone. There is also evidence that three types of brief specific psychotherapy, cognitive, behavioral, and interpersonal psychotherapy, specifically designed to treat depression, can be successfully used in the treatment of mild to moderate depressive disorders. However, learning to become a competent psychotherapist in using one of these forms of psychotherapy, requires considerable training and experience to achieve results comparable to those obtained with the relatively simple administration of an antidepressant. Nevertheless, it is recommended that the nonpsychiatric physician rely primarily on the antidepressants or lithium (depending upon the disorder being treated) in combination with educational and supportive psychotherapeutic approaches in the management of patients with major affective disorders (see Chap. 369).

SCHIZOPHRENIC DISORDERS[2]

Schizophrenic disorders are serious mental illnesses that have a duration of 6 months or more and cause significant social, vocational, and personal disability and suffering. The schizophrenic patient often appears to be bizarre, inappropriate, and mentally impaired. Despite its stereotypic presentation, perhaps no other psychiatric disorder has proved as vexing and difficult to define, identify, and treat.

Schizophrenia has a lifetime prevalence rate of about 1 percent across all cultures. In the United States alone there are perhaps 2 million affected individuals who often become ill in their late teenage years and in the third decade of life. Poor outcome frequently leads to extensive and long-term disability, and schizophrenia accounts for a staggering estimated $20 billion per year of lost productivity in 1975 dollars. Most patients with schizophrenic disorders also cause major perturbations for family and social support systems, adding to the economic losses and the toll of human misery. Cumulatively, these factors make schizophrenia one of the most costly and vexing health problems.

DEFINITION AND CLINICAL MANIFESTATIONS In 1919, Emil Kraepelin first made the distinction between dementia praecox, a psychotic illness with progressive deterioration, and manic depressive psychosis. Kraepelin noted, however, that about 13 percent of patients with dementia praecox did not have an inevitably deteriorating outcome, and this favorable outcome has significantly increased largely due to the development and use of antipsychotic medications. Eugen Bleuler concentrated on the putative underlying psychological splitting of personality functions in his classic paper on the "group of schizophrenias." Bleuler's emphasis was on the "four As" of schizophrenia: *a*utism, flattened *a*ffect, loose *a*ssociations, and *am*bivalence. Other authors have focused on specific symptoms of schizophrenia, such as the sense of being influenced by others and feelings of being controlled by outside forces. To date, research has yet to identify specific and inevitably pathognomonic signs or symptoms of the schizophrenic disorders.

According to DSM-IIIR, after the first and most central criterion of psychotic symptoms is met (see Table 368-4), the schizophrenic individual must show deterioration from a previous level of functioning in such areas as work, social relations, and self-care. The disorder is not attributable to other diagnoses such as mood disorder with psychotic features or organically induced syndromes. Finally, continuous signs of the illness should be present for 6 months at some point during the individual's life with some signs of illness at the time of diagnosis. There may be prodromal, active, and/or residual phases of the illness that are not always clearly demarcated. Prodromal or residual symptoms are somewhat nonspecific and may consist of isolation; marked psychosocial impairment; peculiar behavior; impaired personal hygiene and grooming; blunted, flat, or inappropriate affect; digressive, vague, over-elaborate, circumstantial, or metaphorical speech; odd or bizarre ideation or magical thinking; and unusual perceptual experiences.

TABLE 368-4 Diagnosis of schizophrenic disorders

A Presence of characteristic psychotic symptoms in active phase, either *1*, *2*, or *3* for at least 1 week (unless symptoms are successfully treated):
- *1* Two of the following:
  - Delusions
  - Prominent hallucinations
  - Incoherence or marked loosening of associations
  - Catatonic behavior
  - Flat or grossly inappropriate affect
- *2* Bizarre delusions
- *3* Prominent hallucinations of a voice with content having no apparent relation to depression or elation, or a voice keeping up a running commentary on the person's behavior or thoughts, or two or more voices conversing with each other

B During the course of disturbance, functioning in areas such as work, social relations, and self-care markedly below highest level achieved before onset of disturbance.

C Schizoaffective disorder and mood disorder with psychotic features have been ruled out.

D Continuous signs of disturbance for at least 6 months. This period must include an active phase (of at least 1 week, or less if symptoms have been successfully treated) during which there were psychotic symptoms characteristic of schizophrenia (see *A* above), with or without a prodromal or residual phase.

E It cannot be established that an organic factor initiated and maintained the disturbance.

F If a history of autistic disorder exists, the additional diagnosis of schizophrenia can be made only if prominent delusions or hallucinations are also present.

SOURCE: Adapted from DSM-IIIR.

[2] By David L. Braff.

The DSM-IIIR lists four major types of schizophrenic disorders:

1 *Catatonic.* A relatively rare type with features of stupor, rigidity, excitement, or posturing.
2 *Disorganized.* A type characterized by incoherence and flat or grossly disorganized affect.
3 *Paranoid.* A type featuring preoccupation with suspiciousness and one or more systematized delusions.
4 *Undifferentiated.* A type of disorder with prominent delusions, hallucinations, incoherence, or disorganized behavior, not meeting the criteria for the other three types (see DSM-IIIR for more detailed descriptions).

This emphasis on subtypes carries forward Bleuler's notion of the "group of schizophrenias." There is moderate support for a paranoid/nonparanoid dichotomy as being important in schizophrenia. In an attempt to reduce diagnostic heterogeneity, researchers have identified "type I" schizophrenic patients with a predominance of "positive" symptoms (e.g., hallucinations, paranoid ideation), normal cerebral ventricular size, and symptoms that respond to the hypothesized dopaminergic-blocking effects of antipsychotic drugs. In contrast, "type II" schizophrenic patients seem similar to Kraepelin's dementia praecox patients. Type II patients show a predominance of "negative" symptoms (e.g., anhedonia, social withdrawal, asociality), neuropsychological impairment, and possibly increased cerebral ventricular volume; they do not respond well to antipsychotic medications, but seem to display a "deficit state." The course of the illness is variable, from "in remission" to "chronic."

DIFFERENTIAL DIAGNOSIS Schizophrenic patients have no unique or pathognomonic signs and symptoms; at times, this makes the diagnosis difficult. DSM-IIIR separates psychotic illnesses by a durational criterion into *brief reactive psychoses* lasting 2 weeks or less, *schizophreniform* disorders lasting between 2 weeks and 6 months, and *schizophrenic disorders* lasting more than 6 months. While these distinctions are practical and heuristic, the scientific basis for such a durational criterion is poorly documented. In addition, an acute manic patient may be difficult to distinguish from the schizophrenic patient, especially on a cross-sectional as opposed to longitudinal basis. To complicate matters further, the initial clinical appearance of a patient intoxicated with phencyclidine (PCP) or amphetamines may also be indistinguishable from that of the paranoid schizophrenic patient. It appears then that many functional and organic states may lead to a final common pathway of psychotic symptoms. The diagnosis can only be established reliably by a broad-based multifactorial approach utilizing neurobiologic data (e.g., toxicologic screens, genetic history) and psychosocial data (e.g., premorbid adjustment status) obtained both acutely and over time. Despite these problems, the DSM-IIIR criteria for schizophrenic disorders have undergone extensive and successful field trials for reliability and validity. In general, clinicians using the DSM-IIIR criteria can accurately and consistently diagnose schizophrenia.

PREDISPOSING, PRECIPITATING, AND SUSTAINING FACTORS IN SCHIZOPHRENIA Factors that contribute to the development of schizophrenia can be analyzed in terms of predisposing, precipitating, and sustaining factors. These factors may be analyzed in terms of neuroanatomic and biochemical factors and neurophysiologic, psychophysiologic, intrapsychic, interpersonal, social, and socioeconomic factors. In a complex, multifactorial disorder such as schizophrenia, these neurobiologic and psychosocial factors should be seen as interactive rather than as competing or mutually exclusive. This approach is analogous to comprehensive analyses of diabetes mellitus or hypertension, which also have contributions based on genetics, receptor physiology, and physiologic, familial, psychosocial, and a myriad of other conceptually diverse factors. Within this context, predisposing factors are linked to etiologic variables, precipitating factors are related to the onset of pathophysiology, and sustaining factors are linked to outcome variables.

Etiology GENETIC FACTORS It is clear from twin, family, and adoptive studies that schizophrenia has a significant genetic basis. Monozygotic twins have roughly a 65 percent or greater concordance rate for schizophrenia, whereas dizygotic twins have a 12 percent concordance rate. Other family studies show that the morbid risk for developing schizophrenia is 5 to 10 percent if one parent is schizophrenic. This figure rises to 46 percent or more if both parents are schizophrenics. Second-degree relatives of schizophrenics run a 2 to 4 percent risk of developing the illness compared to a risk of 1 to 2 percent in the general population.

Adoption studies reveal that these risk factors are largely genetically linked and are not primarily due to the "schizophrenogenic" psychosocial environment of certain families. Still, these figures are fraught with methodologic complexities. For example, reflecting the probable complex mode of inheritance, 89 percent of schizophrenics do not have a parent who is schizophrenic. Eighty-one percent of schizophrenics do not have either a schizophrenic sibling or parent. The appropriate model with which to explain these figures is complex and may include a weighted polygenic model or other sophisticated interpretations of genetic theory. Most recently, there has been an explosion of new knowledge about the genetics of schizophrenia, featuring molecular studies and linkages to chromosome 5 and possibly X (see the entire vol. 15, no. 3, of *Schizophrenia Bulletin,* 1989, and Crow et al.).

The *stress-diathesis model* hypothesizes that there is a vulnerability which is inherited in schizophrenia-prone individuals. These vulnerable individuals are at high risk for developing schizophrenia under certain stressful circumstances. Studies of high-risk children with one or two schizophrenic parents indicate that such children may have a significantly increased incidence of morbidity in utero, at birth, and in the perinatal period. In addition, these infants and children may have psychophysiologic lability, attentional dysfunction, and specific motor disturbances. A number of human and animal studies suggest that such labile attentional mechanisms may result partly or largely from instabilities and increased activity of the mesolimbic and mesocortical dopaminergic systems that have significant connections to the frontal cortex. The literature on neurophysiologically labile and vulnerable children seems to tie the genetic, dopaminergic, and attentional dysfunction hypotheses together. According to the stress-diathesis model, a host of stressful factors may precipitate a psychotic state in a high-risk individual. These factors include intoxication with PCP or amphetamines as well as more nonspecific factors such as medical illnesses and psychosocial life events with concomitant general stress. Further, specific hallucinogens such as lysergic acid diethylamide (LSD) may precipitate a psychotic episode that is ultimately indistinguishable from a schizophrenic disorder. Lastly, there have been a number of hypotheses that a viral vector or early developmental abnormalities may be important as etiologic agents in a least some cases of schizophrenic disorders.

PSYCHOSOCIAL FACTORS There are many psychosocial hypotheses concerning the creation of a predisposition or vulnerability to developing schizophrenia. Empirical support for most of these hypotheses is variable and far from definitive.

In the vulnerable individual, schizophrenia is seen as having its onset in a critical developmental period. The teenager may attempt to leave home and separate from family members for school or work reasons. The onset is often, but not invariably, insidious. In terms of psychosocial approaches to schizophrenia, there is felt to be a developmental or intrapsychic deficit in the vulnerable individual. Once set into motion, the psychosis passes through a series of stages leading to the final common pathway of a psychotic state.

Despite much theorizing, there is no inevitable schizophrenia-prone personality type, although at least a small but significant percentage of schizoid, paranoid, and schizotypal personality-disordered individuals do seem to be vulnerable to developing schizophrenic disorders. In the 1960s, a more family-systems-oriented view emerged. An example of this approach is the "double-bind" hypothesis of Bateson and coworkers who analyzed the formal communications patterns in "schizophrenogenic" families. In this view, communications content is less important than the frequently conflicting and self-contradictory form of communications style of schizophrenic patients' families. It remains unclear whether these familial factors are a cause or a result of having a schizophrenic child in the family. As the importance of biologic factors in schizophrenia have become clearer, family psychosocial factors have been seen more as secondary or epiphenomenal factors.

Psychosocial researchers have also examined the importance of socioeconomic factors in schizophrenia. Lower socioeconomic status correlates with a higher incidence of schizophrenia. There are two possible interpretations of these data. First, there may be a "social drift" of vulnerable individuals to lower socioeconomic status. The second hypothesis is more etiologic—socioeconomic stresses may precipitate schizophrenic episodes, especially in vulnerable individuals.

Pathophysiology NEUROTRANSMITTERS AND NEUROPEPTIDES A number of neurobiologic factors have been correlated with schizophrenic episodes. Which neurobiologic systems underlie the acute psychotic symptoms? Currently, the predominant neurotransmitter hypothesis explaining the pathophysiology of schizophrenic disorders involves dopaminergic overactivity. Evidence supporting the *dopamine hypothesis* comes from several sources. First, the potency of all antipsychotic medications can be roughly predicted by their dopaminergic-blocking capacity. Second, mesolimbic dopamine plays a role in attentional mechanisms and stimulus filtering. When stimulus-filtering mechanisms break down, there is a collapse of the information-processing capacity of the individual, with resulting sensory inundation, cognitive fragmentation, and symptoms of thought disorder.

Despite this support, the dopamine theory of schizophrenia is fraught with complexities when compared with the catecholamine theory of the affective disorders. Affective disorders hypothetically (and oversimplistically) reflect a decrease in norepinephrine tone in hypothalamic nuclei leading to a final common pathway of neurovegetative symptoms. In schizophrenia, there seems to be increased dopamine tone in critical subcortical pathways leading to cognitive fragmentation, thought disorder, and clinical impairment; the impairment and the clinical symptoms are quite complex and highly variable. In this framework, affective disorders may be seen as impinging on the diencephalic "core" of the brain, whereas schizophrenia is conceptualized as a disorder of the mesolimbic-frontal cortical mantle. It is doubtful if any "one neurotransmitter" theory of any psychiatric disorder can reflect the interactive complexity of various neurobiologic and psychosocial systems, although such theories may be useful.

The hypothesis of dopamine overactivity in schizophrenia is generally characterized as a static theory. In reality, dopamine tone is related in a dynamic and variable manner to gamma-aminobutyric acid, serotonin, and other neurotransmitters that are functionally arrayed in a cascade of important brain systems, such as the dorsolateral prefrontal cortex, mesial temporal cortex, nucleus accumbens, ventral pallidum, and the hippocampus. Longer-term correlates of schizophrenia may also involve alterations of neuropeptides with their longer latency and response effects on behavior. At an eletrophysiologic level, it has been hypothesized that the initial disturbance in schizophrenia is an aberrant (perhaps excitotoxic-induced) temporal lobe focus that perturbs the homeostasis of the dopamine system. All of these theories are receiving critical experiment scrutiny.

NEUROPATHOLOGIC CHANGES The use of computed tomography (CT) and magnetic resonance imaging (MRI) has been widely employed in studies of schizophrenic patients. Initial reports indicated that a minority of schizophrenic patients had abnormally increased ventricle-brain ratios, reflecting increased ventricular fluid volume associated with brain atrophy. Subsequent studies in identical twins have confirmed increased ventricular size in schizophrenic patients, supporting the contention that schizophrenia is accompanied by brain atrophy. It is quite possible that type II patients have a disorder that is distinct and associated with poor medication response and poor clinical outcome. Positron emission tomography (PET) data reveal patterns of decreased frontal lobe activity in schizophrenia (hypofrontality) that seem important, especially in view of the close relationship of dopamine activity and frontal lobe function. Future PET studies utilizing new ligands will undoubtedly add to the knowledge of dopamine and other neurotransmitters in the schizophrenic disorders.

PSYCHOPHYSIOLOGY AND INFORMATION PROCESSING Important insights into the pathophysiology of schizophrenia have also been generated by psychophysiologic and information-processing studies. Individuals at high risk for developing schizophrenia and patients with a schizophrenic disorder are frequently psychophysiologically labile and vulnerable to being inundated by stimuli. The proposed mechanism for such vulnerability is an impairment in an individual's ability to screen out irrelevant stimuli and an associated inability to habituate to externally and internally generated cues. Ultimately, this dysfunction, which has been linked to dopamine overactivity in humans and animals, leads to an information-processing overload. The affected person becomes inundated with stimuli and displays cognitive fragmentation and thought disorder. Using attentional tasks, skin conductance habituation, and other measures, investigators have increasingly underscored the importance of these dysfunctions in the schizophrenic disorders. New techniques, such as magnetoencephalography, also offer exciting possibilities for specifying the locus and type of brain disturbance characteristic of the various types of schizophrenic disorders.

Treatment and outcome NEUROBIOLOGIC FACTORS Five-year follow-up studies show that 60 percent of schizophrenic individuals have social recovery and half of those are employed. Thirty percent are handicapped and 10 percent remain hospitalized. This pattern of outcome seems still to be generally accurate. Which factors determine the outcome of the schizophrenic disorders are not clear. It is commonly stated that the outcome of schizophrenia is better when disorientation, affective symptoms, and acute onset are present. The outcome of schizophrenic disorders is thought to be poorer when the patient is well-oriented and has fewer affective symptoms and when the onset is insidious.

The outcome of schizophrenic disorders has been greatly improved by the use of potent and efficacious antipsychotic medications, such as the phenothiazines (see Chap. 369). Studies indicate that antipsychotic medications (often expressed in terms of chlorpromazine equivalents) act selectively against specific target symptoms that are similar to the "positive" symptoms of type I schizophrenia, which include hallucinations and psychotic agitation. In contrast to these responsive target symptoms, antipsychotic medications may not necessarily improve "negative" symptoms such as anhedonia and social withdrawal. The primary treatment modalities for the acute schizophrenic disorders are antipsychotic medication along with psychosocial therapies. The typical schizophrenic patient usually requires at least the equivalent of 600 to 800 mg per day of chlorpromazine administered for 4 to 6 weeks, although higher doses are frequently necessary. Maintenance doses of antipsychotic medications in lower doses and given on a continuous or intermittent basis are often required to prevent relapse.

Antipsychotic medications alter dopaminergic-cholinergic balance in nigrostriatal structures (via dopamine blockade) so that acute extrapyramidal side effects are induced (e.g. dystonia, motor restlessness). These side effects can be treated with anticholinergic medications that restore dopaminergic-cholinergic balance. Aliphatic phenothiazines (such as chlorpromazine) with inherent anticholinergic properties cause fewer extrapyramidal side effects but induce more anticholinergic side effects, such as hypotension or blurred vision. Additionally, blood dyscrasias, liver toxicity, and other idiosyncratic reactions can occur. Also, the long-term use of antipsychotic medications may induce nigrostriatal damage and tardive dyskinesia, a long-lasting and potentially disabling motor syndrome (see Chaps. 25 and 369). Thus the search for new antipsychotic medications with more selective (i.e., nonnigrostriatal) sites of action is critically important for the pharmacologic treatment of schizophrenia. Drugs, such as clozaryl, have been postulated (but not proven) to have such selective properties.

PSYCHOSOCIAL FACTORS The outcome of schizophrenic patients can be divided into the semi-independent axes of symptoms, rehospitalization, social function, and vocational function. It is possible to treat the specific psychotic symptoms of a schizophrenic individual (affecting the symptomatic axis of outcome), but the patient may be left with major psychosocial deficits (the social axis of outcome). Antipsychotic medications should thus be combined with sensitive psychosocial management including, where appropriate, individual and group psychotherapy, family counseling, and vocational rehabilitation in order to maximize therapeutic outcome and to restore the patient to the premorbid level of adjustment. For example, returning an acutely treated schizophrenic patient to a home filled with hostility, criticisms, and emotional overinvolvement (the so-called high-expressed-emotion family) without the benefit of family therapy is poor psychosocial management and may lead to relapse and poor outcome. Family counseling is often a critical determinant of therapeutic outcome in the schizophrenic disorders.

ANXIETY DISORDERS[3]

Anxiety is a common emotion and as such is often a normal response to the vicissitudes of life. In its mild forms, anxiety may be adaptive. A little anxiety, for example, helps a student prepare for examinations. In its extreme forms, however, anxiety is incapacitating or terrifying. High anxiety may cause the same student to lose concentration, memory, or even his or her voice.

Physicians observe anxiety most commonly in patients experiencing an acute external stress. Although short-term treatment with antianxiety or sedative drugs, such as benzodiazepines, has a place in the management of such patients, physicians often can offer more help by their presence, reassurances, and attitude. Anxiety states often resolve spontaneously with time, although clinicians should be aware that acute stress can lead to chronic anxiety or posttraumatic stress disorder.

The word *anxiety* has more precise diagnostic meaning in psychiatry. It refers to both *paroxysmal* and *persistent* psychological feelings (dread, irritability, ruminations) and physiologic changes (dyspnea, sweating, insomnia, trembling) which endure over time and impair normal functioning. These are often chronic disorders in which symptoms persist in the absence of obvious contemporaneous external stresses or in which the degree of symptoms seems out of proportion to the degree of external stress. Anxiety disorders were formerly lumped together under the term "anxiety neurosis." It is now recognized that a number of relatively distinct syndromes exist under the general rubric of anxiety disorders (Table 368-5).

TABLE 368-5 Classification of anxiety disorders

Anxiety states:
- Panic disorder
- Generalized anxiety disorder
- Obsessive-compulsive disorder
- Posttraumatic stress disorder

Phobic disorders:
- Agoraphobia (with and without panic attacks)
- Social phobia
- Simple phobia

PANIC DISORDER Definition The cardinal feature of panic disorder is the sudden, unexpected, and often overwhelming feeling of terror and apprehension accompanied by somatic symptoms in multiple organ systems such as dyspnea, palpitations, and faintness. The symptoms and signs of panic disorder are similar to those occurring during intense physical exertion or in a life-threatening situation.

Incidence and epidemiology Panic disorder is estimated to occur in 1 to 2 percent of the population and is equally divided between the sexes. The most frequent age of onset of panic attack is the late teen years and early twenties. Panic disorders tend to be familial, and both panic disorder and affective disorder often coexist in the same family. If an individual has a diagnosed panic disorder, up to 18 percent of first-degree relatives also will have panic disorder. Furthermore, twin studies demonstrate a greater incidence in monozygotic twins, suggesting that panic anxiety may have a genetic basis.

Clinical features A typical panic attack often begins abruptly and without warning while a patient is involved in a relatively nonthreatening and nonstressful activity, like entering a store, driving a car, or sitting at a desk working. The patient becomes flushed, lightheaded, and sweaty and is overwhelmed by feelings of terror, apprehension, and impending doom. Dyspnea may occur with a subjective sense of choking or smothering, and palpitations or chest pain are often so severe that patients believe they are having a heart attack or are dying. The symptoms of panic attacks usually peak in less than 10 min and resolve in 20 to 30 min. Most patients experiencing their first panic attack obtain help, sometimes going to a doctor's office or emergency room, but the fear has usually subsided by this time. Fatigue or exhaustion frequently follows a panic attack, and the patient may sleep.

Patients with panic disorder may constitute as many as 15 percent of patients who consult cardiologists and 5 to 25 percent of patients in outpatient psychiatric settings.

The DSM-IIIR criteria for diagnosis of panic disorder are listed in Table 368-6.

Complications After repeated panic attacks, most patients develop some degree of anticipatory anxiety and try to avoid those situations that have been paired with panic attacks in the past. Many patients, particularly females by a 2:1 ratio to males, develop *agoraphobia*—an irrational fear of being alone or in public places. Without effective treatment, the course of panic attacks and agoraphobia leads to an increasingly restricted life-style marked by preoccupation with avoiding those situations that might trigger an attack. Cases of severe panic disorder with agoraphobia may result

TABLE 368-6 Diagnostic criteria for panic disorder

A At some time during the disturbance, one or more panic attacks (discrete periods of intense fear or discomfort) have occurred that were (1) unexpected, i.e., did not occur immediately before or on exposure to a situation that almost always caused anxiety. and (2) not triggered by situations in which the person was the focus of others' attention.

B Either four attacks, as defined in criterion *A*, have occurred within a 4-week period, or one or more attacks have been followed by a period of at least a month of persistent fear of having another attack.

C At least four of the following symptoms developed during at least one of the attacks:*
- *1* Shortness of breath (dyspnea) or smothering sensations
- *2* Dizziness, unsteady feelings, or faintness
- *3* Palpitations or accelerated heart rate (tachycardia)
- *4* Trembling or shaking
- *5* Sweating
- *6* Choking
- *7* Nausea or abdominal distress
- *8* Depersonalization or derealization
- *9* Numbness or tingling sensations (paresthesias)
- *10* Flushes (hot flashes) or chills
- *11* Chest pain or discomfort
- *12* Fear of dying
- *13* Fear of going crazy or of doing something uncontrolled

D During at least some of the attacks, at least four of the *C* symptoms developed suddenly and increased in intensity within 10 min of the beginning of the first *C* symptom noticed in the attack.

E It cannot be established that an organic factor initiated and maintained the disturbance, e.g., amphetamine or caffeine intoxication, hyperthyroidism.

* Attacks nvolving four or more symptoms are panic attacks; attacks involving fewer than four symptoms are limited symptom attacks.

NOTE: Mitral valve prolapse may be an associated condition, but does not preclude a diagnosis of panic disorder.

SOURCE: Adapted from DSM-IIIR.

[3] By Karen Thatcher Britton, S. Craig Risch, and J. Christian Gillin.

in patients remaining house-bound for one or more decades, convinced that leaving the house will induce an attack.

Other complications of panic disorder include major depressive syndrome, higher death rates from both suicide and cardiovascular disease, and drug and alcohol dependency. Losses from unemployment and health care costs are estimated to exceed $100 million a year.

Laboratory findings Lactate infusions precipitate panic attacks in vulnerable individuals, although at present this is only used as a test in research paradigms. One study employing positron emission tomography demonstrated a decrease rate of blood flow in the left parahippocampus during panic attacks.

Differential diagnosis Many patients with panic disorder complain of chest pain, cardiac extrasystoles, and palpitations. The diagnostic challenge is to differentiate anxiety with cardiovascular symptoms from the organic diseases it mimics. Because there may be an increased prevalence of mitral valve prolapse in patients with panic disorder this condition should be investigated; however, in the vast majority of patients with panic disorder, no significant cardiac pathology is ever found.

Other diagnostic possibilities include both hyperthyroidism and hypothyroidism, a catecholamine-secreting pheochromocytoma, complex partial seizures, and hypoglycemia. Drug ingestions (amphetamine, cocaine, caffeine, sympathomimetic nasal decongestants) and drug withdrawal (alcohol, barbiturates, opiates, minor tranquilizers) may produce symptoms that simulate panic attacks.

Etiology and pathophysiology The etiology of panic disorders is uncertain and involves an interplay of multiple psychological and biologic determinants.

PSYCHOLOGICAL FACTORS In the psychodynamic model, anxiety is considered to be a response to the threatened emergence into consciousness of painful, unacceptable thoughts, impulses, or desires, i.e., psychological conflicts from the past and present. The anxiety response is an attempt to mobilize and ward off danger to the self.

PHYSIOLOGIC FACTORS Clinical and experimental evidence point to the involvement of noradrenergic neurons, particularly those projecting rostrally from the locus coeruleus in the upper brainstem, in the pathophysiology of panic disorder. Three lines of evidence suggest that hyperactivity of noradrenergic pathways may play a role in the pathogenesis of panic. First, the clinical manifestations of panic attacks are similar to those induced by sudden, massive stimulation of beta-adrenergic receptors. Second, isoproterenol hydrochloride, a beta agonist, and yohimbine, an alpha-adrenergic receptor antagonist that increases noradrenergic function, produce signs and symptoms that mimic panic attacks. Third, clinical studies support a role for noradrenergic beta blockers, such as propranolol, in successful treatment of pathologic anxiety.

Another avenue of investigation is based on the finding that infusions of sodium lactate into patients with a history of panic disorder often provoke a panic attack indistinguishable from a spontaneous one. Normal subjects without a history of panic disorder are unaffected. In addition, patients whose panic attacks are controlled by antidepressants are protected against lactate-induced panic attacks. Inhalation of CO_2 by susceptible persons also precipitates anxiety and panic. Although the mechanism of lactate's effect is unclear, the findings appear to have diagnostic usefulness and provide a good model of anxiety for further clinical investigation.

Overall, the evidence suggests that the main contribution to panic disorder may be a genetic vulnerability to a biologic disease state. Over time, panic attacks may become associated with environmental events that by themselves are able to elicit symptoms. The particular constellation of environmental stimuli that precipitate panic attacks may be influenced by past experience or particular psychological conflicts. A full understanding of the etiology of anxiety probably will require knowledge of a combination of genetic, biologic, and psychological factors.

Treatment A comprehensive treatment program combines both pharmacologic and psychotherapeutic approaches. The first step is to block the attacks pharmacologically, usually with tricyclic antidepressants or monoamine oxidase inhibitors (see Chap. 369). These drugs have 80 to 90 percent effectiveness in the treatment and prevention of spontaneous panic attacks. New antianxiety medications such as alprazolam given in high dose are as effective as antidepressants, have fewer side effects, and work within 1 or 2 days. Other benzodiazepines have not proved uniformly efficacious. Antidepressant medication may take 4 to 6 weeks before being effective. Beta blockers, e.g., propranolol or atenolol, may lock the peripheral manifestations of the panic attacks but have proved ineffective in preventing the psychic fear or panic and may also predispose to or worsen depressive symptomatology. Clonidine may also block panic manifestations, but its efficacy is usually only transient. Relapse is common on discontinuance of pharmacotherapy. More recently, claims have been made for the antipanic capacities of the serotonin-uptake inhibitor fluoxetine.

For some patients with panic disorder, particularly those with debilitating agoraphobia, psychotherapy is indicated. The exact form of psychotherapy needed is controversial, but approaches that seek to understand the anxiety and encourage the patient to confront the feared situations are the most effective.

GENERALIZED ANXIETY DISORDER **Definition** Unlike patients with panic disorders whose symptoms come on suddenly, patients with generalized anxiety disorder experience persistent diffuse anxiety, without the specific symptoms that characterize phobic disorders, panic disorders, or obsessive-compulsive disorders. Although the symptoms and signs of anxiety vary from individual to individual, common signs are motor tension, autonomic hyperactivity, apprehensive expectation, and vigilance. Patients with generalized anxiety disorder do not report acute fluctuations in anxiety level and autonomic arousal characteristic of panic disorder.

Incidence and epidemiology The prevalence of generalized anxiety disorder has been estimated at 2 to 3 percent, but precise epidemiologic data are lacking because of variations in definition and case acquisition. In patients who seek professional help for anxiety, women outnumber men by two to one. There is no evidence to support the popular belief that anxiety is related to the stresses of modern society. In contrast to panic disorder, studies showing a familial or genetic basis for generalized anxiety disorder are inconclusive.

The diagnostic criteria for generalized anxiety disorder are listed in Table 368-7.

Complications In contrast to panic disorder, generalized anxiety disorder has a more chronic course and favorable outcome. However, the symptoms are persistent and can lead to secondary depression and alcohol and drug abuse, especially of benzodiazepines.

Differential diagnosis Symptoms and signs resembling anxiety may occur with a number of medical disorders including coronary artery disease, thyroid disease, and drug intoxication or withdrawal. Anxiety may be present in other psychiatric disorders such as depression, schizophrenia, and organic mental states. Diagnosis of these conditions is essential, since the treatment of them is different from that of the anxiety disorders. Because patients with generalized anxiety may abuse alcohol or antianxiety medications to reduce or block anxiety, a careful history of drug use is important. Although the overall degree of psychosocial or occupational impairment is generally less than that noted for the other anxiety disorders, chronic anxiety is an uncomfortable emotion that can restrict a person's ability to enjoy a normal life.

Etiology and pathophysiology One approach to understanding the etiology of anxiety has been to delineate the mechanisms by which antianxiety drugs exert their therapeutic effects. High affinity, stereospecific receptors for benzodiazepines have been discovered that appear to be coupled to the receptor for the inhibitory neurotransmitter GABA. Considerable evidence supports the hypothesis that the anxiolytic actions of the benzodiazepines are mediated through this receptor.

These findings have several implications. First, the characterization of a benzodiazepine receptor complex implies the existence of a

TABLE 368-7 Diagnostic criteria for generalized anxiety disorder

A Unrealistic or excessive anxiety and worry (apprehensive expectation) about two or more life circumstances, e.g., worry about possible misfortune to one's child (who is in no danger) and worry about finances (for no good reason), for a period of 6 months or longer, during which the person has been bothered more days than not by these concerns. In children and adolescents, this may take the form of anxiety and worry about academic, athletic, and social performance.
B If another anxiety disorder is present, the focus of the anxiety and worry in *A* is unrelated to it, e.g., the anxiety or worry is not about having a panic attack (as in panic disorder), being embarrassed in public (as in social phobia), being contaminated (as in obsessive-compulsive disorder), or gaining weight (as in anorexia nervosa).
C The disturbance does not occur only during the course of a mood disorder or a psychotic disorder.
D At least 6 of the following 18 symptoms are often present when anxious (do not include symptoms present only during panic attacks):
Motor tension
1 Trembling, twitching, or feeling shaky
2 Muscle tension, aches, or soreness
3 Restlessness
4 Easy fatigability
Autonomic hyperactivity
5 Shortness of breath or smothering sensations
6 Palpitations or accelerated heart rate (tachycardia)
7 Sweating, or cold clammy hands
8 Dry mouth
9 Dizziness or lightheadedness
10 Nausea, diarrhea, or other abdominal distress
11 Flushes (hot flashes) or chills
12 Frequent urination
13 Trouble swallowing or "lump in throat"
Vigilance and scanning
14 Feeling keyed up or on edge
15 Exaggerated startle response
16 Difficulty concentrating or "mind going blank" because of anxiety
17 Trouble falling or staying asleep
18 Irritability
E It cannot be established that an organic factor initiated and maintained the disturbance, e.g., hyperthyroidism, caffeine intoxication.

SOURCE: Adapted from DSM-IIIR.

natural (endogenous) ligand for the receptor. Conceivably, the levels of this substance might correlate with individual differences in anxiety or emotionality or tolerance to stress. Second, pharmacologic antagonists of this receptor block the effects of benzodiazepines and may induce anxiety, a finding that implicates these mechanisms in pathologic anxiety. Third, new *anxiolytic* compounds that influence benzodiazepine receptor binding are being discovered that have fewer and potentially less serious side effects. The possibility exists that *anxiogenic* substances may also be found in the brain. Though major questions remain to be answered, these advances have opened new avenues for understanding the origins and management of anxiety.

Treatment Because feelings of anxiety are normal human emotions with adaptive value, a decision must be made before any treatment or medication is considered concerning whether or not the manifestations of anxiety are within the normal range. There is no justification for the use of anxiolytic drugs in anxiety if it is considered to be within the normal limits of human experience.

Once a decision is made to treat, consideration should be given first to modalities of nonpharmacologic intervention, including supportive or intensive psychotherapy. These approaches may modify maladaptive life-styles, cognition, and avoidance behaviors. Behavior therapy aims at teaching the patient practical means to reduce anxiety and includes techniques like relaxation training, biofeedback, and desensitization. These techniques are of at least temporary benefit for many people.

When generalized anxiety is severe enough to warrant treatment with drugs, benzodiazepines are the agents of choice. In many patients, short courses of anxiolytic drugs (5 to 7 days) are effective, following which the drug should be discontinued. Patients should be warned about the possibility of dependence with long-term use, and the physician should make regular assessments of the need for continuation of medications. Buspirone, a nonbenzodiazepine anxiolytic, may become a drug of first choice for these patients. Although it has a delayed onset of action, it lacks many of the problems associated with the benzodiazepines, such as psychomotor impairment, physical dependence, or withdrawal symptoms.

POSTTRAUMATIC STRESS DISORDER Definition Acute and chronic psychological distress following traumatic events have long been recognized. The diagnostic criteria for posttraumatic stress disorders (PTSD), according to DSM-IIIR, are listed in Table 368-8.

PTSD is classified as either acute or chronic (or delayed). In the former, onset of symptoms begin within 6 months of the trauma, or the duration of the symptoms persists less than 6 months. In the latter, symptoms persist more than 6 months (chronic) or start more than 6 months after the trauma (delayed).

Etiology Whether or not PTSD develops appears to depend upon the nature of the trauma, the characteristics of the individual, and the context in which these events take place. The trauma can be anticipated or not, acute or chronic, constant or repetitive, due to natural events (e.g., an earthquake) or malevolence (e.g., rape, child abuse, torture). PTSD can develop in individuals who were apparently healthy, successful, and well-adjusted prior to the traumatic experiences. Among the factors which influence the development of PTSD are (1) the extent to which the individual's life-space is affected, (2) the duration of the impact, (3) the extent to which the individual perceives human malevolence behind the traumatic event (e.g., a fire attributed to arson will probably be more traumatic than one attributed to lightning), and (4) social isolation.

TABLE 368-8 Diagnostic criteria for posttraumatic stress disorder

A The person has experienced an event that is outside the range of usual human experience and that would be markedly distressing to almost anyone, e.g., serious threat to one's life or physical integrity; serious threat or harm to one's children, spouse, or other close relatives and friends; sudden destruction of one's home or community; or seeing another person who has recently been, or is being, seriously injured or killed as the result of an accident or physical violence.
B The traumatic event is persistently reexperienced in at least one of the following ways:
1 Recurrent and intrusive distressing recollections of the event (in young children, repetitive play in which themes or aspects of the trauma are expressed)
2 Recurrent distressing dreams of the event
3 Sudden acting or feeling as if the traumatic event were recurring [includes a sense of reliving the experience, illusions, hallucinations, and dissociative (flashback) episodes, even those that occur upon awakening or when intoxicated]
4 Intense psychological distress at exposure to events that symbolize or resemble an aspect of the traumatic event, including anniversaries of the trauma
C Persistent avoidance of stimuli associated with the trauma or numbing of general responsiveness (not present before the trauma), as indicated by at least three of the following:
1 Efforts to avoid thoughts or feelings associated with the trauma
2 Efforts to avoid activities or situations that arouse recollections of the trauma
3 Inability to recall an important aspect of the trauma (psychogenic amnesia)
4 Markedly diminished interest in significant activities (in young children, loss of recently acquired developmental skills such as toilet training or language skills)
5 Feeling of detachment or estrangement from others
6 Restricted range of affect, e.g., unable to have loving feelings
7 Sense of a foreshortened future, e.g., does not expect to have a career, marriage, or children, or a long life
D Persistent symptoms of increased arousal (not present before the trauma), as indicated by at least two of the following:
1 Difficulty falling or staying asleep
2 Irritability or outbursts of anger
3 Difficulty concentrating
4 Hypervigilance
5 Exaggerated startle response
6 Physiologic reactivity upon exposure to events that symbolize or resemble an aspect of the traumatic event (e.g., a woman who was raped in an elevator breaks out in a sweat when entering any elevator)
E Duration of the disturbance (symptoms in *B*, *C*, and *D*) of at least 1 month.

SOURCE: Adapted from DSM-IIIR.

Epidemiology It is difficult to gauge the extent of PTSD following a traumatic event because the studies that have been done have often followed subjects for only a short period of time, and the nature of the events is often so situation-specific. About 15 percent or more of the civilian population may experience mental distress severe enough to require treatment following a major natural disaster. For example, in a study that followed survivors of a shipboard fire for 3½ to 4½ years, one-third were found to be unable to return to sea because of psychological symptoms. Following extreme prolonged harsh conditions such as combat, prisoner-of-war camps, or Nazi death camps, a higher incidence of both acute and delayed PTSD is likely. Some evidence, based on follow-up of World War II veterans 20 years after the war, indicates an increasing incidence of new patients seeking psychiatric care for war-associated symptoms. The vicissitudes of normal aging may unmask a latent traumatic stress disorder.

Complications Anxiety, depression, alcoholism, drug abuse, impaired marital and occupational activities, and perhaps increased physical morbidity and mortality have been blamed on various forms of PTSD.

Differential diagnosis In adjustment disorder, symptoms such as reexperiencing the trauma are absent. Other considerations include major depressive disorder, generalized anxiety disorder, phobic disorder, organic mental disorders, and other conditions such as "compensation neurosis" and "postconcussion sydrome."

Prophylaxis Military experience suggests that PTSD can be prevented partially if soldiers are taught that a degree of fear and anxiety are normal concomitants of battle rather than signs of cowardice or mental illness. Furthermore, the development of chronic PTSD can often be prevented if the soldier with acute PTSD is seen close to the battle front under the principles of immediate treatment, expectancy of return to normal duties, and brevity of treatment contact.

Treatment The treatment goals of PTSD are reduction of target symptoms, prevention of chronic disability, and occupational and social rehabilitation. An important therapeutic issue is the extent to which the victim of acute PTSD should be allowed to leave the traumatic situation, to regress, and to enjoy the secondary gains of the patient role. The caretakers' unthinking natural sympathy, nurturing instincts, admiration, and, indeed, gratitude (for example, in the case of soldiers who are protecting the homeland) may be as detrimental as an unreasonably cynical, suspicious distrust of someone who is seen as trying to get attention and avoid responsibilities or hoping to collect money from the consequences of the traumatic experience. Successful treatment involves a combination of psychosocial support systems, psychotherapy, behavioral and conditioning techniques, and medications. Group therapy with others who have shared similar experiences may be beneficial.

OBSESSIVE-COMPULSIVE DISORDER Definition The major characteristics are recurrent *obsessions* (persistent intrusive thoughts) and *compulsions* (intrusive behaviors) which the patient experiences as involuntary, senseless, or repugnant. The DSM-IIIR diagnostic criteria for obsessive-compulsive disorder are listed in Table 368-9.

Common obsessions include thoughts of violence (e.g., killing a loved one), obsessive slowness, fears of germs or contamination, and doubt (e.g., a priest who worries excessively that he had not said his prayers properly). Examples of compulsions include repeated checking to be assured that something was done properly, hand washing, extreme neatness, and counting rituals, as in numbering steps while walking.

Obsessions and compulsions do not invariably coexist in the same individual. The relationship of the obsessive-compulsive disorder to obsessive or compulsive characterologic traits remains controversial.

Etiology and pathophysiology The etiology of the obsessive-compulsive state is uncertain, but it can be viewed from psychodynamic, psychosocial, and biologic perspectives. Obsessions and compulsions often seem to symbolize unconscious wishes, impulses, and fears and to reflect dynamic adaptations to unwanted aggressive or sexual urges. Biologic factors are suggested by reports of an increased incidence of obsessive-compulsive disorder in monozygotic twins and first-degree relatives of probands, of biologic markers associated with the disorder, and of favorable response to certain tricyclic antidepressants and monoamine oxidase inhibitors.

TABLE 368-9 Diagnostic criteria for obsessive-compulsive disorder

A Either obsessions or compulsions:
  1 Obsessions:
    a Recurrent and persistent ideas, thoughts, impulses, or images that are experienced, at least initially, as intrusive and senseless, e.g., a parent's having repeated impulses to kill a loved child, a religious person's having recurrent blasphemous thoughts
    b The person attempts to ignore or suppress such thoughts or impulses or to neutralize them with some other thought or action
    c The person recognizes that the obsessions are the product of his or her own mind, not imposed from without (as in thought insertion)
    d If another disorder is present, the content of the obsession is unrelated to it, e.g., the ideas, thoughts, impulses, or images are not about food in the presence of an eating disorder, about drugs in the presence of a psychoactive substance use disorder, or guilty thoughts in the presence of a major depression
  2 Compulsions:
    a Repetitive, purposeful, and intentional behaviors that are performed in response to an obsession, or according to certain rules, or in a stereotyped fashion
    b The behavior is designed to neutralize or to prevent discomfort or some dreaded event or situation; however, either the activity is not connected in a realistic way with what it is designed to neutralize or prevent, or it is clearly excessive
    c The person recognizes that his or her behavior is excessive or unreasonable (this may not be true for young children; it may no longer be true for people whose obsessions have evolved into overvalued ideas)

B The obsessions or compulsions cause marked distress, are time-consuming (take more than 1 h/d), or significantly interfere with the person's normal routine, occupational functioning, or usual social activities or relationships with others.

SOURCE: Adapted from DSM-IIIR.

Epidemiology The lifetime prevalence of obsessive-compulsive disorder, based upon interviews of the general population 18 years and older, varies between 1.9 and 3.0 percent. The prevalence tends to be slightly higher in females than males but does not vary significantly by race, education, or urbanization of area of residence.

Clinical manifestations These disorders usually begin in adolescence or young adulthood, with about 65 percent of cases beginning before age 25. They are rarely seen in children. Clear precipitants are reported in up to 60 percent of cases. Long-term prognosis appears to be variable. Some patients (perhaps 10 percent) show a chronic, unremitting course; some show periods of complete remission; the majority show an episodic course with periods of incomplete remission.

Complications Depression is probably the most common secondary problem but anxiety, avoidant behavior, alcoholism, abuse of sleeping pills and tranquilizers, and impairment of social, marital, and occupational life can be marked.

Laboratory findings No pathognomonic pathologic or laboratory abnormalities have been found.

Differential diagnosis Repetitive self-destructive behaviors, such as gambling, drinking, drug abuse, and overeating, should not be diagnosed as "obsessive-compulsive" disorder since the individual normally derives pleasure from the activity. Stereotyped behavior is also common in schizophrenia, Tourette's syndrome, and depression.

Treatment Clomipramine appears to be the most effective pharmacologic treatment for obsessive-compulsive disorder. The beneficial effects may be delayed 6 to 8 weeks, and it is most effective when specific compulsions are present. Recent reports suggest that fluoxetine, which has effects on the serotoninergic neurotransmitter system, is also successful in the treatment of some patients with obsessive-compulsive disorder.

Obsessive-compulsive patients also may respond to psychotherapeutic intervention. However, in the absence of adequate studies of psychotherapy in this disorder, it is hard to make valid generalizations about its effectiveness. Behavioral therapy can be helpful, and desensitization, flooding, implosion therapy, and aversive conditioning have all been used with variable success.

PHOBIC DISORDERS Phobic disorders comprise a group of disorders having in common persistently recurring, irrational severe anxiety of specific objects, activities, or situations with secondary avoidance behavior of the phobic stimulus. Phobias are relatively commonplace, and the diagnosis of a phobic disorder is made only when fear or avoidance behavior is a significant source of distress to the individual or interferes with social or occupational functioning.

The phobic disorders listed in DSM-IIIR include three separate disorders—agoraphobia, social phobia, and simple phobia.

Agoraphobia DEFINITION Agoraphobia, the fear of being alone or in public places (see Table 368-10), may occur rarely in the absence of panic disorder, but it is almost invariably preceded by that condition.

Social phobias DEFINITION Social phobias are persistent irrational fears and the need to avoid any situation where one might be exposed to scrutiny by others and potentially be embarrassed or humiliated. Even the possibility of such a situation evokes anticipatory anxiety. The individual is aware that this fear is excessive. Common examples are excessive fear of public speaking and anxiety induced by eating in restaurants or by any public performance. The resulting anxiety may actually impair performance and thereby potentiate the phobic disorder.

EPIDEMIOLOGY AND PATHOGENESIS Social phobias are relatively rare, and there is no evidence for a genetic or familial transmission. Social phobias presumably arise from stressful life events occurring during early development. The disorder usually begins in late childhood or early adolescence and tends to be chronic and to wax and wane in severity.

COMPLICATIONS Complications are rare and the disorder is not often incapacitating; it may lead to sedative or hypnotic drug and alcohol abuse and addiction, and to problems in professional advancement.

TREATMENT Treatment of social phobia is primarily behavioral, with use of such techniques as relaxation therapy, systematic desensitization, and related techniques. Pharmacotherapy with beta blockers, i.e., propranolol or atenolol and/or alprazolam, may also be helpful.

Simple phobia DEFINITION Simple phobias are persistent irrational fears and avoidance of specific objects or situations.

CLINICAL FEATURES The individuals experiences significant distress when confronted with the phobic stimulus or even the possibility of confrontation with the phobic stimulus and also recognizes this fear and anxiety as irrational and excessive. When confronted with the phobic stimulus the individual may experience symptoms identical to those of panic attacks. Common examples include fear of heights (acrophobia), fear of closed spaces (claustrophobia), and fear of animals. Fear of the possibility of exposure to the phobic stimulus will often cause the individual to attempt to elicit significant information, e.g., if the party or restaurant is at the top of a high-rise building; if they have a dog.

Age of onset is variable, but the disorder often begins in childhood. Simple phobias that begin in childhood may disappear without treatment, but may persist into adulthood. Although phobias are relatively common in the general population, they rarely result in significant impairment and individuals rarely seek treatment. Simple phobias are more common in women. Treatment, if required, is behavioral using relaxation therapy and systematic desensitization.

TABLE 368-10 Diagnosis of agoraphobia

A	The individual has marked fear of and thus avoids being alone or being in public places from which escape might be difficult or help not available in case of sudden incapacitation, e.g., crowds, tunnels, bridges, public transportation.
B	There is increasing constriction of normal activities until the fear or avoidance behavior dominates the individual's life.

PERSONALITY DISORDERS[4]

Personality denotes characteristic ways of thinking, feeling, behaving, and reacting to the environment. When this "psychological signature" strikes a useful balance between consistency and adaptive flexibility, we speak of personality *traits*. A personality *disorder* is said to exist when a person chronically uses certain mechanisms of coping in an inappropriate, stereotyped, and maladaptive fashion.

DIAGNOSIS OF PERSONALITY DISORDERS DSM-IIIR recognizes 11 distinctive personality disorders. These are grouped into three thematic clusters. *Paranoid, schizoid,* and *schizotypal* personality disorders are characterized by oddness or eccentricity. *Histrionic, narcissistic, antisocial,* and *borderline* personality disorders share a dramatic presentation along with self-centeredness, emotionality, and erratic behavior. Anxiety and fear underlie *avoidant, dependent, compulsive,* and *passive-aggressive* personalities.

The DSM-IIIR diagnostic classification scheme stipulates specific inclusion and exclusion criteria for diagnosis of each disorder. Since the number of specific criteria for individual disorders can be extensive, the descriptions in this chapter are highlights rather than complete expositions. The reader is referred to the DSM-IIIR for the detailed listing of the necessary signs and symptoms required to make the diagnosis of the various personality disorders.

Paranoid personality disorder People with this disorder are suspicious and hypersensitive to perceived slights and injuries. They are hypervigilant to the possibility that someone might trick or harm them and tend to be guarded and secretive and to blame others. They may be jealous and concerned with hidden meanings. They tend to exaggerate difficulties, to take offense and become hostile easily, to hold grudges, and to question the loyalty and fidelity of others.

Schizoid personality disorder Schizoid individuals are loners who seem to have little need for others. They appear emotionally cold and aloof and indifferent to praise and criticism; they lack close friendships, and may be social recluses.

In earlier nomenclatures eccentric thinking was sometimes added to the schizoid picture. DSM-IIIR, however, has split off a second category, schizotypal (see below), to describe persons whose principal difficulties are cognitive rather than interpersonal.

Schizotypal personality disorder Schizotypal persons share with schizophrenics certain eccentricities of thinking, perception, speech, and interpersonal interaction; however, the degree and pervasiveness of such "schizophrenic-like" symptomatology is not sufficient to meet diagnostic criteria for schizophrenia. Odd speech (e.g., vague, circumstantial, metaphorical), ideas of reference (inappropriately inferring that neutral events have some special relevance to the person), magical thinking, and suspiciousness can be prominent. Many schizotypal persons are also socially isolated, and this can lead to confusion with schizoid personality (see above).

Borderline personality disorder Borderline persons have been described as having "stable instability," characterized by chronic difficulty in regulating mood and interpersonal attachments and in maintaining a consistent self-image. Borderline persons can manifest impulsive behavior, some of it self-damaging (e.g., self-mutilation, suicidal behavior). Their mood is unpredictable. Some have brief outbursts of anger, irritability, sadness, and fear. Others suffer from a chronic emptiness. Despite having chaotic interpersonal relationships punctuated by intense love and hate, borderline persons generally are intolerant of being alone. The defense mechanism of "splitting" (regarding persons and events either as "all good" are "all bad") can be prominent.

Histrionic personality disorder People with a histrionic personality have seemingly intense but actually superficial relationships.

[4] By Igor Grant.

They present in a dramatic, engaging, but self-centered fashion. There is an exaggerated expression of emotions, attention seeking, craving for excitement, and a tendency to overreact. While superficially warm and charming, even sexually seductive, histrionic persons are generally perceived as shallow, inconsiderate, self-indulgent, vain, demanding, dependent, and manipulative. Some make frequent suicidal threats or attempts.

Narcissistic personality disorder The narcissistic person has an inflated sense of self-importance, and may be preoccupied with being unique, powerful, and gifted. The patient exaggerates his or her talents and contributions, seeks admiration, feels entitled to preferential treatment, and uses others to achieve a better position, while being indifferent to their feelings and needs. A rejection can produce excessive rage, inferiority, shame, or humiliation.

Antisocial personality disorder Antisocial behavior is characterized by unconcern with the rules and expectations of society and repeated violation of the rights of others. The diagnosis is limited to adults (persons under 18 with antisocial features are classified as having conduct disorder) and requires a history of antisocial behaviors that have their onset before age 15. Such behaviors include truancy, delinquency, running away from home, lying, precocious sexuality, troubles with the law, and alcohol or drug abuse. Beyond such historical considerations, the antisocial diagnosis requires current evidence of certain deviant behaviors which include irresponsibility in work, as a parent, in financial matters, and in personal behavior (e.g., recklessness, driving while intoxicated). Additionally, antisocial persons will usually commit multiple illegal acts, lie and deceive, but lack remorse for such behavior. They manifest an inability to maintain a long-term attachment to a sexual partner, and exhibit irritability and aggressiveness. Alcohol or other substance abuse is common.

Avoidant personality disorder People who are inappropriately concerned with rejection or humiliation, and for this reason avoid close ties with others, are classified as having an avoidant personality disorder. Despite being withdrawn, they give evidence for wishing that they did have intimate relations with others. In contrast with the narcissistic individual, the avoidant person tends to manifest low self-esteem and a tendency to exaggerate his or her shortcomings.

Dependent personality disorder Dependent people allow others to assume responsibility for major aspects of their life and decision making. Because they see themselves as helpless or inept, and fear separation, they are willing to subordinate their needs and wishes to those of others in order to avoid taking personal responsibility.

Passive-aggressive personality disorder Passive-aggressive people resent responsibility, either social or work-related. Rather than expressing their opposition directly, they tend to procastinate, dawdle, behave stubbornly, work inefficiently, and "forget." Additional features may include a tendency to be argumentative or sulky when asked to do something they do not want to do, and to resent authority.

Obsessive-compulsive personality disorder This term describes people who tend to be perfectionistic and inflexible, preoccupied with rules, procedures, and detail. They are often stubbornly insistent on certain things being done a particular way, yet at other times may become indecisive to the point of ineffectiveness. Compulsives tend to value their work and possessions more than interpersonal relationships. They have difficulty expressing warm and tender feelings toward others and are sometimes seen as stiff, cold, and awkward.

Other personality disorders The DSM-IIIR has a category "Personality Disorder Not Otherwise Specified" to accommodate disturbances that do not fit neatly into the foregoing categories. In this residual category are the terms, from the old DSM, *mixed personality disorder* and *atypical personality disorder*. Mixed personality disorder indicates that an individual's behavior fulfills the criteria for more than one personality disorder, e.g., passive-aggressive and dependent. Atypical personality disorder is used when a disorder is suspected but there is insufficient information for a clear classification, and for a disturbance not specifically included in DSM-IIIR, e.g., sadistic, masochistic (self-defeating), impulsive, or immature personality (which are concepts from other diagnostic schemes). One increasingly recognized disorder is *adult attention deficit disorder* (ADD), a residual form of childhood ADD (hyperkinesis). As adults, such individuals continue to have problems in attending and manifest labile mood, explosive temper, impulsivity, stress intolerance, and inability to complete tasks. They may also manifest a paradoxical (calming) reaction to central nervous system (CNS) stimulants.

RELIABILITY OF PERSONALITY DISORDER DIAGNOSES Despite continued research efforts to improve interclinician agreement through specification of diagnostic criteria, reliability is problematic for most personality disorder diagnoses. While trained clinicians tend to agree whether or not some form of personality disorder is present, this reliability breaks down when specific diagnoses are attempted. Best agreement is reported for antisocial and paranoid personality disorders.

DIFFERENTIAL DIAGNOSIS Major mental disorders In its early phases, *schizophrenia* can be mistaken for schizoid, schizotypal, paranoid, and borderline personality disorders. *Affective disorders* can mimic some features of borderline, histrionic, and compulsive personality disorders. *Anxiety disorders* can share features with compulsive, histrionic, and avoidant personalities. *Alcohol and substance abuse disorders* may need to be differentiated from antisocial, borderline, and histrionic personalities. *Paranoid disorders* can sometimes be difficult to differentiate from paranoid, schizotypal, and borderline personalities. Differential diagnostic points are that the major mental disorders tend to have a definite time of onset, that the symptomatology is more severe and causes greater disturbance in everyday functioning, and that specific diagnostic features will be present that transcend the criteria for personality disorders.

Additional personality disorders DSM-IIIR criteria for personality disorders sometimes overlap. "Schizophrenic-like" phenomena, including eccentricity and psychotic experiences, can form part of the picture of paranoid, schizoid, schizotypal, and borderline personalities. Dramatic presentation, emotional outbursts, and erratic behavior can lead to confusion among antisocial, borderline, narcissistic, and histrionic personalities. Impulsivity is found in antisocial, borderline, and histrionic personalities; while anxiety and fearfulness can be part of avoidant, passive-aggressive, dependent, and compulsive behavior. Unfortunately, the DSM-IIIR revision of the criteria for some of the personality disorders has worsened the problem of overlap. In one series it was noted that of patients considered by therapists to have a personality diagnosis almost 52 percent met criteria for two separate disorders.

Medical conditions Medical and neurologic conditions can mimic personality disorders. For example, persons with complex partial seizures with foci in the left temporal lobe can present with excessive orderliness, religiosity, and "viscosity" which might be confused with compulsive personality. Alternatively, they can develop paranoid features or fuzzy thinking suggestive of paranoid or schizotypal personality. Rigid, orderly, and ritualistic behavior mirroring compulsive personality can be part of a dementing process or a sequel of head injury, while irritability, dysregulation of affect, and inappropriate interpersonal behavior in such patients can be confused with borderline personality. Beyond these specific examples, virtually any disease affecting the brain can cause behavioral change suggestive of a personality disorder. The key differential points are that there is a relatively sudden onset and that there are neuropsychological changes indicative of compromised brain function.

ETIOLOGY AND PATHOPHYSIOLOGY It was commonly held that the personality disorders reflected the warping effect of adverse early social environment. Now there is mounting evidence that personality is, in great measure, biologically determined. Both genetic and constitutional (i.e., intrauterine and early physical developmental) factors may be important.

Genetic factors Although not all personality disorders have been examined, for the majority there is a severalfold increase in concordance between monozygotic twins compared with dizygotic twins.

Some of the most careful work has been with antisocial personality. Here it is noted that prevalence among men is three- to fourfold higher than in women, and that first-degree relatives of persons diagnosed as antisocial show increased prevalence of antisocial personality, alcoholism, and somatization disorder (Briquet's syndrome). The latter is characterized by intractable multiorgan system complaints in women who often have a histrionic personality. The association of these two disorders in the same pedigrees has led to suggestions that Briquet's syndrome and antisocial disorder are expressions in women and men of a common biogenetic substrate.

The operation of genetic factors in antisocial personality is further demonstrated by the finding that biologic offspring of antisocial and alcoholic parents have a higher risk of developing antisocial personality disorder even if they are raised by adoptive parents who do not have any antisocial traits. The converse has also been demonstrated; children adopted by antisocial parents tend not to develop antisocial disorder themselves unless they have antisocial personality or alcoholism in their blood relatives.

The XYY chromosomal abnormality was once thought to be related to antisocial personality disorder. More recent studies indicate that although XYY might be overrepresented in certain prison populations, the vast majority of XYY men are not antisocial.

The schizotypal, borderline, and schizoid diagnoses evolved originally from the notion that there ought to be a ''preclinical'' form of schizophrenia characterized by lesser severity or fewer numbers of the cognitive and interpersonal symptoms of that disorder. Thus, the schizotypal personality might, theoretically, embody earlier forms of the disturbance in thinking, perception, and attention that occur in schizophrenia; whereas the schizoid personality would represent the interpersonal awkwardness inherent in that disorder. Genetic studies have confirmed that there is some increase in schizotypal (but not schizoid) personality in relatives of diagnosed schizophrenics.

The borderline personality is genetically heterogeneous. Up to 50 percent of borderline patients have a family history of affective disorder. Borderline disorder itself, as well as other personality disorders, are also more common in first-degree relatives of borderline patients, but schizophrenia is not consistently related.

There is increased schizophrenia in the families of patients with paranoid personality. For compulsive disorder, twin studies indicate increased concordance for obsessional traits in monozygotic versus dizygotic twins. There is also some evidence that orderliness and rigidity run in families.

The other personality disorders have been studied carefully from a biogenetic standpoint.

Constitutional factors Although there is good evidence that infants are born with certain temperamental characteristics (e.g., high versus low activity level; long versus short attention span), there is little evidence that these temperamental characteristics persist into adolescence. Infant temperament does not appear to predict later personality disorder with the exception that the ''difficult child'' (irritable, hard to console, irregular rhythms) tends to exhibit more behavioral disturbances. Low intelligence quotient and poor physical health as a child have been noted more frequently in the histories of persons with personality disorders.

Neurophysiologic and neuroendocrine correlates Several neurophysiologic and biochemical changes may be associated with personality disorders. Abnormal slow waves and spikes have been reported in the EEGs of antisocial persons. For borderline patients, patterns suggestive of periodic limbic epileptiform discharges have sometimes been noted.

Some observers suggest that a common neurophysiologic feature of both antisocial and hysterical disorders is reduced cortical arousal to cortical stimulation, secondary to increased inhibition from lower brain regions. This may be coupled with motor disinhibition in antisocial persons and autonomic disinhibition in hysterics.

The schizotypal personality disorder has been associated with disturbance in smooth pursuit eye movement (SPEM). Since many schizophrenics are also poor trackers, it may be that schizotypals share with schizophrenics decreased neural effectiveness in ''centering.'' Some schizophrenics and schizotypals have lowered platelet MAO levels. It has been suggested that lowered MAO activity could be related to inefficient degradation of certain biologically active amines, leading to accumulation of substance with psychotomimetic properties.

Cortisol escape from dexamethasone suppression and shortened REM latency (REM latency is the time between falling asleep and first REM episode) are associated with affective disorder. Both phenomena have also been observed in borderline and obsessive-compulsive personalities, suggesting a link among the affective, borderline, and obsessive-compulsive disorders.

There are no specific data on biologic correlates of the other personality disorders.

Cloninger has postulated that genetically influenced differences in the responsivity and interaction of three chemically coded neural networks—dopaminergic (DA), serotoninergic, and noradrenergic—may explain three broad personality dimensions termed behavioral activation (novelty seeking), behavioral inhibition (harm avoidance), and behavioral maintenance (reward dependence). As an example, someone with DA-dependent high behavioral activation might tend toward the personality characteristics of curiosity, impulsivity, enthusiasm, excitability; those low on activation might tend toward being content, quiet, reserved, slow-tempered, and methodical. Efforts are continuing to validate this ''tridimensional neuroadaptive model'' of personality.

Environmental factors Early social environment has proved to be an inconsistent predictor of late personality disorder. For example, one study found that 30 percent of men with personality disorders who were investigated reported lack of maternal warmth as children, but so did 24 percent of controls. Multiple problems in the early environment were found in 16 percent of personality-disordered men and 10 percent of those without disorders. Being abused as a child is associated with violence in later life.

The relative weakness of both temperamental and environmental factors as predictors of future personality disorder has led to a ''goodness of fit'' hypothesis. This theory suggests that later behavioral disorders are more likely when there is a severe mismatch between a child's temperament and childrearing practices and environmental circumstances.

EPIDEMIOLOGY The prevalence of personality disorders ranges from 5 to 23 percent. Antisocial personality is diagnosed more commonly in men than women, whereas borderline and histrionic personalities are diagnosed more commonly in women.

There is increased prevalence of personality disorder in inner cities, prisons, and areas of social disintegration. Personality disorders are three times as common in the lowest social classes as compared to the highest. These sociodemographic patterns are particularly striking for antisocial personality disorder. Among patients attending psychiatric clinics the rates for personality disorder have ranged from 49 to 86 percent, with some studies noting that 50 percent qualified for more than one personality disorder.

NATURAL HISTORY AND PROGNOSIS Compared to controls, a disproportionate number of persons with personality disorders are found to have emotional problems as children. The prevalence of most personality disorders declines with age, the peak being in the age group 20 to 29. This trend is especially prominent for antisocial personality disorder. It is possible that slowly evolving maturational processes during adulthood account for these age effects.

Although only about 20 percent of persons with personality disorders seek psychiatric treatment, the majority evidence long-standing difficulties in maintaining stable employment, marriages, and friendships.

With regard to psychiatric complications, about one-third of persons with personality disorders have significant depression or anxiety. Alcohol abuse is related to personality disorder, with the association being particularly striking for men, whose rate of alcohol problems approaches 50 percent.

TREATMENT Persons with personality disorders generally do not recognize the inner source of their difficulties. They tend to blame others and their environment and make those around them feel badly. Only 20 percent of persons with personality disorders actually present for psychiatric treatment.

Treatment usually consists of psychotherapy in some form. In some specific instances psychopharmacology has been used. Success has been claimed for various types of psychotherapy. Individual, group, couples, and family treatments all have been employed. Despite differences in techniques and orientations, most psychotherapists emphasize the importance (and initial difficulty) of establishing a trusting relationship. The goals tend to be to identify inner sources of maladaptive behavior. From a psychodynamic standpoint this means that the painful feelings which are being avoided need to be identified and their causes traced. Cognitive-behavioral therapists will try to identify the faulty assumptions, lack of foresight regarding consequences of behavior, and ineffectiveness of the existing coping repertoire, with an eye to teaching more useful behavior.

As a broad generalization patients with "dramatic" presentations (borderline, antisocial, histrionic, narcissistic) tend to require a more intrusive, confrontative, limit-setting posture by the therapist. More specifically, antisocial personality probably cannot be treated in an outpatient setting and requires a containing environment (e.g., prison, inpatient unit). In such a setting groups emphasizing mutual interdependence and confrontation appear to produce some success. Regarding the treatment of borderline persons, psychiatrists are divided as to whether a supportive "here and now" versus intensive exploration works best. In either instance, treatment is often punctuated by prolonged periods in which the patient expresses negative feelings toward the therapist, makes suicide attempts, or undergoes psychotic decompensation requiring hospitalization.

In contrast to this more intrusive posture, patients whose personalities fit into the "fearful" and "odd" clusters may benefit from a more gentle, accepting, and clarifying approach.

Psychotherapy tends to be a long-term enterprise, lasting many years. Therapists can expect to feel frustrated, angry, helpless, and inadequate at times. Clinical reports of major improvements are many, but controlled outcome studies are practically nonexistent. This reflects continuing problems in achieving reliable diagnoses and in general methodologic issues in outcome research, especially in prospective studies spanning many years.

There is increasing evidence that psychopharmacologic intervention may be helpful for some of the personality diagnoses. Borderline patients, particularly those with coexisting mood disorder, have benefited from tricyclic antidepressants and MAO inhibitors. Other groups of borderline patients in whom mood dysregulation and impulsiveness are prominent have responded to lithium. Still others with explosive outbursts have benefited from carbamazepine. A few such patients have had EEG abnormalities suggestive of epileptic foci in limbic structures. Both borderline and schizotypal patients undergoing cognitive disorganization can improve with low doses of neuroleptic drugs.

Persons with obsessive-compulsive personality disorder who have obsessional ruminations may benefit from clomipramine, fluoxetine, or fluvoxamine. These agents have specific antiruminative effects that go beyond antidepressive activity. The utility of other antidepressants for this disorder has not been established, although the MAO inhibitors may be useful in compulsives who also experience anxiety or panic attacks.

Methylphenidate may improve inattention and reduce motor overactivity, affective lability, and impulsivity in persons whose personality difficulties are related to adult attention deficit disorder.

REFERENCES

Major affective disorders

Baldessarini RJ: Biological hypotheses in psychiatry, in *Chemotherapy in Psychiatry*, Cambridge, Mass, Harvard, 1985, pp 9–12

———: *Biomedical Aspects of Depression*. Washington, DC, APA Press. 1982, pp 1–83

Baron M, Risch N: X-linkage and genetic heterogeneity in bipolar-related major affective illness: Reanalysis of linkage data. Ann Hum Genet 46 (pt 2):153, 1982

——— et al: Genetic linkage between X-chromosome markers and bipolar affective illness. Nature 326:289, 1987

Clayton PJ, Barrett JE (eds): *Treatment of Depression: Old Controversies and New Approaches*. New York, Raven, 1983

Diagnostic and Statistical Manual of Mental Disorders (3d edition, revised). Washington, DC, American Psychiatric Association, 1987

Egeland JA et al: Bipolar affective disorders linked to DNA markers on chromosome II. Nature 325:783, 1987

Kelsoe JR et al: Re-evaluation of the linkage relationship between chromosome 11p loci and the gene for bipolar affective disorder in the Old Order Amish. Nature 342:238, 1989

Klerman GL: History and development of modern concepts of affective illness, in *Neurobiology of Mood Disorders*. RM Post, RC Ballenger (eds). Baltimore, Williams & Wilkins, 1984, pp 1–19

Martin JB, Reichlin S: *Clinical Neuroendocrinology*, 2d ed. Philadelphia, Davis, 1987

Post RM, Ballenger JC (eds): *Neurobiology of Mood Disorders*. Baltimore, Williams & Wilkins, 1984, vol 1

———, Weiss SRB: Kindling and manic depressive illness, in *The Clinical Relevance of Kindling*. TB Bolwig, MR Trimble (eds). Chichester, England, Wiley, 1989, pp 209–230

Robins LN et al: Lifetime prevalence of specific psychiatric disorders in three sites. Arch Gen Psychiatry 41:949, 1984

Rosenthal NE et al: Seasonal affective disorder: A description of the syndrome and preliminary findings with light therapy. Arch Gen Psychiatry 41:72, 1984

Stewart AL et al: Functional status and well-being of patients with chronic conditions. Results from the Medical Outcomes Study. JAMA 262(7):907, 1989

Wells KB et al: The functioning and well-being of depressed patients. Results from the Medical Outcomes Study. JAMA 262(7):914, 1989

Schizophrenic disorders

Braff DL: Attention, information processing, and habituation in psychiatric disorders. *Psychiatry III*. Philadelphia, Lippincott, 1985

———, Geyer MA: Sensorimotor gating and schizophrenia. Arch Gen Psychiatry 47:181, 1990

Brown GW et al: Influence of family life on the course of schizophrenic disorders: A replication. Br J Psychiatry 11:241, 1972

Carlson G, Goodwin F: The stages of mania. Arch Gen Psychiatry 28:221, 1973

Christison GW et al: A quantitative investigation of hippocampal pyramidal cell size, shape, and variability of orientation in schizophrenia. Arch Gen Psychiatry 46:1027, 1989

Crow TJ et al: Schizophrenia as an anomaly of development of cerebral asymmetry: A postmortem study and a proposal concerning the genetic basis of the disease. Arch Gen Psychiatry 46:1145, 1989

Docherty JP et al: Stages of onset of schizophrenic psychosis. Am J Psychiatry 135:420, 1978

Jeste DV, Lohr JB: Hippocampal pathologic findings in schizophrenia. Arch Gen Psychiatry 46:1019, 1989

Rosenbaum CP: *The Meaning of Madness*. New York, Science House, 1970

Rosenthal D, Kety S: *The Transmission of Schizophrenia*. New York, Pergamon, 1968

Special issue: Negative symptoms in schizophrenia. Schizophr Bull 11, 1985

Special issue. Schizophr Bull 15(3), 1989

Strauss JS, Carpenter WT: *Schizophrenia*. New York, Plenum Medical Book Company, 1981

Suddath RL et al: Anatomic abnormalities in the brains of monozygotic twins discordant for schizophrenia. N Engl J Med 322:789, 1990

Walker E et al: Environmental factors related to schizophrenia in psychophysiologically labile high-risk males. J Abnorm Psychol 90:313, 1981

Wysowski DK, Baum C: Antipsychotic drug use in the United States, 1976–1985. Arch Gen Psychiatry 46:929, 1989

Anxiety disorders

Charney DS et al: Noradrenergic function in panic anxiety. Arch Gen Psychiatry 41:75, 1984

——— et al: Neurobiological mechanisms of panic anxiety: Biochemical and behavioral correlates of yohimbine-induced panic attacks. Am J Psychiatry 144:1030, 1987

Dubovsky S: Generalized anxiety disorder: New concepts and psychopharmacologic therapies. J Clin Psychiatry 51(suppl):3, 1990

Goldberg J et al: A twin study of the effects of the Vietnam war on posttraumatic stress disorder. JAMA 263:1227, 1990

JENIKE M et al: Obsessive-compulsive disorder: A double-blind, placebo-controlled trial of clomipramine in 27 patients. Am J Psychiatry 146:1328, 1989

LIEBOWITZ MR et al: Lactate provocation of anxiety attacks. Arch Gen Psychiatry 41:764, 1984

MARKOWITZ JS et al: Quality of life in panic disorder. Arch Gen Psychiatry 46:984, 1989

TALLMAN JF et al: Receptors for the age of anxiety: Pharmacology of the benzodiazepines. Science 207:274, 1984

Personality disorders

ALNAES R, TORGERSEN S: DSM-III symptom disorders (Axis I) and personality disorders (Axis II) in an outpatient population. Acta Psychiatr Scand 78:348, 1988

BLUME SB: Dual diagnosis: Psychoactive substance dependence and the personality disorders. *Psychoactive Drugs* 21:139, 1989

CLONINGER CR: A unified biosocial theory of personality and its role in the development of anxiety states: A reply to commentaries. Psychiatr Dev 2:83, 1988

DRAKE RE, VAILLANT GE: A validity study of Axis II of DSM-III. Am J Psychiatry 142:555, 1985

FROSCH JP: The psychosocial treatment of personality disorders, in *Current Perspectives on Personality Disorders.* JP Frosch (ed). Washington, DC, APA Press, 1983, pp 96–112

GRANT I: *Behavioral Disorders: Understanding Clinical Psychopathology.* New York, Spectrum, 1979

GUNDERSON JG: DSM-III diagnoses of personality disorders, in *Current Perspectives on Personality Disorders.* JP Frosch (ed). Washington, DC, APA Press, 1983, pp 68–93

LAHMEYER HW et al: EEG sleep, lithium transport, dexamethasone suppression, and monoamine oxidase activity in borderline personality disorder. *Psychiatry Res* 25:19, 1988

LIEBOWITZ MR: Psychopharmacological intervention in personality disorders. *Current Perspectives on Personality Disorders.* JP Frosch (ed). Washington DC, APA Press, 1983, pp 68–93

LION JR: *Personality Disorders: Diagnosis and Management (Revised for DSM-III)*, 2d ed. Baltimore, Williams & Wilkins, 1981

MILLON T: *Disorders of Personality, DSM-III, Axis II*, New York, Wiley, 1981

MOREY LC: Personality disorders in DSM-III and DSM-III-R: Convergence, coverage, and internal consistency. Am J Psychiatry 145:573, 1988

PERRY JC, VAILLANT GE: Personality disorders, in *Comprehensive Textbook of Psychiatry/V*, HI Kaplan, BJ Sadock (eds). Baltimore, Williams & Wilkins, 1989, pp 1352–1387

PERSE TL et al: Fluvoxamine treatment of obsessive compulsive disorder. Am J Psychiatry 144:1543, 1987

REICH JH: Update on instruments to measure DSM-III and DSM-III-R personality disorders. J Nerv Ment Dis 177:366, 1989

SIEVER LJ et al: Biogenetic factors in personalities, in *Current Perspectives on Personality Disorders*, JP Frosch (ed). Washington, DC, APA Press, 1983, pp 42–65

WENDER PH et al: A controlled study in the treatment of attention deficit disorder, residual type, in adults. Am J Psychiatry 142:547, 1985

WIDIGER TA et al: The DSM-III-R personality disorders: An overview. Am J Psychiatry 145:7, 1988

369 THE THERAPEUTIC USE OF PSYCHOTROPIC MEDICATIONS

LEWIS L. JUDD

Perhaps no other area of pharmacology has experienced the rapid development that has occurred in psychopharmacology during the past several decades. An almost bewildering array of specific and effective psychotropic agents is currently available, with new medications appearing with great frequency. This chapter presents an overview of the major classes of psychopharmacologic drugs to provide the reader with a pragmatic understanding of these potent medications. The most clinically meaningful classification schema is based upon the therapeutic use in patients, as follows: antidepressant medications, lithium and other mood stabilizing medications, anxiolytic or antianxiety medications, and antipsychotic or neuroleptic medications.

ANTIDEPRESSANT MEDICATIONS

The successful search for new and better antidepressant medications has resulted in the two generations of antidepressants that are currently available. The first-generation antidepressants include the tricyclic (TCA) and the monoamine oxidase (MAO) inhibitor antidepressants. To date no newly developed drug has been proven to have greater clinical efficacy than antidepressants in these two major classes. The main benefit of the new generation of antidepressants is that they have provided the physician with an expanded range of pharmacologic options for the treatment of patients who cannot tolerate or who do not respond to the older drugs. The MAO inhibitors are clinically effective and recently have experienced a resurgence in clinical use, but the problems of drug-drug and drug-food interactions have made these the second-line medications in the treatment of depressive disorders. However, the MAO inhibitors appear to be especially effective for depression accompanied by panic attacks or prominent anxiety. The TCAs imipramine and amitriptyline have emerged as the standards for antidepressant efficacy.

No antidepressant is ideal, and currently available drugs have at least one of the following undesirable characteristics: delayed onset of therapeutic action (7 to 28 d), significant anticholinergic side effects, sedation, cardiotoxicity, weight gain, the possible induction of manic or hypomanic episodes in patients with bipolar disorders, or other equally problematic adverse reactions. The search for new medications may yet yield a superior antidepressant, one with a consistently high rate of improvement, rapid onset of action, and fewer side effects.

MECHANISMS OF ACTION TCAs were originally hypothesized to increase synaptic concentrations of central nervous system (CNS) monoaminergic neurotransmitter substances (e.g., norepinephrine, serotonin, and dopamine) by blocking their reuptake by presynaptic monoaminergic neurons. While this assumption is still valid, the focus now is on the regulation of postsynaptic receptor activity of monoaminergic neurons and the down-regulation of neurotransmitter receptors that have been associated with an antidepressant effect. These mechanisms have been hypothesized to account for the activity of most of the established antidepressants, but not of some of the newer antidepressants. At present, therefore, there is a great deal of information available about how antidepressants may ameliorate the pathophysiologic processes associated with depressive disorders, but no precise central mechanism(s) has been identified by which all drugs with antidepressant properties work.

CLINICAL CONDITIONS FOR USE Antidepressants are very effective in treatment of the clinical syndrome of major depression (Chap. 368) but do not affect normal mood changes or make unhappy people into happy ones. Chronic low-grade depression or dysthymic disorders (neurotic depression) generally do not respond well to antidepressants alone, although the combination of antidepressants and psychotherapy has proven effective in some cases. Antidepressants are only rarely prescribed for patients who become temporarily depressed over difficult and stressful life situations (situational depression).

There is growing evidence that antidepressants are effective in the treatment of some anxiety disorders (Chap. 368). TCAs and the MAO inhibitor antidepressants are the drugs of choice for agoraphobia, simple phobias, and panic disorder. Patients with phobic or panic disorders have concomitant anxiety about the recurrence of these attacks; this "anticipatory" anxiety may not respond to antidepressants but may benefit from concomitant treatment with antianxiety medication. There may be a broader role for the antidepressants in the management of pure anxiety disorders, but this possibility requires further study.

CLINICAL USE OF ANTIDEPRESSANTS Table 369-1 lists the more commonly used first-generation antidepressants and the oral doses needed for therapeutic efficacy in the typical patient. Currently imipramine and amitriptyline are the standards for antidepressant potency. Amitriptyline tends to have sedative effects, while imipramine is more energizing. Because of the undesirable side effects observed in these original TCAs, during the past decade growing numbers of experienced clinical psychopharmacologists have gradu-

TABLE 369-1 Commonly used first-generation antidepressants

Antidepressant	Daily oral therapeutic dose range, mg
Tricyclic derivatives:	
Amitriptyline (Elavil, etc.)	150–300
Nortriptyline (Aventyl, etc.)	50–150
Imipramine (Tofranil, etc.)	150–300
Desipramine (Norpramin)	150–250
Doxepin (Sinequan, etc.)	150–300
Monoamine oxidase inhibitors:	
Phenelzine (Nardil)	15–60
Tranylcypromine (Parnate)	20–30
Isocarboxazid (Marplan)	10–30

ally selected the secondary tricyclic amines desipramine and nortriptyline as the antidepressant drugs of choice. Both desipramine and nortriptyline have relatively fewer anticholinergic side effects and are less sedating. Nortriptyline appears to have a clearer relationship between plasma levels and clinical efficacy.

Before antidepressants are prescribed, a patient's physical health must be evaluated by a physical examination. The patient should show normal values on baseline complete blood count (CBC), urinalysis, liver function tests, and (if over 45 years) electrocardiogram (ECG). Patients are started on low doses in a twice daily regimen for a single day (e.g., 25 mg desipramine bid) and checked for side effects (e.g., postural hypotension). The dose is then raised quickly over a few days to that needed for a full therapeutic response. The minimum daily dose for clinical response is the low figure in the ranges listed in Table 369-1, but often higher doses are needed. However, dose schedules in the elderly should be reduced 30 to 50 percent. Physicians inexperienced in psychopharmacology should not exceed the upper dosage limits listed in the table. Treatment from 7 to 28 d is required to achieve a full therapeutic effect. Changes in the depressive symptoms are often noted by friends and family before the patient reports feeling better. A therapeutic trial of an antidepressant requires at least 28 d at the upper end of the dose range. Patients are usually maintained on antidepressants for approximately 9 to 12 months after the depressive symptoms disappear, to reduce the possibility of relapse resulting from premature withdrawal of medication. Highest relapse rates occur during the first 2 months after medication is discontinued, and patients and clinicians should be especially watchful during this time period.

Medications can be given in a single dose an hour before bedtime once an appropriate dose has been established. This procedure improves medication compliance, and sedative side effects are likely to induce sleep in depressed patients, who are often insomniac. Further, if troublesome side effects occur, they do so while the patient is alseep. For patients who cannot tolerate the single bedtime dose, a daytime twice daily or thrice daily schedule is necessary. Tests for plasma levels of the tricyclic antidepressants are routinely available, but unfortunately the relationship of plasma levels to clinical response has been inconsistent. For imipramine, desipramine, and amitriptyline, the relationship is linear, but nortriptyline may have a curvilinear plasma level–response relationship, implying a therapeutic window. Plasma levels may be useful in treatment-resistant patients to evaluate compliance and to see if the dose is sufficient to maintain concentrations above the threshold necessary for response (e.g., imipramine, >180 ng/mL; desipramine, >125 ng/mL; amitriptyline, >95 ng/mL; and nortriptyline, 50 to 150 ng/mL).

After about 10 to 12 months of treatment with an antidepressant, the drug should be withdrawn gradually over a 3- to 4-week period rather than suddenly stopped. Should depressive symptoms reemerge, antidepressant treatment should be restored and maintained for several more months before the withdrawal attempt is repeated.

SIDE EFFECTS AND INTERACTIONS Listed in Table 369-2 are some of the more common side effects from the tricyclic antidepressants. They include dry mouth, sedation, a fine tremor of the hands, and mild constipation. More serious are the effects on the cardiovascular system, of which tachycardia and postural hypotension are the most common. The TCAs, especially imipramine, have a quinidine-like action, can induce cardiac arrhythmias, and have been associated with sudden death in a few patients (see section below on overdose). For patients with preexisting cardiac illness, especially those with heart block, TCAs should be used cautiously; drugs with milder cardiac effects should be considered. The most bothersome symptoms are from the anticholinergic effects; while rarely serious, they do cause discomfort and compliance problems.

Some preexisting medical conditions increase the risks associated with using TCAs in certain depressed patients. Tricyclics can produce tachycardia, which may push some patients from asymptomatic congestive failure into symptomatic heart failure. TCAs also lower the seizure threshold and should be used cautiously in patients with seizures. The anticholinergic effects preclude TCA treatment in patients with glaucoma and pose a problem for men with mild to moderate prostatic hypertrophy, who may develop urinary retention. Finally, the use of tricyclic antidepressants in patients with bipolar disorders may shorten the cycle length between affective episodes, may induce an acute manic episode in some patients, and has been related to the phenomenon of rapid cycling.

The tricyclics, especially amitriptyline, imipramine, and doxepin, potentiate the effects of other CNS-depressant medications (e.g., ethanol, benzodiazepines), and patients should be cautioned about ethanol use while on antidepressants. Patients should either not drink or reduce their usual ethanol dose by one-half during tricyclic treatment. Other drug interactions include the potentiation of other anticholinergic agents (e.g., antihistamines, antiparkinsonian agents), which can result in severe constipation, urinary retention, and even paralytic ileus. This combination in the elderly, which can produce a serious anticholinergic blockade (e.g., paralytic ileus, fecal impaction), often has been the cause of frank delirium and confusional states in geriatric patients. Therefore this combination should be avoided in older patients.

Despite the problems, the risk-benefit ratio is overwhelmingly in favor of the antidepressants, and literally hundreds of thousands of patients have been treated with these compounds safely and effectively.

NEWER ANTIDEPRESSANTS Table 369-3 lists the more prominent second-generation drugs for which some evidence of antidepressant efficacy exists. How these drugs will fare over time under more rigorous scrutiny is unknown. An example of the unforseen problems that arise when promising new drugs are given broader exposure is the experience with zimelidine. This relatively selective serotonin-uptake blocker was originally reported to be an effective antidepressant with milder anticholinergic side effects than others. Increased study has revealed it to be associated with Guillain-Barré syndrome in several patients. Zimelidine has now been withdrawn from the market. Nonetheless, this new generation of psychotropic

TABLE 369-2 Common side effects of tricyclic antidepressants

Anticholinergic (atropine-like) responses:
- Dry mouth
- Nausea and vomiting*
- Constipation
- Urinary retention
- Blurred vision (mydriasis and cycloplegia)

Cardiovascular effects:
- Postural hypotension*
- Tachycardia
- Cardiotoxic side effects—can induce an arrhythmia

Obstructive jaundice—more rare—is reversible when drug is removed

Drowsiness and sleepiness—may want to avoid driving a car until this diminishes*

Fine rapid tremor*

Dizziness, ataxia

Hematologic effects:
- Leukopenia

* Side effects seen most commonly

TABLE 369-3 Selected second-generation antidepressants

Antidepressant	Daily oral therapeutic dose range, mg
Tricyclic derivatives:	
Trimipramine (Surmonil)	100–250
Amoxapine (Asendin)	150–300
Tetracyclic derivatives:	
Maprotiline (Ludiomil)	100–225
Derivatives of other chemical classes:	
Fluoxetine (Prozac)	10–40
Bupropion (Wellbutrin)	200–300
Trazodone (Desyrel)	100–600

medications is very promising and has already expanded the physicians' therapeutic choices in the treatment of depressive disorders.

Amoxapine is a tricyclic derivative with clinical efficacy equal to that of the original antidepressants. An unsubstantiated early onset of action has been claimed by the manufacturer (within the first week), although its clinical efficacy at the endpoint of treatment is identical to that of the original TCAs. One of its metabolites (7-hydroxyamoxapine) is a neuroleptic, which accounts for the unwanted extrapyramidal side effects seen with amoxapine including tardive dyskinesia and parkinsonism. Other side effects from amoxapine appear to be similar to those of the original tricyclics, although a disproportionate number of seizures was found in some retrospective studies.

Clomipramine, a tricyclic that inhibits serotonin reuptake, is commonly used worldwide and is now approved for use in the United States. It has been shown in controlled studies to be an effective drug in the treatment of depression and to be effective in obsessive-compulsive disorders, which are frequently disabling and resistant to treatment.

Fluoxetine is a relatively selective serotonin-uptake inhibitor with antidepressant efficacy comparable to imipramine. Improvement in symptoms has been found as early as 1 week. Side effects similar to those observed with other serotonin-uptake blockers include nausea, diarrhea, tremor, headache, agitation, and weight loss, and range from mild to moderate severity. Patients show few signs of cardiotoxicity or dizziness. Fluoxetine is one of the first of a series of highly specific and potent serotonin-uptake inhibitors to be marketed in the United States (e.g., sertraline, fluvoxamine, indalpine) for the treatment of depression. There are also anecdotal reports of successful treatment of obsessive-compulsive disorder by fluoxetine, but no controlled studies have been reported to date.

Maprotiline is a tetracyclic derivative that is equal in antidepressant potency to the original tricyclics and reportedly has fewer anticholinergic side effects. Originally it was offered as a promising drug for use in patients with cardiovascular problems, but this has not been established and it is not recommended for this purpose. It has been reported to cause seizures at two to four times the rate at which the TCAs induce seizures, and a lower dosage schedule is now recommended. Moreover, its use has been associated with more than the expected incidence of blood dyscrasia.

Nomifensine, a potentially interesting antidepressant related to a nonanalgesic opiate derivative, has now been withdrawn from the market worldwide because of serious hypersensitivity reactions.

Trazodone is a triazolopyridine derivative originally introduced for use as an antidepressant. There remains controversy around whether the drug has significant antidepressant properties. The drug produces a high level of sedation and is useful as a hypnotic. It has few, if any, cardiotoxic effects but is associated with increased risk of priapism.

Alprazolam, a benzodiazepine with anxiolytic efficacy, has been reported to be an effective antidepressant, although it may be less potent than the original TCAs in treating major depressive disorders. It is likely to have a place in the treatment of mixed anxiety and depressive syndromes and has the added advantage of relatively rapid onset. It has no anticholinergic or cardiotoxic effects but causes sedation and lethargy. Since it is a benzodiazepine, withdrawal symptoms, including seizures, may appear after prolonged used so the drug should be withdrawn gradually (i.e., no faster than 0.5 mg every 4 to 5 d; the last milligram should be tapered by 0.25 mg/week) (see Table 369-5 below).

Bupropion was withdrawn from the market because it produced a high rate of seizures in a subpopulation of bulimic patients. It was subsequently re-released when the seizure rate was found to be no greater than that produced by the TCAs (estimated at about 0.4 percent) and is currently used for treating major depression. A role for bupropion in stabilizing patients with rapid-cycling disorders has also been proposed. The mechanism of action may be related to dopamine-reuptake inhibition, although this is not established. Bupropion has energizing properties and consequently is less sedating, with mild side effects including headache, agitation, and some anticholinergic effects.

TRICYCLIC OVERDOSAGE Antidepressants are the fourth most common cause of drug overdose seen in emergency departments in the United States and the third most frequent cause of drug-related death (after alcohol-drug combinations and heroin). Of the antidepressants, tricyclics are the most frequent cause of death. In a California study (Callaham and Kassel) the annual frequency of fatal tricyclic overdose was 1.3 per 100,000 of population; more than two-thirds of the victims were women. Amitriptyline, desipramine, and nortriptyline were the most frequently implicated.

The first 6 h after an overdose of a tricyclic antidepressant are crucial. CNS depression and seizures, respiratory arrest, and cardiovascular arrhythmias are the principal causes of death. ECG changes showing QRS prolongation are early signs of toxicity, and ventricular fibrillation is a common complication. ECG changes are a more sensitive measure for monitoring patients than are blood levels of the drug.

LITHIUM AND OTHER MOOD-NORMALIZING MEDICATIONS

The most important psychotropic medication in this group is lithium. Although lithium possesses some antidepressant properties, it is not, strictly speaking, an antidepressant. Its effectiveness in treating patients with bipolar disorders (see Chap. 368) and other disorders of mood has revolutionized the practice of psychiatry. Lithium's approval by the Food and Drug Administration (FDA) in 1970 for the treatment of acute mania and in 1975 for the maintenance treatment of manic-depressive disorder generated an explosion of basic and clinical research focused on its pharmacologic mechanisms and clinical use.

MECHANISM OF ACTION The central mechanisms by which lithium exerts its clinical effects on extremes of mood are not fully understood. Lithium affects the brain's monoaminergic neurotransmitter concentrations at the synapse, has strong effects on biologic membranes, and intracellularly inhibits the conversion of inositol monophosphate to free inositol. This latter effect may, in turn, reduce neuronal excitability.

CLINICAL CONDITIONS FOR USE Lithium is the drug of choice for treating acute manic/hypomanic episodes and for prevention of recurrent episodes of mania and depression in bipolar illness. Recent studies suggest that the relapse rate among lithium-treated bipolar patients is about one-half that of control patients receiving a placebo. It may also be an effective agent in the prophylaxis of recurrent unipolar depressive disorders. Lithium also has antidepressant properties, especially in depressions seen in bipolar disorders; however, it is not a drug of choice for major depression per se. It has been successfully used in conjunction with neuroleptics in schizoaffective disorders; there may be a subpopulation of schizophrenics responsive to lithium, although most workers feel that such lithium responders are atypical bipolar patients and not schizophrenics. Finally, there are conflicting reports that lithium may be useful in treating alcoholism, a possibility requiring further study.

CLINICAL USE OF LITHIUM Lithium is a very safe drug with an excellent risk-benefit ratio when it is used knowledgeably. The only genuine contraindication to lithium's use is seriously compromised renal function. The following baseline studies should be obtained before prescribing lithium: CBC, routine urinalysis with a concentration test, thyroxine (T_4), free T_4 index, thyroid-stimulating hormone (TSH), serum creatinine, electrolytes, and (for those over 40) an ECG.

Serum lithium levels peak 1 to 3 h after an oral dose, and the biologic half-life, which averages 24 h, varies with age. Elderly patients frequently have a drug half-life over 30 h, often requiring lower doses. Lithium is monitored by serum levels, which are most informative approximately 10 h after the last dose. Therapeutic efficacy in acute mania is achieved at levels between 0.8 and 1.4 mmol/L. Patients rarely require treatment at serum levels above 1.5 mmol/L. Lithium is always administered orally. Dose ranges are from 600 mg to 3000 mg daily, unless the patient is elderly. A general rule of thumb equates a 0.2 mmol/L rise in serum level with each additional 300-mg tablet of lithium. Unless sustained-release tablets are used, lithium is usually administered twice or three times daily, allowing for smooth, sustained 24-h serum levels. Because there is a 7- to 10-d delay in achieving full therapeutic effects, the addition of antipsychotic medications is often needed during the early phase of treating a manic patient. During acute manic episodes patients often tolerate relatively higher doses of lithium, but once the manic episode remits, it is necessary to reduce the dose.

The current maintenance treatment strategy is to prevent future recurrent episodes of mania and depression in patients with bipolar disorders. Clinicians are advised to seek the lowest possible serum levels in the range from 0.6 to 1.0 mmol/L that will prevent relapse. Lithium's excretion rate is very stable within each patient; as a result patients can be maintained on the same dose day in and day out, with relative certainty that stable levels are present. During maintenance patients are seen every 3 to 6 months, and serum lithium, sodium, potassium, T_4, free T_4 index, TSH, and creatinine are monitored along with urinalysis with a concentration test. The lithium excretion pattern is altered by conditions that change sodium concentrations, and patients on thiazide diuretics or low-salt diets should be warned and monitored more frequently.

SIDE EFFECTS AND INTERACTIONS Lithium's side effects are listed in a continuum ranging from those seen relatively commonly to those indicating lithium toxicity (see Table 369-4). Many of these are minor side effects, which appear early and disappear as time passes, but some may persist throughout treatment. Because the rapid escalation of serum levels often induces side effects, especially those involving the gastrointestinal tract, smoother, more gradual serum lithium increases are desirable.

Some of the first signs of lithium toxicity are coarsening of tremor, increases in the deep tendon reflexes, and muscle fasciculations. Unusual degrees of sedation and cognitive disruption also may herald lithium toxicity. Lithium toxicity mimics barbiturate intoxication, and when death occurs it is secondary to respiratory depression and its complications. The treatment of lithium toxicity involves good supportive care and excellent hydration. Since lithium's half-life is 24 h, this treatment sustains the patient until the kidneys eliminate the medication. Various methods to improve the treatment of lithium toxicity, such as increasing lithium excretion by aminophylline or alkalinizing the urine, have all been disappointing. For life-threatening cases, the last resort is renal dialysis, but toxicity does not commonly progress to the point where this intervention is needed.

There is some evidence that lithium is a teratogen, particularly when administered during the first trimester of pregnancy. Cardiovascular and valve abnormalities have been detected in 18-week-old fetuses. While there is little evidence for teratogenesis during the second and third trimesters, alternative treatments in pregnant women should be considered.

TABLE 369-4 Common lithium side effects

Severity	Side effect
SIDE EFFECTS COMMONLY SEEN	
Very mild	Thirst
	Nausea (particularly during first few days of treatment)
	Fine tremor of hand
Mild to moderate	Anorexia
	Vomiting
	Diarrhea
	"Upset stomach" or "abdominal pain"
	Polydipsia and/or polyuria
	Muscular weakness and fatigue
SIDE EFFECTS INDICATING TOXICITY	
	Muscle hyperirritability with twitching, muscle fasciculation, or chronic movements
	Sedation, sluggishness, languidness, drowsiness, giddiness
	Coarse tremor
	Ataxia
Moderate to severe	Hypertonic muscles
	Hyperactive deep tendon reflexes
	Hyperextension of arms and legs with grunts and gasping
	Chorea, athetotic movements
	Impairment of consciousness
	Somnolence, confusion, stupor
	Seizures
	Transient focal neurologic signs
	Dysarthria
	Cranial nerve signs
Very severe	Coma
	Complications of coma
	Death

Lithium's interactions with other drugs primarily involve its reciprocal relationship with the sodium ion. Diuretics, which increase sodium excretion, can increase lithium toxicity. There have also been reports that combined neuroleptic and lithium therapy has resulted in a reversible neurotoxicity in a small number of middle-aged and older patients. Clinical observations indicate that this combination is safe and effective provided that both drugs are used in low to moderate doses, carefully monitored, and discontinued as soon as the lithium effect is sufficiently present for the patient to be managed without the neuroleptic.

MEDICAL SEQUELAE OF LITHIUM'S USE Several medical complications can develop during lithium treatment. Because of its effect on adenylate cyclase activity, lithium inhibits the thyroid gland's secretory function; nontoxic goiters and hypothyroidism can develop, which can be readily corrected during lithium therapy by thyroid supplement. Lithium may induce the following ECG changes especially in older patients: T-wave depression, sinus node dysfunctions, and, very rarely, sinoatrial block and ventricular irritability.

The most important sequelae are the renal complications. About 25 percent of patients develop some degree of vasopressin-resistant nephrogenic diabetes insipidus with polyuria and polydipsia. The lithium inhibition of adenylate cyclase activity is responsible for the disruption of renal tubular transport. These symptoms are usually completely reversible by lithium withdrawal and often can be ameliorated by a reduction in dosage. The most economic and accurate method of monitoring changes in renal function during lithium treatment is by the urine concentration test and serum creatinine level. Consistent urine concentration levels below a specific gravity of 1.025 indicate an early renal effect, and a creatinine clearance test should be obtained. If creatinine clearance is abnormal, the patient's clinical condition should be reevaluated and termination of the lithium treatment considered. There have been reports of renal focal necrosis and interstitial fibrosis in a few long-term lithium patients, and there is evidence, by biopsy, for an increased basal rate of renal pathology among patients with affective disorders. Nonetheless, this nonspecific renal lesion does appear more frequently in patients receiving long-term lithium.

Evidence has emerged linking the more serious renal complications to increased episodes of lithium toxicity and possibly to prolonged combined use of lithium and neuroleptics. While good clinical practice should obviate lithium toxicity, it may be equally important to avoid extremes of high and low serum lithium levels during the day. Despite these concerns, lithium remains one of the most important and effective psychotropic agents and its risk-benefit ratio is excellent.

CARBAMAZEPINE AND OTHER MOOD-STABILIZING MEDICATIONS The anticonvulsant carbamazepine has, in controlled trials, been used successfully in the treatment of manic and, to a lesser extent, depressive episodes in bipolar patients. There is also growing evidence that some bipolar patients (15 to 60 percent) who do not respond to lithium benefit from carbamazepine treatment, and that the combination of lithium and carbamazepine may be therapeutically additive. The drug regimen for bipolar disorders is initiated with 200 mg bid administered orally, increasing to 600 to 1600 mg daily in divided doses and, although not well-correlated with therapeutic response, blood levels may range from 8 to 12 mg/dL.

Carbamazepine is not a completely benign drug; side effects include nausea, blurred vision, and ataxia, and more importantly there have been cases of fatal leukopenia and aplastic anemia reported (incidence $\leq$ 1 in 20,000). Patients treated with carbamazepine must be monitored for renal, liver, and bone marrow functions while they are on the medication. There are also reports of reversible CNS toxicity when this drug is combined with lithium. Therefore patients on this combination should be monitored carefully. Valproic acid, the drug of choice in certain seizure disorders, has also been reported to prevent recurrence of manic episodes in a small number of bipolar patients. The development of this new class of psychotropic compounds is very promising and may herald the future development of a new and useful group of medications.

ANTIANXIETY OR ANXIOLYTIC MEDICATIONS

The development of the benzodiazepines has been a great advance in the pharmacologic management of anxiety. They have also replaced barbiturates as the sedative-hypnotic drugs of choice. The benzodiazepines, unlike the barbiturates, are partial CNS depressants and thus, even at high doses, are rarely associated with lethal respiratory depression or vasomotor collapse. In addition, depending upon the dose, benzodiazepines possess anticonvulsant and muscle relaxant properties.

MECHANISMS OF ACTION There is growing evidence that gamma-aminobutyric acid (GABA), an inhibitory amino acid neurotransmitter, may play a central role in the brain mechanism(s) of anxiety. Benzodiazepines selectively, but indirectly, enhance GABA neurotransmission, possibly by increasing neuronal receptor sensitivity to GABA. Also, a close interaction has been described between GABA and benzodiazepine receptor binding, leading to an increase in neuronal chloride conductance. Despite these observations, the specific mechanism by which benzodiazepines mediate their clinical effects is not completely understood.

CLINICAL CONDITIONS FOR USE The antianxiety medications are most effective in the management of relatively short-lived reactive states of tension and anxiety and are the drugs of choice in the treatment of generalized anxiety disorders (see Chap. 368). Although alprazolam at high doses (4 to 10 mg) can block panic attacks, the TCAs and MAO inhibitors are the drugs of choice for treating panic disorders (see Chap. 368). However, the anxiolytics may have a role in the treatment of anticipatory anxiety, which is almost always present in patients with panic disorders. Sometimes, both a TCA and a benzodiazepine anxiolytic may be necessary in the treatment of panic disorder. The anxiolytics are also useful in treating anxiety symptoms that accompany phobic disorders.

TABLE 369-5 Commonly used benzodiazepines

Benzodiazepine	Daily oral dose range, mg	Half-life, h*
Anxiolytics:		
Chlordiazepoxide (Librium)	20–100†	7–28*
Diazepam (Valium)	5–40†	20–90*
Lorazepam (Ativan)	1–10‡	10–12
Oxazepam (Serax)	30–120‡	3–20
Prazepam (Centrax)	20–60†	40–70*
Alprazolam (Xanax)	0.75–10.0‡	12–15
Sedative-hypnotics:		
Flurazepam (Dalmane)	15–30§	24–100*
Temazepam (Restoril)	30§	8–10
Triazolam (Halcion)	0.125–0.5§	2–5

* Indicates long-acting active metabolites.
† Prescribed in a daily or twice daily regimen.
‡ Prescribed in a three or four times daily regimen.
§ Prescribed in a daily or bedtime regimen.

CLINICAL USE OF ANTIANXIETY MEDICATIONS The benzodiazepines have been most frequently prescribed as anxiolytics. The shorter-acting benzodiazepines, however, are also effective sedative-hypnotics. The more commonly prescribed drugs are listed in Table 369-5 along with the usual oral dose ranges. The pharmacokinetic characteristics of many of the benzodiazepines are complicated by long drug elimination half-lives and the metabolic conversion of parent compounds to active metabolites (see Table 369-5). Diazepam is converted to the active metabolite desmethyldiazepam (nordiazepam) which, in turn, can be hydroxylated to yield oxazepam, also a potent benzodiazepine. This metabolic pathway extends the activity half-life of diazepam threefold. The hypnotic flurazepam is converted to active metabolite *N*-1-desalkylflurazepam, which has a half-life of more than 48 h; hence, repetitive daily doses given in excess of a week or two can result in the accumulation of the active metabolites of the drug. Prazepam has metabolic breakdown products identical to those of diazepam and has a similar drug elimination half-life. Oxazepam and lorazepam, both of which undergo glucuronide conjugation, have no active metabolites and therefore have the advantage of a shorter half-life. The benzodiazepines temazepam, triazolam, and alprazolam also have the advantage of shorter half-lives and to date, no long-acting active metabolites have been identified.

Diazepam has been the standard against which all anxiolytic drugs are measured, and no other anxiolytics have demonstrated better antianxiety efficacy. The newly developed benzodiazepines appear equally effective and have eliminated certain of the undesirable side effects. Specifically, lorazepam, oxazepam, and alprazolam are without active metabolites and, with proper dosage, cumulative effects of daytime sedation are less noticeable.

Treatment regimens usually last 4 weeks or less, and medications are prescribed continually for 7 to 10 d followed by a 2- to 3-d drug holiday; then this sequence is repeated. This schedule helps avoid the development of tolerance to the anxiolytic effects. The shorter-acting medications (e.g., lorazepam, alprazolam) are prescribed in a three or four times daily regimen, and the longer-acting drugs (e.g., diazepam) are given in a single dose or a twice daily regimen. For example, it is common practice to prescribe one dose of diazepam at bedtime, since it will both promote sleep and reduce anxiety levels the following day.

In prescribing the anxiolytic benzodiazepines clinicians should avoid the possibility of habituating patients to chronic benzodiazepine use. One of the earliest signs is the development of tolerance in which the patient repeatedly requests escalations in drug dose. Since benzodiazepines do produce mild euphoria and a sense of well-being, anxious patients often want to preserve this feeling and request additional medication. However, clinical surveys of prescription practices have shown that clinicians are aware of the problems of benzodiazepine habituation and sometimes respond by being too cautious and by unnecessarily undertreating patients. The use of the drug holiday treatment regimen described above and the physician's resistance to repetitively increasing dosage will help to minimize the problem of drug habituation.

In addition to its role as an anxiolytic, diazepam is also the drug of choice in this class for muscle relaxation and for the treatment of alcohol withdrawal syndromes. It is the benzodiazepine of choice for intractable seizures. Oxazepam, because of the nonaccumulation of active metabolites, is a good choice for anxiolysis in the elderly.

SIDE EFFECTS AND INTERACTIONS The most important adverse effect of the benzodiazepines is the discomfort caused by the withdrawal syndrome, which can occur after chronic treatment. There is little risk of debilitating addiction to these drugs when used appropriately. However, physical dependence does occur since withdrawal symptoms are seen in a high percentage of patients after cessation of chronic benzodiazepine treatment. Motivation to sustain mild feelings of well-being and avoid the discomfort of withdrawal symptoms may contribute to psychological dependence. Withdrawal symptoms include muscle aches, agitation, restlessness, insomnia, and generalized anxious dysphoria. In some patients, more commonly those taking short-acting benzodiazepines, more serious CNS withdrawal symptoms may appear, including confusional and delirium states and, more rarely, grand mal seizures. Rebound anxiety can also be seen in patients with anxiety disorders but is less prevalent when benzodiazepines with long-acting metabolites are used and if medication is gradually discontinued. Risk for withdrawal symptoms increases with the length of treatment; they occur with much greater frequency (e.g., more than 90 percent) among patients who have been treated for 1 year or more. Withdrawal symptoms occur within the first 24 to 48 h after treatment with short-acting benzodiazepines ceases, but for those benzodiazepines with long-acting metabolites (e.g., diazepam, chlordiazepoxide) the withdrawal symptoms can occur 4 to 6 d and even longer after drug cessation. With the usual recommended dosage regimens and the gradual withdrawal technique (e.g., over 3 to 4 weeks), the appearance of a withdrawal syndrome in patients can be minimized significantly. While there is little true addiction potential, patients should be on these medication for only as long as necessary.

The most common minor side effects are daytime sedation, mild cognitive impairment, motor clumsiness, and (e.g., lorazepam, triazolam) specific memory decrements. Another rare but troublesome side effect from some benzodiazepines is paradoxical emotional responses, primarily manifested as aggressive and impulsive behavior.

Unlike barbiturates, the benzodiazepines do not noticeably induce hepatic microsomal enzyme activity and therefore do not affect the metabolism of other medications. The benzodiazepines potentiate the CNS depressant effects of other drugs including barbiturates, general anesthetics, and alcohol. The cross-tolerance with ethanol has made the benzodiazepines ideal medications for the treatment of alcohol withdrawal syndromes. Patients should be cautioned that ethanol's effects are potentiated by benzodiazepines and this combination should be avoided.

NEWER ANXIOLYTIC MEDICATIONS It has been established that certain beta-adrenergic blocking agents, such as *propranolol*, can dampen the peripheral physiologic symptoms of anxiety. Initially, it was felt that these drugs might be better nonsedative anxiolytic compounds, but this promise has not been fulfilled in controlled studies. While propranolol does attenuate somatic manifestations of anxiety (e.g., palpitations, tremor), it appears to have lesser effects on the psychological components (e.g., intense fearfulness). Although propranolol has been used for treating patients extremely fearful of speaking or performing in public (oral dose 40 to 320 mg qd), it is not a comprehensively effective anxiolytic. With additional study, other peripheral blocking agents may prove to be more effective.

A new class of anxiolytic drugs, the azaspirodecanediones, has been developed. One of the first compounds studied clinically is *buspirone*. It has no structural similarity to other anxiolytics or even to other psychotropics. It is not anticonvulsant, does not interact with the benzodiazepine receptor, is not cross-tolerant with other CNS depressants, and no abstinence syndrome has yet been described. In several controlled trials it has proved to be an effective anxiolytic with significantly less sedation and decrements in psychomotor performance. Because of the near absence of sedation and motor impairment and the relatively long latency for anxiolytic effects to appear (i.e., days to weeks), patients occasionally report that the drug is ineffective. This is most common in individuals who have previously received benzodiazepines such as diazepam. Numerous studies are currently being conducted with buspirone to determine possible side effects.

In addition to the efficacy of *tricyclic antidepressants* in panic and phobic disorders, there are controlled studies reporting that they are anxiolytics as effective as the benzodiazepines in generalized anxiety disorders. It is possible that continued investigations will identify a broader role for TCAs in the treatment of the full spectrum of anxiety disorders.

ANTIPSYCHOTIC OR NEUROLEPTIC MEDICATIONS

The antipsychotics have the capacity to sedate, tranquilize, blunt emotional expression, attenuate aggressive and impulsive behavior, and cause disinterest in the environment and lack of initiative. Unique features of the drugs are that they leave higher intellectual functions relatively intact yet specifically ameliorate the agitation and bizarre behavior and thinking of psychotic patients. Unfortunately no antipsychotic medication currently available even approaches the criteria for an ideal drug in this group. Virtually all have prominent anticholinergic side effects and produce a wide variety of dystonias and extrapyramidal symptoms. Of greater concern is the fact that long-term administration of these agents can cause tardive dyskinesia in some patients (see Chap. 25), a seriously disabling movement disorder that is often irreversible. Nonetheless, the antipsychotics, primarily used in schizophrenia, have helped to reduce enormously the patient populations in mental hospitals and have allowed chronic mentally ill patients who previously would have been lifelong residents of hospitals to live in the community.

MECHANISM OF ACTION With few exceptions, antipsychotic neuroleptics have notable effects on the brain's dopaminergic neurotransmitter system. Specifically, these medications antagonize the effects of the neurotransmitter dopamine in the basal ganglia and in the limbic portions of the forebrain. Since the central characteristic of neuroleptics is their capacity to block dopaminergic neurotransmission, this has led researchers to postulate that an abnormality in the CNS dopaminergic neurotransmitter system is one of the key pathophysiologic mechanisms in the etiology of schizophrenia. Many effects of antipsychotic medications on the brain have been well-described, but the underlying mechanism by which these drugs achieve their antipsychotic efficacy is not yet fully understood.

CLINICAL CONDITIONS FOR USE Because the overall risk of tardive dyskinesia is estimated at 20 to 40 percent with chronic treatment, antipsychotics should only be used when necessary and in those conditions for which they are the drug of choice: in treating schizophrenic disorders (see Chap. 368); in combination with lithium for acute manic episodes (see Chap. 368); and in combination with antidepressants for psychotic and agitated depressions. They are also used in treating Tourette's syndrome and Huntington's disease. Although the antipsychotics should be used with only a relatively narrow spectrum of mental disorders, patients with these disorders make up a significant majority of all patients with serious and chronic mental illness.

CLINICAL USE OF THE ANTIPSYCHOTICS The more commonly used antipsychotics from each pharmacologic class and their average daily oral doses are given in Table 369-6. Chlorpromazine, one of the first drugs of this class to be developed, is the prototypic antipsychotic drug and the potency standard for the others. Dose equivalence for an antipsychotic drug is calculated in comparison with the effect of 100 mg of chlorpromazine. For example, 5 mg of

TABLE 369-6 Some commonly used antipsychotic medications

	Average daily oral dose range, mg	Potency ratio compared to 100 mg of chlorpromazine
Phenothiazines:		
Aliphatics:		
Chlorpromazine (Thorazine)	400–800	1:1
Piperazines:		
Fluphenazine (Prolixin)	4–20	1:50
Fluphenazine enanthate or decanoate	25–100*	
Perphenazine (Trilafon)	8–32	1:10
Trifluoperazine (Stelazine)	6–20	1:20
Piperidines:		
Thioridazine (Mellaril)	200–600	1:1
Butyrophenones:		
Haloperidol (Haldol)	8–32	1:50
Thioxanthenes:		
Chlorprothixene (Taractan)	400–800	1:1 (approx)
Thiothixene (Navane)	15–30	1:25
Oxoindoles:		
Molindone (Moban, Lidone)	40–200	1:10
Dibenzoxazepines:		
Loxapine (Loxitane, Daxolin)	60–100	1:10

* For intramuscular injection only.

trifluoperazine or 2 mg of haloperidol is equivalent in potency to 100 mg of chlorpromazine. Using this ratio as a reference point, acutely psychotic patients usually require an accumulated dose of 500 to 800 mg orally of a chlorpromazine equivalent during the first 24 to 36 h. Following control of the acute agitation, the oral dose is increased over the next week to the chlorpromazine equivalent of between 600 and 1500 mg a day in divided doses. It is uncommon for therapeutic benefits to be measurably increased by exceeding the daily dose equivalent of 1500 mg of chlorpromazine, although it may be necessary to go to two and three times this level in some patients.

Because schizophrenia is a chronic disorder, patients need long-term maintenance on antipsychotics to prevent relapse. In controlled studies as many as 60 percent of schizophrenics relapse within 6 months after discontinuing drug therapy. Patients are maintained on the lowest dose possible that will prevent reemergence of symptoms. This is usually in the range of 20 percent of the peak dose level needed to ameliorate the acute phase of the psychotic symptoms. Compliance is difficult to achieve in this chronically disordered group of patients, and it is often therapeutically advantageous for the clinician to use parenteral long-acting fluphenazine enanthate or decanoate, which can be administered by injection every week or two. Previously it was recommended that drug holidays be used, but this practice has not prevented tardive dyskinesia, and there are few if any advantages to this technique, which is now rarely used.

SIDE EFFECTS AND INTERACTIONS Initially patients are sedated, lethargic, and drowsy, but within days they develop tolerance to these effects. All of the antipsychotics have anticholinergic action, which may produce dry mouth, cycloplegia, postural hypotension, constipation, and urinary retention. Obstructive jaundice, retinal pigmentation (thioridazine), lenticular opacities, skin pigmentation and hypersensitivity to sunlight, and male impotence are also side effects seen with antipsychotics.

The extrapyramidal side effects are the most troublesome, however. During the first five days of treatment, patients may develop acute muscular dystonic reactions but the extrapyramidal Parkinson-like syndrome is the most common. Both the dystonia and the parkinsonism respond well to antiparkinsonian medications (e.g., benztropine mesylate, 1 to 2 mg bid or tid; trihexyphenidyl, 2 to 5 mg bid or tid). Another common side effect is akathisia, a motor restlessness in which patients feel compelled to move their extremities and to move about. It is not uncommon to mistake akathisia for psychotic agitation and increase the antipsychotic dose, exacerbating the problem. Akathisia may respond to beta blockers (Lipinski et al.) and antiparkinsonian agents but more often requires decreasing the dose of the antipsychotic. It is rarely necessary to continue antiparkinsonian drug treatment beyond the first 3 months of antipsychotic maintenance.

The most serious side effect of the antipsychotics is tardive dyskinesia, which has been seen with virtually every neuroleptic. The specter of tardive dyskinesia has altered the risk-benefit ratio of the antipsychotics; they should only be used for those disorders in which they are clearly the drugs of choice. Usually the symptoms of tardive dyskinesia appear late in treatment and consist of involuntary, repetitive movements of the lips, tongue (e.g., tongue thrusting, lip smacking), and not infrequently of the extremities and trunk. Patients over 60 and those with preexisting CNS pathology are at a higher risk for this disorder (up to 70 percent), but other risk factors have not been confirmed. Although tardive dyskinesia cannot be prevented or reversed once it has developed, newer antipsychotic medications such as clozapine, which can attenuate some of the symptoms, may be substituted for the neuroleptic being used. However, it is too early to determine whether tardive dyskinesia is reduced with some of the newer antipsychotic medications.

The malignant neuroleptic syndrome, a rare complication of neuroleptic drugs, is discussed in Chap. 377.

NEWER ANTIPSYCHOTIC MEDICATIONS Although development of new antipsychotic medications has lagged significantly behind that of the antidepressants and anxiolytic drugs, some promising medications have appeared recently.

Clozapine is a dibenzodiazepine that binds to serotonin and alpha-adrenergic, histaminergic, and dopaminergic receptors. It has been approved by the FDA for use in treatment-refractory psychotic patients and in those who have intolerable side effects with their current medications. Its antipsychotic activity is comparable to the traditional neuroleptics, and it is also effective in attenuating anxiety and tension. Clozapine has proven effective in about 30 percent of treatment-resistant schizophrenics. The drug produces some sedation and muscle relaxation but few extrapyramidal symptoms. It is not known to cause tardive dyskinesia and may, in high doses, attenuate it. Clozapine's side effects include orthostatic hypotension, sinus tachycardia, hypersalivation, temperature elevation, lowered seizure threshold, and constipation. A 1 to 2 percent incidence of potentially fatal agranulocytosis has been reported but this may be considerably higher in eastern European and Jewish subpopulations. Frequent (e.g., weekly) CBCs should be obtained.

Sulpiride, which is available in Europe, is a substituted benzamide that selectively binds to presynaptic, sodium-dependent, D-2 receptors. Its antipsychotic efficacy is comparable to traditional neuroleptics. Moreover, it may cause fewer cases of tardive dyskinesia and extrapyramidal syndrome. This novel structure may herald the development of new classes of safer and better antipsychotics.

REFERENCES

APPLETON WS, DAVIS JM: *Practical Clinical Psychopharmacology,* 2d ed. Baltimore, Williams & Wilkins, 1980

BALDESSARINI RJ: *Chemotherapy in Psychiatry.* Cambridge, Mass, Harvard, 1985

BOEHNERT MT, LOVEJOY FH JR: Value of the QRS duration versus the serum drug level in predicting seizures and ventricular arrhythmias after an acute overdose of tricyclic antidepressants. N Engl J Med 313:474, 1985

CALLAHAM M, KASSEL D: Epidemiology of fatal tricyclic antidepressant ingestion: Implications for management. Ann Emerg Med 14:1, 1985

COOPER TB et al (eds): *Lithium: Controversies and Unresolved Issues.* Amsterdam, Excerpta Medica, 1979

GELENBERG AJ: et al: Comparison of standard and low serum levels of lithium for maintenance treatment of bipolar disorder. N Engl J Med 321:1489, 1989

GILMAN AG et al (eds): *Goodman and Gilman's The Pharmacological Basis of Therapeutics,* 7th ed. New York, MacMillan, 1985

GUZE BH, BAXTER LR JR: Current concepts: Malignant neuroleptic syndrome. N Engl J Med 313:163, 1985

HANESTON PD: *Drug Interactions,* 3d ed. Philadelphia, Lea & Febiger, 1975

HIPPUIS H, WINOKUR G (eds): Part 2, clinical psychopharmacology, in *Psychopharmacology 1.* Amsterdam, Excerpta Medica, 1983

HOLLISTER LE: *Clinical Pharmacology of Psychotherapeutic Drugs.* New York, Churchill Livingston, 1978

IVERSON LL, SNYDER SS (eds): *Handbook of Psychopharmacology*. New York, Plenum, 1977

JARVIK ME: *Psychopharmacology in the Practice of Medicine*. New York, Appleton-Century-Crofts, 1977

KANE J et al (with Clozaril Collaborative Study Group): Clozapine for the treatment-resistant schizophrenic. Arch Gen Psychiatry 45:789, 1988

KLEIN DF et al: *Diagnosis and Drug Treatment of Psychiatric Disorders: Adults and Children*, 2d ed. Baltimore, Williams & Wilkins, 1980

LIEBERMAN JA et al: Clozapine-induced agranulocytosis: Non-cross-reactivity with other psychotropic drugs. J Clin Psychiatry 49(7):271, 1988

LIPINSKI JF JR et al: Propranalol in the treatment of neuroleptic induced akathisia. Am J Psychiatry 141:412, 1984

MELTZER HY (ed): *Psychopharmacology: The Third Generation of Progress*. New York, Raven, 1987

POST RM, BALLENGER JC (eds): Neurobiology of mood disorders, in *Frontiers of Clinical Neuroscience*. Baltimore, Williams & Wilkins, 1984, vol 1

section 2 Alcoholism and drug dependency

370 ALCOHOL AND ALCOHOLISM

MARC A. SCHUCKIT

Ninety percent of people drink alcohol, 40 to 50 percent of men have temporary alcohol-induced problems, and 10 percent of men and 3 to 5 percent of women develop pervasive and persistent alcohol-related problems (alcoholism). The usual alcoholic has a family and a job; only about 5 percent fit the skid row stereotype. Even light drinking may adversely interact with other medications, temporary heavier drinking can exacerbate most medical illnesses, and alcoholism can masquerade as many different medical disorders and psychiatric syndromes. The following sections describe the pharmacology and clinical effects of alcohol and identify circumstances where drinking may cause a major medical or psychiatric problem or exacerbate a preexisting disorder. While these comments apply to the hypothetical "average" person, there is considerable individual variability depending on genetic vulnerability, concomitant drug use, and prior unrelated pathology or disease.

PHARMACOLOGY OF ETHANOL: ABSORPTION AND METABOLISM Ethanol is a weakly charged molecule that moves easily through cell membranes, rapidly equilibrating between blood and tissues. The effects of drinking depend in part on the amount of ethanol consumed per unit of body weight; the level of alcohol in the blood is expressed as milligrams or grams of ethanol per deciliter (e.g., 100 mg/dL or 0.1000 g/dL). In round figures, 340 mL (12 oz) of beer, 115 mL (4 oz) of nonfortified wine, and 43 mL (1.5 oz) (a shot) of 80-proof beverage each contain approximately 10 g of ethanol; 1 pint of 86-proof beverage contains approximately 160 g and 1 L of wine contains approximately 80 g of ethanol. Congeners found in alcohol beverages may contribute to body damage with heavy drinking; these include low-molecular-weight alcohols (e.g. methanol and butanol), aldehydes, esters, histamine, phenols, tannins, iron, lead, and cobalt.

Ethanol is a central nervous system (CNS) depressant that decreases activity of neurons, although some behavioral stimulation is observed at low blood levels. This drug has cross-tolerance and shares a similar pattern of behavioral problems with other brain depressants, including the benzodiazepines, barbiturates, and other sedatives and hypnotics. Alcohol is absorbed from mucus membranes of the mouth and esophagus (in very small amounts), from the stomach and large bowel (in modest amounts), and from the proximal portion of the small intestine (the major site). The rate of absorption *increases* with rapid gastric emptying; the absence of proteins, fats, or carbohydrates (which interfere with absorption); the absence of congeners; dilution to a modest percentage of ethanol (maximum absorption is seen at about 20 percent by volume); and carbonation (champagne).

Between 2 percent (at low blood alcohol concentrations) and about 10 percent (at high blood alcohol concentrations) of ethanol is excreted directly through the lungs, urine, or sweat, but the greater part is metabolized to acetaldehyde in the liver. At least two metabolic routes, each with different optimal concentrations of ethanol (K_m), result in the metabolism of approximately one drink per hour. The *first* and clinically most important pathway occurs in the cell cytosol via alcohol dehydrogenase (ADH) with a K_m of about 2 mmol. This reaction produces acetaldehyde which is then rapidly destroyed by aldehyde dehydrogenase (ALDH) in the cytosol and mitochondria. Each of these steps requires nicotinamide adenine dinucleotide (NAD) as a cofactor, and it is the increased ratio of the reduced cofactor (NADH) to NAD (NADH:NAD) that is responsible for many of the metabolic derangements observed after drinking. *Second,* microsomes of the smooth endoplasmic reticulum (the microsomal ethanol-oxidizing system or MEOS) with a K_m of about 10 mmol may be responsible for 10 percent or more of ethanol oxidation at high blood alcohol concentrations. Increased activity of this system can be induced after repeated exposure to ethanol.

All pathways result in the production of acetaldehyde, which is oxidized to acetate. The specific clinical significance of acetaldehyde is not fully known, but low levels of this substance may cause stimulation and behavioral reinforcement. Accumulation of higher levels in liver, brain, or other body tissues may cause organ damage.

BEHAVIORAL EFFECTS, TOLERANCE, AND DEPENDENCE The behavioral and physiologic effects of any drug depend upon the dose, its rate of increase in plasma, the concomitant presence of other drugs or medical problems, and the past experience with the agent. With alcohol, one must also consider whether observation is during rising (where the effects are more intense) or falling blood alcohol levels.

Even though "legal intoxication" requires a blood alcohol concentration of at least 80 to 100 mg/dL (0.1 g/dL), behavioral, psychomotor, and cognitive changes are seen at levels as low as 20 to 30 mg/dL (i.e., after one to two drinks). Narcosis or deep sleep is induced in many people at twice the legal intoxication level, and even in the absence of concomitant medications, death can occur with levels between 300 and 400 mg/dL. Ethanol, either alone or in combination with agents such as benzodiazepines, is probably responsible for more toxic overdose deaths than any other agent.

The mechanisms of action of ethanol on nervous tissues are not fully understood because even modest doses simultaneously change many neurotransmitters and increase the fluidity of neuronal cell membranes. After repeated exposure to the drug, the body compensates in at least three ways to tolerate higher ethanol levels. *First,* after 1 to 2 weeks of daily drinking the liver can increase the metabolic rate of ethanol in humans by as much as 30 percent; i.e., there is *metabolic or pharmacokinetic tolerance,* an adaptation that disappears almost as rapidly as it develops. *Second,* cellular or *pharmacodynamic tolerance* probably occurs through complex neurochemical adaptations or changes in cell membranes with subsequent altered ion flow—

changes that may contribute to physical dependence. *Third,* even at the same blood alcohol concentrations and neuronal adaptation, organisms can learn to adapt behavior and to function better than expected under drug influence (*behavioral tolerance*). For example, practicing driving while intoxicated might result in a psychomotor performance which (*while still impaired*) is better than that observed before practice.

Once the cells have adapted to chronic ethanol exposure, the structural or biochemical changes may not return to normal for several weeks or more. In the face of these adaptations, the neurons require ethanol to function optimally; i.e., the person is physically addicted or drug-dependent. This physical condition is distinct from psychological dependence, a poorly defined concept indicating that the person is psychologically uncomfortable without the drug.

NUTRITIONAL FACTORS One gram of ethanol has approximately 29.7 kJ (7.1 kcal), and a drink contains between 293.0 and 418.6 kJ (70 and 100 kcal) from ethanol and other carbohydrates. Therefore, 8 to 10 drinks can yield over 4186 kJ (1000 kcal) per day, but these are "empty" of nutrients such as minerals, proteins, and vitamins.

Any vitamin absorbed through the small intestine by active transport or stored in the liver can be deficient in alcoholics. These include folate (folacin or folic acid), pyridoxine (B_6), thiamine (B_1), nicotinic acid or niacin (B_3), and vitamin A. Thiamine deficiency causes Wernicke's and Korsakoff's syndromes (see Chap. 357).

Low blood potassium, magnesium, calcium, zinc, and phosphorus can occur as a consequence of dietary deficiency and acid-base imbalances during excess alcohol ingestion or withdrawal. Hypokalemia can lead to periodic muscle paralysis and areflexia. Deficiencies in magnesium can add to a clouded sensorium and other neurologic symptoms; hypocalcemia can cause tetany and weakness; low levels of zinc are speculated to contribute to gonadal dysfunction, anorexia, problems with wound healing, and immune deficiencies; and low phosphate levels can contribute to myocardial failure, brain dysfunction, weakness of muscles (including those of respiration), and white blood cell and platelet dysfunction.

An ethanol load in a fasting, healthy individual is likely to produce transient hypoglycemia within 6 to 36 h, secondary to the acute actions of ethanol on gluconeogenesis. This impairment is exacerbated by poor diet and by liver and pancreatic disease. As a result, glucose intolerance may be marked until the alcoholic has been abstinent for 2 to 4 weeks. Alcohol ketoacidosis, probably reflecting a decrease in fatty acid oxidation coupled with poor diet or recurrent vomiting, should not be misdiagnosed as diabetic ketosis. With the former, patients show an increase in serum ketones along with a mild increase in glucose but a large anion gap, a mild to moderate increase in serum lactate, and a β-hydroxybutyrate/lactate ratio of between 2:1 and 9:1 (with normal being 1:1).

THE EFFECTS OF ETHANOL ON BODY SYSTEMS

This overview of acute and chronic effects of alcohol on body systems outlines signs and symptoms that can aid in the recognition of the hidden alcoholic. It emphasizes the interactions between drinking and medications and the effects of alcohol on chronic medical conditions, factors that are also important in helping the clinician to understand the effects of alcohol on nonalcoholic patients.

CENTRAL NERVOUS SYSTEM In addition to acute behavioral effects, an evening of heavy drinking can result in an alcoholic "*blackout,*" i.e., an episode of forgetting all or part of what occurred during drinking. This problem is experienced by 30 to 40 percent of men in their late teens and early 20s, most of whom do not go on to develop more serious and pervasive alcohol-related problems. Even after only a few drinks, alcohol acutely decreases *sleep* latency (helping people to fall asleep) and depresses rapid eye movement (REM) sleep early in the night, sometimes followed by later REM rebound associated with bad dreams. The consequence is to "fragment" sleep, causing a more rapid than normal alternation between sleep stages and a deficiency in deep sleep.

Chronic intake of high doses of ethanol can cause *peripheral neuropathy* in 5 to 15 percent of alcoholics (see Chaps. 357 and 363). This syndrome probably results from both thiamine deficiency and direct effects of ethanol and/or acetaldehyde. Patients complain of bilateral limb numbness, tingling, and parasthesias, more pronounced distally than proximally. Although these symptoms can be incapacitating, more often the pain and numbness are mild to moderate in severity. The treatment is abstinence and thiamine supplementation.

Wernicke's and Korsakoff's syndromes are important problems in alcoholics (see Chap. 357). Thiamine deficiency is the major cause in vulnerable individuals (possibly interacting with a genetic transketolase deficiency). Classically, patients with Korsakoff's syndrome present with profound anterograde (unable to learn new material) and retrograde amnesia along with possible impairment in visuospatial, abstract, and conceptual reasoning but with a normal intelligence quotient (IQ). In general, the level of recent memory loss is out of proportion to the global level of cognitive impairment. While most patients demonstrate an acute onset of Korsakoff's syndrome in association with the neurologic stigmata seen with Wernicke's syndrome (e.g., sixth nerve palsy and ataxia), some individuals may have a more gradual development of symptoms probably secondary to repeated bouts of thiamine deficiency. Wernicke's syndrome responds rapidly to oral thiamine replacement of 50 to 100 mg followed by 50 to 100 mg/d. However, only one-quarter of Korsakoff's patients are likely to achieve full recovery, one-half experience partial recovery, and one-quarter show no improvement with thiamine even after many months of supplementation.

About 1 percent of alcoholics with long histories of associated malnutrition develop *cerebellar degeneration,* a syndrome of progressive unsteady stance and gait often accompanied by mild nystagmus (see Chap. 357). Cerebellar atrophy is seen on CT or MRI scan, but the cerebrospinal fluid is usually normal. While ethanol or acetaldehyde might contribute to the problem, the major cause is probably nutritional, and identical symptoms can be seen with some forms of severe malnutrition alone. Treatment consists of abstinence and multiple vitamin supplementation, although improvement is often minimal.

Alcoholics can show severe *cognitive* problems and impairment in recent and remote memory for weeks to months after an alcoholic binge. Cortical functioning (e.g., psychomotor performance and short-term memory) tends to improve with abstinence, but long-term memory problems, perhaps reflecting subcortical damage, may persist. Increased size of the brain ventricles and cerebral sulci are seen in up to 50 percent of chronic alcoholics. These changes are partially reversible, returning toward normal after a year or more of abstinence. Permanent CNS impairment (*alcoholic dementia*) may supervene. Up to 20 percent of chronically demented patients may have had prior alcoholism. There is no single alcoholic dementia syndrome; rather, this label is used to describe patients who have apparently irreversible cognitive changes (possibly from diverse causes) in the midst of chronic alcoholism (see also Chap. 357).

Finally, to borrow a phrase from the past, alcohol could be termed "the great mimicker" because almost every psychiatric syndrome can be seen during heavy drinking or subsequent withdrawal. These include: intense *sadness* lasting for days to weeks in the midst of heavy drinking, a problem that can be viewed as a "normal" effect of alcohol; severe *anxiety* during alcoholic withdrawal, often remaining for many months after cessation of drinking; *psychoses* during the severe form of the alcohol abstinence syndrome; and auditory *hallucinations* and/or *paranoid delusions* in the absence of any obvious signs of withdrawal—a state called alcoholic hallucinosis or alcoholic paranoia. Whatever the cause, the treatment of alcohol-induced psychopathology includes abstinence and supportive care, with the likelihood of full recovery within several days or weeks. Alcohol intake is an important part of the differential diagnosis of *any* patient with one of these psychological symptoms. Another alcohol-related psychiatric syndrome is *pathologic intoxication* or alcohol idiosyncratic intoxication, a state of severe agitation, confusion, and violence lasting minutes to hours which is seen after a very low dose of ethanol (e.g., one to two drinks) and for which the individual is amnestic. This extremely rare phenomenon, seen almost exclusively in individuals with severe preexisting brain damage, is sometimes invoked erroneously for the purposes of legal defense.

THE GASTROINTESTINAL SYSTEM **Esophagus and stomach** Acute alcoholic intake can result in inflammation of the esophagus (possibly secondary to reflux of gastric contents) and stomach (resulting from damage to the gastric mucosal barrier). Esophagitis can cause epigastric distress, and gastritis, the most frequent cause of gastrointestinal bleeding in heavy drinkers, can present with anorexia and abdominal pain. Chronic heavy drinking, if associated with violent vomiting, can produce a longitudinal tear in the mucosa at the gastroesophageal junction—a Mallory-Weiss lesion. Although many gastrointestinal problems are reversible, two complications of chronic alcoholism, esophageal varices secondary to cirrhosis-induced portal hypertension and atrophy of gastric cells, may be irreversible (see Chaps. 237 and 239).

Small bowel The greater part of the ethanol is absorbed from the proximal small bowel, where it may interfere with absorption of B vitamins and other nutrients. Acutely, ethanol can cause hemorrhagic lesions of the duodenal villi and diarrhea secondary to increased small-bowel motility and decreased water and electrolyte absorption. Chronic alcoholism can contribute to diarrhea through its effects on the pancreas (see Chaps. 240 and 260).

Pancreas Alcoholics commonly develop acute or chronic pancreatitis (see Chap. 260).

Liver Ethanol absorbed from the small bowel is carried directly to the liver, where it becomes the preferred fuel; NADH accumulates and oxygen utilization escalates, gluconeogenesis is impaired (with a resulting fall in the amount of glucose produced from glycogen), lactate production increases, and there is a decreased oxidation of fatty acids in the citric cycle with an increase in fat accumulation within liver cells. In the healthy individual taking no medications these changes are reversible, but with repeated exposure to ethanol more severe changes in liver functioning are likely to occur. These include, in overlapping stages, fatty accumulation, alcohol-induced hepatitis, and cirrhosis (see Chap. 254).

Increased cancer risk Cancer is the second leading cause of death in alcoholics (after cardiovascular disease), who have a rate of carcinoma 10 times higher than that expected in the general population. The sites with the greatest increase over expected rates include the head and neck, esophagus, cardia of the stomach, liver, pancreas, and, according to recent data, breast.

HEMATOPOIETIC SYSTEM Ethanol exerts multiple reversible acute and chronic effects on all blood cells. Alcohol alters acutely the production of red blood cells (RBC), which reaches clinical significance after days to weeks of heavy drinking. The most common finding is an increase in RBC size (mean corpuscular volume, MCV) with a mild anemia. If this is accompanied by folic acid deficiency, there can also be hypersegmented neutrophils, reticulocytopenia, and hyperplastic bone marrow. Other forms of anemia, including sideroblastic changes, can occur concomitantly, especially in the presence of severe malnutrition.

Chronic heavy drinking can also decrease production of most white blood cells (WBC), decrease granulocyte mobility and adherence, and impair the delayed hypersensitivity response to new antigens (with a possible false-negative tuberculin skin test). While the changes in WBCs themselves are usually temporary, they may contribute to the risk of infections, liver damage, and perhaps to the increased risk of cancers in alcoholics. Alcohol can also cause toxic granulocytosis.

Many alcoholics present with mild thrombocytopenia (rarely associated with hemorrhage) due to a decrease in platelet survival and altered function; hypersplenism may occur as a complication of cirrhosis. Alcohol may decrease platelet aggregation and inhibit release of thromboxane A_2. These problems usually return toward normal within a week of abstinence.

CARDIOVASCULAR SYSTEM Modest doses of alcohol can have both deleterious and beneficial effects in individuals with normal cardiovascular status who take no medications. Ethanol decreases myocardial contractility and causes peripheral vasodilatation resulting in a mild drop in blood pressure and a compensatory increased heart rate and cardiac output. Exercise-induced increases in cardiac oxygen consumption are higher after alcohol. On the other hand, one to two drinks per day over long periods may decrease the risk of cardiovascular death, perhaps through an increase in high density lipoprotein cholesterol (HDL) or changes in clotting mechanisms.

Although ethanol in low doses causes a mild acute drop in blood pressure, the consumption of three or more drinks per day results in a dose-dependent increase in blood pressure which returns to normal within weeks of abstinence. As a result, heavy drinking is an important contributor to reversible causes of mild to moderate hypertension. Chronic heavy drinking can cause cardiomyopathy with symptoms ranging from unexplained arrhythmias in the presence of left ventricular impairment to heart failure with dilatation of all four heart chambers and hypocontractility of heart muscle. Mural thrombi can form in the left atrium or ventricle, while heart enlargement exceeding 25 percent can cause mitral regurgitation. Finally, there is an association between cerebrovascular accidents and alcoholism, especially within 24 h of heavy drinking. Atrial or ventricular arrhythmias, especially paroxysmal tachycardia, can also occur after a binge in individuals showing no other evidence of heart-disease—a syndrome known as the "holiday heart."

GENITOURINARY SYSTEM CHANGES, SEXUAL FUNCTIONING, AND FETAL DEVELOPMENT Acutely, modest ethanol doses (e.g., blood alcohol concentrations of 100 mg/dL or even less) increase sexual drive in men. However, modest ethanol doses may simultaneously decrease erectile capacity. Even in the absence of liver impairment, a significant minority of chronic alcoholic men may show irreversible testicular atrophy with concomitant shrinkage of the seminiferous tubules and loss of sperm cells (see Chap. 321).

The repeated ingestion of high doses of ethanol by women can result in amenorrhea, a decrease in ovarian size, an absence of corpora lutea with associated infertility, and spontaneous abortions. Heavy drinking during pregnancy results in the rapid placental transfer of both ethanol and acetaldehyde, which may have serious consequences for fetal development. The *fetal alcohol syndrome* can include a mixture of any of the following: facial changes with epicanthal eye folds, poorly formed concha, and small teeth with faulty enamel; cardiac atrial or ventricular septal defects; an aberrant palmar crease and limitation in joint movement; and microcephaly with mental retardation (see Chap. 358). The specific amount of ethanol and/or specific time of vulnerability during pregnancy has not been defined, making it advisable for pregnant women to abstain completely.

OTHER EFFECTS OF ETHANOL Heavy drinking can produce an acute *alcoholic myopathy* characterized by painful and swollen muscles, high levels of serum creatine phosphokinase (CK), and rarely myoglobinemia and myoglobinuria. Effects on the *skeletal system* include alterations in calcium metabolism with an increased risk for fractures and osteonecrosis of the femoral head. *Hormonal* changes include an increase in cortisol levels, which can remain elevated during heavy drinking; inhibition of vasopressin secretion at rising blood alcohol concentrations and the opposite at falling blood alcohol concentrations, with the final result that most alcoholics are likely to be slightly overhydrated; a modest and reversible decrease in serum thyroxine (T_4); and a more marked decrease in serum triiodothyronine (T_3).

ALCOHOLISM

Because many drinkers occasionally imbibe to excess, temporary alcohol-related pathology is common in nonalcoholics. The time of heaviest drinking is usually the late teens to the late twenties when between one-third and one-half of male drinkers experience some isolated (although potentially dangerous) alcohol-related social, occupational, or driving difficulty. These include alcohol-related blackouts, a single drunk driving arrest, arguments with friends, and so on. This prevalent alcohol-related morbidity, however, is temporary and a separate problem from alcoholism. The following sections describe diagnostic criteria for alcoholism, offer suggestions for identifying the usual (i.e., middle-class) alcoholic in everyday medical practice, review evidence that alcoholism is a biologic and genetically influenced disorder, and offer advice on confrontation, detoxification, and rehabilitation of alcoholics.

DEFINITIONS AND EPIDEMIOLOGY The original version of the Third Diagnostic and Statistical Manual of the American Psychiatric Association (DSM-III) and the more recent revision (DSM-IIIR) divide alcoholism into alcohol abuse and alcohol dependence, but this distinction may not be clinically relevant. *Alcohol abuse* indicates psychological dependence, i.e., the need for alcohol for adequate functioning, along with occasional heavy consumption, and continuation of drinking despite social or occupational problems. *Alcohol dependence* encompasses similar impairment *along with* evidence of increased ethanol tolerance or physical signs on withdrawal from alcohol.

A modified approach to a definition of alcoholism is easier to apply in clinical settings. The diagnosis of *alcoholism* is made when an individual ignores the early warning signs that alcohol is causing problems in marriage and goes on to an alcohol-related marital separation or divorce; *or* when alcohol-related problems on the job actually result in the patient being fired or laid off; *or* when there are two or more arrests related to alcohol; *or* when there is physical evidence that alcohol has harmed health (e.g., cardiomyopathy, cirrhosis, alcoholic hepatitis), including signs of alcoholic withdrawal.

It is important to distinguish between *primary and secondary alcoholism*. For example, serious alcohol-related problems occurring during the course of mania or a preexisting antisocial personality disorder (i.e., secondary alcoholism) might be symptomatic of the primary diagnosis, and the course is likely to be that of the primary disorder, not alcoholism. The information on alcoholism offered in this chapter is relevant for *primary alcoholism*. This diagnosis applies to the majority of alcoholics (70 to 80 percent) who develop major life problems from alcohol *before* they fulfill criteria for any other major psychiatric illness.

Using this or similar criteria, the lifetime risk for primary alcoholism in most western countries is about 10 percent for men and 3 to 5 percent for women. When less stringent criteria are used, the rates are substantially higher. Alcoholism is seen in all races, ethnic groups, and socioeconomic strata and, therefore, the average alcoholic (just as the average person) is a blue-collar or white-collar worker or housewife. The homeless or skid row alcoholic represents only 5 percent or less of alcoholics.

GENETICS OF ALCOHOLISM There is strong evidence that alcoholism is a multifactorial disorder in which biologic and genetic factors interact. The importance of genetic factors in alcoholism is supported by family, twin, and adoption studies. Close relatives of primary alcoholics have an approximately fourfold increased risk for the disorder but are not significantly more vulnerable for other psychiatric illnesses. The probability that the familial nature of the problem is in part a consequence of genetic factors is supported by twin research, where the risk for the identical twin of an alcoholic is much higher than for the fraternal twin of an alcohol abuser. Finally, adoption studies reveal that the fourfold increased risk for children of alcoholics is true even if they were adopted away at birth and raised without knowledge of the problems of their biologic parents.

The evidence supporting genetic influences in alcoholism has stimulated numerous studies of children of alcoholics. The goal is to identify possible trait markers of a vulnerability toward the disorder before alcoholism appears. For example, some studies suggest that these children become significantly less intoxicated at a given blood alcohol concentration than do controls, even before alcoholism develops. After modest alcohol doses, the sons of alcoholics report less intense subjective feelings of intoxication, show less alcohol-related impairment in cognitive and psychomotor tests, and have less intense changes in prolactin and cortisol secretion than do controls. These data may indicate that men at high future risk for alcoholism may be less able than controls to tell when they are beginning to become intoxicated. Taken as a whole these data underscore the probability that alcoholism is biologically influenced and not related to a lack of "moral fiber." It is not surprising that the average alcoholic may continue to work, has a family, and may be difficult to identify if the physician persists with old stereotypes.

NATURAL HISTORY For the "average" alcoholic, the age of first drink and first minor problems (e.g., an argument with a friend while drunk or an alcoholic blackout) are similar to those in the general population. However, by the mid to late twenties, most men and women moderate their drinking (perhaps learning from minor problems), whereas difficulties for alcoholics are likely to escalate, with the first major life problem from alcohol appearing in the late twenties to early forties. Once established, the course of alcoholism is likely to be one of exacerbations and remissions; the alcoholic becomes frightened when a problem develops and abstains for a period of days to months before experimenting with controlled drinking; this step almost inevitably results in escalation of drinking and problems. The course is not hopeless because a fifth or more achieve permanent abstinence without formal treatment or aid from self-help groups such as Alcoholics Anonymous (AA). However, should the alcoholic continue to drink, the life span is shortened by an average of 15 years with the leading causes of death, in decreasing order, being heart disease, cancer, accidents, and suicide.

IDENTIFICATION AND CONFRONTATION OF THE ALCOHOLIC The physician should recognize that any patient may have alcoholism and must therefore pay attention to physical findings and laboratory tests that are likely to be abnormal in the alcoholic. These include a high normal or slightly elevated MCV, γ-glutamyl transferase (GGT) (35 to 40 or more units), serum uric acid [greater than 416 μmol/L (7 mg/dL)], and triglycerides [2.0 mmol/L (180 mg/dL) or more]. Mild and fluctuating levels of hypertension (e.g., 140/95), repeated infections such as pneumonia, and otherwise unexplained cardiac arrhythmias all suggest that the patient might be an alcoholic. Certain specific clinical findings also should raise suspicions, including cancer of the head and neck, esophagus, or cardia of the stomach as well as cirrhosis, unexplained hepatitis, pancreatitis, bilateral parotid gland swelling, and peripheral neuropathy.

Once the likelihood of alcoholism is established, only a few moments are needed to gather the history of alcohol-related life problems. The patient *and spouse* should be asked about patterns of accidents, marital difficulties, problems on the job, and driving-related difficulties, after which the role played by alcohol should be identified. All physicians should be able to take the time needed to gather such information. In addition, a simple 25-item form to be answered by the patient, the Michigan Alcohol Screening Test (MAST), is available to aid in identifying the alcoholic.

After an alcoholic is identified, he or she should be confronted with the diagnosis. The presenting complaint can be used as an entrée to the alcohol problem. For instance, the patient complaining of insomnia or hypertension could be told that these are clinically important symptoms and that laboratory tests and physical findings indicate that alcohol appears to have contributed to the complaints and is increasing the risk for further medical and psychological problems. The physician should share information about the course of alcoholism and explore possible avenues of attacking the problem.

The process of confrontation is rarely accomplished in one session. It is helpful to let patients know that they are responsible for their own actions and that the decision to quit drinking rests with them. For the person who refuses to stop drinking at the first confrontation, a logical step is to "keep the door open," establishing future meetings so that help is available as problems escalate. In the meantime the family may benefit from counseling or referral to self-help group such as Alanon (the Alcoholics Anonymous group for family members) and Alateen (for teenage children of alcoholics).

Those patients who refuse to stop but who want to "cut down" should be reminded that the average alcoholic successfully cuts back scores of times but that sooner or later drinking again escalates. The patient who refuses to stop might be offered a guideline of drinking no more than two drinks [115 mL (4 oz) of wine, 340 mL (12 oz) of beer, or 43 mL (1.5 oz) of 80-proof beverage amounts to one drink)] in any 24-h period, but it is very unlikely that this will be effective for an extended period of time. This is another way of keeping the door open in the hope that the patient will return as drinking escalates.

TREATMENT OF THE ALCOHOL-RELATED WITHDRAWAL SYNDROME **The clinical syndrome** In the presence of ethanol-induced cellular tolerance, any sudden decrease in ethanol may lead to symptoms of withdrawal from the CNS-depressant effects. As with most syndromes, most patients do not develop every symptom and the usual clinical picture is mild. Features include a tremor of the hands (shakes or jitters); autonomic nervous sytem dysfunction such as increases in pulse, respiratory rate, and body temperature; insomnia, possibly accompanied by bad dreams; feelings of generalized anxiety or panic attacks; and gastrointestinal upset. Symptoms begin within 5 to 10 h of decreasing ethanol intake (addicted patients are likely to awaken in the morning with some signs of withdrawal), peak in intensity on day 2 or 3, and improve by day 4 or 5. Anxiety, insomnia, and mild levels of autonomic dysfunction may persist for 6 months or more, as a protracted abstinence syndrome that may contribute to the tendency to return to drinking.

About 5 percent of alcoholics show evidence of severe withdrawal symptoms. These include a state of confusion sometimes accompanied by visual, tactile, or auditory hallucinations. These psychotic symptoms are likely to disappear as the mental state becomes clearer over a period of several days and are distinct from the chronic alcoholic auditory hallucinosis with a clear sensorium described earlier in this chapter. A small percentage of alcoholics also demonstrate one or two generalized seizures ("rum fits"), usually within 48 h of stopping drinking. These are rarely focal in nature (unless there is underlying neuropathology) and electroencephalographic abnormalities are mild and usually return to normal within several days. There is no evidence that withdrawal seizures represent "latent" epilepsy.

The diagnosis of delirium tremens (DTs) is made when the course progresses beyond the usual symptoms of withdrawal to include confusion (with associated delusions and hallucinations), severe agitation, and generalized seizures. The likelihood of developing severe withdrawal symptoms increases with concomitant infections or medical problems, a prior history of withdrawal seizures or DTs, and higher quantity and frequency of drinking. Most periods of severe withdrawal begin and end abruptly, rarely lasting longer than 3 to 5 days. The mortality risk for DTs is quite low but increases with preexisting medical illnesses or organ system failure.

Treatment of withdrawal The *first* and most important step is to perform a *thorough* physical examination in all alcoholics who are considering stopping drinking and in those patients who might be undergoing withdrawal. It is necessary to evaluate organ systems likely to be impaired by heavy drinking, including searching for evidence of liver failure, gastrointestinal bleeding, cardiac arrhythmia, and glucose or electrolyte imbalance.

The *second* step in treating withdrawal is to give patients adequate nutrition and rest. All patients should be administered multiple B vitamins, including 50 to 100 mg of thiamine daily for a week or more. Most patients enter withdrawal with normal levels of body water or mild levels of overhydration, and intravenous fluids should be avoided unless there is evidence of hypotension or a history of recent excessive bleeding, vomiting, or diarrhea. Usually medications can be administered orally.

The *third* step in treatment is to recognize the CNS symptoms caused by removal of the brain-depressant effects of ethanol. Symptoms can be alleviated by administering another CNS depressant and gradually decreasing the levels of the drug over a 3- to 5-day period. While many CNS depressants are effective, the *benzodiazepines* have the highest margin of safety and are, therefore, the preferred class of drugs in the treatment of alcohol withdrawal. Benzodiazepines with short half-lives (see Chap. 369) are especially useful for patients with serious liver impairment or evidence of preexisting encephalopathy or brain damage. On the other hand, short half-life benzodiazepines, e.g., oxazepam or lorazepam, result in rapidly changing drug blood levels; administration every 4 h is required to avoid abrupt fluctuations in blood levels that may increase the risk for seizures. Therefore, most clinicians use drugs with longer half-lives, like diazepam or chlordiazepoxide. The goal is to administer sufficient drug on day 1 to alleviate most of the symptoms of withdrawal and then to decrease the dose by 20 percent on successive days over a period of 3 to 5 days. The dose is increased if signs of withdrawal escalate, and the medication is withheld if the patient is sleeping or shows signs of increasing orthostatic hypotension. The average patient requires 25 to 50 mg of chlordiazepoxide or 10 mg of diazepam given orally every 4 to 6 h on the first day.

The most effective treatment of *severe withdrawal* including delirium tremens remains controversial. Most clinicians use benzodiazepines, but despite as much as 300 mg or more per day of chlordiazepoxide the patient may still remain awake and agitated. Since it is probable that the confused, agitated state will persist for 3 to 5 days regardless of the pharmacologic intervention used, drugs are given to control behavior rather than to change the course of the syndrome. Antipsychotic medications like thioridazine or haloperidol have no place in the treatment of mild withdrawal symptoms.

The generalized seizures or "rum fits" rarely require aggressive pharmacologic intervention beyond that given to the usual patient undergoing withdrawal, i.e., adequate doses of benzodiazepines. There is little evidence that phenytoin is effective in drug withdrawal seizures, and the risk of seizures usually has passed by the time effective drug levels are reached. The rare patient with status epilepticus can be treated initially with intravenous diazepam. If anticonvulsants are used for alcohol withdrawal seizures, they should be stopped within 5 to 7 days unless a cause for a persisting seizure disorder is documented.

While alcohol withdrawal is often treated in a hospital, efforts at reducing costs have resulted in experimentation with outpatient detoxification for alcoholics with mild abstinence syndromes. This outpatient approach is appropriate for patients in good physical condition who demonstrate mild signs of withdrawal despite low blood alcohol concentrations and for those without prior history of DTs or withdrawal seizures. Such individuals still require careful physical examination, evaluation of blood tests, and treatment with vitamin supplementation, and appropriate doses of benzodiazepines might also be used. The latter are given *in a 1- to 2-day supply* to be administered to the patient by a spouse four times a day. Patients are asked to *return daily* for evaluation of vital signs, and the patient's family or friends are told to bring him or her to the emergency room if signs and symptoms of withdrawal escalate.

THE TREATMENT OR REHABILITATION OF ALCOHOLICS After completing alcoholic rehabilitation, 60 percent or more of middle-class alcoholics maintain abstinence for at least a year, many for a lifetime. There is no single best way to rehabilitate the alcoholic, and therapeutic approaches center on general supports which meet commonsense guidelines. Considering the lack of evidence for superiority of any specific treatment type, it is best to keep interventions as simple, safe, and inexpensive as possible.

Maneuvers in rehabilitation fall into two general categories. *First* are attempts to help the alcoholic achieve and maintain a high level of motivation toward abstinence. This includes educating the patient about alcoholism, and teaching the family and/or friends to stop protecting the alcoholic from the problems caused by alcohol. The *second* series of maneuvers help the patient to readjust to life without alcohol and to reestablish a functional life-style through personal counseling, vocational rehabilitation, family support, and sexual counseling.

There is no convincing evidence that inpatient rehabilitation is more effective for the average primary alcoholic than is outpatient care. The decision to hospitalize can be made if (1) the patient has medical problems that are difficult to treat outside a hospital; (2) depression, confusion, or psychosis interfere with outpatient care; (3) the patient has such a severe life crisis that it is difficult to get his or her attention as an outpatient; (4) outpatient treatment has failed; or (5) the patient lives too far from the treatment center. If inpatient care is needed, free-standing treatment programs, units that are divisions of general hospitals, and those in psychiatric hospitals are equally effective. The characteristics of the patient predict outcome more than any specific attribute of the program.

Whether the treatment begins in an inpatient or an outpatient setting, subsequent contact should be maintained for a minimum of 6 months after abstinence is achieved. Counseling with an individual physician or through groups focuses on day-to-day living—emphasizing areas of improved functioning in the absence of alcohol (i.e., why it is a good idea to continue to abstain) and helping the patient to deal with free time without alcohol, develop a nondrinking peer group, and handle stresses on the job without alcohol.

The physician serves an important role in identifying the alcoholic, treating medical or psychiatric syndromes associated with alcoholism, carrying out detoxification, referring to rehabilitation programs, and counseling alcoholics in an inpatient or outpatient setting. The physician must also regulate drug treatment during alcoholism rehabilitation. Once acute detoxification is complete (an average of 3 to 5 days), there is *no place* for hypnotics or antianxiety drugs in the treatment of most alcoholics. The patient has already demonstrated an inability to moderate the use of one brain depressant, alcohol, and is at considerable risk for abusing sleeping pills or tranquilizers. Anxiety and insomnia can be treated with behavior modification such as relaxation training, meditation, and exercise or through increased activity in hobbies or religion.

One medication which has been used in alcohol rehabilitation is disulfiram, usually given as 250 mg/d. This drug inhibits aldehyde dehydrogenase, causing very high levels of acetaldehyde to accumulate after alcohol is consumed. The disulfiram ethanol reaction includes tremor, hypertension or hypotension, nausea and possibly severe vomiting, and diarrhea. Disulfiram must not be given to persons for whom such a reaction could be dangerous, including patients with portal hypertension, diabetes mellitus, heart disease, or a history of stroke. All drugs have their dangers, and the physician is advised to read carefully about disulfiram and be fully aware of the potential, although rare, serious adverse reactions that can occur. Unfortunately, there is little convincing evidence from carefully controlled studies that the effectiveness of disulfiram is significantly greater than placebo. As result, this drug should not be routinely prescribed.

Finally, an inexpensive, readily available, and dedicated additional support for all alcoholics is available in almost every community. Alcoholics Anonymous is a self-help group of recovering alcoholics (men and women who have stopped drinking, perhaps many years ago) which offers an effective model showing that abstinence can be achieved, provides a sober peer group, and makes crisis intervention available when the drive to drink escalates. No matter what type of rehabilitation program is planned, the alcoholic should be offered the option of joining Alcoholics Anonymous.

REFERENCES

BAUMGARTNER GR et al: Clonidine vs. chlordiazepoxide in the acute alcohol withdrawal syndrome. Arch Intern Med 147:1223, 1987

BLUM K et al: Allelic association of human dopamine D_2 receptor gene in alcoholism. JAMA 263:2055, 1990

CRIQUI MH: Alcohol consumption, blood pressure, lipids, and cardiovascular mortality. Alc: Clin Exp Res 10:564, 1986

DONAHUE RP et al: Alcohol and hemorrhagic stroke. JAMA 255:2311, 1986

FRANK D, RAICHT RF: Alcohol-induced liver disease. Alc: Clin Exp Res 9:66, 1985

FULLER RK et al: Disulfiram treatment of alcoholism. JAMA 256:1449, 1986

GOLDSTEIN DB: *Pharmacology of Alcohol*. New York, Oxford University Press, 1983

GOODWIN DW, GUZE SB: *Psychiatric Diagnosis*, 4th ed. New York, Oxford University Press, 1989

GRANT I: Alcohol and the brain. JCCP 55:310, 1987

GREENSPON AJ, SCHAAL SF: The "holiday heart": Electrophysiologic studies of alcohol effects in alcoholics. Ann Intern Med 98:135, 1983

HARPER C et al: Are we drinking our neurones away? Br Med H 294:534, 1987

IRWIN M et al: Monitoring heavy drinking. Am J Psychiatry 145:595, 1988

LIEBER C: *Metabolic Aspects of Alcoholism*. Lancaster, England, MTP Press, 1977

———: To drink (moderately) or not to drink? N Engl J Med 310:846, 1984

LISHMAN WA: Cerebral disorder in alcoholism: Syndromes of impairment. Brain 104:1, 1981

LISKOW BI, GOODWIN DW: Pharmacological treatment of alcohol intoxication, withdrawal and dependence. J Stud Alc 48:356, 1987

MEAGHER RC et al: Suppression of hematopoietic-progenitor-cell proliferation by ethanol and acetaldehyde. N Engl J Med 307:845, 1982

MELLO NK, BREE MP: Alcohol self-administration disrupts reproductive function in female macaque monkeys. Science 221:677, 1983

MENDELSON JH, MELLO NK: Biologic concomitants of alcoholism. N Engl J Med 301:912, 1979

MUKHERJEE AB et al: Transketolase abnormality in fibroblasts from chronic alcoholics. J Clin Invest 79:1039, 1987

PFEFFERBAUM A et al: Brain CT changes in alcoholics. Alc: Clin Exp Res 12:81, 1988

POTTER JF, BEEVERS DG: Pressor effect of alcohol in hypertension. Lancet: 1:119, 1984

SCHUCKIT MA et al: A simultaneous evaluation of multiple markers of ethanol response in sons of alcoholics. Arch Gen Psychiatr 45:211, 1988

———: Genetic and clinical implications of alcoholism and affective disorder. Am J Psychiatry 143:140, 1986

———: *Drug and Alcohol Abuse: A Clinical Guide to Diagnosis and Treatment*, 3d ed. New York, Plenum, 1989

SCHUCKIT MA: *Alcohol Patterns and Problems*. New Brunswick, Rutgers Press, 1985

———: Genetics and the risk for alcoholism. JAMA 254:2614, 1985

SELLERS EM, KALANT H: Alcohol intoxication and withdrawal. N Engl J Med 294:757, 1976

STREISSGUTH AP, LANDESMAN-DWYER S: Teratogenic effects of alcohol in humans and laboratory animals. Science 209:353, 1980

VAILLANT GE: *The Natural History of Alcoholism*. Cambridge, Mass., Harvard, 1983

VAN THIEL DH: Gastrointestinal and hepatic manifestations of chronic alcoholism. Gastroenterology 81:594, 1981

VICTOR M, ADAMS RD: *The Wernicke-Korsakoff Syndrome*, 2d ed. Philadelphia, Davis, 1989

371 OPIOID DRUG USE

MARC A. SCHUCKIT / DAVID S. SEGAL

The principal effects of the opioids (opiate-like drugs) are a significant damping of pain perception along with modest levels of sedation and euphoria. Tolerance to any one opioid is likely to generalize to the others (i.e., cross-tolerance is likely), and all share a similar pattern of drug-related problems. Each of these substances is capable of producing physical addiction (and thus they all have some legal restrictions), and the abstinence syndrome from any one of the substances can be treated with administration of any of the others.

PHARMACOLOGY The prototypic opiates, morphine and codeine (3-methoxymorphine), are taken directly from the milky juice of the poppy, *Papaver somniferum*. The semisynthetic drugs produced from the morphine or thebane molecules include hydromorphone, codeine, diacetylmorphine (heroin), and oxycodone. The purely synthetic opioids, sharing many of the basic properties of opium and morphine, include meperidine, propoxyphene, diphenoxylate, methadone, and pentazocine. Despite claims to the contrary, all of these substances (including almost all prescription analgesics) are capable of producing euphoria as well as psychological and physical dependence when taken in high enough doses over prolonged periods of time.

The opioids produce their effects by binding to different types of opioid receptors throughout the body including the central nervous system. Endogenous opioid peptides (i.e., enkephalins, endorphins, dynorphin, and others) have been identified that appear to be natural ligands for opioid receptors. These peptides have a distinct distribution in the CNS. Recent evidence suggests that the receptors with which opioid peptides interact may be differentially engaged in production of the various opiate effects such as analgesia, respiratory depression, constipation, and euphoria. Substances capable of antagonizing one or more of these actions include nalorphine, levallophan, cyclazocine, and pentazocine, each of which has mixed agonist and antagonist properties, as well as naloxone and naltrexone, which are pure opiate antagonists. Mixed agonist-antagonist drugs (for example, pentazocine), if administered to a patient addicted to other narcotics, may precipitate opiate withdrawal symptoms. The availability of relatively specific antagonists has helped identify different receptor subtypes including the μ_1 subtype of the classic morphine receptor μ.

Opiate tolerance, dependence, and withdrawal are considered to be related phenomena with common underlying mechanisms. A number of neurochemical systems and psychological processes appear to be implicated in these effects that emerge with chronic administration of morphine or related opiates. Perhaps reflecting the actions of different classes of receptors, tolerance to various opiate actions may develop at different rates, and these same mechanisms might contribute to the diverse signs and symptoms characteristic of withdrawal. Other biochemical systems that might contribute to the development of tolerance and dependence include changes in intracellular modulators such as adenyl nucleotides, calcium and related substances, as well as alterations in neurotransmitters, including acetylcholine, serotonin, and the catecholamines norepinephrine and dopamine. Evidence also implicates environmental and learning factors. For example, clinical observations suggest that classic conditioning plays a role in maintaining dependence in at least some addicts and that conditioning extinction procedures may be useful when integrated into a comprehensive treatment program for opioid addiction. Further research into these phenomena and efforts to elucidate neurochemical mechanisms could significantly facilitate the development of more effective approaches to treatment and prevention.

All of the opioid drugs are easily absorbed from the gastrointestinal system, the lungs, and the muscles. The most rapid and pronounced effects occur following intravenous administration, and the least intense actions are seen after absorption from the digestive tract, at least in part because some of the oral drug is metabolized before it passes into the general circulation. Most of the metabolism of opiates occurs in the liver, primarily through conjugation with glucuronic acid, and only small amounts are excreted directly in the urine or feces. The plasma half-lives of these drugs range from 2.5 to 3 h for morphine to more than 22 h for methadone and even longer for methadyl acetate.

Street heroin typically contains only 5 to 10 percent of the opiate. The remainder consists of materials such as lactose and fruit sugars, quinine, powdered milk, phenacetin, caffeine, antipyrine, and strychnine which are used to "cut" the drug and increase the margin of profit.

THE ACUTE AND CHRONIC EFFECTS OF OPIOID DRUGS ON BODY SYSTEMS With the exception of overdose conditions and changes associated with physical addiction, most opiate actions are relatively benign and rapidly reversible.

Effects on body systems Acute changes in the *gastrointestinal system* are the result of decreased GI motility with resulting constipation and anorexia. Chronic GI problems in opiate addicts typically occur as a consequence of impaired liver function resulting from concomitant administration of other drugs and from the development of hepatitis B from shared "dirty" needles.

The direct effects on opiate receptors in the *central nervous system* can result in nausea and vomiting (medulla), decreased pain perception (spinal cord, thalamus, and periaqueductal grey region), euphoria (limbic system), and sedation (reticular activating system and striatum). The adulterants added to street drugs may contribute to some of the more permanent nervous system damage, including peripheral neuropathy, amblyopia, myelopathy, and leukoencephalopathy, while use of contaminated needles can produce abscesses in the CNS and transmit AIDS. Acute opiate administration results in decreases in luteinizing hormone (LH), with a subsequent decrease in testosterone which might contribute to the decreased sex drive reported by most opiate addicts. Other hormonal changes include a decrease in the release of thyrotropin as well as increases in prolactin and possibly in growth hormone (see Chap. 313).

Acute changes in the *respiratory system* include respiratory depression, which results from a decreased response of the brainstem to carbon dioxide tension, a component of the drug overdose syndrome described below. At even low drug doses, this effect can be clinically significant in individuals with compromised lung activity. *Cardiovascular* changes tend to be relatively mild with no direct opiate effect on heart rhythm or myocardial contractility, but there is a potential problem from orthostatic hypotension, probably secondary to dilatation of peripheral vessels. Bacterial infections of both the lungs and heart valves can occur from contaminated needles.

The toxic reaction or overdose syndrome High doses of opiates taken intentionally (in a suicide attempt) or by the street user who has misjudged the potency of the injected substance can result in a toxic reaction or overdose syndrome with a potentially lethal consequence. The typical syndrome, which occurs immediately with intravenous (IV) overdose, includes shallow respirations of two to four per minute, pupillary miosis (with mydriasis once brain anoxia develops), bradycardia, a decrease in body temperature, and a general absence of responsiveness to external stimulation. If this medical emergency is not treated rapidly, symptoms can progress to cyanosis, and death can ensue from respiratory depression and cardiorespiratory arrest. Postmortem examination reveals few specific changes except for diffuse cerebral edema. An "allergic-like" reaction to adulterants can also occur and is characterized by decreased alertness, a frothy pulmonary edema, and an elevation in the blood eosinophil count.

The preferred treatment for the typical opiate overdose is the narcotic antagonist naloxone, given in an initial dose of 0.4 mg (1 mL) or 0.01 mg/kg intramuscularly (IM) or IV, which can be repeated in 3 to 10 min if no response occurs. Because the effects of this drug diminish within 2 to 3 h, it is important to monitor the individual for at least 24 h after a heroin overdose and 72 h after an overdose of longer-acting drugs such as methadone. Patients who are also physically addicted to an opioid are likely to experience a precipitous onset of an abstinence syndrome within 2 to 8 h after administration of the opioid antagonist, but aggressive treatment of this syndrome is not appropriate until all vital signs are relatively stable.

As with any drug overdose, treatment of either the typical or the "allergic" type of opiate toxic reaction often requires support of vital signs until the body detoxifies the substance. Patients may require a respirator (especially one using oxygen and positive pressure breathing for the "allergic" type of overdose), IV fluids perhaps accompanied by pressor agents to support blood pressure, and gastric lavage to remove any remaining drug, with care taken to use a cuffed endotracheal tube to prevent aspiration if the patient is not alert. Cardiac arrhythmias and/or convulsions, especially likely to be seen with codeine, propoxyphene, or meperidine, also need to be treated.

THE OPIATE ABUSER The medical abuser Two groups of individuals are at high risk for abusing analgesics. First, evidence suggests that a majority of people with *chronic pain syndromes* (e.g., back, joint, and muscle disorders) may misuse their prescribed drugs at various times. If physical dependence is established, abstinence syndromes can then intensify the pain, promoting continued drug intake. A few precautions can help the physician to avoid contributing to physical dependence in chronic pain patients, particularly those who have demonstrated a propensity to misuse opioids: (1) the goal is to minimize the debilitating effects of pain with the understanding that discomfort may not be completely eliminated (Chap. 15); (2) all possible efforts must be taken to reinforce the need for the patient to become actively involved in and committed to improvement; (3) analgesic medication should be only one component of treatment and limited to oral administration of the least potent analgesic required to take the "edge off" the pain (e.g., propoxyphene); all such drugs should be coordinated through one physician; (4) behavior modification techniques can include muscle relaxation and meditation, while carefully selected exercises can help increase function and decrease pain; (5) nonmedicinal approaches including electrical transcutaneous neurostimulation for muscle and joint disease can be applied (see also Chap. 15).

The second group at high risk are *physicians, nurses, and pharmacists,* primarily because of their easy access to substances of abuse. Physicians may begin to use opiates to help them sleep or to reduce stress or physical aches and pains. A family history of substance abuse (including alcoholism) probably helps to identify the physician at exceptionally high risk. Because of the growing awareness of these problems, impaired physician programs have been established in many hospitals and by most state medical societies. These groups attempt to identify and aid substance-impaired physicians, giving them peer support and education so as to achieve abstinence before problems escalate to the point of licensure revocation. In general, doctors are advised never to prescribe opiates for themselves or for members of their family—physicians deserve the same level of care and protection from future problems as their patients.

The street abuser Some opiate addicts satisfy criteria for the antisocial personality disorder as evidenced by serious antisocial problems beginning prior to age 15 and before the first major life problem from drugs (see Chap. 368). However, the majority of opiate addicts have a relatively high level of premorbid functioning. The usual street abuser begins using opiates occasionally, often after experimenting with tobacco, then alcohol, then marijuana, and then brain depressants or stimulants. Occasional opiate use, or "chipping," might continue for some time, and some individuals probably never escalate their intake to the point of developing serious problems. Another pattern of temporary or intermittent abuse is represented by the experiences of Vietnam soldiers, most of whom had little or no prior experience with opiates and who found themselves in a situation of high stress and readily available drugs. Under these circumstances, as many as one-half tried opiates and, although many became physically addicted, those who had not misused drugs before Vietnam tended to return to drug-free status when back in their home communities.

Once persistent opiate use is established, the outcome is often extremely serious. At least 25 percent of such opiate abusers are likely to die within 10 to 20 years of active abuse, with death from suicide, homicide, accidents, and infectious diseases such as tuberculosis or serum hepatitis. The mortality rate has escalated in recent years in response to the epidemic of AIDS among IV drug abusers (see Chap. 264). As many as 50 percent of male and 25 percent of female addicts turn to alcohol when their primary drug is not available, and many of these people meet the criteria for secondary alcohol abuse. The prevalence of alcohol misuse is higher in drug treatment dropouts than in those who stay with therapy, and abuse is more likely in individuals with a history of alcohol problems before they developed opiate-related difficulties.

PHYSICAL ADDICTION AND THE OPIATE ABSTINENCE SYNDROME **The symptoms of withdrawal** The time to onset as well as the intensity and duration of the acute abstinence syndrome are influenced by a number of factors including the drug's half-life, its dose, and the chronicity of administration. The withdrawal symptoms tend to be opposite to the acute effects of the drug and include nausea and diarrhea, coughing, lacrimation, rhinorrhea, profuse sweating, twitching muscles, and piloerection or "goose bumps"; mild elevations in body temperature, respiratory rate, and blood pressure are also observed. In addition, sensations of diffuse body pain, insomnia, and yawning occur with intense drug craving. Drugs with a short half-life, such as morphine or heroin, cause symptoms typically within 8 to 16 h of the last dose (thus, many addicts awake in mild withdrawal every morning); peak effects are apparent within 36 to 72 h after discontinuation of the drug, and the acute syndrome disappears within 5 to 8 days. However, a protracted abstinence phase of mild symptoms (e.g., slight changes in pupillary size, autonomic dysfunction, changes in sleep pattern) may persist for 6 or more months.

Treatment of the withdrawal syndrome Patients *must* receive a thorough physical examination which includes an assessment of liver and neurologic function as well as identification of local and systemic infections, especially abscesses. Proper nutrition and rest must be initiated as soon as possible.

Effective treatment of withdrawal, however, also requires readministration of sufficient opiate medication on day one to decrease symptoms, followed by a more gradual withdrawal of the drug, usually over 5 to 10 days. Any opiate will work (they all have some level of cross-tolerance) but for ease of administration many physicians prefer to use a long-acting drug like methadone. In estimating the first day's dose from the patient's history, 1 mg of methadone is approximately equivalent to 3 mg of morphine, 1 mg of heroin, or 20 mg of meperidine. Most patients require between 10 and 25 mg of methadone orally given twice on day one, with higher doses given if prominent symptoms of withdrawal are not damped. After several days of a stabilized drug dose, the opiate is then decreased by 10 to 20 percent of the original day's dose each day.

Most states have restrictions on the prescription of opiates to addicts, and in the absence of special permits, detoxification with opiates is usually limited to 1 month or less. One relatively successful nonopiate approach to the treatment of withdrawal is the use of the $alpha_2$-adrenergic agonist clonidine, used in part to decrease sympathetic nervous system overactivity. Given at doses of approximately 5 μg/kg (up to 0.3 mg given two to four times a day), clonidine causes most patients undergoing opiate withdrawal to experience a decrease in autonomic nervous system dysfunction. Opiates, however, are more effective in relieving discomfort and pain, and clonidine is often not well tolerated because it produces high levels of sedation and orthostatic hypotension. Therefore, under most circumstances opiates are the treatment of choice.

A special case of opiate withdrawal is seen in the newborn, passively addicted by the mother's drug misuse during pregnancy. Some level of addiction develops in 50 to 90 percent of children of heroin-dependent mothers, and the withdrawal syndrome carries a mortality of between 3 and 30 percent if not treated when prominent signs are apparent. In distinction to street addicts, as few as 25 percent of infants of methadone-maintenance-addicted mothers show clinically relevant withdrawal symptoms. The syndrome consists of irritability, crying, a tremor (in 80 percent), increased reflexes, increased respiratory rate, diarrhea, hyperactivity (in 60 percent), vomiting (40 percent), and sneezing/yawning/hiccuping (in 30 percent). The child usually has a low birth weight but may be otherwise unremarkable until the second day, when symptoms are likely to begin.

The treatment follows the same general steps used in the treatment of the physically addicted adult. The child must be carefully evaluated to rule out medical problems such as hypoglycemia, hypocalcemia, infections, and trauma; general supports in a warm, quiet environment and regulation of electrolytes and glucose are also required. The infant with moderate to severe symptoms can be treated with any of the following: paregoric (0.2 mL orally every 3 to 4 h); methadone, (0.1 to 0.5 mg/k per day); phenobarbital (8 mg/kg per day); or diazepam (1 to 2 mg/kg every 8 h). Medication should be given in decreasing levels for 10 to 20 days. It is also possible to treat the addicted infants of mothers on methadone maintenance by having them breast feed while the mothers continue to take methadone.

REHABILITATION OF OPIATE ADDICTS Despite some differences in demographics, the same general rules for rehabilitation apply to the opiate abuser and to the alcoholic. The basic strategy includes beginning detoxification and general family support. It is also important to establish realistic patient goals and a program of counseling and education to increase motivation toward abstinence. A long-term commitment to rebuilding a life-style without the substance is essential for preventing recidivism.

Identifying and confronting the patient The first step in treatment requires identification of the opiate abuser—an especially difficult problem with the middle-class street abuser and the medical patient or physician with an iatrogenic addiction. An important step is to gather a clinical history which includes the patterns of opiate usage, information regarding the possible existence of an antisocial personality disorder, or a history of chronic pain. Blood and urine screens can be used to identify opiates in patients in whom misuse is suspected, and clinicians should search for physical stigmata of misuse (e.g., needle marks). One potentially important diagnostic procedure (which should be used carefully because it can precipitate an intense withdrawal) is the opiate antagonist challenge. A 0.4-mg dose of naloxone is given subcutaneously or slowly IV over a 5-min period, and the patient is observed for signs of withdrawal over the next several hours. This challenge test should only be carried out in the presence of a physician and it is important to be prepared to begin treating withdrawal if needed.

After identifying the opiate addict, the next step is confrontation. The need for active treatment of the abstinence syndrome can be presented, and the availability of help in establishing a drug-free life-style can be emphasized. The final decision, of course, rests with the patient.

Rehabilitation Most rehabilitation approaches have common elements. Patients are educated about their responsibility for improving their lives and *motivation for abstinence* is increased by providing information about the medical and psychological problems that can be expected if addiction continues. Patients and families are helped to *establish an opiate-free life-style* by being educated about dealing with chronic pain and developing realistic vocational planning (e.g., this applies to pharmacists, physicians, and nurses). The addict should also be encouraged to establish a drug-free peer group and to participate in self-help groups such as Narcotics Anonymous. Much of this advice and counseling can be given by the physician, but many clinicians refer patients to more formal drug programs, including methadone maintenance clinics, programs using narcotic antagonists, and therapeutic communities. Long-term follow-up of treated patients shows that approximately one-third of addicts are completely drug free in the year before the follow-up interview, and that a total of 60 percent are off opiates, although some may be abusing other substances. Individuals who stay in methadone maintenance or in therapeutic communities show significant decreases in police and social problems and increases in job functioning. In general, the best prognosis for rehabilitation is for those who are employed, who have higher levels of school completion, and who remain in treatment for at least 2 months.

METHADONE MAINTENANCE Methadone and methadyl acetate maintenance should only be used along with education and counseling. It is important to note that drug maintenance is not aimed at "curing" opiate addiction; rather it provides a substitute drug that is legally accessible. The goal is to help the addict who has failed in drug-free programs to improve functioning within the family and job, to decrease legal problems, and to improve health.

Methadone is a long-acting opiate that possesses almost all the physiologic properties of heroin. The addict who has been carefully screened to rule out prior psychiatric disorders may be maintained on a relatively low dose (e.g., 30 to 40 mg/d); a higher dosage schedule (100 to 120 mg/d) can also be used and may be more effective in blocking heroin-induced euphoria. Although the results are not definite, there is some evidence that the higher methadone doses may result in greater retention in treatment and consequently lower levels of arrest and readdiction to street drugs. Methadone is administered in an oral liquid given once a day at the program center, with weekend portions taken by the patient at home. The longer acting analogues, such as methadyl acetate, can be given in lower doses (e.g., 20 to 30 mg) two or three times a week, with levels increased to as high as 80 mg three times a week if needed.

After a period of maintenance (usually 6 months to 1 year or longer), the clinician should work closely with the patient to regulate the rate of drug decrease (by about 5 percent per week). The British have used heroin maintenance with similar goals and following similar guidelines as those used for methadone. There is no evidence that heroin maintenance has any advantages over methadone maintenance, but the heroin approach does add the risk that the drug will be sold on the streets.

OPIATE ANTAGONISTS The opiate antagonists (e.g., naloxone) compete with heroin and other opiates for opioid receptors, reducing the effects of the opiate agonists. Administered over long periods of time in order to block the "high" produced if the patient takes opiates, these drugs can be useful as part of an overall treatment approach that includes counseling and support. Cyclazocine was the first antagonist tested, but its blockade of receptors is incomplete and the level of side effects (including a drunken feeling) are unacceptable. Naloxone is an excellent narcotic antagonist with no agonistic properties, but it has such a short period of action (2 to 3 h) that it is of little use in rehabilitation. The most widely used antagonist in rehabilitation is naltrexone, which is effective for about 24 h with few side effects. A dose of 50 mg of naltrexone per day will block 15 mg of heroin for 24 h, and higher doses (125 to 150 mg) are capable of blocking the effects of 25 mg of IV heroin for up to 3 days. Naltrexone is free of agonist properties, there are no known withdrawal symptoms when the medication is stopped, and side effects tend to be mild. Patients started on this antagonist should be free of opiates for a minimum of 5 days. In addition they must be given a thorough physical examination and should be challenged with 0.4 or 0.8 mg of the shorter-acting naloxone to be certain that they are able to tolerate the long-acting antagonist. Following this procedure, a test dose of 10 mg of naltrexone can be given, with the expectation that any withdrawal symptoms will be seen in $\frac{1}{2}$ to 2 h. Over the next 10 days, the daily dose should be increased to about 100 mg on Mondays and Wednesdays and 150 mg on Fridays. Unfortunately, despite the apparent advantages of this treatment approach, patients demonstrate great resistance to continuing care. In one study, only about 60 percent of the patients completed 6 days of naltrexone induction, and only 10 percent remained in the program at the end of 6 months.

DRUG-FREE PROGRAMS Most existing half-way houses and recovery centers for the opiate abuser utilize the therapeutic community approach. This is an exception to the general preference for short-term inpatient rehabilitation, as care lasts up to a year while the addict is taken out of the street culture and given a new life within the group. In this structure members, including addict leaders, frequently confront participants in an attempt to help them gain insights into more successful life-styles for coping with problems.

REFERENCES

CROWLEY T et al: Naltrexone-induced dysphoria in former opioid addicts. Am J Psychiatry142:1081, 1985

FINNEGAN L: Neonatal abstinence syndrome, in *Neonatal Therapy*, F Rubatelli (ed). New York, Elsevier, 1986, pp 122–146

FRIEDLAND GH et al: Transmission of the human immunodeficiency virus. N Engl J Med 317:1125, 1987

GREENSTEIN RA et al: Naltrexone: A short-term treatment of opiate dependence. Am J Drug Alcohol Abuse 8:291, 1981

JAFFE JH, MARTIN WR: Opiate analgesics and antagonists, in *Goodman and Gilman's The Pharmacological Basis of Therapeutics*, 7th ed, AG Gilman et al (eds). New York, Macmillan, 1985, pp 491–531

JASINSKI D et al: Clonidine in morphine withdrawal. Arch Gen Psychiat 42:1063, 1985

KLEBER HK, RIORDAN CE: The treatment of narcotic withdrawal: A historical review. J Clin Psychiatry 43:30 1982

MCAULIFFE WE et al: Psychoactive drug use among physicians and medical students. N Engl J Med 315:805, 1986

MCCUE JD: The effects of stress on physicians and their medical practice. N Engl J Med 306:458, 1982

O'BRIEN CP, WOODY GE: Long-term consequences of opiate dependence. N Engl J Med 304:1098, 1981

——— et al: Classical conditioning is opiate dependence, in *Problems of Drug Dependence*, LS Harris (ed). NIDA Research, Monograph 49, pp 35–46. Washington, DC, US Government Printing Office, 1984

OLIVERIO A et al: Psychobiology of opioids. Int Rev Neurobiol 25:277, 1984

PASTERNAK GW: Multiple morphine and enkephalin receptors and the relief of pain. JAMA 259:1362, 1988

REDMOND DE JR, KRYSTAL JH: Multiple mechanisms of withdrawal from opioid drugs. Annu Rev Neurosci 7:443, 1984

ROUNSAVILLE BJ et al: Identifying alcoholism in treated opiate addicts. Am J Psychiatry 140:764, 1983
SCHUCKIT MA: *Drug and Alcohol Abuse: A Clinical Guide to Diagnosis and Treatment*, 3d ed. New York, Plenum, 1989
SIMON E: Recent studies on opioid receptors: Heterogeneity and isolation, in *Problems of Drug Dependence*, LS Harris (ed). NIDA Research Monograph 49, pp 5–13. Washington, DC, US Government Printing Office, 1984
SIMPSON DD et al: Six-year follow-up of opioid addicts after admission to treatment. Arch Gen Psychiat 39:1318, 1982
VAILLANT GE: A 20-year follow-up of New York narcotic addicts. Arch Gen Psychiat 29:237, 1973
WALLOT H, LAMBERT J: Characteristics of physician addicts. Am J Drug Alcohol Abuse 10:53, 1984

372 COMMONLY ABUSED DRUGS

JACK H. MENDELSON / NANCY K. MELLO

The prevalence of drug abuse in the United States remained at epidemic levels during 1988 and is believed to exceed that of other industrial nations. The extent of drug abuse problems in the United States is illustrated by a December 1988 report from the Division of Epidemiology and Statistical Analysis of the National Institute on Drug Abuse (NIDA): "More than one-half of the American youth try an illicit drug before they finish high school. The number of people admitted to emergency rooms following cocaine use, as reported by the Drug Abuse Warning Network (DAWN), increased more than fivefold over the past five 12-month periods. Further, the number of people who died following cocaine use increased almost fourfold during the same time period. Drug abuse in the United States clearly remains a major public health problem; it is pervasive in extent, diverse in its manifestations, and constantly changing." During the 1980s, drug abuse was the third most frequently reported psychiatric disorder by men (ages 18 to 65) and the second most frequently reported psychiatric disorder by women (ages 18 to 24).

The adverse health consequences of drug abuse are further complicated by AIDS, and drug abuse also increases the risk for HIV exposure. In 1988, NIDA estimated that 31 percent of all AIDS victims are intravenous drug abusers. Drug abuse contributes to the AIDS epidemic by the transmission of HIV infection through needle sharing by intravenous drug users and by direct immunosuppressive and immunomodulatory effects of abused drugs.

The initiation and continuation of drug abuse is determined by a complex interaction of the pharmacologic properties and relative availability of each drug, the personality and expectancy of the user, and the environmental context in which the drug is used. Polydrug abuse, the concurrent use of several drugs with different pharmacologic effects, is increasingly common among individuals from all socioeconomic strata. There has been an alarming increase in a particularly dangerous form of polydrug abuse, the combined use of both heroin and cocaine intravenously, called "speedballing." DAWN reports, based upon emergency room data, indicate that combined heroin and cocaine use increased almost threefold from 1984 to 1988. Deaths due to concurrent use of heroin and cocaine increased fivefold from 1984 through 1988. There is no simple explanation for this change in polydrug use patterns. Sometimes drug abusers attempt to attenuate one drug effect with another, e.g., heroin or alcohol is used to modulate the cocaine high. Sometimes one drug is used to enhance the effects of another, as with benzodiazepines and methadone, or cocaine plus heroin in methadone-maintained patients. Toxic drug interactions associated with polydrug abuse also contribute to the adverse health consequences of drug abuse. This chapter discusses cocaine, marijuana, two hallucinogens (PCP and LSD), and polydrug abuse. Elsewhere there are discussions of alcohol abuse (Chap. 370) and opioid abuse (Chap. 371).

COCAINE Cocaine is a stimulant and a local anesthetic with potent vasoconstrictor properties. The leaves of the coca plant (*Erythroxylon coca*) contain approximately 0.5 to 1 percent cocaine. The drug produces physiologic and behavioral effects when administered orally, intranasally, intravenously, or via inhalation following pyrolysis (smoking). It is now recognized that cocaine has potent pharmacologic effects on dopamine, norepinephrine, and serotonin neurons in the central nervous system. These effects involve alteration and blockade of cellular membrane transport and prevention of the reuptake of biogenic amines. It has been postulated that cocaine-induced euphoria is due to cocaine effects on dopaminergic neurons, but that chronic cocaine use may cause depletion and destruction of crucial dopaminergic pathways in the brain.

Prevalence of cocaine use Cocaine has become more widely available throughout the United States since its cost (relative to disposable income) has decreased considerably. Cocaine is no longer considered a "status" drug since cocaine abuse occurs in virtually all social and economic strata of our society. In 1985 the NIDA National Household Survey on Drug Abuse revealed that 22 million men and women had used cocaine on at least one occasion. Six million persons reported using cocaine at least once during the month prior to the survey, and 12 million individuals had used the drug at least once during the year prior to the survey. Cocaine-related health problems have continued to increase according to DAWN. The number of hospital emergency room cases associated with cocaine abuse increased from 7155 in 1984 to 39,657 in the 12-month period ending June 1988. The number of cocaine-related deaths in major metropolitan areas increased fourfold from 1984 to 1988. The overall increase in cocaine abuse in the general population has been paralleled by an increase in cocaine abuse by heroin-dependent persons, including those in methadone maintenance programs. Intravenous cocaine is often used concurrently with intravenous heroin (the speedball), a combination that purportedly attenuates the postcocaine crash and substitutes the cocaine "high" for the former heroin "high" blocked by methadone. Intravenous use of cocaine plus heroin may further increase risk for HIV infection, both through needle sharing and through the combined immunosuppressive effects of both drugs.

Acute and chronic cocaine intoxication Although cocaine is commonly self-administered by inhalation (snorting), there has been a dramatic increase in both intravenous administration and inhalation of pyrolyzed material via smoking. Following intranasal administration, changes in mood and feeling states are perceived within 3 to 5 min, and peak effects occur at 10 to 20 min. Duration of cocaine effects rarely exceed 1 h following intranasal administration. Inhalation of pyrolyzed materials includes smoking coca paste, a product produced by extracting cocaine preparations with flammable solvents, and cocaine free-base smoking. Coca paste is frequently contaminated with toxic solvents used in its preparation. Cocaine free-base, including the free-base prepared with sodium bicarbonate (crack), is becoming increasingly popular because of the relative high potency of the compounds and their rapid onset of action (8 to 10 s following smoking).

Cocaine produces a brief, dose-related stimulation and enhancement of mood; cardiac rate and blood pressure also increase in a dose-related manner. An increase in body temperature usually occurs following cocaine administration, and high doses of cocaine may induce lethal pyrexia or hypertension. Because cocaine inhibits reuptake of catecholamines at adrenergic nerve endings, the drug potentiates sympathetic nervous system activity. Cocaine has a short plasma half-life of approximately 1 h. In humans, cocaine is primarily metabolized by plasma esterases, and cocaine metabolites are excreted in urine. The very short duration of euphorigenic effects of cocaine observed in chronic abusers is probably due to both acute and chronic tolerance. Frequent self-administration of the drug (two to three times per hour) is often reported by chronic cocaine abusers. Alcohol is used to modulate both the cocaine "high" and the dysphoria associated with the abrupt disappearance of cocaine's effects.

The prevalent assumption that cocaine use is relatively safe is challenged by reports of death from respiratory depression, cardiac arrhythmias, and convulsions after cocaine snorting and intravenous administration. Severe pulmonary disease may develop in individuals who smoke coca paste; this is attributed both to the direct effects of cocaine and to residual solvent contaminants in the smoked material. Hepatic necrosis has also been reported to occur in coca paste smokers. Although men and women who abuse cocaine may report that the drug enhances libidinal drive, chronic cocaine use causes significant decrements in libido and adversely affects reproductive function. Impotence and gynecomastia have been observed in male cocaine abusers, and these abnormalities have persisted for long periods following drug abstinence. Women who abuse cocaine have reported major derangements in menstrual cycle function including galactorrhea, amenorrhea, and infertility. Chronic cocaine abuse may cause persistent hyperprolactinemia as a consequence of cocaine-induced disorders of dopaminergic regulation of prolactin secretion by the pituitary. Cocaine abuse may also adversely affect pregnancy. Infants exposed to cocaine in utero have an increased risk for congenital malformations as well as perinatal cardiovascular and cerebrovascular disease.

Numerous clinical reports, dating from the late nineteenth century, strongly suggest that protracted cocaine abuse may cause paranoid ideation and visual and auditory hallucinations, a state which resembles alcoholic hallucinosis. Psychological dependence upon cocaine, as manifested by inability to abstain from frequent compulsive use, has also been reported. Although occurrence of withdrawal syndromes involving psychomotor agitation and autonomic hyperactivity remains controversial, severe depression (''crashing'') following cocaine intoxication may be a concomitant of drug withdrawal.

Treatment of cocaine intoxication and abuse Treatment of cocaine overdose is a medical emergency which involves resuscitation in an intensive care unit. Cocaine toxicity produces hypertension, tachycardia, tonic-clonic seizures, dyspnea, and ventricular arrhythmias. Intravenous diazepam in doses up to 0.5 mg/kg administered over an 8-h period has been shown to be effective for control of seizures. The systemic concomitants of a hypermetabolic state produced by cocaine toxicity with concurrent ventricular arrhythmias have been managed successfully by administration of 0.5 to 1.0 mg propranolol intravenously. Since many instances of cocaine-related mortality have also been associated with concomitant use of other illicit drugs (particularly heroin), the physician must be prepared to institute effective emergency treatment for multiple-drug toxicity.

Treatment of chronic cocaine abuse requires combined efforts by family physicians, psychiatrists, and psychosocial care providers. Early abstinence from cocaine use is often complicated by symptoms of depression and guilt, insomnia, and anorexia, which may be as severe as those observed in major affective disorders. Individual and group psychotherapy, family therapy, and peer group assistance programs are often useful for inducing prolonged remission from drug use. Preliminary reports suggest that tricyclic antidepressant medication (desipramine) may be of value in the treatment of cocaine abuse, even when affective disorder or depression are not present. In fact, depressive illness does not appear to be a frequent antecedent of cocaine abuse.

MARIJUANA AND CANNABIS COMPOUNDS *Cannabis sativa* contains over 400 compounds in addition to the psychoactive substance, delta-9-tetrahydrocannabinol (THC). Marijuana cigarettes are prepared from the leaves and flowering tops of the plant, and a typical marijuana cigarette contains 0.5 to 1 g of plant material. Although the usual THC concentration varies between 5 and 20 mg, concentrations as high as 100 mg per cigarette have been detected. Hashish is prepared from concentrated resin of *Cannabis sativa* and contains a THC concentration of between 8 to 12 percent by weight. ''Hash oil,'' a lipid-soluble plant extract, may contain a THC concentration of 25 to 60 percent, and it may be added to marijuana or hashish to enhance their THC concentration. Smoking is the most common mode of marijuana or hashish self-administration. During pyrolysis, over 150 compounds in addition to the THC are released in the smoke. Although most of these compounds do not have psychoactive properties, they do have potential physiologic effects.

THC is quickly absorbed from the lungs into blood and is then rapidly sequestered in tissues. It is metabolized primarily in the liver where it is converted to 11-hydroxy-THC, a psychoactive compound, and more than 20 other metabolites. Most THC metabolites are excreted through the feces at a rate of clearance that is relatively slow in comparison to that of most other psychoactive drugs.

Prevalence of marijuana use The National Institute on Drug Abuse 1985 National Household Survey on Drug Abuse revealed that 62 million persons had used marijuana or hashish at least once in their lifetime and that 18 million individuals reported using the drug at least once during the month prior to the survey. One encouraging datum was a decrease in marijuana use by young persons aged 12 to 17, but 27 percent of persons in this age group reported marijuana use. The DAWN records of marijuana or hashish in emergency room settings increased from 3490 during 1984 to 7934 in 1988. However, the NIDA cautions that ''interpreting the trend of marijuana emergencies is problematic since marijuana is often used in conjunction with other substances such as PCP, alcohol, or heroin. In fact, in 1987, 83 percent of all marijuana emergency room mentions were in combination with another substance.'' Thus, there is a continuing trend for polydrug abuse among young marijuana users, and there are major health hazards associated with this behavior.

Acute and chronic marijuana intoxication Acute intoxication from marijuana and cannabis compounds is related to both THC dose and route of administration. THC is absorbed more rapidly from marijuana smoking than from orally ingesting cannabis compounds. The most frequent form of acute intoxication consists of a subjective perception of relaxation and mild euphoria resembling mild to moderate alcohol intoxication. This condition is usually accompanied by some impairment in thinking, concentration, and perceptual and psychomotor functions. Higher doses of cannabis may produce behavioral effects analogous to severe alcohol intoxication. Although the effects of acute marijuana intoxication are relatively benign in normal users, the drug can precipitate severe emotional disorders in individuals who have antecedent psychotic or neurotic problems. As with other psychoactive compounds, both set (user's expectancy) and setting (environmental context) are important determinants of the type and severity of behavioral intoxication.

As is true of alcoholics, chronic marijuana abusers may lose interest in common socially desirable goals and devote progressively more time to drug acquisition and use. However, it should be emphasized that THC does not cause a specific and unique ''amotivational syndrome.'' The range of symptoms sometimes attributed to marijuana use are difficult to distinguish from mild depression and the maturational dysfunctions often associated with protracted adolescence. Chronic use of marijuana has also been reported to increase the probability of exacerbation of psychotic symptoms in individuals with a past history of schizophrenia.

Physical effects of marijuana Conjunctival injection and tachycardia are the most frequent immediate physical concomitants of smoking marijuana. Tolerance for marijuana-induced tachycardia develops rapidly among regular users; angina may be precipitated by marijuana smoking in persons with a history of coronary insufficiency. Exercise-induced angina may be increased after marijuana use to a greater extent than after tobacco cigarette smoking. Patients with cardiac disease should be strongly advised not to smoke marijuana or use cannabis compounds.

Significant decrements in pulmonary vital capacity have been found in regular daily marijuana smokers. Because marijuana smoking typically involves deep inhalation and prolonged retention of marijuana smoke, marijuana smokers may develop pulmonary disease such as chronic bronchial irritation. Impairment of single-breath carbon monoxide diffusion capacity (DL_{CO}) is greater in persons who smoke both marijuana and tobacco than in tobacco smokers. Despite the well-documented association between tobacco smoking and lung cancer, at present there is no direct evidence that marijuana smoking induces lung cancer. However, it should be emphasized that heavy marijuana use among Americans may be of too brief duration for detection of this problem.

Although marijuana has also been associated with adverse effects on a number of other systems, many of these studies await replication and confirmation. For example, the reported correlation between marijuana use and decreased testosterone levels in males has not been confirmed. Decreased sperm count and motility and abnormalities of morphology of spermatozoa following marijuana use have also been reported. Administration of high doses of marijuana to female rhesus monkeys has revealed significant marijuana-induced suppression of pituitary gonadotropins and gonadal steroids. Carefully conducted prospective studies demonstrated a significant correlation between impaired fetal growth and development and heavy marijuana use during pregnancy. Marijuana also has been implicated in derangements of the immune response system, in chromosomal abnormalities, and in inhibition of DNA, RNA, and protein synthesis, but these findings have not been confirmed or related to any specific physiologic effect of marijuana in humans. One report of cannabis-induced brain atrophy in young adults has not been confirmed in computed tomographic studies of young men who had documented histories of heavy marijuana smoking.

Tolerance and physical dependence Habitual marijuana users rapidly develop tolerance to the psychoactive effects of marijuana, often smoking more frequently and trying to secure more potent cannabis compounds. Tolerance for physiologic effects of marijuana develops at different rates; e.g., tolerance for marijuana-induced tachycardia develops rapidly, but tolerance for marijuana-induced conjunctival injection develops more slowly. Tolerance to both behavioral and physiologic effects of marijuana decreases rapidly upon cessation of marijuana use.

Withdrawal signs and symptoms have been reported in chronic cannabis users, with severity of symptoms related to dosage and duration of use. These include tremor, nystagmus, sweating, nausea, vomiting, diarrhea, irritability, anorexia, and sleep disturbances. Withdrawal signs and symptoms observed in chronic marijuana users are usually relatively mild in comparison to those observed in heavy opiate or alcohol users and rarely require medical or pharmacologic intervention. Somewhat more severe and protracted abstinence syndromes may occur after sustained use of high-potency cannabis compounds for long periods.

LYSERGIC ACID DIETHYLAMIDE The serendipitous discovery of psychedelic effects of LSD in 1947 culminated in an epidemic of LSD abuse during the 1960s. Imposition of stringent legal and regulatory constraints on the manufacture and distribution of LSD (classified as a schedule I substance by the FDA), as well as public recognition that psychedelic experiences induced by LSD were a health hazard, has resulted in a significant reduction in LSD abuse. During 1984, relatively few instances of LSD abuse were reported, but the drug still retains some popularity among adolescents and young adults.

LSD is a very potent drug; oral doses as low as 20 μg may induce profound psychological and physiologic effects. Tachycardia, hypertension, pupillary dilation, tremor, and hyperpyrexia occur within minutes following LSD in oral doses of 0.5 to 2 μg/kg. A variety of bizarre and often conflicting perceptual and mood changes, including visual illusions, synesthesias, and extreme lability of mood, usually occur within $\frac{1}{2}$ h after LSD intake. The action of LSD may persist for 12 to 18 h even though the half-life of the drug is only 3 h.

Tolerance develops rapidly for LSD-induced changes in psychological function when the drug is used one or more times per day over a course of 4 days or more. Abrupt abstinence following continued use does not produce withdrawal signs or symptoms. To date there have been no clinical reports of death caused by the direct effects of LSD.

The most frequent acute medical emergency associated with LSD use is panic episodes which may persist up to 24 h ("the bad trip"). Management of this problem is best accomplished by supportive reassurance ("talking down") and, if necessary, administration of small doses of anxiolytic drugs. Adverse consequences of chronic LSD use include enhanced risk for schizophreniform psychosis and derangements in memory function, problem solving, and abstract thinking. Treatment of these disorders is best carried out in specialized psychiatric facilities.

PHENYCYCLIDINE Phencyclidine, a cyclohexylamine derivative, is widely used in veterinary medicine to briefly immobilize large animals and is sometimes described as a dissociative anesthetic. PCP is easily synthesized and is abused, primarily by young people and polydrug users. The true extent of PCP abuse is unknown, but recent national surveys indicate an increase in frequency of use.

Phencyclidine is taken orally, by smoking, or by intravenous injection. It is also used as an adulterant in illicit sales of THC, LSD, amphetamine, or cocaine. The most common street preparation, "angel dust," is a white granular powder which contains 50 to 100 percent of the drug. Low doses (5 mg) produce agitation, excitement, impaired motor coordination, dysarthria, and analgesia. Users may have horizontal or vertical nystagmus, flushing, diaphoresis, and hyperacusis. Behavioral changes include distortions of body image, disorganization of thinking, and feelings of estrangement. Higher doses of PCP (5 to 10 mg) may produce hypersalivation, vomiting, myoclonus, fever, stupor, or coma. PCP doses of 10 mg or more cause convulsions, opisthotonus, and decerebrate posturing which may be followed by prolonged coma.

The diagnosis of PCP overdose is difficult because the patient's initial symptoms may suggest an acute schizophrenic reaction. Confirmation of PCP use is possible by determination of PCP levels in serum or urine. PCP analysis is currently available at most toxicologic centers. Large quantities of PCP remain in urine for 1 to 5 days following high-dosage PCP intake.

PCP overdose requires prompt life support measures including treatment of coma, convulsions, and respiratory depression in a hospital intensive care unit. There is no specific antidote or antagonist for PCP. PCP excretion from the body can be enhanced by acidification of urine and gastric lavage. Death from PCP overdose may occur as a consequence of some combination of pharyngeal hypersecretion, hyperthermia, respiratory depression, severe hypertension, seizures, hypertensive encephalopathy, and intracerebral hemorrhage.

Acute psychosis associated with PCP use should be considered a psychiatric emergency since patients may be at high risk for suicide or extreme violence toward others. Phenothiazines should not be used for treatment of acute PCP psychosis because these drugs potentiate PCP's anticholinergic effects. Haloperidol (5 mg intramuscularly) has been administered on an hourly basis to induce suppression of psychotic behavior. PCP, like LSD and mescaline, produces vasospasm of cerebral arteries at relatively low doses. Chronic PCP use has been shown to induce insomnia, anorexia, severe social and behavioral changes, and, in some cases, chronic schizophrenia.

POLYDRUG ABUSE Although drug abusers often report a preference for a particular drug, such as alcohol or opiates, the concurrent use of other drugs is common. Multiple-drug use often involves substances which may have different pharmacologic effects from the preferred drug. Concurrent use of such dissimilar compounds as stimulants and opiates or stimulants and alcohol is not unusual. The diversity of reported drug use combinations suggests that achieving some perceptible change in state, rather than any particular direction of change (stimulation or sedation), may be the primary reinforcer in polydrug use and abuse. There is also evidence that intoxication with alcohol or opiates is associated with increased tobacco smoking but marijuana smoking does not increase during alcohol intoxication. At present, there is relatively little systematic information available about drug interactions. However, it is known that the combined use of cocaine, heroin, and alcohol increases the risk for toxic effects and adverse medical consequences over risks associated with use of a single drug.

A practical determinant of polydrug use patterns is the relative availability and cost of the drugs. There are many examples of situationally determined drug use patterns, including the fact that soldiers who became dependent on heroin in Vietnam seldom continued heroin use after separation from military service. However, a significant number of men who were heroin addicts in Vietnam abused alcohol and became alcohol-dependent when they returned to the United States. Alcohol abuse, with its attendant medical complications, is one of the most serious problems encountered in former heroin addicts participating in methadone maintenance programs.

The physician must recognize that perpetuation of polydrug abuse and drug dependence is not necessarily a symptom of an underlying emotional disorder. Neither alleviation of anxiety nor reduction of depression accounts for initiation and perpetuation of polydrug abuse. Severe depression and anxiety are as frequently the consequences of polydrug abuse as they are the antecedents. There is also evidence that some of the most adverse consequences of drug use may be reinforcing and contribute to the continuation of polydrug abuse.

Adequate treatment of polydrug abuse, as well as other forms of drug abuse, requires innovative and eclectic programs of intervention. The first step in successful treatment is detoxification, a process which may be difficult because the patient has abused several drugs with different pharmacologic actions (e.g., alcohol, opiates, and cocaine). Since patients may not recall or may deny simultaneous multiple-drug use, diagnostic evaluation should always include urinalysis for qualitative detection of psychoactive substances and their metabolites. Treatment of polydrug abuse requires hospitalization or inpatient residential care during detoxification and the initial phase of drug abstinence. When possible, specialized facilities for the care and treatment of chemically dependent persons should be used. Outpatient detoxification of polydrug abuse patients is likely to be ineffective and may be dangerous.

As in the treatment of alcohol abuse, no single therapeutic modality has been shown to be uniquely effective in inducing remission. Polydrug abuse is a chronic disorder with an unpredictable pattern of remission and recrudescence. Therapeutic management of chronic disorders such as cardiac or neoplastic disease should serve as a model for helping the person with polydrug abuse problems. Even temporary remissions with attendant physical, social, and psychological improvements are preferable to the continuation or progressive acceleration of polydrug abuse and its related adverse medical and interpersonal consequences. In polydrug abuse, as in most chronic disorders, definitive "cures" rarely occur. The concerned physician should continue to assist polydrug abuse patients throughout the cyclic oscillations of this complex behavior disorder, recognizing that resumption of drug use may be the rule rather than the exception.

REFERENCES

BALSTER RL: The behavioral pharmacology of phencyclidine, in *Psychopharmacology: The Third Generation of Progress*, HY Meltzer (ed). New York, Raven, 1987, pp 1573–1579

CREGLER LL, MARK H: Medical complications of cocaine abuse. N Engl J Med 315:1495, 1986

FISCHMAN MW: Cocaine and the amphetamines, in *Psychopharmacology: The Third Generation of Progress*, HY Meltzer (ed). New York, Raven, 1987, pp 1543–1553

GAWIN FH, ELLINWOOD EH JR: Cocaine and other stimulants. Actions, abuse, and treatment. N Engl J Med 318:1173, 1988

———: Cocaine dependence. Ann Rev Med 40:149, 1989

JAFFE JH: Drug addiction and drug abuse, in *The Pharmacological Basis of Therapeutics*, 7th ed, AG Gilman et al (eds). New York, Macmillan, 1985, pp 532–581

KREEK MJ: Multiple drug abuse patterns and medical consequences, in *Psychopharmacology: The Third Generation of Progress*, HY Meltzer (ed). New York, Raven, 1987, pp 1597–1604

MELLO NK: A behavioral analysis of the reinforcing properties of alcohol and other drugs in man, in *The Pathogenesis of Alcoholism, Biological Factors*, B Kissin, H Begleiter (eds). New York, Plenum, 1983, vol 7, pp 133–198

———: Alcohol abuse and alcoholism: 1978–1987, in *Psychopharmacology: The Third Generation of Progress*, HY Meltzer (ed). New York, Raven, 1987, pp 1515–1520

MENDELSON JH: Marijuana, in *Psychopharmacology: The Third Generation of Progress*, HY Meltzer (ed). New York, Raven, 1987, pp 1565–1571

———, MELLO NK (eds): *The Diagnosis and Treatment of Alcoholism*, 2d ed. New York, McGraw-Hill, 1985

PETERSEN RC, STILLMAN RD (eds): *Phencyclidine (PCP) Abuse: An Appraisal*, NIDA Research Monograph Series no 21, US Department of Health, Education and Welfare Publication (ADM) 78-728, 1978

VAN DYKE C, BYCK R: Cocaine use in man, in *Advances in Substance Abuse, Behavioral and Biological Research*, NK Mello (ed). Greenwich, JAI Press, 1983, vol 3, pp 1–24

WEISS RD, MIRIN SM: *Cocaine*. Washington, American Psychiatric Press, 1987

373 TOBACCO

JOHN H. HOLBROOK

Tobacco smoke is a ubiquitous personal and environmental pollutant. Although tobacco has been used in western culture for more than 400 years, human inhalation of cigarette smoke is a twentieth century phenomenon with major medical and economic consequences. In industrialized nations cigarette smoking is the principal cause of preventable disease, disability, and premature death.

Important changes in smoking trends are occurring in the United States. In general, there is less smoking. For example, annual per capita cigarette consumption in adults declined from its 1963 peak of 4345 cigarettes to a 1987 estimate of 3196 cigarettes. In the United States between 1965 and 1987, the prevalence of smoking among aduts declined from 52 to 32 percent of men and 34 to 27 percent of women. There are 48.8 million current adult smokers and 39.9 million former smokers in the United States; the distribution of smokers between the sexes is approximately equal with 25.0 million men and 23.8 million women. Among teenagers, smoking is slightly more prevalent in females than in males. While consumption of cigar and pipe tobacco has decreased, use of smokeless tobacco, especially snuff, has increased among teenage males.

CIGARETTE SMOKE More than 4000 substances have been identified in cigarette smoke, including some that are pharmacologically active, antigenic, cytotoxic, mutagenic, and carcinogenic; these diverse biologic effects provide a framework for understanding the adverse consequences of smoking.

Cigarette smoke is a heterogeneous aerosol produced by incomplete combustion of the tobacco leaf. It is composed of a gas phase in which particulate matter is dispersed. Mainstream smoke emerges from the mouthpiece during puffing. Sidestream smoke is emitted between puffs at the burning cone and from the mouthpiece. The composition of the smoke is influenced by several factors including type of tobacco, temperature of combustion, length of the cigarette, porosity of the paper, additives, and filters. The major tobacco leaf constituents are carbohydrates, nonfatty organic acids, nitrogen-containing compounds, and resins. Cigarette temperatures vary greatly from 30°C at the mouthpiece to 900°C at the burning cone. In the presence of intense heat some tobacco constituents undergo thermic decomposition (pyrolysis). Volatile substances are distilled directly into the smoke. Unstable molecules recombine to generate new compounds (pyrosynthesis). Concentration of smoke constituents occurs as the smoke is filtered by unburnt tobacco and is redistilled by the burning cone. Some substances found in tobacco pass unchanged into cigarette smoke.

Approximately 92 to 95 percent of the total weight of mainstream smoke is present in the gas phase. Nitrogen, oxygen, and carbon dioxide account for 85 percent of the smoke's weight. The remaining gases and particulate matter are the substances of medical importance (Table 373-1). Mainstream smoke contains 0.3 to 3.3 billion particles per milliliter; the mean particle size is 0.2 to 0.5 μm, which is within the respirable range.

A pack-a-day cigarette smoker puffs more than 70,000 times a year, and the membranes of the mouth, nose, pharynx, and trach-

TABLE 373-1 Selected cigarette smoke constituents

Substance	Effect
PARTICULATE PHASE	
"Tar"*	Carcinogen
Polynuclear aromatic hydrocarbons	Carcinogens
Nicotine	Ganglionic stimulator and depressor
Phenol	Cocarcinogen and irritant
Cresol	Cocarcinogen and irritant
β-Naphthylamine	Carcinogen
N-Nitrosonornicotine	Carcinogen
Benzo[a]pyrene	Carcinogen
Trace metals (e.g., nickel, arsenic, polonium 210)	Carcinogens
Indole	Tumor accelerator
Carbazole	Tumor accelerator
Catechol	Cocarcinogen
GAS PHASE	
Carbon monoxide	Impairs oxygen transport and utilization
Hydrocyanic acid	Ciliotoxin and irritant
Acetaldehyde	Ciliotoxin and irritant
Acrolein	Ciliotoxin and irritant
Ammonia	Ciliotoxin and irritant
Formaldehyde	Ciliotoxin and irritant
Oxides of nitrogen	Ciliotoxin and irritant
Nitrosamines	Carcinogen
Hydrazine	Carcinogen
Vinyl chloride	Carcinogen

* The aggregate of particulate matter in cigarette smoke after subtracting nicotine and moisture.

eobronchial tree are exposed repetitively to tobacco smoke. Some constituents act directly on the membranes, while others are absorbed into the blood or are dissolved in saliva and swallowed.

PHARMACOLOGY Tissue and organ system responses to cigarette smoke inhalation are multiple and complex. Most studies in humans have dealt with exposure to whole smoke or to selected constituents thought to pose the greatest risk to health, such as nicotine and carbon monoxide. Relatively little is known about the individual effects and interactions of other potentially toxic smoke constituents that are present in low concentrations.

Nicotine, the component most characteristic of tobacco, is a highly toxic alkaloid that is both a ganglionic stimulant and depressant. Many of its complex effects are mediated by catecholamine release. Acute cardiovascular responses to nicotine observed in normal smokers include increases in systolic and diastolic blood pressure, heart rate, force of myocardial contraction, myocardial oxygen consumption, coronary artery blood flow, myocardial excitability, and peripheral vasoconstriction. Nicotine has also been shown to increase serum concentrations of glucose, cortisol, free fatty acids, vasopressin, and β-endorphin. Nicotine appears to be the major source of addiction to tobacco.

Carbon monoxide is a toxic gas that interferes with oxygen transport and utilization. Because cigarette smoke contains 2 to 6 percent carbon monoxide, smokers inhale concentrations as high as 400 parts per million (ppm) and develop elevated carboxyhemoglobin (COHb) levels. The range of COHb found in smokers is 2 to 15 percent, while levels for nonsmokers are near 1 percent. The average COHb level of moderate cigarette smokers is 5 percent. Carbon monoxide produces its adverse effects by reducing the amount of available oxyhemoglobin and myoglobin, and by displacing the oxygen-hemoglobin dissociation curve to the left. Chronic, mild elevations of COHb due to smoking are a common cause of mild polycythemia and may produce subtle impairment of central nervous system function.

Cigarette smoke and its condensate are carcinogenic in several species of animals. The major identified carcinogens in cigarette smoke are polynuclear aromatic hydrocarbons, aromatic amines, and nitrosamines (Table 373-1). Cocarcinogens present in cigarette smoke, such as catechol, greatly enhance its carcinogenicity. The sister chromatid exchange rate, a sensitive indicator of mutagenic effects, is higher in the lymphocytes of smokers than in nonsmokers. Cigarette smoke condensate is also mutagenic in a microbial test system.

Potent pulmonary irritants and ciliotoxins are found in cigarette smoke (Table 373-1). These substances increase bronchial mucus secretion and mediate acute and chronic decreases in pulmonary and mucociliary function. Cigarette smoke also increases lung epithelial permeability.

EPIDEMIOLOGY Data from large prospective studies of populations in several countries have shown that cigarette-smoking men have 70 percent higher overall death rates than nonsmokers. The effect on mortality is proportionately greatest in younger age groups. The excess mortality of female smokers has been somewhat less than that of male smokers, but it has increased. Cigarette smoking is the largest single health risk in the United States and is responsible for an estimated 350,000 premature deaths each year; this is equivalent to approximately one-sixth of all deaths. Coronary heart disease (CHD) and lung cancer are the chief contributors to smoking-related excess mortality. In the United States, cigarette smokers also experience more disability due to chronic illness and report significantly more days absent from work than do nonsmokers.

A strong dose-response relationship exists between cigarette smoking and excess mortality, as measured by the age at onset of smoking, the number of cigarettes smoked, the number of years of smoking, and the depth of inhalation. Cessation of smoking is associated with a decrease in the excess mortality. These observations together with clinical, experimental, and pathologic studies indicate that smoking, per se, causes the excess mortality.

CHARACTERISTICS OF SMOKERS Demographic, anthropometric, physiologic, and laboratory features which distinguish cigarette smokers from nonsmokers are due both to baseline differences between these groups and to the effects of smoking. Smokers drink more alcohol, coffee, and tea than do nonsmokers. Their weight and blood pressure are slightly less and their heart rate is slightly faster than those of nonsmokers. In women the menopause comes earlier in smokers than in nonsmokers. Smokers have impaired maximum exercise performance and impaired immune systems compared to nonsmokers. A markedly increased number of pulmonary alveolar macrophages is present in smokers, and the function and metabolism of these cells are abnormal. When compared with nonsmokers, smokers show small increases in the total white blood cell count and serum IgE levels as well as small decreases in leukocyte vitamin C levels, serum uric acid, and albumin. In smokers, the ratio of high-density lipoprotein cholesterol to low-density lipoprotein cholesterol is reduced. Smokers also show reduced levels of prostacyclin (PGI_2).

CLINICAL CORRELATIONS Large population studies have shown a strong association between cigarette smoking and several diseases. Atherosclerotic cardiovascular disease, cancer, and chronic obstructive pulmonary disease account for most of the excess mortality and morbidity due to smoking.

Individual patient risks due to cigarette smoking vary widely. Factors which influence these risks include the duration, intensity, and type of smoke exposure; genetically mediated susceptibility; occupational and environmental exposures; use of medication; and coexisting risk factors and diseases.

Cardiovascular disease Cigarette smoking is a major cause of coronary heart disease (CHD), and premature CHD is one of its most important medical consequences. Approximately 21 percent of the 500,000 CHD deaths occurring each year in the United States is attributable to smoking. Cigarette smoking, hypertension, and hypercholesterolemia are the three major CHD risk factors. Smoking acts both independently of and synergistically with these other CHD risk factors. Two risk factors may produce a fourfold increase in CHD risk and three risk factors may produce an eightfold increase in CHD risk. There is a dose-response relationship between CHD risk and cigarette smoking. These CHD death rates are 60 to 70 percent greater in male smokers than nonsmokers. Sudden death may be the first manifestation of CHD, and it is two to four times more likely to occur in younger male cigarette smokers than in nonsmokers. Women cigarette smokers are also at greater risk of developing CHD than nonsmokers, and the use of both cigarettes and oral contraceptives increases this risk approximately tenfold. Cessation of smoking is associated with decreased CHD mortality, an effect which is measurable within 1 year. Those who continue to smoke after an acute myocardial infarction are more likely to die from CHD than are those who quit smoking. Smokers who undergo coronary artery bypass surgery have increased perioperative mortality compared to nonsmokers. Cigarette smoking may produce an imbalance between myocardial oxygen supply and demand, coronary artery spasm, decrease in the threshold for ventricular fibrillation, a hypercoagulable state, and an increase in platelet aggregation; avoidance of these effects may explain the prompt cardiac benefits of quitting smoking. Cigarette smoking may interfere with the efficacy of medication used to treat CHD, such as propranolol and nifedipine.

Cigarette smoking is an important cause of cerebrovascular disease and accounts for an estimated 18 percent of the 150,000 stroke deaths that occur each year in the United States. Large epidemiologic studies in men and women have shown an increased risk of stroke among smokers compared to nonsmokers, a dose-response relationship between smoking and stroke risk, and a decrease in stroke risk with smoking cessation. Among women, subarachnoid hemorrhage is more likely to occur in smokers than nonsmokers, and the use of both cigarettes and oral contraceptives greatly increases this risk.

Cigarette smoking is the most powerful risk factor for arteriosclerosis obliterans and thromboangiitis obliterans. It also aggravates peripheral ischemia and may adversely affect peripheral bypass grafts. The mortality rate for atherosclerotic aortic aneurysm is greater in male smokers than nonsmokers.

Cigarette smoking is not a risk factor for the development of hypertension; however, hypertensives who smoke are at a greater risk to develop malignant hypertension and to die from hypertension. Cigarette smoking may also interfere with the efficacy of medication used to treat hypertension, such as propranolol. Because of the association with chronic obstructive pulmonary disease, cigarette smoking is an important factor leading to chronic pulmonary heart disease.

Cancer Cigarette smoking is the single most important cause of cancer mortality in the United States, accounting for 30 percent of all cancer deaths. In spite of the well-documented cause-and-effect relationship between cigarette smoking and lung cancer, more Americans continue to die from this cancer than from any other tumor (see Chap. 215). In 1988 an estimated 139,000 lung cancer deaths occurred in the United States; 87 percent of these deaths were attributable to cigarette smoking. The risk of developing lung cancer is quantitatively related to cigarette smoke exposure. Men who smoke one pack a day increase their risk tenfold compared with nonsmokers; men who smoke two packs a day may increase their risk more than 25 times compared with nonsmokers. Asbestos workers who smoke cigarettes are at especially high risk for developing lung cancer. Cigarette consumption by women increased rapidly in the United States during the past 50 years, and lung cancer mortality among smokers is currently increasing at a faster rate in women than in men. Lung cancer has become the leading cause of cancer death among American women. Because 5-year survival rates for lung cancer are less than 10 percent, emphasis must be placed on prevention. Giving up cigarettes is associated with a gradual decline in the risk of developing lung cancer.

Cigarette smoking is a cause of laryngeal, oral, and esophageal cancer in men and women. Alcohol consumption acts synergistically with cigarette smoking to increase the risk for these neoplasms. Cigarette smoking is an important contributory factor for the development of bladder, kidney, and pancreatic cancer; it is also associated with cancer of the stomach and uterine cervix.

Respiratory disease Cigarette smoking is the major cause of chronic obstructive pulmonary disease (COPD), that is, chronic bronchitis and emphysema (see Chap. 210). Of the estimated 70,000 deaths from COPD that occurred in the United States in 1988, 82 percent were attributable to smoking, and many of these deaths were preceded by prolonged respiratory disability. There is a dose-response relationship between COPD death rates and cigarette smoking. Depending upon the extent of smoke exposure, male cigarette smokers experience from 4 to 25 times higher mortality secondary to COPD than do nonsmokers. Although the death rate from COPD among female smokers is somewhat lower than among male smokers, it is increasing much more rapidly in female than in male smokers. Chronic cough, sputum production, and breathlessness are much more common in smokers. Smokers are more likely than nonsmokers to show abnormalities in a number of pulmonary function tests including measurements of elastic recoil, airflow in large and small airways, and diffusing capacity. Mild airflow obstruction in small airways may be present even in teenage smokers. When compared with continuing smokers, ex-smokers experience a decrease in mortality from COPD, a decrease in prevalence of pulmonary symptoms, and a slowing of the rate of decline of lung function to approximately that seen in age-matched nonsmokers. Chronic inhalation of pulmonary irritants and ciliotoxins (Table 373-1) may contribute to the development of COPD. Studies of the pathogenesis of emphysema suggest that smoking results in an excess of pulmonary proteases, which may produce pulmonary damage. The damage is apparently mediated via release of elastase from increased numbers of lung leukocytes and partial inactivation of pulmonary antiproteases by oxidants present in smoke. For most people in the United States cigarette smoking is a more important cause of COPD than are occupational or environmental factors; however, factors such as cotton dust exposure may act independently or conjointly with smoking to produce COPD. In a rare disorder, homozygous α_1-antitrypsin deficiency, smoking greatly accelerates the tendency to panacinar emphysema; furthermore, smoking may play an additive role in individuals heterozygous for this state.

Cigarette smoking has been associated with an increased incidence of respiratory infections and deaths from pneumonia and influenza. Postoperative respiratory complications and spontaneous pneumothorax are also more common in smokers. Because tobacco smoke may increase airway obstruction, asthmatics should be urged not to smoke. Chronic stomatitis and chronic laryngitis occur more frequently in smokers than in nonsmokers.

Pregnancy Smoking may delay conception, and smoking during pregnancy may affect the fetus adversely. Infants whose mothers smoked during pregnancy weigh, on an average, 170 g less than infants whose mothers did not smoke. This effect probably results from impaired uteroplacental circulation. Maternal smoking during pregnancy increases the risk of spontaneous abortion, fetal death, neonatal death, and the sudden infant death syndrome. This increased risk may be much greater in pregnancies already at high risk due to other factors. Smoking by a woman during pregnancy may also adversely affect the long-term physical growth and intellectual development of the child.

Gastrointestinal disorders Gastric and duodenal ulcer disease is more prevalent in male than female cigarette smokers and causes more deaths in male smokers than in nonsmokers. Smoking impairs spontaneous and drug-induced healing of peptic ulcers, increases the likelihood of duodenal ulcer recurrence, inhibits pancreatic bicarbonate secretion, and decreases the pressure of esophageal and pyloric sphincters. Histamine-2-receptor antagonist inhibition of nocturnal gastric secretion is also prevented by smoking.

Involuntary smoke inhalation Indoor atmospheres and other confined spaces are often contaminated by tobacco smoke which is inhaled involuntarily by both smokers and nonsmokers. Most of the atmospheric pollutants arise from sidestream smoke. It contains greater concentrations of many smoke constituents than does mainstream smoke, but since sidestream smoke is diluted in a large volume of air, the smoke exposure from involuntary inhalation is less than that associated with smoking.

Initially, involuntary or passive smoking was thought to cause primarily an irritant effect such as ocular burning. It is now recognized as an important cause of air pollution and a cause of lung cancer in nonsmokers. Parental smoking in the home is associated with an increased risk of acute respiratory illnesses, middle-ear effusions, chronic respiratory symptoms, and slightly impaired lung function in children.

Drug effects Tobacco smoke constituents induce hepatic microsomal enzyme systems that are important in the metabolism of several drugs. For example, cigarette smoking increases the metabolism of propranolol, propoxyphene, and theophylline. Smoking may also decrease the absorption of subcutaneously administered insulin. Hence, changes in smoking behavior may cause significant alterations of serum drug levels that may result in either drug toxicity or failure of drug treatment.

TYPES OF SMOKING During the past 20 years the amount of tar and nicotine delivered by cigarettes made in the United States has decreased by more than 50 percent. Filter-tipped cigarettes and lower-tar and -nicotine cigarettes now account for more than 90 and 50 percent of sales, respectively. Lung cancer and laryngeal cancer are the only tobacco-related diseases for which the use of lower-tar and -nicotine cigarettes has been shown to result in risk reduction, compared with the use of higher-tar and -nicotine cigarettes; however, compared with not smoking or quitting, the benefits are minimal. Consumers who choose lower-tar and -nicotine cigarettes and then smoke a larger number of cigarettes or inhale more frequently or deeply may actually increase their exposure to harmful substances. There is also concern because unidentified flavoring agents are added to these cigarettes to enhance consumer acceptance.

Cigar and pipe smokers usually inhale less smoke than cigarette smokers, presumably because the alkaline pH of cigar and pipe tobacco makes it more irritating to the respiratory tract. The smoke exposure and overall mortality rates of pipe and cigar smokers in the United States are substantially less than those of cigarette smokers; however, death rates of cigarette, cigar, and pipe smokers are approximately equal for carcinoma of the oral cavity, larynx, and esophagus, sites where exposures to cigarette, cigar, and pipe smoke are similar. The mortality rates of most cigar and pipe smokers for cancer at other sites, CHD, and COPD are not greatly elevated above the rates of nonsmokers, but cigar and pipe smokers who inhale consistently may experience adverse health effects comparable with those of cigarette smokers. The use of chewing tobacco and snuff may produce plasma nicotine levels comparable to those of cigarette smokers and lead to nicotine dependence or addiction. The use of such smokeless tobacco products also increases the risk for oral cancer.

CESSATION OF SMOKING Psychosocial forces lead to initiation of smoking, especially among children and teenagers. Later, nicotine addiction and psychological factors help maintain dependence on tobacco. It is estimated that more than 40 million people in the United States have stopped smoking; 95 percent of these succeeded without formal assistance. Smoking cessation reduces the risk of tobacco-related diseases. For example, ten or more years after quitting, the death rate of those who smoked 20 cigarettes a day or less is about the same as that of nonsmokers. For heavier smokers cessation may never reduce the risk to the level of the nonsmoker. Ex-smokers usually experience prompt symptomatic improvement. On the average they also gain approximately 5 lb.

In the United States more than 80 percent of cigarette smokers would like to stop smoking. Many self-care and organized programs are available to assist these individuals. Organized programs employ several techniques including instruction, counseling, withdrawal clinics, behavioral modification, hypnosis, aversive conditioning, self-monitoring, and drug therapy. In these programs 1-year abstinence rates of 20 to 30 percent are common. Relapse usually occurs during the 3-month interval after quitting. Successful programs emphasize maintenance of the nonsmoking state during this critical period. There is a great need for physicians to provide personalized smoking cessation assistance for their patients.

Although less than 10 percent of physicians smoke, a minority of patients report receiving advice from their physician to quit. Controlled trials have shown that physician counseling increases long-term smoking cessation rates. Surveys also show that patients are inadequately informed about the hazards and addictive nature of smoking. All smokers should be encouraged to quit, especially those in high-risk groups. Physicians can help their patients by accepting smoking as a chronic medical problem requiring treatment and by following these guidelines:

1. Obtain a quantitative smoking history.
2. Explain the health risks in a personally relevant fashion.
3. Emphasize the benefits associated with cessation.
4. Assess patient interest in smoking cessation.
5. Assist the patient to quit by setting a target quitting date and by suggesting smoking cessation strategies.
6. Provide self-help reading materials.
7. Support the patient in a maintenance program.

A nicotine-containing chewing gum, which helps alleviate withdrawal symptoms, may be a useful adjunct in medically supervised programs. Preliminary data suggest that clonidine may be of value in a smoking cessation program. Selected patients may benefit from referral to a smoking cessation specialist.

Political, social, and cultural forces play a critical role in the individual decision to start or stop smoking. For this reason, physicians should lead and support efforts to increase tobacco excise taxes, to eliminate all tobacco advertisements and promotional activities, and to ban smoking in public places.

Ultimately, primary smoking prevention in the pediatric and adolescent age groups may be the most effective program. Young people who have been trained to resist social pressures, who understand the consequences of smoking to their health, and who appreciate the difficulty of quitting are less likely to start smoking.

REFERENCES

BENOWITZ NL: Pharmacologic aspects of cigarette smoking and nicotine addiction. N Engl J Med 319:1318, 1988

GRITZ ER: Cigarette smoking: The need for action by health professionals. CA 38:194, 1988

US DEPARTMENT OF HEALTH AND HUMAN SERVICES: *The health consequences of involuntary smoking. A report of the Surgeon General.* DHHS(CDC) Publication no 87-8398, 1987

US DEPARTMENT OF HEALTH AND HUMAN SERVICES: *The health consequences of smoking: Nicotine addiction. A report of the Surgeon General.* DHHS(CDC) Publication no 88-8406, 1988

US DEPARTMENT OF HEALTH AND HUMAN SERVICES: *Reducing the health consequences of smoking: 25 years of progress. A report of the Surgeon General.* DHHS(CDC) Publication no 89-8411, 1989

PART FIFTEEN ENVIRONMENTAL AND OCCUPATIONAL HAZARDS

374 ACUTE POISON AND DRUG OVERDOSAGE

FREDERICK H. LOVEJOY, JR. / CHRISTOPHER H. LINDEN

A poison (toxin) is a chemical substance capable of producing adverse effects in a living organism. Chemicals may be divided into those intended for human use (foods and their additives, pharmaceuticals, toiletries, cosmetics) and those that are not (household products, industrial chemicals, nonfood nondrug botanicals). An overdose implies exposure to excessive amounts of the former and any amount of the latter; it may or may not result in poisoning.

Poisoning may be local (limited to the eyes, skin, lungs, or gastrointestinal tract), systemic, or both, depending on the dose, extent of absorption and distribution, intrinsic potency of the poison, and host susceptibility. Absorption and distribution are influenced by properties of the chemical itself (molecular size, degree of ionization, lipid and water solubility, protein binding) and of the biologic barriers (membrane composition, pore size, chemical transport systems) through which it penetrates.

Local effects are due to nonspecific chemical reactions such as oxidation, protein denaturation, desiccation, and solvent activity. Their severity and reversibility depend on the dose (concentration), contact time, the potency of the chemical, and the type and condition of the exposed surface. The nature (generalized or limited), severity, and reversibility of systemic effects depend on the dose, potency, and metabolic disposition of the chemical, the functional reserve of the individual or affected tissue, and the presence of secondary complications (shock, hypoxia). Other variables that influence toxicity include coexisting illnesses, previous chemical exposure, and individual differences in biologic response, tissue concentration of a chemical (pharmacodynamics), and/or its pharmacokinetics (absorption, distribution, metabolism, elimination).

EPIDEMIOLOGY

In the United States, poison exposures result in an estimated 5 million requests for medical advice or treatment each year. The common routes of exposure are ingestion (79 percent), dermal (7 percent), ophthalmic (6 percent), inhalation (5 percent), bites and stings (3 percent), and parenteral injections (0.3 percent). Pharmaceutical preparations are involved in 40 percent of exposures. Substances most frequently involved are cleaning agents, analgesics, cosmetics, plants, cough and cold preparations, and hydrocarbons. The majority of exposures are acute, accidental, occur in the home, result in minor or no toxicity, and involve children under 6 years of age.

Accidental exposures also result from the improper use of chemicals at work or at play, product mislabeling, label misreading, mistaken identification of unlabeled chemicals, uninformed self-medication, and dosing errors by nurses, parents, pharmacists, physicians, and the elderly. Other unintended poisonings are due to the use of drugs for psychotropic effects (abuse) and excessive self-dosing (misuse). Excluding the recreational use of ethanol, attempted suicide is the most common reason for intentional exposure.

Although only 4 percent of victims of exposure require hospitalization, they account for roughly 5 percent of intensive care unit admissions and up to 30 percent of psychiatric admissions. Suicide attempts account for the majority (60 to 90 percent) of serious or fatal poisonings. Most deaths result from carbon monoxide poisoning and occur prior to arrival at a hospital. Antidepresssants, analgesics, stimulants and street drugs, cardiovascular agents, sedative-hypnotics, and asthma medications are responsible for most drug-related fatalities. Nonpharmaceutical agents implicated in fatal poisoning include inorganic chemicals, alcohols and glycols, cleaning agents, and hydrocarbons.

DIAGNOSIS OF POISONING

Although poisoning can mimic other illnesses, the correct diagnosis can usually be established by the history, physical examination, routine and toxicologic laboratory evaluation, and clinical course. The history should include the time, route, duration, and circumstances (location, surrounding events, intent) of exposure; the name and amount of each drug, chemical, or ingredient involved; the time of onset, nature, and severity of symptoms; the time and type of first aid measures provided; and the past medical and psychiatric history. In many cases the victim is confused, comatose, and unaware of an exposure, or unable or unwilling to admit to one. Suspicious circumstances include unexplained illness in a previously healthy person; a history of psychiatric problems (particularly depression); recent changes in health, economic status, or social relationships; and the onset of illness while working with chemicals or after ingesting food, drink (especially ethanol), or medications. Patients who become ill soon after arriving from a foreign country or after arrest for criminal activity should be suspected of having illicit drugs concealed in body cavities (the GI tract). Family, friends, paramedics, police, pharmacists, physicians, and employers may provide valuable information regarding habits, hobbies, behavior changes, available medications, and antecedent events. A search of the victim's clothes and place of discovery may reveal a suicide note or empty container of drugs or chemicals. The imprint code on pills, the label and manufacturer of chemical products, a text or Physicians Desk Reference, or regional poison control center may be used to identify the ingredients and potential toxicity of a suspected poison.

The physical examination should initially focus on the vital signs and cardiopulmonary and neurologic status to assess the need for immediate supportive treatment. These parameters also provide the most important diagnostic clues in poisoning of unknown etiology (Table 374-1). Although vital signs may sometimes be discordant, the clinical picture can usually be characterized by either physiologic stimulation or depression. Examination of the eyes (for nystagmus, pupil size, and reactivity), abdomen (for bowel activity and bladder),

TABLE 374-1 Differential diagnosis of poisoning based on vital signs and CNS activity

Stimulant poisoning	Depressant poisoning
Sympathomimetic syndrome Amphetamines Caffeine Cocaine Decongestants Ergot alkaloids MAO inhibitors Theophylline	Sympatholytic syndrome Adrenergic blockers Antiarrhythmics Antidepressants (tricyclic) Antihypertensives Calcium channel blockers Digoxin
Anticholinergic syndrome Antidepressants (tricyclic) Antihistamines Anti-Parkinsonian agents Antipsychotics Antispasmodics (GI, GU) Belladonna alkaloids Cyclobenzaprine Mydriatics (topical) Plants/mushrooms	Cholinergic syndrome Bethanecol Carbamate insecticides Organophosphate insecticides Myasthenia gravis drugs (e.g., pyridostigmine) Physostigmine
Hallucinogenic syndrome LSD and synthetic analogues Marijuana Mescaline and synthetic analogues Phencyclidine	Narcotic syndrome Analgesics Antispasmodics (GI)
Withdrawal syndrome Alcohol Antidepressants Beta-blockers Clonidine Narcotics Sedative-hypnotics	Sedative-hypnotic syndrome Alcohol Antiepileptics Barbiturates Benzodiazepines Ethchlorvynol Hydrocarbons Glutethimide Methyprylon

and skin (for burns, bullae, color, warmth, moisture, pressure sores, and puncture marks) often narrow the diagnosis to a particular syndrome. Grading the severity of poisoning (Table 374-2) may be useful for assessing prognosis and for following the clinical course.

The patient should also be examined for evidence of trauma and underlying illnesses. Except with theophylline and drugs that cause hypoglycemia and hypoxia, seizures and neurologic dysfunction due to poisoning are almost never focal. Hence, focal findings should prompt evaluation for a structural CNS lesion. When the history is unclear, all orifices should be examined for the presence of chemical burns and drug packets. The odor of breath or vomitus and the color of nails, skin, or urine may occasionally provide diagnostic clues.

TABLE 374-2 Severity of stimulant and depressant poisoning and drug withdrawal

Severity	Signs and symptoms
STIMULANT POISONING	
Grade 1	Diaphoresis, flushing, hyperreflexia, irritability, mydriasis, tremors
Grade 2	Confusion, fever, hyperactivity, hypertension, tachycardia, tachypnea
Grade 3	Delirium, mania, hyperpyrexia, tachyarrhythmias
Grade 4	Coma, convulsions, cardiovascular collapse
DEPRESSANT POISONING	
Grade 1	Lethargic but arousable; able to answer questions and follow commands
Grade 2	Comatose; withdraws from pain; brainstem and deep tendon reflexes intact
Grade 3	Comatose; no response to pain; most reflexes absent; respiratory depression
Grade 4	Comatose; no response to pain; reflexes absent; respiratory and cardiovascular depression

An increased anion-gap metabolic acidosis is characteristic of methanol, ethylene glycol, and salicylate intoxication, and lactic acidosis may occur in any poisoning that results in hypoxia, hypotension, or seizures. An osmolal gap, the difference between the measured serum osmolality (freezing point depression, not the vapor pressure method) and the calculated osmolality (from the serum sodium, glucose, and BUN), of more than 10 mosmol/kg indicates the presence of a low-molecular-weight solute such as acetone, ethanol, ethylene glycol, isopropyl alcohol, or methanol or an unmeasured electrolyte (magnesium) or sugar (mannitol). An increased anion-gap metabolic acidosis with respiratory alkalosis, ketosis, and tinnitus suggests salicylate poisoning. An increased anion-gap metabolic acidosis and osmolal gap, accompanied by back pain, hypocalcemia, and crystalluria, may be seen with ethylene glycol intoxication, whereas the presence of visual symptoms suggests methanol poisoning. Lists of poisons that cause specific signs, symptoms, and other laboratory abnormalities may be found in the references cited.

Pulmonary edema can occur with carbon monoxide, cyanide, narcotic, paraquat, sedative-hypnotic, and salicylate poisoning; inhalation of irritant gas (chlorine, nitrogen dioxide, metal and polymer fume); or prolonged shock. Aspiration pneumonia is common in patients with coma, seizures, petroleum distillate ingestion, and irritant gas inhalation. Radiopaque densities may be visible on abdominal x-rays following the ingestion of calcium, chloral hydrate, chlorinated hydrocarbons, enteric-coated tablets, heavy metals, phenothiazines, and salicylates.

Bradycardia and AV block may occur in patients poisoned by antiarrhythmic agents, beta blockers, calcium channel blockers, cholinergic agents (carbamate and organophosphate insecticides), digitalis, lithium, phenylpropanolamine, and tricyclic antidepressants. QRS- and QT-interval prolongation may be caused by amantidine, antiarrhythmics, antipsychotics, tricyclic antidepressants, fluorides, heavy metals (arsenic, thallium), lithium, magnesium, or neuroleptics. Ventricular tachyarrhythmias may be seen in poisoning with sympathomimetics and agents that cause QRS and QT prolongation.

Analysis of urine and blood (and occasionally gastric contents and chemical samples) may be useful to confirm or rule out suspected poisoning. Interpretation of laboratory data requires knowledge of the tests used for screening and confirmation (thin layer, gas-liquid, high performance liquid chromatography; colorimetric and fluorometric assays; enzyme-multiplied and radioimmunoassays; gas chromatography; mass spectrometry) and of their sensitivity (limit of detection) and specificity and of the best type and time of sampling of biologic specimens. Personal communication with the laboratory is essential. A negative screen may mean the poison is not detectable at all or its concentration is too low for detection. In such an instance, repeating the test on a sample obtained at a later time will often yield positive results.

Since screening tests require 2 to 6 h for completion, immediate management decisions often must be based on the history, physical examination, and routine ancillary tests. When the patient is asymptomatic or when the clinical picture is consistent with the reported history, qualitative screening is neither clinically useful nor cost-effective. It is of greatest value in patients with severe or unexplained toxicity such as coma, seizures, cardiovascular instability, metabolic or respiratory acidosis, and non-sinus cardiac rhythms. Quantitative analysis is appropriate for acetaminophen, acetone, alcohol (including ethylene glycol), antiarrhythmic, antiepileptic, barbiturate, digoxin, heavy metal, lithium, salicylate, and theophylline poisoning and in carboxyhemoglobinemia and methemoglobinemia. Results are often available within an hour.

Response to antidotes may also be used for diagnostic purposes. Resolution of altered mental status and abnormal vital signs within minutes of intravenous dextrose, naloxone, or flumazenil administration is virtually diagnostic of hypoglycemia, narcotic poisoning, and benzodiazepine intoxication, respectively. The prompt reversal of acute dystonic (extrapyramidal) reactions following an intravenous dose of benztropine or diphenhydramine confirms the diagnosis of benzodiazepine intoxication. *Vin rosé* urine color following a diagnostic dose of deferoxamine can be used to confirm iron poisoning when serum iron and total iron-binding capacity levels are not immediately available. Although reversal of both central and peripheral manifestations of anticholinergic poisoning by physostigmine is diagnostic, physostigmine may cause arousal in patients with central nervous system depression of any etiology.

The absence of signs and symptoms soon after an overdose does not rule out a poisoning. Common poisons whose effects are delayed in onset include acetaminophen, cancer chemotherapeutic agents, carbon tetrachloride, colchicine, digoxin, ethylene glycol, heavy metals, methanol, mushrooms, some plants, narcotics, salicylate, and slow- or sustained-release medications.

TREATMENT

Treatment goals include support of vital signs, prevention of further poison absorption, enhancement of poison elimination, administration of specific antidotes, and prevention of reexposure (Table 374-3). Treatment is based on the identity of the poison, the route and amount of exposure, the time of presentation relative to the time of exposure, and the severity of poisoning. Knowledge of toxin pharmacokinetics and pharmacodynamics is essential.

For patients who present during the preclinical phase, between the time of ingestion and the onset of manifestations, treatment must be based on the history. The maximum potential toxicity based on the greatest possible amount ingested should be assumed. Gastrointestinal decontamination to minimize absorption and decrease the severity of toxicity is the first priority. Since the decontamination is more effective the sooner it is performed, the history and physical examination should initially be brief. It is also advisable to establish intravenous access and initiate cardiac monitoring, particularly in patients with potentially serious ingestions or unclear histories. The choice of decontamination procedure depends on the predicted toxicity; the availability, efficacy, and contraindications of the procedure; and the nature, severity, and risk of complications. For the home management of patients with accidental ingestions, reliable histories, and mild predicted toxicity, emesis can be induced with ipecac syrup. For patients treated in medical facilities, activated charcoal is administered for most poisons. It has comparable or greater efficacy, fewer contraindications and complications, and is less invasive than ipecac or gastric lavage. Alternative methods should be used if the ingested agent is not well-absorbed by activated charcoal. When the reasons are compelling (e.g., witnessed ingestion of a potentially severe overdose) the use of invasive procedures (gastric lavage) may be justified in an asymptomatic patient. Aspiration or esophageal perforation may result from the forcible use of a lavage tube in an uncooperative patient with a trivial ingestion.

TABLE 374-3 Fundamentals of poisoning management

I Supportive care
- *A* Airway protection
- *B* Oxygenation/ventilation
- *C* Treatment of arrhythmias
- *D* Hemodynamic support
- *E* Treatment of seizures
- *F* Correction of temperature abnormalities
- *G* Correction of metabolic derangements
- *H* Prevention of secondary complications

II Prevention of further poison absorption
- *A* Gastrointestinal decontamination
  - *1* Syrup of ipecac–induced emesis
  - *2* Gastric lavage
  - *3* Activated charcoal
  - *4* Whole bowel irrigation
  - *5* Catharsis
  - *6* Dilution
  - *7* Endoscopic/surgical removal
- *B* Decontamination of other sites
  - *1* Eye decontamination
  - *2* Skin decontamination
  - *3* Body cavity evacuation

III Enhancement of poison elimination
- *A* Multiple-dose activated charcoal
- *B* Forced diuresis
- *C* Alteration of urinary pH
- *D* Chelation (see heavy metal section)
- *E* Extracorporeal removal
  - *1* Peritoneal dialysis
  - *2* Hemodialysis
  - *3* Hemoperfusion
  - *4* Hemofiltration
  - *5* Plasmapheresis
  - *6* Exchange transfusion
- *F* Hyperbaric oxygenation

IV Administration of antidotes
- *A* Neutralization by antibodies
- *B* Neutralization by chemical binding
- *C* Metabolic antagonism
- *D* Physiologic antagonism

V Prevention of reexposure
- *A* Adult education
- *B* Child-proofing
- *C* Notification of regulatory agencies
- *D* Psychiatric referral

When an accurate history is not obtainable, a poison causing delayed toxicity or irreversible damage is suspected, or the patient develops severe clinical toxicity, toxicologic screening should be accomplished as soon as possible. Obtaining additional blood and urine samples and saving them for future analysis is often helpful. Due to continuing absorption and distribution, blood levels may be greater than those in tissue and not reflect clinical toxicity or the need for additional treatment. However, high blood levels of agents whose metabolites are more toxic than the parent compound (acetaminophen, ethylene glycol, or methanol) may indicate the need for additional interventions (antidotes, dialysis).

After evaluation and GI tract decontamination, some patients may be sent home because the predicted toxicity is minimal or the time of expected maximal toxicity has passed without incident. Observation for at least 4 to 6 h following GI tract decontamination assures that most patients who remain asymptomatic can be discharged safely. Patients ingesting agents that slow gastric emptying and intestinal motility (anticholinergics, narcotics, sedative hypnotics, salicylates), have slow dissolution and absorption characteristics (carbamazepine, phenytoin, enteric-coated tablets, lithium, salicylate, and sustained-release preparations), or tend to form bezoars or concretions (enteric-coated tablets, meprobamate, salicylate) may require longer observation. In such patients, the passage of a charcoal stool prior to discharge should preclude delayed absorption and subsequent toxicity.

During the toxic phase, from the time of onset to the peak clinical or laboratory evidence of poisoning, management is based on clinical and laboratory findings. Resuscitation and stabilization are the first priority. All symptomatic patients should have an intravenous line, supplemental oxygen, cardiac monitoring, continuous observation, and baseline laboratory, ECG, and x-ray evaluation. Patients with altered mental status, particularly those with coma or seizures, should be given an intravenous bolus of glucose, naloxone, and thiamine and additional antidotes as indicated. Further poison absorption should be limited by administering activated charcoal or gastric lavage. Since aspiration is a hazard, ipecac syrup should be used with caution. Patients may be given charcoal by mouth or by a stomach tube. Administering a dose of charcoal both before and after gastric lavage may be more effective than giving charcoal only after lavage. An initial dose of charcoal can be given by small-bore (no. 18 French or less) nasogastric tube while monitoring and supportive measures are being initiated. Once the patient is stable, lavage with a large-bore orogastric tube can be followed with a second dose of charcoal. The rare patient who deteriorates after this regimen should be lavaged and given another dose of charcoal.

Measures that enhance poison elimination may shorten the duration of toxicity and lessen its severity. However, the risks of poison removal must be weighed against the benefits. Diagnostic certainty (usually via laboratory confirmation) is a prerequisite. Intestinal dialysis using activated charcoal is generally safe and effective. The efficacy of diuresis and chelation therapy is limited to a relatively small number of poisons. Extracorporal removal methods are effective for many but not all poisons, but their use should be limited to patients who would otherwise not have a favorable outcome.

Patients with severe poisoning (coma, respiratory depression, hypotension, cardiac conduction abnormalities, cardiac arrhythmias, hypothermia or hyperthermia, seizures), those needing close monitoring or antidotes or enhanced elimination therapy, those showing progressive clinical deterioration, and those with significant underlying medical problems should be admitted to an intensive care unit. Patients with moderate toxicity can be managed on a general medical service, intermediate care unit, or emergency department observation area depending on the anticipated duration and level of monitoring needed (intermittent clinical observation versus continuous clinical, cardiac, and respiratory monitoring). Suicidal patients sometimes require a particularly high level of care.

During the resolution phase, between peak toxicity and full recovery, supportive care should continue until the patient is alert and laboratory and ECG abnormalities are resolved. Repeat charcoal dosing may prevent rebound toxicity when depressed GI function improves and the poison still in the gut is absorbed or additional active metabolites are formed. Since poison is eliminated from the blood before tissues, blood levels are generally lower than tissue levels during this phase and are not necessarily predictive of toxicity. This is particularly true when extracorporal elimination procedures are used. Because of redistribution of poison, relapse and rebound increase in blood level may occur after the termination of such procedures. When a metabolite is responsible for toxic effects, continued treatment of an asymptomatic patient may be necessary because of a previously toxic blood level (acetaminophen and methanol).

Prior to discharge, patients with accidental ingestions (and/or the caregivers) should be instructed about preventive measures, and suicidal patients should receive appropriate psychiatric assessment, disposition, and follow-up.

SUPPORTIVE CARE

The goal of supportive therapy is to maintain physiologic homeostasis until detoxification is accomplished and to prevent and treat secondary complications such as aspiration, bed sores, cerebral and pulmonary edema, pneumonia, rhabdomyolysis, sepsis, and generalized organ dysfunction due to prolonged hypoxia or shock.

In addition to those needing urgent endotracheal intubation, many poisoned patients require semielective endotracheal intubation for protection of the airway against aspiration of gastrointestinal contents and of the poison itself. The gag reflex alone is not a reliable indicator of the need for intubation. Since patients may maintain airway patency while being stimulated but not if left unattended, those who cannot respond to voice or who are unable to sit and drink fluids without assistance are best managed by prophylactic intubation. Patients with severe excitation may also require intubation for airway protection (due to the risk or existence of seizures) and sedation or paralysis for control of agitation and prevention of hyperthermia, acidosis, and rhabdomyolysis. The need for oxygenation and ventilation is best determined by analyses of arterial blood gases.

Drug-induced pulmonary edema is usually secondary to hypoxia, although myocardial depression may contribute. Measurement of pulmonary artery pressure may be necessary to establish the etiology. Arrhythmias can result from direct cardiotoxicity, abnormal cardiovascular reflexes, or metabolic derangements. Supraventricular tachycardia associated with hypertension and CNS excitation is almost always due to sympathetic, anticholinergic, or hallucinogenic stimulation or to drug withdrawal (Table 374-1). Most cases are mild or moderate in severity and require only observation or nonspecific sedation with a benzodiazepine. If severe or associated with hemodynamic instability, chest pain, or ECG evidence of ischemia, specific therapy is indicated. Hypoxia, hypoglycemia, and other metabolic causes of sympathetic stimulation should be ruled out first. For patients with sympathetic hyperactivity, treatment with a combined alpha and beta blocker (labetalol) or a combination of beta blocker and vasodilator (esmolol and nitroprusside) is preferred. For those with anticholinergic hyperactivity, physostigmine is the treatment of choice. Supraventricular tachycardia without hypertension is generally secondary to vasodilation or hypovolemia and responds to fluid administration.

Ventricular tachyarrhythmias may be caused by sympathetic stimulation, myocardial membrane destabilization, or metabolic derangements. Lidocaine and phenytoin are generally safe, but beta blockers can be hazardous unless the arrhythmia is clearly from sympathetic hyperactivity. In tricyclic antidepressant poisoning, quinidine and procainamide are contraindicated (because of similar electrophysiologic effects), but sodium bicarbonate may be therapeutic. Magnesium sulfate and overdrive pacing (by isoproterenol or a pacemaker) may be useful in patients with torsade de pointes and prolonged QT interval. Magnesium and antidigoxin antibodies should be considered for digoxin poisoning. Without invasive (esophageal or intracardiac) ECG recording, it may be impossible to distinguish the origin (ventricular or supraventricular) of wide-complex tachycardias (see Chap. 185). If the patient is hemodynamically stable, it may be prudent to observe rather than to treat with a potentially harmful cardioactive agent. Arrhythmias may be resistant to drug therapy until underlying acid-base and electrolyte derangements, hypoxia, or hypothermia are corrected.

Bradyarrhythmias associated with hypotension should be treated as described in Chap. 184, and the management of hypotension is described in Chap. 39. If hypotension is unresponsive to volume expansion, norepinephrine or high-dose dopamine may be appropriate.

Drug-induced seizures may be due to direct or indirect CNS neuroreceptor stimulation (or inhibition), neuronal membrane destabilization, ischemia, edema, or metabolic abnormalities. Seizures due to excessive stimulation of catecholamine receptors (sympathomimetic or hallucinogen poisoning and drug withdrawal) or decreased activity of inhibitory receptors mediated by gamma-aminobutyric acid (GABA) (isoniazid poisoning) or glycine (strychnine poisoning) are best treated with GABA agonists such as benzodiazepines or barbiturates. Seizures caused by isoniazid, which inhibits the synthesis of GABA, may not respond to agonist therapy until GABA synthesis is restored, because agonists act, at least partially, by promoting the release of GABA from presynaptic vesicles. High doses of pyridoxine, which is necessary for the synthesis of GABA, are often necessary to terminate seizures resulting from isoniazid intoxication. For poisons with central dopaminergic effects (phencyclidine), an agent with opposing activity, such as haloperidol, may be useful. Seizures resulting from membrane destabilization (beta blocker, cyclic antidepressant poisoning) may require a membrane-active agent such as phenytoin as well as a GABA agonist. In rare cases (anticholinergic or cyanide poisoning), specific antidotal therapy may be necessary.

The treatment of seizures secondary to ischemia, edema, or metabolic abnormalities should include correction of the underlying cause. Since prolonged convulsions can lead to rhabdomyolysis and severe acidosis, neuromuscular paralysis is indicated in refractory cases. Aggressive treatment of seizures is necessary to prevent permanent neurologic damage.

Temperature extremes, metabolic, hepatic, and renal abnormalities, and secondary complications should be treated by standard measures. Invasive interventions, such as extracorporal membrane oxygenation, intraaortic balloon pump counterpulsation, and partial (femoral) cardiopulmonary bypass pump circulatory support, should be considered in severe but reversible poisoning.

PREVENTION OF POISON ABSORPTION

GASTROINTESTINAL DECONTAMINATION *Syrup of ipecac* is administered orally in a dose of 30 mL for adults, 15 mL for children, and 10 mL for small infants. Clear liquids should also be given. Ipecac irritates the stomach and stimulates the central chemoreceptor trigger zone. Vomiting usually occurs approximately 22 min following administration. The dose may be repeated if vomiting does not occur. Ipecac decreases drug or poison absorption by an average of 57 percent (range 28 to 73 percent) if given within 5 min of drug ingestion and about 30 percent (range 2 to 45 percent) if given within half an hour. Because there are no suitable control groups, its efficacy in overdose patients is not established. Side effects include lethargy in children (12 percent) and protracted vomiting (8 to 17 percent). Chronic ipecac use (by patients with anorexia nervosa or bulimia) may cause electrolyte and fluid abnormalities, cardiac toxicity, and myopathy. Except for aspiration, serious complications are rare. Isolated cases of gastric and esophageal tears and perforations and stroke have been reported. Ipecac is contraindicated in patients with recent GI surgery, CNS depression, seizures, and ingestions of corrosives and rapidly acting CNS poisons (camphor, cyanide, tricyclic antidepressants, propoxyphene, strychnine).

Gastric lavage is optimally performed using a no. 28 French orogastric tube in children and a no. 40 French tube in adults with about 5 mL fluid per kg body weight. Except for infants, tap water is acceptable. The patient should be placed in Trendelenburg and left lateral decubitus positions to prevent aspiration (even if an endotracheal tube is in place). Lavage decreases poison absorption by an average of 69 percent (range 54 to 84 percent) if performed within 5 min of poison ingestion, 31 percent (range 26 to 38 percent) if performed at 30 min; and 11 percent (range 8 to 13 percent) if performed at 60 min. Its efficacy is similar to that of ipecac. Significant amounts of ingested drug are recovered in a tenth of patients. As with ipecac, its effect on the clinical outcome of poisoned patients is not known. Aspiration is a common complication (up to 10 percent) especially when lavage is improperly performed. Serious complications (tracheal lavage, esophageal and gastric perforation) occur in approximately 1 percent of patients. For this reason, only a physician should insert the lavage tube, and the patient must be restrained (with pharmacologic sedation if necessary) during the procedure. Gastric lavage is contraindicated in patients with ingestion of corrosives and petroleum distillate hydrocarbons because of the risk of aspiration-induced hydrocarbon pneumonia and gastroesophageal perforation.

Activated charcoal, as a suspension in water alone or with a carthartic, is given orally via a nippled bottle (for infants), glass, straw, or small-bore nasogastric tube (for uncooperative patients). The recommended dose is 1 to 2 g/kg body weight, using 8 mL of diluent per gram of charcoal, if a premixed formulation is not available. Palatability may be increased by adding a sweetener (sorbitol) or a flavoring agent (cherry, chocolate, or coke syrup) to the suspension. Charcoal adsorbs ingested poisons within the gut lumen, allowing the charcoal-toxin complex to be evacuated with stool. The complex can also be removed from the stomach by induced emesis or lavage. In vitro, charcoal adsorbs 90 percent or more of most poisons when given in a ratio 10 times that of the toxin. Superactivated charcoal (SuperChar) is two to three times more effective than standard charcoal. Charged (ionized) chemicals such as mineral acids, alkalis, and highly dissociated salts of cyanide, fluoride, iron, lithium, and other inorganic compounds are not well adsorbed by charcoal. Charcoal decreases the absorption of other poisons by an average of 80 percent when given within 5 min of poison administration, 59 percent when given at 30 min, and 33 percent at 60 min. Charcoal is of equal or greater efficacy than ipecac syrup or gastric lavage. Lavage followed by charcoal is more effective than charcoal alone, and charcoal before and after lavage is more effective than charcoal alone or charcoal after lavage. Although the clinical efficacy of charcoal is not known, the outcome of patients treated with charcoal alone is at least as favorable as of those given ipecac followed by charcoal and those treated with lavage followed by charcoal. In those treated sooner than 1 h, the combination of lavage and charcoal is more effective than charcoal alone. Side effects of charcoal include nausea, vomiting, and diarrhea or constipation. Charcoal may also prevent the absorption of orally administered therapeutic agents. Complications include mechanical obstruction of the airway, aspiration, vomiting, and bowel obstruction by inspissated charcoal. Charcoal is contraindicated in patients with corrosive ingestion because it obscures endoscopy.

Whole-bowel irrigation is performed by administering a bowel cleansing solution containing electrolytes and polyethylene glycol (Golytely, Colyte) orally or by gastric tube at a rate of up 0.5 L/h in children and 2.0 L/h in adults until rectal effluent is clear. The patient must be in a sitting position. Although data are limited, whole-bowel irrigation may be more effective than the previously discussed procedures. It may be of particular benefit in patients with foreign body, drug packet, and slow-release medication ingestions.

Cathartic salts (disodium phosphate, magnesium citrate and sulfate, sodium sulfate) or *saccharides* (mannitol, sorbitol) promote the rectal evacuation of gastrointestinal contents. The most effective cathartic is sorbitol in a dose of 1 to 2 g/kg body weight. Alone, cathartics do not prevent poison absorption, except perhaps for the agents used with whole-bowel irrigation. They are of primary use to prevent constipation following charcoal administration. Abdominal cramps, nausea, and vomiting are occasional side effects. Complications include hypermagnesemia and excessive diarrhea. The agents are contraindicated in patients who have ingested corrosives and in those with preexisting diarrhea. Magnesium-containing cathartics should not be used in patients with renal failure.

Dilution is accomplished by having the patient drink 5 mL/kg body weight of water or other clear liquid as soon as possible after the ingestion of a corrosive (acids, alkali). Dilution may also be used as an adjunct to ipecac syrup. Otherwise, it is not indicated because it may increase the dissolution rate (and hence absorption) of capsules, tablets, and other solids.

Endoscopic or surgical removal of poisons may be useful in rare situations such as ingestion of a potentially toxic foreign body that fails to transit the GI tract, a potentially lethal amount of a heavy metal (arsenic, iron, mercury, thallium), or large concretions of pills. Patients who ingest packets of drugs (cocaine) and then become toxic due to packet leakage or rupture require immediate surgical intervention.

DECONTAMINATION OF OTHER SITES Immediate copious flushing with water, saline, or other available clear drinkable liquid is the initial treatment of topical exposures (particularly with corrosives and solvents). Saline is preferred for eye irrigation. A triple wash (water then soap then more water) may be optimal for dermal decontamination. Inhalational exposures should be initially treated with fresh air or oxygen. The removal of liquid poisons from body cavities such as the vagina or rectum is best accomplished by irrigation. Solid poisons (drug packets, pills) should be removed with visual guidance.

ENHANCEMENT OF POISON ELIMINATION

Although the elimination of most poisons can be accelerated by therapeutic interventions, pharmacokinetic efficacy (removal of drug at a rate greater than that accomplished by intrinsic elimination) and the clinical benefits (shortened duration of toxicity, improved outcome) are often more theoretical than proven. Hence, the decision to use a procedure should be based on the actual or predicted toxicity and the potential efficacy and risks.

MULTIPLE-DOSE ACTIVATED CHARCOAL Repeated oral dosing with charcoal (with sorbitol as needed to enhance gastrointestinal motility) enhances the elimination of some poisons. A dose of 1 g/kg body weight every 2 to 4 h, adjusted downward to avoid regurgitation in patients with decreased gastrointestinal motility, is generally recommended. This treatment enhances the elimination of a variety of drugs (carbamazepine, dapsone, diazepam, digoxin, glutethimide, meprobamate, methotrexate, phenobarbital, phenytoin, salicylate, theophylline, valproic acid). Efficacy approaches that of hemodialysis for some agents (theophylline). Multiple-dose therapy is not effective in accelerating elimination of chlorpropamide or imipramine.

FORCED DIURESIS AND ALTERATION OF URINARY pH Diuresis and ion trapping via alteration of urine pH may prevent the renal reabsorption of poisons that undergo excretion by glomerular filtration and active tubular secretion. Since membranes are more permeable to nonionized molecules than to their ionized counterparts, acidic (low pK_a) poisons are ionized and trapped in an alkaline urine, and basic poisons are ionized and trapped in an acid urine. Alkaline diuresis (a urine pH of 7.5 or greater and a urine output of 3 to 6 mL/kg body weight per hour) enhances the elimination of chlorphenoxyacetic acid herbicides, chlorpropamide, phenobarbital (and probably other long-acting barbiturates), and salicylates. Contraindications include congestive heart failure, renal failure, and cerebral edema. Acid-base, fluid, and electrolyte parameters should be carefully monitored. Saline diuresis may enhance the secretion of bromide, lithium, and isoniazid. Acid diuresis enhances the renal elimination of several poisons (amphetamines, cocaine, phencyclidine, quinidine, quinine, sympathomimetics, strychnine), but its use has been largely abandoned because risks are significant and because clinical efficacy has not been established.

EXTRACORPORAL REMOVAL Peritoneal dialysis, hemodialysis, charcoal or resin hemoperfusion, hemofiltration, plasmapheresis, and exchange transfusion are capable of removing any toxin from the bloodstream. Toxins most amenable to enhanced elimination by dialysis have low molecular mass (<500 Da), high water solubility, low protein binding, small volumes of distribution (<1 L/kg body weight), prolonged elimination (long half-life), and high dialysis clearance relative to total body clearance. The efficacy of the other forms of extracorporal removal is not limited by molecular weight, water solubility, or protein binding. Dialysis should be considered in severe poisoning due to bromide, chloral hydrate, ethanol, ethylene glycol, isopropyl alcohol, lithium, heavy metals, methanol, and salicylate. Although hemoperfusion may be effective in removing some of these poisons, it does not correct associated acid-base and electrolyte abnormalities.

Hemoperfusion should be considered in severe poisoning due to chloramphenicol, disopyramide, and hypnotic sedatives (barbiturates, ethchlorvynol, glutethimide, meprobamate, methaqualone, phenytoin, and theophylline). Both techniques require central venous access and systemic anticoagulation and often result in transient hypotension. Hemoperfusion may also cause hemolysis, hypocalcemia, and thrombocytopenia. Peritoneal dialysis and exchange transfusion are less effective but may be used when other procedures are not available, are contraindicated, or are technically difficult (in infants). Exchange transfusion removes poisons affecting red blood cells (e.g., methemoglobinemia or arsine-induced hemolysis). The efficacy of other extracorporal elimination procedures has not been defined.

Candidates for these invasive treatments include patients with severe toxicity who deteriorate despite aggressive supportive therapy, those with potentially dangerous blood levels of toxins, those who lack the capacity for self-detoxification because of liver or renal failure, and those with serious underlying illnesses or complications that adversely affect recovery.

OTHER TECHNIQUES The enhanced elimination of heavy metals by chelation and urinary excretion of the metal-chelator complex and the accelerated removal of carbon monoxide by hyperbaric oxygenation are discussed with the specific poisons.

ADMINISTRATION OF ANTIDOTES

Antidotes counteract the effects of poisons by neutralizing them (antibody-antigen reactions, chelation, chemical binding) or by antagonizing their physiologic effects (activation of opposing nervous system activity, provision of competitive metabolic or receptor substrate). Antidotes can significantly reduce morbidity and mortality, but most antidotes are potentially toxic. Poisons or conditions with specific antidotes include acetaminophen, anticholinergic agents, anticoagulants, beta blockers, calcium channel blockers, carbon monoxide, cholinergic agents, cyanide, digitalis, drugs that cause dystonic reactions, ethylene glycol, fluoride, heavy metals, hydrogen sulfide, hypoglycemic agents, isoniazid, methemoglobinemia, narcotics, sympathomimetics, and vacor. Since the safe use of antidotes requires correct identification of a specific poisoning or syndrome, antidotal therapy is discussed with the conditions for which they are indicated.

PREVENTION OF REEXPOSURE

Poisoning is a preventable illness. Unfortunately, some adults and children are poison-prone, and recurrences are common. Adults with accidental exposures should be instructed regarding the safe use of medications and chemicals (according to labeling instructions). Confused patients may need assistance with the administration of medications. Errors in dosing by health care providers require special educational efforts. Patients should be advised to avoid circumstances that result in chemical exposure or poisoning. Regulatory agencies and health departments should be notified in cases of environmental or workplace exposure. The best approach with young children and patients with intentional overdose is to limit access to poisons. Indeed, the environment of children must be made poison-proof. Alcoholic beverages, medications, household products (automotive, cleaning, fuel, pet-care, toiletry products), nonedible plants, and vitamins should be kept out of reach or in locked or child-proof cabinets. Depressed or psychotic patients should be given prescriptions for a limited (2 week) supply of drugs and with a limited number of refills. All patients should be monitored for compliance and response to therapy.

SPECIFIC POISONS

The poisons in this section are common, produce life-threatening toxicity, or require unique therapeutic interventions. Poisons not mentioned here are described in the referenced texts. Drug and alcohol abuse are discussed in Chaps. 370 to 372. Heavy metal poisoning is discussed in Chap. 375.

ACETAMINOPHEN At therapeutic doses, acetaminophen is metabolized to sulfate and glucuronide conjugates that are excreted in the urine. Minor amounts are excreted unchanged or as mercapturic acid after conjugation with hepatic glutathione. Following an acute overdose of 140 mg/kg body weight or more, the sulfate and glucuronide pathways become saturated, resulting in an increased fraction of acetaminophen metabolized to mercapturic acid. Once hepatic glutathione is depleted, reactive metabolites are formed that covalently bind to hepatocytes and cause cell lysis. Acetaminophen is rapidly absorbed from the stomach and small bowel and has a volume of distribution of 1 L/kg body weight. Approximately 50 percent is protein bound. The plasma half-life is 1 to 2 h.

Clinical signs Early manifestations of poisoning are nonspecific and not predictive of subsequent hepatotoxicity. Within 2 to 4 h of ingestion, nausea, vomiting, diaphoresis, and pallor develop. Central nervous system depression is absent unless depressant drugs are co-ingested. Within 24 to 48 h, hepatotoxicity is evidenced by right upper quadrant tenderness and mild hepatomegaly and followed by the appearance of jaundice, clotting abnormalities, and hepatic encephalopathy. Laboratory evidence of hepatic toxicity includes elevation in serum transaminase activity (AST, ALT). With severe ingestion, prolongation of the prothrombin time, elevation of serum bilirubin, and ultimately hyperammonemia may occur. A twofold

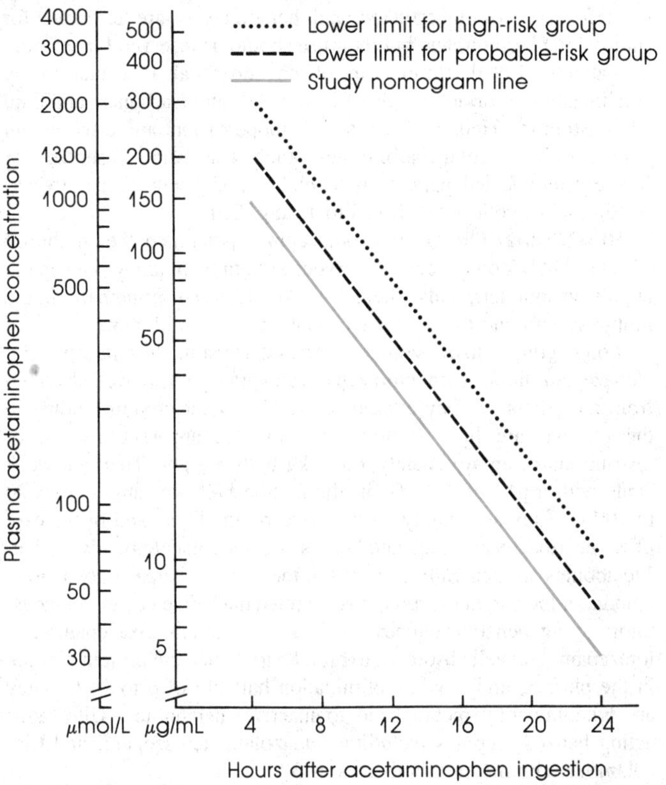

FIGURE 374-1 Nomogram to define risk according to initial plasma acetaminophen concentration. (*After BH Rumack, H Matthew, Pediatrics 55:871, 1975.*)

prolongation of prothombin time and/or serum bilirubin greater than 68 μmol/L (4 mg/dL) on the 3d to 5th day after ingestion indicate severe hepatotoxicity. Histologic evidence of liver damage varies from cytolysis to centrilobular necrosis. Liver histology returns to normal within 3 months. Renal function may also be affected.

Diagnosis A serum acetaminophen level should be determined between 4 and 24 h after ingestion and compared against the Rumack-Matthew nomogram (Fig. 374-1). A level above the two lines on the nomogram is predictive of possible or probable hepatotoxicity. The acetaminophen half-life may be prolonged in patients who develop liver damage.

Treatment Initial treatment involves removal of the ingested product from the gastrointestinal tract. Activated charcoal should be administered. (Charcoal does not significantly interfere with acetylcysteine therapy.) In patients with an acetaminophen level exceeding the lower nomogram line, acetylcysteine therapy is indicated up to 24 h following ingestion. Maximal benefit is achieved if therapy is instituted within 8 to 10 h of the ingestion. Acetylcysteine is given at a loading dose of 140 mg/kg body weight, followed by a maintenance dose of 70 mg/kg body weight every 4 h for 17 doses. Side effects include nausea, vomiting, and epigastric discomfort. If treatment is started prior to availability of the serum level and if the level is subsequently shown to be below the toxic level, therapy may be discontinued. Intravenous acetylcysteine is an investigational drug in this country and requires a protocol for administration. Diuresis has no value.

ACIDS AND ALKALI Burns of the mouth, esophagus, and stomach result from the ingestion of liquid or solid forms of alkali or acids. Common alkaline products include industrial-strength bleach, drain cleaners (sodium hydroxide), surface cleaners (ammonia, phosphates), laundry and dishwasher detergents (phosphates, carbonates), disc batteries, denture cleaners (borates, phosphates, carbonates), and Clinitest tablets (sodium hydroxides). Acids are used in toilet bowl cleaners (hydrofluoric, phosphoric, sulfuric acids), soldering fluxes (hydrochloric acid), antirust compounds (hydrofluoric, oxalic acids), automobile battery fluid (sulfuric acid), and slate cleaners (hydrofluoric acid).

Alkalies produce liquefactive necrosis with rapidly penetrating tissue burns and higher risk of perforation of the esophagus and stomach than do acids. Acids produce coagulative necrosis. Both burn the mouth, esophagus, and stomach. Liquids tend to produce superficial, often circumferential burns over a larger surface area, while solids and tablets cause localized deeper burns. The severity of the burn relates to the contact time, amount ingested, and the pH (especially <2, >12) of the ingested product.

Clinical signs Burns of the mouth result in excess salivation, pain, dysphonia, and dysphagia. Examination of the mouth shows erythema, edema, ulceration, and necrosis. Deep burns may destroy mucosal nerve endings and produce anesthesia. Esophageal symptoms and signs include drooling, painful swallowing, retrosternal pain, and neck tenderness. Vomiting of blood and mucus may occur. Perforation following alkali ingestion is suggested by increasing severity of chest pain, often with respiratory distress. Epigastric pain, vomiting, and tenderness may occur with burns to the stomach. Aspiration of acids and alkalis results in fulminant tracheitis and bronchial pneumonia. In severe cases hypotension, shock, metabolic acidosis, liver and renal dysfunction, hemolysis, and disseminated intravascular coagulation may be seen. Edema, erythema, and ulceration of the esophagus may be followed by fibrosis with stricture formation and obstruction of the esophagus (in the case of alkalis) or of the gastric outlet (in the case of acids).

Diagnosis A careful history will suggest the ingestion of an acid or an alkali. The lack of oral involvement does not rule out esophageal or gastric injury. Endoscopy is safe within 48 h (optimally 12 to 24 h) of the ingestion and will document the anatomic site and often the severity but not the depth of the injury. The endoscope should be advanced to the site of injury but not past it due to risk of producing perforation. Residual effects of the ingestion can be assessed by barium swallow. Chest x-rays may be necessary to confirm aspiration of the ingested product.

Treatment Treatment consists of immediate dilution to wash the product off the mucosal surface. Weak acid or basic solutions should not be used since the heat of neutralization may cause thermal burns and increase tissue injury. Symptomatic patients should be admitted for endoscopy. If alkali burns of the esophagus exist, glucocorticoids should be started within 48 h and given for 3 weeks followed by tapering. Use of prophylactic broad-spectrum antibiotics is controversial. Antacids should be used for burns of the stomach. For acid burns glucocorticoids are not useful. Esophageal stricture or gastric outlet obstruction may require subsequent dilation and bouginage or surgical reconstruction.

ANTIARRHYTHMIC DRUGS Antiarrhythmic drugs can be divided into three classes: class IA (disopyramide, procainamide, and quinidine), class IB (lidocaine, phenytoin, and tocainide), and class IC (encainide and flecainide). These agents are rapidly absorbed (except for disopyramide and sustained-release formulations), have short half-lives (3 to 11 h, somewhat longer for class IC agents), and are predominantly eliminated by hepatic metabolism.

Clinical signs The acute ingestion of more than twice the usual daily dose is potentially toxic. Onset of toxicity occurs within 1 h, and peak effects are demonstrable within several hours. Manifestations include nausea, vomiting, and diarrhea followed by lethargy, confusion, ataxia, bradycardia, hypotension, and cardiovascular collapse. Anticholinergic effects (blurred vision, dry mucosa) may be seen in disopyramide poisoning. Quinidine and class IB agents may cause agitation, dysphoria, and seizures. Nonspecific ECG findings include bradycardia with AV block and QRS-interval prolongation. Ventricular tachycardia, ventricular fibrillation, (including the polymorphous form, torsade de pointes), and QT-interval prolongation are characteristics of poisoning due to class IA and IC drugs. Depressed myocardial contactility and arrhythmias may lead to decreased cardiac output and pulmonary edema. Laboratory findings are nonspecific (metabolic acidosis), except for hypoglycemia and mild hypokalemia, which may be seen with disopyramide and quinidine intoxication, respectively. Toxicology screening will detect most of these agents. Measurement of serum levels may confirm an overdose and indicate the need for monitoring.

Treatment Treatment consists of gastrointestinal decontamination and supportive therapy. Hypotension, bradyarrhythmias, and seizures are treated with standard measures. Patients with persistent hypotension and bradycardia require monitoring of pulmonary arterial pressure. Cardiac pacing, intraaortic balloon pump counterpulsation, and cardiopulmonary bypass may be necessary. Ventricular tachyarrhythmias should be treated with lidocaine, phenytoin, and bretylium. Sodium bicarbonate or sodium lactate may be effective for tachyarrhythmias due to class IA or IC agents. Mild hypokalemia may be protective, and potassium levels that do not fall below 3.0 mmol/L may be best treated by close monitoring. For torsade de pointes (polymorphous or atypical ventricular tachycardia), magnesium sulfate (4 g or 40 mL of a 10% solution intravenously over 10 to 20 min) and overdrive pacing (with isoproterenol or electricity) may be effective. Hemodialysis and hemoperfusion may enhance the elimination of disopyramide and the active procainamide metabolite, *N*-acetylprocainamide. However, clinical experience is inadequate to support routine use.

BARBITURATES Barbiturates are generally classified into long-acting and short-acting. Long-acting barbiturates include mephobarbital, barbital, phenobarbital, and primidone. Short-acting agents include those with intermediate, short, and ultrashort durations of action such as amobarbital, butabarbital, pentobarbital.

Barbiturates exert their effects through depression of the central nervous system. Long-acting barbiturates are well absorbed from the stomach and the small bowel. Peak plasma concentrations occur within 2 to 4 h. Phenobarbital, as an example of a long-acting barbiturate, is a weak acid with a pK_a of 7.2, a volume of distribution of 0.8 L/kg body weight, and 50 percent protein binding in the plasma. Approximately 75 percent of an ingested dose is metabolized by hydroxylation, and 25 percent is excreted unchanged by the kidneys. Other long-acting barbiturates are converted to active metabolites by the liver prior to excretion (primidone to phenobarbital, mephobarbital to barbital). Phenobarbital is eliminated by first-order kinetics with a half life of 80 to 120 h in overdose. Intermediate-, short-, and ultrashort-acting barbiturates are rapidly absorbed with an onset of action within 30 min following ingestion and peak concentrations 1 to 2 h following administration. They are lipid soluble and have an apparent volume of distribution ranging from 0.8 to 1.5 L/kg body weight. They have a pK_a of 8, are partly bound to protein in the plasma, and are mainly metabolized in the liver (up to 99 percent). The mean half-life varies from 4 h for ultrashort- to approximately 35 h for intermediate-acting barbiturates.

Clinical signs Barbiturates in low overdose produce confusion and in large overdose cause CNS depression ranging from lethargy to coma, hypotension, pulmonary edema, and cardiac arrest. Hypothermia is common in acute intoxication. Pupils are generally constricted but may dilate in terminal phases. Bullous skin lesions are seen in severe barbiturate overdose. Signs of toxicity usually appear when serum concentrations of long-acting barbiturates exceed 170 μmol/L (4 mg/dL) and short-acting barbiturates exceed 88 μmol/L (2 mg/dL). Maximal toxicity occurs within 4 to 6 h after short-acting barbiturate but may be delayed 10 h or more after overdosage with long-acting barbiturates. The degree of CNS depression relative to ingested dose is dependent upon prior exposure to the drug.

Treatment Initial management involves prompt gastrointestinal decontamination. Barbiturates are well adsorbed by activated charcoal. In the case of long acting barbiturate poisoning, repetitive administration of activated charcoal every 2 to 4 h enhances elimination threefold and decreases half-life by approximately 50 percent. For all barbiturates, attention should be given to hemodynamic and respiratory support, correction of temperature and electrolyte derangement, and monitoring for pulmonary complications. Since short-acting barbiturates are predominantly metabolized by the liver, diuresis is ineffective. Hemoperfusion and hemodialysis are effective for short-acting barbiturates, but their use should be reserved for severely ill patients. Renal elimination of phenobarbital is enhanced by alkalinization of urine to a pH of 8 with sodium bicarbonate and fluid administration. Hemodialysis and hemoperfusion are effective in removing long-acting barbiturates, their use being reserved for severely intoxicated patients with high blood levels [generally exceeding 430 to 650 μmol/L (10 to 15 mg/dL)].

BENZODIAZEPINES Benzodiazepines potentiate the inhibitory effect of GABA on the central nervous system by binding to receptors at polysynaptic terminals where GABA is released, principally in the limbic system and the reticular formation of the midbrain.

Long-acting benzodiazepines such as diazepam, chlordiazepoxide, clonazepam, flurazepam, clorazepate, and prazepam are well absorbed from the GI tract. They exhibit 85 to 95 percent protein binding in the plasma, are lipid soluble and have an apparent volume of distribution of approximately 1.1 L/kg body weight. They are weak acids with a pK_a of 3.4. Their elimination half-life ranges from 20 to 100 h. They are mainly metabolized by the liver, and in the case of some (diazepam) the metabolites are pharmacologically active. Metabolites are generally excreted in the urine, whereas only a small amount of the parent compound is excreted unchanged by the kidneys. Short-acting benzodiazepines, such as alprazolam, oxazepam, and lorazepam, are well absorbed, exhibit 85 to 95 percent protein binding in the plasma, and have an elimination half-life of 6 to 24 h. They are predominantly metabolized to inactive metabolites. Ultrashort-acting benzodiazepines including midazolam, temazepam, and triazolam have elimination half-lives of 3 to 12 h.

Clinical signs The major effects include weakness, ataxia, drowsiness, and, in severe overdose, coma and respiratory depression. Pupils are generally constricted and unresponsive to naloxone. Respiratory support is rarely needed except in the case of ultrashort-acting agents, massive overdose, or the co-ingestion of other sedative drugs. Ethanol enhances the absorption of benzodiazepine and potentiates the CNS depression. Confirmation of the diagnosis is made by identification of the metabolites in urine.

Treatment Initial management includes prompt gastrointestinal decontamination. Single-dose as well as repeated-dose activated charcoal when metabolites are active (diazepam) is indicated. High protein binding of benzodiazepines limits efficacy of hemodialysis.

BETA-ADRENERGIC BLOCKING AGENTS Beta-adrenergic blocking agents approved for use in the United States include acebutolol, atenolol, esmolol, labetalol, metoprolol, nadolol, pindolol, propranolol, sotalol, and timolol.

Beta blockers act by competitively blocking beta-adrenergic neurohumoral receptors in the bronchial and vascular smooth muscle and myocardium. At therapeutic doses, some beta-blockers act predominantly on $beta_1$ receptors and are "cardioselective" (acebutolol, atenolol, metoprolol), some have partial agonist or sympathomimetic activity (acebutolol, pindolol, timolol), and some have quinidine-like myocardial membrane stabilizing effects (acebutolol, metoprolol, pindolol, propranolol, sotalol). Antiarrhythmic effects are due to a reduction of sodium and calcium influx during membrane depolarization (phase 0) as a consequence of decreased production of cyclic AMP by adenylate cyclase. This activity defines beta blockers as class II antiarrhythmics. Beta blockers decrease cardiac contractility by directly inhibiting the release of calcium from sarcoplasmic reticulum. Following overdose, cardioselectivity is lost, and all beta blockers may cause membrane depressant effects.

Beta blockers are rapidly and well absorbed. They exhibit variable protein binding (5 to 93 percent), low water solubility and variable volumes of distribution (1 to 5.6 L/kg body weight), and are eliminated predominantly by hepatic metabolism (exceptions include nadolol and atenolol).

Clinical signs Manifestations of toxicity usually begin with 1/2 h following an overdose and become maximal within 2 h. Common findings include nausea, vomiting, and diarrhea followed by bradycardia, hypotension, and CNS depression. However, agents with sympathomimetic activity can cause hypertension and tachycardia. Central nervous system effects vary from lethargy and confusion to coma and seizures and tend to be more pronounced with the more lipophilic agents (acebutolol, metoprolol, pindolol, propranol, and timolol). The skin is often pale and cool. Bronchospasm and pulmonary edema may occur in those with a history of asthma, chronic obstructive pulmonary disease, or congestive heart failure. Metabolic abnormalities include hyperkalemia and hypoglycemia (as a direct result of beta-adrenergic receptor blockade) and metabolic acidosis (due to seizures, shock, or respiratory depression). Electrocardiographic manifestations include all degrees of AV block, bundle branch block, prolonged QRS duration, and asystole. Sotalol poisoning may also cause QT-interval prolongation with ventricular tachycardia, ventricular fibrillation, and torsade de pointes. Patients with mild poisoning usually recover within 6 to 12 h whereas those with severe poisoning may be symptomatic for 24 to 48 h. A toxicology screen may identify the presence of beta blockers, but blood levels are not generally available nor helpful in guiding therapy.

Treatment Treatment includes gastrointestinal decontamination, nonspecific supportive measures, and the administration of calcium and glucagon. Because gastric emptying procedures may produce vagal stimulation and exacerbate bradyarrhythmias, monitoring should be instituted first. Treatment of bradycardia and hypotension should begin with atropine, isoproterenol, and dopamine. With severe poisoning these agents may be ineffective, and glucagon, calcium, cardiac pacing (external or internal), and intraaortic balloon pump support may be necessary. Glucagon, which stimulates adenylate cyclase by a nonadrenergic mechanism, should be given at an initial dose of 5 to 10 mg for adults. Patients who respond favorably should then be given an infusion of 1 to 5 mg/L. Calcium, which may reverse nonadrenergic negative inotropic effects, should be given in the same initial dose as described for calcium channel blocker poisoning. Patients with altered mental status or abnormal vital signs should also be given intravenous glucose. Bronchospasm may be treated with inhaled beta agonists, subcutaneous epinephrine, and intravenous aminophylline. Lidocaine or overdrive pacing may be used for sotalol-induced ventricular tachyarrhythmias. Extracorporal elimination procedures are probably not of benefit (exceptions include atenolol, metoprolol, nadolol, and sotalol), but clearcut clinical data are not available.

BLEACH Because of its widespread availability, sodium hypochlorite (bleach, Clorox) is associated with both accidental and purposeful overdose. Bleach solutions for home use generally contain 3 to 6% sodium hypochlorite, and industrial bleaches may have higher concentrations. These solutions have a pH of 10.5 to 11.0, and contain free chlorine, which gives the compound its characteristic odor.

Sodium hypochlorite decomposes rapidly to hypochloric acid on contact with moisture and is irritating but not caustic. Sodium hypochlorite mixed with acid decomposes to chlorine gas and when mixed with ammonia produces chloramine gas. Both chlorine and chloramine gas are highly irritating.

Clinical signs Sodium hypochlorite is irritating to the gastrointestinal mucosa and to mucous membranes of the lips, mouth, and eyes. Household bleach causes superficial injury to the esophagus, but stricture formation does not occur. If the agent is inhaled, chemical pneumonia and pulmonary edema can ensue. Industrial bleaches do cause deep burns of the esophagus with the potential for stricture formation.

Treatment Ingestion of small quantities of sodium hypochlorite should be treated by dilution with milk or water. Neutralization is not necessary, and activated charcoal and cathartics are not indicated. Large ingestions of sodium hypochlorite may require gastric lavage. Care should be taken to prevent vomiting and secondary aspiration. Exposed skin and eyes should be washed.

CALCIUM CHANNEL BLOCKERS Diltiazem, nicardipine, nifedipine, and verapamil are approved for use in the United States. These agents act by decreasing the influx of calcium across slow calcium channels in the membranes of myocardial and vascular smooth muscle cells during phases 2 (plateau) and 4 (spontaneous depolarization) of the action potential (class IV antiarrhythmics). Electrophysiologic effects include decreased cardiac contractility, heart (SA nodal) rate, AV nodal conduction, and vascular tone.

Calcium channel blockers are rapidly absorbed, exhibit high protein binding in the plasma, and have large volumes of distribution (>2 L/kg body weight). They are predominantly eliminated by hepatic metabolism, and their half-lives range from 3 to 8 h.

Clinical signs Toxicity usually develops within $\frac{1}{2}$ to 1 h of ingestion of amounts five to ten times the usual therapeutic dose. Clinical manifestations include bradycardia, hypotension, and cyanosis. Mental status changes range from confusion and drowsiness to coma and seizures and are due both to direct membrane effects and to cerebral hypoperfusion. Depression of cardiac function may lead to pulmonary edema. Electrocardiographic findings include all degrees of AV block, prolonged QRS and QT intervals (mainly with verapamil), evidence of ischemia or infarction, and asystole. Metabolic acidosis (secondary to shock) and hyperglycemia (resulting in the inhibition of insulin release) may be present. Serum calcium levels, however, remain normal.

Treatment Treatment consists of the administration of calcium and glucagon, GI tract decontamination, and supportive measures. Atropine, calcium, isoproterenol, glucagon, and electrical (external or internal) pacing, in order of preference, may be used for symptomatic bradycardia. Calcium, as the 10% chloride or gluconate salt solution, should be given in a dose of 0.2 mL/kg body weight (up to 10 mL) intravenously over 5 min. This dose may be repeated up to four times in patients with a partial, transient, or absent response, provided that serum calcium levels are monitored. A continuous calcium infusion (0.2 mL/kg body weight per hour up to a maximum of 10 mL/h) may be appropriate when relapse occurs after an initial bolus. Although electrical pacing is often required, glucagon, in the same dose as for beta-blocker poisoning, should be tried first. Hypotension that persists despite resolution of bradycardia should be treated with fluids and adrenergic agents. Amrinone, dopamine, dobutamine, glucagon and norepinephrine, alone or in combination, have been used. The benefit of restored perfusion is particularly important in patients with organ ischemia. Intraaortic balloon pump support should be used in patients unresponsive to the above measures. Patients with mild toxicity usually recover within a few hours, whereas those with severe toxicity or overdose with sustained-release preparations may remain symptomatic for 24 h or longer. Extracorporal removal techniques are unlikely to be of benefit.

CARBON MONOXIDE Carbon monoxide is produced in large amounts in industry as well as by gasoline engines, home appliances, and the incomplete combustion of wood, natural gas, and tobacco products. In addition, methylene chloride, a solvent in paint removers, is metabolized to carbon monoxide.

Carbon monoxide is rapidly absorbed through the lungs and binds to hemoglobin (forming carboxyhemoglobin) with an affinity 210 times that of oxygen, resulting in cellular anoxia. This occurs by limiting oxygen-carrying by hemoglobin, by decreasing release of oxygen to tissues (the oxygen dissociation curve shifts to the left), and by binding to various heme proteins (cytochrome oxidase, myoglobin). Once carbon monoxide exposure is discontinued, dissociation of the hemoglobin carbon monoxide complex occurs, and carbon monoxide is excreted through the lungs. At room air this results in a carbon monoxide half-life of 4 to 6 h; the half-life decreases in 100% oxygen to 40 to 80 min and in hyperbaric oxygen to 15 to 30 min. The half-life after methylene chloride exposure is considerably longer.

Clinical signs Manifestations of carbon monoxide poisoning include shortness of breath, dyspnea, tachypnea, headache, emotional lability, confusion, impaired judgment, and clumsiness. Nausea, vomiting, and diarrhea may also occur. Respiratory depression occurs with severe poisoning. Pulmonary edema may result from myocardial failure, and aspiration of vomitus may cause pneumonia. Cardiovascular manifestations include arrhythmias, heart failure, and hypotension. Blisters and bullae may develop over pressure points. The "cherry-red" color of skin and mucous membranes is rare, and cyanosis is usual. Visual field defects, blindness, and venous engorgement with papilledema or optic atrophy may be noted. Neurologic sequelae of acute carbon monoxide poisoning are due to hypoxia.

Sequelae correlate with the level of consciousness on presentation to the hospital. Up to 30 percent of exposed individuals develop multifocal neurologic signs 1 to 3 weeks after initial exposure with varying rates of eventual recovery. While elevated carboxyhemoglobin levels document carbon monoxide exposure, they do not necessarily indicate the severity of the poisoning. Traditionally, levels of 20 to 30 percent are associated with mild symptoms, 30 to 50 percent with moderate symptoms, 50 to 60 percent with severe symptoms, and levels above 60 percent are often fatal. Diffuse slow waves of low voltage on EEG may be noted. Electrocardiographic changes include sinus tachycardia, ST depression, T-wave flattening, premature ventricular contraction, and abnormalities in left ventricular wall function. Serum creatine phosphokinase (CPK) and lactate dehydrogenase (LDH) levels may be elevated. Myoglobinuria, secondary to muscle necrosis, may result in renal failure. Arterial blood gases reveal normal P_{O_2}, decreased oxygen saturation (by direct measurement rather than calculated value), and normal or slightly decreased P_{CO_2}. Metabolic acidosis is generally present.

Treatment The patients should be removed from the site of exposure. Oxygen (100%) should be administered by a tightly fitting mask at 10 L/min until carbon monoxide levels are less than 10 percent and all symptoms have resolved. Infants and pregnant women may require prolonged treatment because fetal hemoglobin has a high affinity for carbon monoxide. Hyperbaric oxygen at 2 to 3 atm decreases the half-life of carbon monoxide to 15 to 30 min and produces sufficient dissolved oxygen to prevent tissue hypoxia. Hyperbaric oxygen shortens the duration of coma and may diminish the sequelae of carbon monoxide poisoning. While its use is limited by availability, hyperbaric oxygen is recommended for comatose patients with carbon monoxide levels over 40 percent, patients with levels above 25 percent who have seizures or intractable arrhythmias, and patients with delayed onset of sequelae.

COCAINE (See Chap. 272).

CYANIDE Hydrogen cyanide is used as a rodenticide and in chemical syntheses. Cyanide salts are used in photography, metallurgy, electroplating, metal cleaning and ore refining. Organic cyanide compounds are used in the synthetic rubber industry as well as in rodenticides. Cyanogenic glycosides are present in the seeds of the chokeberry, cherry, plum, peach, apricot, pear, bean, apple, and crabapple.

Cyanide inhibits mitochondrial ferricytochrome oxidase and other enzyme systems and hence blocks electron transport resulting in decreased oxidative metabolism and oxygen utilization, decreased ATP production, and lactic acidosis. Cyanide is rapidly absorbed from the stomach, lungs, mucosal surfaces, and unbroken skin. In the stomach it reacts with hydrochloric acid, liberating hydrocyanic acid, which is absorbed as cyanide ion. Cyanide is 60 percent protein bound, is concentrated in red cells, and has a volume of distribution of 1.5 L/kg body weight. Cyanide is metabolized by the mitochondrial enzyme rhodanase, which mediates the transfer of sulfur from thiosulfate to the cyanide ion producing thiocyanate, which in turn is excreted in the urine.

Clinical signs The lethal dose of potassium or sodium cyanide is 200 to 300 mg and of hydrocyanic acid is 50 mg. Early effects of cyanide poisoning include headache, faintness, vertigo, excitement, anxiety, burning sensation in the mouth and throat, and dyspnea. Cardiovascular manifestations include tachycardia and hypertension. Nausea, vomiting, and diaphoresis are common. A bitter almond odor may be detected on the breath. Later effects include coma, convulsions, opisthotonus, trismus, paralysis, respiratory depression, pulmonary edema, arrhythmias, bradycardia, and hypotension. Therapeutic intervention must be initiated on the basis of history and consistent clinical and laboratory findings. Variable correlation exists between blood cyanide levels and symptoms: levels less than 8 μmol/L (0.02 mg/dL) are associated with no symptoms, 20 to 40 μmol/L (0.05 to 0.1 mg/dL) with flushing and tachycardia, 40 to 100 μmol/L (0.1 to 0.25 mg/dL) with obtundation, 100 to 200 μmol/L (0.25 to 0.3 mg/dL) with coma and respiratory depression, and levels greater than 120 μmol/L (0.3 mg/dL) with death. Other laboratory abnormalities include lactic acidosis and narrowing of the arteriovenous oxygen saturation difference. Electrocardiographic abnormalities include both tachyarrhythmias and bradyarrhythmias such as nodal or idioventricular rhythm, atrioventricular dissociation, and progressive slowing of heart rate.

Treatment Initial management involves general supportive measures and gastrointestinal decontamination. Amyl nitrite, sodium nitrite, and sodium thiosulfate (the Lilly cyanide antidote kit) coupled with oxygen are the cornerstones of therapy. Amyl nitrite is administered by broken ampul and inhaled by the patient for 30 s of each minute. A new ampul should be used every 3 min. The drug produces 5% methemoglobinemia (by converting ferrous iron to its ferric state). Methemoglobin has a higher affinity for cyanide, thereby promoting release of cyanide from mitochondrial cytochrome oxidase sites and forming cyanomethemoglobin. This process is continued while sodium nitrite is being prepared but may be omitted if sodium nitrite is available. Sodium nitrite is then administered intravenously as a 3% solution at a rate of 2.5 to 5.0 mL per minute up to a total dose of 10 to 15 mL (300 to 450 mg) in an effort to produce a 25% methemoglobin concentration. The dose in children is 0.33 mL/kg body weight (10 mg/kg body weight). Finally, sodium thiosulfate is used to remove and bind circulating cyanide from its methemoglobin sites and produce sodium thiocyanate that is excreted by the kidneys. Sodium thiosulfate is administered intravenously as a 25% solution at a dose of 50 mL (12.5 g) given over 1 to 2 min. The dose in children is 1.65 mL/kg body weight (0.5 g/kg body weight). With recurrent symptoms, half of the initial doses of both sodium nitrite and sodium thiosulfate are administered. Sodium thiosulfate is of low toxicity. Oxygen is a safe and important antidote by reversing binding of cyanide to cytochrome oxidase sites and increasing the delivery of oxygen to tissues. It also enhances the efficacy of sodium nitrite and sodium thiosulfate.

DIGOXIN Cardiac glycoside poisoning occurs most frequently as overdosage during therapeutic use of digitalis preparations and on occasion with plant (oleander) ingestion. Digoxin and other glycosides act by inhibiting the enzyme sodium-potassium ATPase, leading to increased intracellular Na^+ and Ca^{2+} and decreased K^+. Serum levels of digoxin peak 2 to 6 h following ingestion. Digoxin is 25 to 30 percent protein bound in the plasma. Digoxin has a large volume of distribution of 5 to 6 L/kg body weight and is localized in skeletal muscle, liver, and heart. The cardiac-to-plasma ratio for digoxin is approximately 30 to 1; the elimination half-life ranges between 36 and 45 h, is prolonged in renal failure, and may be shortened in overdose. Approximately 60 percent of a dose is excreted unchanged by the kidneys, and the remainder is metabolized by the liver to inactive metabolites. The mean therapeutic serum concentration ranges from 0.6 to 2.5 nmol/L (0.5 to 2.0 ng/mL).

Clinical signs Symptoms of toxicity include vomiting, confusion, delirium, and occasionally hallucinations, blurred vision, photophobia, scotomata, and disturbed color perception. Cardiac manifestations include sinus arrhythmia, sinus bradycardia and all degrees of atrioventricular block. Premature ventricular contractions, bigeminy, ventricular tachycardia, and fibrillation also occur. The combination of supraventricular tachyarrhythmia and atrioventricular block is highly suggestive of digitalis toxicity. While hypokalemia is commonly associated with chronic intoxication, acute overdose produces hyperkalemia [generally with digoxin serum levels above 13 nmol/L (10 ng/mL)]. Clinical toxicity is seen with digoxin levels in excess of 3.8 to 6.4 nmol/L (3 to 5 ng/mL), and levels as high as

64 to 77 nmol/L (50 to 60 ng/mL) have been seen in the overdose setting. Levels measured sooner than 8 h after ingestion may not reflect complete tissue distributions.

Treatment Gastrointestinal decontamination is carried out with care to avoid vagal stimulation which may worsen existing conduction block. Digitalis is adsorbed effectively by activated charcoal, and repeated doses can be administered to absorb active metabolites as they are excreted by the biliary tract. Diuresis, hemodialysis, and hemoperfusion are ineffective because of the large volume of distribution. Hyerkalemia should be managed with oral sodium polystyrene sulfonate, insulin, and glucose. Atropine is effective for sinus bradycardia and for second and third degree heart block. Electrical pacing may be necessary when heart block is unresponsive to atropine, and magnesium sulfate, phenytoin, and lidocaine may be useful in the treatment of arrhythmias. Cardiac glycoside antibodies are also available for the treatment of severe poisoning. These digoxin-specific Fab fragment antibodies are given intravenously in molar equivalency with the estimated ingested overdose to patients with refractory arrhythmias and significantly elevated serum digoxin concentrations. Following their administration, cardiac arrhythmias and hyperkalemia are corrected within hours; digoxin is bound to Fab fragments and excreted with a half-life of 9 h. The antibodies are given intravenously over 30 min, unless cardiac arrest has occurred, in which case the solution is given as a bolus. The dosage (in 40-mg vials to be given) is estimated by dividing the ingested dose in milligrams by 0.6 mg/vial. (Each milligram of Fab fragments binds 0.015 mg digoxin.) Alternatively, the dose (in vials) can be estimated by multiplying the steady-state serum concentration of digoxin by 0.0093 times the patient's weight (in kilograms). If both dose and serum levels are unknown, an initial dose of 5 to 10 vials may be given to adults. The antibodies cross-react with other cardiac glycosides so that larger doses may be needed for toxicity involving digitoxin.

ETHANOL (See Chap. 370)

ETHYLENE GLYCOL Ethylene glycol is a colorless, odorless, sweet-tasting water soluble liquid that is used as a solvent for paints, plastics, and pharmaceuticals and in the manufacture of explosives, fire extinguishers, foams, hydraulic fluids, windshield cleaners, and de-icer preparations. Most cases of poisoning occur as a result of the ingestion of automobile radiator antifreeze, which contains 95 percent ethylene glycol.

Ethylene glycol is rapidly absorbed. Peak levels occur approximately 2 h following ingestion. Ethylene glycol has a volume of distribution of 0.6 to 0.8 L/kg body weight. Ethylene glycol is oxidized by alcohol dehydrogenase to glycoaldehyde, then metabolized to glycolic acid, glyoxylic acid, and oxalic acid. As much as 20 to 50 percent is excreted unchanged in the urine. The half-life ranges from 3 to 8 h. Since alcohol dehydrogenase has a higher affinity for ethanol than ethylene glycol, ethanol is preferentially metabolized when both alcohols are present. Ethanol inhibits metabolism of ethylene glycol and prolongs its half-life to about 17 h. Ethylene glycol produces CNS depression in overdose. Glycoaldehyde also produces CNS depression, but because of rapid metabolism is unlikely to cause signs and symptoms. Glycolic acid is responsible for decreased serum bicarbonate, metabolic acidosis, and increased anion gap and for interstitial and tubular damage to the kidney. Glyoxylic acid is more toxic than glycolic acid, but because it is oxidized so rapidly to oxalic acid, glycolic acid contributes little to the toxicity of ethylene glycol. Oxalic acid may precipitate as calcium oxalate crystals in the brain, heart, kidney, lung, pancreas, and urine. Precipitation of calcium oxalate may result in hypocalcemia.

Clinical signs As little as 120 mg/kg body weight or 0.1 mL/kg body weight of pure ethylene glycol can result in a serum ethylene glycol concentration of 3 mmol/L (20 mg/dL). Hence, one swallow of ethylene glycol is potentially hazardous. Signs and symptoms appear within 30 min following ingestion and include nausea, vomiting, slurred speech, ataxia, nystagmus, and lethargy. A faint, sweet aromatic odor may be detected on the breath. Coma, seizures, respiratory depression, cardiovascular collapse, and death may occur. Ethylene glycol metabolites produce signs and symptoms 4 to 12 h following ingestion. At this stage the patient appears more ill than intoxicated. Manifestations include tachypnea, hypotension, agitation, confusion, lethargy, coma, and seizures. Hypocalcemia occurs in a third of patients. Leukocytosis is present in the majority. In severe cases adult respiratory distress syndrome, cyanosis, pulmonary edema, and cardiomegaly may be seen. In this stage the diagnosis is suggested by metabolic acidosis and an abnormal urinalysis (crystalluria). In patients who survive the early stages, acute tubular necrosis manifested by proteinuria, oliguria, and anuria ensues 12 to 24 h following ingestion. Early in intoxication an elevated osmolality is present. Later, an elevated anion gap and decreased serum bicarbonate and chloride are observed. Signs of alcohol-like intoxication suggest a serum ethylene glycol level greater than 8 to 16 mmol/L (50 to 100 mg/dL). Survival has been reported with levels as high as 100 mmol/L (650 mg/dL).

Diagnosis Diagnosis is suggested by a history of exposure to antifreeze in association with CNS depression, an elevated serum osmolality, and a large anion gap. Levels of ethylene glycol (early) and glycolic acid (late) should be determined. Oxalate crystals in the urine suggest the diagnosis.

Treatment Gastrointestinal lavage and then activated charcoal should be administered. Supportive measures include protection of the airway and ventilatory and circulatory support. Seizures should be treated with phenytoin, a short-acting barbiturate, or a benzodiazepine. Hypocalcemia is treated with intravenous calcium salts at a dose of 7 to 14 mL (a 10% solution diluted 10 to 1 with intravenous fluids and given at a rate of 1 mL/min). Metabolic acidosis should be corrected with sodium bicarbonate. Fluids and diuretics may reverse oligura but do not enhance the elimination rate of ethylene glycol. Indications for ethanol therapy include a history or strong suspicion of ethylene glycol ingestion, an ethylene glycol concentration greater than 3 mmol/L (20 mg/dL), and acidosis regardless of the absolute ethylene glycol concentration. A serum ethanol level of at least 20 mmol/L (100 mg/dL) is required to inhibit alcohol dehydrogenase (higher levels may be needed with very high ethylene glycol concentrations). The loading and maintenance doses of ethanol are the same as for methanol poisoning. Serum ethanol and ethylene glycol concentrations should be monitored frequently. Methypyrazole, a competitive inhibitor of alcohol dehydrogenase, is under study as a nontoxic, experimental alternative to ethanol for ethylene glycol poisoning. Hemodialysis reduces ethylene glycol half-life from 17 h on ethanol therapy to 3 h. Indications for hemodialysis include metabolic acidosis not correctable with bicarbonate and ethanol therapy, failure to improve despite treatment, ethylene glycol concentrations greater than 8 mmol/L (50 mg/dL), or renal failure. Supplemental thiamine and pyridoxine may also be beneficial.

HALLUCINOGENS (See also Chap. 372) Hallucinogens occur in three chemical classes, phenylalkylamines, tryptamines, and ergolines, with mescaline, psilocybin, and lysergic acid (LSD) being the prototype for each. Large numbers of synthetic analogues exist in each class. Mescaline is a derivative of the peyote cactus which grows in the southwestern United States. Psilocybin is derived from mushrooms. Lysergic acid is found in the fungus *Claviceps purpurea,* which grows as a contaminant on rye and wheat, and in morning glory seeds. Synthetic LSD is the common source of the street drug.

Mescaline is well absorbed from the gastrointestinal tract and nasal mucosa. It has an apparent volume of distribution of 2 to 3 L/kg body weight and is eliminated by hepatic metabolism. Psilocybin is also rapidly absorbed from the gastrointestinal tract and converted to an active psilocin. Pharmacokinetics of psilocybin are not well worked out. Lysergic acid is generally taken either by ingestion or inhalation (''snorting'') and is rapidly absorbed by both the nasal mucosa and gastrointestinal tract. Peak levels of LSD are achieved within 1 to 2 h following ingestion. The drug is protein bound (80 to 90 percent) and has an apparent volume of distribution of 0.8 L/

kg body weight. It is concentrated in kidney, spleen, and liver and in the reticular activating system of the brain. It is metabolized to inactive metabolites that are excreted in the feces and urine. The half-life of LSD is 3 h.

Clinical signs The primary effect of these agents is to produce disordered thought, mood changes, and sensory misperceptions (auditory, gustatory, olfactory, and visual dysesthesias). Mescaline is one four-thousandths as potent as LSD. It is associated with a higher incidence of nausea and vomiting but causes only mild physiologic stimulation (Table 374-2). Psilocybin has one two-hundredths the potency of LSD. Its effects are similar to those of LSD with unique features including fever, hypotonia, and seizures. The effects of LSD may last for 4 to 6 h and include mydriasis, conjunctival injection, piloerection, hypertension, tachycardia, tachypnea, anorexia, tremors, and hyperreflexia. Psychological effects include loss of body image, visual illusions, and alteration of the senses. The psychological effects (''trip'') generally last for 6 to 12 h and can be pleasant or alarming. The EEG may show paroxysmal discharges, and seizures may occur. Flashbacks or recurrences of visual images may appear up to 18 months after ingestion.

Diagnosis Identification of LSD in serum is difficult because of its small quantities. In urine, LSD can be detected for up to 5 days following ingestion, and mescaline can be detected for up to 24 h. Psilocybin is usually not detected in the routine toxic screens.

Treatment Gastrointestinal decontamination is not useful once symptoms are present and may lead to further exacerbation of symptoms. The mainstay of therapy is prevention of physical injury by calming in a quiet room with low lights. Physical restraint may cause hyperthermia, rhabdomyolysis, and acute renal failure. Benzodiazepines are effective for acute panic reaction, and butyrephenones (haloperidol in particular) may be indicated for severe psychotic reactions (see Chap. 372).

HYDROCARBONS Hydrocarbons exist in a number of forms including aromatic hydrocarbons, such as xylene and toluene, halogenated hydrocarbons, such as carbon tetrachloride and trichlorethane, and petroleum distillate hydrocarbons, such as gasoline, lacquer thinner, mineral seal oil, kerosene, and lighter fluid.

All hydrocarbons are CNS depressants. Aromatic and halogenated hydrocarbons are rapidly absorbed and distributed into the central nervous system, myocardium, liver, and kidneys. Petroleum distillate hydrocarbons are toxic to the GI tract, central nervous system, and lungs. The lung involvement is predominantly due to aspiration pneumonitis.

Clinical signs Aromatic hydrocarbons and halogenated hydrocarbons produce excitation in low dose and depression of the central nervous system in high dose. Coma and, rarely, seizures may occur. Other target organs include the GI tract (nausea, vomiting, and abdominal pain), the kidneys (renal tubular acidosis), the hematopoietic system (bone marrow suppression), skeletal muscles (rhabdomyolysis), and brain (permanent psychosis and cerebral atrophy). Sudden death due to myocardial irritability and ventricular fibrillation may occur following hydrocarbon sniffing. Petroleum distillate hydrocarbons cause burning of the mouth and throat with subsequent nausea, vomiting, and diarrhea. Respiratory symptoms include cough, dyspnea, tachypnea, hypoxia, and cyanosis. Lethargy is the most prominent CNS manifestation. Coma and convulsions are rare. Laboratory diagnosis of aromatic, halogenated, or petroleum distillate hydrocarbon poisoning is not available at present.

Treatment Aromatic and halogenated hydrocarbons require prompt gastric lavage. Absorption is rapid and complete within 1 to 2 h following ingestion. Activated charcoal is generally not effective. Supportive therapy includes oxygen, respiratory support, and monitoring of liver, renal, and myocardial function. In the case of petroleum distillate hydrocarbons, unless very large amounts (greater than 18 mL/kg body weight) are ingested, gastric lavage and ipecac-induced emesis are contraindicated. Activated charcoal adsorbs petroleum distillate hydrocarbons, but because administration may result in vomiting and subsequent aspiration their use is contraindicated. Pulmonary involvement causes consistent symptoms and x-ray changes. If pneumonia is present, supportive therapy and monitoring for superimposed bacterial infection are indicated. Glucocorticoids are ineffective for hydrocarbon pneumonia. CNS effects are relatively short-lived and require careful monitoring and respiratory support.

HYDROGEN SULFIDE Hydrogen sulfide is encountered in the petroleum and mining industry, tanning of leather, vulcanization of rubber, production of synthetic fabrics, metal refining, production of heavy water for atomic reactors, and glue and felt manufacturing. It is encountered in sewers, sulfur springs, the holds of fishing vessels, and as a by-product of manure storage.

The hydrogen sulfide anion inhibits electron transport in the cytochrome oxidase system, thereby inhibiting aerobic metabolism with resultant cellular anoxia and cell death. Hydrogen sulfide is a highly toxic, malodorous, colorless, highly irritating gas that gains access to the blood through the mucous membranes of the tracheobronchial tree. Hydrogen sulfide is detoxified to sulfate products that are principally excreted by the kidneys.

Clinical signs Hydrogen sulfide has a characteristic odor of ''rotten eggs'' at low concentrations. It is highly irritating, resulting in rhinitis, conjunctivitis, and pharyngitis. Systemic effects include headache, vertigo, nausea, confusion, seizures, and coma. As a respiratory depressant, it also produces hypoventilation, hypoxia, cyanosis, and metabolic acidosis. Pneumonia and pulmonary edema are frequent complications of vomiting. The majority of deaths occur at the site of exposure. There is no readily available laboratory test for immediate diagnosis, and the diagnosis is based on history and clinical features.

Treatment Treatment begins with removal of the victim promptly from the site of exposure. The airway should be cleared, assisted ventilation should be used when indicated, and 100% oxygen should be administered. Nitrites may be given (see ''Cyanide'' section above) to bind the sulfide ion by removing it from cytochrome oxidase sites, thereby forming a sulfide-methemoglobin complex (sulfmethemoglobin). Nitrites also enhance detoxification by acting as a catalyst for sulfide oxidation. Absolute indications for nitrite administration do not exist. For optimal effectiveness they must be utilized immediately in symptomatic patients (sulfide oxidation is so rapid that the amount of sulfide bound to cytochrome is minimal by the time the patient presents for treatment). The dosage schedule for nitrites is the same as for cyanide poisoning. The use of thiosulfate is not necessary in sulfide poisoning. Hyperbaric oxygen should be considered in patients who do not respond to the above measures.

IRON Iron preparations may contain one of three ferrous salts (sulfate, fumarate, and gluconate). Toxicity is based on the amount of elemental iron in the salt (20 percent in the sulfate salt, 33 percent in the fumarate, and 12 percent in the gluconate). Ingestion of more than 20 mg/kg body weight of elemental iron produces gastrointestinal toxicity and of more than 60 mg/kg body weight results in systemic toxicity.

Ferrous iron is absorbed into mucosal cells of the duodenum and jejunum and is oxidized to ferric iron where it is bound to ferritin. It is slowly released from ferritin into the plasma where it is bound to transferrin, an iron-specific binding globulin, and transported to tissues for use in hemoglobin, cytochrome, and myoglobin synthesis. Approximately 70 percent of total body iron is present as hemoglobin, 25 percent is stored in liver and spleen as ferritin and hemosiderin, and 5 percent is present in myoglobin and tissue enzymes. Iron bound to transferrin is nontoxic. Free iron that exceeds the iron-binding capacity is toxic to the vasculature and also leads to the release of vasoactive substances such as serotonin and histamine. In addition, excess quantities of ferritin result in vasodilation. All these mechanisms result in increased permeability and fluid loss through the vasculature, with subsequent hypotension and metabolic acidosis. Finally, free iron injures mitochondria, causes lipid peroxidation, and results in renal, tubular, and hepatic necrosis and on occasion in myocardial and pulmonary injury. Iron can also cause irritation and ulceration of the stomach and small bowel. In overdose, iron is deposited in liver, spleen, and kidneys and causes fatty degeneration and necrosis in hepatocytes, renal tubules, and myocardial cells.

Clinical signs Initial manifestations of iron poisoning include vomiting and diarrhea (often bloody), fever, hyperglycemia, and leukocytosis. Later effects include lethargy, hypotension, and metabolic acidosis and, with severe ingestions, seizures, coma, and vascular collapse. Jaundice, elevated hepatic enzymes, prolongation of prothrombin time, and hyperammonemia are indicative of liver injury. Proteinuria and cells in urine indicate renal injury. Pulmonary edema and hemorrhage are seen with severe overdose. In the recovering patient, gastric outlet scarring may cause obstruction. An overgrowth of *Yersinia enterocolitica* with sepsis is an infrequent complication.

Diagnosis Iron overdosage may be confirmed by x-ray identification of iron tablets in the stomach or small bowel or by measurement of serum iron. A serum iron concentration above the iron-binding capacity [a serum level generally greater than 50 μmol/L (300 μg/dL)] suggests serious poisoning. A positive urine deferoxamine provocative challenge test (a *vin rosé* color) indicating the presence of ferrioxamine (the complex of free iron bound to deferoxamine) is diagnostic and indicates an iron level greater than the iron-binding capacity. The dose used is 50 mg/kg body weight up to 1 g of deferoxamine given intramuscularly or intravenously. In addition, a white count of greater than 15,000 and a blood sugar greater than 7 mmol/L (120 mg/dL) are associated with serum iron levels greater than 50 μmol/L (300 μg/dL).

Treatment Removal of ingested iron is best accomplished with either ipecac-induced emesis or a large orogastric tube to remove the iron tablets. An x-ray film following gastric lavage will define the success of the decontamination procedure. Gastrostomy may be necessary for concretion formation or large quantities of iron tablets. Fifty to 100 mL of 1% bicarbonate may be instilled through the gastric tube following lavage in an effort to form an insoluble ferrous carbonate salt. Activated charcoal is ineffective. Oral deferoxamine will complex iron remaining in the stomach in an iron deferoxamine complex (ferrioxamine) which is insoluble. Since the amount of the deferoxamine to be administered is large and since iron is rapidly absorbed, this therapy is rarely used. Intravenous sodium bicarbonate should be used to correct metabolic acidosis. Hypotension may respond to volume expansion. Coagulation abnormalities should be treated with vitamin K or blood products. When serum iron exceeds the iron-binding capacity, deferoxamine should be administered intravenously. A dose of 1 to 2 g is given at an infusion rate not to exceed 10 to 15 mg/kg body weight per hour. The success of therapy is monitored through measurement of serum iron levels and showing a clearing of the *vin rosé* color in the urine. Once the serum iron is less than the iron-binding capacity, deferoxamine therapy can be discontinued. When iron levels exceed 180 μmol/L (1000 μg/dL), larger doses of deferoxamine can be given and followed by exchange transfusion or plasmapheresis to remove the iron-desferal (ferrioxamine) complex.

ISONIAZID In acute overdose, isoniazid decreases the synthesis of the inhibitory neurotransmitter GABA by inhibiting the pyridoxal phosphate-dependent enzyme glutamic acid decarboxylase. The consequence is CNS stimulation as well as coma. Isoniazid is rapidly absorbed mainly from the small intestine. Peak serum concentrations occur within 1 to 2 h. The volume of distribution is approximately 0.6 L/kg body weight. Serum protein binding is small. Isoniazid is acetylated to acetyl-isoniazid and then hydrolyzed to isonicotinic acid. Approximately 15 percent of an ingested dose of isoniazid is excreted unchanged by the kidneys. The serum half-life of isoniazid in overdose is approximately 1 to 4 h.

Clinical signs Within 30 min of ingestion symptoms include nausea, vomiting, dizziness, and slurred speech. The major manifestations include coma, generalized seizures, and metabolic acidosis. Seizures are protracted and relatively unresponsive to standard anticonvulsant therapy. Acidosis is transiently responsive to bicarbonate therapy and does not occur when seizures are prevented. CNS manifestations vary from obtundation to coma and respiratory depression. Diagnosis is made through identification of isoniazid in urine or blood. Toxicity occurs with concentrations as low as 15 μmol/L (2 mg/L). Significant symptoms are seen with serum concentrations greater than 30 to 35 μmol/L (4 to 5 mg/L).

Treatment Initial therapy consists of prompt gastrointestinal decontamination. Ipecac-induced vomiting should be avoided because of the high incidence of seizures. Isoniazid is well adsorbed by activated charcoal. Pyridoxine (vitamin B6) prevents a decrease in brain GABA concentrations and is efficacious in preventing seizures. Pyridoxine should be given slowly intravenously in weight equivalency with the ingested dose of isoniazid. When the ingested dose is not known, 5 g of pyridoxine should be administered intravenously over 30 min as a 5 to 10% concentration. Cessation of seizures and correction of metabolic acidosis are prompt. Correction of CNS depression occurs more gradually. The dose may be repeated with partial response or when symptoms recur. Diazepam is synergistic with pyridoxine for the control of isoniazid-induced seizures. Due to its low protein binding and small volume of distribution, isoniazid is efficiently removed by hemodialysis, but dialysis is rarely necessary because of the efficacy of pyridoxine.

ISOPROPYL ALCOHOL Isopropyl alcohol is a component of rubbing alcohol, solvents, after-shave lotions, antifreeze, and window cleaners. Its metabolite, acetone, is found in cleaners, solvents, and nail polish removers.

Isopropyl alcohol, a CNS depressant, is rapidly absorbed from the stomach and the lungs but only minimally through skin. It is distributed in body water and has a volume of distribution of 0.6 L/kg body weight. Its half-life ranges from 3 to 6 h. Isopropyl alcohol is metabolized in the liver by the enzyme alcohol dehydrogenase to acetone, which is excreted by the kidneys and lungs with a half-life of 20 to 30 h. Approximately 20 percent of isopropyl alcohol is excreted unchanged through the kidneys.

Clinical signs Symptoms occur within 30 min following ingestion. Gastrointestinal effects include vomiting, abdominal discomfort, and hematemesis. A characteristic smell of rubbing alcohol may be noted. Isopropyl alcohol and acetone are two to three times more potent than ethanol as a CNS depressant. Central nervous system manifestations include headache, dizziness, confusion, and excitation. With severe ingestion, obtundation, coma, respiratory depression, hypothermia, and hypotension may occur. Hypoglycemia may be seen. Isopropyl alcohol can cause a falsely elevated serum creatinine. Myopathy and hemolytic anemias are occasionally present. Concentrations of 8 to 17 mmol/L (50 to 100 mg/dL) produce lethargy, concentrations greater than 25 to 33 mmol/L (150 to 200 mg/dL) are associated with coma, and concentrations greater than 66 to 84 mmol/L (400 to 500 mg/dL) are potentially fatal. Serum acetone levels rise during the first 24 h following ingestion and contribute to the observed toxicity. A small anion gap may be seen as well as an increase in the serum osmolality.

Treatment Gastrointestinal decontamination must be instituted soon following ingestion. Activated charcoal is ineffective in significantly adsorbing isopropyl alcohol. Supportive measures should include intravenous fluids and bicarbonate to correct dehydration, shock, and acidosis. Isopropyl alcohol and acetone are efficiently removed by hemodialysis. The procedure should be considered in patients with levels in the potentially lethal range or in patients inadequately managed by conservative therapy.

LITHIUM Lithium is most commonly available as the carbonate or the citrate salt. Lithium may substitute for cellular cations (K^+ and Na^+), thereby interfering with adenylate cyclase activation, inhibiting neurotransmitter (norepinephrine) release, and reducing sodium potassium ATPase activity.

The drug is rapidly absorbed from the gastrointestinal tract and reaches peak levels within 2 to 4 h of ingestion (and later with sustained-release preparations). It exhibits low plasma protein binding and has a volume of distribution of approximately 0.6 L/kg body weight. Removal from the body is primarily (95 percent) by glomerular filtration with significant reabsorption (80 percent) by the proximal tubules. Lithium clearance is increased by alkalinization of the urine and decreased by hyponatremia. Serum half-life ranges from 18 to 36 h; the therapeutic levels range from 0.6 to 1.2 mmol/L.

Clinical signs Signs and symptoms occur 1 to 4 h after ingestion. Gastrointestinal effects include nausea, vomiting, and diarrhea; neuromuscular effects include weakness, fasciculations, and twitching; CNS effects include ataxia, tremor, myoclonus, choreoathetosis, seizures, confusion, and coma; and cardiovascular effects include ECG changes and hypotension. Laboratory abnormalities include leukocytosis, hyperglycemia, albuminuria, glycosuria, nephrogenic diabetes insipidus, ECG changes (flattened or inverted T waves, atrioventricular block, prolonged QT interval), and ventricular arrhythmias. Death is due to seizures, coma, cardiovascular collapse, or secondary infection. Chronic intoxication is associated with signs and symptoms at lower serum levels than with acute intoxication. In chronic poisoning, concentrations greater than 1.5 mmol/L are associated with nausea and vomiting; levels between 2 and 2.5 mmol/L cause drowsiness, ataxia, and muscle weakness; levels between 2.5 and 3 mmol/L produce choreoathetosis, myoclonus, and coma; levels between 3 and 4 mmol/L cause seizures and cardiac arrhythmias; and levels greater than 4 mmol/L cause hypotension and coma. In acute poisoning, serum levels may exceed 3 to 4 mmol/L with the patient remaining minimally asymptomatic.

Treatment If seen within 2 to 4 h following ingestion, gastrointestinal decontamination is indicated. Serial lithium levels should be measured until the peak level is achieved because both absorption and tissue distribution occur slowly in the overdose setting. Lithium is poorly adsorbed by activated charcoal. Supportive therapy includes standard treatments for seizures, hypotension, and arrhythmias. Symptomatic patients with serum concentrations greater than 2 to 3 mmol/L require diuretics with saline and osmotic or diuretic agents. Sodium bicarbonate enhances renal excretion of lithium. Hemodialysis is the treatment of choice for acute intoxication and is recommended in symptomatic patients with serum levels above 4.0 mmol/L. Hemodialysis may be indicated in the case of chronic ingestion in patients with serum levels less than 4.0 mmol/L. Hemodialysis may need to be repeated or prolonged due to rebound in serum levels upon cessation of hemodialysis.

MONOAMINE OXIDASE (MAO) INHIBITORS MAO inhibitors used in the treatment of endogenous depression include tranylcypromine, phenelzine, and isocarboxazid. MAO inhibitors block monoamine oxidase, thus inhibiting a major pathway for catabolism of neurotransmitters such as dopamine, norepinephrine, and 5-hydroxytryptamine. Toxicity results from accumulation and hence potentiation of neurotransmitter action.

MAO inhibitors are absorbed efficiently from the GI tract. The volume of distribution is not known but is probably large. The drugs are eliminated predominantly by hepatic metabolism, and less than 5 percent is excreted unchanged in the urine. Plasma half-life of phenelzine and tranylcypromine at therapeutic doses is 24 h.

Clinical signs Signs and symptoms begin 6 to 12 h after ingestion and may not reach peak effect until 24 h following ingestion. Early effects are those of CNS stimulation, hyperpyrexia, tachycardia, hypertension, and tachypnea (Table 374-2). Nausea and vomiting are also early manifestations. Pupils are generally dilated, and nystagmus and papilledema may be present. Agitation, hyperactivity, and confusion may be coupled with fasciculations, twitching, tremor, and rigidity. Cardiovascular and CNS depression occurs in severe overdose. The duration of illness is 3 to 5 days. Toxic concentrations of MAO inhibitors have not been established, and no assay methods are commonly available. The diagnosis is clinical.

Treatment Gastrointestinal decontamination should be vigorous and should be followed by activated charcoal and cathartics. Hyperthermia should be treated with external cooling, sedation, and neuromuscular paralysis. Severe hypertension and tachycardia may require treatment with nitroprusside and propranolol respectively. Dantrolene (2.5 mg/kg body weight by mouth or intravenously every 6 h) may be effective for hyperthermia. Hypotension should be treated with volume expanders, and pressor therapy should be administered with caution and at lower than normal doses because of the possibility of producing an exaggerated pharmacologic response. In fact, before any drug is given potential adverse interactions should be investigated. Convulsions and other severe neuromuscular effects should be treated with anticonvulsant agents. Diuresis, hemodialysis, and hemoperfusion are not effective. No specific antidote exists. Because of persistence of MAO inhibition, both drug therapy and diet should be carefully monitored for 7 to 10 days.

METHANOL Methanol is a component of shellacs, varnishes, paint removers, Sterno, windshield-washer solutions, and copy machine fluid. It is also a denaturant to make ethanol unfit for consumption.

Methanol, a mild CNS depressant, is metabolized to formaldehyde and formic acid, which in turn causes metabolic acidosis and injury to the retina.

Methanol is rapidly and completely absorbed from the GI tract, and peak levels occur within 1 to 2 h of ingestion. It is distributed throughout body water with a volume of distribution of 0.7 L/kg body weight. Its protein binding is negligible. Elimination occurs predominantly by hepatic metabolism, and 3 to 5 percent is excreted unchanged by the kidneys. Elimination follows first-order kinetics at low serum levels and converts to zero-order kinetics [approximately 3 mmol/L per hour (8.5 mg/dL per hour)] at higher levels. The rate of elimination at low overdose is approximately 14 to 20 h and at high overdose 24 to 30 h. Inhibition of alcohol dehydrogenase by ethanol [20 to 30 mmol/L (100 to 150 mg/dL)] increases the elimination time to 30 to 35 h.

Clinical signs Onset of illness is variable and may be delayed. Absence of signs and symptoms should not be equated with absence of subsequent toxicity. Early manifestations are caused by methanol, and late manifestations are due to the methanol metabolite formic acid. Methanol produces nausea, vomiting, and abdominal pain. Central nervous system manifestations include headache, vertigo, and confusion at low overdose [levels of approximately 60 mmol/L (200 mg/dL)]. In large overdose [levels greater than 60 mmol/L (200 mg/dL)] obtundation, convulsions, and coma may be seen. Late manifestations include metabolic acidosis and retinal injury. Metabolic acidosis is secondary to accumulation of formic acid, lactic acid (secondary to poor tissue perfusion), and ketones. A serum HCO_3^- below 12 mmol/L is associated with a large anion gap. Opthalmologic manifestations are present 15 to 19 hours following ingestion and include clouding and diminished vision, dancing and flashing spots, dilated or fixed pupils, hyperemia of the disk, retinal edema, and blindness. These changes are potentially reversible with prompt institution of therapy. Respirations are often rapid due to metabolic acidosis. Cardiac manifestations with severe poisoning include myocardial depression, bradycardia, and shock. Anuria predicts a poor prognosis.

Diagnosis Early diagnosis is suggested by ethanol-like signs of intoxication and an elevated serum osmolality and is confirmed by measurement of serum methanol [usually greater than 6 mmol/L (20 mg/dL)] 12 to 48 h following ingestion. The diagnosis of methanol-derived formic acidosis is suggested by a large anion gap, a low serum bicarbonate, an elevated serum formate level, and an elevated blood methanol.

Treatment Gastrointestinal decontamination is indicated soon after ingestion. Activated charcoal is not routinely used because methanol is poorly adsorbed. Cathartics are not effective. Renal clearance is not increased by diuresis. Systemic acidosis should be corrected with sodium bicarbonate. Seizures should be treated with diazepam and phenytoin. Ethanol therapy is indicated in patients with visual symptoms or a methanol level exceeding 6 to 9 mmol/L (20 to 30 mg/dL). The loading dose and subsequent maintenance dose of ethanol are as follows: loading dose—10 mL/kg body weight of 10% ethanol intravenously or 1 mL/kg body weight of 95% ethanol by mouth; maintenance dose—1.5 mL/kg body weight per hour of

10% ethanol intravenously and 3.0 mL/kg body weight per hour of 10% ethanol intravenously during dialysis. Therapy should be continued until the serum methanol level falls below 6 mmol/L (20 μg/dL) and all clinical signs are resolved. Methanol is efficiently cleared by hemodialysis because of its small volume of distribution and low protein binding. Hemodialysis is indicated for patients with methanol levels exceeding 15 mmol/L (50 mg/dL), for patients with visual signs, and for those patients whose acidosis is unresponsive to bicarbonate. For patients seen late (12 to 24 h or later) after ingestion, ethanol should be used to block further conversion of methanol to formic acid, and sodium bicarbonate should be given to correct metabolic acidosis. Elimination of formic acid is enhanced by alkalization of the urine. A formic acid level at which hemodialysis should be instituted has not been established.

METHEMOGLOBINEMIA Methemoglobinemia results from exposure to a wide variety of chemicals that oxidize ferrous hemoglobin (Fe^{2+}) to its ferric (Fe^{3+}) state. Oxidizing agents include sodium nitrite used as a meat preservative; amyl nitrite and nitroglycerin used as medications; nitrates in contaminated well water; aniline in shoe polish, paints, varnish, and inks; medications such as phenacetin, sulfonamides, pyridium, dapsone, primaquine, lidocaine, and benzocaine; and chemicals such as nitrobenzene, nitrophenol, toluidine, and isobutyl nitrate.

Ferric hemoglobin has a decreased oxygen-carrying capacity, and clinical effects are the result of tissue hypoxia. In addition, the shift of the oxygen dissociation curve to the left limits the release of oxygen to tissues. Oxidant inactivation systems include ascorbic acid and sulfhydryl agents such as glutathione, which combine with oxidizing agents and transform them to less toxic compounds. Mechanisms for the reduction of methemoglobin to oxyhemoglobin include NADH-methemoglobin reductase (responsible for 95% of activity), NADPH-methemoglobin reductase, reduced glutathione, and ascorbic acid. In the presence of NADH-methemoglobin reductase, NADH combines with methemoglobin to form oxyhemoglobin and NAD. The NADPH combines with methemoglobin in the presence of NADPH-methemoglobin reductase to produce oxyhemoglobin and NADP.

Clinical signs Cyanosis occurs with methemoglobin levels greater than 15 percent (15 g/L or 1.5 g/dL absolute methemoglobin). Patients are asymptomatic until methemoglobin levels exceed 30 percent, at which point fatigue, headache, tachycardia, dizziness, and weakness develop. At levels greater than 55 percent, dyspnea, bradycardia, hypoxia, acidosis, seizures, coma, and cardiac arrhythmias may occur. At levels greater than 70 percent, death may ensue secondary to hypoxia. Hemolytic anemia may lead to hyperkalemia and renal failure 1 to 3 days after exposure.

Diagnosis The diagnosis should be suspected in the presence of respiratory distress, brown or gray cyanosis unresponsive to oxygen, and absence of significant CNS depression. Cyanosis in conjunction with a normal P_{O_2} and decreased oxygen saturation (measured by oximeter rather than derived) suggests methemoglobinemia. Blood with high levels of methemoglobin is chocolate colored when placed on filter paper and compared to normal blood. The chocolate color does not revert to pink with oxygen but does return to normal when exposed to 10% potassium cyanide. Methemoglobin is identified by its absorption at a frequency of 630 nm on light spectrometry. Finally, the toxic screen on blood or urine may identify the drug or chemical that serves as the oxidizing agent.

Treatment The toxin, if recently ingested, should be removed by gastrointestinal decontamination followed by administration of activated charcoal and cathartics. Most oxidizing agents are metabolized rapidly, making diuresis ineffective. Dialysis may be effective, depending upon the specific compound. Treatment for methemoglobinemia includes methylene blue, packed red blood cells or exchange transfusion, and oxygen. Indications for methylene blue include a methemoglobin level above 30 g/L (cyanosis alone is not an indication for methylene blue therapy) or methemoglobinemia with hypoxia. In the patient with anemia or cardiovascular disease, methylene blue may be indicated at lower levels due to a greater risk from tissue hypoxia. Methylene blue is given at a dose of 1 to 2 mg/kg body weight as a 1% solution over 5 min. If a clinical response is not observed within 1 h, the dose may be repeated. A methemoglobin level of 40 g/L can be expected to decrease by half in 1 to 2 h. As long as the oxidizing agent remains in the body methemoglobin will continue to be generated, and additional doses may be necessary. Side effects of methylene blue include precordial pain, dyspnea, restlessness, apprehension, and tremor; a transient blue color to the skin and urine; and the production of methemoglobin at high doses (greater than 7 mg/kg body weight) of methylene blue. Methylene blue is contraindicated in patients with deficiency of glucose-6-phosphate dehydrogenase. Additional approaches to treatment include transfusion with packed red cells optimally to a hemoglobin of 150 g/L to increase oxygen-carrying capacity and administration of 100% oxygen or hyperbaric oxygen to enhance oxygen delivery to tissues. If the methemoglobin level is very high or the patient is deficient in glucose-6-phosphate dehydrogenase exchange transfusion may be indicated.

MUSCLE RELAXANTS Muscle relaxants include orphenadrine, methocarbamol, baclofen, chlorphenesin, cyclobenzaprine, chlorzoxazone, and carisoprodol. Muscle relaxants exert some direct muscle relaxant activity but predominantly act by causing analgesia and sedation (Table 374-2). They depress synaptic reflexes, prolong synaptic recovery time, and reduce repetitive discharges. They are rapidly and completely absorbed, and peak blood levels occur 1 to 2 h following ingestion. The therapeutic half-lives are variable, with most between 1 to 4 h. The majority are metabolized by the liver to derivatives that are generally inactive and are excreted by the kidneys. Baclofen, an exception, is largely excreted unchanged in the urine but is metabolized in the liver to metabolites that undergo enterohepatic circulation.

Clinical signs Manifestations of excess amounts of carisoprodol, chlorphenesin, chlorzoxazone, and methocarbamol include nausea, vomiting, dizziness, headache, nystagmus, hypotonia, and central nervous system depression. Signs and symptoms of excess cyclobenzaprine, baclofen, and orphenadrine are more severe. Cyclobenzaprine produces anticholinergic effects coupled with agitation, hallucination, convulsions, stupor, coma, and hypotension. Baclofen causes CNS depression, hypothermia, excitability, delirium, myoclonus, seizures, conduction abnormalities, tachycardia, bradycardia, and hypotension. Orphenadrine produces anticholinergic effects, tachycardia, arrhythmias, agitation, and depression. The drugs may be identified in blood or urine by toxic screen.

Treatment Initial management includes prompt gastrointestinal decontamination. Muscle relaxants are well adsorbed by single-dose activated charcoal. Repetitive charcoal may be used for baclofen. Cathartics are also indicated. Diuresis is ineffective. The efficacy of hemodialysis or hemoperfusion is not established. Physostigmine is useful for treatment of the anticholinergic effects of orphenadrine and cyclobenzaprine.

NARCOTICS (See Chaps. 371 and 372)

NONSTEROIDAL ANTI-INFLAMMATORY DRUGS Nonsteroidal anti-inflammatory drugs (NSAIDs) fall into two classes: carboxylic acids such as ibuprofen, indomethacin, naproxen, diflunisal, fenoprofen, and tolmetin and enolic acids including phenylbutazone and piroxicam. NSAIDs inhibit prostaglandin synthesis by blocking cyclooxygenase. They are rapidly absorbed with peak blood concentrations achieved within 1 to 2 h following ingestion. They are tightly bound (greater than 95 percent) to plasma protein and have a small volume of distribution of 1.0 L/kg body weight. The pK_a ranges from 3.5 to 6.3. They are predominantly metabolized by conjugation, oxidation, and hydroxylation. Indomethacin and piroxicam undergo enterohepatic recirculation, but the activity of their metabolites is not established. A small portion (1 to 15 percent) is eliminated unchanged by the kidneys. Half-lives vary from 1 h with tolmetin to 50 to 100 h with phenylbutazone.

Clinical signs All NSAIDs may produce gastroenteritis. Other types of toxicity are variable with the carboxylic acid group. Signs and symptoms of ibuprofen toxicity are mild and include nausea, vomiting, abdominal pain, drowsiness, nystagmus, and obtundation. Diflunisal produces, in addition, hyperventilation, tachycardia, and sweating; fenoprofen is toxic to the kidneys. The enolic acid group produces coma, metabolic acidosis, seizures, and renal failure. Hepatic injury has been reported.

Diagnosis The diagnosis is confirmed by quantification of drug in blood or urine.

Treatment Therapy for NSAID poisoning includes gastrointestinal decontamination followed by activated charcoal and cathartics. Repeated doses of activated charcoal are of benefit for indomethacin, phenylbutazone, and piroxicam. Renal excretion is not increased by diuresis, and protein binding limits efficacy of hemodialysis. Although experience is limited, hemoperfusion can reduce serum half-life and increase clearance. No antidote is available.

ORGANOPHOSPHATE AND CARBAMATE INSECTICIDES Organophosphorus compounds such as malathion, parathion, dichlorvos, diazinon, and chlorothion are used as agricultural and household insecticides and in the treatment of animal ectoparasites and human lice infestations. Carbamate insecticides include carbaryl, aldicarb, and propoxur. Organophosphorus insecticides irreversibly inhibit the acetylcholinesterase and cause accumulation of acetylcholine at muscarinic and nicotinic synapses. The exact mechanism by which organophosphorus compounds affect the central nervous system is unclear. Carbamates reversibly inhibit acetylcholinesterase and cause accumulation of acetylcholine at neurosynapses. Organophosphorus compounds are absorbed through the skin, lungs, and gastrointestinal tract and are distributed widely in tissues. They are metabolized in the liver, and the oxidative metabolites are active (paroxon, maloxone). Subsequent hydrolysis of organophosphorus compounds in the liver produces inactive metabolites. The elimination half-life of organophosphorus compounds has not been determined. Absorption, distribution, and elimination of carbamate insecticides are similar to those of organophosphorus insecticides.

Clinical signs Organophosphorus compounds produce muscarinic, nicotinic, and CNS effects. Carbamates produce a similar picture but have a shorter duration of effect and a lower order of toxicity. Symptoms occur 30 min to 2 h following exposure. Early muscarinic manifestations include nausea, vomiting, abdominal cramps, and urinary and fecal incontinence. Cholinergic stimulation of the respiratory tract produces increased bronchial secretions, cough, and occasionally pulmonary edema. Cholinergic stimulation of sweat, salivary, and lacrimal glands produces sweating, salivation, and lacrimation. Miosis is usual, and blurring of vision may occur. Cholinergic stimulation results in urinary frequency and incontinence. Cholinergic effects on the cardiovascular system include bradycardia, conduction block, and hypotension. In more serious poisoning, nicotinic signs include twitching, fasciculations, weakness, diminished respiratory effort, hypertension, and tachycardia. Central nervous system effects include anxiety, restlessness, tremor, convulsions, confusion, weakness, and coma. Most patients recover within 24 to 48 h, but long-acting agents may cause toxicity for weeks to months. Death is most often due to pulmonary secretions and inadequate ventilation. A reduction of cholinesterase activity in plasma or in red blood cells to less than 50 percent of normal is diagnostic. The activity of red blood cell cholinesterase correlates best with cholinesterase activity in nerve endings and with clinical severity (at least during acute poisoning). Without treatment, return of blood cholinesterase activity to normal may take as long as 4 to 5 weeks.

In the case of carbamate insecticides, depression in plasma or red blood cell cholinesterase levels is rare because of the rapid reversibility of the inhibition. Since cholinesterase assays are not routinely or rapidly available, the initial diagnosis is clinical. Insecticides may be identified in urine on toxic screen.

Treatment The skin should be rapidly washed with soap and water to remove the toxin, and the patient should be removed from the site of inhalation exposure. In the case of ingestion, gastrointestinal decontamination should be followed by activated charcoal. In the case of symptomatic organophosphorus and carbamate poisoning, large doses of atropine should be administered for muscarinic symptoms. A dose of 0.5 to 2 mg atropine is administered intravenously every 15 to 20 min until complete atropinization is achieved (drying of bronchial and mucous membrane secretions). Pupil size and heart rate cannot be used as end points. Once atropinization is achieved repeated doses or a constant atropine drip is necessary for several days to maintain therapeutic effectiveness. Atropine is useful for muscarinic signs, less so for CNS signs, and ineffective for nicotinic effects. Pralidoxime (2-PAM), an oxime, is effective for most nicotonic symptoms in organophosphate insecticide poisoning. The dose is 1 to 2 g intravenously over several minutes. The dose may be repeated every 8 h until nicotinic signs resolve. Reversal of CNS effects is less pronounced, and pralidoxime is ineffective for muscarinic signs. In carbamate poisoning, controversy exists over the use of pralidoxime. It should not be used in carbaryl poisoning, and in overdosage with other carbamate insecticides it should be used in conjunction with atropine.

PHENOTHIAZINE The three major classes of phenothiazines are based on side chain substitutions—aliphatic (chlorpromazine, promethazine, promazine), piperidine (mesoridazine, thioridazine), and piperazine (perphenazine, fluphenazine, prochlorperazine, trifluoperazine) derivatives. Phenothiazines block postsynaptic dopamine receptors, exhibit anticholinergic activity, and inhibit reuptake of norepinephrine and 5-hydroxytryptamine. They also exert peripheral alpha-adrenergic blockade, lower the seizure threshold, and exert a quinidine-like effect on the heart. Peripheral anticholinergic effects result from blockade of cholinergic transmission.

Phenothiazines are efficiently absorbed from the GI tract and are metabolized promptly by the liver. Phenothiazines exhibit 95 percent protein binding, and hence the apparent volume of distribution is large (10 to 20 L/kg body weight). Only 1 percent of the administered dose is excreted unchanged in the urine. The majority of metabolites are inactive. The mean half-life for phenothiazines is generally greater than 24 h.

Clinical signs Phenothiazines are CNS depressants, causing lethargy, obtundation, respiratory depression, and coma. Pupils are often constricted, and hypothermia and hypotension are common. Cardiac effects include hypotension, supraventricular tachycardia, atrioventricular block, and atrial and ventricular arrhythmias. Torsade de pointes, prolonged PR, QRS, and QT intervals, and U- and T-wave abnormalities may be seen especially with thioridazine and its metabolite mesoridazine. The malignant neuroleptic syndrome occurs rarely with the use of phenothiazines. Acute dystonic reactions (extrapyramidal tract signs) are prominent with the piperazine group; signs and symptoms include rigidity, opisthotonus, stiff neck, hyperreflexia, irritability, dystonia, fixed speech, torticollis, tremors, trismus, and oculogyric crisis. The reaction is idiosyncratic rather than dose related.

Diagnosis The diagnosis is established by toxic screen on blood and urine. In the presence of extrapyramidal tract toxicity, a therapeutic response to diphenhydramine or benztropine confirms the diagnosis.

Treatment Phenothiazine overdose should be treated with gastrointestinal decontamination followed by activated charcoal and cathartics. Repeated charcoal is not indicated. Diuresis and dialysis are ineffective. Seizures should be treated with anticonvulsants, hypotension should be managed with volume expanders and alpha agonists, and sodium bicarbonate is administered for acidosis. Quinidine and procainanide should be avoided. For treatment of ventricular arrhythmias see Chap. 185. Dantrolene and bromocryptine may be useful in the treatment of neuroleptic malignant syndrome. Extrapyramidal signs respond rapidly and well to intravenous diphenhydramine (1 to 2 mg/kg body weight per dose to a maximum of 50 mg) given over 2 min. Treatment is generally continued for 24 h to prevent recurrence of symptoms.

SALICYLATES Salicylates increase the sensitivity of respiratory centers in the brain to changes in P_{O_2} and P_{CO_2} resulting in an increased rate and depth of respiration. Salicylates also uncouple oxidative phosphorylation and produce increases in metabolic rate, oxygen consumption, glucose utilization, and heat production. Salicylates inhibit the Krebs tricarboxylic cycle and block carbohydrate and lipid metabolism, resulting in lactic acidosis and ketonemia. Salicylates produce hepatocyte damage, resulting in increased plasma enzyme activity and prolongation of prothrombin time. They also decrease platelet aggregation.

Salicylates are well absorbed both from the stomach and the small bowel. In the plasma, 50 to 80 percent is bound to albumin. Because salicylate is a weak acid with a pK of 3, the unbound portion in the plasma exists in an ionized state. It has a small volume of distribution of 0.2 L/kg body weight which increases with chronic poisoning and with increasing doses. Acidosis increases distribution of salicylate into brain, liver, and other tissues. Salicylates are eliminated by both hepatic metabolism and renal excretion. Saturation of hepatic metabolic pathways partially explains the prolonged half-life (20 to 36 h) in overdose. By alkalinizing the urine to a pH of 8, the drug in the renal tubules is maintained in an ionized state, is not reabsorbed, and is excreted in urine.

Clinical signs Clinical manifestations of mild poisoning include vomiting, tachycardia, hyperpnea, fever, tinnitus, lethargy, and mental confusion. In severe poisoning, convulsions, coma, and respiratory and cardiovascular failure may occur. Vomiting, poor intake, and hyperventilation may cause severe dehydration. Other complications include cerebral and pulmonary edema and myocardial or renal failure. An elevated hematocrit, white blood cell count, and platelet count; hypernatremia; hyperkalemia; and hypoglycemia may be seen. Respiratory alkalosis is commonly coupled with metabolic acidosis (40 to 50 percent), but respiratory alkalosis (20 percent), metabolic acidosis (20 percent), mixed respiratory and metabolic acidosis (5 to 10 percent) may be present. Lactic and other organic acids are responsible for an increased anion gap. Prothrombin time may be prolonged. Salicylates are identified by a positive ferric chloride test on either blood or urine. In the case of an acute single ingestion, a level less than 2.5 mmol/L (35 mg/dL) is associated with no symptoms, 2.5 to 5 mmol/L (35 to 70 mg/dL) with mild to moderate symptoms, 5 to 7 mmol/L (70 to 100 mg/dL) with severe symptoms, and greater than 7 mmol/L (100 mg/dL) with potentially fatal manifestations. In chronic poisoning, symptoms are seen at lower serum levels.

Treatment An ingested dose greater than 150 mg/kg body weight should be removed from the stomach. Concretions may delay absorption, and removal may be helpful up to 12 to 24 h after ingestion. The serum half-life may be shortened and elimination may be increased by repeated administration of activated charcoal. Parenteral fluids should be given to correct fluid losses and to produce a brisk urine flow. Seizures should be controlled with intravenous phenobarbital or diazepam. Myocardial failure should be treated with immediate correction of acidosis, administration of oxygen, and possibly digitalis therapy. Prolongation of prothrombin time should be corrected with intravenous vitamin K. Pulmonary edema should be managed with fluid restriction, osmotic diuresis, and positive end-expiratory ventilation. Cerebral edema requires fluid restriction and often hemodialysis. Sodium bicarbonate should be administered to correct serum pH and thus limit tissue distribution of salicylates. In addition, alkalinization of the urine to a pH of 8 enhances urinary excretion and decreases serum half-life. Potassium losses should be replenished, and sufficient fluids should be given to assure adequate renal perfusion. Salicylates are effectively removed by hemodialysis, which should be considered in severe overdose, cerebral edema, failure of conventional therapy, or compromised renal or hepatic function.

STIMULANTS Amphetamines, phenylpropanolamines, and cocaine are the most commonly used stimulants. Amphetamines have a long record of both abuse and overdose. For cocaine abuse see Chap. 272. Phenylpropanolamine can either be a street drug or a mail-order "legal stimulant." These agents affect both the central and sympathetic nervous systems (Table 374-1).

Amphetamines stimulate alpha- and beta-adrenergic receptors, whereas phenylpropanolamine stimulates only beta-adrenergic receptors. Amphetamines are rapidly absorbed from the GI tract, reaching peak levels 1 to 2 h following ingestion. Amphetamine is a weak base with a pK_a of 8 to 10 and a volume of distribution of 2 to 3 L/kg body weight. The drug is concentrated in brain, lung, and kidneys. Thirty to 40 percent is metabolized by the liver, and the hydroxylated metabolite may be responsible for the psychotic effects. The remainder (60 to 70 percent) is excreted directly by the kidneys. Excretion of amphetamines is enhanced in an acid urine and slowed in an alkaline urine. Plasma half-life is 16 to 31 h at a urine pH greater than 7.5 and falls to 6 to 8 h when the urinary pH is less than 5.0. Phenylpropanolamine is a white crystal powder with a pK_a of 9.4. It is rapidly absorbed from the GI tract. Its apparent volume of distribution is 4.5 L/kg body weight. Only 10 percent of the parent compound is metabolized by the liver, and the bulk is excreted unchanged in the urine. The biologic half-life ranges between 3 h in an acid urine and 6 h in an alkaline.

Clinical signs Effects of amphetamine overdose are seen within 30 to 60 min following ingestion. Gastrointestinal findings include nausea, vomiting, diarrhea, and abdominal cramps. The patient often exhibits excess talkativeness, irritability, confusion, delirium, combativeness, and auditory and visual hallucinations. Tremors and hyperreflexia are common. Hyperpyrexia may precede seizures and rhabdomyolysis. Cardiovascular effects include palpitations, tachycardia, hypertension, and cardiac arrhythmias. Cardiovascular collapse may occur in severe overdose. Sympathomimetic symptoms include dilated pupils, dry mouth, pallor, flushing of the skin, and tachypnea. Fatalities are rare and are usually associated with convulsions, coma, hyperpyrexia, cardiac arrhythmias, cardiovascular collapse, or intracranial hemorrhage. Phenylpropanolamine produces similar clinical findings. Cardiac manifestations include hypertension and reflex bradycardia. Amphetamines and phenylpropanolamine may be identified on toxic screen. Phenylpropanolamine and amphetamine serum levels may be quantitated, but no clear relationship exists between serum level and symptoms.

Treatment Gastric lavage should be followed by administration of activated charcoal and a cathartic. Supportive care includes treatment of seizures with phenytoin or benzodiazepines; hypertension with nitroprusside; hyperpyrexia with cooling blankets, salicylates, and acetaminophen; and agitation with sedatives. Droperidol and haloperidol are particularly effective for acute sedation in the agitated patient. Ventricular tachyarrhythmias should be treated with the appropriate antiarrhythmic drug (see Chap. 185). Seizures may cause myoglobinuria, which in association with an acid urine can lead to acute renal failure. Consequently, acidification of the urine is not recommended. Because of the short duration of effect of phenylpropanolamine, acidification of the urine is not indicated. Extracorporal therapy is of limited value.

THEOPHYLLINE Theophylline causes the release of endogenous catecholamines and prolongs their effects by inhibiting the degradation of cyclic AMP by phosphodiesterase. Theophylline is rapidly and well absorbed from the stomach and upper small bowel. Peak levels are achieved 1 to 2 h after ingestion of liquid preparations and by 2 to 4 h with tablets. Sustained-release preparations reach peak levels 7 to 24 h after ingestion. Theophylline has a pK_a of 9.5. Approximately 60 percent is bound to albumin. Theophylline has a low volume of distribution of 0.6 L/kg body weight, and 95 percent of the parent compound is metabolized by the liver to 1,3-dimethyluric acid, 1-methyluric acid, and 3-methyluric acid. In overdose, the 1-demethylation step of metabolism appears to be saturable. Only 5 percent of the theophylline is excreted unchanged by the kidneys. Theophylline elimination is decreased with impaired liver function, congestive heart failure, viral infections, and concomitantly administered drugs such as cimetidine that interfere with the cytochrome P_{450} system. The serum half-life in overdose is 10 to 12 h.

Clinical signs Vomiting is frequent in overdose, and hematemesis is occasionally seen. Restlessness, irritability, agitation, tachypnea, tachycardia, and muscle tremors are common. Coma and respiratory depression are rare. Generalized tonic-clonic and occasionally focal convulsions occur in severe poisoning. Convulsions are often protracted, repetitive, and resistant to anticonvulsant therapy. Cardiovascular effects include atrial arrhythmias, multifocal premature ventricular contractions, idioventricular rhythms, ventricular tachycardia, and ventricular fibrillation. Rhabdomyolysis with renal failure is occasionally seen. Metabolic abnormalities include ketosis, metabolic acidosis, increased serum amylase, hyperglycemia, and decreased serum potassium, calcium, and phosphorus. Death occurs as a result of cardiovascular collapse or uncontrolled convulsions. Mortality rates are higher after chronic ingestion. Cardiac arrhythmias and seizures may be seen following chronic ingestion with serum levels of 200 to 300 μmol/L (40 to 60 mg/L). With acute ingestions, higher levels are associated with seizures and cardiac arrhythmias. Serial levels should be measured to determine the peak concentration (serving as an important indicator for hemodialysis) and the elimination half-life during recovery.

Treatment Initial therapy involves prompt gastrointestinal decontamination. Theophylline is well adsorbed by activated charcoal. With sustained-release forms of theophylline, removal should be considered up to 6 to 12 h following ingestion, and charcoal may be indicated up to 12 to 24 h following ingestion. When charcoal is administered every 2 to 4 h, serum half-life is shortened by approximately 50 percent. Metaclopramide is useful in controlling theophylline-induced vomiting. Tachycardia should be treated with propranolol or esmolol, and hypotension is treated with volume expansion and propranolol. Benzodiazepines and barbiturates are drugs of choice for convulsions. Phenytoin is ineffective. Arrhythmias should be treated with antiarrhythmic agents, and atropine or epinephrine may be administered for asystole. Diuresis is ineffective for enhancing removal of theophylline. The indication for hemodialysis and hemoperfusion in patients with acute ingestion is a serum level greater than 500 μmol/L (100 mg/L). With chronic ingestion, hemodialysis or hemoperfusion is indicated with serum levels greater than 200 to 300 μmol/L (40 to 60 mg/L). Hemoperfusion should be considered with lower levels in association with refractory seizures or arrythmias, in patients with chronic obstructive lung disease, and in people above age 60.

TRICYCLIC ANTIDEPRESSANTS Commonly available compounds include amitriptyline, imipramine, desipramine, doxepin, and nortriptyline. Tricylic antidepressants block reuptake of synaptic transmitters such as norepinephrine and dopamine in the central nervous system. In addition they have central and peripheral anticholinergic activity, have peripheral alpha-blocking activity, and exert quinidine-like effects on the heart.

Tricyclics are well absorbed from the GI tract, and peak levels are reached within 2 to 4 h of ingestion. In serious overdose, anticholinergic effects may predominate resulting in prolonged absorption and delayed peak levels (6 to 12 h following ingestion). Tricyclics exhibit high protein binding in the plasma. They have large volumes of distribution in the range of 20 to 40 L/kg body weight. Elimination is predominantly by hepatic metabolism with an initial demethylation generating pharmacologically active metabolites. These metabolites generally undergo enterohepatic circulation. Subsequent steps of metabolism result in increasing polarity of metabolites that are then excreted by the kidneys. Less than 5 percent of the parent compound is excreted unchanged in urine. Biliary excretion accounts for up to 15 percent of an ingested dose. The half-life of tricyclics and their demethylated metabolites ranges from 25 to 80 h in the overdose setting.

Clinical signs Symptoms generally develop within 1 to 2 h of ingestion but may be delayed for up to 6 h. In low overdose anticholinergic effects are coupled with agitation and hypertension. In high overdose CNS depression is coupled with depressed myocardial function, seizures, and hypotension. Anticholinergic effects include fever, mydriasis, tachycardia, flushing of the skin, urinary retention, and decreased bowel activity. Central nervous system manifestations include excitation, restlessness, myoclonus, hyperreflexia, disorientation, confusion, and hallucinations. Lethargy, coma, and seizures occur in large overdose. Both hypertension and hypotension are common. Tachycardia (anticholinergic effect) occurs in low overdose, and ventricular tachyarrhythmias with terminal bradycardia and decreased cardiac output are seen in high overdose. Various degrees of cardiac conduction blocks and atrial arrhythmias also occur. Aspiration pneumonia and pulmonary edema may develop. Death occurs usually within the first 2 to 6 h following ingestion. Prolongation of the QRS complex (greater than 100 ms) in severe overdose is correlated with an increased risk of cardiac arrhythmias and seizures. Serum levels are diagnostic and correlate with severity. Levels less than about 1000 nmol/L (300 ng/mL) are considered therapeutic. Levels over 3300 nmol/L (1000 ng/mL) indicate serious poisoning and are associated with QRS complexes wider than 100 ms. The demethylated metabolite as well as the parent compound should be summed to indicate the total serum concentration.

Treatment Ipecac-induced emesis is contraindicated with tricyclic ingestions. Gastric lavage is indicated for recent ingestions, and activated charcoal every 2 to 4 h may interrupt enterohepatic recycling. Cathartics should be alternated with doses of activated charcoal. Appropriate care includes support of respiration, correction of metabolic acidosis with sodium bicarbonate, and volume expansion and norepinephrine or high-dose dopamine for hypotension. Hypertension is generally limited and does not require specific therapy. Seizures should be treated with phenytoin or diazepam. Treatment of arrhythmias may involve sodium bicarbonate (0.5 to 1 mmol/kg body weight), lidocaine, and phenytoin. Beta-adrenergic blockers and class 1A antiarrhythmics (quinidine, procainamide, and disopyramide) should be avoided. Cardiac pacing may be necessary for the severely depressed myocardium and bradycardia. Correction of acidosis is an important component of the treatment of cardiac arrhythmias. Physostigmine reverses anticholinergic signs, mydriatic pupils, tachycardia, and agitation, thereby helping to establish a clinical diagnosis (diagnostic trial). Physostigmine is contraindicated in the presence of coma, ventricular arrhythmias, or seizures because of unproven efficacy, short duration of effect, and potential for worsening cardiac toxicity.

REFERENCES

General aspects

BRANCATA DJ, NELSON RC: Poisoning mortality in the United States 1980. Vet Hum Toxicol 26:273, 1984

LITOVITZ TL et al: 1987 Annual report of the American Association of Poison Control Centers National Data Collection System. Am J Emerg Med 6:479, 1988

MCCARRON MM: Current trends in drug overdose. West J Med 141:98, 1984

Diagnosis

BRETT AS: Implication of discordance between clinical impression and toxicology analysis in drug overdose. Arch Intern Med 148:437, 1988

COUNCIL OF SCIENTIFIC AFFAIRS, AMERICAN MEDICAL ASSOCIATION: Scientific issues in drug testing. JAMA 257:3110, 1987

EMMETT M, NARINS RG: Clinical use of the anion gap. Medicine 56:38, 1977

GLASSER L et al: Serum osmolality and its applicability to drug overdose. Am J Clin Pathol 60:695, 1973

HEPLER BR et al: Role of the toxicology lab in the treatment of acute poisoning. Med Toxicol 1:61, 1986

JAEGER RW et al: Radiopacity of drugs and plants in vivo—limited usefulness. Vet Hum Toxicol 23(Suppl 1):2, 1981

KELLERMANN AL et al: Impact of drug screening in suspected overdose. Ann Emerg Med 16:1206, 1987

MITCHELL AA et al: Drug ingestions associated with miosis in comatose children. J Pediatr 89(2):303, 1977

OLSON KR et al: Physical assessment and differential diagnosis of the poisoned patient. Med Toxicol 2:52, 1987

ROBERTS JR et al: The body stuffer syndrome: A clandestine form of drug overdose. Am J Emerg Med 4:24, 1986

SCHERZ RG: The differential diagnosis of coma due to poisoning and exogenous toxins. Pediatrician 6:190, 1977

SMITHLINE N, GARDNER KD JR: Gaps—anionic and osmolal. JAMA 236:1594, 1976

Treatment

ALBERTSON TE et al: Superiority of activated charcoal alone compared with ipecac and activated charcoal in the treatment of acute toxic ingestions. Ann Emerg Med 18:56, 1989

BRETT AS et al: Predicting the clinical course of intentional drug overdose: Implications for utilization of the intensive care unit. Arch Intern Med 147:133, 1987

BURTON BT et al: Comparison of activated charcoal and gastric lavage in the prevention of aspirin absorption. J Emerg Med 1:411, 1984

CURTIS RA et al: Efficacy of ipecac and activated charcoal/cathartic: Prevention of salicylate absorption in a simulated overdose. Arch Intern Med 144:48, 1984

GOLDBERG MJ et al: An approach to the management of the poisoned patient. Arch Intern Med 146:1381, 1986

GOLDFRANK L et al: Newer antidotes and controversies in antidotal therapy, in *Emergency Medicine Annual,* DA Rund, BW Wolcott (eds). Norwalk, Conn, Appleton-Century-Crofts, 1984, vol 3, pp 223–266.

KING WD: Syrup of ipecac: A drug review. Clin Toxicol 17:353, 1980

KRENZELOK EP et al: Gastrointestinal transit times of carthartics combined with charcoal. Ann Emerg Med 14:1152, 1985

KULIG K et al: Management of acutely poisoned patients without gastric emptying. Ann Emerg Med 14:562, 1985

LITOVITZ TL: The anecdotal antidotes. Emerg Med Clin North Am 2:145, 1984

MANNO BR, MANNO JE: Toxicology of ipecac: A review. Clin Toxicol 10:221, 1977

MCCARRON MM, WOOD JD: The cocaine "body packer" syndrome: Diagnosis and treatment. JAMA 250:1417, 1983

MINOCHA A, SPYKER DA: Acute overdose with sustained-release drug formulations: Perspectives in treatment. Med Toxicol 1:300, 1986

NEUVONEN PJ: Clinical pharmacokinetics of oral activated charcoal in acute intoxications. Clin Pharmacokinet 7:465, 1982

———, OLKKOLA KT: Oral activated charcoal in the treatment of intoxications: Role of single and repeated doses. Med Toxicol 3:33, 1988

PARK GD et al: Expanded role of charcoal in the poisoned and overdosed patient. Arch Intern Med 146:969, 1986

PETERSON RG, PETERSON LN: Cleansing the blood: Hemodialysis, peritoneal dialysis, exchange transfusion, charcoal hemoperfusion, forced diuresis. Pediatr Clin North Am 33:675, 1986

POND SM: Diuresis, dialysis and hemoperfusion: Indications and benefits. Emerg Med Clin North Am 2:29, 1984

ROSENBERG J et al: Pharmacokinetics of drug overdose. Clin Pharmacokinet 6:161, 1981

SHANNON M et al: Carthartics and laxatives: Do they still have a place in management of the poisoned patient? Med Toxicol 1:247, 1986

SPYKER DA, MINOCHA A: Toxicodynamic approach to the management of the poisoned patient. J Emerg Med 6:117, 1988

STEAD AH, MOFFAT AC: A collection of therapeutic, toxic and fatal blood drug concentrations in man. Hum Toxicol 3:437, 1983

STEWART JJ: Effects of emetic and cathartic agents on the gastrointestinal tract and the treatment of toxic ingestion. Clin Toxicol 20:199, 1983

TENEBEIN M: Whole bowel irrigation as a gastrointestinal decontamination procedure after acute poisoning. Med Toxicol 3:77, 1988

——— et al: Efficacy of ipecac-induced emesis, orogastric lavage, and activated charcoal for acute drug overdose. Ann Emerg Med 16:838, 1987

WHEELER USHER DH et al: Gastric emptying: Risk versus benefit in the treatment of acute poisoning. Med Toxicol 1:142, 1986

Reference texts

ARENA JM, DREW RH: *Poisoning: Toxicology, Symptoms, Treatments,* 5th ed. Springfield, Ill., Charles C Thomas, 1986

BASET RC: *Disposition of Toxic Drugs and Chemicals in Man,* 2d ed. Davis, Calif, Biomedical Publications, 1982

BLOCK JB: *The Signs and Symptoms of Chemical Exposure.* Springfield, Ill., Charles C Thomas, 1980

BRYSON PD: *Comprehensive Review in Toxicology.* Rockville, Md, Aspen, 1989

CLAYTON GD, CLAYTON FE (eds): *Patty's Industrial Hygiene and Toxicology,* 3d ed. New York, Wiley, 1978

DANGAARD J: *Symptoms and Signs in Occupational Disease: A Practical Guide,* Copenhagen, Year Book Medical Publishers, 1978

ELLENHORN MJ, BARCELOUX DG: *Medical Toxicology: Diagnosis and Treatment of Human Poisoning.* New York, Elsevier, 1988

FINKEL AJ: *Hamilton and Hardy's Industrial Toxicology,* 4th ed. Boston, John Wright, 1983

GOLDFRANK LR et al (eds): *Goldfrank's Toxicologic Emergencies,* 3d ed. Norwalk, Conn, Appleton-Century-Crofts, 1986

GOSSELIN RE: *Clinical Toxicology of Commercial Products: Acute Poisoning,* 5th ed. Baltimore, Williams & Wilkins, 1984

HADDAD LM, WINCHESTER JF: *Clinical Management of Poisoning and Drug Overdose.* Philadelphia, Saunders, 1983

HAYES WJ: *Pesticides Studies in Man.* Baltimore, Williams & Wilkins, 1982

KLASSEN CD et al (eds): *Casarett and Doull's Toxicology: The Basic Science of Poisons,* 3d ed. New York, Macmillan, 1986

LAMPE KF, MCCANN MA (eds): *AMA Handbook of Poisonous and Injurious Plants.* Chicago, American Medical Association, 1985

RUMACK BH (ed): *Poisindex Information System* (updated quarterly). Denver, Micromedex

Specific poisons

Acetaminophen

FLANAGAN RJ: The role of acetylcysteine in clinical toxicology. Med Toxicol 2:93, 1987

PRESCOTT LF: Paracetamol overdose. Drugs 25:290, 1983

SMILKSTEIN MJ et al: Efficacy of oral *N*-acetylcysteine in the treatment of acetaminophen overdose. N Engl J Med 319:1558, 1988

Acids and alkali

FRIEDMAN EM, LOVEJOY FH JR: The emergency management of caustic ingestions. Emerg Med Clin North Am 2:77, 1984

HOWELL JM: Alkaline ingestions. Ann Emerg Med 15:820, 1986

PENNER GE: Acid ingestion: Toxicology and treatment. Ann Emerg Med 9:374, 1980

Antiarrhythmic drugs

BENOWITZ NL: Quinidine, procainamide, and disopyramide, in *Clinical Management of Poisoning and Drug Overdose,* LM Haddad, JF Winchester (eds). Philadelphia, Saunders, 1983, pp 853–862

FREEDMAN MD et al: Extracorporeal pump assistance—a novel treatment for acute lidocaine poisoning. Eur J Clin Pharmacol 22:129, 1982

HRUBY K, MISSLIVETZ J: Poisoning with oral antiarrhythmic drugs. Int J Clin Pharmacol 23:253, 1985

Barbiturates

HENDERSON LW, MERRILL JP: Treatment of barbiturate intoxication. Ann Intern Med 64:876, 1966

MATTHEW H: Barbiturates. Clin Toxicol 8(5):495, 1975

MCCARRON MM et al: Short-acting barbiturate overdosage: Correlation of intoxication score with serum barbiturate concentration. JAMA 248:55, 1982

Benzodiazepines

DIVOLL M et al: Benzodiazepine overdosage: Plasma concentrations and clinical outcome. Psycho Pharmacol 73:381, 1981

GREENBLATT DJ et al: Acute overdosage with benzodiazepine derivatives. Clin Pharmacol Ther 21:497, 1977

PRISCHL F et al: Value of flumazenil in benzodiazepine self-poisoning. Med Toxicol 3:334, 1988

Beta blockers

HEATH A: β-Adrenoceptor blocker toxicity: Clinical features and therapy. Am J Emerg Med 2:518, 1984

HENRY M et al: Cardiogenic shock associated with calcium-channel and β-blockers: Reversal with intravenous calcium chloride. Am J Emerg Med 3:334, 1985

WEINSTEIN RS: Recognition and management of poisoning with beta-adrenergic blocking agents. Ann Emerg Med 13:1123, 1984

Bleach

GAPAY-GAPANAVICUIUS M: Chloramine—induced pneumonitis from mixing household cleaning agents. Br Med J 288:1086, 1982

GAUDREAULT P et al: Predictability of esophageal injury from signs and symptoms. Pediatrics 71:767, 1983

LANDAU GD, SAUNDERS WH: The effect of chlorine bleach on the esophagus. Arch Otolaryngol 80:174, 1964

Calcium channel blockers

HERRINGTON DM et al: Nifedipine overdose. Am J Cardiol 81:344, 1986

SNOVER SW, BOCCHINO V: Massive diltiazem overdose. Ann Emerg Med 15:1221, 1986

ZARITSKY AL et al: Glucagon antagonism of calcium channel blocker induced myocardium dysfunction. Crit Care Med 16:246, 1988

Carbon monoxide

DOLAN MC: Carbon monoxide poisoning. Can Med Assoc J 133:392, 1985

Symposium—carbon monoxide poisoning—mechanism of damage, late sequelae and therapy. Clin Toxicol 23:247, 1985

WINTER PM, MILLER JN: Carbon monoxide poisoning. JAMA 236:1502, 1976

Cocaine

CREGLER LL, MARK H: Medical complications of cocaine abuse. N Engl J Med 315:1495, 1986

JONSSON S et al: Acute cocaine poisoning. Am J Med 75:1061, 1983

Cyanide

GRAHAM DL et al: Acute cyanide poisoning complicated by lactic acidosis and pulmonary edema. Arch Intern Med 137:1051, 1977

HALL AH et al: Clinical toxicology of cyanide: North American clinical experiences, in *Clinical and Experimental Toxicology of Cyanides,* B Ballantyne, TC Marrs (eds). Bristol, Wright, 1987

Digoxin

EKINS BR, WATANABE AS: Acute digoxin poisonings: Review of therapy. Am J Hosp Pharm 35:268, 1978

SMITH TW: New advances in the assessment and treatment of digitalis toxicity. J Clin Pharmacol 25:522, 1985

——— et al: Treatment of life-threatening digitalis intoxication with digoxin-specific FAB antibody fragments. N Engl J Med 307:1357, 1982

Ethanol

DAVID DJ, SPYKER DA: The acute toxicity of ethanol: Dosage and kinetic nomograms. Vet Hum Toxicol 21:272, 1979
ECKARDT MJ et al: Health hazards associated with alcohol consumption. JAMA 246:648, 1981
HALPERIN ML et al: Metabolic acidosis in the alcoholic: A pathophysiologic approach. Metabolism 32:308, 1983

Ethylene glycol

JACOBSEN D, MCMARTIN KE: Methanol and ethylene glycol poisonings: Mechanism of toxicity, clinical course, diagnosis and treatment. Med Toxicol 1:309, 1986
PARRY MF, WALLACH R: Ethylene glycol poisoning. Am J Med 57:143, 1974

Hallucinogens

BROWN RT, BRADEN NJ: Hallucinogens. Pediatr Clin North Am 34:341, 1987
COHEN S: The hallucinogens and the inhalents. Psych Clin North Am 7:681, 1984
STREICHEN M et al: Syndromes of solvent sniffing in adults. Ann Intern Med 94:758, 1981

Hydrocarbons

ANAS N et al: Criteria for hospitalizing children who have ingested products containing hydrocarbons. JAMA 246:840, 1981
MARKS ME et al: Adrenocorticosteroid treatment of hydrocarbon pneumonia in children—a cooperative study. J Pediatr 81:366, 1972
TRUEMPIER E et al: Clinical characteristics, pathophysiology and management of hydrocarbon ingestion: Case report and review of the literature. Pediatr Emerg Care 3:187, 1987

Hydrogen sulfide

SMITH RP: Management of acute sulfide poisoning. Arch Environ Health 31:166, 1976
STINE RJ et al: Hydrogen sulfide intoxication. Ann Intern Med 85:756, 1976
WHITECRAFT DD et al: Hydrogen sulfide poisoning treated with hyperbaric oxygen. J Emerg Med 3:23, 1985

Iron

PROUDFOOT AT et al: Management of acute iron poisoning. Med Toxicol 1:83, 1986
ROBOTHAM JL, LEITMAN PS: Acute iron poisoning—a review. Am J Dis Child 134:875, 1980
WHITTEN CF et al: Studies in acute iron poisoning: Further observations of desferrioxamine in the treatment of acute experimental iron poisoning. J Pediatr 38:102, 1966

Isoniazid

CHIN L et al: Evaluation of diazepam and pyridoxine as antidotes to isoniazid intoxication in rats and dogs. Toxicol Appl Pharmacol 45:713, 1978
SIEVERS ML, HERRIER RN: Treatment of acute isoniazid toxicity. Am J Hosp Pharm 32:202, 1975
WASON S et al: Single high-dose pyridoxine treatment for isoniazid overdose. JAMA 246:1102, 1981

Isopropyl alcohol

LACOUTURE PG et al: A review of acute isopropyl alcohol intoxication: Diagnosis and management. Am J Med 75:680, 1983
NATOWICZ M et al: Pharmacokinetic analysis of a case of isopropyl intoxication. Clin Chem 31:326, 1985

Lithium

AMDISEN A: Clinical features and management of lithium poisoning. Med Toxicol 3:18, 1988
HANSEN HE, AMDISEN A: Lithium intoxication. Q Med J 47:123, 1978

MAO inhibitors

KAPLAN RF et al: Phenelzine overdose treated with dantrolene sodium. JAMA 255:642, 1986
LINDEN CH: Monoamine oxidase inhibitor overdose. Ann Emerg Med 13:1137, 1984

Methanol

JACOBSEN D, MCMARTIN KE: Methanol and ethylene glycol poisoning: Mechanism of toxicity, clinical course, diagnosis and treatment. Med Toxicol:309, 1986
OSTERLOH JD et al: Serum formate concentrations in methanol intoxication as a criterion for hemodialysis. Ann Intern Med 104:200, 1986
SWARTZ RD et al: Epidemic methanol poisoning: Clinical and biochemical analysis of a recent episode. Medicine 60:373, 1981

Methemoglobinemia

CURRY S: Methemoglobinemia. Ann Emerg Med 11:214, 1982
HALL AH et al: Drug and chemical-induced methaemoglobinaemia. Med Toxicol 1:253, 1986
HARVEY JW, KEITT AS: Studies of the efficacy and potential hazards of methylene blue therapy in aniline-induced methaemoglobinaemia. Br J Haematol 53:29, 1983

Muscle relaxants

DOMINO EF: Muscle relaxants of the mephenesin type. Ann NY Acad Sci 86:238, 1974
VALTONEN EJ: A controlled trial of chlormezanone, orphenadrine, paracetamol and placebo in treatment of painful skeletal muscle spasms. Ann Clin Res 7:85, 1975

Narcotics

CUDDY P: Management of acute opioid intoxication. Crit Care Q 4:65, 1982
FULTZ JM, SENAY EC: Guidelines for the management of hospitalized addicts. Ann Intern Med 82:815, 1975
LAWSON AAH, NORTHRIDGE DB: Dextropropoxyphene overdose. Med Toxicol 2:430, 1987

Nonsteroidal anti-inflammatory drugs

COURT H, VOLANS GN: Poisoning after overdose with nonsteroidal anti-inflammatory drugs. Adverse Drug React Acute Poisoning Rev 3:1, 1984
HALL AH et al: Ibuprofen overdose: 126 cases. Ann Emerg Med 15:1308, 1986
VALE JA, MEREDITH TJ: Acute poisoning due to nonsteroidal anti-inflammatory drugs: Clinical features and management. Med Toxicol 1:11, 1986

Organophosphate and carbamates insecticides

MINTON NA, MURRAY VSG: A review of organophosphate poisoning. Med Toxicol 3:350, 1988
NAMBA T et al: Poisoning due to organophosphate insecticides. Am J Med 50:475, 1971
NATOFF IL, REIFF B: Effect of oximes on the acute toxicity of anticholinesterase carbamates. Toxicol Appl Pharmacol 25:569, 1973

Phenothiazines

BARRY D et al: Phenothiazine poisoning: A review of 48 cases. Calif Med 118:1, 1983
BENOWITZ NL et al: Cardiopulmonary catastrophes in drug-overdosed patients. Med Clin North Am 63:267, 1979

Salicylates

GAUDREAULT P et al: The relative severity of acute vs chronic salicylate poisoning in children: A clinical comparison. Pediatrics 70:566, 1982
MCGUIGAN MA: A two-year review of salicylate deaths in Ontario. Arch Intern Med 147:510, 1987
TEMPLE AR: Acute and chronic effects of aspirin toxicity and their treatment. Arch Intern Med 141:364, 1981

Stimulants

GARY NE, SAIDI P: Methamphetamine intoxication. Am J Med 64:537, 1978
LINDEN CH et al: Amphetamines. Top Emerg Med 7:18, 1985
PENTEL P: Toxicity of over-the-counter stimulants. JAMA 252:1898, 1984

Theophylline

GAUDREAULT P, GUAY J: Theophylline poisoning. Med Toxicol 1:169, 1986
OLSON KR et al: Theophylline overdose: Acute single ingestion versus chronic repeated overmedication. Am J Emerg Med 3:386, 1985
PARK GD et al: Use of hemoperfusion for treatment of theophylline intoxication. Am J Med 74:961, 1983

Tricyclic antidepressants

BOEHNERT MT, LOVEJOY FH JR: Value of QRS duration versus the serum drug level in predicting seizures and ventricular arrhythmias after an acute overdose of tricyclic antidepressants. N Engl J Med 313:474, 1985
CROME P: Poisoning due to tricyclic antidepressant overdose. Med Toxicol 1:261, 1986
FROMMER DA et al: Tricyclic antidepressant overdose; A review. JAMA 257:521, 1987

375 HEAVY METAL POISONING

JOHN W. GRAEF / FREDERICK H. LOVEJOY, JR.

ARSENIC

SOURCE Inorganic arsenic compounds such as arsenic trioxide, arsenic pentoxide, and sodium and potassium arsenite and arsenate are found in insecticides, rodenticides, fungicides, wood preservatives, herbicides, and compounds used in glass manufacturing. Organic arsenic is widely distributed in the environment. Arsine gas is produced in the smelting and refining of metals, in galvanizing and etching, in lead plating, and in making silicon microchips. Historically, organic arsenical compounds have been used in the treatment of syphilis, epilepsy, psoriasis, and amebiasis. Currently, acute toxicity is encountered following accidental ingestion, industrial accidents, or suicidal or homicidal intoxications. Chronic exposures occur most commonly following low-dose exposure in industry or chronic consumption of contaminated food, water, or medications.

METABOLISM Arsenic is absorbed through the skin, lungs, and gastrointestinal tract. Inorganic compounds are absorbed more readily than organic, with greater than 80 percent of an ingested dose absorbed by the gastrointestinal tract. Arsine gas is absorbed through the lungs. Arsenic is distributed from blood to liver, kidney, lung, and spleen within 24 h of ingestion and to skin, hair, and bone within 2 weeks. Inorganic arsenic compounds are found in high concentrations in leukocytes. Inorganic arsenic does not cross the blood-brain barrier but does cross the placenta. Five to ten percent is excreted in feces, and 90 to 95 percent is excreted in the urine. Small amounts are recovered in bile, feces, and saliva. Arsenic may be detected in urine for 7 to 21 days following an overdose and detected in the serum for a shorter period of time.

CLINICAL TOXICOLOGY Arsine gas combines with hemoglobin in red blood cells to produce severe hemolysis with anemia, hemoglobinuria, and hematuria within 3 to 4 h of ingestion. Subsequent jaundice may be severe. Signs and symptoms of toxicity include nausea, vomiting and diarrhea, apprehension and malaise, tachycardia, and dyspnea. Acute renal failure is frequent and often fatal.

The reported lethal dose for arsenic ranges from 130 to 300 mg. Manifestations of acute toxicity include for the gastrointestinal tract—burning in the throat, difficulty swallowing, nausea, vomiting, diarrhea, abdominal pain, and a garlic odor on the breath; for the cardiovascular system—cyanosis, difficulty breathing, and hypotension; for the central nervous system—delirium, coma, and seizures; for the kidneys—acute tubular necrosis; for the hematologic system—hemolysis, eosinophilia, and, rarely, bone marrow depression. Manifestations of chronic arsenic poisoning occur 2 to 8 weeks following ingestion and include for the skin and nails—erythroderma, hyperkeratosis, hyperpigmentation, exfoliative dermatitis, and Aldrich-Mees lines (transverse white striae of the fingernails); for the mucous membranes—laryngitis, tracheitis, and bronchitis; for the central nervous system—polyneuritis (sensory and motor). Basal cell carcinomas, squamous cell carcinomas, Bowen's disease of the skin (see Chap. 59), and lung carcinomas have been associated with chronic arsenic exposure.

Arsenic produces its toxicity by binding with tissue sulfhydryl groups. Arsenic also binds to enzymes in the Krebs tricarboxylic acid cycle, thereby interfering with oxidative phosphorylation. Other effects include capillary injury and direct toxic effects on large organs. Pathologic findings include necrosis of the stomach, small bowel, and vasculature and degenerative changes in the liver and kidneys.

LABORATORY FINDINGS Arsenic is radiopaque and is seen on x-ray of the abdomen. It may also be detected in hair and nails for months following exposure. Specific organ effects include: abnormal liver function tests; anemia, leukocytosis, leukopenia, and hemoglobinemia; proteinuria, hematuria, hemoglobinuria, and cellular casts in the urine. Urine arsenic (As) levels are normally less than 67 nmol (5 μg)/d.

TREATMENT Acute ingestion should be treated by inducing vomiting with ipecac syrup if the patient is alert. Gastric lavage is indicated if the patient is obtunded. Activated charcoal is ineffective, and cathartics are contraindicated. Dimercaprol chelates arsenic by producing an insoluble complex that is excreted by the kidneys. For mild symptoms and elevated serum or urinary levels, 2 to 3 mg/kg body weight per dose is given intramuscularly every 6 h for 24 h and then every 12 to 24 h for 10 days. Adequacy of urinary mobilization of arsenic is confirmed and followed during treatment by measurement of serum and urinary levels. Treatment should be continued until 24-h urine As levels are less than 67 nmol (5 μg)/d. Toxic manifestations of dimercaprol (increased blood pressure, tachycardia, nausea, vomiting, headache, burning sensation in the lips, mucous membrane irritation, coma, and convulsions) occur with increasing doses. For patients with severe symptoms and very high arsenic levels 3 to 5 mg/kg body weight per intramuscular dose of dimercaprol is administered in a similar regime. The water-soluble analogue of dimercaprol, succimer (DMSA), may be more effective and is less toxic than dimercaprol.

Penicillamine has been successfully used in acute and chronic poisoning, administered orally at a dose of 100 mg/kg body weight per day (the maximum dose not to exceed 1 g/d) in four divided doses for 5 days. Side effects of penicillamine include rash, leukopenia, thrombocytopenia, and nephrotoxicity. Hemodialysis removes arsenic (24 to 100 mg in 24 h) with a clearance of 80 to 90 mL/min and is indicated if renal failure occurs. Hemodialysis early in the clinical course in conjunction with dimercaprol may limit arsenic's distribution phase and enhance clearance of free and complexed arsenic.

Exchange transfusion and, if renal failure develops, hemodialysis are the preferred treatments for arsine gas poisoning. Dimercaprol affords no protection against red cell destruction.

CADMIUM

SOURCE Exposure to cadmium is usually occupational or via pollution from mining or smelting operations. Cadmium is produced commercially as a by-product of copper and lead or zinc smelting and is used in the manufacture of batteries, in ceramics, in electroplating, and as a pigment in paints and plastics. In contaminated areas, high concentrations may be found in shellfish.

METABOLISM Absorption occurs via ingestion or inhalation. Normal daily oral intake is up to 200 μg with an estimated mean of 20 to 40 μg/d. Only 5 to 10 percent of this is absorbed, although like lead, absorption may be increased in the presence of calcium and iron deficiency. About 5 percent of inhaled cadmium is absorbed depending on particle size. Small, highly soluble particles are absorbed at a rate of 25 to 50 percent.

About 50 percent of absorbed cadmium is concentrated in the liver and kidneys. In erythrocytes and soft tissues cadmium is bound to metallothionein, a low-molecular-weight polypeptide containing a large number of available sulfhydryl groups that exert a protective effect. With large single-dose cadmium exposures saturation of the protein may result in loss of protective effect. Cadmium does not pass the placenta and gradually accumulates in the body with age. Biologic half-life has been estimated at more than 20 years except in the presence of kidney damage when urinary excretion is increased. In the kidney, metallothionein-bound cadmium is filtered at the glomerulus and is then reabsorbed by the proximal tubules. The urinary excretion rarely exceeds 5 nmol (0.5 μg)/d.

CLINICAL TOXICOLOGY Acute cadmium intoxication may occur after either ingestion or inhalation. Ingestion of water containing concentrations of 15 mg/L or foods containing as little as 30 mg of cadmium can induce vomiting, abdominal pain, and severe diarrhea. Shock may ensue. Acute inhalation of cadmium dust produces dyspnea, weakness, chest pain, shortness of breath, and cough. A chemical pneumonitis produces pulmonary edema and respiratory failure. Clinical symptoms may occur with air exposure as low as 1 mg/m^2 surface area over 8 h. During the same time period inhalation of 5 mg/m^2 surface area may be fatal. A latent period of 4 to 24 h from exposure to onset of symptoms may complicate accurate diagnosis. Death usually occurs in 5 to 10 days. Chemical pneumonitis may continue for several months, and pulmonary function can be abnormal for longer than 1 year after exposure.

Chronic intoxication usually occurs by industrial inhalation and produces emphysema and characteristic renal tubular damage with proteinuria and increased urinary excretion of beta$_2$ microglobulin. Cadmium's inhibitory effect on alpha$_1$ antitrypsin may be responsible for cadmium-induced emphysema. Relatively minor changes in liver function, a microcytic hypochromic anemia unresponsive to iron therapy, and hypertension are associated findings. Chronic oral intake of contaminated rice and drinking water has produced a syndrome in Japan called *itai-itai* (ouch-ouch) disease with manifestations that include renal tubular damage and osteomalacia.

LABORATORY FINDINGS Measurement of blood cadmium levels is not useful. Urinary cadmium excretion exceeding 0.1 μmol

(10 μg)/L is associated with renal tubular damage especially when accompanied by elevated urinary beta$_2$ microglobulin and metallothionein levels. Kidney cadmium content obtained by renal biopsy can be assessed by neutron activation analysis. A renal cadmium concentration exceeding 2 μmol/g (200 μg/g) of wet weight is associated with renal disease.

TREATMENT Treatment is controversial. Although chelating agents bind cadmium, they may effectively shift cadmium to the kidney, where further damage can occur. In acute exposure, ethylenediaminetetraacetic acid (edetate) in a dose of 1 g/m^2 surface area daily can be beneficial. Although dimercaprol is not effective, another oral chelating agent, succimer (DMSA), appears promising. Acute inhalation pneumonitis should be treated with glucocorticoids and diuretics. Itai-itai disease appears to respond to large doses of vitamin D. Long-term sequelae of chronic cadmium exposure include emphysema and chronic renal insufficiency.

LEAD

SOURCE Lead is a normal constituent of the earth's crust and is found throughout nature. The increased use of lead during the Industrial Revolution caused extensive disease among lead workers; the addition of lead salts to paints as coloring agents and stabilizers set the stage for the largest epidemic of lead poisoning in history, that of childhood plumbism. This syndrome, caused by ingestion by small children of lead from paint, soil, household dust, and, infrequently, from drinking water, affects an estimated 2,000,000 preschool children annually in the United States alone. Evidence of permanent neurologic sequelae from levels of lead previously thought to be safe has raised fears of possible damage to the fetus and newborn as well. The nature of this epidemic has forced prohibition against the addition of organic lead salts to gasoline as well as extensive prohibitions against the use of lead in consumer products.

METABOLISM Inorganic lead salts are absorbed through ingestion or inhalation. Organic lead salts may also be absorbed through the skin. Generally, gastrointestinal absorption is about 10 percent of an ingested dose, but in children may be as high as 50 percent. It is enhanced by deficiency of iron, calcium, and zinc. Absorption through the lung varies with tidal volume and particle size. Particles smaller than 1 μm may be absorbed if they reach the alveoli. Adults may ingest up to 0.7 μmol (150 μg)/d of lead from normal exposure to food and drinking water. Positive lead balance may occur at these levels since renal excretion normally does not exceed 0.4 μmol (80 μg)/d. In children, no more than 0.02 μmol (5 μg)/kg body weight is tolerated without increasing the body lead burden.

Under steady state conditions, 5 to 10 percent of ingested lead may be found in blood; 95 percent of that fraction is associated with the erythrocyte. Up to 80 to 90 percent is taken up by bone and incorporated into hydroxyapatite crystals, where it is relatively inactive. The remainder is found in soft tissues, principally the kidneys and brain. The principal route of excretion is stool (80 to 90 percent), and the remainder is found in the urine (10 percent). Small amounts are excreted in hair, nails, sweat, and saliva. Lead passes the placenta and blood-brain barrier and may be found in milk. The half-life of lead in blood and soft tissues is 24 to 40 days, and in bone, 104 days.

Lead is a poison of enzymes, binding to the sulfhydryl groups of proteins. In high concentration, lead alters the tertiary structure of intracellular proteins, denaturing them and causing cell death and tissue inflammation.

CLINICAL TOXICOLOGY The toxic effects of lead differ between children and adults. The adult form is generally characterized by abdominal pain, anemia, renal disease, headache, peripheral neuropathy with demyelination of long neurons, ataxia, and memory loss. Symptoms are usually associated with prolonged elevation of lead levels above 4 to 5 μmol/L (80 to 100 μg/dL) of whole blood. A subclinical form in adults affects primarily the peripheral nervous system and the kidneys. A linear association between hypertension and elevated lead levels [i.e., greater than 1.4 μmol/L (30 μg/dL)] has been reported. Encephalopathy is rare in adults.

Childhood lead poisoning is manifested by abdominal pain and anemia, but the central nervous system effects are most important. As an enzymatic poison, lead affects developing tissues more than tissues with slow turnover. Hence, subclinical lead poisoning is most dangerous to children because its effects emerge without associated symptoms that bring the victim to medical attention. In the acute clinical form, signs and symptoms reflect both the direct effect of high concentrations of lead [(i.e., blood lead greater than 4 μmol/L (80 μg/dL)] and consequent severe alterations in porphyrin synthesis. Signs and symptoms include abdominal pain, irritability followed by lethargy, anorexia, pallor (anemia), ataxia, and slurred speech. In severe cases, convulsions, coma, and death are usually due to severe generalized cerebral edema and renal failure. A history of "high-dose" exposure to lead (usually paint chips), pica (the ingestion of nonfood substances), and malnutrition (iron, calcium, and zinc deficiency) almost always is associated with this syndrome.

The subclinical form of childhood plumbism is associated with elevated blood lead and increased erythrocyte protoporphyrin. However, no symptoms are usually detected. The syndrome is widespread, and its effects on the developing central nervous system are irreversible. These include mental retardation and selective deficits in language, cognitive functions, and behavior, depending on the age and duration of exposure. These latter factors are more important than the height of the lead level.

LABORATORY FINDINGS Laboratory abnormalities include blood lead levels greater than 1.2 μmol/L (25 μg/dL) associated with free erythrocyte protoporphyrin (FEP) greater than 0.6 μmol/L (35 μg/dL). Biochemical and neurodevelopmental abnormalities may occur in association with blood lead levels as low as 0.7 μmol/L (15 μg/dL), particularly in very young children. Although a hemolytic anemia is associated with acute plumbism, chronic plumbism produces a microcytic hypochromic anemia with associated or secondary iron deficiency. Other heme precursors are increased in plasma and urine (e.g., delta aminolevulinic acid).

Renal abnormalities include pyuria, the Fanconi syndrome, and azotemia. In plumbism, urinary excretion of lead exceeds 4 μmol (80 μg)/d. In adults, demyelination of long nerves produces prolonged nerve conduction time and subsequent paralysis of extensor muscles with atrophy (wrist drop or foot drop). While slight prolongation of nerve conduction can be seen in children, it is clinically evident only in those with sickle cell disease. Abnormalities of cardiac, thyroid, and hepatic function occur in adults. In children, a characteristic finding is increased density at the metaphyseal plate of growing long bones, so-called lead lines. These are generally seen in association with levels greater than 2.4 μmol/L (50 μg/dL) of whole blood for a prolonged period. They are not seen in adults.

TREATMENT The *sine qua non* of treatment is removal of the source of exposure. Cases of industrial lead poisoning should be reported to the Occupational Safety Hazards Administration (OSHA). Cases of childhood plumbism should be reported to the local board of health to initiate examination of housing for sources of lead.

Reduction of the body burden of lead is accomplished by use of chelating agents, principally edetate calcium disodium (EDTA), dimercaprol, and penicillamine. The oral chelating agent succimer is undergoing clinical trials and appears to be as effective as parenteral edetate. The lead mobilization test is used to determine the size of the "chelatable" pool of lead. In this test, administration of a calculated dose of chelating agent, usually edetate, induces a lead diuresis that is then compared to the dose of chelating agent. The test is positive when greater than 5 nmol (1 μg) lead is excreted per milligram of chelating agent administered per 24 h. An outpatient modification of this test may be used in which urine is collected for 6 to 8 h. The test is considered positive when greater than 2.5 nmol (0.5 μg) of lead is excreted per milligram of chelating agent. The mobilization test can be useful in determining the utility of chelation therapy in patients with borderline lead levels or in those patients who have been previously treated. The use of x-ray fluorescence of bone to determine the lead burden is under investigation as an alternative to the lead mobilization test.

In acute encephalopathy, double therapy (dimercaprol and edetate) is used until blood lead levels are less than 2 μmol/L (40 μg/dL). Urine flow must be established, and even in the presence of cerebral edema, fluids must be sufficient to produce a lead diuresis. Mannitol and dexamethasone can reduce cerebral edema, but removal of the metal is essential. In symptomatic adults and children, therapy with both dimercaprol and edetate should be used for 5 days at edetate doses of 0.5 to 1 g/m² surface area up to 1.5 g/m² surface area daily and dimercaprol doses of 12 to 24 mg/kg body weight per day. If further chelation is required, a minimum interval of 48 to 72 h should intervene between courses of therapy. The penicillamine dose is 20 to 40 mg/kg body weight per day, not to exceed 1 g/d. Adverse effects, particularly allergy, may be reduced by beginning therapy with one-quarter of the total dose for 1 week, then doubling and redoubling the dose until full dose is reached. Penicillamine can be administered for 3 to 6 months until the body lead burden is depleted. Only penicillamine and, to a lesser extent, edetate remove lead directly from bone. If edetate is indicated, as many separate 5-day courses as are needed may be given provided that the total safe dose is not exceeded and proper intervals between courses are observed.

MERCURY

SOURCE Humans may encounter mercury in an inorganic (elemental or mercuric salt) or an organic (usually methyl) form. All three are toxic, but organic mercury is most widespread and potentially dangerous. Elemental mercury is used in thermometers, sphygmomanometers, and dental amalgams. It is volatile at room temperature and rapidly oxidizes to mercuric mercury when exposed to oxygen. Toxicity usually occurs from inhalation of mercury vapor during industrial exposure. Mercuric salts are found in topical medicines, in catalytic agents in the manufacture of plastics, in cathartics (e.g., Calomel), and in foodstuffs. Toxicity occurs usually as a result of gastrointestinal exposure. Organic mercury is in paints, fungicides, seeds, foods, medicines, and cosmetic agents. Large amounts of methyl mercury are formed by methylation of mercury salt wastes as occurred in the mercury epidemic in Minamata Bay, Japan.

METABOLISM Elemental mercury is poorly absorbed by the gastrointestinal tract but is absorbed efficiently as vapor through the lungs, with 80 to 100 percent of inhaled mercury entering the bloodstream through the alveoli. Absorbed mercury vapor is lipid-soluble and readily crosses the blood-brain barrier and the placenta. It is rapidly oxidized to its mercuric form and combines with sulfhydryl groups. Excretion is via the urine and feces. Small amounts of mercury vapor may be excreted via the lungs. The half-life of elemental mercury is approximately 60 days.

Inorganic mercury salts are absorbed through the gastrointestinal tract and skin. Large overdoses may produce corrosive effects on the gastrointestinal tract with consequent increased absorption. Normal uptake is less than 10 percent of an ingested dose. Mercuric salts accumulate primarily in the kidney, but are distributed to the liver, erythrocytes, bone marrow, spleen, lung, intestine, and skin. Excretion is via the urine and feces. The half-life of inorganic mercury is approximately 40 days.

Organic (methyl) mercury is readily absorbed through the intestines and the skin. Short-chain alkyl and methyl mercury penetrate the erythrocyte membrane and bind to hemoglobin. The ratio of red blood cell to plasma methyl mercury may be as high as 9:1. Because of its high lipid solubility, methyl mercury freely passes the placenta and blood-brain barrier and enters breast milk. Organic mercury also concentrates in the kidneys and the central nervous system. Metallothionein synthesis is induced by mercury, and the augmented concentration of the protein exerts a protective effect against tissue damage. Excretion is complex. About 1 percent of organic mercury is excreted in urine directly. Methyl mercury is acetylated in the liver or may be conjugated with cysteine or glutathione. The *N*-acetylhomocysteine–methyl mercury complex then enters the enterohepatic circulation and is ultimately excreted in the urine. The half-life of organic mercury in humans is about 70 days.

CLINICAL TOXICOLOGY Acute metallic mercury (vapor) poisoning causes inflammation of large and small airways and interstitial pneumonitis. The rapid uptake of mercury vapor into the central nervous system produces tremor and increased excitability. Chronic mercury vapor poisoning primarily affects the central nervous system. Initial symptoms include lassitude, anorexia, weight loss, and gastrointestinal disturbances. Increasing exposure produces the characteristic intention tremor of mercury poisoning and is accompanied by mercurial *erethism* (timidity, memory loss, insomnia, excitability, and, in severe cases, delirium). This neurologic picture in felt-hat workers exposed to mercury vapor and mercuric salts led to the phrase "mad as a hatter."

Chronic inorganic mercury poisoning produces the above neurologic findings as well as excessive salivation, loosening of the teeth, gingivitis, and stomatitis. When applied to the skin, mercuric salts may cause hypersensitivity reactions ranging from mild erythema to exfoliative dermatitis. Acrodynia, or Pink's disease, occurs in young children and may be mistaken for Kawasaki's disease. Symptoms include generalized rash, irritability, photophobia, hypertrichosis, profuse perspiration, and swelling and desquamation of the feet and hands.

Acute inorganic mercury poisoning is characterized by corrosive effects on the gastrointestinal tract, including nausea, vomiting, hematemesis, and abdominal pain followed by tenesmus, bloody diarrhea, and necrosis of intestinal mucosa. Acute fluid redistribution in massive overdose can produce shock and death. Acute inorganic mercury poisoning causes acute tubular necrosis, while chronic inorganic mercury poisoning produces a nephrotic syndrome.

Acute and chronic organic mercury poisoning are indistinguishable. Prenatal poisoning produces cerebral palsy as a result of cortical and cerebellar atrophy. Postnatal poisoning causes paresthesias, headache, pain, visual, hearing, and speech disorders, neurasthenia, loss of memory, incoordination, erethism, spasticity, paralysis, stupor, and coma. These neurologic abnormalities are often permanent.

The daily intake of methyl mercury should not exceed 100 parts per billion. Blood mercury levels above 180 nmol/L (3.5 μg/dL) and urine mercury levels above 0.7 μmol/L (150 μg/L) are abnormal. Symptoms may be seen with blood mercury levels above 1 μmol/L (20 μg/dL) and urine mercury levels above 3 μmol/L (600 μg/L). Clinical findings may be associated with somewhat lower concentrations depending on when exposure occurred.

TREATMENT Treatment is aimed at reducing the absorption of mercury, protecting susceptible tissues, and enhancing elimination. In the case of ingestion of mercuric salts, initial treatment consists of removing mercury from the stomach by inducing emesis or by gastric lavage. Polythiol resins are effective in binding mercury in the gastrointestinal tract. Activated charcoal, however, does not bind metals.

Generally, chelation therapy is indicated when elevated urine or blood mercury levels are present. Chelating agents with active mono- or dithiol groups are most effective. These include dimercaprol and penicillamine. The oral chelating agent succimer shows promise.

In acute inorganic mercury poisoning, dimercaprol should be used at a dose not exceeding 24 mg/kg body weight per 24 h intramuscularly, in divided doses. Generally, therapy should not exceed 5 days at a time but can be reinstituted after a suitable rest period. Penicillamine can be used in the treatment of inorganic mercury poisoning but *N*-acetyl-DL-penicillamine is equally effective, and less toxic. The dose is 30 mg/kg body weight per day in two to three divided doses. Peritoneal hemodialysis have also been used with some success. Neither is as effective as chelation therapy but may be useful in the presence of renal failure.

In chronic inorganic mercury poisoning, dimercaprol is ineffective. Penicillamine is the drug of choice. The investigational drug *N*-acetyl-DL-penicillamine is more effective than either dimercaprol or edetate.

THALLIUM

SOURCE Thallium is used as an insecticide and rodenticide, as a catalyst in fireworks, in manufacturing imitation jewelry and optical lenses, in industry as an alloy, and in cardiac perfusion imaging. Accidental as well as purposeful ingestions of thallium occur. Epidemic poisoning has followed the ingestion of grain impregnated with thallium. Thallium is available as iodide, sulfate, acetate, carbonate, and nitrate salts.

METABOLISM Thallium is absorbed percutaneously, by inhalation, and by oral ingestion. It has a large volume of distribution of 4 to 6 L/kg body weight with distribution to body organs including kidney, pancreas, spleen, liver, lung, muscles, and brain. Thallium is bound to sulfhydryl groups on mitochondrial membranes at intracellular sites. The elimination half-life is variable, ranging from 3 to 15 days. The major pathway of elimination is in the urine, conforming to first-order pharmacokinetics; 3 percent of a dose is eliminated per day, or 75 mL/min total-body clearance.

Thallium interferes with oxidative phosphorylation by inhibition of ATPase and substitutes for potassium in many physiologic reactions. Pathologic findings at postmortem include cerebral edema, loss of myelin in peripheral nerves, fatty infiltration of the liver, and degenerative changes in the myocardium.

CLINICAL TOXICOLOGY Severe poisoning occurs following a single ingested dose greater than 1 g or 8 mg/kg body weight. Death has occurred following an ingested dose of 15 mg/kg body weight.

Immediate signs and symptoms (occurring within 3 to 4 h of ingestion) include nausea and vomiting, abdominal pain, diarrhea, and hematochezia. Intermediate manifestations (within 1 week of ingestion) include involvement of the central nervous system with confusion, psychosis, choreoathetosis, organic brain syndrome, convulsions, and coma. Peripheral neurologic involvement is both motor and sensory and includes paresthesias, myalgias, weakness, tremor, and ataxia. Autonomic manifestations are less common and include tachycardia, hypertension, and salivation. Ophthalmologic abnormalities are neuritis, ophthalmoplegia, ptosis, strabismus, and cranial nerve palsies. Late manifestations (occurring 2 to 4 weeks after ingestion) include diffuse hair loss (with sparing of pubic and body hair and the lateral one-third of the eyebrows) with regrowth occurring as body burden decreases over time. Residual effects include memory loss, ataxia, tremor, and foot drop.

LABORATORY FINDINGS Thallium is radiopaque and is evident on an abdomenal x-ray. Thallium levels with severe ingestion range, in blood, from 1.5 to 10 μmol/L (30 to 200 μg/dL) and, in urine, from 0.05 to 0.1 μmol (10 to 20 μg)/d. The electroencephalogram (EEG) is diffusely abnormal, and peripheral nerve conduction may be delayed.

TREATMENT Therapeutic modalities include gastrointestinal decontamination, enhanced renal excretion, and dialysis. Gastric lavage or ipecac syrup is indicated within 4 to 6 h of acute ingestion. Adequacy of removal of thallium can be documented by follow-up abdominal x-ray. Prussian blue absorbs thallium in the gastrointestinal tract by exchanging potassium for thallium on its crystal lattice network thereby preventing absorption. The oral dose is 250 mg/kg body weight, administered once. Activated charcoal is as effective as Prussian blue in increasing fecal elimination by interrupting the enterohepatic circulation of thallium. Mannitol or magnesium citrate is used as a laxative to enhance gastrointestinal removal.

Forced diuresis is the oldest technique in use, and increases urinary excretion by 50 to 100 percent. Potassium chloride promotes renal excretion of thallium through the exchange of potassium for thallium, thereby releasing thallium from tissue sites into blood and augmenting urinary excretion two- to threefold. This therapy shortens thallium half-life in humans but may aggravate neurologic symptoms by redistributing thallium into the brain. The amount of thallium removed as compared to the total ingested dose of potassium is small. Diuretics (furosemide) also increase urinary elimination of thallium. Peritoneal dialysis removes 15 to 20 mg of thallium per day and hemodialysis 8 mg for each 8 h of dialysis. Prolonged hemodialysis can remove up to 25 mg of thallium per day, the total amount removed being relatively small. Charcoal hemoperfusion achieves average blood clearance values of 100 mL/min at a blood flow rate of 300 mL/min. Thus, the combination of forced diuresis, diuretic therapy, and hemoperfusion will most effectively enhance total-body clearance of thallium. This therapy should be combined with oral administration of Prussian blue or activated charcoal plus cathartics.

Ditiocarb has been advocated for early use in overdose because it leads to increased thallium blood levels and a two- to threefold increase in thallium excretion. However, ditiocarb-thallium complexes diffuse into the brain with subsequent clinical and EEG worsening; therefore, ditiocarb is contraindicated in thallium intoxication.

CHELATING AGENTS

Chelating agents are used to bind toxic metals in stable, cyclic compounds with relatively low toxicity and enhanced renal and fecal excretion.

DIMERCAPROL (BRITISH ANTI-LEWISITE, BAL) Dimercaprol was first developed as an antidote for the arsenical war gas lewisite; its chelating property is due to its four sulfhydryl groups which bind in a complex to polyvalent metal ions. Its affinity for metals is strong enough to reverse a significant portion of toxic metal enzyme binding. Dimercaprol diffuses into erythrocytes and enhances fecal as well as urinary metal excretion. It is given intramuscularly in peanut oil every 4 to 8 h in a dose of 12 to 24 mg/kg body weight per 24 h. Toxicity includes mild febrile reactions, nausea, headache, lacrimation, conjunctivitis, salivation, and rhinorrhea. The drug emits a strong sulfide odor, and patients may complain of metallic taste. Contraindications to dimercaprol include glucose-6-phosphate dehydrogenase deficiency, allergy to peanut oil, and concurrent use of medicinal iron, which forms a toxic complex with dimercaprol. Succimer (DMSA), an oral congener of dimercaprol, is under clinical trials in the United States for the treatment of lead and mercury poisoning. It has not been shown to be effective for other metals, although it may work in copper poisoning as well. Its dosage, effectiveness, and safety appear to be comparable to those of parenteral edetate with the advantage of oral administration and more selective excretion of the heavy metal. Mechanism of action appears to be comparable to that of dimercaprol.

EDETATE (EDTA) Because the sodium salt of edetate can produce profound hypocalcemia, only the calcium disodium salt should be used in therapy of metal poisoning. Calcium edetate forms a complex with divalent cations exchanging one atom of calcium for each metal ion. It enhances urinary excretion of lead twenty- to fiftyfold and also increases excretion of zinc and, to a lesser extent, other metals. It does not enter the erythrocyte but removes metals from the extracellular sites. Oral administration is contraindicated because it is variably absorbed and it enhances absorption of metals from the gastrointestinal tract. The drug is given parenterally either by constant intravenous infusion or intramuscular injection in a dose of 500 to 1000 mg/m^2 surface area per day. The drug can be used safely in conjunction with other chelating agents. Toxicity increases after 4 to 5 days of administration with concomitant reduction in metal excretion; as a consequence, the drug is given for several ''courses'' of from 3 to 5 days each.

Toxicity is principally renal, dose-related, and usually reversible. It can be reduced by maintaining adequate urine flow. During treatment renal function should be carefully monitored.

PENICILLAMINE Penicillamine is the only commercially available oral chelating agent. Not presently approved by the Federal

Drug Administration for treatment of lead poisoning, it is licensed for use in the treatment of rheumatoid arthritis, Wilson's disease, and cystinuria. Nevertheless, there is extensive experience in its use in chelation of other metals. The *N*-acetyl form is particularly helpful in the treatment of inorganic and organic mercury poisoning.

Penicillamine enhances excretion of heavy metals in the urine by an unclear mechanism. The drug is given orally in a dose of 40 mg/kg body weight per day. By initiating therapy at low doses (usually 25 percent of the anticipated maximum dose) and gradually increasing the dose, the frequency of side effects can be reduced substantially.

Side effects may be seen in up to 20 to 30 percent of patients receiving penicillamine and resemble penicillin hypersensitivity, including rash, fever, thrombocytopenia, and leukopenia. Rare side effects include autoimmune hemolytic anemia and Stevens-Johnson syndrome. Anorexia, nausea, sleep disturbances, and urinary frequency may be seen occasionally. Nephrotoxicity is reported in adults receiving large doses and in one case has been reported in a child. Patients receiving penicillamine should, therefore, be carefully monitored for signs of renal, hematologic, or allergic side effects.

REFERENCES

Arsenic

FESMIRE FM et al: Survival following massive arsenic ingestion. Am J Emerg Med 6:602, 1988

FOWLER BA, WEISSBERG JB: Arsine poisoning. N Engl J Med 291:1171, 1974

KLEVAY LM: Pharmacology and toxicology of heavy metals: Arsenic. Pharmacol Ther 1:189, 1976

PETERSON RG, RUMACK BH: D-Penicillamine therapy of acute arsine poisoning. J Pediatr 91:661, 1977

Cadmium

DUNPHY B: Acute occupational cadmium poisoning. J Occup Med 9:22, 1967

FRIBERG L et al: *Cadmium in the Environment*, 2d ed. Cleveland, CRC Press, 1974

——— et al: *Handbook on the Toxicology of Metals*. Amsterdam, Elsevier, 1979

Lead

CARNOW B (ed): *Health Effects of Occupational Lead and Arsenic Exposure, A Symposium*. Chicago, US Department of Health, Education, and Welfare, 1976

NATIONAL ACADEMY OF SCIENCES: *Lead in the Human Environment*. A Report Prepared by the Committee on Lead in the Human Environment, Environmental Studies Board, Commission on Natural Resources, National Research Council, Washington, DC, 1980

KEHOE RA: The metabolism of lead in man in health and disease. The Harben Lectures, 1960. J R Inst Pub Health 24:1, 101; 129; 177, 1961

PIOMELLIS et al: Management of childhood lead poisoning. J Pediatr 105:523, 1984

WALDRON HA, STOFEN D: *Sub-Clinical Lead Poisoning*. New York, Academic, 1974

Mercury

ELHASSANI SB: The many faces of methylmercury poisoning. J Toxicol Clin Toxicol 19:875, 1982–83

FRIBERG L, VOSTAL J (eds): *Mercury in the Environment*. Cleveland, CRC Press, 1972

NATIONAL ACADEMY OF SCIENCES: *An Assessment of Mercury in the Environment*, Washington, DC, 1978

PETERING HG, TEPPER LB: Pharmacology and toxicology of heavy metals: Mercury. Pharmacol Ther 1:131, 1976

WHO Environmental Health Criteria, Mercury. Geneva, World Health Organization, 1976

Thallium

BANK WJ et al: Thallium poisoning. Arch Neurol 26:456, 1972

CHISOLM JJ JR: The use of chelating agents in the treatment of acute and chronic lead intoxication in childhood. J Pediatr 73:1, 1968

DE GROOT G, VAN HEIJST ANP: Toxicokinetic aspects of thallium poisoning. Methods of treatment by toxin elimination. Sci Total Environ 71:411, 1988

——— et al: The evaluation of the efficacy of charcoal hemoperfusion in the treatment of three cases of thallium poisoning. Arch Toxicol 57:61, 1985

Chelating agents

HRUBY R, DONNER A: 2,3-Dimercapto-1-propanesulphonate in heavy metal poisoning, Med Toxicol 2:317, 1987

376 DISORDERS CAUSED BY VENOMS, BITES, AND STINGS

JAMES F. WALLACE

Humans have the propensity to come into contact with a great variety of venomous animals. These contacts occur with many zoologic classes including snakes, lizards, sea animals, spiders, scorpions, and numerous species of insects. In general two types of injuries result: those due to the direct effect of venom on the victim, as exemplified in snakebite, and those due to indirect effects of the poison, of which hypersensitivity reaction to bee stings is an example. Each year in the United States at least 50 persons die as the result of venomous injuries. Three groups of animals—hymenopterous insects, snakes, and spiders—account for over 90 percent of the fatalities. Of even greater public health significance is the loss in economic productivity and human potential resulting from the many serious, nonfatal envenomations that occur annually in otherwise healthy children or working adults.

SNAKE BITE

EPIDEMIOLOGY Fewer than one-tenth of the nearly 3500 known species of snakes are venomous. These poisonous varieties belong to five families or subfamilies: Elapidae (cobras, kraits, mambas, and coral snakes) found in all parts of the world except Europe; Viperidae (true vipers) found in all parts of the world except the Americas; Hydrophidae (sea snakes); Crotalidae (pit vipers) found in Asia and the Americas; and Colubridae (boomslangs, bird snakes) of the African continent. The poisonous varieties of the United States, with the single exception of the coral snake, are pit vipers and include rattlesnakes, the water moccasin, and the copperhead. Although this discussion centers around these species, most of the therapeutic measures outlined are applicable to snakes in all parts of the world.

The number of individuals bitten by poisonous snakes in the United States is estimated to be about 8000 per year, with a relatively large number occurring in the southeastern and Gulf states, particularly Texas. Deaths are not reported separately but are undoubtedly rare, numbering fewer than 20 per year, and most are due to bites of various species of rattlesnake. In many European countries deaths from snakebite have averaged only one every 3 to 5 years for the last half-century. In contrast, the estimate of annual deaths from snakebite throughout the world is between 30,000 and 40,000 with the largest number occurring in the countries of Burma and Brazil, where 2000 deaths are estimated to occur each year.

ETIOLOGY The *coral snake* is found in the southern states from Florida to Arizona. It is usually marked by alternating red and black bands separated by yellow rings; however, black and albino forms exist. Coral snakes are generally nocturnal in their activities, shy and elusive, and rarely bite humans. Their fangs are short and permanently erect; the highly toxic venom is injected into multiple puncture wounds produced by a series of chewing movements.

The *pit vipers* are so named because of a small pit between the eye and the nostril. Large venom glands in the temporal regions give the head a triangular appearance. They are generally aggressive and likely to strike if disturbed. The fangs are long and hinged, folding posteriorly when the mouth is closed. Pit vipers strike suddenly with a forward thrust of the head. The instant that the erect fangs make contact, venom is expressed by sudden muscular contraction.

The *rattlesnakes*, recognized by the horny rattle on the tail, which buzzes when the snake is disturbed, are widely distributed. The diamondbacks (*Crotalus adamanteus* in the southeast and *C. atrox* in the southwest) are the largest and most dangerous snakes in this country. Others include the prairie rattler (*C. confluentus*), the timber rattler (*C. horridus*), and the pigmy rattlers.

The *water moccasin*, or cottonmouth (*Agkistrodon piscivorus*), is found in swampy areas or along the banks of streams. It is a strong swimmer and can bite under water. This snake is notorious for inflicting severe facial bites when disturbed in the branches of small trees. The copperhead, or highland moccasin (*A. mokasen*), is a closely related species. Its bite is painful but rarely fatal.

PATHOGENESIS **Snake venoms** The venoms of most species that have been analyzed have been found to be mixtures of many toxic proteins and enzymes with diversified and complicated pharmacologic effects. As an example, the venom of the Indian cobra (*Naja naja*) contains these distinct and separate substances: a neurotoxin, a hemolysin, a cardiotoxin, a cholinesterase, at least three phosphatases, a nucleotidase, and a potent inhibitor of cytochrome oxidase. Several venoms, including those of the pit vipers, contain hyaluronidase and numerous proteolytic enzymes. Although the exact roles of these components in toxicity are incompletely understood, the venom of a given species is usually predominantly neurotoxic or necrotizing and is frequently associated with hemolysis, abnormalities of blood coagulation, changes in cardiac dynamics, and alterations in vascular resistance. Venoms of elapids, including the coral snake, are neurotoxic, with death resulting from respiratory paralysis probably caused by damage to brain centers and a curariform interference with transmission at the neuromuscular junction. Venoms of crotalid snakes produce local tissue injury, hemorrhage, and hemolysis. Death is often preceded by circulatory collapse associated with a marked fall in circulating blood volume resulting from pooling of blood in the microcirculation, and loss of plasma due to increased capillary permeability. Systemic absorption of venom occurs through the lymphatics, and therapeutic measures designed to reduce lymphatic function are helpful in controlling symptoms.

Factors affecting severity of snake bite Several factors affect the outcome of snake bite:

1 The age, size, and health of the patient. Envenomation in children is usually serious, and a fatal outcome is more likely, since a relatively large dose of poison is injected into a small victim.
2 Location of bite. Bites on extremities or into adipose tissue are less dangerous than those on the trunk, face, or directly into a blood vessel. A direct strike of the fangs is more dangerous than a scratch, a glancing blow, or one hitting a bone. The discharge orifice of a fang is well above its tip so that the point of the fang can penetrate the skin without envenomation; even a thin layer of clothing may afford great protection. Because of the superficial nature of the wound, as many as one-fifth of patients bitten by venomous snakes will have no evidence of envenomation, even though the fangs have penetrated the skin.
3 The size of the snake (a large pit viper can inject over 1000 mg venom, six times a lethal dose for an adult), the extent of its anger or fear (if hurt it may inject a larger amount of venom), the condition of the fangs (broken or recently renewed), and the condition of the venom glands (recently discharged or full). All these factors are important. Contrary to popular belief, the bite of a snake which has recently killed and fed is not necessarily less venomous for humans; the snake usually does not exhaust its venom in a single bite.
4 The presence of various bacteria, particularly clostridia and other anaerobic organisms, in the mouth of the snake or on the skin of the victim. This may lead to serious infection in the necrotic tissues at the local site.
5 Exercise or exertion, such as running, immediately after the bite. This speeds systemic absorption of toxin.

MANIFESTATIONS Following the bite of a pit viper, severe burning pain develops within a few minutes at the site of the wound. Local swelling rapidly develops and spreads in all directions, accompanied by the appearance of ecchymoses and bullae over the involved area. As the edema spreads, serosanguinous fluid oozes from the puncture wounds. Later gangrene of the skin and subcutaneous tissues may develop. Systemic effects resulting from the absorption of venom and local tissue destruction may include fever, nausea and vomiting, circulatory collapse, bleeding into the skin and from all body orifices, low-grade jaundice, neuropathic muscle cramping, pupillary constriction, disorientation, delirium, and convulsions. Death may occur after 6 to 48 h. Survival may be attended by massive local tissue loss from gangrene or secondary infection, or may be complicated by acute renal failure, secondary to disseminated intravascular clotting and cortical necrosis, or by tubular necrosis following circulatory collapse.

The bite of the coral snake causes little pain and local swelling. There are usually multiple fang marks. Within 10 to 15 min numbness and weakness begin in the region of the bite, followed by ataxia, ptosis, pupillary dilatation, palatal and pharyngeal paralysis, slurring of speech, salivation, and occasionally nausea and vomiting. The patient becomes comatose, develops respiratory paralysis and seizures, and dies within 8 to 72 h.

Cobra bites are painful and are often accompanied by severe hemolysis, local necrosis, and sloughing in addition to their neurotoxic effects. There is little pain and no edema at the site of a sea snake bite. Symptoms of systemic envenomation follow a latent period which may vary from 15 min to 8 h. Although the venom is both myotoxic and neurotoxic, the injury to skeletal muscle is most prominent and is characterized by generalized muscle pain, weakness, and myoglobinuria. Hemorrhagic manifestations predominate following envenomation by colubrids (boomslangs and bird snakes) and many pit vipers including certain species of rattlesnake.

LABORATORY ABNORMALITIES In severe cases, laboratory abnormalities may include progressive anemia, polymorphonuclear leukocytosis of 20,000 to 30,000 cells per microliter, thrombocytopenia, hypofibrinogenemia, disordered tests of coagulation, proteinuria, and azotemia.

TREATMENT An attempt should be made to determine with certainty that the patient has been bitten by a poisonous snake. Absence of distinct fang punctures and failure of local pain, edema, numbness, or weakness to appear within 20 min are strong evidence against snake venom poisoning. The approximate size of the snake should be noted since larger snakes usually cause more severe envenomation. If the species of snake is not known, the offending reptile should be killed for the purpose of identification.

First aid This consists of reassuring and calming the victim, instituting measures to retard the absorption of venom and to remove it from the tissues as quickly as possible after the bite, and arranging for transportation to the nearest hospital. The patient should be promptly placed at rest and the bitten extremity immobilized to reduce the rate of spread of the venom. This is best achieved by splinting. If anatomically feasible, a wide constriction band should be placed a few centimeters above the bite and made tight enough to allow one finger to pass beneath with difficulty. The purpose is to impede lymph flow; it is not necessary to obstruct venous return. The band should be loosened and moved proximally when local swelling causes it to tighten. There is no evidence in humans that incision and suction of the wound remove significant amounts of venom or improve outcome. Therefore this procedure is no longer recommended.

In order to help assess the severity of envenomation, the level of swelling should be marked on the skin every 15 min while the patient is being transported to a hospital. Although ice packs relieve pain and slow lymphatic drainage, they do not neutralize venom, and even a small amount of cooling may result in irreparable damage to already injured tissues by causing ischemia. For this reason, it is recommended that no form of cryotherapy be used.

Immediate hospital care This should include appropriate treatment for shock and respiratory difficulty, antivenin, measures to combat infection, and general supportive care. Initial laboratory studies in a patient with obvious crotalid envenomation should include blood typing and cross-matching, a complete blood count, urinalysis, coagulation screening tests, blood urea nitrogen (BUN), blood glucose, and serum electrolytes. In severe envenomations it is also advisable to obtain an electrocardiogram. None of these tests are particularly helpful in the initial evaluation of a patient with a coral snake bite.

Antivenin is the only specific treatment of snake venom poisoning, and its use in severe bites is vital. In the United States polyvalent crotaline antivenin effective against all American pit vipers and antivenin for North American coral snake poisoning are commercially available. Both products are a lyophilized powder of refined horse serum. Kits are available containing antivenin powder (reconstituted by diluting with water to 10 mL per vial), syringe, normal horse serum for prior sensitivity testing of the patient, and detailed instructions. Intravenously administered antivenin leads to the most rapid and effective response. It is not advisable to infiltrate antivenin at the local site. The initial dose should depend upon an estimate of the amount of envenomation. For pit viper bites accompanied by progressive local swelling but no systemic symptoms (minimal envenomation), 5 vials (50 mL) are usually sufficient. When swelling has progressed beyond the site of the bite, and mild systemic symptoms and/or hematologic and coagulation abnormalities are present, moderate envenomation has occurred, and initial treatment should be 5 to 15 vials (50 to 150 mL). For severe poisonings, associated with rapidly progressive and extensive local effects as well as systemic symptoms and evidence of hemolysis or coagulopathy, 15 to 20 vials (150 to 200 mL) or more should be administered. Up to 50 percent greater doses of antivenin should be given to children or small adults to neutralize the relatively higher venom concentrations. Reconstituted antivenin is diluted in 500 mL of intravenous fluid and administered as rapidly as tolerated over 1 to 2 h. Additional infusions containing 5 to 10 vials (50 to 100 mL) should be repeated every 2 h until progressive swelling in the bitten part ceases and systemic signs and symptoms have disappeared. When an adequate dose has been achieved, improvement in the victim's clinical signs is often extremely rapid.

If *any* evidence of envenomation appears during the first several hours following a coral snake bite, antivenin should be given without waiting for systemic manifestations to develop. Four vials of antivenin should be given intravenously for bites associated only with minimal swelling and/or local paresthesias. If evidence of a bite is more definitive, particularly if there was initial pain, 6 to 10 vials of antivenin should be given as soon as possible. Larger doses should be used in severe bites from large snakes, if the snake bite was prolonged for more than a few seconds, or if the victim is a child.

In the patient with severe envenomation who is allergic to horse serum, the relative risk of death from anaphylaxis rather than from venom poisoning should be carefully weighed before undertaking desensitization with small doses of diluted horse serum.

No antivenin for other snakes is manufactured in the United States, but antiserum for various types is usually kept on hand at large zoos all over the world. A national antivenin index is maintained by the Oklahoma Poison Information Center in cooperation with the Oklahoma City Zoo [(405) 271–5454], and provides 24-h telephone consultation service for physicians needing advice in handling snakebite accidents.

Maintaining *respiration* by mechanical or other means is important. In patients bitten by elapid snakes, respiratory failure is usually reversible. *Tetanus toxoid* or *tetanus immune globulin* of human origin should be given (see Chap. 105). If wound infections appear, antibiotics should be used with the knowledge that the predominant microorganisms in the mouths of snakes are gram-negative pathogens. Treatment should be preceded by appropriate aerobic and anaerobic cultures. *Fasciotomy* occasionally may be necessary to prevent further ischemic injury to a massively swollen limb. Whenever possible, intracompartmental tissue pressures should be monitored, with surgical decompression undertaken only if pressure exceeds 30 to 40 mmHg. *Surgical debridement* of vesicles and superficial necrotic tissue should be instituted near the end of the first week following the bite. *Relief of pain* with salicylates or meperidine, moderate sedation, maintenance of fluid balance, measures to combat shock and hemorrhagic diathesis, and appropriate management of coma or convulsions are all important.

The usefulness of glucocorticoids to prevent tissue damage or systemic intoxication has not been convincingly demonstrated. However, these drugs may be of value in the management of severe shock associated with envenomation and for allergic reactions, particularly serum sickness, following the administration of antivenin.

PREVENTION In snake-infested regions long trousers, high shoes, boots, or leggings, and gloves should be worn. Most important of all is to look where one steps or reaches. A constriction band and antiseptic suffice for an emergency kit, and in inaccessible areas, antivenin should also be carried.

POISONOUS LIZARD BITE

Of the nearly 3000 species of lizard in the world, only two are venomous: the Gila monster (*Heloderma suspectum*) of the arid southwestern United States and the closely related Mexican beaded lizard (*H. horridum*) which inhabits the lowland forests of western Mexico. These reptiles are not aggressive, and virtually every instance of their attacking a human has involved teasing or handling the animals in captivity. The venom is elaborated in eight glands in the floor of the mouth and secreted directly into the oral cavity, where it bathes the teeth, which are grooved posteriorly. The lizard clings tenaciously and is often dislodged only after considerable effort; envenomation occurs by contamination of the wound. The venom contains a potent neurotoxin which is undoubtedly responsible for its lethal effect on experimental animals. Death in humans following a bite is extremely rare. Most often, human envenomation results in tissue injury, excruciating pain, massive edema, and patchy erythema. Acute systemic symptoms may last for 3 to 4 days and include nausea, vomiting, hematemesis, blurred vision, dyspnea, dysphonia, and profound weakness. Intense hyperesthesia of the bitten extremity may persist for several weeks. There is no antivenin available. Treatment should consist of constriction band, cooling of the bitten area, measures to prevent or combat infection, including tetanus, and supportive measures. Parenteral meperidine (Demerol) or infiltration of local anesthetic around the bite may be necessary to relieve pain.

SPIDER BITES

The bite of many spiders is locally irritating, and several species can cause severe, even fatal systemic poisoning in humans. In North America, only two types of spiders are of medical importance: the widow spiders (*Latrodectus* species) and the recluse spiders (*Loxosceles* species).

WIDOW SPIDER BITE The most numerous and important of the venomous spiders are members of the genus *Latrodectus,* widely distributed throughout the world. In the United States and Canada, *L. mactans,* the black widow or show-button spider, causes a majority of clinically significant arachnidism. In Florida, *L. bishopi,* the red-legged widow spider, has been reported to produce human poisoning resembling mild black widow bite.

It is the female *L. mactans,* the black widow, that bites humans. She is glossy black with a body 1 cm in diameter, a leg span of 5 cm, and a characteristic red hourglass mark on her abdomen. She spins her web in woodpiles, sheds, basements, or outdoor privies, is very aggressive, and will bite on slight provocation. The venom produces diffuse central and peripheral nervous excitement, autonomic activity, muscle spasm, hypertension, and vasoconstriction.

In the United States, most black widow bites occur between April and October, and many patients are males bitten on the genitalia or buttocks while using a privy. After a momentary sharp pain at the site, there is cramping pain that begins locally within 15 to 60 min and gradually spreads. It may involve all extremities and the trunk. The abdomen is boardlike, and the waves of pain become excruciating, causing the patient to turn, toss, and cry out. Respirations are often labored and grunting. There are also nausea, vomiting, headache, sweating, salivation, hyperactive reflexes, twitching, tremor, paresthesias of the hands and feet, and occasionally, systolic hypertension. A mild polymorphonuclear leukocytosis is usual, and many patients have slight fever. After several hours, the pains subside, although mild recurrences for 2 or 3 days are common. It may be a week before well-being is restored. Deaths due to cardiac or respiratory failure have occurred, mostly in children and the aged.

Because the bite itself is not prominent, patients are often thought to have some abdominal catastrophe such as perforated ulcer, pancreatitis, or appendicitis. Renal colic, myocardial infarction, tetanus, strychnine poisoning, tabetic crisis, lead colic, and porphyria are other conditions to be ruled out. The abdomen is not tender to palpation in arachnidism, and pains in the extremities are not typical of most of these other disorders.

TREATMENT For *Latrodectus* poisoning, treatment consists of measures to relieve pain and administration of antivenin. Initial treatment should include a hot tub bath which affords prompt, although temporary, relief. A vial (10 mL) of 10% calcium gluconate slowly injected intravenously over 10 to 20 min usually produces dramatic, but transient, cessation of cramps. A solution of 10% methocarbamol administered intravenously also may be effective in treatment of muscle spasms. Opiates are sometimes necessary. When symptoms are severe or when the patient is a small child or is at special risk due to other associated medical problems, treatment with *Latrodectus* antivenin is indicated. An intravenous injection of 1 vial (2.5 mL) diluted in 50 mL of saline and administered over a 15-min period is usually quite effective within a few hours and can be repeated if symptoms recur. Since the antivenin is prepared from horse serum, appropriate testing for hypersensitivity should be undertaken prior to its administration.

***LOXOSCELES* SPIDER BITE** During the past 30 years in the United States, there have been increasing numbers of reports of severe necrotizing bites due to *Loxosceles* spiders. Originally thought to be a problem only in the midwestern states and associated only with the brown recluse spider, necrotic arachnidism has now been seen in many of the southern and southwestern states as well as in California and has been attributed to at least six species of *Loxosceles* spider. The bite of these spiders may initially produce only a mild stinging discomfort. In severe bites, intense local pain appears within 2 to 8 h, accompanied by bullae formation and erythema at the site of the wound. Subsequently, ischemic necrosis occurs leaving a deep ulcer with a necrotic base. The pathogenetic mechanism for the local reaction is not completely understood but is thought to involve complement-activated tissue damage. Some patients also experience a systemic reaction characterized by fever, myalgias, and a morbilliform rash 24 to 48 h after the bite. Intravascular hemolysis is seen occasionally, and in severe cases hemoglobinuria and acute renal failure may occur. Fatalities have been reported, mostly in children.

Treatment depends upon the severity of the bite. If bullae formation, intense pain, and signs of rapidly progressing ischemic necrosis do not appear within the first 6 to 8 h, the bite is probably not severe and treatment is unnecessary. When symptoms of more serious local reaction are present, the parenteral use of glucocorticoids within the first 24 h following a bite has been advocated to prevent progression of the lesion, but convincing evidence that this is effective is lacking. Dapsone and/or brown recluse antivenin have been reported to prevent extensive ulceration in rapidly progressing *Loxosceles* spider bites. However, use of these forms of therapy should be considered experimental. Other therapeutic measures consist mainly of local wound care including cool compresses, elevation of the bitten extremity, timely surgical debridement, and treatment of secondary infection, if it occurs. The ulcer usually heals spontaneously, although skin grafting may be required on occasion. Patients with systemic loxoscelism should be hospitalized and monitored closely for signs of hemolysis, disseminated intravascular coagulation, and acute renal failure. Although of unproven efficacy, systemic glucocorticoids are usually given only for the duration of the acute phase of the illness, which lasts 2 to 4 days. Renal failure should be treated as advised in Chap. 223.

SCORPION STING

Scorpions are eight-legged arthropods. Glands in the terminal segment produce venom, which is injected into the victim by a stinger located on the tip of the tail. Scorpions often enter dwellings. During the day they retreat into crevices; emerging at night, they often get into shoes and clothing and even into bedding. They do not deliberately attack humans, but accidental contact results in a sting.

Of about 650 species, roughly 40 occur in the United States, distributed over three-fourths of the nation. They are most numerous in the south from Florida to California, but the only dangerous species, *Centruroides exilicauda,* is limited to Arizona, New Mexico, southern California, parts of Texas, and northern Mexico. This species reaches a maximal length of about 7 cm. Their sting may be fatal to young children or old people, but seldom to a healthy adult.

Most of the nonlethal species of scorpions in the United States cause only minor reactions, like a bee sting. Some in the southwest, however, produce local edema and ecchymosis, with burning pain. In contrast, many species whose venom has potentially lethal systemic effects, including the Arizona *Centruroides,* evoke little or no visible reaction at the site of the sting. There is an immediate burning sensation followed by local paresthesia (''pins and needles''), hyperesthesia, or numbness. These sensations spread to involve the whole extremity, and within an hour or two, malaise, restlessness, neurologic hyperexcitability, lacrimation, rhinorrhea, salivation, perspiration, nausea, and vomiting may appear.

The patient may pass from an agitated state with hyperactive reflexes into coma; convulsions follow. Release of catecholamines may result in tachycardia, various arrhythmias, and hypertension. Myocarditis and pancreatitis have also been reported. Death usually occurs within 12 h, but sometimes as late as 2 days after the sting.

TREATMENT Despite the reputation for lethality associated with envenomation by *C. exilicauda,* most often the symptoms consist only of pain and paresthesias lasting less than 4 h. These patients can be treated at home with cold compresses and mild analgesics. There is no clear consensus on the management of more severe envenomations. Although the use of constriction bands as in the treatment of snake bite has been recommended, the amount of venom is minute; it produces no local necrotizing effect and is absorbed very rapidly.

Specific antivenin, reconstituted from lyophilized goat serum, is available in some areas and should be considered if the victim develops signs of cranial nerve dysfunction and increased involuntary activity in skeletal muscles other than those innervated by cranial nerves. An intravenous injection of 1 or 2 vials (5.0 or 10.0 mL) administered over 15 to 30 min usually reverses the severe neurologic symptoms within minutes following the infusion. Supportive therapy is directed at combating shock and dehydration. Diazepam or phenobarbital are useful in reducing restlessness, and adrenergic blockers in managing symptoms secondary to catecholamine release.

PREVENTION This depends upon alertness in avoiding contact with scorpions in infested areas. Clothing and shoes should be well shaken before being put on in the morning. Towels and bedclothes should be inspected. A house infested with scorpions can in time be rid of them by closing all obvious ways of ingress; picking up debris in the environment, such as piles of brush, logs, stones; introducing a mixture of fuel oil or kerosene, containing a small amount of creosote, between the earth and the house foundation; and spraying with a mixture of 2% chlordane, and 0.2% pyrethrins in an oil base.

HYMENOPTERA STINGS

Each year in the United States, nearly twice as many people die as a result of bites by hymenopterous insects (including bees, wasps, hornets, yellow jackets, and fire ants) as from poisonous snake bites. Occasionally, multiple stings in enormous numbers (500 to 1000) are the cause of death. However, the majority of systemic reactions and deaths are due to allergic reactions to the venoms of these insects.

Hymenoptera venoms contain many nonallergenic amines and peptides such as histamine and various kinins which contribute to the local sting reaction through their inflammatory and vasoactive properties. The allergenic venom proteins, which elicit an IgE antibody response in those who are stung, include phospholipases, hyaluronidases, acid phosphatases, and melittin. Venoms are distinctly different for each of the three genera of hymenoptera capable of causing allergic sting reactions: Apidae (various species of bees), Vespidae (hornets, yellowjackets, and wasps), and *Solenopsis* (fire ants).

The usual reaction to a single bee or wasp sting is sharp pain, which lasts for several minutes, local wheal and erythema, followed by intense itching. All signs of the sting normally subside within a few hours. Only in the rare case when a bee is swallowed or inhaled and edema of the laryngopharynx or glottis develops is there danger. A sting directly into a peripheral nerve can destroy its function for a time, much as does an injection of alcohol. Bell's palsy has followed a sting into the trunk of the facial nerve. Unusual reactions such as optic neuritis, generalized polyneuropathy, and myasthenia gravis may follow a sting. The etiology of these reactions is unknown. Acute renal failure has been reported following multiple bee stings. Nephrotoxicity, due to venom-induced rhabdomyolysis, and renal ischemia are thought to be the probable mechanisms.

In hypersensitive individuals, the response to a single sting may vary from an exaggerated local reaction, unassociated with systemic symptoms, to serious anaphylaxis with urticaria, nausea, abdominal or uterine cramps, bronchospasm, massive edema of the face and glottis, dyspnea, cyanosis, hypotension, coma, and death. These symptoms usually appear within a few minutes of the sting. Other patients may experience delayed reactions of the serum-sickness type occurring 10 to 14 days after envenomation. Sensitization is usually the result of previous stings although many fatalities have occurred in individuals who experienced no apparent allergic reaction to earlier envenomation. It has been estimated that 10 to 15 percent of the general population in this country has hymenoptera venom allergy. Those who have experienced a previous systemic allergic reaction to a sting, such as respiratory difficulty, hypotension, or generalized urticaria, are at greatest risk for serious reactions if stung again by the same type of insect.

Since being accidentally introduced into southern Brazil in 1957, African bees have gradually spread through South and Central America. Within the next decade, their northernmost advance will be achieved and is expected to encompass the southern portion of the United States from North Carolina to southern California. Although widely touted as a human health problem, the actual risk is difficult to estimate because of a lack of reliable medical statistics. African bee venom appears to be qualitatively similar to that of European bees, although the median lethal dose may be smaller. Further research is needed to determine its toxocologic and pathologic characteristics.

Many species of ant can produce stinging bites with local redness and swelling. The most notorious of these are the fire ants (*Solenopsis*), particularly two "imported" South American species (*S. invicta* and *S. richteri*). The *invicta* species is now found in thirteen southern states and has largely supplanted all others, including several domestic species. In addition to being a major agricultural pest, fire ants, whose bites may result in extensive vesiculation and skin necrosis or cause serious hypersensitivity reactions, have become a significant health hazard to humans. Unlike other hymenoptera venoms, fire ant venom is mostly a simple insoluble alkaloid rather than a complex mixture of proteins. Although associated with life-threatening allergic reactions of the type seen with IgE-mediated immediate hypersensitivity, there is limited cross-sensitivity between fire ant venom and the venoms of bees, wasps, hornets, and yellowjackets.

TREATMENT The wound site should be examined for a stinger which, if present, should be carefully removed in order to prevent further envenomation from the attached gland. The local reaction to the usual sting is treated by local cool application and antipruritic lotions or oral antihistamines. Fire ant stings, which are frequently multiple, should be thoroughly cleaned with soap and water. Secondary bacterial infection is common and should be anticipated and treated promptly. Epinephrine, 0.3 to 0.5 mL of a 1:1000 aqueous solution subcutaneously repeated every 20 to 30 min, may be lifesaving in patients with an anaphylactic reaction to a sting. A tourniquet to slow the absorption of venom and ice packs to relieve pain may be used. Oxygen, endotracheal intubation, vasopressors, and other supportive measures should be used as needed. In addition, glucocorticoids should be employed in severe cases, although their maximum effect is not achieved until several hours after administration.

PREVENTION Allergic persons should make every effort to avoid contact with these insects, including wearing shoes when outside and not wearing perfumes or bright colors which may attract them. In addition, they should keep epinephrine readily available for immediate use in case of a sting, without waiting for symptoms to develop. Sting kits containing premeasured doses of 1:1000 epinephrine in disposable syringes, tourniquets, and antihistamine tablets are commercially available. Careful instruction in their use should be provided by the person's physician.

IMMUNOTHERAPY Desensitization by injection of preparations containing venom of the specific insect has long been recommended for any patient who has had a systemic or generalized reaction to hymenopterous insect stings. For many years, the only products available for this purpose were extracts of the crushed whole bodies of the stinging insect. However, skin testing with whole-body extracts was frequently unreliable in identifying persons at risk for systemic reactions, and immunization with these materials did not increase IgG-blocking antibodies to venom proteins, a response felt to be essential for protection against insect allergy. In contrast, purified hymenopterous venoms, which were approved for clinical use in the United States in 1979, have proved to be highly accurate in the diagnosis of sting allergy by skin testing. In addition, venom immunotherapy has been shown consistently to stimulate production of circulating venom specific IgG antibodies, and to provide much better protection than whole-body extracts. The purified venoms have not been associated with a greater number of adverse reactions than treatment with whole-body extracts or with desensitization for pollinosis. These venom antigens are the materials of choice for diagnosis and immunotherapy of high-risk patients, those who have had previous systemic sting reactions and who have positive venom skin tests. The optimal duration of immunotherapy remains to be defined.

TICK BITE

Although ticks may be vectors for such serious diseases as Rocky Mountain spotted fever, Q fever, tularemia, borreliosis, human babesiosis, and Lyme disease, the local reaction to the bite of a tick may be nothing more than an itching papule that subsides within a few days unless there is secondary bacterial infection. However, incomplete removal of a tick, with retention of the mouthparts, may result in the local formation of a nodule that continues to grow and is sometimes annoyingly pruritic. The definitive treatment is surgical excision of the nodule. Histologically, the nodule is a granuloma, but the inflammatory response is sometimes so bizarre and changes in the overlying epithelium are so striking that, in the absence of a history of tick bite, a mistaken diagnosis of malignant tumor may be made.

Ticks should always be removed intact, using gentle, steady traction. Fine tweezers or blunt forceps should be employed if possible. When fingers are used instead, they should be protected with facial tissue and washed afterwards. Application of a drop of oil, petrolatum, nail polish, or other organic solvent may facilitate removal without leaving embedded remnants. However, touching with a hot object such as a glowing cigarette should be discouraged because of the likelihood of injuring the patient.

TICK PARALYSIS A progressive, ascending, flaccid paralysis, acute ataxia, or a combination of both sometimes develops in humans and certain other mammals while a tick is engorging upon them. Human cases have most frequently been reported from the northwestern United States and western Canada, where the wood tick, *Dermacentor andersoni* Stiles, is responsible. The dog tick, *D. variabilis* Say, has been identified in a number of cases occurring in the southeastern states. *Amblyomma americanum*, the Lone Star tick, *A. maculatum*, the Gulf Coast tick, and *Ixodes scapularis*, the black-legged deer tick, have also been incriminated.

This disorder is caused by a neurotoxin secreted in the saliva of the engorging tick which acts upon spinal and bulbar nuclei, slowing motor nerve conduction without affecting neuromuscular transmission. The tick must feed for several days before symptoms develop.

Most human cases occur in children, generally in young girls. The tick is usually attached to the scalp and hidden by the hair, but may be found on any part of the body, especially the ear, axilla, groin, vulva, or popliteal region.

The patient may be irritable or restless for up to 24 h before frank motor involvement appears. Weakness usually is noted first in the distal muscles of the lower extremities, progressing over the next 24 to 48 h to flaccid paralysis, which may extend to involve the trunk, arms, neck, tongue, pharynx, and bulbar centers. Sensory changes are typically absent, and there is little or no fever unless a secondary infection is present. Results of routine laboratory tests including cerebrospinal fluid examination are normal. Nerve conduction studies may reveal decreased velocities and compound action potentials of nerves and their corresponding muscles.

Tick paralysis is apt to be confused with poliomyelitis, the more so because ticks are active in warm weather when poliomyelitis is most prevalent. Among other diseases which might be considered in differential diagnosis are diphtheritic polyneuropathy, transverse myelitis, the Guillain-Barré syndrome, myasthenia gravis, the Eaton-Lambert syndrome, and botulism.

Definitive treatment is removal of the tick, including any mouthparts retained in the skin. After this is done, there is striking improvement of motor function within a few hours and complete recovery within 48 h.

The patient should be observed until the recovery trend is established, because if other ticks or retained mouthparts have been overlooked, the paralysis may progress. When bulbar or respiratory paralysis is present, death may occur if the tick is not removed in time. The mortality rate is 10 percent; nearly all who die are children.

OTHER ARTHROPOD BITES AND ENVENOMATIONS

FLEA BITE There are many fleas that attack humans, including *Pulex irritans* and chicken fleas. In sensitive individuals, the salivary secretion of these bloodsuckers produces large, itching papules. It is thought that much of the papular urticaria of children is probably due to flea bites. Treatment is symptomatic only. Elimination of fleas from the environment may be very difficult, but persistent treatment of animals and of premises with appropriate insecticides is usually successful.

CENTIPEDE BITE The giant desert centipede, which reaches 15 cm in length, is responsible for most centipede bites in the United States. It is capable of inflicting an intensely painful bite, associated with erythema, edema, and sometimes with regional lymphangitis. Rhabdomyolysis and acute renal failure have occurred following the bite of this arthropod. Pain usually disappears within a few hours, but may require oral or parenteral analgesics. The wound should be washed well with soap and water to help prevent secondary infection.

CATERPILLAR RASH Contact with the early larval or caterpillar stage of several species of moth produces irritation of skin and mucous membranes resulting in a pruritic, erythematous rash, occasionally accompanied by urticaria and bullae. Symptoms come on rapidly after direct contact with caterpillars, after handling cocoons, or on being exposed to windblown fuzz. The pathogenesis is thought to be due to the direct irritant effects of insect hairs or appendages, although other mechanisms, including intracutaneous injection of toxins or hypersensitivity to insect antigens, have been suggested. The symptoms usually subside within a few days. Local soaks and oral antihistamines are often indicated.

BEDBUG BITE Members of the genus *Cimex* inflict bites that leave reactions varying from a simple puncture to large urticarial lesions, apparently depending on the sensitivity of the bitten individual. There is no specific treatment.

KISSING BUG BITE Of the many species of true bugs, those in the family Reduviidae are relatively commonly associated with severe bite reactions. The most important reduviid bug in this country is the kissing bug (genus *Triatoma*), which is found throughout the southern crescent of the United States. The bites of this bug, which is a nocturnal feeder, are characteristically inflicted in multiple groups. Reactions which follow are thought to be allergic in nature and may include intensely pruritic and painful papules with a central punctum, grouped vesicles with moderate swelling and redness but no central lesions, giant urticaria, generalized allergic reactions, including systemic anaphylaxis, and hemorrhagic nodular-to-bullous lesions on a hand or foot, appearing several days after the bite. These may be confused with necrotizing spider bites or with erythema multiforme. However, the former are usually single lesions and the latter rarely has a unilateral distribution. The possibility of kissing bug bites should be considered in patients who awaken in the middle of the night with intense itching, hives, and other signs of a systemic allergic reaction.

Treatment of the local reaction is symptomatic. More severe reactions should be managed similarly to other allergic sting reactions. Patients who have had accelerated reactions to reduviid bites should be provided with sting kits and instructions in their use. Immunotherapy with whole body extracts of kissing bugs has been attempted but its value is unproven.

CHIGGERS OR REDBUGS These are tiny mites that are commonly found in foliage or grass in many parts of the world. In the United States, the larval form of *Eutrobicula alfreddugesi* attacks the skin by secreting a substance which digests tissue, creating a red papule that itches intensely. The tiny reddish larva can be seen in the center of the lesion. Treatment is palliative and consists of antipruritic applications. The use of insect repellents, appropriate protective clothing, and prompt bathing after exposure reduce the risk of infestation considerably.

BLOODSUCKING-FLY BITE Many species of flies, particularly the horsefly and the deerfly, viciously attack and feed upon warm-blooded animals, including humans. Occasionally, transmission of diseases such as anthrax, tularemia, loiasis, and trypanosomiasis has been attributed to horseflies and deerflies. More commonly in North America, however, their bites are responsible for painful, intensely pruritic cutaneous lesions which may be followed by delayed localized allergic reactions characterized by erythema, edema, and urticaria. Treatment should include thorough cleaning of the bite sites, topical glucocorticoids, and oral antihistaminics for severe itching. Antibiotics may be necessary if the wounds become secondarily infected.

MARINE ANIMAL VENOM DISEASES

The venoms of certain marine animals are known to cause illness in humans after injection or inoculation under naturally occurring conditions. Information concerning these toxins is limited; most appear to be composed of proteins and peptides as well as other substances that are pharmacologically active. Although probably less complex than the venoms of reptiles, many marine animal venoms are capable of causing several pathologic effects including neurotoxicity as well as local necrosis.

PORTUGUESE MAN-OF-WAR AND JELLYFISH STINGS The burning discomfort induced by contact with sea nettles or jellyfish is familiar to most surf bathers. Contact with the tentacles of the colorful Portuguese man-of-war (*Physalia* species), which is found mainly in or near the Gulf of Mexico, or the more toxic jellyfish (*Chiropsalmus* of the Indian Ocean and *Rhizostoma* of the Atlantic) is followed by burning pain, swelling, and erythema. Severe, generalized muscular cramps, nausea, vomiting, and pulmonary edema may occur. Victims have died as a result of jellyfish stings, sometimes within minutes after contact. In nonfatal cases, systemic symptoms usually subside within several hours. Treatment consists of bathing the wound in salt water, taking care not to rub the area of the sting. Next, any tentacles still clinging to the skin should be scraped off after first inactivating any remaining nematocysts to prevent discharge of additional venom into the victim. This can be done by sprinkling baking soda over the wound to form a slurry for sea nettle stings or by bathing with vinegar for man-of-war stings. Rinsing with fresh water, isopropyl alcohol, or household ammonia, or rubbing with sand are not recommended since these measures may actually cause nematocysts to discharge. Analgesics should be used for pain control, and antihistaminics if there is an accompanying pruritic rash. Severe envenomations may require advanced life-support measures. Glucocorticoids may be helpful in these cases. An antivenin is now available for treatment of stings by the highly lethal Australian sea wasp, *Chironex fleckeri*.

CORAL WOUNDS AND STINGS The colorful structures known as coral are composed of thousands of small marine animals of the coelenterate phylum, surrounded by a stony exoskeleton of calcium carbonate. Several species, including the fire coral, found in many parts of the world, contain microscopic nematocysts capable of producing painful stings similar to those caused by jellyfish. Often more serious are wounds resulting from abrasions and cuts by the sharp edges of the outer skeleton. These frequently contain small pieces of animal protein and skeletal material that act as foreign bodies and may lead to chronic, suppurative wound infections if not promptly and adequately debrided.

SEA ANEMONE STING ("SPONGE DIVER'S DISEASE") Contact with certain sea anemones (especially *Sargatia elegans*) in Mediterranean and African waters produces extensive dermatitis with chronic ulceration. Occasionally, especially during August and September, systemic symptoms of headache, sneezing, nausea, chills, fever, and collapse are noted. Rare fatalities have occurred. Application of vinegar may inactivate nematocyst discharge. No other specific therapy is known; symptomatic treatment with topical steroids or oral antihistaminics may provide temporary relief.

CONE SHELL POISONING The colorful cone shells are highly prized by collectors. However, many species in the Pacific are venomous, a great danger to unwary hobbyists who pick them up. The poison, a neurotoxin, is delivered into a wound inflicted by pointed hollow teeth resembling darts in the long proboscis of the animal. Local manifestations include sudden intense pain, followed by swelling and numbness, which may persist for several days. Symptoms of serious poisoning include muscular incoordination and weakness progressing to respiratory paralysis. Death may occur within 3 to 6 h, but recovery within 24 h is the rule. There is no specific therapy; recommended treatment is the use of tourniquet, incision, and suction and supportive measures which may include artificial respiration and administration of oxygen.

SPONGE DERMATITIS Direct contact with several species of sponge results in a painful dermatitis, which may persist for several weeks. The lesions appear to be caused by mechanical irritation from the exoskeleton of the sponge as well as by toxins within its tissues. Delayed hypersensitivity reactions may also occur. Topical glucocorticoids or oral antihistamines may provide relief from the pruritus; dilute acetic acid ameliorates local pain, while alkali will intensify it. The lesions are self-limited.

SEA URCHIN WOUNDS AND STINGS Contact with the spines of some species of sea urchin results in painful erythema and ulceration, occasionally accompanied by neurotoxic symptoms of weakness and frank paralysis of lips, tongue, and face lasting for several hours. Treatment is purely symptomatic and supportive. The toxins isolated from sea urchins have produced paralysis in animals and are notably resistant to heat. Deaths from paralysis and drowning have been reported. Occasionally, fragments of sea urchin spines may remain in the skin, leading to granulomatous reactions, or they may migrate into a joint or lodge against a nerve, causing intractable pain. Treatment of these complications is surgical.

PARALYTIC AND NEUROTOXIC SHELLFISH POISONING Certain dinoflagellates, which make up part of the marine phytoplankton, elaborate a potent neurotoxin. Occasionally, conditions in coastal waters become favorable for the growth of excessive numbers of these organisms, causing the water to develop an amber appearance termed the "red tide" and killing massive numbers of fish by exhausting their oxygen supply. When humans ingest shellfish which have themselves ingested toxic dinoflagellates, an illness occurs that is characterized by paresthesias of the face and extremities, dysphonia, and generalized muscular weakness, often accompanied by nausea, vomiting, and diarrhea and occasionally by paralysis and respiratory arrest. The more severe syndrome, known as paralytic shellfish poisoning, is encountered along the Pacific northwest and New England coasts. A milder form, not associated with paralysis in humans, is seen along the Gulf and Atlantic coasts of Florida. Treatment should include induced emesis and purgation to remove unabsorbed toxin from the gastrointestinal tract and whatever additional supportive measures are necessary. Spontaneous recovery usually takes place within 24 h. There is a standardized mouse bioassay procedure for demonstrating and quantitating toxin in shellfish but no diagnostic test for detecting toxin in clinical specimens.

VENOMOUS FISH INJURIES The dorsal fins or spines of bullhead sharks, dogfish, and ratfish and the dorsal and other fins of the lionfish, weeverfish, toadfish, and catfish are grooved, and at their bases are found venom glands. Little is known of the venoms involved except that they contain highly unstable proteins of variable molecular weights and are capable of causing toxic as well as allergic reactions.

Envenomation results in immediate, severe local pain and edema which, if untreated, reaches greatest intensity in 60 to 90 min and resolves within 8 to 12 h. Local necrosis with extensive tissue loss may occur, particularly following lionfish and catfish stings. Systemic reactions, including cardiac arrhythmias, hypotension, muscular weakness, seizures, and paralysis, have been reported and attributed to the effects of the venom.

Treatment should be immediate immersion of the wound in water as hot as the patient can stand for at least 1 h or until symptoms subside. The venoms are extremely heat labile, accounting for the usefulness of this procedure. Although rarely needed, an antivenin is available for patients with severe systemic reactions from stonefish envenomation. It can be obtained from the Health Services Department, Sea World of San Diego [(619) 222–0411]. Tetanus prophylaxis should be given as needed. Narcotics may be required to control pain. Secondary pyogenic infection is a frequent complication.

Probably the most frequent type of fish envenomation in the United States is that produced by the lashing tail of the stingray of the California coast (*Urobatis halleri*). The bony spine is encased in a sheath of epithelial cells containing venom which is expressed into the puncture wound. The wound may be several centimeters deep; portions of the bony spine may break off in it, or, more often, the integumentary sheath remains in the wound. The venom is a circulatory depressant in animals, but local injury predominates in humans. Severe pain and blanching followed by erythema and edema occur immediately. Symptoms due to systemic absorption of venom are infrequent but may include salivation, muscle cramps and weakness, cardiac arrhythmias, seizures, and death. Treatment consists of application of a constriction band (the vast majority of these injuries occur on the legs) and copious syringing of the wound with salt water to remove fragments of sheath. Additional therapeutic measures are the same as for other fish envenomations, including immersion of the injured area in hot water for up to 1 h.

REFERENCES

Hymenoptera stings

GOLDEN DBK et al: Discontinuing venom immunotherapy (VIT): Immunologic and clinical criteria. J Allergy Clin Immunol 79:126, 1987

——— et al: Epidemiology of insect venom sensitivity. JAMA 262:240, 1989

LIGHT WC et al: Unusual reactions following insect stings. J Allergy Clin Immun 59:391, 1977

PATTERSON R, VALENTINE M: Anaphylactic and related allergic emergencies including reactions to insect stings. JAMA 248:2632, 1982

PAULL BR: Imported fire ant allergy: Perspectives on diagnosis and treatment. Postgrad Med 76:155, 1984

TAYLOR OR JR: Health problems associated with African bees, editorial. Ann Intern Med 104:267, 1986

Marine animal venoms

AUERBACH PS, HALSTEAD BW: Hazardous marine life, in *Management of Wilderness and Environmental Emergencies*, PS Auerbach, HR Gee (eds). New York, MacMillan, 1983

BURNETT JW, CARLTON GJ: Jellyfish envenomation syndromes updated. Ann Emerg Med 26:1000, 1987

HUGHES JM, MERSON MH: Fish and shellfish poisoning. N Engl J Med 295:1117, 1976

KIZER KW: Marine envenomations. J Toxicol-Clin Toxicol 21:527, 1983–1984

——— et al: Scorpaenidae envenomation: A 5-year poison center experience. JAMA 253:807, 1985

ROSSON CL, TOLLE SW: Management of marine stings and scrapes. West J Med 150:97, 1989

ZERMAN MG: Catfish stings: A report of 3 cases. Ann Emerg Med 18:211, 1989

Other arthropod bites and stings

FRAZIER CA: *Insect Allergy: Allergic and Toxic Reactions to Insects and Other Arthropods*. St Louis, Grace, 1969

HILLIER FF, WARM RP: Caterpillar dermatitis. Br Med J 1:346, 1967

HUNT GR: Bites and stings of uncommon arthropods: 2. Reduviids, fire ants, puss caterpillars, and scorpions. Postgrad Med 70:107, 1981

LOGAN JL, OGDEN DA: Rhabdomyolysis and acute renal failure following the bite of the giant desert centipede *Scolopendra heros*. West J Med 142:549, 1985

SHELLEY ED et al: The diagnostic challenge of non-burrowing mite bites. JAMA 251:2690, 1984

WIRTZ RA: Allergic and toxic reactions to non-stinging arthropods. Ann Rev Entomol 29:47, 1984

Scorpion stings

CURRY SC et al: Envenomation by the scorpian *Centuroides sculpteratus*. J Toxicol-Clin Toxicol 21:417, 1983–84

LIKES K et al: *Centuroides exilicauda* envenomation in Arizona. West J Med 141:634, 1984

Snake and lizard bites

JURKOVICH GL et al: Complications of Crotalidae antivenin therapy. J Trauma 28:1032, 1988

KITCHENS CS, VAN MIEROP LHS: Envenomation by the eastern coral snake (*Micrurus fulvius fulvius*): A study of 39 victims. JAMA 258, 1615, 1987

LOPRINZI CL et al: Snake antivenin administration in a patient allergic to horse serum. South Med J 76:501, 1983

MITRAKUL C, DHAMKRONG A: Clinical features of neurotoxic snake bite and response to antivenom in 47 children. Am J Trop Med Hyg 33:1258, 1984

RUSSELL FE: *Snake Venom Poisoning*. New York, Scholium International, 1983

———, BOGERT CM: Gila monster: Its biology, venom and bite: A review. Toxicon 19:341, 1981

WINGERT WA, CHAN L: Rattlesnake bites in southern California and rationale for recommended treatment. West J Med 148:37, 1988

Spider bites

HUNT GR: Bites and stings of uncommon arthropods: 1 Spiders. Postgrad Med 70:91, 1981

RAUBER A: Black widow spider bites. J Toxicol-Clin Toxicol 21:473, 1983–84

REES R et al: The diagnosis and treatment of brown recluse spider bites. Ann Emerg Med 16:945, 1987

Tick bite and tick paralysis

GOTHE R et al: The mechanism of pathogenicity in the tick paralysis. J Med Entomol 16:357, 1979

NEEDHAM GR: Evaluation of 5 popular methods for tick removal. Pediatrics 75:997, 1985

SPIELMAN A: How to diagnose and treat tick and mite infestations. Drug Therapy 11:77, 1981

377 HYPOTHERMIA AND HYPERTHERMIA

ROBERT G. PETERSDORF

CONTROL OF BODY TEMPERATURE

In health, the body temperature of humans is maintained within a narrow range despite extremes in environmental conditions and physical activity. This is also true for most birds and mammals, and such animals are termed *homeothermic*, or warm-blooded. An almost invariable accompaniment of systemic illness is a disturbance in temperature regulation, usually an abnormal elevation, or *fever*. Even in the absence of a frank febrile response, interference with heat regulation by disease is evident. This may take the form of flushing, pallor, sweating, shivering, and abnormal sensations of cold or warmth, or it may consist of erratic fluctuations of body temperature within normal limits when a patient is at bed rest. The pathogenesis, diagnosis, and treatment of fever are discussed in Chap. 20.

HEAT PRODUCTION The major sources of basal heat production are through thyroid thermogenesis and the action of adenosine triphosphatase (ATPase) on the sodium pump of all membranes. The muscles are most important in promoting increased heat production through increased shivering. Heat production by muscle is of particular importance because the quantity can be varied according to the need. In most circumstances this variation consists of small increases and decreases in the number of nerve impulses to the muscles, causing inapparent tensing or relaxing. When, however, there is a strong stimulus for heat production, muscle activity may increase to the point of shivering, or even to a generalized rigor. During digestion of food, gastrointestinal production of heat is significant.

HEAT LOSS Heat is lost from the body in several ways. Small amounts are used in warming food or drink and in the evaporation of moisture from the respiratory tract. Most heat is lost from the surface of the body by *convection*. Heat loss by convection depends on the existence of a temperature gradient between the body surface and the ambient air. A second mechanism for heat loss is *radiation*, which may be defined as an exchange of electromagnetic energy between the body and the radiant environment. *Evaporation* is the third major mechanism for dissipating heat and is particularly important when the ambient temperature exceeds that of the body, or when core temperatures are increased by vigorous exercise.

The principal method of regulating heat loss is by varying the volume of blood flowing to the surface of the body. A rich circulation in the skin and subcutaneous tissues carries heat to the surface, where it can escape. In addition, sweating increases heat loss by providing water to be vaporized. The sweat, or eccrine, glands are under the control of the sympathetic nerves which, in this instance, mediate cholinergic stimuli. Heat loss by sweating may be tremendous, and as much as 1 L/h of sweat may be evaporated. The amount of heat loss through sweating is also dependent upon the humidity in the air. The greater the humidity, the less the ability to lose heat through sweat.

When there is need for conservation of heat, adrenergic autonomic stimuli cause a sharp reduction in the blood flow to the surface. This causes vasoconstriction and transforms the skin and subcutaneous tissue into layers of insulation.

HEAT TRANSFER WITHIN THE BODY This depends upon *conduction*, i.e., the transfer of heat between adjacent organs, and upon *circulatory convection*, which is governed by bulk movement of body fluids and which is responsible for the transfer of heat between the cells and the bloodstream. It is useful, although oversimplified, to visualize the body as a central core at uniform temperatures surrounded by an insulating shell. The role of the shell as a mediator for heat conservation and heat loss is determined in part by its blood supply and by vasoconstriction or vasodilatation. Although insulation is relatively uniform throughout the body, some parts, such as the digits, are particularly susceptible to cold because of the increased surface-to-volume ratio. Moreover, blood that reaches the digits has already been cooled on the way. Insulation may be enhanced by the addition of clothing.

NEURAL CONTROL OF TEMPERATURE The control of body temperature, integrating the various physical and chemical processes for heat production or heat loss, is a function of cerebral centers located in the hypothalamus. The temperature-regulating system is a negative feedback control system and possesses three elements essential to such a system: (1) receptors that sense the existing central temperatures; (2) effector mechanisms, consisting of the vasomotor, sudomotor, and metabolic effectors; and (3) integrative structures that determine whether the existing temperature is too high or too low and that activate the appropriate motor response. It is a negative feedback system because a rise in central temperature initiates mechanisms for losing heat while a fall in central temperature activates mechanisms for heat production and heat conservation. The activation of these effector responses is governed by a central integrative mechanism that may be compared with a thermostat and that responds to a variety of stimuli, such as the sensory impulses engendered in flushing or sweating, behavioral impulses, exercise, endocrine influences, and probably the temperature of the blood circulating through the hypothalamic centers. In a sense all these stimuli reset the thermostat, thereby activating compensatory heat loss or heat conservation mechanisms.

A classic example of the neuroendocrine influence on temperature is the effect of menstruation. The mean body temperature of women is higher during the second half of the menstrual cycle than it is between the onset of menstruation and the time of ovulation. The sensations of intense heat followed by diaphoresis that characterize the vasomotor instability experienced by some women at the menopause are most likely the result of neuroendocrine imbalance.

NORMAL BODY TEMPERATURE It is not practical to designate an exact upper level of normal body temperature because there are small differences among normal persons. There are rare individuals whose temperatures are always elevated slightly above accepted "normal" levels, and there is considerable variation in temperature in a given individual. In general, however, it is safe to regard an oral temperature above 37.2°C (99°F) in a person at bed rest as probable indication of disease. The temperature may be as low as 35.8°C (96.5°F) in healthy persons. Rectal temperature is usually 0.3 to 0.6°C (0.5 to 1.0°F) above oral temperature. In very hot weather the body temperature may be elevated by the same amounts.

There is a distinct diurnal variation in body temperature in healthy human beings. Oral readings of 36.1°C (97°F) are relatively common on arising in the morning. Body temperature rises steadily through the day, reaches a peak of 37.2°C (99°F) or greater between 6 P.M. and 10 P.M., and then drops slowly to reach a minimum at 2 A.M. to 4 A.M. Although it has been postulated that this diurnal variation is dependent upon increasing activity during the day and rest at night, the pattern is not reversed in individuals who work at night and sleep during the day. The febrile patterns of most human diseases also tend to follow this normal diurnal variation. Fevers tend to be higher, that is, to "spike," in the evening, and many patients with febrile disease have relatively normal temperatures in the early morning hours.

Body temperature is more labile in young children, and transient elevations after relatively slight exertion in warm weather are frequently observed in them.

Severe or prolonged exercise can produce considerable elevation in body temperature. For example, marathon runners may develop temperatures between 39 and 41°C (103.2 and 105.8°F). Although heat loss may be increased by cutaneous vasodilatation and by hyperventilation, these compensatory mechanisms may fail, leading to hyperpyrexia and, if uncontrolled, to heat stroke. Many of the adverse effects of long-distance running can be prevented by holding races only if the ambient temperature is below 27.8°C (82°F), preferably in the early morning or early evening, and by ensuring ample fluid intake both before and during a race.

DISORDERED THERMOREGULATION In exercise, there is a temporary imbalance between heat production and heat loss with prompt reestablishment of normal temperatures at rest due to continuing activation of heat loss mechanisms. In prolonged exercise, cutaneous vasodilatation in response to an increase in central body temperature ceases in order to preserve central temperature. Less adaptation occurs in fever because once a stable body temperature is reached, heat production equals heat loss, but both are greater than in the basal state. Cutaneous blood flow plays a greater role in controlling heat production and heat loss in fever than does sweating. At the beginning of fever, the body temperature as sensed by the thermoreceptors is low, and the individual responds physiologically as if he or she were cold. *Heat production* is increased by shivering, and *heat loss* is decreased by vasoconstriction. These events explain the sensation of cold or chills that characterizes the beginning of fever. Conversely, when the cause of fever is removed, the temperature returns to normal, and the individual responds as if warm. Cutaneous vasodilatation, sweating, and inhibition of shivering are the compensatory responses.

Deviations of 3°C (approximately 5°F) from the normal body temperature do not interfere appreciably with most bodily functions. Convulsions are common at temperatures higher than 41.1°C (106°F) in children, and irreversible brain damage is common when temperatures of 42.2°C (108°F) are reached. Fortunately, when hyperthermia reaches dangerous levels, the mechanisms for heat loss are suddenly activated; consequently, oral temperatures above 41.1°C (106°F) are relatively rare in humans. Conversely, when temperatures are lowered to 32.8°C (91°F) or below, confusion and loss of consciousness occur; at 30°C (86°F) and below slow atrial fibrillation supervenes. Ventricular fibrillation occurs at extremely hypothermic temperatures and is often a terminal event.

Disease of the regulatory centers in the hypothalamus may affect body temperature. Cases have been observed in which there was destruction of the centers controlling heat-conserving mechanisms, with resulting hypothermia. More commonly, cerebral lesions are manifested by hyperthermia; they include tumors, degenerative diseases, vascular accidents, particularly cerebral hemorrhage, or infections involving the hypothalamus, such as encephalitis. Central fever is accompanied by lack of a diurnal variation, absence of sweating, resistance to antipyretic drugs, excessive response to external cooling, and loss of consciousness.

DISORDERS ASSOCIATED WITH HIGH TEMPERATURES

HEAT SYNDROMES Four clinical syndromes are associated with high environmental temperature: *heat cramps, heat exhaustion, exertional heat injury*, and *heat stroke*. Although each of these entities may be separated from the others on clinical grounds, there is considerable overlap between them, and they may be considered as a series of syndromes along a single spectrum. The incidence of heat syndromes is unknown, but during an ordinary summer about 200 cases of heat stroke are reported. During the heat wave of June 1984, there was a 35 percent increase in mortality in New York City almost exclusively due to a rise in deaths in elderly persons living at home. Heat syndromes occur primarily at elevated ambient temperatures [>32°C (>90°F)] and at high relative humidities (>60%) in elderly individuals, particularly those with mental illness or alcoholism or who receive antipsychotic drugs, diuretics, and anticholinergics, or those who reside in poorly ventilated places without air conditioning. Heat syndromes are especially prevalent during the first days of a heat wave before effective acclimatization can occur. Prophylaxis by augmenting fluid intake prior to exposure and by ensuring that susceptible individuals, particularly the elderly or the very young, wear light clothing, take frequent cool baths, remain in a cool environment, and avoid strenuous physical activity can help prevent the full-blown syndrome, especially heat stroke.

Acclimatization The basic mechanism by which humans accommodate to excessive temperatures is unknown. Acclimatization does not increase the threshold for sweating. However, sweating is the most effective natural means of combating heat stress and can occur with little or no change in the core temperature of the body. As long as sweating continues, humans can withstand remarkably high temperatures, provided water and sodium chloride, the most important physiologic constituents of sweat, are replaced. The concentration of sodium chloride varies between very low concentrations up to that of interstitial fluid. The ability to secrete sweat with a low sodium chloride content, or to increase the quantity of sweat, is a major mechanism for salt conservation in hot weather. Dilatation of the peripheral blood vessels in an attempt to dissipate heat is another major way for the body to acclimatize to hot temperatures. Other alterations include a decrease in total circulating blood volume, a decrease in renal blood flow, an increase of antidiuretic hormone (ADH) as well as aldosterone, a decrease in urine sodium, and an increase in respiratory and pulse rates. Ordinarily, acclimatization takes from 4 to 7 days. The hyperaldosteronism may result in potassium loss, which may be aggravated by replacement of sodium without concomitant repletion of potassium. Initially there is an increase in cardiac output, but as heat stress persists, venous return diminishes and cardiac output may fall. If environmental temperatures in excess of the body's temperature persist, heat is retained and hyperpyrexia develops.

Heat cramps Heat cramps are the most benign heat syndrome. They are characterized by brief, intermittent, and often excruciating cramping pain, and usually follow strenuous exercise in the muscles that have been subjected to extensive work. Individuals who develop this syndrome are usually athletes in excellent physical condition who are well acclimatized. External temperatures do not usually exceed the body temperature, and direct exposure to the sun is not necessary. The body temperature is usually normal, and the victim sweats normally or excessively. Heat cramps may even be precipitated by strenuous exercise in cold environments in untrained persons heavily clothed. Muscles of the extremities bear the brunt of physical activity and hence show the highest incidence of cramps. Treatment consists of rest in a cool environment and replacement of sodium, potassium, and fluid. This syndrome may be prevented by liberal salting of food and ample intake of water. Salt tablets and electrolyte solutions are of no particular value.

Heat exhaustion This is also called heat prostration, or heat collapse, and is probably the most common heat syndrome. It represents a failure of the cardiovascular responses to high external temperatures and is common in elderly individuals who are receiving diuretics. Weakness, anxiety, fatigue, thirst, vertigo, headache, anorexia, nausea, vomiting, the urge to defecate, and faintness may precede collapse. There may be hyperventilation, muscular incoordination, agitation, impaired judgment, and confusion. Heat collapse occurs in both physically active and sedentary individuals. The onset is usually sudden and the duration of collapse brief. During the acute stage, the patient looks ashen-gray. The skin is cold and clammy. The pupils are dilated. The blood pressure may be low and the pulse rate elevated. Since prostration develops before exposure to heat is prolonged, body temperature is subnormal or normal. The duration of exposure and the extent to which sweat is lost determine the treatment, which consists of removing the patient to a cool area and placing him or her in the recumbent position. Spontaneous recovery then usually takes place. Intravenous administration of saline solution is rarely necessary, and, for the most part, water and electrolytes, including sodium and potassium, can be replaced orally.

Exertional heat injury This syndrome occurs in individuals who are exerting themselves in hot ambient temperatures [≥27°C (≥ 80°F)] when the relative humidity is high. It is particularly common in runners who enter races with insufficient acclimatization, inadequate conditioning, or improper hydration (before and during the race). Obesity, age, and previous heat stroke; hypertension; ingestion of drugs, including diuretics, anticholinergics, vasodilators, antihistamines, tranquilizers, sedatives, beta-blockers and amphetamines; and alcohol consumption are contributing predisposing factors. In contrast to classic heat stroke, individuals with exertional heat injury usually sweat freely, and their temperatures are lower [38.9 to 40°C (102 to 104°F) as opposed to 41.1°C (106°F) and higher in heat stroke]. Symptoms consist of headache, piloerection (gooseflesh) on the chest and upper arms, chills, hyperventilation, nausea, vomiting, muscle cramps, ataxia, unsteady gait, and incoherent speech. In some individuals, loss of consciousness occurs. Physical examination shows tachycardia, hypotension, and evidence of low peripheral resistance. Laboratory data show hemoconcentration, hypernatremia, abnormal liver and muscle enzymes, hypocalcemia, hypophosphatemia, and, in some instances, hypoglycemia. An occasional patient has thrombocytopenia, hemolysis, disseminated intravascular coagulation, rhabdomyolysis, myoglobinuria, and acute tubular necrosis. Injury to the vascular endothelium may be widespread and contribute to these manifestations as well as to organ failure. These severe complications can be avoided by prompt treatment, which consists of placing the victim under wet cold sheets to lower core temperature to 38°C (100.4°F) as quickly as possible, massaging the extremities to improve blood flow from the core to the periphery, and infusing fluids consisting primarily of hypotonic glucose-saline. Patients should be hospitalized for observation.

Exertional heat injury can be prevented by (1) running races early in the morning (before 8 A.M.) when the temperature and humidity are likely to be low, (2) educating runners to enter a race well hydrated by drinking 300 mL of water 10 min before a race and 250 mL every 3 to 4 km (salt and glucose solutions should be avoided), (3) placing aid stations at 5-km intervals, (4) instructing runners not to increase their pace after most of the race has been run, and (5) avoiding alcohol before a race.

Heat stroke Heat stroke can be divided into "exertional" and "classic." Exertional heat stroke occurs in healthy, young individuals and is generally sporadic. The patient usually sweats. Disseminated intravascular coagulation (DIC), acute renal failure, rhabdomyolysis, and lactic acidosis are common complications. Classic heat stroke occurs in older individuals in epidemic form during heat waves. Patients do not sweat. Acute renal failure, rhabdomyolysis, and lactic acidosis are rare. Most persons with classic heat stroke have preexisting chronic disease, including arteriosclerosis and congestive heart failure (particularly when such patients receive diuretics), diabetes mellitus, alcoholism, or have received one or several of the drugs described above. Skin disorders in which it may be difficult to lose heat such as ectodermal dysplasia, congenital absence of the sweat glands, or severe scleroderma predispose to heat stroke. The vasoconstriction that accompanies heat stroke prevents dissipation of heat from the core, but whether this vasoconstriction is cause or effect is not clear. Direct exposure to the sun is not a necessary prerequisite for the development of heat stroke.

There may be few premonitory symptoms, and loss of consciousness may be the first sign. Other patients may complain of headache, vertigo, faintness, abdominal distress, confusion, or hyperpnea. Delirium may develop in more severe cases. Pyrexia and prostration are the significant findings on physical examination. A rectal temperature greater than 41.1°C (106°F) is common, and internal body temperatures as high as 44.4°C (112 to 113°F) have been recorded. The skin is hot and dry, the pulse rate is rapid, and respirations are rapid and weak. The blood pressure is usually low. The muscles are flaccid, and tendon reflexes may be diminished. Lethargy, stupor, or coma, depending on the severity, is present. Shock is common in fatal cases. Coma, hypotension, disseminated intravascular coagulation, and the necessity of intubation are bad prognostic indicators.

Examination of the blood and urine may show few abnormalities. Hemoconcentration is common. Leukocytosis is characteristic, as are proteinuria, cylindruria, and an elevation in BUN. There is usually a respiratory alkalosis which is followed by a metabolic acidosis.

Lactic acidosis is common in classic heat stroke. Serum potassium is normal or low, and there are usually hypocalcemia and hypophosphatemia. The electrocardiogram may show, in addition to tachycardia and sinus arrhythmia, flattening and subsequent inversion of the T waves and depression of the ST segments. Diffuse myocardial necrosis with ECG evidence of myocardial infarction has been reported. Other major laboratory abnormalities include thrombocytopenia; prolonged bleeding, clotting, and prothrombin times; afibrinogenemia and fibrinolysis; and disseminated intravascular coagulation. All these may be responsible for diffuse bleeding. Liver damage is common; it appears 24 to 36 h after admission and is characterized by clinically apparent jaundice and, often, by abnormalities of hepatocellular enzymes. Renal failure is a common complication of exertional heat stroke.

Patients with heat stroke may die within a few hours after being discovered, or may die of complications such as acute renal failure. However, a number of patients will die several weeks after the acute episode, usually of myocardial infarction, heart failure, renal failure, bronchopneumonia, or complicating bacteremia. In such patients autopsy may show extensive parenchymal damage to various organs, either from hyperpyrexia per se or from petechial hemorrhages in the brain, heart, kidneys, or liver.

TREATMENT Heat stroke is a medical emergency, and immediate heroic emergency measures are required. In hot climates, ambulances should be air-conditioned. Once the patient is in the emergency room, time is of the essence. All clothing should be removed. The patient should be wheeled into a shower on a gurney. A successful protocol consists of vigorous massage of the patient, particularly the torso and neck, to decrease peripheral vasoconstriction. At the same time, ice should be applied to the lateral aspects of the trunk while the patient is sprayed with tepid water from the shower. A fan should be directed on the patient to accelerate heat dissipation by convection. Intravenous solutions should be chilled before administration.

After immediate evaluation and measurement of vital signs, the temperature should be measured with an equilibrated thermocouple. Using these measures, the rectal temperature should fall to 37.8 to 38.9°C (100 to 102°F) within 1 h. While immersion of the patient in an ice-water bath is a time-honored treatment, it appears to be no more effective than the less cumbersome measures described above. Massage of the skin should be employed along with cooling because it stimulates return of the cool peripheral blood to the overheated brain and viscera and aids acceleration of heat loss. A Swan-Ganz catheter may be necessary, and urinary output needs to be monitored. Prompt cooling, massage of the limbs, and vigorous hydration along with establishment of a proper airway, avoidance of aspiration, treating coma and convulsions, and watching for arrhythmias will lead to survival of most patients, particularly if they are young and were previously well. Unfortunately, the poor, ill, and elderly, who are often not discovered until heat hyperpyrexia has been present for some hours, have a much less favorable outcome.

MALIGNANT HYPERTHERMIA Etiology and epidemiology Malignant hyperthermia (MH) consists of a group of inherited disorders that are characterized by a rapid increase in temperature to 39 to 42°C (102.2 to 107.6°F) in response to inhalational anesthetics such as halothane, methoxyflurane, cyclopropane, and ethyl ether or muscle relaxants, notably succinylcholine. In one form of the disease in which the mechanism of inheritance is autosomal dominant, the individuals are normal between attacks although some have an elevation in creatine phosphokinase (CPK), and in 90 percent of such cases, biopsied muscle from susceptible individuals contracts on exposure to caffeine or halothane at concentrations that do not alter normal muscle contraction. The incidence of the autosomal dominant form is 1:50,000 to 1:100,000. MH occurs in one per 40,000 adult and one per 15,000 pediatric surgical cases. Interval CPK screening is not effective in detecting susceptible patients. Muscle biopsy followed by the halothane-caffeine contraction reaction is accurate but tedious. A careful history from the patient, including questioning about abnormal reactions during surgery suggestive of MH in relatives, is the most accurate way to detect and prevent MH. Some anesthesiologists feel that an increase in end-tidal CO_2, unexplained tachycardia, and an increase in core temperature provide early clues.

A second, recessive, form occurs in young boys and, less commonly, girls, with a number of congenital abnormalities including short stature, undescended testes, lumbar lordosis, thoracic kyphosis, pectus carinatum, webbed neck, winged scapulae, small chin, low-set ears, and an antimongoloid obliquity of the palpebral fissures. This form is called the *King syndrome*. MH has also been described in several other myopathies including myotonia congenita, central core disease, and Duchenne's muscular dystrophy.

Pathogenesis The triggering anesthetic releases calcium from the membrane of the muscle cell's sarcoplasmic reticulum, which is defective in storing this ion. The result is a sudden increase in myoplasmic calcium. The calcium activates myosin ATPase, which converts adenosine triphosphate to adenosine diphosphate, phosphate, and heat. There are also inhibition of troponin, uncoupling of oxidative phosphorylation, activation of phosphorylase kinase, and increased glycolysis. Muscular contraction occurs, and it, as well as the chemical events, leads to production of heat.

Manifestations Existence of malignant hyperthermia can be suspected if diminished relaxation is noted during induction of anesthesia and muscle fasciculations become evident when succinylcholine is given. In some patients trismus during intubation is the first sign of a muscle disorder. Although the elevation in temperature is the result of muscular contraction, it may rise very rapidly, and if the temperature is not monitored, the first signs may be a hot skin and tachycardia or a cardiac arrhythmia. In addition to the high fever, muscle rigidity, hypotension, and mottled cyanosis are present.

Early laboratory abnormalities include respiratory and metabolic acidosis, hyperkalemia and hypermagnesemia, and elevation in blood lactate and pyruvate. Late complications include massive skeletal muscle swelling, pulmonary edema, disseminated intravascular coagulation, and acute renal failure.

Treatment Malignant hyperthermia is a medical emergency. The treatment protocol prescribed by the American Society of Anesthesiologists should be followed. It includes prompt interruption of surgery, cessation of the inhalational anesthetic, changing rubber tubing on the anesthesia machine, and external cooling. One hundred percent oxygen should be given, along with sodium bicarbonate (1 to 2 mg/kg), to combat the severe metabolic acidosis. A diuresis should be induced with fluids and diuretics to reduce myoglobinemia and hyperkalemia. Specific treatment consists of dantrolene sodium, 1 mg/kg, by rapid intravenous infusion. The drug should be continued until symptoms have begun to subside or up to a maximum single dose of 10 mg/kg. The regimen can be repeated if symptoms recur. Drugs to combat arrhythmias should be administered under ECG monitoring (see Chap. 185).

Prevention Because of the tendency of this syndrome to run in families, its detection is essential. This can be achieved by monitoring the temperature of all patients under anesthesia; the best way to avert it altogether is to take a thorough family history. Examining patients preoperatively is often not helpful because between attacks persons susceptible to MH are usually entirely normal. In susceptible patients dantrolene should be given prophylactically. The dose is 4 to 8 mg/kg by mouth for 1 to 2 days prior to surgery; the last dose should be administered 3 to 4 h prior to anesthesia. Some favor an additional dose of 2 to 5 mg/kg intravenously immediately prior to induction of anesthesia.

NEUROLEPTIC MALIGNANT SYNDROME (NMS) This syndrome is characterized by autonomic dysfunction, extrapyramidal dysfunction, and hyperthermia. Autonomic dysfunction is characterized by tachycardia, labile blood pressure (range 180 to 40 mmHg systolic), profuse diaphoresis, dyspnea, and urinary incontinence. Extrapyramidal dysfunction is manifested by catatonic behavior, dystonia, generalized muscular rigidity, pseudo-parkinsonism (ptyalism, masked facies, tremors, and brady- or akinesia). The temperature may be as high as 41°C (106°F). Consciousness fluctuates from alertness to coma. Laboratory abnormalities consist of leukocytosis (15,000 to 30,000 per microliter) and elevation in CK. The syndrome occurs after use of potent neuroleptics in therapeutic doses. Most cases have been reported after use of haloperidol, thiothixene, or piperazine phenothiazines. Young adult males with affective disorders predominate. The NMS lasts 5 to 10 days after administration of oral neuroleptics is discontinued, and longer after depot injection. These drugs are not dialyzable, hence the long period necessary for their excretion. The overall mortality is 20 percent and fatalities have occurred as late as 30 days after onset and have been due to renal failure, arrhythmias, pulmonary emboli, or aspiration pneumonia.

The mechanism of action is presumed to be due to blockade of the dopaminic pathways in the basal ganglia and the hypothalamus. Because neuroleptic drugs block dopamine receptors, NMS is attributed to dopamine depletion and this is the rationale for treatment with bromocryptine (a dopamine agonist) in dosage of 7.5 to 60 mg/d divided into 3 daily doses. Dantrolene sodium (as described above for oral prophylaxis of MH) has been successful occasionally, as has amantadine. Supportive measures, including cooling and drug withdrawal, are the *sine qua non* of treatment.

DISORDERS ASSOCIATED WITH LOW TEMPERATURES

HYPOTHERMIA Hypothermia is defined as a central or core temperature of 35°C (95°F) or lower. The central (core) temperature is maintained at the expense of the periphery. During cold weather blood is shunted away from the skin and the extremities to preserve, protect, and maintain core temperatures. Although far less common than is elevation in temperature, hypothermia is of considerable importance because it can represent a medical emergency.

Accidental hypothermia This is a well-known complication of exposure to cold and has been reported frequently during the winter months. It usually occurs after prolonged exposure, not necessarily to excessively low external temperatures. The diagnosis of hypothermia may prove elusive because clinical thermometers do not record temperatures below 35°C (95°F). Whenever a patient presents with a temperature below this level, the true temperature should be determined with an incubator thermometer or a thermocouple. Accidental hypothermia has been found in association with sepsis, hypothyroidism, pituitary insufficiency, adrenal insufficiency, hypoglycemia, cerebrovascular disease, Wernicke's encephalopathy, myocardial infarction, cirrhosis, pancreatitis, and ingestion of drugs—most particularly alcohol. For example, it is not uncommon to find a derelict in a railroad yard or under a bridge following an alcoholic debauch with a core temperature between 28.5 and 32.3°C (85 and 90°F) or lower. From 1976 to 1985, 7450 deaths in the United States were caused by exposure to cold. Most had core temperatures <35°C (<95°F), and individuals older than 60 were at greatest risk. In 428 cases reported from 13 emergency departments, there was a direct correlation between lower body temperatures and outcome.

These patients usually appear cold and pale and, when their temperatures are very low, give the appearance of having rigor mortis, so stiff is their musculature. Patients with temperatures less than 26.7°C (80°F) are usually unconscious. The pupils are usually miotic, respiration tends to be shallow and slow, there is bradycardia, and most patients are hypotensive. Generalized edema is often present. When the temperature falls below 25°C (77°F), coma, areflexia, and lack of pupillary response supervene.

Laboratory data tend to show hemoconcentration, mild azotemia, and metabolic acidosis. The acidosis is due to lactic acidemia, which in turn is a consequence of decreased perfusion and hypoxemia in peripheral tissues. At cold temperatures, the hemoglobin dissociation curve is shifted to the left, and there is decreased unloading of oxygen in the peripheral tissues. Some patients have hypoglycemia while others have hyperglycemia. Thyroid function tests may give results typical of myxedema. Some patients have elevations in serum amylase, and a few show pancreatitis at autopsy. The electrocardiogram is distorted by muscular tremors and may show bradycardia or slow atrial fibrillation and a characteristic J wave (occurring at the junction of the QRS complex and ST segment). Other arrhythmias are common; ventricular fibrillation is usually a terminal event. The mortality rate is five times higher in people over 75.

TREATMENT Hypothermia is a medical emergency, and therapy should be instituted at once. The following steps are indicated:

1. An airway must be established and maintained, and the patient should be well oxygenated. Warmed oxygen may be helpful. Tracheal intubation of these patients poses no undue risk.
2. Blood gases should be monitored and corrected for temperature.
3. Blood volume should be expanded with warmed glucose and saline, low-molecular-weight dextran, or albumin. Maintenance of blood volume is necessary to prevent the infarctions which have been a hallmark in fatal cases and to avert "rewarming shock." If the patient has persistent hypotension, respiratory failure, or unexplained oliguria, hemodynamic monitoring with Swan-Ganz catheterization may be necessary.
4. Because of the tendency to arrhythmias, serum potassium should be monitored carefully; a transvenous pacemaker may be indicated.
5. Sodium bicarbonate should be given if pH is less than 7.25.
6. Although external rewarming with heating blankets or placing the patient in a warm room is appropriate in patients with mild hypothermia, patients who are moderately hypothermic require reestablishment of core temperature. This can be done effectively by placing the patient in a warm bath or a Hubbard tank at 40 to 42°C (104 to 108°F). This maneuver must be carried out cautiously; physiologic monitoring may be difficult, and if an arrhythmia occurs, resuscitation is hampered. Nevertheless, external warming tends to dilate the constricted peripheral blood vessels and to divert blood from the visceral organs. In severely hypothermic patients, this may result in rewarming shock and restoration of the core temperature may be insufficient to warm the myocardium to make it responsive to antiarrhythmic agents. In this situation extracorporeal circulation with externally warmed blood is the method of choice. Peritoneal dialysis, during which the dialysate is warmed to 37°C (98.6°F), and colonic and gastric lavage with warmed fluids are also helpful. It is particularly important to rewarm the myocardium because in cases of ventricular fibrillation defibrillation will not be successful until myocardial temperature is raised to near normal levels.
7. Many of these patients have systemic infections including sepsis (see Chap. 89); cultures of the blood, urine, and other suspected sites should be obtained and broad-spectrum antibiotic therapy initiated and continued until infection has been excluded. Sepsis should be considered strongly in patients on hemodynamic monitoring who are found to have a lowered systemic vascular resistance and elevated cardiac index.
8. Resuscitative efforts should be vigorous and prolonged despite the poor prognosis which is related primarily to advanced age and associated debilitating disease. In younger individuals, some remarkable rescues have been recorded. Authorities agree that hypothermia victims without vital signs (prolonged asystole) should not be pronounced dead until they have been rewarmed to 36°C (96.8°F) and remain unresponsive to CPR at that temperature. "No one is dead until warm and dead." Mild hypothermia [above 32.2°C (90°F)] has a 25 percent mortality; in moderate hypothermia [26.6 to 32.2°C (80 to 90°F)] the mortality is 50 percent; and below 26.6°C (80°C) it is 60 percent.

Hypothermia secondary to acute illness There is a group of patients who develop moderate hypothermia in association with acute diseases including congestive heart failure, uremia, diabetes mellitus, drug overdose, acute respiratory failure, and hypoglycemia. These patients are generally elderly and upon admission to the hospital are found to have temperatures of 33.3 to 34.4°C (92 to 93.9°F). They also have a severe metabolic acidosis, due to increased production of lactic acid, and cardiac arrhythmias. Most of these patients are comatose. This entity differs from accidental hypothermia only in the absence of exposure; these cases have all occurred at normal ambient temperatures. The mechanism appears to be an acute failure of thermoregulation; shivering did not occur in any of these patients. Usually these patients have been rewarmed within a few hours. Upon return to normal temperature, cardiac arrhythmias, which were present in most of these patients, responded to treatment, and the sensorium returned to normal. With the exception that core rewarming is established by external means, other facets of therapy should follow the steps outlined above. In addition, treatment of the underlying disease such as diabetes with insulin, uremia with dialysis, or congestive heart failure with appropriate cardiac drugs and diuretics, is essential. The prognosis is good provided the syndrome is recognized early and treatment is instituted at once. In general, patients under 60 have the most favorable outcome.

Immersion hypothermia Responses to cold-water immersion may be classified as (1) stimulatory, with deep body temperature normal to 35°C (95°F); (2) depressant, with deep body temperature 35 to 30°C (95 to 86°F); and (3) critical, with deep body temperature 30 to 25°C (86 to 77°F).

The long-distance swimmer is able to maintain a normal body temperature for periods of 15 to 25 h or more in water that may plunge skin temperature to 15°C (59°F) or lower, which is some 15.7°C (28°F) below deep body temperature, lending support to the concept of a body core insulated by a body shell. The vasoconstriction operative in cold water greatly reduces heat loss. However, there is great individual variability in heat loss in cold water. The relatively obese swimmer may maintain a normal rectal temperature for 2 h without shivering in 16°C (61°F) water. A lean person under the same conditions, despite violent shivering, may experience a fall in rectal temperature of several degrees and become incapacitated from the rigor. In hypersensitive persons, immersion in cold water may be followed by vascular spasm, vomiting, and syncope. Other compensatory responses include bradycardia, a slight rise in blood pressure, and an early rise in rectal temperature followed by a fall. At 30°C (86°F), atrial fibrillation is common.

Rewarming in warm water has been recommended as the treatment of immersion hypothermia. In severe cases, extracorporeal circulation or peritoneal dialysis should be instituted.

LOCAL COLD INJURIES Mechanisms of freezing injury These can be divided into phenomena that affect cells and extracellular fluids (direct effects) and those that disrupt the function of organized tissues and the integrity of the circulation (indirect effects).

When tissue freezes, ice crystals form and, concomitantly, solutes in the residual liquid become concentrated. The physical dislocation during slow freezing is extreme. Ice crystals many times the size of individual cells form but are confined to the extracellular spaces. Large ice crystals can develop between cells in soft tissue without producing irreversible injury as long as the percentage of water frozen does not exceed a critical amount. A major source of damage to living cells during freezing and thawing appears to be the strong salt solutions which develop during formation and dissolution of ice; changes in the proportions of lipids and phospholipids in the cell membrane are also of great importance.

The fulminating vascular reaction and stasis that supervene are associated with production of histamine-like substances which increase the permeability of the capillary bed. Within blood vessels, cellular elements aggregate. Irreversible occlusion of small blood vessels by cell masses has been demonstrated in thawed tissue following freezing injury. The damaged frozen tissue simulates tissue damage produced by burns.

Manifestations The mildest form of cold injury is called *frostnip* and tends to occur in organs farthest removed from the core of the body such as the earlobes, nose, cheeks, fingers and toes, and hands and feet. Frostnip represents reversible damage that is characterized by blanching of the skin and numbness. It can be prevented by warm clothing and treated with simple rewarming. More consequential local cold injuries may be divided into freezing (frostbite) and nonfreezing (immersion foot) injuries. The two types may be observed in the same extremity or in different extremities in the same individual. The diagnosis of freezing versus nonfreezing injury generally can be made on the basis of the history and clinical manifestations.

Immersion foot is an entity observed in shipwreck survivors or in soldiers (trench foot) whose feet have been wet but not freezing cold for prolonged periods. There is primarily injury to nerve and muscle tissue, but no gross or irreparable pathologic changes occur in the blood vessels and skin. The clinical picture reflects primary hypoxic trauma giving rise to three clearly recognizable states: (1) *ischemia*, denoted by a pale, pulseless extremity; (2) *hyperemia*, characterized by a bounding pulsatile circulation in red, swollen, painful feet; and (3) the *posthyperemic* or recovery period. The initial cold-induced vasoconstriction, increased blood viscosity, and impaired oxygen transport in the ischemic state are aggravated by such factors as malnutrition, general hypothermia, dehydration, and trauma from relatively fixed, pendant extremities. The problem of rewarming is critical in these patients during the stage of ischemia, when overheating of tissue may lead to gangrene. In the state of hyperemia, the red, swollen feet require judicious cooling. Severe cases may show muscular weakness, atrophy, ulceration, and gangrene of superficial areas. Sensitivity to cold and pain on weight bearing, which may cause discomfort for many years, are sequelae even of milder injuries.

Frostbite, in contrast to immersion foot, is primarily a vascular problem because the blood vessels may be severely and irreparably injured. The circulation of blood ceases, and the vascular bed of the frozen tissue is occluded by agglutinated cell aggregates and thrombi. The cutaneous injury consists in part of separation of the epidermal-dermal interface. Early the intravascular clumping is reversible. However, with the passage of time, clumped red blood cells within vessels in injured tissue lose their morphologic identity and take on the appearance of a homogeneous, hyalinaceous plug. It has been shown in some, but not all, experimental studies that much of the intravascular aggregation following freezing injury can be reversed and microcirculatory perfusion improved if low-molecular-weight dextran is given intraveneously shortly after injury, but the data in humans are less convincing. Tissue damage can be aggravated by trauma to insensitive and friable limbs and by refreezing. Moreover, frostbitten tissues are often neglected and with thawing become macerated. It is important, therefore, not to walk, bear weight or put excessive pressure on a thawed frostbitten area. Thawing followed by refreezing is particularly harmful.

The method of rewarming has been a matter of controversy. It seems most rational to warm the core of the body before treating the local area of frostbite. Following restoration of the core temperature to normal, warming of a frostbitten limb should begin in water at 10 to 15°C (50 to 59°F), which is then increased 5°C (9°F) every 5 min to a maximum of 40°C (104°F). Once the frostbitten limb has been rewarmed, treatment of the areas of tissue damage should be conservative and consist of bed rest, elevation of the injured part, tetanus toxoid administration, and use of antibiotics if infection is present; aseptic early drainage of blebs and bullae; daily washes with chlorhexidine or an iodophor; and early institution of physiotherapy. Alcohol and cigarettes are strongly contraindicated. Except for compartment syndromes that may occur as a result of massive swelling in the early post-thaw period, and that may require surgical release, surgical amputation and reconstruction is usually not necessary. In fact, 3 to 6 months may be required to determine the true level of tissue loss, contraindicating aggressive surgery.

Some patients with frostbite have residua consisting of excessive sweating, pain, cold insensitivity, numbness, abnormal color, dry and cracking skin, arthralgias, and degenerative arthritis. The symptoms are generally worse in the winter and following exposure to cold. These patients also often show abnormal nails, discoloration and pigmentation, hyperhidrosis, and, by x-ray, osteoporosis and cystic defects near the joints. These abnormalities tend to be milder in patients who have had sympathetic blockade. Most cold injuries are preventable by graded exposure to cold, as well as appropriate clothing in freezing temperatures.

REFERENCES

General

MITCHELL D, LABURN HP: Pathophysiology of temperature regulation. Physiologist 28:507, 1985

Heat syndromes

KENNEDY LW: Physiological correlates of heat intolerance. Sports Med 2:279, 1985

TUCKER LE et al: Classical heat stroke. Clinical and laboratory assessment. South Med J 78:20, 1985

Malignant hyperthermia

GRONERT GA et al: Aetiology of malignant hyperthermia. Br J Anaesth 60:253, 1988

PAASUKE RT, BROWNWELL AKW: Serum creatine kinase level as a screening test for malignant hyperthermia. JAMA 255:769, 1986

STEENSON AJ, TORKELSON RD: King syndrome with malignant hyperthermia. Am J Dis Child 141:271, 1987

WARD A et al: Dantrolene. A review of its pharmacodynamic and pharmacokinetic properties and therapeutic use in malignant hyperthermia, the neuroleptic malignant syndrome and an update of its use in muscle spasticity. Drugs 32:130, 1986

Neuroleptic malignant syndrome

ADDONIZIO G et al: Neuroleptic malignant syndrome: Review and analysis of 115 cases. Biol Psychol 22:1004, 1987

GIBB WRG, LEES AJ: The neuroleptic malignant syndrome—a review. Q J Med (ns 56) 220:421, 1985

HARSCH HH: Neuroleptic malignant syndrome. Physiological and laboratory findings in a series of 9 cases. J Clin Psychol 48:328, 1987

LEVENSON JL: Neuroleptic malignant syndrome. Am J Psychiatry 142:1137, 1985

Cold injury

CENTERS FOR DISEASE CONTROL: Hypothermia prevention. Morb Mort Week Rep 37:780, 1988

DANZEL DT, PAZOS RF: Multicenter hypothermia survey. Ann Emerg Med 16:1042, 1987

GRACE TG: Cold exposure injuries in the winter athlete. Orthop Related Res 216:55, 1987

MORRIS DL et al: Hemodynamic characteristics of patients with hypothermia due to occult infection and other causes. Ann Intern Med 102:153, 1985

WHITTLE JL, BATES JH: Thermoregulatory failure secondary to acute illness: Complications and treatment. Arch Intern Med 139:418, 1979

378 DROWNING AND NEAR-DROWNING

JAMES F. WALLACE

EPIDEMIOLOGY In the United States, drowning is the third leading cause of accidental death among all age groups and the second among individuals ages 5 to 44 years. In 1984 there were approximately 5400 drowning deaths or 2.3 per 100,000 persons. This represents a substantial decline from 1978 when there were nearly 7000 deaths. Although no national statistics are available, it has been estimated that as many as 48,000 persons annually are near-drowning victims: those who live at least temporarily following an immersion incident. Children and young adults are most often the victims, and nearly 80 percent are males. Other risk factors are epilepsy, mental retardation, alcohol consumption while swimming or boating, lack of proper swimming training, failure to use personal floating devices, increased use of hot tubs and spas, and use of small, open, or high-speed boats. With the increasing popularity of boating and water sports in this country nearly half the population is at risk of drowning each year, especially during the summer months.

PATHOPHYSIOLOGY Ten to twenty percent of drowning victims have no evidence of water aspiration in their lungs at autopsy ("dry drowning"). Death is due to asphyxia secondary to reflex laryngospasm and glottic closure. It is probable that a similar number of near-drowning victims also do not aspirate. If ventilation is reestablished before they sustain irreversible anoxic brain damage, prompt and complete recovery can be anticipated.

When aspiration accompanies drowning ("wet drowning"), the clinical situation is further complicated by the amount of surrounding water that is introduced into the respiratory tract as well as by the solutes and solids contained in it. A severe pulmonary injury often occurs, resulting in persistent arterial hypoxia and metabolic acidosis even after ventilation has been restored.

In the past, an important distinction was made between the pathophysiology of saltwater and freshwater drowning with respect to changes in blood volume, serum electrolyte concentrations, and cardiovascular function. However, it has been established that the most important problem in human near-drowning is hypoxia and that the other disturbances are of considerably less significance in determining survival.

The mechanisms by which hypoxia develops in near-drowning with aspiration are often multiple: laryngospasm, bronchospasm, airway obstruction secondary to aspirated particulate matter, and pulmonary edema following prolonged hypoxia can take place regardless of the composition of the water aspirated, while other types of lung injury causing hypoxia depend upon the osmolar and chemical characteristics of the immersion fluid. Aspiration of seawater, which is hypertonic compared with blood and chemically irritating to the pulmonary alveolocapillary membrane, causes a rapid shift of plasma proteins and water from the circulation into the alveolar lumen. Continued perfusion of these nonventilated, edema-filled alveoli results in an intrapulmonary right-to-left shunt and arterial hypoxia. When hypotonic fresh water is aspirated, fluid is rapidly absorbed from the lung into the circulation. Injury to alveolar lining cells takes place, altering or destroying the property of pulmonary surfactant that maintains surface tension and leading to alveolar collapse. Ventilation-perfusion ratios change in these atelectatic areas of lung, and hypoxia is the result. Metabolic acidosis, which is present in as many as 70 percent of near-drowning victims, is a consequence of tissue hypoxia and may be severe.

Although changes in electrolyte concentrations occur, depending upon the type and volume of fluid aspirated, these disturbances are rarely life-threatening. Most persons who aspirate sufficient quantities to produce marked electrolyte abnormalities do not survive the immersion incident. Similarly, profound changes in circulating blood volume are unusual. However, hypovolemia requiring treatment may be seen in massive saltwater aspiration accompanied by shifts of fluid from the vascular space into the lung.

Although rarely of clinical significance, some hemolysis of red blood cells often takes place, especially with freshwater aspiration. Free hemoglobin may be found in the urine and blood, but the abnormality requires no specific therapy. Disseminated intravascular coagulation has been reported as a complication of freshwater near-drowning. It is thought that with extensive pulmonary injury, "tissue factor" in lung parenchyma and plasminogen activator from pulmonary endothelium are released, triggering the extrinsic clotting and fibrinolytic systems. Other pathophysiologic events in near-drowning include the development of renal failure secondary to acute tubular necrosis, probably due to the combined effects of hypoxia and hypotension, and neurologic deficits secondary to cerebral anoxia. Although the extent of the central nervous system injury tends to correlate with the duration of hypoxia, hypothermia accompanying the incident may be a moderating factor by reducing cerebral oxygen requirements. Complete neurologic recovery has been reported in victims submerged as long as 66 min in water temperatures less than 10°C. However, the mean age of survivors with good neurologic outcomes following ice water submersion accidents is only 10 years.

CLINICAL MANIFESTATIONS The clinical features in near-drowning are variable and depend upon many factors including the amount and type of water aspirated and the promptness and effectiveness of treatment. Pulmonary and neurologic abnormalities usually predominate. Patients may present with mild cough and tachypnea, or with fulminant pulmonary edema. At least a third will require endotracheal intubation and some type of ventilatory therapy for the management of pulmonary injury. Instead of gradual recovery during the first 48 to 72 h of treatment, some patients will develop the adult respiratory distress syndrome, associated with progressive respiratory failure and reduction in lung compliance (see Chap. 218). Other pulmonary complications often include regional atelectasis due to aspirated particulate matter; secondary bacterial pneumonia; lung abscess; empyema; and injuries such as pneumothorax or pneumomediastinum sustained during resuscitation or related to ventilator therapy.

Early neurologic manifestations include seizures, especially during resuscitative efforts, and altered mental status, including agitation, combativeness, or coma. Patients may present with speech, motor, or visual abnormalities or with more diffuse organic brain syndromes. Some of these neurologic deficits will improve gradually and resolve over several months. However, 5 to 20 percent of patients will have permanent sequelae, many of which prove ultimately fatal. Neurologic status usually does not continue to worsen after a near-drowning victim is admitted to the hospital unless there has been a preceding deterioration in pulmonary status. The possibility of unrecognized head trauma coincident with the drowning episode or a subdural hematoma should be considered as well.

Near-drowning victims often require treatment for cardiac as well as respiratory arrest during resuscitation. If this is successfully accomplished, most patients experience few additional cardiovascular problems. Supraventricular arrhythmias are common but usually resolve promptly when acidosis and hypoxia are treated. Heart failure secondary to myocardial ischemia or acutely expanded blood volume is unusual. Instead, pulmonary edema and low cardiac output states are usually due to the pulmonary injury from water aspiration with extravasation of fluid into the lung, resulting in hypovolemia.

Fever, frequently greater than 38°C, is seen in most patients within the first 24 h following significant aspiration. Its appearance later in the hospital course usually indicates a complicating infection. Vomiting is common during and after resuscitation. This often is associated with gastric distention by large quantities of fluid and air swallowed during the near-drowning episode and may result in additional aspiration. Other rare, but clinically important, features which may be encountered include acute renal failure and a severe hemorrhagic diathesis.

LABORATORY FINDINGS Arterial blood gas and pH determinations on admission reveal varying degrees of hypoxia and acidosis; follow-up values are the most reliable indicators of the effectiveness of ventilatory therapy. In 25 percent of near-drowning victims the initial chest x-ray film may be normal; however, this finding does not exclude the possibility that the patient has significant hypoxia. In the remainder of cases, radiologic findings range from fine, symmetric, perihilar infiltrates with relative sparing of apexes, bases, and lateral lung fields to massive bilateral pulmonary edema with little or no areas of sparing. Marked clearing of these abnormalities usually takes place within 72 to 96 h.

Alterations in serum sodium and potassium are generally mild and require no corrective treatment. Leukocytosis up to 40,000 white blood cells per microliter is common during the first 24 to 48 h following near-drowning; significant changes in hematocrit and hemoglobin are rare, irrespective of the type of fluid aspirated. A *falling* hematocrit should raise the possibility of bleeding, not hemolysis, which, if it has occurred, should be apparent at the time of initial evaluation. Thrombocytopenia, prolonged prothrombin and partial thromboplastin times, hypofibrinogenemia, and elevated fibrin degradation products may be seen if disseminated intravascular coagulation takes place (see Chap. 288).

THERAPY The primary objective of therapy is to correct hypoxia and acidosis as rapidly as possible. On-the-scene efforts should include immediate institution of mouth-to-mouth breathing and, if necessary, closed-chest cardiac massage. Time should not be wasted with attempts to drain water from the victim's lungs. However, it is important to establish and maintain a clear airway at the onset of resuscitation in order to avoid accidental overdistention of the stomach, which might result in regurgitation and aspiration. The application of a subdiaphragmatic abdominal thrust (Heimlich maneuver) should be used only if foreign-body obstruction to the airway is suspected and cannot be removed manually or by suction. It is ineffective in removing water from the lower airways and may cause forceful reflux of gastric contents, resulting in aspiration. Victims who are hypothermic may appear dead with no apparent heartbeat or brain function. However, experience from ice-water submersion survivors suggests that full resuscitative efforts can be continued until core body temperature is near normal. One hundred percent oxygen should be administered by inhalation as soon as possible, and other necessary resuscitative efforts continued during evacuation to the hospital. Even if spontaneous ventilation returns and the patient seems coherent, high concentrations of oxygen should be continued, since severe hypoxia and acidosis may be present even in persons who are alert and without cyanosis.

All near-drowning victims should be taken to a hospital for further evaluation. Initial diagnostic studies should include measurement of rectal temperature, arterial blood gas and pH determinations, hemogram, serum electrolytes, and chest x-ray. Patients who are alert, have normal chest x-rays, and show no evidence of hypothermia, hypoxia, or acidosis usually require no further therapy. Nevertheless they should be observed for several hours for evidence of deterioration in blood gas and acid-base status prior to discharge. Hypothermia should be treated as outlined in Chap. 377. Metabolic acidosis should be treated by intravenous administration of sodium bicarbonate ($NaHCO_3$), and hypoxia with supplemental oxygen. If bronchospasm is present, aerosol inhalation of a bronchodilator may be given. Patients with pulmonary edema or hypoxia that fails to respond to increasing inspired oxygen tensions up to 40 percent should be intubated endotracheally and have positive end-expiratory pressure (PEEP) applied to the airways. When respiratory failure is present, lung compliance is markedly reduced, or the patient is unable to breathe spontaneously, mechanical ventilatory support should be used in addition to PEEP. Arterial blood gas tensions and pH should be determined frequently to assess the adequacy of respiratory therapy. Treatment with PEEP should be continued long enough for the lung injury to stabilize before it is withdrawn. This may take 48 to 72 h or even longer. Monitoring the magnitude of the intrapulmonary shunt, the pulmonary wedge pressure, and cardiac output by means of a Swan-Ganz intraarterial catheter is often very helpful in weaning patients from PEEP as well as in managing cases complicated by low cardiac output and hypotension.

Comatose near-drowning victims frequently are found to have elevated intracranial pressure, which is caused by cerebral edema and loss of cerebrovascular autoregulation. Prolonged elevations over 2.0 to 2.7 kPa (15 to 20 mmHg) lead to reductions of cerebral blood flow, adding ischemic injury to already damaged brain tissue. In order to preserve cerebral function in such patients, aggressive therapy termed *cerebral resuscitation,* and including controlled hyperventilation, deliberate hypothermia, and the use of barbiturates, glucocorticoids, and osmotic and loop diuretics, has been advocated while the intracranial pressure is closely monitored via subarachnoid bolts and intraventricular catheters. Although several investigators have reported that there are fewer major neurologic sequelae, particularly in children treated in this manner, these therapeutic interventions are unproven and controversial. Recent studies suggest that neither induced hypothermia, high-dose glucocorticoids, nor barbiturate coma improves survival or neurologic outcome. The need for such aggressive and potentially hazardous therapy requires further study before it can be recommended for all patients in deep coma following near-drowning.

Other therapeutic measures are largely supportive. Patients should be observed closely for evidence of pulmonary infection and treated with appropriate antibiotics on the basis of results of cultures of respiratory secretions. Prophylactic use of antibiotics and glucocorticoids has been of no benefit in near-drowning victims. Fluid and electrolyte balance should be carefully maintained. If hypovolemia is associated with low urinary output or hypotension, plasma expanders may be required. Transfusion with packed red blood cells or whole blood, depending upon circulating blood volume status, may be used for significant anemia. Acute renal failure should be managed as described in Chap. 223.

PROGNOSIS The prognosis depends largely upon the extent and duration of the hypoxic episode. In addition, such factors as the temperature of the submersion medium, the availability and appropriate application of specific treatment, and coexisting medical illness or trauma are often important in determining the outcome. In general, patients who are alert and have normal chest x-rays upon arrival at the hospital can be expected to recover fully. Those who are obtunded but arousable and have normal respirations have nearly as good a prognosis, while approximately two-thirds of those requiring cardiopulmonary resuscitation and who present in coma die or are left with significant neurologic deficits. Prediction of outcome on the basis of other presenting neurologic features or laboratory abnormalities is unreliable. The fact that nearly 90 percent of victims who live long enough to receive definitive hospital care will survive should serve to emphasize that extensive resuscitative efforts are advisable in all cases of near-drowning.

REFERENCES

BOLTE RG et al: The use of extracorporeal rewarming in a child submerged for 66 minutes. JAMA 260:377, 1988

FRATES RC JR: Analysis of predictive factors in assessment of warm-water near-drowning in children. Am J Dis Child 135:1006, 1981

GULAID JA, SATTIN RW: Drownings in the United States, 1978–1984. Morb Mort Week Rep 37(SS-1):27, 1988

MODELL JH: Biology of drowning. Ann Rev Med 29:1, 1978

OAKES DD et al: Prognosis and management of victims of near-drowning. J Trauma 22:544, 1982

ORLOWSKI JP: Drowning, near-drowning, and ice-water drowning (editorial). JAMA 260, 390, 1988

ORNATO JP: The resuscitation of near-drowning victims. JAMA 256:75, 1986

YATSU FM: Cardiopulmonary-cerebral resuscitation (editorial). N Engl J Med 314:440, 1986

379 ELECTRICAL INJURIES

JAMES F. WALLACE

EPIDEMIOLOGY Since the first human fatality from accidental electrocution was reported in 1879, electrical injury has become progressively more common. In recent years, nearly 4000 electricity-related injuries have occurred annually in the United States, and major electrical burns have constituted nearly 5 percent of all admissions to burn centers. There are approximately 1000 deaths each year from electric current accidents, while another 100 persons die as a result of being struck by lightning. Electrical injuries occur most commonly among agricultural workers, utility pole linemen, crane and heavy equipment operators, and construction workers who come into contact with high-tension current, but nearly a third result from accidents in the home or other settings including the hospital with its many electrically powered instruments and appliances.

PATHOGENESIS For an electric current to flow, there must be a closed pathway or circuit, and a difference in potential or voltage must exist between two points in this completed circuit. The flow of current is directly related to the voltage difference and inversely proportional to the electrical resistance between two points in the circuit (Ohm's law). High-resistance paths allow relatively small currents to flow, while low resistances permit large currents to flow. When the voltage is very high, the flow of current will likewise be relatively great, unless the resistance is increased proportionally to the voltage; however, if the potential difference between the two points can be minimized, the current flow can also be minimized regardless of resistance.

Although the end result of passage of an electric current through the human body is unpredictable in the individual case, many factors are known to influence the nature and severity of electrical injuries. Body tissues vary considerably in their resistance to the flow of current, with conductivity being roughly proportional to water content. Bone and skin offer relatively high resistance, while blood, muscle, and nerve are good conductors. The resistance of normal skin can be lowered by moisture, and this factor alone can convert what might ordinarily be a mild injury to a fatal shock. Of importance at the time of contact is grounding which, if effective, can minimize the voltage difference between two points in the electric circuit and lower the intensity of current passing through the body. The pathway of the current through the body is also crucial. An accident involving passage of a current between a point of contact on the leg and the ground is less likely to be injurious than one between the head and the foot, in which the heart lies between the two poles of the circuit. Similarly, a small current leak which would be innocuous when applied to the surface of the intact body may result in a fatal arrhythmia when conducted directly to the heart via a low-resistance intracardiac catheter. Duration of contact also influences the outcome of electrical injury. Alternating current is much more dangerous than direct current, partly because of its ability to produce tetanic muscular contractions, which prevent the victim from being able to release contact with the circuit. The contractions are usually accompanied by sweating, which lowers skin resistance, allowing current of still greater intensity to pass into the body until fatal cardiac arrhythmia results.

In general, when sudden death occurs following low-voltage shock, it is due to the direct effect of relatively small amounts of current upon the myocardium resulting in ventricular fibrillation. With high-tension injury (greater than 1000 V), cardiac asystole and respiratory arrest occur probably as a result of injury to the medullary centers of the brain.

In addition, contact with high-intensity current may cause three types of thermal injuries. Current coursing externally to the body from the contact point to the ground may generate temperatures as high as 10,000°C and cause extensive carbonification of skin and immediately underlying tissues termed *arc* or *flash burns*. Such burns often ignite surrounding clothing or nearby objects which result in *flame burns*. Finally, there is injury due to the *direct heating* of tissues by electric current. As it traverses the skin, energy from current is converted into heat, which produces coagulation necrosis at the points where it enters and exits from the skin as well as in striated muscle and blood vessels through which it passes. The associated vascular injury results in thromboses, often at sites distant from the body surface, and accounts for the observation that a greater amount of tissue destruction characteristically occurs in an electrical injury than is apparent on first inspection.

PATHOLOGY In patients who die immediately, autopsy findings are limited to burns and generalized petechial hemorrhages. If patients survive for a period of days or longer, postmortem examination reveals focal necrosis of bone, large blood vessels, muscle, peripheral nerves, spinal cord, or brain. Renal tubular necrosis may also be seen when acute renal failure follows extensive tissue destruction.

CLINICAL MANIFESTATIONS Immediately after a severe electrical shock, patients are usually comatose, apneic, and in circulatory collapse from ventricular fibrillation or cardiac standstill. If they survive this stage, they often are disoriented, combative, and frequently have seizures. Often they will be found to have fractures of bone caused either by convulsive muscular contractions accompanying the shock or from falls at the time of the accident. Hypovolemic shock often appears soon after high-tension electrical injury and is due to the rapid loss of fluid into areas of tissue damage and from body surface burns. Hypotension, direct injury to the kidneys by the electric current, and renal tubular damage from myoglobin and hemoglobin pigments liberated during massive muscle necrosis and hemolysis may lead to acute renal failure.

Besides the extensive destruction of tissue occurring instantly in electrical burns, additional injury from ischemia produced by swelling of damaged tissues may appear later and is often accompanied by severe metabolic acidosis. Other serious complications are severe ventricular arrhythmias, which typically begin several hours following the burn injury, neurogenic pulmonary edema, gastrointestinal hemorrhage from preexisting or acute Curling-type ulcers, disseminated intravascular coagulation, and both anaerobic and aerobic infections originating in inadequately debrided necrotic muscle masses. Lightning injury may result in cerebral edema with coma lasting from several minutes to several days. Rupture of one or both tympanic membranes is seen in over half of lightning victims.

Late effects include various neurologic disabilities, visual disturbances, and the residual damage left by burns. Nervous system injuries are frequent and include peripheral neuropathies, nerve entrapment syndromes, incomplete transection of the spinal cord, and reflex sympathetic dystrophies, as well as late convulsive disorders and intractable headache. Psychological effects, particularly disturbances in memory and mood, are common in survivors of lightning strikes and may last for several months. The development of cataracts of one or both eyes has been reported to occur up to 3 years following electrical injury.

LABORATORY FINDINGS Immediately following major electrical injury the hematocrit is elevated and the plasma volume reduced, reflecting sequestration of fluid in the wound. Unless extensive flame burns are also present, serial determinations of either of these parameters provide a good means of monitoring the adequacy of fluid replacement therapy. Myoglobinuria is seen frequently in association with severe shocks, and when it persists following establishment of urine flow, usually indicates massive muscle injury. In many patients arterial blood pH determinations will indicate the presence of metabolic acidosis. Lumbar puncture may show elevated pressure associated with cerebral edema or bloody spinal fluid as a result of intracerebral hemorrhage. The electrocardiogram not infrequently shows tachycardia and minor ST-segment alterations, which can persist for several weeks following injury. Unexplained acute hypokalemia leading to respiratory arrest and cardiac arrhythmias has developed in some patients between the second and fourth weeks following injury.

TREATMENT Removal of victims from contact with the current should be accomplished immediately without touching them directly. Rescuers should use a rubber sheet, a leather belt applied as a sling, a wooden pole, or other nonconductive material to detach them, and this should be preceded by cutting off the source of current when possible. If the victim is not breathing, mouth-to-mouth ventilation should be instituted at once. Although most cases who survive develop spontaneous respiration within half an hour, complete recovery after longer periods occurs often enough that respiratory support should be continued for at least 4 h. If there is no evidence of heartbeat, external cardiac massage should accompany ventilatory resuscitation. Persons struck by lightning frequently have cardiac asystole which responds to a manual blow to the chest, or which spontaneously resolves after several minutes of closed-chest cardiac massage and mouth-to-mouth resuscitation, while victims of low-voltage shocks will usually require defibrillation to restore heart action. During cardiopulmonary resuscitation and evacuation to the hospital, attention should be paid to possible broken bones and spinal cord injuries incurred at the time of the accident.

Subsequent hospital management of patients with electrothermal injuries requires considerable specialized care; whenever feasible, they should be referred to an appropriate burn or trauma unit.

Rapid institution of fluid and electrolyte therapy for hypovolemic shock and acidosis is essential, with guidelines being the patient's urine output, hematocrit, osmolality, central venous pressure, and arterial blood gases. Standard burn formulas should not be used to estimate fluid therapy since these are based only upon extent of body surface area injury and do not take into account the extensive damage to muscle which is usually present. Instead, fluid replacement principles used in the treatment of crush injury, which electrical injury closely resembles, should be followed. Large volumes of fluid, preferably lactated Ringer's solution, should be administered in order to maintain urine output greater than 50 mL/h. If myoglobinuria persists after adequate urine flow has been established, the use of furosemide or an osmotic diuretic such as mannitol along with alkalinization of the urine is indicated. Since focal myocardial injury is not uncommon when electrical current has passed through the thorax and since coronary blood flow is decreased in response to burn shock, careful cardiac evaluation should be included in initial hospital care. Even in the absence of diagnostic ECG or enzymatic changes, patients should be monitored electrocardiographically for at least 24 h for significant arrhythmias, which often have a delayed onset. Management of the electrical burn wound should include adequate debridement of necrotic tissue and often will require fasciotomy to prevent further ischemic injury. Tetanus toxoid should be administered to all previously immunized patients. Unimmunized patients who have major burns should be given tetanus antitoxin (3000 units) as well as an initial immunizing dose of toxoid. Topical antimicrobial chemotherapy may be useful in preventing or delaying infections in extensive surface burns. Silver sulfadiazine cream currently is the preferred agent. Systemic antibiotics are poorly delivered to the ischemic areas of the burn wound, therefore their routine use to prevent streptococcal and staphylococcal infections is not recommended. Instead, the patient should be closely monitored, and antimicrobial therapy selected as indicated by the results of routine cultures. Survivors of the acute episode often require extensive treatment for infection, visceral injury, and delayed hemorrhage as devitalized tissues slough. If acute renal failure occurs, it should be managed as described in Chap. 223. Patients who remain comatose after being struck by lightning should undergo monitoring of intracranial pressure and cerebral perfusion and be treated for cerebral edema if it should develop.

PREVENTION Proper installation of appliances, grounding of telephone lines and radio and television aerials, and the use of rubber gloves and dry shoes when working with electric circuits should be routine. Unused wall sockets should be kept plugged and live extension cords not left unattended, particularly in households where there are young children. Electrical appliances used in bathrooms should be disconnected when not in use and never used in wet bathtubs. During a severe thunderstorm, refuge near hilltops, riverbanks, hedges, telephone poles, and trees should be avoided. The safest shelter is the closed house, while a closed automobile, cave, ditch, or even lying on the ground curled up with hands close together is relatively secure. In hospitalized patients, the hazard of ventricular fibrillation precipitated by minute current leaks conducted directly to the myocardium from monitoring equipment via pacemakers or intravascular manometric catheters should be more widely appreciated. Hospital personnel should be aware that, in addition to medical instruments, patient contact with two or more other power line–operated devices such as television sets, radios, electric razors, lamps, and especially electric beds can also result in electrocution if the heart lies within the current path through the patient. These hazards can be minimized by proper grounding of equipment *before* a patient is connected to the instrument, periodic measurement for leakage of current supplied by each device, and by instruction in the principles of electrical safety for hospital personnel who use the complex and dangerous equipment that is so much a part of modern medical practice.

REFERENCES

Amy BW et al: Lightning injury with survival in 5 patients. JAMA 253:243, 1985
Apfelberg DB et al: Pathophysiology and treatment of lightning injuries. J Trauma 14:453, 1974

BAXTER CR: Emergency treatment of burn injury. Ann Emerg Med 17:1305, 1988
HUNT J et al: Acute electrical burns: Current diagnostic and therapeutic approaches to management. Arch Surg 115:434, 1980
JENSEN PJ et al: Electrical injury causing ventricular arrhythmias. Br Heart J 57:279, 1987
ROSENBERG DB, NELSON M: Rehabilitation concerns in electrical burn patients. A review of the literature. J Trauma 28:808, 1988

380 RADIATION INJURY

STUART C. FINCH

Throughout life human beings are continuously exposed to many types of radiation, some harmless and some harmful. The most harmful is *ionizing radiation,* which damages tissue through the action of charged particles. More is known about the acute and late somatic, teratogenic, and genetic effects of ionizing radiation than any other environmental, physical, or chemical agent or force, yet many gaps remain in our knowledge concerning its effects. Most important and least well understood are the late effects of chronic low-dose exposure on humans. There is little reliable direct information, so that it is only possible to estimate such effects by extrapolation from information pertaining to high-dose exposure.

There are two types of ionizing radiation: The first consists of high-frequency electromagnetic waves of relatively short wavelength with particle characteristics, such as naturally occurring gamma rays or machine-made x-rays. These waves are capable of deep tissue penetration and moderate ionization of the tissues along their pathways by indirect mechanisms. Their interactions with the atoms and molecules of tissue structures result in the release of orbital electrons and the formation of ions and reactive radicals that damage cell components and disrupt biologic processes. The second type of ionizing radiation consists of a variety of subatomic particles, the most important of which are electrically charged alpha particles, protons, and electrons and electrically uncharged neutrons. The charged particles densely ionize structures along their pathways in tissues. The depth of penetration is quite limited and varies as a function of particle size, charge, and velocity. Tissue damage is due to the direct ionization of water, oxygen, and other molecules with the formation of free hydroxyl radicals and highly reactive oxygen species. Neutrons penetrate tissues much more deeply than charged particles of equivalent size (such as protons). They indirectly ionize through their interactions with the nuclei of atoms, resulting in the release of protons, alpha particles, and other nuclear fragments that ionize and damage other tissues.

The longer-wavelength waves of the electromagnetic spectrum do not ionize, but some may damage tissues by other mechanisms. For example, ultraviolet light penetrates very little, but it photochemically induces cell damage, some of which may be permanent. Ultrasonic, infrared, radio, and microwave electromagnetic waves are capable of deep tissue penetration with the generation of heat, the effects of which are largely reversible. Weak, low-frequency electromagnetic waves have been shown to modulate ion flow and to interfere with both RNA transcription and DNA synthesis at the cellular level, but the overall effects in humans remain uncertain. This chapter will consider only the acute and late effects of exposure to ionizing radiation.

TERMINOLOGY AND DEFINITIONS Some familiarity with radiation terminology and units is essential for the understanding of radiation effects. An early term for the quantitation of exposure was the *roentgen,* or R, which represents the amount of radiation-induced ionization in a standard volume of air. Much more important is the *rad* (radiation absorbed dose), which represents a unit of absorbed dose in tissue. One rad corresponds to the absorption of one hundred ergs of energy (or about 1 R) in one gram of tissue. Since the same dose in rads of different kinds of ionizing radiation can produce different biologic effects, the term *rem* (roentgen equivalent man) was introduced. It represents the rad multiplied by its RBE (relative biologic effectiveness), which is a quality factor for the biologic effects of the particular type of radiation used in comparison to a radiation standard. The biologic effect of gamma radiation is the usual standard for comparison. Gamma radiation, therefore, has an RBE of 1, and 1 rad of gamma exposure is roughly equal to 1 rem. Most x-rays have an RBE of 1 or slightly higher, whereas neutrons and some charged particles may have an RBE of 5 to 20 or greater. The terms *gray* (Gy), one unit of which is the equivalent of one hundred rads, and *sievert* (Sv), one unit of which is equal to one hundred rems, have been adopted to replace the rad and rem terminologies, respectively. One-thousandth of a gray is written as mGy (0.1 rad), and one-thousandth of an Sv as mSv (0.1 rem).

The density of tissue ionization produced per unit length along the pathway of ionizing radiation is expressed as its *linear energy transfer* (LET). In general, electrically charged particles or particles of relatively high mass (alpha particles, protons, and neutrons) have high energy transfer (high LET), resulting in relatively large amounts of tissue damage. In contrast, electromagnetic forms of ionizing radiation (gamma rays or x-rays) or charged particles of small mass (electrons) transfer less energy per unit length of travel (have low LET) and produce less tissue damage. There is quite a good correlation between LET and RBE.

The *threshold dose* is the minimum radiation dose that will produce a biologic effect. Radiation effects that vary with dose and frequency but not in severity are called *stochastic* effects. Examples of these are radiation-induced carcinogenic, mutagenic, and teratogenic effects. *Nonstochastic* effects vary in severity above a threshold dose depending on the number of cells injured. Examples of such effects are radiation-induced cataracts of the eye or fibrosis of the bone marrow. The interval of time between exposure and the occurrence of a radiation effect is identified as its *latent period.* The *maximum permissible dose* is that dose of ionizing radiation that, in the light of present knowledge, is not expected to cause any appreciable bodily injury to any person at any time during a lifetime.

TYPES AND SOURCES OF IONIZING RADIATION Most of a person's lifetime radiation exposure is from low-dose background radiation. The average annual effective dose for persons in the United States is estimated to be about 3.6 mSv. About two-thirds of this radiation is from natural sources, of which radon, cosmic rays, radionuclides in the earth, and radioactive elements in the body are the major contributors.

Radon now is believed to contribute about 55 percent of a person's total background radiation exposure. This represents about 2 mSv of exposure per year. Radon is a colorless, odorless, and tasteless alpha particle emitting radioactive gas which is derived from naturally occurring uranium deposits in the earth. It seeps up through soil into the air, where it and its decay products attach to dust, aerosols, or droplets which are inhaled and retained in bronchial epithelium and adjacent structures. The greatest exposures occur in certain indoor areas and mines where there are high adjacent rock concentrations of phosphates, granite, and black shale. Radon itself is not particularly harmful, but some of its alpha-emitting polonium radioactive decay products may heavily irradiate bronchial epithelium cells for many months or years.

Cosmic radiation accounts for about 0.3 mSv of background radiation per year at sea level. It is composed of protons, neutrons, and heavy nuclei from galactic sources and low-energy charged particles from the sun which interact with atmospheric nuclei to produce small secondary particles and electrons that enter the body and ionize tissue. The earth's atmosphere acts as a shield, so that the dose is about doubled with every 1500-m increase in altitude. Radioactive potassium and carbon and other radionuclides within the body contribute about another 0.4 mSv to the average person's annual background radiation exposure. Radioactive decay of thorium and uranium radionuclides in the earth's crust constitute the major sources of terrestrial radiation, which, in most areas, is about 0.3 mSv per year. Amounts of terrestrial radiation may vary by a factor of four to six or more in different geographic locations.

The remaining 18 percent of a person's total background radiation exposure is from man-made sources. Diagnostic x-ray and nuclear medicine account for over 0.5 mSv of the estimated annual total of about 0.65 mSv. Exposure from these sources has doubled in the United States and many other countries during the past 20 years.

Most acute or intermittent excessive exposures to ionizing radiation occur in association with radiation therapy, preparation for organ transplantation, nuclear weapon detonations, nuclear reactor accidents, or accidental ingestion of radionuclides. Most of such exposures are to x- or gamma rays, but direct radiation exposure or fallout from nuclear weapon detonations or reactor accidents or radionuclide ingestion, inhalation, or injection may result in significant exposures to high-LET radiation.

PATHOGENESIS OF RADIATION INJURY There are many types of cellular injury following exposure to ionizing radiation. Most important is damage to the genetic apparatus of the nucleus due to structural alterations of DNA and chromosomes.

Many types of DNA damage may occur, but most common with low-LET radiation are single-strand breaks and base alterations. High-LET radiation produces more double-strand breaks and more complex types of DNA base damage. In both instances, free radicals generated by ionizing radiation are largely responsible for the DNA and chromosome alterations. The extent to which damaged DNA will be responsible for cell death or will become a permanent mutation depends upon the ability of the cells to repair the damage. Repair of DNA damage from low-LET radiation is much more efficient than it is from high-LET radiation. This is extremely important because most of the somatic mutational and late neoplastic effects in replicating cells probably are due to the persistence of radiation-induced unrepaired or misrepaired DNA bases.

Chromosome damage of many types as a function of unrepaired DNA constitutes the other major type of radiation-induced injury to the genetic apparatus of the cell. Chromosomal breaks with rearrangements associated with loss of considerable amounts of chromosomal mass usually are responsible for cell death at the first or one of the first few postirradiation mitotic divisions. Consequently the number of chromosome aberrations present at any one time during the postirradiation period will depend on both the number induced and the rate of cell turnover. Balanced chromosomal rearrangements involving little loss of chromosomal material may persist as stable intracellular markers of radiation injury for many years. There is strong evidence that chromosome rearrangements involving breaks near proto-oncogenes play an important role in the process of radiation-induced malignant transformation (see Chap. 10).

Repair of radiation-induced DNA and chromosomal damage is inversely related to the rate at which the radiation is absorbed. This is particularly true for low-LET radiation, where a high rate of radiation absorption may increase residual tissue damage by factors of 2 to 10 times that experienced with a low rate of radiation absorption.

High doses of radiation may produce direct cell death due to membrane or cytoplasmic structural damage. This type of interphase cell death of autonomic nerve cells, lymphocytes, and capillaries is responsible for most of the early clinical manifestations of high-dose acute radiation exposure. Relatively little direct membrane and cytoplasmic damage occurs following exposure to low doses of ionizing radiation.

HISTORY Most of our knowledge concerning the *late* effects of ionizing radiation exposure for humans has been derived from a series of unfortunate accidents and errors during the past 75 years. In the early 1920s and 1930s about 2000 luminous dial workers, mostly young women in the United States, inadvertently ingested large amounts of radium 226 by means of absorption from their tongues and lips. Many later developed carcinomas of the paranasal sinuses and osteosarcomas. In Germany in the mid-1940s a number of children with bone tuberculosis and many adults with rheumatoid arthritis were injected with radium 224. Five to ten years later many of them also developed osteosarcomas. Increased mortality from leukemia and multiple myeloma was reported for radiologists during the early years of use of medical x-ray equipment. In the 1930s and through the early 1950s thorium dioxide (Thorotrast) was employed as a contrast medium in a number of medical clinics throughout the world. Many injected persons developed hepatic tumors, leukemia, or aplastic anemia in later years. Increased rates of thyroid cancer and leukemia have been reported for children treated with x-rays in the 1940s and 1950s for tinea capitis and presumed thymus enlargement. A sizable number of individuals with ankylosing spondylitis in England who received radiation therapy later developed aplastic anemia and leukemia. Increased incidence of lung cancer has been recognized in uranium miners. Fallout from weapons testing in the Marshall Islands has produced an increased occurrence of hypothyroidism and benign thyroid nodules. Studies of the atomic bomb survivors of Hiroshima and Nagasaki, however, have provided the most extensive and reliable information concerning the late effects of exposure to ionizing radiation.

Most information concerning *acute* radiation exposure derives from two sources: the atomic bomb explosions and radiation accidents. There were approximately 110,000 to 120,000 civilian deaths from the atomic bomb explosions of Hiroshima and Nagasaki, about one-third of which are believed to have been caused by radiation exposure. The Radiation Accident Registry at Oak Ridge has identified 305 major worldwide radiation accidents between 1944 and 1989, involving 122,614 people. There were 1871 significant exposures and 101 deaths. Forty-four of the deaths were attributed to the acute radiation syndrome.

CLINICAL EFFECTS OF RADIATION EXPOSURE *Acute, or early, effects* occur within the first few minutes up to 2 to 3 months following exposure to large amounts of radiation over a short period of time and are due to cell killing, impairment of cell function, inflammation, and infection. *Intermediate effects* occur after the first few months up to a few years following exposure. *Late effects* are the diseases and disorders that develop after the first few months or years for which previous ionizing radiation exposure is responsible.

Acute radiation effects The early clinical manifestations of excessive acute whole-body exposure to ionizing radiation constitute the *acute radiation syndrome*. Its time of onset, severity, and duration will depend on the quality, quantity, and distribution of the radiation absorbed.

There are four classic clinical stages of the complete acute radiation syndrome. The earliest phase is the prodrome, which invariably consists of anorexia, nausea, and vomiting but also may include diarrhea, salivation, abdominal cramps, and dehydration. It commences within minutes to hours of exposure and lasts from a few hours to 1 or 2 days. This usually is followed by a relatively asymptomatic second stage of a few days to a few weeks in duration. The third stage usually begins during the second to fifth weeks following exposure with the abrupt onset of moderate to severe gastrointestinal tract disturbances and manifestations of bone marrow depression. The fourth stage involves recovery, which may take weeks to months, or death.

Persons who receive whole-body radiation in the range of 50 Gy or more invariably will die within 24 to 48 h from complications associated with the *neurovascular syndrome*. This is characterized by the rapid onset of apathy, lethargy, and prostration, frequently followed by seizures ranging from muscle contractions to grand mal convulsions, ataxia, and death. The early occurrence of severe central nervous system problems frequently yields to intractable hypotension, arrhythmias, and shock before death occurs. This sometimes is identified as the *cardiovascular syndrome*.

A significant prodrome also will develop rapidly in persons exposed to whole-body radiation in the range of 10 to 50 Gy. Following a latent period of a few days, the *gastrointestinal syndrome* develops as the result of intestinal tract ulceration, infection, and hemorrhage secondary to mucosal cell atrophy and bone marrow depression. Its clinical manifestations are associated with massive fluid, protein, and electrolyte loss, invariably leading to death within a few more days.

Whole-body exposures in the range of 2 to 10 Gy are characterized by manifestations of the *bone marrow syndrome* due to a loss of marrow stem cells. Following a prodrome of 1 to 3 days and a relatively asymptomatic period of 1 to 3 weeks, buccal and pharyngeal ulcerations, localized and systemic forms of infection, cutaneous petechiae, and possibly generalized bleeding may develop secondary to thrombocytopenia and agranulocytosis. Concomitant loss of gastrointestinal epithelium often results in persistent diarrhea, abdominal distention, dehydration, circulatory collapse, and death. Survivors will experience rapid clinical improvement following partial return of peripheral blood granulocytes and platelets in 6 to 8 weeks, but full recovery may take several months. Epilation usually commences 1 to 2 weeks following exposure and is greatest at 5 to 7 weeks. Regrowth of new hair may take 4 to 6 months or more.

Mild gastrointestinal symptoms are experienced by 25 to 75 percent of persons exposed to less than 2 Gy of whole-body radiation. Hematologic complications rarely develop, because there is only moderate depression of the formed blood elements. Complete recovery of almost everyone in this exposure category is expected within 2 to 5 weeks.

Peripheral blood lymphopenia invariably develops during the first 12 to 48 h following any significant exposure. The rate and magnitude of the drop are reasonably related to radiation exposures up to about 5 to 6 Gy. At higher levels of exposure, lymphopenia is extreme, so that correlations with exposure dose are poor. Reduced lymphocyte levels usually persist for 6 to 8 weeks. There often is a modest increase in numbers of peripheral blood granulocytes during the first 1 to 2 days in response to exposure of more than 2 Gy followed by a continual decline to maximum granulocytopenia in 2 to 5 weeks. The rate of granulocyte decline and the severity of granulocytopenia are functions of the bone marrow exposure dose. The peripheral blood platelet count responses are similar to those of the granulocytes except that early thrombocytosis is rare and rates of both decline and recovery usually are slower. Reversible dose-dependent reticulocytopenia and mild anemia may develop up to radiation doses of about 5 to 6 Gy. Higher exposures usually result in irreversible bone marrow damage.

Early radiation-induced chromosome aberrations observed in peripheral blood lymphocytes include dicentrics, rings, deletions, translocations, inversions, and other types of rearrangements. Other dose-related somatic mutations observed following acute whole-body exposure include loss of hypoxanthine-guanine phosphoribosyl transferase (HPRT) from some circulating lymphocytes and alterations in the structure of erythrocyte membrane glycophorin A.

Reproductive system disturbances are other important early clinical sequelae of acute whole-body radiation exposure. Male oligospermia or aspermia usually is temporary for weeks or months following exposures of 1.5 to 4 Gy, but permanent sterility usually develops at exposures of 5 to 9 Gy or greater. Sterility may be temporary in females exposed to 1.5 to 6.5 Gy and permanent at higher levels.

Intermediate and late radiation effects The most important late effect of exposure to ionizing radiation is increased incidence of cancer. An increased incidence of leukemia appeared in the Japanese atomic bomb survivors within 2 to 3 years following exposure. Peak rates occurred about 7 to 8 years after the bombings, followed by a steady decline to near-baseline levels during the next 30 to 35 years. Childhood leukemia rates peaked early and returned to normal 15 years after exposure. The latent period for acute leukemia in adults increased with age at the time of exposure. Most of the radiation-induced childhood leukemias were acute lymphocytic in type, but a high incidence of chronic myeloid leukemia also occurred. Acute and chronic myeloid leukemias predominated in adults, but acute lymphocytic leukemia also appeared to be radiation-related. There is no evidence from any studies of human radiation effects that chronic lymphocytic leukemia is radiation-related. Based on atomic bomb survivor information, the expected excess number of deaths from leukemia from low-LET radiation over a period of 40 years is about 10 cases for every 1000 adults exposed to 1 Sv of radiation.

A significant relationship between radiation exposure and the frequency of death from multiple myeloma and cancers of the female breast, esophagus, stomach, colon, lung, ovary, and urinary bladder has been observed in atomic bomb survivors (Table 380-1). Significant increases in mortality have not been observed for lymphomas, bone tumors, and cancers of the rectum, gallbladder, pancreas, uterus, and prostate in this population. Most of the radiation-induced solid tumors have appeared at their usual ages of occurrence, with minimum latent periods ranging from 15 to 35 years. Since the incidence of most cancers increases with aging, it is likely that the increased risk for cancer from radiation exposure lasts for life. There is a dose-dependent shortening of the latent period and a significant increase in cancer risk for children exposed under the age of 10. Excess deaths for specific radiation-induced cancers are about equal in males and females, except for a significant increase in deaths from leukemia in males. The radiation dose-response relationship for solid tumors is linear, but for leukemia it appears to be more linear-quadratic. The radiation response for the induction of tumors is believed to be stochastic, but organ-absorbed doses in the range of 0.2 to 0.49 Gy for leukemia, lung cancer, and several other cancers are the lowest levels for which a significant increase in cancer mortality has been observed (Table 380-1). Excess lifetime mortality from low-LET radiation in adults for cancers other than leukemia is estimated on the basis of atomic bomb survivor information to be about 47 new cases for every 1000 persons exposed to 1 Sv.

Increased incidence of thyroid cancer, benign thyroid adenomas, and hypothyroidism may occur following either external or internal exposure of the thyroid gland to ionizing radiation. The risk of developing thyroid cancer from external irradiation during childhood is about twice that for exposure during adulthood. The female-to-male ratio for radiation-induced thyroid cancer is about 2:1, with latent periods ranging from 4 to 30 years or longer. Persons of Jewish descent appear to be at higher risk than are those of other ethnic backgrounds who have been studied. Thyroid gland exposures to low-LET radiation in the range of 0.2 to 15 Gy have resulted in the increased late occurrence of thyroid cancer. The absolute risk for low-LET radiation–induced thyroid cancer is quite uncertain and depends on many factors, but probably is in the range of 6 to 12 excess cases per 10^4 persons year Gy. The induction rate for benign adenomas is about 30 to 50 percent greater than that for cancer. Radioiodine therapy with thyroid gland doses greater than 15 to 20 Gy kills parenchymal cells and almost invariably results in hypothy-

TABLE 380-1 Significant radiation-induced cancer information for atomic bomb survivors, 1950–1985 (radiation exposure expressed as organ-absorbed dose)

Type of cancer	Excess relative risk at 1 Gy*	Excess deaths per 10^4 persons/year, Gy*	Minimum dose for increased mortality, Gy	Minimum latent period to death, years
Leukemia	5.2	2.9	0.2–0.5	3–5
Multiple myeloma	2.3	0.3	—	30–34
Ovary	1.3	0.7	0.2–0.3	25–29
Urinary tract	1.3	0.7	—	30–34
Female breast	1.2	1.2	0.5–1.0	20–24
Colon	0.9	0.8	1.0–1.9	30–34
Lung	0.6	1.7	0.2–0.5	20–24
Esophagus	0.6	0.5	—	—
All (except leukemia)	0.4	10.1	0.2–0.5	—
Stomach	0.3	2.4	0.5–1.0	15–19

* Rates from UNSCEAR and Radiation Effects Research Foundation reports have been rounded to the nearest tenth.

roidism rather than cancer. Radioiodine used for diagnostic thyroid studies increases the incidence of benign adenomas but does not increase the incidence of thyroid cancer.

Many types of cancer and other late effects have been related to exposure to ionizing radiation from internally deposited radioisotopes (Table 380-2). The only recognized late effect from excessive radon exposure is lung cancer. The risk of death in the United States from indoor radon exposure is estimated to be 0.4 percent. This would result in the development of 6000 to 25,000 lung cancers per year. The risks of radon exposure and smoking for lung cancer are at least additive.

Bilateral posterior-central dotlike opacities with surrounding granules and vacuoles may develop in the *lens* of the eye within weeks or months following low-LET radiation exposure. The more heavily irradiated persons may have lateral extension of these tiny opacities with central clearing and anterior extension to the anterior surface of the lens. The lesions are defined as cataracts, but they rarely impair vision or progress over the years. Children are more prone to develop radiation-induced lenticular damage than are adults. The lenticular changes induced by radiation are nonstochastic, with a threshold dose of about 0.3 Gy for low-LET radiation.

The early radiation-induced dicentric and ring-form chromosomal aberrations in blood lymphocytes disappear with the first mitosis, so that few remain in later years, but many of the radiation-induced balanced structural rearrangements persist as biologic radiation markers throughout life. Reciprocal translocations and inversions predominate. The radiation dose-response is linear and is not influenced by age at time of exposure. The early radiation-induced structural alterations in erythrocyte membrane glycophorin A persist in later years, but the changes in lymphocyte HPRT disappear with time.

A radiation dose-response relationship for the occurrence of small head size has been observed in newborn infants following in utero exposure of the fetus to atomic bomb radiation during the first 15 weeks of pregnancy. Small head size has been observed in 40 to 50 percent of these infants following exposures of 1 Gy or more. A dose-related risk of mental retardation also has been observed in children following in utero exposure between the eighth and fifteenth weeks of gestation to greater than 0.4 Gy of low-LET radiation. A lower risk for mental retardation exists for exposure between the sixteenth and twenty-fifth weeks of gestation with an apparent threshold at about 0.7 Gy. Prenatal exposure during the eighth to fifteenth weeks of gestation and, to a lesser extent, between the sixteenth and twenty-eighth weeks also is dose-related to an increased incidence of reduced school achievement, lower intelligence test scores, and unprovoked seizures later in life. The crude incidence of cancer 40 years following intrauterine exposure to radiation above 0.3 Gy is three- to nine-fold greater than for unexposed controls.

TABLE 380-2 Late effects of radionuclide exposure

Radionuclide	Route of administration	Late effects
Thorium^{232} dioxide (Thorotrast)	Intravenous	Liver angiosarcoma, hemangioendothelioma, hepatic cell carcinoma, and cirrhosis. Bile duct carcinoma, kidney cancer, leukemia, splenic atrophy and fibrosis, and aplastic anemia.
Radium^{224}	Intravenous	Osteosarcoma, chondroblastic sarcoma, cataracts, leukemia, and renal insufficiency.
Radium^{226,228}	Oral	Osteosarcoma, chondroblastic sarcoma, paranasal and mastoid carcinoma, and colon cancer.
Radon^{222}	Inhalation	Lung cancer.
Iodine^{125,131}	Oral and intravenous	Hypothyroidism, thyroid adenomas, and thyroid cancer.
Strontium^{90}	Topical	Anterior lenticular cataracts from eye applicators; fallout-induced acute beta skin burns may lead to eventual skin necrosis and atrophy.
Phosphorus^{32}	Topical	Fallout-induced acute beta skin burns may lead to eventual skin necrosis and atrophy.

Excessive prenatal or childhood radiation exposure in the range of 1 Gy or more has been shown eventually to result in slight reduction in maximum height. Other late effects of whole-body exposure in atomic bomb survivors include accelerated decline in cell-mediated immunity with aging and an increased occurrence of hyperparathyroidism.

There are few direct data for humans concerning the genetic effects of exposure to ionizing radiation. It is believed, however, that the dose-response relationship is linear without a threshold and that the overwhelming majority of induced mutations are damaging. Atomic bomb survivor studies have failed to demonstrate a statistically significant increase in the genetic effects evaluated in the children of exposed persons, but the data suggest that the amount of acute parental radiation required to double the spontaneous mutation rate (*doubling dose*) is about 2 Sv. The Japanese data also suggest a doubling dose for chronic parental radiation exposure of about 4 Sv, in comparison to other estimates from mouse data ranging from 0.5 to 2.5 Sv. All of these estimates have considerable error.

Local or regional radiotherapy Radiation administered in small intermittent (fractionated) doses is better tolerated by tissue structures than an equivalent amount of radiation given as a single dose. However, since the cumulative total local and regional radiotherapy tissue doses usually are very high, the acute, intermediate, and late effects may be severe and quite different from those due to whole-body exposure. For example, intensive local x-ray therapy to the lung may cause radiation pneumonitis and fibrosis, yet little lung damage will occur following exposure to near lethal amounts of whole-body radiation. Internists should be familiar with the major acute, intermediate, and late effects of radiotherapy, which have been well-documented elsewhere.

TREATMENT There is no specific therapy for tissue radiation injury, but much can be done to reduce the morbitity and mortality for persons who have been acutely exposed to excessive amounts of whole-body ionizing radiation.

Persons with possible surface contamination from radioactive substances must be evacuated promptly, monitored for external contamination, and decontaminated if necessary. It is extremely important to estimate the dose of radiation exposure as early as possible in order to determine the need for various types of therapy. This may be extremely difficult even under the best of circumstances. The most reliable early indicators of dose in the absence of an actual dosimeter measurement are the exposure history, the severity of clinical symptoms, and the frequency of certain radiation-induced biologic markers in blood cells. The severity and rapidity of the development of lymphopenia may give some early index of exposure dose, but much more reliable is the radiation-induced frequency of dicentric chromosome aberrations in mitogen-stimulated and spontaneously dividing peripheral blood lymphocytes. (An emergency service for lymphocyte chromosome aberrations is available from the Radiation Emergency Assistance Center/Training Site in Oak Ridge, Tennessee.) The rate of granulocyte decline also is a very reliable and practical early biologic radiation dosimeter, but it may take 3 to 5 days or more before the rate is determined accurately. Bone marrow aspirations have limited quantitative relationships to exposure, but if performed in various sites, they may indicate the extent of marrow damage. Measurements of radiation-induced loss of HPRT in lymphocytes and glycophorin A mutations in the red cell membrane also show great promise as biologic dosimeters for the early estimation of radiation dose.

Persons with few symptoms probably are exposed to less than 2 Gy and will require little or no therapy, but should be kept under observation for a few days. Persons with estimated exposures in the range of 2 to 5 or 6 Gy require hospitalization for vigorous supportive therapy. Intravenous fluids and broad-spectrum antibiotic coverage should be instituted if either bacterial infection or severe agranulocytosis develops. Other supportive measures may include the administration of immunoglobulins, antifungal and antiviral agents, and antibiotics for the reduction of intestinal tract bacterial flora. Platelet transfusions should be administered for either clinical bleeding due to thrombocytopenia or with platelet counts below 20×10^9/L. Blood transfusions are necessary if anemia develops. Bone marrow transfusions are not indicated for persons in this group, but the early and continuous administration of granulocyte colony stimulating factors may be important adjuncts to the other forms of supportive therapy.

If the level of granulocytes falls during the first week to 0.25×10^9/L or less and the level of platelets to less than 30×10^9/L in 10 days, the total-body exposure probably is in the range of 5 to 15 Gy. Exposure doses in this range usually will irreversibly destroy the bone marrow stem cells. Survival with supportive therapy alone usually is not possible, so that the addition of allogeneic bone marrow transplantation and the concomitant administration of granulocyte colony stimulating factors may offer the best hopes for survival (see Chap. 299). Bone marrow transplantations probably are most effective if performed within the first 3 to 5 days of exposure, so early radiation dose estimates are very important. Peripheral blood lymphocytes should be collected as early as is possible for histocompatibility testing, because they disappear rapidly from circulation. Platelets and blood should be irradiated with about 20 Gy prior to transfusion in order to reduce recipient alloantigen sensitization. Preparatory immunosuppression with chemotherapeutic agents and whole-body irradiation probably are not advisable prior to bone marrow transfusion, as permanent engraftment may not be necessary. Furthermore, they will contribute considerably to the severity of the overall illness. Persons with acute exposure to more than 15 to 20 Gy should be admitted to the hospital for supportive therapy only.

It is recommended that persons exposed to fallout in contaminated areas be treated as early as possible with 130 mg/d of potassium iodide for 10 days in order to prevent the accumulation of radioactive iodine in the thyroid gland.

PROGNOSIS Prognosis for survival from the acute manifestations of whole-body exposure to ionizing radiation depends almost entirely upon tissue dose. Mortality without any therapy is negligible at 1 Gy or less and is virtually 100 percent above 15 Gy despite optimal therapy. About 50 percent of persons exposed to between 2 and 4 Gy will succumb without therapy, but most will survive with vigorous support. There is a very high probability of death, even with vigorous general support therapy, at exposures between 5 and 15 Gy, but it seems likely that some people will survive with allogeneic bone marrow transplantation and other forms of supportive therapy.

There are no known forms of therapy for prevention of the late effects of ionizing radiation exposure. They are influenced by tissue dose, rate of exposure, age at time of exposure, concomitant exposure to other carcinogens or radioprotective agents, inherent repair mechanisms, and many other unknown factors. The clinical course and response to therapy of radiation-induced leukemias and solid tumors are not significantly different from those which are not radiation-related.

REFERENCES

COMMITTEE ON THE BIOLOGICAL EFFECTS OF IONIZING RADIATION, NATIONAL RESEARCH COUNCIL: *Health Risks of Radon and Other Internally Deposited Alpha-emitters (BEIR IV)*. Washington, D.C., National Academy Press, 1988

———: *Health Effects of Exposure to Low Levels of Ionizing Radiation (BEIR V)*. Washington, D.C., National Academy Press, 1990

METTLER JR FA, MOSELY JR RD: *Medical Effects of Radiation*. Orlando, Florida, Grune and Stratton, 1985, pp 1–288

NEEL JV et al: The children of parents exposed to atomic bombs: Estimates of the genetic doubling dose of radiation for humans. Am J Human Gen 46:1053, 1990

SHIMUZU Y et al: Studies of the mortality of A-bomb survivors. 9. Mortality, 1950–85, Part 2. Cancer mortality based on the recently revised doses (DS 86). Radiat Res 121:120, 1990.

UNITED NATIONS SCIENTIFIC COMMITTEES ON THE EFFECTS OF ATOMIC RADIATION: *Sources, Effects and Risks of Ionizing Radiation*. Report No. 88. IX. 7. New York, United Nations, 1988

APPENDIX AND INDEX

APPENDIX LABORATORY VALUES OF CLINICAL IMPORTANCE

INTRODUCTORY COMMENTS

In preparing the Appendix, the editors have taken into account the fact that the system of international units (SI, système international d'unités) is now used in most countries and in virtually all medical and scientific journals including those in the United States.[1] However, many or most clinical laboratories in the United States continue to report values in traditional units. Therefore, in this book we utilize both systems for the Appendix and for the text itself. Values in SI units appear first, and *traditional units appear in parentheses* after the SI units. This dual approach is also used for the large part in the text. In those instances in which the numbers remain the same but only the terminology is changed (mmol/L for meq/L or IU/L for mIU/mL) only the SI units are given. In all other instances the SI unit is followed by the traditional unit in parentheses. The SI base units, SI derived units, other units of measure referred to in the Appendix, and SI prefixes are listed in Tables A-1 to A-3 at the end of the Appendix. Conversions from one system to another can be made as follows:

$$\text{mmol/L} = \frac{\text{mg/dL} \times 10}{\text{atomic weight}}$$

$$\text{mg/dL} = \frac{\text{mmol/L} \times \text{atomic weight}}{10}$$

ASCITIC FLUID

See Table 48-1, p. 270.

BODY FLUIDS AND OTHER MASS DATA

Body fluid, total volume: 50 percent (in obese) to 70 percent (lean) of body weight
- Intracellular: 0.3–0.4 of body weight
- Extracellular: 0.2–0.3 of body weight

Blood:
- Total volume:
  - Males: 69 mL per kg body weight
  - Females: 65 mL per kg body weight
- Plasma volume:
  - Males: 39 mL per kg body weight
  - Females: 40 mL per kg body weight
- Red blood cell volume:
  - Males: 30 mL per kg body weight (1.15–1.21 L/m² body surface area)
  - Females: 25 mL per kg body weight (0.95–1.00 L/m² body surface area)

CEREBROSPINAL FLUID[2]

		Conversion factor (CF) (C × CF = SI)
Osmolality	292–297 mosmol/kg (292–297 mosmol/L)	—
Electrolytes:		
Sodium	137–145 mmol/L (137–145 meq/L)	—
Potassium	2.7–3.9 mmol/L (2.7–3.9 meq/L)	—
Calcium	1–1.5 mmol/L (2.1–3.0 meq/L)	0.5
Magnesium	1–1.2 mmol/L (2.0–2.5 meq/L)	0.5
Chloride	116–122 mmol/L (116–122 meq/L)	—
CO_2 content	20–24 mmol/L (20–24 meq/L)	—
P_{CO_2}	6–7 kPa (45–49 mmHg)	0.1333
pH	7.31–7.34	—
Glucose	2.2–3.9 mmol/L (40–70 mg/dL)	0.05551
Lactate	1–2 mmol/L (10–20 mg/dL)	0.1110
Total protein:	0.2–0.4 g/L (20–40 mg/dL)	0.01
Prealbumin	2–6 percent	—
Albumin	56–75 percent	—
Alpha$_1$ globulin	2–7 percent	—
Alpha$_2$ globulin	4–12 percent	—
Beta globulin	8–16 percent	—
Gamma globulin	3–12 percent	—
IgG	0.01–0.014 g/L (1–1.4 mg/dL)	0.01
IgA	0.001–0.003 g/L (0.1–0.3 mg/dL)	0.01
IgM	0.0001–0.00012 g/L (0.01–0.012 mg/dL)	0.01
Ammonia	15–47 µmol/L (25–80 µg/dL)	0.5872
Creatinine	44–168 µmol/L (0.5–1.9 mg/dL)	88.40
Myelin basic protein	<4 µg/L	—
CSF pressure	50–180 mmH$_2$O	—
CSF volume (adult)	100–160 mL	—
Leukocytes:		
Total	<4 per mL	—
Differential:		
Lymphocytes	60–70 percent	—
Monocytes	30–50 percent	—
Neutrophils	1–3 percent	—

[1] Young DS: Implementation of SI Units for Clinical Laboratory Data. Ann Intern Med 106:114, 1987

[2] Since cerebrospinal fluid concentrations are equilibrium values, measurements of the same parameters in blood plasma obtained at the same time is recommended. However, there is a time lag in attainment of equilibrium, and cerebrospinal levels of plasma constituents that can fluctuate rapidly (such as plasma glucose) may not achieve stable values until after a significant lag phase.

CHEMICAL CONSTITUENTS OF BLOOD

See also "Function Tests," especially "Metabolic and Endocrine."

	Conversion factor (CF) (C × CF = SI)
Acetoacetate, plasma: <100 μmol/L (<1 mg/dL)	97.95
Albumin, serum: 35–55 g/L (3.5–5.5 g/dL)	10
Aldolase: 0–100 nkat/L (0–6 U/L)	16.67
$Alpha_1$ antitrypsin, serum: 0.8–2.1 g/L (85–213 mg/dL)	0.01
Alpha fetoprotein (adult), serum: <30 μg/L (<30 ng/mL)	—
Aminotransferases, serum:	
Aspartate (AST, SGOT): 0–0.58 μkat/L (0–35 U/L)	0.01667
Alanine (ALT, SGPT): 0–0.58 μkat/L (0–35 U/L)	0.01667
Ammonia, whole blood, venous: 47–65 μmol/L (80–110 μg/dL)	0.5872
Amylase, serum: 0.8–3.2 μkat/L (60–180 U/L)	0.01667
Arterial blood gases:	
[HCO_3^-]: 21–28 mmol/L (21–28 meq/L)	—
P_{CO_2}: 4.7–5.9 kPa (35–45 mmHg)	0.1333
pH: 7.38–7.44	—
P_{O_2}: 11–13 kPa (80–100 mmHg)	0.1333
Ascorbic acid (vitamin C), serum: 23–57 μmol/L (0.4–1.0 mg/dL)	56.78
Barbiturates, serum: normal, nondetectable	
Phenobarbital, "potentially fatal" level: approximately 390 μmol/L (9 mg/dL)	43.06
Most short-acting barbiturates, "potentially fatal" levels: approximately 150 μmol/L (35 mg/L)	4.419
Base, total, serum: 145–155 mmol/L (145–155 meq/L)	—
β-Hydroxybutyrate, plasma: <300 μmol/L (<3 mg/dL)	96.05
Bilirubin, total, serum (Malloy-Evelyn): 5.1–17 μmol/L (0.3–1.0 mg/dL)	17.10
Direct, serum: 1.7–5.1 μmol/L (0.1–0.3 mg/dL)	17.10
Indirect, serum: 3.4–12 μmol/L (0.2–0.7 mg/dL)	17.10
Bromides, serum: nondetectable	
Toxic levels: >17 mmol/L (>17 meq/L)	—
Bromsulphalein, BSP (5 mg per kg body weight, intravenously): 5 percent or less retention after 45 min	—
Calciferols (vitamin D), plasma:	
1,25-dihydroxyvitamin D [$1,25(OH)_2D$]: 5–14 nmol/L (20–60 pg/mL)	0.2400
25-hydroxyvitamin D [25(OH)D]: 20–100 nmol/L (8–42 ng/mL)	2.496
Calcium, ionized: 1.1–1.4 mmol/L (2.3–2.8 meq/L; 4.5–5.6 mg/dL)	0.2495
Calcium, plasma: 2.2–2.6 mmol/L (9–10.5 mg/dL)	0.2495
Carbon dioxide content, plasma (sea level): 21–30 mmol/L (21–30 meq/L)	—
Carbon dioxide tension (P_{CO_2}), arterial blood (sea level): 4.7–6.0 kPa (35–45 mmHg)	0.1333
Carbon monoxide content, blood: symptoms with over 20 percent saturation of hemoglobin	
Carotenoids, serum: 0.9–5.6 μmol/L (50–300 μg/dL)	0.01863
Ceruloplasmin, serum: 270–370 mg/L (27–37 mg/dL)	10
Chlorides, serum (as Cl^-): 98–106 mmol/L (98–106 meq/L)	—
Cholesterol: see Table A-4	
Complement, serum:	
C3: 0.55–1.20 g/L (55–120 mg/dL)	0.01
C4: 0.20–0.50 g/L (20–50 mg/dL)	0.01

	Conversion factor (CF) (C × CF = SI)
Copper, serum: 11–22 μmol/L (70–140 μg/dL)	0.1574
Creatine phosphokinase, serum (total):	
Females: 0.17–1.17 μkat/L (10–70 U/L)	0.01667
Males: 0.42–1.50 μkat/L (25–90 U/L)	0.01667
Creatinine, serum: <133 μmol/L (<1.5 mg/dL)	88.40
Digoxin serum:	
Therapeutic level: 0.6–2.8 nmol/L (0.5–2.2 ng/mL)	1.281
Toxic level: >3.1 nmol/L (>2.4 ng/mL)	1.281
Ethanol, blood:	
Mild to moderate intoxication: 17–43 mmol/L (80–200 mg/dL)	0.2171
Marked intoxication: 54–87 mmol/L (250–400 mg/dL)	0.2171
Severe intoxication: >87 mmol/L (>400 mg/dL)	0.2171
Fatty acids, free (nonesterified), plasma: <180 mg/L (<18 mg/dL)	10
Ferritin, serum: 15–200 μg/L (15–200 ng/mL)	—
Fibrinogen, plasma: see "Platelets and Coagulation"	—
Fibrinogen split products: see "Platelets and Coagulation"	—
Folic acid, red cell: 340–1020 nmol/L cells (150–450 ng/mL cells)	2.266
Gastrin, serum: 40–200 ng/L (40–200 pg/mL)	—
Globulins, serum: 20–30 g/L (2.0–3.0 g/dL)	10
Glucose (fasting), plasma:	
Normal: 4.2–6.4 mmol/L (75–115 mg/dL)	0.05551
Diabetes mellitus: >7.8 mmol/L [>140 mg/dL (on more than one occasion)]	0.05551
Glucose, 2 h postprandial, plasma:	
Normal: <7.8 mmol/L (<140 mg/dL)	0.05551
Impaired glucose tolerance: 7.8–11.1 mmol/L (140–200 mg/dL)	0.05551
Diabetes mellitus: >11.1 mmol/L on more than one occasion (>200 mg/dL)	0.05551
Hemoglobin, blood (sea level):	
Male: 140–180 g/L (14–18 g/dL)	10
Female: 120–160 g/L (12–16 g/dL)	10
Hemoglobin A_{1c}: up to 6 percent of total hemoglobin	—
Immunoglobulins, serum:	
IgA: 0.9–3.2 g/L (90–325 mg/dL)	0.01
IgD: 0–0.08 g/L (0–8 mg/dL)	0.01
IgE: <0.00025 g/L (<0.025 mg/dL)	0.01
IgG: 8.0–15.0 g/L (800–1500 mg/dL)	0.01
IgM: 0.45–1.5 g/L (45–150 mg/dL)	0.01
Iron, serum: 14–32 μmol/L (80–180 μg/dL)	0.1791
Iron-binding capacity, serum: 45–82 μmol/L (250–460 μg/dL)	0.1791
Saturation: 0.2–0.45 (20–45 percent)	
Lactate dehydrogenase, serum:	
200–450 units/mL (Wrobleski)	—
60–100 units/mL (Wacker)	—
0.4–1.7 μkat/L (25–100 units/L)	0.01667
Lactic dehydrogenase isoenzymes, serum (agarose):	
Fraction 1 (of total): 0.14–0.25 (14–26 percent)	0.01
Fraction 2: 0.29–0.39 (29–39 percent)	0.01
Fraction 3: 0.20–0.25 (20–26 percent)	0.01
Fraction 4: 0.08–0.16 (8–16 percent)	0.01
Fraction 5: 0.06–0.16 (6–16 percent)	0.01
Lactate, venous plasma: 0.6–1.7 mmol/L (5–15 mg/dL)	0.1110
Lead, serum: <1.0 μmol/L (<20 μg/dL)	0.04826
Lipids: see Table A-4	—
Lipids, triglyceride, serum: see "Triglycerides"	

	Conversion factor (CF) (C × CF = SI)
Lipoprotein: see Table A-4	—
Lithium, serum:	
Therapeutic level: 0.6–1.2 mmol/L (0.6–1.2 meq/L)	—
Toxic level: >2 mmol/L (>2 meq/L)	—
Magnesium, serum: 0.8–1.2 mmol/L (2–3 mg/dL)	0.4114
Osmolality, plasma: 285–295 mosmol per kg serum water	—
Oxygen content:	
Arterial blood (sea level): 17–21 volume percent	—
Venous blood, arm (sea level): 10 to 16 volume percent	—
Oxygen percent saturation (sea level):	
Arterial blood: 0.97 mol/mol (97 percent)	0.01
Venous blood, arm: 0.60–0.85 mol/mol (60–85 percent)	0.01
Oxygen tension (P_{O_2}) blood: 11–13 kPa (80–100 mmHg)	0.1333
pH, blood: 7.38–7.44	—
Phenytoin, plasma:	
Therapeutic level: 40–80 μmol/L (10–20 mg/L)	3.964
Toxic level: >120 μmol/L (>30 mg/L)	3.964
Phosphorus, inorganic, serum: 1.0–1.4 mmol/L (3–4.5 mg/dL	0.3229
Potassium, serum: 3.5–5.0 mmol/L (3.5–5.0 meq/L)	—
Proteins, total, serum: 55–80 g/L (5.5–8.0 g/dL)	10
Protein fractions, serum:	
Albumin: 35–55 g/L [3.5–5.5 g/dL (50–60 percent)]	10
Globulin: 20–35 g/L [2.0–3.5 g/dL (40–50 percent)]	10
Alpha$_1$: 2–4 g/L [0.2–0.4 g/dL (4.2–7.2 percent)]	10
Alpha$_2$: 5–9 g/L [0.5–0.9 g/dL (6.8–12 percent)]	10
Beta: 6–11 g/L [0.6–1.1 g/dL (9.3–15 percent)]	10
Gamma: 7–17 g/L [0.7–1.7 g/dL (13–23 percent)]	10
Pyruvate, venous, plasma: 60–170 μmol/L (0.5–1.5 mg/dL)	113.6
Quinidine, serum:	
Therapeutic range: 4.6–9.2 μmol/L (1.5–3 mg/L)	3.082
Toxic range: 15.4–18.5 μmol/L (5–6 mg/L)	3.082
Salicylate, plasma: 0 mmol/L	—
Therapeutic range: 1.4–1.8 mmol/L (20–25 mg/dL)	0.07240
Toxic range: >2.2 mmol/L (>30 mg/dL)	0.07240
Sodium, serum: 136–145 mmol/L (136–145 meq/L)	—
Steroids: see "Metabolic and Endocrine" under "Function Tests"	—
Triglycerides: <1.8 mmol/L (<160 mg/dL)	0.01129
Urea nitrogen, serum: 3.6–7.1 mmol/L (10–20 mg/dL)	0.3570
Uric acid, serum:	
Men: 150–480 μmol/L (2.5–8.0 mg/dL)	59.48
Women: 90–360 μmol/L (1.5–6.0 mg/dL)	59.48
Vitamin A, serum: 0.7–3.5 μmol/L (20–100 μg/dL)	0.03491
Vitamin B_{12}, serum: 148–443 pmol/L (200–600 pg/mL)	0.7378
Zinc, serum: 11.5–18.5 μmol/L (75–120 μg/dL)	0.1530

FUNCTION TESTS

Circulation

Arteriovenous oxygen difference: 30–50 mL/L
Cardiac output (Fick): 2.5–3.6 L/m² body surface area per min
Contractility indexes:
Maximum left ventricular *dp/dt*: 1650 ± 300 mmHg/s
Maximum (*dp/dt*)/*p*: 44 ± 8.4 s^{-1}
(*dp/dt*)/DP at DP = 40 mmHg: 37.6 ± 12.2 s^{-1} (DP = diastolic press.)
Mean normalized systolic ejection rate (angiography): 3.32 ± 0.84 end-diastolic volumes per second
Mean velocity of circumferential fiber shortening (angiography) 1.66 ± 0.42 circumferences per second
Ejection fraction, stroke volume/end-diastolic volume (SV/EDV):
Normal range: 0.55–0.78; average: 0.67
End-diastolic volume: 75 ± 15 mL/m²
End-systolic volume: 25 ± 8 mL/m²
Left ventricular work:
Stroke work index: 30–110 (g·m)/m²
Left ventricular minute work index: 1.8–6.6 [(kg · m)/m²]/min
Oxygen consumption index: 110–150 mL
Pressures, intracardiac and intraarterial: see Table A-5
Pulmonary vascular resistance: 2–12 (kPa·s)/L [20–120 (dyn·s)/cm⁵]
Systemic vascular resistance: 77–150 (kPa·s)/L [770–1500 (dyn·s)/cm⁵]
Systolic time intervals: see Table A-6

Gastrointestinal See also "Stool."

Absorption tests:
D-Xylose absorption test: After an overnight fast, 25 g xylose is given in aqueous solution by mouth. Urine collected for the following 5 h should contain 33–53 mmol (5–8 g) (or >20 percent of ingested dose). Serum xylose should be 1.7–2.7 mmol/L 1 h after the oral dose (25–40 mg per 100 mL).
Vitamin A absorption test: A fasting blood specimen is obtained and 200,000 units of vitamin A in oil is given by mouth. Serum vitamin A levels should rise to twice fasting level in 3–5 h.
Bentiromide test (pancreatic function): 500 mg bentiromide (chymex) orally; *p*-aminobenzoic acid (PABA) measured in plasma and/or urine
Plasma: >3.6(±1.1) mg/L at 90 min
Urine: >50 percent recovered as PABA in 6 h

	Conversion factor (CF) (C × CF = SI)
Gastric juice:	
Volume:	
24 h: 2–3 L	
Nocturnal: 600–700 mL	
Basal, fasting: 30–70 mL/h	
Reaction:	
pH: 1.6–1.8	
Titratable acidity of fasting juice: 4–9 μmol/s (15–35 meq/h)	0.261
Acid output:	
Basal:	
Females (mean ± 1 SD): 0.6 ± 0.5 μmol/s (2.0 ± 1.8 meq/h)	0.2778
Males (mean ± 1 SD): 0.8 ± 0.6 μmol/s (3.0 ± 2.0 meq/h)	0.2778
Maximal (after subcutaneous histamine acid phosphate 0.004 mg/kg body weight and preceded by 50 mg promethazine or after betazole 1.7 mg/kg body weight or pentagastrin 6 μg/kg body weight):	
Females (mean ± 1 SD): 4.4 ± 1.4 μmol/s (16 ± 5 meq/h)	0.2778
Males (mean ± 1 SD): 6.4 ± 1.4 μmol/s (23 ± 5 meq/h)	0.2778
Basal acid output/maximal acid output ratio: 0.6 or less	

	Conversion factor (CF) (C × CF = SI)
Gastrin, serum: 40–200 ng/L (40–200 pg/mL)	—
Secretin test (pancreatic exocrine function): 1 unit per kg body weight, intravenously	
Volume (pancreatic juice): >2.0 mL/kg in 80 min	—
Bicarbonate concentration: >80 mmol/L (>80 meq/L)	—
Bicarbonate output: >10 mmol in 30 min (>10 meq in 30 min)	—
Metabolic and endocrine	
Adrenocorticotropin (ACTH) plasma, 8 A.M.: <18 pmol/L (<80 pg/mL)	0.2202
Adrenal cortex function tests: see Chap. 317	—
Adrenal medulla function tests: see Chap. 318	—
Adrenal steroids, plasma:	
Aldosterone, 8 A.M.: <220 pmol/L (patient supine, 100 meq Na and 60–100 meq K intake) (<8 ng/dL)	27.74
Cortisol:	
8 A.M.: 140–690 nmol/L (5–25 μg/dL)	27.59
4 P.M.: 80–330 nmol/L (3–12 μg/dL)	27.59
Dehydroepiandrosterone (DHEA): 7–31 nmol/L (2–9 μg/L)	3.467
Dehydroepiandrosterone sulfate (DHEA sulfate): 1.3–6.7 μmol/L (500–2500 μg/L)	0.002714
11-Deoxycortisol (compound S): <30 nmol/L (<1 μg/dL)	28.86
17-Hydroxyprogesterone:	
Women: follicular phase, 0.6–3 nmol/L (0.20–1 μg/L); luteal phase, 1.5–10.6 nmol/L (0.5–3.5 μg/L)	3.026
Men: 0.2–9 nmol/L (0.06–3 μg/L)	3.026
Adrenal steroids, urinary excretion:	
Aldosterone: 14–53 nmol/d (5–19 μg/d)	2.774
Cortisol, free: 55–275 nmol/d (20–100 μg/d)	2.759
17-Hydroxycorticosteroids: 5.5–28 μmol/d (2–10 mg/d)	2.759
17-Ketosteroids:	
Men: 24–88 μmol/d (7–25 mg/d)	3.467
Women: 14–52 μmol/d (4–15 mg/d)	3.467
Angiotensin II, plasma, 8 A.M.: 10–30 nmol/L (10–30 pg/mL)	—
Arginine vasopressin (AVP), plasma:	
Random fluid intake: 2.3–7.4 pmol/L (2.5–8 ng/ L)	0.92
Calcitonin, plasma: <50 ng/L (<50 pg/mL)	—
Catecholamines, urinary excretion:	
Free catecholamines: <590 nmol/d (<100 μg/d)	5.911
Epinephrine: <275 nmol/d (<50 μg/d)	5.458
Metanephrines: <7 μmol/d (<1.3 mg/d)	5.458
Vanillylmandelic acid (VMA): <40 μmol/d (<8 mg/d)	5.046
Glucagon, plasma: 50–100 ng/L (50–100 pg/mL)	—
Gonadal function tests: see Chaps. 321 and 322	—
Gonadal steroids, plasma:	
Androstenedione:	
Women: 3.5–7.0 nmol/L (1–2 ng/ml)	3.492
Men: 3.0–5.0 mmol/L (0.8–1.3 ng/ml)	3.492
Estradiol:	
Women: 70–220 pmol/L (20–60 pg/mL), higher at ovulation	3.671
Men: <180 pmol/L (<50 pg/mL)	3.671
Progesterone:	
Men, prepubertal girls, preovulatory women, and postmenopausal women: <6 nmol/L (2 ng/mL)	3.180
Women, luteal, peak: >16 nmol/L (>5 ng/mL)	3.180

	Conversion factor (CF) (C × CF = SI)
Testosterone:	
Women: <3.5 nmol/L (<1 ng/mL)	3.467
Men: 10–35 nmol/L (3–10 ng/mL)	3.467
Prepubertal boys and girls: 0.17–0.7 nmol/L (0.05–0.2 ng/mL)	3.467
Gonadotropins, plasma:	
Women, mature, premenopausal, except at ovulation:	
FSH: 5–20 IU/L (5–20 mIU/mL)	—
LH: 5–25 IU/L (5–25 mIU/mL)	—
Ovulatory surge:	—
FSH: 12–30 IU/L (12–30 mIU/mL)	
LH: 25–100 IU/L (25–100 mIU/mL)	—
Postmenopausal women:	
FSH: >12–30 IU/L (>12–30 mIU/mL)	—
LH: >50 IU/L (>50 mIU/mL)	—
Men, mature:	
FSH: 5–20 IU/L (5–20 mIU/mL)	—
LH: 5–20 IU/L (5–20 mIU/mL)	—
Children of both sexes, prepubertal:	
FSH: <5 IU/L (<5 mIU/mL)	—
Growth hormone, after 100 g glucose by mouth: <5 μg/L (<5 ng/mL)	—
Human chorionic gonadotropin, β subunit (β-hCG), plasma:	
Men and nonpregnant women: <3 IU/L (<3 mIU/mL)	—
Insulin, serum or plasma, fasting: 43–186 pmol/L (6–26 μU/mL)	7.175
Insulin-like growth factor 1 (somatomedin C, IGF-1/SM-C): see Chap. 314	—
Oxytocin:	
Random: 1–4 pmol/L (1.25–5 ng/L)	0.80
Ovulatory peak in women: 4–8 pmol/L (5–10 ng/L)	0.80
Pancreatic islet function tests: see Chap. 319	—
Parathyroid function tests: see Chap. 340	—
Pituitary function tests: see Chaps. 313 to 315	—
Pregnancy tests: see Chap. 322	—
Prolactin, serum: 2–15 μg/L (2–15 ng/mL)	—
Renin-angiotensin function tests: see Chap. 317	—
Semen analysis: see Chap. 321	—
Thyroid function tests:	
Dynamic tests of thyroid function: see Chap. 316	—
Radioactive iodine uptake, 24 h: 5–30 percent (range varies in different areas due to variations in iodine intake)	
Resin T_3 uptake: 0.25–0.35 (25–35 percent) (varies among laboratories; for calculation of indexes of resin T_3 uptake, see Chap. 316)	0.01
Reverse triiodothyronine (rT_3), plasma: 0.15–0.61 nmol/L (10–40 ng/dL)	0.01536
Thyroid-stimulating hormone (TSH): 0.4–5 mU/L (0.4–5 μU/mL)	—
Thyroxine (T_4), serum radioimmunoassay: 64–154 nmol/L (5–12 μg/dL)	12.86
Triiodothyronine (T_3), plasma: 1.1–2.9 nmol/L (70–190) ng/dL)	0.01536
Pulmonary See Tables A-9 and A-10.	
Renal	
Clearances (corrected to 1.72 m^2 body surface area):	
Measures of glomerular filtration rate:	
Inulin clearance (C1):	
Males (mean ± 1 SD): 2.1 ± 0.4 mL/s (124 ± 25.8 mL/min)	0.01667

	Conversion factor (CF) (C × CF = SI)
Females (mean ± 1 SD): 2.0 ± 0.2 mL/s (119 ± 12.8 mL/min)	0.01667
Endogenous creatinine clearance: 1.5–2.2 mL/s (91–130 mL/min)	0.01667
Urea: 1.0–1.7 mL/s (60–100 mL/min)	0.01667
Measures of effective renal plasma flow and tubular function:	
p-Aminohippuric acid clearance (Cl_{PAH}):	
Males (mean ± 1 SD): 10.9 ± 2.7 mL/s (654 ± 163 mL/min)	0.01667
Females (mean ± 1 SD): 9.9 ± 1.7 mL/s (594 ± 102 mL/min)	0.01667
Concentration and dilution test:	
Specific gravity of urine:	
After 12-h fluid restriction: 1.025 or more	—
After 12-h deliberate water intake: 1.003 or less	—
Protein excretion, urine: <0.15 g/d (<150 mg/d)	0.001
Males: 0–0.06 g/d (0–60 mg/d)	0.001
Females: 0–0.09 g/d (0–90 mg/d)	0.001
Specific gravity, maximal range: 1.002–1.028	—
Tubular reabsorption, phosphorus: 79–94 percent of filtered load	—

HEMATOLOGIC EXAMINATIONS

See also "Chemical Constituents of Blood."

Bone marrow See Table A-12.

Erythrocytes and hemoglobin See also Table A-12.

Carboxyhemoblogin:	
Nonsmoker: 0–0.023 (0–2.3 percent)	0.01
Smoker: 0.021–0.042 (2.1–4.2 percent)	0.01
Erythrocyte "life span":	
Normal survival: 120 days	—
Chromium-labeled, half-life ($t_{1/2}$): 28 days	—
Glucose-6-phosphate dehydrogenase: 12.1 ± 2 IU/gHb (WHO)	—
Ham's test (acid serum): negative	—
Haptoglobin, serum 0.5–2.2 g/L (50–220 mg/dL)	0.01
Hemoglobin, plasma: 0.01–0.05 g/L (1–5 mg/dL)	0.01
Hemoglobin A_2 (HbA_2): 0.015–0.035 (1.5–3.5 percent)	0.01
Hemoglobin, fetal (HbF): <0.02 (<2 percent)	0.01
Hemoglobin H prep: negative	—
Methemoglobin: <0.017 (<1.7 percent)	0.01
Osmotic fragility:	
Slight hemolysis: 0.45–0.39 percent	—
Complete hemolysis: 0.33–0.30 percent	—
Plasma iron turnover: 20–42 mg/d or 0.45 mg/kg body weight per day	—
Protoporphyrin, free erythrocyte (FEP): 0.28–0.64 μmol/L of red blood cells (16–36 μg/dL of red blood cells)	0.0177
Red cell distribution width (Coulter): 13 ± 1.5 percent	
Sedimentation rate:	
Westergren, <50 years of age:	
Males: 0–15 mm/h	
Females: 0–20 mm/h	
Westergren, >50 years of age:	
Males: 0–20 mm/h	
Females: 0–30 mm/h	
Sucrose hemolysis: negative	

Leukocytes See Table A-13.

Platelets and coagulation

	Conversion factor (CF) (C × CF = SI)
$Alpha_2$ antiplasmin: 70–130 percent	
Antithrombin III: 80–120 percent	
Bleeding time:	
Duke method: <4 min	
Simplate: <7 min	
Clot retraction, qualitative: apparent in 60 min, complete <24 h, usually <6 h	
Euglobulin lysis time: >2 h	
Factor II: 60–100 percent	
Factor V: 60–100 percent	
Factor VII: 60–100 percent	
Factor IX: 60–100 percent	
Factor X: 60–100 percent	
Factor XI: 60–100 percent	
Factor XII: 60–100 percent	
Factor XIII: clot stable in urea	
Fibrinogen: 2.0–4.0 g/L (200–400 mg/dL)	0.01
Fibrin split products: <10 mg/L (<10 μg/mL)	—
Plasminogen: 2.4–4.4 CTA U/mL	
Protein C (antigenic assay): 58–148 percent	
Protein S (antigenic assay): 58–148 percent	
Partial thromboplastin time (activated PTT): comparable to control	
Prothrombin time (quick one-stage): control ± 1 s	
Protamine paracoagulation (3P) test: negative	
Platelets: 130,000–400,000 per microliter	
Thrombin time: control ± 3 s	
von Willebrand's antigen: 60–150 percent	

Miscellaneous

Leukocyte alkaline phosphatase (LAP): 0.2–1.6 μkat/L (13–100 U/L)	0.01667
Lysozyme (muramidase), serum: 5–25 mg/L (5–25 μg/mL)	—
Lysozyme, urine: <2 mg/L (<2 μg/mL)	—
Schilling test: excretion in urine of orally administered radioactive vitamin B_{12}: 7–40 percent	—
Viscosity, plasma: 1.7–2.1	—
Viscosity, serum: 1.4–1.8	—

STOOL

Bulk:	
Wet weight: <197.5 (115 ± 41) g/d	—
Dry weight: <66.4 (34 ± 15) g/d	—
$Alpha_1$ antitrypsin: 0.98 (±0.17) mg/g dry weight stool	—
Coproporphyrin: 600–1500 nmol/d (400–1000 μg/d)	1.527
Fat (on diet containing at least 50 g fat): <6.0 (4.0 ± 1.5) g/d when measured on a 3-day (or longer) collection	
Percent of dry weight: <0.30 (<30.4 percent)	0.01
Coefficient of fat absorption: >0.95 (>95 percent)	0.01
Fatty acid:	
Free: 0.01–0.10 (1–10 percent of dry matter)	0.01
Combined as soap: 0.005–0.12 (0.5–12 percent of dry matter)	0.01
Nitrogen: <1.7 (1.4 ± 0.2) g/d	—
Protein content: minimal	—
Urobilinogen: 68–470 μmol/d (40–280 mg/d)	1.693
Water: 0.65 (approximately 65 percent)	0.01

URINE

	Conversion factor (CF) (C × CF = SI)
See also "Metabolic and Endocrine" under "Function Tests."	
Acidity, titratable: 20–40 mmol/d (20–40 meq/d)	—
Ammonia: 30–50 mmol/d (30–50 meq/d)	—
Amylase: 35–260 Somogyi units/h	—
Amylase/creatinine clearance ratio [$(Cl_{am}/Cl_{cr}) \times 100$]: 1–5	—
Bentiromide (pancreatic function): 50 percent excreted in 6 h as *p*-amino benzoic acid (PABA) after 500 mg oral bentiromide	—
Calcium (10 meq/d or 200-mg/d calcium diet): <3.8 mmol/d (<7.5 meq/d)	0.5
Catecholamines: <600 nmol/d (<100 μg/d)	5.911
Copper: 0–0.4 μmol/d (0–25 μg/d)	0.01574
Coproporphyrins (types I and III): 150–460 nmol/d (100–300 μg/d)	1.527
Creatine, as creatinine:	
Adult males: <380 pmol/d (<50 mg/d)	7.625
Adult females: <760 pmol/d (<100 mg/d)	7.625
Creatinine: 8.8–14 mmol/d (1.0–1.6 g/d)	8.840
Glucose, true (oxidase method): 0.3–1.7 mmol/d (50–300 mg/d)	0.5551
5-Hydroxyindoleacetic acid (5-HIAA): 10–47 μmol/d (2–9 mg/d)	5.230
Lead: <0.4 μmol/d (<80 μg/d)	0.004826
Protein: <0.15 g/d (<150 mg/d)	0.1
Porphobilinogen: none	—
Potassium: 25–100 mmol/d [25–100 meq/d (varies with intake)]	—
Sodium: 100–260 mmol/d [100–260 meq/d (varies with intake)]	—
Urobilinogen: 1.7–5.9 μmol/d (1–3.5 mg/d)	1.693
Vanillylmandelic acid (VMA): <40 μmol/d (<8 mg/d)	5.046
D-Xylose excretion: 5 to 8 g within 5 h after oral dose of 25 g	—

TABLE A-1 SI and other units

Quantity	Name of unit	Symbol for unit	Derivation of units
SI BASE UNITS			
Length	meter	m	
Mass	kilogram	kg	
Time	second	s	
Thermodynamic temperature	Kelvin	K	
Amount of substance	mole	mol	
SI DERIVED UNITS			
Area	square meter	m^2	
Force	newton	N	$(m \cdot kg)/g^2$
Pressure	pascal	Pa	$N \cdot m^2$
Work, energy	joule	J	$N \cdot m$
Celsius temperature	degree Celsius	°C	K
OTHER UNITS RETAINED FOR USE			
Time	minute	min	
	hour	h	
	day	d	
Volume	liter	L	

TABLE A-2 Radiation derived units

Quantity	Old unit	SI unit	Name for SI unit (and abbreviation)	Conversion
Activity	curie (Ci)	Disintegrations per second (dps)	becquerel (Bq)	1 Ci = 3.7 × 10^{10} Bq 1 mCi = 37 mBq 1 μCi = 0.037 MBq or 37 GBq 1 Bq = 2.703 × 10^{-11} Ci
Absorbed dose	rad	joule per kilogram (J/kg)	gray (Gy)	1 Gy = 100 rad 1 rad = 0.01 Gy 1 mrad = 10^{-3} cGy
Exposure	roentgen (R)	coulomb per kilogram (C/kg)	—	1 C/kg = 3876 R 1 R = 2.58 × 10^{-4} C/kg 1 mR = 258 pC/kg
Dose equivalent	rem	joule per kilogram (J/kg)	sievert (Sv)	1 Sv = 100 rem 1 rem = 0.01 Sv 1 mrem = 10 μSv

TABLE A-3 SI prefixes and their symbols

Factor	Prefix	Symbol for prefix
10^9	giga	G
10^6	mega	M
10^3	kilo	k
10^2	hecto	h
10^1	deka	da
10^{-1}	deci	d
10^{-2}	centi	c
10^{-3}	milli	m
10^{-6}	micro	μ
10^{-9}	nano	n
10^{-12}	pico	p
10^{-15}	femto	f
10^{-18}	alto	a

TABLE A-4 Classification of total cholesterol and LDL-cholesterol values

	Total plasma cholesterol	LDL-cholesterol	Conversion factor (C to SI)
Desirable	<5.20 mmol/L (<200 mg/dL)	<3.36 mmol/L (<130 mg/dL)	0.02586
Borderline high	5.20–6.18 mmol/L (200–239 mg/dL)	3.36–4.11 mmol/L (130–159 mg/dL)	0.02586
High	≥6.21 mmol/L (≥240 mg/dL)	≥4.14 mmol/L (≥160 mg/dL)	0.02586

SOURCE: The Expert Panel. Report of the National Cholesterol Education Program Expert Panel on Detection, Evaluation, and Treatment of High Blood Cholesterol in Adults. Arch Intern Med 148:36, 1988

TABLE A-5 Hemodynamic values

Pressures (mmHg):	
Systemic arterial:	
Peak systolic/end-diastolic	100–140/60–90
Mean	70–105
Left ventricle:	
Peak systolic/end-diastolic	100–140/3–12
Left atrium (or pulmonary capillary wedge):	
Mean	2–12
a wave	3–10
v wave	3–15
Pulmonary artery:	
Peak systolic/end-diastolic	15–30/4–14
Mean	9–17
Right ventricle:	
Peak systolic/end-diastolic	15–30/2–7
Right atrium:	
Mean	2–6
a wave	2–8
v wave	2–7
Resistances [(dyn·s)/cm^5]:	
Systemic vascular resistance	700–1600
Total pulmonary resistance	100–300
Pulmonary vascular resistance	30–130
Flows:	
Cardiac index (liters per minute per square meter)	2.4–3.8
Stroke index (milliliters per beat per square meter)	30–65
Oxygen consumption (liters per minute per square meter)	110–150
Arteriovenous oxygen difference (milliliters per liter)	30–50

TABLE A-6 Systolic time intervals in normal individuals (in milliseconds)

Regression equation	SD of index
QS_2 (M) = −2.1 HR + 546	14
QS_2 (F) = −2.0 HR + 549	14
PEP (M) = −0.4 HR + 131	13
PEP (F) = −0.4 HR + 133	11
LVET (M) = −1.7 HR + 413	10
LVET (F) = −1.6 HR + 418	10

NOTE: QS_2 = total electromechanical systole, PEP = preejection phase, LVET = left ventricular ejection time, HR = heart rate, M = male, F = female, SD = standard deviation of the systolic time interval index. Systolic ejection period = 220–320 ms per beat; diastolic filling period = 380–500 ms per beat.

SOURCE: AM Weissler, CL Garrard, Mod Concepts Cardiovasc Dis 40:1, 1971.

TABLE A-7 Normal values of echocardiographic measurements in adults*

	Range, cm	Mean, cm	Number of subjects
Age (years)	13 to 54	26	134
Body surface area (m^2)	1.45 to 2.22	1.8	130
RVD—flat	0.7 to 2.3	1.5	84
RVD—left lateral	0.9 to 2.6	1.7	83
LVID—flat	3.7 to 5.6	4.7	82
LVID—left lateral	3.5 to 5.7	4.7	81
Posterior LV wall thickness	0.6 to 1.1	0.9	137
Posterior LV wall amplitude	0.9 to 1.4	1.2	48
IVS wall thickness	0.6 to 1.1	0.9	137
Mid IVS amplitude	0.3 to 0.8	0.5	10
Apical IVS amplitude	0.5 to 1.2	0.7	38
Left atrial dimension	1.9 to 4.0	2.9	133
Aortic root dimension	2.0 to 3.7	2.7	121
Aortic cusps' separation	1.5 to 2.6	1.9	93
Percentage of fractional shortening†	34 to 44%	36%	20
Mean rate of circumferential shortening (Vcf)‡, or mean normalized shortening velocity	1.02 to 1.94 circ/s	1.3 circ/s	38

* RVD = right ventricular dimension; LVID = left ventricular internal dimension; d = end diastole; s = end systole; LV = left ventricle; IVS = interventricular septum.

† $\dfrac{\text{LVIDd} - \text{LVIDs}}{\text{LVIDd}}$

‡ $\dfrac{\text{LVIDd} - \text{LVIDs}}{\text{LVIDd} \times \text{ejection time}}$

SOURCE: From H Feigenbaum, Echocardiography, in *Heart Disease—A Textbook of Cardiovascular Medicine,* E Braunwald (ed), Philadelphia, Saunders, 1980.

TABLE A-8 Amplitude of Q, R, S, and T waves in scalar electrocardiogram of 100 normal adults*

	I	II	III	aV_R	aV_L	aV_F	V_1	V_5	V_6
Patients with Q wave	38%	41%	50%	—	38%	40%	0%	60%	75%
Q amplitude:									
Mean	0.4	0.6	0.9	—	0.4	0.7	0	0.3	0.3
Range	0 to 0.10	0 to 1.6	0 to 2.3	—	0 to 1.1	0 to 1.7	0	0 to 1.8	0 to 1.8
R amplitude:									
Mean	5.6	8.9	4.5	1.3	3.4	6.0	1.9	12.6	10.2
Range	1.0 to 10.0	2.0 to 16.9	1.0 to 12.1	0 to 2.9	0 to 8.2	0 to 13.8	1.0 to 6.0	7.0 to 21.0	5.0 to 18.0
S amplitude:									
Mean	2.0	2.1	2.4	7.0	2.6	—	8.0	2.5	1.3
Range	0 to 5.0	0 to 3.7	0 to 6.4	2.2 to 11.8	0 to 5.8	—	3.0 to 13.0	0 to 5.0	0 to 2.0
T amplitude:									
Mean	1.9	2.3	1.0	—	0.3	1.7	1.0	3.3	1.0
Range	1.0 to 3.0	1.0 to 4.0	−2.0 to 2.0	—	−1.0 to 2.0	0 to 4.0	−2.0 to 2.0	2.0 to 7.0	1.0 to 4.0

* Values of Q, R, S, and T amplitudes are in millimeters (1 mm = 0.1 mv).

SOURCE: From J D Cooksey et al, *Clinical Vectorcardiography and Electrocardiography*, 2d ed, Chicago, Year Book Medical Publishers, 1977. Used by permission.

TABLE A-9 Summary of values useful in pulmonary physiology

	Symbol	Typical values: Men	Women
PULMONARY MECHANICS			
Spirometry—volume-time curves:			
Forced vital capacity	FVC	≥4.0 liters	≥3.0 liters
Forced expiratory volume in 1 s	FEV_1	>3.0 liters	>2.0 liters
FEV_1/FVC	FEV_1%	>60%	>70%
Maximal midexpiratory flow	MMF (FEF 25–27)	>2.0 liters per second	>1.6 liters per second
Maximal expiratory flow rate	MEFR (FEF 200–1200)	>3.5 liters per second	>3.0 liters per second
Spirometry—flow-volume curves:			
Maximal expiratory flow at 50% of expired vital capacity	$\dot{V}_{max}$ 50 (FEF 50%)	>2.5 liters per second	>2.0 liters per second
Maximal expiratory flow at 75% of expired vital capacity	$\dot{V}_{max}$ 75 (FEF 75%)	>1.5 liters per second	>1.0 liters per second
Resistance to airflow:			
Pulmonary resistance	RL (R_L)	<3.0 cmH_2O/s per liter	
Airway resistance	Raw	<2.5 cmH_2O/s per liter	
Specific conductance	SGaw	>0.13 cmH_2O/s	
Pulmonary compliance:			
Static recoil pressure at total lung capacity	Pst TLC	25 ± 5 cmH_2O	
Compliance of lungs (static)	CL	0.2 L/cmH_2O	
Compliance of lungs and thorax	C(L + T)	0.1 L/cmH_2O	
Dynamic compliance of 20 breaths per minute	C dyn 20	0.25 ± 0.05 liters per cmH_2O	
Maximal static respiratory pressures:			
Maximal inspiratory pressure	MIP	>90 cmH_2O	>50 cmH_2O
Maximal expiratory pressure	MEP	>150 cmH_2O	>120 cmH_2O
LUNG VOLUMES			
Total lung capacity	TLC	6–7 liters	5–6 liters
Functional residual capacity	FRC	2–3 liters	2–3 liters
Residual volume	RV	1–2 liters	1–2 liters
Inspiratory capacity	IC	2–4 liters	2–4 liters
Expiratory reserve volume	ERV	1–2 liters	1–2 liters
Vital capacity	VC	4–5 liters	3–4 liters
GAS EXCHANGE (SEA LEVEL)			
Arterial O_2 tension	Pa_{O_2}	95 ± 5 mmHg	
Arterial CO_2 tension	Pa_{CO_2}	40 ± 2 mmHg	
Arterial O_2 saturation	Sa_{O_2}	97 ± 2%	
Arterial blood pH	pH	7.40 ± 0.02	
Arterial bicarbonate	HCO_3^-	24 ± 2 mmol/L	
Base excess	BE	0 ± 2 mmol/L	
Diffusing capacity for carbon monoxide (single breath)	DL_{CO}	25 mL CO/min/mmHg	
Dead space volume	V_D	50 ± 25 mL	
Physiologic dead space: dead space-tidal volume ratio (rest)	V_D/V_T	≤35% V_T	
(exercise)		≤20% V_T	
Alveolar-arterial difference for O_2	A-a D_{O_2}	≤20 mmHg	

TABLE A-10 Prediction equations for spirometric tests, lung volumes, and gas exchange in adults

Variable	Sex	Age (A)	Height (H)	Weight (W)	Constant (C)	Standard deviation (SD)
PULMONARY MECHANICS						
Spirometry—volume-time curves* (H in inches):						
FVC	M	−0.025	+0.148	—	−4.241	0.74
	F	−0.024	+0.115	—	−2.852	0.52
FEV_1	M	−0.032	+0.092	—	−1.260	0.55
	F	−0.025	+0.089	—	−1.932	0.47
MEFR	M	−0.047	+0.109	—	+2.010	1.66
(FEF 200–1200)	F	−0.036	+0.145	—	−2.532	1.19
MMF	M	−0.045	+0.047	—	+2.513	1.12
(FEF 25–75)	F	−0.030	+0.060	—	+0.551	0.80
Spirometry—flow-volume curves† (H in centimeters):						
$\dot{V}_{max}$ 50	M	−0.015	+0.069	—	−5.400	1.422
(FEF 50%)	F	−0.013	+0.035	—	−0.444	1.22
$\dot{V}_{max}$ 75	M	−0.012	+0.044	—	−4.143	1.026
(FEF 75%)	F	−0.014	—	—	+3.042	0.936
Lung volumes‡ (H in meters; W in kilograms):						
TLC	M	—	+6.92	−0.017	−4.30	0.67
	F	−0.015	+6.71	—	−5.77	0.48
FRC	M	+0.015	+5.30	−0.037	−3.89	0.56
	F	—	+5.13	−0.028	−4.50	0.41
RV	M	+0.022	+1.98	−0.015	−1.54	0.38
	F	+0.007	+2.68	—	−3.42	0.32
VC	M	−0.020	+4.81	—	−2.81	0.50
	F	−0.022	+4.04	—	−2.35	0.40
Gas exchange§ (H in meters; W in kilograms):						
DL_{CO}	M	−0.20	+32.5	—	−17.6	5.1
	F	−0.16	+21.2	—	− 2.66	3.6

NOTE: Answer = (A × age) + (H × height) + (W × weight) + C ± 2 SD. Example: The normal value and lower limit for the FEV_1 are sought in a man, age 40 years, height 183 cm, and weight 91 kg. The following equation gives the normal value:
$FEV_1 = (-0.032 \times 40) + (0.092 \times 72) + (-1.260) = 4.08$ liters
The lower limit of normal:
$4.08 - (2 \times SD) = 4.08 - (2 \times 0.55) = 2.98$ liters
Only 2.5% of a normal population will fall below this value (2 SD below the mean).
For other abbreviations, see Table A-9.

* Morris et al, Am Rev Respir Dis 103:57, 1971.
† Knudson et al, Am Rev Respir Dis 113:587, 1976.
‡ Grimby G, Söderholm B, Acta Med Scand 173:199, 1963.
§ Coates JE, *Lung Function and Application in Medicine*, Philadelphia, Davis, 1965.

TABLE A-11 Differential nucleated cell counts of bone marrow

	Normal, mean%*	Range, %†
Myeloid:	56.7	
Neutrophilic series:	53.6	
Myeloblast	0.9	0.2–1.5
Promyelocyte	3.3	2.1–4.1
Myelocyte	12.7	8.2–15.7
Metamyelocyte	15.9	9.6–24.6
Band	12.4	9.5–15.3
Segmented		
Eosinophilic series	3.1	1.2–5.3
Basophilic series	<0.1	0–0.2
Erythroid:	25.6	
Pronormoblasts	0.6	0.2–1.3
Basophilic normoblasts	1.4	0.5–2.4
Polychromatophilic normoblasts	21.6	17.9–29.2
Orthochromatic normoblasts	2.0	0.4–4.6
Megakaryocytes	<0.1	
Lymphoreticular	17.8	
Lymphocytes	16.2	11.1–23.2
Plasma cells	2.3	0.4–3.9
Reticulum cells	0.3	0–0.9

* From MM Wintrobe et al, *Clinical Hematology*, 8th ed, Philadelphia, Lea & Febiger, 1981.
† Range observed in 12 healthy men.

TABLE A-12 Erythrocytes and hemoglobin: Normal values at various ages

Age	Red blood cell count,* 10^{12}/L	Hemoglobin,* g/L (g/dL)	Vol. packed RBCs,* mL/dL	Corpuscular values: MCV, fL	MCH, pg	MCHC, g/L (g/dL)	MCD, μm
Days 1–13	5.1 ± 1.0	195 ± 50 (19.5 ± 5)	54.0 ± 10.0	106–98	38–33	340–360 (36–34)	8.6
Days 14–60	4.7 ± 0.9	140 ± 33 (14 ± 3.3)	42.0 ± 7.0	90	30	330 (33)	8.1
3 months to 10 years	4.5 ± 0.7	122 ± 23 (12.2 ± 2.3)	36.0 ± 5.0	80	27	340 (34)	7.7
11–15 years	4.8	131 (13.14)	39.0	82	28	340 (34)	
Adults:							
Females	4.8 ± 0.6	140 ± 20 (14 ± 2)	42.0 ± 5.0	90 ± 7	29 ± 2	340 ± 20 (34 ± 2)	7.5 ± 0.3
Males	5.4 ± 0.9	160 ± 20 (16 ± 2)	47.0 ± 5.0	90 ± 7	29 ± 2	340 ± 20 (34 ± 2)	7.5 ± 0.3

* The range of values represents almost the extremes of observed variations (93 percent or more) at sea level. The blood values of healthy persons should fall well within these mean ± SD figures.

NOTE: MCV = mean corpuscular volume, MCH = mean corpuscular hemoglobin, MCHC = mean corpuscular hemoglobin concentration, MCD = mean corpuscular diameter.

SOURCE: MM Wintrobe et al, *Clinical Hematology*, 8th ed, Philadelphia, Lea & Febiger, 1981.

TABLE A-13 Normal leukocyte count, differential count, and hemoglobin concentration at various ages

Age	Leukocytes, total	Neutrophils: Total	Band	Segmented	Eosinophils	Basophils	Lymphocytes	Monocytes
12 mo	11.4(6.0–17.5)	3.5(1.5–8.5)	0.35	3.2	0.3(0.05–0.7)	0.05(0–0.20)	7.0(4.0–10.5)	0.55(0.05–1.1)
		31	3.1	28	0.4	0.4	61	4.8
4 yr	9.1(5.5–15.5)	3.8(1.5–8.5)	0.27(0–1.0)	3.5(1.5–7.5)	0.25(0.02–0.65)	0.05(0–0.20)	4.5(2.0–8.0)	0.45(0–0.8)
		42	3.0	39	2.8	0.6	50	5.0
6 yr	4.3(1.5–8.0)	0.25(0–1.0)	4.0(1.5–7.0)	4.0(1.5–7.0)	0.23(0–0.65)	0.05(0–0.20)	3.5(1.5–7.0)	0.40(0–0.8)
		51	3.0	48	2.7	0.6	42	4.7
10 yr	8.1(4.5–13.5)	4.4(1.8–8.0)	0.24(0–1.0)	4.2(1.8–7.0)	0.20(0–0.60)	0.04(0–0.20)	3.1(1.5–6.5)	0.35(0–0.8)
		54	3.0	51	2.4	0.5	38	4.3
21 yr	7.4(4.5–11.0)	4.4(1.8–7.7)	0.22(0–0.7)	4.2(1.8–7.0)	0.20(0–0.45)	0.04(0–0.20)	2.5(1.0–4.8)	0.30(0–0.8)
		59	3.0	56	2.7	0.5	34	4.0

NOTE: Values are expressed as "cells × 10^9/L." The numbers underlined are percentages.

SOURCE: WJ Williams et al (eds), *Hematology*, 3d ed, New York, McGraw-Hill, 1983. By permission.

INDEX

(Page numbers in **boldface** indicate major discussions; numbers preceded by *A* indicate Atlas plates.)

TOPICAL TABLE OF CONTENTS